FOUNDATIONS OF OSTEOPATHIC MEDICINE

Philosophy, Science, Clinical Applications, and Research

Fifth Edition

Published under the auspices of the American Osteopathic Association

FOUNDATIONS OF OSTEOPATHIC MEDICINE

Philosophy, Science, Clinical Applications, and Research

Fifth Edition

Published under the auspices of the American Osteopathic Association

Executive Editors

Kurt P. Heinking, DO, FAAO
Professor and Chair of Osteopathic Manipulative Medicine
Chicago College of Osteopathic Medicine
Midwestern University
Downers Grove, Illinois

Rebecca E. Giusti, DO
Professor, Chair of Neuromusculoskeletal Medicine/
Osteopathic Manipulative Medicine and Family Medicine
College of Osteopathic Medicine of the Pacific and
College of Osteopathic Medicine of the Pacific—Northwest
Western University of Health Sciences
Pomona, California

Kendi L. Hensel, DO, PhD, FAAO
Professor and Vice Chair
Department of Family Medicine and Osteopathic Manipulative Medicine
Texas College of Osteopathic Medicine
University of North Texas Health Science Center
Fort Worth, Texas

Featuring Color Illustrations by William A. Kuchera, DO, FAAO

Wolters Kluwer

Philadelphia • Baltimore • New York • London
Buenos Aires • Hong Kong • Sydney • Tokyo

Acquisitions Editor: Matt Hauber
Development Editor: Deborah Bordeaux
Editorial Coordinator: Bhavani Ganesan
Marketing Manager: Kirsten Watrud
Senior Production Project Manager: Catherine Ott
Manager, Graphic Arts & Design: Stephen Druding
Art Director, Illustration: Jennifer Clements
Manufacturing Coordinator: Margie Orzech
Prepress Vendor: Aptara, Inc.

9 8 7 6 5 4 3 2 1

Printed in Mexico

Library of Congress Cataloging-in-Publication Data

ISBN 978-1-9751-9864-0
Cataloging in Publication data available on request from publisher.

---

shop.lww.com

QUADM1025

DEDICATION

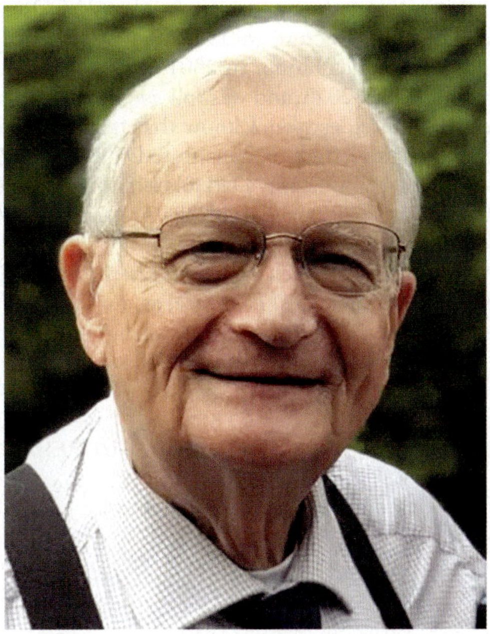

WILLIAM A. KUCHERA, DO, FAAO
1933–2023

Known to most of his patients as "Dr. Bill" and to his students as "Papa Kuch." William A. Kuchera, DO, FAAO was the second of a three-generation osteopathic family. After graduating from the Kirksville College of Osteopathy and Surgery (now ATSU-KCOM) in 1958 and completing his postgraduate training in Kirksville, he joined his father, Louis H. Kuchera, DO (Des Moines 1928) in Albert Lea MN before moving to Davenport/Bettendorf Iowa to continue his general practice with an emphasis on obstetrics. In his nearly 30 years of general practice, he documented use of osteopathic manipulative treatment (OMT) as an integral component in over 75% of his patients.

In 1980, Paul Kimberly, DO, FAAO recruited both "Dr. Bill" and his son, "Dr. Mike," to the osteopathic manipulative medicine (OMM) Department of the Kirksville College of Osteopathic Medicine (KCOM) to teach basic OPP/OMT skills as well as the integration of OMM for care of general/family medicine patients. In 1988, after many years of a shared osteopathic general practice, both were granted their OMM specialty certification from the AOA and earned fellowships from the American Academy of Osteopathy (FAAO). Even as an OMM specialist, Dr. Bill continued to deliver babies and integrate his general practice perspective. Drs. Bill and Mike practiced and taught together for 15 years before Dr. Bill retired as an emeritus professor from KCOM.

Bill was passionate about life—defined in faith, family, and education. He was flawlessly consistent and optimistic in his love and approach to all life, and always curious! Dr. Bill was especially committed to distinctively osteopathic education…in his mentorship, writings, and lectures…but above all, he served as a role model of a compassionate osteopathic physician who treated patients, staff, students, and colleagues equally with the utmost respect. He was instrumental for his representation in the Educational Council on Osteopathic Principles where he was a major contributor in the development of the *Glossary of Osteopathic Terminology* and in formatting *The Osteopathic Core Curriculum.* He is most widely recognized for his coauthorship in *Osteopathic Principles in Practice* and *Osteopathic Considerations in Systemic Dysfunction* (standard osteopathic texts published prior to the first *Foundations for Osteopathic Medicine [FOM]* which were referenced several hundred times by *FOM* chapter authors) and for his uniquely osteopathic diagrams in those and several other osteopathic texts. He served as a sub-editor in *FOM 1–2*, a contributor to *FOM 1–5*, and in addition to his many individual diagrams in all editions, he was selected to illustrate a significant portion of *FOM 4*. Active even after his retirement, he illustrated Michael Seffinger's *Evidence-Based Manual Medicine: A Problem-Oriented Approach* (2007) and coauthored (and illustrated) *Osteopathic Considerations in HEENT Disorders* (translated into Korean in 2021).

Dr. Bill was a humble man; he never sought an office nor recognition for his activities. However, colleagues and students nominated and rewarded his many contributions over the years ranging from KCOM's Gender Equity Award to their A.T. Still Staff Award for Teaching Excellence. Furthermore, his peers at the American Academy of Osteopathy selected him to deliver the TL Northup Memorial Lecture in 1992 and bestowed upon him their highest recognition, the A.T. Still Medallion of Honor in 2001.

Dr. Bill passed gently on June 12, 2023, and was followed 6 months later by his wife, Natalie Kuchera, of nearly 69 years. As his eldest son, I know that family, including his seven children and many grandchildren/great-grandchildren, constituted the most important part of his life and he entertained them with nearly constant "Dad jokes" and other "Kuchera groaners." Upon meeting each new grandchild or great-grandchild, his first instinct was to bond with them while palpating their little heads.

How he conducted his life inspired each of his children to try to be better spouses, better parents, and, generally, better individuals. Likewise, as a role model within his osteopathic family, many whose lives he touched credit him with challenging them to be better osteopathic students, caregivers, teachers, and/or mentors through the integration of OPP/OMT and a sincere, consistent respect of others.

MICHAEL L. KUCHERA, DO, FAAO, FNAOME

DEDICATION

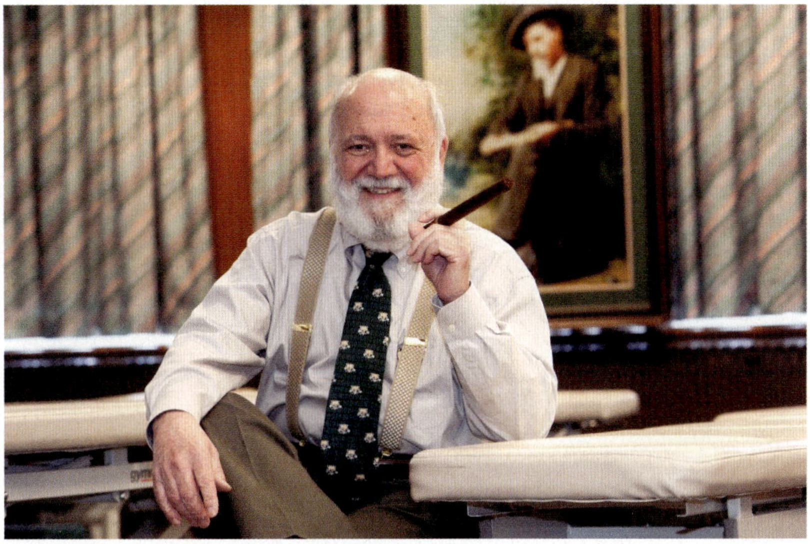

ANTHONY G. CHILA, DO, FAAO, FCA (Dist)
1937–2022

It is with great sadness that I write of the passing of Anthony G. Chila, DO, FAAO, FCA (Dist). As Executive Editor of *Foundations of Osteopathic Medicine,* Third Edition, he is well known to this audience and his absence is greatly mourned.

Dr. Chila was born on December 14, 1937, in Youngstown, Ohio. He was graduated from Youngstown State University in 1960 with a Bachelor of Arts degree, and then received his Doctor of Osteopathy from the Kansas City College of Osteopathic Medicine in 1965. He practiced the full scope of family medicine for 11 years in Ohio, until joining the faculty of Michigan State University College of Osteopathic Medicine. In 1978, he joined the faculty of the newly established Ohio University College of Osteopathic Medicine (now the Ohio University Heritage College of Osteopathic Medicine). He remained faculty until his retirement in 2011, though he continued to see patients in the clinic for some time after that.

Dr. Chila received numerous awards throughout his career, including the Scott, Burns, Northup, Sutherland, and A.T. Still Memorial Lectures. He was the 1995 recipient of the AOA Bureau of Research Gutensohn-Denslow Award. In 1997, he received with the A.T. Still Medallion of Honor by the American Academy of Osteopathy. In 2013, he received the American Osteopathic Foundation Educator of the Year award. Finally, just before his death, he was awarded the James O. Watson Memorial Lecture Award by the Ohio University Heritage College of Osteopathic Medicine, in recognition of years of service to the osteopathic profession, particularly in the State of Ohio.

These many recognitions, though, tell us little of the man himself, his thoughts, or his philosophies. The man, Anthony "Tony" Chila, before anything else, was devoted to his wife, Helen, and his daughter, Annie. They were the light of his life, and it was rare that some reference to one of them was not made. He was devoted to his faith, first as Roman Catholic, then as Greek Orthodox, even serving for a time on the Board of Trustees for St. Vladmir's Orthodox Theological Seminary.

Philosophically, he believed in the application of basic, foundational principles. Osteopathically, he often said there were no techniques, only the application of principles. He tried to pare away all excess, to boil a principle down to its essence. In doing so, he often spoke of things in threes. In osteopathic manipulation, some examples include:

"See no thing," by which he meant, get your head out of the way. Clear yourself of your own preconceptions and biases, what you want to do. Listen to what the body is offering you and work within that.

> *"Look, See. Perceive."* One must first his eyes open, to look at what might be happening. Then he must actually see what is in front of him, what the object is offering of itself. And, finally, to perceive: to be changed by the seeing in oneself, to see the Truth of the interaction between the two.

How many of us are willing to do these things? Very few, as he well knew, but it is what he tried to teach.

Tony could be difficult at times because of these things, but it was the standard to which he held himself, and the standard he expected from others.

Personally, I mourn the passing of dear friend, and mentor, from whom I have learned, and continue to learn, so much. As a profession, we have lost an icon, a dedicated teacher and practitioner. But as any good teacher, he has tried to pass on others what he had learned—and in so doing, we are all improved because of him.

RICHARD G. SCHUSTER, DO

DEDICATION

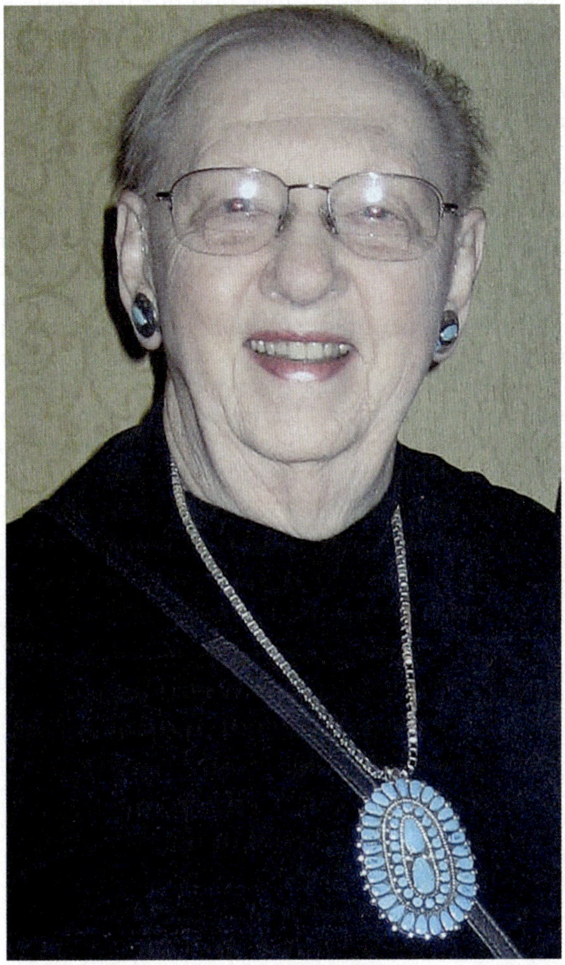

SARA "SALLY" SUTTON, DO, FAAO

1926–2024

It is with deep sadness that we have lost yet another stalwart of our profession in this past year. Sara "Sally" Sutton, DO, FAAO, is a name many may not recognize, but her influence upon the osteopathic profession has been profound.

Dr. Sutton attended the Des Moines Still College of Osteopathy and Surgery, 1949–1953. As one of two women in the class, she was met with resentment by her male colleagues who felt she was taking a seat away from returning veterans. She often heard that seats were wasted on women who would only get married, have children, and never practice. This only added to her determination and motivation. She served as President of the American Academy of Osteopathy, 1969–1970. In 1993, she received the A.T. Still Medallion of Honor, the highest accolade of the AAO. In 2011, she received the AOA Mentor of the Year award. In 2013, she received the Pioneer in Osteopathy Award from the Des Moines University Board of Trustees, on which she served for 25 years. Few others in her class could boast such achievements.

While in her first 2 years of school, she served as personal secretary to Paul Kimberly, DO, FAAO, who became her friend and mentor. He allowed her to see and treat patients with him in his clinic. In the early 1960s, she attended a presentation at the Iowa Osteopathic Association meeting by Fred Mitchell Sr, DO, FAAO, on a technique he termed "muscle energy." She thought this technique suited her better than the high-velocity/low-amplitude techniques she had been trained in. She travelled to Chattanooga several times over the succeeding years, spending

4–5 days with Dr. Mitchell each time, but was frustrated by her inability to make the technique work in her own clinic. Dr. Mitchell, in turn, had become frustrated by his inability to teach others his technique, so when Dr. Sutton suggested he teach a week-long tutorial to a small group, he readily agreed.

The first Muscle Energy Tutorial was taught in 1970, at Dr. Sutton's home in Fort Dodge, Iowa. The week-long course was taught to Sally Sutton, Edward Stiles, Phillip Greenman, John Goodrich, and Roland Miller (each of whom became distinguished in their own right). Unbeknownst to the attendees, Dr. Mitchell had decided that if he could not teach these five individuals, he would never talk about muscle energy again. This tutorial changed the course of osteopathic education and manipulative medicine, the results of which reverberate to this day.

Nineteen-seventy was also the year Dr. Sutton was president of the AAO. Taking advantage of her position, she invited two students to Convocation, the first time any students had been invited to a major professional society meeting. We now can hardly imagine a specialty society meeting that does not include some level of student involvement.

Sara "Sally" Sutton, DO, FAAO, dedicated her life to teaching and practicing osteopathy as a comprehensive system of medicine in which osteopathic manipulation was but a piece. She insisted upon the importance of history, physical examination, and differential diagnosis in every clinical encounter. She continued to practice osteopathic medicine until her late 80s when a series of injuries prevented her from continuing her practice. Despite her limitations, she still invited students into her home to learn and practice osteopathic manipulation, physical examination, clinical reasoning and osteopathic philosophy.

Sally was both friend and mentor to me. Her professional achievements are extensive, but speak little to the woman, the person, she was. She could be a difficult task master, demanding dedication and attention to detail. But she always did so with the intent of making those she instructed the best osteopathic physician they might be. More than anything, though, Sally tried to bring people together, to build community. More than anyone, she recognized that it was not for individual achievement or adulation, but rather that in working together, teaching one another, we could improve the entire profession and the world around us.

Dr. Sutton's last years were plagued by health issues that did not allow her to interact with others as she wished. May you rest in peace, Sally, knowing the legacy of the lives you touched. Your efforts leave an indelible mark upon the entire osteopathic profession.

RICHARD G. SCHUSTER, DO

DEDICATION

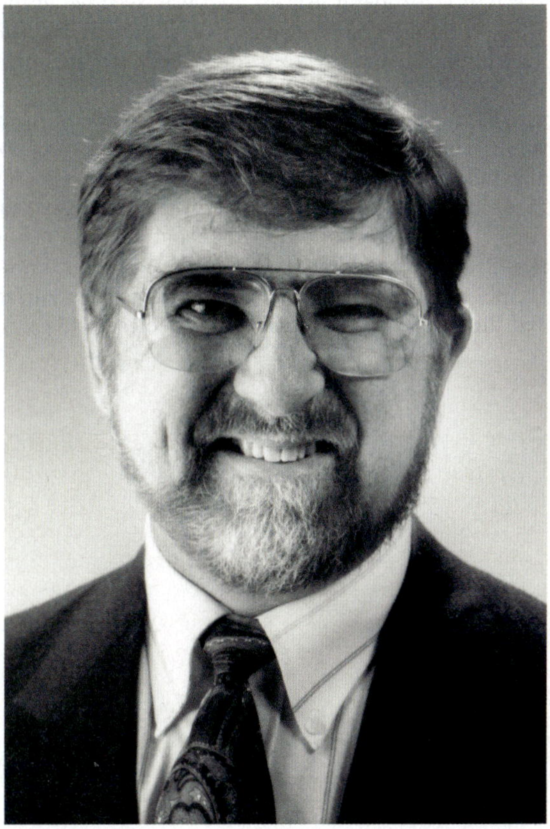

MICHAEL M. PATTERSON, PhD

1942–2022

(Photo courtesy of the American Osteopathic Association)

Michael M. Patterson, PhD (1942–2022) was born with the osteopathic profession in his blood. His father was H.M. Patterson, DO, a small town general practitioner in Mediapolis, Iowa. Michael was born in March 1942 in Muscatine, Iowa and graduated from Mediapolis High School. This was the beginning of a lifelong career in academics which spanned his graduation from Grinnell College in 1964 to receiving his PhD in Experimental Psychology from the University of Iowa in 1969. After completing further research training, he joined the faculty of AT Still University-Kirksville College of Osteopathic Medicine as an assistant professor in the Department of Physiology, where he worked with and was influenced by the legendary I.M. Korr, PhD.

Dr. Patterson made significant contributions to the basic science research foundations of osteopathic medicine, especially in the realm of the neurophysiologic basis of somatic dysfunction. He served as the Director of Research at three Colleges of Osteopathic Medicine from 1977 until retiring in 2008 (Ohio University, Athens, OH, Kansas City University College of Osteopathic Medicine and Nova Southeastern University, Ft. Lauderdale, FL). As his career progressed, he also conducted clinical research related to osteopathic manipulative treatment.

On a national level, Mike was an honorary lifetime member and significant figure in the American Academy of Osteopathy (AAO). He lectured many times at the AAO's annual convocation and served on the Academy's Louisa Burns Osteopathic Research Committee. Michael contributed his considerable editorial skills to the AAO, the American Osteopathic Association (AOA), and to osteopathic publications around the world. Mike was the Chair of the AAO's First International Symposium, "The Central Connection: Somatovisceral and Viscerosomatic Interactions." He was a long-time member of the AOA's Bureau of Research and chaired the

AOA Research Conference on three different occasions. He served as an Associate Editor for the AOA's *Journal of Osteopathic Medicine*, and the Foundations of Osteopathic Medicine textbook.

Dr. Patterson's contributions to osteopathy extended internationally as well. He taught in many countries for many organizations and schools, and also served as a board member for the World Osteopathic Health Organization. He earned many honors and awards, including the AOA's Gutensohn-Denslow Research and Education award, the AOA's Irvin M. Korr Award for Research, the AAO's Academy Award, and was awarded an honorary Diploma in Osteopathy by the College d'Etudes Osteopathiques de Montreal. Michael was also honored to receive the Distinguished Service Award from the American Osteopathic Association (the AOA's highest award) in 2017.

Mike was a dedicated family man, with many activities outside of his professional endeavors. He was an avid camper and loved international travel. He was proud of his distinguished Scouting career, in which he earned his Eagle Scout, was a scout master and earned the Silver Beaver award for distinguished service in scouting. He was an active leader in his church communities and a Rotarian.

Dr. Patterson's tireless dedication and immense contribution to the knowledge and advancement of the Osteopathic philosophy has influenced generations of physicians and will not soon be forgotten. Mike loved the osteopathic profession and dedicated his remarkable career to its success.

BOYD R. BUSER, DO, FACOFP (Dist)

SECTION EDITORS

Mischa Coleman, DO
Discipline Director of Osteopathic Manipulative Medicine
Department of Clinical Sciences
Rocky Vista University College of Osteopathic Medicine
Billings, Montana

Regina K. Fleming, DO
Assistant Dean of OPP/OMM
Associate Professor
Baptist University College of Osteopathic Medicine
Memphis, Tennessee

Chris LaFontano, DO
Assistant Dean of Osteopathic Integration
Department of Osteopathic Principles and Practices
Rocky Vista University College of Osteopathic Medicine
Englewood, Colorado

J'Aimee Lippert, DO
Associate Professor, Associate Department Chair
Department of Osteopathic Manipulative Medicine
College of Osteopathic Medicine
Michigan State University
East Lansing, Michigan

Crystal Martin, DO
Osteopathic Curriculum Director/Assistant Professor of Osteopathic Principles and Practice
Department of Family Medicine and Osteopathic Principles and Practice
Pacific Northwest University of Health Sciences
Yakima, Washington

David Mason, DO, MBA
Assistant Dean of Osteopathic Clinical Education and Professor
Department of Family Medicine and Osteopathic Manipulative Medicine
Texas College of Osteopathic Medicine
University of North Texas Health Science Center
Fort Worth, Texas

Kara Mintier, DO
Associate Professor
Department of Neuromusculoskeletal Medicine/Osteopathic Manipulative Medicine
College of Osteopathic Medicine of the Pacific—Northwest
Western University of Health Sciences
Lebanon, Oregon

Thomas Motyka, DO, MHPE
Associate Professor and Chair
Department of Osteopathic Manipulative Medicine
Jerry M. Wallace School of Osteopathic Medicine, Campbell University
Buies Creek, North Carolina

Nathan Nakken, DO
Chair, Osteopathic Principles and Practice
Department of Osteopathic Principles and Practice
Noorda College of Osteopathic Medicine
Provo, Utah

Kristin Putnam, DO
Assistant Professor, Osteopathic Principles and Practice
Department of Osteopathic Principles and Practice
Rocky Vista University College of Osteopathic Medicine
Aurora, Colorado

Deborah Schmidt, DO
Professor
Department of Osteopathic Principles and Practice
West Virginia School of Osteopathic Medicine
Lewisburg, West Virginia

Eva Shay, DO
Professor of Osteopathic Manipulative Medicine (Retired)
Department of Osteopathic Manipulative Medicine
Wichita, Kansas

Gregory Stevens, DO
Associate Clinical Faculty
College of Osteopathic Medicine
University of New England
Biddeford, Maine

Michael Terzella, DO
Associate Professor
Department of Osteopathic Manipulative Medicine
New York Institute of Technology College of Osteopathic Medicine
Old Westbury, New York

Frank H. Willard, MS, PhD
Professor of Anatomy
Department of Biomedical Sciences
College of Osteopathic Medicine
University of New England
Biddeford, Maine

Marissa Zajac, DO
Assistant Professor
Clinical Applied Science Education Department-Developing Osteopathic Clinical Skills
University of the Incarnate Word School of Osteopathic Medicine
San Antonio, Texas

CONTRIBUTORS

Peter Adler-Michaelson, DO
Private Practice
Sebastian, Florida

Ramey Alfarra, DO
Resident PGY2
Osteopathic Neuromusculoskeletal Medicine Residency
Lake Granbury Medical Center
Granbury, Texas

James S. Aston, DO
Assistant Professor
Department of Family Medicine and Osteopathic Manipulative Medicine
University of North Texas Health Science Center
Fort Worth, Texas

Mary Banihashem, MS, DO
Associate Professor, Director of Osteopathic Medicine Department
Department of Osteopathic Manipulative Medicine
Touro University
Bronxville, New York

Jordan L. Barry, DO
OMS-IV Osteopathic Manipulative Medicine Scholar
Department of Osteopathic Manipulative Medicine
Midwestern University
Downers Grove, Illinois

Ken Baxa, DO, AOBIM Internal Medicine, AOBIM Rheumatology, AOBNM Neuromuscular Medicine, and Osteopathic Manipulative Medicine
Physician
Department of Rheumatology
Clara Barton Hospital
Hoisington, Kansas

Jennifer A. Belsky, DO, MS
Director of Pediatric Lymphoma
Department of Pediatric Hematology/Oncology/BMT
Riley Hospital for Children at Indiana University Health
Indianapolis, Indiana

Amanda Bernett, BS
OMS-IV, Osteopathic Manipulative Medicine Scholar
Department of Osteopathic Manipulative Medicine
Chicago College of Osteopathic Medicine
Midwestern University
Downers Grove, Illinois

Eric Beveridge, DO
Resident Physician
Department of Pediatrics
University of Tennessee, College of Medicine Chattanooga
Chattanooga, Tennessee

Janice U. Blumer, DO, FAAO
Professor of Neuromusculoskeletal Medicine/Osteopathic Manipulative Medicine
Department of Neuromusculoskeletal Medicine/Osteopathic Manipulative Medicine
College of Osteopathic Medicine of the Pacific—Northwest
Western University of Health Sciences
Lebanon, Oregon

Timothy E. Blumer, DO
Child and Adolescent Psychiatrist
Department of Psychiatry
Samaritan Health Services
Corvallis, Oregon

Cameron Braz, MS
OMS-IV Osteopathic Manipulative Medicine Scholar
Department of Osteopathic Manipulative Medicine
Midwestern University
Downers Grove, Illinois

Kristen Brennan, DO
Resident Physician
Department of Osteopathic Manipulative Medicine
Midwestern University
Downers Grove, Illinois

Joseph P. Brindise, DO
Orthopaedic Spinal Surgeon
Orthopaedic Department
Romano Orthopaedic Center
River Forest, Illinois

Per Gunnar Brolinson, DO
Vice Provost for Research
Department of Sports Medicine
Edward Via College of Osteopathic Medicine
Blacksburg, Virginia

Stephanie Z. Brown, DO
Assistant Clinical Faculty
Department of Osteopathic Manipulative Medicine
AZCOM at Midwestern University
Glendale, Arizona

Denise K. Burns, DO, FAAO
Chairperson
Department of Osteopathic Manipulative Medicine
Touro College of Osteopathic Medicine
Middletown, New York

Cassaundra Burt, MD
Physician
Department of Obstetrics and Gynecology
Advocate Aurora Health
Chicago, Illinois

Todd Capistrant, DO, MHA
Physician
Department of Osteopathic Manipulative Medicine
Foundation Health Partners
Fairbanks, Alaska

Donald J. Ciancio III, DPT
Physical Therapist
Department of Orthopedic Physical Therapy
University of Chicago
Chicago, Illinois

Mae J. Ciancio, PhD
Associate Professor
Biomedical Sciences Program
Midwestern University
Downers Grove, Illinois

William Thomas Crow, DO
Physician, Private Practice
Ocoee, Florida

Gilbert E. D'Alonzo Jr, DO, MS
Professor of Thoracic Medicine and Surgery
Department of Thoracic Medicine and Surgery
Lewis Katz School of Medicine, Temple University
Philadelphia, Pennsylvania

Reem Darwish, BS
OMS-IV Osteopathic Manipulative Medicine Scholar
Department of Osteopathic Manipulative Medicine
Chicago College of Osteopathic Medicine
Midwestern University
Downers Grove, Illinois

Brian F. Degenhardt, DO, C-NMM/OMM
Assistant Vice Chancellor for Osteopathic Research
Professor
Department of Osteopathic Manipulative Medicine
A.T. Still University-Kirksville College of Osteopathic Medicine
Kirksville, Missouri

Lisa A. DeStefano, DO
Emeritus Professor
Department of Osteopathic Manipulative Medicine
College of Osteopathic Medicine, Michigan State University
East Lansing, Michigan

William H. Devine, DO
Clinical Professor
Postgraduate Education Program
AZCOM at Midwestern University
Phoenix, Arizona

Stephen E. DiCarlo, PhD
Professor
Department of Physiology
Michigan State University
East Lansing, Michigan

Dennis J. Dowling, DO, MA, FAAO
Attending Physician
Department of Physical Medicine and Rehabilitation
and Family Medicine
Nassau University Medical Center
East Meadow, New York

Robyn L.-F. Dreibelbis, DO
Associate Dean for Graduate Medical Education
Office of Graduate Medical Education
Idaho College of Osteopathic Medicine (ICOM)
Meridian, Idaho

Walter C. Ehrenfeuchter, DO, FAAO
Professor Emeritus
Department of Osteopathic Manipulative Medicine
PCOM Georgia
Suwanee, Georgia

David Eland, DO, FAAO
Professor and Chair
Department of Osteopathic Manipulative Medicine
Marian University College of Osteopathic Medicine
Indianapolis, Indiana

Mitchell L. Elkiss, DO, FACN, CSPOMM
Associate Professor of Neurology
College of Osteopathic Medicine
Michigan State University
East Lansing, Michigan
Emeritus Member Associates in Neurology, PC
Farmington Hills, Michigan
Co-Director of Curriculum Helms Medical Institute
Medical Acupuncture for Physicians
Berkeley, California

Nicholas C. Elwert, DO
Assistant Professor
Department of Physical Medicine and Rehabilitation
University of Kentucky
Lexington, Kentucky

Anna E. Esparham, MD
PGY4 Resident Physician
Department of Osteopathic Manipulative Medicine
A.T. Still University/Still OPTI
Kirksville, Missouri

Hugh M. Ettlinger, DO, FAAO, FCA
Director, ONMM Residency
Department of Osteopathic Manipulative Medicine
St. Barnabas Health System
Ossining, New York

Christian Evans, PT, PhD
Professor
Department of Physical Therapy
Midwestern University
Downers Grove, Illinois

Regina K. Fleming, DO
Assistant Dean of OPP/OMM
Associate Professor
Baptist University College of Osteopathic Medicine
Memphis, Tennessee

William Foley, DO, MSc
Founder and Osteopathic Consultant
Department of Osteopathic Medicine
Boston Osteopathic Health
Newton, Massachusetts

Christian Fossum, DO
Associate Professor
School of Health Sciences
Kristiania University College
Oslo, Norway

Marcel P. Fraix, DO, MBA, FAAPMR
Associate Dean, Admissions & Enrollment
Chair & Professor, Department of Physical Medicine & Rehabilitation
Chief, Section of Health Policy & Management, Department of Population Health Science
College of Osteopathic Medicine of the Pacific
Western University of Health Sciences
Pomona, California

Harry Friedman, DO, FAAO
Clinical Professor
Department of Family Medicine/Osteopathic Manipulative Medicine
Touro University California
Vallejo, California

David B. Fuller, DO, FAAO
Professor
Department of Osteopathic Manipulative Medicine
Philadelphia College of Osteopathic Medicine
Philadelphia, Pennsylvania

Stephen Fung, DO
Assistant Professor
Department of Family Medicine and Osteopathic Manipulative Medicine
University of North Texas Health Science Center
Fort Worth, Texas

John Gimpel, DO, MEd
President and CEO
Executive
National Board of Osteopathic Medical Examiners
Chicago, Illinois

Rebecca E. Giusti, DO
Professor, Chair of Neuromusculoskeletal Medicine/ Osteopathic Manipulative Medicine and Family Medicine
College of Osteopathic Medicine of the Pacific and College of Osteopathic Medicine of the Pacific—Northwest
Western University of Health Sciences
Pomona, California

John C. Glover, MS, DO, FAAO (Dist)
Emeritus Professor
Department of Osteopathic Manipulative Medicine
College of Osteopathic Medicine
Touro University California
Vallejo, California

Adam Grunbaum, DO
Rheumatologist
Department of Rheumatology
HCA Healthcare Florida/USF Morsani College of Medicine GME Consortium
Trinity, Florida

Sharon Gustowski, DO, MPH
Campus Dean
Office of the COM Campus Dean KC
Associate Professor of Osteopathic Manipulative Medicine
Department of Osteopathic Manipulative Medicine
Kansas City University College of Osteopathic Medicine
Kansas City, Missouri

Bill D. Hampton, DO, FACOEP
Emergency Physician
Emergency Department
Midwestern University
Downers Grove, Illinois

Malinda Hansen, DO, MS, CAQSM
Assistant Professor
Department of Family Medicine and Osteopathic Manipulative Medicine
Texas College Osteopathic Medicine
University of North Texas Health Science Center
Fort Worth, Texas

Mary Anne Morelli Haskell, DO
Associate Clinical Professor of Osteopathic Manipulative Medicine and Pediatrics
College of Osteopathic Medicine of the Pacific
Western University of Health Sciences
Pomona, California

Jason Haxton, MA, DO (hc)
Director, Museum of Osteopathic Medicine
University Advancement
A.T. Still University of Health Sciences
Kirksville, Missouri

Kurt P. Heinking, DO, FAAO
Professor and Chair of Osteopathic Manipulative Medicine
Chicago College of Osteopathic Medicine
Midwestern University
Downers Grove, Illinois

Jan T. Hendryx, MS, DO
Clinical Professor and Course Director
Department of Osteopathic Principles and Practice
Lake Erie College of Osteopathic Medicine
Erie, Pennsylvania

Kendi L. Hensel, DO, PhD, FAAO
Professor and Vice Chair
Department of Family Medicine and Osteopathic Manipulative Medicine
Texas College of Osteopathic Medicine
University of North Texas Health Science Center
Fort Worth, Texas

Stephanie Hermann, DO
Family Medicine Resident
Graduate Medical Education
OMIT Graduate Medical Education
Christ Health Family Medicine Residency at St. Vincent's East
Birmingham, Alabama

Natalie Hollick Price, DO
Pediatrician
Children's Primary Care Medical Group
San Diego, California

Robert W. Hostoffer, DO, MBA, MMED
Professor
Department of Pediatric Allergy/Immunology
Lake Erie College of Osteopathic Medicine
Erie, Pennsylvania

Raymond J. Hruby, DO, MS, FAAO (Dist)
Professor
Neuromusculoskeletal Medicine/Osteopathic Manipulative Medicine
College of Osteopathic Medicine of the Pacific
Western University of Health Sciences
Pomona, California

Teodor Huzij, DO
Associate Professor
Department of Osteopathic Principles and Practice
Rocky Vista University College of Osteopathic Medicine
Parker, Colorado

Natalie Hyppolite, DO, MBS
Chair of Department of Osteopathic Manipulative Medicine
College of Osteopathic Medicine
Chicago, Illinois

Annamarie C. Jansky, DDS
Floss Dental Care
Homewood, Illinois

John A. Jerome, PhD
Clinical Psychologist
East Lansing, Michigan

John M. Jones III, DO
Founding Chair and Professor (Retired)
Department of Osteopathic Principles and Practice
William Carey University College of Osteopathic Medicine
Hattiesburg, Mississippi

Alyssa Kampen, MS
OMS-IV Osteopathic Manipulative Medicine Scholar
Department of Osteopathic Manipulative Medicine
Chicago College of Osteopathic Medicine
Midwestern University
Downers Grover, Illinois

Brian E. Kaufman, DO
Physician and Adjunct Professor
College of Osteopathic Medicine
University of New England
Biddeford, Maine

Katie Kerrigan, DO
Assistant Professor
Department of Internal Medicine
Huntsman Cancer Institute
Salt Lake City, Utah

Hollis H. King, DO, PhD
Physician
Center for Integrative Medicine
UC San Diego School of Medicine
San Diego, California

Janice A. Knebl, DO, MBA
DSWOP Endowed Chair and UNT Regents Professor, Interim Chair, Department of Internal Medicine and Geriatrics, HSC Health Chief Medical Officer
Department of Internal Medicine and Geriatrics
University of North Texas Health Science Center
Fort Worth, Texas

Albert J. Kozar, DO, FAOASM, R-MSK
Professor of Sports Medicine and Osteopathic Manipulative Medicine and Program Director of Osteopathic Neuromusculoskeletal Medicine
Department of Sports Medicine and Osteopathic Manipulative Medicine
Edward Via College of Osteopathic Medicine
Blacksburg, Virginia

Samuel L. Krachman, DO
Professor of Medicine
Department of Thoracic Medicine and Surgery
Lewis Katz School of Medicine at Temple University
Philadelphia, Pennsylvania

Janet Krettek, DO
General Surgeon, Osteopathic Manipulative Medicine/Neuromusculoskeletal Medicine, Director of Medical Education/Designated Institutional Official
Surgery and Office of Medical Education
Holy Redeemer Hospital and Medical Center
Meadowbrook, Pennsylvania

Michael L. Kuchera, BA, BS, DO, C-SPOMM, FAAO
Clinical Professor
Department of Osteopathic Manipulative Medicine
Tom and Julie Wood College of Osteopathic Medicine
Marian University
Indianapolis, Indiana

Yein Lee, DO, MMS
Associate Professor
Department of Family Medicine and Osteopathic Manipulative Medicine
Texas College of Osteopathic Medicine
Fort Worth, Texas

Judith Oh Leonor, DO
Pediatrician
Department of Pediatrics
Loma Linda University Health
Loma Linda, California

John Licciardone, DO, MS, MBA
Regents Professor
Department of Family Medicine and Osteopathic Manipulative Medicine
University of North Texas Health Science Center
Fort Worth, Texas

J'Aimee Lippert, DO
Associate Professor, Associate Department Chair
Department of Osteopathic Manipulative Medicine
College of Osteopathic Medicine
Michigan State University
East Lansing, Michigan

Kenneth Lossing, DO
Private Practice
San Rafael, California

Michael Lough, DO
Resident Physician
Department of Anesthesiology and Pain Medicine
Cook County Hospital
Chicago, Illinois

Brian Loveless, DO
Chief Medical Officer and Professor of Neuromusculoskeletal Medicine/Osteopathic Manipulative Medicine
Chief Medical Officer, WesternU Health
Western University of Health Sciences
Pomona, California

Robert G. Lucas, DO
Resident
Osteopathic Neuromusculoskeletal Medicine Residency
Lake Granbury Medical Center
Granbury, Texas

Krista Lund, DO
Assistant Professor
Department of Neuromusculoskeletal Medicine/Osteopathic Manipulative Medicine
College of Osteopathic Medicine of the Pacific
Western University of Health Sciences
Pomona, California

Mary Ann Magoun, DO
Assistant Professor, Pediatrician
Department of Pediatrics, Neuromusculoskeletal Medicine
College of Osteopathic Medicine of the Pacific
Western University of Health Sciences
Pomona, California

Lukas Martincik, DO
Pediatrician
Group Practice,
Riverside, California

Kristina Martinez-Guryn, PhD, RD
Associate Professor
Department of Biomedical Sciences
Midwestern University
Downers Grove, Illinois

Mindy A. Chilman McComb, DO
Assistant Professor
Department of Osteopathic Manipulative Medicine
Michigan State University
East Lansing, Michigan

Christopher Medina, DO
Assistant Professor
Department of Family Medicine and Osteopathic Manipulative Medicine
Texas College of Osteopathic Medicine
University of North Texas Health Science Center
Fort Worth, Texas

Miriam V. Mills, MD, FAAP, FCA
Clinical Professor (Retired)
Department of Osteopathic Manual Medicine
Oklahoma State University Center for Health Sciences
Tulsa, Oklahoma

Veera Motashaw, DO, HMDC
Director of Outpatient University Palliative Care
Core Faculty, Hospice and Palliative Medicine Fellowship
Clinical Professor of Family Medicine
University Palliative Care
The University of Tennessee Medical Center
Knoxville, Tennessee

Nathan Nakken, DO
Chair, Osteopathic Principles and Practice
Department of Osteopathic Principles and Practice
Noorda College of Osteopathic Medicine
Provo, Utah

Meaghan C. Nelsen, DO, MS
Associate Professor
Department of Family Medicine and Osteopathic Manipulative Medicine
The University of North Texas Health Science Center-Texas College of Osteopathic Medicine
Fort Worth, Texas

Natalie A. Nevins, DO, MSHPE
Associate Dean of Graduate Medical Education and Program Development
College of Osteopathic Medicine
Touro University California
West Hollywood, California

Karen J. Nichols, DO, MA, MACOI, FACP, CS-F
Adjunct Clinical Professor (Retired)
Department of Internal Medicine
Chicago College of Osteopathic Medicine
Midwestern University
Mesa, Arizona

Clarence L. Nicodemus, DO, PhD
Professor and Director of the Center for Neuromusculoskeletal Clinical Research
Department of Osteopathic Neuromusculoskeletal Medicine/Osteopathic Manipulative Medicine
College of Osteopathic Medicine
Michigan State University
East Lansing, Michigan

David C. Nieman, DrPH
Professor
Department of Biology
Appalachian State University
Boone, North Carolina

Bobby B. Nourani, DO, FAAO
Associate Professor
Neuromusculoskeletal Medicine/Osteopathic Manipulative Medicine
College of Osteopathic Medicine of the Pacific
Western University of Health Sciences
Pomona, California

Judith A. O'Connell, DO, MHA, FAAO
President, Pain Alternatives, Inc.
Beavercreek, Ohio

Jessica Pelletier, DO
Medical Education Fellow
Department of Emergency Medicine
Washington University School of Medicine
St. Louis, Missouri

Thomas Pentzer, DO
Resident Physician
Department of Family Medicine/Osteopathic Manipulative Tratment
Maine Dartmouth Family Medicine Residency
Augusta, Maine

Kim Pfotenhauer, DO, FACOFP
Assistant Professor, Director of Clerkship Curriculum
Clinical Education and Family Medicine Programs
College of Osteopathic Medicine
Michigan State University
East Lansing, Michigan

Andrew J. Picca, DO, MAEd
Assistant Professor
Department of Pediatrics
Medical University of South Carolina
Charleston, South Carolina

John M. Popovich Jr, PhD, DPT, MS, BS
Assistant Professor
Department of Osteopathic Manipulative Medicine
Michigan State University
East Lansing, Michigan

Kristin Putnam, DO
Assistant Professor, Osteopathic Principles and Practice
Department of Osteopathic Principles and Practice
Rocky Vista University College of Osteopathic Medicine
Aurora, Colorado

Kenneth A. Ramey, DO, FACOFP
President and CEO
Ramey Wellness, Inc.
Parker, Colorado

Paul R. Rennie, DO, FAAO
Professor and Chair
Department of Osteopathic Manipulative Medicine
Touro University Nevada College of Osteopathic Medicine
Henderson, Nevada

Sarah E. Ross, DO, MS
Associate Professor
Department of Internal Medicine and Geriatrics
University of North Texas Health Science Center
Fort Worth, Texas

Maxwell Rouse, DO
Osteopathic Neuromusculoskeletal Medicine Fellow
MSU Health Care Osteopathic Manipulative Medicine
Michigan State University
East Lansing, Michigan

Kelly Rychter, DO
Cardiologist
Department of Cardiology
ProHealth Waukesha
Oconomowoc, Wisconsin

Jesus Sanchez Jr, DO, MSPHE, MA
Clinician, Professor, Researcher
Neuromusculoskeletal Medicine/Osteopathic Manipulative Medicine and Family Medicine
College of Osteopathic Medicine of the Pacific
Western University of Health Sciences
Pomona, California

Hans-Georg Schaible, MD
Senior Professor
Institute of Physiology 1
University Hospital Jena
Jena, Germany

Deborah Schmidt, DO
Professor
Department of Osteopathic Principles and Practice
West Virginia School of Osteopathic Medicine
Lewisburg, West Virginia

Mark D. Schuenke, PhD
Professor of Anatomy
Department of Biomedical Sciences
College of Osteopathic Medicine
University of New England
Biddeford, Maine

Ryan A. Seals, DO
Senior Associate Dean of Academic Affairs
Department of Family Medicine and Osteopathic Manipulative Medicine
Texas College of Osteopathic Medicine
Fort Worth, Texas

Michael A. Seffinger, DO
Professor Emeritus
Department of Neuromusculoskeletal Medicine/Osteopathic Manipulative Medicine
College of Osteopathic Medicine of the Pacific
Western University of Health Sciences
Pomona, California

Frank Serrecchia, DO
Clinical Associate Professor
Osteopathic Manipulative Medicine and Clinical Integration
Midwestern University
Downers Grove, Illinois

Mohamed Shitia, DO
Assistant Professor
Department of Sports Medicine
Edward Via College of Osteopathic Medicine
Blacksburg, Virginia

Anita Showalter, DO, MA, FACOOG (Dist)
Chair, Division Chief and Professor of OBGYN
Specialty Medicine
Proposed Duquesne University College of Osteopathic Medicine
Pittsburgh, Pennsylvania

Jay H. Shubrook, DO, FACOFP, FAAFP
Professor
Primary Care Department
College of Osteopathic Medicine
Touro University California
Vallejo, California

Kent P. Simmonds, DO, PhD
Resident Physician
Physical Medicine and Rehabilitation
University of Texas Southwestern Medical Center
Dallas, Texas

Maureen J. Simmonds, MSc, PT, PhD
Adjunct Professor
School of Public Health
University of Texas at San Antonio
San Antonio, Texas

Turner Slicho, DO, MS
Assistant Professor
Osteopathic Manipulative Medicine
Kansas City University
Kansas City, Missouri

Eric J. Snider, DO
Associate Professor and Chairperson
Department of Osteopathic Manipulative Medicine
A.T. Still University-Kirksville College of Osteopathic Medicine
Kirksville, Missouri

Karen T. Snider, DO, FAAO, FNAOME
Assistant Dean, Osteopathic Principles and Practice Integration
Department of Osteopathic Manipulative Medicine
A.T. Still University-Kirksville College of Osteopathic Medicine
Kirksville, Missouri

Karen M. Steele, DO, FAAO
Professor Emerita
Department of Osteopathic Medical Education
West Virginia School of Osteopathic Medicine
Lewisburg, West Virginia

Sajid A. Surve, DO, FAOCPMR
Assistant Dean of Osteopathic Recognition
Director of Osteopathic Education
Office of Educational Programs
Texas College of Osteopathic Medicine
University of North Texas Health Science Center
Fort Worth, Texas

Julie Swartzendruber, PhD
Associate Professor
Department of Microbiology and Immunology
Midwestern University
Downers Grove, Illinois

Gerald R. Thrush, PhD
Vice Dean, Academic Affairs
Office of Academic Affairs
Western University of Health Sciences
Pomona, California

Jeffrey Tsai, DO
Physician
Department of Anesthesiology
MultiCare Health
Tacoma, Washington

Angela K. Tyson, DO
Assistant Professor of Pediatrics
Department of Neonatology
The University of Rochester
Rochester, New York

Kevin D. Valvano, DO
Physician
Department of Sports Medicine
Private Practice
Parsippany, New Jersey

Richard L. Van Buskirk, DO, PhD, FAAO
President
Van Buskirk Osteopathic
Sarasota, Florida

Jason Vo, BS
OMS-IV Osteopathic Manipulative Medicine Scholar
Department of Osteopathic Manipulative Medicine
Chicago College of Osteopathic Medicine
Midwestern University
Downers Grove, Illinois

J. Michael Wieting, DO, MEd
Senior Associate Dean
Professor of Physical Medicine and Rehabilitation
Professor of Osteopathic Manipulative Medicine
Department of Osteopathic Manipulative Medicine and of Physical Medicine and Rehabilitation
Lincoln Memorial University-DeBusk College of Osteopathic Medicine
Harrogate, Tennessee

Scott Wilkie, DO, MS
Assistant Professor of Osteopathic Principles and Practices
Department of Osteopathic Principles and Practices
Rocky Vista University College of Osteopathic Medicine
Englewood, Colorado

Frank H. Willard, MS, PhD
Professor of Anatomy
Department of Biomedical Sciences
College of Osteopathic Medicine
University of New England
Biddeford, Maine

Adrian L. Woolley, DO
Director of Osteopathic Principles and Practice Education
Department of Osteopathic Clinical Medicine
College of Osteopathic Medicine
Des Moines University Medicine and Health Sciences
Des Moines, Iowa

Shan Shan Wu, DO
Allergist/Immunologist
Allergy/Immunology Associates, Inc.
Pulmonary and Critical Care
University Hospitals Cleveland Medical Center
Mayfield Heights, Ohio

Rajiv L. Yadava, DO
Private Practice
Optimal Medicine
St. Louis, Missouri

Sheldon C. Yao, DO, FAAO
Professor, Chair
Department of Osteopathic Manipulative Medicine
New York Institute of Technology College of Osteopathic Medicine
Old Westbury, New York

Miho Yoshida, DO, MA
Associate Clinical Professor
Department of Family and Community Medicine
University of California San Francisco, Fresno Campus
Fresno, California

FOREWORD

As a testament to the dedicated efforts of the members and governing bodies of the osteopathic profession, the number of students attending osteopathic medical schools has increased 77% over the past decade. Today, 25% of all U.S. medical students are educated at an accredited College of Osteopathic Medicine (COM). As osteopathic physicians, we share a common set of skills and a common vision. The Educational Council on Osteopathic Principles (ECOP) clarifies these commonalities into a shared lexicon—a lexicon that serves as the scaffolding to support the art that is osteopathic medicine. The unified curriculum incorporated within the fifth edition of *Foundations of Osteopathic Medicine* is integral to the continued supported expansion of osteopathic medicine.

The National Board of Osteopathic Medical Examiners (NBOME) was established in 1934, and by 1963, COMs were using the NBOME assessments as a quality assurance standard in preparing their future physicians. In 1969, the six COMs of that time—Kirksville, Des Moines, Philadelphia, Chicago, Kansas City, and Michigan—recognized a need to work together to standardize osteopathic language, curriculum, definitions, and technique standards; they founded the ECOP. The ECOP joined the American Association of Colleges of Osteopathic Medicine as a component council in 1974; the modern iteration of this body includes one OMM content expert representing each COM (most often the OMM department chair).

Working together to create a unified curriculum for all COMs, the ECOP—representing 41 accredited COMs and encompassing 66 teaching locations in 35 states—has created the *Teaching Guide for Osteopathic Manipulative Medicine*—commonly referred to as the "ECOP modules," the *Glossary of Osteopathic Terminology*, and various consensus documents and white papers, which are regularly updated and refined. The ECOP also collaborates with the NBOME to develop standardized osteopathic content and decrease "regionality" in board exam items, ensuring consistent testing for osteopathic students nationwide. Many ECOP members serve as national faculty for the NBOME and as site inspectors for the Commission on Osteopathic College Accreditation. The ECOP has also successfully updated the U.S. Systematized Medical Nomenclature for Medicine (SNOMED) database with osteopathic terms and is currently working on inputting our profession's terms into SNOMED International.

This fifth edition of *Foundations of Osteopathic Medicine* is a truly collaborative long-term effort by a diverse and dedicated group of clinical and biomedical science faculty from around the country. The ECOP members, both past and present, serve as executive editors, section editors, and authors in this text. This edition has incorporated key ECOP consensus documents to create a unified curriculum that faculty at all levels of osteopathic education can rely on to meet the educational needs of their students and residents.

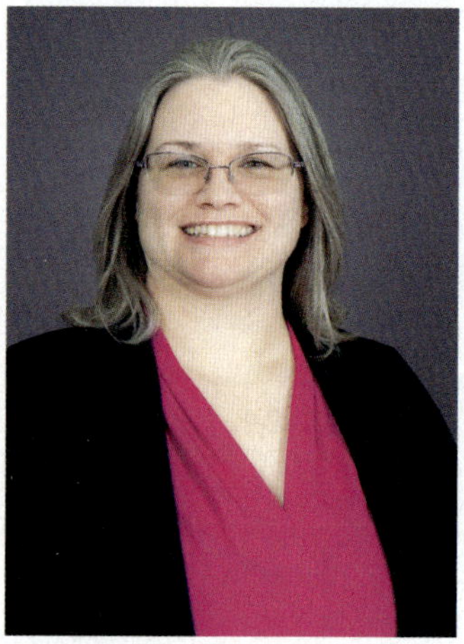

REGINA K. FLEMING, DO

Assistant Dean for Osteopathic Principles and Practice/Osteopathic Manipulative Medicine

Associate Professor, Baptist College of Osteopathic Medicine

Chair, Educational Council on Osteopathic Principles, AACOM

Board Member, American Osteopathic Board of Neuromusculoskeletal Medicine

Chair, Longitudinal Assessment Committee for Osteopathic Continuous Certification Component 4, American Osteopathic Board of Neuromusculoskeletal Medicine

National Faculty, National Board of Osteopathic Medical Examiners

FOREWORD

The year 2024 marks 150 years since Andrew Taylor Still "flung to the breeze the banner of Osteopathy," an auspicious date in the history of medicine in the United States and beyond. It has been nearly 30 years since the publication of the first edition of "*Foundations of Osteopathic Medicine*." Since its inception, this seminal text has been a beacon in the field, guiding students, clinicians, and educators through the principles and practices that define osteopathic medicine. Many things have changed in our profession since that first edition went to press. First and foremost, the number of DOs in the United States has more than tripled, coinciding with the rapid expansion of the number of accredited colleges of osteopathic medicine, a trend which shows no signs of abating. DOs currently comprise more than 11% of the U.S. physician workforce, and 25% of all medical students in the United States are enrolled in a college of osteopathic medicine.

The osteopathic profession has expanded internationally as well. The first osteopathic school outside the United States was established in London in 1915 by one of Dr. Still's students, Dr. J. Martin Littlejohn. Since then, the profession has developed along two distinct practice models, sharing the same principles and philosophical approach. The American Osteopathic Association (AOA) spearheaded the establishment of the Osteopathic International Alliance (OIA), which was formed 20 years ago. At that time, the worldwide profession recognized a need for a unifying international organization to interrelate with the World Health Organization (WHO) and to enhance communication and collaboration between the osteopath and osteopathic physician professional streams. The OIA has achieved the status of "official relations" with WHO, and OIA leadership has influenced WHO and worldwide health care through this relationship. In cooperation with WHO, the OIA is currently developing an international glossary of osteopathic terminology along with other projects important to the expansion of osteopathic health care. Other international advancements of the osteopathic profession include recognition of the status of U.S. trained osteopathic physicians by the United Nations' International Labor Organization, the World Federation for Medical Education, and the International Association of Medical Regulatory Authorities.

As the landscape of osteopathic medicine evolves, so too does our understanding of health and wellness. This edition reflects these advancements, offering updated perspectives on anatomy, physiology, pathology, and osteopathic principles and practices. It serves as a comprehensive resource for students embarking on their journey into osteopathic medicine, providing a solid foundation upon which to build their knowledge and skills.

Importantly, this text honors the legacy of the pioneers who laid the groundwork for osteopathic medicine. Their vision of treating the whole person—mind, body, and spirit—continues to resonate in today's health care environment, reminding us of the profound impact that compassionate, patient-centered care can have on healing.

I extend my gratitude to the authors, editors, and contributors whose tireless efforts have brought this edition to fruition. May "*Foundations of Osteopathic Medicine,*" now in its fifth edition, continue to inspire, educate, and shape the future of osteopathic health care for years to come. The continuing growth of our profession presents a greater opportunity to expand access to that training than ever before and ultimately to increase access to osteopathic medical care; what our patients want, what they deserve, and what all DOs are trained to provide.

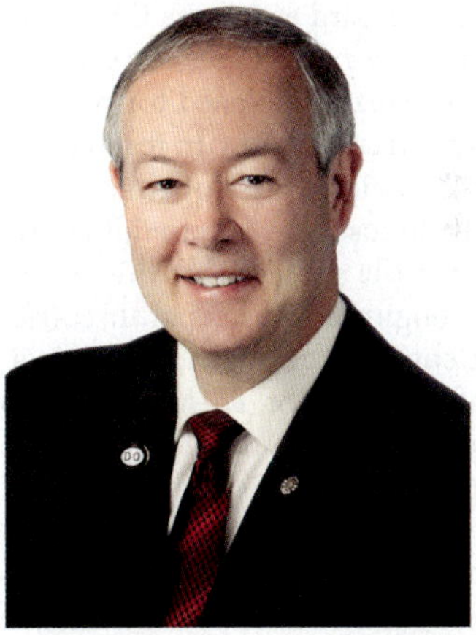

BOYD R. BUSER, DO, FACOFP (DIST)
Board Chair, Osteopathic International Alliance
Past President, American Osteopathic Association

FOREWORD

It is our privilege and honor to be osteopathic physicians and the executive editors of the fifth edition of *Foundations of Osteopathic Medicine*.

The history of this textbook is steeped in the richness and distinctiveness of the profession and has been both supported by and unified the major organizations of the profession today, the AOA, the AAO, AACOM, and the NBOME.

After Andrew Taylor Still passed away in 1917, the American Osteopathic Association (AOA) created the House of Delegates in 1920 to govern and set policies for the profession. They passed a resolution that the A.T. Still Research Institute, headed by Louisa Burns, DO, would publish an updated version of the most popular textbook on osteopathic principles with the addition of the most current scientific knowledge in support of the philosophy. The book was reviewed by all the osteopathic colleges at that time. As indicated by Dr. Buser in the fourth edition of this textbook, in 1922, this consensus-based textbook, *Hulett's Principles*, was published by the A.T. Still Research Institute as a revised edition of the classic textbook by G. D. Hulett, originally written at the turn of the 20th century.

With the advent of all osteopathic students sitting for the National Osteopathic Board exam, the Chairs of the Departments of Osteopathic Principles and Practice (OPP) of the six existing osteopathic schools realized the need for nationally unified osteopathic terminology and curriculum. In response to this, they formed the Educational Council on Osteopathic Principles (ECOP) in 1969. Part of their discussion was providing an updated comprehensive textbook for the profession. This informal proposal as a component of the longitudinal osteopathic curriculum in OPP was brought to the attention of the AOA Bureau of Research. In the late 1980s, the AOA Board of Trustees and House of Delegates provided financial support for the development of this textbook. After several proposals were reviewed, the project was launched in July 1990 under the supervision of the AOA Bureau of Research as the "Osteopathic Principles Textbook Project." Robert C. Ward, DO, FAAO, served as Executive Editor for the first and second editions of this textbook in 1997 and 2003. The third edition, published in 2011 and helmed by Anthony C. Chila, DO, FAAO, FCA (Dist), featured a restructured text demonstrating the osteopathic thought process in clinical practice. Michael Seffinger, DO, who had been involved with the textbook since its initial outline within the ECOP in 1984, became the executive editor of the fourth edition, published in 2018, adding color pictures, easy to use charts, and student-friendly formatting.

The mission statement of the first edition, like the osteopathic tenets, holds true today and indeed will remain timeless as advances in science, medicine, imaging, and technology continue to be incorporated into osteopathic medicine.

> *Osteopathic medicine is a philosophy, a science, and an art. Its philosophy embraces the concept of the unity of the living organism's structure and function in health and disease. Its science includes the biological, behavioral, chemical, physical, and spiritual knowledge related to the maintenance and restoration of health, as well as identification, prevention, cure, and alleviation of disease. Its art is the application of the philosophy in the practice of medicine and surgery in all its branches and specialties.*
>
> —Editorial Board, First meeting, July 1990, Chicago, Illinois

Since its first edition, the purpose of this textbook has been to guide students and physicians alike how to "think osteopathically." The text presents patient care through the distinctive lens of the osteopathic tenets, models of osteopathic care, palpatory diagnosis, and osteopathic manipulative treatment. It encompasses multiple specialties making it an excellent tool for all osteopathic students and physicians regardless of their training. The osteopathic principles and practice hold true for all fields of medicine. Gilbert Alonzo, DO, FACOI, wrote in the second edition of this text:

> *"This text is significant not only for students, but also for osteopathic physicians already in practice…I read portions of the first edition that focused on the etiology and clinical applications relating to somatic dysfunction. I found plausible scientific information that helped me better understand this particular concept in greater depth. The result was that it allowed me to apply osteopathic principles and practices to pulmonology and critical care medicine in ways I had never envisioned before… after reviewing these materials carefully, these special osteopathically oriented relationships became more understandable. As an osteopathic physician, I became much stronger."*

This edition involved the dedication and expertise of numerous DOs, PhDs, residents, and students. Many members of the AACOM-ECOP contributed to the writing of these chapters. As the members of the AACOM-ECOP are Chairs or designees of the Chairs of the NMM/OMM or OPP Departments nationwide, the information presented here will provide the foundational and in-depth material upon which the curriculum is based. As in-seat time continues to be challenged across colleges of osteopathic medicine across the nation, this textbook may provide the invaluable pre- and postread material that will allow students to have a deeper understanding of the interwoven anatomy, physiology, and palpatory diagnosis and treatment that are integral to osteopathic medicine. As education and assessment are closely linked, this textbook has historically served as a primary reference for the NBOME's COMLEX-USA licensure exam series as well as for the AOBNMM and other board certification exams.

Many osteopathic physicians chose this profession knowing that it would furnish them with opportunities that would both challenge them and provide continuous learning throughout their career, whether from patients, colleagues, or self-guided education. This edition offers new and seasoned authors, the latest evidence on underlying mechanisms of action and illumination on our history as new documents and information are uncovered. It is our hope that this edition will provide fresh perspective on the distinctiveness of our profession so that those who read it may gain a broader or different way of thinking that may transform their practice, all with the goal of improving the lives of those we serve, those who trust us, our very reason for choosing this incredible profession, our patients.

Dr. Still asked us to "Dig on," to keep on uncovering, for the betterment of humankind. This updated edition "digs on" in the constant quest to evolve and advance the osteopathic profession.

This book is dedicated to so many knowledgeable osteopathic physicians who came before us, but we would like to take a moment to include our patients, past, present, and future. Thank you for inspiring us, thank you for pushing us, thank you for holding us to a high standard of integrity and knowledge, and for making us use our heads, hands, and hearts to be the best osteopathic physicians possible. Without you, this textbook would not exist.

Sincerely,
Kurt P. Heinking, DO, FAAO
Rebecca E. Giusti, DO
Kendi L. Hensel, DO, PhD, FAAO

PREFACE

Welcome to the fifth edition of *Foundations of Osteopathic Medicine*. The history of this textbook is rich, and its content provides the reader with expert opinions from many outstanding physicians, clinicians, and academics. This textbook represents a body of hard work and dedication by devoted authors, section editors, artists, staff, librarians, and many others. It is a multidisciplinary, interprofessional text that highlights the distinctiveness of the osteopathic profession, with its unique education, skills, and the abilities of osteopathic physicians.

The text "*Foundations for Osteopathic Medicine*" had its beginnings as an outline within the Educational Council of Osteopathic Principles (ECOP) in 1984, leading to its first published edition in 1991. It is now in its fifth edition, some 35 years later, combining ideas and expertise to culminate in a profession-wide textbook. Each successive edition was edited by an expert in osteopathic manipulative medicine (Drs. Ward, Chila, and Seffinger) and has now grown to such a size that three executive editors were necessary to share the workload. Prior editions included new and updated chapters that alternated the focus on specialty or population-based patient care and case-based patient care. The organizational structure changed from edition to edition based on feedback, author, and editor preference. Currently, many historic drawings crafted by William A. Kuchera, DO, FAAO are still utilized for their exceptional utility in making complex topics easy to understand for the reader. In addition, color photos, illustrations, and new images have been added to facilitate clarity and ease of reading.

For many years, this textbook has been crafted and utilized as a primary reference text for the education of osteopathic medical students. It has also been used by residents and physicians in practice looking to review and refresh concepts and skills. One of its goals is to help students, residents, and clinicians grasp how to "think osteopathically" and implement the distinctive osteopathic philosophy into patient care.

For the fifth edition of this book, substantial changes have been made with significant updates and modernization of references. In this undertaking, the editors have utilized many new authors with fresh ideas. While all chapters were reviewed and edited, approximately 23 chapters have been completely rewritten or are brand new topics for this edition. The rewritten and new chapters are listed below:

- Chapter 10: Musculoskeletal Vibration Physiology
- Chapter 19: Role of "Spirit" and Spirituality in the History of Osteopathic Medicine
- Chapter 20: Spirituality and Health Care
- Chapter 23: Microbiome: New Considerations in Clinical Management
- Chapter 25: Medical Professionalism and the Physician–Patient Relationship
- Chapter 38: Functional Anatomy and Diagnosis of the Sacrum
- Chapter 39: Upper Extremity
- Chapter 40: Lower Extremity
- Chapter 63: Fascial Distortion Model
- Chapter 64: Integrated General Osteopathic Technique
- Chapter 71: Osteopathic Considerations in Cardiovascular Medicine
- Chapter 72: Osteopathic Considerations in Pulmonology
- Chapter 85: Osteopathic Considerations in Emergency Medicine
- Chapter 88: An Osteopathic Approach to the Exercise Prescription
- Chapter 90: Performing Arts Medicine
- Chapter 91: Osteopathic Approach to Diagnosing and Treating Somatic Dysfunction in the Extremities
- Chapter 92: Postural Considerations in Osteopathic Diagnosis and Treatment
- Chapter 93: Osteopathic Considerations in the Patient with Low Back Pain
- Chapter 94: Overview of Methods and Evidence Relating to Osteopathic Manipulative Treatment Research
- Chapter 108: COVID-19
- Chapter 111: Case Study: Upper Extremity
- Chapter 112: Case Study: Supination Ankle Sprain
- Chapter 113: Case Study: Endocrinology

A new section of 17 cases has been created to enhance case-based learning in osteopathic medicine. The functional anatomy section has been completely updated and is now called the Functional Anatomy and Diagnosis (FAD) section. It reviews the relevant anatomy and includes the regional diagnosis of somatic dysfunction. The material on sacrum has been completely rewritten, enhanced, and placed in one location. The section on the ECOP treatment modules has been updated with the most recent information from the ECOP module subcommittees. The chapters on somatic dysfunction in the extremities have been completely reworked and updated to help the ECOP reach professional consensus on the described dysfunctions. An updated glossary based upon terms defined by the ECOP has been included. Although the textbook is not specifically a procedure manual, osteopathic manipulative treatment procedures taught at many osteopathic colleges around the country are included as examples.

This fifth edition of FOM has been crafted with the goal of maintaining the historic tradition of the book yet enhancing and updating the material. It was organized with a modified framework, so that educators at the osteopathic schools can more readily find and utilize the content for their educational programs.

It has been an honor to complete this text in service to the osteopathic profession. We hope it serves our ultimate goal: to improve osteopathic medical education for students, and osteopathic medical care for patients.

Sincerely,
Kurt P. Heinking, DO, FAAO
Rebecca E. Giusti, DO
Kendi L. Hensel, DO, PhD, FAAO

ACKNOWLEDGMENTS

The Foundations of Osteopathic Medicine Textbook project has contributed to distinctive osteopathic practice for more than 30 years. It is an enormous undertaking to write, maintain, and update a distinctive, multidiscipline, multigenerational, profession-wide textbook. The success of the project is due to the talented and dedicated people both past and present who contributed their time, effort, and knowledge to this textbook. The FOM5 project has been at the forefront of my professional duties and responsibilities for the past several years. I am thankful and appreciative of many of my students, colleagues, and staff as well as members of the ECOP, who have assisted and supported me through this time.

I would like to acknowledge and thank the Midwestern University/CCOM OMM Department pre-doctoral student scholars for all their writing, editing, formatting, and computer assistance: Kristen Brennan, Sonja Hedblom, Michael Lough, Stephanie Hermann, Emily Daly, Ryan Schultz, Jordan Barry, Cameron Braz, Jason Vo, Aly Kampen, Amanda Bernett, and Reem Darwish.

I would like to acknowledge and thank the Midwestern University/CCOM OMM Department faculty for all their academic support and editing, assistance: Dr. Haley Koth, Dr. Alyssa Hart, Dr. Mark McKeigue, Dr. Kim McKinnon, and Dr. Frank Serrecchia. I would also like to thank our education specialist Ms. Yejide Samuel and senior administrative assistant Laura Trusk for their support and help in managing my busy schedule.

I would like to acknowledge and thank the Midwestern University administration, specifically President Dr. Kathleen Goeppinger and Dean Dr. Tom Boyle for their support during the production of this textbook and for their dedication to the advancement of the osteopathic profession.

Finally, I would also like to thank my wife Laura, son Kyle, and daughter Samantha for allowing me to sit for hours and days at a time feverishly working at the computer—evenings, weekends, and holidays until the project was complete.

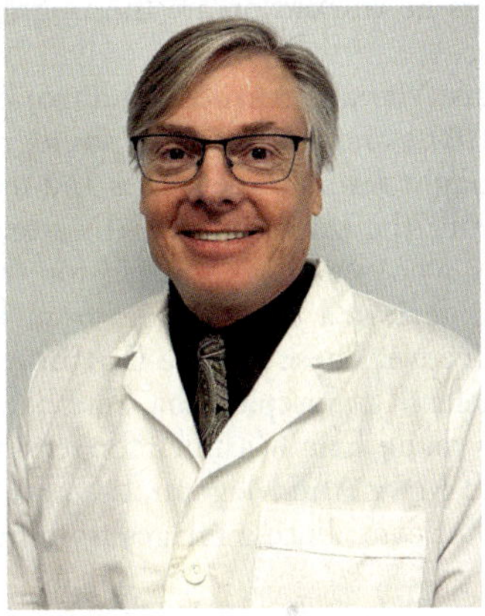

EXECUTIVE EDITOR: KURT P. HEINKING, DO, FAAO

ACKNOWLEDGMENTS

I wish to acknowledge the many contributions of Western University to this edition of *Foundations of Osteopathic Medicine*. First, this edition would not be as complete and thorough without the skills and expertise of our research assistant, Eric Martinez, BS. He has been an invaluable member of the NMM/OMM Department for the past 5 years. He painstakingly ensured that all of the chapters provided to him were referenced appropriately, oftentimes searching out hard to find resources, finding appropriate updated sources, and creating and revising multiple charts and key figures. Thanks to his diligence and attention to detail, the chapters he worked on are thoroughly researched and updated.

I wish to thank Maria (Fernanda) Durazo, BA for her expertise in the Visual Arts and her amazing photography and editing skills. She has brought several experiences and techniques to life.

I wish to thank the numerous Pre-Doctoral NMM/OMM Teaching Fellows who served as models for the images in the edition as well as reviewed the chapters from both an editorial and student perspective. These include Eric Beveridge, Lisa Chik, Keiko Inouye, Kaelen Kay, Joseph Luba, Pete Bae, and Tyler Beale.

I also wish to thank Eric Martinez for serving as a model for several images and Mary Ann Magoun, DO, FAAP for serving as a model and also for contributing images from her practice.

I could not have completed this important project without the support of my amazing NMM/OMM Department faculty, Dr. Ray Hruby, Dr. Mindy A. Chilman McComb, Dr. Krista Lund, Dr. Kara Mintier, Dr. Bobby Nourani, Dr. Brian Loveless, Dr. Jesus Sanchez (all of whom were authors and/or editors for this edition), Dr. David Redding, Dr. Ed Goering, Dr. Bachtuyet Le, and Dr. Megan Smith. I wish to extend a big thank you to the NMM/OMM staff, our amazing Office Manager, Carlos Mendez and our administrative assistants, Christine Ross, Maria (Fernanda) Durazo, and Katherine Olsen and support staff, Tiffany Scott, Shaina Burnett, and Laura Hysell.

I want to thank my patients for putting up with my hectic schedule as I worked on this project and thank you to two of our students, Pallavi Sripathi and Sunjum Singh, who served as the models for the cover of this textbook and are also pictured here.

This project would not have been possible without the blessing and support of the Western University and COMP and COMP-NW leadership; former Interim Dean Dr. David Connett, Dean Warren, Provost Crone, and President Farias-Eisner. Thank you so much for your dedication to the advancement of the osteopathic profession.

And thank you to Dr. Mickey Seffinger for this amazing opportunity. This was not possible without you!

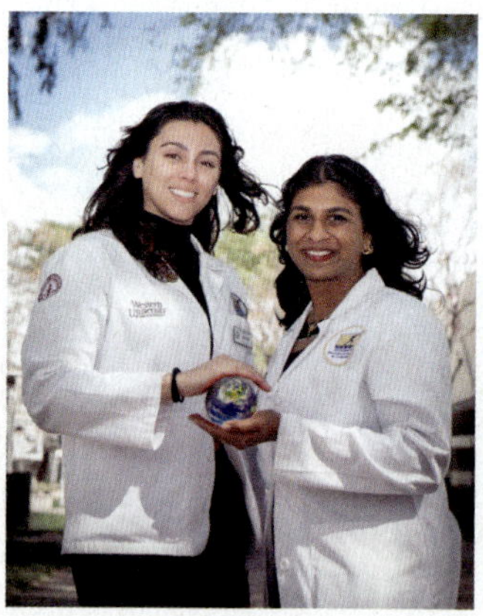

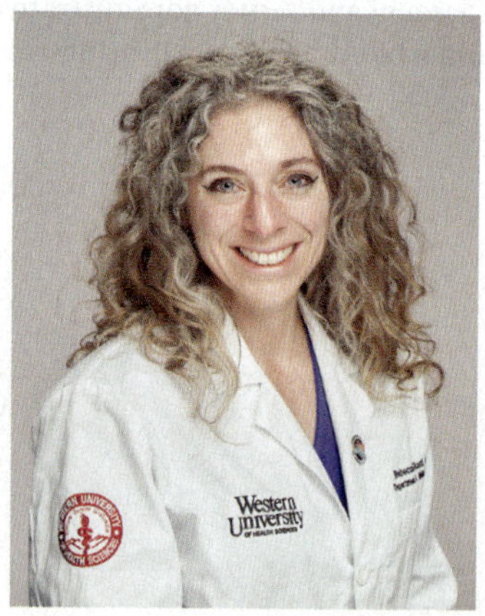

EXECUTIVE EDITOR: REBECCA E. GIUSTI, DO

ACKNOWLEDGMENTS

A project like FOM5 is an incredible undertaking. It involved 113 chapters with lead authors, many secondary or tertiary authors, 16 section editors, 3 executive editors, a team at Wolters Kluwer, and countless others that read bits and pieces, wrote material in previous editions that was carried forward and updated in this edition, or supported in some way. It represents 4 years of work, from conception to print.

I would like to thank the incredible faculty at the Texas College of Osteopathic Medicine for their support, encouragement, and contribution to this edition of Foundations. All our OMM faculty were authors or section editors, including Dr. Malinda Hansen, Dr. Ryan Seals, Dr. Yein Lee, Dr. Sajid Surve, Dr. Meaghan Nelsen, Dr. Stephen Fung, Dr. James Aston, Dr. David Mason, and Dr. Christopher Medina. Two residents from the new Lake Granbury Medical Center ONMM Residency also contributed, Dr. Robert Lucas and Dr. Ramey Alfarra.

A special thank you to a few pinch hitters, that stepped up to rewrite, edit, or review chapters on a short timeline: Dr. Karen Snider, Dr. Sharon Gustowski, Dr. Mindy A. Chilman McComb, Dr. Laura Griffin, and Dr. Lisa DeStefano.

Also, many thanks to ECOP for their support and involvement. Many volunteers for FOM5 were obtained through emails and announcements at ECOP meetings.

My involvement would not have been possible without the support of my department chair, Dr. Curtis Galke, TCOM former dean Dr. Frank Filipetto, TCOM dean Dr. Lisa Nash, UNTHSC Provost Dr. Charles Taylor, and President Dr. Sylvia Trent-Adams.

Finally, I would like to thank my family and friends, namely my late husband Shannon Dyer, daughter Kaylin Dyer, Lisa DeStefano, and Laura Griffin for their encouragement and support through this process. I love you all!

Thank you all for your commitment to advancing osteopathic education.

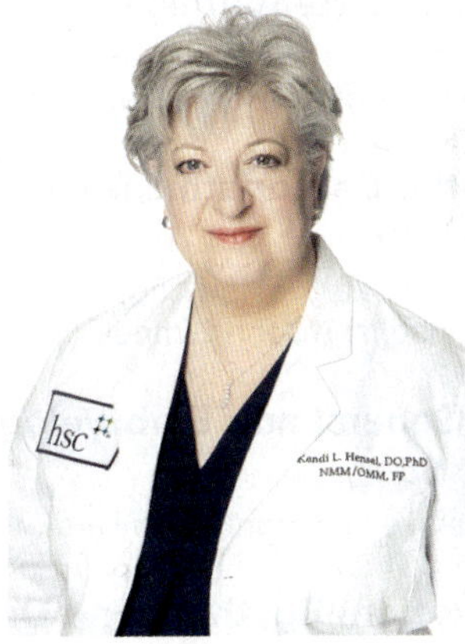

EXECUTIVE EDITOR: KENDI L. HENSEL, DO, PhD, FAAO

CONTENTS

PART ONE

Origins of Osteopathic Medicine and Foundational Concepts

1

Philosophy of Osteopathic Medicine

MICHAEL A. SEFFINGER ▪ RAYMOND J. HRUBY ▪ FRANK H. WILLARD ▪ JOHN LICCIARDONE ▪ JOHN M. JONES III ▪ HOLLIS H. KING

KEY CONCEPTS

- Osteopathic philosophy forms the foundation for the practice of osteopathic medicine, which is a comprehensive and scientifically based school of medicine.
- Classic osteopathic philosophy was articulated by the founder of the profession, Dr. Andrew Taylor Still, and his direct students.
- Classic osteopathic philosophy expresses Dr. Still's understanding of health and disease and his approach to patient care.
- Various aspects of osteopathic philosophy and principles have ancient historical roots, but, as a unified set of concepts, the philosophy represents a unique approach to health and patient care.
- The expression and emphasis of osteopathic philosophy and its tenets continue to evolve over time.
- Irvin M. Korr, PhD, as a professor at several osteopathic colleges throughout the latter half of the 20th century, eloquently expressed the tenets of osteopathic philosophy to generations of osteopathic students, physicians, and scientists.
- The Educational Council on Osteopathic Principles (ECOP) of the American Association of Colleges of Osteopathic Medicine developed a Glossary of Osteopathic Terminology and identified the fundamental osteopathic approaches to patient care.
- Osteopathic principles guide osteopathic physicians toward a health-oriented, patient-centered approach to health care.

INTRODUCTION

Osteopathic philosophy, deceptively simple in its presentation, forms the basis for osteopathic medicine's distinctive approach to health care. The philosophy acts as a unifying set of ideas for the organization and application of scientific knowledge to patient care. Through the philosophy, this knowledge is organized in relation to all aspects of health (physical, mental, emotional, and spiritual). A patient-centered focus, using health-oriented principles of patient care and unique skills, including hands-on manual diagnosis and treatment, guides the application of that knowledge. These concepts form the foundation for practicing osteopathic medicine.

Viewpoints and attitudes arising from osteopathic principles give osteopathic physicians an important template for clinical problem-solving, health restoration and maintenance, and patient education. This viewpoint is particularly useful as practitioners from a wide variety of disciplines confront increasingly complex physical, psychological, social, ethical, and spiritual problems affecting individuals, families, and populations from a wide variety of cultures and backgrounds.

HOW IT ALL BEGAN

Andrew Taylor Still, Physician and Surgeon, DO (Fig. 1.1) (1828–1917), was an American frontier doctor who was convinced that the patient care of his time was severely inadequate. This resulted in an intense desire on his part to improve surgery, obstetrics, and the general treatment of diseases, placing them on a more rational and scientific basis.

As his perspectives and clinical understanding evolved, Still created an innovative system of diagnosis and treatment with two major emphases. The first highlights treatment of physical and mental ailments (i.e., diseases) while emphasizing the normalization of body structures and functions. Its hallmark was a detailed knowledge of anatomy that became the basis for much of his diagnostic and clinical work, most notably palpatory diagnosis and manipulative treatment. The second emphasizes the importance of health and well-being in its broadest sense, including mental, emotional, and spiritual health, and the avoidance of alcohol and drugs and other habits that adversely impact health.

ORIGINS OF OSTEOPATHIC PHILOSOPHY

Historically, Still was not the first to call attention to inadequacies of the health care of his time; Hippocrates (c. 460–c. 377 B.C.E.), Galen (c. 130–c. 200), and Sydenham (1624–1689) were others. Each, in his own way, criticized the inadequacies of existing medical practices while focusing contemporary thinking on the patient's natural ability to heal.

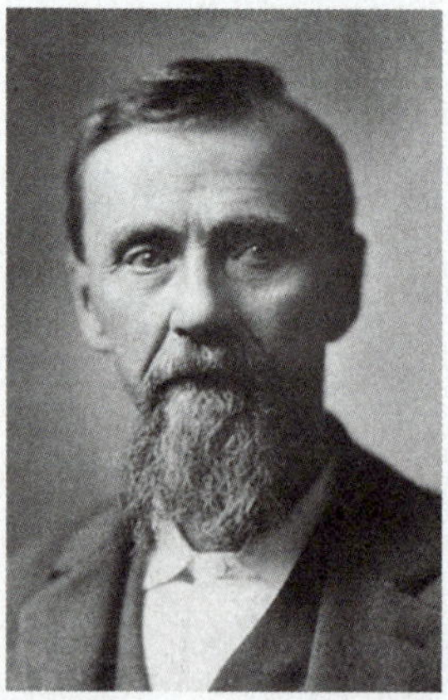

Figure 1.1. A.T. Still, Founder of Osteopathy. (Reprinted with permission from Still National Osteopathic Museum, Kirksville, MO.)

In addition, Still was deeply influenced by a number of philosophers, scientists, and medical practitioners of his time. There is also evidence he was well versed in the religious philosophies and concepts of the Methodist, Spiritualist, and Universalist movements of the period.[1]

Following the loss of three children to spinal meningitis in 1864, Still immersed himself in the study of the nature of health, illness, and disease.[2] His goal was to discover definitive methods for curing and preventing all that ailed his patients. He implicitly believed there was "a God of truth," and that

> *All His works, spiritual and material, are harmonious. His law of animal life is absolute. So wise a God had certainly placed the remedy within the material house in which the spirit of life dwells.*

Furthermore, he believed he could access these natural inherent remedies

> *... by adjusting the body in such a manner that the remedies may naturally associate themselves together, hear the cries, and relieve the afflicted.*[2]

In this quest, he combined contemporary philosophical concepts and principles with existing scientific theories. Always a pragmatist, Still accepted aspects of different philosophies, concepts, and practices that worked for him and his patients. He then integrated them with personal discoveries of his own from in-depth studies of anatomy, physics, chemistry, and biology.[1] The result was the formulation of his new philosophy and its applications. He called it "osteopathy."

Still's moment of clarity came on June 22, 1874. He writes,

> *I was shot, not in the heart, but in the dome of reason.*[2]

> *Like a burst of sunshine the whole truth dawned on my mind, that I was gradually approaching a science by study, research, and observation that would be a great benefit to the world.*[2]

He realized that all living things, especially humans, were created by a perfect God. If humans were the embodiment of perfection, then they were fundamentally made to be healthy. There should be no defect in their structures and functions.

Since he believed that "the greatest study of man is man," he dissected numerous cadavers to test his hypothesis.[2] He believed that if he could understand the construction (anatomy) of the human body, he would comprehend nature's laws and unlock the keys to health. Still found no flaws in the concepts of the body's well-designed structure, proving to himself that his own hypothesis was correct.

A corollary to Still's revelation was that the physician does not cure diseases. In his view, it was the job of the physician to correct structural disturbances so the body works normally, just as a mechanic adjusts his machine. In Research and Practice he wrote,

> *The God of Nature is the fountain of skill and wisdom and the mechanical work done in all natural bodies is the result of absolute knowledge. Man cannot add anything to this perfect work nor improve the functioning of the normal body.... Man's power to cure is good as far as he has a knowledge of the right or normal position, and so far as he has the skill to adjust the bones, muscles and ligaments and give freedom to nerves, blood, secretions and excretions, and no farther. We credit God with wisdom and skill to perform perfect work on the house of life in which man lives. It is only justice that God should receive this credit and we are ready to adjust the parts and trust the results.*[3]

While Still practiced the orthodox medicine of his day from 1853 to 1879, including the use of oral medications, such as purgatives, diuretics, stimulants, sedatives, and analgesics, and externally applied salves and plasters, once he began using his new philosophical system, he virtually ceased using drugs. This occurred after several years where he experimented with combinations of drugs and manipulative treatment. In addition, he compared his results with those of patients who received no treatment at all.[2] After several years' experience, he became convinced that his mechanical corrections consistently achieved the same or better results without using medications.

It was at that point that Still philosophically divorced himself from the orthodox practices of 19th century medicine.[2] He writes,

> *Having been familiar myself for years with all their methods and having experimented with them I became disheartened and dropped them.*[3]

His unerring faith in the natural healing capabilities of the mechanically adjusted body formed the foundation for his new philosophy.

Unsure of what to call his new hands-on approach in the early years, Still at times referred to himself as a "magnetic healer" and "lightning bonesetter."[1,4] In the 1880s, Still began publicly using the term "osteopathy" as the chosen name for his new profession.[1,5] He writes,

> *Osteopathy is compounded of two words, osteon, meaning bone, (and) pathos, (or) pathine, to suffer. I reasoned that the bone, 'Osteon,' was the starting point from which I was to ascertain the cause of pathological conditions, and so I combined the 'Osteo' with the 'pathy' and had as a result, Osteopathy.*[2]

As the name osteopathy implies, Still used the bony skeleton as his reference point for understanding clinical problems and their pathologic processes. On the surface, he was most interested in anatomy. On the other hand, he taught that there is more to the skeleton than 206 bones attached together by ligaments and connective tissue. In his discourses, Still would describe the anatomy of the arterial supply to the femur, for example, trace it back to the heart and lungs, and relate it to all of the surrounding and interrelated nerves, soft tissues, and organs along the way (Fig. 1.2). He would then demonstrate how the obstruction of arterial flow anywhere along the pathway toward the femur would result in pathophysiologic changes in the bone, producing pain or dysfunction.

He writes of his treatment concepts:

> *Bones can be used as levers to relieve pressure on nerves, veins and arteries.*[2]

This can be understood in the context that vascular and neural structures pass between bones or through orifices (foramina) within a bone. These are places where they are most vulnerable to bony compression and disruption of their functions. In addition, fascia is a type of connective tissue that attaches to bones. Fascia also envelops all muscles, nerves, and vascular structures. When strained or twisted by overuse or trauma, myofascial structures not only restrict bony mobility but also compress neurovascular structures and disturb their functions. By using the bones as manual levers, bony or myofascial entrapments of nerves or vascular structures can be removed, thus restoring normal nervous and vascular functions.

As Korr explained,

> *Even at the time of the founding of the osteopathic profession in 1892, the available knowledge in the sciences of physiology, biochemistry, microbiology, immunology, and pathology was meager. Indeed, immunology, biochemistry, and various other neurosciences and biomedical sciences had yet to appear as distinct disciplines. Therefore, these principles could only be expressed as aphorisms, embellished perhaps with conjectures about their biological basis.*[6]

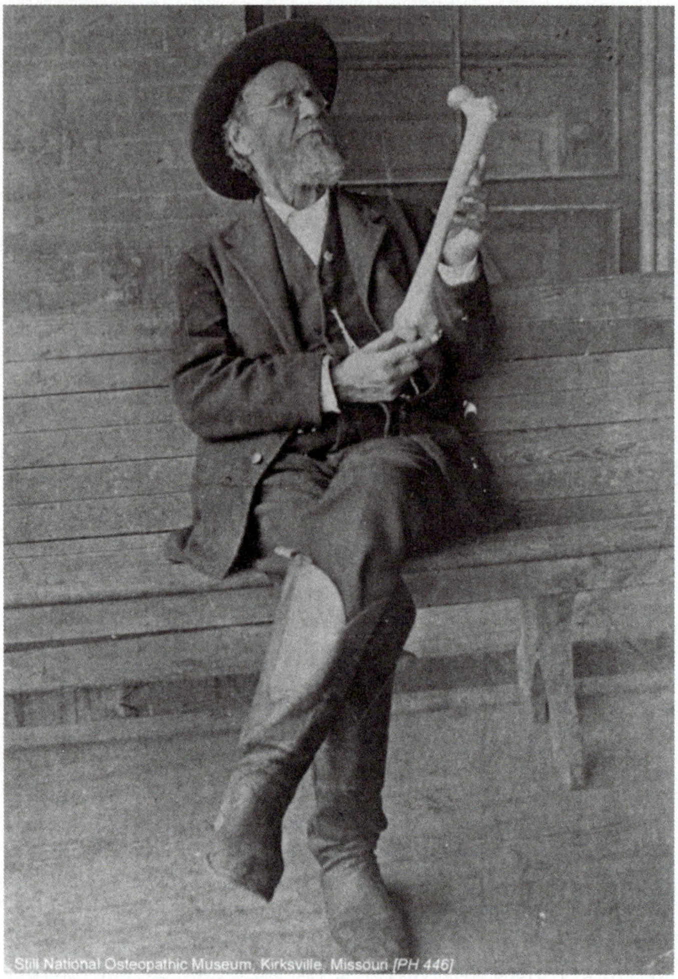

Figure 1.2. A. T. Still analyzing a human femur as he ponders the principles of osteopathy. (Reprinted with permission from Still National Osteopathic Museum, Kirksville, MO.)

Beyond Neuromusculoskeletal Diagnosis and Treatment

The osteopathic medical profession is not only a neuromusculoskeletal-oriented diagnostic and treatment system; it is also a comprehensive and scientifically based school of medicine that is grounded in a philosophy. In answer to the question "What is osteopathy?" Still stated,

> *It is a scientific knowledge of anatomy and physiology in the hands of a person of intelligence and skill, who can apply that knowledge to the use of man when sick or wounded by strains, shocks, falls, or mechanical derangement or injury of any kind to the body.*[7]

Furthermore, osteopathy had a greater calling. In what could be considered a mission statement, Still wrote,

> *The object of Osteopathy is to improve upon the present systems of surgery, midwifery, and treatment of general diseases.*[2]

The primary ideologic components that distinguish one philosophy of healing from another are that system's concepts of what constitutes health, disease, and patient care. The following sections delineate how osteopathic philosophy has evolved and expressed itself regarding these three concepts.

Classical osteopathic philosophy is described in Box 1.1.

BOX 1.1 Classical Osteopathic Philosophy

A.T. Still's fundamental concepts of osteopathy can be organized in terms of health, disease, and patient care.

Health

1. Health is a natural state of harmony.
2. The human body is a perfect machine created for health and activity.
3. A healthy state exists as long as there is normal flow of body fluids and nerve activity.

Disease

1. Disease is an effect of underlying, often multifactorial causes.
2. Illness is often caused by mechanical impediments to normal flow of body fluids and nerve activity.
3. Environmental, social, mental, and behavioral factors contribute to the etiology of disease and illness.

Patient Care

1. The human body provides all the chemicals necessary for the needs of its tissues and organs.
2. Removal of mechanical impediments allows optimal body fluid flow, nerve function, and restoration of health.
3. Environmental, cultural, social, mental, and behavioral factors need to be addressed as part of any management plan.
4. Any management plan should realistically meet the needs of the individual patient.

CLASSIC OSTEOPATHIC PHILOSOPHY OF HEALTH

Health Is a Natural State of Harmony

Still believed health to be the natural state of the human being. In his own words:

> *Osteopathy is based on the perfection of Nature's work. When all parts of the human body are in line we have health. When they are not the effect is disease. When the parts are readjusted disease gives place to health. The work of the osteopath is to adjust the body from the abnormal to the normal, then the abnormal conditions give place to the normal and health is the result of the normal condition.*[3]

Mechanics and Health

Still's concept of a healthy person is insightful. It places his belief of the importance of structural and mechanical integrity within the perspective of a comprehensive view of a human being within society:

> *When complete, he is a self-acting, individualized, separate personage, endowed with the power to move, and mind to direct in locomotion, with a care for comfort and a thought for his continued existence in the preparation and consumption of food to keep him in size and form to suit the duties he may have to perform.*[7]

Still believed that life exists as a unification of vital forces and matter. Since the body is controlled by the mind to exhibit purposeful motion in attaining the needs and goals of the organism, he stated that

> *Osteopathy … is the law of mind, matter and motion.*[2]

Once Still accepted that motion is an inherent quality of life itself, it was a small step to inquire into what is moving and how it moves. Through his in-depth study of anatomy, he could see the interdependent relationships among different tissues and their component parts. He observed that each part developed as the body was moving, growing, and developing from embryo to fetus to newborn and throughout life. Thus, each tissue, organ, and structure is designed for motion.

> *As motion is the first and only evidence of life, by this thought we are conducted to the machinery through which life works to accomplish these results.*[8]

If "life is matter in motion,"[7] then what is the effect on a body part that is not moving? Still reasoned that a lack of motion is not conducive to life or health.

> *[The osteopath's] duties as a philosopher admonish him that life and matter can be united, and that that union cannot continue with any hindrance to free and absolute motion.*[7]

Further, he boldly states that the practice of osteopathy

> *covers all phases of disease and it is the law that keeps life in motion.*[2]

Normal Nerve Activity and Flow of Body Fluids

A machine cannot run without proper lubrication, fuel, and mechanisms to remove the by-products of combustion. In teaching his students, Still identified each component of the body's intricate mechanisms as he knew them. In the process, he discussed various forces that he reasoned create motion and maintain life. He explained how lubricating and nourishing fluids flow through the arteries, veins, lymphatics, and nerves. He also noted that they turn over by-products of metabolism through the venous and lymphatic systems.

> *The human body is a machine run by the unseen force called life, and that it may be run harmoniously it is necessary that there be liberty of blood, nerves and arteries from their generating point to their destination.*[2]

Another component of Still's machine concept was the power source. He identified the brain as the dynamo, the electric battery that keeps the body moving and working:

> *The brain furnishes nerve-action and forces to suit each class of work to be done by that set of nerves, which is to construct forms and to keep blood constantly in motion in the arteries and from all parts back to the heart through the veins that it may be purified, renewed, and re-enter circulation.*[7]

CLASSIC OSTEOPATHIC PHILOSOPHY OF DISEASE

Disease Is an Effect of an Underlying Cause or Causes

From the time of Hippocrates through the first half of the 20th century, diseases were identified primarily through simple and complex descriptions of symptoms and signs. Many afflictions were without clear etiology. In spite of our current greater levels of knowledge and understanding, this is still true in many cases.

Still taught that disease is the effect of an abnormal anatomic state with subsequent physiologic breakdown and decreased host adaptability. Germs were first discovered in the 17th century with the invention of the microscope, but the germ theory of disease was not accepted until Pasteur provided convincing scientific evidence in the mid-19th century. However, experienced clinicians like Still, as well as an emerging group of laboratory scientists, saw germs as opportunists to decreased host function, not as primary causes of disease in themselves. They speculated that infections resulted from an interaction between the degree of virulence and quantity of the infecting agent and the level of host immunity.

Still also realized that there were multifactorial components to disease processes.[9,10] He believed that disease was a combination of influences arising from decreased host adaptability and adverse environmental conditions. He recognized that symptoms often were a manifestation of nerves irritated by pathophysiologic processes commonly created by an accumulation of fluids (congestion and inflammation). This diminished the patient's ability to adapt to the environment.[2] In addition, Still was keenly aware of the deleterious effects of environmentally induced trauma, or abrupt changes in the atmosphere, causing physical or emotional "shock" or inertia and therefore obstructing normal metabolic processes, body fluids, and nerve activity.[3]

Mechanical Impediments to Flow of Body Fluids and Nerve Activity

Still's study of pathology found that in all forms of disease there is mechanical interruption of normal circulation of body fluids and nerve force to and from cells, tissues, and organs.[3]

> *Sickness is an effect caused by the stoppage of some supply of fluid or quality of life.*[2]

He understood that it is the combination of free circulation of wholesome blood, and motor, nutrient, and sensory nerve activity that creates tissues and organs and facilitates their growth, maintenance, and repair. Through cadaver dissection studies, he reasoned that strains, twists, or distortions in fascia, ligaments, or muscle fibers surrounding the small capillaries and nerve bundles could very well be the cause of ischemia and congestion by mechanical obstruction, interruption, or impediment to normal flow of vital fluids.

Still understood that the flow of body fluids was under the control of the nerves that innervated blood vessel walls, adjusting the diameter of the vessels and thus controlling the amount and rate of blood flow to the tissues and organs.

> *While the vascular and nervous systems are dependent upon each other, it must be remembered that the bloodstream is under the control of the nervous system, not only indirectly through the heart, but directly through the vasoconstrictor and vasodilator nerve fibers, which regulate the caliber and rhythm of the blood vessels.*[10]

Still writes,

> *All diseases are mere effects, the cause being a partial or complete failure of the nerves to properly conduct the fluids of life.*[2]

Although he emphasized that

> *the rule of the artery is absolute, universal, and it must be unobstructed, or disease will result.*[2]

He also pointed out the importance of unimpeded flow of lymphatics:

> *[W]e must keep the lymphatics normal all the time or see confused Nature in the form of disease. We strike at the source of life and death when we go to the lymphatics.*[7]

However, even if the blood and the lymph are flowing normally, Still pointed out that

> *the cerebrospinal fluid is the highest known element that is contained in the human body, and unless the brain furnishes this fluid in abundance a disabled condition of the body will remain. He who is able to reason*

will see that this great river of life must be tapped and the withering field irrigated at once, or the harvest of health be forever lost.[8]

Holistic Aspects—Environmental and Biopsychosocial Etiologies

For the most part, Still described the origins of disease and illness as a result of

anatomic disturbances followed by physiologic discord.[2]

However, at the same time, he acknowledged the potential detrimental influences of heredity, lifestyle, environmental conditions, contagious diseases, inactivity and other personal behavior choices, and psychological and social stress on health.[7,9,10]

Still also recognized that all of the following contributed to illness and disease:

- Substance abuse (e.g., alcohol and opium)
- Poor sanitation
- Poor personal hygiene
- Dietary indiscretion
- Lack of exercise or fitness

He lectured passionately against the social forces that promulgated these deleterious behaviors and social situations, including slavery and economic inequities. Indeed, he spoke from personal experience as he and his family members suffered from these challenging social circumstances during the pioneer days of the 19th century Midwest.

CLASSIC OSTEOPATHIC PHILOSOPHY AND PATIENT CARE

The Body Provides Its Own Drug Store

Like many others, Still observed that some people are more susceptible to epidemic diseases than others. It was also recognized that host resistance to disease is more apparent in certain individuals who have so-called natural immunity that is either inherited or acquired.[11–13] Still believed that promoting free flow of arterial blood to an infected area would enable "Nature's own germicide" to eradicate the infectious agent.[3] Still's philosophy places complete trust in the innate self-healing ability of the body. Removing all hindrances to health was not enough, however, as it was incumbent upon the physician to ensure that the body's natural chemicals were able to work effectively in alleviating any pathophysiologic processes.[2]

Medications

On medications, Still writes,

I was born and raised to respect and confide in the remedial power of drugs, but after many years of practice in close conformity to the dictations of the very best medical authors and in consultation with representatives of the various schools, I failed to get from drugs the results hoped for and I was face to face with the evidence that medication was not only untrustworthy but was dangerous.[3]

Initially, Still conceived of osteopathic medicine as

a system of healing that reaches both internal and external diseases by manual operation and without drugs.[2]

Still opposed so-called "materia medica" and did not permit the teaching of the available pharmacology of that era as most only addressed symptoms or abnormal bodily responses to an unknown cause. He believed that in osteopathy, there is no place for injurious medications, whose risks outweigh their benefits, especially if safer and equally effective alternatives exist. However, he did state the following:

To be able to intelligently prescribe any and all drugs, one must first learn the fundamental principles that govern their administrations. Namely: There must exist within the body the physiologic wrong for which a drug is given. Otherwise, it becomes a poison instead of a remedial agent. (Walter, GW. The First School of Osteopathic Medicine: A Chronicle, 1892–1992. Kirksville, Mo. Thomas Jefferson University Press, Northeast Missouri State University: 1992, p. 37)

Specifically, Still was against the irrational use of drugs that:

a. Showed no benefit
b. Had proven to be harmful
c. Had no proven relationship to the cause of disease processes

He accepted the use of anesthetics, poison antidotes, and a few others that had proven beneficial.

Osteopathy has no use for drugs as remedies, but a great use for chemistry when dealing with poisons and antidotes.[14]

Still supports his reasons by listing the life-threatening risks of using drugs commonly employed in the late 19th century, namely, calomel, digitalis, aloe, morphine, chloral hydrate, veratrine, pulsatilla, and sedatives.[2] Still persuasively argued that a detailed physical examination, with focus on the neuromusculoskeletal system, followed by a well-designed manipulative treatment, often removes impediments to motion and function. Where he differed from others was his view that manipulative treatment should always be used before deciding that the body had failed in its own efforts.

Vaccinations

Jenner introduced the smallpox vaccine in the 17th century with considerable success. Still acknowledged this by stating,

I believe the philosophy of fighting one infection with another infectious substance that could hold the body immune by long and continuous possession is good and was good.[7]

Without disrespect to Jenner, he described shortcomings of Jenner's methods, pointing out that there were many patients on whom the vaccine did not work or who became disabled or fatally ill. He stated his belief that there is a less harmful method of vaccination and requested that Jenner's methods be improved.

Still's rejection of drugs and vaccinations was evident in the initial mission statement for the American School of Osteopathy (ASO).[3] However, in 1910, even while he was president, the school changed its stance and accepted vaccinations and serums as part of osteopathic practices.

First and foremost, Still clearly believed that the osteopathic physician should strive to help the patient's body release its own medicine for a particular problem. He writes:

The brain of man was God's drug store, and had in it all liquids, drugs, lubricating oils, opiates, acids, and antacids, and every quality of drugs that the wisdom of God thought necessary for human happiness and health.[14]

The Mechanical Approach to Treating the Cause of Disease

Still reasoned that the cause of most diseases was mechanical; therefore, treatment must follow the laws of mechanics. As a consequence, he used manipulative approaches designed to release bony and soft tissue barriers to nervous and circulatory functions in order to improve chances for healing. He claimed that mobilization of these structures improved the outcomes of his patients.[3] However, manipulation procedures were applied not only to relieve musculoskeletal strains and injuries but to treat internal organ diseases as well. For example, he found characteristic paraspinal muscle rigidity and other abnormal myofascial tensions in patients with infectious diseases. He noted improvement in the health of these patients as well when the musculoskeletal and myofascial impediments to normal physiologic processes were alleviated. In a majority of cases, the patient's condition was seemingly cured, leading him to believe that the mechanical aspects of dysfunction or disease were vitally important.[3] Still thus proposed that in all diseases, mobilization of all the spinal joints not in their proper positional and functional relationships was necessary to ensure proper nerve activity and blood and lymph flow throughout the body. This included everything from the occiput to the coccyx and indicated adjustment of the pelvis, clavicles, scapulae, costal cage, and diaphragm.

Comprehensive Treatment

While heavily committed to the use of palpatory diagnosis and manipulative treatment, Dr. Still continued many other aspects of patient care. He practiced surgery and midwifery (obstetrics), although little is documented about specific activities.

His patient education strategies highlighted moderation. He included advice for removing noxious or toxic substances from the diet and environment and behavioral adjustments such as adding exercises and stopping smoking. He also admonished his patients for abusing alcohol, opium, and heroin.

Mental illness and stress-related problems were also important to Still.[2,3] He wrote about the role the physician can take in providing emotional support and encouragement to patients with end-stage medical problems. He described the importance of giving hope to patients and, at the same time, providing them with a realistic approach to managing their clinical condition.[3]

Individualized Treatment

Each person is treated as a unique individual, not as a disease entity. Still taught that the history and physical evaluation of each person may reveal unhealthy self-care behaviors or circumstances and parts of the body that are not functioning or moving normally. This combination would interfere with the body's natural ability to heal itself. The treatment would then be specifically tailored to each patient's particular needs.

HISTORICAL DEVELOPMENT OF OSTEOPATHIC CONCEPTS

Exactly how much influence previous or contemporary philosophies and practices had on Still is purely speculative since he never discussed specific attachments for any particular philosopher or scientist. The writings of contemporary philosophers of science and biology, like Herbert Spencer (1820–1903) and Alfred Russel Wallace (1823–1913), resonated with those of Still.[1] They promoted theories of evolution and the interdependence of the environment and the organism in all biologic processes, including the origins of disease. They also promoted the concepts of the interdependence of structure and function and the importance of differentiating cause and effect and emphasized the unity of the organism and interrelatedness of its parts. Throughout his life, however, Still maintained that his discoveries and thoughts were based on personal observation, experimentation, applications of factual knowledge, and the power of reasoning. After nearly 50 years of developing his concepts, he stated:

> *I have explored by reading and inquiry much that has been written on kindred subjects, hoping to get something on this great law written by the ancient philosophers, but I come back as empty as I started.*[2]

A number of scholars and educators have attempted to trace both the historical development and the evolution of thoughts and practices that may have influenced Still's thinking.[11–13,15–19] In general, the authors compare Still's ideas with well-known discourses passed on principally through Western cultural ideas. In 1901, Littlejohn, one of Still's students who became a faculty member at the ASO and founder of two osteopathic colleges, wrote,

> *Osteopathy did not invent a new anatomy or physiology or construct a new pathology. It has built upon the foundation of sciences already deeply seated in the philosophy of truth, chemistry, anatomy and physiology, a new etiology of diseases, gathering together, adding to and reinforcing natural methods of treating disease that have been accumulating since the art of healing began.*[11]

However, other students of A.T. Still disagreed with this perspective. C.M.T. Hulett emphatically stated that

> *Osteopathy is a new system of thought, a new philosophy of life.*[20]

Whereas Littlejohn[15] finds the foundation of osteopathy in Greek and Roman medicine, G.D. Hulett[13] and Downing[16] trace the origins of various osteopathic concepts to the philosophy and practice of medicine found in other ancient writings, such as those of the Ptolemies, Brahmins, Chinese, and Hebrews. All agree on the further development of medicine throughout Europe as a precursor to American osteopathic medical practice. Northup compares osteopathy to the concepts of Hippocrates and the Cnidian schools.[19] Korr contrasts the contributions of Asclepian and Hygeian roots.[18] Whereas G.D. Hulett[13] and Korr[18] describe osteopathy as part of an *evolution* of the philosophy of medicine, Lane[12] and Northup[19] consider it a *reformation* of medical theory and practice.

Still's use of spinal manipulation had many precedents. Schiötz and Cyriax[21] and Lomax,[22] among many, document the use of manual treatments for millennia. Hippocrates discussed "subluxations" or minor displacements of vertebra in his treatise "On the Articulations" and the manual adjustments used to correct them.[23] In the 18th and 19th centuries, many American and European practitioners acknowledged that there are relationships among displaced or "subluxed" vertebrae and "irritated" spinal nerves in relation to both musculoskeletal and visceral disorders.[24]

EVOLUTION OF OSTEOPATHIC PHILOSOPHY

In his unique way, Still integrated many of these concepts into his new system and molded it into a distinctive medical school curriculum that continues to evolve to this day. Still was adamant that he did not expect his students and colleagues to take what he advocated as dogma. He taught,

> *You must reason. I say reason, or you will finally fail in all enterprises. Form your own opinions, select all facts you can obtain. Compare, decide, then act. Use no man's opinion; accept his works only.*[7]

He urged his students to study, test, and improve upon his ideas.

An example of this evolution is a shift from Still's early, and virtually exclusive, emphasis on anatomy to a more inclusive stress on primary physiologic functions that strengthen his concepts. Initially, Littlejohn[15] and, later, Burns,[25] Cole,[26,27] Denslow,[28] and

BOX 1.2 Irvin Korr, PhD

Irvin Korr, PhD, received his physiology degree from Princeton University. Most of his teaching and research career was spent at the Kirksville College of Osteopathic Medicine in Missouri, with later appointments at both Michigan State University College of Osteopathic Medicine and The Texas College of Osteopathic Medicine (University of North Texas Health Science Center). A multitalented individual, Korr was an accomplished violinist, sometimes playing chamber music with Albert Einstein, who was in residence at the time of his postgraduate training. He published extensively with several colleagues, including J.S. Denslow, A.D. Krems, Martin J. Goldstein, Price E. Thomas, Harry M. Wright, and Gustavo S.L. Appeltauer. In 1947, Korr's initial publication, with Denslow and Krems, focused on facilitation of neural impulses in motoneuron pools. Original research papers followed this on dermal autonomic activity, electrical skin resistance, and trophic function of nerves.[29] As Korr gained insight into Still's concepts, he lectured widely and published a number of important treatises tying osteopathic concepts together with proven physiologic models that emphasized the important roles played by the neuromusculoskeletal system. Whereas Still emphasized a focus on bones as the starting place from which he was to discern the cause of pathology, Korr expanded this concept to include the integrative activity of the spinal cord and its relationships with the musculoskeletal and the sympathetic nervous systems.[29] Similar to Still, however, Korr often referred to the neuromusculoskeletal system as the "Primary Machinery of Life."

For 50 years, Irvin M. Korr, scientist, philosopher, and humanist, led and inspired several generations of osteopathic physicians and educators. His final treatise on osteopathic philosophy was written for the first edition of this text published in 1997. Upon reflection on the osteopathic principles, Korr stated "It is to the credit and honor of the osteopathic profession that it contributed cogent elaboration of the principles, developed effective methods for their implementation, built a system of practice upon those principles, and disclosed much about their basis in biologic mechanisms through research.[6]"

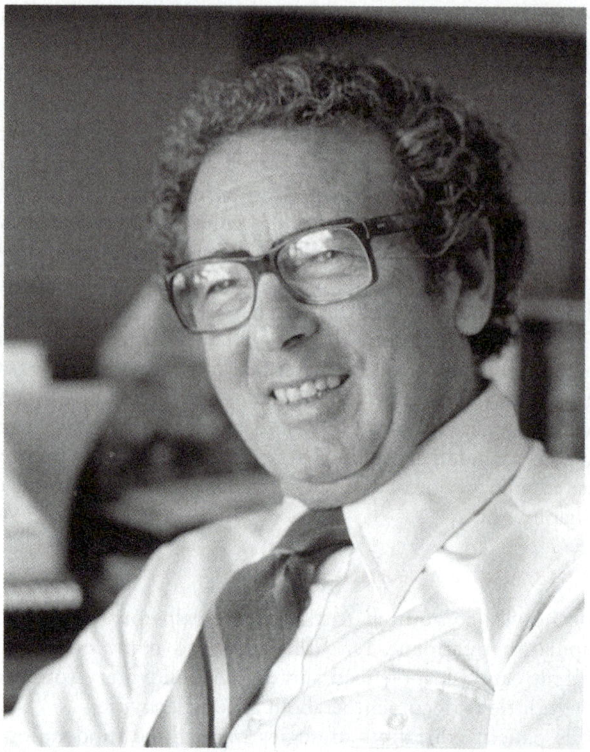

Figure 1.3. Irvin M. Korr, PhD (1909–2004), "The second great osteopathic philosopher."

Korr[29,30] promoted integrative neurophysiologic and neuroendocrine concepts.

Whereas Littlejohn interpreted Still's concepts in light of 19th century physiologic theories, Burns, Cole, Denslow, and Korr pioneered distinctive osteopathic approaches to physiologic investigations, making significant scientific contributions. Korr was particularly influential in interpreting osteopathic concepts in light of the rapidly developing science of physiology in the 20th century (Box 1.2). He has been referred to as "the second great osteopathic philosopher"[31] (Figs. 1.3 and 1.4).

The Definition of Osteopathy

Osteopathic philosophy has been defined in various ways over the years. To get a better sense of the evolution of the osteopathic philosophy since its inception, it is instructive to follow how it has been defined over time. In his autobiography, Still gave a "technical" definition as follows:

> *Osteopathy is that science which consists of such exact, exhaustive, and verifiable knowledge of the structure and functions of the human mechanism, anatomical, physiological, and psychological, including the chemistry and physics of its known elements, as has made discoverable certain organic laws and remedial resources, within the body itself, by which nature under the scientific treatment peculiar to osteopathic practice, apart from all ordinary methods of extraneous, artificial, or medicinal stimulation, and in harmonious accord with its own mechanical principles, molecular activities, and metabolic processes, may recover from displacements, disorganizations, derangements, and consequent disease, and regain its normal equilibrium of form and function in health and strength*[2] (Fig. 1.5).

Besides Still, several other American osteopathic scholars wrote treatises on osteopathic philosophy and principles.[12,13,16,17,26,27,32–38] Each author had their own definition and explanation of osteopathic philosophy. There have been several attempts over the past century to obtain consensus, or agreement, on a unifying definition and clearly stated tenets or principles that govern the practice of osteopathic medicine.

According to Littlejohn, the first consensus definition of osteopathy, among multiple faculty members representing several osteopathic medical schools, was published in 1900.[11] After Still passed away in 1917, the first American Osteopathic Association (AOA) House of Delegates convened in 1920 and soon thereafter passed a resolution that the A.T. Still Research Institute, under the direction of Louisa Burns, DO at the time, would publish an updated version of the most popular textbook on osteopathic principles in print, adding current scientific knowledge in support of the philosophy.[39] The eight osteopathic colleges funded, reviewed, contributed to, and consented on the content.[40] In 1922, this consensus-based textbook was published by the A.T. Still Research Institute as a revised edition of the classic textbook by G. D. Hulett initially written at the turn of the 20th century.[13] By this time in

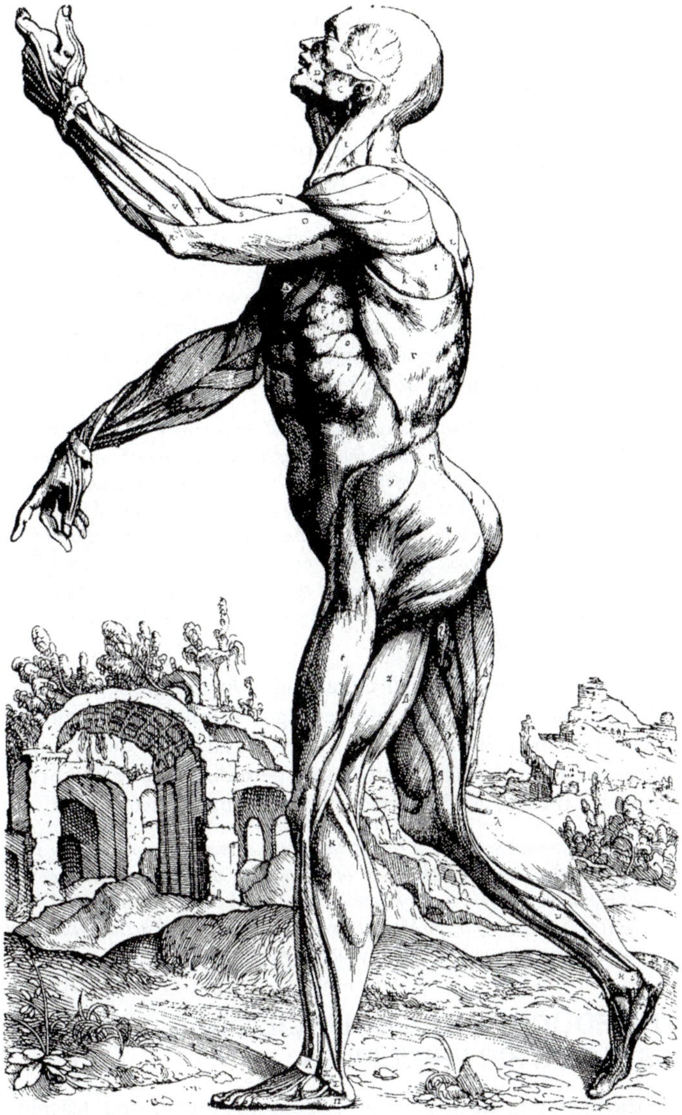

Figure 1.4. I.M. Korr, PhD, like A.T. Still, MD, DO, emphasized the role of the musculoskeletal system as the primary machinery of life. This is a drawing by the renowned anatomist, Vesalius (1514–1564), depicting the muscles of the body in a dramatic pose. (Vesalius, Andreas De humani corporis fabrica plate 25 [Liber I] Basileae, [Ex officina Joannis Oporini, 1543]. Courtesy of the National Library of Medicine.)

medical thought, it was widely accepted that cellular level activity was a strong determinant of health or disease states. In an attempt to update osteopathic philosophy in light of emerging concepts in cellular biology, the authors applied Still's mechanistic viewpoint to cellular physiology. The following passage not only illustrates this approach but also demonstrates the desire of the profession to state osteopathic philosophy and principles in terms of concise tenets based on contemporary scientific knowledge:

The osteopathic view of the cell…is largely covered by the following statements:

- Normal structure is essential to normal function.
- Normal function is essential if normal structure is to be maintained.
- Normal environment is essential to normal function and structure, though some degree of adaptation is possible for a time, even under abnormal conditions.

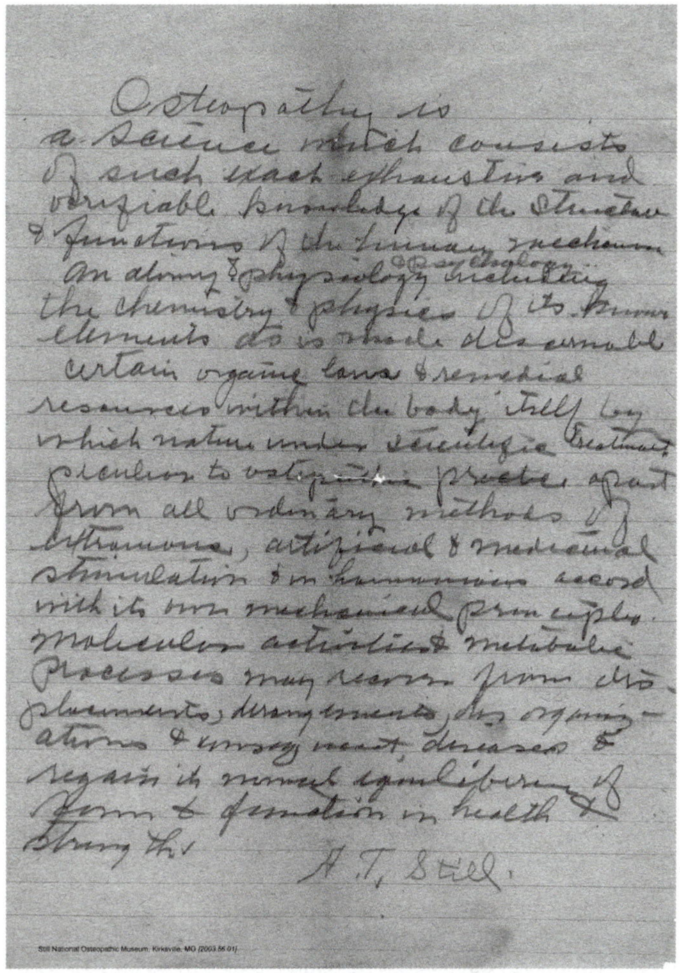

Osteopathy is
a Science which consists
of such exact exhaustive and
verifiable knowledge of the Structure
& functions of the human mechanism
anatomy & physiology & psychology including
the chemistry & physics of its known
elements as is made discoverable
certain organic laws & remedial
resources within the body itself by
which nature under scientific treatment
peculiar to osteopathic practice apart
from all ordinary methods of
extraneous, artificial & medicinal
stimulation & in harmonious accord
with its own mechanical principles,
molecular activities & metabolic
processes may recover from dis-
placements, derangements, disorganiz-
ations & consequent diseases &
regain its normal equilibrium of
form & function in health &
strength.
A.T. Still.

Figure 1.5. Handwritten definition of osteopathy by A. T. Still, MD, DO. (Reprinted with permission from Still National Osteopathic Museum, Kirksville, MO.)

In the human body, with its diversified functions, we may add also:

- The blood preserves and defends the cells of the body.
- The nervous system unifies the body in its activities.
- Disease symptoms are due either to failure of the organism to meet adverse circumstances efficiently, or to structural abnormalities.
- Rational methods of treatment are based upon an attempt to provide normal nutrition, innervation, and drainage to all tissues of the body, and these depend chiefly upon the maintenance of normal structural relations.[13]

The addition of medications in the practices of osteopathic physicians and surgeons over the years affected how the philosophy was stated. For example, in 1948, the faculty at the College of Osteopathic Physicians and Surgeons in Los Angeles added the following phrase to their basic osteopathic principles statement: "Like a machine, the body can function efficiently only when in proper adjustment and when its chemical needs are satisfied either by food or medical substances".[41] Further evolution occurred in 1953 when the faculty of the Kirksville College of Osteopathy and Surgery agreed on the following:

Osteopathy, or Osteopathic Medicine, is a philosophy, a science, and an art. Its philosophy embraces the concept of the unity of body structure and function in health and disease. Its science includes the chemical, physical, and biological sciences related to the maintenance of health and the prevention, cure, and alleviation of disease. Its art is the application of the philosophy and the science in the practice of osteopathic medicine and surgery in all its branches and specialties.

Health is based on the natural capacity of the human organism to resist and combat noxious influences in the environment and to compensate for their effects—to meet, with adequate reserve, the usual stresses of daily life, and the occasional severe stresses imposed by extremes of environment and activity. Disease begins when this natural capacity is reduced, or when it is exceeded or overcome by noxious influences.

Osteopathic medicine recognizes that many factors impair this capacity and the natural tendency toward recovery, and that among the most important of these factors are the local disturbances or lesions of the musculoskeletal system. Osteopathic medicine is therefore concerned with liberating and developing all the resources that constitute the capacity for resistance and recovery, thus recognizing the validity of the ancient observation that the physician deals with a patient as well as a disease.[42]

They then combined several concepts and restated them as four principles:

The osteopathic concept emphasizes four general principles from which are derived an etiological concept, a philosophy and a therapeutic technic that are distinctive, but not the only features of osteopathic diagnosis and treatment.

The body is a unit.

The body possesses self-regulatory mechanisms.

Structure and function are reciprocally inter-related.

Rational therapy is based upon an understanding of body unity, self-regulatory mechanisms, and the inter-relationship of structure and function.[42]

Over the ensuing 40 years, advances in the biologic sciences elucidated many mechanisms in support of the concept that optimal health calls for integration of countless functions ranging from the molecular to the behavioral level. When this integration breaks down, dysfunction and disease commonly follow. Infectious and metabolic diseases, as well as diseases of aging and genetics, are frequent examples. Interdisciplinary fields of study have been developed to investigate and delineate the complex interactions of numerous coordinated body functions in health and disease. Psychoneuroimmunology, for example, provides substantial evidence linking mind, body, and spiritual activities with a wide variety of biologic observations.[43–46]

Clinical applications of the advances in molecular, cellular, neurologic, and behavioral sciences, combined with the decreased emphasis on mechanical factors within osteopathic medical practice, demanded a new consensus statement. Using the 1953 Kirksville faculty statement as a beginning, the associate editors of the first edition of this text (1997) stated:

Health is the adaptive and optimal attainment of physical, mental, emotional, and spiritual well-being. It is based on our natural capacity to meet, with adequate reserves, the usual stresses of daily life and the occasional severe stresses imposed by extremes of environment and activity. It includes our ability to resist and combat noxious influences in our environment and to compensate for their effects. One's health at any given time depends on many factors including his or her polygenetic inheritance, environmental influences, and adaptive response to stressors.[47]

The editors modified the four key principles of osteopathic philosophy as follows:

1. The body is a unit; the person is a unit of body, mind, and spirit.
2. The body is capable of self-regulation, self-healing, and health maintenance.
3. Structure and function are reciprocally interrelated.
4. Rational treatment is based upon an understanding of the basic principles of body unity, self-regulation, and the interrelationship of structure and function.[47]

In July 2008, the AOA House of Delegates adopted a policy statement accepting these four tenets as stated. They reaffirmed them in 2013 and 2018 and adopted them in 2023.

The Osteopathic International Alliance (OIA) was formed in 2003 to ensure that osteopathy and osteopathic medicine were formally recognized by the World Health Organization (WHO) as a distinct profession. The OIA collects and disseminates information about the state of the osteopathic profession worldwide.[48] In its description of osteopathic care, elements of the tenets are clearly evident:

Osteopathic care... incorporates a broad range of approaches to the maintenance of health and the management of disease. It embraces the concept of the unity of the individual's structure (anatomy) and function (physiology); recognizes that each patient's clinical signs and symptoms are the consequences of the interaction of multiple physical and non-physical factors; and emphasizes the importance of the patient-practitioner relationship in the therapeutic process. Osteopathy and osteopathic medicine are person-centered approaches (rather than disease-centered) to healthcare.

In order to represent an increasingly diverse group of osteopathic physicians, the AOA adopted a general statement regarding osteopathic medicine. Since 1991, the official AOA definition of *osteopathic medicine* has been reviewed periodically. The latest rendition, adopted in 2023, define osteopathic medicine:

The preferred term for a complete system of medical care with a philosophy that combines the needs of the patient with the current practice of medicine, surgery and obstetrics; that emphasizes the concept of body unity, the interrelationship between structure and function; and that has an appreciation of the body's ability to heal itself.

THE EDUCATIONAL COUNCIL ON OSTEOPATHIC PRINCIPLES

In the contemporary era, the evolution, growth, and teaching of osteopathic philosophy have been coordinated through the Educational Council on Osteopathic Principles (ECOP). This Council was originally formed by the six osteopathic schools in existence in 1969. With the emergence of the new National Board Exam, the schools of osteopathic medicine realized that consistent terminology of the profession was needed as well as a core curriculum for all of the schools. They set out to accomplish three goals; create a glossary of osteopathic terminology, create a core osteopathic curriculum, and generate a textbook for the profession. Eventually, the ECOP became a council of the American Association of Colleges of Osteopathic Medicine consisting of the chairs of the departments of osteopathic principles and practice from each osteopathic medical school or their designee. This council is considered the "expert panel" in the osteopathic medical profession with regard to osteopathic manipulative medicine, osteopathic philosophy, and principles and training students in the osteopathic philosophy, principles, and practice, including osteopathic manipulative treatment (OMT). These osteopathic physicians are regarded as leading-edge thinkers in terms of osteopathic philosophy and principles.

One of the ECOP's charges was to obtain consensus on the usage of terms within the profession. *The Glossary of Osteopathic Terminology* was first published in 1981[49] and is updated annually. The latest edition is available through the American Association of Colleges of Osteopathic Medicine and the AOA websites and is included as a Glossary of Osteopathic Terminology in this textbook. The Glossary includes the following definition of the philosophy of osteopathy:

A framework of health care supported by expanding scientific knowledge that embraces the interconnectedness and unity of the living organism's structure (anatomy) and function (physiology). This philosophy emphasizes the following osteopathic principles.

1. The body is a unit; the person is a unit of body, mind, and spirit.
2. The body is capable of self-regulation, self-healing, and health maintenance.
3. Structure and function are reciprocally interrelated.
4. Rational treatment is based upon an understanding of the basic principles of body unity, self-regulation, and the interrelationship of structure and function.

One of the products of ECOP's work was the development of a uniquely osteopathic curriculum for medical education that was founded upon a health-oriented, patient-centered perspective and focused on restoration, enhancement, and maintenance of normal physiologic processes.[50] When utilizing a health-oriented perspective, it is crucial to restrain from focusing solely on that which is dysfunctional or impeding function but to also acknowledge the physiologic adaptive response pattern that can be facilitated to enhance the patient's capacity to maintain or restore optimal function and health. Physiology texts (e.g., Vander) describe 10 basic coordinated body functions, namely:

1. Control of posture and body movement
2. Respiration
3. Circulation
4. Regulation of water and electrolyte balance
5. Digestion and absorption of nutrients and elimination of wastes
6. Metabolism and energy balance
7. Protective mechanisms
8. The sensory system
9. Reproduction
10. Consciousness and behavior

The ECOP group combined these into five basic integrative and coordinated body functions and coping strategies that were considered in a context of healthful adaptation to life and its circumstances:

1. Posture and motion, including fundamental structural and biomechanical reliability
2. Gross and cellular respiratory and circulatory factors
3. Metabolic processes of all types, including endocrine-mediated, immune-regulatory, and nutritionally related biochemical processes
4. Neurologic integration, including central, peripheral, autonomic, neuroendocrine, and neurocirculatory and their reflex relationships
5. Psychosocial, cultural, behavioral, and spiritual elements

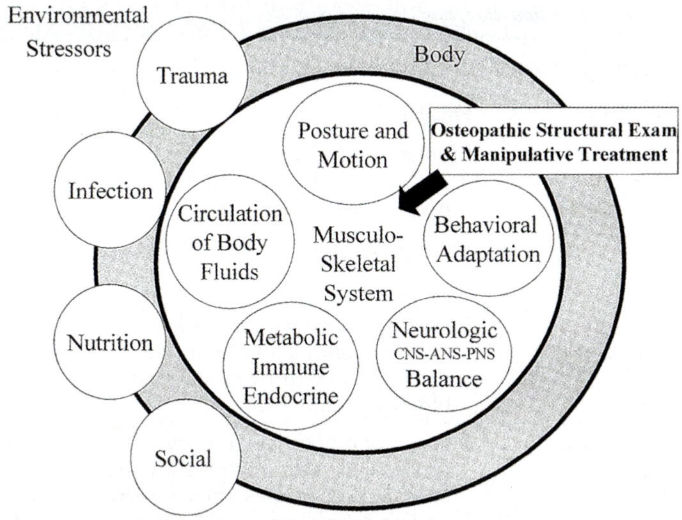

Figure 1.6. Osteopathic philosophy of health displayed as the coordinated activity of five basic body functions, integrated by the musculoskeletal system, adapting to environmental stressors. Evaluation and treatment of the musculoskeletal system is performed in light of its ability to affect not only the five functions but also ultimately the person's own ability to adapt to internal and external stressors.

These formed the foundation for what is called the "Five Models of Osteopathic Care" (see Fig. 1.6, Table 1.1, and Chapter 26).

The applicability of these concepts to patient care scenarios is demonstrated in the case presentations in Chapter 28.

The classical philosophy of osteopathic medicine formed the foundation upon which contemporary osteopathic patient care is based (Box 1.1). The contemporary "Five Models of Osteopathic Care" can be understood in the context of the classical osteopathic philosophy of health, disease, and patient care, as depicted in Table 1.2.

TABLE 1.1

Osteopathic Approaches to Patient Care

Model	Anatomical Correlates	Physiologic Functions
Biomechanical	Postural muscles, spine, and extremities	Posture and motion
Respiratory–Circulatory	Thoracic inlet, thoracic and pelvic diaphragms, tentorium cerebelli, costal cage	Respiration, circulation, venous, and lymphatic drainage
Metabolic–Energy	Internal organs, endocrine glands	Metabolic processes, homeostasis, energy balance, regulatory processes; immunologic activities and inflammation and repair; digestion, absorption of nutrients, removal of waste; reproduction
Neurologic	Head (organs of special senses), brain, spinal cord, autonomic nervous system, peripheral nerves	Control, coordination, and integration of body functions; protective mechanisms; sensation
Biopsychosocial/behavioral	Brain	Psychological and social activities, e.g., anxiety, stress, work, family; habits, e.g., sleep, drug abuse, sexual activities, exercise; values, attitudes, beliefs

TABLE 1.2

Osteopathic Five Models in the Context of the Three Domains of a Philosophy of Medicine

Models	Health	Disease	Patient Care[a]
Biomechanical	Efficient and effective posture and motion throughout the musculoskeletal system	Somatic dysfunction; inefficient posture; joint motion restrictions or hypermobility; instability	Alleviate somatic dysfunction utilizing osteopathic palpatory diagnosis and osteopathic manipulative treatment (OMT) to restore normal motion and function throughout the body
Respiratory–Circulatory	Efficient and effective arterial supply, venous and lymphatic drainage to and from all cells; effective respiration	Vascular compromise, edema, tissue congestion; poor gas exchange	Remove mechanical impediments to respiration and circulation and relieve congestion and edema by improving venous and lymphatic drainage
Neurologic	Efficient and effective sensory processing, neural integration and control, autonomic balance, central and peripheral nervous functions	Abnormal sensation, imbalance of autonomic functions, central and peripheral sensitization/malfunction; pain syndromes	Restore normal sensation, neurologic processes, and control; alleviate pain
Metabolic–Energy	Efficient and effective cellular metabolic processes, energy expenditure and exchange, endocrine and immune regulation and control	Energy loss, fatigue, ineffective metabolic processes, toxic waste buildup, inflammation, infection, poor wound healing, poor nutrition; adverse response to medication; loss of endocrine control of vital functions	Restore efficient metabolic processes and bioenergetics, alleviate inflammation and infection, restore healing, and repair functions and endocrine control
Biopsychosocial/Behavioral	Efficient and effective mental, emotional, and spiritual functions; healthy lifestyle choices and activities; good social support system	Ineffective function due to drug abuse, environmental chemical exposure or trauma, poor lifestyle choices (i.e., inactivity, dietary indiscretions); inability to adapt to stress or environmental challenges	Assess and treat the whole person—physical, psychological, social, cultural, behavioral, and spiritual aspects; collaborative partnership; individualized patient care and self-responsibility for healthy lifestyle choices

[a]Utilizing combinations of osteopathic manipulative medicine, medications, surgery, and education as appropriate.

OSTEOPATHIC PRINCIPLES AS PRACTICE

The contributions of A.T. Still and the osteopathic medical profession affect many aspects of general patient care. First, irrespective of diagnoses or practitioner, the patient is of central importance. Second, a competent differential diagnosis is essential. This includes all aspects of the person (body, mind, and spirit), as shown in Box 1.3. Third, clinical activities integrate realistic expectations with measurable outcomes. Finally, and ideally, patient-oriented educational efforts pragmatically address both personal and family-related concerns. The patient is ultimately responsible for long-term self-health care. Emphasis is on health restoration and disease prevention.

In 2002, an ad hoc interdisciplinary task force of osteopathic educators, philosophers, and researchers proposed osteopathic principles for patient care[51]:

1. **The Patient Is the Focus for Health Care**—All osteopathic physicians, irrespective of the specialty of the practitioner, are trained to focus on the individual patient. The relationship between clinician and patient is a partnership in which both parties are actively engaged. The osteopathic physician is an advocate for the patient, supporting their efforts to optimize the circumstances to maintain, improve, or restore health.
2. **The Patient Has the Primary Responsibility for Their Health**—While the physician is the professional charged with the responsibility to assist a patient in being well, the physician can no more impart health to another person than they can impart charm, wisdom, wit, or any other desirable trait. Although the patient–physician relationship is a partnership, and the physician has significant obligations to the patient due to their knowledge base and skill, ultimately the patient has primary responsibility for their own health. The patient has

BOX 1.3 Health Restoration and Disease Prevention

Although osteopathically oriented medical care emphasizes competent comprehensive patient management, it also places importance on restoration of well-being appropriate for the patient's age and health potential. This includes addressing:

- Physical, mental, and spiritual components
- Personal safety
- Sufficient rest and relaxation
- Proper nutrition
- Regular aerobic, stretching, and strengthening exercises
- Maintaining rewarding social relationships
- Avoidance of tobacco and other abused substances
- Eliminating or modifying abusive personal, interpersonal, family, and work-related behavior patterns
- Avoidance of environmental radiation and toxins

inherent healing powers and must nurture these through proper diet and exercise as well as adherence to appropriate stress management, sleep, body weight, and avoidance of abuse.

3. **An Effective Treatment Program for Patient Care**—An effective treatment program for patient care is founded on the osteopathic tenets and incorporates evidence-based guidelines, optimizes the patient's natural healing capacity, addresses the primary cause of disease, and emphasizes health maintenance and disease prevention. The emphasis on the musculoskeletal system as an integral part of patient care is one of the defining characteristics of osteopathic medicine.

When applied as part of a coherent philosophy of the practice of medicine, these principles represent a distinct and necessary approach to health care. Evidence-based guidelines should be used to encourage those treatments with proven efficacy and to discourage those that are not beneficial, or even harmful. Osteopathic medicine embraces the concept of evidence-based medicine as part of a valuable reformation of clinical practice.

Andrew Taylor Still told his students "the object of the doctor is to seek health; anyone can find disease." This precept provides a useful orientation in patient care. An emphasis on health rather than disease helps to promote optimism. It may facilitate efforts to engage the patient as an active participant in recovery from illness. It may also encourage the realization that no single treatment approach is successful for every patient. Rather, optimal approaches will use diet, exercise, medications, manipulative treatment, surgery, or other modalities according to the needs and wishes of the patient and the skill and aptitude of the practitioner.[51]

In end-stage conditions, it is recognized that treatment may be only palliative, remedial, and supportive. The AOA position paper on end-of-life care promotes compassionate and humanistic care tailored to the needs of each individual patient and their family.

Osteopathically oriented problem-solving and treatment plans help guide the application of osteopathic principles in medical, behavioral, and surgical care. In 1987, ECOP developed guidelines for use by osteopathic physicians in developing an osteopathic management plan.[50] The extent to which palpatory diagnosis and manipulative treatment are specifically useful interventions for a wide variety of neuromusculoskeletal problems continue to be explored through research. However, since many clinical presentations commonly interfere with a patient's ability to meet the requirements of normal daily activities (including appropriate exercise), it stands to reason that improving the efficiency of the neuromusculoskeletal system would benefit each patient. "There is a somatic component in all clinical situations. The somatic component is addressed to the extent that it influences patient well-being. Conceptually, OMT is designed to address both structural abnormalities and self-regulatory capabilities".[50]

SUMMARY

Osteopathic medicine is based on a health-oriented and patient-centered philosophy. The osteopathic physician's primary roles are to:

- Address primary cause(s) of disease using available evidence-based practices
- Enhance the patient's healing capacity
- Individualize patient management plans with an emphasis on health restoration and disease prevention
- Use palpatory diagnosis and manipulative treatment to focus on and affect somatic signs of altered structural, mechanical, and physiologic states

Osteopathic philosophy is meant to guide osteopathic physicians in the best use of scientific and clinical knowledge to optimize health and diminish disease processes. Upon founding his profession and school, Still expressed the hope that "the osteopath will take up the subject and travel a few miles farther toward the fountain of this great source of knowledge and apply the results to the relief and comfort of the afflicted who come for counsel and advice".[7]

In this spirit, the authors of this textbook hope to present current medical, scientific, and clinical knowledge through the universal truths of the osteopathic philosophy and tenets. Osteopathic medicine is a complete system of medical care grounded in a distinct philosophy and practice. This lens will provide a road map for the osteopathic student and physician alike to further the study of the science of osteopathic medicine and practice the highest-quality, patient-centered health care possible.

FINAL THOUGHTS

Korr's Explication of Osteopathic Principles

For the first edition of the *Foundations of Osteopathic Medicine* textbook, Korr wrote an "Explication of Osteopathic Principles," which was his last published work. Soon after submitting it for publication, his health declined and no further editorial changes were made. It is included here to demonstrate how he was able to use the osteopathic philosophy and tenets to organize and apply 20th century scientific knowledge to patient care. It was written informally, as if he was giving a lecture, and captures the style and ease with which he was able to communicate osteopathic philosophy to several generations of osteopathic physicians. His teachings are as pertinent today as they were in his day:

> *At this stage of your medical training, you have become familiar with osteopathic principles and can recite them in their usual brief, maxim form. The purpose of this section is to explore more fully the meaning, biologic foundations, and clinical implications of the founding principles of osteopathic medicine.*

Remember that these principles began to evolve centuries ago, even before the time of Hippocrates. However, their basis in animal and, more specifically, human biology did not begin to become evident through research until late in the 19th century. The origin of these principles, therefore, was largely empirical; that is, they were the product of thoughtful and widely shared observations of ill and injured people. For example, it could hardly escape notice, even in primitive societies, that people (and animals) recovered from illness and wounds healed without intervention, and therefore, some natural indwelling healing power must be at work.

Even at the time of the founding of the osteopathic profession in 1892, the available knowledge in the sciences of physiology, biochemistry, microbiology, immunology, and pathology was meager. Indeed, immunology, biochemistry, and various other neurosciences and biomedical sciences had yet to appear as distinct disciplines. Therefore, these principles could only be expressed as aphorisms, embellished perhaps with conjectures about their biologic basis. It is to the credit and honor of the osteopathic profession that it contributed cogent elaboration of the principles, developed effective methods for their implementation, built a system of practice upon those principles, and disclosed much about their basis in biologic mechanisms through research.

In view of the enormous amount of biomedical knowledge recorded throughout the 20th century, it is timely to examine the principles that guide osteopathic practice in the light of that knowledge and to explore their relevance to clinical practice and to current and future health problems. What follows is an effort in that direction, without detailed reference to individual research.

THE PERSON AS A WHOLE

The Body

The principle of the unity of the body, so central to osteopathic practice, states that every part of the body depends on other parts for maintenance of its optimal function and even of its integrity. This interdependence of body components is mediated by the communication systems of the body: exchange of substances via circulating blood and other body fluids and exchange of nerve impulses and neurotransmitters through the nervous system.

The circulatory and nervous systems also mediate the regulation and coordination of cellular, tissue, and organ functions and thus the maintenance of the integrity of the body as a whole. The organized and integrated collaboration of the body components is reflected in the concept of homeostasis, the maintenance of the relative constancy of the internal environment in which all the cells live and function.

In view of this interdependence and exchange of influences, it is inevitable that dysfunction or failure of a major body component will adversely affect the competence of other organs and tissues and, therefore, one's health.

The Person

Important and valid as is the concept of body unity, it is incomplete in that it is, by implication, limited to the physical realm. Physicians minister not to bodies but to individuals, each of whom is unique by virtue of their genetic endowment, personal history, and the variety of environments in which that history has been lived.

The person, obviously, is more than a body, for the person has a mind, also the product of heredity and biography. Separation of body and mind, whether conceptually or in practice, is an anachronistic remnant of such dualistic thinking as that of the 17th century philosopher–scientist René Descartes. It was his belief that the body and mind are separate domains, one publicly visible and palpable and the other invisible, impalpable, and private. This dualistic concept is anachronistic because, while it is almost universally rejected as a concept, it is still acted out in much of clinical practice and in biomedical research.

Clinical and biomedical research (as well as everyday experience) has irrefutably shown that body and mind are so inseparable, so pervasive to each other, that they can be regarded—and treated—as a single entity. It is now widely recognized (whether or not it is demonstrated in practice) that what goes on (or goes wrong) in either body or mind has repercussions in the other. It is for reasons such as these that I prefer unity of the person to unity of the body, conveying totally integrated humanity and individuality.

The Person as Context

Phenomena assigned to the mind (consciousness, thought, feelings, beliefs, attitudes, etc.) have their physiologic and behavioral counterparts; conversely, bodily and behavioral changes have psychological concomitants, such as altered feelings and perceptions. It must be noted, however, that it is the person who is feeling, perceiving, and responding, not the body or the mind. It is you who feels well, ill, happy, or sad, and not your body or mind. What goes on in body and mind is conditioned by who the person is and their entire history.

In short, the person is far more than the union of body and mind, in the same sense that water is more than the union of hydrogen and oxygen. Nothing that we know about either oxygen or hydrogen accounts for the three states of water (liquid, solid, and gas), their respective properties, the boiling and freezing points, viscosity, and so forth. Water incorporates yet transcends oxygen and hydrogen. To understand water, we must study water and not only its components. In the same way, at an enormously more complex level, the person comprises yet transcends body and mind.

Moreover, once hydrogen and oxygen are joined to form water, they become subject to the laws that govern water. In the same but infinitely more complex sense, it is you who makes up your mind, changes your mind, trains and enriches your mind, and puts it to work. It is you who determines from moment to moment whether and in what way you will express, through your body, what is in or on your mind.

Thus, the person is the context, the environment, in which all the body parts live and function and in which the mind finds expression. Everything about the person—genetics, history from conception to the present moment, nutrition, use and abuse of body and mind, parental and school conditioning, physical and sociocultural environments, and so on—enters into determining the quality of physical and mental function. The better the quality of the environment provided by the person for the mental and bodily components, the better they will function. For example, someone who has a peptic ulcer is not ill because of the ulcer. The ulcer exists because of an unfavorable internal environment.

In conclusion, just as the proper study of mankind is man (Alexander Pope), so is the study of human health and illness also man. As will become evident, the principle of the unity of the person leads us naturally to the next principle.

THE PLACE OF THE MUSCULOSKELETAL SYSTEM IN HUMAN LIFE

The Means of Expression of Our Humanity and Individuality

Structure determines function, structure and function are reciprocally interrelated, and similar aphorisms have traditionally represented another osteopathic principle. That principle recognizes the special place of the musculoskeletal system among the body systems and its relation to the health of the person. We examine now the basis for the osteopathic emphasis on the musculoskeletal system in total health care.

Human life is expressed in human behavior, in humans doing the things that humans do. And whatever humans do, they do it with the musculoskeletal system. That system is the ultimate instrument for carrying out human action and behavior. It is the means through which we manifest our human qualities and our personal uniqueness—personality, intellect, imagination, creativity, perceptions, love, compassion, values, and philosophies. The most noble ethical, moral, or religious principle has value only insofar as it can be overtly expressed through behavior.

That expression is made possible by the coordinated contractions and relaxations of striated muscles, most of them acting upon bones and joints. The musculoskeletal system is the means through which we communicate with each other, whether it be by written, spoken, or signed language or by gesture or facial expression. Agriculture, industry, technology, literature, and the arts and sciences—our very civilization—are the products of human action, interaction, communication, and behavior, that is, by the orchestrated contractions and relaxations of the body's musculature.

Relation to the Body Economy

The musculoskeletal system is the most massive system in the community of body systems. Its muscular components are collectively the largest consumer in the body economy. This is true not only because of their mass but because of their high energy requirements. Furthermore, those requirements may vary widely from moment to moment according to what the person is doing, with what feelings, and in what environments.

The high and varying metabolic requirements of the musculoskeletal system are met by the cardiovascular, respiratory, digestive, renal, and other visceral systems. Together, they supply the required fuels and nutrients, remove the products of metabolism, and control the composition and physical properties of the internal environment. In servicing the musculoskeletal system in this manner, these organ systems are at the same time servicing each other (and, of course, the nervous system).

The nervous system is also, to a great degree, occupied with the musculoskeletal system, that is, with behavior and motor control. Indeed, most of the fibers in the spinal nerves are those converging impulses to and from the muscles and other components of the musculoskeletal system. In addition, the nervous system, its autonomic components, and the circulatory system mediate communication and exchange of signals and substances between the soma and the viscera. In this way, visceral, metabolic, and endocrine activity is continually tuned to moment-to-moment requirements of the musculoskeletal system, that is, to what the person is doing from moment to moment.

Consequences of Visceral Dysfunction

Impairment or failure of some visceral function or of communication between the musculoskeletal system and the viscera is reflected in the musculoskeletal system. When the resulting dysfunction is severe and diffuse, motor activity and even maintenance of posture are difficult or impossible and automatically imposed.

The Musculoskeletal System as Source of Adverse Influences on Other Systems

In view of the rich afferent input of the musculoskeletal system into the central nervous system and its rich interchange of substances with other systems through the body fluids, it is inevitable that structural and functional disturbances in the musculoskeletal system will have repercussions elsewhere in the body.

Such structural and functional disturbances may be of postural, traumatic, or behavioral origin (neglect, misuse, or abuse by the person). Further, it must be appreciated that the human framework is, compared with other (quadruped) mammals, uniquely unstable and vulnerable to compressive, torsional, and shearing forces, because of the vertical configuration, higher center of gravity, and the comparatively small, bipedal base.

The human musculoskeletal system, therefore, is the frequent source of aberrant afferent input to the central nervous system and its autonomic distribution, with at least potential consequences to visceral function. Which organs, blood vessels, etc. are at risk is determined by the site of the musculoskeletal dysfunction and the part(s) of the central nervous system (e.g., spinal segments) into which it discharges its sensory impulses.

When a dysfunction or pathology has developed in a visceral organ, that disturbance is reflected in segmentally related somatic tissues. Viscus and soma become linked in a vicious circle of afferent and efferent impulses, which sustain and exacerbate the disturbance. Appropriate treatment of the somatic component reduces its input to the vicious circle and may even interrupt that circle with therapeutic effect.

Importance of the Personal Context

Whether or not visceral or vasomotor consequences of somatic dysfunction occur, and with what consequences to the person, depends on other factors in the person's life, such as the genetic, nutritional, psychological, behavioral, sociocultural, and environmental. As research has shown, however, the presence of somatic dysfunction and the accompanying reflex and neurotrophic effects exaggerate the impact of other detrimental factors on the person's health. Effective treatment of the musculoskeletal dysfunction shields the patient by reducing the deleterious effects of the other factors. Such treatment, therefore, has preventive as well as therapeutic benefits.

Such treatment directed to the musculoskeletal system assumes even greater and often crucial significance when it is recognized that the other kinds of harmful factors, such as those enumerated above, are not readily subject to change and may even require social or governmental intervention. The musculoskeletal system, however, is readily accessible and responsive to OMT. I view these considerations as the rationale for OMT and its strategic role in total health care.

Finally, the osteopathic philosophy and the unity of the person concept enjoin the physician to treat the patient as a whole and not merely the affected parts. Hence, appropriate corrective attention should also be given to other significant risk factors that are subject to change by both patient and physician.

OUR PERSONAL HEALTH CARE SYSTEMS

The Natural Healing Power

Appreciation, even in ancient times, of our inherent recuperative, restorative, and rehabilitative powers is reflected in the Latin phrase vis medicatrix naturae (nature's healing force). We recover from illnesses, fevers drop, blood clots and wounds heal, broken bones reunite, infections are overcome, skin eruptions clear up, and even cancers are known to occasionally undergo spontaneous remission. But miraculous as is the healing power (and appreciated as it was until we became more impressed by human-made miracles and breakthroughs), the other, more recently revealed components of the health care system with which each of us is endowed are no less marvelous.

The Component System That Defends Against Threats from Without

This component includes, among others, immune mechanisms that defend us against the enormous variety and potency of foreign organisms that invade our bodies, wreaking damage and even bringing death. These same immune mechanisms guard us against those of our own cells that become foreign and malignant as the result of mutation. Included also are the mechanisms that defend against foreign and poisonous substances that we may take in with our food and drink or that enter through the skin and lungs, by disarming them, converting them to innocuous substances, and eliminating them from the body. They defend us (until overwhelmed) even against the toxic substances that we ourselves introduce into the atmosphere, soil, water, or more directly into our own bodies.

Mechanisms That Defend Against Changes in the Internal Environment

We humans are exposed to, and adapt to, wide variations in physical and chemical properties of our environment (e.g., temperature, barometric pressure, oxygen, and carbon dioxide concentrations) and sustain ourselves with chemically diverse food and drink. But the cells of our body can function and survive only in the internal environment of interstitial fluids that maintain body functions within relatively narrow limits as regards variations in chemical composition, temperature, tissue, osmotic pressure, pH, etc.

This phenomenon, called homeostasis, is based on thousands of simultaneously dynamic equilibria occurring throughout the body. Examples include rates of energy consumption and replenishment by the cells. Homeostasis constancy and quick restoration of constancy must be accomplished regardless of the variations in the external environment, composition of food and drink, and the moment-to-moment activities of the person. It is accomplished by an enormously complex array of regulatory mechanisms that continually monitor and control respiratory, circulatory, digestive, renal, metabolic, and countless other functions and processes. Maintenance of optimal environments for cellular function is essential to health. The homeostatic mechanisms may, therefore, be viewed as the health maintenance system of the body.

Commentary

These, then, are the three major components of our indwelling health care system, each comprising numerous component systems. In the order in which humans became aware of them, they are (a) the healing (remedial, curative, palliative, recuperative, rehabilitative) component; (b) the component that defends against threats from the external environment; and (c) the homeostatic, health-maintaining component. These major component systems, of course, share subcomponents and mechanisms.

When the internal health care system is permitted to operate optimally, without impediment, its product is what we call health. Its natural tendency is always toward health and the recovery of health. Indeed, the personal health care system is the very source of health, upon which all externally applied measures depend for their beneficial effects. The internal health care system, in effect, makes its own diagnoses, issues its own prescriptions, draws upon its own vast pharmacy, and, in most situations, administers each dose without side effects.

Health and healing, therefore, come from within. It is the patient who gets well and not the practitioner or the treatment that makes them well.

THE THREE PRINCIPLES AS GUIDES TO MEDICAL PRACTICE

The Unity of the Person

In caring for the whole person, the well-grounded osteopathic physician goes beyond the presenting complaint, beyond relief of symptoms, and beyond identification of the disease and treatment of the impaired organ, malfunction, or pathology, important as they are to total care. The osteopathic physician also explores those factors in the person and the person's life that may have contributed to the illness and that, appropriately modified, compensated, or eliminated, would favor recovery, prevent recurrence, and improve health in general.

The physician then selects that factor or combination of factors that are readily subject to change and that would be of sufficient impact to shift the balance toward recovery and enhancement of health. The possible factors include such categories as the biologic (e.g., genetic, nutritional), psychological, behavioral (use, neglect, or abuse of body and mind; interpersonal relationships; habits; etc.), sociocultural, occupational, and environmental. Some of these factors, especially some of the biologic, are responsive to appropriate clinical intervention, some are responsive only to social or governmental action, and still others require changes by patients themselves. Osteopathic whole-person care, therefore, is a collaborative relationship between patient and physician.

The Place of the Musculoskeletal System in Human Biology and Behavior: The Strategic Role of Osteopathic Manipulative Treatment

It is obvious that some of the most deleterious factors are difficult or impossible for patient and physician to change or eliminate. These include (at least at present) genetic factors (although some inherited predispositions can be mitigated by lifestyle change). They include also such items as social convention, lifelong habits (e.g., dietary and behavioral), widely shared beliefs, prejudices, misconceptions and cultural doctrines, attitudes, and values. Others, such as the quality of the physical or socioeconomic environments, may require concerted community, national, and even international action.

Focus falls, therefore, upon those deleterious factors that are favorably modifiable by personal and professional action and that, when appropriately modified or eliminated, mitigate the health-impairing effects of the less changeable factors. Improvement of body mechanics by OMT is a major consideration when dealing with these complex interactions.

OUR PERSONAL HEALTH CARE SYSTEMS

This principle has important implications for the respective responsibilities of patient and physician and for their relationship. Since each person is the owner and hence the guardian of their own personal health care system, the ultimate source of health and healing, the primary responsibility for one's health is each individual's. That responsibility is met by the way the person lives, thinks, behaves, nourishes themselves, uses body and mind, and relates to others and the other factor usually called lifestyle. Each person must be taught and enabled to assume that responsibility.

It is the physician's responsibility, while giving palliative and remedial attention to the patient's immediate problem, to support each patient's internal health care system, to remove impediments to its competence, and, above all, to do it no harm. It is also the responsibility of physicians to instruct patients on how to do the same for themselves and to strive to motivate them to do so, especially by their own example.

The relationship between patient and osteopathic physician is therefore a collaborative one, a partnership, in maintaining and enhancing the competence of the patient's personal health care system. The maintenance and enhancement of health is the most effective and comprehensive form of preventive medicine, for health is the best defense against disease. As stated by Still, "To find health should be the object of the doctor. Anyone can find disease."

Relevance to the Current and Future Health of the Nation

The preventive strategy of health maintenance and health enhancement, intrinsic to the osteopathic philosophy, is urgently needed by our society today. One of the greatest burdens on the nation's health care system and on the national economy is in the care of victims of the chronic degenerative diseases, such as heart disease, cancer, stroke, and arthritis, which require long-term care.

The incidence of these diseases has increased and will continue to increase well into the next century as the average age of our population continues to increase. The widely accepted (but usually unspoken) assumption that guides current practice (and national policy) is that the chronic degenerative diseases are an inevitable aspect of the aging process; that is, that aging is itself pathologic. It is now increasingly apparent, however, that the increase of their incidence with age is because the longer one lives, the greater the toll taken by minor, seemingly inconsequential, inconspicuous, treatable impairments, and modifiable contributing factors in and around the person. They are, therefore, largely the natural culmination of less-than-favorable lifestyles, and hence, they are largely preventable.

The great national tragedy is that, while the nation's health care system is so extensively and expensively absorbed in the care of millions of older adult victims of chronic disease (at per capita cost 3.5 times that of persons under the age of 65 years), tens of millions of younger people and children are living on and embarking on life paths that will culminate in the same diseases. The health care system simply must move upstream to move people from pathogenic to salutary paths. And the osteopathic profession can show the way.

The osteopathic profession has a historic opportunity to make an enormous contribution to the enhancement of the health of our nation. It can do this by giving leadership in addressing this great tragedy by bringing its basic strategy of whole-person, health-oriented care to bear on the problem and demonstrating its effectiveness in practice.

Having reviewed and enlarged on the principles of osteopathic medicine, their meaning, biologic foundations, and clinical implications, it seems appropriate to propose a definition of osteopathic medicine. The author offers the following: Osteopathic medicine is a system of medicine that is based on the continually deepening and expanding understanding of (a) human nature; (b) those components of human biology that are centrally relevant to health, namely, the inherent regulatory, protective, regenerative, and recuperative biologic mechanisms, whose combined effect is consistently in the direction of the maintenance, enhancement, and recovery of health; and (c) the factors in and around the person that both favorably and unfavorably affect those mechanisms.

The practice of osteopathic medicine is, essentially, the potentiation of the intrinsic health-maintaining and health-restoring resources of the individual. The methods and agents employed are those that are effective in enhancing the favorable factors and diminishing or eliminating the unfavorable factors affecting each individual. Osteopathic medical practice necessarily includes the application of palliative and remedial measures but always on the condition that they do no harm to the patient's own health-maintaining and health-restoring resources. This stipulation governing the choice of methods and agents is based on the recognition that all therapeutic methods depend on the patient's own recuperative power for their effectiveness and are valueless without it and that health and the recovery of health come from within.

The art and science of osteopathic medicine are expressed in the identification and selection of those factors in each individual that are accessible and amenable to change and that, when changed, would most decisively potentate the person on health-supporting resources.

Osteopathic physicians give special emphasis to factors originating in the musculoskeletal system, for the following reasons:

The vertical human framework (a) is highly vulnerable to compressive (gravitational), torsional, and shearing forces, and (b) encases the entire central nervous system.

Since the massive, energy-demanding system has rich two-way communication with all other body systems, it is, because of its vulnerability, a common and frequent source of impediments to the functions of other systems.

These impediments exaggerate the physiologic impact of other detrimental factors in the person's life, and, through the central nervous system, focus it on specific organs and tissues.

The musculoskeletal impediments (somatic dysfunctions) are readily accessible to the hands and responsive to the manipulative and other methods developed and refined by the osteopathic medical profession.

ACKNOWLEDGMENTS

The authors and editors of this chapter would like to acknowledge the scholarly contributions of Dr. Felix R. Rogers to prior editions of this chapter.

REFERENCES

1. Trowbridge C. *Andrew Taylor Still 1828–1917.* Thomas Jefferson University Press; 1991:95–140.
2. Still AT. *Autobiography of Andrew T. Still With a History of the Discovery and Development of the Science of Osteopathy.* The Author, American Academy of Osteopathy; 1908.
3. Still AT. *Osteopathy Research and Practice.* Eastland Press; 1992. Originally published by the author; 1910.
4. Still CE Jr. *Frontier Doctor Medical Pioneer: The Life and Times of A.T. Still and His Family.* Thomas Jefferson University Press, Northeast Missouri State University; 1991.
5. Hildreth AG. *The Lengthening Shadow of Dr. Andrew Taylor Still. Privately published; 1942. Reprinted and distributed:* Osteopathic Enterprises, Inc.
6. Korr IM. An explication of osteopathic principles. In: Ward RC, exec ed. *Foundations for Osteopathic Medicine.* Williams & Wilkins; 1997:7–12.
7. Still AT. *The Philosophy and Mechanical Principles of Osteopathy.* Author; 1892. Osteopathic Enterprises; 1986.
8. Still AT. *Philosophy of Osteopathy.* Author; 1899. Reprinted, Academy of Applied Osteopathy; 1946.
9. Booth ER. Summation of causes in disease and death. *J Am Osteopath Assoc.* 1902;2(2):33–41.
10. Lyne ST. Osteopathic philosophy of the cause of disease. *J Am Osteopath Assoc.* 1904;3(12):395–403. Reprinted in *J Am Osteopath Assoc.* 2000;100(3): 181–189.
11. Littlejohn JM. Osteopathy: an independent system co-extensive with the science and art of healing. *J Am Osteopath Assoc.* 1901;1. Reprinted in *J Am Osteopath Assoc.* 2000;100(1):14–26.
12. Lane MA. *Dr. A.T. Still. Founder of Osteopathy.* The Osteopathic Publishing Co.; 1918.
13. Hulett GD. *A Text Book of the Principles of Osteopathy.* 5th ed. A.T. Still Research Institute; 1922.
14. Schnucker RV, ed. *Early Osteopathy: In the Words of A.T. Still.* Thomas Jefferson University Press, Northeast Missouri State University; 1991.
15. Littlejohn JM. The physiological basis of the therapeutic law. *J Am Osteopath Assoc.* 1902;2:42–60.
16. Downing CH. *Osteopathic Principles in Disease.* Ricardo J. Orozco; 1935. Reprinted and published, American Academy of Osteopathy; 1988.
17. Page LE. *Principles of Osteopathy.* Academy of Applied Osteopathy; 1952.
18. Korr IM. The osteopathic role in medical evolution. The DO. November 1973.

19. Northup GW. *Osteopathic Medicine: An American Reformation*. American Osteopathic Association; 1979.
20. Hulett CMT. Relation of osteopathy to other systems. *J Am Osteopath Assoc*. 1901;1:227–233.
21. Schiötz EH, Cyriax J. *Manipulation: Past and Present*. William Heinemann Medical Books Ltd; 1975.
22. Lomax E. Manipulative therapy: a historical perspective from ancient times to the modern era. In: Goldstein M, ed. *The Research Status of Spinal Manipulative Therapy*. U.S. Dept. of Health, Education and Welfare; 1975:11–17.
23. Adams F. *The Genuine Works of Hippocrates*. Williams & Wilkins; 1939.
24. Harris JD, McPartland JM. Historical perspectives of manual medicine. In: Stanton DF, Mein EA, eds. *Phys Med Rehabil Clin N Am*. 1996;7(4): 679–692.
25. Burns L. *Pathogenesis of Visceral Disease Following Vertebral Lesions*. American Osteopathic Association; 1948.
26. Beal MC, ed. *The Cole Book of Papers Selected From the Writings and Lectures of Wilbur V. Cole, D.O., F.A.A.O.* American Academy of Osteopathy; 1969.
27. Hoag JM, Cole WV, Bradford SG, eds. *Osteopathic Medicine*. McGraw-Hill; 1969.
28. Beal MC, ed. *Selected Papers of John Stedman Denslow, DO*. American Academy of Osteopathy; 1993.
29. Korr IM. *The Neurobiologic Mechanisms of Manipulative Therapy*. Plenum Press; 1977.
30. Peterson B, ed. *The Collected Papers of Irvin M. Korr*. The American Academy of Osteopathy; 1979.
31. Jones JM. Osteopathic philosophy. In: Gallagher RM, Humphrey FJ, eds. *Osteopathic Medicine: A Reformation in Progress*. Churchill Livingstone; 2001.
32. McConnell CP, Teall CC. *The Practice of Osteopathy*. 3rd ed. The Journal Printing Co.; 1906.
33. Tasker D. *Principles of Osteopathy*. Baumgardt Publishing Co.; 1903.
34. Burns L. *Studies in the Osteopathic Sciences: Basic Principles*. Vol 1. Occident Printery; 1907.
35. Downing CH. *Principles and Practice of Osteopathy*. Williams Publishing Co.; 1923.
36. Barber E. *Osteopathy Complete*. Hudson-Kimberly Publishing; 1898.
37. Booth ER. *History of Osteopathy and Twentieth Century Medical Practice*. Jennings and Graham; 1905.
38. Hildreth AG. *The Lengthening Shadow of Andrew Taylor Still*. Privately published by Mrs. AG Hildreth and Mrs. AE Van Vleck; 1942.
39. Gaddis CJ. Hulett's principles, editorial. *J Am Osteopath Assoc*. 1923; Feb:344.
40. Kjerner SH. Report of the committee on book revision. *J Am Osteopath Assoc*. 1923;Oct:89.
41. College of Osteopathic Physician and Surgeons documents, 1948. *University of California at Irvine, Library Archives, Special Collections*.
42. Special Committee on Osteopathic Principles and Osteopathic Technic, Kirksville College of Osteopathy and Surgery. An interpretation of the osteopathic concept. Tentative formulation of a teaching guide for faculty, hospital staff and student body. *J Osteopath*. 1953;60(10):7–10.
43. Felton DL. Neural influence on immune responses: underlying suppositions and basic principles of neural-immune signaling. *Prog Brain Res* 2000;122:381–389.
44. Pert CB. *Molecules of Emotion: The Science Behind Mind-Body Medicine*. Touchstone, Simon and Schuster; 1997.
45. Damasio A. *The Feeling of What Happens: Body and Emotion in the Making of Consciousness*. Harcourt; 1999.
46. Dossey L. *Prayer Is Good Medicine: How to Reap the Healing Benefits of Prayer*. HarperCollins; 1996.
47. Seffinger MA. Development of osteopathic philosophy. In: Ward RC, exec ed. *Foundations for Osteopathic Medicine*. Williams & Wilkins; 1997:3–7.
48. Osteopathic International Alliance. *Osteopathy and Osteopathic Medicine. A Global View of Practice, Patients, Education and the Contribution to Healthcare Delivery*. OIA; 2013.
49. Ward R, Sprafka S. Glossary of osteopathic terminology. *J Am Osteopath Assoc*. 1981;80(8):552–567.
50. Educational Council on Osteopathic Principles. *Core Curriculum Outline*. American Association of Colleges of Osteopathic Medicine; Approved by the Council of Deans; 1987.
51. Rogers FJ, D'Alonzo GE, Glover J, et al. Proposed tenets of osteopathic medicine and principles for patient care. *J Am Osteopath Assoc*. 2002;102(2):63–65.

2 History of the Osteopathic Medical Profession

JOHN M. JONES III ▪ KURT P. HEINKING ▪ JASON HAXTON ▪ REBECCA E. GIUSTI ▪ JOHN GIMPEL

KEY CONCEPTS

- Osteopathic medicine originated from a search for improvement in the system of health care.
- Growth of the osteopathic profession followed a philosophy enunciated by Andrew Taylor Still.
- The osteopathic philosophy quickly began to spread in the United States and other countries.
- Andrew Taylor Still did not initially intend to establish a separate profession for the practice of medicine but sought acceptance of his ideas within teaching programs of traditional medicine.
- Concerted resistance from conventional medical organizations, as well as patient response and outcomes with care from DOs early on, made it clear that osteopathic medicine would emerge as a distinctive profession within the house of medicine.
- The emergence of professional self-regulation and continued demonstration of strength and growth by the osteopathic profession led to recognition by state and federal governments. This included the development of the National Board of Osteopathic Medical Examiners (NBOME) in 1934 and recognition of the American Osteopathic Association (AOA) (later delineated to the AOA's Commission on Osteopathic College Accreditation [COCA]) as the official accrediting body for osteopathic medical education in 1957.
- Expanded teaching of osteopathic theory, methods, and practice led to the development of osteopathic hospitals, postgraduate specialty training programs, and primary care emphasis.
- The merger between the California Osteopathic and Medical Associations in 1961 led to recruitment and acceptance of DOs into Accreditation Council for Graduate Medical Education (ACGME) postgraduate training programs nationwide, specialty and membership medical organizations, and positions of leadership within the greater medical community; it also sparked a rapid increase in the number of osteopathic colleges and graduates, which ultimately led to a shortage of osteopathic-accredited postgraduate training positions by the end of the 20th century.
- To maintain its membership and sovereignty, the AOA mandated that all osteopathic postgraduate training programs be affiliated with an osteopathic educational institution and that all members of osteopathic specialties be members of the AOA.
- Research in osteopathic principles, patient care, and osteopathic manipulative treatment (OMT) has historically been underfunded; however, significant basic science and clinical research has demonstrated the efficacy of this unique approach to health care.
- Since its inception, osteopathic medicine has promoted cultural diversity, equal opportunity for women and minorities, and health care outreach to patients in underserved communities.
- Rapid expansion of colleges of osteopathic medicine (COMs) and DO students from 2000 to the present time and closure of many community-based hospitals with osteopathic postgraduate training programs created challenges for the future residency training for DO graduates.
- While related health care professions with limited practice rights, most often referred to as osteopathy, emerged from early in the profession's history in the United Kingdom, Australia, New Zealand, Germany, France, and around the globe, US-trained osteopathic physicians were increasingly granted full scope of practice rights in many other countries.
- In 2014, helping to facilitate access to residency and fellowship training for the increasing number of DO graduates, the AOA agreed to participate with the ACGME in a unified pathway for postgraduate training. By 2020, eight DOs were added to the ACGME Board of Directors and over 250 residency programs had achieved osteopathic recognition status. Record numbers of DO graduates were matching each year in most specialties, though challenges to match into highly selective specialties for applicants and to remain distinctive and meet new ACGME requirements for some smaller, community-based former AOA programs ensued.
- Legal challenges in 2018 resulted in a settlement that decoupled the AOA membership requirement for DOs to maintain board certification, and this threatened the profession's osteopathic distinctive board certification process in numerous specialties.
- The profession has successfully navigated the many challenges of its first 130 years by continuing to build on opportunities to provide the type of health care in the places that it is most needed in the United States and also around the globe. By 2022, with 37 COMs, operating at over 60 campus locations, and with 178,000 DOs and DO students working nationally and around the world, the osteopathic profession has expanded its impact in providing the type of "body–mind–spirit" patient-focused health care that is needed in numerous underserved communities and to more patients than ever before.

INTRODUCTION

Osteopathic medicine was and is based on ideas and tenets that were considered revolutionary and controversial at the time of its inception, more than a century ago.[1–4] It is striking that these ideas, still quoted extensively today,[5] came not from universities or medical centers but from the creative problem-solving of an informally educated American frontier doctor named Andrew Taylor Still. The history of osteopathic medicine reveals multiple struggles internally and externally to maintain its identity based upon those ideas presented in the previous chapter. Highlighting the life of Dr. Still may help current and future osteopathic physicians appreciate the distinctive osteopathic approach to health and healing.

ANDREW TAYLOR STILL

Life in the Frontier

Andrew Taylor Still was born in 1828 in a humble log cabin near Jonesville, Virginia, to Reverend Abram and Martha Still (Fig. 2.1). Still's family farmed for their livelihood, but his father was also a Methodist circuit rider and physician. As they came of age, Reverend Abram taught his five sons to be doctors in the frontier apprentice system of the time.

Reverend Abram's career as a missionary mandated that the family frequently relocate. The family left Virginia in 1834 for Tennessee and then Missouri, prior to moving to Kansas in 1851.

Still had the inconsistent education of a frontier child,[3] but he was inventive and liked to read. Eventually, he would become familiar with many of the major practical and ideologic trends of his time. Learning to survive had to come first; Missouri and Kansas were true frontiers, fraught with dangers for settlers including extreme weather, isolation and skirmishes with Native Americans. Indeed James Moore Junior, A.T. Still's maternal grandfather was captured by the Shawnee and was eventually traded for goods with a Canadian named John Bateeste Ariome, who took James Moore to Canada for several years[6] (p. 24). While James Moore was in Canada, he learned from Ariome that the Shawnee had killed most of his family, but his sister Mary had been taken captive and was now not far from him in Canada[6] (pp. 31–34). Eventually, James and Mary returned to the United States.[6]

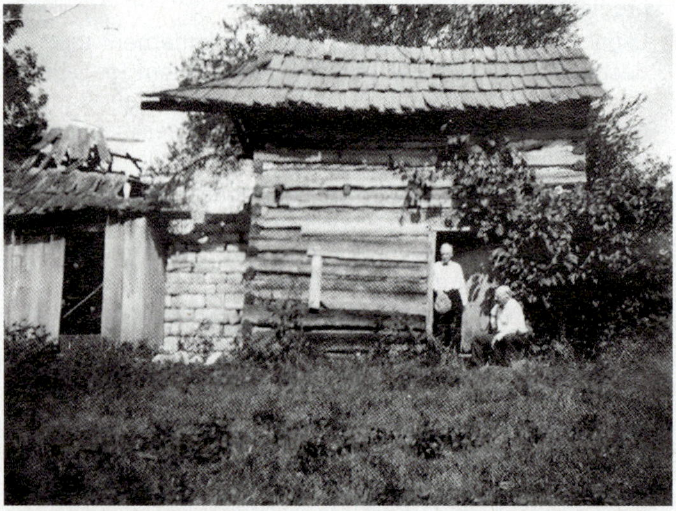

Figure 2.1. Dr. A.T. Still's birthplace: a one-room log cabin near Jonesville, Virginia. Preserved and displayed at the A.T. Still Museum on the campus of A.T. Still University in Kirksville, MO. (Reprinted with permission from A.T. Still Pension File. Still National Osteopathic Museum, Kirksville, MO.)

As pioneers, the Stills first eked out a living by hunting for food and making some of their clothes from animal skins. The family plowed their land claim and established a farm while Abram Still rode a circuit among scattered settlers, ministering to others in body, mind, and spirit. It was a lifestyle that gave substance to the word "survivor" during this time period.[7]

A.T. Still hunted for his family's food and cleaned and processed the game himself. He would later say how important animal dissection had been as a preparation for the study of human anatomy. He also recorded another prophetic childhood experience in his autobiography:

> *One day, when about ten years old, I suffered from a headache. I made a swing of my father's plow-line between two trees; but my head hurt too much to make swinging comfortable, so I let the rope down to about eight or ten inches of the ground, threw the end of a blanket on it, and I lay down on the ground and used the rope for a swinging pillow. Thus, I lay stretched on my back, with my neck across the rope. Soon I became easy and went to sleep, got up in a little while with the headache gone. As I knew nothing of anatomy at this time, I took no thought of how a rope could stop headache and the sick stomach which accompanied it. After that discovery I roped my neck whenever I felt one of those spells coming on.*[3]

To the end of his life, Still continued to "rope his neck" (Fig. 2.2). In his old age, he would lie down daily with his neck on a "saint's rest"—a wooden frame with a leather strap suspended across it—giving the same effect as a plow rope suspended between two trees. In his middle years, he discovered other crude but effective methods for self-treatment that typically involved biomechanical and structure–function relationships, including a croquet ball upon which he would lie down at the correct point when the problem seemed related to his back rather than his neck (Mrs. J.S. Denslow [Dr. Still's granddaughter], personal communication with Barbara Peterson, 1972).

Medical Education on the Frontier

In the 1840s, the issue of slavery divided the Methodist church, and the Stills sided with the northern (abolitionist) branch. After a hailstorm destroyed his crops and his realization that he was not satisfied with a teaching career, A.T. Still decided to assume a medical apprenticeship with his father, Rev. Abram Still, a trained MD. "In May, 1853, my wife and I moved to the Wakarusa Mission, Kansas, occupied by the Shawnee tribe....Then with my father I doctored the Indians all fall"[3] (pp. 60–61). This was a legitimate form of medical training for the time. America's frontier lands in the mid-1850s were former territories that had only recently become states and lacked opportunities for a formal medical education, especially as the Federal government had no laws funding education. As a result, physician licensing was purposely lax due to the need for doctors with any skill to help the sick and dying. Dr. A.T. Still described the frontier as a daily struggle between life and death. "Death was the rule, recovery was the exception"[3] (p. 282). When the student achieved the necessary level of competence, the mentoring physician would take the student to the local courthouse, pay a fee, and receive a physician and surgeon license.[8]

The few trained doctors in the region could make a good income creating proprietary schools that ran a term of 6 to 9 months. These small schools opened and closed rapidly, gave no degree, had few books, limited equipment, no cadaveric training, and no opportunity for clinical training. Topics of education included bleeding, blistering, and drug dosing as standard treatments. According to his son-in-law, Dr. George "Geo" M. Laughlin, A.T. Still hoped to broaden his medical tutelage from his father's apprenticeship and sought out a proprietary medical school.

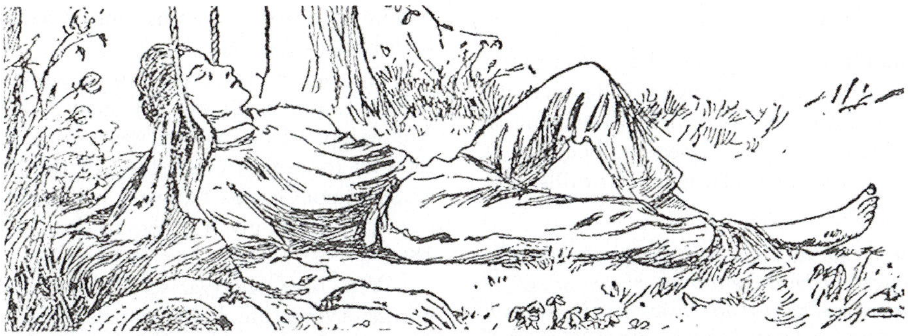

Figure 2.2. Headache and the Rope: Like many physicians before and after him, Dr. A.T. Still applied his new philosophy first to himself and then to his patients. In a famous early anecdote, he stopped a headache by suspending his neck across a low-lying rope swing. He later applied self-adjustments of spinal joint dysfunction to abate an attack of "flux" (bloody dysentery). After he was successful at curing 17 children of the same affliction by adjusting their spinal joint dysfunctions, he realized he was onto something worthwhile. (From Still AT. Autobiography of Andrew T. Still. Rev Ed. Published by the author; 1908. Distributed: American Academy of Osteopathy.)

"He attended there one full term and finished up the work but did not get his diploma. He says he was so disgusted with the whole outfit he never went back after it."[9] However, A.T. Still remained vague about the school he enrolled in and the dates he attended.[10] Failing to officially graduate and pick up his diploma, Dr. A.T. Still would not be an MD despite receiving the full training of the day. Nonetheless, Still was a legitimate physician and surgeon as his Missouri license states from his apprenticeship experience. He was registered as number 71 in the Missouri Roll of Physician and Surgeons dated July 28, 1883.

A.T. Still and the Native American Community He Served

It is important to note that on the frontier there existed very complex and fluid relationships between the Native Americans and the settlers. The communities were often interconnected by marriage and blood relations. Wilson Hobbs, a doctor who lived with the Shawnee from 1850 to 1852 at the same time as Rev. Abram and A.T. Still, observed: "At the time of my residency…The Parkses (Joe and William), the Blue-jackets (Charles Henry, and George), the Fishes (Paschal and John), the most noted and influential men of their tribe…" were of mixed ancestry.[11]

A.T. Still himself was descended from the Cheraw/Lumbee tribe according to the census through his great grandmother Sarah Anna (Wilkenson) Davis, and grandmother Mary Lyda (Abram Still's mother). According to this lineage, Andrew Taylor Still was 1/8 or 12.5% Native American.[12]

At the time that A.T. Still moved to the Wakarusa Mission, Kansas in 1853, Paschal Fish Jr. was the Shawnee tribal leader.[13]

He was descended from Paschal Fish Sr., a White man originally named William Jackson but who took the name "Paschal," the Latin word for "Easter." Paschal Fish Sr. was born about 1760 and was taken from his White family in the Ohio River Valley to be the adopted son of Black Fish (of the Shawnee) before 1778. He was educated at a mission school in Ohio. He married Elizabeth Bishop, a White woman, around 1789 and became the tribal leader upon the death of Black Fish. Paschal Fish Sr. later took a Shawnee wife and then married Polly Rogers, the granddaughter of Black Fish, who was half-Shawnee. He had several children, including Paschal Fish Jr., a child with his Shawnee wife. Paschal Fish Sr. died at the Shawnee Indian Mission in 1834.

Paschal Fish Jr. was the Shawnee tribe leader, and was also an innkeeper, a ferry operator, and a Methodist minister. At age 33, Paschal Fish Jr. (also spelled "Pascel," "Pascal," "Paschall," "Pasqual," and "Pescel") assumed leadership of the Fish Tribe, also known as the Jackson tribe. In 1837, he worked as a blacksmith and gunsmith assistant at Fort Leavenworth, according to Indian Department employment records.[11]

The Fish Tribe with Fish Jr. moved to the Wakarusa area in the early 1840s. On 1854 Indian census rolls, Fish Jr. was listed as being 50 years of age with a wife, Martha, age 40. His children were Obadiah, 12; Eudora (Udora), 9; and Leander Jackson.[11]

A.T. Still's sister, Morovia further detailed in her autobiography, "our truest and best friend was Paschal Fish [Jr.], and brother of Charles. Charles Fish was my father's interpreter. My father [Abram Still] would preach and he [Charles] would interpret into the Indian language. He [Paschal Fish Jr.] came over to see us nearly every day as he lived only a few hundred yards from the Mission. Father had built a small smoke house so that he could sit there, rest, and read when he came in from his work and he and Mr. Fish would sit there and related their experiences and surely if anyone enjoyed a hearty laugh he did."[14]

At this time, Still had begun practicing medicine with his father. Abram Still and the Shawnee chief, Paschal Fish, built the Wakarusa Mission together[13] and it was here that A.T. Still and his father administered medical care to the Shawnee, providing "such drugs as white men used [and] cured most of the cases [they] met."[3] Unfortunately, several years after the Still family moved to Kansas, the community experienced a deadly outbreak of cholera, resulting in the rapid burial of the dead. The Shawnee were particularly susceptible and experienced a high mortality rate. In an attempt to further understand this deadly disease (the source of cholera, *vibrio cholerae* was not discovered until 1883)[15] and to aid his living patients of the Wakarusa Mission and beyond, A.T. Still desperately studied the bodies of deceased Native American Indians, searching for a cure.

While the tribe had sold its land holdings to the German Immigrant Settlement Company (with the stipulation that the town site be called Eudora in honor of Paschal Fish Jr.'s daughter) and moved to Miami, Oklahoma (where they reside today), it seems that Chief Fish and the Shawnee community were aware of A.T. Still's search for a cure and may have even granted Still permission to study the deceased due to the horrific circumstances of the outbreak where hundreds of their community had died.[13]

Abolition and Pre–Civil War

In addition to the devastation caused by the cholera outbreak, political factors soon caused further violence.[13] The Kansas–Nebraska Act of 1854 turned Kansas into a virtual war zone as both abolitionists and proslavery settlers rushed in. The fate of Kansas as a free state depended on a popular vote. The Stills were active abolitionists. Still recalled,

> *I could not do otherwise, for no man can have delegated to him by statute a just right to any man's liberty, either on account of race or color. With these truths before me I entered all combats for the abolition of slavery at home and abroad, and soon had a host of bitter political enemies, which resulted in many thrilling and curious adventures.*[3]

The Stills knew John Brown and fought under the command of Jim Lane, two of the abolitionist leaders active on the Western frontier. Numerous dangerous encounters occurred between the abolitionists and proslavery partisans during the pre–Civil War days.[13,16,17] The struggle lasted, said Still, "until Abraham Lincoln wrote the golden words: 'Forever free, without regard to race or color.' I will add—or sex."[3] The territorial political situation was volatile and confusing, with even the elections seemingly decided by gun battles, as both sides struggled for supremacy in "Bloody Kansas." Still was a proud representative in the Free State Legislature elected in 1857 to develop a constitution and apply for statehood.[18]

Amid the violence and political turmoil, Still experienced further tragedy when his first wife, Mary Margaret Vaughn Still, died in September 1859 following a complicated pregnancy which also resulted in the death of their newborn. This left Still alone with their three children. In November 1860, he married a young schoolteacher, Mary Elvira Turner Still, who had learned to mix prescriptions for her physician father. She accepted Still's medical and spiritual speculations[13] and supported her husband and family through the long period of doubt and criticism that preceded the successful establishment of the osteopathic profession and through the heady days of unexpected success.

War and Medicine

When the Civil War officially began (April 12th, 1861), Still served the Union. This included both organized unofficial and recognized state militias, rather than the US Army. He enlisted in the cavalry division of a force assigned to Jim Lane.

Later, he organized a company of Kansas militia, which was in turn consolidated with other militia battalions. Still was commissioned a Major and saw active combat with several close calls; some experiences are recounted in his autobiography.[3] He also served as a military surgeon, though he had been listed as a hospital steward on the official record.[19]

Since he was serving in state militias rather than directly in the Union Army, not all his time was spent on active duty. He experienced profound loss during his leave in February 1864. Two of his children from his first marriage (Abraham, 11, and Susan, 7) and an "adopted girl," 9, died on successive days of cerebrospinal meningitis, despite the best efforts of the physicians (including Still's brother James, a graduate of Rush Medical College in Chicago) and the standard medical treatment available.[20] Within 3 weeks, his 13-month-old daughter (Marcia) died of pneumonia leaving Mary Elvira childless as she had lost her firstborn infant son shortly after his birth.

Despite this devastation to his family, Still was summoned back into service in September and commissioned a Major in the 21st Regiment, Kansas State Militia, to combat the Army of Missouri (Confederate) under Major General Sterling Price, who had invaded from Arkansas, crossed Missouri, and now threatened to cross into Kansas.

The Battle of Westport, on October 23 to 24, 1864, in what is now Kansas City, was the largest Civil War battle west of the Mississippi River, involved more than 30,000 men and has been referred to as the "Gettysburg of the West." After Union forces under Major General Samuel Curtis triumphed, and Price retreated south, Still was given orders to disband his unit on October 29, 1864.

With his Civil War service over, Still went home to resume normal civilian life. It was not exactly a joyful homecoming. Aside from the fact that he had lost four children all within weeks of each other, Still returned to find that many veterans and others had become addicted to alcohol or morphine, and considered that these were "habits, customs, and traditions no better than slavery in its worst days."[3]

Mainstream Civil War medicine still depended heavily on purging, bloodletting, and an armamentarium of medicines that could only be characterized as highly toxic. On both sides, there were many more casualties from sickness than from battle injuries.[21] A history of American medicine recounts:

> *Even the most erudite and experienced physician had few effective medicines at his command. Some of those which were effective were unknown to the poorly educated practitioner; others he knew not how to use. The short list of effective agents in the 1870s included the anesthetics (ether, chloroform, and nitrous oxide); opium and its alkaloids (morphine was first used extensively during the Civil War to ease the pain of the wounded); digitalis, which was used chiefly for cardiac edema [congestive heart failure]; ergot, to stimulate uterine contractions and to control postpartum hemorrhage; mercury in the form of an injunction for syphilis and in the form of calomel to purge and salivate; various cathartics of botanical origin; iron, usually in the form of Blaud's pills for anemia; quinine for malaria; amyl nitrite, which was first recommended for the relief of angina pectoris by Sir Thomas Lauder Brunton in 1867 but was still not well known in 1876; sulfur ointment for the itch (scabies); green vegetables or citrus fruit for the prevention or treatment of scurvy. These various medicines were administered either by mouth, by rectum, by inhalation, or by application to the skin. The hypodermic syringe had been introduced by the French surgeon Pravaz in 1851. He employed it to inject "chloride of iron" into vascular tumors to coagulate their contents. Although it was subsequently used for other restricted purposes, the danger of infection limited its use until the physician had learned how to prevent infections by the preparation of sterile solutions.*[22]

This description of the best of the medical armamentarium available was recorded about a decade after the Civil War. Though urban populations benefited from breakthroughs, frontier doctors and their patients were very much worse off. In a quote from his autobiography, Still is in agony over the current state of affairs and recalls his anatomical studies of the cholera victims, determined to find a way to alleviate his patients' pain and free them from addiction:

> *My sleep was well-nigh ruined; by day and night I saw legions of men and women staggering to and fro, all over the land, crying for freedom from habits of drugs and drink; I dreamed of the dead and dying who were and had been slaves of habit. I sought to know the cause of so much death, bondage, and distress among my race; I who had had some experience in alleviating pain found medicine a failure. Since my early life I had been a student of nature's book. In my early days in windswept Kansas, I had devoted my attention to the study of anatomy. I became a robber in the name of science. Indian graves were desecrated, and the bodies of the sleeping dead exhumed in the name of science. Yes, I grew to be one of those vultures with the scalpel, and studied the dead that the living might be benefited. I had printed books but went back to the great book of nature as my chief study.*[3]

Still was speaking in the language of the day. The public thought of doctors who disinterred and dissected bodies as grave robbers, but sources indicate that Still actually had permission to study the deceased Shawnee from the Chief during the cholera epidemic.[13]

The Search for a Better Way

In the years following the Civil War, Still explored his spirit of innovation and mechanical inclination as evidenced by his invention of a butter churn and a version of a grain reaper. He and Mary Elvira had several more children, sons and a daughter who would become prominent in the profession that he would eventually found. However, a blight on his life was the estrangement of his oldest daughter from his first marriage who had survived the bouts of cerebral meningitis and blamed her father for the death of her mother and for the inability to save her siblings. It was perhaps this very personal loss combined with the suffering of his patients that led Still in this next decade (1865–1875) to devote himself to search for a better way to find, restore and maintain health.

The post–Civil War period was a time of great diversity in the healing professions, including how one became identified as a physician and how one approached the practice.[23] As previously alluded to, in the mid-19th century, there were no licensing boards and only scattered state laws governing medical practice. There were a few medical schools, but no standard curricula. Schools generally required lectures only a few hours a day, for a single term of less than 6 months, with patient treatment left until after graduation. Most physicians, especially on the frontiers, were trained as apprentices, reading books and serving alongside a physician for an unstated length of time.

Physicians, heavily influenced by the "heroic medicine" of Benjamin Rush, followed the proverb that desperate diseases required desperate remedies. Rush said that "there is but one disease in the world" and that it was treatable by "depletion," which translated into bloodletting, blistering, and purging. One influential textbook writer, John Esten Cooke, wrote that:

> *All diseases, particularly fevers, arose from cold or malaria, which weakened the heart and thus produced an accumulation of blood in the vena cavae and in the adjoining large veins of the liver. Consequently, calomel and other cathartics which acted on that organ were the cure. 'If calomel did not salivate and opium did not constipate, there is no telling what we could do in the practice of physic.'*[23]

Calomel and other mercury compounds were still listed as late as 1899 in the first Merck Manual, along with opium and morphine and many alcohol-based compounds.[25] The practice of "heroic" dosing was well established and highly defended by the medical community of the time. By the time of the Civil War, this standard system of medicine as taught in the medical schools was called *allopathy*.

Allopathy is defined as "that system of therapeutics in which diseases are treated by producing a condition incompatible with or antagonistic to the condition to be cured or alleviated."[26] Samuel Hahnemann created the term allopathy to describe standard medicine in contrast with the system he originated, *homeopathy*.

The damage caused by the "heroic" techniques was obvious to thinkers before Still. They created alternative systems of medicine used by some physicians and lay people.

- Home remedies and Native American herbal preparations were a basic choice, and this lore was substantial and widely used.[24] Numerous resources for botanic preparations, such as Thomson's New Guide to Health; or Botanic Family Physician (1822), were available as well; many of these manuals were widely circulated.
- Homeopathy was a major influence in the 19th century. Developed by Samuel Hahnemann (1755–1843), it was a system of therapy in which "diseases are treated by drugs which are capable of producing in healthy persons symptoms like those of the disease to be treated, the drug being administered in minute doses,"[26,27] or, most commonly, doses that contained no remaining active ingredient due to the successive dilution used to prepare them.
- Eclecticism was another choice, described as "a once popular system of medicine which treats diseases by the application of single remedies to known pathologic conditions, without reference to nosology, special attention being given to developing indigenous plant remedies."[23]
- Magnetic healing "combined spiritualism and healing by seeking to restore the balance of an invisible magnetic fluid circulating throughout the body."[23] Variations attempting to use electrical current to restore health were also employed.
- Hydropathy (the water cure) emphasized hygiene, anti-alcoholism or temperance, fresh air and sunlight, nutritional programs, and physical education.
- Mental diagnosis and healing techniques included hypnotism, spiritualism (table rapping), and phrenology.
- *Bonesetting* was an uncommon traditional lay practice (primarily in Europe) used to reset joints and to set fractures, with few local practitioners.

Still initially linked his name to two of these methods for a time: *magnetic healing* and *bonesetting*.

In 1875, he briefly advertised himself in Kirksville as a *magnetic healer*,[20] possibly persuaded by "the metaphor of the harmonious balance of the interaction of body parts and the unobstructed flow of body fluids."[23] Still had traveled to Ottumwa, Iowa, to investigate the methods of Paul Caster, a self-professed magnetic healer, who felt that Still had the same ability. A farm girl, who fell off a horse and temporarily lost her vision, said that whenever Still touched her, she felt as if a kind of magnetic power went throughout her whole body. She regained her vision after several weeks of treatments.[20]

Still was using manipulation of the bones and soft tissue to achieve unobstructed flow of blood, lymph and neurotrophic elements, and his goal was to lead the body back to healthy physiologic function. But he realized that *magnetic healing* was not describing his methods. He dropped that term rapidly and continued his quest for a word that would identify his methods accurately. After a Kansas City newspaper designated him as a *bonesetter* when reporting on his cure of a young woman's dislocated hip,[20] Still had professional cards printed, which identified him as a "lightning bonesetter."

The Banner of Osteopathy

After a decade of study, Still states in his Autobiography that he "flung to the breeze the banner of osteopathy" in 1874.[3] However, it seemed that this represented his feelings of being "divorced from allopathy"[3] (p. 318), and his feelings that the "machinery He (God) put in man is perfect"[3] (p. 304). Indeed, the term osteopathy would not be officially adopted until 1889.[20]

In an attempt to promulgate his new approach, Still applied to present a public lecture on his ideas at Baker University, in now Baldwin City, Kansas, a Methodist institution that he and his family had helped build by donating land, purchasing a sawmill, and sawing lumber for the building.[28] The Baker University president accused Still of trying to imitate Christ by using the hands to achieve miraculous cures and would not let him speak.[20] In addition, a Baldwin Methodist preacher ranted and raved about him (while his wife and two children sat in the pews) to the point that people in the town thought him a heretic, misled by the devil and possibly insane.[20] Still's description of the treatments that provoked these reactions makes it clear that his "laying on of hands" was therapeutic manipulation.

In August 1874, the town of Baldwin, Kansas suffered a plague of locusts that destroyed all of their crops. Still went to Macon, Missouri, to collect donations of food and clothing for the beleaguered Kansans. After delivering the supplies in Baldwin, he returned to Macon to help his brother Ed[20] rid himself of his morphine addiction, acquired through his self-prescribed medical treatment. This experience solidified in Still not only the inability of the medications of the day to save lives, such as those of his family, but also highlighted the dangers they posed. It roused in Still a hatred for the indiscriminate, excessive use of opiates and other toxic medications of the day. His polarization sometimes appeared to be nearly absolute, even when the armamentarium of drugs began to move from harmful toward helpful.[1–4,29]

However, Still's own writings reveal that he sometimes used home remedies (e.g., the chewing of willow bark which contains salicin, a similar chemical to that found in aspirin, learned from the Native Americans), topical solutions or ointments, and other medications. He washed the wounds of snakebites with spirits of ammonia, the areas bitten by a rabid dog with a diluted sulfuric acid solution, and a spasmodic tetanic joint with alcohol.[4] He used glycerin to help free or dissolve granules under the eyelid.[30] His son Charles (also a DO) provided an affidavit about his father's further practices using analgesics including opiates when nothing else would work (Fig. 2.3).

Late in 1875, Still moved from Kansas to Kirksville, Missouri, his home for the rest of his life. For several years, Still used Kirksville as a base to conduct a marginal itinerant practice in northern Missouri.[31] His methods evolved with additional experience, becoming more specific as his anatomical knowledge and palpatory skills increased. Although he had investigated the traditions of magnetic healing and identified himself for a short time as a lightning bonesetter, he continued the natural progression of his own ideas. His hands-on treatments emphasized detailed knowledge of anatomy and body mechanics so that the treatment could restore normal function, motion, and movement of fluids.

In Still's book *Philosophy of Osteopathy*, Chapter 1 describes the foundational principles of the philosophy and its evolution. Essentially, his system was based on the following precepts:

- The body is an efficient chemical laboratory that makes all the "drugs" it naturally needs when in a state of good health.[3]
- The object of treatment is to discover what caused the sickness and remove the interference so that the body can heal itself.[2]

STATE OF MISSOURI)
) SS.
COUNTY OF ADAIR)

CHARLES E. STILL, being first duly sworn, on oath deposes and says:

1. That he is a son of Dr. Andrew Taylor Still, late of Kirksville, Missouri, and was born in January 7, 1865

2. That from an early age he was acquainted with the osteopathic practice of his father, the said Andrew Taylor Still; that he was associated with his said father in the practice of osteopathy and was taught osteopathy by precept and by example by his father; that he assisted his father, Andrew Taylor Still, in the organization of the American School of Osteopathy in 1892; that he was active in the administration of the said college from its origin and was instrumental in organizing its curriculum and in formulating the policies of the osteopathic education of the college, all of which was done under the guidance and supervision of and in full and complete cooperation with said Andrew Taylor Still, in pursuance of the plan and design of the said Andrew Taylor Still, to teach the principles and practice of the osteopathic school of the healing art.

3. That from 1865 until the death of his father, the said Andrew Taylor Still, in 1917 your affiant was closely associated with said Andrew Taylor Still in the development and practice of osteopathy and in the administration of the American School of Osteopathy which was devoted to the teaching of the principles of the osteopathic school of the healing art.

4. That his father, the said Andrew Taylor Still, from the time when he first enunciated and applied the principles and practice of osteopathy always considered surgery and the administration of anaesthetics and narcotics in connection therewith to be a part of the practice of osteopathy.

5. That he personally witnessed his father, the said Andrew Taylor Still, personally perform a large number of surgical operations and administer anaesthetics and narcotics in connection therewith, all of which the said Andrew Taylor Still believed to be and expressed to be an integral part of the practice of osteopathy.

6. That immediately upon the original organization of the American School of Osteopathy in 1892 there was taught therein the principles and practice of osteopathy as developed and practiced by said Andrew Taylor Still and that the curriculum of the said college included careful and extensive training in surgery and in the administration and uses of anaesthetics and narcotics in connection therewith as a part of its teaching of the practice and principles of osteopathy.

7. That this affidavit is made for the purpose of establishing that Andrew Taylor Still, as evidenced by his expressions and acts, considered surgery and the use of anaesthetics and narcotics in connection therewith to be a part of the practice and principles of the osteopathic school of the healing art.

C E Still

Subscribed and sworn to before me this 4th day of Sept., 1940.

Notary Public.

Figure 2.3. Charles Still's affidavit concerning his father's stance on pharmaceuticals and surgery. (Reprinted with permission from A.T. Still Pension File. Still National Osteopathic Museum, Kirksville, MO.)

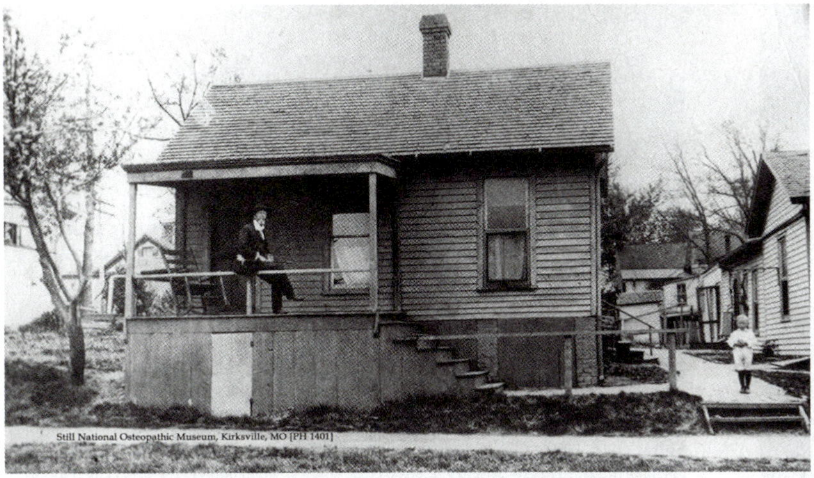

Figure 2.4. The American School of Osteopathy in the 1890s with Dr. A.T. Still sitting on a rail on the porch. (Reprinted with permission from A.T. Still Pension File. Still National Osteopathic Museum, Kirksville, MO.)

- To cure disease, the abnormal parts must be adjusted back to normal.[4]

By 1887, enough patients were arriving in Kirksville seeking his method of treatment that Still could stop his itinerant practice. His health-focused philosophy using manual medicine and stories of dramatic successful outcomes had spread via the newspapers and word of mouth. This drew literally hundreds of patients to him weekly and his practice quickly became overwhelmed. Still began to think about teaching others his methods; unlike many alternative practitioners of his day, he never intended to keep therapeutic secrets to himself or to grow rich from his methods.

He attempted to train apprentices and then to teach a group of interested individuals including some of his adolescent children to assist in the practice of osteopathy. These attempts were largely unsuccessful because the students lacked Still's detailed knowledge of anatomy and bodily function.

While Still may have used the term *osteopathy* earlier, it was officially adopted in 1889.[20] When challenged that this word was not in the dictionary, Still replied, "We are going to put it there."[32] The word became for Still and his followers a symbol for medical reform, for a science that would refocus medicine on the restoration of normal function. Osteopathy aimed to *work with and facilitate* the natural physiologic mechanisms of the body for normal and reparative function. The contemporary standard purgatives, emetics, bloodletting, and addictive drugs seemed to be *working against* the body's own mechanisms. To solidify this new way of thinking, and to ensure its continuation, A.T. Still realized he would have to establish formal osteopathic training.

PROFESSIONAL EDUCATION AND GROWTH

First School

To meet the patient demands for his unique medical approach to health care and to continue to grow osteopathy, Dr. A.T. Still founded the American School of Osteopathy (ASO). It was chartered in May of 1892[33] and opened that October with 18 students present on the first day. Enrollment increased early in the term to 16 men and 5 women, including members of Still's family and other local people (Figs. 2.4 and 2.5). There were two faculty members: Still and Dr. William Smith, a physician who graduated in 1889 from the University of Edinburgh, Scotland, and taught anatomy in exchange for learning osteopathy (Fig. 2.6).

The revised (1894) charter for the school reiterated that the goal of the school was "to improve our present system of surgery, obstetrics, and treatment of diseases generally, and [to] place the same on a more rational and scientific basis, and to impart information to the medical profession."

The charter could have granted the Doctor of Medicine (MD) degree, but Still insisted on a distinctive recognition for graduates, DO, for Diplomate in Osteopathy[33] (later Doctors of Osteopathy,

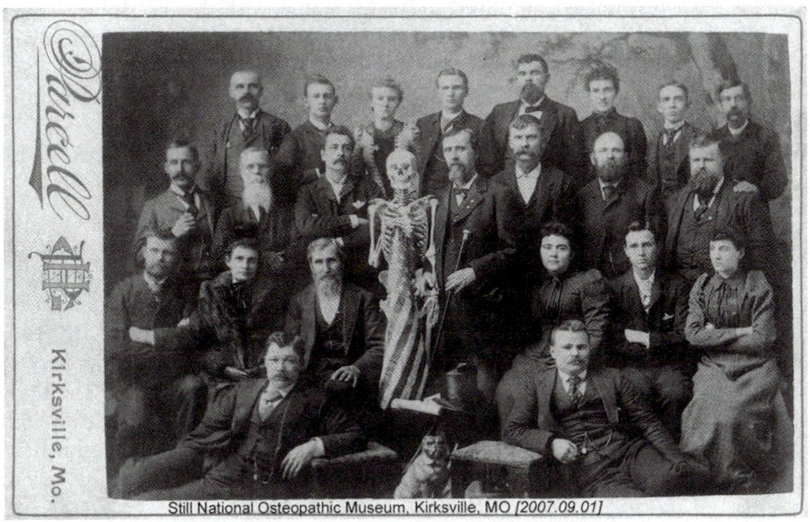

Figure 2.5. The first class of the American School of Osteopathy included five women (1892). (Reprinted with permission from A.T. Still Pension File. Still National Osteopathic Museum, Kirksville, MO.)

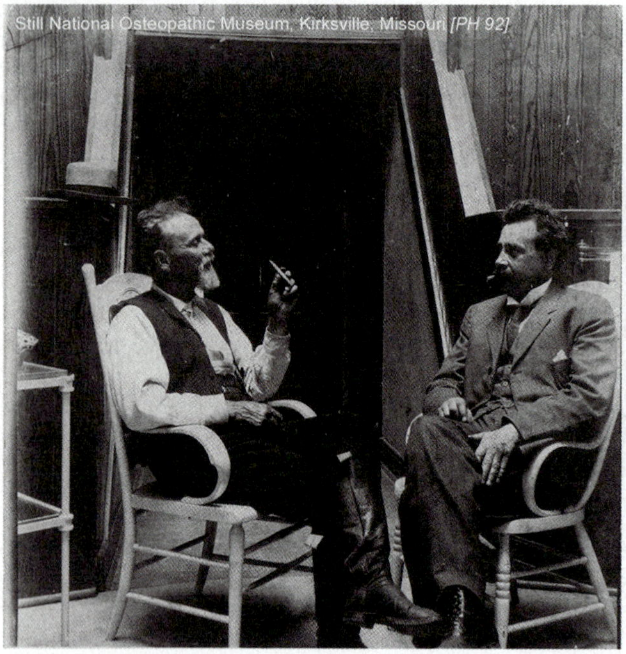

Figure 2.6. Shown here at the ASO hospital, A. T. Still, Physician and Surgeon (left), and William Smith, MD, were the inaugural faculty of the newly founded American School of Osteopathy in 1892. (Reprinted with permission from A.T. Still Pension File. Still National Osteopathic Museum, Kirksville, MO.)

then Doctors of Osteopathic Medicine). William Smith, MD, received the first handwritten DO diploma in February, 1893 and left to practice in Kansas City.[33] Graduates were finally considered to be legal physicians in Missouri on March 4, 1897. Up to that point their practice had been tolerated but they were not considered to be legally practicing and were diplomates, not physicians. On this date, Governor Lon Stephens passed a bill making them osteopathic physicians, legal doctors equivalent to MDs. "The people of Missouri were for giving the friends of osteopathy the protection of our state laws. The Science of Osteopathy, as far as it has come under my observation, assists in relieving suffering humanity, and I do not think I have erred in signing the bill."[34]

Some have questioned whether or how A.T. Still himself received an official DO degree, since when he issued the first Diplomate of Osteopathy degrees, there was no one with the authority to issue the degree to him. The Trustees of the ASO settled that point on June 22, 1897, when they voted to grant diplomas under the school's new charter to 25 "former graduates." The first name on the list is Dr. A.T. Still.[35]

Jeanette "Nettie" Hubbard Bowles, DO, a graduate of the first class, became the new anatomy professor. Smith returned as faculty from 1896 to 1899 when Bolles moved to Colorado to establish an osteopathic school there along with her husband Alden Bolles, also an ASO graduate.

The first course was from October through February; all but a few of the students voluntarily returned for a second year of additional training. The program became officially 2 years long, two terms of 5 months each. In addition to their study of anatomy, students worked in the clinic under Still and his new graduates.

During the last 5 years of the 19th century, the growth of both the clinic and the school was spectacular. Patients came from near and far, having heard by word of mouth or by printed accounts of near-miraculous cures. There were enough such "miracles" that the osteopathic profession was widely promoted by grateful patients.

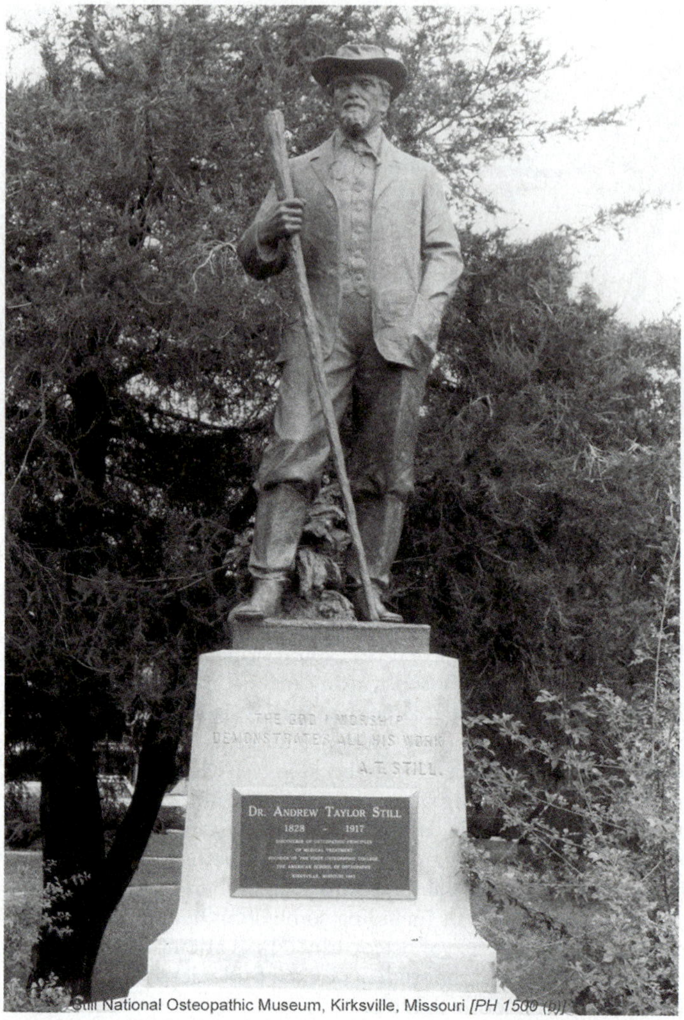

Figure 2.7. The statue dedicated in 1917 to Dr. A.T. Still in Kirksville, MO, still stands today in the town square. (Reprinted with permission from A.T. Still Pension File. Still National Osteopathic Museum, Kirksville, MO.)

A significant number of early DOs were either former patients or family members of patients, who based on their own or others' recoveries came to their studies with a kind of evangelical fervor. The town of Kirksville prospered and came to regard Still, once ridiculed, as a citizen of immense importance. He was lavishly praised, and lived to see his statue, with the inscription "The God I Worship Demonstrates All His Work," erected in the town square[36,37] (Fig. 2.7).

Data on numbers of enrolled students illustrate the school's dramatic growth:

- October 1895: 28 students
- Summer, 1896: 102 students
- 1900: Over 700 students and 18 faculty[33] (Fig. 2.8)

At the turn of the century, there were about 23 "daughter" schools founded by graduates of the original school.[38] Some of the schools were well organized under the model established by Still; others were criticized as "diploma mills," anticipated to generate large revenues for the founders. Still considered many of these to be for training "engine wipers" who were incapable or inexperienced in the practice of osteopathy. As standards were established by the AOA and state licensure boards, many closed; only seven remained open by 1915.[39]

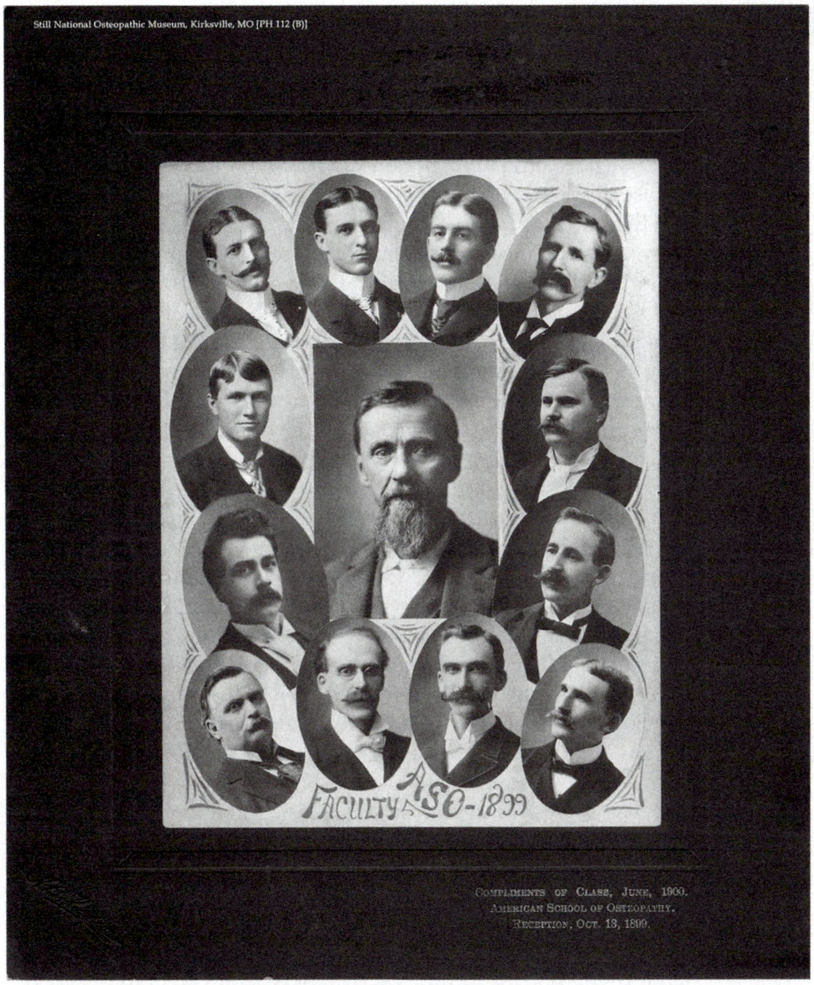

Figure 2.8. The faculty of the American School of Osteopathy in 1899. Several soon thereafter became leaders in the profession and founded new osteopathic colleges. (Reprinted with permission from A.T. Still Pension File. Still National Osteopathic Museum, Kirksville, MO.)

Rapid Medical Education Changes in the Early 20th Century

Medical education in the late 19th century was not well regulated. Many schools—allopathic, eclectic, homeopathic, and osteopathic—had virtually no entrance requirements except tuition payments and were for-profit institutions. Licensing laws had not yet reached a stage where they were effective in setting educational standards.

The American Medical Association (AMA), founded in 1847 and later a powerful influence on raising educational standards, was weak and in need of reorganization in the 1890s.

The reorganized AMA observed that there were too many doctors, including a significant number with questionable education. Revising its constitution, the organization made the regulation of medical education its first order of business. Its Council on Medical Education was formed in 1904, with a charge to improve the academic requirements for medical schools. Medical schools were rated as Class A (approved), B (probation), or C (unapproved), and the findings were made available to state licensing boards.[40] Osteopathic schools were not included in the first AMA survey.

Even before the AMA formed its Council on Medical Education, the young AOA had adopted standards of its own for approval of osteopathic colleges (1902) and began inspections (1903).[41] In addition, some larger osteopathic institutions, seeking to limit competition for both students and patients, bought out some of the smaller "daughter" schools subsequently closing them and admitting their students. By 1915, the number of osteopathic institutions had fallen from 23 to 7. The Flexner Report, published in 1910,[42] harshly condemned many medical schools including many osteopathic schools. State licensing boards began to enforce stricter requirements, which was an even more decisive influence on increasing standards than the Flexner Report.[23,43] Fallout from these processes included the closure of marginal medical schools, with surviving schools converting to a not-for-profit status. Few schools established for training Black physicians survived,[44] and all but two or three schools for women were closed.[45,46]

Curriculum

Many early 20th century medical schools gained both experienced science faculty and stable funding by forming affiliations with universities. This was not an option for osteopathic institutions at that time, and they faced a difficult dilemma: either raise entry standards and lose a major portion of their only source of income (tuition) or adopt a "go slow" attitude. Choosing the latter, their medical educational reforms lagged by about two decades.[39]

AOA standards increased the required length of osteopathic curricula to 3 years in 1905 and to 4 years in 1915.[36]

The profession responded officially to external criticism by pointing out the differences between osteopathic and orthodox medical education, and raised general standards in the 1930s when the opportunity arose again. By the mid-1930s, osteopathic colleges required at least 2 years of college before matriculation. In 1954, 3 years were required; by 1960, over 70% of students had either baccalaureate or advanced degrees prior to entry.[39] Today,

TABLE 2.1

Description of Course of Study by Term

American School of Osteopathy, 1899–1900

Term	Topics
1	• Descriptive anatomy, including osteology, syndesmology, and myology • Lectures on histology, illustrated by microstereopticon • Principles of general inorganic chemistry, physics, and toxicology
2	• Descriptive and regional anatomy with demonstrations • Didactic and laboratory work in histology • Physiology and physiologic demonstrations • Physiologic chemistry and urinalysis • Principles of osteopathy • Clinical demonstrations in osteopathy
3	• Demonstrations in regional anatomy • Physiology and physiologic demonstrations • Lectures on pathology illustrated by microstereopticon • Symptomatology • Bacteriology • Physiologic psychology • Clinical demonstrations in osteopathy and osteopathic diagnosis and therapeutics
4	• Symptomatology • Surgery • Didactic and laboratory work in pathology • Psychopathology and psychotherapeutics • Gynecology • Obstetrics • Hygiene and public health • Venereal diseases • Medical jurisprudence • Dietetics • Clinical demonstrations • Osteopathic and operative clinics

virtually all students enter COMs with at least baccalaureate degrees, and many have advanced degrees.

Curriculum content grew and evolved with the times. The 1899–1900 Kirksville catalog described a 2-year course of study, divided into four terms of 5 months each, as shown in Table 2.1.[47] The major differences between this curriculum and that of an allopathic medical school of the same period were that unique osteopathic content was included, while *materia medica* (pharmacology) was excluded.

Differences appeared with respect to scope of practice between the so-called "lesion" osteopaths and "broad" osteopaths early in osteopathic history.

- Lesion osteopaths limited their therapeutic practice essentially to manipulation.
- Broad osteopaths utilized all the tools available to medicine, including *materia medica.*

Still practiced midwifery (obstetrics) and surgery; both were taught under his guidance. Though Still remained skeptical about using or teaching pharmaceutical therapy, he was not opposed to using anesthetics or opiates with surgical patients, and may have used opiates with terminal patients. Charles Still, Sr.'s affidavit that his father used anesthetics and opiates in surgical cases is included earlier in this chapter (Fig. 2.3).[48]

Still's general opposition to drugs did not prevent early DOs from using them for treatment. A few had been trained as MDs before they entered osteopathic schools. Others went on to earn MD degrees after they became DOs. Some DOs simply decided to use all the adjunctive treatments available. Most "broad" osteopaths felt that incorporating the new safer medications as they were developed was consistent with osteopathic practice.

The most direct early confrontation came in 1897, when a DO–MD opened the short-lived Columbian School of Osteopathy in Kirksville, with the intention of offering DO and MD degrees from a course in manipulation, surgery, and *materia medica.* The competitive and personal issues in this case extended beyond the academic questions, and the school closed after graduating only three classes.[33] The issue remained professionally divisive for over two more decades.

Adjunctive treatments became a major subject of extended debate within the AOA and the Associated Colleges of Osteopathy (now the American Association of Colleges of Osteopathic Medicine [AACOM]). The question finally was resolved in favor of the "broad" osteopaths, not by consensus over the idea but by recognizing that state licensing laws required fuller training. In 1916, against the direct protest of Still,[49] the trustees revoked a previous year's action condemning individuals and colleges that taught drug therapy, effectively opening the way for the colleges to form their own curricula.

The profession's great success in using manipulative treatment during the 1918 influenza epidemic[50] probably slowed the integration of *materia medica* into the osteopathic curriculum. In 1927, the Associated Colleges of Osteopathy voted to include instruction about medications[33] as part of the courses in "comparative therapeutics," of which pharmacology was one subheading.[39] By the mid-1930s, the integration was complete at all osteopathic schools, prior to use of most modern medications.

More recently developed medications demonstrated efficacy and improved safety, yielding pharmaceutical treatment with benefits outweighing risks. To give historic context to the adoption of pharmaceuticals by the osteopathic profession, most medications in the last decade of the 19th century and at the beginning of the 20th were toxic, based on tradition and without proven benefit. That was Still's original objection to contemporary *materia medica.* Scientific research slowly replaced tradition, providing better options and production methods. Smallpox vaccine had become increasingly purified, decreasing its danger. Arsphenamine (the first modern antimicrobial agent) was marketed as Salvarsan in 1910 for treatment of syphilis. It worked but had significant side effects and was hard to store. Insulin became widely available in the western world in the 1920s, and sulfa drugs in the 1930s. Penicillin became available to the public in 1945, after wartime (WWII) production methods were developed to permit its significant use on soldiers by the invasion of Normandy in June 1944. As two generations of scientific development replaced *materia medica* with modern pharmacology, DOs included the use of medications in their curricula and increasingly integrated them in treatment.

Curricular Improvement

Teaching facilities improved, and more full-time faculty were hired, particularly in the biomedical sciences. Instruction by physicians in active practice was an advantage for students who were developing clinical skills, but the biomedical sciences and laboratory-based research required faculty who could give these interests their full attention and laboratories to support them. All the colleges had established and expanded full-time biomedical science faculty by the middle of the century. The first new osteopathic medical school since 1915 was founded as a private school in 1969 but became public and affiliated with a major American university in 1971 (Michigan State University College of Osteopathic Medicine [MSUCOM]). Similar affiliations had been the route by which allopathic schools had strengthened their basic science teaching and research programs earlier in the 20th century.

The AOA became the accrediting agency recognized by the US Department of Education for predoctoral osteopathic education in 1957.[36] By the end of the 1930s, osteopathic and allopathic medical schools had very similar curricula; however, osteopathic medical schools also included didactics in osteopathic philosophy and principles, and unique training in osteopathic diagnostics and manipulative treatment. The osteopathic manipulative techniques taught were similar at the schools but generally based on individual school traditions; a more standardized approach started to include new treatment systems due to their representation on licensure exams and when the number of schools began to increase again in 1969.

Educational Council on Osteopathic Principles (AACOM-ECOP): Standardizing OPP Instruction

In 1968, a small intercollegiate group of osteopathic principles professors met to discuss the new initiative of uniform medical coding and a movement to change the term *osteopathic lesion* to *somatic dysfunction*. The group was organized in 1969 as the Educational Council on Osteopathic Principles (ECOP) under the leadership of Ira Rumney, DO, and Norm Larson, DO. The ECOP consists of the Chairs (or their designees) of the osteopathic college departments that oversee the teaching of osteopathic philosophy, structural diagnosis, and OMT. In 1974, the council became affiliated with AACOM in order to work more closely with the Board of Deans. The ECOP has steadily worked to develop common osteopathic terminology, best practices in the unique aspects of osteopathic education, and a standard curriculum for osteopathic principles and practice (OPP). Consensus documents toward standardization were first produced in 1981 and continue to be updated. These include the following:

- 1981 *Glossary of Osteopathic Terminology* (first edition; a current copy is in this text)
- 1987 *Core Curriculum for Osteopathic Education* for the AACOM colleges
- 1997 *Foundations for Osteopathic Medicine* (members have performed vital roles as organizers, authors, editors, and peer reviewers for each edition of the AOA reference book [1997, 2003, 2010, 2018 to current])
- 2002 *Clinically Osteopathically Integrated Learning Scenarios* (COILS)
- 2018 and 2025 *A Teaching Guide for Osteopathic Manipulative Medicine, 2nd and 3rd editions* (updated about every 5 years)
- Position papers regarding types of OPP and their teaching (e.g., safety, faculty:student ratios)
- Recommendations for standardized test content for the NBOME's Comprehensive Osteopathic Medical Licensing Examination of the United States (COMLEX-USA) licensing examinations

The ECOP also generated a definition of a US-trained osteopathic physician for accurate and easy reference by osteopathic students, members of the profession, and the general public. The definition consists of four essential points:

- A fully qualified and licensed physician who has graduated from a COCA accredited college of osteopathic medicine
- Educated within a context of a distinct patient-centered, health-oriented philosophy
- Who is trained to combine specialized diagnostic and therapeutic hands-on skills (OMT) with the latest advances in the science and practice of medicine
- To offer comprehensive health care to patients

Curriculum Delivery

The Colleges of Osteopathic Medicine (COMs, used as a generic term but including some which are titled Schools of Osteopathic Medicine) developed several strategies for curriculum delivery in the latter 20th and early 21st centuries. All schools had a 4-year curriculum divided into didactic (classroom and laboratory) and clinical (hospital and clinic) portions. Comparing the MD and DO undergraduate clinical training approaches, each had advantages and disadvantages:

- Most MD schools became academic medical centers and presented 2 years of biomedical science didactics, followed by 2 years of clinical rotations (2+2 model), which incorporated clinical science didactics at tertiary care hospitals.
  - Pros:
    - Residents were offered excellent training with scope and variety of complex cases rarely seen in less densely populated areas.
    - Many excellent lecturers and physician trainers in specialties were available.
    - Tertiary care programs have a higher proportion of rare cases (zebras/horses) seen than in most primary care medicine.
  - Cons:
    - The medical postgraduate training hierarchy often delayed student or even intern hands-on training on procedures, as often the more senior trainees performed most of them.
    - A high number of urban, academic medical center residents entered practice in specialties and subspecialties; the number of primary care physicians produced decreased.
    - Urban-trained physicians preferred to stay in urban areas to practice; the geographic maldistribution of physicians increased.
- COMs with few and limited exceptions had a 2+2 model, but most relied on a community-based model for the 2 clinical years, rather than tertiary care facilities. Many clinical rotations were in widely dispersed community hospitals, as well as small town and rural clinics.
  - Pros:
    - Students in a community-based system worked directly under experienced attending physicians most of the time.
    - Without a hierarchical system where procedural training opportunities were more reserved for fellows, residents, and interns, students (and interns) obtained more rapid and additional training in procedural skills.
    - More experience with primary care medicine was provided.
    - Students and postgraduates, especially those who had grown up in small towns and rural settings, often maintained their preference for small town living, returning to practice in similar locations.
    - Students and residents were granted the opportunity to do more elective clinical rotations at other (including tertiary care) institutions.

- Cons:
  - A more limited number of faculty physicians, practicing at smaller hospitals with fewer doctors, were often busy with their practices and unlike those at academic medical centers, did not have much release time to prepare and deliver clinical lectures or engage in research.
  - The smaller hospitals were less likely to have all the subspecialties represented on-site; to compensate, students and residents were allowed to do those rotations off-site at tertiary care institutions.

New Curricular Models and Technologies

Active learning strategies were introduced in the latter 20th century to supplement or replace the standard lecture format of the first two didactic school years. These required students to prepare for class and actively engage during seat time. Problem-based learning (PBL), case-based learning (CBL), and team-based learning (TBL) curricula were designed with a focus on the most common clinical problems. Integration of biomedical science instruction with clinical information increased relevance of biomedical didactics while helping students to begin to "think like a clinician." No one method was proven to have been superior once the students had been on clinical rotations for several months. In the 21st century, the "flipped classroom" model took advantage of instant polling possibilities by assigning students readings or exercises and utilizing class time for problem solving and higher participation in discussion. In many cases, the *sage on the stage* was replaced by the *guide by the side* as students were assigned more responsibility for learning, rather than simple absorption of delivered information.

New information and communication technology encouraged additional approaches.

- Simultaneous distance learning increased the possibilities of off- and on-site education.
- Asynchronous delivery of information and feedback allowed students autonomy in setting a personal learning schedule.
- Simulation training increased hands-on engagement, and likely decreased student anxiety in initial patient encounters. Students were able to practice under supervision with critique before performing procedures on living patients thereby accomplishing an additional goal of improving safety for patients.
- Objective Structured Clinical Examination (OSCE) experiences prepared students for their encounters with real patients by practicing with trained surrogate patients and incorporating training in their emotional intelligence or bedside manner.
- Preclinical training in skills such as diagnostic ultrasound enhanced diagnostic skill and accuracy of treatment.
- A wide variety of self-training materials became available which helped to promote self-directed learning with the new technologies.

Both osteopathic and allopathic schools have fully or partly incorporated many of these educational strategies in curricular delivery. In addition, students are likely to participate in interprofessional education, learning with other health care profession students, promoting a more team-based approach and collaboration in hospitals and clinics. According to COCA standards from 2023, each COM must have in place a body that exercises collective responsibilities to an education program, and has a responsibility for the development, management, evaluation, and enhancement of the curriculum.[51] This body or committee must include student and faculty representation of all preclinical and clinical education years. The committee must also include representation from any additional campus locations. The curriculum must ensure that students have the opportunity to attain the skills, including osteopathic core competencies, interprofessional education, and humanistic skills, necessary to demonstrate Graduate Medical Education readiness and meet the mission of the COM. In addition, all students must successfully pass COMLEX-USA Level 1, and COMLEX-USA Level 2-CE prior to graduation from an osteopathic medical school.

The COVID-19 Pandemic caused massive changes to osteopathic education in the early and mid-phases of the pandemic (2020–2022). As these changes were related to the social and workplace distortions induced by the pandemic and measures to combat it, they will be discussed in the section on the pandemic.

Growth of the Profession's Schools

EARLY DAYS

By the end of 1915, only seven osteopathic schools were still in operation. Six of these survived into the new millennium, some with complicated charter histories, name changes, relocations, expansion, mergers, and affiliations with other educational institutions. Five remained osteopathic, as osteopathic medical schools, and one became an MD granting school of medicine. The five original schools still accredited by the COCA[38] are:

- Kirksville College of Osteopathic Medicine at Andrew Taylor Still University [from the original ASO] (1892)
- Philadelphia College of Osteopathic Medicine (1898)
- Chicago College of Osteopathic Medicine at Midwestern University (1900)
- College of Osteopathic Medicine at Des Moines University (1905) (There had been a prior osteopathic college in Des Moines as early as 1898.)
- College of Osteopathic Medicine at Kansas City University (1916) (There had been a prior osteopathic college in Kansas City as early as 1895.)

The College of Osteopathic Physicians and Surgeons (1896) in Los Angeles, California, survived as the University of California at Irvine School of Medicine after a brief period as an independent MD granting institution following the temporary "California Merger" of allopathic and osteopathic professions in the state of California in the 1960s. This merger—described below and briefly in the section on State Licensure—resulted not only in the change of an osteopathic college to an allopathic college, but also in igniting exponential growth in the osteopathic profession around the country.

1960s

In 1964, the Michigan Association of Osteopathic Physicians and Surgeons committed itself to developing a new, independently funded college of osteopathic medicine.

- More than 1,000 osteopathic physicians practiced in the state, representing about 5% of the state's physician total and estimated to be providing care (most did primary care) for about 20% of the state's patients. Yet, none of these DOs had received their education in the state.
- In 1969, 18 students enrolled in the first class at a new campus in Pontiac, Michigan.
- Within 2 years, it was clear that a program of such complexity could not survive financially as a freestanding institution.
- Strong supporters in the Michigan legislature, plus Michigan's governor, were willing to support a bill for state funding with one major stipulation: the college had to be integrated with an existing, accredited university program. After complex negotiations, the program transferred to the campus of Michigan State

University in 1971, where it became the first university-based osteopathic college.

Michigan was able to set up a new medical school without the great expense of the startup costs of a new MD school. As this affiliation proved successful, rural state legislatures paid attention. Many states suffered from both a shortage and maldistribution of physicians (new doctors primarily established their practices in urban areas). The osteopathic profession became suddenly notable:

- DOs tended to go into primary care.
- Many of them practiced in small towns, which often served as hubs for rural areas.
- In 1961 to 1962, the State of California, with support from the California Medical Association (CMA), had decided that DOs were equally qualified and were able to exchange their DO degree for an MD degree (only recognized in California), becoming eligible for ACGME-accredited postgraduate training, and service in the armed forces.[39]
- By 1969, DO graduates, without having to exchange their degrees, were being accepted as members of the AMA, trained in ACGME residencies, and conscripted into service as physicians in the armed forces.[39]

In less than a decade, Texas, Oklahoma, West Virginia, Ohio, and New Jersey quickly assumed funding responsibility for, or created new state-funded public COMs in their university systems.

1970s

The loss of the original California school in the 1960s inspired osteopathic physicians in states with physician shortages to work together with legislators, patients, and community leaders to create more COMs. Ten new osteopathic medical colleges (public and private) were founded or chartered between 1969 and 1979, one being in Pomona, California, the College of Osteopathic Medicine of the Pacific, once the California Supreme Court ruled that osteopathic licensure should resume in the state. This tripled the number of schools in a short time and challenged the profession's educational infrastructure, creating a tremendous need for more professors, administrators, and postgraduate education positions.

1980s

The 1980s saw a landmark antitrust case for the osteopathic profession, with Dr. Malcolm Weiss, DO, versus York Hospital (Pennsylvania) when he was denied staff privileges. Generally, a physician can admit and treat patients only at hospitals where they have staff privileges. If a patient desires to receive medical treatment at a hospital for which that patient's doctor does not have staff privileges (either because the patient prefers the reputation of that hospital or because that hospital is the only available hospital with equipment that is necessary for the patient's treatment) then the patient's doctor will have to refer the patient to another physician who has staff privileges at the hospital in question.[52]

At that time, York Hospital had significant market dominance and "testimony at trial established that certain complex, highly technical tertiary care services and facilities are, for a number of reasons, only available at York... therapeutic radiology, open heart surgery, cardiac catheterization, renal dialysis, neo-natal intensive care, short-term acute psychiatric care, monitored stroke treatment, audiology, burn care, cardiopulmonary laboratory, cardiopulmonary rehabilitation, electroencephalography, genetic counseling, prosthetic service, speech therapy, computerized axial tomography (CAT scan), and infusion aspirator."[52]

The gravamen of Weiss' lawsuit is that, although allopaths (medical doctors or MDs) and osteopaths (DOs) are equally trained and qualified to practice medicine, his application for staff privileges at York hospital was turned down solely because of his status as an osteopathic physician.[52] Dr. Weiss brought this suit, both individually and as representative of the class of all osteopathic physicians in the York Medical Service Area (York MSA), against York Hospital ("York"), the York Medical and Dental Staff, and 10 individual physicians who served on the York Medical Staff Executive Committee and the York Judicial Review Committee.[52]

In 1984, the court sided with Dr. Weiss. This case and its outcome in effect ended the discrimination of osteopathic physicians at allopathic hospitals that had been ongoing for almost a century. No longer could DOs be kept from practicing and gaining staff privileges at allopathic institutions. While this represented a victory for osteopathic equality and recognition it also diminished the perceived need for separate osteopathic hospitals. Dr. Malcom Weiss felt that gaining equality came at the cost of losing some of the unique aspects of osteopathic philosophy that was part of the osteopathic hospital system.

The 1980s also marked a change in osteopathic educational institutions. Beginning in the 1980s, and with the process accelerating in the 1990s and 2000s, a few COMs (e.g., those in Des Moines, Florida, California, and Missouri) expanded into free-standing health science universities. Other COMs followed these successful prototypes, so that in the 21st century many institutions included schools for physician assistants, masters, and doctoral degrees in the health professions (e.g., dentistry, health science education, nursing and nurse practitioners, occupational therapy, optometry, pharmacy, physical therapy, podiatry, public health, and veterinary medicine).

1990–2000s

In 1992, a slower third wave of new schools began, expanding the number of colleges but this time through novel development of COMs by groups who seemed to differ from the earlier college movement which seemed to be primarily motivated by the secular, nonprofit ideals of osteopathic medicine. Some of these institutions founded more than one COM, while others opened branches after establishing a base campus.

- Jewish, Baptist, Catholic, and Evangelical Protestant religious universities (Touro University, William Carey University, Campbell University, Marian University, University of the Incarnate Word, Liberty University) created COMs as part of their own university systems.
- Rocky Vista University in Colorado, the first for-profit medical school in the United States since 1910, was founded by an entrepreneur in 2006. This radical departure from the nonprofit model universally used for both DO and MD schools in the United States after the Flexner Report caused considerable debate in both branches of the medical profession. Additional campuses were opened in Utah and Montana years later.
- Entrepreneurs started multiple COMs/campuses through their personal foundations.
  - Edward Via College of Osteopathic Medicine at Virginia Tech (not-for-profit)
- Burrell College of Osteopathic Medicine in New Mexico (for-profit)
- Idaho College of Osteopathic Medicine (for-profit, Burrell Group)
- Southeast Alabama Medical Center, a regional hospital, founded the Alabama College of Osteopathic Medicine (ACOM).

- Several public and private existing colleges either built branch campuses or secondary educational sites.

2023

By June of 2023, the AOA Committee on Osteopathic College Accreditation website reported that for the 2023–2024 academic year, COCA accredited 41 COMs educating at 66 different sites in 35 states with projected enrollment of over 36,000 students for the 2023–2024 academic year.[53]

- Between 2009 and 2021, COM matriculants grew from 4,936 to 8,511.
- Forecasted growth is predicted to be 11,389 by 2030 and 12,995 by 2035.
- COMs grew from 26 (2012) to 40 (2023).
- As a result, the number of osteopathic physicians in the United States increased by 30% from 2018 to 2023.[53]
- As of 2023, there were almost 149,000 DOs in the United States.[54]
- There are numerous schools currently in the planning or pre-accreditation stage, as new schools and sites are being developed to meet the need for additional physicians, particularly in primary care specialties and small-town or rural areas.
- The statistics for this rapidly changing educational scene are best surveyed by consulting the AOA (Osteopathic.org) and AACOM (AACOM.org) websites for up-to-date information, including links to school websites.

STATE LICENSURE AND PROFESSIONAL SELF-REGULATION

Medical licensure in the United States is a right administered by the individual states, not the federal government. Educational standards are closely related to state licensure laws. In the early 1900s as state medical boards became increasingly strict, legislative recognition and professional regulation for a growing profession was necessary.

- The first legislative recognition of osteopathic practice came from Vermont in 1896[55] where graduates of the ASO, Kirksville, were accorded the right to practice in that state.
- Missouri had a successful bill as early as 1895, but it was vetoed by the governor; what was hailed as a better bill was passed and signed into law in March 1897.[29,56]

Greeted triumphantly as the dawn of a new profession which would become national, these laws allowed the osteopathic profession to rapidly expand into states where legislation provided a friendly welcome. Osteopathic history includes numerous stories about legal action against DOs for practicing without a valid license, David-and-Goliath encounters of DOs with MD-dominated legislatures, and testimony or influence offered by prominent people who were osteopathic patients (e.g., Presidents Teddy Roosevelt and Taft, Buffalo Bill Cody, Mark Twain, and later, Vice President Nelson Rockefeller). These colorful tales were the war stories of an energetic first generation of DOs who managed to secure legislative rights to at least limited practice in most states.

Early leaders of the profession at the AOA recognized that educational standards and professional self-regulation were necessary to earn the public's trust and to safeguard patients. More states (but not all) were beginning to require physicians to pass tests on basic science knowledge to show they had minimal mastery of subjects necessary for practicing medicine on a scientific (rather than traditional) basis. Discussions toward forming a national (osteopathically based) testing standard can be traced back to 1910. The increase in a variety of (and concurrent lack of) state basic science board examinations galvanized the founding of the NBOME (first called the National Board of Examiners for Osteopathic Physicians and Surgeons) in 1934. Asa Willard, AOA President in 1925 and the first secretary-treasurer of the new national board, said "Independence in regulation is the vital factor essential to maintenance of our professional identity and our numerical expansion."[57]

Registration and licensure were related (but often different) matters. The profession's growth was limited while the whole state medical licensure issue was being debated and established. States used three different approaches to osteopathic physician licensure:

- Formation of separate osteopathic medical licensing boards
- Adding an osteopathic representative to an existing or composite state board of medicine
- Permitting DOs to apply through a state medical licensing board without osteopathic representation

The roles of these state boards were not immediately clear at the time of their formation. There was opposition on ideologic grounds even to the idea of licensure. Some populists, not partisan to either osteopathic or allopathic physicians, said that medical licensure was discriminatory. Others said that licensing would interfere with freedom of medical research. Some social Darwinists went so far as to say that if the "poor" died of their own foolishness in choosing bad medical practitioners, the species would improve.[44]

By 1901, however, every state had some form of legislation requiring at least registration, with a diploma from an accepted school, or a state examination of some type. When the Missouri board began to function in 1903, the first certificate it issued was to Still.[58] Licensure to practice a full scope of medicine was another matter, and in most places, it was related first to the content of the osteopathic curriculum and later to the results of state-developed examinations.

- At the ASO, by 1897, the subjects taught had expanded to include:
  - ☐ Anatomy
  - ☐ Chemistry
  - ☐ Histology
  - ☐ Midwifery
  - ☐ Pathology
  - ☐ Physiology
  - ☐ Surgery
  - ☐ Symptomatology
  - ☐ Toxicology
  - ☐ Urinalysis

Everything was included except *materia medica* and academic consciences were temporarily satisfied. In 1934, the chartering of the nonprofit assessment organization, the National Board of Examiners for Osteopathic Physicians and Surgeons, now known as the NBOME (National Board of Osteopathic Medical Examiners), produced the first national standardized assessments for licensure, an important milestone in defensibility for the qualifications of DOs and professional self-regulation for the profession. By 1937, however, only 26 states had any provision to provide unlimited licenses to DOs.

In some states, DOs were ineligible to apply for state licenses because their education did not meet specific criteria.

- In 1937, osteopathic standards did not meet preprofessional college requirements in 16 states; in 8 states, a year's internship was needed.

- DOs in those early years who took state-based examinations under state medical or composite boards showed a much lower pass rate. This was not surprising due to test construction bias (assessments constructed to align with the MD degree pathway) and administered, often with oral exams, by MDs.

Over time, the curricula were altered, and the pass rates increased, and more and more states began to accept national standardized exams for licensure for DOs and MDs. Osteopathic exams were better aligned with the distinctive practice of osteopathic medicine and the curricular model and content used at the schools. The major changes were the addition of more basic science courses, more faculty, larger clinical facilities, and osteopathic standardized assessments.[39] After World War II, a major effort was made to change the old, limited practice laws. These efforts, along with major changes in all medical education including in osteopathic medical education, enabled the enactment of new practice laws for DOs and MDs in all 50 states.[59]

Brief History of the California Merger

A dramatic chapter in the American licensing story of the osteopathic profession came when the California Osteopathic Association (COA) began negotiations in 1960 to merge with the California Medical Association (CMA). The AOA revoked the charter of the COA and approved a new state association, the Osteopathic Physicians and Surgeons of California (OPSC). The COA then officially merged with the CMA in 1961. The COA leadership next successfully lobbied the Board of Trustees of the College of Osteopathic Physicians and Surgeons to change from a DO school to an accredited MD school of medicine. This led to a referendum on the state ballot to prevent new licensure of DOs in the state. OPSC battled against the referendum, but the citizens of California voted in favor of the proposition, nearly annihilating the osteopathic profession in California. As a result of the activities of the COA–CMA merger and the state legislature:

- The College of Osteopathic Physicians and Surgeons (COP&S), Los Angeles, became the California College of Medicine[39] and soon thereafter the University of California College of Medicine (1964)[51] and now University of California, Irvine (UCI).[60]
- DOs who applied were conferred MD degrees by the California College of Medicine beginning in March 1962, as preparation for the referendum.[51]
- No additional training, education, or competency assessment was required to be granted the MD degree.[39,51]
- There was an administrative charge of $65 assessed for processing and investigating the diplomas, certificates of training, and licensure status of the ex-DOs, now new MDs, in preparation for oversight by the state MD licensing board.[51,61]
- Of 2,696 DOs who were granted the MD degree, 1,953 were COP&S graduates.[51]
- About 400 DOs refused to change their degree; 250 were members of OPSC.[51]
- Proposition 22 was approved by voters in 1962.[51]
- The new licensure of DOs in California was discontinued.[39,51]

Continuing the battle in 1968, OPSC backed Ted D'Amico and other out-of-state DOs who were commissioned medical officers in the military. D'Amico et al. sued the Attorney General of the State of California, as well as the medical and osteopathic licensing boards, alleging civil rights infraction and restriction of trade.[51] The California Supreme Court rendered a decision on March 19, 1974 that licensure of DOs must be resumed.[39,51,61,62] Symbolically, to the OPSC leadership, that date also happened to be the same date that the swallows annually return to San Juan Capistrano, California, from their southern winter homes.[61] That year, California licenses were granted to over 340 qualified DOs from out of state.[51] Osteopathic professional continuity was restored in 1982 when the College of Osteopathic Medicine of the Pacific (founded in 1977 in Pomona, CA) graduated its first class of osteopathic medical students.[61,62]

LICENSURE

In 1973, Mississippi became the last state to grant DOs full scope of medical practice rights and with the court order for resumption of licensure in California, it was possible by the end of 1974 for DOs to obtain an unlimited license in all 50 states. Thirteen states maintain separate osteopathic and allopathic licensing boards; most states and other US jurisdictions have composite state medical boards. Graduate medical education is required for new licenses (for DOs and MDs) yet varies state to state with most requiring 1 or 2 years of residency training.

During the 1970s and 1980s, most states moved away from state-developed examinations for licensure and began to accept national standardized comprehensive assessments for licensure. By this time, oral examinations and essay exams were replaced with more objective multiple-choice exam formats. Most DOs began to be licensed based on NBOME examinations designed for state licensure, and most MDs took one of several different national licensing exams designed for MDs. As the 20th century ended, most states were now requiring valid and reliable national standardized exams. To address this, MDs took the new 3-part USMLE exam developed by the Federation of State Medical Boards (FSMB) and the National Board of Medical Examiners (NBME), and DOs took the 3-part COMLEX-USA designed specifically for osteopathic medical practice. While the FSMB and the NBME periodically attempted to amalgamate all physician licensure exams several times in the 1990s and early 2000s, the AOA and the NBOME withstood challenges to their validity and professional self-regulation. In 2005, the State of Louisiana became the final state to accept DOs for licensure with COMLEX-USA. This made a significant difference, relative to DOs choosing to practice in the state, helping to reduce physician shortage areas in underserved regions.

To compare and contrast, in the mid-1800s when Still became a physician, a frontier physician in Missouri with limited formal medical school training was able to register at the county courthouse if local physicians would vouch for him. In some territories and states, practice was by tolerance (no registration laws existed).

However, 21st century state license requirements currently include:

- Graduation from an accredited medical school
- Postgraduate training (1 to 3 years)
- Passage of a standardized national licensure exam (COMLEX-USA for DOs, USMLE for MDs)
- Additional requirements (e.g., criminal background checks, attestations of character, review of the physician data bank, letters of reference, licensure fee)

State-based licensure is for a specific period (typically 1 to 2 years) and must be periodically renewed with (in most states) evidence of continued education and capacity to practice, as specified by individual states. Hospitals and other organizations (such as third party/health insurance companies) determine and grant the privileges a physician is allowed within their systems (e.g., hospital admission and the right to perform procedures, reimbursement for services).

A physician's credentials include official records of:

- Educational history
- Degrees
- Awards
- Residency completion
- Licensure and national licensure assessments
- Board certification
- Activity logs (to demonstrate experience and currency with diagnostic and medical or surgical procedures)

Licensing boards, specialty societies, and privileging organizations also have the prerogative to specify amounts and types of continuing medical education (CME) required to keep physicians eligible and current. This includes osteopathic specific requirements for DOs, and physicians who achieve specialty board certification status who often have the most rigorous CME and assessment requirements for continuous certification or maintenance of certification. This demonstration of competency remains an important component of a profession's self-regulation, ensuring trust and quality care for the public.

OSTEOPATHIC PROFESSIONAL ORGANIZATION

Every profession needs organizations for its multiple facets that coordinate and monitor activities for the greater good of the group and its members. Osteopathic organizations were developed beginning in the first decade of the profession. Many independent and interdependent organizations related to the osteopathic medical profession play local, state, and national roles. These include government licensing groups such as state boards, nongovernment not-for-profit foundations, and professional and health care organizations. The three primary national organizations for the American osteopathic profession are the:

- American Osteopathic Association (AOA) (osteopathic.org)
- American Association of Colleges of Osteopathic Medicine (AACOM) (aacom.org)
- National Board of Osteopathic Medical Examiners (NBOME) (nbome.org)

American Osteopathic Association (AOA)

The AOA began in 1897 as a student organization in Kirksville, Missouri under the name American Association for the Advancement of Osteopathy. This evolved into the regulatory group of the profession as the graduates took control. The current name was adopted in 1901.[63] Among other accomplishments, the AOA played a vital role in encouraging and supporting early osteopathic research. In 1907, the first organization devoted to osteopathic research began, though the first recorded osteopathic research was performed almost a decade earlier.[64]

A major early effort of the AOA was to produce a code of ethics in 1904. A participant in those deliberations observed that the problem was not because anyone really wished to practice unethically, but rather that on some points, it was difficult to agree upon what was ethical.[65] To put this in perspective, the issue of advertising was a hard-fought question among all professionals at that time. The question was resolved by declaring advertising unethical except for brief professional card listings. By the 1990s, advertising by professionals was ultimately considered ethical, though not of course to condone unfounded claims.

State (divisional) and local (district) osteopathic organizations were established to serve DOs in their own localities. When the AOA grew too large for general membership meetings, in 1920 state societies began to name representatives to serve in an AOA House of Delegates (HOD), the chief policy-making group for the osteopathic profession. A Board of Trustees elected by the HOD oversees the implementation of those policies. Students participate as voting members of delegations from the states in which their schools are located, are appointed to AOA boards (including the Board of Trustees [BOT]), bureaus, and committees, and have their own organizations.

The AOA has been the umbrella group that recognizes and coordinates many of the efforts on behalf of the profession. All organizations recognized by the AOA accept ongoing controls such as approval of any changes in basic documents and designation of how many representatives (if any) are sent to the AOA HOD as a voice and to vote in professional policy affairs. A current guide to all AOA-recognized osteopathic organizations is available online and updated annually.[66]

The AOA staff, directed by elected officers and the Board of Trustees, provide:

- Professional services
- Public and legislative education
- Member services including maintenance of central records for members
- Management and certification for educational meetings and activities, OMED (the annual AOA conference), and CME
- Publication of position papers (approved by the HOD) defining the profession's position on questions of public health and professional interest
- Coordinated special efforts on a variety of concerns

Through its bureaus, councils, and committees, the AOA has been the osteopathic accrediting organization through the early 21st century for undergraduate, graduate, and CME. The central organization organizes, recognizes, and at least partially regulates a network of:

- AOA Bureaus and Councils
- Specialty boards
- Specialty colleges, distinct from the certifying boards, that conduct educational affairs and recognize their own members' achievements through fellowships and other awards
- AOA-supported programs
- Research grants and related projects
- Divisional and affiliate societies
    - State and local district societies
    - Colleges, with student and alumni groups, clubs, and special interest groups
    - Auxiliary organizations, including for spouses
    - Nonpractice affiliates

American Association of Colleges of Osteopathic Medicine (AACOM)

The second national association was the Associated Colleges of Osteopathy (now AACOM), formed in 1898. The Associated Colleges became a discussion and consensus group for faculty and officers of the schools. This organization independently focused on (and cooperated with the AOA, and later COCA) the goals of protecting and raising standards for osteopathic education. AACOM:

- Is nongovernment and not-for-profit
- Is guided by a Board of Deans

- Has a large number of councils and committees working on educational standards, organization, and teaching methods
- Facilitates communications, collaboration, and innovation as a community to create and enhance progress in all areas of osteopathic medical education
- Collects and analyzes educational data to provide evidence as a basis for action
- Operates the system through which students apply to osteopathic medical schools, the American Association of Colleges of Osteopathic Medicine Application Service (AACOMAS)
- Publishes an annual report with updated information on all its activities (accessible at aacom.org)

National Board of Osteopathic Medical Examiners (NBOME)

As states initially developed basic science examinations as a qualification for licensure, not all had adequate resources for development and security of high-quality tests. There was a great deal of variance in quality of those which existed, and some states accepted others' examinations. The shared goal was to secure the safety of the public, with all applicants for medical licensure meeting minimum knowledge standards. Based upon this need and professional self-regulation, the NBOME was founded as an independent, nonprofit organization in 1934. The NBOME has as its main goal the protection of the public, ensuring that all physicians eligible to apply for state licenses to practice medicine have demonstrated competence for the practice of osteopathic medicine and to a national standard. Development and administration of and reporting on the following rigorous examinations is the primary means by which the NBOME fulfills this goal:[67]

- COMLEX-USA three-level licensure assessment
- Comprehensive Osteopathic Medical Achievement Tests (COMAT) in clinical subjects as well as foundational biomedical sciences used by DO schools
- Providing assessment services for numerous professional societies and organizations, including for board certification, resident in-training assessment, and continuous certification

The COMLEX-USA is a three-level, national standardized licensure examination designed for licensure for the practice of osteopathic medicine. The COMLEX-USA Examination Series is designed to assess osteopathic medical knowledge, knowledge fluency, clinical skills, and other competencies essential for practice as an osteopathic generalist physician. It is also a graduation requirement for attaining a DO (Doctor of Osteopathic Medicine) degree from COMs in the United States, and for entry into and promotion within graduate medical education (residency) training programs.

From 2002 to 2020, COMLEX-USA included a Level 2-Performance Evaluation that assessed osteopathic clinical skills including doctor–patient communication skills and professionalism; medical interview skills, data gathering, and physical exam skills; OMT, clinical problem-solving, and osteopathic medical documentation. This examination was discontinued when COVID-19 pandemic conditions persisted, and the NBOME implemented enhanced attestation requirements for clinical skills proficiencies at the schools. The NBOME, working with the licensing community, the AOA and the COCA, the osteopathic medical education community, and others, has continued to study the impact and alternatives for longer term ways to ensure that each DO graduate has demonstrated osteopathic clinical skills competencies for safe and effective patient care.

Additional independent organizations related to the osteopathic medical profession that play major local, state, and national roles include government licensing groups such as state boards, nongovernment not-for-profit foundations, and health care organizations.

FEDERAL GOVERNMENT RECOGNITION

The first major attempt by the AOA to obtain federal government recognition was during World War I, in an attempt to gain commissions for DOs as military physicians.[50] This effort was unsuccessful in spite of active support by such prominent advocates as the former President of the United States, Theodore Roosevelt.[68]

At that time, a federal general medical examination was set, and it was understood that if DOs (along with MDs) took this and passed it, they could be commissioned as medical officers.

- About 25 DOs took the examination and were recommended for commissions.
- The Surgeon General unilaterally ruled that only MDs were eligible.
- Bills were then introduced (1917) in both the US House of Representatives and the US Senate to correct this inequity.
  - The bills were referred to the Military Affairs Committees, which held hearings.
  - The committee then referred the issue to the Surgeon General. His statement of opposition claimed that regular physicians would withhold their services if DOs were allowed to serve.
  - The bills remained in committee without resolution until the end of the war.
- DOs served as regular soldiers, unable to use their medical training.

The situation remained uncorrected when World War II began. Again, there were efforts to obtain commissions for DOs, this time emphasizing regulatory rather than legislative barriers.[50,69] DOs were deferred rather than drafted, waiting for the possibility to serve in a medical capacity that never came. Ironically, the DOs remaining stateside became family physicians to many thousands of patients left unattended by the MDs who served their country in the military. This exposure to a broader patient population enhanced the public's view of DOs as full-service physicians.

Pressure for federal recognition continued after World War II ended. Nearly every advance for DOs came after a long and difficult fight. A progression of milestones followed.[39,41]

- 1951: The US Public Health Service first awarded renewable teaching grants to each of the six osteopathic colleges.
- 1956: Federal law provided for the appointment of DOs as commissioned officers in the nation's military medical corps. However, implementation of that law was blocked for another 10 years until the Vietnam conflict created greater need for military physicians.
- 1957: US Office of Education, Department of Health, Education, and Welfare (DHEW) recognized the AOA as the accrediting body for osteopathic education.
- 1963: US Civil Service accepted DOs as medical officers, enabling public careers.
- 1963: The Health Professions Educational Assistance Act included a provision for matching construction grants for osteopathic colleges and loans to osteopathic students.

- 1966: Harry J. Walter, DO, was sworn in as a First Lieutenant in the US Air Force on July 13, 1966,[50] becoming the first DO commissioned as an officer in the Armed Forces Medical Corps.
- 1966: The Department of Health and Human Services (DHHS, the new name for DHEW) designated the AOA as the official accrediting body for osteopathic hospitals under Medicare.
- 1967: The AMA withdrew its long-standing opposition, and DOs were included in the doctor draft. Serving as generalists and specialists in Vietnam, a number of DOs also helped locals, and some were decorated for their service, including both purple hearts and bronze stars.[70] Edward M. Feldman, DO, was nominated for the Medal of Honor.[71]
- 1967: The National Commission of Accrediting recognized the AOA as the accrediting agency for all facets of osteopathic education (undergraduate and postgraduate).
- 1972: The US Postal Service commemorated a stamp in honor of the 75th anniversary of the founding of the AOA. It was also the 80th anniversary of the first osteopathic medical school and nearly a century since Still "flung to the breeze the banner of osteopathy" in 1874 (Fig. 2.9).
- 1977: Association of Military Osteopathic Physicians and Surgeons (AMOPS) is established.
- 1983: The first osteopathic flag officer in the US military was appointed.[41]
- 1996: Ronald R. Blanck, DO, was appointed the first osteopathic Surgeon General of the US Army.

The AMOPS serves and has represented thousands of osteopathic physicians in the Uniformed Services (DOs comprise approximately 10% of the physicians in the Armed Forces). AMOPS also represents the interests of former Medical Corps DOs who have retired or separated from the military, private practice physicians serving in the Guard or Reserve, osteopathic medical students in the Health Professions Scholarship Program and federally employed physicians.

By the end of the 20th Century, integration of the osteopathic medical profession had been accomplished at all levels. To continue this, the AOA maintains an office presence in Washington, DC, where it represents the profession, monitoring, networking, lobbying, and ensuring protection of practice rights and inclusion of DOs and osteopathic institutions as active partners in all relevant legislative and regulatory initiatives. AACOM has likewise enhanced legislative efforts in recent decades, along with the advocacy efforts of many other osteopathic state and specialty affiliates.

Figure 2.9. In 1972, an osteopathic medicine commemorative stamp was issued by the US Postal Service. (Reprinted with permission from A.T. Still Pension File. Still National Osteopathic Museum, Kirksville, MO.)

During the Second Persian Gulf War, the March 20, 2006 cover of Newsweek Magazine featured a military DO. Richard Jadick was credited with saving 30 lives in the Battle for Fallujah, including running and crawling onto the battlefield under fire to drag numerous soldiers back to safety and providing medical care. However, the Newsweek cover showed that journalists, editors, and many of the public were still often unaware of the osteopathic medical profession, as the magazine cover read "Hero MD." A correction was issued a day later.[72]

The American Osteopathic Foundation (AOF) established The Distinguished Military Service Recognition Award in 2019.[73] It is based on major achievements in the nominee's primary medical field, contributions to enhancing the role of osteopathic medicine in the military, and recognition of leadership ability (exceptional leader, teacher, clinician, or mentor).

The 21st century continues the profession's representation in American medical leadership and the benefits of its unique skills in neuromusculoskeletal diagnosis and hands-on treatment. Two DOs (CMDR Sean Conley, DO, and Colonel Kevin O'Connor, DO) have served as White House Physician or Physician to the President.[74] Military DOs who have mastered the skills have the advantage of using OMT to help pilots maintain flight status when somatic dysfunction or medication would bar them from flying.[75] J.D. Polk, DO, is NASA's Chief Health and Medical Officer, helping the team prepare for the latest manned moon mission and the voyage to Mars.[76]

SPECIALTIES AND HOSPITALS

Specialties

Perhaps the first osteopathic medical specialty (as general practice transformed and differentiated) began in 1898, only 3 years after Wilhelm Roentgen announced the discovery of radiographs.

- The second x-ray machine west of the Mississippi River (a skiagraph) was installed in Kirksville in 1898. With it, Dr. William Smith formulated a method to inject a radiopaque substance in cadaveric veins and arteries to demonstrate the normal pattern of circulation.
- The Journal of Osteopathy, a Kirksville journal associated with the ASO, and the fledgling American X-Ray Journal each published an article on x-rays in 1898. (These were reprinted for modern reference in AOA publications in 1974).[77] When formal certifying boards for osteopathic specialties were organized, radiology was the first in 1939.[41]

The development of osteopathic hospitals and specialties, with their standards, examinations, certifying boards, and specialty colleges or academies, promoted postgraduate educational programs (internships, residencies, CME). A full complement of specialties was well established in the osteopathic profession by the 1990s, including a board recognizing osteopathic manipulative medicine, the American Osteopathic Board of Neuromusculoskeletal Medicine and Manipulation (AOBNMM, established in March 1990).

As specialization increased, the profession was maintaining and improving what would come to be the most needed type of practice by the 1990s, primary care. The United States was suffering from a shortage and growing maldistribution of practitioners. By the last decade of the 20th century, the osteopathic profession found itself in the enviable role of adviser on how to replicate its educational processes for those seeking to increase production of primary care physicians.

Osteopathic clinical education has historically taken place in primary care settings, including community hospitals and clinics. Training within community settings was now considered to be an advantage for success in producing primary care physicians, including many willing to work in underserved (primarily rural but including some inner city) communities. Among many influences on the choice of practice specialties and locations, undergraduate experiences and role models factor heavily.[78]

- Medical students trained in academic medical centers tend to have subspecialists as role models and are more likely to choose specialties themselves.
- Osteopathic medical students do a significant amount of their training in community clinics and hospitals, with many primary care physicians as faculty role models.
- Rural clinics, long a mainstay of clinical education at the Kirksville college and later for other osteopathic schools, have become a model for primary care education.[79]
- Many of the COMs developed after 1969 were started in states seeking to specifically address the rural and small-town shortage of physicians, particularly primary care physicians.

From the time that the AOA began approving specialty boards, certification through them was only open to AOA members. The AOA HOD regularly reaffirmed this practice when it came up for a vote every 5 years. The policy boosted the percentage of practicing DOs who maintained AOA membership, adding strength to the AOA as a national organization. In February 2016 the AOA BOT voted to decouple the specialty board certification process from AOA membership for several reasons, including marketing board certification separately from membership. Four AOA members brought a class action lawsuit against the AOA in 2016 over the requirement before the change was implemented (which would have required AOA HOD approval in July). When the AOA settled the lawsuit in 2018, the AOA membership requirement for board certification was dropped. The lawsuit may have actually delayed the process.[80]

Currently 16 AOA certifying boards offer certifications in 27 primary specialties and 48 subspecialties. The individual boards are administered by the AOA's Department of Certifying Board Services.[81]

Hospitals

As with medicine in general, hospitals had their share of developmental problems in the 19th century. Inadequate facilities and staff, hospital ownership, disagreement over who should get patient fees, social stigma, and infection all played roles. Public hospitals were generally for those of limited financial means, and families often had to provide some of the nursing care for their relatives. Early small private institutions owned by surgeons furnished hotel services and nursing for their own patients.

By the early 1900s, things were changing.

- Hospitals became safer with the expansion of an educated nursing profession and modern sanitation practices.
- As technology and antiseptic (later, aseptic) surgical technique became the norm, and intravenous medications and fluids were developed, new general hospitals began to appeal to patients other than those with limited means.
- Patient fees began to help with hospital development.[43]

When Flexner's inspection took place in the first decade, the osteopathic profession was very small and only 5 osteopathic hospitals were listed[39]:

- Kirksville, 54 beds
- Chicago, 20 beds
- Pacific College, 15 beds
- Boston, 10 beds
- Philadelphia, 3 beds

Eventually, the numbers and size of osteopathic hospitals grew, but few reached the size and diversity of specialties that characterized the academic medical centers associated with contemporary university medical schools. An exception was the separate building devoted (from 1928 on) to osteopathic medicine at the Los Angeles County Hospital.[51] With the increase in hospitals, the osteopathic profession set hospital standards, first for the training of interns and residents and then for accreditation of the hospitals themselves. The growth of osteopathic hospitals was especially marked in the period during and after World War II, when MD-run hospitals did not permit DOs to join their medical staff.

- When US government programs were approved to help with construction of hospitals, osteopathic institutions participated. Many community teaching hospitals were constructed during those years.
- In 1950, with the leadership of State Senator Stephen Teale, DO, Mark Twain Hospital was built in San Andreas, California, using state bond funds that prohibited discrimination against DOs who wanted to admit and care for patients.[51]
- In 1954, a landmark court decision in Audrain County, Missouri, made it illegal for public hospitals to deny staff membership and admitting privileges to qualified DOs. This initiated a series of changes in other states.
- Most public hospitals were open to DOs by the 1960s.
- Most private hospitals began giving DOs hospital privileges by the 1980s especially after the landmark case of Weiss versus York Hospital.

As many ACGME medical residencies accepted DOs in the 1990s, the development of a separate network of osteopathic hospitals for training purposes was significantly reduced. The AOA adopted mechanisms to recognize training that took place in MD institutions as acceptable for osteopathic board certification, through affiliation of the MD institution with an accredited osteopathic college or by direct AOA accreditation of the training institution.[65] By 1999, Osteopathic Post Graduate Training Institutes (OPTI) became standard for accrediting all osteopathic medical residencies, linking resources through required hospital-college consortiums.

Reorganization of the health care system itself dictated changes.

- Third party payment and medical business reorganization led to the formation of large networks of health care providers such as health maintenance organizations (HMOs) and preferred provider organizations (PPOs).
- Outpatient facilities, extended or long-term care, home care, and hospice care took over some of the work formerly done by hospitals or by patients' families.
- Many community hospitals—including many osteopathic institutions—merged with larger groups or simply closed.
- Differences between osteopathic and allopathic hospitals blurred as both came under the umbrella of managed care organizations.
- The American Osteopathic Hospital Association (AOHA) faded out of the picture and ceased operating as economic changes and mergers eliminated or absorbed all but a few of the distinctly osteopathic hospitals which had been built for a time when DOs were not allowed on hospital medical staffs.

- The Single GME Accreditation System under the ACGME was fully implemented by the ACGME and AOA in 2020 and the OPTIs were replaced by the ACGME program requirements.

Economic and political factors have dominated control of US medical education and training, health care access, and delivery in different ways than in countries with national health services. The profit motive is a major factor for pharmaceutical companies, insurance companies, hospitals, health care organizations, and educational institutions. The government's role in medicine has expanded enormously over the past 60 years and is now a major issue in presidential and congressional elections.

To achieve meaningful high-quality sustainable, universally accessible medical care and education, corporate and government stakeholders must participate with patients, physicians, health care workers, business experts, and educators. Providing excellence in affordable patient care and physician education is something physicians need to champion. This is due to a complex and competitive society that balances limited resources with providing equity, safety, progress, and efficiency. Attaining and maintaining good health in the maximum number of individual citizens is a strong component of a society seeking to reach its highest potential.

SINGLE GME ACCREDITATION SYSTEM UNDER THE ACGME FOR POSTGRADUATE MEDICAL TRAINING

Osteopathic medical graduate education programs were initially created in the early 20th century due to a need for more structured postgraduate training and the recognition that MD postgraduate programs at the time did not accept DO graduates. MD programs also did not incorporate OPP or manipulation.

A demographic shift in postgraduate medical education occurred in the 1970s. The rapid expansion of the number of osteopathic medical schools beginning in 1969 increased the number of graduates. Osteopathic postgraduate programs did not expand sufficiently to accommodate the number of graduates. AOA programs were also concentrated in certain regions of the country, limiting geographic options for graduating students. Challenges were exacerbated by the establishment of new COMs in regions of the United States sparsely populated by DOs. Students recruited locally were often most interested in programs in that region, which were often ACGME programs. Increasing specialization of the physician workforce led to the development of residencies and fellowships not always provided in osteopathic programs. An increasing number of graduates began to choose their training based on the perception that quality ACGME programs would allow training in their own regions, or perhaps allow them to be more competitive for postgraduate subspecialty fellowships.

ACGME programs demonstrated an increased willingness to accept DOs. The ACGME reorganized its programs in 2009, including educational outcomes based on six core competencies. It announced in 2011 that beginning in 2016, moving from a non-ACGME program to an ACGME program would be restricted (e.g., from an AOA or Canadian internal medicine residency to an ACGME nephrology fellowship). This restriction was partly precipitated by residents who were being assessed using these new core competencies. Fellows who themselves had not been trained in those competencies and who came from residency programs outside of the ACGME system were sometimes their trainers.

- The new ACGME rules would exclude graduates who went through a non-ACGME postgraduate program from entering ACGME programs beyond an entry-level residency position.
- After discussions beginning in 2012, the AOA and AACOM signed a letter of intent with ACGME in 2014 to create a unified single pathway for postgraduate medical education programs.[82] While many identified risks for the profession including the potential for some dilution of osteopathic graduate medical education,[83] the growth of the schools and closure of some osteopathic hospitals appeared to require a solution to ensure GME opportunities for the increasing number of DO graduates.

Over half of osteopathic graduates were already in ACGME programs, an accrediting system without any osteopathic input. It was also argued that unified accreditation would create a stronger combined political presence in government funding and support for new and existing programs. The time frame for development and implementation was from July 1, 2015 to June 30, 2020.

The AOA and AACOM had significant concerns regarding the need to have OPP included for the DOs in the ACGME postgraduate programs and obtained agreements on how this would be accomplished.

- Osteopathic Recognition (OR) was created by ACGME expressly for the purpose of providing a mechanism to recognize an additional osteopathic focus and training in a specific program.
- AACOM would maintain a list of programs with OR.[84] Programs in any specialty were eligible to apply for OR.
- Physicians training in these programs would receive additional training in osteopathic principles and manipulation.
- Non-DOs could be part of the OR programs, but prerequisite education in OPP is required.
- The ACGME would establish the Osteopathic Neuromusculoskeletal Medicine Review Committee to set standards and accredit programs, preserving this specialty (which had no ACGME equivalent).
- The ACGME board initially added four directors, two from the AOA and two from the AACOM. A ramp-up schedule added more AOA and AACOM nominated directors until at the conclusion of the implementation of the single system, all seven member organizations had four directors each.
- AOA board certification is an equivalent outcome measure to board certification from an American Board of Medical Specialties (ABMS) specialty board examination and process.
- The COCA is the accreditor of COMs, and COMLEX-USA is the national standardized licensure assessment for DOs.

With these safeguards, a single pathway for postgraduate medical education was recommended by the AOA leadership and ultimately approved by the AOA HOD. The AACOM board also voted to approve the new system. Both AOA and AACOM represented constituencies that paralleled those entities that were already member organizations of the ACGME, so both osteopathic organizations had to approve the new single GME system to move the new system forward. Approval was not without significant controversy. Multiple concerns were raised.

- How many osteopathic medical graduates would choose to pursue OR in residencies with the new additional requirements?
- Would osteopathic graduates be able to enter specialties in the same proportions that existed prior to full implementation of the single pathway, especially in highly competitive fields (e.g., emergency medicine, surgical specialties)? Loss of programs

open only to DO graduates, accredited solely by the AOA Council on Postdoctoral Training (COPT) and its Program and Trainee Review Committee (PTRC) might impact demographic outcomes.

- Would osteopathic GME programs in rural and other community-based health centers be able to meet quantitative-focused ACGME requirements for accreditation?
- Would there be enough trainers available for those OR programs?
- Would future graduates apply for AOA board certification?
- Would residency and fellowship programs be allowed to discriminate based on their lack of familiarity with DOs or DO educational pathways or credentials?
- Considering that not all residents plan to become educators, would there be enough residencies in osteopathic neuromusculoskeletal medicine to provide sufficient professors to teach this core material in the expanding number of osteopathic medical schools?

The AOA HOD requested that numerous aspects of the single pathway be monitored for the 5-year duration of the implementation of the new single system, to ensure the preservation of OPP.[82] The new single pathway effectively eliminated the osteopathic profession's autonomous control of osteopathic medical education beyond the undergraduate years but included safeguards and representation. It also provided participation and input into the ACGME system that, by 2015, was training most of the osteopathic residents.

The impact of this decision remains uncertain to some and there have certainly been some challenges, both predictable and unpredictable. It preserves the ability of osteopathic medical school graduates to be accepted into ACGME postgraduate training programs including subspecialty fellowship training. The results of DO graduates matching both into pipeline ACGME residency training programs as well as fellowship programs in most specialties have continued to increase significantly from 2014 to 2024, where match and placement rates remain at historic highs year after year. Challenges include the increasing competitiveness for all applicants in surgical fields and smaller specialties (e.g., dermatology), continued bias in certain GME programs against DO applicants, and the resultant professional identity formation and insecurities heightened in the learners entering the profession, reminiscent of California in 1962.

Some of the challenges were furthered by the COVID-19 pandemic in 2020 and continued competitiveness for residency programs for DO students, MD students, and international MDs, MBBSs, and other physician designations. Challenges for DO students worsened in the pandemic in procuring visiting student/audition clinical rotation experiences as well as GME programs shifting to virtual video interviews for residency programs exacerbated the insecurities of being in a minority position. Virtual instruction necessitated by the pandemic further limited professional identity formation for DO students entering the profession. Indeed, COMs had grown so much that osteopathic medical students received training by significantly more MD and PhD medical educators and role models than DOs.[85] Osteopathic organizations such as the AOA, the NBOME, and the AACOM continued to strengthen their advocacy initiatives for DO students, the DO educational pathway, and their validated credentials. As active participants in the Coalition for Physician Accountability[86] (physicianaccountability.org), AOA, NBOME, and AACOM have positioned themselves well to continue to advocate for parity and inclusion and share the many benefits to patients of the distinctive osteopathic medical education pathway and profession.

CHANGING DEMOGRAPHICS

An ardent abolitionist, Andrew Taylor Still and his family were friends with John Brown and his sons. Having fought in the Civil War for the freedom of African Americans, Still invited the African American laborers who helped build his school to attend the dedication of a new ASO building, which was not the custom in Missouri at the time. He explained to surprised guests that they had helped to construct it and had just as much right to be there as anyone.[3]

Still was a suffragist, supporting women's causes and admitting five women in the first class at the ASO.

One thing that did please the Old Doctor was that women as well as men were enrolled in his first class. He had watched his well-educated wife struggle when they needed money and the most she could do was sell magazines and get odd jobs. Even women who were teachers were paid very little. It had always been one of his goals to establish osteopathy as a career open to women, too. He could envision that osteopathy would offer a good livelihood and he made a point to see that women had every opportunity to have the same access to this career as the men. As further incentive to women, he had lowered their tuition to about half that of men.[87]

A significant number of the women graduates who offered leadership in the late 19th and early 20th century were educators and researchers specifically interested in the original osteopathic concepts, rather than AOA officials or college administrators.

Two of the women who attended the inaugural class at the ASO, Jeanette "Nettie" Bowles, DO, and Still's daughter Blanche Still, DO, (m. Laughlin) filled roles as leaders at the profession's beginning. Bowles became the second anatomy professor when William Smith left in March 1893 for private practice after getting his diploma in February. She was the founding editor of the Journal of Osteopathy in May 1894. After teaching at the ASO, she left for Colorado and helped found an osteopathic school there.[33] She was the founding president of the American Colleges of Osteopathy in 1898 and was the vice president for the American Association for the Advancement of Osteopathy (now the AOA) in 1897 and 1905.[88,89]

Blanche Still attended at least part of the first year of class at the ASO at the age of 16, though she did not receive her degree until 1895. She was listed as a member of the Board of Trustees of the ASO when its new Articles of Incorporation were filed in October 1894. She became editor in chief of the Journal of Osteopathy in January 1895. She never actively practiced. In 1900, she married George M. Laughlin, DO, who was to become a renowned surgeon and the President of two osteopathic medical schools including the ASO, as well as owner of a hospital in Kirksville and a sanatorium in Arkansas. Her supportive efforts in all these endeavors were noted.[33]

Edythe Ashmore, DO, a 1901 graduate of the S.S. Still College of Osteopathy in Des Moines, wrote and published *Osteopathic Mechanics: A Textbook*, while she was the head of the Department of Osteopathic Technique at the ASO from 1914 to 1916. This was the first official textbook on osteopathic mechanics used at the school.[90]

Charlotte Weaver, DO, FACN was directed by Still to focus her studies on circulation from the head through the spinal cord. Her research began in the second decade of the 20th century and focused on the anatomy, diagnosis and treatment of the cranial region, its systemic effects in general and neurologic conditions in particular. She published numerous articles in the Journal of the American Osteopathic Association (JAOA) from 1936 to 1938 and was later cited by Sutherland. Her methods did not survive because she did not train successors in her diagnostic and treatment techniques. She was elected to the American College of Neuropsychiatry (an MD organization) in 1940, an unusual achievement in that era, and became a Fellow.[91]

Beryl Arbuckle, DO, a board-certified pediatrician, conducted anatomical dissections at Angus Cathie's anatomy lab at what is now the Philadelphia College of Osteopathic Medicine, and participated in extensive autopsies at the college hospital in the 1940s and 1950s. Her area of interest was cranial anatomy, including the stresses of the dura and cranium.[92] Her works supported W.G. Sutherland's cranial concepts. She founded the first cerebral palsy clinic in Philadelphia in 1947.

Louisa Burns, DO, was a schoolteacher who contracted spinal meningitis and suffered debility. When osteopathic treatment restored her health, she attended the Pacific College of Osteopathy (PCO) and graduated in 1903. After receiving a Master of Science degree from the Borden Institute (where she had previously received her bachelor's diploma) and a Doctor of Science degree from PCO, she began a research career. Using animal models, she investigated the anatomical and physiologic characteristics and impact of the osteopathic lesion (somatic dysfunction). She published numerous papers and a series of books, and became head of the A.T. Still Research Institute (ATSRI) from 1917 to 1935.[93] She continued research until her retirement in 1958 and is primarily known for elaborating viscerosomatic and somatovisceral reflexes.

Although most medical schools at the beginning of the 20th century were not only segregated, but also had few female students, the ASO *June Class of 1902* graduation picture shows that 74 of 192 graduates were women (framed picture owned by Jones). The number of female students decreased in virtually all-American medical schools after 1910 and did not begin to rise again until the 1960s.

Grace B. Bell, DO, became the first female dean of any American medical school that was not strictly a women's college[51] when she became Dean of the College of Osteopathic Physicians and Surgeons at Los Angeles (COP&S) in 1956.[59]

Changing demographics, culture, and the growing diversity in the osteopathic profession through its history have matched American trends. The six osteopathic medical colleges at the beginning of the 1960s were all private, free-standing tuition-driven institutions, with limited if any endowment, and had only a few small scholarships. Recruiting minority students was difficult when scholarships were easier to obtain with affirmative action programs at state universities and private schools with large endowments. Knowledge of osteopathic medicine was not widespread in minority communities; most DOs practiced in small-town and rural areas of the Midwest, where four of those colleges were located.

Ethnic and cultural changes shifted American population, educational, and workplace demographics through the latter half of the 20th and early 21st centuries. The proportion of European ethnic heritage diminished greatly, the Black proportion increased mildly, and the Latin and Asian American populations increased greatly.[94] In addition, the increasing number of American women being educated and within the workforce led to a huge change in the proportion of female physicians. Increasing DO diversity mirrored general societal shifts and was reflected over time in AOA members, as well as in the demographics of state associations, colleges, hospitals and osteopathic physician leadership in general.

Meta L. Christy, DO, a 1921 graduate of Philadelphia College of Infirmary and Osteopathy (PCIO), later Philadelphia College of Osteopathic Medicine, was the first African American doctor of osteopathic medicine. After practicing briefly in Indiana, she started a practice Las Vegas, New Mexico. According to historian Joseph Lordi, "Dr. Christy's medical practice catered to African Americans who, because of discrimination at that time, were denied service at the local hospital. There were about 100 African Americans and no one to treat them. She also treated white patients."[95]

In the 1940s, Dr. Christy served on the board of directors of the New Mexico Osteopathic Medical Association, which awarded her a certificate of merit in 1955 and its Distinguished Service Award in 1956. She was also active with the Southwestern Osteopathic Association.[95]

Upon her death in 1968, Dr. Christy, a "widely known osteopathic physician" according to her obituary, was serving on the Health Fact-Finding Committee to which New Mexico Governor David F. Cargo had appointed her. In 1995, PCOM's Student National Medical Association paid tribute to the world's first African American osteopath by establishing the Meta L. Christy Award, their top honor, in recognition of exemplary practice of osteopathic medicine, service to the community, and inspiration to future doctors of osteopathic medicine.[95]

Marcelino Oliva, Jr., DO, FACOFP (Fig. 2.10), was the first Latino president of the AOA. Born in Cuba, his love of medicine developed while observing his uncle, who was a physician, care for his mother, whom he lost at age 8. His father moved the family to Tampa, Florida to start a new life.

- Dr. Oliva graduated from Kansas City College of Osteopathic Medicine (now Kansas City University) in 1964, and did his internship in Tulsa, Oklahoma.
- He joined his mentor for a number of years, later buying the family practice and 9-bed hospital he owned in Dade City, Florida (rural at the time).
- He delivered approximately 3,000 babies through his career of mid-20th century general practice, which included office visits, surgery, house calls, and weekends at the hospital emergency room.
- He became Chief of Staff at a larger hospital that initially denied him and other DOs privileges, and was a board and executive committee member at other local hospitals.

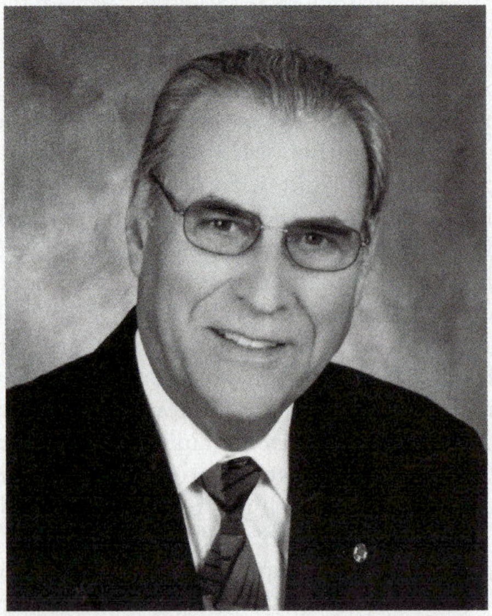

Figure 2.10. Marcelino Oliva, Jr., DO, FACOFP. First Latino President of the AOA (1988). (Photo courtesy of the American Osteopathic Association and Natalie Nevins.)

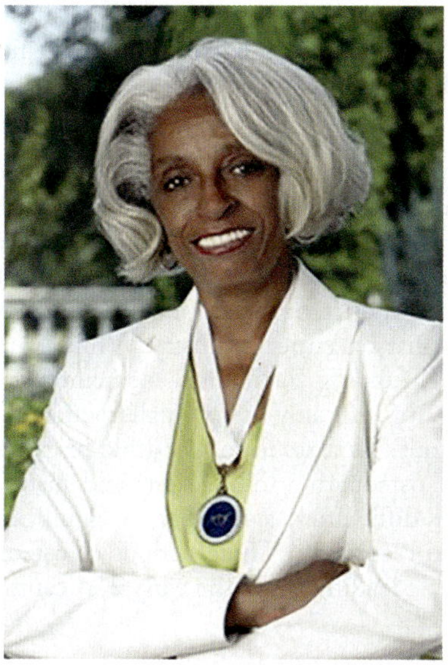

Figure 2.11. Barbara Ross-Lee, DO, FACOFP. First female African American Dean of an American Medical School, the Ohio University College of Osteopathic Medicine (1993).

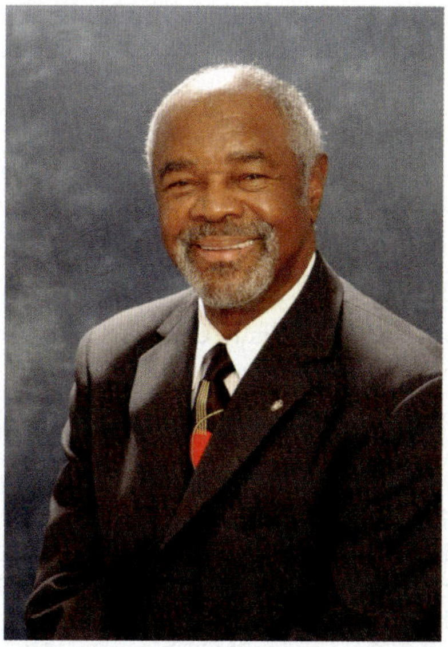

Figure 2.12. William G. Anderson, DO, FACOS. First African American President of the AOA (1994).

- He was President of the Florida Osteopathic Medical Association, and a Founding Trustee of Nova-Southeastern College of Osteopathic Medicine.
- After his term as the first minority President of the AOA in 1988-1989, Dr. Oliva continued serving the profession nationally as Chair of the AOA Bureaus for Federal Health Programs and Legislative Affairs for many years, and in 2007 was the ACOFP Physician of the Year.[96,97]

Barbara Ross-Lee, DO, FACOFP (Fig. 2.11) made history in 1993 as the first female African American dean of any American medical school, when she became Dean of the Ohio University College of Osteopathic Medicine.

- Ross-Lee later joined the New York Institute of Technology as Vice President of Health Sciences and Medical Affairs, serving also at various times as Dean of Allied Health and Life Sciences and Dean of the New York College of Osteopathic Medicine.
- An advocate of medical care in underserved communities, she followed up being the first DO to be awarded a health policy fellowship with the Robert Wood Johnson Foundation by founding and supervising the AOA Health Policy Fellowship.

William G. Anderson, DO, FACOS, was elected as the first African American president of the AOA in 1994[98] (Fig. 2.12).

- He graduated in Des Moines in the early 1950s.
- After internship, he and his wife moved back to the state of his birth, Georgia, to begin a general practice in 1957.

Anderson founded the Coalition for Desegregation in Albany, Georgia (*The Albany Movement*).

- Members, including William and his wife, Norma Anderson, were jailed multiple times for protesting segregation.
- He called his good friend, Martin Luther King Jr., to visit Albany and announced in church (to King's surprise) that Dr. King would lead a march the next day.
- Jailed together, King chose to remain incarcerated while Dr. Anderson was released so that he could appear on national television and explain the situation.
- Charged with Felony Obstruction of Justice (for trying to overturn what he rightly considered an unconstitutional law), Anderson had a hung jury from an all-White jury in the first trial in Albany, then left Georgia to do a surgical residency in Michigan. Since he had clearly committed the offense, he knew that meant at least one juror refused to convict him (likely, he thought, out of conscience).
- At his second trial, in Federal Court in Detroit, he was judged guilty and sentenced to 20 years, suspended sentence, with unsupervised probation for a year.
- He completed a general surgery residency, became a general surgeon, and served on the AOA Board of Trustees for 20 years before becoming the AOA President.
- In addition to ongoing service to the AOA, Dr. Anderson continued working as a surgeon, hospital medical education director and as an Associate Dean for ATSU-KCOM[98] and was a long-standing board member of the NBOME.

Karen J. Nichols, DO, MACOI (Fig. 2.13), an internal medicine specialist from Arizona became the first female AOA

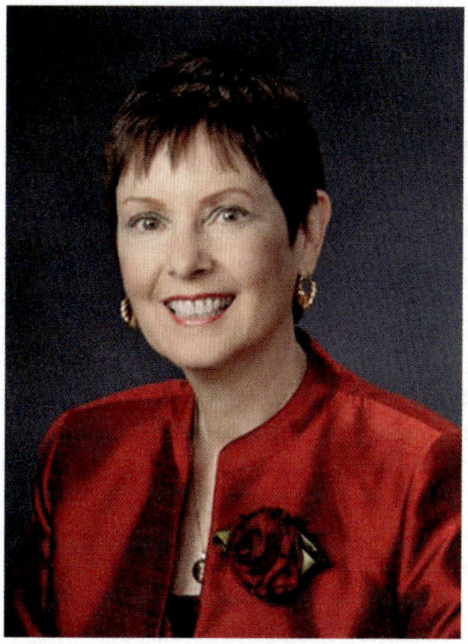

Figure 2.13. Karen J. Nichols, DO, FACOI. First female President of the AOA (2010).

President in 2010. Well-known for her leadership style, dynamism, mentorship, and ability to forge consensus, Nichols has also served as:

- Arizona Osteopathic Medical Association President
- American College of Osteopathic Internists President
- President of the Institute of Medicine of Chicago and the first DO to be elected to the position
- Member of the Board of Directors of the Osteopathic International Alliance
- Dean of Midwestern University/Chicago College of Osteopathic Medicine
- Member of the Board of Directors of the ACGME and the first DO to be elected Chair of the ACGME Board of Directors

In 2020, the Cherokee Nation and the Oklahoma State University College of Osteopathic Medicine opened the first tribally associated medical school in the country. While the school is located on the Cherokee Nation Reservation, over 11 federally recognized tribes are represented within the student body.

As of 2024, 42 accredited COMs exist, having numerous additional branches or locations from north to south and coast to coast, most of which have established some form of diversity, equity, and inclusion program, policies, offices, or officers to address these issues. Likewise, the AOA,[99] AACOM,[100] the NBOME and virtually every osteopathic organization have produced organized responses, policies and offices to meet these needs.

LGBTQ+ civil rights gains and redefinition of the concept of gender in the United States and western world increased equal rights and proportionate representation for previously underrepresented and sometimes invisible population segments. Most of these changes involved community and national civil debate. This cultural shift created considerable social and political polarization as people's rights (including public educational changes) continued to be adjudicated up to the highest levels.

The AOA and AACOM track various diversity issues. Consult their websites for the most recently compiled statistics and news demonstrating the historic slow but steady growth of diversity in the matriculants, graduates, and osteopathic physicians over the past decades. Currently the majority of matriculating first-year osteopathic medical students are women, which first occurred in the academic year 2003-2004 and has now been the norm since 2019-2020.[54]

OSTEOPATHIC RESEARCH

Introduction

The osteopathic philosophy and osteopathic manipulation developed as an experimental approach to clinical conditions that did not respond to the conventional treatments in the mid to late 1800s. The practical success of osteopathic manipulation became the empirical research results that led to the "why" and "what if" appropriate for laboratory study. Medical research in the 20th century paralleled medical education as both developed new methods, traditions, controls, and better equipment.

As the original schools matured and university-based schools were founded from 1971 forward, biomedical scientists recruited to teach wished to continue their own lines of research. DO specialists also began to conduct research related to their specialties that did not involve osteopathic manipulation. That raised the question: what defines osteopathic research?

Most of the original research performed in the profession up through the 1960s concerned the unique elements of the profession:

- OPP
- Osteopathic manipulative medicine (OMM) (including unique neuromusculoskeletal diagnosis)
- OMT

Financial and practical challenges limited the study of the scientific questions raised by osteopathic manipulative practice. Most medical research has been paid for by companies seeking financial gain, or by the government. Research on methods that might decrease the need for their product, or the amount sold, are not likely to elicit funding by the pharmaceutical industry. While National Institutes of Health (NIH) funding for manual medicine has increased over the past decades, it is still only a very small fraction of the total available research funds. As a result, osteopathic research has primarily been funded by osteopathic foundations and institutions. Despite these and other difficulties, a number of significant accomplishments have been recorded.[56] Three periods of osteopathic research are distinguishable leading up to the early 21st century.

Development Preceded Research

A.T. Still conducted his own personal study, as opposed to modern organized research, but it was in line with what still forms the basis of almost all medical research. He followed a continual process of making observations that led to questions; he constructed testable hypotheses and then tried new therapeutic interventions; he refined his hypotheses and altered his practice in ways expected to improve outcomes. What new approaches seemed to give a good patient response, he incorporated into his methods of treatment.

With the idea that structure and function are always interrelated, Still studied anatomy in depth, developed finely tuned palpatory skills, and devised techniques to improve blood and lymphatic flow, movement capabilities, and neurologic function.

Still told his students that if they knew their anatomy, they were free to develop their own techniques as long as they could achieve the same results. He personally encouraged or directed some of the early students to investigate specific regions. Charlotte Weaver was one whom he directed to study the cranium. Though she published her anatomic studies and theory, her techniques were lost because other physicians did not learn and preserve her techniques. Another early student was F. P. Millard, whom Still encouraged to investigate the lymphatic system.

Still's techniques were often accompanied by a little click, but on rare occasion had a popping sound. Some of his earliest students increased the speed and used more force over a short range of motion, later known as high velocity/low amplitude (HVLA) technique. Taught and practiced student-to-student, this variant came to dominate the curriculum when early students became the new professors. Professor Edyth Ashmore, in charge of teaching osteopathic methods, commented that it was different from what the earlier osteopaths did but easier to teach.

Early osteopaths created techniques on a pragmatic basis, but in most cases were not researchers. Through the 20th century, DO developers followed Still's principles as they studied, observed, and assembled new methods into systems of diagnosis and treatment. They published their thoughts, theories and methods in local, state or occasionally national journals. At the request of their peers, they began to teach these new methods to fellow graduates, often against resistance.

In the first half of the 20th century, William Garner Sutherland developed osteopathy in the cranial field. Because osteopathic physicians found his system useful, they studied, organized, taught and researched it. Over the next fifty years, what is today called *osteopathic cranial manipulative medicine* (OCMM) became a component of standard osteopathic curricula.

In the second half of the century, Fred Mitchell, Sr. developed the Muscle Energy system. Lawrence Jones, DO developed Strain/Counterstrain. Robert Ward, John Peckham and Anthony Chila modified earlier fascial approaches to include muscle release techniques as they originated Myofascial Release (MFR). Stan Schiowitz based a new system on a few techniques he had been taught, expanding them into Facilitated Positional Release (FPR). Everything came full circle as Richard Van Buskirk searched the early literature and began teaching Still's original techniques. The history of these developments is expanded in the technique chapters.

Sutherland: An Early Developer

Sutherland was an early developer who expanded Still's philosophy and theories into practical diagnosis and treatment of the cranium, sacrum and other parts of the body. From an early age he worked in the newspaper printing industry, before matriculating at the ASO in 1898 at the age of 25.

His work as a compositor, laying out type cases and working on proofs required great dexterity, fine motor skills, and a high level of sensitive haptic perception. Proprioception, visual discrimination and coordination were inherent to this work. This often required work that was upside down and backward[101] (p. 73). As a primer, he worked on the printing presses mechanically with adjustments and repairs, giving him an appreciation for mechanical principles that easily translated into osteopathic principles[101] (p. 98).

The invention of the linotype when he was 10 or 11 years old meant that this type of work would be replaced by technology, obviating the need for this level of finely dexterous manual skill. He also wrote for the newspaper, developing journalistic skills. When he visited the ASO with a friend who was attending, the administration offered him a full scholarship for the fall of 1898.

Sutherland's fascination with a Beauchene (exploded) skull at the ASO gave him the sudden thought that the articulations of the sphenoid and temporal bones were "beveled like the gills of a fish, indicating articular mobility for a respiratory mechanism."[102] But standard teaching said that the bones of the skull were fused after childhood, devoid of motion. Clinical experience with head-injury patients forced him to revive his long-suppressed thoughts. Palpating carefully, he perceived subtle motion. He disarticulated skulls to study the cranial joints. Observing and describing the motion he felt in his patients, he attempted to gently disimpact compressed tissues and restore normal physiologic function. Using homemade devices, he compressed different parts of his own skull, noted the effects, and experimented with correcting the distortions he had created. This led to successful patient care.

He described his theories and cases in local osteopathic publications, and presented them at the AOA Convention in 1932. Though only seven physicians attended, interest grew and he began teaching a small group his methods. By 1946, the Osteopathic Cranial Association was formed as an affiliate of the Academy of Applied Osteopathy to promote his theories and methods, which eventually became part of the standard osteopathic curriculum.

Early Research: The First Period of Osteopathic Research (1874–1939)

Still's early students began formally studying the anomalies that they called the osteopathic lesion (somatic dysfunction).

- Skiagraphy (a crude initial form of x-ray) was used by William Smith, MD, DO, before 1900 in search of evidence.
- Laboratory studies began among osteopathic physicians almost as soon as an organized osteopathic school was established[64] (pp. 24–26).
- Animal models were used to determine the physiologic effects of the palpatory findings that created the "lesion."[103]

HARRISON FRYETTE, DO

In 1918, at the AOA convention in Boston MA, H.H. Fryette presented the principles of physiologic motion of the spine to the osteopathic profession. Influenced by R.W. Lovett, MD, Dr. Fryette came to his own conclusions after years of careful study and general practice and analysis in anatomic dissection labs.[104]

E.A. HOSKINS, DO, W.A. SCHWAB, DO

Another significant contribution to the osteopathic concept came from Drs. W.A. Schwab and E.R. Hoskins. Working together they developed the standing postural x-ray in 1921 and applied it to osteopathic concepts.[105] It was through this methodology in the early 20th century that Dr. Fryette's spinal principles were demonstrated radiographically.[105]

BERYL ARBUCKLE, DO

Beryl Arbuckle, DO, was one of Sutherland's first students. She did extensive research on cranial anatomy from the 1940s–1960s, including the dura and other structures inside the head, finding dural and connective tissues that transmitted stress in the cranium along the lines that Sutherland had described. She performed or participated in over 1,500 autopsies and dissections of preterm and infant skulls, publishing articles and books on her research.

A.T. Still Research Institute

Research at several osteopathic schools[106] during the first third of the 1900s produced small studies on basic neural and physiologic mechanisms underlying somatic dysfunction and the effects of osteopathic treatment on symptoms and immune function. Much of this research would only be considered suggestive by today's standards but formed the conceptual basis for evolving lines of study. Examination of early osteopathic research suggests that it was comparable to medical research of that era and included a small number of large-scale projects.

The AOA founded the A.T. Still Postgraduate College of Osteopathy (renamed 3 years later as the A. T. Still Research Institute) and requested donations to fund it. $16,000 was raised from private donations (about half a million dollars in 2023). About 1913, the institute opened in a dedicated building in Chicago with Wilborn J. Deason directing research. Louisa Burns, the next director, battled many challenges to the institute's survival and pioneered a "bench-to-bedside" model consistent with modern translational research.

LOUISA BURNS, DO

Through the early 1950s, Burns investigated the effects of spinal "lesions" primarily in a rabbit model.[107,108] Her studies indicated that artificially produced strains of specific vertebral segments produced a somewhat reproducible constellation of functional changes in organs and tissues innervated from the area of strain. Wilbur Cole, who worked with Louisa Burns in the 1940s, substantiated this using various neural strains.[109] Cole[110] acknowledged the difficulty Burns had in describing the "boney lesion" in operationally defined terms, which are now routine through the application of technology.[111] Dr. Burns also described the impact of OMT on humans and its effect on heart rate and blood pressure.[107] She published four books,[111–115] a collected work,[116] and several reports from the institute that still contain information of value to the modern researcher.

A few early studies had relatively large sample sizes and comparison groups for the time. These studies may have lacked the rigor of modern research design but were at or above the standards of the day.

L.M. WHITING, DO

Whiting[117] in 1911 reported on the impact of OMT on labor and delivery outcomes.

- In a sample of 223 women, average labor times of both primiparous and multiparous women who received prenatal OMT were dramatically shorter than women who did not (primiparous women: 9 hours 54 minutes, compared with 21 hours 6 minutes, and multiparous women: 6 hours 19 minutes, compared with 11 hours 41 minutes, respectively).[118]

S.V. ROBUCK

S.V. Robuck in 1933 reported a chart analysis of 13,816 women who received OMT during pregnancy and found the maternal mortality rate to be much lower (one-third of the maternal mortality reported in "government bulletins").[119]

SMITH

Smith[120] reported an observational study with 110,120 influenza patients in 1918 to 1919 who received OMT and suffered a much lower mortality rate than the general population. While caution is advised in the interpretation of the data,[121] it was collected in similar ways to MD patient data collection.

Kirksville: The Second Period of Osteopathic Research (1940–1969)

I.M. KORR AND J.S. DENSLOW

In 1938, John Stedman Denslow, DO, became a faculty member at what is now Kirksville College of Osteopathic Medicine (ATSU-KCOM) and began a renaissance in osteopathic research, using electromyography to study the *osteopathic lesion*. In the immediate post–World War II era, technology advanced and was affordable; KCOM was able to produce significant research describing the concept of the osteopathic lesion, now known as *somatic dysfunction*.[122–126]

- Irvin M. Korr, PhD (Physiology) (Fig. 2.14), joined Denslow's team in 1945.

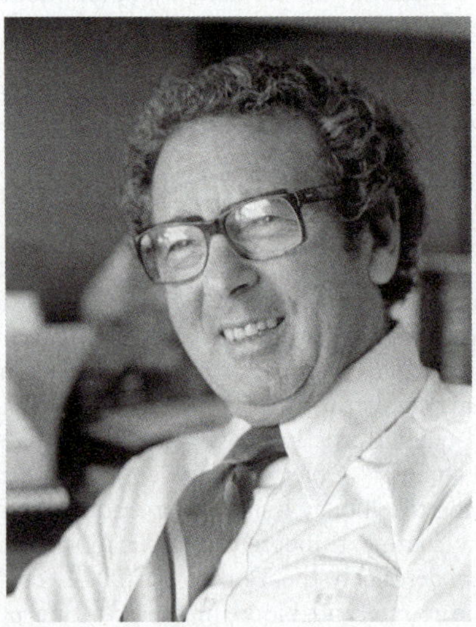

Figure 2.14. Irvin M. Korr, PhD (1909–2004). "The second great osteopathic philosopher."

- Denslow and Korr oversaw the hiring of faculty with the goal of building a research team.
- The Kirksville group published research articles in journals outside the osteopathic profession to spread the findings of uniquely osteopathic research to the larger medical/scientific community. They focused on a conceptual framework that has dominated osteopathic thinking about the basis for palpation and treatment to the present day:
  - Basic characteristics of muscle activity related to palpatory diagnosis
  - The activity of the nervous system in somatic dysfunction
  - The concept of the facilitated segment[124,127,128]

Funding for the Kirksville group's research was primarily from the AOA, the A.T. Still Osteopathic Foundation, and KCOM. Starting in 1958, federal funding came from the Public Health Service and Office of Naval Research.[126,129] Through the 1960s and 1970s, funding initially came from the NIH[130,131] and, later, the National Institutes of Neurological Diseases and Stroke.[132,133]

The expansion of the NIH, with its emphasis on biomedical research and its funding of new laboratories and programs, fueled an explosive growth of the biomedical research community in the United States. Unfortunately, the small number of researchers in the osteopathic profession was not able to benefit from it (the focus remained on producing physicians that would directly care for the US population). Although several additional studies were published, such as those on joint mechanics,[134] research progressed slowly as the profession was busy training a flood of returning soldiers and adjusting to the new postwar world.

Expanding Schools: The Third Period of Osteopathic Research (1970–2000)

MICHIGAN STATE UNIVERSITY COLLEGE OF OSTEOPATHIC MEDICINE

Though only five of the original osteopathic schools remained in the late 1960s, 15 existed in the early 1980s. New university-based schools were founded, and the original schools expanded in the 1970s, hiring more research-trained faculty. The new MSUCOM formed a Department of Biomechanics devoted to osteopathic research. In the early 1970s, NIH research funding was awarded at an osteopathic school for the first time in many years.

AMERICAN OSTEOPATHIC ASSOCIATION

Activities that fostered additional research included:

- AOA funding and activities through the Bureau of Research and the annual Research Conference
- COCA requirements for accreditation
- Joint DO and PhD degree programs
- Research requirements instituted in residency programs
  - When the COCA required schools to include research, many COMs began to provide funds from their operating budgets to seed programs and encouraged faculty and students to engage in projects.

AMERICAN ACADEMY OF OSTEOPATHY

- AAO Louisa Burns Research Committee (LBORC) activities
- AAO International Symposia
  - 1989 Somatovisceral/Viscerosomatic Interaction[135]
  - 1992 Nociception and the Neuroendocrine-immune Connection[136]
- Research awards were established to honor:
  - Louisa Burns (1969)

- □ Max Gutensohn (1984)
- □ John Denslow (1984)
- □ Irvin M. Korr (1999)
- □ John and Mary Burnett

W.L. JOHNSTON, M. BEAL, A.F. KELSO

William L. Johnston, DO, and Myron C. Beal, DO, at MSUCOM, and Albert F. Kelso, PhD, at the Chicago College of Osteopathic Medicine (Midwestern University), kept up the momentum of OMM-related research through the 1980s and 1990s with funding primarily from the AOA and their own institutions. They provided important leadership at conferences and worked to:

- Develop/promote essential osteopathic terminology such as *TART* (tissue texture abnormalities, asymmetry, restriction of motion, and tenderness) and *somatic dysfunction*
- Perform studies on interexaminer and intraexaminer reliability of palpatory assessment[137–140]
- Review and explore viscerosomatic and somatovisceral reflex interactions[141,142]
- Describe the impact of OMM on systemic disorders[143–146]

M.M. PATTERSON

Michael M. Patterson, PhD (Fig. 2.15) functioned as a bridge spanning the last three decades of the 20th century and the first two decades of the 21st century. Patterson maintained continuity and focus on uniquely osteopathic research through his own laboratory research, teaching, mentorship, and leadership at national and international research meetings and conferences. He served on many grant and thesis review committees and as Associate Editor of the *JAOA*. His outstanding devotion, service and invaluable contributions to the profession during his 45-year career were recognized by the AOA in 2017 as recipient of their highest honor, the AOA Distinguished Service Award.

21st Century Osteopathic Research (2001–Present)

Research programs of the osteopathic profession had not yet matured sufficiently by the 1980s and 1990s to support a center of excellence like the NIH was sponsoring in those decades. By 1999, changes in NIH funding meant the profession would have to commit funds from its own resources.

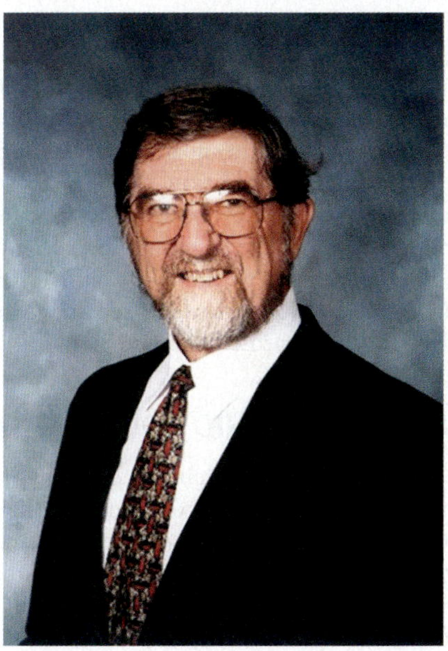

Figure 2.15. Michael M. Patterson, PhD, DO (HON). 2017 AOA Distinguished Service Award Recipient, in recognition of over 45 years of outstanding contributions in all areas of osteopathic research.

R.E. KAPPLER

A landmark study for the osteopathic profession was published in 1999 in the New England Journal of Medicine.[147] This study on low back pain was one of the first major research studies on the clinical effectiveness of osteopathic care. It was very important for the profession as it provided *evidence of the efficacy of OMT in one of the top medical journals in the world.* It was a randomized, controlled trial that involved patients who had had low back pain for at least 3 weeks but less than 6 months. A total of 178 patients were randomized to usual care and OMT, or to usual care only. The OMT protocol allowed for individualized treatment approaches, including thrust, muscle energy, counterstrain, articulation, and myofascial release techniques. Although the results indicated that the OMT and usual care groups did not differ in the primary outcome measures (pain relief, function, and satisfaction), the authors reported that patients in the osteopathic-treatment group required significantly less medication (analgesics, anti-inflammatory agents, and muscle relaxants) ($P < .001$) and used less physical therapy (0.2% vs. 2.6%).[147] The historical impact of this study was extremely beneficial to the osteopathic profession, and its overall impact transcends specific findings of the study.

The Louisa Burns Research Committee

The LBORC of the AAO, the AOA Bureau of Research, and the AACOM were leading discussions about forming an osteopathic research center by 1997, and funds were committed by 2000. One of five schools that submitted plans for a center for osteopathic research, the Texas College of Osteopathic Medicine (University of North Texas Health Science Center) was awarded the funding in 2001.

Osteopathic Research Center (UNTHSC), J.C. Licciardone

The Osteopathic Research Center, under the direction of Executive Director John C. Licciardone, DO, MS, MBA (Fig. 2.16),

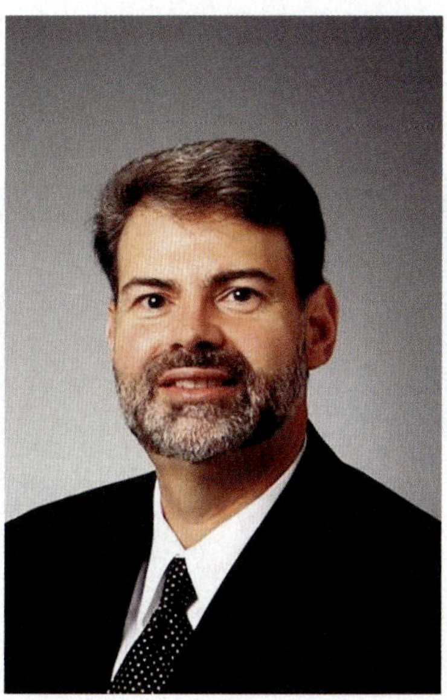

Figure 2.16. John C. Licciardone, DO, MS, MBA. Executive Director, Osteopathic Research Center at UNT HSC, Fort Worth, Texas.

functioned as an early coordinating and centralizing force in the early 21st century, fostering collaboration within the osteopathic research community.

- Numerous clinical trials were successfully conducted, including the use of OMT in pregnant patients.[148]
- OMT effects in animal models[149] were studied.
- A meta-analysis of OMT randomized clinical trials for patients with low back pain was published.[150]
- In a randomized, double-blind, sham-controlled trial, Licciardone showed that OMT has medium to large treatment effects in subgroups of patients with certain baseline levels of low back pain intensity and back-specific functioning.[151]

Osteopathic Research Center (UNTHSC), L. Hodge

Continuing in line with the animal-based research that Louisa Burns initiated a century ago, Lisa M. Hodge, PhD, (Fig. 2.17), Basic Science Research Chair for the Osteopathic Research Center (UNTHSC), developed unique inquiries examining the role of osteopathic manual lymphatic pump procedures in modulating lymph flow and function in the face of infectious diseases, such as pneumonia and cancer.

American Osteopathic Association

In 2005, the AOA Research Task Force released a report, *Research Strategic Direction for the American Osteopathic Association*.[152] The report recognized the value of all areas of biomedical research but recommended that the AOA focus its limited funding on investigating "...the unique aspects of osteopathic medicine with an emphasis on OMM." That focus includes but is not limited to:

- Mechanisms of action of OMM
- Clinical efficacy of OMM
- Interexaminer and intraexaminer reliability of palpatory assessment
- Osteopathic physician and patient interactions
- Cost-effectiveness of osteopathic health care
- Methods of teaching palpation and OMM

See Chapter 94 for the current strategic research plan.

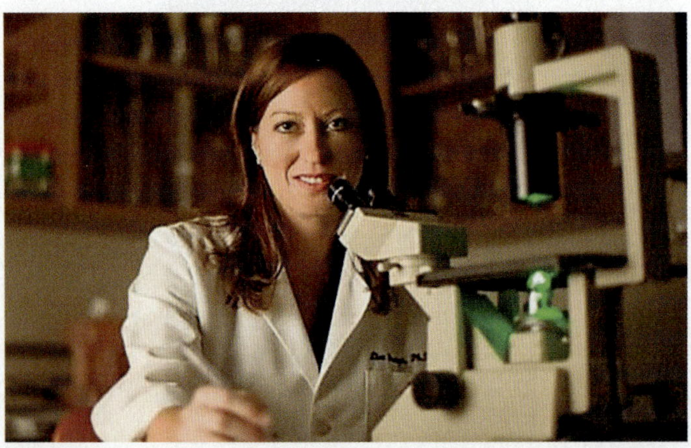

Figure 2.17. Lisa M. Hodge, PhD. Basic Science Research Chair, Osteopathic Research Center at UNT HSC, Fort Worth, TX.

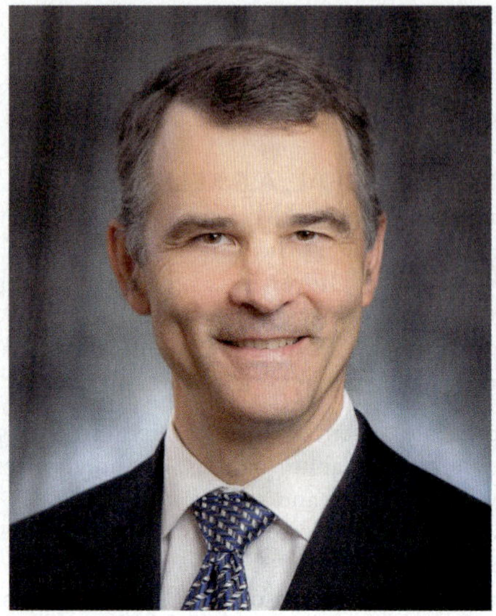

Figure 2.18. Brian F. Degenhardt, DO. Director, A. T. Still Research Institute at ATSU, Kirksville, MO.

The A.T. Still Research Institute (ATSRI)

The ATSRI uses both local researchers and a network of DOs in numerous states under the leadership of Director Brian F. Degenhardt, DO (Fig 2.18). It is funded internally (A.T. Still University) and with help from foundations. Since 2004, the institute sponsored numerous successful research efforts and published a large, multicenter trial, the Multicenter Osteopathic Pneumonia Study in the Elderly (MOPSE)[153] (see Chapter 72). The ATSRI also developed the DO-Touch.NET practice-based nationwide research network of DOs (as well as some international practitioners), to assess practice outcomes, safety, and adverse events after OMT.

Osteopathic Heritage Foundations

Current research funding trends mirror the pattern started in the last half of the 20th century but with significant funds added from foundations derived from and supportive of osteopathic medicine. Between 1999 and 2017, under the visionary and exceptional leadership of President/CEO Richard A. Vincent, the Osteopathic Heritage Foundations in Ohio approved over $230 million in funding awards including research, educational, and community health programs[154] with the goal of continuing osteopathic traditions in health care. In addition to their major support of osteopathic research at both the Osteopathic Research Center at UNTHSC and the ATRSI, the foundations granted transformative funding of $105 million to the Ohio University College of Osteopathic Medicine, which renamed itself the Ohio University Heritage College of Osteopathic Medicine.[154]

AMERICAN OSTEOPATHIC FOUNDATION

Evidence-based osteopathic research began with Still's observations and clinical experience; what constitutes sufficient evidence and the appropriate methodology to collect and analyze it have changed over time. Funding for osteopathic research has grown but still remains a challenge.

The AOF is a national 501(c)(3) charitable foundation that has been serving the osteopathic profession since 1949 through five funding priorities—educational scholarships, community service, scholarly research, international mission trips, and OR. Since its inception, the Foundation has been supporting programs and initiatives that align with the mission of advancing osteopathic tenets and principles and has provided numerous grants, scholarships, and awards to the osteopathic community.

Current and Future Directions

Considering the current identified opioid overuse epidemic, osteopathic manipulative medicine provides a reasonable alternative having been shown to be less likely to induce harmful side effects or create addiction in patients with chronic low back pain (exactly as Still had demonstrated in the post–Civil War era).[3] Another study demonstrates that OMT, in combination with traditional pharmacology, was associated with reduction of somatic pain, higher success with medication-assisted treatment, and lower costs.[155]

Challenges in Osteopathic Research

STUDY DESIGN, SHAM TREATMENTS, AND BLINDING

The basis of osteopathic care is individualized to each patient and their distinct structural, emotional, and biopsychosocial components. Therefore, it can be challenging to 'fit" osteopathic medicine into current research protocols that inherently do not consider the patient as a unique individual entity.

Practical considerations for clinical studies to align with scientific standards included the following:

- Double Blind: How can both the physician performing OMT and the patient receiving it be blinded to the fact that OMT is being used, if double-blind studies are the gold standard?
- Placebo: What can be used as a placebo in place of manipulation? Touch by itself is a form of treatment and is not generally considered to be neutral. A treatment sham using touch generally compares nonspecific relaxation accompanying the comfort of human touch against touch imparting a more specific treatment. Improper use of sham control can therefore seriously weaken a study, resulting in no significant outcomes, when the comfort of human touch is involved in both sham and treatment.
- Osteopathic treatment study or manual technique study:
  - Technique study: The same reproducible technique is performed on each patient.
  - Treatment study: Discovering the patient and tissue condition through observation and palpation, the physician then performs a treatment. This is done by selecting and modifying techniques thought to both address what is found and be best suited for the patient's condition. (Most osteopathic treatments rely on the cumulative and integrated effects of multiple techniques, specifically chosen to address one or more diagnosed anatomic–physiologic problems.)
- Treatment Sequence: Using a series of identical techniques with a particular diagnosis, is the sequence significant?
  - Different ordering of techniques may alter the way mechanical force distribution occurs through musculoskeletal tensegrity, modifying physiologic changes in blood/lymphatic circulation and the nervous system in a dynamical fashion.
  - Incremental changes may interact differently through complex adaptive systems (involving multilevel feedback and feed-forward mechanisms).
  - Is the wrong sequence doomed to ineffectiveness because it's analogous to turning a door handle before unlocking it?
- What are the best pre- and postmeasures, and what technology is required to demonstrate and document that change has or has not taken place?

Community Based Education Model

The current challenge presented by the osteopathic community-based education model is creating the network of clinicians and bioscientists needed to perform bench-to-bedside translational studies. Technologic improvements continue to assist this process. It may be further improved as researchers use artificial intelligence to analyze large data from enhanced collecting networks yet to be developed. Providing evidence of efficacy, cost-effectiveness, and the mechanisms of osteopathic treatment, as well as osteopathic principles that may or may not focus on OMT (e.g., physician empathy, nutrition and exercise, preventive care) should assist the osteopathic medical profession in helping the country and the world to re-establish and maintain health. Research on extending the health span as far as possible through the lifespan will guide osteopathic physicians to go beyond the diagnosis of disease and maximize human potential by *seeking health in patients*.

INTERNATIONAL DEVELOPMENT OF THE PROFESSION OF OSTEOPATHIC MEDICINE AND OSTEOPATHY

As osteopathy evolved into osteopathic medicine in the United States, osteopathic concepts spread worldwide along different developmental paths.

- Early graduates of the ASO and other schools returned to their homelands or went to new countries, initially from the United States to the United Kingdom, Canada, and Australia.
- They established schools and independent professions with practice limited to osteopathic manipulation. Graduates practiced osteopathy by tolerance rather than legal rights.
- The British School of Osteopathy (BSO), founded by John Martin Littlejohn, DO, PhD, MD, had the most widespread international influence (Box 2.1).
- After World War II, a few American osteopathic physicians visiting other countries taught osteopathic diagnosis and treatment to both physicians with full practice rights and physiotherapists or other individuals with limited or no practice rights.
- Beginning in the 1980s, American DOs were represented in the Federation Internationale de Medicine Manuelle (FIMM), an umbrella organization for physicians around the world who specialized in treating musculoskeletal conditions with manual techniques.
- Forums conducted by the AAO beginning in 1989 channeled information on international groups (primarily but not exclusively nonphysicians) to the AOA.
- The AOA established the Council on International Osteopathic Medical Education and Affairs (CIOMEA) in 1998, later renamed the Bureau of International Osteopathic Medicine (BIOM)[162] (Box 2.2).

Two organizations arose to help establish standardization on common issues within the international osteopathic community and worked together to promote training and practice rights of osteopathic physicians and osteopaths. Both groups helped develop the World Health Organization's (WHO) *Guidelines for the Training and Practice of Osteopathy*, which defines a shared core curriculum and core competencies.

- World Osteopathic Health Organization (WOHO) (2003–2011). WOHO was founded by individual practitioners, educators, and researchers, most of whom had participated in the AAO's late-century International Forum programs.[163]

BOX 2.1 John Martin Littlejohn, DO, PhD (1865–1947)

John Martin Littlejohn was born in 1865 and educated at Glasgow University, Scotland, in divinity, law, oriental languages, and political history.[156]

- He immigrated to the United States for health-related reasons in 1892.
- His PhD thesis was published at Columbia University.[156–157]
- In 1894, he accepted the position as President of the liberal arts Amity College in College Springs, IA.
- In 1897, Littlejohn began traveling to Kirksville, MO, to receive treatment from Still for a throat condition. Impressed with the results, he decided to study osteopathy.[158]
- While still a student, he was appointed Professor of Physiology, Psychology, and Dietetics and eventually in 1898 as the ASO Dean of Faculty.[156,158,159]
- Within a year of his appointments, he wrote and published three textbooks about physiology and inaugurated two osteopathic journals.
- After graduating from the ASO in 1900, Littlejohn left for Chicago where he and his brother established the American College of Osteopathic Medicine and Surgery; the name represented the founders' belief that osteopathy was a system of medicine and should be recognized as such.[160] This may have been the first time the term "osteopathic medicine" was officially used.

Littlejohn introduced osteopathy in the United Kingdom through a series of talks to the Society of Science, Letters, and Arts in London in 1898, 1899, and 1900.[158]

- Although he held talks in 1903 with other ASO graduates, it was not until he returned to the United Kingdom for good in 1913 that the BSO was incorporated in London (1917) as a nonprofit organization.
- Neither the degree nor the profession was recognized by legislation.
- Its 4-year curriculum, excluding pharmacology and surgery, was completed in 1921.[161]
- Access to hospitals, dissection laboratories, and other aspects of physician training was denied.
- Without national regulation, the osteopathic profession in the United Kingdom was practiced by tolerance until Parliament passed the Osteopaths Act in 1993 and the General Osteopathic Council (GOsC) was formed.

- Osteopathic International Alliance (OIA) (2004–present). The OIA was founded after the AOA invited representatives of various national organizations to Chicago in 2003 to create an international organization to ensure that the WHO recognized osteopathic medicine and osteopathy as distinctive from other manual medicine professions including chiropractic[162] (Box 2.3).

The AOA has had a long-standing concern that US-trained DOs should have the same practice right possibilities internationally that MDs enjoy if they want to practice in another country and wish to apply for licensure there. A list of countries in which DOs can get full licensure is maintained by the AOA, and it changes from year to year. A map is also provided demonstrating what rights are available. Individuals should consult the website for up-to-date information regarding any country in which they have interest (osteopathic.org).[165]

Many U.S. COM students or prospective students are interested in exploring international medicine and osteopathy. Most US COMs have international educational opportunities for their

BOX 2.2 Osteopath or Osteopathic Physician: What's the Difference?

Still called his original graduates osteopaths, and the ASO diplomas in 1893 read Diplomate in Osteopathy. This was almost immediately changed to Doctor of Osteopathy.

- The American osteopathic profession continued Still's medical reformation by incorporating pertinent scientific discoveries as they occurred.
- The AOA favored osteopathic physician as a more accurate description of the scope of practice, and by the latter 20th century, the colleges redefined the DO degree as Doctor of Osteopathic Medicine.

American osteopathic medical colleges are recognized by the World Health Organization (WHO) as medical schools.

- In other countries, graduates of schools of osteopathy were not granted (and many did not desire) full scope medical practice rights.
- The profession of osteopathy in other countries provides a less broad scope of practice typically limited to osteopathic manual treatment.

As a result, osteopathic physician and osteopath are now defined differently.

- Osteopathic physician: a person with full, unlimited medical practice rights who has achieved the nationally recognized academic and professional standards within the country to diagnose and provide treatment, based upon the principles of osteopathic philosophy.
- Osteopath: a person with limited practice rights who has achieved the nationally recognized academic and professional standards within the country to independently practice diagnosis and treatment, based upon the principles of osteopathic philosophy.

Both osteopathic physicians and osteopaths use manual treatment, including OMT. Significant differences in education, clinical competencies, and scope of practice exist between the two recognized groups.

- American Doctors of Osteopathic Medicine (osteopathic physicians) are trained in osteopathic medical philosophy and have unlimited practice rights including medicine, surgery, obstetrics, and OMT.
- International Diplomats of Osteopathy (osteopaths) are trained in osteopathic philosophy and OMT and have limited practice rights.
- In some countries in which osteopathy and osteopathic medicine are not legally regulated, some individuals using OMT and the osteopathic philosophy do so under the scope of practice regulated by another profession (e.g., Japan).

BOX 2.3 Osteopathic International Alliance (OIA)[162]

In June 2003, 34 individuals representing 10 countries and 17 international organizations traveled to Chicago, Illinois, USA, to attend the 1st Invitational Conference to Organize an International Osteopathic Association. Those in attendance exchanged information about the state of the related professions of osteopathic medicine and osteopathy in their home countries and decided that it was important to convene the professions for collaborative efforts to advance the osteopathic philosophy of patient care worldwide.

- The OIA was officially incorporated in the state of Illinois in the United States, in December 2004.
- In July 2005, the OIA held its Inaugural Conference in Washington DC, USA, with 45 attendees from nearly a dozen countries, representing more than thirty different international organizations.
- Today, the OIA represents more than 75 organizations of osteopathic physicians and osteopaths from 20 countries on 5 continents and more than 120,000 osteopathic practitioners.
- In 2018 the OIA was admitted into official relations with the WHO. This official relationship was renewed in 2021 and then again in 2024, making the OIA the primary international organization advocating for high-quality osteopathic health care and the leading representative of osteopathic professionals worldwide.
- Building on previous collaboration, the OIA will support the strategic objectives of the WHO Traditional Medicine Strategy 2025–2034 via these three agreed-upon collaborative projects: Updating Benchmarks in Training for Osteopathy, Update on the Global Profession (Global Survey) and the Glossary of Osteopathic Terms. The OIA will also continue to support the WHO on an ad hoc basis as requested.[164]

students. These may include clinical rotations or medical mission work. The AOA maintains a detailed report of college international activities at its website.[166]

PANDEMIC!

In modern times, there have been two worldwide pandemics separated by a century.

- 1918–1920 Great Influenza Pandemic (H1N1 Influenza A)
- 2019–2021 COVID-19 Pandemic (SARS-CoV-2)

The two pandemics had striking similarities and differences in the medical establishment, media, government, health care workers, and public response. In both pandemics, uncertainty and misinformation enhanced morbidity and mortality, but the statistics from both pandemics continue to be argued by proponents of multiple points of view—many of whom claim that the basis of their point of view is science.

These few paragraphs will not attempt to cover the science, debates, politics, or conspiracy theories regarding the recent COVID-19 pandemic. Many research papers, articles, and books are and will be written about the most recent pandemic, just as they were (and still are) about the Great Influenza Pandemic.

This discussion will be limited to the effects of the health crisis on osteopathic medical practice, the osteopathic educational system, and the profession's organizations, physicians, and students.

Response of the Osteopathic Medical Profession

Unlike the 1918–1919 Influenza Pandemic, the treatment offered by the osteopathic medical profession was not distinctively different from the allopathic approach. In the influenza pandemic a century earlier, there were no antiviral medications, no vaccines, no effective antibiotics for secondary infections, no intravenous fluids for dehydration, no oxygen usage or effective breathing treatments, almost none of the medications now available, and the hospital structures and equipment were vastly different. Most victims who did not recover died at home, some succumbing to secondary bacterial infections or lung damage up to months later (e.g., Sir William Osler). The virulence of the disease was also strikingly different, particularly in the second wave of the influenza pandemic, which was far more deadly than the first wave, and often rapidly so.

This contrasted with higher contagiousness but weaker virulence of successive variants of COVID-19.

Effects on Health Care Workers, Medical Practices, and Hospitals

Although some states and regions suffered earlier, by the end of 2020, hospitals and other health care facilities such as nursing homes around the country were overwhelmed with caring for COVID-19 patients as the world struggled. A few of the related issues and effects included:

- Inadequate supplies of Personal Protection Equipment (PPE) for health care workers, support staff and other front-line workers such as custodians, housekeepers, and lab personnel due to foreign supply chains was problematic and likely contributed to fatalities.
- Physicians, nurses, and other health care workers were accosted and even verbally or physically attacked by distraught people with opposing political views regarding vaccines or the wearing of masks.
- Some health care workers who were exposed to patients or others who did not follow isolation procedures suffered illness or died.
- Some private practice physicians were overwhelmed by numbers in their practices while others had to close them, change their practices, or even declare bankruptcy due to lack of PPE or patients putting off care out of fear of exposure.
- Burnout and mental health problems accompanied long shifts with physical and emotional exhaustion mounting as the pandemic seemed to go on interminably.
- Hospital services prioritized COVID patients as needed, overwhelming some hospital services, and leaving others lacking.
- Telemedicine became utilized rapidly, creating infrastructure problems as well as some issues with drug prescription.
- Retired physicians (even with inactive licenses) were in some cases asked or permitted to volunteer to give inoculations or participate with a team doing so once vaccines were available, as state governments rushed to obtain them.

Effects on the COMs

The 2019–2023 COVID-19 pandemic caused a radical departure from the norm and vast modifications to medical education delivery, evaluation, and admission processes. Osteopathic and allopathic medical schools put most of the two didactic years of instruction online as remote study became the norm. Not all schools had equal platforms or equipment to support this immediately and schools did their best to deliver curriculum safely, meet requirements, and provide appropriate evaluation.

Pre-clerkship students found themselves suddenly assigned to a virtual curriculum. While many schools were already recording all lectures (which facilitated the transformation), this was not true of all classes and at all schools. Social distancing meant students had to work on the materials at home, and without the IT Department down the hall for immediate help if they needed it. The same was true of professors, who were generally accustomed to presenting their lectures at the classroom podium and now found themselves doing this from home. Not all guest lecturers were prepared for this, and the increased delivery platform traffic—particularly for real-time participatory learning activities—caused problems and sometimes breakdowns which had to be rapidly fixed. Schools rapidly adapted the best they could, with IT Departments facing unique challenges. So did the students who needed immediate help and found it largely unavailable due to the overload.

Not all classes could be delivered virtually. Physical examination, diagnostic practice, OSCEs, and osteopathic diagnostic and manipulation training could not be done virtually—yet, for periods of time when there was insufficient PPE, an attempt at instructional continuity demanded a certain level of isolated viewing of demonstrations or videos and mental skill practice in place of actual hands-on participation. Curricula in these topics were modified and truncated in many cases. Evaluation became an issue, with less formative evaluation while modified summative evaluation was maintained as best as could be done. Again, social distancing issues and PPE were determining factors.[167]

Effect on Clerkships

The same challenges faced students on clerkships who often found themselves excluded from physical participation at the clinics and hospitals because they simply did not have enough PPE even for their own physicians, nurses, and other vital frontline personnel such as custodians, housekeepers, aides, lab workers, and many others. Clinical preceptors suffered as well. Awareness of the heroic efforts and risks of mentors bravely working while at risk due to insufficient PPE, being aware of illness and fatalities in mentors, patients, family members, coworkers, and students plus isolation and fear of illness took a toll on medical students, training faculty, and all of society. Fear of inadequate board scores due to lack of experience or missing class time affected students as well.

Pandemic Disruption to Licensure Examinations

As the COVID-19 pandemic emergency quarantine laws shut down professional testing centers, COMLEX-USA administrations were disrupted for several months during the busiest times of the annual testing cycles. Students and residents were faced with frequent exam cancellations and rescheduling often due to changing local laws and the need for physical distancing at test centers. The NBOME worked with the testing vendor on safety protocols to both deliver the examinations to the students and to mitigate risks of COVID-19 exposure in testing centers. The clinical skills component to COMLEX-USA, the Level 2-Performance examination, was suspended for several months at a time in 2020 as this examination was administered at two national centers,[168] potentially requiring travel and also close contact with standardized patients. The NBOME expanded contingency planning and invested in opening a third national clinical skills testing center on the West Coast to assist with built-up demand, should testing be determined safe to resume. Ultimately, and after an announcement completely terminating the MD counterpart exam (USMLE Step 2-Clinical Skills) in early 2021, and resultant mounting pressures from stakeholders, the NBOME announced permanent suspension of the Level 2-PE.[169] It was temporarily replaced with an attestation process of clinical skills competencies by each COM dean, allowing students in impacted graduation years to progress to graduation and proceed to take COMLEX-USA Level 3 as residents, preventing disruptions in training, licensure, or the physician workforce.

The NBOME created a Special Commission that included stakeholder representation from the AOA, the AACOM, the GME, and licensure communities, students and residents, and patient representatives. After extensive review, the commission generated a final report that emphasized the importance of clinical skills testing in professional self-regulation to protect the public, and recommended exploration of a new clinical skills competency assessment to a national graduation standard but delivered in partnership with the COM campuses. This model could potentially reduce travel and related expenses for most, as well as continue to assess fundamental competencies for DOs that include interviewing patients and communication skills, hands-on physical exam skills, and OMT. This new "Core Competency Capstone for DOs" ("C3DO") initiative was piloted by NBOME and four COMs in 2023, and eight are scheduled to pilot the competency-based assessment in 2024. The future of C3DO and any role that it could play in licensure is scheduled to be determined by July 2025. In the interim, the NBOME has extended the temporary clinical skills attestation requirement.

Effect on Research

Following the COVID pandemic, research on OMT for patients suffering respiratory distress has been ongoing. In a 2022 study of hospitalized patients with COVID and respiratory distress it was found that[170]:

- OMT for hospitalized COVID-19 patients in respiratory distress is well accepted by patients, who perceived value in OMT treatments and experienced no adverse events.
- OMT for hospitalized COVID-19 patients in respiratory distress showed marginally significant reductions in length of hospital stay.
- OMT for hospitalized COVID-19 patients in respiratory distress appears to have better effect on patients with more comorbidities.
- OMT for hospitalized COVID-19 patients in respiratory distress did not have an impact on mortality of or hospital disposition for patients.

Effects on the AOA

As in many organizations, a great deal of work by the office personnel was done remotely. Committee and bureau meetings were accomplished on videotelephony software such as Zoom. In addition, CME requirements for board certification were suspended or delayed as needed for a time to provide time for infrastructure and new habits to catch up. Telehealth updates were provided for physicians, including videos and other information to keep physicians updated on the latest recommendations, resources, and research.

Information regarding the new vaccines and dealing with vaccine hesitancy was distributed.[171] The AOA also took a stand with other health care organizations promoting the requirement of vaccine mandates for health care workers.[172]

Remote delivery of OMED (the annual conference of the AOA) allowed participants to attend from home, and the AOA certifying boards also offered both oral and written exams remotely.[173]

Pandemic Lessons

A black swan is an unexpected disruptive event, often with extreme consequences. Such is a pandemic. The COVID-19 pandemic called upon students, physicians, nurses, other front-line workers, colleges, clinics, hospitals, and professional organizations to adapt and make do with what was available, demonstrate resilience, and maintain processes as functional and normal as possible in delivery of health care, education, CME, and licensing as well as many other issues. Fortunately, technology was available to continue modified educational programs and provide telemedicine visits. As time progressed, rapid IT infrastructure development and response by IT workers helped continue programs and allow progress as normally or adaptive as possible. The nation, the world, and the osteopathic profession rose to the occasion.

SUMMARY

Osteopathic medicine began as a reform movement, at a time when most medications were toxic or ineffective, antibiotics would not be developed for decades, and surgery was extremely dangerous. A single pioneer physician, Andrew Taylor Still, DO, developed a medical model that examined the whole person, analyzed structure and function, and used OMT as his primary treatment method to promote the body's self-healing capabilities. He encouraged his followers to base their practice on science.

Still elaborated his theories in 1874 and founded the ASO in 1892. In the 150 years since his announcement, the new osteopathic medical profession has grown from the base he formed with his students in Kirksville, Missouri.

- A medical education system was developed de novo, expanding to more than 40 COMs today, with almost a third of all American medical students currently enrolled in them.
- Research programs were developed starting with the original students, but the profession's focus stayed on producing practicing physicians and primary care.
- Practice rights were obtained state by state, from Vermont to Mississippi.
- Organizations were developed to promote the profession and regulate it internally.
- Government recognition and inclusion was obtained step by step.
- Specialties evolved; osteopathic hospitals were built, staffed, and regulated until DOs were universally integrated in public and private hospitals nationwide by the 1980s.
- As the country became more diverse and inclusive, so did the profession.
- Mutual respect built as physicians with both DO and MD degrees combined efforts on many issues, including in 2020, the implementation of the single GME accreditation system.
- Recognizing that Still's ideas had spread or generated interest internationally, the profession connected both with MDs and osteopathic practitioners around the world to create co-operative health care and educational efforts.[174–176]
- Two pandemics bracketing 100 years reminded the world and health care professions that a health care crisis is a disruptive event whose challenges demand perseverance and resilience.

At the start of the 21st century, the *parallel and distinctive* osteopathic medical profession has achieved respect with its emphasis on primary care and whole-person philosophy. The unique contribution of osteopathic diagnosis and treatment started a reform movement that continues today.

An outstanding osteopathic leader, writer, and editor, George W. Northup, wrote in 1988:

> "Today, the practice of medicine needs as never before the guiding light of a fundamental philosophy. It needs to recognize the action and interaction of all body systems. It should apply known truths and explore new frontiers founded on the osteopathic profession's basic philosophy....Dr. Still did not say he was giving the world a philosophy that should act as a guide to the future. Rather, in his book, The Philosophy of Osteopathy, he stated his desire was '...to give the world a start in a philosophy that may be a guide to the future.'"[177]

ACKNOWLEDGMENTS

The author and editors would like to acknowledge review and contributions by the following people and thank them for their support: First, Barbara Peterson, who wrote the original chapter for the first three editions of FOM. The current lead author revised Peterson's work, expanding the chapter to cover progress of the last three decades and developing additional topics of interest by the fourth edition. History of research materials by Michael Patterson and Brian Degenhardt were also condensed and modified for inclusion in this chapter by the fourth edition, and are expanded by the lead author for this edition. Individuals who contributed or modified material on the following topics include: Jason Haxton (early history, illustrations); John Gimpel (NBOME); Karen Nichols (Single GME Accreditation system); Kurt Heinking (editing and references); and Rebecca Giusti (editing and international osteopathy).

REFERENCES

1. Still AT. *The Philosophy and Mechanical Principles of Osteopathy*. Hudson-Kimberley Publishing Co.; 1892, 1902.
2. Still AT. *Philosophy of Osteopathy*. Author; 1899.
3. Still AT. *Autobiography of Andrew T. Still with a History of the Discovery and Development of the Science of Osteopathy*. Rev ed., Kirksville, MO: Published by the author; 1908.
4. Still AT. *Osteopathy, Research and Practice*. Published by the author; 1910.
5. Gallagher RM, Humphrey FJ II, Micozzi MS, eds. *Osteopathic Medicine: A Reformation in Progress*. Churchill Livingstone; 2001.
6. Brown JM, Woodworth RB. *The Captives of Abb's Valley; a Legend of Frontier Life*. New ed. Printed for the author by the McClure Co.; 1942.
7. Dick E. *The Sod-House Frontier*. Johnsen Publishing Co.; 1954.
8. *Dr. AT Still Medical License*. Andrew Taylor Still Papers. No. 2009.10.973. Located at: Museum of Osteopathic Medicine.
9. Asks if A.T. Still ever was a real doctor. *The Osteopathic Physician*. 1909;15(1):8.
10. Gevitz N. A degree of difference: the origins of osteopathy and first use of the "DO" designation. *J Am Osteopath Assoc*. 2014;114(1):30–40.
11. Higgins C. Where the Wakarusa Meets the Kaw: The History of Eudora, Kansas. Accessed March 1, 2024. https://eudorakshistory.com/a-1
12. AT Still Genealogy Reference Sheet, Museum of Osteopathic Medicine. Accessed December 11, 2024. https://www.atsu.edu/museum-of-osteopathic-medicine/research
13. Trowbridge C. *Andrew Taylor Still, 1828–1917*. Thomas Jefferson University Press, Northeast Missouri State University; 1991.
14. Clark MS. *Memoirs of Morovia Still Clark*. Museum of Osteopathic Medicine; 1920.
15. The etiology of cholera. *Nature*. 1885;33:97–98.
16. Thomas JL, ed. *Slavery Attacked: The Abolitionist Crusade*. Prentice-Hall; 1965.

17. Monaghan J. *Civil War on the Western Border, 1854–1865.* Bonanza Books; 1965.
18. Eldridge SW. First free-state legislature. In: *Recollections of Early Days in Kansas: Publications of the Kansas State Historical Society.* Vol 2. Kansas State Printing Plant; 1920:149–158.
19. A.T. Still Pension File. *Still National Osteopathic Museum, Kirksville, MO.*
20. Lewis J. *A T. Still: From the Dry Bone to the Living Man.* Dry Bone Press; 2012.
21. Duffy J. *From Humors to Medical Science: A History of American Medicine.* 2nd ed. University of Illinois Press; 1993.
22. Bordley J, Harvey AM. *Two Centuries of American Medicine, 1776–1976.* WB Saunders Co.; 1976:97.
23. Osborn GG. The beginning: nineteenth century medical sectarianism. In: Humphrey RM, Gallagher FJ, eds. *Osteopathic Medicine: A Reformation in Progress.* Churchill Livingstone; 2001:3–26.
24. Pickard ME, Buley RC. *The Midwest Pioneer; His Ills, Cures & Doctors.* R.E. Banta; 1945.
25. *Merck's 1899 Manual of the Materia Medica, Together with a Summary of Therapeutic Indications and a Classification of Medicaments: A Ready-Reference Pocket Book for the Practicing Physician.* Merck & Co.; 1899. Reprinted in facsimile by Merck & Co.; 1999.
26. Dorland WAN. *Dorland's Illustrated Medical Dictionary.* 26th ed. WB Saunders Co.; 1981.
27. Danciger E. *The Emergence of Homeopathy: Alchemy into Medicine.* Century Hutchinson Ltd; 1987.
28. Ebright HK. *The History of Baker University.* Baker University; 1951.
29. Schnucker RV, ed. *Early Osteopathy in the Words of A.T. Still.* Thomas Jefferson University Press, Northeast Missouri State University; 1991.
30. Hildreth AG, ed. *The Lengthening Shadow of Dr. Andrew Taylor Still.* Author; 1938.
31. Still CE. A.T. Still: the itinerant years. In: From the Archives. *The DO.* 1975;(Mar):27–30.
32. Riley GW. Following osteopathic principles. In: Hildreth AG, ed. *The Lengthening Shadow of Dr. Andrew Taylor Still.* Author; 1938:411–435.
33. Walter GW. *The First School of Osteopathic Medicine; a Chronicle, 1892–1992.* Thomas Jefferson University Press, Northeast Missouri State University; 1992.
34. Booth ER. *History of Osteopathy and Twentieth-Century Medical Practice.* Press of Jennings and Graham; 1905:103.
35. *Dr. A.T. Still D.O. receives diploma. ASO Board of Trustees Minutes 1894-1898.* No. 1987.1226.01 p. 15 Located at: Museum of Osteopathic Medicine.
36. Violette EM. *History of Adair County.* Denslow History Co.; 1911:253.
37. Still CE Jr. *Frontier Doctor, Medical Pioneer: The Life and Times of A.T. Still and His Family.* Thomas Jefferson University Press, Northeast Missouri State University; 1991.
38. Anonymous. Historic reference of osteopathic colleges. American Osteopathic Association. 2009. Accessed December 20, 2009. http://history.osteopathic.org/collegehist.shtml
39. Gevitz N. *The D.O.s: Osteopathic Medicine in America.* 2nd ed. Johns Hopkins University Press; 2004:75–87.
40. Johnson V, Weiskotten HG. *A History of the Council on Medical Education and Hospitals of the American Medical Association.* American Medical Association; 1960.
41. Anonymous. *Important Dates in Osteopathic History.* 2009. Accessed December 20, 2009. http://history.osteopathic.org/timeline.shtml.
42. Flexner A. *Medical Education in the United States and Canada: A Report to the Carnegie Foundation for the Advancement of Teaching.* Merrymount Press; 1910.
43. Starr P. *The Social Transformation of American Medicine.* Basic Books; 1982.
44. Morais HM. *The history of the Negro in medicine. International Library of Negro Life and History.* Vol 4. *The Association for the Study of Negro Life and History.* Publishers Co.; 1968.
45. Lopate C. *Women in Medicine.* Johns Hopkins Press; 1968. Published for the Josiah Macy Jr. Foundation.
46. Walsh MR. *Doctors Wanted: No Women Need Apply. Sexual Barriers in the Medical Profession.* Yale University Press; 1977.
47. Catalogue of the American School of Osteopathy, Session of 1899–1900. Kirksville, MO: American School of Osteopathy; Seventh Annual Announcement. Published 1899. Accessed December 11, 2024. https://www.atsu.edu/museum-of-osteopathic-medicine/wp-content/uploads/2019/04/1899-1900ASO.pdf.
48. Peterson B. The memoirs of Dr. Charles Still; IV. A postscript. In: From the Archives. *The DO.* 1975;(Jun):25–26.
49. Booth ER. *History of Osteopathy and Twentieth-Century Medical Practice.* Printed for the author by the Caxton Press; 1924.
50. Gevitz N. The sword and the scalpel— the osteopathic 'war' to enter the Military Medical Corps: 1916–1966. *J Am Osteopath Assoc.* 1998;98(5): 279–286.
51. Reinsch S, Seffinger MA, Tobis JS. *The Merger: M.D.s and D.O.s in California.* Xlibris Press; 2009.
52. Weiss V. York Hosp., 548 F. Supp. 1048 (M.D. Pa. 1982). Accessed December 11, 2024. https://law.justia.com/cases/federal/district-courts/FSupp/548/1048/1651009/.
53. Commission on Osteopathic College Accreditation. *American Osteopathic Association.* Accessed April 3, 2024. https://osteopathic.org/accreditation/
54. American Osteopathic Association. Osteopathic Medical Profession Report 2023. Accessed October 3, 2023. https://osteopathic.org/about/aoa-statistics/.
55. Peterson B. A Vermont story and Contacts with the law. In: From the Archives. *The DO.* 1972;(Nov):46–50.
56. Cole WV. Historical basis for osteopathic theory and practice. In: Northup GW, ed. *Osteopathic Research: Growth and Development.* American Osteopathic Association; 1987:57.
57. Burnett B. *In the Public Trust: The National Board of Osteopathic Medical Examiners 1934–2009.* National Board of Medical Examiners; 2010. Accessed April 2, 2024. https://www.nbome.org/Content/NBOME/History_of_NBOME.pdf
58. The Old Doctor gets first certificate. *J Osteopathy.* 1904;11:28.
59. Ross-Lee B, Wood DL. Osteopathic medical education. In: Sirica CM, ed. *Osteopathic Medicine: Past, Present and Future.* Josiah Macy, Jr. Foundation; 1996.
60. History of UCI School of Medicine. Accessed March 29, 2024. https://medschool.uci.edu/about/history
61. Seffinger MA, Reinsch S, Melvin-McCann J, et al. *Resurgence: Osteopathic Physicians and Surgeons of California.* Samjill Publishing Company; 2011. Accessed August 8, 2017. https://cdn.ymaws.com/www.opsc.org/resource/resmgr/media/resurgence%20final%20edit%20v2%20 8.27.12%20henley.pdf.
62. Frymann VM. Alexander Tobin, 1921–1992. In: King HH, ed., *The Collected Papers of Viola M. Frymann, DO.* American Academy of Osteopathy; 1996.
63. Anonymous. Students form association in American Osteopathic Association. 2009. Accessed December 20, 2009. http://history.osteopathic.org/aoa.shtml
64. Peterson B. How old is osteopathic research? In: Time Capsule. *The DO.* 1978;(Dec):24–26.
65. Evans AL. The beginnings of the AOA (1928 manuscript). In: From the Archives. *The DO.* 1972;(Sep):34–38.
66. American Osteopathic Association. Accessed December 20, 2009. http://www.osteopathic.org
67. National Board of Osteopathic Medical Examiners. Accessed June 19, 2017. nbome.org
68. Peterson B. They passed the exam, but they could not serve: the DO doughboys. In: From the Archives. *The DO.* 1975;(Aug):39–40, 42, 47–48.
69. How Dos gained commissions. In: Time Capsule. *The DO.* 1980;(Apr): 25–32.
70. Boose B. A door, and a war: drafted D.O.s pave their profession's way. Des Moines University Medicine & Health Sciences. November 3, 2016. Updated November 8, 2016. Accessed April 1, 2024. https://www.dmu.edu/blog/2016/11/a-door-and-a-war
71. The DO Staff. In memoriam: Edward M. Feldman, DO, trailblazing military physician. *The DO.* October 13, 2017. Accessed April 1, 2024. https://thedo.osteopathic.org/2017/10/memoriam-edward-m-feldman-trailblazing-military-physician/

72. Newsweek Magazine. Hero M.D. The amazing story of the war's most fearless doctor. March 20, 2006. https://www.newsweek.com/call-hell-106161
73. Orthopedic traumatologist receives 2019 AOF Distinguished Military Service Award. American Osteopathic Foundation. October 24, 2019. Accessed April 1, 2024. https://aof.org/news/orthopedic-traumatologist-receives-2019-aof-distinguished-military-service-award
74. Esteemed veterans in medicine: KCU military professor applauds colleague appointed as white house physician. Kansas City University. March 2, 2021. Accessed April 1, 2024. https://www.kansascity.edu/blog/awards-and-recognition/kcu-military-professor-applauds-colleague-appointed-as-wh-physician
75. Semano K. OMT: the military pilot's drug-free treatment option. *The DO*. February 17, 2017. Accessed on April 1, 2024. https://thedo.osteopathic.org/2017/02/omt-the-military-pilots-drug-free-treatment-option/
76. Palikuca S. NASA's top doc: a DO is helping launch the first human journey to Mars. *The DO*. May 1, 2019. Accessed April 1, 2024. https://thedo.osteopathic.org/2019/05/nasas-top-doc-a-do-is-helping-launch-the-first-human-journey-to-mars/
77. Peterson B. 1898: radiology in Kirksville. *J Am Osteopath Assoc*. 1974; 74(2):167–172.
78. Rodos JJ, Peterson B. *Proposed Strategies for Fulfilling Primary Care Manpower Needs: A White Paper Prepared for the National Advisory Council, National Health Service Corps, U.S. Public Health Service*. National Health Service Corps; 1990.
79. Blondell RD, Smith IJ, Byrne ME, Higgins CW. Rural health, family practice, and area health education centers: a national study. *Fam Med*. 1989;21(3):183–186.
80. AOA Staff. AOA settles class-action lawsuit. *The DO*. July 27, 2018. Accessed April 2, 2024. https://thedo.osteopathic.org/2018/07/aoa-settles-class-action-lawsuit/
81. Specialties and Subspecialties. American Osteopathic Association. April 2, 2024. https://certification.osteopathic.org/specialties-and-subspecialties/.
82. Buser BR, Swartwout MA, Gross C, Biszewski M. The single graduate medical education accreditation system *J Am Osteopath Assoc*. 2015; 115(4):251–255.
83. Gevitz N. The transformation of osteopathic medical education. *Acad Med*. 2009;84(6):701–706.
84. Programs with osteopathic recognition. American Association of Colleges of Osteopathic Medicine. Updated February 22, 2024. Accessed April 2, 2024. https://www.aacom.org/gme/osteopathic-recognition/programs-with-osteopathic-recognition
85. American Association of Colleges of Osteopathic Medicine. Accessed April 2, 2024. https://www.aacom.org/programs-events/programs-initiatives/interprofessional-education
86. Coalition for Physician Accountability. Accessed April 2, 2024. https://physicianaccountability.org/
87. Still CE. *Frontier Doctor Medical Pioneer: The Life and Times of A.T. Still and his Family*. The Thomas Jefferson University Press at Northeast Missouri State University; 1991:140.
88. Booth ER. *History of Osteopathy and Twentieth-Century Medical Practice*. Printed for the author by the Caxton Press; 1924:252.
89. Blumer JU. *Strong Medicine: Honoring the Women Pioneers of Osteopathy*. Independently published; 2021.
90. Ashmore, E. *Osteopathic Mechanics: A Textbook*. Journal Printing Company; 1915.
91. Margaret S, ed. *Charlotte Weaver: Pioneer in Cranial Osteopathy*. The Cranial Academy; 2010:294.
92. Arbuckle BE. *The Selected Writings of Beryl E. Arbuckle, D.O., F.A.C.O.P.* National Osteopathic Institute and Cerebral Palsy Foundation; 1977.
93. Burns L. *Studies in the Osteopathic Sciences; Basic Principles. Vol 1 and 2*. The Occident Printery; 1907.
94. U.S. Census Bureau. Washington, DC: U.S. Department of Commerce. Accessed April 2, 2024. https://www.census.gov/
95. Perloff CB. Meta L. Cristy, DO. The first African American osteopathic physician. Philadelphia College of Osteopathic Medicine. February 16, 2021. Accessed April 2, 2024. https://www.pcom.edu/about/departments/marketing-and-communications/digest-magazine/digest-featured-stories/meta-christy-do-first-african-american-osteopathic-physician.html
96. Tampa Bay Times. Marcelino Oliva Obituary. July 10, 2011. Accessed April 2, 2024. https://www.legacy.com/us/obituaries/tampabaytimes/name/marcelino-oliva-obituary?id=11227728
97. Oliva M. Interview by ACOFPT Archival & Historical Committee. *Interview with Marcelino Oliva, DO, FACOFP, American Osteopathic Association President–1999-2000*. March 7, 2009. Accessed December 11, 2024. https://imis.acofp.org/ACOFPIMIS/acofporg/PDFs/About/Mission_History/M_Oliva.pdf.
98. Anderson N, Grauer P, Anderson W. Autobiographies of a Black couple of the greatest generation, Norma and William Anderson. Self Published; 2004.
99. Scheid D. What the AOA is doing to promote diversity, equity and inclusion. *The DO*. February 26, 2021. Accessed on April 2, 2024. https://thedo.osteopathic.org/2021/02/what-the-aoa-is-doing-to-promote-diversity-equity-and-inclusion/
100. Shapiro J, DeCarlo C. Nation's colleges of osteopathic medicine unanimously commit to addressing systemic inequity. American Association of Colleges of Osteopathic Medicine. October 4, 2021. Accessed April 2, 2024. https://www.aacom.org/news-reports/news/2021/10/04/nation-s-colleges-of-osteopathic-medicine-unanimously-commit-to-addressing-systemic-inequity
101. Stark JE. *Journeyman: William Garner Sutherland, the Formative Years (1873-1900)*. Roe House Press; 2020.
102. Sutherland William G. Transcript of lecture—Philosophy of Osteopathy; and: It's Application by Cranial Concept. Second Annual Convention of the Osteopathic Cranial Association, Boston Mass July 8, 1948. P. 6. Artifact: # 1981.639.04.
103. Smith WA. Skiagraphy and the circulation. *J Osteopath*. 1899;5(8): 365–384.
104. Fryette HH. Physiologic movements of the spine. *J Am Osteopath Assoc*. 1918;18:1–2.
105. Beilke M. Roentgenological spinal analysis and the technique for taking standing X-Ray plates. *Journal of the AOA*. 1936:414–418.
106. Kelso AF, Townsend AA. The status and future of osteopathic research. In: Northup GW, ed. *Osteopathic Research: Growth and Development*. American Osteopathic Association; 1987:93–117.
107. Burns L. Viscero-somatic and somato-visceral spinal reflexes. 1907. *J Am Osteopath Assoc*. 2000;100(4):249–258.
108. Burns L. The immediate effects of boney lesions. *J Am Osteopath Assoc*. 1910;9:469–475.
109. Northup GW, ed. *Osteopathic Research: Growth and Development*. American Osteopathic Association; 1987.
110. Cole WV. Louisa Burns memorial lecture. *J Am Osteopath Assoc*. 1970; 69:1005–1017.
111. Kawchuk GN, Fauvel OR, Dmowski J. Ultrasonic indentation (UI): a procedure for the non-invasive quantification of force-displacement properties of the lumbar spine. *J Manipulative Physiol Ther*. 2001;24(3): 149–156.
112. Burns L. *The Nerve Centers*. Vol 2. Monfort and Company; 1911.
113. Burns L. *Basic Principles*. Vol 1. The Occident Printery; 1907.
114. Burns L. *The Physiology of Consciousness*. Vol 3. Monfort and Company; 1911.
115. Burns L. *Cells of the Blood*. Vol 4. A. T. Still Research Institute; 1931.
116. Burns L, ed. *Pathogenesis of Visceral Disease Following Vertebral Lesions*. American Osteopathic Association; 1948.
117. Whiting LM. Can length of labor be shortened by osteopathic treatment? *J Am Osteopath Assoc*. 1911;11:917–921.
118. Lavelle JM. Osteopathic manipulative treatment in pregnant women. *J Am Osteopath Assoc*. 2012;112(6):343–346.
119. Jones M. Osteopathy and obstetrical mortality and stillbirth and infant mortality: symposium on osteopathy in obstetrics chaired by S.V. Robuck, DO. *J Am Osteopath Assoc*. 1933;33:350–353.
120. Smith RK. One hundred thousand cases of influenza with a death rate of one-fortieth of that officially reported under conventional medical treatment. *J Am Osteopath Assoc*. 1920;20:172–175. Reprinted in: *J Am Osteopath Assoc*. 2000;100:320–323.

121. D'Alonzo GE. Influenza epidemic or pandemic? Time to roll up sleeves, vaccinate patients, and hone osteopathic manipulative skills. *J Am Osteopath Assoc.* 2004;104(9):370–371.
122. Denslow JS, Hassett CC. The central excitatory state associated with postural abnormalities. *J Neurophysiol.* 1942;5(5):393–400. doi:10.1152/jn.1942.5.5.393.
123. Korr IM. The neural basis of the osteopathic lesion. *J Am Osteopath Assoc.* 1947;47:191–198.
124. Denslow JS, Korr IM, Krems AD. Quantitative studies of chronic facilitation in human motoneuron pools. *Am J Physiol.* 1947;105:229–238.
125. Korr IM, Thomas PE. The automatic recording of electrical skin resistance patterns on the human trunk. *Electroencephalogr Clin Neurophysiol.* 1951;3:361–368.
126. Thomas PE, Korr IM. Relationship between sweat gland activity and electrical resistance of the skin. *J Appl Physiol.* 1957;10(3):505–510.
127. Korr IM. The neural basis of the osteopathic lesion. *J Am Osteopath Assoc.* 1947; 46:191–198.
128. Korr IM. The emerging concept of the osteopathic lesion. *J Am Osteopath Assoc.* 1948;Nov:1–8.
129. Korr IM, Wright HM, Thomas PE. Effects of experimental myofascial insults on cutaneous patterns of sympathetic activity in man. *Acta Neuroveg (Wien).* 1962;23:329–355.
130. Wright HM, Korr IM. Neural and spinal components of disease: progress in the application of "thermography". *J Am Osteopath Assoc.* 1965;64: 918–921.
131. Korr IM, Appletauer GSL. The time-course of axonal proteins to muscle. *Exp Neurol.* 1974;43:452–463.
132. Appletauer GSL, Korr IM. Axonal delivery of soluble, insoluble and electrophoretic fractions of neuronal proteins to muscle. *Exp Neurol.* 1975; 46:132–146.
133. Appletauer GSL, Korr IM. Axonal migration of some particle-bound proteins in the hypoglossal nerve and their failure to enter the styloglossus muscle. *J Am Osteopath Assoc.* 1978;77:479–481.
134. Beckwith CG. Thoracic vertebral mechanics. *J Am Osteopath Assoc.* 1944;43:436–439.
135. Patterson MM, Howell JN, eds. *The Central Connection: Somatovisceral Viscerosomatic Interaction.* American Academy of Osteopathy; 1992.
136. Willard FW, Patterson MM, eds. *Nociception and the Neuroendocrine-Immune Connection.* American Academy of Osteopathy; 1994.
137. Johnston WL. Interexaminer reliability studies; spanning a gap in medical research. Louisa Burns Memorial Lecture. *J Am Osteopath Assoc.* 1982;81(2):43–53.
138. Johnston WL, Elkiss ML, Marino RV, Blum GA. Passive gross motion testing Part II. A study of interexaminer agreement. *J Am Osteopath Assoc.* 1982;81(5):65–69.
139. Johnston WL, Beal MC, Blum GA, Hendra JL, Neff DR, Rosen ME. Passive gross motion testing Part III: examiner agreement on selected subjects. *J Am Osteopath Assoc.* 1982;81(5):309–313.
140. Friedman HD, Johnston WL, Kelso AF, Schwartz FN, Beal MC, Seffinger MA. Standardization of the hospital record for osteopathic structural examination. *J Am Osteopath Assoc.* 1996;96(9):529–536.
141. Beal MC. Viscerosomatic reflexes: a review. *J Am Osteopath Assoc.* 1985; 85(7):786–801.
142. Johnston WL. Osteopathic clinical aspects of somatovisceral interaction. In: Patterson MM, Howell JN, eds. *The Central Connection: Somatovisceral/Viscerosomatic Interaction.* American Academy of Osteopathy; 1989.
143. Beal MC, Kleiber GE. Somatic dysfunction as a predictor of coronary artery disease. *J Am Osteopath Assoc.* 1985;85(5):302–307.
144. Kelso AF, Grant RG, Johnston WL. Use of thermograms to support assessment of somatic dysfunction or effects of osteopathic manipulative treatment: a preliminary report. *J Am Osteopath Assoc.* 1982;82(3): 182–188.
145. Johnston WL, Kelso AF, Hollandsworth DL, Karrat JJ. Somatic manifestations in renal disease: a clinical research study. *J Am Osteopath Assoc.* 1987;87(1):61–74.
146. Johnston WL, Kelso AF. Changes in presence of a segmental dysfunction pattern associated with hypertension: Part II. A long-term longitudinal study. *J Am Osteopath Assoc.* 1995;95(5):315–318.
147. Andersson GBJ, Lucente T, Davis A, Kappler RE, Lipton JA, Leurgans S. A comparison of osteopathic spinal manipulation with standard care for patients with low back pain. *N Engl J Med.* 1999;341(19):1426–1431.
148. Hensel K, Carnes M, Stoll S. Pregnancy research on osteopathic manipulation optimizing treatment effects: the PROMOTE study protocol. *J Am Osteopath Assoc.* 2016;116:716–724.
149. Schander A, Padro D, King HH, Downey HF, Hodge LM. Lymphatic pump treatment repeatedly enhances the lymphatic and immune system. *Lymphat Res Biol.* 2013;11(4):219–226.
150. Licciardone JC, Brimhall AK, King LN. Osteopathic manipulative treatment for low back pain: a systematic review and meta-analysis of randomized controlled trials. *BMC Musculoskelet Disord.* 2005;6:43.
151. Licciardone JC, Gatchel RJ, Aryal S. Targeting patient subgroups with chronic low back pain for osteopathic manipulative treatment: responder analyses from a randomized controlled trial. *J Am Osteopath Assoc.* 2016;116(3):156–168.
152. AOA Research Task Force Report. Research Strategic Direction for the American Osteopathic Association. January 2005.
153. Noll D, Degenhardt B, Johnson J. Multicenter osteopathic pneumonia study in the elderly: subgroup analysis on hospital length of stay, ventilator-dependent respiratory failure rate, and in-hospital mortality rate. *J Am Osteopath Assoc.* 2016;116:574–587.
154. Osteopathic Heritage Foundation. Accessed June 19, 2017. http://osteopathicheritage.org/
155. Shmuts R, Soled H, Patel S, Abend D. The Virtues of osteopathic manipulative treatments in patients with opioid use disorder. *Osteopathic Family Physician.* 2023;15(1):20–24.
156. Collins M. *Osteopathy in Britain: The First Hundred Years.* BookSurge Publishing; 2005.
157. Littlejohn LM. *The Political theory of the Schoolmen and Grotius.* Current Press; 1895.
158. Hall T. The Littlejohn memorial. *Osteopath Q.* 1952;5:101–107.
159. Booth E. *History of Osteopathy and Twentieth Century Medical Practice.* 2nd ed. Press of Jennings and Graham; 1924.
160. Littlejohn JM. Osteopathy in Great Britain. *The Reflex.* 1923:96–97.
161. McKone L. *Osteopathic Medicine—Philosophy, Principles, and Practice.* Blackwell Science; 2001.
162. International Osteopathic Medicine. American Osteopathic Association. Accessed March 13, 2017. http://www.osteopathic.org/inside-aoa/development/international-osteopathic-medicine/Pages/default.aspx
163. World Osteopathic Health Organization (WOHO). Union of International Associations (UIA) Yearbook Profile. Accessed April 1, 2024. https://uia.org/s/or/en/1100055125
164. We are the Osteopathic International Alliance. *Osteopathic International Alliance.* Accessed April 2, 2024. https://oialliance.org/
165. International Licensure. American Osteopathic Association. Accessed April 1, 2024. https://osteopathic.org/life-career/medical-licensure/international-licensure/
166. College of Osteopathic Medicine: International Activities Report 2022. American Osteopathic Association. 2022. Accessed on April 2, 2024. https://osteopathic.org/index.php?aam-media=/wp-content/uploads/COM-International-Activities-Report.pdf
167. Dalisay J. How 2 osteopathic medical schools navigated the challenges of COVID-19. *The DO.* April 1, 2022. Accessed April 2, 2024. https://thedo.osteopathic.org/columns/how-2-osteopathic-medical-schools-navigated-the-challenges-of-covid-19/
168. Frellick M. Thanks to COVID, clinical skills testing will never be the same. *Medscape.* August 12, 2022. Accessed April 2, 2024. https://www.medscape.com/viewarticle/979143
169. Joint Statement from the Osteopathic Community. *National Board of Osteopathic Medical Examiners.* February 27, 2021. Accessed April 2, 2024. https://www.nbome.org/news/joint-statement-osteopathic-community/
170. Lennon RP, Dong H, Zgierska AE, et al. Adjunctive osteopathic therapy for hospitalized COVID-19 patients: A feasibility-oriented chart review study with matched controls. *Int J Osteopath Med.* 2022;44: 3–8.
171. Facts on Vax. *American Osteopathic Association.* Accessed on April 2, 2024. https://osteopathic.org/practicing-medicine/providing-care/factsonvax/

172. AOA Media Team. AOA supports legislation aimed at bolstering vaccination education efforts. *American Osteopathic Association*. February 18, 2021. Accessed April 2, 2024. https://osteopathic.org/2021/02/18/aoa-supports-legislation-aimed-at-bolstering-vaccination-education-efforts/
173. Speed, innovation drive AOA board certification strategy. *American Osteopathic Association Board Certification*. December 13, 2021. Accessed on April 2, 2024. https://certification.osteopathic.org/news/speed-innovation-drive-aoa-board-certification-strategy/
174. Svoboda J. C'mon, take your medicine—global. *The DO*. 2000;(12):56–58.
175. Vitucci N. Healing hands around the world. *The DO*. 2002;(3):36–40.
176. Vitucci N. Finding common ground. *The DO*. 2002;(3):42–45.
177. Northup GW. Mission accomplished? *J Am Osteopath Assoc*. 1988;88(9):1077, 1080. Reprinted in Beal MC ed. 1995–96 Yearbook: Osteopathic Vision. Indianapolis, IN: American Academy of Osteopathy; 1996:124.

3 Anatomy: General and Embryologic Concepts

MARK D. SCHUENKE ▪ FRANK H. WILLARD

KEY CONCEPTS

- Knowledge of anatomy facilitates the physician's ability to accurately assess the patient's condition using the Five-Model Concept.
- Anatomical knowledge is contingent on understanding embryologic events; major events in the embryo establish patterns that are still present in the adult.
- A fundamental step in embryogenesis is the development of the nervous system out of the ectodermal layer and the musculoskeletal system out of the mesodermal layer.
- The segmentation of the somatic mesoderm is reflected in the formation of segmental (spinal) nerves and serves to map the body onto the spinal cord.
- A specific region of the spinal cord, through the spinal nerve, represents all components of the somite—dermatome, myotome, and sclerotome.
- Sensory and motor representation of visceral organs in the spinal cord, viscerotomes, overlap with representation of the somatic sensory systems, thus providing a bidirectional neural link between the musculoskeletal system and the visceral organs.
- Limb buds develop laterally out of an interaction between apical ectoderm and underlying somatic mesoderm.
- The musculoskeletal system impacts all components of the Five-Model approach to the patient.
- Movement, as generated by the musculoskeletal system, is a sustaining feature of health by facilitating the fluid dynamics of the vasculature and lymphatic systems.
- The fascial system of the body provides support for muscles, tendons, ligaments, aponeuroses, and bones as well as all visceral organs thereby contributing to the unity of body structure and function.

INTRODUCTION

> "You begin with anatomy, and you end with anatomy, a knowledge of anatomy is all you want or need ..." (A.T. Still Philosophy of Osteopathy, 1899).[1] Although Dr. Still was clearly being hyperbolic and did not truly believe anatomical knowledge alone makes a qualified physician, his implication is clear—anatomy is foundational to osteopathy. Structure elucidates function, and by extension, atypical structure often explains dysfunction. After all, "an Osteopath reasons from his knowledge of anatomy. He compares the work of the abnormal body with the work of the normal body." (A.T. Still Osteopathy Research and Practice).[2]

From the above statement, it is clear that an in-depth understanding of anatomy is fundamental to the rational practice of osteopathic medicine.

- To assess health and disease, physicians must have a detailed knowledge of the structures of the body.
  - This knowledge must include macrostructure and microstructure of the tissues and organs as well as their ontogeny.
- A physician's comprehensive anatomical knowledge may be restricted to the particular body area or functional system used in a specialized practice.
  - However, effective physicians, even those in specialized practices, have and use a working knowledge of the reciprocal, interactive nature of the body's structure and function.
- Osteopathic physicians require sufficient knowledge of body structure, function, and development to understand how focal destructive causes may not only lead to localized effects but also contribute to more subtle, widespread, or distant degenerative, morbid events.
- The reward for mastering anatomy and embryology is the ability to practice medicine—especially osteopathic medicine—in a more intelligent, predictable, and effective manner.
  - Specifically, it facilitates the physician's ability to accurately assess the patient's condition using the Five-Model Concept of coordinated body function and, from this assessment, to design the best approach for helping that patient's body restore its optimal health (see Chapter 26 The Five Models of Osteopathic Patient Care for further explication of this approach).

This chapter does not attempt to thoroughly review all the anatomy that is necessary for medical practice. Numerous excellent books and programs are available on human anatomy and embryology (see selected list in the references), and the effective methods of teaching anatomy vary from school to school. The purpose of this chapter is to provide the beginning osteopathic student with an overview of basic anatomic concepts, including embryology, histology, and basic neuromusculoskeletal anatomy, and to integrate this information with the five conceptual models of body function used in the practice of osteopathic medicine.

DEVELOPMENTAL ANATOMY

Understanding the developmental history of the body is the first topic that truly assists the learning of gross anatomy. The principles of gross anatomy are grounded in the following; the general rules of where structures are and how they relate to other structures is predicated on the rules of embryologic developmental. Thus, understanding general developmental events will greatly enhance the comprehension and retention of the anatomy of the mature form.

The basic body plan for the developing individual is established in the first few days following fertilization.

- Beginning within the first 30 hours postfertilization, a zygote undergoes its first mitotic division.
- Over the course of the next approximately 40 hours, the zygote will continue to grow in cell number via mitosis.

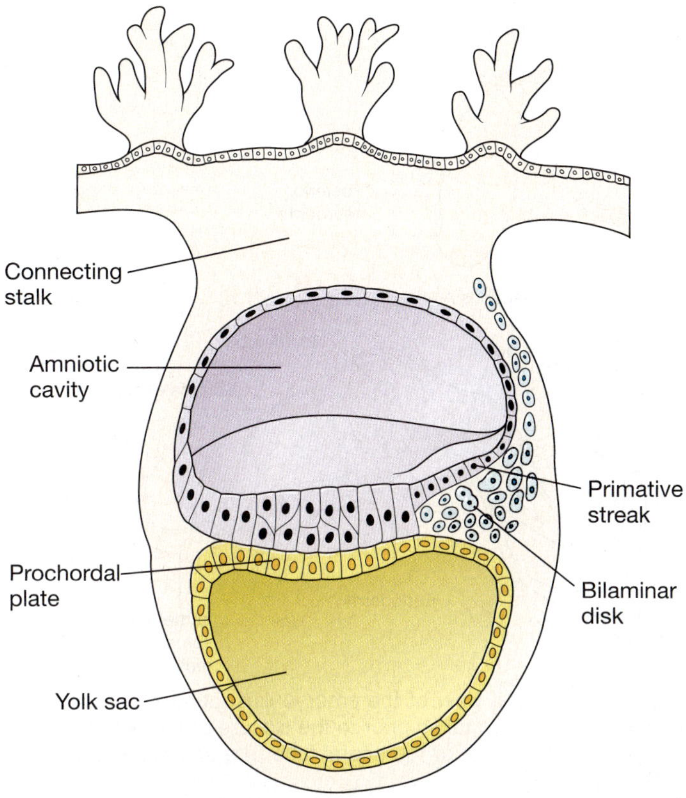

Figure 3.1. A schematic drawing of a 15-day-old human embryo illustrating the bilaminar disk with the primitive streak starting to develop and the upper surface of the disk. The lower space (outlined in *yellow*) will become the yolk sac. (Redrawn from Hamilton WJ, Boyd JD, Mossman HW. *Human Embryology: Prenatal Development of Form and Function.* 2nd ed. Williams & Wilkins Company; 1952.)

- By the third day, the dividing cell mass becomes spherical, now named a morula.
- Within the next 24 to 48 hours, the morula cavitates, producing a fluid-filled cavity, termed blastocoele, and prompting a name change to blastocyst.
- An inner cell mass then develops within the blastocoele, which will give rise to the developing human.
- Trophoblasts grow outside of the blastocoele and contribute to the placenta.
- The inner cell mass segregates into:
  1. A bilaminar disk, consisting of a simple columnar epiblast oriented dorsal to the basement membrane.
  2. A simple cuboidal hypoblast, oriented ventral to the basement membrane.

Early in the third week, an elongated groove (the primitive streak) develops on the dorsal, midsagittal aspect of the epiblast (Fig. 3.1).

- Then, in a process known as epithelial–mesenchymal transition (EMT), cells from the primitive streak migrate between the epiblast and hypoblast layers to create a trilaminar embryonic disk.
- During EMT, the epiblast cells of the primitive streak dissociate from the basement membrane and assume a mesenchymal cell phenotype.
  - The newly formed mesenchymal layer is dubbed the mesoderm.
  - The epiblast is renamed the ectoderm.
  - The hypoblast is renamed the endoderm.

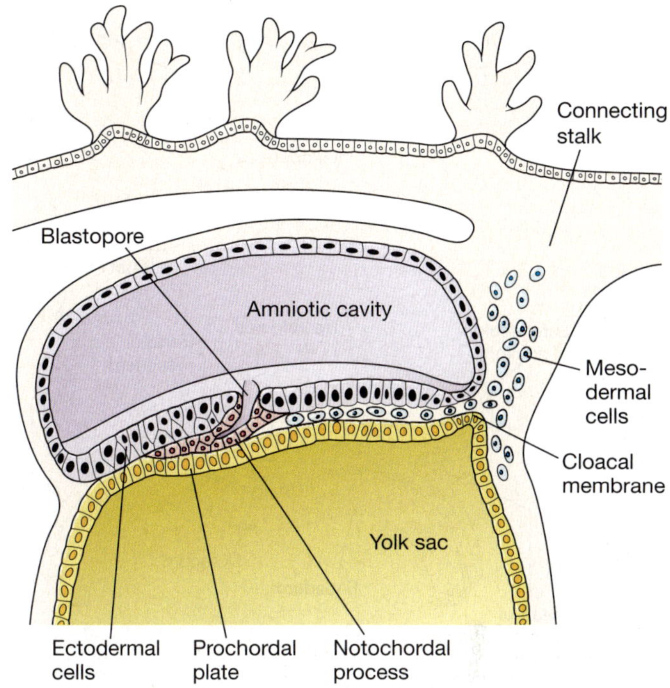

Figure 3.2. This is a reconstruction of an embryo early in the third week. The ectodermal cells have black nuclei, the endodermal cells have yellow nuclei, the mesodermal cells have blue nuclei, and the cells forming the notochord have red nuclei. Cells migrating downward from the epiblast form the notochordal process. (Redrawn from Hamilton WJ, Boyd JD, Mossman HW. *Human Embryology: Prenatal Development of Form and Function.* 2nd ed. Williams & Wilkins Company; 1952.)

- Of particular note are the cells that invaginate into the primitive streak on the midline.
  - They migrate forward, forming a specialized tubular column of cells termed the notochord (Figs. 3.2 and 3.3).

At this point in time:

- The plan of the embryo has been formulated through induction.
- The central axis of the future body has been determined (notochord).
- Left–right patterning has begun to develop in the embryonic disk.

For a more detailed description of the events occurring during embryogenesis, see Moore et al.[3]

MUSCULOSKELETAL SYSTEM: EMBRYOLOGY

Development of the Trunk

Once the embryonic disk has formed a primitive streak and polarized, the growth of the musculoskeletal system can begin. The development of the musculoskeletal system centers primarily on the mesoderm, with neural and epithelial contributions from the ectoderm.

- The mesenchymal tissue of the mesoderm is composed of stellate, multipotent mesenchymal cells, and a fibrous extracellular matrix (ECM).
- The mesenchymal cells are capable of differentiating a myriad of cell types, including:
  - Fibroblasts
  - Adipoblasts
  - Chondroblasts
  - Osteoblasts
  - Myoblasts

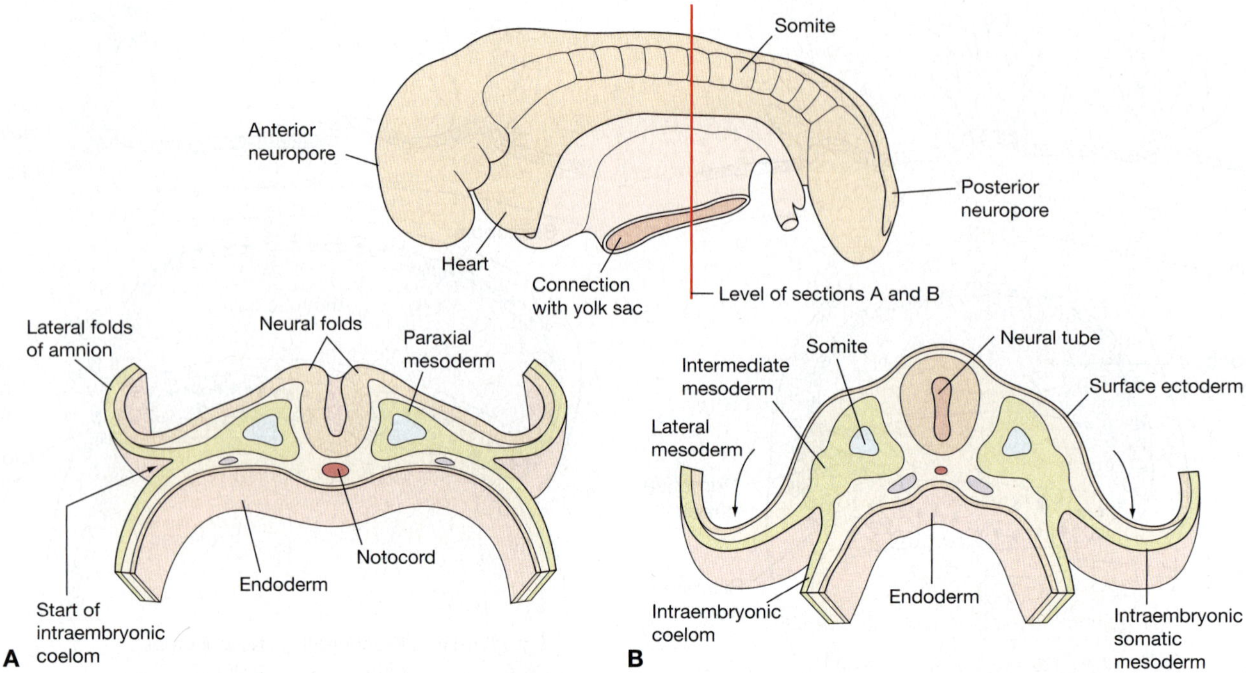

Figure 3.3. Formation of a neural tube and somites. The top image is a lateral view of the embryo illustrating a series of somites forming lateral to the neural tube. **A.** An axial plane section of an embryo taken prior to the closure of the neural tube. **B.** An axial plane section of an embryo taken immediately following the closure of the neural tube. The somite, intermediate mesoderm, and lateral mesoderm can be clearly seen in **B.**

Throughout the third week, the mesoderm gives rise to three bands of cells on either side of the notochord (see Fig. 3.3):

1. The paraxial mesoderm, which gives rise to the somites of the body.
2. The intermediate mesoderm, which contributes to the urogenital system.
3. The lateral mesoderm, which contributes to the formation of somatic and visceral fascia as well as the fascia of the limbs as described below.

The lateral plate mesoderm then subdivides into somatopleuric and splanchnopleuric mesoderms, separated by an intraembryonic coelom.

- The splanchnopleuric mesoderm:
  - Provides the corresponding viscera for each cavity.
  - Gives rise to the visceral fascia that lines body cavities.
- The somatopleuric mesoderm:
  - Gives rise to the parietal layers of the mesothelium, the transversalis fascia, and the anterolateral abdominal wall.
  - Contributes the connective tissue elements to the developing limb buds.
- The coelom:
  - Further subdivides into pericardial, pleural, and peritoneal cavities.

Concurrently in the developing trunk region, a process of segmentation commences as the mesenchymal cells of the paraxial mesoderm condense into discrete blocks, called somites (Box 3.1).

- Somitogenesis progresses from cranially to caudally, driven by a biologic segmentation clock mechanism that is well conserved across phylogeny.
- On day 20, the first pair of somites is visible, and a new pair is added approximately every 90 minutes until 42 to 44 pairs have formed.
- Many of the somites in the caudal eminence will disappear, resulting in a total of 33 to 37 paired somites in the human embryo.

As somites form in the middle layer of embryonic cells, related developmental events are taking place in the overlying ectoderm.

- The ectoderm becomes grooved in the midline, and the edges of the groove then move together until a tube is formed.
  - The tube—now called the neural tube—is the embryonic precursor of the spinal cord and is oriented along the long axis of the future embryo, parallel to the axis of the primitive streak and the underlying notochord (see Figs. 3.3 and 3.4).
- Ectodermal tissue adjacent to the neural tube is called the neural crest.
  - As the two walls of the neural tube approach each other on the midline, the crest cells squeeze out through another process of epithelial-to-mesenchymal cell transformation.
  - These crest cells are the precursor of elements of the peripheral nervous system, such as the dorsal root ganglia and the autonomic ganglia.

BOX 3.1 Segmentation Clock

- An oscillator network of genes governs the periodic pattern of somite formation.
- Fibroblast growth factor, Delta-Notch, and Wnt are implicated in the cyclic nature of segmentation.
- Segmentation is described as a "clock and wave front" mechanism to explain the periodicity (clock) and anteroposterior progression (wave front).[4]

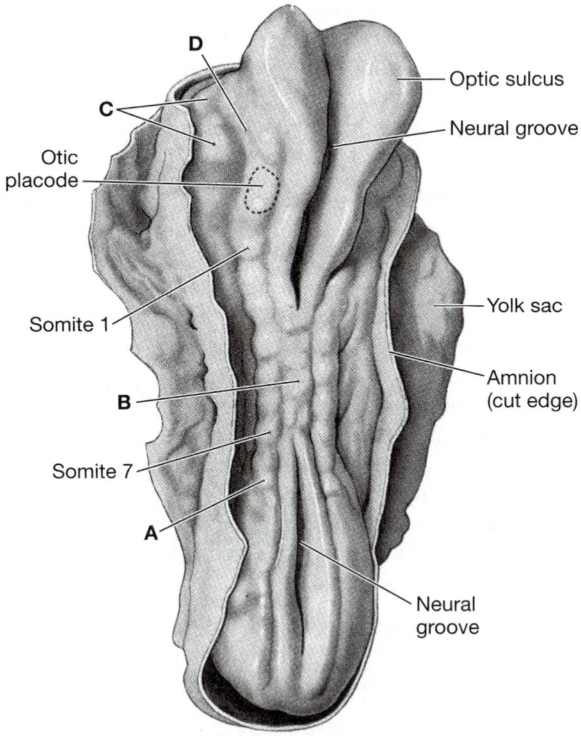

Figure 3.4. This is a dorsal view of a reconstruction of a 7-somite embryo. A. Partially segmented paraxial mesoderm. **B.** Roof of the neural tube. **C.** Pericardial area. **D.** Branchial arch region. (Redrawn from Hamilton WJ, Boyd JD, Mossman HW. *Human Embryology: Prenatal Development of Form and Function.* 2nd ed. Williams & Wilkins Company; 1952.)

Surrounding the nascent neural tube, the somites compartmentalize into three main components (Fig. 3.5):

1. The myotome, which gives rise to skeletal muscle.
2. The dermatome, which gives rise to the dermis portion of the skin.
3. The sclerotome, which gives rise to the hard connective tissues.

Early in the fifth week, the myotome will divide in two:

1. A smaller epaxial myotome (or epimere), which becomes the intrinsic back musculature.
2. A larger hypaxial myotome (or hypomere), which gives rise to the extrinsic back and ventral body wall, as well as the appendicular (extremity) musculature (Fig. 3.6).

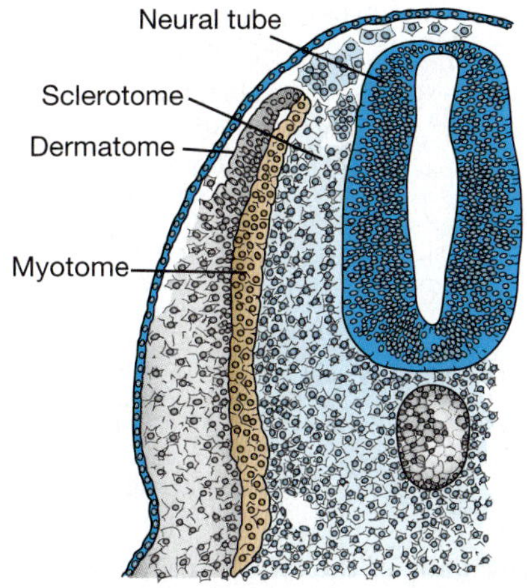

Figure 3.5. Formation of a somite. The somite is divided into a dermatome, myotome, and sclerotome. Recently, the concept of a viscerotome, more midline mesoderm, has been added to the somite. (Reprinted with permission from Sadler TW. *Langman's Medical Embryology.* 13th ed. Wolters Kluwer; 2015.)

At that point, the developing spinal nerve splits into dorsal and ventral primary rami that subsequently innervate the epimere and hypomere, respectively. Two small subportions of the dorsal aspect of the sclerotome can also be recognized:

1. The syndetome, on the dorsal aspect of the sclerotome, gives rise to cells within tendons.
2. The arthrotome, the innermost aspect of the sclerotome, gives rise to a portion of the zygapophyseal joints and the intervertebral disks.

The spinal nerve grows into the somite, and through this connection, each newly formed somite is mapped to a specific region of the neural tube.

- Each spinal nerve is composed of dorsal (sensory) rootlets and ventral (motor) rootlets.
  - The rootlets unite into dorsal and ventral roots, which then merge into a spinal nerve that enters the somite.
- Upon entering the somite, each spinal nerve divides to form a posterior primary ramus and an anterior primary ramus (Fig. 3.7).
  - Each ramus contains both sensory and motor nerve fibers.
  - The posterior (dorsal) primary rami are distributed to the deep ("true") back muscles; the joints, which the muscles functionally move; and the skin over these muscles.

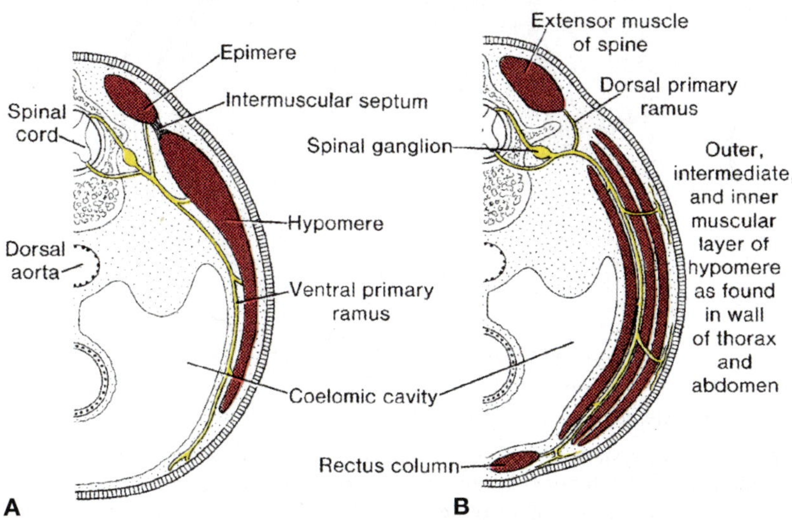

Figure 3.6. Division of a somite into epimere and hypomere. A. Transverse section taken through the body of a 5-week-old embryo. **B.** Transverse section taken through the body of an embryo at approximately 5 and a half weeks' gestation. The epimere is innervated by the dorsal primary ramus, while the hypomere is innervated by the ventral primary ramus. (Reprinted with permission from Sadler TW. *Langman's Medical Embryology.* 9th ed. Lippincott Williams & Wilkins; 2003.)

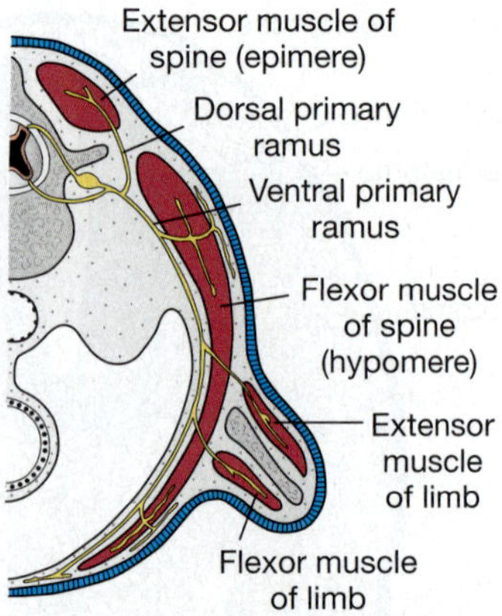

Figure 3.7. Ontogeny of the limb bud. The dorsal primary ramus is seen innervating the epaxial muscles (the epimere). The ventral primary ramus is seen innervating the hypaxial (hypomere) muscles. In addition, branches from the ventral ramus continue into the limb bud to innervate the limb. In doing so, some of these branches segregate into those innervating the flexor compartment and those innervating the extensor compartment. (Reprinted with permission from Sadler TW. *Langman's Medical Embryology*. 13th ed. Wolters Kluwer; 2015.)

- The anterior (ventral) primary ramus in the thoracic and lumbar regions innervates the muscles of the body wall (i.e., intercostal and abdominal muscles) and the skin of the thorax and abdomen (Fig. 3.8).

- The pattern of thoracic and lumbar nerve distribution is clinically demonstrated as the dermatomes—restricted areas of the skin, served by individual spinal nerves, and recognizable on a neurologic exam (see Fig. 3.10).
  - Thus, a close correspondence is maintained between the developing segments of the body wall and the central nervous system (CNS).

While the close coherence between the spinal cord and the truncal musculoskeletal system is maintained by these developmental events, anticipating the visceral–somatic relationships to be discussed below, it is useful to note that there is also a relationship between the developing thoracic and abdominopelvic organs and the spinal cord.

- Each spinal nerve in the thoracic and lumbar region of the body provides innervation to a region of the developing splanchnopleure, termed "viscerotomes."
- It is from the splanchnopleure that the visceral organs will develop, enveloped in fascia also derived from the splanchnopleure.
- Through overlapping somatic and visceral sensory projections into the spinal cord, the nervous system provides the link between the somatic tissue of the trunk (i.e., bones and muscles) and the viscera (i.e., heart or gastrointestinal system).
- This segmental relationship between the body wall and internal organs is hypothesized to be the underlying mechanism for referred pain—perceiving pain on the body wall (i.e., chest pain) when the tissue damage is in an internal organ (i.e., cardiac ischemia).

As will be typical throughout the body, there is also a segmentation of blood supply to the thoracic and abdominal wall that is similar to segmentation of muscles and nerves.

- For example:
  - In the thoracic region, the aorta gives rise to right and left posterior intercostal arteries, which supply the thoracic and abdominal walls segmentally (see Fig. 3.8B).
  - Structures supplied by posterior intercostal arteries include the skin, superficial and deep fascia, intercostal and abdominal musculature, ribs, vertebrae, and paravertebral musculature.
- This parallel segmentation of nerves and vessels is readily seen on the inferior surface of each rib where a neurovascular

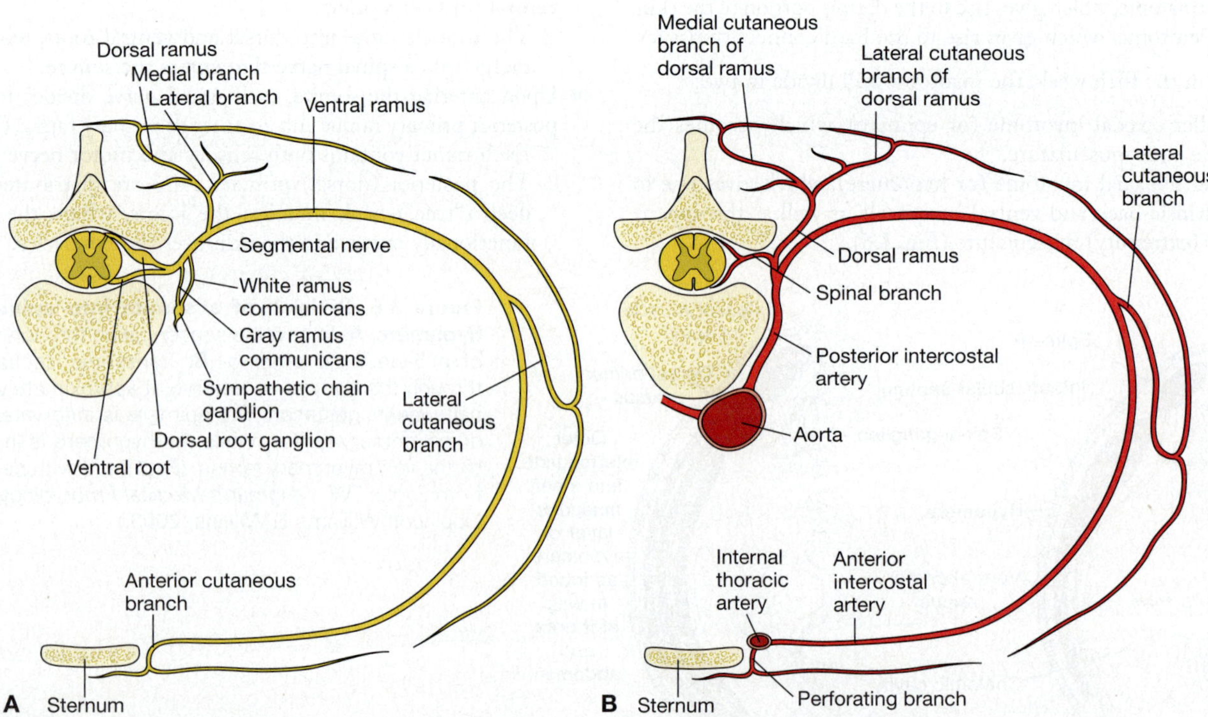

Figure 3.8. Segmental innervation and arterial supply. A. Intercostal nerve. **B.** Intercostal artery. The posterior (dorsal) primary ramus innervates the (epaxial) paraspinal muscles, while the anterior (ventral) primary ramus innervates the hypaxial muscles such as the scalene muscles, intercostal muscles, and abdominal muscles.

bundle, which includes the intercostal nerve, artery, and vein (as well as segmental intercostal lymphatics) is located (see Fig. 3.8A).

- These structures supply and drain the muscle, connective tissue, and skin within and over the thorax and abdomen.

- The segmental pattern of neurovascular distribution in the thorax and abdomen is an example of developmental segmentation the body maintains into adulthood.
  - However, this segmental pattern is significantly modified in the limbs by differential growth and development.

Development of the Limbs

The segmentation events, readily seen in the development of the torso, are not as apparent in the adult limbs. Nevertheless, keeping the original segmentation pattern in mind will aid in understanding the overall anatomy of the limbs.

- The anatomy of the upper and lower limbs is comparable.
- The limbs are divided into four major parts.
  - The upper limb is divided into the:
    1. Shoulder (shoulder girdle)
    2. Arm
    3. Forearm
    4. Hand
  - The lower limb is divided into four parts:
    1. Pelvic girdle
    2. Thigh
    3. Leg
    4. Foot
- Each region of the limb typically can be divided into anterior and posterior fascial compartments.
- Functionally related groups of muscles tend to be contained within a given compartment and to be innervated by a specific nerve.
  - For example, the flexor muscles of the arm are contained within the anterior compartment of the arm and are innervated by the musculocutaneous nerve.

The section on fascia will return to this concept. For a more detailed overview of limb structure, see Hollinshead.[5]

The development of the limbs begins early in the fourth week of gestation, whereby portions of mesenchyme from the somatopleuric mesoderm begin condensing into four limb buds.

- The mesenchymal cells of the bud push laterally into, and become covered by, the overlying ectoderm (Fig. 3.9).
- A thickened ridge of ectoderm at the leading edge of the limb bud, termed the apical ectodermal ridge, promotes growth and development of the limb.
- The mesenchymal cells of the limb bud begin differentiating into several mature connective tissues of the limb, such as the dermis, cartilage (including the fetal cartilaginous skeleton), fascia, and eventually bone.
- However, under normal developmental conditions, the mesenchymal tissue of the somatopleuric mesoderm does not produce skeletal muscle. Instead, near the end of the fifth week, myoblasts from the hypaxial myotome in the trunk will migrate outward to enter the limb bud mesenchyme (see Fig. 3.7).

As the limb bud expands laterally, it is invaded by the peripheral nerves derived from the region of the neural tube. Whereas the muscles in the limb arise from the mesoderm, the axons of the peripheral nerve derive from the ectoderm of the neural tube and the neural crest.

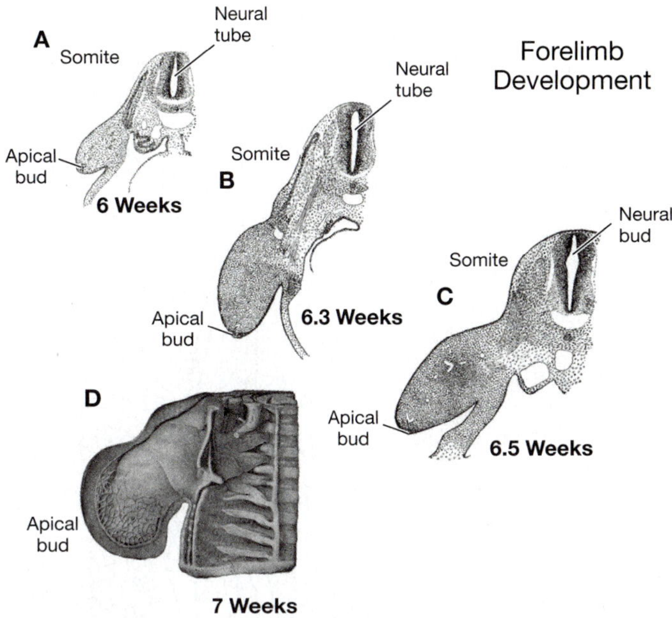

Figure 3.9. The development of the limbs. These drawings are taken from embryos in the 6th to 7th weeks of development. The apical limb bud is seen on the leading edge of the limb as the limb grows in length. (Images modified from Bailey FR, Miller AM. *Textbook of Embryology*. 3rd ed. William Wood and Company; 1916.)

- Sensory neurons develop from neural crest and reside in the dorsal root ganglion.
  - Each sensory neuron sends a central process into the spinal cord over the dorsal root and a peripheral process that joins the spinal nerve.
- Motor axons develop from the ventral portion of the neural tube.
  - Within the ventral neural tube, motor neurons destined to supply similar targets are organized into columns—the medial column for axial musculature, the lateral motor column for appendicular musculature.

Axonal growth for these motor neurons is directed by a growth cone capable of lengthening or withdrawing in response to guiding stimuli released by the somite, such as ephrins, netrins, and semaphorins.

- Receptors on the growing axons derived from the medial column differ from the receptors of axons from the lateral motor column. Thus, axons from each column are drawn toward their respective targets.
- Boundary cap cells located at the entry and exit points of the spinal cord, prevent the motor neuron somas from migrating along with the axons.
- Because axonal growth outside the neural tube is directed by the somite, predictable cutaneous innervation patterns (dermatomes) are formed (Fig. 3.10).

For a detailed discussion of the growth of spinal nerves and the innervation of limb muscles, see Martin et al.[6]

Spinal levels in the cervical and lumbosacral regions send spinal nerves toward the appropriate limb buds.

- At the base of developing limb buds, fascicles from several spinal nerves converge into a complex formation, termed a plexus (e.g., fascicles from C5 to T1 segments merge into a brachial plexus; Fig. 3.11).

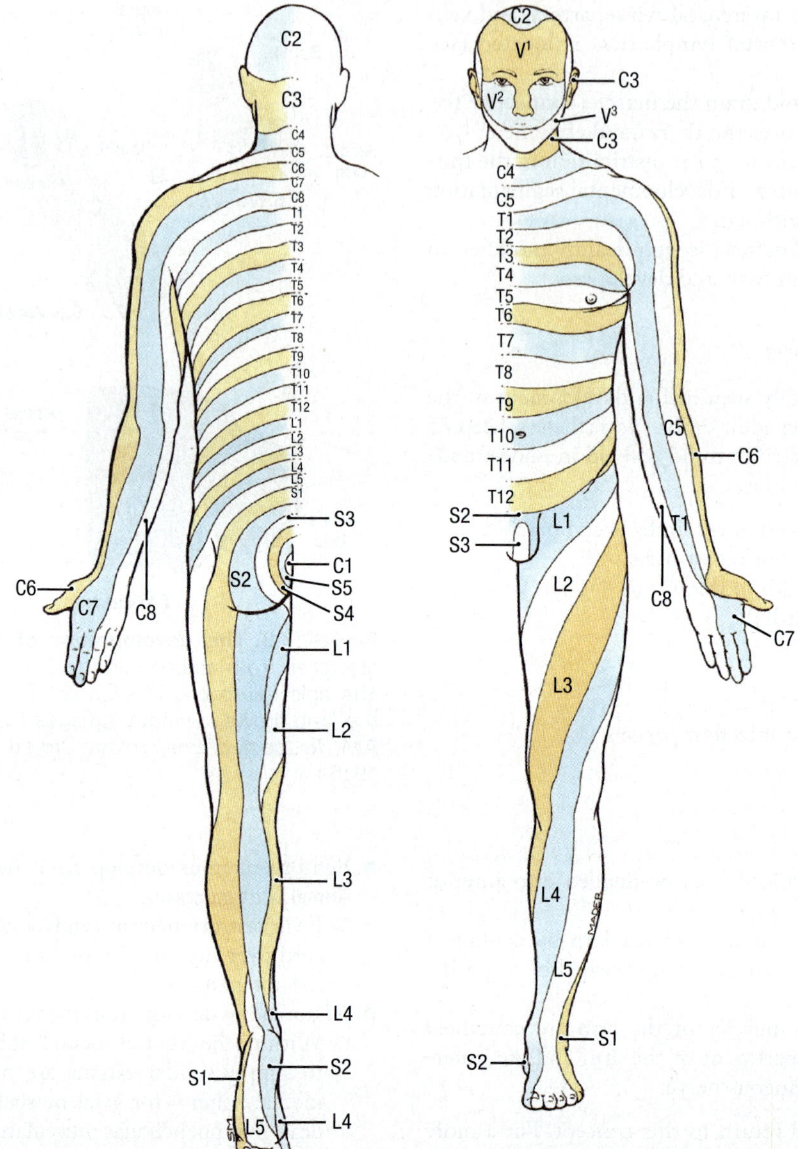

Figure 3.10. Dermatome map. Dermatomes represent an orderly mapping of spinal cord segments onto the skin.

- These fascicles divide into two fundamental groups that follow two separate routes into the limb:
  1. A ventral route leading into the flexor compartment of the limb.
  2. A dorsal route leading into the extensor compartment of the limb.

These groupings create the anterior and posterior division of the brachial plexus, respectively (see Fig. 3.7).

- Within the plexus, axons are exchanged from one spinal nerve to another, such that the exiting peripheral nerves are carrying axons representing a rich mixture of spinal levels.
- As growing axons approach the plexus, axonal growth cones expand and diverge from each other.
  - □ This divergence appears to involve an increase in Neural Cell Adhesion Molecules (NCAM) polysialic acid, which inhibits axon–axon adherence.
- Divergent axons are able to take a tangential course through the plexus, ultimately joining a different axonal grouping, resulting in the creation of mixed peripheral nerves, each carrying axons from multiple, different spinal cord levels.

For a landmark study on the formation of a plexus, see Landmesser.[7]

The limb bud mesenchyme appears to play a role in directing the migration and patterning of myogenic masses in the limbs.

- Fascial precursors of the limb bud mesenchyme express the *hox11* gene and transcription factor 4 (Tcf4).
  - □ If expression of either of these factors is disrupted, limb muscle mass will be absent or malformed.
- However, in models for which myoblasts are experimentally ablated, the positioning of fascial precursor cells into investing fascial layers in the limb is unaffected.
  - □ This preservation of fascial superstructure suggests that even in the absence of muscles, some semblance of epi-, peri-, and endomysial layers, the fascial skeleton of the muscle, would exist.
- Thus, it appears that the precursors of the fascial tissue are involved in establishing the model for the development of individual muscles.

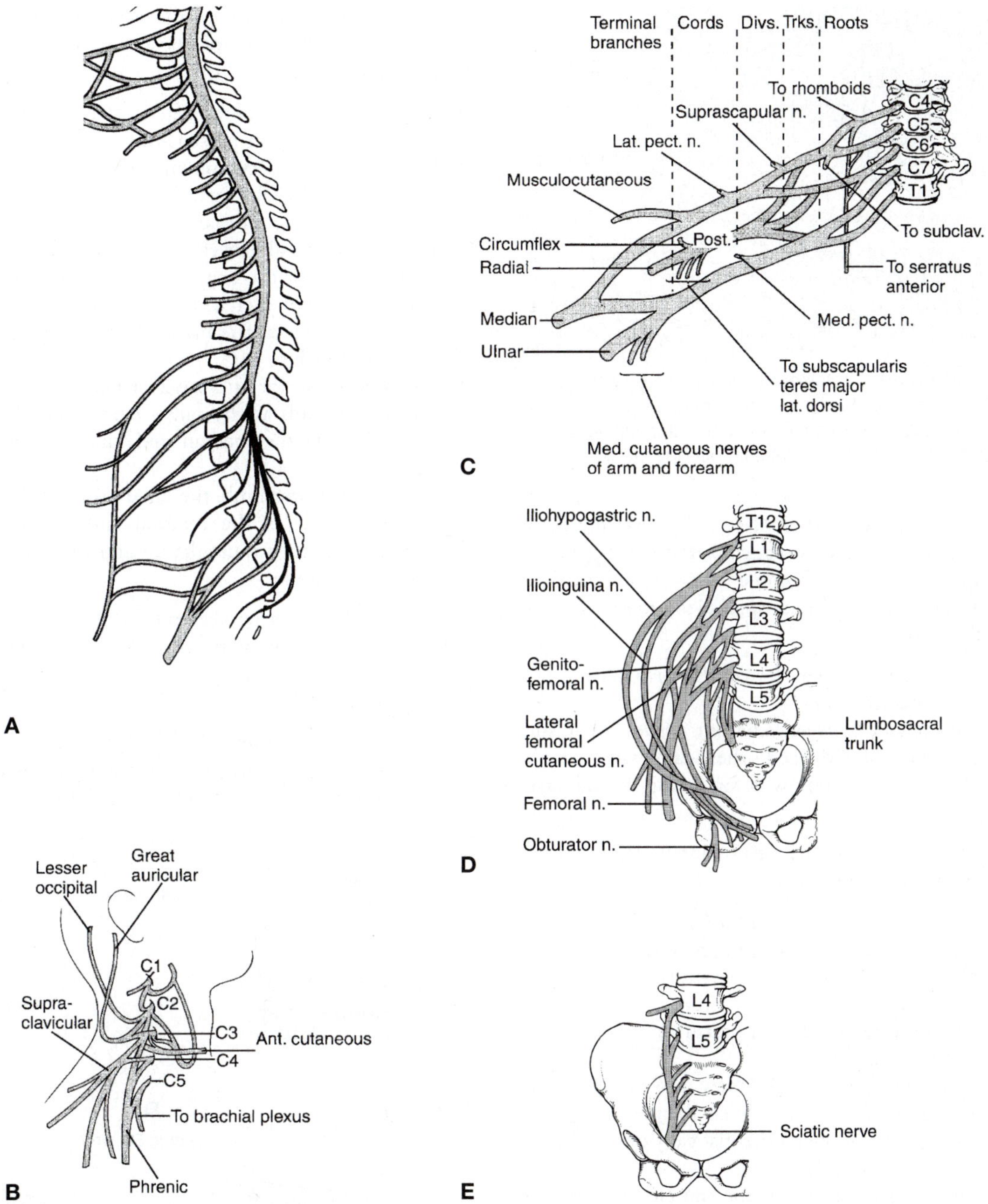

Figure 3.11. The plexuses of the body. A. This schematic illustrates the upper (brachial) and lower (lumbosacral) extremity plexuses as they combine different levels of the spinal cord. **B.** The cervical plexus contains input from spinal levels C1 to C4 and innervates the muscles of the neck. **C.** The brachial plexus contains input from spinal levels C5 to T1 and innervates the muscles of the upper extremity. **D, E.** The lumbosacral plexus contains input from spinal levels L3 to S3 and innervates the lower extremity.

The bones of the upper and lower limbs arise from mesenchymal cells in situ in the developing limb buds.

- Within the limb, a portion of somatopleuric mesenchymal cells passes through several differentiation stages:
  1. A condensation of mesenchymal cells in the site of the future bone.
  2. Chondrogenesis and the formation of a cartilaginous model of the bone.
- Osteogenesis and the conversion of the cartilaginous model to bone occurs by a process of endochondral ossification.[8] Simultaneously, the associated myogenic mass is divided into dorsal and ventral masses around the developing bone.
- As this occurs, a portion of Tcf4-positive mesenchymal cells continue to surround each myogenic mass and developing bone, destined to become the investing fascial and periosteal layers, respectively.
- Furthermore, as the myogenic masses divide into individual muscles, Tcf4-positive cells continue to envelop each muscle, as presumed precursors to the epimysium.
- In addition, more Tcf4-positive cells continue to infiltrate the growing mass, contributing to the peri- and endomysial layers.
- For a detailed discussion of bone development, see Karaplis.[9]

In a similar fashion to the process seen in muscle and bone, the development of tendons, ligaments, and aponeuroses involves the condensation of mesenchymal cells into a dense mass. Here, however, the

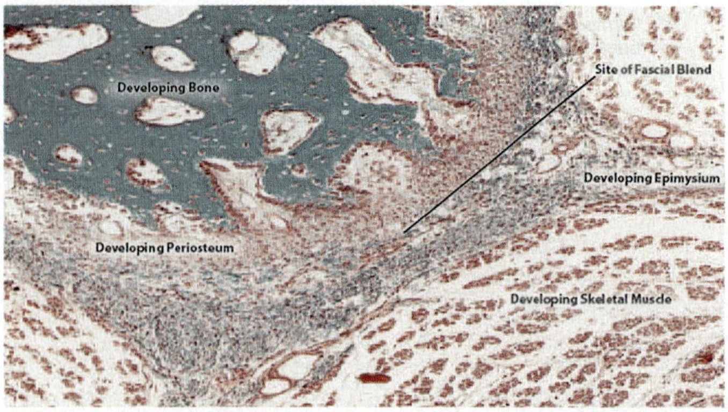

Figure 3.12. Fascial blend. Histologic preparation of developing forearm; note the seamless blend of the developing periosteal and epimysial fascial layers. (Image taken from the University of Michigan image collection on the Virtual Microscopy Database.)

mesenchymal cells differentiate into fibroblasts rather than myoblasts or osteoblasts and begin laying down oriented bands of collagen.

Mesenchymal cells destined to become fascia (peritenon, perichondrium, periosteum) surround each specialized matrix such as muscle, bone, cartilage, or tendon.

- Regardless of the tissue being enveloped, the surrounding fasciae exhibit similar characteristics.
- Thus, in areas of contact between adjacent tissues, their surrounding fasciae will blend with each other seamlessly.
- This creates a continuous, body-wide investing fascial layer (Fig. 3.12).[10]

The process of angiogenesis may also contribute to muscle mass partitioning and fascial bundling.

- Platelet-derived growth factor-B (PDGF-B) is released by endothelial cells as they enter a developing region.
  - □ PDGF-B inhibits myoblasts, thereby producing cleavage planes in muscle masses.
  - □ PDGF-B also stimulates the fascial precursor mesenchymal cells to fill in the cleavage planes.
- By this mechanism, blood vessels gain entry into intramuscular fascial planes, through which the muscle can be perfused.
- In a similar fashion, nerves develop synergistically on the framework of developing blood vessels.
  - □ Therefore, they too gain access to the muscle by following fascial planes.
- The close developmental association of nerves with growing blood vessels creates the neurovascular bundles seen during surgical or cadaveric dissection.

All fasciae derive from similar mesenchymal origins, and often, this origin is different from that of the tissue it invests.

- Therefore, in addition to forming a global connective tissue network, each fascial layer may provide beneficial services (growth and repair) to neighboring tissues. For example:
  - □ Cells of the peritenon exhibit a faster proliferation rate, migration speed, and osteogenic potential, relative to the neighboring tenocytes.
  - □ Epimysial cells express transcription factors associated with pluripotency and self-renewal.
  - □ In particular, epimysial cells demonstrate great potential for differentiation to a chondrogenic lineage.
- Fasciae have also demonstrated the capacity for inflammatory reactions associated with cellular proliferation and adhesion.

As previously described, the growing ventral primary ramus of the spinal nerve splits into posterior and anterior branches (see Figs. 3.6 and 3.7).

- Posterior branches enter extensor musculature while anterior branches enter flexor musculature.
- With continued development, multiple posterior and anterior branches from each ventral primary ramus unite with those from surrounding primary rami to form large posterior and anterior peripheral nerves.
  - □ This union of the original segmental posterior and anterior branches from each anterior primary ramus is the basis for the formation of the brachial and lumbosacral plexuses (see Fig. 3.11A–E).
- The large posterior and anterior nerves are represented in the adult upper limb as the radial nerve supplying extensor musculature, while the median and ulnar nerves innervate flexor musculature.
- In the adult lower limb, the large posterior and anterior nerves are represented as the femoral and common fibular nerves supplying extensor musculature and the tibial nerve supplying flexor musculature.

Contact between nerves and differentiating muscle cells is a prerequisite for complete functional muscle differentiation.

- The segmental spinal nerves also provide sensory innervation of the limb dermatomes.
  - □ The original segmental dermatomal pattern is modified with growth of the limbs, yet remnants of this orderly sequence remains present in the adult (Fig. 3.13).

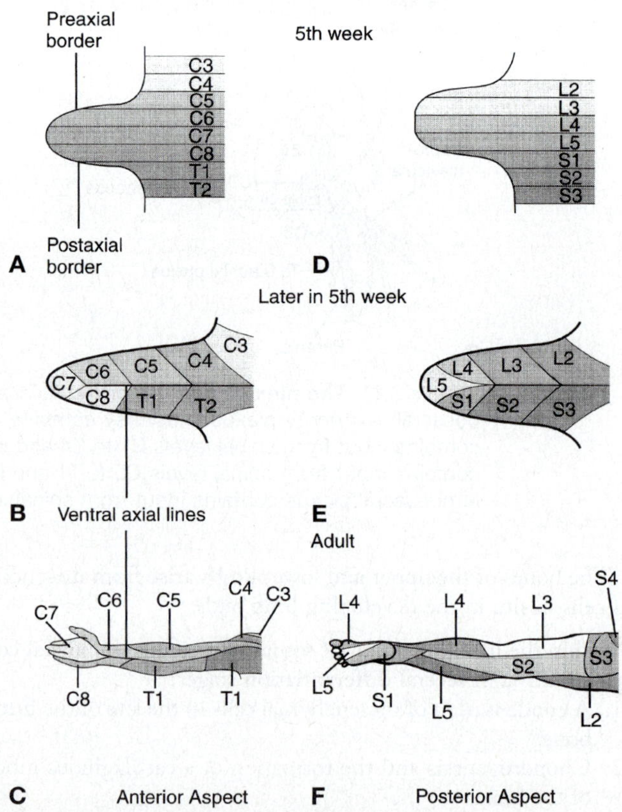

Figure 3.13. Developing dermatome pattern. A–C are from the upper extremity; D–F are from the lower extremity. A, D. The initial pattern of dermatomes in the limbs. B, E. With growth, the initial pattern becomes modified. C, F. The adult pattern of dermatomes.

- Finally, the orderly exchange of axons between spinal nerves leading to the formation of peripheral nerves, containing mixed spinal levels, means that almost all muscles in a limb receive input from more than one spinal level.
  - □ This arrangement may have a protective value, since the loss of function in a spinal nerve will tend to weaken a limb muscle but not paralyze the muscle, allowing for the retention of some movement.

While the development of the upper and lower limbs is similar, there is one major difference: the limbs rotate in opposite directions.

- The upper limb rotates 90 degrees laterally so that:
  - □ The elbow points posteriorly.
  - □ The extensor musculature lies on lateral and posterior surfaces, while the flexor musculature lies on anterior and medial surfaces.
  - □ The thumb lies laterally on the anterior-facing palm.
- The lower limb rotates 90 degrees medially so that:
  - □ The knee points anteriorly.
  - □ The extensor muscles are on the anterior surface, while the flexor muscles are on the posterior surface.
  - □ The big toe is medial.

In the limbs, deep fascia and intermuscular septa connecting with bone separate or compartmentalize groups of muscles. The arrangement is very orderly; typically, the muscles in each compartment share similar functions, developmental histories, nerve and arterial supply, and venous and lymphatic drainage.

- For additional information on the development of vertebrate limbs, see Tickle and Eichele.[11]

Development of the Head and Neck

The head and neck region is highly specialized for cognition, integration, and rapid reactions as well as other specialized functions such as phonation and mastication. As such, it is also unique in embryologic development. The neuroanatomy of the head is beyond the scope of this introductory summary, so the following is a brief overview of only the musculoskeletal aspects of head and neck development. For additional details concerning the development of the head, see Moore et al.[3]

At 3 weeks of development, the head region of the embryo is divided into two compartments, dorsal and ventral, by a thickened membrane.

- The dorsal compartment will go on to become bulbous in shape and contain the developing brain.
- The ventral compartment will form the oral cavity, pharynx, and larynx.
- The dividing membrane will initially chondrify and then ossify, forming the future basicranium (Fig. 3.14).

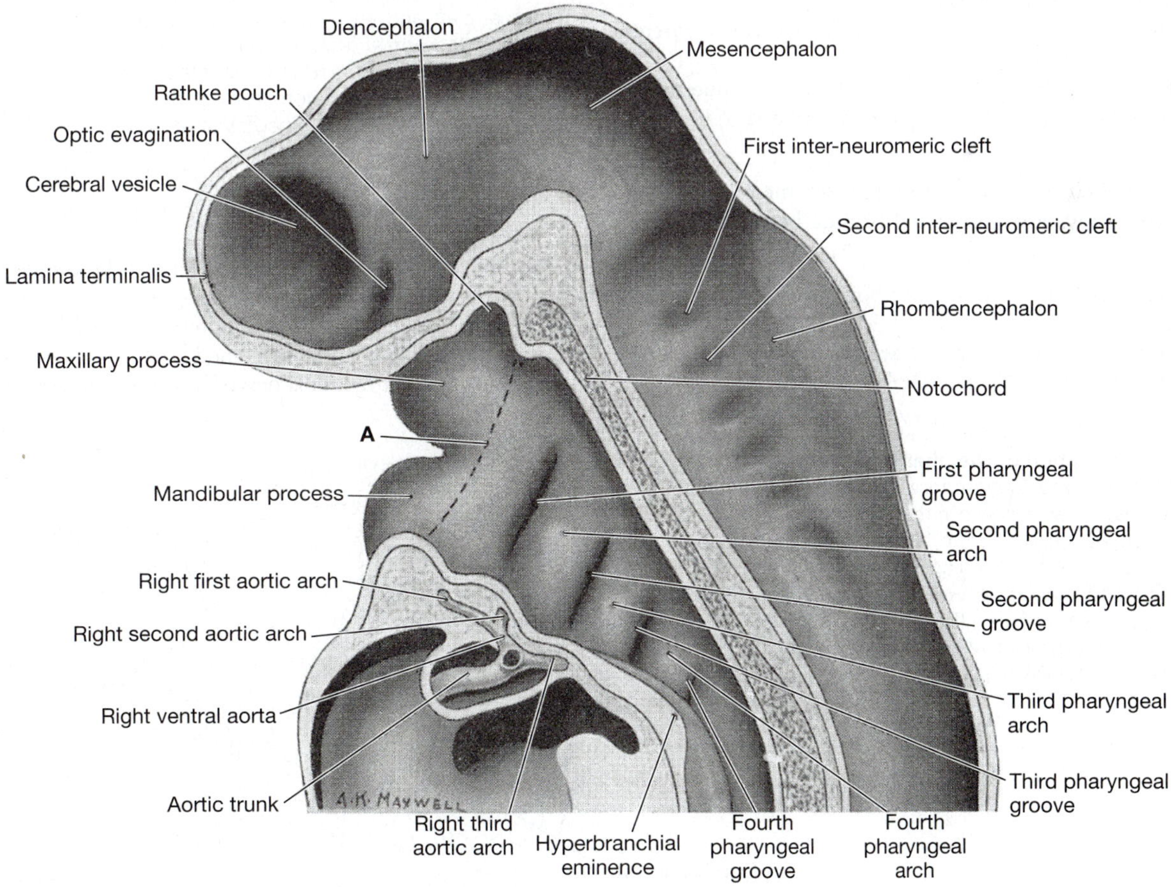

Figure 3.14. A sagittal section of the head of an embryo in the 6th week of development. The basicranium is seen as a rostral extension of the notochord, separating the dorsally positioned neural tube from the ventrally positioned oropharynx. The oropharyngeal region is seen below the basicranium, while the cavity for the brain, the neurocranium, is seen above the basicranium. The dashed lined marked **A** denotes the location of the buccopharyngeal membrane. (From Hamilton WJ, Boyd JD, Mossman HW. *Hamilton, Boyd and Mossman's Human Embryology: Parental Development of Form and Function.* 4th ed. W. Heffer & Sons Ltd; 1972.)

When compared to bones of somite origin, those of the cranium demonstrate significantly more phylogenetic variation, possibly associated with the rapid development of brain size in the vertebrates, especially primates.

- These extensive changes in the size and shape of the neurocranium have a major impact on the shape of the human face, forcing it to elongate in the vertical axis and slide under the enlarging frontal bones.
- Some of the uniqueness of cranial structure is due to the interaction between the mesenchyme of the head region and a particularly large influx of neural crest cells into this region.[12]
- The uniqueness of the developmental history of the cranial bones may underlie the ability of skilled physicians to effect change in cranial bone relationships, at least in newborns and young children.

For detailed information on the development of the cranium, see Lieberman.[13]

Four weeks into embryogenesis, the six branchial arches begin emerging from the ventral compartment of the head and neck region.

- Ectoderm lines the exterior surface of each arch and forms the pharyngeal clefts between the arches.
- Endoderm lines the interior surface of each arch and forms the oral cavity.
- The pouches are formed by the outward (lateralward) growth of the oral cavity wall between each arch.
- Thus, ectoderm and endoderm approach each other where a cleft meets a pouch (Fig. 3.15).
- In the first cleft, the close approximation of ectoderm and endoderm serves to form the tympanic membrane of the external ear.

Mesenchymal tissue, derived from paraxial mesoderm, lateral plate mesoderm, and neural crest cells, reside between the ectoderm and endoderm.

- Neural crest cells give rise to most bones and cartilages from the arches.
  - □ However, laryngeal cartilages, as well as the vasculature components, derive from the lateral plate mesoderm.

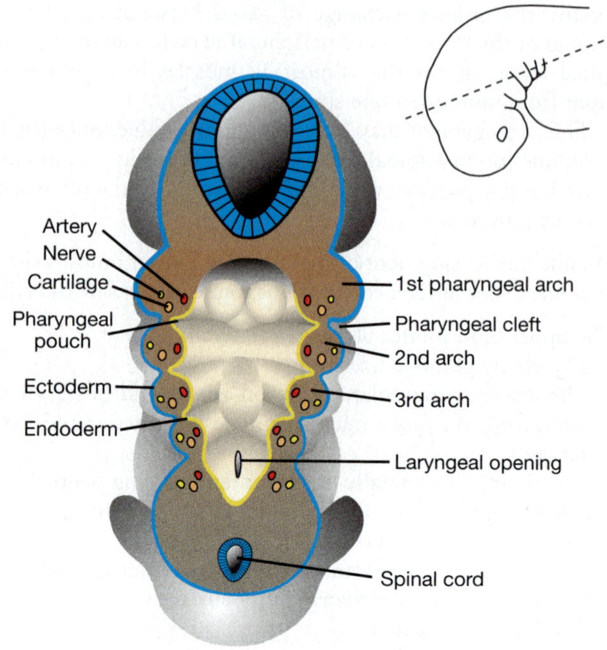

Figure 3.15. Development of the head. This is a coronal section taken through the developing head of a 4-week-old embryo (the *dashed line* in the **inset** represents the plane of section). At 4 weeks of development, the walls of the oral cavity are parsed into a series of six pharyngeal arches, with each arch separated by an external cleft and an internal pouch. Only five of the pouches are visible in the above image. Each arch contains a cartilaginous bar, an artery, and a vein, and is innervated by a specific cranial nerve. (Reprinted with permission from Sadler TW. *Langman's Medical Embryology*. 10th ed. Lippincott Williams & Wilkins; 2006.)

- As in other body regions, muscle derives from the paraxial mesoderm, but in the cranial region, paraxial mesoderm does not segment into discrete somites.
  - □ Nevertheless, paraxial mesodermal cells migrate into each arch as it is developing.
- As each arch is supplied by a different cranial nerve, the derivation of a muscle can be discerned by its innervation (Fig. 3.16).
  - □ First arch—trigeminal nerve (CN V)—muscles of mastication

Figure 3.16. Innervation of the pharyngeal arches. Cranial nerves V, VII, IX, and X provide innervation to the pharyngeal arches in the head. Cranial nerve V, the trigeminal, innervates the first arch; cranial nerve VII, the facial, innervates the second arch; cranial nerve IX, the glossopharyngeal, innervates the third arch; and cranial nerve X, the vagus, innervates the remaining three arches. (Reprinted with permission from Sadler TW. *Langman's Medical Embryology*. 10th ed. Lippincott Williams & Wilkins; 2006.)

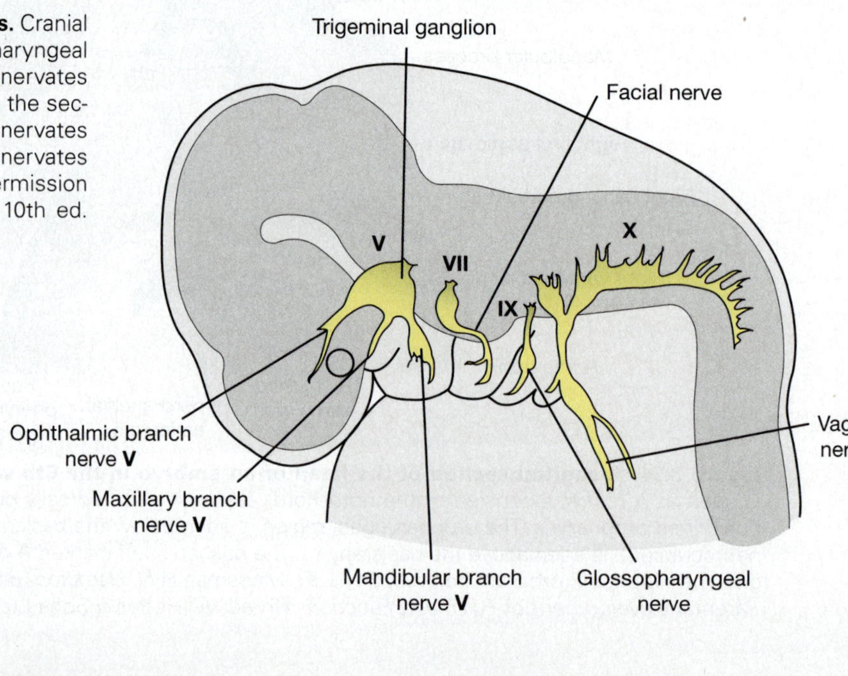

- Second arch—facial nerve (CN VII)—muscles of facial expression
- Third arch—glossopharyngeal nerve (CN IX)—stylopharyngeus muscle
- Fourth arch—vagus nerve (CN X)—pharyngeal muscle
- Fifth arch—rudimentary in a human
- Sixth arch—vagus nerve (CN X)—laryngeal muscles

- The muscles of a given arch have not only a common innervation but also a common function.
  - This arrangement of branchial or pharyngeal arches is considered to be "special" and differs from the development of muscle derived from somites.
- Components of these pharyngeal arches have recently been found as far into the torso as the heart and roots of the great vessels in the thorax.[14]

MUSCULOSKELETAL SYSTEM: FUNCTIONAL ANATOMY

Understanding the function of the musculoskeletal system remains at the heart of osteopathic medical practice and, so, constitutes a significant portion of most anatomy courses taught in Colleges of Osteopathic Medicine.

- The musculoskeletal system is approximately 75% of the body mass; this vast system:
  - Provides mobility, a feature which is known to improve general health.
  - Provides diagnostic clues to dysfunction and disease.
  - Offers a mode of treatment to support the patient who is experiencing disease or stress.
- The **biomechanical model**, one of the five conceptual models used in the osteopathic approach to the patient, in large part focuses on an understanding of the musculoskeletal system structure and function, along with the pervasive effects of musculoskeletal pathology.

Traditional use of the term "musculoskeletal" is misrepresentative of the system to which osteopathic physicians refer when using the phrase.

- As the name implies, the musculoskeletal system is composed of skeletal muscle and the bones they move.
- However, the system also includes tendons, ligaments, cartilage, and fascia that serve to integrate the muscles and skeletal framework.
- Furthermore, it is difficult to discuss this system without any acknowledgment of neurovascular supply.

Finally, understanding the rules that govern function in the musculoskeletal system leads inevitably to a series of questions predicated on more complex structural and functional interrelationships:

- How might dysfunction of the muscle (or other musculoskeletal component) affect total body efficiency and health?
- How might dysfunction of some visceral element degrade the structural or functional integrity of the musculoskeletal system?
- How are these dysfunctions segmentally related to other tissues and organ systems?

These questions form the core of rational osteopathic medical practice and the basis for the Five-Model Concept in the osteopathic approach to helping the patient find health.

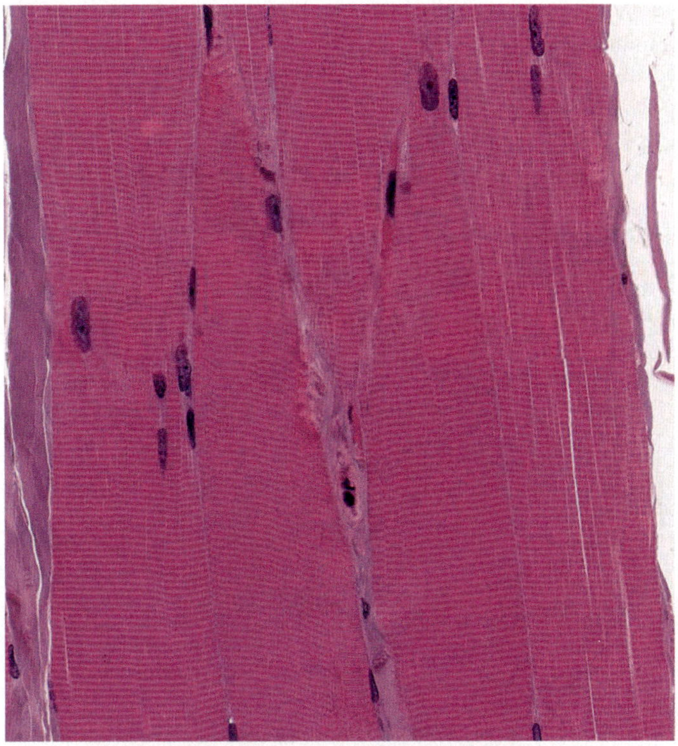

Figure 3.17. A histologic section of skeletal muscle. Note the striated pattern of myofibrils and the position of the nuclei along the outer margin of each myocyte.

Skeletal Muscle

The name skeletal muscle derives from the tissue's ability to produce forces conferred, via tendon, to bones.

- Skeletal muscle (e.g., latissimus dorsi) is composed of many elongated, multinucleate cells called muscle fibers or myofibers (Fig. 3.17).
  - A collection of these fibers can be classified as a fascicle (a bundle surrounded by a fascial perimysium).
  - All fibers innervated by a single motor neuron are classified as a motor unit.
- Embryologically, muscle fibers or myocytes derive from the fusion of uninucleate myoblasts into one elongated, multinucleated fiber, encased in a plasma membrane (sarcolemma).
  - Each nucleus governs a portion of the cytoplasm, known as a myonuclear domain.
- Hypertrophy of the fiber through exercise requires fusion of muscle-specific stem cells, called satellite cells, in order to reestablish the appropriate myonuclear domain.
- Similarly, myofiber atrophy may result in myonuclear apoptosis.
- A glance at a histologic section of skeletal muscle quickly reveals the precision in the organization of fibers present in each myocyte.
  - The highly differentiated cytoarchitecture of muscle tissue relates closely to the inability of the muscle tissue to heal following injury.

The ultrastructure of a muscle fiber (cell) is extremely well organized.

- Each muscle fiber is filled with myofibrils (see Fig. 3.17).
- Each myofibril is composed of sarcomeres aligned in series.
- The sarcomeres are functional units of skeletal muscle and are composed primarily of myosin and actin myofilaments (Fig. 3.18).

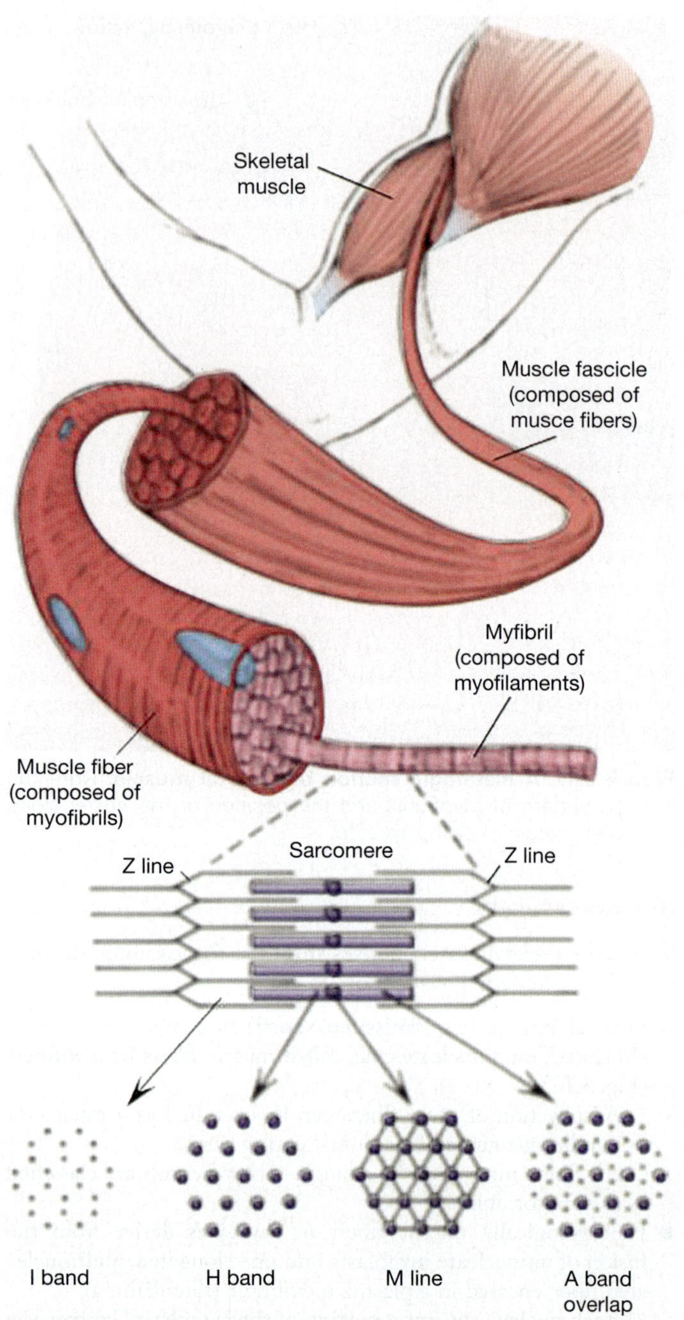

Figure 3.18. The structure of skeletal muscle. The muscle belly is seen at the top of the figure. An individual fascicle of the muscle has been pulled out, from which a myofibril has been isolated. The arrangement of myofilaments within the myofibril is then demonstrated. (Reprinted with permission from Ross MH, Pawlina W. *Histology: A Text and Atlas with Correlated Cell and Molecular Biology*. 6th ed. Wolters Kluwer Health/Lippincott Williams & Wilkins; 2011.)

- The myofilaments are held in a highly organized register, resulting in a striated appearance.

During muscle contraction, myosin pulls actin toward the center of the sarcomere, resulting in a shortening of the sarcomere.

- Simultaneous shortening of sarcomeres in series results in rapid reduction in muscle fiber length.
- The force produced by sarcomeric shortening causes tension in tendons, in turn pulling on bones to produce movement.[8]

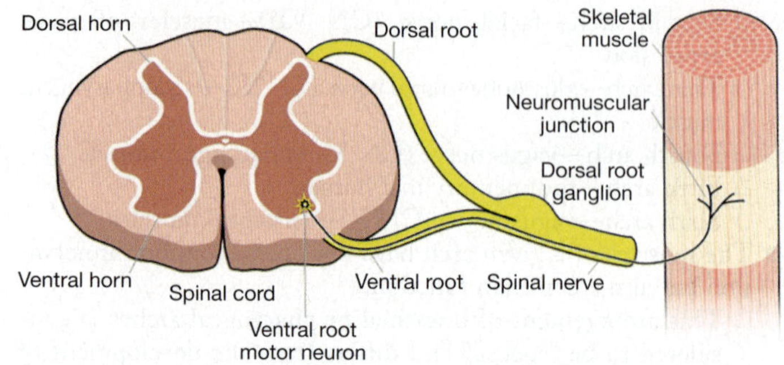

Figure 3.19. The motor unit. The spinal cord is illustrated above; the cell body of an alpha-motor neuron is seen in the ventral horn with its axon passing through the ventral root to reach the spinal nerve. Ultimately, the motor axon makes contact through neuromuscular synapses with several fascicles of the muscle. The ratio of fascicles to axons varies between muscles and is an index of the function of the muscle. Low ratios are more typical of muscles with precise, delicate tasks, while high ratios are seen in large muscles required to produce significant power in movement. (Courtesy of Oran Suta.)

A muscle normally contracts because it is stimulated by a motor nerve.

- A single motor nerve fiber innervates more than one skeletal muscle fiber.
- Motor units (one motor neuron and all muscle fibers that it innervates; Fig. 3.19) are scaled in size based on the delicate nature of the task it accomplishes.
  - Small muscles that react quickly (e.g., extraocular muscles) typically have 10 or fewer muscle fibers innervated by a single nerve fiber.
  - Large muscles that do not require fine CNS control (e.g., deep back muscles) may have up to 1,000 muscle fibers in a motor unit.
  - In the event of damage to a motor nerve fiber that results in loss of innervation to a motor unit, an adjacent nerve fiber will branch to take over the innervation duties. This increases the size, and decreases the precision, of the newly formed motor unit.
- When a muscle is resting, some motor units are always discharging. However, it may not be the same motor units at each instance in time.
  - This type of motor activity (muscle tone) is the background for muscular contraction in the performance of a purposeful movement.

When most muscles contract, their fibers act through tendons attached to moveable bones to obtain the desired action (Fig. 3.20).

- Most movements require the combined action of several muscles.
- The term prime mover is used for those muscles that act directly to bring about the desired movement.
- Movement results from the activation of motor units in prime movers, also called the agonist, and the simultaneous relaxation of motor units in opposing muscles, termed the antagonists. For example:
  - When considering flexion of the elbow:
    - The biceps brachii and brachialis facilitate flexion and are termed the agonist muscles.
    - The triceps brachii, an extensor muscle, is termed the antagonist muscle.

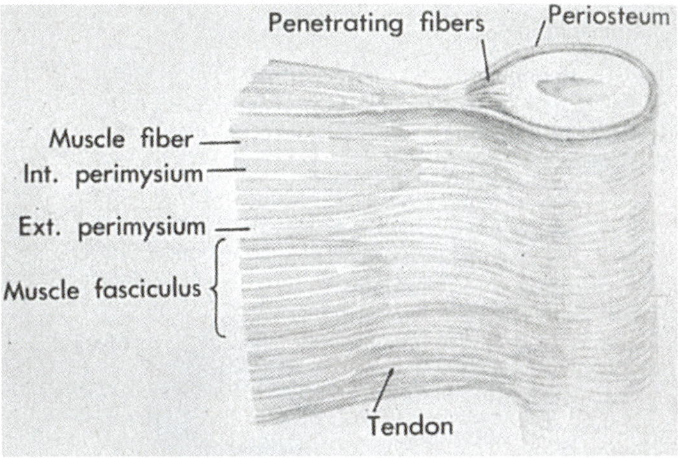

Figure 3.20. The muscle–tendon–bone junction. The myofibrils of the muscle are embedded into the tendon, and the collagenous fibers of the tendon fuse with the periosteum of the bone and can insert into the matrix of the bone as well. The complex junction between the tendon and the bone is termed the enthesis.

- The role of these two muscles will reverse when considering the extension of the elbow:
  - The triceps brachii is the agonist of extension, while the biceps brachii and brachialis are the antagonists of this movement.

Joint movement that comes about from muscle contraction will result in a change in length of the contracting muscles.

- However, during any such movement around a joint, both agonists and antagonists are contracting:
  - The agonist contracts more forcefully to produce movement.
  - The antagonist maintains some tonus that does not significantly block the action of the agonist.
- In this manner, the antagonist helps to stabilize the movement, reducing unwanted movements in the joint.
- When this occurs, tension created within the contracting muscles remains constant and the resulting contraction is termed isotonic.
  - Isotonic contractions may be concentric (shortening of the muscle) or eccentric (lengthening of the muscle).
- If the agonist and the antagonist contract equally, movement does not occur as a result of muscle contraction, and muscle length stays constant with elevated tension generated within the muscles; this type of contraction is termed isometric (e.g., posterior compartment muscles of the leg in standing).
- Agonist–antagonist muscle pairs that cocontract against each other are termed fixators.
  - This type of contraction occurs to stabilize a joint or hold a part of the body in an appropriate position.

Muscles that contract at the same time as the agonist–antagonist pair and that aid in the performance of a specific movement are termed synergists.

- Although these muscles are not the prime movers of the joint in a specified action, they can prevent unwanted movement that would be counterproductive to that action.
- A synergist muscle in one movement of a specific joint may become the prime mover in a different motion of that same joint.

Finally, individual muscles should not always be considered as isolated units with a single function, and different parts of the same muscle may have different, even antagonistic, actions (e.g., the trapezius).

- The upper portion of the trapezius elevates the scapula (shoulder).
- The lower portion of the trapezius depresses the scapula.

Any complex movement such as running or throwing a baseball will require a multitude of differing forms of muscle contractions happening throughout the body simultaneously. Coordination of this activity is derived from patterns of neural activity in the brain and spinal cord that are then relayed in a highly specific order to the muscles via peripheral nerves.

Peripheral Nerves

Nerves supply vital components to every portion of the body.

1. First, nerves provide control.
   - They are a major component of the body's homeostatic mechanisms.
   - Nerve cell bodies in the CNS send nerve fibers to control contraction of smooth (involuntary) muscles and skeletal (voluntary) muscles and to control secretion of glands.
2. Second, nerves also transmit sensory input.
   - They convey either exteroceptive input concerning physical forces that impinge on the body or interoceptive feedback about the status of the internal milieu.
3. Third, nerve fibers also deliver chemical materials from the CNS to the periphery and vice versa.
   - Through the mechanism of axoplasmic transport, trophic (growth promoting) chemicals are manufactured in the neuron cell body and carried to target muscles or organs where, after release into the synaptic space, they are taken into the target tissue to promote healthy function.
   - These chemical substances can be:
     - Small molecules (e.g., amino acids)
     - Neurotransmitters such as acetylcholine and serotonin
     - More complex molecules such as substance P, calcitonin gene-related peptide, somatostatin, glucagon, and vasoactive intestinal peptide that are associated with other physiologic functions.

Passing in the opposite direction, chemicals (messenger molecules) from the muscle or organ can cross the synapse, be taken up into the axon terminal, and be retrograde transported to the neuron cell bodies where the chemicals can then alter basic neuronal function.

- A bidirectional communication is established, fostering the exchange of information between the nervous system and the somatic and visceral tissues of the body.
- This communication between nerve and muscle is necessary to maintain the muscle.
  - Loss of the nerve will result in the eventual atrophy and loss of the muscle. Thus, the nerve is said to provide trophic substances maintaining the vitality of the muscle.[8]

Nerves are not synonymous with neurons.

- Neurons are cells capable of conducting an impulse either toward (afferent) or away from (efferent) the CNS.
  - Neurons consist of:
    - A cell body (soma, perikaryon).
    - One or more dendrites to deliver impulses to the soma.
    - A singular axon to convey an impulse toward an effector organ.
  - A neuron can be located either in the CNS or in a ganglion positioned along a nerve in the peripheral nervous system.

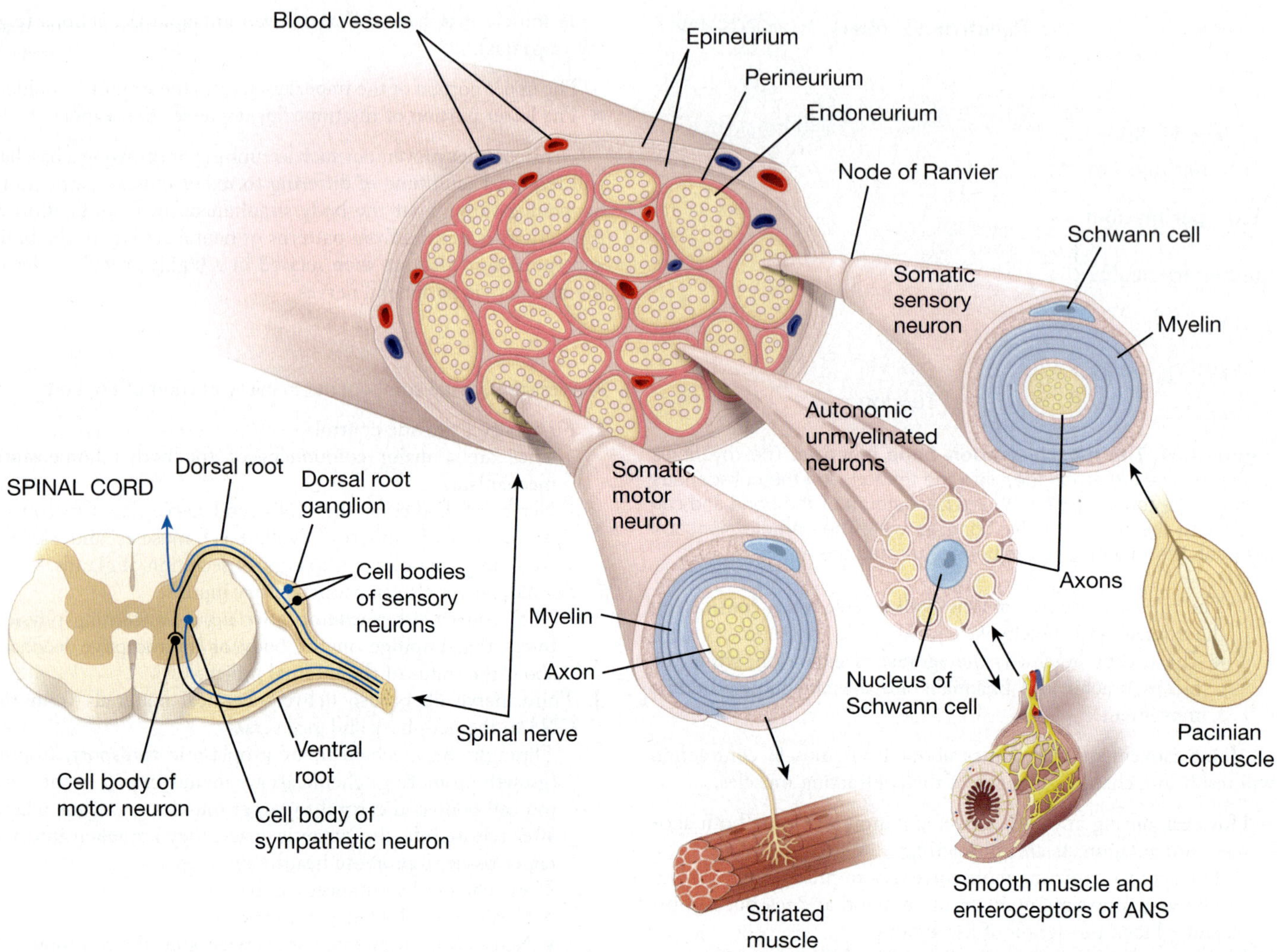

Figure 3.21. The spinal nerve. The spinal nerve is composed of the axons of many neurons. Sensory neurons have peripheral receptors with axons leading back to the spinal cord; their cell bodies are located in the dorsal root ganglion. Motor neurons have a cell body located in the ventral horn and an axon that exits the spinal cord on the ventral root passing through the spinal nerve to reach the appropriate muscle. Finally, not shown in this diagram, the spinal nerve will also carry the axons of ganglionic neurons of the autonomic nervous system. (Reprinted with permission from Pawlina W. *Histology: A Text and Atlas with Correlated Cell and Molecular Biology*. 7th ed. Wolters Kluwer; 2016.)

- A nerve, on the other hand, is located only in the peripheral nervous system and is a collection of axons and dendrites traveling within a series of fascial sheaths (endo-, peri-, and epineurium; Fig. 3.21).

Dendrites provide an important function: gathering information through numerous synaptic connections or receptor organs. The number of dendrites on a given neuron varies significantly depending on the function of the neuron.

- Multipolar neurons typically have many dendrites delivering impulses toward the soma and one axon conveying the impulse away.
  - Efferent (somatic and visceral) neurons and interneurons are multipolar.
- Bipolar neurons have exactly one axon and one dendrite.
  - Bipolar neurons are only located in the retina (cranial nerve II) and in the ganglia of the vestibulocochlear nerve (cranial nerve VIII).
- Pseudounipolar neurons (occasionally, erroneously termed unipolar) have a singular axon that bifurcates functionally into a process that conveys impulses toward the soma and a process that conveys impulses away from the soma.
  - Typically, these neurons carry sensory impulses, and their somas reside in either dorsal root ganglia or cranial nerve ganglia.
- Their cell body is located in the dorsal root ganglion.
- Their central process, termed an axon, extends through the dorsal root carrying information away from the cell body to the spinal cord.
- Their peripheral process, termed a dendrite, passes through a peripheral nerve to gather information from target tissue somewhere in the body, and carry that information toward the cell body.
- However, upon histologic examination, the peripheral and the central process appear to be the same and behave in the same way upon electrophysiologic study.
  - Thus, although the peripheral process is functioning as a dendrite by carrying information toward the cell body, it appears similar to an axon in its structure and physiology.
  - For this reason, axons and dendrites traveling in peripheral nerves are often simply termed fibers.

The impulse carried in neurons is a wave of depolarization, called an action potential.

- The speed at which an action potential is propagated in many axons is augmented by myelination.
  - Myelin is a sheath of insulation created by several wraps of the plasma membrane of Schwann cells (or oligodendrocytes in the CNS).
  - The myelin prevents transcellular ion exchange, thereby forcing the action potential to "jump" to a gap in the myelination, known as a node of Ranvier.
- The process of jumping from node to node is called saltatory conduction and increases propagation speed while reducing energy requirements.
- As this action potential reaches the axon terminal, it stimulates the release of neurotransmitters that cross a synaptic cleft and bind receptors on a postsynaptic cell (e.g., another neuron, muscle fiber, gland) (for additional details, see Boron and Boulpaep[15]).

Between the spinal cord and the peripheral target tissue, nerve fibers travel through numerous different components of the peripheral nervous system. Each component is important since it can manifest with a differential clinical presentation when damaged.[16]

- Beginning with the spinal cord, numerous rootlets are formed both dorsally and ventrally; these rootlets combine within the spinal canal to form 31 pairs of dorsal and ventral roots.
- Spinal nerves are then formed by the convergence of dorsal and ventral roots within the intervertebral foramen. Although the dorsal and ventral roots are segregated functionally (sensory and motor), once they combine, the resulting spinal nerve is mixed, containing both sensory and motor fibers.
- After leaving the intervertebral foramen, the spinal nerve diverges into dorsal and ventral primary rami, heading toward the epaxial and hypaxial masses, respectively.
- Peripheral nerves are formed from the subsequent branching of these dorsal and ventral primary rami and are composed of axons from both sensory and motor neurons (see Fig. 3.21).

Peripheral nerves carry somatic motor and sensory fibers along with axons from neurons associated with the autonomic nervous system. The location of cell bodies varies with the function of the neuron:

- The bodies of somatic motor neurons reside in the ventral horns of the spinal cord.
- The bodies of sensory neurons reside in the dorsal root ganglion.
- The preganglionic cell bodies of autonomic nervous system neurons reside in the lateral horn of the spinal cord or in the brain stem.
- The postganglionic cell bodies of autonomic nervous system neurons predominantly reside in the sympathetic trunk (sympathetic) or in mural ganglia (parasympathetic) (see Chapter 6 Autonomic Nervous System for further discussion).

As described above, individual peripheral nerves have a specific segmental relationship to the CNS and, therefore, to the entire body. The segmental origin of nerves is pertinent to three general targets of innervation:

1. Skin
2. Muscles
3. Internal organs

The dermatomal (skin) innervation pattern is relatively straightforward (see Fig. 3.10).

- Pain or sensory loss over some specific dermatomal zone leads the physician to infer about the integrity of restricted areas of the CNS or of nerves near their origin.
- Innervation of the skin of the limbs becomes a bit more complicated because the sensory nerves from specific spinal cord segments are drawn together into specific cutaneous nerves that contain sensory fibers from more than one spinal cord segment.
- A specific peripheral nerve, such as the medial cutaneous nerve of the forearm, will contain fibers from two or more segments, in this case C8 and T1, although those fibers will distribute at their termination in the skin in a dermatomal pattern.
- Here, the notion is that the examining physician must have sufficient understanding of anatomy to be able to differentiate sensory disturbances that arise in a particular peripheral nerve, termed peripheral neuropathy, as opposed to an entire segmental level as occurs when a spinal nerve or root is damaged, termed radiculopathy.

The innervation pattern of muscles is particularly pertinent to osteopathic medicine because changes in the tone, texture, or function of a muscle may be related to the dysfunction of the segmental source of nerve supply to that muscle.

- The innervation of muscles of the trunk is relatively simple and follows a pattern similar to that of the dermatomes.
- Nerve fibers to the muscles of the limbs, on the other hand, arise from the spinal cord and are woven through complex networks (the brachial plexus and lumbosacral plexus; see Fig. 3.11) that combine fibers from several spinal cord segments into motor nerves that typically serve functional groups of muscles.
- A physician must understand innervation of limb muscles well enough to reconstruct those nerve fibers from their termination, through the plexus to their spinal cord origin.
- As with the sensory nerves, the goal for the physician is to be able to differentiate motor losses due to compromise of a distal, peripheral nerve versus losses associated with a lesion of one or more spinal cord segments or associated spinal nerves.

The internal viscera receive abundant autonomic nerve supply. The sensory innervation to the internal viscera that signals functional status, distention, and pain typically accompanies the autonomic innervation to the target organ (Fig. 3.22).

- The various patterns by which this autonomic and sensory nerve supply arises from the spinal cord or brain stem and passes to the target tissue are presented in Chapter 6 Autonomic Nervous System.
- The key point to be made, however, is that because of developmental and maturational events, an organ in the adult may come to be relatively distant from its embryonic, segmental origin having pulled its nerve supply with it during the developmental period. For this reason:
  - Pathologic changes in a specific organ will be sensed by nerve fibers that report to the part of the developed neural tube (i.e., the spinal cord or brainstem) that was adjacent to that organ's embryonic, segmental origin.
  - Pathologic changes in a particular visceral organ may appear as pain to the body surface some distance from the organ.
  - The painful or altered input from an organ can alter the somatic and autonomic outflow from that part of the spinal cord.
- For example, aberrant sensory feedback from a diseased organ can produce changes in muscle tonus or sympathetic function at a seemingly unrelated site.
- Conversely, painful sensory input from localized musculoskeletal misalignment may produce alteration in autonomic outflow

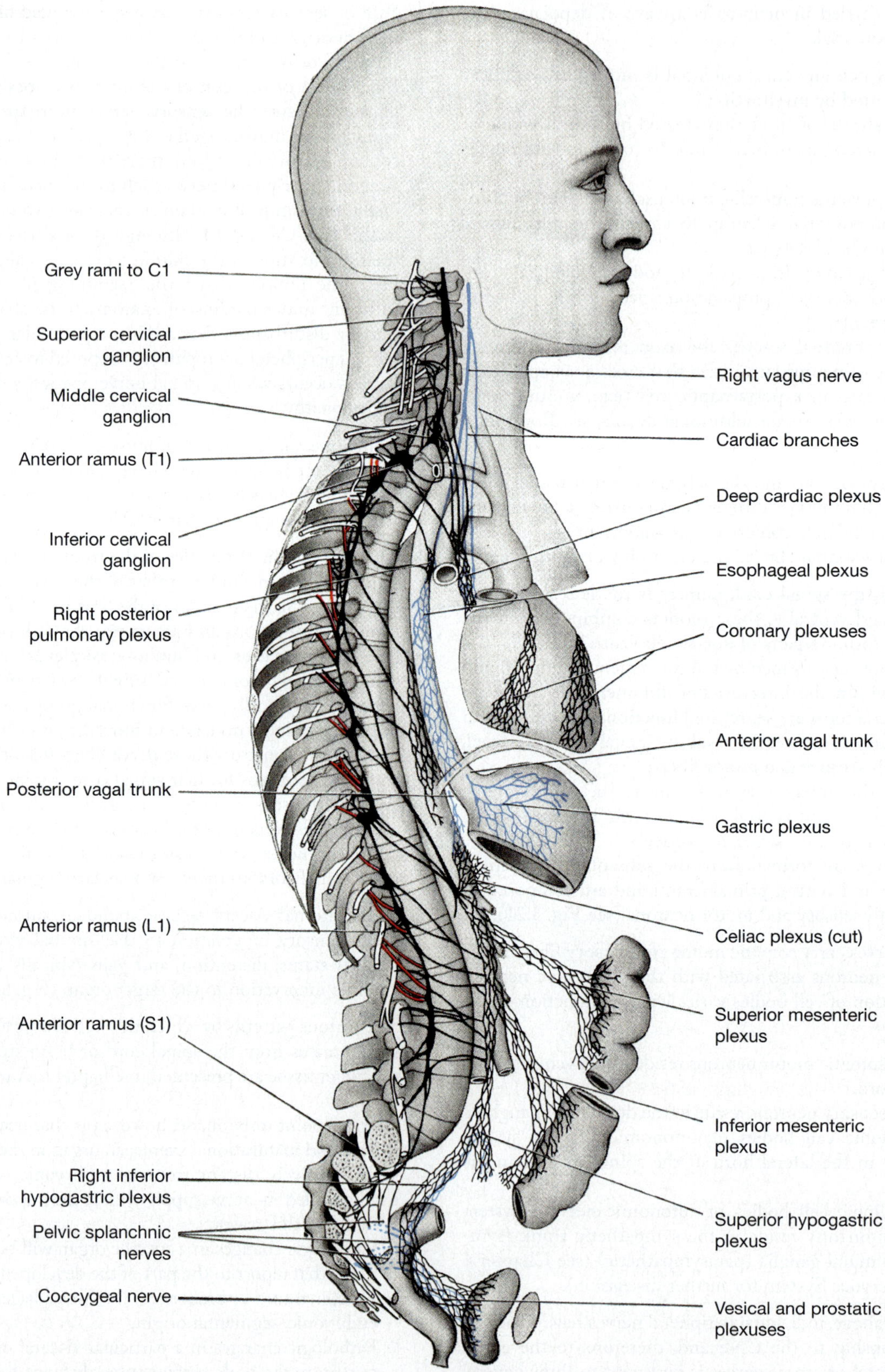

Figure 3.22. The autonomic nervous system of the thorax, abdomen, and pelvis. A dense plexus of autonomic fibers is seen extending from the thoracic region, through the diaphragm, into the abdominopelvic cavity. (Used with permission of Elsevier Science & Technology Journals from Warwick R, Williams PL. *Gray's Anatomy*. 35th ed. Churchill Livingstone; 1973:1071; permission conveyed through Copyright Clearance Center, Inc.)

from the related segmental zone of the spinal cord and may disturb function in an internal organ some distance away from that segment.

- In a very general way, internal organs map to the body surface and vice versa, through shared spinal cord segments.
- Therefore, to make accurate diagnoses, the osteopathic physician must:
  - Understand both the general segmental origin and the anatomical pathway by which autonomic nerve fibers and the accompanying sensory nerve fibers pass to the various internal organs.
  - Be alert to the implications of pain and musculoskeletal changes as diagnostic clues and treatment options.

Nerves supply important functional and trophic control to all parts of the body. An important aspect of osteopathic medical practice is to recognize and treat conditions that alter nerve supply to a region or organ.

- How well the physician understands the route that nerves take from their origin to their destination directly affects:
  - The success of palpation and treatments in recognizing and relieving compression or irritation to nerves.
  - The effectiveness of maintenance of nerve traffic by healthy lifestyles.
- This arrangement is the basis for the **neurologic model**, one of the five models used in the osteopathic approach to the patient.

Finally, the peripheral nervous system and the spinal cord are under the control of neurons located in the forebrain and brain stem.

- Forebrain regions that are particularly sensitive to emotions and stress can significantly affect the peripheral somatic and autonomic nervous system, altering skeletal muscle and organ system functions. These regions include the
  - Ventral aspect of the prefrontal cortex
  - Medial aspect of the temporal cortex
  - Ventral aspect of the insular cortex
- This is the underlying basis of the **behavioral or psychosocial model**, one of the five conceptual models used in the osteopathic approach to the patient.

Vasculature and Lymphatics

STRUCTURE

Two structural entities, arteries and nerves, are important for the health and maintenance of any organ or area.

- Arteries supply nutrients, oxygen, and a variety of immune and endocrine regulatory substances to the area of their distribution.
- Nerves provide ongoing neural control of skeletal and smooth muscle and glandular tissue as well as deliver trophic or regulatory factors to the muscles or organs that they innervate.
- A.T. Still[1] noted the importance of having appropriate vascular supply to maintain the normal health of the tissue as stated in his "Rule of the Artery."
- The movement of fluid in and out of tissues everywhere in the body forms the basis for the **circulatory–respiratory model**, one of the five conceptual models used in diagnostic and treatment protocols by osteopathic physicians.

This discussion of vasculature includes blood vessels and lymphatic vessels.

- During blood circulation, arteries and arterioles typically carry oxygen-rich blood, under high pressure, to capillaries.
- Venules and veins return poorly oxygenated blood to the heart under low pressure.
- These functional distinctions dictate microstructural variation.
- The walls of most blood vessels contain three distinct tunics, but the thickness and composition of these layers vary among the types of vessels (Fig. 3.23):
  1. Tunica intima
  2. Tunica media
  3. Tunica adventitia

The tunica intima is nearest the vessel lumen and consists of a simple squamous (single, scalelike) endothelial cell layer and an underlying subendothelial layer of loose connective tissue.

- Larger vessels contain a visible layer of fenestrated elastin fibers called an internal elastic membrane.
- The elastin of the internal elastic membrane accommodates for changes in blood pressure while the fenestrae allow for diffusion to the outer layers of the vessel wall.

The tunica media consists primarily of concentric smooth muscle layers (Fig. 3.24).

- Gap junctions between the endothelial cells and these smooth muscles cells allow the tunica intima and tunica media to maintain a close functional relationship.
- In addition to functioning in vasoconstriction, smooth muscle of the tunica media produces the ECM (collagen and elastic fibers, ground substance) for this layer.
- Larger arteries contain high quantities of elastic fibers in the tunica media, and an external elastic lamina is often visible histologically separating the tunica media from the tunica adventitia.
- The tunica media is the thickest layer in arteries and arterioles.[8]

Tunica adventitia is composed of dense connective tissue that follows the contours of the vessel.

- Elements of the tunica adventitia blend with neighboring connective tissue, allowing unimpeded distension of the vessels.
- In large, thick-walled vessels, the tunica adventitia contains its own collection of arteries and veins, termed the vasa vasorum, that perfuse the tissue within its walls along with its own collection of nerves, termed the nervi vasorum.
- The tunica adventitia is the thickest layer in veins.

Beginning with the aorta, the continuum of vessels starts with elastic arteries containing a thick, elastin-rich tunica media and many vasa vasorum in the tunica adventitia (Box 3.2).

- As arteries branch from the aorta, their tunica media will progressively lose most of their elastin content and become predominated by smooth muscle.
- As the number of smooth muscle cell layers decreases to two, the vessel becomes known as an arteriole.
  - Arterioles will continue to give off branches of smaller lumen caliber and thinner walls.
- When the lumen diameter reaches approximately 8 µm and the tunica media and adventitia layers become indiscernible, then the vessel becomes known as a capillary.
  - It is through the thin walls of these capillaries that most gas and fluid exchange occur.
- Distal to the capillary, lumen size will increase in venules (Fig. 3.25).
  - Larger venules will have a layer or two of smooth muscle but are discernible from arterioles by a much larger lumen size and larger tunica adventitia.
  - Venules deliver blood to progressively larger veins—identified by their larger tunica adventitia to tunica media ratio.

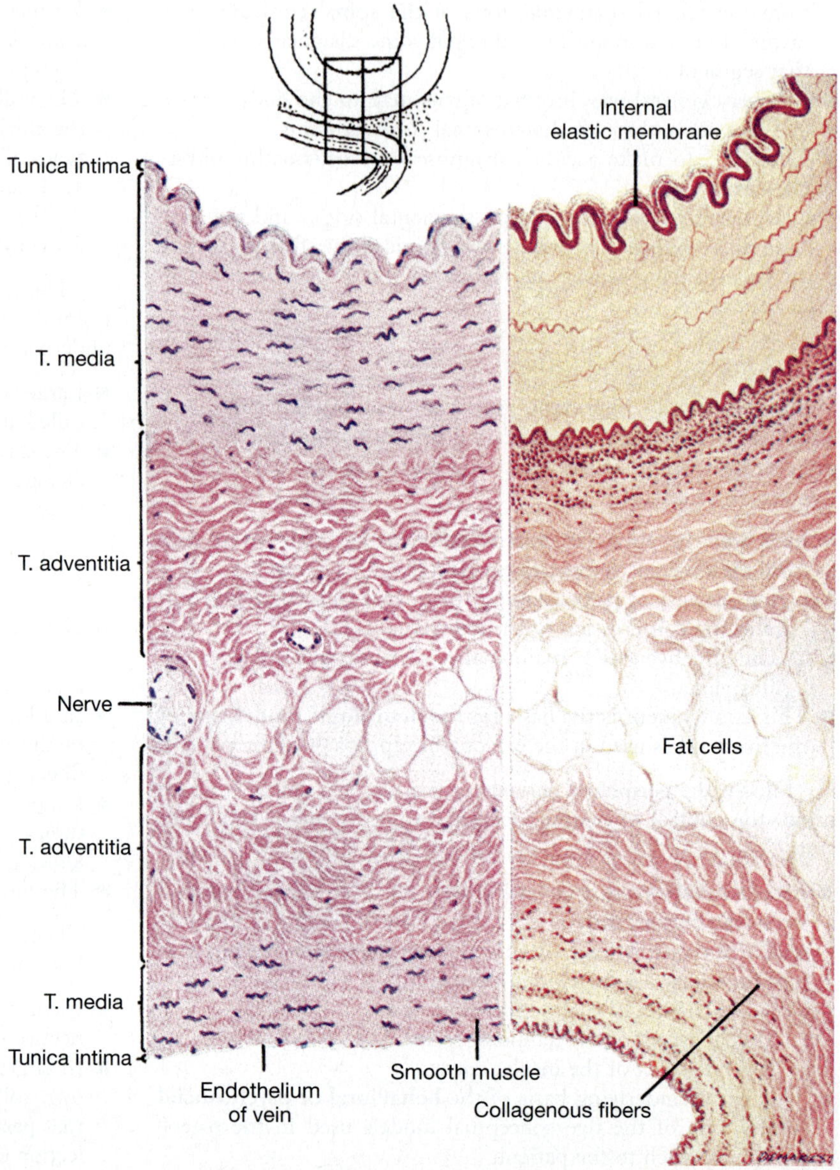

Figure 3.23. The layered wall of blood vessels. A cross-sectional view of an artery and vein illustrates the three layers present in the wall: the three tunics are intima, media, and adventitia. Although present in most large vessels, their composition and thickness vary greatly between arteries, veins, and lymphatic vessels. The artery is on the right and the vein on the left. (Reprinted with permission from Kelly DE, Wood RL, Enders AC. *Bailey's Textbook of Microscopic Anatomy*. 18th ed. Williams & Wilkins; 1984.)

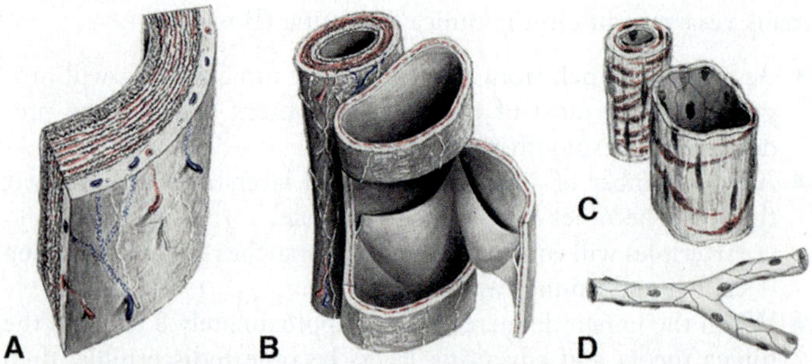

Figure 3.24. Vascular wall structure. A. The aorta illustrating elastic fibers in the tunica media. The vasa vasorum and nervi vasorum are seen on the wall of the aorta. **B.** A muscular artery and large vein with smooth muscle in the tunica media and valves in the tunica intima of the vein. **C.** An arteriole and venule with a thin layer of smooth muscle in the arteriole and scattered slips of smooth muscle in the venule. **D.** A capillary composed of just endothelial cells. (Reprinted with permission from Lockhart RD, Hamilton GF, Fyfe FW. *Anatomy of the Human Body*. J.B. Lippincott Company; 1960.)

BOX 3.2 High- Versus Low-Pressure Systems

- Blood is forced along the circulatory system by a cardiac pump, creating a high pressure system on the arterial side.
- Arterial pressure is reduced with successive branching of the vasculature, approaching 35 mm Hg at the arteriolar end of the capillary, and continuing to decline to approximately 5 to 10 mm Hg at the venular end of the capillary.
- If blood pressure is higher than osmotic pressure, fluid and some plasma proteins filter into the extracellular space as interstitial fluid.
- Conversely, if blood pressure is lower than osmotic pressure, interstitial fluid is reabsorbed.
- Pressure in venous and lymphatic vessels is low, relying on the contraction of neighboring muscles to force fluid through valves.

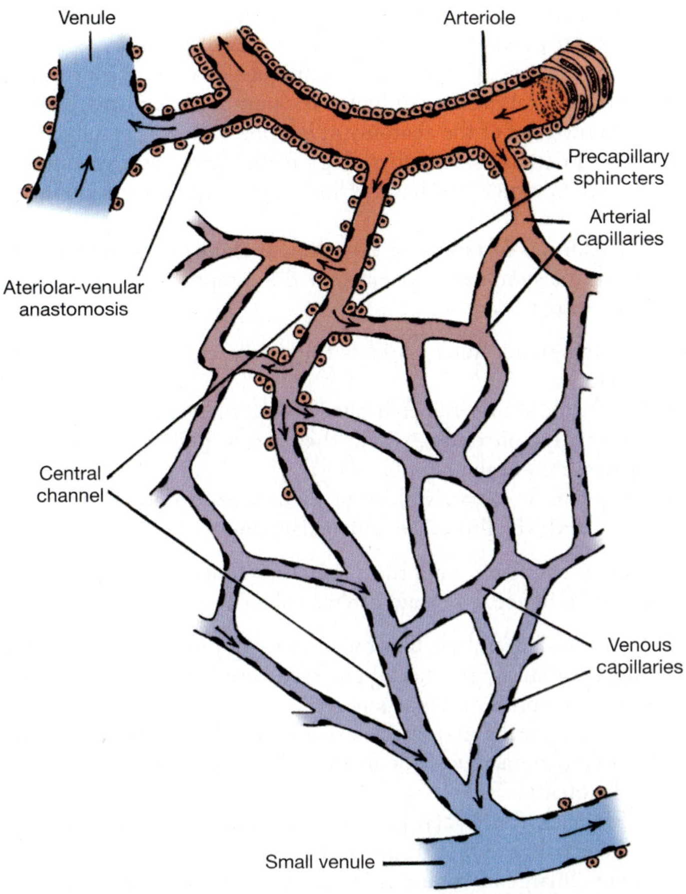

Figure 3.25. The capillary bed. This diagram illustrates the arterial flow into a capillary bed and its subsequent venous drainage. Arterioles have a thin layer of smooth muscle. Precapillary sphincters have isolated slips of smooth muscle. Capillaries have no smooth muscle layer. Small veins (venules) have only isolated slips of smooth muscle in their wall. (Reprinted with permission from Kelly DE, Wood RL, Enders AC. *Bailey's Textbook of Microscopic Anatomy*. 18th ed. Williams & Wilkins; 1984.)

As blood passes through the capillaries, fluid passes through the capillary wall from the lumen to the ECM.

- Nearer the arteriolar end of the capillary, more plasma filtrate passes out of the capillary than can be taken up by the venule-associated end of the capillary.
- Lymphatic vessels are responsible for removing most of this fluid, as well as proteins and particulate matter, from the ECM.
  - In a 24-hour span, approximately 3 L of lymph is removed.
- If the lymphatic system fails to remove lymph from the ECM, osmotic pressures will rise above the physiologic range. This leads to the clinical result of edema, the collection of fluid in tissue.
- Understanding the role of lymphatic tissue in maintaining fluid homeostatic balance is a critical component of the circulatory–respiratory model.

Lymphatic capillaries, consisting of little more than a collection of overlapping endothelial cells oriented around a blindly ending lumen, reside in the connective tissue.

The endothelial cells blend into the surrounding connective tissue via anchoring filaments. Pressure in the lymph capillaries is low (1 mm Hg or less).

- As pressure rises in the ECM, the anchoring filaments come under tension.
- At that time, the overlapping borders of endothelial cells open like valves and allow fluid to enter the capillary.
- Lymph capillaries merge into a plexus that is drained by larger afferent vessels.
- Once in the vessel, lymph will flow toward lymph nodes, as dictated by unidirectional valves, driven by:
  - Contraction of scattered slips of smooth muscle in the vessel walls
  - Contraction of surrounding skeletal muscle
  - The movements of the body
- Within the lymph node, lymph is filtered and immune responses are mounted against foreign antigens.
- Lymph is then carried away from the node via efferent lymphatic vessels. Approximately 30% of lymph in a lymph node is returned to venous circulation via high endothelial venules.
  - Larger lymphatic vessels contain oblique slips of smooth muscle between the valves that contract at an intrinsic rhythm.
- Eventually, these large lymphatic vessels flow into a duct (thoracic duct or right lymphatic duct) that will return the lymph to venous circulation.

For additional details on the histology of the lymphatic system, see Pawlina.[8]

FUNCTION

Few statements are more cogent than A.T. Still's insightful dictum, "the rule of the artery is supreme."

- An adequate blood supply during varying physiologic conditions is a prerequisite for health of any organ or body region.
- Conversely, compromise to the blood supply often leads to diminished functional capacity, cascading, in turn, toward disease both locally and systemically.
- In this sense, the osteopathic physician must work to ensure continued blood supply in the healthy state and, when treating injury or disease, should attempt to enhance arterial supply to affected regions.
- The recognition of ischemia or anoxia in the tissue requires both knowledge of the blood supply and knowledge of metabolic processes.
- These two content areas form the basis of the respiratory–circulatory model and the **metabolic energy model** used by the osteopathic physician in the approach to the patient.

The mainstay of the osteopathic approach involves:

1. Optimizing the flow of blood into and out of a region of tissue.
2. Ensuring adequate oxygenation of the blood through a well-functioning respiratory movement.
3. Providing sufficient nutrients for maintaining appropriate energy metabolism.

It is designed to help the patient's body return to the most healthful state possible for that individual.

One of the goals of an osteopathic approach to medical treatment is, first, to recognize which aspect of surrounding tissue might be compressing an artery and, having visualized the mechanical impediment to blood flow, adopt appropriate treatment to relieve the compression and thereby restore normal flow. Similarly, the osteopathic physician works to recognize in the healthy individual those areas or organs that might be at risk for reduced blood flow caused by lifestyle, activities, posture, obesity, etc., and adopt a treatment plan to maintain health in zones that may be at risk.

While the arterial supply is the only means by which fluid and blood cellular components are taken to an area, two pathways remove fluids and blood cells from a region.

1. The venous network collects the deoxygenated blood from the capillary bed.
2. The lymphatic channels drain the relatively cell-free extracellular fluid that accumulates outside the vascular system.

Compromise to either of these return channels leads to edema in the affected area: simply put, more fluid goes in to the tissue than comes out.

To alleviate edema, a protocol may be chosen to enhance venous and/or lymphatic return.

- The selected strategy will depend on the medical condition of the patient and a thorough knowledge of the anatomy and physiology of the venous and lymphatic systems.
- As with the arterial system, the knowledge of anatomy places venous and lymphatic channels into the context of surrounding organs, muscles, bones, fascia, etc., usually by appreciating those structures on the basis of subtle palpable or surface landmarks.

Peripheral venous channels tend to be somewhat variable, with considerable anastomoses. For general medical application, it is acceptable to understand the overall pattern of peripheral venous drainage and to concentrate effort on the larger, more predictable central veins.

- Understanding the anastomoses of peripheral venous channels is useful in the treatment of tissue fluid imbalance. For example, venous anastomoses offer therapeutic strategies for the physician as alternate routes of venous drainage are established.
- Understanding the routes of venous anastomoses is critical to correctly diagnosing pathology as significant venous blood flow through some anastomoses is unusual and may indicate a pathologic condition.

The rule of venous drainage is to know:

1. By which veins an area is typically drained of blood.
2. By what routes blood drains if the typical route is blocked.
3. Where the veins lie relative to the surrounding structures.

This knowledge can assist in designing a plan for restoration of normal function in a patient suffering with edematous conditions.

Lymphatic channels are typically even more variable than veins in their gross morphology; knowing general patterns and spatial relations of lymph drainage is usually sufficient.

- Although they are less well defined anatomically, they are important to understand.
- As with venous return, selecting osteopathic approaches to treatment of edema assumes a working knowledge of the location of lymph channels and how to augment lymphatic flow.[8]

As the lymphatic system has no centrally located, intrinsic pump, as that seen in the cardiovascular system, fluid is moved from peripheral to central regions by:

- Osmotic pressure differentials
- Skeletal muscular contractions
- External pressure differentials
- Thoracoabdominal pressure differentials
- Contraction of mural smooth muscle

There are various techniques to increase lymphatic return; however, simply restoring normal movement to the musculoskeletal system in that portion of the body, thus allowing the patient to perform daily activities of living, can be very helpful in regaining fluid homeostasis. When using techniques of muscle contraction or applying local pressure or lymphatic pump mechanisms, prerequisite knowledge of the anatomy of lymphatic flow is required. For additional details on the physiology of the lymphatic system, see Hall[17] and Chapter 14 Anatomy and Physiology of the Lymphatic System.

In addition to returning extracellular fluid to the general circulation, the lymphatic system and the lymph nodes may often indicate disease.

- The lymphoid system houses important cells of the immune system.
- As a result of infection, lymphocytes proliferate and are sequestered in lymph nodes, where they attack pathogens (bacteria, viruses, etc.) in the lymph.
- Cancer in an organ will often metastasize to adjacent lymph nodes and will also cause node enlargement.

Because of this important immune function, lymph nodes draining an infected area are often swollen and palpable.

- It is crucial, therefore, that the examining physician understand the potential significance of enlarged lymph nodes and the pattern of lymph flow. For example:
  - Breast cancer may metastasize to the lymph nodes on the lateral thoracic wall or in the axilla that drain lymph from the breast.
  - Stomach cancer can present as an enlarged node above the clavicle in the root of the neck.
- When enlarged lymph nodes are detected, the examining physician can use knowledge of the anatomical pattern by which lymph drains to infer the source of a disease process.

Connective Tissue

Of the basic tissue types, connective tissue is unique in that it is not composed exclusively of cells.

- Connective tissue is composed of three components, in varying proportions:
  1. Cells
  2. Fibers
  3. Ground substance (glycosaminoglycans [GAGs], proteoglycans, and glycoproteins)
- The most common cell types in connective tissue (e.g., fibroblasts, mast cells, macrophages) are described in this chapter.
  - However, other cell types (e.g., lymphocytes) may also infiltrate the fascia, under pathologic conditions.
- Fibers and ground substance together are commonly referred to as ECM.
  - The ECM creates a structural network while also generating an environment for transient cell migration and nutrient/waste exchange.
  - The ECM also participates in growth factor sequestration and the ECM–cell interface facilitates mechanotransduction.[18]

Several types of connective tissue are described. Based on the orientation of collagenous fibers, connective tissue can be termed regular or irregular.

- In regular connective tissue, the collagenous fibers have a definitive pattern of arrangement, such as is seen in tendons, ligaments, and aponeuroses (Fig. 3.26).

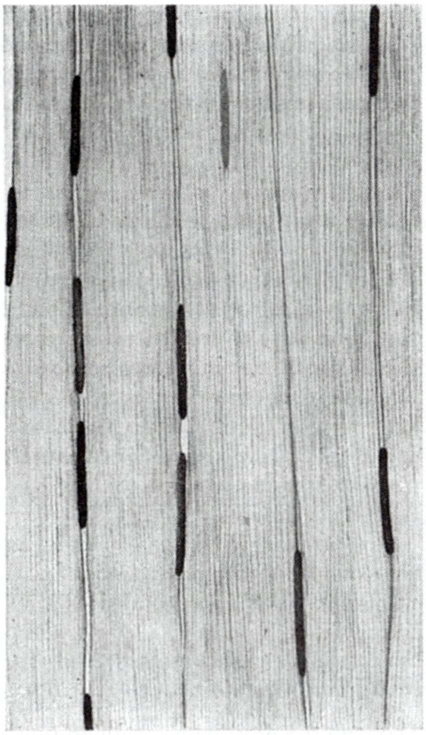

Figure 3.26. The distribution of fibrocytes and collagen fibers in dense regular connective tissue, such as a tendon or ligament. Note the common alignment of the collagenous fiber bundles in this tissue. (Reprinted with permission from Kelly DE, Wood RL, Enders AC. *Bailey's Textbook of Microscopic Anatomy.* 18th ed. Williams & Wilkins; 1984.)

- Conversely, connective tissue with an irregular arrangement of collagenous fibers is typically termed fascia.
  - If the ratio of cells to fibers is high, the tissue is termed loose connective tissue (Fig. 3.27).
  - If the ratio of cells to fibers is low, it is termed dense connective tissue.

Fibroblasts

The fibroblast is the primary cell type in basic connective tissue (see Figs. 3.27 and 3.28).

- Although quiescent fibroblasts are fusiform, active fibroblasts assume a stellate form.
- The dendritic processes of adjacent fibroblasts often bind through gap junctions, thus contributing to a three-dimensional network within the connective tissue.[19]

Fibroblasts produce most of the ground substance and fibrillar content of the ECM.

- Fibroblasts also help to regulate the interstitium.[8]
- They monitor the ECM for altered tension or chemical composition that may be produced in neighboring tissues (e.g., muscle contraction, local inflammation) or externally (e.g., osteopathic manipulation).
- In response to these tissue changes, fibroblasts may release growth factors, interleukins, and matrix metalloproteases.
- They may also produce minute smooth muscle–like contractions to modify tissue tone.

In response to more extreme mechanical strain, fibroblasts can differentiate into myofibroblasts.

- Myofibroblasts retain a resemblance to fibroblasts, but express smooth muscle α-actin (α-SMA).
  - The α-SMA can sustain contractions for long durations.
- The myofibroblasts form stress fibers that attach to extracellular fibers and elements of the ground substance via cadherins, thereby passing the tension they produce through the local environment.
- The myofibroblasts may continue to produce components of the ECM.
- These functions continue as long as the mechanical strain persists.
  - Conversely, if the strain is resolved, the myofibroblasts remove themselves from the connective tissue through a process involving apoptosis.

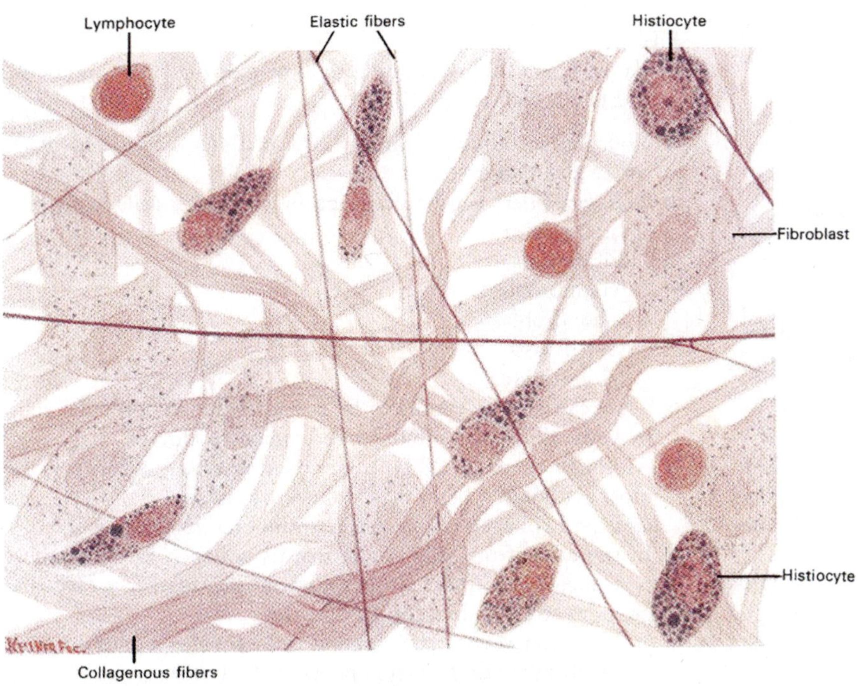

Figure 3.27. The cellular and fibrous components of loose connective tissue. Note the irregular weave of collagenous fibers present in this tissue. (Reprinted with permission from Kelly DE, Wood RL, Enders AC. *Bailey's Textbook of Microscopic Anatomy.* 18th ed. Williams & Wilkins; 1984.)

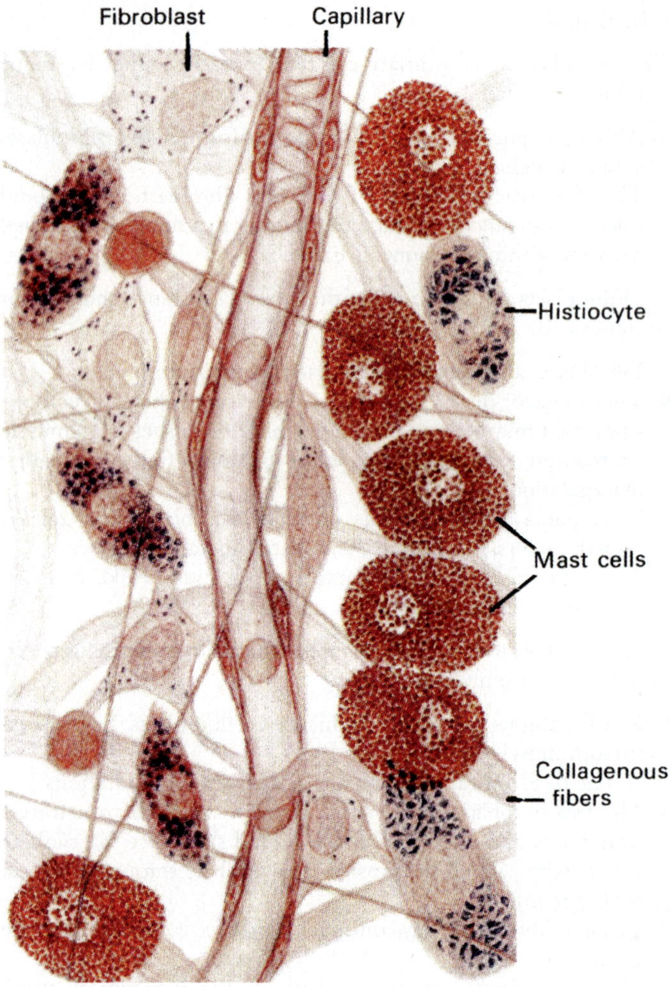

Figure 3.28. The cells of connective tissue. This is a section of loose connective tissue demonstrating the presence of mast cells, macrophages (histiocytes), and fibroblasts. (Reprinted with permission from Kelly DE, Wood RL, Enders AC. *Bailey's Textbook of Microscopic Anatomy*. 18th ed. Williams & Wilkins; 1984.)

The location, function, and adaptability of fibroblasts enable them to respond well to both injury and manipulation of soft tissue. Research suggests that osteopathic manipulation may:

- Increase tissue hydration
- Rearrange collagen cross-links
- Alter mechanical forces of the fibroblasts
- See Chapter 7 The Fascial System of the Body for additional information on myofibroblasts.

MACROPHAGES

Macrophages (histiocytes) are large resident cells in basic connective tissue (see Figs. 3.27 and 3.28). Believed to be derived from circulating monocytes, they perform important immune functions in the ECM.

- Macrophages phagocytose foreign material and cellular debris.[8]
- Epitopic peptide fragments from the foreign matter are then loaded onto major histocompatibility complex II molecules, allowing the macrophages to act as antigen-presenting cells.
- Macrophages are classified into either M1 or M2 macrophages.
  - M1 releases proinflammatory cytokines, reactive oxygen intermediates, and nitric oxide as a protective mechanism against bacteria and some viruses.
  - M2 releases anti-inflammatory cytokines, such as TGF-β and IL-10. They also participate in wound repair by stimulating fibroblast proliferation and collagen deposition. They may also promote myofibroblast differentiation.

These functions promote tissue healing but in chronic conditions may result in fibrosis and scarring.

- For more details on macrophage function, see Delves et al.[20]

MAST CELLS

Like macrophages, mast cells are of the myeloid lineage and enter circulation prior to maturation. They take up residence in connective tissue (see Fig. 3.28) where they complete their development.

- Two subtypes of mast cell have been identified based on location:
  - Mucosal mast cells
  - Connective tissue mast cells
- Both are integral in coordinating immune function.
- The predominate subtype found in basic connective tissue produces proteases (chymase and tryptase), proinflammatory cytokines (e.g., tumor necrosis factor-α, interleukin-4), and eicosanoids (e.g., prostaglandin D2).

Mast cells migrate into injured or inflamed tissue where they can exacerbate the inflammatory process as well as perform phagocytosis.

- These cells contain receptors with a high affinity for immunoglobulin E (IgE).
- The IgE isotype is active in parasitic reactions and allergic reactions.
- Upon binding to the receptor, mast cells degranulate, releasing heparin, histamine, and several enzymes including tryptase, carboxypeptidase, and acid hydrolase.
- The release of histamine and heparin into connective tissue gives mast cells an active role in[21]:
  - The normal healing process
  - Host defense mechanisms
  - Acute and chronic inflammation
  - Angiogenesis
- Mast cells also participate in fibroblast activity and potentially facilitate fibrosis through the release of tumor necrosis factor-α.

FIBERS

Collagen fibers are present in both loose (see Fig. 3.27) and dense connective tissue (see Fig. 3.26).

- Collagen accounts for almost 20% of tissue volume in dense connective tissue.
- Collagen fibers can be produced by numerous cells of mesenchymal origin:
  - Fibroblasts
  - Myofibroblasts
  - Chondroblasts
  - Osteoblasts
  - Monocytes
- They can also be produced by certain types of epithelial cells; however, fibroblasts are the predominant producers.
- Although there are 28 types of collagen, type I collagen is the most abundant type in most connective tissues.
  - Type I collagen resists tensile strain unidirectionally.
- In the case of irregular connective tissues such as fascia, these type I collagen fibers are oriented in an irregular weave that provides strength in multiple directions.
  - This interwoven configuration also provides a scaffold upon which other ECM components are laid down.

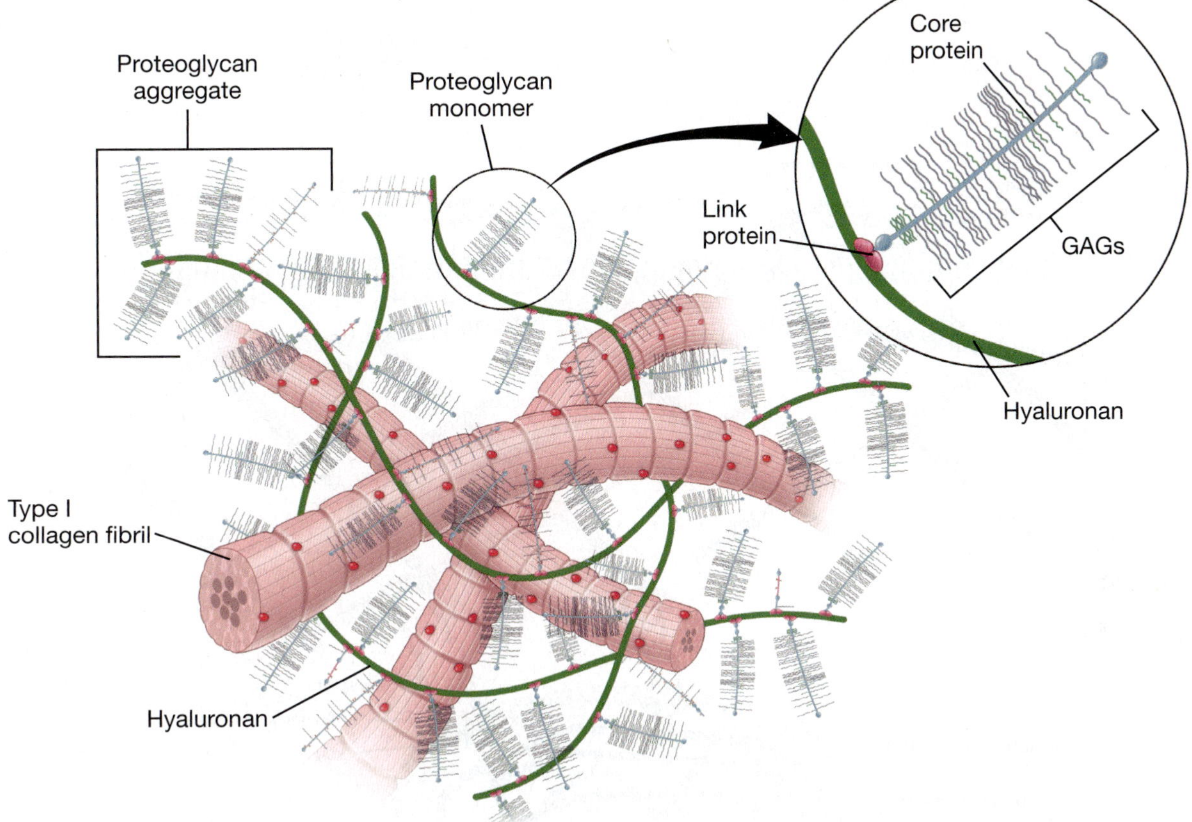

Figure 3.29. Composition of the ECM. The glycosaminoglycans (GAGs) are seen attached to proteoglycans that are woven around collagen fibers. GAGs are hydrophilic and attach water to the matrix. (Reprinted with permission from Pawlina W. *Histology: A Text and Atlas with Correlated Cell and Molecular Biology*. 7th ed. Wolters Kluwer; 2016.)

ELASTIC FIBERS

Elastic fibers provide resilience to tissue distension. Fibroblasts produce tropoelastin (a precursor to the amorphous elastin) and fibrillin. In the ECM, fibrillin forms a scaffold that invests elastin molecules to produce elastic fibers. These account for approximately 1% of the overall tissue volume.

GROUND SUBSTANCE

The ECM is also rich with a mixture of:

- GAGs
- Proteoglycans
- Glycoproteins

Collectively, these substances are known as ground substance.

GAGs are unbranched polysaccharide chains and are often sulfated (e.g., heparin sulfate), conferring a negative charge that attracts sodium.

- Water follows the sodium and hydrates the tissue.
- GAGs often bind to large core proteins to create proteoglycans.
- Given the large number of GAGs, these proteoglycans contain tremendous ability to draw fluid into the tissue.

Glycoproteins are adhesive molecules with binding domains for:

- Cell surface receptors
- Collagen
- Elastic fibers
- GAGs

These connections allow the glycoproteins to link together all of the components of the ECM as well as the resident cells of connective tissue (Fig. 3.29).

MECHANOTRANSDUCTION

The components of ECM create a rich interconnected network capable of transmitting tension from the fibers into the cell, potentially impacting nuclear activity (Fig. 3.30).

- Fibronectin is a common glycoprotein in fascial ECM and it possesses binding domains for connective tissue fibers, proteoglycans, and transmembrane cell receptors (e.g., integrins, syndecans).
- Fibronectin also contains cryptic self-polymerization sites.
    - Under tension, these cryptic sites are exposed, transforming many fibronectin molecules into massive fibronectin fibrils that couple several cells to one another and to the ECM.
- Fibronectin is capable of directing fibroblast proliferation and collagen deposition.[18]

The cellular portion of the transmembrane receptor binds to elements of the actin cytoskeleton.

- This cytoskeleton is composed of globular (G) actin polymerized into filaments.
- The filamentous (F) actin is capable of changing its length by addition or subtraction of G actin, a process known as treadmilling.
- F-actin also interacts with nonmuscle myosin to form contractile "stress fibers."

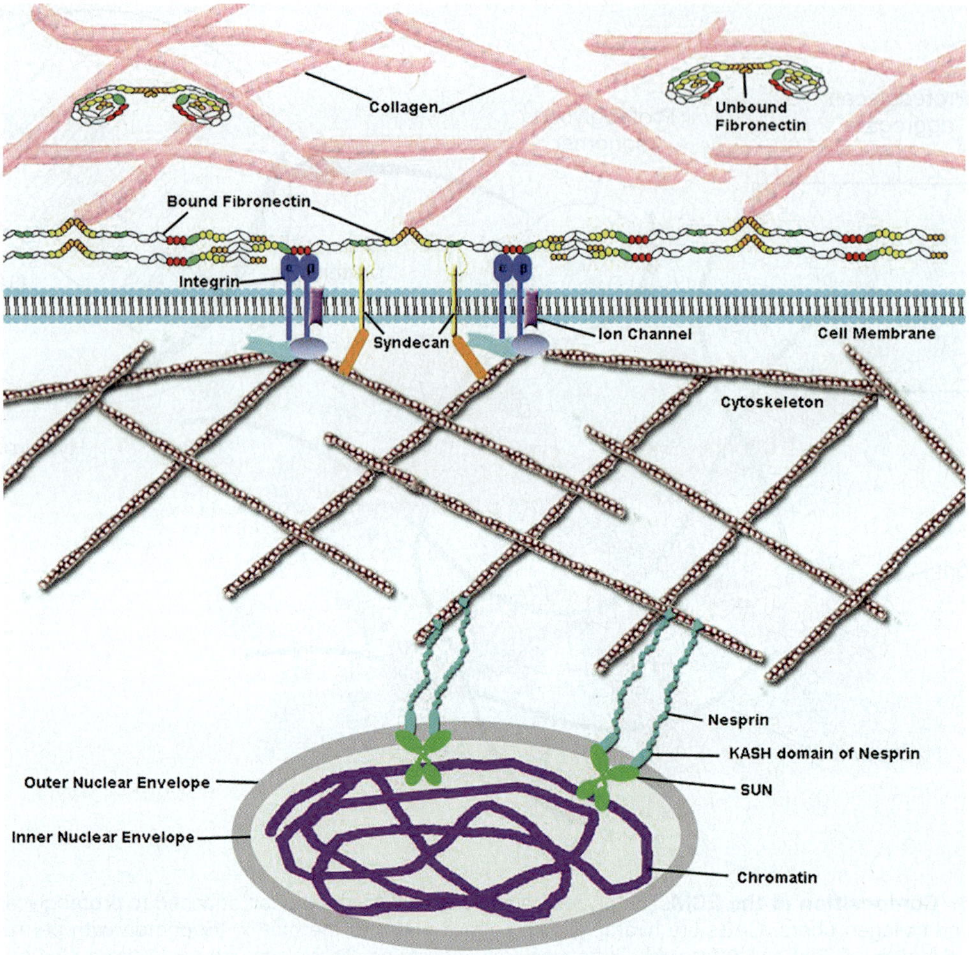

Figure 3.30. The molecular architecture of mechanotransduction (see text for explanation). (Courtesy of Mark Schuenke.)

- The contractile and treadmilling capabilities of the cytoskeleton allow the cell to assess and modify the stability of the ECM.

Under homeostatic conditions, a transient group of transmembrane receptors (integrins), called a focal complex, couples fibronectin to cytoskeletal actin.

- However, when the cell encounters consistent stress, the focal complexes will mature into larger, more stable focal adhesions and fibrillar adhesions.
- These adhesions tightly couple the ECM to the cytoskeleton.

The integrins of these large adhesion complexes impact formation of additional cytoskeletal F-actin.

- Stress from the extracellular environment triggers a chain reaction:
  1. Activation of focal adhesion kinase (FAK)
  2. FAK regulates RhoA, a small GTPase
  3. RhoA then regulates cytoskeletal dynamics
- Under stress, RhoA directs the organization of F-actin and junctional complexes.
- This cascade is also involved in actin treadmilling and the cell's ability to produce tension.

In addition to their role in activating FAK, integrins create calcium channels in the cell membrane.

- When the integrins encounter an external stress, there is an influx of calcium from the ECM.
- The downstream impact of the stress-induced calcium influx is not yet fully understood, but it appears to be a conversion of extracellular tension into an intracellular signaling mechanism.

As the cytoskeleton is altered, those changes impact the nuclear position and state of the chromatin.

- Within the cell:
  - Nesprin binds to both actin and SUN, a protein of the nuclear envelope.
  - SUN then binds to nuclear lamina, which has continuity with the chromatin.
- If tension is passed through this chain, chromatin will unravel, making the genetic material available for transcription.
- At the same time, there is a direct correlation between integrin tension and recruitment of ribosomes and mRNA to the area of tension (see Fig. 3.30).
- Thus, mechanical forces delivered to the tissue as a whole may be transferred through the ECM, eventually reaching the cellular level and influencing genetic function; this process is termed mechanotransduction.

Mechanotransduction is known to play a role in the remodeling of such hard connective tissue as bone and is also thought to be involved in normal and pathologic changes in soft connective tissue such as fascia. Understanding mechanotransduction and its effects on tissue function and dysfunction is important for the future of osteopathic medicine.

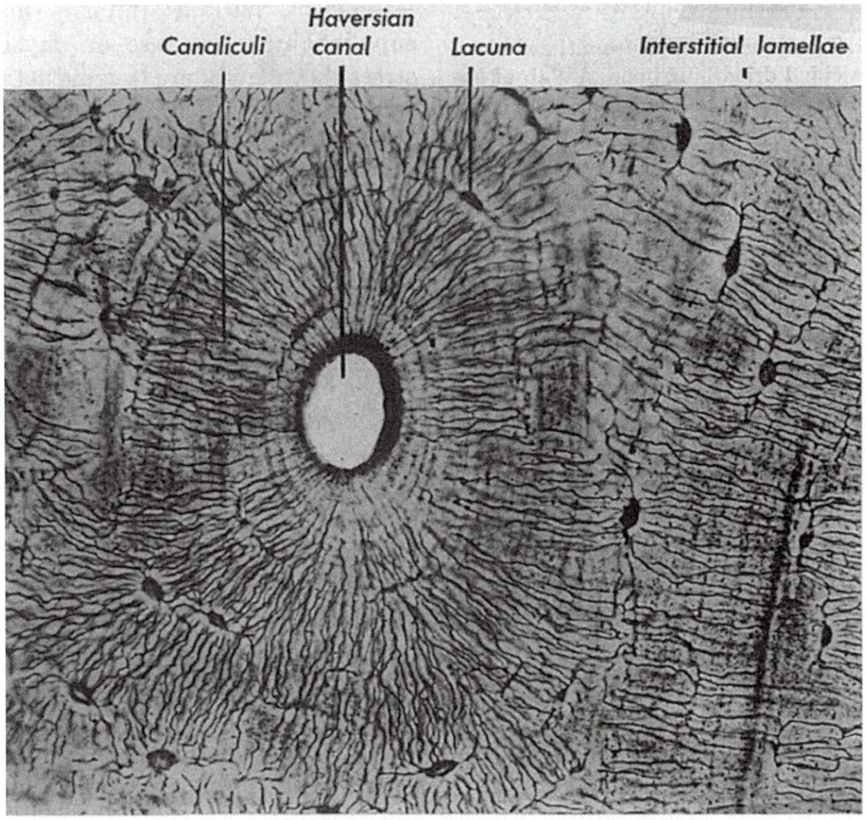

Figure 3.31. Transverse section illustrating the cellular elements of bone.

Types of Specialized Connective Tissue in Musculoskeletal Anatomy

BONE

As with all forms of connective tissue, bone contains:

- Cells
- Fibers
- Ground substance

However, the ECM of bone is highly specialized for support and protection.

- The predominant fiber type is type I collagen, and the ECM is rich in calcium and phosphate.
- These minerals are organized into hydroxyapatite crystals [$Ca_{10}(PO_4)_6(OH)_2$] to resist compression.

The osteocytes of bone are maintained in a rigid matrix, which is calcified and reinforced by connective tissue fibers produced by the osteoblasts.

- The structural unit of bone is the osteon (Haversian system).
  - The osteon is formed by concentric lamellae of bone surrounding a microscopic neurovascular bundle in the Haversian canal.
  - The osteocytes are located within microscopic small spaces (lacunae) between the concentric bone matrix lamellae.
  - The process of osteocytes extends into the matrix in small canaliculi (Fig. 3.31).
- The concentric rings of bony matrix provide great strength to the bone.

Bone can be organized into:

1. Cortical (compact)
2. Trabecular (spongy, cancellous)

Cortical bone:

- Is located on the outer surface of bones
- Provides protection and support (Fig. 3.32)
- Is oriented into osteons

The ECM of bone is too dense to allow for diffusion; small channels (canaliculi) pass through the concentric layers.

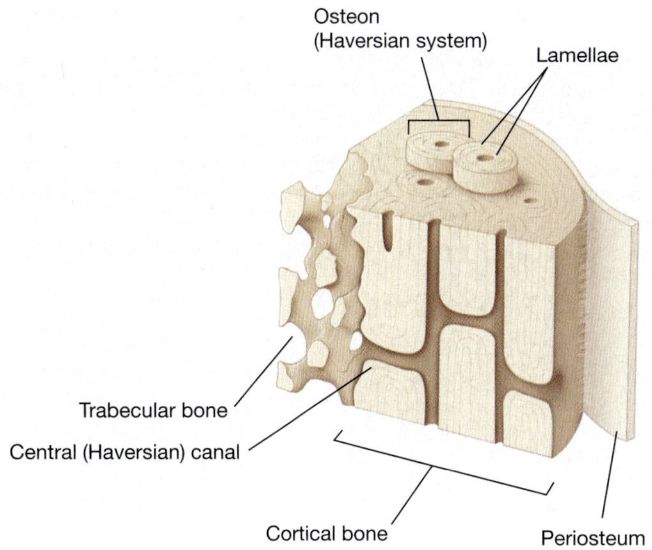

Figure 3.32. The structure of bone. This is a section of a long bone illustrating the outer wall of cortical bone surrounded peripherally by periosteum and internally by trabeculated bone. (Reprinted with permission from Golan DE, Tashjian AH, Armstrong EJ, Armstong AW. *Principles of Pharmacology: The Pathophysiologic Basis of Drug Therapy*. 3rd ed. Wolters Kluwer Health/Lippincott Williams & Wilkins; 2012.)

- Cytoplasmic processes of the osteocytes reside in the canaliculi and transfer nutrients and wastes via gap junctions.
- This cell-to-cell connectivity is thought to underlie the mechanotransduction that occurs in bone and is responsible for stress-induced shape changes in bone.

Cancellous bone creates open spaces in the bone marrow cavity.

- It contains small trabeculae (spicules) of bone in no discernible pattern.
  - The trabeculae are composed of a hydroxyapatite-rich matrix and osteocytes in lacunae.
- The trabeculae are surrounded by osteoblasts and osteoclasts.
  - Osteoblasts lay down bone matrix, whereas osteoclasts resorb bone.
  - This relationship allows for tight regulation of blood calcium levels.

CARTILAGE

Cartilage is another specialized connective tissue with a high GAG:fiber ratio.

- The hydrophilic nature of GAGs increases the tissue's turgidity, thereby making cartilage resistant to compression.
- The high water content in cartilaginous ECM also encourages diffusion in the avascular tissue.

The chondroblast is responsible for producing the ground substance and fibers of the three types of cartilage:

1. Hyaline (articular; found in synovial joints)
2. Elastic (found in the external ear, auditory tube, larynx, and epiglottis)
3. Fibrous (found in intervertebral disks and the pubic symphysis)

These three cartilage types are avascular and vary in histologic makeup on the basis of their ground substance and predominant fiber type (collagen or elastin) and are avascular (Figs. 3.33 to 3.35).

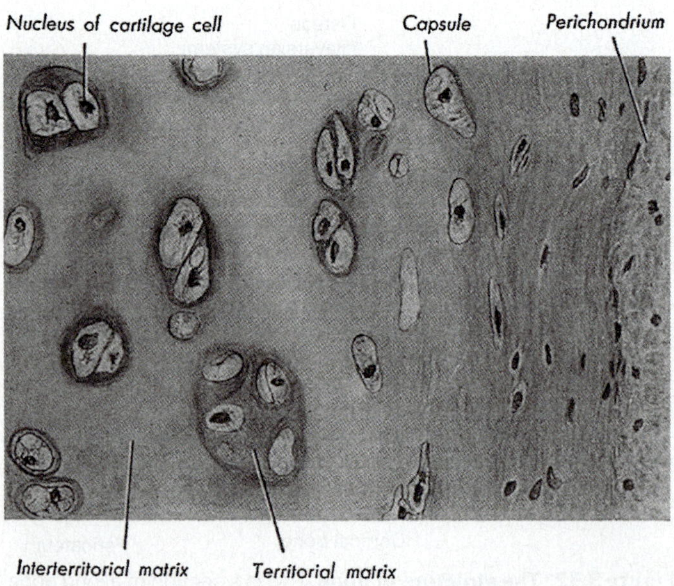

Figure 3.33. Cellular elements of hyaline cartilage. The chondrocytes are located in lacunae. There is no communication between lacunae or between chondrocytes and a blood supply. Initially, each lacuna has one chondrocyte. The lacuna divides, forming two chondrocytes. Each chondrocyte can then divide a second time, resulting in as many as four cells in each lacunae.

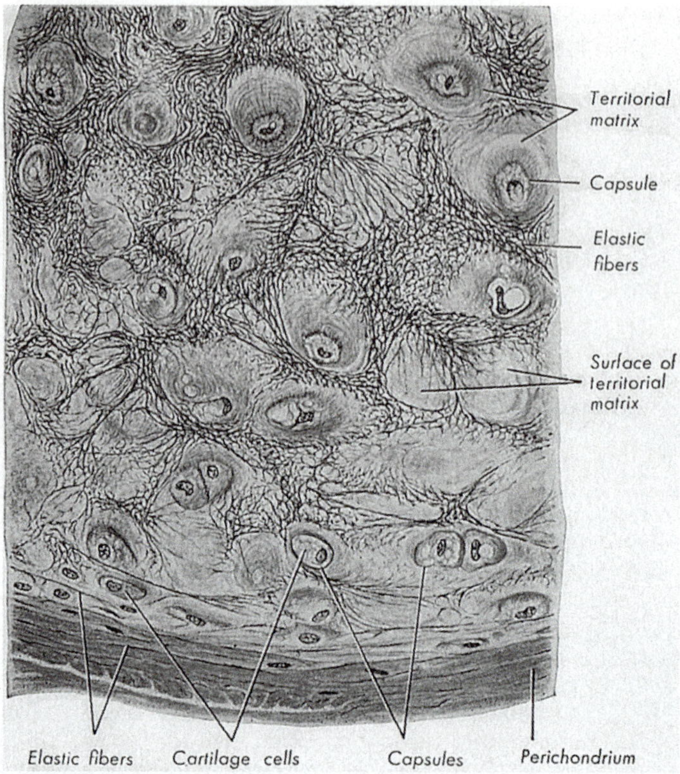

Figure 3.34. Cellular elements of elastic cartilage. Structurally, elastic cartilage appears similar to that of hyaline cartilage, with the exception of the dense distribution of elastic fibers woven around the lacunae.

Within the matrix, chondrocytes reside in lacunae. Chondrocytes are generally quiescent but are capable of undergoing mitosis and producing cartilage matrix to grow the tissue. Once formed, there is little possibility for chondrocytes to participate in tissue repair, thus damaged cartilage is typically replaced by fibrosis.

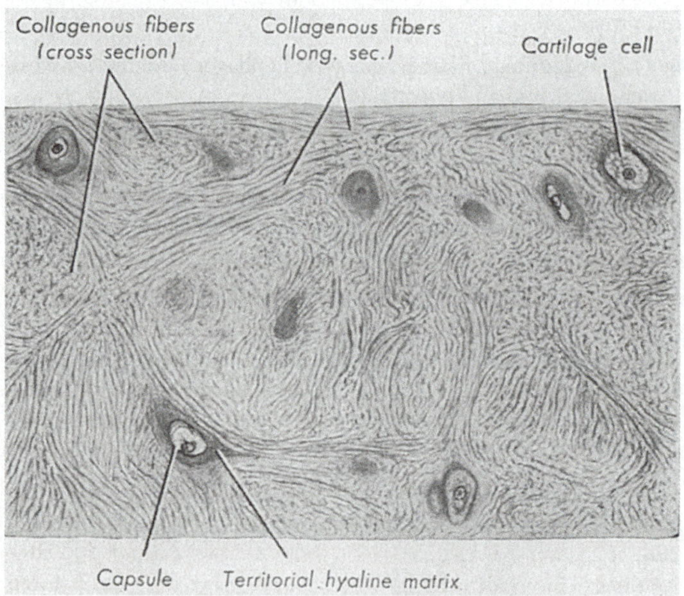

Figure 3.35. Cellular elements of fibrocartilage. Although looking much like dense connective tissue, fibrocartilage is distinctive because of the presence of lacunae containing chondrocytes.

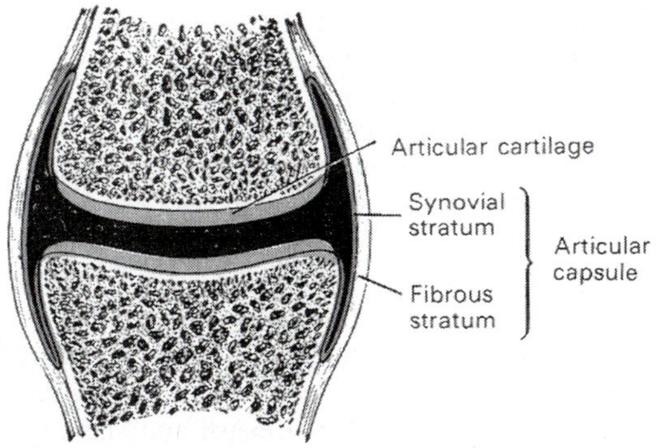

Figure 3.36. Schematic drawing of a typical synovial joint without an articular disk.

Synovial Joints

The aforementioned components of the musculoskeletal system would not be well suited for locomotion, were it not for synovial joints.

- Synovial joints allow contiguous bones to move with relative freedom. The "typical" synovial joint is exemplified in Figure 3.36.
- The shape of the corresponding bones dictates the degrees of freedom the joint will have. For example:
  - A hinge joint is generally capable of movement in only one plane.
  - A ball-and-socket joint allows movement in multiple planes.

JOINT STRUCTURE

The outermost component of a synovial joint is the joint capsule.

- The joint capsule is composed of dense connective tissue that anchors to the periosteum of the articulating bones.
  - The collagen fibers of the capsule are organized into sheets.
  - Within a sheet, the fibers have a regular orientation, but the sheets are positioned at angles to one another, creating a robust weave.
- The joint capsules are well innervated:
  - Free nerve endings provide for nociception.
  - Large encapsulated nerve endings provide for proprioception.

For additional information on joint structure, see Standring,[22] and for joint function, see Nordin and Frankel.[23]

The fibrous capsule encloses a joint space that is lined by a synovial membrane (Fig. 3.37).

- This membrane produces a serous fluid to reduce friction.
- The synovial membrane consists of:
  - A subintimal layer that is rich in blood vessels, adipocytes, and fibroblasts.
  - An intimal layer that lines the lumen of the joint cavity.
- The intimal layer is composed of macrophage-like synoviocytes and fibroblast-like synoviocytes for cleaning the cavity and producing synovial fluid, respectively.

The articulating surfaces of bones in synovial joints are lined by articular cartilage. Articular cartilage matrix is of a similar consistency to hyaline cartilage but has a much more distinct orientation. Several distinct layers of articular cartilage can be identified:

- A region of calcified cartilage is closest to the articular bone.
- Moving toward the joint space, a distinct "tide mark" signifies the transition from calcified cartilage to the deepest layer of articular cartilage.
  - This deepest layer of noncalcified articular cartilage contains collagen fibers that radiate from the tide mark.
  - Chondrocytes in this layer are large and the matrix is plentiful for resisting compression.
- An intermediate layer displays collagen fibers in transition from the radiant orientation of the deep layer toward a more tangential orientation.
- The superficial layer of articular cartilage (closest to the lumen of the joint cavity) lines the synovial cavity lumen and is specialized to resist shear stress.
  - The superficial layer is subdivided into:
    1. A cellular sublayer
    2. An acellular sublayer called lamina splendens

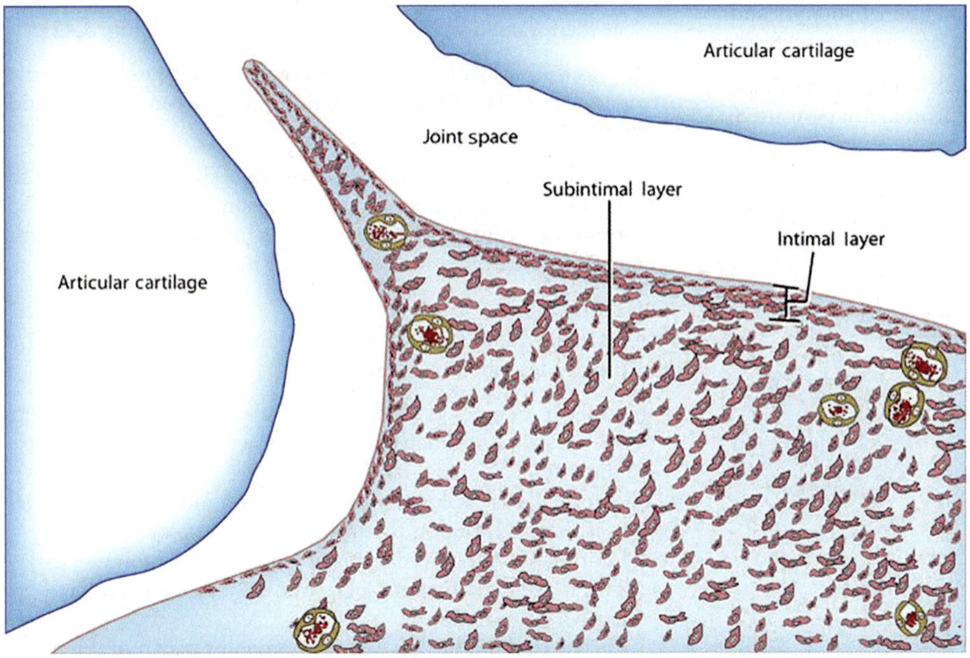

Figure 3.37. The synovial membrane. The synovial membrane is seen extending from the inside of the joint capsule to insert between two articular surfaces. This membrane is made up of connective tissue forming an oily structure that can massage the articular surfaces, providing lubrication.

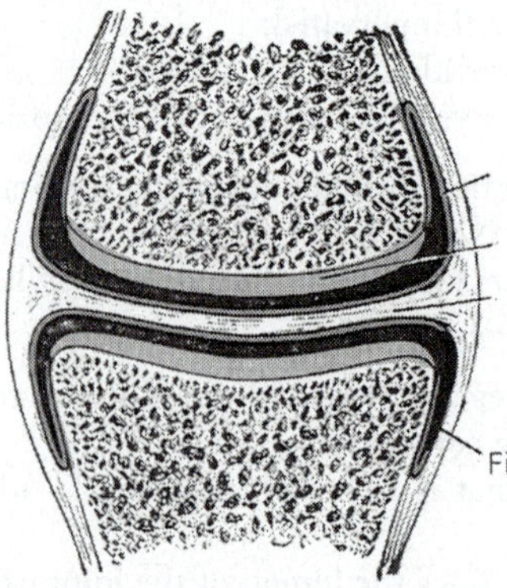

Figure 3.38. A schematic diagram of a synovial joint with an articular disk.

- ☐ Both sublayers consist of collagen fibers oriented parallel to the articulating surface.
- ☐ The chondrocytes in the cellular sublayer are flattened relative to the chondrocytes in the underlying layers, and they secrete the specialized lubricating glycoproteins, lubricin, and superficial zone protein.
- ☐ This superficial layer is the first damaged in osteoarthritis. Because it is highly specialized to resist shear stress and produce lubrication, the loss of this superficial layer can lead to rapid deterioration of the articulating cartilage.

Each synovial joint is stabilized by specific ligaments.

- Ligaments may be classified as:
  1. Capsular ligaments, which are a part of the fibrous outer layer of the joint capsule
  2. Accessory ligaments, which are located either within the joint cavity (intracapsular) or outside the joint capsule, separated from the fibrous outer layer (extracapsular)
- All ligaments are histologically composed of dense regular fibrous connective tissue and have microscopic, structural, and functional continuity with the periosteum of adjacent bone.
- Some joints (e.g., temporomandibular joint or knee joint) are even more specialized as they have the unique feature of either a disk or a meniscus (incomplete disk) within the joint cavity (Fig. 3.38).
- The fibrocartilaginous disk provides for additional support and stability as it separates the two hyaline cartilage articular surfaces.

Synovial joints are commonly classified according to the shape of the articular surfaces and/or the movements that are permitted.

- None of the articular surfaces are truly flat.
- Biomechanically, these joint surfaces permit motion (Fig. 3.39):
  1. Spin, which represents rotation about the longitudinal axis of a bone
  2. Roll, which is the result of decreasing and increasing the angle between the two bones at an articulation
  3. Slide, which is the result of a translatory motion of one bone gliding/sliding on the other at the joint
- Specific details regarding the classification system and individual synovial joints can be found in any anatomy textbook.[24]

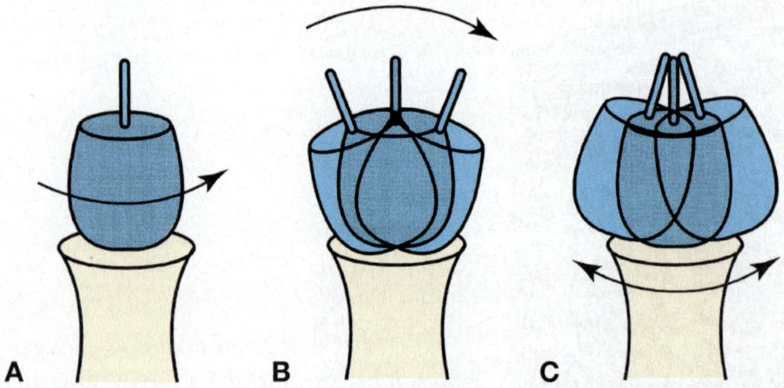

Figure 3.39. Motion at a synovial joint. A. Spin. **B.** Roll. **C.** Slide.

Nonsynovial joints are subdivided into fibrous and cartilaginous types.

- These joints, where the articulating bones are directly connected by either fibrous tissue or cartilage, have no free surface for movement, but provide for strength and stability between adjacent bones.
- The fibrous joints include:
  - ☐ The sutures of the skull (Fig. 3.40)
  - ☐ The teeth in the mandible and maxilla
  - ☐ The distal tibiofibular joint
- The cartilaginous joints include:
  - ☐ The fibrocartilaginous intervertebral disks between adjacent vertebral bodies and the pubic symphysis (Fig. 3.41)

The sutures of the skull provide a classic example of the interrelationship between structure and function.

- Each suture (joint) between adjacent cranial bones uniquely provides support and mobility.
- Unlike the freely moveable synovial joints, the sutures are highly restricted to slight gliding motion.
- However, motion loss/restriction is the clinically significant factor in describing somatic dysfunction of the joint.
- Ossification of many cranial sutures occurs with advancing age.

Cranial bone motion is also influenced by the tension of the cranial dura mater, which covers the brain and forms the internal lining of the skull.

- Cranial dura mater consists of two layers:
  1. Periosteal (outer dura): The periosteal layer is the periosteal lining of the cranium, and there is histologic continuity of this layer with the fibrous tissue (sutural ligament) at each cranial suture (see Fig. 3.40).
  2. Meningeal (inner dura): The meningeal layer of cranial dura mater has continuity with the spinal dura mater (thecal sac) at the foramen magnum of the occipital bone (Fig. 3.42).

In summary, synovial and nonsynovial joints exemplify the osteopathic concept of the interrelationship between structure and function.

- Synovial joints, which are freely moveable, allow for the body to have mobility and greater range of motion.
- Nonsynovial joints (fibrous and cartilaginous) provide strength and stability within a limited range of motion.

JOINT PLAY

The voluntary movement of synovial joints is accommodated by joint play as described by Mennell.[25]

- Joint play is defined as a small but precise amount of movement (<1/8 in), which is independent of the action of voluntary muscle function.
- The normal, easy, voluntary range of active motion at a synovial joint is dependent upon the integrity of joint play:
  - ☐ Joint play is only present in the living synovial joint.
  - ☐ The movement of joint play can only be demonstrated by passive examination.
  - ☐ Each synovial joint has one or more joint play movements.

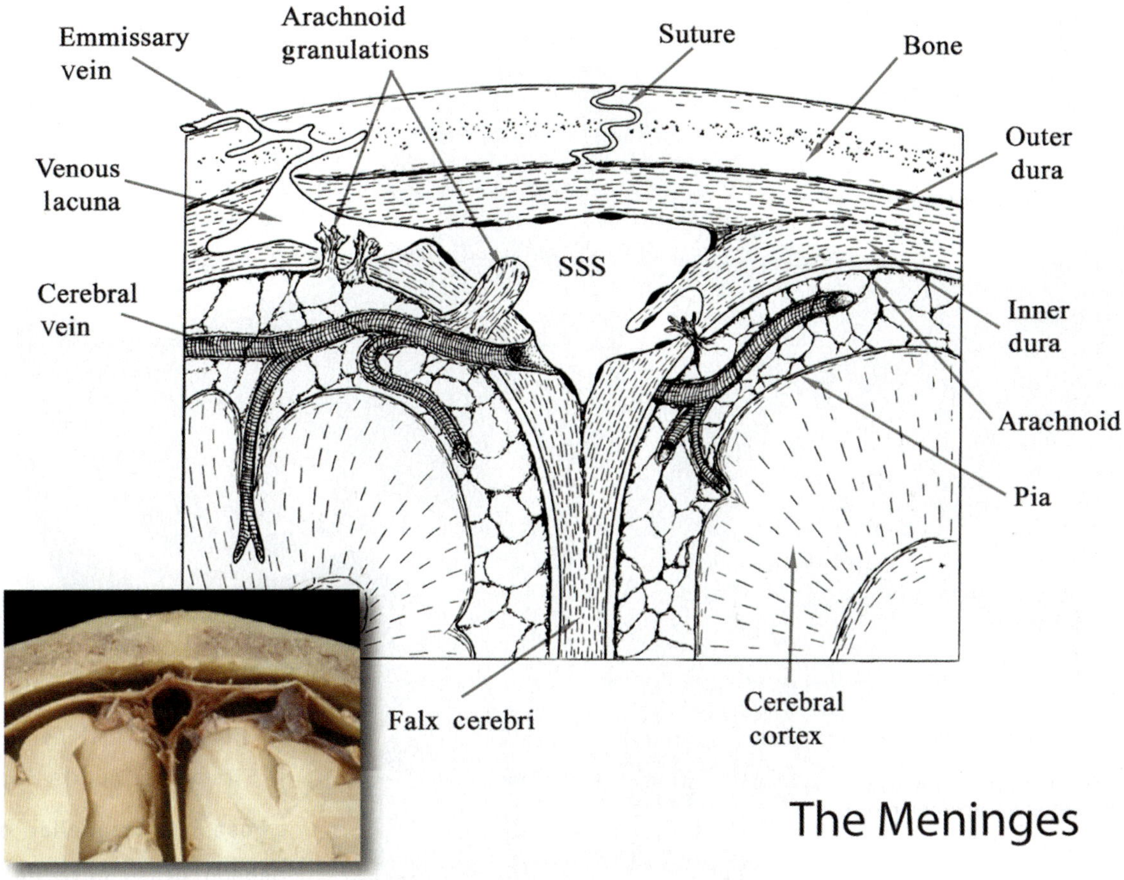

Figure 3.40. **Sutures of the skull.** This is a cross section taken through a cranial suture. The two cranial bones are covered with dense connective tissue, termed periosteum on the external surface, and dura mater on the internal surface. The dura mater is divided into a periosteal layer and a meningeal layer. At the suture, the bones align with each other, and the connective tissue of the periosteum and periosteal dura fuse together. (Reprinted with permission from Willard FH, Perl DP. *Medical Neuroanatomy: A Problem-Oriented Manual with Annotated Atlas.* J.B. Lippincott; 1993.)

- Joint dysfunction is defined as the loss of joint play and therefore a limitation of the voluntary range of motion at a synovial joint.
  - Joint dysfunction is a component of somatic dysfunction (acute or chronic), which is diagnosed in the evaluation of the neuromusculoskeletal system.
- The restoration of joint play appears to be the basis for the success of synovial joint mobilization using direct or indirect action treatment techniques in osteopathic manipulation.
- The evaluation of joint play and the restoration of normal joint movement is a major component of the **biomechanical model**, one of the five conceptual models used in the evaluation of a patient.

So far, it has been pointed out that specific features of anatomy and function apply to a given model system in the osteopathic approach to the patient. It is important to understand that all five models are interconnected and interrelate with each other when considering the presentation of illness. For example:

- The loss of joint function and joint play reduces motion (biomechanical model) about a joint but is well known to reduce motion about joints at a distance as well.
- Increased resistance to motion in a joint or group of joints increases the amount of energy consumed when attempting to move the joint. This can be seen in the increased energy required (metabolic energy model) for ambulation in patients with a fixed (casted) joint.
- Lack of motion in tissue reduces the movement of fluids from the tissue, facilitating edema (respiratory–circulatory model) and furthering the retention of metabolic wastes (metabolic–energetic model) in the tissue.
- Changes in acidity, alteration in stiffness, and reduced motion all result in increased pain and discomfort when attempting motion (neurologic model).
- Ultimately, these factors can summate, resulting in altered perception of oneself and a change in psychological well-being (behavioral/psychosocial model).

All of these are factors that must be considered when attempting to help a patient seek health. This leads to the concept of body unity.

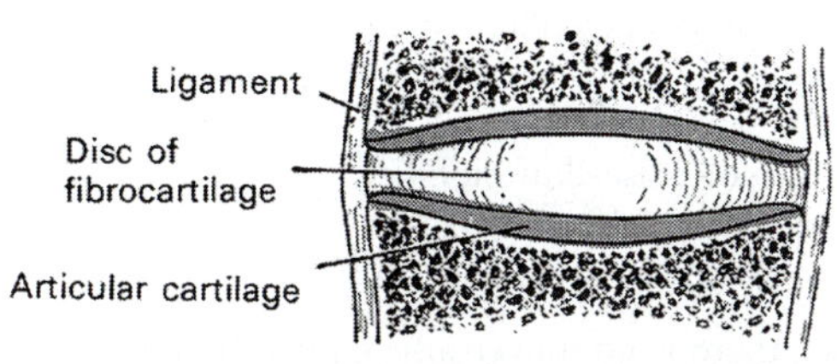

Figure 3.41. **The intervertebral disk of the vertebral column.** A symphysis is an example of a cartilaginous joint.

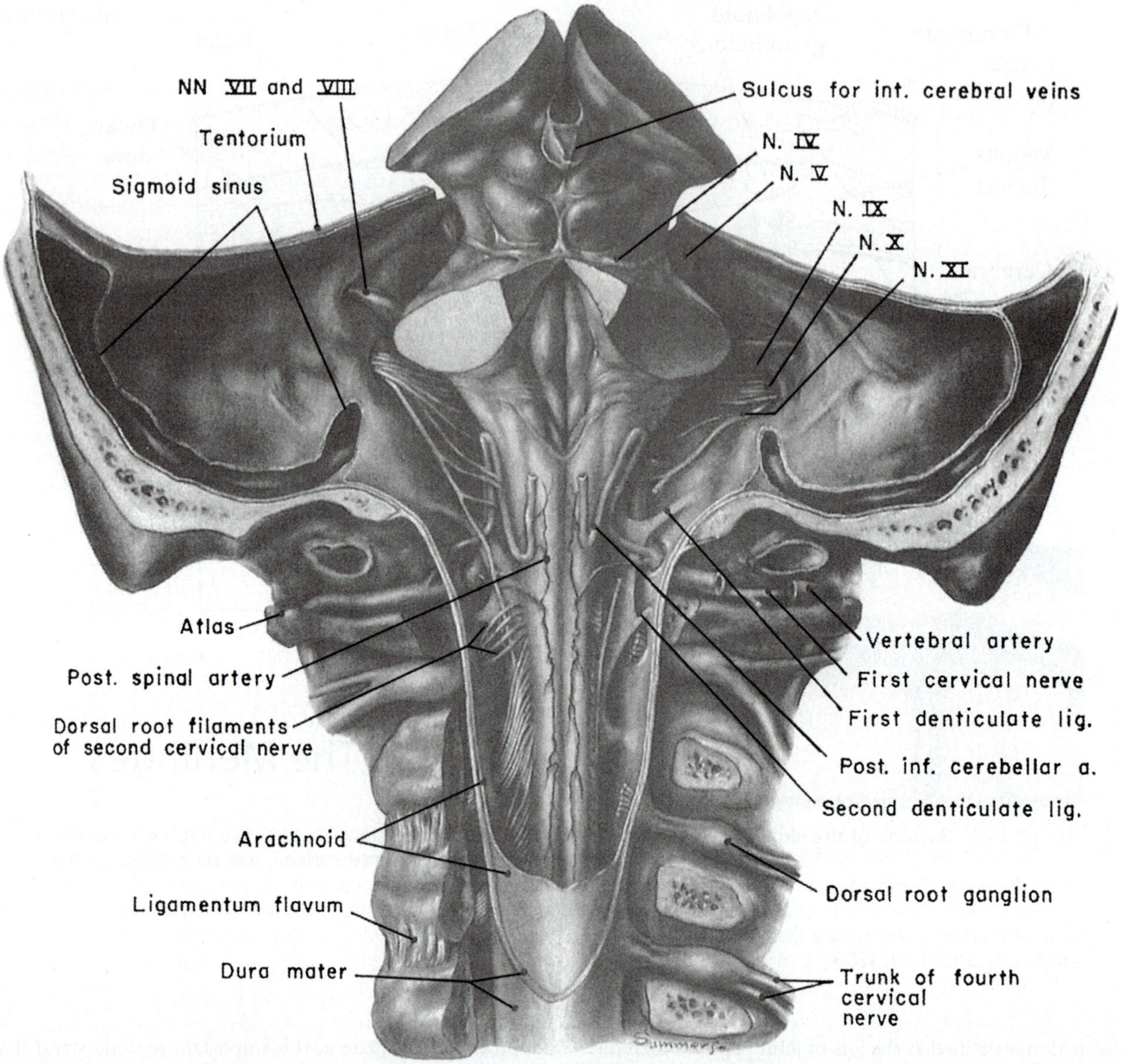

Figure 3.42. Area of the foramen magnum. Cranial dura mater lines the internal surface of the cranium, is continuous with the fibrous tissue of the sutures, and is continuous with the spinal dura of the foramen magnum.

BODY UNITY

Although to this point, this text has emphasized the segmental and cellular nature of the human body, in reality, the body is one unified structure.

- The various regional anatomical and cellular components of the neuromusculoskeletal system—derived embryologically from somites and associated neural precursors—are bound together and unified into a functional whole by:
  - Arteries
  - Veins
  - Lymphatics
  - Nerves
  - Circulating factors
  - Fasciae
- This observation forms the basis for the Five-Model Concept used in performing osteopathic diagnosis and in designing appropriate treatment protocols.

The common feature interconnecting all of these systems is the fascial network of the body, into which these systems are embedded. This network is composed of irregular connective tissue that supports and integrates all components of the body into a functioning whole.

Fascia

Fascia is a rather generalized term for sheets or layers of connective tissue that envelop specific structures and segregate one structure, organ, or area from another.

- For example, throughout the body, there is a subcutaneous layer of loose connective tissue called the superficial fascia (Fig. 3.43).
  - It contains collagen fibers that connect the skin to underlying structures as well as variable amounts of fat.
- Superficial fascia:
  - Serves to increase skin mobility
  - Acts as a thermal insulator
  - Stores energy for metabolic use[10]

To date, there is no universally agreed-upon definition of fascia. An effective definition of fascia would allow its reader to easily identify fascia upon finding it in the body. This chapter will use

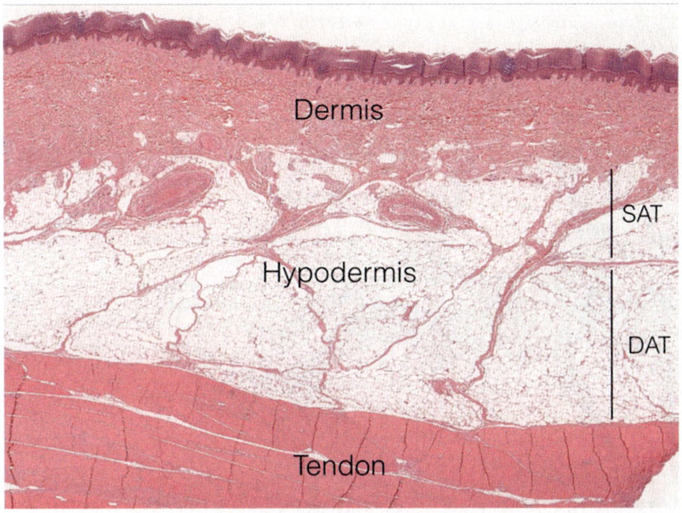

Figure 3.43. This is a cross section of tissue taken through the superficial fascia of the foot. The superficial adipose tissue (SAT) and deep adipose tissue (DAT), along with the thin septa of collagenous fibers, constitute the superficial fascia seen covering most parts of the body.

the definition described in several older texts—an irregular weave of collagen with variable density.[26]

- This irregular arrangement implies:
  - Equal resistance to tensile strain
  - Potential for mechanotransduction in any direction
- The irregularity of the collagenous weave also includes packing material as a potential function of fascia and excludes tendons, ligaments, and aponeuroses from its definition.

For more anatomical details on fascia, see Stecco.[10]

TYPES OF FASCIA

Fascia is generally divided into four categories that can be conceived as concentric tubes enveloping the trunk:

1. Pannicular
2. Investing
3. Meningeal
4. Splanchnic

A more comprehensive description of fascia is provided in Chapter 7 The Fascial System of the Body.

Pannicular or Superficial Fascia

In brief, the pannicular fascia, or more colloquially the superficial fascia, is the outermost layer that envelops the body. Many clinicians and scientists consider the pannicular fascia to be analogous to the hypodermis. This layer is divided into three sublayers:

1. The most superficial sublayer consists of adipocytes and the retinaculum cutis superficialis (see SAT in Fig. 3.43).
2. The middle sublayer is membranous, with fibers primarily oriented parallel to the skin's surface.
3. The deepest sublayer fascia (see DAT in Fig. 3.43) consists primarily of adipocytes and the retinaculum cutis profundus.

Deep Investing Fascia

The investing, or deep, fascia is located internal to the pannicular fascial layer.

- The investing fascia is denser than the pannicular fascia and has a reduced number of adipocytes when compared to superficial fascia.
- The irregular arrangement of collagen confers a "feltlike" texture and whitish appearance to the fascia.

As the name implies, investing fascia encase organs of the musculoskeletal system.

- The investing fascia can be seen as forming compartments into which the muscles are inserted (Fig. 3.44).
- In the extremities, the muscle compartments themselves are grouped into functional compartments by large fascial septa.
  - An example would be the flexor and extensor compartments of the upper extremity (Fig. 3.45).
- Similar functional compartments are seen in the torso:
  - A fascial compartment surrounds the anterior (hypaxial) muscles.
  - A fascial compartment surrounds the posterior (epaxial) muscles.
  - Both compartments are united laterally by a fascial connection that fuses to the transverse processes of the vertebral column (Fig. 3.46).
  - Anteriorly, the intercostal and abdominal muscles in the hypaxial compartment contribute flexion and side bending of the torso and posteriorly, the paraspinal muscles in the epaxial compartment function in extension of the torso.

The investing fascia of skeletal muscles is the epimysium.

- This investing fascia becomes:
  - Periosteum around bones
  - Perichondrium around cartilages
  - Periligamentum of ligaments
  - Peritenon of tendons
- There is also a similar association with aponeuroses, broad, flat sheets of regularly arranged dense connective tissue that joins muscle to bone, similar to a tendon.
- A continuity exists between the periosteum of bone and the peritenon of tendons attached to the bone.
- Similarly, the peritenon of the tendon is continuous with the epimysium of the muscle attached to the tendon.
- In this fashion, the entire musculoskeletal system is joined into a continuous fascial network.

Finally, the investing fascia is subdivided, based on embryology, into:

- Axial investing fascia, around the muscles of the thoracoabdominopelvic region
- Appendicular investing fascia, enveloping the limb musculature

The appendicular investing fascia, when approaching the torso, passes external to the axial fascia of the torso extending to the midline, where it can attach to the spinous processes posteriorly and the sternum anteriorly.

Meningeal Fascia

The meningeal fascia includes the dura, arachnoid, and pia mater layers that envelop the brain and spinal cord.

- Although each layer is continuous from the cranial vault to the vertebral canal, the mesodermal origins are regionally distinct:
  - The neural crest gives rise to the meninges of the telencephalon.
  - The cephalic mesoderm gives rise to the brain stem meninges.
  - The somatic mesoderm gives rise to the meninges of the spinal cord.[27]
- The meningeal fascia is continuous with the epineurium of peripheral nerves.

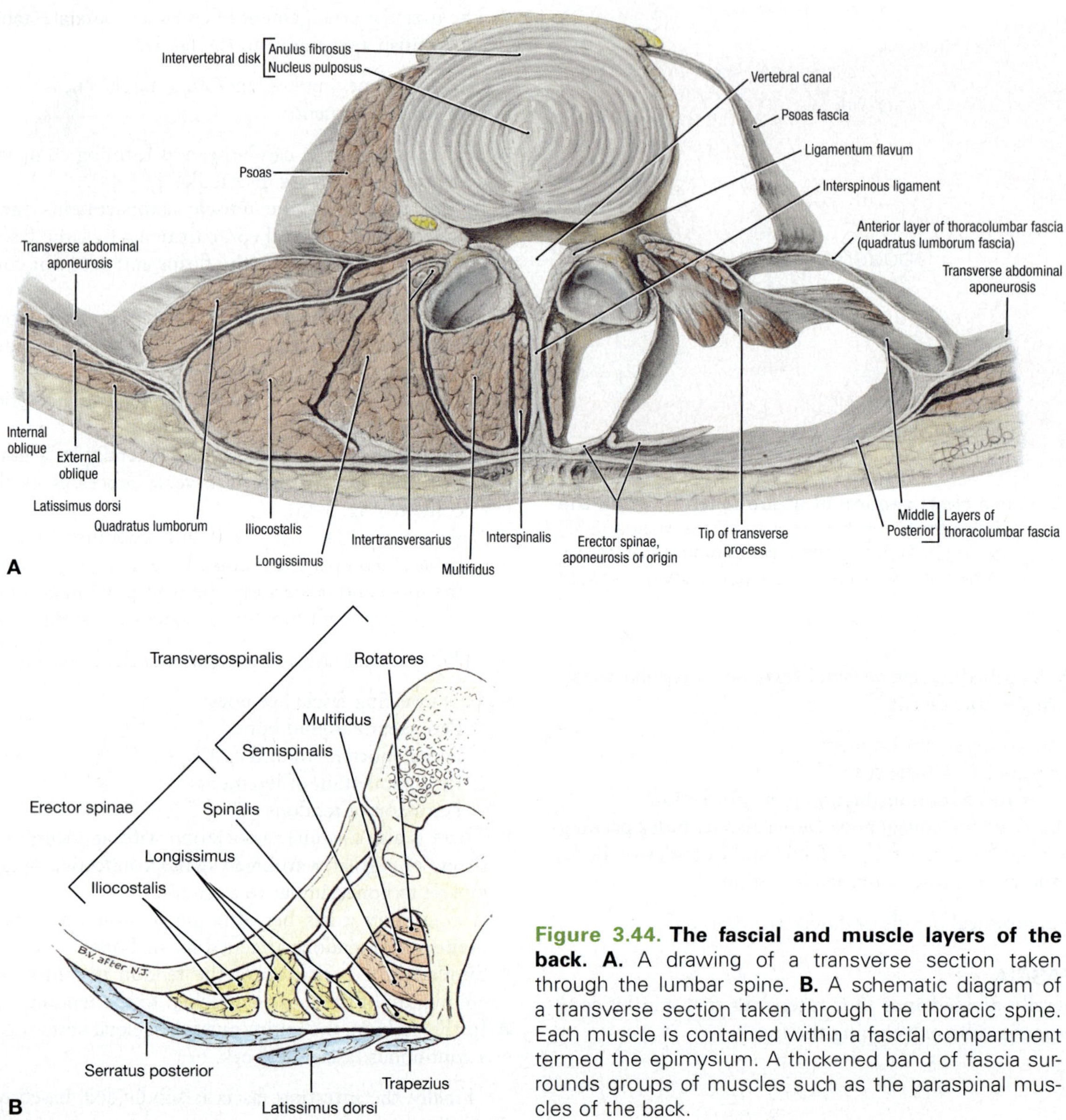

Figure 3.44. The fascial and muscle layers of the back. A. A drawing of a transverse section taken through the lumbar spine. **B.** A schematic diagram of a transverse section taken through the thoracic spine. Each muscle is contained within a fascial compartment termed the epimysium. A thickened band of fascia surrounds groups of muscles such as the paraspinal muscles of the back.

Splanchnic or Visceral Fascia

Splanchnic or visceral fascia extends from the cranial base to the pelvic diaphragm and provides the surface of the superior most pelvic organs.

- Splanchnic fascia is specified regionally, with the prefix "endo-" followed by the cavity (e.g., endothoracic fascia in the thoracic cavity); however, the anterior portion of the endoabdominal fascia may also be referred to as the transversalis fascia.
- The splanchnic fascia envelops the body cavities (e.g., pleural, pericardial, and peritoneal) and their contained organs.
- The splanchnic fascia serves as a conduit for neurovascular and lymphatic bundles and also as a shock-absorptive packing material.
- The visceral fascia of the pelvic cavity and the pannicular fascia of the ischiorectal fossa are separated by the levator ani muscle.

THE FUNCTION OF FASCIA IN BODY CONTINUITY

At a basic anatomical level, these fasciae define the individual muscles and muscle groups.

- For example, each of the muscles in the anterior compartment of the leg has its own investing fascia.
- The entire group is bounded:
  - □ Laterally by a wall of fascia, the anterior crural septum
  - □ Medially by fascia that is continuous with the periosteum of the tibia
  - □ Anteriorly by the encasing deep fascia of the leg
- As is typical, the blood and nervous supply to these muscles, as well as venous and lymphatic return, are principally contained within this fascial compartment.
- These fasciae collectively define the anterior compartment.
- More importantly, they enhance the extensor functions of the muscles while simultaneously providing protection, support, and separation from other muscle groups.
- The fasciae define the normal, healthy limit of the group; they tend to constrain destructive states and prevent the spread of bleeding, infection, tumor growth, etc., into adjacent compartments.

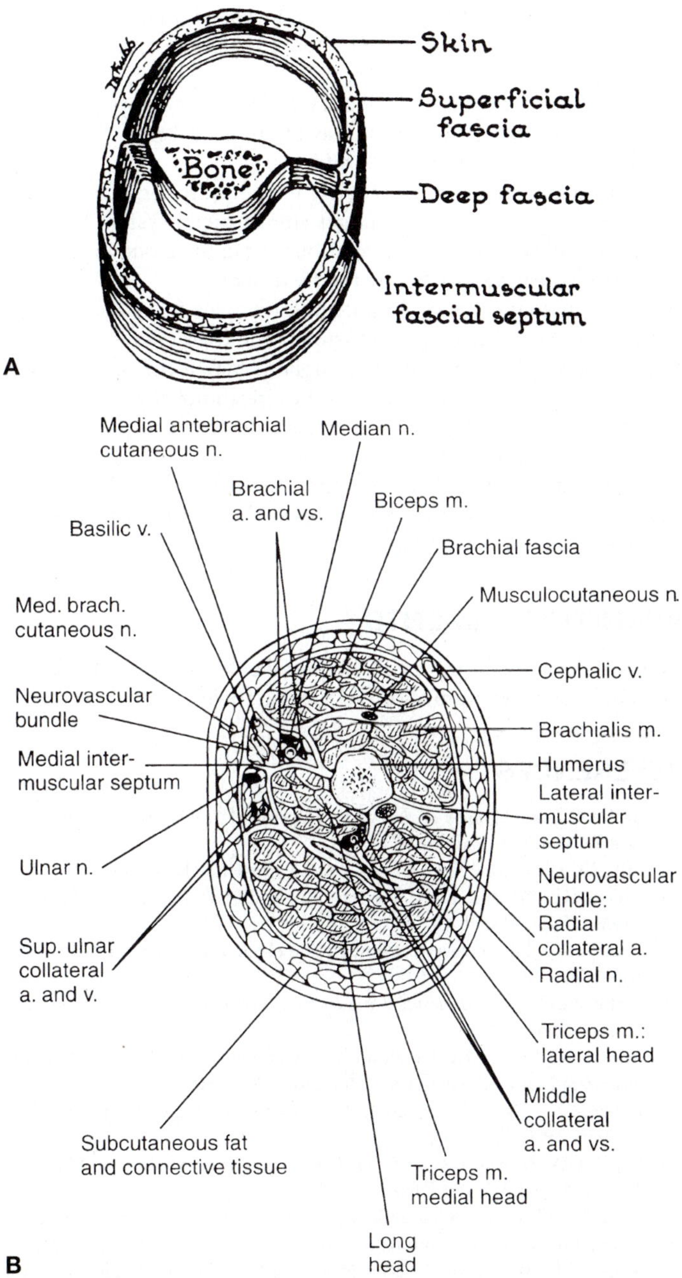

Figure 3.45. The functional compartments of the extremity. **A.** A schematic diagram of the fascial compartment. **B.** A cross section of a fascial compartment in the arm. Each extremity is divided into an anterior compartment and a posterior compartment by a fascial septum that communicates with the bones of the extremity. Within a compartment, each muscle is surrounded by a fascial layer termed the epimysium.

Fascial compartments also separate muscles of the trunk.

- The muscles of the anterior abdominal wall, for example, are easily divided into planes and groups by tough enveloping fascia.
- The following are delineable as a group and from one another not only by their attachments and orientations but also by the tight-fitting sheets of fascia that enclose them:
  - □ External oblique
  - □ Internal oblique
  - □ Transversus abdominis
  - □ Rectus abdominis

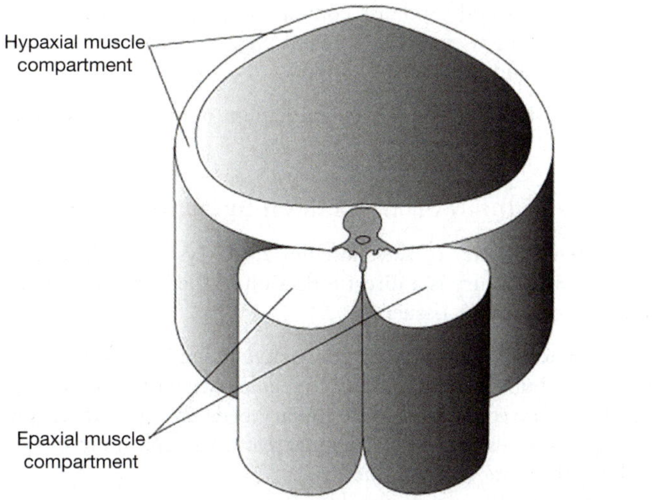

Figure 3.46. The functional fascial compartments of the torso. An anterior fascial compartment surrounds the hypaxial muscles innervated by the ventral primary ramus. A posterior fascial compartment surrounds the epaxial muscles innervated by the dorsal primary ramus. The epaxial compartment is divided into two parts by the spinous process of the vertebrae. These fascial compartments contribute to the structural stability of the torso.

- Planes of fascia are also found in the subcutaneous space, external to the deep fascia that bounds the surfaces of the muscles.
- Understanding the placement of these fasciae is important in a variety of medical and surgical settings.

Peripheral nerves, blood, and lymph vessels lie in loose connective tissue located between muscles.

- This fascia serves to bind these nerves and vessels together and collectively the components form the neurovascular bundle (see Fig. 3.45).
- Also, being loose in its arrangement allows for sliding movements of the neurovascular bundle as the surrounding muscle contract.

While fascia tends to separate and isolate groups of muscles of similar location and function, many of the layers of fascia, whether subcutaneous or investing, merge together and/or have common points of attachment.

- The fascia that separates and ensheathes the external and internal abdominal obliques merge posteriorly with the thick, connective tissue of thoracolumbar fascia; they are continuous superiorly, encasing and separating the deep muscles of the back.
- Anteriorly, the fasciae of the abdominal muscles merge, split, and are reflected to contribute to the inguinal anatomy and abdominal aponeurosis surrounding the rectus abdominis.
- These fasciae are continuous with connective tissue sheets that flow over the crest of the pelvis and become the fascia lata of the thigh.
- The fascia of the thigh is continuous, in turn, with the crural fascia of the leg.
- As a consequence of the widespread continuity of fascia, distortion, damage, or inflammation in one region of the body can have effects in a distant, seemingly unrelated area.

The importance of the two-faceted aspect of fascia, that it separates and segregates but is also continuous structure to structure and area to area, should not be overlooked.

- This pervasive connector (along with muscle and bone) helps to regionalize the body and also connects region to region.
- Such a dualism is apparent in many physical manifestations of both health and disease.

For more details on the possible functions of fascia in the body, see Schleip.[28]

Response of the Musculoskeletal System to Injury

The inherent capacity of the musculoskeletal system to heal and repair following injury is a direct reflection of the histologic organization of connective tissue.

- At the macroscopic level, the connective tissue invests the neurovascular bundles, which supply specific parts of the body.
- At the microscopic level, the capillary beds are located within the open meshwork of loose connective tissue and nourish the cellular elements of the tissue.

These cells in turn produce the ground substance and fibers of the connective tissue.

Following injury, a complex biochemical reaction results in stimulating the inherent capacity of healing and repair.

- In general, the more differentiated any tissue is (i.e., the less it resembles the embryonic tissue from which it was derived), the less capable that tissue is of cell division and, therefore, the less able the tissue is to heal via mitotic addition of new cells following injury.
  - Because of its highly differentiated nature, skeletal muscle and cartilage often repair as a scar mainly composed of irregular dense connective tissue.
- Bone represents a major exception to this rule. Since bone is actively remodeling in the living state, it will rapidly form a scar following injury and then gradually remodel the scar into the normal architecture of the adult bone.
- A corollary of this principle on differentiation can be seen in cancerous tissue.
  - Generally, differentiated cells have to dedifferentiate in order to become a malignancy.
  - The more undifferentiated a cell becomes, the more potential it has to divide; thus, some of the most dangerous malignancies are anaplastic lesions in which cells appear to return to a primitive, embryonic-looking state.

SUMMARY

The body, so often represented as a group of discrete regions or functional systems, is in reality an integrated whole.

- The integration of the body region to region and system to system is accomplished by a series of connectors.
- Some of these connectors, the endocrine and immune systems, are more commonly included in the context of physiology, biochemistry, or immunology.
- The nervous system, the vascular system, and the lymphatics are also important connectors, the structural components of which are part of anatomical disciplines.
- Finally, the visible connective tissues of the body, and particularly the fascia, are great physical connectors that bind organs or muscles into larger groups.

Coherent medical practice requires attention to the connected nature of the unified human organism.

- Typically, one disturbing force (a localized injury, lesion, or infection) causes a cascade of altered structural and functional changes in other areas or systems.
- Similarly, the treatment of localized disease or injury must not only be localized but must also attempt to bring the whole organism into healthy equilibrium.
- Planned treatments must account for not only the effect of the treatment protocol on the target site or organ system but also the so-called side effect alterations brought about in distant, relatively healthy systems by the treatment.
- These anatomical and physiologic principles form the basis of the Five-Model Concept in Osteopathic Medicine.
- Although the patient's chief complaint may focus on one issue alone, that issue has numerous ramifications throughout the individual's body, all of which act as a deterrent to the patient's ability to regain health.
- Use of the five models in analyzing the patient's health, as discussed in this chapter, helps to assess the multifold manifestations of the focal disorder.

ACKNOWLEDGMENTS

The authors and editors of this chapter would like to acknowledge the scholarly contributions of Dr. Lex C. Towns.

REFERENCES

1. Still AT. *Autobiography of A.T. Still.* (Reprint of 1899 edition). American Academy of Osteopathy; 1977.
2. Still AT. *Osteopathy: Research and Practice.* Eastland Press; 1992.
3. Moore KL, Persaud TVN, Torchia M. *The Developing Human.* 11th ed. Elsevier Saunders; 2020.
4. Pourquie O. The vertebrate segmentation clock. *J Anat.* 2001;199(Pt 1–2): 169–175.
5. Hollinshead WH. *Anatomy for Surgeons: The Back and Limbs.* 2nd ed. Hoeber-Harper; 1969.
6. Martin R, Brown DA, Diamond ME, Cattaneo A, DeMiguel FF. *From Neuron to Brain.* 6th ed. Oxford University Press; 2020.
7. Landmesser L. The generation of neuromuscular specificity. *Ann Rev Neurosci.* 1980;3:279–302.
8. Pawlina W. *Histology: A Text and Atlas with Correlated Cell and Molecular Biology.* 9th ed. Wolters Kluwer; 2024.
9. Karaplis AC. Embryonic development of bone and regulation of intramembranous and endochondral bone formation. In: Bilezikian JP, Raisz LG, Martin TJ, eds. *Principles of Bone Biology.* 3rd ed. Elsevier Academic Press; 2008:53–84.
10. Stecco C. *Functional Atlas of the Human Fascial System.* Churchill Livingstone Elsevier; 2015.
11. Tickle C, Eichele G. Vertebrate limb development. [Review]. *Annu Rev Cell Biol.* 1994;10:121–152.
12. Gans C, Northcutt RG. Neural crest and the origin of vertebrates: a new head. *Science.* 1983;220(4594):268–273.
13. Lieberman DE. *The Evolution of the Human Head.* Belnap Press of Harvard; 2011.
14. Diogo R, Kelly RG, Christiaen L, et al. A new heart for a new head in vertebrate cardiopharyngeal evolution. *Nature.* 2015;520(7548):466–473.
15. Boron WF, Boulpaep EL. *Medical Physiology.* 3rd ed. Elsevier; 2016.
16. Brazis PW, Masdeu JC, Biller J. *Localization in Clinical Neurology.* 6th ed. Lippincott Williams & Wilkins; 2011.
17. Hall JE. *Guyton and Hall Textbook of Medical Physiology.* Saunders Elsevier; 2015.
18. Graham DM, Burridge K. Mechanotransduction and nuclear function. *Curr Opin Cell Biol.* 2016;40:98–105.
19. Langevin HM. Connective tissue: a body-wide signaling network? *Med Hypotheses.* 2006;66(6):1074–1077.

20. Delves PJ, Martin SJ, Burton DR, Roitt IM. *Roitt's Essential Immunology*. 12th ed. Wiley-Blackwell; 2011.
21. Gruber BL, Kaplan AP. Mast cells and rheumatic disease. In: Koopman WJ, eds. *Arthritis and Allied Conditions. A Textbook of Rheumatology*. 14th ed. Lippincott Williams & Wilkins; 2001:393–423.
22. Standring S. *Gray's Anatomy: The Anatomical Basis of Clinical Practice*. Elsevier Churchill Livingston; 2020.
23. Nordin M, Frankel VH. *Basic Biomechanics of the Musculoskeletal System*. Wolters Kluwer; Lippincott Williams & Wilkins; 2021.
24. O'Rahilly R. *Gardner–Gray–O'Rahilly Anatomy: A Regional Study of Human Structure*. 5th ed. W.B. Saunders Comp.; 1986.
25. Mennell J. *Joint Pain*. Little Brown Co.; 1964.
26. Clemente CD. *Gray's Anatomy of the Human Body*. Lea & Febiger; 1985.
27. Catala M. Embryonic and fetal development of structures associated with the cerebro-spinal fluid in man and other species. Part I: the ventricular system, meninges and choroid plexuses. *Arch Anat Cytol Pathol*. 1998;46(3):153–169.
28. Schleip R, Findley TW, Chaitow L, Huijing PA. *Fascia: The Tensional Network of the Human Body*. Churchill Livingston; 2012.

4 Inherent Motion, Rhythms and Oscillations

DEBORAH SCHMIDT

KEY CONCEPTS

- Since the days of the early students of Dr. Still, oscillatory physiologic motion within the structure of the human body has been observed by the osteopathic profession and used to diagnose and treat somatic dysfunctions.
- Waveforms are complex phenomenon that show periodicity in both time and space and can communicate properties of energy through matter and space.
- Waves communicate via a specialized form of energy transfer using properties that enhance or alter their interaction with other waves. These properties include resonance or synchronization, modulation by amplitude or frequency, and phase modulation. Waves can lock frequency and phase with other waves through a phenomenon called entrainment.
- The coherence of several waveforms can be evaluated to determine the degree of similarity in either time or frequency domain. Time domain waveforms can be converted mathematically into frequency domain spectrum by a formula called a fast Fourier transform (FFT).
- Our physical world is regulated by oscillatory wave patterns coupled to oscillators greater and smaller than ourselves, that allow the waveforms of different organisms to communicate, or entrain, with other oscillators.
- The anatomic locus of the central clock that organizes circadian rhythm was mapped within the suprachiasmatic nucleus of the brain. The central clock is regulated by a transcription-translation feedback loop involving the phosphorylation of specific genes that autoregulate by feedback of their own protein products to form autonomous oscillations.
- Oscillatory ranges are being mapped for many human physiologic functions including cardiac oscillatory rhythms, muscle sympathetic nerve activity, brain waves/EEGs, fMRI brain networks, and inherent motion monitoring that may correlate to the cranial rhythmic impulse (CRI).

"As motion is the first and only evidence of life, by this thought we are conducted to the machinery through which life works to accomplish the results as witnessed in ***motion.****"*[1]

—*Andrew Taylor Still, MD, DO*

One of the goals of a living organism is the maintenance of homeostasis of form and function in the face of an ever-changing environment. Oscillations serve as a form of equilibrium, or return to balance, in a wave form that can change in space and time. Biologic rhythms are attempts to restore and maintain homeostasis and appear in all physiologic systems to regulate function. Examples include heart rate variability (HRV), respiratory rate (RR) variability, brain waves, peristalsis, endocrine secretion, and the global function of the autonomic nervous system.

The human body contains multiple cells that perform as time cues, or zeitgebers, and are termed "clocks" that set the reference point in the fluctuation of a biologic system to an equilibrium or "normal." They have been studied in the central nervous system (central clocks) within the suprachiasmatic nucleus (SCN) of the hypothalamus and in the peripheral nervous system (peripheral clocks), like the cardiac-related pacemaker cells, the pancreatic secretory cells, and gluconeogenic cells of the liver. These cells perform specific physiologic functions repeatedly over periods of time. As further study evolves, central and peripheral clocks have been found in most cells and have the ability to shift or fluctuate their function based upon the demands of their environment and needs. The living organism has the ability to self-regulate.

The time cue generators, or zeitgebers, have been found to contain specific biochemical and DNA translational processes that occur in sequence over a set period of time, thus setting the "clock" of that biologic rhythm. These rhythms have properties that all waves or oscillations possess, namely that they can synchronize with each other based on influence via a phenomenon called entrainment, they can provide interference to each other and inhibit or augment each other, and they can perform in specific recurrent intervals in a form or harmonic interaction called resonance. The set cues respond to environmental changes, the most studied being the light/dark cycle, sleep, temperature control/thermoregulation, food availability/metabolism, and many others that have yet to be discovered.

The influence of the environment on the living organism reaches from the local (immediate vicinity) to the global (geologic rhythms, seasonal rhythms, magnetic rhythms) to the cosmologic (sun spots, gamma radiation). Homeostatic mechanisms depend upon a set reference point of optimal function with the flexibility to adjust to new environmental challenges, which is found in oscillatory behavior.

OSTEOPATHIC MEDICINE AND THE IMPORTANCE OF BIOLOGIC RHYTHMS

The concept of the observation of oscillatory physiologic motion in humans is not new to osteopathic medicine, nor is the use of oscillations/vibrations to treat somatic dysfunction. Zachary Comeaux, DO,[2] describes how the philosophical influences of the time influenced the early progression of osteopathic thought in regard to vibration/oscillation. Dr. Still was influenced by English philosopher/scientist Herbert Spencer, whose integrated approach to evolutionary biology and cosmology lent well to the concept of the reciprocity of structure and function and integration of the whole person into diagnosis and treatment.

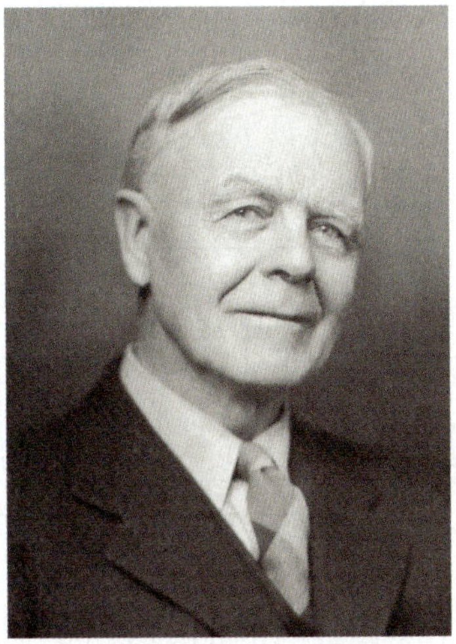

W.G. Sutherland, DO
(Courtesy of Sutherland Cranial Teaching Foundation.)

W. G. Sutherland, DO, an early student of Dr. Still, went through a lifelong evolution of thought in regard to the concepts of freedom and restriction of motion in the human structure. Sutherland first discovered the concept of the articular mobility of the cranial bones indicating repetitive motion, then by careful palpation, uncovered the vital rhythmic potency of what he termed "the Tide" which he defined as the organizing concept behind the Life Force. In *Teachings in the Science of Osteopathy*, he describes a sequence of lymphatic mobilization:

> *"The physiologic emptying requires a gentle and rather unique siphoning process in the thoracic duct. This process can be assisted or facilitated by the use of feeling, seeing, thinking, and knowing fingers. This guidance varies from manual manipulation. During the application, fingers of one hand establish a contact over lymph nodes while a transmitted vibration is initiated through the other hand, which is placed on top of it. A quiet pause-rest should occur between applications. The first application is to the upper left thorax near the axilla. The second is done with a lift to the area above the receptaculum chyli. The third is at the great omentum, with a lift. The transmitted vibration initiates the siphoning process."*[3]

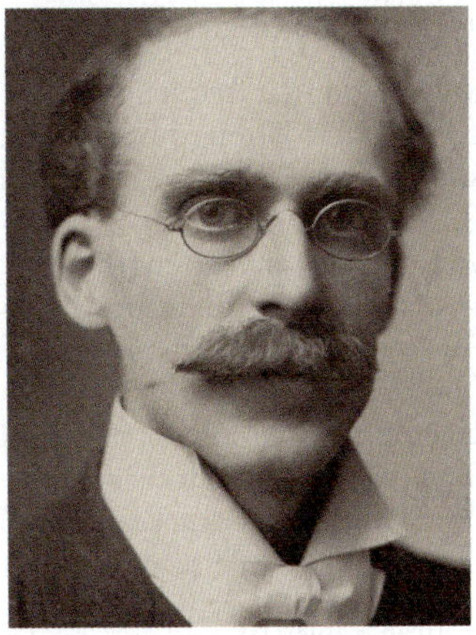

J.M. Littlejohn, DO
(From https://johnwernhamclassicalosteopathy.com/. Used by kind permission of The John Wernham College of Classical Osteopathy [UK]).

J.M. Littlejohn, DO, was another of Stills' early students and co-lecturer at the American School of Osteopathy in Kirksville who went on to found the American College of Osteopathic Medicine with his brother in Chicago. Ten years later he founded the British School of Osteopathy in London. Littlejohn recognized the importance of vibrational motion in the preparation of tissues for articular correction.

In 1902, Littlejohn stated the following regarding biologic oscillations: *"The vital cycle depends upon vibration. Waves of vibration pass along the tissues, especially from the nerves and the brain to and along the muscle tissues. There is no function of the body that does not have peristaltic or rhythmic vibrations…the power of osteopathic treatment occurs from its effect upon physiologic oscillations."*[4]

As the muscle energy model evolved, the role of oscillatory manipulation as a part of the treatment sequence to restore normal neurologic balance and therefore muscle tone was introduced. T.J. Ruddy, DO, an early pioneer in muscle energy technique, used a rhythmic muscular contraction by the patient to restore normal muscle tone. Fred Mitchell, Jr., DO, used an active oscillatory motion against constant patient contraction to overcome the myotatic reflex of tight scalene muscles.

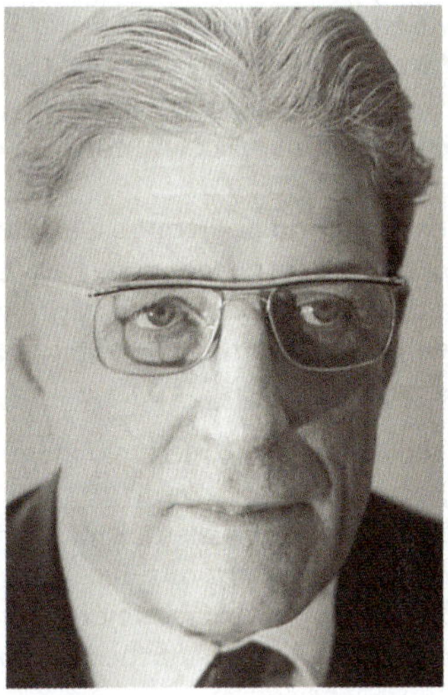

Robert Fulford, DO
(Photo courtesy of Sara Saxton, DO.)

Robert Fulford, DO, another student of Sutherland, through intuitive study embraced the concept of health as a dynamic system in which restriction of the dynamic process was responsible for loss of health, motion, and comfort.[2] He developed the concept of a fluctuating "breath of life" that sustained health in the physical, emotional, and spiritual being and could be restricted physically, emotionally (through trauma), and spiritually. He developed the use of the Foredom Percussion Vibrator as an augmentation tool to effectively transmit his therapeutic intention to treat not just the physical but the energetic (etheric) body.

Many students evolved from these osteopathic physicians and have helped to expand the concept of oscillatory motion as a diagnostic and therapeutic tool in the osteopathic approach to a patient. They include Carlisle Holland, DO, Richard Koss, DO, Rajiv Yadava, DO, John McPartland, DO, Eric Mein, MD, James Jealous, DO, and Zachary Comeaux, DO.

WAVE CHARACTERISTICS AND PROPERTIES

Oscillations are periodic motions or vibrations relative to an equilibrium point. Waves are oscillations that propagate in space, so they transfer energy. Waves are complex phenomena that show periodicity in both time and space.

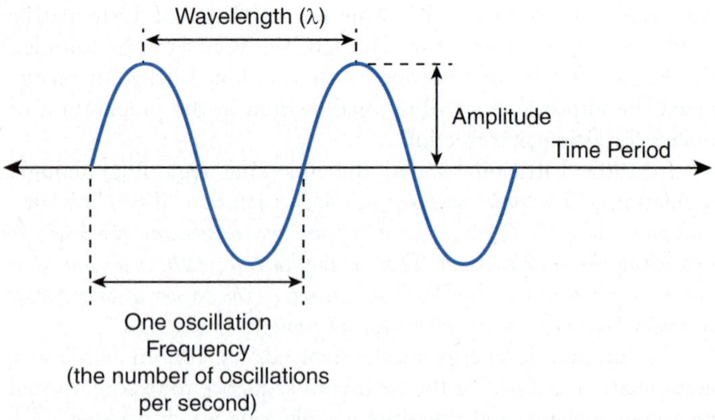

Figure 4.1. **Wave characteristics.**

Mechanical waves require a medium (water or air molecules) to propagate and can form in two ways. When particles of the medium move in a *perpendicular direction* to the wave propagation they are called *transverse waves*, as in musical instruments, light waves, and water waves. When particles of the medium vibrate *parallel to the direction* of wave propagation they are called *longitudinal waves*. These waves slink back and forth, like sound waves or P-waves in earthquakes.

Nonmechanical waves do not require a medium and can travel through a vacuum, like electromagnetic waves. Living organisms propagate both mechanical and nonmechanical waves.

All waves have a wavelength, frequency, speed, periodicity (time period), and amplitude (Fig. 4.1).

Wavelength: the distance between two identical points (crests or troughs) on a wave.

Frequency: the number of oscillations passing a fixed point on the wave in a given amount of time.

The standard unit (SU) of frequency is a **Hertz (Hz)** which is the number of oscillations of the waveform in 1 second.

1 Hertz (Hz) = 1 cycle per second (or 60 cycles per minute [cpm])

When comparing waveform frequency, care must be taken to use the same standard unit (Hertz) to describe each wave. Waves are typically described within a range of frequencies, for example, 0.05 to 0.1 Hz would represent 3 to 6 cpm.

In music, middle C is 262 Hz. If we could see the waves passing when someone played middle C, we would see about 262 waves pass our eyes in each second. The wavelength of middle C is 132 cm. Human hearing ranges 20 to 20,000 Hz, depending on age. The frequency of a sound is referred to as its pitch. High-frequency notes are high notes and low-frequency notes are low notes. Frequency in light describes the color of the light. Red light has a relatively low frequency and violet light has a high frequency. Frequency and wavelength are inversely proportional to each other. The longer the wavelength, the lower the frequency.

Speed: for a wave, speed is the distance traveled by a particular point on the wave in the given interval of time. Speed is measured in meters per second. Speed is related to frequency and wavelength through the equation:

Speed = wavelength × frequency

Each wave travels at a particular speed. Water waves travel at variable speeds. Electromagnetic waves always travel at the same speed (300 million meters per second). Sound waves travel at the same speed in a given medium (about 340 meters per second in air).

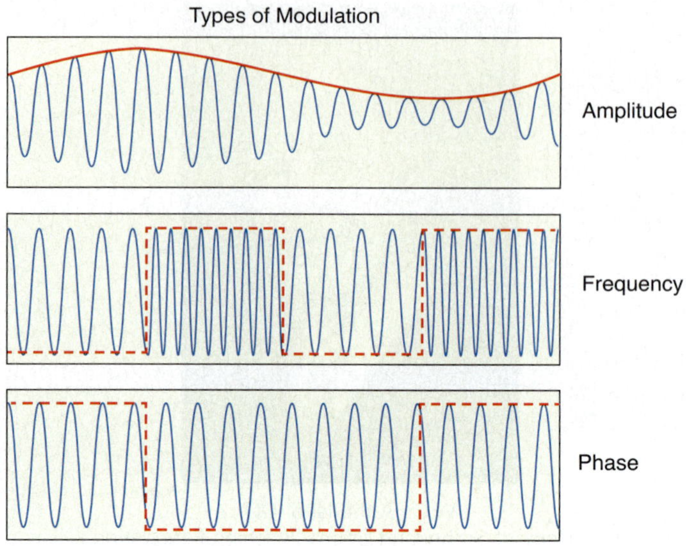

Figure 4.2. **Types of wave modulation.**

Period/periodicity: the time period required for a complete oscillation or vibration.

Amplitude: the maximum displacement of a wave crest from its equilibrium position, or height, of the waveform.

Period and **frequency** define the cycle and **amplitude** defines the strength (or power) of the cycle.

As a specialized form of communication by energy transfer, a wave can have properties that enhance or alter their interaction with other waves.

One such property is **resonance,** or the phenomenon that occurs when an object experiences an oscillating force that is close to one of its own natural frequencies. This causes an object to vibrate **in step** or **in phase** with that externally applied oscillatory force. In sound, it is the reinforcement of a sound by another vibrating body at nearly the same frequency. Another word for resonance is **synchronization.**

Modulation is the change over time in an oscillating periodic wave that can convey a message or information. A few of the common modulation methods are (Fig. 4.2):

Amplitude modulation: the frequency of the carrier waveform does not change but its strength varies with the modulating signal. Example: Arterial pressure is modulated (amplified or reduced) by the RR interval.

Frequency modulation: the strength of the carrier waves remains constant but the frequency of the carrier wave is changed. For example, the variation of blood flow velocity with HRV over time.

Phase modulation: modulation of the timing of the onset of a waveform with respect to a second waveform of the same amplitude and frequency. For example, jet lag, when a rhythm resets the phase of circadian rhythm (phase shift).

In 1665, the Dutch physicist and inventor of the pendulum clock, Christiaan Huygens, was confined to his room by a minor illness. With nothing to do, he observed two of his clocks that were suspended by a common support and noted that they were locked in perfect synchrony and remained that way. Even if one was stopped and restarted out of phase with the other, synchrony would be regained shortly. Only if they were relocated to opposite sides of the room could the lockstep of their pendulums be disrupted.

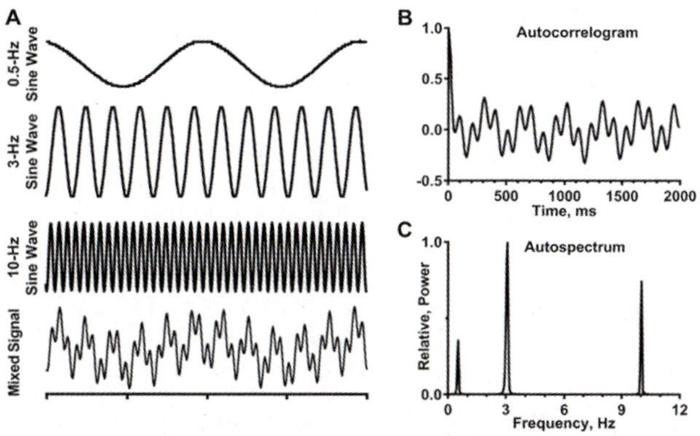

Figure 4.3. Comparison of time and frequency-domain analysis. Comparison of **time**- and **frequency-domain analyses** to quantify the characteristics of a complex analog signal. **A.** Outputs of three sine-wave generators are shown separately (0.5, 3.0, and 10 Hz), as well as in combination (mixed signal). Time scale = 1 s/division. **B.** Autocorrelogram is the **time-domain analysis** of a 5-minute recording of the mixed signal; 5-ms bin resolution. **C.** Autospectrum is the **frequency-domain analysis** of the same 5-minute recording of the mixed signal; it is based on 29 20-s windows with 50% overlap and frequency resolution of 0.04 Hz per bin. A Digidata 1322A digitizer (Axon Instruments, Union City, CA) was used to acquire data. (Reprinted with permission from Barman SM. 2019 Ludwig Lecture: rhythms in sympathetic nerve activity are a key to understanding neural control of the cardiovascular system. *Am J Physiol Regul Integr Comp Physiol.* 2020;318(2):R191–R205. Copyright © 2020 the American Physiological Society.)

This began the **study of coupled oscillators** and demonstrates the locking of frequency and phase of waves which is called **entrainment.** Different amounts of energy transferred between moving bodies due to the asynchronous movement periods cause negative feedback, which drives an adjustment process in which the different energy amounts are gradually eliminated to zero until both moving bodies move in resonant frequency or synchrony. The stronger oscillator locks the weaker into its frequency. When both oscillating bodies have equally strong energy, both systems move toward each other, the faster system slows down and the slower system speeds up until they lock into a common movement period.[6]

In order to **analyze periodic waveforms for coherence,** they need to undergo mathematical manipulation to assess the degree of similarity/quantification they have within either the **time domain** or **frequency domain.** Figure 4.3 demonstrates the comparison of three separate sine waves (0.5, 3.0, and 10 Hz) as well as a mixed signal of all three. B shows the **time-domain analysis** of the mixed signal with autocorrelogram and the variation in time becomes obvious, but the frequency quantities are more difficult to assess. C shows the **frequency-domain analysis** of the mixed signal using autospectrum and the quantity and frequency of each sine wave becomes much more apparent and easier to compare (Fig. 4.3).[7]

FAST FOURIER TRANSFORM (FFT)

If over a given time there is more than one periodic pattern mixed with aperiodic activity, or irregular activity, frequency-domain analysis is useful to identify the different wave form frequencies. A time-domain wave form can be converted mathematically into a frequency-domain spectrum by a formula called a **fast Fourier transform (FFT),** which decomposes an analog signal into its frequency components by matching the signal to sine waves within a broad range of frequencies. This is much more useful to delineate the population proportion of each specific frequency in order to identify it within a physiologic recording.

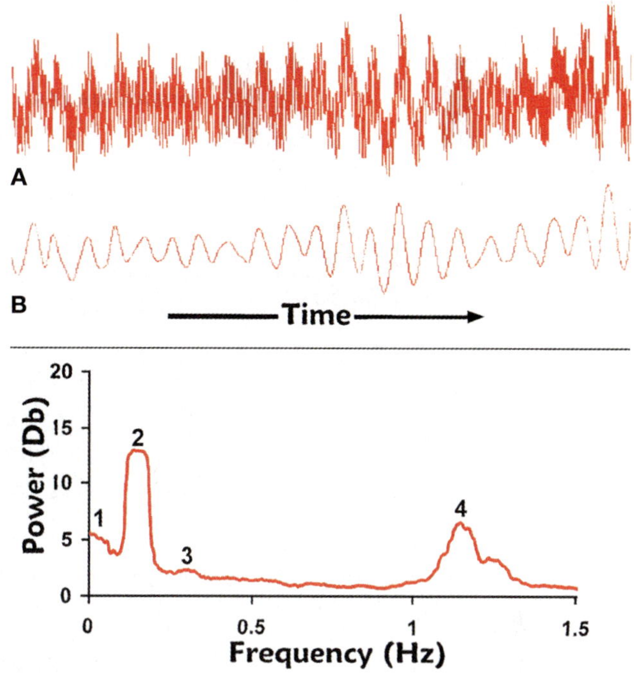

Figure 4.4. **(A)** Waves upon waves upon waves; the time-domain record of a complete blood flow velocity record, demonstrating the heart rate waveform upon the low-frequency baroreflex waveform upon the very–low-frequency waveform. (**B**) Filtered record showing respiratory, low-, and very–low-frequency components only. **Bottom spectrum:** The FT, frequency-domain spectrum of waveform (**A**), demonstrating (1) very–low-frequency signal component, (2) low-frequency signal component, (3) higher-frequency respiration signal, and (4) the heart rate spectral component. (From Glonek T, Sergueef N, Nelson KE. Inherent motion, rhythms, and oscillations. In: Seffinger MA, ed. *Foundations of Osteopathic Medicine: Philosophy, Science, Clinical Applications, and Research.* 4th ed. Wolters Kluwer; 2018:135–166. Figure 6-1.)

Figure 4.4 provides an example of a recording of blood flow velocity that demonstrates a mixed signal of HRV wave at 1.4 Hz, RR wave at 0.35 Hz, low-frequency baroreflex wave at (0.2 Hz), and very–low-frequency wave at (0.1 Hz) (Fig. 4.4).

Entrainment of oscillating waveforms is how most biologic systems regulate themselves. Some examples of biologic coupled oscillators include circadian cycles, digestive/metabolic cycles, pulsatile waves of low arterial pressure (Traube–Hering), and neurons communicating action potentials.

John McPartland, DO, termed **entrainment** as the integration or harmonization of oscillators. A **frequency-selective entrainment** is such a harmonic frequency that incorporates rhythms of multiple biologic oscillators into a single, dominant frequency. He suggests that the cranial rhythmic impulse (CRI), which has been measured by palpatory means by the Woods in 1961, Magoun in 1976, and Upledger in 1983, may be the result of entrainment of many other oscillations that are being measured within the body's physiologic systems.[5]

OUR PHYSICAL WORLD is regulated by oscillatory wave patterns that are coupled to oscillators greater than and smaller than themselves. Each phenomenon has its own defined frequency and wavelength yet entrains, or communicates, with other oscillatory rhythms (Fig. 4.5).

Humans exist within a myriad of oscillatory patterns, cosmologic, atmospheric, geologic, seasonal, societal, personal, cellular, and molecular. Each of these waveforms is governed by the characteristics and properties just discussed (Fig. 4.6).

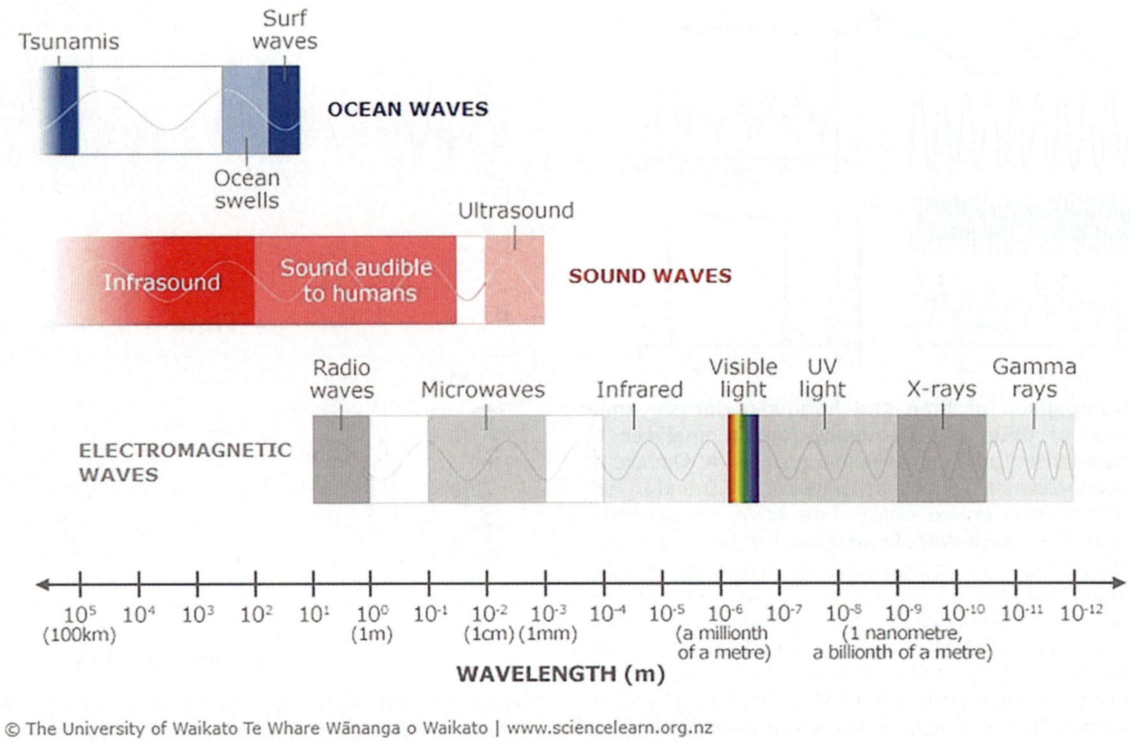

Figure 4.5. Geophysical spectrum. (From https://www.sciencelearn.org.nz/images/112-wavelengths-of-different-wave-types. Reprinted with permission from The University of Waikato Te Whare Wānanga o Waikato.)

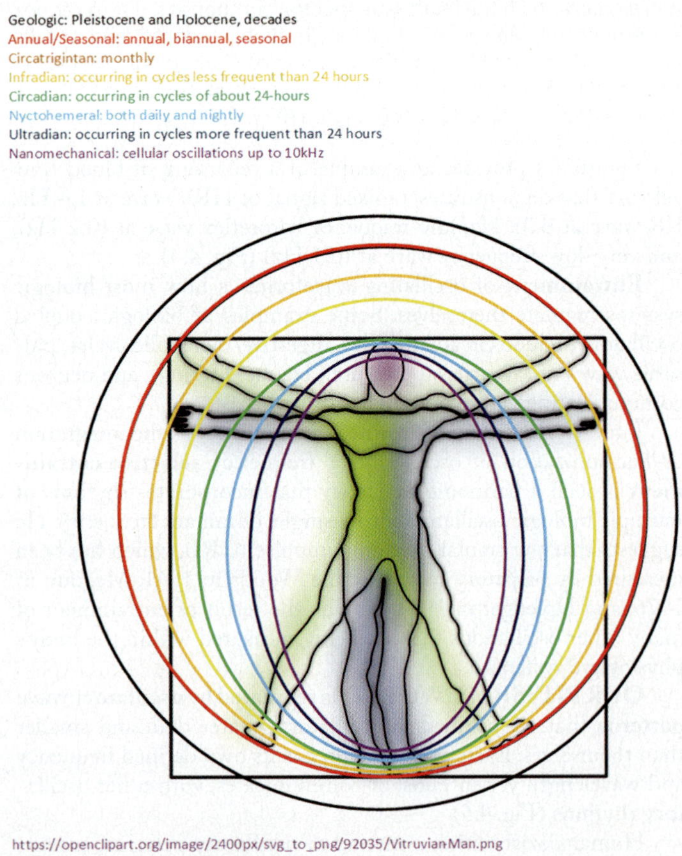

Figure 4.6. ViruvianMan. (From Adrienne Kania, DO; 2023. https://openclipart.org/image/2400px/svg_to_png/92035/VitruvianMan.png.)

BIOLOGIC RHYTHMS have distinct advantages in the regulatory function of living organisms over randomly occurring events. Periodic oscillations of all frequency ranges are critical for the regulation of many physiologic behaviors. Some rhythms are the result of environmental changes, like alterations in cardiovascular variables and others are bidirectional, and allow highly branched communication patterns, like within the central nervous system. Rhythmicity allows a **dynamic response** to the environment by constantly returning to a point of reference (normal). The biologic system is **stabilized** and any drift of function is mitigated. Thus, an organism is better able to **maintain homeostasis** and accommodate repetitive events leading to more efficient behavior for normal function. It is **energy efficient**, particularly in living organisms that have multiple oscillatory systems each with their own equilibrium that are able to regulate energy expenditure by modulation of each other. Oscillations allow **communication** between systems because waves can influence each other through the processes of entrainment, modulation, and phase coherence.[7]

Human physiologic oscillations include seasonal, circatrigintan (monthly), infradian (less frequent than every 24 hours), circadian (roughly 24 hours), nyctohemeral (diurnal), and nanomechanical (cellular) rhythms. The **circatrigintan rhythm,** which roughly occurs monthly and is often lunar, includes the estrous/menstrual cycle which dictates fertility. The most familiar pattern of **nyctohemeral** oscillations includes the diurnal rhythms of corticosteroid release (Fig. 4.7).

Circadian rhythms are the near 24-hour oscillations found in essentially every physiologic process in the human brain and body.[8] Oscillatory rhythms require a **time-cue**, or **zeitgeber** (time-giver) that is an external or environmental cue that synchronizes an organism's biologic rhythm. This zeitgeber is usually naturally occurring and serves to entrain the organism to the Earth's 24-hour light/dark and 12-month cycles. These time cues are capable of

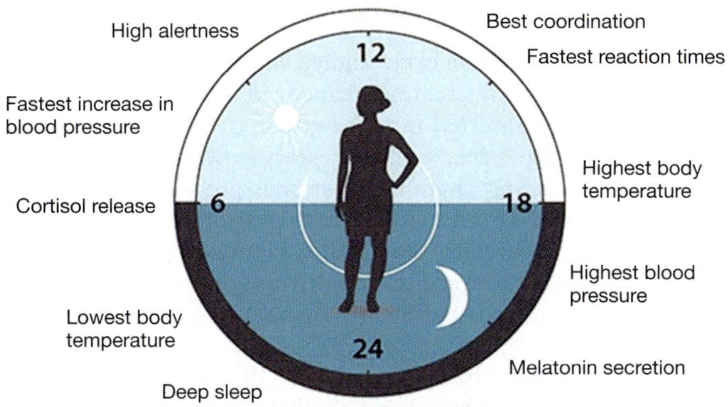

Figure 4.7. A 24-hour day. (Illustration: © The Nobel Committee for Physiology or Medicine. Illustrator: Mattias Karlén.)

entraining circadian (and other) rhythms and can establish the phase of an oscillating wave and synchronize a system of wave phenomenon. The time cues may include sleep (light-dark cycle), activity (thermal/temperature), food availability, and other cues yet to be determined. This endogenous 24-hour "clock" contributes to the regulation of sleep, locomotor activity, body temperature, metabolism, and endocrine release.

The Central Clock—the Suprachiasmatic Nucleus

In 1994, the neurochemical organization of the circadian rhythm of the **suprachiasmatic nucleus** (SCN) was mapped. The SCN, or the **central clock**, is located bilaterally above the optic chiasm on opposite sides of the third ventricle in the anterior basal hypothalamus. It serves as the master pacemaker that sets the timing of rhythms by regulating neuronal activity, body temperature, and hormonal signals. The SCN has a period of roughly 24.18 hours.[9]

The discovery of a mutant gene that was responsible for alterations in the normal 24-hour circadian cycle of a fruit fly, Drosophila, occurred in 1971. This mutation was found to involve a gene that was later named ***period***. A decade later, the ***period*** gene was isolated and molecularly characterized but its mechanism of action in circadian cycles was elusive. In 2017, Hall, Rosbash, and Young were awarded the Nobel Prize in Medicine/Physiology for their elucidation of the molecular feedback loops that regulate the circadian clock.[10] They describe a mechanism of transcription-translation feedback loop (TTLF) where transcription of the gene, ***period***, and its partner gene, ***timeless***, are repressed by their own gene products, the PERIOD (PER) and TIME-LESS (TIM) proteins, which generate autonomous oscillation. Further studies revealed a series of interlocked TTLFs, together with a complex network of reactions that involved regulated protein phosphorylation and degradation of TTFL components, protein complex assembly, nuclear translocation, and other posttranslational modifications that generate oscillations with a period of about 24 hours.[11] These TTFLs have been demonstrated in the SCN central clock and peripheral clocks through a series of negative and positive feedback loops. This discovery has led to an explosion of research in the field of chronobiology (Fig. 4.8).

Afferent input to the SCN begins as light enters the organism through specialized melanopsin-producing intrinsically photosensitive retinal ganglion cells (ipRGCs) in the eye. These specialized retinal ganglion cells are involved in non–image-forming visual processes such as the pupillary light reflex and circadian entrainment but also contribute to the perception of vision. They are particularly sensitive to the absorption of short-wavelength (blue) visible light. The afferent input then travels directly to the SCN via a retinohypothalamic tract (RHT), which uses glutamate as the primary neurotransmitter. The SCN then secretes vasoactive intestinal peptide (VIP) and gastrin-releasing peptide (GRP) in the retinorecipient core of the SCN and arginine vasopressin (AVP) expressing cells in the shell of the SCN.

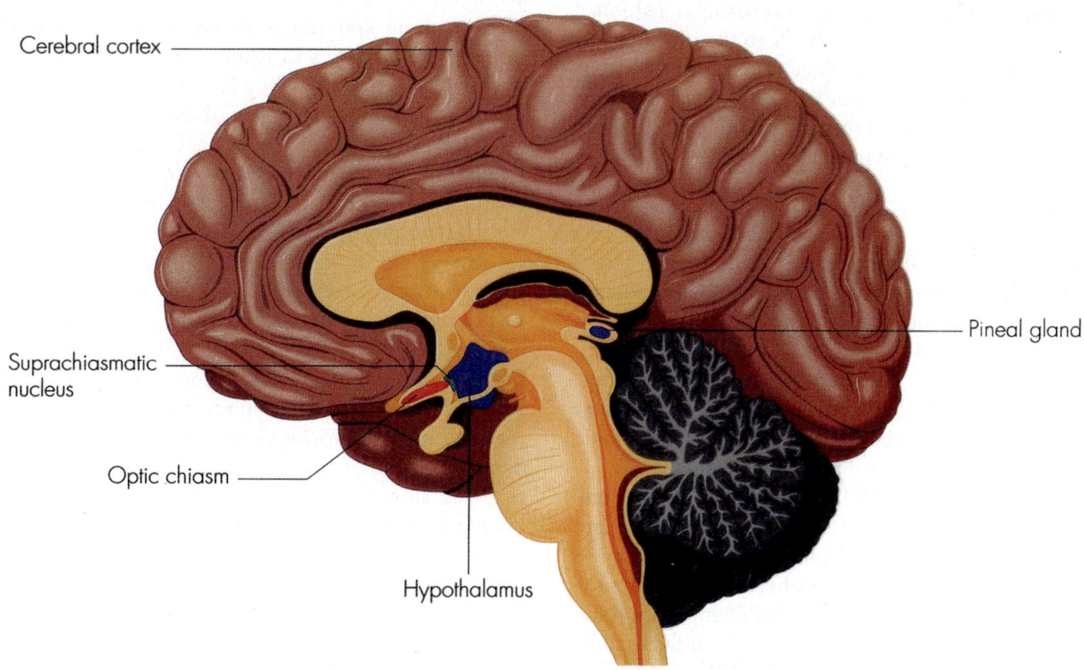

Figure 4.8. The suprachiasmatic nucleus, optic chiasm, and pineal gland. (From https://upload.wikimedia.org/wikipedia/commons/thumb/8/80/Suprachiasmatic_Nucleus.jpg/1920px-Suprachiasmatic_Nucleus.jpg. https://creativecommons.org/licenses/by-sa/3.0/deed.en)

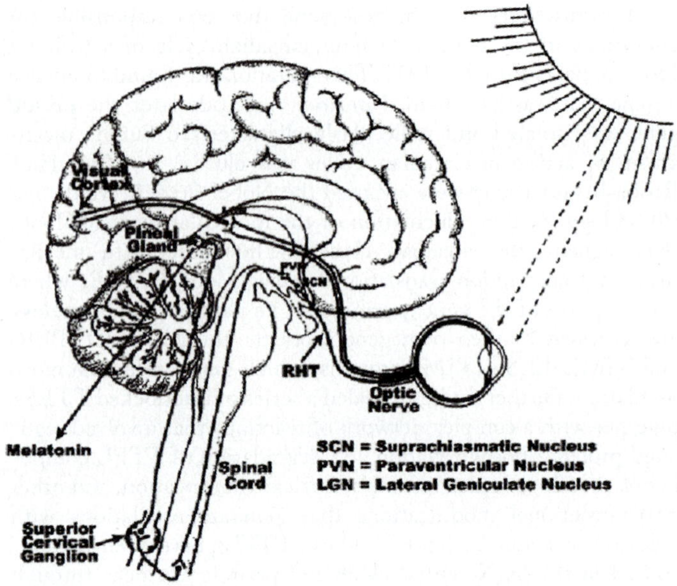

Figure 4.9. **Pathway of output from SCN>>paraventricular nucleus (PVN)>>preganglionic sympathetic neurons (intermediolateral nucleus of thoracic spinal cord)>>noradrenergic neurons of superior cervical (stellate) ganglia>>pineal gland>>melatonin secretion.** (Used with permission of Springer Nature BV from Jasser SA, Blask DE, Brainard GC. Light during darkness and cancer: relationships in circadian photoreception and tumor biology. *Cancer Causes Control.* 2006;17(4):515–523; permission conveyed through Copyright Clearance Center, Inc.)

These transmitters help coordinate circadian feeding and thirst rhythms.[12]

Efferent output of the SCN includes both humoral (vasopressin release) and neural mechanisms via the peripheral autonomic nervous system. One of the most studied outputs of the SCN is the regulation of melatonin synthesis by the pineal gland, which occurs in a diurnal rhythm regulated by light in a daily and seasonal fashion.[13] The course of neuronal stimulus from the SCN to the pineal gland would be expected to be relatively short since they are both within the diencephalon, but they are not. Instead, these pathways make a long detour from the hypothalamus via the spinal cord before returning as sympathetic innervation to the pineal gland (Fig. 4.9).

The Peripheral Clocks

Other pathways of SCN autonomic control of hormonal secretion include SCN>>PVN>>sympathetic nervous system>>adrenal gland axis that controls corticosterone release, SCN regulation of glucose metabolism by circadian modulation of insulin sensitivity, and hepatic glucose productions. The SCN sends neural information to the pancreas, the liver and the adipose (white and brown) tissue, the heart, and the kidney via sympathetic/parasympathetic pathways.[14]

Thus, the master oscillator, the SCN, uses **humoral** and **neuronal input** to coordinate peripheral circadian clocks that are located in lung, liver, pancreas, kidney, heart, muscle, and adipose tissue (both white and brown). These peripheral organs all produce circadian gene expression based on the combination of photic input to the SCN and nonphotic input from behavioral factors like food intake availability and locomotor activity.[15] SCN can be regulated by metabolic feedback loops of the products of the peripheral clocks but only the SCN has light-dark regulatory control (Fig. 4.10).

PHYSIOLOGIC RHYTHMS

Physiologic rhythms have been studied since 1733 when Stephen Hale monitored the fluctuating changes in arterial pressure in a vertical glass pipe inserted into the crural artery of a "mare tied down alive on her back."[15] In the 19th century, Carl Ludwig confirmed fluctuating rhythms of arterial pressure, and Traube and Hering documented the relationship of the arterial pressure rhythms with respiration (the Traube–Hering wave). Cyon and Mayer documented arterial pressure rhythms that were slower than respiration (Mayer wave) although the nature of these waves was unclear.[7]

Because studies have reproduced the frequency-domain mappings of various physiologic rhythms, we now can identify oscillatory ranges for some human physiologic functions. We can monitor arterial pressure changes, R-R interval patterns, intrathoracic pressure changes, and muscle sympathetic nerve activity (mSNA) waves and study their variability via FT. The HRV activity (R-R interval) is now an acceptable surrogate for human vagal-cardiac nerve activity (VCNA) or parasympathetic activity to the heart.

Respiratory control seems to have a physiologic "gate" that opens with expiration (frequency increases) and closes during inspiration (frequency decreases). Respiratory phases seem to gate mSNA and VCNA, indicating a control over these autonomic functions with breathing. Human muscle SNA can be directly measured to predict SNA tone to the heart, kidney, and muscle vascular beds. VCNA is gated by respiration, so there is more vagal firing in expiration than inspiration.

Autonomic oscillations seem to range between very–low-frequency (0.015 to 0.05 Hz) to low-frequency ranges (0.05 to 0.1 Hz) to high-frequency ranges (0.2 to 0.3 Hz). Autonomic nerve activity rates reflect the influence of the respective neurotransmitter on each organ. For instance, mSNA rates seem to reflect the length of time it takes for norepinephrine to influence peripheral vascular tone and return to base state. Vagal/parasympathetic tone seems dictated by the time constraints of acetylcholine action on the target organs. Traube–Hering–Mayer (THM) waves seem to occur spontaneously (without overt stimulation) and are slower than cardiac and respiratory cycles, and can be modulated by drugs or pathology. They have been used as a basis for the fMRI functional connectivity maps of the brain.[16,17]

The central sympathetic network is capable of generating oscillatory activity at various frequencies that work in modulatory relationships with each other. Barman and Gebber have studied barbiturate-anesthetized, paralyzed, and artificially ventilated cats to observe the functional oscillations of the SNA and relationship of various oscillatory waves. A respiratory-related frequency was demonstrated at 0.25 Hz that strongly correlated to phrenic nerve activity (PNA), a 3.80-Hz frequency strongly correlated to the arterial pulse (AP) confirming it was cardiac-related SNA and second SNA 10-Hz frequency was also identified. They ablated the carotid sinus, aortic depressor, and vagus nerves (baroreceptor denervation) and saw the cardiac-related SNA replaced by a 2- to 6-Hz slow wave band plus the 10-Hz frequency band. They observed that when there was a spontaneous transition in SNA from a prominent cardiac-related rhythm to a dominant 10-Hz rhythm there was a marked increase in arterial blood pressure (ABP). Similarly, elimination of the 10-Hz rhythm by chemical inactivation of brainstem excitatory amino acids caused a significant reduction in ABP.[16] Malpas suggests that different frequency patterns in the SNA may not simply modulate the degree of vasoconstriction but may reflect distinct functional responses as a result of the release of specific neurotransmitters.[18] So different

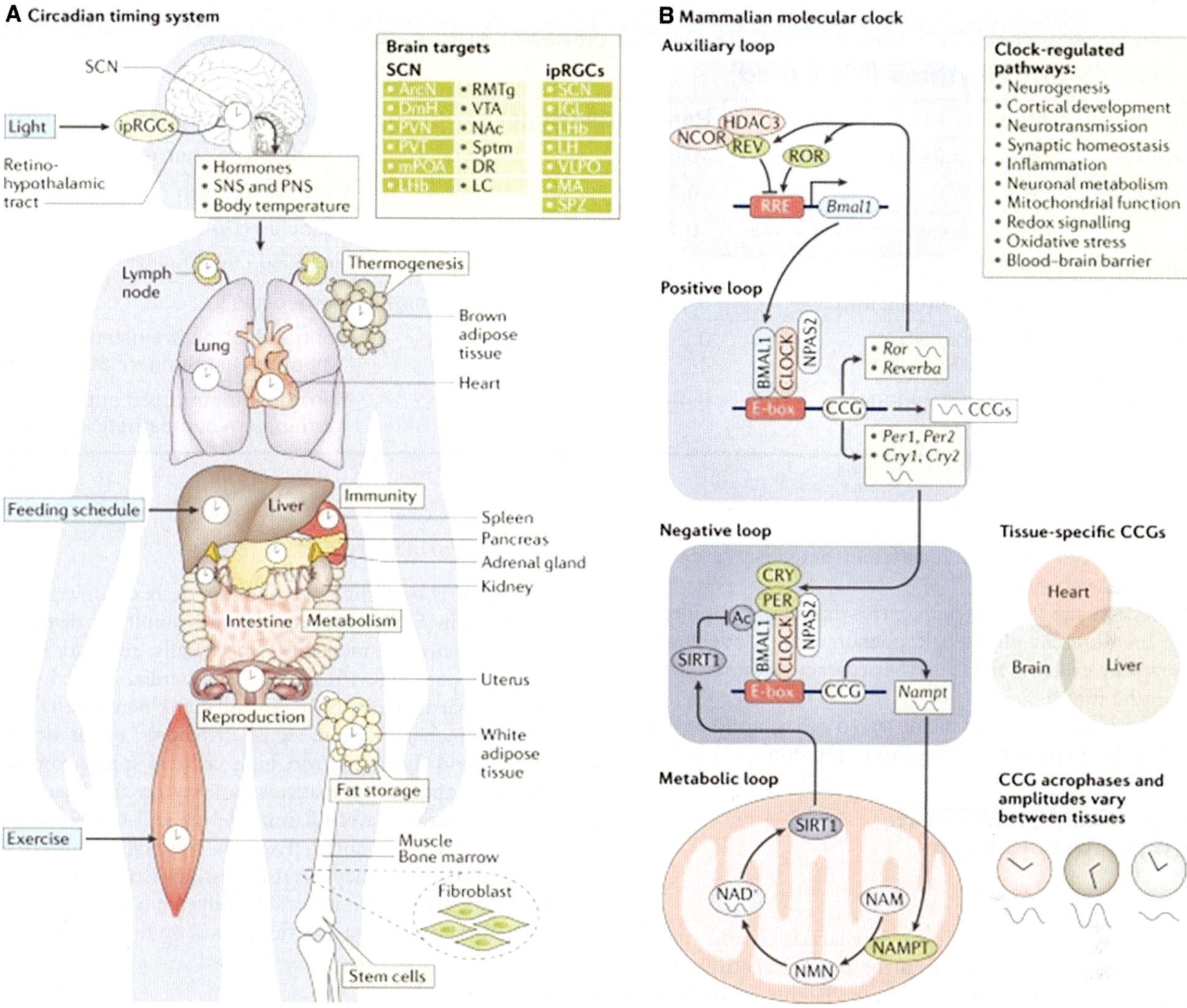

Figure 4.10. Circadian timing system/molecular clock. A. The circadian timing system synchronizes clocks across the entire body to adapt and optimize physiology to changes in our environment. Light is received by specialized melanopsin-producing photoreceptive retinal ganglion cells (ipRGCs) in the eye. These ipRGCs project through the retinohypothalamic tract to the suprachiasmatic nucleus (SCN), among other brain regions. The SCN relays timing information to other areas of the brain via direct projections (*dark green boxes*) and indirect projections (*light green boxes*). Humoral signals and the peripheral nervous system (i.e., the sympathetic nervous system [SNS] and parasympathetic nervous system [PNS]) convey information from the SCN to orchestrate peripheral clocks. Feeding schedules and exercise can also entrain central and peripheral clocks. Circadian rhythms are key regulators of thermogenesis, immune function, metabolism, reproduction, and stem cell development. **B.** The mammalian molecular clock is composed of transcriptional and translational feedback loops that oscillate with a near-24-hour cycle. The positive loop is driven by the heterodimerization of either circadian locomotor output cycles protein kaput (CLOCK) or neuronal PAS domain-containing protein 2 (NPAS2) with brain and muscle ARNT-like 1 (BMAL1) in the nucleus. The resulting heterodimers bind to enhancer boxes (E-boxes) in gene promoters to regulate the transcription of clock-controlled genes (CCGs), including those encoding period (PER) proteins and cryptochrome (CRY) proteins. PER and CRY proteins accumulate in the cytoplasm during the circadian cycle, eventually dimerizing and shuttling to the nucleus to inhibit their own transcription, thus closing the negative-feedback loop. The auxiliary loop includes the nuclear retinoic acid receptor-related orphan receptors (RORα and RORβ) and REV-ERBs (REV-ERBα and REV-ERBβ), which are also transcriptionally regulated by CLOCK–BMAL1 heterodimers. REV-ERBα (REV in the figure) and RORα repress and activate the transcription of *Bmal1*, respectively, by inhibiting and activating the ROR or REV-ERB response elements (RREs). CLOCK–BMAL1 complexes also control the expression of nicotinamide phosphoribosyltransferase (NAMPT), which is the rate-limiting enzyme of NAD^+ biosynthesis from nicotinamide (NAM). NAM is modified by NAMPT to produce nicotinamide mononucleotide (NMN), which in turn is converted to NAD^+ by several adenyltransferases. Thus, NAMPT oscillations control circadian fluctuations in NAD^+ levels, which in turn modulate sirtuin 1 (SIRT1) activity and signaling. High levels of NAD^+ promote SIRT1 activation. SIRT1 interacts directly with CLOCK–BMAL1 to deacetylate BMAL1 and inhibit CLOCK-driven transcription. Between tissues and cell types, CCGs and other molecular and cellular rhythms may be expressed with different acrophases (phase of peak expression), amplitudes, and even periodicities. ArcN, arcuate nucleus; DmH, dorsomedial hypothalamus; DR, dorsal raphe; IGL, intergeniculate leaflet; LC, locus coeruleus; LH, lateral hypothalamus; LHb, lateral habenula; MA, medial amygdala; mPOA, medial preoptic area; NAc, nucleus accumbens; PVN, paraventricular nucleus of the hypothalamus; PVT, paraventricular nucleus of the thalamus; RMTg, rostromedial tegmental nucleus; Sptm, septum; SPZ, subparaventricular zone; VLPO, ventrolateral preoptic nucleus; VTA, ventral tegmental area. (Reprinted by permission from Nature: Logan RW, McClung CA. Rhythms of life: circadian disruption and brain disorders across the lifespan. *Nat Rev Neurosci.* 2019;20(1):49–65. Copyright © 2018 Springer Nature.)

TABLE 4.1

Observed Oscillatory Rhythms (Measured)

Oscillation	Type	Range or Average	Proposed Function
Very-low frequency	Thermo-reflex (beta) wave	~0.02 Hz	Temperature control[7]
Very-low frequency	SNA	~0.04 Hz	Vascular smooth muscle oscillation[7]
	Arterial pressure/Mayer wave	~0.1 Hz	Associated with baroreflex[15]
Low frequency	Cardiac-vagal reflex	0.08–0.12 Hz	Heart rate variability[7]
Inherent motion	Cranial rhythmic impulse	0.17–0.23 Hz (10–14 cycles/min)	Homeostasis
High frequency	Respiratory/SNA	0.2–0.3 Hz	Central SNA on brainstem respiratory neurons and lung inflation afferents[7]
Sympathetic nerve activity	Cardiac-related/SNA	0.4–0.7 Hz in humans	Baroreceptor-induced entrainment of brainstem sympathetic network[7]

Compiled by D. Schmidt (2023).

neurotransmitters may be elicited at different frequency levels in this complex neural network.

Table 4.1 reflects the range of frequencies that have been identified to date for different physiologic phenomenon. Understand that this is a rapidly evolving field and the accuracy of these values may change in the future.

Inherent motion is defined as the observed other motion after cessation of heartbeat and is not related to respiration.

SPECIFIC SYSTEMS: CARDIAC OSCILLATORY RHYTHMS[19]

Anatomic Sources (Known)

Cardiac rhythmicity is the spontaneous depolarization and repolarization of cardiac muscle cells within the heart. Repetitive and stable rhythmicity is consistent with health. Variability in the heart rate rhythm is also consistent with health. When there is a reduction in the variability, it often precedes cardiac distress and is an indicator of increased mortality.

Cardiac automaticity occurs because of pacemakers within the myocardium. Heart rate and rhythm are under control of the autonomic nervous system. Parasympathetic activity is mediated by muscarinic receptors responding to a release of acetylcholine. Sympathetic control is executed via epinephrine and norepinephrine acting on adrenergic receptors.

Under resting conditions, parasympathetic activity predominates via the vagus nerve. Afferent vagal stimulation leads to increased reflex excitation of vagal efferent activity and inhibits sympathetic efferent activity. The opposite reflex also exists. These efferent reflex activities direct the sinus node to discharge and initiate the heartbeat. The respiratory and vasomotor centers, changes in arterial pressure, and respiratory movements modulate the firing of the sinus node.

Measurement of Electrical Rhythms

HVR is a measure of the variation in time between each heartbeat. This is typically measured via time-domain, geometric, or frequency-domain methods. Time-domain methods analyze the difference in time between beats, typically measuring the normal-to-normal or NN (beat-to-beat) intervals. Geometric methods sample density distribution of NN intervals. Frequency-domain methods count the number of NN intervals within an assigned band of frequency. This is the preferred method when evaluating short-term recordings of a minute or less.

Heart Rate Variability

Reduced HRV is thought to be due to a decrease in vagal activity. This decrease in HRV has been noted in multiple disease states and is a predictor of mortality. Specifically, reduced HRV has been noted in patients with an acute myocardial infarction, diabetes mellitus (particularly those with diabetic neuropathy), cardiac transplantation, heart failure, sepsis, cirrhosis, major depression, and other mood disorders, and high cervical spinal cord lesions. The predominance of sympathetic activity on the heart leads to increased circulating catecholamine levels and cardiac irritability with increased ectopy noted. Exercise training has been shown to increase HRV and may decrease cardiovascular mortality and sudden death. This is thought to modify the balance between the parasympathetic and sympathetic reflexes on heart activity.

Pulse Pressure[20]

Pulse pressure (PP) is the calculated difference between systolic blood pressure (SBP) and diastolic blood pressure (DBP). It can be used as an index of arterial compliance, as long as the cardiac systolic volume is constant, and a gauge of cardiac function. It is more reliable as an index of arterial compliance in elastic (aorta and central arteries) rather than muscular (peripheral) arteries. PP increases with aging because of a decrease in arterial compliance. The Framingham Heart Study has shown that PP is a stronger predictor of CAD than SBP or DBP.

SPECIFIC SYSTEMS: BRAIN WAVES/ EEGS/FMRI BRAIN MAPPINGS[33]

Since 1875, neurons have been known to communicate via electrical brain waves in sheep. The first recording of human brain waves occurred in 1925 and was published in 1929 by Hans Berger. By the late 1930s electroencephalogram (EEG) monitoring had become a key diagnostic and research tool. The early studies using EEG were of small deflections in EEG tracing that occur within a few hundred milliseconds after an auditory, visual, or motor event, called event-related potentials (ERPs). The EEG is recorded by affixing 10 to 20 small electrodes on the scalp in specific pattern and recording the electrical activity of the brain within the location of the brain under the electrode. The initial wave patterns show time-domain data, which is difficult to interpret, so FFT is applied to an EEG tracing to deconstruct raw EEG recordings into specific frequencies. Thus, physiologically relevant frequencies can be studied.

TABLE 4.2

Brain Waves Frequencies and Properties[32]

Brain Waves	Characteristic	EEG Frequency Range	Attributes
Gamma waves	Will	>35–100 Hz	Actively engaged, extreme focus, energy, ecstasy, learning, high cognitive function
Beta waves	Thought	12–38 Hz	Awake, alert, perception, focusing, sustained attention dominant state
Sensorimotor waves	Focused	12–15 Hz	Mental alertness, physical relaxation
Alpha waves	Consciousness	8–12 Hz	Aware of the body, quiet, contemplative, alert and peaceful, reading
Theta waves	Emotion	3–8 Hz	Drives, feelings, creativity, deeply relaxed, meditative, sleep
Delta wave	Instinct	0.5–4 Hz	Dreamless sleep survival, coma, complex problem solving

The billions of neurons in our brain have now been found to communicate via electrochemical events. The electric potential of a large number of neurons (specifically in the pyramid cells of the cortex) can be measured and related to functional brain states. Changes in the electrical activity in the brain depend upon the type of activity being done by the person. Brain waves measured by EEG are traditionally classified into five categories by their frequency bands (Table 4.2). Each frequency band/waveform occurs predominantly during specific brain states and is relative to the location of the EEG electrode placement on the head.

In addition to the five wave categories per traditional EEG, a baseline oscillatory "idle" rhythm of synchronized electric brain activity has been identified as the sensorimotor rhythm (SMR). The frequency of the SMR for most individuals is in the range of 13 to 15 Hz. The SMR amplitude is stronger when the brain is idle and decreases in amplitude when the sensory or motor cortex is activated.

The study of brain neural connectivity has blossomed recently with the use of resting-state functional MRI (R-fMRI) imaging. This reveals large-amplitude spontaneous low-frequency (<0.1) fluctuations in fMRI signal that are temporally correlated across functionally related areas. This is called a *functional connectome* and yields a detailed map of complex neural systems/connectivity in an individual. Using brain mapping, we should see exponential increases in knowledge regarding brain frequencies, function, and interconnectivity in the next few years.[17]

SPECIFIC SYSTEMS: INHERENT MOTION STUDIES[21–25]

THM waves are oscillations noted in ABP due to oscillations in the baroreceptor and chemoreceptor reflex control systems. These waves are noted in continuous blood pressure recordings and in ECG recordings and have a frequency of 0.10 Hz. Low-frequency THM waves have been observed in blood pressure, HRV, pulmonary blood flow, and cerebral blood flow recordings, as well as movement of the cerebral spinal fluid and sympathetic tone of muscle recordings.

The search for a physiologic source of the inherent motion termed the primary respiratory motion (PRM) has been elusive to the osteopathic profession. It has been noted that the CRI, which is the palpation of the PRM on the head described by Dr. Sutherland, has the same frequency range as THM waves. This correlation has been studied by multiple authors, including Nelson, Glonek, and Sergueef who used peripheral PP monitoring to assess blood flow velocity oscillations and correlated them with cranial palpation by experienced practitioners. Their study looked at several protocols using mathematical analysis (Fourier transforms and spectral analysis) to assess the change in blood flow velocity created by the CRI and osteopathic cranial manipulative techniques.

The first protocol compared low-frequency blood flow velocity waves with cranial palpation by assessing the effect of the flexion/extension motion of the SBS on blood flow velocity. This was measured via a clip on the subject's earlobe. The CRI and low-frequency (0.10 to 0.20 Hz) blood flow velocity waves occurred concurrently.

The second protocol assessed the effect of an individually determined cranial manipulative treatment compared with monitoring the cranium (sham) on blood flow velocity waves. There was a significant decrease in the very–low-frequency signal and an increase in the low-frequency signal during and immediately after the cranial manipulative treatment. This indicates a sympathetic baroreflex activity induced by the cranial manipulative treatment.

A third protocol evaluated the effect of the incitant technique of bitemporal rocking on the THM waves. The subjects underwent evaluation of this technique and an increase in very–low-frequency and low-frequency wave forms were noted during the active cranial manipulation. The subjects' heart rate also increased by 18%.

The fourth protocol evaluated the effect of the CV-4 technique on low-frequency blood flow velocity waves. During the application of the CV-4 technique, the occipital bone was held in extension which dampened the low-frequency waves. These disappeared when the technique achieved a still point or absence of the flexion-extension motion of the SBS. The low-frequency oscillations increased in amplitude which is consistent with an increase in the amplitude of the CRI noted after the still point created by the application of the CV-4 technique.

A fifth protocol was performed to assess the normative values of the CRI. The rate of the CRI has been classically reported as 10 to 14 cpm. A review of various studies reveals a different range, with those using palpation yielding a rate of 4 to 6 cpm or 10 to 14 cpm. Studies using instrumentation to determine the CRI yield rates in the 6 to 14 cpm range. The difference is thought to be due to which waves are being tracked by the palpating clinicians. Some clinicians track very–low-frequency waves while others track the low-frequency waves consistent to what instrumentation records.

The sixth protocol to measure the rate of the CRI was performed using a variety of individuals as examiners and participants. These were osteopathic medical students or physicians with 1-year, 2-year, or 1-to-25-years' experience with osteopathic cranial manipulative medicine. The mean rate was reported as 6.88 ± 4.45 cpm. The examiners with the greatest experience palpated a rate of 4.78 ± 2.57 cpm (0.08 Hz, range 0.04 to 0.12 Hz).

Conclusions from the Above Six Protocols

From the protocols described, the following conclusions can be drawn:

1. Palpation of the CRI tracks identifiable frequencies in blood flow velocity (Protocol 1).
2. The very–low-frequency (0.003 to 0.05 Hz, 0.18 to 3.0 cpm) and low-frequency (0.10 to 0.20 Hz, 6.0 to 12 cpm) components of the flowmetry record, respectively, are remarkably consistent with the "slow tide" (six cycles in 10 minutes) and the "fast tide" (8 to 12 cpm) of the PRM as described by Becker.[26] (Protocol 1).
3. Cranial palpation alone may be employed as sham treatment for research into the clinical impact of cranial manipulation (Protocol 2).
4. Cranial manipulation appears to exert effects upon baroreflex physiology (Protocols 2, 3, and 4).
5. Cranial manipulation affects the low-frequency 0.10- to 0.20-Hz signal and to a lesser extent the very–low-frequency 0.003- to 0.05-Hz signal in blood flow velocity and does so in a manner consistent with the type of manipulative procedure being employed (Protocols 2, 3, and 4).
6. A signal of frequency 0.08 Hz (0.04 to 0.11 Hz) has been identified in the flowmetry record that is closely related to the 0.10- to 0.20-Hz signal. Both are demonstrated to be affected by cranial manipulation, in this case, by CV-4 (Protocol 4).
7. Although not all physicians appear to be palpating the CRI at the same frequency, everyone tracks the 0.10- to 0.20-Hz signal with the majority tracking at 0.04 to 0.11 Hz or one CRI cycle to two low-frequency blood flow velocity waves (Protocol 5).
8. The nearly identical palpated rates for the CRI of 4.54 ± 2.08 cpm (Protocol 5) and 4.78 ± 2.57 cpm (Protocol 6) appear to indicate that the majority of experienced physicians are tracking the 0.08-Hz (4.5 cpm) minor signal (Protocol 4).
9. A new normative range for the CRI of 2 to 7 cpm, as palpated by experienced physicians, has been identified (Protocols 5 and 6).

Recent Studies in Inherent Motion

Recent studies have utilized methods combining replications of older studies with newer physiologic monitoring technologies. In 1971, Dr. Viola Frymann performed studies on human subjects in which she directly measured physical movements of the head independent of respiration. Dr. Frymann affixed pressure–strain gauges onto the parietal bones of subjects in order to measure lateral displacement of the cranium while monitoring cardiac and respiratory rates. Using oscillograph recording, she found a third, slower rhythm of the cranium that persisted throughout breath-holding and was independent of cardiac rate in her subjects, but the apparatus was too uncomfortable for subjects to tolerate further studies.[27]

In 2019, Rasmussen, et al.,[28] developed a more comfortable and precise method to obtain real-time sampling data of direct physical movements of the living head. He used two servo actuators (sensors with sensitivity to detect physical movements of 1 micrometer) positioned on the skin at the level of the temporal mastoids that kept a persistent contact of 10 g at all measure times to measure lateral movement (displacement) of the cranium. Respiration was measured by a mouse trapper sensor placed on the upper abdomen anterior to the respiratory diaphragm and a Fitbit pulse wristlet measured the AP. Software was designed and independently validated by the Danish National Metrology Institute to track any rhythmic movements of 20 measure points per second, then isolated using Fourier transformations. In 50 healthy individuals, rhythmic oscillations of the head were measured in real-time for 42 minutes in a supine resting state without any intervention while respiratory and cardiac cycles were also measured.

In all individuals, a third rhythm of the cranium was distinguished as separate from the arterial and respiratory rhythm. The third rhythm was observed as a dynamic physiologic phenomenon with a narrow range in resting healthy individuals with a mean of 0.1 Hz or 6.16 cycles per minute (cpm) with range of (4.25 cpm–7.07 cpm). The third rhythm differed in the periodic wave function from the respiratory movement, which showed a sigmoid curve form with head expansion and contraction (Fig. 4.11C). The third rhythm showed a wave within wave movement with a "shoulder" in the wave movement halfway from maximum expansion to maximum retraction (Fig. 4.11D). The significant contributions to the amplitude of the measured movements were (1) the respiratory breathing and (2) this third slower rhythm, whereas the contribution from the arterial pulsing was minor (Fig. 4.11A–D).

The third rhythm was observed in all 50 subjects and the level of fluctuation in the third rhythm was shown to be individual, with a higher variance (0.53) in individuals with a high rate third rhythm (7.07 cpm) compared to the subjects shown with a lower rate third rhythm (5.42 and 4.25 cpm, respectively) having a lower variance (0.10 and 0.14, respectively). There was a significant ($p < .001$) and moderate positive correlation ($r = 0.52$) between the third rhythm rate and third rhythm variance in this group of healthy individuals (Fig. 4.12). This begs the question of whether variability of this third rhythm may be a predictor of health or disease much like HRV. Future studies using this method are warranted to further evaluate and validate this phenomenon.

Use of Oscillations in Osteopathic Treatment

"Vibration is an accepted fact in science. Solid bodies are composed of atoms which are vibrating at almost infinite velocities. One substance differs from another mainly in the modulus of vibratility, the different planes of substance representing the planes of gradually increasing vibratility.

The higher vibratility governs and molds the lower, just as the sun centralizes [our] solar system. The most refined vibrations that mean life and light with all their accompaniments to the planets in the solar system. In man this vibratile characteristic also predominates, for within [our bodies we combine] the higher and lower grades of vibratility in connection with mind, brain, bone, muscle, blood. So long as these combined vibratilities are in harmony the organism enjoys life and health."[4]

— Littlejohn, 1902

The use of oscillations in osteopathic treatment is not a new concept. A treatment known as General Osteopathic Technique in today's parlance was referred to as "rhythmic treatment" by Dr. Littlejohn.[29] It is a method of gentle oscillations to create a fluid wave that acts in a spiral fashion to resolve somatic dysfunction. It can be used to treat somatic dysfunction throughout the body. A spiral motion is introduced via a rhythmic rocking of a distal part of the body (leg or pelvis) to send a fluid wave to the level of the somatic dysfunction. Typically, five to eight oscillations are sufficient to resolve somatic dysfunction. The cranium is not treated by this method, but frequently somatic dysfunction present in the cranium will resolve as somatic dysfunction elsewhere in the body resolves.

In addition, Dr. Littlejohn wrote extensively about using a common technique using vibratory activation over inflamed lymph nodes for the treatment of infectious diseases.

The earlier discussion of the research on how cranial manipulative techniques affect THM waves and the CRI, and affect somatic dysfunctions in the cranium, is another example of an oscillatory approach to osteopathic treatment.

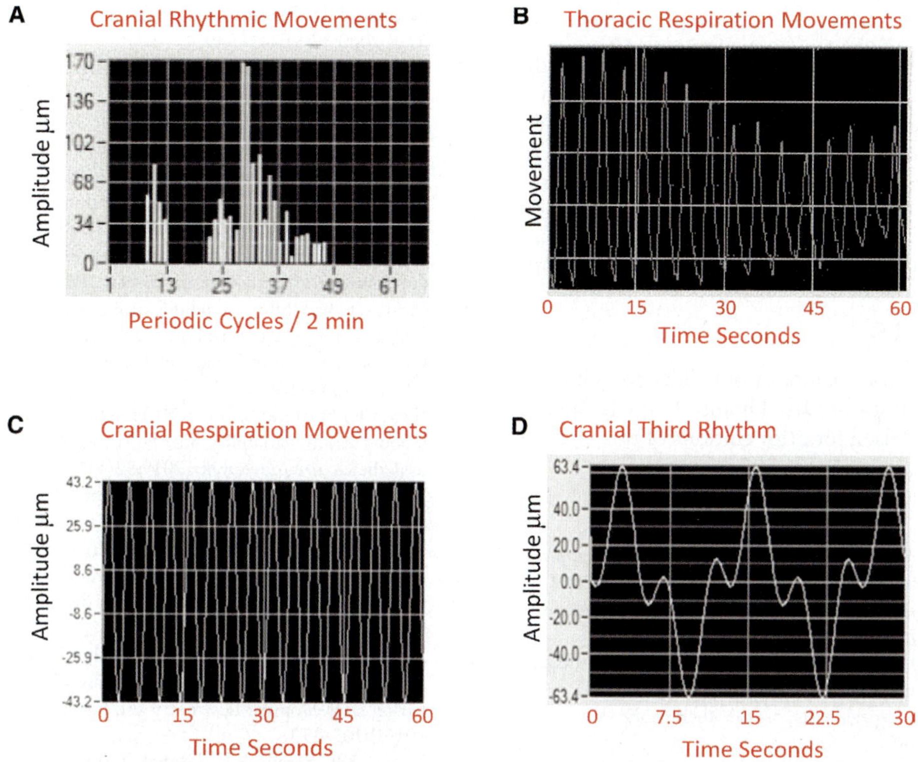

FIGURE 4.11. Measure of cranial rhythmic movements and separating a third rhythm from the movement of the head with respiratory breathing. A. The x-axis in Figure 1A is the frequency of movement in relation to time (note that the scale in **A** is cycles per 2 min). The frequency is obtained by converting the fast Fourier transformation analysis to frequency/2 min. The height of a signal on the y-axis in **A**, is the maximum distance in µm between the servo actuator signals, for the periodic movement identified in the Fourier transformation. A window of possible rhythmic movements with frequencies from up 35 cpm is shown (70/2 cycles/min). A narrow cluster of rhythmic head movements was identified at 4 to 6 cpm, and a broader cluster of movements from 9 to 24 cpm. **B.** A time window of 1 minute of respiratory movement measured at the respiratory diaphragm with a respiratory frequency of 16 cpm was observed for the illustrated person. The y-axis is a movement without a specific scale, and the mouse trapper is only to detect the rate of the movement. **C.** The rhythmic movement in the broad cluster (9–24 cpm) identified in **A** is shown. A sigmoid curve with an average cpm of 16 is identified. **D.** The rhythmic movement in the narrow cluster of 4 to 6 cpm identified in **A** is shown. The movement identified is wave within a wave function with a "shoulder" about halfway between maximum and minimum amplitude. This movement is referred to as the third rhythm. (Reprinted with permission from Rasmussen TR, Meulengracht KC. Direct measurement of the rhythmic motions of the human head identifies a third rhythm. *J Bodyw Mov Ther.* 2021;26:24–29.)

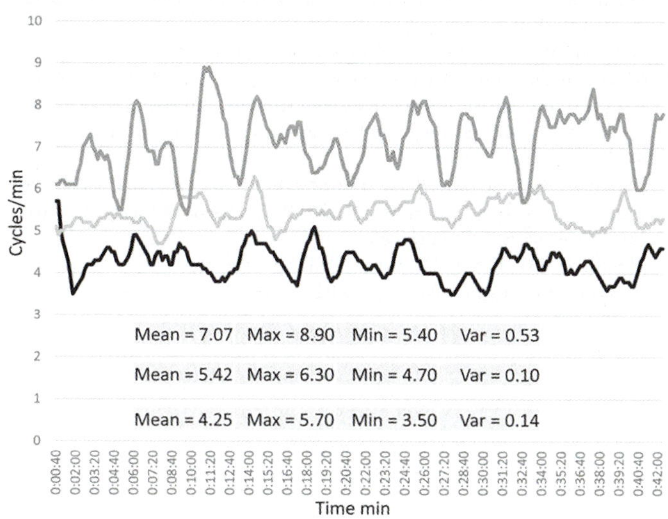

Figure 4.12. Dynamic nature of the third rhythm during rest as measured in all participants (n = 50). Shown is the third rhythm measured in three healthy individuals lying supine over a time of 42 minutes. The three persons represent the highest, lowest, and midrange third rhythm. Mean, max, min, and variance are given for each person. (Reprinted with permission from Rasmussen TR, Meulengracht KC. Direct measurement of the rhythmic motions of the human head identifies a third rhythm. *J Bodyw Mov Ther.* 2021;26:24–29.)

Jean-Pierre Barral, DO, studied motion of abdominal organs via fluoroscopy and noted inherent motion (motility) present in the organs. He named the motion as *inspir* and *expir*[30] as it occurs with the cycles of flexion and extension of the cranial base (sphenobasilar symphysis). Visceral manipulative techniques address the mobility and motility of organs to resolve somatic dysfunction present in them.

Working with the awareness of faster and slower oscillations within the body and environment[31] is the approach to osteopathic treatment discussed in the "Rule of the Artery" courses. This approach utilizes the awareness that the boundary of the phenomena is not limited to the space between your hands. It requires a refinement of perception and palpation beyond the basic palpatory techniques taught in the first 2 years of osteopathic medical instruction.

In contradistinction, another awareness of oscillations can be the presence of an oscillating somatic dysfunction. Dr. Fred Mitchell, Jr., DO, FAAO, reported this phenomenon in his text, The Muscle Energy Manual. This type of oscillation occurs as a response to a fixed structure about which another structure moves in an oscillatory manner. This is commonly found with an innominate bone rotating anteriorly and posteriorly about the other, nonmoving innominate.

CONCLUSION

Awareness of the properties underlying the oscillations within the physical world allows us to explore phenomena within the human body. Research evaluating any of the oscillatory patterns sheds new light on how the human body functions. As we learn more about these phenomena, we can utilize those properties to effect therapeutic change through appropriate use of osteopathic manipulative medicine and gain greater understanding of how osteopathic medicine supports a patient to regain their homeostasis and enjoy better health.

ACKNOWLEDGMENTS

The author and editors of this chapter would like to acknowledge the scholarly contributions of Drs. Thomas Glonek, Nicette Sergueef, and Kenneth E. Nelson for prior editions of this chapter.

REFERENCES

1. Truhlar RE, Doctor AT. *Still in the Living: His Concepts and Principles of Health and Disease.* (quote from 1950) Literary Licensing, LLC; 2012.
2. Comeaux Z. The role of vibration or oscillation in the development of osteopathic thought. *AAO J.* 2000:19–24.
3. Sutherland WG. *Teachings in the Science of Osteopathy.* The Sutherland Cranial Teaching Foundation; 1990:136–138.
4. Littlejohn JM. The physiological basis of the therapeutic law. *J Am Osteopath Assoc.* 1902;2:42–60.
5. McPartland JM, Mein EA. Entrainment and the cranial rhythmic impulse. *Altern Ther Health Med.* 1997;3(1):40–45.
6. Pantaleone J. Synchronization of metronomes. *Am J Phys.* 2002;70: 992–1000.
7. Barman B. Chapter 27: Rhythms in sympathetic nerve activity. In: Biaggioni I, Browning K, eds. *Primer on the Autonomic Nervous System.* 4th ed. Academic Press/Elsevier; 2023:157–160.
8. Reppert SM, Weaver DR. Coordination of circadian timing in mammals. *Nature.* 2002;418:935–941.
9. Czeisler CA, Diffy JF, Shanahan TL, et al. Stability, precision and near-24-hour period of the human circadian pacemaker. *Science.* 1999;284(5423): 2177–2181.
10. *MLA style: Press release. NobelPrize.org. Nobel Prize Outreach AB 2023.* Accessed February 22, 2023. https://www.nobelprize.org/prizes/medicine/2017/press-release
11. Ibanez C. *Scientific Background Discoveries of Molecular Mechanisms Controlling the Circadian Rhythm.* The Nobel Assembly at Karolinska Institutet; 2017.
12. Hastings MH, Maywood ES, Brancaccio M. Generation of circadian rhythms in the suprachiasmatic nucleus. *Nat Rev Neurosci.* 2018;19(8): 453–469.
13. Golombek D, Vigo D. Chapter 28: Circadian rhythms and autonomic function. In: Biaggioni I, Browning K, eds. *Primer on the Autonomic Nervous System.* 4th ed. Academic; 2023:160–163.
14. Ma M, Morrison E. *Neuroanatomy, Nucleus Suprachiasmatic.* StatPearls-NCBI Bookself/StatPearls Publishing; 2022.
15. Eckberg DL. Physiological basis for human autonomic rhythms. *Ann Med.* 2000;32(5):341–349.
16. Barman SM. 2019 Ludwig Lecture: Rhythms in sympathetic nerve activity are a key to understanding neural control of the cardiovascular system. *Am J Physiol Regul Integr Comp Physiol.* 2020;318(2):R191–R205.
17. Schmidt SH. *Bandwidth-specific functional connectivity of physiological low frequency oscillations in fMRI.* Medizinische Fakultät Charité—Universitatsmedizin Berlin (Dissertation in English). 2009:70. http://www.diss.fu-berlin.de/diss/receive/FUDISS_thesis_000000008598
18. Malpas SC. Sympathetic nervous system overactivity and its role in the development of cardiovascular disease. *Physiol Rev.* 2010;90:513–557.
19. Heart rate variability: standards of measurement, physiological interpretation, and clinical use: Task Force of the European Society of Cardiology and the North American Society of Pacing and Electrophysiology. *Circulation.* 1996;93:1043–1065.
20. Narita K, Hoshide S, Kario K. Hemodynamic stress, pulse pressure, and blood pressure variability may be strong triggers of cardiovascular events in diabetes. *Am J Hypertens.* 2019;32(11):1045–1047.
21. Sergueef N, Nelson KE, Glonek T. The effect of cranial manipulation on the Traube-Hering-Mayer oscillation as measured by laser-Doppler flowmetry. *Altern Ther Health Med.* 2002;8(6):74–76.
22. Nelson KE, Sergueef N, Glonek T. Cranial manipulation induces sequential changes in blood flow velocity on demand. *Amer Acad Osteop J.* 2004; 14(3):15–17.
23. Nelson KE, Sergueef N, Lipinski CM, Chapman AR, Glonek T. Cranial rhythmic impulse related to the Traube-Hering-Mayer oscillation: comparing laser-Doppler flowmetry and palpation. *J Am Osteopath Assoc.* 2001; 101(3):163–173.
24. Nelson KE, Sergueef N, Glonek T. The effect of an alternative medical procedure upon low-frequency oscillations in cutaneous blood flow velocity. *J Manip Physiol Ther.* 2006;29(8):626–636.
25. Guinn KK, Rodriguez C, Bucheli D, et al. Reproducibility assessment of the response to CV4 as measured by the laser Doppler flowmeter and electrocardiogram. *J Am Osteopath Assoc.* 2007;107(8; Abs. P7):332–EOA.
26. Becker RE. Chapter 3: Life in motion. In: Brooks RE, ed. *The Cerebrospinal Fluid Tide.* Rudra Press; 1997:10.
27. Frymann VM. A study of the rhythmic motions of the living cranium. *J Am Osteopath Assoc.* 1971;70:928–945.
28. Rasmussen RT, Meulengracht KC. Direct measurement of the rhythmic motions of the human head identified a third rhythm. *J Bodyw Mov Ther.* 2021;26:24–29.
29. Wernham J. *Notes on Dr. J.M. Littlejohn's Principles of Osteopathy.* 1910;1(3):61.
30. Barral JP, Mercier P. *Visceral Manipulation.* Eastland Press; 2005.
31. Muehsam D, Ventura C, Life rhythm as a symphony of oscillatory patterns: electromagnetic energy and sound vibration modulates gene expression for biological signaling and healing. *Glob Adv Health Med.* 2014;3(2): 40–55.
32. Sorkin J. *Getting into Brain Waves: History and Resources.* Wu Tasi Neurosciences Institute. April 18, 2016; Accessed February 22, 2023. https://neuroscience.stanford.edu.
33. Hyndman BW, Kitney RI, Sayers BM. Spontaneous rhythms in physiological control systems. *Nature.* 1971;233:339–341.

5 Tissue Respiration and Circulation

STEPHEN E. DICARLO ▪ MINDY A. CHILMAN MCCOMB

KEY CONCEPTS

- The respiratory and circulatory systems provide cells with a lifeline to the outside world.
- Oxidative phosphorylation is the primary source of energy production in the form of adenosine triphosphate (ATP). Cells therefore require a steady supply of oxygen.
- The respiratory system obtains the required oxygen for energy production and releases a major byproduct of cellular metabolism, carbon dioxide.
- Gas exchange involves three primary processes: ventilation, perfusion, and diffusion.
- The circulatory system transports substrates to and waste products from metabolizing cells.
- The lungs, heart, vasculature, and red blood cells (RBCs) play essential roles in oxygen and carbon dioxide transport.
- Blood flow is locally regulated by three mechanisms: metabolic, myogenic, and paracrine.
- Four processes involving those general mechanisms modulate local blood flow: active hyperemia, reactive hyperemia, autoregulation, and the vascular response to injury.
- Myocardium is an example of a tissue in which blood flow is primarily determined by metabolic demand.
- Skin is an example of a tissue with low metabolic demand, but it plays an important role in thermoregulation. Control of cutaneous blood flow reflects this critical function.

INTRODUCTION

A major role of the physician is to encourage the normal physiologic processes responsible for the maintenance of a favorable environment for each cell of the body, and if necessary, to intervene when pathologic events disrupt this environment.[1] Cellular energy production, in the form of ATP, is vital for life as energy is required for cellular metabolism and biochemical reactions throughout the body. Each cell must meet its energy needs by producing ATP in sufficient quantities. In most cells, oxidative phosphorylation is the primary means of ATP production. Oxidative phosphorylation requires a cellular environment that provides a steady supply of oxygen and substrate and a route for the disposal of the byproducts of cellular respiration, such as carbon dioxide.

The respiratory and circulatory systems work together in a complex and tightly coordinated manner to maintain this cellular environment (Fig. 5.1).

The respiratory system is responsible for gas exchange—obtaining oxygen and releasing carbon dioxide—while also maintaining blood pH. The circulatory system is responsible for transport. By supplying oxygen and substrates and removing metabolic waste products, circulation is the cell's connection to the outside world.

This chapter discusses the regulation of tissue respiration and mechanisms that modulate tissue circulation to maintain an optimal internal environment.

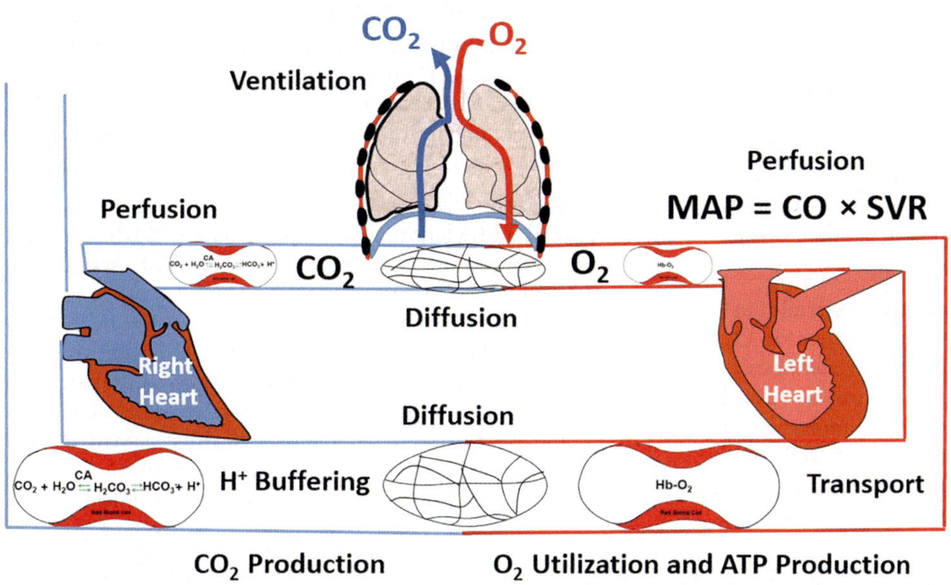

Figure 5.1. **The lungs, heart, vasculature, and red blood cells play essential roles in oxygen and carbon dioxide transport.**

REGULATION OF TISSUE RESPIRATION

A brief review of the complete process of respiration is foundational in understanding the regulation of tissue respiration. This includes external respiration, internal respiration, and cellular respiration. External respiration is the exchange of gases between the lungs and pulmonary blood. Internal respiration is the exchange of gases between capillary blood and metabolizing tissues. Cellular and tissue respiration are sometimes used interchangeably, but tissue respiration refers to the collective oxygen utilization and energy production by cells within a tissue whereas cellular respiration refers to the use of oxygen in biochemical processes to produce energy within the cell.

Cellular Metabolism

ATP is the common intermediate that provides chemical energy for cellular function. Motility, pumping of ions, muscle contraction, and metabolic pathways all use ATP as a source of energy.[1] The cell makes use of ATP by enzymatically transforming ATP to adenosine diphosphate (ADP) and inorganic phosphate (Pi), capturing the chemical energy released in the process.

All cells need a continuous supply of ATP calibrated to meet their needs at a given time. Very little ATP is stored for direct energy transformation; instead, the cell has elaborate metabolic pathways for synthesizing ATP. These bioenergetic synthesizing processes are finely calibrated to meet cellular needs on demand. Several energy-sensing mechanisms have evolved in mammalian tissues to maintain a constant ratio of ATP: ADP + Pi. In a recent review by Britton and Koch, it has even been postulated that all of evolution may have revolved around ATP-generating mechanisms.[2]

In some cells, such as muscle fibers, energy requirements may vary greatly in just a few seconds as the cells go from resting to high activity.[3] When ATP is rapidly broken down, it must be promptly resynthesized from ADP. In many cells, including skeletal and cardiac muscle, phosphocreatine (PCr, also known as creatine phosphate) provides a quick source of ATP by the following reaction: ADP + PCr ↔ ATP + Cr.[4] The equilibrium constant for this reaction favors the formation of ATP so that PCr falls to approximately 10% of its maximal value before a physiologically significant decrease in ATP occurs. Although PCr is a rapid means to replenish ATP, the amount of ATP available via this pathway is limited. Cells must turn to other pathways for a more sustained supply of ATP.

Cellular respiration is a series of chemical reactions that break down glucose to form ATP. Glycolysis, the breakdown of glucose into pyruvate, is the first step in cellular respiration. It captures only a small fraction of the energy available in the glucose molecule for the formation of ATP (two molecules of ATP per molecule of glucose), but it does this quickly and without requiring oxygen (O_2).

Glycolysis occurs under both aerobic and anaerobic conditions; the resulting pyruvate is metabolized differently depending on the presence or absence of O_2 in the cell.

- During intense physical activity such as sprinting, skeletal muscle cells rely on anaerobic respiration. In the absence of O_2, pyruvate is converted to lactic acid in order to regenerate nicotinamide adenine dinucleotide (NAD^+), which can be reused in ongoing glycolysis. This nets an additional two molecules of ATP per molecule of glucose. The consequence of lactic acid accumulation, however, is attenuation or loss of muscle contraction, so anaerobic respiration can only be sustained for a short period of time.
- During prolonged physical activity such as running a marathon, skeletal muscle cells utilize aerobic respiration. Pyruvate is converted to acetyl-CoA which serves as the substrate for the tricarboxylic acid (TCA) cycle (also called the citric acid cycle or Krebs cycle). This allows for oxidative phosphorylation via the electron transport chain and ATP synthase. These processes require O_2, but net significantly more ATP—altogether, up to an additional 36 molecules per molecule of glucose. The byproducts are carbon dioxide (CO_2) and water (H_2O).

The mitochondrion is the intracellular site of the events that make use of O_2, substrate, ADP, and Pi to produce ATP, CO_2, and H_2O.

In a few cell types, including RBCs (which have no mitochondria), glycolysis is the sole source of ATP. In most cells, glycolysis serves to provide ATP for a few seconds before oxidative phosphorylation begins to meet the ongoing need for ATP. When short bursts of energy are needed, or when the supply of oxygen is limited, glycolysis is a significant source of ATP.[5]

Under most circumstances, in most cells, oxidative phosphorylation is the mainstay for the synthesis of ATP from ADP and Pi. Oxidative phosphorylation can supply ATP for a wide range of cellular energy requirements. As the rate of oxidative phosphorylation increases, the respiratory and circulatory systems must deliver an increasing supply of oxygen and substrates.

How this delivery is regulated will be discussed later in this chapter. For now, it is assumed that oxygen and substrate are available. If that is the case, ATP supply from oxidative phosphorylation exactly matches ATP utilization. How is oxidative phosphorylation regulated?

REGULATION OF CELLULAR RESPIRATION

While the cellular controls that match ATP supply to ATP demand are not fully understood, three independent variables are involved in regulating oxidative phosphorylation.[6]

1. Oxygen concentration within the cell: A shortage of oxygen reduces ATP production.
2. Intramitochondrial redox status, that is, the ratio of NAD^+ to NADH: NADH is formed at several steps in the metabolism of substrates, some from glycolysis but most importantly in the TCA cycle. NADH is a thermodynamic driving force increasing the rate of oxidative phosphorylation.[7] Accumulating concentrations of NAD^+ act allosterically to stimulate dehydrogenases of the TCA cycle to increase production of electron-carrying redox substrates such as NADH. This increases electron delivery to the electron transport chain, stimulating oxidative phosphorylation and ATP production.
3. The rate of ATP utilization of the cell: Increased rates of ATP utilization require more ATP production by oxidative phosphorylation.

These variables affect the energy state of the cell, that is, ratios of ATP, ADP, and adenosine monophosphate (AMP). Feedback regulation of the energy state ensures that ATP synthesis is matched to ATP utilization.

Additionally, an increase in cytosolic calcium ion (Ca^{2+}) concentration raises the effectiveness of NADH in driving oxidative phosphorylation. This observation raises the possibility that, in the presence of increased calcium concentration, minimal changes in ADP, Pi, and NADH may be adequate to drive oxidative phosphorylation. This view is compatible with the available information from the study of oxidative phosphorylation in intact hearts.[8]

- The view that Ca^{2+} is integral to the normal regulation of oxidative phosphorylation puts this ion in a central role in both the synthesis and the use of ATP. For example, in cardiac muscle, increased cytosolic Ca^{2+} concentration stimulates actomyosin cross-bridge cycling and contraction. This dramatically increases the utilization of ATP. At the same time, the increase in cytosolic Ca^{2+} concentration stimulates oxidative phosphorylation. In this scenario, the same stimulus (increased Ca^{2+} concentration) is responsible for increasing both ATP synthesis and utilization.[8]

The need for a constant supply of oxygen in cells is clear, so how does it get there? The next section discusses how atmospheric oxygen enters the blood and how carbon dioxide is eliminated.

External Respiration: Gas Exchange between the Atmosphere and Pulmonary Blood

Gas exchange between the atmosphere and pulmonary blood involves three primary processes: ventilation, perfusion, and diffusion. These three processes must be coordinated for optimal exchange. Ventilation exchanges air in the alveoli, providing a constant supply of oxygen and releasing carbon dioxide waste into the atmosphere. Perfusion delivers blood to the lungs and capillaries surrounding alveoli. Diffusion is the passive means by which gases move between alveoli and capillary blood. Demand for oxygen in the body, however, exceeds the amount that can be simply dissolved in blood plasma. Hemoglobin (Hb) and RBCs are therefore utilized to increase blood's oxygen-carrying capacity and meet the demands of living tissue.

VENTILATION

Pulmonary ventilation is the process by which air is delivered to and removed from the alveoli by alternating inflation and deflation of the lungs. This is commonly referred to as breathing. The main gases of interest are oxygen (O_2) and carbon dioxide (CO_2), as nitrogen is biologically inert. Nevertheless, nitrogen is the most abundant constituent of both ambient and alveolar air and is important in maintaining inflation of the alveoli.

Air is delivered to the gas exchange sites of the lung by bulk flow due to contractions of inspiratory muscles, primarily the diaphragm and external intercostals. Relaxed normal expiration is passive, resulting from elastic recoil.

When a person is upright, ventilation is greater at the base of the lung than at the apex.[9] This is partially due to the gradient of pleural pressure resulting from gravity, but ongoing research suggests this is not the only factor.[10] Regardless, alveoli are less expanded and more compliant at the lung base in upright postures. With inspiration, lung volume increases more substantially in the base for greater ventilation. Voluntary changes in breathing movements and diaphragm activity can also influence regional ventilation of the lung.[11,12] This understanding helps the physician in interpreting signs and symptoms of respiratory pathology and guides rational treatment.

The respiratory control system is designed to closely regulate physically dissolved CO_2. Since CO_2 readily reacts with water to yield hydrogen ions (H^+) and bicarbonate (HCO_3^-), the control of dissolved CO_2 by ventilation helps to maintain a stable acid–base environment in the body which is essential for enzymatic function. Thus, the respiratory control system is tailored first towards the regulation of dissolved CO_2 and pH, while the maintenance of adequate blood oxygenation is secondary. When ventilation is sufficient to maintain proper CO_2 levels and blood pH, oxygenation is, in most instances, also adequate. Had the respiratory control system been designed to regulate arterial O_2 levels within narrow limits, it would be of minimal benefit to blood O_2 content and result in less fine control of acid–base balance.

PERFUSION

Blood gases are delivered to and transported from lung alveoli by pulmonary blood flow, or perfusion. In the lungs, deoxygenated blood from the rest of the body (via the right side of the heart) flows through pulmonary capillaries surrounding alveoli. This allows blood O_2 to be replenished and CO_2 to be released before blood returns to the heart for transport back to the rest of the body.

In normal adult circulation, the output of the right and left ventricles (for pulmonary and systemic flow, respectively) must be equal to maintain normal physiologic function. Otherwise, blood would pool either in the lungs or systemic vasculature.

As with ventilation, when a person is upright, lung perfusion is greater at the base of the lung than at the apex.[9] Again, gravity plays a part, but research suggests other factors, likely structural, play a greater role.[10,13,14] Interestingly, when recumbent, lying prone results in greater lung perfusion than lying supine. This appears to be due to the heart and adjacent structures compressing the central posterior portions of the lung while supine more so than central anterior portions while prone.[15] These concepts have important implications for the treatment of patients with respiratory compromise.

The regulation of tissue perfusion is complex and will be discussed later in the chapter.

DIFFUSION

Diffusion is the passive movement of a molecule from an area of higher concentration to an area of lower concentration. The driving force is the concentration gradient; diffusion requires no additional energy. In alveoli, O_2 and CO_2 move by simple diffusion into and out of pulmonary capillary blood. The design of the alveolar capillary bed is nearly ideal for optimal gas diffusion. No artificial device approaches the efficiency of the lungs for gas exchange.

The factors that govern the rate of exchange or diffusion for the lung are described by Fick's laws of diffusion and may be summarized as follows:

- Substances diffuse from areas of higher concentration to areas of lower concentration.
- The rate of diffusion increases with:
  - Increased surface area for exchange
  - Decreased membrane thickness
  - Higher pressure gradients
  - Better solubility of the substance (e.g., CO_2 is more soluble in blood and therefore diffuses more rapidly than O_2)

The concentration gradient driving diffusion at the level of the alveolus is the difference in the partial pressure of each gas in alveolar air versus capillary blood. Oxygen will be discussed in greater detail as an example.

Oxygen diffuses into pulmonary capillary blood because the partial pressure of oxygen (PO_2) in the atmosphere and alveoli is greater than that of pulmonary capillary blood. The PO_2 in inspired ambient air at sea level is about 159 mm Hg. This decreases to 149 mm Hg as water vapor dilutes inspired air in the upper airway. The alveolar PO_2 is only about 104 mm Hg because inspired air mixes with alveolar air.[16] This is equilibrated with capillary blood by diffusion. There is, however, a further decline in PO_2 between the alveolus and systemic arterial blood, where the PO_2 is normally between 96 and 100 mm Hg. This difference is called the alveolar–arterial gradient (A-a gradient). The A-a gradient is due, in part, to differences in apical and basilar ventilation and perfusion, and has clinical implications in determining the cause of hypoxemia.

Diffusion of CO_2 occurs in the opposite direction. The concentration of CO_2 in alveoli is lower than that of pulmonary capillary blood, so CO_2 diffuses from the blood to the lungs for exhalation.

Internal Respiration: Gas Exchange between Capillary Blood and Metabolizing Tissues

Simple diffusion drives O_2 exchange between tissue interstitial fluid and tissue capillary blood just as it drives O_2 exchange between alveolar air and pulmonary capillary blood. However, the pressure gradient in metabolizing tissues is reversed from what is seen in the lungs. Higher PO_2 in tissue capillary blood relative to PO_2 in tissue interstitial fluid means O_2 diffuses from the blood into the tissue for use in cellular respiration.

Oxygen is relatively insoluble in blood plasma and dissolved blood O_2 would be insufficient to meet the body's energy demand. Transport of O_2 within blood is therefore largely dependent on Hb present in RBCs. Most O_2 carried by the blood binds chemically, but reversibly, with Hb and is transported by blood flow to the tissue capillaries. Lower PO_2 in tissue interstitial fluid drives dissolved oxygen out of the blood and into the tissue interstitium. Hb then releases bound O_2 for use in metabolizing tissues.

Diffusion of CO_2 within metabolizing tissues again occurs in the opposite direction of O_2. Carbon dioxide is formed as a waste product of cellular respiration and diffuses from tissue interstitial fluid (higher concentration of CO_2) into tissue capillary blood (lower concentration of CO_2).

RBCs are also important in CO_2 transport. Carbonic anhydrase, an enzyme present mainly in RBCs, facilitates the hydration of CO_2 to HCO_3^- and H^+ such that most CO_2 carried to the lungs for excretion is in the form of HCO_3^-.

Blood flow is the transport link between external respiration in the lungs and internal respiration in metabolizing tissues. The next section discusses factors that influence blood flow within metabolizing tissues. Maintaining the balance of supply and demand for oxygen in tissues is necessary for cells to generate the energy needed to carry out their vital functions.

REGULATION OF TISSUE CIRCULATION

The function of the circulatory system is to provide blood flow (perfusion) to tissues in amounts adequate to meet tissue needs over a wide range of varying conditions. To accomplish this function, the human body has developed a system of pumps and distribution vessels of various types that provide adequate blood flow to supply cells with nutrients and remove waste products.

The energy for transport of blood throughout circulation is provided by the beating of the heart (cardiac output) and constriction or dilation of blood vessels (systemic vascular resistance) in the form of arterial blood pressure: blood pressure = cardiac output × systemic vascular resistance. With each cardiac contraction, the right ventricle of the heart ejects a volume of blood (stroke volume) into the pulmonary artery, and the left ventricle ejects an equal stroke volume into the aorta. The resulting arterial pressures in the pulmonary artery and in the aorta represent potential energy that propels blood flow through the pulmonary and systemic blood vessels, respectively.

- Cardiac output is defined as the total blood volume pumped per minute by one ventricle: cardiac output = stroke volume × heart rate.
- Systemic vascular resistance is mainly determined by constriction or dilation of arterioles, which regulate how rapidly blood leaves the arterial system.

The volume of flow through tissues is determined by the pressure gradient across a tissue (i.e., perfusion pressure) and resistance within the tissue. Vasculature plays an important role in pressure gradients and resistance and will be discussed next. Given an adequate blood pressure, tissue blood flow is regulated by local mechanisms that allow precise regional adjustment of blood flow. These mechanisms will be discussed later in the chapter.

Structure and Function of Vasculature

Blood flows in response to a pressure gradient. Pumping of the heart raises the pressure of blood contained within the arterial system, resulting in forward flow. Tissue blood flow is determined by the pressure difference between the arterial and venous sides of its circulation and the resistance to flow offered by its own vasculature. The structure and function of the various types of blood vessels impact tissue circulation and will be discussed next.

ELASTIC ARTERIES

Blood flows into arteries from the heart. The aorta and large arteries (elastic arteries) are strong, elastic vessels that can withstand high pressure. The walls of elastic arteries have a large amount of elastin and collagen. The tunica media is broad with concentric fenestrated sheets of elastin. It also contains collagen and a lesser amount of smooth muscle fibers.

During contraction of the heart (systole), blood surges into elastic arteries which stretch to accommodate, thereby storing potential energy in vessel walls. During relaxation of the heart (diastole), the walls of elastic arteries recoil, maintaining arterial blood pressure and forward flow.

Elastic arteries are therefore said to function as the "pressure reservoirs" of circulation. Elastic arteries allow blood to be distributed with a minimal drop in pressure while reducing pulsatility, which is especially important when blood arrives in delicate vascular beds.

MUSCULAR ARTERIES

Muscular arteries are still sizeable, but smaller than large elastic arteries. Muscular arteries are also called distributing arteries because they branch to distribute blood to the vast network of arterioles.

These arteries are farther from the heart where the surge of blood has dampened. Their tunica media is thick with a large amount of smooth muscle and less elastin. The thick tunica media allows muscular arteries to play a role in vasoconstriction, but the decrease in elastin limits their ability to expand.

ARTERIOLES

Smaller arteries and arterioles are the main sites of resistance to blood flow. This is because their walls are primarily smooth muscle without significant elastin.

Arterioles can adjust their resistance by contracting the smooth muscle in their walls, causing vasoconstriction, or relaxing the smooth muscle, causing vasodilation. This allows arterioles to locally control the amount of blood flow directed downstream into tissue capillaries.

CAPILLARIES

Capillaries connect arterioles to venules. Capillaries and small venules are the sites of exchange in tissues. The exchange of gases and other substances occurs in the capillary bed between blood, interstitial fluid, and the surrounding cells.

The diameter of a capillary lumen ranges from 5 to 10 micrometers; the smallest are just wide enough for an erythrocyte (RBC) to squeeze through. The wall of a capillary consists of the endothelial layer surrounded by a basement membrane. There is some variation in wall structure depending on size. In a large capillary, several endothelial cells bordering each other may line the lumen; in a small capillary, there may only be a single cell layer that wraps around to contact itself.

For capillaries to function, their walls must allow substances to pass through. Capillaries are categorized into three types which differ in their degree of "leakiness": continuous, fenestrated, and discontinuous. Continuous capillaries are most common and have small gaps between endothelial cells. Fenestrated capillaries are "leakier" and contain small pores in addition to small gaps between endothelial cells, allowing the exchange of larger molecules in tissues that require a lot of exchange. Discontinuous capillaries (also called sinusoidal capillaries) are the most permeable but least common. They are "leakiest" due to large gaps between endothelial cells, in addition to pores and small gaps, allowing large molecules and even cells to pass through.

VENULES

Postcapillary venules join multiple capillaries exiting from a capillary bed. A venule is an extremely small vein, generally 8 to 100 micrometers in diameter. The walls of venules consist of endothelium, a thin middle layer with a few muscle cells and elastic fibers, plus an outer layer of connective tissue fibers that constitute a very thin tunica externa.

VEINS

Venules empty into veins, which return blood to the heart. Compared with arteries, veins are thin-walled vessels with large and irregular lumens. Venous walls are stretchy and compliant making veins capacitance vessels that readily expand to store a high volume of blood at low pressure.

Veins are therefore said to function as the "volume reservoirs" of circulation. Systemic veins contain approximately 70% of blood volume at any given time.[17]

Because they are low-pressure vessels, larger veins often have valves to prevent backflow due to gravity. Unidirectional flow of venous blood toward the heart is important for normal physiologic function since backflow would cause congestion in tissue capillary beds.

Local Regulation of Tissue Perfusion

The local regulation of blood flow precisely controls how much blood flows through tissue capillary beds. After a discussion of the general mechanisms governing the local regulation of blood flow, two contrasting vascular beds will be considered in some detail: coronary blood flow and cutaneous blood flow.

- Regulation of coronary blood flow is dominated by the need to balance myocardial oxygen supply with myocardial oxygen demand.
  - The coronary vascular bed will serve as an example of local regulation of blood flow in a tissue that undergoes large changes in cellular respiration and ATP production.
- In contrast, regulation of cutaneous blood flow reflects its importance in thermoregulation of the body.
  - The oxygen demand of skin is relatively low and cutaneous blood flow is typically sufficient to meet its metabolic needs.
  - Skin is the site of heat loss to the external environment and the control of its blood flow reflects this.
  - Skin interfaces with the external environment and is frequently injured, so changes in cutaneous blood flow in response to injury will also be discussed.

GENERAL MECHANISMS GOVERNING LOCAL REGULATION OF BLOOD FLOW

Local regulation of blood flow occurs by means of three basic regulatory mechanisms:

1. Metabolic regulation
2. Myogenic regulation
3. Paracrine regulation

The control of blood flow in any one tissue can be understood as an interplay of these mechanisms.[18]

Metabolic Regulation

Metabolic regulation of blood flow is the most important local control mechanism. Metabolic regulation refers to changes in blood flow that occur in response to alterations in the ratio of blood flow (supply) to the metabolic requirements (demand) of tissues.[19] An increased metabolic rate of a tissue increases the consumption of oxygen. Increased consumption of oxygen increases the production of metabolic products, including carbon dioxide, adenosine, and lactic acid. Thus, as the metabolism of a tissue increases, the interstitial concentration of oxygen decreases and the interstitial concentrations of metabolic byproducts increase.

If blood flow is inadequate to meet metabolic demand, the production and accumulation of metabolites by ischemic tissue initiates vasodilation. This increases blood flow in the tissue so that it can match the metabolic rate of the tissue.

Metabolic regulation is mediated by vasodilator metabolites, including adenosine, potassium ions (K^+), CO_2, and H^+ released from parenchymal cells. These vasodilators relax the smooth muscle of nearby arterioles. Vasodilation results in reduced resistance to flow and, in the presence of a constant arterial pressure, increased blood flow. Increased blood flow supplies more O_2 and other nutrients.

The stimulus for release of vasodilator metabolites can be either increased metabolic activity of parenchymal cells or decreased tissue PO_2 resulting from reduced O_2 supply relative to utilization (see Fig. 5.2).

In this feedback loop, a decrease in arterial pressure reduces blood flow and oxygen delivery. The mismatch between O_2 supply and utilization lowers tissue PO_2. Lowered tissue PO_2 limits the

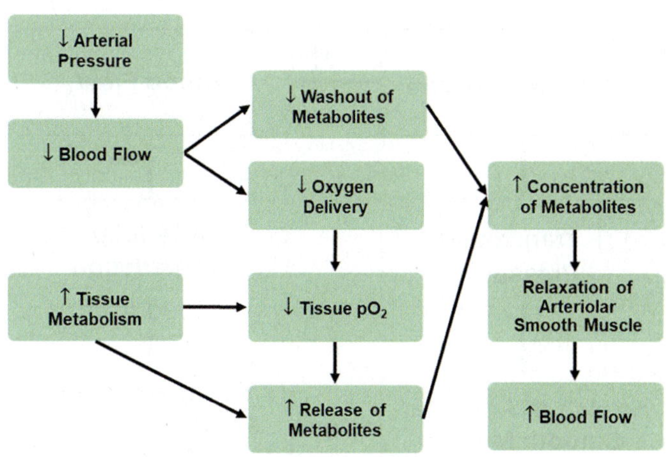

Figure 5.2. Metabolic regulation of blood flow. Either reduced arterial pressure or increased tissue metabolism reduces tissue PO_2. This leads to release of vasodilator metabolites, relaxation of arteriolar smooth muscle, and decreased vascular resistance. In the case of decreased arterial pressure, blood flow returns toward the original value (autoregulation). In the case of increased metabolism, blood flow increases (active hyperemia). Metabolic regulation of blood flow also plays a role in reactive hyperemia.

formation of ATP and results in the release of vasodilator metabolites: adenosine, for example. Vasodilator metabolites relax arteriolar smooth muscle, increasing blood flow to match demand.

Alternatively, increased tissue metabolism leads to increased O_2 use and lowers tissue PO_2. Lowered PO_2 limits the formation of ATP from ADP and increases the same vasodilator metabolites, resulting in increased blood flow to restore tissue PO_2.

In Figure 5.2, tissue PO_2 is used as the error signal in the negative feedback loop. However, some metabolites are not ordinarily released in response to lowered tissue PO_2. A good example is K^+, which is released with each action potential of the tissue. K^+ acts as a *feed-forward mechanism*, initiating vasodilation before the action potentials that release it can trigger cellular events that will ultimately result in increased O_2 use.

The relative importance of the various metabolic vasodilator mechanisms depends on the parenchymal cell in question, the mix of tissue activity, and blood supply.

Myogenic Regulation

Myogenic regulation refers to changes in the tone of resistance vessels in response to alterations in their transmural pressure. It occurs when a change in transmural pressure results in increased or decreased stretch of the vascular smooth muscle of those resistance vessels (Fig. 5.3). Increased transmural pressure leads to increased stretch of vascular smooth muscle, prompting the muscle to contract.

The myogenic response counteracts the influence of increased or decreased transmural pressure on resistance vessel diameter. For example, in order for a person to stand, transmural pressure increases dramatically in the resistance vessels of the legs and feet. These resistance vessels are stretched and their response is to constrict. This response has at least two beneficial effects:

1. It prevents the dilation that would otherwise occur as a result of the increased transmural pressure. Vasoconstriction helps to buffer the fall in arterial pressure that occurs upon standing.
2. Constriction of the resistance vessels lessens the hydrostatic pressure transmitted to the capillaries of the legs and feet as a result of standing.

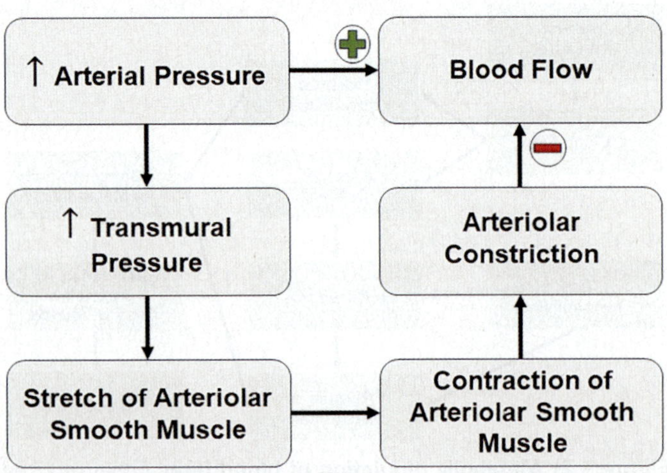

Figure 5.3. Myogenic regulation of blood flow results from a change in arteriolar tone in response to a change in stretch of arteriolar smooth muscle. Increased transmural pressure (typically due to increased arterial pressure) stretches the vascular wall, which causes contraction of arteriolar smooth muscle, arteriolar constriction, and a decrease in blood flow. Myogenic regulation plays a role in autoregulation of blood flow and reactive hyperemia.

The error signal for myogenic regulation is stretch of vascular smooth muscle cells within the wall of resistance vessels.[20] Stretch of vascular smooth muscle causes opening of stretch-activated cation channels that carry Ca^{2+} and initiate contraction.[21] Stretch also activates signaling pathways involving phospholipase C and protein kinase C.[22]

Paracrine Regulation

Paracrine regulation refers to the local release of chemical mediators that cause vasodilation or vasoconstriction. Only a small fraction of these mediators will be discussed. Many paracrine agents have effects on smooth muscle growth and/or apoptosis, but only effects on vascular smooth muscle tone will be considered here.

Endothelial cells and platelets release mediators that influence vascular smooth muscle tone.[23] In some cases, endothelial cells modify the effects of substances released by platelets so that intact blood vessels respond differently than damaged vessels. For example, serotonin, ADP, and thrombin released from platelets cause vascular relaxation in the presence of endothelium, but these agents act directly on vascular smooth muscle to cause contraction.

Perhaps the most significant interaction is between thromboxane A_2 (TxA_2) and prostacyclin (PGI_2). Platelets release TxA_2, a vasoconstrictor, and this effect predominates when the endothelial layer of the blood vessel is damaged. Normal endothelium releases PGI_2, a vasodilator, and this has the dominant effect on intact blood vessels.[24]

Figure 5.4 shows two other phenomena that are not strictly paracrine but are of significance. Flow-induced dilation[25] plays an important role in producing high flows in the heart during metabolic hyperemia and depends on endothelial signaling. The axon reflex is also shown in this figure and will be described later in the discussion of cutaneous blood flow.[26]

Even under resting conditions, mechanisms of local blood flow regulation precisely match flow with tissue metabolism.

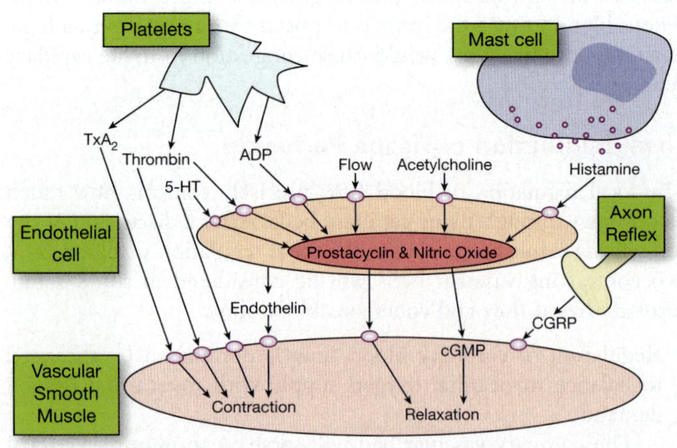

Figure 5.4. Paracrine regulation of blood flow results from mediators released from blood elements and endothelial cells. Platelets release thromboxane A_2, thrombin, and serotonin that, in the absence of intact endothelium, cause contraction of the underlying vascular smooth muscle. Thrombin, serotonin, and ADP cause release of nitric oxide and/or prostacyclin from endothelial cells, which results in vascular smooth muscle relaxation. Thus, activated platelets cause vasoconstriction only in the presence of locally disrupted endothelium. Histamine released from mast cells also causes vasodilation via endothelial cells. Two elements of local control that are not paracrine are flow-induced vasodilation and vasodilators released from collaterals of axons mediating nociception.

PROCESSES CONTROLLING LOCAL BLOOD FLOW

The three regulatory mechanisms (metabolic, myogenic, and paracrine) underlie in varying degrees four processes which control local blood flow:

1. Active hyperemia (metabolic and paracrine mechanisms)
2. Reactive hyperemia (metabolic, myogenic, and paracrine mechanisms)
3. Autoregulation (metabolic and myogenic mechanisms)
4. Vascular response to injury (paracrine mechanisms)

Active Hyperemia

Active hyperemia occurs when tissue metabolism is increased. The local vasodilation responsible for active hyperemia is caused by metabolic and paracrine regulatory mechanisms.

An increase in tissue metabolism leads to release of vasodilator metabolites in proportion to the level of activity of the tissue. Paracrine factors such as prostaglandins are also released during increased metabolic activity. The result is that as metabolic activity increases, so does tissue blood flow.

In many tissues, including cardiac muscle, skeletal muscle, brain, and gut, there is a linear relationship between oxygen consumption and blood flow. In this way, oxygen supply, oxygen demand, and oxygen consumption are matched.

The precise mix of metabolites and paracrine factors depends on the conditions of the increased metabolism, how well oxygen supply meets oxygen demand, and the type of tissue involved.

Reactive Hyperemia

Reactive hyperemia occurs when blood flow resumes after being stopped due to occlusion of the artery supplying a region. The occlusion may be caused by compression of the artery by external pressure or by thrombus formation in the lumen. In the case of reactive hyperemia, the duration of the occlusion is short enough that there is no sustained cell injury or death, although there may be metabolic adjustments in the tissue in response to a lack of oxygen. When the occlusion is removed, flow increases well above the level observed before the occlusion. It then returns to baseline with a time course dependent on the duration of the occlusion: the longer the occlusion, the longer the duration of reactive hyperemia.

The local vasodilation responsible for reactive hyperemia is regulated by metabolic, myogenic, and paracrine mechanisms. The occlusion of the artery supplying a region of tissue lowers transmural pressure in the resistance vessels beyond the occlusion. This reduces stretch of the vascular smooth muscle and results in its relaxation. Vasodilator metabolites, paracrine hormones, and cytokines are released when flow to the affected region is stopped and tissue PO_2 drops. They accumulate in the tissue because there is no blood flow to wash them out. In time, they completely dilate the resistance vessels.

In general, the myogenic response dominates in occlusions of short duration when there is little time for the build-up of metabolites and paracrine factors. The paracrine and metabolic responses gain importance in occlusions of longer duration.

Autoregulation

Autoregulation of blood flow refers to the ability of tissues to maintain flow within a narrow range despite changes in arterial pressure. Most tissues, including the brain, heart, kidney, skin, and gut, display autoregulation. Autoregulation depends on metabolic and myogenic regulatory mechanisms.

The reduction in flow accompanying a decrease in perfusion pressure allows the buildup of locally released metabolic vasodilators. These vasodilators relax arteriolar smooth muscle, decreasing vascular resistance and restoring flow. The converse happens when perfusion pressure is elevated.

A fall in perfusion pressure also reduces transmural pressure in resistance vessels. The myogenic response leads to a reduction in vascular smooth muscle tone and a decrease in resistance, restoring blood flow. Again, the converse happens when perfusion pressure is elevated.

Both mechanisms aim to restore blood flow to its original level in response to a change in arterial pressure, maintaining steady flow through the tissue.

The Vascular Response to Injury

The vascular response to injury refers to the constellation of vascular changes after local tissue injury. In general, paracrine factors such as histamine, bradykinin, and prostanoids are released and cause dilation of resistance and capacitance vessels as well as increased leakiness of exchange vessels to plasma proteins. Cutaneous circulation demonstrates the prototypical vascular response to injury and will be discussed later in the chapter.

Systemic Control of Tissue Perfusion

Local blood flow control mechanisms primarily modulate tissue perfusion, but also influence systemic circulation. Likewise, systemic circulation affects tissue perfusion.

Local control of vascular resistance impacts venous blood return. Venous blood return determines stroke volume which is the most important factor regulating cardiac output in the normal heart.

- An increase in tissue metabolism results in increased tissue oxygen consumption. This reduces tissue PO_2 and increases the production and release of vasodilator metabolites leading to decreased vascular resistance and increased blood flow, venous return, and cardiac output.
- Myogenic mechanisms in response to local vascular pressures and paracrine factors released in response to the local environment also affect vascular resistance. Dilation of arterioles reduces vascular resistance and increases local blood flow. As a result, venous return to the heart increases, increasing stroke volume and cardiac output.

The circulatory system adjusts cardiac output, or blood flow supply, to match the metabolic activity, or blood flow demand, of all the organs of systemic circulation.

If cardiac output cannot be increased enough to fully meet the metabolic demands of all tissues, the circulatory system will selectively reduce or ration blood flow to some tissues in order to prioritize tissues and organs that are critical for moment-to-moment body function and survival.

The organs that are most responsive to this increased sympathetic drive are those whose arterioles are primarily under neurohormonal control rather than local (metabolic, myogenic, and paracrine) control. Generally, these organs are noncritical in the sense that they can tolerate temporary reductions in blood flow without jeopardizing survival of the body. These organs include the splanchnic organs, kidneys, and resting skeletal muscle.

In contrast, local (metabolic, myogenic, and paracrine) control predominates over neurohormonal control in the brain, myocardium (cardiac muscle), and exercising skeletal muscle. These critical organs must have adequate blood flow to match their metabolism on a minute-to-minute basis to ensure survival.

The skin is a special case because under thermal stress, brisk blood flow to the skin is critical to dissipate metabolically produced heat. In the absence of heat stress, blood flow to the skin is not critical and can be reduced to help maintain arterial pressure.

The net effect of vasoconstriction in noncritical organs is to increase systemic vascular resistance, which helps to keep arterial blood pressure high enough to perfuse critical organs.

Thus, generally, the most important function of neurohormonal control mechanisms is to regulate blood pressure and blood volume in such a way that the heart can deliver adequate blood flow to all organs of the body. When that's not possible, these control mechanisms ensure adequate blood flow to critical organs at the expense of blood flow to noncritical organs.

An understanding of the general mechanisms of blood flow regulation and the processes controlling local blood flow provides the foundation for deeper exploration of blood flow in two contrasting vascular beds: myocardium and skin. The following sections explore these in greater detail.

Blood Flow in the Myocardium

CORONARY BLOOD FLOW

The heart comprises only 0.5% of body weight, yet under resting conditions receives about 5% of cardiac output.[27] Almost the entire blood supply is provided by the right and left coronary arteries. These vessels originate from the root of the aorta; the two coronary ostia are located behind the aortic cusps in the sinus of Valsalva. Coronary artery perfusion pressure is therefore determined by the pressure generated from the left ventricle. The larger distributing coronary arteries run over the epicardial surface of the heart. Transmural branches penetrate the myocardium and deliver blood flow throughout the thickness of the wall. After perfusing the myocardial tissue, blood returns to the heart via the coronary sinus, which drains about 90% of the left ventricle. Other coronary veins and Thebesian vessels also drain various portions of the myocardium.

OXYGEN EXTRACTION

At rest, 60% to 70% of oxygen is extracted from coronary arterial blood as it flows through myocardial capillaries.[27] Coronary sinus (venous) oxygen levels approach the minimal level attainable by tissues. Since oxygen extraction cannot increase significantly, increased oxygen demand can only be met by increases in coronary blood flow.

REGULATION OF CORONARY BLOOD FLOW

Coronary blood flow is determined by the interaction of multiple factors and regulatory mechanisms, including:

1. Extravascular compressive forces (tissue pressure)
2. Coronary perfusion pressure
3. Local blood flow (metabolic, myogenic, and paracrine) regulatory mechanisms
4. Neurohormonal control

Together, these modulate myocardial vascular resistance in order to ensure that blood flow meets myocardial oxygen demand.[28]

Extravascular Compression and the Coronary Blood Flow Cycle

During systole and diastole, the coronary arteries are subject to marked changes in extravascular pressures. The transmural vessels and their branches within the myocardium are subject to the compressive forces of each cardiac contraction.

With contraction of the left ventricle (systole), extravascular compression causes flow in vessels supplied by the left coronary artery to fall to zero, or even transiently become retrograde. During early diastole, relaxation of the left ventricle results in a large inflow into these vessels such that most flow to the myocardium of the left ventricle occurs during diastole. The high flow during diastole can be viewed as reactive hyperemia in response to the cessation of flow with each systole. Flow parallels aortic pressure during the remainder of the cycle.

Conversely, in arteries supplying the myocardium of the right ventricle, maximal flow occurs during systole because extravascular pressures in this structure do not exceed systolic aortic pressure. The flow profile in the right ventricular myocardium closely resembles the pressure profile in the aorta.

Increases in heart rate, which increase cardiac work, restrict left coronary inflow because rate increases occur primarily at the expense of the diastolic interval. The increased cardiac metabolism, however, causes coronary resistance vessels to dilate, overriding the effect of extravascular compression. The net result is that coronary blood flow increases as heart rate increases, allowing oxygen delivery to meet demand.

In hearts with limited blood flow, as may occur with coronary arterial disease, an increased heart rate may cause chest pain (angina) because flow cannot increase adequately to meet the increased oxygen demand.

Coronary Perfusion Pressure

Recall that perfusion pressure is the pressure gradient across a tissue vascular bed. Coronary veins of the left ventricle are usually compressed by the relatively high extravascular pressure (i.e., tissue pressure), even during diastole. Pressure upstream builds until the vessels are forced open and flow proceeds to the coronary sinus. This is known as the waterfall phenomenon.[29] When considering the perfusion pressure of the left coronary vascular bed, the upstream pressure is diastolic arterial pressure while the downstream pressure is just above tissue pressure, the minimum necessary to keep coronary veins from collapsing.

Myocardial tissue pressure is close to diastolic ventricular cavity pressure. This number is ordinarily low compared with diastolic arterial pressure, and its effect can be ignored. However, in the presence of elevated diastolic ventricular cavity pressure (as occurs with decreased diastolic ventricular compliance), the downstream pressure can become a significant factor in limiting coronary flow. This occurs, for example, with myocardial hypertrophy.

Local (Metabolic, Myogenic, and Paracrine) Mechanisms and Neurohormonal Control

The remaining mechanisms will be discussed together due to their complex interactions.

Physiologic increases in myocardial metabolism are almost always the result of increased sympathetic nerve activity to the heart. Heart rate and contractility increase in response to sympathetic drive, which leads to an increase in oxygen demand. This leads to active hyperemia, which is the main determinant of coronary blood flow.[19,28]

The primary mechanism causing increased coronary blood flow during active hyperemia is dilation of arterioles by local metabolites and paracrine factors, and the full development of active hyperemia is dependent on normal endothelial cell function.

Flow-induced dilation of distributing arteries in the heart is necessary to maintain the full pressure gradient across the wall of the heart. An increase in local blood flow results in higher flow velocities upstream. If the coronary endothelium is normal, increased flow velocity in distributing arteries causes the release of nitric oxide from endothelial cells. Nitric oxide diffuses to vascular smooth muscle where it causes relaxation by elevating smooth muscle cyclic guanosine monophosphate (cGMP). The resulting increase in the diameter of distributing arteries is sufficient to minimize the drop in pressure that would otherwise result from increased blood flow associated with active hyperemia.[30]

If the distributing arteries in the heart do not dilate in response to increased flow velocities, the result is an increased pressure drop along their length. This means that the pressure available to drive blood flow across the wall through transmural vessels is reduced. This occurs when endothelial communication with vascular smooth muscle is impeded by atherosclerosis, hypertension, and other conditions.

Coronary endothelium also plays an important role in protecting vascular smooth muscle from the constrictor effects of several agonists in the blood. These include platelet-derived serotonin and thrombin.[23,31] These substances cause vascular relaxation in the presence of endothelium but act directly on vascular smooth muscle to cause contraction. Endothelial dysfunction is one of the mechanisms that can lead to coronary artery spasm, along with oxidative stress and low-grade chronic inflammation.[32]

MYOCARDIAL RESPONSE TO ALTERED CORONARY BLOOD FLOW

Stenosis of coronary arteries occurs in individuals with coronary atherosclerosis. Stenosis increases total coronary resistance and therefore reduces maximal coronary blood flow. Until stenosis becomes quite severe, however, it has little or no effect on resting coronary blood flow due to autoregulation.

Figure 5.5 shows coronary flow as a function of coronary perfusion pressure downstream from stenosis of a major coronary artery. The region of the curve where changes in pressure are accompanied by small changes in flow is the result of autoregulation.

When coronary circulation is within the autoregulatory range: (1) Reactive hyperemia can be elicited by briefly stopping flow; and (2) Infusion of a vasodilator, such as adenosine, causes increased flow. Both responses require that the resistance vessels downstream from the stenosis are able to dilate. Resistance vessels can only respond to an added vasodilator stimulus to the extent that they are not already maximally dilated to maintain resting flow in the face of an upstream stenosis. The remaining ability for resistance vessels to dilate in the face of an upstream stenosis is called *coronary reserve*. The magnitude of the increase in flow observed with

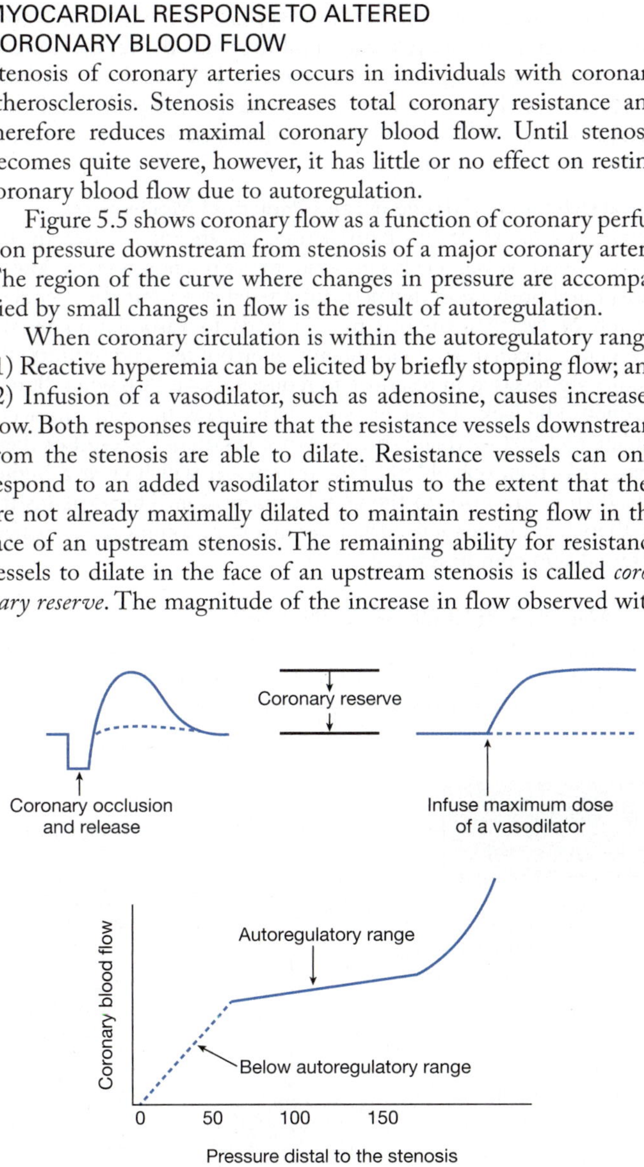

Figure 5.5. Coronary reserve refers to the ability of vessels downstream from a stenosis to dilate. It is manifested in the autoregulatory range by reactive hyperemia and/or increased flow in response to a vasodilator. Below the autoregulatory range, vessels downstream from a stenosis are completely dilated and so a vasodilator stimulus such as reactive hyperemia or a drug does not increase flow. Within the autoregulatory range, the magnitude of coronary reserve depends on how much downstream dilation is necessary to compensate for an upstream stenosis; that is, more coronary reserve is found when the pressure distal to the stenosis is 100 mm Hg than when it is 75 mm Hg.

reactive hyperemia or drug infusion provides an estimate of the coronary reserve.

If pressure distal to a stenosis falls below the autoregulatory range (Fig. 5.5) flow decreases in proportion to the drop in pressure. This is because the ability of the resistance vessels to dilate (coronary reserve) has been completely exhausted. At this point, reactive hyperemia and increased flow in response to a vasodilator can no longer occur.

An estimate of coronary reserve can also be made by measuring the pressure drop across the stenosis during infusion of a vasodilator.[33] This method relies on the assumption that the resistance across the stenosis does not change. In this situation, if increased flow occurs because of downstream resistance vessel dilation, the pressure drop across the stenosis increases. If no change in the pressure drop across the stenosis is observed, the conclusion is that no increase in flow is possible and that coronary reserve is exhausted.

The issue of reduced flow caused by coronary stenosis is made more complex by the fact that if coronary flow is reduced, the myocardium quickly adjusts to this new situation. During a period of reduced flow that results in a reduced oxygen supply relative to myocardial demand, a rapid decrease in myocardial contractility is found in the region impacted by the reduced flow.

After one or more periods of reduced oxygen supply relative to demand, myocardial contractility may be reduced for minutes to hours, despite a return to normal resting coronary blood flow. This is called *myocardial stunning*.[34] The reduction in the supply/demand ratio that causes myocardial stunning may be the result of either periods of reduced coronary blood flow or increased myocardial oxygen consumption. The cause of myocardial stunning appears to involve the release of oxygen free radicals and a decrease in the sensitivity of the contractile machinery to calcium ions.[35]

After repeated bouts of myocardial stunning or after a sustained period of suboptimal blood flow, a chronic depression in myocardial contractility may ensue. This is called hibernation.[34,36,37] It is not the result of infarction of myocardium. At first, during *functional hibernation*, the causes may be similar to those of myocardial stunning. A more severe and/or longer period is referred to as *structural hibernation* and involves rarefaction of contractile proteins, reduced mitochondria, and other later changes, including apoptosis. If normal flow is restored by coronary artery bypass or angioplasty, hibernating myocardium can return to normal function.[38]

The myocardium is protected from stunning, hibernation, and infarction by previous short bouts of ischemia. This is called *ischemic preconditioning*.[39] Ischemic preconditioning occurs in many organs in addition to the heart, including the brain, lung, liver, and skeletal muscle.

The discussion of blood flow in the myocardium illustrates how local blood flow regulatory mechanisms interact to supply oxygen in a tissue with high oxygen demands. The following section discusses a contrasting vascular bed: the skin. As metabolic needs in the skin are lower, oxygen demand is not the major determinant of blood flow. Cutaneous blood flow is primarily influenced by other stimuli.

Blood Flow in the Skin

Skin has a low metabolic rate that remains constant, so its nutrient requirements are typically met unless severe pathologic reductions in blood flow occur. Skin comprises 16% of total body weight[40] but typically receives ~5% of cardiac output.[41] Because of its proximity to the external environment, cutaneous blood flow plays an important role in temperature regulation of the body by modulating heat dissipation.

STRUCTURAL CONSIDERATIONS

The vasculature of the skin is arranged in two plexuses within the dermis that run parallel to the skin, one in the superficial layer and one in the deep layer. The majority of vessels are in the superficial plexus, 1 to 2 mm below the epidermis. This plexus is a major determinant of heat exchange with the environment. The deeper plexus contains arterioles that ascend to the upper plexus and other skin structures such as hair follicles and sweat glands.

The ability to control cutaneous blood flow for heat dissipation or conservation at rest is in part due to a particular vascular structural feature in the deep plexus of glabrous skin: the arteriovenous anastomosis (AVA). AVAs are short vessel segments with a large inner diameter, thick wall, and low resistance, allowing for high flow rates directly from arterioles to venules.

- Glabrous, or apical, skin, which is free of hair (palms, soles, lips), has many AVAs. Opening or closing AVAs can cause substantial changes in glabrous skin blood flow.
- Nonglabrous, or nonapical, skin, which is hairy, has few if any AVAs.

REGULATION OF CUTANEOUS BLOOD FLOW

Blood flow in the skin is determined by a combination of factors and mechanisms, including:

1. Neurohormonal control
2. Body and environmental temperatures
3. Local blood flow (metabolic, myogenic, and paracrine) regulatory mechanisms

Neurohormonal Control

Human cutaneous circulation is unique in that it is controlled by two populations of sympathetic nerves: (1) sympathetic adrenergic vasoconstrictor nerves, and (2) sympathetic vasodilator nerves. Glabrous skin has only sympathetic vasoconstrictor nerves, which richly innervate the numerous AVAs. Nonglabrous skin is innervated by both sympathetic vasoconstrictor and sympathetic vasodilator nerves.

Sympathetic vasoconstrictor nerves release norepinephrine which interacts with postsynaptic alpha 1- and alpha 2-adrenergic receptors on cutaneous arterioles and AVAs. In addition, sympathetic vasoconstrictor nerves release cotransmitters that further contribute to vasoconstriction, including neuropeptide Y (NPY)[42] and ATP.[43]

Body and Environmental Temperatures

The vasoconstrictor system in human skin is tonically active in thermoneutral environments. Subtle changes in vasoconstriction are responsible for maintenance of normal body temperature in response to slight changes in activity or ambient temperature. This is possible because small changes in skin blood flow can cause relatively large changes in heat dissipation. The vasoconstrictor system is also responsible for the decrease in skin blood flow that occurs with cold exposure.

As core body temperature increases, cutaneous blood flow rises.[44,45] This is a result of at least two events[46]: (1) the withdrawal of sympathetic vasoconstrictor tone; and (2) the activation of sympathetic vasodilator nerves. When body temperature is elevated (hyperthermia), withdrawal of the activity of sympathetic vasoconstrictors only accounts for 10% to 20% of cutaneous vasodilation. The large increases in skin blood flow are mediated primarily (80% to 90%) by activation of sympathetic vasodilator nerves in the skin.[44,47]

The sympathetic vasodilator system in humans is not tonically active in normothermia and is only activated during increases in internal temperature, such as those that occur during exercise or environmental heat exposure. Active vasodilation is mediated by cotransmission from sympathetic cholinergic nerves. In this state, skin blood flow can increase to as much as 60% of cardiac output (7 to 8 L/min).[48]

Skin temperature both influences and is influenced by blood flow.[49] At a given core temperature, placing skin in a warmer local temperature increases blood flow. This is because increased local temperature reduces sensitivity of cutaneous vessels to norepinephrine.

At extremely low or high temperatures, other mechanisms come into play. At local temperatures below 10 °C, cold-induced vasodilation may be observed.[50] Initially, vascular smooth muscle contraction fails due to the low temperature, resulting in cutaneous vasodilation. This leads to increased blood flow, warming vascular smooth muscle until function resumes and the muscle can contract. Vasoconstriction reduces blood flow and the temperature of the vascular smooth muscle drops again. This results in periodic oscillations of skin blood flow at lower temperatures. At local temperatures over 45 °C, tissue can be damaged and the cutaneous response to injury occurs.

Local (Metabolic, Myogenic, and Paracrine) Mechanisms

Cutaneous blood vessels demonstrate significant reactive hyperemia. Blood vessel occlusion due to skin compression lowers transmural pressure in downstream resistance vessels. The reduced stretch of vascular smooth muscle leads to vasodilation by the myogenic mechanism. Vasodilator metabolites and endothelial factors are released in response to reduced tissue PO_2 when flow is stopped. The lack of flow prevents washout, so these factors accumulate and further dilate the resistance vessels. The result of these changes is that, once blood flow resumes, it will flow at a higher rate than it had prior to the vessel compression. This explains the erythema and increase in surface temperature commonly seen after external skin compression.

CUTANEOUS RESPONSE TO INJURY

The cutaneous response to injury (Fig. 5.6) is seen following various stimuli ranging from mechanical and thermal damage to insect bites and allergic reactions.[51]

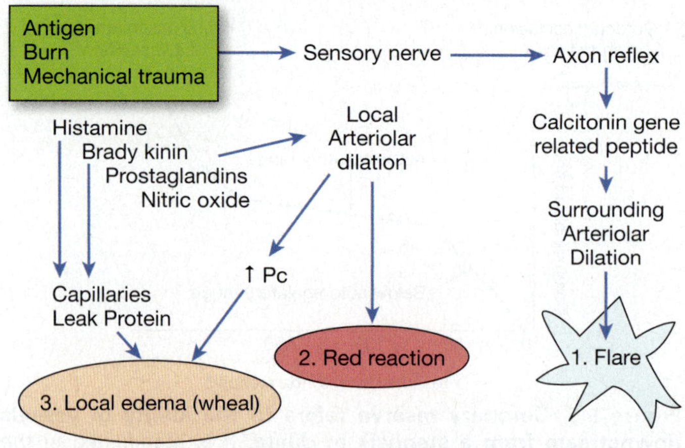

Figure 5.6. The cutaneous response to injury consists of three elements. Local dilation at the site of the injury (red reaction) results from local release of a number of vasodilators, including histamine, bradykinin, prostaglandins, and nitric oxide. Edema results from a combination of increased transport of proteins across the capillary wall stimulated by histamine and bradykinin, and increased capillary hydrostatic pressure resulting from arteriolar dilation. Collaterals of nociceptive C fibers that release calcitonin gene-related peptide and other vasodilators cause the flare around an injury.

Following mechanical injury, a red reaction appears at the site of the insult. This is due to the local release of several vasodilators including histamine, bradykinin, prostaglandins, and nitric oxide. These vasodilators increase filling of the subcutaneous venous plexus resulting in localized erythema.

Noxious stimuli also activate sensory nerves. Nociceptive C fibers (a type of pain fiber) have additional collaterals which innervate the region near their sensory nerve endings.[52] Collaterals arise directly from the sensory nerve axon without passing through a synapse. When activated, collaterals release several peptides in the region including substance P and calcitonin gene-related peptide (CGRP). This is known as an *axon reflex*. CGRP causes vasodilation around the site of the injury, resulting in a flare. Substance P, histamine, and bradykinin increase transport of plasma proteins into the interstitial space while vasodilators increase capillary hydrostatic pressure. This combination causes local edema formation, resulting in a wheal.

SUMMARY

The primary functions of the circulatory and respiratory systems can be summarized in two words: transport and exchange. These systems obtain and transport oxygen and other substances necessary for normal cellular function, delivering them to the interstitial fluid that bathes each cell of the body. Likewise, they remove carbon dioxide and other waste products, transporting them to the lungs or other excretory organs for elimination.

Tissue respiration is matched to cellular requirements for generating ATP. Most cells rely primarily on oxidative phosphorylation for energy production. This requires a consistent and adaptable supply of oxygen and substrates. Local blood flow regulatory mechanisms (metabolic, myogenic, and paracrine) adjust tissue blood flow to meet tissue metabolic demand. These basic mechanisms underlie the processes of active hyperemia, reactive hyperemia, autoregulation, and the vascular response to injury.

Coronary blood flow provides an excellent example of a tissue in which local regulation of blood flow is primarily concerned with matching oxygen supply to the demand generated by oxidative phosphorylation.

Skin blood flow is a counterexample in which matching of metabolism and blood flow is not typically of great significance. Instead, regulation of skin blood flow is primarily determined by temperature regulatory needs.

ACKNOWLEDGMENTS

The authors and editors of this chapter would like to acknowledge the scholarly contributions of Dr. Harvey V. Sparks Jr. for prior editions of this chapter.

REFERENCES

1. Boyer PD. The ATP synthase—a splendid molecular machine. *Annu Rev Biochem*. 1997;66:717–749.
2. Koch LG, Britton SL. Biology: motion is function. *Function (Oxf)*. 2022;3(4):zqac030.
3. Korzeniewski B. Regulation of ATP supply in mammalian skeletal muscle during resting state to intensive work transition. *Biophys Chem*. 2000;83:19–34.
4. Sahlin K, Tonkonogi M, Söderlund K. Energy supply and muscle fatigue in humans. *Acta Physiol Scand*. 1998;162(3):261–266.
5. Hardie DG. Metabolic control: a new solution to an old problem. *Curr Biol*. 2000;10:R757–R759.
6. Wilson DF. Oxidative phosphorylation: regulation and role in cellular and tissue metabolism. *J Physiol*. 2017;595(23):7023–7038.
7. Moreno-Sánchez R, Hogue BA, Hansford RG. Influence of NAD-linked dehydrogenase activity on flux through oxidative phosphorylation. *Biochem J*. 1990;268:421–428.
8. Territo PR, Mootha VK, French SA, Balaban RS. Ca^{2+} activation of heart mitochondrial oxidative phosphorylation: role of the F0/F1-ATPase. *Am J Physiol Cell Physiol*. 2000;278:C423–C435.
9. Petersson J, Rohdin M, Sánchez-Crespo A, et al. Regional lung blood flow and ventilation in upright humans studied with quantitative SPECT. *Respir Physiol Neurobiol*. 2009;166(1):54–60.
10. Galvin I, Drummond GB, Nirmalan M. Distribution of blood flow and ventilation in the lung: gravity is not the only factor. *Br J Anaesth*. 2007;98(4):420–428.
11. Sampson MG, Smaldone GC. Voluntary induced alterations in regional ventilation in normal humans. *J Appl Physiol Respir Environ Exerc Physiol*. 1984;56(1):196–201.
12. Roussos CS, Fukuchi Y, Macklem PT, Engel LA. Influence of diaphragmatic contraction on ventilation distribution in horizontal man. *J Appl Physiol*. 1976;40(3):417–424.
13. Glenny RW, Robertson HT. Fractal modeling of pulmonary blood flow heterogeneity. *J Appl Physiol (1985)*. 1991;70(3):1024–1030.
14. Hakim TS, Lisbona R, Dean GW. Gravity-independent inequality in pulmonary blood flow in humans. *J Appl Physiol (1985)*. 1987;63(3):1114–1121.
15. Prisk GK, Yamada K, Henderson AC, et al. Pulmonary perfusion in the prone and supine postures in the normal human lung. *J Appl Physiol (1985)*. 2007;103(3):883–894.
16. Ortiz-Prado E, Dunn JF, Vasconez J, Castillo D, Viscor G. Partial pressure of oxygen in the human body: a general review. *Am J Blood Res*. 2019; 9(1):1–14.
17. Rothe CF. Reflex control of veins and vascular capacitance. *Physiol Rev*. 1983;63(4):1281–1342.
18. Clifford PS. Local control of blood flow. *Adv Physiol Educ*. 2011;35(1):5–15.
19. Laughlin MH, Korthuis RJ, Duncker DJ, et al. Control of blood flow to cardiac and skeletal muscle during exercise. In: Rowell LB, Shepherd JT, eds. *Handbook of Physiology Section 12: Exercise: Regulation and Integration of Multiple Systems*. Oxford University Press; 1996.
20. Davis MJ, Hill MA. Signaling mechanisms underlying the vascular myogenic response. *Physiol Rev*. 1999;79:387–423.
21. Jackson WF. Ion channels and vascular tone. *Hypertension*. 2000;35:173–178.
22. Bakker EN, Kerkhof CJ, Sipkema P. Signal transduction in spontaneous myogenic tone in isolated arterioles from rat skeletal muscle. *Cardiovasc Res*. 1999;41(1):229–236.
23. Vanhoutte PM. Endothelial dysfunction and inhibition of converting enzyme. *Eur Heart J*. 1998;19(Suppl J):J7–J15.
24. Ware JA, Heistad DD. Platelet-endothelium interactions. *N Engl J Med*. 1993;328:628–635.
25. Bevan JA. Shear stress, the endothelium and the balance between flow-induced contraction and dilation in animals and man. *Int J Microcirc Clin Exp*. 1997;17:248–256.
26. Owman C. Peptidergic vasodilator nerves in the peripheral circulation and in the vascular beds of the heart and brain. *Blood Vessels*. 1990;27:73–93.
27. Deussen A, Ohanyan V, Jannasch A, Yin L, Chilian W. Mechanisms of metabolic coronary flow regulation. *J Mol Cell Cardiol*. 2012;52(4):794–801.
28. Goodwill AG, Dick GM, Kiel AM, Tune JD. Regulation of coronary blood flow. *Compr Physiol*. 2017;7(2):321–382.
29. Downey JM. Extravascular coronary resistance. In: Sperelakis N, ed. *Physiology and Pathophysiology of the Heart*. 2nd ed. Kluwer Academic Publishers; 1989.
30. Sparks HV, Wangler RD, Gorman MW. Control of the coronary circulation. In: Sperelakis N, ed. *Physiology and Pathophysiology of the Heart*. 2nd ed. Kluwer Academic Publishers; 1989.
31. Fleming I, Busse R. NO: the primary EDRF. *J Mol Cell Cardiol*. 1999;31:5–14.
32. Yasue H, Mizuno Y, Harada E. Coronary artery spasm - clinical features, pathogenesis and treatment. *Proc Jpn Acad Ser B Phys Biol Sci*. 2019;95(2):53–66.
33. Pijls NH, De Bruyne B. Coronary pressure measurement and fractional flow reserve. *Heart*. 1998;80:539–542.
34. Camici PG, Dutka DP. Repetitive stunning, hibernation, and heart failure: contribution of PET to establishing a link. *Am J Physiol Heart Circ Physiol*. 2001;280(3):H929–H936.
35. Bolli R, Marban E. Molecular and cellular mechanisms of myocardial stunning. *Physiol Rev*. 1999;79(2):609–634.

36. Canty JM Jr, Fallavollita JA. Chronic hibernation and chronic stunning: a continuum. *J Nucl Cardiol.* 2000;7(5):509–527.
37. Heusch G, Schulz R. The biology of myocardial hibernation. *Trends Cardiovasc Med.* 2000;10(3):108–114.
38. Rahimtoola SH. Concept and evaluation of hibernating myocardium. *Annu Rev Med.* 1999;50:75–86.
39. Ferrari R, Ceconi C, Curello S, Percoco G, Toselli T, Antonioli G. Ischemic preconditioning, myocardial stunning, and hibernation: basic aspects. *Am Heart J.* 1999;138:S61–S68.
40. D'Orazio J, Jarrett S, Amaro-Ortiz A, Scott T. UV radiation and the skin. *Int J Mol Sci.* 2013;14(6):12222–12248.
41. Low DA, Jones H, Cable NT, Alexander LM, Kenney WL. Historical reviews of the assessment of human cardiovascular function: interrogation and understanding of the control of skin blood flow. *Eur J Appl Physiol.* 2020;120(1):1–16.
42. Stephens DP, Saad AR, Bennett LA, Kosiba WA, Johnson JM. Neuropeptide Y antagonism reduces reflex cutaneous vasoconstriction in humans. *Am J Physiol Heart Circ Physiol.* 2004;287(3):H1404–H1409.
43. Lang JA, Krajek AC, Smaller KA. Evidence for a functional vasoconstrictor role for ATP in the human cutaneous microvasculature. *Exp Physiol.* 2017;102(6):684–693.
44. Rowell LB. *Human Circulation Regulation during Physical Stress.* Oxford University Press; 1986:177–178.
45. Rowell LB. *Human Cardiovascular Control.* Oxford University Press; 1993.
46. Joyner MJ, Halliwill JR. Sympathetic vasodilatation in human limbs. *J Physiol.* 2000;526(Pt 3):471–480.
47. Francisco MA, Gibson BM, Simmons GH, Halliwill JR, Minson CT. Cholinergic nerve contribution to cutaneous active vasodilation during exercise is similar to whole body passive heating. *J Appl Physiol (1985).* 2023;134(4):933–940.
48. Chou TH, Coyle EF. Cardiovascular responses to hot skin at rest and during exercise. *Temperature (Austin).* 2022;10(3):326–357.
49. Minson CT, Berry LT, Joyner MJ. Nitric oxide and neurally mediated regulation of skin blood flow during local heating. *J Appl Physiol.* 2001;91(4):1619–1626.
50. Lewis T. Observations upon the reaction of the vessels of the human skin to cold. *Heart.* 1930;15:177–208.
51. Borici-Mazi R, Kouridakis S, Kontou-Fili K. Cutaneous responses to substance P and calcitonin gene–related peptide in chronic urticaria: the effect of cetirizine and dimethindene. *Allergy.* 1999;54:46–56.
52. Sann H, Pierau FK. Efferent functions of C-fiber nociceptors. *Z Rheumatol.* 1998;57(Suppl 2):8–13.

6 Autonomic Nervous System

FRANK H. WILLARD

KEY CONCEPTS

- The two major efferent components of the peripheral nervous system (PNS) are somatic and autonomic. The somatic component provides innervation of the skeletal muscle, while the autonomic component is seen on almost all other tissues in the body such as smooth muscle, glands and the immune system.
- Organization of the autonomic nervous system is similar to the somatic nervous system, including the following roles: receiving afferent fibers, processing information in central circuits, and forming an output (efferent fibers).
- A major distinctive feature of the autonomic nervous system is the two-step output pathway, involving centrally located preganglionic neurons and peripherally located ganglionic neurons that form postganglionic axons.
- There are two anatomically, biochemically, and functionally distinct divisions of the peripheral autonomic nervous system: sympathetic and parasympathetic, although this distinction becomes a little less clear in the distal end of the spinal cord.
- The great midline thoracoabdominopelvic autonomic plexus is supplied with parasympathetic fibers from the vagus and pelvic splanchnic nerves and sympathetic fibers from the thoracic, lumbar, and sacral splanchnic nerves.
- All sympathetic and parasympathetic nerves in the body are supplied with a significant complement of sensory axons.
- The primary afferent (sensory) innervation of organ systems is instrumental in controlling the output of the autonomic nervous system.

INTRODUCTION

The daily existence of humans depends on the coordinated activities of their internal organ systems. A major factor in orchestrating the diverse functions of these internal structures is the autonomic nervous system.

- Through an extensive network of connections, the autonomic nervous system helps maintain the normal rhythm of activity in the visceral organs, adjusting their output to accommodate both internal and external challenges.
- Although the term "autonomic" is used to describe the system, it is by no means independent of the cerebral influences. Not only do the older, more midline (limbic or emotional) structures of the forebrain brain exert direct control of the autonomic nervous system through the hypothalamus, but the cognitive areas of the neocortex also have a significant influence on its workings.[1,2]
- In addition, the hypothalamus itself is closely integrated into a complex network involving the endocrine and immune systems. This conglomerate of interlocking systems, with its pervasive influence on our physiology and psychology, is called the neuroendocrine–immune network.

The terminology used to describe that part of the nervous system usually not under voluntary control varies widely. Since the 18th century, different terms have been used by researchers in different countries.

- None of these terms refer to the exact same group of structures or functions; examples include
  - ☐ vegetative nervensystem
  - ☐ grand sympathique
  - ☐ ganglionic nervous system
  - ☐ visceral nervous system
- The two most commonly used terms are
  - ☐ vegetative nervous system
  - ☐ autonomic nervous system

For a thorough discussion of the history of terminology concerning this system, see Clarke and Jacyna.[3]

- The present chapter uses the term autonomic nervous system to refer to all components of the nervous system using preganglionic and ganglionic neurons as an efferent pathway.
- This definition was strongly proposed by James Langley in the early 1900s[4] and later by Kuntz[5] in the mid-1900s.
- In terms of efferent pathways in the PNS, this definition excludes only the neuromuscular junctions between the ventral horn of the spinal cord (and a few cranial nuclei) and the skeletal muscle.
- The above definition also includes the innervation of the adrenal medulla since the target cells in the adrenal medulla are derived from neural crest cells and function similar to sympathetic ganglionic neurons by producing catecholamines.

Defining the central components of the autonomic nervous system is much more difficult, and it may not be possible to formulate a completely exclusive definition.

- This is due to the fact that many regions of the forebrain, not just the "limbic system" exert influence over output to the vasculature, glands, viscera organs, and the immune system.
- Recently, a complex "Central Autonomic Network" has been described involving such regions as the insular cortex, anterior cingulate cortex, amygdala, and hypothalamus plus several regions in the brainstem.[1]

The clinical importance of understanding the circuits of the autonomic nervous system cannot be overstated.

- Almost all communication between neurons in these circuits occurs via synaptic transmission; this process depends on the production, distribution, and recognition of specific neurochemicals.
- Most pharmaceutical agents, either as a desired first action or as an undesired side effect, influence these metabolic and stereologic events.

- Knowledge of nervous system structure, function, and chemistry is a necessity for the educated use of these substances and the intelligent approach to the maintenance of health.
- Disorders of the autonomic nervous system are numerous and can have wide-ranging systemic manifestations, grossly interfering with normal body homeostasis and general health.[6,7]

The autonomic nervous system is sensitive to events occurring in somatic tissue, such as cutaneous and musculoskeletal systems.

- The autonomic and somatic nervous systems are interlocked through numerous somatovisceral and viscerosomatic reflexes.
- Inflammation and nociception as well as physiologic and emotional stressors can be strong drives on the central autonomic network.
- Visceral symptoms may be the primary manifestations of somatic dysfunction and vice versa.[8]
- The output of the autonomic nervous system not only influences smooth muscle and glands, but also forms a bidirectional relationship with the cells of the immune system.[9]
- This chapter examines the organization of the autonomic nervous system and its afferent component; it places emphasis on the:
  - innervation of the peripheral vasculature
  - pattern of innervation reaching the major organs of the core of the body
  - segmental representation of these organs in the spinal cord

Finally, most systemic diseases have an impact on the autonomic functions.

- Thus, it is through the systemic manifestations of altered autonomic activity, such as elevated sympathetic output, that such diseases can influence the overall health of the individual.
- This concept is especially germane to the osteopathic approach that focuses on helping the patient's body seek a return to health.

ORGANIZATION OF THE AUTONOMIC NERVOUS SYSTEM

The autonomic nervous system has components in both the central nervous system (CNS) and the PNS (Fig. 6.1).

- The major autonomic components of the CNS include[1]
  - forebrain regions such as the anterior cingulate and insular cortex, amygdala and hippocampal formation
  - hypothalamus
  - several brainstem nuclei
  - intermediolateral cell column of the spinal cord
- The autonomic components of the PNS include
  - numerous ganglia (collections of neuron cell bodies located outside of the CNS)
  - a network of fibers distributed to all tissues of the body, with the exception of the hyaline cartilages
  - the centers of the intervertebral disks
  - the parenchymal tissues of the CNS

This chapter focuses on the peripheral distribution of the autonomic nervous system and its influence on health.

Peripheral Nervous Systems

The axons from neurons located in the CNS enter the periphery through spinal and cranial nerves. The peripheral portion of the

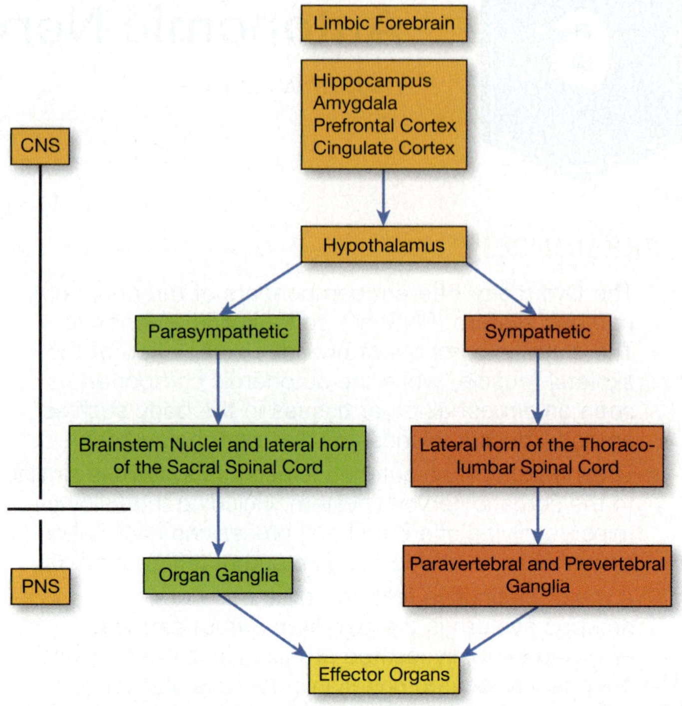

Figure 6.1. The general organization of the autonomic nervous system. The sympathetic (*brown*) and parasympathetic (*green*) components are seen as parallel pathways, bridging between the CNS and PNS, to reach the effector organs. They are controlled by a series of forebrain regions classically described as the limbic system.

nervous system can be divided into two fundamental parts based on the structures targeted by efferent fibers (see Fig. 6.1).

1. Axons derived from the somatic component of the PNS innervate exclusively skeletal muscle.
2. Axons derived from the autonomic component of the PNS enter the periphery and form complex interwoven plexuses containing clusters of cell bodies, termed ganglia. Neurons in these ganglia innervate all other targets, including:
   - smooth muscle
   - glands
   - connective tissue
   - cells in the immune system

This fundamental division in the PNS also reflects differential methods in cellular communication.

- The mechanism of transmission in the neuromuscular junction of the somatic system involves ionotrophic principles.[10]
- This mechanism uses the ion-gated channels to quickly depolarize the cell membrane, a process referred to as fast transmission.
- Conversely, chemical signaling in the autonomic PNS typically relies on metabotrophic principles and volume transmission, the diffusion of transmitter substance away from axonal vesicles, as well as fast synaptic transmission seen in the somatic nervous system.
- The metabotrophic methods of signaling usually involve a neuromodulator that binds to a membrane receptor, activating second-messenger pathways within the target cell.
- These methods are also called slow transmission and often lead to altered gene expression.[10]
- To further understand the distinction between somatic and visceral PNS, compare the typical neural circuitry present in reflex arcs seen in Figures 6.2 and 6.3.[5,11–14]

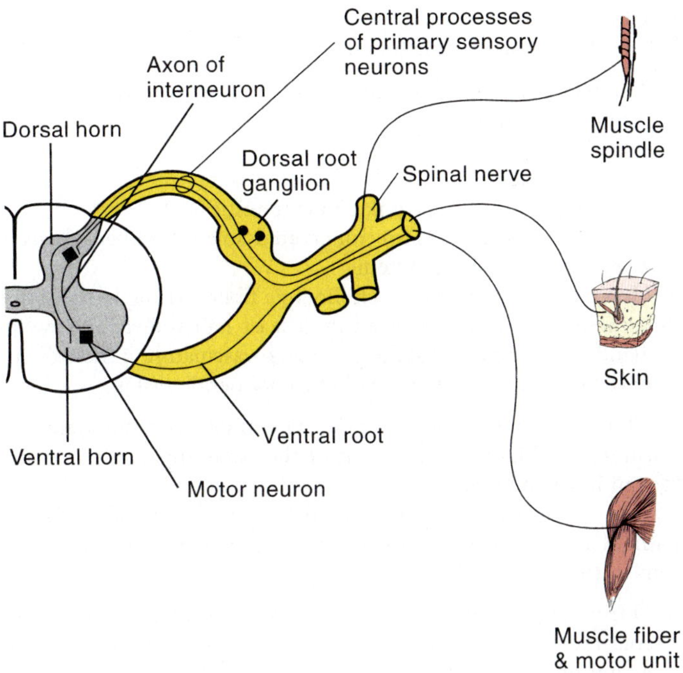

Figure 6.2. The somatic reflex arc. The somatic reflex arc consists of afferent neurons with cell bodies located in the dorsal root ganglia and efferent neurons with cell bodies located in the ventral horn of the spinal cord. As shown here, interneurons with cell bodies located in the spinal gray matter may intercalate between the central process of the afferent fiber and the efferent cell body or associated dendrites.

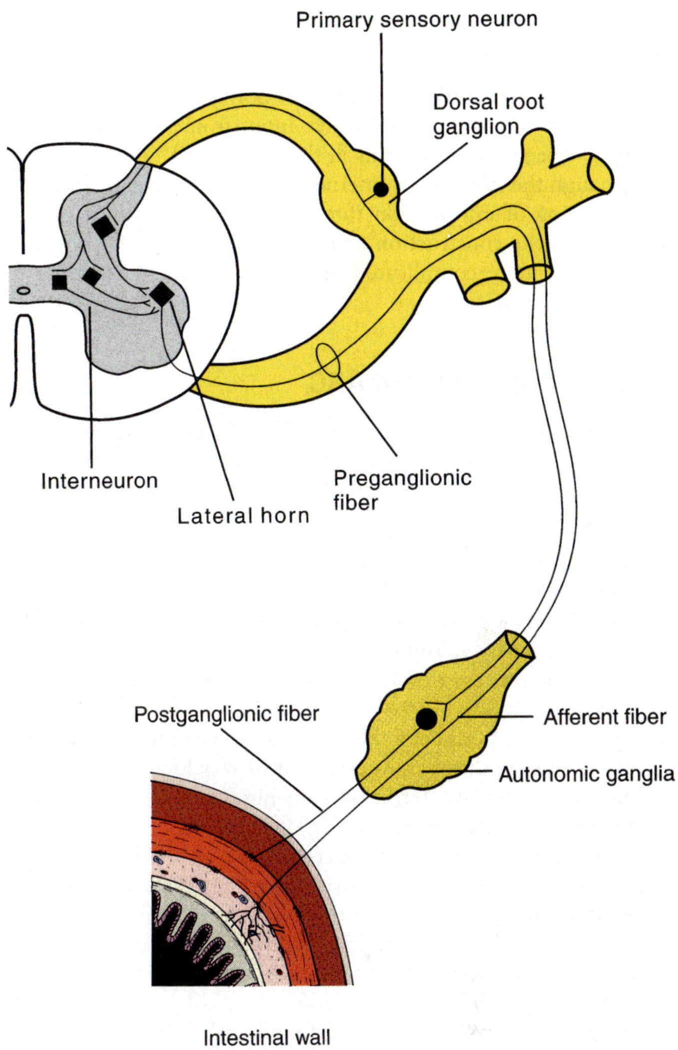

Figure 6.3. The autonomic reflex arc. The autonomic reflex arc consists of primary afferent neurons with cell bodies in the dorsal root ganglion, interneurons in the spinal gray matter, and efferent neurons located in the intermediolateral nucleus of the spinal cord. In addition, the efferent pathway features a second set of efferent neurons located in a peripheral ganglion. This pattern is modified in the brainstem to place the afferent neuron in a cranial nerve ganglion and the interneurons and efferent neurons in brainstem nuclei.

SOMATIC REFLEX ARC

Input and output for the peripheral somatic nervous system occur through spinal and cranial nerves. Figure 6.2 diagrams a typical spinal nerve, illustrating the basic circuitry of the somatic reflex arc.

- In its simplest form, the reflex arc contains a primary afferent neuron in a sensory ganglion and a centrally located motor neuron connected by a synaptic junction; since only one synapse separates the input from the output, this circuit is called a monosynaptic reflex.
- The pseudounipolar cell body of the primary sensory neuron is typically located in the dorsal root ganglia or in the peripheral sensory ganglia of a cranial nerve such as the trigeminal nerve.
- The peripheral process of the sensory neuron is directed outward along a spinal or cranial nerve to reach its target in the peripheral tissue. This process either acts as a receptor end organ itself or is attached to one located in skin, muscle, or connective tissue.
- Each sensory neuron also has a central process (axon) that extends into the dorsal horn of the spinal cord or into sensory nuclei located in the brainstem.

Two fundamental types of primary afferent neurons are present in sensory ganglia.[15,16]

1. One class of sensory neuron features a large cell body with a myelinated process; this kind of cell:
   - □ Typically forms the large-caliber fiber system
2. Is involved in proprioception or discriminative mechanoreception
3. Conversely, other sensory neurons have small cell bodies, with lightly myelinated or unmyelinated processes. These cells:
   - □ Typically form the A-delta and C-fiber small-caliber fiber systems
   - □ Are involved in crude touch and nociception (see Chapters 9 and 11 for additional discussion of this concept)

- There are a few large cells present in the dorsal root ganglia that have been shown to behave electrophysiologically as small cells.

The second component of the monosynaptic reflex arc, the motor neuron, has a multipolar cell body in the ventral horn of the spinal cord or in a brainstem nucleus.

- Motor neuron axons leave the CNS in the ventral root of a spinal nerve or in a cranial nerve, eventually innervating its effector organ, skeletal muscle, through a neuromuscular synaptic junction.
- These monosynaptic reflex connections occur between the largest sensory neurons, typically A-alpha fibers, and ventral horn motor neurons, innervating skeletal muscle.
- This concept is well reviewed in most textbooks in neuroscience.[17]

All other somatic reflexes involve the presence of interneurons situated between the central processes of the sensory neuron and the motoneurons; several synaptic connections must be traversed to complete the arc.

- Such circuits are called disynaptic or polysynaptic reflex arcs.
- The polysynaptic reflexes involve input from A-beta, A-delta, and C-fibers to interneurons in the spinal cord.
- Although the addition of interneurons into the circuit slows the conducting of information through these reflex arcs, it greatly facilitates the construction of more complex circuits and, consequently, more complicated behavior patterns in response to sensory information.

AUTONOMIC REFLEX ARC

Input and output for the peripheral autonomic nervous system occur via spinal, cranial, and splanchnic (visceral) nerves.[18] Figure 6.3 is a diagram of a typical spinal nerve and its connections with a splanchnic nerve.

- The visceral afferent neuron has:
  - a peripheral process ending in a visceral organ or a blood vessel
  - a cell body located in the dorsal root ganglia morphologically indistinguishable from those of the somatic reflex arcs
  - a central process that terminates in the dorsal horn of spinal cord
- Typically, the peripheral fiber has a naked ending; however, encapsulated endings are present but in very low numbers.
- This central process terminates on interneurons that, in turn, innervate the effector neurons (motorneurons or premotoneurons) in the gray matter of the spinal cord or brainstem.
- The effector neurons, also termed preganglionic neurons, are found in the intermediate portion and lateral horn of the spinal cord gray matter, or in specific brainstem nuclei; their myelinated preganglionic axons terminate on ganglionic neurons located in the PNS.
- These peripheral neurons are found either in encapsulated ganglia in the fascia of the body wall or in (mural) ganglia embedded in the fascia surrounding a specific organ.
- Unmyelinated, postganglionic axons travel from peripheral ganglia to cellular targets located in visceral organs.
- The presence of two sequential neurons in the output pathway is a critical feature distinguishing the autonomic from somatic components of the PNS. For a well-organized review of fundamental autonomic nervous system organization, see Jänig.[11]
- The sensory neurons of these two systems, somatic and autonomic, are very similar in morphology and function.

DIVISIONS OF THE AUTONOMIC NERVOUS SYSTEM

The peripheral autonomic nervous system can be separated into three major divisions based on structure, chemistry, and function[4,5,11,18,19]:

- Sympathetic nervous system
- Parasympathetic nervous system
- Enteric nervous system
  - The enteric nervous system is a special division involved in regulating the gastrointestinal system and will be considered later.[20]

In general, each organ receives innervation from the sympathetic and parasympathetic divisions. Although often stated in texts that these two divisions are antagonistic, generally they work in coordination with each other to regulate organ function in a balanced and homeostatic manner.

- The major exception to this rule of dual or two-system innervation is found in the:
  - peripheral vasculature
  - hair follicles
  - sweat glands of the trunk and extremities
- These latter structures are innervated solely by fibers derived from the sympathetic system.
- However, in this situation, cholinergic fibers arising in the sympathetic ganglia are involved in at least hair follicle and sweat gland innervation, if not the peripheral vasculature[21]; these fibers have been termed the sympathetic cholinergic system.

The general distribution of the sympathetic nervous system is illustrated in Figure 6.4 and that of the parasympathetic nervous system in Figure 6.5.

An initial distinction between the sympathetic and parasympathetic systems is seen in the location of their preganglionic neurons in the CNS.

- During development of the nervous system, a longitudinal, discontinuous cell column arises close to the sulcus limitans of the neural tube.
- This column differentiates into the preganglionic neurons of the autonomic nervous system (Fig. 6.6).
- The rostral portion of the column forms several clusters of parasympathetic preganglionic neurons, which become associated with cranial nerves III, VII, IX, and X, and this portion of the parasympathetic system has been termed the cranial autonomic system.[4,18]
- The thoracic and upper lumbar portions of the column establish the lateral horn of the spinal cord and give rise to thoracolumbar sympathetic preganglionic neurons.
- Finally, in the sacral region of the spinal cord, again in the region of the sulcus limitans, a cluster of preganglionic neurons develops.
- Although these neurons share similarities with the sympathetic preganglionic neurons in terms of transcription factor expression,[22] their connectivity and functional properties most closely resemble parasympathetic neurons and thus have been classified as such.
- Their axons form the pelvis splanchnic nerves and contribute to the sacral autonomic system.[11,18]

Thus, although the preganglionic neurons all arise from a common embryologic column of cells in the neural tube, sympathetic and parasympathetic preganglionic neurons differ significantly in their location along the longitudinal axis of the CNS.

- Another morphologic distinction between sympathetic and parasympathetic systems is seen in the arrangement of their ganglia.
- Ganglionic neurons of the sympathetic nervous system exist outside of the CNS and generally are found clustered primarily in three locations (see Fig. 6.4):
  - The paravertebral ganglia or sympathetic trunk lying along the side of the spinal cord.
  - The prevertebral sympathetic ganglia or collateral ganglia scattered in several clusters associated with the large vessels of the abdominal cavity.
  - Isolated sympathetic ganglia, termed hypogastric ganglia are embedded in the adventitial tissue of specific visceral organs of the pelvis.
- Parasympathetic ganglia are more likely to be found intercalated into the walls of an organ hence their collective term, mural ganglia.

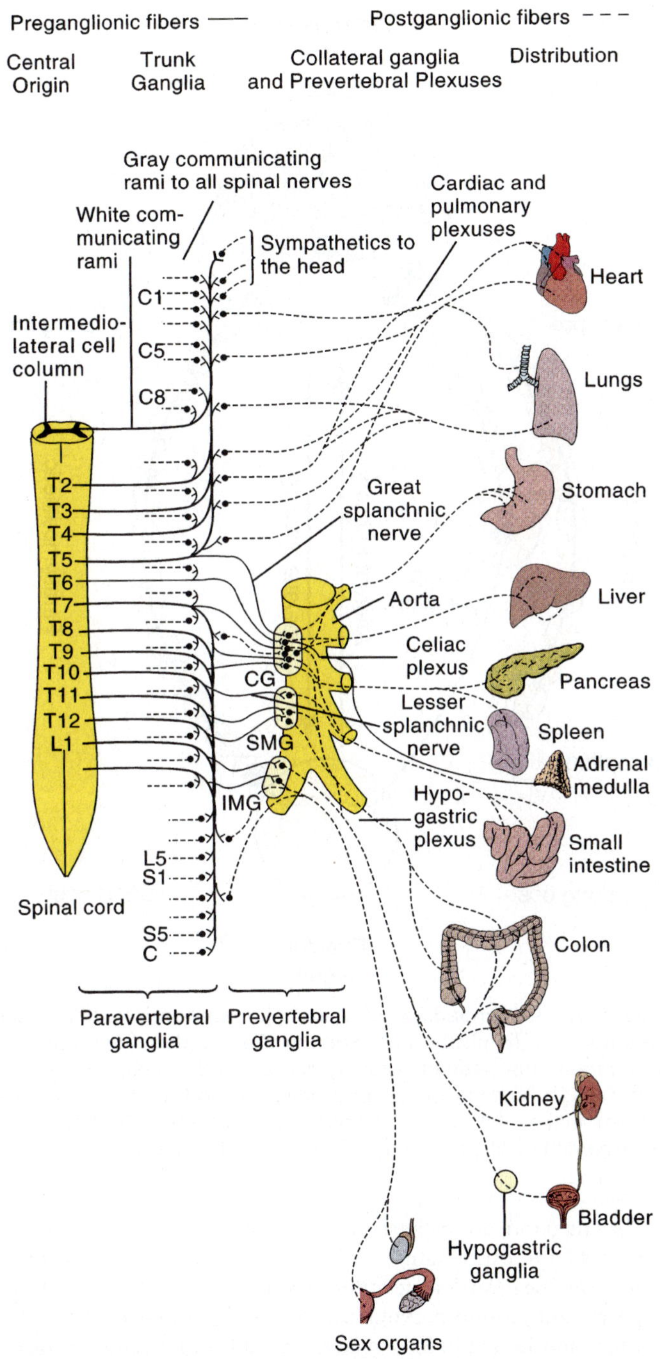

Figure 6.4. The peripheral distribution of the sympathetic nervous system. (CG, celiac ganglion; SMG, superior mesenteric ganglion; IMG, inferior mesenteric ganglion.) (Modified with permission from Chusid JG. *Correlative Neuroanatomy & Functional Neurology*. 19th ed. Lange Medical Publications; 1985:163. Figure 8-1. Copyright © 1985 Lange Medical Publications.)

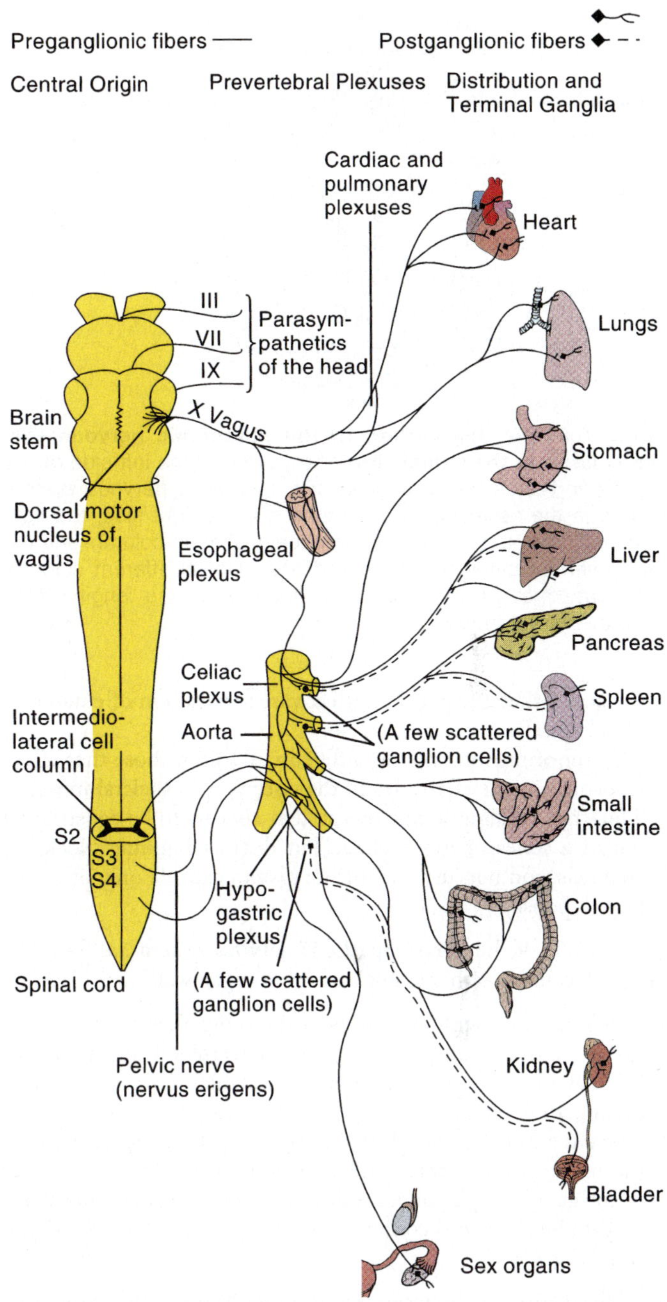

Figure 6.5. The peripheral distribution of the parasympathetic nervous system. (Modified with permission from Chusid JG. *Correlative Neuroanatomy & Functional Neurology*. 19th ed. Lange Medical Publications; 1985:164. Figure 8-2. Copyright © 1985 Lange Medical Publications.)

- The enteric ganglia of the gastrointestinal system are very complex compared to sympathetic and parasympathetic ganglia and have therefore been given a separate designation of their own.

These autonomic ganglia contain a variety of chemically differentiated neurons producing numerous neuroregulators.

- The ratio between pre- and postganglionic neurons has been reported to range from 1:2 to 1:196 for sympathetic ganglia and from 1:1 to 1:6,000 for parasympathetic ganglia.[23]
- This arrangement of a few central neurons, influencing effector organs through a large battery of chemically distinct, postganglionic neurons is divergent in nature.
- As such, it allows for a limited number of input channels on the preganglionic side to initiate numerous, complex motor and secretomotor responses in the peripheral tissue.
- Although divergent in nature, the output pathways are discrete entities and function as separate units.[11]

Pronounced differentiation in function exists within the sympathetic ganglia.

- A unique set of preganglionic neurons in the thoracolumbar spinal cord control a functional set of ganglionic neurons in

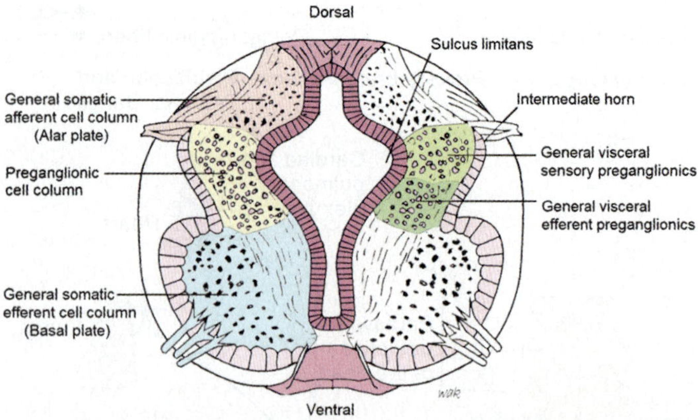

Figure 6.6. The distribution of the autonomic nervous system column in the spinal cord. The *yellow* on the left side of the diagram indicates the location of the autonomic nervous system column in the developing neural tube. On the right side, the light green indicates the location of the visceral afferent column, and the *dark green* indicates the location of the visceral efferent column. Appreciate that these columns of neurons course longitudinally along the neural tube.

the sympathetic trunk that affect vasoconstriction of cutaneous blood vessels.

- This set of neurons can be differentiated from those that affect vasoconstriction of arteries in the viscera or in skeletal muscle.
- Thus, the autonomic nervous system appears to be constructed out of a series of inter-related but distinct building blocks or channels, and not just one diffuse system capable only of a unitary response.[11]

Neurons of the parasympathetic nervous system are found in ganglia located in either cranial nerves or organ walls (see Fig. 6.5).

- While the preganglionic axons of the sympathetic system tend to be short, reaching only to the paravertebral and prevertebral ganglia, the postganglionic axons, which reach the visceral organs, are longer.
- The situation is reversed in the parasympathetic system where the preganglionic axons tend to be long (extending all the way to the ganglia in the organ wall), while the postganglionic axons tend to be short and confined to a distribution along the organ wall (Fig. 6.7).

This distinction between the major divisions of the autonomic nervous system is reflected in their chemistry.

- The sympathetic system arises from cholinergic preganglionic neurons located in the lateral horn of the thoracic and lumbar spinal cord; it is also called the thoracolumbar system.
  - In general, the postganglionic neurons of the sympathetic system are adrenergic and secrete norepinephrine.
  - However, there are important exceptions; for example, some cholinergic ganglionic neurons contribute to the innervation of the hair follicles and sweat glands as well as possibly innervating the vasculature in skeletal muscle.[21]

The parasympathetic system arises from cholinergic preganglionic neurons located in either cranial nerve nuclei of the brainstem or the lateral horn of the sacral spinal cord, and has therefore been called the craniosacral system.

- The postganglionic neurons of the parasympathetic system secrete acetylcholine and a wide variety of other neuron modulators such as the neuropeptides.

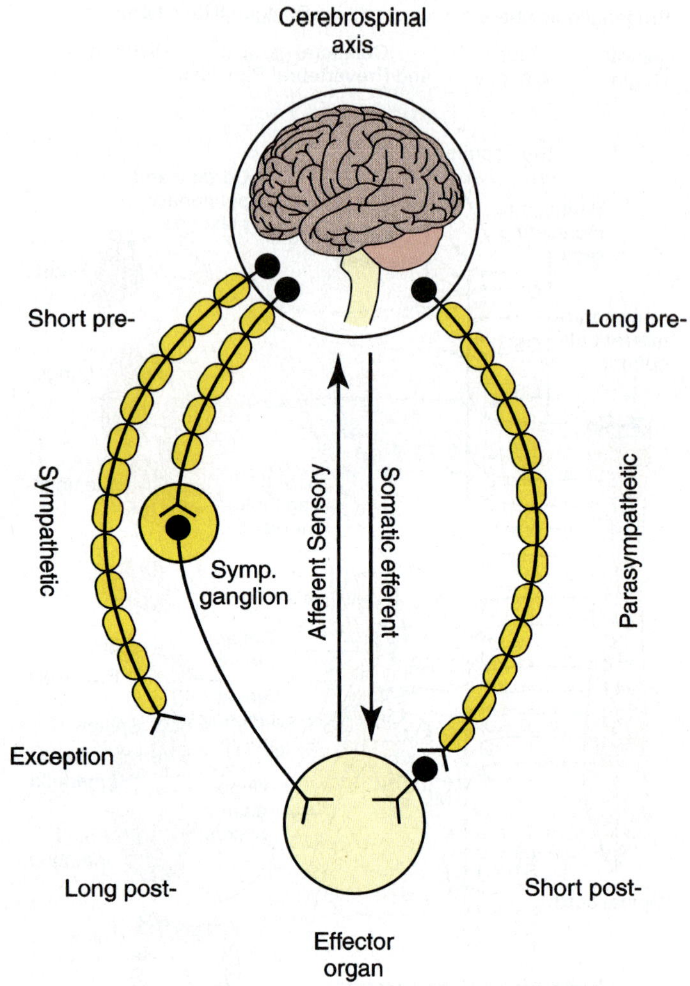

Figure 6.7. A comparison of the major anatomical differences between the distribution of axons in the peripheral sympathetic and parasympathetic nervous systems. (Modified with permission from Harati Y. Anatomy of the spinal and peripheral autonomic nervous system. In: Low PA, ed. *Clinical Autonomic Disorders: Evaluation and Management*. Little, Brown and Company; 1993:17–37.)

- Recent publications based on molecular studies of transcription factor expression[22] and on a review of catecholamine neuron location[24] have questioned the organization of the pelvic autonomic nervous system as described by Langley[4]; these studies are based on anatomical findings and not physiologic events, thus at this time it does not appear meritorious of reorganizing the description of the autonomic nervous system.

Many of the peripheral ganglia, especially in the gastrointestinal system, also contain sensory neurons that do not communicate with the CNS; instead, their axons terminate on ganglionic efferent cells or on interneurons located in the ganglia.[25]

- Local reflex arcs are established that do not communicate with the CNS.
- In the gastrointestinal system, the visceral autonomic ganglia act as small brains.[20]
- These ganglia can maintain some visceral organ functions even when all communications with the CNS are severed.
- In such cases, even though the gastrointestinal organ responds to changing internal stimuli, it is not able to respond to changes in external stimuli.

Sympathetic Nervous System

The sympathetic autonomic nervous system has two major components: peripheral vasculature and visceral.

1. The vascular component is associated with the spinal nerves and innervates:
   - □ Fascia
   - □ Smooth muscle of vasculature
   - □ Smooth muscle of hair follicles
   - □ Secretory cells in the sweat glands of the skin
2. The visceral component innervates:
   - □ Smooth muscle
   - □ Cardiac nodal tissue muscle
   - □ Glandular organs of the thoracic, abdominal, pelvic, and perineal viscera

The ganglionic neurons of the sympathetic nervous system are located in the following ganglia: paravertebral and prevertebral (see Fig. 6.4).

1. The paravertebral ganglia form bilateral long chains termed the sympathetic trunks located on either side of the vertebral column (Figs. 6.8 and 6.9).
   - □ Each sympathetic trunk extends from the cranial base down the anterior aspect of the upper cervical vertebrae, along the heads of the ribs in the thorax, on the sides of the lumbar vertebral bodies in the abdomen, and along the ventromedial aspect of the sacroiliac joint in the pelvis.
   - □ Inferiorly, the two trunks can terminate in some individuals by uniting to form the ganglion impar, a small neural structure on the ventral aspect of the coccygeal vertebrae; otherwise, they may end by fusing without a ganglion involved or by ending separately.
2. The three major prevertebral ganglia are found in clusters, embedded in the abdominal plexuses that surround the anterior branches of the aorta; additional small clusters of prevertebral ganglia are found scattered in the autonomic plexus of the pelvic basin.

The detailed organization of the sympathetic system is illustrated in Figure 6.4. The following features are critical:

1. Most preganglionic cell bodies are located in the lateral horn of spinal cord segments primarily between T1 and L2; however, they can extend as high as C7 and scattered neurons have been found in the lower lumbar spinal cord.
   - □ Their axons leave the spinal cord through ventral roots T1–L2 and course along the corresponding spinal nerves to reach white communicating rami (see Figs. 6.8 and 6.9).
   - □ The white rami carry these myelinated, preganglionic fibers from the spinal nerve directly into the paravertebral ganglia; they also carry sensory fibers that will enter the spinal nerve.
2. The paravertebral ganglia are present on both sides of the spinal cord in the following distribution[26]:
   - □ Often the upper thoracic and lower cervical ganglia are fused to form the stellate ganglion, in this case there will be:
     - Three cervical ganglia
     - Ten to twelve thoracic ganglia
     - Four lumbar ganglia
     - At least four or five sacral ganglia
   - □ Only the ganglia between T1 and L2-L3 receive white rami because preganglionic fibers arise only from these segments.
3. Neurons in paravertebral ganglia located either above T1 or below L2 receive their innervation from preganglionic fibers arising in spinal segments T1–L2.

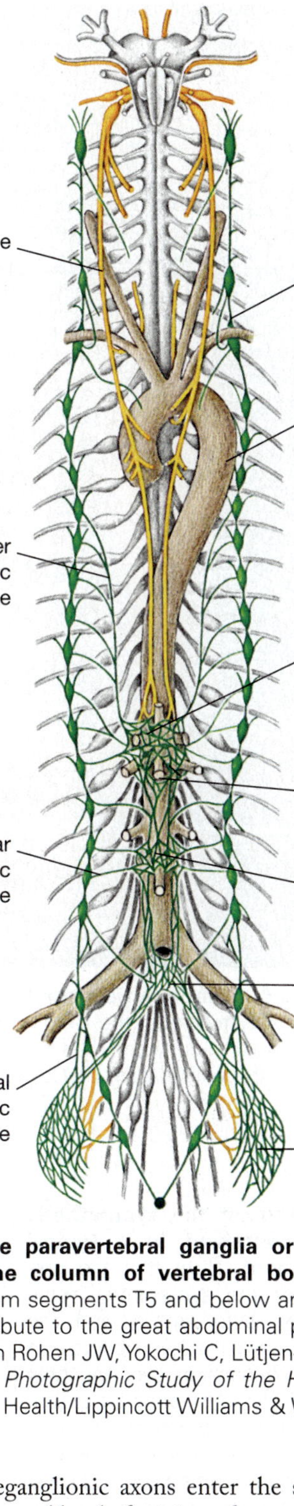

Figure 6.8. The paravertebral ganglia or sympathetic trunk lying along the column of vertebral bodies. The splanchnic nerves arise from segments T5 and below and course inferior and medial to contribute to the great abdominal plexus. (Adapted with permission from Rohen JW, Yokochi C, Lütjen-Drecoll E. *Color Atlas of Anatomy: A Photographic Study of the Human Body.* 7th ed. Wolters Kluwer Health/Lippincott Williams & Wilkins; 2011.)

   - □ These preganglionic axons enter the sympathetic trunk at their segmental level of origin and ascend or descend through the trunk to reach ganglia positioned above or below T1–L2.
4. Ganglionic neurons destined to innervate blood vessels, smooth muscles, and glands of the skin are found in all the paravertebral ganglia.
   - □ Their postganglionic axons gain access to spinal nerves by passing over gray rami (Fig. 6.10).
   - □ All paravertebral ganglia give rise to gray rami; each spinal nerve receives at least one gray ramus.
   - □ The postganglionic axons follow the spinal nerves distally before shifting to assume a position in the fascia along the wall of a blood vessel.[12]

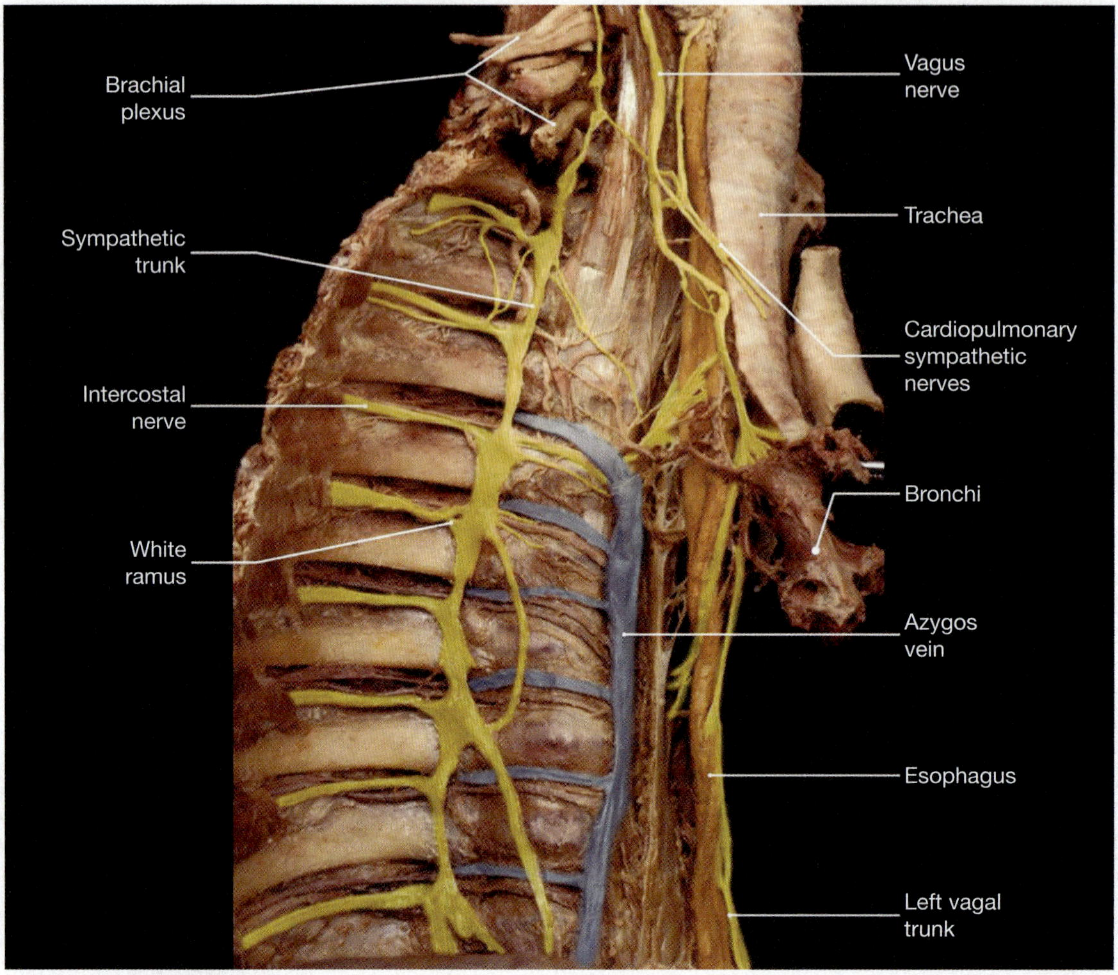

Figure 6.9. Sympathetic trunk in the upper thoracic region. This is a lateral view of the right side of the pleural cavity following the removal of the heart, lungs, and parietal pleural lining to expose the sympathetic trunk. The nervous system has been highlighted in *yellow*, and the venous system in *blue*. (Used with permission from the Willard/Carreiro Collection, University of New England.)

Figure 6.10. A diagram of the sympathetic neuronal circuitry contained in a typical thoracic spinal segment. Note that the preganglionic axons reach the sympathetic trunk by passing over the white ramus, and the postganglionic axons leave the ganglion to join the peripheral nerve by passing over the gray ramus. Once in a ganglion, a preganglionic axon can ascend or descend multiple levels to reach ganglionic neurons in the cervical or lower lumbar and sacral regions. (Modified with permission from Harati Y. Anatomy of the spinal and peripheral autonomic nervous system. In: Low PA, ed. *Clinical Autonomic Disorders: Evaluation and Management*. Little, Brown and Company; 1993:17–37.)

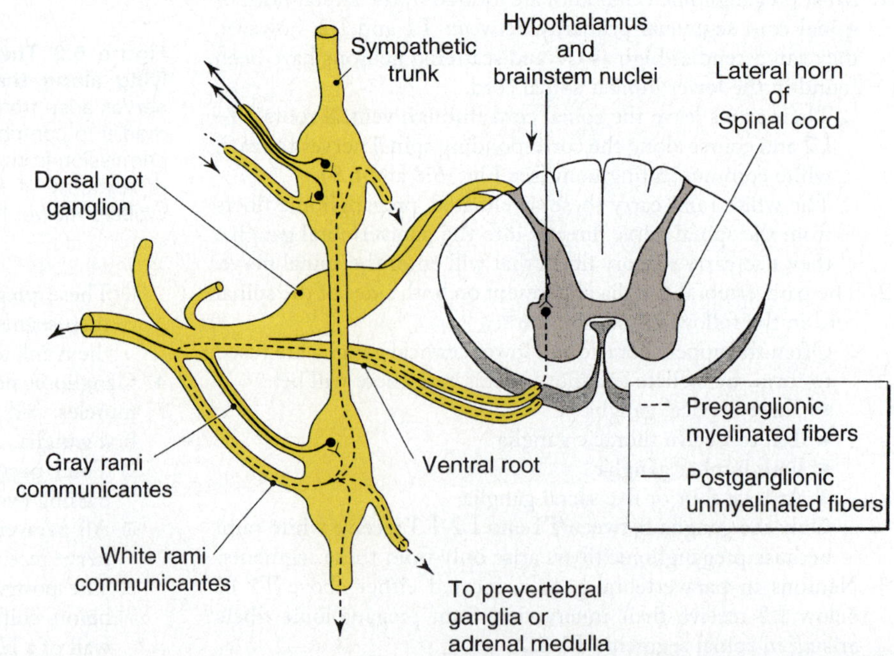

5. Ganglionic neurons with axons innervating thoracic, abdominal, and pelvic viscera are found in the three cervical ganglia, the upper five thoracic paravertebral ganglia, and the abdominal prevertebral ganglia.
   - The latter are the celiac and the superior and inferior mesenteric ganglia, as well as small scattered ganglia in the pelvic plexus.
   - Prevertebral ganglia receive their preganglionic axons through thoracic, lumbar, and sacral splanchnic (visceral) nerves.
   - The term splanchnic refers to the viscera; thus splanchnic nerves are simply visceral nerves.
   - Thoracic, lumbar, and sacral splanchnic nerves carry preganglionic sympathetic fibers, and pelvic splanchnic nerves carry preganglionic parasympathetic fibers.

The sympathetic ganglia receive information from the CNS through the axons of the preganglionic neurons.

- A preganglionic axon of the sympathetic system has a number of options after passing through a white ramus between T1 and L2 to enter a paravertebral ganglion[11]:
  1. It can innervate a ganglionic neuron in the paravertebral ganglion at its spinal cord level of entry.
  2. It can pass either up or down in the sympathetic trunk to innervate ganglionic neurons located at levels not serviced by white rami.
  3. It can proceed through the paravertebral ganglia without forming synaptic contacts, join a thoracic, lumbar, or sacral splanchnic nerve, and subsequently innervate neurons in one of the retroperitoneal prevertebral ganglia.

These options are diagrammed in Figure 6.10, which illustrates a typical thoracic spinal segment and its accompanying spinal nerve and associated paravertebral ganglia. The significance of these innervation patterns is further considered as the innervation of specific organs is examined.

Parasympathetic Nervous System

The parasympathetic autonomic nervous system, unlike its sympathetic counterpart, innervates only visceral organs in the:

- head and neck
- thorax
- abdomen
- pelvis

The parasympathetic nervous system lacks a division innervating the peripheral vasculature of the extremities, trunk, neck, and head. Based on the location of its preganglionic neurons, the parasympathetic nervous system is divided into two portions:

1. Cranial
2. Sacral (see Fig. 6.5)

CRANIAL

The cranial portion consists of several brainstem nuclei and their preganglionic nerves. Cranial nerves III, VII, and IX give rise to parasympathetic preganglionic fibers that innervate ganglia located in the:

- orbit (ciliary ganglion; CN III)
- sphenopalatine fossa (sphenopalatine ganglion; CN VII)
- inferior temporal fossa (otic ganglion; CN IX)
- floor of the mouth (submandibular and sublingual ganglia; CN VII)

Cranial nerve X, the vagus nerve, innervates ganglia in the organs of the cervical, thoracic, and superior portions of the abdominal viscera.

- The vagus nerve is a significant source of parasympathetic innervation to the thoracic and upper abdominal viscera (Fig. 6.11).
- It enters the thoracic cavity along the upper portion of the mediastinal wall and passes posterior to the root of the lung to gain a position on the walls of the esophagus.
- Vagal branches are given off to the cardiac and pulmonary plexuses and to the esophageal plexus.
- Through the upper portion of the vagus, the nucleus ambiguous of the medulla contributes innervation to the pharynx, larynx, and skeletal muscle portions of the upper esophagus.
- Preganglionic vagal fibers, arising from the dorsal motor nucleus of the medulla, terminate in ganglia on the walls of each organ beginning in the upper esophagus and extending to the splenic flexure of the colon.
- From these ganglia, postganglionic fibers arise and course in and around the smooth muscle layers and glands of the organ.
- In the organs of the gastrointestinal system, starting with the midportion of the esophagus, the ganglionic neurons are essentially included in the enteric nervous system rather than being termed parasympathetic in nature. The rationale behind this classification and nomenclature will be presented with the gastrointestinal system.

The left and right trunks of the vagus rotate around the esophagus (due to the fetal rotation of the gut), forming the anterior and posterior trunks of the vagus, respectively.[27]

- At the distal end of the esophagus, these two trunks slip through the esophageal hiatus of the diaphragm, riding in the fatty adventitial fascia of the esophageal walls (Fig. 6.12).
- Although the identity of the vagus nerve as a structure is lost as its axons join the celiac plexus, its preganglionic fibers continue in the celiac and superior mesenteric plexus (SMP), eventually reaching the full extent of these two corresponding neurovascular territories.
- Thus vagal preganglionic axons reach only as far inferiorly as the splenic flexure of the colon.

SACRAL

The lower portion of the gastrointestinal tract located distal to the splenic flexure, as well as the pelvic viscera, receives parasympathetic innervation from the pelvic splanchnic nerves. These latter nerves form the sacral component of the parasympathetic nervous system.[5,18]

- The preganglionic neurons are located in the intermediate region of spinal cord segments S2–S4, approximately where the lateral horn would be in the thoracolumbar portion of the spinal cord.
- Their axons exit the spinal cord by traveling in the ventral roots of the sacral nerves.
- As these roots pass through the endopelvic fascia, small pelvic splanchnic nerves branch off.
- These branches quickly join the inferior hypogastric plexus (pelvic plexus), which is also located in the endopelvic fascia.
  - Through this plexus, the preganglionic axons can reach the visceral organs of the pelvic basin such as the urinary bladder, the internal reproductive organs, as well as the rectum.
  - By ascending along the hypogastric plexus, these axons also enter the inferior mesenteric plexus of the abdomen.
- From the inferior mesenteric plexus, preganglionic axons follow the vascular branches of the inferior mesenteric artery to innervate the descending and sigmoid colon.

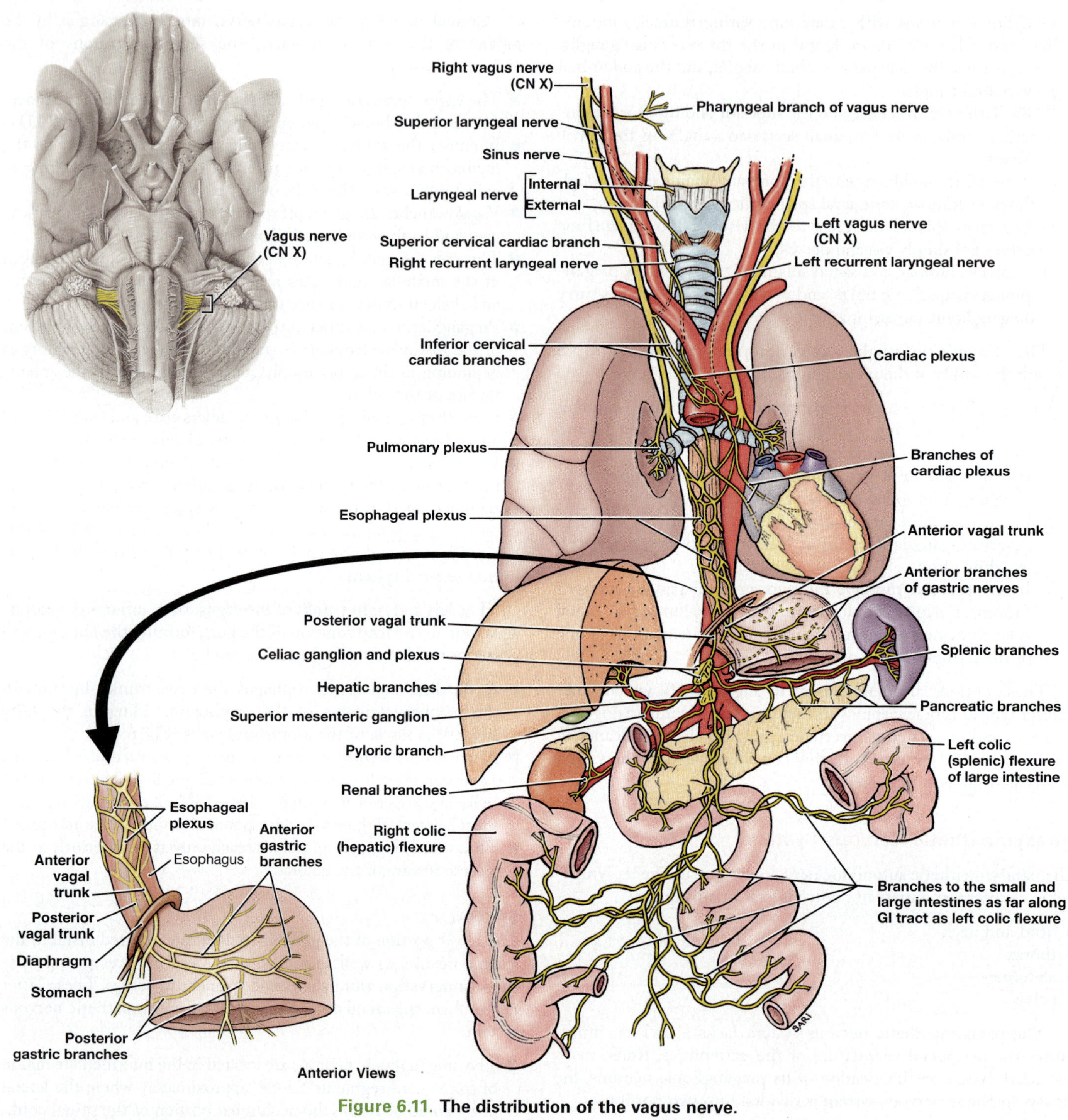

Figure 6.11. The distribution of the vagus nerve.

- The preganglionic axons of the vagus and of the pelvic splanchnic nerves terminate in ganglia located in the walls of the abdominopelvic viscera.
- Short, postganglionic axons invade the organ to terminate in layers of smooth muscle and in surrounding glands.
- The pattern of parasympathetic innervation of the visceral organs continues in an uninterrupted manner through the abdominopelvic cavity, even though the source of this innervation shifts from cranial origins to sacral origins at the splenic flexure of the large bowel.
- Recent studies have also found catecholamine-positive fibers in the hypogastric plexus and documented synaptic relationships with neurons in parasympathetic ganglia.[24]

Primary Visceral Afferent Fibers

The autonomic nervous system is not strictly an efferent system.[28] All nerves containing autonomic efferent axons also carry primary afferent fibers, typically termed visceral afferents fibers.

- Note that although many of the sensory fibers course along sympathetic nerves to reach the spinal cord, use of the term "sympathetic afferent fibers" is to be discouraged.
- The rationale behind this comes from the fact that these fibers, once in the spinal cord, affect much more than just the sympathetic preganglionic neurons.
- Therefore, the term sympathetic afferent fibers would be far too restrictive a description.[29]

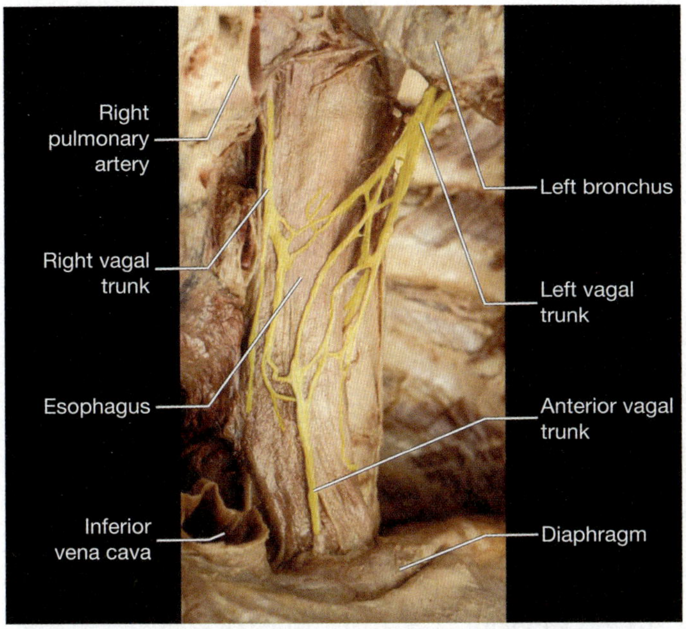

Figure 6.12. The esophageal plexus of the vagus nerve. (Used with permission from the Willard/Carreiro Collection, University of New England.)

The principal autonomic targets of these primary afferent fibers are the:

- dorsal horn of the spinal cord from approximately T1–L2 and S2–S4
- solitary nucleus of the vagal complex in the medulla

Although the majority of primary afferent fibers in autonomic nerves are of the small-caliber variety, a few larger, myelinated fibers are also present.

In general, the input over visceral afferent fibers to the medullary brainstem involves the non-noxious regulation of organ function. Conversely, many of the primary afferent fibers targeting the spinal cord have the characteristics of nociceptive fibers.

- They produce neuropeptides such as substance-P and calcitonin gene–related polypeptide and respond to nociceptive stimuli.
- In addition, some are capable of eliciting a neurogenic inflammatory response in the surrounding tissue.[30,31]
- Nociceptive input from these fibers to the spinal cord can facilitate spinal segments. This:
  - □ Initiates vasomotor changes and alters the output to somatic musculature (viscerosomatic reflexes)
  - □ Refers pain to the somatic structures[32,33]

In summary, through its sympathetic and parasympathetic divisions, the autonomic nervous system provides input and receives afferent fibers from the following:

- vasculature (and therefore fascias) throughout the body
- visceral organs of the head and neck
- visceral organs of the thoracoabdominopelvic cavity
- spleen
- thymus
- bone marrow
- lymph nodes

The remainder of the chapter focuses on the regional distribution of the autonomic nervous system.

REGIONAL DISTRIBUTION OF THE AUTONOMIC NERVOUS SYSTEM

Head and Neck

The glands and smooth muscle of the vasculature and the eye receive a parasympathetic innervation from four cranial nerves:

1. Cranial nerve III, the oculomotor nerve
2. Cranial nerve VII, the facial nerve
3. Cranial nerve IX, the glossopharyngeal nerve
4. Cranial nerve X, the vagus nerve

In addition, a sympathetic innervation derived from the superior cervical ganglion of the sympathetic trunk also reaches the head (Fig. 6.13).

These nerves play a role in numerous disorders of the head and neck. The precise details of the pathways taken by these nerves to reach their targets in the head are very complex and well described in standard texts of anatomy.[34,35] This chapter will focus on an overview of the cranial autonomic system.

PARASYMPATHETIC INNERVATION OF THE HEAD

Four circumscribed parasympathetic ganglia exist in the head along with numerous scattered clusters of ganglionic neurons embedded in cranial nerves (Fig. 6.14).

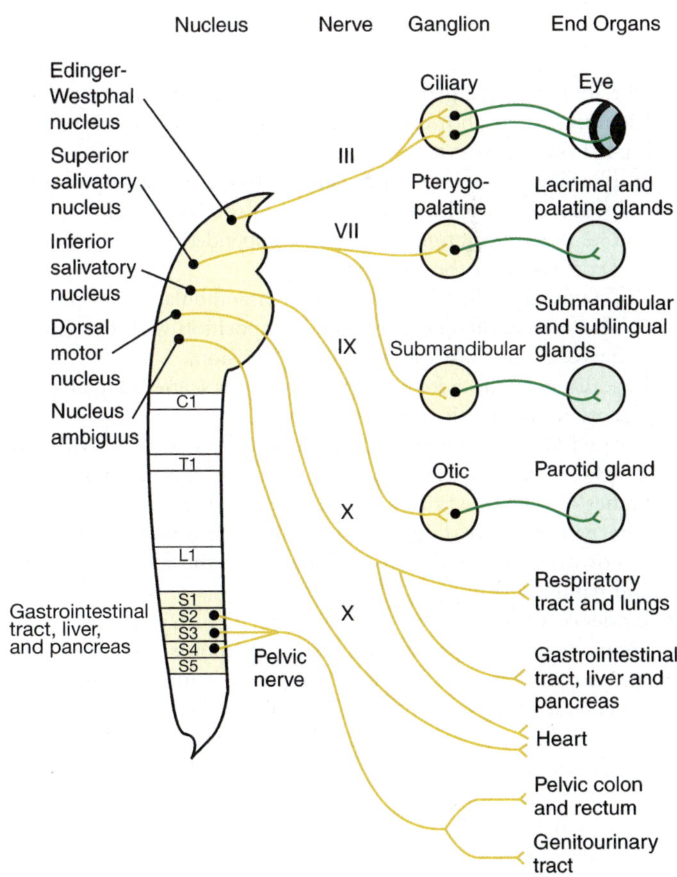

Figure 6.13. A summary of the distribution of parasympathetic nervous system, emphasizing the connections to the ganglia present in cranial nerves III, VII, IX, and X. (Modified with permission from Barron KD, Chokroverty S. Anatomy of the autonomic nervous system: brain and brainstem. In: Low PA, ed. *Clinical Autonomic Disorders: Evaluation and Management*. Little, Brown and Company; 1993:3–15.)

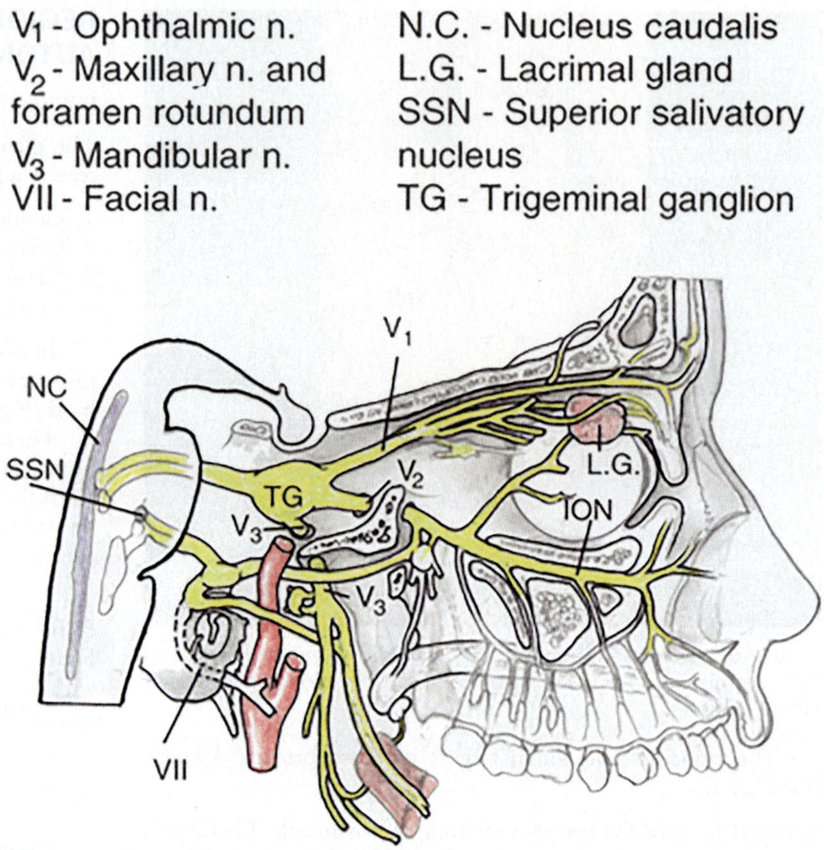

Figure 6.14. Trigeminal nerve. V1, ophthalmic nerve; V2, maxillary nerve and foramen rotundum; V3, mandibular nerve; VII, facial nerve; NC, nucleus caudalis of the spinal trigeminal complex; LG, lacrimal gland; SSN, superior salivatory nucleus; TG, trigeminal ganglion; ION, infraorbital nerve. (Reprinted with permission from Johnson JT, Rosen CA. *Bailey's Head and Neck Surgery: Otolaryngology.* 5th ed. Wolters Kluwer Health/Lippincott Williams & Wilkins; 2013. Figure 19-1.)

- The four main ganglia are all closely related to branches of the trigeminal nerve; however, none of them appear to receive direct input from this nerve.
  - The ciliary ganglion is associated with the nasociliary nerve, a branch of the ophthalmic division of the trigeminal.
  - The pterygopalatine ganglion is suspended from the maxillary division of the trigeminal.
  - The otic ganglion is related to the mandibular division.
  - The submandibular is in close juxtaposition with the lingual nerve, a branch of the mandibular division.
- In addition to these four ganglia, numerous scattered microganglia are found within the cranial nerves.
- Isolated ganglionic neurons, not specifically associated with any ganglion, are also seen scattered about in the mucous membranes of the oral cavity walls and the tongue.[29]
- The parasympathetic ganglia provide secretomotor and sudomotor drive to vasculature and glands of the face, oral cavity, and nasal cavity.
- Evidence to date, based on the neurochemistry of these ganglionic neurons, suggests that the secretomotor and sudomotor systems are separate and under a separate central control[29]; the concept that separate populations of ganglionic neurons perform differing functions based on the chemistry of their neurotransmitters is termed "neurochemical coding."[11]

Ciliary Ganglion

The ciliary ganglion is located deep in the orbit near the supraorbital fissure. It is in close association with the:

- nasociliary nerve
- optic nerve
- lateral rectus muscle (Fig. 6.15)

Typically, three roots composed of sensory, motor (parasympathetic), and sympathetic fibers, reach the ciliary ganglion.[18,36]

- The sensory roots or long ciliary nerves are multiple in number and are derived from the nasociliary nerve (ophthalmic division of the trigeminal).
  - These nerves carry trigeminal sensory fibers destined to innervate the cornea and sclera.
- The motor (parasympathetic) root, the shortest, is derived from the inferior division of the oculomotor nerve.
  - It carries preganglionic axons from the Edinger–Westphal nucleus, a cluster of neurons located in the rostral pole of the oculomotor nuclear complex in the midbrain.
- The sympathetic root is variable in location, but it constantly carries postganglionic sympathetic fibers from the carotid plexus.
  - These sympathetic fibers gain access to the ophthalmic, oculomotor, trochlear, and abducens nerves in the cavernous sinus.
  - While these fibers do reach the ciliary ganglion, they do not form synapses; instead, they pass through the ganglion to gain access to the short ciliary nerves, a series of nerves passing from the ganglion to the globe.
- Some accessory ganglionic neurons have been noted to be embedded in the long ciliary and nasociliary nerves, as well as in the choroid layer of the globe.[29]

The output from the ciliary ganglion consists of the short ciliary nerves.

- These nerves pass forward from the ganglion to penetrate the sclera and course in the perichoroid space.
  - Along with the postganglionic parasympathetic fibers from neurons from the ciliary ganglion, these nerves contain:
    - Trigeminal sensory fibers from the long ciliary nerves
    - Postganglionic sympathetic fibers from the carotid plexus
- The ciliary parasympathetic fibers provide excitatory drive to the pupillary constrictor muscles and the ciliary muscle located in the ciliary body. The latter muscle is involved in the accommodation reflex.

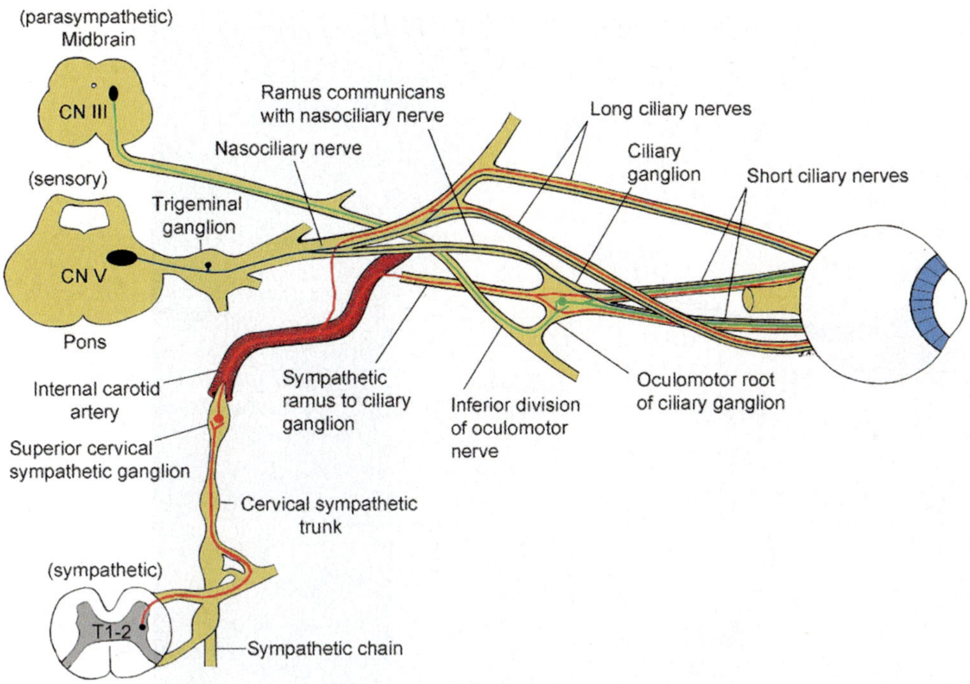

Figure 6.15. The autonomic innervation of the orbit and of the ciliary ganglion. Parasympathetic input is shown approaching the ciliary ganglion on the inferior division of the oculomotor nerve. Sympathetic input reaches the ciliary ganglion either directly from the internal carotid or indirectly via the long ciliary nerves. (Modified with permission from Hollinshead WH. *Anatomy for Surgeons: The Head and Neck.* Hoeber-Harper; 1954.)

- The central pathways controlling these two reflexes are most likely different since they can occur separately.[29]
- The tarsal muscles (smooth muscle) in the upper and lower eyelid are innervated by postganglioninc sympathetic axons; their course through the orbit is not fully known, however, it is thought that they gain access to the branches of the ophthalmic nerve in the cavernous sinus and follow that nerve into the eyelids.[37]

Sphenopalatine (Pterygopalatine) Ganglion

The sphenopalatine or pterygopalatine ganglion, the largest ganglion of the cranial autonomic system, lies in the pterygopalatine fossa in the posterolateral corner of the nasal cavity near the sphenopalatine foramen (Figs. 6.16 to 6.18).

- The ganglion is in close association with the maxillary division of the trigeminal nerve, but it is not innervated by any trigeminal fibers.

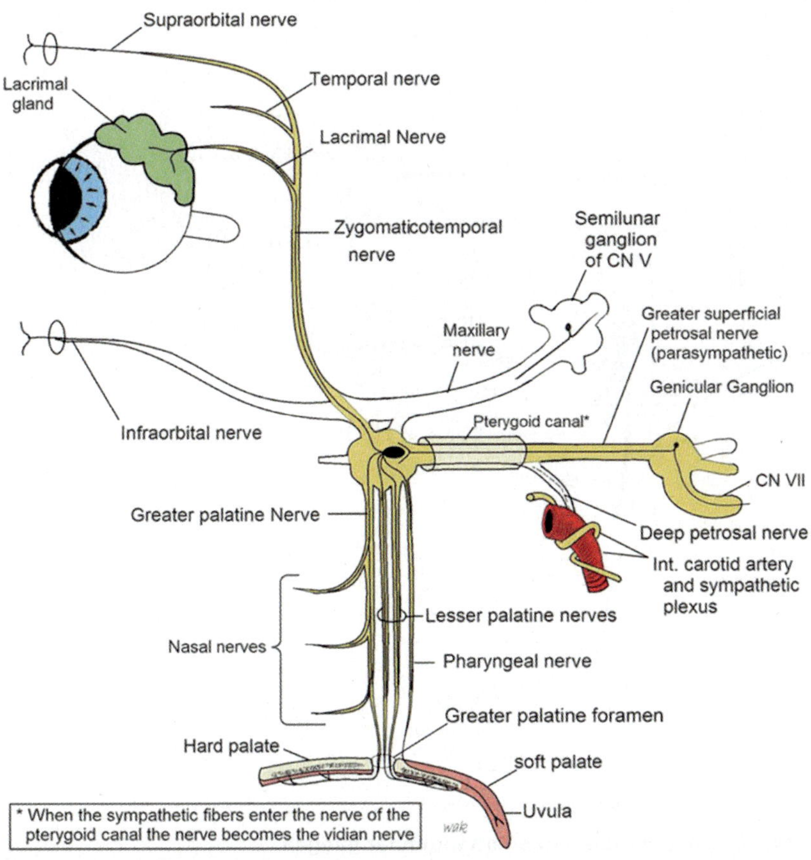

Figure 6.16. The innervation of the sphenopalatine ganglion. The superficial and deep petrosal nerves are seen uniting together to innervate the sphenopalatine ganglion. Branches from the ganglion join the greater and lesser palatine nerves to innervate the nasal mucosa and superior oral mucosa. These branches also join the zygomaticotemporal nerve to reach the lacrimal gland. (Modified with permission from Hollinshead WH. *Anatomy for Surgeons: The Head and Neck.* Hoeber-Harper; 1954.)

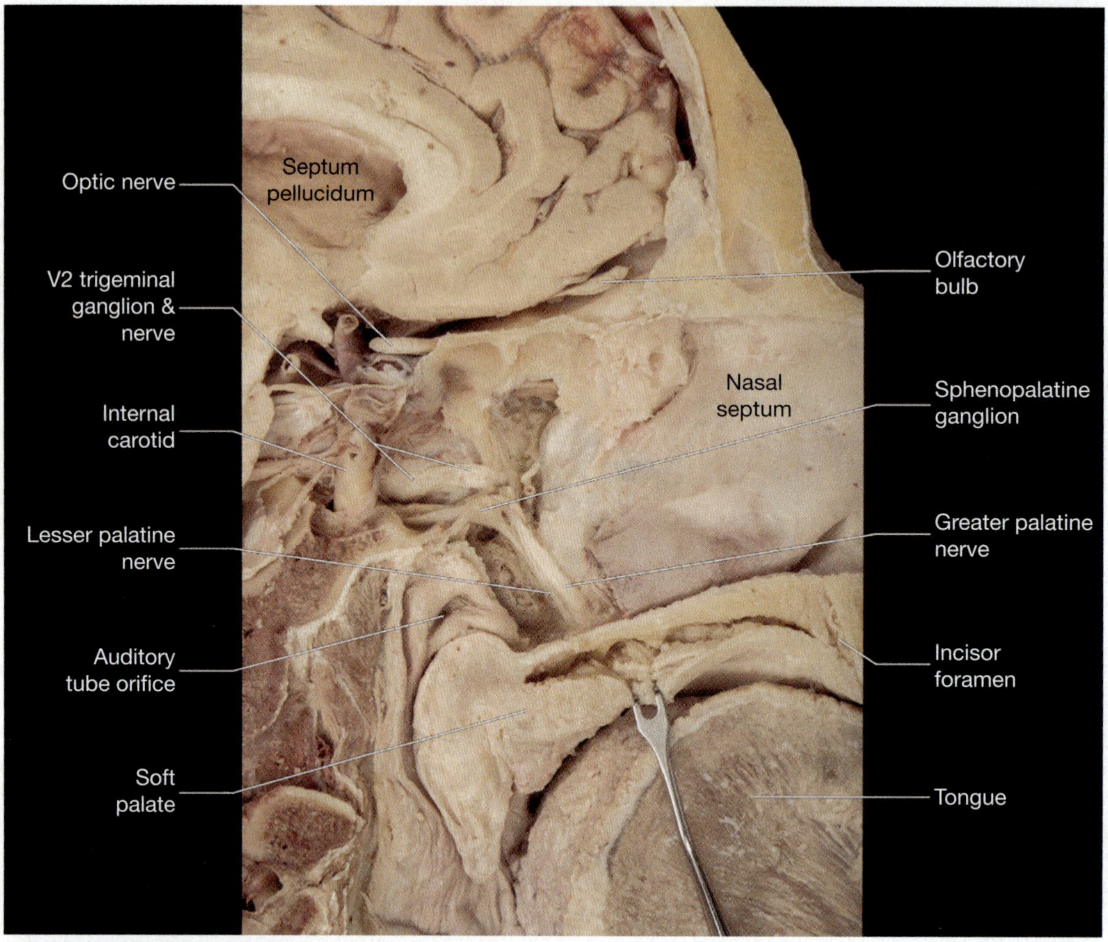

Figure 6.17. **This is a medial view of the pterygopalatine fossa following the removal of the nasal mucosa and underlying bone to expose the sphenopalatine ganglion and palatine nerves.** (Used with permission from the Willard/Carreiro Collection, University of New England.)

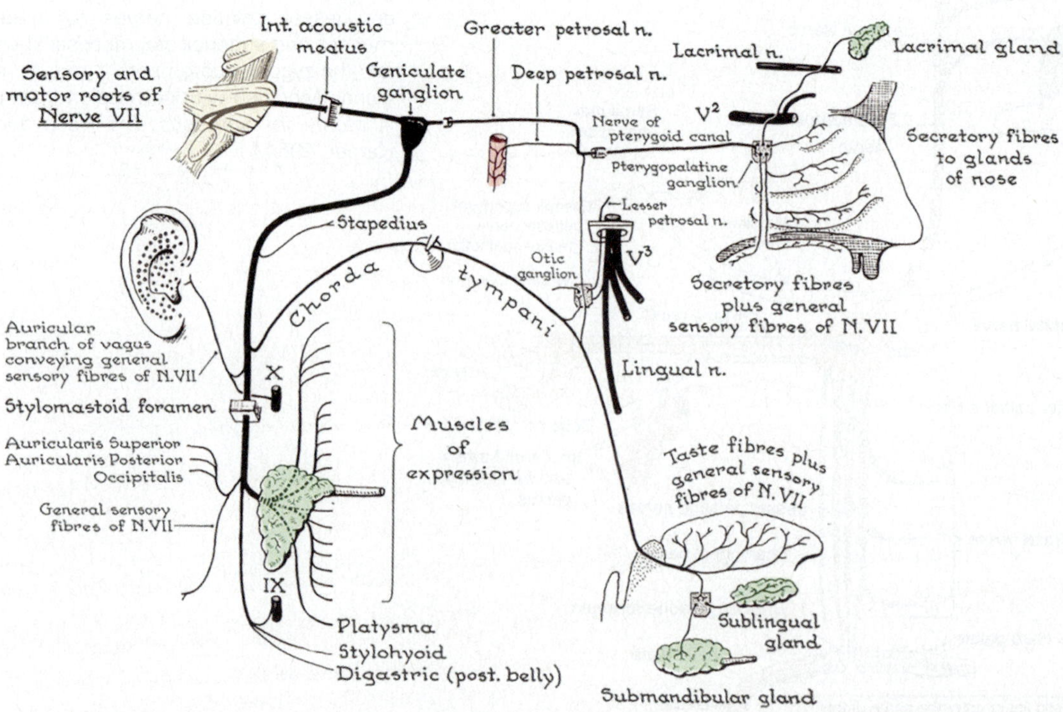

Figure 6.18. **The innervation of the sphenopalatine and submandibular ganglia.**

- The ganglion uses the maxillary nerve branches to access the face from the roof of the mouth to the roof of the orbit, targeting the:
  - □ lacrimal gland
  - □ glands in the nasal mucosa
  - □ glands on the under surface of the palate.

Input to the ganglion comes from two sources:

- The greater superficial petrosal nerve (motor root) carries preganglionic parasympathetic axons derived from the superior salivatory nucleus in the pons and traveling in the facial nerve.
- The deep petrosal nerve (sympathetic root) carries postganglionic sympathetic fibers derived from the carotid plexus.

These two nerves unite in the pterygoid (Vidian) canal before entering the ganglion as the nerve of the pterygoid canal or Vidian nerve.

- Fibers from the maxillary nerve (sensory root) pass along the lateral side of the ganglion to form the:
  - □ nasopalatine nerve
  - □ posterior superior nasal nerves
  - □ palatine nerves
  - □ pharyngeal nerve
- Each of these trigeminal branches represents an output channel for the postganglionic parasympathetic fibers of the sphenopalatine ganglion, as well as a conduit for the sympathetic fibers from the Vidian nerve.
- Thus, the sphenopalatine ganglion supplies vasodilator fibers to the blood vessels and sudomotor fibers to:
  - □ the glands of the nasal mucosa
  - □ the mucosa of the sphenoid and posterior ethmoid paranasal sinuses
  - □ the mucosa of the palate and pharynx
- In addition, parasympathetic fibers from the ganglion and sympathetic fibers from the Vidian nerve pass over the infraorbital nerve to reach the zygomatic and zygomaticotemporal nerve and then transfer to the lacrimal nerve (from the ophthalmic division) to ultimately innervate the lacrimal gland.
- Conversely, some of the parasympathetic postganglionic fibers remain on the infraorbital nerve through the infraorbital foramen to access the inferior orbit and the inferior palpebral tarsal muscles; these muscles respond to sympathetic drive by contracting, and their response to parasympathetic activity is unknown at this time.
- Sympathetic fibers to the inferior tarsal muscles most likely course from the cavernous sinus onto the maxillary division of the trigeminal nerve located in the trigeminal (Meckel's) cave from which they can reach the infraorbital nerve as well.

Submandibular Ganglion

The submandibular ganglion is located in the floor of the oral cavity in close association with the lingual nerve (see Fig. 6.18); however, this ganglion is not innervated by any trigeminal axons in this nerve.[18]

- Instead, the input to the submandibular ganglion is derived from the preganglionic axons that arise in the superior salivatory nucleus of the pons, exit the brainstem in the facial nerve, and then join the chorda tympani deep in the facial canal.
- These autonomic fibers become associated with the lingual nerve when the chorda tympani joins this nerve deep in the infratemporal fossa.
- Sympathetic fibers also join the ganglion from the plexus surrounding the facial artery or its branches.

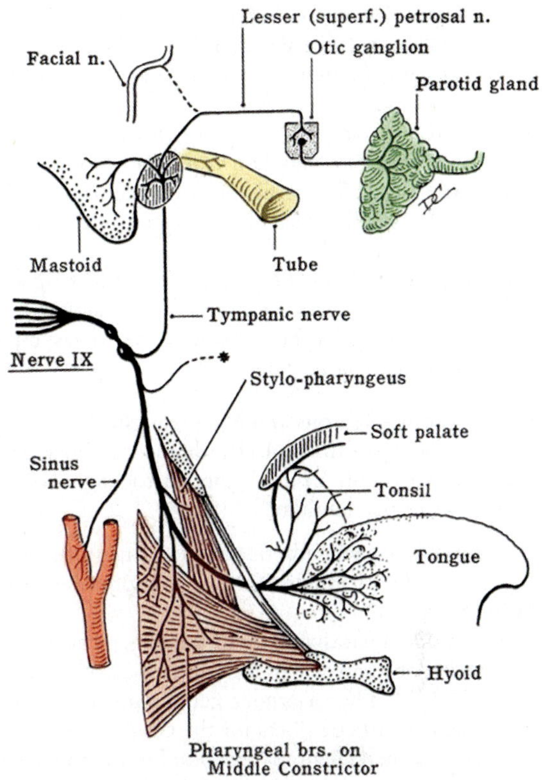

Figure 6.19. A summary diagram illustrating the parasympathetic innervation of the otic ganglion, by the tympanic branch of the glossopharyngeal nerve. (Modified with permission from Grant JCB. *An Atlas of Anatomy.* 6th ed. Williams & Wilkins; 1972.)

- The submandibular ganglion is the source of postganglionic secretomotor and sudomotor fibers for blood vessels and glands in the face, below the opening for the mouth.
- Major contributions from the ganglion target the submandibular and sublingual glands.

Otic Ganglion

The otic ganglion is located in the retromandibular space in close association with the medial aspect of the mandibular division of the trigeminal nerve (see Figs. 6.13 and 6.19); however, despite this close proximity, the ganglion receives no known trigeminal fibers.[18]

- This ganglion is much smaller than the submandibular ganglion, and it may be present as a series of ganglionic clusters rather than a single entity.
- The sudomotor postganglionic output is directed to the parotid gland over the auriculotemporal nerve, a branch of the mandibular division.
- Secretomotor fibers also pass onto the vasculature in the vicinity of the gland as well as to the those of the cerebral circulation.[29]

Control over the otic ganglion is typically said to arise from preganglionic neurons in the inferior salvatory nucleus of the medulla; their axons exit the brainstem with the glossopharyngeal nerve.

- A small tympanic branch from this nerve carries the fibers through the tympanic canaliculus into the temporal bone, where it joins the tympanic plexus in the walls of the middle ear cavity.
- From there, the lesser superficial petrosal nerve, carrying preganglionic parasympathetic fibers, passes rostrally through a bony hiatus, especially for that nerve, and enters into the middle cranial fossa.

- It courses laterally, parallel to the greater superficial petrosal nerve, to reach the mandibular division of the trigeminal and passes through the foramen ovale to gain access to the otic ganglion.
- However, there also appears to be a contribution of preganglionic fibers to the otic ganglion from the greater superficial petrosal nerve as well. These fibers reach the otic ganglion by passing through a small branch of the greater superficial petrosal nerve (Fig. 6.18).
- Sympathetic postganglionic fibers access the otic ganglion from the middle meningeal nerve,[5] although not thought to synapse in the ganglia, they join the postganglionic parasympathetic fibers leaving the ganglion.

Scattered Ganglionic Neurons and Microganglia

In addition to the four anatomically defined ganglia described above, scattered ganglionic neurons and microganglia are located in numerous sites in the cranium.[29]

- Small clusters of parasympathetic ganglionic neurons are located in the nerve to the pterygoid canal as it approaches the sphenopalatine fossa.
- Recently, additional parasympathetic ganglia, termed cavernous ganglia, located on the walls of the internal carotid artery, have been described.[38–40] The cavernous ganglia possibly represent a source of parasympathetic fibers for the cerebral vasculature.
- Other parasympathetic neurons are found in the tongue around the von Ebner glands and in the choroid of the eye.

The autonomic innervation of the cranial viscera, the function of these nerves, and the neurology of their dysfunction are amply described elsewhere.[2,35,41–43]

SYMPATHETIC INNERVATION OF THE HEAD

The sympathetic innervation of the head and neck derives from the superior cervical ganglia, the largest of the ganglia in the sympathetic trunk.[12,18]

- The ganglion is located on the anterior prevertebral surface lying on the longus colli muscle at approximately the level of the second to fourth cervical vertebral body.
- Its control arises from preganglionic axons derived from white rami in the uppermost thoracic region; these axons ascend in the trunk to reach the superior cervical ganglion.
- A few small twigs from the upper cervical nerves also join the ganglion.
- Following synaptic connections in the ganglion, postganglionic fibers leave the apical pole of the ganglion in the internal carotid nerve and form a plexus on that artery; other branches from the ganglion reach anteriorly to form a plexus on the external carotid.
- Fibers in the periarterial internal carotid plexus follow that artery to the cavernous sinus from which they can reach the cerebral vasculature and gain access to the divisions of the trigeminal nerve.
- Additional ganglia and sympathetic plexus can be found on the vertebral artery.
- Sympathetic fibers use the nasociliary nerve to enter the orbit and the globe.
- Sympathetic postganglionic fibers from the external carotid plexus may also gain access to the cranial vault by following the maxillary artery to the middle meningeal plexus and subsequently the meningeal arteries into the cranial fossa.

The targets of the postganglionic sympathetic fibers in the head are numerous (Box 6.1).

BOX 6.1 Innervation of the Cranial Vasculature

The superior cervical ganglion provides postganglionic sympathetic fibers for the internal and external carotid nerves.

The stellate and middle cervical ganglia provide postganglionic sympathetic axons for the vertebral nerves.

The cavernous ganglia on the walls of the internal carotid in the cavernous sinus may represent a source of parasympathetic fibers for the cerebral vasculature.

- The superior cervical ganglion provides sympathetic fibers to the upper portion of the common carotid and the stellate ganglion to the lower portion; the midportion of artery, is poorly innervated.[12]
- Some sympathetic fibers from the superior cervical plexus contribute to the innervation of the carotid body and sinus, along with its sensory innervation, which is derived from the glossopharyngeal and vagal fibers.[12]
- The extra- and intracranial vasculatures receive sympathetic fibers from the periarterial plexuses, surrounding the external and internal carotids, respectively.
- Sympathetic fibers on the internal carotid access the cranium through the cavernous sinus, those on the external carotid can gain access to the cranium by following the meningeal arteries.
- For the most part, the postganglionic sympathetic fibers on the internal carotid appear to be vasoconstrictive in nature.
- However, those on the external carotid are both vasomotor, sudomotor, and pilomotor controlling the vasculature, sweat glands, and hair follicles of the face (Box 6.2).
- Typically facial sympathetic fibers are vasoconstricting except under stress or elevated heat, when they can vasodilate.[44]
- In the eye and orbit, sympathetic fibers:
  - excite the pupillary dilator and tarsal muscles of the eyelid
  - inhibit the pupillary sphincter muscles
- Of the major glands in the head, all but the sublingual receive postganglionic sympathetic fibers.
- Similar sympathetic fibers reach the mucus glands in the nasal mucosa.
- Most of these fibers reach their targets by coursing along blood vessels derived from the carotid system.

The vertebral artery also carries a periarterial plexus of postganglionic sympathetic fibers.

- The origin of these fibers lies in the stellate and middle cervical ganglia of the neck.

BOX 6.2 Mapping the Vascular System onto the Spinal Cord

Preganglionic sympathetic input to the cranial vasculature and dura arises in the upper thoracic spinal segments.

Those controlling the vasculature of the brain and meninges are located in segments T1–T2, and those involved with the vasculature of the face and neck are located in T2–T4.[1]

- In addition, a vertebral ganglion is often located between the stellate and middle ganglia on the sympathetic trunk at a level just opposite the vertebral artery as it enters the intertransverse foramen (see figures 100 and 101 in Mitchell[12]).
- The vertebral ganglion contributes to the sixth and seventh cervical nerves as well as giving fibers to the vertebral nerves.
- At least two identifiable vertebral nerves, posterior and anterior, are seen coursing on the vertebral artery.
- Segmental level branches from the vertebral nerves contribute to the innervation of the cervical intervertebral disks and ligaments surrounding the vertebral bodies.[45–47]
- Distally, the sympathetic periarterial plexus extends into the cranium to innervate the vasculature of the vertebrobasilar circulation, possibly including the posterior cerebral artery.[12]

The cranial dura and its associated vasculature receive a rich innervation, consisting of both postganglionic sympathetic fibers and small-caliber, primary afferent fibers.[48–50]

- Ganglionic neurons are located in the superior cervical sympathetic ganglion and in small ganglia embedded in the fibers of the internal carotid nerve.[51]
- Their axons course along the carotid arteries; those going to the cerebral vessels and dura form the well-developed internal carotid nerve.
- Within the dura, the adrenergic fibers diverge away from the vasculature to form a dense plexus within the connective tissue substrate of the dura itself.[49]
- The extensive autonomic innervation may play a role in regulating the metabolic activity of the dural tissue.

Parasympathetic axons innervating the cerebral vasculature arise in these ganglia: sphenopalatine, otic, and internal carotid.[39,52–54]

- Axons from these ganglia contain acetylcholine and neuropeptides such as vasoactive intestinal polypeptide and neuropeptide-Y, among others.[40,55]
- The axons form a delicate plexus wrapped around cerebral arteries as they travel through the subarachnoid space.
- Primary afferent fibers containing neuropeptides such as substance-P and calcitonin gene–related polypeptide are also present in the plexus surrounding the cerebral vessels.
  - ☐ These fibers arise in the ophthalmic and maxillary divisions of the trigeminal ganglion[56] and constitute the "trigeminovascular system."[57]
- Similar primary afferent fibers of trigeminal origin and containing substance-P and calcitonin gene–related polypeptide have been described in the dura mater.[48,49]
  - ☐ Some of these fibers form free endings and are postulated to have trophic relationships with the connective tissue cells in the dura, such as the fibroblast and mast cells.
  - ☐ Release of these proinflammatory peptides has been indicated in the pathogenesis of inflammatory vascular headaches, such as migraine.[58]

Trunk and Limbs

PERIPHERAL VASCULATURE

The vascular tree of the somatic body is divided into four different types of vessels based on their distinctive architecture and function of their walls[59]:

1. Conduit vessels comprise the arterial system proximal to the arterioles.
2. Resistance vessels represent precapillary arterioles.
3. Exchange vessels are capillaries.
4. Capacitance vessels consisting of the venous system.

Most aspects of the vascular tree receive an innervation that controls the resistance of these vessels to blood flow.[21,59,60]

- Different types of axons in these vascular nerves can be identified by their neurochemistry.
- Sensory fibers, coursing in the vascular nerves, typically contain neuropeptides such as substance-P and calcitonin gene–related polypeptide.
- Efferent axons in the peripheral autonomic nerves can be identified as[59]:
  - ☐ adrenergic
  - ☐ cholinergic
  - ☐ histaminergic
  - ☐ purinergic

In general, the adrenergic sympathetic fibers function as constrictors, contracting smooth muscle in the tunica media and increasing the resistance in the peripheral vasculature.

- These norepinephrine-containing fibers arise from the paravertebral ganglia of the sympathetic nervous system, and they innervate all vasculature of the body.
- Cholinergic fibers are much fewer in number in most tissues and are typically vasodilating in nature.
- These nerves are of mixed origin and most often arise from the parasympathetic ganglia innervating the vasculature in the head and neck, and the visceral organs of the thorax, abdomen, and pelvis.
- Cholinergic vasodilator fibers, innervating blood vessels in the extremities, arise in the sympathetic trunk of some mammals; however, the importance of this system in humans is not well understood at this time.[11,61]
- Purinergic and histaminergic axons also mediate relaxation of vascular wall smooth muscle, but their origin and role in vasodilation are not clear.[59]

The sympathetic innervation of blood vessels in muscle and skin is accomplished by preganglionic neurons located in the lateral horn of spinal segments T2 through L2–L3.[12]

- Their axons leave the spinal cord in the ventral roots and pass through white rami to innervate neurons located in the paravertebral ganglia (see Figs. 6.10 and 6.20).
- Vasomotor neurons present in the paravertebral ganglia give rise to axons that leave the ganglia over the gray rami to rejoin the spinal nerves.
- In this way, the postganglionic axons reach the somatic peripheral tissue where they innervate blood vessels, sweat glands, and hair follicles.

A topographic map of the vasculature in the body is contained within paravertebral ganglia such that[51,59]:

- The vasomotor fibers to the head and neck come from spinal segments T1–T4.
- Their axons travel superiorly in the sympathetic trunk to reach the cervical ganglia.
- Postganglionic axons from the superior cervical ganglion follow the carotid vascular tree to reach the head and neck; those from the middle and stellate ganglia joint the vertebral artery and ascend to the head.
- Spinal segments T1–T2 provide innervation for the brain and meninges; T2–T4 provides innervation to the vasculature of the face and neck (Box 6.3).

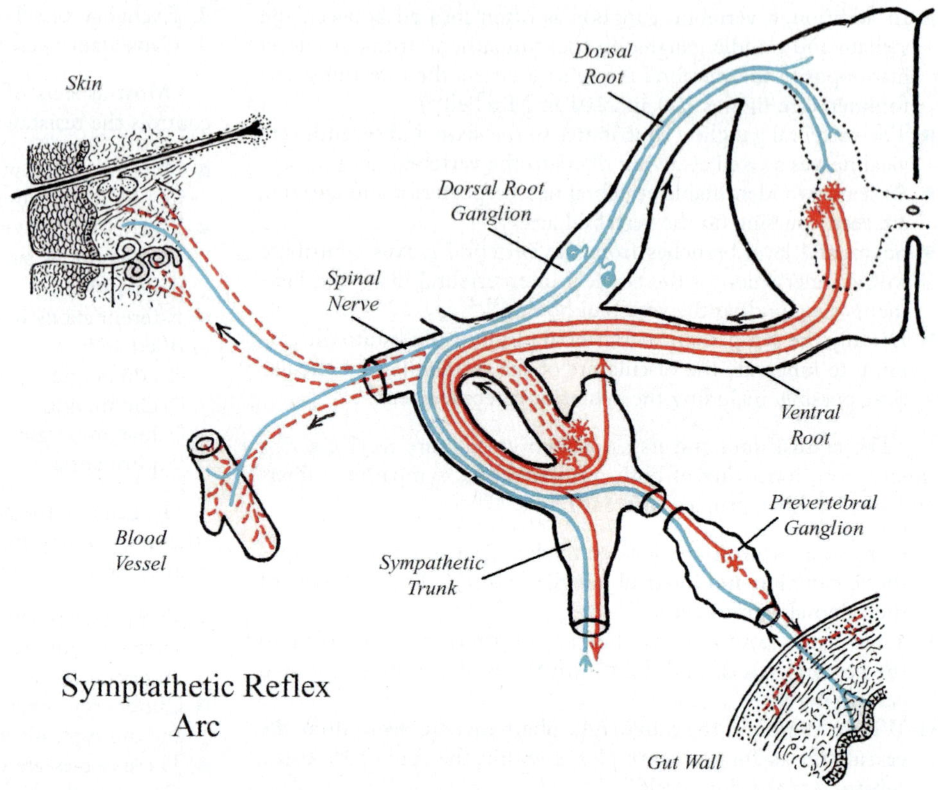

Figure 6.20. This is a schematic diagram illustrating the innervation of hair follicles, sweat glands, and blood vessels by axons from the sympathetic trunk (paravertebral ganglia). The *solid red* axons are preganglionic fibers; the *dashed red* fibers are postganglionic fibers; and the *blue* axons are primary afferent fibers. (Illustration modified with permission from Carpenter MB, Sutin J. Human Neuroanatomy. 8th ed. Williams and Wilkins; 1983.)

The vasomotor fibers to the upper extremity originate in spinal segments T5–T7.

- Their axons course superiorly in the sympathetic trunk to reach the upper thoracic and lower cervical ganglia, specifically the stellate ganglion.
- Postganglionic axons join the spinal nerves of the brachial plexus to reach the vasculature of the upper extremity.

Vasomotor fibers supplying the thorax and upper abdomen arise segmentally from the lateral horn, enter the spinal nerve through the ventral root, and use a white ramus to access a paravertebral ganglion (see Fig. 6.20).

- Postsynaptic fibers from the ganglion pass over the gray rami to regain access to the spinal nerve and distribute to peripheral arteries.[12]

The vasomotor fibers to the lower extremity arise from spinal segments T10 through L2–L3.

- Their axons descend in the sympathetic trunk to reach the lower lumbar and sacral ganglia.
- Postganglionic axons join the spinal nerves of the lumbosacral plexus to reach the vasculature of the lower extremity.

Sympathetic fibers course along the outer border of the tunica media of the artery and secrete their neuroregulators into the extracellular fluids surrounding the vascular smooth muscle.

BOX 6.3 Cutaneous Autonomic Innervation

Primary functions are:

- Thermoregulation
- Vasoregulation

- Most sympathetic fibers release norepinephrine from small swellings along the terminal distribution of the axon.
- This neuromodulator interacts with its specific receptors on the vascular smooth muscle cell membranes.

Both α- and β-adrenergic receptors are present on these plasma membranes.[62]

- Typically, activation of α-adrenoceptors leads to contraction of the smooth muscle cells and vasoconstriction, while activation of the β-adrenoceptors mediates relaxation of the muscle cell, resulting in vasodilatation.
- In general, the α-adrenoceptors predominate on the smooth muscle of resistance vessels; therefore, adrenergic stimulation yields vasoconstriction in skeletal muscle, even in actively contracting muscle.

Additional control of skeletal muscle resistance arteries is accomplished through numerous endothelium-derived substances such as the vasodilator nitric oxide or the vasoconstrictors prostacyclin, endothelin, and angiotensin.[63]

- The tone in the vessel wall is the product of a complex interaction of these vasoactive substances.[64]
- Neurally mediated, active vasodilation of cutaneous capillary bed is well established in the literature.[61]
- Sympathetic cholinergic fibers do not appear to innervate the cutaneous vascular tree; instead, a nonadrenergic, noncholinergic vasodilatory mechanism exists for these vessels.[11,65]
- In 1903, Langley discussed the problem of the origin of the vasodilators in the peripheral tissue and made the remarkable suggestion that it might arise from the afferent fibers with naked nerve endings.[4]
- Recent work has strongly pointed to the retrograde activity, termed dorsal root reflexes, and the resulting release of vasodilating peptides from small-caliber, primary afferent fibers as the sources of the vasodilation counterbalancing the constricting forces of the sympathetic fibers.[29,66]

- Neurally mediated, active vasodilation of skeletal muscle vascular beds appears to be doubtful and has been questioned.[61]

Along with the efferent innervation of the vascular tree, afferent or sensory fibers also course in the walls of the blood vessels.

- Little is known of the sensory feedback to the spinal cord provided by these fibers.
- The nomenclature of these afferent fibers is confusing because it is not clear whether they are somatic or visceral afferent fibers.
- Jinkins et al.[67] have termed the vascular afferent fibers found in somatic tissue "somatosympathetic fibers" because they course through somatic tissue but are related to the autonomic nervous system.
- The use of the term "sympathetic afferent fibers" is to be discouraged since it implies that the fibers act only on reflexes concerning control of the sympathetic outflow, and this is certainly not the case. These afferent fibers influence both sympathetic and somatic reflexes at the spinal cord, brainstem, and forebrain levels, as pointed out by Gibbins.[29]
- However, because these afferent fibers are generally small caliber and contain an array of neuropeptides such as substance-P, much of the information they carry is most likely also related to nociceptive stimuli.
- The normal, baseline release of neuropeptides such as substance-P from these fibers may play an important role in maintaining vascular tone.[68]
- Thus, as described in the preceding paragraph, the small-caliber, primary afferent fibers appear to have additional homeostatic functions in the peripheral tissue beyond that of nociception.

When irritated, some of these small-caliber, sensory axons can secrete quantities of substance-P (a proinflammatory, vasodilatory neuropeptide) into the surrounding tissue.

- This release of an inflammatory agent from a peripheral nerve terminal is involved in initiating the processes of neurogenic inflammation and edema.[69]
- Neurogenic inflammation is a critical component in inflammatory joint disease, which suggests an important role for the small-caliber, primary afferent fibers in these rheumatologic diseases.[70]

An interaction between sensory axons and sympathetic neurons appears to occur in the peripheral tissues.

- Sympathetic adrenergic terminals often end in close association with the peripheral processes of sensory neurons.
- Secretion of norepinephrine can increase the levels of prostaglandins E2 and I2 in the tissue.[71]
- Prostaglandins are irritating to many small-caliber, primary afferent fibers.
- Sufficient sympathetic discharge therefore can result in a nociceptive input to the spinal cord.
- In addition, evidence strongly suggests that small-caliber, primary afferent fibers can become sensitized to sympathetic nervous system activity.[71]
- This interaction between sympathetic efferent axons and primary afferent neurons is a possible mechanism for sympathetically dependent hyperalgesia, such as that present in complex regional pain syndromes.[72]

SWEAT GLANDS AND CONNECTIVE TISSUE

Along with innervating the vasculature, the peripheral autonomic fibers also provide innervation to sweat glands and fascia (see Fig. 6.20).

- Sweat glands receive an exclusively cholinergic sudomotor innervation from the sympathetic trunk ganglia; these fibers are termed the "sympathetic cholinergic system."[60]
- The cholinergic fibers stimulate secretory activity in the gland.

Small-caliber, neuropeptide-containing, primary afferent fibers innervate all forms of connective tissue.

- These fibers often course in close association with adrenergic sympathetic axons and blood vessels.
- A close relationship between these small-caliber fibers and the connective tissue components of the fascia is seen in such tissue as the:
  - ☐ cranial dura[49,50]
  - ☐ gastrointestinal tract[73]
  - ☐ synovium of diarthrodial joints[74]
- In several locations, such as joints, these fibers have been demonstrated to play a role in modulating the cellular components (mast cells) of the connective tissue and contribute to the maintenance of tissue integrity.[74,75]

Finally, the interaction of these two fiber types, sympathetic efferents and small-caliber afferents, appears to play an important role in the maintenance of normal vascular tone in connective tissue.[68]

THORAX AUTONOMIC NERVOUS SYSTEM

A large autonomic plexus of fibers extends from the superior mediastinum inferiorly through the posterior mediastinum (Fig. 6.21).

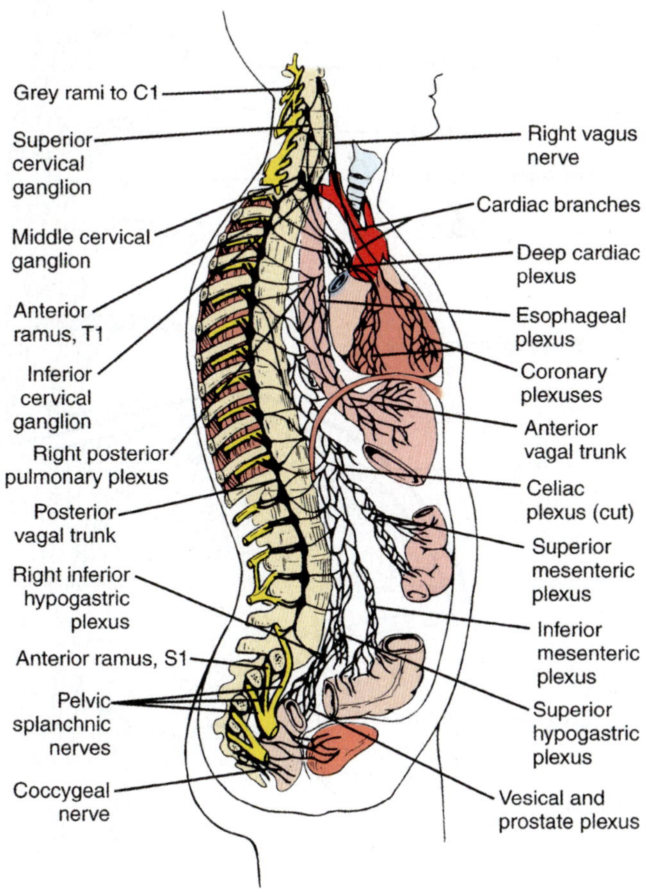

Figure 6.21. Great plexus of autonomic fibers in the thorax, abdomen, and pelvis. (Modified with permission of Elsevier Science & Technology Journals from Bannister LH, Williams PL. *Gray's Anatomy: The Anatomical Basis of Medicine and Surgery*. 38th ed. Churchill Livingstone; 1995:1301; permission conveyed through Copyright Clearance Center, Inc.)

In total, this complex arrangement of fibers is best termed the thoracic plexus, although it has several regionally named components. Distally, the thoracic plexus is continuous with the great abdominopelvic plexus that is located under the abdominal diaphragm.

The thoracic plexus is derived from the (Fig. 6.22):

- Branches of the vagus nerve in the cervical and thoracic region (parasympathetic source)
- Branches from the cervical and upper thoracic sympathetic trunk (sympathetic source)
- All branches of this plexus will contain afferent fibers traveling to the spinal cord with the sympathetic nerves or the brainstem with the vagal fibers[18]

The two vagal nerves enter the thorax asymmetrically.[76]

- The left vagus enters the thorax by passing through the thoracic inlet coursing between the left common carotid and the left

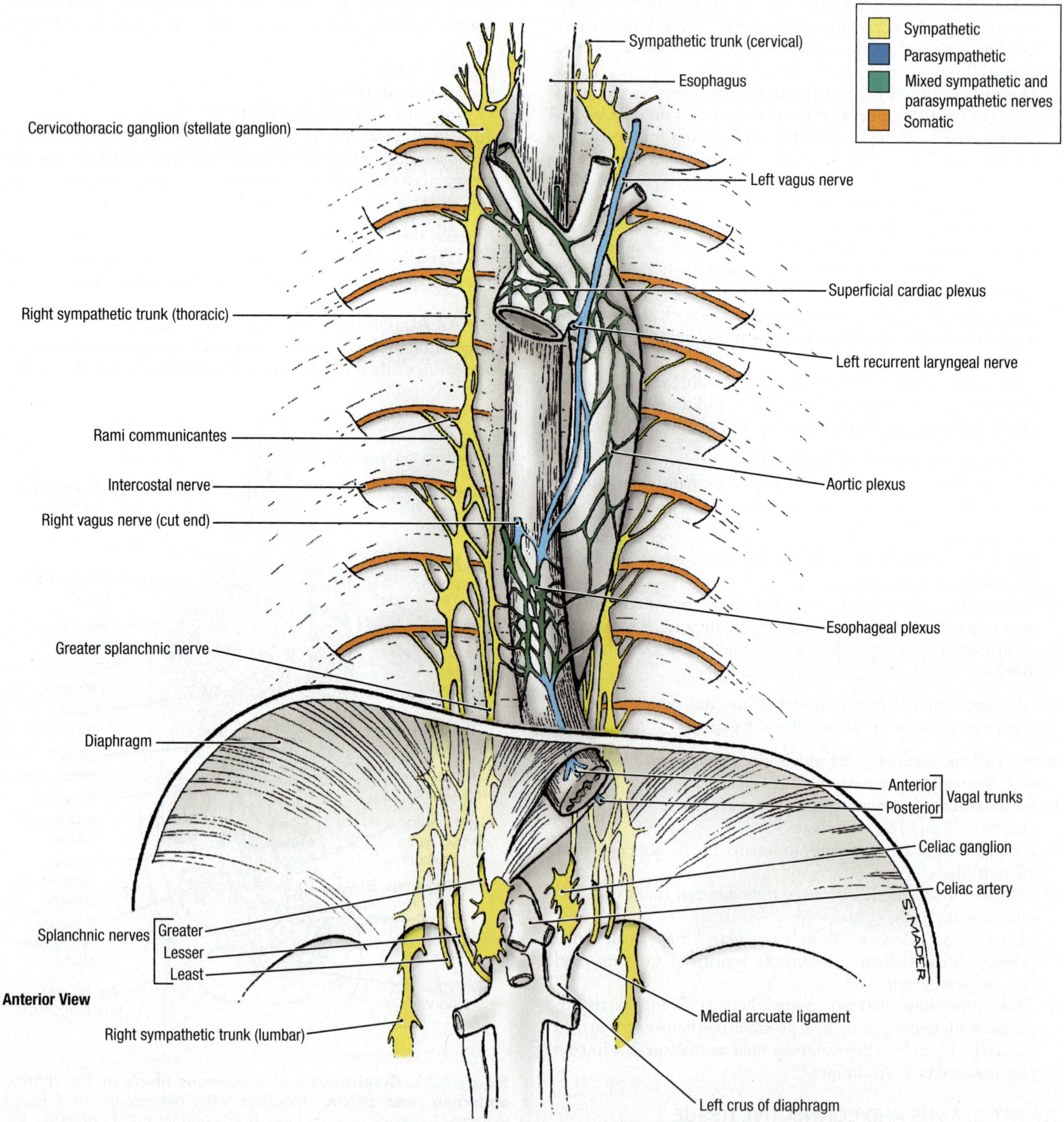

Figure 6.22. An anterior view of the thoracic plexus. The sympathetic trunk and splanchnic nerves are seen in *orange*; the vagus is *green*; and the mixed fibers (sympathetic and parasympathetic) are *blue*. (Reprinted with permission from Agur AMR, Dalley AF II. *Grant's Atlas of Anatomy*. 12th ed. Wolters Kluwer Health/Lippincott Williams & Wilkins; 2009.)

subclavian artery. It passes anterolaterally in front of the arch of the aorta giving off the left recurrent laryngeal branch before moving posterior to the root of the lung to take up a position on the left side of the esophagus.
- The right vagus enters the thorax by passing through the thoracic inlet coursing with the right common carotid, it passes anterior to the right subclavian artery giving off the right recurrent laryngeal before passing posterior to the root of the lung to reach the right aspect of the esophagus.

The sympathetic trunk follows the longus colli through the thoracic inlet.[18]

- In the upper and middle thorax, it courses along the heads of the ribs.
- In the lower thorax it passes more medially under the lumbar leaflet of the diaphragm to follow the medial contour of the psoas major attachment to the lumbar vertebral bodies.
- In some individuals, the trunk is overlapped by the fibers of the psoas.
- Throughout the thorax the ganglia of the trunk are segmentally arranged, however, the first ganglion is often fused with the lower cervical to form the stellate ganglion and the last can fuse with the first lumbar ganglion.

The thoracic plexus is located near the midline in the superior and posterior mediastinum; it is divided approximately into two parts: superior and inferior.

- Superiorly, this complex arrangement of fibers contains the interwoven cardiac and pulmonary plexuses that are distributed around the great vessels of the heart and the large airways.
- Inferiorly, it contains the esophageal plexus wrapped around the esophagus as it courses through the posterior mediastinum.

Figure 6.23 is a schematic diagram illustrating the thoracic plexus.

Branches from the autonomic plexus in the thorax supply the following with afferent and efferent nerves:

- Heart
- Trachea
- Bronchi
- Lungs
- Esophagus
- Thoracic duct

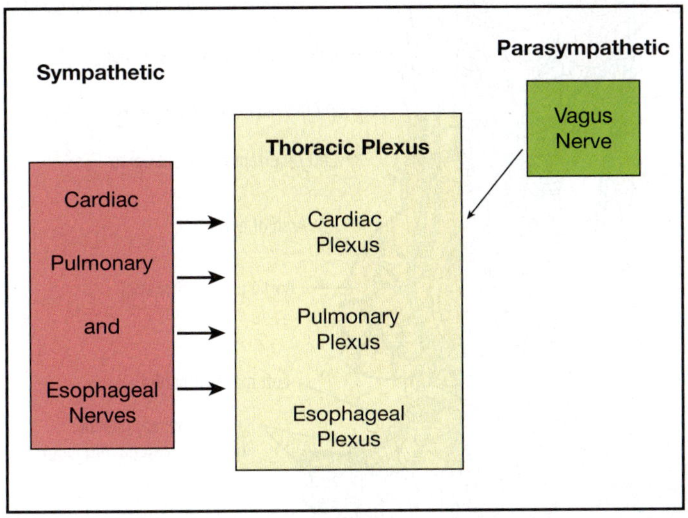

Figure 6.23. A schematic diagram of the thoracic plexus. All input to this plexus is in the form of postganglionic axons.

Sympathetic innervation of the thoracic viscera arises from preganglionic neurons located in the lateral horn of spinal cord segments T1 through T5 or T6.

- Axons from preganglionic neurons located in these segments synapse with ganglionic neurons in the superior, middle, and inferior cervical ganglia, as well as in the sympathetic trunk ganglia of the upper thorax.
- Sympathetic postganglionic axons from these paravertebral ganglia join the thoracic plexus via a series of small, delicate cardiac, pulmonary, and esophageal nerves.
- Within the thoracic plexus, sympathetic cardiac and pulmonary nerves descend through the superior mediastinum, joining with similarly named parasympathetic branches from the vagus and recurrent laryngeal nerves. They form the complex cardiopulmonary plexus of fibers surrounding the great vessels of the heart (Fig. 6.24), along with the vasculature and airway structures of the lungs (Fig. 6.25).
- The individual superior, middle, and inferior cardiac nerves of the sympathetic trunk and vagus are extremely inconsistent in actual form.[19]
- The esophageal sympathetic nerves arise from the thoracic paravertebral ganglia and course diagonally downward across the thoracic vertebral bodies to reach the adventitial fascia, surrounding the esophagus in the posterior mediastinum. Here, they join with the main trunks of the vagus nerve (parasympathetic) to form the esophageal plexus.

The mixing of parasympathetic and sympathetic axons begins in the most superior aspect of the thoracic autonomic plexus as it extends upward into the cervical region.

- Scattered communicating branches unite the vagus and recurrent laryngeal nerves with the sympathetic trunk.
- Therefore, even at the most superior aspect of the plexus, there are no pure sympathetic or parasympathetic nerves.
- Also, all fibers in the plexus contain a mixture of afferent and efferent axons, so the plexus cannot be considered a purely efferent structure either.[18]

CARDIOVASCULAR PLEXUS

The cardiac plexus represents a region of the thoracic plexus closely related to the innervation of the heart.

- The cardiac plexus consists of a mixture of sympathetic and parasympathetic fibers (as well as afferent fibers) woven around the great vessels of the heart (see Fig. 6.24).
- Sympathetic input to the cardiac plexus arises from preganglionic neurons located in the nucleus intermediolateralis of the lateral horn of the spinal cord, extending from segments T1 to T4–T5. This column of spinal cord neurons contains a topographic map of the heart.
- The ventricular innervation is represented in the higher thoracic segments, while the atrial representation is found in the lower segments.[12] This inverted cardiac map results from the embryologic origin of the heart; the ventricular system forms superior to the atrial system.[27]

The preganglionic axons of the spinal cord neurons enter the sympathetic trunk by passing over white rami in the upper thoracic segments.

- Once in the trunk, most of these fibers ascend to reach their ganglionic neurons, located primarily in the upper two to three cervical ganglia.

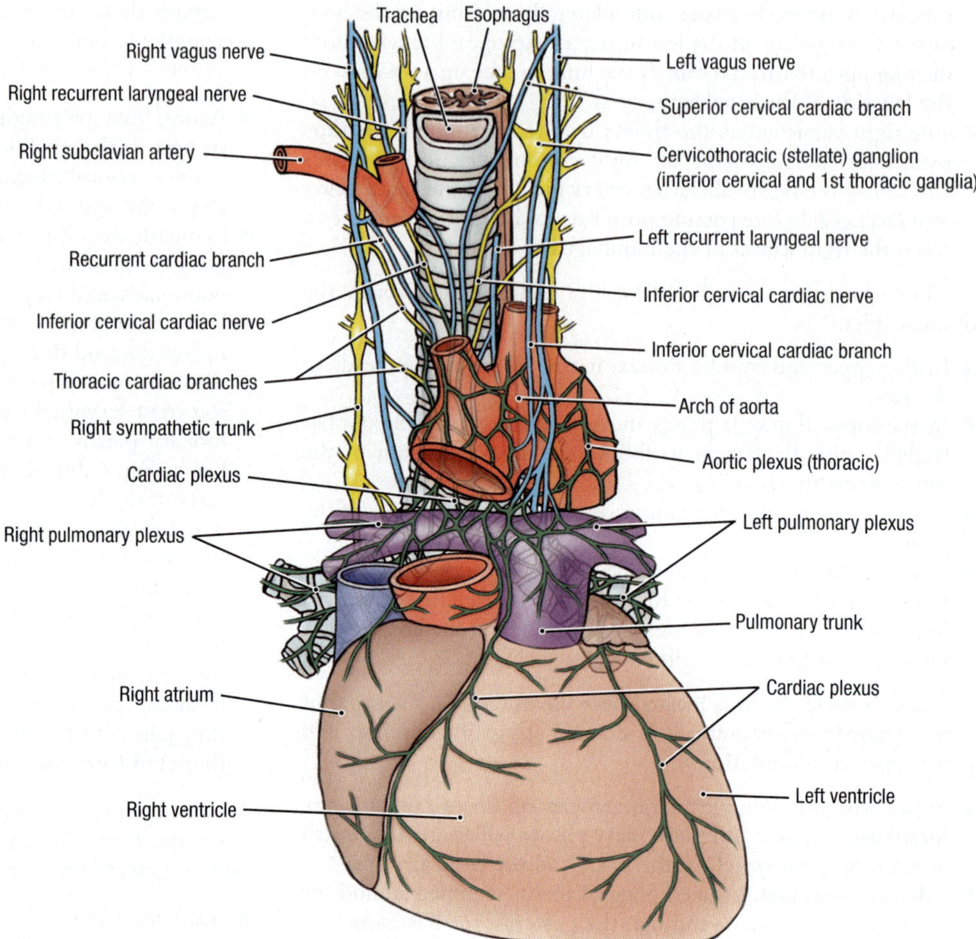

Figure 6.24. The cardiac plexus. The sympathetic trunk is *yellow*; the vagus and its branches are *blue*; and the mixed fibers of the plexus are *green*. (Reprinted with permission from Agur AMR, Dalley AF II. *Grant's Atlas of Anatomy*. 12th ed. Wolters Kluwer Health/Lippincott Williams & Wilkins; 2009.)

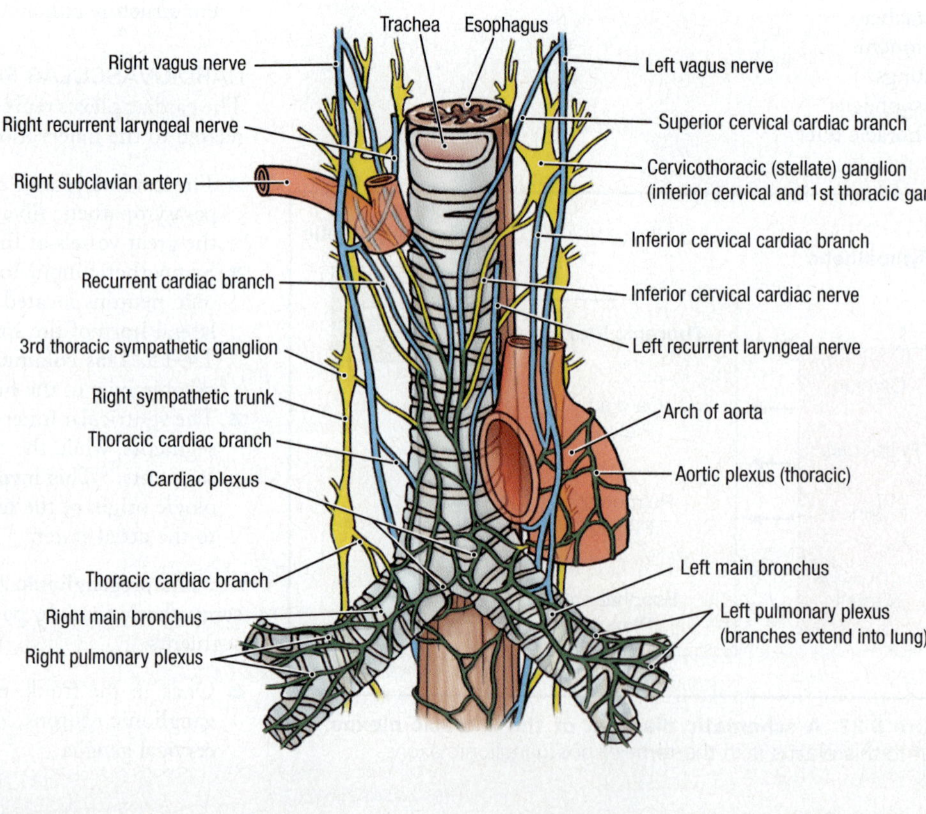

Figure 6.25. The pulmonary plexus. The sympathetic trunk is *yellow*; the vagus and its branches are *blue*; and the mixed fibers of the plexus are *green*. (Reprinted with permission from Agur AMR, Dalley AF II. *Grant's Atlas of Anatomy*. 12th ed. Wolters Kluwer Health/Lippincott Williams & Wilkins; 2009.)

- Cardiac sympathetic nerves arise mainly from the stellate and middle cervical ganglia, the superior cervical ganglion has only a minor contribution to the cardiac plexus.[77]
- Variable numbers of cervical and thoracic sympathetic cardiac nerves leave the cervical and upper thoracic ganglia, course through the fascia of the mediastinum, and join the cardiac branches of the vagus to form the cardiac plexus; these nerves have been described as superior, middle, and inferior cardiac nerves.
- The cardiac plexus is primarily located on the walls of the pulmonary arterial tree.[78]
- A superficial and deep division of the cardiac plexus has been described.[5] The superficial division, located in front of the aortic arch, is made up of fibers primarily from the left superior cardiac sympathetic nerve and the left inferior cervical cardiac branch of the vagus.
- All of the remaining sympathetic and vagal cardiac nerves contribute to the deep cardiac plexus, located posterior to the aortic arch.

The parasympathetic input to the cardiac plexus arises from preganglionic neurons in the dorsal motor nucleus of the vagus and the nucleus ambiguous of the medulla.[79,80]

- These preganglionic axons leave the vagus nerve over its variable (one to three) cardiac branches, beginning in the neck and extending into the superior mediastinum.
  - □ The axons target a parasympathetic ganglion embedded in the cardiac plexuses, termed the Wristberg ganglion.
- Short cholinergic axons from these ganglia reach the sinoatrial (SA) and atrioventricular (AV) nodes and course in the myocardium of the ventricles.
  - □ The parasympathetic innervation of the ventricular wall is much less dense than that of the sympathetic fibers.[81]

From the cardiac plexus, sympathetic adrenergic and parasympathetic cholinergic, postganglionic axons form a rich network of fibers distributed along the coronary vasculature, coursing throughout the myocardium of the atria and ventricles and reaching the SA and AV nodes.[81]

- The innervation of the intrinsic nodal system of the heart is bilaterally asymmetric; the right side of the plexus favors the SA node, but the left side of the plexus tends to target the AV node. Thus, stimulation of the sympathetic fibers on the left side accelerates cardiac output but is arrhythmogenic because it is directed to the AV node.[82]
- A similar reaction is obtained by cooling the right sympathetic fibers, indicating that cardiac activity is influenced by the balance of activity between the two bilateral sympathetic inputs.[82]
- Stimulation of the parasympathetic vagal fibers tends to stabilize heart rate. It appears that the balance of tonic neural activity occurring in the vagus and sympathetic systems influences, in part, heart rate and volume output.

Cardiac afferent nerves are an important consideration in understanding:

- Reflex control of the heart
- Patterns of referred cardiac pain
- Patterns of cardiac-facilitated segments

Small-caliber, primary afferent fibers are distributed throughout the[83–85]:

- myocardium
- coronary vasculature
- roots of its great vessel
- parietal pericardium

There are at least two different pathways for these cardiac sensory fibers.[86,87]

1. Those visceral afferents coursing with the sympathetic nerves have their cell bodies located in dorsal root ganglia extending from approximately C6 to T7 and their central processes that terminate in the dorsal horn of the spinal cord.
2. Sensory axons coursing with the parasympathetic nerves have cell bodies located in the nodose ganglion of the vagus nerve and central processes that terminate in the solitary nucleus of the medulla.

In addition to the autonomic nerves supplying an afferent innervation of the pericardium, afferent fibers reach this structure over the phrenic nerve as well.

- These phrenic afferent fibers enter the spinal cord over segments C3–C5.
- The phrenic nerve pierces the diaphragm and communicates with the autonomic plexus in the abdomen.[88]
- Catecholamine fibers have been documented in the phrenic nerve and were thought to originate in the celiac ganglion.[89]
- Little is known concerning the function of this communication. However the phrenic nerve most likely is providing a conduit for sympathetic fibers to reach the vascular system of the diaphragm and the "caval bodies" in the walls of the inferior vena cava.[89]
- Sensory fibers, in the phrenic nerve, reaching organs in the upper abdominal cavity could explain the occurrence of referred pain from the upper abdominal gastrointestinal system to the base of the neck.[90]

Along with the dual origin of sensory nerves, there is a differential distribution of these two sensory pathways in the cardiovascular system.[84,85]

- The afferent fibers of the vagus nerve terminate in the:
  - □ ascending aorta
  - □ aortic arch
  - □ pulmonary trunk
  - □ arterial walls
  - □ atrial walls
  - □ atrioventricular valve
  - □ ventricular walls
- The afferent fibers from the sympathetic nerves reach the:
  - □ atrial walls
  - □ pulmonary arteries
  - □ atrioventricular and aortic valves

Afferent fibers from both systems reach the coronary arteries.

- Those from the vagus extend to a more distal level of the vasculature, closer to the apex of the heart, than do afferent fibers associated with the sympathetic nervous system.
- Both Aδ- and C-afferent fibers are present in the heart.[91]
- Many of these fibers contain neuropeptides such as substance-P or calcitonin gene–related polypeptide that are typical of small-caliber, primary afferent fibers.
- At least one population of these cardiac C-fibers has the physiologic properties of nociceptive axons.

In general, the afferent fibers coursing with the sympathetic nerves are involved with cardiac nociception, and those following the parasympathetic nerves are mainly involved in reflexogenic regulation of heart functions through their brainstem connection.[86]

- Transection of the sympathetic nerves to the heart can relieve cardiac pain in the chest, arms, and neck.[92] These cardiac afferent fibers enter the spinal cord over a range of segments from C6 to T7, but the influence of these nerves can extend at least two segments below T7.[93]

- The signs of segmental facilitation due to cardiac disease can present in the vicinity of the cervicothoracic junction and extend downward through at least T9.[94] Importantly, the nociceptive afferent fibers reaching the dorsal horn of the spinal cord influence neurons with concomitant somatic receptive fields.
- This viscerosomatic convergence of nociceptive information provides an explanation for the referral of pain from cardiac structures to the body wall and extremity.[95]
- Spinal afferent fibers responding to noxious stimuli in the heart can also explain the palpatory finds that occur in the fourth and fifth thoracic vertebral region in the setting of anginal pain.[96]

The viscerosomatic convergence of primary afferent fibers in the dorsal horn of the spinal cord leads to the formation of cardiosomatic and somatocardiac reflexes. Studies of these reflexes have demonstrated the following:

- The somatic fibers of cutaneous origin that have the greatest influence on visceral organ function are the small-caliber unmyelinated or C-fibers; activity in large cutaneous myelinated fibers has little or no influence on visceral organ function.[97]
- Stimulation of either cutaneous (C-fibers) or muscle (group IV fibers) can significantly elevate heart rate.[98]
- Painful movement of inflamed joints can stimulate elevation in both heart rate and blood pressure.[99]
- Somatocardiac reflexes involve at least two separate pathways, local level reflexes related to the segment of input (propriospinal reflexes) are seen best when stimulating a segment close to the cardiac sympathetic outflow (T1–T5), and ascending pathways to the brainstem (supraspinal reflexes) can be evoked regardless of the level of input.[100]

Cardiosomatic reflexes can be demonstrated by triggering small-caliber cardiac sensory fibers (placing capsaicin into the pericardial sac) and recording electromyographic activity from the paraspinal muscles.

- These reflexes are modified by the rostroventral medulla,[101] an area well known to be involved in regulation of the cardiovascular functions.
- Studies focused on viscerosomatic integration support the concept that noxious somatic stimuli can trigger changes in sympathetic outflow at both spinal and medullary levels resulting in altered, typically increased, cardiac output and elevation in blood pressure.
- Conversely, noxious visceral stimuli involving the heart can alter the muscle tone expressed in portions of the somatic system, typically the paraspinal muscles of the back.

RESPIRATORY PLEXUS

The respiratory airways receive their innervation through the large pulmonary plexus that surrounds the pulmonary artery and extends onto the posterior surface of the trachea and bronchi (see Fig. 6.25).

- Sympathetic preganglionic neurons that contribute to this plexus are located in the lateral horn of spinal segments approximately T2–T6(T7), and their ganglionic neurons are located in the cervical and first four thoracic ganglia.[18]
- Postganglionic axons from these ganglia course through cardiac and esophageal nerves from the sympathetic trunk to reach the pulmonary plexus. These adrenergic axons primarily target the glandular tissue surrounding the bronchi and bronchioles; little direct adrenergic innervation of the bronchial musculature has been noted.
- β-Adrenergic receptors are present in the glandular cells and bronchial smooth muscle cells. Stimulation of the β-adrenergic, sympathetic nervous system leads to bronchial dilation and the release of a more viscous secretion.[102]

The vagus nerve is the source of parasympathetic innervation for the respiratory airways.

- After entering the thorax, the vagus shifts posteriorly in the mediastinum to pass behind the root of the lung.
- Anterior and posterior pulmonary branches are given off that contribute to the pulmonary plexus.
- Parasympathetic (mural) ganglia located in the walls of the airways receive preganglionic fibers from these vagal branches.
- Postganglionic parasympathetic fibers course in the arteriobronchial tree to terminate around bronchial smooth musculature, mucosal glands, and blood vessels. Stimulation of these cholinergic fibers causes[102]:
  - ☐ bronchoconstriction
  - ☐ hypersecretion of a serous secretion
  - ☐ vasodilation

Anterior and posterior pulmonary plexuses are recognized.[76]

- The anterior pulmonary plexus lies between the aorta and pulmonary trunk anteriorly and the trachea and carina and primary bronchi posteriorly, it is derived from several branches of the vagus that pass anterior to the bronchi as well as twigs from the sympathetic trunk.
- The larger posterior plexus lies on the posterior aspect of the mainstem bronchi and is derived from the two vagal trunks, bilaterally, and receives twigs from the sympathetic trunk bilaterally.

The pulmonary plexus and ganglia contain intrinsic neurons, that is, cells whose processes remain in the peripheral tissue and do not innervate the CNS. Such cells are called interneurons.

- Some of these cells produce a variety of neuropeptides, among which is vasoactive intestinal polypeptide, a potent bronchodilator.
- In addition, several neuropeptides co-release with norepinephrine from sympathetic terminals and with acetylcholine from parasympathetic terminals.
- These ubiquitous neuropeptides have recently gained considerable interest due to their role in controlling the diameter of the bronchial lumen and the initiation of bronchial wall inflammation.[103]

The parasympathetic system is the main source of neural control in the airway.[104]

- Vagal parasympathetic fibers bronchoconstrict the airway smooth musculature, stimulate glandular secretion, and vasodilate arteries.
- Little if any sympathetic fibers reach the airway smooth muscle, however, these muscle cells have a rich display of beta-adenoreceptors on their surfaces; most likely these receptors are responding to circulating catecholamines rather than sympathetic innervation.[105]

Small-caliber, primary afferent fibers are also present in the pulmonary plexus. These fibers provide sensory information to the brainstem via the vagus and to the spinal cord via the sympathetic trunk. This information is involved in reflex arcs related to:

- sneezing
- coughing

- bronchospasms
- pulmonary congestion

Many of these fibers, and particularly the smallest of them, contain neuropeptides such as substance-P and calcitonin gene–related polypeptide, among others.

- Irritation of these sensory fibers results in the release of proinflammatory substances, leading to neurogenic edema and inflammation in the lung.
- Substance-P, released from these sensory axons into the pulmonary parenchyma, is a potent:
  - bronchoconstrictor
  - vasodilator
  - secretagogue[106]

Activation of these primary afferent nociceptors can also facilitate segments in the spinal cord, extending from the cervical region into the low thoracic cord.[94]

- The extended range of activation most likely relates to the wide distribution of the central processes of these primary afferent fibers.
- Changes in spinal cord activity are seen in response to pulmonary afferent stimulation.
- Electrical stimulation of inflamed tracheobronchial mucosa produces a decrease in electrical skin resistance in the T2–T5 dermatomes, followed by cutaneous hyperalgesia hours later.[92]

Unlike the heart, pain from the airway is carried in the vagal fibers as well as in the spinal afferent fibers.

- Lung tumors can refer pain to the skin around the ear,[106] which is a region of the head innervated by small cutaneous branches of the vagus nerve.
- Electrical stimulation of the laryngeal and tracheal mucosa refers pain to the neck, and similar irritation of the bronchial tree refers pain to the anterior chest wall.
- Section of the vagus nerve below the recurrent laryngeal branch ameliorates the pain,[107] suggesting that the nerve is the conduit for this referred pain.

The costal parietal pleura receives an afferent innervation derived from the intercostal nerves of the thorax.

- The mediastinal pleura is innervated by sensory fibers from the phrenic nerve.
- The diaphragmatic pleura is innervated by twigs from the intercostal nerves.[106]
- The parietal plural membrane is sensitive to noxious stimuli.
- The visceral pleura of the lungs receives sympathetic and sensory fibers from the autonomic plexuses surrounding the bronchi but is insensate to pain.[106]

ESOPHAGEAL PLEXUS

The esophagus extends from an upper sphincter, the cricopharyngeus, located at the inferior border of the pharynx to a lower sphincter region located at the border of the stomach. Along its route, the body of the esophagus is lodged in the visceral fascia (loose connective tissues) of the superior and posterior mediastinum (Fig. 6.26).

- The upper esophageal sphincter is composed of skeletal muscle derived mainly from the cricopharyngeus and thyropharyngeus muscles (together they compose the inferior pharyngeal constrictor), which receive their innervation from the pharyngeal plexus composed of the superior laryngeal and pharyngeal branches of the vagus nerve.[108]
- The body of the esophagus is surrounded by a plexus of autonomic nerves derived from the inferior laryngeal branch of the vagus, direct branches of the vagus, and esophageal branches of the sympathetic trunk.[109]
- The superior portion of the esophagus is a mixture of skeletal and smooth muscle, although the lower portion is composed of smooth muscle only.
- The preganglionic parasympathetic innervation to the superior portion of the esophagus (skeletal muscle portion) is derived mainly from the nucleus ambiguous in the medulla of the brainstem.[18]
- Innervation of the smooth muscle of the esophagus is derived primarily from the dorsal motor nucleus of the vagus nerve,[110] also located in the medulla.
- The left and right vagal trunks approach the esophagus at the root of the lung
  - The recurrent laryngeal branches take up a position between the esophagus and the trachea, supplying both with an innervation.
  - An elaborate plexus is formed by the left and right vagus extending from the midpoint of the organ downward to the diaphragm (see Fig. 6.12).
  - The vagus and its branch, the inferior laryngeal, are joined by esophageal branches from the sympathetic trunk.

The postganglionic parasympathetic neurons are contained in two intrinsic ganglia in the walls of the esophagus:

- Auerbach, or the myenteric plexus
- Meissner, or the submucosal plexus

Sympathetic preganglionic neurons are located in the intermediolateral nucleus of spinal cord segments.

- Controversy exists concerning their location along the spinal cord range from:
  - T4–T6[18]
  - T2–T7[111]

The preganglionic axons synapse mainly in the stellate and upper thoracic sympathetic ganglia.

- Small esophageal branches, derived from the cervical to fourth and fifth thoracic ganglia and carrying postganglionic sympathetic fibers from these ganglia, join the vagal plexus along the walls of the esophagus.[112]
- At rest, the cricopharyngeus and thyropharyngeus muscles maintain a tonic contraction driven by the vagal fibers from the nucleus ambiguous.[107]
- During swallowing, the tonic vagal drive is inhibited and the upper esophageal sphincter relaxes.
- Peristalsis in the upper portion (skeletal muscle portion) of the esophagus is driven by the nucleus ambiguous of the vagus nerve, although that in the body and lower portion of the esophagus is driven by the dorsal motor nucleus of the vagus.[108]
- The relaxation of the lower esophageal sphincter is accomplished by the nitric oxide–producing neurons located in the myenteric (Auerbach) plexus and driven by the dorsal motor nucleus of the vagus nerve.[113]

Afferent fibers from the esophageal walls follow the vagus nerve back to the solitary nucleus of the medulla.

- Sensory fibers also follow the sympathetic fibers back to the dorsal horn of the upper segment of the spinal cord.[114]
- Dorsal horn neurons from T2 to T7 respond to stimulation of the esophagus using balloon distension.[111]

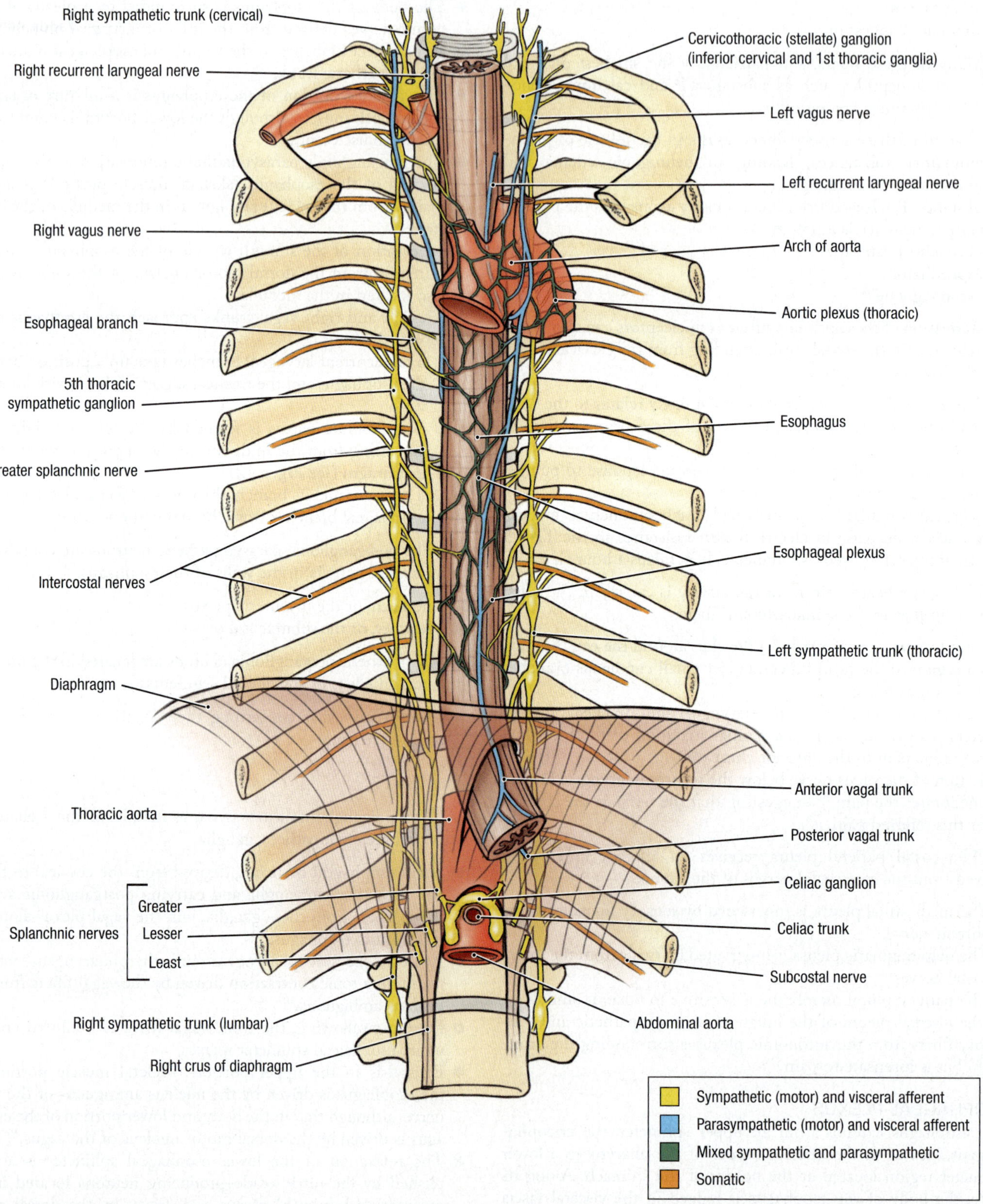

Figure 6.26. The esophageal plexus. The sympathetic trunk is in *yellow*; the vagus and its branches are in *blue*; and the mixed fibers of the plexus are in *green*. (Reprinted with permission from Agur AMR, Dalley AF II. *Grant's Atlas of Anatomy*. 12th ed. Wolters Kluwer Health/Lippincott Williams & Wilkins; 2009.)

- Vagal afferent fibers ending in the solitary nucleus of the medulla contribute to a viscerovisceral reflex arc by synapsing on premotor neurons of the nucleus ambiguous and preganglionic neurons of the dorsal motor nucleus of the vagus nerve.[108]
- The premotor neurons subsequently innervate the motor neurons of the nucleus ambiguous.
  - The premotor neurons form the central pattern generator for organized movements of the esophagus, such as the peristaltic waves involved in swallowing.[113]
- The spinal afferent fibers from the esophagus contribute to the referral of pain. These afferent fibers innervate spinal segments that also receive afferent information from the:
  - heart
  - pulmonary tree
  - chest
  - upper back and torso

Esophageal pain can refer substernally (heartburn) or posteriorly through the back into the area of the scapula.[115]

- Referred pain from the esophagus has numerous patterns, the more common of which involve a gripping, pressing, boring, or stabbing painful feeling.[116]
- The distribution of afferent fibers along the length of the spinal cord is difficult to estimate, pain of esophageal origin ranges from mandible dentation, the neck, the retrosternal region, upper midline back, and into the upper abdominal region.[117,118]

AORTIC PLEXUS

The thoracic aorta has an intimate relationship with both divisions of the autonomic nervous system.[92,119]

- The superior thoracic aorta receives sympathetic input as well as sensory fibers through cardiac nerves, as well as by following direct aortic branches from the sympathetic trunk (Fig. 6.27).
- The inferior thoracic aorta receives branches of the thoracic splanchnic nerves and small branches from the thoracic ganglia.
- The preganglionic sympathetic axons arise in the upper five thoracic spinal segments, and the postganglionic fibers arise from the upper five or six thoracic paravertebral ganglia.
  - From the trunk, these fibers spread medially and anteriorly to wrap around the walls of the aorta (Fig. 6.28).
  - Once on the wall of the aorta, these fibers form an adrenergic plexus in the adventitial tissue.
  - Afferent fibers from this large, elastic artery follow the sympathetic nerves back to the upper five thoracic spinal segments.[92]
  - This observation accounts for the referral of pain from the wall of the thoracic aorta to the thoracic spinal segments, resulting in their subsequent segmental facilitation of the spinal cord.
- Vagal cardiac nerves traverse the walls of the aorta as they descend toward their targets. Small twigs from these branches provide afferent as well as parasympathetic efferent innervation to the thoracic aorta.

THORACIC DUCT INNERVATION

The thoracic duct, located in the posterior mediastinum near the esophagus, receives an innervation similar to the vascular innervation elsewhere in the trunk.

- Its muscular walls receive cholinergic innervation from the vagus nerve and sympathetic adrenergic innervation from branches of the intercostal nerves in a segmental pattern.

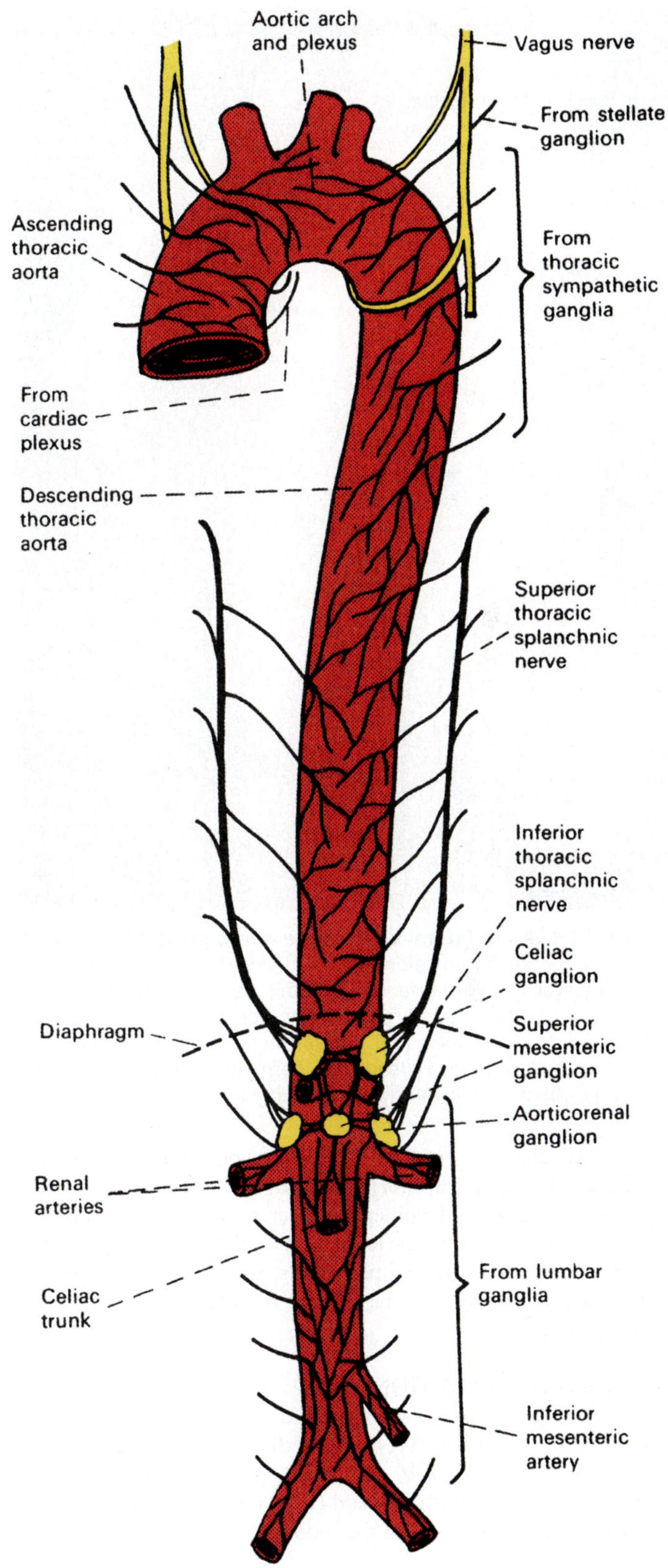

Figure 6.27. The aortic plexus. Fibers from the splanchnic nerves are seen approaching the wall of the aorta. This vessel also receives contributions directly from the sympathetic trunk as shown in Figure 6.28. (Reprinted with permission from Bonica JJ. General considerations of pain in the chest. In: Bonica JJ, ed. *The Management of Pain*. 2nd ed. Lea & Febiger; 1990:959–1000.)

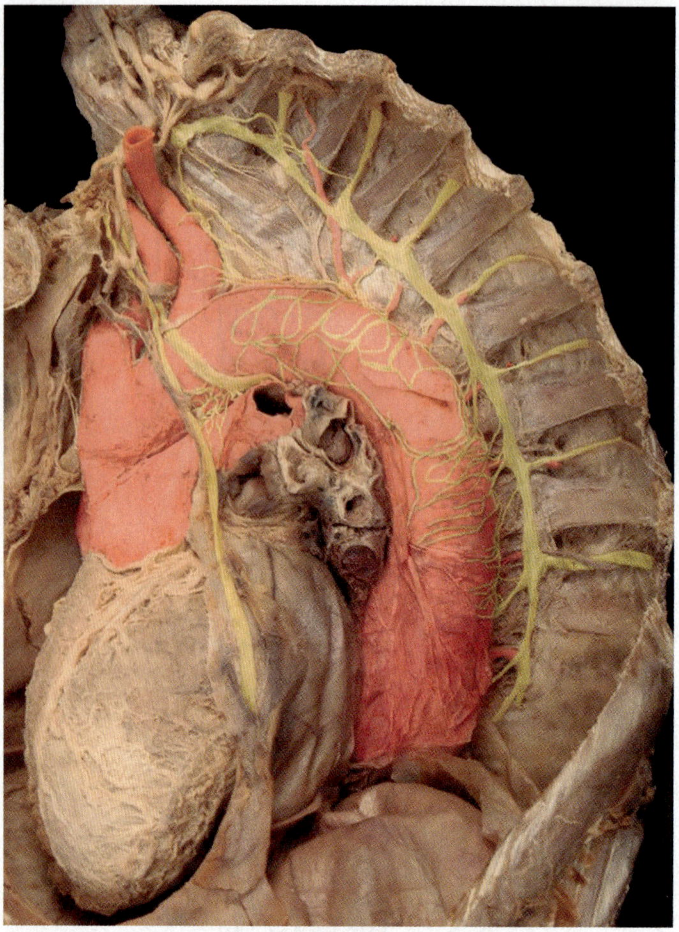

Figure 6.28. A left lateral view of the aortic plexus. The sympathetic trunk is seen lying along the rib heads. Many small branches reach the walls of the aorta. The vagus is seen passing anterior to the aortic arch, and the left recurrent laryngeal nerve passes under the aortic arch. The aorta and the surrounding nerves were highlighted with Photoshop. (Used with permission from the Willard/Carreiro Collection, University of New England.)

- The 11th thoracic ganglion and the left splanchnic nerve innervate the cisterna chyli, which is the origin of the thoracic duct.[120]
- Norepinephrine and epinephrine act to increase the flow of lymph through the thoracic duct.[121] The effect of these adrenergic compounds on lymph vessels appears to be mediated through α-receptors on the smooth muscle cells of the lymph vessel wall.[122]

ABDOMINOPELVIC AUTONOMICS

The thoracic plexus passes through the diaphragm to continue inferiorly in the abdominopelvic cavity as the abdominopelvic (aortic) plexus (see Figs. 6.22, 6.26, and 6.29). This massive network of fibers lies embedded in the visceral fascia along the midline, astride the aorta, and extending from the abdominal diaphragm to the pelvic diaphragm.[76]

At the level of the abdominal diaphragm, the plexus has two major components: parasympathetic and sympathetic.

- The two vagal trunks and their associated branches, representing the parasympathetic component, enter the abdomen riding on the walls of the esophagus.
- The sympathetic component (or thoracic splanchnic nerves) passes directly through the crura of the diaphragm or posterior to the medial arcuate ligament to enter the abdomen.
- Once in the abdominal cavity, the vagal trunks and thoracic splanchnic nerves unite around the aortic prevertebral ganglia.
- The resultant abdominopelvic plexus of fibers descends along the lateral aspect of the aorta and inferior vena cava, eventually uniting into one mass of fibers, the superior hypogastric (presacral) plexus, anterior to the midline vasculature, at around the level of the 4th or 5th lumbar vertebral body.
- The superior hypogastric plexus descends to the level of the sacral promontory where it bifurcates into the two inferior hypogastric (pelvic) plexuses that sweep laterally around the pelvic organs (see Fig. 6.29).

Throughout the abdomen, the plexus contains both sympathetic and parasympathetic axons and also is heavily endowed with numerous afferent fibers.

- Preganglionic sympathetic fibers join the plexus from the sympathetic trunk at all levels, these nerves are termed splanchnic nerves and are designated by the level from which they leave the trunk, thus there are thoracic, lumbar and sacral splanchnic nerves.
- Preganglionic parasympathetic fibers join the plexus from above in the form of the vagus nerve and from below in the form of the pelvic splanchnic nerves (nervi erigentes) derived from sacral roots S2–S4.

Like the thoracic plexus, the abdominopelvic plexus can be divided into several geographical regions.

- Along the abdominal aorta, the major prevertebral ganglia mark out differing territories:
  - □ Celiac
  - □ Superior mesenteric
  - □ Inferior mesenteric
- The celiac plexus contains the celiac ganglia and surrounds the arterial trunk of its namesake, and spreads laterally along the renal artery as well (see Fig. 6.29). This latter portion has been termed the aorticorenal ganglia and plexus by some authors.
- The celiac plexus fuses imperceptibly with the SMP surrounding its namesake artery.

Descending fibers from the SMP reach a few ganglia at the level of the inferior mesenteric artery before descending toward the pelvic brim to form the superior hypogastric plexus.

- The superior hypogastric plexus lies between the inferior mesenteric plexus and the sacral promontory.
- Below the sacral promontory, the plexus splits to pass laterally around the pelvic organs. This region is called the inferior hypogastric plexus or, simply, the pelvic plexus.
- Frequently, the fibers of the superior hypogastric plexus unite into a few large cords in the region directly over the sacral promontory and just prior to bifurcation into the two inferior hypogastric plexuses. These cords are referred to in the surgical literature as the presacral nerve.[123]

Although the abdominal autonomic nervous system has regional names, in reality, the components blend together to form one massive structure: the great abdominopelvic plexus.

- The abdominal portion of this great plexus supplies efferent and afferent nerves to the organs of the abdominal cavity, including the:
  - □ gastrointestinal organs
  - □ spleen
  - □ kidneys

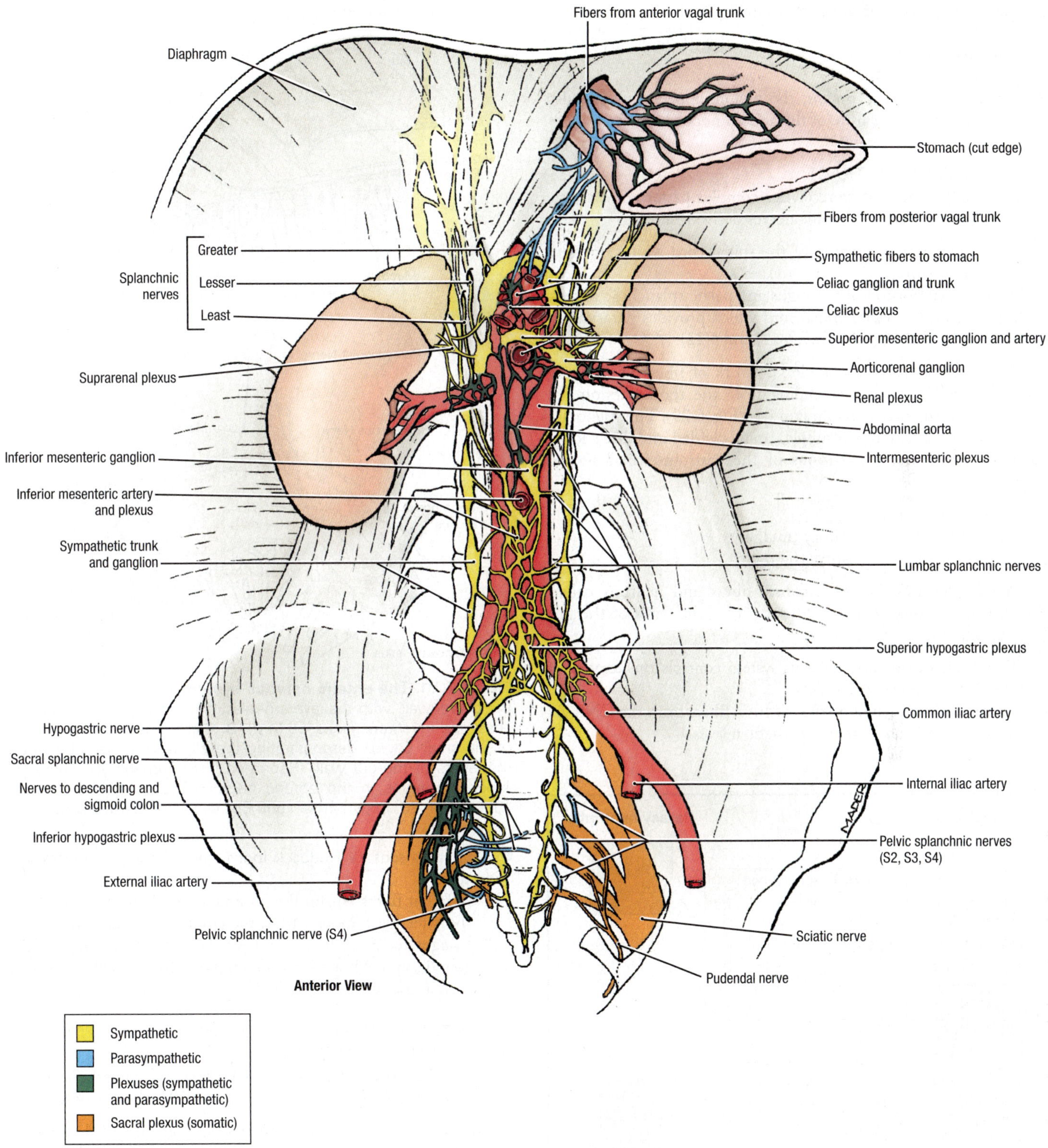

Figure 6.29. Abdominopelvic plexus. This diagram illustrates the location of the great abdominopelvic plexus in the midline fascia surrounding the abdominal aorta. The sympathetic trunk and associated sympathetic nerves are in *yellow*; the vagus and its branches are in *blue*; and the mixed fibers of the plexus are in *green*. The aorta and its branches are shown in *red*. (Reprinted with permission from Agur AMR, Dalley AF II. *Grant's Atlas of Anatomy*. 12th ed. Wolters Kluwer Health/Lippincott Williams & Wilkins; 2009.)

- The pelvic portion of this plexus supplies the:
  - rectum
  - urinary organs
  - reproductive organs
- In addition to these organs, the abdominopelvic plexus also innervates the vasculature of the abdominopelvic cavity.

GASTROINTESTINAL TRACT

The gastrointestinal system receives a complex pattern of extrinsic innervation involving splanchnic nerves derived from:

- The thoracolumbar portion of the spinal cord which provides sympathetic input.
- The terminal portion of the vagus and pelvic splanchnic nerves, derived from the sacral spinal cord which provides parasympathetic input (see Figs. 6.4, 6.5, 6.11, and 6.22).

These nerves form a complex network of fibers lying along the abdominal aorta and extending from the thoracoabdominal diaphragm to the pelvic diaphragm (see Fig. 6.29). This elaborate plexus, like its visceral blood supply, can be divided into three zones based on embryologic partitions of the gastrointestinal system (Fig. 6.30):

1. Celiac territory (foregut)
2. Superior mesenteric territory (midgut)
3. Inferior mesenteric territory (hindgut)

A complex network of intrinsic fibers and neurons called the enteric nervous system is found within the walls of the gut (Fig. 6.31).[124]

- The enteric or intrinsic nervous system controls the activity of gut smooth muscle and glands.
- In turn, it is modulated by the extrinsic fibers from the CNS via the sympathetic and parasympathetic nerves.

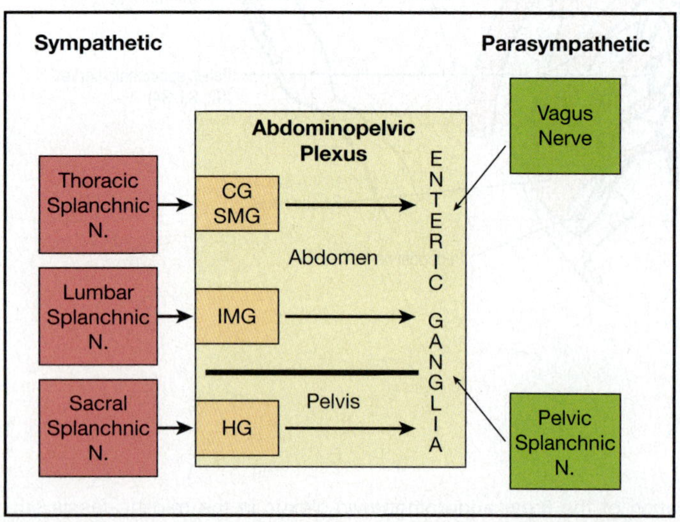

Figure 6.30. A schematic diagram of the great abdominopelvic plexus. Thoracic, lumbar, and sacral splanchnic nerves for the sympathetic trunk carry sympathetic preganglionic fibers to the paravertebral ganglia located in the plexus. Postganglionic axons from the par paravertebral ganglia target the intrinsic enteric ganglia of the organ walls. Parasympathetic fibers arise in the vagus nerve superiorly and in the pelvic splanchnic nerves inferiorly. These fibers also target the intrinsic enteric ganglia located on the organ walls. (CG, celiac ganglion; SMG, superior mesenteric ganglion; IMG, inferior mesenteric ganglion; HG, hypogastric ganglion.)

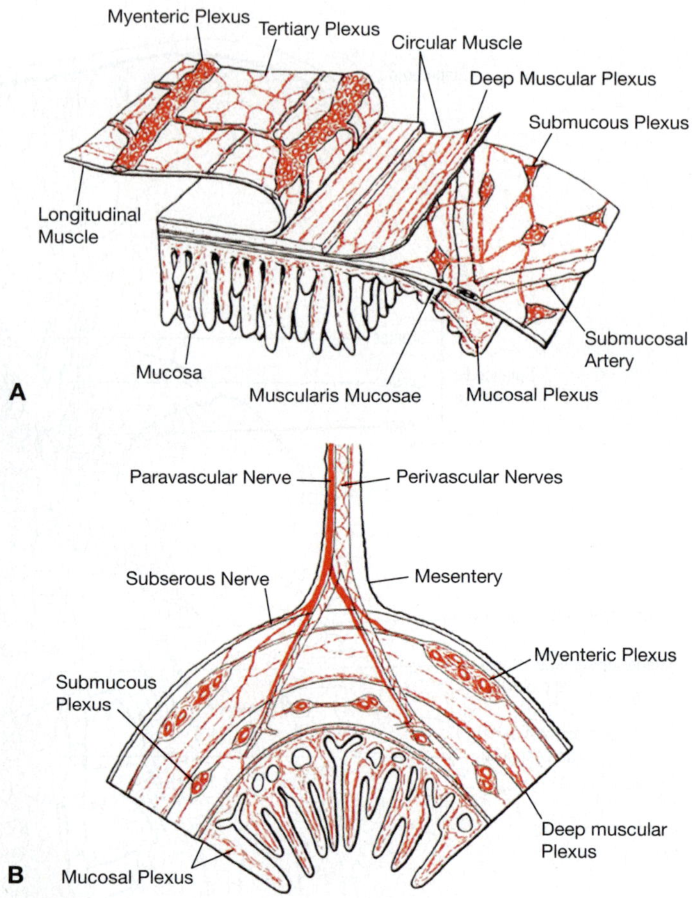

Figure 6.31. The enteric nervous system. A. A small section of the bowel wall, with the layers peeled open to expose the submucosal and myenteric plexuses (*red*). **B.** A cross-section of a portion of the small bowel, demonstrating the plexuses lying in between the layers of the gut wall. (Reprinted from Furness JB, Costa M. Types of nerves in the enteric nervous system. *Neuroscience*. 1980;5(1):1–20. Copyright © 1980 Elsevier. With permission.)

- Numerous sensory feedback loops exist in the gastrointestinal system.
  - Afferent fibers within the luminal surface and gut wall form short feedback loops within the enteric nervous system.
  - Longer feedback loops connect the gut to the prevertebral ganglia, and still longer loops connect the gut with the spinal cord and brainstem (Fig. 6.32).

SYMPATHETIC INNERVATION OF THE GASTROINTESTINAL TRACT

The gastrointestinal tract has a special pattern of sympathetic innervation that differs significantly from that of the thoracic viscera.

- Preganglionic fibers arise in the lateral horn of spinal segments T9–L2, but they do not terminate in the paravertebral ganglia.
- Instead, they pass through a series of thoracic, lumbar, and sacral splanchnic nerves (medially-directed branches off of the sympathetic trunk) to reach the prevertebral sympathetic ganglia on the anterior wall of the abdominal aorta (see Figs. 6.22, 6.29, and 6.30).

The major prevertebral ganglia are distributed around the three abdominal arteries:

1. Celiac
2. Superior mesenteric
3. Inferior mesenteric

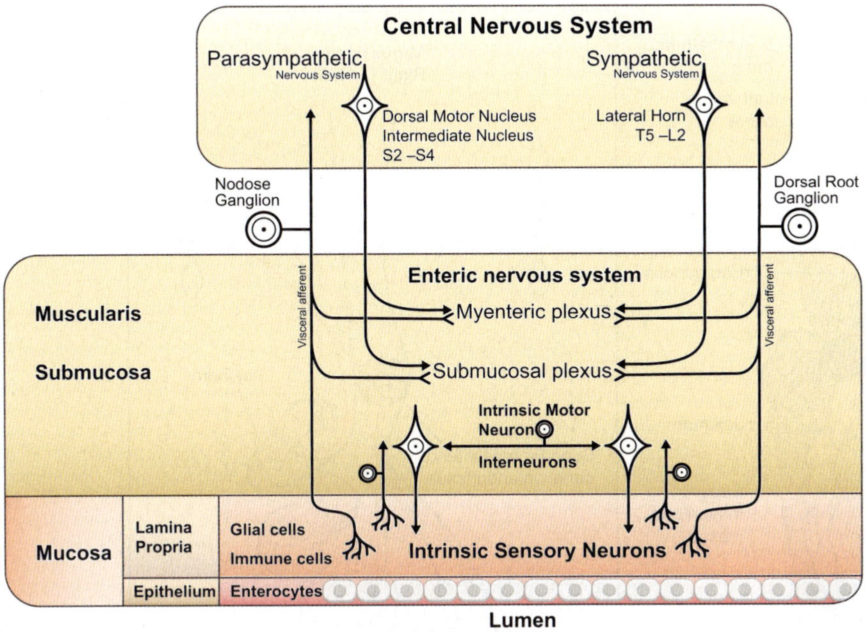

Figure 6.32. This schematic diagram illustrates the relationship between the central nervous system, the parasympathetic (PSNS) and sympathetic (SNS) nervous systems and the enteric nervous system (ENS). The PSNS and SNS have central neurons in the brainstem and spinal cord. These autonomic regions are under control of forebrain structures. In addition, the autonomic regions receive sensory information from the alimentary tract through visceral afferent fibers. The PSNS and SNS innervate the motor neurons in the myenteric and submucosal plexuses of the ENS. Also contained within these two plexuses are intrinsic sensory neurons and intrinsic interneurons. The intrinsic interneurons contain the patterns for specific gut activities. Glial cells, immune cells, and enterocytes interact with the intrinsic neurons of the ENS to regulate and modify the patterns of gut activity.

Numerous subdivisions of the ganglia have been described that are beyond the scope of this chapter.[5]

- The celiac and superior mesenteric ganglia are often fused together into an inseparable mass surrounding the trunks of their two arteries. An older term for this arrangement was the solar plexus.
- Additional clusters of sympathetic ganglia neurons are found scattered in the hypogastric plexus as it enters the pelvic basin.

Neurons in each prevertebral ganglion give rise to postganglionic fibers that innervate abdominal and pelvic viscera.

- These axons travel to their target organs by hitchhiking on abdominal and pelvic vascular bundles.
- Thus, each prevertebral ganglion innervates a different region of the viscera based on the vascular territory with which it associates.

1. Celiac Ganglia

The celiac ganglionic mass surrounds the celiac trunk. It is often fused to the superior mesenteric ganglia to form one large, complex mass. When carefully dissected, the precise shape of the ganglion complex is very irregular and defies meaningful classification.[19] The celiac ganglia receive afferent fibers from the thoracic splanchnic nerves, typically T5–T9.[18] In turn, it supplies postganglionic sympathetic axons to the vascular territory of the celiac artery including the (Fig. 6.33):

- distal esophagus
- stomach
- proximal duodenum
- liver
- gall bladder
- spleen
- portions of the pancreas

2. Superior Mesenteric Ganglia

This ganglion is found wrapped around the superior mesenteric artery. As mentioned above, it is often fused with the celiac ganglia. The superior mesenteric ganglia also receive preganglionic axons from the thoracic splanchnic nerves, typically T9–T11 or T12.[18] Its distribution of postganglionic axons reaches the territory supplied by the superior mesenteric artery including the (Fig. 6.34):

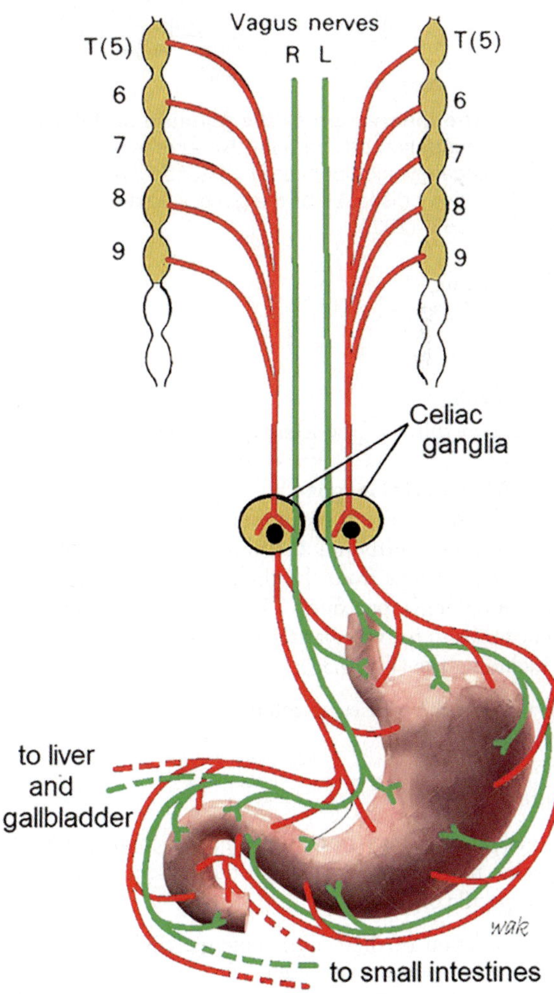

Figure 6.33. The celiac plexus and upper GI innervation. The sympathetic innervation (*red*) arises from spinal levels T(5) 6–9, and the sympathetic ganglionic nervous are located in the celiac ganglia. The parasympathetic innervation is derived from the vagus (*green*). Generally, autonomic fibers reach the gastric wall by following along the vasculature. Thus, the greater and lesser curvatures represent the route into the stomach.

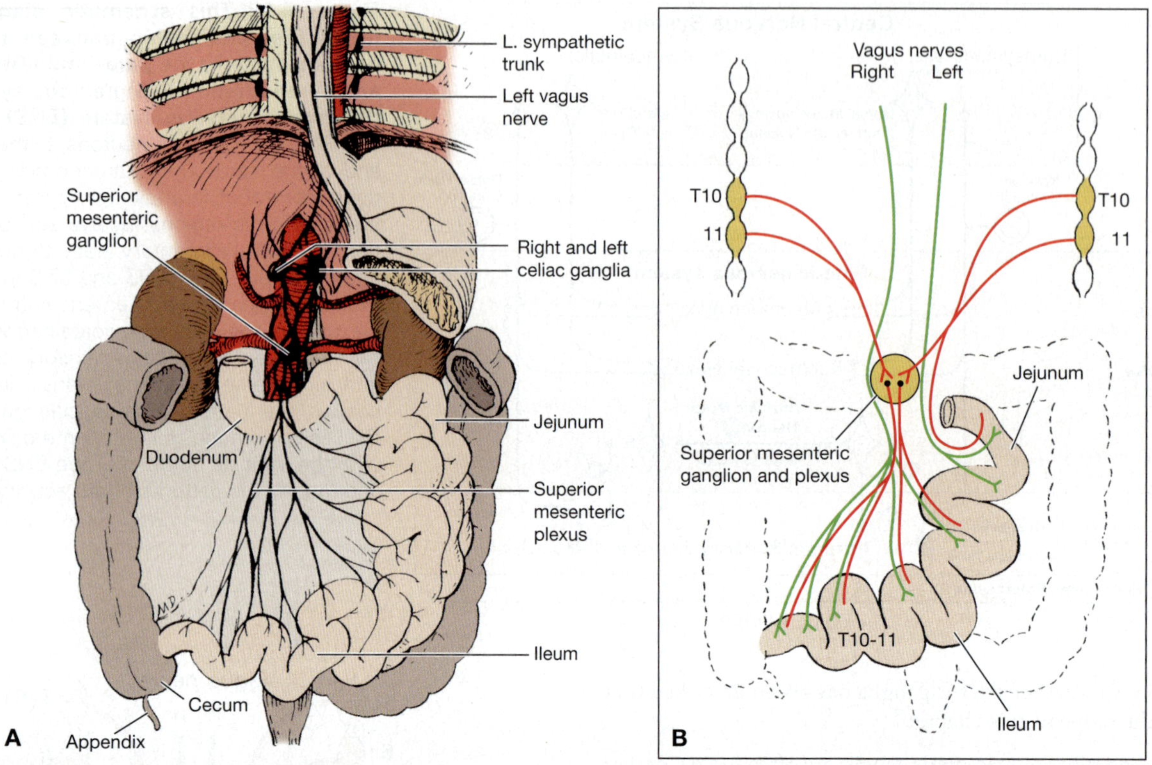

Figure 6.34. The innervation of the jejunum and ileum. The illustration on the left (**A**) represents the efferent fibers associated with the SMP. The illustration on the right (**B**) represents the afferent fibers associated with the SMP. Preganglionic fibers are represented by *solid lines*; postganglionic fibers are by *dashed lines. Fine dotted lines* indicate sensory fibers. (Reprinted with permission from Tobin RW, Kimmey MB. Painful diseases of the gastrointestinal tract. In: Loeser JD, ed. *Bonica's Management of Pain.* 3rd ed. Lippincott Williams & Wilkins; 2001:1269–1292.)

- distal duodenum
- portions of the pancreas
- jejunum
- ileum
- ascending colon
- proximal two-thirds of the transverse colon

3. Inferior Mesenteric Ganglia

The most ventral of the three prevertebral ganglia, the inferior mesenteric ganglia, surrounds the abdominal artery of the same name. It receives axons from the three lumbar splanchnic nerves, typically containing input from L1 and L2[18], and supplies postganglionic axons to the vascular territory of the inferior mesenteric vessels including the (Fig. 6.35):

- distal third of the transverse colon
- descending colon
- sigmoid colon
- rectum

Postganglionic fibers from these prevertebral ganglia follow their specific blood supplies through the mesenteric ligaments to reach the specific organs.

- The termination of these noradrenergic fibers is primarily on the neurons in the enteric ganglia.[125]
- Sympathetic fibers also terminate in the muscular coat of blood vessels, and an abundance of these fibers reaches the muscular sphincters of the enteric wall.
- Only scattered sympathetic fibers are present in the muscularis externa and submucosa of the gastrointestinal tract.[126]
- There are almost no adrenergic cell bodies in the enteric plexus; therefore, most enteric adrenergic fibers are of external origin.
- In general, stimulation of the sympathetic fibers inhibits the activity of cholinergic neurons of the parasympathetic system and slows peristalsis and motility.

PARASYMPATHETIC INNERVATION OF THE GASTROINTESTINAL TRACT

The parasympathetic innervation of the organs located below the thoracoabdominal diaphragm has a dual origin, which like the sympathetic input, also segregates along vascular and embryologic divisions.[76]

- The organs of the foregut and midgut, serviced by the celiac and superior mesenteric arteries, receive parasympathetic preganglionic fibers from the vagus nerve (see Figs. 6.33 to 6.35).
- The vagus nerve follows the esophagus through the diaphragm to enter the abdominal cavity on the walls of the stomach.
- The esophageal hiatus of the diaphragm is the last place the vagus can be identified as a distinct entity.
- Vagal axons, however, continue into the abdominal cavity, joining those of the sympathetic system in the celiac and superior mesenteric ganglia and forming mixed nerves, which pass along celiac and superior mesenteric blood vessels eventually to reach the abdominal viscera.
- Vagal fibers are plentiful in the walls of the stomach and small bowel, and a few reach as far distally in the enteric plexus as the splenic flexure of the large colon.

The preganglionic vagal axons terminate on neurons in enteric ganglia.

- Short postganglionic fibers from these neurons innervate the glands and course within the layers of smooth muscle of the alimentary canal.

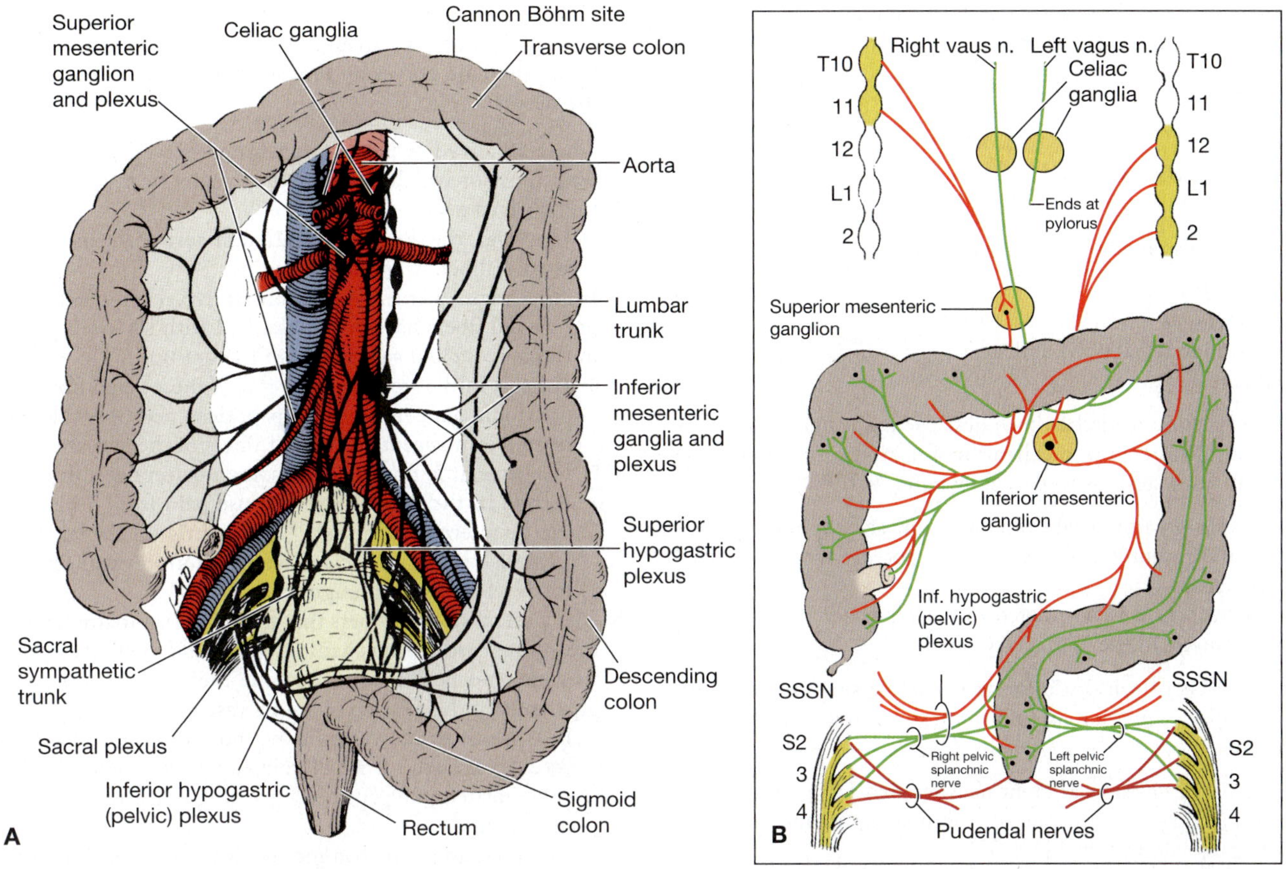

Figure 6.35. The innervation of the large bowel. The illustration on the left (**A**) is an anterior view illustrating the distribution of the superior and inferior mesenteric plexus to the large bowel. The schematic diagram on the right (**B**) summarizes the innervation of the large bowel. The ascending and transverse colon are innervated by postganglionic fibers derived from the superior mesenteric ganglion. The descending colon and sigmoid colon are innervated by postganglionic fibers from the inferior mesenteric ganglion. (Reprinted with permission from Tobin RW, Kimmey MB. Painful diseases of the gastrointestinal tract. In: Loeser JD, ed. *Bonica's Management of Pain*. 3rd ed. Lippincott Williams & Wilkins; 2001:1269–1292.)

- Cholinergic stimulation increases glandular secretions and peristaltic activity.

The organs of hindgut origin (transverse colon to anus) receive parasympathetic preganglionic innervation from the pelvic splanchnic nerves (see Figs. 6.29 and 6.35).

- These nerves arise in the lateral horn of the S2, S3, S4, and a few fibers from S5 spinal cord segments and exit the spinal canal with the sacral nerve roots.[18]
- As the roots pass along the pelvic wall on their way to the greater sciatic foramen, they give off the delicate pelvic splanchnic nerves.
- These thin nerves course through the endopelvic fascia to reach the inferior hypogastric plexus surrounding the walls of the rectum.
- Once in the hypogastric plexus, these parasympathetic preganglionic fibers can ascend to the origin of the inferior mesenteric artery.
- By hitchhiking along the branches of this artery, they reach upward to the splenic flexure of the large colon.
- Not all parasympathetic axons from the pelvis follow this route to reach the inferior abdominal organs. Some preganglionic fibers in the inferior hypogastric plexus gain access to the enteric plexus in the wall of the rectum and ascend along the colon to reach more proximal levels of the hindgut.
- The preganglionic axons of the pelvic splanchnic nerves eventually terminate on the neurons of the enteric nervous system.
- Stimulation of the parasympathetic fibers increases gut peristalsis and mobility.

The Enteric Nervous System

The enteric ganglia and plexus within the walls of the gut form a highly complex and elaborate network, often referred to as the third division of the autonomic nervous system or the "Second Brain" (see Figs. 6.31 and 6.32). It exerts a major influence over all activities in the gut.[20]

- The enteric nervous system is estimated to possess as many neurons as are found in the entire length of the spinal cord.[127]
- The enteric system is divided into two layers:
  - The external layer is the myenteric plexus (Auerbach) controlling the muscularis externa.
  - The internal layer is the submucosal (Meissner) controlling the glandular and immune components of the submucosal layers.
- Both layers receive input from the sympathetic and parasympathetic systems (see Fig. 6.32); in addition, afferent fibers from the gut wall innervate the two ganglionic layers as well as the spinal cord and brainstem.[25]
- A full understanding of these structures requires the knowledge of gastrointestinal histology and is beyond the scope of this review.[128–130]

Numerous neurotransmitters and neuromodulators are found within enteric neurons, for example:

- acetylcholine
- serotonin
- purines
- gamma-amino butyric acid
- histamine

There are also many peptides such as:

- substance-P
- somatostatin
- vasoactive intestinal polypeptide
- enkephalins

Recently, nitric oxide has been described as a significant noncholinergic, nonadrenergic mechanism of neurotransmission in the enteric nervous system, as well as elsewhere.[124,131,132]

- Nitric oxide is synthesized from the amino acid arginine by neurons in the myenteric plexus and is a potent smooth muscle–relaxing factor.
- For this reason, it is postulated to be important in dilation of smooth muscle in the alimentary canal.

Three levels of sensory information processing are necessary for the proper regulation of gastrointestinal tract function[25,133] (Box 6.4).

- The first-level features afferent neurons that form a short loop interconnecting the gut mucosa, submucosa, or muscle to the enteric ganglia only (see Fig. 6.32).
  - □ These neurons are responsible for local reflexes along the gut wall.
- The second level of sensory information processing is arranged in a longer loop, involving afferent neurons from the mucosa that project to the prevertebral ganglia along the aorta.
  - □ These sensory neurons participate in intra-abdominal reflex arcs coordinating various regions of the gastrointestinal system.
  - □ Neither of these two sensory levels can reach consciousness; thus, one is generally unaware of the normal reflex control activity occurring in the gut wall.
- The third level of sensory feedback loops involves afferent neurons that project from the gut wall to the brainstem via the vagus nerve, or to the spinal cord via the thoracic, lumbar, and pelvic splanchnic nerves.
  - □ These visceral afferent neurons assist the CNS in integrating the activity of the alimentary canal with that of external environmental conditions.
  - □ Information in this third sensory level can, on occasion, reach consciousness.

BOX 6.4 Visceral Afferent Fibers

The sensory fibers that course alongside the sympathetic and parasympathetic efferent fibers are best termed visceral afferent (sensory) fibers.

Use of the term sympathetic or parasympathetic afferent fibers is discouraged since these afferent fibers target much more than sympathetic or parasympathetic nuclei in the brainstem and spinal cord.

There are significant differences in distribution, morphology, and neurochemistry between the visceral afferent fibers associated with sympathetic nerves and those coursing with the parasympathetic nerves.

- There are very few large, encapsulated nerve endings in the gut wall, most of which are related to axons from the parasympathetic vagus nerve.
  - □ However, the majority of afferent terminals in the gut are small-caliber, naked nerve endings.[133]
- In the vagus nerve, mechanoreceptive, chemoreceptive, and polymodal fibers have been described with their receptive fields in the mucosa and submucosa of the gut wall.
  - □ At least in the stomach, very few of these vagal fibers contain calcitonin gene–related polypeptide, a neuropeptide typically related in nociceptive afferent fibers of the somatic tissue.
  - □ However, it is possible that some nociceptive information is carried in the vagus nerve because pain from a hiatal hernia can be referred to the face[134] apparently via the vagus nerve.
  - □ Little is known of nociceptive function in vagal fibers below the level of the diaphragm.
- The visceral afferent fibers that follow the sympathetic nerves to the spinal cord are mechanoreceptive and chemoreceptive, and they tend to be distributed to the mesenteries and peritoneal ligaments of the gut and along its vascular system.
  - □ In contrast to the vagal fibers, those projecting to the spinal cord are mostly of small caliber and are rich in calcitonin gene–related polypeptide, suggesting that they have a role in nociception.
  - □ Their endings are commonly distributed within the mesentery and supporting ligaments of the abdominal organs.[135]
  - □ These nerve endings are frequently present near the branch points for the vasculature in the peritoneal lining. Few small-caliber nerve endings are present within the visceral organs themselves.

Physiologic[95] and clinical studies support the general separation of regulatory information into the vagal system and nociceptive information into the spinal cord.

- Stimulating the greater thoracic splanchnic nerve at surgery elicits severe pain; while, blockade of the splanchnic nerve relieves pain.[136]
- In addition, applying local anesthetic to the greater thoracic splanchnic nerve after abdominal surgery prevents the endocrine metabolic responses such as increased plasma cortisol and urinary adrenaline levels that are usually present in the early stages of recovery.[137]

The projection of the viscera afferent fibers through the sympathetic system creates a nociceptive map of the abdominopelvic organs on the dorsal horn of the spinal cord.

- This map has been demonstrated in humans by sectioning the white rami commicans during the surgical treatment of visceral pain (White and Sweet, as cited in Jänig and Morrison[135]). A summary of the organotopic map of the human viscera is presented in Table 6.1.
- The position of a specific organ in the visceral afferent organotopic map of the spinal cord coincides approximately with the origin of the sympathetic efferent system to that specific organ.
- The nociceptive input to the spinal cord over these visceral afferent fibers is not precisely mapped; instead, input from any one organ overlaps considerably with that from surrounding organs.

TABLE 6.1

Summary of Autonomic Nervous System Distribution

Structure	Preganglionic Neuron	Postganglion Neuron	Pathway	Function	Reference
Eye and eyelids	T1–T2 cord segments	Superior cervical and cavernous ganglia	Internal carotid to cavernous sinus to orbit on nasociliary and ciliary nerves	Pupillary dilation, vasoconstriction, partial lid elevation	Mitchell (1953)[18]
Parotid salivary gland	T1–T2 cord segments	Superior cervical ganglion	External carotid to maxillary artery; middle meningeal plexus, auriculotemporal nerve	Vasoconstriction and small flow but rich in protein	Mitchell (1953)[18]
Submandibular and sublingual salivary glands	T1–T2 cord segments	Superior cervical ganglion	External carotid to facial plexus, lingual nerve	Vasoconstriction and small flow but rich in protein	Mitchell (1953 [18]
Facial skin	T1–T2 cord segments	Superior cervical ganglion	Branches of the external carotid, facial, and maxillary arteries	Vasoconstriction, sudomotor, and pilomotor effects; Vasodilation under stress and heat	Drummond (1994)[44]
Cranial vasculature	T1–T2 (T3) cord segments	Superior cervical, internal carotid and vertebral ganglia	Perivascular plexuses following branches of the carotids and vertebral arteries	Vasoconstriction	Mitchell (1953)[18]
Upper limbs	T2 (T3)–T6 (T7) cord segments	Stellate and upper thoracic ganglia	Gray rami to the roots of the brachial plexus	Vasoconstriction, sudomotor, and pilomotor effects	Mitchell (1953)[18]
Heart	T1–T4(T5)	All cervical and uppermost thoracic ganglia	Superior, middle, and inferior cardiac sympathetic nerves	Increase heart rate; balance metabolic vasodilation	Sato et al. (2024)[188]
Airway	T2(T3)–T6(T7) cord segments	Stellate, middle, and, to a lesser extent, superior cervical ganglia	Pulmonary cardiac sympathetic branches from upper thoracic sympathetic trunk	Bronchodilation	Mitchell (1953)[18]
Esophagus	(T2)T4–T6(T7)	Cervical and thoracic ganglia	Esophageal branches of the sympathetic trunk	Diminish peristalsis	Mitchell (1953)[18], Sengupta (2000)[111]
Stomach	T6–T9	Celiac ganglion and plexus	Greater thoracic splanchnic nerve to celiac plexus; celiac vessels to organs	Diminish peristalsis and secretion; vasoconstriction; contraction of the pylorus	Mitchell (1953)[18]
Gall bladder and biliary tree	T4(T5)–T9(T10)	Celiac ganglion and plexus	Greater thoracic splanchnic nerve to celiac plexus; celiac vessels to organs	Diminish peristalsis	Mitchell (1953)[18]
Liver	T6(T7)–T9(T10)	Celiac ganglion and plexus	Greater thoracic splanchnic nerve to celiac plexus; celiac vessels to organs	Vasoconstriction; Increase the secretion of glucose	Mitchell (1953)[18], Jarhult et al. (1979)[189], Zsombok et al. (2024)[190]
Pancreas	T6–T10	Celiac ganglion and plexus	Greater thoracic splanchnic nerve to celiac plexus; celiac vessels to organs	Vasoconstriction; increase secretion of glucagon and decrease secretion of insulin	Mitchell (1953)[18], Faber et al. (2020)[191]

(*continued*)

TABLE 6.1 (*Continued*)

Summary of Autonomic Nervous System Distribution

Structure	Preganglionic Neuron	Postganglion Neuron	Pathway	Function	Reference
Small bowel	(T8)T9–T10(T11)	Celiac and superior mesenteric ganglia	Greater and lesser thoracic splanchnic nerves to the celiac and superior mesenteric ganglia	Diminution of peristalsis and secretions; allows for a reduction in luminal alkalinization	Mitchell (1953)[18], Nylander et al. (2022)[192]
Cecum and appendix	T10–T12	Celiac and superior mesenteric ganglia	Greater and lesser thoracic splanchnic nerves to the celiac and superior mesenteric ganglia	Diminution of peristalsis and secretion	Mitchell (1953)[18]
Descending colon	L1–L2	Inferior mesenteric ganglion	Lumbar and sacral splanchnic nerves and the hypogastric plexus	Diminution of peristalsis and secretion; contraction of the internal anal sphincter	Mitchell (1953)[18]
Adrenal gland	T10–L1(L2)	Adrenal medulla	Greater, lesser, and least thoracic and first lumbar splanchnic nerves	Secretion of catecholamines	Mitchell (1953)[18]
Kidneys	(T11)T12–L1(L2)	Aorticorenal ganglia in celiac plexus	Last two thoracic and first lumbar splanchnic nerves	Secretion of renin and increased glomerular filtration rate	Mitchell (1953)[18], Burnstock and Loesh (2016)[138]
Ureters	L1–L2	Aorticorenal, superior, and inferior mesenteric ganglia	Lumbar and sacral splanchnic nerves and the hypogastric plexus	Alpha-adenoreceptors and tachykinins elicit contraction; beta-adenoreceptors relax ureteral smooth muscle	Mitchell (1953)[18], Canda et al. (2007)[139]
Uterus	(T11)T12–L1(L2)	Inferior hypogastric (uterine) ganglia	Lumbar and sacral splanchnic nerves and the hypogastric plexus	Vasoconstriction and uterine muscle contraction	Mitchell (1953)[18], Sato et al. (1996)[193]
Lower limbs	(T10)T11–L2	Lumbar and sacral paravertebral ganglia	Gray rami to the roots of the lumbar and sacral plexuses	Vasoconstriction, sudomotor, and pilomotor effects	Mitchell (1953)[18]

The understanding of the afferent or sensory role of the vagus nerve, in transmitting information from the gastrointestinal system and abdominal cavity, has recently undergone significant change.[140]

- The immune system acts as a diffuse sensory system (immunosensory system), detecting potentially dangerous substances in the gut.
- Dendritic cells, the sentinel cells of the immune system, release proinflammatory cytokines in response to pathogens or their products.
- Dendritic cells, capable of expressing interleukin-1, are present within the fibers of the vagus nerve and with the paraganglia.
- Interleukin-1 can activate vagal afferent fibers through receptors located on the membrane of the peripheral process of the vagal fiber.
- As a result, a signal is sent into the brainstem and hypothalamus initiating physiologic and psychological responses, termed sickness behavior.
- The only nerve where this has been demonstrated is the vagus.
- Interruption of the vagus nerve can block the induction of pathogen-mediated acute phase responses, such as fever in experimental paradigms.
- This is an excellent example of how the immune system, with its ability to detect a wide array of diverse pathogenic stimuli, can combine with a neural system to affect physiologic and psychological adaptations for survival.

HEPATOBILIARY TREE AND PANCREAS

The vasculature and parenchyma of the liver and pancreas, as well as their associated ducts, receive innervation from both divisions of the autonomic nervous system (Fig. 6.36). In addition, these two organs have an abundant supply of visceral afferent fibers that course in the vagus and thoracic splanchnic nerves.

- Preganglionic sympathetic innervation to these organs arises in thoracic segments at approximately T6 to T9–T10 and

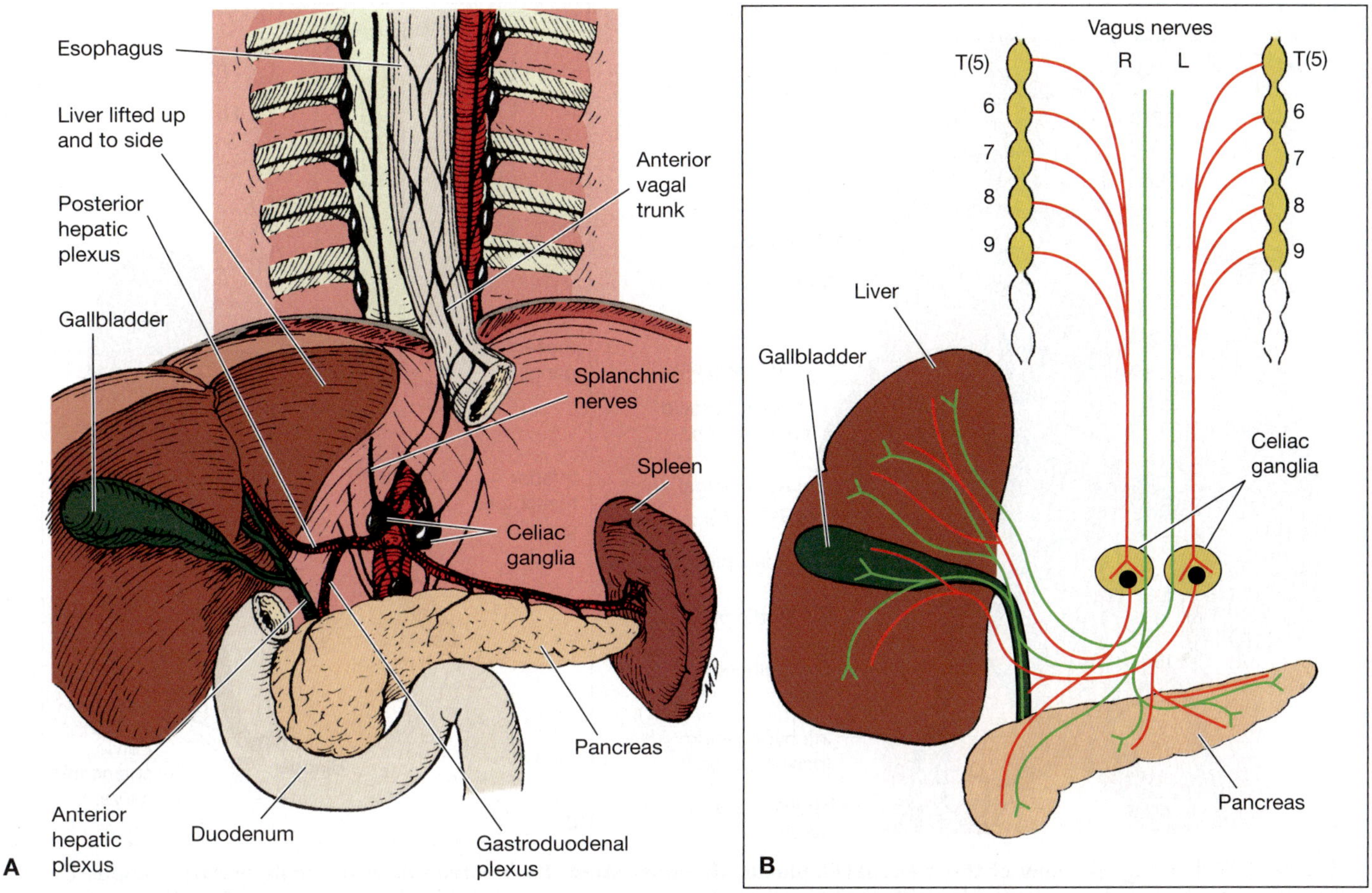

Figure 6.36. Innervation of the hepatobiliary tree and pancreas. The illustration on the left (**A**) represents the efferent fibers associated with the celiac plexus. The illustration on the right (**B**) represents a summary diagram. (Figure compiled with permission from Tobin RW, Kimmey MB. Painful diseases of the gastrointestinal tract. In: Loeser JD, ed. *Bonica's Management of Pain.* 3rd ed. Lippincott Williams & Wilkins; 2001:1269–1292 and Graham DD, Bonica JJ. Painful diseases of the liver biliary system and pancreas. In: Loeser JD, ed. *Bonica's Management of Pain.* 3rd ed. Lippincott Williams & Wilkins; 2001:1293–1308.)

approaches the abdomen through the thoracic splanchnic nerves.[18]

- Sympathetic ganglionic neurons are located in the celiac ganglia. Their postganglionic axons reach the liver and pancreas by hitchhiking on the hepatic and pancreatic branches of the celiac trunk.
- Preganglionic parasympathetic axons, derived from the vagus nerve, pass through the fascia of the celiac region and follow the vasculature to the target organs.
- Sympathetic activation increases the output of glucose from the liver.[141]
- Liver sympathetic overactivity has been associated with increasing hyperglycemia.[142]
- Percutaneous endovascular denervation of the common hepatic artery, a rich supply of sympathetic fibers, has been suggested as a novel treatment for type 2 diabetes.[143]

A significant adrenergic innervation of the interlobular bile ducts, bile ductules, and canals of Hering has been demonstrated.[144]

- Direct innervation of the cholangiocytes has been observed.

A significant percentage of the axons in the vagus and thoracic splanchnic nerves traveling to the liver and pancreas are sensory in nature. Approximately 90% of the vagal axons and 50% of the splanchnic axons to the liver are visceral afferent fibers.[145] These two afferent systems perform different functions.[32]

- Those afferent axons traveling with the vagus nerve have cell bodies located cranially in the nodose ganglion and respond to such stimuli as:
  - plasma glucose concentration
  - portal venous blood osmotic pressure
  - temperature changes
- The visceral afferent fibers associated with the splanchnic nerves have cell bodies located in the dorsal root ganglia of spinal nerves.
  - These afferent fibers tend to be high-threshold mechanoreceptors and chemoreceptors with peripheral processes located in the walls of the biliary system, among other places, and are responsive to stretch and bradykinin concentration.
  - The evidence available to date suggests that pain sensation from the liver and biliary tree is transmitted via the splanchnic nerves and not the vagus nerve.

KIDNEY AND URINARY TRACT

Kidney

Although the kidney is primarily controlled by endocrine mechanisms, it does receive significant innervation from the sympathetic adrenergic system regulating, in part, the glomerular filtration rate, retention of sodium, and release of renin (Table 6.1).[146]

- In addition, the renal nerves interact with cells from the immune system to regulate inflammation in the kidney, which is now thought to be a significant source of hypertension.[147]

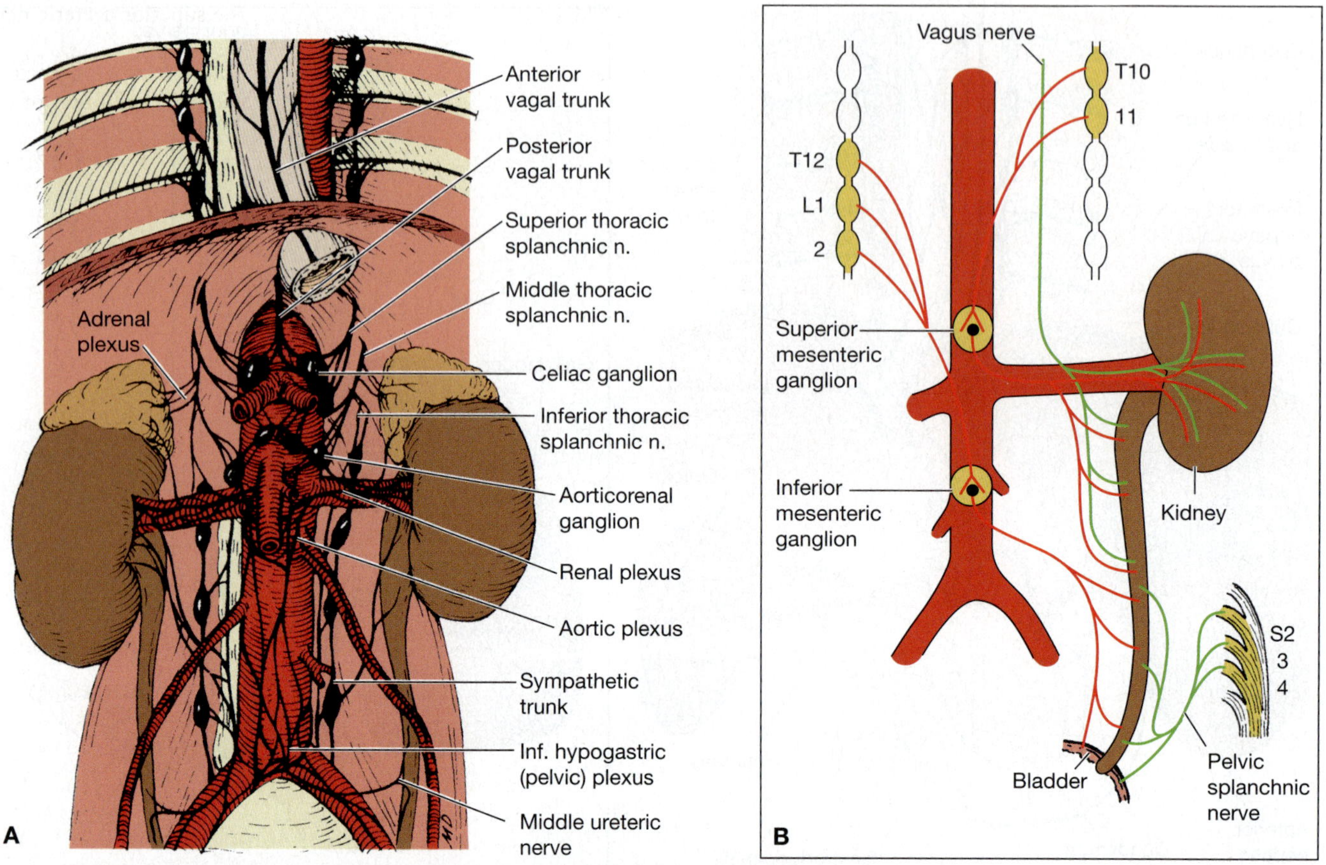

Figure 6.37. Parasagittal view of the male pelvic plexus, demonstrating the innervation of the male urinary bladder. The illustration on the left (**A**) represents the efferent fibers associated with the renal plexus. The illustration on the right (**B**) represents the afferent fibers associated with renal plexus. (Reprinted with permission from Gee WF, Ansell JS. Pelvic and perineal pain of urologic origin. In: Bonica JJ, ed. *The Management of Pain*. 2nd ed. Lea & Febiger; 1990:1368–1394.)

The kidney receives a rich innervation, most of which is derived from the thoracolumbar spinal cord.

- Preganglionic sympathetic neurons regulating the kidney are located in the lateral horn of the spinal cord, extending approximately from segments (T11)T12 to L1(L2) (Fig. 6.37).[18]
- Their axons enter the abdominopelvic plexus over the lower thoracic and first lumbar splanchnic nerves (see Table 6.1) and proceed to the renal hilum where they contribute to a renal plexus of fibers.
- Nerves are also seen joining the renal plexus from the intramesenteric plexus as well as from the superior hypogastric plexus.[18]

The postganglionic sympathetic adrenergic fibers are derived from laterally positioned aorticorenal ganglia, a subdivision of the celiac and SMPs.

- These ganglia are microscopic in size; their postganglionic fibers course into the hilum of the kidney along the renal artery more so than the renal vein.[5]
- Postganglionic sympathetic fibers have been traced to the intrarenal vasculature such as the afferent and efferent arterioles, the juxtaglomerular apparatus as well as the proximal and distal renal tubular system, and the collecting duct system.[138,148]

The adrenergic axons of the mammalian kidney terminate on the[149]:

- afferent and efferent glomerular arterioles
- proximal and distal renal tubules
- ascending limb of the Henle loop
- juxtaglomerular apparatus

All portions of the cortical tubular nephron are under neural influence.

- The relative density of adrenergic fibers is greatest around the ascending limb of the loop of Henle, followed by decreasing relative density by the distal convoluted tubule and the proximal convoluted tubule.[150,151]
- α-Adrenoceptors have been located on the proximal convoluted tubule[152] as well as on the smooth muscle of the vasculature.

Sympathetic innervation of the kidney is involved in the normal regulation of sodium retention, both by increasing the transport of sodium across the tubule walls and by directly increasing the release of renin from the juxtaglomerular apparatus and subsequently the renin–angiotensin–aldosterone system.[146]

- Activation of the sympathetic nervous system outflow to the kidneys increases the reabsorption of sodium and water from the renal tubular system.[148]
- Studies have also shown that there is increased activity in the renal sympathetic nervous system in essential hypertension in humans.[153]

The renal plexus is joined by fibers from the vagus; however, very little vagal parasympathetic (cholinergic) input to the kidney has been reported.

The kidney does, however, receive neuropeptide-containing, primary afferent fibers that course along with the adrenergic fibers (see Fig. 6.37).

- A dual sensory innervation of the kidney exists:
  - Afferent fibers follow the thoracic and lumbar splanchnic nerves back to the spinal cord
  - Afferent fibers follow the vagus nerve back to the brainstem[18]
- Within the kidney, peripheral endings of both mechanoreceptors and chemoreceptors are found in close association with ureteric blood vessels (arteries and veins) and in the walls of the pelvis of the ureter.[154]
- Their cell bodies are in the dorsal root ganglia, located mainly in segments at the thoracolumbar junction (T10 to L3), and their central processes terminate in the dorsal horn of the spinal cord.
- These afferent axons are classified as A-delta and C-fibers.

Vagal afferent fibers, both mechanoreceptors and chemoreceptors, play a role in renorenal reflexes.

- The mechanoreceptors are also involved in modulating cardiovascular reflexes, thus regulating blood pressure.[154]

Pain is the only detectable sensory perception that can be elicited from the kidney.[17]

- This modality is carried in the visceral afferent fibers of the thoracic splanchnic nerves to reach the spinal cord and in the spinothalamic tracts to reach the forebrain.
- In a study of the sympathetic renal afferent fibers in the primate, all spinothalamic tract cells excited by renal afferent fibers were also excited by somatic afferent fibers from the body wall, indicating a powerful somatovisceral convergence on these cells.[154]
- This convergence has been suggested as a mechanism to explain the referral of pain from the kidney to somatic structures, such as the flank of the body.
- In addition, this relationship may explain the palpable changes in the tone of muscle innervated by the segments T10–L1 that accompany renal infection or inflammation.

Ureter

The primary function of the ureter is the unidirectional flow of urine from the kidney to the urinary bladder.

- Although it is richly invested with nerves,[155] peristalsis in the ureter is primarily myogenic in nature, driven by specialized pacemaker cells located in its walls.[156]
- The course of the ureter is retroperitoneal, lying along the posterior abdominal body wall and embedded in the endoabdominal and endopelvic fascia.
- The walls of the ureter consist of interlacing bundles of smooth muscle fibers woven into a theca muscularis.
- Individual smooth muscle cells interconnect via numerous gap junctions, making the muscularis a functional syncytium.[157]
- Modified smooth muscle cells within the muscular layer serve as pacemakers, initiating peristaltic contractions.[158]
- A plexus of efferent and afferent nerve fibers that are capable of regulating the pacemaker cells is wrapped around the muscularis.
- The plexus is rich in peptide-containing neurons and gains in density as it progresses from the renal pelvis to the ureterovesical junction in the pelvis.[159]

The ureter receives its innervation from three different sources, termed superior, middle, and inferior ureteric nerves.[18]

- The upper portion is innervated by the superior ureteric nerves derived mainly from the renal plexus.
  - This plexus contains nerve fibers from the lower thoracic and upper lumbar splanchnic nerve (L1 or L2) and fibers of vagal origin as well.
  - Ganglionic neurons are located in the celiac and associated renal and gonadal (testicular or ovarian) ganglia.
- The middle ureteric nerves supply the intermediate portion of the ureter; they arise from the ipsilateral superior hypogastric plexus.
  - The origin of these fibers is from the lower lumbar splanchnic nerves (L1–L2) most likely these nerves also contain some vagal fibers as well.
  - The middle ureteric nerves are closely associated with the plexus of gonadal nerves.
- The lower portion of the ureter is innervated by the inferior ureteric nerves derived from the inferior hypogastric plexus and is associated with ganglia located in the inferior hypogastric plexus (see Table 6.1 and Fig. 6.37).
  - At this level, the sympathetic innervation from lumbar and sacral splanchnic nerves (L1–L2) contribute to ganglia located in the superior and inferior hypogastric plexus.[160]

The wall of the ureter contains a dense distribution of several types of nerve fibers.

- Sympathetic fibers containing tyrosine hydroxylase and neuropeptide-Y, are present in the outer muscle layers and the surrounding adventitia of the human ureter.[159,161,162]
- Activation of α-adrenergic receptors increases ureter peristalsis and elevates luminal pressures; in contrast, activation of β-adrenergic receptors decreases ureter peristaltic frequency and lowers intraureter pressures.[139,163]
- The actual role of the noradrenergic system in human ureter peristalsis has been questioned, and it appears that control over the surrounding vascular system is the dominant theme for the ureteric nerves.[156]
- Parasympathetic innervation for the upper portion of the ureter arises in the vagus nerve and reaches the ureter through the celiac and SMP.
- The ureteral wall in the pelvic region receives its cholinergic innervation from spinal segments S2 to S4; these pelvic splanchnic nerves communicate with the ureter via the inferior hypogastric plexus.

Acetylcholine-containing neurons are present in the mural ganglia of the ureter, and fibers containing acetylcholine are present in the mammalian ureter.[163,164]

- These fibers are of the greatest density as the ureter enters the vesicle wall.
- Stimulation of the ureter wall with acetylcholine results in an increased contractile activity and an increased basal tone of the mural smooth muscle.
- Acetylcholine also relaxes the ureter resistance arteries using a mechanism involving endothelium-derived nitric oxide.

Much of the peristaltic action present in the ureter is of myogenic origin with pacemaker cells being present in the upper portions of the ureter[139]; however, neurogenic activity is also important in controlling contractions in this organ.

- Ureteral smooth muscle contractions are enhanced by both cholinergic and noradrenergic mechanisms, the noradrenergic being dependent on the ratio of α-adrenergic receptors to β-receptors.
- Generally, neuropeptides facilitate contractions, and nitric oxide will relax the ureteral smooth muscle.

Afferent fibers to the ureter are derived from dorsal root ganglia ranging from the lower thoracic to upper lumbar segments[5]; they have also been demonstrated to arise in the sacral segments, S1–S2, in nonhuman species.[165]

- Two classes of mechanoreceptors have been described in the ureter walls[166]:
  - One class has low thresholds and is responsive to peristaltic-type contractions of the ureteric smooth muscle.
  - The other class of mechanoreceptor has higher thresholds of activation and is most likely related to nociception.
- Many of these primary afferent fibers contain neuropeptides such as substance-P and calcitonin gene–related polypeptide, thereby suggesting that they are involved in nociceptive activities.

Pain, presumably from these nociceptors, is the only sensory perception obtainable from the human ureter.[33]

- In the thoracolumbar dorsal horn of the spinal cord, input from the ureter converges with somatic input from thoracolumbar spinal segments.
- Pain from distention of the ureter is often referred to the somatic body wall over a range of body segments.
  - From the upper ureter, pain refers to the area from the anterior superior spine of the ilium anteriorly to the border of the rectus abdominis muscle (T11–T12).
  - From the middle ureter, pain refers to the area from the inguinal ligament anteriorly to the rectus abdominis muscle (T12–L1).
  - From the lower ureter, pain refers to the suprapubic area (L1) and below into the scrotum or labia (L2), as described by Gee and Ansell.[167]
- This descending segmental pattern of primary afferent fibers from the ureter is responsible for the clinically detectable, descending movement of facilitated segments as any obstructing material moves through the ureteric lumen.

Urinary Bladder

The muscular components of the urinary bladder can be divided into two anatomical and functional parts: the body (or detrusor urinae muscle) and the base (or the trigone muscle).

- The detrusor urinae muscle is the larger of the two parts and is active during expulsion of urine from the bladder.
- The trigone muscle surrounds the openings of the ureter in the base and the opening of the urethra in the neck of the bladder. It acts as an internal sphincter and, when contracted, helps to prevent the flow of urine from the bladder.

The detrusor and the trigone tend to oppose each other in activity.

- Both detrusor and trigone muscles comprise multiple layers of smooth muscle fibers and receive an efferent innervation from the large autonomic pelvic plexus.

A third muscle related to bladder function is located inferior to the trigone in the layers of the perineum.

- It is the deep transverse perineal muscle; the portion of this muscle that surrounds the urethra that is called the sphincter urethra.
- Unlike the detrusor and trigone, this component of the perineal diaphragm is composed of skeletal muscle and innervated by terminal branches of the pudendal nerve, a somatic nerve (S2–S4).

The autonomic innervation of the urinary bladder is accomplished through the hypogastric plexus, which is embedded in endopelvic fascia (Fig. 6.38).

- Parasympathetic preganglionic (cholinergic) fibers from the intermediolateral nucleus of spinal segments S2–S4 enter the hypogastric plexus via the pelvic splanchnic nerves.
- These axons continue anteriorly into the vesicle plexus to terminate on ganglionic neurons located in the walls of the bladder.
- Their postganglionic (cholinergic and purinergic) axons supply motor innervation to all portions of the bladder wall.
- Stimulation of the parasympathetic system, which occurs during voiding, is excitatory to the detrusor muscle and inhibitory to the trigone muscle.[168]

Sympathetic tone facilitates contraction of the trigone muscles and relaxation of the detrusor urinae muscle, which is necessary to allow expansion of the bladder while it is in the filling phase.[167,169]

- Sympathetic preganglionic fibers arise in the intermediolateral nucleus of spinal segments T11–L2 (see Fig. 6.38).
- These fibers leave the sympathetic trunk coursing on both lumbar and sacral splanchnic nerves to enter the inferior hypogastric plexus, eventually targeting prevertebral ganglia.
- Sympathetic postganglionic (adrenergic) axons pass anteriorly through the inferior hypogastric plexus and ultimately contribute to the vesicle plexus in the bladder adventitia.
- Their major target is the smooth muscle cells of the trigone muscle, with a much smaller contribution to the smooth muscle of the detrusor urinae.

The vesicle plexus, a component of the pelvic plexus, contains many ganglionic neurons traditionally associated with the parasympathetic system.[5]

- However, it is now clear that these neurons also receive input from adrenergic axons in the sympathetic system.
- Thus, the sympathetic system can influence the activity of the parasympathetic system by modulating the activity of the ganglion cells.
- The ganglion cells innervating the trigone muscle have α-adrenoceptors on their membranes and respond to sympathetic stimulation by driving contractions.
- Conversely, ganglion cells innervating the detrusor muscle have β-adrenoceptors on their membranes and respond to sympathetic stimulation by driving relaxation.
- It is through this differential distribution of adrenoceptors that the sympathetic nervous system is capable of increasing the tone in the trigone while simultaneously relaxing the detrusor urinae.[170]

The sphincter urethrae muscle, or external urethral sphincter, at the base of the bladder, is skeletal muscle; it receives its innervation from the perineal branches of the pudendal nerve (see Fig. 6.38).

- This is a somatic nerve containing axons from motoneurons located in the ventral horn of the spinal cord (S2–S4). The release of urine from the bladder requires an integrated viscerosomatic reflex involving:
  - Excitation of the parasympathetic system to activate the detrusor urinae muscle.
  - Inhibition of the sympathetic system to relax the trigone and internal sphincteral muscles.
  - Subsequent inhibition of the pudendal nerve to relax the external sphincteral muscles.

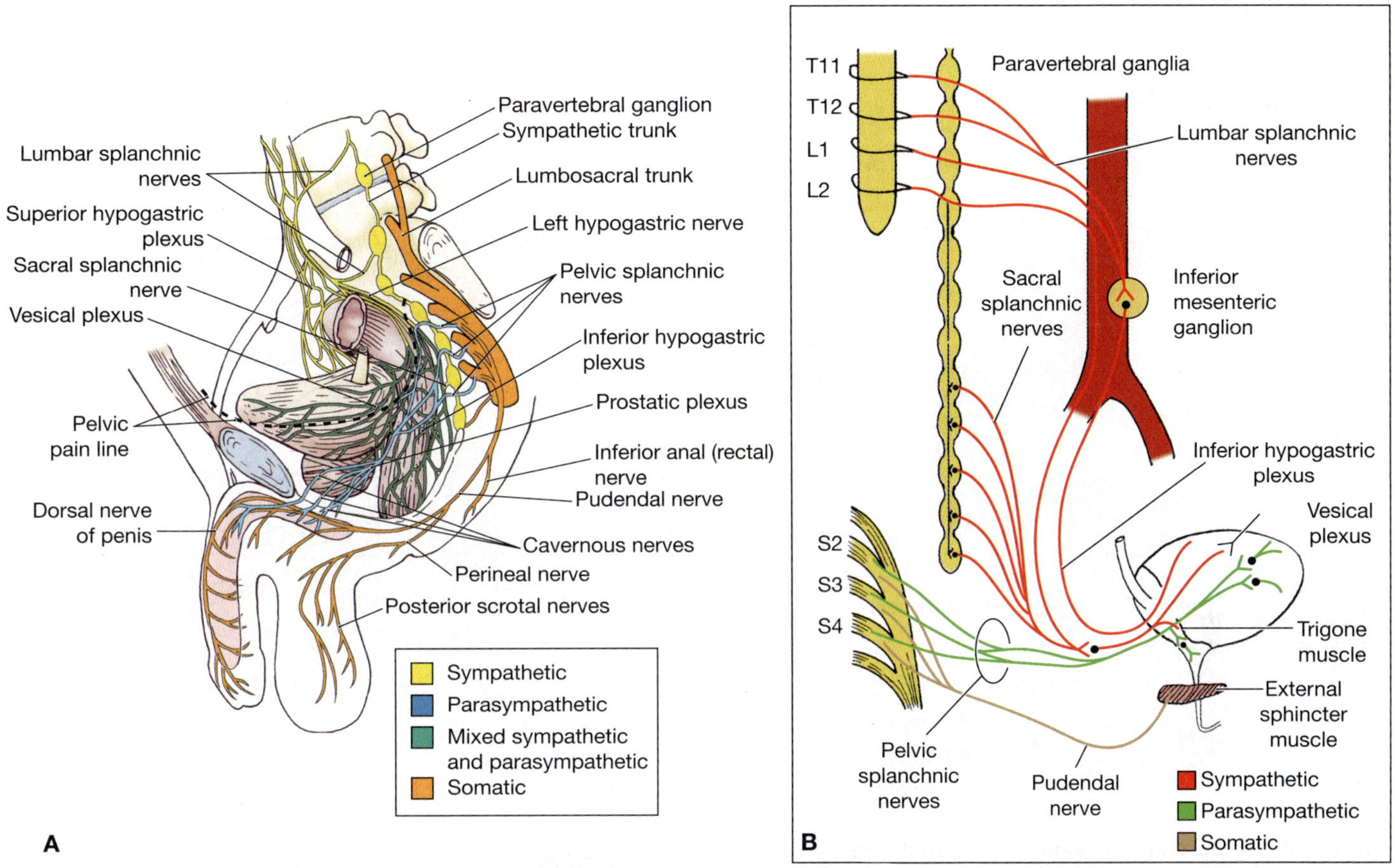

Figure 6.38. A parasagittal view of the male pelvic plexus, demonstrating the innervation of the male reproductive organs. The illustration on the left (**A**) represents the efferent fibers associated with the male pelvic plexus. The illustration on the right (**B**) represents the afferent fibers associated with the male pelvic plexus. (Reprinted with permission from Gee WF, Ansell JS. Pelvic and perineal pain of urologic origin. In: Bonica JJ, ed. *The Management of Pain*. 2nd ed. Lea & Febiger; 1990:1368–1394.)

Vesicle afferent fibers arise from mechanoreceptor endings in the connective tissue and epithelium of the vesicle mucosa.

- These fibers travel over the lumbar and pelvic splanchnic nerves and pudendal nerves to reach the cord at the L1–L2 and S2–S4 levels.
- Cell bodies for the nerves are present in the associated dorsal root ganglia.
- Many of these fibers contain neuropeptides such as those represented in the small-caliber, primary afferent fiber systems.[171]
- The afferent fibers reach primarily the dorsal horn of the spinal cord near their segmental level of entry; however, a small number of these fibers enter the spinal cord and follow the ascending tracts rostrally to terminate in the lower regions of the medulla.

Sensory information from distension of the bladder initiates the reflexes involved in voiding.

- Initial filling of the bladder triggers low-level afferent volleys allowing the bladder to serve as a reservoir for urine, such that:
  - □ The tone in the trigone muscle and external sphincter muscles is increased
  - □ The tone in the detrusor urinae muscle is inhibited
- After a certain level of filling is reached, approximately 200 cc in the average male, a higher intensity of afferent volleys from the bladder wall reverses these reflexes, which prepares the bladder for voiding, such that:
  - □ the detrusor urinae muscle tone is enhanced
  - □ the tone of the trigone and external sphincter is inhibited
- The last step, relaxation of the external sphincter, requires coordination of the suprasegmental control of the bladder musculature, allowing volitional control of voiding.[169]

Central control of the lower urinary tract reflexes involves regions in the spinal cord at the thoracolumbar and sacral, as well as regions in the pons and midbrain.[169]

- This system appears to be sensitive to intense, painful somatic afferent activity.
- Essentially, painful somatic stimulation was excitatory to the relaxed bladder, causing the initiation of peristalsis.
- Conversely, a similar painful stimulus was inhibitory to a bladder that was expanded and actively contracting.[172]
- To be effective, bladder stimuli needed to be in the range required to activate somatic nociceptive fibers.
- Stimulation of the tissue in the perineum gave the most effective response.
- However, stimulation of other regions of the body such as the neck, chest, or abdomen gave an effective inhibitory response in a contracting bladder but not in a relaxed bladder.
- These findings suggest an interesting application for osteopathic manipulative medicine (OMM) in the treatment of postsurgical or post-traumatic injury bladder dysfunctions.

Reproductive Tract

The pelvic and perineal organs of the male and female reproductive systems receive both sympathetic and parasympathetic

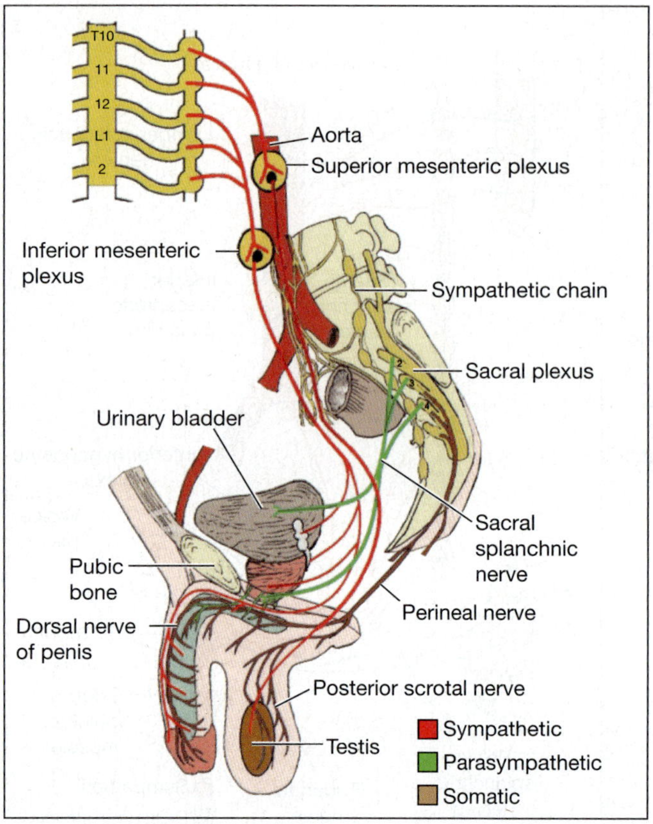

Figure 6.39. A parasagittal view of the male pelvic plexus demonstrating the innervation of the urinary bladder. (Reprinted with permission from Gee WF, Ansell JS. Pelvic and perineal pain of urologic origin. In: Bonica JJ, ed. *The Management of Pain*. 2nd ed. Lea & Febiger; 1990:1368–1394.)

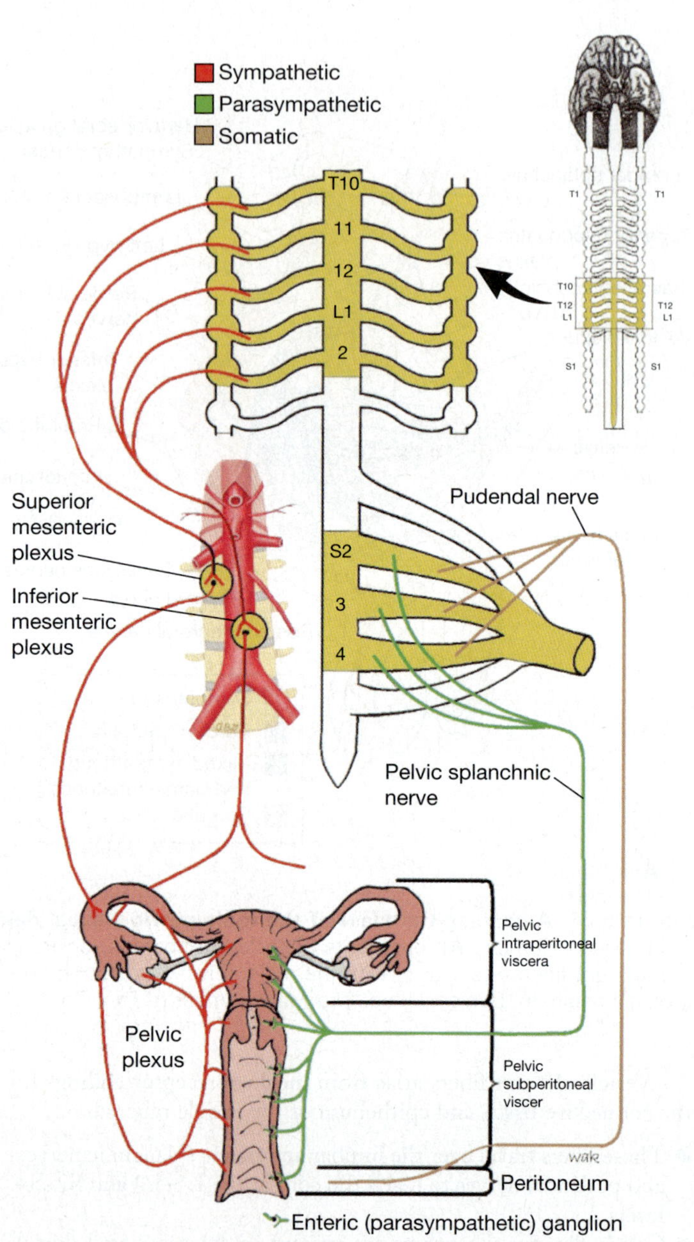

Figure 6.40. Innervation of the female reproductive system. (Modified with permission from Agur AMR, Dalley AF II. *Grant's Atlas of Anatomy*. 12th ed. Wolters Kluwer Health/Lippincott Williams & Wilkins; 2009.)

innervation through the complex abdominopelvic plexus (Figs. 6.39 and 6.40).[5,18,171,173,174]

- This innervation targets the glandular cells and smooth muscle of the vasculature, as well as the mural smooth muscle present in the tubular portions of these organs.
- The origin of this innervation varies according to the embryonic origin of the specific organs.
- The testis and the ovary, which arise in the gonadal ridge of the posterior abdominal wall, receive their efferent supply from the upper abdominal portions of the abdominopelvic plexus.
- The remaining pelvic organs of reproduction are innervated from the lower abdominal and pelvic portion of the plexus.
- Afferent fibers are present in each of these organs, and their input to the spinal cord, either in the thoracolumbar junction or in the sacral region, is a key feature in the presentation of pelvic pain.

TESTIS AND OVARY

The gonadal (testicular and ovarian) arteries are surrounded by a plexus of autonomic nerve fibers.[18,175]

- Preganglionic axons are located in the T10 and T11 segments of the spinal cord, and postganglionic nerves reaching toward the organs are found in three regions:
  - ☐ A superior group of fibers arise from the renal ganglia.
  - ☐ A middle group arises from ganglia in the superior hypogastric plexus and upper portion of the inferior hypogastric nerve.
  - ☐ A third group of fibers arise in the lower portion of the inferior hypogastric plexus.
- In females, the gonadal (ovarian) plexus follows the ovarian artery to innervate the ovary, with twigs extending outward to reach the uterine tubes (see Fig. 6.40).
- In males, the gonadal (spermatic) plexus joins the spermatic cord at the level of the vas deferens in the pelvis and proceeds through the inguinal canal to reach the scrotum (see Fig. 6.39).
- Adrenergic fibers in the testis are present around blood vessels and interstitial cells of the seminiferous tubules and also in the tubules of the epididymis.[163]
- Stimulation of the sympathetic nervous system initiates strong peristaltic waves in the vas deferens, and these are responsible for the propulsion of sperm.
- Parasympathetic innervation of the gonadal tissue is less dense than that of the sympathetic fibers.
- The testis receives mostly sympathetic fiber input, while the epididymis receives both sympathetic and parasympathetic inputs.[5]

- Cholinergic fibers arise from the vesical plexus and join the gonadal plexus as it passes through the pelvis.
- These parasympathetic fibers primarily target the epididymis, vas deferens, and seminal vesicles.

Afferent fibers from the testis, epididymis, and vas deferens extend through the gonadal plexus to reach the thoracolumbar spinal cord (see Fig. 6.39).

- Fibers arising in the testis target segment T10 and above can possibly reach as high up as T6. Fibers from the epididymis enter the spinal cord at T11 and T12, although those from the vas deferens enter at T10–L1.[5,167]

Afferent fibers from the ovary also ascend in the gonadal plexus to enter the spinal cord around the T10 level (see Fig. 6.40).

- The passage of afferent axons from the gonadal tissue to the lower thoracic level of the spinal cord is responsible for the referral of pain to the thoracolumbar junction and the facilitation of segments in this area, consequent to irritation of the gonadal tissue.

PELVIC BASIN REPRODUCTIVE ORGANS

In males and females, the distal portion of the abdominopelvic plexus from each side of the body unites on the midline around the L4 vertebral body to form the superior hypogastric plexus or presacral nerve.[76]

- This unpaired, midline structure descends over the sacral promontory and bifurcates as it enters the pelvic basin forming the bilateral inferior hypogastric plexuses both of which are positioned laterally between the midline pelvic organs and the fascia of the levator ani (Figs. 6.41 to 6.44).
- A contribution to the inferior hypogastric plexus arises from the sacral splanchnic nerves derived from the sacral sympathetic trunk, especially S2.[176]
- Finally, the distal end of the inferior hypogastric plexus receives the pelvic splanchnic nerves, parasympathetic fibers from the sacral nerve roots S2 through S4 and sometimes S5.
- This deep pelvic portion of the inferior hypogastric plexus, uniting the inferior hypogastric nerves with parasympathetic nerves, is often termed the pelvic plexus.[76]
- Organ-specific regions of the pelvic plexus can be identified such as the prostatic, rectal, or uterine plexuses.

PROSTATE

In the male, a prostatic plexus takes the place of the uterine plexus of the female (see Fig. 6.38).

- A dense supply of autonomic fibers has been reported around the human prostate.[177,178]
- Noradrenergic fibers are described as providing an innervation of the stromal tissue, but not the glandular epithelium of the organ.
- These sympathetic fibers arise in the prostatic plexus and, in humans, mediate the prostatic alpha-adrenergic contractile response, an event necessary for normal ejaculation.
- Evidence also supports the role of the adrenergic fibers in stimulating the growth of the prostate in the adult.

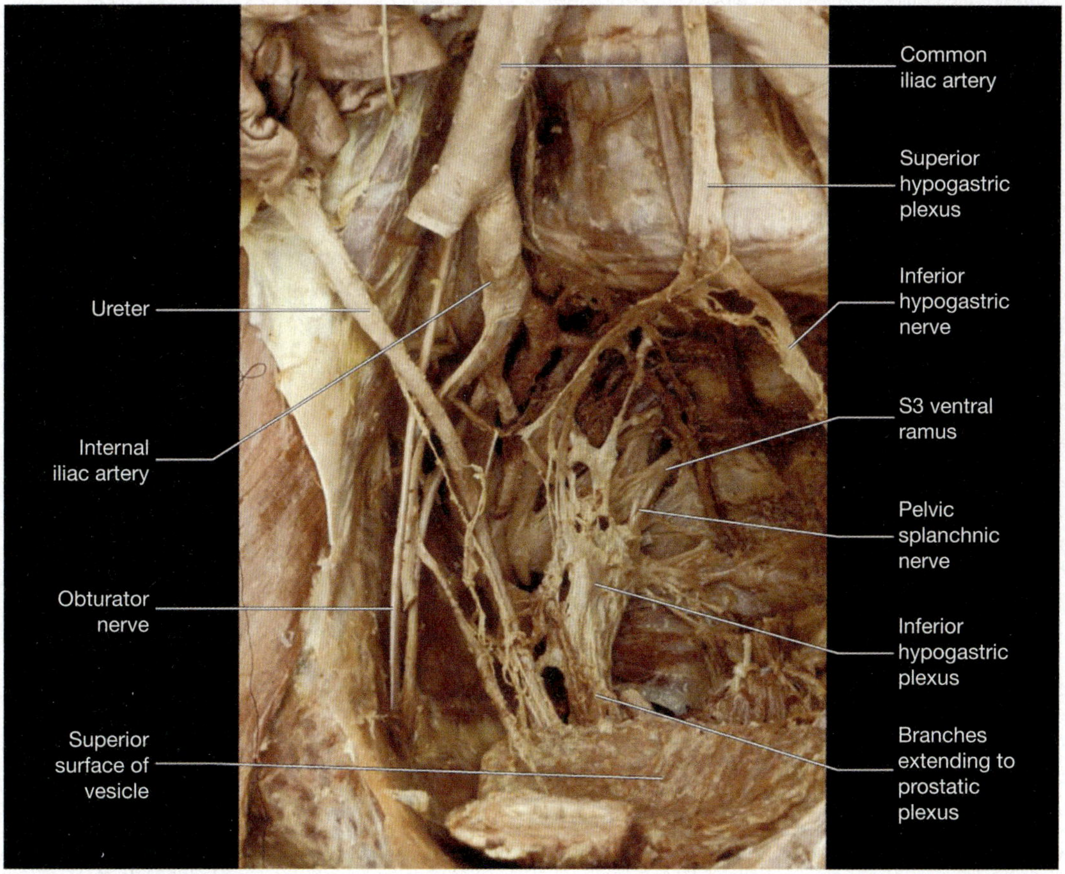

Figure 6.41. Innervation of the male pelvis. This is an anterior view of the male pelvis illustrating the pelvic plexus. The pelvic fascia and rectum have been removed to expose the pelvic plexus. (Used with permission from the Willard/Carreiro Collection, University of New England.)

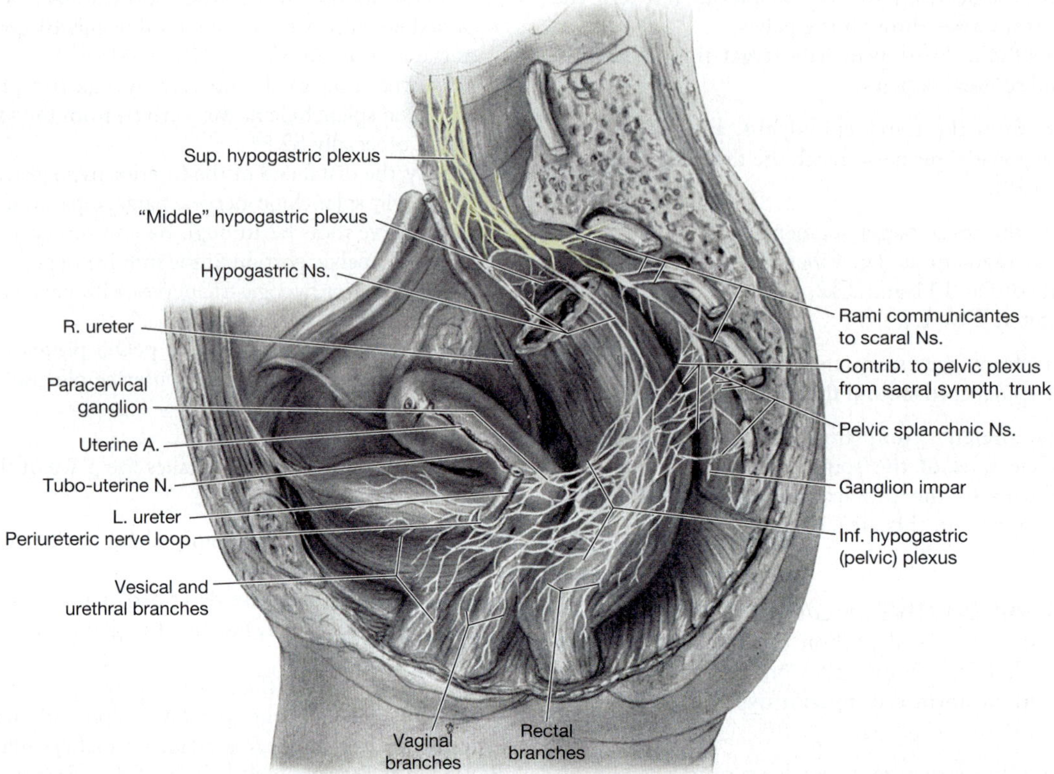

Figure 6.42. Innervation of the female reproductive system. Sympathetic efferent fibers arise in large part from the sacral splanchnic nerves and parasympathetic efferent fibers from the pelvic splanchnic nerves. (From Anatomical Chart Company. *Nervous System Anatomical Chart.* Lippincott Williams & Wilkins; 2003.)

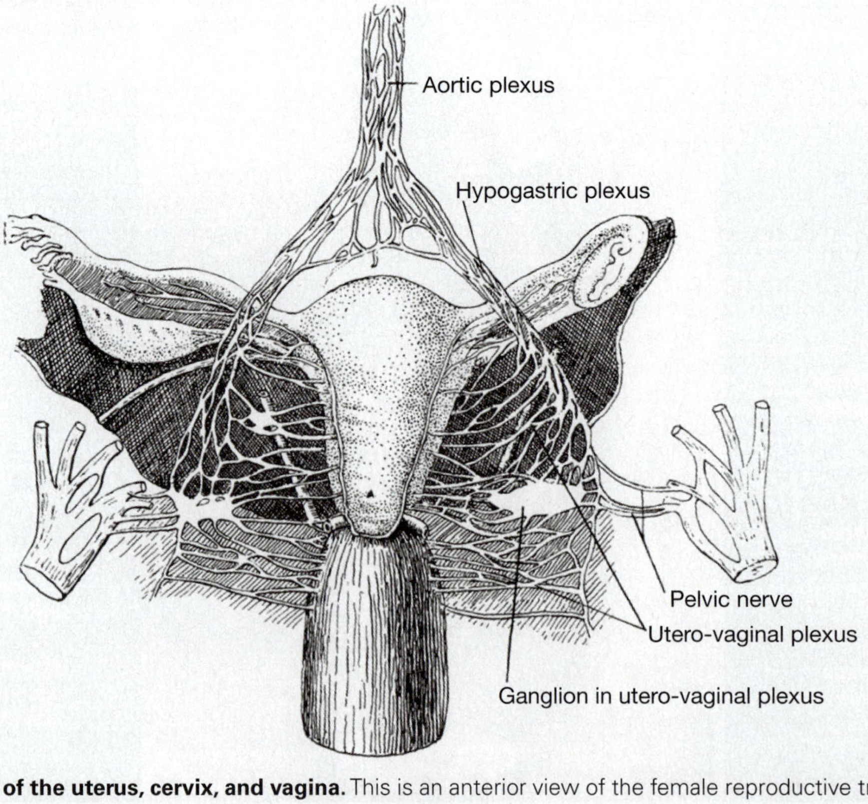

Figure 6.43. Innervation of the uterus, cervix, and vagina. This is an anterior view of the female reproductive tract following the removal of the anterior layer of broad ligament. The ganglion depicted in the figure is situated in between the layers of the broad ligament and lies embedded in the transverse cervical (cardinal) ligament. Pelvic splanchnic fibers are seen joining the plexus from the roots of the sacral nerves. Most of the fibers that enter the hypogastric plexus are sensory in function and will return to the spinal cord by passing over white rami at the T12–L2 level. (Modified with permission from Kuntz A. *The Autonomic Nervous System.* 3rd ed. Lea & Febiger; 1945.)

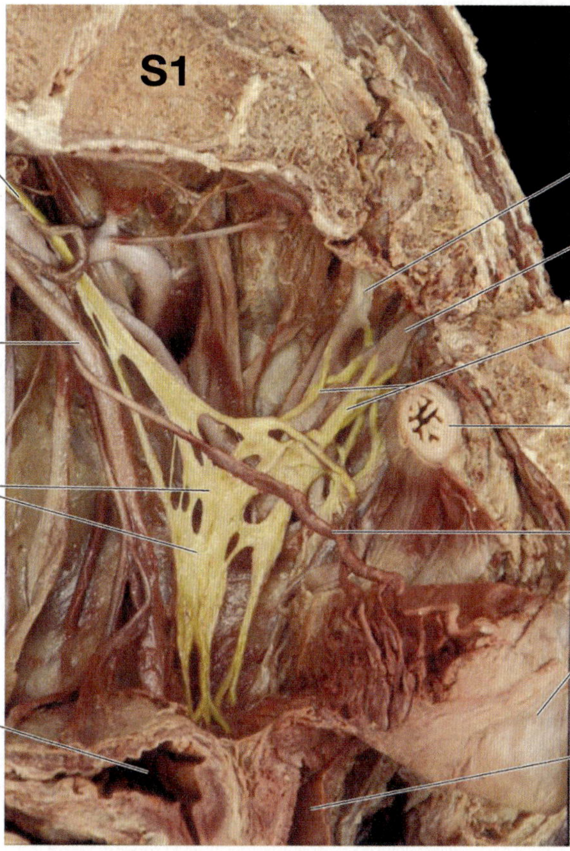

Figure 6.44. A midsagittal section of the female pelvis demonstrating the pelvic plexus. The large masses seen in the pelvic plexus are ganglia. Parasympathetic fibers enter the plexus through the pelvic splanchnic nerves (seen to the right of the plexus). Sensory fibers innervating pelvic organs located at the cervical level and above pass upward from the inferior hypogastric plexus eventually forming the presacral nerve. (Used with permission from the Willard/Carreiro Collection, University of New England.)

- Cholinergic fibers and nonadrenergic, noncholinergic fibers are also seen in the gland, especially around the epithelium, an observation supporting a primary secretory function for these systems.

UTERUS, UTERINE TUBE, CERVIX, AND VAGINA

A dense collection of sympathetic and parasympathetic fibers, derived from the inferior hypogastric plexus, situated on the transverse cervical ligament is termed the uterine or vaginouterine plexus.

- The inferior hypogastric plexus, a complex network of ganglia and fibers, sweeps laterally along the pelvic walls to surround the midline organs of the female pelvis, deep in the pelvis, it acquires branches of the pelvic splanchnic nerves to become the pelvic plexus, a portion of the inferior hypogastric plexus.[76]
- As these fibers cross over the transverse cervical ligament, its fibrous network thickens to form the elaborate plexus of Frankenhuser or uterine plexus (a regional subset of the pelvic plexus; see Figs. 6.43 and 6.44).
- Numerous ganglia are embedded within this plexus.
- From here, autonomic axons accompany the uterine vessels medially along the transverse cervical ligament, they approach the uterus at the level of the cervix
  - Descending branches to the vaginal wall
  - Ascending branches climb up the lateral aspect of the uterus
  - Small branches extend outward to reach the uterine tubes
- The remainder of the pelvic plexus extends anteriorly to surround the urinary bladder (this collection of fibers is often referred to as the vesical plexus).
- Additional branches will extend anteroinferiorly to reach the perineum.

The uterine tubes receive an innervation derived from the uterine and ovarian plexuses as well as a few fibers from the superior hypogastric plexus.[5]

- The uterine plexus is the portion of the pelvic plexus located beneath the broad ligament and situated on the transverse cervical ligament as illustrated in Figures 6.43 and 6.44.
- It is reported that parasympathetic efferent fibers reach the uterine tubes through the uterine plexus, while sympathetic efferent fibers approach primarily through the ovarian and superior hypogastric route.[5]
- Afferent fibers from the uterine tubes accompany the hypogastric plexus to reach the T12, L1, and L2 levels of the spinal cord.

Sympathetic preganglionic neurons capable of influencing the uterus and cervix are located in intermediolateral nucleus of the (T11)T12–L1(L2) spinal segments (see Fig. 6.42).[18]

- Their axons course in the superior and inferior hypogastric plexus to eventually reach a position on the transverse cervical ligament under the broad ligament.
- A particularly large ganglion in this plexus is located near the cervix and is termed the cervical ganglion.[5]
- Postganglionic fibers from the pelvic ganglia enter the walls of the uterus, cervix, and vagina.

For the most part, these adrenergic fibers end on the vasculature of the uterus.

- Some axons terminate in the smooth muscle of the myometrium, particularly in the longitudinal layer[179] and among the glands of the endometrium.

- The parasympathetic input to the uterus and cervix arises in the intermediolateral nucleus of spinal segments S2–S4.
  - These axons target ganglia located in the plexus of Frankenhuser; in turn, postganglionic (cholinergic) axons extend from this plexus into the uterus following the uterine artery.
  - Most of the cholinergic fibers to the uterus are confined to the vascular supply with a small amount reaching the glands of the endometrium and only a few fibers in the circular muscle layer of the myometrium.[179,180]
  - Beyond regulation of the vasculature, the function of this elaborate autonomic innervation of the uterus is not well known.
- Evidence suggests that stimulation of the adrenergic and cholinergic inputs can enhance the contraction of mammalian uterine myometrium.[181]
  - The number and size of adrenergic nerves appear to increase in the uterus during pregnancy,[182] further suggesting a role for these fibers in the uterine contractions of labor and delivery.

The uterus, cervix, and vagina receive an afferent innervation that influences the referral of pain during parturition.[183]

- Experimental studies in cats demonstrate that afferent fibers from the uterus and cervix enter the spinal cord over a range of levels, ranging from T12 to S3[184]; however, in humans, the range appears to be closer to T11 to L1(2).[18]
- The majority of fibers from the fallopian tubes have cell bodies in the dorsal root ganglia of the lumbar segments, whereas the majority of fibers from the cervix have cell bodies in the dorsal root ganglia of the sacral segments.
- Clinical studies suggest that the afferent fibers from the human uterus may project to even higher levels of the spinal cord, such as T10, and that the majority of pain fibers from the uterus enter the thoracolumbar spinal cord.[183,185]
- Nociceptive fibers from the uterus pass upward through the superior hypogastric plexus and lumbar splanchnic nerves to enter the spinal cord over the white rami of the lower thoracic and lumbar segments. For this reason, the white ramus at the thoracolumbar junction can be particularly large.
- The pathways handling sensory information from the female reproductive tract are split.
  - Input from above the cervix ascends through the superior hypogastric plexus to the thoracolumbar junction.
  - Afferent fibers from the cervix and below descend into the sacral spinal cord.[95]
- This arrangement of primary afferent fibers is responsible, in part, for the presentation of low-back pain late in pregnancy as well as accompanying facilitation of spinal segments around the thoracolumbar junction.

ERECTILE TISSUE OF THE PENIS AND CLITORIS

The sympathetic innervation of the vasculature and erectile tissue in the penis and clitoris has its origin in the intermediolateral cell column of spinal cord segments T11 to L2 (see Figs. 6.39 and 6.40). At least two routes exist through which these fibers reach the penis.

- One route involves preganglionic axons that arise in the thoracolumbar spinal cord and synapse in the associated paravertebral ganglia. From these ganglia, adrenergic postganglionic fibers join the hypogastric plexus to pass into the pelvic basin, through the prostatic plexus and eventually enter the penis at its root on the perineal diaphragm.
- The second route comprises sympathetic preganglionic axons from thoracolumbar segments that pass inferiorly into the pelvic basin on the sympathetic trunk.
- They leave the paravertebral trunk through sacral splanchnic nerves to terminate in pelvic ganglia, located deep in the pelvic plexus.
- Postganglionic adrenergic axons from these ganglia pass through the prostatic plexus to reach the root of the penis or clitoris by following the associated perineal vasculature.

Parasympathetic innervation of the vasculature and erectile tissue arises in the sacral (S2 to S4) spinal cord.

- Postganglionic axons from neurons in the scattered ganglia of the pelvic plexus join the sympathetic axons entering the penis or clitoris over its root.
- Nonadrenergic, noncholinergic axons, presumably from cells located in the pelvic ganglia, also innervate the erectile tissue.

The prostatic plexus is located in the fascia between the prostate gland and the levator ani.

- Mixed fibers from the prostatic plexus coalesce along the inferior and lateral border of the gland to form a definitive neurovascular bundle (of Walsh) that sweeps anteriorly into the perineum to innervate the vasculature of the erectile tissue of the male.[186,187]
- In the female, the erectile tissue is innervated by anteriorly directed fibers from the uterine plexus.

Somatic motor innervation of the skeletal muscle associated with the clitoris and penis arises in the Onuf nucleus of the ventral horn of spinal cord segments S2–S4. Their axons travel the course of the pudendal nerve to the perineum where they innervate the following structures, all of which are composed of skeletal muscle:

- Bulbocavernosus muscles
- Ischiocavernosus muscles
- Superficial and deep perineal muscles
- External urethral sphincters
- Anal sphincters

The sex act requires coordinated viscerosomatic reflexes involving the organs and musculature of the pelvic and perineal region.[171]

- Initially, somatic and/or emotional stimuli activate parasympathetic outflow from the sacral cord to the vasculature of the erectile tissue.
- The cholinergic fibers activate the release of nitric oxide from endothelial cells, which relax the vessel walls and result in increased perfusion of the tissue.
- Once the erectile tissue is engorged, additional stimuli initiate a sympathetic barrage from the thoracolumbar junction of the cord. This output results in contraction of smooth muscle in the vas deferens in the male and in the walls of the vagina in the female.
- Coordinated reflex activation of the pudendal nerve subsequently results in contraction of the bulbospongiosus, ischiocavernosus, and transverse perineal muscles. The rhythmic contraction of these muscles assists in forcing the ejaculate along the urethra in the male and constricts the vestibule of the vagina in the female.
- Integration of these three efferent pathways (parasympathetic, sympathetic, and somatic) occurs in the circuitry of the sacral spinal cord segments and is necessary for successful completion of the sex act.

CONCLUSION

The autonomic nervous system plays a major role in orchestrating the diverse functions of our *internal milieu*. Through an extensive network of connections, this diverse system helps maintain the normal rhythm of activity in visceral organs throughout the body, as well as adjusting their output to accommodate external challenges.

The mapping of the autonomic nervous system to the spinal cord provides one avenue through which the visceral efferent system communicates with the somatic nervous system.

- This visceral somatic integration facilitates the occurrence of somatic reactions to visceral disease and visceral reactions to somatic disease.
- The presence of palpable somatic changes can represent diagnostic clues to the underlying visceral issues.

Finally, although the autonomic nervous system is often presented as an efferent system, its nerves throughout the body carry numerous visceral afferent fibers.

- These sensory neurons can adjust both the visceral output to the internal organs and vascular system as well as many of the somatic reflexes.
- Along with the reflexogenic activities, much of what is carried on these visceral afferent fibers is related to the perception of pain.
- The overlap in the spinal territories of the visceral afferent distribution and the somatic afferent distribution provides an explanation for the common occurrence of referred pain of visceral origin into a somatic perception.

ACKNOWLEDGMENTS

Artwork by William A. Kuchera.

REFERENCES

1. Benarroch EE. Central autonomic network. In: Low PA, Benarroch EE, eds. *Clinical Autonomic Disorders*. 3rd ed. Wolters Kluwer Lippincott Williams & Wilkins; 2008:17–28.
2. Bonica JJ. General considerations of pain in the head. In: Bonica JJ, ed. *The Management of Pain*. Lea & Febiger; 1990:651–675.
3. Clarke E, Jacyna LS. *Nineteenth-Century Origins of Neuroscientific Concepts*. University of California Press; 1987.
4. Langley JN. The autonomic nervous system. *Brain*. 1903;26:1–26.
5. Kuntz A. *The Autonomic Nervous System*. Lea & Febiger; 1945.
6. Bannister R, Mathias CJ. *Autonomic Failure*. Oxford Medical Publications; 1992.
7. Low PA, Benarroch EE. *Clinical Autonomic Disorders*. Wolters Kluwer/Lippincott Williams & Wilkins; 2008.
8. Pottenger FM. *Symptoms of Visceral Disease*. Mosby Comp.; 1922.
9. Shouman K, Benarroch EE. Peripheral neuroimmune interactions: selected review and some clinical implications. *Clin Auton Res*. 2021;31:477–489.
10. Nestler EJ, Hyman SE, Malenka RC. *Molecular Pharmacology: A Foundation for Clinical Neuroscience*. McGraw Hill Medical; 2009.
11. Jänig W. *The Integrative Action of the Autonomic Nervous System*. Cambridge University Press; 2022:408.
12. Mitchell GAG. *Cardiovascular Innervation*. E.S. Livingstone; 1956.
13. Parent A. *Carpenter's Human Anatomy*. Williams & Wilkins; 1996.
14. Ropper AH, Samuels MA, Klein JP, Prasad S. *Adams and Victor's Principles of Neurology*. McGraw-Hill; 2019.
15. Prechtl JC, Powley TL. B-afferents: a fundamental division of the nervous system mediating homeostasis? *Behav Brain Sci*. 1990;13:289–331.
16. Willis WD, Coggeshall RE. *Sensory Mechanisms of the Spinal Cord*. Springer Science+Business Media; 2004.
17. Kandel ER, Schwartz JH, Jessell TM, Siegelbaum SA, Hudspeth AJ. *Principles of Neural Sciences*. McGraw-Hill Medical; 2013.
18. Mitchell GAG. *Anatomy of the Autonomic Nervous System*. E. & S. Livingstone Ltd.; 1953.
19. Pick J. *The Autonomic Nervous System*. J.B. Lippincott Comp.; 1970.
20. Gershon MD. The enteric nervous system: a second brain. *Hosp Pract (1995)*. 1999;34(7):31–52.
21. Renkin EM. Control of microcirculation and blood-tissue exchange. In: Renkin EM, Michel CC, eds. *Handbook of Physiology*. Sect. 2, Vol. IV. 1984:627–687.
22. Espinosa-Medina I, Saha O, Boismoreau F, et al. The sacral autonomic outflow is sympathetic. *Science*. 2016;354:893–897.
23. Wang FB, Holst MC, Powley TL. The ratio of pre- to postganglionic neurons and related issues in the autonomic nervous system. *Brain Res Rev*. 1995;21:93–115.
24. Verlinden TJM, Lamers WH, Herrler A, Kohler SE. The differences in the anatomy of the thoracolumbar and sacral autonomic outflow are quantitative. *Clin Auton Res*. 2024;34:79–97.
25. Goyal RK, Hirano I. The enteric nervous system. *N Engl J Med*. 1996;334:1106–1115.
26. Harati Y. Anatomy of the spinal and peripheral autonomic nervous system. In: Low PA, ed. *Clinical Autonomic Disorders*. Little, Brown and Comp.; 1993:17–37.
27. Moore KL, Persaud TVN, Torche M. *The Developing Human: Clinically-Oriented Embryology*. Elsevier; 2020.
28. Freire-Maia L, Azevedo AD. The autonomic nervous system is not a purely efferent system. *Med Hypothesis*. 1990;32:91–99.
29. Gibbins I. Peripheral autonomic pathways. In: Paximos G, Mai JK, eds. *The Human Nervous System*. 2nd ed. Elsevier Academic Press; 2004:134–189.
30. Dockray GJ, Sharkey KA. Neurochemistry of visceral afferent neurones. *Prog Brain Res*. 1986;67:133–148.
31. Schott GD. Visceral afferents: their contribution to "sympathetic dependent" pain. *Brain*. 1994;117:397–413.
32. Cervero F. Mechanisms of acute visceral pain. *Br Med Bull*. 1991;47:549–560.
33. Cervero F. Sensory innervation of the viscera: peripheral basis of visceral pain. *Physiol Rev*. 1994;74:95–138.
34. Clemente CD. *Gray's Anatomy of the Human Body*. Lea & Febiger; 1985.
35. Standring S. *Gray's Anatomy: The Anatomical Basis of Clinical Practice*. Elsevier Limited; 2021.
36. Hollinshead WH. *Anatomy for Surgeons: The Head and Neck*. Hoeber-Harper; 1954.
37. Manson PN, Lazarus RB, Morgan R, Iliff N. Pathways of sympathetic innervation to the superior and inferior (Muller's) tarsal muscles. *Plast Reconstr Surg*. 1986;78:33–40.
38. Hardebo JE. Activation of pain fibers to the internal carotid artery intercranially may cause the pain and local signs of refuced sympathetic and enhanced parasympathetic activity in cluster headache. *Headache*. 1991;31:314–320.
39. Suzuki N, Hardebo JE. Anatomical basis for a parasympathetic and sensory innervation of the intracranial segment of the internal carotid artery in man. Possible implication for vascular headache. *J Neurol Sci*. 1991;104:19–31.
40. Suzuki N, Hardebo JE. The cerebrovascular parasympathetic innervation. *Cerebrovasc Brain Metab Rev*. 1993;5:33–46.
41. Haerer AF. *DeJong's The Neurologic Examination*. J.B. Lippincott; 1992.
42. Spalding JMK, Nelson E. The autonomic nervous system. In: Joynt RJ, ed. *Clinical Neurology*. Vol. 4, Chap. 57. Lippincott Williams & Wilkins; 1986:1–58.
43. Wilson-Pauwels L, Stewart PA, Akesson EJ. *Autonomic Nerves*. B.C. Decker; 1997.
44. Drummond PD. Sweating and vascular responses in the face: normal regulation and dysfunction in migraine, cluster headache and harlequin syndrome. *Clin Auton Res*. 1994;4:273–285.
45. Bogduk N, Windsor M, Inglis A. The innervation of the cervical intervertebral discs. *Spine*. 1988;13:2–8.
46. Groen GJ, Baljet B, Drukker J. Nerves and nerve plexuses of the human vertebral column. *Am J Anat*. 1990;188:282–296.
47. Stilwell DL Jr. The nerve supply of the vertebral column and its associated structures in the monkey. *Anat Rec*. 1956;125:139–169.
48. Bove GM, Moskowitz MA. Primary afferent neurons innervating guinea pig dura. *J Neurophysiol*. 1997;77:299–308.
49. Keller JT, Marfurt CF. Peptidergic and serotonergic innervation of the rat dura mater. *J Comp Neurol*. 1991;309:515–534.

50. Keller JT, Marfurt CF, Dimlich RVW, Tierney BE. Sympathetic innervation of the supratentorial dura mater of the rat. *J Comp Neurol.* 1989;290:310–321.
51. Mitchell GAG. The cranial extremities of the sympathetic trunks. *Acta Anat (Basel).* 1953;18:195–201.
52. Ruskell GL. The orbital branches of the pterygopalatine ganglion and their relationship with internal carotid nerve branches in primates. *J Anat.* 1970;106:323–339.
53. Suzuki N, Hardebo JE, Skagerberg G, Owman C. Central origins of preganglionic fibers to the sphenopalatine ganglion in the rat. A fluorescent retrograde tracer study with special reference to its relation to central catecholaminergic systems. *J Auton Nerv Syst.* 1990;30:101–109.
54. Walters BB, Gillespie SA, Moskowitz MA. Cerebrovascular projections from the sphenopalatine and otic ganglia to the middle cerebral artery of the cat. *Stroke.* 1986;17:488–494.
55. Hardebo JE, Suzuki N, Ekblad E, Owman C. Vasoactive intestinal polypeptide and acetylcholine coexist with neuropeptide Y, dopamine-beta-hydroxylase, tyrosine hydroxylase, substance P or calcitonin gene-related peptide in neuronal subpopulations in cranial parasympathetic ganglia of rat. *Cell Tissue Res.* 1992;267:291–300.
56. Suzuki N, Hardebo JE, Owman C. Origins and pathways of cerebrovascular nerves storing substance P and calcitonin gene-related peptide in rat. *Neuroscience.* 1989;31:427–438.
57. Moskowitz MA. The neurobiology of vascular head pain. *Ann Neurol.* 1984;16:157–168.
58. Edvinsson JCA, Vigano A, Alekseeva A, et al; European Headache Federation School of Advanced Studies (EHF-SAS). The fifth cranial nerve in headaches. *J Headache Pain.* 2020;21:65.
59. Vanhoutte PM, Shepherd JT. Autonomic nerves of the systemic blood vessels. In: Dyck PNPJ, Thomas PK, eds. W.B. Saunders Company; 1993:208–227.
60. Burnstock G. Cholinergic and purinergic regulation of blood vessels. In: Bohr DF, Somlyo AD, Sparks HW, Geiger SR, eds. *Handbook of Physiology: Section 2, The Cardiovascular System: Volume II, Vascular Smooth Muscle.* American Physiology Society; 1980:567–612.
61. Joyner MJ, Halliwill JR. Sympathetic vasodilatation in human limbs. *J Physiol.* 2000;526:471–480.
62. Bevan JA, Bevan RD, Duckles SP. Adrenergic regulation of vascular smooth muscle. In: Bohr DF, Somlyo AP, Sparks HV, Geiger SR, eds. *Handbook of Physiology: Section 2, The Cardiovascular System: Volume II, Vascular Smooth Muscle.* American Physiology Society; 1980:515–566.
63. Shepherd RFJ, Shepherd JT. Control of blood pressure and the circulation in man. In: Bannister R, Mathias CJ, eds. *Autonomic Failure.* 3rd ed. Oxford Medical Publications; 1992:78–93.
64. Joyner MJ, Shepherd JT. Autonomic control of circulation. In: Low PA, ed. *Clinical Autonomic Disorders.* Little, Brown and Company; 1993:55–67.
65. Kawarai M, Koss MC. Neurogenic cutaneous vasodilation in the cat forepaw. *J Auton Nerv Syst.* 1992;37:39–46.
66. Rees H, Sluka KA, Westlund KN, Willis WD. Do dorsal root reflexes augment peripheral inflammation? *Neuroreport.* 1994;5:821–824.
67. Jinkins JR, Whittermore AR, Bradley WG. The anatomic basis of vertebrogenic pain and the autonomic syndrome associated with lumbar disk extrusion. *AJR Am J Roentgenol.* 1989;152:1277–1289.
68. Yonehara N, Chen JQ, Imai Y, Inoki R. Involvement of substance P present in primary afferent neurons in modulation of cutaneous blood flow in the instep of the rat hind paw. *Br J Pharmacol.* 1992;106:256–262.
69. Basbaum AI, Levine JD. The contributions of the nervous system to inflammation and inflammatory disease. *Can J Physiol Pharmacol.* 1991; 69:647–651.
70. Kidd BL, Gibson SJ, O'Higgins F, et al. A neurogenic mechanism for symmetrical arthritis. *Lancet.* 1989;334:1128–1130.
71. Gonzales R, Sherbourne CD, Goldyne ME, Levine JD. Noradrenaline-induced prostaglandin production by sympathetic postganglionic neurons is mediated by 2-adrenergic receptors. *J Neurochem.* 1991;57:1145–1150.
72. Levine JD, Fields HL, Basbaum AI. Peptides and the primary afferent nociceptor. *J Neurosci.* 1993;13:2273–2286.
73. Stead RH, Dixon MF, Bramwell NH, Riddell RH, Bienenstock J. Mast cells are closely apposed to nerves in the human gastrointestinal mucosa. *Gastroenterology.* 1989;97:575–585.
74. Levine JD, Coderre TJ, Covinsky K, Basbaum AI. Neural influences on synovial mast cell density in rat. *J Neurosci Res.* 1990;26:301–307.
75. Levine JD, Dardick SJ, Roizen MF, Helms C, Basbaum AI. Contribution of sensory afferents and sympathetic efferents to joint injury in experimental arthritis. *J Neurosci.* 1986;6:3423–3429.
76. Hollinshead WH. *Anatomy for Surgeons: The Thorax, Abdomen and Pelvis.* Hoeber-Harper; 1956.
77. Chen HS, van Roon L, Ge Y, et al. The relevance of the superior cervical ganglion for cardiac autonomic innervation in health and disease: a systematic review. *Clin Auton Res.* 2024;34:45–77.
78. Mizeres NJ. The cardiac plexus in man. *Am J Anat.* 1963;112:141–141.
79. Standish A, Enquist LW, Escardo JA, Schwaber JS. Central neuronal circuit innervating the rat heart defined by transneuronal transport of pseudorabies virus. *J Neurosci.* 1995;15:1998–2012.
80. Standish A, Enquist LW, Schwaber JS. Innervation of the heart and its central medullary origin defined by viral tracing. *Science.* 1994;263:232–234.
81. Levy M, Martin PJ. Neural control of the heart. In: *Handbook of Physiology, Section 2: The Nervous System.* Vol. 1. OUP Australia and New Zealand; 1979:581–620.
82. Talman WT. The central nervous system an cardiovascular control in health and disease. In: Low PA, ed. *Clinical Autonomic Disorders.* Little, Brown and Comp. 1993;39–53.
83. Baluk P, Gabella G. Some intrinsic neurons of the guinea-pig heart contain substance-P. *Neurosci Lett.* 1989;104:269–273.
84. Quigg M. Distribution of vagal afferent fibers of the guinea pig heart labeled by anterograde transport of conjugated horseradish peroxidase. *J Auton Nerv Syst.* 1991;36:13–24.
85. Quigg M, Elfvin LG, Aldskogius H. Distribution of cardiac sympathetic afferent fibers in the guinea pig heart labeled by anterograde transport of wheat germ agglutinin-horseradish peroxidase. *J Auton Nerv Syst.* 1988; 25:107–118.
86. Hopkins DA, Armour JA. Ganglionic distribution of afferent neurons innervating the canine heart and cardiopulmonary nerves. *J Auton Nerv Syst.* 1989;26:213–222.
87. Malliani A, Lombardi F, Pagni M. Sensory innervation of the heart. *Prog Brain Res.* 1986;67:39–48.
88. Loukas M, Du Plessis M, Louis RG Jr, Tubbs RS, Wartmann CT, Apaydin N. The subdiaphragmatic part of the phrenic nerve—morphometry and connections to autonomic ganglia. *Clin Anat.* 2016;29:120–128.
89. Verlinden TJM, van Dijk P, Herrler A, de Gier-de Vries C, Lamers WH, Kohler SE. The human phrenic nerve serves as a morphological conduit for autonomic nerves and innervates the caval body of the diaphragm. *Sci Rep.* 2018;8:11697.
90. Oliva-Pascual-Vaca A, Gonzalez-Gonzalez C, Oliva-Pascual-Vaca J, et al. Visceral origin: an underestimated source of neck pain. A systematic scoping review. *Diagnostics (Basel).* 2019;9:186.
91. Foreman RD, Blair RW, Ammons WS. Neural mechanisms of cardiac pain. *Prog Brain Res.* 1986;67:227–243.
92. Bonica JJ. General considerations of pain in the chest. In: Bonica JJ, ed. *The Management of Pain.* Lea & Febiger; 1990:959–1000.
93. Ammons WS. Cardiopulmonary sympathetic afferent excitation of lower thoracic spinoreticular and spinothalmic neurons. *J Neurophysiol.* 1990; 64:1907–1916.
94. Beal MC. Viscerosomatic reflexes: a review. *J Am Osteopath Assoc.* 1985; 85:786–801.
95. Ruch TC. Pathophysiology of pain. In: Ruch TC, Patton HD, Woodbury JW, Towe AL, eds. *Neurophysiology.* 2nd ed. W.B. Saunders Comp.; 1965:345–363.
96. Cox JM, Gorbis S, Dick LM, Rogers JC, Rogers FJ. Palpable musculoskeletal findings in coronary artery disease: results of a double-blind study. *J Am Osteopath Assoc.* 1983;82:832–836.
97. Sato A, Schmidt RF. Somatosympathetic reflexes: afferent fibers, central pathways, discharge characteristics. *Physiol Rev.* 1973;53:916–947.
98. Sato A, Sato Y, Schmidt RF. The effects of somatic afferent activity on the heart rate. In: Brooks C, ed. *Integrative functions of the Autonomic Nervous System.* Elsevier; 1979:275–282.
99. Sato A, Sato Y, Schmidt RF. Changes in blood pressure and heart rate induced by movements of normal and inflamed knee joints. *Neurosci Lett.* 1984;52:55–60.

100. Kimura A, Ohsawa H, Sato A, Sato Y. Somatocardiovascular reflexes in anesthetized rats with the central nervous system intact or acutely spinalized at the cervical level. *Neurosci Res.* 1995;22:297–305.
101. Sun N, Liu XH, Du JQ, Zhu JX, Tang JS, Li Q. Rostroventral medulla-mediated biphasic modulation of the rat cardiosomatic motor reflex. *Neuroscience.* 2011;185:174–182.
102. Thurlbeck WM, Miller RR. The respiratory system. In: Rubin E. Farber JL, eds. *Pathology*. J.B. Lippincott; 1988:542–627.
103. Barnes PJ, Baraniuk JN, Belvisi MG. Neuropeptides in the respiratory tract. *Am Rev Respir Dis.* 1991;144:1187–1198.
104. Canning BJ. Reflex regulation of airway smooth muscle tone. *J Appl Physiol (1985).* 2006;101:971–985.
105. Kistemaker LEM, Prakash YS. Airway innervation and plasticity in asthma. *Physiology (Bethesda).* 2019;34:283–298.
106. Drazen JM, Gaston B, Shore SA. Chemical regulation of pulmonary airway tone. *Annu Rev Physiol.* 1995;57:151–170.
107. Morton DR, Klassen KP, Curtis GM. Clinical physiology of the human bronchi: I. Pain of tracheobronchial origin. *Surgery.* 1950;28:669–669.
108. Sivarao DV, Goyal RK. Functional anatomy and physiology of the upper esophageal sphincter. *Am J Med.* 2000;108(Suppl 4a):27S–37S.
109. Richards WG, Sugarbaker DJ. Neuronal control of esophageal function. *Chest Surg Clin N Am.* 1995;5:157–171.
110. Collman PI, Tremblay L, Diamant NE. The central vagal efferent supply to the esophagus and lower esophageal sphincter of the cat. *Gastroenterology.* 1993;104:1430–1438.
111. Sengupta JN. An overview of esophageal sensory receptors. *Am J Med.* 2000;108(Suppl 4a):87S–89S.
112. Hightower NC. Applied anatomy and physiology of the esophagus. In: Bockus HL, ed. *Gastroenterology.* W.B. Saunders Comp.; 1974:127–142.
113. Goyal RK, Padmanabhan R, Sang Q. Neural circuits in swallowing and abdominal vagal afferent-mediated lower esophageal sphincter relaxation. *Am J Med.* 2001;111(Suppl 8A):95S–105S.
114. Collman PI, Tremblay L, Diamant NE. The distribution of spinal and vagal sensory neurons that innervate the esophagus of the cat. *Gastroenterology.* 1992;103:817–822.
115. Pope CE. Heartburn, dysphagia, and chest pain of esophageal origin. In: Sleisenger MH, Fordtran JS, eds. *Gastrointestinal Disease: Pathophysiology, Diagnosis, Management.* W.B. Saunders Comp.; 1983:145–148.
116. Bennett J. ABC of the upper gastrointestinal tract: oesophagus: atypical chest pain and motility disorders. *BMJ.* 2001;323:791–794.
117. Myers DE. Review of visceral throat and chest disorders causing nonodontogenic orofacial pain. *J Am Dent Assoc.* 2022;153:769–775.
118. Pope CE. Chest pain of esophageal origin. In: Loeser JD, Butler SH, Chapman CR, Turk DC, eds. *Bonica's Management of Pain.* Lippincott Williams & Wilkins; 2001.
119. Stelmakh GY, Khmara TV, Lukashevych IV, Vizniuk VV, Kiiun ID, Knut RP. The source of innervation of the aortic arch and thoracic aorta in human fetuses. *Arch Balkian Med Union.* 2021;56:468–476.
120. Bulloch K. Neuroanatomy of lymphoid tissue: a review. In: Guillemin R, Cohn M, Melnechuk T, eds. *Neural Modulation of Immunity.* Raven Press; 1985:111–141.
121. McHale NG. Innervation of the lymphatic circulation. In: Johnston MG, ed. *Experimental Biology of the Lymphatic Circulation.* Elsevier Scientific Pub.; 1985:121–140.
122. Benoit JN. Effects of alpha-adrenergic stimuli on mesenteric collecting lymphatics in the rat. *Am J Physiol.* 1997;273:R331–R336.
123. Elaut L. The surgical anatomy of the so called presacral nerve. *Surg Gynecol Obstet.* 1932;55:581–589.
124. Sharkey KA, Mawe GM. The enteric nervous system. *Physiol Rev.* 2023;103:1487–1564.
125. Wood JD. Physiology of the enteric nervous system. In: Johnson LR, ed. *Physiology of the Gastrointestinal Tract.* Vol. 1. Raven Press; 1981:1–37.
126. Gabella G. Structure of muscles and nerves in the gastrointestinal tract. In: Johnson LR, ed. *Physiology of the Gastrointestinal Tract.* Raven Press; 1981:197–241.
127. Ottaway CA. Neuroimmunomodulation in the intestinal mucosa. *Gastroenterol Clin North Am.* 1991;20:511–529.
128. Bloom W, Fawcett D. *A Textbook of Histology.* W.B.Saunders Comp.; 1968.
129. Pawlina W. *Histology: A Text with Atlas: With Correlated Cell and Molecular Biology.* Lippincott Williams & Wilkins; 2021.
130. Schofield GC. Anatomy of muscular and neural tissues in the alimentary canal. In: Code C, ed. *Handbook of Physiology: Section 6, Alimentary Canal: Volume IV, Motility.* American Physiology Society; 1968:1579–1627.
131. Sanders KM, Ward SM. Nitric oxide as a mediator of nonadrenergic noncholinergic neurotransmission. *Am J Physiol.* 1992;262:G379–G392.
132. Stark ME, Szurszewski JH. Role of nitric oxide in gastrointestinal and hepatic function and disease. *Gastroenterology.* 1992;103:1928–1949.
133. Mayer EA, Raybould HE. Role of visceral afferent mechanisms in functional bowel disorders. *Gastroenterology.* 1990;99:1688–1704.
134. Blau JN, MacGregor EA. Migraine and the neck. *Headache.* 1994;34:88–90.
135. JänigW, Morrison JFB. Functional properties of spinal visceral afferents supplying abdominal and pelvic organs, with special emphasis on visceral nociception. *Prog Brain Res.* 1986;67:87–114.
136. Cervero F. Neurophysiology of gastrointestinal pain. *Baillieres Clin Gastroenterol.* 1988;2:183–199.
137. Shirasaka C, Tsuji H, Asoh T, Takeuchi Y. Role of the splanchnic nerves in the endocrine and metabolic response to abdominal surgery. *Br J Surg.* 1986;73:142–145.
138. Burnstock G, Loesch A. Sympathetic innervation of the kidney in health and disease: emphasis on the role of purinergic cotransmission. *Auton Neurosci.* 2016;204:4–16.
139. Canda AE, Turna B, Cinar GM, Nazli O. Physiology and pharmacology of the human ureter: basis for current and future treatments. *Urol Int.* 2007;78:289–298.
140. Goehler LE, Gaykema RP, Hansen MK, Anderson K, Maier SF, Watkins LR. Vagal immune-to-brain communication: a visceral chemosensory pathway. *Auton Neurosci.* 2000;85:49–59.
141. Nonogaki K, Iguchi A. Role of central neural mechanisms in the regulation of hepatic glucose metabolism. *Life Sci.* 1997;60:797–807.
142. Silva A, Caron A. Pathophysiological mechanisms that alter the autonomic brain-liver communication in metabolic diseases. *Endocrinology.* 2021;162:bqab164.
143. Tzafriri AR, Garcia-Polite F, Keating J, et al. Morphometric analysis of the human common hepatic artery reveals a rich and accessible target for sympathetic liver denervation. *Sci Rep.* 2022;12:1413.
144. Zanchi A, Reidy J, Feldman HJ, et al. Innervation of the proximal human biliary tree. *Virchows Arch.* 2020;477:385–392.
145. Mulholland MW, Debas HT. Diseases of the liver, biliary system, and pancreas. In: Bonica JJ, ed. *The Management of Pain.* Lea & Febiger; 1990:1214–1231.
146. Osborn JW, Tyshynsky R, Vulchanova L. Function of renal nerves in kidney physiology and pathophysiology. *Annu Rev Physiol.* 2021;83:429–450.
147. Gauthier MM, Hayoz S, Banek CT. Neuroimmune interplay in kidney health and disease: role of renal nerves. *Auton Neurosci.* 2023;250:103133.
148. DiBona GF. Physiology in perspective: the wisdom of the body. Neural control of the kidney. *Am J Physiol Regul Integr Comp Physiol.* 2005;289:R633–R641.
149. DiBona GF, Kopp UC. Neural control of renal function. *Physiol Rev.* 1997;77:75–197.
150. Barajas L, Powers K. Innervation of the renal proximal convoluted tubule of the rat. *Am J Anat.* 1989;186:378–388.
151. Barajas L, Powers K, Wang P. Innervation of the renal cortical tubules: a quantitative study. *Am J Physiol.* 1984;247:F50–F60.
152. Insel PA, Snavely MD, Healy DP, Munzel PA, Potenza CL, Nord EP. Radioligand binding and functional assays demonstrate postsynaptic alpha2-receptors on proximal tubules of rat and rabbit kidney. *J Cardiovasc Pharmacol.* 1985;7:S9–S17.
153. Hollenbreg NK. Renal vascular tone in essential and secondary hypertension. *Medicine (Baltimore).* 1975;54:29–44.
154. Ammons WS. Electrophysiological characteristics of primate spinothalamic neurons with renal and somatic inputs. *J Neurophysiol.* 1989;61(6):1121–1130.
155. Nemeth L, O'Briain DS, Puri P. Demonstration of neuronal networks in the human upper urinary tract using confocal laser scanning microscopy. *J Urol.* 2001;166:255–258.

156. Santicioli P, Maggi CA. Myogenic and neurogenic factors in the control of pyeloureteral motility and ureteral peristalsis. *Pharmacol Rev.* 1998;50: 683–722.
157. Tahara H. The three-dimensional structure of the musculature and the nerve elements in the rabbit ureter. *J Anat.* 1990;170:183–191.
158. Weiss RM. Physiology and pharmacology of the renal pelvis and ureter. In: Walsh C'sUPC, Gittes RF, Perlmutter AD, Stamey TA, eds. W.B. Saunders Comp.; 1986;94–128.
159. Edyvane KA, Trussell DC, Jonavicius J, Henwood A, Marshall VR. Presence and regional variation in peptide-containing nerves in the human ureter. *J Auton Nerv Syst.* 1992;39:127–137.
160. Ansell JS, Gee WF. Diseases of the kidney and ureter. In: Bonica JJ, ed. *The Management of Pain.* Lea & Febiger; 1990:1232–1249.
161. Edyvane KA, Smet PJ, Trussell DC, Jonavicius J, Marshall VR. Patterns of neuronal colocalisation of tyrosine hydroxylase, neuropeptide Y, vasoactive intestinal polypeptide, calcitonin gene-related peptide and substance P in human ureter. *J Auton Nerv Syst.* 1994;48:241–255.
162. Smet PJ, Edyvane KA, Jonavicius J, Marshall VR. Colocalization of nitric oxide synthase with vasoactive intestinal peptide, neuropeptide Y, and tyrosine hydroxylase in nerves supplying the human ureter. *J Urol.* 1994;152:1292–1296.
163. Stewart JD. Autonomic regulation of sexual function. In: Low PA, ed. *Clinical Autonomic Disorders.* Little, Brown and Comp; 1993:117–123.
164. Prieto D, Simonsen U, Martin J, et al. Histochemical and functional evidence for a cholinergic innervation of the equine ureter. *J Auton Nerv Syst.* 1994;47:159–170.
165. Semenenko FM, Cervero F. Afferent fibres from the guinea-pig ureter: size and peptide content of the dorsal root ganglion cells of origin. *Neuroscience.* 1992;47:197–201.
166. Cervero F, Sann H. Mechanically evoked responses of afferent fibres innervating the guinea-pig's ureter: an in vitro study. *J Physiol.* 1989;412:245–266.
167. Gee WF, Ansell JS. Pelvic and perineal pain of urologic origin. In: Bonica JJ, ed. *The Management of Pain.* Lea & Febiger; 1990:1368–1394.
168. De Groat WC. Anatomy and physiology of the lower urinary tract. *Urol Clin North Am.* 1993;20:383–401.
169. De Groat WC, Yoshimura N. Anatomy and physiology of the lower urinary tract. *Handb Clin Neurol.* 2015;130:61–108.
170. Ochodnicky P, Uvelius B, Andersson KE, Michel MC. Autonomic nervous control of the urinary bladder. *Acta Physiol (Oxf).* 2013;207:16–33.
171. De Groat WC, Booth AM. Autonomic systems to the urinary bladder and sexual organs. In: Dyck PJ, Thomas PK, eds. *Peripheral Neuropathy.* 3rd ed. W.B. Saunders Company; 1993:198–207.
172. Sato A, Sato Y, Schmidt RF. Somatic afferents and their effects on bladder function. In: Brooks CM, Koizumi K, Sato A, eds. *Integrative Functions of the Autonomic Nervous System.* University of Tokyo Press; 1979:309–318.
173. Gillilan LA. *Clinical Aspects of the Autonomic Nervous System.* Little, Brown and Company; 1953.
174. Krier J, Adams T. Autonomic and somatic systems to the anorectum and pelvic floor. In: Dyck PNPJ, Thomas PK, eds. *Gastroenterology and Hepatology.* W.B. Saunders Comp.; 1993;187–197.
175. Gerendai I, Banczerowski P, Halasz B. Functional significance of the innervation of the gonads. *Endocrine.* 2005;28:309–318.
176. Baader B, Herrmann M. Topography of the pelvic autonomic nervous system and its potential impact on surgical intervention in the pelvis. *Clin Anat.* 2003;16:119–130.
177. Benoit G, Merlaud L, Meduri G, et al. Anatomy of the prostatic nerves. *Surg Radiol Anat.* 1994;16:23–29.
178. White CW, Xie JH, Ventura S. Age-related changes in the innervation of the prostate gland: implications for prostate cancer initiation and progression. *Organogenesis.* 2013;9:206–215.
179. Taneike T, Miyazaki H, Nakamura H, Ohga A. Autonomic innervation of the circular and longitudinal layers in swine myometrium. *Biol Reprod.* 1991;45:831–340.
180. Thilander G, Rodriguez-Martinez H. Distribution of adrenergic and cholinergic nerves in the porcine myometrium during the oestrous cycle. A histochemical investigation. *Zentralbl Veterinarmed A.* 1989;36: 276–284.
181. Bulat R, Kannan MS, Garfield RE. Studies of the innervation of rabbit myometrium and cervix. *Can J Physiol Pharmacol.* 1989;67:837–844.
182. Thilander G. Adrenergic and cholinergic nerve supply in the porcine myometrium and cervix. A histochemical investigation during pregnancy and parturition. *Zentralbl Veterinarmed A.* 1989;36:585–595.
183. Bonica JJ, McDonald JS. The pain of childbirth. In: Bonica JJ, ed. *The Management of Pain.* Lea & Febiger; 1990:1313–1343.
184. Kawatani M, Takeshige C, De Groat WC. Central distribution of afferent pathways from the uterus of the cat. *J Comp Neurol.* 1990;302: 294–304.
185. Bonica JJ, Chadwick HS. Labor pain. In: Wall TPPD, Melzack R, eds. Churchill Livingstone; 1989:482–499.
186. Park YH, Jeong CW, Lee SE. A comprehensive review of neuroanatomy of the prostate. *Prostate Int.* 2013;1:139–145.
187. Schlegel PN, Walsh PC. Neuroanatomical approach to radical cystoprostatectomy with preservation of sexual function. *J Urol.* 1987;138: 1402–1406.
188. Sato T, Hanna P, Mori S. Innervation of the coronary arteries and its role in controlling microvascular resistance. *J Cardiol.* 2024;84:1–13.
189. Jarhult J, Falck B, Ingemansson S, Nobin A. The functional importance of sympathetic nerves to the liver and endocrine pancreas. *Ann Surg.* 1979;189:96–100.
190. Zsombok A, Desmoulins LD, Derbenev AV. Sympathetic circuits regulating hepatic glucose metabolism: where we stand. *Physiol Rev.* 2024;104:85–101.
191. Faber CL, Deem JD, Campos CA, Taborsky GJ, Jr., Morton GJ. CNS control of the endocrine pancreas. *Diabetologia.* 2020;63:2086–2094.
192. Nylander O, Sjoblom M, Sedin J, Dahlgren D. Effects of alpha2-adrenoceptor stimulation on luminal alkalinisation and net fluid flux in rat duodenum. *PLoS One.* 2022;17:e0273208.
193. Sato Y, Hotta H, Nakayama H, Suzuki H. Sympathetic and parasympathetic regulation of the uterine blood flow and contraction in the rat. *Journal of the Autonomic Nervous System.* 1996;59:151–158.

7 The Fascial System of the Body

FRANK H. WILLARD ▪ CHRISTIAN FOSSUM

KEY CONCEPTS

- Fascia is a unitary body system with a function that can be described as supportive, protective, and healing in nature.
- Fascia is composed of irregular connective tissue that can have varying densities.
- Four fundamental layers of fascia can be described: a layer of pannicular fascia covering the body, a continuous layer of dense investing fascia surrounding the musculoskeletal system of the axial and appendicular body, a complex series of meningeal fascial layers surrounding the central nervous system, and a fatty layer of visceral fascia surrounding the body cavities and organ systems.
- Fascia has a dynamic aspect imparted by its cellular components, especially by the fibroblast and the myofibroblast.

INTRODUCTION

Definition

Fascia is a form of connective tissue that unites all aspects of the body. While by definition fascia functions as packing tissue and as a system for organ protection,[1,2] its cellular composition suggests that it is also critical for metabolic activity and immune surveillance[3] (also see Chapter 3).

- Unfortunately, there is much confusion in the literature concerning the components of fascia, in regard to its architecture and distribution within the body (see discussion in Fasel et al.).[4]
- Recently, a detailed atlas has been published[5] describing the fascias of the somatic systems, but it did not cover those of the body cavities.
- The lack of precision in a definition poses a problem when trying to decide which tissues actually belong to fascia and which are really part of another organ system such as a tendon, ligament, or joint capsule.
- Early writings described fascia in a broad sense as being everywhere, interconnected, and serving a packing function[6]; however, more recent studies, performed to solve surgical issues, have taken a more fractionated approach[7]
- Henry Gray's Textbook of Human Anatomy describes fascia as the "dissectable, fibrous connective tissue of the body, other than the specifically organized structures tendons, aponeuroses, and ligaments."[8]
  - This definition of fascia was introduced under C.M. Goss as editor of the American version of *Gray's Anatomy* in 1948, and it was retained in the most recent edition.[1]
  - This definition is relatively clear in its exclusion of tendons, ligaments, and aponeurosis from the term *fascia*; it also goes on to describe the investing nature of most fascia, in providing a packing substance around muscles, tendons, ligaments, and aponeuroses as well as visceral organs.
  - The exclusion of tendons, ligaments, and aponeuroses from the category of fascia makes sense since these structures are themselves, in turn, covered with thin layer of deep investing fascia as described in *Gray's Anatomy*[1]
- A similar definition of fascia is offered in the English version of *Gray's Anatomy*,[2] where fascia is described as having collagenous fibers that are generally interwoven, as opposed to the parallel array of fibers seen in tendons, ligaments, and aponeuroses.

This chapter will offer an expanded definition of fascia, as a system:

1. Complete with blood supply, fluid drainage, and innervations and is thus the largest organ system in the body
2. Composed of irregularly arranged fibrous elements of varying densities
3. Involved in tissue protection and healing of surrounding systems

- As consistent with the definition in *Gray's Anatomy*, tendons, ligaments, and aponeuroses are excluded from the term *fascia* based on their histologic composition.
- The cells and extracellular substance that constitute fascia will then be examined.
- The chapter will conclude with a discussion of the dynamics of fascia, its role in tissue repair (Box 7.1), and the pathologic spread of fascia leading to fibrosis.

Previous Studies of Fascia

Recently, there has been a strong resurgence of interest in both basic and applied science research in fascia.[9] Traditionally, fascias had been relegated to a supportive role and were considered inconsequential residues that were less important than the tissues with which they were associated.[10]

- The term *fascia*, derived from Latin for *band* or *bandage (bound together)*, emerged in its anatomical and medical usage in the 16th and 18th centuries.
- The sometimes vague and inconsistent descriptions of fascia in anatomy and across languages resulted in the publication of two anatomy texts in the 1930s solely devoted to the anatomy of the fascial planes.[11,12]

BOX 7.1 Definition of Fascia

The term fascia is best defined as connective tissue with an irregular weave of collagenous fibers, unlike the regular arrangement seen in

- Tendons
- Ligaments
- Aponeuroses

- Subsequently, based on developmental approaches involving studies of the sequential development of visceral changes, as observed in closely graded series of human embryos, fetuses, newborn infants, and adults, a detailed investigation of the adult fascia was performed.[13]
  - □ It highlighted the process of development and organ migration that produces different types of fascia in a predictable and confirmable pattern, referring to it as *migration fascia*.
  - □ It also described the fascia resulting from fusion of the primitive mesenteries as *fusion fascia* and the *parietal fascia* as intrinsic to the structures in the wall of the developing abdominopelvic cavity.
  - □ This was one of the first attempts at linking embryologic development and growth to the anatomy of the adult fascia.
- Innervation of the deep fascia in both human and animals, in the form of nerve terminations consisting of free endings and simple small encapsulated endings, was described around the same time,[14] and it was proposed that they may have a kinesthetic function as well as contribution to pain transmission.
- Based on such observations and experimentations, it became more obvious that the fascia, rather than being an inert structure with a passive function, is a very active tissue playing an important role in the economy of the body and in health and disease.[15]

Despite the advancement in the anatomical knowledge of the fascia, some confusion still remains on the proper terminology.

- Efforts have been made in recent years to standardize anatomical terminology with the introduction and constant revision of the *Nomina Anatomica*, but despite this, adequate descriptions of fascial structures from an anatomical point of view are still lacking.[16,17]
- Most recently,[5] an atlas was published on the fascias of the somatic body, including the extremities and torso but not considering those of the splanchnic tissues. This excellent text examines the superficial and deep fascia of the extremities and the somatic portions of the torso, demonstrating the interconnected nature of these fascia layers.
- Interestingly, Stecco classified fascia as dense regular connective tissue and then divided all fascia into two basic types:
  1. Those with parallel construction of their collagen fibers.
  2. Those with multilayered construction of their collagen fibers. The latter category was then further divided into *aponeurotic* fasciae and *epimysial* fasciae.
- The reclassification of fascia as regular connective tissue awaits general verification and agreement among anatomists; however, the subdivision of fascia into aponeurotic and epimysial may yet prove to be very helpful in the understanding of this tissue.

Overview of Fascia

Tendons, ligaments, and joint capsules are generally composed of dense connective tissue, with regularly arranged fibrous elements designed to meet specific functional requirements such as to resist pull, shear, or compressive stress in a given direction (Fig. 7.1). These elements typically have definable anatomical borders where tendons, ligaments, or joint capsules attach to surrounding structures.

- Conversely, by its very nature, fascia lacks this specificity in design; it packs the spaces around organ systems, and interconnects between systems seemingly without providing specific functions (Fig. 7.2).
  - □ This lack of specificity is best suited by an irregular arrangement of fibrous elements capable of resisting pull or stretch in multiple different directions.

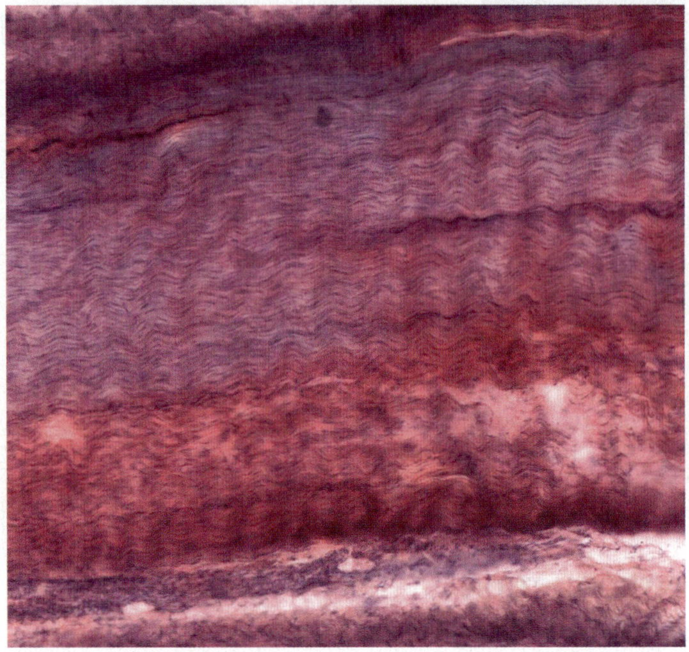

Figure 7.1. This is a longitudinal section taken through a tendon. The *wavy lines* represent thick bundles of collagenous fibers. The thin dark spots are the nuclei of fibrocytes embedded in the layers of collagenous fibers. This is an example of regularly arranged dense connective tissue. This structure is built to resist stress in one direction only.

  - □ The irregular or multiplanar construction of fascial tissue also facilitates its continuity from one region of the body to another without forming the precise borders seen with such structures as tendons and ligaments of joint capsules (Box 7.2).
- Thus, the *epimysium* (fascia matrix into which skeletal muscle is embedded) is anatomically continuous with a sheath covering the tendon or ligament, termed the *epitenon* (18); also termed peritenon, which is anatomically continuous with the *fibrous layer of periosteum* surrounding bone.[18]
  - □ Outside of the epitenon, there lies a delicate layer of loose connective tissue that has been termed the *paratenon*[19]; this layer represents an adventitia and can grade into surrounding fasciae.
  - □ Similar adventitial layers are present on most musculoskeletal components.
- Thus, tendons, ligaments, aponeuroses, skeletal muscles, and bones are surrounded by a thin, protective fascial sheath of typically dense connective tissue, typically named in relation to the structure it surrounds (epimysium, epitenon, periosteum).
  - □ These sheaths grade into each other establishing a fascial continuity among musculoskeletal elements.

BOX 7.2 Deep Investing Fascias

The following are covered with an investing fascia termed epimysium, epitenon, or periosteum:

- Muscles
- Tendons
- Ligaments
- Aponeuroses
- Bone

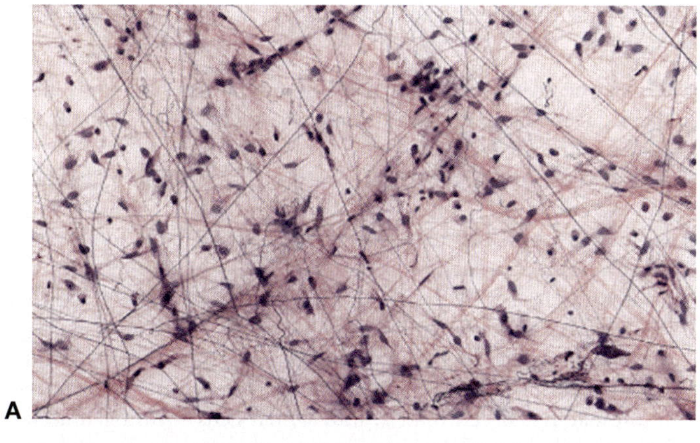

Figure 7.2. Forms of connective tissue typically found in fascia. A. This is a loose connective (areolar) tissue spread, demonstrating a fairly random arrangement of collagenous and elastic fibers. (Courtesy of the University of New England, Histology Site.) **B.** This is a cross section taken through mesentery, demonstrating a thin layer of dense, irregular collagenous fibers underlying the mesothelium with a central core of adipose tissue surrounding several vessels and lymph nodes. Note the thickened tunica adventitia of the vessels. (University of Michigan Histology Site, http://histology.sites.uofmhosting.net/. Copyright © 2015 The Regents of the University of Michigan.) **C.** This is a magnified view of the mesentery border showing the thin layer of dense irregular collagenous fibers underlying the single cell layer of mesothelium.

  - Each sheath is surrounded by an adventitia composed of loose connective tissue (also fascia) that grades outward into the fascia surrounding any nonmusculoskeletal structures such as neurovascular bundles.
  - The lack of precise borders seen in the fascial tissue allows it to form long planes, spanning multiple organ systems or compartments, surrounding one or more muscles.
- Each of the investing fascial sheaths forms inner septae that penetrate the organ (muscle, tendon, ligament) forming an internal skeleton.
  - For example, the epimysium forms internally directed perimysia that lobate the belly of the muscle into fascicles.
  - Within each fascicle, delicate fibers, termed endomysium, form a matrix around individual muscle fibers (cells).
- When entering fascial compartments, neurovascular bundles—which themselves are surrounded by irregular dense connective tissue fascial wrappings—course along or through fascial planes that would otherwise represent obstacles if composed of highly organized, regularly arranged fibrous elements, such as seen in an aponeurosis, tendon, ligament, or joint capsule.
- Lymphatic flow, which would be quickly interrupted if forced through tissue with precise boundaries, can flow easily through lymphatic vessels distributed in the irregular tissue of the fascial plane.

As with any other organ system, fascia has an innervation (see the Section "Innervation of the Fascia").

- As vessels course through fascial planes, they are typically accompanied by small-caliber nerve fibers.
- Some of these fibers contain catecholamines and belong to the autonomic nervous system,[20,21] whereas others are somatic nerve fibers,[22] many of which contain neuropeptides[23] and belong to sensory systems (also see Chapter 11 Nociception and Pain).
- Endings from these fibers have a basal release of catecholamines and neuropeptides into the vessel wall and surrounding tissue.
- These compounds may exert trophic control over the vasculature and determine, in part, the texture of the tissue and the trafficking of white blood cells through the tissue.[24]

Finally, like any other organ system of the body, fascia has definitive functions and capabilities.

- Most organ systems, including both musculoskeletal and visceral organs, are surrounded by a fascial capsule from which septa arise and penetrate into the organ, often subdividing it into functionally distinct regions; this imparts fascia with a packing function in addition to providing access routes for metabolic channels (Box 7.3).
- In essence, fascial septa are acting as the skeleton for the specific organ system. As the body moves, so does its organs; to avoid friction and injury, healthy fascial layers distort easily, tolerating stretch in planes and thereby providing a distensible cushion that allows organs to glide by each other while protecting more delicate fluid channels.
- Where organs are exposed in the body cavity and/or in contact with each other, the fascial capsule is covered by a thin layer of squamous mesothelial cells termed a visceral epithelium; in a similar manner, the body cavities are lined with a thin layer of fascia and the exposed surface is covered with thin layer of squamous mesothelial cells, termed a parietal epithelium.
- Mesothelial cells are flattened squamous secretory cells that can produce a veneer of fluid that facilitates the sliding movements of organs.[25]
- Each organ is supplied with one or more neurovascular bundles and numerous lymphatic drainage routes, which communicate with the organ through its fascial layers; in this way, fascia is providing a movable conduit through which the neurovascular lifeline for the metabolic activity of the organ system can pass.

BOX 7.3 Functional Definition of Fascia

The irregular weave present in fascial tissue allows it to resist stress or strain in multiple directions, unlike the unidirectional resistance seen in tendons and ligaments.

Generally, all layers of fascia are themselves supplied with a well-organized blood supply and fluid drainage routes through venous and lymphatic channels (see Chapter 14 Anatomy and Physiology of the Lymphatic System).

- Given the irregular arrangement of the fibrous nature of fascia, it is quick to initiate repair following injury and often will rapidly form a scar or callus.
    - Thus, fascia plays an important role in wound healing and tissue repair.
- Although it has been long thought to be relatively motionless—one prominent textbook of histology defined fascia as "noncontractile connective tissue"—recent evidence is beginning to demonstrate a slow contractile nature to fascial tissue[26,27]
    - This contractile nature appears to be closely related to the tissue repair process and will be discussed at the end of this chapter.

Architecture of Fascia

GENERAL APPROACH

Several attempts at describing the fascias of the body have been published.[5,10–12]

- Numerous discrepancies exist concerning which layers are considered fascia and how many subdivisions exist for each layer.
- Unfortunately, the lack of a clear definition of fascia has prevented any resolution of such arguments.[4,17,28]
- Since all tissues of the body derive from an embryologic basis, any description of fascia should be grounded in developmental sequences.
- This chapter, using irregular connective tissue as a histologic definition, will describe an embryologically based system of four primary layers that cover the axial portion of the body. Modification of this fundamental plan will allow accommodation of the head and limbs.

The four primary layers in the torso are arranged as a series of concentric tubes. Starting with the outermost layer of fascia, it is best termed the *superficial fascia*, *panniculus*, or *panniculus adiposus* (Box 7.4).

- The latter terms were used by Singer[12] in his treatise on fascia and strongly urged for general usage by Last in his textbook.[29]
- This is an overall layer of fascia that covers the entire body and also is present directly under the epidermis.
- The superficial layer often contains much embedded adipose tissue and is partitioned by numerous thin septa,[5] termed the *retinaculi cutis*.
- Although this can be subdivided into a superficial and deep component, this is not consistent throughout the body.

BOX 7.4 Fundamental Layers of Fascia

Essentially, four layers of fascia can be identified in the body:

1. Superficial fascia
2. Deep investing fascia
3. Meningeal fascia
4. Visceral fascia

The development of these layers can be traced from their embryonic origins in the primitive mesenchyme.

Deep to the superficial or pannicular layer is the *axial fascia* of the torso.

- This layer gives rise to the investing fascia that surrounds all of the axial muscles, tendons, bones, ligaments, and aponeuroses of the body.
- It is also continuous with the appendicular (investing) fascia in the extremity.
- It may be possible to subdivide this layer into aponeurotic (sheetlike) fascia, such as:
    - The fascia lata of the thigh and crural fascia of the leg that surround multiple structures.
    - The epimysial fascia that intimately surrounds the individual structures.[5] The epimysial fascia derives from the primitive mesenchymal cell matrix, into which cells forming muscles, bones, ligaments, and aponeuroses develop during embryogenesis.[30]

Internal to the axial fascia are two additional layers:

1. The first surrounds the neural structures and is termed *meningeal fascia*.
2. The second surrounds all body cavities and is best termed *visceral fascia*.

In considering the limbs:

- The superficial layer extends outward, covering the entire surface of the limb.
- Under the superficial layer, a fascial layer of similar composition to the axial fascia is present surrounding the muscles of the extremity and can be termed *appendicular investing fascia*; it lies deep to the superficial fascia and invests the appendicular muscles. Regional names often relate the fascia to a specific muscle, such as deltoid or clavipectoral fascia.
- Internal to the appendicular fascia is the intramuscular septum housing the neurovascular bundles; this septal layer is thought to be derived developmentally from the axial fascia at the base of the limb, as the limb bud grows distally.

FOUR PRIMARY LAYERS OF FASCIA

Superficial or Pannicular Fascia

The outermost layer is the superficial or pannicular layer of fat and fascia,[1,2] and it includes the dermis and hypodermis.

- Numerous studies employing dissection, histology, and radiology have demonstrated the intrinsic structure of this fascial layer but have used varying terminology.[31]
- The superficial layer is derived from the somatic mesenchyme (dermatomyotome) and surrounds the entire body with the exception of its orifices such as the orbits, nasal passages, and the oral and aboral openings.
- Although numerous regional variations in composition exist, the hypodermal portion is typically divided into a superficial and deep compartment by a thin septum of irregular connective tissue termed the stratum membranosum (SM), but has also been referred to as superficial fascia[31] (Fig. 7.3).

The thin band of irregular connective tissue forming the SM is present throughout the extremities and torso as well as continuous with the superior musculoaponeurotic system present over portions of the face.[32]

- The SM courses parallel to the dermis and underlying musculoskeletal tissues; sometimes dividing into two or more layers.

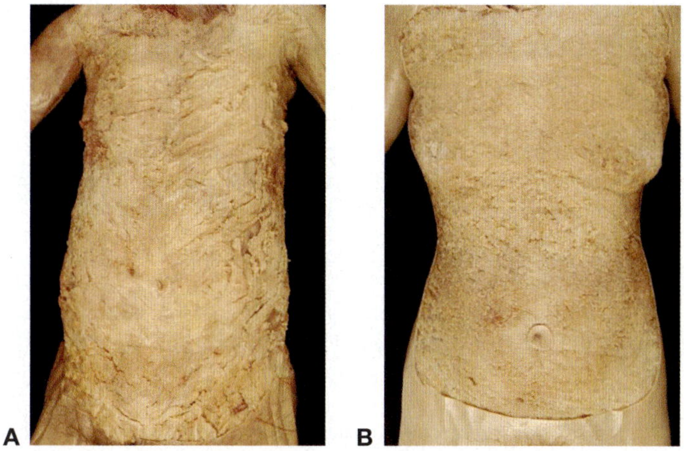

Figure 7.3. The superficial or pannicular layer of fascia. This is an anterior view of the thorax and abdomen of a 54-year-old male cadaver (**A**) and a 54-year-old female cadaver (**B**). Both specimens have had the dermis removed to reveal the superficial layer of fascia. (Used with permission from the Willard/Carreiro Collection, University of New England.)

- The adipose tissue above the SM is termed the superficial adipose tissue (SAT) layer, and that which is located under the SM is the deep adipose tissue (DAT) layer.[31]
- The SM is anchored by numerous perpendicular and diagonal septae, termed the retinaculum cutis (RC), that extend between the SM and the dermis and the SM and underlying musculoskeletal tissues.
- These bands have also been termed fibrous trabeculae[33] and are described as forming major networks for neurovascular bundles and lymphatic vessels.
- The superficial RC anchor into the reticular dermis, while the deep RC anchor to the investing fascias of the underlying musculoskeletal tissue, such as the epimysium of underlying muscle
- As such, the RC create numerous compartments or lobules filled with adipocytes.
- The arrangement and thickness of the RC demonstrate considerable regional variation being nonexistent over portions of the cranium to extremely thick and elongated in the axilla, ischiorectal fossa, and the female breast (Fig. 7.4).
- In the region of the head and neck, humans have several thin muscles embedded in the SM; these are the platysma (Fig. 7.5) and associated muscles of facial expression (or pannicular muscles) innervated by the facial nerve (CN VII).
- The RC of the hypodermis, in combination with the SM, make up a complex retaining connective network (RCN) that stabilizes the adipose tissue located between the RC and determines the outward appearance of the skin[34]; it also creates a dynamic matrix that allows for movement of the dermal layer against the underlying musculoskeletal tissue.[5]
- Neurovascular bundles course through the RC and SM to reach targets in the dermis.

In the extremities, RCN demonstrates significant regional variation.

- Over much of the upper and lower extremity, the three compartments of the hypodermis,SAT, SM, and DAT are clearly discernable; however, their thicknesses may vary considerably.
- Over regions where the skin is tightly adhered to underlying bone, the entire hypodermis can be reduced to a thin layer of connective tissue on the deep surface of the dermis.
- In regions such as the perineum and ischiorectal fossa, the RCs of the deep adipose layer can become extremely elongated and thickened.

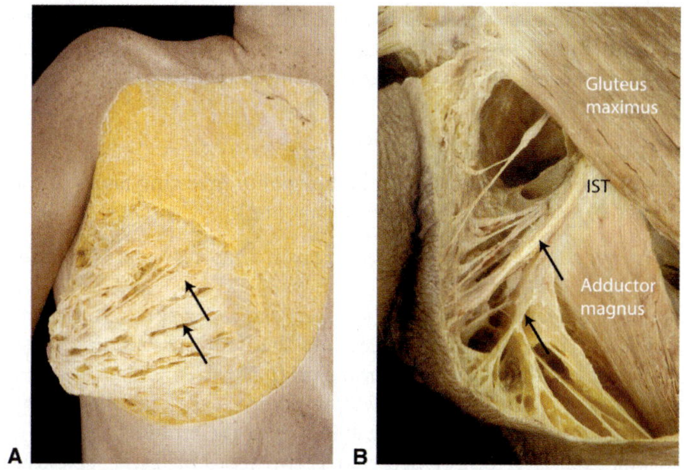

Figure 7.4. Specialized regions of the retinaculum cutis in a 42-year-old female. A. This is an anterior view of a female left mammary gland following the removal of the dermis and the adipose tissue from the area between retinacula cutis of the underlying hypodermis. Note how the bands of fascia are thickened in the breast tissue (indicated by the *arrows*). **B**. This is a posterior view into the right ischiorectal fossa following the removal of the overlying dermis and the adipose tissue present in the hypodermis sparing the retinacula cutis. Note the length of the retinacula in the depths of the fossa (indicated by the *arrows*). IST denotes ischial tuberosity.

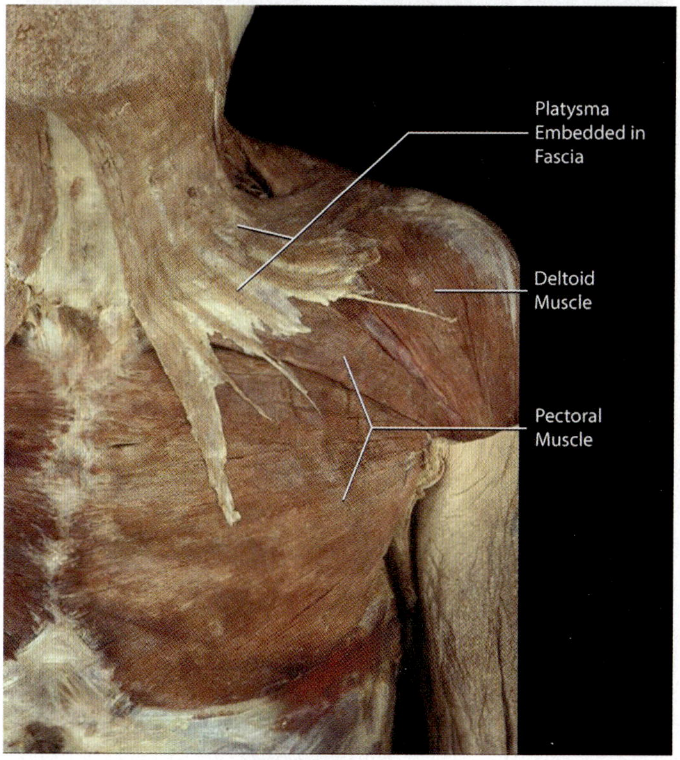

Figure 7.5. This is an anterior view of the upper thorax and neck of an adult male illustrating the platysma, a pannicular muscle, embedded in the superficial (pannicular) fascia and separated from the underlying muscles. The deltoid and pectoral muscles are extremity muscles and are normally embedded in fascia derived from the extremity. The investing fascia of the extremity has been cleaned off of the deltoid and pectoral muscles. (Used with permission from the Willard/Carreiro Collection, University of New England.)

- On the plantar surface of the foot, the RCs thicken and become more numerous, creating the plantar fascia, their deep RCs anchor to the fascia covering the plantar aponeurosis.

Axial and Appendicular Investing Fascia

Internal to the superficial layer is the axial or investing fascia of the torso (*deep fascia* as described in Clemente.).[1]

- As with the superficial fascial layer, it is also derived from somatic mesenchyme.
- The axial layer is fused to the superficial fascia through the retinacula cutis and extends deep into the body, surrounding muscles of both hypaxial and epaxial origin.
- This layer contributes to the epimysium of skeletal muscle, the periosteum of bone, and the epitenon of the tendons.
- The axial layer can be depicted as two tubes of fascia separated centrally by the vertebral column (notochord in the embryo; see Fig. 7.6):
  1. The anterior tube surrounds the hypaxial muscles and attaches to the vertebral column at the transverse process. The hypaxial muscles include the longus and scalene muscles in the cervical region, the intercostal muscles in the thoracic region, and the oblique and rectus muscles in the abdominal region.
  2. The posterior tube of axial fascia surrounds the epaxial muscles and is attached to the transverse processes. At each level, the vertebral spinous process divides the epaxial fascial tube into two "half-tubes" (Fig. 7.6). The paraspinal muscles of the back are contained in the "half-tube" of the epaxial fascia (Box 7.5).

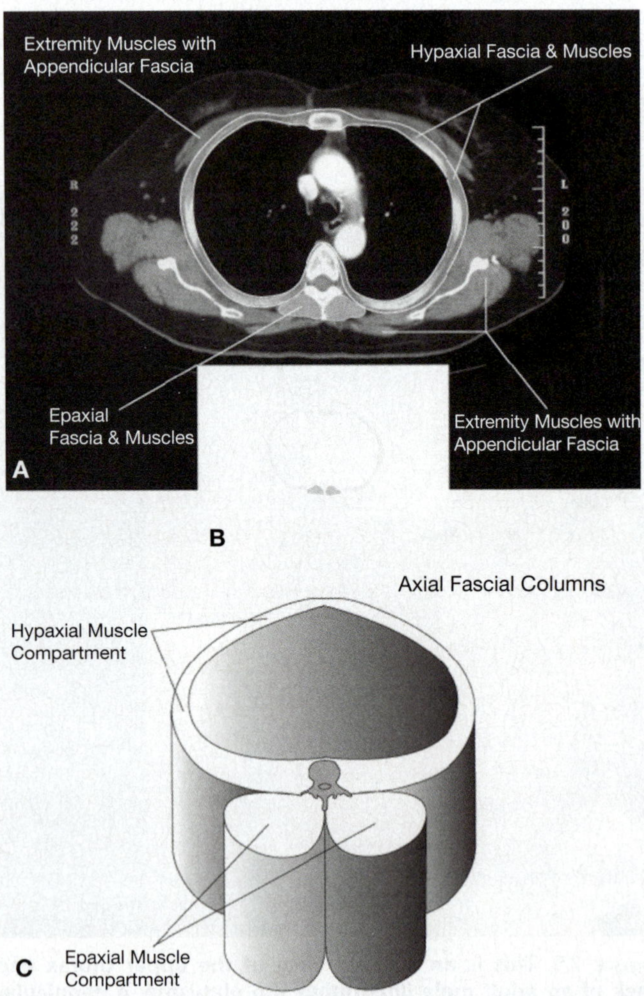

Figure 7.6. The construction of the torso. A. This is an axial plane spiral CT taken through a male thorax. The *white outline* surrounding the axial muscles—hypaxial and epaxial—marks the course of the axial fascia. **B.** This is an outline of the hypaxial and epaxial compartments. **C.** This is a schematic diagram demonstrating the cylinder-like arrangement of the torso. (Used with permission from the Willard/Carreiro Collection, University of New England.)

BOX 7.5 Fascial Construction of the Torso

The torso of the body can be conceptualized as two cylinders lined with investing fascia. The two cylinders are joined together about the vertebral column.

1. The ventral column or hypaxial musculature surrounds the body cavity.
2. The dorsal or epaxial compartment is split into two halves by the spinous processes of the vertebral column.

Axial fascia extends into the extremities forming an investing layer surrounding individual muscles.

- The appendicular investing fascia has been divided into two components, aponeurotic fascia and epimysial fascia[31]
- Aponeurotic fascia forms a membrane that surrounds the musculoskeletal components of the extremity similar to a support stocking, while the epimysial fascia is said to surround individual muscles and other structures such as tendons, retinacula, ligaments, and bones.
- The fascial sheath that surrounds the neurovascular bundles, such as the brachial plexus and lumbosacral plexus, is termed the tunica adventitia and it extends outward to form the intermuscular septum of the limb, in which branches of the neurovascular bundle will course as they progress distally in the extremity.
- The neurovascular layer of adventitial fascia fuses to the surrounding epimysial fasciae in the extremity.

The arrangement of fascias within the body wall is made very complex by the attachment of the limbs.

- The muscles of the upper extremity, such as the pectoralis, trapezius, serratus anterior, and latissimus dorsi muscles, form long winglike expansions that wrap over the torso, superficial to the paraspinal muscles, to attach to the midline of the body or to structures that ultimately attach to the midline such as the thoracolumbar fascia (Fig. 7.7).
- These extremity muscles pass internal to the pannicular fascia but external to the axial fascia as they embrace the axial body wall.
- Each muscle is surrounded by its own layer of investing or appendicular fascia, where the extremity muscles come in contact with the axial muscles, their dense connective tissue investing fascial layers are typically joined by a thin layer of loose connective tissue.[31,35]

The arrangement of these fascial sheets (of investing or appendicular fascia) is visualized in the two dissections, illustrated in Figures 7.8 to 7.12.

- In Figure 7.8, the epidermis and dermis have been removed to expose the underlying hypodermal portion of the superficial fascia. An elongated rectangular window (outline) was opened into

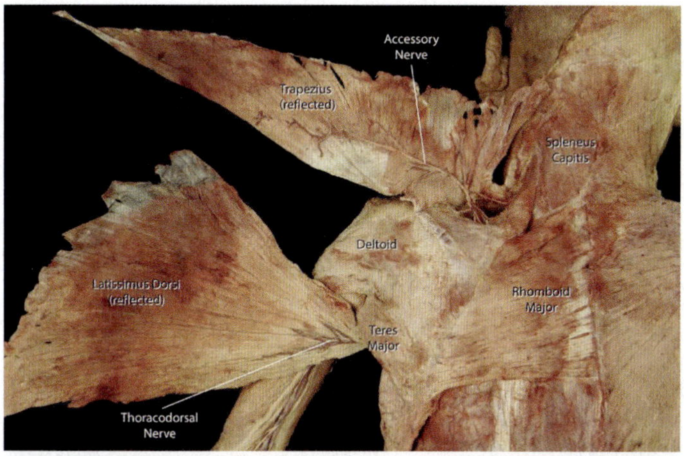

Figure 7.7. Winglike arrangement of the trapezius and latissimus dorsi. (Used with permission from the Willard/Carreiro Collection, University of New England.)

the superficial fascia to expose the investing fascia (appendicular fascia) of the pectoral muscles.

- In Figure 7.9, the window was enlarged and divided into two portions. The medial portion still has appendicular fascia covering the muscle, but in the lateral portion, the investing appendicular fascia has been removed to expose the pectoralis muscle.
- With the inferolateral border of the pectoral muscle elevated (see Fig. 7.10), the investing (appendicular) fascia separating it from the serratus anterior can be visualized. Developmentally,

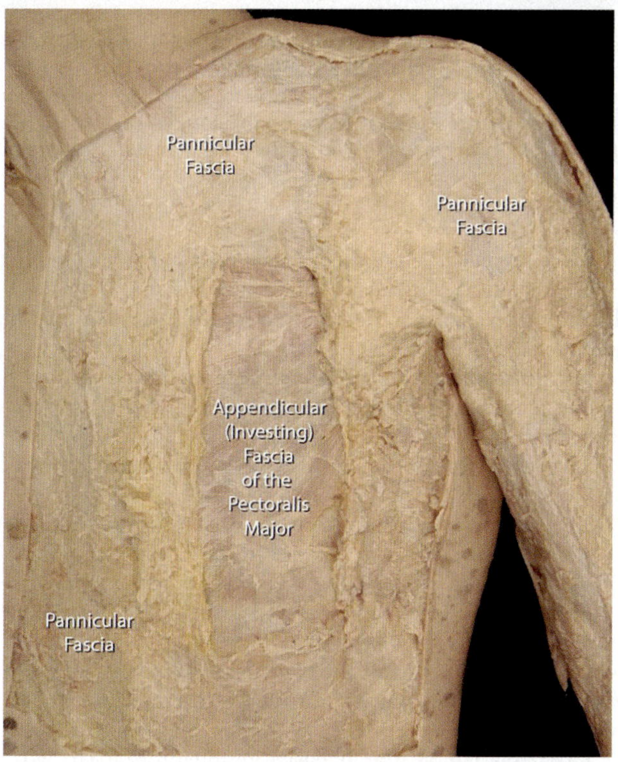

Figure 7.8. This is a photograph of a male with the epidermis and dermis removed to expose the pannicular fascia on the chest wall. A vertical window has been cut in the pannicular fascia to expose the underlying appendicular fascia. (Used with permission from the Willard/Carreiro Collection, University of New England.)

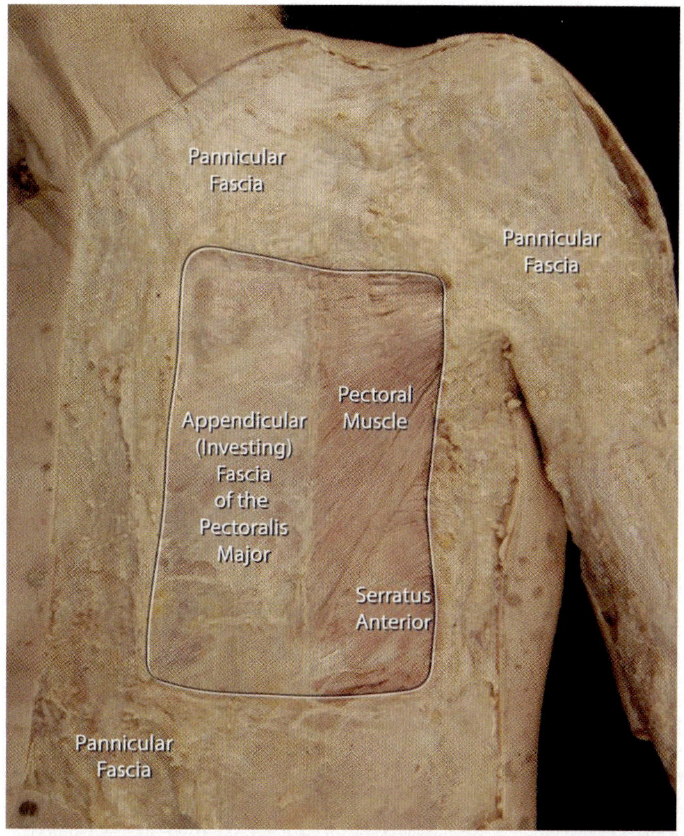

Figure 7.9. The fascia of the anterior chest wall. A window has been cut in the pannicular fascia. On the left side of the window, the appendicular fascia investing the pectoralis major is seen. On the right side of the window, this fascia has been removed to demonstrate the muscle. (Used with permission from the Willard/Carreiro Collection, University of New England.)

this fascial sheet begins as two separate layers that fuse together during life: the posterior investing fascia of the pectoralis major and the anterior investing fascia of the serratus anterior.

- To expose the axial investing fascia of the intercostal muscles, the pectoral major and serratus anterior muscles and their investing appendicular fascia must be removed (see Fig. 7.11). In this figure, the pectoralis major and serratus anterior muscles have been removed to expose the intercostal muscles and their thin layer of investing axial fascia (note that the pectoralis minor muscle is still attached).
- Finally, Figure 7.12 shows the exposed intercostal muscles by carefully dissecting away all axial fascia.

Meningeal Fascia

The third fascial layer is meningeal fascia, which surrounds the nervous system (Fig. 7.13).

- This layer, including the dura and the underlying leptomeninges, derives from the primitive meninx that surrounds the embryonic nervous system.
- Specifically, the spinal meninges are most likely derived from the somatic mesoderm, while the brain stem meninges are derived from cephalic mesoderm, and the telencephalic meninges from the neural crest.[36]
- Meningeal fascia terminates just distal to the dorsal root ganglion, with the development of the epineurium that surrounds the peripheral nerve.

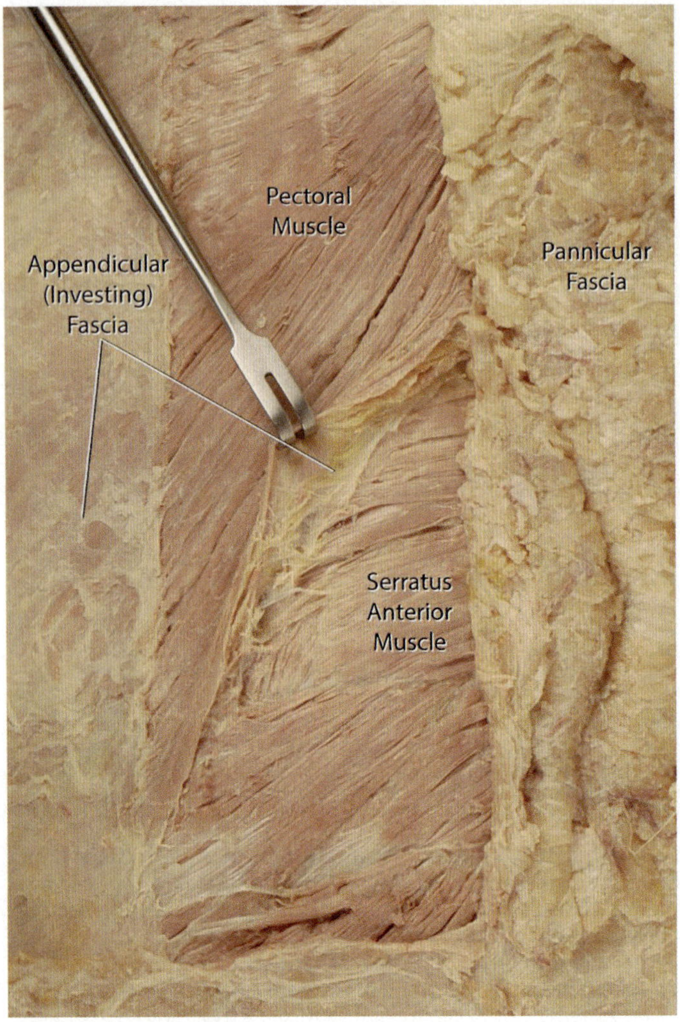

Figure 7.10. The fascia of the anterior chest wall. A window has been cut in the pannicular fascia as described in Figure 7.8. The inferolateral border of the pectoralis major muscle has been elevated to reveal the investing appendicular fascia separating this muscle from the underlying anterior serratus. (Used with permission from the Willard/Carreiro Collection, University of New England.)

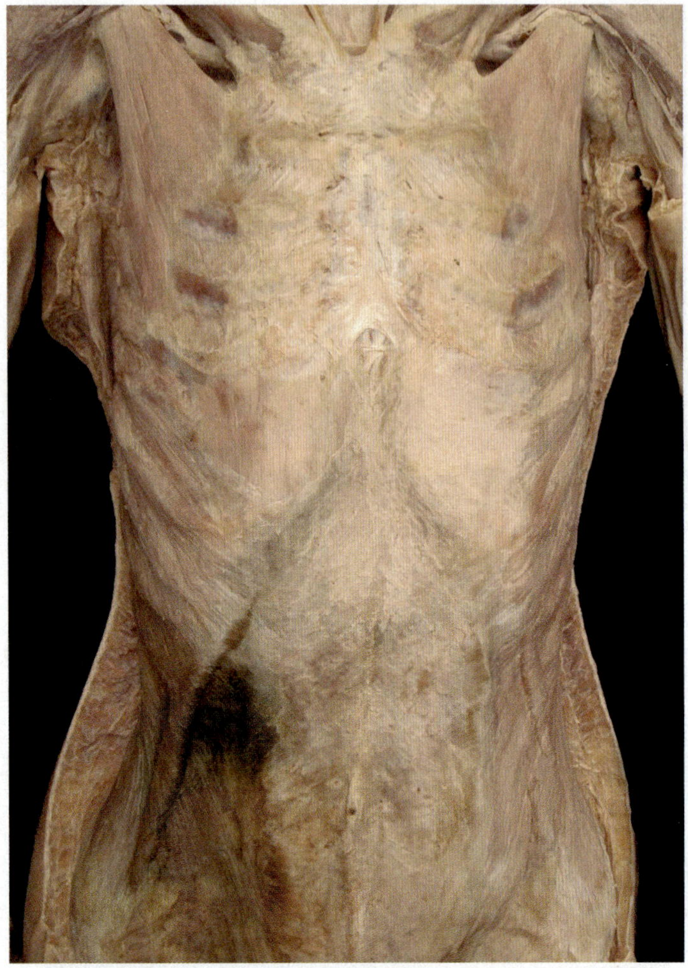

Figure 7.11. This is an anterior view of a 54-year-old female following the removal of her pectoralis major. The axial fascia surrounding the sternum, ribs, and intercostal muscles is exposed. The pectoralis minor is still in place on this female specimen. (Used with permission from the Willard/Carreiro Collection, University of New England.)

Visceral Fascia

The fourth fascial layer is visceral fascia and is by far the most complex of the four main layers of fascia.

- Embryologically, this layer is derived from the splanchnic mesodermal layer (Box 7.6).
- In the third week of development, the neural tube becomes surrounded on both sides by the paraxial mesoderm, which subsequently begins dividing into more than 40 segments, termed somites.[37]
  - Each somite has a dorsolateral layer termed the dermomyotome from which the skin and muscles will arise, and a ventromedial layer termed the sclerotome from which the hard connective tissues of the body will form.
- Lateral to the paraxial mesoderm is a solid layer of lateral plate mesoderm.
  - Just prior to week 4, the lateral plate mesoderm divides into dorsal and ventral layers by a cleavage plane that creates the primitive body cavity.
  - The cavity walls become lined with a simple squamous cell lining termed the parietal mesothelium.
  - The dorsal layer is termed the somatic mesoderm (somatopleure) and it gives rise to the fascial components of the body wall, while the ventral layer is termed the visceral mesoderm (splanchnopleure) and is the origin of the visceral fascia (Fig. 7.14).
- At the medial junction of the two lateral mesoderm layers, close to the somite, a third layer, termed the intermediate strata,[38] is seen to form.
  - From this region, the extensive retroperitoneal fat pads are derived, which forms the bed of the kidney (pararenal fascia) and surrounds the renal capsule (perirenal fascia).

> **BOX 7.6 Visceral Fascia**
>
> Visceral fascia arises from the visceral mesoderm (splanchnopleure), derived from the lateral plate mesoderm.

The visceral mesoderm (splanchnopleure) is in immediate contact with the developing visceral organs (Box 7.7).

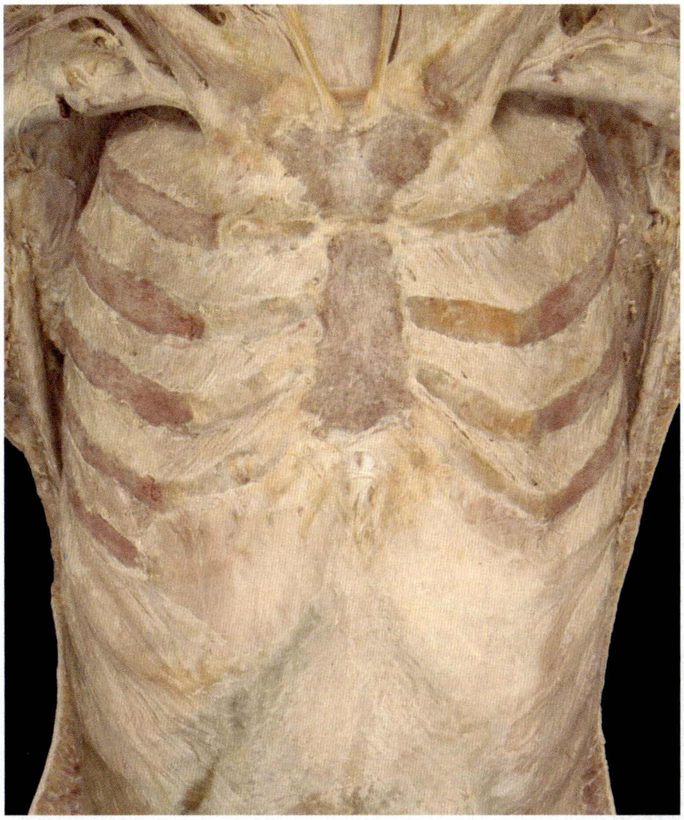

Figure 7.12. **On the previous specimen, the axial fascia has been removed to expose the sternum, ribs, and intercostal muscles.** (Used with permission from the Willard/Carreiro Collection, University of New England.)

- As an organ moves off the body wall and into the abdominal cavity, it carries a layer of the visceral fascia with it, covered by a blanket of mesothelium.
- Where the mesothelium directly covers the organ, it is termed the visceral peritoneum.
- These suspensory structures become the root of the lung in the pleural cavity, as well as the mesenteries and mesocolons of the peritoneal cavity and the broad ligament of the uterus in the pelvic cavity.
- The visceral fascia contained within these structures acts as a conduit for the passage of neurovascular bundles between the body wall and the organ.

In the cranial region, visceral fascia surrounds the pharynx and its attachment to the cranial base.

- Superiorly, visceral fascia includes the pharyngobasilar and pharyngobuccal fascia and, as such, fuses to the cranial base surrounding the attachments of the superior constrictor muscles.[29]

BOX 7.7 Mesenteries and Mesocolons

The mesenteries and the mesocolons of the abdominal cavity are composed of a sheet of visceral fascia with a serous (mesothelial) lining on both sides, one end continuous with the body cavity and the other end in contact with the organ.

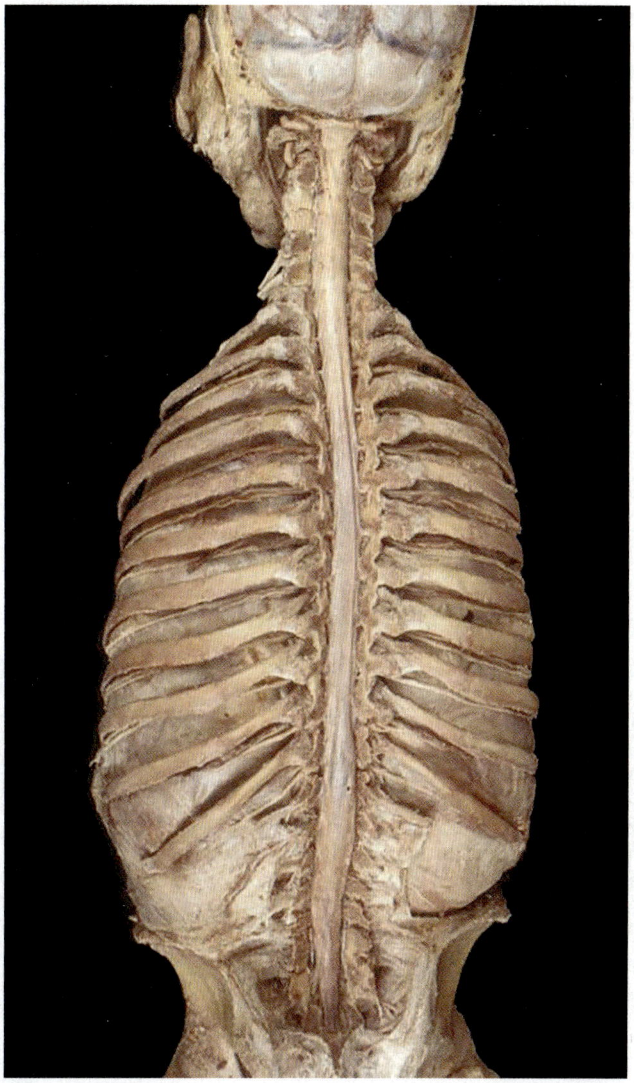

Figure 7.13. **The paraspinal muscles have been removed and a total laminectomy has been performed to expose the spinal dural sac.** In addition, the occipital bone was removed to demonstrate the cranial dura. (Used with permission from the Willard/Carreiro Collection, University of New England.)

- Cervical visceral fascia extends inferiorly into the neck surrounding the nasopharynx, oropharynx, and remaining cervical viscera.
- Thus, at the cranial base, cervical fascia has a flared opening, expanding to encompass the nasal passageways and the mouth (Fig. 7.15).

In the neck, visceral fascia incorporates such regional fascias as pretracheal, retropharyngeal, and alar (carotid sheath) fascias, as well as the fascia surrounding the thyroid cartilage and thyroid gland (Fig. 7.15).

- Thus, visceral fascia can be conceived of as a continuous vertical sleeve lying internal to the hyoid muscles, anterior to the longus muscles, and extending into the thorax (Fig. 7.16).
- As such, it is continuous from the cranial base into the thorax.

Upon entering the thorax, the visceral fascia, derived from the visceral mesoderm (splanchnopleure), is forced medially by the two pleural cavities.

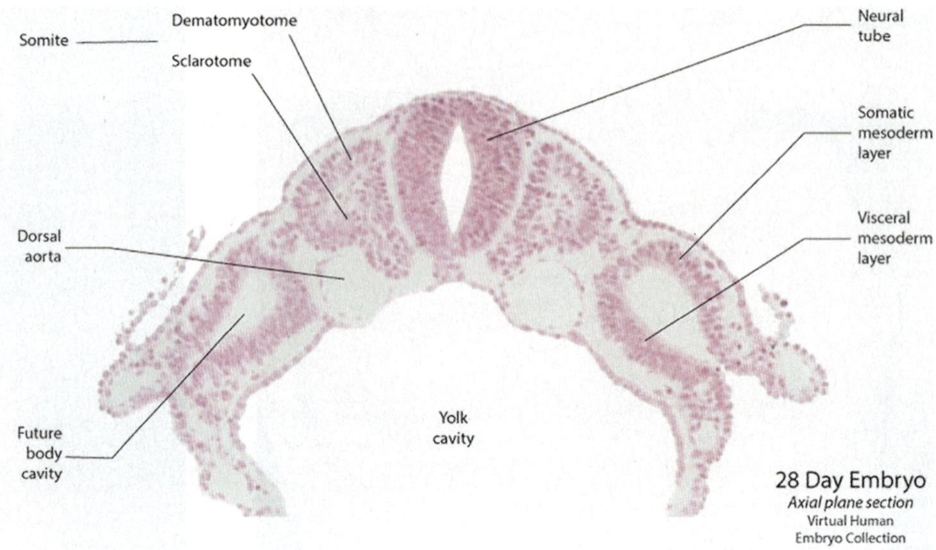

Figure 7.14. This is an axial section through the torso of a 28-day human embryo. The neural tube is seen in the center of the section. A somite is located on either side of the neural tube, and the dorsal aorta appears on the ventrolateral margin of the somite. The lateral plate mesoderm has been cleaved into two layers by the development of the future body cavity. The dorsal layer is the somatic mesoderm (somatopleure), and the ventral layer is the visceral mesoderm (splanchnopleure).

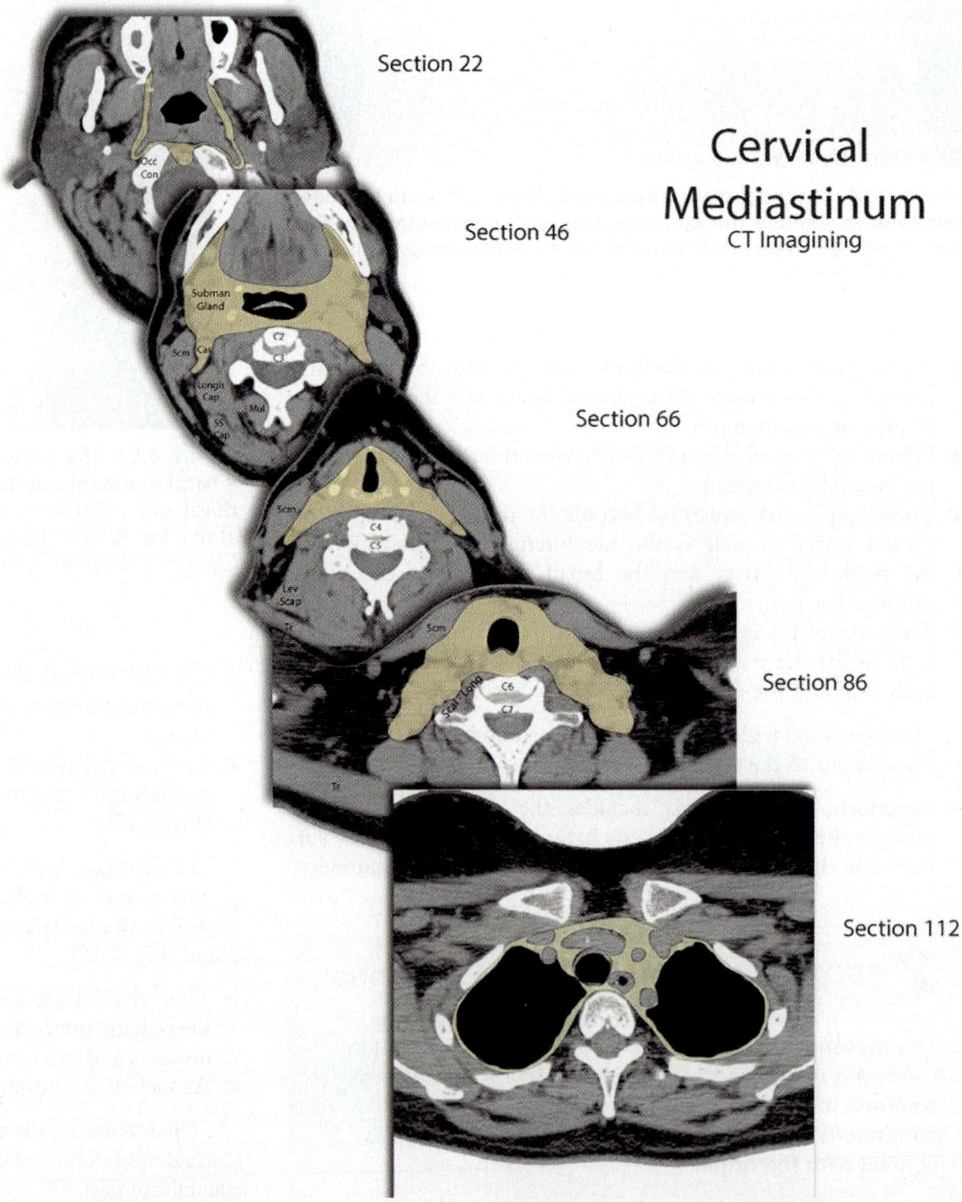

Figure 7.15. Cervical visceral fascia. These images are a series of four cervical CT sections from one individual with the visceral fascia indicated by shading. This fascia begins as a flared opening (Sections 22 and 46) attached to the cranial base, and consolidates into a continuous column of irregular connective tissue as it descends through the neck (Sections 66 and 86).

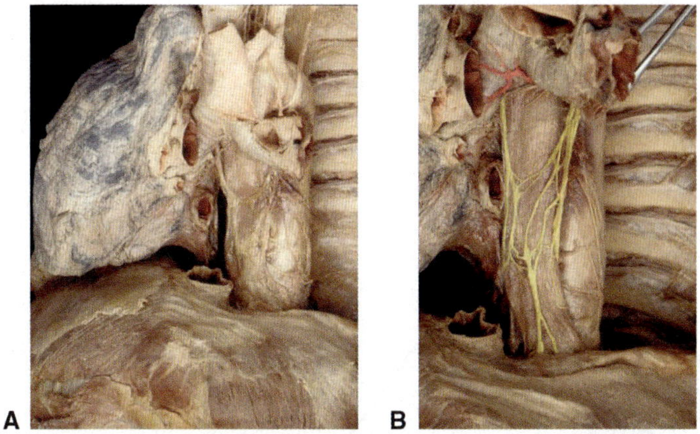

Figure 7.16. The mediastinum: visceral fascia. In (**A**), the esophagus, vagus nerve, and aorta are still embedded in the visceral fascia, while in (**B**), the visceral fascia has been removed to expose these organs. (Used with permission from the Willard/Carreiro Collection, University of New England.)

- The pleural cavities are formed from the cleavage plane that separates the dorsal and ventral layers of the lateral plate mesoderm.
- Thus, a centrally located column of visceral fascia, termed the thoracic mediastinum, is created from the cervical visceral fascia.
- This fascia forms a loose matrix surrounding the:
  - Aorta
  - Esophagus
  - Trachea
  - Primary bronchi
  - Azygos venous system
  - Thoracic duct (see Fig. 7.16)
- This matrix is very loose to allow distension of the esophagus upon swallowing.
- Importantly, there are no significant condensations of fascia present in the region posterior to the pericardial sac or esophagus.[39,40]
- Finally, visceral fascia surrounds the bronchi as they pass through the root of the lung; this fascia is continuous with the stroma surrounding the airways in the lung.

Developmentally, a thin layer of fascia also surrounds the posterior, lateral, and anterior aspects of the pleural cavity. This fascia is derived from the somatic mesoderm (somatopleure) and has been termed the endothoracic fascia or *fascia parietalis*.[38]

- Visceral fascia also accompanies the esophagus into the abdominal cavity. Here, the visceral layer spreads outward to surround the peritoneum where it is termed *fascia parietalis* or *endoabdominal fascia*, an anterior region of which has been termed the *transversalis fascia*.[17,41]
- The endoabdominal fascia, which is similar in composition and continuous in nature with the endothoracic fascia, thickens significantly along the posterior midline and forms a column analogous to the mediastinum of the thoracic cavity (Fig. 7.17).
- As in the thorax, the abdominal mediastinum contains the major neurovascular channels.
  - Extensions of the abdominal mediastinal fascia pass into the ligaments derived from the mesogastrium, the mesenteries, and the mesocolon to reach the associated visceral organs of the abdomen.
  - The fascia of the mesenteries and mesocolons is continuous from stomach to rectum and all organs of the gastrointestinal system are contained within this fascia[42]
  - The abdominal mediastinum forms a pathway through which the blood supply, lymphatic drainage, and nerves reach the intraperitoneal organs.
  - This situation is remarkably similar to that seen with the thorax where the mediastinum is a conduit for neurovascular bundles reaching the root of the lung and passing into the lung tissue.
- A specialized fascial pad, the pararenal fascia lies on the quadratus lumborum, forming the bed of the kidney. In this bed, the kidney lies wrapped in an additional layer of adipose tissue termed the perirenal fat pad or *Gerota fascia*[43,44] (Fig. 7.18).

In the pelvic basin, the endoabdominal fascia becomes continuous with the endopelvic fascia, which surrounds the inferior region of the peritoneum.

- The inferior border of the endopelvic fascia lies in the inner surface of the pelvic diaphragm, composed of the levator ani and coccygeus muscles.
- Inferior to the pelvic diaphragm is the ischiorectal (ischioanal) fossa; it is packed with pannicular fascia derived from the fascia of the gluteal region (see Fig. 7.19).
- The anterior and inferior border of the endopelvic fascia fills the retropubic space surrounding the base of the urinary bladder.
- As in the thorax and abdomen, the endopelvic fascia thickens on the midline where it again forms a mediastinum surrounding the rectum, reproductive organs, and urinary bladder.
- Similar to the mediastinum in the thorax and abdomen, the endopelvic fascia serves as a conduit through which the major organ systems in the pelvic basin receive their blood supply and innervations as well as their lymphatic drainage.
- In the female, extensions of the pelvic mediastinal component of the visceral fascia form the core of the broad ligament, and condensations of this visceral fascia form the transverse cervical ligament of the uterus.
- In addition, there are thickening in various regions of the pelvic fascia of surgical importance that have received specific or regional names such as the fascia of Denonvillier, a thickened band lying between the rectum and the prostate[45]

On the midline of the body, the visceral fascia forms a thickened mediastinum that extends from the cranial base into the pelvic cavity, although it is typically only named as such in the thorax (Box 7.8).[1,2]

- This column of visceral fascia can be traced through Figures 7.15, 7.17, and 7.19.
- Although the column is named only in the thorax where it is termed the mediastinum, it truly forms a mediastinum from the cranial base to the pelvic floor.
- The visceral fascia contained within this middle column of the torso lines the root of the lung and the mesenteries, providing a conduit for neurovascular bundles to reach the internal organs.

In summary, visceral fascia can be traced from the cranial base into the pelvic cavity. It forms the packing surrounding the visceral

BOX 7.8 Mediastinum of the Body

A vertical ridge of visceral fascia extends from the cranial base to the pelvic floor, lying along the midline of the torso. This fascial construct represents a mediastinum. It contains the major neurovascular system of the body.

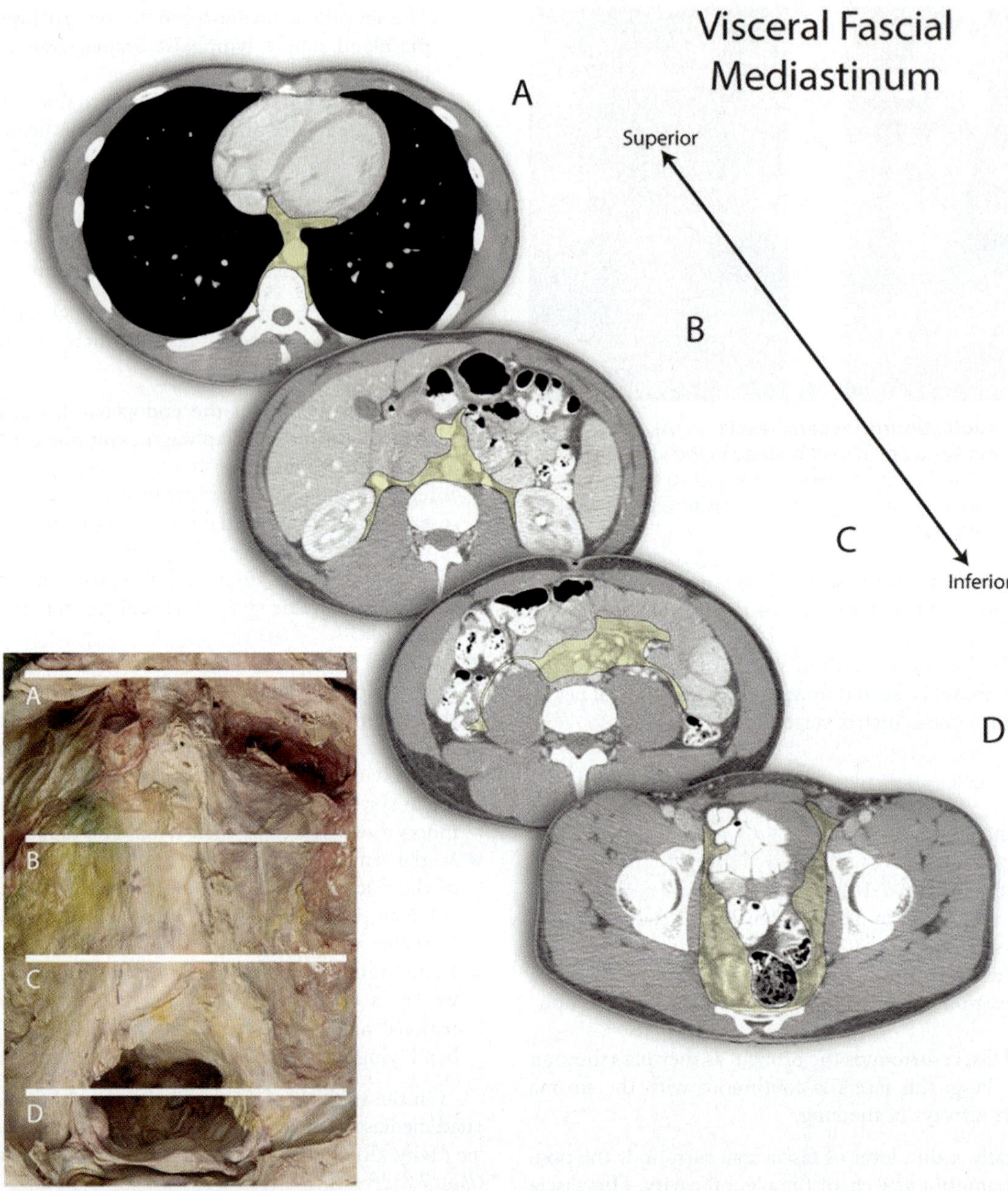

Figure 7.17. This is a series of four axial plane CT scans taken through the thorax, abdomen, and pelvis of a patient. The visceral fascia has been outlined and faintly shaded in each image.

organs, many of which it reaches by passing along the suspensory ligaments, such as the mesenteries.

- This fascia also functions as a conduit for the neurovascular and lymphatic bundles as they radiate outward from the thoracic, abdominal, and pelvic mediastinum to reach the specific organs.

Visceral Ligaments

A note here is necessary concerning the use of the word *ligament* when referring to structures found in the body cavity. Visceral ligaments are in no sense of the word similar to the ligaments seen in the somatic region of the body.

- Ligaments in the somatic portion of the body are structures that join bone to bone and are composed of dense, regular connective tissue, which itself is surrounded by a thin epitenon of investing fascia, typically part of the axial or appendicular fascia.
- The word *ligament* used for structures found in body cavities refers to a loose condensation of visceral fascia (irregular connective tissue of varying density) in some cases surrounded by a thin serous membrane, such as:
  - ☐ Pulmonary ligaments
  - ☐ Treitz ligament
  - ☐ Transverse cervical ligament
  - ☐ Broad ligament
- Visceral ligaments generally cannot bear as much strain as somatic ligaments nor are they as clearly defined on dissection.
  - ☐ Unlike ligaments in somatic tissue, visceral ligaments typically function to carry blood supply and innervations to an organ system or to loosely anchor an organ in the body cavity.
  - ☐ Visceral ligaments also need to be distinguished from the fibrotic adhesions that typically develop secondary to irritation and inflammation.[46]

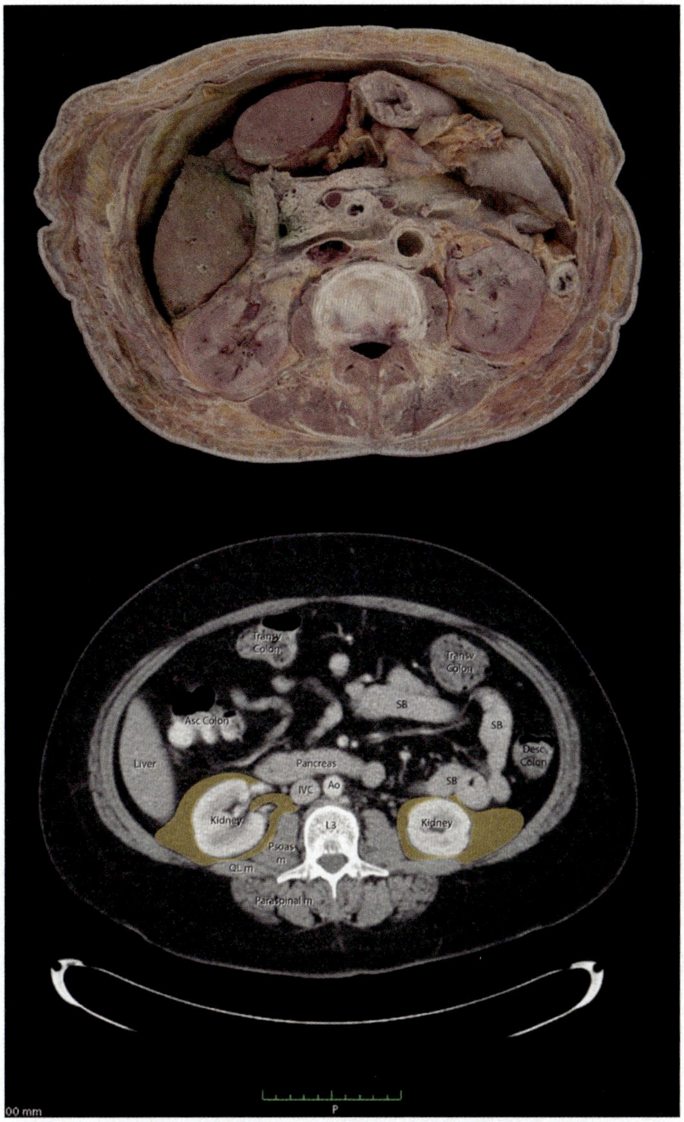

Figure 7.18. The perirenal fascia. The perirenal pad of fat and fascia has been outlined and faintly shaded.

Adhesions

Fibrotic adhesions derive from areas of chronic inflammation.[47]

- Irritation or infection of the mesothelium, either on the body wall or covering an organ system, results in the release of proinflammatory cytokines from immune cells and the subsequent activation of fibroblasts.
  - ☐ Fibrinogen is produced and converted to fibrin.
  - ☐ Fibroblasts then lay down collagen and extracellular matrix.
- Myofibroblasts, derived from surrounding fibroblasts and other mesenchymal cells, increase collagen production as well as contract to compress the newly formed tissue into thickened bands.[48]
  - ☐ The collagen laid down is irregular in arrangement and is thus similar to fascia in its construction.
  - ☐ When excessive, these bands of increased collagen can form adhesions that can reach pathologic proportions.
- Adhesions can occur in any region of the body either visceral or somatic (Box 7.9).
  - ☐ In the abdomen and pelvis, adhesions can envelope the tubular bowel and be strong enough to obstruct movement within its lumen or interfere with reproductive organ functions.
  - ☐ Similarly, adhesions forming in and around synovial sheaths in the carpal tunnel can interfere with movement of the digital flexor tendons.

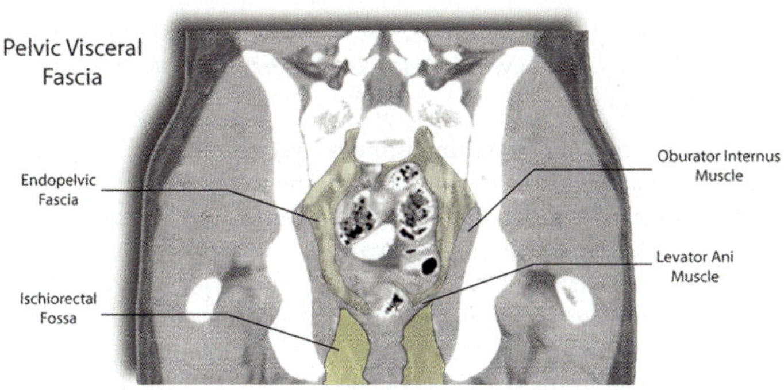

Figure 7.19. The fascias of the pelvis. The levator ani separates the endopelvic fascia (*lighter shading*) that surrounds the pelvic viscera from the pannicular fascia of the ischiorectal fossa (*darker shading*). (Used with permission from the Willard/Carreiro Collection, University of New England.)

BOX 7.9 Visceral Ligaments and Fascial Adhesions

Visceral ligaments and fascial adhesions are different entities.

- Visceral ligaments are present since birth and are considered normal structures.
- Adhesions occur subsequent to tissue irritation and inflammation. Adhesions are not considered normal tissue.

Innervation of the Fascia

It has been proposed that the fascia plays an important role in:

- Musculoskeletal biomechanics
- Peripheral motor coordination
- Proprioception
- Regulation of posture
- Acting as a potential pain generator.[49–51]

Central to these roles is the innervation and the cellular-mediated contractility of the fascia.

- Reports suggest that the fascia is richly innervated.
- Abundant free and encapsulated nerve endings have been described at a number of anatomical sites,[10,52–58] such as the:
  - ☐ Thoracolumbar fascia
  - ☐ Bicipital aponeuroses
  - ☐ Crural fascia
- These nerve endings are particularly numerous around vessels but are also distributed homogeneously throughout the fibrous components of the fascia.[59]
- Beside the identified Ruffini, Pacini, and Golgi–Mazzoni corpuscles and their possible proprioceptive role,[58,60,61] some of the nerve fibers associated with the fascia are adrenergic and likely to be involved in controlling local blood flow.[10] This is supported by reports that when intrafascial nerve fibers were subjected to morphologic evaluation, they exhibited characteristics typical of autonomic nerve fibers.[59,61]

As for the proposed proprioceptive role, the fascia should be considered in close association with its related muscles.

- When muscles contract, their tension is transmitted to the fascia causing traction of it, possibly activating nerve terminals embedded in the fascia.[59,61]
- The degree of innervation may also change in patients with chronic pain, as described in thoracolumbar fascia in patients with back pain.[62]
- Following excessive stimulation, or when the mechanoreceptors are stretched beyond their physiologic limit, they have the ability of becoming nociceptors.[61]
- It has also been suggested that manual loading of fascia as in various manual medicine modalities may cause changes through activation of these receptors.[60,63,64]
- Despite the recent advances in knowledge concerning the innervation of the fascia, the understanding of it is still very incomplete.[10,65]

COMPONENTS OF FASCIA

Fascia is composed of connective tissue with varying densities of irregularly arranged collagenous fibers. As such, the components of fascia are the items typically found in irregular connective tissue.

Cellular Elements

FIBROCYTES

Fascia supports biochemical, and biophysical associations between its own components and underlying muscles, bones, and organs.[66]

- Fibrocytes are the principal cell type of fascia; they synthesize and secrete:
  - Cytokines (e.g., interleukins [ILs], interferons, growth factors, etc.)
  - Connective tissue extracellular matrix proteins (ECMPs), such as collagen, fibronectin, and others
- Fibrocytes also secrete and maintain connective tissue ground substance containing glycosaminoglycans, proteoglycans, hyaluronic acid, and glycoproteins.
  - This ground substance provides the medium through which exchange of molecules between blood, lymph, and tissue cells takes place, thereby making fibroblast secretions deliverable both locally and systemically.
- Within the tissue, fibrocytes have long, wavy dendritic processes that establish connections with surrounding cells and the fibrous matrix (Fig. 7.20).

The shape of the fibroblast is dependent upon the environment in which it is located.

- Elongate or fusiform cell shapes are seen when the cell is at rest, such as occurs in mature connective tissue where the cell is typically entangled in thick bundles of collagen fibers.
- The stellate cell shape is seen when fibroblasts are grown in tissue culture or are present either in immature or healing tissue or in a fibrotic tissue.[67]

Fibroblast shape is also sensitive to the tension in the tissue.

- In the quiescent state, cells have spindle shapes with long dendritic process.
- However, when mechanically stressed, these cells round up becoming stellate in shape.[68,69]

Some fibroblasts are of mesenchymal origin, similar to osteocytes and chondrocytes; however, other fibroblasts, particularly those found in the connective tissue layers of visceral organs such as lung, liver, and kidney, can arise from a process of transformation from epithelial cells.[70]

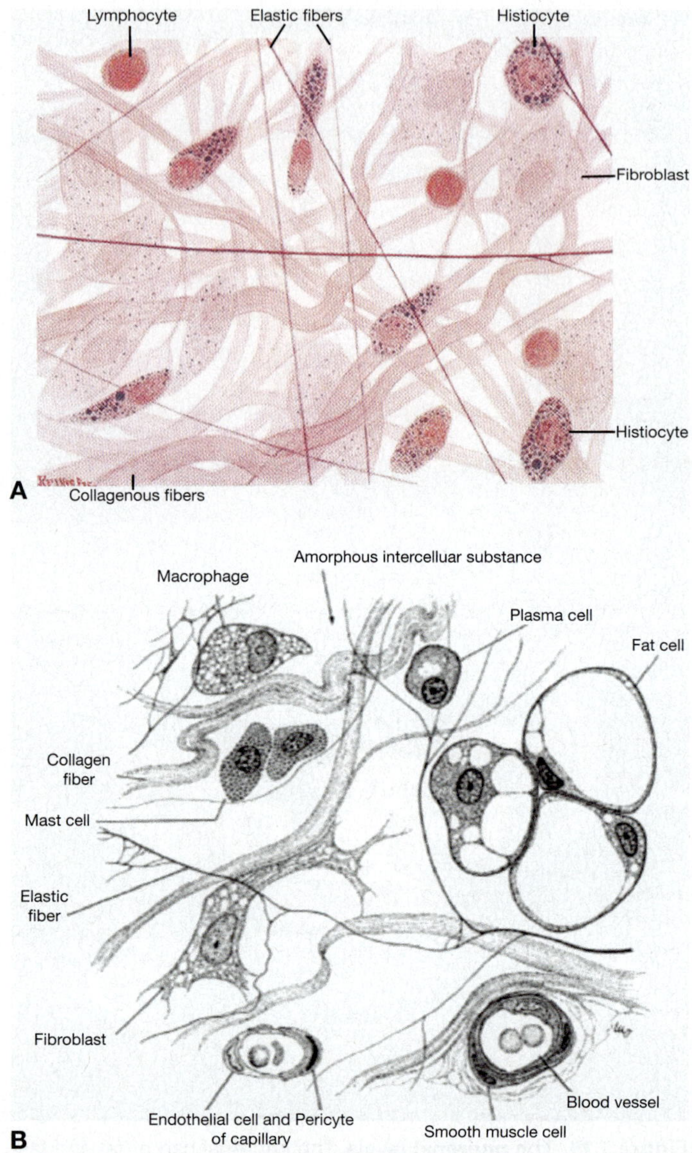

Figure 7.20. Histologic sections of loose connective tissue demonstrating the fibrous and cellular components. (Figure A reprinted with permission from Kelly DE, Wood RL, Enders AC. *Bailey's Textbook of Microscopic Anatomy*. 18th ed. Williams & Wilkins; 1984. Figure B reprinted with permission from Cormack DH. *Ham's Histology*. 9th ed. J.B. Lippincott; 1987.)

- This metamorphosis occurs through a process termed *epithelial–mesenchymal transition*, which allows the polarized cells located in a sheet of epithelium to transition into highly motile cells inside the connective tissue matrix.[71]
- The formation of fibroblasts from epithelial cells is currently thought to be a significant event in normal developmental processes and to play a critical role in such pathologic processes as tissue repair, fibrosis, and oncogenesis.[72–74]

Regardless of their origin, fibroblasts are charged with maintenance of homeostasis in the matrix of the connective tissue through the production and remodeling of both fibers and the extracellular matrix.[75]

- Part of this task also involves monitoring and maintaining the appropriate degree of tension in the connective tissues[76,77] and the chemical quality of the tissue.
- Thus, fibroblasts are capable of both mechanoreception (responsive to tension) and chemoreception (responsive to growth factors).

Fibroblasts exist in the extracellular matrix of the fascia.

- A primary role of the fascia and its ECMPs is to endow cells and tissues with their specific mechanical and physiochemical properties.
- As such, the extracellular matrix represents a three-dimensional scaffolding that supports cellular adhesion and tissue-specific functions.
- Since imposed mechanical loads physically affect the fascia, it plays important simultaneous roles of a force sensor and a transmitter of force input generated by muscle contractions and by external forces.
- Fibroblasts can detect the change in tension, convert to myofibroblasts, and generate an adaptive response, which can involve contraction and the secretion of large quantities of collagen[78,79]
  - Thus, fascia itself may also be capable of smooth muscle–like contractions, thereby influencing underlying musculoskeletal dynamics and displaying the existence of true (i.e., skeletal muscle–independent) fascial tone.[80,81]
  - OMT is hypothesized to mediate corrections of such fascial hypertonicity and/or abnormal tissue collagen cross-linking,[82] which may occur post injury or during prolonged immobilization.
- Therefore, fibroblasts have been thought to be uniquely poised to be targets of soft tissue injuries, myofascial release (MFR), and other OMT[83,84] due to their:
  - Location within the ground substance
  - Ability to secrete ECMPs and mediators of pain and inflammation
  - Ability to generate and transduce force input

Along with changing tension, fibroblasts also respond to growth factors and inflammatory substances secreted into the matrix from epithelial cells, mast cells, macrophages, and lymphocytes.

- Numerous cell types found in connective tissue produce transforming growth factor-beta (TGF-β),[75] such as:
  - Macrophages
  - Mast cell
  - Epithelial cells
  - Fibroblasts
- Similar to physical stress, activation of fibroblasts by TGF-β or inflammatory compounds leads to the expression of as many as 150 genes.[75]
- An end result of this process is the:
  - Production of collagen
  - Differentiation of the fibroblast into a myofibroblast with focal cellular adhesions to the matrix and a contractile ability (see the Section "Myofibroblasts" and Boxes 7.10 and 7.11)

Fibroblasts form a distinct network in connective tissue.

- The long thin processes of the cell make contact with those of other fibroblasts, creating a three-dimensional network within the tissue.[85]
- Control of the formation of dendritic processes and their coupling with other fibroblast processes appears to lie with the balance of growth factors in the tissue.
  - These factors, such as platelet-derived growth factor and lysophosphatidic acid, act on the fibroblast through a family of small G-proteins involving Rho and Rac.[76]
- The gap junction protein, connexin 43, has been detected at points where fibroblast processes make contact.[85,86]
- Yet, to date, gap junctions, as seen with electron microscopy, have not been visualized at these points of contact between fibroblast processes.
  - However, the presence of the connexin protein on these processes raises the interesting possibility that the fibroblasts have an interconnected communications network throughout connective tissue that functions through the membrane-bound connexin proteins.
- The concept of an interconnected cellular network among fibroblasts would not be out of context, since similar networks are seen between mature osteocytes (mesenchymal-derived cells) located in bone, as well as between fibroblasts located around bundles of collagen fibers in tendons.
  - In both bone and tendon, these cellular networks function to detect mechanical stress and orchestrate an adaptive response by the tissue.[87]

BOX 7.10 Fibroblast-to-Myofibroblast Conversion

Activated fibroblasts can convert to myofibroblasts. These cells:

- Express smooth muscle actin
- Have the capability to contract
- Can produce collagen and extracellular matrix components

Myofibroblasts play an important role in tissue healing, but can also be a factor in the formation of scars and adhesions.

MYOFIBROBLASTS

Myofibroblasts can differentiate from fibroblasts as well as numerous other cell types.

- In their fully developed state, they share many cellular and biochemical similarities with smooth muscle cells.
- Although myofibroblasts typically arise in response to injury (Fig. 7.21),[88] they also can be derived from epithelial cells or endothelial cells through a transformation process.
- In addition, a circulating fibroblast-like bone marrow stem cell capable of forming myofibroblasts has been described,[47] and in the liver, stellate cells along the margins of the sinusoids transform into myofibroblasts.

BOX 7.11 Myofibroblasts

- Can derive from fibroblasts
- Can produce smooth muscle actin
- Can have contractile properties during wound repair
- Can be removed from tissue either through apoptosis or deactivation
- Can produce fibrosis if their activity is prolonged

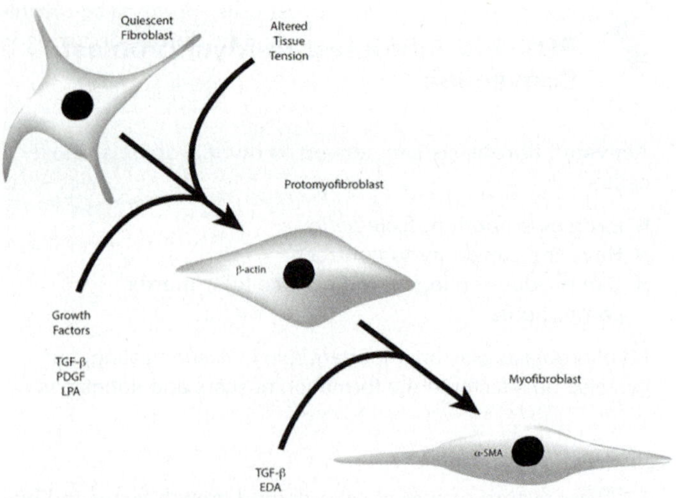

Figure 7.21. The stages in the transformation of a fibroblast into a myofibroblast.

Myofibroblasts have a well-developed endoplasmic reticulum, suggesting that they are secretory cells.

- Histochemically, myofibroblasts express a number of specific markers used to differentiate them from undifferentiated fibroblasts. These include:
  - □ Alpha smooth muscle actin (αSMA)
  - □ Cadherin II[89]
  - □ Paladin 4lg[90]
- In some tissues, myofibroblasts play long-standing resident roles of support and immunology.
  - □ For example, myofibroblasts normally function to maintain and regulate the shape of crypts and villi in the alimentary tract, but can also act as stem cells and as atypical antigen-presenting cells.
  - □ They lend structural support to tissues and perform paracrine/endocrine functions.
- In most other tissues, myofibroblasts exist in the short term to facilitate wound healing. After injury, myofibroblasts resemble many aspects of a smooth muscle cell and, when activated, migrate to sites of damaged tissues and synthesize cytokines and ECMPs to facilitate healing.[91]

Myofibroblasts have been described as the "construction workers" of the wound healing process.[79]

- Signals for fibroblast to myofibroblast differentiation include biomechanical strain and a variety of cytokines, most notably TGF-β (see Fig. 7.21; Box 7.11).
- In response to mechanical strain, fibroblasts acquire contractile stress fibers composed of cytoplasmic actins.[92]
- At this stage, a unique phenotype, the protomyofibroblast, appears to exist. These cells begin the process connecting to ECMPs via stress fibers and to other cells via N-cadherin–type adherens junctions.[80]
- Increased interstitial fluid flow increases:
  - □ Fibroblast to myofibroblast differentiation
  - □ Collagen production
  - □ Alignment and fibroblast proliferation
- These observations lead to the speculation that enhanced lymphatic drainage may play a role in fibrogenesis and fascial repair by promoting interstitial fluid flow.[80]

Expression of αSMA allows for significant contractile ability.[93]

- This process appears to be irreversible and regulated at the level of Rho/Rho kinase–mediated inhibition of myosin light-chain phosphatase.[94]
- If this occurs throughout the fascia, then the hypothesis that fascia is capable of contraction may have its origin in the recruitment and/or differentiation of fibroblasts to myofibroblasts.[81]
- Since myofibroblasts express gap junctions, cell-to-cell communication is facilitated, and potential syncytial behavior, such as coordinated contraction of large sheets of myofibroblasts,[95] lends further support that fascia has the capacity for myofascial-mediated contraction that is propagated and reinforced cell to cell.
- Normally, at the conclusion of tissue repair, the reconstructed ECMPs (produced by matured myofibroblasts) take over the mechanical load, leading to the lack of further need for resident myofibroblasts.[77]

Myofibroblasts either remove themselves through apoptosis or become deactivated; however, persistent activation of myofibroblasts can lead to excessive deposition of collagenous fibers, termed fibrosis.[88,96]

MACROPHAGES

Several types of cells typically found in connective tissue appear to have the ability to activate fibroblasts, enhance fibrosis, and most likely increase the transformation of these cells into myofibroblasts.

- The first of these cell types is the fixed macrophage or histiocyte (see Fig. 7.20); these cells represent the major link between the fascial system and the immune system.
- Macrophages are derived from circulating monocytes that have migrated into the tissue.
- Once in the tissue, monocytes differentiate into one of the three main lineages:
  - □ Tissue macrophages (histiocytes such as is seen in fascia, Kupffer cells in the liver, and microglia in the central nervous system)
  - □ Myeloid dendritic cells[97]
  - □ Osteoclasts in bone
- Cellular debris or proinflammatory cytokines in the surrounding extracellular matrix activate tissue macrophages.
  - □ Activation increases macrophage phagocytic capabilities and their secretory activity, producing additional cytokines.
  - □ Taken together, macrophages and monocytes are the largest producer of tumor necrosis factor-α (TNF-α).[98]
  - □ In addition, activated macrophages express more class II major histocompatibility complex (MHC) molecules and are more potent antigen-presenting cells than resting macrophages.
- Migration of additional macrophages into injured tissue is further enhanced by proinflammatory substances.
- Importantly, activated tissue macrophages release TGF-β1, which promotes the proliferation and differentiation of collagen-producing cells such as fibroblasts and myofibroblasts[99]; these processes predispose increased fibrosis and scar or adhesion formation.

MAST CELLS

Histamine-containing mast cells are scattered throughout connective tissue and typically associated with neurovascular bundles (see Fig. 7.21).

- The precursors of these histamine-containing cells are generated by hematopoietic stem cells in bone marrow.[100]

- Contrary to histamine-containing basophils, the precursors of the mast cell enter the circulation in an immature form and do not complete their maturation until they enter the peripheral tissue.
- Mast cells are heterogeneous with at least two populations identifiable by staining[100]:
  - □ One group contains tryptase and favors visceral organs in their distribution.
  - □ The other group contains multiple protease enzymes and is more often found in connective tissue, such as the dermis.
- Commonly associated with the response to parasite invasion, mast cells are known to have other functions in connective tissue as well. These granule-laden cells are capable of:
  - □ Phagocytosis
  - □ The production of proinflammatory cytokines
- Mast cells express FcεRI, a receptor that binds the Fc portion of the IgE antibody.
- When IgE binds to the cell, a degranulation process is initiated, resulting in the release of a host of biologically active agents such as[101]:
  - □ Histamine
  - □ Heparin
  - □ Chondroitin sulfates
  - □ Neutral proteases (tryptase)
  - □ Acid hydrolases
  - □ Cathepsin G
  - □ Carboxypeptidase

The location of the mast cell in connective tissue facilitates the delivery of its active agents to fibroblasts.

- Connective tissue mast cells have been identified as carrying prefabricated stores of TNF-α, a potent proinflammatory compound that stimulates fibroblasts and results in fibrosis.[101]
- Mast cells have been reported in increased numbers in tissue undergoing fibrosis,[100] but their role in tissue healing is not yet clarified.
- Thus, along with macrophages, mast cells appear to be capable of activating fibroblasts and enhancing the fibrosis occurring in and about an inflammatory event.

Extracellular Matrix Components

Connective tissue is composed of two major extracellular components[102]:

1. The first is a fibrous component responsible for the toughness of connective tissue.
2. The second is the gel-like ground substance into which the cells and fibers are embedded.

The most prevalent of the fibers present in connective tissue are those constructed of collagen molecules.

COLLAGEN FIBERS

Collagen is an insoluble fibrous protein, each fibrous molecule of which is made up of three pro-α-chains of amino acids woven together in a triple helix.

- The collagen molecules are woven together in a periodic manner as illustrated in Figure 7.22.
- Variations in the types of amino acids utilized in the α-chains create at least 27 described variants of collagen.[103]
- Differing collagens types are found in diverse tissues reflecting their various functions (Table 7.1).
- Major forms in the human body are types I, II, and III.

Although individual collagen molecules are synthesized intracellularly, the fibrils are assembled in the extracellular medium surrounding the cell.

- Collagen is produced by fibroblasts and myofibroblasts as well as by some forms of epithelial cells.[104] Activated monocytes also act as a potential source of collagen.
- Common factors that can enhance the production of collagen include:

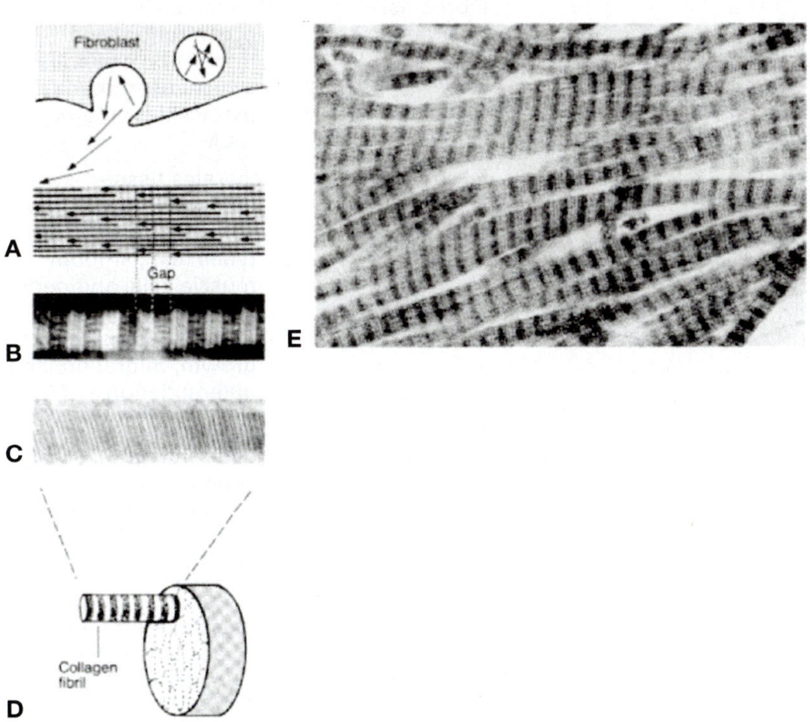

Figure 7.22. A diagram summarizing the formation and periodic nature of collagen fibrils. (Reprinted with permission from Cormack DH. *Ham's Histology*. 9th ed. J.B. Lippincott; 1987.)

TABLE 7.1

Summary of Collagen Types Along with Their Structure and Function

Classes of Collagen	Collagen Type	Tissue Distribution	Ultrastructure	Site of Synthesis	Function
Fibril-forming collagens	I	Dermis, bone, tendon, teeth, fascia, sclera, organ capsules, fibrous cartilage	Densely packed thick fibrils with marked variation in diameter	Fibroblast, osteoblast, odontoblast	Resistance to tension
	II	Hyaline and elastic cartilage, intervertebral disk, vitreous humor	No fibers, very thin fibrils embedded in ground substance	Chondroblast	Resistance to tension
	III	Bone, skin, smooth muscle, arteries, uterus, kidney, lung, tendon, periosteum, endoneurium	Loosely packed thin fibrils with more uniform diameter	Fibroblast, smooth muscle cells, Schwann cells, hepatocytes, mesenchymal cells	Structural maintenance in expansile organs, wound healing, mediate attachments of tendon, ligament, and periosteum to bone cortex
	V	Skin, bone, tendon, synovial membrane, liver, vascular tissue, placenta, teeth	Form quarter staggered fibrils	Fibroblasts, osteoblasts	Control of fiber diameter
	XI	Cartilaginous tissue	Form quarter staggered fibrils	Chondrocytes	Control of fiber diameter
Fibril-associated collagens	IX	Uniform throughout cartilage matrix, vitreous humor	Covalently cross-linked to type II collagen fibrils	Chondrocytes	Contributor of mechanical stability and resistance to swelling of type II collagen framework
	XII	Ligament, tendon, perichondrium, periosteum, periodontal ligament, reticular dermis	Covalently cross-linked to type I collagen fibrils	Fibroblast, myoblast	Control of fiber diameter and interaction of proteoglycans
	XIV	Codistributed with type I	Covalently cross-linked to collagen fibrils	Fibroblast, myoblast, osteoblasts, endoneural and perineural cells	Control of fiber diameter and interaction or proteoglycans
	XVI	Skin and cartilage		Fibroblasts, keratinocytes	Maintenance, organization, and interaction of fibrillar structures in the extracellular matrix (ECM)
Network-forming collagens	IV	Basement membranes		Fibroblasts	Separates tissue compartments, surrounds many cell types (e.g., smooth muscle cells and nerve cells), plays a role in regulation of cell growth, migration, and differentiation
Filamentous collagens	VI	Ubiquitous in connective tissue, concentrated in particular and adjacent to basement membranes of myofibers, blood vessels, and intramuscular nerves		Fibroblasts, macrophages	Cell attachment, differentiation, suppression of apoptosis, and as an anchoring meshwork for ECM structures
Short-chain collagens	VIII	Cornea and vascular tissue		Smooth muscle cells	Stimulates smooth muscle cell migration, invasion, and binding in vascular tissue

TABLE 7.1 (Continued)

Summary of Collagen Types Along with Their Structure and Function

Classes of Collagen	Collagen Type	Tissue Distribution	Ultrastructure	Site of Synthesis	Function
	X	Hyaline cartilage		Chondrocytes	Possibly endochondral ossification and indirectly hematopoiesis
	XIII	Blood vessel wall, glomeruli of the kidney, myotendinous junction		Fibroblasts, osteoblasts	
Long-chain collagens	VII	Skin basement membrane		Keratinocytes, fibroblasts	Secures basement membrane to adjacent connective tissue matrix

- Acetaldehyde
- Radiation
- Ascorbic acid
- Glucose (type III collagen only)

- Growth factors such as TGF-β and platelet-derived growth factor (PDGF) increase collagen synthesis, while TNF-α (originally named *cachexin*) suppresses collagen synthesis.
- Minerals such as calcium and hormones such as estrogen enhance collagen synthesis, while parathyroid hormone decreases collagen synthesis.[103]

ELASTIC FIBERS

Similar to collagen, elastin is a water-insoluble protein molecule, derived from tropoelastin.[102]

- This precursor protein is synthesized in the cell and assembled into fibrils in the extracellular matrix.
- However, unlike collagen, tropoelastin is an amorphous substance.
- An additional molecule, a microfibril, also has to be produced and secreted in order for elastic fibers to form.
- The microfibril acts as scaffolding into which the tropoelastin molecules are placed.[105]
- Elastic fibers are distensible and will rebound when released from a stressor; thus, as the percentage of elastin increases, the connective tissue becomes more resilient.
- Examples include the ligamentum flavum in the spine and the elastic layers present in the larger arteries.

LAMININ AND FIBRONECTIN

To maintain healthy and responsive connective tissue, there must be a mechanism for linking its cellular components to the surrounding environment.

- This involves several glycoprotein molecules, of which laminin and fibronectin are key representative examples.[102]
- These molecules function, in part, to link the cytoskeleton of the cell to the fibrous skeleton—collagenous and elastic—of the surrounding connective tissue.
- Laminin and fibronectin are secreted from fibrocytes and bind with integrins (adhesion molecules) located on the membranes of cells, as well as with matrix components such as collagen, fibrin and heparin sulfate proteoglycans.
- In this manner, the cell attaches to the surrounding extracellular matrix and the resulting complex:
  - Determines cell shape
  - Facilitates cell migration through the matrix
  - Enhances the cells' responsiveness to stressors within the matrix

Integrins initiate cell signaling processes leading to changes in cell function.[106]

- Thus, integrins, by transmitting force across the cell membrane, represent a major link between external mechanical force applied to the extracellular matrix and the cell and the initiation of movement and metabolic changes within the cell.[107]
- This process has been termed *mechanotransduction* and is a feature of:
  - Fibroblasts
  - Chondrocytes
  - Osteoblasts
- Importantly, stress and strain placed on the connective tissue can be transferred, through its fibrous component, to the cell membrane and cell cytoplasm. The time frame on this response is relatively rapid; changes in integrin composition can be noted in stressed cells within tens of seconds to tens of minutes after the onset of the stressor.

Mechanotransduction leading to intracellular signal transduction plays numerous roles in normal development, the maintenance of health and the ontogeny of disease, and particularly in the aging process.[108]

- Aging can impair the ability of skeletal muscle to respond to altered load and tension; the pathophysiologic causes of these changes appear to involve intracellular signaling transduction pathways sensitive to mechanotransduction at the cell surface.[109]
- Similarly, synovial joints respond best to cyclic stimulation; this quality is mediated by mechanotransduction and is diminished in the aging joint.
- Additional age-related changes in mechanotransduction in the cardiovascular and respiratory systems underlie the onset of the loss of compliance in the heart as well as endothelial cell and smooth muscle dysfunction in the vasculature.
- Age-related loss in control of smooth muscle cell contraction, leading to airway hypersensitivity and hyperreactivity, is possibly

related to a decreased sensitivity to tension in the airway walls, a result of the slow loss of mechanotransduction in the airway smooth muscle.

- Age-related loss of contact between fibroblast processes and collagen fibers in the dermis results in diminishing mechanotransduction and is thought to be related to decreasing resilience of skin with age.[109]
- Finally, mechanotransduction provides an interface between external environmental forces and the nucleus of the cell through mechanical stresses which can alter gene function.[110]

Growth Factors Associated with Fibrosis

TRANSFORMING GROWTH FACTOR-β

Extensive cell-to-cell communication is necessary in all tissues in order to maintain normal homeostatic activities and to respond appropriately to any allostatic challenge.[111,112]

- Cytokines represent a group of soluble mediators intimately involved in regulating cell function in health and disease.
- The transforming growth factor (TGF) family is a major group of cytokines regulating[113]:
  - The growth and differentiation of cells
  - Cellular response to stress and injury, including programmed cell death
- TGF-β, one of several members of the TGF family, is a protein secreted in an inactive form, which is subsequently activated through proteolysis.
- Numerous cell types produce TGF-β; however, a very significant reserve of TGF-β in tissue comes from blood platelets.
- The receptors for TGF-β are members of a kinase family and initiate signal transduction pathways in the receiving cell.[113]
- TGF-β plays a significant role in:
  - The normal development and maturation of tissues
  - Tissue healing subsequent to injury
  - Tissue remodeling leading to fibrosis and oncogenesis[114–117]

The function of TGF-β is dependent on the specific tissue in which it is located and the surrounding extracellular milieu (Box 7.12).

- Thus, activated TGF-β can either inhibit or stimulate cell proliferation based on environmental factors; however, in most situations, it appears to repress cell division and enhance differentiation.[113]
- It is also chemoattractive to immune cells and enhances the deposition of extracellular matrix by activating fibroblasts.[115]
- Interestingly, TGF-β is capable of autoinduction of its own production from connective tissue cells such as macrophages.
- In inflamed tissue, TGF-β can inhibit the production of TNF-α and IL-1 and suppress free radical production by macrophages, giving it an anti-inflammatory role.

TGF-β is extensively involved in wound repair and overproduction of TGF-β is a key feature in tissue fibrosis.[118]

BOX 7.12 Transforming Growth Factor-β1

- Typically inhibits cellular proliferation
- Stimulates cellular differentiation
- Is a key controlling feature for differentiation and activation of myofibroblasts

- Acute injury presents with a transient increase in TGF-β; however, chronic reinjury results in overproduction of TGF-β and subsequent tissue fibrosis.
- Elevated levels of TGF-β are seen in disease states and during chemotherapy and are thought to be responsible for the resulting tissue fibrosis in the liver and lung.[99]
- The connection between TGF-β and fibrosis appears to lie in the induction of myofibroblasts; most other factors known to induce myofibroblasts appear to achieve this action by stimulation of TGF-β.[88]

TISSUE DYNAMICS: FIBROSIS AND TISSUE REPAIR

Fibrosis involves the proliferation of extracellular matrix material replacing or overgrowing the parenchymal tissue, resulting in the scarring and hardening of the organ.

- Typically, it develops from a chronic inflammatory state and can occur in such organs as the kidney, liver, and lung as well as in muscle and tendon.[47]
- In acute tissue injury, transient expression of TGF-β leads to the development of myofibroblasts and the synthesis of collagen; both processes are beneficial to normal wound repair.
- However, persistent irritation of the tissue sustains the production of growth factors such as TGF-β, leading to the persistence of myofibroblasts and the excessive secretion of collagen; such processes foster the buildup of fibrotic scars.

The fact that myofibroblasts normally disappear from newly repaired sites support its role in wound repair, and this process is one of spontaneous and widespread myofibroblast apoptosis—also termed *programmed cell death*.[119]

- Therefore, proapoptotic molecules such as nitric oxide (NO) signal the end of the reparative stage, and their premature presence could lead to incomplete repair by premature loss of load-bearing myofibroblasts and the ECMP they secrete.
- In cases where normal apoptosis does not occur, fibroblasts as well as myofibroblasts proliferate, leading to fibrosis. The increased secretion of ECMPs by these cells, while affording tissue repair, also potentiates tensile strength and may ultimately restrict the very structures it aims to repair and protect.
- In fact, fascial restrictions, palpable by clinicians, are the very sites targeted by several modalities of OMT including direct and indirect MFR techniques.

Proliferative fasciitis is associated with activated pericytes (fibroblast-like cells found lying along blood vessels), which appear to act as additional sources of fibroblasts and/or myofibroblasts.[120]

- Presence of additional myofibroblasts, in turn, would perpetuate enhanced fascial tension and exacerbate inflammatory cytokine production.
- In addition to ECMPs, myofibroblasts also express and secrete numerous cytokines including the ILs and others.
- Given that fascia has been shown to support blood cell flow through channels (fascial extensions of inferiorly based fasciocutaneous flaps that exhibit erythrocyte flow in vascular channels of the deep fascia),[121] it is theorized that fascia-derived cytokines have the ability to be delivered systemically by hematogenous movement.
- Prostaglandin E2 and prostaglandin F2 alpha have been identified in association with nodular myofibroblasts in the fascia of patients with Dupuytren disease.[122]

- Therefore, molecules such as these with vasoactive capacity may also play key roles in the recruitment and/or differentiation of myofibroblasts as well as distribution of myofibroblast-derived cytokines to distant tissues such as the brain, lung, heart, or kidney.
- If true, this could be a mechanism by which osteopathic manipulative treatment targeting fascia in specific anatomical locations could effect change at distant sites.[83,84]

Clinically, anti-inflammatory cytokines may play cardinal roles in the efficacy of osteopathic manipulative treatment as they:

1. Reduce edema
2. Increase range of motion (ROM)
3. Decrease analgesic requirements[84,123–125]

- Relevant to this notion, equibiaxial strain of tendon fibroblasts (3.5% beyond resting length) for 2 hours resulted in increased ATP release and inhibition of IL-1β expression.[126]
- Since IL-1β is proinflammatory, such fibroblast strain may set in motion a cascade of events to attenuate proinflammatory as well as stimulate anti-inflammatory signaling pathways.
- Other reports have shown that biophysical perturbation (in the form of shear stress) decreased expression of a number of inflammatory biomarkers (e.g., IL-1α, IL-14, IL-15, IL-16, and the IL-13 receptor) in endothelial cells,[127] a process that may be attributed to upregulation of the transcription factors NF-κB and activator protein-1 (AP-1).[128]

Fascial Response to Stress

The mechanisms by which the fascia generates and responds to biomechanical strain are not clearly elucidated and are likely multifaceted.

- Mechanosignaling could result from:
  - Normal movements
  - Injury
  - OMT as well as other stimuli
- Mechanosignaling appears to rely on:
  - Ion channel gating
  - Integrins
  - Focal adhesions
  - α smooth muscle actin itself[129]
- Mechanical deformation of cell shape stretches cells in one or more axes.
- Types of stretch range from:
  - Pressure that can be positive (e.g., increased blood vessel flow) or negative (e.g., hypertonic extracellular fluid [ECF]-induced cell shrinking)
  - Flow over a cell surface (e.g., shear forces such as seen in vascular endothelial cells)
  - Cell elongation (e.g., as seen in muscle cells and various fibroblasts)
  - Cell bending (e.g., as seen in normal bone cells)[130]

Fibroblasts and myofibroblasts respond in multiple ways to a wide variety of biophysical perturbations.

- While integrins and their receptors appear to be critical for some aspects of "outside-in signaling" as reported for ligamentous fibroblasts,[131,132] strain is sensed at the cellular level by integrin-independent alterations in membrane ion conductances.[133]
- Mechanogated ion channels have been reported, and a subset that conducts calcium and that is blocked by the lanthanide gadolinium (Gd) has been termed stretch-activated calcium channels (SACCs) (see Gupta et al.[82]).

BOX 7.13 Mechanotransduction

Mechanotransduction is the conversion of mechanical forces, such as linear stress, into an electrochemical signaling code that can modify cellular activity.

Mechanical forces acting on the cell membrane can alter gene activity within the cell.[110]

- Potential roles for calcium in strain-regulated fibroblast function have been reported.
  - For example, palmar fascia responded to mechanical stress by significantly increasing tissue intracellular free calcium concentration.[82]
  - In other studies, gingival fibroblasts were stretched in vitro to 1% or 2.8% beyond resting length. While the 1% group showed no intracellular free calcium changes, the 2.8% group displayed a significant increase in free calcium followed by calcium oscillations with a frequency of 2,000/s.
  - These oscillations appear to involve extracellular calcium flux through SACCs in a process that required intact actin scaffolding.[134]

A Role for Actin in Mechanotransduction

Disruption of polymerized actin, whose expression is greatly elevated upon fibroblast differentiation into myofibroblasts, inhibit strain-induced intracellular Ca^{2+} release, as reported in several studies[134–136] (Box 7.13).

- These data highlight the potential importance of the actin cytoskeleton in cosensing biophysical strain and perhaps themselves being responsible for changes in SACC conductance observed with strain.
- The precise role of actin in mediating these responses is unclear, but it likely involves the ability of mechanically activated Src (a nonreceptor tyrosine kinase[136]).
  - Specifically, when actin (by cytochalasin D) or microtubules (by the antineoplastic agent nocodazole) were disrupted, force-induced changes in endothelial cell Src activation were blocked.
  - The directional Src activation observed (i.e., pointing in the direction opposite the applied stretching of the cell) may aid in the release of cell tension, thus serving as a feedback mechanism for cells to adapt to mechanical perturbations.
- Others have shown SACC activation to be dependent upon an intact actin cytoskeleton,[134,135,137] which suggests that injuries and therapeutic forces or strains induced when performing osteopathic manipulative treatment could be mechanotransduced cellularly by actin/SACC association.

Direction of the Strain

In addition to strain frequency, magnitude, and duration, recent in vitro data suggest that strain direction differentially regulates fibroblast growth, ion conductance, and gene expression (Box 7.14).

BOX 7.14 Fibroblast Response to Strain

Strain frequency, magnitude, duration, and direction can influence the nuclear-mediated response of fibroblasts to the stimulus.

- For example, human dermal fibroblasts strained multiaxially caused cellular alignment in a manner perpendicular to the strain vector. However, uniaxial shear stress did not affect cells in this regard.[138]
  - Cultured fibroblasts also responded to uniaxial strain with increased thymidine incorporation (signifying DNA replication) and collagen incorporation of labeled proline.
  - Importantly, both these measures *decreased* significantly in fibroblasts strained biaxially.[139]
  - Fibroblasts depolarized (by increasing nonspecific inward cation current) when compressed, but hyperpolarized when stretched uniaxially between two patch pipettes.[140]
- Others reported that smooth muscle responded to hyposmotic ECF-induced cell stretch (yielding multiaxial strain) with increased inward calcium current within one minute.
  - This response was not, however, repeatable if cells were stretched uniaxially between two electrodes.[141]
  - When C2C12 myotubes were strained multiaxially, ribosomal S6 kinase phosphorylation increased significantly, a response found to be actin dependent since cytochalasin D blocked it.
  - Interestingly, this study also reported that myotubes stretched multiaxially responded with increased p70 signaling, and this was Gd (and therefore SACC) insensitive.
  - Conversely, uniaxial strain of these cells increased protein kinase B expression, a response that was Gd sensitive.[142]
- Taken together, these data strongly suggest that fascial fibroblasts and myofibroblasts are capable of discerning among various strain directions and responding accordingly with differential SACC signaling.
- Data from these studies suggest mechanisms by which uni- and multiaxial fascia-directed OMT might yield distinct clinical outcomes.

Cyclic stretch of aortic tissue cultures increased mitogen-activated protein kinase (MAPK) phosphorylation.

- This process led to extracellular signal-regulated kinase-1 and kinase-2 transfer to the nucleus, where they phosphorylated transcription factors including NF-κB and AP-1.[143]
  - Since these factors are responsible for IL-6 and IL-8 expression,[123] they may be involved in strain regulation of fibroblast IL and other cytokine secretion.
  - These data further suggest a mechanism (i.e., MAPK) by which strain stimulates fibroblast proliferation.[139,144,145]
- Fibroblast proliferation, while often thought of as contributing to tissue congestion, edema, and other proinflammatory processes, could also serve as a mechanism by which MFR and other manual medicine techniques result in long-term positive treatment outcomes (Box 7.14).
  - This would be accomplished by further (and potentially sustained) enhancement of cytokine pools from actively proliferating fascial fibroblasts and correction of dysfunctional ECMP cross-linking, as has been postulated by others.[82]
  - Alternatively, long-term efficacy could result from MFR-induced release of apoptotic cytokines (e.g., NO) (see Dodd et al.[146]) causing selective fibroblast death from injury sites and removal of fibrotic materials responsible for pain and attenuated ROM.
- It has been reported that fibroblasts themselves respond to various strain types by increasing secretion of several ILs while decreasing secretion of others.[83,84]
  - In fact, in vitro modeling of repetitive motion strains on cultured human fibroblasts increases inflammatory IL secretion, while a modeled form of counterstrain on similar cultures actually decreased proinflammatory cytokine secretion.
  - Whether this process involves fibroblast to myofibroblast differentiation has not been reported.
- Clinically, activation of anti-inflammatory cytokines (and/or attenuation of proinflammatory ones) could account for:
  - Increased ROM of injured tissues and joints
  - Decreased edema
  - Decreased need for analgesics in manners dependent upon fibroblast growth responses

SUMMARY

Fascia is defined as irregular connective tissue that plays a role in surrounding and protecting the organ systems of the body.

- Four distinct layers of fascia were presented:
  - Pannicular
  - Axial (appendicular)
  - Meningeal
  - Visceral
- The components of fascia were presented with particular emphasis placed on the fibroblasts and their transformation into myofibroblasts.
- Cultured fibroblasts are sensitive, via mechanotransduction, to strain intensity and direction; these forces can alter cellular proliferation as well as the secretion of proinflammatory cytokines.
- Possible correlations between fibroblast strain sensitivity and influence of manual medicine techniques are presented.

ACKNOWLEDGMENTS

The authors and editors of this chapter would like to acknowledge the scholarly contributions of Paul R. Standley for prior editions of this chapter.

REFERENCES

1. Clemente CD. *Gray's Anatomy of the Human Body.* Lea & Febiger; 1985.
2. Standring S. *Gray's Anatomy; The Anatomical Basis of Clinical Practice.* Elsevier Limited; 2021.
3. Cormack DH. *Ham's Histology.* J.B. Lippincott Co; 1987.
4. Fasel JH, Dembé JC, Majno PE. Fascia: a pragmatic overview for surgeons. *Am Surg.* 2007;73:451–453.
5. Stecco C. *Functional Atlas of the Human Fascial System.* Elsevier Health Sciences; 2015.
6. Anderson W, Makins GH. The planes of subperitoneal and subpleural connective tissue, with their connections. *J Anat Physiol.* 1890;25:78–86.
7. García-Armengol J, García-Botello S, Martinez-Soriano F, Roig JV, Lledó S. Review of the anatomic concepts in relation to the retrorectal space and endopelvic fascia: Waldeyer's fascia and the rectosacral fascia. *Colorectal Dis.* 2008;10:298–302.
8. Goss CM. *Gray's Anatomy of the Human Body.* Lea & Febiger; 1948.
9. Huijing PA, Hollander P, Findley T, Schleip R. *Fascia Research II: Basic Science and Implications for Conventional and Complementary Health Care.* Urban & Fischer; 2009.
10. Benjamin M. The fascia of the limbs and back–a review. *J Anat.* 2009; 214:1–18.
11. Gallaudet BB. *A Description of the Planes of Fascia of the Human Body with Special Reference to the Fascias of the Abdomen, Pelvis and Perineum.* Columbia University Press; 1931:76.
12. Singer E. *Fascia of the Human Body and Their Relations to the Organs They Envelop.* Williams and Wilkins; 1935.
13. Hayes MA. Abdominopelvic fascia. *Am J Anat.* 1950;87:119–161.
14. Stilwell DL Jr. The innervation of tendons and aponeuroses. *Am J Anat.* 1956;100:289–317.

15. Snyder G. *Fasciae—Applied Anatomy and Physiology.* Academy of Applied Osteopathy Yearbook; 1956.
16. Ercoli A, Delmas V, Fanfani F, et al. Terminologia Anatomica versus unofficial descriptions and nomenclature of the fasciae and ligaments of the female pelvis: a dissection-based comparative study. *Am J Obstet Gynecol.* 2005;193:1565–1573.
17. Skandalakis PN, Zoras O, Skandalakis JE, Mirilas P. Transversalis, endoabdominal, endothoracic fascia: who's who? *Am Surg.* 2006;72:16–18.
18. Bisseret D, Kaci R, Lafage-Proust MH, et al. Periosteum: characteristic imaging findings with emphasis on radiologic-pathologic comparisons. *Skeletal Radiol.* 2015;44:321–338.
19. Jozsa L, Kannus P. *Human tendons: Anatomy, Physiology and Pathology.* Human Kinetics; 1997.
20. Bevan JA, Bevan RD, Duckles SP. Adrenergic regulation of vascular smooth muscle. In: Bohr DF, Somlyo AP, Sparks HV, Geiger SR, eds. *Handbook of Physiology: Section 2, The Cardiovascular System: Volume II, Vascular Smooth Muscle.* American Physiological Society; 1980:515–566.
21. Burnstock G. Cholinergic and purinergic regulation of blood vessels. In: Bohr DF, Somlyo AP, Sparks HV, Geiger SR, eds. *Handbook of Physiology, Section 2: The Cardiovascular System. Vol. II. Vascular Smooth Muscle.* American Physiological Society/Waverly Press; 1980:567–612.
22. Stilwell DL Jr. The nerve supply of the vertebral column and its associated structures in the monkey. *Anat Rec.* 1956;125:139–169.
23. Walsh DA, McWilliams F. Tachykinins and the cardiovascular system. *Curr Drug Targets.* 2006;7:1031–1042.
24. Gold MS, Caterina MJ. Molecular biology of the nociceptor/transduction. In: Basbaum AI, Bushnell MC, ed. *Science of Pain.* Amsterdam; 2009:43–73.
25. Mutsaers SE. The mesothelial cell. *Int J Biochem Cell Biol.* 2004;36:9–16.
26. Hoppe K, Schleip R, Lehmann-Horn F, Jager H, Klingler W. Contractile elements in muscular fascial tissue – implications for in-vitro contracture testing for malignant hyperthermia. *Anaesthesia.* 2014;69:1002–1008.
27. Schleip R, Gabbiani G, Wilke J, et al. Fascia is able to actively contract and may thereby influence musculoskeletal dynamics: a histochemical and mechanographic investigation. *Front Physiol.* 2019;10:336.
28. Wendell-Smith CP. Fascia: an illustrative problem in international terminology. *Surg Radiol Anat.* 1997;19:273–277.
29. Last RJ. *Anatomy: Regional and Applied.* Churchill Livingstone; 1978.
30. Arey LB. *Development Anatomy.* 7th ed. Philadelphia, PA: W.B. Saunders Company; 1965.
31. Stecco C, Tiengo C, Stecco A, et al. Fascia redefined: anatomical features and technical relevance in fascial flap surgery. *Surg Radiol Anat.* 2013; 35:369–376.
32. Macchi V, Tiengo C, Porzionato A, et al. Histotopographic study of the fibroadipose connective cheek system. *Cells Tissues Organs.* 2010;191: 47–56.
33. Ackerman AB. *Histological Diagnosis of Inflammatory Skin Disease.* Lea & Febiger; 1978.
34. Herlin C, Chica-Rosa A, Subsol G, et al. Three-dimensional study of the skin/subcutaneous complex using in vivo whole body 3T MRI: review of the literature and confirmation of a generic pattern of organization. *Surg Radiol Anat.* 2015;37:731–741.
35. Catala M. Embryonic and fetal development of structures associated with the cerebro-spinal fluid in man and other species. Part I: the ventricular system, meninges and choroid plexuses. *Arch Anat Cytol Pathol.* 1998;46:153–169.
36. Catala M, Teillet MA, De Robertis EM, Le Douarin NM. A spinal cord fate map in the avian embryo: while regressing, Hensen's node lays down the notochord and floor plate thus joining the spinal cord lateral walls. *Development.* 1996;122:2599–2610.
37. Moore KL, Persaud TVN, Torche M. *The Developing Human: Clinically-Oriented Embryology.* Elsevier; 2020.
38. Mirilas P, Skandalakis JE. Surgical anatomy of the retroperitoneal spaces—part I: embryogenesis and anatomy. *Am Surg.* 2009;75:1091–1097.
39. Hollinshead WH. *Anatomy for Surgeons: The Thorax, Abdomen and Pelvis.* Hoeber-Harper; 1956.
40. Popa GT, Lucinescu E. The mechanostructure of the pericardium. *J Anat.* 1932;67:78–107.
41. Bendavid R, Howarth D. Transversalis fascia rediscovered. *Surg Clin North Am.* 2000;80:25–33.
42. Byrnes KG, Walsh D, Dockery P, McDermott K, Coffey JC. Anatomy of the mesentery: Current understanding and mechanisms of attachment. *Semin Cell Dev Biol.* 2019;92:12–17.
43. Amin M, Blandford AT, Polk HC Jr. Renal fascia of Gerota. *Urology.* 1976;7:1–3.
44. Liang JT, Huang J, Chen TC, Hung JS. The Toldt fascia: a historic review and surgical implications in complete mesocolic excision for colon cancer. *Asian J Surg.* 2019;42:1–5.
45. Chen Z, Zhang XJ, Chang HD, et al. From basic to clinical: anatomy of Denonvilliers' fascia and its application in laparoscopic radical resection of rectal cancer. *World J Gastrointest Surg.* 2023;15:2108–2114.
46. Duron JJ. Postoperative intraperitoneal adhesion pathophysiology. *Colorectal Dis.* 2007;9(Suppl 2):14–24.
47. Wynn TA. Cellular and molecular mechanisms of fibrosis. *J Pathol.* 2008;214:199–210.
48. Beyene RT, Kavalukas SL, Barbul A. Intra-abdominal adhesions: anatomy, physiology, pathophysiology, and treatment. *Curr Probl Surg.* 2015; 52:271–319.
49. Langevin HM. Potential role of fascia in chronic musculoskeletal pain. In: Audette JF, Bailey A, ed. *Integrative Pain Medicine: The Science and Practice of Complementary and Alternative Medicine in Pain Management.* Humana Press; 2008:123–132.
50. Langevin HM, Sherman KJ. Pathophysiological model for chronic low back pain integrating connective tissue and nervous system mechanisms. *Med Hypotheses.* 2007;68:74–80.
51. Stecco C, Gagey O, Belloni A, et al. Anatomy of the deep fascia of the upper limb. Second part: study of innervation. *Morphologie.* 2007;91:38–43.
52. Palmieri G, Panu R, Asole A, Farina V, Sanna L, Gabbi C. Macroscopic organization and sensitive innervation of the tendinous intersection and the lacertus fibrosus of the biceps brachii muscle in the ass and horse. *Arch Anat Histol Embryol.* 1986;69:73–82.
53. Sanchis-Alfonso V, Roselló-Sastre E. Immunohistochemical analysis for neural markers of the lateral retinaculum in patients with isolated symptomatic patellofemoral malalignment. A neuroanatomic basis for anterior knee pain in the active young patient. *Am J Sports Med.* 2000;28:725–731.
54. Staubesand J, Li Y. Zum feinbau der fascia cruris mit Besonderer Berucksichtigung epi- und intrafasziale Nerven. *Manuelle Medizin.* 1996; 34:196–200.
55. Stecco C, Porzionato A, Macchi V, et al. Histological characteristics of the deep fascia of the upper limb. *Ital J Anat Embryol.* 2006;111:105–110.
56. Stilwell DL Jr. Regional variations in the innervation of deep fasciae and aponeuroses. *Anat Rec.* 1957;127:635–653.
57. Tanaka S, Ito T. Histochemical demonstration of adrenergic fibers in the fascia periosteum and retinaculum. *Clin Orthop Relat Res.* 1977;(126): 276–281.
58. Yahia L, Rhalmi S, Newman N, Isler M. Sensory innervation of human thoracolumbar fascia. An immunohistochemical study. *Acta Orthop Scand.* 1992;63:195–197.
59. Stecco C, Porzionato A, Lancerotto L, et al. Histological study of the deep fasciae of the limbs. *J Bodyw Mov Ther.* 2008;12:225–230.
60. Schleip R. Fascial plasticity—a new neurobiological explanation: Part 1. *J Bodyw Mov Ther.* 2003;7:11–19.
61. Stecco C, Gagey O, Macchi V, et al. Tendinous muscular insertions onto the deep fascia of the upper limb. First part: anatomical study. *Morphologie.* 2007;91:29–37.
62. Bednar DA, Orr FW, Simon GT. Observations on the pathomorphology of the thoracolumbar fascia in chronic mechanical back pain: a microscopic study. *Spine (Phila Pa 1976).* 1995;20:1161–1164.
63. Lundon K. The effect of mechanical load on soft connective tissues. In: Hammer WI, ed. *Functional Soft-Tissue Examination and Treatment by Manual Methods.* Bartlett and Jones Publishers; 2007;15–30.
64. Schleip R. Fascial plasticity—a new neurobiological explanation: part 2. *J Bodyw Mov Ther.* 2003;7:104–116.
65. Suarez-Rodriguez V, Fede C, Pirri C, et al. Fascial innervation: a systematic review of the literature. *Int J Mol Sci.* 2022;23(10):5674.
66. Pawlina W. *Histology, A Text and Atlas: With Correlated Cell and Molecular Biology.* Wolters Kluwer; 2016.
67. Rhee S, Grinnell F. Fibroblast mechanics in 3D collagen matrices. *Adv Drug Deliv Rev.* 2007;59:1299–1305.

68. Grinnell F. Fibroblast biology in three-dimensional collagen matrices. *Trends Cell Biol.* 2003;13:264–269.
69. Langevin HM, Bouffard NA, Badger GJ, Iatridis JC, Howe AK. Dynamic fibroblast cytoskeletal response to subcutaneous tissue stretch ex vivo and in vivo. *Am J Physiol Cell Physiol.* 2005;288:C747–C756.
70. Neilson EG. Mechanisms of disease: fibroblasts–a new look at an old problem. *Nat Clin Pract Nephrol.* 2006;2:101–108.
71. Yang J, Weinberg RA. Epithelial-mesenchymal transition: at the crossroads of development and tumor metastasis. *Dev Cell.* 2008;14: 818–829.
72. Coyte PC, Croxford R, McIsaac W, Feldman W, Friedberg J. The role of adjuvant adenoidectomy and tonsillectomy in the outcome of the insertion of tympanostomy tubes. *N Engl J Med.* 2001;344:1188–1195.
73. Hadpech S, Thongboonkerd V. Epithelial-mesenchymal plasticity in kidney fibrosis. *Genesis.* 2024;62:e23529.
74. Mottais A, Riberi L, Falco A, Soccal S, Gohy S, De Rose V. Epithelial-mesenchymal transition mechanisms in chronic airway diseases: a common process to target? *Int J Mol Sci.* 2023;24:12412.
75. Laurent GJ, Chambers RC, Hill MR, McAnulty RJ. Regulation of matrix turnover: fibroblasts, forces, factors and fibrosis. *Biochem Soc Trans.* 2007;35:647–651.
76. Grinnell F, Ho CH, Tamariz E, Lee DJ, Skuta G. Dendritic fibroblasts in three-dimensional collagen matrices. *Mol Biol Cell.* 2003;14:384–95.
77. Tomasek JJ, Gabbiani G, Hinz B, Chaponnier C, Brown RA. Myofibroblasts and mechano-regulation of connective tissue remodelling. *Nat Rev Mol Cell Biol.* 2002;3:349–363.
78. Fernandes MG, da Silva LP, Cerqueira MT, et al. Mechanomodulatory biomaterials prospects in scar prevention and treatment. *Acta Biomater.* 2022;150:22–33.
79. Schuster R, Younesi F, Ezzo M, Hinz B. The role of myofibroblasts in physiological and pathological tissue repair. *Cold Spring Harb Perspect Biol.* 2023;15:1–39.
80. Hinz B, Pittet P, Smith-Clerc J, Chaponnier C, Meister JJ. Myofibroblast development is characterized by specific cell-cell adherens junctions. *Mol Biol Cell.* 2004;15:4310–4320.
81. Schleip R, Klingler W, Lehmann-Horn F. Active fascial contractility: fascia may be able to contract in a smooth muscle-like manner and thereby influence musculoskeletal dynamics. *Med Hypotheses.* 2005;65:273–277.
82. Gupta R, Allen F, Tan V, Bozentka DJ, Bora FW, Osterman AL. The effect of shear stress on fibroblasts derived from Dupuytren's tissue and normal palmar fascia. *J Hand Surg Am.* 1998;23:945–950.
83. Eagan TS, Meltzer KR, Standley PR. Importance of strain direction in regulating human fibroblast proliferation and cytokine secretion: a useful in vitro model for soft tissue injury and manual medicine treatments. *J Manipulative Physiol Ther.* 2007;30:584–592.
84. Meltzer KR, Standley PR. Modeled repetitive motion strain and indirect osteopathic manipulative techniques in regulation of human fibroblast proliferation and interleukin secretion. *J Am Osteopath Assoc.* 2007; 107:527–536.
85. Langevin HM, Cornbrooks CJ, Taatjes DJ. Fibroblasts form a body-wide cellular network. *Histochem Cell Biol.* 2004;122:7–15.
86. Wan L, Jiang D, Correa-Gallegos D, et al. Connexin43 gap junction drives fascia mobilization and repair of deep skin wounds. *Matrix Biol.* 2021;97:58–71.
87. Banes AJ, Tsuzaki M, Yamamoto J, et al. Mechanoreception at the cellular level: the detection, interpretation, and diversity of responses to mechanical signals. *Biochem Cell Biol.* 1995;73:349–365.
88. Hinz B. Myofibroblasts. *Exp Eye Res.* 2016;142:56–70.
89. Ehrlich HP, Allison GM, Leggett M. The myofibroblast, cadherin, alpha smooth muscle actin and the collagen effect. *Cell Biochem Funct.* 2006;24:63–70.
90. Ronty MJ, Leivonen SK, Hinz B, et al. Isoform-specific regulation of the actin-organizing protein palladin during TGF-beta1-induced myofibroblast differentiation. *J Invest Dermatol.* 2006;126:2387–2396.
91. Hinz B. Formation and function of the myofibroblast during tissue repair. *J Invest Dermatol.* 2007;127:526–537.
92. Werner S, Grose R. Regulation of wound healing by growth factors and cytokines. *Physiol Rev.* 2003;83:835–870.
93. Hinz B, Celetta G, Tomasek JJ, Gabbiani G, Chaponnier C. Alpha-smooth muscle actin expression upregulates fibroblast contractile activity. *Mol Biol Cell.* 2001;12:2730–2741.
94. Tomasek JJ, Vaughan MB, Kropp BP, et al. Contraction of myofibroblasts in granulation tissue is dependent on Rho/Rho kinase/myosin light chain phosphatase activity. *Wound Repair Regen.* 2006;14:313–320.
95. Gabbiani G, Ryan GB, Majne G. Presence of modified fibroblasts in granulation tissue and their possible role in wound contraction. *Experientia.* 1971;27:549–550.
96. Bomb R, Heckle MR, Sun Y, et al. Myofibroblast secretome and its auto-/paracrine signaling. *Expert Rev Cardiovasc Ther.* 2016;14:591–598.
97. Lipscomb MF, Masten BJ. Dendritic cells: immune regulators in health and disease. *Physiol Rev.* 2002;82:97–130.
98. Papadakis KA, Targan SR. Tumor necrosis factor: biology and therapeutic inhibitors. *Gastroenterology.* 2000;119:1148–1157.
99. Kisseleva T, Brenner DA. Mechanisms of fibrogenesis. *Exp Biol Med (Maywood).* 2008;233:109–122.
100. Metcalfe DD, Baram D, Mekori YA. Mast cells. *Physiol Rev.* 1997;77: 1033–1079.
101. Galli SJ. New concepts about the mast cell. *N Engl J Med.* 1993;328: 257–265.
102. Pawlina W. *Histology: A Text with Atlas: With Correlated Cell and Molecular Biology*. Lippincott Williams & Wilkins; 2021.
103. Kavitha O, Thampan RV. Factors influencing collagen biosynthesis. *J Cell Biochem.* 2008;104:1150–1160.
104. Tabata T, Kawakatsu H, Maidji E, et al. Induction of an epithelial integrin alphavbeta6 in human cytomegalovirus-infected endothelial cells leads to activation of transforming growth factor-beta1 and increased collagen production. *Am J Pathol.* 2008;172:1127–1140.
105. Wagenseil JE, Mecham RP. New insights into elastic fiber assembly. *Birth Defects Res C Embryo Today.* 2007;81:229–240.
106. Schwartz MA, DeSimone DW. Cell adhesion receptors in mechanotransduction. *Curr Opin Cell Biol.* 2008;20:551–556.
107. Katsumi A, Orr AW, Tzima E, Schwartz MA. Integrins in mechanotransduction. *J Biol Chem.* 2004;279:12001–12004.
108. Silver FH, DeVore D, Siperko LM. Invited review: role of mechanophysiology in aging of ECM: effects of changes in mechanochemical transduction. *J Appl Physiol.* 2003;95:2134–2141.
109. Wu M, Fannin J, Rice KM, Wang B, Blough ER. Effect of aging on cellular mechanotransduction. *Ageing Res Rev.* 2009;10:1–15.
110. Graham DM, Burridge K. Mechanotransduction and nuclear function. *Curr Opin Cell Biol.* 2016;40:98–105.
111. Morikawa M, Derynck R, Miyazono K. TGF-beta and the TGF-beta family: context-dependent roles in cell and tissue physiology. *Cold Spring Harb Perspect Biol.* 2016;8:a021873.
112. Roberts AB, Flanders KC, Kondaiah P, et al. Transforming growth factor beta: biochemistry and roles in embryogenesis, tissue repair and remodeling, and carcinogenesis. *Recent Prog Horm Res.* 1988;44:157–197.
113. Massague J. The transforming growth factor-beta family. *Annu Rev Cell Biol.* 1990;6:597–641.
114. August P, Suthanthiran M. Transforming growth factor beta signaling, vascular remodeling, and hypertension. *N Engl J Med.* 2006;354:2721–2723.
115. Border WA, Noble NA. Transforming growth factor beta in tissue fibrosis. *N Engl J Med.* 1994;331:1286–1292.
116. Kitisin K, Saha T, Blake T, et al. Tgf-Beta signaling in development. *Sci STKE.* 2007;2007: cm1.
117. Sporn MB, Roberts AB, Wakefield LM, Assoian RK. Transforming growth factor-á: biological function and chemical structure. *Science.* 1986;233:532–534.
118. Barrientos S, Stojadinovic O, Golinko MS, Brem H, Tomic-Canic M. Growth factors and cytokines in wound healing. *Wound Repair Regen.* 2008;16:585–601.
119. Carlson MA, Longaker MT, Thompson J. Wound splinting regulates granulation tissue survival. *J Surg Res.* 2003;110:304–309.
120. Chou Y-H, Pan S-Y, Shih H-M, Lin S-L. Update of pericytes function and their roles in kidney diseases. *J Formos Med Assoc.* 2024;123(3): 307–317.

121. Bhattacharya V, Watts RK, Reddy GR. Live demonstration of microcirculation in the deep fascia and its implication. *Plast Reconstr Surg.* 2005;115:458–463.
122. Badalamente MA, Hurst LC, Sampson SP. Prostaglandins influence myofibroblast contractility in Dupuytren's disease. *J Hand Surg Am.* 1988;13(6):867–871.
123. Andoh A, Zhang Z, Inatomi O, et al. Interleukin-22, a member of the IL-10 subfamily, induces inflammatory responses in colonic subepithelial myofibroblasts. *Gastroenterology.* 2005;129:969–984.
124. Glover JC, Rennei PR. Strain and counterstrain techniques. In: Ward R, ed. *Foundations for Osteopathic Medicine.* Lippincott, Williams & Wilkins; 2003:1002–1016.
125. Nemet D, Hong S, Mills PJ, Ziegler MG, Hill M, Cooper DM. Systemic vs. local cytokine and leukocyte responses to unilateral wrist flexion exercise. *J Appl Physiol.* 2002;93:546–554.
126. Tsuzaki M, Bynum D, Almekinders L, Yang X, Faber J, Banes AJ. ATP modulates load-inducible IL-1beta, COX 2, and MMP-3 gene expression in human tendon cells. *J Cell Biochem.* 2003;89:556–562.
127. Chen BP, Li YS, Zhao Y, et al. DNA microarray analysis of gene expression in endothelial cells in response to 24-h shear stress. *Physiol Genomics.* 2001;7:55–63.
128. Resnick N, Gimbrone MA Jr. Hemodynamic forces are complex regulators of endothelial gene expression. *FASEB J.* 1995;9:874–882.
129. Goffin JM, Pittet P, Csucs G, Lussi JW, Meister JJ, Hinz B. Focal adhesion size controls tension-dependent recruitment of alpha-smooth muscle actin to stress fibers. *J Cell Biol.* 2006;172:259–268.
130. Brown TD. Techniques for mechanical stimulation of cells in vitro: a review. *J Biomech.* 2000;33:3–14.
131. Hannafin JA, Attia EA, Henshaw R, Warren RF, Bhargava MM. Effect of cyclic strain and plating matrix on cell proliferation and integrin expression by ligament fibroblasts. *J Orthop Res.* 2006;24:149–158.
132. Khalsa PS, Ge W, Uddin MZ, Hadjiargyrou M. Integrin alpha2beta1 affects mechano-transduction in slowly and rapidly adapting cutaneous mechanoreceptors in rat hairy skin. *Neuroscience.* 2004;129:447–459.
133. Yang G, Crawford RC, Wang JH-C. Proliferation and collagen production of human patellar tendon fibroblasts in response to cyclic uniaxial stretching in serum-free conditions. *J Biomech.* 2004;37:1543–1550.
134. Arora PD, Bibby KJ, McCulloch CA. Slow oscillations of free intracellular calcium ion concentration in human fibroblasts responding to mechanical stretch. *J Cell Physiol.* 1994;161:187–200.
135. Mohanty MJ, Li X. Stretch-induced Ca(2+) release via an IP(3)-insensitive Ca(2+) channel. *Am J Physiol Cell Physiol.* 2002;283:C456–C462.
136. Wang Y, Botvinick EL, Zhao Y, et al. Visualizing the mechanical activation of Src. *Nature.* 2005;434:1040–1045.
137. Ko KS, Arora PD, Bhide V, Chen A, McCulloch CA. Cell-cell adhesion in human fibroblasts requires calcium signaling. *J Cell Sci.* 2001; 114:1155–1167.
138. Neidlinger-Wilke C, Grood ES, Wang JHC, Brand RA, Claes L. Cell alignment is induced by cyclic changes in cell length: studies of cells grown in cyclically stretched substrates. *J Orthop Res.* 2001;19:286–293.
139. Berry CC, Cacou C, Lee DA, Bader DL, Shelton JC. Dermal fibroblasts respond to mechanical conditioning in a strain profile dependent manner. *Biorheology.* 2003;40:337–345.
140. Kamkin A, Kiseleva I, Isenberg G. Activation and inactivation of a non-selective cation conductance by local mechanical deformation of acutely isolated cardiac fibroblasts. *Cardiovasc Res.* 2003;57:793–803.
141. Xu WX, Li Y, Wu LR, Li ZL. Effects of different kinds of stretch on voltage-dependent calcium current in antrial circular smooth muscle cells of the guinea-pig. *Sheng Li Xue Bao.* 2000;52:69–74.
142. Hornberger TA, Armstrong DD, Koh TJ, Burkholder TJ, Esser KA. Intracellular signaling specificity in response to uniaxial vs. multiaxial stretch: implications for mechanotransduction. *Am J Physiol Cell Physiol.* 2005;288:C185–C194.
143. Lehoux S, Esposito B, Merval R, Loufrani L, Tedgui A. Pulsatile stretch-induced extracellular signal-regulated kinase 1/2 activation in organ culture of rabbit aorta involves reactive oxygen species. *Arterioscler Thromb Vasc Biol.* 2000;20:2366–2372.
144. Standley PR, Obards TJ, Martina CL. Cyclic stretch regulates autocrine IGF-I in vascular smooth muscle cells: implications in vascular hyperplasia. *Am J Physiol.* 1999;276:E697–E705.
145. Standley PR, Stanley MA, Senechal P. Activation of mitogenic and antimitogenic pathways in cyclically stretched arterial smooth muscle. *Am J Physiol Endocrinol Metab.* 2001;281:E1165–E1171.
146. Dodd JG, Good MM, Nguyen TL, Grigg AI, Batia LM, Standley PR. In vitro biophysical strain model for understanding mechanisms of osteopathic manipulative treatment. *J Am Osteopath Assoc.* 2006;106:157–166.

8 Biomechanics

CLARENCE L. NICODEMUS ▪ JOHN M. POPOVICH JR.

KEY CONCEPTS

- Biomechanics describes the relationship between structure and function and applies the principles of mechanics to the human body.
- Motion and forces in three-dimensional space can be divided into components with a magnitude of action in each dimension.
- Stress, strain, and force moments are terms used to describe how forces act on objects and how objects respond to those forces.
- The biomaterial properties of tissues, such as bone, cartilage, muscles, tendons, and ligaments, are based on a hierarchy of biomechanical properties from the molecular, cellular, tissue, and gross anatomic levels.
- Tissues are constantly remodeling in response to the stresses placed upon them.
- Excessive stresses or inadequate responses to them (loss of homeostasis) result in injury or disease in tissues.
- The basic biomaterial properties and remodeling capacity (adaptability) of tissues change with age, generally rendering them more vulnerable to stresses and injury.
- The gross biomechanical properties of the skeleton are defined by bony structure and the attachment of muscles and tendons that produce forces across joints.
- The primary motions at the surfaces of articulations are gliding (translation), rotation, rolling, compression, and distraction.
- Basic properties of joint kinetics can be described by measuring the forces produced by muscles and the length of moment arms acting across joints.
- The elastic properties of muscles, tendons, and ligaments allow them to store energy in some phases of movements for release during others.
- All tissues of the body exhibit viscoelastic properties.
- Normal movement in the spinal column is a composite of smaller motions of individual vertebrae. Restrictions of movement in one area can result in a compensatory increased mobility in others.
- The orientation of intervertebral joint facets in the spine, in association with the direction of spinal muscle contraction, produces a motion coupling of vertebral movement. These coupling relationships differ over areas of the spine.
- It is necessary to consider the biomechanical relationships of the body as a whole when attempting to define the consequences of injury or altered function of a body segment.

CHAPTER OVERVIEW

The interrelationship of structure and function in the body is one of the basic principles of the osteopathic medical profession.

- The science of biomechanics is dedicated to describing this relationship more generally in biologic systems. This can apply to the organism as a whole (as with kinesiology) or even on a subcellular level (as with microtubular transport mechanisms).
- The approach to the mechanics of biologic systems is similar to the mechanics of inanimate objects and consists largely of how they respond to forces applied to them.
  - When struck with a hammer, an object may shatter or absorb the force and be accelerated into movement.
  - The response will depend upon a variety of factors including the material comprising the object, the object's shape, internal structure, where and how the force is applied, and so forth.
  - The response of the human body to either externally or internally applied forces can be described similarly, as it must obey the same basic laws of physics.
  - However, the human body and other biologic systems have extremely intricate structural arrangements of highly variable materials down to the molecular level.
  - This can make the accurate biomechanical modeling of even simple movements very challenging.
  - Additionally, the body also has the essential biologic ability to adapt and structurally remodel itself according to the stresses placed upon it.
    - Some of these adaptations, as in the mechanical properties of tissues, can occur relatively rapidly.
    - This "moving target" property can add an additional layer of difficulty for accurate description.

The capacity of the body to adapt appropriately to environmental stress can be the difference between health and disease.

- One goal of the osteopathic physician is to assist the body in regaining a balance with the stressors of the patient's environment, usually at multiple levels of consideration.
- From a biomechanical standpoint, this may involve the correction of somatic dysfunction or to break cycles of inappropriate responses that have produced them.
- In doing so, the primary biomechanical considerations for the osteopathic physician must include broad characteristics encompassing both biomaterial characteristics of tissues and the primary mechanical operation of the body as a unit.
- As opposed to other medical disciplines, this must include a literal "feel" for the characteristics of tissues in addition to a figurative "feel" for the understanding of body mechanics derived from knowledge of anatomy.

The primary goal of this chapter is to assist the reader in obtaining this latter knowledge. For this reason, an emphasis will be placed on basic biomaterial and biomechanical concepts rather than mathematical modeling of properties. As with other chapters in this volume, this chapter is intended to be a summary of biomechanical concepts that are of particular relevance to those who study osteopathic medicine. More comprehensive discussions may be readily obtained from texts on particular topics. It will be assumed that the reader has a basic working knowledge of gross anatomy and the concepts relating anatomy to function.

There are many daily examples of the relationship between anatomy (structure) and function. Consider a simple ankle sprain obtained during an impromptu basketball game or volleyball game at the beach. For a period of 6 to 8 weeks, the individual will reduce the full weight bearing of the involved leg secondary to pain and thus alter the biomechanics of their gait. Normally, this will be a temporary condition that corrects as healing occurs and the ankle pain reduces; however, at times, the compensatory altered mechanics of walking persist once the sprain has healed and is no longer painful. This compensatory change in the use of pelvic, hip, lower thoracic, and leg muscle coordination will alter the forces placed on the spine, sacrum, and hip joints and may result in such conditions as chronic low back pain, premature disk or hip joint degeneration, etc. There are many such examples that relate to structural changes and function (or dysfunction). Indeed, diagnosis and treatment of this relationship are much of the stock and trade of osteopathic medicine.

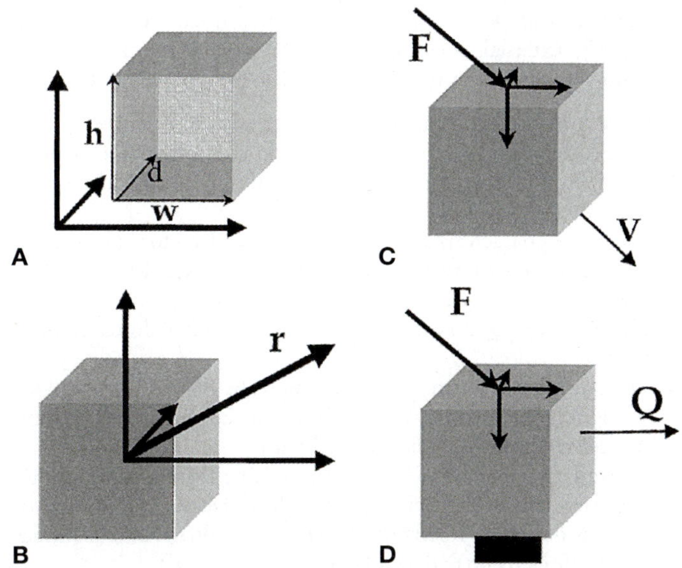

Figure 8.1. **A.** An object in three-dimensional space (axes) can be described by the length vectors (height [*h*], width [*w*], depth [*d*]). **B.** The motion of an object can be described as three separate primary vectors of velocity. The actual movement of the object is represented by the resultant vector (*r*). **C.** A force (*F*) that is applied to an object may also be represented by separate force vectors in each dimension directed into the object. The object may be moved in a direction (*v*) by the force. **D.** If one component of the accelerating force is resisted, the object will move in a new direction (*Q*), determined by the magnitude of the remaining vector components.

MOTION AND FORCES

The strategy for describing the mechanics of biologic materials begins with the same terms and methods employed to describe inanimate objects. The process of interest is broken down into components that can be measured and characterized. These components and their properties are then incorporated into models (often mathematical) that can be used to describe the system and predict its reaction to defined stresses. The terminology used is common to areas of mechanical engineering and can be categorized into terms related to:

- Dimensions and movement in three-dimensional space
- The nature of applied forces
- Properties of biomaterials

Dimensions and Movement in Three-Dimensional Space

Objects and movements in three-dimensional space can be described as magnitudes and components in each of the three dimensions of space.

- A coordinate system is used to define the position and motion of rigid bodies in space or with respect to one another. For musculoskeletal biomechanics, the rectangular or Cartesian system is most commonly used, with *x-y-z* directions mutually perpendicular (orthogonal) to one another.
- An object can be described by the magnitude of its size in each of its dimensions (length, width, height; Fig. 8.1).
- Similarly, simple movement (translation) of an object in three-dimensional space can be described as three different components (*vectors*) of movement (up and down, back and forth, in and out relative to the page) that can occur simultaneously.
    - Vectors will have a magnitude and direction and can be used to represent a force (newtons) or a velocity (meters per second).
    - Vector components are shown on a coordinate system (Fig. 8.1) that is used to model three-dimensional space.
    - By describing the velocity vectors in each of these three dimensions, the motion of the object can be characterized.
    - The actual magnitude and direction of the object movement is referred to as the *resultant velocity vector*.
    - Biomechanical analysis uses similar vector systems to describe most parameters in space, including velocity, acceleration, and force.

Beyond simple models, the properties of each component of a resultant vector can become increasingly complex. For example, an object of irregular shape will require more than a simple length measurement in each dimension to describe it. Similarly, an object moving in space may also rotate about an axis. Because of this, even relatively simple movements of body segments may require sophisticated mathematical modeling to describe the movement.

The Nature of Applied Forces

Applied forces can also be expressed as three-dimensional vectors.

- Applied *forces*, such as a manipulative thrust, are essentially *pressure* (force per unit area) over an area (usually by the hand) applied to an object. By Newton laws, forces act to accelerate an object of a given mass.
- Accordingly, an object at rest must have a force applied to it in order to achieve movement through acceleration.
- An object moving at a constant velocity will require no forces to sustain movement, unless other forces (e.g., friction) are acting to resist the movement.
- The object's resistance to change of velocity (*inertia*) is also described as the force required to accelerate it from rest (zero velocity) or to decelerate it from movement.

The magnitude of forces and associated force vectors are used to describe external forces applied to the body and internal forces like those generated in muscles to achieve limb movement.

- Force magnitudes are expressed as the mass of the object times the acceleration ($F = ma$). The metric unit of force is a newton (N) or 1 kg accelerated to a velocity of 1 m/s each second ($kg \times m/s^2$).
- Forces are characterized as a combination of vector components of a certain magnitude in each of the three axes defining space (Fig. 8.1).
- The *resultant force* is the sum of the individual force components.
- The manner in which the object might be moved or mobilized by the force will depend upon which of the vector components are resisted and which are not (Fig. 8.1).
  - Similarly, a resultant force vector arising from a manipulative procedure would be characterized by describing force components not only directly into the body but also in lateral surface directions (cephalad, caudal, medial, or lateral).

Mobilization of body segments by a force will depend upon which components of the procedure meet with direct resistance and obviously how the body is positioned. In biomechanics, it is important to characterize the different components that a force may have in order to understand the reaction of the tissue or body structures.

- Moments are forces that act at a distance to produce rotation of an object or apply a rotational force to an object.
- Forces that act to produce rotation of an object about an axis (in three dimensions), or in two-dimensional models, a center point (Fig. 8.2), are called *force moments* (also *moment* or *torque*).
- The magnitude of a moment is the product of the force applied and the perpendicular distance between the line of action of the force and the center of rotation (force × distance).
- The latter perpendicular distance is referred to as the *moment arm*.

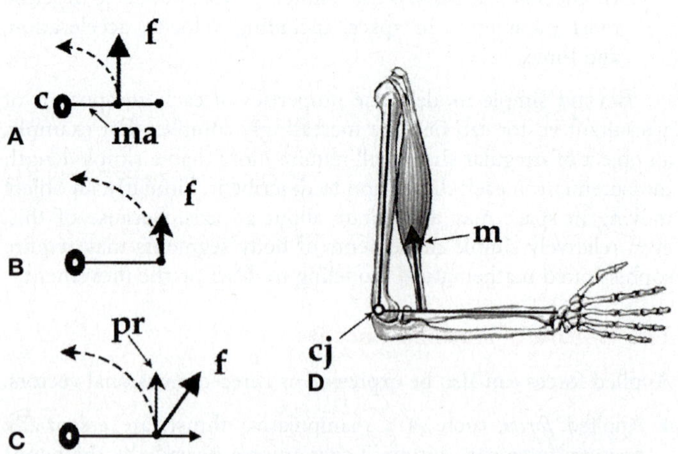

Figure 8.2. Force moments on an object such as a door. A. A force (*f*) applied at a distance (moment arm, *ma*) in the middle of the door can produce rotation (*dotted arrow*) around a center or axis (*c*) located at the hinge. The moment is the force applied times the distance (*d*) from the center (*f* × *d*). **B.** A smaller force acting on a longer moment arm at the doorknob will produce the same moment (*f* × *d*). **C.** If the force is applied in a direction other than directly against the moment arm, only part (*pr*) of the force will be used to produce the rotation. **D.** In the body, force moments are generated by muscle contraction forces (*m*) that produce rotation of a mobile body segment about a center in the joint (*cj*).

- This is essentially a process of using a lever to produce rotation about an axis.
- Because of this relationship, it is important to note that moments of the same magnitude may be produced by increasing the force applied while proportionately reducing the moment arm or vice versa (Fig. 8.2).
- A common example of the properties of force moments can be obtained from pushing open a door (Fig. 8.2).
  - Pushing the door open at the handle usually is relatively easy (low force), because of the long distance (moment arm) between the handle and the center of rotation at the hinge.
    - Note, however, that opening the door at the handle requires a relatively large distance of movement (large displacement).
    - Attempting to push the door open at a point near the hinge (short moment arm) is much more difficult (greater force) but requires less displacement to open the door.
    - Note also that the direction or angle at which the push is applied to the door will determine how much of the force applied is actually used to push the door open. This rotation component of the applied force is at a right angle (perpendicular) to the surface of the door (directly into the door) at any instant.
    - The remaining force component will be in a direction along the surface of the door.
    - For the same opening force to be maintained, the direction of the applied force must change constantly to move in a circle with the door.

The strategy of changing the force or the length of the moment arm and the direction in which forces are applied is often employed in body mechanics and in manipulation techniques, depending upon the need for more or less force at the cost of greater or lesser displacement.

Moments are used in the biomechanical modeling of body motion because most movements are composites of rotational movements of individual body segments around joints.

- Moments are generated from the contraction of muscles attached between two body segments causing the movement of the more mobile segment around a center of rotation (Fig. 8.2). Figure 8.2 shows the biceps applying a force to the forearm, resulting in a moment that rotates the forearm around the elbow.
- The center of rotation is usually near the articulation surface in the less mobile segment.
- The moment arm of the contracting force is related to the distance of the muscle insertion on the mobile segment from the center of rotation.
- In simple biomechanical models of body movement, this center of rotation in the joint is usually shown as stationary. In actual movements, both segments may be mobile and relative motions between joint surfaces within the joint may also occur to change the center of rotation.

A force applied over an area of an object is defined as *stress (force per unit of area)* (Fig. 8.3).

- The magnitude of stress is described as the force applied over a defined unit of object surface area. Stress that is perpendicular to an area is called normal stress. Pressure is an example of such a stress.
- Stress has units of pounds per square inch (psi) or in the metric form, Pascal's (N per meter squared).
- Particular types of stress are identified to describe their relationship to the object acted upon (Fig. 8.3).

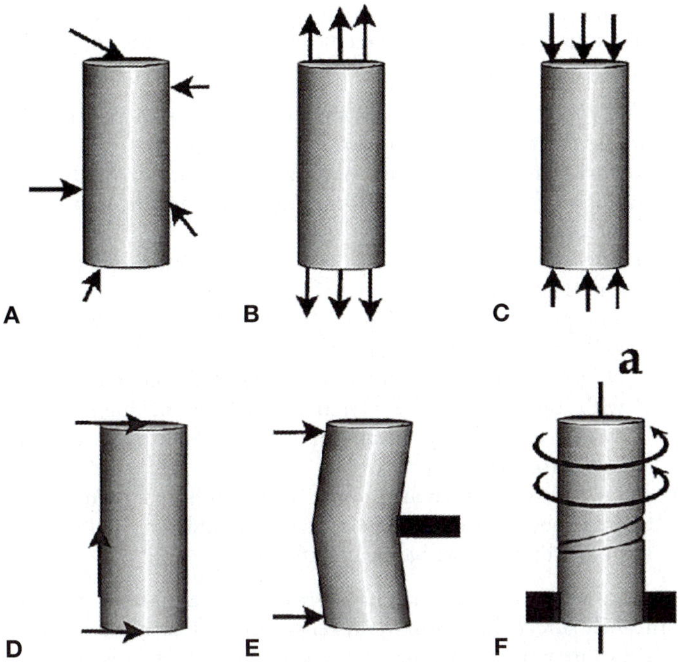

Figure 8.3. **A.** Stresses are forces acting from various orientations relative to the object. Stresses are named according to their action upon the object. **B.** Tensile stresses act to stretch an object. **C.** Compressive stresses compact the object. **D.** Shear stresses act parallel to the surface of an object. **E.** Bending stress acts to fold an object about an axis. **F.** Torsion stresses twist an object about an axis.

- For convenience, stress is usually described as an object that is immobilized or constrained, such that the object must resist the stress and movement other than deformation (see "The Relationship between Stress and Strain," later in the chapter).
- *Tensile* stress is defined as being the result of a force applied perpendicularly outward from the surface of an object (pull), such that the object would be elongated or stretched.
- *Compressive* stress is defined as being the result of a force applied perpendicularly inward (push) to the surface of an object, such that the object would be shortened or compressed.
- *Shear* stress is defined as being the result of forces applied parallel to the surface of an object.
- *Torsion* is a rotational force or moment, which, on a constrained object, acts to twist it about a neutral axis (i.e., an axis that would not be translated or moved by the force). Some refer to the stress resulting from this twisting force as torsional stress. It results in a combination of shear, tensile, and compressive stress in the constrained object.
- *Bending* is also technically a rotation-like force (moment) (or coupled coactive forces) that acts to fold or bend an appropriately constrained object along a neutral axis. Some refer to the stresses resulting from bending as the bending stress. Bending results in compressive stress on the inside of the bend and tensile stress on the outside of the bend.

General Properties of Biomaterials

The behavior of an object or material may be isotropic (material behavior is the same regardless of direction) or anisotropic (material behavior depends on the direction being examined). While stresses may originate from external forces applied to an object's surfaces, they are also transmitted from the area of contact through the entire substance comprising the object.

The primary factors affecting the transmission of forces through an object are its shape and material composition including infrastructure.

- The shape of an object may dramatically affect the manner in which it responds to stresses exerted in different places on the object.
  - An object, such as a sphere of homogenous composition, will respond in the same way to a particular type and magnitude of stress applied to any point on its surface. This type of object is referred to as *isotropic* in relation to stresses.
  - Objects having a nonuniform surface shape (such as an irregular cube) or heterogeneous composition will respond to the same stress differently depending upon the point of application. These objects or materials are referred to as *anisotropic*. Most biologic structures fall into this category.
- The characteristics of the material composition of the object will determine if the object can be accelerated or rotated by a stress of sufficient magnitude or if it will be physically broken by it. As with surface characteristics, the internal structure or composition of an object will also determine its response characteristics to stresses.
  - The response of biologic materials to stresses is determined by structural properties layered down to the subcellular level.
    - In objects that have an anisotropic internal composition, such as biologic materials, the fiber and cellular composition in a given direction is a primary determinant of the resistance of the material to applied stresses.
    - Mechanical models describing nonbiologic materials are difficult to apply directly to biologic systems, due in part to the complicated structure of biologic materials.

THE RELATIONSHIP BETWEEN STRESS AND STRAIN

As discussed subsequently, bone, muscle, tendons, and ligaments are composed of cellular/molecular structures that cause dramatically differing responses depending upon the orientation of the applied stress.

Strain is deformation produced by stress.

- As muscles contract, they apply primary localized tensile stress to the bone in order to accelerate a mobile segment(s) or to stabilize an immobile segment(s).
  - Under this condition, the applied stress produces a change in the shape of the bone or object (*deformation*).
- The magnitude of deformation produced by stress is referred to as *strain*.
- The actual deformation of an object will depend upon the same factors defining stress distribution (internal composition and infrastructure) and is characterized as a sum of different strain vectors.
  - These vectors are usually named for the type of stress producing them (e.g., tensile strain, compressive strain, etc.) and are formulated in directions that match the x, y, z coordinate system, similar to the forces.
- Many different strain vectors may be produced within an object by a particular type of stress.
  - A simple example is a bending stress that produces tensile strain on the side of the object opposite the neutral axis and compressive strain in the direction of bending (Fig. 8.4).
  - A similar condition exists with strain on a spinal disk with bending between segments.
  - Muscle stretch, or elongation of a muscle, is a type of strain.

While it can generally be assumed that increases in stress on an object will produce an increase in strain, the relationship

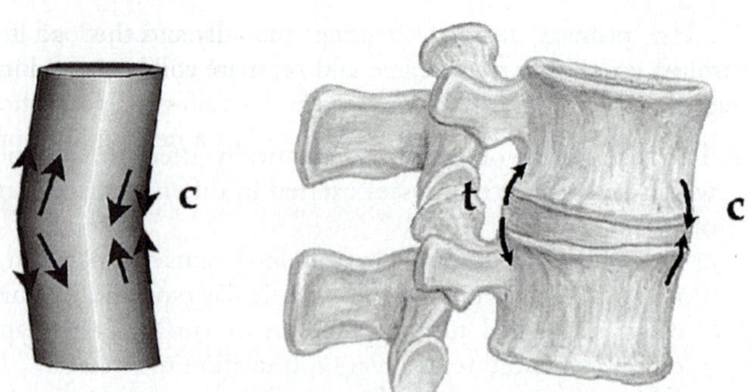

A B

Figure 8.4. **A.** Bending strain produces tensile stress (*t*) on one side of an object and compressive stress (*c*) on the other. **B.** This same principle applies directly to biologic materials, such as spinal disks.

is not direct, particularly for biologic materials. The relationship between the amount of a particular stress applied to an object and the resulting deformation or strain is shown by a stress/strain curve (Fig. 8.5). In this instance, a material is subjected to a defined stress such as tension.

- In this model, the strain may be quantified as the change in length of the object (as with a tendon or ligament) under tensile or compressive stress loads.
- A similar result could be obtained by bending an object, which creates both tensile and compressive stresses (as with a bone).
- Stress/strain relationships for most materials have a linear region (elastic behavior) in which increasing stress produces a corresponding amount of deformation (Fig. 8.5).
- Reducing the stress or unloading of the object will allow it to return to its former shape without a permanent change in shape.
- In this elastic area of the stress/strain curve, the slope of the line (stress/strain) is termed the *elastic modulus*.
  - The elastic modulus is also a quantitative description of *stiffness*, a term commonly associated with the amount of force necessary to produce deformation of an object.

When an applied stress is greater than that defined by the elastic area (Fig. 8.5), a permanent deformation of the material or plasticity will result;

- The plastic behavior area of the curve ends with the material *failure* or breaking of the object.
- Materials may also be described as *brittle* or *ductile* depending upon the amount of deformation they can undergo before failure.
- *Brittle* objects such as glass will undergo little deformation before they break (fail).
  - The pieces after breaking retain their shape such that pieces will fit together to produce a puzzle-like reproduction of the object with little deformation. A similar phenomenon occurs with bone under the extreme condition of high-velocity impact as with a projectile or vehicle, resulting in comminuted fractures.
- *Ductile* materials such as a copper wire will have a permanently altered shape beyond their elastic region and after failure. The same is true for most biologic materials.

Many factors other than basic structure of a material may significantly affect the stress/strain relationship. The most common of these are temperature and the rate at which a stress is applied.

VISCOELASTICITY

The rate at which a stress is applied is an important determinant in the response of materials that exhibit a combination of both elastic and viscous behavior in response to an applied stress. All biologic tissues fall under the category of having viscoelastic properties.

- Viscous behavior can be described as resistance to flow, such as that observed with cold syrup.
- Viscosity in biologic materials arises largely, but not completely, from the resistance of their water content to flow into and out of the material with applied stress.
  - For example, spaces between molecules of collagen in ligaments contain a large amount of water with salts and other small relatively mobile molecules.

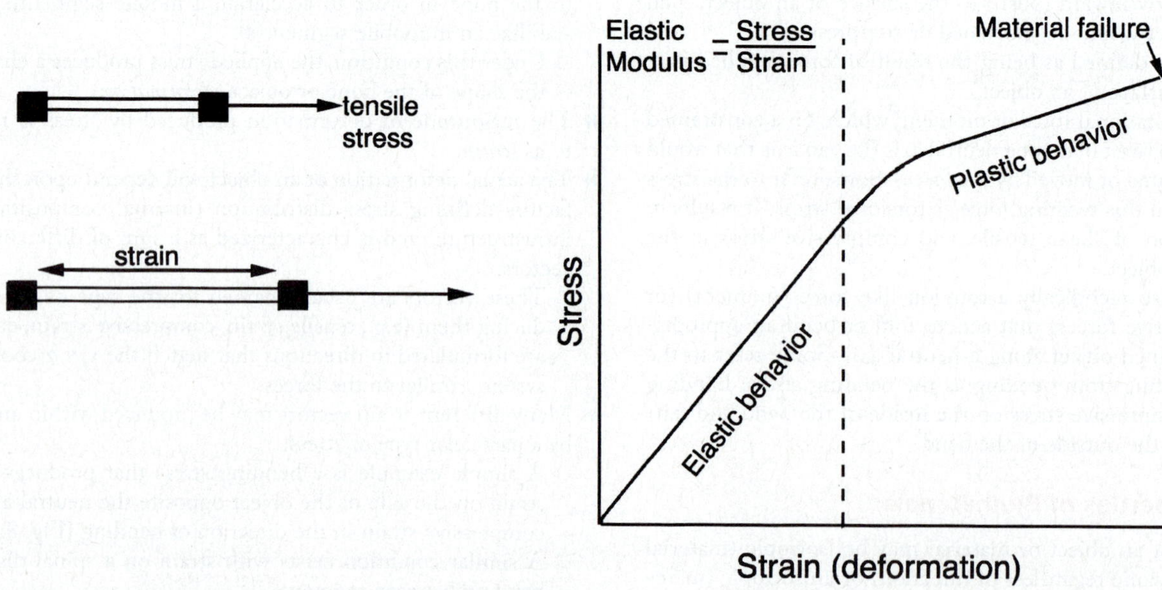

Figure 8.5. A stress/strain curve (right) of an object undergoing increasing tensile stress (left). The change in length can be used as a measure of strain. The curve has an area of elastic behavior, in which a release of stress will allow the object to return to its original shape. In this area, the stress/strain relationship can be expressed as elastic modulus. With increasing stress, the material has permanent deformation or plastic behavior, followed by material failure.

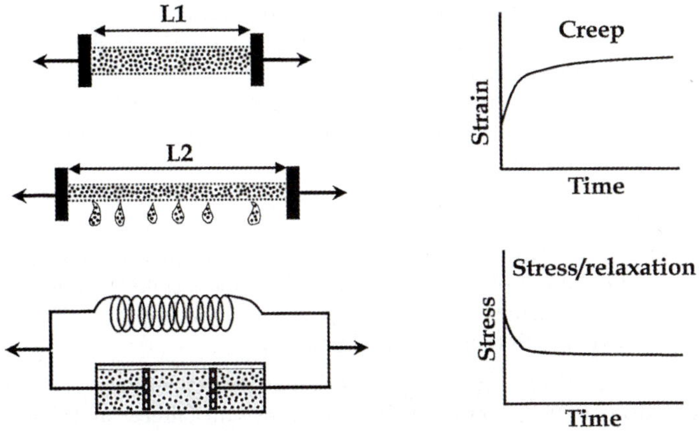

Figure 8.6. Left. Viscoelastic behavior occurs when a material containing a mobile fluid phase is stretched (or compressed) from a resting length (*L1*) to force fluid out of an elastic matrix similar to a sponge to a greater length (*L2*). This can be modeled schematically (**bottom**) as a spring in parallel with a fluid-containing resistance compartment with porous baffles. **Right.** Time-dependent viscoelastic behavior of a material under tensile stress. Creep (**top**) is a measure of deformation (strain) over time with stress (stretch force) held constant. Stress/relaxation (**bottom**) is a measure of stress over time with strain held constant. (Portions of this figure have been adapted with permission from Carlstedt CA, Nordin M. Biomechanics of tendons and ligaments. In: Nordin M, Frankel VH, eds. *Basic Biomechanics of the Musculoskeletal System*. 2nd ed. Lea & Febiger; 1989:59–74.)

- □ Tensile stress (stretching) of the ligament will decrease the available space between collagen molecules, forcing the fluid between them out of the ligament. This process is similar to stretching a wet sponge (Fig. 8.6).
- □ If the structure is stretched rapidly, there is an increasing resistance to fluid movement out of (and into) these spaces, since this requires time. The time required for fluids to move out of intermolecular spaces acts to slow the rate of deformation of an elastic material. This alters the elastic and plastic regions of the stress/strain curve and the material is said to become more stiff.
- □ In combination with the elastic properties of the material, this behavior is described as *viscoelasticity*. This property is usually modeled as a spring acting in parallel to a resistance provided by a fluid compartment (Fig. 8.6).

Besides the flow of small molecules from intermolecular spaces, frictional resistance due to molecular movement and ionic interactions between molecules also contributes to the viscosity in a material. These molecular interactions, along with the elastic properties of the material, are important in the return of water and other small molecules back into the matrix, again much as a sponge reabsorbs fluid after being squeezed. This recovery process is important if the biomaterial properties of the tissue are to be maintained under repeated loading. Additionally, since viscoelastic behavior involves the movement of small molecules and the interaction between molecules, temperature can significantly affect this property.

- Viscoelastic properties can produce significant alteration of material behavior when the rate of loading is too fast for the fluid exchange to occur.
  - □ Under these conditions, a material may exhibit a higher elastic modulus (i.e., appear stiffer) under faster loading rates (short time period), as compared to the same load applied over a longer period of time.
- If a viscoelastic material is stretched rapidly and the load is sustained after the initial loading period, there will be a rapid initial deformation of the material followed by a slower deformation as the remaining fluid in the matrix reaches a new equilibrium at a slower rate (Fig. 8.6).
  - □ Two types of measurements are used to describe this property.
    - First, if the material is subjected to an initial load, such as tensile stress (Fig. 8.6), which is then maintained, the material will stretch to an initial length and then more slowly increase in length as the more resistant fluid in the matrix effuses. The slower phase after the initial stretch is called *creep*.
    - Another measurement looks at the load necessary to maintain a constant deformation or, in the case of Figure 8.6, the length of the material. As the matrix reaches equilibrium, the load necessary to maintain the length will decrease. This property is referred to as *stress/relaxation*.

Because of their high water and solute content, bone, muscle, ligament, tendon, and other biologic materials have viscoelastic properties that are specific to their function. Due to the differences in the cellular structure and the matrix between cells in these materials, the actual viscoelastic properties of these tissues differ markedly.

FATIGUE

Fatigue is a multifaceted term that is used to describe material failure after repeated application of stresses that, if applied individually over a long duration, would not produce failure.

- In nonbiologic materials such as metals, a significant part of fatigue failure can result from the accumulated breakdown of crystalline structure as the result of repeated stress, such as breaking a steel or copper wire by repeated bending.
- In biologic systems, the process of fatigue failure becomes more complicated, because of the ability to repair and adapt materials to repeated stress.
  - □ For example, bone under repeated stress may undergo microfractures in its structure (see the following section). Depending upon the frequency of the stress and the ability of the bone to repair these microfractures, the bone may suffer a fatigue fracture or adapt to the stress by increasing its mass.

PROPERTIES OF BIOLOGIC MATERIALS

Bone

Bone is an anisotropic material. Still, the material properties of bone structure as a whole are clearly traceable from tissue structure.[1]

- Bone consists of connective tissue cells organized and embedded in a highly mineralized extracellular matrix.
  - □ Although lower than other tissues, this matrix also contains significant amounts of water and other small molecules, giving bone viscoelastic material properties.
- The basic unit of organization is the osteon or Haversian system.
  - □ These systems consist of concentric rings of bone cells or osteocytes around a central cavity (the Haversian canal) through which the blood vessels and nerves supplying the bone travel (Fig. 8.7).
- The osteons are arranged in a dense, regular pattern around the shaft of long bones to form cortical or compact bone.
  - □ The border between osteons is the *cement line*.
- The cement line is structurally weaker than the substance of the circularly oriented osteons and can often be identified microscopically as the site of failure of bone tissue under high stresses.[2]

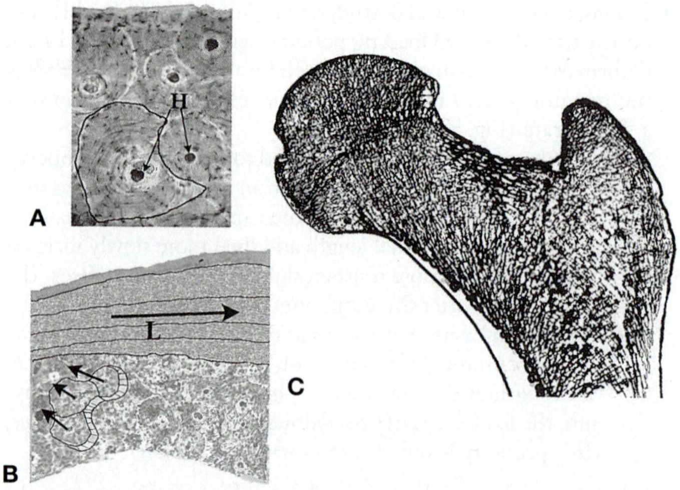

Figure 8.7. Histologic and structural properties of bone. **A.** Compact bone structure is organized into cylinder-shaped osteons with Haversian canals (*H*) that are separated by a cement line (*outline*). **B.** In long bones, osteons are oriented longitudinally along the axis of the bone and surrounded by circumferentially oriented lamellar bone (*L*). Both surround a marrow space that contains marrow and cancellous bone. **C.** The organization of cancellous bone is not random in structures such as the femur, where the trabeculae (*black*) help to distribute stresses through the internal structure of the bone.

- Osteocyte lacunae may also be a site of structural weakness.[3]
- Beneath the cortical layer of compact bone is a central core of more porous bone (termed cancellous, trabecular, or spongy bone), with lacunae comprising the marrow space.

BONE STRUCTURE AND STRESSES

While the structure of cancellous bone may initially appear as a random mesh of thin bone, it can be readily shown that areas of organization do exist and contribute to the structural stability of the bone as a whole by distributing stresses internally in the bone structure[4] (Fig. 8.7).

Bone structure resists primary functional stresses. As might be expected, the highly organized cellular and gross structure of bone causes it to behave in an anisotropic manner to applied stresses. The outward structure and infrastructure of bones are organized to resist the major stresses to which they are subjected under normal physiologic conditions.

For the structure of a long bone such as the tibia, the compressive loading lengthwise will require much higher stress before failure compared to a stress of similar magnitude applied perpendicularly to the long axis. In this manner, from the subcellular to gross structure, bone represents one of the most obvious examples of the structure-to-function relationship. This anisotropic behavior also defines the manner in which bones will undergo material failure when excessive stresses are placed upon them.

DIFFERENT STRESS VECTORS PRODUCE VARYING TYPES OF BONE FAILURE (FRACTURE)

The material failure (fracture) of bone can be observed clinically for all major categories of stresses, with the mechanism of material failure varying with the type of loading.[1] Also, the viscoelastic behavior of bone gives it sensitivity to loading rate.

- At rapid loading rates, bone appears stiffer as the movement of fluid and molecular friction increasingly resists deformation.
  - This causes bone to store more energy before failure.
- When bone does fail at high loading rates, its more brittle behavior makes it more likely to fragment, much like shattering glass (comminuted fracture).[5]
- Accordingly, fractures can also be categorized into different types according to the energy absorbed with the resulting failure:
  - Low energy
  - High energy
  - Very high energy
- Higher-energy fractures (automobile accidents, gunshot wounds) are typically accompanied by bone fragmentation and soft-tissue damage, as the energy stored under rapid loading is dissipated with biomaterial failure.

Under physiologic conditions, bones will experience a combination of stress vectors at the same time and failures may result from the combination rather than a particular stress type. However, fractures do begin in the stress component direction most prone to failure according to the material properties of the bone. This allows the description of some types of fracture resulting from particular stress categories.

- Muscles pulling on bone typically generate tensile stress fractures.
  - The tensile fracture of the calcaneus adjacent to the Achilles tendon insertion is a frequent example (Fig. 8.8).
- Compression fractures are most commonly found in the vertebral column, which is subject to high compressive load and a weakening of the bones with age.
- Shear forces act parallel to bone surfaces, typically at articulations, where bones are in contact.
- Shear fractures can occur under conditions of compression loading of a joint, coupled with a shear or a lateral force across the articulation with a failure of the joint bony plateau.
- Bending and torsional loading produce multiple types of material stresses on bone depending upon the direction of the loading.
  - As described earlier, bending of an object produces tensile stress on one side of an object and compression on the other (Fig. 8.4).

Bone is weaker in tension than compression, so bone material failure begins upon the tensile stress side (Fig. 8.8).

- Immature bone, which is less calcified and more ductile, may be more sensitive to compression and fractures may occur on the compressive side first.

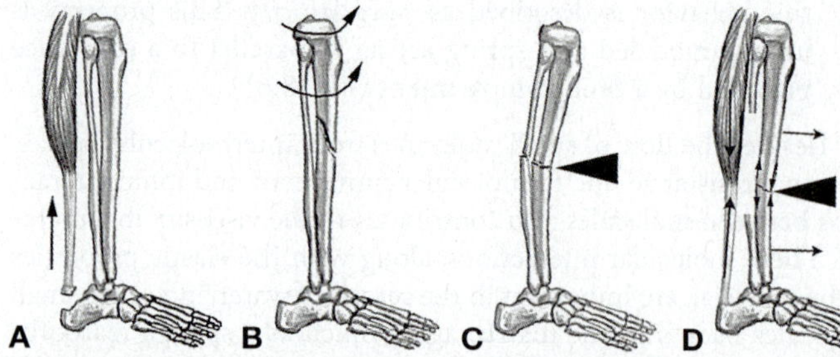

Figure 8.8. Examples of fracture types resulting from a material failure due to a primary stress component. **A.** Tensile fracture of the calcaneus. **B.** Spiral fracture from torsional stress of the tibia. **C.** Bending stress fracture. **D.** Example of how muscle contraction forces can act to counter bending stress. Bending stress produces tensile forces on one side of the tibia and compressive stress on the other (see Fig. 5.4). Muscle contraction can act to counter the tensile component by producing a compressive moment. (Portions of this figure have been adapted from Gollnick PD, Matoba H. The muscle fiber composition of skeletal muscle as a predictor of athletic success. An overview. *Am J Sports Med.* 1984;12(3):212–217. Copyright © 1984 American Orthopaedic Society for Sports Medicine. Reprinted by permission of SAGE Publications, Inc.)

- Torsional loading (Fig. 8.8), or usually twisting around the long axis of bones, produces shear stresses around the neutral axis while compression and tension loading are diagonal to the axis.
  - The resulting failure (spiral fracture) is initially due to shear stress followed by tensile stress failure along a diagonal axis at the surface of the bone.

As should be expected, if there are weaknesses in the bone structure, such as during rehabilitation after injury, failure will occur at the weakest point or at the site of bony defect loads.

The biomaterial failure of bone under stress is greatly influenced by the attachment and contraction of muscles.

- Muscle activity can decrease or counter stresses produced on the bone by altering the direction of the resultant stress vectors to a direction which the bone may tolerate better.
- Figure 8.8 shows how muscle activity may alter a bending or tensile stress to produce compression stress.
- As bone is very resistant to compressive stress (such as weight on the long axis of the tibia), this redistribution of stress can be important to avoiding stress fracture.
- The physiologic tiring of muscle during strenuous exercise can contribute significantly to fractures because the protective mechanism is lost.
- While sudden, large stresses are usually associated with bone fracture, failure of the material itself can result from repetitive loading over a period of time.
- Fatigue-type fracture of bone involves an accumulation of smaller failures within the bony microstructure and is dependent upon the:
  - Magnitude
  - Frequency
  - Rate of loading

Even low-level repetitive loads may produce fatigue microfractures in the bone.[6] In living bone, these microfractures will be repaired by cellular reactions to the injury. If the fatigue process outpaces the repair, failure will eventually occur as a repetitive stress fracture. A common example of this is the fatigue fracture of metatarsal bones in long-distance runners.[7]

In the presence of stresses, bone can alter size, shape, and structure to withstand stresses placed upon it. The unusual corollary to this property is that bone must be subjected to stress in order to maintain its biomaterial properties. The underlying principle of this process in bone has been expressed as Wolff law, which states that bone is increased where needed and resorbed where not needed.[8]

- The resorption of bone under conditions of reduced usage or immobilization[9] is of particular concern clinically, since mechanical stress on bone is reduced during casting or in more limited conditions, such as weightlessness in space travel.[10]
- Immobilization results in the resorption of periosteal and subperiosteal bone[11] and a decrease in bone strength and stiffness.[12]
- Conversely, the hypertrophy[13,14] and increase in density of bone[15] may be observed in normal bones in response to strenuous exercise.
- Both hypertrophy and resorption of bone may be observed around implant screws and plates used to surgically stabilize bone defects or to attach prosthetic joints.[16]

Bone properties also are altered with aging, with a progressive loss of bone density and size.[17,18] This is independent of the condition of osteoporosis. The result is a decrease in bone strength and stiffness and altered stress/strain properties, including an increase in brittleness and a reduction in energy storage capacity. These properties make bones more susceptible to material failure under high-stress conditions with increasing age.

Articular Cartilage

There are three identified primary types of cartilage in the human body:

- Hyaline cartilage
- Fibrocartilage
- Elastic cartilage

HYALINE CARTILAGE

Hyaline cartilage covers the surface of the articulations of almost all diarthrodial joints and will be the focus of our description of basic biomaterial properties of cartilage.

- Cartilage has some similarity to bone in that it consists of cells (chondrocytes) surrounded by an extensive extracellular matrix that they secrete.
- Cartilage is avascular, lacking blood vessels, lymph channels, or nerves within its matrix, and the matrix secreted is not calcified as in bone.

The extracellular matrix of cartilage consists primarily of a network type II collagen (COLII) and an interlocking mesh of fibrous proteins and proteoglycans (PGs), hyaluronic acid (HA), chondroitin sulfate, and water.[19,20]

The collagen and PGs form the major structural elements of cartilage, and these interact extensively on a molecular level with the smaller molecules, including water. The interaction of these elements with each other within cartilage and their interaction with the water in the matrix determine the primary biomaterial properties of cartilage.

The major collagen and PG structural element on the cartilage of articular surfaces is not randomly organized and can be divided into histologic zones that differ in cellular organization from the surface to the underlying subchondral bone[20] (Fig. 8.9).

- The orientation of collagen fibril bundles within the matrix differs between the layers (Fig. 8.9). There are three types of orientation:
  - A tangential orientation at the surface
  - Random organization in the middle zone
  - Radial orientation near the subchondral bone surface

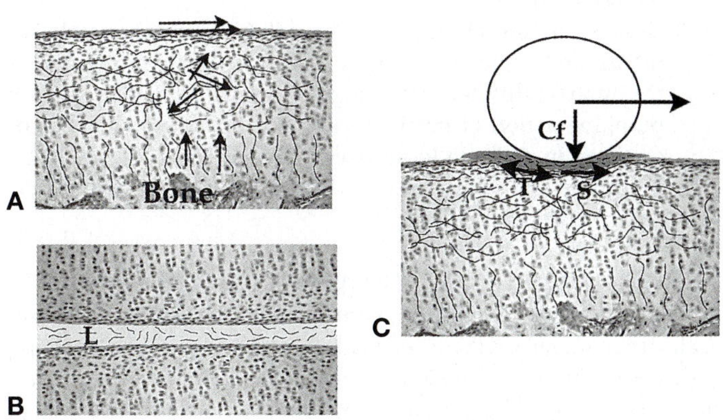

Figure 8.9. **A.** Schematic of the orientation (*arrows*) of collagen fibrils (*drawn lines*) in articular cartilage. The orientation varies from the articular surface to the bone interface. **B.** Representation of cartilage surface separated by a thin layer of lubricating fluid (*L*) that prevents direct surface contact. **C.** With a compressive force on the surface (*cf*), additional fluid is exuded and the matrix is compressed. Lateral movement produces tensile (*t*) and shear (*s*) stress on the cartilage surface and matrix components.

This orientation provides the basic structural framework for the cartilage and resistance to the loads placed upon it. Depending upon the particular joint function, the primary stresses may be compression, which, as the joint moves, contributes to shear and tensile stresses on the cartilage surfaces (Fig. 8.9).

The collagen and PG structural elements of cartilage have spaces between them filled with water, salts, and other small molecules, forming a matrix with viscoelastic properties as previously described.

- The structural elements contain molecules such as HA and have ionically charged groups throughout their structure.
- This property allows them to strongly bind water and inorganic salt within the cartilaginous matrix.
- The cartilage matrix has properties of flexibility from a pliable, porous collagen superstructure containing small molecules that can be forced out, but with some molecular and ionic interaction–based resistance to the efflux.
  - The properties of this matrix allow a viscoelastic behavior in which the cartilage allows rapid, but declining deformation (cushioning) in response to compressive loads followed by creep or stress/relaxation[21] (Fig. 8.6).
  - The slower deformation will continue until equilibrium is reached between the load and the forces resisting it within the matrix.
  - The differing mechanical properties of the layers of articular cartilage interact dynamically to reach equilibrium in response to a sustained compressive force.[22]

On a tissue level more closely related to normal function, the viscoelastic response of cartilage can be explained by a compressive stress that produces a rapid efflux of fluid forced out of the extracellular matrix directly beneath it and in areas immediately adjacent to it (Fig. 8.9).

- The resistance to this efflux of fluid is dependent upon the effective porosity or space available in the cartilage matrix for fluid to move.
- Other resistance to matrix deformation includes the internal friction generated by movement between long polymer molecules such as collagen and attached PGs and the ionic binding of these chains to the water and other small molecules.
  - The time required for the fluid phase to reach a full equilibrium between cartilage layers under the applied load may require hours.[21]
  - Because of the elasticity of the collagenous structural elements and ionic interactions with the small molecules of the matrix, this fluid exchange is reversible and supplies a pumping action of nutrients into and waste products out of cartilage in addition to normal diffusion.
    - This action is particularly important because of the avascular nature of cartilage.

ARTICULAR CARTILAGE AND WEAR DAMAGE

Under physiologic conditions, cartilage surfaces of joints contact each other under a variety of loading conditions while showing little wear. This occurs in spite of the fact that joint surfaces are not perfectly smooth. The prevention of wear is due in part to a system of lubrication of synovial articular surfaces provided by synovial fluid and the properties of the cartilage itself.

- Fluids lubricate surfaces by preventing their direct contact (Fig. 8.9).
- The first level of lubrication of joint surfaces is the absorption of lubricin, a glycoprotein in synovial fluid that is absorbed onto articular surfaces.
  - This provides a thin boundary of lubricant on the joint surface.
- The synovial fluid itself also provides a thin film of fluid between the joint surfaces that can be redistributed under loading conditions.
- During loading, the fluid extruded as a result of the compressive deformation of the cartilage will provide a fluid layer to separate the opposed surfaces.[23]

Under normal conditions, the fluid-lubricating properties of the joint will prevent the direct contact of uneven sections or asperities of joint surfaces to contact each other. If contact does occur, wear of the joint surfaces or interfacial wear (mechanical removal of material from a solid surface) may occur.

- This may consist of abrasion of the joint surface because of contact of uneven elements of the surface or small fragments of joint surfaces may adhere to each other and be dislodged.
- The efficient lubricating properties of normal joint usually preclude interfacial wear, but it may occur in damaged or degenerated joints.[22]

INTRINSIC CHANGES WITH AGING

While cartilage can be damaged as a result of traumatic injury as in shearing stress applied to the meniscal cartilage of the knee, the mechanisms of abnormal wear are not as clear. Hypotheses of the mechanism of cartilage wear include the disruption of the structural molecules of the cartilage matrix through repeated stress[24,25] and the alteration of the matrix content under the same conditions.

- As with bone, rapid loading of a viscoelastic matrix increases the stiffness of cartilage, and the loss of the fluid component of the matrix will also increase stiffness.
  - This loss of fluid may include soluble PGs from the cartilage surface that are important in the maintenance of its properties.
- Under conditions of rapidly repeated high-impact loading, the fluid forced from the matrix that would normally provide a cushioning effect cannot be reabsorbed in time to cushion subsequent impacts.
  - This may also produce plastic deformation of cartilage surfaces that does not sufficiently recover for smooth surface contact upon subsequent loading.
- The increased stiffness and deformation of the matrix increases the likelihood of mechanical wear in addition to rendering the subchondral bone surface more vulnerable to damage.

Cartilage wear may also be complicated by the limited capacity of cartilage to repair or regenerate. This property gives it a limited capacity to adapt to stress. In conjunction with repeated stresses and minor injuries, a cycle of damage, wear, and insufficient recovery may occur, leading to joint degeneration and/or osteoarthritis.

- The inability of cartilage to recover during repeated high-stress loads may be one source of macroscopic structural defects observed in cartilage[26] and responsible for the high incidence of specific joint degeneration and the development of osteoarthritis in persons with certain occupations (football players and dancers).
- The intrinsic composition and properties of cartilage also change with age.[27]
- The matrix composition changes and permeability increases, decreasing cartilage stiffness and rendering it less resistant to rapid loading.
- With the accumulation of injuries from which the tissue cannot recover, these age-related changes may contribute to the increased incidence of joint degeneration with age.

Ligaments and Tendons

Ligaments and tendons, along with joint capsules, surround the articulations of the skeletal system. Their functions are, in the case of ligaments and joint capsules, to structurally connect, stabilize, and guide the bones forming the articulation.[28] They may also act as a sensor for joint position and strain affecting the joint.

- Tendons connect muscle to bone and transmit forces from muscle to bone to produce motion.
- Both tendons and ligaments are classified as dense, regular connective tissues.
- They have sparse cellular elements and abundant extracellular matrix in a highly organized array.
- The extracellular matrix is rich in collagen and water with a small amount of elastin.
  - This produces a viscoelastic behavior under stress.
  - The collagen molecules are linked together in lengthwise overlapping arrays to microfibrils.
    - Combined in similar overlapping arrays to form fibrils, then fibers, and bundles of fibers to form the macroscopic tendon (Fig. 8.10).
- This successive parallel linkage down to the molecular level makes ligaments and tendons capable of handling high tensile loads.
- The arrangement of fibrils in ligament tissue is less parallel than tendons and accounts for its higher resistance to tensile loading in orientations other than along the tissue axis.
- The collagen molecules are also linked to each other by cross links.

While there are some important biomechanical differences between ligaments and tendons, most of their properties are similar and will be described together here.

CHARACTERISTICS OF LIGAMENTS AND TENDONS

The primary stress response characteristics of ligaments and tendons are described by their modulus of elasticity properties. Under tensile loading (stretch), ligaments and tendons exhibit a modulus of elasticity that is variable with load (Fig. 8.10).

- Under low loading, there is a relatively large increase in length in response to the load applied (low elastic modulus).

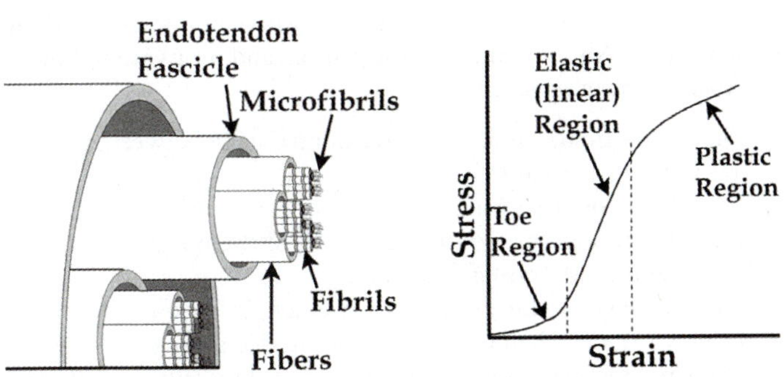

Figure 8.10. **Left.** Schematic view of the structural organization of tendon. Microfibrils are the smallest component consisting of collagen molecules. Microfibrils are organized into fibrils that are grouped into fibers. Fibers are grouped into fascicles that comprise the tendon. **Right.** Idealized version of a stress/strain curve for tendon under tensile stress. The toe region is a nonlinear behavior attributed to the "slack" between collagen molecules. The elastic region has a linear relationship between stress and strain. In the plastic region, permanent deformation occurs, eventually resulting in failure.

  - This is attributed to lengthening as the result of macromolecular "slack" within the collagen fiber structure that offers less resistance to an imposed load.
  - As the slack is taken up, fibers slide relative to each other and fluid is extruded from the matrix.
  - The elastic modulus then increases (stiffness increases) gradually with increasing load and shows a linear response up to the point where failure begins.

The behavior of tendons and ligaments is similar except for ligament tissue such as the ligamentum flavum of the spinal column, where a high elastic content produces a different pattern of the elastic modulus.

The extracellular matrix of tendons and ligaments between the collagen fibrils has PGs, with high water content, and other small ionically charged molecules that can interact with structural elements.

- The matrix is comparatively more porous than cartilage or bone and is structured to resist tensile rather than compressive stresses.
- The viscoelastic properties become evident at high loading rates, where the tissue will demonstrate increased stiffness and offer increased resistance to tensile stress (stretch).
- As with cartilage, repeated tensile loading in cycles can result in a slow increase in elastic stiffness due to plastic deformation.[29,30]
  - This plastic deformation is presumably due to molecular deformation in the fibrous structural elements of the tendon or ligament and also to the inability of fluid and small charged molecules to re-equilibrate within the molecular structure.

Ligaments and tendons also demonstrate the viscoelastic properties of stress or load relaxation and creep. To characterize these properties, the tissue is placed under a tensile load (stretch) within the linear region of the elastic modulus and maintained at a constant length (stress relaxation) or a constant load (creep).

- Ligament and tendon tissue adjusts its molecular structure and fluid distribution to the load primarily within the first 6 to 8 hours but will continue over a period of months.
- The creep phenomenon is used clinically as plaster casts or braces are employed to place a constant load to correct a soft-tissue deformity, such as some spinal curvatures.[31]

MATERIAL FAILURE OF LIGAMENTS AND TENDONS

Overall failure of the ligament or tendon is usually sudden and preceded by the microfailure of the attachments between collagen fibers within the tissue and loss of the ability of the tendon or ligament to recover its length.

- With tendons and ligaments, it is also important to distinguish eventual failure due to a sustained load (creep failure) from sustained cyclic loading and unloading (fatigue failure).
  - Both are important biomaterial properties for tendons and ligaments.
- As with bone, a smaller degree of microfailure may occur within the range of physiologic loading, suggesting that repeated stress may lead to declining strength or fatigue over time.[32]
- There may be a range of damage depending upon the total deformation and extent of partial failure. Inflammation resulting from such damage is associated with tendonitis.[32]

Failure of both tendons and ligaments may also occur at the bone interface. The site of failure may depend upon the loading rate.[33] Tendons, with their attached muscles, typically have a higher tensile strength than muscle, and rupture of muscle is more common than tendon. The instability of the joint that may result from tendinous or ligamentous damage can contribute to and be complicated by damage to the joint capsule. This damage and associated abnormal loading patterns may contribute to osteoarthritis.[31]

LIGAMENTS AND TENDONS CAN ADAPT TO STRESSES

Like other tissues, ligaments and tendons structurally remodel in response to the stresses placed upon them within the limits of damage.[32]

- They become stronger and stiffer with increased stress and weaker and less stiff with a reduction in stress.[34]
- Physical training can increase the strength of tendons and ligaments along with the ligament–bone interface.[35,36]
- Immobilization (such as from casting) can decrease the strength and stiffness of ligaments. While reconditioning can occur, it can require a considerable length of time.[34,37]

THE PROPERTIES AND STRUCTURE OF LIGAMENTS AND TENDONS CHANGE WITH AGE

During maturation, the number and quality of cross-links increases in the collagen of ligaments and tendons and fibril diameter increases as well,[38] producing increased tensile strength.

- The mechanical properties of collagen reach a maximum with maturation and begin to decrease with age.[39]
- The collagen content of ligaments and tendons decreases.
  - □ This loss of collagen results in a decrease in strength, stiffness, and the amount of deformation required to produce failure.[40]
- The overall biomechanical properties of tendons remain reasonably constant with age.[41]
- The amount of time required for tissue repair and reconditioning (discussed previously) will also increase.
- Other physiologic factors, such as pregnancy, can also affect the biomechanical properties of ligaments and tendons.[31,40]

Skeletal Muscle and Body Movement

Since a more complete description of muscle is given elsewhere in this volume, only those elements essential to understanding the biomechanical aspects of muscle tissue will be given here. Of the three types of muscle tissue, skeletal muscle is the most abundant tissue in the body, accounting for 40% of body weight.[42]

- The forces necessary to provide movement to the body are provided by the contraction of skeletal muscles acting across joints.
  - □ These contractions may produce dynamic work or participate in static maintenance of posture.
- Subcellular units known as *sarcomeres* are the source of muscle contraction.
- The basic contractile unit of skeletal muscle as a tissue is the *muscle fiber*.
  - □ The fiber may range in size from 10 to 100 μm in diameter and between 1 and 30 cm in length.[43]
  - □ The metabolic and contractile properties of muscle fibers may differ according to the physiologic demands placed upon them as described subsequently.

CONTRACTILE ELEMENTS AND CONNECTIVE TISSUE

Muscles may be histologically and mechanically described as bundles of contractile elements in a series of connective tissue sheaths (Fig. 8.11).

- The *endomysium* is the basic unit of the contractile/connective tissue; individual muscle fiber surrounded by a connective tissue sheath.

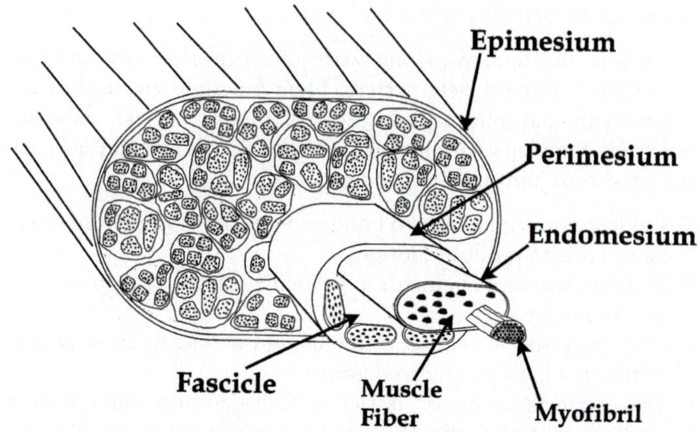

Figure 8.11. Schematic of the structural organization of a muscle. The basic subcellular unit of the muscle is the myofibril. Collections of myofibrils are present in muscle cells (muscle fibers). Muscle fibers are organized into fascicles and groups of fascicles make up the muscle. The connective tissue coverings of the muscle include the endomysium that surrounds muscle fibers, the perimysium surrounding muscle fascicles, and the epimysium surrounding the entire muscle.

- This basic unit of skeletal muscle is then organized into fascicles or groups of fibers by a thicker connective tissue sheath, the *perimysium*.
- Groups of muscle fascicles are organized into the entire muscle itself and covered by the epimysium, which surrounds the entire structure.
  - □ *Epimysium* and loose connective tissue form the fascial planes between muscles.
  - □ The connective tissue sheaths are continuous with each other and the muscle tendon and/or attachments to bone.
    - Both connective tissue and the contractile elements contribute to the biomechanical properties of muscle.
    - The contractile elements provide active energy-expending forces with some elastic and viscoelastic properties, while the connective tissue contributes passive elastic and viscoelastic influences on the pattern of force transduction to the skeleton.

THE MOTOR UNIT

Muscle fibers contract in response to acetylcholine released by motor nerves. An individual motor neuron, and its associated muscle fibers forms a *motor unit*.

- The size of motor units may vary dramatically between muscles and within the muscle itself.
- The motor neuron generates an action potential lasting 1 to 2 ms that produces a contraction of all of the muscle fibers in a motor unit in an "on–off" fashion.
- The response of the motor unit to a single action potential is termed a *twitch*, the basic unit of recordable muscle activity.
- The time required for a motor unit to fully contract and then return to resting length is variable (from 10 to 100 ms) according to fiber type but in all cases much longer than a nerve action potential.
- If additional nerve stimulation occurs before the contraction phase of the twitch has ended, contraction can be maintained and increased in a process called *summation*.
  - □ The limit of summation, such that contraction is maintained and does not increase with a greater frequency of stimulation, is called *tetanic contraction* or *tetany*.

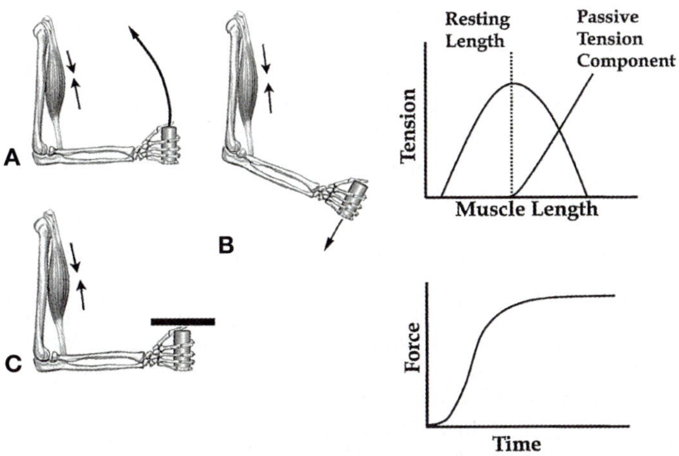

Figure 8.12. Left. Types of muscle contraction. **A.** Concentric. **B.** Eccentric. **C.** Isometric. **Right. Top**—Muscle tension relationship to muscle length. The greatest active tension is near the muscle-resting length. The passive tension component from the stretch of connective tissue increases beyond the resting length. **Bottom**—Force–time relationship of muscle contraction. The time lag in reaching maximum force is related to the elasticity of tissue components.

- The force of contraction of the muscle as a whole may be further regulated by increasing or decreasing the number of motor units used to produce the contraction, a process termed *recruitment*.
  - In this way, the nervous system may control the force of muscle contraction by the size and number of motor units employed to produce the contraction and the frequency of activation of motor units.

TYPES OF MUSCLE CONTRACTIONS

Dynamic muscle contractions in the processes of producing movement can be classified as *concentric* and *eccentric*.

- *Concentric contractions* produce movement in the direction of muscle contraction (Fig. 8.12).
- *Eccentric contractions* act to decelerate or resist movement, as in slowly placing an object down rather than letting it fall.
- Muscles also produce contractions without substantial movement, as in static posture against gravity.
  - This type of contraction is termed *isometric*, as no change in muscle length occurs during contraction.
  - *Isotonic* contraction refers to muscle contraction with a change in length under constant tension.

MUSCULOTENDINOUS UNIT

The force production characteristics of a muscle as a whole are a combination of the material properties of its contractile components, the connective tissue that surrounds them (and the whole muscle), and the tendon of its insertion. From a mechanical viewpoint, this combination is a *musculotendinous unit*.[44]

- The contractile elements add a rapid tensile load on the connective tissue elements and in turn respond according to their elastic and viscoelastic properties.
- As with ligaments and tendons alone, this will mean that there is rapid component to stretch, produced in this case by contraction, followed by a slower change in length as the connective tissue elements reach equilibrium with the contracting force (Fig. 8.12).

The connective tissues surrounding the muscle and its tendon have elastic properties that can store energy with stretch like a rubber band. In the process of muscle contraction, the tendon and connective tissue are stretched. The energy is released by moving a body segment or by stretching the contractile elements as the muscle relaxes.

- Elasticity helps to keep the muscle prepared for contraction by reducing the slackening of contractile elements.
  - Prevents passive overstretch of muscle fibers, thereby reducing the danger of injury.
  - This energy storage also occurs as muscles are stretched under load.
  - The muscle contractile elements may also have some elastic-like properties of energy storage.[45,46]

The sum of the interaction of the contractile elements and elastic elements of muscle contraction can be demonstrated in the force–time curve of muscle contraction (Fig. 8.12). While the tension or force of contraction of the muscle fibers may reach maximum within a relatively short time, a much longer time is required for this tension to be transferred through the elastic components. Because of this time lag, the active contraction process must be long enough in time for the full transfer of tension to occur.

LENGTH, LOAD, AND TEMPERATURE

The force of muscle contraction can be affected by various mechanical factors including:

- Force–time properties[43]
- Length–tension relationships
- Load-velocity
- Muscle fatigue
- Prestretching
- Temperature

The length–tension property of a muscle as a whole (Fig. 8.12) involves both the active contractile elements and the passive connective tissue elements.[47]

- The maximum force or tension produced by contractile elements, such as the muscle fiber, is obtained near its resting length.
- Contraction at lengths beyond or smaller than the resting length results in reduced tension production by the muscle fiber.
  - This is a result of intrinsic properties of muscle fiber sarcomeres.
- For the muscle as a whole, reducing or increasing the muscle length from its resting position will reduce the tension produced by contractile elements.
- Increasing muscle length will also produce a passive tension as a result of stretching the connective tissue elements, although the contractile force is reduced.
- The passive component of stretch, which is readily detectable by passively stretching a relaxed limb, will eventually become the dominant source of resistance or tension as muscle length increases, effectively protecting the muscle from overstretch (Fig. 8.12).

APPLIED LOADS AFFECT THE VELOCITY OF MUSCLE CONTRACTION

The relationship of the load applied to a muscle and the velocity with which it contracts defines the load–velocity property of muscle contraction. The shortening of muscles contracting concentrically is most rapid with no external load and progressively slows with increasing external loads.[48]

- The shortening velocity will reach zero as the load reaches the maximum contraction force of the muscle (isometric contraction) and then reverses to a lengthening velocity with eccentric contraction.

- Eccentric contraction lengthening velocity increases with increasing external load.

TEMPERATURE AND MUSCLE CONTRACTION

In the process of contraction, muscle efficiency is usually no more than 20% to 25% in the translation of chemical energy into useful work, with the majority of the energy being dissipated as heat.[42]

- Heat dissipation can have positive effects on muscle contraction properties by increasing temperature.
- Temperature increases usually arise from increased blood flow and the production of heat by the muscle itself from metabolic reactions and friction generated by the sliding of molecules past each other in the contractile and elastic elements.
  - Within physiologic ranges, increases in temperature will increase the conduction velocity across the muscle fiber membrane (sarcolemma),[48] which increases the rate of contraction and the rate at which the muscle can be stimulated.
  - This can result in an increase in the production of muscle force.
- A rise in temperature can also increase enzymatic activity related to muscle metabolism and increase the efficiency of muscle contraction.
- The viscoelastic properties of the musculotendinous unit are also affected by rises in temperature.
  - This may result in increased elasticity of the collagen, decreased stiffness, and enhance the extensibility of the unit.
- While these basic biomechanical properties of muscle tissue change with temperature to enhance the contractile properties of the musculotendinous unit, the effects from stretching or "warming up" prior to activity are much more complex and not completely understood.[49,50]

The physiologic aspects of stretch (or release) involve highly significant neural components and reflexes beyond the biomechanical properties of the tissues alone.

MUSCLE FATIGUE PROPERTIES

Fatigue of muscle with prolonged contraction activity results from the depletion of the nutrients and oxygen required to produce adenosine triphosphate (ATP) as an energy supply from either aerobic or anaerobic glycolysis.

- The result is a decrease in force production by the muscle eventually to total cessation.[42]
- The rate at which a muscle will reach fatigue can vary according to the types of muscle fibers it contains.
- Muscle fiber types are distinguished by the rate at which ATP can be made available to the sarcomeres for contraction and the metabolic pathways through which ATP is generated.
- The rate of availability of ATP directly affects the rate of contraction or twitch time of a muscle fiber.
- Muscle fiber types can be classified as *slow* or *fast twitch*.
- Two primary metabolic pathways involved in generating ATP (oxidative or glycolytic) further divide these two basic types of contractile behavior.
- Using these properties, three primary muscle fiber types are distinguished including;
  - Type I or slow-twitch oxidative fibers
  - Type IIA, fast-twitch oxidative-glycolytic fibers
  - Type IIB, fast-twitch glycolytic fibers.
  - These different fiber types have varying degrees of contraction time, resistance to fatigue, and a dependence on aerobic or anaerobic metabolism.
  - As their names suggest, type I fibers have slower contraction rates, and, with a metabolism directed toward aerobic pathways, are more resistant to fatigue.
    - They are relatively small in diameter and produce a relatively low amount of tension per fiber.
    - These properties make this fiber type well-suited for prolonged low-intensity work.[51]
- Type IIA fibers are fast contracting and rich in aerobic and anaerobic (glycolytic) enzymes with a moderate resistance to fatigue.
  - They appear to be intermediate between type I and type IIB in their capacity for contractile force and resistance to fatigue.
- Type IIB fibers are fast contracting, rely primarily on glycolytic pathways, and may fatigue rapidly.
  - They have a large fiber diameter and can produce relatively large amounts of tension.

MUSCLE FIBER TYPES ACCORDING TO DEMAND

Most muscles are of mixed fiber types with the proportion of fiber types determined by the nerve innervating the muscle.[52,53] The overall distribution of muscle fiber types in the muscles of the body appears to have a strong genetic component.[42,51,54]

- The fiber type can be changed with nerve stimulation,[55] suggesting that patterns of activity may alter fiber metabolism.
- Some changes in fiber types may also occur with physical training, but much of this change is a result of increases in the cross-sectional area of the fiber type corresponding to the activity rather than an actual change in fiber type.[54,56]
- The extent to which actual alterations in the type of muscle fiber occur as a result of activity demand therefore remains unclear.

MUSCLE ADAPTS TO PHYSIOLOGIC DEMANDS

Although the extent of fiber type change under physiologic conditions is unclear, muscle will clearly remodel according to the stresses placed upon it.

- Muscle atrophies with disuse and hypertrophies with increased use.

Studies of muscle atrophy in both animal and clinical studies suggest that early dynamic motion after debilitating injury may be important in the minimization of atrophy, particularly of type I muscle fibers.[57,58]

- Electric stimulation may also prevent some of this fiber loss.[56]
- Hypertrophy of muscle with physical training is generally the result of increases in the cross-sectional area of all muscle fibers.[58,59]

MUSCULOSKELETAL BIOMECHANICS

Primary Biomechanical Musculoskeletal Models

Biomechanical aspects of the skeleton involve contributions from all of the biomechanical aspects of the tissues described in the process of producing movement. As a simplistic model, it is easiest to consider the body as a series of segments (bones) containing muscles that are attached across the segments. Joints form the junctions between segments or bones and transfer the forces generated by muscles or from external sources between the segments. In the following simple models of movement, joints will be regarded as simple pivot points, moving in one plane (coplanar). The more complex considerations of joint movement and shape of articulation will be addressed in subsequent sections.

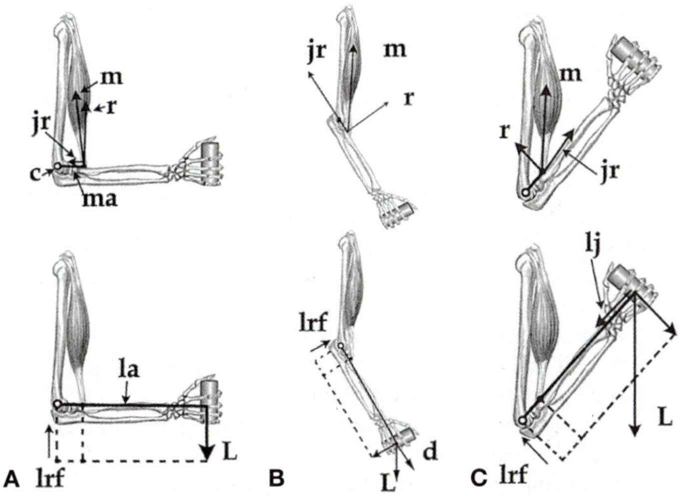

Figure 8.13. Schematic of basic joint moments and their variation with movement. Sections on top represent muscle contraction moments. Figures on the bottom show moments generated by the load. **A.** Right angle resistance to a load (*l*). **Top.** Moments about the joint center (*c*) include the moment arm of the muscle (*ma*) that is moved by a resisting component (*r*) of the muscle contraction force (*m*); this is resisted by the load (**bottom**) acting on a load moment arm (*la*). Joint reaction forces include the portion of the muscle force directed into the joint (*jr*) and a moment generated from the load into the joint with a center of rotation about the muscle insertion (*lrf, dotted lines displaced*). **B.** At extension, the angle of muscle pull directs more of the muscle force into the joint (**top**) and a portion of the load force (*l*) moment pulls out on the joint as a distracting force (*d*). **C.** In a flexed position, the muscle moment (**top**) is divided into the resisting component (*r*) and a joint reaction distracting force away from the joint (*jr*). A portion of the load force (**bottom**) now is directed into the joint (*lj*).

MOMENTS ARE USED TO DESCRIBE MODELS OF MUSCULOSKELETAL MOVEMENT

Using the simple model used for the descriptions of moments earlier in the chapter, a joint, such as the elbow (Fig. 8.13), becomes a rotation system with the flexor system and the extensors using the joint as a center of rotation to move the distal limb and any load on the limb.

- In mathematical modeling of joint function, the description of such movements is a system of balanced moments produced by the load on the limb and muscle contraction forces.
- Characterizing movement in this way becomes particularly important as other aspects of joint function (noncoplanar movement, movement within the joint) and more mechanically complicated joint types are modeled.

As a distal segment moves relative to a more proximal segment, the distal segment will rotate about the instant center of the joint or center of rotation (*c*, Fig. 8.13).

- The effective distance from the center of the joint's rotation to where the force is acting (muscle insertion) is the *moment arm* (*ma*) for the muscle.
- The product of the force applied from the muscle and the moment arm (force × distance) is the *moment* (or torque) used to resist a load on the distal limb.
- For concentric contraction to occur, this moment of resistance must exceed the moment produced by the load (distance to the load from *c* × weight).
- In a more complete model, the weight of the limb must also be considered.
- Note also that if the load moment is resisted by the pull of the muscle, there is also a center of rotation created at the point of muscle insertion about which the load exerts a moment into the joint (*lrf*, Fig. 8.13).
- Together with the portion of the muscle contraction force directed into the joint (discussed subsequently), this becomes part of the *joint reaction force* that applies a stress to the joint during movement.

MUSCLE MOMENTS NECESSARY TO RESIST A LOAD VARY WITH JOINT POSITION

As can be seen from Figure 8.13, although the length moment arm does not change, the proportion of muscle contraction force (*vector*) that is applied to resist the load will vary as the limb is flexed. With the joint fully extended, most of the muscle contraction force vector is directed into the joint.

- This muscle component force also contributes to the joint reaction force and may be particularly important in the stabilization of load-bearing joints, such as the knee.
- The relative size of the joint reaction and load-resistive forces can be expressed by simple trigonometric functions in mathematical models, but it is sufficient here to be aware of how these forces change with joint position.
- In this model, the portion of the muscle contraction vector used to resist the load increases as the angle of tendon is closer to a right angle (Fig. 8.13A, orthogonal) to the forearm.
- Beyond this point, a portion of the load vector becomes directed into the joint (Fig. 8.13C) reducing the effective load on the muscle, but placing stress on the joint and more proximal segments.
- In the flexed position, the angle of pull by the muscle directs a portion of the muscle contraction force against this load into the joint.

MUSCLE MOMENTS ARE ALSO TRANSFERRED ACROSS JOINTS BY TENDONS

Muscle forces are also conveyed to distal segments across joints by tendons. In joints associated with the knee, hands, and feet, tendons cross the joint(*s*) to produce a "pulley" effect (Fig. 8.14). In this arrangement, as in the knee, the distance between the center of rotation of the joint and the tendon defines the moment arm for the contracting muscle.

The wheel and axle mechanism[60] is an instructive related model used to achieve rotary movements (Fig. 8.14). In this case, muscle contraction forces are applied to the opposite sides of a segment to produce rotation about an axis.

- The length moment arm in this case is the distance to the center of rotation.
- This mechanism is used widely throughout the body to achieve rotation of limbs and the body, as in rotation of the head, torso, or shoulder.
- As with simple flexors and extensors, muscles producing rotational components work in pairs and significant clinical problems may arise from imbalances that result in dysfunction of a pair.

MUSCLE MOMENTS GENERALLY HAVE A LOW MECHANICAL ADVANTAGE

As suggested in the examples that have been given, the lever arrangement of muscle insertions and joints in limbs is such that a comparatively small distance of muscle contraction can produce a large displacement of the load at the expense of needing large muscle contraction forces.

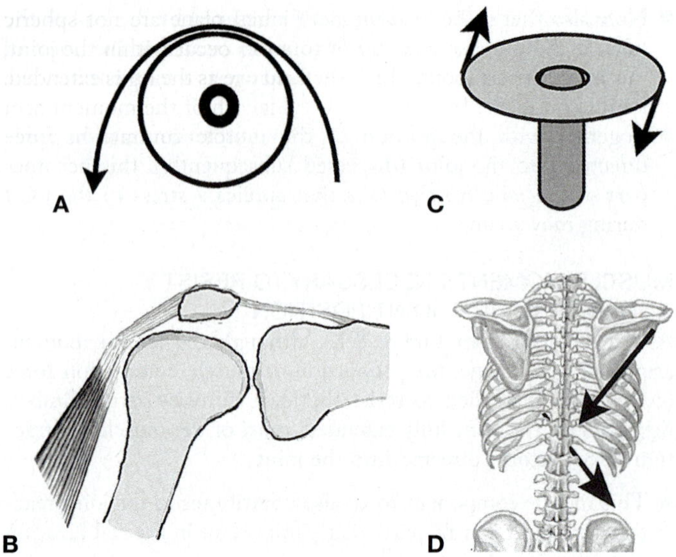

Figure 8.14. Strategies of muscles and tendons pulling across joints. A. A pulleylike mechanism in which the direction of pull is changed. **B.** A similar mechanism is used in knee extension. **C.** A wheel and axle mechanism in which coactive forces act to rotate an axle, such as the shoulders (**D**) relative to the spine.

- This is described as having a *low mechanical advantage.*
- The *relative mechanical advantage* is a function of the position of the muscle origin and insertion on the two bony segments relative to the joint.
  - Because both the moment arm (distance, d) and the contraction force (f) equally contribute to the moment ($f \times d$) producing the movement or resistance, small differences in the moment arm can produce significant changes in the amount of muscle contraction required.
  - As origins and insertions of muscles and segment lengths vary markedly between individuals, the ability to produce different types of movement using the same muscle contraction force will also differ.

While muscles must create large forces to produce movements at a low mechanical advantage, distally applied loads, such as to the hand acting through the elbow, have a comparatively large moment arm (Fig. 8.13) and require less force to produce large moments about the joint. This will be true of manipulative forces placed distally for purposes of applying passive stretch to muscles and joints. It is a useful principle but must be approached with caution since large, potentially damaging force moments can be generated.

Joint Structure and Movement

Beyond movement models that regard joints as simple pivot points for the transfer muscle forces between body segments, the next level of modeling must consider the structure of these intersegmental contacts. In fact, the directions of movement that can occur between body segments are largely defined by the structure of the joints between them.

- Joints are classified according to the type of tissue they contain and their structure.
- On a tissue level, joints are classified into three primary types:
  - Fibrous
    - *Fibrous joints* are located in areas such as the articulations of the skull.
  - Cartilaginous
    - *Cartilaginous joints* include the disks between vertebrae.
  - Synovial
    - *Synovial joints* are located in the articulations of the limbs.
- The vast majority of body motion occurs across synovial and cartilaginous joints.
  - The primary cartilaginous articulations will be described subsequently, with considerations of the spinal column.
- The remaining synovial joints have been divided into several categories according to the primary types of movements that occur across them.
  - Anatomically, the major types are[61]:
    - Ball and socket (e.g., glenohumeral [shoulder] joint and femoroacetabular [hip] joint)
    - Condyloid (e.g., metacarpophalangeal joints, metatarsophalangeal joints)
    - Gliding (e.g., acromioclavicular joint)
    - Hinge (e.g., tibiofemoral [knee] joint)
    - Pivot (e.g., atlantoaxial joint, radioulnar joint)
    - Saddle (e.g., trapeziometacarpal joint [base of thumb])

Other than the joints described later in this chapter, more detailed descriptions of these joint structures and their limitations on range of motion can be found in general anatomic texts.

RANGE OF MOTION

Movements are usually described as occurring in one of the primary body planes (coronal/frontal, sagittal, or transverse). The extent of joint motion in a plane defines its *range of motion* in that plane, usually in degrees.

- Although all synovial joints may have some minor range of motion in all three planes, most joints in the extremities have a primary degree of freedom in one plane, such as in the following:
  - Knees
  - Elbows
  - Fingers
- Shoulder and hip joints are an exception, as they have significant ranges of motion in all three planes.
- Joints may also have a significant rotational component, usually expressed as range of motion of the distal rotated element, as in pronation and supination of the hand.
- In general, there is a trade-off between intrinsic structural stability of joints and range of motion, depending upon the physiologic demands placed upon the joint.

JOINT SURFACES AND TYPES OF RELATIVE MOVEMENT

As body segments are moved through their range of motion, surfaces within the joint will also move relative to each other. This movement may contribute to various aspects of the motion produced.

- The relative motion of joint surfaces may include (Fig. 8.15):
  - Gliding
    - *Gliding* (also referred to as translation or sliding) represents a movement of one surface relative to another without a rotational component.
  - Rolling
    - In *rolling,* one surface of the articulation rolls over the other, like a ball rolling over a surface
  - Rotation
    - *Rotation* (spinning) consists of one joint surface spinning on the surface of the other without a translational component.

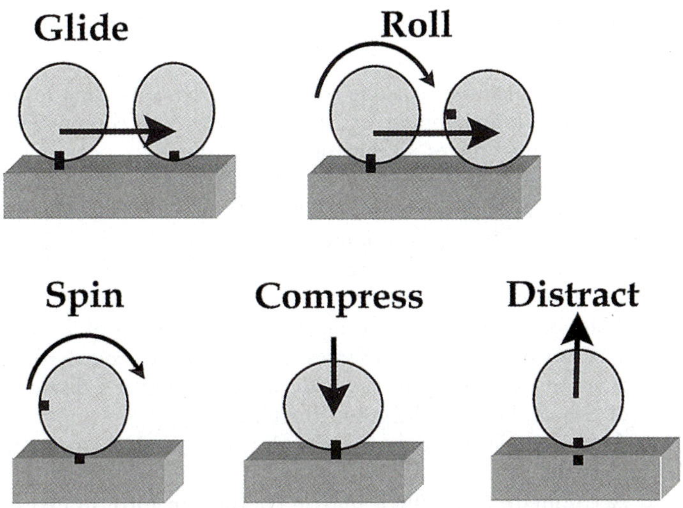

Figure 8.15. Intra-articular movement of joint surfaces relative to each other. In gliding (also referred to as "sliding" or "translation"), surfaces move without rotation. In rolling, one surface rotates and translates over the other at a distance equal to the arc of the rotating surface. In spinning, one surface rotates on the other without translation. Compression and distraction are opposing vertical forces on the joint.

- □ Compression
  - *Compression* represents force pushing the joint surfaces together.
- □ Distraction
  - *Distraction* tends to pull the surfaces apart.

- Or a combination of these movements can occur.
- This can also be termed "traction" on the joint or "tension" in the joint.

Movements between articular surfaces in a joint can occur in consistent combinations (coupled) such that one type of motion is always accompanied by another. This motion coupling can occur for movements within the same articulation (see the upcoming example given under "The Knee") or in another joint that is part of an articulation complex (see the example given with "The Elbow" later in the chapter).[62]

- A disruption of one part of a coupled motion will affect the other and can produce dysfunction of the joint or joint complex.
  - □ An example of this is the elbow complex where there is a coupling of the intra-articular motions of humeroulnar and humeroradial joints during flexion/extension movements (see "The Elbow").
- Coupling of articular surface motions within the joint also depends upon which segment of the joint is mobile.[62]
  - □ An example of this difference is the articular surface movement of the knee during weight bearing versus swing phase (see "The Knee").
- Significant alterations in the relative movements of joint surfaces can produce problems in joints, including abnormal wear and dislocation.

THE INSTANT CENTER

In order to study movement within a joint during functional movement, both the motion of the surfaces relative to each other and the shape of the articulating surfaces must be considered. As one segment moves in a joint such as the knee, the center of rotation located within the joint at any instant will have zero velocity.

- Because the femoral condyles and tibial plane are not spheric surfaces and translational movement can occur within the joint, the center of rotation of the leg will change as the leg is extended.
- To determine properties such as the length of the moment arm under these circumstances, the center of rotation must be redefined as *instant center* of rotation joint at any given time.[63]
- The instant center can be defined clinically from sequential roentgenograms or other pictures of movement using the intersection of lines from defined points from the joint segments.
  - □ This technique can be important for identifying abnormal joint movement. It should be noted, however, that displacement of the instant center can occur in all three dimensions simultaneously.
  - □ Roentgenograms or other planar depictions of joint motion can be misleading. From a functional point of view, changes in the location of the instant center will change the relative magnitude of the contraction-force vectors of the muscle tendon acting across a joint. This can result in weakness or abnormal stresses within the joint.

SOME PROPERTIES OF SPECIFIC JOINT ARTICULATIONS

The previous discussions in this chapter have focused on the biomechanical properties of tissues and models of forces acting to create movements or stresses on body segments. Now consider how these properties apply to some of the primary articulation systems in the body. The biomechanical aspects to be considered are not intended to be comprehensive.

The Knee

The knee joins two of the body's longest moment arms (the proximal and distal lower extremity) in a joint consisting of two primary articulations, the tibiofemoral joint, and the patellofemoral joint (Fig. 8.16). Because of its location and weight-bearing properties,

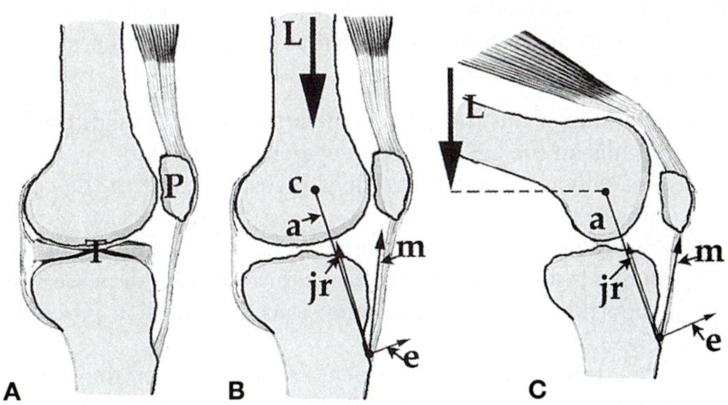

Figure 8.16. A. The knee joint consists of the tibiofibular (*t*) and patellofibular joints (*p*). **B.** Moments produced by the load (*L*) of body weight require little muscle activity with the knee extended but are maintained by a muscle contraction force through the patellar tendon (*m*), which produces moments through a moment arm (*a*) to the instant center of rotation of the joint (*c*). The moment is divided by the angle of muscle pull into a joint reaction force (*jr*) and an extending component (*e*). **C.** With the knee flexed, the body weight produces a moment through the joint (*c*) that must be resisted by the extending component (*e*). In this instance, the patella increases the distance of the tendon from the femur to provide a more advantageous angle for the muscle contraction force on the tibia. This increases the proportion of the extension moment. Note that the position of the center of rotation (*c*) has changed slightly.

the knee sustains relatively high load forces and is particularly susceptible to injury.

- Stability of the knee is obtained from the following structures:
  - Internal and external ligaments.
  - Joint capsule.
  - Muscles acting across the joint.
  - The cartilage menisci distributing the compressive stresses between the condyles of the femur and the tibial plateau.

RANGE OF MOTION IN THE SAGITTAL PLANE

Although the knee joint itself has some range of motion in all three planes of motion, its primary range of motion is in the sagittal plane where a range from full extension to full flexion is approximately 140 degrees.[63]

- Motion in the transverse plane (internal and external rotation) and frontal planes (abduction and adduction) is dependent upon the positioning of the tibia relative to the femur.
  - In the transverse and frontal planes, full extension of the knee precludes almost all motion due to an interlocking of the femoral and tibial condyles, while range of motion increases as the knee is flexed.
- Maximal internal and external rotation is possible with the knee flexed at approximately 90 degrees ranging from a neutral position to 45 degrees of external rotation and 30 degrees of internal rotation.
- In the frontal plane, passive adduction and abduction are obtained at approximately 30 degrees of flexion, but it is only a few degrees in either direction.[63]

THE HAMSTRINGS AND THE PATELLAR TENDON

The primary muscle forces through the joint occur through the quadriceps tendon and hamstrings. The hamstrings use the knee joint as a primary lever in flexing, while the quadriceps use the patellar tendon system as a pulley in extension with the center of rotation within the femoral condyles (Fig. 8.16). As with other hinge-type joints, in a basic biomechanical model, muscle contraction forces are divided primarily into a joint reaction force directed into the joint and a force moment that acts to move the mobile segment.

- In extension of the knee, the moment that acts to straighten the knee pulls on the leg through the patella and tendon.
  - This will act to rotate the tibial plateau relative to the condyles of the femur.
  - Presuming a constant muscle force, this component of moment decreases or mechanical advantage decreases in proportion to the joint reaction force as extension proceeds (Fig. 8.16).
  - This decrease is to some extent compensated by the movement of the patella and the shape of the femoral condyles as described subsequently.
- With flexing a straightened knee, the opposite is true; the proportion of the flexor moment increases relative to the joint reaction force as the movement proceeds.

HIGH JOINT REACTION STRESS FORCES

In a load- or weight-bearing model of the knee, the leg is considered stable, and muscle contraction forces and joint structure are used to resist gravity. The force exerted through the knee from the weight of the body is termed the *ground reaction force* (body mass × the acceleration of gravity). Note that both the ground reaction force and muscle contraction forces contribute to produce the *joint-reaction force* or total force directed into the joint as described previously.

- These combined forces, along with the impact of landing from activities such as jumping, can produce very high compressive and other stress forces on the knee joint surfaces.
- If the knee is fully extended, most of the ground reaction force is directed through the bone structure of the femur and tibia (a moment arm through the joint of almost zero), and minimal or no muscle contraction force is required to resist the ground reaction force.
  - This changes as the knee is bent, and at 90 degrees of flexion, extensor muscle reaction forces must resist the ground reaction force consisting of the body weight acting at a distance of almost the entire length of the femur.
  - At this angle, the extensor muscles have a relatively small moment arm.
  - Accordingly, a very high muscle contraction force in excess of body weight must be exerted to resist a moment of this magnitude. The knee joint has several mechanisms to help compensate for the rather low mechanical advantage of muscle contraction forces in this situation.

STRUCTURAL PROPERTIES OF THE JOINT

Beyond the basic segment model, there are basic structural properties of the knee that change the mechanical advantage muscles across the joint.

- These primary structural properties include the patellofemoral joint and the shape and movement of the femoral condyles.
- The patella and tendon act to increase the moment arm for the quadriceps by increasing the effective distance of the tendon from the center of rotation of the joint.
  - This increases the component of the muscle contraction force vector acting to straighten the joint (Fig. 8.16).
  - This adds mechanical advantage to the extensor muscle contraction forces in a partially flexed knee.
  - The gliding (sliding) motion of the patella between the medial and the lateral femoral facets also alters the moment arm over the range of motion of the knee.
  - Additionally, the patella acts to distribute this force over the surface of the femoral condyles.

The primary properties of the femoral condyles that affect the mechanics of movement include:

- The noncircular shape of the condyles and their movement on the tibial plateau (Fig. 8.16).
- The shape of the femoral condyles is such that the center of rotation of the joint changes through the knee's range of motion, giving a greater moment arm to extensor forces as the knee is flexed.
  - This can be important in resisting the high forces such as body weight with a partially flexed knee.

In addition to a noncircular shape, the femoral condyles also have differences in their effective diameters with the medial being larger.

- This produces a coupling of flexion and extension with a rotational component to the knee (called the *screw-home mechanism*), such that flexion is accompanied by an internal rotation component and extension is accompanied by external rotation of the femoral condyles relative to the tibial plateau.[64]
  - This provides additional stability to the joint in certain circumstances.

MOVING AND LOAD BEARING

The femoral condyles also glide (slide, translate) on the tibial plateau as the knee is moved (described previously). These structural properties of the femoral condyles can act to change the center of rotation as the joint progresses through its range of motion and alters the effective moment arm length through which the muscle contraction forces are acting.

- The relative movements of the joint surfaces in the knee give an example of how motion coupling can depend upon the load status of the joint and which joint surface is mobile.[62]
- In walking, as the leg swings forward (swing phase), the femoral condyles and tibial plateau are not under the compressive load of the body.
  - ☐ The movement is a gliding motion of the tibial plateau coupled with a rolling of the tibia on the femoral condyles in the same direction.
- When the leg is placed on the ground with the knee partially flexed and then extended as the body is moved forward (see "Normal Locomotion (Gait) Employs the Entire Body for Efficiency of Movement" later in the chapter), the tibial plateau is stable relative to the femoral condyles.
  - ☐ The motion of the joint surfaces now consists of gliding and rolling of the femoral condyles on the tibia in opposite directions.
    - This is an example of how compressive forces and segment stabilization change articular surface motion. This can have important implications in surface damage and dysfunction.

EFFICIENCY OF MOVEMENT

Through their structure and interaction during movement, the patellofemoral joint and femoral condyles contribute to the efficient use of muscle contraction forces for movement and joint stability by changing the moment arm (mechanical advantage) of the contracting muscles in the process of extending or flexing the knee.

- This has important consequences for movement through the knee and load bearing.
- The effective use of these structural properties is dependent upon internal joint movement and the joint stability provided by soft tissues.
  - ☐ For this reason, soft-tissue injury or changes producing either a lack of or excess of internal "play" in the knee joint can contribute to serious problems with joint function.

The Hip

THE HIP IS A LOAD-BEARING BALL-AND-SOCKET JOINT

The relatively rigid ball-and-socket arrangement of the hip joint between the head of the femur and the acetabulum provides greater intrinsic stability compared to joints such as the knee. In addition to stability, the ball-and-socket structure of the hip allows greater range of motion in all three planes of body movement.

- Motion in the sagittal plane is greatest with approximately 140 degrees of flexion and 15 degrees of extension from a neutral position.
- The range of abduction is approximately 30 degrees and adduction 25 degrees.
- External rotation from a flexed position is approximately 90 degrees.
- Internal rotation is approximately 70 degrees.
- Rotation decreases with extension due to soft-tissue restrictions.[65]

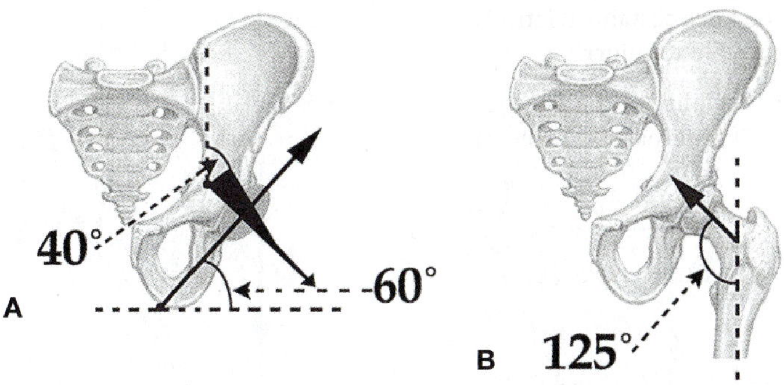

Figure 8.17. A. Angle of the opening of the acetabulum. The opening is oriented 60 degrees lateral to a transverse plane and 40 degrees posterior to a sagittal plane. **B.** The angle between the femoral neck and the shaft is approximately 125 degrees.

ANGULAR ALIGNMENT OF THE ARTICULAR COMPONENTS

The angular structure of the joint relative to the pelvis, femoral shaft, and knee joint can vary significantly between individuals and have a great influence on the biomechanics of the lower limb.

- In the relationship of the joint surface to the pelvis, the location of the acetabulum places the plane of its opening angled 40 degrees posterior to a sagittal plane and 60 degrees lateral to a transverse plane (Fig. 8.17).
- Both the femoral head and the acetabulum have roughly spherical surfaces of contact.
- The relationship of the femoral head through its neck with the femoral shaft is important in the biomechanics of hip function and load-bearing stress on the neck.
- It is an important determinant of the effective moment arms of the muscles producing movement across the joint. The angle of inclination of the neck to the shaft (Fig. 8.17) is approximately 125 degrees, but may vary between 90 and 135 degrees.
  - ☐ This angle offsets the femoral shaft from the pelvis laterally.
- The angle in a transverse plane between lines drawn through the femoral head and greater trochanter and between the medial and the lateral condyles (angle of anteversion) determines the normal relationship of the primary plane of movement of the knee to the hip.
  - ☐ It is normally about 12 degrees but can vary widely.[65]
  - ☐ An angle of greater than 12 degrees tends to produce internal compensatory rotation of the leg during gait, while an angle of less than 12 degrees produces an external rotation.
    - These compensations are made to maintain the stability of the hip. They are common in children and usually outgrown.[65]

BALANCE, GROUND REACTION, JOINT, AND MUSCLE CONTRACTION FORCES

Biomechanical models of the hip can be used to illustrate some of the important aspects of the structure–function relationship of the joint. Stability of the hip joint is maintained through the alignment of the body over the joint (Fig. 8.18), the joint capsule, and capsular ligaments and muscle contraction to counteract remaining ground force moments.

- The relative magnitude of forces applied into and across the hip joint can be considered through a model of a single leg stance with the body center of mass (or gravity) balanced (i.e., located on an axis of alignment) over one hip joint (Fig. 8.18).
- In this balanced condition, little or no muscle contraction forces are necessary to maintain equilibrium, as in the knee.

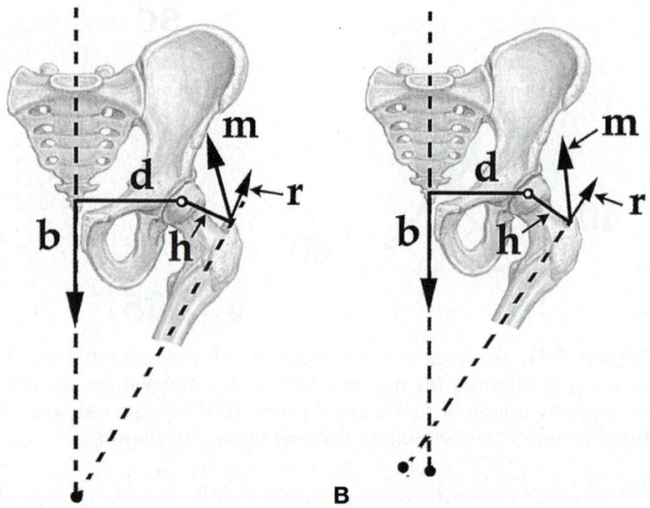

Figure 8.18. A simple coplanar model of a single leg stance moment in balance. A. In the balanced state, the body weight (*b*) is balanced over the foot (not shown), which would be at the intersection of the *dotted lines*. In this balance, the body weight (*b*) acts as a force applied on a moment arm (*d*) through the center of rotation in the femoral head to produce a body moment ($b \times d$). This is balanced by the rotational component (*r*) of the muscle contraction force (*m*) acting over a moment arm through the femur (*h*) to produce a muscle contraction moment ($r \times h$). For balance to be maintained ($b \times d$) = ($r \times h$). **B.** The balanced condition can be disturbed by a shift of the body and a slight change of the angle of pull by the muscle (*m*). To restore balance, the moment (*r*) must be increased or altered so that the moments can be rebalanced.

- The joint reaction force or force directed into the joint will equal the ground reaction force produced by the weight of the body above the hip.
- In an unbalanced state, the body's center of mass is no longer directly over the bony structure and produces an unbalanced moment about the center of rotation of the hip joint.
- To restore equilibrium, the force of the contracting joint activator muscles must generate an equal force moment across the hip in the direction opposite of the moment generated by the body weight.
- By measuring the length of the moment arms for muscle contraction in the body and knowing the body weight, the approximate resisting moment of muscle contraction can be calculated along with the joint reaction component produced.

Note that in this model, the angle of the femoral neck will affect the relative lengths of the moment arms (or the angle of pull) by muscles. This will directly influence the muscle contraction forces required to resist the body weight moment and the proportion of the contraction force directed into the joint. This is why an abnormal angle of the femoral neck can adversely affect hip function and the stresses on the joint.

HIGH JOINT REACTION FORCES

As with the knee, it can be seen that hip stability under load-bearing conditions can require high muscle contraction forces because of a relatively short moment arm through which the muscle forces are applied. As a combination of ground reaction force and the portion of the muscle contraction forces directed into the joint, the joint reaction forces are also high relative to the body weight.

- Calculations suggest that under these conditions, the muscle contraction force is approximately twice the body weight and the joint reaction force almost three times the body weight.[66,67]
- Joint reaction forces are important in consideration of stresses on the hip joint itself in replacement or repair.
- Strategies to minimize the joint reaction force can also be important in subjects with arthritic pain in the hip joint.
- A reduction in joint reaction forces may be achieved by altering the angle of the hip by increasing the muscle moment arms.
    - This can also be accomplished by using a support device, such as a cane on the opposite side, to reduce the opposing body weight moment.

The Elbow

THE ELBOW IS COMPLEX

The upper limb analogue of the knee is the elbow, which has adapted for increased mobility of the upper limb and a reduced load-bearing requirement. In achieving this, the joint has become a complex of three articulations, including (Fig. 8.19):

- Humeroulnar
- Humeroradial
- Proximal radioulnar joints
- The joint complex allows two primary ranges of motion: flexion/extension and pronation–supination.
    - Flexion and extension occur across the humeroulnar and humeroradial joints, which act as a hinged joint.
    - The normal range of motion in flexion/extension is approximately 140 degrees, with limits established by the angular characteristics of the bony components.[68]
    - The axis of motion passes through the middle of the trochlea and is principally a gliding motion[69] up to the last 5 to 10 degrees of flexion, where rolling occurs.
    - Pronation and supination occur at the humeroradial and proximal radioulnar joints.
    - The reported normal range of motion varies between studies[68] with the American Academy of Orthopaedic Surgeons[70] reporting an average of 70 degrees of pronation and 85 degrees of supination.
    - The range of motion required for typical daily activities of both flexion/extension and pronation–supination can be performed between a much more limited range.[71]

Much of the elbow joint's stability during normal use is supplied by the shape of the articulating surfaces. Of the three articulations, the humeroulnar articulation supplies the primary anterior–posterior stability, although the radiohumeral articulation can contribute to stability from posterior dislocation at flexion of 90 degrees or more. Beyond the bony stability of the joint, the ligaments and joint capsules around the elbow provide remaining stability, and the interosseous membrane binds the radial and ulnar shafts together.

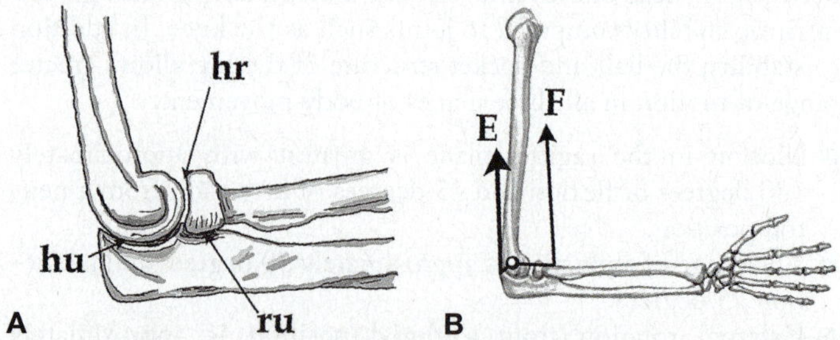

Figure 8.19. A. The elbow joint complex consists of the humeroulnar (*hu*), humeroradial (*hr*), and proximal radioulnar joints. **B.** The primary flexor (*F*) and extensor (*E*) moments across the joint.

SIMPLE JOINT MOMENTS

The basic biomechanics of the elbow can be described largely as a system of simple levers or joint moments as suggested earlier in the section on basic mechanics of joint systems (Figs. 8.13 and 8.19).

- Muscle forces act at a low mechanical advantage to achieve a large movement.
- Due to disadvantageous vector angles through some of their range, relatively high muscle contraction forces are required.
  - These muscle contraction forces typically generate large joint reaction force components that act through the bony elements to stabilize the elbow.
  - These joint reaction forces may exceed body weight even during normal activities.

DYSFUNCTIONS FROM THE COUPLING OF INTRA-ARTICULAR MOTION

As a joint complex, the elbow provides a reasonably simple example of coupling relationships of intra-articular joint motions that, when disrupted, can produce dysfunction.

- During flexion/extension movements, the humeroulnar joint has a primary gliding motion that is accompanied by a movement of the head of the radius on the capitulum of the humerus.
  - This produces a smaller proximal and distal gliding of the proximal radius in the radial notch of the ulna.[62]
  - The extent of this latter movement is greatest when the joint is half-flexed.
  - Although this motion is not a primary component of the segmental motion, its disruption can produce pain and dysfunction in the joint during movement.
  - It is therefore important to understand the coupled movements of the complex as well as the individual articulations. More complicated examples can occur in more extensive joint chains such as in the spine and feet.

The Shoulder

THE SHOULDER IS A COMPLEX OF FOUR JOINTS WITH DIFFERENT PROPERTIES

The shoulder consists of a complex of four articulations:

1. Glenohumeral
2. Acromioclavicular
3. Sternoclavicular
4. Scapulothoracic articulations (Fig. 8.20)

Of these, the scapulothoracic articulation is not a true articulation, but an indirect attachment of the scapula to the thoracic wall indirectly through muscles.

- The shoulder complex acts in concert with contributions from each joint resulting in a summative greater range of motion of this complex.
- The glenohumeral joint is a basic ball-and-socket joint but has much less intrinsic stability than its lower limb analog at the hip.
- The reduced stability is reflected by the structure of the articulating surfaces of the joint.
- The area of the glenoid fossa that contacts the humerus is only one-third to one-fourth the size of the joint surface of the humeral head.[72]

This allows a more circular range of motion relative to the scapula but at the cost of intrinsic structural stability of the joint. Although some vertical structural support may be derived from the overlying acromion process and attached clavicle, the glenohumeral joint is reliant, to a great degree, on soft-tissue structures (ligaments, tendons, joint capsules, and muscles) for stability.[73] During function, the glenohumeral joint primarily rotates, but rolling and translation may also take place. This translation may increase substantially with soft-tissue injury or dislocation.

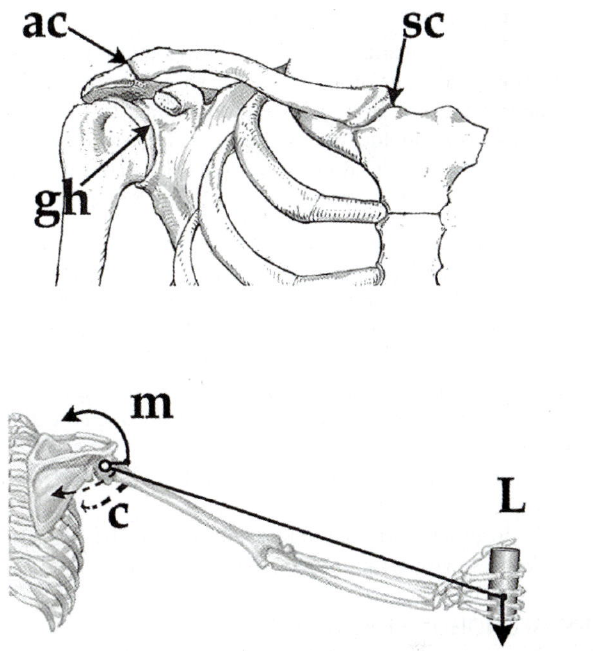

Figure 8.20. Top. Front view of the shoulder complex consisting of the glenohumeral (*gh*) acromioclavicular (*ac*) and sternoclavicular (*sc*) articulations. The scapulothoracic junction is not a true articulation, but describes the relationship of the scapula and thorax as can be seen in the lower figure. **Bottom.** An example of the differences in the moment arms of shoulder muscles (*m*) and a load (*L*) in a lift with the shoulder abducted and arm extended. Cocontracting muscles (*c, dotted arrows*) are important to stabilize the shoulder complex during such tasks.

- The scapula attaches to the thoracic skeleton through a chain of two articulations, the acromioclavicular and sternoclavicular joints.
- The acromioclavicular joint between the clavicle and the proximal acromion of the scapula has a meniscus of cartilage, a thick fibrous capsule, and supporting ligaments that stabilize the joint and allows the scapula motion in three planes.[74]
  - These planes include a vertical axis (protraction and retraction) and transverse axes in the frontal and sagittal planes.
- The proximal end of the clavicle (sternoclavicular joint) is stabilized by a fibrocartilage, meniscus-containing, articulation capsule, and ligaments to the sternum and first rib.
- The concept of a scapulothoracic articulation involves a description of the movement of the scapula relative to the thorax as limited by its muscular attachments and the clavicular chain.
  - This structural arrangement allows a wide range of motion of the scapula including protraction retraction, elevation, depression, and rotation.
- Movement of the scapula involves the translocation of the entire glenohumeral joint, contributing substantially to the range of motion of the arm.
  - A simple example is the contribution of scapular motion to the elevation of the arm. In this circumstance, the scapula rotates to elevate the shoulder and the glenohumeral joint as the arm is raised.

SHOULDER RANGE OF MOTION

Due to the intricate and multi-faceted interactions of its individual articulations, the range of motion of the shoulder complex is usually described as a whole. From a resting position at the side, the range of motion in the shoulder complex is typically described in the context of the range of elevation of the shoulder or movement of the humerus away from the thorax in any of the three primary planes.

- Forward flexion and abduction are approximately 180 degrees and in the plane of the scapula, may exceed 180 degrees.
- Backward elevation or extension is approximately 60 degrees.
- Adduction of the humerus in front of and in the plane of the body across the midline is approximately 75 degrees.[70]
- Horizontal flexion in a transverse plane at 90 degrees of abduction is approximately 135 degrees, with horizontal extension of 45 degrees.
- Rotation about the long axis of the humerus varies with the degree of arm elevation.
- Both internal and external rotation can be approximately 90 degrees, with a total range of 180 degrees.[74]

THE GLENOHUMERAL JOINT

Because of the relative lack of structural stability of the glenohumeral joint, soft-tissue connections through the joint must play a greater role in its stability. In addition to the joint capsule and ligamentous connections, muscle contraction forces that essentially hold the joint together become more important in resisting the loads placed on the distal upper limb.

- The use of force-coupling arrangements in the muscles of the rotator cuff is particularly important in this process.
- In force coupling, muscles of the rotator cuff act in concert to produce offsetting moments (a net joint reaction force) to stabilize the joint (Fig. 8.20) as elevation is produced.
- The actual calculations of joint reaction forces under these circumstances are difficult due to the large numbers of muscles involved in arrangements that vary according to the plane of motion.
- Estimates of these forces suggest magnitudes near body weight.[75]
- It is also important to note that the low mechanical advantage of muscles in the shoulder compared to the moment arm of a load in the hand of an extended arm requires very high contraction forces (Fig. 8.20).
- The low mechanical advantage of shoulder muscles under loading and the dependency of the joint on soft tissues for stability make the shoulder particularly vulnerable to injury.

The Spine

The spine as a whole represents an extremely complicated system of articulations and bony segments that act to protect the spinal cord while providing a basic support axis for the upper body. The structure and motion of spinal segments differ substantially over the spinal column. The spine consists of 24 bony elements, generally placed into 4 groups: cervical (generally 5 typical vertebrae and 2 atypical vertebrae), thoracic (generally 12 vertebrae), lumbar (generally 5 vertebrae), and the sacrum (generally described as a single element). Due to this complexity and variation, only some basic principles of spinal biomechanics can be covered here. The cervical segments and the sacrum will be discussed because of their unique roles and complexities.

SPINAL MOTION SEGMENTS

The *functional unit of the spine* or motion segment consists of two vertebrae, the intervertebral disk in between them and their associated soft tissues (Fig. 8.21). The segment is functionally and physically divided into anterior and posterior segments.

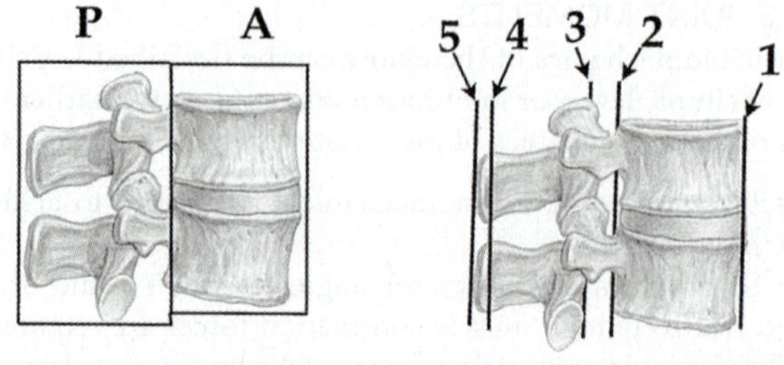

Figure 8.21. Left. A basic motion segment of the lumbar spine divided into anterior (*A*) and posterior (*P*) portions. The anterior portion contains the vertebral bodies, the spinal disk, and the anterior longitudinal (1) and posterior longitudinal (2) ligaments (**right**). The posterior portion contains the vertebral canal, the bony segments associated with it, and associated ligaments including the ligamentum flavum (3) the interspinous ligament(4), and the supraspinous ligament (5). Capsular ligaments are not shown.

- The anterior portion consists of the vertebral body, the disk between them, and the longitudinal ligaments (Fig. 8.21).
  - □ The anterior segment of the unit is the primary load-bearing section, with the vertebral bodies and the intervening disk increasing in size in the lower segments to sustain greater loading stress.
- The posterior segment is more designed for motion, consisting of the vertebral arches, the articulations between the facets, the transverse and spinous processes, and the ligaments that bind them together.
  - □ Besides containing the spinal cord and associated structures, the architecture of the posterior segment acts to guide and limit the motion that can occur between the vertebrae of the segment.
  - □ Load bearing in the posterior segment can be significant when the spine is hyperextended[76] and during forward bending coupled with rotation.[77]

THE BONY STRUCTURE OF THE SPINE

The soft-tissue support for the spinal column consists of the ligaments, joint capsules, and muscles that connect to the transverse and spinous processes of the vertebrae as part of the posterior motion segments.

- The primary ligaments, all of which provide intrinsic support for the spinal column, include (Fig. 8.21):
  - □ Anterior longitudinal ligaments
  - □ Posterior longitudinal ligaments
  - □ Ligamentum flavum
  - □ Supraspinous ligaments
  - □ Interspinous ligaments
  - □ Intertransverse ligaments
- The capsular ligaments for the facet articulations also contribute to stability and limitation of motion.
- The ligaments have a high collagen content except for the ligamentum flavum, which has a high elastin content.
- The ligaments add stability and store energy during movement of the spinal column. For example:
  - □ Flexion primarily stretches the interspinous ligaments, capsular ligaments, ligamentum flavum, and the posterior longitudinal ligaments.
  - □ Extension stretches the anterior longitudinal ligaments and the capsular ligaments.

- □ These store energy like an elastic band and can be used for subsequent recovery to a neutral position.
- □ Other ligaments similarly participate in lateral bending and rotation.

INTERVERTEBRAL DISKS

The intervertebral disks sustain and distribute primarily compressive loading of the vertebrae and restrict excessive motion.

- The disk consists of:
  - □ A tough outer covering of fibrocartilage
  - □ The *annulus fibrosus*, bounded above and below by a plate of hyaline cartilage adjacent to the vertebrae.
    - The collagen fibers of the annulus fibrosus are arranged in concentric layers and differing orientations to the vertical axis of ±30 degrees in a cross-hatched arrangement.
  - □ This covering encloses a gelatinous inner core, the *nucleus pulposus* that acts to distribute and redirect stresses and store energy, similar to a partially inflated ball.
    - The nucleus pulposus contains a water-binding glycosaminoglycan gel (80% to 88% water)[78] that becomes progressively less hydrated with age.[79]
    - This change can reduce the elasticity, ability to store energy, and stress-loading distribution properties of the disk and make it less capable of resisting loads.

In the unloaded condition, longitudinal ligaments and the ligamenta flava exert pressure on the disk to create a prestress condition.[80] Compressive stress on the disk through the vertebral bodies creates a circumferential tensile stress that is resisted by the annular fibers of the annulus fibrosus.

- During motions such as flexion bending, the vertebrae rotate forward, creating compression stress and some strain (bulging) on the anterior disk and tensile stress on the posterior portion of the disk (Fig. 8.4).
- Rotation produces torsional stress on the disk, which is also redistributed through its structure.
- These strain patterns allow vertebral movement under load, and redistribution of forces across the vertebral–disk interface, to minimize localized extremes in stress.

THE BONY STRUCTURE OF THE POSTERIOR PORTION OF THE MOTION SEGMENT

Aside from their connection through the vertebral bodies and the intervening disk, the vertebrae interact structurally through the facets of intervertebral joints in the posterior portion of the motion segment. Under most circumstances, vertebral movement is restricted by the orientation of these facets relative to the vertebral column and each other (Fig. 8.22).

- Exceptions include particular regions of the spinal column, where articulations with structures such as the skull, ribs, or sacrum may add additional constraints on vertebral movement.
- The orientation of intervertebral facets changes throughout the spinal column[81] and the actual angle of the facets may vary significantly between individuals.
- The orientation of intervertebral facets also acts to produce additional directional components (motion coupling, as described in the next section) in vertebral motion during basic movement, such as flexion, extension, rotation, and lateral flexion.

The primary variation in facet orientation can be defined in the transverse and frontal planes. A positive angle deviation from the transverse plane indicates that the facets are oriented above a horizontal (transverse) plane through the body (Fig. 8.22).

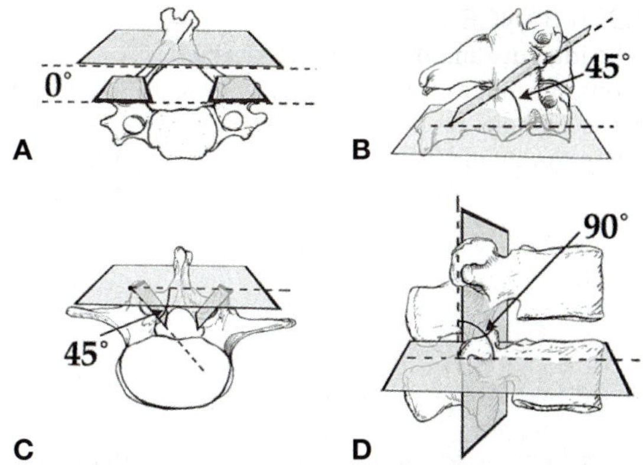

Figure 8.22. The orientation of intervertebral joint facets in the frontal and transverse planes relative to the spinal column. In the cervical vertebrae (**A** and **B**), the surfaces of the facets on either side are parallel to each and to a frontal plane (**A**) but inclined at 45 degrees above a transverse plane through a vertebra as viewed from the side (**B**). In the lumbar spine (**C** and **D**), the surfaces of the facets are oriented at 45 degrees to the frontal plane (**C**) and 90 degrees above a transverse plane as shown from the side (**D**). The facet orientations restrict the mobility of intervertebral movement and define the motion-coupling characteristics.

- Positive deviation in the frontal plane effectively describes the orientation of the facet surfaces on each side of the vertebra relative to each other, although the angle is defined relative to a frontal plane (Fig. 8.22).
- The atlas and axis have facets that are almost parallel to the transverse plane, with the remaining facets of the cervical vertebrae oriented at a 45-degree angle to the transverse plane and parallel to the frontal plane (Fig. 8.22).
- The alignment of the C3–C7 vertebrae allows flexion, extension, lateral flexion, and rotation.[82]
  - □ This can be compared to the facets of thoracic vertebrae that are oriented 60 degrees from the transverse plane and 20 degrees from the frontal plane.
  - □ This allows lateral bending, rotation, and some flexion and extension.
- The lumbar vertebrae have facets oriented 90 degrees to the transverse plane and 45 degrees to the frontal plane.
  - □ This allows for flexion, extension, and sidebending but very little rotation.
  - □ The lumbosacral joints do allow more rotation,[83] with facets oriented more obliquely to the transverse plane.

SPINAL MOTION

The kinematic and kinetic considerations of spinal movements are particularly complicated, since overall movements are a composite of comparatively small movements of each vertebral segment.

- Each vertebra has some degree of rotation or translation in each of its transverse, sagittal, and longitudinal axes (or 6 degrees of freedom in movement).
  - □ This movement is largely limited by the intervertebral joint facet orientations.
  - □ These orientations vary markedly at the different regions of the spinal column.[81]
- Flexion/extension movements are greatest in the cervical, lower thoracic, and lumbar spine;
  - □ Rotation is greatest in the cervical and upper thoracic spine (Boxes 8.1 to 8.6).
  - □ Lateral bending is greatest in the cervical spine and more evenly distributed over remaining vertebrae.

BOX 8.1 Lower Extremity

Region	Joint	Movement plane	Qualifier	Normal ROM
	Hip	Sagittal plane	Flexion	100–120
			Extension	15–30
		Coronal plane	Abduction	45–50
			Adduction	20–30
		Transverse plane	Internal rotation	30–40
			External rotation	40–60
	Knee	Sagittal plane	Flexion	135–155
			Extension	0
		Transverse plane	Internal (medial) rotation	10
			External (lateral) rotation	10
	Talocrural joint	Sagittal plane	Dorsiflexion	10–20
			Plantar flexion	40–50
	Subtalar joint	Coronal plane	Inversion	5
			Eversion	5
	Forefoot	Transverse plane	Abduction	20
			Adduction	10
	MTP joint	Sagittal plane	Flexion	70–90
			Extension	45

Compiled in part from: Hoppenfeld S. *Physical Examination of the Spine & Extremities*. Appleton & Lange; 1976 and Standring S. *Gray's Anatomy, The Anatomical Basis of Clinical Practice*. Elsevier Churchill Livingston; 2015.

BOX 8.2 Upper Extremity

Region	Joint	Movement plane	Qualifier	Normal ROM
	Shoulder	Coronal plane	Abduction	180
			Adduction	45
		Sagittal plane	Flexion	180
			Extension	45
		Transverse plane	Medial rotation	45
			Lateral rotation	55
	Elbow	Sagittal plane	Flexion	135
			Extension	0–5
		Transverse plane	Supination	90
			Pronation	90
	Wrist	Sagittal plane	Flexion	80
			Extension	70
		Coronal plane	Abduction (radial deviation)	20
			Adduction (ulnar deviation)	30
	Fingers	Sagittal plane	Flexion	90
			Extension	30–45
		Coronal plane	Abduction	20
			Adduction	0

Compiled in part from: Hoppenfeld S. *Physical Examination of the Spine & Extremities*. Appleton & Lange; 1976 and Standring S. *Gray's Anatomy, The Anatomical Basis of Clinical Practice*. Elsevier Churchill Livingston; 2015.

BOX 8.3 Cervical Spine

Region	Joint	Movement plane	Qualifier	Normal ROM	Range
	C0–C1	Sagittal plane	Combined flexion–extension	25	
		Coronal plane	Lateral bending (one side)	5	
		Transverse plane	Axial rotation (one side)	5	
	C1–C2	Sagittal plane	Combined flexion–extension	20	
		Coronal plane	Lateral bending (one side)	5	
		Transverse plane	Axial rotation (one side)	40	
	C2–C3	Sagittal plane	Combined flexion–extension	10	5–16
		Coronal plane	Lateral bending (one side)	10	11–20
		Transverse plane	Axial rotation (one side)	3	0–10
	C3–C4	Sagittal plane	Combined flexion–extension	15	7–26
		Coronal plane	Lateral bending (one side)	11	9–15
		Transverse plane	Axial rotation (one side)	7	3–10
	C4–C5	Sagittal plane	Combined flexion–extension	20	13–29
		Coronal plane	Lateral bending (one side)	11	0–16
		Transverse plane	Axial rotation (one side)	7	1–12
	C5–C6	Sagittal plane	Combined flexion–extension	20	13–29
		Coronal plane	Lateral bending (one side)	8	0–16
		Transverse plane	Axial rotation (one side)	7	2–12
	C6–C7	Sagittal plane	Combined flexion–extension	17	6–26
		Coronal plane	Lateral bending (one side)	7	0–17
		Transverse plane	Axial rotation (one side)	6	2–10
	C7–T1	Sagittal plane	Combined flexion–extension	9	4–7
		Coronal plane	Lateral bending (one side)	4	0–17
		Transverse plane	Axial rotation (one side)	2	0–7

Reprinted with permission from White AA III, Panjabi MM. *Clinical Biomechanics of the Spine*. 2nd ed. Lippincott Williams & Wilkins; 1990.

BOX 8.4 Thoracic Spine

Region	Joint	Movement plane	Qualifier	Normal ROM	Range
	T1–T2	Sagittal plane	Combined flexion–extension	4	3–5
		Coronal plane	Lateral bending (one side)	5	5
		Transverse plane	Axial rotation (one side)	9	14
	T2–T3	Sagittal plane	Combined flexion–extension	4	3–5
		Coronal plane	Lateral bending (one side)	6	5–7
		Transverse plane	Axial rotation (one side)	8	4–12
	T3–T4	Sagittal plane	Combined flexion–extension	4	2–5
		Coronal plane	Lateral bending (one side)	5	3–7
		Transverse plane	Axial rotation (one side)	8	5–11
	T4–T5	Sagittal plane	Combined flexion–extension	4	2–5
		Coronal plane	Lateral bending (one side)	6	5–6
		Transverse plane	Axial rotation (one side)	8	5–11

(*continued*)

BOX 8.4 Thoracic Spine (*Continued*)

Region	Joint	Movement plane	Qualifier	Normal ROM	Range
	T5–T6	Sagittal plane	Combined flexion–extension	4	3–5
		Coronal plane	Lateral bending (one side)	6	5–6
		Transverse plane	Axial rotation (one side)	8	5–11
	T6–T7	Sagittal plane	Combined flexion–extension	5	2–7
		Coronal plane	Lateral bending (one side)	6	6
		Transverse plane	Axial rotation (one side)	7	4–11
	T7–T8	Sagittal plane	Combined flexion–extension	6	3–8
		Coronal plane	Lateral bending (one side)	6	3–8
		Transverse plane	Axial rotation (one side)	7	4–11
	T8–T9	Sagittal plane	Combined flexion–extension	6	3–8
		Coronal plane	Lateral bending (one side)	6	4–7
		Transverse plane	Axial rotation (one side)	6	6–7
	T9–T10	Sagittal plane	Combined flexion–extension	6	3–8
		Coronal plane	Lateral bending (one side)	6	4–7
		Transverse plane	Axial rotation (one side)	4	3–5
	T10–T11	Sagittal plane	Combined flexion–extension	9	4–14
		Coronal plane	Lateral bending (one side)	7	3–10
		Transverse plane	Axial rotation (one side)	2	2–3
	T11–T12	Sagittal plane	Combined flexion–extension	12	6–20
		Coronal plane	Lateral bending (one side)	9	4–13
		Transverse plane	Axial rotation (one side)	2	2–3
	T12–L1	Sagittal plane	Combined flexion–extension	12	6–20
		Coronal plane	Lateral bending (one side)	8	5–10
		Transverse plane	Axial rotation (one side)	2	2–3

Reprinted with permission from White AA III, Panjabi MM. *Clinical Biomechanics of the Spine*. 2nd ed. Lippincott Williams & Wilkins; 1990.

BOX 8.5 Lumbar Spine

Region	Joint	Movement plane	Qualifier	Normal ROM	Range
	L1–L2	Sagittal plane	Combined flexion–extension	12	5–16
		Coronal plane	Lateral bending (one side)	6	3–8
		Transverse plane	Axial rotation (one side)	2	1–3
	L2–L3	Sagittal plane	Combined flexion–extension	14	8–18
		Coronal plane	Lateral bending (one side)	6	3–10
		Transverse plane	Axial rotation (one side)	2	1–3
	L3–L4	Sagittal plane	Combined flexion–extension	15	6–17
		Coronal plane	Lateral bending (one side)	8	4–12
		Transverse plane	Axial rotation (one side)	2	1–3
	L4–L5	Sagittal plane	Combined flexion–extension	16	9–21
		Coronal plane	Lateral bending (one side)	6	3–9
		Transverse plane	Axial rotation (one side)	2	1–3
	L5–S1	Sagittal plane	Combined flexion–extension	17	10–24
		Coronal plane	Lateral bending (one side)	3	2–6
		Transverse plane	Axial rotation (one side)	1	0–2

Reprinted with permission from White AA III, Panjabi MM. *Clinical Biomechanics of the Spine*. 2nd ed. Lippincott Williams & Wilkins; 1990.

BOX 8.6 Cervical Spine Age-Related ROM

Motion	20–29 ys	30–39 ys	40–49 ys	50–59 ys
Flexion	60	58	59	53
Extension	75	69	66	64
Left sidebending	46	43	41	38
Right sidebending	45	42	40	38
Left rotation	78	79	79	71
Right rotation	79	79	78	71

Reprinted with permission from Swinkels RA, Swinkels-Meewisse IE. Normal values for cervical range of motion. *Spine (Phila Pa 1976)*. 2014;39(5):362–367.

- Flexion, extension, rotation, sidebending, and translation refer to actions at the joint. So it is proper to say that L4 moves anteriorly relative to L5 when the L4–L5 joint flexes rather than saying that L4 flexes on L5.

It should be noted here that the convention in osteopathic medicine is to describe rotation of a vertebra as the direction in which the anterior part of the vertebral body or anterior segment rotates, consistent with the anatomical position. In some biomechanical texts, rotation of the vertebra is described as the direction in which the posterior segment or spinous process rotates. Even though these conventions describe the same rotary motion, they are on opposite sides of the center of rotation and therefore the inverse of each other.

This difference can become particularly confusing in relation to descriptions of motion coupling between vertebrae over the spine (discussed subsequently). The osteopathic convention will be used here, unless specific reference is made to the spinous process. Another caveat of the descriptions of vertebral movements given is that active, muscle contraction-based movement characteristics may or may not be similar to movements produced by external forces (e.g., manipulations). This should be taken into account in comparisons of these characteristics as described in the chapters on manipulation.

Physiologically, normal movements of the spinal column in any of the primary directions (flexion–extension, lateral bending, rotation) produce additional motion vectors in the vertebrae as a consequence of the orientation of the intervertebral facets and other articulations (Fig. 8.23).

- This coupling may include motions of lateral bending (sidebending), rotation, and translation in several axes simultaneously, although only major coupling relationships are typically noted as clinically significant.
- The coupling can differ markedly over the spine and only a limited description will be given here.
    - In the thoracic region, rotation is coupled with sidebending.
        - This is greatest in the upper thoracic region, with the vertebrae rotating toward the same side as the sidebending.[81]
- In the lumbar spine, rotation is also coupled with sidebending, but the vertebrae generally rotate in a direction opposite the sidebending.

Additional motion coupling in the cervical spine and sacrum are described subsequently.

VARIABILITY OF SPINAL MOTION

Motion of the spine varies widely between individuals. The composite nature of spinal movements along with individual structural and soft-tissue differences help to explain the great variation in range of motion in individuals. There are also significant variations in spinal range of motion with age and sex.[84] This makes the listing of normal values without specification of these factors of little clinical significance.

- Difficulties in defining normal ranges of motion (Box 8.7) also derive from a large capacity of the spine to produce compensatory changes in movement to achieve a similar net movement.
- In this strategy, a limitation of movement that exists in the structural aspects of one area of the spinal column can be alleviated by a compensatory greater mobility in other areas.[85]
    - For example, the movement of the spinal column is also accompanied by motion in the pelvis. In body flexion, the initial 50 to 60 degrees of motion occurs in the lumbar spine

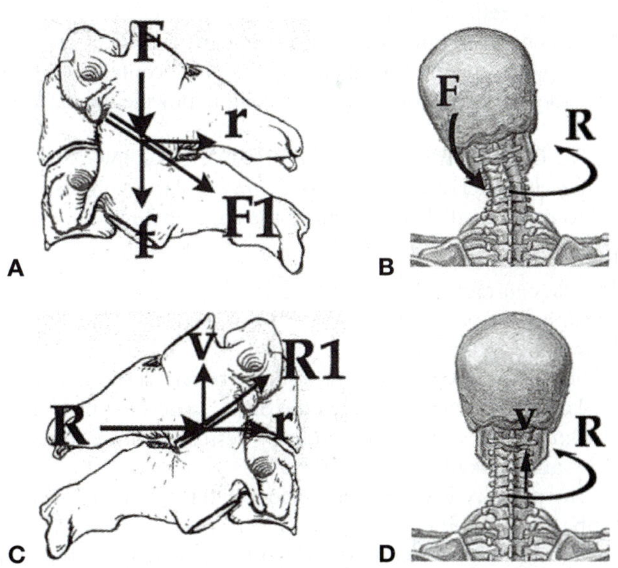

Figure 8.23. Motion coupling as influenced by the orientation of intervertebral facets in cervical vertebrae. A. A lateral flexing force (*F*) on the side of the vertebrae acting to move the upper vertebrae relative to the bottom will be redirected by the facets in a new direction (*F1*). The divided moment will have a remaining flexing component (*f*) and a rotational component (*r*) that will add (couple) rotation (*R*) of the vertebrae to the flexing movement (**B**). **C.** A rotational force (*R*) on one vertebra is redirected by the facets to glide in a new direction (*R1*). R1 has both a vertical (*v*) and a remaining rotational component (*r*) (vectors). The vertical component will cause the side of the vertebra to lift upward and produces lateral flexion on the opposite side (**D**). However, in isolated rotation movements, this flexing moment is restricted to produce vertical translation (telescoping) of the cervical spine, particularly at the C1–C2 joint.

BOX 8.7 Spinal Regional Normal Ranges of Motion

		Flexion	Extension	Rotation	Lateral Bending
Cervical Spine	*Entire C-spine*	45–90	45–90	70–90	30–45
Thoracic Spine	*T1–T4*				5–25
	T5–T8				10–30
	T9–T12			70–90	20–40
	Total			70–90	35–95
Lumbar Spine	*Entire L-spine*	70–90	30–45		

Adapted from Luttgens K, Hamilton NP. *Kinesiology: Scientific Basis of Human Motion.* 9th ed. Brown & Benchmark. 1997; Windle WF. *The Spinal Cord and Its Reaction to Traumatic Injury: Anatomy, Physiology, Pharmacology, Therapeutics.* New York, NY: M Dekker. 1980: xi, 384; Geelhoed MA, McGaugh J, Brewer PA, Murphy D. A new model to facilitate palpation of the level of the transverse processes of the thoracic spine. *J Orthop Sports Phys Ther.* 2006;36(11):876–881; Yukawa Y, Matsumoto T, Kollor H, et al. Local sagittal alignment of the lumbar spine and range of motion in 627 asymptomatic subjects: Age-related changes and sex-based differences. *Asian Spine J.* 2019;13(4):663–671. Published 2019 Mar 26.

with little contribution from the thoracic vertebra due to the orientation of the facets and the rib cage.
  - Additional flexion is accomplished by the tilting of the pelvis.
- Restriction of movement in the lumbar spine can be replaced, to some extent, by greater and earlier tilting of the pelvis.
- The movement of the pelvis also contributes to sidebending and rotation of the trunk and may be used similarly to compensate for restrictions.
- As in other multiple-articulation chains, movements of the spine are accomplished through complex interactions of agonist and antagonist muscle groups.
- Movement aspects are accomplished through the cooperative actions of antagonistic trunk and spinal muscles, some contracting to produce the movement, others cocontracting to provide stabilization.

KINETIC CONSIDERATIONS OF SPINAL LOADING

Loading characteristics of the spine are similarly complex compared to movement. The loading of the spine includes:

- Body weight
- Muscle contraction
- Ligamentous prestressing
- Externally applied loads
  - The natural kyphosis and lordosis of the spine add to the elastic resistance to load of the disks, again by redistributing compressive stress into bending stresses that can be resisted by muscle contraction (Fig. 8.24).
  - The primary load-bearing region of the spinal column is in the lumbar spine.
  - During normal standing, the center of gravity of the trunk passes near the center of the body of the third lumbar vertebra.[86]
    - This distribution and the static load on the spine can be altered appreciably by the angle of the pelvis.
    - Tilting the pelvic angle (sacral angle) forward from its normal 30 degrees to the transverse plane accentuates the lumbar lordosis.
    - Tilting backward from the normal angle flattens the lumbar lordosis.
    - Both movements affect the lever arm of the body weight on the spine and require compensatory muscle activity to resist.
      - This also creates greater loads on the lumbar spine during sitting versus relaxed standing.[87]
      - Reorientation of the spine from its normal curvature also produces stresses on the disks by changing the alignment of the vertebrae.

THE ORIENTATION OF THE SPINE DURING LIFTING

Lifting an object places added stress on the spine by creating an added load at a distance (moment) from the center of support in the spine (Fig. 8.24). The stress on the lumbar vertebrae by the load is primarily a function of the distance of the load from the vertebrae (moment arm or lever arm) and the weight of the load, counteracted by contraction of the activator muscles of the lumbar spine in the back.

- Bending the body forward adds distance from the body, whether or not the knees are bent.[82]
- Contraction of back muscles and to some degree intra-abdominal pressure must counterbalance the forward-bending forces.
- In consideration of posture in lifting, the lumbar spine has less resistance to bending compared to direct compressive forces[88] and sidebending or flexion combined with axial rotation[87] increases pressure on lumbar disks.
  - This further suggests that a vertical lifting position of the spine is preferred to reduce pressures on lumbar disks.

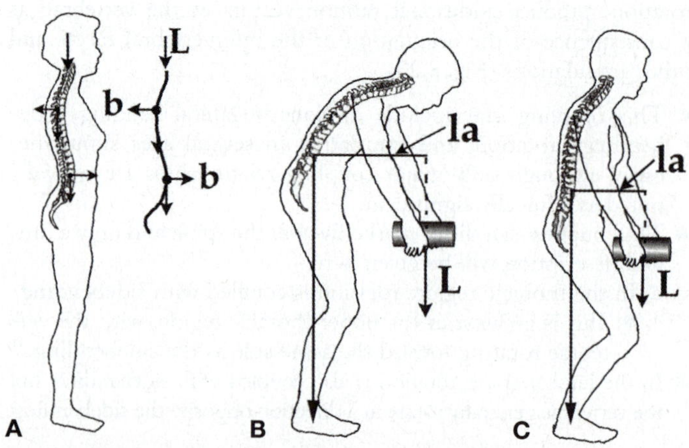

Figure 8.24. A. The normal curvatures of the spine in situ and in a model **(right)** will split vertical compression components into bending forces (*b*) that can be counteracted with muscle contraction. **B.** Force moments on the back are larger if an object is further from the vertebrae being compressed. The force moment is a product of the load (*L*) and the load arm (*la*). This compressive force alone is not dependent upon the bending of the knees **(C)**, but bending of the knees can help to shorten the load arm.

THE CERVICAL SPINE'S STRUCTURAL AND BIOMECHANICAL PROPERTIES

The cervical spine and its articulation with the skull have some unique biomechanical and structural properties that require special consideration.

- It has five of seven vertebrae that are described as more or less typical, except for the presence of the transverse foramen for the vertebral artery in C3–C6.
- The grooving of the transverse process for the exit of the cervical nerves lends to further structural weakness.
- Both the presence of the vertebral artery and the comparative structural weakness of the transverse process suggest reason for caution with high-velocity manipulations of this region.
    - This is particularly true for older adults in whom both soft tissue and bone biomechanical properties add weakness to this region.
- Other structural differences in the C3–C6 vertebrae include more prominent uncinate processes and thinner intervertebral disks.
    - Because of this, uncinate processes may also play a role in guiding and limiting cervical motion.[89]

THE ATLAS AND AXIS HAVE ADDITIONAL STRUCTURAL PROPERTIES

The atypical vertebrae (C1 and C2) have unique bony structures that limit their mobility.

- The atlas (C1) has no true vertebral body or disk, but an anterior arch with an articulating surface for the dens of the axis (C2).
- The atlas articulates with the skull in two superior facets that have a semicircular shape.
    - This limits the motion of the skull relative to the atlas to almost no rotation.
    - The inferior facets of the atlas articulate with C2 almost parallel to the transverse plane.
- The axis, with its superior protrusion, the dens, provides an axis of rotation for C1.
- Posterior translation of the dens within the vertebral foramen is prevented by ligamentous support from the cruciform ligament.
    - It also contains two superior, convex-shaped facets for articulation, with two slightly convex-shaped articulations[62] of the atlas that affect motion coupling in rotation.

These structural properties help to make the cervical region the most mobile region of the spine. The range of motion at the atlanto-occipital articulation is approximately 10 to 15 degrees of flexion/extension and 8 degrees of sidebending.[81,89] Axial rotation is largely precluded by the structure of the articulation and is transferred to the C1–C2 articulation. The C1–C2 interface is the most mobile segment of the spine with about 47 degrees of axial rotation, or almost 50% of the axial rotation capability of the entire cervical spine.[90] Flexion/extension is limited to 10 degrees, and little or no lateral bending occurs. Throughout the cervical spine, the combined range of motion is approximately 145 degrees of flexion–extension, 180 degrees of axial rotation, and 90 degrees of lateral flexion.[89]

MOTION COUPLING OF THE CERVICAL SPINE

Motion coupling of the cervical spine also has some important characteristics in addition to those mentioned earlier due to its unique anatomy.

- Flexion/extension is coupled with transverse translation, particularly at the C1–C2 interface.[89,91]
- Sidebending tends to cause rotation in the same direction (rotation of the spinous process away [vertebral body toward] from the direction of bending) (Fig. 8.23).[81]
- Isolated rotation produces a vertical translation, or telescoping, of the cervical spine due to the orientation of the facets and restriction of flexor moments (Fig. 8.23).

INCREASED MOBILITY OF THE CERVICAL SPINE

The high range of motion in the cervical spine is accompanied by a lower intrinsic stability but reduced load compared to the lumbar spine. This makes the cervical spine and associated soft-tissue support particularly vulnerable to excessive dynamic loading, with flexion/extension injuries being the most common.

- Restriction of movement in the cervical spine usually results in an increased compensatory mobility of other areas to achieve a functional range of motion.
- As a result, restriction of motion at one level, due to injury or a brace, may produce increased motion (and increased stress) at other levels.[83,92]
    - This consideration can be important in the determination of symptom–cause relationships in the diagnosis of spinal dysfunction.

THE SACRUM

The sacrum is formed by the fusion of five sacral elements of the spine during ages 15 to 30.

- The sacrum is triangular shaped and has joints with L5 superiorly, with the ilia on both sides and with the coccyx inferiorly. The superior portion, which joins with L5, is called the base and the lower portions, which join with the coccyx, on either side are called the ala of the sacrum.
- The sacrum provides support for the spine as a whole (when vertical) and serves to protect the sacral nerves that extend from the spinal cord.
- The sacrum is held in place between the ilia by a network of ligaments:
    - The iliolumbar ligaments extend from the iliac crests to the transverse process processes of L4 and L5 bilaterally.
    - The thick anterior and posterior sacral ligaments of the SI joint itself.
    - In addition, this network continues inferiorly with attachments to the spinous process (sacrospinous ligament) and to the ischial tuberosity of the ilium (sacrotuberous ligament).
- The lateral surfaces of the sacrum are in the form of an undulating "L" shape that serves as the sacral aspect of the joint with the ilium (SI joint) on both sides.

MOTION OF THE SACRUM

The sacrum is a key element in the spine in that it serves as the base of support for the entire spine and upper body. In a way, the sacrum acts as a distribution center for static and dynamic loads between the upper body from above and the lower body from below. Lumbosacral motion is complex because at times it is appropriate to refer to the sacrum as part of the spine and at other times the sacrum is described independently of spinal motion in relation to the SI joints or to the ilia.

- When the spine extends as a whole, the sacrum acts in a consistent manner with all lumbar vertebrae; in extension, the superior element of the lumbosacral joint, L5, moves posterior relative to the sacrum and thus (by Glossary definition) the lumbosacral joint is said to extend.
- At other times, when concerned with SI joint motion, sacral motion is studied in relation to the ilia. In this case, when the

spine extends generally, the sacral base is observed to move anteriorly within the SI joint or it is said to *nutate.* Clearly, the opposite terms apply when considering spinal flexion with regard to sacral motion and when the spine flexes generally, the sacrum is said to *counter nutate.* This is simple sacral motion.

- Some clinicians use the terms sacral flexion or extension to indicate this nutation and counter-nutation motion, respectively, even though the terms seem contradictory.
- Conversely, the Osteopathic Cranial Academy and Sutherland Cranial Teaching Foundation maintain that the sacrum mechanics related to primary respiratory motion are linked to motion at the sphenobasilar symphysis (SBS) and use the terms sacral flexion (when the SBS rises into flexion) and extension (when the SBS falls into extension) to indicated counter nutation and nutation motion, respectively. See Chapter 53 Osteopathic Cranial Manipulative Medicine.

- Sacral mechanics are more difficult to analyze precisely when the body is performing more complex activities such as during gait with the opposite motions between the upper and the lower extremities or in flexing and rotating the spine during a lifting maneuver.
  - During gait movements, the sacrum moves in what is called a forward torsion pattern.
  - During spinal flexion and rotation as in lifting an object and moving it to the side, the sacrum will move into a backward torsion.
  - These concepts are discussed in detail later in chapters on diagnosis and treatment of the pelvis and sacrum.

BIOMECHANICAL CONSIDERATIONS OF THE BODY AS A UNIT

Low Back and Sacroiliac Joint Pain and Spinal Stability

While this chapter primarily focuses on biomechanical principles, it is necessary to consider the role of the neuromusculoskeletal system when attempting to define the biomechanical relationships of the body as a unit. Afterall, lifting, bending, and walking all require the coordination of the entire neuromusculoskeletal system. An example of the biomechanical relationship that incorporates the whole body can be illustrated through the concept of spinal stability and low back and sacroiliac joint pain.

The lumbosacropelvic region is one of the most important structural and functional regions of the human body. The anatomical and functional relationship of the pelvis and lumbar regions influence each other and together provide structure and support, facilitate movement between other body regions, and provide protection of the spinal cord and nerve roots. Considering the osteoligamentous spine can only withstand 20N[93]–90N[94] of compressive load before buckling, it is apparent that the basic biomechanical functions of the lumbosacropelvic region are the result of the coordinated effort of the neuromusculoskeletal system which include the stabilizing effects of the ligamentous system as well as the muscles and their control. In fact, Panjabi[85] described the spinal stabilizing system as a system that functions to provide stability in response to changes in spinal posture, as well as static and dynamic loads. The spinal stabilizing system is conceptualized as three separate, yet interdependent, subsystems (Fig. 8.25). The passive subsystem is made up of tissues that do not actively generate spinal movements (e.g., vertebrae, sacrum, intervertebral disks, ligaments). The active subsystem is comprised of the musculotendinous tissues (e.g., lumbosacropelvic muscles) that generate forces to produce movement and provide spinal stability. And finally, the

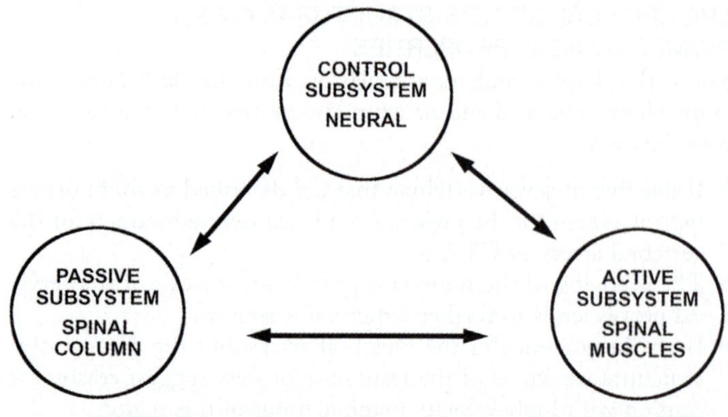

Figure 8.25. The passive, active, and neural control subsystems of the spinal stabilizing system as proposed by Panjabi (1992). (Reprinted with permission from Panjabi MM. The stabilizing system of the spine. Part I. Function, dysfunction, adaptation, and enhancement. *J Spinal Disord.* 1992;5(4):383–397.)

control subsystem (i.e., nervous system) communicates with the active and passive subsystems through afferent and efferent neural pathways.

For these subsystems to work effectively, feedback control (i.e., afferent/sensory feedback) is necessary. In fact, feedback control is necessary for many biologic systems to function and maintain homeostasis (as discussed in subsequent chapters). To understand the concept of feedback control, a common example is how room temperature is controlled by a thermostat. In the case of an air-conditioned room, a thermostat is set to a desired temperature and the actual room temperature is constantly monitored (i.e., temperature sensor or thermometer). If the desired room temperature is surpassed, the air conditioning unit will turn on to cool the room until the desired temperature is achieved.

The concept of feedback control can be applied to understanding how the human body executes movements, provides stability to the lumbosacropelvic region, and, in turn, affects the biomechanics of the system. In the case of lifting an object from the floor, to execute the desired movement (e.g., proper lifting biomechanics) efferent input from the control subsystem (i.e., neural controller/nervous system) is sent to the active subsystem (i.e., muscles) which is passed through to the passive subsystem (i.e., skeleton/spinal column) to execute the movement. Sensory/afferent information is sent back (i.e., feedback) to the CNS to allow for adjustments to be made to facilitate the achievement of the desired state of lifting (input).

However, there are situations (e.g., injury, joint dysfunction, or when pain is present) when sensory feedback may be impaired, which introduces "noise" into the system. Impairment in sensory feedback may lead to poor control and execution of the desired movement, thus resulting in maladaptive motor control strategies often observed in individuals with low back and sacroiliac joint pain. These maladaptive strategies may lead to biomechanical changes such as increased delayed muscle responses,[95–97] muscle coactivation,[98–102] increased spinal loading,[103–106] and reduced movement (i.e., decreased ROM, increased stiffness).[107–111] Alterations in sensory feedback and the resulting biomechanical sequela could also explain the reorganization of the sensory and motor cortices in individuals with low back pain,[112–118] While this example focuses on the feedback control of the lumbosacropelvic region, these concepts can be further extrapolated to other joints of the body.

Understanding the interactions between the different systems in the human body and the resulting biomechanics is complex but is fundamental to the osteopathic approach of treating neuromusculoskeletal conditions. As with numerous diseases and medical conditions, the magnitude of factors and the interaction amongst factors substantially increases their complexity. Low back pain and sacroiliac joint dysfunction are prime examples of conditions comprised of many biopsychosocial factors and result in an enormous level of complexity. That is, although biomechanical factors are part of the complex models of low back and sacroiliac joint dysfunction, other factors spanning the entire biopsychosocial spectrum contribute to the complexity of such conditions. Thus, when integrating the biomechanical considerations of the body as a unit into clinical practice, it is imperative to recognize the complexity of neuromusculoskeletal conditions, which may be reflected in the osteopathic approaches to patient care (i.e., five models of osteopathic approaches to patient care described in Chapter 1).

Gait

NORMAL LOCOMOTION (GAIT) EMPLOYS THE ENTIRE BODY FOR EFFICIENCY OF MOVEMENT

Motions of the body incorporate the individual biomechanical properties of soft and hard tissues and kinematic aspects of the individual articulations into complicated movement processes. A particularly good example of this integration can be found in normal ambulation or gait (Fig. 8.26).

- Gait may be described as a controlled falling with propulsion.
  - In this process, the center of mass of the body is subjected to relatively small vertical displacements.
  - The actual energy expended is distributed over many muscle groups beyond the legs and by subtle but significant movements.
- In normal gait, one leg is moved forward while the weight of the body is supported by the opposing leg (swing phase) (Fig. 8.26).
  - In the swing phase of the leg, the foot goes from plantar flexion to dorsal flexion.
  - The knee is flexed and then extended; the hip moves from extension to flexion.
  - The pelvis rotates and changes its tilt as muscles of the lower spine and trunk are used to generate power.

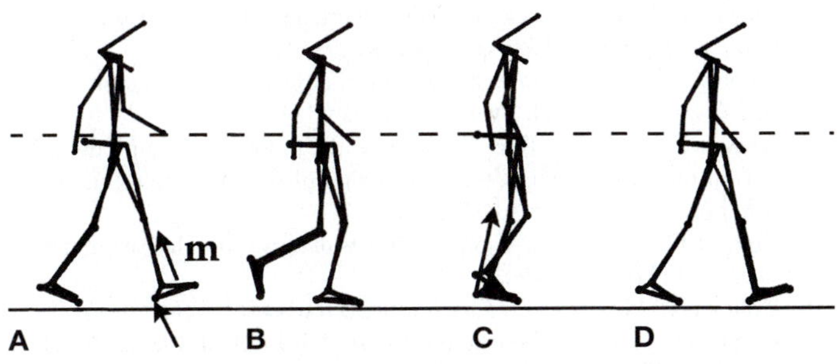

Figure 8.26. Basic gait patterns using computer-generated (Peak Performance Technologies, Inc., Englewood, CO) stick figures of an individual in normal gait. A. The gait cycle arbitrarily begins with the contact of one heel with the floor. The force of the body weight and motion on the heel (*arrow*) is decelerated by the anterior muscle group of the leg (*m, arrow*) through the ankle. **B.** Body weight is transferred to the supporting leg, which supports the body with slight knee flexion. **C.** The moving leg is swung forward and the supporting leg is slightly extended (*arrow*) to raise the body's center of mass to its high point (*dotted line*). **D.** The body is propelled forward by plantar flexion of the supporting leg to be "caught" with the heel strike of the moving leg and the cycle begins for the opposite side.

Swinging the opposing arm will assist in compensating balance and rotation moments through the trunk. The body is propelled forward and its center of mass moved slightly upward and then forward and down to be "caught" by the heel strike of the extended leg.

- As the heel hits a surface, the foot rocks down and is decelerated by the anterior muscle groups of the leg.
- The knee, which initially is almost completely extended, begins to flex and becomes progressively loaded as the body weight is transferred from the opposing leg.
- The opposing hip and pelvis are then rotated forward to begin the process for the opposite side.
- Small adjustments, such as increasing the tilt of the trunk and head in the direction of progression, bring the center of mass of the body forward and assist in increasing the rate of movement.

This basic process, grossly simplified here, can reflect one of the most frequently encountered examples of the ability of the body to adapt to injury or degenerative processes. Compensatory gait patterns can vary widely according to the underlying cause but always have an underlying biomechanical rationale, even though these adaptations may themselves produce problems. In a typical example, an injury to the knee or foot on one side may produce a compensatory shift of the body center of mass over the opposing limb.

- This will produce pain, stress injuries, or palpable dysfunctions in the opposite knee, back, hip, or even neck, if body posture has been significantly affected.
- Some aspects of these compensatory adjustments may survive the healing of the original injury, particularly if the recuperative process has been lengthy.

This emphasizes the importance of the subject's history and careful observation and knowledge of mechanical body function in the diagnosis and treatment of somatic dysfunctions.

ACKNOWLEDGMENTS

The authors and editors of this chapter would like to acknowledge the scholarly contributions of Dr. Michael R. Wells for prior editions of this chapter.

REFERENCES

1. Nordin M, Frankel VH. Biomechanics of bone. In: Nordin M, Frankel VH, eds. *Basic Biomechanics of the Musculoskeletal System*. 2nd ed. Lea & Febiger; 1989:3–27.
2. Dempster WT, Coleman RF. Tensile strength of bone along and across the grain. *J Appl Physiol.* 1961;16:355–360.
3. Reilly GC. Observations of microdamage around osteocyte lacunae in bone. *J Biomech.* 2000;33:1131–1134.
4. Siffert RS, Levy RN. Trabecular patterns and the internal architecture of bone. *Mt Sinai J Med.* 1981;48:221–229.
5. Sammarco J, Burstein A, Davis W, Frankel VH. The biomechanics of torsional fractures: the effect of loading on ultimate properties. *J Biomech.* 1971;4:113–117.
6. Carter DR, Hayes WC. Compact bone fatigue damage. A microscopic examination. *Clin Orthop Relat Res.* 1977;127:265–274.
7. Korpelainen R, Orava S, Karpakka J, Siira P, Hulkko A. Risk factors for recurrent stress fractures in athletes. *Am J Sports Med.* 2001;29:304–310.
8. Wolff J. *The Law of Bone Remodeling*. In: Maquet P, Furlong R, trans. Springer-Verlag; 1986, originally published in 1870.

9. Schneider VS, McDonald J. Skeletal calcium homeostasis and counter measures to prevent disuse osteoporosis. *Calcif Tissue Int.* 1984;36(suppl 1): 5141–5144.
10. Zerath E. Effects of microgravity on bone and calcium homeostasis. *Adv Space Res.* 1998;21:1049–1058.
11. Jenkins DP, Cochran TH. Osteoporosis: the dramatic effect of disuse of an extremity. *Clin Orthop.* 1969;64:128–134.
12. Kazarian LE, vonGierke HE. Bone loss as a result of immobilization and chelation. Preliminary results in Macaca mulatta. *Clin Orthop Relat Res.* 1969;65:67–75.
13. Huddleston AL, Rockwell D, Kulund DN, Harrison RB. Bone mass in lifetime tennis athletes. *JAMA.* 1980;244:1107–1109.
14. Woo SL, Kuei SC, Amiel D, et al. The effect of prolonged physical training on the properties of long bone: a study of Wolff's law. *J Bone Joint Surg Am.* 1981;63(5):780–787.
15. Morris FL, Naughton GA, Gibbs JL, Carlson JS, Wark JD. Prospective ten-month exercise intervention in premenarchal girls: positive effects on bone and lean mass. *J Bone Miner Res.* 1997;12(9):1453–1462.
16. Burstein AH, Currey J, Frankel VH, Heiple KG, Lunseth P, Vessely JC. Bone strength. The effect of screw holes. *J Bone Joint Surg Am.* 1972;54: 1143–1156.
17. Smith EL, Gilligan C. Physical activity effects on bone metabolism. *Calcif Tissue Int.* 1991;49(suppl):S50–S54.
18. Wilmore JH. The aging of bone and muscle. *Clin Sports Med.* 1991;10: 231–244.
19. Gao Y, Liu S, Huang J, et al. The ECM-cell interaction of cartilage extracellular matrix on chondrocytes. *Biomed Res Int.* 2014;2014:648459, 8 pages.
20. Poole AR, Kojima T, Yasuda T, Mwale F, Kobayashi M, Laverty S. Composition and structure of articular cartilage: a template for tissue repair. *Clin Orthop Relat Res.* 2001;391(suppl):S26–S33.
21. Mow VC, Kuei SC, Lai WM, Armstrong CG. Biphasic creep and stress relaxation of articular cartilage in compression: theory and experiments. *J Biomech Eng.* 1980;102:73–84.
22. Mow VC, Proctor CS, Kelly MA. Biomechanics of articular cartilage. In: Nordin M, Frankel VH, eds. *Basic Biomechanics of the Musculoskeletal System.* 2nd ed. Lea & Febiger; 1989:31–58.
23. Mansour JM, Mow VC. The permeability of articular cartilage under compressive strain and at high pressures. *J Bone Joint Surg.* 1976;58: 509–516.
24. Freeman MAR. The fatigue of cartilage in the pathogenesis of osteoarthritis. *Acta Orthop Scand.* 1975;46:323–328.
25. Weightman B, Kempson G. *Load carriage.* In: Freeman MAR, ed. *Adult Articular Cartilage.* 2nd ed. Pitman Medical; 1979:291–329.
26. Meachim G, Fergie IA. Morphological patterns of articular cartilage fibrillation. *J Pathol.* 1975;115:231–240.
27. Inerot S, Heinegård D, Audell L, Olsson SE. Articular-cartilage proteoglycans in aging and osteoarthritis. *Biochem J.* 1978;169:143–156.
28. Frank CB, Shrive, NG. Ligament. In: Nigg BM, Herzog W, eds. *Biomechanics of the Musculoskeletal System.* 2nd ed. John Wiley & Sons; 1999:107–126.
29. Viidik A. Elasticity and tensile strength of the anterior cruciate ligament in rabbits as influenced by training. *Acta Physiol Scand.* 1968;74: 372–380.
30. Schatzmann L, Brunner P, Stäubli HU. Effect of cyclic preconditioning on the tensile properties of human quadricep tendons and patellar ligaments. *Knee Surg Sports Traumatol Arthrosc.* 1998;6(suppl 1):556–561.
31. Carlstedt CA, Nordin M. Biomechanics of tendons and ligaments. In: Nordin M, Frankel VH, eds. *Basic Biomechanics of the Musculoskeletal System.* 2nd ed. Lea & Febiger; 1989:59–74.
32. Herzog W, Gal J. Tendon. In: Nigg BM, Herzog W, eds. *Biomechanics of the Musculoskeletal System.* 2nd ed. John Wiley & Sons; 1999:127–147.
33. Noyes FR, Grood ES. The strength of the anterior cruciate ligament in humans and Rhesus monkeys. Age-related and species-related changes. *J Bone Joint Surg.* 1976;58A:1074–1082.
34. Noyes FR. Functional properties of knee ligaments and alterations induced by immobilization: a correlative biomechanical and histological study in primates. *Clin Orthop Relat Res.* 1977;123:210–242.
35. Hayashi K. Biomechanical studies of the remodeling of knee joint tendons and ligaments. *J Biomech.* 1996;29:707–716.
36. Kannus P, Józsa L, Natri A, Järvinen M. Effects of training, immobilization and remobilization on tendons. *Scand J Med Sci Sports.* 1997;7: 67–71.
37. Yasuda K, Hayashi K. Changes in biomechanical properties of tendons and ligaments from joint disuse. *Osteoarthritis Cartilage.* 1999;7: 122–129.
38. Parry DAD, Barnes GRG, Craig AS. A comparison of the size distribution of collagen fibrils in connective tissues as a function of age and a possible relation between fibril size distribution and mechanical properties. *Proc R Soc Lond B Biol Sci.* 1978;203:305–321.
39. Viidik A, Danielsen CC, Oxlund H. On fundamental and phenomenological models, structure and mechanical properties of collagen, elastic and glycosaminoglycan complexes. *Biorheology.* 1982;19:437–451.
40. Zernicke RF, Judex S. Adaptation of biological materials to exercise, disuse, and aging. In: Nigg BM, Herzog W, eds. *Biomechanics of the Musculoskeletal System.* 2nd ed. John Wiley & Sons; 1999:189–204.
41. Johnson GA, Tramaglini DM, Levine RE, Ohno K, Choi NY, Woo SL. Tensile and viscoelastic properties of human patellar tendon. *J Orthop Res.* 1994;12:796–803.
42. Guyton AC, Hall JE. *Textbook of Medical Physiology.* 9th ed. WB Saunders Co.; 1996.
43. Pitman MI, Peterson L. Biomechanics of skeletal muscle. In: Nordin M, Frankel VH, eds. *Basic Biomechanics of the Musculoskeletal System.* 2nd ed. Lea & Febiger; 1989:89–111.
44. Hill AV. *First and Last Experiments in Muscle Mechanics.* Cambridge University Press; 1970.
45. Cavanagh PR, Komi PV. Electromechanical delay in human muscle under concentric and eccentric contractions. *Eur J Appl Physiol Occup Physiol.* 1979;42:159–163.
46. Ciullo JV, Zarins B. Biomechanics of the musculotendinous unit: relation to athletic performance and injury. *Clin Sports Med.* 1983;2:71–86.
47. Crawford GNC, James NT. The design of muscles. In: Owen R, Goodfellow J, Bullough P, eds. *Scientific Foundations of Orthopaedics and Traumatology.* William Heinemann; 1980:67–74.
48. Phillips CA, Petrofsky JS. *Mechanics of Skeletal and Cardiac Muscle.* Charles C Thomas Publisher; 1983.
49. Stanish WP. Neurophysiology of stretching. In: D'Ambrosio I, Drey O, eds. *Prevention and Treatment of Running Injuries.* Chas B Leach; 1982.
50. Taylor DC, Dalton JD Jr, Seaber AV, Garrett WE Jr. Viscoelastic properties of muscle-tendon units. The biomechanical effects of stretching. *Am J Sports Med.* 1990;18:300–309.
51. Gollnick PD, Matoba H. The muscle fiber composition of skeletal muscle as a predictor of athletic success. An overview. *Am J Sports Med.* 1984;12:212–217.
52. Buller AJ, Eccles JC, Eccles RM. Differentiation of fast and slow muscles in the cat hind limb. *J Physiol.* 1960;150:399–416.
53. Dubowitz V. Change in enzyme pattern after cross-innervation of fast and slow skeletal muscle. *Nature.* 1967;214:840–841.
54. Jansson E, Sjodin B, Tesch P. Changes in muscle fibre type distribution in man after physical training. A sign of fiber type transformation. *Acta Physiol Scand.* 1978;104:235–237.
55. Munsat TL, McNeal D, Waters R. Effects of nerve stimulation on human muscle. *Arch Neurol.* 1976;33:608–617.
56. Eriksson E, Häggmark T, Kiessling KH, Karlsson J. Effect of electrical stimulation on human skeletal muscle. *Int J Sports Med.* 1981;2:18–22.
57. Häggmark T, Eriksson E. Cylinder or mobile cast brace after knee ligament surgery: a clinical analysis and morphologic and enzymatic study of changes in the quadriceps muscle. *Am J Sports Med.* 1979;7:48–56.
58. Häggmark T, Eriksson E. Hypertrophy of the soleus muscle in man after Achilles tendon rupture Discussion of findings obtained by computer tomography and morphologic studies. *Am J Sports Med.* 1979;7: 121–126.
59. Arvidsson I, Eriksson E, Pitman, M. Neuromuscular basis of rehabilitation. In: Hunter E, Funk J, eds. *Rehabilitation of the Injured Knee.* CV Mosby; 1984:210–234.
60. Schafer RC. *Clinical Biomechanics: Musculoskeletal Actions and Reactions.* 2nd ed. Williams & Wilkins; 1987:54–55.
61. Van De Graaff KM. *Human Anatomy.* 4th ed. William C Brown; 1997: 197–200.

62. Warwick R, Williams PL. Arthrology. In: Williams PL, ed. *Gray's Anatomy*. 35th ed. WB Saunders Co.; 1973:389–471.
63. Nordin M, Frankel VH. Biomechanics of the knee. In: Nordin M, Frankel VH, eds. *Basic Biomechanics of the Musculoskeletal System*. 2nd ed. Lea & Febiger; 1989:115–133.
64. Helfet AJ. Anatomy and mechanics of movement of the knee joint. In: Helfet A, ed. *Disorders of the Knee*. JB Lippincott Co.; 1974:1–17.
65. Nordin M, Frankel VH. Biomechanics of the hip. In: Nordin M, Frankel VH, eds. *Basic Biomechanics of the Musculoskeletal System*. 2nd ed. Lea & Febiger; 1989:135–161.
66. Rydell NW. Forces acting on the femoral head prosthesis. A study on strain gauge supplied prostheses in living persons. *Acta Orthop Scand*. 1966;88:1–132.
67. English TA, Kilvington M. In vivo records of hip loads using a femoral implant with telemetric output (a preliminary report). *J Biomed Eng*. 1979;1:111–115.
68. Zuckerman JD, Matsen FA. Biomechanics of the elbow. In: Nordin M, Frankel VH, eds. *Basic Biomechanics of the Musculoskeletal System*. 2nd ed. Lea & Febiger; 1989:249–260.
69. London JT. Kinematics of the elbow. *J Bone Joint Surg Am*. 1981;63: 529–535.
70. American Academy of Orthopaedic Surgeons. *Joint Motion. Method of Measuring and Recording*. American Academy of Orthopaedic Surgeons; 1965. Reprinted by the British Orthopaedic Association; 1966.
71. Morrey BF, Askew LJ, An KN, Chao EY. A biomechanical study of normal elbow motion. *J Bone Joint Surg*. 1981;63:872–877.
72. Saha AK. Dynamic stability of the glenohumeral joint. *Acta Orthop Scand*. 1971;42:491–505.
73. Bigliani LU, Kelkar R, Flatow EL, Pollock RG, Mow VC. Glenohumeral stability. Biomechanical properties of passive and active stabilizers. *Clin Orthop Relat Res*. 1996;330:13–30.
74. Zuckerman JD, Matsen FA. Biomechanics of the shoulder. In: Nordin M, Frankel VH, eds. *Basic Biomechanics of the Musculoskeletal System*. 2nd ed. Lea & Febiger; 1989:225–247.
75. Poppen NK, Walker PS. Forces at the glenohumeral joint in abduction. *Clin Orthop Relat Res*. 1978;135:165–170.
76. King AI, Prasad P, Ewing CL. Mechanism of spinal injury due to caudocephalad acceleration. *Orthop Clin North Am*. 1975;6:19–31.
77. El-Bohy AA, King AI. Intervertebral disc and facet contact pressure in axial torsion. In: Lantz SA, King AI, eds. *Advances in Bioengineering*. American Society of Mechanical Engineers; 1986:26–27.
78. Gower WE, Pedrini, V. Age-related variations in protein-polysaccharides from human nucleus pulposus, annulus fibrosus and costal cartilage. *J Bone Joint Surg*. 1969;51:1154–1162.
79. Urban JPG, McMullin JF. Swelling pressure of the intervertebral disc: influence of proteoglycan and collagen contents. *Biorheology*. 1985;22:145–157.
80. Nachemson A. Lumbar intradiscal pressure. *Acta Orthop Scand Suppl*. 1960;43:1–140.
81. White AA, Panjabi MM. *Clinical Biomechanics of the Spine*. JB Lippincott Co.; 1978.
82. Lindh M. Biomechanics of the lumbar spine. In: Nordin M, Frankel VH, eds. *Basic Biomechanics of the Musculoskeletal System*. 2nd ed. Lea & Febiger; 1989:183–207.
83. Lumsden R, Morris JM. An in vivo study of axial rotation and immobilization at the lumbosacral joint. *J Bone Joint Surg*. 1968;50:1591–1602.
84. Moll JMH, Wright V. Normal range of spinal mobility. An objective study. *Ann Rheum Dis*. 1971;30:381–386.
85. Panjabi MM. The stabilizing system of the spine. Part I. Function, dysfunction, adaptation, and enhancement. *J Spinal Disord*. 1992;5(4): 383–389; discussion 397.
86. Legaye J, Duval-Beaupere G. Gravitational forces and sagittal shape of the spine. Clinical estimation of their relations. *Int Orthop*. 2008;32(6):809–816.
87. Andersson GBJ, Örtengren R, Nachemson A. Intradiskal pressure, intra-abdominal pressure and myoelectric back muscle activity related to posture and loading. *Clin Orthop Relat Res*. 1977;129:156–164.
88. Lin HS, Liu YK, Adams KH. Mechanical response of the lumbar intervertebral joint under physiological (complex) loading. *J Bone Joint Surg*. 1978;60:41–55.
89. Shapiro I, Frankel VH. Biomechanics of the cervical spine. In: Nordin M, Frankel VH, eds. *Basic Biomechanics of the Musculoskeletal System*. 2nd ed. Lea & Febiger; 1989:209–224.
90. Crisco JJ III, Panjabi MM, Dvorak J. A model of the alar ligaments of the upper cervical spine in axial rotation. *J Biomech*. 1991;24:607–614.
91. Oda T, Panjabi MM, Crisco JJ III. Three-dimensional translational movements of the upper cervical spine. *J Spinal Disord*. 1991;4:411–419.
92. Norton PL, Brown T. The immobilizing efficiency of back braces; their effect on the posture and motion of the lumbosacral spine. *J Bone Joint Surg*. 1957;39-A:111–139; passim.
93. Lucas DB, Bressler B. *Stability of the ligamentous spine*. 1961. *Technical Report No. 40*.
94. Crisco JJ, Panjabi MM, Yamamoto I, Oxland TR. Euler stability of the human ligamentous lumbar spine. Part II: Experiment. *Clin Biomech (Bristol, Avon)*. 1992;7(1):27–32.
95. Cholewicki J, Silfies SP, Shah RA, et al. Delayed trunk muscle reflex responses increase the risk of low back injuries. *Spine*. 2005;30(23):2614–2620.
96. Hungerford B, Gilleard W, Hodges P. Evidence of altered lumbopelvic muscle recruitment in the presence of sacroiliac joint pain. *Spine*. 2003; 28(14):1593–600.
97. Silfies SP, Mehta R, Smith SS, Karduna AR. Differences in feedforward trunk muscle activity in subgroups of patients with mechanical low back pain. *Arch Phys Med Rehabil*. 2009;90(7):1159–1169.
98. D'Hooge R, Hodges P, Tsao H, Hall L, Macdonald D, Danneels L. Altered trunk muscle coordination during rapid trunk flexion in people in remission of recurrent low back pain. *J Electromyogr Kinesiol*. 2013; 23(1):173–181.
99. Nelson-Wong E, Callaghan JP. Is muscle co-activation a predisposing factor for low back pain development during standing? A multifactorial approach for early identification of at-risk individuals. *J Electromyogr Kinesiol*. 2010;20(2):256–263.
100. Radebold A, Cholewicki J, Panjabi MM, Patel TC. Muscle response pattern to sudden trunk loading in healthy individuals and in patients with chronic low back pain. *Spine*. 2000;25(8):947–954.
101. Schinkel-Ivy A, Nairn BC, Drake JD. Investigation of trunk muscle co-contraction and its association with low back pain development during prolonged sitting. *J Electromyogr Kinesiol*. 2013;23(4):778–786.
102. van Dieën JH, Cholewicki J, Radebold A. Trunk muscle recruitment patterns in patients with low back pain enhance the stability of the lumbar spine. *Spine*. 2003;28(8):834–841.
103. Heidari E, Arjmand N, Kahrizi S. Comparisons of lumbar spine loads and kinematics in healthy and non-specific low back pain individuals during unstable lifting activities. *J Biomech*. 2022;144:111344.
104. Marras WS, Davis KG, Ferguson SA, Lucas BR, Gupta P. Spine loading characteristics of patients with low back pain compared with asymptomatic individuals. *Spine*. 2001;26(23):2566–2574.
105. Marras WS, Ferguson SA, Burr D, Davis KG, Gupta P. Spine loading in patients with low back pain during asymmetric lifting exertions. *Spine J*. 2004;4(1):64–75.
106. Nyayapati P, Booker J, Wu PI, et al. Compensatory biomechanics and spinal loading during dynamic maneuvers in patients with chronic low back pain. *Eur Spine J*. 2022;31(7):1889–1896.
107. Freddolini M, Strike S, Lee RY. Stiffness properties of the trunk in people with low back pain. *Hum Mov Sci*. 2014;36:70–79.
108. Hodges P, van den Hoorn W, Dawson A, Cholewicki J. Changes in the mechanical properties of the trunk in low back pain may be associated with recurrence. *J Biomech*. 2009;42(1):61–66.
109. Laird RA, Gilbert J, Kent P, Keating JL. Comparing lumbo-pelvic kinematics in people with and without back pain: a systematic review and meta-analysis. *BMC Musculoskelet Disord*. 2014;15:229.
110. Rowley KM, Smith JA, Kulig K. Reduced trunk coupling in persons with recurrent low back pain is associated with greater deep-to-superficial trunk muscle activation ratios during the balance-dexterity task. *J Orthop Sports Phys Ther*. 2019;49(12):887–898.
111. Varrecchia T, Conforto S, De Nunzio AM, Draicchio F, Falla D, Ranavolo A. Trunk muscle coactivation in people with and without low back pain during fatiguing frequency-dependent lifting activities. *Sensors (Basel)*. 2022;22(4):1417.

112. Brumagne S, Diers M, Danneels L, Moseley GL, Hodges PW. Neuroplasticity of sensorimotor control in low back pain. *J Orthop Sports Phys Ther*. 2019;49(6):402–414.
113. Corti EJ, Marinovic W, Nguyen AT, Gasson N, Loftus AM. Motor cortex excitability in chronic low back pain. *Exp Brain Res*. 2022;240(12):3249–3257.
114. Flor H. The modification of cortical reorganization and chronic pain by sensory feedback. *Appl Psychophysiol Biofeedback*. 2002;27(3):215–227.
115. Flor H, Braun C, Elbert T, Birbaumer N. Extensive reorganization of primary somatosensory cortex in chronic back pain patients. *Neurosci Lett*. 1997;224(1):5–8.
116. Goossens N, Janssens L, Brumagne S. Changes in the organization of the secondary somatosensory cortex while processing lumbar proprioception and the relationship with sensorimotor control in low back pain. *Clin J Pain*. 2019;35(5):394–406.
117. Schabrun SM, Elgueta-Cancino EL, Hodges PW. Smudging of the motor cortex is related to the severity of low back pain. *Spine*. 2017;42(15): 1172–1178.
118. Tsao H, Danneels LA, Hodges PW. ISSLS prize winner: smudging the motor brain in young adults with recurrent low back pain. *Spine*. 2011;36(21):1721–1727.

9 The Physiology of Touch

FRANK H. WILLARD ▪ JOHN A. JEROME ▪ MITCHELL L. ELKISS

KEY CONCEPTS

- The brain derives much of its perception of the external world through the activity of receptors in the skin, and particularly from the skin of the hands.
- Touch is a perception that is emergent from neural activity in a complex network that includes the somatic sensory cortex as well as numerous other regions of the cerebrum.
- While touch has long been understood for its role in localization of physical contact, new data concerning the somatic sensory system suggests that touch also includes a separate channel directed at the emotional component of the forebrain.
- Touch is paramount to osteopathic physicians with respect to connecting with, diagnosing, treating, and optimizing patients and their integrated components of body, mind, and spirit.

INTRODUCTION

Touch as a Primary Sensation

The sense of touch plays an important role in the awareness of the world.

- From the moment of waking in the morning, the hands contact the surrounding objects and communicate such information as to where a person is and what they are doing.
- The skin is the largest sensory organ in the body, throughout the day, touch from the skin provides a focal point for orientation and communication between the individual and the environment, as well as between the individuals in the world.
- The brain derives much of its perception of the world through the activity of receptors in the skin, and particularly from the skin of the hands. Contact and exploration of surrounding objects and individuals using the somesthetic sense is generated by touch with the hands.
- Texture, shape, weight, and size as well as friend, foe, harmless, or dangerous can all be determined, in part, through palpation.
- The response to touch is filtered by the highly individualistic and personal emotional axes of the brain.
- Thus, whether the touch evokes kindness and trust or hatred and anger all depend on the context of the environment in which the touch occurs, and the background and prior experiences of the individual being touched.
- Finally, touch is a dynamic process, adapting to use or disuse, differing between sexes,[1] varying across lifespan[2] and varying with culture.[3]

Touch as a Primary Mechanism for Communicating with Patients

Touch can be a primary diagnostic tool.

- The physician touches the patient; the patient, in many ways, touches the physician. The dynamics of this contact between individuals are essential to the establishment of a trusting, respectful relationship (Fig. 9.1).
- The communication developed through the touch of the physician in the physical and structural exam is the first step in helping the patient retrace the steps back to a healthy state of body, mind, and spirit.
- What begins as a palpatory examination quickly becomes a tactile conversation. The physician gains greater proprioceptive awareness of the structural impediments underlying physical as well as emotional and behavioral dysfunctions.

Significance of Touch to an Osteopathic Physician

Students begin to develop discriminative palpatory skills by touching other students, gradually transferring these abilities to the examination of patients. Through repeated practice, palpation progresses into deeper layers of the body—skin, fascia, muscle, bone, joint, and finally viscera—slowly unmasking the health of the tissue to the physician.

- Palpation of tissue may tell the skilled physician much more about the state of the patient's health than the patient can put into words.

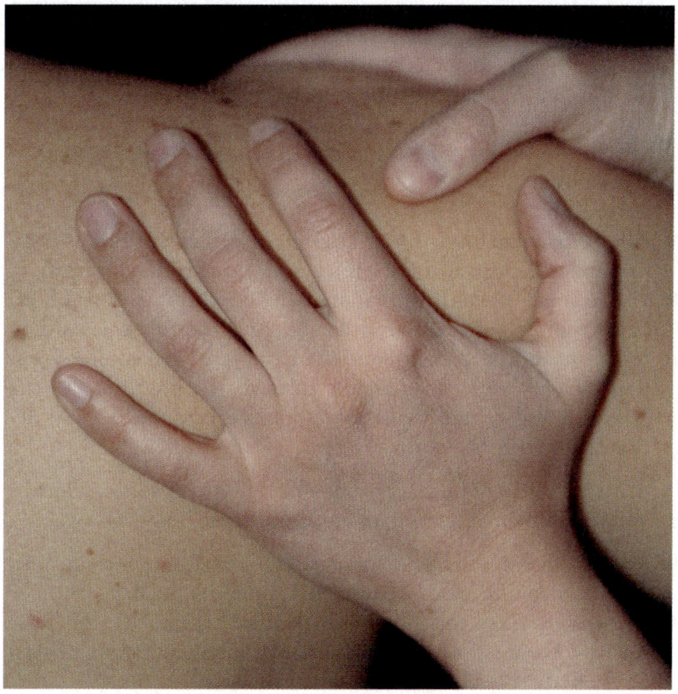

Figure 9.1. Touch in osteopathic medicine. (Used with permission from the Willard/Carreiro Collection, University of New England.)

- Being put at ease while being diagnostically touched by the physician includes an explanation of intention and nature of the touching, its purpose, and what the patient is likely to experience.
- This dialogue enhances confidence and trust. Meaningful touch, skillful palpation, and communication forge a deep verbal and tactile relationship between the physician and the patient.
- Gradually, the skilled osteopathic physician develops tactile memories of tissue dysfunctions both within a patient and across multiple patients.
- With time, palpatory skills may be used to monitor the patient's progress in the return to a healthy state.
- Even with chronic illness where complete healing and a cure are unlikely, there is a reestablished human connection based upon compassionate touch and careful attention to the dialogue; this is the osteopathic path to restore function and self-healing.
- This chapter explores the biophysical mechanisms involved when the contact between the skin of the examining physician and the skin of the patient is converted into touch in the minds of both individuals.
- See Chapter 29 Palpatory Skills and Exercises for Developing the Sense of Touch for clinical applications.

TOUCH: ANATOMY AND PHYSIOLOGY

Overview

It has been said that humans do not see with the eyes, do not hear with the ears, nor touch with the hands; instead, seeing, hearing, and touch are accomplished when the brain interacts with the information provided by sensory epithelia located in the eyes, ears, and hands. While a little less romantic, this neural-based process is integral to understanding the perception of touch.

- Touch is a perception that is emergent from neural activity in a complex network that includes the somatic sensory system, as well as portions of many additional cortical regions in the cerebrum.
- This activity begins with the formation of a stimulus code in the peripheral process of primary afferent neurons, distributed in the dermis and epidermis throughout the extremities, body, and head. The characteristic features encoded by these sensory neurons are stimulus:
  - □ Quality
  - □ Intensity
  - □ Duration
  - □ Location
- The primary neurons bring the touch-initiated stimulus code to the dorsal aspect of the spinal cord or medullary brainstem.
- While some of this information is delivered to the dorsal horn of the spinal cord, a significant amount ascends the cord to reach the dorsal column nuclei in the caudal medulla. From these nuclei, projections ascend through the brainstem to the posterior and ventral thalamus and are relayed on to the postcentral gyrus of the parietal cortex.

The entrance of primary axons into the spinal cord is done in an orderly fashion, reflecting their origin in the body.

- Thus, afferent fiber addition to the spinal tracts creates an orderly map of the body—termed a somatotopic map.
- In essence, these maps, composed of central nuclei and fiber tracts, contain information based on the segmentation pattern of the body.
- This orderly arrangement is preserved in the following:
  - □ Spinal cord
  - □ Medulla
  - □ Thalamus
  - □ Postcentral gyrus of the cerebrum

From the postcentral gyrus, the sensorineural code is mapped to several somatic sensory regions in the parietal cortex as well as to areas associated with the processing of emotions.

- These codes are modified and distributed across a large network of neural connections involving the following lobes of the cerebral cortex:
  - □ Parietal
  - □ Insular
  - □ Occipital
  - □ Temporal
  - □ Frontal
- It is within this cortical network that the somesthetic input becomes integrated with that from the other senses, such as vision and hearing.
- The perceptions of touch represent emergent properties derived from extraction of the activity of these complex neural networks on the surface of the cerebrum.
- Several regions of the cerebrum associated with the emotional systems of the brain receive input from the ascending somatic sensory system; this somatic component is responsible for the social aspects or affective nature of touch.
- This chapter will discuss the details of somatic sensory processing at multiple levels of the peripheral nervous system, spinal cord, brainstem, and forebrain.

Peripheral Processing: From Physical Stimulus to Neural Code

THE PRIMARY AFFERENT NEURONS HAVE PERIPHERAL PROCESSES IN THE SKIN, DEEP TISSUE, AND CENTRAL PROCESSES IN THE SPINAL CORD

Most of the sensation of touch arises from mechanical energy generated as an object makes contact with and deforms the skin.

- In the dermis underlying the epidermis, one can identify two major groups of primary afferent nerve endings:
  - □ Free endings that ramify in the surrounding connective tissue
  - □ Encapsulated endings that are surrounded by specialized structures (Fig. 9.2)

Free nerve endings are typically associated with unmyelinated or lightly myelinated axons and are further discussed in Chapter 11 Nociception and Pain.

- Cell bodies for these sensory fibers are present in the dorsal root ganglion.
- The central processes of these small fibers terminate in the dorsal horn of the spinal cord.
- Many of the free nerve endings have high thresholds for activation suggesting that they respond to tissue damaging forms of energy.
- However, a class of unmyelinated fibers sensitive to low levels of mechanical energy have been described,[4] these axons have been named C-tactile (CT) fibers and are found in hairy skin and, as of yet, have not been reported in glabrous skin.

The peripheral processes of the encapsulated cutaneous endings are illustrated in Figure 9.2; in general, they include the following:

- □ Merkel disks
- □ Meissner corpuscles
- □ Pacinian corpuscles
- □ Ruffini endings

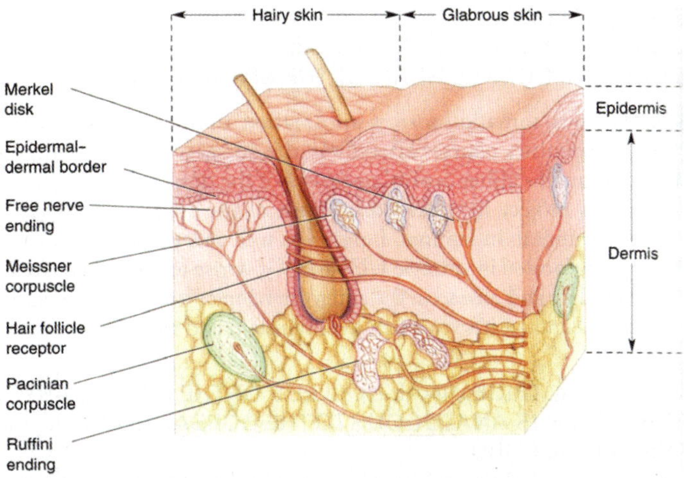

Figure 9.2. The sensory endings typically involved in tactile sensation. (Reprinted with permission from Bear MF, Connors BW, Paradiso MA. *Neuroscience: Exploring the Brain.* 2nd ed. Lippincott Williams & Wilkins; 2001. Figure 12.1.)

- However, additional specialized receptors are also found innervating the bases of follicles in hairy skin and elsewhere.
- Typically, the encapsulated endings are associated with well-myelinated (A-beta) axons.
- The cell bodies for these fibers are large and are found in the dorsal root ganglia or the trigeminal ganglion.

Central processes of all somatic sensory neurons course in the dorsal root or trigeminal nerve root to enter the spinal cord through the dorsal root entry zone or the trigeminal entry zone (Fig. 9.3).

- The central process of the large, myelinated fibers can either synapse on neurons in the ventral horn or ascend in the spinal cord tracts to nuclei located in the medulla.
- Conversely, the central process of the small, unmyelinated axons generally will terminate on cells locally in the spinal gray matter or in the spinal trigeminal nucleus.

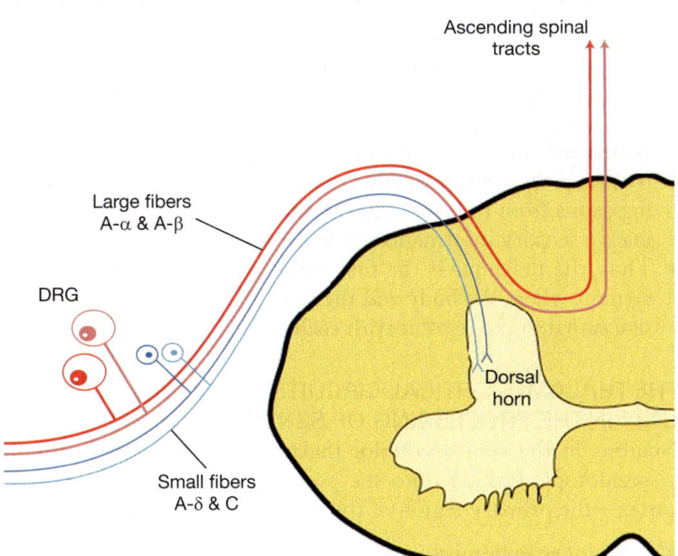

Figure 9.3. The dorsal root entry zone. The fibers of the dorsal root segregate prior to entering the dorsal horn of the spinal cord. (Used with permission from the Willard/Carreiro Collection, University of New England.)

THE PRIMARY AFFERENT NEURONS DETECT PHYSICAL (MECHANICAL) STIMULI IN THE PERIPHERAL TISSUE, DEVELOP A SENSORINEURAL CODE BASED ON ENERGY CONTAINED IN THE STIMULUS, AND CONDUCT THIS INFORMATION TO THE SPINAL CORD AND BRAINSTEM

Primary afferent fibers detect various aspects of mechanical energy in the skin and encode this information into a series of discharge patterns that are conducted to the spinal cord.

- Concerning the encapsulated endings, four general patterns of activity have been cataloged based on the response properties and general position of each sensory neuron in the dermis.
- Two types of receptors have rapidly adapting endings and quickly change discharge patterns to a static stimulus; these are the Meissner and Pacinian corpuscles, both with elaborate encapsulations. These rapidly adapting receptors are much better at recording a dynamic or moving stimulus than a static stimulus.
- The other two receptors, Merkel disks and Ruffini endings, demonstrate slowly adapting discharge patterns, much better designed to detect a static stimulus.
- Of these four types of receptors, the Meissner corpuscles and Merkel disks are located superficially at the epidermal–dermal junction, while the Pacinian corpuscle and Ruffini ending are located in the deeper portion of the dermis and hypodermis.
- Each of these receptors is capable of encoding a specific characteristic of the physical stimulus presented to the skin; therefore, for any given object touching the skin in any specific manner, a unique sensorineural code will be generated. This sensorineural code is conducted into the spinal cord by the central processes of the primary neurons.

The small-caliber, unmyelinated fibers that have free nerve endings in the periphery, they are typically involved in nociceptive or warning type of information.

- Many of these small fibers have high thresholds of activation and respond to noxious or potentially damaging energy with a high-frequency intense burst of activity.
- However, a group of these small fibers, termed the C-tactile fibers, are found in hairy skin and respond with high-frequency discharges to innocuous stimuli such as slow, light stroking of the skin.[4]
- Contrary to nociceptive fibers, the evidence suggests that individuals generate a pleasant feeling to activation of the C-tactile fiber system.[5]

THE POSITION OF THE SENSORY AXON IN THE DORSAL ROOT ENTRY ZONE IS RELATED TO ITS FUNCTION

The dorsal root entry zone; this zone is segregated based on fiber size.

- The small fibers move laterally in the root and enter directly into the dorsal horn. Many of these fibers encode nociceptive stimuli and activate appropriate defensive reflexes (see Chapter 11 Nociception and Pain).
- Conversely, the large myelinated fibers shift medially, passing over the dorsal horn and gain entrance to the more medially located dorsal columns of the spinal cord.
- The large-fiber system, composed of A-alpha and A-beta fiber, is associated with precise localization, proprioception, and discriminative touch.
- As large fibers add to the dorsal columns, they do so in an orderly manner, thus preserving the topographic representation of the body.
- The dorsal columns ascend the full length of the spinal cord to reach the dorsal column nuclei located at the cervicomedullary junction.

THE SMALL-FIBER SYSTEM CAN BE DIVIDED INTO TWO SEPARATE INPUT CHANNELS BASED ON THEIR THRESHOLDS FOR ACTIVATION

One channel is composed of small, unmyelinated or lightly myelinated fibers associated with nociception and the feelings of discomfort such as pain.

- These slowly conducting fibers typically have high thresholds of activation, thus it requires potentially tissue-damaging levels of energy to alter their discharge rate; perception of their activity is typically unpleasant in nature.
- The fibers of this first channel have been termed C-fiber mechanoheat–sensitive (CMH) nociceptors, many of which also respond to chemical stimulation and have therefore been termed **polymodal nociceptors**.

The second small-fiber channel is also composed of unmyelinated or lightly myelinated fibers but these fibers have a low threshold of activation and can thus respond to very light touch.[4]

- They have been termed low-threshold mechanosensitive C-fibers (CLTMs) or C-fiber tactile (CT fibers), most commonly in the literature they are referred to as **C-tactile fibers**.
- In humans, C-tactile fibers are found in hairy skin but have yet to be documented in the skin of the palms or the soles (glabrous skin).
- Perception of their activity has been tentatively associated with pleasantness.[5]
- The C-tactile channel has been associated with the emotional or affective nature of touch.[6]
- Although some small-caliber fiber types belong to an exteroceptive system as their afferent neurons detect external stimuli impacting on our bodies, many of them also belong to an interoceptive system that reacts to the chemical quality of our tissues.[7]

Central Processing: From Spinal Cord to Cerebral Cortex

MYELINATED AXONS OF CUTANEOUS TOUCH CORPUSCLES ENTER THE DORSAL COLUMN NUCLEI

Neurons in the dorsal column nuclei receive the large myelinated, group II afferent fibers in an orderly (somatotopic fashion) reflecting a map of the torso and extremities.

- Within the dorsal column nuclei, each ascending axon synapses on a limited number of neurons, thereby maintaining the high fidelity of the information.
- These synapses are large and secure to ensure transmission of the information to the target neurons.

In addition, the neurons of the dorsal column nuclei also receive the synaptic endings of corticonuclear fibers arising in the parietal cortex; thus, central processing of the sensorineural code really begins at this point.

THE CHIEF SENSORY NUCLEUS OF THE TRIGEMINAL SYSTEM IN THE BRAINSTEM IS ANALOGOUS IN FUNCTION TO THE DORSAL COLUMN NUCLEI

Primary afferent neurons innervating touch corpuscles in the face have their cell bodies in the trigeminal ganglion.[8]

- Central projections from these ganglionic neurons reach the chief sensory nucleus in the trigeminal complex, which is located in the pontine portion of the brainstem (see Fig. 9.3).
- The chief sensory nucleus is similar in function to the dorsal column nuclei; thus, the chief nucleus represents the first relay for discriminative information from the face.
- Projections from the chief sensory nucleus cross the midline and ascend to the contralateral thalamus.

SMALL-CALIBER, LIGHTLY MYELINATED OR UNMYELINATED SENSORY FIBERS FROM THE BODY ENTER THE DORSAL HORN OF THE SPINAL CORD

- Cutaneous somatic sensory information from the neck, torso, and extremities courses laterally in the dorsal root entry zone.
- These small-caliber central processes of the dorsal root ganglion neurons project into the dorsal horn of the spinal cord where they terminate in laminae I and II as well as laminae IV and V.
- Neurons located in laminae I, IV, and V give rise to axons that cross the midline and ascend in the anterolateral tract (spinoreticular and spinothalamic tracts) to reach the brainstem and thalamus.

THE SPINAL TRIGEMINAL NUCLEUS OF THE MEDULLARY BRAINSTEM IS ANALOGOUS TO THE DORSAL HORN OF THE SPINAL CORD

Small-caliber, lightly myelinated or unmyelinated sensory fibers from the region of the face enter the brainstem through the root of the trigeminal nerve.

- The spinal trigeminal nucleus receives many of the unmyelinated sensory fibers from the face.
- Neurons in this nucleus project axons to brainstem targets as well as to the thalamus
- In essence, the dorsal horn of the cervical spinal cord continues rostrally as the spinal trigeminal nucleus of the medulla, both structures are involved in processing nociception.

THE POSTERIOR THALAMUS RECEIVES THE ASCENDING SENSORY TRACTS FROM THE DORSAL COLUMN NUCLEI AND TRIGEMINAL SYSTEM

Axons from the dorsal column nuclei cross the midline and ascend to the posterior thalamus in a large, well-organized fiber tract termed the medial lemniscus.

- Above the pons, the medial lemniscus is joined in its course by the ascending trigeminal fibers from the chief sensory nucleus of the trigeminal system, which form the dorsal trigeminothalamic lemniscus.
- These combined sensory pathways, from the face and the body, enter the posterior aspect of the thalamus to terminate in the ventroposterior nucleus (see Fig. 9.3).
- Laterally, the ventroposterior thalamic nucleus receives axons from the medial lemniscus in a structured, orderly fashion, thus preserving the topographic map of the body (feet laterally positioned and arms more medially located).
- Medially, the ventroposterior thalamic nucleus receives ascending axons from the chief sensory nucleus, representing discriminative sensory information from the face.
- Thus, the thalamus is the first region in the ascending sensory systems where the body and the face are represented in a cohesive somatotopic register with each other.

THE THALAMOCORTICAL CIRCUITRY FUNCTIONS AS A UNIT IN THE PROCESSING OF SENSORY INFORMATION

Neurons in the ventroposterior thalamic nuclei project axons in a somatotopic fashion onto the postcentral gyrus of the parietal cortex—the primary region of the somatic sensory system.

- The upper extremity is represented laterally on the convexity of the cortical hemisphere while the lower extremity is located on the medial aspect of the hemisphere.
- The ventroposterior medial nucleus, representing the face, projects to the lateralmost portion of the hemisphere on the upper border of the lateral sulcus.

- Precisely mapped reciprocal connections from primary somatic sensory cortex to ventroposterior thalamus mean that the thalamocortical circuitry acts as an interlocked functioning unit.
- The reciprocal connections between the thalamus and the overlying cortex establish a strong oscillating rhythm, through which information is transferred to the cerebral cortex.

THE NEOCORTEX IS PARTITIONED INTO FUNCTIONAL REGIONS BASED ON ITS DISTINCT CYTOARCHITECTURE AND CONNECTIVITY

The human cerebral neocortex is partitioned in several domains principally associated with motor or sensory functions; these domains are surrounded by significantly larger cortical regions, termed association cortex, which are given over to the integration of cortical information between multiple sensory and motor areas[9] (Fig. 9.4).

- The primary somatic sensory cortex is located along the postcentral gyrus and is directly posterior to the somatic motor cortex located on the precentral gyrus (Figs. 9.5 and 9.6).
- Although these cortical areas were originally defined by their distinct cytoarchitecture, they have been confirmed and elaborated based on their connections and physiology.

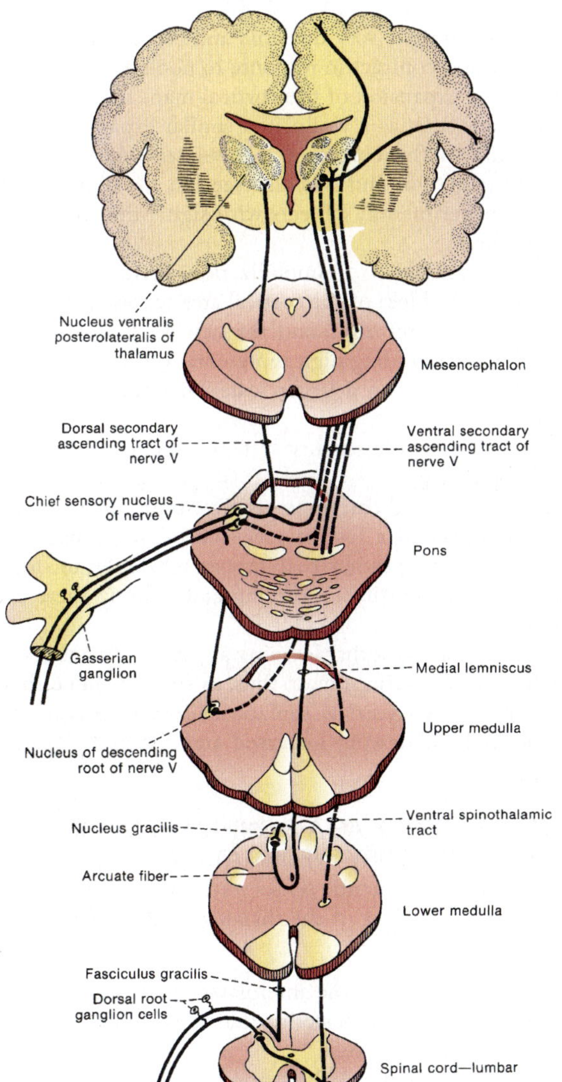

Figure 9.4. The spinal cord and brainstem pathways involved in tactile sensation. (Reprinted with permission from Campbell WW. *DeJong's The Neurologic Examination.* 6th ed. Lippincott Williams & Wilkins; 2005. Figure 32.4.)

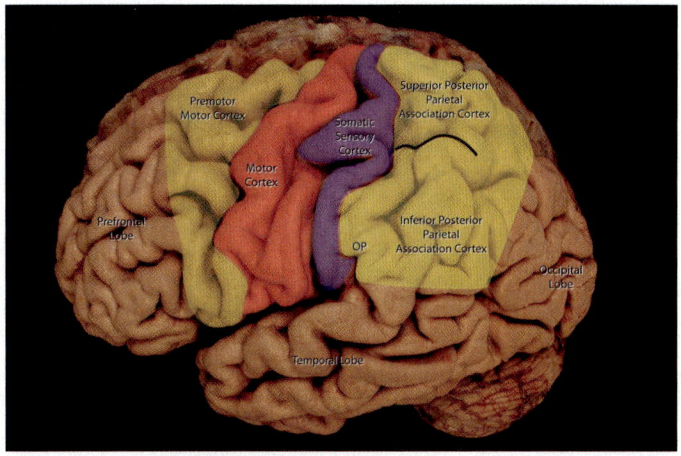

Figure 9.5. The location of the somatic sensory cortex on the convexity of the cerebral hemisphere. The primary somatic sensory cortex (areas 3, 1, and 2) is illustrated in *blue*; posterior to the primary somatic sensory area lies the large posterior parietal association cortex. It is divided into superior and inferior regions by the intraparietal sulcus (*black line*). (Used with permission from the Willard/Carreiro Collection, University of New England.)

- Three distinct regions are present in the primary somatic sensory cortex—from anterior to posterior across the postcentral gyrus these are areas 3, 1, and 2—with area 3 further subdivided into 3a and 3b.
- Each of these areas is further organized into a somatotopic map of the body including the hand, neurons in each of these areas receive a different type of input from the periphery.

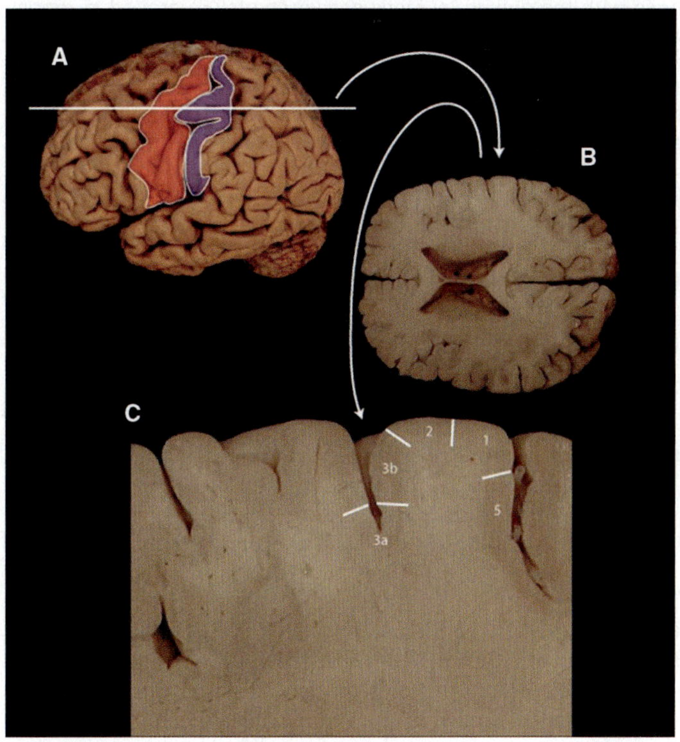

Figure 9.6. Primary somatic sensory cortex. A. A lateral view of the brain that demonstrates the primary somatic sensory cortex in *blue* and the primary motor cortex in *red*. The *white line* illustrates the plane of section for the cut demonstrated in (**B**). **C.** Magnification of the postcentral gyrus illustrating the approximate locations of areas 3a, 3b, 1, and 2. (Used with permission from the Willard/Carreiro collection, University of New England.)

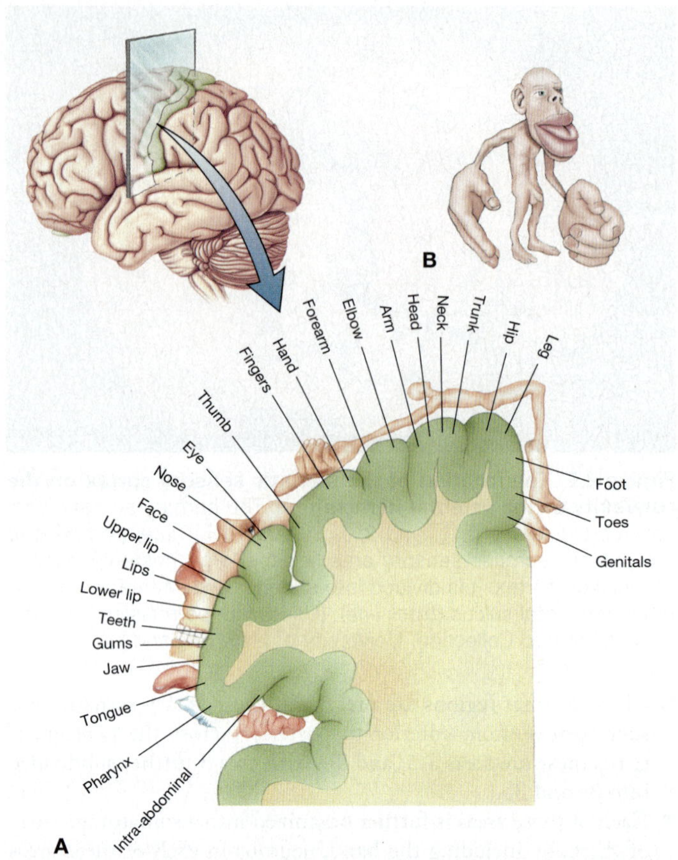

Figure 9.7. The somatotopic organization of the primary somatic sensory cortex. The *upper left corner* presents a lateral view of the brain with the primary somatic sensory cortex illustrated in *green*. **A.** A section parallel to the postcentral gyrus demonstrating the approximate location of the body map. **B.** A figurine demonstrating the distortion in the sensory map; areas of the body such as the hands and the mouth with increased density of sensory receptors receive a disproportionally large representation in the cortical sensory map. (Reprinted with permission from Bear MF, Connors BW, Paradiso MA. *Neuroscience: Exploring the Brain.* 2nd ed. Lippincott Williams & Wilkins; 2001.)

- This map is arranged by body segments proceeding from the face (trigeminal nerve) through the cervical segments, located laterally on the convexity of the cortex and eventually extending medially to the sacral segments, with the sacral segments located on the medial aspect of the cortex just above the corpus callosum.
- There is a disproportional representation of hands and mouth, which is reflective of increased density of sensory receptors; this arrangement translates into increased sensitivity and sensory discrimination for the hand and oral regions of the body (Fig. 9.7).

PRIMARY SOMATIC SENSORY CORTEX RECEIVES HIGH-FIDELITY SENSORY INFORMATION

The somatic sensory cortex is divided into a series of elongated stripes arranged parallel to the central sulcus; each stripe is designated an area and receives input from differing sensory receptor sources (see Fig. 9.6).[9]

- Area 3a is targeted by input from muscle stretch organs such as the muscle spindle apparatuses and the Golgi tendon organs.
- Area 3b receives input from group II slow and rapidly adapting superficial cutaneous receptors.
- Area 1 receives input from rapidly adapting receptors, both superficial and deep in the skin.
- Area 2 neurons are very complex; they receive input from joint receptors, periosteum, and deep fascias but respond more to movement than to individual stimuli.
- Area 5 active touch.

Unlike areas 3a, 3b, and 1 where digit representation is relatively discrete, digit representation is overlapping in area 2, thus creating a more complex pattern of neural activity.[10]

- The regions of the cerebrum posterior to the primary somatic sensory cortex are lacking in precise topography and the neuronal response properties are very complex.
- This arrangement is in keeping with regions involved in higher cortical functions.

REPRESENTATION OF BODY SCHEMA ON THE PRIMARY SOMATIC SENSORY CORTICAL SURFACE IS PLASTIC AND CAN BE INFLUENCED BY THE ENVIRONMENT

Often, the impression given in descriptions of cerebral sensory maps is that these systems are relatively hardwired from birth, but this is far from true.

- Cortical mapping is very dynamic and can expand in response to exercise and contract in response to nonuse.[11–13]
- Witness the expansion of the cortical maps for the digits seen in musicians such as a violinist; a similar expansion undoubtedly occurs in the cortex of a physician when training the hands in palpation and was also seen in the digital representation of experimental subjects with sight who were taught to read Braille.
- Conversely, anesthesia, immobilization, or removal of a digit results in a rapid loss of the cortical area representing the anesthetized or missing digit, and the newly available territory is claimed by surrounding digit representations. Such reallocation of territory occurs on a larger scale when an entire extremity is lost.
- Abuse of the somatic sensory system can also alter the cortical somatotopic maps.
- Studies that created chronic repetitive strain injury in primates have demonstrated a loss in precision of the somatic sensory cortical maps, suggesting that proper rehabilitation following such injury may involve reforming and refining these cerebral projection maps.[14]
- These studies suggest that learning any type of manual skill will alter the cortical surface map; thus, as students hone their palpatory skills, their cortical somatic sensory map is most likely responding by allocating increased area for the representation of digits.

THE INSULA CORTEX AS A SIGNIFICANT TARGET OF SOMATIC SENSORY INFORMATION

A component of the somatic sensory system input relays through the ventromedial nucleus of the thalamus and reaches the insular cortex.

- The ascending fibers in the anterolateral system target a ventromedial nucleus in the posterior thalamus, which, in turn send axons to the insular cortex.[15]
- Some of this input involves nociceptive information from high-threshold fibers however, also contained in this system is the input from small, unmyelinated, but low-threshold mechanoreceptors (C-tactile fibers) located in hairy skin.[16,17]

- Our perception of activity in C-tactile fiber component of the small-fiber system is related to our emotions, thus it is said to provide social or affective touch.[5]

Central Processing: Converting a Neural Code into Perception

PRIMARY SOMATIC SENSORY CORTEX IS INVOLVED IN A HIGH-SPEED FEEDBACK PATHWAY FOR PRIMARY MOTOR CORTEX

The dorsal column–medial lemniscus pathway is a high-speed pathway carrying touch and proprioceptive sensory information to the primary somatic sensory cortex.

- Intracortical connections map these data onto the primary motor cortex where it can act as a feedback system regulating discrete movements of the hands and feet.
- Motor cortex can control the actions of individual muscles in the distal extremities through the corticospinal tracts and their connections in the ventral horn of the spinal cord.[9]
- The osteopathic physician utilizes this somatomotor feedback system while learning to adjust the depth of palpation accomplished by the fingers.

INTEGRATION WITH SURROUNDING AREAS OF ASSOCIATION CORTEX PROVIDES THE COMPLEXITY OF THE SENSORY EXPERIENCE

Although the primary somatic sensory cortex has the tactile world mapped in a high-fidelity Cartesian system of intersecting body segments and receptor types as previously described, the individual does not feel specific receptor types or specific segmental boundaries; instead, what are felt are objects, textures, and shades of firmness, often colored by emotions; clearly, this cannot happen solely within the primary somatic sensory cortex.

- Rather, data from the Cartesian map on primary somatic sensory cortex are projected outward to surrounding cortical regions termed association cortex; typically, these are located in the posterior parietal cortex, the parietal operculum, and the inferior temporal cortex.
- The association cortices establish complex interconnections with numerous surrounding cortical regions as well as the primary somatic sensory areas.
- In addition, portions of these association cortices also map to other major sensory systems such as the visual system and auditory system; thus, neurons in these areas are often polysensory in nature.
- What emerges is a complex neuronal network involving high-fidelity data representation in the primary cortex, and numerous network activity nodes spread across the posterior association cortex of the brain.
- The sustainability of activity in these nodes depends on the power contained in the thalamocortical circuitry; each region of the node is mapped to a unique region in the thalamus in the underlying thalamic nuclei.
- Repeated thalamocortical oscillations augment the intracortical connections and contribute to network sustainability, thus fostering the formation of a memory.
- In addition to repetitive thalamic input, dense connections from the prefrontal cortex serve to augment and reinforce the activity occurring in this network.
- It is currently believed that sensations such as touch, sight, and audition as well as emotions are a result of the summated activity of this complex neuronal interaction.

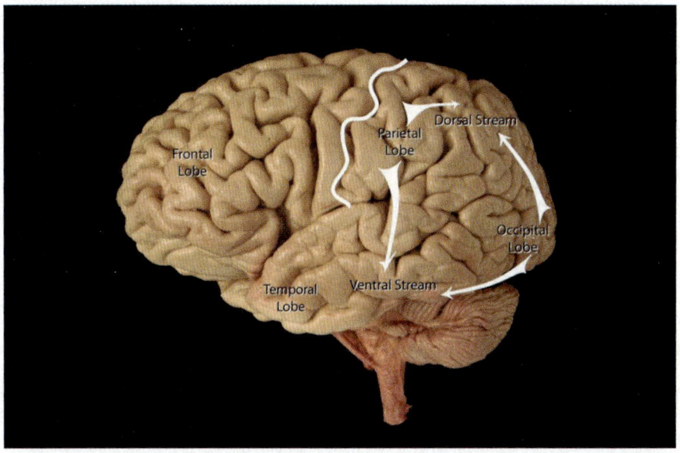

Figure 9.8. The information processing streams in the posterior association cortex. A dorsal stream arises from the visual and somatic sensory cortex termed the "where" pathway. A ventral stream arises from the visual and somatic sensory cortex and is termed the "what pathway." (Used with permission from the Willard/Carreiro Collection, University of New England.)

TWO MAJOR PROCESSING STREAMS THROUGH THE CEREBRAL CORTEX HELP INTEGRATE SOMATIC SENSORY INPUT WITH OTHER SENSORY SYSTEMS TO RENDER THE COMPLEX TEXTURES OF TOUCH

The somatic sensory parietal cortex has a dorsally directed projection that appears to participate in the "where pathway," while ventrally directed projections contribute to the "what pathway."[18] This cortical organization affords humans the ability to integrate visual and somesthetic senses into coherent images.

- The dorsal stream, or "*where pathway*," involves occipital and parietal cortical projections to the superior posterior parietal lobule (Fig. 9.8).
- This stream processes information involved with attention to, as well as location of, the stimulus.
- Activity in this information stream helps in fitting the stimulus into a three-dimensional map of extra-personal space.
- The ventral stream or "*what pathway*" involves occipital and parietal cortical projections to the inferior temporal lobe.
- This stream provides information useful in recognizing, cataloging, and naming a stimulus.

Central Processing: From Perception to Cognition

THE PREFRONTAL CORTEX IS INVOLVED IN REENFORCING THE NETWORK ESTABLISHED IN THE POSTERIOR ASSOCIATION CORTEX CONTRIBUTING TO THE FORMATION OF TACTILE MEMORIES

Dorsolateral prefrontal cortex is richly interconnected with the posterior parietal cortex and the inferior temporal cortex. These prefrontal cortex connections function to integrate information between the dorsal and the ventral information streams in the posterior association cortex.[19]

- Through this integration of multiple distributed cortical networks, the prefrontal cortex helps to create tactile memories.
- Thus, the prefrontal cortex uses the same information streams in parietal and temporal cortical areas that initially process tactile information to create the working memory of the experience.[20]
- Tactile memory is used to compare tissue feelings; from this memory, the student develops a sense of normal and abnormal tissue texture.

REPRESENTATION OF BODY SCHEMA IS COMPLEX AND OCCURS IN HIERARCHICAL PROCESS OF LAYERS

The thalamic projections to the primary somatic sensory cortex are highly organized by body segment and by receptor type; this represents the first level in a hierarchy of body maps.

- The topography of body representation in this portion of the somatic sensory cortex is distorted by sensitivity; areas of skin having the greatest sensitivity, such as the hand, have a disproportionally larger representation in the primary somatic sensory cortex; yet this distortion in sensory representation is not perceived by the mind.
- A second level of representation based on topography is necessary to accurately register stimulus location regardless of the density of innervations and tissue sensitivity.[21]
- This map must be updated temporally to account for age-related changes in body habits.
- Such updating occurs slowly; witness the clumsiness seen in pubescent individuals experiencing a "growth spurt."[22]
- A third level of representation is required to adjust the body map dependent on body posture.[12]
- Finally, an additional level of processing is postulated to involve the mapping of the conscious body image; evidence suggests that this process may be located in the posterior parietal cortex.[22]

Central Processing: From Perception to Emotion

INTEGRATION WITH LIMBIC AREAS OF THE CEREBRAL CORTEX PROVIDES THE EMOTIONAL CONTEXT OF THE SENSORY EXPERIENCE

The somatic sensory pathways discussed so far in this chapter all involve input from heavily myelinated systems with elaborate encapsulated sensory endings.

- An additional nonmyelinated sensory system arising from fibers with naked nerve endings also provides input through the thalamus to the cerebral cortex.
- This latter system targets a portion of the insular cortex in a region that represents an extension of the somatic sensory cortex around the operculum into the lateral fissure.
- This system, composed of C-tactile fiber input, is postulated to play a significant role in modulating the body's response to touch through its influence on the limbic-related regions of cortex.[6]
- This input also appears to influence the individual's emotional state through its projections to the insular cortex, orbital prefrontal gyrus, and the anterior cingulate gyrus.[23]
- These regions of the brain are associated with what many researchers have termed the limbic system—a loosely defined system that is believed to strongly regulate emotions.[24]

Activity in the orbital prefrontal cortex affects a strong reinforcement system, augmenting the individual's positive or negative impressions of the particular tactile stimuli.[25,26]

- Thus, tactile stimuli, using high-speed myelinated pathways, gain access to a discriminative and cognitive cortical system based in the somatic sensory cortex, allowing analytical evaluation of touch such as the osteopathic physician might use in physical and structural diagnosis.
- However, there is an additional component of the tactile information, which employs slower, unmyelinated or lightly myelinated C-tactile fibers that percolate through a strong cerebral emotional filter in the insular and orbitofrontal cortical regions and play a large role in the individual's final impression of touch.[27]
- Psychophysiologic studies support the notion that the feelings and emotions arising from touch may be a cross product of an interaction between the two systems.[5]

Numerous recent publications have explored the possible ramifications of the C-tactile afferent system in health, disease, and treatment.

- Pharmacologic activation of the C-fiber, low-threshold, mechanoreceptive neurons in mice (equivalent to the C-tactile fibers in humans) results in a preference for the region paired with the activation, suggesting a pleasurable experience.[28]
- The gentle stroking frequency for pleasant sensations in humans matches the optimum stroking frequency for activating C-tactile fibers.
- C-tactile afferent fibers appear to be related to the *affective touch* expressed in family and other intimate relationships.[29]
- Use of light touch, in the range that would activate C-tactile fibers has shown weak but encouraging results in the treatment of patients with atopic dermatitis or burns and scars and the treatment of patients undergoing conventional therapy for cancer.[30]
- It is well known that sensory systems and the surrounding environment play a significant role in the normal development of the brain.[31]
- A strong positive influence of affective touch, such as licking and grooming, on early brain and social development in rodents has been documented to modify DNA methylation and thus gene expression in the off-spring.[31]
- Finally, a possible role for touch-evoked activation of C-tactile fibers in osteopathic medicine has been explored using hospital-bound neonates[32]; a twice-a-week osteopathic treatment routine was effective in reducing the hospital stay of preterm infants.

SUMMARY

The processing of somatic sensory information, such as touch, in the nervous system is extremely complex.

- Initial input from skin is fractionated into several different channels that pass through the spinal cord and brainstem to target the thalamus.
- Thalamocortical systems map this information on to the cortical surface in a high-fidelity format.
- Extensive corticocortical connections integrate the somatic sensory input into diffuse neuronal networks incorporating both other sensory information plus past experiences ultimately facilitating the brain's ability to develop cognitive, reflexive, and emotional responses.
- These cortical networks are dynamic and can be modified and expanded by training or damaged by abusive or repetitive motion activities.
- Within the ascending pathways from skin to cerebral cortex, there are at least two somatic sensory systems involved in touch: one is high-speed network providing discriminative touch and localization, the other is a much slower system, supplying the emotional aspect of touch.
- As can be seen in this chapter, touch is one of the most basic forms of communication between human beings, it can be very informative as well as evoke significant emotions, the clinical value of touch cannot be overestimated.

REFERENCES

1. Russo V, Ottaviani C, Spitoni GF. Affective touch: a meta-analysis on sex differences. *Neurosci Biobehav Rev.* 2020;108:445–452.
2. Cascio CJ, Moore D, McGlone F. Social touch and human development. *Dev Cogn Neurosci.* 2019;35:5–11.
3. Muliira JK, Muliira RS. Teaching culturally appropriate therapeutic touch to nursing students in the Sultanate of Oman: reflections on observations and experiences with Muslim patients. *Holist Nurs Pract.* 2013;27:45–48.
4. Olausson H, Wessberg J, Morrison I, McGlone F, Vallbo A. The neurophysiology of unmyelinated tactile afferents. *Neurosci Biobehav Rev.* 2010; 34:185–191.
5. Vallbo AB. Pleasant touch. In: Squire LR, ed. *Encyclopedia of Neuroscience.* Academic Press; 2009:741–748.
6. McGlone F, Wessberg J, Olausson H. Discriminative and affective touch: sensing and feeling. *Neuron.* 2014;82:737–755.
7. Craig AD. *How Do You Feel? An Interoceptive Moment with Your Neurobiological Self.* Princeton University Press; 2015; 343.
8. Terrier LM, Hadjikhani N, Destrieux C. The trigeminal pathways. *J Neurol.* 2022;269:3443–3460.
9. Kandel ER, Schwartz JH, Jessell TM, Siegelbaum SA, Hudspeth AJ. *Principles of Neural Sciences.* McGraw-Hill Medical; 2013.
10. Young JP, Herath P, Eickhoff S, et al. Somatotopy and attentional modulation of the human parietal and opercular regions. *J Neurosci.* 2004;24:5391–5399.
11. Buonomano DV, Merzenich MM. Cortical plasticity: from synapses to maps. *Annu Rev Neurosci.* 1998;21:149–186.
12. Medina J, Coslett HB. From maps to form to space: touch and the body schema. *Neuropsychologia.* 2010;48:645–654.
13. Tommerdahl M, Favorov OV, Whitsel BL. Dynamic representations of the somatosensory cortex. *Neurosci Biobehav Rev.* 2010;34:160–170.
14. Byl NN, Merzenich MM, Jenkins WM. A primate genesis model of focal dystonia and repetitive strain injury: I. Learning-induced dedifferentiation of the representation of the hand in the primary somatosensory cortex in adult monkeys. *Neurology.* 1996;47:508–520.
15. Craig AD How do you feel? Interoception: the sense of the physiological condition of the body. *Nature Reviews Neuroscience.* 2002;3:655–666.
16. Bjornsdotter M, Loken L, Olausson H, Vallbo A, Wessberg J. Somatotopic organization of gentle touch processing in the posterior insular cortex. *J Neurosci.* 2009;29:9314–9320.
17. Olausson H, Lamarre Y, Backlund H, et al. Unmyelinated tactile afferents signal touch and project to insular cortex. *Nat Neurosci.* 2002;5:900–904.
18. Prather SC, Votaw JR, Sathian K. Task-specific recruitment of dorsal and ventral visual areas during tactile perception. *Neuropsychologia.* 2004;42:1079–1087.
19. Rao SC, Rainer G, Miller EK. Integration of what and where in the primate prefrontal cortex. *Science.* 1997;276:821–824.
20. Gallace A, Spence C. The cognitive and neural correlates of tactile memory. *Psychol Bull.* 2009;135:380–406.
21. Serino A, Haggard P. Touch and the body. *Neurosci Biobehav Rev.* 2010; 34:224–236.
22. Longo MR, Azañón E, Haggard P. More than skin deep: body representation beyond primary somatosensory cortex. *Neuropsychologia.* 2010;48: 655–668.
23. Olausson H, Lamarre Y, Backlund H, et al. Unmyelinated tactile afferents signal touch and project to insular cortex. *Nat Neurosci.* 2002b;5: 900–904.
24. Morgane PJ, Mokler DJ. The limbic brain: continuing resolution. *Neurosci Biobehav Rev.* 2006;30:119–125.
25. Rolls ET. The functions of the orbitofrontal cortex. *Brain Cogn.* 2004; 55:11–29.
26. Rolls ET. *Emotion Explained.* Oxford University Press; 2005.
27. Rolls ET. The affective and cognitive processing of touch, oral texture, and temperature in the brain. *Neurosci Biobehav Rev.* 2010;34:237–245.
28. Watkins RH. Slow touch in non-human species: translational research into C-tactile (CT) afferent system. *Curr Opin Behav Sci.* 2022;43:193–199.
29. Walker SC, Marshall A, Pawling R. Psychophysiology and motivated emotion: testing the affective touch hypothesis of C-tactile afferent function. *Curr Opin Behav Sci.* 2022;43:131–137.
30. Ferreira BR, Aguirre CC, Rapoport-Hubschman N, et al. The skin-brain connection and pleasant touch as supportive care for psychocutaneous disorders. *Skin Health Dis.* 2024;4:e310.
31. Kaffman A, Meaney MJ. Neurodevelopmental sequelae of postnatal maternal care in rodents: clinical and research implications of molecular insights. *J Child Psychol Psychiatry.* 2007;48:224–244.
32. McGlone F, Cerritelli F, Walker S, Esteves J. The role of gentle touch in perinatal osteopathic manual therapy. *Neurosci Biobehav Rev.* 2017;72: 1–9.

10 Musculoskeletal Vibration Physiology

MALINDA HANSEN

KEY CONCEPTS

- This chapter provides an overview of the current physiologic understanding of mechanoreceptors (specifically muscle spindles and Golgi tendon organs [GTOs]) and how the mechanical and proprioceptive feedback integrated within the muscle, spinal cord, and higher motor cortex centers in the brain can respond to a local muscle vibratory/percussive stimulus.
- Local muscle vibration (LMV) involves a very targeted application of vibration to a muscle–tendon unit by imposing repetitive rapid length changes which represents a potent stimulus for activating muscle spindles—mainly the Ia-afferents.
- LMV has gained popularity as a cost-effective treatment modality for a wide range of clinical conditions. There is growing evidence that it may improve muscle activation, improve peak muscle torque after anterior cruciate ligament reconstruction (ACLR), improve function and gait parameters in the elderly, assist in muscle recovery, improve sarcopenia, improve blood flow, assist in sexual dysfunction of patients with spinal cord lesions and improve arthrogenic inhibition.

INTRODUCTION

Local and whole-body vibration have been utilized since the 1880s when the French neurologist Jean-Martin Charcot noticed that patients suffering from Parkinson's experienced a reduction in their resting tremor after a train carriage ride or after horseback riding.[1] His understudy, Georges Gilles de la Tourette extended the observations and fashioned a helmet that vibrated the head on the premise that the brain responded directly to these pulsations.[2,3] In the past 15 years, local muscle vibration (LMV) has gained popularity as a cost-effective modality, with growing evidence that it has been shown to improve muscle activation, improve peak muscle torque after anterior cruciate ligament reconstruction (ACLR), improve function and gait parameters in the elderly, assist in muscle recovery, improve sarcopenia, improve blood flow, and improve arthrogenic inhibition.[1,4–11]

Vibrometry is an exceptionally potent stimulus on muscle spindles, the motor neuron pool in the spinal cord, the motor cortex of the brain, and subsequent corticospinal tracts. The contributions of proprioceptive feedback from muscle spindles and Golgi tendon organs (GTOs) have often been classically discussed in circuit elements like the stretch reflex,[12] reciprocal inhibition,[13] or the inverse myotatic reflex mechanism.[14] The musculoskeletal system and the myriad mechanical and proprioceptive pathways constitute incredibly complex circuitry that is difficult to understand as a set of independent modules. These feedback pathways function to promote and control interjoint coordination and regulate the mechanical properties of the limb that govern the response to any external perturbation[15] (Fig. 10.1).

The goal of this chapter is to review the current physiologic understanding of mechanoreceptors (specifically muscle spindles and GTOs) and how the mechanical and proprioceptive feedback is integrated within the muscle, spinal cord, and higher motor cortex centers in the brain in response to a local muscle vibratory/percussive stimulus.

PHYSIOLOGY OF MUSCLE SPINDLES

Mammalian muscle spindles are found in almost all skeletal muscles of mammals.[17] They lie in parallel with muscle fascicles, their ends attaching to the connective tissues within a muscle and responding to changes in length of the fascicle rather than length of the muscle–tendon unit.[15,18–20] Motor end plates are located at the ends of each intrafusal fiber and provide a mechanism for inducing the intrafusal fiber to shorten or place tension on the center of the muscle fiber. This increased tension triggers action potentials in the sensory endings (Ia) afferent fibers. The afferent Ia fibers project to the spinal cord, contacting motor neurons that project back to that muscle.

Each spindle consists of a bundle of intrafusal fibers enclosed within a fluid-filled capsule, all receiving terminations of the Ia afferent fiber.[17,21] The Ia are *exceptionally* sensitive to small length changes (~30 μm)[20] and have been shown be the most responsive receptors to muscle stretch, while type II fibers signals absolute muscle length[22–24] (Figs. 10.2 to 10.4).

The muscle spindle is the only sensory receptor known to possess its own motor supply, the γ-motoneuron. Stimulation of the γ-motoneuron produces no overt tension in the muscle, but does result in considerable excitation of the primary and secondary spindle afferents.[25] During extrafusal muscle contraction the muscle shortens, which unloads the spindle, thus reducing its spontaneous discharge. The γ-motoneuron is then co-activated, which restores the tension of the muscle spindle by contracting the polar ends of the intrafusal fibers. In this way, the γ-motoneurons control the sensitivity of the muscle spindle afferents as length detectors.[25]

Stretching a muscle leads to increased activity of the Ia afferents which then communicate with α-motoneurons (α-M) in the ventral horn of the spinal cord. This has been well defined as the monosynaptic stretch reflex. This synaptic connection between the Ia afferents and the motoneurons within the ventral horn is highly selective. The motoneurons supplying a particular muscle are grouped together in the spinal cord.[26] Higher neural centers at the cortical level are also activated in response to muscle stretching and voluntary contraction.[27] Overall, this leads to inhibition of the antagonistic muscle and contraction of the agonist muscle (Figs. 10.5 and 10.6).

PHYSIOLOGY OF GOLGI TENDON ORGANS

GTOs are found between muscle tissue, in the aponeuroses of origin and insertion, and in the musculotendinous junctions[28,29]

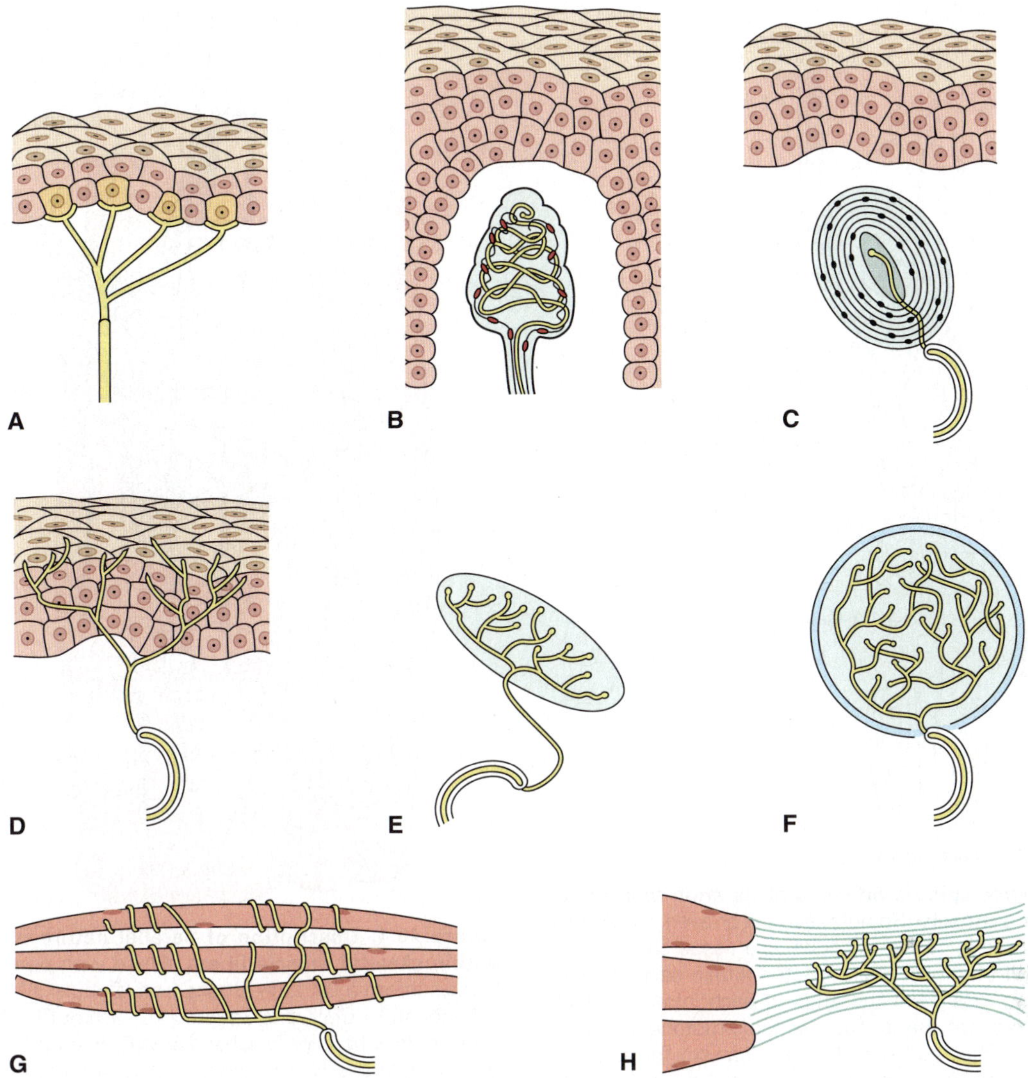

Figure 10.1. Various types of specialized receptors. A. Merkel disk—slowly adapting (points, edges, curvature, tactile stimulus). **B.** Meissner corpuscle—insensitive to static skin deformation; rapid adapting 20 to 40 Hz[2] (skin motion, low-frequency vibration). **C.** Pacinian corpuscle—rapid adapting (pressure, vibration) highest sensitivity at 100 to 300 Hz.[2,16] **D.** Free nerve endings, nociceptors, and thermoreceptors. **E.** Ruffini corpuscle—slowly adapting (stretch). **F.** Krause end bulb (cold receptor). **G.** Neuromuscular spindle. **H.** Golgi tendon organ. (Reprinted with permission from Gartner LP. *BRS Cell Biology and Histology*. 8th ed. Wolters Kluwer; 2019. Figure 19-1.)

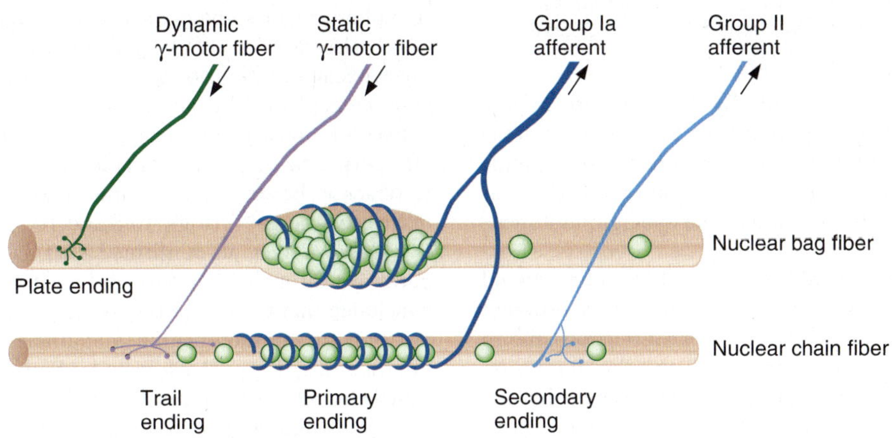

Figure 10.2. Organization of the muscle spindle. (Modified with permission from Matthews PBC. Muscle spindles and their motor control. *Physiol Rev*. 1964;44:219–288. Copyright © 1964 the American Physiological Society.)

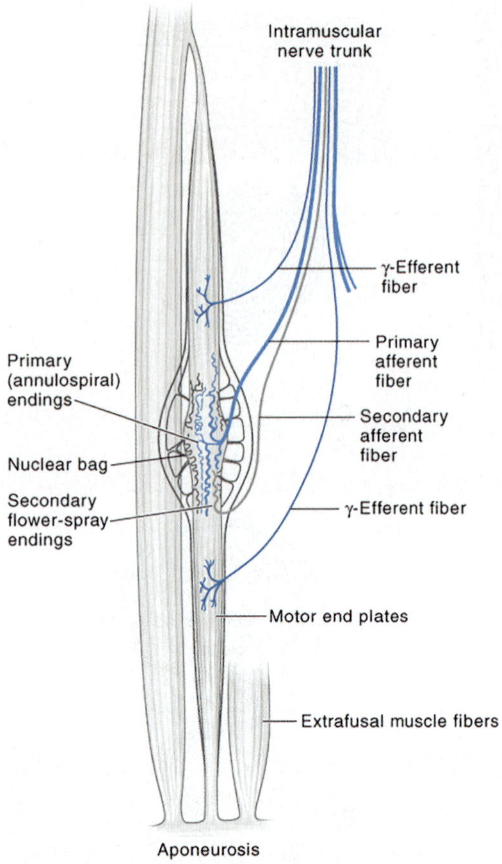

Figure 10.3. A muscle spindle attaches at its ends to connective tissues within a muscle. Sometimes two or even three spindles are interconnected in series. A connective tissue capsule surrounds three to eight intrafusal fibers located within each spindle. Motor end plates are located at the ends of each intrafusal fiber. These endplates represent the junction of the γ-motoneuron with the intrafusal muscle fiber and provide a mechanism for inducing the intrafusal fiber to shorten or place tension on the center of the muscle fiber. This increased tension triggers action potentials in the sensory endings—that is, annulospiral (primary) and flower spray (secondary) afferent fibers. These endings also can be activated by passively stretching the muscle and therefore the spindles. The afferent input projects to the spinal cord making synaptic contact on most motoneurons that project to that muscle. This input also projects to some motoneurons that innervate synergistic muscles, as well as to interneurons that inhibit motoneurons innervating antagonistic muscles. (Modified with permission from Ross MH, Romrell LJ, Kaye GI. *Histology: A Text and Atlas.* 3rd ed. Williams & Wilkins; 1995:227.)

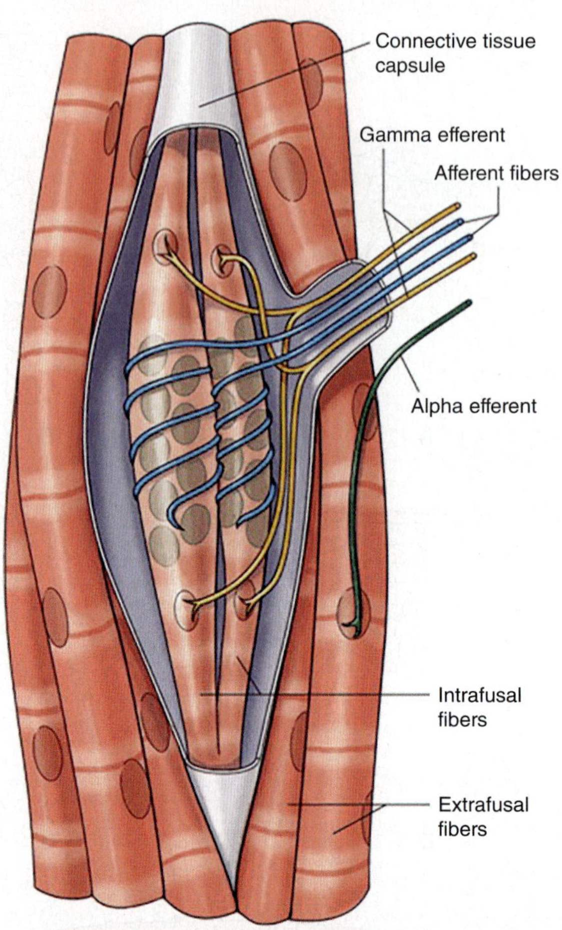

Figure 10.4. Description of parallel nature of muscle spindles within skeletal muscle fibers. (Used with permission of Taylor & Francis Informa UK Ltd—Books from Coburn JW, Beck TW, deVries HA, Housh TJ, Cochrane-Snyman KC, Schick EE. The neuromuscular system. In: Chandler TJ, Chandler WB, Bishop C, eds. *Conditioning for Strength and Human Performance.* 4th ed. Routledge; 2025:58. Figure 3.2; permission conveyed through Copyright Clearance Center, Inc.)

and are therefore connected mechanically in-series with muscle fascicles. They are most effectively stimulated by active contractile forces and can detect forces as low as those exerted by a single muscle fiber.[15,19,20,30] The Ib afferent fiber acts on motoneurons as an autogenic inhibition of homonymous and synergic motoneurons[14,20] (Fig. 10.7).

Inhibitory connections attributed to GTOs were found between muscles within synergistic groups that cross different combinations of joints.[18,31,32] During voluntary contractions, the Ib inhibition of these motoneurons is depressed, and this depression increases with the strength of the contraction. This shows that the gain of the Ib force feedback varies during active, voluntary contractions. Functionally, GTOs smooth the progression of muscular contraction and curb the recruitment of further motor units (MUs) based on the demand placed upon them.

INTEGRATED PHYSIOLOGY OF MUSCLE SPINDLES AND GTOs

Although muscle spindles respond during the relaxation (stretch) phase of the twitch and GTO afferents respond during the contraction phase, many spindles are active during a voluntary contraction which also recruits GTOs and motor axons.[25] The integration of mechanical and proprioceptive feedback described could in principle be explained by summation at the motoneuron membrane, between monosynaptic Ia input and multisynaptic input from Ib afferents. The segmental circuitry that mediates proprioceptive feedback is, however, more complex, as illustrated by a long series of investigations[33–35] (Figs. 10.8 and 10.9).

Jankowska et al. confirmed that Ia and Ib afferents share pathways through inhibitory and excitatory interneurons.[35] They concluded that the integration of length and force feedback occurs not only at the motoneuron membrane but also in the relevant interneurons; the feedback includes both inhibitory and excitatory signals from both receptors. It was shown further that interneurons receiving oligosynaptic excitation from group I afferents receive the feedback from several muscles. The convergence of these pathways further indicates that the regulation of limb mechanics is not localized to single muscles or groups of muscles.[15,18]

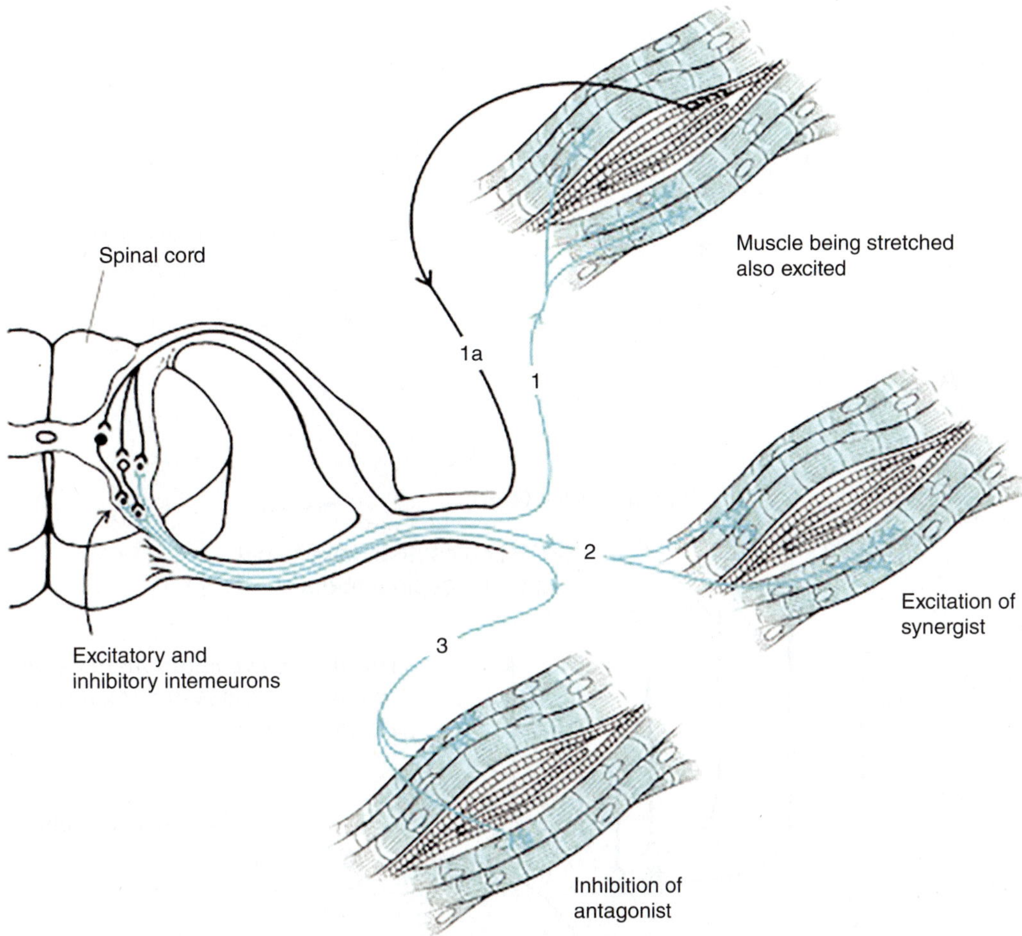

Figure 10.5. Order of spindle signaling to the motor neuron pool. (Reprinted with permission from Hamill J, Knutzen K, Derrick T. *Biomechanical Basis of Human Movement.* 5th ed. Wolters Kluwer; 2022:132. Figure 4-18.)

In spite of differences in morphology, location, measured input, effect and other characteristics, these two mechanoreceptors share the ability to respond to mechanical changes in their local muscle, initiate a rapid response in their respective sensory afferent fibers, and ultimately modulate local muscle tension through segmental and longer monosynaptic and polysynaptic reflexes (see Table 10.1).

VIBRATION PHYSIOLOGY

LMV involves a very targeted application of vibration to a muscle–tendon unit by imposing repetitive rapid length changes which represents a potent stimulus for activating muscle spindles—mainly the Ia-afferents.[36,37] The projection of the Ia excitatory afferents to both the spinal cord and higher cortical structures seems to allow the Ia afferents to facilitate neural activation during voluntary contractions.[24,38] These contractions can enhance the force of contraction with added excitatory input onto α-M.[25,39,40] When 100 to 105 Hz vibrations are applied to a belly or tendon of a muscle, Ia afferent activation elicit an excitatory input on the alpha motor neuron (α-M), resulting in a muscle-spindle–based polysynaptic spinal reflex called the tonic vibration reflex (TVR).[41]

TABLE 10.1

Differences between Muscle Spindles and GTOs

Muscle Spindles	Golgi Tendon Organs
In parallel with muscle fascicles	In series with muscle fascicles
Monitor stretch	Monitor contraction
Active with stretch	Active with active contraction
Quiet with active contraction	Quiet with stretch
Ia afferent fibers	Ib afferent fibers
Has inhibitory and excitatory signals	Has inhibitory and excitatory signals
Communicate with α-motoneurons	Inhibits homonymous and synergistic motoneurons

The TVR, a reflexive contraction following vibration stimulation, causes repetitive excitation of the primary Ia afferent neuron of the muscle spindle.[6,42,43] Eklund and Hagbarth found that vibration of a relaxed tendon caused a gradual increase in the agonist activity (contraction) and concomitant relaxation of the antagonist due to reciprocal inhibition.[43,44] Through the Ia afferents, the TVR has a very short-lived response. The increased potency of vibration to the tendon has been shown to have a greater effect on corticospinal excitability (CSE).[43,45–53] Any stimulation given for more than 10 seconds could reduce the firing frequency of the muscle spindle, resulting in reduced muscle activation.[54] This reduction in muscle activation is the nidus for neuromodulation.

While the TVR can increase muscle contraction during the first seconds of LMV, prolonged exposure leads to an impairment in neural drive evidenced by decreased α-M activity as the Ia input is dampened. This spinal neuron excitability of the α-M pool is

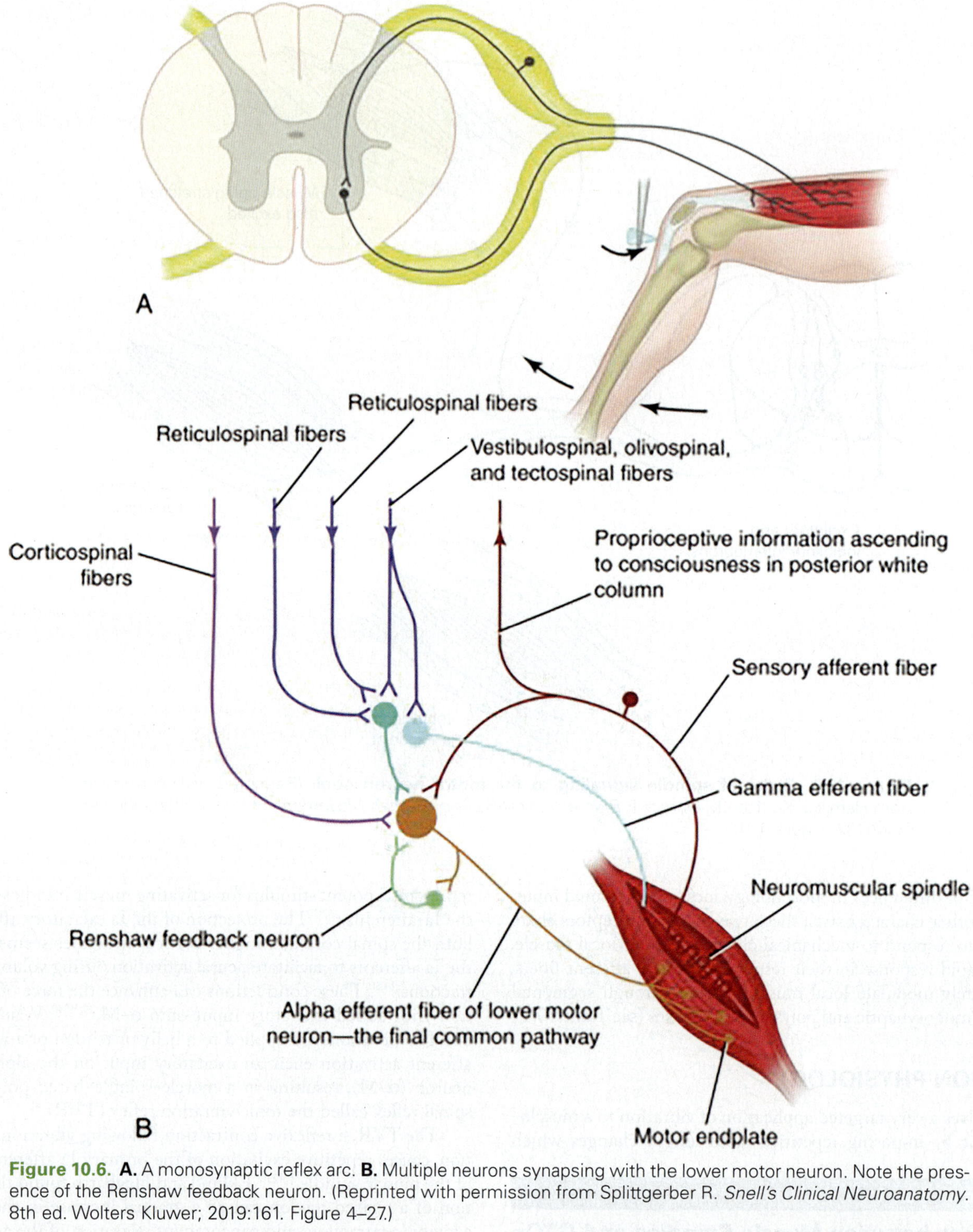

Figure 10.6. **A.** A monosynaptic reflex arc. **B.** Multiple neurons synapsing with the lower motor neuron. Note the presence of the Renshaw feedback neuron. (Reprinted with permission from Splittgerber R. *Snell's Clinical Neuroanatomy*. 8th ed. Wolters Kluwer; 2019:161. Figure 4–27.)

commonly evaluated through the Hoffman reflex (H-reflex), which has been likened to the stretch reflex albeit circumventing the muscle spindle.[36,37,44,55] The H-reflex depends on α-M excitability and the efficiency of the Ia-alpha pathway which in turn, depends on the level of presynaptic inhibition.[56] When vibration of Ia afferents activates Ia afferents and α-Ms, it is associated with a depression of the H-reflex during LMV application. This is called the vibration paradox as originally described by Desmedt and Godaux[49,57,58] (Table 10.2).

Type Ia afferents are particularly sensitive to low-amplitude, high-frequency mechanical vibrations (0.1 to 3 mm) and have a very potent stimulus response between 80 and 120 Hz of frequency.[23] Prolonged vibration (>10 minutes)[24,45,46,59–63] creates a reduction in the neural command, resulting in a decrease in force generation capacity. This has been demonstrated by a decrease in maximal EMG amplitude on the soleus, gastrocnemius, knee extensor, and first dorsal interossei.[38,64–67]

Because some of the effects of prolonged vibration exposure include muscle fatigue, reduction in muscle contraction force, reduction in motor firing rate, and delay in nerve conduction velocity,[36,68–71] this vibration paradox and its resultant effects on MU excitability creates a potential for neuromodulation, neural

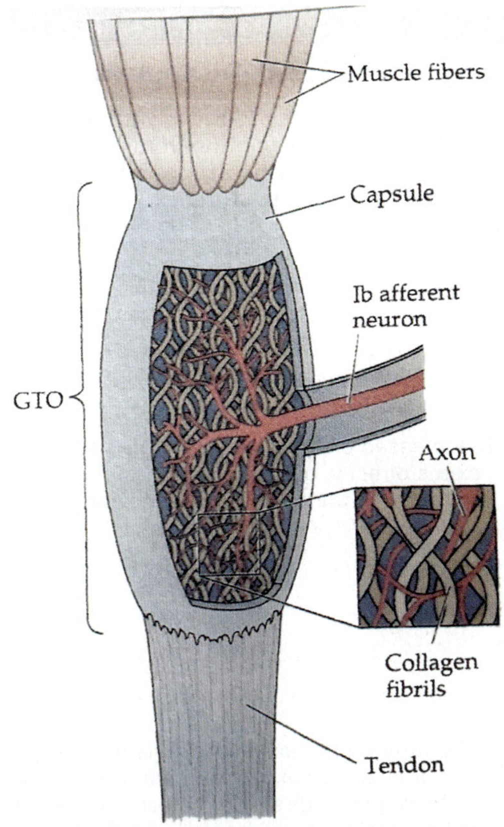

Figure 10.7. Golgi tendon organ anatomy. (From Purves D, Augustine GJ, Fitzpatrick D, et al., eds. *Neuroscience*. 3rd ed. Sinauer Associates; 2004:383. Figure 15.11. Reproduced with permission of the Oxford Publishing Limited through PLSclear.)

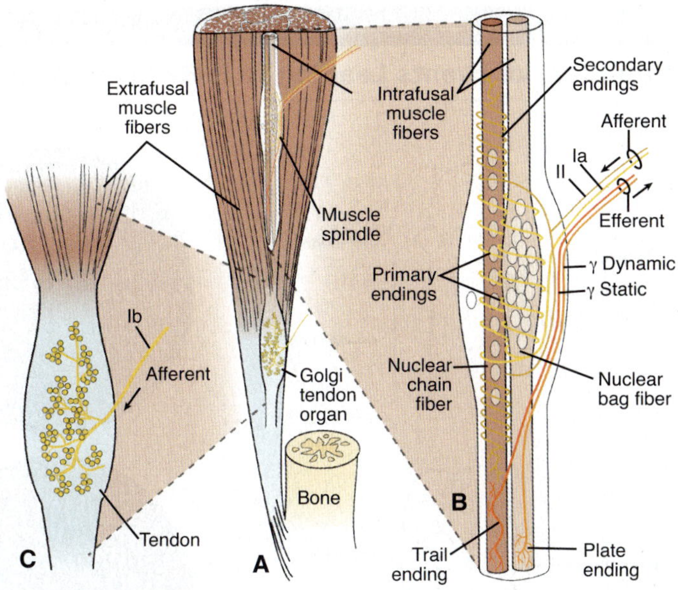

Figure 10.9. Muscle spindle location compared to Golgi tendon location. (Reprinted with permission from Rhoades RA, Bell DR. *Medical Physiology: Principles for Clinical Medicine*. 6th ed. Wolters Kluwer; 2023:96. Figure 5.4.)

patterning, and adaptation. According to Henneman's size principle, MUs are both recruited and inactivated in a linear fashion in which they were activated.[72] Theoretically then, if muscles are activated in a given pattern with concomitant LMV, the recruitment of MUs will follow Henneman's principle in establishing a particular motor pattern. As a result, prolonged LMV exposure at rest (i.e., 20 to 60 minutes) has been found to induce acute neural

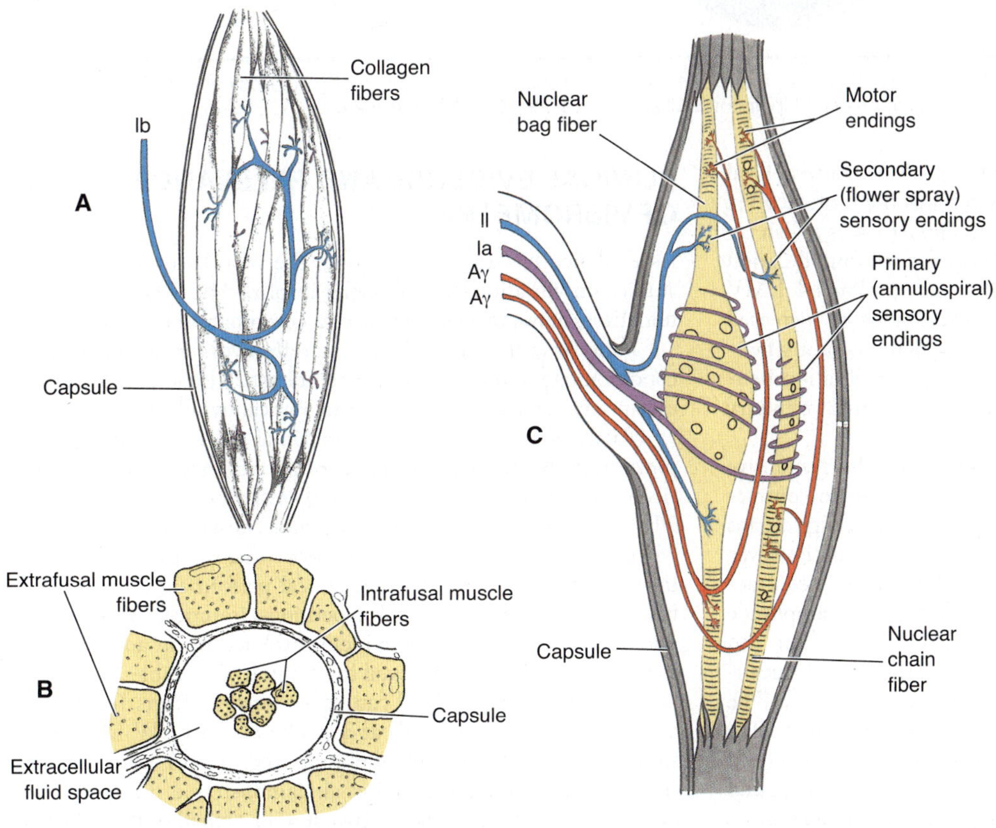

Figures 10.8. Specialized sensory endings in skeletal muscle and tendon. Sensory axons are shown in shades of *blue*, fusimotor axons in *red*, muscle fibers in *yellow*, and connective tissue in *black and gray*. **A.** A Golgi tendon organ. **B.** Neuromuscular spindle in transverse section. **C.** Innervation of a muscle spindle. (Reprinted with permission from Kiernan JA, Rajakumar N. *Barr's the Human Nervous System: An Anatomical Viewpoint*. 10th ed. Wolters Kluwer Lippincott Williams & Wilkins; 2014:39. Figure 3-4.)

TABLE 10.2

Summary of Events Leading to H-Reflex Appearance, M-Wave, and H-Reflex Disappearance

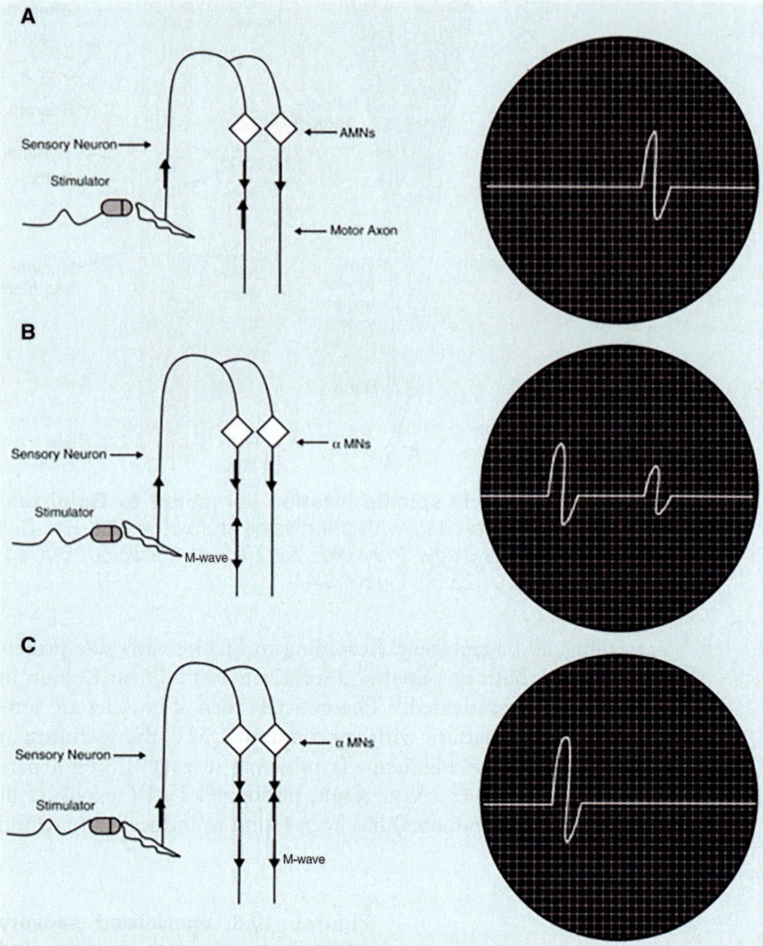

(A) Electrical stimulus selectively activates sensory 1a fibers, causing an orthodromic (traveling in a normal direction) response, firing alpha-motoneurons and the H-reflex.

(B) Increased electrical stimulus also activates motor axons directly, but not all antidromic firings will collide with the orthodromic activity. H-reflex and M-wave both present.

(C) Continuing to increase stimulation intensity will recruit all motor axons, and antidromic (traveling in the opposite direction) collision will eradicate all orthodromic activity created and the H-response will disappear.

Reprinted with permission from Padberg AM, Raynor BL, Thuet ED, Bolon SM. Spinal cord and nerve root monitoring. In: Bridwell KH, Dewald RL, eds. *The Textbook of Spinal Surgery*. 3rd ed. Wolters Kluwer Health/Lippincott Williams & Wilkins; 2011:17. Figure 2.6.

modulations in many populations. Essentially, LMV creates a local weakness or instability which ultimately reaches the motor cortex which subsequently recruits more motor units to reestablish an appropriate firing pattern. This is the basis for neuromodulation with LMV. Therefore, when chronically used, prolonged LMV exposure can in turn trigger long-term adaptations of increased strength.[61] There have been numerous studies demonstrating benefit of LMV (improving spasticity poststroke, rehabilitation benefits after ACLR, blood flow parameters, and maximal voluntary contractions [MVCs])[4,24,48,53,59,73–88] (Fig. 10.10).

The Golgi organ, or type Ib afferent fibers, are also responsive to LMV with the effect likely occurring during muscle contraction.[22,23,89,90] In the absence of any tonic activity, the Golgi organs are very difficult to activate with low-amplitude vibrations, however, their discharge frequency increases as a function of muscle contraction.[23] After about 20 minutes of a high-frequency, low-amplitude vibration, the Ia threshold rises above that of the Ib fibers for 5 to 15 minutes. A weak stimulation (1.2 to 1.3 times the group I threshold) applied to the motoneuron will only recruit Ib fibers.[20] The secondary endings do not respond much to frequencies beyond 10 to 20 Hz.[23] The GTOs level the progression of muscular contraction and control the recruitment of further MUs based on the demand placed upon them and thereby, aid in the fine-tuning of force production.

CLINICAL EVIDENCE AND RELEVANCE OF VIBROMETRY

As evidence has accumulated over the past 15 to 20 years from studies on vibration, the following information is taken from systematic reviews, meta-analyses, or a combination of both.

Fattorini et al. reviewed LMV as an effective intervention for motor conditioning for inducing persistent (at least 24 hours post-treatment) enhancements of conditional abilities in healthy subjects.

Analysis revealed that the maximal muscular strength and power were the more investigated motor parameters, and the quadriceps muscle was the most commonly tested muscle. In this regard, MVC increased up to 30% in young subjects, whereas, in the elderly, MVC improvements of 40% and 50% were reported, respectively, in males and females. The mechanical performance, evaluated by the number of the motor task repetitions, improved by about 40% and 30%, whereas the fatigue index, explored by an analysis of the myoelectrical signals, improved by about 20%[86] (Table 10.3).

The stimulus of LMV can cause lasting effects for 2 weeks and return to baseline levels at 3 weeks. Using LMV for one session of 30 minutes at low amplitude (0.05 to 0.1 mm) and high frequency (100 Hz), Marconi et al. demonstrated increased cortical excitability for 2 weeks.[91] Two studies extended the follow-up

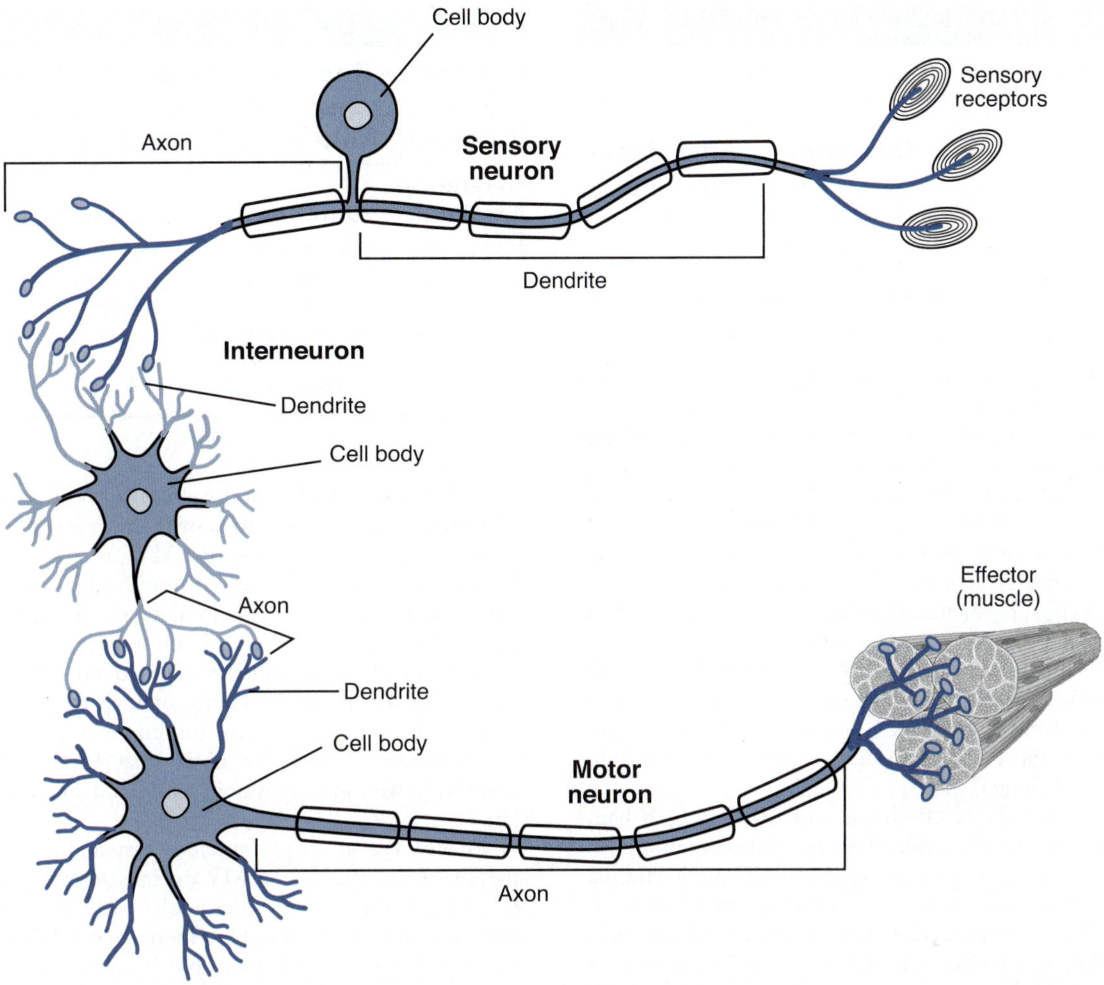

Figure 10.10. Motor, sensory, and interneurons. Sensory neurons arise from sensory endings and converge onto the spinal cord where they make connections with interneurons, motor neurons, and other sensory neurons. Lower motor neurons are shown originating from the spinal interneurons and exiting out of the spinal cord to the muscles. Not shown are upper motor neurons descending out of the brain and connecting to interneurons and lower motor neurons. (Reprinted with permission from Ives JC. Motor *Behavior: Connecting Mind and Body for Optimal Performance.* 2nd ed. Wolters Kluwer; 2019:26. Figure 2.2.)

and a surprisingly long persistence of focal vibration treatments (FVT) after-effects was evidenced by Brunetti's group, up to 240 and 360 days. This data seemed to be confirmed by other authors, who showed the absence of any significant decay of the after-effect throughout the follow-up period which ranged between 15 days and 16 weeks[86] (Table 10.4).

Many studies have examined the clinical benefits of poststroke use of vibration for improved function[84] reviewed 22 studies evaluating LMV for stroke rehabilitation, specifically, protocols that have been tested.

The most frequently used combination was 100 Hz and 0.2 to 0.5 mm, followed by 120 Hz and 0.01 mm and 99.5 Hz and 1 mm. The focal muscle vibration (FMV) frequency ranged from 30 to 300 Hz and the amplitude ranged from 0.01 to 2 mm. The frequency of treatments ranged from a single session to two, three, or five times per week. The duration of the treatment protocol was 1 day, 3 days, 2 weeks, 4 weeks, 6 weeks, or 8 weeks. The vibration durations were 14 to 20 seconds, 5 minutes, 30 minutes, or 60 minutes. One study did not specify the duration of the vibration. Instead, the participants received repeated FMV for 35 seconds after a 15-second rest until they felt better (Tables 10.5 and 10.6).

The review by Wang et al. agreed with the findings that FMV therapy may reduce spasticity in both upper and lower extremities and improve function in individuals with stroke. The positive effect

TABLE 10.3

Motor Coordination[86]

Frequency/Amplitude	Duration	Outcomes	After-Effects
100 Hz/0.1–2 mm	Single session 10 consecutive minutes repeated 3×/day for 3 days 15, 30, or 60 min once daily 3×/wk	↑ Max voluntary contraction ↑ motor task repetitions ↑ fatigue index	15 days–16 wk Seem to favor the shorter, more concentrated protocol

TABLE 10.4

Sarcopenia/Aging[9]

Frequency/ Amplitude	Duration	Outcomes	After-Effects
300 Hz/amp not given	15 min, 1–3×/wk Duration 8–12 wk	Lower limb muscle strength ↑ by 43%	Maintained for 12 wk

of FMV in inhibiting hemiplegic upper and lower extremity spasticity in patients with strokes was confirmed with other reviews.[84]

The incidence of anterior cruciate ligament (ACL) injuries among sport-playing youth athletes has been steadily increasing, particularly among female athletes, with the most recent estimate at over 400 tears per 100,000 persons in adolescents.[93]

Maghbouli et al. performed a systematic review and meta-analysis of the effectiveness of LMV on postural control in individuals with ACL reconstruction (ACLR). This meta-analysis evaluated a total of 407 patients. The sample size for each study ranged from 20 to 56. Overall, 175 (42.7%) of studied patients were women, with the mean age ranging from 20 to 31 years for all participants.[10] A recent study from Coulondre et al. also demonstrated efficacy in the early postoperative period of ACLR for quadriceps strengthening.[61]

The pooled data indicate effectiveness of LMV in both hamstring and quadriceps muscles strengthening, with more prominent results for the hamstring. The hamstring can limit anterior translation and rotation of the tibia on the femur, which compensates for the function of the ACL. Therefore, these two muscle imbalances lead to more functional disability following ACL injury and reconstruction. This analysis indicates the effectiveness of LMV, especially LMV type with vibration frequency higher than 100 Hz, for rehabilitation of patients who have undergone ACLR. Although improvement in peak torque of hamstring and quadriceps muscles was seen, there was no significant improvement in postural control, especially closed eye, in comparison with conventional rehabilitation[10] (Table 10.7).

There have also been studies evaluating the effects of LMV in healthy adults. Various researchers have examined the effects of vibration applied locally to the target muscle and found increased muscle performance. Couto et al. reported increased muscle performance following the application of local vibration (8 Hz and 26 Hz) directed to the target muscle.[94,95] Pamukoff et al. reported significant effects of 30 Hz of LMV on quadriceps muscle activation.[48–50]

TABLE 10.5

Stroke Upper Limb[53] on Contracting Wrist Flexor

Frequency/ Amplitude	Duration	Outcomes	After-Effects
100 Hz/0.05–1 mm	30 min		↑ Corticospinal excitability ×2 wk; returned to baseline after 3 wk Improved/faster movements in a reaching task

TABLE 10.6

Poststroke Recovery[92] Upper Limb Flexor Muscles, Lower Limb Extensor Muscles. Both with Mild Tonic Contraction

Frequency/ Amplitude	Duration	Outcomes	After-Effects
70–120 Hz/ 10 μ–1 mm	10–30 min in repetitive sessions Sessions varied from 3–20 sessions	Various functional tests	N/A

Alghadir et al. looked at the effect of LMV on muscle strength in healthy adults.[54] The results of their systematic review provide evidence that the application of LMV can affect muscle strength. As most of the studies involved untrained or moderately trained healthy adults, the effect of local vibration on muscle strength appears to be advantageous for these populations. However, an examination of the included studies found a lack of robustness and consistency in methodology, making it difficult to establish an optimal vibration protocol for improving muscle strength in healthy adults. It was also noted that LMV enhances muscle strength, power, joint position sense, and blood flow under the skin.[54]

Finally, Wu et al. performed a systematic review and meta-analysis of the effects of LMV on muscle mass, muscle strength and physical function in older adults with sarcopenia. Of the six available studies to review, they found that LMV may not have a notable effect on muscle mass, but it has a significant impact on muscle strength and physical function in older adults with sarcopenia[9] (Table 10.8).

The physiologic pathways of local muscle vibration have been explored, and continue to be elucidated. In 1996, Dr. Frost proposed a theory of "minimum effective strain" which morphed into the mechanostat theory that describes the adaptation of bones to their mechanical environment by a simple feedback loop.[96–102] The essence of the theory is a threshold for which vibration is essential for bone structure to be maintained as well as a threshold for which vibration would start to break bone down.[96–103] Elements of vibration are part of everyday activities such as walking, riding a bike, driving a car, flying on an airplane, etc. and muscle dampens the everyday vibration of walking, running, etc. Once consistent parameters of frequency and amplitude are found, LMV has the potential to be a potent clinical tool in neuromuscular reeducation.

TABLE 10.7

ACLR Systematic Review and Meta-Analysis of Clinical Trials[10]

Frequency/ Amplitude	Duration	Outcomes	After-Effects
≥100 Hz/ 2–9 mm Ranged b/t 10 Hz and 300 Hz	4–12 wk 3–24 sessions Up to 16 repetitions for up to 60 sec	↑ peak torque of quadriceps and hamstrings ↑ muscle strength in quadriceps and hamstrings	N/A

TABLE 10.8

Muscle Strength Healthy Adults[53]

Frequency/ Amplitude	Duration	Outcomes	After-Effects
8–38 Hz/ 2.5–6 mm	Ranges: 5–6-min single session; 10-min single session; 20-min single session; 72 sec, 4 wk	↑ muscle strength; ↑ motor control	N/A

SUMMARY

The use of vibration/percussion exogenously has been shown to have significant potential for clinical benefit. Data is still lacking, however, for the amplitude and frequency of dosage for specific conditions. What is becoming clear, however, is the neurophysiology of how the human neuromusculoskeletal system responds and how clinical parameters are beginning to take shape. Vibration/percussion is quickly becoming a tool that has potential to positively influence structure and function.

REFERENCES

1. Charcot JM. Vibratory therapeutics.–The application of rapid and continuous vibrations to the treatment of certain diseases of the nervous system. 1892. *J Nerv Ment Dis.* 2011;199(11):821–827.
2. Saggini R. *The Mechanical Vibration: Therapeutic Effects and Applications.* Bentham Science Publishers; 2017.
3. Anonymous. Vibratory therapeutics. *Sci Am.* 1892;67(17):265.
4. Alashram AR, Padua E, Romagnoli C, Annino G. Effectiveness of focal muscle vibration on hemiplegic upper extremity spasticity in individuals with stroke: a systematic review. *NeuroRehabilitation.* 2019;45(4):471–481.
5. Zaidell LN, Mileva KN, Sumners DP, Bowtell JL. Experimental evidence of the tonic vibration reflex during whole-body vibration of the loaded and unloaded leg. *PLoS One.* 2013;8(12):e85247.
6. Pujari AN, Neilson RD, Cardinale M. Effects of different vibration frequencies, amplitudes and contraction levels on lower limb muscles during graded isometric contractions superimposed on whole body vibration stimulation. *J Rehabil Assist Technol Eng.* 2019;6:2055668319827466.
7. Blackburn JT, Pamukoff DN, Sakr M, Vaughan AJ, Berkoff DJ. Whole body and local muscle vibration reduce artificially induced quadriceps arthrogenic inhibition. *Arch Phys Med Rehabil.* 2014;95(11):2021–2028.
8. Cidem M, Karacan I, Cakar HI, et al. Vibration parameters affecting vibration-induced reflex muscle activity. *Somatosens Mot Res.* 2017;34(1):47–51.
9. Wu S, Ning HT, Xiao SM, et al. Effects of vibration therapy on muscle mass, muscle strength and physical function in older adults with sarcopenia: a systematic review and meta-analysis. *Eur Rev Aging Phys Act.* 2020;17:14.
10. Maghbouli N, Khodadost M, Pourhassan S. The effectiveness of vibration therapy for muscle peak torque and postural control in individuals with anterior cruciate ligament reconstruction: a systematic review and meta-analysis of clinical trials. *J Orthop Traumatol.* 2021;22(1):28.
11. Pietrangelo T, Mancinelli R, Toniolo L, et al. Effects of local vibrations on skeletal muscle trophism in elderly people: mechanical, cellular, and molecular events. *Int J Mol Med.* 2009;24(4):503–512.
12. Houk JC. Regulation of stiffness by skeletomotor reflexes. *Annu Rev Physiol.* 1979;41:99–114.
13. Lloyd DP. Integrative pattern of excitation and inhibition in two-neuron reflex arcs. *J Neurophysiol.* 1946;9(6):439–444.
14. Laporte Y, Lloyd DP. Nature and significance of the reflex connections established by large afferent fibers of muscular origin. *Am J Physiol.* 1952;169(3):609–621.
15. Nichols TR. Distributed force feedback in the spinal cord and the regulation of limb mechanics. *J Neurophysiol.* 2018;119(3):1186–1200.
16. Johnson KO. The roles and functions of cutaneous mechanoreceptors. *Curr Opin Neurobiol.* 2001;11(4):455–461.
17. Barker D. The morphology of muscle receptors. In: *Muscle Receptors.* Springer; 1974:1–190.
18. Nichols TR. Receptor mechanisms underlying heterogenic reflexes among the triceps surae muscles of the cat. *J Neurophysiol.* 1999;81(2):467–478.
19. Blecher R, Heinemann-Yerushalmi L, Assaraf E, et al. New functions for the proprioceptive system in skeletal biology. *Philos Trans R Soc Lond B Biol Sci.* 2018;373(1759):20170327.
20. Jami L. Golgi tendon organs in mammalian skeletal muscle: functional properties and central actions. *Physiol Rev.* 1992;72(3):623–666.
21. Arthur C. Guyton JEH, Hall M. *Guyton and Hall Textbook of Medical Physiology.* 14th ed. Elsevier; 2021.
22. Fallon JB, Macefield VG. Vibration sensitivity of human muscle spindles and Golgi tendon organs. *Muscle Nerve.* 2007;36(1):21–29.
23. Roll JP, Vedel JP, Ribot E. Alteration of proprioceptive messages induced by tendon vibration in man: a microneurographic study. *Exp Brain Res.* 1989;76(1):213–222.
24. Souron R, Besson T, Millet GY, Lapole T. Acute and chronic neuromuscular adaptations to local vibration training. *Eur J Appl Physiol.* 2017;117(10):1939–1964.
25. Macefield VG, Knellwolf TP. Functional properties of human muscle spindles. *J Neurophysiol.* 2018;120(2):452–467.
26. Chen HH, Hippenmeyer S, Arber S, Frank E. Development of the monosynaptic stretch reflex circuit. *Curr Opin Neurobiol.* 2003;13(1):96–102.
27. Goodwin GM, McCloskey DI, Matthews PB. Proprioceptive illusions induced by muscle vibration: contribution by muscle spindles to perception? *Science.* 1972;175(4028):1382–1384.
28. Golgi C. Golgi C. Sui nervi dei tendini dell'Uomo et di altri vertebrati e di un nuovo organo nervoso terminale musculo-tendineo. *Mem R Acad Sci Torino.* 1880;(32):359–385.
29. Golgi C. Intorno alla distribuzione e terminazione dei nervi nei tendini dell'uomo e di altri vertebrati. *Rend R 1st Lomb Sci Lett.* 1878;(B11):445–453.
30. Houk J, Henneman E. Responses of Golgi tendon organs to active contractions of the soleus muscle of the cat. *J Neurophysiol.* 1967;30(3):466–481.
31. Eccles JC, Eccles RM, Lundberg A. The convergence of monosynaptic excitatory afferents on to many different species of alpha motoneurones. *J Physiol.* 1957;137(1):22–50.
32. Eccles JC, Eccles RM, Lundberg A. Synaptic actions on motoneurones caused by impulses in Golgi tendon organ afferents. *J Physiol.* 1957;138(2):227–252.
33. Jankowska E, McCrea D, Mackel R. Oligosynaptic excitation of motoneurones by impulses in group Ia muscle spindle afferents in the cat. *J Physiol.* 1981;316:411–425.
34. Jankowska E, Hammar I. Interactions between spinal interneurons and ventral spinocerebellar tract neurons. *J Physiol.* 2013;591(22):5445–5451.
35. Jankowska E, McCrea DA. Shared reflex pathways from Ib tendon organ afferents and Ia muscle spindle afferents in the cat. *J Physiol.* 1983;338:99–111.
36. Škarabot J, Mesquita RNO, Ansdell P. Elucidating the neurophysiology of local vibration: changes in neuromodulatory drive rather than presynaptic inhibition? *J Physiol.* 2019;597(24):5753–5755.
37. Cakar HI, Cidem M, Kara S, Karacan I. Vibration paradox and H-reflex suppression: is H-reflex suppression results from distorting effect of vibration? *J Musculoskelet Neuronal Interact.* 2014;14(3):318–324.
38. Mosier EM, Herda TJ, Trevino MA, Miller JD. The influence of prolonged vibration on motor unit behavior. *Muscle Nerve.* 2017;55(4):500–507.
39. Gandevia SC. Neural control in human muscle fatigue: changes in muscle afferents, motoneurones and motor cortical drive [corrected]. *Acta Physiol Scand.* 1998;162(3):275–283.

40. Ellaway PH, Taylor A, Durbaba R. Muscle spindle and fusimotor activity in locomotion. *J Anat.* 2015;227(2):157–166.
41. Kalaoglu E, Bucak OF, Kokce M, et al. Whole body vibration activates the tonic vibration reflex during voluntary contraction. *J Phys Ther Sci.* 2023; 35(6):408–413.
42. Guang H, Ji L, Shi Y. Focal vibration stretches muscle fibers by producing muscle waves. *IEEE Trans Neural Syst Rehabil Eng.* 2018;26(4):839–846.
43. Eklund G, Hagbarth KE. Normal variability of tonic vibration reflexes in man. *Exp Neurol.* 1966;16(1):80–92.
44. Eklund G, Hagbarth KE. Motor effects of vibratory muscle stimuli in man. *Electroencephalogr Clin Neurophysiol.* 1966;19:619.
45. Farabet A, Souron R, Millet GY, Lapole T. Changes in tibialis anterior corticospinal properties after acute prolonged muscle vibration. *Eur J Appl Physiol.* 2016;116(6):1197–1205.
46. Souron R, Oriol M, Millet GY, Lapole T. Intermediate muscle length and tendon vibration optimize corticospinal excitability during knee extensors local vibration. *Front Physiol.* 2018;9:1266.
47. Costantino C, Galuppo L, Romiti D. Short-term effect of local muscle vibration treatment versus sham therapy on upper limb in chronic post-stroke patients: a randomized controlled trial. *Eur J Phys Rehabil Med.* 2017;53(1):32–40.
48. Pamukoff DN, Ryan ED, Blackburn JT. The acute effects of local muscle vibration frequency on peak torque, rate of torque development, and EMG activity. *J Electromyogr Kinesiol.* 2014;24(6):888–894.
49. Pamukoff DN, Pietrosimone B, Lewek MD, et al. Immediate effect of vibratory stimuli on quadriceps function in healthy adults. *Muscle Nerve.* 2016;54(3):469–478.
50. Pamukoff DN, Pietrosimone B, Lewek MD, et al. Whole-body and local muscle vibration immediately improve quadriceps function in individuals with anterior cruciate ligament reconstruction. *Arch Phys Med Rehabil.* 2016;97(7):1121–1129.
51. Kossev A, Siggelkow S, Schubert M, Wohlfarth K, Dengler R. Muscle vibration: different effects on transcranial magnetic and electrical stimulation. *Muscle Nerve.* 1999;22(7):946–948.
52. Poenaru D, Cinteza D, Petrusca I, Cioc L, Dumitrascu D. Local application of vibration in motor rehabilitation – scientific and practical considerations. *Maedica (Bucur).* 2016;11(3):227–231.
53. Mortaza N, Abou-Setta AM, Zarychanski R, Loewen H, Rabbani R, Glazebrook CM. Upper limb tendon/muscle vibration in persons with subacute and chronic stroke: a systematic review and meta-analysis. *Eur J Phys Rehabil Med.* 2019;55(5):558–569.
54. Alghadir AH, Anwer S, Zafar H, Iqbal ZA. Effect of localised vibration on muscle strength in healthy adults: a systematic review. *Physiotherapy.* 2018;104(1):18–24.
55. McNeil CJ, Butler JE, Taylor JL, Gandevia SC. Testing the excitability of human motoneurons. *Front Hum Neurosci.* 2013;7:152.
56. Mazevet D, Meunier S, Pradat-Diehl P, Marchand-Pauvert V, Pierrot-Deseilligny E. Changes in propriospinally mediated excitation of upper limb motoneurons in stroke patients. *Brain.* 2003;126(Pt 4):988–1000.
57. Desmedt JE, Godaux E. Mechanism of the vibration paradox: excitatory and inhibitory effects of tendon vibration on single soleus muscle motor units in man. *J Physiol.* 1978;285:197–207.
58. Desmedt JE. Mechanisms of vibration-induced inhibition or potentiation: tonic vibration reflex and vibration paradox in man. *Adv Neurol.* 1983;39:671–683.
59. Souron R, Zambelli A, Espeit L, Besson T, Cochrane DJ, Lapole T. Active versus local vibration warm-up effects on knee extensors stiffness and neuromuscular performance of healthy young males. *J Sci Med Sport.* 2019;22(2):206–211.
60. Souron R, Farabet A, Féasson L, Belli A, Millet GY, Lapole T. Eight weeks of local vibration training increases dorsiflexor muscle cortical voluntary activation. *J Appl Physiol (1985).* 2017;122(6):1504–1515.
61. Coulondre C, Souron R, Rambaud A, et al. Local vibration training improves the recovery of quadriceps strength in early rehabilitation after anterior cruciate ligament reconstruction: a feasibility randomised controlled trial. *Ann Phys Rehabil Med.* 2022;65:101441.
62. Souron R, Besson T, Lapole T, Millet GY. Neural adaptations in quadriceps muscle after 4 weeks of local vibration training in young versus older subjects. *Appl Physiol Nutr Metab.* 2018;43(5):427–436.
63. Souron R, Baudry S, Millet GY, Lapole T. Vibration-induced depression in spinal loop excitability revisited. *J Physiol.* 2019;597(21):5179–5193.
64. Yoshitake Y, Shinohara M, Kouzaki M, Fukunaga T. Fluctuations in plantar flexion force are reduced after prolonged tendon vibration. *J Appl Physiol (1985).* 2004;97(6):2090–2097.
65. Ushiyama J, Masani K, Kouzaki M, Kanehisa H, Fukunaga T. Difference in aftereffects following prolonged Achilles tendon vibration on muscle activity during maximal voluntary contraction among plantar flexor synergists. *J Appl Physiol (1985).* 2005;98(4):1427–1433.
66. Shinohara M, Moritz CT, Pascoe MA, Enoka RM. Prolonged muscle vibration increases stretch reflex amplitude, motor unit discharge rate, and force fluctuations in a hand muscle. *J Appl Physiol (1985).* 2005; 99(5):1835–1842.
67. Jackson SW, Turner DL. Prolonged muscle vibration reduces maximal voluntary knee extension performance in both the ipsilateral and the contralateral limb in man. *Eur J Appl Physiol.* 2003;88(4–5):380–386.
68. Adamo DE, Martin BJ, Johnson PW. Vibration-induced muscle fatigue, a possible contribution to musculoskeletal injury. *Eur J Appl Physiol.* 2002; 88(1–2):134–140.
69. Necking LE, Lundborg G, Friden J. Hand muscle weakness in long-term vibration exposure. *J Hand Surg Br.* 2002;27(6):520–525.
70. Bongiovanni LG, Hagbarth KE, Stjernberg L. Prolonged muscle vibration reducing motor output in maximal voluntary contractions in man. *J Physiol.* 1990;423:15–26.
71. Dupuis H, Jansen G. Immediate effects of vibration transmitted to the hand. In: Bianchi G, Frolov KV, Olędzki A, eds. *Studies in Environmental Science.* Vol 13. Elsevier; 1981:76–86.
72. Henneman E, Clamann HP, Gillies JD, Skinner RD. Rank order of motoneurons within a pool: law of combination. *J Neurophysiol.* 1974; 37(6):1338–1349.
73. Cochrane DJ. The acute effect of direct vibration on muscular power performance in master athletes. *Int J Sports Med.* 2016;37(2):144–148.
74. Pournot H, Tindel J, Testa R, Mathevon L, Lapole T. The acute effect of local vibration as a recovery modality from exercise-induced increased muscle stiffness. *J Sports Sci Med.* 2016;15(1):142–147.
75. Peer KS, Barkley JE, Knapp DM. The acute effects of local vibration therapy on ankle sprain and hamstring strain injuries. *Phys Sportsmed.* 2009;37(4):31–38.
76. Kent P, Williams G, Kester RC. Altered sensitivity of digital blood flow to acute vibration in patients with vasospastic disease. *J Biomed Eng.* 1991;13(3):269–271.
77. Bovenzi M, Lindsell CJ, Griffin MJ. Duration of acute exposures to vibration and finger circulation. *Scand J Work Environ Health.* 1998;24(2): 130–137.
78. Liao F, Zhang K, Zhou L, Chen Y, Elliott J, Jan YK. Effect of different local vibration frequencies on the multiscale regularity of plantar skin blood flow. *Entropy (Basel).* 2020;22(11):1288.
79. Zhu T, Wang Y, Wang X, Liao F, Liu Y, Jan YK. Effect of local vibrations on plantar skin blood flow responses during weight-bearing standing in healthy volunteers. *Wound Manag Prev.* 2020;66(8):7–14.
80. Aboutorabi A, Arazpour M, Bahramizadeh M, Farahmand F, Fadayevatan R. Effect of vibration on postural control and gait of elderly subjects: a systematic review. *Aging Clin Exp Res.* 2018;30(7):713–726.
81. Mukhtar AM, Abid AK, Mohd F. Effects of different vibration therapy protocols on neuromuscular performance. *Muscles Ligaments Tendons J (MLTJ).* 2021;11(1):161–177.
82. Ayvat F, Özçakar L, Ayvat E, Aksu Yıldırım S, Kılınç M. Effects of low vs. high frequency local vibration on mild-moderate muscle spasticity: ultrasonographical and functional evaluation in patients with multiple sclerosis. *Mult Scler Relat Disord.* 2021;51:102930.
83. Zhu X, Wu FL, Zhu T, Liao F, Ren Y, Jan YK. Effects of preconditioning local vibrations on subsequent plantar skin blood flow response to walking. *Int J Low Extrem Wounds.* 2021;20(2):143–149.
84. Wang H, Chandrashekhar R, Rippetoe J, Ghazi M. Focal muscle vibration for stroke rehabilitation: a review of vibration parameters and protocols. *Applied Sciences.* 2020;10(22):8270.
85. Rice D, Lewis G, McNair P. Impaired regulation of submaximal force after ACL reconstruction: role of muscle spindles. *Int J Sports Med.* 2021; 42(6):550–558.

86. Fattorini L, Rodio A, Pettorossi VE, Filippi GM. Is the focal muscle vibration an effective motor conditioning intervention? A systematic review. *J Funct Morphol Kinesiol.* 2021;6(2):39.
87. Burke D, Andrews CJ, Lance JW. Tonic vibration reflex in spasticity, Parkinson's disease, and normal subjects. *J Neurol Neurosurg Psychiatry.* 1972;35(4):477–486.
88. Bovenzi M, Griffin MJ, Ruffell CM. Vascular responses to acute vibration in the fingers of normal subjects. *Cent Eur J Public Health.* 1995; 3 Suppl:15–18.
89. Burke D, Hagbarth KE, Löfstedt L, Wallin BG. The responses of human muscle spindle endings to vibration of non-contracting muscles. *J Physiol.* 1976;261(3):673–693.
90. Hayward LF, Nielsen RP, Heckman CJ, Hutton RS. Tendon vibration-induced inhibition of human and cat triceps surae group I reflexes: evidence of selective Ib afferent fiber activation. *Exp Neurol.* 1986;94(2):333–347.
91. Marconi B, Filippi GM, Koch G, et al. Long-term effects on cortical excitability and motor recovery induced by repeated muscle vibration in chronic stroke patients. *Neurorehabil Neural Repair.* 2011;25(1):48–60.
92. Celletti C, Fattorini L, Camerota F, et al. Focal muscle vibration as a possible intervention to prevent falls in elderly women: a pragmatic randomized controlled trial. *Aging Clin Exp Res.* 2015;27(6):857–863.
93. Bram JT, Magee LC, Mehta NN, Patel NM, Ganley TJ. Anterior cruciate ligament injury incidence in adolescent athletes: a systematic review and meta-analysis. *Am J Sports Med.* 2021;49(7):1962–1972.
94. Couto BP, Silva HR, Filho AG, et al. Acute effects of resistance training with local vibration. *Int J Sports Med.* 2013;34(9):814–819.
95. Couto BP, Silva HR, Barbosa MP, Szmuchrowski LA. Chronic effects of different frequencies of local vibrations. *Int J Sports Med.* 2012;33(2): 123–129.
96. Frost HM. Bone "mass" and the "mechanostat": a proposal. *Anat Rec.* 1987;219(1):1–9.
97. Frost HM. A determinant of bone architecture. The minimum effective strain. *Clin Orthop Relat Res.* 1983;(175):286–292.
98. Frost HM. Perspectives: a proposed general model of the "mechanostat" (suggestions from a new skeletal-biologic paradigm). *Anat Rec.* 1996; 244(2):139–147.
99. Frost HM. Skeletal structural adaptations to mechanical usage (SATMU): 2. Redefining Wolff's law: the remodeling problem. *Anat Rec.* 1990;226(4):414–422.
100. Frost HM. Skeletal structural adaptations to mechanical usage (SATMU): 3. The hyaline cartilage modeling problem. *Anat Rec.* 1990;226(4): 423–432.
101. Frost HM. Strain and other mechanical influences on bone strength and maintenance. *Current Opinion in Orthopaedics.* 1997;8(5):60–70.
102. Frost HM. Wolff's Law and bone's structural adaptations to mechanical usage: an overview for clinicians. *Angle Orthod.* 1994;64(3):175–188.
103. Frost HM. From Wolff's law to the mechanostat: a new "face" of physiology. *J Orthop Sci.* 1998;3(5):282–286.

11 Nociception and Pain

FRANK H. WILLARD ▪ JOHN A. JEROME ▪ MITCHELL L. ELKISS ▪ HANS-GEORG SCHAIBLE

KEY CONCEPTS

- Tissue injury activates small primary afferent fibers in a process termed nociception.
- Nociceptive information from these afferent fibers passes through the dorsal horn of the spinal cord to reach the brain stem and thalamus.
- In the brain stem, reflexes are initiated that can modify the individual's homeostatic mechanisms in a protective manner.
- From the thalamus, numerous cortical areas are engaged, creating a matrix of activity in the cerebrum, contributing to the emergence of feelings of pain.
- Based on the nociceptive input, protective physiologic and psychological reflexes are initiated by the individual.
- Acute injury typically results in acute pain, a process which should resolve as the tissues heal; this is termed **nociceptive pain**.
- However, each level in the system is capable of sensitizing to the nociceptive activity, thereby enhancing both physiologic and psychological responses to the noxious event.
- Descending projections from forebrain and brain stem nuclei can modify the activity of neurons in the spinal cord suppressing or enhancing the processing of nociception.
- Excessive modification (plasticity) in the neural circuitry involved in processing nociception can lead to altered activity that outlasts the inciting event, this process has recently been termed **nociplastic pain**.
- Frank damage to the nervous system itself can give rise to a very intense pain termed **neuropathic pain**.
- In these chronic pain patterns, protective physiologic and psychological reflexes now become pathologic, such dysfunction will affect the individual's overall health and well-being.
- Continued obsession with the pain further facilitates the involved forebrain circuitry, creating a progressively worsening downward cycle of dysfunctional ideation, carrying the individual into despair and depression.
- It is the role of the osteopathic physician to identify the physical (somatic and visceral) as well as behavioral factors contributing to these chronic dysfunctional patterns; it is the philosophy and practice of the osteopathic physician to assist the patient in seeking ameliorative and restorative strategies in the quest to regain health.

INTRODUCTION: THE NOCICEPTIVE SYSTEM AND PAIN

Every organism requires some form of a protective system to avoid potential external and internal environmental threats and to craft the behavioral expression of defensive behaviors.

- An ideal warning system would activate just prior to tissue damage and arrest when the threat has remitted.
- In addition to protective reflexes, this system should also trigger a strong learning experience that sensitizes the organism to future situations and helps foster avoidance behavior.
- Humans are endowed with just such a system; it is composed of small, slowly conducting peripheral nerve fibers that can trigger rapid defensive responses at spinal cord and brain stem levels; it can elicit slower, longer-lasting defensive changes involving neural, endocrine, and immune adaptations orchestrated from complex forebrain circuits.
- Accompanying these physiologic and behavioral adaptations, there can also be a hard-to-define feeling of discomfort or unpleasantness that is often termed "pain."
- The electrochemical activity generated in the nervous system by a dangerous or potentially dangerous stimulus is not pain as such; it is best termed nociception, a mechanical and neurochemical process that is similar in physiology and intensity regardless of the individual concerned (Box 11.1 and Box 11.2).
- The term nociception is therefore not synonymous with pain; indeed, pain is the perception placed on neural activity occurring in the brain; thus, the feeling of pain emerges from activity occurring in the thalamus and cerebral cortex and represents both a protective and defensive response as well as a learning experience.
- Pain arises not from the small, primary afferent fibers in the periphery detecting a noxious stimulus, but from the response of complex interacting systems contained in the forebrain, reacting to the barrage of nociceptive peripheral input.
- Along with the response to noxious stimulus, the "feeling of pain" also involves the integration of many previous situations in the context of the individual's current emotional status; for this reason, painful feelings may vary tremendously in intensity and quality from individual to individual, as well as within an individual over time.

This chapter will examine the small-fiber systems in the periphery that respond to potentially damaging stimuli and their initial short-loop reactions in the gray matter of the spinal cord.

- Next, a treatment of longer-loop reflexes, generated in the brain stem and forebrain, will be developed.

BOX 11.1 Definition of Nociception

Nociception is a mechanical, thermal or chemical event activation of small-caliber primary afferent fibers.

Pain is a perception place on neural activity located in the circuits of the forebrain.

> **BOX 11.2 The Nature of the Nociceptive System**
>
> The nociceptive system uses feed-forward principles to evoke rapid responses to noxious or potentially noxious stimuli.

- This will be followed by the integration of nociceptive input into the other defensive systems, such as the endocrine response and the immune response, to create an elaborate supersystem sculpting the organism's overall physiologic and behavioral adaptations.
- In an effort to understand normal individual adaptations, emphasis will be placed on the role of integrating the emotional circuitry of the brain into the defensive response, along with the pathologic responses associated with chronic pain scenarios.
- As with any physiologic system, the central processes can regulate the peripheral systems; therefore, this chapter will also explore the descending neuronal and endocrine systems that influence the operation of the input systems, both at the peripheral level and in the spinal cord and brain stem.

Finally, as with any complex system, failures can and do occur frequently resulting in pathology.

- Complete loss of the small-fiber system, which can occur in certain familiar disorders, has catastrophic consequences for the affected individual.
- Lack of a warning system allows for self-mutilation and the eventual demise of the musculoskeletal system.[1]
- Conversely, gain-of-function mutations in sodium channels, such as Nav 1.8, can underlie the rapid formation of action potentials in a nociceptive fiber and the excessive responses to non-noxious stimuli resulting in the generation of a painful feeling in the absence of nociceptive activity.[2]
- From the study of such patients, it is clear that the normal activity of a nociceptive system is necessary for the maintenance of the individual's health; however, the seeds for destruction are contained within the power of that same system.

Since Nociception and Pain Are Separate But Related Entities, They Can Be Disassociated from Each Other

During injury, small primary afferent fibers are activated that carry action potentials to the spinal cord, which are capable of initiating protective reflexes.

- The activation of small-caliber primary afferent fibers is termed nociception and can be initiated through mechanical, chemical, or thermal stimuli; however, this event does not necessarily result in a sensation of pain.
- Through the small-caliber primary afferent fibers, the spinal cord can become activated and relay these nociceptive signals to the brain stem, where other reflexes concerning the autonomic nervous system and endocrine system may then be initiated; however, these events still do not necessarily result in a sensation of pain.
- In fact, all of these subcortical events can occur without conscious awareness of the situation (Box 11.3).
- Projections from the spinal cord and trigeminal brain stem nuclei also reach the thalamus, triggering thalamocortical circuitry and generating a network of activity on the cerebral cortex.
- Various regions of the cortex are involved in stimulus localization, as well as orchestrating the autonomic nervous system responses, emotions, and affectation.

> **BOX 11.3 The Nature of Pain**
>
> The feeling of pain appears to involve the activity of a complex neural matrix on the surface of the cerebral cortex.

- These regions become interconnected in a network, thus constituting a large matrix of activity from which pain is an emergent feeling.[3]

Thus, the feeling of pain, which is defined as an unpleasant sensation, does not arise from any one region in the cerebrum but instead from a complex and variable network colored by the individual's past physical and emotional experiences.

- Since nociception and pain are separate but related entities, they can be disassociated from each other; people can experience physical trauma and not feel pain.
- Conversely, patients can experience much pain but lack any physical evidence of ongoing nociception in peripheral tissue.
- Many of the patients encountered in clinical practice fall into this latter category.
- This chapter will focus on the mechanisms of nociception first and then consider the experience of pain and its impact on the patient's health.

Distinction between Acute and Chronic Pain

Fundamentally, pain can be divided into two major categories:

- Pain that is good for the individual (protective), termed eudynia
- Pain that is not good for the individual (maladaptive), termed maldynia

Eudynia is commonly designated as acute pain or, more recently, nociceptive pain.

- It is an expected symptom of tissue damage.
- It is protective in nature.
- Acute pain lessens in intensity with time and eventually ceases as the tissue returns to normal.

Chronically recurring or unremitting pain is not a normal experience; it is a pathology indicating that something has gone seriously wrong with the nociceptive system either peripherally, centrally or both.

- Either tissue is very abnormal in its composition (chronic inflammation leading to granulation tissue) and thus a constant nociceptive signal is being generated or the neural pathways of the spinal nociceptive system and the cerebral cortex have become facilitated and, as such, have suffered a significant change in organization and are malfunctioning.
- Alternatively, the tissue has healed normally. However significant changes have occurred in the circuitry of the nervous system leading to abnormal discharges triggering the perception of pain.
- Finally, combination of both peripheral tissue and central system dysregulation is also possible.
- Ultimately, this abnormal activity can result in the system overresponding to noxious stimuli (hyperalgesia) or even non-noxious stimuli (allodynia); in some cases, the system can simply generate spontaneous activity that the patient's brain then interprets as continuous pain (Box 11.4).

BOX 11.4 Acute vs. Chronic Pain

Acute pain is a normal and very protective experience. Chronic pain is a pathology generated by changed activity in the peripheral tissue or in the central nervous system.

- Chronic pain, that is pain persisting past a reasonable, acute period of time after the tissue has healed (2 to 4 months typically), is often associated with a wide array of biopsychosocial reactions[4] and is a pathologic state.
- Recently, chronic pain has been divided into two categories:
  - ☐ Neuropathic pain which results from damage to neural tissue
  - ☐ Nociplastic pain which arises from a modification in the circuitry of the nervous system typically through a process of sensitization.

THE PERIPHERAL NERVOUS SYSTEM

Compartments of the Peripheral Nervous System

The peripheral nervous system of the body can be divided into three major compartments:

- The **somatic afferent system** that innervates the skin, dermis, fascias, and deep tissues such as muscle, bone, tendon, and enthesis as well as joint capsules.
- The **visceral afferent system** that provides sensory innervation to the organs of the body located in the thoracic, abdominal, and pelvic cavities.
- **Vascular afferent system** that courses along the neurovascular bundles and provides innervation to the vascular system, both in the somatic and the visceral locations.

Primary Afferent Neurons Innervate Peripheral Tissue

Most peripheral nerves in the body contain a mixture of afferent (sensory) and efferent (motor) axons along with a complement of autonomic efferent fibers; this section will focus on the afferent fiber system.

- The sensory cells of the peripheral nervous system are termed primary afferent neurons.[5]
- Their cell bodies are located in a dorsal root ganglion.
- Their peripheral process extends into the tissues of the body where they form sensory endings for the transduction of stimuli.

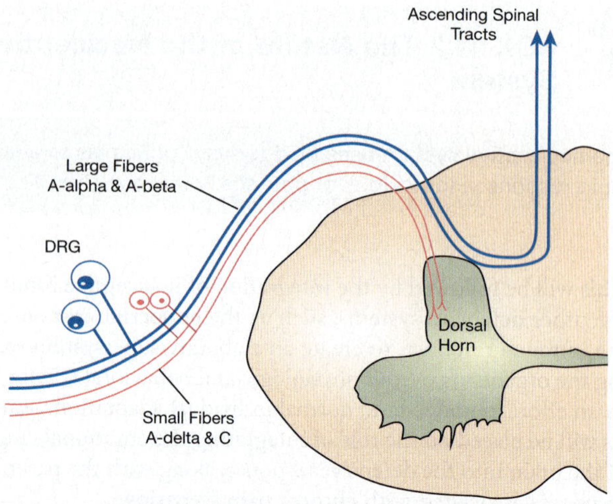

Figure 11.1. The termination of primary afferent fibers in the spinal cord. Large myelinated fibers with large cell bodies in the dorsal root ganglion (DRG) can be seen passing dorsal to the dorsal horn to enter the dorsal columns, while small laterally positioned fibers with small cell bodies in the DRG are shown entering the dorsal horn laterally. (Used with permission from the Willard/Carreiro Collection, University of New England.)

- The central processes of these primary afferent neurons terminate in the spinal cord or brain stem (Fig. 11.1).
- In general, these primary afferent neurons are divided into four fundamental types of fibers based on the size of their axon and the type of peripheral ending (Table 11.1).
- The four sensory fiber types of the peripheral nervous system can be grouped into roughly two general categories:
  - ☐ Large-caliber myelinated fibers with encapsulated endings and small-caliber lightly myelinated or unmyelinated fibers with naked nerve endings
  - ☐ Although this division, based on size is not perfect, it is supported by evidence that suggests:
- The cell bodies of the two types differ in size.
  - ☐ The development of the two groups occurs on differing timetables.
  - ☐ They can be differentiated by their immunohistochemistry[6,7]

THE LARGE-FIBER SYSTEM

The large-fiber system involves large diameter fibers and is mainly concerned with discriminative touch, vibratory sense, and proprioception.

TABLE 11.1

Classification of Fiber Types in the Peripheral Nervous System

Classification	Fiber Size and Velocity	Myelin	Origin	Receptor Organ	Effective Stimulus
Group Ia (A-alpha)	12–20 µm; 70–120 m/s	Yes	Muscle	Annulospiral	Stretch–low threshold
Group Ib (A-alpha)	2–20 µm; 70–120 m/s	Yes	Muscle	Golgi tendon organs	Active contraction of muscle
Group II (A-beta)	5–12 µm; 30–70 m/s	Yes	Muscle	Flower spray	Stretch–low threshold
		Yes	Skin	Touch corpuscles	Mechanical deformation of the skin
Group III (A-delta)	2–5 µm; 12–30 m/s	Yes	Muscle and skin	Nociception	Mechanical deformation of the skin; heat; cold; chemical stimulation
Group IV (C fibers)	0.5–1 µm; 0.5–2 m/s	No	Muscle and skin	Nociception	Mechanical deformation of the skin; heat; chemical stimulation

- The large-fiber system also plays a significant role in modulating the nociceptive system.[8]
- In addition, a few of the fibers in this system have been demonstrated to terminate in nociceptive endings.

The Large-Fiber System Is Mainly Involved with Discrimination and Proprioception

The large-fiber sensory system is composed of heavily myelinated, rapidly conducting A-alpha and A-beta fibers.

- The A-alpha fibers are the largest, they are connected to muscle spindle and Golgi tendon organs at their distal endings.
- The A-beta fibers are slightly smaller in diameter, generally their peripheral endings are typically attached to cutaneous touch corpuscles or related endings located in deeper tissues, such as joint capsules.
- Table 11.1 compares the properties of these two rapidly conducting fiber systems.

Typically, members of the largest fibers are easily activated, being sensitive to low levels of mechanical energy, and have the fastest conduction velocities.

- The ascending projections of the large-fiber system travel in both the dorsal column–medial lemniscus system and the spinocerebellar systems to reach the thalamus, from which they are relayed onto the somatic sensory cortex (Fig. 11.2).
- Along with their ascending fibers in the dorsal columns, these fibers can also project to the segmental dorsal horn (lamina III) and form synapses on neurons of the anterolateral quadrant (e.g., spinothalamic tract).
- The mapping of these fibers is fairly precise and supports high-fidelity representation of the homunculus on the postcentral gyrus of the cerebral cortex (reviewed in Kandel[9]) (Box 11.5).
- Collectively, the large-fiber system provides the sensory modalities of vibratory sense, discriminative touch, and proprioception.
- Individual fibers of this system are said to be line-labeled in so much as they represent a specific modality; varying the intensity of the stimulus for these fibers does not significantly alter the modality that they represent.
- Thus, an A-beta fiber associated with a Pacinian corpuscle, when activated, gives the individual a sense of vibration regardless of the intensity of the activation; this consistency in sensory perception contributes to the accuracy and precision of the system.
- An additional property, prominent in the large-fiber system, is the ability of many of its endings to undergo adaptation to repetitive stimuli.
- In these fibers, repetitive stimuli initially activate the fiber ending, which then adapts to the stimulus by altering its shape in such a way that it becomes nonresponsive to that particular stimulus.

> **BOX 11.5 The Large Fiber System**
>
> The large-fiber system:
>
> - Is mainly involved in discriminative touch, vibratory sense, and proprioception.
> - Plays a role in modulating the nociceptive system.
> - Typically adapts to a repetitive stimulus.

- This adaptation can be very rapid, as seen in the Pacinian and Meissner's corpuscle or very slow as seen in the Ruffini and Merkel's endings.
- Adaptation of these fibers facilitates the detection of novel stimuli in the environment.

The Large-Fiber System Is Active in Pain Control

Although the major target of A-beta fibers is the dorsal column nuclei of the brain stem, as they enter the spinal cord, many of these fibers give collateral branches that invade the dorsal horn as well.

- These collateral branches, through an inhibitory mechanism, can modulate the transmission of information in the small-fiber system in the dorsal horn and thereby prevent nociceptive information from ascending in the spinal cord tracks.
- The mechanism of small-fiber gating has been termed the *gate control theory of pain modulation* and appears to play a significant role in controlling the activity of the small-fiber system.[10]
- Conversely, under situations of intense peripheral stimuli involving inflammation, some members of the large-fiber system have been observed to undergo a phenotypic change, such that they can now activate dorsal horn neurons and produce a neuropeptide such as substance P (SP), a marker for the small-fiber system.[11]
- This type of alteration in fiber function would have profound effects on the amplification of signal in the dorsal horn and the patient's perception of pain.

THE SMALL-FIBER SYSTEM

The small-fiber sensory system is composed of A-delta and C fibers; collectively, these fibers have been referred to as primary afferent nociceptors (PANs).

- The A-delta fibers have a thin myelin sheath, whereas the C fibers only have a thin wrapping derived from the Schwann cell membrane but no myelin.
- A common feature of these small-fiber types is their termination as an exposed or naked axon ending, also termed free nerve ending, embedded in the extracellular matrix of the surrounding tissue.
- Many of these fibers have high thresholds and are associated with the sensation of itch or the initial feelings of sharp pain.
- However, there are some A-delta fibers with thresholds of activation in the same range as the large-fiber systems previously described.[12]
- A few of these myelinated nociceptors are known to contain neuropeptides that can be released into the surrounding peripheral tissue.
- A characteristic feature of many, but not all, unmyelinated nociceptors in the C-fiber range is the secretion of neuropeptides, such as SP or calcitonin gene–related peptide, from their distal terminals into the surrounding tissue.
- In general, many of these small-caliber fibers have high thresholds of activation, requiring tissue-damaging or potentially tissue-damaging levels of energy before generating action potentials.
- These small fibers can act as nociceptors detecting tissue damaging stimuli.
- Many of the small fibers can function as thermoreceptors for innocuous warmth.
- Small fibers, often located in the knee joint, skin viscera, may not respond to damage initially, however, as the tissue chemistry changes following the injury, these fibers can develop a latent but very strong response and have been dubbed "silent nociceptors."[13]

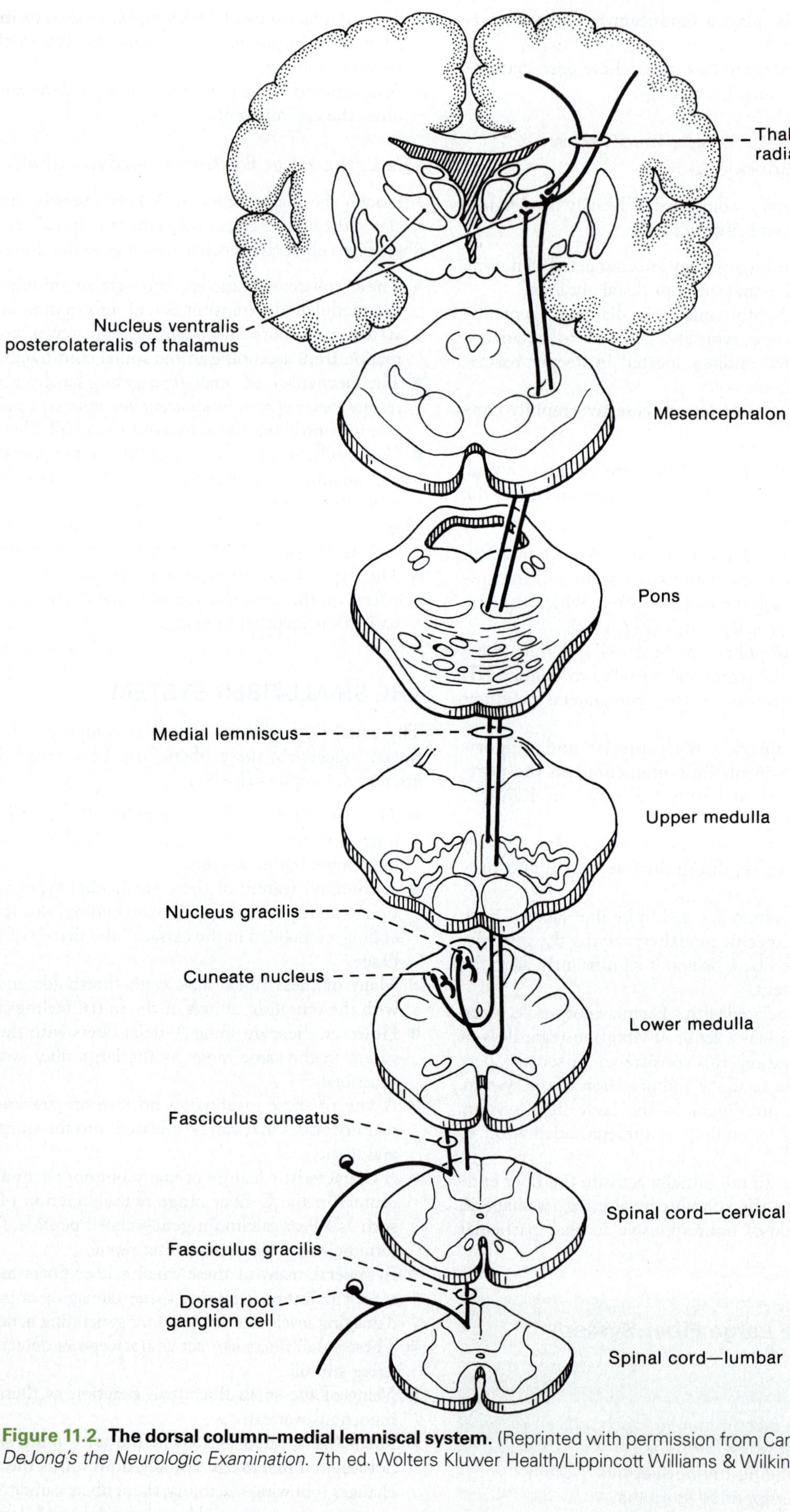

Figure 11.2. The dorsal column–medial lemniscal system. (Reprinted with permission from Campbell WW. *DeJong's the Neurologic Examination.* 7th ed. Wolters Kluwer Health/Lippincott Williams & Wilkins; 2013.)

- In addition, recent research has documented a group of small-caliber fibers, termed C-tactile fibers, that have low threshold for activation and, surprisingly, appear to carry a pleasant sensation.[14]

The Small-Fiber System Targets the Dorsal Horn

The central process of the small-caliber fibers terminates in the ipsilateral dorsal horn of the spinal cord (see Fig. 11.1), or if the fiber arises in the trigeminal territory of the face, its central process terminates in the spinal trigeminal nucleus of the medullary brain stem.

- Specifically, these small-diameter afferent fibers reach laminae I, II, and V of the dorsal horn, as well as the central portion of the gray matter around lamina X.
- Ascending projections from neurons in the dorsal horn cross the midline in the anterior white commissure of the spinal cord and course upward in the anterolateral tract or system to reach the brain stem and thalamus (Fig. 11.3).

The Output of the Small-Fiber System Is Protective in Nature

In addition to warning signals such as pain sensation, the small-caliber system activates a complex response from the brain stem, termed the general adaptive response by Hans Selye.[15]

- This response involves alterations in the autonomic nervous system and the hypothalamic–pituitary–adrenal axis, both which contribute to the inherent ability of the body for self-regulation and the re-establishment of health.
- These concepts will be further discussed toward the end of the chapter.

An additional distinctive property of the small-caliber system is its ability to sensitize to repetitive stimuli.

- Unlike the large-fiber system, which tends to adapt to a stimulus, many of the components in the small-fiber system—either at the level of the peripheral neuron, spinal cord neurons, or even higher in the CNS—will increase their sensitivity to the stimulus (Box 11.6).
- This enhanced activity secondary to sensitization of neurons has significant implications for the small-fiber system in the pathology of chronic pain.[16]

Summary

Both small- and large-fiber systems can play a role in the human perception of pain.

- However, typically, the small-caliber system has by far the greatest impact.
- In normal tissue, small fibers typically transmit nociceptive information, and their activity is perceived as pain.

BOX 11.6 C and A-delta Fibers

The small-fiber system:

- Plays a significant role in generating protective responses.
- Such responses can involve simple avoidance or more complex activation of a neuroendocrine response.
- Can sensitize to a stimulus.

- The large-fiber system helps to gate the activity of the small-fiber system and thereby control the amount of nociceptive information gaining access to the spinal cord neurons.
- However, in injured tissue, the situation changes dramatically.
- The large-fiber system can become a player in generating the perception of pain.
- The next section of this chapter will be focused on the anatomical organization and functional properties of the small fibers and their interaction with the large-fiber system in pathologic situations.

SMALL-FIBER LOCATION

PANs terminate with naked nerve endings in numerous tissues throughout the body. The specific locations in which these fibers are important for understanding clinical patterns of pain presentation.

Skin and Fascia

PANs are present in the dermis and underlying fascia throughout the body.[17]

- Cutaneous PANs can be divided into several subtypes by the molecular structure of their membrane.[18]
- Upon entering the dermis, much branching of these fibers occurs before their termination.
- A few of the PANs in the dermis have small terminal branches that actually penetrate the epidermis and embed between cells of the squamous epithelium; these are termed intraepithelial endings, their interaction with keratinocytes is thought to facilitate nociceptive mechanisms.[19]
- The PANs in the deep fascia are mostly associated with blood vessels.
- PANs also reach the specializations of the integument such as the nail beds, tympanic membrane, and cornea.

Muscle

Muscle nerves can be composed of as much as 50% small fibers.[20]

- Within the muscle, PANs are seen to course in the connective tissue surrounding the vasculature.
- While PANs do not directly innervate myocytes, they do remain in the surrounding connective tissue, termed the perimysium, and are thought to play a major role in regulating the vascular dynamics of the muscle.
    - Many of these small fibers contain vasodilating neuropeptides such as SP and calcitonin gene–related peptide, consistent with their role as sensory fibers and neurosecretory fibers.
    - In addition, many of the neuropeptide-containing fibers also express acid-sensitive ion channels known to be involved in the detection of reduced tissue pH.[21]
- Thresholds energies for activation muscle PANs are usually somewhat lower than the energy level necessary to actually damage the surrounding muscle tissue.
- Muscle PANs appear to be sensitive to inflammatory substances and to the breakdown products resulting from intense muscle activity.
- The peripheral distribution of the PANs is complex; many of these fibers have more than one receptive field in the peripheral tissue, and often the two fields are not contiguous.
- One receptive field may be normally active and the other silent until an injury, then both fields can become active thereby causing the sensation of pain to spread.[22]

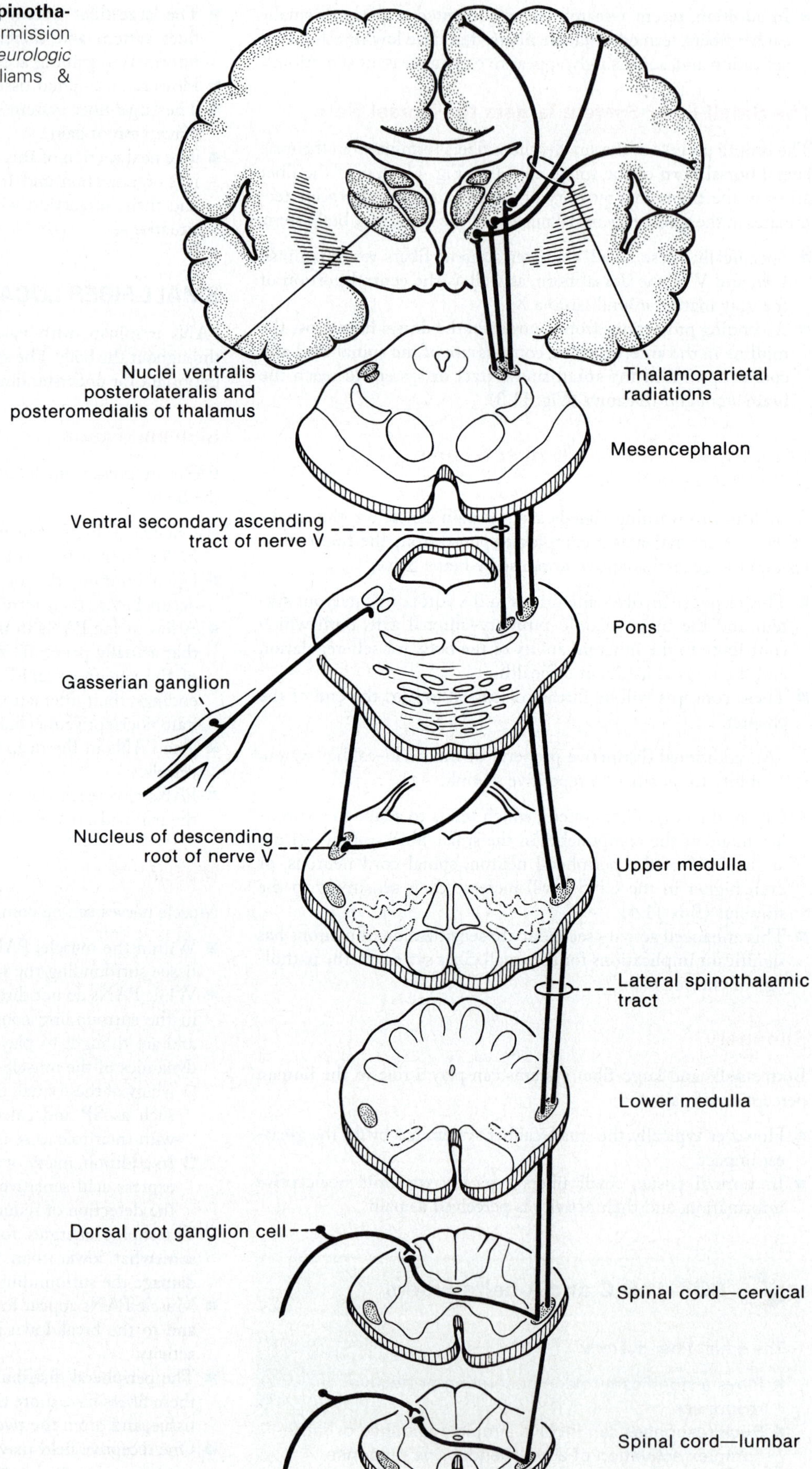

Figure 11.3. The anterolateral or spinothalamic system. (Reprinted with permission from Campbell WW. *DeJong's The Neurologic Examination*. 6th ed. Lippincott Williams & Wilkins; 2005.)

- Muscle PANs are also well noted for their ability to increase activity in the spinal cord, leading to sensitization of the dorsal horn neurons.[20,23]

Tendon

The PANs present in tendons are not very well characterized at this time.

- Small sensory fibers have been described in the peritendineum and in the enthesis, but are very scant in the body of the tendon.[20]
- Although a network of nerve fibers extending the length of the human bicep tendon has been described[24]; most studies find few nerve fibers in the body of a tendon, but a rich supply of nerves in the soft, investing peritendinous fascial tissue surrounding the tendon.
- Many of the small fibers in these neural networks contain several neuropeptides typically associated with sensory fibers such as PANs, other fibers are tyrosine kinase positive suggesting they are sympathetic fibers.[25]
- Although small, peptide containing fibers are found in the investing fascial sheath of the tendon, few fibers are seen in the tendon or enthesis itself.[26,27]
- The concentration of these nerve fibers at the tissue surrounding the enthesis could be related to the notably painful presentation of enthesitis.[25]

Blood Vessels

Control of vessel diameter is normally dominated by intrinsic, endothelial cell–derived factors such as endothelin-1 and nitric oxide; however, somatic and visceral blood vessels receive an ample supply of small-caliber sensory fibers as well as a sympathetic innervation.

- PANs follow the sympathetic nervous system coursing in the tunica adventitia of these blood vessels.
- These small vascular afferent fibers release vasodilatory neuropeptides and can act as a counterregulatory force to the vasoconstrictive nature of the sympathetic system.
- This is especially interesting in light of the fact that the somatic peripheral vessels do not receive a parasympathetic innervation; thus, the PANs could be providing some, if not most, of the external dilatory signals to the vasculature.[28]

Nerves

The epineural connective tissue sheath surrounding most nerves contains a PAN innervation.[29,30]

- Where it has been studied, these fibers contain and release proinflammatory neuropeptides and have high thresholds of activation, similar to nociceptors.
- It is possible that some of the pain arising from chronic injury of a nerve could be arising from the PANs in the connective sheath surrounding the nerve, rather than from the discharge of axons contained within the nerve itself.

Joints

Joints, especially those of the synovial type, typically receive multiple articular nerves.

- In general, this includes all structures in the joint such as the capsule, internal and external ligaments subchondral bone, articular cartilage and synovial membrane.
- These nerves have been demonstrated to contain as much as 80% small-caliber (C-fiber range) axons; of these small fibers, there is approximately an even split between those of the sympathetic nervous system and PANs.[31]
- Fibers of all calibers innervate the joint capsule, ligaments, menisci, and surrounding periosteum; however, only small-caliber, peptide-containing fibers are typically seen in the synovial membranes.
- Neuropeptides released from the PANs can interact with immune cells in the synovial membrane of the joint to produce a significant inflammatory response.
- Although the density of small-caliber afferent fibers has been shown to increase in the bone and even appear *de novo* in the cartilage of osteoarthritic joints in other species,[32] these fibers have been reported to drop in density in the synovial lining of such joints in humans[33]; this suggests that pain in osteoarthritic joints may be coming from irritation of the joint capsule, subchondral bone or articular cartilage rather than the synovial lining.

Viscera

The axons entering viscera are typically small in size, being in the A-delta and C-fiber range.[34,35]

- Afferent fibers enter the thoracic–abdominal–pelvic cavity either with the vagus nerve or with the splanchnic nerves derived from the sympathetic trunk.
- These sensory fibers are distributed via suspensory ligaments (mesenteries and mesocolons) to the hollow viscera.
- Sensory innervation of tissue can be found in the suspensory ligament, as well as in the muscular wall and mucosa of the organ.
- Solid organs, such as the liver, are primarily innervated in the region of the fibrous capsule with very little projecting into the organ parenchyma.
- Many fibers are mechanoinsensitive, responding only to inflammatory compounds in the tissue.
- As such, they have been termed silent nociceptors to denote the lack of initial response to mechanical deformation,[34] for example, during surgery.
- However, within the time period following the insult, the inflammation in the tissue ripens and these silent nociceptors become active.[13]
- Although the total number of visceral afferent fibers is marginal compared to the somatic afferent system, the visceral system compensates for this by heavy branching and ramification of the central terminals in the spinal cord and brain stem.[35]
- Visceral nociceptive fibers are also known to be highly plastic in nature and can significantly change their response properties consequent to events occurring early in development.[36]

Meninges

Small-caliber fibers innervate the dura and extracerebral blood vessels surrounding the brain.

- These small fibers are components of the trigeminovascular system.
- The cell bodies of these sensory neurons are located in the trigeminal ganglion and their peripheral processes follow the cerebrovascular system until it penetrates the brain.
- Many of the small fibers found in the trigeminovascular system are rich in neuropeptides.[37]
- Inflammatory irritation of these fibers plays a crucial role in migraine and other vascular head pains.[38]
- Recent evidence suggests that some of these sensory fibers reach the arachnoid and pial surface of the brain.[39]

BOX 11.7 Distribution of PANs

PANs are found in carrying densities in most tissues of the body, with the exception of the solid internal organs such as the brain and liver.

Annulus Fibrosis

In a normal intervertebral disk, PANs penetrate approximately one-third of the way into the structure, reaching most of the annulus fibrosis, but normally do not extend into the nucleus pulposus.[40,41]

- These fibers are derived from the sinuvertebral (recurrent meningeal) nerve posteriorly and from the prevertebral plexus (somatosympathetic nerves) anteriorly.[42]
- Many of these fibers contain neuropeptides typical of small-caliber primary afferent fibers and are involved in diskogenic pain.
- A branch of the sinuvertebral nerve, termed the basivertebral nerve, penetrates the body of the vertebra posteriorly and, once inside spreads out to innervate the inner surfaces of the cartilaginous end plates; this small nerve is strongly associated with low back pain of disrupted disk origin.[43,44]
- In addition, PANs are found in the anterior and posterior longitudinal ligaments, in the facet joint capsules, and in other ligaments of the vertebral column.
- This network of small-caliber fibers surrounding the vertebral column is involved in the axial pain syndromes.[45]

Summary

- PANs have an almost universal distribution in the body.
- A few areas such as solid organs, such as brain, liver and lung, have been demonstrated to be completely devoid of PANs; they are also absent in articular cartilage and the nucleus pulposus of the intervertebral disks (Box 11.7).
- The density of small-fiber distribution is not uniform throughout the tissue of the body, being greatest in the dermis and more scattered in distribution through the visceral organs.
- There also appears to be some differential distribution of neuropeptides within various regions of the body.
- The widespread and plentiful nature of these small-caliber primary afferent fibers forms the basis of the interoceptive system and is a testament to their important role in the maintenance of our health.

BOX 11.8 Primary Afferent Nociceptior Cell Membranes

Three main forms of membrane complexes are present on the terminals of PANs:

- Ion channels
- G-coupled proteins
- Growth factor receptors

SMALL-FIBER ACTIVATION AND SENSITIZATION

PANs can respond to mechanical, thermal (heat), and chemical irritation.

- Activation of a PAN implies that the stimulus evokes action potentials directly by opening ion channels on the membrane of the axon.
- Several different forms of membrane-bound receptor mechanisms and ion channels are present and a variety of events can activate or sensitize these fibers (see Table 11.1).
- To accomplish this feat, the terminal membranes of PANs have three general classes of signal transduction mechanisms[18] (Box 11.8):
  - □ Ion channels—These structures are opened by stimuli and allow the influx of ions, usually calcium and sodium which depolarize the neuron.
  - □ G-coupled protein receptors—these membrane receptors activate second messenger cascades and sensitize neurons. Note that they are particularly strong sensitizers.
  - □ Growth factor (tyrosine kinase or cytokine) receptors. Note that they are particularly strong sensitizers (Table 11.2).
- However, not all PANs have the same constellation of receptors.
- Mechanical distortion of tissue can force open mechanosensitive ion channels of some PANs and initiate depolarization of the sensory fiber.
- Thermal stimuli can also open thermal-sensitive ion channels on some PAN fiber membranes.
- These heat-sensitive channels have been identified and were originally described as vanilloid receptors (V1) or, as more recently termed, "transient receptor potential channels" (TRPV1).
- Substances released in the environment of the chemoreceptive PANs, during tissue injury or inflammation, can engage receptors located on the exposed membrane of these sensory fibers (Fig. 11.4).

TABLE 11.2

PAN Receptors and Their Activating Substances

PAN Receptor Class	Activating Substances	Examples	Function
Ion channels	Heat; mechanical force	Transient receptor potential channels (vanilloid receptors); proton-gated channels; sodium channels; potassium channels; calcium channels; serotonin (5-HT3) channels	Na^{++} and Ca^{++} influx into the axon
G-Protein	Bradykinin, prostaglandin; endocannabinoids	BK-1, BK-2, DP, EP, FP, IP, TP	Initiate second-messenger cascades in the axon
Cytokine receptors	Growth factors and cytokines	Trk-A, Trk-B, Trk-C, NT-4/5.NT-3, IL-1RI, sIL-6R, TNFR1	Modify surrounding ion channel activity

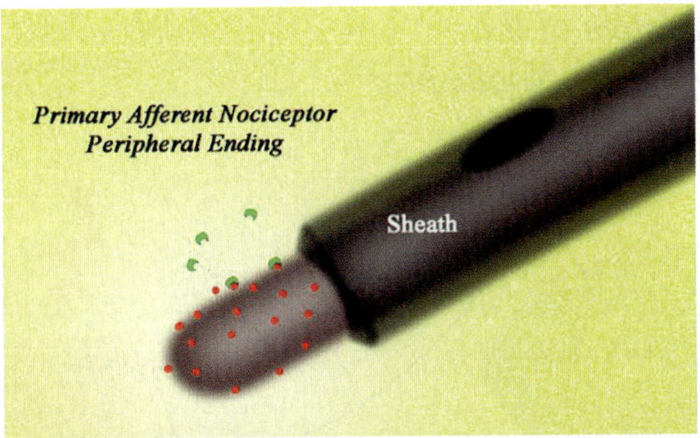

Figure 11.4. Primary afferent fiber ending. Primary afferent nociceptors (PANs) are covered with a Schwann cell sheath containing little or no myelin. At the end of the fiber, the sheath terminates to expose the naked end of the axon. The membrane of the axon has receptors that can detect chemicals in the surrounding extracellular fluids. (Used with permission from the Willard/Carreiro Collection, University of New England.)

- Rather than directly activating the axon, most proinflammatory compounds sensitize the axon by acting through second messenger cascades. Although they do not directly result in the formation of action potentials, they do lower the threshold for activation.
- Many different substances (called allodynogens) can activate PANs directly or sensitize the PAN, making it much more responsive to physical touch or temperature.
- Thus, chemoreceptive PANs are responsive to a wide range of modifications in the chemical milieu of the surrounding tissue.[46]

There is a growing list of allodynogens capable of activating PANs; some of the better-known examples are listed in Table 11.3.

- Most of these substances are present either in a blocked form or are sequestered in cells or the extracellular matrix, to be activated or released in the face of tissue injury.
- Histamine is contained in the granules of mast cells, which are situated along neurovascular bundles in fascia.
- Injury disrupts the mast cell thereby releasing histamine into the tissue.
- Similarly, disruption of vascular endothelial cells releases prostaglandins into the surrounding tissue.
- Finally, bradykinin, a plasma protein produced in the liver, is present in circulation in a blocked form termed preprobradykinin.
- Tissue damage activates enzymes in a fashion similar to the clotting cascade that ultimately results in the release of bradykinin in the surrounding tissue.

TABLE 11.3

The Allodynogens and Their Receptors

Allodynogen	Receptor	Origin
Bradykinin	BK1 and BK2	Plasma protein from the liver
Histamine	H1	Mast cells
Serotonin	5-HT2A	Blood platelets
Prostaglandins	DP, EP, FP, IP, TP	Vascular endothelial cells
ATP	Purine	Local cell rupture
Protons	Vanilloid receptor (VR1)	Local cell rupture

BOX 11.9 Allodynogens

Common inflammatory allodynogens include:

- Bradykinin
- Histamine
- Prostaglandins
- Cytokines

Inflammation releases a cascade of chemicals, many of them bactericidal and capable of helping cleanse the tissue and stimulate wound repair in short-term exposure; however, most of these substances are also well-known allodynogens.[47]

- PANs have receptors for many of these chemicals and can record their release into the tissue by depolarization and action potential formation in local PANs (Box 11.9).
- Peripheral release of neuropeptide allodynogens from PANs can initiate or exacerbate an inflammatory response (Fig. 11.5).
- Some of these same substances are also used as neurotransmitters or neuromodulators, released from the central process of the PAN in the dorsal horn.
- PAN activation serves as a warning and initiates spinal cord and brain stem level reflexes to protect the injured area.
- In addition, exposure to some of these proinflammatory compounds activates G-protein–signaling cascades capable of sensitizing the PAN.
- Examples include prostaglandins, released from endothelial cells, which activate E-type prostanoid (EP) receptors as well as proinflammatory cytokines capable of activating the tyrosine kinase receptors on the PAN membrane.
- In essence, the PANs are interoceptors, sensitive to the quality of the tissue, and can inform the central nervous system of tissue health.

PANs Contribute to a Feed-Forward Allostatic Process Involved in Somatic Dysfunction and Tissue Repair

When activated, certain PANs can secrete potent, proinflammatory neuropeptides that enhance the release of histamine, prostaglandins, and cytokines[48]

- A feed-forward loop is established, with the PANs releasing substances that ultimately provoke additional activity from the same fiber.
- Importantly, this loop has no established end point or set point.
- These types of feedforward reactions, rapidly fulminating, epitomize a process characterized by the term allostasis (reviewed in Schulkin[49]).
- In allostatic processes, rapid change in the tissue chemistry is protective and contributes to the long-term survival of the individual.
- This is contrary to homeostasis, in which inhibitory feedback control establishes boundary parameters that oscillate around a defined set point.
- Allostatic processes lack immediate boundaries or set points; thus, this inflammatory process can potentially run out of control and become a chronic issue.
- Eventually, the increasing systemic levels of norepinephrine and glucocorticoids, due to long-loop inhibitory feedback systems, should aid in suppressing the inflammatory response.

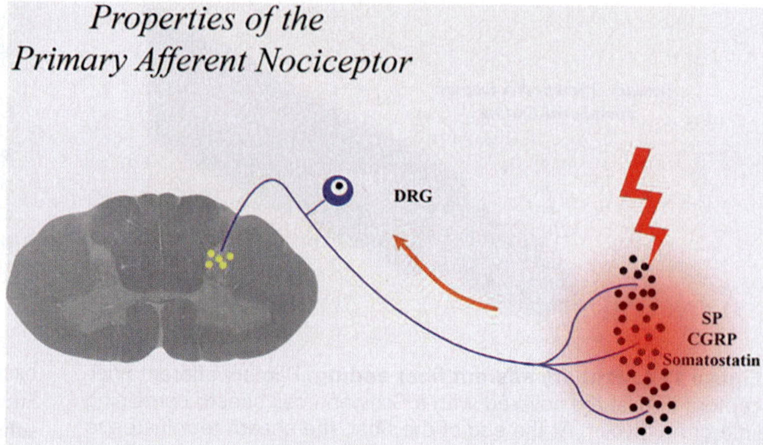

Figure 11.5. Activation of a PAN and the release of proinflammatory compounds into the surrounding tissue. Tissue irritation results in the release of proinflammatory compounds from the distal ends of some PANs. Interactions with compounds from immune cells, mast cells, and platelets result in an inflammatory soup that sensitizes the PAN leading to the increased release of neurotransmitters and neuromodulators in the dorsal horn of the spinal cord. (Used with permission from the Willard/Carreiro Collection, University of New England.)

- Acute exposure to an allostatic process can be very protective, initiating protective reflexes and creating an area of increased sensitivity to mechanical stimulation (allodynia), and an increased response to a stimulus, which is normally painful (hyperalgesia).
- In uninjured tissue, the uncontrolled release of inflammatory peptides from PANs can create an inflammatory response *de novo*, this event has been referred to as a **neurogenic inflammation**.
- When controlled, a neurogenic inflammatory event can be a normal component of the healing process, when uncontrolled it can be a pathologic event.

Most likely, the allostatic condition involving the release of allodynogens and the enhancement of the inflammatory soup of chemicals in the tissue environment, resulting in sensitization of the PANs, epitomizes the diagnostic conditions found in somatic dysfunction (Box 11.10).

- The potentiated PANs would generate a condition of hyperalgesia.
- The surrounding inflammatory cocktail would produce edema giving the tissue a boggy texture upon manual palpation, such as occurs in a neurogenic inflammation.
- Increased sensitivity to touch and tissue texture changes are two of the cardinal manifestations of somatic dysfunction.[50]

Nerve Damage and the Feelings of Pain

Acute damage to a peripheral nerve fiber is usually relatively painless and, when done experimentally, rarely produces more than a few seconds of rapid axonal discharges typically felt as paresthesias.

- Acute damage to the dorsal root ganglion can produce long periods of excitation and rapid firing lasting 5 to 25 minutes; thus, the ganglion appears to be the most sensitive part of the normal nerve to compressive injury.
- However, acute compression of a chronically injured, inflamed nerve represents a different situation and will produce several minutes of repetitive firing; it has been suggested that this long-duration rapid firing is the basis for radicular pain.[51]

BOX 11.10 Allostasis vs. Homeostasis

- Homeostasis involves feedback control about a set point.
- Allostasis involves feed-forward control without a set point.

- Injury to a nerve can facilitate sprouting from the peripheral terminal of fibers within the nerve; this can be accompanied by the invasion of sympathetic axons into the dorsal root ganglion.
- Although these nascent sympathetic axons do not form synapses with the sensory fibers, the inappropriate release of catecholamines from these fibers into the extracellular space can activate adrenergic receptors on the membranes of sensory neurons, as such these receptors are known to be upregulated following nerve injury, these events have also been associated with abnormal sprouting of the central process of sensory neurons in the dorsal horn.[52–54]
- All of these scenarios can contribute to the development of an intense chronic pain condition, termed ***neuropathic pain***, which is pain initiated or caused by a primary lesion or dysfunction in the nervous system.[55]

The Spinal Cord and Pain

When PANs become active, they transmit action potentials to the dorsal horn of the spinal cord via their central process (see Fig. 11.5), releasing transmitters such as the amino acid glutamate, and neuromodulators such as the peptides SP, CGRP and others into the dorsal horn.

- Various cells, including both neurons and glia in the dorsal horn, are influenced by this chemical milieu.
- Interestingly, the response of the dorsal horn cells can outlast the activity of the PAN.
- The sustainability of this activity pattern among neurons in the dorsal horn represents central sensitization and is believed to be a major factor influencing numerous pain syndromes.
- The interaction in the spinal cord of the central process of PANs from various regions in the body can substantially alter acute pain patterns (referral and association patterns), as well as states of chronic pain.

PANs Terminate in the Dorsal Horn of the Spinal Cord

The central process of the PANs enters the spinal cord by coursing in the lateral aspect of the dorsal root entry zone, entering the dorsal most aspect of the dorsal horn, and extending inward to terminate generally in laminae I, II, and V of the dorsal horn.[56]

- Conversely, collateral branches of low-threshold, mechanoreceptive fibers tend to terminate deep in laminae III through VI.
- The organization of the PANs in the dorsal horn is orderly, forming a somatotropic body map extending approximately from

BOX 11.11 The Dorsal Horn

The central processes of PANs terminate in the dorsal horn of the spina cord.

Dorsal horn neurons respond to PAN activation, but their activity may outlast the activity of the PAN.

Sustained dorsal horn neuron activation is thought to play a major role in some chronic pain situations.

medial to lateral across the dorsal horn[57]; however, much overlap in receptor territories exist allowing for referral of activity patterns to associated regions of the somatotropic map (Box 11.11).

PANs represent a heterogeneous population of fibers; thus, not all PANs are the same in terms of anatomy and neurochemistry.

- Beyond the size difference seen between A-delta fibers and C fibers, the C fibers divide into two functionally and chemically differentiated groups:
  - Those that contain neuropeptides such as calcitonin gene–related peptide or SP.
  - Those that do not contain neuropeptides,[58,59] typically they can be identified by their reaction with isolectin on their membrane surface.[60]
- The neuropeptide-containing fibers seem to terminate principally in laminae I, while the non–peptide-containing fibers terminate in laminae II.
- This dichotomy of fiber types and distributions suggests that differing aspects of nociception could be carried by specialized PANs. Specifically:
  - The peptidergic PANs terminating in lamina I are thought to be involved in localization of the injury.
  - The nonpeptidergic fibers in lamina II are thought to be more associated with the affective nature of the pain.[61]

Dorsal Horn Neurons and PAN Central Synapses

The three anatomical types of dorsal horn neurons are

1. Projection cells
2. Interneurons
3. Propriospinal cells

- Projection cells, the best studied of the three types, send their axons upstream in the ascending tracts of the spinal cord to reach the brain stem and the thalamus.
- Local circuit interneurons confine their projections to the segment that their cell body is located within, while propriospinal cells represent a combination of the first two types; their axons ramify interconnecting the various spinal segments, but do not extend out of the spinal cord.
- Several different forms of projection cells exist in the spinal cord[62]: each form of these cells receives synaptic endings from the PANs.
- Projection cells in the superficial layer of the dorsal horn are relatively specific to PAN input and have been termed nociceptor-specific cells, however, the interaction of PANs with the superficial dorsal horn neurons is complicated and still not well understood.[63]
- A class of projection cells, located throughout the dorsal horn, but more typically in the deeper layers, respond to a wide range of inputs, including A-beta fibers, A-delta fibers, and C fibers, and have therefore been termed wide dynamic range (WDR) neurons.[64,65]
- Although gentle mechanical stimulation can activate a WDR neuron, maximal response from these cells can be obtained from noxious stimuli[66] or repetitive innoxious stimuli.[64]
- Evidence does support the concept that the affective perception of pain is related to the activity of the WDR neuron, while the perception of the pain location may be due to the activity of the nociceptor-specific cells[67]; however, these concepts still remain a controversial area in perceptual neuroscience.

EXAMINATION OF A PAN CENTRAL SYNAPSE

Central Pan Synaptic Terminals Contain at Least Two Types of Neurotransmitters

The central process of the neuropeptide-containing PANs forms terminals on the dendrites of dorsal horn neurons.

- A closer look at the neurochemistry of these PAN synapses will help in understanding the central sensitization of dorsal horn neurons.
- Neuropeptide-containing PAN synaptic terminals produce excitatory amino acids (EAAs), such as glutamate or aspartate, and neuropeptide neurotransmitters such as SP or calcitonin gene–related peptide.[68]
- The different forms of transmitters are co-released from the same terminal.
- However, while the amino acid is released during any sufficient depolarization of the ending, neuropeptide release requires more prolonged summation of depolarizations, such as would occur during tonic discharges.[69]

Excitatory Amino Acid

The most common EAA in the PAN central terminal is glutamate.

- Release of glutamate activates the alpha-amino-3-hydroxy-5-methyl-4-isoxazolepropionic acid (AMPA) receptors on the postsynaptic surface.
- AMPA receptors are ion channels that allow sodium to enter the cell when open, as such, these channels can cause a rapid depolarization of the postsynaptic process when activated.
- This type of excitatory amino acid transmission is relatively quick, involving milliseconds at most, and has thus been termed fast transmission.
- Most neurons in the dorsal horn express AMPA receptors on their membranes.
- In addition to AMPA receptors, glutamate release–activated kainate and *N*-methyl-D-aspartate (NMDA) receptors are also found on dorsal horn neurons.
- Little is known about the kainate receptor, conversely the NMDA receptor has been well studied.
- Although the NMDA receptor responds to glutamate, it is normally blocked by a large divalent cation such as magnesium.
- Strong depolarization of the neuron by the action of glutamate on AMPA receptors can expel the magnesium ion from the NMDA receptors allowing an influx of calcium ion into the cell.
- Calcium can act as a second messenger system sensitizing the AMPA receptors and lowering the threshold or activation for the neuron, a process termed central sensitization (see Woolf and Salter[70]).
- NMDA receptors are key for neuronal sensitization and neuroplasticity. If NMDA receptors are blocked, for example by ketamine, central sensitization can be prevented.

> **BOX 11.12 PAN Neurotransmitters**
>
> Both EAAs and neuropeptides can be released from the central terminals of PANs.
>
> Whereas amino acids are fast acting, neuropeptides require the accumulation of volume to create and effect change and thus require more time.
>
> Neuropeptide effects can be longer lasting, resulting in a change in response properties of the dorsal horn neurons.

Neuropeptide

A specific population of PAN central terminals contain neuropeptides as well as EAAs (Box 11.12).

- Upon release, these peptides diffuse onto receptors located on the postsynaptic membrane, but not necessarily into the synaptic cleft.
- Tonic or repeated activation of the PAN is required to cause enough peptide release to activate the peptide receptors, this is termed **volume transmission** as opposed to synaptic transmission.
- Thus, the time required to obtain adequate volume of peptide release and the longer diffusion route to a more distant receptor complex combine to increase the time required for a response.[69]
- When activated by attachment to the peptide, the peptide–receptor complex internalizes into the postsynaptic neuron through a process of endocytosis.[71]
- Thus, the peptide is acting on the postsynaptic neuron in a way that is similar to some hormones, in that it physically enters the postsynaptic cell to effect changes at the cytosolic and nuclear levels.
- Once across the cell membrane, the peptide–receptor complex can act as an enzyme and initiate second-messenger cascades leading to the phosphorylation of the AMPA receptor and surrounding NMDA receptors.
- Phosphorylation of the NMDA receptors opens its channel allowing calcium ions to enter the cell, thereby facilitating the activity of the dorsal horn neuron.
- This type of transmission requires seconds to minutes and has thus been termed slow or volume transmission since it is dependent on the volume of transmitter available.
- The result of this cascade of events is a potentiation of the responsiveness of dorsal horn cells that contributes to central sensitization, that is, the response properties of these dorsal horn neurons undergoing a leftward shift on the stimulus–response curve.
- Interestingly, excessive activation of the PANs can lead to the spread of neurons expressing receptors for SP in the dorsal horn[72]; this change would also facilitate the response of the dorsal horn neurons to afferent stimuli.

BEHAVIOR OF NOCICEPTIVE NEURONS IN THE DORSAL HORN

Transient Change in Dorsal Horn Circuitry: Activity-Dependent Plasticity

Neurons in the dorsal horn demonstrate a plasticity in their response properties that is directly related to the afferent activity to which they are exposed.[72]

> **BOX 11.13 Neural Plasticity in the Dorsal Horn**
>
> Neuronal plasticity, the ability of a neuron to alter its response properties depending on the type and intensity of the input it receives, can be very protective in the short term and very damaging if prolonged or made permanent.

- This type of plasticity is characteristic of any biologic system that is adaptive in nature.
- Through these plastic changes, afferent activity involving PANs can result in sensitization of the dorsal horn circuitry.
- These rapid changes in sensitivity represent a form of allostasis, similar to that already described in the peripheral nervous system, and as such can be very protective in the short term (Box 11.13).

Numerous cellular mechanisms contribute to the plasticity of the dorsal horn system.[16]

- Initially, dorsal horn cells show a progressive increase in activity to a train of constant stimuli, an event termed windup, which will cease when the stimulus ceases; this is dependent on the NMDA receptor activity.
- Prolonged exposure to the stimulus leads to the development of a classic form of central sensitization, where the heightened central neural response outlasts that of the peripheral stimulus by tens of minutes.
- High-frequency PAN stimulation of dorsal horn neurons, working through and dependent on the NMDA receptor, can result in a much longer-lasting response termed long-term potentiation (LTP); in fact, the duration of the response exceeds that of most experimental studies.
- Within the postsynaptic neurons, protein kinase activation with subsequent phosphorylation events can lead to the induction of numerous genes; this form of sensitization is referred to as *transcription-dependent* and can be very long lasting in nature.
- While the large projection neurons are undergoing an excitatory form of sensitization, their surrounding inhibitory neurons can also be changing activity characteristics.
- Long-term depression can occur in inhibitory interneurons located in the dorsal horn, resulting in reduced inhibition on the projection neurons and, thus, more information traveling upstream to the brain stem, thalamus, and cerebral cortex.
- Finally, two additional events can lead to a permanent form of sensitization: inhibitory cell loss[73] and rearrangement of synaptic connections.[72,74]

Central Sensitization and Secondary Hyperalgesia

Sensitization of dorsal horn neurons can alter their response properties, typically shifting the response versus stimulus intensity curve to the left.

- An additional prominent feature of sensitization is the expansion of the neuron's receptive field.
- The area involving the injury will develop a sensitivity termed *primary hyperalgesia*.
- Expansion of the cell's receptive field outside the area of immediate injury will contribute to the formation of *secondary hyperalgesia*.[75,76]

- In other words, noninjured tissue contiguous with the primary site of injury will develop increased sensitivity to mechanical stimuli.
- In addition to receptive field expansion, some dorsal horn neurons, particularly those driven by skeletal muscle afferent fibers, can develop new, noncontiguous receptive fields.[77]
- Irritation of the noncontiguous receptor fields results in the sensation of pain occurring outside of the area of primary and secondary hyperalgesia.[20,78]
- While the expansion of the receptive field contributes to the phenomena of secondary hyperalgesia, the development of new, noncontiguous receptive fields could contribute to the expression of either tender points or trigger points.

Central Sensitization and Glial Cell Activation

The classic notion is that a neuronal synaptic chain extends from periphery to cerebral cortex representing the pathways for processing nociception and generating the sensation of pain.

- However, recent evidence has forced a revisal of this concept to include other cells, such as glia, that can modify the information processing in the neuronal chain.[79]
- Glial cells form a matrix surrounding all dorsal horn neurons and central neurons in general.
- Multiple types of glia are present, but the ones most associated with immune responses are the astrocytes and microglia.
- In the dorsal horn (and to date only in this region), these two glial cell types express receptors for SP.
- Interaction with SP can activate these two forms of glia.
- Activated glial cells release proinflammatory cytokines such as tumor necrosis factor-α and interleukins 1 and 6.
- Although at this time it is not clear how proinflammatory cytokines work in the dorsal horn, it is certain that they contribute to increasing spinal facilitation and hyperalgesia.
- Activated glia also increase the production of NO and PGE2 in the dorsal horn; both substances are known to increase spinal facilitation and the resulting hyperalgesia.
- Interestingly, these glial cells also increase the release of SP from the central terminals of the PANs, thus creating another feed-forward loop in the interoceptive system pathways.
- Neurons in the dorsal horn have been demonstrated to express receptors for proinflammatory cytokines, and IL-1 is known to increase the influx of calcium ions through the NMDA receptor, thereby also increasing spinal facilitation.
- Thus, multiple factors occurring within the dorsal horn are combining to create plastic changes in the dorsal horn neurons.
- Finally, glial cell–neuron interaction can explain the formation of mirror-image pain, that is, pain that occurs contralateral to injured tissue[80] (Box 11.14).
- Spinal cord glial cells are interconnected with each other by gap junctions, thereby constructing a large and complex syncytial matrix that extends across the midline in the spinal cord.

> **BOX 11.14 PANs and Dorsal Horn Glial Cells**
>
> A relatively new finding suggests that dorsal horn glial cells, acting through the release of proinflammatory cytokines, play an important role in the sensitization of dorsal horn neurons and, possibly, in the development of some chronic pain patterns.

- Blocking the spread of information through these glial gap junctions prevents the development of mirror-image pain in experimental models.
- From all of this, it is clear that glia cell activity in the dorsal horn can rapidly modify the processing of nociceptive information and increase the sensation of pain.
- While protective in the short term, such a response, if uncontrolled, has the potential to fulminate and become part of a chronic problem.

PERMANENT CHANGE IN THE DORSAL HORN CIRCUITRY

All of the changes in dorsal horn circuitry discussed so far appear to be reversible; however, excessive PAN stimulation or peripheral nerve injury can also result in a permanent alteration in the dorsal horn; two irreversible mechanisms have been proposed.

- The smallest neurons in the dorsal horn, typically GABA-ergic neurons, appear to undergo an apoptotic cell death following excessive activation.[73]
- This loss of small neurons can be prevented by blocking the NMDA receptor in the dorsal horn.[81]
- Loss of these neurons would diminish the inhibition in the spinal cord circuitry, thus creating a more easily excited segment, possibly one that displays spontaneous activity.
- Although questionable, a second method of permanent change in the dorsal horn may involve the sprouting of A-beta afferent fibers following peripheral nerve injury.[82]
- The normal distribution of the A-beta afferent fibers is focused on the deeper layers of the dorsal horn.
- In animal models, following nerve injury, the terminals of the A-beta afferent fibers can be seen in the superficial layers replacing sites occupied typically by PANs.
- Both of the above alterations in the dorsal horn circuitry would create permanent change and could contribute to chronic pain scenarios.

Dorsal Horn Involvement in Modified Pain Presentation Patterns

DORSAL HORN ALTERATION IN CHRONIC PAIN STATES

Normal plasticity in the dorsal horn circuitry is necessary to insure adequate warning information and protective reflexes during the healing process (Box 11.15).

- To be protective, these changes have to occur rapidly; they typically involve numerous feed-forward events without an immediate set point, thus fitting the definition of an allostatic process.[49]

> **BOX 11.15 Dorsal Horn Neuroplasticity**
>
> Changes in dorsal horn circuitry involving the following may contribute to the development of chronic pain patterns:
>
> - Increased expression of receptors for neuropeptides
> - Expansion of neuronal receptive fields
> - Loss of inhibitory interneurons
> - Sprouting and expansion of afferent fiber terminal fields

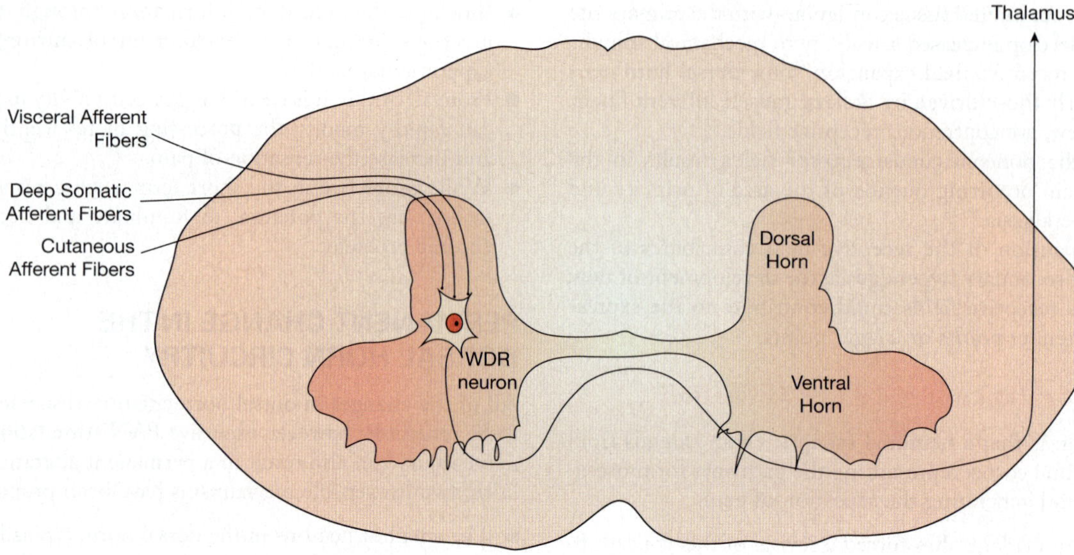

Figure 11.6. The convergence of PANs for cutaneous, deep somatic, and visceral sources on the WDR neurons in the dorsal horn of the spinal cord. Primary afferent fibers from visceral, deep somatic, and cutaneous sources are shown converging on a WDR neuron in the dorsal horn of the spinal cord. (Used with permission from the Willard/Carreiro Collection, University of New England.)

- However, excessive activation of the dorsal horn or inadequate control mechanisms (to be discussed below) can turn the normal plasticity into a pathologic response that leads to the development of a chronic pattern of abnormal neuronal activity, underlying the onset of chronic pain in the patient, recently this type of pain scenario has been termed **nociplastic pain**[83]
- Adaptive changes that can become pathologic include the:
  - ☐ Spread of neurons expressing receptors for SP[72]
  - ☐ Expansion of dorsal horn neuron receptive fields
  - ☐ Possible loss of GABA-ergic inhibitory interneurons
  - ☐ Possible sprouting of A-beta fibers into the superficial layer of the dorsal horn
- Thus, the chronic pain state can be considered as a failure of normal allostatic mechanisms leading to a pathologic condition, similar to other chronic stress-related diseases such as:
  - ☐ Depression[84,85]
  - ☐ Type 2 diabetes mellitus[86]
  - ☐ Cardiovascular disease[87]

CLINICAL EXPRESSIONS OF SENSITIZATION

Following the onset of central sensitization, the activity pattern of neurons in the dorsal horn is altered.

- Expanding receptive fields of dorsal horn neurons create a zone of increased sensitivity that surrounds the initial injury site, which is termed secondary hyperalgesia.
- Many dorsal horn neurons have axonal projections or at least collateral axons that terminate on ventral horn neurons.
- Sensitization of dorsal horn neurons can then alter the activity patterns of the large ventral horn alpha-motoneurons.[88,89]
- The ventral horn output can produce muscle spasms and, when prolonged, increased muscle tone and hyperreflexia akin to that seen in spasticity.
- Changes in muscle tone can result in the anatomic asymmetry seen in somatic dysfunction.
- Patients with this condition may feel pain but lack a peripheral lesion that can be identified as the causal factor for nociceptive pain and at the same time also lack any obvious damage to the nervous system that could result in neuropathic pain; these individuals now fall into the category of nociplastic pain, the result of plastic changes to the nociceptive system.[83,90]

Convergence of Visceral and Somatic Input in the Dorsal Horn

Visceral afferent fibers from thoracoabdominal and pelvic organs enter the spinal cord through the dorsal root and terminate in the lateral aspect of the deep dorsal horn (Fig. 11.6; also, see Chapter 13 Somatic Dysfunction, Spinal Facilitation, and Viscerosomatic Integration).

- Visceral PAN input overlaps with the somatic PAN input, and many cells in the dorsal horn can be driven by both visceral and somatic inputs.[91,92]
- In fact, it appears that all dorsal horn neurons that receive visceral inputs also receive somatic input.[93,94]
- Somatic input can sensitize dorsal horn neurons eliciting specific reflexes.
- Subsequent visceral input can activate the previously facilitated circuit, eliciting a similar pain pattern and some of the same reflexes.
- The reverse situation is also often seen clinically, as pointed out by Sir Henry Head many years ago[95]: that is, visceral input first sensitizes the dorsal horn circuitry and subsequent somatic injury elicits the previous visceral pain pattern and its associated reflexes.[96]

Influence of Primary Afferent Fibers along the Spinal Cord

As PANs enter the spinal cord through the dorsal root entry zone, they undergo a trifurcation.

- Typically, one branch innervates the dorsal horn at the segment of entry, of the two other branches, one ascends and the other descends along the dorsal margin of the dorsal horn in a bundle of fibers termed Lissauer tract.[97]

- Older diagrams of PAN termination clearly indicated this branching pattern,[98] although it has been removed from most modern text for simplification.
- The division of the PAN is important since it can result in the spreading of nociceptive information up and down the spinal cord to reach distant segmental levels.
- It is unclear how far this information can spread. Cutaneous PANs spread out at least two to three segments within the spinal cord, while visceral PANs have reported distributions involving greater than five segments[99]; however, even greater distances are possible.[100]
- The three-dimensional distribution of PAN information in the spinal cord allows for the interpretation of otherwise confusing pain patterns.
- For example, a patient could have an existing area of spinal facilitation in the midthoracic region consequent to a remote disease process, such as an inflamed gallbladder.
- A recent revival of this old pain pattern, despite the prior removal of the gallbladder, could indicate the new onset of another disease process such as myocardial ischemia or gastric ulcer.
- The visceral PANs from the myocardium or the stomach enter the spinal cord in the upper thoracic region.
- Early in the disease processes, their input may be present in lower thoracic segments due to segmental spread of afferent input, but below the threshold of detection by the patient.
- However, spread of neural activity in the inferior direction could subsequently activate the portion of the spinal cord originally sensitized by the remote history of gallbladder disease.
- The patient perceives the gallbladder-associated pain pattern; however, this time, the etiology of the nociception lies in the myocardium and not in the gallbladder.
- In general, the recent and otherwise unexplained revival of an old pain pattern should be considered the harbinger of new disease until proven otherwise.

The Dorsal Horn and Dorsal Root Reflexes (DRRs)

Normally, the dorsal root is considered as a strictly afferent system, carrying action potentials from the peripheral tissue into the spinal cord only.

- However, it is now known that under appropriate conditions, the dorsal root can act as an efferent pathway from the spinal cord.
- When this type of antidromic activity occurs in an intact sensory nerve, it has been termed a **dorsal root reflex**.[101]

Centrifugally conducted activity on dorsal rootlets has been known since the late 19th century but was not really examined in detail until the middle of the 20th century.[102]

- Dorsal root reflexes are present in both large myelinated and in small myelinated and unmyelinated fibers (see Willis[102] for a discussion of the difficulties in recording DRRs from the smallest fibers).
- This review will focus on those reflexes present in the small fibers, such as PANs.

To trigger these reflexes in PANs, the initial input stimulus to the spinal cord must be in the range required to activate the PANs (C-fiber range).

BOX 11.16 Dorsal Root Reflexes

Intense PAN input to the spinal cord can result in widespread depolarization and the activation of surrounding central terminals of other PANs, a process termed "dorsal root reflex."

The antidromic conduction of an action potential into the peripheral process of a PAN can result in the release of neuropeptides and the initiation of a neurogenic inflammatory process in otherwise normal tissue.

Such a mechanism could account for "cross-sensitization," whereby disease in one organ influences the function of surrounding organs.[115,162]

- When such an afferent barrage reaches the dorsal horn, a wave of depolarization, termed primary afferent depolarization (PAD), occurs and spreads both upward and downward for several segments in the dorsal horn of the spinal cord.
- Interestingly, dorsal horn depolarization is facilitated by central sensitization of dorsal horn neurons; thus, past experience involving intense PAN activation can influence the magnitude of this depolarization event.
- When an area of the dorsal horn depolarizes, the central terminals of surrounding primary afferent fibers contained within this area also depolarize.
- This mechanism is most likely a spin-off event of presynaptic inhibition.
- It is known to involve GABA-a receptors and GABA released by local interneurons and is influenced by serotonin receptors.[103]
- Significant depolarization of the central terminals of primary afferent fibers can result in the generation of action potentials within these fibers that move antidromically (outward) to invade the peripheral terminals of this PAN (Box 11.16).
- The resulting antidromic output from the dorsal horn can be recorded as a compound action potential, termed dorsal root potential (DRP) on adjacent dorsal rootlets.
- Truncating these adjacent rootlet does not affect the DRP, thus the activity is generated from within the spinal cord.
- In the peripheral terminals of these PANs, the antidromic action potentials act similar to those involved in a classic axon reflex.
- In this reflex, injury to tissue that depolarizes a branch of an axon will spread to all branches of the axon resulting in the release of proinflammatory substances outside the bounds of the primary injury.
- The clinical manifestation of the classic axon reflex is the erythematous wheal of swollen tissue surrounding the primary injury.
- Similarly, the DRP triggers a dorsal root reflex that results in the release of neuropeptides into the peripheral tissue (Fig. 11.7), thus either initiating or exacerbating an inflammatory reaction.
- Antidromic activity over dorsal roots (dorsal root reflex) can occur both ipsilateral and contralateral to the input root.[104]
- Dorsal root reflexes have been demonstrated to play a significant role in the spread of **neurogenic inflammation**.[105]
- Finally, recent studies have revealed that dorsal root reflexes can be enhanced by stimulation of the periaqueductal gray region of the midbrain[106]; this finding has significant implications with respect to the generation of diffuse pain patterns and will be reconsidered in the section on descending pain control mechanisms.

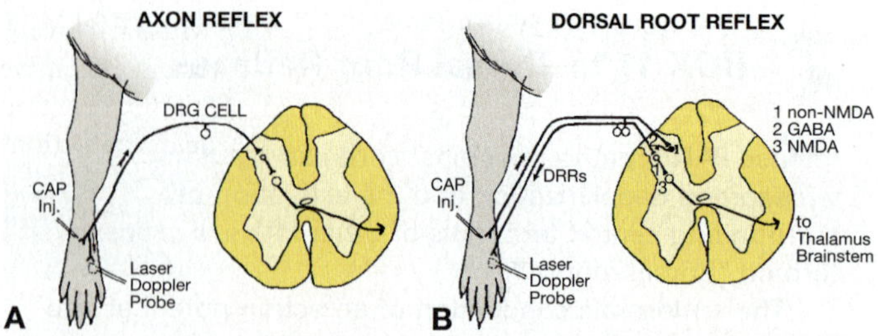

Figure 11.7. Comparison of an axon reflex to a dorsal root reflex. A. Diagram of an axon reflex. **B.** Diagram of a dorsal root reflex. Note that the dorsal root reflex simply involves the conduction of an action potential to the spinal cord, depolarization of surrounding fibers in the dorsal horn, and the conduction of an action potential out to the periphery on a depolarized sensory fiber. (Reprinted by permission from Springer: Willis WD Jr. Dorsal root potentials and dorsal root reflexes: a double-edged sword. *Exp Brain Res.* 1999;124(4):395–421. Copyright © 1999 Springer-Verlag Berlin Heidelberg.)

ASCENDING PATHWAYS INVOLVED IN THE PERCEPTION OF PAIN

The Anterolateral System in the Spinal Cord and Brain Stem

Neuronal activity in the dorsal horn is projected upstream to the brain stem and thalamus, via dorsal horn neurons with long ascending axons (Fig. 11.8).

- These projection neurons, arising mainly in laminae I, IV to V, and VII to VIII in the dorsal horn, send their axons contralaterally to reach the anterior and lateral quadrant of the spinal cord.[107]
- Most of the projection neurons represent either nociceptive-specific cells located in lamina I or WDR cells located in the deeper laminae of the dorsal horn.
- Axons from these neurons leave the dorsal horn to ascend diagonally, crossing the midline of the spinal cord in the anterior white commissure.
- The tract formed by these axons has been termed the anterolateral system (ALS).
- Within the ALS, axons are arranged such that the cervical fibers are positioned most medially and the sacral fibers are most laterally.
- Also, anterolateral segregation of axons occurs within the tract, such that:
  - The anterior portion of the ALS contains fibers activated by light touch.
  - The lateral portions of the ALS contain more of the pain and temperature-responsive fibers.
- Finally, based on target site, two basic components of the anterolateral system can be identified:
  - The spinoreticular tracts—targeting the reticular formation of the brain stem
  - The spinothalamic tracts—targeting the thalamus

Spinoreticular Tracts

The spinoreticular fibers arise from neurons located in the dorsal horn and terminate in nuclei of the medulla, pons, and midbrain.

- Specific sites targeted by the spinoreticular fibers include the:
  - Catecholamine cell groups (A1 to A7)
  - Subnucleus reticularis dorsalis

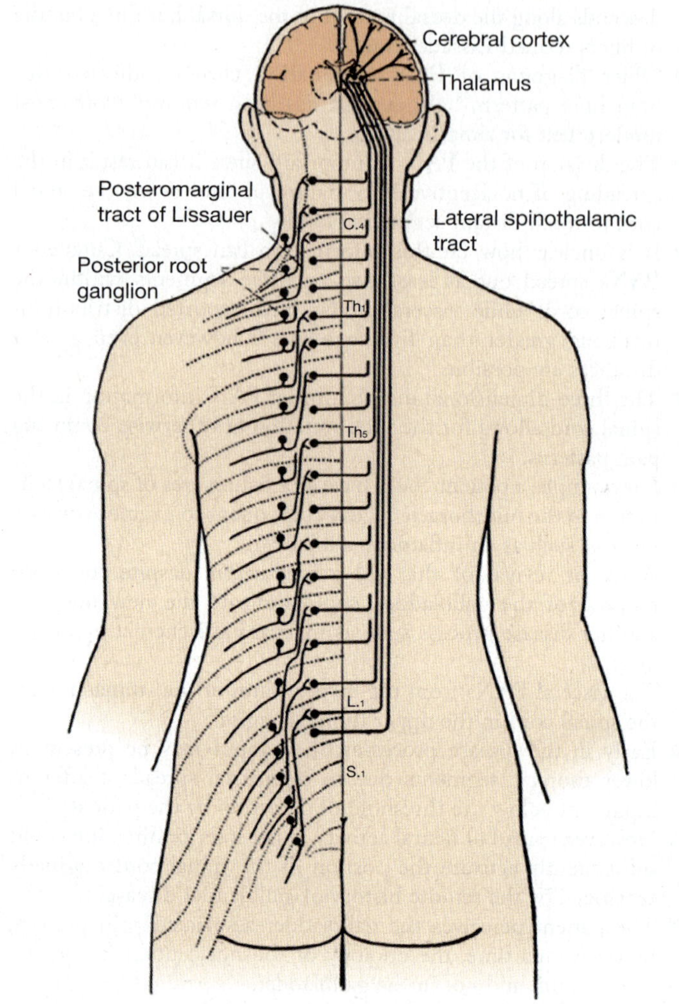

Figure 11.8. Anterolateral system of the spinal cord. The entry of spinal nerves is shown on the left with their synapse on a dorsal horn neuron. The spinothalamic axons arise in the dorsal horn, decussate over the midline, and ascend to the brain stem and thalamus in the anterolateral tract, also termed spinothalamic tract. (Modified with permission from Larsell O. *Anatomy of the Nervous System.* 2nd ed. Appleton-Century Crofts, Inc.; 1951:244. Figure 205. Copyright © 1951 Appleton-Century Crofts, Inc.)

  - Ventrolateral medulla
  - Parabrachial nucleus
  - Periaqueductal gray
  - Anterior pretectal area[107,108]
- Since these areas are thought to regulate much of the descending brain stem–spinal cord projections, they therefore could play a significant role in the modulation of pain.
- It is also known that most of these regions play a significant role in central control of the autonomic nervous system[109]; thus, ascending activity of nociceptive origin in the spinoreticular tracts can trigger changes in peripheral autonomic functions such as increased heart rate or blood pressure.
- Of these two tracts contained within the anterolateral system, the spinoreticular appears to have the most direct role in regulating the arousal system of the brain stem, however, collateral branches from the spinothalamic tract axons may also be involved.

Spinothalamic Tract

Axons from dorsal horn neurons project to the thalamus forming the spinothalamic tract, in its ascent, the spinothalamic fibers course along with spinoreticular axons that target the brainstem, in a quadrant of the spinal white matter termed the anterolateral system.

- In fact, some of the brain stem terminals can be collateral branches of the spinothalamic fibers.
- Spinothalamic axons located in the lateral most portion of the ALS tend to be most responsive to noxious and thermal stimuli.
- At the rostral end of the spinothalamic tract, a division occurs; the larger fibers in the tract remain laterally positioned to enter the thalamus, terminating in the vicinity of the ventroposterior and ventromedial thalamic nuclei, while the finer fibers in the tract segregate and enter the medial thalamus and terminate in the intralaminar nuclei.
- This arrangement underlies the creation of medial and lateral pain systems in the thalamus.[110]
- Many of the ascending fibers entering the medial thalamus appear to be of brain stem origin rather than of spinal cord origin.
- In general, the lateral pain system is thought to be a phylogenetically newer system involved more with localization of the noxious stimulus, while the medial system is an older system more likely involved in arousal and affectation of event.[111]

Thalamic Representation of Pain

Until this point, the chapter has been focused on a nociceptive system, that is, a system that can generate a signal in response to tissue-damaging or potentially tissue-damaging energy.

- At the level of the thalamus, a transition occurs; a strictly nociceptive system no longer exists, having become a system that can precipitate the uncomfortable feeling of pain and its associated emotions, such as anxiety and depression.
- Neural activity below the thalamus can occur without perception of pain, resulting in reflexes as well as certain defensive behaviors; however, the thalamus and cerebral cortex function as a unit and it is at the level of the thalamocortical connections that perception of pain is initiated.
- While the spinal cord and brain stem can initiate primitive, withdrawal-type reflexes to nociceptive stimuli, the thalamocortical system is required to initiate more elaborate evasive movements, along with the complicated psychological responses to painful situations.

The thalamus is a major target for ascending information from the spinal cord and brain stem to the cerebral cortex.

- As mentioned, two pain systems, medial and lateral, can be identified in the thalamus, separated from each other anatomically and having differing functions[110,112–116]; also, see Figure 11.9.
- From the thalamus, projections that are responsive to nociception radiate to numerous areas of the cerebral cortex such as the insular cortex (IC), cingulate cortex, and sensorimotor cortices as well as to subcortical regions such as the amygdala. In this way an elaborate "pain connectome" is established in the forebrain.

Lateral Thalamic Pain System

The spinothalamic tract (also termed the neospinothalamic tract) innervates laterally and ventrally positioned nuclei of the thalamus, including the:

- ☐ Ventroposterior lateral nucleus
- ☐ Ventromedial nucleus
- ☐ Portions of the posterior nuclear group
- ☐ Portions of the ventrolateral nucleus (Fig. 11.9)

- These structures rapidly relay information to the somatic sensory and insular cortex and play a role in localizing the qualities and intensity of pain perception.[117]

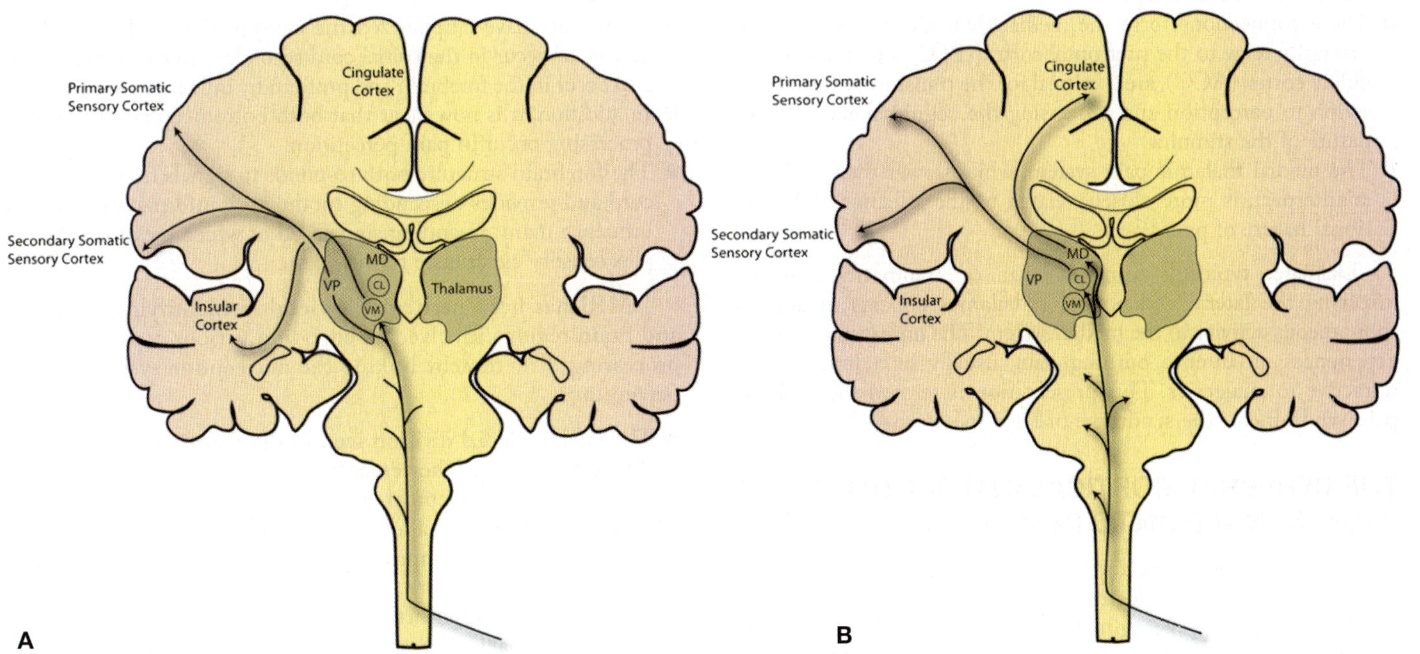

Figure 11.9. The ascending nociceptive systems in the thalamus. A. This figure demonstrates the projection of spinothalamic axons to the ventroposterior (ventral caudal) and ventromedial nuclei of the lateral thalamus and their relationship with primary and secondary somatic sensory cortex and in the insular cortex. **B.** Other spinothalamic and spinoreticulothalamic axons terminate in the central lateral and dorsomedial nuclei of the medial thalamus. Their cortical representation involves the cingulated cortex as well as the major somatic sensory areas.

BOX 11.17 Ascending Pathways for Nociception

There are two fundamental ascending systems involved in the processing of nociceptive information:

1. A phylogenetically new lateral system composed of neospinothalamic fibers that localizes the site of nociceptive activity.
2. An older medial system, composed of both paleospinothalamic and spinoreticular fibers that initiates the affective nature of the nociceptive event and triggers the autonomic and endocrine responses.

- In one published case of a patient with a lesion involving the postcentral gyrus of the cerebral cortex (a significant target of the lateral pain system of the thalamus), the individual lost the ability to accurately localize painful stimuli, but retained the ability to experience the affective nature of the pain.[118]

Medial Thalamic Pain System

The medial fibers of the spinothalamic tract (often termed the paleospinothalamic fibers) enter the thalamus medially (see Fig. 11.9) to innervate the:

- ☐ Centromedian nucleus
- ☐ Centrolateral nucleus
- ☐ Dorsomedial nucleus
- ☐ Nucleus submedius
- ☐ Intralaminar nuclei[114]
- ☐ Paraventricular nucleus (in the hypothalamus) (Box 11.17)

- Included in this ascending system would be projections from lower brain stem areas that have themselves been innervated by the spinoreticular axons.
- These connections form the medial thalamic pain system and primarily relay to the prefrontal cortex (PFC) and anterior cingulate cortex (ACC), areas critical for the transformation of sensation to perception and processing the cognitive and affective nature of the stimulus.
- The medial thalamic pain system, while slower than its lateral counterpart, is more closely related to the affective and emotional nature of pain.[111]

Damage, typically from vascular or traumatic accidents, involving the lateral and posterior thalamus appears to unmask spontaneous activity in the medial system. The unfortunate patient experiences an intense burning pain, usually in a limb, that is refractive to analgesics. This presentation is termed the thalamic pain syndrome or the syndrome of Dejerine–Roussy.[119]

THE CEREBRAL CORTICAL INTERACTIONS: FROM SENSATION TO PERCEPTION

An understanding of the forebrain's role in pain processing was limited to animal and electrophysiologic studies, until sophisticated human brain imaging methodologies were refined and complex meta-analysis of study results were performed.[120,121]

- Appreciation of brain involvement in pain perception was also slowed by the state of physiology at the turn of the century,[122] which questioned the participation of the cerebral cortex in human pain perception.
- In fact, in the 1970s, Ronald Melzack even proclaimed at one point that neuroscientists were "scooping out the brain" and ignoring the fact that a person could have, for example, a pain in their foot and not have a foot as illustrated with phantom limb pain.[123]

Fortunately, there has been a flood of refined scientific data that have visualized the brain in processing nociception.[124,125]

- These studies were driven by recent technologies such as:
  - ☐ Positron emission PET scan
  - ☐ Functional MRI (fMRI)
  - ☐ Single-photon computed tomography (SPECT)
  - ☐ Magnetoencephalography (MEG)
  - ☐ Electroencephalography (EEG)
- The listed studies measure such factors as:
  - ☐ Perfusion
  - ☐ Metabolism
  - ☐ Glucose
  - ☐ Oxygen utilization
- The resulting data explain how a painful experience can occur in the forebrain without a concurrent primary nociceptive input in the peripheral nerve such as in the foot.[113,126–128]
- The shift in mindset that considers pain that is unrelated to or out of proportion with the nociceptive stimulus as being a disease state, rather than a symptom, has accelerated treatment paradigms.
- When examining a patient with a chronic pain pattern, it is now necessary to consider the whole person and their environment, rather than just the presenting signs and symptoms; this is an approach that is quite consistent with the osteopathic philosophy.

With the brain now available for direct examination with sophisticated imaging, there has been a virtual revolution in accessing the role of forebrain structures in the formulation of a neural matrix used in the perception of pain.[125,129,130]

- These data have emphasized the concept that facilitation, long known to occur in the spinal cord secondary to tissue injury, can also occur in the forebrain and profoundly influence perception.[120]
- In addition, it is now clear that both bottom-up and top-down processing occur in pain perception.
- The forebrain structure both responds to signals from the spinal cord and provides descending modulatory information that can influence many ascending signals, all of which creates the complex sensory experience termed pain.

fMRI has been particularly useful in identifying pathways and brain regions involved in encoding various aspects of pain processing,[121,131] thereby linking the nociception system to pain perception.

- The lateral–medial division seen in the thalamus is reflected in the organization of the cerebrum.
- The lateral component of the nociceptive pathway is involved in pain localization and in recording pain intensity, while the medial system appears to encode the more emotional–motivational component.
- This latter system is further tempered by powerful escape and avoidance behaviors,[132] sculpting the biopsychosocial modulation of pain.
- Pain is a conscious perception and an emergent property of a complex array of connections, termed a *connectome*, through which the brain transforms a nociceptive input into a disagreeable perception.[110,133,134]

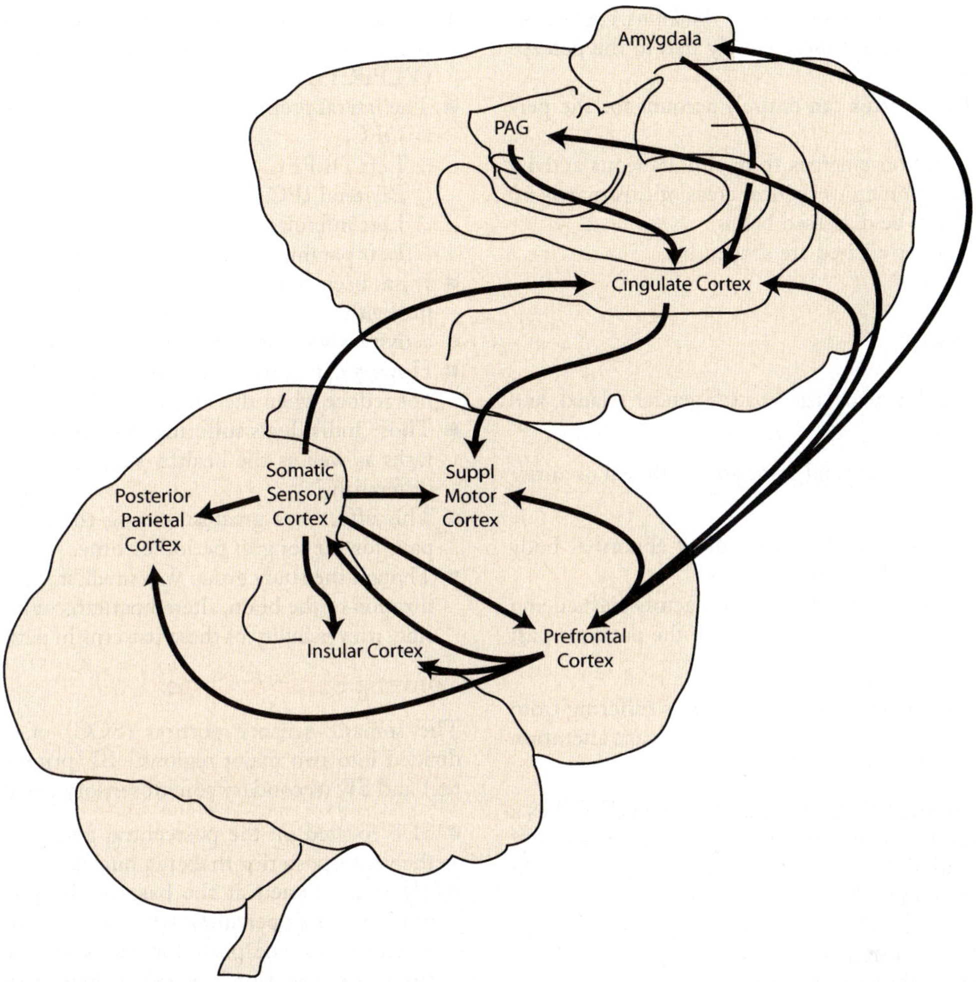

Figure 11.10. Cerebral cortical interactions. Numerous regions of the cerebral cortex are interconnected and function to process nociceptive information. From this matrix emerges our complex feelings of pain. (Used with permission from the Willard/Carreiro Collection, University of New England.)

- Based on functional imaging studies, the areas involved with the pain connectome include the:
  - Somatic sensory cortex
  - Insula
  - ACC
  - PFC
  - Amygdala (Fig. 11.10)
- Use of the term connectome implies that there are a myriad of possible connections on the cerebral cortex that can give rise to the emergent feeling of discomfort termed pain, as opposed to only one specific combination of connections.
- The ability to follow changes in cortical activity over time has allowed the analysis of cerebral mechanisms in the processing of nociceptive signs and given rise to the concept of a Dynamic Pain Connectome.[131]

Cortical level activity does appear to be related to pain perception.

- Coghill and coworkers found a significant correlation between the intensity of the patient's feelings of pain and the amount of cortical activity detectable with functional imaging[135] (Box 11.18).
- Specifically, the neural activity was present primarily in the somatic sensory cortex, ACC, and PFC.

BOX 11.18 The Pain Connectome

There is no one locus in the cerebral cortex that is responsible for the perception of pain.

Instead, there exists a complex, parallel distributed network, termed the pain connectome, involving numerous regions of the cortex that contribute to the perception of pain.

The general forebrain areas involved in this connectome include region such as the:

- Somatic sensory cortex
- IC
- Parietal cortex
- PFC
- Amygdala
- Hippocampal formation
- Thalamus and basal ganglia

Evidence of altered brain structure and function in chronic pain patients has been detected with functional imaging studies.

- A similar correlation was not found in the thalamus, suggesting that cortical level processing is more closely tied to the perception of pain.
- No one portion of the cortex can entirely account for the perception of pain.
- Conversely, the perception emerges from simultaneous activity and the interaction of numerous cortical areas of this matrix.[3]
- Each of these areas will be discussed below.
- The behavioral responses elicited are shaped by:
  - Previous learning
  - Stress levels
  - Attention and arousal
  - Memories
  - Cognitive, emotional, genetic, age-related, gender-related, and sociocultural factors

Pain is inherently unpleasant and associated with real or anticipated tissue damage.

- Its presentation can be masked in a cloud of abnormal body function, chronic pain, and suffering.
- What has become very clear is that many factors influencing the pain experience are centrally mediated by the patient's past experiences.

Recent studies raise the possibility that patients suffering from chronic pain scenarios may have undergone a significant alteration in the base mechanism of brain function.

- In 2001, Raichle proposed a default mode network (DMN) as a means of understanding the baseline activity of the cerebrum.[136]
- The DMN represents the resting state of connected activity in representative cortical and subcortical structures.
- These structures show basal activity when the person is conscious and relaxed, not focused on any one thing.
- The activity of the DMN is typically greatest at rest and decreases during cognitive processing.
- Using fMRI, blood oxygen level–dependent (BOLD) analysis and *f*unctional *c*onnectivity MRI (fc-MRI), signal fluctuations of various regions of interest and their temporal relationship are being explored.[137]
  - In areas of increased neuronal activity, oxygen consumption is also increased which in turn triggers increased perfusion.
  - The oxygen content in the activated regions actually increases due to the strong increase in perfusion.
  - The effect of increased perfusion is so strong that the oxygen content increases in spite of metabolic deoxygenation induced by elevated neuronal activity.
  - Recent evidence suggests that BOLD imaging is dependent on a neuronal-astrocyte-vascular pathway exists, coupled by calcium signaling.[138]

The default mode network includes prominently the structures of the posterior cingulate cortex (PCC) and the ventral–anterior cingulate cortex (ACC). In addition, the ventromedial prefrontal cortex (VMPFC) and the left inferior parietal cortex (LIPC) are involved.

- The ventral ACC is linked to limbic and subcortical structures of the orbitofrontal cortex (OFC), nucleus accumbens, hypothalamus, and midbrain.
- These connections represent an emotional-affective functional link in the brain.
- The PCC is mainly related to cortical structures that suggest a role in consciousness.
- These areas all show a decrease in activity on fMRI, in healthy subjects, when they are asked to perform a simple task.
- At the same time, with task performance, attention, and cognition, there is an increase in activity in the ventrolateral prefrontal cortex (VLPFC) and in the dorsolateral prefrontal cortex (DLPFC).
- The lateral prefrontal regions include the:
  - OFC
  - Left DLPFC
  - Bilateral IPC
  - Left inferolateral temporal cortex
  - Left parahippocampal gyrus (PHG)[139]
- It has been confirmed with fMRI that the DMN activity at rest in healthy subjects reveals an equilibrium that shows a decrease in activity when they are asked to pay attention or perform a task.[140]
- However, in chronic back pain subjects, the DMN activity does not reduce when the subjects are asked to perform simple tasks.
- Those individuals suffering from pain were able to perform the tasks as well as the healthy subjects, but they used their brains differently.
- This effect was greatest among the patients who had been in pain for the longest period of time.
- Though the study group was small, it suggests functional reorganization of the brain, altered patterns of brain activity, and a possibly irreversibility of these patterns in patients with chronic pain.

Somatic Sensory Cortex

The somatic sensory portion (SCC) of the cerebral cortex is divided into two major regions—SI (primary somatosensory cortex) and SII (secondary somatosensory cortex) (Fig. 11.11).

- SI is located on the postcentral gyrus and receives input from the ventroposterior thalamic nuclei.
- SII is positioned at the base of the postcentral gyrus, wrapping over the operculum (the cortex adjacent to the insula) and reaching into the posterior insula lobe. It receives input from the ventroposterior inferior nucleus, a small thalamic nucleus closely related to the VP complex.[141]
- SI has a high-fidelity representation of the contralateral body, while SII contains a less well-defined representation of the body bilaterally.[69,142]
- Although considerable question has existed in the older literature as to how much, if any, nociception is represented in the somatic sensory cortex, functional mapping studies have shed much light on this situation.[139]
- SI appears to be involved in the localized discrimination of a painful stimulus.

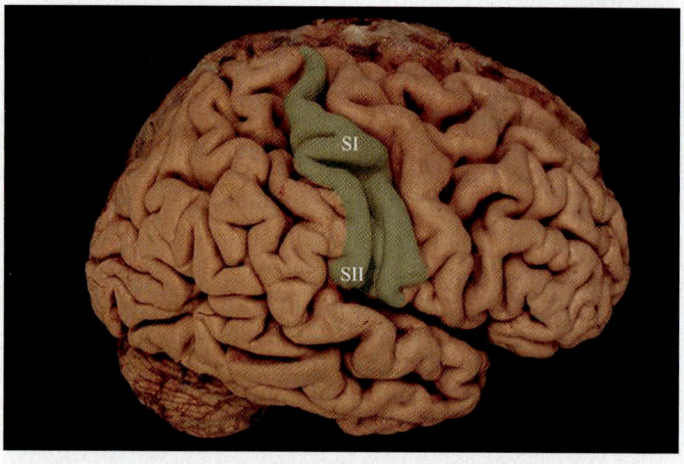

Figure 11.11. Areas I and II of the somatic sensory cortex. (Used with permission from the Willard/Carreiro Collection, University of New England.)

- At least one carefully documented case of a parietal stroke involving SI in a human diminished the patient's ability to localize a painful stimulus, but left him with a strong unpleasant feel induced by the stimulus.[118]

Visceral sensory information is also represented on the surface of the parietal cortex.

- Visceral afferent fibers from the thoracic and upper lumbar spinal cord ascend in the dorsal columns to reach the ventral and medial thalamic nuclei, from which they are relayed to both SI and SII cortices.
- Although SI can be activated by some noxious visceral stimuli, SII appears to function as a primary cortex for a variety of visceral sensory information.
- From SII, connections are established with the ACC and the IC.
- Ramping up the delivery of visceral noxious stimuli will result in the spread of the activation outward, from SII, into the region of the anterior cingulate and insular areas.
- Thus, SII has been depicted as a gateway into the paralimbic regions of the cortex.
- The differential processing between visceral and somatic nociceptive stimuli at the cortical level may underlie the difference in feeling that characterizes visceral and somatic pains.[139]

Insular Cortex (IC)

Located in the depths of the lateral sulcus, between the frontoparietal cortex above and the temporal cortex below (Fig. 11.12), the insula is a major area in the cortical pain connectome.[143]

- This region of cortex receives thalamic projections from the ventromedial nucleus and posterior nuclei,[141] areas that are innervated by the spinothalamic tract (reviewed in Craig[144]).
- The insula also receives cortical projections from adjacent somatic sensory areas.
- In primates, SI and SII project to the anterior and posterior portions of the insula.[145]
- The same regions of IC that receive pain-related projections feed this information into the limbic forebrain, including such structures as the:
  - □ Hypothalamus
  - □ Amygdala
  - □ ACC
  - □ Medial PFC[146,147]

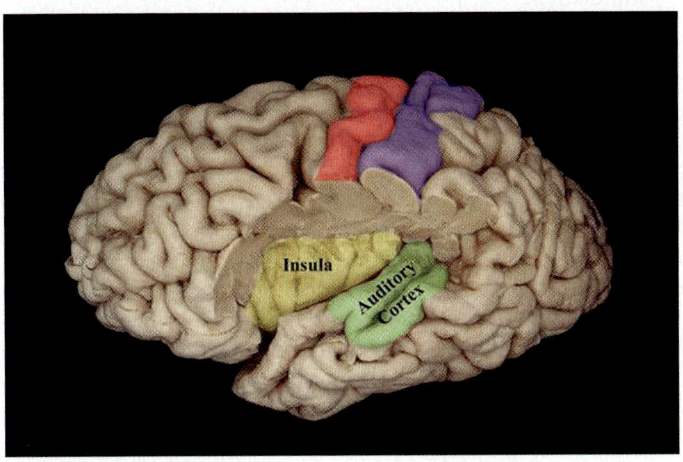

Figure 11.12. The insular cortex. (Used with permission from the Willard/Carreiro Collection, University of New England.)

Recent findings concerning the connectivity of the insula have demonstrated that:

- The anterior portions of the insula project to limbic and paralimbic forebrain regions as well as to the inferior frontal gyrus.
- The posterior portion of the insula projects to the parietal and temporal cortex.[149]

Finally, the insula also has descending projections to the brain stem, through which it exerts control over aspects of the autonomic nervous system[147] and appears to regulate the descending pain control systems.

- Studies have documented the presence of opioids such as dynorphin and enkephalin in the IC and suggested a role for these opioid systems in the generation of cortically mediated analgesia.[150]

The IC activity is anatomically heterogeneous,[151] and processing in its posterior portion may be more related to sensory aspects of pain.

- The anterior IC is anatomically more continuous with PFC, and as a result, it may be more important in the emotional, cognitive, and memory-related aspects of pain perception.
- One possible interpretation of this neurologic arrangement is that the insula, working through the autonomic nervous system, helps to orchestrate physiologic response to pain, including pain control or enhancement depending on the situation.[146]
- Interestingly, disruption of the deep white matter at the caudal border of the insula can produce an intense central pain, similar in quality to thalamic pain, an event termed pseudothalamic pain syndrome.[152]
- Conversely, a tumor compressing the posterior aspect of the insula altered tactile perception and the perception of mechanical and thermal pain by raising pain thresholds.[153]
- Finally, damage to the insula, or disconnection of the somatic sensory areas of parietal cortex from the insula, has been proposed as the mechanism for the presentation of asymbolia for pain[154] (Box 11.19).
- In asymbolia, patients can localize the painful stimulus but do not experience the normal emotional or affective nature of the pain.
- In this state, it is proposed that the link between the somatic sensory system and the limbic system has been interrupted.

Besides interoceptive (somatic and visceral) input (containing information concerning tissue chemistry), the insula also is the target of olfactory, gustatory, and vestibular information[155] and has been thought of as forming a chemical map of the body (Box 11.20).

BOX 11.19 Asymbolia and the Insular Cortex

Asymbolia is a postinjury state in which patients can still sense and localize pain, but the pain does not have the expected emotional or affective quality.

Recent evidence has related asymbolia to lesions of the insular cortex. The posterior region of the insula is involved in pain intensity and localization while the anterior portion is innvolved in emotional mediation. Lesions of the insular cortex have been demonstrated to produce asymbolia. These findings support the concept that localization of pain and emotional responses to pain are processed in different regions of the forebrain.[148]

BOX 11.20 The Interoceptive System

Interoception is a termed coined by Sherrington in the early part of the last century, to indicate an awareness of the condition of one's body tissues: a system that detects the state of homeostasis in one's own body.

More recently, the pathways involved in interoception have become better understood.[144] Typically, these pathways begin with C-fiber axons and involve the:

- Dorsal horn
- Anterolateral system of ascending tracts
- Components of the reticular formation of the brain stem
- Specific thalamic nuclei
- Portions of the IC

In essence, what is often described as a "pain pathway system" is in fact a subset of the interoceptive system that develops a state of "feeling" for the body tissue, the sensing of body-related afferent information. Pain, therefore, represents the extreme feeling related to abnormal tissue homeostasis; possibly in the other direction, a euphoric feeling may represent normal or well-balanced tissue homeostasis.[157,158,159]

- Studies suggest that the anterior IC plays a significant role in forming a short-term memory of an acute pain[156] and possibly in integrating the response into a balanced homeostatic mechanism.
- Thus, the insula could be pooling a wide range of information concerning the condition of tissues in the body and integrating this information into the limbic system as well as regulating autonomic response patterns.[110]
- To this extent, the main function of IC has been described as a "cortical hub," receiving and integrating external and internal signals as well as cognitive activity, assigning a salience to the information, and directing output to behavioral streams that can modulate the autonomic nervous system, attention, and cognitive processing thereby regulating homeostasis.[149]

Anterior Cingulate Cortex (ACC)

A common feature of almost all studies that use functional imaging to examine the cerebral processing of pain is the engagement of ACC.

- The ACC is traditionally considered part of the limbic system and, as such, is located on the medial aspect of the cerebral hemisphere, wrapped around the genu of the corpus callosum (Fig. 11.13).
- A major afferent contribution to the ACC arises in the dorsomedial nucleus of the thalamus and constitutes a significant portion of the medial pain system.
- Other contributions arise in the intralaminar nuclei of the thalamus and, thus, also involve the medial thalamic pain system.

Activation of the ACC has been repeatedly reported in PET studies of somatic or visceral pain and is linked to the emotional response to pain.[160,161]

- Lesions of the ACC do not destroy the ability to perceive or localize acute pain or reduce pain-related behaviors; however, they do blunt the affective nature of the pain.[110,162,163]

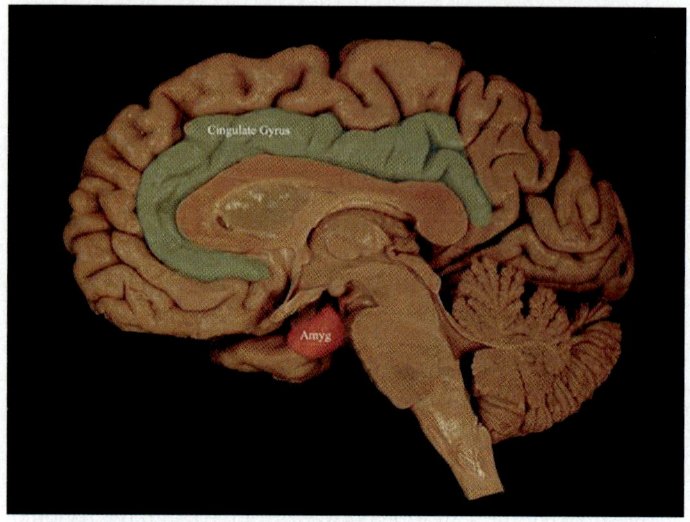

Figure 11.13. The cingulate cortex and the amygdala. (Used with permission from the Willard/Carreiro Collection, University of New England.)

The ACC is also associated with the anticipatory emotional aspects of pain.[111,164]

- Anticipation can be a particular problem for patients with chronic pain, because such patients are already in varying degrees of distress.
- Researchers have used imaging techniques to characterize brain activation related to the intensity of expected pain and experienced pain, finding that pain-related brain activation partially overlapped with expectation-related activation, in regions including anterior insular cortex and the ACC.[165]
- The ACC is not only involved in the actual perception of pain but also in imagined pain experience and in the (empathic) observation of another human receiving a painful stimulus.[166]
- When expected pain decreased, activation in this portion of the cerebral cortex also diminished.

The relationship between activity in the ACC and the anticipation and expectation of pain feelings is very strong.

- Anticipation and expectation have a powerful influence on the eventual perception of pain.
- Directing attention away from a painful stimulus is known to reduce the perceived pain intensity and results in decreased activation of ACC subregions responsive to painful stimulation.[167,168]
- The placebo response in pain seems to be mediated, at least in part, by the ACC,[164,169] as does the response to hypnosis[113,170] and numerous other pain distracting techniques.

The feeling of pain can be acquired or enhanced through the conditioned process of operant learning, possibly involving processing in the ACC.

- In some instances, for example, individuals might receive positive reinforcement for the expressions of pain.
- In studies of patients with chronic back pain who were given a painful electrical stimulation, those with a "solicitous" spouse present had an exacerbated pain response compared with those in the company of a nonsolicitous spouse.
- Imaging showed that the brain of patients with a solicitous spouse had increased activity in the ACC.[171]

Anticipation of pain can lead to the development of avoidance pain behaviors.[172]

- Animal studies have strongly indicated the ACC in mediating escape–avoidance behavior associated with painful stimuli.[173]
- These behavioral patterns represent powerful reflexive activity initiated in an attempt to minimize or avoid triggering a painful pattern.
- Such behaviors can also be learned, are fairly automatic, and are not always in the patient's conscious awareness.

The anticipation of pain can cause patients to avoid movement, tense muscles, or move in aberrant patterns, thereby disrupting mechanisms for posture and balance.

- These biomechanical imbalances may:
  - □ Affect dynamic function
  - □ Increase energy expenditure
  - □ Alter proprioception
  - □ Change joint structure
  - □ Impede neurovascular function
  - □ Alter metabolism
- Osteopathic manipulative treatment can be employed to not only restore posture and function but to also reduce fear of movement and the experience of anticipatory pain.

Prefrontal Cortex (PFC)

It has been known since the early 1990s that pain is represented in multiple areas of the cerebral cortex and that these areas included portions of the PFC.[174]

- In humans, the PFC is formed by the very prominent rostral pole of the frontal lobe (Fig. 11.14).
- This region of the frontal cortex receives extensive afferent projections from the medial thalamus including the rostral portion of the large dorsomedial nucleus; however, unlike the other regions involved in the processing of pain, the PFC does not receive input from any portion of a thalamic nucleus known to receive ascending nociceptive information.
- Instead, the PFC is activated in response to nociceptive stimuli via other regions in the cerebral cortex such as the ACC[175] (also, see Fig. 11.10).

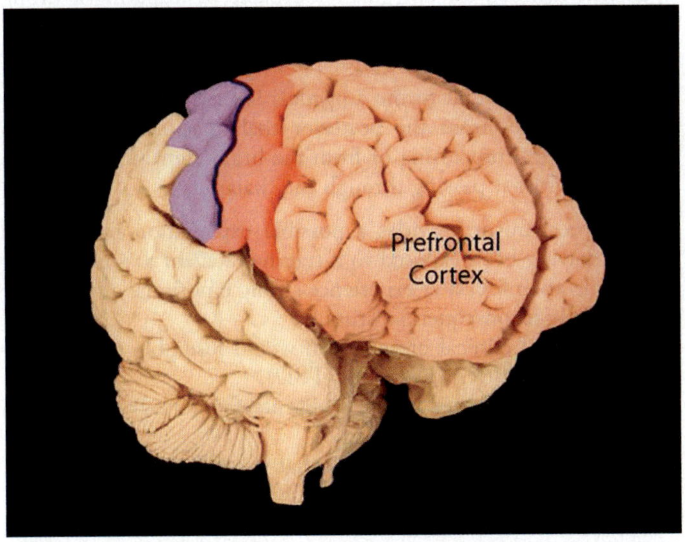

Figure 11.14. The prefrontal cortex. The darker *red* and *blue* stripes represent the precentral and postcentral gyri, respectively. (Artwork by Rachel Milner; Used with permission from the Willard/Carreiro Collection, University of New England.)

The PFC can be divided into two major regions.[176]

- The PFC proper, usually termed *dorsolateral prefrontal cortex* (DLPFC), represents the convex surface of the frontal lobe.
- The *orbitofrontal prefrontal cortex* (OFC), involving the inferior or orbital surface and the medial surface of the frontal lobe.
- In most fMRI studies, the use of the term OFC also includes the anterior region of the cingulated cortex (ACC).

The PFC is activated in some but not all studies of brain representation of nociceptive events.

- In addition, when the PFC does demonstrate neuronal activity, it is not necessarily proportional to the intensity of the painful stimulus.[175,177]
- The DLPFC is thought to be involved with executive functions and appears to play a significant role in the attentive and cognitive aspect of pain.[178]
- The distinction in functional activity between the OFC and ACC is still not clear in the literature; however, it has been suggested that:
  - □ The strong affective–motivational character of pain develops from activity in this region.[116]
  - □ The ACC is specifically involved in the unpleasantness of some painful stimuli.
  - □ The orbitofrontal cortex, with its massive limbic system connections, may process some of the secondary effects of pain, such as emotional feelings and suffering.

Although the precise role of the DLPFC in the forebrain pain matrix is not known at this time, there is a strong suggestion that it is intimately involved in regulating the perception of pain.

- Consistent with this concept is the observation that, in a paradigm using a thermal probe to sensitize skin, increased activity in the DLPFC correlated with suppression of activity in the medial thalamus and midbrain.[178]
- This phenomenon suggests that given the proper conditions, the DLPFC can initiate a source of descending inhibition on the ascending nociceptive pathways.

A significant problem encountered when attempting to assign specific pain processing functions to anatomically defined regions of the PFC relates to the alteration in cortical activity patterns with temporal sequence (acute vs. chronic).

- In a metastudy reviewing published functional imaging studies of acute and chronic pain patients, it was concluded that the thalamic–somatic sensory cortical pathways leading to activation of the IC and ACC are strongly involved in acute pain patients.
- However, in chronic pain patients, these same pathways appeared somewhat reduced in activity.
- Conversely, in these latter patients, the DLPFC area imaged demonstrated increased activity.[120]
- The shift in brain activity between acute and chronic pain states strongly suggests that:
  - □ Plasticity exists in the forebrain processing.
  - □ The chronic pain state is a pathology representing uncontrolled or dysregulated activity in certain forebrain areas.

The role of the DLPFC in the pathology of long-term pain states is further suggested by the observation that a significant alteration in brain chemistry[179] and an accompanying loss of neural tissue[180] occur in this region, in patients suffering from various forms of chronic pain.[181]

- The loss in gray matter from the DLPFC was related to the duration of the chronic pain scenario, thereby suggesting some type of fulminating process.

BOX 11.21 Cerebral Plasticity in Chronic Pain

Acute and chronic pain patterns appear to involve differing aspects of the pain connectome.

The feeling of pain can be enhanced contextually and even be a learned response in some situations.

The ACCs and PFCs are important regions involved in the affective and cognitive aspects of the perception of pain and can play a significant role in the development of chronic pain patterns.

The approach to treatment of chronic pain patterns involves both an understanding of the pain etiology and an appreciation of the role of the biopsychosocial factors that influence the patient and their desire or will to participate in the treatment strategy.

- Since the loss of gray matter volume has been seen in numerous different forms of chronic pain,[182] it therefore does not appear related to the origin of the pain, but rather to its chronicity (Box 11.21).

Interestingly, since the DLPFC is not directly involved in recording the intensity, quality, or location of pain, it may instead play a more general role in attending to, or not attending to, pain.

- This concept would fit well with the generally accepted role of the DLPFC in working memory, controlling attention to stimuli, and the decision to act or not act on neuronal information processed in other regions of cerebral cortex.
- Studies have pointed to the DLPFC as playing a significant role in attention to painful stimuli.[178]
- The amount of activity imaged in the midbrain and thalamus—representing ascending information—triggered by a noxious stimulus was inversely proportional to the activity imaged in the DLPFC.
- This suggests that the DLPFC functions to modulate activity in the ascending pathways and the amount of pain the individual feels.
- Thus, pathologic mechanisms occurring in DLPFC could manifest as increased activity in cortical pain connectome (see below), even in the absence of noxious peripheral stimuli.
- In such a situation, a patient could be feeling significant amounts of pain, even though there is no obvious peripheral source for the pain.

Like the dorsolateral PFC, the ventrolateral PFC does not receive direct input from regions of the thalamus responding to spinothalamic tract activity. Therefore, it also relies on activation to nociceptive stimuli via other cortical areas.

- Functional imaging studies have provided data linking the activity of VLPFC to descending pain modulation systems in the brain stem.[183]
- There is evidence that has tied VLPFC to pain modulation, consequent to specific religious beliefs.
- Such context-dependent pain modulation specifically involved the right (nondominant) VLPFC and engaged the ventral midbrain.
- This suggests that the initiation of activity in the descending pain modulation systems creates increased tolerance to painful stimuli.[184]

All of these observations, taken together, strongly suggest that the PFC plays a major role in:

- □ Determining attention to a painful stimulus
- □ The patient's ability to modulate the intensity of pain

The importance of these observations cannot be overstated in:

- □ Developing a sound strategy for pain management in chronic pain patients
- □ Obtaining the patient's buy-in to accept the treatment strategy

- Total lack of confidence in the strategy and obsession over the pain state can initiate a downward spiral that results in pain management failure, along with magnification of the perceived pain on the part of the patient

Amygdala

The amygdala is located on the medial aspect of the temporal lobe, forming a prominent enlargement on the cortical surface termed the uncus (see Fig. 11.13).

- This collection of nuclei is central for emotional fear and for organizing the emotional motor, visceral autonomic and neuroendocrine response to threatening (noxious) stimuli; they therefore play a key role in the emotional response to pain.
- The amygdala receives numerous projections from the most associative portions of the cerebral cortex—particularly the orbitofrontal cortex—as well as a set of subcortical projections from the parabrachial region of the pontomesencephalic border of the brain stem termed the spino–parabrachio–amygdaloid pathway.[147]
- Intensely painful stimuli, acting through the spino–parabrachio–amygdaloid pathway, not involving cortical structures, exert a strong drive on portions of the amygdala.[185]
- This aspect of the medial temporal lobe is well known for its ability to facilitate (a form of central sensitization), and through this process, to form memories of fear-provoking stimuli.[186]
- Efferent fibers from the amygdala provide a strong drive on the hypothalamic and brain stem areas involved in control of the sympathetic–adrenal system.
- In this manner, the amygdala is capable of initiating a strong arousal response to a painful stimulus or to the threat of a painful stimulus.[187]

Some of the input to the amygdala is subcortical in nature—that is, it passes from the posterior thalamus to the amygdala without cortical processing or from the brain stem directly to the amygdala without passing through the thalamus.

- This mechanism provides a possible explanation for patients who, having been exposed to a traumatic event at some earlier point in their life, later experience strong emotional arousal over seemingly inconsequential stimuli.
- This type of clinical presentation would resemble that seen in posttraumatic stress disorder (PTSD).
- The initial traumatic event or events facilitated areas in the medial temporal lobe.
- Subsequently, innocuous stimuli that might only tangentially be related to the initial event can now evoke a major protective response from the amygdala.
- Given its plasticity, it is possible that the amygdala is a junction point between chronic pain states and those of depression and anxiety,[188] along with the concomitant physiologic responses.[189]

Cerebellum and Basal Ganglia

Functional imaging of an individual exposed to various pain states has frequently demonstrated the involvement of the cerebellum and basal ganglia in the central processing nociceptive information.[175,190]

- The cerebellum is often seen to contain neural activity in pain imaging studies of pain states.[191]
- Nociceptive events have also been demonstrated to alter neuronal activity in the cerebellar vermis and portions of the hemispheres.
- Descending pathways from the deep cerebellar nuclei reach several brain stem locations that contribute to the control of nociceptive activity.
- Nociceptive-related cerebellar activity could relate to the coordination of motor programs necessary to control the individual's pain-related movements.
- The cerebellum is very clearly involved in learning and memory related to the motor system, and recent studies have suggested that the cerebellum can control large areas of the cerebral cortex, extending much beyond pure motor function.[192,193]
- Supporting this assertion is the observation that patients suffering from cerebellar damage can present with cognitive and behavioral deficits as well as the expected ataxic movements.[194,195]
- Thus, it is possible that the cerebellar activity evoked by pain is involved in cognitive learning processes.

The basal ganglia are located in the deep white matter of the cerebrum and have well-described connections with much of the cerebral cortex.[176]

- This collection of nuclei represents an integral part of a recurrent pathway, linking various regions of the cerebral cortex.
- Like the cerebellum, the basal ganglia function to regulate the output of the cerebral cortex.
- A fairly consistent finding in most broad-based functional imaging studies is the involvement of the putamen, a portion of the basal ganglia, in the processing of nociceptive information.
- As a functional unit, the basal ganglia are known to exert significant influence on the thalamocortical circuitry.
- Thus, in processing nociceptive input, the basal ganglia may be modulating the amount of activity in the medial thalamocortical circuits that are critical to the perception of pain.[196]
- In support of this concept are the observations that diseases of the basal ganglia can interfere with pain thresholds and pain sensitivity.

THE PAIN CONNECTOME

The current understanding of supraspinal pain mechanisms is based on recent neuroimaging studies and meta-analyses.

- Such data show a nociceptive system, from primary afferent fibers through the cerebral cortex, strongly modulated by the interactions of the ascending and descending pathway.[110,122]
- At the level of the forebrain, it has become apparent that the interaction of multiple different regions of the cerebrum is responsible for feeling of discomfort that is referred to as pain.
- Thus, a complex network of reciprocally interconnected regions of the cerebrum responds to noxious stimuli.
- From this distributed neural network, feelings and emotions related to pain are an emergent property.
- Originally termed the **pain neuromatrix**,[197] this network has more recently been termed a dynamic connectome[133] to emphasize the fact that the myriad of connections can vary considerably in organization yet still produce a sensation of extreme discomfort (Fig. 11.15).

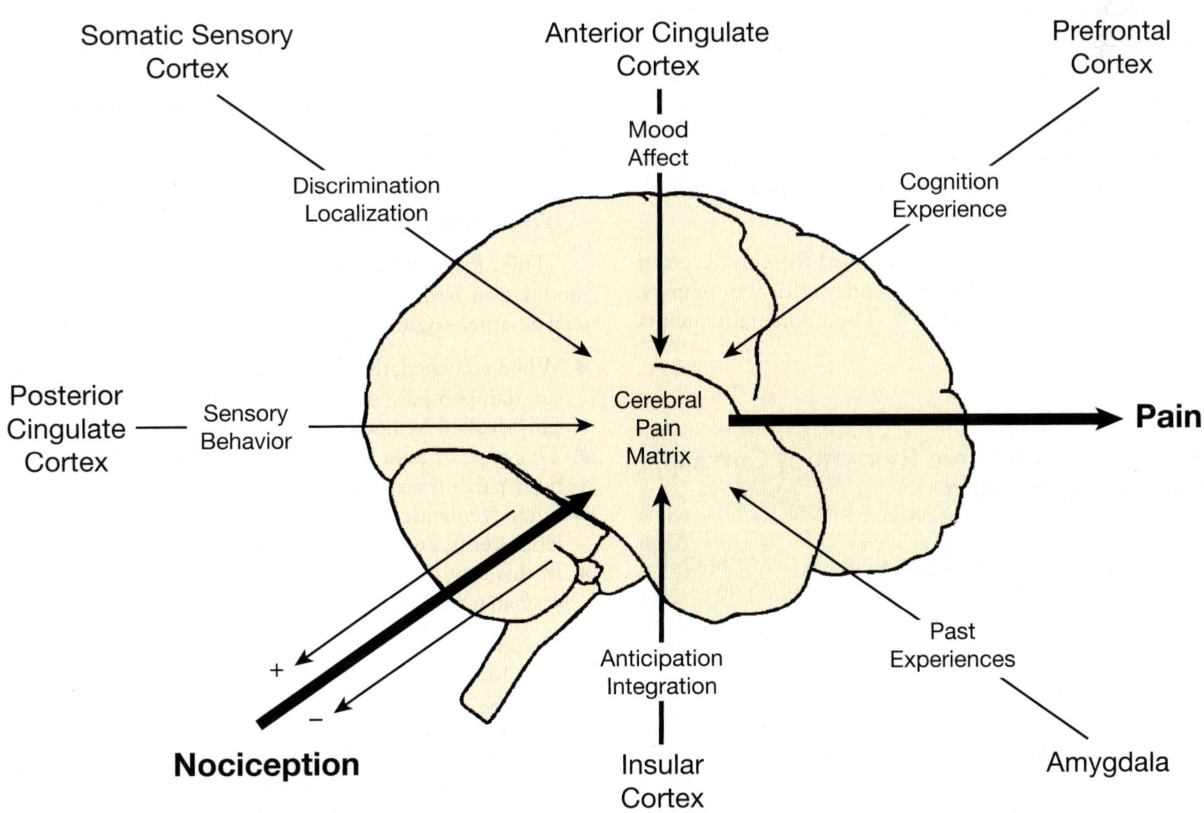

Figure 11.15. The pain connectome transforms nociceptive input into thoughts, emotions, and behaviors. (Used with permission from the Willard/Carreiro Collection, University of New England.)

- It is important to consider that each area involved in pain perception has various other tasks as well, thus while portions of the anterior cingulate may contribute to the perception of pain, this region of the brain has numerous additional functions.
- There is no specific set of cortical connections solely dedicated to the perception of pain, instead, the feeling of pain emerges from the combined activity of numerous multitasking cortical areas in the brain, which can vary from situation to situation and between individuals.
- Based on the construction of the connectome, it can be appreciated that the feeling of pain, to a given stimulus, will vary between individuals based on the contextual setting and the individual's prior experiences.

Three separate but interconnected systems for generating the emergent feelings of pain have been defined in this distributed network[116,198,199]:

- A *sensory-discriminative system* that codes pain location and intensity.
- An *affective–motivational system* that encodes the suffering associated with the feelings of pain.
- A *cognitive–behavioral system* that encodes the conscious behavior to a painful stimulus or to an ongoing painful experience.

The somatosensory cortices on the postcentral gyrus are involved in encoding intensity, temporal, and spatial aspects of nociception and thereby function mainly in the sensory-discriminative zone.

- Conversely, the ACC plays a role in the affective–emotional component, as well as in pain-related anxiety and attention.
- The insula, through its interaction with the autonomic nervous system, appears to be mediating both affective–motivational and sensory-discriminative aspects of pain perception.
- The PFC, while not having intensity-coding properties, devotes significant amount of processing to the cognitive and emotional introspections and planning strategies underlying efforts to cope with the pain.
- Finally, the amygdala has emerged as the junction point for anxiety and depression, the negative aspects of pain, sensitizing to past pains and coloring the reception of future painful stimuli (Box 11.22).

Pain perception is now clearly distinguished from nociception by the significant engagement of brain circuitry critical to sensory, affective, and evaluative assessments.[200,201] These forebrain circuits involve:

- Selectively reviewing all information at the onset of pain.
- Retaining various aspects of the information to be analyzed and organized into meaningful patterns.
- Comparing this noxious stimulus information to pain information already catalogued in short- and long-term memory.
- Transmitting recognized pain patterns to specific brain appraisal systems, including those responsible for attaching affect and meaning to the experience and those responsible for translating the pain experience into behaviors, musculoskeletal reactions, and problem-solving routines.
- Selecting and executing various problem-solving strategies in an effort to adapt and cope with pain.
- Importantly, these pain strategies both influence and are influenced by the patient's neuromusculoskeletal environment.
- For example, evidence suggests that exercise has a significant impact on the way in which individuals process information in the nociceptive system.[202]

BOX 11.22 The Three System of Cortical Processing for Pain

Three separate but interconnected systems in the forebrain are responsible for processing nociceptive stimuli and generating the feelings of pain:

1. A sensory-discriminative system that codes pain location and intensity.
2. An affective–motivational system that encodes the suffering associated with the feelings of pain.
3. A cognitive–behavioral system that encodes conscious behavior to a painful stimulus or to an ongoing painful experience.

The Endogenous Pain Control Systems

In response to injury, the body can suppress the transmission of nociceptive information through the spinal cord, thus facilitating the ability to focus on escape and survival. Then, when safe to do so, reverse the situation by enhancing nociceptive transmission, thereby facilitating protective guarding of the injured structure.

- To accomplish this control, the brain has the ability to modulate activity in the spinal cord, by regulating the amount of information that is allowed to rise into consciousness.
- Descending pathways of brain stem origin, involving neurotransmitters such as serotonin and norepinephrine among others, perform modulation of the dorsal horn and spinal trigeminal nucleus.[203,204]
- As such, these pathways form an endogenous and powerful antinociceptive system.[205,206]
- Ascending nociceptive information reaches areas in the medulla, rostral pons, and midbrain; in turn, these areas can initiate a complex descending pain control system capable of significantly modifying signal transmission in the dorsal horn.
- This descending system is named for its major nuclei in the brain stem: the periaqueductal gray–rostral medulla–dorsal horn (PAG–RM–DH) system.

This PAG–RM–DH system is under dynamic top-down modulation by brain mechanisms associated with anticipation, as well as other cognitive and affective factors.

- When activated, the descending brain stem pain control systems can dampen pain sensation and inhibit behavior reactions typically evoked by nociception.[207]
- This type of pain suppression can permit the use of an injured body part on an emergency basis.
- Such events are reported in combat situation, competitive athletic events, and other high-stakes crisis situations.
- In this way, the endogenous pain control system can represent a very adaptive behavior (Box 11.23).

In addition to its descending control, the PAG–RM–DH system is also capable of enhancing sensitivity to pain, an event that can also be protective in some situations.[206]

- By promoting activities that limit aggravation of the painful area, through immobilization or other protective measures, these systems may have a positive effect on healing.
- Therefore, enhancing the neurotransmission of nociception and the associated perception of pain may serve an adaptive role.

BOX 11.23 Endogenous Pain Control Systems

Endogenous pain control pathways arise in the brain stem and project downward into the spinal cord.

These pathways can suppress ascending nociceptive information, thus reducing or blocking the feeling of pain for a given stimulus.

Conversely, existing data also suggest that these pathways can facilitate activity in the spinal cord, thus increasing the perception of pain to a given stimulus.

Control of these descending pathways is derived from the hypothalamus and from forebrain systems involved in emotion, motivational behavior, and cognition.

- Unfortunately, an extended period of pain facilitation or diminished pain inhibition may no longer be serving an obvious adaptive function, and may, in fact, be creating excess suffering.

An additional descending pain control system has been identified, termed diffuse noxious inhibitory controls (DNIC).[208,209]

- Unlike the PAG–RM–DH system, when this system is activated by primary afferent fiber discharge, it provides a diffuse blanket of inhibition over the entire spinal cord, with the exception of the segment that is stimulated.
- Once DNIC has been initiated, a second nociceptive stimulus, at a distance in the body from the first, is blunted in its effect on the spinal cord.
- The neural pathways utilized in DNIC are separate from those of the PAG–RM–DH and involve the subnucleus reticularis dorsalis in the medulla.
- However, like the PAG–RM–DH system, DNIC is modulated by multiple supraspinal mechanisms.
- DNIC has been demonstrated in humans and appears to have similar effects in males and females,[210] despite the fact that men generally have a higher threshold for pain than women.
- In women, DNIC was demonstrated to vary somewhat during the menstrual cycle, being most effective during the ovulatory phase.[211]

The DNIC system appears to be a key player in what has recently been termed "**conditioned pain modulation**"[212] or CPM, a clinically important procedure that is thought to test the integrity of the descending pain modulation systems.

- The test is based on the fact that an ongoing nociceptive event will trigger a body-wide inhibition of other nociceptive input.
- In this procedure, a conditioning stimulus is employed to test inhibition on a test-stimulus.
- The conditioning stimulus is a noxious event, such as exposure of the upper extremity to ice-water, it prevents the test-stimulus from registering as a noxious event.
- When successful it demonstrates that the individuals endogenous pain control systems are working; if it does not elicit inhibition, it suggests that the individual has a defect in the function of the endogenous pain control pathways.
- This test has been used to better understand the pathology found in chronic pain patients.[213]

The following discussion gives rise to some very intriguing possibilities:

- The observation that at least some of the pain modulation system can facilitate nociceptive transmission as well as inhibit it at the spinal or trigeminal level.
- The knowledge that multiple forebrain areas, especially those long felt to be located in the limbic system, exert a strong regulation over these pathways.

Complex supraspinal networks, influenced by emotions and hormones, could be responsible for enhancing or suppressing feeling of pain from a noxious stimulus. Thus, the way that an individual ultimately responds to a noxious stimulus may have a lot to do with:

- The social and psychological context of the injury
- The degree of anticipation and anxiety
- The individual's past experience with similar or related stimuli
- The individual's current body physiology

Finally, it is important to note that what has been described as "descending endogenous pain control pathways" may only be a specific function of a much more broad-based system controlling numerous aspects of the spinal cord.

- It has been long known that areas in the brain stem, closely related to those involved in pain modulation, control the functions of the spinal components of the autonomic nervous system as well as the activity of motoneurons in the ventral horns.[214]
- Thus, the so-described pain control system may be an integral component of a larger brain stem system controlling spinal cord facilitation in general.

Pain Perception

There is a significant distinction between nociception and pain perception.

- Nociception occurs at the peripheral nerve, spinal cord, and brain stem level.
- It facilitates spinal cord and brain stem circuits, triggering reflexes and unconscious adaptive behavior.
- Conversely, pain perception begins with the activation of thalamocortical circuitry.
- From the thalamus there is simultaneous involvement of the primary and secondary somatic sensory cortical areas, the insula, anterior cingulate, amygdala, and PFC as previously described.

The perception of pain is a construct[3] that emerges from the sum total of activity in this matrix and is not a specific property of any one region.

- The brain scans a pain threat or the potentially painful event for recognizable patterns, in an effort to attach meaning and emotions and to generate problem-solving strategies.
- Each component of the cortical pain connectome provides aspects of the physiologic, emotional, and cognitive response.
- The native activity in each of these cortical regions is strongly colored by the sum total of previous experience, such as past pains and emotional events—in essence—the baggage of life.
- It follows then that the experience of a given pain and the subsequent emotional reactions that it generates may differ significantly between individuals.

At this point, it is important to distinguish between what is termed acute pain and the more ominous state termed chronic pain.

- Acute pain, also termed physiologic pain or eudynia (good pain), occurs when a noxious stimulus is present, it has also been termed *nociceptive pain*.

- Peripheral nerve and central systems in the spinal cord, brain stem, and forebrain can sensitize and ramp-up activity, but acute pain will remit with the natural course of tissue repair.
- In contrast, chronic pain, also termed surgical pain or maldynia (bad pain), is pain that is still present 3 to 6 months following the expected natural healing of the injured tissue.
- In some diseases, such as rheumatoid arthritis, healing may not be completed and may represent a nerve ending mixture of acute and chronic pain mechanisms summating in the patient.
- In this way, chronic pain represents dysregulation in the normal sensitization systems either at a peripheral nerve, spinal cord, brain stem, or forebrain level, a more recent term for this type of event is *nociplastic pain*.[90]
- From these observations, two significant conclusions can be made.
  - First, chronic pain is a pathology representing altered neuronal activity—such as neuronal cell death or altered morphology such as a loss of dentritic spines or unnatural sprouting of new terminals—in multiple areas of the brain, possibly including the PFC, thus chronic pain is more than simply prolonged nociceptive activity triggered by peripheral generators[215,216]
  - Second, the longer patients are exposed to chronic pain, the more sensitization mechanisms are stressed and falter, leading to greater pain scenarios.
- Clinically, this means that the longer patients experience chronic pain patterns, the more intense these patterns will become, and the harder it will be to ameliorate these pain syndromes.

Pain and Stress

The neural and endocrine linkage between the nociceptive system and the stress response system is very strong[49] (Box 11.24).

BOX 11.24 Interoceptive System and Addictive Behavior

There is a strong correlation between the corticolimbic circuits of the forebrain involved in pain perception and the circuits involved in behaviors such as reward–antireward, motivation, emotions, attention and cognition, and arousal. Evidence to date suggests that in specific circumstances, acute pain and euphorigenic drugs will activate the dopaminergic systems (reward effects), whereas prolonged periods of pain or drug consumption will suppress the dopaminergic system (antireward effects), producing hypodopaminergic state.[217,218]

The common feature of these systems appears to be their integration with the interoceptive system through various connections with the insular cortex. Thus, the activity of the interoceptive system appears to contribute to drug addiction, possibly through the following arrangement: The current internal state of the individual, based on somatic and visceral afferent fiber systems, as processed in the insular cortex is integrated in the forebrain systems for recall of past experiences and the generation of predicted body states (IC and amygdala). This information modulates the generation of approach or avoidance behavior in any given situation.[219] The integration of the interoceptive and reward systems in the shaping of approach and aversive behaviors opens a role for osteopathic medicine in the treatment of drug addiction.

- Both systems operate on a feed-forward mechanism that is adaptive in nature.
- Neither the stress response axis nor the pain response system has an established set point around which it operates; thus, when activated, both are open-ended responses that meet the current definition for an allostatic event.
- Both systems offer mechanisms that are protective in the short-term or acute response.
- Acute pain and acute stress are symptoms of a problem that has occurred, and that will typically resolve.
- Both systems can become pathologic (disease) when prolonged.
- Chronic pain and chronic stress represent diseases that are no longer responding to a triggering stimulus, but have taken on a life of their own in the patient.
- This can be further exacerbated in the patient who is suffering from other chronic diseases such as colitis or rheumatoid arthritis; the diseased tissue is continually provoking the acute nociception system that is constantly driving a sensitized chronic nociceptive system ultimately resulting in more stress for the patient.
- Both the pain response system and the stress response system have long-loop, slow feedback control system that attempt to re-establish the normal homeostatic rhythms of the body once the nociceptive event or the stressor remits.
- Destruction of these long-loop control systems through excitotoxic pathologic mechanisms is known to occur, such as seen in the loss of glucocorticoid-expressing hippocampal neurons when exposed to elevated glucocorticoids.[220]
- This breakdown in control results in an inability to downregulate either the pain response or the stress response or both,[49,221,222] in essence, both systems are stuck in the "on" position.
- In addition, long-term exposure to activity in either or both chronic pain and chronic stress system can result in the onset of depression, indeed, there is strong crossover between each system.
- Patients with chronic pain repeatedly activate the stress response system, often resulting in the onset of depression, while those caught in a chronic stress response are also more inclined to develop chronic pain.[223]

Allostatic Mechanisms

Pain—and the stress it creates in the body and brain—is, in essence, an allostatic process influenced by a complex network of cortical and subcortical brain structures.

- All levels of the nociceptive system are capable of an allostatic (feed-forward) response to noxious stimuli.
- At the level of PANs, peripheral sensitization can occur, in a feed-forward process, enhancing the activity of the afferent fiber.
- In the spinal cord, central sensitization can occur, again in a feed-forward process, creating regions of segmental facilitation.
- Similar facilitation also occurs, again using feed-forward mechanisms, in the forebrain areas such as the amygdala.
- At this level, emotional experiences surrounding the painful event can facilitate amygdaloid activity, resulting in enhanced fear memories and increased drive on the neuroendocrine systems of the hypothalamus and midbrain.
- These systems increase the production and release of norepinephrine and cortisol, resulting in an enhanced protective response to arousal-provoking stimuli, such as pain.
- While such a response may be highly protective in the short-term situation, long-term exposure to allostatic mechanisms is known to be pathologic to numerous body systems, thus

predisposing one to physiologic dysregulation[224] and psychological states such as depression and anxiety.

- Viewed in this light, chronic pain is the end product or disease that occurs in the nociceptive system, when a normal allostatic response, such as acute pain, exceeds its control systems and becomes fixed in a pathologic state.

Thorough understanding of pain, from the peripheral generation of a nociceptive signal to its conversion into a painful feeling in the forebrain, is necessary to provide a framework for managing somatic dysfunction.

- The patient in pain is more than a biologic event; the patient is a thinking, feeling individual capable of sophisticated problem-solving.
- Such a person, when confronted with chronic pain, actively:
  - Seeks information
  - Makes decisions
  - Attempts to put forth their best effort possible in adapting to the painful condition
- The approach to the patient in pain by the osteopathic physician is aimed at taking the patient beyond the symptom of pain by exploring and addressing factors in the patient's life, that, when appropriately modified, will:
  - Facilitate recovery
  - Prevent the reoccurrence of chronic pain
  - Improve their health and inherent recuperative and restorative powers

REFERENCES

1. Nagasako EM, Oaklander AL, Dworkin RH. Congenital insensitivity to pain: an update. *Pain*. 2003;101:213–219.
2. Garrison SR, Weyer AD, Barabas ME, Beutler BA, Stucky CL. A gain-of-function voltage-gated sodium channel 1.8 mutation drives intense hyperexcitability of A- and C-fiber neurons. *Pain*. 2014;155:896–905.
3. Chapman CR. Psychological aspects of pain: a consciousness studies perspective In: M Pappagallo, ed. *The Neurological Basis of Pain*. McGraw-Hill; 2005:157–167.
4. Gatchel RJ, Garofalo JP, Ellis E, Holt C. Major psychological disorders in acute and chronic TMD: an initial examination. *J Am Dent Assoc*. 1996;127:1365–1370, 72, 74.
5. Willis WD, Coggeshall RE. *Sensory Mechanisms of the Spinal Cord*. Springer Science+Business Media; 2004.
6. Fitzgerald M. The development of nociceptive circuits. *Nat Rev Neurosci*. 2005;6:507–520.
7. Prechtl JC, Powley TL. B-afferents: a fundamental division of the nervous system mediating homeostasis? *Behav Brain Sci*. 1990;13:289–331.
8. Wall PD. The gate control theory of pain mechanisms. A re-examination and re-statement. *Brain*. 1978;101:1–18.
9. Kandel ER, Schwartz JH, Jessell TM, Siegelbaum SA, Hudspeth AJ. *Principles of Neural Sciences*. McGraw-Hill Medical; 2013.
10. Melzack R, Wall PD. Pain mechanisms: a new theory. *Science*. 1965; 150:971–979.
11. Neumann S, Doubell TP, Leslie T, Woolf CJ. Inflammatory pain hypersensitivity mediated by phenotypic switch in myelinated primary sensory neurons. *Nature*. 1996;384:360–364.
12. Meyer RA, Ringkamp M, Campbell JN, Raja SN. Peripheral mechanisms of cutaneous nociception. In: SB McMahon, M Koltzenburg, eds. *Wall and Melzack's Textbook of Pain*. Elsevier Churchill Livingston; 2006:3–34.
13. Michaelis M, Habler HJ, Jäenig W. Silent afferents: a separate class of primary afferents? *Clin Exp Pharmacol Physiol*. 1996;23:99–105.
14. Olausson H, Wessberg J, Morrison I, McGlone F, Vallbo A. The neurophysiology of unmyelinated tactile afferents. *Neurosci Biobehav Rev*. 2010;34:185–191.
15. Selye H. The general adaptive syndrome and the diseases of adaptation. *J Clin Endocrinol*. 1946;6:117–173.
16. Ji RR, Kohno T, Moore KA, Woolf CJ. Central sensitization and LTP: do pain and memory share similar mechanisms? *Trends Neurosci*. 2003; 26:696–705.
17. Munger BL, Ide C. The structure and function of cutaneous sensory receptors. *Arch Histol Cytol*. 1988;51:1–34.
18. Julius D, Basbaum AI. Molecular mechanisms of nociception. *Nature*. 2001;413:203–210.
19. Stucky CL, Mikesell AR. Cutaneous pain in disorders affecting peripheral nerves. *Neurosci Lett*. 2021;765:136233.
20. Mense S, Simons DG. *Muscle Pain: Understanding Its Nature, Diagnosis, and Treatment*. Lippincott, Williams & Wilkins; 2001.
21. Abdelhamid RE, Sluka KA. ASICs mediate pain and inflammation in musculoskeletal diseases. *Physiology (Bethesda)*. 2015; 30:449–459.
22. Hoheisel U, Mense S. Long-term changes in discharge behaviour of cat dorsal horn neurones following noxious stimulation of deep tissues. *Pain*. 1989;36:239–247.
23. Wall PD, Woolf CJ. Muscle but not cutaneous C-afferent input produces prolonged increases in the excitability of the flexion reflex in the rat. *J Physiol*. 1984;356:453–458.
24. Alpantaki K, McLaughlin D, Karagogeos D, Hadjipavlou A, Kontakis G. Sympathetic and sensory neural elements in the tendon of the long head of the biceps. *J Bone Joint Surg Am*. 2005;87:1580–1583.
25. De Lorenzis E, Natalello G, Simon D, Schett G, D'Agostino MA. Concepts of entheseal pain. *Arthritis Rheumatol*. 2023;75:493–498.
26. Andersson G, Danielson P, Alfredson H, Forsgren S. Nerve-related characteristics of ventral paratendinous tissue in chronic Achilles tendinosis. *Knee Surg Sports Traumatol Arthrosc*. 2007;15:1272–1279.
27. Danielson P, Alfredson H, Forsgren S. Distribution of general (PGP 9.5) and sensory (substance P/CGRP) innervations in the human patellar tendon. *Knee Surg Sports Traumatol Arthrosc*. 2006;14:125–132.
28. Premkumar LS, Raisinghani M. Nociceptors in cardiovascular functions: complex interplay as a result of cyclooxygenase inhibition. *Mol Pain*. 2006;2:26.
29. Bove GM, Light AR. CGRP-like immunoreactivity of fine afferents innervating peripheral nerve sheaths. *Soc Neuosci Abstr*. 1993;19:324–324.
30. Bove GM, Light AR. Calcitonin gene-related peptide and peripherin immunoreactivity in nerve sheaths. *Somatosens Mot Res*. 1995;12:49–57.
31. Schaible HG, Grubb BD. Afferent and spinal mechanisms of joint pain. *Pain*. 1993;55:5–54.
32. Fortier LA, Nixon AJ. Distributional changes in substance P nociceptive fiber patterns in naturally osteoarthritic articulations. *J Rheumatol*. 1997;24:524–530.
33. Eitner A, Pester J, Nietzsche S, Hofmann GO, Schaible HG. The innervation of synovium of human osteoarthritic joints in comparison with normal rat and sheep synovium. *Osteoarthr Cartil*. 2013;21:1383–1391.
34. Cervero F, Jänig W. Visceral nociceptors: a new world order? *Trends Neurosci*. 1992;15:374–378.
35. Cervero F. Mechanisms of acute visceral pain. *Br Med Bull*. 1991;47:549–560.
36. Christianson JA, Bielefeldt K, Altier C, et al. Development, plasticity and modulation of visceral afferents. *Brain Res Rev*. 2009;60:171–186.
37. Tajti J, Szok D, Majlath Z, Tuka B, Csati A, Vecsei L. Migraine and neuropeptides. *Neuropeptides*. 2015;52:19–30.
38. Sanchez del Rio M, Moskowitz MA. The trigeminal system In: J Olesen, P Tfelt-Hansen, KMA Welch, eds. *The Headaches*. Lippincott, Williams and Wilkins; 2000:141–150.
39. Terrier LM, Fontaine D. Intracranial nociception. *Rev Neurol (Paris)*. 2021;177:765–772.
40. Groen GJ, Baljet B, Drukker J. Nerves and nerve plexuses of the human vertebral column. *Am J Anat*. 1990;188:282–296.
41. Stilwell DL. The nerve supply of the vertebral column and its associated structures in the monkey. *Anat Rec*. 1956;125:139–169.
42. Jinkins JR, Whittermore AR, Bradley WG. The anatomic basis of vertebrogenic pain and the autonomic syndrome associated with lumbar disk extrusion. *AJR Am J Roentgenol*. 1989;152:1277–1289.
43. Bailey JF, Liebenberg E, Degmetich S, Lotz JC. Innervation patterns of PGP 9.5-positive nerve fibers within the human lumbar vertebra. *J Anat*. 2011;218:263–270.
44. Fields AJ, Ballatori A, Liebenberg EC, Lotz JC. Contribution of the endplates to disc degeneration. *Curr Mol Biol Rep*. 2018;4:151–160.

45. Willard FH. The muscular, ligamentous, and neural structure of the lumbosacrum and its relationship to low back pain. In: Vleeming A, Mooney V, Stoeckart R, eds. *Movement, Stability & Lumbopelvic Pain*. Churchill Livingstone Elsevier; 2007:5–45.
46. Levine JD, Fields HL, Basbaum AI. Peptides and the primary afferent nociceptor. *J Neurosci*. 1993;13:2273–2286.
47. McMahon SB, Bennett DLH, Bevan S. Inflammatory mediators and modulators of pain In: SB McMahon, M Koltzenburg, eds. *Wall and Melzack's Textbook of Pain*: Elsevier Churchill Livingston; 2006:49–72.
48. Mantyh PW, Clohisy DR, Koltzenburg M, Hunt SP. Molecular mechanisms of cancer pain. *Nat Rev Cancer*. 2002;2:201–209.
49. Schulkin J. *Rethinking Homeostasis*. The MIT Press; 2003.
50. Denslow JS. Pathophysiologic evidence for the osteopathic lesion: the known, unknown, and controversial. *J Am Osteopath Assoc*. 1975;74:415–421.
51. Howe JF, Loeser JD, Calvin WH. Mechanosensitivity of dorsal root ganglia and chronically injured axons: a physiological basis for the radicular pain of nerve root compression. *Pain*. 1977;3:25–41.
52. Amir R, Devor M. Chemically mediated cross-excitation in rat dorsal root ganglia. *J Neurosci*. 1996;16:4733–4741.
53. McLachlan EM, Jänig W, Devor M, Michaelis M. Peripheral nerve injury triggers noradrenergic sprouting within dorsal root ganglia. *Nature*. 1993;363:543–546.
54. Ramer MS, Bisby MA. Rapid sprouting of sympathetic axons in dorsal root ganglia of rats with a chronic constriction injury. *Pain*. 1997;70:237–244.
55. Merskey H, Bogduk N. *Classification of Chronic Pain: Descriptions of Chronic Pain Syndromes and Definitions of Pain Terms*. International Association for the Study of Pain Press; 1994.
56. Todd AJ, Koerber R. Neuroanatomical substrates of spinal nociception. In: SB McMahon, M Koltzenburg, eds. *Wall and Melzack's Textbook of Pain*: Elsevier Churchill Livingston; 2006:73–90.
57. Wilson P, Kitchener PD. Plasticity of cutaneous primary afferent projections to the spinal dorsal horn. *Prog Neurobiol*. 1996;48:105–113.
58. Hunt SP, Rossi J. Peptide- and non-peptide-containing unmyelinated primary afferents: the parallel processing of nociceptive information. *Philos Trans R Soc Lond B Biol Sci*. 1985;308:283–289.
59. Todd AJ. Anatomy and neurochemistry of the dorsal horn. *Handb Clin Neurol*. 2006;81(3rd Series):61–76.
60. Stucky CL, Lewin GR. Isolectin B(4)-positive and -negative nociceptors are functionally distinct. *J Neurosci*. 1999;19:6497–6505.
61. Braz JM, Nassar MA, Wood JN, Basbaum AI. Parallel "pain" pathways arise from subpopulations of primary afferent nociceptor. *Neuron*. 2005;47:787–793.
62. Cervero F. Pain and the spinal cord. *Handb Clin Neurol*. 2006;81 (3rd Series):77–92.
63. Graham BA, Brichta AM, Callister RJ. Moving from an averaged to specific view of spinal cord pain processing circuits. *J Neurophysiol*. 2007;98:1057–12063.
64. Le Bars D, Cadden SW. What is a wide-dynamic-range cell? In: AI Basbaum, M Bushnell, eds. *Science of Pain*. Elsevier; 2009:331–338.
65. Mendell LM. Physiological properties of unmyelinated fiber projection to the spinal cord. *Exp Neurol*. 1966;16:316–332.
66. Willis WD. Physiology of dorsal horn and spinal cord pathways related to pain. In: RF Beers, EG Bassett, eds. *Mechanisms of Pain and Analgesic Compounds*. Raven Press; 1979:143–156.
67. Mayer DJ, Price DD, Becker DP. Neurophysiological characterization of the anterolateral spinal cord neurons contributing to pain perception in man. *Pain*. 1975;1:51–58.
68. Basbaum AI. Distinct neurochemical features of acute and persistent pain. *P Natl Acad Sci USA*. 1999;96:7739–7743.
69. Millan MJ. The induction of pain: an integrative review. *Prog Neurobiol*. 1999;57:1–164.
70. Woolf CJ, Salter MW. Plasticity and pain: role of the dorsal horn. In: SB McMahon, M Koltzenburg, eds. *Wall and Melzack's Textbook of Pain*. Elsevier Churchill Livingston; 2006:91–105.
71. Mantyh PW, Allen CJ, Ghilardi JR, et al. Rapid endocytosis of a G protein-coupled receptor: substance P evoked internalization of its receptor in the rat striatum in vivo. *Proc Natl Acad Sci*. 1995;92:2622–2626.
72. Abbadie C, Trafton J, Liu HT, Mantyh PW, Basbaum AI. Inflammation increases the distribution of dorsal horn neurons that internalize the neurokinin-1 receptor in response to noxious and non-noxious stimulation. *J Neurosci*. 1997;17:8049–8060.
73. Scholz J, Broom DC, Youn DH, et al. Blocking caspase activity prevents transsynaptic neuronal apoptosis and the loss of inhibition in lamina II of the dorsal horn after peripheral nerve injury. *J Neurosci*. 2005;25:7317–7323.
74. Doubell TP, Mannion RJ, Woolf CJ. Intact sciatic myelinated primary afferent terminals collaterally sprout in the adult rat dorsal horn following section of a neighbouring peripheral nerve. *J Comp Neurol*. 1997;380:95–104.
75. Grubb BD, Stiller RU, Schaible HG. Dynamic changes in the receptive field properties of spinal cord neurons with ankle input in rats with chronic unilateral inflammation in the ankle region. *Exp Brain Res*. 1993;92:441–452.
76. Koerber HR, Mirnics K. Plasticity of dorsal horn cell receptive fields after peripheral nerve regeneration. *J Neurophysiol*. 1996;75:2255–2267.
77. Mense S. Physiology of nociception in muscles. *J Man Med*. 1991;6:24–33.
78. Hoheisel U, Mense S, Simons DG, Yu XM. Appearance of new receptive fields in rat dorsal horn neurons following noxious stimulation of skeletal muscle: a model for referral of muscle pain? *Neurosci Lett*. 1993;153:9–12.
79. Watkins LR, Wieseler-Frank J, Hutchinson MR, et al. Neuroimmune interactions and pain: the role of immune and glial cells In: R Ader, ed. *Psychoneuroimmunology*. Vol. 1. Elsevier Academic Press; 2007:393–414.
80. Wieseler-Frank J, Maier SF, Watkins LR. Immune-to-brain communication dynamically modulates pain: physiological and pathological consequences. *Brain Behav Immun*. 2005;19:104–111.
81. Inquimbert P, Moll M, Latremoliere A, et al. NMDA receptor activation underlies the loss of spinal dorsal horn neurons and the transition to persistent pain after peripheral nerve injury. *Cell Rep*. 2018;23:2678–2689.
82. Neumann S, Woolf CJ. Regeneration of dorsal column fibers into and beyond the lesion site following adult spinal cord injury. *Neuron*. 1999;23:83–91.
83. Kosek E, Cohen M, Baron R, et al. Do we need a third mechanistic descriptor for chronic pain states? *Pain*. 2016;157:1382–1386.
84. McEwen BS. Mood disorders and allostatic load. *Biol Psychiatry*. 2003;54:200–207.
85. Schulkin J, McEwen BS, Gold PW. Allostasis, amygdala, and anticipatory angst. *Neurosci Biobehav Rev*. 1994;18:385–396.
86. Stumvoll M, Tataranni PA, Stefan N, Vozarova B, Bogardus C. Glucose allostasis. *Diabetes*. 2003;52:903.
87. McEwen BS, Seeman T. Protective and damaging effects of mediators of stress. Elaborating and testing the concepts of allostasis and allostatic load. *Ann NY Acad Sci*. 1999;896:30–47.
88. Grigg P, Schaible HG, Schmidt RF. Mechanical sensitivity of group III and IV afferents from posterior articular nerve in normal and inflamed cat knee. *J Neurophysiol*. 1986;55:635–643.
89. He X, Proske U, Schaible HG, Schmidt RF. Acute inflammation of the knee joint in the cat alters responses of flexor motoneurons to leg movements. *J Neurophysiol*. 1988;59:326–340.
90. Trouvin AP, Perrot S. New concepts of pain. *Best Pract Res Clin Rheumatol*. 2019;33:101415.
91. Sato A. Somatovisceral reflexes. *J Manipulative Physiol Ther*. 1995;18:597–602.
92. Sato A, Sato Y, Schmidt RF, Torigata Y. Somato-vesical reflexes in chronic spinal cats. *J Auton Nerv Syst*. 1983;7:351–362.
93. Foreman RD. Mechanisms of cardiac pain. *Annu Rev Physiol*. 1999;61:143–167.
94. Little JM, Qin C, Farber JP, Foreman RD. Spinal cord processing of cardiac nociception: are there sex differences between male and proestrous female rats? *Brain Res*. 2011;1413:24–31.
95. Head H. *Studies in Neurology*. Vol. I. Henry Frowde and Hodder & Stoughton, Ltd; 1920.
96. Henry JA, Montuschi E. Cardiac pain referred to site of previously experienced somatic pain. *Br Med J*. 1978;2:1605–1606.
97. Carpenter MB, Sutin J. *Human Neuroanatomy*. Williams and Wilkins; 1983.

98. Ramon y Cajal S. *Histologie du Systeme Nerveux de l'Homme et des Vertebres (L. Azoulay, trans)*. Instituto Ramon y Cajal del C.S.I.C; 1909.
99. Sugiura Y, Terui N, Hosoya Y. Difference in distribution of central terminals between visceral and somatic unmyelinated (C) primary afferent fibers. *J Neurophysiol.* 1989;62:834–840.
100. Wall PD, Bennett DL. Postsynaptic effects of long-range afferents in distant segments caudal to their entry point in rat spinal cord under the influence of picrotoxin or strychnine. *J Neurophysiol.* 1994;72:2703–2713.
101. Rees H, Sluka KA, Westlund KN, Willis WD. Do dorsal root reflexes augment peripheral inflammation? *Neuroreport.* 1994;5:821–824.
102. Willis WD. Dorsal root potentials and dorsal root reflexes: a double-edged sword. *Exp Brain Res.* 1999;124:395–421.
103. Peng YB, Wu J, Willis WD, Kenshalo DR. GABA(A) and 5-HT(3) receptors are involved in dorsal root reflexes: possible role in periaqueductal gray descending inhibition. *J Neurophysiol.* 2001;86:49–58.
104. Rees H, Sluka KA, Lu Y, Westlund KN, Willis WD. Dorsal root reflexes in articular afferents occur bilaterally in a chronic model of arthritis in rats. *J Neurophysiol.* 1996;76:4190–4193.
105. Lin Q, Wu J, Willis WD. Dorsal root reflexes and cutaneous neurogenic inflammation after intradermal injection of capsaicin in rats. *J Neurophysiol.* 1999;82:2602–2611.
106. Peng YB, Kenshalo DR, Gracely RH. Periaqueductal gray-evoked dorsal root reflex is frequency dependent. *Brain Res.* 2003;976:217–226.
107. Dostrovsky JO, Craig AD. Ascending projection systems. In: SB McMahon, M Koltzenburg, eds. *Wall and Melzack's Textbook of Pain.* Elsevier Churchill Livingston; 2006:187–203.
108. Westlund KN. Neurophysiology of pain. In: M Pappagallo, ed. *The Neurological Basis of Pain.* McGraw-Hill; 2005:3–19.
109. Benarroch EE. Central autonomic network. In: PA Low, EE Benarroch, eds. *Clinical Autonomic Disorders.* Wolters Kluwer Lippincott Williams & Wilkins; 2008:17–28.
110. May A. Neuroimaging: visualising the brain in pain. *Neurol Sci.* 2007; 28(Suppl 2):S101–S107.
111. Sewards TV, Sewards MA. The medial pain system: neural representations of the motivational aspect of pain. *Brain Res Bull.* 2002;59:163–180.
112. Albe-Fessard D, Berkley KJ, Kruger L, Ralston HJ, 3rd, Willis WD, Jr. Diencephalic mechanisms of pain sensation. *Brain Res.* 1985;356: 217–296.
113. Derbyshire SW, Whalley MG, Stenger VA, Oakley DA. Cerebral activation during hypnotically induced and imagined pain. *Neuroimage.* 2004; 23:392–401.
114. Dostrovsky JO. Brainstem and thalamic relays. *Handb Clin Neurol.* 2006; 81 127–139.
115. Jones AKP, Derbyshire SWG. Cerebral mechanisms operating in the presence and absence of inflammatory pain. *Ann Rheum Dis.* 1996;55: 411–420.
116. Treede RD, Kenshalo DR, Gracely RH, Jones AK. The cortical representation of pain. *Pain.* 1999;79:105–111.
117. Ma Q. A functional subdivision within the somatosensory system and its implications for pain research. *Neuron.* 2022.
118. Ploner M, Freund HJ, Schnitzler A. Pain affect without pain sensation in a patient with a postcentral lesion. *Pain.* 1999;81:211–214.
119. Ropper AH, Samuels MA. *Adams and Victor's Principles of Neurology.* 9th ed. McGraw Hill Medical; 2009.
120. Apkarian AV, Bushnell MC, Treede RD, Zubieta JK. Human brain mechanisms of pain perception and regulation in health and disease. *Eur J Pain.* 2005;9:463–484.
121. Tracey I, Mantyh PW. The cerebral signature for pain perception and its modulation. *Neuron.* 2007;55:377–391.
122. Head H, Holmes G. Sensory disturbances from cerebral lesions. *Brain.* 1911;34:102–254.
123. Melzack R. The gate control theory 25 years later: New perspectives on phantom limb pain. *Proceedings of the 6th World Congress on Pain.* 1991.
124. Davis K. Brain imaging of pain In: M Pappagallo, ed. *The Neurological Basis of Pain.* McGraw-Hill; 2005:151–156.
125. Martucci KT, Mackey SC. Imaging pain. *Anesthesiol Clin.* 2016;34: 255–269.
126. Casey KL. Central pain: distributed effects of focal lesions. *Pain.* 2004; 108:205–206.
127. Eisenberger NI, Lieberman MD. Why rejection hurts: a common neural alarm system for physical and social pain. *Trends Cogn Sci.* 2004;8:294–300.
128. Singer T, Seymour B, O'Doherty J, Kaube H, Dolan RJ, Frith CD. Empathy for pain involves the affective but not sensory components of pain. *Science.* 2004;303:1157–1162.
129. Tracey I. Functional connectivity and pain: how effectively connected is your brain? *Pain.* 2005;116:173–174.
130. Tracey I. Nociceptive processing in the human brain. *Curr Opin Neurobiol.* 2005;15:478–487.
131. Necka EA, Lee IS, Kucyi A, Cheng JC, Yu Q, Atlas LY. Applications of dynamic functional connectivity to pain and its modulation. *Pain Rep.* 2019;4:e752.
132. Price DD. Psychological and neural mechanisms of the affective dimension of pain. *Science.* 2000;288:1769–1772.
133. Kucyi A, Davis KD. The dynamic pain connectome. *Trends Neurosci.* 2015;38:86–95.
134. Melzack R. From the gate to the neuromatrix. *Pain.* 1999;(Suppl 6): S121–S126.
135. Coghill RC, McHaffie JG, Yen YF. Neural correlates of interindividual differences in the subjective experience of pain. *P Natl Acad Sci USA.* 2003;100:8538–8542.
136. Raichle ME, Macleod AM, Snyder AZ, Powers WJ, Gusnard DA, Shulman GL. A default mode of brain function. *P Natl Acad Sci USA.* 2001;98:676–682.
137. Ogawa S, Lee TM, Kay AR, Tank DW. Brain magnetic resonance imaging with contrast dependent on blood oxygenation. *Proc Natl Acad Sci USA.* 1990;87:9868–9872.
138. Tesler F, Linne ML, Destexhe A. Modeling the relationship between neuronal activity and the BOLD signal: contributions from astrocyte calcium dynamics. *Sci Rep.* 2023;13:6451.
139. Aziz Q, Schnitzler A, Enck P. Functional neuroimaging of visceral sensation. *J Clin Neurophysiol.* 2000;17:604–612.
140. Baliki MN, Geha PY, Apkarian AV, Chialvo DR. Beyond feeling: chronic pain hurts the brain, disrupting the default-mode network dynamics. *J Neurosci.* 2008;28:1398–1403.
141. Friedman DP, Murray EA. Thalamic connectivity of the second somatosensory area and neighboring somatosensory fields of the lateral sulcus of the macaque. *J Comp Neurol.* 1986;252:348–373.
142. Casey KL, Tran TD. Cortical mechanisms mediating acute and chronic pain in humans. *Handb Clin Neurol.* 2006;81 159–177.
143. Hofbauer RK, Rainville P, Duncan GH, Bushnell MC. Cortical representation of the sensory dimension of pain. *J Neurophysiol.* 2001;86:402–411.
144. Craig AD. *How Do You Feel? An Interoceptive Moment with Your Neurobiological Self.* Princeton University Press; 2015:343.
145. Friedman DP, Murray EA, O'Neill JB, Mishkin M. Cortical connections of the somatosensory fields of the lateral sulcus of macaques: evidence for a corticolimbic pathway for touch. *J Comp Neurol.* 1986;252:323–347.
146. Augustine JR. Circuitry and functional aspects of the insular lobe in primates including humans. *Brain Res Rev.* 1996;22:229–244.
147. Jasmin L, Burkey AR, Granato A, Ohara PT. Rostral agranular insular cortex and pain areas of the central nervous system: a tract-tracing study in the rat. *J Comp Neurol.* 2004;468:425–440.
148. McBenedict B, Petrus D, Pires MP, et al. The role of the insula in chronic pain and associated structural changes: An integrative review. *Cureus.* 2024; 16:e58511.
149. Borsook D, Veggeberg R, Erpelding N, et al. The insula: a "hub of activity" in migraine. *Neuroscientist.* 2016;22:632–652.
150. Evans JM, Bey V, Burkey AR, Commons KG. Organization of endogenous opioids in the rostral agranular insular cortex of the rat. *J Comp Neurol.* 2006;500:530–541.
151. Mesulam MM, Mufson EJ. Insula of the old world monkey. I: architectonics in the insulo-orbito-temporal component of the paralimbic brain. *J Comp Neurol.* 1982;212:1–22.
152. Schmahmann JD, Leifer D. Parietal pseudothalamic pain syndrome. Clinical features and anatomic correlates. *Arch Neurol.* 1992;49:1032–1037.
153. Greenspan JD, Winfield JA. Reversible pain and tactile deficits associated with a cerebral tumor compressing the posterior insula and parietal operculum. *Pain.* 1992;50:29–39.

154. Geschwind N. Disconnection syndrome in animals and man. Part I. *Brain.* 1965;88:237–294.
155. Shipley MT, Geinisman Y. Anatomical evidence for convergence of olfactory, gustatory, and visceral afferent pathways in mouse cerebral cortex. *Brain Res Bull.* 1984;12:221–226.
156. Albanese MC, Duerden EG, Rainville P, Duncan GH. Memory traces of pain in human cortex. *J Neurosci.* 2007;27:4612–4620.
157. Koob GF, Buck CL, Cohen A, et al. Addiction as a stress surfeit disorder. *Neuropharmacology.* 2014;76 (Pt B):370–382.
158. Borsook D, Linnman C, Faria V, Strassman AM, Becerra L, Elman I. Reward deficiency and anti-reward in pain chronification. *Neuroscience and Biobehavioral Reviews.* 2016;68:282–297.
159. Paulus MP, Stewart JL. Interoception and drug addiction. *Neuropharmacology.* 2014;76 (Pt B):342–350.
160. Hsieh JC, Hannerz J, Ingvar M. Right-lateralised central processing for pain of nitroglycerin- induced cluster headache. *Pain.* 1996;67:59–68.
161. Rosen SD, Paulesu E, Frith CD, et al. Central nervous pathways mediating angina pectoris. *Lancet.* 1994;344:147–150.
162. Johansen JP, Fields HL, Manning BH. The affective component of pain in rodents: direct evidence for a contribution of the anterior cingulate cortex. *P Natl Acad Sci USA.* 2001;98:8077–8082.
163. Rainville P, Duncan GH, Price DD, Carrier B, Bushnell MC. Pain affect encoded in human anterior cingulate but not somatosensory cortex. *Science.* 1997;277:968–971.
164. Wager TD, Rilling JK, Smith EE, et al. Placebo-induced changes in fMRI in the anticipation and experience of pain. *Science.* 2004;303:1162–1167.
165. Koyama T, McHaffie JG, Laurienti PJ, Coghill RC. The subjective experience of pain: where expectations become reality. *Proc Natl Acad Sci USA.* 2005;102:12950–12955.
166. Devinsky O, Morrell MJ, Vogt BA. Contributions of anterior cingulate cortex to behaviour. *Brain.* 1995;118:279–306.
167. Frankenstein UN, Richter W, McIntyre MC, Remy F. Distraction modulates anterior cingulate gyrus activations during the cold pressor test. *Neuroimage.* 2001;14:827–836.
168. Petrovic P, Petersson KM, Ghatan PH, Stone-Elander S, Ingvar M. Pain-related cerebral activation is altered by a distracting cognitive task. *Pain.* 2000;85:19–30.
169. Rainville P, Duncan GH. Functional brain imaging of placebo analgesia: methodological challenges and recommendations. *Pain.* 2006;121: 177–180.
170. Faymonville ME, Roediger L, Del FG, et al. Increased cerebral functional connectivity underlying the antinociceptive effects of hypnosis. *Brain Res Cogn Brain Res.* 2003;17:255–262.
171. Hampton T. Pain and the brain: researchers focus on tackling pain memories. *JAMA.* 2005;293:2845–2846.
172. Fordyce W. *Beavioral Methods for Chronic Pain and Illness.* Mosby; 2009.
173. Fuchs PN, Peng YB, Boyette-Davis JA, Uhelski ML. The anterior cingulate cortex and pain processing. *Front Integr Neurosci.* 2014;8:35.
174. Talbot J, Marrett S, Evans A, Meyer E, Bushnell M, Duncan G. Multiple representations of pain in human cerebral cortex. *Science.* 1991;251: 1355–1358.
175. Bushnell MC, Apkarian AV. Representation of pain in the brain. In: SB McMahon, M Koltzenburg, eds. *Wall and Melzack's Textbook of Pain.* Elsevier Churchill Livingstone; 2006:107–124.
176. Parent A. *Carpenter's Human Anatomy.* Williams & Wilkins; 1996.
177. Coghill RC, Sang CN, Maisog JM, Iadarola MJ. Pain intensity processing within the human brain: a bilateral, distributed mechanism. *J Neurophysiol.* 1999;82:1934–1943.
178. Lorenz J, Minoshima S, Casey KL. Keeping pain out of mind: the role of the dorsolateral prefrontal cortex in pain modulation. *Brain.* 2003; 126:1079–1091.
179. Grachev ID, Fredrickson BE, Apkarian AV. Abnormal brain chemistry in chronic back pain: an in vivo proton magnetic resonance spectroscopy study. *Pain.* 2000;89:7–18.
180. Apkarian AV, Sosa Y, Sonty S, et al. Chronic back pain is associated with decreased prefrontal and thalamic gray matter density. *J Neurosci.* 2004;24:10410–110415.
181. Obermann M, Nebel K, Schumann C, et al. Gray matter changes related to chronic posttraumatic headache. *Neurology.* 2009;73:978–983.
182. May A. Chronic pain may change the structure of the brain. *Pain.* 2008;137:7–15.
183. Wiech K, Farias M, Kahane G, Shackel N, Tiede W, Tracey I. An fMRI study measuring analgesia enhanced by religion as a belief system. *Pain.* 2008;139:467–476.
184. Wiech K, Ploner M, Tracey I. Neurocognitive aspects of pain perception. *Trends Cogn Sci.* 2008;12:306–313.
185. Neugebauer V, Li W. Processing of nociceptive mechanical and thermal information in central amygdala neurons with knee-joint input. *J Neurophysiol.* 2002;87:103–112.
186. Schafe GE, LeDoux JE. The neural basis of fear. In: MS Gazzaniga, ed. *The Cognitive Neurosciences.* A Bradford Book, MIT Press; 2004: 987–1003.
187. Gauriau C, Bernard JF. Pain pathways and parabrachial circuits in the rat. *Exp Physiol.* 2002;87:251–258.
188. McEwen BS. Glucocorticoids, depression, and mood disorders: structural remodeling in the brain. *Metabolism.* 2005;54:20–23.
189. Neugebauer V, Li W, Bird GC, Han JS. The amygdala and persistent pain. *Neuroscientist.* 2004;10:221–234.
190. Bingel U, Glascher J, Weiller C, Buchel C. Somatotopic representation of nociceptive information in the putamen: an event-related fMRI study. *Cereb Cortex.* 2004;14:1340–1345.
191. Saab CY, Willis WD. The cerebellum: organization, functions and its role in nociception. *Brain Res Brain Res Rev.* 2003;42:85–95.
192. Barinaga M. The cerebellum: movement coordinator or much more? *Science.* 1996;272:482–483.
193. Fiez JA. Cerebellar contributions to cognition. *Neuron.* 1996;16:13–15.
194. Schmahmann JD. Disorders of the cerebellum: ataxia, dysmetria of thought, and the cerebellar cognitive affective syndrome. *J Neuropsychiatry Clin Neurosci.* 2004;16:367–378.
195. Schmahmann JD, Sherman JC. The cerebellar cognitive affective syndrome. *Brain.* 1998;121 (Pt 4):561–579.
196. Chudler EH, Dong WK. The role of the basal ganglia in nociception and pain. *Pain.* 1995;60:3–38.
197. Ingvar M. Pain and functional imaging. *Philos Trans R Soc Lond B Biol Sci.* 1999;354:1347–1358.
198. Neugebauer V, Galhardo V, Maione S, Mackey SC. Forebrain pain mechanisms. *Brain Res Rev.* 2009;60:226–242.
199. Ohara PT, Vit JP, Jasmin L. Cortical modulation of pain. *Cell Mol Life Sci.* 2005;62:44–52.
200. Jerome JA. Transmission or transformation? Information processing theory of chronic human pain. *Am Pain Soc J.* 1993;2:160–171.
201. Turk DC, Melchenbaum D, Genest M. *Pain and Behavior Medicine: A Cognitive Behavioral Perspective.* Guilford Press; 1993.
202. Rice D, Nijs J, Kosek E, et al. Exercise-induced hypoalgesia in pain-free and chronic pain populations: state of the art and future directions. *J Pain.* 2019;20:1249–1266.
203. Fields HL, Basbaum AI. Brainstem control of spinal pain-transmission neurons. *Annu Rev Physiol.* 1978;40:217–248.
204. Mayer DJ, Price DD. Central nervous system mechanisms of analgesia. *Pain.* 1976;2:379–404.
205. Basbaum AI, Fields HL. Endogenous pain control mechanisms: review and hypothesis. *Ann Neurol.* 1978;4:451–462.
206. Ren K, Dubner R. Descending control mechanisms In: AI Basbaum, MC Bushnell, eds. *Science of Pain.* Academic Press Elsevier; 2009:723–762.
207. Fields HL, Basbaum AI, Heinricher MM. Central nervous system mechanisms of pain modulation. In SB McMahon, M Koltzenburg, eds. *Wall and Melzack's Textbook of Pain.* Elsevier Churchill Livingston; 2006: 125–142.
208. Le Bars D. The whole body receptive field of dorsal horn multireceptive neurones. *Brain Res Brain Res Rev.* 2002;40:29–44.
209. Le Bars D, Willer JC. Diffuse noxious inhibitory controls (DNIC). In C Basbaum, MC Bushnell, eds. *Science of Pain.* Academic Press Elsevier; 2009:763–773.
210. France CR, Suchowiecki S. A comparison of diffuse noxious inhibitory controls in men and women. *Pain.* 1999;81:77–84.
211. Tousignant-Laflamme Y, Marchand S. Excitatory and inhibitory pain mechanisms during the menstrual cycle in healthy women. *Pain.* 2009; 146:47–55.

212. Piche M. Mechanistic perspective on conditioned pain modulation. *Pain.* 2023;164:e1–e2.
213. Ramaswamy S, Wodehouse T. Conditioned pain modulation-A comprehensive review. *Neurophysiol Clin.* 2021;51:197–208.
214. Mason P. Deconstructing endogenous pain modulations. *J Neurophysiol.* 2005;94:1659–1663.
215. Mannion RJ, Doubell TP, Coggeshall RE, Woolf CJ. Collateral sprouting of uninjured primary afferent A-fibers into the superficial dorsal horn of the adult rat spinal cord after topical capsaicin treatment to the sciatic nerve. *J Neurosci.* 1996;16:5189–5195.
216. Moore KA, Kohno T, Karchewski LA, Scholz J, Baba H, Woolf CJ. Partial peripheral nerve injury promotes a selective loss of GABAergic inhibition in the superficial dorsal horn of the spinal cord. *J Neurosci.* 2002;22:6724–6731.
217. Dagher M, Alayoubi M, Sigal GH, Cahill CM. Unveiling the link between chronic pain and misuse of opioids and cannabis. *J Neural Transm.* 2024;131:563–580.
218. Taylor AMW, Becker S, Schweinhardt P, Cahill C. Mesolimbic dopamine signaling in acute and chronic pain: implications for motivation, analgesia, and addiction. *Pain.* 2016;157:1194–1198.
219. Paulus MP, Stewart JL. Interoception and drug addiction. *Neuropharmacology.* 2014;76 (Pt B):342–350.
220. Sapolsky RM, Krey LC, McEwen BS. Prolonged glucocorticoid exposure reduces hippocampal neuron number: implications for aging. *J Neurosci.* 1985;5:1222–1227.
221. Lee AL, Ogle WO, Sapolsky RM. Stress and depression: possible links to neuron death in the hippocampus. *Bipolar Disord.* 2002;4:117–128.
222. Schulkin J. Allostasis: a neural behavioral perspective. *Horm Behav.* 2003;43:21–27.
223. Magni G, Moreschi C, Rigatti-Luchini S, Merskey H. Prospective study on the relationship between depressive symptoms and chronic musculoskeletal pain. *Pain.* 1994;56:289–297.
224. Chapman CR, Tuckett RP, Song CW. Pain and stress in a systems perspective: reciprocal neural, endocrine, and immune interactions. *J Pain.* 2008;9:122–145.

12 The Role of Inflammation in Healing and Homeostasis

GERALD R. THRUSH

KEY CONCEPTS

- The osteopathic approach to inflammation and tissue repair views the body as a self-regulatory, self-healing, and structurally integrated unit of function.
- The inflammatory response is made up of several interacting cellular and molecular events that lead to homeostasis. These events result in defenses, repair mechanisms, and adaptive responses that serve to protect individuals from internal and external stressors.
- Disease leading to illness results when the natural capacity to maintain homeostasis becomes overwhelmed.
- An inflammatory reaction results in changes in metabolic, endocrinologic, neurologic, and immunologic functions.
- In response to external and internal stressors, humans have several protective adaptive responses including physical barriers, alternation in body temperature, activation of phagocytic cells, chemical detoxification systems, and stimulation of inflammation, coagulation, complement cascade, and adaptive immune responses.
- In order to restore physiologic homeostasis, the stress response includes a series of interactive responses resulting in the activation of molecular, cellular, physiologic, and behavioral pathways.
- The inflammatory reaction is a nonspecific response to both local and systemic tissue damage.
- The hallmark signs/symptoms of the inflammatory response are redness, swelling, increased local temperature, and pain. In addition, loss of function can occur.
- Much of the signs of inflammation are due to vasodilation, increased vascular permeability, edema, and tissue damage.
- Proinflammatory cytokines, including interleukin 1 (IL-1), interleukin 6 (IL-6), and tumor necrosis factor-α (TNF-α) and various chemokines are central in stimulating and modulating the inflammatory response.

CHAPTER OVERVIEW

The inflammatory response plays a critical role in health and disease, both as a mechanism to bring one back to homeostasis or potentially, to further exacerbate a particular pathologic condition. In the first edition of this textbook, Eugene Mochan, PhD, DO wrote,[1] "Osteopathic philosophy is centered on the unity of structure and function in health and disease. This unity allows us homeostasis and maintenance of our structural integrity, functional capabilities and allow for normal growth and development. Should anything disrupt our natural order, our body has the capacity for healing. Nowhere is this more evident than with the inflammatory response."[2,3] In-depth reviews on the topic of inflammation have been published, and this chapter will detail the major concepts related to healing via inflammation.[4–6] This chapter will address the answer to the question: "What is the molecular basis of the inflammatory process that protect individuals from internal and external disturbances, and their osteopathic significance?"

As humans, homeostasis is based on our ability, through various regulatory biochemical reactions, to achieve a steady state.[7] Our body recognizes disturbances and via various regulatory and biochemical adaptations, typically the return to a normal state ensues. If our body is not able to return to homeostasis, disease and illness often results. Unfortunately, in some individuals, one's responses to an imbalance in homeostasis can result in disease (see Box 12.1).[8]

Health and Disease: Osteopathic Approach

Quoting E. Mochan, "Health reflects a state of equilibrium between a person and their physical, emotional, and social environment that is compatible with full functional activity of the person (Fig. 12.1)." The balance between health and illness is impacted by various factors including the source of illness or the stressor (e.g., infection, trauma, etc.) and factors related to the individual.[1–3] Regarding the stressor, the type, intensity, timing, and duration play important roles in whether or not disease results. The condition of the individual, including their genetics, age, and their nutritional and environmental status are but a few factors that can play an important role in this balance.

A.T. Still stated that: "When all parts of the human body are in line we have health."[9] It seems clear that health is a dynamic state between the stressor and the host. At one end of the spectrum is a high level of wellness, the optimal state of well-being of a person and at the other extreme is complete disabling illness.

BOX 12.1 Clinical Correlate: Immune Reaction Can Stress the Body More Than the Infection

The body's reaction to a streptococcal infection can be much worse than the infectious disease itself. It is because of the immune reaction that "strep throat," once diagnosed, is treated with antibiotics which prevent the associated immune response that can result in much more serious and lasting effects such as seizures and rheumatic heart disease.

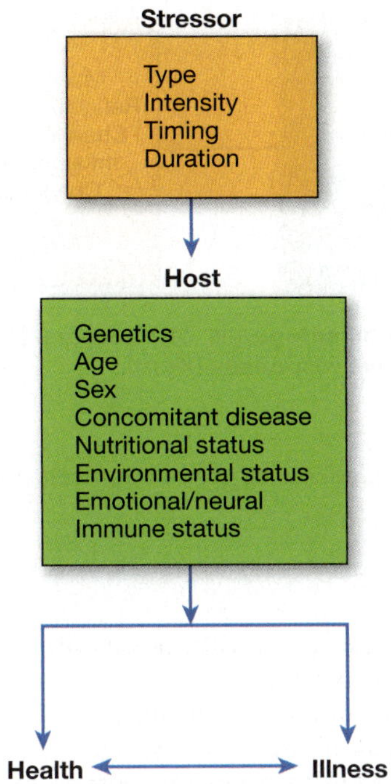

Figure 12.1. Stress response in health and disease.

In the first edition of this textbook, E. Mochan wrote: "Impaired body function due to disease is manifested by a characteristic set of signs and symptoms. Alterations in body structure and/or the composition of body fluids is the manifestation of disease resulting in impaired function and thus leading to illness. Likewise, it is the return of normal function that usually marks recovery from illness."[1] He went on to state that: "osteopathic medicine has emphasized the whole person and that the individual's health and wellness is due to a combination of factors, including physical, emotional, and environmental factors. Therapies have been developed based on established anatomical and physiological concepts."[1] Most recently, we have realized that integrative physiology not only must be viewed in terms of the interrelationships of the physiologic regulatory mechanisms that occur within the organism but also must incorporate the understanding that these mechanisms appear to be influenced by mental and emotional stimuli. Therefore, osteopathic physicians are trained to appreciate that to maintain health, one must take a holistic approach and consider all factors impacting an individual's health and wellness and give each of these factors specific consideration in the prevention, diagnosis, and treatment of illness.

Host Defense Systems

Human beings are constantly being threatened with bodily injury from biologic, chemical, and physical agents from the environment. Through the process of natural selection, humans have evolved mechanisms by which we are able to survive and function which include:

- Innate defenses:
  - Physical and chemical barriers (e.g., skin, stomach acid, mucous membranes)
  - Inflammation
  - Coagulation
  - Chemical detoxification (e.g., liver functions)
  - Phagocytic cells
- Adaptive defenses:
  - Immune responses

The host, rather than using these modalities independently, often responds to stressors/injuries at the molecular level with a concerted combination of host responses referred to collectively as the *stress response*.[10] This response is most commonly seen in people following a number of inflammatory stimuli including:

- Infection
- Trauma and tissue damage
- Burns
- Surgery

After stimulating a stress response that induces an inflammatory reaction, impacts on metabolic, endocrinologic, neurologic, and immunologic changes occur. Most of these changes are observed within hours or days after the onset of injury. They represent a series of local and systemic responses designed to aid survival by neutralizing the offending agent and restoring normal tissue function (Fig. 12.2). In most cases, the magnitude of the stress response is related to the severity of the injured state. When there are cases of major injury, survival occurs if these interactive defense responses are sufficient to compensate for the imposed stresses. An optimal defense response is contingent upon a variety of host factors and can play a role in determining individual survival, including:

- Age
- Sex
- Nutritional status
- Immune status
- Concomitant disease

In many cases, the return to the normal steady state may be unsuccessful and a return to a normal homeostasis is not achieved. Stress response changes can persist that cause further damage (e.g., chronic inflammatory disease such as rheumatoid arthritis). Outside of the molecular cascade of the stress response and return to homeostasis, the interrelationship of the inflammatory and immune responses can change our well-being, and conversely, our well-being can also impact the effectiveness of our host defense response.[11] The importance of maintaining a holistic state of well-being is critical for proper functioning of our physiology.

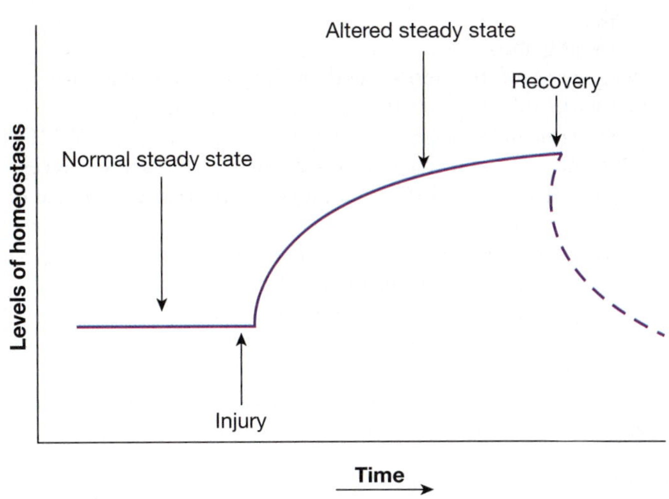

Figure 12.2. Effects of internal and external stressors on homeostasis.

Overview of Stressors and Human Defense Systems

Humans have developed selective survival advantages by acquiring molecular regulatory devices that neutralize threatening stressors. When it comes to stimulation of the inflammatory reaction, there are essentially two types of stressors:

1. Environmental
2. Physical

Environmental stressors can be:

- Physical:
  - Trauma
  - Radiation
  - Temperature extremes
- Chemical:
  - Carcinogens
  - Teratogens
  - Mutagens
  - Toxins in various forms—Liquid, Gas, Air, Metal, Soil
- Infectious disease:
  - Bacterial (e.g., tuberculosis [TB])
  - Viral (e.g., hepatitis)
  - Fungal and parasitic (e.g., toxoplasmosis, malaria)
- Psychological:
  - Terrorism
  - Emotional abuse
  - Isolation

Physiologic stressors can be:

- Hypoxia
- Hypoglycemia
- Fever
- Hemorrhage
- Anemia

Humans adapt to external and internal stressors. The major categories of protective adaptive responses to stressors include:

- Physical and chemical barriers to prevent entry of microbes into the body:
  - Skin
  - Mucous membranes
  - Gastric acidity
- Maintenance of internal body temperature to allow for optimal enzymatic and biologic activity:
  - Skin
  - Sweat glands
- Phagocytes of the reticuloendothelial system which play an important role in responding to stressors including:
  - Recognizing pathogen-associated molecular patterns (PAMPs) on the surface of microbes via the pattern recognition receptors (PRR, e.g., toll-like receptors [TLRs]) on the surface of phagocytes[6]
  - "Ingesting" and "digesting" the microbe
  - Three examples of phagocytic cells are:
    - neutrophils (polymorphonuclear leukocytes)
    - monocytes/macrophages
    - dendritic cells
- Chemical detoxification systems to break down xenobiotics into forms that are not able to cause biologic damage to our body/cells
- Inflammatory reactions:
  - Enable recognition of a foreign invader
  - Recruit cells to respond to the invader
  - Stimulate the release of proinflammatory cytokines, including:
    - IL-1
    - IL-6
    - TNF-α
  - Enable extravasation of white blood cells (WBCs) to the site of tissue injury resulting in:
    - Destruction of the foreign entity
    - Tissue repair to the site of damage
- Coagulation system to begin the clotting cascade to prevent blood loss as well as walling off the damaged tissue
- Complement system to assist in the destruction of microbes that may be at the site of tissue damage via:
  - Cell lysis
  - Opsonization
  - Further stimulation of inflammation
- Immune system recognition of antigens (nonhuman foreign molecules) via the activation of adaptive responses (T and B lymphocytes)
- Stress response to trigger the body's cellular response to tissue damage/injury and activation of mechanisms to repair the damage. See Figure 12.3.

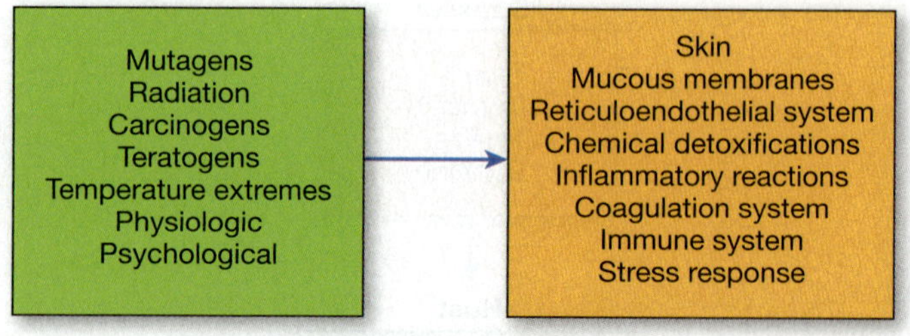

Figure 12.3. Major categories of stressors (*left*) and human protective/adaptive responses (*right*).

HUMAN STRESS RESPONSE

Inflammatory Mediators

As referenced by E. Mochar,[1] our body's responses to challenge can be specific to the stressor or can be generalized and nonspecific.[7,12–14] Responses of the latter type appear to occur only if the magnitude of the stressor to homeostasis exceeds a certain threshold. In humans and other mammals, this response is referred to as the stress response or general adaptation response.

- In order to restore physiologic homeostasis, the stress response includes a series of interactive responses including:
  - Molecular
  - Cellular
  - Physiologic
  - Behavioral
- Depending on the nature of the stressor, one aspect of the stress response is activation of the inflammatory reaction and potentially the immune response. Stimulation of inflammation requires significant energy; therefore, the counterregulatory hormones enable the body to dedicate needed energy to the inflammatory response.

Inflammation is one of the fundamental defense reactions to various stressors, including infections.[4–6,15,16] It is basically nonspecific and is often a systemic as well as local response to tissue damage. The inflammatory response can be activated due to an

BOX 12.2 Clinical Correlate: Examples of Sterile Inflammation

- Gout, due to accumulation of monosodium urate in the joints, is a painful disease of the joints due in large part to the acute inflammatory reaction to these crystals.
- Cholesterol deposits in the arteries and the resultant inflammation plays an important role in atherosclerosis.[17–19]
- Connections between periodontal inflammation and systemic diseases, including cardiovascular disease, are gaining much attention in health care and somewhat blurs the lines between infectious and sterile causes of the inflammatory reaction.[20–22]
- The important role of the inflammatory reaction in neurologic diseases, including Alzheimer disease, is still under investigation in efforts to control the neurologic damage seen in this disorder.[23,24]
- Tissue necrosis has been shown to be a potent stimulator of the acute inflammatory response.[25] Efforts to inhibit this type of inflammation may prevent surrounding tissue damage.

infection or due to noninfectious stimuli (also called the sterile inflammatory response).

- Sterile inflammation is key in responding to damage due to irritant chemicals (e.g., protein aggregates, crystals, etc.).[5]
- For clinical correlates, see Box 12.2.

Altogether, the inflammatory reaction, whether initiated due to infection or sterile irritants, results in a cascade of similar events.[5] Unfortunately, inflammation can be a double-edged sword. On one side, it is an important mechanism to get rid of the body of a foreign invader, and on the other side, bystander tissue damage can be severe.

Cell or tissue injury evokes an acute reaction frequently referred to as the *acute phase response*. If no complications occur, homeostasis is usually restored within a week. If the process continues, *chronic inflammation* occurs, a characteristic of many diseases. Over the years, evidence has accumulated that most, if not all, features of inflammation are directly caused by the action of host-derived substances, rather than the accompanying environmental/infectious perturbation. Changes in the vasculature at the site of injury are key in this process.[4] First described in ancient times, inflammation is characterized by the four cardinal signs:

- Redness (rubor)
- Swelling (tumor)
- Increased local temperature (calor)
- Pain (dolor)

In addition, loss of function can be another hallmark of inflammation. Ultimately, the goal of the inflammatory response is to deliver the innate defense mediators to the site of tissue damage, respond to the root cause of the damage, and initiate the repair process to bring the body back to homeostasis. These inflammatory symptoms are collectively due to:

- Vasodilation
- Increased vascular permeability
- Edema
- Tissue damage

Upon tissue injury/insult:

1. Blood vessel transiently constricts and dilates due to the release of nitric oxide (NO), histamine, and other soluble mediators (e.g., TNF proteins).
2. Increased vascular permeability allows blood and cells to access the damaged tissue.
3. Kinins, the complement cascade, and the clotting cascade are activated, further increasing vascular permeability.
4. Neutrophils arrive to the site of tissue damage and begin to attack the damaged components.
5. Once the offending agent is removed, tissue repair/healing can commence.

CELLS OF INFLAMMATION

The inflammatory reaction/inflammation is a complex interplay between a number of cells and chemicals in response to some type of tissue damage.[4,26] WBCs (leukocytes) are the major players in this response and include participation by:

- Neutrophils
- B and T lymphocytes
- Monocytes/macrophages
- Eosinophils
- Basophils
- Mast cells
- For clinical correlates, see Box 12.3.

While each cell type plays its part in inflammation, there is significant overlap in their roles. One of the early innate cells to arrive at the site of tissue damage are the *neutrophils* or polymorphonuclear leukocytes (PMNs).[27]

- Neutrophils are in the highest concentration of all WBCs, and they can rapidly localize to the site of damage.
- Neutrophils are phagocytic, and they produce a number of factors that play a role in antimicrobial functions, attracting/activating macrophages and dendritic cells, and recruiting T lymphocytes. Another important cell type of the inflammatory reaction is the *endothelial cell*.
- Upon production of various chemical mediators, the endothelial cells allow for extravasation of WBCs from the blood into the tissues.
- Endothelial cells produce arachidonic acid–derived factors that ultimately form oxygen radicals to assist in smooth muscle contraction as well as direct antimicrobial effects.

BOX 12.3 Clinical Correlate: WBCs Associated with Infectious Disease

In clinical practice, the relative increase in the type of WBCs can imply the etiology of symptoms, whether for example, bacterial, viral, fungal, parasitic, allergic, autoimmune, or cancerous. For infections and contingent upon the signs and symptoms, an increase in neutrophils is often indicative of a bacterial infection whereas an increase in lymphocytes is often indicative of a viral infection.[27]

BOX 12.4 Major Histocompatibility Complex I and II

- MHC class I is involved in presenting cytosolic-derived proteins.
- MHC class II presents extracellular proteins.
- A mnemonic to remember this is "one comes before two, and c comes before e."

- Endothelial cells produce IL-1, IL-6, TNF-α, and NO.
  - All play a very important role in the proinflammatory response (the role of these factors is detailed below).
- In order to assist in the inflammatory response, endothelial cells have an impact on the clotting cascade including the release of:
  - Anticoagulants
  - Fibrinolytic factors
  - Prothrombotic agents
- Activation of endothelial cells by IL-1 and TNF-α leads to the vascular changes associated with tissue injury and inflammation.
- Important events include release of the vasodilators, prostacyclin I2 (PGI2, also called prostaglandin I2) and prostaglandin E2 (PGE2), and alterations in endothelial surface adhesion molecules to enhance adherence of neutrophils, monocytes, and lymphocytes.
- The combination of these events initiates vascular congestion, clot formation, and cellular infiltration.

Monocyte/macrophages as well as *tissue dendritic cells* are potent phagocytic cells. In addition, because of their expression of the major histocompatibility complex II antigens (MHC class II), each cell type plays an important role as a bridge between the innate defenses and the adaptive responses. Processing and presentation of foreign antigens via the MHC class II molecules can activate antigen-specific CD4 positive T helper lymphocytes, which, in turn, produce cytokines to further activate the immune response (e.g., stimulate cytotoxicity, inflammation, and/or humoral immune responses due to activation of T and B lymphocytes). See Box 12.4.

INFLAMMATORY MEDIATORS

A number of inflammatory cytokines have been identified that are responsible for the inflammatory response (Table 12.1).

The fact that there are many different types of mediators points to the complexity and coordinated activity involved with the localized inflammatory process. A schematic of the inflammatory reaction can be viewed in Figure 12.4.[4] Individuals lacking in the ability to mount an effective inflammatory response are susceptible to recurrent infections.

Cytokines play a central role in the systemic effects of inflammation.[28–33] Table 12.2,[1] summarizes the classes of cytokines, and Table 12.3,[1] details the common characteristics of these proteins.

- Cytokines are groups of polypeptide cell regulators produced by WBCs, especially by monocytes/macrophages and lymphocytes, for example:
  - Lymphokines (cytokines made by lymphocytes)
  - Interleukins (IL) (cytokines made by one leukocyte and act on other leukocytes)
  - Interferons (a broad class of cytokines divided into three classes; Type I, II, and III)[34]
  - Monokines (cytokines made by monocytes)[35]
  - Colony-stimulating factors (CSF) (homodimeric cytokines)[36]

TABLE 12.1

Inflammatory Mediators and Biologic Role[1]

Major Inflammatory Effect	Mediator
Vasodilation	Prostaglandins
Increased vascular permeability	Vasoactive amines C3a and C5a (complement cascade enzymes through their stimulation of liberating amines) Bradykinins Leukotriene C4, D4, E4, platelet-aggregating factor (PAF)
Chemotaxis	C5a Leukotriene B4 Other chemotactic lipids Bacterial products
Fever	IL-1, TNF-α Prostaglandins
Pain	Prostaglandins Bradykinin
Tissue damage	Neutrophil and monocyte/macrophage lysosomal enzymes Oxygen metabolites

- Collectively, cytokines play an important role in many physiologic responses.
- They are critical in the immune response.
- They regulate activation, growth, and functional activities of all immune cellular components.
- They are involved in the pathophysiology of many diseases and are also used therapeutically.
- Individual cytokines have multiple overlapping cell regulatory actions.
- Current evidence suggests that the response of a cell to a given cytokine depends on the local concentration of the cytokine and other cell modulators as well as the cell type.

TABLE 12.2

Classes of Cytokines[1]

Class
I. Interleukins (ILs) IL-1 → IL-41
II. Interferons (IFN) IFN-α, IFN-β, IFN-γ
III. CSF Granulocyte (G-CSF) Granulocyte–monocyte (GM-CSF) Monocyte (M-CSF)
IV. Tumor necrosis factor TNF-α, TNF-β
V. Chemokines
VI. Growth factors

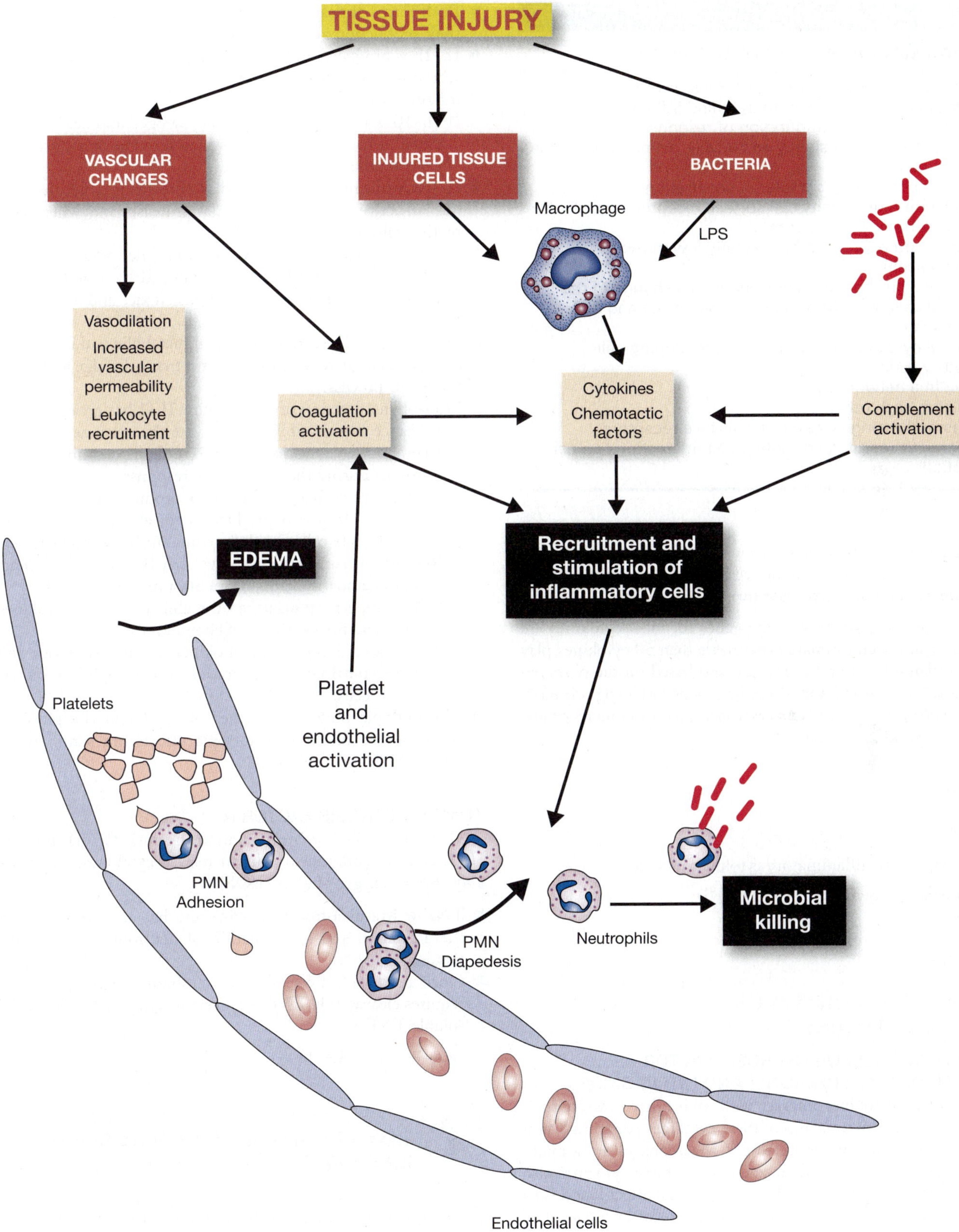

Figure 12.4. The inflammatory response to injury.[4] (Reprinted with permission from Lovitch SB. Inflammation. In: Strayer DS, Saffitz JE, eds. *Rubin's Pathology: Mechanisms of Human Disease*. 8th ed. Wolters Kluwer; 2020:60. Figure 2-1.)

TABLE 12.3

Common Characteristics of Cytokines[1]

- Low molecular mass (<80 kDa) secreted proteins, often glycosylated, involved in immunity and inflammation
- Regulate amplitude and duration of response
- Usually produced transiently and locally, acting in paracrine or autocrine manner
- Extremely potent at picomolar concentrations
- Interact with high-affinity cell surface receptors specific for each cytokine or cytokine group
- Receptors are expressed at relatively low number (10–10,000/cell)
- Cell surface binding ultimately leads to a change in the pattern of cellular RNA and protein synthesis and altered cell behavior
- Individual cytokines have multiple overlapping cell regulatory actions
- Interact in a network by:
  - Inducing each other
  - Transmodulating cytokine cell surface receptors
  - Synergistic, additive, or antagonist interactions on cell function

- Cytokines appear to interact in a network by inducing each other and modulating cytokine receptors. Their impact on cell function can be synergistic, additive, or antagonistic.

During physiologic stresses, the genes for most cytokines are expressed. It has been estimated that more than 50 cytokines play a role in inflammation and immunity, and based on the observed biologic activities, the cytokines may be grouped as being primarily *proinflammatory* or *anti-inflammatory molecules*. Prominent proinflammatory cytokines include:

- IL-1
- TNF-α
- IL-6
- IFN-γ

The major anti-inflammatory cytokines include:

- Transforming growth factor-β (TGF-β)
- IL-4
- IL-10
- Interferons

Key Biology Modulators of the Inflammatory Reaction

INTERLEUKIN-1, TUMOR NECROSIS FACTOR-α, INTERLEUKIN-6, INTERFERON-γ, AND NITRIC OXIDE

Although many cytokines interact with each other to exert their functional roles, the partnership of these cytokines plays important roles in the inflammatory process.[6,31–39] Macrophages are a major source of both IL-1 and TNF-α and both of these cytokines also mediate fever, impact muscle cell catabolism, and affect blood flow during inflammation.[4,39,40] IL-6 can also be produced by monocytes/macrophages as well as by T helper cells, B-cells and endothelial cells.[39–41] NO is produced by macrophages among other cells.

INTERLEUKIN-1

IL-1 is a protein that exists in two molecularly distinct forms, IL-1α and IL-1β.[37]

- Both forms appear to have similar biologic activities; however, their production and activation are different.
- IL-1β is produced and released as an inactive protein that, after secretion from cells, is activated by caspase-1 associated with the inflammasome.[5,37,40]
  - ☐ IL-1β is a powerful endogenous pyrogen and has been implicated in tissue damage and systemic symptoms of sepsis and several inflammatory diseases.[40]
- IL-1α, while initially translated as a precursor molecule, matures into an active form by intracellular proteases and, when released by the cells, is biologically active.
- IL-1 is produced primarily by monocytes and macrophages but has been reported to be synthesized by a wide variety of cell types in response to infectious, toxic, and inflammatory stimuli.
- Once formed, IL-1 induces several metabolic and immunologic changes that guard against excessive tissue damage and enhance the repair process.
- Probably no function of the cytokine IL-1 has greater defensive significance than its ability to activate the immune system.
  - ☐ Lymphocyte activation by IL-1 enhances immunoglobulin synthesis during the acute phase response.
  - ☐ IL-1 activates helper T-cells to produce IL-2 and IFN-γ, and macrophages to produce IL-6, all of which influence B-lymphocyte cell stimulation and antibody production.
  - ☐ Recently, it has also been shown that IL-1 and TNF-α act as potent chemoattractants for neutrophils and T-cells.
    - This appears to occur via the ability of these cytokines to stimulate the synthesis of chemokines.
    - Increased levels of chemokines at sites of tissue injury likely contribute to infiltration of neutrophils, monocytes, and T-cells.
- The multiple biologic activities of IL-1 and the physiologic consequences of these pleiotropic effects are summarized in Figure 12.5, and Table 12.4.[1]

TUMOR NECROSIS FACTOR-α

TNF-α (also called *cachexin* or tumor necrosis factor), along with IL-1, activate endothelial cells to release cytokines, chemokines, and reactive oxygen species (ROS).[39]

- TNF-α is a pleiotropic cytokine and has an important role in the activation and accumulation of neutrophils to the site of tissue damage.[38]
- Once produced, TNF-α is a membrane-bound protein that requires cleavage via TNFα-converting enzyme to release active, soluble TNF-α.

See Box 12.5 for clinical correlate.

BOX 12.5 Medications Now Target Inhibiting TNF-α

- Medications targeting the action of TNF-α have been approved for ameliorating the inflammation seen in the following conditions:
  - ☐ Rheumatoid arthritis
  - ☐ Inflammatory bowel disease
  - ☐ Psoriasis and others

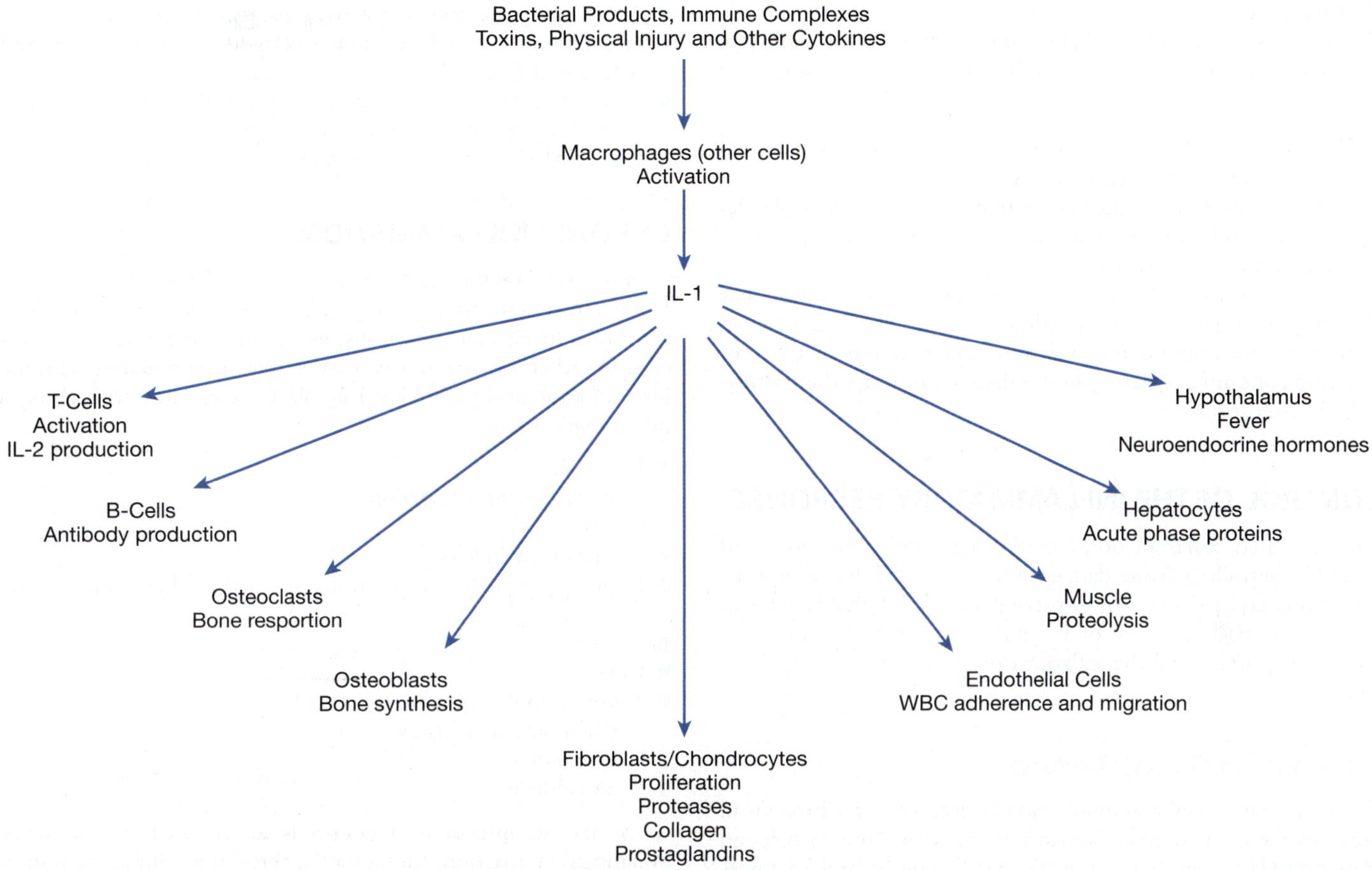

Figure 12.5. Multiple biologic activation of IL-1.

INTERLEUKIN-6

IL-6 is produced by a variety of cell types and was initially cloned for its B-cell–stimulatory role.[39,41]

- IL-6 has multiple roles, including being involved in the inflammatory reaction.
- Engagement of *TLRs* leads to a signaling cascade producing IL-6 as well as IL-1 (both cytokines initiate the inflammatory reaction).
- IL-6 has a variety of actions including the induction of the acute-phase response by the liver, producing C-reactive protein among other molecules in response to bacterial infection.

INTERFERON-γ

Another important molecule in the inflammatory response is IFN-γ.[4,42]

- IFN-γ is produced by T helper cells and natural killer cells (NK cells).
- IFN-γ is a potent stimulator of macrophage activation and cytokine production in response to intracellular pathogens (e.g., viral infections, intracellular bacteria, etc.).
- IFN-γ can further amplify the inflammatory reaction initiated by IL-1, TNF-α, and IL-6.

TABLE 12.4

Biologic Effects of IL-1[1]

Metabolic	Physiologic	Hematologic	Immunologic
↑ **ACTH**	Fever	Neutrophilia	T-cell activation
↑ **Corticosteroids**	Sleep	↑ Colony stimulating factors (CSFs)	B-cell activation
↑↓ **Insulin**	↓ Appetite	Interferon	↑ Natural killer (NK) cell binding
↓ **Plasma, zinc, and iron**	Hypotension	↑ Endothelial procoagulant	Adjuvant
↑ **Hepatic protein**	↑ Sodium excretion	↑ Resistance to infection	↑ Cytokine production
↓ **Albumin**		Radioprotection	
↓ **Cytochrome P-450**			
↓ **Lipoprotein lipase**			
Weight loss			

NITRIC OXIDE

NO is produced by macrophages, among other cells, and plays an important role in killing microbes during the inflammatory reaction.[43,44]

- NO is produced by the macrophage upon the expression of inducible nitric oxide synthase (iNOS).
- NO is an intracellular messenger that helps to prevent platelet adherence and aggregation at sites of tissue injury and also plays a role in production of ROS.
- The importance of NO in the inflammatory reaction has been investigated as to whether exhaled NO could be an effective measure of the inflammatory reaction in cases of asthma and inflammatory bowel disease, among other pathologic conditions.[45,46]

CONTROL OF THE INFLAMMATORY RESPONSE

Once initiated, inflammation can effectively fight infections and assist in controlling tissue damage. Once initiated, however, control of this process is critical to prevent significant and permanent damage to our body. One of the major anti-inflammatory protein helping to control the inflammatory reaction is the cytokine, TGF-β.

Transforming Growth Factor-β

Extensive cell-to-cell communication is necessary in all tissues in order to maintain normal homeostatic activities and to respond appropriately to any allostatic challenge.[47] To revert back to a normal homeostasis after an inflammatory reaction, factors are produced and the TGF family is one of the major groups of cytokines regulating the growth and differentiation of cells as well as the cellular response impacting stress and injury.[48,49] These molecules also play a role in programmed cell death.[41]

- TGF-β, one of several members of the TGF family, is a protein secreted in an inactive form which is subsequently activated through proteolysis.
- Numerous cell types produce TGF-β; however, a very significant reserve of TGF-β in tissue comes from blood platelets.
- The receptors for TGF-β are members of a kinase family and initiate signal transduction pathways in the receiving cell.[49–52]
- TGF-β plays a significant role in the normal development and maturation of tissues and in tissue healing subsequent to injury as well as in tissue remodeling leading to fibrosis and oncogenesis.[49,53–56]
- The function of TGF-β is dependent on the specific tissue in which it is located and the surrounding extracellular milieu. Thus, activated TGF-β can either inhibit or stimulate cell proliferation based on environmental factors; however, in most situations it appears to repress cell division and enhance differentiation.[51,57]
- TGF-β is chemoattractive to immune cells and enhances the deposition of extracellular matrix by activating fibroblasts.[49,54]
- Interestingly, TGF-β is capable of autoinduction of its own production from connective tissue cells such as macrophages.
- In inflamed tissue, TGF-β can inhibit the production of TNF-α and IL-1 and suppress free radical production by macrophages, giving it an anti-inflammatory role.
- TGF-β is extensively involved in wound repair, and overproduction of TGF-β is a key feature in tissue fibrosis.[49,58]
- Acute injury presents with a transient increase in TGF-β; however, chronic reinjury results in overproduction of TGF-β and subsequent tissue fibrosis.
- Elevated levels of TGF-β are seen in disease states and during chemotherapy are thought to be responsible for the resulting tissue fibrosis in the liver and lung.[59]

CHRONIC INFLAMMATION

Chronic inflammation is defined as a prolonged response in which tissue repair and tissue injury coexists. While some infections develop into chronic infections, especially if the microbe is not cleared, other mediators can play a role in stimulating chronic inflammation and pathology. Key players associated with chronic inflammation are:

- Infection
  - □ Parasitic worm infections
  - □ TB
- Apoptosis of PMNs
- Improper regulation of proinflammatory cytokines and signaling
- Trauma
- Cancer
- Autoimmune disease
  - □ Rheumatoid arthritis
  - □ Psoriasis
  - □ Sarcoidosis

When an infectious organism is not cleared by the acute inflammatory reaction, the potential for chronic inflammation is present. Typically, neutrophils clear the invading organism; unfortunately, in diseases such as TB, the *Mycobacterium tuberculosis* microbe is not cleared. The body attempts to isolate the microbe and eventually forms a granuloma, a protective response due to chronic inflammation. While TB is a classic example of an infection that can cause granuloma formation, other infectious agents (e.g., fungi) and persistence of foreign material (e.g., suture, parasitic worm eggs) can also incite a granuloma to form.[4,60,61]

During chronic inflammation, cells become hyperplastic along with cell death resulting in scar formation and potential loss of organ function.[4] Chronic inflammation plays a major role in a variety of diseases that are not directly associated with infections, including:

- Chronic lung disease
- Autoimmune disease
- Ulcerative colitis and Crohn disease
- Chronic kidney disease

A hallmark of chronic inflammation is increased production and activation of tissue macrophages and proinflammatory cytokines, especially IL-6. As depicted in Figure 12.6, macrophages play a central role in the development of chronic inflammation.[4] Lymphocytes are also typically found at the site of chronic inflammation. See Box 12.6 for clinical correlates regarding chronic inflammation.

TISSUE REPAIR

The body's attempt to heal damage induced by local injury involves a series of coordinated activities.[2,4,72] The final successful outcome involves the repair and replacement of damaged and/or dead cells by healthy cells. Once this process is complete, restoration to the normal homeostasis state is feasible.

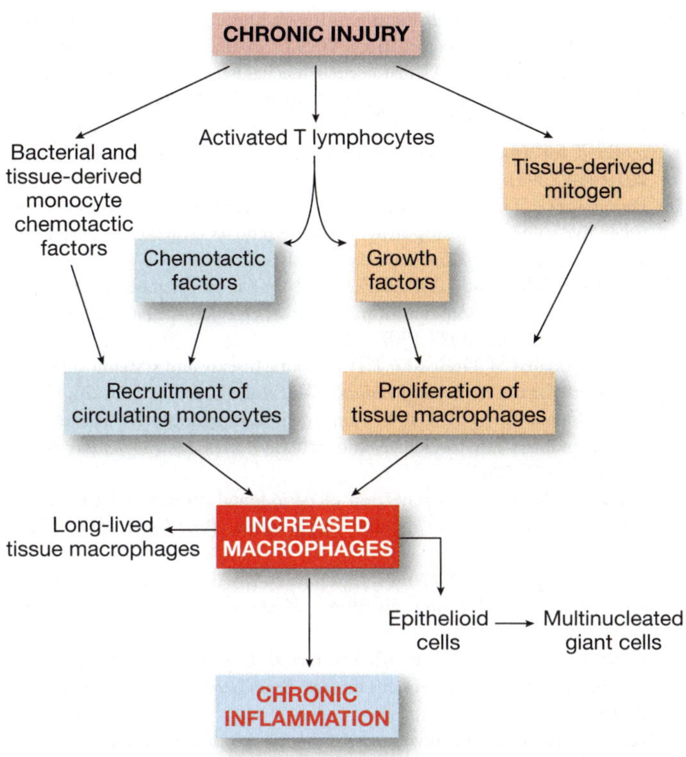

Figure 12.6. Accumulation of macrophages is central to development of chronic inflammation.[4] (Reprinted with permission from Lovitch SB. Inflammation. In: Strayer DS, Saffitz JE, eds. *Rubin's Pathology: Mechanisms of Human Disease*. 8th ed. Wolters Kluwer; 2020:89. Figure 2-34.)

Although the mechanistic details of this important process are not completely understood, four stages appear to be necessary:

1. New capillary growth
2. Fibroblast growth and proliferation
3. Collagen deposition
4. Scar tissue formation

Several growth factors (e.g., platelet-derived growth factor, fibroblast growth factor) and inflammatory mediators (e.g., IL-1, and TNF-α) appear to be involved in these various steps.

BOX 12.6 Clinical Correlate: Chronic Inflammation

- Chronic inflammation and chronic infection, which can stimulate the production of C-reactive protein, IL-6, and lipoprotein-associated phospholipase A2, have been associated with stroke risk and prognosis.[62,63]
- Chronic inflammatory diseases show shifts in the microbiota towards chronic inflammation and the activation of an immune response contributing to disease.[64]
- Tumors have been shown to stimulate inflammatory cascades that play a role in tumorigenesis.[65,66]
- Autoimmune psoriasis has been associated with T helper cell subset activation, which contributes to chronic inflammatory skin disease.[67–69]
- Patients with the autoimmune disease, rheumatoid arthritis, have an increased risk of cardiovascular disease.[70,71]

CYTOKINE INTERACTION WITH IMMUNE AND CENTRAL NERVOUS SYSTEMS

The stress response, inflammation, and the neuroendocrine system are mechanistically linked.[7,12,13,73–77] The interrelationship between these systems is bidirectional. IL-1 produced by the peripheral immune system not only exerts proinflammatory and immunostimulatory effects at the inflammatory site but also acts at the level of the hypothalamus to stimulate corticotropin-releasing hormone (CRH) production. Therefore, IL-1 appears to participate in a negative feedback loop that ultimately leads to the production of cortisol, which in turn depresses peripheral IL-1 production as well as other inflammatory mediators. These relationships are summarized in Figure 12.7.

Acute Phase Protein Response

Another important aspect of the varied metabolic changes after infection and/or tissue injury is known as the *acute phase protein response*. It involves increased production of hepatic protein synthesis that includes:

- Serum amyloid A
- C-reactive protein
- Haptoglobin
- Protease inhibitors
- Complement cascade
- Ceruloplasmin
- Fibrinogen

Other aspects of this response include a decrease in:

- Albumin synthesis
- Leukocytosis
- Hypergammaglobulinemia

The roles that these proteins play in host defense systems are not completely understood. Since some acute phase proteins bind to lipids or directly to bacterial surfaces, it has been speculated

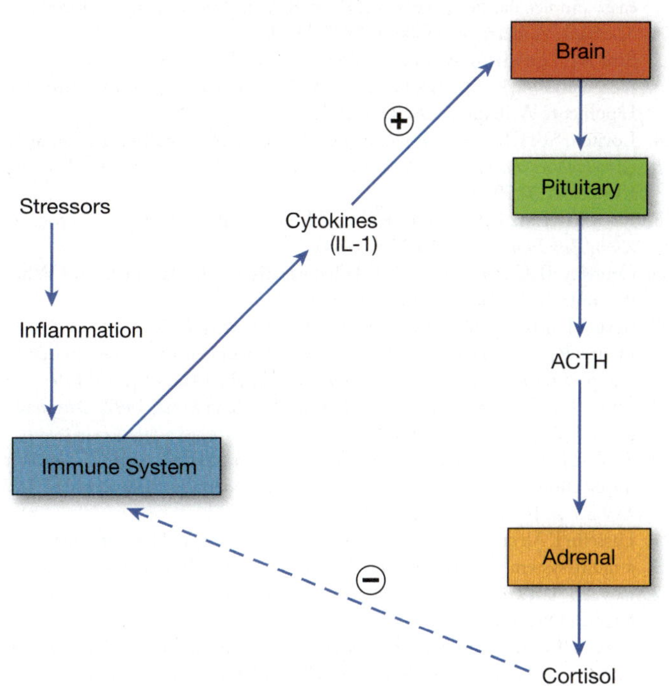

Figure 12.7. Interrelationships between neuroendocrine and immune systems.

that they may function as a nonspecific opsonin to help stimulate phagocytosis. It also has been speculated that other acute phase proteins function as oxygen scavengers. The antiproteinases could function to neutralize destructive effects of proteolytic enzymes from tissue damage and/or bacterial infection. Induced metalloproteins that bind and remove iron and zinc from tissue fluids may inhibit bacterial or tumor cell replication.

CONCLUSION

As written by E. Mochan: "...the study of the inflammatory response and how we respond to tissue damage via stressors is complex and not completely understood. Suggestions have been made that a significant percentage of diseases prevalent in Western society today are related to abnormalities in these responses."[1] Most recently, the role of the host response, including inflammation, has been shown to be complex in its response to COVID-19 (SARS-CoV-2) infection.[62] The disease severity and pathogenesis seem linked to an individual's host defense response. Investigations to allow fully understanding the mechanism by which the human body maintains health and recovers from illness is ongoing. It is important for the osteopathic physician to be actively involved in helping to define and promote the use of these concepts in practice. The implications for the profession, and most importantly for health care, are potentially immense.

ACKNOWLEDGMENTS

This chapter is based on the foundations written by Eugene Mochan, PhD, DO in his chapter on "Human Regulatory Adaptations in Health and Disease" published in the 1st edition of this textbook.

REFERENCES

1. Mochan E. Chap. 8: Human regulatory adaptations in health and disease: a molecular perspective. In: Ward RC, ed. *Foundations for Osteopathic Medicine*. Williams & Wilkins; 1997:99–106.
2. Still AT. *Osteopathy: Research and Practice*. The Pioneer Co.; 1910.
3. DeStefano LA. *Greenman's Principles of Manual Medicine*. 5th ed. Lippincott Williams & Wilkins; 2016.
4. Lovitch, SB. Chapter 2: Inflammation. In: Strayer DS, Saffitz JE, Rubin E, eds. *Rubin's Pathology: Mechanisms of Human Disease*. 8th ed. Wolters Klower; 2020:59–94.
5. Rock KL, Latz E, Ontiveros F, Kono H. The sterile inflammatory response. *Annu Rev Immunol.* 2010;28:321–342.
6. Oronsky, B, Caroen, S, Reid, T. What exactly is inflammation (and What it is not?). *Int J Mol Sci.* 2022;23(23):14905.
7. Seyle H. *Stress in Health and Disease*. Butterworths; 1976.
8. Henrie R, Cherniawsky H, Marcon K, et al. Inflammatory diseases in hematology: a review. *Am J Physiol Cell Physiol.* 2022;323(4):C1121–C1136.
9. Still AT. *Osteopathy: Research and Practice*. Eastland Press; 1992. Originally published by the author; 1910.
10. Su K-H, Dai C. Metabolic control of the proteotoxic stress response: implications in diabetes mellitus and neurodegenerative disorders. *Cell Mol Life Sci.* 2016;73(22):4231–4248.
11. Lasselin J, Alvarez-Salas E, Grigoleit J-S. Well-being and immune response: a multi-system perspective. *Curr Opin Pharmacol.* 2016;29:34–41.
12. Lovallo WR. *Stress and Health: Biological and Psychological Interactions*. Sage Publications; 2016.
13. Cryer PE. Adrenaline: a physiological metabolic regulatory hormone in humans? *Int J Obes Relat Metab Disord.* 1993;17(suppl 3):S43–S46.
14. Saltiel AR. Insulin signaling in the control of glucose and lipid homeostasis. *Handb Exp Pharmacol.* 2016;233:51–71.
15. Colaco HG, Moita LF. Initiation of innate immune responses by surveillance of homeostasis perturbations. *FEBS J.* 2016;283(13):2448–2457.
16. Leifer CA, Medvedev AE. Molecular mechanisms of regulation of Toll-like receptor signaling. *J Leukoc Biol.* 2016;100(5):927–941.
17. Duewell P, Kono H, Rayner KJ, et al. NLRP3 inflammasomes are required for atherogenesis and activated by cholesterol crystals. *Nature.* 2010;464(7293):1357–1361.
18. Paquissi FC. The role of inflammation in cardiovascular diseases: the predictive value of neutrophil-lymphocyte ratio as a marker in peripheral arterial disease. *Ther Clin Risk Manag.* 2016;27:851–860.
19. Engelen SE, Robinson AJB, Zurke YX, Monaco C. Therapeutic strategies targeting inflammation and immunity in atherosclerosis: how to proceed? *Nature Rev Cardiol.* 2022 19(8):522–542.
20. John V, Alqallaf H, DeBedout T. Periodontal disease and systemic diseases: an update for the clinician. *J Indiana Dent Assoc.* 2016;95(1):16–23.
21. Kurita-Ochiai T, Jia R, Cai Y, Yamaguchi Y, Yamamoto M. Periodontal disease-induced atherosclerosis and oxidative stress. *Antioxidants (Basel).* 2015;4(3):577–590.
22. Hajishengallis G. Interconnection of periodontal disease and comorbidities: evidence, mechanisms, and implications. *Periodontol 2000.* 2022; 89(1):9–18.
23. Calsolaro V, Edison P. Neuroinflammation in Alzheimer's disease: current evidence and future directions. *Alzheimers Dement.* 2016;12(6): 719–732.
24. Whitson HE, Colton C, El Khoury J, et al. Infection and inflammation: new perspectives on Alzheimer's disease. *Brain Behav Immun Health.* 2022; 22:100462.
25. Rock KL, Kono H. The inflammatory response to cell death. *Annu Rev Pathol.* 2008;3:99-126.
26. Margraf A, Lowell CA, Zarbock A. Neutrophils in acute inflammation: current concepts and translational implications. *Blood.* 2022;139(14):2130–2144.
27. Buonacera A, Stancanelli B, Colaci M, Malatino L. Neutrophil to lymphocyte ratio: an emerging marker of the relationships between the immune system and diseases. *Int J Mol Sci.* 2022;23(7):3636.
28. Dinarello CA, Wolff SM. The role of interleukin-1 in disease. *N Engl J Med.* 1993;328(2):106–113.
29. Tracey KJ, Cerami A. Tumor necrosis factor, other cytokines and disease. *Ann Rev Cell Biol.* 1993;9:317–343.
30. Kushner I. Regulation of the acute phase response by cytokines. *Perspect Biol Med.* 1993;36(4):611–622.
31. Fietta P, Costa E, Delsante G. Interleukins (ILs), a fascinating family of cytokines. Part I: ILs from IL-1 to IL-19. *Theor Biol Forum.* 2014;107(1–2): 13–45.
32. Fietta P, Costa E, Delsante G. Interleukins (ILs), a fascinating family of cytokines. Part II: ILs from IL-20 to IL-38. *Theor Biol Forum.* 2015; 108(1–2):19–40.
33. Roe K. An inflammation classification system using cytokine parameters. *Scand J Immunol.* 2021;93(2):e12970.
34. Negishi H, Taniguchi T, Yanai H. The Interferon (IFN) class of cytokines and the IFN Regulatory Factor (IRF) transcription factor family. *Cold Spring Harb Perspect Biol.* 2018;10(11):a028423.
35. Zhang JM, An J. Cytokines, inflammation, and pain. *Int Anesthesiol Clin.* 2007;45(2):27–37.
36. Trapnell BC, Abe S. Colony stimulating factors. In: Laurent GJ, Shapiro SD, eds. *Encyclopedia of Respiratory Medicine*. Academic Press; 2006:540–546. https://www.sciencedirect.com/science/article/abs/pii/B0123708796000934
37. Palomo J, Dietrich D, Martin P, Palmer G, Gabay C. The interleukin (IL)-1 cytokine family–balance between agonists and antagonists in inflammatory disease. *Cytokine.* 2015;76(1):25–37.
38. Kalliolias GD, Ivashkiv LB. TNF biology, pathogenic mechanisms and emerging therapeutic strategies. *Nature Rev Rheumatol.* 2016;12(1): 49–62.
39. Kany S, Vollrath JT, Relja B. Cytokines in inflammatory disease. *Int J Mol Sci.* 2019;20(23):6008.
40. Mantovani A, Dinarello CA, Molgora M, Garlanda C. IL-1 and related cytokines in the regulation of inflammation and immunity. *Immunity.* 2019;50(4):778–795.
41. Schaper F, Rose-John S. Interleukin-6: biology, signaling and strategies of blockade. *Cytokine Growth Factor Rev.* 2015;26(5):475–487.

42. Ivashkiv LB. IFNγ: signalling, epigenetics and roles in immunity, metabolism, disease and cancer immunotherapy. *Nat Rev Immunol.* 2018;18(9):545–558.
43. Robinson MA, Baumgardner JE, Otto CM. Oxygen-dependent regulation of nitric oxide production by inducible nitric oxide synthase. *Free Radic Biol Med.* 2011;51(11):1952–1965.
44. Cinelli MA, Do HT, Miley GP, Silverman RB. Inducible nitric oxide synthase: regulation, structure, and inhibition. *Med Res Rev.* 2020;40(1):158–189.
45. Lundberg JO, Lundberg JM, Alving K, Weitzberg E. Nitric oxide and inflammation: the answer is blowing in the wind. *Nat Med.* 1997;3(1):30–31.
46. Amer M, Cowan J, Gray A, Brockway B, Dummer J. Effect of inhaled β2-agonist on exhaled nitric oxide in chronic obstructive pulmonary disease. *PLoS One.* 2016;11(6):e0157019.
47. Xin T, Greco V, Myung P. Hardwiring stem cell communication through tissue structure. *Cell.* 2016;164(6):1212–1225.
48. Batlle E, Massagué J. Transforming grown factor-β signaling in immunity and cancer. *Immunity.* 2019;50(4):924–940.
49. Lodyga M, Hinz B. TFG-β1–A truly transforming growth factor in fibrosis and immunity. *Semin Cell Dev Biol.* 2020;101:123–139.
50. Morikawa M, Derynck R, Miyazono K. TGF-β and the TGF-β family: context-dependent roles in cell and tissue physiology. *Cold Spring Harb Perspect Biol.* 2016;8(5):a021873.
51. Okamura T, Morita K, Iwasaki Y, et al. Role of TGF-β3 in the regulation of the immune responses. *Clin Exp Rheumatol.* 2015;33(suppl 92):S63–S69.
52. Massagué J. TGFβ signaling: receptors, transducers, and mad proteins. *Cell.* 1996;85(7):947–950.
53. August P, Suthanthiran M. Transforming growth factor beta signaling, vascular remodeling, and hypertension. *N Engl J Med.* 2006;354(25):2721–2723.
54. Border WA, Noble NA. Transforming growth factor beta in tissue fibrosis. *N Engl J Med.* 1994;331(19):1286–1292.
55. Kitisin K, Saha T, Blake T, et al. TGF-Beta signaling in development. *Sci STKE.* 2007;2007(399):cm1.
56. Sporn MB, Roberts AB, Wakefield LM, Assoian RK. Transforming growth factor-beta: biological function and chemical structure. *Science.* 1986;233(4763):532–534.
57. Massague J. The transforming growth factor-beta family. *Annu Rev Cell Biol.* 1990;6:597–641.
58. Barrientos S, Stojadinovic O, Golinko MS, Brem H, Tomic-Canic M. Growth factors and cytokines in wound healing. *Wound Repair Regen.* 2008;16(5):585–601.
59. Kisseleva T, Brenner DA. Mechanisms of fibrogenesis. *Exp Biol Med.* 2008;233(2):109–122.
60. Amaral EP, Vinhaes CL, Oliveira-de-Souza D, Nogueira B, Akrami KM, Andrade BB. The interplay between systemic inflammation, oxidative stress, and tissue remodeling in tuberculosis. *Antioxid Redox Signal.* 2021;34(6):471–485.
61. Sia JK, Rengarajan J. Immunology of *Mycobacterium tuberculosis* infections. *Microbiol Spectr.* 2019;7(4).
62. Merad M, Blish CA, Sallusto F, Iwasaki A. The immunology and immunopathology of COVID-19. *Science.* 2022:375(6585):1122–1127.
63. Esenwa CC, Elkind MS. Inflammatory risk factors, biomarkers and associated therapy in ischaemic stroke. *Nat Rev Neurol.* 2016;12(10):594–604.
64. Endres M, Moro MA, Nolte CH, Dames C, Buckwalter MS, Meisel A. Immune pathways in etiology, acute phase, and chronic sequelae of ischemic stroke. *Circ Res.* 2022:130(8):1167–1186.
65. Hand TW, Vujkovic-Cvijin I, Ridaura VK, Belkaid Y. Linking the microbiota, chronic disease, and the immune system. *Trends Endocrinol Metab.* 2016;27(12):831–843.
66. Murata M. Inflammation and cancer. *Environ Health Prev Med.* 2018:23(1):50.
67. Atretkhany K-SN, Drutskaya MS, Nedospasov SA, Grivennikov SI, Kuprash DV. Chemokines, cytokines and exosomes help tumors to shape inflammatory microenvironment. *Pharmacol Ther.* 2016;168:98–112.
68. Diani M, Altomare G, Reali E. T helper cell subsets in clinical manifestations of psoriasis. *J Immunol Res.* 2016;2016:7692024.
69. Chiang CC, Cheng WJ, Korinek M, Lin CY, Hwang TL. Neutrophils in psoriasis. *Front Immunol.* 2019;10:2376.
70. Liao KP. Cardiovascular disease in patients with rheumatoid arthritis. *Trends Cardiovasc Med.* 2017;27(2):136–140.
71. Dijkshoorn B, Raadsen R, Nurmohamed MT. Cardiovascular disease risk in rheumatoid arthritis. *J Clin Med.* 2022;11(10):2704.
72. Wilkinson HN, Hardman MJ. Wound healing: cellular mechanisms and pathological outcomes. *Open Biol.* 2020;10(9):200223.
73. Bellinger DL, Lorton D, Romano TD, Olschowka JA, Felten SY, Felten DL. Neuropeptide innervation of lymphoid organs. *Ann NY Acad Sci.* 1990;594:17–33.
74. Karalis K, Sano H, Redwine J, Listwak S, Wilder RL, Chrousos GP. Autocrine or paracrine inflammatory actions of corticotropin-releasing hormone in vivo. *Science.* 1991;254(5030):421–423.
75. Taylor MK, Carpenter J, Stone M, et al. Genetic and environmental modulation of neurotrophic and anabolic stress response: counterbalancing forces. *Physiol Behav.* 2015;151:1–8.
76. Habib KE, Gold PW, Chrousos GP. Neuroendocrinology of stress. *Endocrinol Metab Clin North Am.* 2001;30(3):695–728.
77. Zhao JL, Baltimore D. Regulation of stress-induced hematopoiesis. *Curr Opin Hematol.* 2015;22(4):286–292.

13 Somatic Dysfunction, Spinal Facilitation, and Viscerosomatic Integration

J'AIMEE LIPPERT

KEY CONCEPTS

- The "osteopathic lesion" was historically conceived as one of the primary factors influencing body economy and the root of many diseases.
- Louisa Burns and her colleagues performed many studies on the effects of somatic dysfunction on visceral function, thus showing many somatovisceral influences well before they were recognized by the scientific and medical communities.
- Reflexes have an afferent arm bringing impulses to the central nervous system (CNS), a central arm within the CNS, and an efferent arm taking impulses to peripheral structures.
- While usually thought of as simple hardwired pathways, reflexes are actually complex interconnections influenced by factors such as ascending messages, descending influences from higher centers, and general CNS excitability.
- Somatovisceral and viscerosomatic reflexes are two of the main integrating mechanisms of body function, closely linking somatic structures and viscera to achieve integrated function.
- In general, sympathetic control from the brain is often localized to specific visceral organs, suggesting that the brain, through the sympathetic nervous system, can selectively influence specific organ function.
- Manipulative treatment of somatic structures can influence sympathetic function and hence visceral function through the somatovisceral reflex networks.
- Sensitization is a process that occurs in spinal gray matter neurons (interneurons) and results in an increased excitability of the involved neurons, thus increasing the gain of the input pathway.
- Long-term sensitization is a prolonged form of excitability in the reflex pathways that can last for hours and often occurs with the same stimuli as sensitization.
- Permanent changes in reflex excitability may occur in reflex pathways with inhibitory cell death and new synapse formation.
- Neurons exhibit a continuous flow of intra-axonal substances both away from and toward the cell body. This flow has been shown to include transport of proteins across the synapse from nerve cell to nerve cell and from nerve cell to end organ.

INTRODUCTION

This chapter presents the neurophysiologic basis for viscerosomatic and somatovisceral interactions, vital to the function of the body and utilized in the diagnostic assessment and treatment of the patient, which includes the use of osteopathic manipulative medicine concepts.

The historical research of Denslow and Korr on spinal excitability laid the foundation for the osteopathic profession's modern views of somatic dysfunction, formerly referred to as the osteopathic lesion. Spinal cord excitability underlies chronic and neuropathic pain syndromes and relates to the physical examination findings of somatic dysfunction.

The foundations of the osteopathic profession, laid by Andrew Taylor Still, D.O., recognize that the state of health is a continuum from perfect function to complete breakdown. One of Still's basic beliefs about function was that the body is a totally integrated unit, its structures working together harmoniously to produce a state of health. In the presence of factors that hinder or obstruct that harmonious function, the body produces conditions contributing to loss of health, or disease.

Implicit in these assumptions is the idea that the various parts of the body are functionally interconnected, allowing for necessary adaptations when demands on the body change. This includes the concept that the viscera are functionally connected with the primary energy consumer of the body, the musculoskeletal system. The communicating systems of the body, including the immune, endocrine, and neural systems, provide this interconnectedness. When a problem develops in the integrating systems of the body, function is compromised, setting the stage for alteration in health, and eventually disease, to occur.

The field of neurophysiology is important to the osteopathic physician, and a thorough knowledge of anatomy and structural relationships within the body is vital. The physician must know how structures function and relate to each other and have a basis for providing the patient with a rational course of treatment, which may include osteopathic manipulative treatment. Through astute palpation, the physician gains deeper understanding of the underlying state of the health in the body.

This chapter focuses on the integration of somatic and visceral function through reflex pathways and relates these interactions to their specific neural basis. Functional alterations in reflex pathways that can disrupt integration are reviewed, along with the non–impulse-based or trophic function of the nervous system, and how this provides a means of two-way communication within the body that is not dependent on the better-understood neural impulse–based communication. These aspects of the integrative activity of the nervous system are important in the osteopathic clinical experience and the role of osteopathic manipulative treatment in health care. As Still recognized before the turn of the century, proper function necessitates the free interaction and integration of all body systems. Rational treatment of functional problems likewise requires an understanding of how these interactions occur and what can alter their function.

NEUROPHYSIOLOGY IN THE OSTEOPATHIC PROFESSION

The search for mechanisms underlying the efficacy of osteopathic methods began with the founding of the osteopathic profession. Although Still did not perform research as it is done today, he constantly questioned his observations and searched for better ways to find health and ameliorate disease. His early students at the American School of Osteopathy actively investigated the scientific foundations for the treatments they were developing. Their observations resulted in the formulation of the concept of the osteopathic lesion, now known as the somatic dysfunction. The osteopathic lesion was a set of palpatory cues and signs indicating a functional disturbance in the body that predisposed it to disease. Early osteopathic pioneers believed that somatic dysfunctions were primary causes of clinical breakdowns, resulting in the many manifestations of disease, either by themselves or by allowing microorganisms to overwhelm the body's defenses. Still stated "...all diseases are mere effects, the cause being a partial or complete failure of the nerves to properly conduct the fluids of life."[1]

Still believed that various diseases were not entities unto themselves but were the result of the body's efforts to regain optimal function in the face of adverse influences. He reinforced that the events that led to the disruption of the body's normal function should be the primary focus for the osteopathic physician, and efforts to remove the influences that resulted in clinical illness were emphasized. The osteopathic lesion was viewed as one of the primary factors influencing body function and was amenable to physical manipulations. In addition, Still and his students realized that the body was an integrated unit; the visceral systems were intimately connected to the somatic systems. They learned that visceral disturbances would cause manifestations in the somatic structures and that somatic disturbances would cause visceral dysfunctions. This reciprocal relationship became very important in the profession's philosophy, clinical practice, and research endeavors.

Early research efforts in the profession were largely aimed at providing evidence for the somatic problems identified as the osteopathic lesion and the effects these dysfunctions had on various aspects of physiology.[2] In their efforts to find objective measures of the osteopathic lesion, researchers at the American School of Osteopathy used skiagraphy, an early form of x-ray, to look at bony placement and circulatory function as early as 1898. Another early research focus examined the effects of somatic disturbances on visceral function. Louisa Burns began this research in the early 1900s with studies on dogs showing that stimulation of the lower dorsal region increased muscle contraction in the stomach and intestines, but that steady pressure tended to inhibit such contractions.[3]

Burns eventually became head of the A.T. Still Research Institute in Chicago and produced a body of research suggesting that strains produced in the vertebral column would, over time, have definite and reproducible effects on visceral function and morphology. Aided later by Wilber Cole, effects of somatic strains on neural end plate function controlling visceral organs were found and documented by neural stains. In addition, Cole[3] was able to delineate the pathways for the effects of somatic influences on visceral function. The early research efforts of the osteopathic profession were attempts to describe the effects of somatic disturbances on visceral function and the effects of manipulative treatment on immune and general function, among other things. They established a firm interest in the profession on the interrelationships between somatic and visceral function.

Beginning in the late 1930s, a new era of research in osteopathic medicine began. In an effort to enhance the profession's reputation, J.S. Denslow began a program of research at the Kirksville College of Osteopathy and Surgery that would span 40 years and add much to the understanding of the methods of manipulative treatment. With his colleagues, Denslow[4] used then cutting-edge electromyography (EMG) to obtain objective evidence of specific alterations in somatic function that correlated almost exactly to palpatory findings. Joined by Irvin M. Korr[5] in 1945, Denslow used EMG to show that one of the underlying causes of palpatory findings was altered muscle excitability. Korr then interpreted these findings in terms of neural function, and the concept of the facilitated segment was developed as an underpinning of the osteopathic lesion. The research of the Kirksville group, discussed later in this chapter, placed the interactions between somatic and visceral structures in the forefront of osteopathic clinical practice and philosophy. It became obvious that the interactions between visceral and somatic structures were important in health maintenance and disease processes. These interactions also provided an explanatory framework for the impact of manipulative treatment as not only influencing somatic function but also having an important effect on visceral function.

The interactions between visceral and somatic structures are foundational to learning the osteopathic approach to health, as are the alterations in spinal cord function that can occur with somatic input and its influence on visceral function. These interactions and alterations, beginning with the organization of the basic reflex arc, are important in understanding the value of osteopathic treatment techniques and the neural basis of health.

THE NEUROLOGIC REFLEX

In 1905, Charles Sherrington[6] published *The Integrative Action of the Nervous System* which explored the fundamental aspects of how the nervous system handled and integrated information. Since that time, considerably more has been learned about the function of the nervous system and how it integrates the many functions of the body. The basic structural unit of the nervous system, the neuron, interacts with other cells through synaptic structures and the release of neurotransmitters and neuromodulators. The billions of neurons and glial cells that make up the nervous system are organized into functional groups, often with widely differing structural and functional characteristics. Many neuron networks respond to stimuli impinging on or even originating in the body, which results in commands to muscles and glands that produce activity or secretions.

These networks, the reflexes, have been more fully analyzed in recent years. What were previously considered to be almost autonomous units of function are actually complex and interactive aspects of an organizational whole. The reflex has been found to be anything but a static unit of input/output relationships; rather, it is an active and ever-changing mosaic. The characteristics of reflex function are modulated by messages from other areas of the nervous system and by activity of the endocrine and immune systems. Reflexes are not separate entities but rather parts of various programs that control motor and secretory actions. Thus, an individual reflex may serve differing functions depending on which control program is operating.[7]

Structure

The common concept of the reflex is basically one of a relationship between an input stimulus to the body and an output action to either a muscle or a secretory organ. Sherrington[6] viewed the reflex as an input/output relationship between information coming into the body and a response to that information. He considered a reflex as always inherited and innately given.

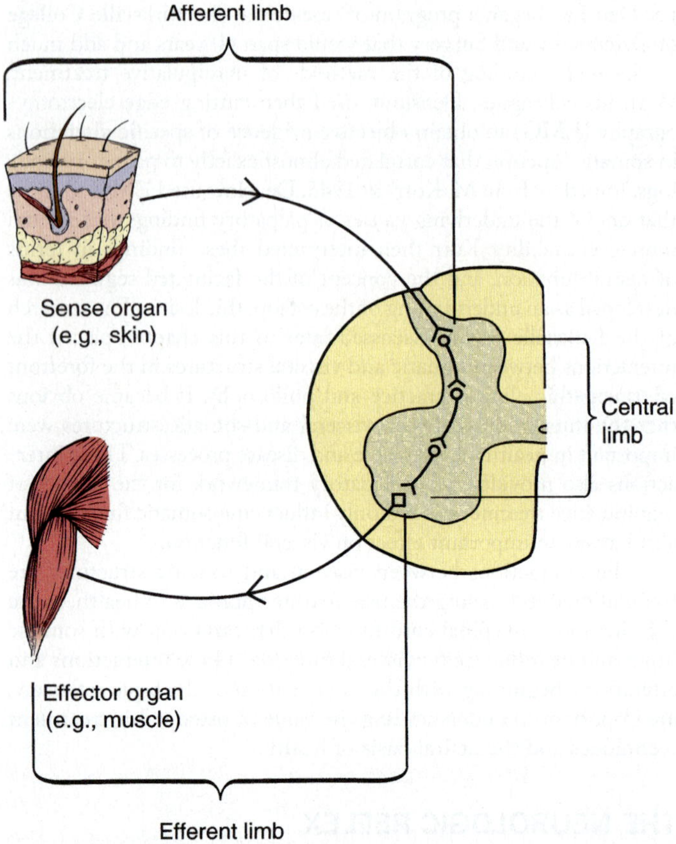

Figure 13.1. Schematic of reflex as it is usually envisioned, with afferent, central, and efferent limbs.

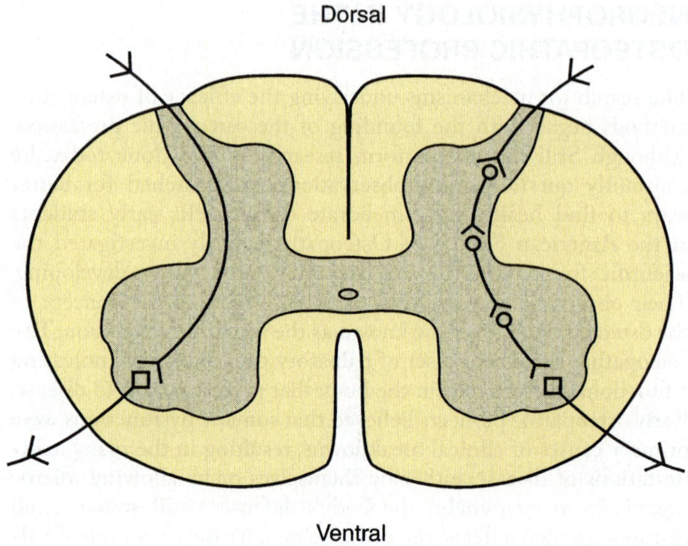

Figure 13.2. A common, mistaken concept of how a reflex is constructed. Afferent limb simply connects with central limb, which activates efferent limb. *Left*, monosynaptic reflex; *right*, polysynaptic reflex. Actual complexity is better represented in Figure 13.3.

The concept of a reflex includes an afferent or incoming limb from a sensory receptor, which is a central component in the spinal cord or brain. It also includes an output (efferent) limb that is usually a motor component to either somatic (musculoskeletal) or visceral structures terminating in synaptic connections that may either activate or inhibit activity in these structures (Fig. 13.1).

The usual concept of the reflex suggests that the reflex limbs are fairly well defined and limited primarily to one input and one output channel, with little interaction with other reflex networks (Figs. 13.2 and 13.3).

Almost all reflex networks can be influenced by a wide variety of other excitatory and inhibitory signals, including those coming from higher or lower levels of the CNS. For example, the picture of a reflex as a simple message pathway from the patellar tendon that causes the quadriceps femoris muscle to contract, resulting in a knee jerk, is a vast oversimplification of the interactions that occur when a stimulus causes a response. This myotatic, or muscle stretch, reflex, exemplified by the patellar tap/knee jerk reflex, is a prime example of the simplest reflex structure.

The myotatic reflex is a monosynaptic reflex. It is the only monosynaptic reflex present in humans. The stimulus of a tap to a tendon stretches the muscle attached to the tendon, which in turn stretches the muscle spindle organs in the muscle. Neural signals, or action potentials, are sent from the spindle organs to the spinal cord on the incoming, or afferent, limb of the reflex. In this case, the signals travel through the spinal cord on the axons from the spindles directly to the motor neurons that innervate the muscle that was stretched. They make synaptic contact with the motor neurons causing them to generate action potentials that travel over the efferent, or outgoing, limb of the reflex network back to the muscle, causing it to contract.

It would be a simple picture if this were all that happened. However, the incoming axons have branches that go to other neurons in the spinal cord that then send axons to the motor neurons of the antagonist of the stretched muscle. These axons provide signals that inhibit the motor neurons innervating the antagonist muscle. When the stretched muscle contracts, the antagonist muscle is inhibited to allow a smooth movement to occur. In addition, other branches from the incoming axons travel up the spinal cord to other spinal areas (e.g., to the arms if the patellar reflex was stimulated), to the brain stem, and down the spinal cord to lower spinal centers.

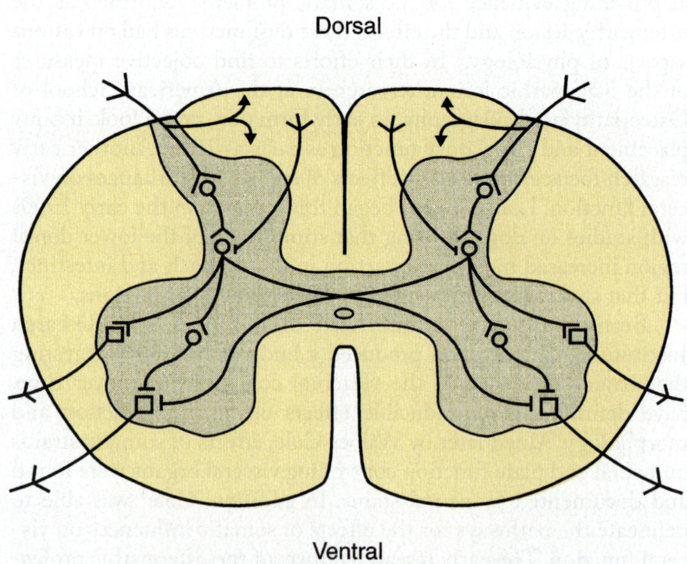

Figure 13.3. Schematic of neural interactions at the spinal level, indicating the complexity of even simple reflexes. Input to the spinal cord sends collaterals up and down the cord and is acted on by ascending and descending influences, as well as input from the opposite side of the cord. Input courses through several synapses and interneurons before acting (in the thoracolumbar cord) on both somatic and sympathetic motoneurons. In cervical and sacral cord areas, parasympathetic pathways are involved.

What appeared to be a simple reflex network has become a complex set of pathways within the spinal cord and brain stem. In addition, pathways from both above and below the level of the input axons can directly influence the basic excitability of the motor neurons involved and, hence, alter the reflex activity observed when the tendon is tapped. When elicited clinically, the myotatic reflex is a window into the nervous system to determine its overall general functioning. Clinically, the main purpose of the myotatic reflex is to test the excitability of motor neurons, as a function of both local and distant influences.

Somatosomatic

Although the myotatic reflex is used a great deal clinically, the most familiar of the spinal reflexes are the defensive reflexes, such as the withdrawal movements of a limb to a noxious stimulus. These somatosomatic reflexes occur when some stimulus is applied to a somatic structure. This initiates a volley of neural activity (often nociceptive) through the afferent limb of the reflex to the spinal cord. The afferent input activity flows through synapses into the interneurons of the spinal cord central gray matter and finally into the ventral horn motor neurons. These motor neurons then cause somatic muscle contraction. The reflexes have at least one interneuron between the sensory input in the dorsal horn of the cord and the motor neurons of the ventral horn (see Fig. 13.3). Their names are derived from the origin of the information and the locus of action, both of which are somatic.

Many somatosomatic reflexes have been documented and studied. The simple somatosomatic reflexes are exemplified by defensive withdrawal actions such as when accidentally touching a hot object and the hand jerks back. Very complex activities, such as the righting reflexes that occur when a cat is dropped upside down and lands on its feet, are also found, but even these reflexes do not occur in isolation; as with the myotatic reflexes, they are accompanied by a spread of activity throughout the nervous system.

Viscerovisceral

Another type of reflex is the viscerovisceral reflex, in which sensory input from a visceral structure causes visceral activity. These reflexes are involved, for example, in distention of the gut that results in increased contraction of the gut muscle. Viscerovisceral reflexes involve afferent activity flowing from the receptors to the spinal cord through interneurons to produce efferent or outflow activity within the sympathetic and/or parasympathetic motor neurons.

Reflex Interactions

Afferent input from somatic structures might be expected to have some influence on visceral organs and input from visceral structures to have some effect on somatic organs. Somatovisceral and viscerosomatic reflexes have been known for many years and are gaining more recognition by the research and medical community. These types of reflex interactions are very important in health and body function integration and for the practice and understanding of osteopathic palpatory diagnosis and treatment.

A familiar example of a viscerosomatic reflex is pain and muscle tightness in the left shoulder with onset of a myocardial infarction (MI). The nociceptive input from the compromised myocardium (a visceral structure) not only is exciting the pathways that are interpreted as shoulder pain (a somatic structure) but is also causing the motor neurons supplying the shoulder muscles to become active. In a classic study, Eble[8] showed several such reflexes by stimulating visceral structures and recording somatic muscle activity. He demonstrated that stimulation of various visceral structures produced somatic muscle activity.

Conversely, activity in a somatic structure can alter visceral function. In a number of studies, Sato[9] demonstrated the effect of somatic stimulation on various visceral functions, ranging from heart rate to adrenal output. These studies have also shown that some of these reflex interactions occur directly in the spinal cord. With others, the afferent activity from the somatic stimulation travels up the spinal cord to the brain stem, resulting in a cascade of activity from the brain stem back down to the spinal autonomic motor neurons.

In both viscerosomatic and somatovisceral reflex networks, activity resulting from the stimulation of a structure can have either an excitatory or an inhibitory influence on the motor neurons involved. For example, stimulation of the skin overlying the abdomen usually results in inhibition of gut activity (a somatovisceral reflex) but increases heart rate.

In daily life, the body's somatic system is active. The skeletal muscles are the machines that carry out activities; the visceral organs are the means by which the energy demands and maintenance of the muscles are met and by which waste is disposed. Without a continuous and highly integrated communication between these two systems, the body could not continue to achieve a balance between its energy needs and supply. The neural connectivity represented by these reflex systems is one of the primary ways this integration is achieved.

For the osteopathic physician, the viscerosomatic and somatovisceral reflexes are of great importance. When using palpatory diagnosis to detect subtle problems in function, whether it is tissue texture changes, motion characteristics, or temperature variations of the body, the physician senses clues from the skin and musculoskeletal system. These clues reflect not only aspects of these tissues but also functional characteristics of the underlying visceral organs and tissues through the viscerosomatic reflex networks. When the physician uses osteopathic manipulative treatment to correct somatic dysfunctions, underlying visceral function is affected through the somatovisceral reflex networks. Thus, for both palpation and treatment, an understanding of reflex function is necessary.

NEURAL BASIS FOR REFLEX INTERACTIONS

Evidence describes the neural basis of viscerosomatic and somatovisceral interactions. When a stimulus is applied, afferent input from either visceral or somatic structures flows into the spinal cord along the dorsal roots and enters the upper areas of the spinal gray matter. The spinal gray matter is commonly divided into 10 layers, first documented on cytoarchitectural evidence by Rexed[10] and are referred to as the Rexed laminae (Fig. 13.4). Large-diameter, cutaneous afferent input that signals nonnociceptive stimuli enters the spinal gray of the dorsal horn and terminates primarily in layers III and IV.

Nociceptive afferents from both somatic and visceral structures enter the cord and send branches rostrally and caudally in Lissauer's tract that runs along the apex of the dorsal horn. Branches of this nociceptive input then terminate in layers I, II, V, VII, and X. Layers I and V display an especially tremendous overlap of the input from somatic and visceral nociceptors.[11]

It appears that in most areas of the spinal cord, a large number of interneurons that receive input from a visceral nociceptor also receive input from a somatic source. It also appears that most interneurons that receive input from somatic structures also receive visceral input. This raises the question of how an individual can distinguish visceral from somatic pain or sensation at all. In many

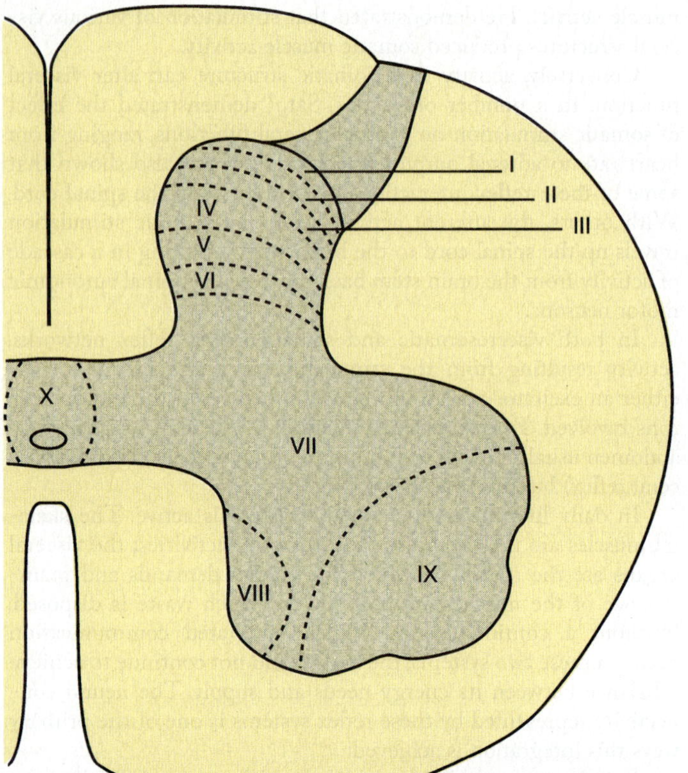

Figure 13.4. Rexed layers. Laminae at the L7 segment of a cat spinal cord. (From Rexed B. The cytoarchitectonic organization of the spinal cord in the cat. *J Comp Neurol.* 1952;96(3):414–495. Copyright © 1954 The Wistar Institute of Anatomy and Biology. Reprinted by permission of John Wiley & Sons, Inc.)

cases, visceral pain is felt as a diffuse and poorly localized sensation and is referred to somatic structures. The overlap of somatic and visceral input explains the referral of visceral pain to somatic structures, which is also called referred pain. In 2015, Luz et al. studied this concept and found evidence for monosynaptic convergence of somatic and visceral C-fiber afferents on neurons in lamina I. This work found that the first site in the CNS where somatic and visceral pathways directly converge is lamina I of the spinal cord. Also, the mechanism of somatovisceral convergence demonstrated a complex functional integration of monosynaptic and polysynaptic excitatory and inhibitory input in specific groups of neurons. This research confirms the complex pattern of convergence between visceral and somatic afferents that contribute to referred pain.[12]

Impulses arriving from visceral structures and converging onto interneurons also receiving somatic afferents activate ascending pathways to the brain that result in the perception of pain in the somatic structure. In addition, more somatic than visceral input occurs because the viscera are much more sparsely innervated with sensory receptors. This suggests that visceral input has much more diffuse functional effects than the corresponding somatic afferents do. Only about 10% of the inflow into the thoracolumbar spinal cord comes from visceral structures.[13] This sparse innervation but wide distribution of visceral afferents may be the basis for the diffuse nature of most visceral pain.

The evidence indicates that the widespread effects of visceral input are due more to spread of activity through networks than collateral branches (functional vs. anatomic divergence).[14] Figure 13.5 shows the afferent terminations of somatic and visceral afferent fibers in the various levels of the spinal cord.

The overlap of input onto common interneurons within the gray matter of the spinal cord is also the basis for the activation of somatic muscle activity seen with visceral disturbances. The excitatory drive provided onto common interneurons by visceral input activates not only sympathetic outflow back to visceral structures but also motor neurons (both alpha and gamma) that innervate skeletal musculature. The result is a tonic activation of skeletal muscles in the referral area of visceral input. This is the viscerosomatic reflex manifestation or splinting that is seen, for example, in appendicitis.

These relationships also underlie the reverse phenomenon of the somatovisceral reflex, in which somatic input alters sympathetic and parasympathetic outflow. The data on the convergence of somatic and visceral input are beginning to explain the interrelations between visceral and somatic structures, especially when nociceptive input is activated.

There are descending influences on the activity of both somatic and visceral reflex pathways. In many of the reflex loops

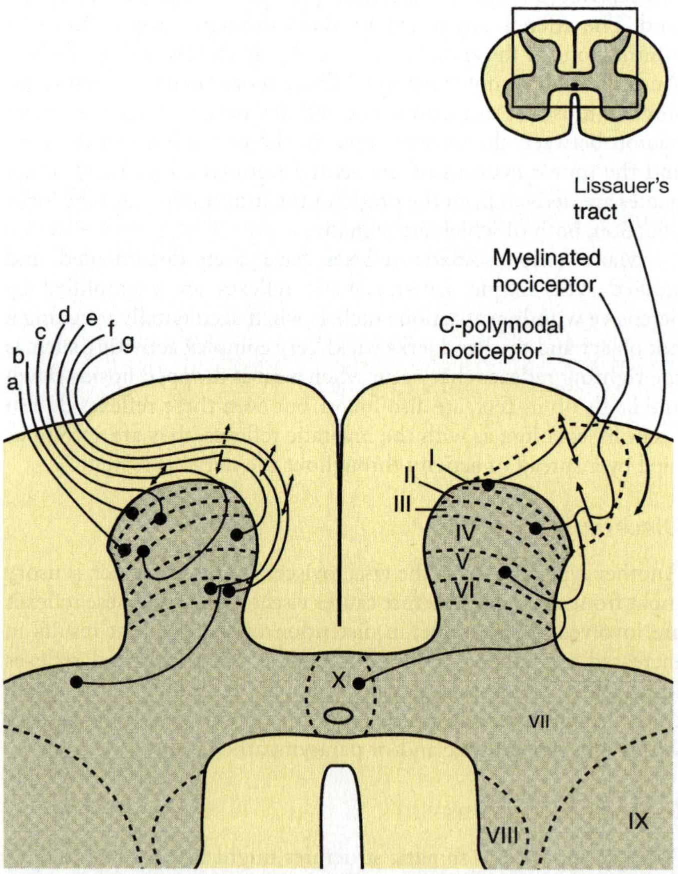

Figure 13.5. Terminal patterns of primary afferent collaterals in the transverse plane of the spinal cord. *Left.* Primary afferent terminations of axons not associated with nociception. *a,* C low-threshold mechanoreceptor; *b,* innocuous cooling receptor; *c,* a hair afferent; *d,* G-1 and G-2 hair receptors; *e,* slowly adapting type I and II afferents; *f,* primary and secondary muscle spindle afferents; *g,* Golgi tendon organ. The *arrow* indicates that the parent axon bifurcates, ascends, and descends the spinal cord for 17 segments, giving off collaterals along this course. *Right.* Nociceptor afferents from both somatic and visceral structures. Both visceral and somatic A and C fiber nociceptor afferents terminate in Rexed lamina I, II, V, and to some extent in VII and X. Lamina are indicated on the right and outlined by *dotted lines.* (From Light AR. *The Initial Processing of Pain and Its Descending Control: Spinal and Trigeminal Systems.* S. Karger; 1992:88. Figure 5-1. Copyright © 1992 S. Karger AG, Basel, Switzerland. Reprinted by permission.)

driven by both visceral and somatic input, there is a strong effect of descending pathways on the long-lasting excitability of the reflex outflow. These descending influences can maintain the excitability of the reflex for extended periods. They may account for some of the long-term increases in sensitivity, muscle contractions, and hyperexcitable sympathetic output seen especially with visceral disturbances.

Likewise, the long-lasting descending influences can be inhibitory, resulting in lowered somatic or autonomic outflow. For example, the effects of rib-raising techniques (a somatic stimulation) on sympathetic outflow seem to be primarily inhibitory through the descending brain influences, resulting in decreased vasoconstriction and better fluid flow in the thoracic area.[15]

Although much of the information on the activation of sympathetic afferents by skeletal input has come from nociceptive input, there is evidence that sympathetic output can also be strongly driven independent of nociception by muscle proprioceptors. For example, Kaufman et al.[16] have shown large effects on sympathetic outflow driven by alteration of proprioceptive input from muscles.

Pickar and his colleagues found evidence for somatosympathetic reflex interactions from the lower back.[17] Thus, the evidence for activation and control of sympathetic activity by somatic input strongly suggests a basis for musculoskeletal activity in the regulation of body function through somatovisceral reflexes.

Likewise, research by Jou et al.[18] has shown that cardiac efferents can have dramatic influences on muscle activity, supporting the role of viscerosomatic reflex connections as underlying the effectiveness of palpatory diagnosis in visceral disease states.

However, the direct interactions through the spinal cord of visceral and somatic inputs are not the only important means of interactions. Goehler and her colleagues have delineated a strong vagal-to-brain input that is primary in signaling pathogenic disturbances in the gut.[19–21] The vagus is a very potent signaler for the very short latency first immune response to impending infections. The total response to vagal signals involves autonomic, somatic, and psychological responses that prepare the body to fight the infection. Called the bottom-up response, it prepares the whole system for defense. Interestingly, the same response can occur from the "top-down" being triggered by psychological stress.[20] The complexity of visceral, somatic, and psychological interactions is an ongoing area of research.

CARDIAC CONTROL

Neural input from somatic structures may affect neural activity in both somatic and visceral structures. A good example of the interaction between somatic afferents and autonomic outflow is the control of the heart, providing an illustration of viscerosomatic and somatovisceral interactions. As with most visceral structures, the heart receives its autonomic innervation from both sympathetic and parasympathetic nerves.

Sympathetic Innervation of the Heart

Excitation of the cardiac sympathetic nerves (Fig. 13.6) causes the following effects:

- Increased heart rate
- Increased atrial and ventricular contractility
- Decreased conduction time from the atrium to the ventricle

The heart's spinal innervation is associated with spinal cord levels from T1 to about T5, with T2 suggested as contributing the most (Fig. 13.7).

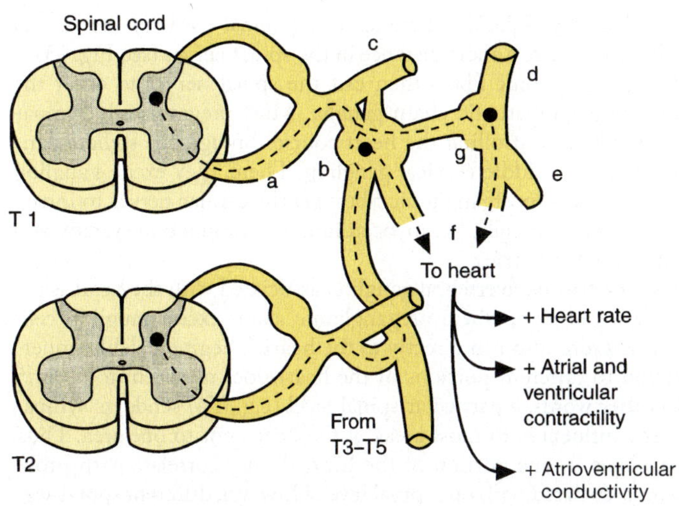

Figure 13.6. Sympathetic innervation of the heart. *a*, ventral root; *b*, stellate ganglion; *c*, spinal nerve; *d*, vagosympathetic trunk; *e*, vagus nerve; *f*, cardiac nerves; *g*, middle cervical ganglion.

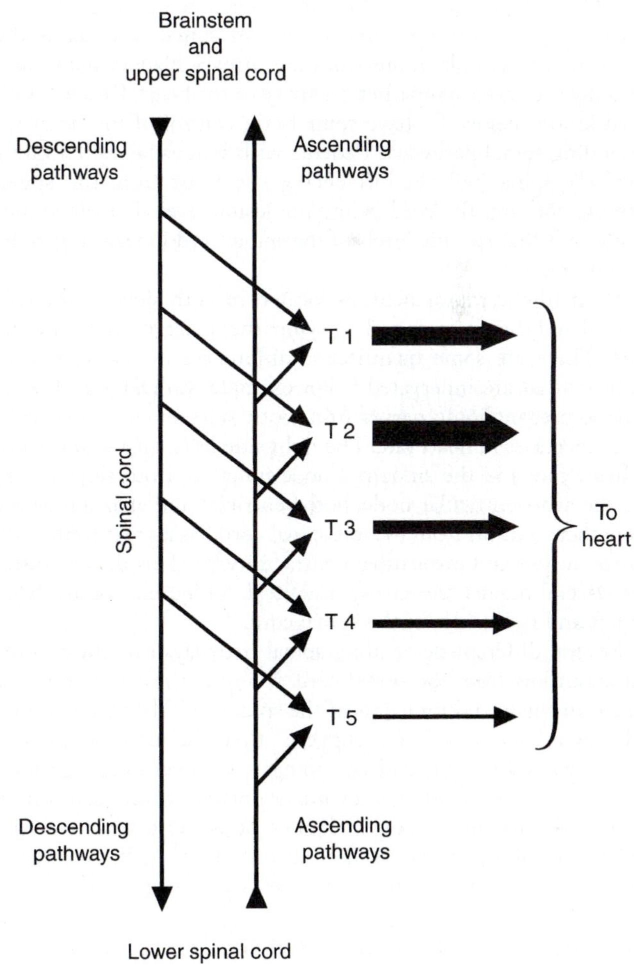

Figure 13.7. Spinal sympathetic innervation of the heart and related ascending and descending pathways. The heart receives spinal cord control via T1–T5 spinal cord levels with T2 making the largest functional contribution. Lesions above T1 and below T5 block brain control of cardiac sympathetic activity and reflex responses to ascending afferent activation, respectively.

The preganglionic fibers leave the spinal cord via the ventral roots and course a short distance in the spinal nerves (see Fig. 13.6). The preganglionic fibers then exit the spinal nerves to enter the adjoining sympathetic chain ganglia. Most preganglionic sympathetic fibers controlling the heart course through the stellate ganglion to the middle cervical ganglion. There, they excite ganglion cells that send postganglionic fibers via the cardiac nerves to innervate pacemaker cells, the myocardium, the conduction system, and the coronary arteries.

The first paravertebral ganglion associated with the heart is the stellate ganglion, where preganglionic axons excite ganglion cells whose axons also run directly to the heart.[22] Segmental-like innervation to different portions of the heart does not seem to occur.[23] In other words, a particular spinal level (e.g., T4) sends its sympathetic influences to most areas of the heart, not to one area. Thus, problems in one portion of the heart do not correlate with problems associated with one spinal level. However, different spinal segmental levels innervate different organs, for example, heart versus lungs, and some degree of segmental-like innervation does occur.

Understanding the spinal cord levels that control the heart is helpful in understanding responses in patients with spinal cord injuries (see Fig. 13.7).[24,25] With spinal cord lesions above T1, the brain has no control of the heart via the spinal cord and sympathetic nerves, but it can still activate the parasympathetic pathways. However, marked cardiac alterations may occur via reflexes mediated by sensory input that enters the spinal cord below the C8 level. For example, input from the urinary bladder may cause markedly increased sympathetic activity to the heart. Patients with spinal lesions below T1 have some brain control of the heart via descending spinal pathways. Patients with lesions below T5 rarely show any spinal reflexes influencing the heart from the spinal afferents entering the cord below the lesion level. This illustrates the concept that specific levels of the spinal cord innervate specific visceral organs.

Sympathetic motor neurons located in both sides of the spinal cord and their corresponding sympathetic nerves innervate the heart. There are some quantitative differences in the regions of the heart that are innervated.[23] For example, stimulation of sympathetic preganglionic nerves from both sides of the spinal cord causes increases in heart rate. The right side has a greater influence on heart rate and the sinoatrial node function. Both sides innervate the atrioventricular node, both ventricles and atria. However, sympathetic output from the left spinal cord has a greater effect on cardiac output and myocardial contractility.[23,25] This demonstrates that visceral organs receive asymmetrical autonomic control from the left and right sides of the spinal cord.

Several different descending spinal pathways can affect autonomic outflow from the spinal cord. Many of these pathways are located in the lateral funiculus of the spinal cord. Both anatomic[26] and physiologic[27] evidence suggests that the descending spinal pathways are organized according to a viscerotropic pattern. Localized lesions of the spinal cord, or portions of the descending spinal pathways, may result in loss of brain control of one particular visceral organ, which also suggests that the brain has the potential to separately control different visceral organs (Fig. 13.8).

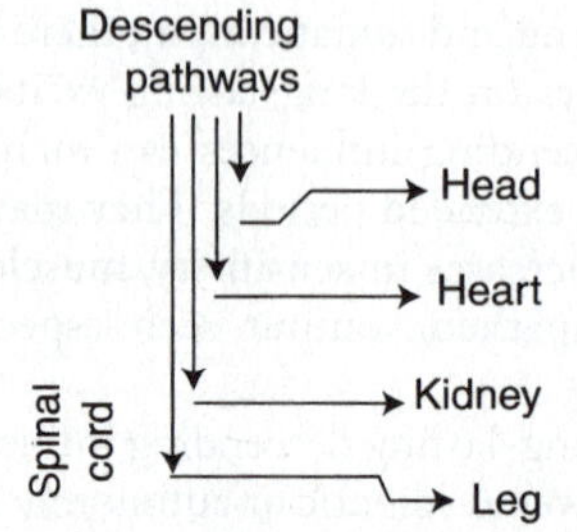

Figure 13.8. Viscerotropic organization of the descending spinal pathways controlling autonomic outflow.

Parasympathetic Innervation of the Heart

Parasympathetic innervation of the heart via the vagus nerve causes the following (Fig. 13.9):

- Decreased heart rate
- Decreased atrial contraction
- Limited decrease of ventricular contractility

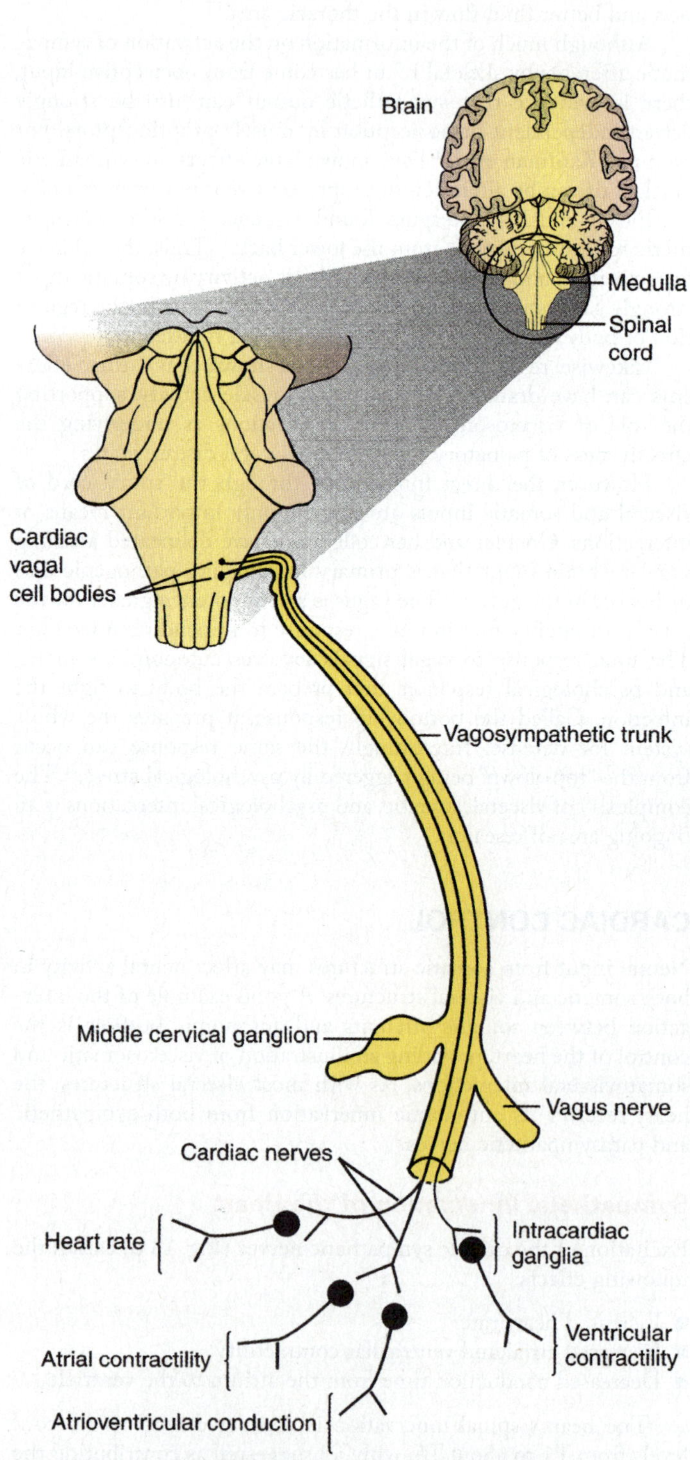

Figure 13.9. Parasympathetic innervation of the heart.

The cardiac vagal fibers travel in the cervical vagus nerve (vagosympathetic trunk) into the thorax where they separate from the vagus nerve to form the cardiac nerves. These cardiac vagal nerves have their cell bodies in the medulla, that is, the nucleus ambiguus and the dorsomotor nucleus.[28–32] These two medullary regions may subserve different cardiac functions. For example, the nucleus ambiguus may mediate heart rate, while the dorsomotor nucleus regulates ventricular contractility.[31] Not only are there regions of the brain stem controlling cardiac function that seem to be distinct from those controlling gastrointestinal function and other visceral organs, but different brain stem regions may also control separate cardiac functions.

Visceral Function Control

Cardiovascular function can be reflexively controlled by somatic afferents via the somatosympathetic reflexes. These reflexes may be mediated at the spinal cord level or via suprasegmental connections. The spinal somatosympathetic reflexes depend on segmental organization. These sympathetic reflex responses at one segmental level are larger if the somatic afferent activity enters at the same spinal level than if it enters at adjoining levels.[32–34] These reflexes also demonstrate laterality because they are larger for ipsilateral reflexes than for contralateral reflexes (Fig. 13.10).

Visceral afferents can also influence somatic reflexes, and muscle tone may be altered by visceral input. These reflexes are very important for osteopathic palpatory diagnosis and treatment because they provide mechanisms for the use of muscle tone as an indicator of visceral disturbances. The work by Eble[8] showed activation of skeletal muscles with stimulation of visceral structures, and Schoen and Finn[35] reported EMG activity in shoulder muscles in feline models following experimental MI. The cardiac viscerosomatic reflex has an influence on somatic musculature.[18]

Not only can there be activity from somatic or visceral structures that influences the opposite structures, but another type of activity, independent of the brain or spinal cord, may also occur. Neural activity has been recorded from in vitro sympathetic ganglion cells and intracardiac ganglion cells, demonstrating considerable action potential activity even when the neuronal connections to the CNS are severed.[28,30–32] These observations suggest that the autonomic ganglia may function as "little brains" within the peripheral ganglia and the heart. These ganglia may have the neural circuitry to act almost independently and have the ability to integrate intrinsic cardio-cardiac reflexes as well as information from the CNS.

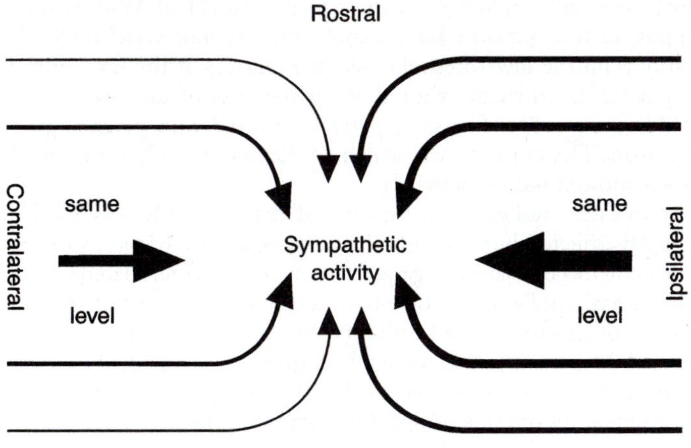

Figure 13.10. Laterality of cardiac sympathetic control and segmental organization of spinal sympathetic reflexes.

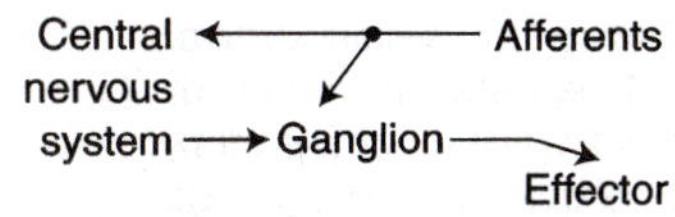

Figure 13.11. Afferent reflex control of autonomic effectors may be mediated via reflexes within peripheral autonomic ganglia, as well as via CNS connections.

However, the functional roles of these peripheral nervous system interactions are not yet fully understood (Fig. 13.11).

The possibility of "little brains" within the autonomic ganglia presents many more possibilities. If visceral afferents have reflexes within the autonomic ganglia, somatic afferents could also have reflex connections within them. Some somatic afferent fibers pass through the autonomic ganglia. It is possible that somatic afferents influence sympathetic activity not only to the somatic structure but also to visceral structures such as the heart. Activation of somatic afferents might cause reflex alteration of cardiac function via direct ganglionic reflexes as well as via the CNS-mediated reflexes. Likewise, visceral afferents might activate sympathetic ganglion cells with axons supplying somatic structures.[36–41] These concepts point toward therapeutic implications of reflexes within autonomic ganglia.

Interactions of Somatic Afferents and Baroreceptor Control of Autonomic Activity

Blood pressure and cardiac function are reflexively controlled through alteration of autonomic activity; this is mediated by arterial blood pressure afferent receptors, called baroreceptors. Increased arterial blood pressure excites baroreceptor activity, which is carried to the brain stem via the glossopharyngeal and vagus nerves. In the brain stem, the baroreceptor afferent activity leads to excitation of the medullary cardiac vagal cell bodies and inhibition of the sympathetic activity to the cardiovascular system via descending brain stem/spinal pathways.[42] Baroreceptor reflexes involving the cardiac vagus nerves have parallel inhibitory effects on the sinoatrial node (slowing heart rate) and atrioventricular node (slowing atrioventricular conduction).[43]

Although these baroreceptor reflexes have powerful influences on cardiovascular function, they also interact with other spinal reflexes, especially from small, high-threshold, afferent fibers. With activation of these spinal afferents, reflex changes in sympathetic activity (somatosympathetic reflexes) occur at the spinal cord level and through suprasegmental reflexes, involving ascending and then descending pathways to and from the brain stem.[44,45]

Baroreceptor reflexes inhibit both spinal- and supraspinal somatosympathetic reflexes.[46] Presumably, other visceral afferents that mediate sympathetic reflexes are also inhibited by these powerful baroreceptor reflexes.

Somatic afferent activity can modulate baroreceptor reflex vagal control of the heart. Somatic afferents and baroreceptors compete for control of autonomic activity. Baroreceptor activation excites the cardiac vagus nerve activity. However, somatic afferent stimulation attenuates or blocks the baroreceptor influence of vagal cardiac nerves. The ascending and descending pathways for these reflexes have been localized in the dorsal portion of the lateral funiculus of the spinal cord.[47–49]

SUMMATION OF CHARACTERISTICS OF SOMATOVISCERAL REFLEXES

Somatovisceral reflexes demonstrate temporal and spatial summation as indicated by the windup phenomenon and the effect

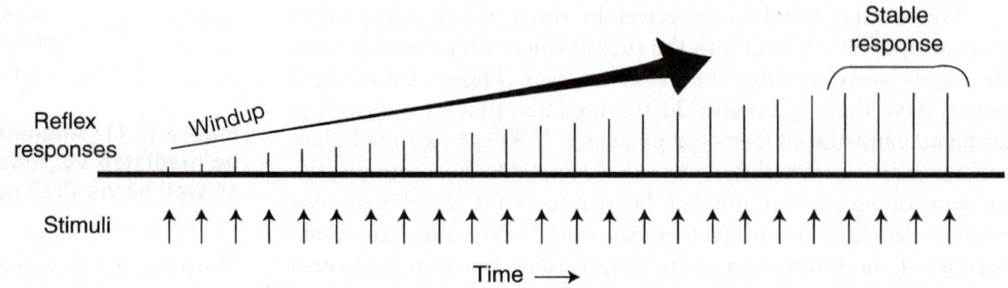

Figure 13.12. Windup or sensitization. When a stimulus is repeated at a rate of once every second or two, response to stimulus may continue to grow for 20 seconds or more. Finally, a stable response level is reached that can continue at an increased level as long as the stimulus is continued.

of input from different parts of the body. These somatovisceral reflexes do not reach their maximal activity immediately.[50] Rather, when stimulated at a slow repetition rate, these reflexes exhibit windup. With each repetition of the stimulation up to about 20 times, the autonomic response increases in size (Fig. 13.12).

The windup, also termed the sensitization phenomenon, suggests that maximal effectiveness of therapeutic procedures involving somatic afferent influences on autonomic control may require frequent repetitions of the procedure to allow the response to build to its maximum. Furthermore, afferent input from different portions of the body can summate to activate autonomic responses.[51] Accordingly, one would expect that a subliminal or noneffective stimulus to one part of the body might actually have an effect if combined with stimulation to another area (Fig. 13.13).

The reflex system is a complex integrating network. Importantly for the osteopathic physician, that somatic input can and does influence visceral function, just as input from the viscera causes changes in output to the somatic structures. This can often be felt as altered tissue tensions or changes in motion characteristics of joints. Maps have been published listing somatic areas that become abnormal to palpation with various visceral disturbances.[52]

A corollary of this is that osteopathic manipulation of the somatic structures can alter the function of visceral structures through the same pathways. The reflexes are not simple systems with only local influences but interconnected networks that receive input from many sources and process that information for distribution to both local and distant areas of the body.

ALTERATION OF INTEGRATIVE FUNCTION

Input from each area of the body and descending brain regions interact on a highly overlapping and integrated neural network in the spinal interneurons. Afferent input from any source influences both visceral and somatic structures. These complex and interacting networks within the nervous system must act in concert for normal functioning of organs, muscles, fluid motion, and other body activities. If any area of the neural network responds either more or less than normal, the finely tuned balance necessary for optimal physiologic function will be disturbed. Not only must the control mechanisms from the brain be normal for proper reflex function,

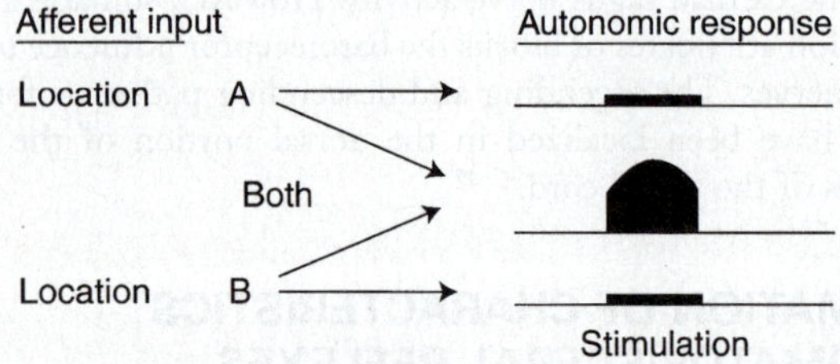

Figure 13.13. Summation of autonomic responses. Input from two different locations adds together to produce a larger autonomic response than either input produces when it occurs alone.

but the networks of neurons that make up the reflexes must also be acting normally. Unfortunately, these networks themselves can be altered, resulting in a loss of proper function.

Evidence is accumulating that the function of reflex networks can be influenced by many factors. They are subject to both short- and long-term changes that can have consequences for the health of the individual.

In the early and mid-1940s, Denslow et al.[53–55] were among the first to show the results of changes in the integrative function of reflex networks in humans. They performed a series of studies on normal, young adult volunteers to determine whether the reflex excitabilities at various spinal levels of the body were stable and comparable. They measured how much stimulation it took to evoke muscle activity (EMG) in the paraspinal muscles of the back at several levels of the thoracic spine.

They found that, on average, reflex excitability to pressure on the spinous processes was highest in the upper thoracic area and lowest in the midlumbar area. Although decreased excitability from the upper thoracic to the lower lumbar areas was seen overall in the subjects studied, practically all individuals studied had areas that were very highly excitable, responding to small amounts of pressure on the spinous process at that spinal level. In contrast, even fairly heavy pressure on the spinous processes in normal areas did not produce any activity in the associated muscles. The highly excitable areas were characterized by both increased muscle activity to pressure on the spinous process and often pain and tenderness in the area. The areas of increased sensitivity to stimulation were not uniform from individual to individual and were long-lasting (some cases remaining almost the same for years). In most cases, the individual did not realize that any change was present.

These long-lasting, low-threshold areas to afferent input could be activated not only by stimulating tissues at the same level of the spinal cord but also by stimulating other areas of the back or even by providing a psychological stress to the individual. With remote input, such as pressure on a spinous process four vertebral levels away from the low-threshold area, the muscles at the level of the input remained silent, while those at the level of the low threshold became active. The same pattern occurred with psychological stressors. The normal areas remained silent, but the low-threshold areas showed muscle activity.

In later studies,[56,57] it was found that not only was muscle activity affected but through altered sympathetic output, so were the activities of visceral organs. Here, again, the interrelatedness of the somatic and visceral portions of the body was shown. Although many otherwise normal subjects had low-threshold or high-excitability areas, it became evident that the excitability changes were not a normal state and further data suggested that increases in excitability often accompanied injury and disease. They represented areas of neural function that were operating out of synchrony with other areas of the neural system, causing the organs served by those neural supplies to be likewise affected with respect to the overall body function.

Korr[5] suggested that these low-threshold spinal reflexes represented pathways held in a hyperexcited state, perhaps by continued bombardment of input. He termed these areas "facilitated segments," as the areas rarely follow dermatomal boundaries. Korr postulated that facilitated segments magnify input to the area from any source and cause a magnified outflow to the organs innervated by that level of the spinal cord. Thermographic studies[56,57] showed that not only did the skeletal muscles respond in an exaggerated fashion in the low-threshold areas, but the sympathetic outflow also increased, suggesting a decrease in the overall integration of body function. No matter the source of input to a facilitated spinal area, the neural outflow would be exaggerated relative to the same response at other spinal levels. Such a situation lasting over time can have only undesirable consequences for overall body function.

Beginning and Maintenance of Reflex Facilitation

The finding that facilitated low-threshold areas could continue for long periods of time, and the fact that these areas were not the same between individuals, suggested that some process could occur that would establish these chronically hyperactive areas. Initial speculation suggested that the hyperexcitability was maintained by tonic afferent input. Most input from either somatic or visceral structures, however, decreases dramatically with activities such as sleep or other forms of relaxation. Why should the hyperexcitability continue even with the loss of afferent activity? What is the nature of the neural processing within the reflex pathways to afferent stimuli that might explain the appearance of regions of hyperexcitability? Additional studies provided some answers regarding how changes in reflex excitability can at times be an adaptive process and at times a detrimental one.

Alteration of Reflex Excitability

The concept of the reflex as a simple, unchanging, static input/output relationship is oversimplified. Although he characterized reflex function as innately given, even Sherrington recognized that reflex excitability could be momentarily altered by influences such as signals from higher brain structures or by rapid and repeated use, which, he noted, caused reflex fatigue. The notion that reflexes are fundamentally unchanging, static input/output relationships is still widespread, despite the fact that it is now clear that the excitability of spinal reflex pathways can be altered by many influences. These changes can range from short-lasting, fleeting changes to very long-lasting ones that may even become permanent. Such long-lasting alterations may well be the basis for the changes shown by Denslow in his studies of human motor neuron excitability and for the facilitated state hypothesized by Korr. These threats to functional integration of the body may be related to the effects of nociceptive stimuli at the periphery.

Alteration of Nociceptive Input

Inflammation from strong stimulation of the skin or other peripheral somatic or visceral structures produces changes in the sensory receptors of the organ that dramatically alter the amount of neural activity sent to the spinal cord.[58] Most tissues are innervated by various sensory receptors, such as touch, temperature, stretch, and nociceptors.

The nociceptors are composed primarily of unmyelinated nerve endings that respond to potentially tissue-damaging stimuli. In the hollow visceral organs, they respond to stretch or dilation of the organ, for example. These receptors send impulses through thin myelinated (group III or A) or unmyelinated (group IV or C) fibers into the spinal gray matter, where they synapse primarily in Rexed layers I and V. When activity occurs in these pathways, the resulting sensation is usually discomfort or pain, although the input may be blocked (by other neural activities) from reaching the areas of the brain stem where they are appreciated as pain. However, even though a nociceptive input to the spinal cord does not reach the conscious level, it may affect the dynamics of the spinal pathways.[59]

Once a stimulus sufficiently strong to activate nociceptive input begins, impulses travel into the spinal cord via the dorsal roots. At the branches of the peripheral neurons, the afferent impulses invade the afferent branches and are conveyed back out to the nerve terminals, where they cause release of various peptides into the surrounding tissues. The sites of peptide release may be some distance from the original stimulus. This starts a cascade of events that leads to involvement of the sympathetic postganglionic nerve terminals and to the release of serum from the surrounding capillaries. Prostaglandins discharged from the sympathetic nerve terminals continue the serum release that leads to local inflammation. These events initiate the healing process, although it may be sufficiently severe that the healing process is impaired.[60]

The inflammation also produces dramatic changes in the characteristics of the local nociceptors in the area. Schmidt[58] demonstrated in the cat knee joint that the number of nociceptors responding to a stretch stimulation may be between 3,000 and 4,000 after inflammation. In contrast, even severe stretch of the normal joint may cause only 400 nociceptors to fire. Also, the receptive fields of the active nociceptors enlarge dramatically in the inflamed area, and the threshold to activation significantly decreases. The result of an inflammatory process (or a strong stimulus that produces tissue damage) will be to lower nociceptor thresholds and dramatically increase input to the spinal cord. Peripheral events can lead to dramatic changes in the amount of stimuli caused by changes in the peripheral receptors.

What happens to spinal reflex networks when stimulus input changes? In the normal reflex pathway, repeated activation of the pathway by a weak afferent input results in a temporary decrease in the output of the network. Sherrington described this short-term decrease in reflex pathway excitability as reflex fatigue. This process, now termed habituation, has been studied extensively and is a characteristic of polysynaptic reflex pathways in the spinal cord and brain stem.

Habituation is characterized by a decrease in output from a neural pathway that has repeated stimulus input of a mild to moderate intensity. A stimulus may initially produce a response of a certain magnitude, but if the stimulus is repeated several times, the response decreases. If the stimulus is then terminated, the response returns to its initial level in a matter of seconds to minutes.[61] The process of habituation is a ubiquitous phenomenon, occurring in almost all animals and in all mammalian reflex pathways except the monosynaptic myotatic reflex. It is a necessary part of the neural integration because it allows nonessential stimuli to be muted in their effects on the nervous system.

The opposite of habituation is an increase in reflex excitability. Earlier, the phenomenon of windup was described, in which a stimulus repeated several times causes an increased number of neural firings. Windup has also been called sensitization in earlier studies (see Fig. 13.12). In this process, a repetitive stimulus can cause an increase in output rather than a decrease. A stimulus causing habituation can cause sensitization simply by increasing its intensity. This causes more nociceptors to become active or the same nociceptors to produce more impulses. Like habituation, sensitization can occur within a matter of seconds, and it can also dissipate in a matter of seconds when the stimulus is terminated.[61]

Habituation and sensitization have been extensively studied at the cellular level. In the mammal, both occur within the spinal central gray matter in the interneuron pathways. They are probably subserved by two different sets of interneurons, which then synapse on the motor neurons of both the sympathetic and the somatic systems.

Sensitization and habituation are apparently presynaptic processes that either inhibit (habituation) or enhance (sensitization) the release of neurotransmitters with each activation of the presynaptic terminal.[62] Both are independent of descending influences from higher nervous centers and can be demonstrated in humans with spinal cord transections.

Habituation and sensitization are different processes but occur at the synaptic level and can occur over a few seconds of sensory input. Although the process of sensitization may not be a unitary one (because there may be more than one form of sensitization), when the initiating stimulus is terminated, both processes do appear to dissipate in a fairly short time. Habituation allows the organism to dampen the response to nonthreatening stimuli, while sensitization allows the individual to respond more forcefully to a stimulus that is stronger and thus threatens tissue damage.

These two processes are valuable in maintaining the organism in its everyday existence. Under normal conditions, the opposing processes of habituation and sensitization function to maintain a balance between overreaction and underreaction to normal stimuli. When the inflammation process occurs, whether minor or severe, the balances of habituation and sensitization are disrupted. The normal damping effects of habituation are shifted toward the sensitization process. This is caused by the larger and more extreme responses of the peripheral receptors to what would usually be a nonthreatening stimulus. The result is a larger-than-normal motor output to both the visceral and the somatic structures innervated by the affected reflex pathways and, thus, to an overresponse to stimuli.

The process disrupts the normal integration of physiologic function.

Once the process of sensitization has begun, often over a few seconds of strong input, a secondary process begins to occur. Sensitization dissipates a few seconds or minutes after the stimulus is gone. A longer-lasting process, termed long-term sensitization, begins to develop in the reflex pathways once sensitization has been in place for several minutes. This process precludes the excitability of the neural pathways from returning to normal for some time, often hours.

The effects of this process can often be seen in laboratory experiments testing the responsiveness of the reflex system, when bursts of stimulation are given, followed by an occasional stimulus pulse. After initial sensitization and the rapid decrease of reflex excitability after stimulus termination, the response being tracked does not return to its prestimulation baseline but remains a small but significant amount above the base level. This hyperexcitability does not decay for varying amounts of time depending on the time and strength of the stimulus. Unlike sensitization, long-term sensitization is thought to be a postsynaptic event, possibly involving the elaboration of proteins in the postsynaptic neuron that remain active for some time after the initiating event.

Mantyh et al.[63] showed dramatic changes in the substance P receptors and even structural reorganization of the dendrites of spinal interneurons after nociceptive input. These changes could be the basis for long-term sensitization. Long-term sensitization involves a different mechanism than the short-term process and can have effects that far outlast the originating stimulus.

Once a stimulus has acted on a reflex network for a longer period, the results can be even more dramatic. For many years, a process known as spinal fixation has been known but not fully recognized. First shown in anesthetized animals, spinal fixation was demonstrated as sustained leg flexion secondary to a cerebellar lesion 3 to 4 hours after the lesion was induced. The lesion produced disrupted outflow from the postural centers in the cerebellum, resulting in sustained flexion of a leg. When the spinal cord was sectioned immediately after the lesion, the limb dropped to the usual flaccid paralysis of the animal. However, if the spinal cord was allowed to remain intact for 3 to 4 hours after the lesion and then transected, the limb remained flexed to some extent. The explanation was that the strong outflow from the injured cerebellum caused a hyperexcitability to develop in the target interneurons of the cord that remained active after spinal transection and resulted in continued motor activity.

In the mid-1960s, research showed that the minimal time necessary for the fixation of this excitability was approximately 45 minutes. Animals receiving the spinal transection within 35 minutes showed no remaining flexion, but those having 45 minutes between lesion and transection showed remaining flexion.[64] This effect has been shown to occur not only as a result of a cerebellar lesion but also with stimulation of the skin of the hind limb. It has further been demonstrated in either intact or animals with spinal transection.[65–67] The change in the spinal reflexes produced by the cerebellar lesion was caused not by pain or nociceptive input but by changes in outflow from the postural centers.

This and subsequent studies show that changes in the reflex functions can occur with both nociceptive and nonnociceptive input, although nociceptive input produces the changes more quickly than nonnociceptive input does. Reflex excitability changes can be influenced by many factors, including stress prior to stimulation, length and severity of stimulation, and whether the spinal cord is intact or sectioned. The changes have been traced for 3 days to 3 weeks after only 45 minutes of fairly intense nociceptive stimulation and may last even longer. With intense stimulus input, the effect is seen after as little as 20 minutes of stimulation.[68] Obviously, strong input, especially nociceptive in nature, can have rapid and long-lasting effects on the excitability of reflex circuits.

Although the locus of the changes seen in fixation is not yet known, it seems likely that the alterations observed are processes akin to long-term sensitization, but which last a much longer time. It appears that the fixation process is also dependent on the elaboration of proteins in the postsynaptic cells and that it would affect the responsiveness of those cells not only to the original input but also to all input to the cell.

Long-lasting reflex excitability is also seen in studies of peripheral inflammation that show peripheral effects of inflammation on afferent input and receptive fields. Continued afferent input from peripheral inflammation produces dramatic changes in the responsiveness of spinal interneurons. Interneurons, on which afferent fibers from affected nociceptors synapse, begin to respond much more easily to input from a variety of sources, such as touch, pressure, and even the movement of distant muscles. These dramatic changes in excitability also last for long periods (days and weeks) and develop during the initial inflammatory episode.[69,70]

Understanding the mechanisms of the changes may allow the physician to restore more normal function. Dubner, Ruda, and Gold[71,72] summarized a series of intracellular changes that are linked to the excitability alterations seen with the inflammation process. The cells activated by nociceptive input from inflamed peripheral structures begin to show enhanced activation of specific parts of the postsynaptic cell membrane called *N*-methyl-D-aspartate receptors. When these receptors become more active, the excitability of the cell is increased.

If cellular activation further continues, changes in the activity of genes within the neuron are seen. A class of genes called immediate-early genes, c-fos, and c-jun become more active, causing increased dynorphin release within the cell. Dynorphin is a substance that causes increased cell excitation. With more of it being produced, the cell is then held in a hyperexcitable state.

Wolpaw[73] provided strong evidence that alterations in excitability can be produced not only by nociceptive input to the spinal circuits but also by nonnociceptive input. In these studies, both increased and decreased spinal reflex excitation was produced by nonnociceptive long-term input. This suggests that spinal circuits can be altered rapidly by nociceptive input and more slowly by nonnociceptive input.

Other studies have begun to show that a fourth type of spinal circuit excitability alteration can occur. With heightened excitability over several days, a process begins in the interneuron cell body that finally destroys the cell. Although both inhibitory and excitatory interneurons should theoretically be affected by this process, it appears that inhibitory interneurons are affected primarily.[74] Thus, after the long-term fixation excitability increases are established, continued activation of the pathways may result in the loss of inhibitory interneurons. This is certainly an almost permanent event. However, it is apparently not the end of the story. In some cases where inhibitory interneurons have been lost, new excitatory synapses may actually be formed to replace the lost inhibitory synapses.[75] These two additional processes would further shift the balance of excitation in the spinal cord toward enhanced excitability, perhaps permanently.

Four steps have been shown to occur in the spinal cord reflex circuitry to alter the excitability of those pathways:

- Sensitization
- Long-term sensitization
- Fixation
- Loss of inhibitory interneurons/new excitatory synapse formation

These four overlapping and progressive stages in spinal excitability alterations are supported by different neural processes, ranging from simple synaptic transmission alterations to complex changes in the genetic function of the cell. With increased understanding of the underlying processes involved, it may be possible to find ways to stop or even reverse them and, hence, reestablish normal excitability in an affected region. In addition, the restoration of normal input to an affected spinal area would have an ameliorative effect on the function. However, at present, little is known about how to reverse the effects of these excitability alterations.

These four steps are a progression from short term to long term and even permanent alterations of spinal excitability. It seems almost certain that these steps underlie the changes recorded by Denslow et al.[53] and interpreted by Korr[5] as the facilitated segment. They saw these alterations as having widespread and often grave consequences for the patient. Although they had no way to understand the basis of the facilitated segment at that time, they rightly viewed these alterations in function as a real threat to the health and function of the patient.

An area of spinal reflex pathways that are either temporarily or permanently in a state of increased excitability would respond to all input in an exaggerated way, with the result that the organs or tissues innervated by those areas of the spinal cord would receive exaggerated neural drive. Thus, the affected tissues, somatic or visceral, would be driven to respond in a fashion that was not in harmony with the rest of the body. Over time, this increased drive on the tissues would be expected to take a toll on the functional ability of the tissues and could result in premature breakdown or loss of normal function.

It is also evident that areas of increased spinal excitability would respond to central commands in an inappropriate way. This could be the reason why some people respond to stress with heart palpitations, while others respond with gastric distress. The abnormally excitable area of the cord would be the one to respond with abnormal drive onto the innervated tissues, resulting in clinical manifestations not seen in other tissues. Thus, a clinical problem may be the result of a long-standing facilitated area of the spinal cord.

In addition to spinal circuit changes, it is apparent that nociceptive input may cause changes in the brain stem and even in the cortical areas; this may account for many of the usual symptoms seen with chronic pain. Indeed, there is evidence that in the prefrontal cortex, cortical neurons analogous to the spinal inhibitory interneurons may be destroyed with some types of pain input.[76] The probable result of these changes in the brain stem, and even cortex that may be analogous to those seen in the spinal cord, will be to alter the ability of the system to respond to environmental stress and may predispose to disease, altered immune function, and depressive states.

Thus, the spinal excitability alterations first seen by Denslow and Korr seem to be supported by a series of progressively longer-lasting spinal circuit alterations that result in altered outflow to central brain areas and to both somatic and visceral tissues innervated by that area. Thus, given an altered reflex network, that area can no longer respond in concert with other networks, producing diminished functional integration and beginning the loss of health associated with disease. The restoration of normal input to the area from somatic and visceral tissues may help normalize the function of the affected areas in all but extreme cases. Osteopathic manipulative procedures aimed at improving tissue function would be expected to help restore normal function in the spinal circuits.

NON–IMPULSE-BASED INTEGRATION

Neurons not only convey impulses throughout the body to integrate function, but they are also conduits of anterograde flow (a steady stream of material flowing from the neural cell body out to the axon and dendrites) and retrograde flow (flow of materials from the periphery of the nerve back to the cell body). This is referred to as axoplasmic flow. Anterograde flow transports materials from where they are manufactured in the cell body down a complex microtubular structure within the axon. Materials to supply rebuilding of the axon walls and to resupply the transmitter substances are transported via this system.

The most common clinical effects of the loss of this transport system can be seen when neural contact is withdrawn from an end organ, such as when a muscle is denervated by cutting its motor nerve (a relatively common occurrence). Not only does the muscle cease to contract, but unless the nerve regrows again to contact the muscle, the muscle fibers eventually lose their ability to contract. They change their structure to that of noncontractile connective tissue. Likewise, if an end organ is damaged, its nerve supply often retracts, and the synapses are lost. The end organ supplies something to the nerve that allows the synapses to remain viable.

A great deal of study has been performed on the uptake of substances supplied by the end organ to nerve terminals. A family of substances known as nerve growth factor (NGF) is essential to continued nerve contact with an end organ and for continued viability of contacts between nerves higher up the chain. If the end organ does not supply NGF, the synaptic contact is lost. This factor is also essential in development, allowing appropriate nerves to reach and establish contact with the appropriate end organs. Loss of appropriate NGF causes deterioration of the nerve and its contacts. NGF is elaborated in the end organ and taken up by the presynaptic membranes, where it is transported up the axon to the cell body (retrograde transport). There, it regulates the function of the nerve and the nerve's ability to maintain synaptic contacts.

Many other substances can be taken up and transported to the cell body, but not all of them are helpful to nerve function. The tetanus toxin, tetanospasmin, is made in peripheral structures after infection by the *Clostridium tetani* bacterium. The toxin is taken up by nerve terminals and transported to the CNS, where it affects neural function, causing the clinical signs of tetanus.

Many common nerve-tracing techniques rely on the ability of the neuron to take up substances and transport them from the periphery of the nerve to the cell body. For example, horseradish peroxidase is used as a nerve tracer by injecting it into the area of nerve terminals, where it is taken into the cell and transported up the axon, eventually filling the cell body and even dendrites. A fixative can then be used to turn the horseradish peroxidase a dark brown-black, providing an easily visualized portrait of the cell. Many other dyes and materials are commonly used in this way to visualize nerve cells.

Much is known about the NGF family and some other substances and about the actual transport mechanisms within the axon. However, less is known about the delivery of substances to end organs through transport from cell body to axon (anterograde flow), such as what is delivered to keep a muscle functional. In 1967, Korr et al.[77] published the results of a study that showed that amino acids placed on the cell bodies of the hypoglossal nucleus on the floor of the fourth ventricle were incorporated into the cell body and transported down the axon to tongue muscle cells.

Later work showed that not only was the material transported, but it was also transported at several different rates of flow. That study and others since have shown that flow rates within an axon vary from as slow as 0.5 mm/d to as fast as 400 mm/d. The observed rates are[78]:

- Slow (0.52 mm/d)
- Medium (25 mm/d)
- Fast (up to 400 mm/d)
- Very fast (up to 2,000 mm/d)

While his work on transsynaptic flow of proteins was at first not taken seriously, in 1971, Grafstein,[79] previously a critic of Korr's work, published data supporting protein transport across synapses in the optic system. There is much research supporting both anterograde and retrograde transport of materials across synapses throughout the nervous system.[80–83]

Although materials transported via anterograde flow are related to support the neuron and synaptic functions (such as supply of neurotransmitter components), materials delivered by the nerve to its end organ are necessary for either its function or continued existence.[84] Thus, the nervous system is not only the network for rapid communications within the body, but it also serves as a vast network for a far slower two-way communication between the central nervous structures and every part of the body.

Disruption of this slow transport of materials has consequences for continued function that may not be immediately evident but range from subtle to disastrous. Complete withdrawal of NGF or of the materials delivered by the nerve to its end organ may result in loss of function. Disturbance of the flow of materials in either direction results in less-than-optimal function of the organs involved.[85]

Many questions remain about the two-way communication of axoplasmic flow.

- What substances are being delivered?
- How necessary are they?
- How do the materials transported from the periphery to the nerve cell bodies impact the function of the cell and the entire CNS?
- Are there crucial times for delivery of nerve factors to end organs for proper development?

However, these questions are answered; it is important to recognize the vast integrating nature of the non–impulse-based transport systems of the nervous system and the importance of proper function of this system.

Many factors have been shown to affect the material flow within the nerve cells. Even small pressure on axons can impede proper axoplasmic flow. A sustained increased number of impulses carried by the neuron (as in those originating in facilitated areas of the cord) may decrease flow rates. Improper supplies of nutrients and oxygen to the cell body or axon alter the flow. The occurrence of tissue tension and fluid flow disturbances often associated with somatic dysfunctions can be factors in altering axoplasmic flows. Treating somatic dysfunction with osteopathic manipulation would be expected to have a positive effect on the flow of materials in axons of the area and, hence, improve body function and integration.

CONCLUSION

In the normal, integrative function of the nervous system, a great number of influences act on any neural pathway. Afferent input activates reflex outflow. Descending activities from higher nervous centers modulate excitability of interneurons. Ascending influences from lower spinal areas increase or decrease activity. Psychological effects influence all levels of the CNS. The nerves deliver the materials necessary for normal function to their end organs, while the end organs send the substances necessary for continued synaptic viability to the nerves.

These influences come together to determine the moment-to-moment excitability of any area of the CNS and to determine overall outflow to both somatic and visceral structures. If all of these influences are working in harmony, optimally integrated function can be expected from the collective organs. If, however, one area is in a hyperexcitable state, optimal function is disrupted and the individual becomes increasingly prone to loss of function and disease.

The long-term alterations in spinal reflex excitability seem to underlie the alterations demonstrated by Denslow and his colleagues. These breaks in the normal integration of the nervous system were shown to affect both visceral and somatic structures. The interaction between visceral and somatic input in the spinal cord provides the basis for that common effect. The changes shown in response to nociceptive input can account for the long-lasting nature of the facilitation identified in those studies. The facilitation was hypothesized by Korr to be the basis for the somatic dysfunctions long recognized by the osteopathic profession.

Because the neurons involved in the altered excitability are interneurons (the neurons on which a variety of different pathways synapse), the data also support the effects of excitability changes on both somatic and autonomic outflow. Input from both visceral and somatic structures end on common interneurons. When the excitability of those interneurons is altered, the outflow to all structures innervated by motor neurons to which those interneurons connect is affected.

The reflex networks of the nervous system are not at all static, genetically determined entities. They are a vast network of highly interconnected pathways that are continually changing to meet local needs and to maintain integration of function. These dynamic processes allow the delicate moment-to-moment integration that characterizes optimal functional capacity.

The integration, however, can be turned against the very system it serves. When abnormal or very strong input occurs, the result can be a long-term disruption of the normal excitatory/inhibitory balances and a shift to excessive excitability (or, in some cases, to excessive inhibition). The result, in either case, is the loss of functional integration and a decrease in functional capacity of the individual.

There are many factors that influence the total function of the individual, including the accumulated effects of life, habits, living environment, nutrition, and psychological and spiritual elements. The status of the nervous system is but one of the factors influencing the total health of the person. Because it affects all organs and structures with which it communicates, an area of central excitation or facilitation delivers the effects of all other stressors on the individual to the end organs. In essence, it is the final common factor in communicating with the end organ. Most of the other stressors in life may be difficult to change, and the osteopathic physician has little impact on or control over them. However, the physician can directly affect the course of the facilitation and its effects by recognizing that it occurs and by applying various therapeutic modalities, especially osteopathic manipulative treatment, to alter it.

Rational therapy dictates the normalization of afferent input as quickly as possible to restore the normal balance of excitation and inhibition. Osteopathic manipulative treatment may be instrumental in accomplishing this, thereby optimizing a patient's functional balance and health.

ACKNOWLEDGMENTS

The author and editors of this chapter would like to acknowledge the scholarly contributions of Dr. Michael M. Patterson and Robert D. Wurster for prior editions of this chapter.

REFERENCES

1. Still AT. *Autobiography of A. T. Still.* Author; 1897.
2. Northup GW, ed. *Osteopathic Research: Growth and Development.* American Osteopathic Association; 1987.
3. Cole WV. The osteopathic lesion syndrome. In: Page LE, ed. *American Academy of Osteopathy Yearbook.* American Academy of Osteopathic Medicine; 1951:149–178.
4. Denslow JS. *The Early Years of Research at the Kirksville College of Osteopathic Medicine.* Kirksville College of Osteopathic Medicine Press; 1982.
5. Korr IM. The neural basis of the osteopathic lesion. *J Am Osteopath Assoc.* 1947;46:191–198.
6. Sherrington CS. *The Integrative Action of the Nervous System.* Yale University Press; 1905.
7. Wurster RD. Program control of circulatory behavior. *Behav Brain Sci.* 1986;9:305.
8. Eble JN. Patterns of response of the paravertebral musculature to visceral stimuli. *Am J Physiol.* 1960;198(2):429–433.
9. Sato A. Reflex modulation of visceral functions by somatic afferent activity. In: Patterson MM, Howell JN, eds. *The Central Connection: Somatovisceral/Viscerosomatic Interaction.* American Academy of Osteopathic Medicine; 1992:53–72.
10. Rexed B. The cytoarchitectonic organization of the spinal cord in the cat. *J Comp Neurol.* 1952;96:415–495.
11. DeGroat WC. Spinal cord processing of visceral and somatic nociceptive input. In: Patterson MM, Howell JN, eds. *The Central Connection: Somatovisceral/Viscerosomatic Interaction.* American Academy of Osteopathic Medicine; 1992:47–71.
12. Luz L, Fernandes E, Sivado M, Kokai E, Szucs P, Safronov B. Monosynaptic convergence of somatic and visceral C-fiber afferents on projection and local circuit neurons in lamina I: a substrate for referred pain. *Pain.* 2015;156(10):2042–2051.
13. Cervero R, Foreman RD. Sensory innervation of the viscera. In: Loewy AD, Spyer KM, eds. *Central Regulation of Autonomic Functions.* Oxford University Press; 1990.
14. Cervero F. Visceral and spinal components of viscero-somatic interactions. In: Patterson MM, Howell JN, eds. *The Central Connection: Somatovisceral/Viscerosomatic Interaction.* American Academy of Osteopathic Medicine; 1992:77–85.
15. Sato A. The somatosympathetic reflexes: their physiological and clinical significance. In: Goldstein M, ed. *The Research Status of Manipulative Therapy.* National Institutes of Health; 1975:163–172.
16. Hill JM, Adreani CM, Kaufman MP. Muscle reflex stimulates sympathetic postganglionic efferents innervating *triceps surae* muscles of cats. *Am J Physiol.* 1996;271(1 pt 2):H38–H43.
17. Kang Y, Kenney M, Spratt K, Pickar JG. Somatosympathetic reflexes from the low back in the anesthetized cat. *J Neurophysiol.* 2003;90(4): 2548–2559.
18. Jou JC, Farber JP, Qin C, Foreman RD. Afferent pathways for cardiac-somatic motor reflexes in rats. *Am J Physiol Regul Integr Comp Physiol.* 2001;281(6):R2096–R2102.
19. Goehler LE, Gaykema RP, Hansen MK, Anderson K, Maier SF, Watkins LR. Vagal immune-to-brain communication: a visceral chemosensory pathway. *Auton Neurosci.* 2000;85(1–3):49–59.
20. Goehler LE. Vagal complexity: substrate for body-mind connections? *Bratisl Lek Listy.* 2006;107(8):275–276.
21. Maier SF, Goehler LE, Fleshner M, Watkins LR. The role of the vagus nerve in cytokine-to-brain communication. *Ann N Y Acad Sci.* 1998; 840:289–300.
22. Hopkins D, Armour J. Localization of sympathetic postganglionic and parasympathetic preganglionic neurons which innervate different regions of the dog heart. *J Comp Neurol.* 1984;229:186–198.
23. Norris JE, Foreman RD, Wurster RK. Responses of the canine heart to stimulation of the first five ventral thoracic roots. *Am J Physiol.* 1974; 227:912.
24. Wurster RD, Randall WC. Cardiovascular responses to bladder distension in patients with spinal transection. *Am J Physiol.* 1975;228:1288–1292.
25. Wurster R. Spinal sympathetic control of the heart. In: Randall WC, ed. *Neural Regulation of the Heart.* Oxford University Press; 1976:157–186.
26. Chung K, Chung JM, LaVelle FW, Wurster RD. The anatomical localization of descending pressor pathways in the cat spinal cord. *Neurosci Lett.* 1979;15:71–75.
27. Barman SM, Wurster RD. Visceromotor organization within descending spinal sympathetic pathways. *Circ Res.* 1975;37:209–214.
28. Geis GS, Kozelka JW, Wurster RD. Organization and reflex control of vagal cardiomotor neurons. *J Auton Nerv Syst.* 1981;3:437–450.
29. Geis GS, Wurster RD. Horseradish peroxidase localization of cardiac vagal preganglionic somata. *Brain Res.* 1980;182:19–30.
30. Geis GS, Wurster RD. Cardiac responses during stimulation of dorsal motor nucleus and nucleus ambiguus in the cat. *Circ Res.* 1980;46:606–611.
31. Kalia M, Mesulam MM. Brainstem projections of sensory and motor components of the vagus complex in the cat. II: Laryngeal, tracheobronchial, pulmonary, cardiac, and gastrointestinal branches. *J Comp Neurol.* 1980;193:467–508.
32. Hopkins DA, Armour JA. Medullary cells of origin of physiologically identified cardiac nerves in the dog. *Brain Res Bull.* 1982;8:359–365.
33. Beacham WS, Perl ER. Background and reflex discharge of sympathetic preganglionic neurons in the spinal cat. *J Physiol.* 1964;172:400–416.
34. Beacham WS, Perl ER. Characteristics of a spinal sympathetic reflex. *J Physiol.* 1964;173:431–448.
35. Schoen RE, Finn WE. A model for studying a viscerosomatic reflex induced by myocardial infarction in the cat. *J Am Osteopath Assoc.* 1978; 78(1):122–123.

36. Amour JA. Activity of in situ stellate ganglion neurons of dogs recorded extracellularly. *Can J Physiol Pharmacol.* 1986;64(2):101–111.
37. Amour JA. Activity of in situ middle cervical ganglion neurons in dogs, using extracellular recording techniques. *Can J Physiol Pharmacol.* 1985;63:704–716.
38. Boznjak Z, Kampine J. Intracellular recordings from the stellate ganglion of the cat. *J Physiol.* 1982;324:273–283.
39. Gagliardi M, Randall WC, Bieger D, Wurster RD, Hopkins DA, Armour JA. Activity of in vivo canine cardiac plexus neurons. *Am J Physiol.* 1988; 255(4 Pt 2):H789–H800.
40. Morris JL, Gibbins IL, Jobling P. Post-stimulus potentiation of transmission in pelvic ganglia enhances sympathetic dilatation of guinea-pig uterine artery in vitro. *J Physiol.* 2005;566(Pt 1):189–203.
41. Jänig W. Non-nicotinic transmission in autonomic ganglia revisited–an important physiological function? *J Physiol.* 2005;566(Pt 1):1–2.
42. Terui N, Koizumi K. Responses of cardiac vagus and sympathetic nerve to excitation of somatic and visceral nerves. *J Auton Nerv Syst.* 1984;10: 73–91.
43. O'Toole MF, Wurster RD, Phillips JG, Randall WC. Parallel baroreceptor control of sinoatrial rate and atrioventricular conduction. *Am J Physiol.* 1984;246(2 Pt 2):H149–H153.
44. Koizumi K, Brooks CM. The integration of autonomic system reactions: discussion of autonomic reflexes, their control and their association with somatic reactions. *Ergeb Physiol.* 1972;67:1–68.
45. Sato A, Schmidt RF. Somatosympathetic reflexes: afferent fibers, central pathways, discharge characteristics. *Physiol Rev.* 1973;53:916–947.
46. Barman S, Wurster RD. Interaction of descending sympathetic pathways and afferent nerves. *Am J Physiol.* 1978;234:H223–H229.
47. Geis GS, Wurster RD. Localization of ascending inotropic and chronotropic pathways in the cat. *Circ Res.* 1981;49:711–717.
48. Kozelka J, Christy G, Wurster R. Somato-autonomic reflexes in anesthetized and unanesthetized dogs. *J Auton Nerv Syst.* 1982;5:63–70.
49. Kozelka J, Chung J, Wurster R. Ascending spinal pathways mediating somato-cardiovascular reflexes. *J Auton Nerv Syst.* 1981;3:171–175.
50. Chung JM, Webber CL Jr, Wurster RD. Ascending spinal pathways for the somatosympathetic A and C reflex. *Am J Physiol.* 1979;237:H342–H347.
51. Chung JM, Wurster RD. Neurophysiological evidence for spatial summation in the CNS from unmyelinated afferent fibers. *Brain Res.* 1978;153: 596–601.
52. Te Poorten BA. Spinal palpatory diagnosis of visceral disease. *Osteopath Ann.* 1979:52–53.
53. Denslow JS, Korr IM, Krems AD. Quantitative studies of chronic facilitation in human motoneuron pools. *Am J Physiol.* 1947;105(2):229–238.
54. Denslow JS. The central excitatory state associated with postural abnormalities. *J Neurophysiol.* 1942;5(5):393–402.
55. Denslow JS. An analysis of the variability of spinal reflex thresholds. *J Neurophysiol.* 1944;7:207–215.
56. Korr IM, Thomas PE, Wright HM. Patterns of electrical skin resistance in man. *Acta Neuroveg (Wien).* 1958;17:77–96.
57. Wright HM, Korr IM, Thomas PE. Local and regional variations in cutaneous vasomotor tone of the human trunk. *Acta Neuroveg (Wien).* 1960; 22:34–52.
58. Schmidt RF. Neurophysiological mechanisms of arthritic pain. In: Patterson MM, Howell JN, eds. *The Central Connection: Somatovisceral/ Viscerosomatic Interaction.* American Academy of Osteopathic Medicine; 1992:130–151.
59. Schmidt RF. Nociception and pain. In: Schmidt RF, Thews G, eds. *Human Physiology.* Springer-Verlag; 1987.
60. Payan DG. Peripheral neuropeptides, inflammation, and nociception. In: Willard FH, Patterson MM, eds. *Nociception and the Neuroendocrine-Immune Connection.* American Academy of Osteopathic Medicine; 1994: 34–42.
61. Groves PM, Thompson RF. Habituation: a dual-process theory. *Psychol Rev.* 1970;77(5):419–450.
62. Kandel ER, Brunelli M, Byrne J, Castellucci V. A common presynaptic locus for the synaptic changes underlying short-term habituation and sensitization of the gill-withdrawal reflex in aplysia. *Cold Spring Harb Symp Quant Biol.* 1976;40:465–482.
63. Mantyh PW, DeMaster E, Malhotra A, et al. Receptor endocytosis and dendrite reshaping in spinal neurons after somatosensory stimulation. *Science.* 1995;268(5217):1629–1632.
64. Chamberlain TJ, Halick P, Gerard RW. Fixation of experience in the rat spinal cord. *J Neurophysiol.* 1963;26:662–673.
65. Steinmetz JE, Cervenka J, Robinson C, Romano AG, Patterson MM. Fixation of spinal reflexes in rats by central and peripheral sensory input. *J Comp Psychol.* 1981;95:548–555.
66. Steinmetz JE, Patterson MM. Fixation of spinal reflex alterations in spinal rats by sensory nerve stimulation. *Behav Neurosci.* 1985;99(1):97–108.
67. Patterson MM, Steinmetz JE. Long-lasting alterations of spinal reflexes: a potential basis for somatic dysfunction. *J Am Osteopath Assoc.* 1986;2:38–42.
68. Patterson MM. Spinal fixation: long-term alterations in spinal reflex excitability. In: Patterson MM, Grau JW, eds. *Spinal Cord Plasticity: Alterations in Reflex Function.* Kluwer Academic Publishers; 2001:77–100.
69. Willis WD. Mechanisms of central sensitization of nociceptive dorsal horn neurons. In: Patterson MM, Grau JW, eds. *Spinal Cord Plasticity: Alterations in Reflex Function.* Kluwer Academic Publishers; 2001:127–162.
70. Coderre TJ. Noxious stimulus-induced plasticity in spinal cord dorsal horn: evidence and insights on mechanisms obtained using the formalin test. In: Patterson MM, Grau JW, eds. *Spinal Cord Plasticity: Alterations in Reflex Function.* Kluwer Academic Publishers; 2001:163–184.
71. Dubner R, Ruda MA. Activity-dependent neuronal plasticity following tissue injury and inflammation. *Trends Neurosci.* 1992;15(3):96–103.
72. Dubner R, Gold M. The neurobiology of pain. *Proc Natl Acad Sci U S A.* 1999;96:7627–7630.
73. Wolpaw JR. Spinal cord plasticity in the acquisition of a simple motor. In: Patterson MM, Grau JW, eds. *Spinal Cord Plasticity: Alterations in Reflex Function.* Kluwer Academic Publishers; 2001:101–126.
74. Mayer DJ, Mao J, Holt J, Price DD. Cellular mechanisms of neuropathic pain, morphine tolerance, and their interactions. *Proc Natl Acad Sci U S A.* 1999;96:7731–7736.
75. Woolf CJ, Saler MW. Neuronal plasticity: increasing the gain in pain. *Science.* 2000;288:1765–1768.
76. Grachev ID, Fredrickson BE, Apkarian AV. Abnormal brain chemistry in chronic back pain: an in vivo proton magnetic resonance spectroscopy study. *Pain.* 2000;89(1):7–18.
77. Korr IM, Wilkinson PN, Chornock FW. Axonal delivery of neuroplasmic components to muscle cells. *Science.* 1967;155(760):342–345.
78. Korr IM, ed. *The Neurobiologic Mechanisms in Manipulative Therapy.* Plenum Publishing; 1978.
79. Grafstein B. Transneuronal transfer of radioactivity in the central nervous system. *Science.* 1971;172(979):177–179.
80. Schwab ME, Thoenen H. Retrograde axonal and transsynaptic transport of macromolecules: physiological and pathophysiological importance. *Agents Actions.* 1977;7(3):361–368.
81. Regalado MP, Terry-Lorenzo RT, Waites CL, Garner CC, Malenka RC. Transsynaptic signaling by postsynaptic synapse-associated protein 97. *J Neurosci.* 2006;26(8):2343–2357.
82. Vizzard MA, Brisson M, de Groat WC. Transneuronal labeling of neurons in the adult rat central nervous system following inoculation of pseudorabies virus into the colon. *Cell Tissue Res.* 2000;299(1):9–26.
83. Banati RB. Brain plasticity and microglia: is transsynaptic glial activation in the thalamus after limb denervation linked to cortical plasticity and central sensitisation? *J Physiol Paris.* 2002;96(3–4):289–299.
84. Korr IM. The spinal cord as organizer of disease process: axonal transport and neurotrophic function in relation to somatic dysfunction. *J Am Osteopath Assoc.* 1981;80(7):451–459.
85. De Vos KJ, Grierson AJ, Ackerley S, Miller CC. Role of axonal transport in neurodegenerative diseases. *Annu Rev Neurosci.* 2008;31:151–173.

14 Anatomy and Physiology of the Lymphatic System

HUGH M. ETTLINGER ▪ FRANK H. WILLARD

KEY CONCEPTS

- The lymphatic system plays a critical role in health and disease.
- It removes extravasated fluid and protein from the interstitium maintaining an osmotic balance in the tissue.
- Lymphatic vessels conduct extracellular fluids, filtered proteins, and absorbed lipids through a sequence of lymph nodes for immune surveillance.
- Activated immune cells from lymph nodes are distributed throughout the body using the lymphatic channels and the venous system.
- Virtually all vascularized tissues have lymphatic capillaries that provide lymph drainage and all lymphatic fluid is subjected to intense immune surveillance prior to return to systemic circulation.
- Inflammation is the generalized response of the body to injury or infection; pro- and anti-inflammatory cells as well as signals are transported in the lymphatic system.
- Movement of fluid in the lymphatic vessels is dependent on two mechanisms: an intrinsic system of contractile units, termed lymphangions, driven by smooth muscle and an extrinsic system of mechanical forces such as muscular contractions, arterial pulse, peristalsis, respiration, and manipulative procedures.
- An imbalance in the amount of fluid removed from local tissue can result in lymphedema; the inability to remove fluid from the tissues of the body can be life threatening.

INTRODUCTION

Throughout the body, the vascular system provides fluid for the extracellular spaces.

This extracellular fluid is the environment in which cellular exchange of gases and nutrients takes place.

- Within these confines, intrinsic homeostatic mechanisms operate to maintain concentration gradients for cellular exchange.
- The lymphatic vasculature and associated lymph nodes represent a unidirectional, low-pressure system that plays an integral role in this process, removing from the interstitium:
  - □ Excess fluid
  - □ Particulate matter
  - □ Proteins
- It is estimated that in humans approximately 8 L of fluid per day passes from capillaries, through the interstitium and into the lymphatic system for return to circulation.[1]
- Not only does this removal of extravasated material serve to maintain osmotic balance between the extracellular, intracellular, and intravascular fluids (Fig. 14.1) but it also facilitates immune surveillance of the tissue insuring early warning in the event of invasion by foreign substances.

Overall, approximately 10% of intravascular protein and fluid volume "leaks" out into the interstitial space each day and must be returned to the circulation via the lymphatics.

- Contrary to previous long-held beliefs, little or no extravasated fluid appears to be returned directly to the venous portion of the capillary bed (Fig. 14.1).
- Instead, this extravasated fluid is processed by lymph nodes in the lymphatic system and returned into circulation through the venous system following its surveillance of lymphatic tissues.
- Acute inflammation disrupts the homeostatic process in the interstitium and dramatically increases the burden on the lymphatic system.
- Damage involving the lymphatic vessels can lead to chronic inflammation[2]

Despite the importance of the lymphatic system to the maintenance of homeostasis, it remains one of the least studied biologic systems.[3]

- This chapter will review the anatomy and physiology of the lymphatic system, its specific role in inflammation, and the general role of the lymphatic system in health and disease.

ANATOMY OF THE LYMPHATIC SYSTEM

General Aspects

Virtually all vascularized tissues have lymphatic capillaries that provide unidirectional lymph drainage, the only exceptions being the following:

- Central nervous system
- Bone
- Bone marrow
- Maternal placenta
- Endomysium surrounding muscle fibers

In these tissues, other forms of lymphatic drainage appear to exist.

Tissues without any blood supply lack any form of lymphatic drainage; examples include the following:

- Cartilage
- Lens and cornea of the eye
- Epidermis
- Inner portion of the walls of large blood vessels

The lymphatic system begins in the interstitial space of tissues with initial lymphatics, also termed terminal lymphatics, or lymph capillaries (Fig. 14.1).

- Lymph is an ultrafiltrate of plasma generated by passing circulating fluids through capillary walls and into interstitial spaces.
- Recent studies have demonstrated that all or almost all of the extravasated fluids are reclaimed through thin-walled initial

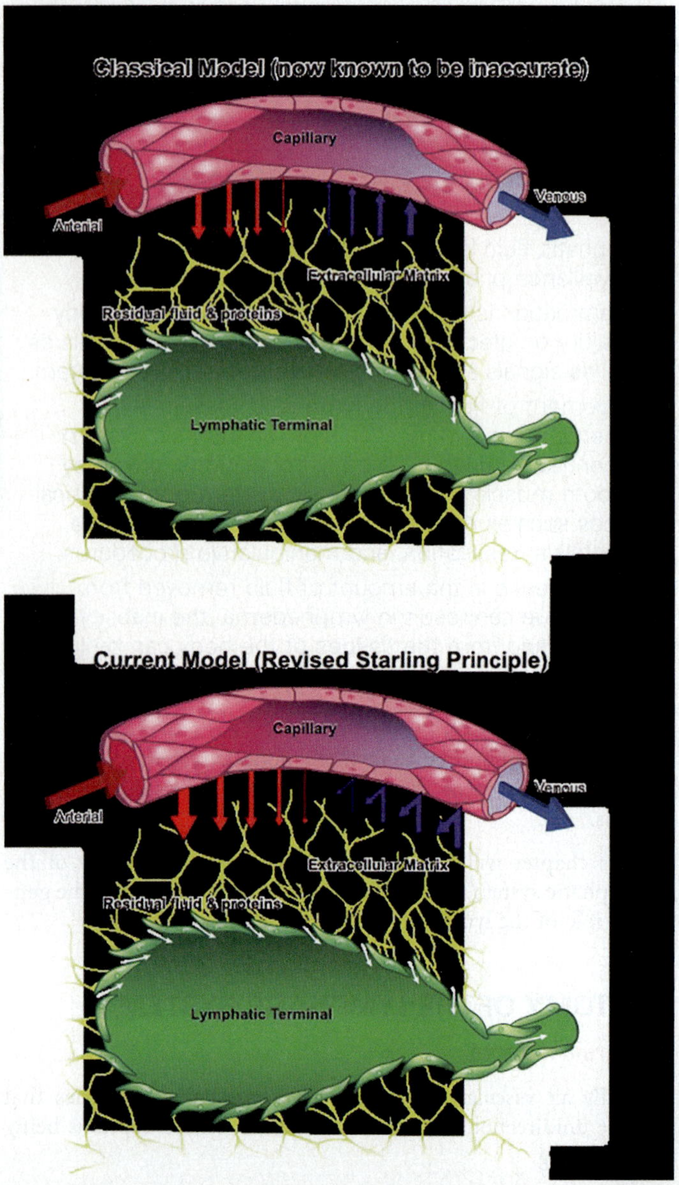

Figure 14.1. Fluid is driven out of capillaries (*red*) on the arterial side of the bed and leached into terminal lymphatics capillaries (*green*) through a series of one-way valves. The classical model (upper model) of Starling forces predicted that extravasated fluid (*red arrows*) would be partially reclaimed by the rising oncotic forces as the plasma became more concentrated toward the venous end of the capillary bed (*blue arrows* returning into the capillary). Recently analysis has found that a thin glycocalyx layer lying on the endothelium of the vessels prevents the oncotic pressure from rising to the level that will reclaim extravasated fluid (reflected *blue arrows* in the lower illustration). Thus most, if not all extravasated fluids are reabsorbed via the initial lymphatic capillaries.

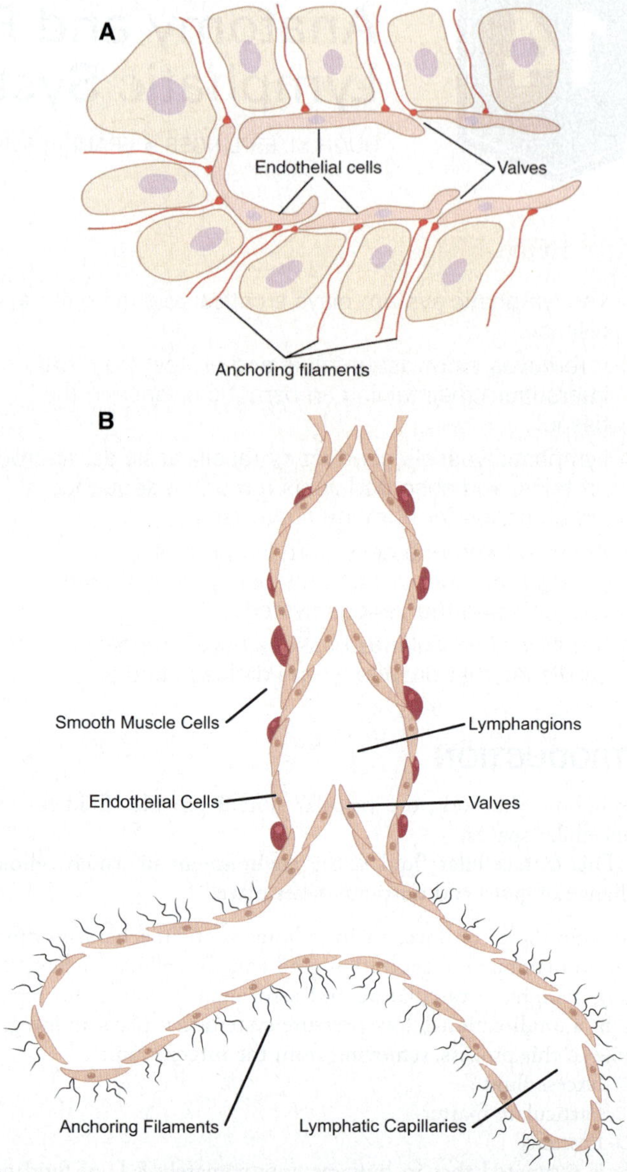

Figure 14.2. The cytoarchitecture of the terminal lymphatics. A. The terminal lymphatics or lymphatic capillaries are seen as endothelial-lined cul-de-sacs anchored into the surrounding extracellular matrix by small filaments. The endothelial cells overlap, creating one-way valves allowing fluid in the ECM to leech into the terminal lymphatic but preventing back drainage. The terminal lymphatics lack smooth muscle walls. (Used with permission of Elsevier Science & Technology Journals from Hall JE, Guyton AC. *Guyton and Hall Textbook of Medical Physiology*. 12th ed. Saunders/Elsevier; 2011:187. Figure 16-8; permission conveyed through Copyright Clearance Center, Inc.) **B.** The collecting vessels begin at the first valve and have both smooth muscle walls and periodic valves derived from the endothelium.

lymphatic vessels, located in the interstitial tissue. Lymph is gathered from the tissue and then coalesced into collecting channels, which drain into progressively larger prenodal or afferent lymph vessels (Fig. 14.2).

- All afferent lymph vessels then pass through one or more lymph nodes, which filter and alter the lymph in a variety of ways.
- As much as 30% of the lymphatic fluid will enter venous circulation through each lymph node.
- Efferent or postnodal lymph vessels drain the remaining fluid from the nodes into larger efferent lymphatic trunks.
- These trunks ultimately return lymph to the venous system at the cervicothoracic junction either via the thoracic duct on the left or the right lymphatic duct (see Clemente[4] for an extensive review of the lymphatic system anatomy).
- Note that all lymphatic vessels bringing lymph into a given node are referred to as "afferent vessels"; all vessels carrying lymph away from a lymph node are termed "efferent vessels"; since the lymph nodes are arranged in chains, an afferent lymphatic vessel to a given node may also be an efferent vessel from a previous node.

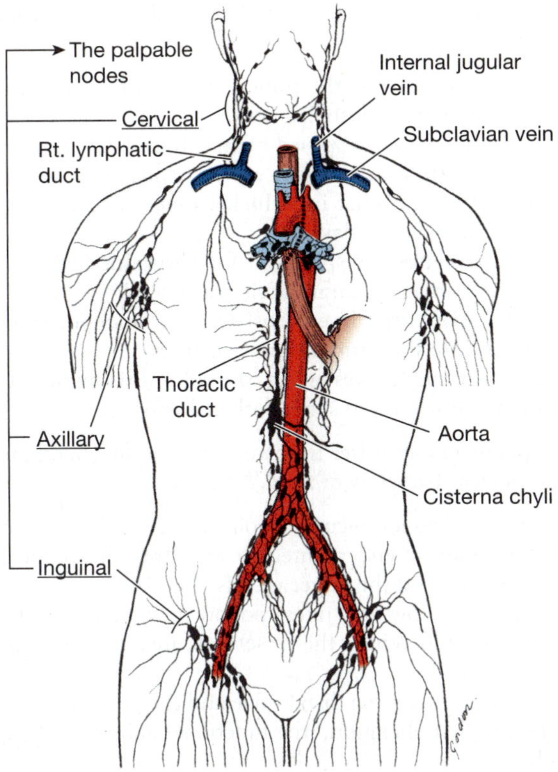

Figure 14.3. The lymphatic system scheme. This diagram illustrates the overall distribution and flow patterns of the lymphatic system. (Reprinted with permission from Basmajian JV. *Grant's Method of Anatomy: By Regions, Descriptive and Deductive.* Williams & Wilkins; 1975.)

Two major routes for lymphatic return into venous circulation are described (Fig. 14.3). Lymph returning to the thoracic duct comes from the:

- Lower extremities, abdominal cavity
- Left thorax and part of the left lung
- Left aspect of the thoracoabdominal diaphragm
- Left arm
- Left side of the head and neck

While lymph returning to the right lymphatic duct originates in the:

- Heart
- Right lung
- Right arm
- Right side of the head and neck
- Right aspect thoracoabdominal diaphragm

Finally, a significant amount of lymphatic fluid is returned directly into venous circulation from each lymph node.

ANATOMY OF THE LYMPH VESSELS

Initial Lymphatics

Lymphatic capillaries are blind-ended terminals located in interstitial spaces of most tissues (see Fig. 14.2). They comprise endothelial cells arranged in a single layer containing no tight junctions and are therefore permeable to large particles and proteins. Although their morphology varies in different tissues, there are notable similarities in anatomic microstructure that are critical to the function of these capillaries in lymph formation (for a description of the histology of the lymphatic system, see Pawlina[5]).

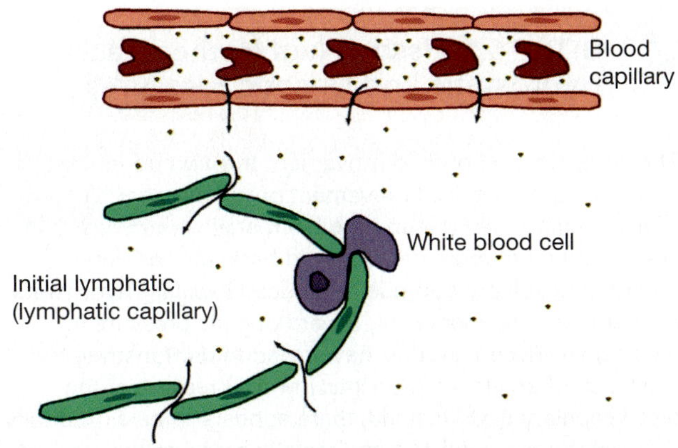

Figure 14.4. The mechanics of the terminal lymphatic vessel. An endothelial cell–lined blood vessel is seen above and a terminal lymphatic below. Fluid, particulates, and protein diffuse out of the vessel and into the extracellular matrix. From the matrix, these items can enter the terminal lymphatic vessel by passing through the small gaps in the endothelial lining. Due to the overlapping nature of these endothelial cells, backflow from the lymphatic vessel into the matrix cannot occur. (Reprinted from Swartz MA. The physiology of the lymphatic system. *Adv Drug Deliv Rev.* 2001; 50(1–2):3–20. Copyright © 2001 Elsevier. With permission.)

Initial lymphatics lie in close juxtaposition with capillaries and postcapillary venules.[6]

- These lymphatic terminals consist of overlapping endothelial cells, arranged on a discontinuous basement membrane and lacking tight junctions but contain anchoring filaments.
- Anchoring filaments are collagenous fiber bundles that attach to the external aspect of the lymphatic endothelium and imbed into the interstitial matrix (see Figs. 14.1 and 14.2).
- Expanding interstitial fluids will increase lymphatic drainage.[7]
- In the setting of edema, anchoring filaments prevent the collapse of the initial lymphatics as interstitial pressure rises.
- These filaments also cause the lymphatic vessel to change shape and volume in response to tissue movement (Fig. 14.4).
- The overlapping endothelial cells are theorized to act as a "primary valve system" that allows entry into the vessel but prevents reflux of fluid into the interstitium from the initial lymphatic.[8–10]
- It is known that the valves can open large enough to let tissue dendritic cells enter the initial lymphatic terminal.

Several morphologic features of the lymphatic capillaries are key to their function, a recent study demonstrated the lack of adhesion molecules at the junctional borders of the endothelial cells of the initial lymphatic.[11]

- The basement membrane of the terminal lymphatic is discontinuous, thereby facilitating the movement of fluid into the vessel.[12]
- This arrangement provides for a one-way flow of lymphatic fluids from the extracellular space into the initial lymphatic vessels.
- It is important to note that these valves do not act as filters; thus, fluid moving into the lumen of the terminal lymphatic vessel has the approximate composition of extracellular fluid.
- The discontinuous basement membrane, open interendothelial junctions, and the anchoring filaments all help to distinguish the terminal lymphatic from a vascular capillary bed.[12]
- Finally, lymphatic capillaries lack smooth muscle cells in their walls; thus, they are dependent on outside forces to both fill the terminal vessel and then expel lymph into the collecting vessels.

Classically, the equation of Starling forces stated that blood entering the capillary bed lost fluid but not large proteins to the

BOX 14.1 Tissue Fluid Homeostasis: Hydrostatic and Oncotic Pressures

The classic model of fluid movement through peripheral tissue features net fluid movement out of the arteriole end of the capillary bed due to high hydrostatic pressure in the vessel and a net movement of fluid back into the venous end of the capillary bed due to reduced capillary hydrostatic pressure and the increasing inward oncotic pressure in the vessels. Recent studies have failed to demonstrate the existence of an elevated oncotic inward pressure at the distal capillary bed.[3] Instead, there appears to be a gradually diminishing but persistent hydrostatic pressure throughout the entire length of the capillary bed. This arrangement suggests that the lymphatic system is the critical means for removing extravasated fluid from peripheral tissue.

Mortimer PS, Rockson SG. New developments in clinical aspects of lymphatic disease. *J Clin Invest.* 2014;124(3):915–921.

surrounding interstitium, gradually, the increasing oncotic pressure in the capillary due to the concentration of protein was high enough to draw some of the fluid back into the capillary; this has since been proven inadequate to explain fluid movement in local tissue[3,13] (Box 14.1).

- A more comprehensive examination of fluid dynamics in tissue finds that little if any of the ultrafiltrate that leaves the vascular capillary to enter the interstitial spaces returns directly into circulation at the venous end of the capillary bed.[14]
- Instead, all fluid in the interstitium appears to be recycled through lymphatic channels at least to the level of the lymph nodes.
- Failure of the vascular capillaries to reclaim extravasated fluid seems to be due to a thin glycocalx layer lining the inner surface of the capillary endothelium and a very narrow sub-glycoclax space separating the glycocalx layer and the endothelial cell membrane.
- The sub-glycoclax space lacks large protein content thereby preventing the oncotic pressure near the endothelium for rising high enough to draw fluids back into the vessel.
- This concept is known as the revised Starling equation.[15]
- Based on this revised equation, it appears that little if any extravasated fluid directly re-enters the capillary bed, instead it is entirely drained off through the lymphatic system facilitating its exposure to immune surveillance in the associated lymph nodes.

COLLECTING VESSELS

Initial lymphatics can end directly into a collecting lymphatic vessel or form a complex hexagonal network with compartments that eventually gives way to the collecting vessels.[7]

- The transition from the initial lymphatic vessel to collecting vessels is marked by the appearance of the first bicuspid valve (see Fig. 14.2).
- Collecting vessels develop a thin connective tissue layer to support the endothelial lining, and a few slips of smooth muscle, which are arranged in a woven fashion surrounding the vessel and concentrated near the valves.
- The smooth muscle layer progressively thickens in a proximal direction, and eventually the vessels develop a three-layer arrangement much like a small vein, with a tunica intima, media, and adventitia.

Thus, collecting lymphatic vessels typically have three layers of tissue in their walls.[16]

- The innermost layer is the tunica intima composed of monolayer of lymphatic endothelial cells.
- The tunica media is composed of an extracellular matrix of collagen and elastin into which is woven bands of smooth muscle cells arranged somewhat in a thicker inner circular layer and a thin longitudinal outer layer.
- The tunica media is responsible for peristaltic activity in the vessel and is driven by an intrinsic pacemaker.
- The outer adventitial layer consists of loose connective tissue that blends into the surrounding structures.
- A vasa vasorum is present in the adventitia with arterioles extending inward to the subendothelial region.

Lymphatic vessels differ from veins in that they have far more valves to prevent backflow of fluid.[16]

- Lymphatic valves are bicuspid, collagenous, and attach so as to have their narrow end pointed in the direction of the lymph flow, that is toward the larger vessels (Fig. 14.5).
- They operate at low flow rates and low pressures, since the valve flaps that are adherent to the vessel wall, are closed by retrograde fluid pressure.
- The region between the distal valve and the proximal valve constitutes the "lymphangion," the functional unit of the lymphatic vessel.
- Each lymphangion is wrapped by several slips of smooth muscle fibers, the smooth muscle cells appear to be the pacemaker initiating contraction of the lymphangion.
- The region of the valve is typically free of smooth muscle fibers.
- Transmural pressure can influence both inotropic (strength) activity and chronotropic (timing) activity.[17]
- Lymphangions exhibit both a filling (diastolic) stage and a contractile (systolic) stage[7] (Fig. 14.6).

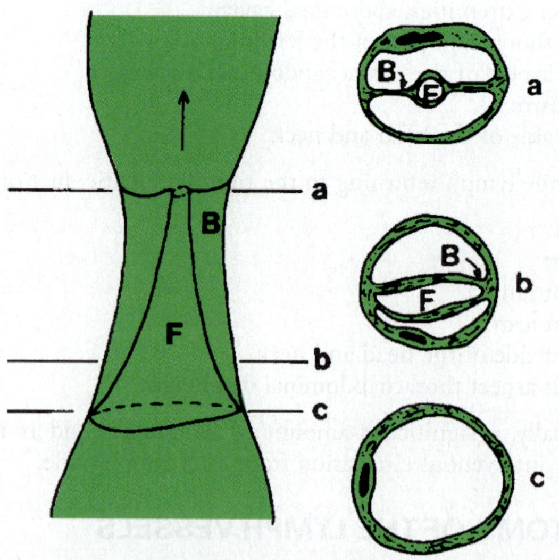

Figure 14.5. The collecting vessel valves. On the *left* is a longitudinal view of the valve in a collecting vessel. On the *right* are cross sections taken through the valve at three separate levels indicated by the horizontal lines. The leaflets of the valve are fused to each other and to the wall of the vessel. As one progresses up the valve, the fusion of the leaflets moves closer to the midline, making it impossible for the valve to invert and thus producing a one-way flow. (Reprinted with permission from Schmid-Schönbein GW. Microlymphatics and lymph flow. *Physiol Rev.* 1990;70(4):987–1028. Copyright © 1990 the American Physiological Society.)

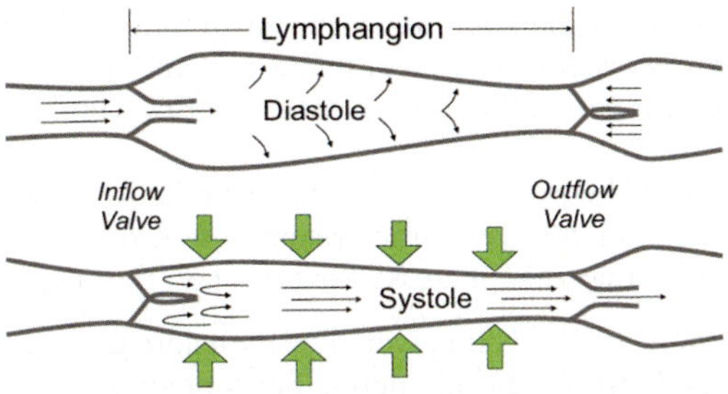

Figure 14.6. Collecting lymphatic phasic contractions. Like the heart, collecting lymphatics have a period of brisk contraction (systole) and a period of relaxation (diastole) between each phasic contraction. Each lymphangion, defined as the segment between two unidirectional valves, can typically exhibit systole and diastole. When a lymphangion is relaxed, the inflow (or upstream) valve will open (given sufficient inflow pressure) for filling of the lymphangion to occur. During systole, the phasic contraction pushes the lymph both upstream and downstream, but the inflow valve closes, so that lymph is forced forward through the outflow valve. The exact valve gating and phasic contraction frequency and force depend heavily on the outflow pressure (afterload), inflow pressure (preload), and the flow of lymph (shear stress). (Reprinted from Breslin JW. Mechanical forces and lymphatic transport. *Microvasc Res.* 2014;96:46–54. Copyright © 2014 Elsevier. With permission.)

Lymph is passed sequentially through multiple lymph nodes before draining into larger postnodal vessels, typically termed lymphatic trunks.

- The collecting vessels prior to the lymph nodes are termed the afferent or prenodal vessels.
- Those draining the node are termed the efferent or postnodal vessel (Fig. 14.7).
- Lymph nodes are encapsulated and contain sinusoids that allow the lymph to "percolate" through a large surface area of cells and vessels, it is here that immune surveillance of the tissue fluids occurs.

Lymph from the afferent vessels first enters into the subcapsular sinus, portions of this fluid are siphoned off into a conduit system of tubules which channel this fluid to the area of the high endothelial venules (HEVs) in the paracortex of the gland.[18]

- This channeled fluid is returned to the blood stream via the HEV; in addition, signaling molecules such as chemokines are used by the endothelial cells in the HEVs to attract lymphocytes to the gland, thus the HEVs are a two-way street.
- The filtration system of the lymph nodes is the means through which small antigens in the lymphatic fluid are trapped, immunocytes are drawn to the node and an immune response is generated.
- Larger foreign particles (<70 kDa) are also removed by nodal macrophages in the subcapsular and trabecular sinuses.
- Lymph nodes have been shown to significantly alter the protein composition of lymph, and are capable of transferring large quantities of fluid to the venous system.[19]
- Approximately 30% of the fluid in the afferent lymph vessel is removed as the lymph passes through the node.[5,20]
- Passage of lymph through a series of nodes significantly concentrates the fluid before entry into the lymphatic trunks.
- Increased venous pressure or congestion in the area of the nodes will interfere with this process, thereby increasing the resistance to lymph flow.[21,22]

Osteopathic treatment to decongest areas around lymph nodes, such as the popliteal spread or pectoral lift, may help maintain the

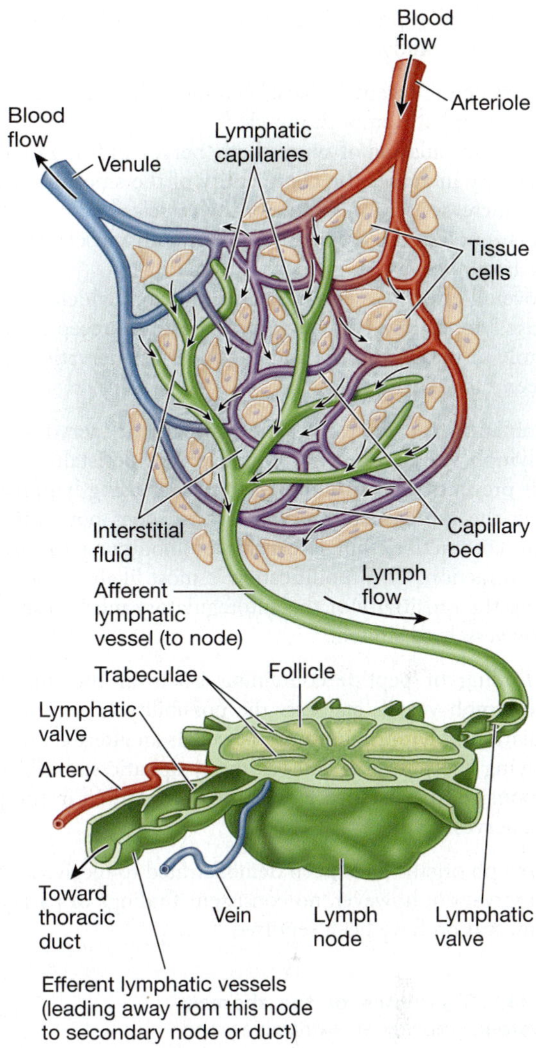

Figure 14.7. The lymphatic system. This figure illustrates the afferent lymphatic collecting vessels arising in the tissue between the arterial and venous system and extending to the lymph nodes. The efferent vessels arise in the capsule of the lymph node and progress toward the thoracic duct. (Reprinted with permission from Agur AMR, Dalley AF II. *Grant's Atlas of Anatomy.* 12th ed. Wolters Kluwer Health/Lippincott Williams & Wilkins; 2009.)

downward hydrostatic gradient between the lymphatic and the venous systems.

- Postnodal or efferent vessels follow fascial planes, progressively moving toward the midline of the body, where they enter the mediastinum in the abdomen, thorax, or cervical region.
- Postnodal or efferent vessels have thicker, more muscular walls, capable of peristaltic action (see Pawlina[5]).
- Eventually, the large postnodal vessels, also termed trunks, drain into the right lymphatic duct or left thoracic duct.
- These large lymphatic ducts, such as the thoracic duct, are organized histologically like a medium-sized vein, except for the greater amount of smooth muscle and valves.

INNERVATION OF LYMPHATIC VESSELS

The smooth muscle in the wall of the lymph vessel contains adrenergic, cholinergic, purinergic, and peptidergic nerves,[12,23] although a sympathetic innervation has been more consistently observed.[24] Chemical stimulation in vitro of the adrenergic receptors causes contraction of the lymphatic smooth muscle[25]; the effect of cholinergic stimulation has been variable and has been questioned by a more recent study.

- Beta-adrenergic receptors have been identified that cause relaxation of lymphatic smooth muscle.[26]
- Electrical stimulation of sympathetic nerves and/or ganglia also consistently increases the contractility of the smooth muscle as well as increases stroke volume of the vessels.[27–29]
- Innervation, like the distribution of smooth muscle, is greatest in the larger vessels.
- The overall effect of sympathetic stimulation, which appears to increase lymph flow, is mediated via the alpha-receptors.
- The role of beta-receptors and cholinergic innervation has not yet been fully elucidated.

Eliminating the effects of the sympathetic nervous system on the lymph vessels does not eliminate the peristaltic contractions but prevents field stimulation from increasing lymph flow,[30] indicating the sympathetic nervous system does not initiate the peristaltic contractions but is capable of modifying the intrinsic rate of contraction. This modification is most likely accomplished by varying the sensitivity of the autoregulatory mechanism in the lymphatic vessels to stretch.[12]

- The finding of peptide-containing fibers in the innervation of the lymph vessels suggests the possibility of sensory reflex modulation of lymph pumping, as well as an alternate means of modifying the pumping rate, as the lymphatic smooth muscle is responsive to substance P, which was identified in the peptidergic nerves.[31]

All lymph organs have been demonstrated to receive a sympathetic innervation; however, no consistent findings of parasympathetic innervation have been reported.[32]

- Sympathetic stimulation has been shown to modify lymphocyte activity,[33] as well as cause contraction of the lymph node capsule, resulting in an increase in the output of lymphocytes from nodes.[24,34–36]
- It has been theorized that the primary role of the sympathetic innervation of the lymphatic system is to modify the immune response, rather than increase flow through the vessels.[37]

The thoracic duct is innervated by both adrenergic and cholinergic fibers; however, the adrenergic fibers predominate.

- Spontaneous, peristaltic contractions have been consistently observed in the thoracic duct of various species; the rate of these spontaneous contractions can be modulated by the sympathetic nervous system.[38]
- Stimulation of adrenergic release results in contraction of the human thoracic duct tissue.[39]
- Cajal-like cells (pacemaker cells) have been detected in the walls of the human thoracic duct.[40]
- In summary, the sympathetic nervous system innervates the thoracic duct and is involved in its regular contractions.

REGIONAL LYMPH DRAINAGE

The movement of lymphatic fluids progresses from the peripheral tissues toward the midline of the body and, once at the midline, toward the cervicothoracic junction where these fluids are returned to systemic circulation through the jugular or subclavian veins.

- Lymph from the two lower extremities, pelvic basin, abdomen, left thorax, left upper extremity, and left side of the head targets the thoracic duct for return to the venous compartment (Fig. 14.8).

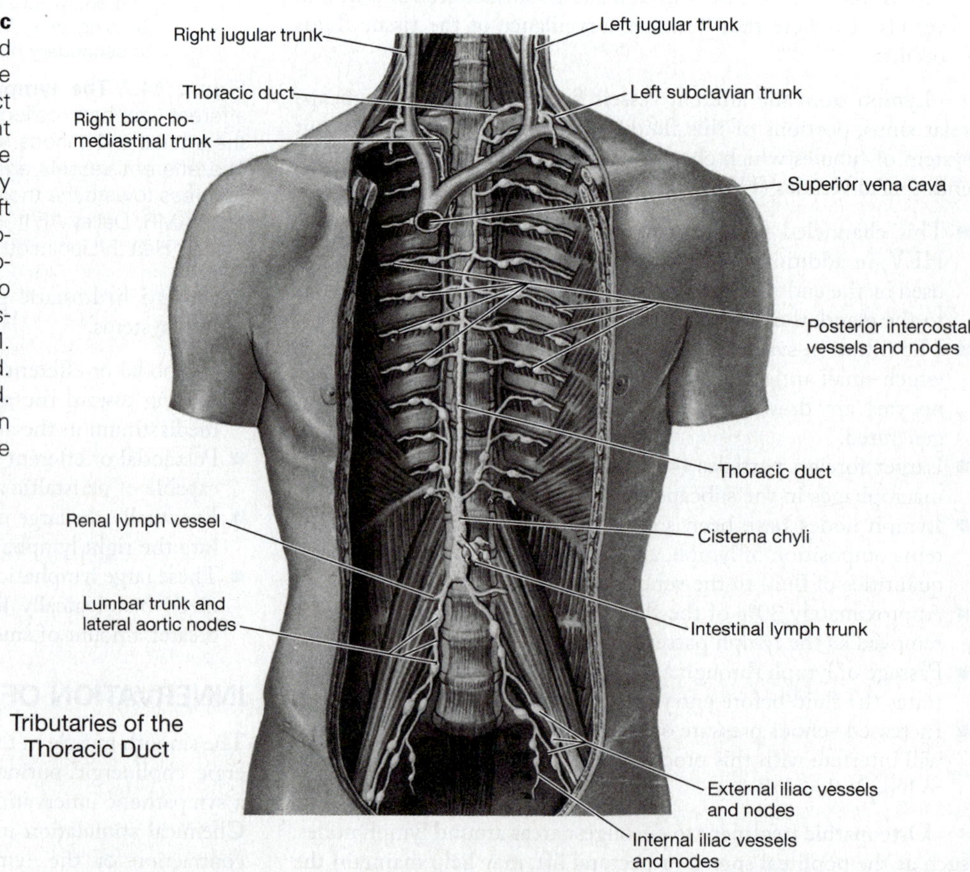

Figure 14.8. Tributaries of the thoracic duct system. The lower extremities and the abdominopelvic cavity drain into the cisterna chyli from which the thoracic duct arises. The cisterna chyli may be absent in which case all of these trunks coalesce directly into the thoracic duct. The left body wall, the left upper extremity, and the left side of the head will also drain into the thoracic duct, leaving the right side of the thorax, upper extremity, and head to drain into a right lymphatic duct. (Used with permission of Springer Nature BV from Yoffey JM. Cardiovascular System. In: Hamilton WJ, ed. *Textbook of Human Anatomy*. 2nd rev. ed. Palgrave Macmillan; 1982:283; permission conveyed through Copyright Clearance Center, Inc.)

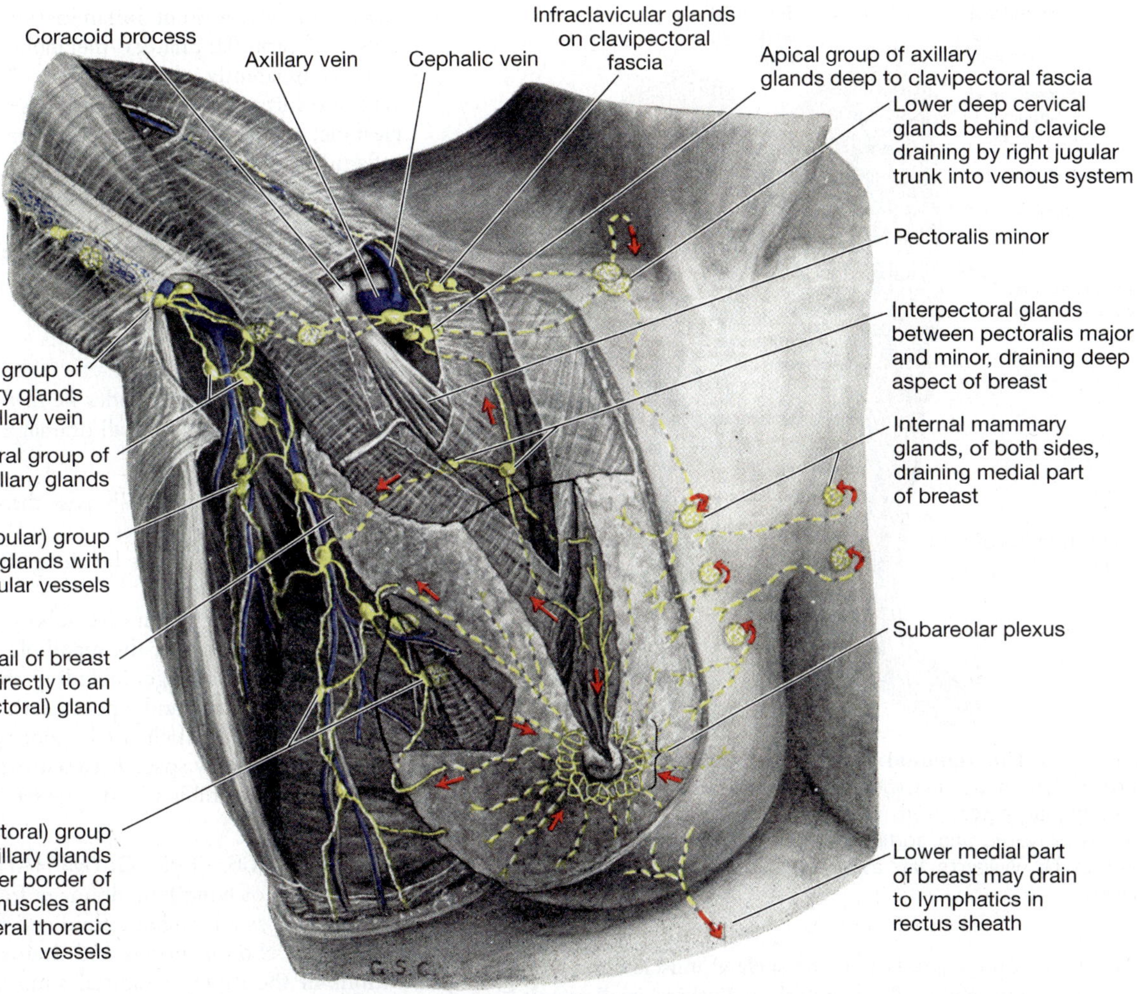

Figure 14.9. Regional lymphatic drainage of the upper extremity. The lymphatic drainage of the upper extremity is seen entering the axillary region where it merges with that of the anterior chest wall including the breast tissue in the female. (Reprinted with permission from Lockhart RD, Hamilton GF, Fyfe FW. *Anatomy of the Human Body*. J.B. Lippincott Company; 1960.)

- Lymphatic vessels draining the right thorax, right upper extremity, and right side of the head flow into the right lymphatic duct before entering the venous system.
- There are slight variations in the structure and of initial lymphatics and collecting channels in various organs and tissues that offer insight into the physiology of lymph formation and propulsion. Some of those differences, as well as the main pathways of drainage of the lymph system, will be described here. For a detailed description of lymphatic drainage, see Anson[41] for a detailed review.

Peripheral Tissues of the Extremities

There is a superficial and deep drainage of the upper and lower extremities.

- The superficial drainage follows subcutaneous routes to proximal nodes at the axilla and inguinal areas.
- Superficial drainage is divided into a dermal plexus and a deeper plexus located at the outermost portion of the investing fascia of the muscles.
- The deep plexus drains joints, bones, tendons, ligaments, and muscles; it follows the neurovascular structures to the same ultimate endpoint and has various nodes at intermediary sites.
- The upper limb lymph exits the axilla via a somewhat vulnerable route through the thoracic outlet, exiting the limb beneath the pectoralis minor muscle, and entering the thorax through the costoclavicular space (Fig. 14.9).
- The upper extremity lymph channels join with those from the anterior thoracic wall including the breast tissue in females (Fig. 14.9).
- The lower extremity drainage enters the abdomen through the femoral triangle, in close proximity to where the iliopsoas tendon crosses the hip joint (Fig. 14.10).
- The deep drainage of the lower extremity passes into the popliteal space between the two heads of the gastrocnemius and exits the popliteal space between the heads of the hamstrings.
  - The small, pliant lymph vessels are most vulnerable to tissue tension as they pass through narrow spaces.
  - When sufficient tension is present, it can limit the lymphatic drainage of the respective extremity.
  - Increasing outflow pressure has been shown to reduce lymph flow in vitro.[42]

The small collecting vessels draining skeletal muscle have been shown to have significantly less smooth muscle.

- The smooth muscle wall of the lymphatic vessels does not appear until the vessel is relatively large in size.

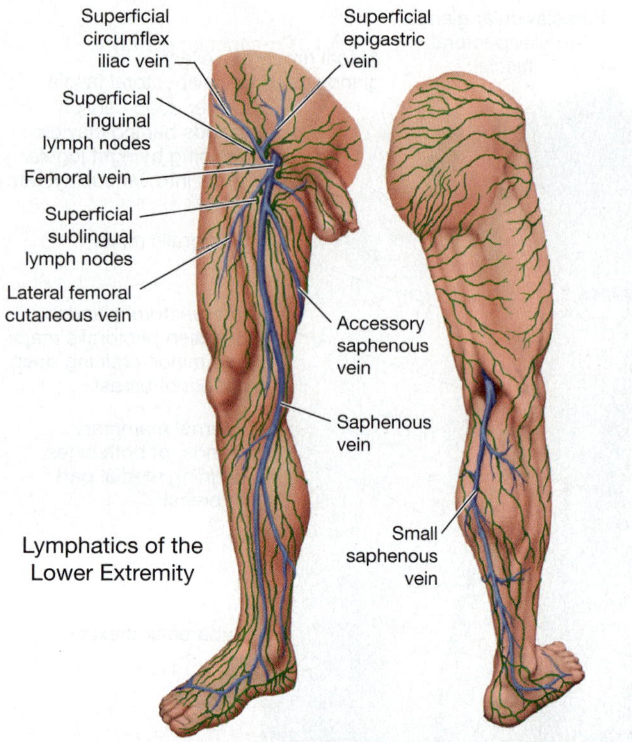

Figure 14.10. The regional lymphatic drainage of the lower extremity. Lymphatic drainage from the lower extremity is directed to the inguinal region, from which it passes along iliac nodes to reach the preaortic and aortic nodes. (Courtesy of Oran Z. Suta, as part of Dr. Willard's lab at the UNE College of Osteopathic Medicine.)

- This observation suggests that the skeletal muscle contraction is effective in propelling the lymph through these small vessels.[6]

The synovial fluid of large joints is drained via the lymphatic system.

- Radiolabeled tracer placed into the synovial space of the knee joint of a pig could be followed as it was removed through the lymphatic channels and entered the thoracic duct.
- The synovial tracer was estimated to have a half-life of approximately 8.3 hours, suggesting that synovial clearance via lymphatics is relatively quick from the large joints of the extremities.[43]
- Proinflammatory compounds have been detected in the lymphatic fluid draining from inflamed joints.[44]

The drainage of synovial fluid through the lymphatic system is one method for ridding the joint of proinflammatory compounds in the presence of inflammatory arthritis.

- Animal studies have demonstrated that enhanced lymph drainage can be protective to joints with chronic inflammatory arthritis[45] and inhibition of lymphatic drainage can worsen the inflammation in the joint.[46]
- However, models of rheumatoid arthritis have demonstrated a complex relationship between the initiation of an inflammatory disorder and the lymphatic drainage network.[47]
    - In the initial prearthritic inflammatory stage of the disease, local lymph nodes expand in size, this is termed the *expansion phase* of the disease.
    - This expansion is associated with lymphangiogenesis resulting in a significant increase in lymphatic drainage of the joint; inhibition of the lymphatics at this stage will hasten the arthritic stage of the disease.
    - Resolution of the joint inflammation brings inflammatory cells and proinflammatory metabolites into the lymphatic system apparently damaging the lymphatic endothelial cells and initiating a "collapsed phase" where the lymphatic clearance markedly decreases resulting in lymphatic stasis of inflammatory fluids within the joint.
    - The collapsed phase leads to enhanced joint pathology characteristic of rheumatoid arthritis.
    - Developing mechanisms to re-establish lymphatic drainage from inflamed joints are at the forefront of treatment.

Head and Neck

The deep cervical vessels and nodes lie in the carotid sheath, and this is the terminal pathway for all drainage of the head and neck (Fig. 14.11).

- Superficial drainage will usually pass through superficial nodes before entering the deep nodes.
    - Many of these deep nodes lie along the borders of the sternocleidomastoid muscle.
    - Other deep nodes lie in the suboccipital space, over the parotid gland, and under the mandible.
- Much of the deep drainage, including that of the ear, sinuses, pharynx, upper larynx, and upper teeth, drain via the upper nodes through the jugulodigastric node, which opens into the deep chain in a narrow space between the mastoid process and the angle of the mandible (for details see Anson[41]).

BRAIN LYMPHATICS—THE "GLYMPHATIC SYSTEM"

The classic model of lymphatic drainage from the brain suggests that the CSF acts as a lymphatic fluid and that most of the CSF is formed in the choroid plexus and drained through arachnoid granulations in the superior sagittal sinus or into spinal arachnoid granulations located just dorsolateral to each dorsal root ganglia.[48–50]

However, a potentially new pathway for fluid movement in the brain has been described[51] involving the possible drainage of the extracellular tissue fluids through the perivascular spaces for direct entry into the venous return (Fig. 14.12).

This pathway is thought to involve the following[48]:

- Movement of CSF into the periarterial (Virchow–Robin) spaces that exist between the pia and the penetrating small arteries of the brain.[52]
- These spaces are visible with heavily T2-weighted sequences, and course parallel to the predominant vascular system.[53]
- At the depths of the perivascular spaces, in the region of capillary beds, the CSF exchanges with brain intracellular fluids.[52]
- The aquaporin 4 channels on the astrocytic end-feet surrounding the vessel have been proposed to facilitate the movement of CSF into the interstitial tissue.[54]
- Drainage from the interstitial spaces appears to be along white matter tracts and perivenous spaces.[52]
- This pathway was named the "glymphatic system" to emphasize the combined activity of the water channels on the glial cells and its functional similarities to the lymphatic system.[54]
- The glymphatic system appears to be more efficient during sleep than wakefulness.[52]
- It is still unclear what the driving forces are that are involved in moving fluid and particles along these narrow spaces[55] but explanations for these observations continue to be offered.[56]

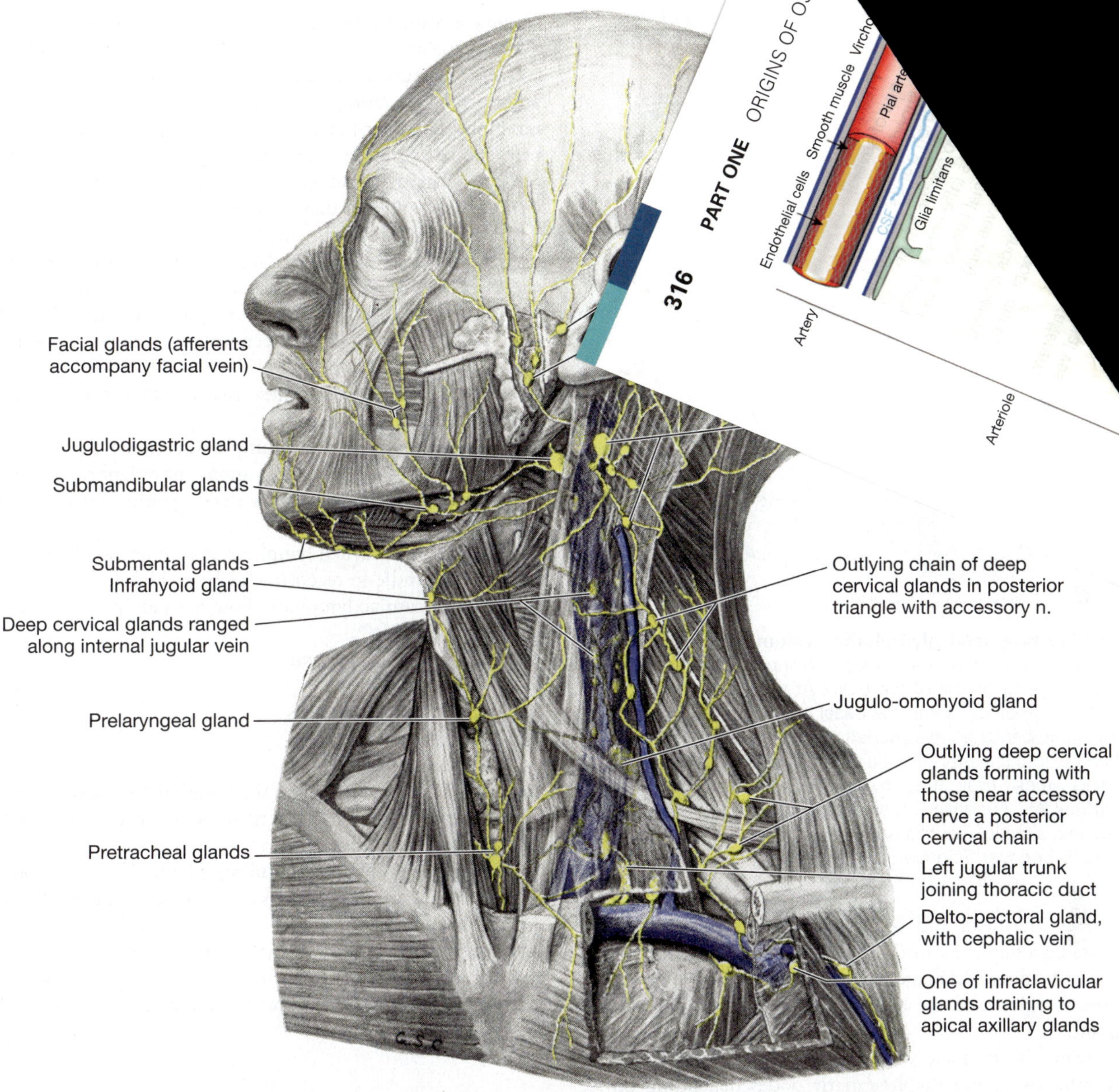

Figure 14.11. The regional lymphatic drainage from the head and neck. Lymphatic channels in the neuro- and visceral cranium converge on the carotid sheath, from which lymph passes downward to join the right lymphatic duct or the thoracic duct on the left. (Reprinted with permission from Lockhart RD, Hamilton GF, Fyfe FW. *Anatomy of the Human Body*. J.B. Lippincott Company; 1960.)

In essence, many of the details of the glymphatic system still remain to be elucidated, however this much can be stated:

- It is evident that the glymphatic system does not replace the drainage of CSF through arachnoid villi into the venous sinuses.
- It may serve to augment and accelerate the clearance of waste products, especially proteins and other large molecules from the brain.
- The rapid removal of waste protein from the brain suggests that dysfunction of the glymphatic system may play a role in the protein deposition diseases such as Alzheimer disease and others.[57]

Along with fluid drainage via arachnoid granulations and through a glymphatic system, several other routes for the removal of cerebrospinal fluid from the cranium have been documented.

- An extensive network of lymphatic vessels has been documented in the meninges of the brain, the precise drainage of these vessels is still uncertain, but it appears that the meningeal lymphatic vessels eventually reach the deep cervical lymph nodes.[48,58]
- CSF is absorbed in the paraneural sheaths of cranial and spinal nerves and removed by lymphatic vessels that run in close juxtaposition to the initial segments of the nerves.
- Drainage of the CSF via the nasal passageways begins along the olfactory tract leading to the olfactory nerve in the cribriform plate, from here fluid enters the lymphatics in the nasal mucosa and eventually arrives at the deep cervical lymph nodes.

Thorax

The thoracocervical junction represents a convergence point for the great lymphatic trunks draining the various regions of the body.[4,59]

- Drainage from the upper extremities enters the thorax through the lymphatic channels in the axilla.

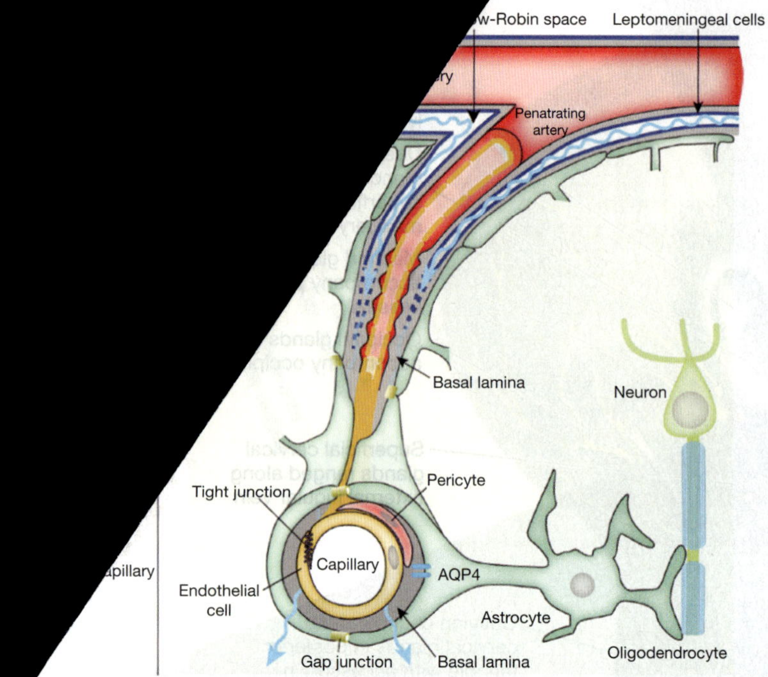

Figure 14.12. The proposed glymphatic system. CSF is shown flowing in the Virchow–Robin spaces surrounding pial arteries and extending into the parenchyma of the brain. At the approach of the capillary bed, the CSF diffuses into the basal lamina from which it is withdrawn by aquaporin channels (AQP4) located in astrocytic endfeet. Here it enters into the interstitial fluid of the brain and is removed via surrounding veins. (Reprinted by permission from Springer: Jessen NA, Munk AS, Lundgaard I, Nedergaard M. The glymphatic system: a beginner's guide. *Neurochem Res.* 2015;40(12):2583–2599. Copyright © 2015 Springer Science Business Media New York.)

- Drainage from the head and neck enters the thoracocervical junction passing along the carotid sheath.
- Superficial ascending drainage routes retrieve lymph from the mammary region and the anterior chest wall and anterior mediastinum.
  - Lymph from the thoracic wall can pass through the parasternal, intercostal, and diaphragmatic nodes depending on its location.
- Deeper routes, draining the thoracic viscera, ascend to the thoracocervical junction along the great vessels and trachea to drain the heart, pericardial sac, and the lungs.
  - Lymph from the thoracic viscera passes through the anterior mediastinal, posterior mediastinal, and the tracheobronchial nodes
- On the right side, these drainage routes converge to form the right lymphatic duct that can empty into the confluence of the internal jugular and the subclavian vein.
- On the left side, these drainage routes converge to form the thoracic duct that can empty into the confluence of the internal jugular and the subclavian vein similar to the right side.
- Rupture of the thoracic duct can result in lymphatic fluid build-up in the pleural space termed chylothorax.[60]

The heart has lymphatic plexuses located in the endocardium, myocardium, and epicardium (Fig. 14.13). The vessels involved have little smooth muscle and appear to depend on myocardial activity for lymphatic flow.

- The flow of lymphatic drainage is from the subendocardium plexus into the myocardial plexus and then to the subepicardial plexus.
- Drainage from the heart features two major routes.[4,61–63]
- The subepicardial channels from much of the ventricular tissue converge on several large lymphatic ducts, which course in the anterior and posterior intraventricular septae, these vessels combine into the major (left) lymphatic trunk in the coronary sulcus near the left coronary artery, this lymphatic trunk ascends near the pulmonary trunk to reach the right superior tracheobronchial lymph nodes and eventually drains into the right lymphatic duct.
- The subepicardial plexus on the right (atrial) side of the heart drains into large collecting vessels, located in the coronary sulcus associated with the right coronary artery, eventually these vessels unit to form a right (minor or lesser) lymphatic trunk that ascends in front of the ascending aorta to reach the anterior mediastinal lymph nodes.
- Communication between these two trunks can occur near the origin of the ascending aorta.
- The pericardium drains in multiple directions.
  - Inferiorly pericardial lymph drains into diaphragmatic nodes or through the inferior vena caval opening into the subdiaphragmatic region.
  - Superiorly pericardial lymph drains along the phrenic neurovascular bundle to reach tracheobronchial nodes.
- Blockage of cardiac lymphatic flow is thought to be associated with the following[64]:
  - Cardiac valvular deformities
  - Coronary arterial injury
  - Conduction disturbances
  - Myocardial injury
  - Poor cardiac performance
- In patients with heart failure, the lymphatic system can increase fluid removal from peripheral tissue well in excess of 10-fold the normal amount of drainage.[1]
  - In the setting of long-standing edema, it appears that the superficial lymphatic vessels dilate widely and leak fluid back into the tissue.
  - It is suggested that the lymphatic vessels have undergone pathologic changes with the increasing afterload experienced as central venous pressure increases secondary to heart failure.

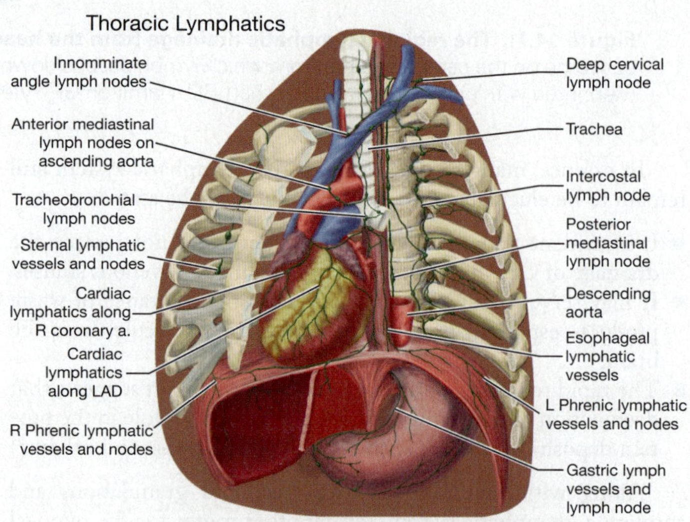

Figure 14.13. Region lymphatic drainage of the thorax. Lymph from the heart and pericardial sac drains into pretracheal and tracheal nodes located at the bifurcation of the trachea. (Courtesy of Oran Z. Suta, as part of Dr. Willard's lab at the UNE College of Osteopathic Medicine.)

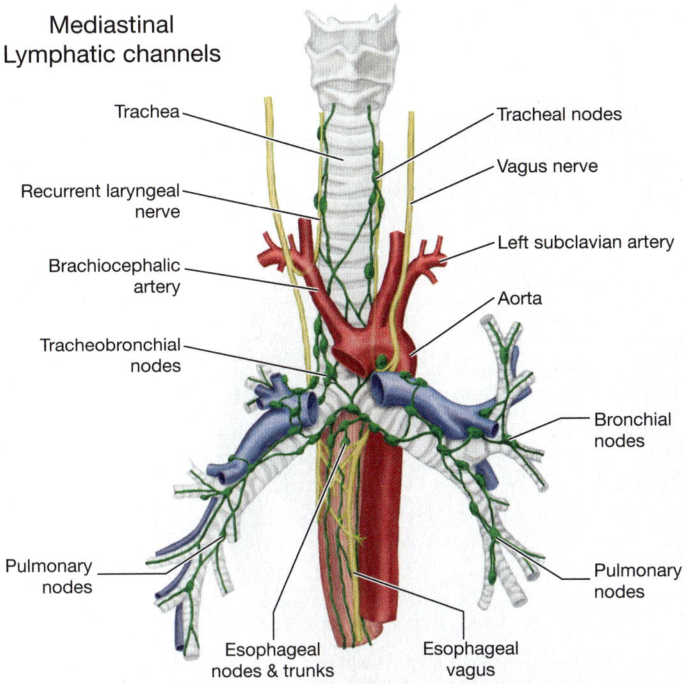

Figure 14.14. Regional lymphatic drainage of the lung. The deep pulmonary plexus surrounding the airways drains upward into the bronchopulmonary nodes. These nodes drain into the tracheobronchial nodes, which then drain into the tracheal nodes. Ultimately, drainage will be into the right lymphatic duct or into the thoracic duct depending on the side of the lymphatic chain. (Courtesy of Oran Z. Suta, as part of Dr. Willard's lab at the UNE College of Osteopathic Medicine.)

- □ The alteration in lymphatic function appears to be part of a feedforward sequence worsening the imbalance in fluid homeostasis in this disorder.

The lymphatics of the lung drain the pulmonary vasculature as well as the bronchial airways (Fig. 14.14).

- Lymph channels extend deep into the lung parenchyma, coursing in the interlobular septae in association with the bronchovascular bundles.[65]
- Recent studies employing immunohistochemical staining for lymphatic endothelial markers have demonstrated lymphatic capillaries in the walls of respiratory bronchioles extending into the walls of the alveolar septae.[65–67]
- These lymphatic vessels are thought to play a significant role in maintaining a relatively dry, narrow alveolar interstitium to optimize the air-blood barrier for gas diffusion.[65,68]
- Pulmonary lymph is formed by the expansion of the lungs during respiratory excursions.
- Lymphatic collecting vessels lack the smooth muscle wraps seen in collecting vessels in most other organ systems and are thus most dependent on alternating surrounding pressures to move fluids.[69]
- Lymphatic vessels follow the bronchovascular channels to eventually drain out of the lung at the hilum into the tracheobronchial nodes and into the right lymph trunk and thoracic duct.
- Intact lymphatic drainage is critical to the normal fluid homeostasis of the lung parenchyma, lymphatic dysfunction is thought to play an important role in numerous pulmonary diseases.[69]
- Diffuse alveolar damage, common in the pathophysiology of ARDS, including ARDS produced by COVID-19, significantly widens the interalveolar space as it fills with fluid, fibrin, and inflammatory mediators resulting in significantly altered gas diffusion.[70–72]

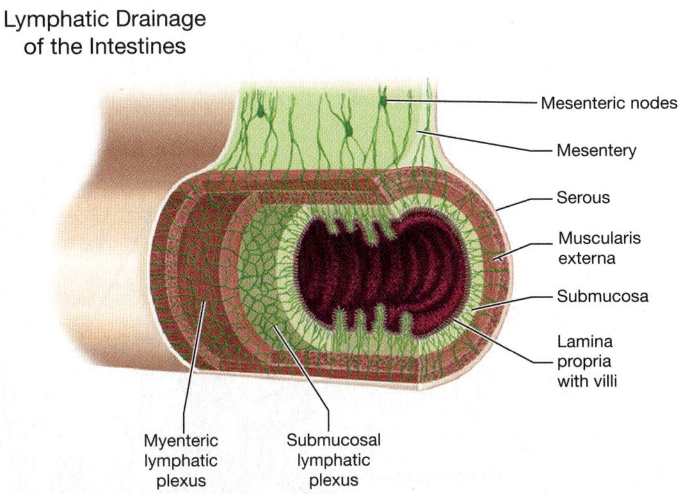

Figure 14.15. The lymphatic drainage of the intestines. This represents a cross section of the small intestines with a portion of its wall removed. The lymphatic drainage begins in the lacteals in the villi of the lumen of the intestine and moves outward through successive plexuses to reach an afferent lymph vessel. This vessel enters the mesenteries where it will drain into a mesenteric lymph node. (Courtesy of Oran Z. Suta, as part of Dr. Willard's lab at the UNE College of Osteopathic Medicine.)

Abdomen

There is a rich lymphatic system draining the gut tube, abdominal viscera, and mesenteries. The lymphatics of the intestines have lacteals for the unique purpose of absorbing fat (chyle) as part of the digestive process, giving abdominal lymph the characteristic milky color and consistency.

- The collecting lymphatics of the gut tube are similar to those of skeletal muscle, lacking smooth muscle for an unusually long distance, indicating the ability of peristalsis to propel lymph in this area.[6,68]
- The lymphatic drainage of the gastrointestinal organs follows the vascular structures back through the mesenteric roots, where they join the iliac and preaortic nodes on route to the cisterna chyli and thoracic duct (Figs. 14.15 to 14.17).
- The preaortic and aortic nodes are clustered around the three large unpaired arteries on the anterior aspect of the aorta, the celiac, superior mesenteric, and inferior mesenteric arteries.

The lymphatic drainage of the tubular gut passes through the mesenteries to reach the posterior body wall (Fig. 14.18).

- Lymph from the two lower extremities enters the abdominal cavity by passing deep to the inguinal ligament in the femoral canal.
- The chain of lymph nodes extends upward along the iliac vessels to reach the lumbar (para-aortic) trunks that pass upward along the lateral margins to the abdominal aorta (Fig. 14.19).
- As these lymphatic vessels follow the iliac vessels, they receive additional contributions from the pelvic basin.

Pelvic Cavity and Perineum

Extensive lymphatic drainage routes exist in the pelvic cavity. In essence, these routes radiate away from the pelvic organs, climb the walls of the pelvic basin, and enter the iliac lymphatic channels that are coursing along the brim of the pelvis toward the sacral

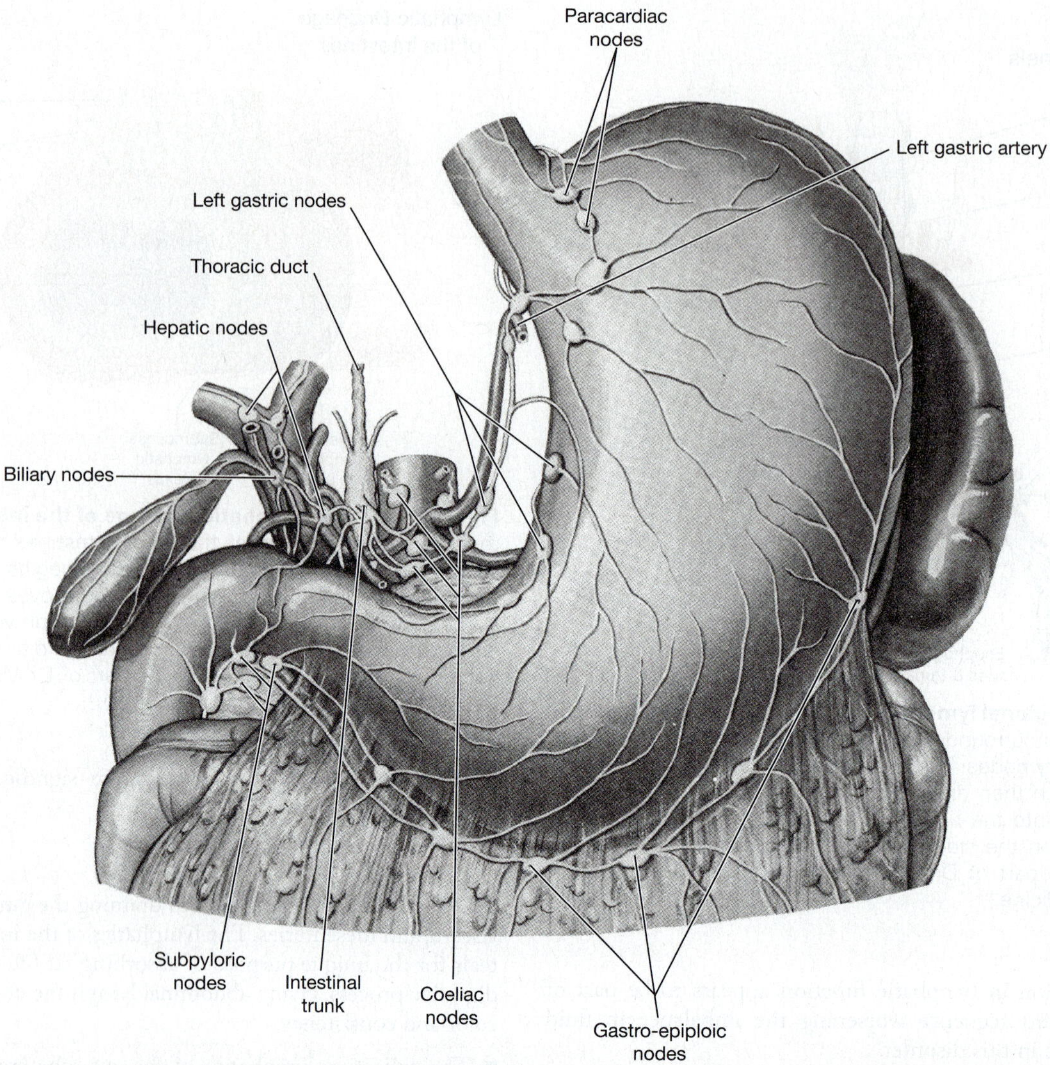

Figure 14.16. Regional lymphatic drainage of the celiac area. Lymphatic trunks are seen coursing parallel to the vascular system eventually reaching the area of the celiac artery where these lymphatic vessels drain into celiac preaortic nodes. Here they mix with lymphatics from the liver and biliary tree. Ultimately, celiac drainage is into the thoracic duct, often by passing through the cisterna chyli. (Used with permission of Springer Nature BV from Yoffey JM. Cardiovascular system. In: Hamilton WJ, ed. *Textbook of Human Anatomy*. 2nd rev. ed. Palgrave Macmillan; 1982:286; permission conveyed through Copyright Clearance Center, Inc.)

promontory (Fig. 14.20). A typical example of this organization is seen with the urinary bladder.

- The anterior and superior portions of the bladder drain superiorly to the hypogastric nodes.
  - The middle of the bladder drains superiorly to the external iliac trunks.
  - The posterior and inferior portion of the bladder have drainage routes that pass posteriorly and superiorly to the common iliac trunks.

In males, lymphatic vessels drain the external and internal reproductive organs in several different directions.[41]

- From the shaft of the penis, lymph drains into the deep inguinal nodes, the nodes of the femoral canal, and the external iliac nodes (Fig. 14.21).
- From the vas deferens, lymph flows superiorly to the external iliac nodes and inferiorly to the hypogastric nodes in the pelvic basin (Fig. 14.22).
- From the prostate gland, lymph radiates superiorly to the external iliac and common iliac nodes as well as inferior and posterior to pass around the rectum and up the sacrum to the lumbar para-aortic nodes.
- In its course, prostatic lymph anastomoses with that of the bladder, vas deferens, and rectum.

In females, lymphatic drainage from the pelvis and perineum also passes through several divergent channels to reach the para-aortic nodes.[41]

- From the perineum and external genitalia, lymphatic drainage is lateral to the superficial and deep inguinal nodes with some drainage anastomosing across the midline anterior to the labia (Fig. 14.23).
- From the ovary, a rich plexus ascends along the suspensory ligament to reach the lumbar para-aortic nodes (Fig. 14.24).
- From the fallopian tubes, lymph flows either superiorly along the lymphatic vessels of the suspensory ligament of the ovary or inward to the uterine lymphatic vessels.

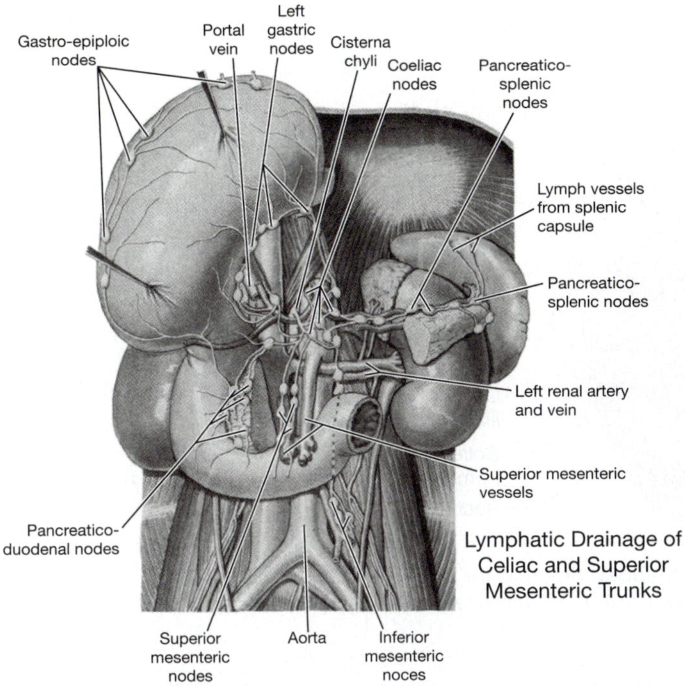

Figure 14.17. Regional lymphatic drainage of the superior mesenteric nodes. Celiac and superior mesenteric nodes drain into preaortic nodes and then into the thoracic duct, typically by passing through the cisterna chyli. (Used with permission of Springer Nature BV from Yoffey JM. Cardiovascular system. In: Hamilton WJ, ed. *Textbook of Human Anatomy*. 2nd rev. ed. Palgrave Macmillan; 1982:287; permission conveyed through Copyright Clearance Center, Inc.)

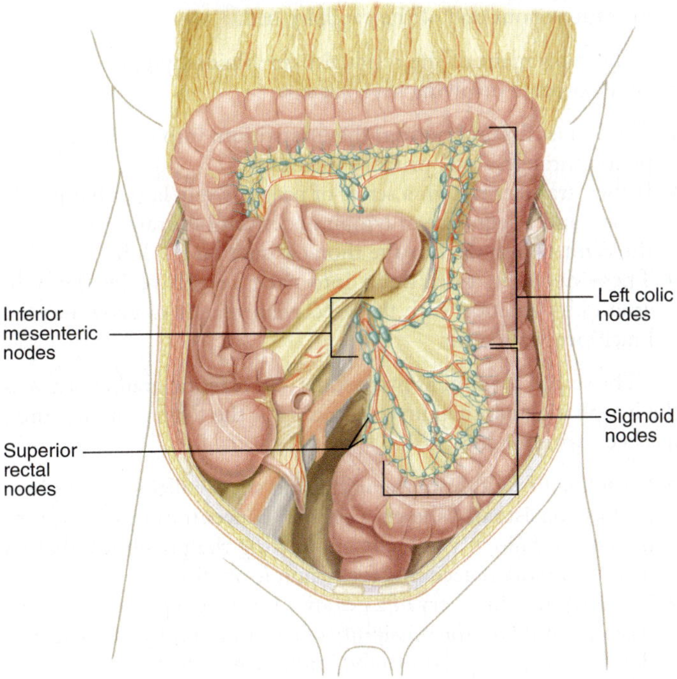

Figure 14.18. Regional lymphatic drainage of the large bowel. Afferent lymph vessels leave the bowel wall and course into mesenteric lymph nodes. Proximal to the splenic flexure, the drainage leads into the superior mesenteric nodes and trunk while distal to the splenic flexure drainage is into the inferior mesenteric nodes and trunk. (Reprinted with permission from Pansky B, Gest TR. *Lippincott Concise Illustrated Anatomy*. Wolters Kluwer Health/Lippincott Williams & Wilkins; 2013. Figure 2-47B.)

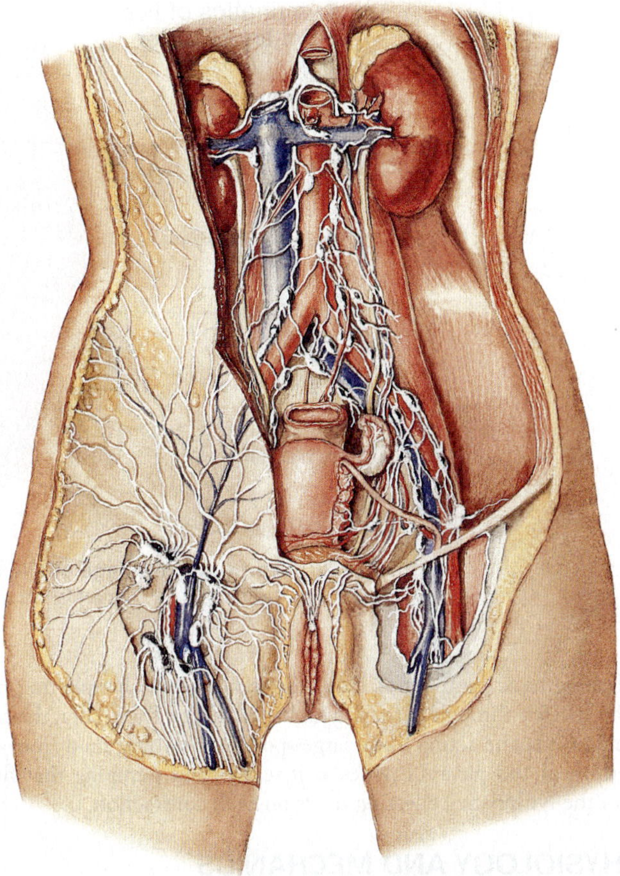

Figure 14.19. Regional lymphatic drainage from the posterior body wall. Iliac lymph nodes drain into the right and left lumbar trunk nodes (also termed para-aortic nodes). Drainage along the aorta enters the cisterna chyli seen as a sac lying to the right of the aorta as this vessel enters the crura of the diaphragm. (From Anatomical Chart Company. Lymphatic System Anatomical Chart. Lippincott Williams & Wilkins; 2001.)

- A complex plexus of lymphatic vessels exists in the uterus (Fig. 14.25) with drainage over three routes: (a) superiorly along the suspensory ligament of the ovary, (b) laterally toward the iliac nodes, and (c) a small set of vessels following the round ligament to reach the superficial inguinal nodes.
- Superficial and deep plexuses of lymphatic channels are found in the wall of the vagina (Fig. 14.26). Drainage from the upper region is into the cervical and uterine system, from the middle portion into the hypogastric nodes, and from the inferior portion into the perineum and inguinal nodes.

Peritoneal and Pleural Fluid

Diaphragmatic stomata have been discovered on the inferior and, to a lesser degree, the superior surfaces of the diaphragm that are open to the peritoneal and pleural cavities, respectively.[73–75]

- These stomata are believed to act as "prelymphatics," connecting to the diaphragmatic lymphatic channels and represent a major pathway for the drainage of peritoneal and pleural fluid.

Of radiolabeled tracer absorbed out of the abdomen of a sheep, 42% returned into circulation via the diaphragm and the remainder passed through other routes that include the organ walls and somatic body wall.[76] Another study[77] found three routes for the removal of radiolabeled tracer from the peritoneum: 55% passed through the

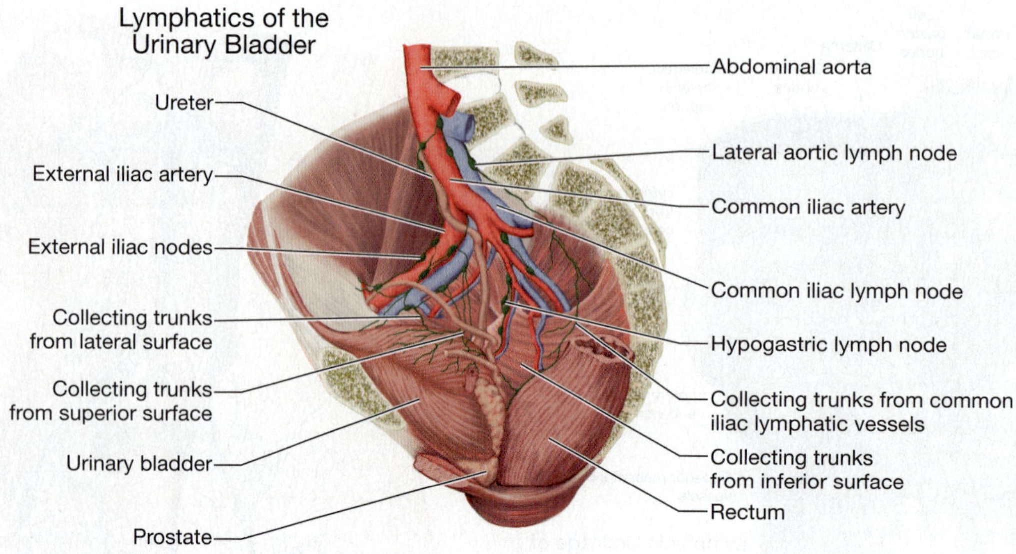

Figure 14.20. Lymphatic drainage of the urinary bladder. See text for an explanation. (Courtesy of Oran Z. Suta, as part of Dr. Willard's lab at the UNE College of Osteopathic Medicine.)

diaphragmatic lymphatics, 30% through visceral lymphatics, and 10% to 15% through parietal lymphatics. Given these data, the diaphragm may be acting like a large sponge, absorbing fluid from the peritoneal and pleural cavities as it relaxes and pumping that fluid into the lymphatic collecting ducts on each contraction.

PHYSIOLOGY AND MECHANICS OF LYMPH FLOW

Lymph formation involves the movement of fluid across a permeable membrane typically in a capillary bed.

- Fluids move in the direction determined by the sum of the hydrostatic and osmotic gradients across the membrane (see Fig. 14.1).

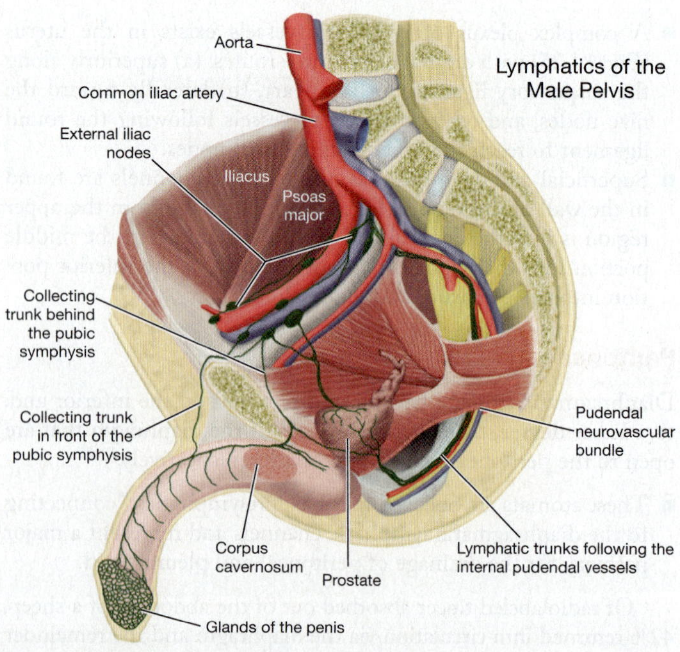

Figure 14.21. Lymphatic drainage of the male erectile tissue. See text for an explanation. (Courtesy of Oran Z. Suta, as part of Dr. Willard's lab at the UNE College of Osteopathic Medicine.)

- Capillaries generally have a hydrostatic gradient that moves fluid out at their arterial end.
- Although traditional thinking described an osmotic gradient that returned fluid to the capillary at the venous end (Box 14.1) this concept has been recently significantly revised.[3,15]
- Due to a thin layer between the glycocalyx and the capillary cell membrane that remains relatively free of macromolecules, the oncotic pressures never reach a level that will draw fluid back into the venous end of the capillary bed.[78]

The movement of the residual tissue fluids (lymph) is a fairly complex process involving several steps.

- Fluid must first move from the interstitium into the initial lymphatic through small primary valves.
- It then travels through a series of progressively larger lymphatic vessels and a sequence of lymph nodes until it drains into either the right lymph duct or the thoracic duct on the left.
- These ducts, in turn, drain into their respective jugular vein around its junction with the subclavian vein or directly into the brachiocephalic vein.

The search for similar hydrostatic and osmotic gradients across the lymphatic endothelium to account for the formation of lymph has been without success.

- Sampling of fluid from the initial and small collecting lymphatics has consistently shown a protein concentration identical to interstitial fluid,[79,80] virtually eliminating the possibility that an osmotic gradient accounts for lymph formation.[22]
- Similarly, the discovery of a negative interstitial pressure in most tissues eliminates the possibility of a continuous hydrostatic gradient from the capillary to the initial lymphatic.[22,81]
- Although a negative pressure has also been found in the initial lymphatic, there appears to be a small uphill gradient between the interstitium and the lymphatics.[22]
- Without a net osmotic or hydrostatic gradient to account for the formation of lymph, one is naturally led to consider mechanical forces.
- The anatomical design of the initial lymphatic vessel allows it to respond to a variety of forces in its environment.

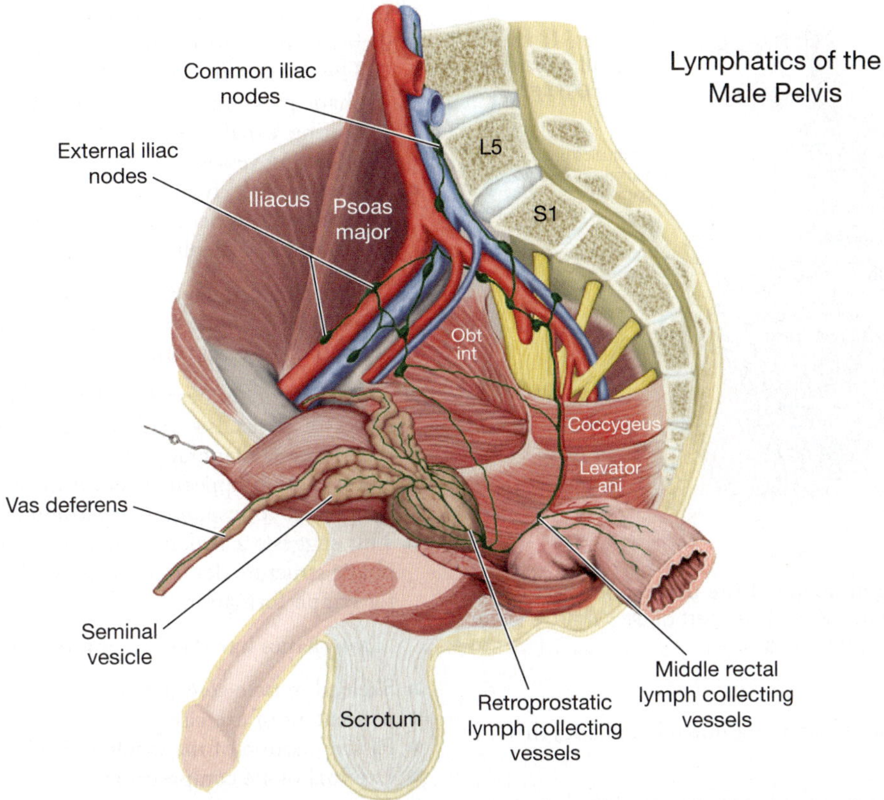

Figure 14.22. Lymphatic drainage of the male internal organ of reproduction. See text for an explanation. (Courtesy of Oran Z. Suta, as part of Dr. Willard's lab at the UNE College of Osteopathic Medicine.)

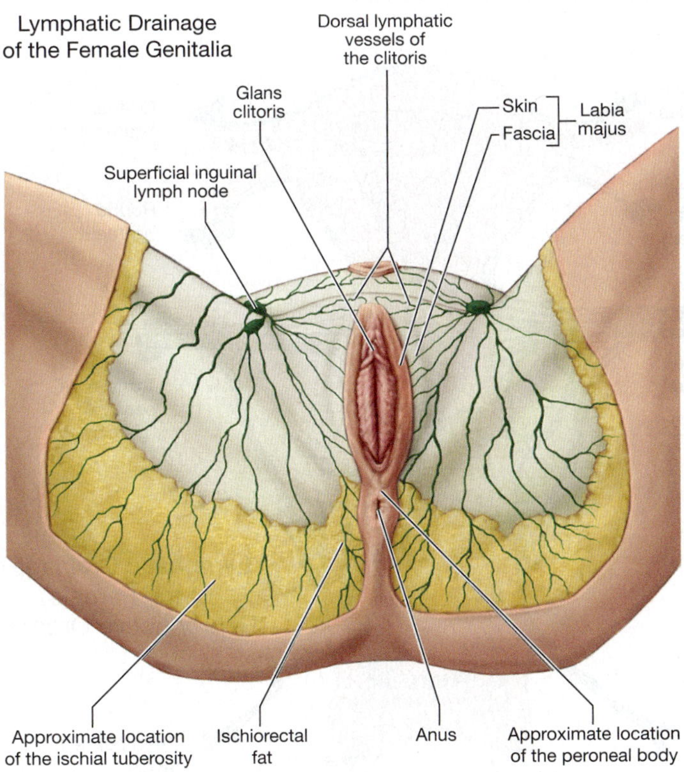

Figure 14.23. Lymphatic drainage of the female perineum. See text for an explanation. (Courtesy of Oran Z. Suta, as part of Dr. Willard's lab at the UNE College of Osteopathic Medicine.)

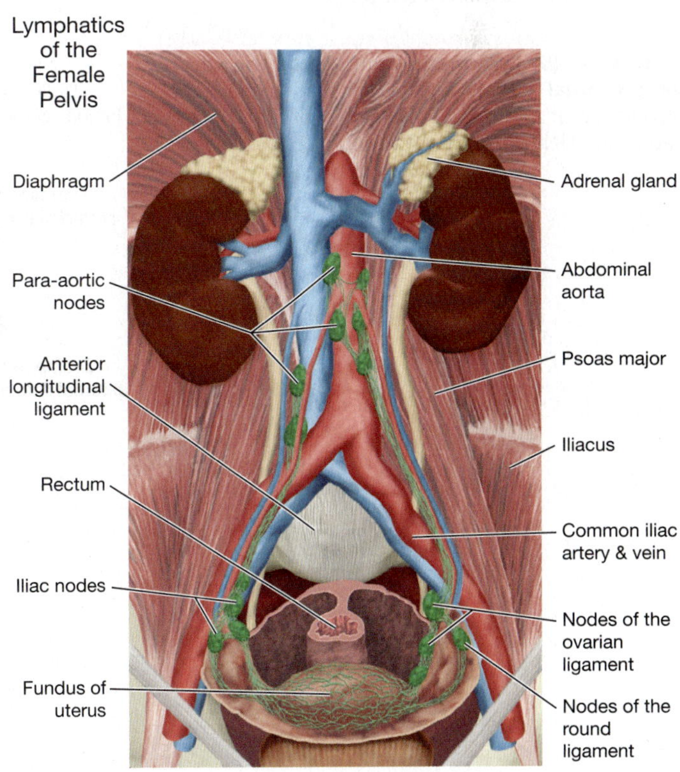

Figure 14.24. Lymphatic drainage of the female pelvic basin. See text for an explanation. (Courtesy of Oran Z. Suta, as part of Dr. Willard's lab at the UNE College of Osteopathic Medicine.)

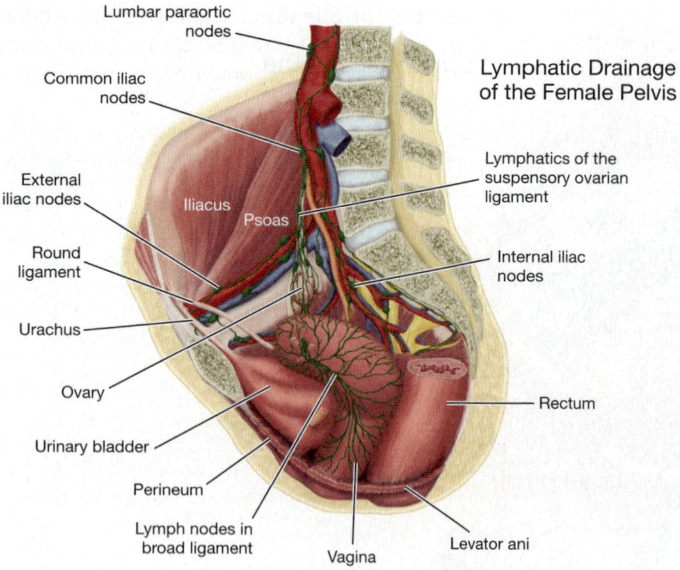

Figure 14.25. Lymphatic drainage of the uterus. See text for an explanation. (Courtesy of Oran Z. Suta, as part of Dr. Willard's lab at the UNE College of Osteopathic Medicine.)

There are two anatomical features of initial lymphatics that are crucial in this regard.

- The anchoring filaments that tether the outside of the lymphatic endothelial cells to the collagen of the interstitium cause the vessel to change shape and volume in response to tissue movement.
  - □ Alternating movements create alternating volume changes in the initial lymphatic.
  - □ These produce intermittent pressure gradients that move fluid into the initial lymphatic.
- In the lung, movements of inhalation and exhalation alternately increase and decrease intralymphatic volume.
  - □ The increased volume during inhalation lowers intralymphatic pressure and produces a gradient for the influx of fluid.
  - □ During exhalation, the fluid is propelled forward into the collecting vessel.
- In the intestine, lymphatics lie between layers of muscle where they respond to peristalsis as well as the movement of the thoracoabdominal diaphragm during breathing.

Interestingly, the resting position of the abdominal lymphatics appears to be an open position, that is, anchoring filaments hold the endothelial cells apart.

- This position is best suited for response to the compressive forces of peristalsis and the inferior movement of the thoracoabdominal diaphragm.[6,68]
- The situation appears reversed in the lungs, which allows the lymphatics to respond to expansion during exhalation.
- This suggests a structure/function relationship, where the lymphatic structure develops to best utilize the local forces available for lymph formation.

Lymphatics have been shown to respond to a variety of forces:

- Skeletal muscle contraction[82]
- Movement of exercise[83]
- Passive motion of the extremities[26,84,85]
- External tissue compression[86]
- Arterial pulse
- Arteriolar vasomotion[87]

Lymphatics are oriented in tissue to maximize their exposure to the various external forces in their environment.

- Many lymphatics closely follow the arterial system, where they can respond to the pulse and vasomotion.

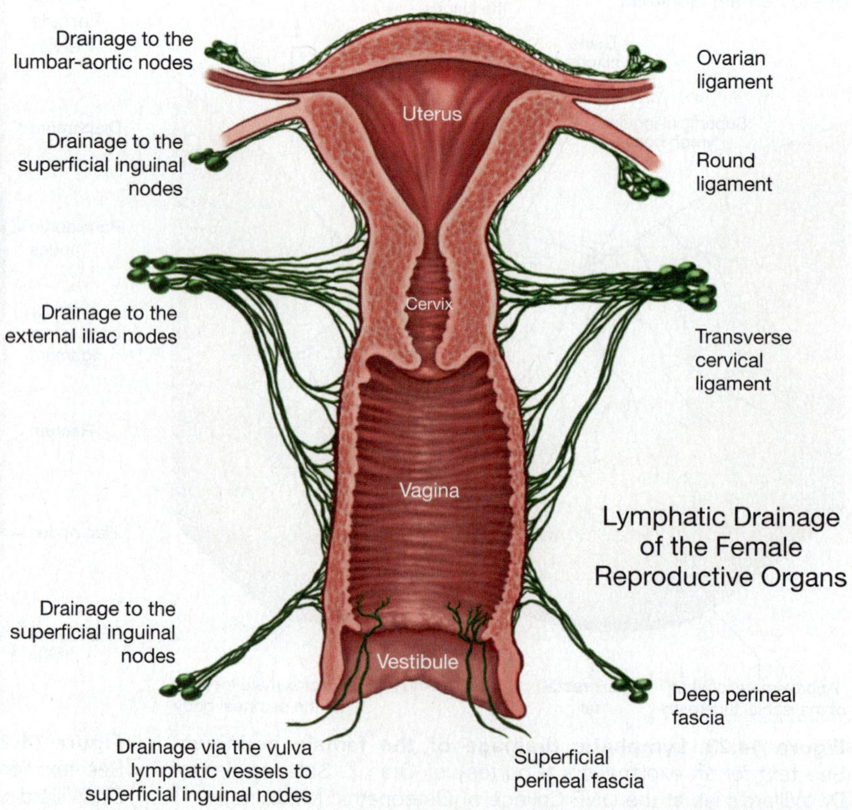

Figure 14.26. Lymphatic drainage of the cervix and vaginal canal. See text for an explanation. (Courtesy of Oran Z. Suta, as part of Dr. Willard's lab at the UNE College of Osteopathic Medicine.)

- Those in muscle are situated between layers, where they are effectively compressed. Although the forces that form lymph are varied, all involve movements that alternately expand and compress the initial lymphatics, creating oscillatory, dynamic pressure gradients between the interstitium and the initial lymphatic.

At the terminal lymphatic, passive motions could play an important role in loading the vessel with extracellular fluids.[12]

- Alternating passive movements could not effectively form lymph if bidirectional flow across the lymphatic endothelium were possible.
- This is prevented by the overlapping endothelial cells in the initial lymphatic.
- These cells form a valve mechanism that allows the movement of fluid into the initial lymphatic but prevents movement out.[9]
- Coupled with the anchoring filaments, this allows the lymphatic to utilize alternating tissue motion to create unidirectional movement of fluid from the interstitium into the lymph system.
  - This feature also allows the initial lymphatic to respond to fluctuations of fluid in the interstitium.
  - A fluid pulse creates a pressure wave in the interstitial fluid.
    - As the pulse approaches the lymphatic, a gradient is produced that opens the endothelial cells and permits fluid to enter.
    - After the pulse crosses, the cells close preventing backflow out of the lymphatic.
- Arteriolar vasomotion appears to create a fluctuant displacement of interstitial fluid, which may influence lymph movement.[87]
  - Fluid fluctuation may account for the movement and exchange of fluid within the interstitium.
  - Capillary hydrostatic gradients dissipate quickly and do not account for the movement of fluid within the interstitial spaces.[22]
- After moving into the initial lymphatic, fluid is propelled through the collecting channels.
  - These channels contain bicuspid valves that ensure unidirectional flow of lymph.
- An intrinsic myogenic pump has been identified that accounts for significant lymph propulsion.
  - This pump consists of smooth muscle in the wall of the lymph vessel and the valves.
- Lymphatic smooth muscle exhibits spontaneous contractions that are peristaltic, traveling distal to proximal at a rate of 4 to 5 mm/s.[88]
  - Evidence suggests that the contraction wave migrates retrogradely along the lymphatic vessels.[89]
    - A pacemaker initiates the spontaneous contractions.[37,88,90–93]
      - The pacemakers are situated in the wall of the lymphatic vessel between the endothelial cell layer and the surrounding smooth muscle; they begin just beyond the first valve.[88,94]
      - The impulses are then coupled to the smooth muscle along the vessel in order to propagate a wave of contraction, producing a peristaltic action.
        - Hogan proposed a mechanical coupling, based on the finding of stretch receptors in the lymphatic wall distal to the valve that initiated a smooth muscle contraction of the lymphangion.[95]
      - The initial pacemaker, located just proximal to the first valve near the initial lymphatic capillary, is also responsive to vessel distention and is stimulated by the distension created by lymph formation.
        - The contraction of this distal segment propels fluid beyond the valve where stretch receptors continue to stimulate smooth muscle contraction, and the peristaltic wave is propagated.
          - In this model then, lymph propulsion is dependent on filling of the terminal lymphatic, or lymph formation.

More recent studies have demonstrated electrical coupling of smooth muscle cells most likely mediated by calcium.[96]

- This, combined with a spontaneously contracting pacemaker, would allow a completely independent, electrically coupled peristaltic wave.
- Zawieja and colleagues[97] found both upstream and downstream propagation of the contractions, supporting the idea of electrical coupling, since a volume-dependent mechanism should only propagate contraction centrally.

Crowe's study[98] suggests that both electrical and mechanical coupling contribute to the propagation and coordination of the intrinsic lymph pump.

- They found that without a minimum amount of filling, no contractions occurred.
- They also found that, in more than half of the specimens studied, the contractions were preceded by a transient dilatation of the vessel and that the propagation of the wave occurred relatively slowly, consistent with mechanical coupling.
- A minority of lymph specimens[9,22] demonstrated characteristics of electrical coupling, bidirectional propagation at a more rapid speed.
- Crowe's group also found that perfusion-induced contractile activity was present in most lymphangions, regardless of how the contraction was propagated, and that the contraction frequency was dependent on the rate of perfusion.
- Lymph formation then appears to be capable of initiating propulsion in some cases and significantly modifying it in others.

Currently, there continues to be debate as to the relative importance of these two mechanisms in the functioning of the intrinsic lymph pump, but little debate about the relative importance of this pumping mechanism in the propulsion of lymph through the lymph vessel.[12,99,100]

- Ohhashi gives evidence of two separate pacemaker mechanisms, one near the valve that responds to filling, and one near the middle of the lymphangion that responds to adrenergic stimulation, which may represent the source of the electrical pacemaker.

Lymph propulsion is also modified by a variety of other factors:

- Lymphatic smooth muscle responds to both adrenergic and humoral influences.
- Adrenergic stimulation has been shown to increase contractility and stroke volume of lymphatic smooth muscle.[99]
- Humoral influences are important in lymph propulsion during inflammation.
- An experimentally induced inflammatory process caused an increase in the stroke volume of the lymphatic vessels and an increase in lymph drainage.[101]
- Endotoxin, on the other hand, has a strong negative effect on lymph pumping and may explain some of the hemodynamic consequences of septic shock.[102]

- In vitro, IL-1 and prostaglandin E_1 reduced lymph contractile activity.[103]
- Bradykinin, PGH_2, and NO increased lymph,[104–106] as did substance P.[107]
- Neurogenic and humoral influences appear less important in the myogenic pump than volumetric displacements.[22]

The effect of external forces of lymph propulsion is somewhat controversial.

- Lymphatic vessels lack anchoring filaments that would allow them to respond to the various forces that form lymph.
- The anatomical design of a thin-walled vessel with valves is consistent with propulsion from external compression.
- This is supported by the finding that lymphatics in the intestine and skeletal muscle have an absence of smooth muscle for a much greater distance from their origin than those from other tissues,[68] presumably because compression from muscle contraction provides the necessary propulsive forces.

Most studies on the effect of external forces on lymph flow do not distinguish the effect of these forces on lymph formation and propulsion. A study by McGeown and colleagues[86,108] attempted to distinguish the effects of external compression on lymph formation versus propulsion.

- They created an inflammatory process on the hoof of a sheep, and then applied compressive forces to the hoof, directly over the area of lymph formation, and compared that to compression over the metatarsal area, where the larger collecting vessels are found.
- The study demonstrated a fourfold increase in flow when the forces were applied to the hoof, the area of lymph formation, and virtually no change when applied to the metatarsal area, where the collecting vessels were found.
- Although this study by itself does not exclude the possibility that external forces contribute to the propulsion of lymph, it provides compelling evidence that external forces are most effective in promoting formation of lymph.

A further study demonstrated that the ability of external pressure to increase lymph flow was both rate and amplitude dependent.[108]

- This carries significant clinical implications for osteopathic approaches to lymph drainage and should be considered in the design of osteopathic treatment plans to promote lymph drainage, especially those using "lymphatic pump" techniques.

Since lymph formation has been shown to initiate and/or strongly increase lymph propulsion, treatment to enhance lymph formation may increase lymph drainage in a number of important ways.

- Postnodal lymph continues to move centrally, eventually draining into the right lymphatic duct or left thoracic duct before reentering the venous circulation at the subclavian vein.
- The smooth muscle in the thoracic duct exhibits spontaneous contractions similar to other lymphatic smooth muscle.[38]
- Respiration has been shown to have a consistent effect on the flow and pressures within the thoracic duct.[109]
  - Although these studies do not exclude the effect of respiration on the formation of lymph in the thorax and abdomen, and its contribution to thoracic duct flow, pressure changes associated with respiration are considered important in central lymph flow.[22]

Osteopathic treatment has been directed toward improving lymph drainage since the time of A.T. Still. Early writing by Millard focused on removing obstruction to the flow of lymph by treating somatic dysfunction along the course of fluid return.[110] Although this concept has not been studied experimentally, it stands to reason that tissue strain in the area of lymph vessels will increase the resistance to lymph flow through those vessels. Earlier descriptions of lymph drainage pathways attempted to identify areas where compression might be likely. Experimentally increasing resistance to lymph flow has reduced lymph flow in distal lymphatics.[22]

Lymph pump techniques (Box 14.2), directed at actually moving lymph, have also been part of the osteopathic approach to the lymphatic system. McGeown's studies about the effects of external compression[86,108] and the discovery of the intrinsic peristaltic contractions of lymphatic smooth muscle responsible for a considerable proportion of lymph propulsion (reviewed in Bridenbaugh et al.[111]) suggest that specific treatment to pump lymph should be directed toward lymph formation at the site of inflammation or lymphedema. Stimulation of the myogenic pacemaker by increasing lymph formation may also increase lymph propulsion. More recent studies on the movement of lymph in the thoracic duct following the application of a lymphatic pump technique have suggested that these procedures can increase the drainage of lymphatic fluid from peripheral tissue.[112]

BOX 14.2 Lymph Movement and Osteopathic Manipulative Medicine

Osteopathic medicine has used osteopathic manipulative treatment (OMT) in an effort to improve fluid movement and lymphatic drainage from tissue for well over a hundred years. Provocative experimental evidence has been reported providing support for the use of these techniques. Using experimental paradigms in rats, dogs, and rabbits, Hodge and colleagues applied lymphatic pump techniques and monitored lymph flow in the thoracic duct and in the cisterna chyli. Results demonstrated a significant increase in the flow of lymph in the duct secondary to the application of the OMT. In addition, specific features of the lymphocytes in circulation were also examined. In this process, it was possible to show an increased outflow of lymphocytes directly from the gut-associated lymphatic tissue (GALT) when the lymphatic pump techniques were applied to the abdomen.

Creasy C, Schander A, Orlowski A, Hodge LM. Thoracic and abdominal lymphatic pump techniques inhibit the growth of *S. pneumoniae* bacteria in the lungs of rats. *Lymphat Res Biol.* 2013;11(3):183–186; Hodge LM, Bearden MK, Schander A, et al. Lymphatic pump treatment mobilizes leukocytes from the gut associated lymphoid tissue into lymph. *Lymphat Res Biol.* 2010;8(2):103–110; Hodge LM, Creasy C, Carter K, Orlowski A, Schander A, King HH. Lymphatic pump treatment as an adjunct to antibiotics for pneumonia in a rat model. *J Am Osteopath Assoc.* 2015;115(5):306–316; Huff JB, Schander A, Downey HF, Hodge LM. Lymphatic pump treatment augments lymphatic flux of lymphocytes in rats. *Lymphat Res Biol.* 2010;8(4):183–187; Schander A, Padro D, King HH, Downey HF, Hodge LM. Lymphatic pump treatment repeatedly enhances the lymphatic and immune systems. *Lymphat Res Biol.* 2013;11(4):219–226.

THE LYMPHATIC SYSTEM AND INFLAMMATION

Inflammation is the generalized response of the body to injury or infection.

- It is a hallmark of most acute illnesses.
- Inflammation is perhaps most accurately viewed as part of a process by which the body defends against injury or infection and repairs the injured tissue.
- This process involves the vascular system, the immune system, and the nervous system, as well as the surrounding connective tissues.
- Numerous chemical mediators, produced locally and systemically, communicate between the cells of these three systems to affect the progression of inflammation and healing.
- Continuous production and removal of these inflammatory mediators is essential for smooth and efficient progression and resolution of inflammation and healing.
- Delay in the removal of inflammatory mediators and exudates early in the process may result in prolonged inflammation with poor or delayed healing.
- Delayed removal of mediators later in the process may lead to a prolonged healing process, eventually leading to adhesions and/or fibrosis.
- The tissue drainage provided by the lymphatics offers an escape route for many of these mediators, as well as the inflammatory exudate, and plays a role in virtually every aspect of the inflammatory process.
- Understanding the factors that influence lymph formation and its removal from tissue is critical to the osteopathic diagnosis and treatment of any patient with an acute or chronic inflammatory process.

Vasodilatation and increased capillary permeability occur early in the inflammatory process and together are responsible for the tremendous influx of fluid and plasma protein into the interstitium of the inflamed tissue.

- This leaves a preponderance of red blood cells in the intravascular space, greatly increasing its viscosity and potentially creating stasis of venules and capillary beds.[113]
- The lymphatic system, therefore, becomes responsible for virtually all fluid drainage from inflamed tissues.
- The rate of blood supply, and the delivery of antibodies, centrally produced mediators, medications, and the oxygen and nutrients necessary to fuel cellular activities will be limited, or even determined, by the rate of lymph flow.

Normal venous drainage will be restored when capillary permeability returns to normal and the osmotic gradient between the interstitium and the vascular system permits sufficient fluid return to reduce the viscosity of capillary blood.

- Capillary permeability is controlled by a variety of endogenous vasoactive mediators, including the following:
  - ☐ Histamine
  - ☐ Bradykinin
  - ☐ Prostaglandin E

Although these mediators can be inactivated locally, there is evidence that lymph drainage also provides a means by which they are removed and/or inactivated.

- Adequate pulmonary lymphatic drainage is required for the resolution of an experimental model of adult respiratory distress syndrome.[114]
- Bradykinin has been shown to be inactivated systemically by plasma.[115]
- Histaminase, responsible for 30% of histamine breakdown, has been identified in high levels in the thoracic duct.[116]
- Prostaglandin E has been identified in the lymph effluent draining from inflamed tissues.[113]

The relative importance of tissue drainage and other mechanisms in the inactivation of these mediators has not been fully elucidated.

- The osmotic pressure in the interstitium will change when proteins and other osmotically active particles are removed.
- Extravasated protein and large particulates cannot return via the venous system, even when capillary permeability is maximally increased,[115] nor is there any evidence that protein is catabolized in the interstitium.[22]
- It is therefore evident that the removal of protein from tissue depends heavily on the lymphatic drainage of the tissues.
- Recent evidence demonstrates that pulmonary lymphatic drainage is required for the resolution of inflammation in adult respiratory distress syndrome.[114]

Inflammation generates both local and central immune responses.

- Locally, chemotactic mediators draw neutrophils and monocytes to the area.
- Neutrophils release lysosomal enzymes into the interstitium that can kill bacteria but can also be destructive to local tissues.
- They are responsible for much of the tissue damage that accompanies acute and chronic inflammatory processes (Box 14.3).
- The tissue damage created by neutrophilic lysosomes can be similar to that caused by pancreatic enzymes.

As the inflammation progresses, the polymorphonuclear leukocytes (also termed PMNs) undergo apoptosis and the remains are ingested by macrophages in a manner that does not release lysosomal enzymes or provoke proinflammatory responses.[117]

- If the PMNs are not phagocytized, they eventually undergo secondary necrosis, releasing their damaging lysozymes into the tissue.
- The ingesting macrophages must then either be removed from the tissue or undergo apoptosis themselves.
- Bellingan et al.[118] found that most macrophages are removed from inflamed tissue via lymphatic drainage. This implies that lymph drainage is an important aspect in the resolution of the inflammatory process.

Lymph drainage has been shown to dramatically reduce the tissue-damaging effects of pancreatic enzymes with obstruction of the main pancreatic duct in dogs.[119]

- Neutrophilic lysosomes have been identified in lymph draining from inflamed tissues.[113]
- Drainage of these enzymes may be important in limiting their destructive effects on tissues.

Central immune responses involve stimulation of T cells and B cells by antigen in lymph nodes and other lymph organs.

- Delivery of antigen to these lymphoid organs occurs entirely by lymphatic drainage of antigen and antigen-containing macrophages from the site of injury.
- Weakening of antigenic stimulation has been demonstrated in chronic lymph stasis and lymphedema.[119]
- Conversely, the B-cell response to immunization in medical students was increased by manipulating the rate of lymph drainage using the lymphatic pump technique.[120]

BOX 14.3 Neutrophilic Extracellular Traps (NETs)

Neutrophils are the most common of the granulocytes, having a life span of 24 to 48 hours and terminating their existence through a process of apoptosis. They contain three forms of granules (Pawlina, 2016):

1. Azurophilic or primary granules contain myeloperoxidase, acid hydrolases, defensins, and cathelicidin.
2. Specific or secondary granules contain collagenases, gelatinases, phospholipases, complement activators, and antimicrobial peptides.
3. Tertiary granules contain phosphatases or metalloproteinases.

Using these substances, neutrophils have long been described as having two major forms of killing power:

1. Engulfing of microbes, a process termed phagocytosis
2. Secretion of antimicrobials derived from their granules

A third process whereby neutrophils provide antimicrobial protection has been described. Contact with microbes, their cell wall products, or certain cytokines can activate neutrophils resulting in the evagination from the granulocyte of a sticky fibrous net composed of DNA and embedded antimicrobial enzymes (Wartha et al., 2007). This net entraps microorganisms, exposing them to the antimicrobials and attracting macrophages to phagocytose the residual.

As positive as this microbicidal action may seem, it has its downsides as well (Sorensen and Borregaard, 2016). NETs may trigger the formation of autoantibodies initiating or enhancing autoimmune disorders, inflammatory disorders, and cancer.

Pawlina W. *Histology, A Text and Atlas with Correlated Cell and Molecular Biology*. 7th ed. Wolters Kluwer; 2016; Sorensen OE, Borregaard N. Neutrophil extracellular traps—the dark side of neutrophils. *J Clin Invest*. 2016;126(5):1612–1620; Wartha F, Beiter K, Normark S, Henriques-Normark B. Neutrophil extracellular traps: casting the NET over pathogenesis. *Curr Opin Microbiol*. 2007;10(1):52–56.

Systemic responses to inflammation occur in the liver and brain.

- The proinflammatory cytokine interleukin-1 (IL-1) is involved in the stimulation of both of these organs.
- IL-1 stimulates the production of acute-phase reactant proteins from the liver.[113]
  - ☐ IL-1 is produced by monocytes and macrophages locally during an inflammatory process.
  - ☐ Although there are systemic sources of IL-1 production, locally produced IL-1 has been shown to produce fever and stimulate acute-phase protein production.[113]
  - ☐ Locally produced IL-1 gains access to the systemic circulation via lymphatic drainage.
  - ☐ It has also been shown to reach circumventricular organs in the ventricular system of the brain, where it produces fever and stimulates the hypothalamic–pituitary axis.[121]

The lymphatic network of vessels plays a significant role in the removal of proinflammatory compounds from tissue.

- Both prostaglandins and leukotrienes have been found in lymphatic drainage of inflamed tissues.
- There is evidence that lymphatic drainage is involved in the removal and inactivation of bradykinin and histamine.
- A variety of inflammatory mediators can stimulate primary afferent nociceptors,[122] potentially resulting in hyperalgesia of the surrounding tissue. These include the following:
  - ☐ Bradykinin
  - ☐ Prostaglandins
  - ☐ Leukotrienes
  - ☐ IL-1
  - ☐ Histamine
- As these mediators are dissipated, the rate of depolarization of the primary nociceptors will remit, and inflammatory pain will be reduced.

The repair of injured or infected tissue proceeds as the acute inflammatory process resolves.

- Fibroblasts, which lay down the matrix of the scar tissue, are stimulated by the inflammatory exudate, as well as several complement factors and cytokines.
- As the balance between proinflammatory and profibroblast forces shifts, the inflammatory process shifts to the healing phase.
- By continually clearing the interstitium of exudate, including inflammatory mediators, the lymphatics can allow this shift to occur more rapidly and smoothly.
- Should proinflammatory mediators remain in the interstitium, acute inflammation will persist, and healing will be delayed.
- The healing process resolves when the inflammatory exudate is removed, and fibroblast activity decreases.

Persistence of the inflammatory exudate in peripheral tissue will lead to excess local scarring and fibrosis.

- Plasma proteins, when trapped in the interstitium, attract monocytes.
- Platelets, extravasated into the tissue, release growth factors such as epidermal growth factor, platelet-derived growth factor, and transforming growth factor β (TGF-β).
- TGF-β helps in the conversion of monocytes to macrophages.
- These cells also release numerous growth factors including fibroblast growth factor (FGF) and TGF-β, which attract and stimulate fibroblasts, eventually leading to fibrogenesis, which can contribute to tissue repair in the acute state as well as fibrosis of tissue in the chronic state[119]; also see Chapter 7 The Fascial System of the Body for further details.

Repeated experimental injection of plasma into soft tissue produced both chronic inflammation and scar formation.[119]

- The lymphatics are the predominant means by which the inflammatory exudate is removed.
- Thus, lymphatics are intimately involved in the progression and resolution of the healing phase of the inflammatory process.

The process of inflammation and healing is the body's response to injury and infection.

- The lymphatics play a role in every aspect of this process.
- In essence, the lymphatic system is responsible for maintaining an interstitial environment conducive to the rapid, unimpaired progression and resolution of this complex process.

- See Chapter 12 The Role of Inflammation in Healing and Homeostasis for further details.

There are several categories of disease processes, which warrant a focus on the lymphatic system:

1. ***Chronic inflammatory diseases:*** These range from smoldering, subclinical infections such as osteomyelitis to autoimmune and collagen vascular diseases such as rheumatoid arthritis. Although most chronic inflammatory diseases are attributed to persistent inflammatory stimuli, there are suggestions that reduced lymph drainage may play a role.
   - Weak antigenic stimulation of regional lymphocytes was found in experimental lymphedema.[119] This finding was implicated in the susceptibility to infection that often complicates lymphedema. Increased lymph drainage from the site of infection should improve immune response and local circulation.
   - Rheumatoid arthritis is thought to occur as a response to immune complexes. These complexes, and the inflammatory exudate they produce, are removed by lymphatic drainage. The inflammatory exudate is responsible for pain and tissue destruction associated with this disease. Increased lymph production and drainage from ankles affected by rheumatoid arthritis has been demonstrated in humans; in addition, this drainage contained elevated levels of proinflammatory cytokines.[44,123]
2. ***Fibrotic diseases:*** Progressive interstitial fibrosis is a characteristic of chronic lymphedema.
   - The pattern and time course of the fibrosis produced by experimental lymphedema is strikingly similar to a variety of diseases, including cirrhosis, interstitial lung diseases such as silicosis, regional ileitis, and even atherosclerosis.[119] Each of these diseases involves repeated inflammatory events with a progressive build-up of protein-rich tissue fluid, influx of leukocytes, release of proinflammatory cytokines, and fibroblast stimulation, eventually leading to fibrosis.
   - Secondary lymphedema, produced by parasitic infections or, more commonly, iatrogenic means, for example, surgery for breast cancer, results in a cycle of stasis, inflammation and fibrosis.[124] Evidence suggests that chronic inflammatory processes such as the production of the smooth muscle relaxant nitric oxide in the tissue, helps to maintain the lack of adequate lymphatic drainage, playing a sentinel role in this process.
   - Postoperative adhesions, common in abdominal surgeries with peritonitis, or other massive inflammatory processes, may result from inadequate drainage of the abdominal exudates. Similarly, surgeries involving lymph node dissections or disruption of lymphatics, such as a modified radical mastectomy, may result in lymphedema from fibrosis and adhesions.

The use of OMT to promote lymph drainage early in these diseases may help prevent the development of these long-term problems.

LYMPHATIC SYSTEM IN HEALTH AND DISEASE

The removal of interstitial fluids from tissue and the trafficking of the immune cells facilitated by the lymphatic system are necessary for the maintenance of normal homeostasis.[16]

- Slight overproduction of tissue fluids that is not met by fluid removal very quickly results in edema
- Long-term edema results in significant changes in the tissue such as fibrosis
- Evidence now suggests that the lymphatic system may not be an innocent bystander in the long-term changes.
- Dilated lymphatic vessels go through a cycle of increasing mural smooth muscle cells and decreasing luminal diameter reducing flow which eventually culminates in fibrosis and occlusion of the vessel.
- Failures in the developmental sequences involved in forming lymph vessels and valves lead to primary lymphedema.
- Infection or surgical reduction can facilitate the formation of secondary (acquired) lymphedema.

Beyond the formation of primary or secondary edema, the lymphatic system is thought to play a role in the manifestation of other systemic disorders as well.[125]

- Lymph nodes play an essential role in both the containment of foreign antigen as well as the containment of the cells reacting to the foreign antigen, failure of containment can lead to sepsis or disseminated intravascular coagulation (DIC).
- The role of lymphatic vessels in the metastatic spread of tumor cells is still an area of debate. Although evidence supports the growth of specific tumors, in some lymph nodes it does appear that the promotion of lymphangiogenesis and the enhancement of T-cell mediated immunity may represent a powerful method for preventing tumor progression.
- A link between obesity and leaky lymphatic vessels has been demonstrated in mouse models leading to the theory that leakage of chyle is adipogenic. A reverse effect has also been demonstrated in that increasing adiposity fosters inflammation increasing the leakage of chyle from the lymphatic vessels.
- Blood vessels have lymphatic drainage from the tunica adventitia, faulty lymphatic drainage is suspected in contributing to the build-up of cholesterol and formation of atherosclerotic plaques in the vessel wall.
- The human heart has a robust lymphatic network throughout the cardiac wall. Lymphangiogenesis following myocardial infarction is critical to the repair process and the reduction of edema in the cardiac tissue including the reduction in the formation of fibrotic scar tissue.
- Finally, significant drainage of cerebrospinal fluids may be occurring through a network of meningeal lymphatics surrounding the brain, experimental manipulation of these lymphatics suggests that this drainage route plays a role in immune function and could impact the course of protein deposition disorders such as Alzheimer and Parkinson diseases as well as inflammatory diseases such as multiple sclerosis.

SUMMARY

The lymphatic system plays a key role in several areas:

- The removal of extravasated fluid and macromolecules from the interstitium and its return to venous circulation.
- The surveillance of this fluid for foreign antigens and the transport of activated immunocytes throughout the body.
- The transport of dietary lipids from their absorption in the intestine to systemic circulation via the venous system.
- Adequate lymphatic circulation is important in the removal of proinflammatory cells and substances from damaged tissue.

Failure of the lymphatic system leads to the build-up of tissue fluids.

- This edema can be either primary due to failure of the lymphatic vessels or secondary due to acquired damage.
- In addition to edema, failure of the lymphatic system has been related to such diseases as obesity, atherosclerosis, myocardial repair following infarction, and several neurologic diseases.

The vessels of the lymphatic system are endowed with one-way valves and an intrinsic pumping system composed of smooth muscle

- This pumping mechanism is enhanced through internal forces such as skeletal muscle contraction, rhythmical beating to the cardiovascular system, and respiratory motions.
- External forces such as osteopathic manipulative procedures have been demonstrated to assist in the movement of lymphatic fluids.

REFERENCES

1. Aronson D. The interstitial compartment as a therapeutic target in heart failure. *Front Cardiovasc Med.* 2022;9:933384.
2. Reno F, Sabbatini M. Breaking a vicious circle: Lymphangiogenesis as a new therapeutic target in wound healing. *Biomedicines.* 2023;11:656.
3. Mortimer PS, Rockson SG. New developments in clinical aspects of lymphatic disease. *J Clin Invest.* 2014;124:915–921.
4. Clemente CD. *Gray's Anatomy of the Human Body.* Lea & Febiger; 1985.
5. Pawlina W. *Histology: A Text with Atlas: With Correlated Cell and Molecular Biology.* Lippincott Williams & Wilkins; 2021.
6. Schmid-Schönbein GW. Microlymphatics and lymph flow. *Physiol Rev.* 1990;70:987–1028.
7. Breslin JW. Mechanical forces and lymphatic transport. *Microvasc Res.* 2014;96:46–54.
8. Mendoza E, Schmid-Schönbein GW. A model for mechanics of primary lymphatic valves. *J Biomech Eng.* 2003;125:407–414.
9. Schmid-Schönbein GW. The second valve system in lymphatics. *Lymphat Res Biol.* 2003;1:25–29.
10. Trzewik J, Mallipattu SK, Artmann GM, Delano FA, Schmid-Schönbein GW. Evidence for a second valve system in lymphatics: endothelial microvalves. *FASEB J.* 2001;15:1711–1717.
11. Murfee WL, Rappleye JW, Ceballos M, Schmid-Schönbein GW. Discontinuous expression of endothelial cell adhesion molecules along initial lymphatic vessels in mesentery: the primary valve structure. *Lymphat Res Biol.* 2007;5:81–89.
12. Witte MH, Jones K, Wilting J, et al. Structure function relationships in the lymphatic system and implications for cancer biology. *Cancer Metastasis Rev.* 2006;25:159–184.
13. Levick JR, Michel CC. Microvascular fluid exchange and the revised Starling principle. *Cardiovasc Res.* 2010;87:198–210.
14. Levick JR. Revision of the Starling principle: new views of tissue fluid balance. *J Physiol.* 2004;557:704.
15. Woodcock TE, Woodcock TM. Revised Starling equation and the glycocalyx model of transvascular fluid exchange: an improved paradigm for prescribing intravenous fluid therapy. *Br J Anaesth.* 2012;108:384–394.
16. Weber E, Agliano M, Bertelli E, Gabriele G, Gennaro P, Barone V. Lymphatic collecting vessels in health and disease: a review of histopathological modifications in lymphedema. *Lymphat Res Biol.* 2022;20:468–477.
17. Gashev AA. Physiologic aspects of lymphatic contractile function: current perspectives. *Ann N Y Acad Sci.* 2002;979:178–187; discussion 188–196.
18. Roozendaal R, Mebius RE, Kraal G. The conduit system of the lymph node. *Int Immunol.* 2008;20:1483–1487.
19. Adair TH, Moffatt DS, Paulsen AW, Guyton AC. Quantitation of changes in lymph protein concentration during lymph node transit. *Am J Physiol.* 1982;243:H351–H359.
20. Ohtani O, Ohtani Y. Structure and function of rat lymph nodes. *Arch Histol Cytol.* 2008;71:69–76.
21. Adair TH, Guyton AC. Modification of lymph by lymph nodes. II. Effect of increased lymph node venous blood pressure. *Am J Physiol.* 1983;245:H616–H622.
22. Aukland K, Reed RK. Interstitial-lymphatic mechanisms in the control of extracellular fluid volume. *Physiol Rev.* 1993;73:1–78.
23. Alessandrini C, Gerli R, Sacchi G, Ibba L, Pucci AM, Fruschelli C. Cholinergic and adrenergic innervation of mesenterial lymph vessels in guinea pig. *Lymphology.* 1981;14:1–6.
24. McHale NG. Lymphatic innervation. *Blood-Vessels.* 1990;27:127–136.
25. Thornbury KD, McHale NG, McGeown JG. Alpha-and beta-components of the popliteal efferent lymph flow response to intra-arterial catecholamine infusions in the sheep. *Blood Vessels.* 1989;26:107–118.
26. Ikomi E, Zweifach BW, Schmid-Schönbein GW. Fluid pressures in the rabbit popliteal afferent lymphatics during passive tissue motion. *Lymphology.* 1997;30:13–23.
27. Benoit JN. Effects of alpha-adrenergic stimuli on mesenteric collecting lymphatics in the rat. *Am J Physiol.* 1997;273:R331–R336.
28. McGeown JG, McHale NG, Thornbury KD. The effect of electrical stimulation of the sympathetic chain on peripheral lymph flow in the anaesthetized sheep. *J Physiol.* 1987;393:123–133.
29. Thornbury KD, Harty HR, McGeown JG, McHale NG. Mesenteric lymph flow responses to splanchnic nerve stimulation in sheep. *Am J Physiol.* 1993;264:H604–H610.
30. Hollywood MA, McHale NG. Mediation of excitatory neurotransmission by the release of ATP and noradrenaline in sheep mesenteric lymphatic vessels. *J Physiol.* 1994;481:415–423.
31. Hukkanen M, Konttinen YT, Rees RG, Gibson SJ, Santavirta S, Polak JM. Innervation of bone from healthy and arthritic rats by substance P and calcitonin gene related peptide containing sensory fibers. *J Rheumatol.* 1992;19:1252–1259.
32. Nance DM, Burns J, Klein CM, Burden HW. Afferent fibers in the reproductive system and pelvic viscera of female rats: anterograde tracing and immunocytochemical studies. *Brain Res Bull.* 1988;21:701–709.
33. Felten DL, Livnat S, Felten SY, Bellinger DL, Yeh P. Sympathetic innervation of lymph nodes in mice. *Brain Res Bull.* 1984;13:693–699.
34. McGeown JG. Splanchnic nerve stimulation increases the lymphocyte output in mesenteric efferent lymph. *Pflugers Arch.* 1993;422:558–563.
35. McHale NG, Thornbury KD. Sympathetic stimulation causes increased output of lymphocytes from the popliteal node in anaesthetized sheep. *Exp Physiol.* 1990;75:847–850.
36. Thornbury KD, McHale NG, Allen JM, Hughes G. Nerve-mediated contractions of sheep mesenteric lymph node capsules. *J Physiol.* 1990; 422:513–522.
37. McHale NG, Meharg MK. Co-ordination of pumping in isolated bovine lymphatic vessels. *J Physiol.* 1992;450:503–512.
38. Reddy NP, Staub NC. Intrinsic propulsive activity of thoracic duct perfused in anesthetized dogs. *Microvasc Res.* 1981;21:183–192.
39. Telinius N, Baandrup U, Rumessen J, et al. The human thoracic duct is functionally innervated by adrenergic nerves. *Am J Physiol Heart Circ Physiol.* 2014;306:H206–213.
40. Briggs Boedtkjer D, Rumessen J, Baandrup U, et al. Identification of interstitial Cajal-like cells in the human thoracic duct. *Cells Tissues Organs.* 2013;197:145–158.
41. Anson BJ. *Morris' Human Anatomy: The Blakiston.* Division McGraw-Hill Book Comp; 1966.
42. Eisenhoffer J, Elias RM, Johnston MG. Effect of outflow pressure on lymphatic pumping in vitro. *Am J Physiol.* 1993;265:R97–R102.
43. Jensen LT, Henriksen JH, Olesen HP, Risteli J, Lorenzen I. Lymphatic clearance of synovial fluid in conscious pigs: the aminoterminal propeptide of type III procollagen. *Eur J Clin Invest.* 1993;23:778–784.
44. Olszewski WL, Pazdur J, Kubasiewicz E, Zaleska M, Cooke CJ, Miller NE. Lymph draining from foot joints in rheumatoid arthritis provides insight into local cytokine and chemokine production and transport to lymph nodes. *Arthritis Rheum.* 2001;44:541–549.
45. Benaglio F, Vitolo B, Scarabelli M, et al. The draining lymph node in rheumatoid arthritis: current concepts and research perspectives. *Biomed Res Int.* 2015;2015:420251.
46. Guo R, Zhou Q, Proulx ST, et al. Inhibition of lymphangiogenesis and lymphatic drainage via vascular endothelial growth factor receptor

3 blockade increases the severity of inflammation in a mouse model of chronic inflammatory arthritis. *Arthritis Rheum*. 2009;60:2666–2676.
47. Cain EL Jr, Dugas JR, Wolf RS, Andrews JR. Elbow injuries in throwing athletes: a current concepts review. *Am J Sports Med*. 2003;31:621–635.
48. Louveau A, Plog BA, Antila S, Alitalo K, Nedergaard M, Kipnis J. Understanding the functions and relationships of the glymphatic system and meningeal lymphatics. *J Clin Invest*. 2017;127:3210–3219.
49. Spector R, Keep RF, Robert SS, Smith QR, Johanson CE. A balanced view of choroid plexus structure and function: focus on adult humans. *Exp Neurol*. 2015;267:78–86.
50. Spector R, Robert SS, Johanson CE. A balanced view of the cerebrospinal fluid composition and functions: focus on adult humans. *Exp Neurol*. 2015;273:57–68.
51. Iliff JJ, Lee H, Yu M, et al. Brain-wide pathway for waste clearance captured by contrast-enhanced MRI. *J Clin Invest*. 2013;123:1299–1309.
52. Bohr T, Hjorth PG, Holst SC, et al. The glymphatic system: current understanding and modeling. *iScience*. 2022;25:104987.
53. Wardlaw JM, Benveniste H, Nedergaard M, et al; Colleagues from the Fondation Leducq Transatlantic Network of Excellence on the Role of the Perivascular Space in Cerebral Small Vessel Disease. Perivascular spaces in the brain: anatomy, physiology and pathology. *Nat Rev Neurol*. 2020;16:137–153.
54. Nedergaard M. Neuroscience. Garbage truck of the brain. *Science*. 2013;340:1529–1530.
55. Faghih MM, Sharp MK. Is bulk flow plausible in perivascular, paravascular and paravenous channels? *Fluids Barriers CNS*. 2018;15:17.
56. Faghih MM, Keith Sharp M. Mechanisms of tracer transport in cerebral perivascular spaces. *J Biomech*. 2021;118:110278.
57. Weller RO, Djuanda E, Yow HY, Carare RO. Lymphatic drainage of the brain and the pathophysiology of neurological disease. *Acta Neuropathol*. 2009;117:1–14.
58. Raper D, Louveau A, Kipnis J. How do meningeal lymphatic vessels drain the CNS? *Trends Neurosci*. 2016;39:581–586.
59. McVay CB. *Anson & McVay Surgical Anatomy*. W.B. Saunders Company; 1984.
60. Bhatnagar M, Fisher A, Ramsaroop S, Carter A, Pippard B. Chylothorax: pathophysiology, diagnosis, and management-a comprehensive review. *J Thorac Dis*. 2024;16:1645–1661.
61. Johnson RA, Blake TM. Lymphatics of the heart. *Circulation*. 1966;33:137–142.
62. Loukas M, Abel N, Tubbs RS, Grabska J, Birungi J, Anderson RH. The cardiac lymphatic system. *Clin Anat*. 2011;24:684–691.
63. Ratajska A, Gula G, Flaht-Zabost A, et al. Comparative and developmental anatomy of cardiac lymphatics. *Scientific World Journal*. 2014;2014:183170.
64. Cui Y. The role of lymphatic vessels in the heart. *Pathophysiology*. 2010;17:307–314.
65. Weber E, Sozio F, Borghini A, Sestini P, Renzoni E. Pulmonary lymphatic vessel morphology: a review. *Ann Anat*. 2018;218:110–117.
66. Kambouchner M, Bernaudin JF. Intralobular pulmonary lymphatic distribution in normal human lung using D2-40 antipodoplanin immunostaining. *J Histochem Cytochem*. 2009;57:643–648.
67. Sozio F, Rossi A, Weber E, et al. Morphometric analysis of intralobular, interlobular and pleural lymphatics in normal human lung. *J Anat*. 2012;220:396–404.
68. Schmid-Schönbein GW. Mechanisms causing initial lymphatics to expand and compress to promote lymph flow. *Arch Histol Cytol*. 1990;53 Suppl:107–114.
69. Trivedi A, Reed HO. The lymphatic vasculature in lung function and respiratory disease. *Front Med (Lausanne)*. 2023;10:1118583.
70. Konopka KE, Nguyen T, Jentzen JM, et al. Diffuse alveolar damage (DAD) resulting from coronavirus disease 2019 infection is morphologically indistinguishable from other causes of DAD. *Histopathology*. 2020;77:570–578.
71. Sweeney RM, McAuley DF. Acute respiratory distress syndrome. *Lancet*. 2016;388:2416–2430.
72. Upadhya S, Rehman J, Malik AB, Chen S. Mechanisms of lung injury induced by SARS-CoV-2 infection. *Physiology (Bethesda)*. 2022;37:88–100.
73. Negrini D, Mukenge S, M. Del Fabbro, Gonano C, Miserocchi G. Distribution of diaphragmatic lymphatic stomata. *J Appl Physiol*. 1991;70:1544–1549.
74. Tsilibary EC, Wissig SL. Absorption from the peritoneal cavity: SEM study of the mesothelium covering the peritoneal surface of the muscular portion of the diaphragm. *Am J Anat*. 1977;149:127–133.
75. Wang NS. The preformed stomas connecting the pleural cavity and the lymphatics in the parietal pleura. *Am Rev Respir Dis*. 1975;111:12–20.
76. Abernethy NJ, Chin W, Hay JB, Rodela H, Oreopoulos D, Johnston MG. Lymphatic removal of dialysate from the peritoneal cavity of anesthetized sheep. *Kidney Int*. 1991;40:174–181.
77. Zakaria ER, Simonsen O, Rippe A, Rippe B. Transport of tracer albumin from peritoneum to plasma: role of diaphragmatic, visceral, and parietal lymphatics. *Am J Physiol*. 1996;270:H1549–H1556.
78. Weinbaum S, Cancel LM, Fu BM, Tarbell JM. The glycocalyx and its role in vascular physiology and vascular related diseases. *Cardiovasc Eng Technol*. 2020;12:37–71.
79. Benoit JN, Zawieja DC, Goodman AH, Granger HJ. Characterization of intact mesenteric lymphatic pump and its responsiveness to acute edemagenic stress. *Am J Physiol*. 1989;257:H2059–H2069.
80. Zawieja DC, Barber BJ. Lymph protein concentration in initial and collecting lymphatics of the rat. *Am J Physiol*. 1987;252:G602–G606.
81. Guyton AC, Barber BJ. The energetics of lymph formation. *Lymphology*. 1980;13:173–176.
82. Mazzoni MC, Skalak TC, Schmid-Schönbein GW. Effects of skeletal muscle fiber deformation on lymphatic volumes. *Am J Physiol*. 1990;259:H1860–H1868.
83. Desai P, Williams AG Jr, Prajapati P, Downey HF. Lymph flow in instrumented dogs varies with exercise intensity. *Lymphat Res Biol*. 2010;8:143–148.
84. Gnepp DR, Sloop CH. The effect of passive motion on the flow and formation of lymph. *Lymphology*. 1978;11:32–36.
85. Ikomi F, Hunt J, Hanna G, Schmid-Schönbein GW. Interstitial fluid, plasma protein, colloid, and leukocyte uptake into initial lymphatics. *J Appl Physiol*. 1996;81:2060–2067.
86. McGeown JG, McHale NG, Thornbury KD. The role of external compression and movement in lymph propulsion in the sheep hind limb. *J Physiol*. 1987;387:83–93.
87. Intaglietta M, Gross JF. Vasomotion, tissue fluid flow and the formation of lymph. *Int J Microcirc Clin Exp*. 1982;1:55–65.
88. Ohhashi T, Azuma T, Sakaguchi M. Active and passive mechanical characteristics of bovine mesenteric lymphatics. *Am J Physiol*. 1980;239:H88–H95.
89. Macdonald AJ, Arkill KP, Tabor GR, McHale NG, Winlove CP. Modeling flow in collecting lymphatic vessels: one-dimensional flow through a series of contractile elements. *Am J Physiol Heart Circ Physiol*. 2008;295:H305–H313.
90. Beckett EA, Hollywood MA, Thornbury KD, McHale NG. Spontaneous electrical activity in sheep mesenteric lymphatics. *Lymphat Res Biol*. 2007;5:29–43.
91. Benoit JN. Relationships between lymphatic pump flow and total lymph flow in the small intestine. *Am J Physiol*. 1991;261:H1970–H1978.
92. Van Helden DF. Pacemaker potentials in lymphatic smooth muscle of the guinea-pig mesentery. *J Physiol*. 1993;471:465–479.
93. Van Helden DF, Hosaka K, Imtiaz MS. Rhythmicity in the microcirculation. *Clin Hemorheol Microcirc*. 2006;34:59–66.
94. McCloskey KD, Hollywood MA, Thornbury KD, Ward SM, McHale NG. Kit-like immunopositive cells in sheep mesenteric lymphatic vessels. *Cell Tissue Res*. 2002;310:77–84.
95. Hogan RD, Unthank JL. Mechanical control of initial lymphatic contractile behavior in bat's wing. *Am J Physiol*. 1986;251:H357–H363.
96. Hollywood MA, Cotton KD, Thornbury KD, McHale NG. Tetrodotoxin-sensitive sodium current in sheep lymphatic smooth muscle. *J Physiol*. 1997;503:13–20.
97. Zawieja DC, Davis KL, Schuster R, Hinds WM, Granger HJ. Distribution, propagation, and coordination of contractile activity in lymphatics. *Am J Physiol*. 1993;264:H1283–H1291.
98. Crowe MJ, von der Weid PY, Brock JA, Van Helden DF. Co-ordination of contractile activity in guinea-pig mesenteric lymphatics. *J Physiol*. 1997;500:235–244.

99. McHale NG. The lymphatic circulation. *Ir J Med Sci.* 1992;161:483–486.
100. Ohhashi T, Mizuno R, Ikomi F, Kawai Y. Current topics of physiology and pharmacology in the lymphatic system. *Pharmacol Ther.* 2005;105:165–188.
101. Benoit JN, Zawieja DC. Effects of f-Met-Leu-Phe-induced inflammation on intestinal lymph flow and lymphatic pump behavior. *Am J Physiol.* 1992;262:G199–G202.
102. Johnston MG, Elias RM, Hayashi A, Nelson W. Role of the lymphatic circulatory system in shock. *J Burn Care Rehabil.* 1987;8:469–474.
103. Hanley CA, Elias RM, Movat HZ, Johnston MG. Suppression of fluid pumping in isolated bovine mesenteric lymphatics by interleukin-1: interaction with prostaglandin E_2. *Microvasc Res.* 1989;37:218–229.
104. Johnston MG, Gordon JL. Regulation of lymphatic contractility by arachidonate metabolites. *Nature.* 1981;293:294–297.
105. Shirasawa Y, Ikomi F, Ohhashi T. Physiological roles of endogenous nitric oxide in lymphatic pump activity of rat mesentery in vivo. *Am J Physiol Gastrointest Liver Physiol.* 2000;278:G551–G556.
106. Yokoyama S, Benoit JN. Effects of bradykinin on lymphatic pumping in rat mesentery. *Am J Physiol.* 1996;270:G752–G756.
107. Zawieja DC. Lymphatic microcirculation. *Microcirculation.* 1996;3:241–243.
108. McGeown JG, McHale NG, Thornbury KD. Effects of varying patterns of external compression on lymph flow in the hindlimb of the anaesthetized sheep. *J Physiol.* 1988;397:449–457.
109. Browse NL, Lord RS, Taylor A. Pressure waves and gradients in the canine thoracic duct. *J Physiol.* 1971;213:507–524.
110. Millard FP. *Applied Anatomy of the Lymphatics.* The Journal Printing Company; 1922.
111. Bridenbaugh EA, Gashev AA, Zawieja DC. Lymphatic muscle: a review of contractile function. *Lymphat Res Biol.* 2003;1:147–158.
112. Cueni LN, Detmar M. The lymphatic system in health and disease. *Lymphat Res Biol.* 2008;6:109–122.
113. Movat HZ, Wasi S. Severe microvascular injury induced by lysosomal releasates of human polymorphonuclear leukocytes. Increase in vasopermeability, hemorrhage, and microthrombosis due to degradation of subendothelial and perivascular matrices. *Am J Pathol.* 1985;121:404–417.
114. Zhang PH, Zhang WW, Wang SS, et al. Efficient pulmonary lymphatic drainage is necessary for inflammation resolution in ARDS. *JCI Insight.* 2024;9:e173440.
115. Hurley JV. Inflammation. In: Staub NC, Taylor AE, eds. *Edema.* Raven Press; 1984:463–488.
116. Atkinson TP. Histamine and serotonin. In: *Inflammation: Basic Principles and Clinical Correlates.* Raven Press; 1994:196.
117. Lawrence T, Gilroy DW. Chronic inflammation: a failure of resolution? *Int J Exp Pathol.* 2007;88:85–94.
118. Bellingan GJ, Caldwell H, Howie SE, Dransfield I, Haslett C. In vivo fate of the inflammatory macrophage during the resolution of inflammation: inflammatory macrophages do not die locally, but emigrate to the draining lymph nodes. *J Immunol.* 1996;157:2577–2585.
119. Witte CL, Witte MH. Lymphatics in the pathophysiology of edema. In: Johston MG, ed. *Experimental Biology of the Lymphatic Circulation.* Elsevier; 1984:167–188.
120. Measel JW Jr. The effect of the lymphatic pump on the immune response: I. Preliminary studies on the antibody response to pneumococcal polysaccharide assayed by bacterial agglutination and passive hemagglutination. *J Am Osteopath Assoc.* 1982;82:28–31.
121. Dinarello CA. Role of interleukin-I and tumor necrosis factor in systemic responses to infection and inflammation. In: Gallen JI, ed. *Inflammation: Basic Principles and Clinical Correlations.* Raven Press; 1992:211–232.
122. Levine JD, Reichling DB. Peripheral mechanisms of inflammatory pain. In: Wall PD, Melzack R, eds. *Textbook of Pain.* 4th ed. Churchill Livingstone; 1999:59–84.
123. Zhou S, Zhao G, Chen R, et al. Lymphatic vessels: roles and potential therapeutic intervention in rheumatoid arthritis and osteoarthritis. *Theranostics.* 2024;14:265–282.
124. Brown S, Dayan JH, Kataru RP, Mehrara BJ. The vicious circle of stasis, inflammation, and fibrosis in lymphedema. *Plast Reconstr Surg.* 2023;151(2):330e–341e.
125. Oliver G, Kipnis J, Randolph GJ, Harvey NL. The lymphatic vasculature in the 21st century: novel functional roles in homeostasis and disease. *Cell.* 2020;182:270–296.

15 Anatomy, Mechanics, and Physiology of Pulmonary Respiration

FRANK H. WILLARD ▪ GILBERT E. D'ALONZO JR ▪ SAMUEL L. KRACHMAN ▪ MARK D. SCHUENKE

KEY CONCEPTS

- Proper respiratory function depends on a delicate harmony with other systems, notably, but not exclusively, the cardiovascular, neuromuscular, and skeletal systems.
- Thoracic cage mechanics are involved in not only respiratory functions but also circulatory, biomechanical, metabolic, neurologic, behavioral, and venous and lymphatic drainage functions.
- Optimal performance of respiratory system mechanics is largely dependent on the neuromusculoskeletal system, the dysfunctions of which are amenable to osteopathic manipulative medicine.
- The thoracoabdominal wall is a fibroelastic cylinder controlled by the respiratory muscles; fixation of the upper border of the ribs facilitates inhalation while fixation of the lower border of the ribs enhances exhalation.
- The thoracoabdominal diaphragm is a dome-shaped muscle; its function is greatly facilitated by its vertical component, termed the zone of apposition.
- The abdominal muscles play a role in fixing the lower border of the ribs as well as compressing the abdominal viscera and thereby expanding the zone of apposition to support the actions of the diaphragm.
- Structural changes in some respiratory muscles are seen at the molecular, cellular, and gross structural levels in disease states such as chronic obstructive pulmonary disease (COPD), kyphosis, and obesity; these changes decrease motion, ultimately decreasing the ability of the respiratory mechanism to supply adequate pumping activity.
- An emphasis is placed on having sufficient motion in the respiratory musculature and thoracic cage to ensure adequate ventilation of the tissues; an important role of the osteopathic physician is to improve the quality and range of motion in the respiratory mechanism.
- Ventilation and pulmonary gas exchange are largely dependent on proper function of the neuromusculoskeletal system.

INTRODUCTION

The Respiratory System

The respiratory system includes:

- All of the components of the upper airway–nasal and oral cavities, nasopharynx, oropharynx, laryngopharynx, and larynx
- The tracheobronchial tree extending deep into the lung and ending with the alveoli
- The lungs and the pulmonary circulation, which are enclosed in the thoracic cage
- The diaphragm, scalene, intercostal and abdominal muscles along with numerous accessory muscles
- The central nervous system with its peripheral connections

The central nervous system performs as a system controller, regulating the activity of the respiratory muscles and the thoracic cage, which functions as a pump.

- Central pattern generators (CPGs) in the brainstem guide the pumping activity of the respiratory muscles.
- The pumping action of this organ system is essential for the lung's mechanism to exchange oxygen for CO_2, but it also assists in the return of venous and lymphatic fluids to the heart.
- Peripheral sensory systems provide feedback to the CPG from the chemoreceptors exposed to the O_2, CO_2 and pH of the blood and stretch receptors in the walls of the airway as well as the chest walls.
- Unimpeded physiologic motion of the thoracic cage is important to maintain:
  - □ Sufficient arterial supply
  - □ Adequate venous drainage
  - □ Efficient lymphatic drainage
  - □ Sensitive and responsive neural regulatory influences on the respiratory system

Besides providing adequate oxygenation vital to end-organ function, the respiratory system also:

- Releases at least one major end product of metabolism, CO_2
- Participates in the homeostasis of acid–base metabolic balance on a moment-to-moment basis
- Helps to move fluid in the low-pressure systems such as the venous and lymphatic vessels

The lungs, upper airway, and chest walls are also involved in the:

- Elimination of various toxins and drugs
- Vocalization
- Pressurization of the abdomen for:
  - □ Defecation
  - □ Micturition (urination)
  - □ Parturition
  - □ Emesis
  - □ Physical work (e.g., lifting, muscular activity)

In addition, the lungs are organs that interface with the environment through the exchange of air that occurs with each breath.

- Each day, the lungs are exposed to more than 10,000 L of ambient air that may contain microorganisms, dusts, and chemicals.
- The exposure to these noxious substances is likely responsible in part for a wide variety of diseases, including:
  - □ Infections
  - □ Inflammatory conditions
  - □ Malignancies

- Most of the conducting portion of the airway focuses on defense mechanisms that reduce the likelihood that injury and disease will develop. (See Chapter 12 The Role of Inflammation in Healing and Homeostasis.)

Proper respiratory function depends on a delicate harmony with other systems, notably, but not exclusively, the cardiovascular, neuromuscular, and skeletal systems.

- However, for optimal mechanical performance, the respiratory system is largely dependent on the neuromusculoskeletal system.
- The neuromusculoskeletal components of respiratory function are easily evaluated through palpatory diagnostic procedures and treatable using osteopathic manipulative methods.

Disease cannot occur in one system without affecting other body systems. The eventual extent of pathology generally depends on the severity of the initial disruption.

- Malfunction of an individual component of any system, or in the respiratory system itself, or alterations of the relationships among various components, can lead to disturbances in end-organ function and, eventually, in total body performance.
- The effect of common diseases on thoracic respiratory system mechanics will be addressed briefly in this chapter, and the effectiveness of osteopathic manipulative medicine to help improve pulmonary function will be addressed in various chapters within the Osteopathic Considerations for the Specialties section. Cranial and sacral region mechanics related to respiratory function will be addressed in Chapter 53 Osteopathic Cranial Manipulative Medicine.

Definition of Thoracic Respiratory Mechanics

The thorax is a flexible fibroelastic cylinder, rhythmically distorted by the action of numerous respiratory muscles that are located both within the thorax and abdomen and extremities (Fig. 15.1).

- The changing shape of this cylinder creates the alternating inhalation and exhalation events necessary for perfusing the lung with air; these movements constitute the mechanics of breathing.
- Diseases that alter the shape of the thorax or its compliancy can have a substantial impact on the mechanics of respiration and, consequently, on the health of the individual.

BIOMECHANICAL FUNCTIONS

The thoracic cage acts as a pump coordinated by a complex central controller mechanism and influenced by coordinated neural reflex activity. When the thorax acts as a pump, it involves:

- Contraction
- Complex muscular relaxation
- Motion of fascial planes
- Movement of nearly 150 joints of the body

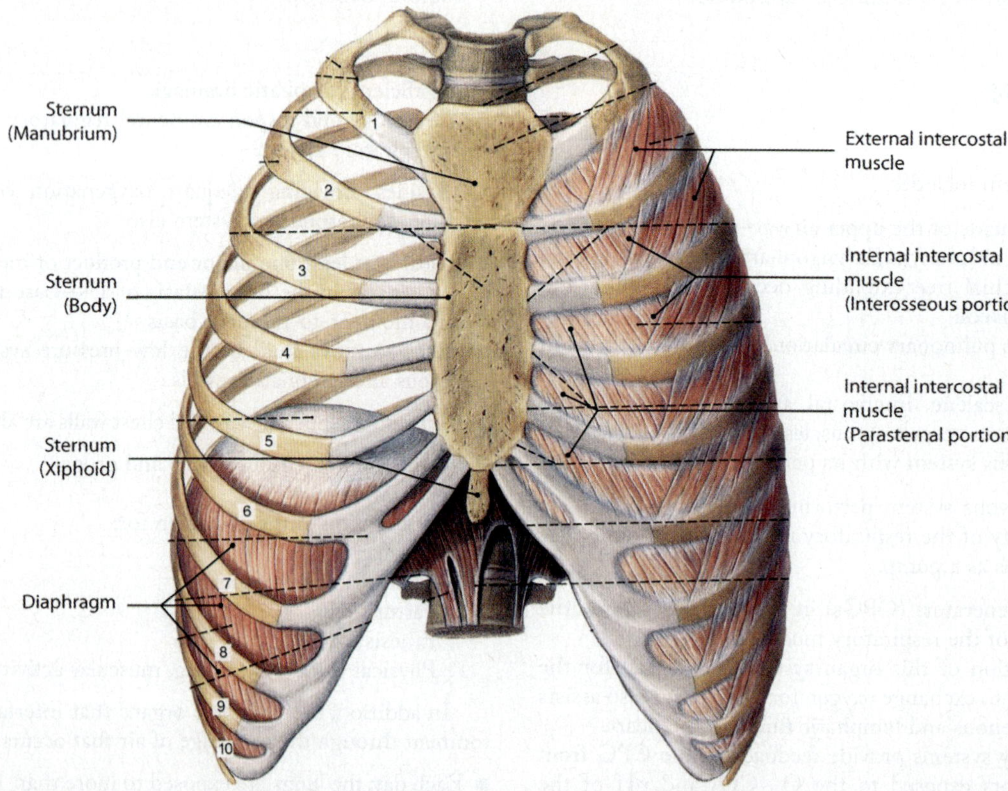

Figure 15.1. The intercostal muscles. On the left side of the thorax, the external intercostal muscles are seen oriented from superoposterior to inferoanterior. These muscles are not present in the most anterior intercostal spaces. The parasternal portion of the internal intercostal muscles is seen occupying the anterior intercostal spaces. Its orientation is opposite that of the external intercostal. The diaphragm is seen on the right side. (Reprinted with permission from Clemente CD. *Anatomy: A Regional Atlas of the Human Body.* 4th ed. Williams & Wilkins; 1997.)

It is clear that the thoracic viscera affect its musculoskeletal pump. Likewise, the thoracic pump, when dysfunctional, negatively affects the thoracic viscera.

- Maintaining normal respiratory motion during inhalation and exhalation inherently tends to create a healthy environment for the thoracic viscera.
- Therefore, dysfunction of the thoracic cage has a negative influence.
- In addition, respiratory motion and function are influenced by the activity of somatic structures in the upper and lower extremities, head and neck regions, and the abdominopelvic regions.

RESPIRATORY AND CIRCULATORY FUNCTIONS

Breathing is a dynamic process involving moment-to-moment active gas exchange at the level of the lungs.

- While alternating thoracoabdominal pressures are critical for the aeration of the pulmonary alveoli, this movement is also an important influence on the redistribution of fluid in the lymphatic system as well as the movement of blood in the venous network of the body and is associated with the drainage of the epidural venous plexus of Batson located in the spinal canal. (See Chapter 14 Anatomy and Physiology of the Lymphatic System for more details.)
- The excursion of the diaphragm is largely responsible for the pumping motion that governs proper pulmonary function.
- With inhibition of diaphragmatic motion, there is marked disruption in pulmonary gas exchange secondary to lung parenchymal atelectasis.

Reduction or impairment of thoracic cage mobility influences lymphatic drainage.

- A reduction in lymphatic drainage from the thoracic viscera may help contribute to the development of pulmonary congestion and a higher likelihood of lung inflammation and infection.
- Osteopathic medicine uses manipulative treatments, for example, rib raising, diaphragm relaxation, and thoracic inlet release, to enhance thoracic cage movement and lymphatic drainage, with both preventive and curative influences on disease. (See Chapter 50 Lymphatic Drainage Procedures for further details.)

In addition, the rhythmic pumping action of the diaphragm with respiration is likely to favorably affect abdominal organ function.

- The rhythmic motion of the diaphragm may have a positive influence on gastrointestinal function and perhaps even enhances venous drainage of other visceral organs such as the liver and spleen.
- Inhibition of diaphragmatic movement is known to reduce lymphatic fluid movement in the thoracic duct.

NEUROLOGIC FUNCTIONS

The phrenic nerves (C3–C5) are responsible for the neuroregulation of the diaphragm.

- The autonomic nerves found in the diaphragm are probably vasomotor afferents.
- Branches from the vagus nerves, containing both afferent and efferent components, make up the parasympathetic innervation of pulmonary structures, particularly the airways.
- The principal vagal effects are mainly secretory and bronchoconstrictive in character.

The autonomic innervation of the airway is derived from the pulmonary plexus. This plexus is divided into an anterior and posterior part by the root of the lung.

- An anterior pulmonary plexus, the smaller of the two, exists in front of the root of the lung
- The posterior pulmonary plexus, a significantly larger structure, is found behind the root of the lung.

The sympathetic supply to the lungs originates in the first to the fifth thoracic spinal cord segments.

- The postganglionic fibers, although not well documented, appear to arise from the second to the sixth thoracic paravertebral ganglia.[1]
- Postganglionic fibers join both the anterior and posterior pulmonary plexuses.
- The sympathetic innervation supplies vasomotor fibers to the trachea, bronchi, and pulmonary blood vessels.

The parasympathetic innervation of the airway arises from the vagus nerve.[2]

- Vagal cardiopulmonary nerves enter the pulmonary plexus.
- Acetylcholine in the lung acts through muscarinic receptors to (reviewed in Buels and Fryer[3]):
    - Contract airway smooth muscle thus facilitating bronchoconstriction
    - Relax vascular smooth muscle thus facilitating vasodilation and fluid extravasation
    - Enhance mucus secretion and ciliary activity enhancing airway protection

Visceromotor reflexes from the lungs express themselves in the somatic area of the upper thoracic region and occasionally extend into the cervical area.

- Viscerosensory reflexes can be found in the same region.
- Viscerosomatic reflexes, emanating from either the lungs or pleura, will affect movement of the thoracic cage.
- This restrictive movement process could induce a splinting effect, asymmetric movement of the chest, and intercostal hyperalgesia.
- It could also induce pain on palpation.
- In severe cases, pain is induced on voluntary motion.
- This reduced thoracic cage motion can also influence gas exchange by the induction of lung parenchymal atelectasis or by altering lung volumes, such as functional residual capacity (FRC) and total lung capacity (TLC), and distributive airflow.
- The most common clinical response to enhanced reflex activity is muscle rigidity in the upper thoracic area, involving mainly the paravertebral musculature.
- This response is also experienced in the cervical area, involving the sternocleidomastoid, scalene, and diaphragm muscles.

METABOLIC FUNCTIONS

The more efficient the respiratory system mechanics are, the more efficient will be the functions that relate to metabolic processes:

- Gas exchange
- Elimination of waste and toxins
- Expulsion of environmental irritants or vectors of disease through coughing and sneezing
- Mucus production and protection from potentially infectious agents
- Metabolism of molecules involved in vital processes, such as blood pressure and control of emboli

BEHAVIORAL FUNCTIONS

Optimal respiratory system mechanics support essential behavioral functions such as:

- Sleep
- Vocalization
- Emotional expression
- Physical activity and exercise
- Elimination of waste from the gastrointestinal and urinary systems
- Parturition

These facts emphasize the importance of striving for smooth continuous respiratory movements in the thoracoabdominal wall regardless of the etiology of the particular disease processes. This chapter will examine the anatomy and function of the muscles involved in respiration. It will also consider the alteration of these movements in specific diseases that involve structural changes in the thoracic wall. In addition, consideration will be given to the influence of respiratory activity on the movement of fluids in the low-pressure systems of the torso.

MUSCLES OF THE THORACIC CYLINDER

Intercostal, Scalene, and Abdominal Muscles

ANATOMY OF THE INTERCOSTAL, SCALENE, AND ABDOMINAL MUSCLES

The intercostal muscles form a distensible fibroelastic sheet surrounding the rib cage (Fig. 15.1).

- The sheet is divided into three incomplete layers.
- These layers are arranged in loose helical spirals (Fig. 15.2).
- Each layer has a different pitch or angle at which the spiral is occurring within the helix.
- Together, these layers act to both protect and alter the structural geometry of the thoracic wall and thus the volume of the pleural sacs.
- This fibromuscular tube is anchored from above by the scalene muscles that attach to the first and second ribs and below by the abdominal muscles that attach to the subcostal margin (Fig. 15.3).

The Scalene Muscles

Three scalene muscles—anterior, middle, and posterior—extend from the transverse processes of the cervical vertebrae (anterior C3–C6, medius C1–C7, and posterior C4–C6) to reach the first rib and, to a lesser extent, the second rib (reviewed in Gardner et al.[4]; see Figs. 15.2 to 15.4).

- Occasionally, a scalenus minimus is found descending from the sixth and seventh cervical transverse process to reach the inside of the first rib with an extension of its investing fascia to fuse with the fascia of the apical pleural of the thoracic cavity (Sibson fascia).
- With the neck fixed in position by tonic contraction of the longus and paraspinal muscles, contraction of the scalene muscles elevates the first and second ribs, an important first step in inhalation.
- The scalene muscles are innervated by branches from the C2 to C7 cervical ventral rami.
- Activity in the scalene muscles is obligatory even in quiet respiratory movements.[5]

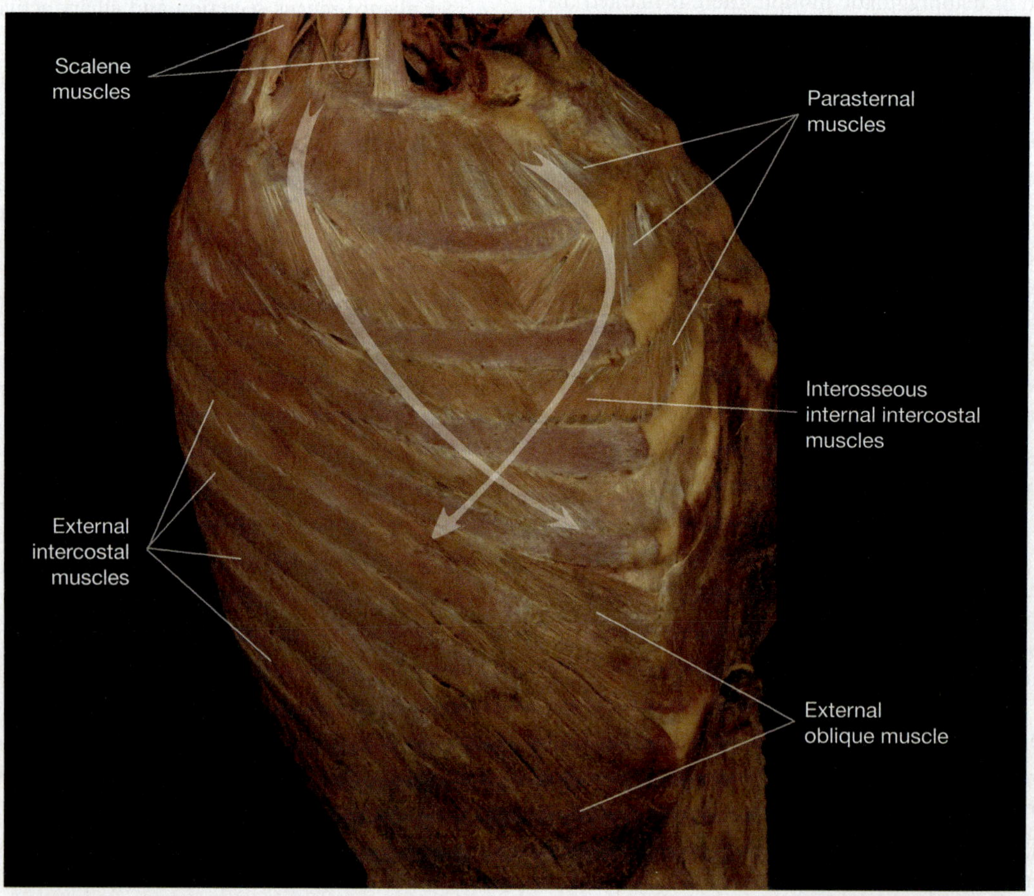

Figure 15.2. This is a lateral view of the thorax, demonstrating the helical spirals established by the external and internal intercostal muscles. The *arrow* that starts on the left represents the pitch of the spiral of the external intercostal muscle, while the *arrow* beginning on the right represents the same for the internal intercostal muscle. (Used with permission from the Willard/Carreiro Collection, University of New England.)

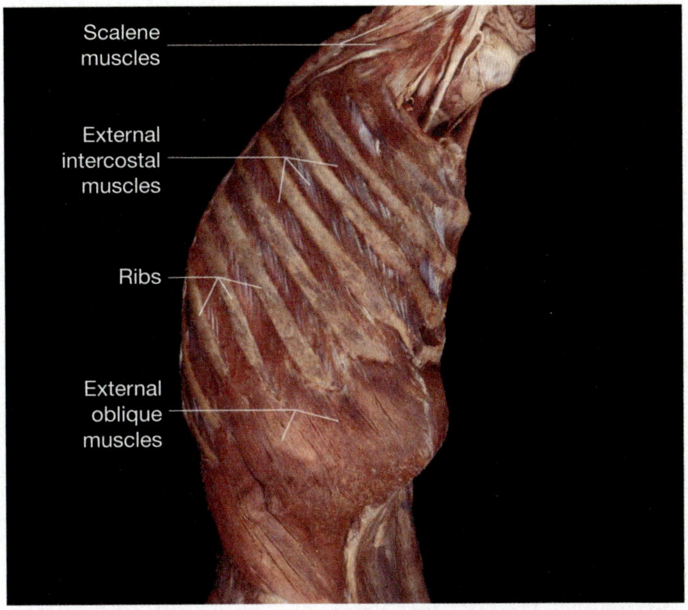

Figure 15.3. This is a lateral view of a male thorax and upper abdomen. The skin and superficial fascia have been removed to reveal the external intercostal and external oblique muscles. (Used with permission from the Willard/Carreiro Collection, University of New England.)

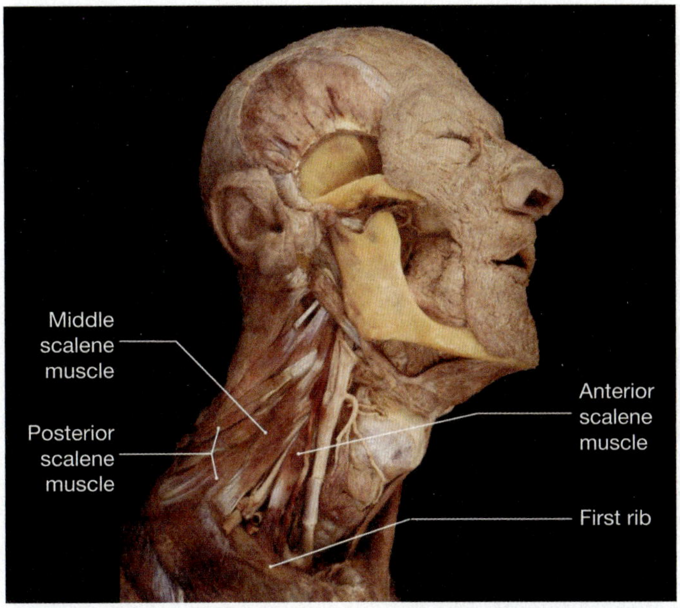

Figure 15.4. This is an oblique view of a male head and neck with the skin, superficial fascia, and upper extremity removed to display the three scalene muscles. A deep dissection was done into the temporal region for other purposes. (Used with permission from the Willard/Carreiro Collection, University of New England.)

External Intercostal Muscle

This thin sheet of muscle extends from the costotransverse ligaments posteriorly at the level of the tubercle of the rib, around the intercostal space, tapering to become a membrane anteriorly at the level of the costochondral junction.

- In the upright position, the orientation of the muscle fibers is close to vertical (see Figs. 15.1 to 15.3, 15.5, and 15.6).
- Throughout its course in each interspace, the muscle is attached to the lower margin of the rib and costal cartilage above and to the upper margin of the rib and costal cartilage below.[6]

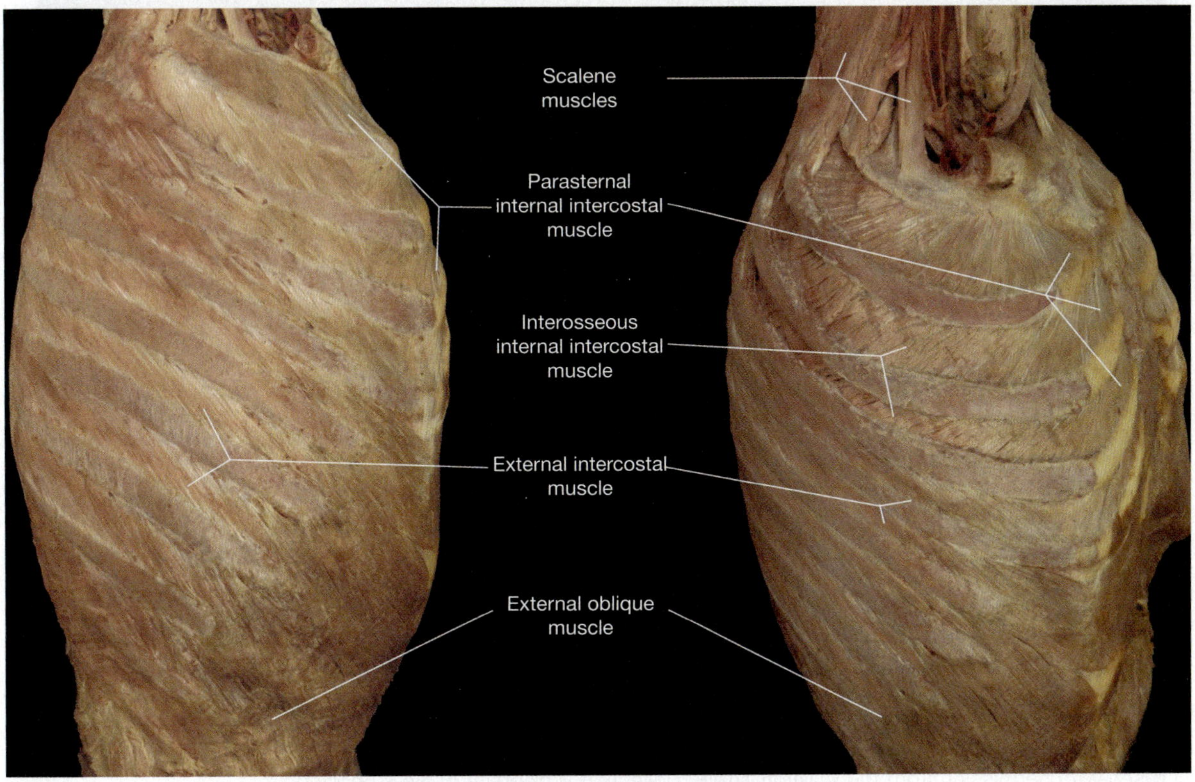

Figure 15.5. These are lateral views of the thorax to illustrate the distribution of the intercostal muscles. In the dissection on the left, the external intercostal muscle is exposed. In the dissection on the right, the external intercostal muscle in the first three interspaces has been removed to expose the internal intercostal muscle. (Used with permission from the Willard/Carreiro Collection, University of New England.)

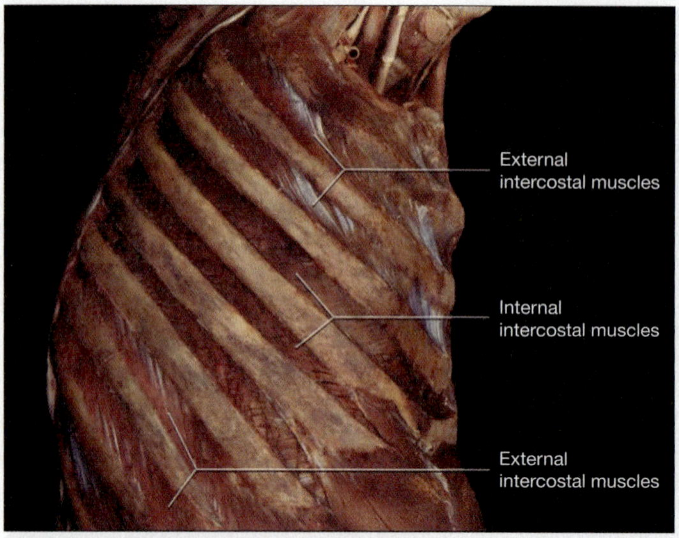

Figure 15.6. A lateral view of the thorax. In this dissection, the skin, superficial fascia, and upper extremity were removed. The external intercostal muscle is seen in the first two interspaces. This muscle was removed in the next three interspaces to reveal the internal intercostal muscles. The external intercostal is seen in the remaining interspaces. (Used with permission from the Willard/Carreiro Collection, University of New England.)

- The external intercostal muscle is thickest in the superior and posterior aspect of the thorax and thinnest inferior and medial aspect of the rib cage.[5]
- The pitch of its helical spiral is from superoposterior to inferoanterior (Fig. 15.2).
- Based on its geometry, thickness, and data from electromyography (EMG) studies, the external intercostal is a powerful muscle of inhalation in the human with the exception of its most anteromedial border, where the muscle is thinnest.
- This latter region, located in the anterior and ventral portions of spaces 6 to 8, appears to represent a weak muscle of exhalation.[5]
- The external intercostal muscles are innervated by branches from the intercostal nerves derived from the thoracic ventral primary rami.

Internal Intercostal Muscles

The internal intercostal muscles are found deep to the external intercostals (see Figs. 15.1 to 15.3 and 15.5 to 15.7). These thin muscles extend from the lateral border of the sternum and wrap around the ribs to eventually become a thin membrane in the posterior intercostal spaces (Fig. 15.5).

- Like the external intercostal muscles, the internal intercostal is attached to the lower margin of the rib and costal cartilage above and to the upper margin of these structures below.

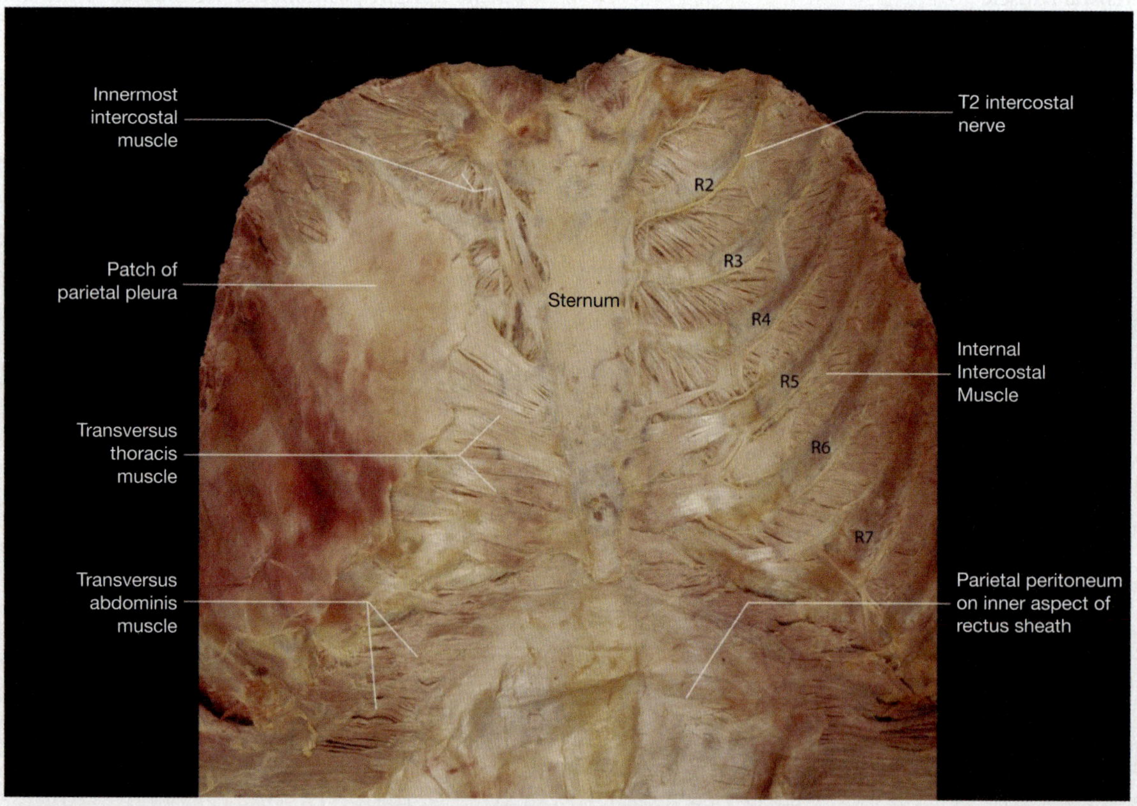

Figure 15.7. This is a posterior view of the anterior thoracic wall. The anterior wall was removed by sectioning the ribs laterally. The parietal pleura was removed from the right side of the wall but has been retained on the left side. The transversus thoracis muscle is seen radiating away from the inferior portion of the sternum. Note the asymmetry of this muscle. Slips of the innermost intercostal muscle can be seen in the upper interspaces. (Used with permission from the Willard/Carreiro Collection, University of New England.)

- The muscle is thickest in the anterior and superior portions and tapers as it passes toward the back.[6]
- The resulting spiral pitch of its muscle fibers is oriented from superoanterior to inferoposterior.
- The muscle is divided into two functionally distinct components.
- The parasternal portion exists between the costal cartilages.
- The interosseous intercostal muscle exists between the bony ribs.[7]
- Analysis of geometry, thickness, and EMG data supports the contention that the interosseous portion is strictly involved in exhalation, while the parasternal portion represents a significant muscle of inhalation.[5,8]
- The internal intercostal muscles are innervated by branches from the intercostal nerves derived from the thoracic ventral primary rami.

Innermost Intercostal Muscles

The innermost intercostal muscles are oriented orthogonal to the ribs (Fig. 15.7). In most individuals, these muscles are very thin and inconsistent in their presence.

- When present, the internal investing fascia of the innermost intercostal muscle is intimately adhered to the endothoracic fascia lining the external surface of the pleural cavity.
- Given this muscle's close geometric relationship with the rib, contraction of the muscle is most likely to assist in moving the ribs closer to each other. Functional analysis of the innermost internal intercostal muscle by EMG analysis is currently lacking.
- The muscle is related embryologically to the transversus thoracis and transversus abdominis muscles.
- The innermost intercostal muscles are innervated by branches from the intercostal nerves derived from the thoracic ventral primary rami.

Transversus Thoracis

The transversus thoracis muscle, also termed sternocostalis or triangularis sterni muscle, arises from the inner surface of the lower sternum, xiphoid process, and lower costal cartilages (Fig. 15.7).

- It radiates outward to attach to the inner borders of the costal cartilages of ribs 2 through 6.[6]
- Only rarely is the muscle symmetric in disposition; often, additional slips of the muscle can be found scattered in the 2nd through 4th interspace as seen in the specimen displayed in Figure 15.7.
- Developmentally, the muscle appears to be most closely related to the innermost intercostal group of muscles and the transversus abdominis muscle.
- In Figure 15.7, the transversus thoracis muscle is seen blending with the superior border of the transversus abdominis muscle; this is most apparent on the left side of the specimen.
- The transversus thoracis muscle is active typically on forced exhalation.
- Quiet, restful breathing in humans does not appear to use the muscle.
- However, exhalation below FRC such as in speech and forceful exhalation such as in coughing, expectoration, and laughing, can utilize the power of this muscle.[5,9]
- The transversus thoracis is innervated by branches from the intercostal nerves derived from the thoracic ventral primary rami.

Subcostal Muscles

The subcostal muscles are typically present on the inner walls of the lower segments of the thorax.

- These muscles arise from the inner aspect of the rib near its angle and descend two to three ribs below to find an attachment to the upper margin of a rib.[6]
- The subcostal muscles run in the same plane as the innermost intercostals and appear to be an embryologic derivative of that layer.
- The subcostal muscles are most prominent in the upper 4 segments or in the inferior portion of the thorax rib (9–11) and with the exception of the 12th rib and remain lateral to the angle to the rib at all levels.
- Most commonly, the bands of the subcostal muscle span two segments; however some bands can span as many as five segments and reach to the attachments on the body of the lower vertebrae.
- The common orientation of these muscles with the internal intercostal suggests a possible function in exhalation.
- The subcostal muscles are innervated by branches from the intercostal nerves derived from the thoracic ventral primary rami.

Levatores Costarum

The levatores costarum (LC) are a group of small muscles located deep to the paraspinal muscles and attached to the ribs on their posterior aspect.

- These muscles arise from the transverse process at the level of the costotransverse joint and extend downward diagonally to attach to the rib or ribs below (Fig. 15.8).
- The short head (LC brevis) of the muscle attaches one rib below its origin while the long head (LC longus) attaches two ribs below.
- Given the position of these muscles on the rib, it is evident that they contribute to elevating the rib on inhalation[5] but have not received extensive physiologic examination to date.
- Unlike the intercostal and abdominal muscles, the levatores costarum are uniformly innervated by small branch from the dorsal primary rami.[10]

The External Oblique Muscle

The outermost abdominal muscle arises from the external and lower borders of the lower eight ribs. The attachment of this muscle interdigitates with the slips of the serratus anterior and latissimus dorsi, both of which are extremity muscles, as well as fuses with the external intercostal muscle of the lower eight ribs (Fig. 15.9).

- The muscle fibers form a broad thin sheet passing anterior and inferior, similar to those of the external intercostals, to reach their attachment to a medially positioned aponeurosis, which extends from the xiphoid process superiorly to the pubic symphysis inferiorly.
- The inferior border of this aponeurosis participates in the formation of the inguinal ligament, and its medial border contributes to the rectus sheath.[6]
- The muscle fibers of the external oblique rarely extend below a line drawn between the umbilicus and the anterior superior iliac spine, the remainder of the sheet below this line being aponeurotic in composition.
- Contraction of the external oblique muscle is capable of distorting the human rib cage.[11]
- The external oblique is quiet during restful breathing but engaged during forceful exhalation functioning to displace the ribs inferiorly.[12]
- The external oblique is innervated by the thoracoabdominal nerves (T7–T11) and the subcostal nerve (T12).

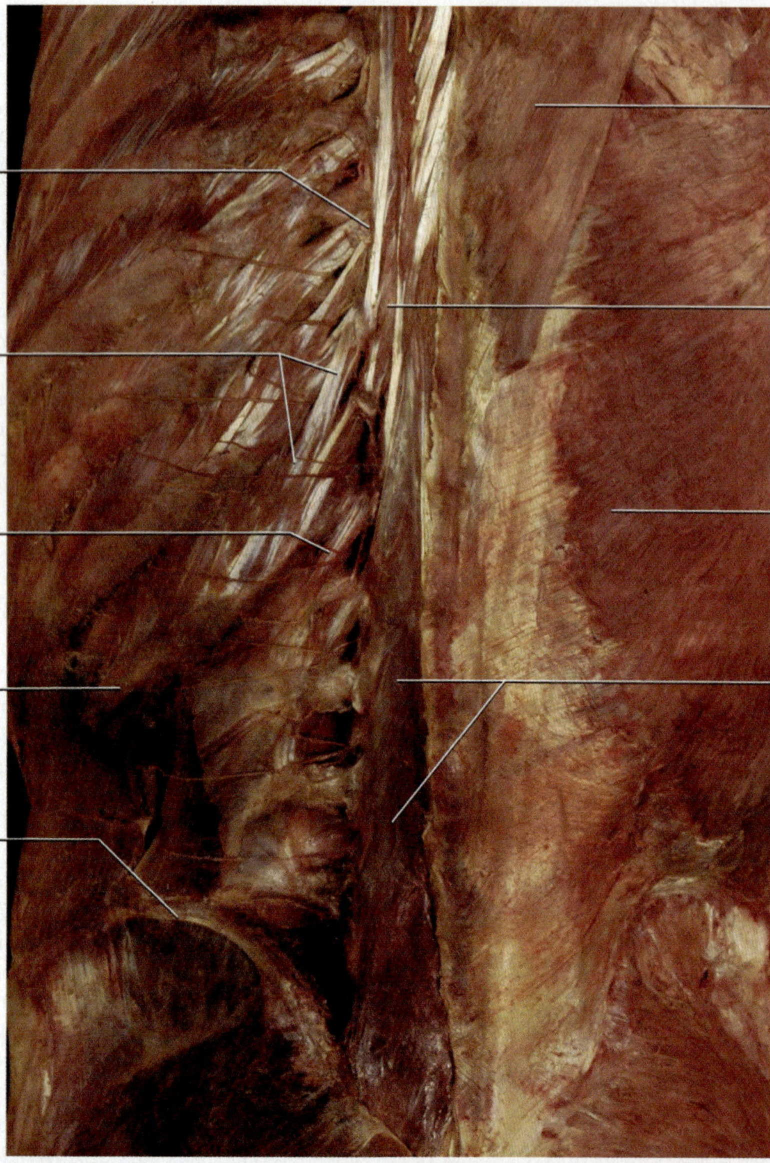

Figure 15.8. Posterior view of the back, with the paraspinal muscles on the left side removed to display the levatores costarum muscles. Levatores costarum longus spans two segments while brevis spans one segment. (Used with permission from the Willard/Carreiro Collection, University of New England.)

Internal Oblique Muscle

The internal oblique muscle has a radiate shape (Fig. 15.10), emanating from the region of the iliac crest and low back and attaching along a line from the pubic symphysis superiorly along the rectus sheath and posteriorly along the subcostal margin to reach the thoracolumbar fascia.

- Specifically, the broad sheet of muscle takes its origin from a curved line involving
  - The upper portion of the inguinal ligament anteriorly
  - The iliac crest centrally
  - The thoracolumbar fascia posteriorly
- From this line, the fibers of the muscle radiate inferiorly to reach the conjoint tendon and pubic symphysis; in doing so, they help form the falx inguinalis under which the spermatic cord or round ligament of the uterus will pass.
- Superiorly, this muscle radiates vertically upward where fibers attach to the inferior margin of the subcostal cartilage as well as interdigitate with the internal intercostal muscles.
- The middle fibers of the muscle pass anteriorly around the curve of the abdomen to join a medially positioned aponeurosis, which eventually splits to house the rectus abdominis muscle.[6]
- Quiet respiration does not appear to engage the internal oblique muscle; however, it will become active on forced exhalation, helping to displace the ribs inferiorly.[12]
- The internal intercostal muscle is innervated by lower branches of the thoracoabdominal nerves, the subcostal nerve, and, in some cases, the ilioinguinal and iliohypogastric may contribute branches to this muscle.

Transversus Abdominis Muscle

Internal to the abdominal obliques lies a third muscle with a predominant horizontal fiber orientation (Fig. 15.11).

- The transversus abdominis arises from the lateral portion of the inguinal ligament, the iliac crest, the thoracolumbar fascia, and the inferior margin of the lower costal cartilages.

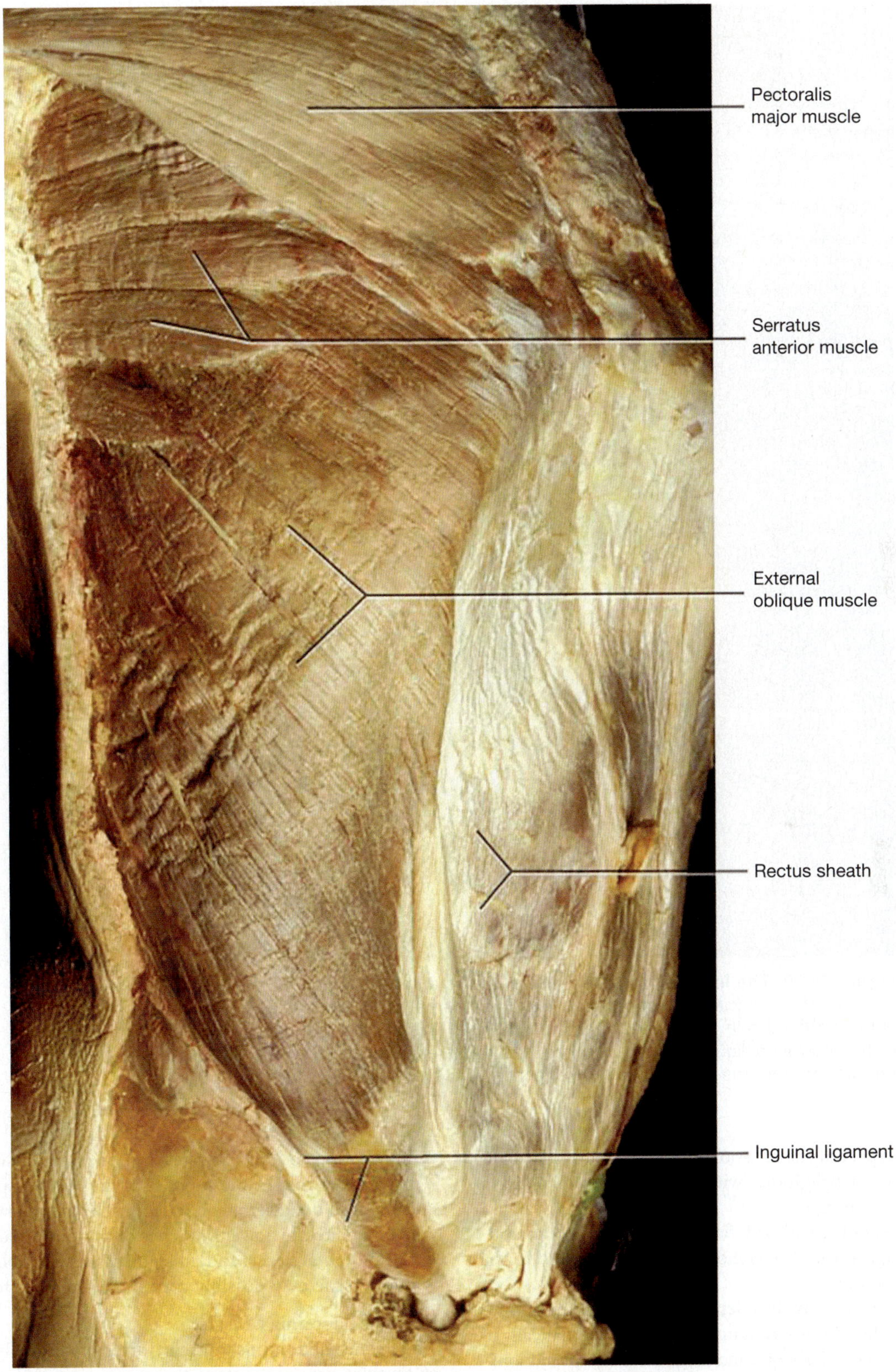

Figure 15.9. Lateral view of the torso, illustrating the external oblique muscle and its attachment to the rectus sheath and the inguinal ligament. Note the interdigitation of the external intercostal muscle with the finger-like attachments of the serratus anterior. In addition, the most inferior fibers of the pectoralis major also blend into the superomedial attachment of the external oblique. (Used with permission from the Willard/Carreiro Collection, University of New England.)

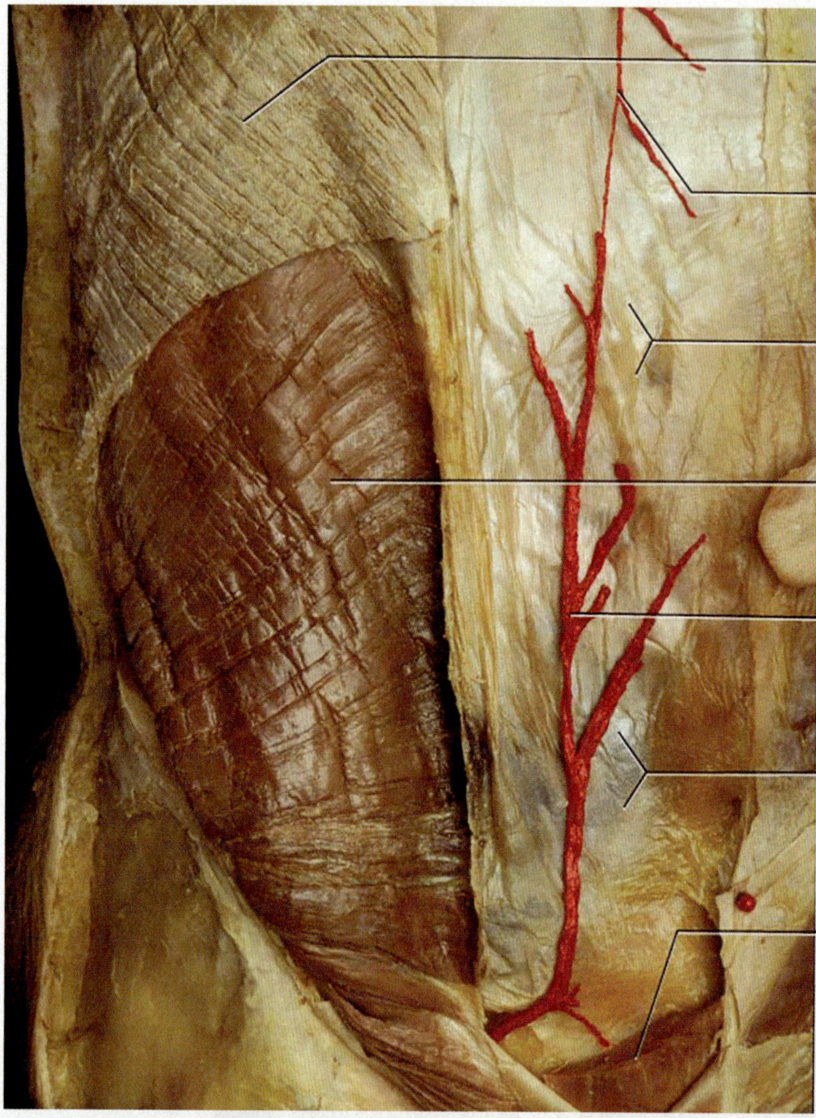

Figure 15.10. The internal oblique muscle. This is an anterior view of the abdominal wall. The skin and superficial fascia have been removed. The external oblique muscle was cleaned and a window cut into the muscle to expose the internal oblique. This photograph demonstrates the middle fibers of the internal oblique as they arise from the iliac crest and attach to the rectus sheath. (Used with permission from the Willard/Carreiro Collection, University of New England.)

- On the internal aspect of the anterior abdominal wall, the transversus abdominis interdigitates with slips of the diaphragm along the subcostal margin.
- Medially, the fibers of this broad, flat muscle attach to an aponeurosis that extends from the xiphoid process superiorly to the conjoint tendon inferiorly.[6]
- All muscle fibers are horizontally oriented except for the most inferior border where the muscle bands turn downward dramatically to joint those of the internal oblique and form the conjoint tendon.
- The horizontal orientation of the muscle fibers allows this muscle to act as a retinaculum, pulling the rectus sheath toward the posterior body and increasing the intra-abdominal pressure.
- This mechanical action has the effect of raising the diaphragm in the thoracic cavity.[7]
- EMG studies have demonstrated that the transversus thoracis is an obligatory muscle of respiration and is active in both exhalation and inhalation, ceasing its activity only as it approaches the portion of maximum inhalation.[5]
- In addition to its role in respiration, the transversus abdominis plays a key role in the support of the lumbar spine.[13]
- Similar to the internal oblique muscle, the transversus abdominis is innervated by lower branches of the thoracoabdominal nerves, the subcostal nerve, and, in some cases, the ilioinguinal and iliohypogastric may possibly contribute branches to this muscle.

Rectus Abdominis Muscle

The rectus abdominis muscle forms a vertically oriented band of muscles extending from the pubic crest and symphysis to the xiphoid process and medial subcostal margin (Fig. 15.12).

- The muscle is typically divided into four plates by three tendinous horizontal bands.
- The rectus abdominis is housed in a dense fibrous connective tissue wrapping termed the rectus sheath.
- Essentially, the sheath is composed of anterior and posterior plates derived from the splitting of the aponeurosis of the internal oblique.

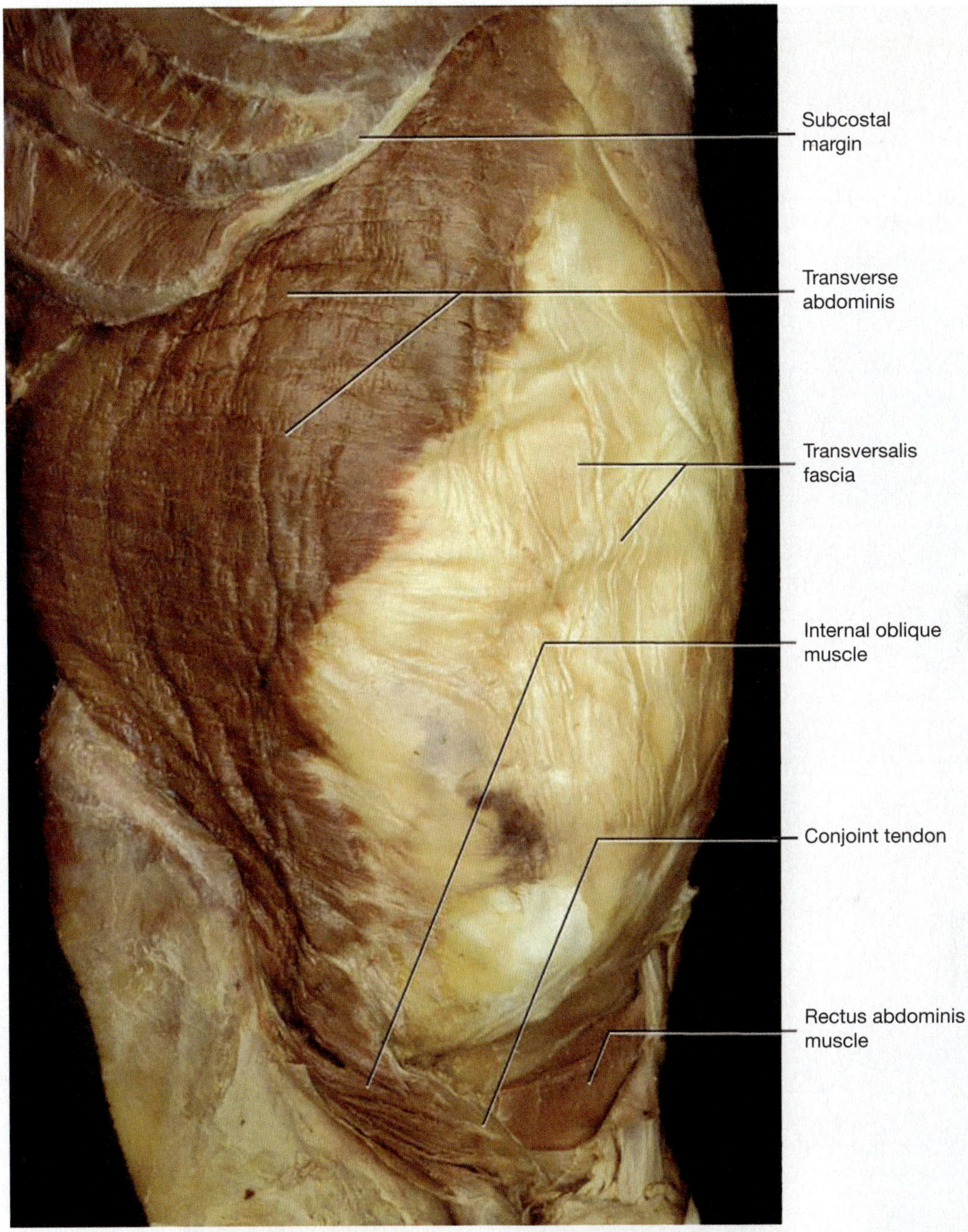

Figure 15.11. This is a lateral view of a male abdomen. The skin, the superficial fascia, and the external and internal oblique muscles have been removed to reveal the transversus thoracis (abdominis) muscle. The rectus sheath has also been removed. The whitish material is the transversalis fascia. Cotton has been placed in the abdominal cavity to expand the transversus abdominis muscle to its full extent. (Used with permission from the Willard/Carreiro Collection, University of New England.)

- This sheath completely surrounds the muscle with the exception of the posterior wall inferior to the umbilicus; here, a defect in the posterior wall of the fibrous sheath transmits the rectus abdominis muscle.
- Inferior to this line, termed the arcuate line, the posterior wall is composed primarily of the transversalis fascia.
- Major functions of the rectus abdominis are:
  - Flexion of the torso
  - Counterbalancing the paraspinal muscle of the back
  - Exhalation
- In addition, the rectus abdominis muscle, in combination with the other abdominal muscles, particularly the transversus abdominis, functions as a corset trussing the abdominal organs in place and pushing them superiorly to make a fulcrum (see section on the diaphragm) over which the thoracoabdominal diaphragm is draped.[7]

Combined Function of the Intercostal, Scalene, and Abdominal Muscles

The various intercostal muscles have differing functions in respiratory movements.

- The external intercostal muscle and the parasternal muscle are key players in inhalation, while the interosseous portion of the

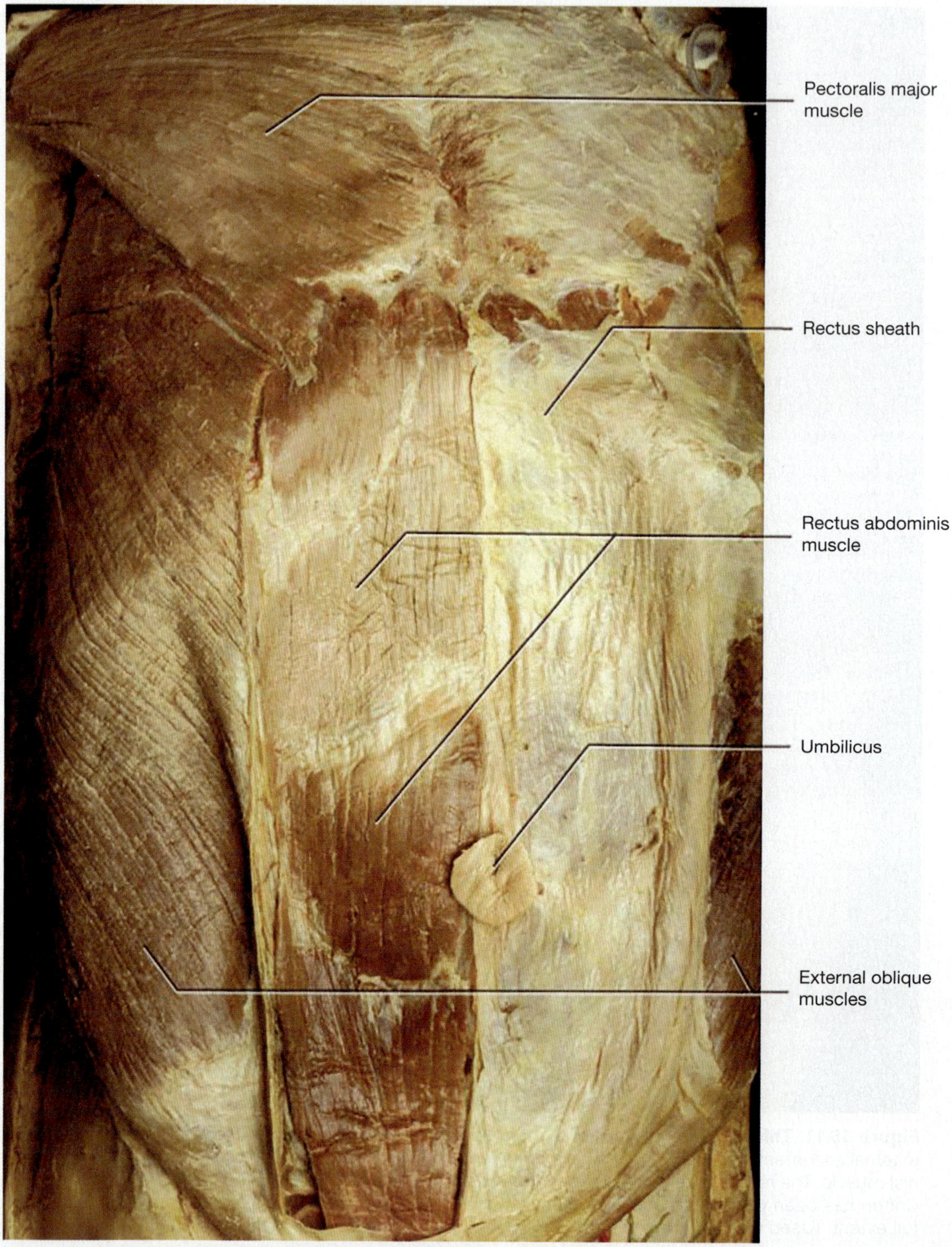

Figure 15.12. This is an anterior view of the anterior abdominal wall. The skin and superficial fascia have been removed to reveal the rectus sheath. The sheath has been removed on the right side of the individual to reveal the rectus abdominis muscle. (Used with permission from the Willard/Carreiro Collection, University of New England.)

internal intercostal muscle has significant involvement in forced exhalation.

- Despite the association of these muscles with different stages of respiration, electrical stimulation of any isolated intercostal muscle will approximate the ribs regardless of its location; thus, the factors differentiating the action of the external intercostal and parasternal muscle from the remainder of the internal intercostal muscle must reside outside the geometry of these muscles alone.[7]

The actions of the intercostal muscles are dependent on the resistance to motion at either end of the thoracic cylinder. This resistance is dependent on the state of contraction of the muscles attached to the cylinder ends. To further explain:

- The contraction of the intercostal muscles is coordinated with the activity of the scalene and abdominal muscles.
- Fixation of the first rib at the superior aspect of the cylinder supports inhalation.
- To initiate inhalation, the scalenes contract fixing the first and second rib which then causes a ripple-like effect of contraction of the superior external intercostal and parasternal muscles in a sequence-like wave down the thoracic wall to the eleventh intercostal rib to draw the ribs superiorly.
- A reverse or ascending wave is seen following contraction of the abdominal muscles and leads to lowering of the ribs and exhalation.[7,5] The contraction of the abdominal muscles fixes the lower ribs and subcostal margin, thus facilitating the lowering of the ribs during exhalation.

Control over the sequential contraction of the intercostal muscles has been shown to reside in the pattern of connectivity regulating ventral horn interneuron activity.[5]

- These cells regulate the discharges of the ventral horn motor neurons, which in turn innervate the intercostal muscles.
- The spinal cord interneurons are modulated by input coming from both the medullary portion of the brain stem and peripheral input from muscle spindles.
- However, this combined input is relatively weak compared to that of the central respiratory drive potential present in the ventral horn, thus suggesting that the spinal interneurons of the ventral horn are dominant.
- As with the control of individual muscle contractions in such repetitive actions as locomotion, there is a central pattern generator (CPG) formed by the interneuronal pool in the ventral horn.
- This group of cells generates repetitive patterns of activity for the motor neurons to deliver to the appropriate skeletal muscles.
- These patterns can be influenced by both the descending activity from the medullary brain stem and the peripheral activity from the muscle afferent fibers; ultimate control however appears to reside in the spinal cord.

The Pumphead in the Thoracic Cylinder

THE THORACOABDOMINAL DIAPHRAGM

The diaphragm is often described as a dome-shaped structure composed of skeletal muscle and tendinous attachments that partially close the passage from thorax to abdomen (Fig. 15.13). However, if the diaphragm is removed from the body and spread on a flat surface, it takes on a shape resembling that of a large butterfly with the central tendon as the body and the leaflets resembling head, wings, and tail. Each of the diaphragm's leaflets is named by its attachments.

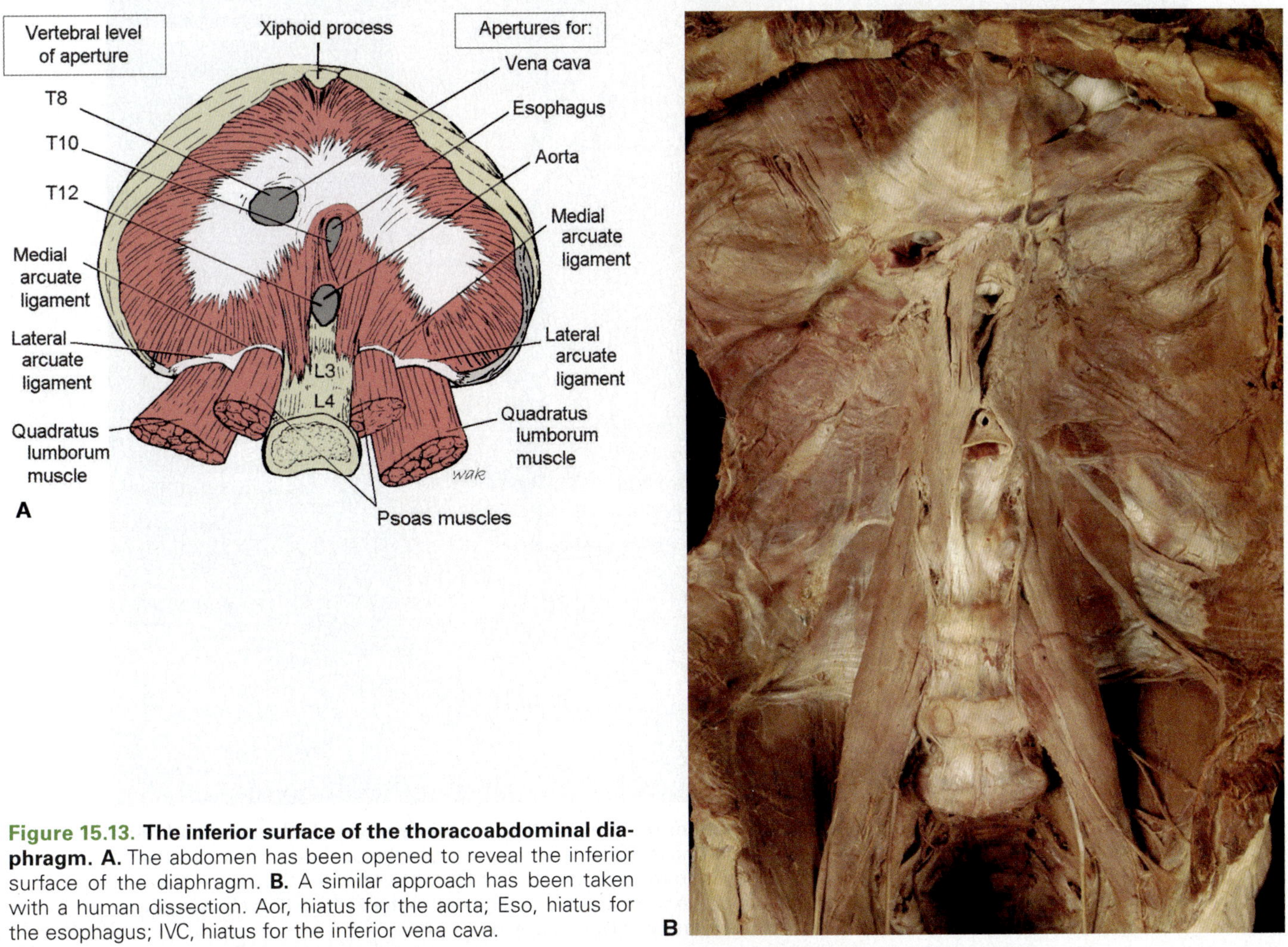

Figure 15.13. **The inferior surface of the thoracoabdominal diaphragm. A.** The abdomen has been opened to reveal the inferior surface of the diaphragm. **B.** A similar approach has been taken with a human dissection. Aor, hiatus for the aorta; Eso, hiatus for the esophagus; IVC, hiatus for the inferior vena cava.

- The sternal leaflets (head of the butterfly) are small and attach to the posterior aspect of the xiphoid process; occasionally, they are missing.
- The costal leaflets (wings of the butterfly) are the largest and attach to the lower six ribs where their muscle fibers interdigitate with muscular slips from the transversus abdominis.
- These two leaflets form the broad sheet of diaphragmatic muscle that courses vertically along the internal margin of the ribs.
- Finally, the lumbar leaflets (tail of the butterfly) extend from the medial borders of the central tendon inferiorly to form two aponeurotic arches, as well as the crura of the diaphragm.

The arcuate ligaments attach to the musculoskeletal structures in the posterior body wall.

- The medial arcuate ligament of the diaphragm is attached to the body of L1 or L2 medially; it then arches over the psoas muscle to attach to the tip of the anterior surface of that vertebra's transverse process laterally.
- The lateral arcuate ligament is attached to the anterior aspect of the same transverse process medially and crosses over the quadratus lumborum muscle to anchor laterally to the tip of the 11th or 12th rib near its midpoint (Fig. 15.14).

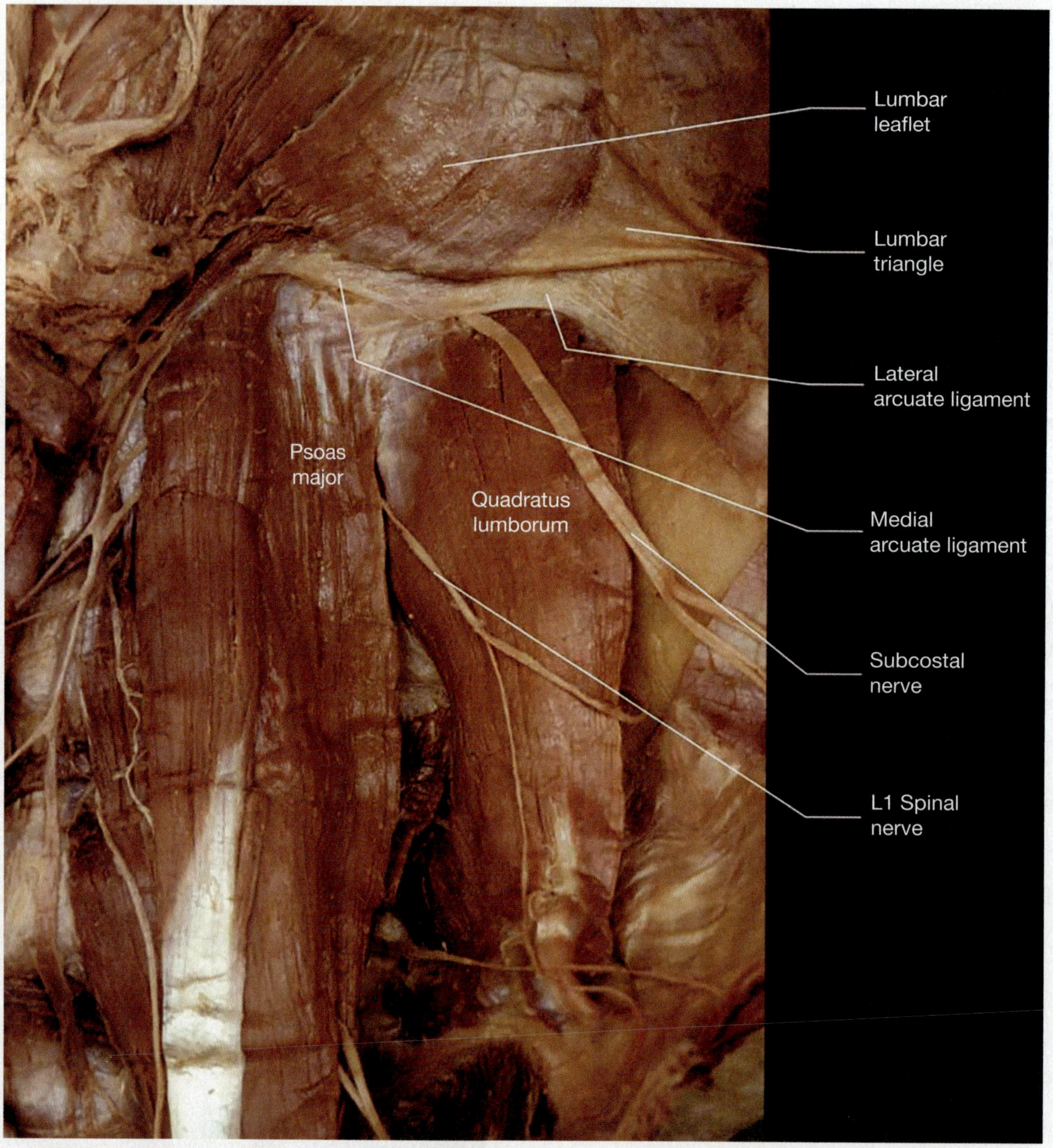

Figure 15.14. This is an anterior view of the posterior body wall following the removal of all organs and renal fat pads. It demonstrates the location of the medial and lateral arcuate ligaments on the posterior–inferior margin of the diaphragm. The medial arcuate ligament extends from the body of L1 or L2 to the tip of its transverse process. The lateral arcuate ligament extends from the tip of the same transverse process to the 11th or 12th rib. (Used with permission from the Willard/Carreiro Collection, University of New England.)

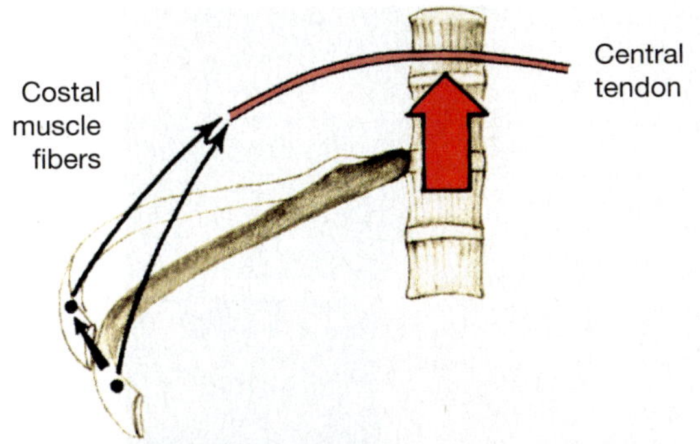

Figure 15.15. Mechanics of the diaphragm. The abdominal viscera (*arrow*) act as the fulcrum of the diaphragm, allowing it to elevate the ribs. (Reprinted from De Troyer A, Estenne M. Functional anatomy of the respiratory muscles. *Clin Chest Med.* 1988;9(2):175–193. Copyright © 1988 Elsevier. With permission.)

- The midline portion of the lumbar leaflets forms the crura of the diaphragm. Both crura arise from the medial most portion of the central tendon and sweep inferiorly, attaching to the anterior longitudinal ligament on the bodies of the upper three lumbar vertebrae.
- The right crus of the diaphragm is larger than the left.
- The medialmost fibers of each crus unite on the midline to form the median arcuate ligament that surrounds the aorta as it passes from thorax to abdomen.

Motor innervation of the diaphragm is accomplished by the phrenic nerve (C3–C5), sensory innervation is accomplished through the phrenic and from twigs derived from the lower intercostal nerves. (For a detailed review of diaphragm anatomy, see Anson and McVay, pp. 365–384.[14])

FUNCTION OF THE DIAPHRAGM

The contents of the abdominal cavity are forced superiorly into the central tendon of the diaphragm by the abdominal musculature (Fig. 15.15), the muscle most responsible for this is the transversus abdominis.[15]

- The dome shape of the diaphragm is created by a piston of viscera including the liver, stomach, and spleen.
- Much of the costal leaflet passes vertically along the wall of the rib cage to reach the subcostal margin and their attachment.
- This dome-shaped arrangement creates an elongated "zone of apposition" between the diaphragmatic muscle and the thoracic wall.[7]
- In this zone, the diaphragm is positioned directly against the costal wall, with no lung tissue in between.

The length of the zone of apposition proves crucial to the function of the diaphragm.

- With the visceral piston placed in the full upright position, contraction of the costal leaflets will pull superiorly on the subcostal margin while attempting to force the visceral piston inferiorly.
- If the visceral piston is adequately buttressed by the abdominal musculature, the central tendon only descends a short distance, less than two segmental interspaces, and the subcostal margin of the ribs is elevated.
- Since the lower ribs are attached by movable joints anteriorly and posteriorly, the body of the rib rotates outward and upward (referred to as "bucket-handle" motion).
- Thus, a function of the abdominal viscera can be considered to be the formation of a fulcrum over which the diaphragm is bent.
- The motion occurring across this visceral fulcrum greatly increases the volume of the thorax while minimizing the amount of descent required by the central tendon (reviewed in De Troyer and Estenne[7]).

It is important to realize that for the diaphragm to maximally lift the ribs during respiration, it has to maintain its vertical zone of apposition along the costal wall.

- Structural changes that alter this arrangement can significantly impair the ventilatory mechanics of the diaphragm.
- Structural changes that impact ventilatory mechanics can include such things as kyphosis, scoliosis, and morbid obesity.

ACCESSORY MUSCLES OF RESPIRATION

Abdominal Muscles

EXTERNAL AND INTERNAL OBLIQUE MUSCLES

Neither the external nor the internal oblique is active on quiet respiration. However, both muscles will become involved in respiratory movements during forced exhalation (reviewed in Epstein[12]).

- These muscles exert an inferior pull on the subcostal margin, thus sliding the thoracic walls over the diaphragm and visceral organs, in essence seating the piston higher in the cylinder.
- This gloving motion helps to decrease the volume of the pleural cavities in the thorax and thus facilitates exhalation.
- The gloving motion is also important in recreating the large zone of apposition preceding the next respiratory cycle.

Limb Girdle Muscles

SERRATUS ANTERIOR MUSCLE

The serratus anterior is a powerful limb muscle capable of influencing the movement of the ribs when the scapula is fixed.

- This broad sheet of muscle arises from the fleshy attachments to the anterior surface of the first eight or nine ribs (Fig. 15.16).
- Each band of the muscle wraps around the thorax passing between the posterolateral thoracic wall and the scapula to reach the medial border of this bone.[6]
- If the upper extremity is fixed by grasping an immovable external object, the serratus anterior can assist in raising the ribs.
- Thus, the serratus anterior can become an accessory muscle of respiration in stressful situations.

Use of this muscle to assist in respiration can be observed in cases involving hyperinflation of the chest such as COPD.

- The patient may grasp the bed rails, fixing the scapula, in an effort to recruit the serratus and assist in respiratory movements.
- The serratus anterior is innervated by the long thoracic nerve (C5–C7) derived from the supraclavicular portion of the brachial plexus.

Oropharyngeal Muscles and Respiratory Movements

PROTECTING AIRWAY PATENCY

The upper airway (the larynx and above) is a collapsible fibromuscular tube attached to the cranial base and extending into the cervical region.

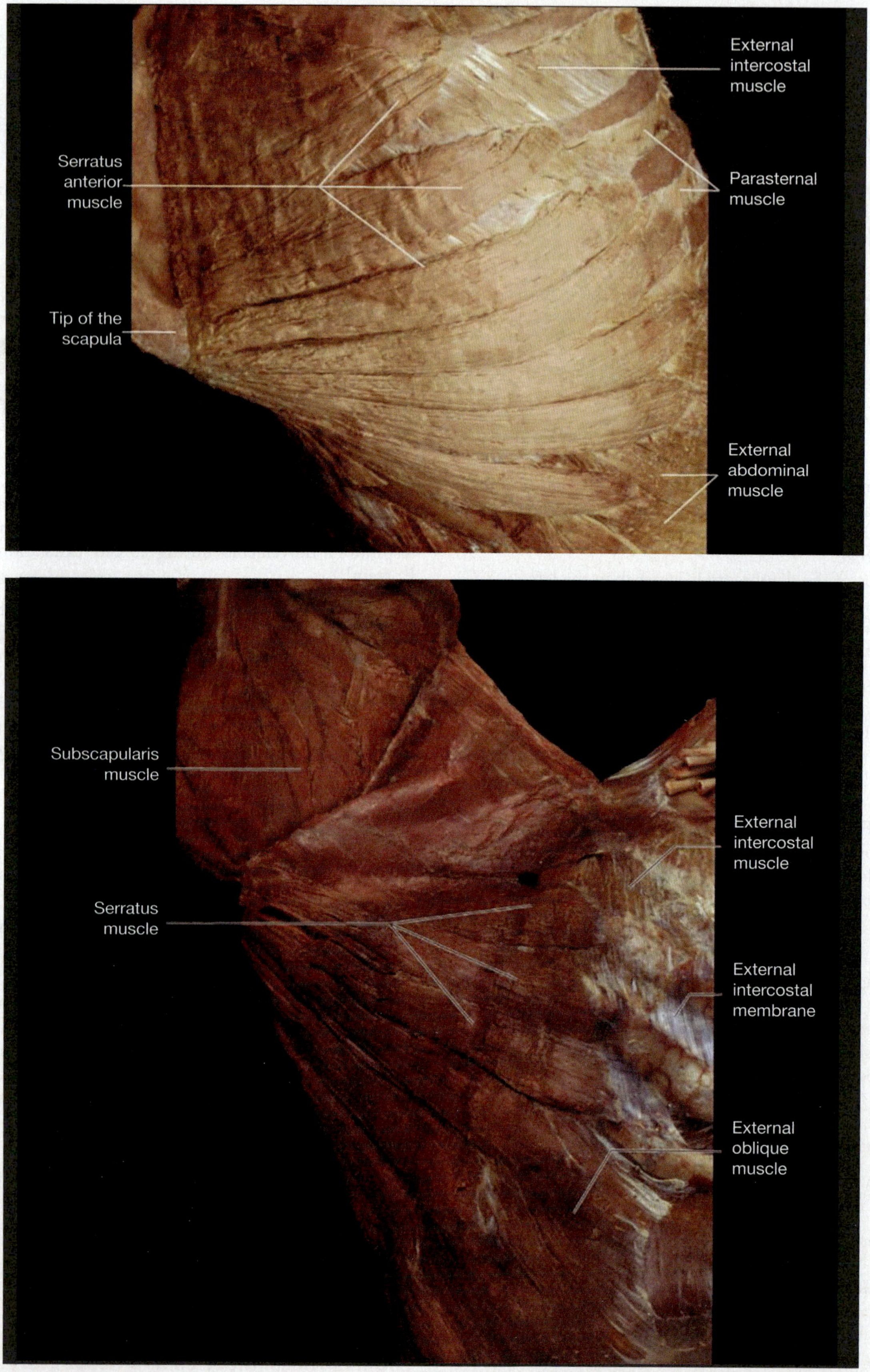

Figure 15.16. The upper illustration is a lateral view of the serratus anterior in a specimen where the scapula has been freed from the body wall by sectioning the latissimus dorsi, trapezius, and rhomboid muscles and cutting the clavicle. The scapula was then abducted as far laterally as possible to stretch the serratus anterior to its full length. The lower illustration is an anterior view of a specimen prepared in a similar manner. The scapula has been fully abducted to expose the serratus anterior muscle. (Used with permission from the Willard/Carreiro Collection, University of New England.)

- Compromise of the airway lumen can occur during inspiration and neonates are especially vulnerable to this event.
- Several muscles act in concert to protect the patency of the air; these are the muscles of the (reviewed in Lee et al.[16]):
  - Tongue such as the genioglossus
  - Those of the hyoid such as the:
    - Geniohyoid
    - Sternohyoid and sternothyroid
    - Thyrohyoid (reviewed in Lee et al.[16]; also see Thach[17])

Bursts of activity in phase with inspiration have been recorded from these muscles (reviewed in Thach[17]).

- An especially important muscle for opening the airway is the posterior cricoarytenoid muscle since it is the only abductor of the vocal folds.
- Although little is known concerning the respiratory-related activity of the posterior cricoarytenoid muscle in humans, work in other species has confirmed an inspiratory rhythm in the muscle.

Contraction of all of these upper airway muscles functions to increase airway rigidity and protect the patency of the lumen (Fig. 15.17).

- The neural pathways underlying the presence of a respiratory rhythm in the upper airway muscles have not been fully elicited.
- However, this activity may be in part due to pressure changes in the lumen of the airway detected by trigeminal afferent fibers and relayed to the hypoglossal nucleus through the trigeminal complex of the medullary brainstem.[18]

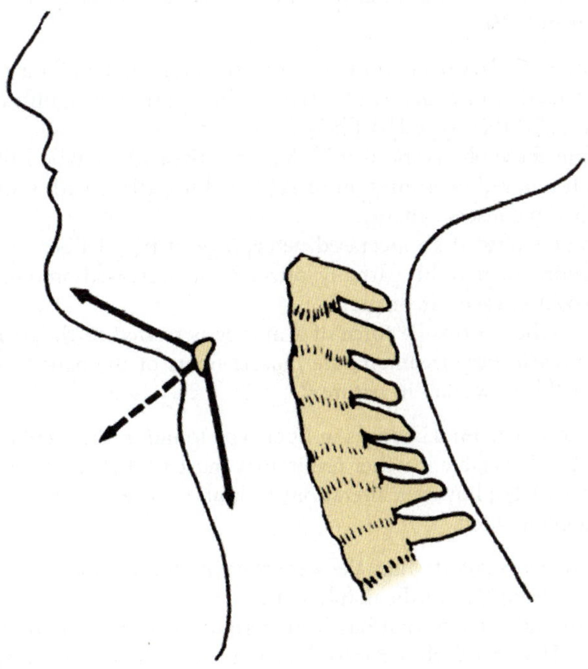

Figure 15.17. This is a schematic view of the muscles supporting the hyoid bone. Simultaneous contraction of these muscle pulls the hyoid anteriorly (*dashed vector arrow*), opening the airway. (Reprinted with permission from Van de Graaff WB, Gottfried SB, Mitra J, van Lunteren E, Cherniack NS, Strohl KP. Respiratory function of hyoid muscles and hyoid arch. *J Appl Physiol Respir Environ Exerc Physiol*. 1984;57(1):197–204. Copyright © 1984 the American Physiological Society.)

THORACIC LYMPHATIC DRAINAGE

The maintenance of proper lymphatic fluid production and drainage has been demonstrated to significantly influence the normal homeostasis and health of the pulmonary tissue.[19] Also see Chapter 14 Anatomy and Physiology of the Lymphatic System and Chapter 50 Lymphatic Drainage Procedures for further discussion.

- Pulmonary edema is the result of a mismatch between production and drainage of lymphatic fluid.
- The edematous condition compromises the integrity of lung tissue by forcing fluids into the interstitial and alveolar spaces, diminishing the ability of pharmaceuticals to access alveolar tissue.

Normally, contraction of the diaphragm and thoracic cage movement during respiration produce substantial pressure gradients between the thoracic and abdominal cavities, resulting in effective lymphatic drainage and venous return to the heart.

- Proper movement and lymphatic drainage throughout the lungs are considered important for the maintenance of normal function and a disease-free existence.
- In addition, proper movement is essential for fighting infection and for reducing healing time.
- Tissue congestion is thought to decrease the effectiveness of medical treatment since both leukocytes and medication have more difficulty getting to the target tissues.
- Tissue congestion also increases the risk of inefficient toxin and waste removal.
- To this end, the use of manual medicine techniques has been demonstrated to reduce the length of hospital stay and the length of time on antibiotics in randomized-controlled trials.[20]

RESPIRATORY MUSCLE PATHOLOGY

Airway Diseases

STRUCTURAL CHANGES IN CHRONIC OBSTRUCTIVE PULMONARY DISEASE

COPD includes patients with chronic bronchitis or emphysema, or both disorders.

- It currently is the third most common cause of death in the United States[21] and has recently become the third most common cause of death worldwide based on World Health Organization statistics.
- These diseases are most often related to tobacco smoking although they can be caused by exposure to any noxious gas including poorly ventilated cooking fumes and biomass heating sources.

Functionally COPD involves the increased resistance to airflow, typically expressed as a reduction in forced ventilation rate with air trapping in the lungs at end-stage exhalation.

- At a tissue level, COPD involves loss of alveolar architecture and narrowing of the small airways either through thickening of the wall from chronic inflammation or plugging with mucus secretions.
- Structurally, air trapping in the lungs at full exhalation results in hyperinflation with enlargement of the A-P dimension of the chest as is typically seen on clinical and radiographic examination of the patient with COPD.[22]
- The hyperinflation is due to either loss of static recoil in the parenchymal tissue or to dynamic hyperinflation, for example,

the presence of residual air in the lung at the end point of exhalation (reviewed in Fitting[23]).

- In essence, the narrowing of the distal end of airway allows air to be drawn into the alveoli but impedes movement of the air out of the lung.
- In hyperinflation, the diaphragm is typically lower in the thoracic cavity and shorter in length with a slightly increased radius of curvature, thus flattening the domed surface of the diaphragm.

Structurally, the flattened diaphragm in the patient with COPD creates a straighter line between the subcostal margins at a lower level in the thorax, thereby significantly reducing the zone of apposition[24] as well as the overall surface area of the muscle (Fig. 15.18).

- Normally, the zone of apposition represents 60% of the muscle's length, but that can be reduced to 40% in COPD.
- This structural change significantly decreases the efficiency of the diaphragm as a muscle of inhalation.
- In addition, the reduced length of the muscle alters the length–tension relationship for the muscle fibers; this reduction in length–tension relationship further compromises the diaphragm's efficiency.
- In the physically lowered state, contraction of the diaphragm can, in fact, become an expiratory action in nature.

An example of this expiratory conversion of the diaphragm is seen when attempting deep inhalations from the flattened state with a marked reduction in the zone of apposition.

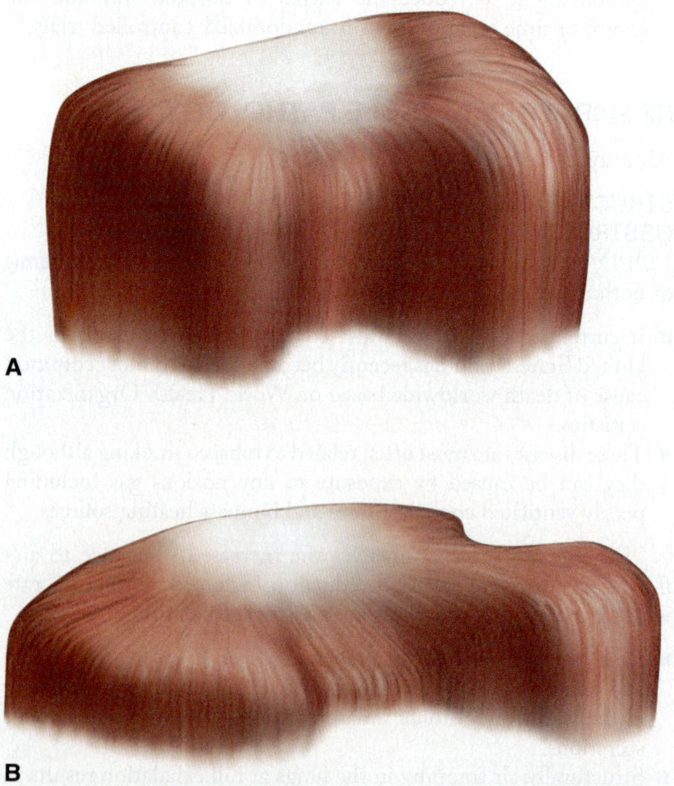

Figure 15.18. This figure illustrates a comparison of the shape of the diaphragm in a normal individual (A) and in a patient with COPD (B). Tracings represent three-dimensional reconstructions derived from a spiral CT imaging study. (Courtesy of Oran Z. Suta, as part of Dr. Willard's lab at the UNE College of Osteopathic Medicine.)

- The subcostal margin is drawn inward at the end stage as the flattened diaphragm pulls in the transverse plane; this is a paradoxical motion termed Hoover sign.[8]
- However, it appears that not all of the inward motion of the subcostal margin during attempted inhalation can be blamed on the loss of the zone of apposition.
- Additional inward force is most likely derived from the large negative intrathoracic pressure against which the diaphragm is pulling in a patient with COPD.[25]

Biochemical Changes in Respiratory Muscles in COPD

Along with the structural changes seen in the diaphragm of patients with COPD, significant histologic and biochemical changes result in adaptations aimed at increasing the efficiency of the muscle.

- A significant change involves the fiber types present in the muscle of the diaphragm.
- Current estimates of respiratory muscle histologic composition in the normal adult human diaphragm indicate:
  - 55% of the fibers are of the slow type (type I fibers)
  - 21% fast oxidative (type IIA fibers)
  - 24% fast glycolytic (type IIB and IIX fibers)
  - Histology of normal intercostal muscles finds greater than 60% are slow fibers.[26]
  - This relatively high percentage of slow twitch fibers present is thought to represent an adaptation imparting the respiratory muscles a fatigue-resistant quality.[27]

The diaphragm muscle of patients with COPD demonstrated a further increase in the slow twitch fibers with a shift to the slow isoforms of the myofibrillar proteins (reviewed in Polla et al.[26] and Levine et al.[28]).

- Since type IIA fibers contract faster than type I, then for a given contraction of equal length, type I fibers consume significantly less ATP than type IIA fibers.
- From these observations it is clear that the shift to type I fibers with reduced consumption of ATP in the patient with COPD helps to conserve energy.
- The benefits of an increased percentage of type I fibers in the diaphragm may be partially offset by a decreased amount of myosin in each sarcomere.
- Since the contractile force of a muscle is related to the density of myosin per sarcomere, the muscle fibers of the patient with COPD are weaker in nature.[29]

These structural changes in fiber type found in the diaphragm were not detectable in other respiratory muscles such as the intercostal muscles; however, alterations in limb muscle fiber type have been documented.

- Evidence suggests that the extremity muscles suffer a reverse effect from that of the diaphragm.
- Histologic observation has demonstrated a shift from type I to type II fibers with a concordant reduction in the diameter of both type I and II fibers that is proportional to the severity of the COPD as measured by a reduction in forced expiratory volume (FEV_1).[30]
- Atrophy, fatty replacement, and fibrosis were enhanced in the extremity muscles of patients with COPD when compared to control subjects.
- Other metabolic and microstructural changes in extremity muscles of those with COPD have been reviewed recently.[29]

- All of these alterations in muscle anatomy and chemistry contribute to significantly increased weakness in patients with COPD, a weakness and muscle mass loss that can be exacerbated by glucocorticoid therapy, and reduced motion such as seen in a sedentary existence.

SYSTEM INFLUENCES

COPD however is much more than a pulmonary system disorder; widespread systemic effects have been documented in patients with this disease.

- Systemic proinflammatory cytokines, such as tumor necrosis factor-α (TNF-α) and interleukin-6 (IL-6), result in cardiovascular effects and generalized muscle wasting[31] secondary to muscle and bone loss (reviewed in Balasubramanian and Varkey[29]).
- The weight loss seen in COPD most likely is associated with cachexia—selective muscle loss and protein degradation—not malnutrition, which is more generalized.[32]
- The cachexia is secondary to elevated proinflammatory cytokines such as TNF-α in circulation.
- In essence, in COPD, the body has entered a negative energy balance state.
- In addition to the musculoskeletal system, cardiovascular, renal, and nervous system dysfunctions have been documented in COPD.[33]

DOWNWARD METABOLIC CASCADE ASSOCIATED WITH COPD

The structural alterations in the diaphragm muscle geometry and fiber type make rapid breathing movements more difficult; thus, a sedentary lifestyle is common with COPD.

- It is well demonstrated that extremity muscle wasting is also a common feature of COPD associated with both a sedentary lifestyle and the systemic release of rhabdomyolytic proinflammatory cytokines.[30]
- Proinflammatory cytokines also have a stimulatory effect on the activity of osteoclasts, thereby enhancing the loss of bone.
- Principal areas of bony regression involve the proximal femur and the end plates of the vertebral bodies (reviewed in Balasubramanian and Varkey[29]).
- These changes increase the patient's susceptibility to femoral neck fractures and vertebral body collapse.
- Chronic hypoxemia, a condition involving low blood oxygen levels, is ubiquitous in the later stages of COPD.
- Inability to deliver sufficient oxygen to the tissue will exacerbate many of the previously noted changes in musculoskeletal system.[31]
- Diminished protein synthesis secondary to hypoxemia leads to diminished production of myosin in muscle sarcomeres and lower production of oxidative enzymes in mitochondria (reviewed in Balasubramanian and Varkey[29]).

Thus, in COPD a downward spiral is established; compromised respiratory muscle function leads to reduced motion as well as hypoxia and inflammatory reactions.

- All these results culminate in loss of muscle and bone mass with further reduction of motion in the patient.
- Lack of activity favors the stagnation of proinflammatory substances in the tissue further exacerbating the process.
- Although movement and exercise cannot restore the damage that has occurred in the lung, it can help arrest the downward spiral and improve the quality of life for the patient.

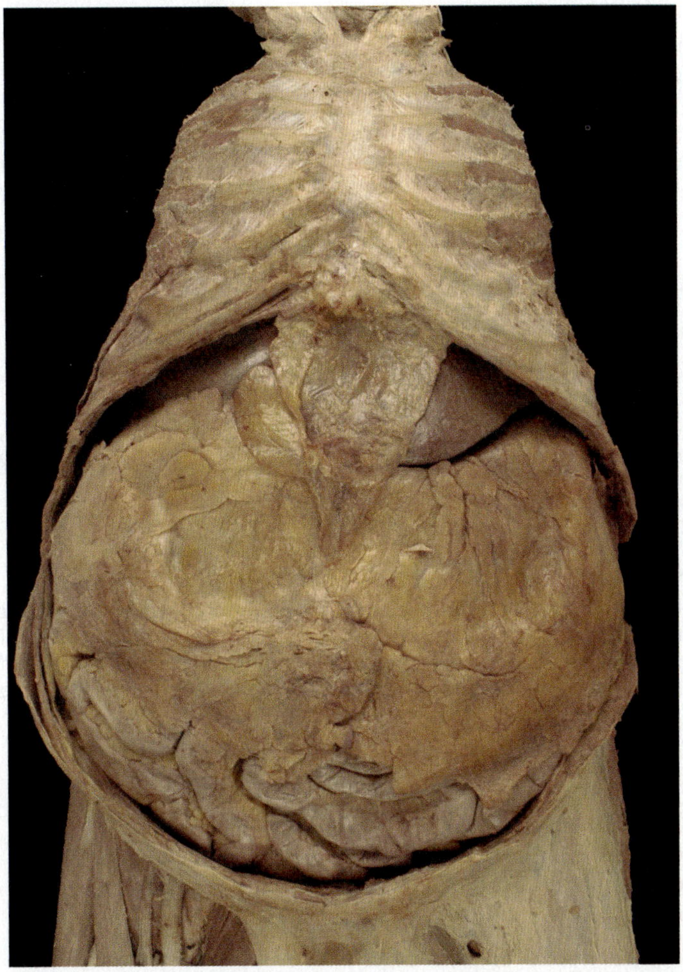

Figure 15.19. The torso of an obese female illustrating the flared, bell-shaped subcostal border. The lateral extensions of the subcostal margin would have the effect of flattening the diaphragm. Contraction of the diaphragm in this configuration would pull the subcostal margins inward, reducing the space available in the thoracic cavity. (Used with permission from the Willard/Carreiro Collection, University of New England.)

- The osteopathic approach to COPD should include consideration of the overall body structure and function in an effort to enhance the patient's ability to increase motion.

Structural Changes Exacerbating Ventilatory Compromise

OBESITY

Abdominal obesity expands the subcostal margins of the rib cage without necessarily altering the superior margin.

- With the expanding subcostal margin, the rib cage takes on a more bell-shaped appearance (Fig. 15.19).
- When this occurs without raising the apex of the diaphragm, the entire muscle becomes more flattened in shape.
- In essence, the lateral margins are moving outward and upward, getting closer to the level of the apex of the diaphragm, and thereby reducing the zone of apposition.
- Attempted deep respiratory excursions of the diaphragm result in lowering the apex closer to the level of the subcostal margin, potentially converting the diaphragm into a muscle of exhalation (Fig. 15.20).

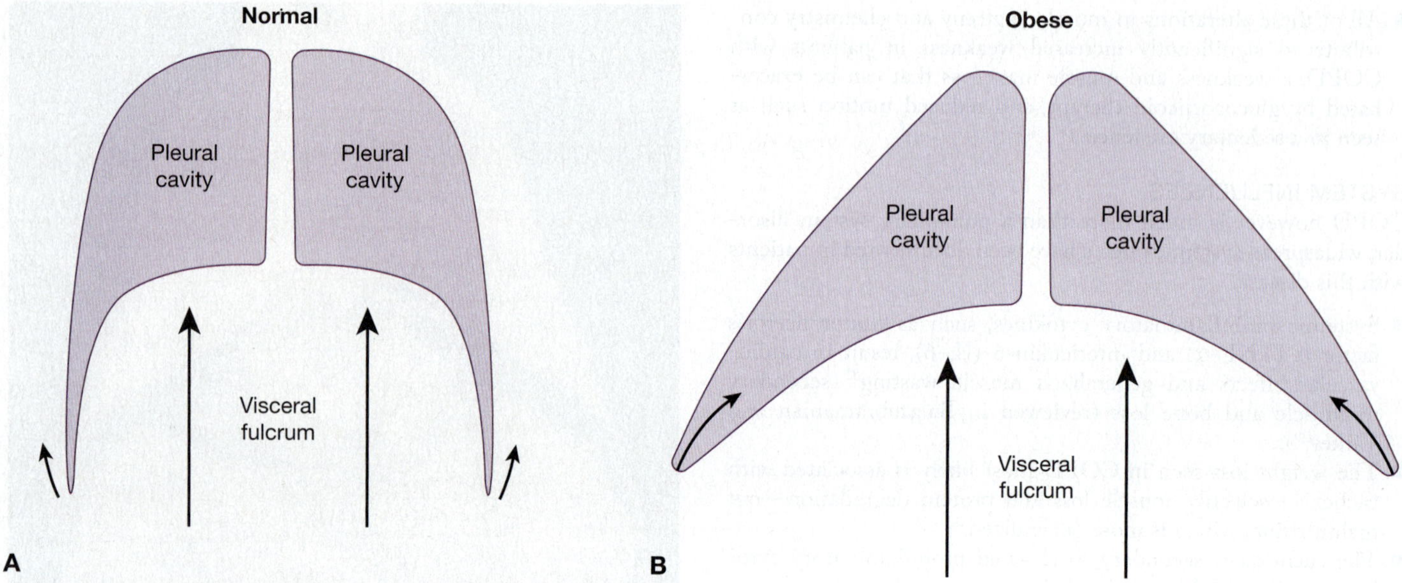

Figure 15.20. Change in pleural space configuration with abdominal obesity. A. The outline of a normal pleural cavity, featuring an elongated zone of apposition between the vertical portion of the diaphragm and the costal wall. **B.** The outline of the pleural cavity in an individual with abdominal obesity. The inferior and lateral margins of the pleural have been forced outward and upward. The diaphragm no longer has a vertical component. Contraction of the diaphragm in this individual would draw the costal walls inward, diminishing the volume of the pleural cavity, thus forcing exhalation.

In an effort to maintain consistent minute volume of oxygen to the lung in the face of reduced amplitude of rib motion, the frequency has to rise; thus, a high-frequency, low-amplitude panting results.

- The hypoxia that associates with reduced respiratory muscle capacity, in a manner similar to that described for COPD, may be a partial cause of the systemic inflammatory response seen in morbidly obese patients.

KYPHOSIS

Individuals with decreased bone density can suffer either acute or progressive loss of height in the anterior aspect of the vertebral bodies.

- In such cases, the vertebral column diminishes in length and slumps anteriorly creating a kyphotic posture in the thorax with enhanced lordotic curvature of the cervical spine as compensation.
- The kyphotic curvature allows the ribs to move inferiorly effectively diminishing, and in many cases completely eliminating, the intercostal spaces.
- Loss of the intercostal muscles prevents the superior and lateral movement of the ribs on inhalation, thereby compromising the depth of the respiratory excursion and the efficacy of respiratory movements.
- Again, a downward spiral of health ensues; compromised respiration yields hypoxia and reduced motion.
- Restricted movements lead to increased bone loss, furthering kyphosis and loss of thoracic motion.

SCOLIOSIS

Scoliosis represents a lateral deformation of the spine in the coronal plane creating a Cobb angle greater than 10 degrees.

- This disorder typically involves the thoracic and lumbar spine.[34]
- Scoliosis is often complexed by kyphosis resulting in the term kyphoscoliosis.
- Of the chest wall disorders, it is a leading cause of respiratory compromise.
- Initially, scoliosis involves a vertebral rotation causing a load imbalance across the vertebral body, it culminates in the development of a lateral curve.
- Lung volume and chest wall movements can be altered by the change in geometry of the thoracolumbar spine.
- These changes manifest as a reduction in lung volume and a restriction of rib movement.
- Respiratory muscle weakness has also been documented.

RESPIRATORY FUNCTION

Ventilation

Ventilation consists of the movement of air from outside the body through the upper air passages and the subdivisions of the conducting airways into the terminal respiratory units and back out again. The amount of inspired air that reaches the sites of gas exchange is determined by many factors, including:

- Lung parenchymal distensibility and the way in which air moves or flows through the tracheobronchial tree.
- A pumping action, requiring a neuromuscular and skeletal effort, is necessary to expand the lungs and to cause air to flow through the respiratory system.
- Therefore, ventilation chiefly depends on the capabilities of the following:
  - ☐ Thoracic cage including the respiratory muscles.
  - ☐ Properties of the airways.
  - ☐ Lung parenchymal respiratory units.
- Respiration occurs at the level of the terminal respiratory unit, which includes the alveoli, and it is defined as the process of gas exchange between the body and its environment.

- This exchange of gases depends on:
  - Volume and distribution of blood flow through the pulmonary circulation.
  - Volume and distribution of ventilation within the lungs.
  - Diffusion characteristics of oxygen and CO_2 across the air–blood barrier.
  - Regulation of breathing influenced by a variety of neurologic and metabolic factors.
- The mechanics of normal ventilation of the lung have already been described (see above).
  - However, it is important to note that the cervical and thoracic spinal column and the cervical fascia, which is continuous with fascia in the thoracic region, diaphragm, and eventually the musculature of the lumbar spine, act as the foundation for this entire respiratory movement process.
  - Gross changes in the organization of the spine, as seen with kyphosis and scoliosis, as just mentioned, can significantly impact the process of mechanical ventilation of the lungs.
  - In addition, somatic dysfunction at any spinal segmental level, whether due to a primary structural disturbance or neurologic or visceral disease, disrupts proper function.
    - An example of this concept is found in a patient who has an acute myocardial infarction and experiences dyspnea or shortness of breath.
    - The dyspnea could be due to associated heart failure, but it could also be due to upper thoracic viscerosomatic dysfunction from the infarction with associated restriction of rib cage movement. (See Chapter 13 Somatic Dysfunction, Spinal Facilitation, and Viscerosomatic Integration for further discussion.)

The interconnection and organization of the major muscles employed in respiratory movements are described above; however, it is important to note that axial (investing) fascia surrounding the neuromusculoskeletal elements in the thoracic region is continuous with the axial fascia present in the abdominal and pelvic region, including the fascia of the mesentery, retroperitoneum, and peritoneum.

- Respiration, therefore, affects viscera via fascial attachments and the resultant changes in thoracic and abdominopelvic pressure gradients and lymphatic and venous drainage from these regions, centrally to the heart.
- These movements are synchronous and interdependent.
- Osteopathic manipulative treatment (OMT) is aimed at enhancing all respiratory mechanics, and conversely, respiratory motion may be utilized to optimize OMT.
- In order to accomplish this, OMT should be directed at somatic dysfunctions of the entire spine, rib cage, thoracic inlet, diaphragm, and all muscles of respiration.

The lungs have a continual elastic tendency to collapse, pulling away from the chest wall, whereas the chest wall tends to recoil outward. These movements in opposite directions are responsible for the development of negative pleural pressure when the respiratory system functions in the intact state.

- The expandability of the lungs and thoracic cage is called compliance.
- Compliance is expressed as the volume increase in the lungs for each unit increase in alveolar pressure or for each unit decrease in pleural pressure.

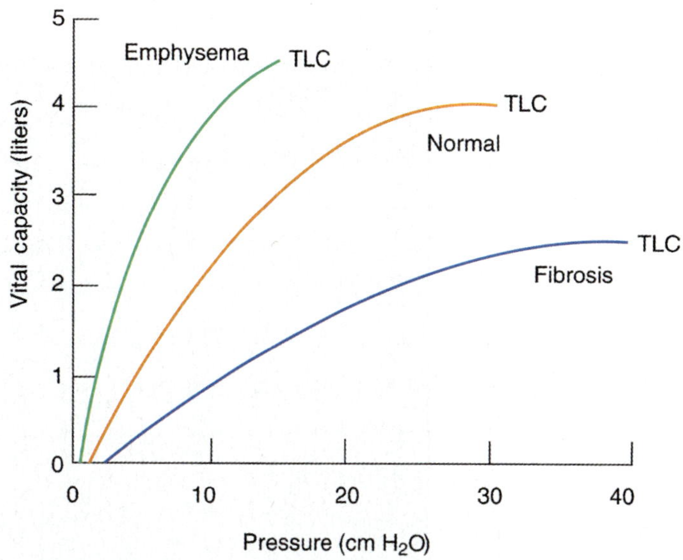

Figure 15.21. Representative volume–pressure curves from adult subjects of same age, sex, and body size showing changes caused by emphysema and pulmonary fibrosis compared with normal lungs.

- Because compliance is an expression of the distensibility of the elastic respiratory system, measured values of compliance depend on the elastic recoil properties of the lungs and chest wall.

The distensibility of the lungs varies significantly based on the patient's pulmonary disease.

- Patients with COPD, such as emphysema, have more distensible lungs.
- Patients with diffuse lung fibrosis or other infiltrative inflammatory diseases have less distensible, or stiffer, than normal lungs.
- Three volume–pressure curves from adults are shown in Figure 15.21; the orange cure is from a normal individual, the green cure from a patient with emphysema and the blue cure, a patient with interstitial fibrosis.

All three patients are assumed to be of similar age and body builds, so they would have thoracic cages with similar vital capacities.

- Note that emphysematous lungs are larger than normal and fibrotic lungs are smaller than normal.
- The curve from the patient with emphysema is shifted to the left and above that of the normal curve.
- The curve from the patient with fibrosis is flatter and shifted downward.
- When expressed at any given lung volume as a percent of the vital capacity (VC), compliance is lower with fibrosis.
- There is also chest wall compliance to consider since every lung disease adversely affects the thoracic cage.
- Total thoracic compliance involves both lung and chest wall components.
- Again, spinal somatic dysfunction can negatively disturb chest wall and lung compliance and, hence, lung ventilatory function.

Another factor that must be considered during breathing is resistance to airflow in the respiratory system.

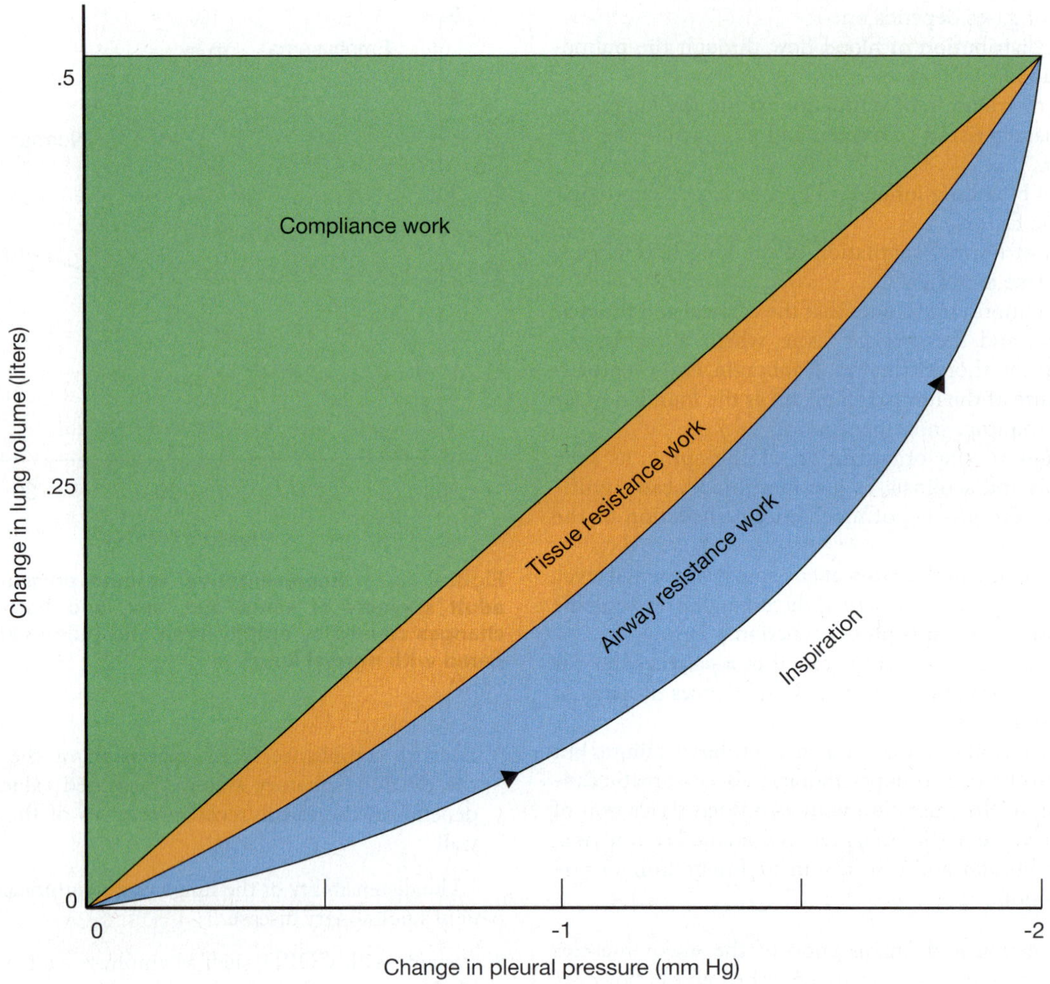

Figure 15.22. **Representation of three different types of work accomplished during inhalation: (1) compliance work, (2) tissue resistance work, and (3) airway resistance work.**

- Resistance is computed from simultaneous measurements of the airflow and the pressure difference causing the airflow.
- Measuring the pressure differences that cause air to flow requires specialized equipment.

The flow resistance properties of individual components of the respiratory system can be analyzed separately (e.g., the airways and the tissues of the lungs and chest wall).

- Figure 15.22 illustrates three types of work that are associated with the inspiratory effort:
  - □ Compliance
  - □ Tissue resistance
  - □ Airway resistance

During normal quiet breathing, most of the work performed by the respiratory muscles is used simply to expand the lungs. Conversely, during heavy breathing when air movement must flow through the respiratory passages at very high velocity, the greater proportion of work is then used to overcome airway and tissue resistance.

- In pulmonary disease, all three of the different work components can be vastly increased.
- Compliance work and tissue resistance work are especially increased by diseases that diffusely involve the lung parenchyma and/or involve the chest wall.
- Airway resistance work is especially increased in diseases that obstruct the airways, such as asthma and other forms of COPD.
- However, even diseases that do not involve the airways, often with increasing severity, affect tissue resistance work.
- In advanced obstructive airway diseases, the presence of malnutrition, respiratory muscle deconditioning, and somatic dysfunction can enhance tissue resistance work.
- During normal quiet breathing, no muscle work is performed during exhalation, which results from passive elastic recoil of the lungs and chest.
- In heavy breathing or when airway and tissue resistances are increased, expiratory muscle work does occur and at times can be greater than inspiratory work.

Normally, the lungs sit within the chest wall and diaphragm. The pressures and forces acting on these structures are interrelated. At the end of normal exhalation, during quiet breathing, the lungs are partially inflated. This is measured as the functional residual capacity (FRC).

- The elastic recoil of the lungs exerts a force that tends to empty the lungs.
- Chest wall volume is such that its elastic recoil promotes outward expansion.

- The lung volume at which the tendency of the lungs to collapse in an inward direction is matched by the equal and opposite tendency of the chest wall to expand is termed FRC.

For the lungs to achieve a volume other than the FRC, the respiratory muscles must actively oppose the tendency of the lungs and the chest wall to return to FRC.

- During inhalation to volumes above FRC, the inspiratory muscles must actively overcome the tendency of the lungs to decrease volume back to FRC.
- During active exhalation below FRC, expiratory muscle activity must overcome the tendency of the chest wall to increase volume back to FRC.
- At peak inhalation or total lung capacity (TLC), the force applied by the inspiratory muscles to expand the lungs is balanced by the inward recoil of the lungs.
- The major determinants of TLC are compliance and inspiratory muscle strength.
- If the lungs become stiffer or less compliant, such as in patients with lung fibrosis, the TLC decreases.
- If the lungs become more compliant, such as in patients with emphysema, the TLC increases.
- If the inspiratory muscles are significantly weakened or impaired, such as is seen with somatic dysfunction, they are less able to overcome the inward elastic recoil of the lungs and the TLC is reduced.

At the end of a maximal exhalation (residual volume, or RV), the force exerted by the expiratory muscles to decrease lung volume is further balanced by the outward recoil of the chest wall. The wall becomes extremely stiff at low lung volumes. The volume of gas found within the lungs at RV is influenced by two factors:

- The ability of the subject to exert a prolonged expiratory effort.
  - This is often related to thoracic skeletal muscle strength and performance and the ability of the patient to override certain sensory stimuli from the chest wall.
  - These stimuli create a sensation that tends to stop the expiratory effort.
- The ability of the lungs to empty to a smaller volume.
  - In lungs with diseased airways, flow limitation or dynamic airway closure can limit the amount of gas that is exhaled.
  - Thoracic cage dysfunction, including muscle weakness or airflow obstructive disease, can result in an elevated RV or air trapping, which disturbs ventilation.

From this discussion, it is easy to appreciate how the respiratory system is an ideal example of structure–function interdependence involving a musculoskeletal–visceral relationship. Somatic dysfunction at any spinal segmental level can adversely affect any of the previously described relationships through several potential mechanisms involving:

- Somatovisceral
- Somatosomatic
- Nociceptive reflexes

PULMONARY CIRCULATION

The principal function of pulmonary circulation is to deliver blood in a thin film to terminal respiratory units so that the exchange of CO_2 for oxygen can occur. Other functions occur besides gas exchange.

- This circulation acts as a filter of the venous drainage from virtually the entire body, removing or inactivating vasoactive substances as they pass through the lung.
- Pulmonary circulation provides nutritional substrates to the lung parenchyma that are important for the synthesis of lung surfactant, which is essential for maintaining alveolar integrity.
- The blood present in the lungs serves as a reservoir or sump for the left ventricle.
- Finally, pulmonary circulation modifies a variety of circulating hormones by biochemical transformation.[35]

The pulmonary vasculature must normally accommodate the entire output of the right ventricle.

- The thin-walled pulmonary vasculature has minimal resistance to blood flow and is capable of handling large volumes of blood at low perfusion pressures compared with that of the systemic circulation.
- The distribution of blood flow throughout the lungs principally depends on hydrostatic forces.
- With an increase in blood flow during exercise, the pulmonary vasculature is capable of recruiting and distending under-perfused vessels.
- Therefore, the pulmonary vasculature is capable of handling large increments in blood flow with a minimal change in vascular resistance and pressure.

Neurogenic, humoral, and chemical stimuli such as norepinephrine, acetylcholine, nitric oxide, and others cause active pulmonary vasomotor reactions.[36]

- Pulmonary arteries and veins are innervated with nerve fibers from the sympathetic trunks and the vagus nerves.
- The endothelial cells lining the pulmonary vessels can produce and release vasoconstricting peptides such as endothelin-1 and vasodilating gases such as nitric oxide.

The degree of influence that the autonomic nervous system exerts over the pulmonary circulation in the normal human adult is uncertain.

- Humoral influences, on the other hand, are likely to be more important.
- Several naturally occurring humoral agents can cause either vasoconstriction (e.g., catecholamines, angiotensin, prostaglandins) or vasodilation (e.g., prostacyclin, acetylcholine) of the pulmonary vascular bed.
- Alveolar hypoxia, at a local level, induces pulmonary vasoconstriction.
- Therefore, a close relationship between ventilation and perfusion is evident.
- A synergistic relationship exists between the effects of alveolar hypoxia and acidosis on pulmonary vascular resistance (Fig. 15.23).
- In the presence of blood or tissue acidosis, as hypoxia becomes more significant, the increase in pulmonary vascular resistance accelerates.
- Regardless of the etiology, thoracic somatic dysfunction adversely affects the lung's circulation, gas exchange, and immunology via substantial negative autonomic and humoral influences.

Pulmonary vascular resistance also increases if thrombi or vascular proliferation diminishes the intraluminal cross-sectional area of the pulmonary circulation.

- Pulmonary vascular resistance can also increase in any disease state in which the small pulmonary vessels are obliterated.

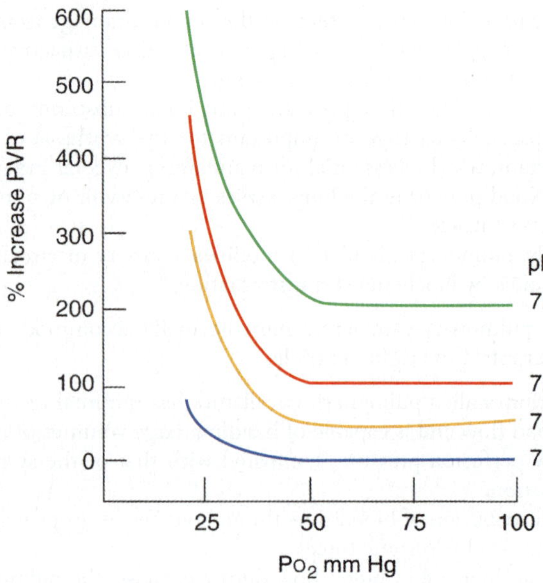

Figure 15.23. Effect of changes in inspired PO_2 on pulmonary vascular resistance (PVR) under conditions of different arterial blood pH. As inspired Po_2 is decreased, pulmonary vascular resistance increases; this effect becomes exaggerated and occurs at progressively higher Po_2.

- Over time, the pulmonary arterial pressure rises, and cardiac output eventually decreases as the right ventricle fails.
- Pulmonary hypertension may be the result of respiratory or cardiovascular disease and may complicate the course and management of the primary disorder responsible for its development.
- Pulmonary hypertension may also result from certain hematologic, infectious, and inflammatory conditions not solely involving the cardiorespiratory system, or it may occur in the absence of an identifiable precipitating disorder.

Regardless of the cause of the pulmonary hypertension, this pathophysiologic alteration usually remains clinically silent until the process is advanced.

- Patients then often present with signs of right-sided heart failure.
- Extrapulmonary diseases, such as severe kyphoscoliosis and fibrothorax, produce distortion of the chest cavity, mechanical compression of lung parenchyma, and alveolar hypoventilation.
- These changes often lead to substantial degrees of pulmonary hypertension.

These structural maladies may be amenable to OMT and other structural corrective interventions, thus the potential for positive influences on the pulmonary circulation by improving lung gas exchange relationships exists.

- Furthermore, OMT may affect certain autonomic and hormonal influences and reduce pulmonary vascular resistance in a more direct way.
- Bronchial, intercostal, internal thoracic, superior epigastric, subclavian, and musculophrenic vessels supply the lungs, chest wall, and diaphragm.
- The venous and lymphatic drainage systems are complex, numerous, and closely associated with the musculoskeletal system of the thorax.
- Increased movement in the thoracic walls enhances the movement of fluids in the venous and lymphatic systems.[37]

PULMONARY GAS EXCHANGE

The primary function of the respiratory system is to remove the appropriate amount of CO_2 from blood entering the pulmonary circulation and to provide adequate oxygen to the blood leaving the pulmonary vascular bed. Therefore, an adequate supply of fresh air to the alveoli and an appropriate degree of ventilation to remove CO_2 from the lungs and, hence, from the circulation, must be available. For these functions to occur, there must be:

- Adequate ventilation or delivery of oxygen to the alveoli and removal of CO_2 from the alveoli.
- Adequate circulation in terms of both perfusion and distribution of blood flow through the lung vascular bed.
- Adequate gas movement across the membranes that make up the alveoli and pulmonary capillaries.
- Appropriate matching of lung ventilation and perfusion.

Hypoxemia is associated with a variety of diseases that affect the lungs or other components of the respiratory system. The four basic mechanisms of hypoxemia are:

- Decrease in the inspired concentration of oxygen
- Hypoventilation
- Right-to-left shunt
- Ventilation–perfusion inequality

Diffusion impairment contributes to hypoxemia in only select clinical circumstances, which are generally extreme in character and uncommon in occurrence.

- The most common cause of hypoxemia is ventilation–perfusion inequality.
- Lung regions with low ventilation–perfusion ratios are most important for the development of arterial hypoxemia.

The essential mechanism underlying hypercapnia is inadequate alveolar ventilation for the amount of CO_2 that is being produced. The causes of arterial hypercapnia include:

- Increased CO_2 production
- Decreased ventilatory drive
- Disease of the respiratory pump
- Increased airway resistance making it difficult to sustain adequate ventilation
- Inefficiency of gas exchange resulting from an increase in dead space and/or excessive ventilation–perfusion inequality

For many patients with disease, more than one mechanism is responsible for the hypercapnia. Different clinical situations are generally associated with a certain mechanism that is responsible for hypoxemia.

- Hypoventilation as a cause of hypoxemia is always associated with an elevated arterial Pco_2.
- A loss of respiratory drive and a variety of neuromuscular diseases are associated with this mechanism of hypoxemia.
- A cardiac shunt as a cause of hypoxemia can result from the movement of blood from the right to the left side of the heart without entering the pulmonary circulation, as occurs with intracardiac shunts.
- Shunting of blood through the pulmonary parenchyma can also occur and is most often the result of disease in which there is an absence of ventilation in areas of lung that remain perfused.
- Atelectasis and alveolar filling diseases, such as pneumonia, respiratory distress syndrome, and pulmonary edema, often increase the shunt fraction of blood that goes through lung parenchyma.

As mentioned, ventilation–perfusion inequality is the most common clinical cause of hypoxemia.

- Lung airway and parenchymal diseases, including asthma, emphysema, chronic bronchitis, and interstitial lung diseases, including all of the infiltrative diseases, demonstrate hypoxemia by this mechanism.
- All of these diseases are associated with thoracic somatic dysfunction, which could influence lung function and further complicate gas exchange.
- A low mixed venous oxygen saturation can also influence the arterial blood in patients with an increased shunt fraction and/or ventilation–perfusion inequality made worse by hypoxemia.

VENTILATORY CONTROL

The many influences that affect breathing and gas exchange are mediated by a control system that incorporates peripheral and central receptors in a complex network of nerve pathways and integrating centers in the brain and spinal cord.

- The neurologic respiratory control system contains three principal interconnecting components:
  - □ A controller located within the central nervous system that initiates signals of its own, in addition to integrating information from sensing units
  - □ A group of effectors in the lungs, airways, and muscles of respiration that carry out commands from the controller
  - □ Different central and peripheral sensors that monitor the adequacy of breathing

Control of respiration by the central nervous system is functionally and anatomically partitioned.

- The brain stem regulates automatic respiration, whereas the cerebral cortex affects voluntary breathing.
- The cerebral cortex is involved in breath-holding complex behaviors, such as:
  - □ Talking
  - □ Crying
  - □ Laughing
  - □ Respiratory responses to pain
  - □ Apprehension
  - □ Excitement
  - □ Exercise
- Integrating neurons in the spinal cord possess efferent information from both upper and lower respiratory centers in the brain as well as afferent information from peripheral proprioceptors.
- Efferent autonomic impulses also travel in the vagus nerves from the central nervous system to the airways and lung parenchyma.
- Branches from the vagus nerves make up the parasympathetic innervation of the airways and with stimulation produce secretory and bronchoconstrictive influences.
- The medulla is the center for spontaneous respiration.
- Inspiratory neurons are found in the dorsal medulla, whereas expiratory neurons are in the ventral medulla.
- The respiratory activity found in the pons serves to smooth the transition from inhalation to exhalation.
- The pons also contains two important regulatory centers:
  - □ The apneustic center
    - The apneustic center appears to contain the normal inspiratory inhibitory mechanism.
  - □ The pneumotaxic center
    - The pneumotaxic center is believed to act as a fine tuner of the pattern of breathing by influencing the response to afferent stimuli generated during hypoxia, hypercapnia, and lung inflation.
  - □ Both of these centers also play a role in modulating respiratory activity.

Stimulation of respiratory components of the cerebral cortex inhibits respiratory movements and, in other areas, increases respiratory frequency.

- Whether the signal to breathe originates from the cortex or medulla, the phrenic nerves must eventually be stimulated.
- Certain behavior-related activities may override autonomic control (which responds chiefly to chemical stimuli and to changes in lung inflation) and cause marked changes in ventilation such as:
  - □ Breathing
  - □ Talking
  - □ Swallowing
  - □ Crying
  - □ Laughing

The descending neurologic tracts that originate in the cortical breathing centers and control voluntary breathing are separate from those that originate in the brain stem that involve involuntary breathing.

- The neurologic influence in these descending tracts is integrated with local reflex information at the level of the spinal cord from which the segmental motoneurons that innervate respiratory muscles emerge.
- These interrelated processes at the segmental level are complex and might differ in various respiratory muscles.

The main effectors of breathing are the muscles of respiration. Other central neuromechanisms regulate both the participation in breathing by skeletal muscle in the upper airway and the response of smooth muscle and mucous glands of the tracheobronchial tree.

- Inspiratory neurons and the medulla receive input from:
  - □ Chemoreceptors
  - □ Peripheral receptors
  - □ Thermoreceptors
  - □ Cerebral cortex
- Facilitatory central neural feedback circuits involving the
  - □ Hypothalamus
  - □ Pons
  - □ Reticular activating system

The respiratory system must be responsive to a wide variety of needs for ventilation. Therefore, it is desirable to have suitable sensors to initiate changes and to monitor whether any correction that occurs in ventilation is appropriate.

- Four sets of well-defined sensors have been described.[38]
  - □ Peripheral chemoreceptors include those found in the arterial aortic bodies and the carotid bodies.
    - The carotid bodies at the bifurcation of the common carotid arteries
    - The aortic bodies along the aortic arch function as chemoreceptors, monitoring the chemical composition of the arterial blood.
  - □ Central chemoreceptors, sensitive to changes of pH in the blood are found in the medulla oblongata.
  - □ Pulmonary stretch receptors located in the tissue of the airway and lung
    - Rapidly adapting stretch receptors (myelinated fibers)
    - Slowly adapting stretch receptors (myelinated fibers)

- Juxtacapillary (J) receptors (unmyelinated fibers)
- Bronchial C-fiber receptors (unmyelinated fibers)

□ Intercostal muscle and rib cage joint receptors

- Muscle spindle apparatus
- Golgi-tendon organs
- Joint receptors

Immediate hyperventilation is one of the principal compensatory responses to sudden hypoxemia.

- A decrease in arterial Po_2, an increase in arterial Pco_2, or a decrease in arterial pH increases chemoreceptor activity from the carotid bodies and/or the aortic bodies.
- Stimulation of the carotid body with signal transmission via the glossopharyngeal nerve to the medulla causes bradycardia and hypotension.
- Stimulation of the aortic body activates the medulla via the vagal nerve resulting in tachycardia and hypertension.

Certain central receptors work to maintain acid–base balance in the central nervous system.

- Chemoreceptors near the medulla respond to changes in bicarbonate and hydrogen ion concentrations in the blood and the Pco_2 in the cerebrospinal fluid.
- The lungs and upper airways are equipped with a multitude of receptors that, when stimulated, have profound effects on breathing as well as on the circulation of other visceral and somatic systems.
- Receptors in the skeletal muscles of respiration help regulate muscle behavior at the spinal segmental level.
- Afferent impulses that originate from these sensors and go to the brain in the ascending spinal tract likely have some influence on the control of breathing.
- Muscle sensors have been linked to the sensation of dyspnea.
- Nociceptor influence at a spinal segmental level could easily influence not only respiratory muscle function and the sensation of dyspnea but also lung function including gas exchange and hemodynamics.
- The nociceptive reflex can be initiated by diseases of either visceral or somatic origin.
- Located in the walls of the airways throughout the lungs are stretch receptors that transmit signals through the vagal system into the central nervous system when the lungs become overstretched.
- These signals affect inhalation in a similar way as signals from the pneumotaxic center (i.e., they limit the duration of inhalation).
- This breathing control process is called the Hering–Breuer inflation reflex.
- This reflex helps protect the lungs from overinflation and from the development of barotrauma.

SUMMARY

The anatomy of mandatory and selected accessory muscles of respiration has been reviewed. The structure of these muscles has been related to their specific functions in the respiratory movements. Dysfunction of these muscles occurs in a number of disorders such as COPD, obesity, and kyphosis. The implications of these structural changes on the respiratory movements have been examined and their resulting systemic effect considered. Each disorder leads to a vicious downward spiral involving motion restriction, hypoxia, inflammation, and further motion restriction. The role of the osteopathic physician is to help the patient restore homeostasis by facilitating motion in the thoracic cage, spine, and the extremities in an effort to arrest the vicious cycle. In addition, thoracic and pulmonary physiology has been reviewed with a focus on the importance of the neuromusculoskeletal system to pulmonary gas exchange and ventilation.

REFERENCES

1. Standring S. *Gray's Anatomy. The Anatomical Basis of Clinical Practice.* Elsevier Limited; 2021.
2. Belvisi MG. Overview of the innervation of the lung. *Curr Opin Pharmacol.* 2002;2:211–215.
3. Buels KS, Fryer AD. Muscarinic receptor antagonists: effects on pulmonary function. *Handb Exp Pharmacol.* 2012;317–341.
4. Gardner ED, Gray DJ, O'Rahilly R. *Anatomy: A Regional Study of Human Structure.* W.B. Saunders Company; 1975.
5. De Troyer A, Kirkwood PA, Wilson TA. Respiratory action of the intercostal muscles. *Physiol Rev.* 2005;85:717–756.
6. O'Rahilly R. *Gardner-Gray-O'Rahilly Anatomy: A Regional Study of Human Structure.* W.B. Saunders Comp; 1986.
7. De Troyer A, Estenne M. Functional anatomy of the respiratory muscles. *Clin Chest Med N Am.* 1988;9:175–193.
8. De Troyer A, Legrand A, Gevenois PA, Wilson TA. Mechanical advantage of the human parasternal intercostal and triangularis sterni muscles. *J Physiol.* 1998;513:915–925.
9. De Troyer A, Ninane V, Gilmartin JJ, Lemerre C, Estenne M. Triangularis sterni muscle use in supine humans. *J Appl Physiol.* 1987;62:919–925.
10. Morrison AB The levatores costarum and their nerve supply. *J Anat.* 1954;88:19–24.
11. Mier A, Brophy C, Estenne M, Moxham J, Green M, De Troyer A. Action of abdominal muscles on rib cage in humans. *J Appl Physiol.* 1985;58: 1438–1443.
12. Epstein SK. An overview of respiratory muscle function. *Clin Chest Med N Am.* 1994;15:619–639.
13. Vleeming A, Schuenke MD, Danneels L, Willard FH. The functional coupling of the deep abdominal and paraspinal muscles: the effects of simulated paraspinal muscle contraction on force transfer to the middle and posterior layer of the thoracolumbar fascia. *J Anat.* 2014;225:447–462.
14. Anson BJ, McVay CB. *Surgical Anatomy.* W.B. Sunders & Co.; 1984.
15. De Troyer A, Estenne M, Ninane V, Van Gansbeke D, Gorini M. Transversus abdominis muscle function in humans. *J Appl Physiol.* 1990; 68:1010–1016.
16. Lee KZ, Fuller DD, Lu IJ, Lin JT, Hwang JC. Neural drive to tongue protrudor and retractor muscles following pulmonary C-fiber activation. *J Appl Physiol.* 2007;102:434–444.
17. Thach BT. Neuromuscular control of upper airway patency. *Clin Perinatol N Am.* 1992;19:773–788.
18. Hwang JC, StJohn WM, Bartlett D Jr. Afferent pathways for hypoglossal and phrenic responses to changes in upper airway pressure. *Respir Physiol.* 1984;55:341–354.
19. Murray JF. Pulmonary edema: pathophysiology and diagnosis. *Int J Tuberc Lung Dis.* 2011;15:155–160.
20. Yao S, Hassani J, Gagne M, George G, Gilliar W. Osteopathic manipulative treatment as a useful adjunctive tool for pneumonia. *J Vis Exp.* 2014;50687.
21. Pahal P, Avula A, Sharma S. Emphysema. In: *StatPearls*; 2023.
22. Celli BR. Pathophysiology of chronic obstructive pulmonary disease. *Chest Surg Clin N Am.* 1995;5:623–634.
23. Fitting JW. Respiratory muscles in chronic obstructive pulmonary disease. *Swiss Med Wkly.* 2001;131:483–486.
24. Cassart M, Pettiaux N, Gevenois PA, Paiva M, Estenne M. Effect of chronic hyperinflation on diaphragm length and surface area. *Am J Respir Crit Care Med.* 1997;156:504–508.
25. Laghi F, Tobin MJ. Disorders of the respiratory muscles. *Am J Respir Crit Care Med.* 2003;168:10–48.
26. Polla B, D'Antona G, Bottinelli R, Reggiani C. Respiratory muscle fibres: specialisation and plasticity. *Thorax.* 2004;59:808–817.
27. Ottenheijm CA, Heunks LM, Dekhuijzen RP. Diaphragm adaptations in patients with COPD. *Respir Res.* 2008;9:12.
28. Levine S, Kaiser L, Leferovich J, Tikunov B. Cellular adaptations in the diaphragm in chronic obstructive pulmonary disease. *N Engl J Med.* 1997;337:1799–1806.

29. Balasubramanian VP, Varkey B. Chronic obstructive pulmonary disease: effects beyond the lungs. *Curr Opin Pulm Med.* 2006;12:106–112.
30. Gosker HR, Kubat B, Schaart G, van der Vusse GJ, Wouters EF, Schols AM. Myopathological features in skeletal muscle of patients with chronic obstructive pulmonary disease. *Eur Respir J.* 2003;22:280–285.
31. Chamberlain JS. Cachexia in cancer–zeroing in on myosin. *N Engl J Med.* 2004;351:2124–2125.
32. Debigare R, Cote CH, Maltais F. Peripheral muscle wasting in chronic obstructive pulmonary disease. Clinical relevance and mechanisms. *Am J Respir Crit Care Med.* 2001;164:1712–1717.
33. Agusti AG, Noguera A, Sauleda J, Sala E, Pons J, Busquets X. Systemic effects of chronic obstructive pulmonary disease. *Eur Respir J.* 2003;21: 347–360.
34. Al-Qadi MO. Disorders of the chest wall: clinical manifestations. *Clin Chest Med.* 2018;39:361–375.
35. Erdos EG. Conversion of angiotensin I to angiotensin II. *Am J Med.* 1976;60:749–759.
36. Barnes PJ, Liu SF. Regulation of pulmonary vascular tone. [Review]. *Pharmacol Rev.* 1995;47:87–131.
37. Downey HF, Durgam P, Williams AG Jr, Rajmane A, King HH, Stoll ST. Lymph flow in the thoracic duct of conscious dogs during lymphatic pump treatment, exercise, and expansion of extracellular fluid volume. *Lymphat Res Biol.* 2008;6:3–13.
38. Jacono FJ, Soler X, Malhotra A. Chapter 11: control of ventilation. In: MA Grippi, ed. *Fishman's Pulmonary Diseases and Disorders.* McGraw-Hill Education; 2015.

16 Psychoneuroimmunology

SCOTT WILKIE ▪ TEODOR HUZIJ

KEY CONCEPTS

- The field of psychoneuroimmunology (PNI) is a relatively new area of study.
- Psychoneuroimmunology describes the interplay between the central nervous system (CNS), psychological/behavioral elements, immune system, and the endocrine system.
- Identified neuroimmune reflexes allow fast interactions between the neurologic and immune systems.
- Neuroendocrine pathways, such as the hypothalamic–pituitary–adrenal axis (HPA), respond to stressors systemically.
- Psychological factors, including depression and anxiety, have been associated with negative comorbid cardiovascular outcomes and immune system suppression.
- Approaching the field of psychoneuroimmunology through the lens of osteopathic philosophy reveals significant insights for the practice of osteopathic medicine.

INTRODUCTION

The disciplines of neurology and immunology have historically been separate studies due to the technically challenging concepts and specific scientific jargon. However, the conceptual interplay between the two disciplines has been noted frequently throughout history. The first discussion of Multiple Sclerosis appears in notes and diaries from around the year 1200 in an Icelandic woman, with significantly more discussion from detailed personal diaries of Sir Augustus d'Esté, born in 1794 (grandson of King George III of England) and the British writer W. N. P. Barbellion (1889–1919). Advances were made from the 1600s (myasthenia gravis), 1800s (Parkinson disease, Huntington disease, Charcot–Marie Tooth disease), and the 1900s (Alzheimer disease, encepahalitis lethargica, and numerous advances in the basic sciences). However, the *Journal of Neuroimmunology* was not created until 1981, and the term neuroimmunology only first appears on PubMed in 1982. Since then, the field has developed from antibody-mediated disease into numerous areas of special investigation, such as investigations into neurogenic inflammation outside of the brain and spinal cord.[1]

With the expansion of neuroimmunology in the 1970s and early 1980s, the discipline of psychoneuroimmunology (PNI) was developed through the work of Ader and Cohen, who found that the immune response could be behaviorally conditioned like Pavlov's studies in canines.[2] The idea that the central nervous system (CNS) may exhibit regulation over the immune system and that the immune system may communicate with the nervous system led to a surge of new scientific advancements. The field of PNI now describes the interplay between the CNS, psychological/behavioral elements, immune system, and the endocrine system.[3,4]

NEUROIMMUNOLOGY CONCEPTS

The Neuroimmune Reflex

Immune homeostasis was historically described as a largely humoral and cellular (T-cell) response. The humoral regulation was provided by glucocorticoid hormones and anti-inflammatory cytokines, while the cellular regulations were mostly performed by T cells and activated macrophages. However, the communication between these mechanisms has inherent limitations. First, communication largely relies on intercellular mechanisms, such as cytokines, and cell-to-cell contact. This means that their response time to changes in their environment is relatively slow. Second, this makes integrating responses to multiple inputs throughout the immunologic environment both challenging and inefficient. Finally, these mechanisms rely on the circulatory system for distribution, making the response inherently systemic, and thus lacking tissue-specific responses.[5]

The neuroimmune reflex addresses these limitations. Neural signaling is fast, unidirectional, exhibits specificity, and can integrate both excitatory and inhibitory signals from a variety of different inputs. Thanks to the explosion of research in Neuroimmunology and PNI, we now know that the nervous system and the immune system interact extensively.

The basic concept of the muscle stretch reflex was established by Sherrington in the early 1900s on the patellar tendon. He noted that tapping the patellar tendon activated stretch receptors, which sent afferent information via action potentials back toward the CNS, where these action potentials were processed and activated an efferent motor neuron to contract the extensor muscle group. Importantly, Sherrington recognized that the sensory information also activated an interneuron response, which inhibited the other flexor muscles. He thought of this as a homeostatic response that stabilized the mechanism.[6] This set the foundation for exploration of the deep tendon reflex mechanism.

Further research on reflex mechanisms demonstrated reflex control of organ systems. For example, reflex mechanisms on the heart were demonstrated in early studies. It was shown that the vagus nerve (the major cholinergic regulatory input to the heart) provides an inhibitory effect on heart rate. In other words, stimulation of the vagus nerve decreases heart rate. In contrast, adrenergic inputs stimulate the heart rate. Thus, the controlling mechanisms of the cardiac cycle began to be understood. Sensory nerves would monitor heart rate and send the information to the brain, where the information regarding heart rate would be processed. Based on a heart rate "set point," either a cholinergic or adrenergic output would be determined by interneurons in the brainstem nuclei, which would maintain heart rate homeostasis. Our understanding of the heart and its regulatory systems has continued to advance, but the basic reflex principles of organ homeostasis had been established.[7]

Once established, researchers sought to understand the reflex mechanisms that maintain homeostasis in other organ systems. One fortuitous observation led to the discovery that the innate immune system, like the heart, was regulated by a reflex of the vagus nerve. The discovery illustrated that the information carried by the vagus nerve regulated the systemic release of tumor necrosis factor (TNF), an inflammatory cytokine of the innate immune system.[7] This finding led to significant advances in understanding the reflex regulation of the vagus nerve on inflammation.

A brief summary of the basic principles of the neuroimmune reflex is provided below. However, the detailed scientific mechanisms are beyond the scope of this chapter. Consider the review articles by Andersson and Tracey,[5] and Pavlov, Chavin, and Tracey,[2] for an introductory explanation on the mechanisms of vagal neuron regulation of inflammation via the following receptors and transcription factors.

- α7 nicotinic acetylcholine (ACh) receptors (α7 nAChR) (associated with a cholinergic anti-inflammatory pathway in the brain)
- Toll-like receptors (TLRs) (important mediators of inflammatory pathways in the gut)
- NF-κB (a transcription factor that induces the expression of various proinflammatory genes)

Numerous cytokines and other molecules that were thought to be specific to regulating the immune system have been discovered on sensory neurons, such as TLRs, TNF, and many interleukins (IL-1β, etc.). Similarly, many molecules thought to be solely for neural communication have been identified to play a role in regulating the immune system. Monocytes, macrophages, T and B cells, endothelial cells, and dendritic cells have been found to display muscaricinic and nicotinic ACh receptors, as well as α- and β-adrenergic receptors.[2]

- Nociceptors are known to express several different types of voltage-gated sodium channels and transient receptor potential (TRP) ion channels, which mediate depolarization to "noxious" stimuli. These noxious stimuli can come in a variety of different forms, such as thermal changes, mechanical changes, chemical sensitivities, or other forms of tissue stressors.[8] These same sensory neurons also exhibit receptors for numerous immune cell cytokines, lipids, and growth factors (TNF, ILs, prostaglandins, etc.). The combined interactions lead to increased sensitivity of these sensory nerves, similar to what would be seen in somatic dysfunction. These features encourage feedback and modification between the two systems. Tissue stress (oxidative strain, damage, infection, etc.) brings about an immune inflammatory response, which facilitates sensory nerves, which is then modified in the CNS, and the CNS creates a feedback mechanism to regulate the immune system inflammatory response.
- As previously mentioned through the vagus nerve, the autonomic nervous system plays a regulatory role in modulation of the immune system. Norepinephrine and epinephrine mediate changes in neutrophils, macrophages, T cells, monocytes, and numerous other immune cells. Signaling in the β2-adrenergic receptor is thought to be anti-inflammatory.[9] Catecholamines acting through this pathway leads to increases in IL-10 and TGF-β (anti-inflammatory). As expected, similar signaling through the α-adrenergic pathway results in increased production of TNF and other cytokines.[10] This simplified signaling mechanism describes the basics of autonomic modification of immune response and potentially explains the inflammatory role in certain emotional states (chronic stress, anxiety, depression, etc.).

ENDOCRINE IMPACTS ON NEUROIMMUNOLOGY

The CNS modifies the immune system in numerous ways. In addition, there are two major endocrine routes that play a regulatory role on the neuroimmune reflex: the autonomic nervous system with norepinephrine, and the hormonal stress response with glucocorticoid production.

Hypothalamic–Pituitary–Adrenal Axis and Sympathetic Nervous System Control

An extensive and convincing array of research has been performed on the endocrine impacts of neuroimmunology. The most extensive research likely lies within the hypothalamic–pituitary–adrenal (HPA) axis, along with the sympathetic nervous system (SNS), and their impact on the neuroimmune reflexes. The fundamental basics will be presented below, but an in-depth analysis is outside of the scope of this chapter. For those interested, consider the review article by Charmandari, Tsigos, and Chrousos.[11]

To review the basic principles of the HPA axis and SNS on neuroimmunology, it is logical to begin with sensory information. Sensory signals traverse the spinal cord to be processed in the paraventricular nucleus of the hypothalamus and the locus coeruleus noradrenergic center. When stressors are present, the hypothalamus releases arginine vasopressin (AVP) and corticotropin-releasing hormone (CRH). The neurons of the paraventricular nucleus (which contain CRH) have efferent pathways to the median eminence and to the noradrenergic centers in the brainstem and spinal cord. This CRH release then acts on the HPA axis, leading to a release of peptides from the pituitary and the cleavage of pro-opiomelanocortin, which increases adrenocorticotropic hormone (ACTH), enkephalins, and endorphins. ACTH release encourages the adrenal cortex to release glucocorticoids. As mentioned in the neuroimmunology basics, CRH and the noradrenergic neurons in the CNS interface, stimulating each other. Once these noradrenergic pathways are activated by CRH, norepinephrine is secreted by the SNS, and both norepinephrine and epinephrine are released from the adrenal medulla. Once the SNS is involved, we have activated and engaged the neuroimmune reflex that can mediate immune function and inflammation. It is also worth noting that T cells express immunoreactive protein or messenger RNA for hormones (especially for CRH, AVP, and prolactin)[3] (Fig. 16.1).

The Stress Response

One definition of a stressor is "a stimulus that activates the HPA axis and/or the sympathetic nervous system to help an organism to adapt physiologically to deal with a threat."[12,13] Another definition describes stress as psychological "demands that exceed an individual's perceived ability to respond."[13,14] Regardless of the definition, these stressor responses activate either the sympathetic–adrenal–medullary axis and/or the HPA axis. The stress hormones (glucocorticoids, substance P, neuropeptide Y, CRH, prolactin, growth

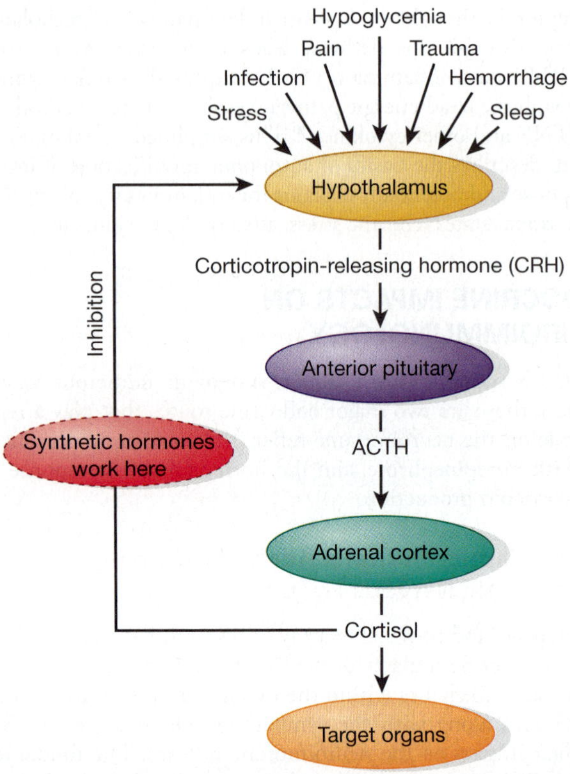

Figure 16.1. HPA axis. (Reprinted with permission from Aschenbrenner DS, Venable SJ. *Drug Therapy in Nursing.* 4th ed. Wolters Kluwer Health/Lippincott Williams & Wilkins; 2012:1012. Figure 48.1.)

hormone, epinephrine, norepinephrine, serotonin, etc.) that act in some manner on a variety of immune cells. Immune modulation by these stress hormones typically occurs via direct binding of the hormone to the cell or by indirect impacts on cytokine levels.[13]

Stressors impact the hypothalamus and lead to a surge of CRH, impacting the pituitary gland. The pituitary releases ACTH, prolactin, and growth hormone in response. The ACTH impacts the adrenal gland, which modifies glucocorticoid release and norepinephrine/epinephrine. Together, these impact our immune cells (T cells, B cells, NK cells, monocytes, etc.), which release and modify the cytokines, like IL-1. The prolactin and growth hormone also impact the immune cells and alter the levels of cytokine production and release.[13] These alterations in SNS and cytokine production bring us back to our neuroimmune reflex and alter immunity, inflammation, healing, and many other systems.

Stress and the impact on the neuroimmune reflex also plays an important role in wound repair and healing. In early healing, the inflammatory load (which is high due to tissue stressors that have induced the neuroimmune reflex) leads to release of platelet-derived growth factors (PDGFs) and other chemo attractants. Cytokines and chemokines (like the ILs, TGF-β, vascular endothelial growth factor, etc.) promote migration of phagocytes.[13] The ILs and TGF-β act as proinflammatory cytokines in this cascade that starts wound healing. However, under chronically stressful conditions, the body produces large amounts of glucocorticoids to deal with the additional stressors. These glucocorticoids alter the levels of the local proinflammatory cytokines, which delay wound healing.[13]

In addition to the role of IL-1 in wound healing, stress plays an important role in inflammation through IL-6. The proinflammatory IL-6 plays an important role in the acute-phase response.[12] IL-6 is an inducer of C-reactive protein in the liver. As discussed above, chronic stressors increase glucocorticoid production, which downregulates IL cytokine responses. Thus, chronic stressors can decrease levels of IL-6 and impact the acute-phase response. This becomes important below, as several psychiatric disease processes, like depression and anxiety can impact levels of IL-6.[13] Again, this links to the neuroimmune reflex and addresses facilitation of inflammatory states in chronically stressed populations, as well as numerous psychiatric conditions.

PSYCHOLOGICAL IMPACT ON THE NEUROIMMUNE REFLEX

Patients with depression have been found to have reduced functional activity and number of circulating immunocompetent cells[15] and subsequently higher rates of infection.[16] The presence of depression in patients appears to stimulate proinflammatory cytokines such as IL-6.[17] The presence of depression can negatively impact patients' nonpsychiatric diseases. Comorbid depression has been associated with an increased risk of cardiovascular and cerebrovascular disease and mortality, which may be mediated by depression influencing physiologic effects including inflammation of vessels, increased platelet activation, hypercoagulability, decreased heart rate variability, increased QT, and increased plasma cortisol levels.[18–20]

In patients with diabetes, depression may contribute less adherence to medications with subsequent poorly controlled blood glucose levels and diabetes progression. Depression has been associated with a cytokine-mediated inflammatory response, possibly because of HPA axis dysregulation, which can promote insulin resistance.[21]

Anxiety symptom severity in patients with generalized anxiety disorder was correlated with immune system suppression, including decreased NK cell activity, and increased disability from upper respiratory infection.[17,22] In patients with asthma, worse asthma was correlated with worse anxiety and depression symptoms as well as reduced globus pallidum size having an association with greater anxiety symptoms in response to a stressor.[23] Psychological stress has been associated with elevated systemic inflammation, which in turn is a risk factor for cardiovascular disease, type II diabetes, and metabolic syndrome.[24]

Low vitamin D levels have been identified as a risk factor for numerous medical conditions including autoimmune diseases, vascular disease, infectious diseases, osteoporosis, obesity, diabetes, cardiovascular disease, and certain cancers.[25] Additionally, low vitamin D levels have been associated with Alzheimer disease, Parkinson disease, major depressive disorder, bipolar disorder, and schizophrenia, which may be mediated through immunomodulation.[25–27]

The emerging links between gut microbiota and the CNS has led to a proposed brain–gut–microbiota axis suggesting that the gut microbiota can modulate brain development, function, and behavior by immune, endocrine, and neural pathways.[28] At this time evidence is derived primarily from animal studies warranting replication with human subjects to further elucidate the proposed brain–gut–microbiota axis as well as etiology and future therapeutic interventions.

OSTEOPATHIC CONSIDERATIONS IN PSYCHONEUROIMMUNOLOGY

Osteopathic philosophy emphasizes a human being as a dynamic unity, including body, mind, and spirit elements. A person's structure and function are reciprocally interrelated, within and between each of the unit's elements. This dynamic unit possesses self-regulatory mechanisms that are self-healing in nature. Approaching the field of PNI through the lens of osteopathic philosophy reveals significant insights for the practice of osteopathic medicine.

First, each person's dynamic unit, including body, mind, and spirit elements are involved in PNI relationships. The body element houses the neurologic, immunologic, and endocrine components such as the CNS, autonomic nervous system, T and B cells, TNF, ILs, and the HPA axis. Each of these components can influence and be influenced by one another, a form of reciprocal interrelatedness. The mind and spirit elements are also relevant to PNI. Psychological, social, and even spiritual stressors can activate interrelated neurologic, immunologic, and endocrine pathways. Alternatively, healthy psychological, social, and spiritual factors can provide beneficial responses, through some of these same pathways, that promote coping, resiliency, and health.

Second, reciprocally interrelated structure and function is evident in each aspect of PNI systems, from the microscopic to the macroscopic. The structure of the CNS and SNS provides innervation (motor, sensory, adrenergic, cholinergic, etc.) throughout the body in discrete tracks and locations, yet synaptic transmission can have a varied effect (function) on even more varied systems (nervous, immunologic, endocrine, psychological, etc.). The structure of specific immunologic elements, such as T or B cells, determines which foreign agent (antigen) will be targeted. (function). The structure of each component of the HPA axis influences its production, storage, transport, and site of action throughout the body. The structural and functional elements of the previously described systems, among others, interface with both internal and external factors to produce the human experience of mind.

Third, the intrinsic self-regulatory mechanisms of each person are self-healing in nature, which underscores the essential understanding of PNI. Whether considering homeostatic or allostatic processes to regulate internal states (such as pH, body temperature, or blood pressure), immune system fluctuations (such as circulating levels of antibodies or rapid cellular response), or endocrine cascades (such as thyroid or corticoid pathways), each is regulated within parameters to maintain function of the dynamic unit.

CONCLUSION

When approaching the field of PNI through the osteopathic principles, it is unsurprising to find the interaction of psychological (thoughts and emotions), neurologic (neurons and transmitters), immunologic (T cells and TNF), and endocrine (CRH and AVP) components manifesting those same principles inherently.

ACKNOWLEDGMENTS

The authors and editors of this chapter would like to acknowledge the scholarly contributions of Drs. Yadi Fernandez-Sweeny, David Baron, Rose Julius, and Frank Willard for prior editions of this chapter.

REFERENCES

1. Nutma E, Willison H, Martino G, Amor S. Neuroimmunology—the past, present and future. *Clin Exp Immunol.* 2019;197(3):278–293.
2. Pavlov V, Chavan S, Tracey K. Molecular and functional neuroscience in immunity. *Annu Rev Immunol.* 2018;36:783–812.
3. Tausk F, Elenkov I, Moynihan J. Psychoneuroimmunology. *Dermatol Ther.* 2008;21:22–31.
4. Venes D. *Taber's Cyclopedic Medical Dictionary.* 22nd ed. F. A. Davis Company; 2013.
5. Andersson U, Tracey K. Reflex principles of immunological homeostasis. *Annu Rev Immunol.* 2012;30:313–335.
6. Sherrington C. *The Integrative Action of the Nervous System.* Yale University Press; 1906.
7. Borovikova L, Ivanova S, Nardi D, et al. Role of vagus nerve signaling in CNI-1493-mediated suppression of acute inflammation. *Auton Neurosci.* 2000;85:141–147.
8. Pinho-Ribeiro F, Verri W, Chiu I. Nociceptor sensory neuron-immune interactions in pain and inflammation. *Trends Immunol.* 2017;38:5–19.
9. Sternberg E. Neural regulation of innate immunity: a coordinated nonspecific host response to pathogens. *Nat Rev Immunol.* 2006;6:318–328.
10. Grisanti L, Woster A, Dahlman J, Sauter E, Combs C, Porter J. α1-Adrenergic receptors positively regulate Toll-like receptor cytokine production from human monocytes and macrophages. *J Pharmacol Exp Ther.* 2011;338:648–657.
11. Charmandari E, Tsigos C, Chrousos G. Endocrinology of the stress response. *Annu Rev Physiol.* 2005;67:259–284.
12. Black P. The inflammatory response is an integral part of the stress response: implications for atherosclerosis, insulin resistance, type II diabetes and metabolic syndrome X. *Brain Behav Immun.* 2003;17:350–364.
13. Glaser R, Kiecolt-Glaser J. Stress-induced immune dysfunction: implications for health. *Nature Reviews Immunology.* 2005;5:243–251.
14. Cohen S, Tyrrell D, Smith A. Psychological stress and susceptibility to the common cold. *N Engl J Med.* 1991;325:606–612.
15. Schleifer S, Keller S, Siris S, et al. Depression and immunity. *Arch Gen Psychiatry.* 1985;42:129–133.
16. Kemeny M, Cohen F, Zegens L. Psychological and immunological predictors of genital herpes recurrence. *Psychosom Med.* 1989;51:195–208.
17. Kiecolt-Glaser J, McGuire L, Robles B, et al. Psychoneuroimmunology and psychosomatic medicine: back to the future. *Psychosom Med.* 2002;64: 15–28.
18. Evans D, Charney D, Lewis L, et al. Mood disorders in the medically ill: scientific review and recommendations. *Biol Psychiatry.* 2005;58:175–189.
19. Frasure-Smith N, Lesperance F, Irwin M, et al. Depression, C-reactive protein, and two-year major adverse cardiac events in men after acute coronary syndromes. *Biol Psychiatry.* 2007;62(4):302–308.
20. Arbelaez J, Ariyo A, Crum R, et al. Depressive symptoms, inflammation and ischemic stroke in older adults: a prospective analysis in the cardiovascular health study. *J Am Geriatr Soc.* 2007;55:1825–1830.
21. Moulton C, Pickup JC, Ismail K. The link between depression and diabetes: the search for shared mechanisms. *Lancet Diabetes Endocrinol.* 2015;3(6):461–471.
22. La Via M, Munno I, Lydiard R, et al. The influence of stress intrusion on immunodepression in generalized anxiety disorder patients and controls. *Psychosom Med.* 1996;58:138–142.
23. Caulfield J. Anxiety, depression, and asthma: New perspectives and approaches for psychoneuroimmunology research. *Brain Behav Immun Health.* 2021;18:100360.
24. Jaremka L, Lindgren ME, Kiecolt-Glaser JK. Synergistic relationships among stress, depression, and troubled relationships: Insights from psychoneuroimmunology. *Depress Anxiety.* 2013;30(4):288–296.
25. Hoang M, Defina LF, Willis BL, Leonard DS, Weiner MF, Brown ES. Association between low serum 25-hydroxyvitamin D and depression in a large sample of healthy adults: The Cooper Center Longitudinal Study. *Mayo Clin Proc.* 2011;86(11):1050–1055.
26. Cereda G, Enrico P, Ciappolino V, Delvecchio G, Brambilla P. The role of vitamin D in bipolar disorder: Epidemiology and influence on disease activity. *J Affect Disord.* 2021;278:209–217.
27. Cui X, McGrath JJ, Burne THJ, Eyles DW. Vitamin D and schizophrenia: 20 years on. *Mol Psychiatry.* 2021;26:2708–2720.
28. Kelly JR, Kennedy PJ, Cryan JF, Dinan TG, Clarke G, Hyland NP. Breaking down the barriers: the gut microbiome, intestinal permeability and stress-related psychiatric disorders. *Front Cell Neurosci.* 2015;9:392.

17 Mind–Body Medicine

TEODOR HUZIJ

KEY CONCEPTS

- Mind–body medicine (MBM) focuses on the interactions among the brain, mind, body, and behavior and on the powerful influence of emotional, mental, social, spiritual, and behavioral factors on physical symptom manifestation and overall health and well-being.
- An osteopathic understanding of mind–body medicine is grounded in the osteopathic principles.
- The body can affect the mind as well as the mind affects the body.
- The possible mind–body medicine interventions are quite diverse.
- Osteopathic management of mind–body conditions is guided by the osteopathic principles, comprehensively addressing a patient's body, mind, and spirit elements.

INTRODUCTION

Behavioral medicine is the integrative study of behavioral, psychosocial, and biomedical sciences, and their effects on health and disease. When Dr. A.T. Still founded osteopathy in 1874, behavioral medicine was yet to be developed as a discipline. Nevertheless, Dr. Still emphasized health physically, mentally, and spiritually, as well as the role of the body in both physical and mental illness. One of Dr. Still's early students and faculty at the American School of Osteopathy, J. Martin Littlejohn, taught lectures on psychophysiology. Osteopathic medicine has long appreciated the interface of body, mind, and soul in both health and disease.

MIND–BODY MEDICINE (MBM)

Mind–body medicine (MBM) focuses on the interactions among the brain, mind, body, and behavior and on the powerful influence of emotional, mental, social, spiritual, and behavioral factors on physical symptom manifestation and overall health and well-being.[1] The experience of illness has a powerful effect on individuals and, for some patients, may become the determining factor in the eventual outcome. In addition, factors such as social support, stable living situations, and personality factors have been shown to play important roles in health outcomes.[2] The state of a patient's mind plays a significant role in treating disease. Ayurveda and Traditional Chinese Medicine identified this relationship more than 2,000 years ago.[3] It was not until the early 20th century that western medicine started to identify neuroendocrine responses to stress in animals.[4] Hans Selye, MD, integrated observations in rats that supported connections between psychological and physiologic processes as stress and a general adaptation syndrome.[5]

MBM emerged from the interaction of psychiatry, specifically psychosomatic medicine now called consultation-liaison psychiatry, humanistic psychology and complimentary/alternative medicine, in response to studies revealing mind–body interactions.[6,7] Four hypothesis or principles of MBM have been proposed[6]: the mind and body are a unity; psychosocial stress gets transduced into cellular stress; cellular oxidative stress is what uncovers disease vulnerability; the MBM equation which calculates the propensity of disease from ratios of oxidative to antioxidative stress factors (Fig. 17.1).

An osteopathic understanding of MBM is grounded in the osteopathic principles, specifically the human being is a dynamic unit of function (including body, mind, and spirit elements), structure and function being reciprocally interrelated as well as self-regulating systems that are self-healing in nature.[8] Considering that a human being is a dynamic unit, this suggests that the different elements of body mind and spirit can both draw from and support one another. Reciprocal interrelation is not exclusively related to structure and function but is also an inherent reality of the dynamic unit elements. As one element, say the body, is struggling with dysfunction, the other elements of mind and spirit can offer healthy resources in support to the dysfunctional element. This reciprocal interrelation of the body unit elements also manifests the body's inherent self-regulatory systems that are self-healing in nature.

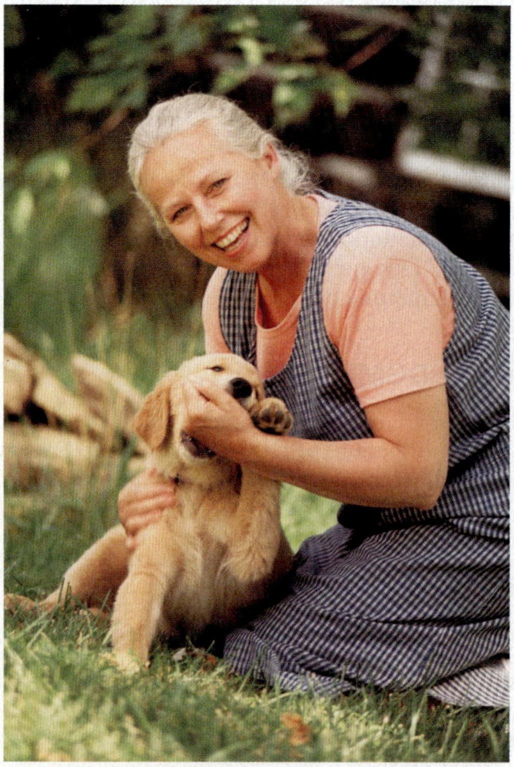

Figure 17.1. Mind–Body–Medicine. (Reprinted with permission from Eliopoulos C. *Gerontological Nursing*. 9th ed. Wolters Kluwer; 2018:93. Figure 7-2.)

EXAMPLES OF MIND–BODY INTERACTIONS

The mind has an ability to affect the body.

- In the late 1800s, psychoanalysis proposed that unconscious mental processes could impact psychological and physical aspects of a person. This interaction was described in the case of "Anna O," a patient with hysteria arising from an unconscious conflict manifesting as neurologic symptoms.[9]
- The Canadian Health Study found that an individual's perception of health was more highly correlated with longevity than other more objective factors, such as the number of chronic diseases.[10]
- Depression is an independent risk factor for death 5 years after an acute myocardial infarction. Even minor depression is associated with an increased risk.[11]
- Personal experiences of feeling hostile and angry have been associated with an increased likelihood of developing myocardial infarctions and higher mortality rates later in life.[12]
- The Alameda study found that individuals with higher levels of social support (defined as being married, being involved in religious or social groups, or having close friends) had 50% lower mortality.[13]
- Emotional reactions to stress have been shown to alter a variety of markers that are associated with poor health outcomes, including cortisol, tissue necrosis factor, interleukin-6, and C-reactive protein.[2,14]
- Several categories of adverse childhood experiences (such as abuse, living with mentally ill household members or maternal violence) have been associated with the later development of adult diseases including ischemic heart disease, cancer, chronic lung disease and liver disease.[15]

The body also has the ability to affect the mind.

- Patients with posttraumatic stress disorder (PTSD) have been found to have higher circulating levels of catecholamines, such as cortisol, as well as reduced hippocampal volume.[16,17] Increased cortisol levels may reduce hippocampal size and therefore impair function, specifically in memory.[18] Additionally, hippocampal activation levels have been identified as a predictive factor in developing PTSD following trauma exposure.[19] Together this evidence suggests that abnormal structure or function of the hippocampus can contribute to the development of PTSD and some of the condition's symptoms including memory impairment.
- Pain perception is modulated by the anterior cingulate cortex as well as the dorsolateral prefrontal cortex.[20–22] Through these neuroanatomic structures a person's mental experience of pain can be physiologically or pathologically regulated.

MIND–BODY MEDICINE INTERVENTIONS

There are several commonly practiced MBM interventions, including biofeedback, guided imagery, hypnosis, relaxation techniques, massage, and therapeutic writing.[1,23–25] However, the possible interventions are quite diverse and may include but are not limited to autogenic training, meditation, tai chi, qi gong, yoga, acupuncture, mindfulness, dance or art therapy, nutritional/dietary supplements, and manual medicine (including osteopathic manipulative treatment).[6,7] Clinical studies have shown varying levels of MBM efficacy for the treatment of arthritis, chronic pain, headache, cancer, incontinence, cardiovascular disease, multiple sclerosis, epilepsy, mild cognitive impairment, and infertility.[1,26–29] It is beyond the scope of this chapter to discuss the variety of interventions for MBM and readers are encouraged to review the references for further information.

OSTEOPATHIC MANAGEMENT OF MIND–BODY CONDITIONS

Considering the multifactorial etiologies of most diseases and the dynamic unity experience of human beings, most illnesses or diseases therefore can be considered mind–body conditions (chronic pain, migraine, arthritis, diabetes, obesity, depression, anxiety, etc.). A rational osteopathic treatment is based on osteopathic principles, as stated previously.[8] Since a human being is a dynamic unit of function, the osteopathic approach to patients with mind–body conditions should include a comprehensive assessment and treatment of the whole person, including body, mind, and spirit elements. In fact, the osteopathic principles can serve as a lens for the physician, through which the patient is perceived and assessed as well as treatment is selected and applied.

Osteopathic assessment begins with a thorough history, especially inquiry of medical comorbidities and any other physical, mental, social, or spiritual factors that may be contributing to the patient's current presentation. Being alive involves exposure to stressors both externally and internally. An osteopathic history should include inquiry of any significant stressors remotely or presently for the patient. Homeostatic and allostatic mechanisms can positively or negatively affect a patient's ability to cope with these stressors. A comprehensive physical exam follows, guided by the insights gained from the patient's history. The osteopathic structural exam should assess for the presence of somatic dysfunction which is present in every disease process and is often associated with autonomic system imbalance. Further laboratory and diagnostic studies may be required and are selected based on suspected etiologies considered most likely. The goal of an osteopathic assessment is to identify, as specifically as possible, the cause of the patient's presenting condition. This cause, which is commonly multifactorial, is then addressed through a comprehensive osteopathic treatment approach. As the osteopathic profession's slogan stated several years ago, osteopathic physicians are DOs treating causes not symptoms.

An osteopathic approach understands that a patient's health is ultimately the responsibility of the patient, who partners and cooperates with the osteopathic physician in the treatment plan, seeking optimal health body, mind, and soul. Osteopathic treatment can address each of the elements of the patient's dynamic unit. Treatment for the body element may involve dietary and fitness changes; supplements; osteopathic manipulative treatment and other manual modalities; medications; and other condition-specific interventions (e.g., specialist referral, IV immunoglobulin, transcranial magnetic stimulation, or surgery). Treatment of the mind element may involve patient education regarding health and disease factors; support groups; meditation; and psychotherapy. Treatment of the spirit element may involve discussion of a patient's value system and worldview as it relates to the patient's health and condition; if applicable for the patient, a referral to a chaplain or other spiritual/religious support may be necessary (please see Chapters 19 and 20 on spirituality in Osteopathic health care). Together, the patient and physician can work to attain a healthy balance of body, mind, and spirit. In doing so, overall wellness is optimized including financial, social, and environmental aspects (Fig. 17.2).

SUMMARY

- Origins of MBM span from ancient eastern medicine through to the present day and emerged from the interaction of psychiatry, specifically psychosomatic medicine now called consultation-liaison psychiatry, humanistic psychology, and complimentary/alternative medicine.

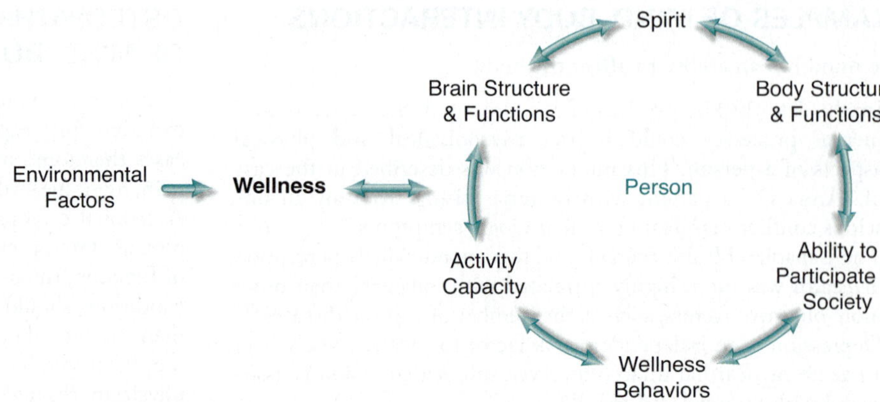

Figure 17.2. The Wellness Interactions Model. (Reprinted with permission from Andrade C-K. *Outcome-Based Massage: Across the Continuum of Care.* 4th ed. Wolters Kluwer; 2023:10. Figure 1-3.)

- The four hypotheses of MBM are both similar to and more specific when compared to the principles of the osteopathic philosophy.
- Osteopathic evaluation of mind–body conditions includes a comprehensive osteopathic assessment, including inquiry of stressors and an osteopathic structural exam.
- Osteopathic treatment of mind–body conditions can provide recommendations and interventions specific to each of the dynamic unit's elements, body, mind, and spirit.

ACKNOWLEDGMENTS

The author and editors of this chapter would like to acknowledge the scholarly contributions of Drs. Yadi Fernandez-Sweeny and Howard Schubiner for prior editions of this chapter.

REFERENCES

1. Kerna NA, Holets HM, Pruitt KD, et al. A practical review of mind-body medicine (MBM): Descriptions of prevalent MBM therapies, indications, contraindications, and efficacy. *EC Psychol Psychiatr*. 2021;10(6):86–98.
2. Kiecolt-Glaser JK, McGuire L, Robles TF, et al. Psychoneuroimmunology: psychological influences on immune function and health. *J Consult Clin Psychol*. 2002;70(3):537–547.
3. Barnes PM, Bloom B, Nahin RL. Complementary and alternative medicine use among adults: United States, 2002. *Seminars in Integrative Medicin*. 2004;2(2):54–71.
4. Cannon WB. *The Wisdom of the Body*. Norton and Co; 1967.
5. Selye H. Stress and the General Adaption Syndrome. *Br Med J*. June 17 1950:1384–1392.
6. Owusu M. Chapter 40. Mind body medicine. In: Stern T. *Massachusetts General Hospital Psychiatry*. 7th ed. Elsevier; 2018.
7. Mind and Body Practices. NIH National Center for Complimentary and Integrative Health https://www.nccih.nih.gov/health/mind-and-body-practices
8. Giusti R. *Glossary of osteopathic terminology*. 3rd ed. American Association of Colleges of Osteopathic Medicine; 2017.
9. Breur J, Freud S. *Studies on Hysteria*. Basic Books. 1891.
10. Mossey JM, Shapiro E. Self-rated health: a predictor of mortality among the elderly. *Am J Public Health*. 1982;72:800–808.
11. Carney RM, Freedland KE, Steinmeyer B, et al. Depression and five-year survival following acute myocardial infarction: a prospective study. *J Affect Disord*. 2008 Jul;109(1–2):133–138.
12. Barefoot J, Williams RB, Mark DB, et al. Hostility as a predictor of survival in patients with coronary artery disease. *Psychosom Med*. 1983;45:59–63.
13. Berkman LF, Syme SL. Social networks, host resistance, and mortality: a nine-year follow up study of Alameda County residents. *Am J Epidemiol*. 1979;109:186–204.
14. Steptoe A, Willemsen G, Owen N, Flower L, Mohamed-Ali V. Acute mental stress elicits delayed increases in circulating inflammatory cytokine levels. *Clin Sci (London)*. 2001;101(2):185–192.
15. Felitti VJ, Anda RF, Nordenberg D, et al. Relationship of childhood abuse and household dysfunction to many of the leading causes of death in adults: the Adverse Childhood Experiences (ACE) Study. *Am J Prev Med*. 1998;14(4):245–258.
16. Ben-Zion Z, Korem N, Spiller TR, et al. Longitudinal volumetric evaluation of hippocampus and amygdala subregions in recent trauma survivors. *Mol Psychiatry*. 2023;28:657–667.
17. Pitman R. Post-traumatic stress disorder, hormones, and memory. *Biol Psychiatry*. 1989;26:221–223.
18. Acheson DT, Gresack JE, Risbrough VB, et al. Hippocampal dysfunction effects on context memory: Possible etiology for posttraumatic stress disorder. *Neuropharmacology*. 2012;62:674–685.
19. Sanne J, Stevens JS, Ely TD, et al. The role of the hippocampus in predicting future posttraumatic stress disorder symptoms in recently traumatized civilians. *Biol Psychiatry*. 2018;84:106–115.
20. Baliki MN, Chialvo DR, Geha PY, et al. Chronic pain and the emotional brain: specific brain activity associated with spontaneous fluctuations of intensity of chronic back pain. *J Neurosci*. 2006;26:12165–12173.
21. deCharms RC, Maeda F, Glover GH, et al. Control over brain activation and pain learned by using real-time functional MRI. *Proc Natl Acad Sci U S A*. 2005;102:18626–18631.
22. Schmahl C, Bohus M, Esposito F, et al. Neural correlates of antinociception in borderline personality disorder. *Arch Gen Psychiatry*. 2006;63:659–667.
23. Astin JA, Shapiro SL, Eisenberg DM, Forys KL. Mind-Body Medicine: State of the science, implications for practice. *J Am Board Fam Pract*. 2003;16(2):131–147.
24. Plews-Ogan M, Owens JE, Goodman M, et al. A pilot study evaluating mindfulness-based stress reduction and massage for the management of chronic pain. *J Gen Intern Med*. 2005;1136–138.
25. Broderick JE, Junghaenel DU, Schwartz JE. Written emotional expression produces health benefits in fibromyalgia patients. *Psychosom Med*. 2005;67:326–334.
26. Duan L, Xu Y, Li M. Effects of mind-body exercise in cancer survivors: a systematic review and meta-analysis. *Evid Based Complement Alternat Med*. 2020;2020:7607161.
27. Greenberg J, Singh T, Popok PJ, Kulich RJ, Vranceanu AM. Sustainability of improvements in physical and emotional function following a mind–body physical activity program for chronic pain. *J Altern Complement Med*. 2021;27:360–364.
28. Zou L, Loprinzi PD, Yeung AS, Zeng N, Huang T. The beneficial effects of mind-body exercises for people with mild cognitive impairment: a systematic review with meta-analysis. *Arch Phys Med Rehabil*. 2019;100:1556–1573.
29. Gaitzsch H, Benard J, Hugon-Rodin J, Benzakour L, Streuli I. The effect of mind-body interventions on psychological and pregnancy outcomes in infertile women: a systematic review. *Arch Womens Ment Health*. 2020;23:479–491.

18 Stress Management

TEODOR HUZIJ ▪ KRISTIN PUTNAM

KEY CONCEPTS

- Stress is a condition experienced when the physical, mental, emotional, or social environment impacts the dynamic unit of a person.
- The various proposed stages of stress can be osteopathically understood through the physiologic mechanisms of homeostasis, allostasis, allostatic load, and overload.
- Neuroendocrine pathways, including the hypothalamic–pituitary–adrenal (HPA) axis and the autonomic nervous system, mediate the systemic response to stress.
- An osteopathic understanding and approach to stress should be guided through the lens of the osteopathic principles.

DEFINITION OF STRESS

Historically, stress theory and terminology has been varied and obfuscatory, possibly resulting from nonspecific conceptual understandings.[1] Efforts to focus the conceptual definition of stress have included a proposal to restrict the term "stress" to "conditions where an environmental demand exceeds the natural regulatory capacity of an organism, in situations that include unpredictability and uncontrollability."[2] This effort to specify the understanding of stress may be overly narrow as it excludes the human reality of regular exposure to stressors routinely in everyday living. Other efforts have defined stress as "a physiological response that serves as a mechanism of mediation linking any given stressor to its target-organ effect."[3] However, this proposed definition is biologically reductionistic and does not honor the complete human experience of stress, physically, psychologically, and spiritually.

A genuinely osteopathic understanding of stress should derive from the principles of the osteopathic philosophy. As a dynamic unit of reciprocally related structure and function, each person inherently possesses self-regulatory processes that are self-healing in nature. Stressors occur daily in human existence and the body unit is designed to manage the vast majority of this routine stress in a healthy manner. A person's response to stress may be appropriate and physiologic, or unhealthy and pathologic. Stress is a condition experienced when the physical, mental, emotional, or social environment impacts the dynamic unit of a person. Some of these demands can exceed resources and create a sense of powerlessness and inability to control the stressor or effect change. The person under such a stress responds as a unit (i.e., mind, body, and spirit) and coordinates an adaptive systemic response to the stressor (i.e., allostasis).

STAGES OF STRESS

General adaptation syndrome, as described by Selye,[4] included three phases of stress response: general alarm reaction, adaptation, and exhaustion (see Fig. 18.1). His experiments, although widely published and accepted by the public, have been challenged by the research community. His research has been determined to be too narrow in focus, focusing on the hypothalamic–pituitary–adrenal (HPA) axis to the exclusion of all other stress-responsive neuroendocrine systems.[5] Walter Cannon was another researcher who was dedicated to the study of stress, but he focused on the importance of the body system to maintain homeostasis and was the first to coin the "flight or fight" response as part of the sympathetic nervous system (SNS). He was also interested in the role of emotions in the stress response. His research was incomplete, yet the Cannon-Bard theory of emotions provided an important step toward the current understanding of stress response.[6]

Although there are many theories to describe the stages of stress, this section will focus on the theory of homeostasis, allostasis, allostatic load, and overload[7] (see Table 18.1). Homeostasis refers to the ability of an organism to maintain an internal environment conducive to life, including the organism's ability to self-regulate and defend itself through innate and acquired immunity. Allostasis refers to the process that maintains homeostasis with the recognition that control may change with the environment. The primary mediators of allostasis include the HPA axis, autonomic nervous system (sympathetic and parasympathetic), and pro- and antiinflammatory cytokines. Allostatic systems allow the organism to respond to its physical state and to cope with stressors in its environment.

An allostatic state refers to the "altered and sustained activity levels of the primary mediators, for example, glucocorticoids, that integrate energetic and associated behaviors in response to changing environments, challenges such as social interactions, weather, disease, predators, pollution, etc. An allostatic state results in an imbalance of the primary mediators reflecting excessive production of some and inadequate production of others."[7]

Allostatic load and overload refer to the cumulative result of an allostatic state (see Fig. 18.2). A normal allostatic response should include initiation of a response to a stressor, sustained response for an appropriate interval, and then resolution of the response. Repeated exposure to the same stressor should result in adaptation and a weakening in the response with each exposure. However, multiple experiences can result in an abnormal allostatic response. These include repeated "hits" from multiple stressors, lack of adaptation to the same stressor, prolonged response due to delayed shut-down, or inadequate response that leads to compensatory hyperactivity of other mediators.[7] The overburdening of a system from allostatic load can result in allostatic overload, which results in a pathophysiologic condition. In addition to environmental stressors, internal behavioral stressors, such as anticipation and worry, can also contribute to allostatic overload. Anticipatory anxiety can drive the output of mediators such as adrenocorticotropic hormone (ACTH), cortisol, and epinephrine.[8] An individual's coping mechanisms,

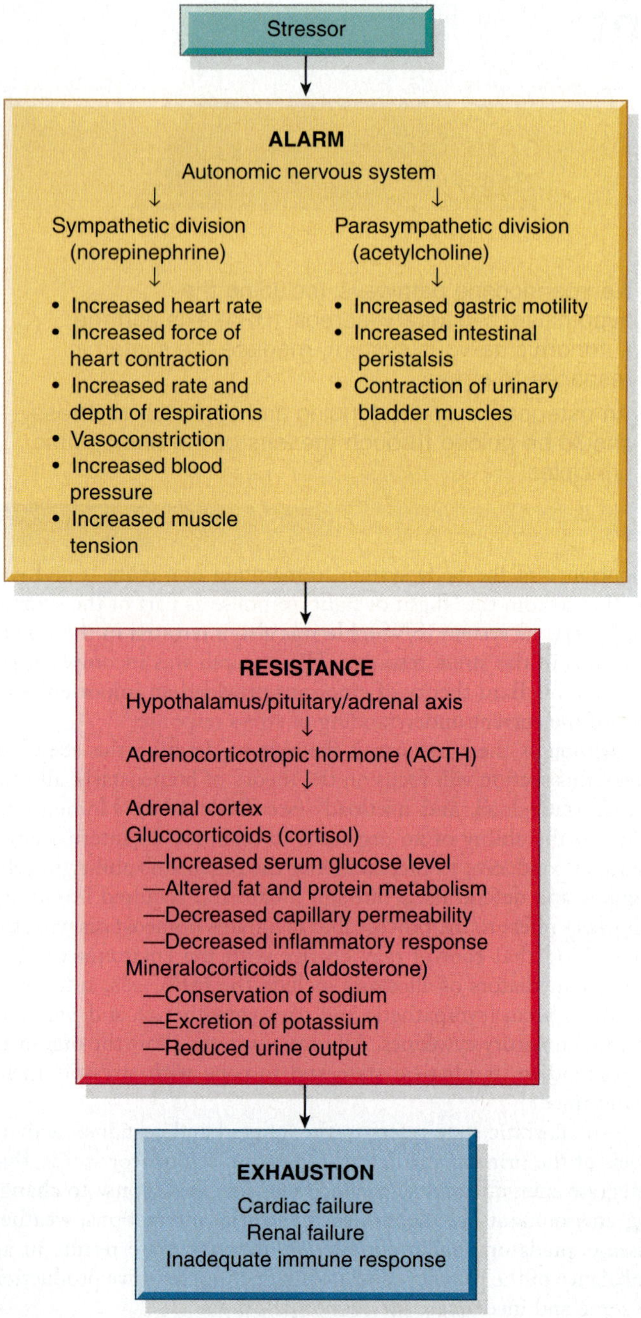

Figure 18.1. General adaptation syndrome. (Reprinted with permission from Timby BK, Smith NE. *Introductory Medical-Surgical Nursing*. 12th ed. Wolters Kluwer; 2018:1249. Figure 67-3.)

including both internal and external behaviors, may also contribute to the increasing or decreasing of allostatic overload.[7]

PHYSIOLOGIC RESPONSE

Hans Selye defined stress as the "nonspecific response of the body to any demand."[4]

However, more recent research has shown that the neuroendocrine system produces a specific response to stressors in both the pathways involved and the intensity of the response.[9,10]

Those responses tend to be driven primarily by the HPA axis and the sympathetic arm of the autonomic nervous system (SNS). Stressors are perceived and processed by the brain which triggers the release of glucocorticoids from the HPA axis and catecholamines (epinephrine and norepinephrine) from the SNS. The brain evaluates and compares the current state of the organism, the stressor it is facing, and compares the current stressor with previous stress experiences. Glucocorticoid response in the brain is mediated by two distinct receptors: mineralocorticoid receptors (MRs) and glucocorticoid receptors (GRs). GRs are more broadly located and have a lower affinity than MRs. However, both are heavily concentrated in the limbic areas responsible for the modulation of the stress response. MRs are considered part of the appraisal process and onset of the stress response, while GRs are responsible for stress-induced behavioral changes and mobilization of energy substrates[9] (see Table 18.2). Once the stressor has been recognized and processed in the brain, the central nervous system then simultaneously activates the SNS and the HPA axis response with the release of catecholamines. Systemic catecholamines and glucocorticoids act synergistically to raise blood glucose levels, increase cardiac output, and shunt blood to the skeletal muscles to facilitate the fight or flight response.[9]

TABLE 18.1

Theories of Stress

Homeostasis	Maintenance of an internal environment conducive to life
Allostasis	Control mechanisms that respond to environmental changes to sustain homeostasis
Allostatic load	Physiologic adaptation to stressors, with expected adaptation maintained by allostasis
Overload	Excess burdening of allostasis with lack of adaptation to the prolonged stressor causing pathophysiologic states

Although the two primary neuroendocrine pathways tend to be the focus of research surrounding stress, neuroimaging and research in the biochemical pathways has broadened our understanding of the brain's response to stress. For example, the amygdala is a prime target of the neurochemical and hormonal mediators of stress, suggesting a key role in the evaluation of emotional events and formation of fearful memories. It also provides a link between the stress response and emotional disorders such as anxiety.[9] In addition, the corticotropin-releasing factor (CRF) peptide family are central neurochemical neurotransmitters that have been implicated as a possible orchestrator of the stress response.[11–13] The locus coeruleus (LC), which is the central nucleus to produce norepinephrine, is sensitive to CRF. CRF promotes a shift in the normal glutamatergic influence, to a high tonic firing state, which creates a sustained excitatory influence over the brain and brainstem in response to stress.[9] The development of central CRF receptor antagonist medications to treat this response system is an area of continued research in multiple central nervous system mediated disease processes.[14–16]

ASSESSING STRESS

Sources of stress and possible impacts are highly variable and require a variety of screening measures. One of the earliest measures developed include Holmes and Rahe's Social Readjustment Rating Scale, in 1967. This measure correlated higher stress scores with a greater probability of illness occurring within the next

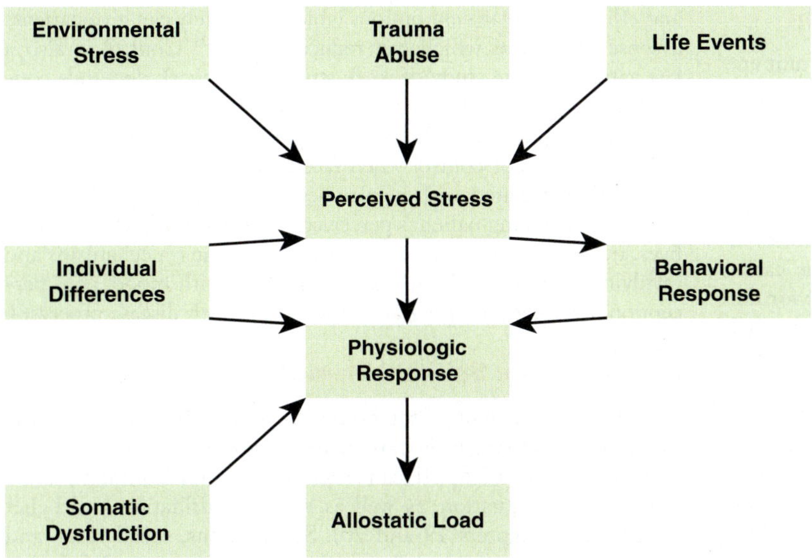

Figure 18.2. Allostatic load. (From Noll DR, Kaufman BE. Osteopathic Considerations in General Internal Medicine. In: Seffinger MA, ed. *Foundations of Osteopathic Medicine: Philosophy, Science, Clinical Applications, and Research.* 4th ed. Wolters Kluwer; 2018:1181. Figure 42C.5.)

2 years.[17] Other measures assessing diverse sources of stress include the Profile of Mood States and the Impact of Events Scale.[18] More specific life events can be assessed with the Survey of Recent Life Experiences.[18] Workplace stress can be assessed with the Job Content Questionnaire or the Effort-Reward Imbalance Questionnaire, while the Stockholm Marital Stress Scale assesses marital stress, and general relationship stress can be assessed with the Bergen Social Relationships Scale.[18]

OSTEOPATHIC APPROACHES

A rational osteopathic approach to stress management should optimally proceed through the osteopathic tenets or principles.

Stress Affects Body, Mind, and Spirit

First, each person is a dynamic unit of function that includes body, mind, and spirit elements. Stress can affect each of these elements specifically. Physical load and stress of the body element can result in somatic dysfunction as in the case of a processing plant employee who performs repetitive hand motions leading to wrist dysfunction and carpal tunnel symptoms. An osteopathic approach for this patient's presentation could include osteopathic manipulative treatment of the wrist somatic dysfunction, a wrist splint to be worn during specific times, and possible occupational modifications such as shorter durations of exacerbating activities or occupational rehabilitation for a different job task. Psychological stress of the mind element can result in cognitive or emotional symptoms as in the case of an employee who is worrying about being fired and is subsequently experiencing tension headaches as well as problems concentrating and sleeping. An osteopathic approach for this patient's presentation could include osteopathic manipulative treatment for any cervical or thoracic dysfunction, coping or job skills training, and formal psychotherapy. Stress of the spiritual element can result in distress about existential or eternal factors as in the case of a patient experiencing severe guilt of having violated a religious precept and subsequently having insomnia and gastroesophageal reflux. An osteopathic approach for this patient's presentation could include osteopathic manipulative medicine to address the autonomic system function and consultation with a chaplain or respective religious supports for the patient. It is worth noting that each of the dynamic unit elements support and reinforce each other in efforts to optimize the health of the whole person.

TABLE 18.2

Glucocorticoid Stress Response Receptors in the Brain

Glucocorticoid Receptors (GRs)	Mineralocorticoid Receptors (MRs)
• More broadly located • Lower affinity *Function:* stress-induced behavioral changes and mobilization of energy substrates	• Less broadly located • Higher affinity *Function:* onset of stress response

Stress Affects the Body's Self-Regulation/Self-Healing

Each person's dynamic unit possesses self-regulatory mechanisms that are self-healing in nature. The concept of homeostasis and allostasis in response to stressors wonderfully illustrate this osteopathic principle. These mechanisms can be functional and beneficial mechanisms such as preferential blood flow to essential areas of need including specific muscle groups or brain regions in the short term to maintain homeostasis. However, these mechanisms may be inadequate or deleterious if required long term for chronic stressors (in the case of high cortisol states) or are unable to meet the level of demand for an acute stressor (hemorrhagic injury). The self-regulatory role of homeostasis involves the nuanced adjustment of isolated essential parameters such as heart rate or blood pH. The role of allostasis involves regulating systemic processes to compensate for the impact of stress on the system. Both mechanisms can respond to and impact the autonomic nervous system. As patients have increasing dysfunction and comorbid medical conditions the self-regulatory and self-healing mechanisms can reach a functional limit in supporting the dynamic unit, this would be considered an example of allostatic overload. An osteopathic approach to such a patient's presentation could include osteopathic manipulative treatment for dysfunction and disease-relevant sympathetic and parasympathetic supply levels, with a goal of supporting systemic compensatory mechanisms.

Stress Affects the Body's Structure and Function

Third, the structure and function of each person's dynamic unit are reciprocally interrelated. This means that structure determines function, and that function determines structure in a dynamic way. This is true for the healthy and functional system just as much as it is for the unhealthy and dysfunctional system. For example, the structure of the knee's bony elements and stabilizing ligaments maximizes flexion and extension with little motion in other planes. However, in the event of overuse, even within the sagittal plane, the cartilage may be injured resulting in a loss of function. Similarly for the knee, a significant force laterally to medially may disrupt the medial stabilizing structures which subsequently results in the dysfunction of joint instability. Additionally, just as the dynamic unit elements support and draw from one another, the structure and function of the dynamic unit elements are reciprocally interrelated as well. This is evident when a person has an injured knee and must bear greater weight and stride duration on the healthy knee as well as consciously change routine behaviors considering acute limitations imposed by the dysfunction. Such a patient could also develop somatic dysfunction in the healthy knee which would limit the ability to compensate for the originally injured knee. An osteopathic approach to such a patient's presentation could include osteopathic manipulative treatment for any somatic dysfunction in both lower extremities, pelvis, and sacrum with a goal of restoring function of the structures to permit ongoing compensation for the originally injured knee.

The brain's response to stress is an example of the relationship between structure and function. Plasticity of the adult differentiated brain allows the individual to respond to and learn from new environments and stressors. Recent research has shown that neuroplastic changes induced by stress may lead to imbalances in neural networks of the central nervous system, however, these changes appear to be reversible.[19] This is particularly relevant in the changes in cognition seen because of stress. Acute stress can have both beneficial and detrimental cognitive influence; however, cognition is predominately undermined with prolonged stress exposure.[20] The use of medication and therapy to help reverse and ameliorate any of the negative side effects of these changes is an area of continued study. Biofeedback teaches a patient to use physiologic parameters to identify and influence responses to various disorders including hypertension, chronic pain, and headaches.[21–23] From an osteopathic perspective, biofeedback makes it possible to extend voluntary control over some elements of somatic dysfunction by decreasing arousal responses affecting somatic and viscerosomatic reflex activities. Learning to master these responses helps develop a sense of control and improves confidence in one's self-healing abilities.

Finally, rational treatment approaches should be based on the aforementioned tenets. A rational osteopathic approach will often include interventions beyond osteopathic manipulative medicine.

Behavioral and Perceived Control of Stress

The connectivity of the mind, body, and spirit is crucial in the treatment of stress in patients. An example of this concept of body unity is the mind's ability to alter the organism's physiologic response to stressors through the perception of control. Control over aversive experiences can influence an individual's stress response. Control can be categorized as direct behavioral control (the availability of direct actions that can modify stress stimulation); perceived control (the sense that one has control over events); cognitive control (the capacity to control one's reactions to events); and self-control (the ability to regulate emotions and delay gratification).[24] Patient education provides a patient with information about their condition and efficacious treatment options which ultimately can give patients a sense of control which can reduce stress.[25,26] Control is also a key variable in the study of work stress. High work demands coupled with low control, especially in the context of an effort-reward imbalance,[27] have been shown to be particularly detrimental to an individual. Loss of control when faced with a chronic condition is frequently associated with helplessness, hopelessness, passivity, and distress. Enhancing patient's perceived control at work, in their daily lives, and in their medical care by providing coping mechanisms and involving them in decision-making can help with mood, pain perception, rehabilitation programs, and coping with disease processes.

Stress and the Spiritual Element

The spiritual element of the body unit and its interplay with the mind and body system is particularly important in the treatment approach to stress. Spirit can refer to one's environment, community, social situation, as well as religious affiliation and belief system (see Chapters 19 and 20). Social status, social roles, and the ambient environment all contribute to environmental determinants of stress.[28] Working with patients to provide resources within their communities can help to reduce their allostatic load and provide more appropriate coping mechanisms to increase their resiliency and overall stress response. Individuals are more likely to seek out and use resources to help with stress when their basic survival needs are met. Those that exhibit connection to their community, whether through their family, culture, or physical community, are also more likely to be more resilient and display less risky coping behaviors in the face of resource loss and stress.[29] Social and spiritual support networks address expanded elements of a patient's dynamic unit. Osteopathic physicians can maintain a resource list for patients including support groups (such as substance use recovery or grief groups) as well as chaplain referral options to offer patients to support the whole person presenting for care.

CONCLUSIONS

The concept of stress has multiple proposed definitions however an osteopathic understanding would best describe stress as a condition experienced when the physical, mental, emotional, or social environment impacts the dynamic unit of a person. The physiologic mechanisms involved in stress response include neuroendocrine pathways such as the HPA axis and autonomic nervous system. The dynamic unit of each person addresses the stress experience through multiple physiologic processes including homeostasis and allostasis. A unique osteopathic understanding and approach to stress for each patient can be guided through the lens of the osteopathic philosophy's principles.

ACKNOWLEDGMENTS

The authors and editors of this chapter would like to acknowledge the scholarly contributions of Drs. Yadi Fernandez-Sweeny, John A. Jerome, and Gerald Guy Osborn for prior editions of this chapter.

REFERENCES

1. Mason JW. A historical view of the stress field. *J Human Stress*. 1975; 1(2):22–36.
2. Koolhaas JM, Bartolomucci A, Buwalda B, et al. Stress revisited: a critical evaluation of the stress concept. *Neurosci Biobehav Rev*. 2011;35(5): 1291–1301.

3. Everly GS, Lating JM. The anatomy and physiology of the human stress Response. *A Clinical Guide to the Treatment of the Human Stress Response.* Springer; 2019. https://doi.org/10.1007/978-1-4939-9098-6_2
4. Selye H. A syndrome produced by diverse nocuous agents. *Nature.* 1936;(138):32.
5. McCarty R. The alarm phase and the general adaptation syndrome: two aspects of Selye's inconsistent legacy. In: Fink G, ed. *Stress: Concepts, Cognition, Emotion, and Behavior.* Vol 1. Academic Press; 2016:13–19. http://dx.doi.org/10.1016/B978-0-12-800951-2.00002-9
6. McCarty R. The fight-or-flight response: a cornerstone of stress research. In: Fink G, ed. *Stress: Concepts, Cognition, Emotion, and Behavior.* Vol 1. Academic Press; 2016:33–37. http://dx.doi.org/10.1016/B978-0-12-800951-2.00004-2
7. McEwen BS. Central role of the brain in stress adaptation: allostasis, biological embedding, and cumulative change. In: Fink G, ed. *Stress: Concepts, Cognition, Emotion, and Behavior.* Vol 1. Academic Press; 2016:39–55. http://dx.doi.org/10.1016/B978-0-12-800951-2.00005-4
8. Schulkin J, McEwen BS, Gold PW. Allostasis, amygdala, and anticipatory angst. *Neurosci Biobehav Rev.* 1994;(18):385–396.
9. Fink G. Stress, definitions, mechanisms, and effects outlined: lessons from anxiety. In: Fink G, ed. *Stress: Concepts, Cognition, Emotion, and Behavior.* Vol 1. Academic Press; 2016:3–11. http://dx.doi.org/10.1016/B978-0-12-800951-2.00001-7
10. Pacak K, Palkovits M. Stressor specificity of central neuroendocrine responses: implications for stress-related disorders. *Endocr Rev.* 2001;(22):502–548.
11. Winsky-Sommerer R, Yamanaka A, Diano S, et al. Interaction between the corticotropin-releasing factor system and hypocretins (orexins): a novel circuit mediating stress response. *J Neurosci.* 2004;24(50):11439–11448.
12. Bale TL, Vale WW. CRF and CRF receptors: role in stress responsivity and other behaviors. *Annu Rev Pharmaol Toxicol.* 2004;44:525–557.
13. Sztainberg Y, Chen A. Neuropeptide regulation of stress-induced behavior: insights from the CRF/urocortin family. In: Fink G, Pfaff DW, Levine JE, eds. *Handbook of Neuroendocrinology.* Academic Press, Elsevier; 2012:355–376.
14. Curley D, Webb A, Sheffler D, Haass-Koffler CL. Corticotropin releasing factor binding protein as a novel target to restore brain homeostasis: Lessons learned from alcohol use disorder research. *Front Behav Neurosci.* 2021:15.
15. Dunlop BW, Binder EB, Iosifescu D, et al. Corticotropin-releasing factor receptor 1 antagonism is ineffective for women with posttraumatic stress disorder. *Biol Psychiatry.* 2017;82(12):866–874.
16. Vandael, D, Gounko, NV. Corticotropin releasing factor-binding protein (CRF-BP) as a potential new therapeutic target in Alzheimer's disease and stress disorders. *Transl Psychiatry.* 2019;9:272.
17. Holmes TH, Rahe RH. The social readjustment rating scale. *J Psychological Res.* 1967;11:213–218.
18. Kopp P, Thege BK, Balog P, et al. Measures of stress in epidemiological research. *J Psychosom Res.* 2010;69(2):211–225.
19. Czeh B, Fuchs E. Remodeling of neural networks by stress. In: Fink G, ed. *Stress: Concepts, Cognition, Emotion, and Behavior.* Vol 1. Academic Press; 2016:117–126. http://dx.doi.org/10.1016/B978-0-12-800951-2.00014-5
20. Calvo MG, Gutierrez-Garcia A. Cognition and stress. In: Fink G, ed. *Stress: Concepts, Cognition, Emotion, and Behavior.* Vol 1. Academic Press; 2016:139–144. http://dx.doi.org/10.1016/B978-0-12-800951-2.00016-9
21. Ferraccioli G, Ghirekki L, Scita F, et al. EMG-biofeedback training in fibromyalgia syndrome. *J Rheumatol.* 1987;14:820–825.
22. Mur E, Drexler A, Gruber J, Hartig F, Günther V. Electromyography biofeedback therapy in fibromyalgia. *Wiener Medizinische Wochenschrift.* 1999;149:561–563.
23. Scott J, Gade G, McKenzie M, Venohr I. Cooperative health care clinics: a group approach to individual care. *Geriatrics.* 1998;53:68.
24. Steptoe A, Poole L. Control and stress. In: Fink G, ed. *Stress: Concepts, Cognition, Emotion, and Behavior.* Vol 1. Academic Press; 2016:73–80. http://dx.doi.org/10.1016/B978-0-12-800951-2.00008-X
25. Brody H. The biopsychosocial model, patient-centered care, and culturally sensitive practice. *J Fam Pract.* 1999;48:585–587.
26. Rosekind MR. The epidemiology and occurrence of insomnia. *J Clin Psychiatry.* 1992;53(suppl 6):4–6.
27. Siegrist J. Effort-reward imbalance model. In: Fink G, ed. *Stress: Concepts, Cognition, Emotion, and Behavior.* Vol 1. Academic Press; 2016:81–86. https://www.sciencedirect.com/science/article/abs/pii/B9780128009512000091
28. Avison WR. Environmental factors. In: Fink G, ed. *Stress: Concepts, Cognition, Emotion, and Behavior.* Vol 1. Academic Press; 2016:87–94. http://dx.doi.org/10.1016/B978-0-12-800951-2.00010-8
29. Hobfoll SE, Tirone V, Holmgreen L, Gerhart J. Conservation of resources theory applied to major Stress. In: Fink G, ed. *Stress: Concepts, Cognition, Emotion, and Behavior.* Vol 1. Academic Press; 2016:65–71. http://dx.doi.org/10.1016/B978-0-12-800951-2.00007-8

19 Role of "Spirit" and Spirituality in the History of Osteopathic Medicine

DAVID B. FULLER

KEY CONCEPTS

- The concepts of spirit and spirituality have played a role throughout the history of osteopathic medicine, from its inception in 1874 through today.
- Andrew Taylor Still (1828–1917), the founder of osteopathic medicine, established and taught osteopathic philosophy that included a spiritual aspect.
- Andrew Taylor Still described the human spirit as an active life force that powers and governs the material body in a harmonious union of body, mind, and spirit.
- This continues to be recognized today in the first tenet of osteopathic medicine, "The body is a unit; the person is a unit of body, mind, and spirit."
- The concepts of spirit and spirituality in osteopathic medicine were developed further by later osteopathic physicians, including J. Martin Littlejohn, William L. Grubb, William G. Sutherland, and Robert C. Fulford.
- The concepts of spirit and spirituality in osteopathic medicine continue to be taught in osteopathic continuing medical education courses and written about in published osteopathic literature.

OVERVIEW

"Spirit" and spirituality have played roles in osteopathic medicine since the beginning of the profession in the late 19th century and continue to play roles today. Andrew Taylor Still, the founder of osteopathic medicine, taught topics related to spirit and spirituality in his teaching and discussed them further in his writings. Related topics have been important to osteopathic physicians that followed, some of whom made unique contributions to the profession in this area. Recognizing that each person is a unit of body, mind, and spirit remains a primary tenet of osteopathic medicine.[1]

The role of spirituality in the history and development of osteopathic medicine has varied over time, taking on different forms and having different influences throughout the development of the profession and into the current day. This chapter will focus on the role that "spirit" and spirituality have played in the founding, history, and development of osteopathic medicine.

ANDREW TAYLOR STILL (FIG. 19.1)

Andrew Taylor Still developed the guiding philosophy and practice of osteopathic medicine during the latter half of the 19th century. In the 1850s, he started to question the paradigms and practice of the conventional, heroic medicine of his day.[2,119,120] Over the next two decades, he developed his own approach that became known as osteopathy, which was the basis for modern osteopathic medicine.[3,121,122] While Still was influenced by different streams of thought and individuals, including those of Spiritualism (a popular metaphysical movement of the middle 19th century), Emanuel Swedenborg (an 18th-century Swedish scientist, philosopher, and theologian), and magnetic healing, to name a few, by 1874 he had developed his own unique, distinct philosophy and practice that he would name osteopathy.[4,53,123,124]

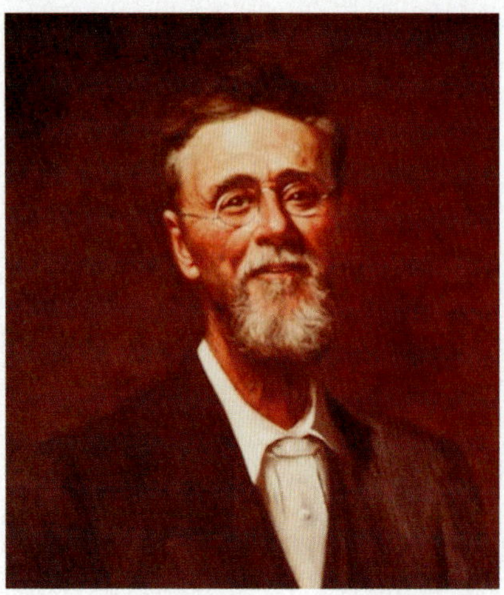

Figure 19.1. Andrew Taylor Still (1828–1917).

A. T. Still adamantly declared that osteopathic medicine is based on philosophy and reason; he understood osteopathic philosophy to be the cornerstone of the successful practice and application of osteopathic medicine.[5] Still also recognized osteopathy as both a philosophy and a science; that is, a science guided by an underlying philosophy that gives greater meaning and insight to the human body and form.[6]

Still did not separate spirituality and material science; his philosophy embraced both.[7] Another view of this is that Still's science included both the material and nonmaterial aspects of the human form and existence.[8,125,126] The underlying philosophy and foundation of early osteopathic medicine integrated and encompassed body, mind, and spirit.[9,121] This continues to be recognized today in the first tenet of osteopathic medicine, "The body is a unit; the person is a unit of body, mind, and spirit."[10]

A. T. Still had a profound interest in the spiritual aspect of humanity, yet he was not tied to any single spiritual or religious tradition.[11,132] He encouraged osteopathic students and physicians to explore such matters and welcomed people from all backgrounds.[12,127–129] In his philosophy and cosmology, Still saw all of creation as reflecting the intelligence and wisdom of a loving and wise Creator. He placed great importance on God as the Architect, Author, and Builder of creation, referring to God by many names, including as the Universal Architect, Grand Architect, and Nature's Architect.[13,130]

Still perceived the entirety of reality as containing eternal wisdom displayed in the laws of all life and form, permeating both natural and spiritual levels.[14] He understood these laws to systematically apply to every level, from astronomical down to the organs and fluids of the human body.[15,130] Still understood the study of natural science in general, and the human body in particular, to be a path toward learning higher truths.[16,133] He saw osteopathy as the application of the understanding of these laws and truths to the human form.[17]

He perceived a unity, a "connected oneness", of the body.[18] Just as body, mind, and spirit are parts of every single human being, so the different parts of the body also form a single entity.[19,121] Still described a "universal harmony" within the body, as each part worked with the rest to form the whole.[20] He saw this oneness and this harmony as manifestations of the ideal, original nature of each individual.[21,134,135]

Still recognized this structure of laws and principles applying to the material and nonmaterial/spiritual aspects of humanity.[22,131] He described material, natural life as being vivified by a spiritual life force.[23,136–138] He saw the human spirit as the active force which powers and governs the material body, as a harmonious union.[24,26] Still sometimes used the terms "life" and "spirit" interchangeably.[24]

He appreciated that this life force is manifested individually, in every person, and that in the body, life and matter are united in motion, manifested throughout all anatomy and physiology.[25] He saw the duty of the osteopathic physician as being to remove any hindrance that might interfere with that union of life and matter in motion.[26] Still described a unity, a "connected oneness" and a "universal harmony" when body, mind, and spirit are working together to manifest in health.[21,27,135] He saw harmony as health and the role of the osteopathic physician to be one of pursuing that harmony for each individual.[20,28,139]

Still recognized that nature has placed within the human body that which is needed for ideal health.[29] He saw the role of the osteopathic physician to be one of facilitating the inherent ability of the body to heal itself, to assist nature to do its own mending.[30] When an osteopathic physician treats the human body, removing obstructions to flow and facilitating motion, then health is the result. This includes addressing structure and function related to the nervous system and circulation, as well as lymphatics, cerebrospinal fluid, and fascia.[31,140–142] Then the ideal normal of perfect health can be realized.[29,32,143] This allows full manifestation and expression of the vital life energy, the spirit, of each person. At the same time that Still worked to resolve diseases and treat conditions, he also endeavored to maximize health and well-being.

The nervous system was very important to Still. He described the brain as supplying a vital nerve force, conveyed by the cerebrospinal fluid and the nervous system to the entire body.[33,144] This vital nerve force has fluid, nutritive, and functional aspects that it delivers to the tissues supplied by the nerves, maintaining the body and guiding the circulatory system as well as controlling the actions of all the organs and somatic structures.[19,34]

The circulatory system was also very important to Still. He recognized that it served as a vehicle to convey the life force into the body.[35] He emphasized that the flow of healthy blood to all structures of the body was foundational to good health.[36,135,145] He also reinforced the importance of appropriate venous return of blood.[37]

There was an axiomatic statement about "the rule of the artery" attributed to Still, after his death, which became well known.[146] While Still did not write that axiom he did write about "the rule of the artery and vein." Still also valued the integration of the circulatory and nervous systems stating, "What is harmony but health? It takes a perfect harmony of every nerve, vein and artery in every part of the body."[38,147]

Still taught that the lymphatic system played an additional role in conveying life force to the body. He described the "spirit of life" as dwelling abundantly in the lymphatics and reinforced how the lymphatic, nervous, and circulatory systems are integrated.[39,41,148]

Still recognized the important role that fascia and related structures played in the health distributions of these "fluids of life."[40] In fact, he saw fascia as a key area of the spirit life force residing in everyone.[40,149]

Furthermore, Still saw the entire musculoskeletal system as of paramount importance to osteopathic diagnosis and treatment. He recognized that this system serves as the point of contact for the osteopathic physician and as a means for affecting improvements throughout the body, not only in the actual bony joints or muscle dysfunctions locally, but also as a means of improving activity throughout the body.[19,150]

The role of the osteopathic physician, according to Still, is to recognize the body as a machine run by the unseen force called life and to ensure that there is proper activity and flow of the nervous, arterial, venous, lymphatic, fascial, and musculoskeletal systems throughout the body so that this life force can manifest in the form of ideal health.[41,151] He saw blockage to flow, or lack of healthy activity, of these life-powered systems as a cause of sickness and poor health.[42]

Still described the structural basis of osteopathic treatment as identifying and addressing any restrictions or impediments to healthy flow and function of these systems, especially in the form of normalizing motion of the spine and all parts affected in any patient's given challenged state.[7,152]

Still also appreciated that the spirit is integrated into a triunity of body, mind, and spirit and a psychological application of this is important in the care of patients.[43,153] The attitude of osteopathic physicians and how they treat patients during times of challenge and crisis have a tremendous impact on patients, affecting their mind, spirit, and body, including the vital life force within each individual.[44]

Still focused osteopathic diagnosis and treatment on the mechanical aspects of the body, while appreciating the inherent ability for it to heal, in the context of a spirit life force powering the entire mechanism, according to inherent wisdom of its structure and function.

Still viewed osteopathic medicine as a science guided by a philosophy, based on reason, that included ideas of the human body vivified by the life force of the spirit as a harmonious oneness, with an innate ability to heal, which could be facilitated by an osteopathic physician using a hands-on structure-and-function approach to treating disease and enhancing wellness that included addressing the nervous system, circulatory system, lymphatic system, as well as the fascial and musculoskeletal systems. His goal was to bring each patient to a balanced and harmonious function throughout the body, recognizing that the body is powered by the life force of the spirit. Still's approach involved simultaneously treating disease and improving overall health.

Still focused on the body, while appreciating that people are more than simply physical machines. He recognized the material body as the matrix housing a spirit, a life force, that powered the various systems of the body and provided a context for his developing the paradigms of osteopathic medicine.

J. MARTIN LITTLEJOHN (FIG. 19.2)

John Martin Littlejohn was an interesting figure who played an important role in the early years of osteopathic medicine, both in the United States as well as in the United Kingdom and Europe. He taught alongside A. T. Still in Missouri and then went on to help start osteopathic schools in both Chicago, Illinois and London, England.

J. Martin Littlejohn was born and raised in Scotland and attended the University of Glasgow, where he studied a wide range of disciplines and earned three degrees—a master of arts, a bachelor of divinity, and a bachelor of laws.[45] While there he received multiple awards in Divinity and Law, as well as the

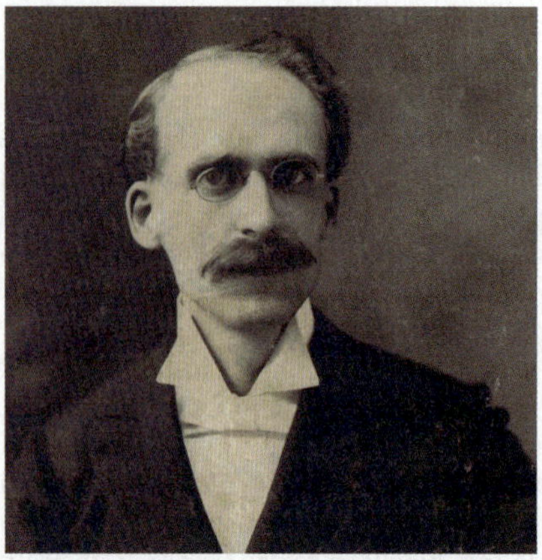

Figure 19.2. J. Martin Littlejohn (1865–1947).

William Hunter Medal for Forensic Medicine.[46] He continued his studies in America, earning a PhD in political science from Columbia University in New York, in 1894.[47,53] He went on to become president of Amity College at College Springs, Iowa, in 1895, which was the same year that he met A. T. Still.[47,53] His relationship with Still eventually led to Littlejohn joining the faculty of the first osteopathic school, the American School of Osteopathy (ASO) (founded by A. T. Still in 1892).[48,53] By 1899 Littlejohn had earned his DO degree, was a professor of physiology, and had been appointed the Dean of Faculty at the ASO.[49]

Littlejohn then moved to Chicago, where he started the school that would become the Chicago College of Osteopathic medicine.[50] In 1913, Littlejohn moved to England and became one of the founding members of the British School of Osteopathy (BSO), which was founded 4 years later.[51] He remained a guiding force at the BSO, until his death in 1947.[52] Littlejohn played a significant role in osteopathic medicine in the United Kingdom and as it spread across Europe and other continents.

Littlejohn followed A. T. Still's philosophy and practice of osteopathic medicine. He did differ slightly with his focus on physiology and his background of university training.[53] However, his overall approach to osteopathy was certainly in the tradition of Still.[54]

Littlejohn described his paradigm of osteopathy as emphasizing certain key points including: a vital force in the body resulting from the union of spirit and matter that originates in the nervous system, flowing out from the brain to the periphery in a vibratile fashion, maintaining the healthy interaction of nervous and circulatory systems and overall structure and function of the body.[55,154] He saw uninterrupted, balanced nerve and blood supply as the foundation of health. Disease, he wrote, starts as obstruction to flow of this vital life force as it moves out to the periphery and surface of the body, which leads to structural changes in the body, in turn leading to inflammation, infection, and abnormal growths.[56,155]

Littlejohn described this vital force as a something that originates and remains in the body, a result of the union of spirit with matter. This vital force plane serves a connection between the material plane and the nonmaterial plane of the spirit.[57]

Littlejohn saw the role of the osteopathic physician as being to restore a balanced healthy flow of vital life force through improved structure and function by osteopathic means.[58] Littlejohn described the goal of osteopathic treatment as the uninterrupted arterial blood supply and unimpeded nerve activity, so that the body vibrates and pulsates in harmonious cycles ("pulsates in the rhythm of life") including the master systems of nervous and circulatory systems.[59,156]

Littlejohn's paradigm of using osteopathic treatment to bring each patient to a balanced, uninterrupted, harmonious function throughout the body, appreciating the fact that the body is powered by the life force of the spirit, is in line with Still's teachings on the same subject.

WILLIAM L. GRUBB (FIG. 19.3)

William L. Grubb was an osteopathic physician who graduated from the Still College of Osteopathy in Des Moines, Iowa in 1906. He practiced as an Osteopathic Eye and Nerve Specialist in Pittsburgh until his death, on August 16, 1930 (Personal communication, Still National Osteopathic Museum, April 10, 2007).[60] Today, he is known mostly for the articles that he wrote in osteopathic journals of his time.

In 1909, Grubb wrote an article in *The Osteopathic Physician* discussing the importance of recognizing the unity of body and psyche, matter, and spirit, in complete care of patients.[61] Grubb described the osteopathic system as a complete system of medicine, one that includes structure, physiology, and psychology, as well as recognizing a vital energy, a life force that powers all of these.[61]

In 1921, Grubb wrote a letter to the editor of *The Western Osteopath* discussing similarities between A. T. Still's writings and those of Emanuel Swedenborg, including the potential interaction of spirit and body, especially in regard to the central nervous system, particularly the cerebrospinal fluid.[60]

Emanuel Swedenborg was an 18th century scientist, philosopher, and theologian who wrote on a wide range of topics over many decades. While he wrote comprehensively on anatomy, his writings also dealt extensively on the concept of humankind having a body and spirit that coexisted, with the life force of the spirit vivifying the body, not only in general, but in every particular aspect, including the cerebrospinal fluid, nervous system, circulatory system, fascia, and lymphatics.[62,157,158] Swedenborg taught extensively on body, mind, and spirit.[63,159] The 1921 article by Grubb praised Swedenborg's anatomical facts as well as his insight into spirit–body coexistence and co-respondence, comparing Swedenborg's ideas to Still's, especially the ideas found in Still's book, *Philosophy and Mechanical Principles*.[60] There is evidence to suggest that Still and later William Garner Sutherland were both influenced by the ideas contained in Swedenborg's writings, from the 1700s.[4,64,160]

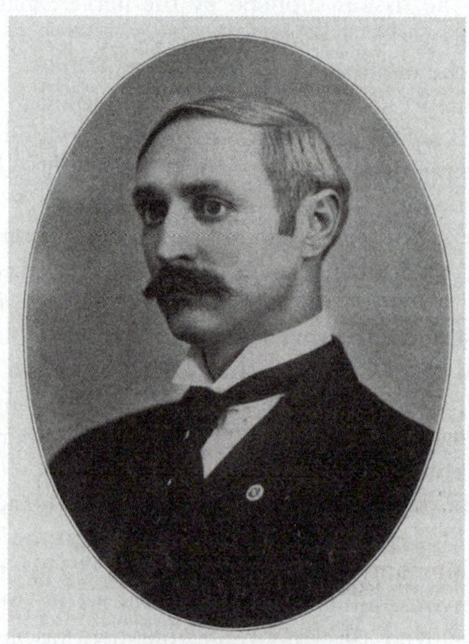

Figure 19.3. William L. Grubb (n.d.–1930).

Grubb's final contribution to the osteopathic literature was a series of 15 articles published in *The Osteopath* from September, 1923 through June, 1925.[65–79] These articles cover 54 pages of the journal, discussing ideas such as soul-body interaction and how the brain and central nervous system might play a role in this, and the importance of osteopathic physicians treating patients in a holistic fashion, mind and body.[65–79] He included many ideas and quotes from Swedenborg's 18th century writings, comparing them to A. T. Still's writings. The editor of *The Osteopath* wrote adulatory introductions to these articles, demonstrating significant support for conversations and writings on these topics.[65–79]

Grubb's articles in osteopathic journals reinforced A. T. Still's concepts of body, mind, and spirit to the osteopathic profession, especially during the 1920s.

WILLIAM G. SUTHERLAND (FIG. 19.4)

William Garner Sutherland left his career as a newspaper editor to attend the ASO in 1898.[80] During his years attending the school, earning his DO degree, Sutherland studied with the ASO faculty of that time, including A. T. Still and J. Martin Littlejohn, graduating in 1900.[81]

While a student at the ASO, Sutherland had an insight about the bones of the cranium that would later change his life and lead to the development of a new application of osteopathic manipulative medicine. This insight came like a "bolt from the blue" that the sutures of the cranial bones were, "beveled like the gills of a fish; indicating articular mobility for a respiratory mechanism."[82] This idea of the bones of the skull moving, especially as part of a greater primary respiratory mechanism, was a radical idea. Sutherland let the idea gestate until about 20 years later, when he picked it up again and began to seriously explore this concept and its ramifications, developing a comprehensive approach to diagnosing and treating patients.[83] He would go on to teach many osteopathic physicians until his death in 1953.[84]

There is a good chance that Sutherland was exposed to the articles published by William L. Grubb, since both physicians read and published articles in osteopathic journals in the same decades.[85] Sutherland certainly learned from both A. T. Still and J. Martin Littlejohn. It is important to realize that Sutherland always credited Still's teaching as his inspiration and his guiding philosophy for developing the cranial concept.[86]

Sutherland described, in tremendous anatomic detail, the effects and manifestation of this mechanism in the motion of the membranes and bones related to the central nervous system and sacrum. He also described that this underlying, important mechanism had an inherent motion and was powered by an initiative spark, a potency, carried by the Breath of Life.[87] The first edition of *Osteopathy in the Cranial Field* discussed a Life Principle that manifested in motion and energy of the elements of the primary respiratory mechanism.[88]

This concept became steadily more important to Sutherland during the last decade of his life.[89] It continued to be taught by Sutherland's students, such as Roland Becker and others.[90]

Dr. Sutherland described this Breath of Life as different than the breath of air, something not material, something that cannot be seen, but that did seem congruous with Still's life force that powered the mind and body.[91,165] Sutherland praised the spiritual aspect of Still's osteopathy, acknowledging that it functioned in accordance with physiologic laws, and lamented the loss of that spiritual aspect of osteopathic medicine over the half century following Still's death.[92] Dr. Sutherland encouraged current and future osteopathic physicians to pursue the spiritual aspect of humanity, including spirituality inherent in the living human body.[93]

Ironically, the later editions of *Osteopathy in the Cranial Field* focused on the mechanical aspects of the primary respiratory mechanism and did not mention a Life Principle, just as generations following Still developed a more mechanical approach to osteopathic medicine.

A. T. Still's recognition that the material human body served as a matrix housing a spirit, with a life force that powered the various systems of the body, was a paradigm that continued to be reflected and interpreted in the osteopathic profession and is evident in the written works of J. Martin Littlejohn, William L. Grubb, and William Garner Sutherland. It is also reflected in the teachings of another influential osteopathic physician, Robert C. Fulford. Each of these osteopathic physicians treated the material aspect of each person, while recognizing that there is something more than material—the spirit.

ROBERT C. FULFORD (FIG. 19.5)

In 1937, Robert C. Fulford left his work at Union Carbide to enroll in the Kansas City College of Osteopathic Medicine and Surgery.[94,161] In 1939, while a student at that school, he first met William G. Sutherland and become intrigued with the cranial concept.[95] After graduating and going into practice, Fulford participated in the early, formal cranial osteopathic manipulative medicine courses with Dr. Sutherland, studying with him for about

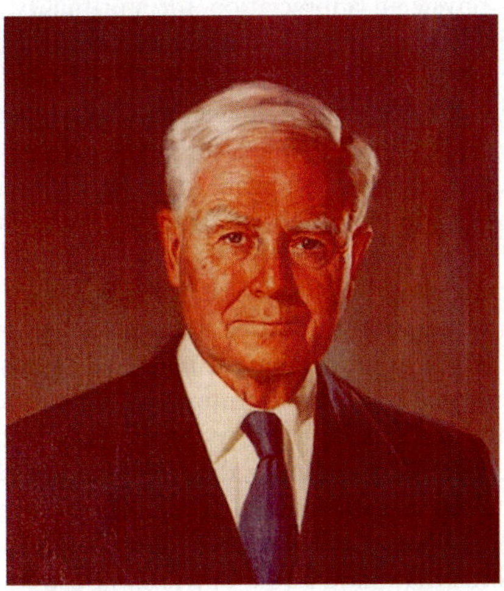

Figure 19.4. William Garner Sutherland, D.O. (1873–1954).

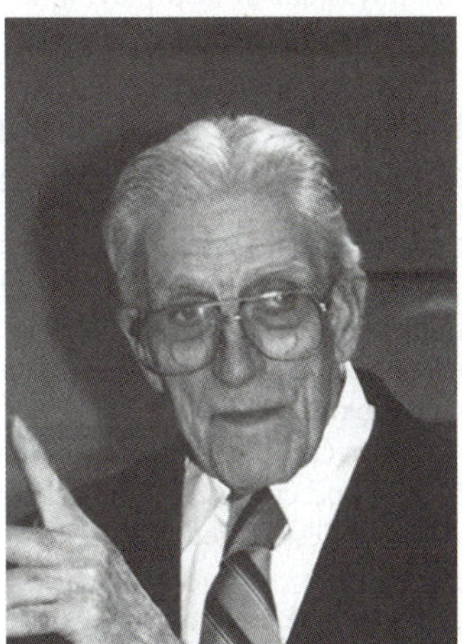

Figure 19.5. Robert C. Fulford, D.O. (1905–1997).

8 years.[96] He then went to study the cranial concept further with one of the faculty who taught with Sutherland, an osteopathic physician named Beryl Arbuckle.[97]

Fulford was eclectic in his studies, bringing in ideas from a wide range of sources and incorporating them into his practice of osteopathic medicine. He developed new ways to apply osteopathic principles and practice, including the use of the percussion vibrator as a tool for osteopathic manipulative medicine, as well as an appreciation for long fascial connections and the power of healthy breathing. He also taught that the attention and intention of the doctor, while treating patients, is vitally important.[98,162] Fulford continually looked to A. T. Still's ideas as his guiding reference and philosophical touchstone.[99,163]

Just as Still described body, mind, and spirit, Fulford taught that every person consists of a spiritual being, a mental being, and a material body.[97,164] Fulford challenged modern medicine in general, and osteopathic medicine in particular, to recognize humankind as a whole once more, recognizing each individual as a being of spirit, mind, and body, without abandoning science.[100,166] He saw matter as the physical carrier for psychic or spiritual substances and influences.[101] He stated that while science can measure matter and physical phenomena, there will always be aspects to humanity that science will never be able to explain, such as morality, love, the spirit, and the soul.[101] Fulford noted that these are worthy of study and should be included in our paradigms for health and healing.[101]

Fulford described the life force inherent in each person as manifesting as an energetic life field immediately surrounding the body.[102] He taught that much of this life force is regulated by the mind and the mind controls the body.[103] Fulford also taught that there is a vibrational quality to the human body, including the life field.[104] He explained that each person has a vibrational aspect to their life force and health and that if this is lacking in part of the body, or the person as a whole, then that can lead to dysfunction and disease.[105,162] When a person's life field has synchronized with the material body, then that presents as wellness that can be perceived by individuals.[105] He treated dysfunctions with osteopathic manipulative treatment, including the use of a percussion hammer, adjusting the vibrational frequency and vectors of force to match what was needed to treat each person, as well as working with proper therapeutic attention and intention.

Up until his death, in 1997, Fulford continued to teach in the tradition of Still and Sutherland that there is a spirituality in people that includes a life force that powers the material body.[106] Like Still, Fulford also reinforced the importance of the appropriate intention of the physician as also playing a significant role in interactions with patients.

RECENT OSTEOPATHIC PROFESSION TEACHING AND PUBLISHING ON SPIRITUALITY

A. T. Still, J. Martin Littlejohn, William G. Sutherland, and Robert C. Fulford all taught widely during their times. The ideas they presented continue to be revisited in the osteopathic profession.

Organizations such as the American Academy of Osteopathy (AAO) and The Osteopathic Cranial Academy (OCA) have been around for many decades (the AAO was founded in 1937 and the OCA founded in 1947) and continue to have annual meetings that occasionally touch on topics related to the spirit aspect of osteopathic medicine.

For example, the theme of the 1997 Annual Convocation of the AAO was titled, "Body, Mind, & Spirit" consisting of a 4-day program of lectures and OMT workshops.[107] This included presentations on related research, practice, and other applications to osteopathic medicine.

In 1998, the AAO dedicated the Annual Convocation to Fulford's work and included lectures and workshops on topics that touched on the "spirit" aspect of osteopathic medicine.[108]

In 2010, the title of the program at the OCA Annual Conference was, "Spirit and Matter: Osteopathic Reflections of Functions, Fluid, and Fascia."[109] This included a presentation on "W. G. Sutherland on Spirit and Matter."[110] The chairman of this course, R. Paul Lee, has written an in-depth book titled, *Interface: Mechanisms of Spirit in Osteopathy*.[111] This book reviews the ideas and writings of A. T. Still, W. G. Sutherland, and is dedicated to Robert C. Fulford. It explores ideas related to these concepts.

There is another area of osteopathic manipulative medicine, developed by James Jealous, DO, that takes the ideas of Sutherland's osteopathic cranial manipulative medicine further into the more-than-material direction. This is known as the biodynamic approach. It also recognizes a more-than-material aspect to each individual that is manifest in the material operations of the body, powered by a life force leading to optimum health.[112]

Osteopathic literature continues to include articles that touch on the spirit aspect of osteopathic medicine.

The Northrup Memorial Lecture given at the 1992 American Osteopathic Association (AOA) Convention was published in the *AAO Journal* and titled, "The Triune Profession."[113] The lecture was given by William A. Kuchera and covered topics that included a paradigm of body-mind-soul (spirit) applied to patients, the development of the osteopathic physician, and the status of the osteopathic profession.[113]

Other articles in the osteopathic literature touch on topics such as "Spirituality in history taking."[114] This article reinforces the importance of including spirituality-related topics in the history portion of patient care.

Current osteopathic textbooks have chapters on topics related to the spirit aspect of osteopathic medicine. Chapter 19C in the *Foundations of Osteopathic Medicine,* 4th edition (2018), is "Spirituality and Healthcare", written under the auspices of the AOA. The second chapter in *Somatic Dysfunction in Osteopathic Family Medicine,* 2nd edition (2015), is "The Triune Nature of Humanity: Body, Mind, and Spirit," written under the auspices of the American College of Family Physicians.[115]

Spirituality in osteopathic medicine is taught in many osteopathic medical schools. This has become more so since the 1990s.[116,167] Structured courses range from 2 to 20 hours on spirituality-related topics.[116]

Recently, physician appreciation for spirituality is coming to play a role throughout medicine, not just within the osteopathic profession.[117,168]

However, osteopathic medicine has the distinction of including an approach that has included a component of hands-on medical care and an appreciation for "spirit" that has played an important role in the formation, development, and current practice of osteopathic medicine for over a century.

The modern application of these ideas will vary according to individual interpretations, practice settings, and applications to patient care. While approaching each patient on a material level, with an emphasis on the complex interplay of the different systems of the body and the inherent ability to heal, osteopathic medicine has a long history of appreciating that there is something more to each person. These ideas played a role in early osteopathic medicine, such as the material body serving as a matrix housing the spirit, a life force that plays a role in health and well-being. These concepts still play a role today.

Various osteopathic physicians have offered fresh perspectives on the spirit aspect of osteopathic medicine for over a century. The future is ripe for new applications and interpretations of spirit and spirituality in osteopathic medicine. This is reinforced by the first tenet of osteopathic medicine, "The body is a unit; the person is a unit of body, mind, and spirit."[118]

REFERENCES

1. Tenets of osteopathic medicine. AOA Governance Documents. Accessed October 16, 2024. https://osteopathic.org/about/leadership/aoa-governance-documents/tenets-of-osteopathic-medicine/
2. Booth ER. *History of Osteopathy and Twentieth-Century Medical Practice.* Classic Osteopathic Medical Works; 1905:46.
3. Booth ER. *History of Osteopathy and Twentieth-Century Medical Practice.* Classic Osteopathic Medical Works; 1905:45, 46.
4. Fuller DB. *Osteopathy and Swedenborg: The Influence of Emanuel Swedenborg on the Genesis and Development of Osteopathy, Specifically on Andrew Taylor Still and William Garner Sutherland.* Bryn Athyn, PA: Swedenborg Scientific Association. 2012;243–277, 405–514.
5. Still AT. *Autobiography of Andrew T. Still: With a History of the Discovery and Development of the Science of Osteopathy.* 1908. Revised edition. 2nd reprint (Original edition 1897). Newark, Ohio: American Academy of Osteopathy, 1989:162.
6. Still AT. *Osteopathy: Research & Practice.* 1910. Reprinted. Seattle: Eastland Press, 1992:6, 11, 20.
7. Still AT. *The Philosophy and Mechanical Principles of Osteopathy.* 1902. Reprinted. Kirksville, Missouri: Osteopathic Enterprises, 1986:250.
8. Still AT. *The Philosophy and Mechanical Principles of Osteopathy.* 1902. Reprinted. Kirksville, Missouri: Osteopathic Enterprises, 1986:48.
9. Still AT. *The Philosophy and Mechanical Principles of Osteopathy.* 1902. Reprinted. Kirksville, Missouri: Osteopathic Enterprises, 1986:16–17.
10. Tenets of osteopathic medicine. American Osteopathic Association. Accessed June 9, 2022. https://osteopathic.org/about/leadership/aoa-governance-documents/tenets-of-osteopathic-medicine/#:~:text=The%20Tenets%20of%20Osteopathic%20Medicine%2Dhealing%2C%20and%20health%20maintenance
11. Still AT. *Osteopathy: Research & Practice.* 1910. Reprinted. Seattle: Eastland Press, 1992:281.
12. Still AT. "*Body and Soul, of Man.*" A. T. Still Papers 5.1.52, Still National Osteopathic Museum, Kirksville, MO. Page 6.
13. Still AT. *Autobiography of Andrew T. Still: With a History of the Discovery and Development of the Science of Osteopathy.* 1908. Revised edition. 2nd reprint (Original edition 1897). Newark, Ohio: American Academy of Osteopathy, 1989:120, 204, 228, 304, 330.
14. Still AT. *Autobiography of Andrew T. Still: With a History of the Discovery and Development of the Science of Osteopathy.* 1908. Revised edition. 2nd reprint (Original edition 1897). Newark, Ohio: American Academy of Osteopathy, 1989:202, 287, 295.
15. Still AT. *Autobiography of Andrew T. Still: With a History of the Discovery and Development of the Science of Osteopathy.* 1908. Revised edition. 2nd reprint (Original edition 1897). Newark, Ohio: American Academy of Osteopathy, 1989:148, 149, 199, 202.
16. Booth ER. *History of Osteopathy and Twentieth-Century Medical Practice.* Classic Osteopathic Medical Works; 1905:490–491.
17. Still AT. *Autobiography of Andrew T. Still: With a History of the Discovery and Development of the Science of Osteopathy.* 1908. Revised edition. 2nd reprint (Original edition 1897). Newark, Ohio: American Academy of Osteopathy, 1989:226, 233, 234.
18. Still AT. *The Philosophy and Mechanical Principles of Osteopathy.* 1902. Reprinted. Kirksville, Missouri: Osteopathic Enterprises, 1986:73.
19. Still AT. *The Philosophy and Mechanical Principles of Osteopathy.* 1902. Reprinted. Kirksville, Missouri: Osteopathic Enterprises, 1986:38, 44.
20. Still AT. *The Philosophy and Mechanical Principles of Osteopathy.* 1902. Reprinted. Kirksville, Missouri: Osteopathic Enterprises, 1986:299.
21. Still AT. *Autobiography of Andrew T. Still: With a History of the Discovery and Development of the Science of Osteopathy.* 1908. Revised edition. 2nd reprint (Original edition 1897). Newark, Ohio: American Academy of Osteopathy, 1989:184.
22. Still AT. *Autobiography of Andrew T. Still: With a History of the Discovery and Development of the Science of Osteopathy.* 1908. Revised edition. 2nd reprint (Original edition 1897). Newark, Ohio: American Academy of Osteopathy, 1989:87, 88, 148, 149, 153, 249.
23. Still AT. *The Philosophy and Mechanical Principles of Osteopathy.* 1902. Reprinted. Kirksville, Missouri: Osteopathic Enterprises, 1986:101, 251.
24. Still AT. *The Philosophy and Mechanical Principles of Osteopathy.* 1902. Reprinted. Kirksville, Missouri: Osteopathic Enterprises, 1986:249, 251, 255.
25. Still AT. *Osteopathy: Research & Practice.* 1910. Reprinted. Seattle: Eastland Press, 1992:279, 280.
26. Still AT. *Osteopathy: Research & Practice.* 1910. Reprinted. Seattle: Eastland Press, 1992:280.
27. Still AT. *The Philosophy and Mechanical Principles of Osteopathy.* 1902. Reprinted. Kirksville, Missouri: Osteopathic Enterprises, 1986:73, 299.
28. Still AT. *The Philosophy and Mechanical Principles of Osteopathy.* 1902. Reprinted. Kirksville, Missouri: Osteopathic Enterprises, 1986:44.
29. Still AT. *Osteopathy: Research & Practice.* 1910. Reprinted. Seattle: Eastland Press, 1992:14.
30. Still AT. *Osteopathy: Research & Practice.* 1910. Reprinted. Seattle: Eastland Press, 1992:xxiii.
31. Still AT. *Osteopathy: Research & Practice.* 1910. Reprinted. Seattle: Eastland Press, 1992:260.
32. Still AT. *The Philosophy and Mechanical Principles of Osteopathy.* 1902. Reprinted. Kirksville, Missouri: Osteopathic Enterprises, 1986:14, 15, 70, 250.
33. Still AT. *Autobiography of Andrew T. Still: With a History of the Discovery and Development of the Science of Osteopathy.* 1908. Revised edition. 2nd reprint (Original edition 1897). Newark, Ohio: American Academy of Osteopathy, 1989:184, 202, 233.
34. Still AT. *Osteopathy: Research & Practice.* 1910. Reprinted. Seattle: Eastland Press, 1992:36.
35. Still AT. *The Philosophy and Mechanical Principles of Osteopathy.* 1902. Reprinted. Kirksville, Missouri: Osteopathic Enterprises, 1986:52.
36. Still AT. *The Philosophy and Mechanical Principles of Osteopathy.* 1902. Reprinted. Kirksville, Missouri: Osteopathic Enterprises, 1986:10–12.
37. Still AT. *Osteopathy: Research & Practice.* 1910. Reprinted. Seattle: Eastland Press, 1992:149, 256.
38. Still AT. *Autobiography of Andrew T. Still: With a History of the Discovery and Development of the Science of Osteopathy.* 1908. Revised edition. 2nd reprint (Original edition 1897). Newark, Ohio: American Academy of Osteopathy, 1989:248.
39. Still AT. *Philosophy of Osteopathy.* 1899. 6th reprint. Newark, Ohio: American Academy of Osteopathy, 1986:104.
40. Still AT. *The Philosophy and Mechanical Principles of Osteopathy.* 1902. Reprinted. Kirksville, Missouri: Osteopathic Enterprises, 1986:60, 61.
41. Still AT. *Autobiography of Andrew T. Still: With a History of the Discovery and Development of the Science of Osteopathy.* 1908. Revised edition. 2nd reprint (Original edition 1897). Newark, Ohio: American Academy of Osteopathy, 1989:184, 194–195, 202.
42. Still AT. *Autobiography of Andrew T. Still: With a History of the Discovery and Development of the Science of Osteopathy.* 1908. Revised edition. 2nd reprint (Original edition 1897). Newark, Ohio: American Academy of Osteopathy, 1989:252.
43. Still AT. *The Philosophy and Mechanical Principles of Osteopathy.* 1902. Reprinted. Kirksville, Missouri: Osteopathic Enterprises, 1986:16, 17.
44. Still AT. *Osteopathy: Research & Practice.* 1910. Reprinted. Seattle: Eastland Press, 1992:79.
45. Gevitz N. The "Diplomate in Osteopathy": From "School of Bones" to "School of Medicine". *Journal of Osteopathic Medicine.* 2014;114(2):114–124.
46. Wernham J. *The Life and Times of John Martin Littlejohn.* JWCCO: 9–12.
47. Wernham J. *The Life and Times of John Martin Littlejohn.* JWCCO: 13–15.
48. Wernham J. *The Life and Times of John Martin Littlejohn.* JWCCO: 16–17.
49. Wernham J. *The Life and Times of John Martin Littlejohn.* JWCCO: 19.
50. Wernham J. *The Life and Times of John Martin Littlejohn.* JWCCO: 47, 52, 53.
51. Wernham J. *The Life and Times of John Martin Littlejohn.* JWCCO: 80, 81.
52. Wernham J. *The Life and Times of John Martin Littlejohn.* JWCCO: 77.

53. Trowbridge C. *Andrew Taylor Still, 1828–1917*. The Thomas Jefferson University Press; 1991:106, 122, 129–131, 139.
54. Fuller DB. *Osteopathy and Swedenborg: The Influence of Emanuel Swedenborg on the Genesis and Development of Osteopathy, Specifically on Andrew Taylor Still and William Garner Sutherland*. Swedenborg Scientific Association; 2012:279–286.
55. Wernham J. *The Life and Times of John Martin Littlejohn*. JWCCO: 96–104.
56. Wernham J. *The Life and Times of John Martin Littlejohn*. JWCCO: 99–104.
57. Littlejohn JM. The physiological basis of the therapeutic law. *J Sci Osteopath*. 1902;8–9.
58. Wernham J. *The Life and Times of John Martin Littlejohn*. JWCCO: 118.
59. Wernham J. *The Life and Times of John Martin Littlejohn*. JWCCO: 102, 118.
60. Grubb WL. "Still College of Osteopathy Announcement"; Letter to the Editor; Still College of Osteopathy. Personal communication, Still National Osteopathic Museum, April 10, 2007.
61. Grubb WL. Is psychology a legitimate part of the osteopathic system of medicine and should we use it? *The Osteopathic Physician*. 1909; 15(1).
62. Swedenborg E. *Divine Love and Wisdom*. New Century Edition; 1889:184, 195, 205, 209.
63. Swedenborg E. *Survey: Soul Body Interaction*. New Century Edition; 2022:8, 12.
64. Sutherland WG. *Contributions of Thought*. Sutherland Cranial Teaching Foundation; 1998:163–164, 210–211.
65. Grubb WL. The Cerebro-Spinal Liquid. *The Osteopath* no. 95 (September 1923):23–25.
66. Grubb WL. The Cerebro-Spinal Liquid: II-The Combination and Distribution of the Juices. *The Osteopath* no. 96 (October 1923): 20–23.
67. Grubb WL. The Cerebro-Spinal Liquid: III-The Laws of Motion of the Cerebro-Spinal Liquid. *The Osteopath* no. 97 (1923): 33–35.
68. Grubb WL. The Cerebro-Spinal Liquid: IV-The Various Species and Degrees of the Cerebro-Spinal Liquid. *The Osteopath* no. 98 (December 1923): 35–37.
69. Grubb WL. The Cerebro-Spinal Liquid: IV-The Various Species and Degrees of the Cerebro-Spinal Liquid. *The Osteopath* no. 99 (January 1924): 29–31.
70. Grubb WL. The Cerebro-Spinal Liquid: IV-The Various Species and Degrees of the Cerebro-Spinal Liquid. *The Osteopath* no. 100 (February 1924): 31–32.
71. Grubb WL. The Cerebro-Spinal Liquid: IV-The Various Species and Degrees of the Cerebro-Spinal Liquid. *The Osteopath* no. 100 (February 1924): 35–37.
72. Grubb WL. The Cerebro-Spinal Liquid: VI-The Universal Circulation of the Cerebro-Spinal Liquid. *The Osteopath* no. 101 (February 1924): 36–40.
73. Grubb WL. The Chymical Laboratory of the Brain: But What Is Truth? *The Osteopath* no. 103 (June 1924): 23–26.
74. Grubb WL. The Chymical Laboratory of the Brain: II-The Corpus Callosum, Its Uses and Functions. *The Osteopath* no. 104 (July 1924): 20–24.
75. Grubb WL. The Chymical Laboratory of the Brain: IV-Septum Lucidum, Its Uses. *The Osteopath* no. 105 (August 1924): 31–32.
76. Grubb WL. The Chymical Laboratory of the Brain: The Functions of the Lateral Ventricles. *The Osteopath* no. 106 (September 1924): 34–36.
77. Grubb WL. The Chymical Laboratory of the Brain: VIII-The Functions of the Pineal Gland. *The Osteopath* no. 109 (June 1924): 29–34.
78. Grubb WL. The Chymical Laboratory of the Brain: VII-The Functions of the Corpora Quadrigemina. *The Osteopath* no. 108 (November 1924): 32–34.
79. Grubb WL. The Chymical Laboratory of the Brain: VI-The Functions of the Choroid Plexuses. *The Osteopath* no. 107 (July 1924): 34–36.
80. Sutherland WG. *Contributions of Thought*. Sutherland Cranial Teaching Foundation; 1998:xxiii.
81. Sutherland AS. *With Thinking Fingers: The Story of William Garner Sutherland*. Cranial Academy; 1962:11.
82. Sutherland WG. *Contributions of Thought*. Sutherland Cranial Teaching Foundation; 1998:146.
83. Sutherland AS. *With Thinking Fingers: The Story of William Garner Sutherland*. Cranial Academy; 1962:18.
84. Sutherland AS. *With Thinking Fingers: The Story of William Garner Sutherland*. Cranial Academy; 1962:41, 58, 62.
85. Stark J. Sutherland's signature. *AAO Journal*. 2011;21(3):25–29.
86. Sutherland WG. *Contributions of Thought*. Sutherland Cranial Teaching Foundation; 1998:xxii, 143, 188, 214.
87. Sutherland WG. *Contributions of Thought*. Sutherland Cranial Teaching Foundation; 1998:137, 142, 204, 209.
88. Magoun HI, ed. *Osteopathy in the Cranial Field*. Sutherland Cranial Teaching Foundation; 1951, reprinted 1997, SCTF: 15.
89. Sutherland WG. *Contributions of Thought*. Sutherland Cranial Teaching Foundation; 1998:299.
90. Brooks RE, ed. *The Stillness of Life: The Osteopathic Philosophy of Rollin E. Becker, DO*. Stillness Press, LLC: xv, xvii, 6, 7, 124.
91. Sutherland WG. *Contributions of Thought*. Sutherland Cranial Teaching Foundation; 1998:137, 147, 209.
92. Sutherland WG. *Contributions of Thought*. Sutherland Cranial Teaching Foundation; 1998:293, 300.
93. Sutherland WG. *Contributions of Thought*. Sutherland Cranial Teaching Foundation; 1998:293.
94. Fulford RC. *Fulford's Touch of Life*. Gallery Books; 1997:15.
95. Goodman HD. *Robert C. Fulford, DO: a personal appreciation*. In: Cisler TA, ed. *Are We On the Path? The Collected Works of Robert C. Fulford*. The Cranial Academy; 2003:xii.
96. Goodman HD. *Robert C. Fulford, DO: a personal appreciation*. In: Cisler TA, ed. *Are We On the Path? The Collected Works of Robert C. Fulford*. The Cranial Academy; 2003:xiv–xvi.
97. Goodman HD. *Robert C. Fulford, DO: a personal appreciation*. In: Cisler TA, ed. *Are We On the Path? The Collected Works of Robert C. Fulford*. The Cranial Academy; 2003:xv–xvii.
98. Fuller DB. *Fulford, Percussion Vibrator Course, class notes*. American Academy of Osteopathy; 1994.
99. Comeaux Z. *Robert Fulford. DO and the Philosopher Physician*. Eastland Pr; 2002:8, 9.
100. Fulford RC. *Fulford's Touch of Life*. Gallery Books; 1997:4–7.
101. Fulford RC. *Fulford's Touch of Life*. Gallery Books; 1997:4–7; Fulford, Percussion Vibrator Course, class notes; Fulford, Advanced Percussion Vibrator Course, class notes.
102. Fulford RC. *Fulford's Touch of Life*. Gallery Books; 1997:29–34.
103. Fulford RC. *Fulford's Touch of Life*. Gallery Book; 1997:30–31.
104. Fulford RC. *Fulford's Touch of Life*. Gallery Book; 1997:34–36.
105. Fulford RC. *Fulford's Touch of Life*. Gallery Book; 1997:36–37.
106. Goodman HD. Robert C. Fulford, DO: a personal appreciation. In: Cisler TA, ed. *Are We On the Path?: The Collected Works of Robert C. Fulford*. The Cranial Academy; 2003:96–97.
107. Fuller D. American Academy of Osteopathy "Body, Mind, & Spirit" 1997 Annual Convocation manual and personal notes, March 19–22, 1997, Colorado Springs, CO.
108. Comeaux Z. *Robert Fulford, DO and the Philosopher Physician*, Eastland Press; 2002:9.
109. Fuller DB. Spirit and matter: osteopathic reflections of function, fluid and fascia. *The Cranial Academy Annual Conference;* 2010.
110. Fuller DB. "W. G. Sutherland on Spirit and Matter" lecture at course entitled, "Spirit and Matter: Osteopathic Reflections of Function, Fluid and Fascia." *The Cranial Academy Annual Conference;* 2010.
111. Lee RP. *Interface: Mechanisms of Spirit in Osteopathy*. Stillness Press; 2006.
112. Jealous J. Biodynamics phase one workbook, 7, 8, 13, 15, 18, 72, 73, 101. Dr. Jealous' Publications. biodynamicsofosteopathy.com
113. Kuchera W. The Triune Profession. *AAOJ*. 1993;3(2):9–14, 27.
114. Spaeth DG. Spirituality in history taking. *JAOA*. 2000;100(10):641–644.
115. Fuller RC. The triune nature of humanity: body, mind, and spirit. Chapter 2. In: *Somatic Dysfunction in Osteopathic Family Medicine*. 2nd ed. Lippincott Williams and Wilkins; 2014:6–10.
116. McClain EK, McClain RL, Desai GJ, Pyle SA. Spirituality and medicine: prevalence of spirituality-in-medicine instruction at osteopathic medicine schools. *JAOA*. 2008;108(4):197–202.
117. Balboni TA, VanderWeele TJ, Doan-Soares SD, et al., Spirituality in serious illness and health. *JAMA*. 2022;328(2):184–197.

118. Tenets of osteopathic medicine. American Osteopathic Association. Accessed June 9, 2022. https://osteopathic.org/about/leadership/aoa-governance-documents/tenets-of-osteopathic-medicine/#:~:text=The%20Tenets%20of%20Osteopathic%20Medicine,%2Dhealing%2C%20and%20health%20maintenance
119. Still AT. *The Philosophy and Mechanical Principles of Osteopathy*. Hudson-Kimberly Pub. Co.; 1902:9.
120. Fuller DB. Osteopathy and Swedenborg: The Influence of Emanuel Swedenborg on the Genesis and Development of Osteopathy, Specifically on Andrew Taylor Still and William Garner Sutherland. Bryn Athyn, PA: Swedenborg Scientific Association. 2012:186–189.
121. Still AT. *Philosophy of Osteopathy*. A.T. Still; 1899:13–14, 25, 26.
122. Still AT. *Osteopathy, Research and Practice*. Museum of Osteopathic Medicine; 1910:148–149.
123. Still AT. *Autobiography of Andrew Taylor Still*. Vol. Ia. OsteoLib, Museum of Osteopathic Medicine; 2006:94–95, 304.
124. Still AT. *Osteopathy, Research and Practice*. Museum of Osteopathic Medicine; 1910:90.
125. Still AT. *Autobiography of Andrew Taylor Still*. pgs 259, 276, 277, OsteoLib, Vol. Ia, Kirksville; 2006:162.
126. Still AT. "*Body and Soul, of Man*." A. T. Still Papers 5.1.52, Still National Osteopathic Museum, Kirksville, MO. Page 5.
127. Still AT. *The Philosophy and Mechanical Principles of Osteopathy*. Hudson-Kimberly Pub. Co.; 1902:258.
128. Booth ER. *History of Osteopathy and Twentieth-Century Medical Practice*. Classic Osteopathic Medical Works; 1905:462–463.
129. Still AT. *Autobiography of Andrew Taylor Still*. Vol. Ia. OsteoLib, Museum of Osteopathic Medicine; 2006:174.
130. Still AT. *Osteopathy, Research and Practice*. Museum of Osteopathic Medicine; 1910:13, 14, Dedication.
131. Still AT. *Osteopathy, Research and Practice*. Museum of Osteopathic Medicine; 1910:13.
132. Pickler EC. Early impressions of Dr. Still. *J Am Osteopath Assoc*. 20(5), January, 1921: 245.
133. Still AT. *Early Osteopathy in the Words of A. T. Still*. Thomas Jefferson University Press; 1991:23–24.
134. Still AT. *The Philosophy and Mechanical Principles of Osteopathy*. Hudson-Kimberly Pub. Co.; 1902:20, 73, 299.
135. Still AT. *Philosophy of Osteopathy*. A.T. Still; 1899:60.
136. Still AT. *The Philosophy of Osteopathy*. A.T. Still; 1899:179.
137. Still AT. *Early Osteopathy in the Words of A. T. Still*. Thomas Jefferson University Press; 1991:374–375.
138. Still AT. *Osteopathy, Research and Practice*. Museum of Osteopathic Medicine; 1910:11.
139. Still AT. *Autobiography of Andrew Taylor Still*. Vol. Ia. OsteoLib. Museum of Osteopathic Medicine; 2006:247–248.
140. Still AT. *The Philosophy and Mechanical Principles of Osteopathy*. Hudson-Kimberly Pub. Co.; 1902:44, 45, 65, 66, 121.
141. Still AT. *Philosophy of Osteopathy*. A.T. Still; 1899:69, 105.
142. Still AT. *Autobiography of Andrew Taylor Still*. Vol. Ia. OsteoLib, Museum of Osteopathic Medicine; 2006:190, 191, 202.
143. Still AT. *Autobiography of Andrew Taylor Still*. Vol. Ia. OsteoLib, Museum of Osteopathic Medicine; 2006:230.
144. Still AT. *Osteopathy, Research and Practice*. Museum of Osteopathic Medicine; 1910:15.
145. Still AT. *Osteopathy, Research and Practice*. Museum of Osteopathic Medicine; 1910:154.
146. Gevitz N. A degree of difference: the origins of osteopathy and the first use of the "DO" designation. *J Osteopath Med*. 2014;114(1):30–40.
147. Still AT. *Osteopathy, Research and Practice*. Museum of Osteopathic Medicine; 1910:187.
148. Still AT. *The Philosophy and Mechanical Principles of Osteopathy*. Hudson-Kimberly Pub. Co.; 1902:66.
149. Still AT. *Philosophy of Osteopathy*. A. T. Still; 1899:22–23.
150. Still AT. *Osteopathy, Research and Practice*. Museum of Osteopathic Medicine; 1910:138.
151. Still AT. *The Philosophy and Mechanical Principles of Osteopathy*. Hudson-Kimberly Pub. Co.; 1902:10.
152. Still AT. *Osteopathy, Research and Practice*. Museum of Osteopathic Medicine; 1910:149.
153. Still AT. *Philosophy of Osteopathy*. A. T. Still; 1899:25–26.
154. Littlejohn JM. The physiological basis of the therapeutic law. *J Sci Osteopath*. 1902;11.
155. Littlejohn JM. The physiological basis of the therapeutic law. *J Sci Osteopath*. 1902;13.
156. Littlejohn JM. The physiological basis of the therapeutic law. *J Sci Osteopath*. 1902;9–14.
157. Swedenborg E. *Universal Human and Soul-Body Interaction*, Paulist Press; 1984:16–18.
158. Swedenborg E. *The Brain*. Vol. 1. Swedenborg Scientific Association; 2005:41, 46, 59, 80, 81, 84, 97, 104, 191.
159. Swedenborg E. *Conjugial Love*. Swedenborg Foundation; 2009:158.
160. Sutherland WG. *Talk Given by Dr. Sutherland*. Sutherland Cranial Teaching Foundation; 1967:3, 18.
161. Goodman HD. *Robert C. Fulford, DO: a personal appreciation*. In: Cisler TA, ed. *Are We On the Path?: The Collected Works of Robert C. Fulford*. The Cranial Academy; 2003:xi–xii.
162. Fuller DB. *Advanced Percussion Vibrator Course, class notes*. American Academy of Osteopathy; 1995.
163. Goodman HD. *Robert C. Fulford, DO: a personal appreciation*. In: Cisler TA, ed. *Are We On the Path?: The Collected Works of Robert C. Fulford*. The Cranial Academy; 2003:xx–xxi.
164. Fulford RC. *Fulford's Touch of Life*. Gallery Book; 1997:4–7; Fulford, Percussion Vibrator Course, class notes.
165. Sutherland. Teachings in Science of Osteopathy, (2003), p. 15, Sutherland, Cranial Bowl: Extracts, Pamphlet, (1944), p. 6.
166. Fuller DB. *Fulford, Percussion Vibrator Course, class notes*. American Academy of Osteopathy; 1994.
167. Reeves RR, Beazley AR. Spirituality is fundamental to osteopathic medicine. *JAOA*. 2008;108(8):468.
168. Academy of Integrative Health and Medicine. Accessed September 10, 2022. https://www.aihm.org/

20 Spirituality and Health Care

MINDY A. CHILMAN MCCOMB ▪ VEERA MOTASHAW ▪ STEPHANIE HERMANN

KEY CONCEPTS

- The osteopathic profession has a rich history of embracing spirituality in both the physician and patient.
- Osteopathic physicians recognize that human beings have complex needs, including those in the spiritual domain.
- Spirituality involves an individual's sense of meaning, purpose, and connectedness. This may or may not be expressed through religious affiliation and practice.
- While some physicians are hesitant to discuss a patient's spiritual needs, patients often desire this discussion and feel it enhances the doctor–patient relationship.
- Taking a spiritual history allows the osteopathic physician to address this domain when relevant to an individual patient, thereby improving patient care and outcomes.

INTRODUCTION

Spirituality is a critical albeit insufficiently addressed component of patient-centered care.[1] Spirituality and health have been intertwined for centuries. Yet as medicine moved toward science and evidence-based practice, the importance of spirituality in patient care fell out of favor. This was seen not only within the osteopathic profession but also within American medical practice and health care more generally.[2]

It is intuitive that spiritual health is interrelated with physical and mental health; anecdotal evidence abounds. A patient in hospice hopes to live long enough to see the birth of their grandchild—and does so, defying all odds. A seemingly healthy patient is diagnosed with metastatic cancer and, devastated by the diagnosis, passes within a few days. A patient with complex mental health issues finds God and rapidly turns their life around. Anecdotal evidence alone, however, does not warrant changes to medical practice in the age of evidence-based medicine.

Fortunately, in recent decades there has been an increase in research regarding the role of spirituality and religion in health and health care. In 1995, the World Health Organization identified "spirituality/religion/personal beliefs" as one of six domains of quality of life following multiple focus groups across varied cultural settings.[3] This prompted more research regarding spiritual well-being such that spiritual health is sometimes referred to as the fourth dimension of health (along with physical health, mental health, and social well-being).

Acknowledging the spiritual needs of a patient in the health care setting does not negate or conflict with the scientific underpinnings of the practice of medicine; rather, it prevents the careless reduction of a human being to an inanimate machine. Instead of dismissing spirituality, evidence should be the guide in providing osteopathic care that is comprehensive, patient-centered, and culturally sensitive.

DEFINING SPIRITUALITY

Spirituality and religion were historically discussed as a dual construct in science literature. Only recently has spirituality begun to be considered as a distinct construct, and admittedly a lack of consensus persists in the understanding of what spirituality is within the context of health care research.[4] While this lack of clarity poses difficulties in conducting research, it is likely helpful in communicating with patients. Inclusive language is beneficial in addressing the needs of patients from varied social, cultural, and religious backgrounds. A term as broad as spirituality allows patients to interpret meaning within the context of their own lives.[5]

Recognizing that spirituality may include, but is not limited to, religion, the following is a frequently cited definition of spirituality in health care literature:

> Spirituality is the personal quest for understanding answers to ultimate questions about life, about meaning, and about relationship to the sacred or transcendent, which may (or may not) lead to or arise from the development of religious rituals and the formation of community.[6]

Another commonly cited definition was developed during a palliative care consensus conference in 2009:

> Spirituality is the aspect of humanity that refers to the way individuals seek and express meaning and purpose and the way they experience their connectedness to the moment, to self, to others, to nature, and to the significant or sacred.[7]

Regardless of the exact definition, it's clear that spirituality is inherently personal and an individual's experience within this domain will undoubtedly be unique as it relates to that individual's perception and interpretation of purpose and meaning in life (Fig. 20.1). This is true even for individuals with similar backgrounds or religious affiliations. It is therefore critical to avoid making assumptions regarding a patient's spiritual life, well-being, and/or suffering. Rather, osteopathic physicians must engage in conversations with their patients in order to address this component of health.

SPIRITUALITY AND THE PATIENT

Spiritual suffering often accompanies serious physical and mental health challenges. These experiences may lead to deep existential suffering, soul searching, and ultimately transformation, for better or worse. As medical science has progressed and human life has been prolonged, it has simultaneously led to prolonged suffering in some cases—further increasing the importance of addressing spirituality in the health care setting.

Just as physical and mental health impact spiritual health, spiritual health impacts physical and mental health (Fig. 20.2). Spiritual suffering can have profound physical consequences.

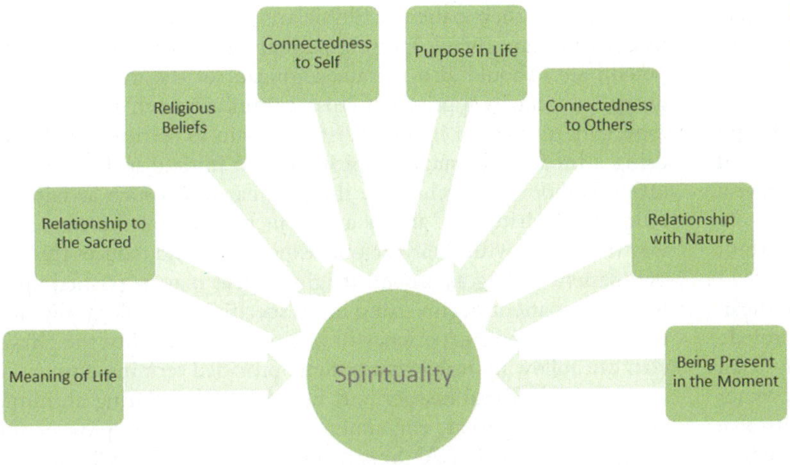

Figure 20.1. An example of the elements contributing to an individual's experience of spirituality. The significance of each to the whole is unique to an individual. Other elements may also be included.

One example is Takotsubo cardiomyopathy, a transient left ventricular apical ballooning typically triggered by an intense emotional stress, inspiring the name "broken heart syndrome." This causality is universally recognized and remains undisputed despite the lack of clarity in understanding the underlying pathophysiology because the evidence speaks for itself.

Fortunately, there is ever-increasing evidence that spirituality can positively impact patients' physical and mental health as well. Patients with stronger religious beliefs have been shown to have fewer complications and shorter hospital stays after heart surgery.[8] A meta-analysis in 2000 showed that patients' religious involvement correlated with lower all-cause mortality.[9] A more recent study of women showed that "frequent attendance at religious services was associated with lower risk of all-cause, cardiovascular and cancer mortality."[10]

Research has consistently shown spirituality and religiosity to have a protective factor against major depressive disorder,[11,12] and frequent religious service attendance was associated with a significantly lower rate of suicide.[13]

For many patients with cancer, spirituality plays a role in coping with illness and spiritual support correlates with improved quality of life. Unfortunately, the spiritual needs of many advanced cancer patients are not supported by religious communities or the medical system.[14] Failure to meet the spiritual needs of cancer patients also correlates with lower perceived quality of care.[15]

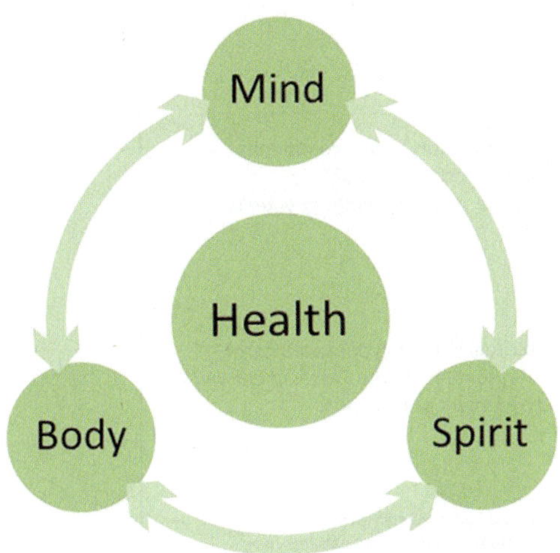

Figure 20.2. There is a complex interplay between body, mind, and spirit that must be considered when providing osteopathic care.

It is important to acknowledge that not all studies regarding spirituality and religion demonstrate correlations with patient health and outcomes. Religious practices were found to have no impact on postdischarge survival in patients with an acute coronary syndrome.[16] Multiple studies exploring the impact of prayer on various health outcomes have been done with mixed results; a Cochrane review in 2009 concluded there is no correlation, though it is unlikely to be harmful.[17]

Perhaps more concerning than null results is the finding that patients with newly diagnosed, invasive colon cancer who scored higher on scales measuring externalizing religious and spiritual beliefs (i.e., attributing responsibility for health outcomes to their god; belief in miraculous healing) presented with later stage disease.[18] This raises the question whether targeted interventions may allow the health care system to identify these patients earlier and ultimately provide better care for these individuals.

SPIRITUALITY AND THE PHYSICIAN

Spirituality can also be a component of well-being for osteopathic physicians as reflected in the previous chapter. It has been suggested that spirituality may even help prevent burnout in physicians, though this warrants dedicated research.[19] Among osteopathic and allopathic medical students, however, a recent study demonstrated that those who consider themselves to be active participants in their religion may be at a lower risk of developing burnout, regardless of the faith they practice, or the actual amount of time spent doing so.[20]

Yet physicians are often reluctant to discuss spirituality with patients in the clinical setting. This is not a reflection of physicians' individual beliefs: 65.2% of physicians believe in God and 16.5% believe in a universal or higher power other than a god. Most physicians also identify as either religious (51.2%) or spiritual (24.8%), while 12.4% identify as agnostic.[21]

So why don't physicians initiate these conversations? Many cite insufficient time during the patient encounter and a lack of training regarding these discussions. Some feel it is outside their area of expertise, while others are concerned that they may have differing beliefs from their patients. There is also concern regarding the power dynamics of the physician–patient encounter. Some physicians would prefer the patient raise the topic because they don't want to be perceived as forcing beliefs on patients. Interestingly, patients are also reluctant to raise the topic due to power dynamics.[22,23]

But many patients want to have these conversations. A majority of patients surveyed felt it was appropriate for physicians to ask about spiritual needs in at least some settings, and patient interest in this discussion increased with severity of illness.[24] Further, patients reported that doctors engaging in spiritual discussion enhanced their doctor–patient relationship.[25]

Helping a patient achieve optimal health–body, mind, and spirit—can be a transcendent experience for both the patient and physician. For the patient, it may allow for a sense of peace or reveal an understanding of what is possible despite that which cannot be changed. For the osteopathic physician, it may be an important reminder of why they dedicated their life to this profession.

To be clear, discussing a patient's spiritual needs does not mean the osteopathic physician must or even should be the one to provide spiritual guidance. Rather, these discussions can help the physician to better understand a patient's individual experience and partner with the patient to enhance their well-being. This may involve referral to a chaplain or another spiritual guide when warranted.

INTEGRATING SPIRITUALITY INTO PATIENT CARE

While more research is needed, the current evidence base warrants that osteopathic physicians put into practice the first tenet of osteopathy and consider body, mind, and spirit in addressing the health of their patients. Physicians aiming to provide quality osteopathic care (whole-person, patient-centered, culturally competent, etc.) should also remain cognizant of the nuance of language and remain apprised of cross-cultural research and findings, especially in such an individualistic domain as spirituality. Again, using a broad term such as spirituality to initiate such a conversation is more comprehensive than similar terms such as faith or religion.[5] "Spirituality" allows a patient to interpret the term in a way that aligns with their personal experiences and reduces the risk of a patient feeling as though religious ideas may be pushed upon them. If a patient begins using more specific terminology aligning with their personal experience or practice of spirituality, the physician can follow up using that patient-provided terminology.

A brief spiritual history may be taken either during an initial visit or a later patient encounter, whether in the hospital or the office setting. The FICA© Spiritual History Tool (Fig. 20.3) utilizes questions regarding a patient's faith/beliefs/meaning, the importance of spirituality in the patient's life and health or well-being, whether a patient is a member of a spiritual community or finds a community to be a source of support, and how the patient would like spiritual issues to be addressed by the health care provider.[26] It may be helpful to think of this in the same context as taking a medical, surgical or family history—each of these components carries

THE GW INSTITUTE FOR
SPIRITUALITY & HEALTH

GWish

FICA Spiritual History Tool©*

The acronym FICA© can help to structure questions for healthcare professionals who are taking a spiritual history.

***

F – Faith, Belief, Meaning

"Do you consider yourself to be spiritual?" or "Is spirituality something important to you?"
"Do you have spiritual beliefs, practices, or values that help you to cope with stress, difficult times, or what you are going through right now?" (contextualize to visit)
"What gives your life meaning?"

I – Importance and Influence

"What importance does spirituality have in your life?"
"Has your spirituality influenced how you take care of yourself, particularly regarding your health?"
"Does your spirituality affect your healthcare decision making?

C – Community

"Are you part of a spiritual community?"
"Is your community of support to you and how?" For people who don't identify with a community consider asking "Is there a group of people you really love or who are important to you?"
(Communities such as churches, temples, mosques, family, groups of like-minded friends, or yoga or similar groups can serve as strong support systems for some patients.)

A - Address/Action in Care

"How would you like me, as your healthcare provider, to address spiritual issues in your healthcare?"
(With newer models, including the diagnosis of spiritual distress, "A" also refers to the "Assessment and Plan" for patient spiritual distress, needs and or resources within a treatment or care plan.

* Adapted from: Puchalski, C., & Romer, A. L. (2000). Taking a spiritual history allows clinicians to understand patients more fully. *Journal of palliative medicine, 3*(1), 129-137.

Figure 20.3. FICA© Spiritual History Tool.

TABLE 20.1

Functional Assessment of Chronic Illness Therapy-Spiritual Well-Being Scale (FACIT-Sp)[27]

FACIT-Sp
Individual items 1. I feel peaceful. 2. I have a reason for living. 3. My life has been productive. 4. I have trouble feeling peace of mind. 5. I feel a sense of purpose in my life. 6. I am able to reach down deep into myself for comfort. 7. I feel a sense of harmony within myself. 8. My life lacks meaning and purpose. 9. I find comfort in my faith or spiritual beliefs. 10. I find strength in my faith or spiritual beliefs. 11. My illness has strengthened my faith or spiritual beliefs. 12. I know that whatever happens with my illness; things will be okay.
Factors Faith (items 9, 10, 11) Peace (items 1, 4, 6, 7, 12) Meaning (items 2, 3, 5, 8)

a different weight for a given individual, but failing to ask the questions in a case where that component is critical will inevitably lead to subpar patient care. An organized approach prevents missing what may be a key component for an individual patient, and spirituality should be included in that organized approach. This approach to history-taking can also lower the barrier for patients who would like to discuss this topic with their physicians.[21]

More extensive scales have also been developed to assess spiritual well-being. A validated tool that can be used to assess a patient's spiritual well-being is the 3-factor structure of the Functional Assessment of Chronic Illness Therapy-Spiritual Well-Being Scale (FACIT-Sp).[27] The FACIT-Sp is a 12-item questionnaire scored on a 5-point Likert scale (Table 20.1). This can be used in clinical and palliative care settings for patients with severe or life-limiting medical illnesses to inform interventions aimed at improving quality of life and spiritual well-being.

While spirituality can play a role in all aspects of health care and patient well-being, it is essential in palliative and end-of-life care. A patient approaching the end of life may experience changing views on spirituality and spend more time reflecting on their life and beliefs. This may either deepen a patient's spirituality or cause spiritual distress.

Assessing a patient's spiritual well-being allows for integration of spiritual care into the treatment plan when appropriate. This will look different for each patient depending on the elements contributing to that individual's spirituality (Fig. 20.1). A useful phrase when offering spiritual resources to a patient is, "Would it be helpful if...?" For example, "Would it be helpful to have a chaplain come by?" This allows a patient to easily decline when no spiritual care is desired. A patient may feel comforted just by being able to be open and honest about their beliefs. In other cases, a patient may desire the integration of spiritual care into their treatment plan. In the inpatient setting, this may include referral to a chaplain or a request to be visited by the patient's own spiritual leader. In the outpatient setting, this may also involve referral to a spiritual leader, but it could additionally include a plan for the patient to engage with nature, utilize meditation techniques, reconnect with friends and loved ones, or interact more with their spiritual community.[28]

CONCLUSION

Addressing the spiritual component of health can be challenging in today's health care system, but doctors must embrace this complexity. The osteopathic physician should assess a patient's spiritual well-being and acknowledge and address spiritual deficits as they would acknowledge and address mood in a patient with depression or glycemic control in a patient with diabetes. Remember, this is not limited to religious affiliation and practice. While religion and spirituality may overlap and are sometimes studied together, they are indeed distinct, and a physician need not identify as religious or practice religion to acknowledge and address a patient's spiritual health. Some physicians may still feel uncomfortable discussing spiritual needs with patients. In those cases, self-reflection and introspection on behalf of the physician may be the first step on the path to addressing their patients' spiritual needs.[29]

Partnering with patients and guiding them to optimal health—body, mind, *and spirit*—is the crux of the osteopathic profession. To do this successfully, the osteopathic physician must be willing to navigate any perceived boundary between science and spirituality in pursuit of providing the best care possible to each individual patient. Let evidence be the guide.

A CLINICAL PERSPECTIVE OF SPIRITUALITY IN HEALTH CARE

In order to recognize, respect, and respond to spiritual care, the practitioner must begin to understand the depth and breadth of spirituality and spiritual suffering in relationship to patient care. In a clinical context, the word "spirit" can be viewed as the "animating principle giving life to physical organisms,"[30] often referred to as the breath of life, or a force within a human being thought to give the body life, energy, and power.[31] "Spiritual perspectives help patients because they attend to the inner world of people suffering physical challenges."[32]

Suffering can be defined as a loss of wholeness. Spiritual suffering occurs when the sense of self has lost its relationship with the greater whole. This may be described as a sense of loss with the relationship of normal, given current circumstances. It may manifest in the patient encounter as purpose, productivity, peace, harmony, anger, sadness, faith, comfort, strength, anxiety, knowing, physical distress, pride, or hundreds of other ways. Patients will describe spiritual distress in many different ways. It is our duty as physicians to attempt to recognize suffering and the loss of wholeness. In this recognition, we can begin to respond by finding the Health within the suffering, nourishing the withering fields in those who need it most.

Because a person's sense of self must have a relationship with the greater whole for the parts to fully function, the whole must always be in the back of the practitioner's mind. The whole serves as a place of orientation during spiritual suffering, and the Health is the fulcrum which the whole can orient around. The parts are never separate from the whole. Each moment of a patient encounter, from nonverbal communication to history taking and physical exam, is a part of therapeutic spiritual care. As therapeutic conversations arise and symptom management occurs, each action must take place within the context of the whole and with great care to recognize the effects on the whole. If this seems daunting or incomprehensible, consider approaching each patient and conversation with the Health in mind. After all, Dr. Still taught, "To find Health should be the object of the doctor. Anyone can find disease."[33]

While screening for spiritual well-being, consider using a validated tool. For example, the FACIT-Sp-12, (3-factor structure) tool focuses on three major components. The tool focuses on measuring a sense of meaning, peace, and assessing the role of faith in illness. The tool is specific to a patient's current spiritual state and is the most validated instrument for this purpose.[27,34] During time-limited encounters, as information is gathered through history taking, consider adding the following question, "What matters to you most?" This question stays within the health and further allows for an open-ended exploration of a patient's current spiritual state. Patients may answer in many ways. Remember, even an answer of physical distress can reflect spiritual distress. Even physical distress must be addressed within the context of the whole in order to minimize spiritual suffering. Let's walk through the following case.

A 62-year-old male with newly diagnosed metastatic gastric cancer presents to your office with fatigue, shortness of breath, and sadness. He is with his daughter and states he is exhausted and though he has only had one treatment of chemotherapy he wants to stop treatment. What do you do?

- After finding a neutral space within your mind and being, work to meet the patient in the space where they are currently present. Do so by acknowledging current emotions and/or distress. Recognize that the patient has lost their normal after a new diagnosis of cancer and that loss is grief and may manifest as a number of reactions.
- Next, work to explore the patient's sentiments within context of the whole. Ask what is most distressing at this moment and what matters to them the most.

He describes that after his first treatment, he started to have trouble breathing and hiccups which are precluding him from sleep or any day-to-day activities. At this moment, what matters to him most is his ability to sleep. He would be amenable to further treatment if he had hope that his symptoms would be better managed, and he could spend quality time with his family.

- You discuss with him medical management of changing medications to alleviate hiccups, which you confirm have been initiated through his oncologist with minimal to no relief. You discuss hands-on treatment and introduce an osteopathic approach and philosophy. The patient states, "I'm so desperate, I'll try anything you say doc."
- As you perform a supine structural exam, you find the patient's diaphragm has minimal movement, spasmodic in nature. You note his tentorium cerebelli, thoraco-abdominal diaphragm, Sibson fascia in the thoracic inlet, and his pelvic floor diaphragm are all restricted in motion and lack coordination with each other during the inspiratory phase of primary respiration. You treat the patient using balanced membranous tension and gentle indirect myofascial release. At the end of your treatment, the patient is resting comfortably on the table and his daughter is in tears. She tells you this is the first time her father has slept comfortably in the last 2 weeks.
- When the patient awakens from his treatment, you discuss rest and a follow-up visit. You remind him he does not need to decide today to discontinue or continue chemotherapy, but that what matters most at this moment is his ability to rest. You recognize if he is able to rest, he can reconnect with his family, his whole.

In subsequent visits, the patient opens up to share his most vulnerable dreams. He brings his family members to visits and they each share in difficult conversation. He praises (and his family affirms) his drastic improvement in quality of life. The family expresses their gratitude and sentiments for the "miracle" that happened during the first visit. The patient requests further osteopathic treatment. Over the next few visits, he notices improvement in function, energy, sleep, and his respirations remain normal. He begins to have more faith in his vitality, and you explore what brings him joy. With your support, he is able to take two out-of-state trips with his family and finds motivation to work on legacy projects with friends. He continues chemotherapy with good success and sets longer-term goals with increased faith in his ability to accomplish them. He goes on to live over a year and dies peacefully, at home, approximately 2 months after accomplishing his last major goal, meeting his third great-grandchild.

When patients' sense of self is lost in relation to circumstances, spiritual suffering is at risk of occurring, if not already present. In the above case, the patient's larger spiritual joy came from time with family and connection to his loved ones. As his physical suffering began, it directly influenced his spiritual suffering. As a practitioner, keeping in mind why you are working on an immediate goal with a patient (in context of the whole) will allow for deeper connection to patients, greater success with symptom management, and ultimately better patient care.

In this encounter, space was intentionally created for trust, empathy, and vulnerability. This same space proceeds with fluid boundaries allowing the patient and family members to proceed into spaces they did not know existed. As a practitioner, the first step to creating space is remembering your physician neutral. Prior to any encounter, you must find your own neutral. Try the exercise below:

- Feel your feet on the ground. Put aside your preconceived notions and judgments of anything you may be experiencing at the moment. Put aside anything you have read, heard, seen, or experienced with this patient previously. Each encounter is unique. Feel your diaphragm and recognize the breath that goes through your diaphragm is the very same breath that nourishes the patient in front of you, their loved ones, and all the things they are connected to. This recognition allows you to enter the space with an awareness of the patient's wholeness. Remember this feeling, it is wholeness. This wholeness will anchor encounters and patients.

Once you have found your neutral and acknowledged the greater whole, if you remain present in this space, even if you do not know what to say, you will find success. At times tension may grow in an encounter, emotions may heighten, a patient may express grief, pain, anger, denial, guilt, or any unexpected emotion. As you listen to their story, remember that it is merely a part of their larger story. Anchor yourself in the whole.

When it comes to the art of medicine and compassionate care for the complex patient, there is no separation between spirituality and medicine. Comprehensive medical care must always consider the patient in front of the physician as a human, a child of a parent, possibly the parent of a child, a grandchild, or a great-grandchild that has come to you in a time of vulnerability, for your expertise. Yet this interaction is not isolated. It is connected to all that the individual brings and has experienced until this moment. The patient is somehow experiencing a loss of normal, causing them to seek help. Loss is grief. Spiritual suffering occurs when a sense of self has lost its orientation to the greater whole. As osteopathic physicians, we are trained to recognize the whole. Incorporating spirituality into patient care is simply remembering your osteopathic roots.

ACKNOWLEDGMENTS

The authors and editors of this chapter would like to acknowledge the scholarly contributions of Drs. Yadi Fernandez-Sweeny and Felix J. Rogers for prior editions of this chapter.

REFERENCES

1. Best M, Butow P, Olver I. Doctors discussing religion and spirituality: a systematic literature review. *Palliat Med.* 2016;30:327–337.
2. Koenig HG. Religion and medicine I: historical background and reasons for separation. *Int J Psychiatry Med.* 2000;30:385–398.
3. The World Health Organization Quality of Life Assessment (WHOQOL): position paper from the World Health Organization. *Soc Sci Med.* 1995; 41:1403–1409.
4. Sena MAB, Damiano RF, Lucchetti G, Peres MFP. Defining spirituality in healthcare: a systematic review and conceptual framework. *Front Psychol.* 2021;12:756080.
5. Koenig HG. Concerns about measuring "spirituality" in research. *J Nerv Ment Dis.* 2008;196:349–355.
6. Koenig HG, McCullough ME, Larson DB, eds. *Handbook of Religion and Health.* 1st ed. Oxford University Press; 2001.
7. Puchalski C, Ferrell B, Virani R, et al. Improving the quality of spiritual care as a dimension of palliative care: the report of the consensus conference. *J Palliat Med.* 2009;12:885–904.
8. Contrada RJ, Goyal TM, Cather C, Rafalson L, Idler EL, Krause TJ. Psychosocial factors in outcomes of heart surgery: the impact of religious involvement and depressive symptoms. *Health Psychol.* 2004;23: 227–238.
9. McCullough ME, Hoyt WT, Larson DB, Koenig HG, Thoresen C. Religious involvement and mortality: a meta-analytic review. *Health Psychol.* 2000;19:211–222.
10. Li S, Stampfer MJ, Williams DR, VanderWeele TJ. Association of religious service attendance with morality among women. *JAMA Intern Med.* 2016;176:777–785.
11. Miller L, Wickramaratne P, Gameroff MJ, Sage M, Tenke CE, Weissman MM. Relgiosity and major depression in adults at high risk: a ten-year prospective study. *Am J Psychiatry.* 2012;169:89–94.
12. Miller L, Bansal R, Wickramaratne P, et al. Neuroanatomical correlates of religiosity and spirituality: a study in adults at high and low familial risk for depression. *JAMA Psychiatry.* 2014;71:128–35.
13. VanderWeele TJ, Li S, Tsai AC, Kawachi I. Association between religious service attendance and lower suicide rates among US women. *JAMA Psychiatry.* 2016;73:845–851.
14. Balboni TA, Vanderwerker LC, Block SD, et al. Religiousness and spiritual support among advanced cancer patients and associations with end-of-life treatment preferences and quality of life. *J Clin Oncol.* 2007;25: 555–60.
15. Astrow AB, Wexler A, Texeira K, He MK, Sulmasy DP. Is failure to meet spiritual needs associated with cancer patients' perceptions of quality of care and their satisfaction with care? *J Clin Oncol.* 2007;25:5753–5757.
16. Abu HO, Lapane KL, Waring ME, et al. Religious practices and long-term survival after hospital discharge for an acute coronary syndrome. *PLoS ONE.* 2019;14:e0223442.
17. Roberts L, Ahmed I, Davison A. Intercessory prayer for the alleviation of ill health. *Cochrane Database Syst Rev.* 2009;2:CD000368.
18. Polite BN, Cipriano-Steffens TM, Hlubocky FJ, et al. Association of externalizing religious and spiritual beliefs on stage of colon cancer diagnosis among black and white multicenter urban patient populations. *Cancer.* 2018;124:2578–2587.
19. Marin DB, Sharma V, Powers R, Fleenor D. *Spiritual Care and Physicians: Understanding Spirituality in Medical Practice.* Spiritual Care Association; 2017. Accessed August 2, 2023. https://members.spiritualcareassociation.org/Files/docs/hccn_whitepaper_spirituality_and_physicians.pdf
20. Haghnegahdar M, Sharma P, Hubbard KP, White WA. The influence of religious belief on burnout in medical students. *Mo Med.* 2021;118:63–67.
21. Robinson KA, Cheng M-R, Hansen PD, Gray RD. Religious and spiritual beliefs of physicians. *J Relig Health.* 2017;56:205–225.
22. Balboni MJ, Sullivan A, Amobi A, et al. Why is spiritual care infrequent at the end of life? Spiritual care perceptions among patients, nurses, and physicians and the role of training. *J Clin Oncol.* 2013;31:461–467.
23. Koenig HG. Religion, spirituality, and medicine: research findings and implications for clinical practice. *South Med J.* 2004;97:1194–1200.
24. Best M, Butow P, Olver I. Do patients want doctors to talk about spirituality? A systematic literature review. *Patient Educ Couns.* 2015;98: 1320–1328.
25. Best M, Butow P, Olver I. Spiritual support of cancer patients and the role of the doctor. *Support Care Cancer.* 2014;22:1333–1339.
26. Puchalski CM. The FICA spiritual history tool: a guide for spiritual assessment in clinical settings. *GWish.* 1996. Updated 2022. Accessed August 29, 2023. https://gwish.org/sites/g/files/zaskib1011/files/2022-08/v2_fica_pdf_2_final_updated_6.29.22.pdf
27. Ahmad N, Sinaii N, Panahi S, et al. The FACIT-Sp spiritual wellbeing scale: a factor analysis in patients with severe and/or life-limiting medical illnesses. *Ann Palliat Med.* 2022;11:3663–3673.
28. Anadarajah G. Doing a culturally sensitive spiritual assessment: recognizing spiritual themes and using the HOPE questions. *Virtual Mentor.* 2005;7:371–374.
29. Best M, Butow P, Olver I. Creating a safe space: a qualitative inquiry into the way doctors discuss spirituality. *Palliat Support Care.* 2016;14:519–531.
30. Lemley WW. A discussion of spirituality and the teaching of spirituality in an osteopathic medical curriculum. *AAOJ.* 2002;12:15–23.
31. *Spirit.* Merriam-Webster. Merriam-Webster. Accessed June 25, 2023. https://www.merriam-webster.com/dictionary/spirit
32. Hilsman GJ. Why record the intangible in healthcare. In: *Spiritual Care in Common Terms—How Chaplains Can Effectively Describe the Spiritual Needs of Patients in Medical Records.* Jessica Kingsley Publishing, Ltd; 2016:26–27.
33. Still AT. *The Philosophy and Mechanical Principles of Osteopathy.* Reprinted Osteopathic Enterprise; 1986. Originally published Hudson-Kimberly Pub Co; 1902.
34. Monod S, Brennan M, Rochat E, Martin E, Rochat S, Bula C. Instruments measuring spirituality in clinical research: a systematic review. *J Gen Intern Med.* 2011;26:1345.

21 Lifestyle Medicine—Osteopathic Perspectives

REBECCA E. GIUSTI ▪ DAVID C. NIEMAN ▪ MARCEL P. FRAIX

KEY CONCEPTS

- The current burden of chronic diseases reflects the cumulative effects of unhealthy lifestyles and risk factors over the lifespan of people.
- The social conditions in which people are born, live, and work are the single most important determinant of their health status.
- Diet consisting of nutritious choices, adequate doses of exercise, fluids, sleep, and control of stress are all important considerations when incorporating Lifestyle Medicine into the care of patients.

INTRODUCTION

The World Health Organization (WHO) defines health as "a state of complete physical, mental, and social well-being and not merely the absence of disease and infirmity."[1]

- A lifestyle of unhealthy living involving the following will most likely lead to disease:
  - Tobacco use
  - Lack of regular physical activity
  - Diets rich in highly saturated fats, sugars, and salt
- This is a lifestyle that results in higher levels of risk factors that act independently and synergistically to cause disease, such as:
  - Cancer
  - Diabetes
  - Dyslipidemia
  - Hypertension
  - Obesity
- These risk factors are frequently undiagnosed or inadequately managed in health services designed to treat acute conditions.[2,3]

The current burden of chronic diseases reflects the cumulative effects of unhealthy lifestyles and risk factors over the lifespan of people.

- Some of these influences are present from before a child is born.
- The social conditions in which people are born, live, and work are the single most important determinant of their health status.[3]
- Even in individuals with chronic disease, systematic participation in physical activities enhances physical function.[4]

A balanced, nutritious diet, adequate exercise, sleep, fluids, and stress management are the cornerstones of the foundation for a healthy lifestyle. Elimination of harmful habits and chemicals (e.g., tobacco and street drugs) as well as environmental toxic exposures is also essential.

DIET AND NUTRITION

The adequate intake of all essential nutrients is necessary for the proper functioning of the body. For many years, the Food and Nutrition Board of the National Academy of Sciences has been reviewing nutrition research and defining nutrient requirements for healthy people.

- Of the nutrient intake requirement guidelines, the Recommended Dietary Allowances (RDAs), which were created in 1941 to prevent diseases caused by vitamin and mineral deficiencies, have historically been highly referenced.[5]
- Since the development of the RDAs, scientists have discovered that certain vitamins and minerals may also be important in the prevention of chronic diseases, including heart disease, osteoporosis, and cancer.[6]
- However, because the RDAs were not designed to consider common chronic diseases, the Food and Nutrition Board sought to revise the RDAs through the creation of new standards known as the Dietary Reference Intakes (DRIs), which include intakes for optimal health based on the prevention of both deficiencies and chronic diseases.[7]
- The RDA/DRI is defined as "the average daily dietary nutrient intake level sufficient to meet the nutrient requirement of nearly all healthy individuals."
- The new DRIs also include the Tolerable Upper Intake Level (UL), defined as the highest average daily nutrient intake level that is likely to pose no risk of adverse health effects to most individuals. The RDA/DRI and UL levels for key nutrients are summarized in Table 21.1.

Dietary Guidelines for Health and Disease Prevention

Regardless of whether an individual is sedentary or very active, a balanced diet should be consumed in order to enhance health and prevent disease.

- This can be a diet that is in alignment with the 2020–2025 *Dietary Guidelines for Americans*,[8] developed by the U.S. Department of Agriculture (USDA), as well as the nutrition recommendations from the American Heart Association and the American Cancer Society.[9,10]
- The guidelines provide four general recommendations that encourage healthy eating patterns and food and beverage choices:
  1. Follow a healthy dietary pattern at every life stage.
  2. Customize and enjoy nutrient-dense food and beverage choices to reflect personal preferences, cultural traditions, and budgetary considerations.
  3. Focus on meeting food group needs with nutrient-dense foods and beverages, and stay within calorie limits.
  4. Limit food and beverages higher in added sugars, saturated fat, and sodium, and limit alcoholic beverages.
- The primary focus of the 2020–2025 *Dietary Guidelines for Americans* is a healthy eating pattern with nutrient-dense foods

TABLE 21.1

Recommended Intakes and Food Sources of Vitamins and Minerals

Nutrient (Other Names)	Recommended Dietary Allowance (RDA)	Daily Value (DV)	Good Sources	Upper Level (UL)	Selected Adverse Effects
Vitamins					
Vitamin A (retinol)	Women: 700 μg Men: 900 μg	5,000 IU[a] (1,500 μg)	Liver, fatty fish, fortified foods (milk, breakfast cereals, etc.)	10,000 IU (3,000 μg)	*Liver toxicity, birth defects.* Inconclusive: bone loss
Carotenoids (alpha-carotene, beta-carotene, beta-cryptoxanthin, lutein, lycopene, zeaxanthin)	None. (NAS advises eating more carotenoid-rich fruits and vegetables)	None	Orange fruits and vegetables (alpha- and beta-carotene), green leafy vegetables (beta-carotene and lutein), tomatoes (lycopene)	None. Panel said don't take beta-carotene, except to get RDA for vitamin A	Smokers who took high doses of beta-carotene supplements (33,000–50,000 IU a day) had higher risk of lung cancer
Thiamin (vitamin B_1)	Women: 1.1 mg Men: 1.2 mg	1.5 mg	Breads, cereals, pasta, and foods made with "enriched" or whole-grain flour; pork	None	None reported
Riboflavin (vitamin B_2)	Women: 1.1 mg Men: 1.3 mg	1.7 mg	Milk, yogurt, foods made with "enriched" or whole-grain flour	None	None reported
Niacin (vitamin B_3)	Women: 14 mg Men: 16 mg	20 mg	Meat, poultry, seafood, foods made with "enriched" *or* whole-grain flour	35 mg[b]	*Flushing (burning, tingling, itching redness), liver damage*
Vitamin B_6 (pyridoxine)	Ages 19–50: 1.3 mg Women 50+: 1.5 mg Men 50+: 1.7 mg	2 mg	Meat, poultry, seafood, fortified foods (cereals, etc.) liver	100 mg	*Reversible nerve damage (burning, shooting, tingling pains, numbness, etc.)*
Vitamin B_{12} (cobalamin)	2.4 μg	6 μg	Meat, poultry, seafood, dairy foods, fortified foods (cereals, etc.)	None	None reported
Folate (folacin, folic acid)	400 μg	400 μg (0.4 mg)	Orange juice, beans, other fruits and vegetables, fortified cereals, foods made with "enriched" or whole-grain flour	1,000 mg[b] (1 mg)	*Can mask or precipitate a B12 deficiency,* which can cause irreversible nerve damage
Vitamin C (ascorbic acid)	Women: 75 mg Men: 90 mg (smokers: add 35 mg)	60 mg	Citrus and other fruits, vegetables, fortified foods (cereals, etc.)	2,000 mg	*Diarrhea*
Vitamin D	Ages 19–50: 200 IU[b] Ages 51–70: 400 IU[c] Over 70: 600 IU[b]	400 IU	Sunlight, fatty fish, fortified foods (milk, breakfast cereals, etc.)	2,000 IU	*High blood calcium,* which may cause kidney and heart damage
Vitamin E (alpha-tocopherol)	15 mg (33 IU—synthetic) (22 IU—natural)	30 IU synthetic	Oils, whole grains, nuts	1,000 mg[b] (1,100 IU synthetic) (1,500 IU natural)	*Hemorrhage:* May lower risk of hemorrhagic stroke
Vitamin K (phylloquinone)	Women: 90 μg[b] Men: 120 μg[c]	80 μg	Green leafy vegetables, oils	None	Interferes with Coumadin and other anticlotting drugs
Calcium	Ages: 19–50: 1,000 mg Over 50: 1,200 mg	1,000 mg	Dairy foods, fortified foods, leafy green vegetables, canned fish (eaten with bones)	2,500 mg	*High blood calcium,* which may cause kidney damage, kidney stones

(continued)

TABLE 21.1 (*Continued*)

Recommended Intakes and Food Sources of Vitamins and Minerals

Nutrient (Other Names)	Recommended Dietary Allowance (RDA)	Daily Value (DV)	Good Sources	Upper Level (UL)	Selected Adverse Effects
Chromium	Women: 25 µg Men: 35 µg	120 µg	Whole grains, bran cereals, meat, poultry, seafood	None	Inconclusive: kidney or muscle damage
Copper	900 µg	2 mg (2,000 µg)	Liver, seafood, nuts, seeds, wheat-bran, whole grains, chocolate	10 mg (10,000 µg)	*Liver damage*
Iron	Women 19–50: 18 mg Women 50+: 8 mg Men: 8 mg	18 mg	Red meat, poultry, seafood, foods made with "enriched" or whole-grain flour	45 mg	*Gastrointestinal effects (constipation, nausea, diarrhea)*
Magnesium	Women: 320 mg Men: 420 mg	400 mg	Green leafy vegetables; whole-grain breads, cereals, etc.; nuts	350 mg[b]	*Diarrhea*
Phosphorus	700 mg	1,000 mg	Dairy foods, meat, poultry, seafood, foods made with phosphate additives (processed cheese, colas, etc.)	Ages 19–70: 4,000 mg Over 70: 3,000 mg	*High blood phosphorus*, which may damage kidneys and bones
Selenium	55 µg	70 µg	Seafood, meat, poultry, grains (depends on levels in soil)	400 µg	Nail or hair loss or brittleness
Zinc	Women: 8 mg Men: 11 mg	15 mg	Red meat, seafood, whole grains, fortified foods (cereals, etc.)	40 mg	*Lower copper levels,* HDL ("good") cholesterol, and immune response

Note: Recommended dietary allowance (RDA). RDAs for adults only.
Daily value (DV). These levels appear on food and supplement labels. Unlike the RDAs, there's only one daily value for everyone over age 4.
Tolerable upper intake level (UL). These levels are safe daily upper limits. ULs for adults only.
Selected adverse effects. What happens if you take too much. *The UL is based on the adverse effect(s) listed in italics.* "Inconclusive" adverse effects are based on inconsistent or weak evidence.

Other tolerable upper intake levels.

Boron: 20 mg	Manganese: 11 mg
Choline: 3.5 g	Molybdenum: 2,000 µg (2 mg)
Fluoride: 10 mg	Nickel: 1 mg
Iodine: 1,100 µg (1.1 mg)	Vanadium: 1.8 mg

[a]We get vitamin A both from retinol and carotenoids, but this number assumes that all of the vitamin A comes from retinol.
[b]From supplements and fortified foods only.
[c]Adequate intake (AI). The National Academy of Sciences (NAS) had too little data to set an RDA.
Source: Food and Nutrition Information Center, www.nal.usda.gov/fnic

and beverages, which will require shifts in food and beverage choices by many individuals[8] (Fig. 21.1). More than 80% have dietary patterns that are low in vegetables, fruits, and dairy, and more than half of the population is meeting or exceeding total grain and total protein foods recommendations, but are not meeting the recommendations for the subgroups within each of these food groups.

- About half of all American adults or 117 million individuals have one or more preventable chronic diseases, many of which are related to poor quality eating patterns and physical inactivity. These diseases include:
  - ☐ Cardiovascular disease (CVD)
  - ☐ Some cancers
  - ☐ Hypertension
  - ☐ Poor bone health
  - ☐ Type 2 diabetes

Key Elements of Healthy Eating Patterns

A primary goal of the 2020–2025 *Dietary Guidelines for Americans* is that individuals throughout all stages of the lifespan have eating patterns that promote good health, a healthy body weight, and disease prevention.[8]

An underlying tenet of the *Dietary Guidelines* is that nutritional needs should be met primarily from foods and beverages—specifically, nutrient-dense foods and beverages. Nutrient-dense foods provide vitamins, minerals, and other health-promoting components and have no or little added sugars, saturated fat, and

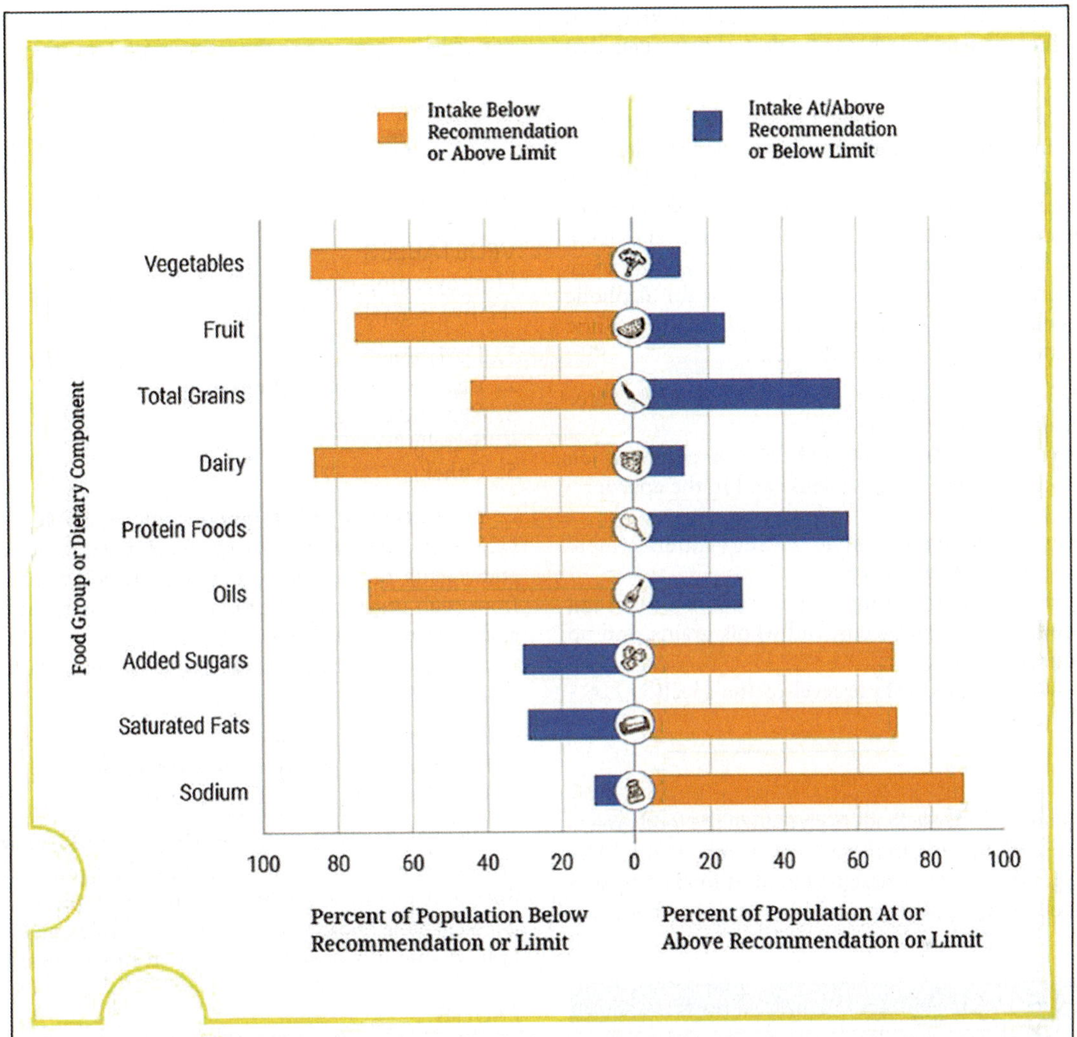

The center (0) line is the goal or limit. For most, those represented by the orange sections of the bars, shifting toward the center line will improve their eating pattern.
Figure from the 2015–2020 Dietary Guidelines for Americans (www.health.gov/dietaryguidelines/2015).

DATA SOURCES: What We Eat in America, NHANES 2007-2010 for average intakes by age-sex group. Healthy U.S.-Style Food Patterns, which vary based on age, sex, and activity level, for recommended intakes and limits.

Figure 21.1. American Dietary Consumption of Nutrients, Added Sugars, Saturated Fat, and Salt. The typical American food intake is too low in most types of vegetables, fruits, whole grains, low-fat dairy products, and seafood. At the same time, intake of refined grains and meats is too high.

sodium. A healthy dietary pattern consists of nutrient-dense forms of foods and beverages across all food groups, in recommended amounts, and within calorie limits. The core elements that make up a healthy dietary pattern include:

- Vegetables of all types—dark green; red and orange; beans, peas, and lentils; starchy; and other vegetables
- Fruits, especially whole fruit
- Grains, at least half of which are whole grain
- Dairy, including fat-free or low-fat milk, yogurt, and cheese, and/or lactose-free versions and fortified soy beverages and yogurt as alternatives
- Protein foods, including lean meats, poultry, and eggs; seafood; beans, peas, and lentils; and nuts, seeds, and soy products
- Oils, including vegetable oils and oils in food, such as seafood and nuts

Physicians and patients alike should try to follow these important principles when making decisions about nutrient dense food and beverage choices to achieve a healthy dietary pattern.

1. **Meet Nutritional Needs Primarily from Foods and Beverages**
   The *Dietary Guidelines* are designed to meet the RDAs and Adequate Intakes for essential nutrients, as well as Acceptable Macronutrient Distribution Ranges, all set by the National Academies. An underlying premise of the Dietary Guidelines is that nutritional needs should be met primarily from foods and beverages—specifically, nutrient-dense foods and beverages. In some cases, when meeting nutrient needs is not otherwise possible, fortified foods and nutrient-containing dietary supplements are useful.
2. **Choose A Variety of Options from Each Food Group**
   Enjoy different foods and beverages within each food group. This can help meet nutrient needs and also allows for flexibility so that the Dietary Guidelines can be tailored to meet cultural and personal preferences. All forms of foods, including fresh, canned, dried, frozen, and 100% juices, in nutrient-dense forms, can be included in healthy dietary patterns.
3. **Pay Attention to Portion Size**
   Portion size is a term often used to describe the amount of a food or beverage served or consumed in one eating occasion. It

is important to pay attention to portion size when making food and beverage choices, particularly for foods and beverages that are not nutrient dense.

Most of the calories a person needs to eat each day—around 85%—are needed to meet food group recommendations healthfully, in nutrient-dense forms. The remaining calories—around 15%—are calories available for other uses, including for added sugars or saturated fat beyond the small amounts found in nutrient-dense forms of foods and beverages within the pattern, to consume more than the recommended amount of a food group, or for alcoholic beverages. This equates to 250 to 350 remaining calories for calorie patterns appropriate for most Americans.

- The 2020–2025 *Dietary Guidelines for Americans* focus on three examples of healthy eating patterns[8,11]:
  1. The Healthy U.S.-Style Eating Pattern (an emphasis on American foods that are nutrient-dense and in the appropriate amounts)
  2. The Healthy Mediterranean-Style Eating Pattern (more fruits and seafood, and less dairy)
  3. The Healthy Vegetarian Eating Pattern (more beans and peas, soy products, nuts and seeds, and whole grains, and no meats, poultry, or seafood)
- Table 21.2 shows the 2,000-calorie level of the Healthy U.S.-Style Eating Pattern.

Food Groups

Eating a variety of nutrient-dense foods from each of the food groups at an appropriate calorie level is important for health. The USDA Food Patterns (e.g., Table 21.2) are designed to meet food group and nutrient recommendations while staying within calorie needs and are based on consuming foods in their nutrient-dense forms (i.e., without added sugars and in the leanest and lowest fat forms).

The calories indicated as "limits on calories for other uses" can be used when counting calories from foods that are not in nutrient-dense forms (e.g., desserts, some snack food products). Calories from alcoholic beverages should also be accounted for within this limit.

TABLE 21.2

Healthy U.S.-Style Eating Pattern at the 2,000-Calorie Level, with Daily or Weekly Amounts from Food Groups, Subgroups, and Components

Food Group	Amount in the 2,000-Calorie-Level Pattern
Vegetables	2½ c-eq/d
Dark green	1½ c-eq/wk
Red and orange	5½ c-eq/wk
Legumes (beans and peas)	1½ c-eq/wk
Starchy	5 c-eq/wk
Other	4 c-eq/wk
Fruits	2 c-eq/d
Grains	6 oz-eq/d
Whole grains	≥3 oz-eq/d
Refined grains	≤3 oz-eq/d
Dairy	3 c-eq/d
Protein Foods	5½ oz-eq/d
Seafood	8 oz-eq/wk
Meats, poultry, eggs	26 oz-eq/wk
Nuts, seeds, soy products	5 oz-eq/wk
Oils	27 g/d
Limit on Calories for Other Uses (% of calories)	270 kcal/d (14%)

VEGETABLES

Healthy eating patterns include a variety of vegetables from all of the five vegetable subgroups:

1. Dark green
2. Legumes (beans and peas)
3. Red and orange
4. Starchy
5. Other

The recommended amount of vegetables in the Healthy U.S.-Style Eating Pattern at the 2,000-calorie level is 2½ cup-equivalents of vegetables per day. In addition, weekly amounts from each vegetable subgroup are recommended to ensure variety and meet nutrient needs.

Vegetables are important sources of many nutrients, including:

- Dietary fiber
- Folate, thiamin, and niacin
- Potassium, magnesium, copper, iron
- Vitamin A, B_6, C, E, K

Dark-green vegetables provide the most vitamin K, red and orange vegetables the most vitamin A, legumes the most dietary fiber, and starchy vegetables the most potassium.

Vegetable choices should vary over time and be consumed with limited amounts of salt, butter, or creamy sauces.

FRUITS

Healthy eating patterns include whole fruits (fresh, canned, frozen, dried) and 100% fruit juice. The recommended amount of fruits in the Healthy U.S.-Style Eating Pattern at the 2,000-calorie level is 2 cup-equivalents per day.

- One cup of 100% fruit juice counts as 1 cup of fruit.
  - Although fruit juice can be part of healthy eating patterns, it is lower than whole fruit in dietary fiber and when consumed in excess can contribute extra calories.
  - When juices are consumed, they should be 100% juice, without added sugars.
- At least half of the recommended amount of fruits should come from whole fruits.
- Also, when selecting canned fruit, choose options that are lowest in added sugars.
- One-half cup of dried fruit counts as one cup-equivalent of fruit.
- Fruits provide dietary fiber, potassium, and vitamin C.

GRAINS

Healthy eating patterns include whole grains (e.g., brown rice, quinoa, and oats) and whole grain products (e.g., some breads, cereals) that contain the entire kernel, including the endosperm, bran, and germ.

- Intake of refined grains and products made with refined grains, especially those high in saturated fats, added sugars, and/or sodium, such as cookies, cakes, and some snack foods should be limited.
  - Refined grains have been processed to remove the bran and germ, which removes dietary fiber, iron, and other nutrients.

  - Most refined grains are enriched, a process that adds back iron and four B vitamins (thiamin, riboflavin, niacin, and folic acid).
- The recommended amount of grains in the Healthy U.S.-Style Eating Pattern at the 2,000-calorie level is 6 oz-equivalents per day. At least half of this amount should be whole grains.

Whole grains are a source of nutrients, such as:

- Copper
- Dietary fiber
- Folate
- Iron
- Magnesium
- Manganese
- Niacin
- Phosphorus
- Riboflavin
- Selenium
- Thiamin
- Vitamin A
- Vitamin B6
- Zinc

DAIRY

Healthy eating patterns include fat-free and low-fat (1%) dairy, including:

- Milk, yogurt, and cheese
- Soy beverages fortified with calcium, vitamin A, and vitamin D (commonly known as "soy milk"). They are included as part of the dairy group because they are similar to milk based on nutrient composition and their use in meals.

The recommended amounts of dairy in the Healthy U.S.-Style Pattern are based on age rather than calorie level and are:

- 2 cup-equivalents per day for children ages 2 to 3 years
- 2½ cup-equivalents per day for children ages 4 to 8 years
- 3 cup-equivalents per day for adolescents ages 9 to 18 years and for adults

The dairy group contributes many nutrients, including:

- Calcium, phosphorus, potassium
- Magnesium, selenium, zinc
- Protein
- Riboflavin, choline
- Vitamin A, D, B_{12}

PROTEIN FOODS

Healthy eating patterns include a variety of protein foods in nutrient-dense forms, from both animal and plant sources, including:

- Eggs
- Meats
- Nuts
- Poultry
- Seafood
- Seeds
- Soy products

Legumes (beans and peas) may also be considered part of the protein foods group as well as the vegetables group. Protein also is found in some foods from other food groups (e.g., dairy). The recommendation for protein foods in the Healthy U.S.-Style Eating Pattern at the 2,000-calorie level is 5½ oz-equivalents of protein foods per day.

Protein foods are important sources of nutrients in addition to protein, including:

- B vitamins
  - Niacin (B_3)
  - Riboflavin (B_2)
  - Vitamin B_6
  - Vitamin B_{12}
  - Selenium, copper, zinc
  - Vitamin D, E

Depending on the source of protein, the nutritional content can also be different.

- Meats provide the most zinc
- Poultry provides the most niacin
- Seafood provides the most vitamin B_{12}
- Eggs provide the most choline
- Nuts and seeds provide the most vitamin E

When selecting protein foods, nuts and seeds should be unsalted and meats and poultry should be consumed in lean forms.

- Meats, poultry, and seafood provide heme iron, which is more bioavailable than the nonheme iron found in plant sources.
- Processed meats and processed poultry are sources of sodium and saturated fats.
- Eating patterns that include lower intake of meats, as well as processed meats and processed poultry, are associated with reduced risk of:
  - CVD
  - Some types of cancer
  - Obesity
  - Type 2 diabetes

OILS

Oils are fats that contain a high percentage of monounsaturated and polyunsaturated fats and are liquid at room temperature.

- Oils are a major source of essential fatty acids and vitamin E.
- Commonly consumed oils extracted from plants include the following:
  - Canola and corn
  - Olive and peanut
  - Safflower and soybean
- Oils are also naturally present in:
  - Nuts and seeds
  - Olives and avocados
  - Seafood
- The fat in some tropical plants, such as coconut oil, palm kernel oil, and palm oil, are not included in the oils category because they contain a higher percentage of saturated fats.
- The recommendation for oils in the Healthy U.S.-Style Eating Pattern at the 2,000-calorie level is 27 g or about five teaspoons per day and should replace solid fats such as butter, lard, and shortening.
- All dietary fats are composed of a mix of polyunsaturated, monounsaturated, and saturated fatty acids, in varied proportions.

Other Dietary Components

At every life stage, meeting food group recommendations—even with nutrient-dense choices—requires most of a person's daily calorie needs and sodium limits. A healthy dietary pattern doesn't have much room for extra added sugars, saturated fat, or sodium—or for alcoholic beverages. A small amount of added sugars, saturated fat, or sodium can be added to nutrient-dense foods and beverages to help meet food group recommendations, but foods and beverages high in these components should be limited. Limits are:

- Added sugars—Less than 10% of calories per day starting at age 2. Avoid foods and beverages with added sugars for those younger than age 2.
- Saturated fat—Less than 10% of calories per day starting at age 2.
- Sodium—Less than 2,300 mg/d—and even less for children younger than age 14.
- Alcoholic beverages—Adults of legal drinking age can choose not to drink or to drink in moderation by limiting intake to 2 drinks or less in a day for men and 1 drink or less in a day for women, when alcohol is consumed. Drinking less is better for health than drinking more. There are some adults who should not drink alcohol, such as women who are pregnant.

ADDED SUGARS

Added sugars total 270 calories or more than 13% of calories per day in the U.S. population.

- About half of the added sugars come from beverages such as:
  - ☐ Alcoholic beverages
  - ☐ Energy drinks and flavored waters
  - ☐ Fruit drinks
- Soft drinks, sweetened coffee, and tea
- Snacks and sweets provide 31% of the added sugar consumed by Americans.
- Naturally occurring sugars, such as those in fruit or milk, are not added sugars and come packaged with many beneficial nutrients.
- When sugars are added to foods and beverages to sweeten them, they add calories without contributing essential nutrients, making it difficult to meet nutrient needs while staying within calorie limits.

Healthy eating patterns limit added sugars to less than 10% of calories per day.[11]

- Examples of added sugars that can be listed as an ingredient include the following:
  - ☐ Corn syrup and sweetener
  - ☐ Dextrose, fructose, and sucrose
  - ☐ High-fructose corn syrup
  - ☐ Malt syrup and maltose
  - ☐ Molasses
  - ☐ Raw and brown sugar

Strategies for lowering added sugar intake include choosing beverages low in added sugars and drinking more:

- 100% fruit or vegetable juices
- Low-fat or fat-free milk
- Water

The food additive listings for six sweeteners that have been approved and are considered safe by the U.S. Food and Drug Administration (FDA) include the following:

- Acesulfame potassium (Ace-K)
- Aspartame
- Saccharin
- Sucralose
- Neotame
- Advantame
- As a note, at the time of the completion of this chapter, the FDA supports the generally recognized as safe (GRAS) conclusions about certain Steviol Glycosides from the leaves of Stevia rebaudiana (Bertoni), extracts from Siraitia gosvernorii (monk fruit), or thaumatin. However, the use of stevia leaf and crude stevia extracts are not considered GRAS and import into the United States is not permitted for use as sweetners.[12]

Replacing added sugars with high-intensity sweeteners may reduce calorie intake in the short term but may not be an effective long-term weight management strategy.

SATURATED FATS

Intake of saturated fats should be limited to less than 10% of calories per day by replacing them with polyunsaturated and monounsaturated fats.

- Doing so will:
  - ☐ Lower blood levels of total cholesterol and of low-density lipoprotein cholesterol (LDL cholesterol)
  - ☐ Reduce the risk of CVD
- Strong and consistent evidence shows that replacing saturated fats with polyunsaturated fats is associated with a reduced risk of cardiovascular events (i.e., heart attacks) and CVD related deaths.

Current average intakes of saturated fats are 11% of calories, just above the 10% recommendation.

- The main sources of saturated fats in the U.S. diet include mixed dishes containing cheese and meat.
- Strategies to lower saturated fat intake include the following:
  - ☐ Consuming smaller portions of foods high in saturated fats
  - ☐ Reading food labels
  - ☐ Substituting with fat-free or low-fat milk, low-fat cheese, and lean cuts of meat
- In place of some of the fatty meat and/or regular cheese in mixed dishes, the ingredients can be changed to increase the amounts of:
  - ☐ Lean meat
  - ☐ Low-fat or fat-free cheese
  - ☐ Vegetables
  - ☐ Whole grains
- Additional strategies include the following:
  - ☐ Preparing foods using oils that are high in polyunsaturated and monounsaturated fats, rather than solid fats, which are high in saturated fats.
  - ☐ Using oil-based dressings and spreads on foods instead of those made from solid fats (e.g., butter, stick margarine, cream cheese).

SODIUM

Healthy eating patterns limit sodium to less than 2,300 mg/d for adults and children ages 1 year and older. 2,300 mg sodium is equivalent to 1 teaspoon of table salt.

- Sodium is essential but is needed by the body in relatively small quantities.
- A clear relationship exists between increased sodium intake and increased blood pressure (BP).
- Sodium is primarily consumed as salt (sodium chloride).
- As shown in Figure 21.2, average intake of sodium is substantially higher than recommended for health.
- For all adult men, the average intake is 4,240 mg.
- For adult women, the average is 2,980 mg/d.

Only a small proportion of total sodium intake is from sodium inherent in foods or from salt added in home cooking or at the table.

- Most sodium consumed in the United States comes from salts added during commercial food processing and preparation.

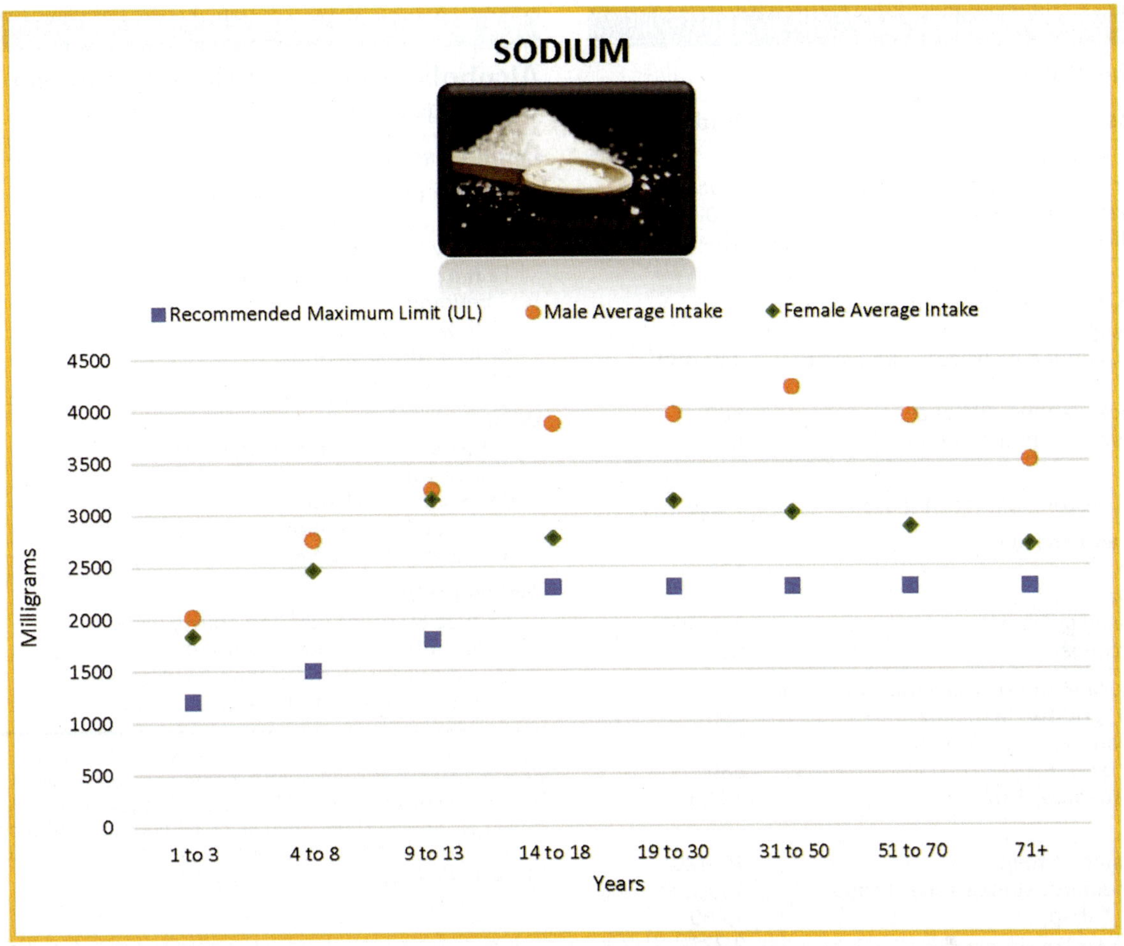

DATA SOURCES: What We Eat in America, NHANES 2017-March 2020 Prepandemic for average intakes by age-sex group, Institute of Medicine Dietary Reference Intakes for Tolerable Upper Intake Levels (UL).

Figure 21.2. American Sodium Consumption in Diet.

- Sodium is found in foods from almost all food categories.
- Mixed dishes (e.g., burgers, pasta dishes, pizza, meat dishes, soups) account for almost half of the sodium consumed in the United States.
- Table 21.3 lists the sodium content for various foods.

Strategies to lower sodium intake include the following:

- Reading food labels
- Choosing products with less sodium
- Using fresh or frozen vegetables
- Choosing fresh poultry, seafood, or pork
- Using lean meat, rather than processed meat and poultry
- Eating at home more often
- Cooking foods from scratch
- Limiting sauces
- Flavoring foods with herbs and spices instead of salt

ALCOHOL

If alcohol is consumed, it should be in moderation (up to one drink per day for women and up to two drinks per day for men) and only by adults of legal drinking age.[8]

- Table 21.4 lists alcoholic drink-equivalents of select beverages, with one alcoholic drink-equivalent described as containing 14 g (0.6 fl oz) of pure alcohol.
- Moderate alcohol consumption can be incorporated into most healthy eating patterns, but the calories from alcohol should be accounted for so that the limits on calories for other uses and total calories are not exceeded.

The Dietary Guidelines does not recommend that individuals who do not drink alcohol start drinking for any reason. There are also many circumstances in which individuals should avoid alcohol, such as during pregnancy.

High-risk drinking is the consumption of:

- For women:
  - ☐ 4 or more drinks on any day
  - ☐ 8 or more drinks per week
- For men:
  - ☐ 5 or more drinks on any day
  - ☐ 15 or more drinks per week

Binge drinking is the consumption within about 2 hours of 4 or more drinks for women and 5 or more drinks for men.

- Excessive alcohol intake has no health benefits and is responsible for 88,000 deaths in the United States each year, including 1 in 10 deaths among working-age adults (ages 20 to 64 years).
- Binge drinking accounts for over half of deaths due to excessive drinking.

TABLE 21.3

Where's the Salt?

Food Groups	Sodium, mg
Bread, cereal, rice, and pasta	
Cooked cereal, rice, pasta, unsalted, 1/2 cup	Trace
Ready-to-eat cereal, 1 oz	100–360
Bread, 1 slice	110–175
Vegetable	
Vegetables, fresh or frozen, cooked without salt, 1/2 cup	<70
Vegetables, canned or frozen with sauce, 1/2 cup	140–460
Tomato juice, canned, 3/4 cup	660
Vegetable soup, canned, 1 cup	820
Fruit	
Fruit, fresh, frozen, canned, 1/2 cup	Trace
Milk, yogurt, and cheese	
Milk, 1 cup	120
Yogurt, 8 oz	160
Natural cheeses, 1½ oz	110–450
Processed cheeses, 2 oz	800
Meat, poultry, fish, dry beans, eggs, and nuts	
Fresh meat, poultry, fish, 3 oz	<90
Tuna, canned, water pack, 3 oz	300
Bologna, 2 oz	580
Ham, lean roasted, 3 oz	1,020
Other	
Salad dressing, 1 tbsp	75–220
Ketchup, mustard, steak sauce, 1 tbsp	130–230
Soy sauce, 1 tbsp	1,030
Salt, 1 tsp	2,330
Dill pickle, 1 medium	930
Potato chips, salted, 1 oz	130
Corn chips, salted, 1 oz	235
Peanuts, roasted in oil, salted, 1 oz	120

Source: U.S. Department of Agriculture.

- Excessive drinking increases the risk of many chronic diseases and violence and can impair short- and long-term cognitive function.
- Binge drinking is associated with a wide range of health and social problems, including:
  - Accidental injuries
  - Sexually transmitted diseases
  - Unintended pregnancy
  - Violent crime

Mixing alcohol and caffeine is not GRAS by the FDA. People who mix alcohol and caffeine may drink more alcohol and become more intoxicated than they realize, increasing the risk of alcohol-related adverse events.

Many individuals should not consume alcohol, including:

- Individuals who are taking certain over-the-counter or prescription medications or who have certain medical conditions.
- Those who are recovering from alcoholism or are unable to control the amount they drink.
- Anyone younger than 21 years of age.
- Individuals who are driving, planning to drive, or are participating in other activities requiring skill, coordination, and alertness.
- Women who are or who may be pregnant, as no safe level of alcohol consumption during pregnancy has been established.

TABLE 21.4

Alcoholic Drink-Equivalents[a] of Select Beverages

Drink Description	Drink-Equivalents
Beer, beer coolers, and malt beverages	
12 fl oz at 4.2% alcohol (includes many light beers)	0.8
12 fl oz at 5% alcohol (reference beverage)	1
16 fl oz at 5% alcohol	1.3
12 fl oz at 7% alcohol	1.4
12 fl oz at 9% alcohol	1.8
Wine	
5 fl oz at 12% alcohol (reference beverage)	1
9 fl oz at 12% alcohol	1.8
5 fl oz at 15% alcohol	1.3
5 fl oz at 17% alcohol	1.4
Distilled spirits	
1.5 fl oz 80 proof distilled spirits (40% alcohol) (reference beverage)	1
Mixed drink with more than 1.5 fl oz 80 proof distilled spirits (40% alcohol)	>1

[a]One alcoholic drink-equivalent is defined as containing 14 g (0.6 fl oz) of pure alcohol. The following are reference beverages that are one alcoholic drink-equivalent: 12 fluid oz of regular beer (5% alcohol), 5 fluid oz of wine (12% alcohol), or 1.5 fluid oz of 80 proof distilled spirits (40% alcohol). Drink-equivalents are not intended to serve as a standard drink definition for regulatory purposes.

When ingested, alcohol passes from the stomach into the small intestine, where it is rapidly absorbed into the blood and distributed throughout the body.

- Peak blood alcohol levels are reached in fasting people within 30 minutes to 2 hours.
- As a rule of thumb, one standard alcoholic drink consumed within 1 hour will produce a blood alcohol level or content (called BAL or BAC) of 0.02 in a 150-lb male.
  - This varies depending on body size, gender, food taken along with the alcohol, and tolerance (i.e., less responsive to alcohol because of long-term use).
  - Five beers consumed within 1 hour will cause the BAC to rise on average to 0.10, which violates the drinking and driving laws of all states. (In 2024, the limit is 0.08 in all states except Utah, where it is 0.05.)
- The liver enzyme system takes 3 hours on average to clear the body of alcohol from two to three drinks.

Encouraging Healthy Eating Patterns

Americans make food and beverage choices in a variety of settings at home, at work, and at play.[8]

- About two-thirds of the calories consumed by the U.S. population are purchased at a store and consumed in the home, with one-third consumed away from home.
- Concerted efforts among professionals within communities, businesses and industries, organizations, governments, and other segments of society are needed to support individuals and families in making lifestyle choices that align with the *Dietary Guidelines*.

BOX 21.1 Aligning with the Dietary Guidelines for Americans: What Does this Mean in Practice?

The *Dietary Guidelines* describes adaptable eating patterns that can help promote health and reduce risk of chronic disease across the lifespan, and presents an array of options that can be tailored to income levels and that can accommodate cultural, ethnic, traditional, and personal preferences.

All segments of society—individuals, families, communities, businesses and industries, organizations, governments, and others—can and should "align with the Dietary Guidelines." In practice, the goal is to take the following actions in their entirety and maintain them over time:

1. Make food and beverage choices that meet the Key Recommendations for food groups, sub-groups, nutrients, and other components in combination to contribute to overall healthy eating patterns.
2. Meet nutritional needs primarily through foods. Foods provide an array of nutrients and other components that are associated with beneficial effects on health. Individuals should aim to consume a diet that achieves the most recent DRIs, which consider many factors, including the individual's age, life stage, and sex. In some cases, fortified foods and dietary supplements may be useful in providing one or more nutrients that otherwise may be consumed in less than recommended amounts or that are of particular concern for specific population groups.
3. Establish and maintain settings (e.g., homes, schools, worksites, restaurants, stores) that support and encourage food and beverage choices that help individuals make shifts to meet the Key Recommendations for healthy eating patterns.
4. Ensure that food is kept safe to eat by using the principles of clean, separate, cook, and chill.
5. Establish and maintain sectors and settings that support and encourage regular physical activity as part of a healthy lifestyle.

All of these actions are important individually, but they are intended to be taken together. Aligning with the Dietary Guidelines by taking these actions is powerful because it can help change social norms and values and ultimately support a new prevention and healthy lifestyle paradigm that will benefit the U.S. population today as well as future generations.

- Professionals have an important role in leading disease prevention efforts to enhance healthy eating and regular physical activity.
- Box 21.1 summarizes what can be done to integrate the *Dietary Guidelines* into the daily lifestyles of Americans.

MYPLATE

MyPlate is used by professionals to help individuals become more aware of and educated about making healthy food and beverage

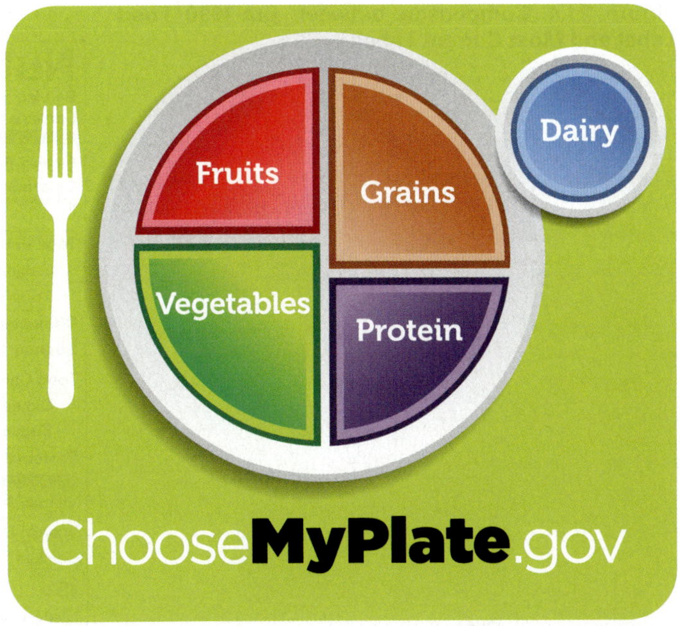

Figure 21.3. ChooseMyPlate.gov website provides information on a balanced, nutritious diet.

choices over time. The MyPlate symbol (Fig. 21.3) and its supporting consumer resources at *ChooseMyPlate.gov* bring together the key elements of healthy eating patterns, translating the *Dietary Guidelines* into key consumer messages that are used in educational materials and tools for the public.

THE FOOD LABEL

In 1990, the FDA approved a new procedure for nutrition labeling of processed foods and authorized appropriate health claims (Fig. 21.4).

- While the old food label emphasized vitamin and mineral content, as of 1990, the food label focused on the real nutritional shortcomings of Americans:
  - Cholesterol
  - Dietary fiber
  - Saturated fat
  - Sodium
  - Sugars
  - Total fat
- The Nutrition Facts food label used the daily values to help consumers plan healthy diets. They serve as the nutrient reference values on the food label, combining information from the RDA/DRI and the *Dietary Guidelines for Americans*.
  - The daily values are based on a 2,000-calorie diet, close to the average American intake.
  - A daily value of 20% for total fat means that a serving of this particular food provides 20% of the total fat allowed for the average adult.

An important feature of the FDA's 1990 mandate to improve food labels was the regulation of nutrient content claims and health claims.

- Nutrient content claims describe the amount of nutrients in foods such as:
  - Cholesterol free
  - Lean

Figure 21.4. Comparison between pre-1990 Food Label and Most Current Label.

1990

Nutrition Facts

Serving Size 2/3 cup (55g)
Servings Per Container About 8

Amount Per Serving	
Calories 230	Calories from Fat 72
	% Daily Value*
Total Fat 8g	12%
Saturated Fat 1g	5%
Trans Fat 0g	
Cholesterol 0mg	0%
Sodium 160mg	7%
Total Carbohydrate 37g	12%
Dietary Fiber 4g	16%
Sugars 1g	
Protein 3g	
Vitamin A	10%
Vitamin C	8%
Calcium	20%
Iron	45%

* Percent Daily Values are based on a 2,000 calorie diet. Your daily value may be higher or lower depending on your calorie needs.

	Calories:	2,000	2,500
Total Fat	Less than	65g	80g
Sat Fat	Less than	20g	25g
Cholesterol	Less than	300mg	300mg
Sodium	Less than	2,400mg	2,400mg
Total Carbohydrate		300g	375g
Dietary Fiber		25g	30g

Current

Nutrition Facts

8 servings per container

Serving size 2/3 cup (55g)

Amount per 2/3 cup

Calories 230

% DV*	
12%	**Total Fat** 8g
5%	Saturated Fat 1g
	Trans Fat 0g
0%	**Cholesterol** 0mg
7%	**Sodium** 160mg
12%	**Total Carbs** 37g
14%	Dietary Fiber 4g
	Sugars 1g
	Added Sugars 0g
	Protein 3g
10%	Vitamin D 2 mcg
20%	Calcium 260 mg
45%	Iron 8 mg
5%	Potassium 235 mg

* Footnote on Daily Values (DV) and calories reference to be inserted here.

  - □ Light
  - □ Low fat
- These nutrient content claims are now based on precise definitions and specific portion sizes to avoid consumer confusion when comparing one food brand with another. For example:
  - □ "Cholesterol free" indicates less than 2 mg of cholesterol per serving.

"Low fat" means 3 g of fat or less per serving. Health claims that link foods with prevention of certain diseases must be scientifically based.

- The FDA has authorized about a dozen health claims allowed on the labels of food products and dietary supplements to show that a food or food component may reduce the risk of a disease or health-related condition, including:
  - □ Fiber with heart disease and cancer
  - □ Diets low in saturated fat and cholesterol with heart disease
  - □ Fruits and vegetables with cancer
  - □ Low-sodium foods with high BP
  - □ Noncariogenic sweeteners with dental caries

Recently, the FDA updated the Nutrition Facts label found on most food packages in the United States.[13] Some of the key changes include (see Fig. 21.4):

1. Required information about added sugars.
2. Updated daily values for nutrients including:
   - □ Calcium
   - □ Dietary fiber
   - □ Potassium
   - □ Iron
   - □ Sodium
   - □ Vitamin D
   - □ *Note—vitamins C and A are no longer required to be listed as these deficiencies are rare today in the United States.
3. Updated serving size requirements to reflect how people eat and drink today.
4. Refreshed the design to make calories and serving sizes more prominent and to emphasize parts of the label that are important in addressing current public health concerns such as CVD, diabetes, and obesity.
5. Shifted the percent daily value to the left of the label.
6. Calories are now larger and bolder.
7. The footnote at the bottom better explains the meaning of % Daily Value (DV), thus providing the consumer with information on nutrition in the context of a total daily diet.
8. The "calories from fat" has been removed as research is showing that the type of fat consumed is more important than the amount.[14]

An important goal is to choose meals and snacks that are high in nutrients but low to moderate in energy content (calories).

- At the same time, limit:
  - □ Added sugars
  - □ Cholesterol
  - □ Saturated and trans fats
  - □ Salt
- An additional premise of the *Dietary Guidelines* is that the nutrients consumed should come primarily from foods.
- Foods contain not only the vitamins and minerals that are often found in supplements but also hundreds of naturally occurring substances, including (Box 21.2).
  - □ Carotenoids
  - □ Flavonoids
  - □ Isoflavones
  - □ Protease inhibitors that may protect against chronic health conditions

BOX 21.2 Plant-Based Diets are Essential for Good Health

One of the strongest and most consistent findings from research conducted around the world in the last two decades is that a high dietary fiber intake from whole grains, fruits, and vegetables improves health and aids in weight management. These foods bring more to the table than just dietary fiber—they also provide many essential nutrients, antioxidants, and phytochemicals that reduce risk for a wide spectrum of chronic diseases.

Here is a sample of research reports that demonstrate the vital importance of a high-fiber diet based on a variety of plant-based foods:

- A diet rich in whole grains helps reduce abdominal fat while lowering the risk of heart disease. A study in the American Journal of Clinical Nutrition showed people who followed a weight loss program incorporating whole-grain breads, cereals, and other foods lost more body fat from the abdominal area than those who ate only refined grains like white bread and rice. In addition, subjects on the whole-grain diet experienced a 38% drop in C-reactive protein (CRP), an indicator of inflammation in the body linked to heart disease.
- Research on 21,000 physicians during a 19-year period showed that consumption of whole-grain breakfast cereals lowered risk of developing type 2 diabetes. Physicians consuming seven or more breakfast cereal servings a week compared to one or none experienced a 38% lowered risk for type 2 diabetes.
- The Mediterranean diet is high in vegetables, legumes, fruits, nuts, whole grains, olive oil, wine, and fish. A large study of 400,000 men and women showed that high conformity to the Mediterranean diet reduced death rates in heart disease and cancer, as reported in the Archives of Internal Medicine. The linkage between the Mediterranean diet and reduction in overall death rates from chronic disease was related (in order of importance) to moderate alcohol intake, low consumption of meat, high vegetable, fruit, and nut intake, high dietary monounsaturated (olive oil) to saturated (butter, red meat) lipid ratio, and high legume consumption.
- In another study of 130,000 men and women followed for 16 years by researchers from the Harvard School of Public Health, adherence to the Mediterranean diet reduced the risk of developing Parkinson Disease by 25%. These researchers reasoned that a high consumption of fruit, vegetables, legumes, and cereals and a low consumption of meats provided plenty of dietary antioxidants and folate and a limited amount of saturated fat. Together, this dietary profile may have lowered oxidative stress, a major contributor to the development of Parkinson Disease.
- High fruit intake, especially apples and pears, lowered risk of lung cancer, according to German researchers who followed nearly 500,000 people for 6 years. Among current smokers, a high intake of root vegetables was linked to decreased lung cancer risk. Quercetin, a pigment in berries, onions, and the peels of apples, is a strong antioxidant and anti-inflammatory, and tends to accumulate in the lungs when regularly consumed. Additional reports from the German study support a protective effect of high fruit and vegetable consumption against colon cancer.
- Vegetarians compared to nonvegetarians live about 3.6 years longer, and have lower rates of obesity, high blood pressure, type 2 diabetes, heart disease, and certain types of cancer. Physically active vegetarians have a lower risk for chronic disease than inactive vegetarians, and vegetarians who run have a better disease risk profile than nonvegetarian runners.
- Pooled data from 12 studies involving 280,000 individuals showed that an intake of five or more servings of fruits and vegetables per day compared to less than three servings was linked to a 17% reduction in heart disease risk.
- A high intake of broccoli and cauliflower (cruciferous vegetables) in a 4-year study of 30,000 men was associated with a 40% lowered risk of prostate cancer, according to Canadian researchers reporting in the Journal of the National Cancer Institute.

These are just a few of the many health benefits linked to high-fiber, plant-based diets. A diet rich in fruit, vegetables, whole grains, nuts, and seeds (the so-called "rainbow diet") not only provides high amounts of dietary fiber but also contributes antioxidants, folate, potassium, carbohydrate, and healthy types of fats, all of which are important for both athletic endeavor and disease prevention.

Fruits, nuts, and vegetables, reports the U.S. Department of Agriculture, play a significant role in human nutrition, and as a group makes significant contributions to overall U.S. diet intake, including 91% of total vitamin C, 48% of vitamin A, 30% of folacin, 27% of vitamin B6, 17% of thiamin, and 15% of niacin. Fruits and vegetables also supply 16% of magnesium, 19% of iron, and 9% of calories. Nuts are a good source of essential fatty acids, fiber, vitamin E, and minerals.

Despite the proven health and nutrition benefits of fruits and vegetables, only 20% of men and 30% of women eat five or more servings a day, according to a report from the Centers for Disease Control and Prevention. This proportion has decreased from 42% of adults eating five or more fruits and vegetables a day in 1988. The average American has only one fruit serving and two vegetable servings per day. Do all you can to add color and fiber to your diet by ingesting fruits, vegetables, and whole grains at each and every meal.

EXERCISE AND PHYSICAL ACTIVITY

In regard to exercise and physical activity, there are two simple mottos that physicians can impart onto their patients:

- "Move more, sit less"[15]
- "Some physical activity is better than none"[16]

Reassure patients that they do not need to be triathletes to gain health benefits from exercise. It may actually be as simple as parking a little farther from their entrance to work. Once a day, they can also walk down their driveway or up a flight of stairs, where they would normally take an elevator.

Important Terms for Discussion of Physical Activity with Patients

When discussing physical activity with patients, physicians should be aware of the following terms and definitions from the Centers for Disease Control and Prevention (CDC).[17]

- **Exercise:** A type of physical activity that involves planned, structured, and repetitive bodily movement done to maintain or improve one or more components of physical fitness.
- **Light-moderate physical activities:** These activities might include moderately paced or leisurely walking or bicycling, slow swimming or dancing, and simple gardening.
- **Occupational activity:** Activity undertaken as part of one's employment. This does not include exercise or physical activities engaged in at employer sponsored gyms or other facilities.
- **Perceived physical activity level:** Self-perceptions of one's own physical activity level compared with: (a) other persons the same age; (b) one's own activity level at an earlier point in time; and (c) the amount of physical activity considered desirable for health.
- **Physical activity:** Any bodily movement that is produced by the contraction of skeletal muscle and that substantially increases energy expenditure.
- **Physical fitness:** A set of attributes that people possess or achieve that relates to the ability to perform physical activity and is comprised of skill-related, health-related, and physiologic components.
- **Strengthening activities:** Activities that require strenuous muscular contractions such as weight lifting, resistance training, push-ups, sit-ups, etc.
- **Transportation-related activity:** Physical activity undertaken for the purpose of getting from place to place, which may include walking, jogging, biking, or any other physically active method of getting from one place to another.
- **Vigorous physical activities:** These activities might include fast walking, fast bicycling, jogging, strenuous swimming or sports play, vigorous aerobic dance, or strenuous gardening.

World Health Organization Guidelines

For patients and physicians alike, the WHO provides a valuable online resource with the most current exercise guidelines, in terms of the recommended levels of physical activity and modifications of physical activity.[16] The WHO defines physical activity and exercise as the following for adults aged 18 and above:

"Physical activity is any bodily movement produced by skeletal muscles that require energy expenditure…Exercise is a subcategory of physical activity that is planned, structured, repetitive, and purposeful in the sense that the improvement or maintenance of one or more components of physical fitness is the objective. 'Exercise' and 'exercise training' frequently are used interchangeably and generally refer to physical activity performed during leisure time with the primary purpose of improving or maintaining physical fitness, physical performance, or health."[16]

The WHO recommends that adults between the ages of 18 to 64 should engage in physical activity as follows:

Adults should do at least 150 to 300 minutes of moderate-intensity aerobic physical activity; or at least 75 to 150 minutes of vigorous-intensity aerobic physical activity; or an equivalent combination of moderate- and vigorous-intensity activity throughout the week, for substantial health benefits.

Adults should also do muscle strengthening activities at moderate or greater intensity that involve all major muscle groups on 2 or more days a week, as these provide additional health benefits.

Adults may increase moderate-intensity aerobic physical activity to more than 300 minutes; or do more than 150 minutes of vigorous-intensity aerobic physical activity; or an equivalent combination of moderate- and vigorous-intensity activity throughout the week for additional health benefits.

Adults should limit the amount of time spent being sedentary. Replacing sedentary time with physical activity of any intensity (including light intensity) provides health benefits.

Doing some physical activity is better than doing none.

- If adults are not meeting these recommendations, doing some physical activity will benefit their health.
- Adults should start by doing small amounts of physical activity, and gradually increase the frequency, intensity and duration over time.[16]

The same recommendations hold true for adults aged 65 and over. However, the WHO further states that:

> As part of their weekly physical activity, older adults should do varied multicomponent physical activity that emphasizes functional balance and strength training at moderate or greater intensity, on 3 or more days a week, to enhance functional capacity and to prevent falls.

In children aged 5 to 17, physical activity includes the following:

- Chores
- Games
- Planned exercise in the context of daily, family, and community activities
- Play
- Physical education
- Recreation
- Sports
- Transportation

The WHO recommends for children:

- Children and adolescents should do at least an average of 60 minutes per day of moderate to vigorous-intensity, mostly aerobic, physical activity, across the week.
- Vigorous-intensity aerobic activities, as well as those that strengthen muscle and bone, should be incorporated at least 3 days a week.
- It is important to provide all children and adolescents with safe and equitable opportunities and encouragement to participate in physical activities that are enjoyable, offer variety, and are appropriate for their age and ability.[16]

American Health Association and American College of Cardiology Recommendations

In their 2019 Guideline on Lifestyle, the American Health Association and American College of Cardiology (AHA/ACC) advised adults to engage in at least 150 minutes per week of accumulated moderate-intensity or 75 minutes per week of vigorous-intensity aerobic physical activity to reduce atherosclerotic cardiovascular disease (ASCVD).[9]

Dosage

MINIMUM AMOUNT OF PHYSICAL ACTIVITY FOR REDUCED MORTALITY

Despite the WHO and AHA/ACC guidelines, many Americans and populations of other countries have difficulty meeting these requirements, which essentially entails 30 minutes of exercise, 5 days a week. This may be due to:

- Time constraints (perceived or real)
- Misconceptions about exercise
- Uncertainty about how to engage in exercise, what type of exercise to engage in and how much exercise is actually needed to benefit their health

A study involving 416,175 individuals in Taiwan over 8 years showed that participants engaging in low-volume activity, averaging 92 minutes a week or 15 minutes a day, had a reduced risk of all-cause mortality by 14% and a longer life expectancy of 3 years, compared to those in the inactive group.

- Each 15 minutes of daily exercise, in addition to the 15 minutes minimum, further reduced all-cause mortality by 4% and all cancer mortality by 1%.
- If inactive individuals engage in low-volume exercise for 15 minutes a day, it appears that one in six deaths could be delayed.
- Individuals who performed an average of 15 minutes of moderate-intensity exercise daily had significant health benefits, compared to those who were inactive.[18]
- Therefore, for previously inactive patients, half of the WHO-recommended 150 minutes of exercise a week may lead to marked health improvements.

It is also interesting to note that the largest risk reduction or the greatest health benefits occur when an inactive individual becomes active with low to moderate exercise intensity. Research from clinical populations and/or the elderly population have shown that health benefits can be achieved at low volumes of exercise.[19]

Physical activity must also be considered in special populations. For example, the Canadian Association of Cardiovascular Prevention and Rehabilitation promotes an exercise program of about 40 minutes a week, for patients in cardiac rehabilitation programs, which is well below the 150 minutes a week recommendation.[20]

Research still needs to be done to determine the optimum dosage of exercise for each medical condition, and of course, for the patient as a whole, taking into consideration their environment, support system, and resources.

DURATION VERSUS CALORIES EXPENDED

Some studies have focused not on the duration of exercise but on the amount of calories expended.

- It seems that minimal adherence to current or previous physical activity recommendations, which will generate energy expenditure on the order of 1,000 kcal/wk, results in decreased all-cause mortality rates with risk reductions on the order of 20% to 30%. An even lower volume of physical activity may be associated with benefit.
- An increase in energy expenditure from physical activity of 1,000 kcal/wk, or an increase in physical fitness of 1 metabolic equivalent task (MET), was associated with a mortality benefit of about 20%.[21]

TYPE OF ACTIVITY

Vigorous-intensity activities appear to generate higher levels of calorie expenditure than moderate-intensity activity.

- However, it is not clear whether vigorous-intensity activity provides additional benefit as compared to moderate activity.
- There are no data on the duration and frequency of physical activity in relation to all-cause mortality rates, after controlling for volume of physical activity.[21]

Resources for Physicians on Patient Physical Activity

Physicians may provide detailed and individualized musculoskeletal exercise prescriptions for patients living with chronic medical conditions.

- Warburton's article "Prescribing exercise as preventative therapy" may serve as a useful guide for physicians regarding:
  - Energy expenditure of daily activities
  - Examples of training ranges
  - Rate of perceived exertion scale[22]

Many physicians know that they should recommend physical activity to patients. However, for certain patients who do not have specific health conditions, such as CVD or musculoskeletal conditions, that would qualify them for prescribed physical therapy sessions, physicians may be at a loss for appropriate recommendations on frequency and type of exercise in order for the patient to safely become more active.

- Gyms, personal trainers, and fitness professionals may be of varying quality. Currently, there is little standardization and credentialing within the fitness industry.
- A physician recommending a patient with fibromyalgia to take an aqua class at a nearby gym may be unaware that the pool is an inadequate temperature for the patient.
- A physician may recommend an overweight, deconditioned patient to hire a personal trainer who may have little experience training this type of client. Such a trainer could push the patient too far too fast, either resulting in injury or in the patient becoming averse to exercise.

To remedy this situation, the Coalition for the Registration of Exercise Professionals (CREP®) developed a registry of certified fitness professionals who have met a set of criteria and who maintain their specific certifications. The mission of CREP® is to secure recognition of registered exercise professionals for their distinct roles in medical, health, fitness, and sports performance fields. Physicians and patients alike can view usreps.org where CREP® maintains the United States Registry of Exercise Professionals® (USREPS®), an internationally recognized registry of exercise professionals in the United States. There they can find exercise professionals who hold National Collegiate Athletic Association (NCAA) accredited or International Organization for Standardization (ISO) 17024 compliant exercise certification on issues that pertain to regulation, access and scope of work. Current exercise certifications of member organizations listed in USREPS® include Certified Personal Trainer, Certified Group Fitness Instructor, Certified Pilates Teacher, Advanced Health and Fitness Specialist, Exercise Specialist, Registered Clinical Exercise Physiologist, and Certified Strength and Conditioning Specialist.[23]

Mortality of the Fit Versus Nonfit Patient

Increased physical activity and exercise are associated with reduced chronic disease risk. Most physiologic systems in the body benefit positively from physical activity and exercise by primary disease prevention and secondary disease prevention and treatment.[24]

The implementation of daily physical activity and exercise prevention interventions support an 80% reduction in CVD risk,[25] 90% reduction in type 2 diabetes risk,[26] 33% reduction in cancer risk,[27] and in some cases reductions in all-cause mortality.[28]

Patients who participated in exercise-based cardiac rehabilitation programming had greatly reduced cardiac mortality,[29–31] reduced need for percutaneous transluminal coronary angioplasty as compared to the control group, reductions in nonfatal myocardial infarctions, and reduction in hospital readmission.[24] Other studies showed that patients who had experienced a myocardial infarction who were enrolled in 3 to 6 months of cardiac rehabilitation programming experienced an 11% to 36% increase in aerobic functional capacity, improved quality of life, and decreased risk for subsequent cardiac events.[25,32]

After becoming physically active, patients with type 2 diabetes improved their overall insulin sensitivity and positively altered skeletal muscle proteins and enzymes associated with glucose metabolism and insulin signaling.[33]

Depression and anxiety symptoms are also improved with daily physical activity and exercise.[34] Daily physical activity and exercise enhance bone health by increasing bone mineral density reducing the incidence of osteoporosis and the risk of future bone fractures.[35,36] Physical activity and exercise also improve the immune system, enabling the body to fight infectious diseases and resulting in less overall susceptibility to sickness.[37]

Community Efforts

Physicians may opt to reach a larger number of patients by becoming involved in or by suggesting worksite behavioral lifestyle interventions.

- Certain studies have shown these to be feasible and effective in significantly improving risk factors for type 2 diabetes and CVD, by positively affecting:
  - BMI
  - HbA1c
  - Peripheral artery disease[38,39]
  - Systolic BP
  - Waist circumference
- In one study, those assigned to the U.S. Diabetes Prevention Program Group Lifestyle Balance (DPP-GLB) had significantly greater improvements in weight, physical activity, and other risk factors for DM and CVD at 6 months than those in the delayed group.
  - After completing 12 months of the intervention, participants responded to a satisfaction survey and reported that it was beneficial (96%) to offer the program at the worksite.
  - Furthermore, 99.5% indicated that they would recommend this program to their coworkers.
- Potential benefits of workplace programs include improved:
  - Absenteeism
  - Health care costs for employers
  - Productivity
  - Retention of employees
- Furthermore, in a recent study, findings suggest that for adults with traumatic brain injury (TBI) who are overweight or obese, participation in the GLB-TBI significantly reduced weight and metabolic risk factors and increased self-reported habits for diet and exercise.[40]

Benefit of Physical Activity in Patients with Diabetes

Many osteopathic physicians are aware that exercise is beneficial to patients with diabetes.

- It appears that in the acute phases, physical activity leads to increased insulin-stimulated glucose uptake into active skeletal muscle, accounting for about 80% of insulin-stimulated glucose disposal.

Long-term effects of physical activity include improved fat oxidation and storage in skeletal muscle, glycemic control, and insulin action.

- Physical activity also seems to:
  - Lessen the risk of obesity, a strong predictor of type 2 diabetes mellitus (T2DM)
  - Modulate body fat distribution
  - Prevent long-term weight gain
  - Promote energy expenditure
  - Specifically decrease visceral fat, which is linked to insulin resistance

RESEARCH RELATED TO LIFESTYLE MEDICINE

In a large prospective study, each increase of 500 kcal in energy expenditure a week was associated with a 6% decrease in the incidence of type 2 diabetes.[27]

In a smaller study, a lifestyle intervention that included moderate physical activity for at least 150 minutes a week proved more effective than metformin alone in reducing the incidence of diabetes.[22]

In insulin-treated subjects with type 2 diabetes, supervised exercise with both aerobic exercise and four resistance exercises was shown to be safe and effective in improving glycemic control and markers of adiposity and inflammation, thus countering the adverse effects of insulin on those parameters.

- Each supervised exercise session was 75 minutes twice weekly for 12 months and included structured exercise counseling versus a control group of counseling alone.
- In the exercise group, the total physical activity volume was significantly higher than the control group.
- The following were also significantly lower in the exercise group than the control group:
  - Coronary heart disease (CHD) risk scores
  - HgbA1C
  - hs-CRP (high-sensitivity CRP)
  - LDL
  - Systolic and diastolic BP
  - Waist circumference
- Only total cholesterol was decreased significantly in the control group.[41]

In a follow-up study of this same group, improved muscular fitness predicted improvements in cardiovascular risk factors in subjects with type 2 diabetes independently of weight loss.

- The authors hypothesize that this may be the result of an improved muscle fuel supply and storage, thus increasing insulin sensitivity.
- It may also be due to myokines, which act in a paracrine fashion, improving metabolism and reducing inflammation.
  - Patients exhibited improvements in: HDL cholesterol, HbA1c, homeostasis model assessment for insulin resistance (HOMA-IR), hs-CRP, insulin and waist circumference.
- The reduction of both diabetic factors and CHD risk score indicate the importance of introducing and maintaining fitness in this patient population.[42]

Increasing physical activity appears to lower the risk for progression of gestational diabetes mellitus (GDM) to T2DM. Additionally, sedentary behaviors like watching TV are positively associated with risk of obesity and type 2 diabetes.

- Bao et al. found a significantly lower risk of T2DM among women who met the recommended minimum level of total physical activity (≥7 MET-h/wk), compared to those who did not.
- The inverse association between total physical activity and T2DM risk persisted across different categories of: age, BMI, family, history of diabetes, time since GDM pregnancy.
- It was concluded that women in the highest quartile of total physical activity, who spent 10 h/wk or less watching TV, had a 62% lower risk of T2DM than women in the lowest quartile of total physical activity, who spent more than 10 h/wk watching TV.
- Engaging in physical activity over the minimum level recommended by the U.S. federal guideline was related to an approximately 45% lower risk for progression from GDM to T2DM.
- Walking and vigorous activity were associated with a lower risk of T2DM.
- Prolonged TV watching was associated with a higher risk for developing T2DM.[43]

Benefits of Physical Activity in Patients with Coronary Heart Disease

Many studies demonstrate physical activity is associated with a decrease in CHD.

In an aggregate data meta-analysis of epidemiologic studies investigating physical activity and primary prevention of CHD, it was found that individuals engaging in 150 min/wk of moderate-intensity leisure-time physical activity had a 14% lower CHD risk compared to inactive individuals.

- Those who performed 300 min/wk of moderate-intensity leisure-time physical activity had a 20% lower risk. Thus, at higher levels of physical activity, relative risks were lower.
- Those who engaged in physical activity lower than the minimum recommended amount also had significantly lower risk of CHD. This demonstrates that "some physical activity is better than none."[19]

There is a graded inverse relationship in women between physical activity and the risk of CVD-related death. The protective effects were seen with as little as 1 hour of walking per week.[44]

Researchers have attempted to elucidate a preferred exercise modality for decreasing cardiovascular risk in patients with metabolic syndrome.

- One study focused on visceral fat accumulation as a primary risk factor for CVD.
- Increased intensity, high-volume training appeared to improve visceral fat loss and carotid–intima–media thickness.
- High-intensity resistance training induced a faster visceral fat loss, once again emphasizing the importance of adding weight training to a patient's fitness regime.
- Many participants in the study did have difficulty maintaining the prescribed 15 to 20 hours of exercise a week.
- However, even those who were able to perform only 8 to 10 hours of exercise a week demonstrated metabolic benefits.[45]

Additionally, there is moderate strength evidence that shows that aerobic physical activity lowers LDL cholesterol by 3 to 6 mg/dL on average, compared to control interventions.[9]

Benefits of Physical Activity in Patients with Elevated Blood Pressure (BP)

Arterial stiffness is related to cardiovascular mortality. It is also a major contributing factor to the development of CVDs, including myocardial infarction and heart failure.

Per the 2017 updated ACC/AHA guidelines (first comprehensive set since 2003) BP categories are:

- Normal: Less than 120/80 mm Hg;
- Elevated: Systolic between 120 and 129 *and* diastolic less than 80;
- Stage 1: Systolic between 130 and 139 *or* diastolic between 80 and 89
- Stage 2: Systolic at least 140 *or* diastolic at least 90 mm Hg.

The guidelines eliminate the category of prehypertension, categorizing patients as having either Elevated (120 and 129 and less than 80) or Stage 1 hypertension (130–139 or 80–89). While previous guidelines classified 140/90 mm Hg as Stage 1 hypertension, this level is classified as Stage 2 hypertension under the new guidelines.

High BP should be treated earlier with lifestyle changes and in some patients with medication—at 130/80 mm Hg rather than 140/90—based on the new ACC/AHA guidelines for the detection, prevention, management, and treatment of high BP.[46]

- Both resistance (strength) and endurance (aerobic) exercise alone reduce peripheral arterial stiffness and central BPs in prehypertensive participants, aged 18 to 35 years old.[47–49]
- A 2019 umbrella review of 18 meta-analyses and systematic reviews including 594,129 adult participants provided strong evidence to support the role of physical activity in preventing hypertension in individuals with normal BP, as well as in reducing BP among individuals with prehypertension or hypertension.[48]
- A meta-analysis of longitudinal studies suggested that individuals who meet the minimum physical activity levels recommended by international guidelines have a 6% lower risk of hypertension than individuals with inactive lifestyles.[50]
- Additionally, isometric exercise, such as handgrip training, may also contribute to lowering BP.[51–53]

Benefits of Physical Activity in Patients with Cancer

There appear to be numerous benefits of physical activity on different aspects of patients with cancer. There is an association between greater physical activity and reduced mortality in colorectal, breast and prostate cancer patients, with 40% to 50% risk reductions observed among individuals undertaking physical activity.[54]

A patient's mental health can likewise be impacted. Physical activity improves physical and social quality of life, reduces anxiety and depression in patients with cancer, and provides positivity in their daily life.[55–57]

With respect to recurrence of cancer, combined aerobic and resistance exercise reduces the incidence of metabolic syndrome in cancer survivors, particularly breast cancer survivors. As metabolic syndrome is a risk factor for breast cancer recurrence, this is significant for patients.[58,59]

Additionally, physical activity reduces the levels of lactate, a factor in promoting tumor growth,[60,61] and improves immune function, thereby providing a better response to immunotherapy.[62,63] It also reduces such side effects of cancer treatment as fatigue, a benefit which persisted one year after the intervention.[55]

Benefits of Physical Activity in Elderly Populations

Musculoskeletal fitness appears to be of paramount importance to the elderly population. Many activities of daily living, such as going from sitting to standing and climbing stairs, require more musculoskeletal fitness as opposed to aerobic fitness.

- Two systematic reviews show that increased musculoskeletal fitness is associated with improved bone health, functional independence, glucose homeostasis, mobility, overall quality of life, psychological well-being, and decreased risk of falls, illness, and premature death.[9,27]

Physicians are encouraged to recommend activities to healthy elderly patients that tax the musculoskeletal system, such as resistance training and flexibility exercises, at least twice a week. This promotes functional independence and appears to maintain or improve overall quality of life.[41] Depending on the patient, the physician might also encourage a total of 30 minutes of moderate-intensity exercise on most days of the week,[22] but even 10-minute bouts of activity throughout the day may prove beneficial.

Sedentary Behavior

It is important to note that sedentary behavior is a separate distinct phenomenon from physical inactivity.

A highly active person can also engage in high levels of sedentary behavior. Sedentary behavior has been defined by the Sedentary Behavior Research network in 2012[64] as waking behavior conducted in a seated or reclined position, with an energy expenditure of less than 1.5 METs, such as:

- Driving a car (commuting)
- Playing computer/video games
- Reading
- Sitting
- Watching television

High levels of physical activity may counteract sedentary behavior, but it is best to avoid sitting for long intervals.

Large amounts of sedentary behavior are linked to several chronic medical conditions.

- The greatest risk for premature mortality is associated with inactive patients that have a high degree of sedentary behavior.[22]
- Prolonged sitting increases colorectal, endometrial, ovarian, and prostate cancer risks, and it has been reported to increase cancer mortality, particularly in women.[65]
- Increased sedentary behavior is also linked to increased total and abdominal body fat and waist circumference.[66]
- Furthermore, increased body fat seems to create a dangerous feed-forward circuit, in which patients with higher body fat exhibit decreased levels of exercise and more sedentary time,[67] which in turn further increases body fat.[68]
- Patients are at greater risk for dyslipidemia, CVD, and diabetes mellitus. Sedentary behaviors induce metabolic dysfunction characterized by elevated blood triglyceride levels, reduced HDL cholesterol levels, and diminished insulin sensitivity.
- Physical inactivity decreases bone mineral density[69] making patients potentially more susceptible to fractures.

However, physicians should be aware of the following to assist their patients in decreasing sedentary behavior:

- A reduction of daily sedentary time by 1.5 h/d was associated with a 1.4-kg body weight reduction over the course of 1 year.
- An increase of 16.8 minutes a day of moderate-to-vigorous activity resulted in a 0.5-kg weight loss in 1 year and a decrease of fat mass of 1.2 kg over 7 years.[70]
- Physicians should also encourage "breaking sedentary time." Interrupting intervals of sedentary behavior with light-intensity activity may have a positive effect on C-peptides, help control adiposity and postprandial glycemia, and reduce insulin levels.[71]

Further encouraging news for patients is that while increased sedentary time increases the mortality among people who engage in little physical activity, adequate physical activity seems to offset the impact of increased sedentary time on mortality.[72]

MENTAL AND EMOTIONAL WELL-BEING

According to the WHO, mental health is a state of mental well-being that enables people to cope with the stresses of life, realize their abilities, learn well and work well, and contribute to their community.[73]

The CDC states: "Mental health includes our emotional, psychological, and social well-being. It affects how we think, feel, and act. It also helps determine how we handle stress, relate to others, and make healthy choices.[74]

A mental disorder is characterized by a clinically significant disturbance in an individual's cognition, emotional regulation, or behavior. It is usually associated with distress or impairment in important areas of functioning. Mental disorders may also be referred to as mental health conditions. The latter is a broader term covering mental disorders, psychosocial disabilities, and (other) mental states associated with significant distress, impairment in functioning, or risk of self-harm. These include anxiety disorders, depression, bipolar disorder, posttraumatic stress disorder, schizophrenia, eating disorders, disruptive behavior and dissocial disorders, and neurodevelopmental disorders.[75]

As per the first osteopathic tenet: the person is a unit of body, mind, and spirit. Osteopathic physicians can have a profound impact on the health of their patients by being equipped to recognize mental health conditions in their patients and help manage and alleviate them.

Stress

Stress is defined as any action or situation (stressor) that places special physical or psychological demands on a person.[76] In other words, stress is anything that unbalances an individual's mental, emotional, and physical equilibrium. There are at least three different types of stress:

1. Routine stress related to the pressures of work, family, and other daily responsibilities.
2. Stress brought about by a sudden negative change, such as losing a job, divorce, or illness.
3. Traumatic stress experienced in an event like a major accident, war, assault, or a natural disaster where one may be seriously hurt or in danger of being killed.

Stress that is poorly managed or overwhelming to the individual can place the person at risk for sleep disturbances, mental health disorders, and substance abuse and have a negative impact on immune function, cognition and memory, and cardiovascular, respiratory, endocrine, and gastrointestinal health.[77]

STRESS MANAGEMENT

Stress management revolves around four major principles[78]:

1. Controlling stressors: Although stressors are omnipresent, they can be modified, reduced in number, avoided, or controlled.
2. Managing stress reactions: The mind can choose a more positive response to any particular stressful event, avoiding the negative health effects of the stress response.
3. Seeking social support: Seeking the social support of others and sharing emotional, social, physical, financial, and other types of comfort and assistance improves stress management.

4. Keeping healthy: Stressors have less of a negative impact when the body is healthy from adequate sleep, exercise, relaxation, and a balanced diet.

PHYSICAL ACTIVITY AND STRESS MANAGEMENT

Individuals who exercise regularly report feeling more relaxed, less tired, having greater self-confidence, and a sense that life is more satisfying and interesting.[79,80]

- Most studies show that psychological mood state is more favorable for active people and can be improved with regular exercise training, especially when mood state is unfavorable.
- People who avoid exercise are at much higher risk for feeling fatigue and depression than those who are physically active.
- Acute exercise appears to have a positive effect on cognitive performance. Most adults should experience improved cognition during and for some time after moderate physical activity bouts lasting 20 minutes or longer.

Sleep

Per the American Academy of Sleep Medicine, adults are recommended to get 7 hours or more of sleep per night.[81]

There are two phases of sleep, rapid eye movement (REM) and non-rapid eye movement (NREM) sleep. NREM sleep is further divided into three stages,N1 to N3. Each phase and stage of sleep includes variations in muscle tone, brain wave patterns, and eye movements. The body cycles through all stages approximately 4 to 6 times each night, averaging 90 minutes for each cycle.[82]

Stages of sleep:

- Wake
- N1 (stage 1) to light sleep (5%)—lightest stage of sleep lasting about 1 to 5 minutes
- N2 (stage 2) to deeper sleep (45%)—characterized by having sleep spindles and K-complexes on EEG recordings
    - Sleep spindles are brief, powerful bursts of neuronal firing in the superior temporal gyri, anterior cingulate, insular cortices, and thalamus, inducing calcium influx into cortical pyramidal cells. They are thought to be essential to synaptic plasticity and several studies indicate that they are needed for memory consolidation, specifically procedural and declarative memory.[83]
    - K-complexes are long delta waves that last approximately one second and may also function in maintaining sleep and memory consolidation.[84]
    - Stage 2 sleep lasts around 25 minutes in the first cycle and lengthens with each successive cycle, eventually comprising about 45% of total sleep. This stage of sleep is when bruxism (teeth grinding) occurs.
- N3 (stage 3) to deepest NREM Sleep (25%)
    - This is known as slow-wave sleep (SWS) and is considered to be the deepest stage of sleep, and therefore the most difficult to wake from. This is the stage when the body repairs and regrows tissues, builds bone and muscle, and strengthens the immune system.
    - It is also when sleepwalking, night terrors, and bedwetting occur.[85]
    - As individuals age, less time is spent in N3 and more time is spent in N2 sleep.
    - If someone is woken from this stage, they will experience transient mental fogginess called sleep inertia. Cognitive tests during this time have shown that they will have moderately impaired mental performance for 30 minutes to 1 hour.[86]
- REM (25%)
    - REM is associated with dreaming and is not considered a restful sleep stage. It usually starts 90 minutes after the onset of sleep, and each cycle of REM increases throughout the night. The first cycle typically lasts 10 minutes, with the final cycle lasting up to 1 hour.[87]
    - REM is when dreaming, nightmares, and penile/clitoral tumescence occur.

Using data from the 2020 National Health Interview Survey (NHIS), the CDC reports that 14.5% of adults had trouble falling asleep most days or every day in the past 30 days and 17.8% of adults had trouble staying asleep.[88] According to the third edition of the International Classification of Sleep Disorders (ICSD-3), insomnia is characterized by difficulty in either initiating sleep or maintaining sleep continuity, or poor sleep quality.

- Consequences of insufficient sleep include and have been linked to the following[89]:
    - Hypertension and anxiety
    - Impaired decision-making and motor vehicle accidents
    - Impaired glucose tolerance, insulin resistance, and obesity
    - Increased mortality

Elements that may help prevent insomnia include regular moderate-intensity aerobic exercise,[80] appropriate sleep hygiene, relaxation therapy, cognitive behavioral therapy for insomnia (CBTi), and, if needed, pharmacologic intervention.

SUMMARY

Diet and nutrition, exercise and physical activity, mental and emotional well-being, and sleep are all important considerations when incorporating Lifestyle Medicine into the care of patients.

- Chronic disease is oftentimes the result of an unhealthy lifestyle over the lifespan of a patient.
- Poor nutrition and lack of physical activity has been linked to a number of diseases, including some cancers, hypertension and CVD, osteoporosis, and type 2 diabetes.
- Focusing on a healthy eating pattern versus specific food or nutrients may be more beneficial in terms of creating better long-term health. This can include the following:
    - Incorporating a variety of nutrient-dense foods that are high in vitamins, minerals, polyphenols, and fiber
    - Considering a patient's sociocultural and personal eating preferences
    - Limiting intake of added sugars, saturated fats, sodium, and alcohol
    - Utilizing dietary guidelines and educational tools such as *MyPlate*
- Encouraging exercise and physical activity can be as simple as having patients "move more, sit less." This can include the following:
    - Using resources such as the WHO Guidelines to recommend age and condition-appropriate levels of physical activity
    - Making the distinction between physical inactivity and sedentary behavior
    - Considering a patient's community and exercise preferences

Reminding patients that "some physical activity is better than none"

- Optimizing a patient's mental, emotional, and social well-being not only addresses potential mental and behavioral disorders but also includes the following:

- ☐ Recognizing routine stressors in a patient's life and encouraging the use of fundamental stress management principles, including social support and positive social connections
- ☐ Recognizing the importance of adequate sleep in overall health

- By incorporating Lifestyle Medicine into the care of patients, the osteopathic physician:
  - ☐ Recognizes how nutrition and exercise can potentially treat disease and promote health by means of the osteopathic metabolic model of care.
  - ☐ Is able to better approach the person as a unit of body, mind, and spirit when considering a patient's mental, emotional, and social well-being.

REFERENCES

1. World Health Organization. Constitution. Accessed October 26, 2024. https://www.who.int/home/search-results?indexCatalogue=genericsearchindex1&searchQuery=health&wordsMode=AnyWord
2. Lloyd-Jones DM, Hong Y, Labarthe D, et al; American Heart Association Strategic Planning Task Force and Statistics Committee. Defining and setting national goals for cardiovascular health promotion and disease reduction: the American Heart Association's strategic Impact Goal through 2020 and beyond. *Circulation*. 2010;121(4):586–613.
3. Fang N, Jiang M, Fan Y. Ideal cardiovascular health metrics and risk of cardiovascular disease or mortality: A meta-analysis. *Int J Cardiol*. 2016; 214:279–283.
4. van Halewijn G, Deckers J, Tay HY, van Domburg R, Kotseva K, Wood D. Lessons from contemporary trials of cardiovascular prevention and rehabilitation: A systematic review and meta-analysis. *Int J Cardiol*. 2017;232: 294–303.
5. Harper AE. Origin of recommended dietary allowances: an historic overview. *Am J Clin Nutr*. 1985;41:140–148.
6. Food and Nutrition Board, National Research Council. *Recommended Dietary Allowances*. 10th ed. National Academy Press; 1989.
7. Otten JJ, Hellwig JP, Meyers LD, eds. *Dietary Reference (intakes: the Essential Guide to Nutrient Requirements*. National Academy Press; 2006.
8. U.S. Department of Agriculture and U.S. Department of Health and Human Services. *Dietary Guidelines for Americans, 2020–2025*. 9th ed. 2020. Accessed October 26, 2024. https://www.dietaryguidelines.gov/download PDF
9. Arnett DK, Blumenthal RS, Albert MA, et al. 2019 ACC/AHA guideline on the primary prevention of cardiovascular disease: A report of the American College of Cardiology/American Heart Association task force on clinical practice guidelines. *Circulation*. 2019;140(11):e596–e646.
10. Kushi LH, Doyle C, McCullough M, et al; American Cancer Society 2010 Nutrition and Physical Activity Guidelines Advisory Committee. American Cancer Society Guidelines on nutrition and physical activity for cancer prevention: reducing the risk of cancer with healthy food choices and physical activity. *CA Cancer J Clin*. 2012;62(1):30–67.
11. Van Horn L, Carson JA, Appel LJ, et al; American Heart Association Nutrition Committee of the Council on Lifestyle and Cardiometabolic Health; Council on Cardiovascular Disease in the Young; Council on Cardiovascular and Stroke Nursing; Council on Clinical Cardiology; and Stroke Council. Recommended dietary pattern to achieve adherence to the American Heart Association/American College of Cardiology (AHA/ACC) guidelines: A scientific statement from the American Heart Association. *Circulation*. 2016;134(22):e505–e529.
12. U.S. Food and Drug Administration. Generally Recognized as Safe (GRAS). Updated March 22, 2023. Accessed May 28, 2024. https://www.fda.gov/food/food-ingredients-packaging/generally-recognized-safe-gras
13. U.S. Food and Drug Administration. Food. Accessed May 28, 2024. https://www.fda.gov/food
14. U.S. Food and Drug Administration. What's on the nutrition facts label. Updated March 24, 2020. Accessed May 28, 2024. https://www.fda.gov/food/nutrition-facts-label/whats-nutrition-facts-label
15. U.S. Department of Health and Human Services. *Physical Activity Guidelines for Americans*. 2nd ed. U.S. Department of Health and Human Services; 2018.
16. World Health Organization. *WHO Guidelines on Physical Activity and Sedentary Behavior*. World Health Organization; 2020. License: CC BY-NC-SA 3.0 IGO.
17. Centers for Disease Control and Prevention. Physical activity glossary. Updated June 3, 2011. Accessed May 28, 2024. https://www.cdc.gov/nchs/nhis/physical_activity/pa_glossary.htm
18. Wen CP, Wai JP, Tsai MK, et al. Minimum amount of physical activity for reduced mortality and extended life expectancy: a prospective cohort study. *Lancet*. 2011;378(9798):1244–1253.
19. Sattelmair J, Pertman J, Ding EL, Kohl HW 3rd, Haskell W, Lee IM. Dose response between physical activity and risk of coronary heart disease: a meta-analysis. *Circulation*. 2011;124(7):789–795.
20. Warburton DE, Bredin SS. Reflections on physical activity and health: What should we recommend?. *Can J Cardiol*. 2016;32(4):495–504.
21. Lee IM, Skerrett PJ. Physical activity and all-cause mortality: what is the dose-response relation? *Med Sci Sports Exerc*. 2001;33(6 Suppl):S459–S494.
22. Warburton DE, Nicol CW, Bredin SS. Prescribing exercise as preventive therapy. *CMAJ*. 2006;174(7):961–974.
23. US Registry of Exercise Professionals® (USREPS®). Employee verification. Accessed May 28, 2024. https://usreps.org/employee-verification
24. Anderson E, Durstine JL. Physical activity, exercise, and chronic diseases: A brief review. *Sports Med Health Sci*. 2019;1(1):3–10.
25. Ades PA, Balady GJ, Berra K. Transforming exercise-based cardiac rehabilitation programs into secondary prevention centers: a national imperative. *J Cardiopulm Rehabil*. 2001;21(5):263–272.
26. Hamman RF, Wing RR, Edelstein SL, et al. Effect of weight loss with lifestyle intervention on risk of diabetes. *Diabetes Care*. 2006;29(9):2102–2107.
27. Warburton DE, Nicol CW, Bredin SS. Health benefits of physical activity: the evidence. *CMAJ*. 2006;174(6):801–809.
28. Fogelholm M. Physical activity, fitness and fatness: relations to mortality, morbidity and disease risk factors. A systematic review. *Obes Rev*. 2010;11(3):202–221.
29. Anderson L, Oldridge N, Thompson DR, et al. Exercise-based cardiac rehabilitation for coronary heart disease: Cochrane systematic review and meta-analysis. *J Am Coll Cardiol*. 2016;67(1):1–12.
30. Sagar VA, Davies EJ, Briscoe S, et al. Exercise-based rehabilitation for heart failure: systematic review and meta-analysis. *Open Heart*. 2015; 2(1):e000163.
31. Powell R, McGregor G, Ennis S, Kimani PK, Underwood M. Is exercise-based cardiac rehabilitation effective? A systematic review and meta-analysis to re-examine the evidence. *BMJ Open*. 2018;8(3):e019656.
32. Wenger NK, Froelicher ES, Smith LK, et al. Cardiac rehabilitation as secondary prevention. Agency for Health Care Policy and Research and National Heart, Lung, and Blood Institute. *Clin Pract Guidel Quick Ref Guide Clin*. 1995;(17):1–23.
33. Kirwan JP, Sacks J, Nieuwoudt S. The essential role of exercise in the management of type 2 diabetes. *Cleve Clin J Med*. 2017;84(7 Suppl 1): S15–S21.
34. Dudgeon WD, Phillips KD, Bopp CM, Hand GA. Physiological and psychological effects of exercise interventions in HIV disease. *AIDS Patient Care STDS*. 2004;18(2):81–98.
35. Xu J, Lombardi G, Jiao W, Banfi G. Effects of exercise on bone status in female subjects, from young girls to postmenopausal women: An overview of systematic reviews and meta-analyses. *Sports Med*. 2016;46(8): 1165–1182.
36. Daly RM. Exercise and nutritional approaches to prevent frail bones, falls and fractures: an update. *Climacteric*. 2017;20(2):119–124.
37. Simpson RJ, Kunz H, Agha N, Graff R. Exercise and the regulation of immune functions. *Prog Mol Biol Transl Sci*. 2015;135:355–380.
38. Ganesan AN, Louise J, Horsfall M, et al. International mobile-health intervention on physical activity, sitting, and weight: The stepathlon cardiovascular health study. *J Am Coll Cardiol*. 2016;67(21):2453–2463.
39. McDermott MM, Guralnik JM, Criqui MH, et al. Home-based walking exercise in peripheral artery disease: 12-month follow-up of the GOALS randomized trial. *J Am Heart Assoc*. 2014;3(3):e000711.
40. Driver S, McShan E, Swank C, et al. Efficacy of the Diabetes Prevention Program Group Lifestyle Balance Program Modified for Individuals with TBI (GLB-TBI): Results from a 12-month randomized controlled trial. *Ann Behav Med*. 2023;57(2):131–145.

41. Balducci S, Zanuso S, Cardelli P, et al; Italian Diabetes Exercise Study (IDES) Investigators. Supervised exercise training counterbalances the adverse effects of insulin therapy in overweight/obese subjects with type 2 diabetes. *Diabetes Care*. 2012;35(1):39–41.
42. Balducci S, Zanuso S, Cardelli P, et al; Italian Diabetes Exercise Study (IDES) Investigators. Changes in physical fitness predict improvements in modifiable cardiovascular risk factors independently of body weight loss in subjects with type 2 diabetes participating in the Italian Diabetes and Exercise Study (IDES). *Diabetes Care*. 2012;35(6):1347–1354.
43. Bao W, Tobias DK, Bowers K, et al. Physical activity and sedentary behaviors associated with risk of progression from gestational diabetes mellitus to type 2 diabetes mellitus: a prospective cohort study. *JAMA Intern Med*. 2014;174(7):1047–1055.
44. Oguma Y, Shinoda-Tagawa T. Physical activity decreases cardiovascular disease risk in women: review and meta-analysis. *Am J Prev Med*. 2004;26(5):407–418.
45. Dutheil F, Lac G, Lesourd B, et al. Different modalities of exercise to reduce visceral fat mass and cardiovascular risk in metabolic syndrome: the RESOLVE randomized trial. *Int J Cardiol*. 2013;168(4):3634–3642.
46. American College of Cardiology. 2017 AHA Blood Pressure Guideline. Updated November 13, 2017. Accessed May 28, 2024. https://www.acc.org/latest-in-cardiology/articles/2017/11/08/11/47/mon-5pm-bp-guideline-aha-2017
47. Beck DT, Martin JS, Casey DP, Braith RW. Exercise training reduces peripheral arterial stiffness and myocardial oxygen demand in young prehypertensive subjects. *Am J Hypertens*. 2013;26(9):1093–1102.
48. Pescatello LS, Buchner DM, Jakicic JM, et al; 2018 Physical Activity Guidelines Advisory Committee. Physical activity to prevent and treat hypertension: A systematic review. *Med Sci Sports Exerc*. 2019;51(6):1314–1323.
49. Naci H, Salcher-Konrad M, Dias S, et al. How does exercise treatment compare with antihypertensive medications? A network meta-analysis of 391 randomised controlled trials assessing exercise and medication effects on systolic blood pressure. *Br J Sports Med*. 2019;53(14):859–869.
50. Liu X, Zhang D, Liu Y, et al. Dose-response association between physical activity and incident hypertension: A systematic review and meta-analysis of cohort studies. *Hypertension*. 2017;69(5):813–820.
51. Cornelissen VA, Fagard RH, Coeckelberghs E, Vanhees L. Impact of resistance training on blood pressure and other cardiovascular risk factors: a meta-analysis of randomized, controlled trials. *Hypertension*. 2011;58(5):950–958.
52. Smart NA, Way D, Carlson D, et al. Effects of isometric resistance training on resting blood pressure: individual participant data meta-analysis. *J Hypertens*. 2019;37(10):1927–1938.
53. Jin YZ, Yan S, Yuan WX. Effect of isometric handgrip training on resting blood pressure in adults: a meta-analysis of randomized controlled trials. *J Sports Med Phys Fitness*. 2017;57(1-2):154–160.
54. McTiernan A, Friedenreich CM, Katzmarzyk PT, et al; 2018 Physical Activity Guidelines Advisory Committee. Physical activity in cancer prevention and survival: A systematic review. *Med Sci Sports Exerc*. 2019; 51(6):1252–1261.
55. Carayol M, Ninot G, Senesse P, et al. Short- and long-term impact of adapted physical activity and diet counseling during adjuvant breast cancer therapy: the "APAD1" randomized controlled trial. *BMC Cancer*. 2019;19(1):737.
56. Singh B, Hayes SC, Spence RR, Steele ML, Millet GY, Gergele L. Exercise and colorectal cancer: a systematic review and meta-analysis of exercise safety, feasibility and effectiveness. *Int J Behav Nutr Phys Act*. 2020;17(1):122.
57. Liska TM, Kolen AM. The role of physical activity in cancer survivors' quality of life. *Health Qual Life Outcomes*. 2020;18(1):197.
58. Dieli-Conwright CM, Courneya KS, Demark-Wahnefried W, et al. Aerobic and resistance exercise improves physical fitness, bone health, and quality of life in overweight and obese breast cancer survivors: a randomized controlled trial. *Breast Cancer Res*. 2018;20(1):124.
59. Dieli-Conwright CM, Courneya KS, Demark-Wahnefried W, et al. Effects of aerobic and resistance exercise on metabolic syndrome, sarcopenic obesity, and circulating biomarkers in overweight or obese survivors of breast cancer: A randomized controlled trial. *J Clin Oncol*. 2018;36(9): 875–883.
60. Hojman P, Gehl J, Christensen JF, Pedersen BK. Molecular mechanisms linking exercise to cancer prevention and treatment. *Cell Metab*. 2018;27(1):10–21.
61. Song M, Chan AT. The potential role of exercise and nutrition in harnessing the immune system to improve colorectal cancer survival. *Gastroenterology*. 2018;155(3):596–600.
62. Derakhshani A, Hashemzadeh S, Asadzadeh Z, et al. Cytotoxic T-lymphocyte antigen-4 in colorectal cancer: Another therapeutic side of capecitabine. *Cancers (Basel)*. 2021;13(10):2414.
63. Gustafson MP, Wheatley-Guy CM, Rosenthal AC, et al. Exercise and the immune system: taking steps to improve responses to cancer immunotherapy. *J Immunother Cancer*. 2021;9(7):e001872.
64. Tremblay MS, Aubert S, Barnes JD, et al; SBRN Terminology Consensus Project Participants. Sedentary Behavior Research Network (SBRN)—Terminology Consensus Project process and outcome. *Int J Behav Nutr Phys Act*. 2017;14(1):75.
65. Lynch BM. Sedentary behavior and cancer: a systematic review of the literature and proposed biological mechanisms. *Cancer Epidemiol Biomarkers Prev*. 2010;19(11):2691–2709.
66. Healy GN, Wijndaele K, Dunstan DW, et al. Objectively measured sedentary time, physical activity, and metabolic risk: the Australian diabetes, obesity and lifestyle study (AusDiab). *Diabetes Care*. 2008;31(2): 369–371.
67. Ohlsson C, Gidestrand E, Bellman J, et al. Increased weight loading reduces body weight and body fat in obese subjects—A proof of concept randomized clinical trial. *EClinicalMedicine*. 2020;22:100338.
68. Levine JA, Lanningham-Foster LM, McCrady SK, et al. Interindividual variation in posture allocation: possible role in human obesity. *Science*. 2005;307(5709):584–586.
69. Zerwekh JE, Ruml LA, Gottschalk F, Pak CY. The effects of twelve weeks of bed rest on bone histology, biochemical markers of bone turnover, and calcium homeostasis in eleven normal subjects. *J Bone Miner Res*. 1998;13(10):1594–1601.
70. Golubic R, Wijndaele K, Sharp SJ, et al. Physical activity, sedentary time and gain in overall and central body fat: 7-year follow-up of the ProActive trial cohort. *Int J Obes (Lond)*. 2015;39(1):142–148.
71. Chastin SF, Egerton T, Leask C, Stamatakis E. Meta-analysis of the relationship between breaks in sedentary behavior and cardiometabolic health. *Obesity (Silver Spring)*. 2015;23(9):1800–1810.
72. Stamatakis E, Gale J, Bauman A, Ekelund U, Hamer M, Ding D. Sitting time, physical activity, and risk of mortality in adults. *J Am Coll Cardiol*. 2019;73(16):2062–2072.
73. World Health Organization. Mental health: Strengthening our response. Updated June 17, 2022. Accessed May 28, 2024. https://www.who.int/news-room/fact-sheets/detail/mental-health-strengthening-our-response
74. Centers for Disease Control and Prevention. About mental health. Updated April 16, 2024. Accessed May 28, 2024. https://www.cdc.gov/mentalhealth/learn/index.htm
75. World Health Organization. Mental disorders. Updated June 8, 2022. Accessed May 28, 2024. https://www.who.int/news-room/fact-sheets/detail/mental-disorders
76. Habib KE, Gold PW, Chrousos GP. Neuroendocrinology of stress. *Endocrinol Metab Clin North Am*. 2001;30(3):695–728, vii–viii.
77. Yaribeygi H, Panahi Y, Sahraei H, Johnston TP, Sahebkar A. The impact of stress on body function: A review. *EXCLI J*. 2017;16:1057–1072.
78. Seward BL. *Managing Stress: Principles and Strategies for Health and Well-Being*. 8th ed. Jones & Bartlett Learning; 2014.
79. Nieman DC. *Exercise Testing and Prescription: A Health-Related Approach*. 7th ed. McGraw-Hill; 2011.
80. U.S. Department of Health and Human Services. 2008 physical activity guidelines for Americans. Accessed May 28, 2024. https://health.gov/paguidelines.
81. Watson NF, Badr MS, Belenky G, et al. Recommended amount of sleep for a healthy adult: a joint consensus statement of the American Academy of Sleep Medicine and Sleep Research Society. *Sleep*. 2015;38(6): 843–844.
82. Memar P, Faradji F. A novel multi-class EEG-based sleep stage classification system. *IEEE Trans Neural Syst Rehabil Eng*. 2018;26(1): 84–95.

83. Antony JW, Schönauer M, Staresina BP, Cairney SA. Sleep spindles and memory reprocessing. *Trends Neurosci.* 2019;42(1):1–3.
84. Cash SS, Halgren E, Dehghani N, et al. The human K-complex represents an isolated cortical down-state. *Science.* 2009;324(5930):1084–1087.
85. El Shakankiry HM. Sleep physiology and sleep disorders in childhood. *Nat Sci Sleep.* 2011;3:101–114.
86. Hilditch CJ, McHill AW. Sleep inertia: current insights. *Nat Sci Sleep.* 2019;11:155–165.
87. Della Monica C, Johnsen S, Atzori G, Groeger JA, Dijk DJ. Rapid eye movement sleep, sleep continuity and slow wave sleep as predictors of cognition, mood, and subjective sleep quality in healthy men and women, aged 20–84 years. *Front Psychiatry.* 2018;9:255.
88. Adjaye-Gbewonyo D, Ng AE, Black LI. Sleep difficulties in adults: United States, 2020. *NCHS Data Brief.* 2022;(436):1–8.
89. Grandner MA, Patel NP, Gehrman PR, Perlis ML, Pack AI. Problems associated with short sleep: bridging the gap between laboratory and epidemiological studies. *Sleep Med Rev.* 2010;14(4):239–247.

22 Energy Balance: Nutrition, Exercise, and the Metabolic Model

MARCEL P. FRAIX ▪ DAVID C. NIEMAN ▪ ROBYN L.-F. DREIBELBIS ▪ REBECCA E. GIUSTI

KEY CONCEPTS

- The Metabolic Model encompasses the balance of energy, both in terms of its production and expenditure.
- Foods provide the nutrients needed by the body for energy production and maintenance of cells, tissues, and organ systems.
- Exercise requires the expenditure of energy and causes both acute and chronic physiologic adaptive responses.

INTRODUCTION

Since its inception with Dr. Andrew Taylor Still, the osteopathic philosophy has evolved and, at the same time, its fundamental principles have remained relevant.

- The following notions have become better defined as research has uncovered the mechanisms that underlie these fundamental tenets, upon which the osteopathic profession is founded:
  - That each human being is a dynamic unit of function
  - The body possesses self-regulatory mechanisms that are self-healing in nature
  - That structure and function are interrelated
- From a physiologic perspective, the Educational Council on Osteopathic Principles (ECOP) recognized the importance of the body's ability to maintain homeostasis, both in terms of maintaining health as well as restoring it in times of illness and disease. In doing so, ECOP created the Five Models of Osteopathic Patient Care, which includes the:
  - Biomechanical Model
  - Respiratory Circulatory Model
  - Neurologic Model
  - Metabolic-Nutritional Model
  - Behavioral Model
- The osteopathic physician utilizes each one of these models individually to assess the health of the patient as well as how these key physiologic processes are working and interacting, as the body adapts to stressors and recovers from illness and disease.

The use of essential nutrients allows the body to produce energy and function at the cellular, tissue, and organ level.

- The Metabolic Model recognizes that the body's capacity for energy production can be influenced by various factors, including:
  - Inflammation and repair
  - Toxic burden
  - Infectious disease
  - Nutrition
- Similarly, exercise has a major influence on energy expenditure and the body's homeostasis. The Metabolic Model acknowledges that exercise not only impacts energy balance, but that it has the capacity to create new set points for physiologic parameters such as:
  - Heart rate
  - Cardiac output
  - Blood flow
- Understanding how nutrition and exercise influence the systems of the body is important in seeing how the Metabolic Model can be applied to the patient, both in terms of health and disease.

NUTRITION

Nutrition is the science that examines how the food consumed affects the functioning and health of the body. The science of nutritional biochemistry is clear in the processes that occur with eating and what happens to the components of food once ingested, but there is also an important consideration of "why do humans eat?"

- The need to eat to support the body's metabolic requirements is clear, and it is driven through a complex interplay between the body and the brain that leads to a feeling of hunger and satiety.
- The act of eating is in part mechanical, biochemical, and metabolic, but it must also consider the psychological and cultural components of eating. Eating is a social act and that drives much of the ability to answer the question of "why do humans eat?"
- This portion of the chapter will focus on the metabolic processes of nutrition rather than the psychology of eating.

Food consumed is made up of a variety of compounds that provide energy, as well as build and maintain cells, organs, and tissues. It also helps regulate several life-sustaining body functions.

- The energy in food is measured in *kilocalories*, with one *kilocalorie* representing the amount of heat needed to raise 1 kg of water from 14.5 °C to 15.5 °C.
- The term *calorie* is used in place of *kilocalorie* to represent the amount of energy in food, even though a *calorie* is actually a much smaller unit of energy.
- Most American adults consume between 1,600 and 2,500 *calories* per day.

NUTRIENTS

For proper functioning and optimal health, the body requires more than 40 essential nutrients that are known currently, yet the research continues to evolve on this issue. The nutrients that the body cannot make on its own must be obtained from foods; these nutrients are classified into six main categories:

1. Carbohydrates
2. Fats
3. Proteins
4. Vitamins
5. Minerals
6. Water

Carbohydrates, fats, and proteins are responsible for supplying energy for the body and are also called macronutrients.

CARBOHYDRATES

Carbohydrates are compounds composed of carbon, hydrogen, and oxygen. They are a main source of energy for the body, providing 4 calories/g.

- Carbohydrates are found in:
  - Grains
  - Fruits
  - Vegetables
  - Milk

It is interesting to note that milk is the only animal-derived food that contains any form of carbohydrate (lactose, also known as milk sugar).

- Carbohydrates are typically classified into two groups:
  1. Simple sugars are composed of one (monosaccharide) or two (disaccharide) basic sugar units.
  2. Complex carbohydrates, or starches, are composed of longer chains of sugar units (polysaccharide).
- Though not often considered a carbohydrate in terms of providing usable energy for the body, dietary fiber does indirectly supply on average 2 calories/g.
  - Intestinal bacteria, collectively referred to as the "gut microbiota," break down dietary fiber and excrete short-chain fatty acids (SCFA) as a waste product of that process.[1–4] Beyond the many known benefits of these SCFA including gut barrier function, glucose homeostasis, and immunomodulation,[2–4] they can also be utilized by the intestinal lumen cells, called enterocytes, as a source of energy.
  - Fiber's main function is to feed the intestinal microbiome ("gut microbiota") as well as to provide bulk to the stool for normal transit through the intestine. Fiber may also be an important dietary component for the prevention of cardiovascular disease (CVD), including coronary heart disease (CHD).[1,3,5,6]
  - The gut microbiota has direct impact on the health of the gastrointestinal tract as well as on the overall health of every cell, tissue, and organ system in the body, in part through its effect on the immune system[2,4] of which it is estimated that approximately 60% lies within our gastrointestinal tract. Total lymphatic fluid production is approximately 1 to 4 L/d most of which is formed in the GI tract (>50%).[2,3] See Chapter 23 Microbiome: New Considerations in Clinical Management for further details.

FATS

Fats are the most energy-rich nutrients, providing 9 calories/g.

- They are present in:
  - Animal tissue
  - Grains
  - Nuts
  - Seeds
  - Some plants
- In addition to providing energy, fats:
  - Enhance the aroma and flavor of foods
  - Contribute to feeling of fullness (also known as satiety)
  - Transport vitamins
  - Are the precursors for cholesterol and sex hormone synthesis
  - Cushion the body's vital organs and are an essential component of cell membranes
- There are two essential fatty acids[7]:
  1. Linoleic acid
  2. Alpha-linolenic acid (ALA)

These essential fatty acids cannot be synthesized by the body and, therefore, must be obtained from the food we eat.

- Linoleic acid is the parent compound of the omega-6 fatty acid group.
  - Linoleic acid is found in:
    - Animal products
    - Most vegetable oils
    - Nuts
    - Seeds
    - Human breast milk[4]
  - Arachidonic acid is a major derivative of linoleic acid and serves as an abundant structural component of the central nervous system and has a significant role in the repair and growth of skeletal muscle during and following exercise.[5]
- ALA is the parent compound of the omega-3 fatty acid group.
  - ALA is present in:
    - Dark green leafy vegetables
    - Some vegetable oils
    - Nuts (especially walnuts)
    - Flax seed
    - Some animal fat (especially in grass fed animals)
  - Eicosapentaenoic acid (EPA) and docosahexaenoic acid (DHA) are derivatives of ALA but the conversion process within the body is slow. EPA and DHA are also found in:
    - Fatty, cold-water fish
    - Shellfish
    - Human breast milk
- The ratio of omega-6 to omega-3 fatty acids in our overall diet is important.
  - The western diet tends to provide excessive amounts of omega-6 and not enough omega-3 fatty acids.
  - It is estimated that humans evolved by eating an omega-6: omega-3 ratio close to 1:1, but the current western diet is closer to 15:1 to 16.7:1 and even up to 50:1 in other research.[6] This is because the western diet is predominated by processed foods which are replete in corn, canola, safflower, sunflower, and canola oils from which much of the omega-6 fats originate.
  - The body stores significant amounts of omega-6 fatty acids in the adipose tissue whereas it stores only small amounts of ALA, EPA, and DHA.
- Omega-3 fatty acids are extremely important to human health. Here are a few known functions of these compounds:
  - They are an integral part of cell membranes throughout the body.
  - They affect the function of the cell receptors in the cell membranes.
  - They are the backbone of the structure for the hormones that regulate blood clotting, contraction and relaxation of artery walls, and inflammation.
  - They bind to receptors in cells that regulate genetic function, both turning on anti-inflammatory genes and turning off proinflammatory genes.
  - Likely due to these collective effects, omega-3 fats:
    - Have been shown to help prevent heart disease, stroke, and arrhythmias.[7,8]
    - May help control autoimmune conditions such as lupus, eczema, and rheumatoid arthritis.
  - Have been shown to enhance the activity of the tumor suppressor genes BRCA1 and BRCA2 (breast cancer gene 1 and 2)

whose function helps to repair DNA damage, and thereby may play a protective role in cancer development, particularly breast and prostate cancer.[9]

PROTEINS

Proteins are compounds composed of carbon, hydrogen, oxygen, and nitrogen. Like carbohydrates, they are a main source of energy, providing 4 calories/g.

- They are found in:
  - Animal foods
  - Legumes
  - Nuts
  - Grains
  - Vegetables
  - Fruits (to a lesser degree)
- The component parts of a protein are amino acids; there are 20 total amino acids that are incorporated into the body's proteins, 9 of which are considered "essential amino acids" because they cannot be manufactured by the body and must be obtained from our food.
  - The nine essential amino acids are:
    1. Histidine
    2. Isoleucine
    3. Leucine
    4. Lysine
    5. Methionine
    6. Phenylalanine
    7. Threonine
    8. Tryptophan
    9. Valine
  - A chain of amino acids linked together is called a polypeptide.
  - One or more polypeptide chains folded and configured in a particular way to perform a specific function is called a protein.
    - Proteins provide structural integrity for tissues and organs.
    - They also help comprise enzymes, hormones, and immune cells and are therefore integral in the proper functioning of the endocrine and immune systems.
- The recommended dietary allowance (RDA) for protein intake is 0.8 g of protein for every kilogram of body weight (or 0.36 g of protein per pound of body weight).[10]
  - For example, a 175-pound-male would have calorie needs of approximately 2,500 calories per day.
    - His protein needs would equate to 175 pounds × 0.36 g/pound = 63 g of protein per day.
    - 63 g of protein × 4 calories/g of protein = 252 calories from protein. 252 divided by 2,500 calories = 10.08% of calories from protein.
  - On average, vegans obtain 10% to 12% of their calories from protein,[11] whereas nonvegetarians' protein intake is closer to 14% to 18% of their total daily calories.

Although they do not provide energy, the other classes of essential nutrients perform other critical functions for the body; these are called micronutrients. These include:

1. Vitamins
2. Minerals

Vitamins

Vitamins are organic carbon-containing substances that are present in minute amounts in foods.

- They are essential in terms of promoting specific chemical reactions in cells, which are key in processes such as:
  - Digestion
  - Muscle contraction
  - Energy production
  - Wound healing
- Vitamins are classified as water or fat soluble, and their solubility affects how they are absorbed, transported, and stored within the body.
  - The fat-soluble vitamins are vitamins A, D, E, and K.
  - The water-soluble vitamins are vitamin C and the B-complex vitamins.

MINERALS

Minerals are inorganic non–carbon-containing substances that represent a small but important fraction of total body weight.

- They are a part of various cells and tissues, including bones, teeth, and nails.
- Like vitamins, minerals can also promote chemical reactions and regulate processes within the body.
- Major minerals present in the body include:
  - Calcium
  - Phosphorus
  - Magnesium
  - Sodium
  - Chloride
  - Potassium
- Trace minerals are those minerals that are found in amounts less than 5 g in the body and include iron and zinc, among many others.

WATER

Water comprises approximately 60% of the body's weight and is integral in many essential processes.

- It acts as a solvent and provides a medium for chemical reactions.
- Water aids in the controlling of body temperature and its balance is critical for health maintenance and exercise performance.
- It is found in fruits, vegetables, and other liquids.

Nutrition's Importance in Health and Disease

When considering the very basic components of human health and leaning on the guiding principles of the osteopathic profession, it is important to recognize that the body has the inherent ability to heal itself, if given the opportunity.

- That "opportunity" can be defined very simply through the "Lifestyle Determinants of Health," those being:
  - Nutrition
  - Physical activity
  - Hydration
  - Sleep
  - Stress reduction
  - Social connectedness
- Adequacy in each of these categories has been shown to lead to human health and longevity[1] (see Chapter 21 Lifestyle Medicine—Osteopathic Perspectives)

Regarding nutrition, it is important to fuel the body with real food to carry out the multitude of macro- and microscopic processes that the human body is expected to perform every second of every day. A balanced, nutritious diet is depicted in Figure 22.1.

- Much like the osteopathic view that each person is a whole unit—body, mind, and spirit—the same consideration must be given to

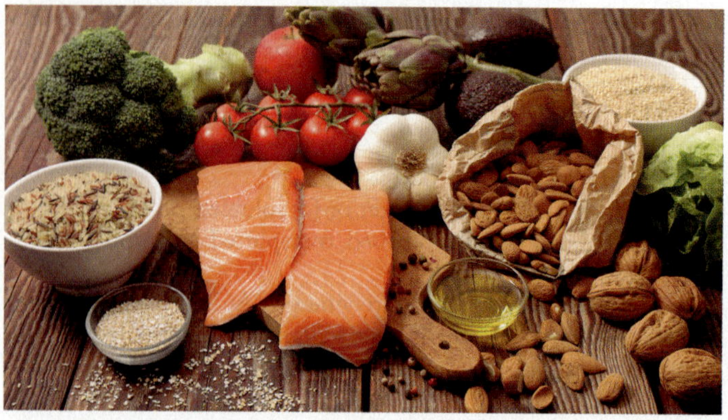

Figure 22.1. Elements of a balanced, nutritious diet. (Margouillat photo/Shutterstock.)

define food; food should be seen not just as individual nutrients but, rather, whole foods eaten mostly as grown (not processed).
- Each whole food not only brings measurable and known components of macro- and micronutrients, but also components yet-to-be-discovered that work in concert and synergistically[1] to eventually become part of the human body at the cellular level—such is the saying "you are what you eat." That statement is indeed true since every component of food will become integrated in the very makeup of the cells.

The assimilation of these macro- and micronutrient components into the body for energy, building, and repair of tissues requires that they are absorbed not as whole foods, but instead in their component parts.

- This occurs through the interface between the external environment of the gastrointestinal lumen, through which food travels after ingestion and the surface cells of the intestine, called enterocytes.
- This complicated process involves:
  - Digestion
  - Absorption
  - Internal transport
  - Integration of these individual nutrients into cells

Simply, metabolism is the balance in the body between reactions that build things up (anabolism) and reactions that break things down (catabolism).

- When it comes to the energy that is obtained from foods, digestion must first occur to gain access to those macronutrients (carbohydrates, fats, and proteins).
- Once the food is broken down by mechanical and chemical processes into its component parts (carbohydrate → glucose; fats → fatty acids; protein → amino acids), each single unit is then absorbed through the intestinal cells.
- Depending on the needs of the body, each undergoes further processing for one of the following:
  - Creation of the energy currency (adenosine triphosphate or ATP) used by the cells of the body
  - Support of the anabolic needs through muscle development/repair
  - Storage in tissues for future energy needs

NUTRITION AND HUMAN HEALTH

According to the World Health Organization, health is defined as "[a] state of complete Physical, Mental, and Social well-being, and not merely the absence of disease and infirmity."

- For millennia, food and medicine were viewed as one in the same as stated succinctly in the words of Hippocrates, often referred to as the father of western medicine, "let food be thy medicine and medicine be thy food."
- From the standpoint of nutrition as it pertains to the Metabolic Model, humans must nourish their bodies with adequate calories for their energy needs while, obtaining adequate amounts of the micronutrients needed to perform the many biochemical processes in their cells.
- The body has the innate ability to garner the necessary nutrients for optimal health from ingested whole food; it does this through an intricate array of feedback mechanisms that involve nearly every organ system in the body.

NUTRITION AND HUMAN DISEASE

In decades and centuries past, and in industrialized and developing countries alike, there has been a significant struggle with undernutrition, regarding both calorie as well as nutrient malnutrition, mostly due to lack of access to nutritious food.

- Certainly, in the industrialized world, the issue continues to this day but has shifted towards a critical, yet evolving situation of malnutrition as seen through a different lens.
- With many adults and children being overfed with regard to calories and macronutrients, yet undernourished with regard to micronutrients there is an alarming trend of overweight and obesity in the face of malnutrition; this dilemma is encapsulated in the words "calorie-rich, nutrient-poor."
- To understand the current situation, much of this can point to the over-reliance on processed foods, which tend to be calorie-rich and nutrient-poor.

According to the most recent data gathered by "the STATE of OBESITY," a project of the Trust for America's Health and the Robert Wood Johnson Foundation, and the Behavioral Risk Factor Surveillance System (BRFSS) (updated 2022):

> *"...adult obesity rates now exceed 35% in 19 states. West Virginia has the highest adult obesity rate at 40.6% and the District of Columbia has the lowest at 24.7%. Between 2020 and 2021, the adult obesity rate increased in 17 states: Kentucky, Maryland, Massachusetts, Minnesota, Missouri, Montana, Nebraska, New Mexico, New York, North Carolina, Ohio, Oklahoma, Oregon, South Carolina, Utah, Vermont, and Virginia."*

- According to 2017–2018 data from the National Health and Nutrition Examination Survey (NHANES) data[13,14]:
  - Nearly 1 in 3 adults (30.7%) are overweight.
  - More than 2 in 5 adults (42.4%) have obesity.
  - About 1 in 11 adults (9.2%) have severe obesity.
- According to 2017–2018 NHANES data:
  - About 1 in 6 children and adolescents ages 2 to 19 (16.1%) are overweight.
  - Almost 1 in 5 children and adolescents ages 2 to 19 (19.3%) have obesity.
  - About 1 in 16 children and adolescents ages 2 to 19 (6.1%) have severe obesity.
- An estimated 129 million people in the United States have at least one major chronic disease, such as heart disease, cancer, diabetes, obesity, or hypertension, as defined by the U.S. Department of Health and Human Services.[15] Five of the top ten leading causes of death in the United States are either chronic diseases or strongly associated with preventable and treatable chronic conditions.[15] Over the past two decades, the prevalence of chronic diseases has increased steadily, and this trend is expected to continue. An increasing proportion of Americans are dealing

with multiple chronic conditions; 42% have two or more, and 12% have at least five.[15] While many chronic diseases are partly the result of individual health behaviors, such as excessive drinking, smoking, sedentary lifestyles, and poor nutrition, structural socioeconomic and environmental factors also play a significant role in their development, prevention, and management.[15]

- To paraphrase David Katz, MD, MPH, "If this is viewed with a positive spin, that means that 80% of the chronic disease is reversible by:
  - What individuals choose to do with their 'forks., fingers, and…feet'
  - What they eat
  - Whether or not they smoke
  - How much physical activity they get"

NUTRITION AS RESTORATIVE MEDICINE (RESTORATION OF HEALTH)

Replacement in deficiency syndromes: There are as many deficiency syndromes as there are macro and micronutrients. Some are common and others are rare.

- In general, they are categorized based on the specific nutrient in the diet that is deficient, though most do not occur as a singular deficiency but instead in concert with other nutrient deficiencies.
- To thwart chronic issues that may arise due to the ongoing lack of nutrients for cellular processes, these nutrient deficiencies must be replaced in the short term, and the cause of the deficiency must be prevented in the long term.
- All can be caused by one or more of the following:
  - Inadequate intake
  - Impaired digestion
  - Inadequate absorption
  - Inadequate utilization

Macronutrient Deficiencies

Protein: In a diet that is calorie replete, it is difficult to become protein deficient.

- There are two main types of protein deficiency:
  - Kwashiorkor: Lack of adequate protein in food despite adequate calories.
  - Marasmus: Severe malnutrition in both protein and calories.
- Because protein is integral in every cell and function of the body, deficiency can affect both the structure and function of the body, at a global and cellular level.
- Common symptoms of protein malnutrition can be seen in any system of the body, but the symptoms that are most noticeable include[16]:
  - Anxiety
  - Depression
  - Lethargy
  - Muscle weakness
  - Growth retardation in children
  - Skin rashes and flaking
  - Poor wound healing
  - Weight loss
  - Edema
- These can be reversed in large part by replacing both high-quality, complete proteins in the diet as well as total calories.

Fat: Since fat is the most calorie-dense macronutrient, diets limited in fat can lead to total body weight loss if the person is unable to maintain calorie needs of the body, as well as fat-soluble vitamin deficiencies (vitamins A, D, E, and K).

- Common symptoms of essential fatty acid deficiency include:
  - Visual problems
  - Nervous system function abnormalities (both psychological and neurologic)
  - Skin rash
  - Growth retardation in infants and children
  - Poor immune function causing increased susceptibility to infection, and poor wound healing.[17]
- These can be reversed by replacing both total fat calorie intake as well as essential fatty acids in the diet.

Carbohydrate: Carbohydrates are the primary source of calories for most people.

- The Institute of Medicine recommends that carbohydrates constitute 45% to 65% of total daily calorie intake. In a standard 2,000-calorie-per-day diet, this amounts to 225 to 325 g every day.
- In the western diet, most carbohydrates are ingested in the form of refined grains and added sugars rather than complex carbohydrate foods.
- Glucose is the preferred energy source for most cells of the body but is virtually the sole source of energy for the brain.
  - The brain lacks the ability to store fuel and therefore requires a continuous supply of glucose.
  - In the resting state, the brain consumes about 120 g daily, which corresponds to an energy input of about 480 calories, accounting for approximately 60% of the body's daily utilization of glucose.
- If carbohydrate intake is insufficient for total body metabolic needs (<50 g/d), gluconeogenesis must occur, and is largely dependent upon the breakdown of amino acids in the diet and body protein stores.
  - A less efficient pathway of glucose production is the utilization of the backbone of triglycerides—glycerol.
- Fatty acids in plasma are bound to albumin; they do not serve as a fuel source for the brain when glucose is unavailable.
  - Under starvation circumstances, ketone bodies generated by the liver from fatty acid degradation partly replace glucose as fuel for the brain.[18]
- Carbohydrate malnutrition and total calorie malnutrition have historically gone hand-in-hand.
  - Low-carbohydrate, high protein diets have become a popular means of weight loss.
  - In the past decade, there has been a purposeful and specific reduction in carbohydrate calorie intake in some people that have the unavoidable side effect of ketosis.
- In the face of adequate total calorie intake from fat and protein, common symptoms of carbohydrate deficiency include:
  - Lethargy
  - Constipation
  - Nausea
  - Headache
  - Bad breath
- These symptoms can be reversed by increasing carbohydrate intake to an estimate greater than 50 g/d (preferably closer to the Institute of Medicine's recommended 45% to 65% of total calories required based on the unique needs of the individual).

Fiber: By definition, fiber is only found in plants. There is no fiber in any animal product and is found only in scant amounts in "junk foods."[19]

- Based on NHANES 2009 to 2010 data, the average daily intake of fiber across the U.S. population is approximately 16 g/d; 97% of the U.S. population does not meet Institute of Medicine

Adequate Intake recommendations (25 g/d for women, 38 g/d for men).[20,21]

- The 2010 Dietary Guidelines for Americans identified dietary fiber as a nutrient of concern.[22] The benefits of dietary fiber are numerous and likely are due to the many beneficial components of foods that are naturally high in fiber. Dietary fiber appears to significantly:

> *"Lower risk for developing coronary heart disease, stroke, hypertension, diabetes, obesity, and certain gastrointestinal diseases. Increasing fiber intake lowers blood pressure and serum cholesterol levels. Increased intake of soluble fiber improves glycemia and insulin sensitivity in non-diabetic and diabetic individuals. Fiber supplementation in obese individuals significantly enhances weight loss. Increased fiber intake benefits a number of gastrointestinal disorders including the following: gastroesophageal reflux disease, duodenal ulcer, diverticulitis, constipation, and hemorrhoids. Prebiotic fibers appear to enhance immune function."*[23]

Consequently, a diet deficient in fiber confers widespread detrimental effects impacting nearly every system of the body.

- Increasing whole plant foods including beans, whole grains, vegetables, and fruits is necessary to obtain the Institute of Medicine Adequate Intake recommendations (25 g/d for women, 38 g/d for men).

Water: The human body is comprised of approximately 60% water, though the exact percentage varies by age, body composition, and gender.

- Water is integral in both the structure and function of every tissue in the human body.
- Loss of total body water is called dehydration, and the severity is considered mild, moderate, or severe based on the percentage of water lost.
  - It is further characterized as isonatremic (130 to 150 mEq/L), hyponatremic (<130 mEq/L), or hypernatremic (>150 mEq/L) dehydration based on the loss of water compared to the concentration of serum sodium.
  - Isonatremic dehydration is the most common (80%).
  - Hypernatremic and hyponatremic dehydration each comprise 5% to 10% of cases.
- Clinical symptoms and signs of dehydration are because of both intracellular and extracellular dehydration with most being attributable to intravascular fluid contraction.
- Rehydration is best accomplished via the oral route.
  - With more severe dehydration or with the inability to tolerate oral rehydration, the intravenous route of fluid rehydration may be preferred.

There can be dangers with rehydration when considering sodium and water balance in the body, due to fluid shifts associated with rehydration.

Micronutrient Deficiencies

Vitamins: Initially, "vitamins" were named by combining "vital" meaning life and "amine," because they were initially thought to include a nitrogen-containing amine group.

- They are organic compounds (carbon containing), which are considered "essential" due to the body's inability to synthesize most vitamins.
- There are 13 currently known vitamins, which are either fat-soluble (vitamins A, D, E, and K) or water-soluble (vitamins C and the B-complex vitamins). See Table 22.1 for specific vitamins.

BOX 22.1

All "B complex" vitamins are integral in conversion of carbohydrates into glucose for energy metabolism affecting the growth, development, and function of cells, as well as to help maintain normal blood glucose levels.

  - Fat-soluble vitamins are absorbed through the gastrointestinal tract; their absorption is facilitated by fat-containing foods. Fat stores of the body serve as a repository for these vitamins with reserves of days to months.
  - Water-soluble vitamins are not stored in the body in large amounts, are excreted in the stool and urine depending on their absorption and must be ingested through foods on an ongoing basis.
- Vitamin deficiencies are rare in isolation and usually occur as a global nutrient deficiency in the diet along with other vitamin deficiencies.

1. Vitamin A
   - Deficiency disease is called xerophthalmia; vitamin A deficiency is one of the main causes of preventable blindness in children.
   - Essential functions:
     - Vision.
     - Immune function.
     - Integrity of the epithelial cells lining the gastrointestinal, respiratory, and urinary tracts.
     - Gene expression.
2. Vitamin B_1
   - Deficiency disease is called beriberi.
   - Thiamine diphosphate (TDP) is the active form of vitamin B_1 and is an essential cofactor for five enzymes involved in glucose, amino acid, and lipid metabolism.
   - Essential functions:
     - All "B-complex" vitamins are integral in conversion of carbohydrates into glucose for energy metabolism, affecting the growth, development, and function of cells (Box 22.1).
3. Vitamin B_2
   - Deficiency disease is called ariboflavinosis.
   - Absorbed in the proximal small intestine.
   - Single ingestion of doses beyond 27 mg cannot be absorbed and are excreted in the stool.
   - Only small amounts of vitamin B_2 and other water-soluble vitamins are stored in the body, so ongoing dietary ingestion is needed to meet the body's needs.
   - It is light sensitive, so excessive light exposure can inactivate it.
   - Since vitamin B_2 is needed for energy production, vegetarian athletes are at increased risk of deficiency due to the limitation of animal products that tend to be good sources of this vitamin, but also because the stresses on the metabolic pathways that utilize vitamin B_2.
   - Essential functions:
     - As above.
     - In addition, it serves as an essential component of various coenzymes, which catalyze numerous cellular processes important in amino acid and other vitamin conversions and homeostasis.
4. Vitamin B_3
   - Deficiency disease is called pellagra.
   - The niacin form of vitamin B_3, when taken in supplement form (usually in doses of >50 mg) can cause a common side effect called "red man syndrome" that involves red flushing on the skin.

TABLE 22.1

Vitamins

Vitamin	Discovered	Also Known as	Solubility	Essential Functions	Symptoms in Deficiency	Food Sources	Interesting Facts
A	1913	Retinols (pre-formed vitamin A) and carotenoids (provitamin A)	Fat-soluble	Vision, immune function, integrity of the epithelial cells lining the gastrointestinal, respiratory, and urinary tracts, as well as gene expression	Night blindness, skin disorders such as dry hair and dry skin, and infectious susceptibility	Retinols (liver, fish, milk); Carotenoids (oranges, carrots, pumpkin, squash, yams, leafy green vegetables)	Deficiency disease is called *xerophthalmia;* vitamin A deficiency is one of the main causes of preventable blindness in children.
B_1	1910	Thiamine	Water-soluble	All "B complex" vitamins are integral in conversion of carbohydrates into glucose for energy metabolism affecting the growth, development, and function of cells, as well as to help maintain normal blood glucose levels.	Peripheral neuropathy, muscle wasting, memory loss, heart failure with sequelae, Wernicke-Korsakoff syndrome usually seen in chronic alcoholism.	Whole grains, meat (especially pork), and fish. Thiamine is also added to foods including breads and cereals.	Deficiency disease is called *beriberi.* Thiamine diphosphate (TDP) is the active form of vitamin B_1 and is an essential cofactor for five enzymes involved in glucose, amino acid, and lipid metabolism.
B_2	1920	Riboflavin	Water-soluble	As above. In addition, it serves as an essential component of various coenzymes which catalyze numerous cellular processes important in amino acid and other vitamins conversion and homeostasis.	Skin disorders, hair loss, hyperemia (excess blood) and edema of the mouth and throat, angular stomatitis (lesions at the corners of the mouth), cheilosis (swollen, cracked lips), reproductive problems, sore throat, itchy and red eyes, anemia, and cataracts.	Eggs, lean meats, kidneys, liver, milk, and green vegetables. Riboflavin is also added to foods including breads and cereals.	Deficiency disease is called ariboflavinosis. Absorbed in the proximal small intestine. Single ingestion of doses beyond 27 mg cannot be absorbed and are excreted in the stool. Only small amounts of this and other water-soluble vitamins are stored in the body so ongoing dietary ingestion is needed to meet the body's needs. It is light sensitive so excessive light exposure can inactivate Riboflavin. Since Riboflavin is needed for energy production, vegetarian athletes are at increased risk of deficiency due to the limitation of animal products that tend to be good sources of this vitamin but also because the stresses on the metabolic pathways that utilize Riboflavin.

(*continued*)

TABLE 22.1 (Continued)

Vitamins

Vitamin	Discovered	Also Known as	Solubility	Essential Functions	Symptoms in Deficiency	Food Sources	Interesting Facts
B_3	1936	3 different forms: Niacin, Niacinamide, Inositol hexaniacinate	Water-soluble	As above. In addition, it helps in the generation of sex and stress hormones and is important in regulating circulation. Niacin also helps to lower LDL ("bad") cholesterol and triglycerides in the blood.	Fatigue, mouth sores, glossitis (burning, swollen, and bright red tongue), dry and cracking skin, indigestion, vomiting, diarrhea, poor circulation, depression, and even dementia if the deficiency is severe.	Beets, beef organ meats (liver, kidney), nutritional yeast, brewer's yeast, fish (salmon, tuna, swordfish), sunflower seeds, and peanuts.	Deficiency disease is called *pellagra.* Niacin taken in supplement form (usually when taking doses of >50 mg) can cause a common side effect called "red man syndrome" that involves red flushing on the skin.
B_5	1931	Pantothenic Acid	Water-soluble	As above. In addition, it helps in the generation of sex and stress hormones and cholesterol. It is important in red blood cell production.	Fatigue, insomnia, depression, irritability, vomiting, stomach pains, burning feet, and upper respiratory infections.	Wide variety of animal foods, vegetables, and whole grains.	Pantothenic acid gets its name from the Greek root "pantos," meaning "everywhere," because it is available in a wide variety of foods. Is the universal precursor of Coenzyme A (CoA), an essential cofactor that is required in the metabolism of carbohydrates and fatty acids.
B_6	1934	Pyridoxine	Water-soluble	Involved in >100 enzyme reactions, mostly involved with protein metabolism. Also involved in amino acid, carbohydrate, and lipid metabolism. In addition, vitamin B_6 is important in the synthesis of neurotransmitters, gluconeogenesis, glycogenolysis, immune function, and hemoglobin formation.	Fatigue (often related to microcytic anemia), dermatitis with cheilosis (scaling on the lips and cracks at the corners of the mouth), glossitis (swollen tongue), depression, symptoms of peripheral neuropathy (including numbness and tingling), confusion, and weakened immune function.	Fish, beef liver and other organ meats, potatoes and other starchy vegetables, and onocitrus fruit. Pyridoxine is also added to foods including cereals.	Absorbed in the jejunum in large amounts but most is eliminated in the urine if the body is replete. Not stored in significant amounts in the body. Both deficiency and excess can cause peripheral neuropathy.

B_7	1931	Biotin	Water soluble	All "B-complex" vitamins are integral in conversion of carbohydrates into glucose for energy metabolism affecting the growth, development and function of cells, as well as to help maintain normal blood glucose levels. Also important in the metabolism of fat. Biotin is a cofactor in many enzyme processes.	Hair loss, skin rashes (a scaly red rash around the eyes, nose, mouth, and genital area). Neurologic symptoms can include depression, lethargy, hallucination, and numbness and tingling of the extremities.	Animal sources (Organ meats, brewer's yeast, chicken, fish, egg yolks, milk, cheeses, pork) and plant sources (barley, corn, soy, wheat bran, avocado, broccoli, cauliflower, legumes, mushrooms, nuts, potatoes, spinach).	The protein in raw egg whites binds biotin which impairs absorption and can lead to a deficiency.
B_9	1941	Folate, folic acid	Water soluble	Folate functions as a coenzyme or cosubstrate in single-carbon transfers in the synthesis of nucleic acids (DNA and RNA) and metabolism of amino acids. One of the most important folate-dependent reactions is the conversion of homocysteine to methionine. Folate is required for proper cell division.	Fatigue due to the classic megaloblastic anemia that can occur in deficiency (fatigue, shortness of breath, muscle weakness, difficulty concentrating, and headache), ulcers in the mouth, and changes in skin pigmentation. In the developing fetus, folate deficiency can cause neural tube defects and low birth weight babies.	Though found naturally in a wide variety of animal and vegetable foods, the foods with the highest levels of folate include spinach, liver, yeast, asparagus, and Brussels sprouts. Folic acid is also added to foods including breads and cereals.	Homocysteine levels rise when the body cannot convert homocysteine to methionine due to a 5-methyl-THF deficiency; homocysteine levels are often used to determine long-term folate adequacy in the body, though this is a nonspecific measure. Due to the risks of neural tube defects in the developing fetus and because cereals and grains are widely consumed in the United States, in January 1998, the U.S. Food and Drug Administration (FDA) began requiring food manufacturers to add folic acid to enriched breads, cereals, flours, cornmeals, pastas, rice, and other grain products to prevent deficiency.

(*continued*)

TABLE 22.1 (Continued)

Vitamins

Vitamin	Discovered	Also Known as	Solubility	Essential Functions	Symptoms in Deficiency	Food Sources	Interesting Facts
B_{12}	1948	Cobalamin	Water soluble	Essential for red blood cell formation, neurologic function, and DNA synthesis. Similar to folate, vitamin B_{12} serves as a cofactor in critical processes that are required for proper formation of nucleic acids (DNA, RNA), hormones, proteins, and lipids.	Symptoms due to the classic megaloblastic anemia that can occur in deficiency (fatigue, shortness of breath, muscle weakness, difficulty concentrating, headache), constipation, loss of appetite, weight loss, numbness and tingling in the hands and feet, difficulty maintaining balance, depression, confusion, dementia, poor memory, and soreness of the mouth or tongue.	Found almost exclusively in animal foods (fish, meat, poultry, eggs, milk, and dairy products). Can also be found in nutritional yeast, which is a dietary source for vegetarians. Vitamin B_{12} is also added to foods including breads and cereals.	Vegetarians (particularly vegans) are at increased risk of vitamin B_{12} deficiency. Contains the mineral cobalt. vitamin B_{12} is bound to protein in food. The acidic environment of the stomach is required to separate and allow the free vitamin B_{12} to combine with intrinsic factor that is released by the parietal cells of the stomach. This complex is then absorbed in the distal ileum. Deficiency disease of vitamin B_{12} can result from an autoimmune disease that affects the gastric mucosa called Pernicious Anemia and, therefore, causes a decreased amount of intrinsic factor. Large amounts of folate ingestion can mask a vitamin B_{12} deficiency due to the correction of the megaloblastic anemia.
C	1920	Ascorbic acid	Water soluble	Required for the synthesis of collagen, the essential component of connective tissue, which is important in wound healing. Also important in protein metabolism, synthesis of L-carnitine, and certain neurotransmitters. Serves a significant role of antioxidant in the body which has important implications in the delay in development of cancers and cardiovascular disease. Helps in the absorption of plant-derived nonheme iron.	Fatigue, connective tissue laxity (including capillary fragility which can cause petechiae, ecchymosis, purpura), joint pain, poor wound healing, hyperkeratosis, corkscrew hairs, depression, swollen and bleeding gums, and loosening or loss of teeth due to tissue and capillary fragility.	Fruits and vegetables including citrus fruits, tomatoes, potatoes, red and green peppers, kiwifruit, broccoli, strawberries, Brussels sprouts, and cantaloupe.	Deficiency disease is called *scurvy*. Signs of *Scurvy* can be appear in as little as 1 mo of inadequate vitamin C intake (<10 mg/d). Humans are unable to synthesize Vitamin C so it is an essential nutrient.

D	1920	Cholecalciferol, calcidiol, calcitriol	Fat soluble	Promotes calcium absorption from the gastrointestinal tract and is important in maintaining balance between calcium and phosphate in the blood which are important in the formation of bone. Vitamin D has important genetic function by modulating many genes encoding proteins that regulate cell proliferation, differentiation, and apoptosis.	Bone pain and skeletal abnormalities related to Rickets. "A committee of the Institute of Medicine concluded that persons are at risk of vitamin D deficiency at serum 25(OH) D concentrations <30 nmol/L (<12 ng/mL). Some are potentially at risk for inadequacy at levels ranging from 30 to 50 nmol/L (12–20 ng/mL). Practically all people are sufficient at levels ≥50 nmol/L (≥20 ng/mL); the committee stated that 50 nmol/L is the serum 25(OH)D level that covers the needs of 97.5% of the population."	Naturally present in very few foods. The fatty fish (such as salmon, tuna, and mackerel) and fish liver oils are among the best sources. Fortified foods provide most of the vitamin D in the American diet.	Deficiency disease can lead to rickets. Naturally present in very few foods, vitamin D is produced when ultraviolet rays from sunlight strike the skin and trigger vitamin D synthesis. Vitamin D obtained from sun exposure, food, and supplements is biologically inert and must undergo multiphasic processing to become active (the first occurs in the liver and the second in the kidney to form active 1, 25-dihydroxyvitamin D [1, 25(OH) 2D], also known as calcitriol). There are many factors that affect vitamin D synthesis from UVB exposure including season of the year, time of day, length of day, cloud cover, smog, skin melanin content, and sunscreen use.
E	1922	Alpha-, Beta-, Delta-, Gamma-tocopherol; Alpha-, Beta-, Delta-, Gamma-tocotrienol	Fat soluble	Global antioxidant activity through their effect on free radicals which may, in turn, protect against cardiovascular disease and cancer. Also involved in immune function, gene expression, and various metabolic processes. In addition, vitamin E helps with blood vessel dilatation and inhibition of platelet aggregation through its effect on two different enzymes.	Peripheral neuropathy (numbness, tingling), ataxia, muscle weakness, retinal degeneration leading to blindness, and impairment of the immune response.	Seeds, nuts, vegetable oils, and green leafy vegetables.	Alpha-tocopherol is the only form currently known to meet human needs yet most vitamin E in the American diet is gotten through Gamma-tocopherol from the various oils (soybean, canola, and corn) used in processed foods.

(*continued*)

TABLE 22.1 (Continued)

Vitamins

Vitamin	Discovered	Also Known as	Solubility	Essential Functions	Symptoms in Deficiency	Food Sources	Interesting Facts
K	1929	Vitamin K1 (phylloquinone), vitamin K2 (menaquinones)	Fat-soluble	Vitamin K functions as a coenzyme in blood clotting and bone mineralization.	Bleeding (due to effect on prothrombin), osteoporosis.	Vitamin K1 (green leafy vegetables), vitamin K2 (meat, dairy, eggs, and some fermented foods but are mainly produced by bacteria in the human GI tract).	Originally named for its function, coagulation, vitamin K comes from the German name "Koagulationsvitamin." Because blood clotting is largely a vitamin K–dependent process, those patients who are on Warfarin must have a constant level of vitamin K–containing foods in their diet in order to maintain predictable anticoagulation. Due to the limited transport of vitamin K across the placenta and the minimal amounts present in human breast milk, newborns are routinely given a single IM injection of vitamin K1 at birth to prevent vitamin K deficiency bleeding (VKDB).

- Essential functions:
  - As above.
  - Helps in the generation of sex and stress hormones.
  - Is important in regulating circulation.
  - The niacin form also helps to lower LDL ("bad") cholesterol and triglycerides in the blood.

5. Vitamin B_5
   - Also called pantothenic acid, which gets its name from the Greek root "pantos," meaning "everywhere," because it is available in a wide variety of foods.
   - Is the universal precursor of Coenzyme A (CoA), an essential cofactor that is required in the metabolism of carbohydrates and fatty acids.
   - Essential functions:
     - As above.
     - Helps in the generation of sex and stress hormones and cholesterol.
     - Is important in red blood cell production.
6. Vitamin B_6
   - Absorbed in the jejunum in large amounts, but most is eliminated in the urine if the body is replete.
   - Not stored in significant amounts in the body.
   - Both deficiency and excess can cause peripheral neuropathy.
   - Essential functions:
     - Involved in:
       - More than 100 enzyme reactions, mostly involved with protein metabolism
       - Amino acid, carbohydrate, and lipid metabolism
     - Important in:
       - The synthesis of neurotransmitters
       - Gluconeogenesis
       - Glycogenolysis
       - Immune function
       - Hemoglobin formation
7. Vitamin B_7
   - The protein in raw egg whites binds vitamin B_7, which impairs absorption and can lead to a deficiency.
   - Essential functions:
     - Also important in the metabolism of fat.
     - Is a cofactor in many enzyme processes.
8. Vitamin B_9
   - Homocysteine levels rise when the body cannot convert homocysteine to methionine due to a 5-Methyltetrahydrofolate (5-MTHF) deficiency; homocysteine levels are often used to determine long-term folate adequacy in the body, though this is a nonspecific measure.
   - Due to the risks of neural tube defects in the developing fetus and because cereals and grains are widely consumed in the United States, in January 1998, the U.S. Food and Drug Administration (FDA) began requiring food manufacturers to add folic acid to enriched breads, cereals, flours, cornmeal, pastas, rice, and other grain products to prevent deficiency.
   - Essential functions:
     - Functions as a coenzyme or cosubstrate in single-carbon transfers in the synthesis of nucleic acids (DNA and RNA) and metabolism of amino acids.
       - One of the most important vitamins. B_9-dependent reactions assist with the conversion of homocysteine to methionine.
       - Is required for proper cell division.
9. Vitamin B_{12}
   - Vegetarians (particularly vegans) are at increased risk of vitamin B_{12} deficiency.
   - Contains the mineral cobalt.
   - Vitamin B_{12} is bound to protein in food.
   - The acidic environment of the stomach is required to separate and allow the free vitamin B_{12} to combine with intrinsic factor that is released by the parietal cells of the stomach. This complex is then absorbed in the distal ileum.
   - Deficiency disease of vitamin B_{12} can result from an autoimmune disease that affects the gastric mucosa called pernicious anemia and, therefore, causes a decreased amount of intrinsic factor.
   - Large amounts of vitamin B_9 ingestion can mask a vitamin B_{12} deficiency due to the correction of the megaloblastic anemia.
   - Essential functions:
     - Essential for:
       - Red blood cell formation
       - Neurologic function
       - DNA synthesis
     - Like vitamin B_9, vitamin B_{12} serves as a cofactor in critical processes that are required for proper formation of:
       - Nucleic acids (DNA, RNA)
       - Hormones
       - Proteins
       - Lipids
10. Vitamin C
    - Deficiency disease is called scurvy. Signs of scurvy can appear in as little as 1 month of inadequate vitamin C intake (<10 mg/d).
    - Humans are unable to synthesize vitamin C, so it is an essential nutrient.
    - Essential functions:
      - Required for the synthesis of collagen, the essential component of connective tissue, which is important in wound healing.
      - Important in protein metabolism, synthesis of L-carnitine, and certain neurotransmitters.
      - Serves a significant role of antioxidant in the body, which has important implications in the delay in the development of cancers and CVD.
      - Helps in the absorption of plant-derived nonheme iron.
11. Vitamin D
    - Deficiency disease can lead to rickets.
    - Naturally present in very few foods.
    - Vitamin D is produced when ultraviolet rays from sunlight strike the skin and trigger vitamin D synthesis.
    - Vitamin D obtained from sun exposure, food, and supplements is biologically inert and must undergo multiphasic processing to become active (the first occurs in the liver and the second in the kidney to form active 1,25-dihydroxyvitamin D [1,25(OH)2D], also known as calcitriol).
    - "A committee of the Institute of Medicine concluded that persons are at risk of vitamin D deficiency at serum 25(OH) D concentrations <30 nmol/L (<12 ng/mL). Some are potentially at risk for inadequacy at levels ranging from 30 to 50 nmol/L (12 to 20 ng/mL). Practically all people are sufficient at levels ≥50 nmol/L (≥20 ng/mL); the committee stated that 50 nmol/L is the serum 25(OH)D level that covers the needs of 97.5% of the population."[24]
    - There are many factors that affect vitamin D synthesis from UVB exposure including:
      - Season of the year
      - Time of day
      - Length of day
      - Cloud cover
      - Smog

- Skin melanin content
- Sunscreen use

□ Essential functions:

- Promotes calcium absorption from the gastrointestinal tract and is important in maintaining balance between calcium and phosphate in the blood, which are important in the formation of bone.
- Has an important genetic function by modulating many genes encoding proteins that regulate cell proliferation, differentiation, and apoptosis.

12. Vitamin E

□ The alpha-tocopherol form of vitamin E is the only form currently known to meet human needs, yet most vitamin E in the American diet is gotten through gamma-tocopherol from the various oils (soybean, canola, and corn) used in processed foods.

□ Essential functions:

- Global antioxidant activity through their effect on free radicals may, in turn, protect against CVD and cancer.
- Involved in:
  - Immune function
  - Gene expression
  - Various metabolic processes
- Helps with blood vessel dilatation and inhibition of platelet aggregation through its effect on two different enzymes.

13. Vitamin K

□ Originally named for its function, coagulation, vitamin K comes from the German name "Koagulationsvitamin."

□ Because blood clotting is largely a vitamin K–dependent process, those patients who are on warfarin must have a constant level of vitamin K–containing foods in their diet in order to maintain predictable anticoagulation.

□ Due to the limited transport of vitamin K across the placenta and the minimal amounts present in human breast milk, newborns are routinely given a single intramuscular injection of vitamin K1 at birth to prevent vitamin K deficiency bleeding (VKDB).

□ Essential functions:

- It is a coenzyme in blood clotting and bone mineralization.

Minerals: See Table 22.2 for specific Minerals.

1. Calcium

□ Most abundant mineral in the body.

□ Less than 1% of total body calcium is needed to support the critical metabolic functions of calcium.

□ Serum calcium does not fluctuate with changes in dietary intakes; the body uses bone as a reservoir for and source of calcium to maintain constant concentrations of calcium in blood, muscle, and intercellular fluids.

□ Essential functions:

- Vasoconstriction
- Vasodilation
- Muscle function
- Nerve impulse transmission
- Intracellular signaling
- Hormonal secretion

2. Magnesium

□ Magnesium is stored in bone and soft tissues.

□ Normal serum concentrations are regulated by the kidneys.

□ Excessive amounts of magnesium are usually from medications or supplements (not from diet).

□ Essential functions:

- Serves as a cofactor in more than 300 biochemical processes in the body.
- Important in:
  - Protein synthesis
  - Muscle function
  - Nerve impulse propagation
  - Blood glucose control
  - Blood pressure regulation
- Magnesium is required for:
  - Energy production
  - Glycolysis
  - Synthesis of nucleic acids (DNA, RNA) and the antioxidant glutathione
- It contributes to the structural development of bone
- Magnesium also plays a role in the active transport of calcium and potassium ions across cell membranes, which is important for:
  - Nerve impulse conduction
  - Muscle contraction
  - Normal heart rhythm

3. Sodium

□ The U.S. Institute of Medicine set its Tolerable Upper Intake Level for sodium at 2.3 g/d, but the average person in the United States consumes 3.4 g/d.

□ Essential functions:

- Regulates:
  - Blood volume
  - Blood pressure
  - Osmotic equilibrium
  - PH of the blood

4. Potassium

□ Most of the total body potassium resides intracellularly.

□ Essential functions:

- Important in:
  - Contraction in smooth and skeletal muscle
  - Propagation of nerve impulses

5. Chloride

□ The major anion that lives in the blood and extracellular fluid.

□ Essential functions:

- Important in:
  - Maintaining acid/base balance in body
  - Propagation of nerve impulses
  - Regulating fluid balance in combination with other electrolytes

6. Phosphorus

□ Present in a wide variety of cola drinks in the form of phosphoric acid.

□ Phosphorus is absorbed in the small intestine and excess amounts are excreted by the kidneys.

□ 85% of the body's total phosphorus is stored in the bones and teeth.

□ Phosphate homeostasis is a tightly regulated along with calcium through the actions of:

- Parathyroid hormone
- Active vitamin D
- Fibroblast growth factor-23

□ Essential functions:

- Important in the structure of cell membranes and nucleic acids.
- Involved in several biologic processes, including:
  - Bone mineralization
  - Energy production
  - Cell signaling through phosphorylation reactions
  - Regulation of acid–base homeostasis

TABLE 22.2

Minerals

Mineral	Also Known as	Normal Serum Levels	Essential Functions	Symptoms in Deficiency	Symptoms in Toxicity	Food Sources	Interesting Facts
Calcium	Ca++	8.5–10.2 mg/dL	Vasoconstriction, vasodilation, muscle function, nerve impulse transmission, intracellular signaling and hormonal secretion.	Numbness and tingling in the extremities, muscle cramps, convulsions, lethargy, and abnormal heart rhythms.	Constipation, kidney stones, risk of kidney injury, soft tissue calcifications.	Dairy foods, broccoli, kale, cabbage.	Most abundant mineral in the body. Less than 1% of total body calcium is needed to support the critical metabolic functions of calcium. Serum calcium does not fluctuate with changes in dietary intakes; the body uses bone as a reservoir for, and source of calcium, to maintain constant concentrations of calcium in blood, muscle, and intercellular fluids.
Magnesium	Mg++	1.7–2.2 mg/dL	Serves as a cofactor in >300 biochemical processes in the body. Important in: protein synthesis, muscle function, nerve impulse propagation, blood glucose control, and blood pressure regulation. Magnesium is required for energy production, glycolysis, synthesis of nucleic acids (DNA, RNA), as well as the antioxidant glutathione. It contributes to the structural development of bone. Magnesium also plays a role in the active transport of calcium and potassium ions across cell membranes, which is important to nerve impulse conduction, muscle contraction, and normal heart rhythm.	Mild: loss of appetite, nausea, vomiting, fatigue, and weakness. Moderate: numbness, tingling, muscle cramping, seizures, personality changes, abnormal heart rhythms, and coronary spasms. Severe: disruption in mineral homeostasis (hypocalcemia and hypokalemia which involve other symptoms listed in this table).	Excessive amount of magnesium is usually from medications or supplements (not from diet). Progressive symptoms of toxicity can include diarrhea, abdominal cramping, hypotension, nausea, vomiting, facial flushing, urinary retention, ileus, depression, fatigue, muscle weakness, difficulty breathing, irregular heartbeat, and cardiac arrest.	Green leafy vegetables (spinach), legumes, nuts, seeds, and whole grains. In general, foods containing dietary fiber (plant foods) provide magnesium. Some mineral waters contain magnesium.	Magnesium is stored in bone and soft tissues. Normal serum concentrations are regulated by the kidneys.

(continued)

TABLE 22.2 (Continued)

Minerals

Mineral	Also Known as	Normal Serum Levels	Essential Functions	Symptoms in Deficiency	Symptoms in Toxicity	Food Sources	Interesting Facts
Sodium	Na^+	135–145 mmol/L	Regulates blood volume, blood pressure, osmotic equilibrium, and pH of the blood.	Mild (nausea, fatigue); moderate (decreased level of consciousness, headache; severe (seizures, coma, death). Significant neurologic symptoms most commonly are seen with very low serum sodium levels (<115 mEq/L), resulting in intracerebral osmotic fluid shifts and brain edema.	Mild (thirst, headache); moderate (muscle cramps, headache, lethargy); severe (seizures, intracranial hemorrhage, coma, death).	Sodium chloride is the main source of sodium in the diet and is present naturally in some foods but most is obtained through processed foods.	The U.S. Institute of Medicine set its Tolerable Upper Intake Level for sodium at 2.3 g/d but the average person in the United States consumes 3.4 g/d.
Potassium	K^+	3.5–5.0 mEq/L	Important in contraction in smooth and skeletal muscle, propagation of nerve impulses.	Muscle weakness, muscle cramps, fatigue, nausea, vomiting, irregular heartbeat.	Mild (diarrhea, abdominal pain, nausea); moderate (muscle weakness, bradycardia); severe (arrhythmia, chest pain, death).	Present in animal foods (meats, fish, dairy). Plant foods depend upon the soil that the plants are grown in (fruits, vegetables, and legumes).	The majority of total body potassium resides intracellularly.
Chloride	Cl^-	96–106 mEq/L	Important in maintaining acid/base balance in body, propagation of nerve impulses, and regulating fluid balance in combination with other electrolytes.	Loss of appetite, muscle weakness, fatigue.	Thirst, fluid retention, high blood pressure.	Sodium chloride is the main source of sodium in the diet and is present naturally in some foods, but most is obtained through processed foods. Chloride can also be found naturally in foods like seaweed, olives, rye, celery, lettuce, tomatoes.	The major anion that lives in the blood and extracellular fluid.

Phosphorus		2.5–4.5 mg/dL	Important in the structure of cell membranes and nucleic acids. Involved in several biologic processes, including bone mineralization, energy production, cell signaling through phosphorylation reactions, and regulation of acid–base homeostasis.	Loss of appetite, muscle weakness, bone fragility, numbness in the extremities, and rickets.	Tetany, dehydration, hypotension, tachycardia, fever, cardiac arrest, and coma.	Present in many animal and plant foods due to the global presence of phosphorus in a wide variety of foods.	Present in a wide variety of cola drinks in the form of phosphoric acid. Phosphorus is absorbed in the small intestine and excess amounts are excreted by the kidneys. 85% of the body's total phosphorus is stored in the bones and teeth. Phosphate homeostasis is tightly regulated along with Calcium through the actions of parathyroid hormone, active vitamin D, and fibroblast growth factor-23.
Iron	Fe++	Serum Ferritin is reflective of total body iron stores (but can be affected by inflammation since it is an acute phase reactant). Men: 12–300 ng/mL. Women: 12–150 ng/mL.	Integral in many iron-dependent proteins and enzymes involved in oxygen transport, electron transfer, energy production, iron storage, and DNA replication and repair.	Most symptoms of iron deficiency are related to the resulting anemia. Those include shortness of breath, fatigue, increased heart rate, palpitations, and exercise intolerance. As the iron deficiency worsens, other symptoms/signs may arise including pica (consumption of nonfood items), nail changes (brittle and spoon-shaped), angular cheilitis (skin breakdown at the corners of the mouth), and restless leg syndrome.	Toxicity due to excessive intake is rare and usually involves the pediatric population; symptoms can include nausea, vomiting, abdominal pain, dark stools, lethargy, weak pulse, tachycardia, low blood pressure, fever, difficulty breathing, and coma. Toxicity may result from a hereditary disease (Hereditary Hemochromatosis, among others) related to a defect in iron metabolism and can lead to iron accumulation in various tissues and organs of the body. Symptoms vary but most commonly affect the cardiovascular, kidney, liver, hematologic, and central nervous systems.	Heme iron: ingested in the form of hemoglobin and myoglobin from the meat, fish, and poultry and is more bioavailable for absorption and is less affected by other dietary factors than is nonheme iron. Nonheme iron: raisins, prunes, spinach, and other green leafy vegetables, beans, lentils, tofu, quinoa, cashews, and hazelnuts.	The body is efficient in recycling iron and excretes very little. The majority of iron found in the body is found in the circulating red blood cells. The storage form of iron is ferritin. Nonheme iron absorption is markedly increased with concomitant intake of vitamin C.

(*continued*)

TABLE 22.2 (*Continued*)

Minerals

Mineral	Also Known as	Normal Serum Levels	Essential Functions	Symptoms in Deficiency	Symptoms in Toxicity	Food Sources	Interesting Facts
Zinc		70–100 μmol/L	Zinc plays a vital role on human metabolism and cellular function in numerous ways. Catalytic role: over 300 enzymes are zinc dependent. Structural role: zinc plays a significant role in both the structure of proteins and cell membranes and in wound healing. Zinc-dependent proteins play a role in gene expression, hormone release, nerve impulse transmission, and apoptosis.	Marginal zinc deficiency can manifest as impaired physical and neuropsychological development and increased susceptibility to life-threatening infections. As the deficiency becomes more severe the following complications may arise: slowing or cessation of growth and development, delayed sexual maturation, skin rashes, diarrhea, immune system deficiencies, impaired wound healing, diminished appetite, impaired taste sensation, night blindness, swelling and clouding of the corneas, and behavioral disturbances.	Most commonly GI-related symptoms of abdominal pain, nausea, vomiting, and diarrhea.	Animal foods: Shellfish (oysters and crab, in particular), beef, and other red meats. Plant foods: Nuts and legumes. Zinc bioavailability is higher in animal foods compared with many plant foods due to the relative absence of compounds that inhibit zinc absorption (phytic acid) and the presence of sulfur-containing amino acids (cysteine and methionine) that improve zinc absorption.	The major consequence of long-term consumption of excessive zinc is copper deficiency. The RDA for zinc (8 mg/d for adult women and 11 mg/d for adult men) appears sufficient to prevent zinc deficiency in most individuals. Intranasal zinc preparations, most commonly used for the short term treatment of common cold symptoms, can cause irreversible loss of the sense of smell (anosmia) so zinc-containing intranasal gels and sprays should be avoided. Currently, there is not a sensitive and specific biomarker to detect zinc deficiency in humans.

7. Iron
   - □ The body is efficient in recycling iron and excretes very little.
   - □ Most of the iron in the body is found in the circulating red blood cells.
   - □ The storage form of iron is ferritin.
   - □ Nonheme iron absorption is markedly increased with concomitant intake of vitamin C.
   - □ Essential functions:
     - Integral in many iron-dependent proteins and enzymes involved in:
       - Oxygen transport
       - Electron transfer
       - Energy production
       - Iron storage
       - DNA replication and repair
8. Zinc
   - □ The major consequence of long-term consumption of excessive zinc is copper deficiency.
   - □ The RDA for zinc (8 mg/d for adult women and 11 mg/d for adult men) appears sufficient to prevent zinc deficiency in most individuals.
   - □ Intranasal zinc preparations, most commonly used for the short-term treatment of common cold symptoms, can cause irreversible loss of the sense of smell (anosmia), so zinc-containing intranasal gels and sprays should be avoided.
   - □ Currently, there is no sensitive and specific biomarker to detect zinc deficiency in humans.
   - □ Essential functions:
     - Zinc plays a vital role in human metabolism and cellular function in numerous ways.
       - Catalytic role: over 300 enzymes are zinc dependent.
       - Structural role: zinc plays a significant role in both the structure of proteins and cell membranes and in wound healing.
     - Zinc-dependent proteins play a role in:
       - Gene expression
       - Hormone release
       - Nerve impulse transmission
       - Apoptosis

Dehydration and Rehydration Principles[25,26]

Dehydration is defined as a negative fluid balance which can result from decreased intake, increased output, or intravascular/extravascular fluid shifts.

- Most of the clinical manifestations of dehydration are related to intravascular fluid depletion, such as:
  - □ Tachycardia
  - □ Hypotension
  - □ Decreased capillary refill
  - □ Skin turgor changes ("tenting" of the skin)
- To appropriately treat dehydration, the underlying cause must be identified.
- Successful and safe rehydration addresses not only total body water depletion, but also:
  - □ Sodium
  - □ Potassium
  - □ Glucose
  - □ Osmolality
  - □ pH
- If able to tolerate, oral rehydration may be preferable in mild to moderately dehydrated individuals.
- In severe dehydration (fluid deficit of 10% to 15% of body weight in infants), intravenous fluid replacement is necessary to replace the total fluid deficit over a 24-hour period of time in two phases.
  - □ Total fluid deficit + daily maintenance fluid requirements are added together. The total is then divided in half.
  - □ Phase 1 is replacing the first half over the first 8 hours.
  - □ Phase 2 is replacing the remainder over the subsequent 16 hours.
- Depending on the severity and the clinical presentation, there may be a need to begin replacement with boluses of fluids in the emergency setting.
- In certain circumstances, too rapid rehydration can lead to serious complications, including cerebral edema and death.

Starvation and Refeeding Principles[27,28]

Severe malnourishment can occur due to lack of macronutrients and micronutrients in situations of famine, forced starvation, fasting, or severe illness.

- During this fasting state, the main fuel source of the body switches from carbohydrates to fatty acids and amino acids, and this lack of total caloric intake can lead to weight loss and body wasting.
  - □ Intracellular vitamin and mineral concentrations decrease over time because of lack of intake and the need to continue necessary cellular metabolic processes.
  - □ Insulin secretion decreases, and glucagon secretion increases in an attempt to maintain glucose levels.
- During refeeding, insulin levels increase, which results in an increase in glycogen as well as fat and protein synthesis, all of which require the presence of micronutrients (phosphate, magnesium, and potassium among others).
  - □ These processes further stress the already depleted intracellular micronutrients, which can lead to cellular dysfunction and a shift of electrolytes from the extracellular to the intracellular space in an attempt to support the micronutrient-dependent intracellular processes.
  - □ This shift of electrolytes and fluids from extracellular to intracellular can lead to cardiac arrhythmias and death, among other sequelae.
  - □ These patients require close monitoring and support during the refeeding phase of treatment.

Fluids and Electrolytes in Surgical and Hospitalized Patients (Basic Needs)[29,30]

The role of the kidney is critical in maintaining fluid volume and electrolyte balance under normal circumstances as well as instances of physiologic stress.

- There is significant interplay between:
  - □ Daily water needs
  - □ Kidney function
  - □ Sodium concentration
  - □ The thirst mechanism
  - □ Antidiuretic hormone (ADH)
- The following information assumes normal kidney function and expected, but not excessive, water losses from urine, skin, lungs, and stool.
- The choice of fluid ultimately depends on the type of fluid lost from the body, the serum electrolyte concentration, and the need for glucose in the IV fluid.
  - □ For maintenance fluids, this may translate into an isotonic or half-isotonic solution with added dextrose and electrolytes

as needed (D5 Normal Saline with 20 mEq KCl/L or D5½ Normal Saline with 20 mEq KCl/L).
  - Ongoing laboratory testing is needed to make decisions about the need to change IV fluid concentration and components.

Maintenance Fluids[31]

"The goal of maintenance fluid therapy is to preserve water and electrolyte balance and to provide (short term) nutrition among patients who are not able to eat or drink."[30]

- Normal, healthy adults are considered to have a minimal obligatory water intake or generation of approximately 1,600 mL/d, composed of the following:
  - Ingested water—500 mL
  - Water in food—800 mL
  - Water from oxidation—300 mL
- The sources of obligatory water output in normal adults are composed of the following:
  - Urine—500 mL
  - Skin—500 mL
  - Respiratory tract—400 mL
  - Stool—200 mL

Replacement Fluids

"The goal of replacement fluid therapy is to correct existing abnormalities in volume status and/or serum electrolytes."[31]

- There is no steadfast formula to accurately determine total body fluid deficit.
  - An estimate can be made if a predeficit weight is known, which can be compared to the current weight of the patient.
  - If this information is not known, then the following can be used to estimate the severity of the deficit:
    - Physical exam signs (blood pressure, jugular venous pressure, mucous membrane hydration, skin tenting, urine output, etc.)
    - Laboratory data (urine sodium concentration)
- With mild to moderate fluid deficit, there is generally no need to give bolus doses of intravenous fluids.
- To treat the fluid deficit and avoid continued worsening, the fluid replacement rate must be greater than the calculated maintenance requirement and continued losses. As a general rule, IV fluid infusion at a rate of 50 to 100 mL/h greater than estimated fluid losses is common.

Processed Foods

Food additives, toxins, and preservatives are not nutritional substances. They are recognized by the immune system as foreign.

- When the body does not recognize something as food (e.g., food additive, a toxin, and a preservative of some sort) there is a profound inflammatory reaction that occurs causing the immune system globally and locally in the gastrointestinal tract to be activated.
- If this occurs often, for instance, with the ingestion of processed foods for breakfast, lunch, and dinner, then the system is under assault from ongoing chronic inflammation, which has significant and lasting effects.
- This chronic inflammatory state is directly involved in the process of atherosclerosis, which may lead to the downstream effects of heart attack and stroke, currently two of the top three causes of death in the United States. A diet high in unprocessed plant foods, particularly fruits and vegetables, maybe the best defense against chronic inflammation.[32,33] This is indeed true for chronic disease regardless of organ system.

EXERCISE BASICS[34]

Acute Physiologic Adaptive Response to Exercise

There are several immediate adaptive responses to exercises, including change in:

- Heart rate
- Stroke volume
- Cardiac output
- Blood pressure and blood flow
- Maximal oxygen uptake

These responses create increased metabolic demands as the body expends more energy during exercise.

- The body must draw upon the resources of the essential nutrients discussed earlier, in order to achieve a short-term homeostatic adaptive response.
- In addition, the acute effects of exercise can be influenced by a variety of factors. These include:
  - Internal factors, such as the nutritional, fitness, and psychological status of the individual exercising.
  - External factors, such as ambient temperature.
- It is useful to interpret the acute physiologic adaptive responses to exercises in light of these factors.

HEART RATE

Heart rate increases in direct proportion to the intensity of exercise being performed. Figure 22.2 summarizes several important points relative to the way heart rate responds to increasing levels of exercise, such as during a graded treadmill exercise test (e.g., the Bruce protocol).

At exhaustion, the rise in heart rate will flatten out. This is called the maximal heart rate.

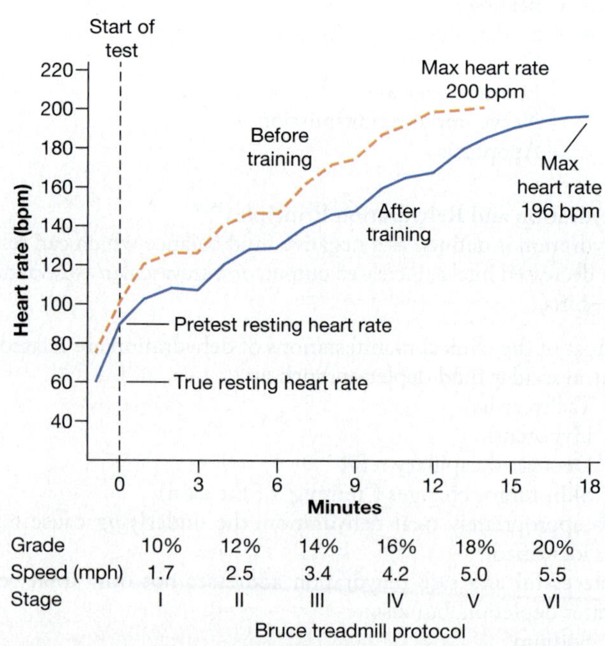

Figure 22.2. Heart rate results during the graded exercise test of a 20-year-old before and after exercise training. Notice that his pretest exercise heart rate is much higher than his true resting heart rate. The exercise heart rate increases in a linear fashion with increase in workload until the maximal heart rate is reached, when it plateaus. (From Nieman DC. *Exercise Testing and Prescription: A Health-Related Approach*. 6th ed. McGraw-Hill; 2006. Reprinted with permission from David C. Nieman, DrPH, FACSM.)

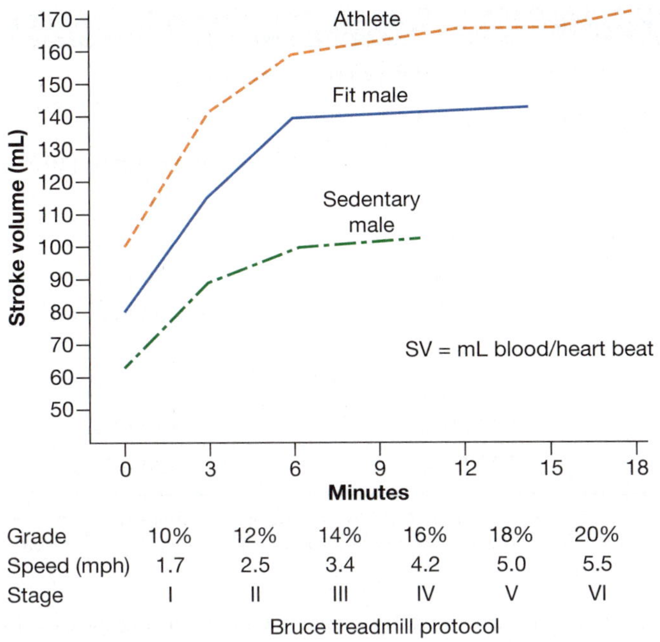

Figure 22.3. Stroke volume represents the amount of blood pumped per beat of the heart. Instead of rising linearly with increase in workload, stroke volume increases strongly up to a workload of 40% to 60% of $\dot{V}O_{2max}$. There is little change beyond this level, despite the increasing workload. (From Nieman DC. *Exercise Testing and Prescription: A Health-Related Approach.* 6th ed. McGraw-Hill; 2006. Reprinted with permission from David C. Nieman, DrPH, FACSM.)

- When the heart rate increases, little if at all after a stage change during a graded exercise test, this is a good indication that the maximal heart rate has been reached.
- The average maximal heart rate is equal to 220 minus the individual's age (in years).
  - This equation, however, is the average found in large groups of people.
  - People of a given age vary widely, with a standard deviation of 10 to 12 beats per minute.
- At submaximal levels of exercise, when the workload is held steady, the heart rate will increase for 1 to 3 minutes and then level off at a steady-state value.
  - The harder the submaximal workload, the longer the heart rate will take to level off.

STROKE VOLUME

Stroke volume is the quantity of blood pumped out of the heart per heartbeat and is regulated by several factors, including the:

- Amount of venous blood returned to the heart
- Capacity to enlarge the ventricle
- Force of contraction of the heart muscle
- Sympathetic nervous stimulation

Figure 22.3 summarizes several important points regarding the change in stroke volume, from rest to exercise exhaustion.

The change in stroke volume during graded exercise does not follow the pattern of change in the heart rate.

- Stroke volume increases strongly only up to a workload of 40% to 60% of maximal oxygen uptake ($\dot{V}O_{2max}$) and beyond this intensity level, increasing workload brings only small increases.[34,35]
- Resting stroke volume values for sedentary people range between 60 and 70 mL of blood per heartbeat, and those who are highly trained may have resting stroke volumes as high as 100 to 120 mL of blood per heartbeat.[34,35]

CARDIAC OUTPUT

Cardiac output (Q) is equal to the stroke volume (SV) times the heart rate (HR) (Q = SV × HR).

- In other words, cardiac output represents the quantity of blood pumped out of the heart each minute.
- At rest, the average cardiac output is approximately 5 L/min and it can rise to 20 to 40 L/min during maximal exercise, depending on individual fitness status and size of the individual. Figure 22.4 summarizes several important points regarding the change in cardiac output during exercise.[34,35]
- The cardiac output rises linearly with increasing workload and plateaus slightly at exercise exhaustion. During the initial stages of exercise, the increase in cardiac output is due to increases in both heart rate and stroke volume.

BLOOD PRESSURE

Systolic blood pressure increases in direct proportion to the increase in aerobic exercise intensity, with resting values of 120 mm Hg, often rising to 200 mm Hg or greater at exhaustion.

Diastolic blood pressure changes little if any during aerobic exercise. The exercise-induced increase in systolic blood pressure is related to the increase in cardiac output.

- The increase in blood pressure would be much higher, except that arterial blood vessels in the active muscles dilate, reducing peripheral resistance, which is the sum of all the forces that oppose blood flow in the body's blood vessel system.
- Cycling with the arms (arm ergometry) increases systolic and diastolic blood pressures 15%, compared to cycling with legs. This probably occurs because of the smaller muscle mass in the arms, which offers a greater resistance to blood flow than the larger muscles in the legs.
- Weight-lifting or isometric contractions cause large increases in both systolic and diastolic blood pressures.

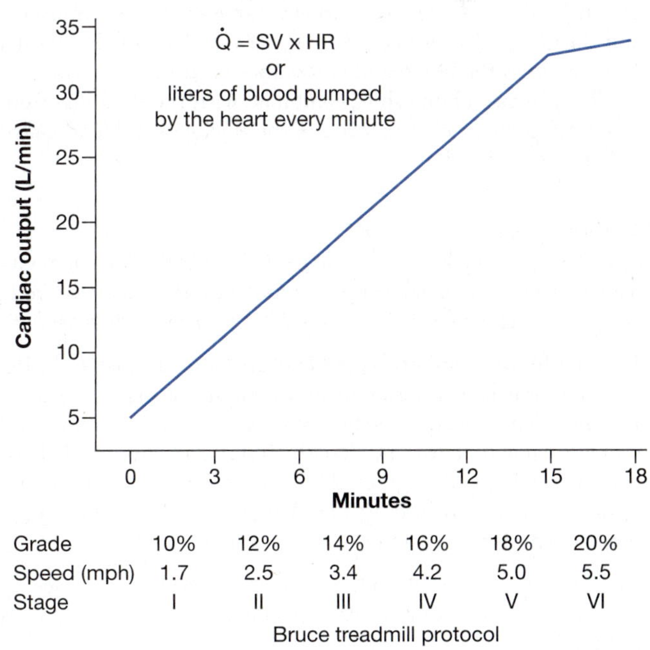

Figure 22.4. Cardiac Output follows a pattern like that of the heart rate. With increasing workload, cardiac output rises linearly and plateaus slightly at exercise exhaustion. (From Nieman DC. *Exercise Testing and Prescription: A Health-Related Approach.* 6th ed. McGraw-Hill; 2006. Reprinted with permission from David C. Nieman, DrPH, FACSM.)

TABLE 22.3

Distribution of Cardiac Output During Rest and Light, Moderate, and Maximal Exercise

	Cardiac Output (mL min⁻¹)			
Vascular Region	**At Rest (6%)**	**Light Exercise (30%)**	**Heavy Exercise (75%)**	**Maximal Exercise (100%)**
Cardiac output	6,000	12,000	24,000	30,000
Cerebral	720 (12%)	720 (6%)	720 (3%)	720 (2%)
Myocardial	240 (4%)	480 (4%)	960 (4%)	1,200 (4%)
Muscle	1,260 (21%)	5,760 (48%)	17,280 (72%)	26,400 (88%)
Renal	1,320 (22%)	1,200 (10%)	720 (3%)	300 (1%)
Hepatosplanchnic	1,560 (26%)	1,440 (12%)	960 (4%)	300 (1%)
Skin	540 (9%)	1,920 (16%)	2,640 (11%)	900 (3%)
Other	360 (6%)	480 (4%)	720 (3%)	180 (<1%)

From Nieman DC. *Exercise Testing and Prescription: A Health-Related Approach.* 6th ed. McGraw-Hill; 2006. Reprinted with permission from David C. Nieman, DrPH, FACSM. Data from Shephard RJ, Åstrand P-O. *Endurance in Sport: The Encyclopedia of Sports Medicine.* Vol 2. Blackwell Scientific Publications; 1992.

BLOOD FLOW

Blood flow is redirected away from areas where it is not needed (e.g., organs) and to the muscles during exercise. At rest, only 21% of the cardiac output goes to the muscles, compared with as much as 88% during exhaustive exercise (see Table 22.3).

As the body temperature increases, blood is directed to the skin in order to conduct heat away from the body core.

- The primary means by which the body loses heat during exercise is through evaporation of sweat on the skin.
  - Sweat glands will use fluid from the cells and from the blood to produce the sweat, which can reach 2 to 3 L/h during hard exercise in humid heat.
  - If the sweat rate is high, blood volume will decrease, ultimately to the point of heat injury.
- During endurance exercise, plasma volume shifts to the muscles, and during graded exercise testing, 12% to 16% of the plasma volume leaves the blood and enters the active muscle tissue.[34]
  - This plasma volume shift, combined with the fluid loss from sweating, leads to an increase in the thickness of blood called hemoconcentration.

MAXIMAL OXYGEN UPTAKE

Maximal oxygen uptake $\dot{V}O_{2max}$, can be defined as the "maximal rate at which oxygen can be taken up, distributed, and used by the body in the performance of exercise that utilize a large muscle mass."[35,36]

- It is the highest rate of oxygen consumption attainable during maximal or exhaustive exercise and with increasing workload.
- During graded exercise, active muscle tissue needs more and more oxygen to burn the carbohydrates and fats needed for energy production. Figures 22.5 to 22.7 summarize several important points regarding the change in $\dot{V}O_{2max}$ and oxygen metabolism during exercise.

With increasing workload, oxygen consumption increases up to the last stage of exercise. At this point, $\dot{V}O_2$ plateaus and is called the $\dot{V}O_{2max}$.

- Oxygen debt refers to the volume of oxygen consumed during the recovery period following exercise, in excess of the volume normally consumed at rest (see Fig. 22.7).
- This debt pays back the oxygen deficit built up during the initial minutes of exercise, on account of the body adjusting to the exercise, plus other metabolic factors built up during the exercise activity.

Chronic Physiologic Adaptive Response to Exercise

The persistent changes in the structure and function of the body following regular exercise training are called chronic adaptations to exercise.[36]

- Several of the cardiorespiratory and metabolic responses of exercise adapt very rapidly to exercise training.[37,38]
  - Within the first 1 to 3 weeks of intensive cardiorespiratory training by young healthy college students (e.g., 40 to 60 minutes per session, six sessions per week, 70% to 90% of $\dot{V}O_{2max}$), significant improvements in $\dot{V}O_{2max}$, submaximal

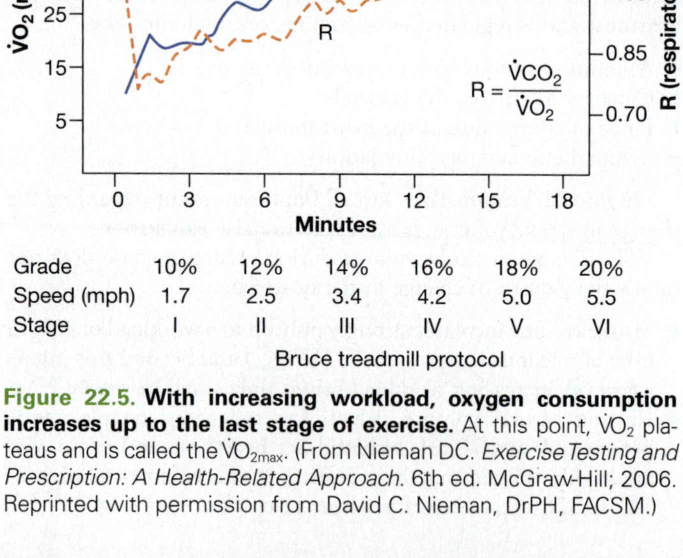

Figure 22.5. With increasing workload, oxygen consumption increases up to the last stage of exercise. At this point, $\dot{V}O_2$ plateaus and is called the $\dot{V}O_{2max}$. (From Nieman DC. *Exercise Testing and Prescription: A Health-Related Approach.* 6th ed. McGraw-Hill; 2006. Reprinted with permission from David C. Nieman, DrPH, FACSM.)

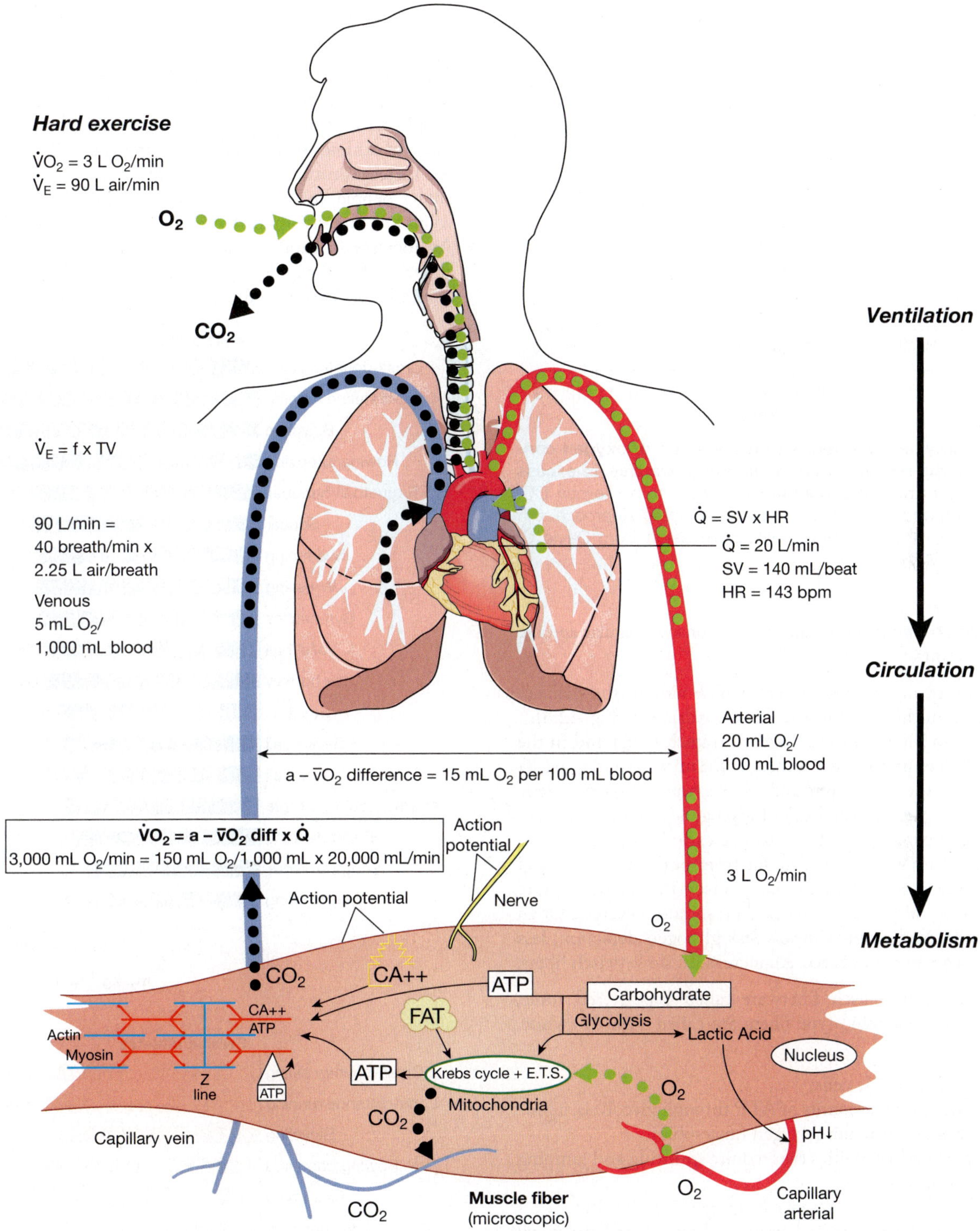

Figure 22.6. A summary of the acute effects of exercise. The body coordinates ventilation, circulation, and metabolism to meet the demands of exercise. If the cardiac output and a-$\dot{V}O_2$ are known, oxygen consumption can be calculated using this formula: $\dot{V}O_2 = \dot{Q} \times$ a–$\dot{V}O_2$ (From Nieman DC. *Exercise Testing and Prescription: A Health-Related Approach.* 6th ed. McGraw-Hill; 2006. Reprinted with permission from David C. Nieman, DrPH, FACSM.)

exercise heart rate, and lactate responses and ventilation can already be measured.

- Some adaptations to aerobic exercise, however, take longer.
  - For example, the increase in number of capillaries per muscle fiber may take several months or years.[38]
- Interestingly, exercise-induced changes are lost just as rapidly as they are gained.
- The magnitude of the chronic adaptations of regular exercise training depends on several factors, including the following:
  - Frequency
  - Intensity
  - Duration of training
  - Mode of activity
  - Initial fitness status

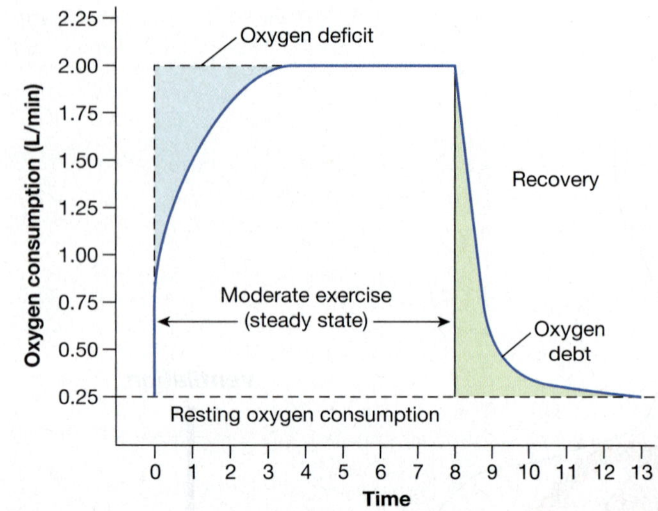

Figure 22.7. Oxygen debt refers to the volume of oxygen consumed during the recovery period following exercise, in excess of the volume normally consumed at rest. (From Nieman DC. *Exercise Testing and Prescription: A Health-Related Approach.* 6th ed. McGraw-Hill; 2006. Reprinted with permission from David C. Nieman, DrPH, FACSM.)

MUSCLES

Muscles undergo significant changes in response to regular aerobic training, including:

- An increase in myoglobin content, which aids in the delivery of oxygen from the blood to the mitochondria (see Fig. 22.6).
- An increase in the number and size of mitochondria and in the concentration of important enzymes in the mitochondria, specifically those of the Krebs cycle and the electron transport system.
- An increase in both the amount of glycogen stored in the muscle and the maximal capacity to oxidize carbohydrates.
- An increased capacity to oxidize fat from both muscle fat and adipose tissue stores.[39,40] The trained person thus oxidizes more fat and less carbohydrate during cardiorespiratory exercise (at an absolute workload), which means less glycogen depletion, less fatigue, and greater endurance. An increase in slow-twitch fibers.

The aerobic-type muscle fibers are called Type I (red, tonic, slow twitch); the anaerobic-type fibers are called Type II (white, glycolytic, fast twitch).

- The fast-twitch muscle cells:
  - Can produce high amounts of ATP through glycolysis, a process that does not require oxygen (anaerobic)
  - Are important in activities that require sprinting and jumping
- Slow-twitch muscle cells:
  - Generate ATP in the presence of oxygen (aerobically)
  - Have high numbers of mitochondria and a good capillary supply
- Endurance athletes usually have a high proportion of slow-twitch muscle fibers, whereas sprinters have a high proportion of fast-twitch muscle fibers.

HEART RATE

Heart rate at rest decreases approximately one beat per minute for every 1 to 2 weeks of aerobic training, for about 10 to 20 weeks.

- Further decreases are possible if training volume and intensity are increased.
- The decrease in resting heart rate is attributable to an increase in parasympathetic control (through the vagus nerve, which slows the heart rate).[35]

Other aerobic training effects on resting physiologic variables include[34,35]:

- An increase in stroke volume, with more blood pumped per beat, with a corresponding decrease in rate. For example, sedentary people have stroke volumes at rest of about 60 mL, whereas those of athletes often measure greater than 100 mL.
- An increase in the total blood volume from about 5 L in sedentary people, to 6 or 7 L in athletes. This increase in plasma volume is directly linked to the increase in stroke volume.
- An increase in capillary density. Untrained human muscle has about 1.5 to 2.0 capillaries per muscle fiber, whereas elite endurance athletes have two to three times this number.

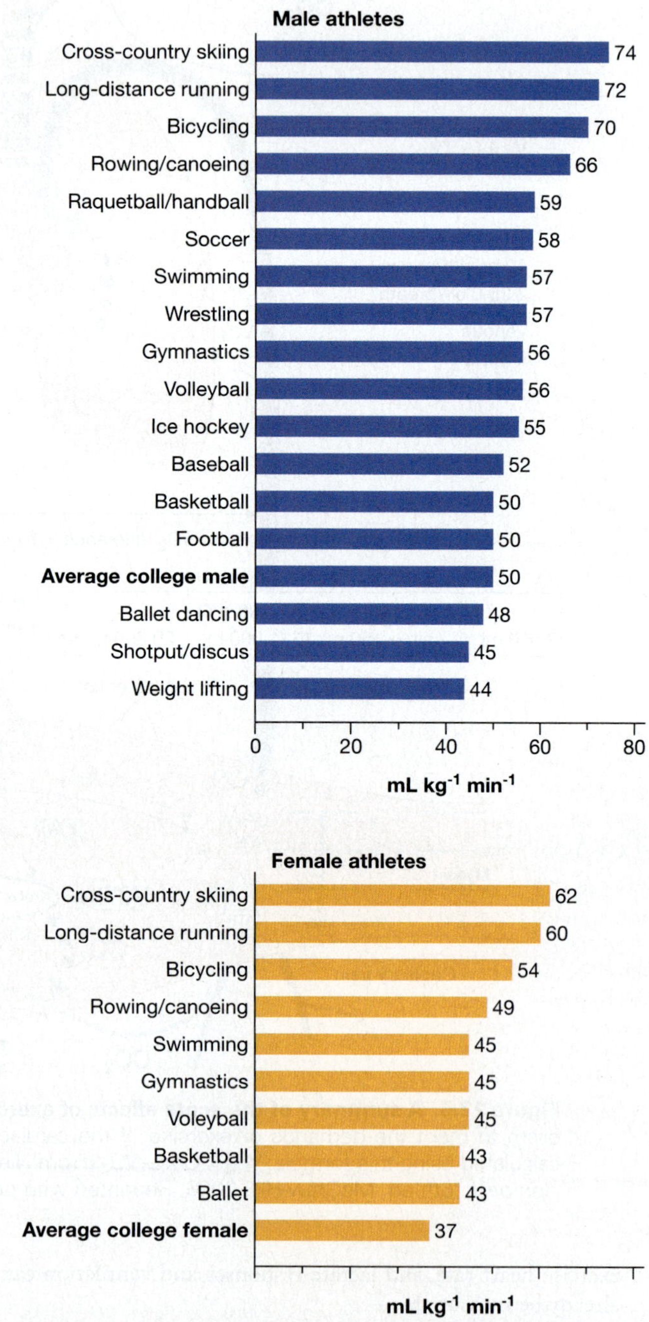

Figure 22.8. Maximal oxygen uptake. Endurance athletes have the highest $\dot{V}O_{2max}$ values for both males and females. (From Nieman DC. *Exercise Testing and Prescription: A Health-Related Approach.* 6th ed. McGraw-Hill; 2006. Reprinted with permission from David C. Nieman, DrPH, FACSM.)

TABLE 22.4

Differences between Sedentary and Trained Males during a Balke Treadmill Graded Exercise Test (Resting and Maximal Exercise Parameters)

Parameter	Sedentary Males (*n* = 9)	Trained Males (*n* = 11)
Age (years)	44.2	42.7
Weight (lb)	185	171
Percent body fat (%)	24.5	12.5
Resting heart rate (bpm)	66.8	52.5
$\dot{V}O_{2max}$ (mL kg^{-1} min^{-1})	33.3	54.2
Ventilation, max (L min^{-1})	119	165
Heart rate, max (bpm)	188	177

From Nieman DC. *Exercise Testing and Prescription: A Health-Related Approach.* 6th ed. McGraw-Hill; 2006. Reprinted with permission from David C. Nieman, DrPH, FACSM. Data from Nieman DC, Tan SA, Lee JW, Berk LS. Complement and immunoglobulin levels in athletes and sedentary controls. *Int J Sports Med.* 1989;10(2):124–128.

MAXIMAL OXYGEN UPTAKE

Maximal oxygen uptake ($\dot{V}O_{2max}$) is higher in trained athletes. This means that trained people can ventilate more air during maximal exercise, and their maximal tidal volume and frequency are also higher.

- Lung diffusion capacity also improves with training. In other words, oxygen can diffuse from the lung alveoli to the blood more readily.
- During maximal graded exercise testing, subjects are taken to complete exhaustion.
  - □ The changes during maximal exercise that can be expected are shown in Table 22.4.
- Training provides a significantly higher maximal aerobic power $\dot{V}O_{2max}$, meaning that a greater amount of oxygen can be consumed during maximal exercise.
  - □ Figure 22.8 outlines an increase in $\dot{V}O_{2max}$ that can be expected in response to increasing levels of training and compares $\dot{V}O_{2max}$ among different athletes.[41] Cross-country skiers generally have the highest $\dot{V}O_{2max}$ because almost all the major muscle groups in the body are activated.[37]

TABLE 22.5

Summary of Changes in Cardiorespiratory Parameters with Endurance Training

Cardiovascular Parameter	Resting	Submax Exercise	Maximal Exercise
Oxygen consumption	No change	No change	Increase
Heart rate	Decrease	Decrease	No/slight change
Stroke volume	Increase	Increase	Increase
Cardiac output	No change	No change	Increase
Active muscle blood flow	No change	Increase	Increase
Ventilation	No change	Decrease	Increase
a – $\dot{V}O_2$ difference	No change	Slight increase	Increase
Lactic acid levels	No change	Decrease	Increase

From Nieman DC. *Exercise Testing and Prescription: A Health-Related Approach.* 6th ed. McGraw-Hill; 2006. Reprinted with permission from David C. Nieman, DrPH, FACSM.

  - □ Table 22.5 summarizes the changes in cardiorespiratory parameters that occur during rest, submaximal exercise, and maximal exercise following endurance training.
  - □ Table 22.6 compares typical values in sedentary, trained, and elite individuals.

TABLE 22.6

Comparison of Hypothetical Physiologic and Body Composition Changes from an Endurance Training Program for a Sedentary, Normal Person, and a World-Class Endurance Runner of the Same Age

Variable	Sedentary Normal Pre-[a]	Sedentary Normal Post-[a]	World-Class Athlete
Cardiovascular			
Resting HR (bpm)	71	59	36
Max HR(bpm)	185	183	174
Resting SV (mL)	65	80	125
Max SV (mL)	120	140	200
Resting $\dot{Q}$ (L/min)	4.6	4.7	4.5
Max $\dot{Q}$ (L/min)	22.2	25.6	34.8
Heart volume (mL)	750	820	1,200
Blood volume (L)	4.7	5.1	6
Resting systolic BP (mm Hg)	135	130	110
Resting diastolic BP (mm Hg)	78	76	70
Respiratory			
Resting $\dot{V}_E$ (L/min)	7	6	6
Max $\dot{V}_E$ (L/min)	110	135	195
Resting F (breaths/min)	14	12	12
Max F (breaths/min)	40	45	55
Resting TV (L/breath)	0.5	0.5	0.5
Max TV (L/breath)	2.75	3.0	3.5
Vital capacity (L)	5.8	6.0	6.2
Residual volume (L)	1.4	1.2	1.2
Metabolic			
a – $\dot{V}O_2$ difference (mL/dL)	6	6	6
Max a – $\dot{V}O_2$ difference (mL/dL)	14.5	15	16
$\dot{V}O_{2max}$ (mL kg^{-1} min^{-1})	40.5	49.8	76.7
Max lactate (mmol/L)	7.5	8.5	9
Body composition			
Weight (lb)	175	170	150
Fat weight (lb)	28	21.3	11.3
Lean weight (lb)	147	148.7	138.7
Relative fat (%)	16	12.5	7.5

[a]6-month training program, jogging 3 to 4 times per week, 30 min/d, at 75% VO_{2max}.

HR, heart rate; SV, stroke volume; $\dot{Q}$, cardiac output; BP, blood pressure; V_E, ventilation; F, frequency; TV, tidal volume.

From Nieman DC. *Exercise Testing and Prescription: A Health-Related Approach.* 6th ed. McGraw-Hill; 2006. Reprinted with permission from David C. Nieman, DrPH, FACSM; From Wilmore JH, Norton AC. *The Heart and Lungs at Work.* Beckman Instruments; 1974.

OTHER ADAPTIVE RESPONSES

Other adaptive responses that occur because of regular aerobic exercise include:

- A small decrease in total body fat and a slight increase in lean body weight.
- An increase in HDL cholesterol, a decrease in triglycerides, but little or no change in total serum or LDL cholesterol.
- A greater ability to exercise in the heat.
- An increase in the density and breaking strength of bones, ligaments, and tendons, and an increase in the thickness of cartilage in the joints.
- Improved insulin sensitivity in skeletal muscle.[42]

SUMMARY

Nutrition and exercise are fundamental considerations when approaching the patient with the Metabolic Model in mind.

- What the body receives in terms of nutrition is important for energy production as well as for its ability to heal and recover from disease and illness.
- For proper functioning and optimal health, the body requires more than 40 essential nutrients. Nutrients are classified into six groups:
  1. Carbohydrates
  2. Fats
  3. Proteins
  4. Vitamins
  5. Minerals
  6. Water
- Adequate nutrition allows for the proper function of the immune system and the ability to defend against infections.
- Proper nutrition is important in the function of multiple systems, including the endocrine, gastrointestinal, and cardiovascular systems.
- Furthermore, improper, or inadequate nutrition can impair the function of these systems and set the stage for the development of diseases, including:
  - □ Type II diabetes mellitus
  - □ Obesity
  - □ CVD
  - □ Cancer

Just as the essential nutrients are key in the production of energy, exercise is a major contributor in its expenditure.

- Adaptive responses to exercise can be both acute and chronic in nature depending on the intensity and duration of activity being performed.
- Exercise has the capacity to alter fundamental physiologic processes, such as resting heart rate and maximal oxygen uptake. In doing so, exercise can have a substantial impact in how the body utilizes energy and its overall energy homeostasis.
- Understanding the fundamental tenets of nutrition and exercise is key to understanding the Metabolic Model, and how it can be applied for both the treatment of disease and promotion of health.

REFERENCES

1. Morrison DJ, Preston T. Formation of short chain fatty acids by the gut microbiota and their impact on human metabolism. *Gut Microbes.* 2016; 7:189–200.
2. Chambers ES, Preston T, Frost G, Morrison DJ. Role of gut microbiota-generated short-chain fatty acids in metabolic and cardiovascular health. *Curr Nutr Rep.* 2018;7:198–206.
3. Veronese N, Solmi M, Caruso MG, et al. Dietary fiber and health outcomes: an umbrella review of systematic reviews and meta-analyses. *Am J Clin Nutr.* 2018;107(3):436–444.
4. Portincasa P, Bonfrate L, Vacca M, et al. Gut microbiota and short chain fatty acids: implications in glucose homeostasis. *Int J Mol Sci.* 2022;23(3):1105.
5. Wu Y, Qian Y, Pan Y, et al. Association between dietary fiber intake and risk of coronary heart disease: A meta-analysis. *Clin Nutr.* 2015;34(4):603–611.
6. Threapleton DE, Greenwood DC, Evans CE, et al. Dietary fibre intake and risk of cardiovascular disease: systematic review and meta-analysis. *BMJ.* 2013;347:f6879.
7. Di Pasquale MG. The essentials of essential fatty acids. *J Diet Suppl.* 2009; 6(2):143–161.
8. Balta I, Stef L, Pet I, Iancu T, Stef D, Corcionivoschi N. Essential fatty acids as biomedicines in cardiac health. *Biomedicines.* 2021;9(10):1466.
9. Bernard-Gallon DJ, Vissac-Sabatier C, Antoine-Vincent D, et al. Differential effects of n-3 and n-6 polyunsaturated fatty acids on BRCA1 and BRCA2 gene expression in breast cell lines. *Br J Nutr.* 2002;87(4):281–289.
10. Wolfe RR, Cifelli AM, Kostas G, Kim IY. Optimizing protein intake in adults: interpretation and application of the recommended dietary allowance compared with the acceptable macronutrient distribution range. *Adv Nutr.* 2017;8(2):266–275.
11. https://www.cdc.gov/obesity/php/data-research/adult-obesity-facts.html
12. https://www.tfah.org/report-details/state-of-obesity-2024/
13. https://www.niddk.nih.gov/health-information/health-statistics/overweight-obesity#prevalence
14. Fryar CD, Carroll MD, Afful J. Prevalence of overweight, obesity, and severe obesity among adults aged 20 and over: United States, 1960–1962 through 2017–2018. *NCHS Health E-Stats, Centers for Disease Control and Prevention.* 2020.
15. Benavidez GA, Zahnd WE, Hung P, Eberth JM. Chronic disease prevalence in the US: sociodemographic and geographic variations by Zip Code tabulation area. *Prev Chronic Dis.* 2024;21:230267.
16. Balint JP. Physical findings in nutritional deficiencies. *Pediatr Clin North Am.* 1998;45(1):245–260.
17. Jeppesen PB, Hoy CE, Mortensen PB. Essential fatty acid deficiency in patients receiving home parenteral nutrition. *Am J Clin Nutr.* 1998; 68(1):126–133.
18. Berg JM, Tymoczko JL, Stryer L. *Biochemistry.* 5th ed. W H Freeman; 2002.
19. Greger M. Where do you get your fiber? *NutritionFacts.org.* http://nutritionfacts.org/2015/09/29/where-do-you-get-your-fiber/. Updated September 29, 2015. Accessed February 9, 2017.
20. Dietary fiber: Usual intakes from food and water, 2003–2006, compared to adequate intakes. U.S. Department of Agriculture, Agricultural Research Service. www.ars.usda.gov/Services/docs.htm?docid=22659. Updated October 4, 2016. Accessed February 9, 2017.
21. Food and Drug Administration. Code of federal regulations, title 21, volume 2. Subpart D – Specific requirement for nutrient content claims. http://www.accessdata.fda/gov/scripts/cdrh/cfdocs/cfcfr/CFRSearch.cfm?fr=101.54. Updated April 1, 2016. Accessed February 9, 2017.
22. U.S. Department of Agriculture and U.S. Department of Health and Human Services. *Dietary Guidelines for Americans, 2010.* 7th ed. U.S. Government Printing Office; 2010.
23. Anderson JW, Baird P, Davis RH Jr, et al. Health benefits of dietary fiber. *Nutr Rev.* 2009;67(4):188–205.
24. Institute of Medicine, Food and Nutrition Board. *Dietary Reference Intakes for Calcium and Vitamin D.* National Academy Press; 2010.
25. Colletti JE, Brown KM, Sharieff GQ, Barata IA, Ishimine P; ACEP Pediatric Emergency Medicine Committee. The management of children with gastroenteritis and dehydration in the emergency department. *J Emerg Med.* 2010;38(5):686–698.
26. Goldman RD, Friedman JN, Parkin PC. Validation of the clinical dehydration scale for children with acute gastroenteritis. *Pediatrics.* 2008;122(3): 545–549.
27. Mehanna HM, Moledina J, Travis J. Refeeding syndrome: what it is, and how to prevent and treat it. *BMJ.* 2008;336(7659):1495–1498.
28. Webb GJ, Smith K, Thursby-Pelham F, Smith T, Stroud MA, Da Silva AN. Complications of emergency refeeding in anorexia nervosa: case series and review. *Acute Med.* 2011;10(2):69–76.

29. Rose BD, Post TW. *Clinical Physiology of Acid-Base and Electrolyte Disorders*. 5th ed. McGraw-Hill; 2001:285.
30. Shafiee MAS, Bohn D, Hoorn EJ, Halperin ML. How to select optimal maintenance intravenous fluid therapy. *QJM*. 2003;96(8):601–610.
31. Sterns RH. Maintenance and replacement fluid therapy in adults. www.uptodate.com/contents/maintenance-and-replacement-fluid-therapy-in-adults. Updated September 23, 2015. Accessed February 9, 2017.
32. Root MM, McGinn MC, Nieman DC, et al. Combined fruit and vegetable intake is correlated with improved inflammatory and oxidant status from a cross-sectional study in a community setting. *Nutrients*. 2012;4(1):29–41.
33. Mozaffarian D, Appel LJ, Van Horn L. Components of a cardioprotective diet: new insights. *Circulation*. 2011;123(24):2870–2891.
34. Brooks GA, Fahey TD, Baldwin KM. *Exercise Physiology: Human Bioenergetics and Its Applications*. 4th ed. McGraw-Hill; 2004.
35. American College of Sports Medicine. *ACSM's Resource Manual for Guidelines for Exercise Testing and Prescription*. 4th ed. Lippincott Williams & Wilkins; 2005.
36. McArdle WD, Katch Fl, Katch VL. *Exercise Physiology: Energy, Nutrition, and Human Performance*. 5th ed. Lippincott Williams & Wilkins; 2001.
37. Smith TP, McNaughton LR, Marshall KJ. Effects of 4-wk training using Vmax/Tmax on VO_{2max} and performance in athletes. *Med Sci Sports Exerc*. 1999;31(6):892–896.
38. Hickson RC, Hagberg JM, Ehsani AA, Holloszy JO. Time course of the adaptive responses of aerobic power and heart rate to training. *Med Sci Sports Exerc*. 1981;13(1):17–20.
39. Spina RJ, Chi MM, Hopkins MG, Nemeth PM, Lowry OH, Holloszy JO. Mitochondrial enzymes increase in muscle in response to 7–10 days of cycle exercise. *J Appl Physiol*. 1996;80(6):2250–2254.
40. Jansson E, Kaijser L. Substrate utilization and enzymes in skeletal muscle of extremely endurance-trained men. *J Appl Physiol*. 1987;62:999–1005.
41. National Center for Health Statistics, Drury EF, ed. Assessing physical fitness and physical activity in population-based surveys. DHHS Pub. No. (PHS) 89–1253. Public Health Service. U.S. Government Printing Office; 1989.
42. Rabøl R, Petersen KF, Dufour S, Flannery C, Shulman GI. Reversal of muscle insulin resistance with exercise reduces postprandial hepatic de novo lipogenesis in insulin resistant individuals. *Proc Natl Acad Sci U S A*. 2011;108(33):13705–13709.

23

Microbiome: New Considerations in Clinical Management

MAE J. CIANCIO ▪ KRISTINA MARTINEZ-GURYN ▪ JULIE SWARTZENDRUBER ▪ KRISTEN BRENNAN ▪ CHRISTIAN EVANS ▪ ANNAMARIE C. JANSKY ▪ CASSAUNDRA BURT ▪ DONALD J. CIANCIO III

KEY CONCEPTS

- To truly understand the whole person, it is imperative to consider the trillions of microbes living in and on our body and how they influence our health.
- Microorganisms populate unique habitats in the nose, oral cavity, respiratory tract, gastrointestinal tract, urogenital tract, skin, and eyes.
- The health and composition of the microbial community are influenced by the host's genetics, lifestyle and environment, and the collection of microbes influences the health of the individual in a mutualistic relationship.
- Detrimental changes or eliminations of microorganisms can result in neurologic impairments, immune dysfunction, and systemic diseases.
- Antibiotics can eliminate pathogenic bacteria, but also impact the quality and quantity of healthy microbiomes.
- Probiotics, prebiotics, and fecal microbiota transplantation can promote or restore a healthy intestinal microbiome.
- The type of sample collected, method of collection, and analysis of its content influence the quality and quantity of clinically impactful information.
- Including the microbiomes' influence on an individual's overall mental and physical health adheres with the clinical tenets of osteopathic medicine.
- Identifying the body's natural and pathogenic microbial inhabitants is a key piece in treating illnesses. Optimization and modification of the microbiome may be curative, correlating with the osteopathic tenet stating, "The body has the inherent capacity to heal."

INTRODUCTION

There are multiple ways the body's immune system fights to maintain homeostasis by attacking and eliminating foreign stressors through inflammatory responses. However, the body harbors specific microbial communities, called microbiota, that foster health, prevent disease, and are recognized by the host's immune cells as "friendly cohabitants." The microbiome is defined as the content of microbiota, including bacteria, fungi, viruses, archaea, and protists, as well as their genetic machinery. Their symbiotic function with the host promotes health and prevents disease (Fig. 23.1). This chapter will highlight the composition of the microbiomes across different body sites, accepted technologies used for the identification and characterization of the microbial components, factors that influence changes to the composition, diseases resulting from an imbalance in these microcommunities, and therapeutic modalities to restore homeostasis and health.

The breadth of literature in this area of basic science and clinical research is profound. Since Antonie van Leeuwenhoek's first report of microorganisms in the late 1600s, scientific interest in their role in animal, plant, and environmental health has piqued dramatically. Since 1956, over a hundred thousand studies have been published on the "microbiome." Much of the research in this area, with specific reference to human health and disease, has been more recent. Many factors have advanced clinicians' knowledge and have fostered new ideas regarding the contribution of microbes to maintaining health and preventing disease. These include identification of specific microbial inhabitants, use of "omics" technologies to understand microbial content and functional responses, absence of microbiota under experimental "germ-free (GF) conditions," and elimination of microbes by specific antibiotic treatments.

Chronic diseases such as obesity, diabetes, inflammatory bowel disease (IBD), cardiovascular disease (CVD), and cancer are being reexamined in relation to changes in the intestinal microbiome and the influence of microbe composition on disease risk.[1,2] Heightened immune responses secondary to changes in the intestinal microbiota are associated with psoriasis, allergies, and rheumatoid arthritis.[3–10] Neuro-development and signaling through the gut–brain axis are influenced by changes in host microbial balance: alterations in the production of gut-derived neurotransmitters can influence neural development and contribute to neurologic disorders such as anxiety, depression, autism spectrum disorders (ASDs), Alzheimer disease, and Parkinson disease (PD).[11–13] By understanding the structural and compositional organization of the microbiome within its respective niches and its function in relation to health and disease, it will provide novel modalities for optimizing organ function and preventing disease, which aligns with the osteopathic medicine tenets that structure and function are reciprocally interrelated.

WHAT IS THE MICROBIOME?

Terminology and Localization

Table 23.1 provides a general overview of common terms used in human and experimental microbiome research.

In early reports, the terms *microflora* and *flora* were used to describe the microorganisms that colonize the host.[14] *Microbiota* is a more appropriate term to describe the collection of microorganisms, including bacteria, archaea, fungi, viruses/phages, and microbial eukaryotes which inhabit unique anatomical locations, such as the eyes, nose, mouth, respiratory, gastrointestinal and urogenital tracts, and skin.[15–18] These communities of microorganisms are unique in their composition and relative abundance, each poised to protect the host from pathogenic organisms and to prime the immune system.[19,20] The term *microbiome* is used to define the microbiota and their "theatre of activity," which includes microbial structural elements (DNA, RNA, proteins/peptides, lipids, polysaccharides), internal and external structural elements (mobile genetic elements including viruses, phages, and relic DNA), microbial metabolites (signaling molecules, toxins, organic molecules), and environmental conditions.[21]

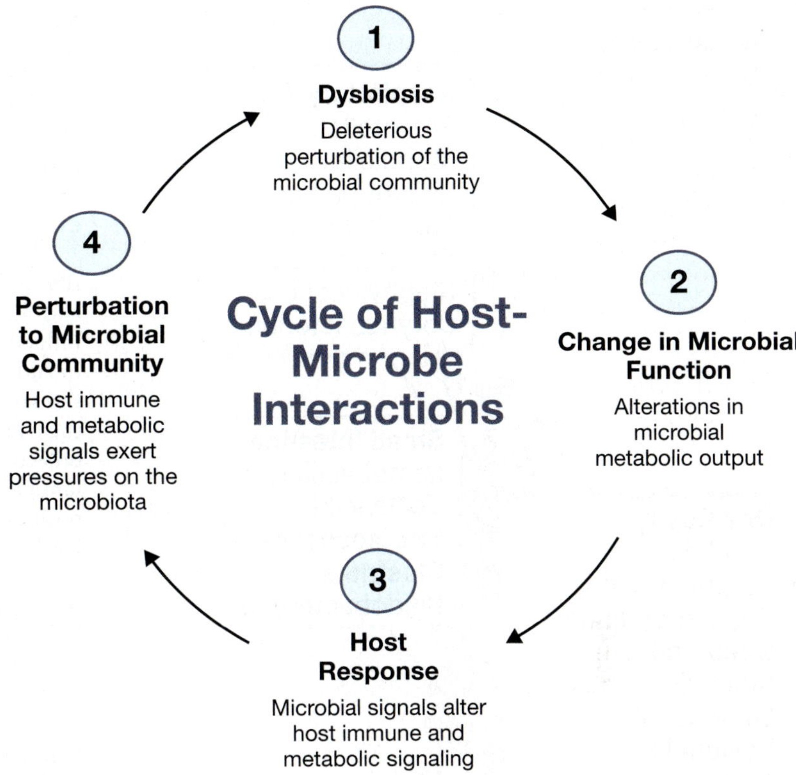

Figure 23.1. Cycle of host–microbe interactions. (1) Dysbiosis ensues upon deleterious restructuring of community composition that may include the outgrowth of pathogenic microorganisms. (2) Within a dysbiotic community, the functional potential of the microbiome changes leading to alterations in microbial metabolic output. (3) These changes in metabolic function can then directly influence the host response through altering host immune and metabolic signaling. (4) Finally, the altered immune and host function of the host can cause changes in the microbial community, thus reinforcing dysbiosis and perpetuating the cycle of host–microbe interactions.

Within the gastrointestinal tract alone, 100 trillion (10^{14}) microbes reside in the colon.[22] Based on their location within the intestines, microbes can influence nutrient extraction and utilization, vitamin formation, nondigestible carbohydrate breakdown (fermentation), drug detoxification, neurologic signaling, and intestinal hormone functions.[23] These microorganisms are influenced by method of birth, diet, environment, genetics, age, pH, hygiene, exercise, and use of supplements such as pre- and probiotics.[23–25] As shown in Figure 23.2, the relative content of identified microorganisms varies based on anatomical location.[26]

TABLE 23.1

Definitions of Important Terms

Terms	Definition
Microbiome	Collective microbial genes in an ecosystem.
Microbiota	Collective microbial cells in an ecosystem, including bacteria, fungi, archaea, viruses and protists.
Microflora	An older term used to describe the microbiota.
Eubiosis	Healthy balance of species in the microbiome.
Dysbiosis	Deleterious reorganization of the microbiome.
Richness	Number of different species in a sample.
Evenness	Distribution of species in a sample.
Alpha Diversity	Number of different species and their distribution within a sample.
Beta Diversity	Similarity and dissimilatory of microbial communities between samples.
Holobiont	Mammalian and microbial cells in their physical location.
Taxonomic classifications	Kingdom, phylum, class, order, family, genus, species, strains
Operational taxonomic units (OTU)	Sequences that have a sequence identity greater than a threshold of 97%.
Niche/habitat	Role of an organism in its community.
Germ-free (GF)	Lacking microbial communities; sterile.
Specific-pathogen free (SPF)	Free of a particular pathogen(s).
Gnotobiotic	Intestinal colonization with known, specific bacteria.

This table provides a general overview of common terms used in human and experimental microbiome research. Information was compiled using references 13–16.

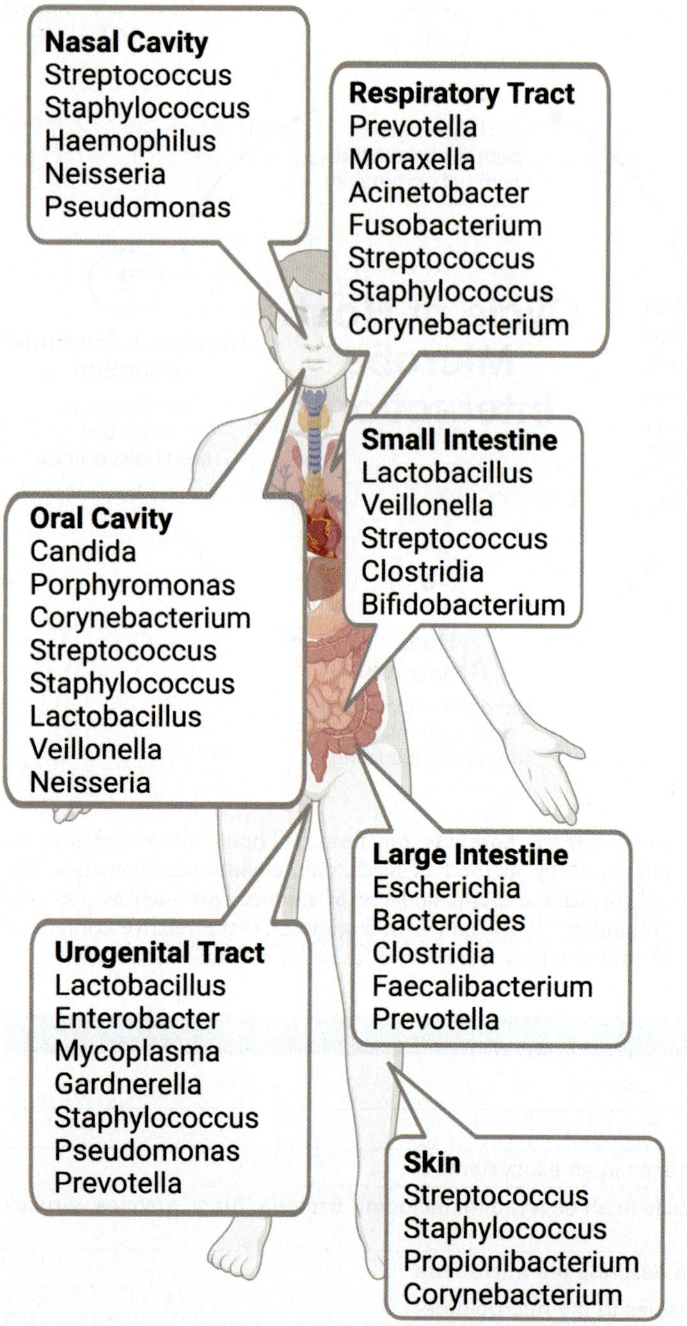

Figure 23.2. Microbial community composition differs among different body sites. Key microbes associated with the nasal cavity, oral cavity, respiratory tract, small and large intestines, urogenital tract and skin are highlighted. Information compiled from references 27–37. (Created with BioRender.com.)

Microbial abundance varies within each anatomical microbial niche, with robust colonization in the oral cavity and colon (10^{12} colony forming units (CFU)/mL) and a drastic reduction in the stomach ($10^{1\text{-}2}$ CFU/mL) due to the acidic environment. Microbe content increases in the small intestines, rising to $1 \times 10^{1\text{-}3}$ CFU/mL in the duodenum, $1 \times 10^{3\text{-}4}$ CFU/mL in the jejunum, and $1 \times 10^{7\text{-}9}$ CFU/mL in the ileum. Functional redundancy exists within the communities, allowing for subtle changes to occur in the host without drastic metabolic consequence.[22,26] Within each niche, alterations in the relative balance of these organisms are linked with function; imbalance or disturbance in their relative abundance, termed *dysbiosis*, is associated with dysfunction within their community and the potential for disease.

With the development of culture-independent, molecular biology techniques designed to analyze the genetic content of samples, such as stool, punch biopsies, bronchial lavage fluids, buccal and vaginal swabs, the capacity to identify specific microorganisms within each anatomical niche has become more sensitive and less expensive.

Listed in Table 23.2 are common techniques used to identify and characterize the contents and function of the bacterial and fungal communities that inhabit the host.[13–16] Several factors influence the quality of information gained with these methods, including how the samples were collected and stored, time of day the samples were collected, and the sample source.[18] For instance, the bacterial species identified in a stool sample do not necessarily reflect the bacterial communities in the mucosal layer lining the luminal epithelial cells of the intestine. Intestinal bacterial composition in adults is relatively stable across individuals at the phyla level; however, unique individual signatures are evident at the species and subspecies levels, with members of the same household having more similarities than individuals from different households or geographical location.[25] The small differences in microbial inhabitants are the focus of studies to identify biomarkers and predictors of disease. Identifying the composition and frequency of unique microbial signatures requires sensitive tools and extensive bioinformatic analyses.

METHODS FOR IDENTIFICATION

Technologic advances have dramatically improved the ability to identify and characterize microorganisms and their functionality.[18,38] Based on the clinical question, the methodology for sample collection and sample analysis can vary considerably, as will the type of information that is retrieved (Fig. 23.3).

Sequencing 16S ribosomal RNA (rRNA) genes directly from samples using polymerase chain reaction (PCR) primers targeted to select regions in the 16S rRNA gene, called hypervariable regions (V1–V3, V4–V5), are used to identify bacterial components present in a community. This non–culture-based method for microbial identification has provided a broad understanding of the phylogenetic inhabitants of a particular microbiome to the genus level, with species identification proving to be more challenging. QIIME/Qiita, BioBakery, and PhyloSeq are statistical tools most appropriate for 16S rRNA sequencing data analyses.[39–41]

Shotgun metagenomic sequencing is a popular method to identify the microbes (bacteria, fungi, and viruses), their relative abundance, and their potential functionality based on genome sequencing. Second-generation sequencing produces billions of short DNA sequences in a single run; the Illumina sequencing systems are one of the most widely used platforms.[42] However, more recent studies employing longer DNA sequences, called third-generation sequencing, are gaining popularity for quantitative metagenomic information, especially for complex microbial communities that colonize the host.[42] Metagenomics involves the sequencing of all genomes captured in a sample in addition to the bacterial 16S rRNA gene, providing an understanding of the functional potential of the particular microbial communities. Metagenome-assembled genomes (MAGs) can be constructed to examine complete strain-level genomes,[43] which can be used for targeting isolation of specific species of interest or pangenome analyses for the direct comparison of genomes across species. While this methodology is more expensive than genome sequencing, the technology is advancing rapidly, allowing the relative cost per sample to be more affordable.

TABLE 23.2

Summary of Techniques Used to Study the Microbiota's Composition and Function

Terms	Goal	Information Provided	Platform Used	Cost
16S rRNA sequencing	Analysis of microbial community composition.	Who's there and how many in proportion to others	Illumina MiSeq Ion Torrent	$
18S rRNA sequencing	Analysis of microbial community composition.	Who's there and how many in proportion to others	Illumina MiSeq	$
Metagenomics	Whole-genome sequencing of entire microbial community. Sample may include host content.	Who's there and what are they doing	Illumina HiSeq	$$
Metatranscriptomics	Sequencing of microbial transcripts in a community.	What they're upregulating	Illumina NovaSeq 6000	$$$
Proteomics	Untargeted screening of proteins in a sample.	What they're making	Mass Spec	$$$
Metabolomics	Untargeted or targeted screening of metabolites and small molecules.	Metabolic activity of a community	GC-MS (SCFAs) LC-MS (Bile Acids)	$$
Lipidomics	Untargeted or targeted screening of lipid species.	Microbe-derived lipid species (e.g. CLA)	LC-MS	$$

This table summarizes common techniques used to identify the microbial content of a particular community as well as its function. The relative cost of each technique is provided for reference.

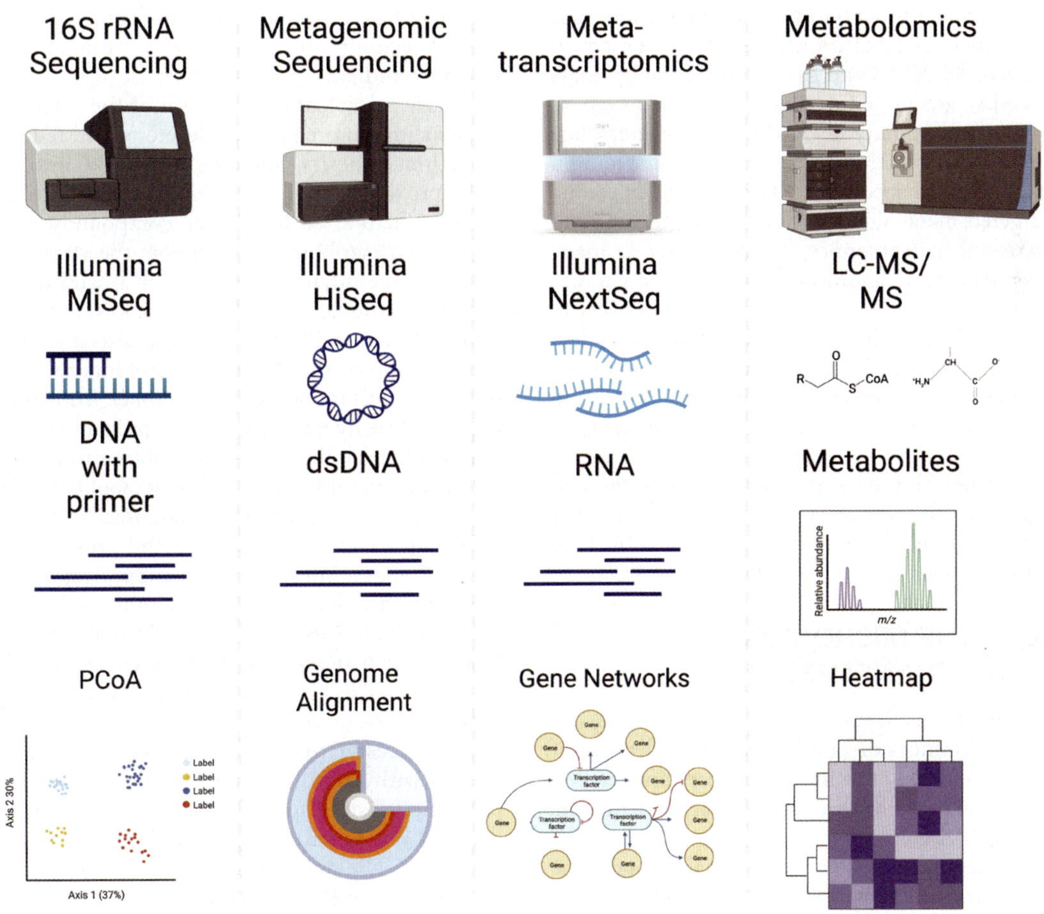

Figure 23.3. Workflow for key techniques used to study the microbiome are displayed. 16S rRNA amplicon sequencing is employed to characterize membership and relative abundances of bacteria. Metagenomic sequencing is based on sequencing and characterizing the collective genome of a microbial community and allows for the complete reassembly of microbial genomes and pangenomic analyses. Metatranscriptomics involves sequencing of all bacterial transcripts of a community. Metabolomics involves targeted and untargeted approaches to measure bacteria-derived small molecules and metabolic by-products from a community using liquid chromatography (LC)–mass spectrometry (MS) or gas chromatography (GC)-MS depending on the nature of the molecules being measured. Example figure types for each methodology are shown but are not limited to those shown. Figure created from information in references 38–59. (Created with BioRender.com.)

Metagenomic data is commonly analyzed using Anvi'o and MG-RAST.[44,45] Limitations to this technique include contamination by human DNA; biases imposed by DNA isolation procedures, sample collection, and amplification primers; the inability to distinguish isolated DNA from live bacteria versus dead bacteria; as well as the inability to discriminate between innate colonizers and transient bacterial inhabitants.[46]

Metatranscriptomics and metaproteomics are the next levels of analysis, and detect transcribed RNA and proteins, respectively, in the samples, with a focus on the potential function of the microbiome as a primary endpoint as compared to content.[47–49] These techniques are limited by the short-lived nature of bacterial transcripts, potential saturation by abundant, but unimportant transcripts, and reports that the correlation between RNA transcripts and protein expression may not be strong.[48] Metaproteomics uses high-resolution mass spectrometry to measure expressed proteins. The use of metaproteomic data processing tools, such as MetaLab, MetaproteomeAnalyzer, Galaxy P, and MetaPro-IQ have advanced the characterization and identification of microbiome and host proteins in a given biologic sample.[49–51] As identified previously, sample saturation by highly expressed, but limited functional proteins, may potentially obscure identification of more important, less expressed proteins.[48,49]

Metabolomics, however, is gaining momentum in this field. By identifying small nonprotein molecules in a sample, it provides a snapshot of microbial function in the specific anatomical location and time. Which metabolites are detected is based on the analytical approach: ^1H NMR and gas chromatography–mass spectrometry (GC-MS) are used for small molecules, such as amino acids, and short-chain fatty acids (SCFAs) whereas liquid chromatography–mass spectrometry (LC-MS) is required for detecting long-chain lipid species.[52–54] These methods can be employed using targeted metabolomics for detecting metabolites of interest or untargeted metabolomics for identifying as many small metabolites as possible, in addition to detecting new molecules.[18,54] Controlling confounders that can impact the sensitivity and specificity of the results is critical.[55] Coupling multiomics data with machine learning may change the clinical approach to maintaining health and preventing diseases, allowing for identification of specific metabolites and microbes that can alter the response to intervention.[56–59] The need for such sensitive and sophisticated equipment to better understand these microbial communities and their impact on overall homeostasis is a signal to physicians that we yet do not fully understand the extent or power held in these small microbial communities.

ACQUISITION OF THE MICROBIOME: MATERNAL–FETAL TRANSMISSION

Maternal–fetal transmission is a major route for colonization of the infant's microbiota. Mother's diet and body mass index, use of antibiotics, method and location of an infant's delivery, and feeding method (breast vs. formula feeding) are factors that influence the neonate's microbial colonization.[60–64]

While traditional dogma and use of GF animals support the existence of a sterile environment during fetal development,[65] recent studies suggest that the womb may provide the infant's first exposure to microorganisms[66–69] without causing gestational infection or inflammation which could severely impact the health of the pregnancy. Mode of delivery significantly influences the initial colonization of the infant's microbiome. During vaginal delivery, the infant is colonized predominantly with the mother's vaginal and fecal bacteria,[68,70] often swallowing these microbes during delivery.[67] However, intrapartum antibiotic use is a confounder in accurately characterizing the impact of the maternal vaginal microbiome in colonizing the infant.[71] *Lactobacillus*, *Prevotella*, or *Sneathia* spp. predominate in vaginally born infants, whereas skin surface microbes, such as *Staphylococcus*, *Corynebacterium*, and *Propionibacterium* spp. dominate in C-section delivered infants.[63,70]

Composition of an infant's microbiota closely resembles the microbiota of their respective mother rather than the particular mode of delivery, supporting the model that vertical transmission of microbiota from mother to infant is responsible for the initial colonization of the infant's microbiota.[63,70,72] Risk of childhood diseases, such as otitis media and allergies within the early years of life, are elevated in infants born by cesarean section compared to nonoperative vaginal delivery; the extent of the association is impacted by the study design.[73–75] Operative vaginal deliveries are reported to increase an infants' potential for infection hospitalizations before age 5 compared to infants born by nonoperative vaginal delivery, supporting the role of other contributing pathways in addition to method of bacterial transfer during delivery to the child's overall health in the first 5 years.[76] Vaginal microbial transfer from mothers to their respective infants delivered by C-section, called *vaginal seeding*, can promote colonization of the infant's microbiota with populations present in their mother's vaginal fluids.[77] However, due to potential safety concerns and insufficient clinical data supporting the clinical efficacy of vaginal seeding,[78] its current use is confined to controlled clinical research studies.

Early microbial colonization of the infant's gut is important to their immunoregulatory development, reducing the incidence of asthma, obesity, allergies, and food intolerances.[79,80] Breast milk provides important digestive and antioxidative enzymes, growth factors, antimicrobial compounds, immunoglobulin A (IgA), and cytokines that support the structural and functional health of the infant's intestines.[81,82] In addition, breast milk is an important source of microbiota, known as human milk microbiota. Human milk microbiota is also a source for the vertical transmission of the mother's microbiota to the infant.[83] Transfer of this important source of microbes from the mom by breastfeeding directly or indirectly by milk microbiota transplant via donor human milk actively contributes to the colonization of the intestinal microbiome and the metabolic and immune health of the infant.[83–85] Nondigestible oligosaccharides known as human milk oligosaccharides enhance the growth of specific bacteria in the infant's intestines, thus supporting intestinal health and digestion. Studies conducted examining the occurrence of acute otitis media (AOM) demonstrated that breastfeeding, especially in the first 6 months of an infant's life, was beneficial in preventing AOM.[86–89] Exclusive breastfeeding provided greater protection from AOM compared to nonexclusive breast feeding.[87,88] Greater than 40% reduction in AOM was reported for infants with exclusive breastfeeding in the first 6 months, with protection lasting for 2 years.[87] Beyond 2 years of age, the evidence is not as strong regarding breastfeeding's protection from AOM.[87,88] The exact mechanisms are unclear, however colonization by the mother's microbiota as well as the presence of IgA found in breast milk are protective against the infectious agents that cause AOM. Furthermore, the act of breastfeeding opens the eustachian tube, preventing build-up of serous fluid in the middle ear, which is a common feature of AOM.

During the neonate's first year, their intestinal microbiota is a very dynamic environment, maturing in content and diversity with the cessation of breastfeeding and the introduction of solid foods.

By 3 years of age, the infant's intestinal microbiota is relatively stable until adulthood, barring any changes in dietary habits, environment, or use of antibiotics.[61] Metagenomic studies highlight the changes in the relative proportion of metabolism genes in the infant's gut during the first 12 months of life, commensurate with changes in the infant's diet. For instance, greater lactose-specific transporters are present in the first 4 months of life, consistent with preferential milk consumption and early colonization of the infant's intestines with lactic acid bacteria that degrade lactose, including *Lactobacillus, Staphylococcus,* and *Bifidobacterium.*[90–92] Formula-fed infants have preferential colonization of *Roseburia, Clostridium,* and *Anaerostipes,*[63] while breastfed infants' microbiota are predominated by *Clostridiales* and *Lactobacillales.* In addition, the IgA profile differs between breast- and formula-fed infants.[93] By 12 months of age, the microbiome is more abundant in genes involved in the metabolism of complex sugars and starch, with an associated increase in the relative abundance of *B. thetaiotamicron.*[63,94] The infant's intestinal microbiota continues to develop during the first 2 years of the infant's life, with an increase in alpha diversity and decrease in beta diversity, supporting a more complex community of microorganisms required to metabolize a more diverse diet.[63,95,96]

In addition to responding to changes in diet, the intestinal microbiota influences the normal development of lymphoid structures and resistance to pathogens.[60] The resultant dysbiosis that can result from early antibiotic use in children may lead to an impaired immune system or susceptibility to infection for the remainder of their lives. As physicians, when parents inevitably request antibiotics for viral infections, you can educate them on (1) why that is unnecessary and that (2) by interfering with the growth and presence of normal organic colonizers of their child's body there may be longstanding complications that manifest in more subtle or chronic ways.

MICROBIOME AND IMMUNE REGULATION

While the host's microbiome is influential in the development of the immune system, the primary function of immune cells is to eliminate "invaders" such as bacteria, viruses and fungi. So how does the immune system learn to not destroy the microbiota that is so important for health? The answer to this is complex and not completely understood but there are several processes that appear to be important. These factors include IgA, antimicrobial products, immunoregulatory cells, and metabolites (Fig. 23.4). How these

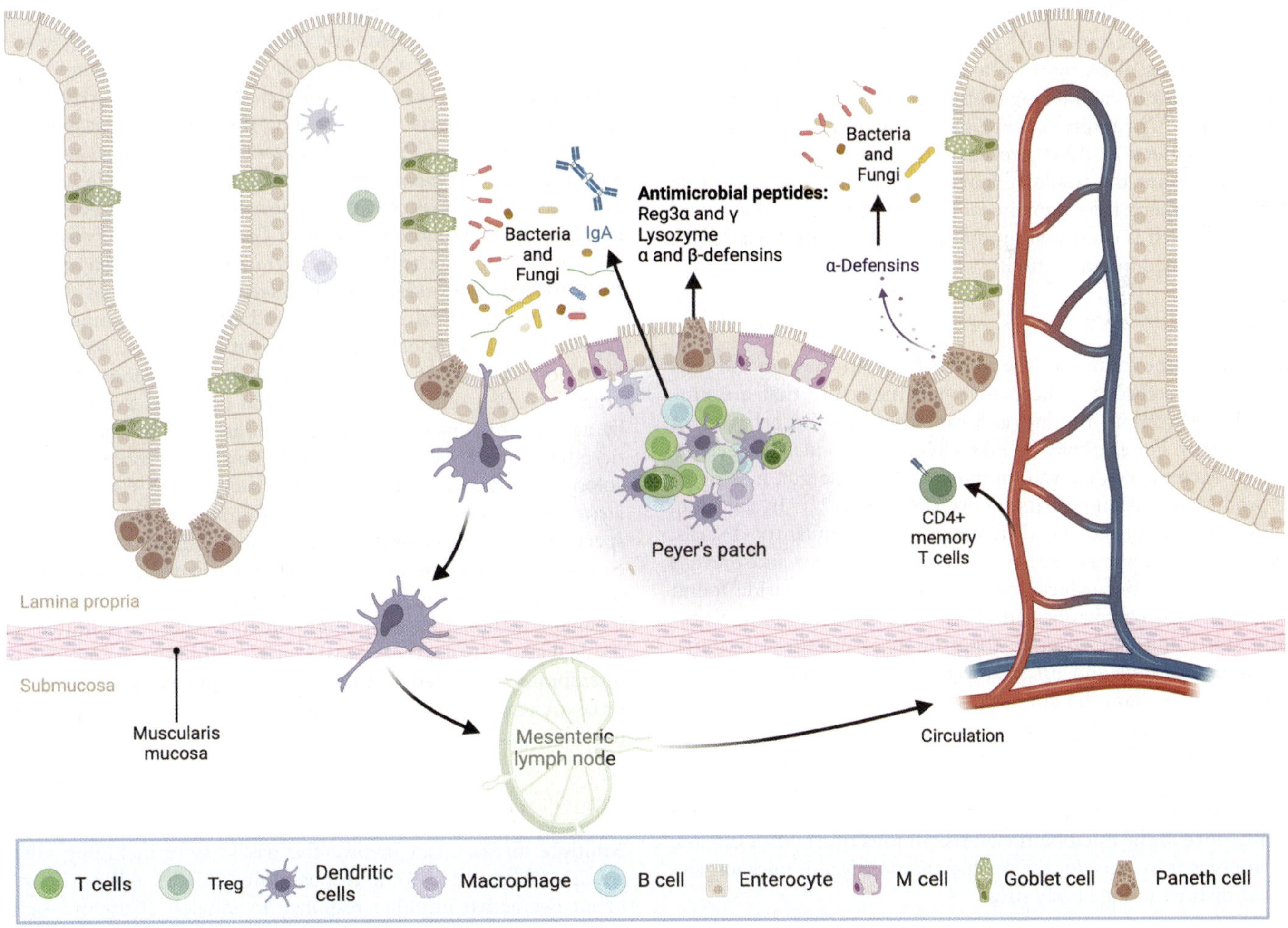

Figure 23.4. Microorganisms in the gut including bacteria and fungi trigger a host immune response that in turn controls gut microbial communities. Peyer patches in the gut house numerous immune cell types including B cells; T cells, including T regulatory cells and proinflammatory T cells such as Th17 cells; macrophages; and dendritic cells. Dendritic cells migrate to the mucosa and sample the luminal environment and upon entry into the mesenteric lymph and circulation, trigger the infiltration of CD4+ memory T cells. Concurrently, Paneth cells abundant in the ileum release antimicrobial peptides such as Reg3 gamma, lysozyme, as well as alpha- and beta-defensins. IgA is also secreted by plasma B cells. Collectively, the host immune system controls the local microbiota, protects the integrity of the gut epithelium and prevents bacterial translocation. (Created with BioRender.com.)

factors influence the homeostasis between the immune system and host microbiome is briefly discussed below.

Immunoglobulin A

IgA is an antibody that plays a critical role in the mucosal immune system, which is the first line of defense against pathogens that enter the body through mucosal surfaces such as the respiratory tract, urogenital tract, and gastrointestinal tract. The microbiome can influence the production and function of IgA in several ways. For example, certain strains of bacteria in the gut have been shown to stimulate the production of IgA in the intestines, which can help protect against pathogenic bacteria and viruses.[97] Conversely, disturbances to the intestinal microbiome, such as those caused by antibiotics or a poor diet, can lead to a reduction in IgA levels and increased susceptibility to infections.[98,99] In addition, bacterial metabolites, such as SCFAs have been shown to enhance the production of IgA and improve gut barrier function.[100,101]

Antimicrobial Products

Antimicrobial products, such as antimicrobial peptides (AMPs), are produced by host defenses to help destroy bacteria and fungi by disrupting cell membranes, cell walls and other components of the microorganism.[102] Commensal bacteria such as *Bacteroides thetaiotamicron* are resistant to AMPs due to differences in their cell wall components, allowing them to evade destruction.[103] There is a growing interest in capitalizing on the use of AMPs as alternatives to antibiotics.[104] In addition, there is a growing list of diseases associated with defects in AMP production. Crohn disease, for example, is sometimes the result of mutations in the gene nucleotide binding oligomerization domain containing 2 (NOD2), the consequence of which is decreased production of the AMP β-defensins and uncontrolled inflammation.[105]

Metabolites

The microbiome influences the immune system through the production of metabolites. These are small molecules that are produced by bacteria in the gut and can influence the behavior of immune cells. For example, SCFAs, which are produced by certain types of bacteria, can activate immune cells in the gut, leading to the production of anti-inflammatory cytokines.[106,107] In addition, SCFAs also influence the differentiation of regulatory T cells, which help to suppress excessive immune responses and prevent inflammation.[108] Beta-glucans are a type of polysaccharide found in the cell walls of microbes and have been shown to have a prebiotic effect and can promote the growth of beneficial bacteria, such as *Lactobacillus* and *Bifidobacterium*.[109,110] Additional benefits of β-glucans include the ability to expand regulatory T cells and suppress intestinal inflammatory disease, such as colitis.[111]

Overall, the interaction between the microbiome and the immune system is complex, with both having important roles in protecting against infections (Fig. 23.4). To completely understand the influence of the microbiome on risk of infection and/or disease, it is important to consider the unique composition of microorganisms at distinct unique body sites.

NASAL MICROBIOME

The nasal cavity is lined with various types of epithelia that provide unique anatomical niches to house microbial communities, from the relatively dry anterior nares lined with nonkeratinized skin-like epithelium to the pseudostratified columnar epithelial cells of the middle meatus that are bathed in warm, nutrient-rich mucous drained from the anterior ethmoids, maxillary and frontal sinuses.[112,113] Most studies exploring the nasal microbiome sample from the anterior nares, the middle meatus, and the nasopharynx, each containing a unique niche of microorganisms. Factors such as method of delivery, age, humidity, seasons, lifestyle, and antibiotic use impact the composition and health of the nasal microbiome.[114–116]

Major bacterial phyla include Firmicutes, Actinobacteria, and Proteobacteria.[116,117] *Corynebacterium, Propionibacterium, Staphylococcus,* and *Moraxella* genera are common nasal bacterial residents. Similar to the oral cavity, the microbe composition of the nose is defined by seven community state types (CSTs), each with its own unique preferential bacteria colonization.[118] CST4 is most common, about 29% prevalence, and is dominated by *Propionibacterium* spp., in particular, *Cutibacterium acnes*, formerly called *Propionibacterium acnes*. *Staphylococcus epidermidis* (CST3) and *S. aureus* (CST1) are the second and third most abundant CSTs, with a combined prevalence of approximately 35%. CST2 is comprised of *Enterobacteriaceae*, in particular *Escherichia* spp., *Proteus* spp., and *Klebsiella* spp. *Corynebacterium* dominates CST5 and the least prevalent is CST6, which is dominated by *Moraxella* spp. *Dolosigranulum pigrum* dominates CST7.

In healthy adults, the anterior nares are colonized by commensal bacteria as well as opportunistic pathogens, including *Staphylococcus aureus, S. epidermidis, Cutibacterium acnes, Dolosigranulum pigrum, Finegoldia magna, Corynebacterium* spp., *Moraxella* spp., *Peptoniphilus* spp., and *Anaerococcus* spp.[119,120] The middle meatus is populated by *Corynebacterium, Propionibacterium, Prevotella, Dolosigranulum, Staphylococcus, Streptococcus, Moraxella,* and *Escherichia shigella*.[121] Similar colonization is reported in the nasopharynx as detected in the middle meatus, with the exception of *Dolosigranulum, Moraxella,* and *E. shigella* which are replaced by *Bifidobacterium, Sphingobacterium, Faecalibacterium, Pseudomonas,* and *Haemophilus*.[121]

Unique microbial interactions and effector mechanisms influence microbial composition and prevent pathogenic bacterial colonization. Release of specific proteins or small molecules by one organism often impacts the health and potential for colonization by another organism(s). This is demonstrated by the antagonistic effects of *Corynebacterium accolens* on *Streptococcus pneumoniae* colonization[122] and the cooperative support of *Corynebacterium accolens* on *S. aureus* colonization.[123] Immune system activation by specific microorganisms may impact the colonization or removal of competing organisms, as in the case of *Haemophilus influenzae* colonization stimulating the phagocytic removal of *S. pneumoniae*.[124] Characterization of the inherent microbiome communities that reside within the nasal cavity will enable clinicians to employ novel microbiome-modulating interventions to prevent pathogenic bacteria colonizers, such as *S. aureus*, and promote healthy, protective, microbiome communities.

Allergic and Chronic Rhinosinusitis

Multiple diseases can involve the nasal cavity including allergic rhinitis (AR) and chronic rhinosinusitis (CRS). AR is the result of an overactive immune response to inhaled allergens, such as pollen, dust mites, and animal dander. The pathogenesis of AR is mediated by allergen-specific immunoglobulin E (IgE) that triggers an immune response characterized by mucus production, nasal congestion, and sneezing. Children with limited exposure to environmental microbes are at increased risk of developing AR.[125] Beyond the influence of microbes on disease development, there is emerging evidence that the composition of microbes may influence

BOX 23.1 Allergic Rhinitis and Chronic Rhinosinusitis: Clinical OMM Pearl

Patients benefit from these Osteopathic Manipulative Techniques with flares[132]:

- Sinus Inhibitory Pressure of the Trigeminal Nerve
- Suboccipital Release—Targeting autonomic nervous system regulation for symptom relief.
- Sinus Percussion—Mobilizes and promotes drainage of fluid and mucous buildup in the sinuses.

disease outcomes, particularly with polyp formation and recurrence in patients with CRS.

CRS is a complicated disease with multiple risk factors contributing to the pathogenesis of disease, including a history of allergic disease, impaired epithelial barrier, and defects in immune function.[126–128] In adults, CRS is an inflammatory reaction in the nose and paranasal sinuses presenting with two or more of the following symptoms: facial pain or pressure; loss or reduction of smell; nasal blockage, obstruction, or congestion; and either anterior or posterior nasal drip for a minimum of 12 consecutive weeks.[128,129] In children, CRS is associated with a cough rather than loss of smell. Corticosteroid sprays and nasal saline irrigation are clinically accepted first lines of treatment with antibiotics prescribed if an underlying infection is suspected. The impact of these treatments with respect to the nasal microbiome are varied.[130] Increasing mucociliary clearance, improving sinus drainage and outflow, eradicating infection, reducing inflammation, and improving access for topical medications are the goals of treatment. When this clinical management fails, endoscopic sinus surgery may be effective. Colonization with certain bacteria, such as *Enterobacteria,* has been linked to recurrence of polyp formation after surgery (Clinical Correlations Box 23.1).[131]

ORAL MICROBIOME

The oral microbial community is a highly diverse population of organisms, second only in content and diversity to the microbial composition of the gastrointestinal tract.[133–135] Various factors impact the assemblage of microbes in the oral cavity, including the surface structure, oxygen levels, nutrient exposure, and shedding. For example, increased oxygen levels promote the expansion of aerobes and facultative anaerobes. Hard and soft tissues including the teeth, gingiva, tongue, hard and soft palatal mucosa, and tonsils are colonized by distinct and highly structured microbiomes.[136,137]

Inhaled and ingested microbes populate the oral mucosa and distribute into unique biofilms along the palate, cheeks, tongue, buccal mucosa, teeth, gingival sulcus, and tonsils.[133,137–139] Biofilm microbial communities are organized within an extracellular polymeric matrix which provides structural stability and gradients of nutrient availability for the microbes to coexist.[140] Healthy biofilms balance pH and suppress pathogenic bacterial growth. Through physical and metabolic processes, these niche-specific microbes communicate and enable horizontal transfer of select genes, including antibiotic resistance genes.[138] Oxygen content, diet, gender, age, oral hygiene, use of medications, systemic, and immune health influence the organization, colonization, and stability of these unique communities.[141]

Bacteroidetes, Firmicutes, Proteobacteria, Fusobacteria, Actinobacteria, and *Spirochaetes* comprise approximately 96% of the oral bacteria taxa.[133] The remaining 4% of the taxa are attributed to the phyla *Euryarchaeota, Chlamydiae, Choroflexi*, SR1, *Synergistetes, Tenericutes*, and *TM7*.[133] Over 770 bacterial species reside in the oral cavity, a finding that will change as technologies and sampling procedures advance.[142] Of these bacterial species, 58% are named, 16% are unnamed but cultivated, and 26% are identified as uncultivated phylotypes.[142] Sampling method and location of sampling impact microbe identification, for each niche within the oral cavity hosts a unique microbial community.[138] Identification of endogenous bacterial species inhabiting the oral cavity compared to transient species identified due to environmental influence is critical to distinguishing healthy microbial colonization from pathogenic insult.[143–146] Next-generation sequencing techniques have identified numerous fungal genera, including *Candida, Cryptococcus, Fusarium, Aspergillus/Emericella/Eurotium*.[147,148]

Using combinatorial labeling and spectral imaging (CLASI)–fluorescence in situ hybridization (FISH), it was visualized that *Corynebacterium* sets the foundation of supragingival plaque creating "hedgehog" structures that form outward facing filaments (due to their resistance to physical disruption), while those in the perimeter are aerobic microorganisms including *Streptococcus*, *Haemophilus/Aggregatibacter*, and *Porphyromanas*.[137] The filament-rich annulus contains *Fusobacerium*, *Leptotrichia*, and *Capnocytophaga* making up the filamentous portion of the hedgehog structures. It was proposed that *Streptococcus* supported the growth of *Fusobacerium* and *Leptotrichia*, through CO_2, lactate, and acetate production. In another study, *Capnocytophaga gingivalis* was reported to carry and aid in the movement of nonmotile bacteria.[149] Therefore, in addition to the highly structured order of bacteria in the oral cavity, these bacteria work in concert to facilitate their propagation in ecologic niches.

Dental caries, malodor, perio- and endodontal diseases, osteitis, and tonsillitis are caused by dysbiosis of the oral microbiota.[135,147,150–152] Host protective measures, such as saliva, salivary IgA, lysozyme, and lactoferrin prevent pathogenic bacteria from colonizing the oral cavity. An imbalance in immune surveillance and disturbance in bacterial colonization can promote tissue inflammation and permanent tissue damage, as demonstrated with untreated periodontal disease.[150,153]

Periodontal disease and dental caries are prevalent microbially mediated diseases worldwide. Anaerobic bacteria, *Porphyromonas gingivalis, Treponema denticola, Tannerella forsythia, BS,* and *TM7* are the major bacterial contributors to periodontitis,[154,155] an inflammation in the subgingival space around the tooth, which can cause destruction of the supporting tissue, bone resorption, and tooth loss. Non–culture-based methods have identified additional potential contributors, including species in the genera *Prevotella*, *Desulfobulbus*, and *Synergistes* as well as *Filifactor alocis*, *Peptoanaerobacter stomatis*, *Dialister* spp., *Megasphaera* spp., and *Selenomonas* spp.[150,156,157] *Veillonella*, *Streptococcus*, and *Granulicatella gingiva* were shown to increase the production of antimicrobial peptides and promote inflammatory cytokine secretion, thus protecting epithelial barrier function and mucosal thickness.[158]

Sugar-driven microbial growth and acidic pH facilitate the demineralization of the tooth enamel and the creation of carious lesions, commonly called cavities. *Streptococcus mutans* and *Lactobacillus* species are the well-recognized microbes associated with caries development.[159] With the advent of newer molecular biology techniques, other microbes have been identified as contributors to the microenvironment associated with carious lesions, including *Bifidobacterium* spp., *Scardovia* spp., and *Actinomyces* spp., as well as the fungi *Candida albicans*.[156,159,160] Localization on the tooth impacts the biofilm organization and microbe content.[161] Studies support a dysbiosis of the biofilm surrounding the tooth rather than an infection caused by an opportunistic pathogen as the mechanism for these pathologies.[147,155]

Enhancing the oral immune function by promoting a healthy oral microbiome prevents deleterious biofilm formation and dental maladies. For instance, breastfeeding seeds the infant's oral microbiota with the mother's human milk microbiota, including bacterial, fungal, viral, and archaeal components.[162] According to the World Health Organization, human milk is recommended as the primary nutritional source for the infant's first 6 months.[163,164] Duration and exclusivity of breastfeeding, as well as the mother's awareness of risk factors for carious lesions, are important in assessing the infant's risk for early childhood caries.[163,165–167] Breastfed infants are reported to have a lower alpha diversity in their oral cavity compared to formula-fed infants.[163] Infants primarily breastfed in the first year had reduced risk of dental caries, however the risk for caries increased in children breastfed for more than 12 months.[166] Nocturnal breastfeeding, especially longer than 1 year, and the progressive emergence of deciduous teeth, increase the risk for caries development.[166]

A healthy, disease-resistant oral microbiome is influenced by host factors as well as microbe-to-microbe communication. Regular brushing, flossing, and eating a healthy diet rich in vegetables and fruits will support a healthy microbiome that protects against oral and systemic diseases.

Oral Candidiasis

The fungus *C. albicans* is a microorganism that is commonly found within the oral cavity.[168] In most healthy individuals, *C. albicans* exists in a nonpathogenic state, being one of the many different species that contribute to the human oral microbiota.[169] In fact, up to 80% of the general population harbor *C. albicans* in their oral microbiota without *C. albicans* over-proliferating and becoming pathogenic.[170] However, in an immunocompromised or susceptible host, where *C. albicans* can over-proliferate, oral candidiasis can occur. There are many reasons why the environment in the oral cavity can change and favor an overgrowth of *C. albicans*. Examples include individuals who wear removable oral devices which prevent sloughing of normal tissue, allowing *C. albicans* to better adhere to tissues[171]; individuals on antibiotics creating decreased microbial competition from normal oral microbiota[172]; immunosuppressed individuals[173,174]; and smokers suffering from reduced salivary production leading to a more favorable environment for *C. albicans* growth.[175]

The clinical presentation of oral candidiasis can vary. For example, pseudomembranous candidiasis (also known as thrush), acute erythematous candidiasis, chronic erythematous candidiasis, and chronic hyperplastic candidiasis can each lead to an oral candidiasis diagnosis.[176] However, the main determinant of such a diagnosis depends on the causal agent. A thorough medical history and clinical exam are necessary to find the causal agent causing the oral candidiasis. Once the causal agent is identified, the correct antifungal therapy can be initiated. For example, the common culprit for pseudomembranous candidiasis is removable oral devices. Poor oral hygiene combined with improper cleaning of the removable oral device provide an ideal environment for overgrowth of *C. albicans*. The first line of treatment for pseudomembranous candidiasis is a nystatin oral rinse combined with disinfecting the oral device.[177]

C. albicans is a pathogen of opportunity. Understanding the different ways it can present, the underlying cause(s), and the appropriate therapy are essential for effective patient care. Addressing the underlying cause and educating your patient are imperative to prevent an oral candidiasis recurrence.

Dental Health and Systemic Diseases

Oral health impacts systemic health and systemic diseases are often first recognized by tangible changes in oral health. Systemic diseases, such as diabetes, metabolic syndrome, obesity, rheumatoid arthritis, preterm childbirth, CVD, Alzheimer disease, and cancer are associated with measurable changes in the oral microbiome.[178,179] Changes in the oral microbiota may serve as potential biomarkers of underlying systemic diseases or may contribute to the progression of these diseases by modulating the host's systemic inflammatory and immune responses. Factors such as lifestyle (smoking, high-fat diet [HFD], processed foods), genetics, medications, immune insufficiency, and microbial dysbiosis can impact the host's defense mechanisms and susceptibility to oral as well as systemic diseases. For instance, studies have reported that *Porphyromonas gingivalis* (*P. gingivalis)*, a major pathogen in periodontal disease, is a risk factor for Alzheimer disease.[180,181] Impaired cognitive function, compromised motor function, medication side-effects, and lack of adequate patient awareness regarding continual oral care contribute to the incidence of periodontal disease in the elderly. Ongoing studies investigating the cooperative relationship between oral health and systemic inflammatory diseases hold promise in revealing new avenues for the prevention and treatment of these debilitating conditions (Fig. 23.5).

RESPIRATORY TRACT MICROBIOME

Healthy Respiratory Tract Microbiome

The respiratory tract includes a range of environments and microbes, with the upper respiratory tract being heavily populated with microbes and the lower respiratory tract housing fewer microbes. When bacteria that normally colonize the upper respiratory tract are displaced into the lower respiratory tract, either through defects in immunity or clearance mechanisms, an individual is at increased risk of developing infections, such as pneumonia. As discussed earlier in this chapter, mother-to-fetus transfer of microbes is important for the initial seeding of the neonate's respiratory tract. Infants born via vaginal delivery have a respiratory tract enriched with *Ureaplasma*, a known commensal of the vaginal microbiome.[182] Conversely, infants delivered via caesarean have an increased presence of common skin bacteria such as *Staphylococcus*.[182] The adult respiratory tract microbiome is shaped by these early life exposures and by the gastrointestinal microbiome, through the gut–lung axis. The gut–lung axis describes the observation that factors that influence the intestinal microbiome, such as diet, can contribute to changes in the lungs.[183] This connection is driven largely by metabolites of the intestinal microbiota, such as SCFAs, that influence the homeostasis and immune response to bacteria in the respiratory tract.[184] The healthy adult respiratory tract microbiota includes *Bacteroidetes, Firmicutes, Streptococcus, Prevotella,* and *Veillonella*.[185] Eubiosis of the respiratory tract microbiota is a constant balance between inhaled environmental exposures and microbial clearance. Defects in microbial clearance either through breakdown in the mucociliary transport system or improper education of the immune system can result in microbial dysbiosis and contribute to disease.

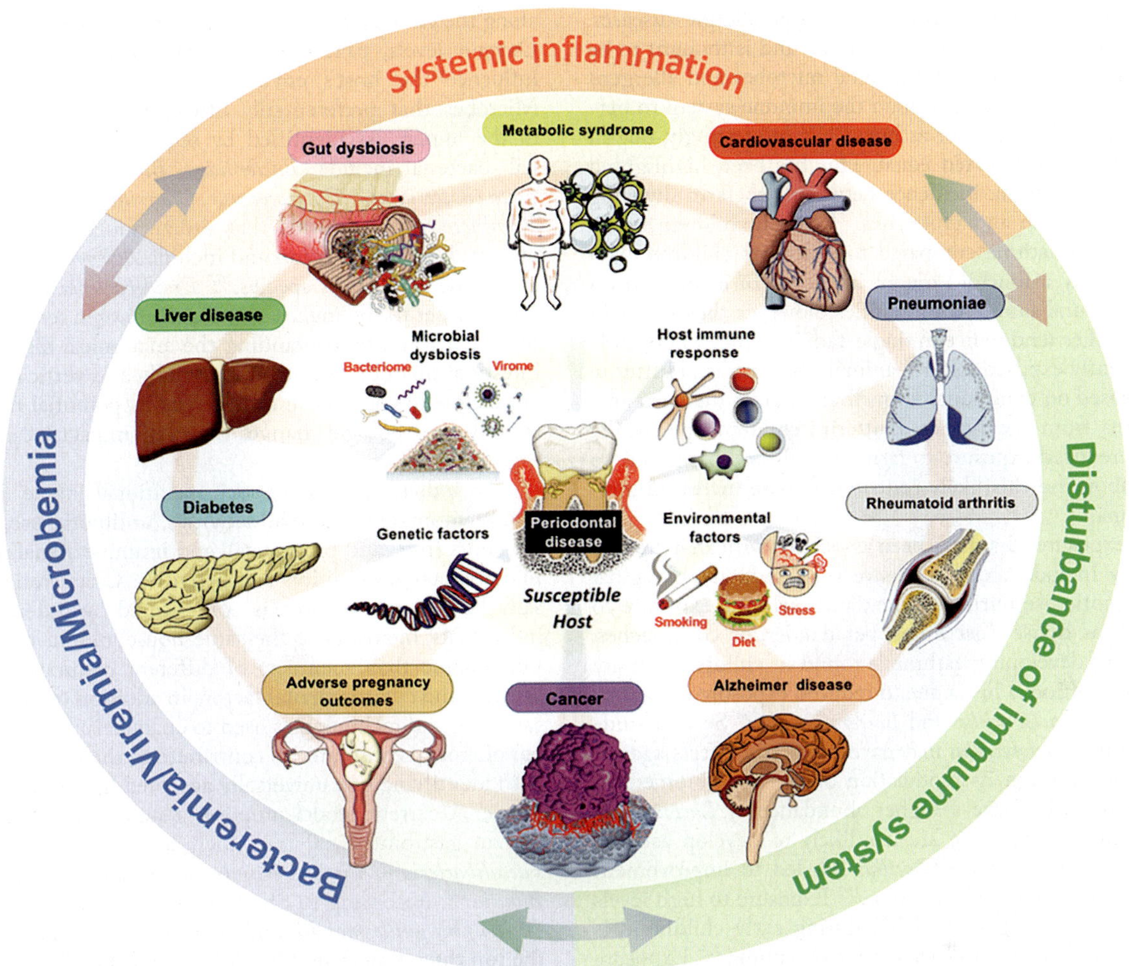

Figure 23.5. Oral microbiome and systemic health. Dysbiosis of the oral microbiome associated with periodontal disease is linked to systemic diseases, such as diabetes, obesity, cardiovascular disease, cancer, adverse pregnancy outcomes, arthritis, and respiratory illnesses. Host microbial colonization, lifestyle, and immune responsiveness are important factors in preventing oral and systemic diseases. (From Kapila YL. Oral health's inextricable connection to systemic health: special populations bring to bear multimodal relationships and factors connecting periodontal disease to systemic diseases and conditions. *Periodontol 2000*. 2021;87(1):11–16. Courtesy of Dr. Ryutaro Kuraji.)

Cystic Fibrosis

The origin of cystic fibrosis (CF) is well-defined as the result of mutations in the CF transmembrane conductance regulator (CFTR) gene. CFTR encodes a chloride channel protein that is expressed by epithelial cells. Mutations associated with CF result in impaired transport of chloride across the epithelium contributing to dysfunction in multiple organs, including the lungs, pancreas, gastrointestinal tract, kidney, liver, and reproductive organs. Defects in chloride transport result in thickened mucus, increased acidity, and defects in epithelial integrity. Thickened mucus in the respiratory tract due to loss of mucociliary clearance creates an ideal environment for dysbiosis. Compromised epithelial integrity and microbial dysbiosis put CF patients at increased risk of microbial infections. Treatment goals include obtaining drainage, improving the dysbiosis, thinning the secretions, and maintaining optimal pulmonary function. Osteopathic manipulative treatments (OMTs) can help loosen the secretions and enhance lymphatic clearance of the lungs and bronchi.[186] Some patients are put on long-term antibiotics to prevent infection, however this is not recommended in the United States due to the risk for antimicrobial resistance, as well as increased risk of infection with *Pseudomonas aeruginosa*.[187] CF patients experience changes to their intestinal pH, dehydrated mucus, and nutrient malabsorption, due to defects in ion channel function. These defects in the host environment, in addition to increased exposure to antibiotics, contribute to an altered gut microbiome in CF patients. The CF gut microbiome has reduced bacterial species diversity; specifically, it has reductions in beneficial bacteria, including *Bacteroidota,* and has elevated levels of pathogenic bacteria, including *Enterococcus* and *Bacillota*.[188,189] There is growing evidence that probiotics may benefit CF patients to reduce respiratory exacerbations and, when used in combination with CFTR modulators to restore CFTR function, are an exciting prospect for the future.[190]

Asthma

Asthma is a chronic respiratory condition characterized by airway inflammation and hyperreactivity, which can cause wheezing, coughing, and difficulty breathing. While the exact causes of asthma are multifactorial, research has suggested that the microbiome influences the development and progression of this disease. Support for microbial influence comes from several observations including that children raised in farming communities have reduced risk of developing asthma and other allergic diseases. This has been referred to as the "farm effect" and is thought to be due to exposure to diverse environmental microbes and allergens during early life, which may help train the immune system to better tolerate potential triggers of asthma.[191,192] Interestingly, not all farm environments are created equal. This has been highlighted in comparisons of asthma incidence between two farm dwelling populations, the Amish and Hutterites.[193] Amish children have a lower incidence of asthma compared to Hutterite children, who have approximately a fourfold higher incidence of asthma. Both populations are rural family communities, however they differ in that Amish families tend to live in single-family homes where children are frequently exposed to farm animals. In contrast, Hutterite children are raised on communal farms that separate the farm animals and barns from the homes. Hutterite children, specifically females, have reduced exposure to farm animals and barns due to divisions of labor, and this likely contributes to an increased incidence of asthma.[193]

Early life exposures that have been associated with an increased risk of asthma include mode of delivery (C-section vs. vaginal delivery), antibiotic use during infancy, and early-life exposure to allergens, such as house dust mites, pet dander, or cockroaches. Increased risk of developing asthma is found in children that are delivered via C-section. This is due to reduced exposure to vaginal microbes, such as *Lactobacillus* and *Bacteroides*.[194–196] Several studies have suggested *Lactobacillus* may have protective effects against asthma, possibly through its modulation of the microbiome. For example, children who have a higher abundance of *Lactobacillus* in their intestinal microbiome are less likely to develop asthma, and supplementation with *Lactobacillus* has led to improvement in asthma symptoms and lung function.[197] Exposure to high levels of house dust mite allergens (HDM) during early childhood is associated with an increased development of asthma.[125] Exposure to HDM can trigger the development of IgE antibodies that can stimulate the allergic immune response and airway inflammation. In addition, HDM-specific allergies are known to influence both the gut and airway microbiome, suggesting crosstalk between the two microbial communities.[7]

Interestingly, a microbiome that consists of parasites, such as helminth worms, may reduce the risk of developing allergic diseases such as asthma.[198–200] This is thought to be due to the role of helminths in training the immune system to establish a strong regulatory network of immune cells.[199] It has been observed that populations with a high prevalence of helminth infections tend to have lower rates of asthma.[200,201] It is important to note that helminth infections are not without their own risks and complications, and there is a need to better understand how genetics and environmental exposures influence the development of asthma.

GASTROINTESTINAL MICROBIOME

Healthy Intestinal Microbiome

The intestinal microbiome is a rich and diverse community. The microbial content of the gut increases exponentially from the stomach (10^1 CFU/g of content) to the colon, culminating in 10^{12} CFU/g of content.[114] Over 50 different bacteria phyla inhabit the intestines, the major phyla being Bacteroidetes, Firmicutes, Actinobacteria, and Proteobacteria, followed by less abundant Fusobacteria and Verrucomicrobia.[61,202,203] Pathogenic bacteria, such as *Campylobacter jejuni*, *Salmonella enterica*, *Vibrio cholera*, *Escherichia coli*, and *Bacteroides fragilis* are harbored in the colon, but in a very small percentage, less than 0.01%.[26] Bacterial colonization along the gut changes longitudinally as well as horizontally.[61,204–206] Oxygen levels, pH, nutrient availability, and immune activity influence the host's environment and microbial colonization. Microbes that preferentially utilize nutrients and starch reside in the lumen. As identified by sequencing stool samples, luminal bacteria include *Bacteroides*, *Bifidobacterium*, *Streptococcus*, *Enterobacteriacae*, *Enterococcus*, *Clostridium*, *Lactobacillus*, and *Ruminococcus*. Organisms that utilize mucin reside in the outer mucous layer of the colon and include *Akkermansia*, *Ruminococcus*, and some *Bacteroides* species.[207] *Proteobacteria* and *Actinobacteria* reside closer to the mucosa, where the oxygen tension is greater.[208] Identifying and understanding the anatomical distribution of the intestinal microbiota both horizontally and vertically are important factors to consider in discovering its potential function locally as well as pathologic changes that may impact local and systemic organ functions.

An individual's age, gender, nutritional intake, neural signaling, environment, lifestyle activities, antibiotic use, dietary supplements (pre- and probiotics), and immune signaling impact the microbiota's composition and activities. Characterizing a universally healthy microbiome is complicated by differences between individuals; members of the same household have a more similar microbiome than members of different communities. Identified lifestyle and environmental factors in addition to differences in the sampling and technologies used to characterize the various intestinal microbial communities contribute to the difficulties associated with identifying one universally accepted human intestinal microbiome. A current model proposes a stable core microbiota in the human gastrointestinal tract including *Bacterioides*, *Eubacterium*, *Faecalibacterium*, *Alistipes*, *Ruminococcus*, *Clostridium*, *Roseburia*, and *Blautia*.[209] According to Shetty et al., *Faecalibacterium prausnitzii*, *Oscillospira guillermondii*, and *Ruminococcus obeum* are reported as the top three taxa shared by all healthy adults.[209]

The gastrointestinal tract is lined by columnar epithelial cells that create a barrier between the luminal contents and the host. This compartmentalization is maintained by tight junctions between adjoining epithelial cells, which prevent luminal bacteria and bacterial antigens from activating the underlying immunosurveillance cells in the mucosa. Pattern recognition molecules, such as toll-like receptors, provide cell-specific signaling and immune activation by luminal microorganisms. Defensins and IgA contribute to the host's innate protection against luminal bacterial entry and pathogenic colonization. Disturbances in this environment can result in compromise to tight junction integrity, migration of bacteria or bacterial cell components such as lipopolysaccharide (LPS), and activation of local immune cells, causing local and potentially systemic inflammation.

Healthy gut motility helps to maintain a healthy microbial balance and prevents bacterial overgrowth by potentially pathogenic bacteria. The intestinal microbiome is important to nutrient digestion, production of SCFAs, bile acid metabolism, vitamin production, oral tolerance, and immune activation. The small intestines, a rich source of simple sugars and amino acids, are preferentially colonized by facultative anaerobic, proteolytic bacteria, including *Proteobacteria* and *Lactobacillaceae*.[210] Duodenal microbial colonization is more similar to the oral microbiome whereas the microbiota in the ileum demonstrate similarities to the colonic colonization.[204] Human jejunum is populated with *Streptococcus*, *Prevotella*, *Veillonella*, *Fusobacterium*, *Escherichia*, *Klebsiella*, and *Citrobacter* genera but devoid of *Alistipes*, *Ruminococcus*, *Faecalibacterium* genera found in the colon.[211] In the colon, where digestion of non-digestible carbohydrates occurs, anaerobic, saccharolytic bacteria predominate, including *Bacteroidales* and *Clostridiales* orders.[212]

SCFAs, including acetate, butyrate, and propionate, are produced in the colon. They significantly impact host physiology. Age-dependent changes in SCFA production have been demonstrated.[213] Acetate is preferentially produced at an early age (0 to 3 years of age) by *Bifidobacteria,* including *B. bifidum, B. infantis, and B. breve.* In adulthood, butyrate and propionate are produced by *Lactobacillaceae, Ruminococcaceae, and Lachnospiraceae.* Butyrate is important in maintaining intestinal tight junction integrity and epithelial cell health.[214] As one continues to age, production of butyrate and propionate decreases, and there is an increase in the relative abundance of *Enterbacteriaceae.*

In addition to the production of SCFAs, intestinal microbes can produce neuroactive compounds that influence neural development, mood, cognition, and neuropathologies via the microbiota–gut–brain (MGB) axis, which will be described in the following section. Host microbes, such as specific strains of *Bifidobacteria,* produce important B vitamins, including biotin, cobalamin, folate, niacin, pantothenic acid, pyridoxine, and riboflavin.[215,216] Osteopathic physicians are focused on person-centered care rather than disease-centered care. The future of medicine markets itself heavily on individualized therapies and treatment plans that will be made possible because of increasing technologic sophistication and the ability to identify microscopic "players" in the patient's macroscopic presentation. The importance of an individualized and holistic approach has been what osteopathic educators have been encouraging physicians to utilize since the founding of osteopathy; it is the ideologic backbone of these scientific endeavors (Fig. 23.6).

Microbiota–Gut–Brain Signaling

Gut–brain communication has been well-accepted since the early studies performed by William Beaumont demonstrating the impact of stress on digestion. Investigations into the bidirectional communication between the gut and the brain initially focused on satiety and digestion. However, investigators, and clinicians' awareness that the intestinal microbiome may influence gut–brain signaling through the production and release of neural modulatory agents gave rise to recognition of the MGB axis: a multi-directional communication between the microbiota in the intestines and their metabolites, the brain, and the autonomic and enteric nervous systems.[217]

Experimental and clinical models reveal the microbiome's impact on gut–brain signaling. Several different experimental and clinical modalities have been useful in identifying and teasing out the microbiome and its impact on CNS development and function. These models include use of GF mice; treatments with nonabsorbable antibiotics such as vancomycin, neomycin, and

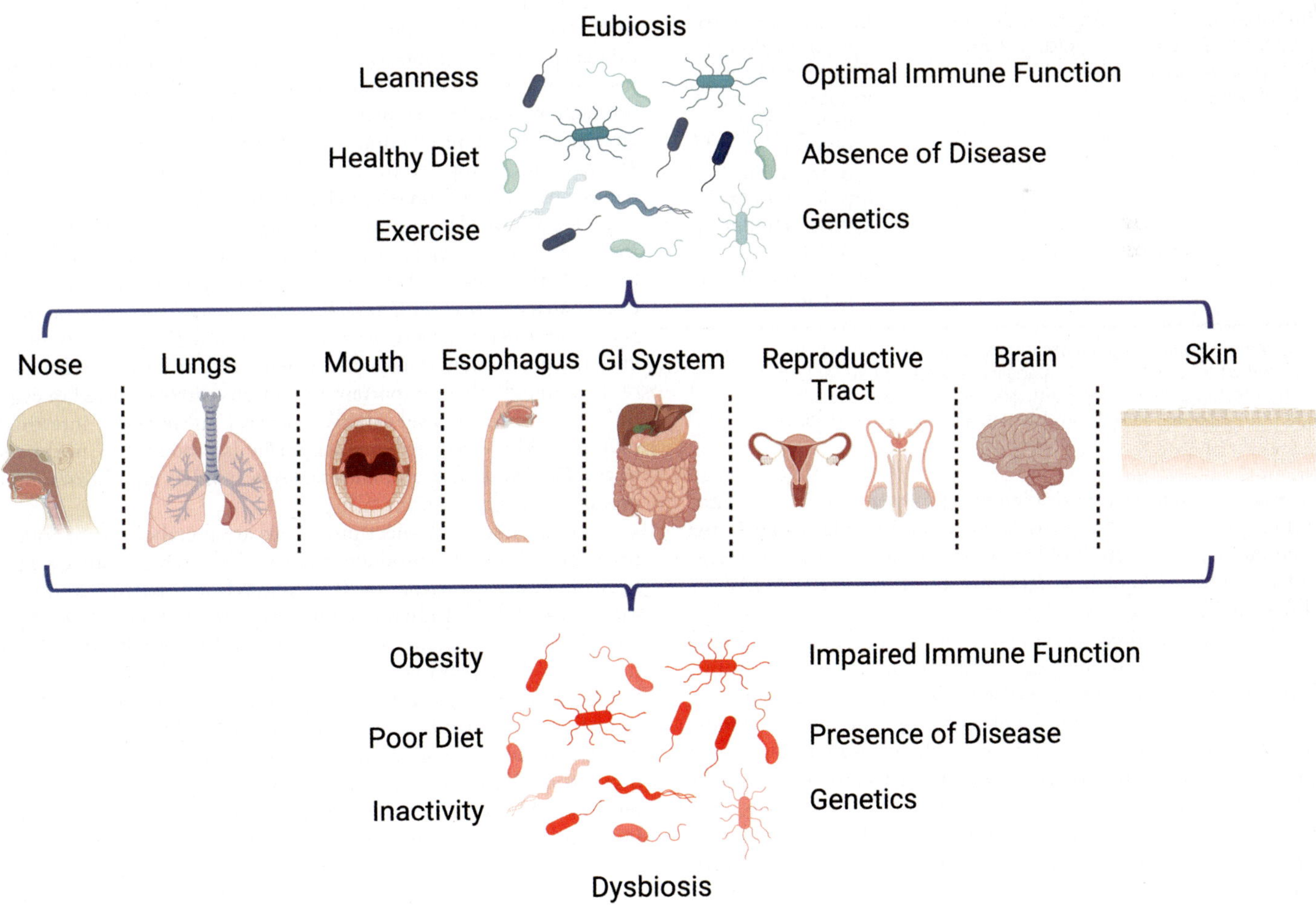

Figure 23.6. Human microbial niches. Microbial communities reside in the healthy nose, respiratory tract, mouth, gastrointestinal and urogenital tracts, and skin. Neuromodulators released from the gastrointestinal tract influence neural development, cognition, and mood. Healthy microbial balance, eubiosis, is important in nutrient extraction, optimal immune function, and health. Factors that distort or deplete the microbiome can result in dysbiosis, which contributes to clinical conditions such as obesity, impaired immune function, and clinical disease. (Created with BioRender.com.)

TABLE 23.3

Microbiota-Gut-Brain Signaling

Microbiota	Signaling Molecule	Biologic Activity
Candida spp. *Streptococcus* spp. *Escherichia* spp. *Enterocossus* spp.	Serotonin (5-HT)	Intestinal motility Hemostasis Mood, Sleep Wound healing
Lactobacillus spp. *Bifiobacterium* spp.	Gamma-aminobutyric acid (GABA)	Reducing anxiety and depressive behaviors Visceral pain
Bacillus clausii Prevotella Bacteriodes Lactobacillus Bifidobacterium Clostridium Enterococcus Ruminococcus	Dopamine	Cognition Reward response Satiety Voluntary movements Intestinal motility and secretions
Bacillus *E. coli* *Saccharomyces* spp.	Norepinephrine	Neurotransmitter Hormone
Lactobacilli	Acetylcholine	Neurotransmitter
Bifidobacteria *Lactobacillaceae* *Ruminococcaceae* *Lachnospiraceae*	Short-chain fatty acids (SCFA)	Energy source for colonocytes Tight junctions Influence lipid, energy and vitamin production Impact appetite Cardiovascular health Mental health and mood

Intestinal microbiota significantly impact gut–brain signaling through the production of neuroactive signaling agents. These factors contribute to neurodevelopment, depression, anxiety, autism spectrum disorder, Parkinson disease, and Alzheimer disease.

bacitracin; administration of dietary supplements such as psychobiotics (pre- and probiotics that induce a measurable change in the microbiome); and transfer of feces from a healthy donor to a recipient in a process known as fecal microbial transfer (FMT)[217–221] (Table 23.3).

Direct and indirect communication occurs along the MGB axis. Direct firing of the vagal efferent and autonomic spinal fibers facilitates moment-to-moment changes in the gastrointestinal tract required to control nutrient digestion and absorption, impacting the richness and diversity of the microbiota. Vagal and spinal afferents activated by gastrointestinal distention trigger CNS processing and release of satiety signals. Enteric nerve complexes coordinate the necessary motility and digestive responses triggered by central and peripheral receptors. Reduced intestinal motility promotes microbial overgrowth and production of microbial metabolites which, when released into the intestinal mucosa, may indirectly influence CNS signaling. Stress-induced release of cortisol by activation of the hypothalamic–pituitary–adrenal axis, can compromise intestinal tight junction integrity and activate mucosal immune cells through a "leaky gut" mechanism,[222,223] fostering cytokine production and release which, in turn, influence CNS signaling as well as microbiome balance.

The relative abundance and composition of the intestinal microbiota can influence CNS function through the production of bacteria-generated intermediaries, such as SCFAs, secondary bile acids, tryptophan metabolites, gamma-aminobutyric acid (GABA), dopamine, and norepinephrine, as well as immunomodulatory cytokines. Mood, cognition, and emotion are influenced by neurotransmitters produced by the intestinal bacteria and released into the systemic circulation to impact CNS function.[224] Neurologic disorders, including anxiety, depression, PD, Alzheimer disease, and ASDs are associated with measurable changes in the microbiome.[224] Many migraine-sufferers also have gastrointestinal disorders such as IBD, irritable bowel syndrome, or celiac disease, supporting that inflammation-associated leaky gut can impact CNS function.[225] Targeting the microbiota in the treatment or prevention of psychiatric disorders may provide a more natural approach to patient care.[226]

Microbiota are capable of producing a host of bioactive agents in vitro, including catecholamines, dopamine, serotonin, and GABA.[227] The intestinal microbiota have enzymes that regulate tryptophan metabolism to serotonin (5-HT), indole, or kynurenine derivatives. Gastrointestinal 5-HT production from dietary tryptophan accounts for most of the body's 5-HT. *Candida* spp., *Streptococcus* spp., *Escherichia* spp., and *Enterococcus* spp. produce bacterial metabolites that influence the enterochromaffin cells' 5-HT production.[228–230] Serotonin acting locally will influence intestinal motility, however, peripheral activities include hemostasis, mood, sleep, and wound healing. Microbiota impact production of the 5-HT precursor, tryptophan, which impacts the amount of 5-HT production in the brain.[231] *Lactobacillus* spp. and *Bifidobacterium* spp. produce GABA which has been shown to reduce anxiety and depressive behaviors as well as visceral pain.[232–237] Studies performed using GF mice suggest that GABA influences the brain via the vagus nerve rather than acting directly in the brain.[238] However, GABA transporters are present in the blood–brain barrier.[239] *Bacillus clausii, Prevotella, Bacteroides, Lactobacillus, Bifidobacterium, Clostridium, Enterococcus*, and *Ruminococcus* influence the production, transporter activity, and/or binding efficiency of dopamine,[240,241] an important neurotransmitter involved in cognition, reward response, satiety, voluntary movements, intestinal motility, and secretions. Norepinephrine is produced by members of the *Bacillus*, *E. coli*, and *Saccharomyces* families and *Lactobacillus* produces acetylcholine.[218,230,242]

Dietary fiber and select probiotics are metabolized by intestinal microbiota to produce SCFAs,[217,220] which up-regulate tight junction proteins in the blood–brain barrier and the intestines.[214,224,243] Individual responses to prebiotics are variable, however, reduced stress, anxiety, and depressive behaviors have been demonstrated.[220,244–246] Bile acids are produced in the liver and upon release into the intestines can undergo modifications to secondary bile acids by inherent microbial species. These changes include deconjugation of glycine or taurine, and dehydroxylation, dehydrogenation, and epimerization of the cholesterol core.[247] Recent studies suggest that the intestinal microbiota may actively conjugate amino acids to bile acids, creating a new class of conjugatively altered bile acids.[248] Dysbiosis of the gut microbiome can significantly alter bile acid metabolism and contribute to IBD.[249] Since the gut–brain signaling involves modulatory agents, and the autonomic and enteric nervous systems, local palpatory viscerosomatic reflexes may be found along the midline of the abdominal wall (Fig. 23.7A,B and Clinical Correlations Box 23.2).

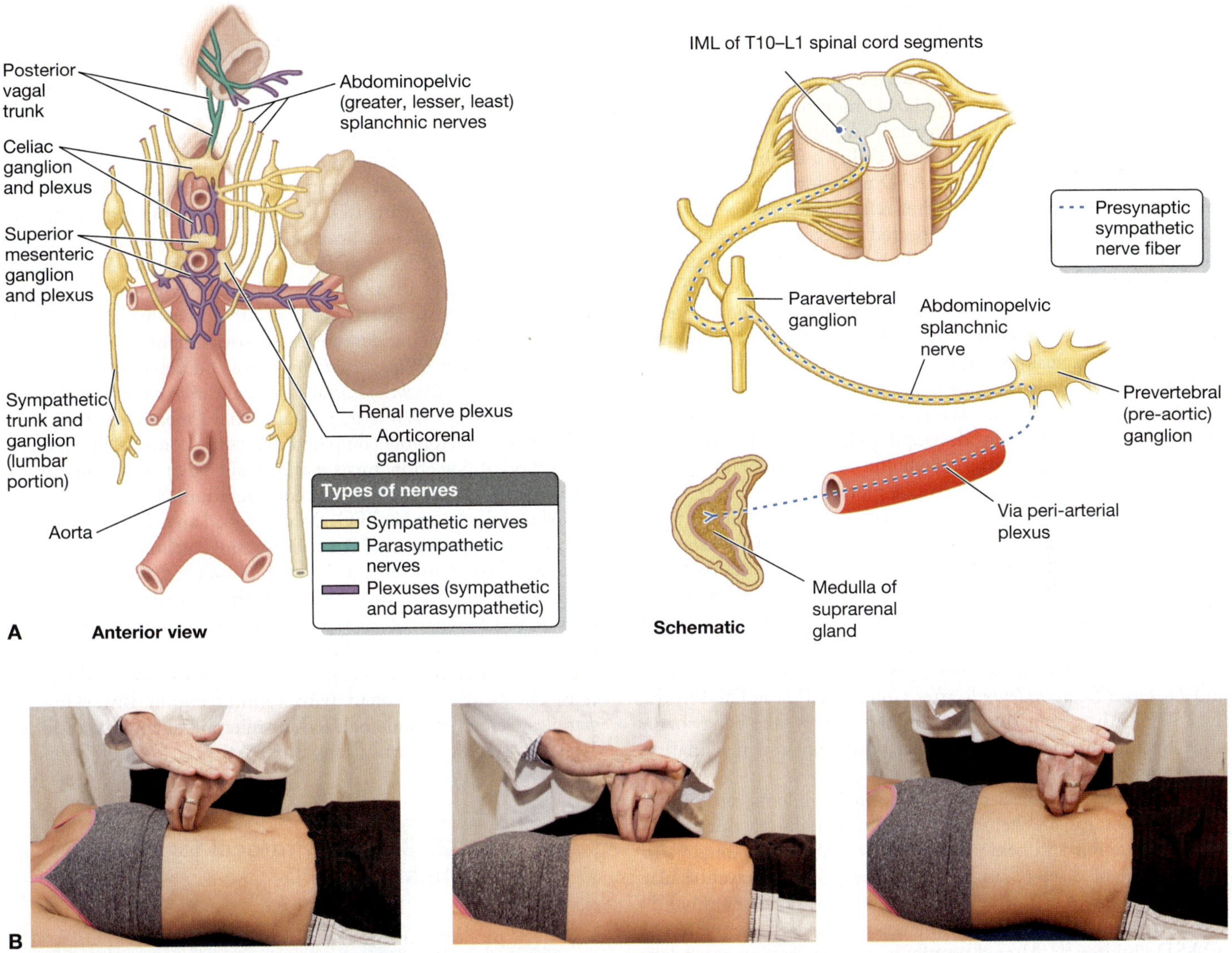

Figure 23.7. A, B. Palpation of abdominal visceral ganglion for diagnostic clues with possible subsequent treatment. Osteopathic palpatory evaluation can provide important diagnostic tools for active inflammatory processes in the gastrointestinal tract. (Reprinted with permission from Moore KL, Dalley AF II, Agur AMR. *Clinically Oriented Anatomy*. 7th ed. Wolters Kluwer Health/Lippincott Williams & Wilkins; 2014. Figure 2.87.)

BOX 23.2 Abdominal Palpatory Findings: Clinical OMM Pearl

Palpatory tissue texture changes and myofascial tension occurs along the midline of the abdomen in discrete areas associated with visceral disease, including dysbiosis. It is thought that these findings relate to abnormal viscerosomatic dysfunction of the GI tract. Each local area represents its respective ganglion (celiac, greater splanchnic, or lesser splanchnic). These palpable findings can be used for diagnostic purposes by indicating macroscopic/microscopic disease and/or dysfunction. OMT may be used to treat these external areas with the goal of altering the abnormal reflexes.

CLINICAL CONDITIONS AND THE MICROBIOME

Neurologic Disorders/Diseases

AUTISM SPECTRUM DISORDERS

ASDs are a group of developmental disabilities characterized by social deficits, narrow interests, stereotyped behaviors such as repetitive motions, as well as verbal and nonverbal communication difficulties. The incidence of ASD is increasing, perhaps caused by improved methodologies to identify ASD behaviors and overall awareness. While the pathogenesis of ASD is unclear, clinicians agree that ASD is caused by genetic factors that impact brain development, especially neural connectivity. Gastrointestinal symptoms, such as diarrhea, constipation, and abdominal pain are more likely in pediatric patients with ASD than healthy children, as well as aversion to wheat and dairy products.[250,251] In a case study reported in 2015, a father noticed significant improvement in his son with ASD after a 10-day course of amoxicillin for strep throat,[252] suggesting that alterations in the microbiome may contribute to the behavior patterns of ASD via the MGB axis. Overall, the microbiota composition of children with ASD is different from non-ASD children.[253] ASD children with hypersensitivity to gluten or casein respond favorably to an exclusionary diet, with a reduction in pain and bowel movements, and measurable changes in gut microbial content.[254] A gluten-free, casein-free (GFCF) diet reduced intestinal permeability, a finding reported in ASD children.[255] The severity of ASD behavior is correlated with the severity of GI symptoms.[251,256] A relative increase in *Clostridia* and decrease in *Bacteroidia* are reported in feces of ASD children compared to healthy controls.[257] Clinical use of Bimuno galactosaccharides (B-GOS), a digestive supplement, with a GFCF diet for 6 weeks improved social behavior scores[254] and demonstrated a significantly higher abundance of *B. longum* in the B-GOS treated children on an exclusionary diet.

Differential levels of microbial-derived phenolic metabolites have been identified in the plasma, urine, and feces of ASD children compared to typically-developing children.[258] For instance, elevated levels of the toxic metabolite 4-methylphenol (*para*-cresol) and its sulfated derivative, 4-methylphenyl sulfate, have been measured in the urine and feces of ASD children.[259,260] Para-cresol is a metabolite produced by intestinal *Clostridiaceae, Lachnospiraceae,* and *Ruminococcaceae.*[261,262] Elevated plasma levels of the phenolic metabolite 4-ethylphenyl sulfate (4-EPS),which is structurally similar to para-cresol sulfate, have been measured in a cohort of ASD children.[258] 4-ethylphenol (4-EP) is produced by intestinal metabolism of dietary tyrosine by *Bacteroides ovatus* and *Lactobacillus plantarum*,[12] after which 4-EP is sulfated in the liver. 4-EPS has been shown to induce anxiety-like behavior in mice by influencing oligodendrocyte function and myelination patterning.[12]

Nonhuman primates, domestic animals, rodents, birds, fish, and invertebrates are being used experimentally to mimic the social interaction and behavior patterns of ASD symptoms.[263] In a rat model of disease, animals administered an intraventricular injection of the SCFA, propionic acid, demonstrated several antisocial behaviors and neurologic changes similar to those measured in ASD children.[263] Altered propionic acid production secondary to changes in the intestinal microbiome suggests that ASD may be related to intestinal dysbiosis impacting neurodevelopment and behavior.[264] Modulation of the gut microbiome by selective use of psychobiotics and fecal microbiota transplantation (FMT) demonstrated measurable improvement.[265] Overall, if there is even a small improvement in the quality of life for patients with ASD secondary to optimization of the gut microbiome, it is worthy of clinical consideration. Autistic individuals and their families have increased barriers to interacting with daily life on every level. These stressors decrease the strength of their body, mind, and spirit on a daily basis.

PARKINSON DISEASE AND APPLICATION OF OMT

While investigators are rapidly developing greater insights into the impact of the microbiome on the rest of the body, research and data investigating the effect of OMT on the human microbiome is scarce. This disparity offers an exciting and important area of novel research for osteopathic physicians. A recent study examined changes in the gut microbiome secondary to a targeted OMT protocol for chronic constipation in patients with PD.[266]

PD is defined as a progressively-worsening neurodegenerative disorder with both motor and nonmotor manifestations.[267] Chronic constipation often predates development of PD and is present in up to 80% of patients with PD.[268] Aside from the decreased quality of life caused by chronic constipation, treatment efficacy varies and can be quite expensive with an estimated annual cost of $1,912 to $7,522 per patient, per year.[269]

Patterns between the normalized abundance of certain microbiota and PD have led researchers to investigate if these bacteria can serve as prospective biomarkers for PD and potential targets for therapeutic intervention. Dysbiotic changes in the intestinal microbiome can result in compromised gut permeability, reduced SCFA production, and intestinal inflammation, all of which have been reported with PD. For example, when comparing PD patients to age-matched healthy control patients, it was found that a relative abundance of *Prevotellaeceae* less than 6.5% had an 86.1% sensitivity and 38.9% specificity for concurrent presence of PD.[270] A meta-analysis report of 10 studies using specifically 16S rRNA sequencing demonstrated enrichment of *Lactobacillus, Akkermansia,* and *Bifidobacterium* genera and depletion of bacteria belonging to the *Lachnospiraceae* family and *Faecalibacterium* genus in PD patients.[271] While investigators have measured changes in PD patients' microbiota compared to healthy controls, factors such as method of detection, treatment, mobility, diet, and ethnicity are important cofactors that require consideration.[272]

Mancini et al. at NYITCOM developed an OMT protocol for chronic constipation in PD patients using techniques previously established to significantly assist in stool transit.[266] Six PD patients (over 40 years old) with chronic constipation (defined by Rome III criteria) underwent 10 weekly visits: visits 1 to 4 served as a control period; visits 5 to 8 involved a weekly OMT provided by a licensed osteopathic physician; and visits 9 and 10 assessed for long term-effects after treatment, with no intervention. Biweekly stool samples were taken and analyzed for microbiota abundance for all 10 weeks (Clinical Correlations Box 23.3).

BOX 23.3 OMM Protocol for Chronic Constipation in PD

OMT Protocol: During weeks 5 to 8, patients received a once weekly, 30 minute OMM sequence performed by an osteopathic physician. Each technique was applied for 2 minutes. Subjects were supine for all interventions except for sacral rock and sometimes mesenteric release was performed in the lateral recumbent position. The osteopathic protocol included the following techniques in this sequence:

Step 1: Suboccipital release
Step 2: Respiratory diaphragm release
Step 3: Celiac, superior mesenteric, and inferior mesenteric ganglion inhibition
Step 4: Bilateral T10–L2 paraspinal inhibition
Step 5: Bilateral sacroiliac joint decompression
Step 6: Sacral rock
Steps 7–8: Mesenteric release of ascending and descending colon
Step 9: Colonic stimulation.

Steps 1, 3, 4, 5, and 6 were chosen to target and treat the autonomic nervous system; Steps 7 to 9 were chosen to target and treat the enteric nervous system; and Step 2 was employed to target diaphragmatic restrictions and promote thoracic excursion. Steps 5 and 6 had the specific aim of treating pelvic floor muscle imbalance and dystonia.

Qualitative improvements in patient constipation and quality of life were found post-OMT intervention along with quantitative changes in the normalized abundance of microbiota in fecal stool samples. Significant changes in the mean abundance of gut microbiota were demonstrated. These changes included, but were not limited to the following:

- A decrease in the mean number of bacterial families within the Firmicutes phylum
- Significant changes in normalized abundance of the phyla Actinobacteria and Verrucomicrobia
- Changes in the normalized abundance of genera *Roseburia* and *Intestimonas*
- Bacteria positively and negatively correlated with the Unified Parkinson's Disease Rating Scale Pre- and Post-OMM, signifying that there may be quantities of bacteria that can be predictive of and possibly contributing to the severity of PD.

As physicians, it is crucial to analyze the risk–benefit ratio before prescribing any intervention to patients, as the goal is always to "do no harm." The subjects in this study reported no adverse side effects from treatment and none of them had worsening constipation. The minimal risk intervention of OMM was proven to improve patient quality of life, target and treat the specific symptom of constipation, and modify the relative abundance of fecal microbiota. The power of OMM is clear in this study as its impact was demonstrated on a macro "quality of life" level as well as a micro "bacterial composition" level. This study demonstrated the micromolecular impact that the noninvasive and nonpharmacologic application of OMM can have on the microbiome.

Gastrointestinal Disorders/Diseases

EOSINOPHILIC ESOPHAGITIS

Eosinophilic esophagitis (EoE) is a disorder in which eosinophils, a type of white blood cells, are recruited to the esophagus promoting inflammation in response to food, seasonal allergies, or acid reflux. Males are three times more likely to have EoE than females.[273] In adults, EoE can cause dysphasia, heart burn, and food impaction, and prolonged inflammation may lead to fibrostenosis. In children, EoE can cause nausea, vomiting, and failure to thrive. Treatments include esophageal dilations for fibrotic patients, proton pump inhibitors, corticosteroids, and exclusion of dietary triggers. Patients with EoE display increased microbial load in their esophagus including increased abundance of *Aggregatibacter* and *Haemophilus*, along with a decrease in the phyla Firmicutes.[273] In a recent study, the esophageal microbiota was assessed in 93 EoE patients, 17 esophageal gastritis (EoG) patients, and 29 controls. It was found that *Streptococcus* and *Gemella* genera were associated with EoE while *Leptotrichia* was associated with EoG.[274] It is unknown whether the changes in gut microbiota composition in EoE are causative. Description of the gut microbiota in this GI region is the first step in understanding whether the microbiota in EoE can be modulated through diet or supplementation, for example, in alleviating the condition.

CELIAC DISEASE

Celiac disease develops in genetically-susceptible individuals in response to dietary proteins from wheat, barley, and rye. The aberrant immune response to dietary gluten and similar prolamins leads to villus atrophy and crypt hyperplasia ultimately leading to severe gastrointestinal symptoms and nutrient malabsorption.[275] Gliadin peptides that are absorbed are converted to highly immunogenic peptides due to transglutaminase activity that converts glutamate residues to glutamine, making them negatively charged allowing for increased binding to the positively-charged binding pockets of the major histocompatibility complex class II (MHC Class II) receptors HLA-DQ2 and DQ8 on antigen presenting cells that then activate $CD4^+$ T cells, initiating an immune response.

Individuals that express the human leukocyte antigen (HLA) receptors DQ2 and DQ8 are susceptible to the development of celiac disease. While 40% of the population express a combination of the genes that encode these receptors, only 1% of the U.S. population develops celiac disease, suggesting that additional factors likely contribute to its development. In addition to the dietary trigger of prolamins including gluten from wheat, hordein from barley, and secalin from rye, other factors have been implicated in the development of celiac disease, such as repeated rotovirus infection and lack of breastfeeding. The latter, however, has been the subject of controversy in recent years.[276] Another factor that is better supported by the literature is the gut microbiome. Individuals with celiac disease display altered gut microbial composition compared to healthy individuals.[277] For example, an entero-adherent *E. coli* strain isolated from a celiac disease patient initiated an immune response to gluten in specific-pathogen free (SPF) mice.[278] Similarly, human patients exhibit an increased abundance of Proteobacteria including *E. coli* and decreased abundance of *Bifidobacteria* and *Lactobacillus* species.[279,280] Gastrointestinal infections increase the likelihood of celiac disease.[281] For example, *Helicobacter pylori*, *C. difficile*, and *Streptococcus pneumoniae* have been associated with celiac disease. *Candida albicans* has also been linked to celiac disease and has been shown to bind to host receptors through host transglutaminase activity.[282] A causative role of microorganisms in celiac disease development has been established in vitro and in animal models. For example, Bifidobacteria was shown to be protective by directly digesting gluten peptides.[283,284]

INFLAMMATORY BOWEL DISEASES: CROHN DISEASE AND ULCERATIVE COLITIS

Crohn disease (Crohn's) and ulcerative colitis (UC) are inflammatory bowel diseases that have increased in prevalence over recent years. While there is a strong genetic component, exemplified by the concordance rate in monozygotic versus dizygotic twins, genetic susceptibility does not fully explain the etiology of the disease. Recent studies from mice and humans have revealed an intimate link between the gut microbiota and the host immune response in Crohn's and UC. Dietary triggers have been found as well. For example, it was demonstrated by Devkota et al. that genetically susceptible $IL10^{-/-}$ mice fed a diet high in saturated milk fat exhibited earlier and more severe development of UC than mice fed low-fat control or a diet high in polyunsaturated fat that was mediated by the pathogen, *Bilophila wadsworthia*.[285] Interestingly, this species, from the Proteobacteria phylum, is bile-loving hence the name, *Bilophila*. It was found that the saturated milk fat content of the diet promoted the abundance of taurine-conjugated bile acids that facilitated the bloom in *Bilophila wadsworthia* that led to worsening disease outcome.[285] This study provided a direct link between dietary intake and changes in the microbiome that result in disease. *Bilophila wadsworthia* has also been found to be increased in abundance in human participants after consuming diets rich in animal protein and cheese products.[24] Other microbes implicated in the development of UC include *Clostridioides difficile*, *Campylobacter jejuni*, and *H. hepaticus*. It is well recognized now that loss of beneficial bacteria is also contributory to the development of UC. Those that have been shown to be decreased in abundance in UC include *F. prausnitzii*, *Roseburia inulinivorans*, and *Blautia faecis*.[286]

Microbes that have been implicated in the development of Crohn disease include adherent invasive *E. coli* and *Ruminococcus gnavus*.[287] Fungi, specifically, *Candida albicans* has been implicated in Crohn disease as well. For example, Crohn disease patients were found to have a greater abundance of *Candida albicans* and less *Saccharomyces cerevisiae* in their gut compared to healthy controls.[288] Similarly, UC patients were found to have a significantly altered gut mycobiome and decreased *Saccharomycopsis*.[289] Further, a toxin produced by *C. albicans* called candidalysin was identified that triggered the production of the inflammatory cytokine interleukin-1β (IL-1β) and expansion of Th-17 cells.[289] While fecal microbiota transplantation for *C. difficile* colitis will be discussed in greater detail later, it is worth noting here that FMT has been shown effective against IBD for some Crohn's and UC patients.[290] For example, in one study, UC patients received pooled donor FMT and were compared to those receiving autologous FMT (from their own stool) for 1 week. Of the 38 participants receiving donor FMT, 32% achieved remission compared to 9% for those that received autologous FMT.[291] In a more recent study, the combination of pooled donor FMT and anti-inflammatory diet (AID) was tested in comparison to standard medical treatment. It was found that the FMT and AID resulted in long-term remission (up to 1 year) in 25% of patients compared to 0% for standard treatment and 60% of patients achieved remission at 8 weeks versus 32.3% receiving standard care.[290] A recent meta-analysis including 324 patients from randomized controlled trials also reported remission success after FMT in UC patients.[292] Another meta-analysis conducted in 228 Crohn disease patients specifically reported remission in 57% of patients after 4 weeks.[291,293] Taken together, gut microorganisms of bacterial and fungal origin are capable of promoting inflammatory bowel diseases, and FMT or restoration of the gut microbial composition may be effective in combating IBD.

NECROTIZING ENTEROCOLITIS

Necrotizing enterocolitis (NEC) is an IBD that is most prevalent in premature infants. It causes deterioration of intestinal tissue that eventually results in the need for resection and can lead to death in infants. Research has focused on improving nutrition and minimizing tissue damage. More recently, investigators are evaluating the potential role of dysbiosis causing disease and restoration of eubiosis in resolving and preventing disease.[294] In addition, alterations in the MGB axis have been suggested for the increased risk of neurodevelopmental outcomes after NEC.[295]

Initial signs and symptoms of NEC include feeding intolerance, abdominal distention, and bloody stools about 8 to 10 days after birth, with a host of other systemic changes.[296,297] If not treated early with medical and surgical interventions, it can cause intestinal perforation, peritonitis, and systemic shock with high morbidity and mortality.[297] Studies examining the fecal microbiome of NEC patients demonstrated reduced diversity as well as significant changes in microbial colonization.[298,299] *Gammaproteobacteria*, specifically *Enterobacteriaceae*, is associated with an increased risk for NEC.[299,300] Probiotics, such as *Lactobacillus* and *Bifidobacteria* species have a beneficial impact, reducing the incidence of NEC.[301–304] Breast milk is protective against NEC, containing important oligosaccharides and IgA that participate in a healthy microbiome.[305–308]

Metabolic Disorders/Diseases

Gut microbes have been intimately linked to metabolic diseases including obesity, type 2 diabetes mellitus (T2DM), non-alcoholic fatty liver disease before the acronym (NAFLD) (more recently termed metabolic dysfunction–associated steatotic liver disease [MASLD]), and CVD (Fig. 23.8).

OBESITY

Direct associations between microbes and metabolic disorders have been documented widely in both humans and animals based on several lines of evidence including: (1) alterations in gut microbiota composition and function in obesity and upon weight loss such as through bariatric surgery[309–312]; (2) changes in gut microbiota composition in response to western-style HFDs[313–316]; (3) changes in metabolic phenotype following antibiotic treatment or through use of GF mice[317]; and (4) physiologic effects of FMT.[318,319] Early observations implicating a role of gut microbes in obesity were discovered by assessing gut microbiota composition in obese versus lean twins.[311,320] The general feature describing the difference

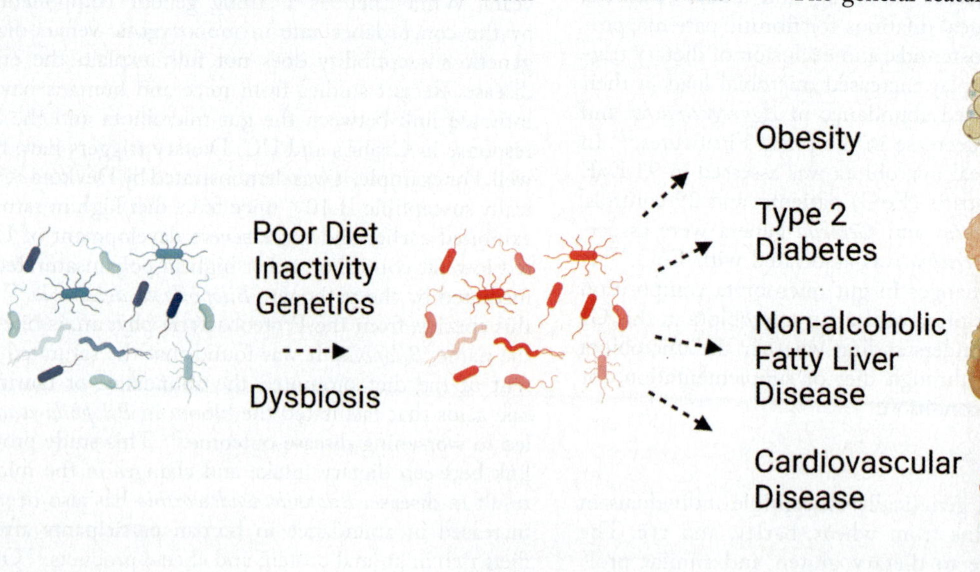

Figure 23.8. Gut dysbiosis directly contributes to the development of metabolic diseases. Gut dysbiosis, mediated by poor dietary habits including consumption of Western-style diets, physical inactivity, and genetic predisposition, have been intimately linked with the progression of obesity, type 2 diabetes, nonalcoholic fatty liver disease, and cardiovascular disease. (Created with BioRender.com.)

between obese and lean subjects was a change in the Bacteroidetes/Firmicutes ratio, where lean subjects displayed greater abundance of microbes belonging to the Bacteroidetes compared to Firmicutes phylum, and obese individuals displayed a higher ratio of Firmicutes to Bacteroidetes.[320] This has long been a metric used for assessing the microbiome in terms of obesity or metabolic dysfunction. It should be noted, however, that this is a grossly generalized assessment. It should not be assumed that all bacteria belonging to the Firmicutes phylum are detrimental. For example, Clostridium cluster XIV strains are SCFA producers that have beneficial metabolic effects.[321,322] Regardless, in both obesity and in those consuming a western diet (WD), Firmicutes and species belonging to this phylum (as well as those belonging to Proteobacteria) are increased in abundance. More recent research has also identified microbe-derived small molecules that are capable of eliciting negative metabolic effects on the host. For example, delta-valerobetaine was identified as an obesogenic microbial metabolic that not only drove obesity in mice but also was elevated in the plasma of obese individuals.[323]

Microbiota with an obese signature changes its composition following weight loss achieved via exercise or bariatric surgery. For example, it was shown that the microbiota composition shifted significantly in mice that underwent Roux-en-Y gastric bypass compared to sham controls and exhibited increases in the abundance of Bacteriodetes and Verrucomicrobia, phyla commonly associated with leanness and metabolic health.[309] Conversely, obese men with metabolic syndrome were given FMT from lean donors and displayed improved symptoms including better glucose tolerance.[319] Specific microbes have been identified that may have protective effects against obesity such as *Akkermansia muciniphila* which belongs to the phyla Verrucomicrobia. Interestingly, individuals undergoing a calorie-restricted diet exhibited increased levels of *Akkermansia muciniphila* in their gut. Further, either live *Akkermansia* or purified protein was found to improve metabolism in obese mice. Clinical trials are underway to determine if *Akkermansia* will be useful as a treatment against obesity and cardiometabolic disease.[324]

Evidence of a causal role of microbes in obesity development has been established using GF mice, that are raised devoid of all microorganisms. Interestingly, GF mice fed an HFD remain resistant to weight gain and remain lean.[313,314] Similar findings have been reported in antibiotic-treated mice.[317] Once GF animals are "conventionalized" or given microbiota via oral gavage (FMT), these animals then gain weight. Using the aforementioned model systems (such as diet-induced obesity models, GF mice), several mechanisms by which microbes promote obesity have been explored including: (1) increasing intestinal macronutrient absorption[314,325–327]; (2) increasing energy acquisition through SCFA production[320]; (3) controlling circadian rhythms and activity levels[328,329]; (4) directly altering metabolic rate; 5) regulation of bile acid composition; and (6) decreasing angplt4/Fiaf that controls fat storage.[330]

Osteopathic physicians care for the patients by diagnosing their illness and, in conjunction with the patient, forming a treatment plan to best suit their recovery goals considering their own medical history, their belief system, and their overall ability to respond to treatment. The abundance of new information regarding gut health and the beneficial metabolic impact that optimizing their gut microbiome may have on an individual is something all physicians need to be educated on in order to combat the obesity epidemic in America.

DIABETES MELLITUS

Gut microbes have been implicated in the development of and protection against type 2 diabetes (T2D). Mechanisms that regulate T2D development by gut microbes include: (1) inflammatory signaling induced by bacterial by-products such as LPS; (2) regulation of intestinal glucose transporters such as GLUT-2; and (3) alterations in SCFA levels that regulate incretin hormone levels such as GLP-1. HFD impairs epithelial barrier function allowing for elevated circulating LPS levels leading to metabolic endotoxemia associated with poor glucose regulation.[331] In human patients, higher endotoxin levels were associated with higher serum blood glucose.[332] Further, GF mice transplanted with obese microbiota from human subjects displayed poor glucose tolerance.[333] A positive association between glucose levels and several members of *Clostridiales* belonging to the Firmicutes phylum was identified.[333]

METABOLIC DYSFUNCTION-ASSOCIATED FATTY LIVER DISEASE

Metabolic dysfunction–associated fatty liver disease (MAFLD) is a newly proposed term for NAFLD with the more advanced stage termed MASLD. These terms have been suggested to describe the pathophysiology of the disease more accurately. MASLD patients exhibit a unique gut microbiota community membership relative to healthy controls[334–336] characterized by reduced *Bifidobacterium*, *Coprococcus*, *Faecalibacterium prausnitzii*, along with increases in *Blautia*, *Dorea*, *Escherichia coli*, and *Klebsiella pneumoniae*.[337] However, a high degree of heterogeneity exists that depends on comorbidities, race/ethnicity, and stage of liver fibrosis. Interestingly, fecal gut microbiota signatures and associated metabolites accurately distinguished patients with advanced MASLD from mild/moderate disease, while fecal taxonomic and metabolomic profiles coupled with the clinical indicator aspartate transferase (AST) distinguished MASLD-cirrhosis patients from non-MASLD controls.[338] Microbial metabolic pathways that were up-regulated in MASLD-cirrhosis patients included those for fatty acid, phospholipid, and cholesterol-related biosynthesis. While diet as a contributor to these alterations was not considered in these studies, gut microbes have been shown to be exquisitely sensitive to WD. Murine studies using high fat (HF), high simple sugar, and high cholesterol (HC) diets reveal that diet-induced microbiota imbalances contribute to MASLD pathogenesis.[339] Conventional or SPF mice fed a WD high in fat, simple sugar, and increasing levels of cholesterol revealed increased onset and severity of nonalcoholic steatohepatitis (NASH) scores compared to LF control mice. Mice fed high-fat very high–cholesterol (HFVHC) diets exhibited increased abundance of *Bilophila wadsworthia* that was also significantly positively associated with NAS score, while *Bifidobacteria* abundance was negatively associated with NAS scores.[340] GF mice, devoid of all microorganisms, were protected from HF, HC–induced NASH.[340] Further, FMT from donor mice harboring microbes with MASLD and hepatocellular carcinoma (HCC) into GF recipient mice demonstrated that microbes transfer donor phenotypes, highlighting a causal role.[341,342] Importantly, FMT in mice and humans has been shown to improve fatty liver.[343] In one study, lean human participants with NAFLD displayed greater improvement following FMT compared to obese participants with NAFLD.[343] In another study utilizing FMT in NAFLD patients, it was found that NAFLD patients receiving lean donor microbiota exhibited decreased small intestinal permeability but not improvement in insulin resistance or degree of fatty liver.[344] While some support for FMT in MAFLD and MASLD patients exist, further studies examining the effectiveness of FMT in MASLD are needed. Recently, a microbial metabolite of dietary polyphenols, namely the flavonoid catabolite, 4-hydroxyphenylacetic acid (4-HPAA), was found to protect against NAFLD in mice.[345] A meta-analysis consisting of 1,252 patients showed that probiotic formulations largely containing Lactobacillus and Bifidobacteria strains improved markers of NAFLD.[346]

ENERGY MALNUTRITION

While the gut microbiota contributes to development of metabolic disease, these same properties may be beneficial in other conditions such as environmental enteropathy and failure to thrive. Microbes have been demonstrated to be critical for growth and recovery from protein-energy malnutrition. First, Smith et al. showed that in twins discordant for Kwashiorkor, a severe acute malnutrition, and fed the same ready-to-eat therapeutic food (RUTF), twins that developed Kwashiorkor developed a distinct microbiome compared to their healthy twin control.[347] An altered immature microbiome in Bangladeshi children[348] and altered DNA virome in Malawian twins have also been described.[349] Blanton et al. demonstrated that FMT from healthy or undernourished infants transferred the respective phenotypes in GF mice where the mice receiving undernourished microbiota exhibited delayed growth.[350] Micronutrient deficiencies also result in an altered microbiome.[351] It is suspected that standard meal replacement is not sufficient to promote improved nutritional status. Gehrig et al aimed to define microbiota-directed complementary food (MDCF) prototypes for better restoration of nutritional status in malnourished Bangladeshi children. Upon defining the microbiota of malnourished Bangladeshi children, this microbiota was used as a transplant in gnotobiotic mice and piglets to identify an effective MDCF.[352] One of these prototypes, MDCF-2, was used in a cohort of Bangladeshi children with mild to moderate malnutrition and it was found that after 3 months of treatment followed by 1 month of monitoring that MDCF-2 was associated with positive effects on overall growth.[353] Therefore, a focus on harnessing the capabilities of one's own microbiome with directed nutritional supplementation may be effective in treating malnutrition.

Cardiovascular Disease

Work by Stanley Hazen's group nicely demonstrated that dietary components from red meat and eggs such as L-carnitine and phosphatidylcholine, respectively, led to the production of trimethylamine (TMA) in the gastrointestinal tract upon metabolism by certain microbes. TMA upon delivery to the liver is converted into trimethylamine N-oxide (TMAO) by flavin monooxygenase that then causes atherosclerosis and plaque development, thus establishing a clear connection between diet, microbes, and metabolic consequences for the host.[354–356] Since these early discoveries, further evidence for a causative role of TMAO in cardiovascular pathology has been reported.

Osteoarthritis

Roughly a quarter of the adult population suffers from osteoarthritis (OA), a degenerative joint disease. There is growing evidence that OA is caused by low-level inflammation and not mechanical wear.[357] In individuals with knee OA there is an uptick in activation of the complement cascade resulting in proinflammatory cytokine production and increased joint erosion when compared to healthy individuals.[358] Recent findings suggest a correlation between dysbiosis of the intestinal microbiome and the detection of proinflammatory markers associated with OA; a consequence of the gut–joint axis.[359,360] Nutraceuticals, such as glucosamine or undenatured type II collagen (UT2C), used as nutritional support for joint health, induce measurable changes in the intestinal microbiota. In an experimental model of trauma-induced OA, degenerative changes in injured joints were decelerated in mice provided diets supplemented with either glucosamine or UT2C.[361] Using bacterial DNA extracted from fecal pellets of the nutraceutical-supplemented mice compared to the vehicle control mice, a relative increase in Bacteroidetes and decrease in Firmicutes were measured, consistent with a potential anti-inflammatory intestinal microbiota profile. Although multiple differences were detected at the individual operational taxonomic units, glucosamine and UTC2 supplementation both increased the relative abundance of *S24-7* and decreased the amount of *Oscillospira* in the feces.[361] In a clinical study characterizing the fecal microbiota of OA patients using whole meta-genome shotgun sequencing compared to healthy controls, relative differences in 279 bacterial species, 10 fungal species, and 627 viral OTUs were identified.[362] These microbial differences were profound to differentiate OA patients from healthy controls. A systematic review of 24 preclinical and 14 clinical studies demonstrated reduced inflammation and a decrease in OA symptoms in response to the probiotic Lactobacillus in some of the studies.[360] Further evidence needs to be developed that strengthen the causal role of gut health on OA onset, severity, and pain. Using next-generation sequencing technologies, Zhao et al. revealed the presence of bacterial nucleic acids in the synovial fluid and synovial tissues isolated aseptically from OA patients.[363] These findings raise the question of potential localized bacterial infection in the articular cavity of OA patients. While the authors admit that detection of bacterial nucleic acids does not prove that viable bacteria were present in the synovial joints or tissues of OA patients, it does prompt further investigations. From a clinical standpoint, understanding the impact of diet and activity on the microbiome and its impact on the gut–joint axis in the prevention and/or treatment of OA is important in providing evidence that can be used to educate the patient. In addition, providing the patient reassurance that joint degeneration is not a by-product of daily mechanical stress but due to low-level inflammation can be helpful to encourage their participation in exercise and thereby help restore microbial balance and potentially reduce systemic inflammation.

UROGENITAL TRACT MICROBIOME

Vaginal Microbiome

Maintaining a healthy balance of vaginal microbes is important to female reproductive health. More than 170 species of bacteria, 10^{10} to 10^{11} bacteria, reside in the vagina.[36] *Lactobacilli* are the most prominent bacteria in the healthy vagina.[36,364,365] Estrogen promotes glycogen storage in the lining epithelial cells, which *Lactobacilli* metabolize into lactic acid, thus fostering a low vaginal pH ($pH < 4.5$) which prevents bacterial overgrowth.[366] *Lactobacilli* also produce bacteriocins, AMPs, that protect the vaginal environment from nonindigenous microorganisms.[367] Inherent characteristics, such as race, ethnicity, genetics, and reproductive age influence the vaginal microbial composition.[364–366,368] Lifestyle factors, such as pregnancy, sexual behavior, hygiene methods, contraceptive use, smoking, stress, and obesity may also impact the innate vaginal microbiome.[369–373]

In the healthy vagina, the relative abundance of *Lactobacilli* fluctuates during the normal menstrual cycle and with biologic age.[364,366,368] Prepubertal girls and postmenopausal women have the lowest levels of *Lactobacillus* species compared to newborn infants, women of reproductive age, and pregnant women.[366,370] These relative changes in *Lactobacilli* content correlate with the relative abundance of estrogen during those phases of a female's life. In women of reproductive age, five major groups of bacterial community-state types (CSTs) have been identified, each group demonstrating a specific prevalent strain of *Lactobacilli*.[365] Vaginal bacteria community groups CST-I, II, III, and V are dominated by *Lactobacillus* species *L. cripatus*, *L. iners*, and *L. jensenii*, respectively, whereas CST-IV has more diversity and a relatively high proportion of anaerobes, but is still considered healthy.[365] Group IV-A has moderate levels of *L. cripatus, L. iners,* or other *Lactobacillus* spp., and low levels of strictly anaerobic bacteria such as *Anaerococcus, Corynebacterium, Finegoldia, or Streptococcus*; IV-B has high abundance of *Atopobium*, and *Prevotella*, *Parvimonas*, *Sneathia*, *Gardnerella*, *Mobiluncus,* and *Peptoniphilus*.[368] However, Group IV-B contains some taxa associated with bacterial vaginosis (BV).[374]

Pregnancy significantly impacts the microbiota of the female reproductive tract. Overall bacterial diversity and richness are reduced with pregnancy and the vaginal microbiome's stability is enhanced.[375,376] Metagenomic and metatranscriptomics analyses of the vaginal microbiomes in a cohort of pregnant women demonstrated the greatest change in the functional microbiome during the first trimester of pregnancy, with significant changes identified in women of African and Hispanic ancestry compared to European ancestry.[376]

Investigators are exploring the potential causal role of microbial dysbiosis in the vagina with clinical conditions such as infertility, preterm birth, sexually transmitted infections (STIs), and gynecologic cancers.[377–380] Because of the multifactorial nature of intrinsic and extrinsic influences on host microbial balance, and the potential for transient alterations in "normal" content that can occur without manifesting disease, these investigations will require continued validation and substantiation before a clear cause and effect can be concluded.

BACTERIAL VAGINOSIS

The vagina has a complex microbiome that changes throughout the menstrual cycle and a woman's life. This microbiome is dominated by *Lactobacillus* species, which leads to lactic acid production and an acidic pH, providing innate host protection from pathogens. A disruption in the vaginal microbiota can lead to a decrease in *Lactobacilli* and a change in the vaginal microbiome; dysbiosis. This change is known as BV and is characterized by an increase in the diversity and taxonomic richness of the vaginal microbiome.[381] Overgrowth of anaerobic bacteria, such as *Gardnerella vaginalis*, *Bacteroides* spp., *Peptostreptococcus* spp., *Fusobacterium* spp., *Prevotella* spp., *Atopobium vaginae*, and several *Clostridium* strains have been documented.[374,381–383]

BV impacts approximately 30% of the female population, 14 to 49 years of age, with many women being asymptomatic.[384] It is the most common cause of abnormal vaginal discharge in reproductive aged women, commonly presenting as thin, off-white, or gray vaginal discharge with a fishy odor.[383] Risks factors for BV include race, ethnicity, age, sexual activity, presence of another STI, douching, and cigarette use.[384–391] It can be diagnosed by microscopy using the Amsel criteria or Gram stain with Nugent scoring or by commercial assays that detect the presence of *G. vaginalis*, the most commonly identified organism in BV.[383]

BV has been associated with adverse reproductive health outcomes. In nonpregnant individuals, the presence of BV increases susceptibility to other STIs, pelvic inflammatory disease, postprocedural gynecologic infections, and may have associations with infertility.[386,392,393] In pregnant individuals, BV has been associated with increased risk of preterm birth.[394] In pregnant and symptomatic nonpregnant individuals, BV is typically treated with a course of antibiotics such as oral or intravaginal metronidazole or intravaginal clindamycin.[395,396] In recurrent or refractory cases, different therapeutic approaches may be used. Prevention strategies include condom use, hormonal contraception, and smoking cessation[395,397]; additional strategies, including use of probiotics, are under investigation.[372,398,399] The vaginal microbiome is complex and necessary for maintaining a balanced vaginal ecosystem.

Urinary Tract Microbiome

The urinary tract (UT) has a unique microbiome, the urobiome, that originally was undetectable by standard culture methods but is now realized with the use of non–culture-based methodology, such as 16S rRNA gene sequencing.[400,401] Dysbiosis of the urobiome secondary to age, use of antibiotics, insufficient contraction of the bladder or flushing of urinary content, in-dwelling catheters, immune dysfunction, nerve damage, vaginal infections, or barrier contraceptive use can lead to colonization of the UT by pathogenic organisms.[402,403] A majority of the studies done to identify a healthy urobiome have been performed in females, since they are disproportionately affected by urinary tract infections (UTIs).[404] In general, the four major phyla of bacteria, Firmicutes, Bacteroidetes, Proteobacteria, and Actinobacteria are detected in the urobiome.[405] As shown in Figure 23.9, the healthy urobiome consists of *Lactobacillus, Prevotella, Corynebacterium, Gardnerella*, and *Shigella. Lactobacillus* and *Corynebacterium* are dominant in the female and male urobiomes, respectively.[402]

Improvements in clinical urine sample collections, processing, and analyses with identification of microbial imbalance may provide more targeted approaches to treating and preventing UTIs.[406,407]

URINARY TRACT INFECTION

UTIs are reported to be the most common outpatient infections in the United States, contributing to substantial healthcare visits and medical costs.[404,408–411] While UTIs impact both sexes, they are a significant cause of morbidity in females, infant boys, and older

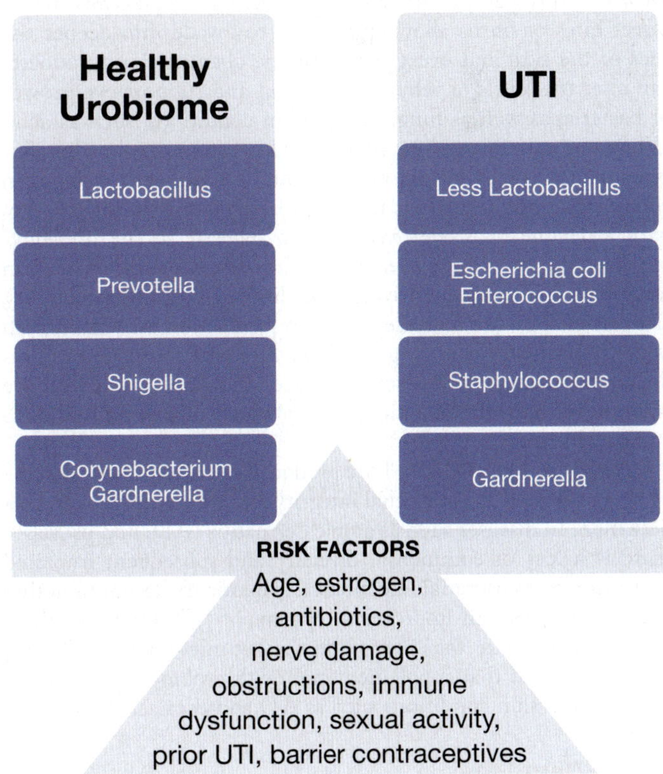

Figure 23.9. Microbial inhabitants of a healthy urobiome and dysregulation with disease. A healthy urobiome is important to preventing bacterial overgrowth with opportunistic pathogens. Risk factors for urinary tract infections (UTIs) include age, estrogen, antibiotics, nerve damage, obstructions, immune dysregulation, sexual activity, previous infections, and barrier contraceptives.

males.[404,411] Clinical symptoms may include urgency, frequency, and dysuria; suprapubic, vaginal, and urethral tenderness; and hematuria.[412] Individuals may be positive for bacteriuria and be asymptomatic.[404,413] Symptomatic patients with bacteriuria can be classified as uncomplicated or complicated, based on the presence of risk factors for UTIs, which include UT structural abnormalities, diabetes mellitus, age, catheterization, spinal cord injury, sexual intercourse, family history, and comorbidities in pediatric patients.[410,413] The opportunistic pathogen, uropathogenic *Escherichia coli* (UPEC), is the most common causative agent for UTIs.[413–417] *Klebsiella pneumoniae, Proteus mirabilis, Enterococcus faecalis*, and *Staphylococcus* spp. also cause UTIs.[404,413,414,418] Appreciating the impact of the urobiome and factors that can alter its homeostasis provide a new paradigm for optimizing patient care for individuals who suffer from recurrent UTIs.[37,419,420]

SKIN MICROBIOME

The most superficial layer of the skin, the epidermis, provides innate host protection against pathogens. Additional protection is provided by commensal bacteria that colonize the surface of the skin.[29] The composition and quantity of microbes on the skin varies at different sites of the body with bacteria that efficiently metabolize lipids, such as *Propionibacterium*, elevated at body sites with increased sebaceous glands, such as hair follicles, while areas of the skin predominated by sweat glands, and therefore increased salt levels, are predominated by halophiles like *Staphylococci* and *Corynebacteria*.[114,421] The skin is also home to fungi, predominately *Malassezia* spp., which can be found the most ubiquitously.[422] Changes in the skin environment increase risk of microbial overgrowth and disease. Examples include damaged epidermis due to insect bites or burns allowing bacteria to invade into deeper tissues of the skin and overgrow; hormone changes during puberty can alter the levels of sebum production and support overgrowth of bacteria, as well as fungi, resulting in conditions, such as acne. While the gut microbiota achieves homeostasis in the first few years of life, the skin microbiome exhibits significant changes in composition not only in the first few years, but also during puberty, with a decline in *Streptococcus* and an increase in the lipid-loving bacteria *Propionibacterium* and *Corynebacterium*.[423] The skin microbiome is uniquely driven by its limited nutrient availability, as evidenced by the increase in sebum production associated with puberty drastically changing the skin's microbial composition. This dependence on limited resources places the skin in a distinctive position for both therapeutic and prophylactic use of probiotics to combat disease.[424]

AMPs and interleukin-1 are produced by skin resident macrophages to defend the epithelial integrity and prevent pathogen colonization. In diseases such as atopic dermatitis (AD) and psoriasis, there is a loss of commensal diversity and subsequent impaired protection from bacterial infections. Antibiotic treatment targeting *S. aureus* overgrowth improves symptoms of AD. However, there is growing evidence that changes to the gut microbiome influence skin disease and that supplementation with probiotics can protect from clinical skin conditions such as AD and psoriasis.[424]

Atopic Dermatitis

AD is a chronic inflammatory skin condition involving pruritis, redness, and inflammation. Risk factors for developing AD include genetic predisposition, immune system and skin barrier dysfunction, environmental factors, and dysbiosis of the skin and intestinal microbiome. Reductions in skin microbial diversity and increased levels of pathogenic bacteria like *Staphylococcus aureus* have been associated with AD.[425] *S. aureus* produce virulence factors that disrupt the skin barrier and exacerbate inflammation. *Staphylococcus epidermidis* is a commensal bacterium that contributes to skin health by competing with pathogenic bacteria for nutrients and space as well as producing AMPs. *S. epidermidis* is also a source of ceramides that help strengthen the skin barrier. However, in AD patients, *S. epidermidis* levels are sometimes abnormally high and begin to contribute to AD pathology.[426]

While it is unlikely that targeting the intestinal microbiome is sufficient to prevent the development of AD, probiotics have been shown to reduce skin inflammation and improve symptoms by enhancing the intestinal barrier and preventing intestinal colonization by pathogenic bacteria.[427] For example, in a randomized clinical trial, administration of *Lactobacillus salivarius* LS01 and *Bifidobacterium breve* BR03 for 12 weeks reduced gut permeability and improved AD.[428] Whether used alone or as adjuvant therapy, probiotics improve quality of life and reduce the severity score for patients with AD.[427]

Psoriasis

Psoriasis is characterized by red, scaly plaques on the skin and, like AD, is associated with microbial dysbiosis. Gut as well as skin microbiome changes have been identified.[429,430] Psoriatic lesions contain a higher bacterial load compared to unaffected skin, with a greater proportion of *Corynebacterium* and smaller proportion of *Propionibacterium* compared to unaffected skin. Dysbiosis in the intestinal and skin microbiomes contribute to proinflammatory conditions and compromised skin barrier integrity. Probiotic supplementation with *Lactobacillus* and *Bifidobacterium* has demonstrated efficacy in patients by reducing psoriatic lesions.[431,432] Other successful treatments for psoriasis target the immune response, including tumor necrosis factor-alpha (TNF-α) and interleukin-17 (IL-17) antagonists. Recent work identified that these biologic therapies can also impact the gut microbiome, specifically by reducing microbial diversity.[433] These findings highlight the need to better understand how the microbiomes of the host are influenced by local and systemic treatments designed to specifically target inflammatory processes.

MECHANISMS TO MODULATE HOST MICROBIAL BALANCE

Probiotics

Probiotics are defined as "live microorganisms that, when administered in adequate amounts, confer a health benefit on the host," according to the International Scientific Association for Probiotics and Prebiotics.[434] Various probiotic products, in the form of dietary supplements or foods, are on the market targeted to improved digestive and gut health for irritable bowel syndrome, antibiotic-associated or infection-induced diarrhea, colic and eczema in infants, and NEC. Probiotics have also been reported to aid in conditions outside the gastrointestinal tract such as those affecting the oral cavity, skin, and the vaginal and urinary tracts. Probiotics targeting the gut typically consist of *Lactobacillus* and *Bifidobacteria* species as well as yeast, such as *Saccharomyces boulardii*. A concern with probiotic supplements is they are unable to sufficiently colonize the human gastrointestinal tract. Therefore, daily use of probiotic supplements is required. Despite this limitation, probiotic supplementation can improve health outcomes related to both gastrointestinal health and metabolism. Probiotics should be used with caution in at-risk populations.[435,436] Consultation with a healthcare provider prior to using probiotics is strongly advised.

Prebiotics, Synbiotics, and Postbiotics

Prebiotics are defined as "a substrate that is selectively utilized by host microorganisms conferring a health benefit" and include soluble fibers consisting of fructans (fructooligosaccharides [FOS] and inulin) and galactans (glucooligosaccharides [GOS]).[437] These are nondigestible carbohydrates that can be metabolized by bacterial enzymes β-fructanosidase and β-galactosidase, specific for FOS and GOS, respectively. *Bifidobacteria*, which are known to have beneficial health effects, express these enzymes. Synbiotics are defined as "a mixture comprising live microorganisms and substrate(s) selectively utilized by host microorganisms that confers a health benefit on the host."[438] Postbiotics are defined as "a preparation of inanimate microorganisms and/or their components that confers a health benefit on the host."[439] Use of these "biotics" may improve intestinal microbial balance and overall health.

Fermented Foods

Fermented foods are defined as "foods made through desired microbial growth and enzymatic conversions of food components."[440] Fermentation of foods is facilitated by either lactic acid bacteria or bacteria that produce acetic or propionic acids. Lactic acid bacteria are used in the fermentation of dairy, cheese, and meat products, as well as sourdough bread and vegetables like kimchi. Yeast, such as Brewer's yeast or *Saccharomyces cerevisiae*, are also used for baking, brewing of beer, and wine production. Kombucha is another example of a common fermented food with purported health benefits. Fermented foods provide an accepted dietary source for bacteria with potential health benefits.

Exercise

Exercise is widely acknowledged as a crucial component of a healthy lifestyle and is endorsed by professional medical associations and societies for preventing and managing obesity, CVD, and other chronic conditions.[441–443] Research suggests that a portion of the benefits of exercise are mediated by the gut microbiota, influencing a broad range of body systems and functions.[444,445] However, the effects of exercise vary based on the type, duration, and intensity. For example, analyzing the gut microbiota before and after acute aerobic exercise shows a more variable, yet similar change compared to the impact of long-term aerobic exercise training.[446,447] Moreover, despite numerous reported health benefits associated with exercise training and linked to changes in the gut microbiota,[445] there is evidence that exercise contributes to exercise-induced gastrointestinal syndrome ("runner's gut"), characterized by bloating, diarrhea, and abdominal distress, in athletes undergoing intense endurance training. Various types of exercise, dietary factors, and other variables likely determine how exercise alters the gut microbiota and how this influences energy balance, body weight, neurologic, metabolic, and immune function, and overall health.[448,449]

Specific effects of exercise on metabolism are linked to changes in the gut microbiota. Evans et al. found that aerobic exercise (voluntary running) prevented weight gain, reduced fat mass, and lowered fasting blood glucose in mice on an HFD, and these changes correlated with a shift in the gut microbiota.[450] Comparable results were found in studies involving lean and obese human adults.[451,452] A systematic review of human studies revealed variable increases in alpha and beta diversity, decreased levels of the *Proteobacteria* phylum, and variable changes in the *Bacteroidetes*:*Firmicutes* ratio.[452] Similar to the situation described in the Obesity section above, changes in the *Bacteroidetes*:*Firmicutes* ratio were not universal and were only found in a subset of studies.[452] Systematic reviews by Boytar et al. and Silva et al. found that exercise increased genera involved in SCFA production, especially butyrate, and that microbiota changes were dose-dependent, with longer duration and greater intensity exercise exerting a greater effect.[444,452] A study in lean and obese humans with a controlled diet found that while exercise helped reduce body weight, it altered the gut microbiota and increased butyrate more in lean than in obese subjects.[451] To determine whether the gut microbiota played a causative role, an animal study transplanted the gut microbiota from exercised mice into antibiotic-treated sedentary mice and found that the benefits of exercise, such as reduced body weight and improvement in indicators of metabolic health and skeletal muscle function, were transferable.[453] Likely, the gut microbiota plays a role in determining other responses to exercise training as well. Animal and human studies in healthy and neurologically-impaired subjects have linked the gut microbiota to the beneficial effect of exercise on cognitive and neurologic function.[454–458] For example, the beneficial effect of exercise on depression is linked to changes in the gut microbiota.[454,455,457] However, these studies only examine the association between exercise, gut microbial makeup, and cognitive or neurologic functioning and cannot determine a cause-and-effect relationship.

One of the most exciting areas where exercise exerts an effect through the gut microbiota is athletic performance. The gut microbiota plays a role in harvesting energy from the diet, producing metabolites, stimulating the release of gut-derived neurotransmitters, maintaining water balance, and modulating free radicals. All of these effects impact endurance, muscle strength, and psychological factors related to athletic performance.[458,459] Studies involving chronic aerobic exercise training on the gut microbiota are complicated by dietary and lifestyle factors (in human studies) and also suggest both benefits and potential pathologic effects.[459,460] A review focused on studies of athletes found no standard athletic gut microbiota.[460] Many different taxa were enriched in different studies, depending on the mode, duration, and intensity of exercise, as well as the age of subjects, diet, location, and other factors.[460] *Akkermansia muciniphila* was the one species that was most commonly identified as enriched, and this microbe is associated with many benefits, such as the protection of the intestinal mucus layer and reduced gut inflammation.[460] Findings suggested exercise confers a gut microbiota profile consistent with lean phenotype and increased production of SCFAs, particularly butyrate, and related KEGG pathways. In the Uchida et al. study mentioned above, gut microbiota transplant confirmed that the "exercise gut microbiota" was the mechanism for improved endurance and exercise tolerance.[453] Nevertheless, the role of the gut microbiota in exercise-induced gastrointestinal syndrome is still unclear. Intense exercise shifts blood flow away from the gut, leading to ischemia and the release of free radicals, inflammation, and leaky gut barrier function.[448] Whether exercise training helps prevent or limit ischemia and these complications, or is the cause, likely depends on duration, intensity, diet (both long-term and prior to exercise), and other factors. The benefits of strength training may also be modulated through the gut microbiota, but this is less well-studied, and human studies often involve changes in diet that confound results.[461] Overall, both animal and human studies support that beneficial effects of exercise are mediated by the gut microbiota and promote increased exercise capacity, and a lean, metabolically healthy phenotype.

Antibiotics

Antibiotics are a powerful treatment to mitigate the pathology caused by infectious diseases. However, their impact on the gastrointestinal microbiota can create an environment for pathogenic bacterial overgrowth by reducing the diversity and colonization of healthy bacteria, altering bacterial metabolite production, and/or increasing the proportion of bacteria possessing drug-resistant genes. It is imperative, therefore, that physicians be judicious in explaining the appropriate use of any prescribed antibiotic and the necessity to take it as prescribed for the duration of the treatment. Educating and empowering the patient concerning the appropriate use of this powerful treatment aligns with the osteopathic philosophy.

Oral consumption of antibiotics may cause dysbiosis of the intestinal microbiota. Broad-spectrum antibiotics can reduce gastrointestinal microbial content as well as diversity.[462,463] As shown in Table 23.4, the various classes of antibiotics can impact the intestinal microbiota, causing transient elevations and eliminations of specific bacteria.[464] The duration of these changes varies based on dosing, type of antibiotic administered, and the health of the host.

Clostridioides difficile (formerly *Clostridium difficile*; *C. difficile*) infection (CDI) is an opportunistic infection caused secondarily by antibiotic use. It is the most frequently diagnosed healthcare and community-acquired infection in the United States.[465] Transmission is from person-to-person by oral–fecal route, direct person-to-person contact, and exposure to contaminated surfaces. Clinical symptoms include diarrhea (≥3 loose stools/24 hours), abdominal pain, nausea, vomiting, and fever. There is the potential for dehydration and in extreme cases, death. Young children and elderly adults are most susceptible to the detrimental effects of CDI. Certain antibiotics and longer courses of antibiotics or use of multiple antibiotics increase the risk of CDI. Clindamycin, fluoroquinolones, as well as third- and fourth-generation cephalosporins and carbapenems are associated with CDI.[466,467]

Ironically, antibiotic therapy is recommended to eradicate this pathogen. Usually, vancomycin or fidaxomicin is recommended for an initial bout of infection. Metronidazole is recommended as a third option.[465] However, when recurrent infections occur due to the development of antibiotic resistance, FMT may be the best therapeutic intervention. FMT is approved for pediatric and adult patients with recurrent, antibiotic-resistant CDI.[468]

FECAL MICROBIOTA TRANSPLANTATION

The power and influence that the gut microbiome has on every organ system in the body has been outlined throughout this chapter. In understanding these effects, physicians and researchers have developed a therapy in which the robust self-regulatory properties of the gut microbiome are provided in the concentrated treatment called fecal microbiota transplantation.

FMT is a treatment option for patients in which stool is harvested from an established healthy donor and is transplanted into a recipient with dysbiosis.[469] The main goal of physically transferring healthy microbial contents is to repopulate the patient's gastrointestinal tract with diverse and well-balanced microbiota to restore eubiosis in the host (Fig. 23.10). This treatment method, also known as a type of bacteriotherapy, is a forced reintroduction of a naturally-produced microbial ecosystem. As defined by the American College of Gastroenterology, bacteriotherapy is the term used to depict the use of microbes and their products to treat an illness. Probiotics and FMT are examples of bacteriotherapy. This therapy highlights the beauty of modern medicine and is osteopathic at its core.

Fecal Microbiota Transplantation Indications and Clinical Implications

FMT was first documented in the medical literature in 1958 for the successful treatment of pseudomembranous colitis,[470] but similar bacteriotherapies and anecdotal evidence of using FMT for food poisoning and severe diarrhea date back to 4th-century China.[471] The delivery methods of this therapy have evolved from "yellow soup" oral preparations and fecal enemas to a variety of sophisticated modalities including but not limited to colonoscopic syringes, nasogastric placement, oral capsules, and retention enemas.[472–474] There is an even newer product called Reboyta which is a rectally

TABLE 23.4

Impact of Antibiotics on Intestinal Microbiota

Antibiotic Class	Penicillin	Lincomycin	Cephalosporins	Macrolides	Quinolone Fluoroquinolones	Carbapenems
Increased with Antibiotic	Enterobacteria *Bacteroidaceae*	*Enterobacteriaceae*	Clostridia; *Bacteroides* spp.	Bacteroidetes; Proteobacteria; Resistant Enterobacteria; Streptococci; Enterococci	Resistant *E. coli*	*Enterococci*
Decreased with Antibiotic	Gram-positive aerobic coci; Lactobacilli; Bifidobacteria; Eubacteria *Lachnospiraceae*	Bacteroides; *Blautia*	*E. coli;* Bifidobacteria; *Enterobacteriaceae*	Actinobacteria; *Lachnospiraceae; Veillonella; Clostriales; Erysipelotrichaceae*	*Lachnospiraceae; Coprococcus;* Gram negative aerobes; *Enterobacteriaceae*	Enterobacteria; Streptococci; Clostridia; Bacteroides; Bifidobacteria; Lactobacillus; Eubacteria

Multiple classes of antibiotics can impact the intestinal microbiota, increasing some bacteria and reducing others. The consequences of these changes can directly impact the microbial communities in the gut as well as cause systemic changes secondary to production of metabolic intermediates. Growth of opportunistic pathogens, such as *C. difficile* secondary to antibiotic therapy–induced dysbiosis can cause significant gastrointestinal stress. Image reconfigured from reference 431.

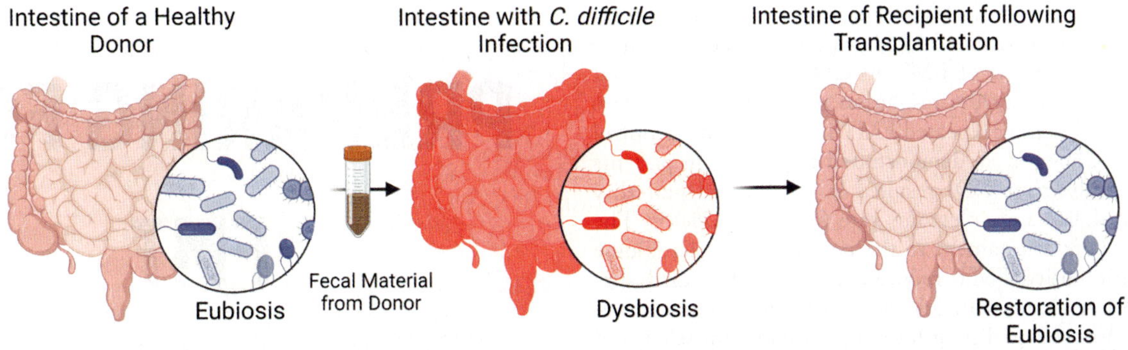

Figure 23.10. Fecal microbiota transplantation at the macro and micro level in the setting of a *C. difficile* infection. Stool containing healthy microbiota isolated from an optimal stool donor (1) is transferred to a patient with *C. difficile* infection (2) restoring eubiosis and healthy microbial balance (3). (Created with BioRender.com.)

administered liquid fecal suspension that can be performed without anesthesia or bowel prep in the outpatient setting.[475]

Patients are often averse to the idea of FMT with the liquid formulation, which makes capsule delivery so appealing. In addition, capsule delivery is a much more convenient delivery method that does not require anesthesia or carry the risks of endoscopy and colonoscopy. Data thus far has indicated that there is no difference in cure rate between capsule delivery and colonoscopy. Studies performed by Kahn et al, revealed that patients with IBD are ambivalent about receiving donor stool as a treatment modality; their main concern is to relieve their symptoms and improve their quality of life.[476]

While recurrent CDIs (rCDI) carry a higher morbidity in adults, children are infected at the same rate. With FMT carrying such a high cure rate in adults,[477] it is important to know that this therapy is also offered to children with rCDI.[478,479] Long-term side effects from prolonged antibiotic therapy compared to FMT therapy have not yet been analyzed but societal guidelines currently advise FMT to be considered in the treatment algorithm for the pediatric population.

The field of research dedicated to understanding and elucidating the impact the gut microbiome has on the human body is rapidly growing. Scientists have been able to establish connections between the composition of the gut microbiome and common disease processes such as obesity, chronic fatigue syndrome, PD, and CVD.[472,480] In identifying these patterns, involved microorganisms, genetic predispositions, and environmental stressors (such as antibiotics, diet, pollutants, mental health, injury), researchers have opened a world of novel treatment target possibilities in the human microbiome.

Recurrent CDIs plague healthcare systems and patients as one of the most common complications of being hospitalized.[481] While there are many organizations and patient safety initiatives that collect this data and provide prevention guidelines to minimize these risks, doctors are still tasked with deciding how to most effectively treat these patients that succumb to a CDI. Provided below is an algorithm outlining the standard of care treatment for CDI. It is important to note that in the instance of recurrent CDI, FMT is not looked at by physicians as an alternative or experimental therapy option, but rather as a routine and superior treatment for patients that have access to it (Fig. 23.11).

The efficacy of FMT therapy can be highlighted by looking at the data when using it as a treatment for CDI. In 2017, Quraishi et al. published a meta-analysis of seven randomized control trials and 30 case studies that compared outcomes of CDI patients treated with the standard antibiotic of care, vancomycin,

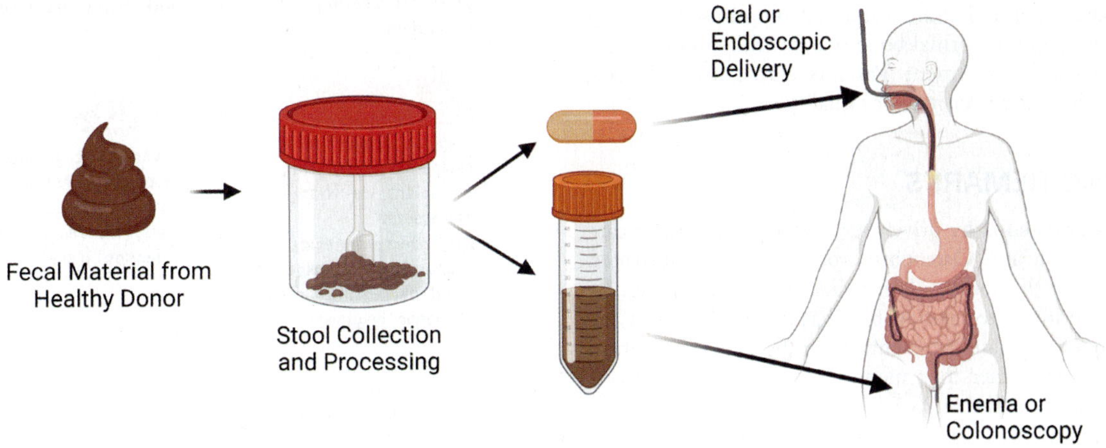

Figure 23.11. Fecal transplant therapy. Donor feces undergo filtration and processing into a liquid suspension or a freeze-dried capsule prior to administration. Fecal matter is typically mixed with normal saline and spun into a homogenized solution which is then poured over a grate/sieve to filter out particulate matter, undigested food, and large undesired contents. The filtered product containing live bacteria is then either administered within 6 hours of emission or preserved in liquid or capsule form via freezing. FMT can be administered via endoscopy, colonoscopy, oral capsules, and retention enemas. (Created with BioRender.com.)

compared to FMT.[482] With FMT boasting resolution rates as high as 92%, the review deemed FMT superior to vancomycin.[482] Another systematic review of FMT in CDI patients carried out by Rossen et al. found a 90% resolution of diarrhea and a 94% resolution of diarrhea after repeated FMT in a randomized control trail.[483] Finally, Cheng et al. demonstrated that FMT in patients with severe or fulminant CDI resulted in a decreased mortality rate (10.2% to 4.4%) and colectomy rate (6.8% to 2.7%).[477] The previous studies are a testament to the power of the microbiome as a therapeutic entity. FMT reduced mortality, decreased surgical intervention along with additional surgical complications, significantly improved quality of life through symptom relief, and resolved rCDI when employed as therapy. Efficacy of FMT in treating rCDI provides evidence for and encourages further treatments to be developed that alter or utilize the gut microbiome as therapy in both gastrointestinal and nongastrointestinal diseases.

Identifying a Stool Donor

Extensive screening and testing standards are in place to ensure safe selection of stool donors (Fig. 23.12). These include: screening questions to eliminate candidates with risk of transmitting dangerous viral or bacterial infections; screening questions similar to those of potential blood donors; testing for blood-borne diseases such as syphilis, hepatitis, and HIV; testing for parasites, *C. difficile*, and other viruses, including Covid-19.[469,472] Individuals who have taken antibiotics within the last 3 months or who have gastrointestinal diseases such as IBD, irritable bowel syndrome, or chronic constipation should not be donors. Ideal stool donors are adult males, in excellent health, who regularly exercise and eat a healthy diet.

POTENTIAL RISKS

Overall, FMT is considered to be safe. Most common side-effects include abdominal discomfort and diarrhea that self-resolves. A possible side effect includes weight gain. Potential procedural complications include perforation, irritation, and aspiration pneumonia secondary to endoscopy. Transmission of infection due to dangerous microbes is rare, due to extensive donor screening. As with any medical intervention, it is the responsibility of the physician and healthcare team to have a transparent and educated conversation with the patient about risks, benefits, treatment options, and patient goals. Patients that are immunocompromised or using medications that suppress normal bone marrow function may not be good candidates for treatment. Patients with advanced HIV, AIDS, or cirrhosis of the liver may not qualify.

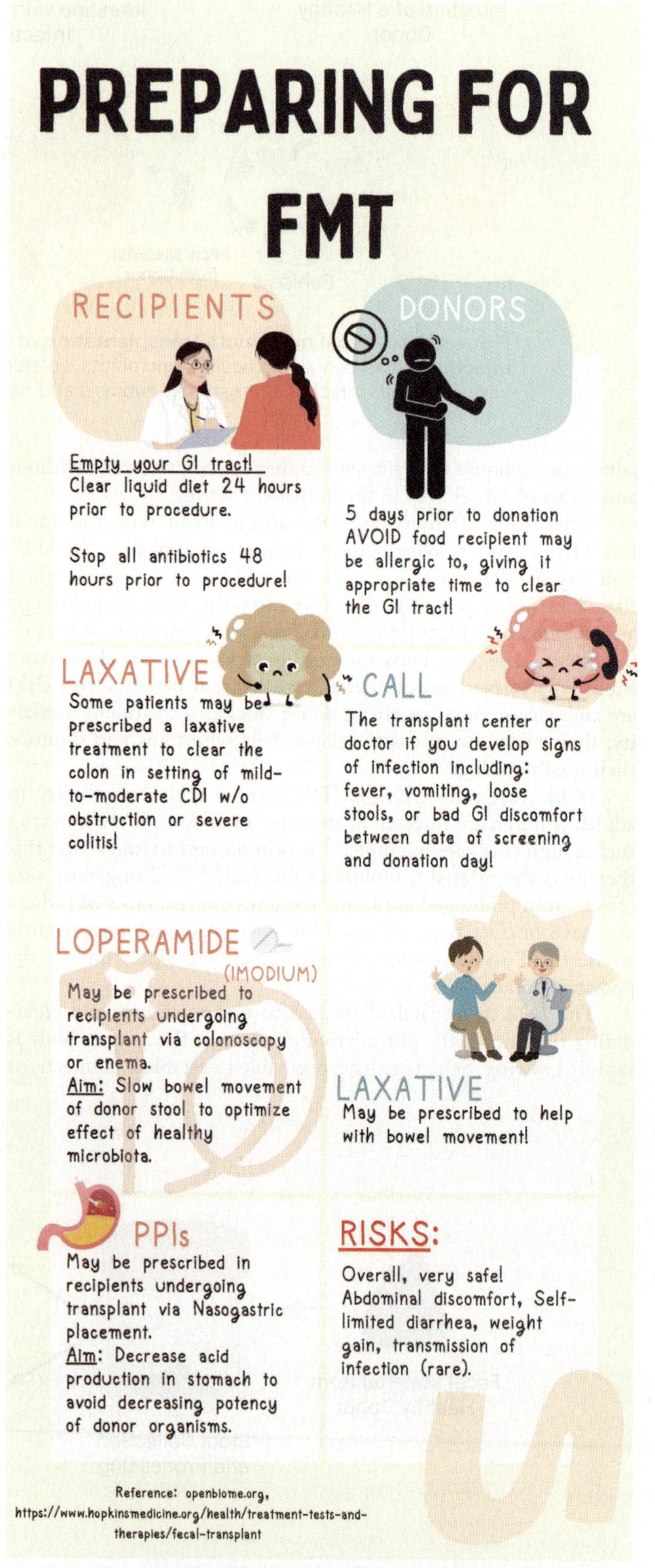

PREPARING FOR FMT
RECIPIENTS
DONORS
Empty your GI tract! Clear liquid diet 24 hours prior to procedure.
Stop all antibiotics 48 hours prior to procedure!
5 days prior to donation AVOID food recipient may be allergic to, giving it appropriate time to clear the GI tract!
LAXATIVE
Some patients may be prescribed a laxative treatment to clear the colon in setting of mild-to-moderate CDI w/o obstruction or severe colitis!
CALL
The transplant center or doctor if you develop signs of infection including: fever, vomiting, loose stools, or bad GI discomfort between date of screening and donation day!
LOPERAMIDE (IMODIUM)
May be prescribed to recipients undergoing transplant via colonoscopy or enema.
Aim: Slow bowel movement of donor stool to optimize effect of healthy microbiota.
LAXATIVE
May be prescribed to help with bowel movement!
PPIs
May be prescribed in recipients undergoing transplant via Nasogastric placement.
Aim: Decrease acid production in stomach to avoid decreasing potency of donor organisms.
RISKS:
Overall, very safe! Abdominal discomfort, Self-limited diarrhea, weight gain, transmission of infection (rare).
Reference: openbiome.org, https://www.hopkinsmedicine.org/health/treatment-tests-and-therapies/fecal-transplant

Figure 23.12. Recipient and donor preparations for fecal microbiota transplantation. General guidelines and expectations set for recipients and donors leading up to FMT donation and reception. (From openbiome.org, https://www.hopkinsmedicine.org/health/treatment-tests-and-therapies/fecal-transplant. Reprinted with permission.)

CONCLUDING REMARKS

The four tenets of osteopathy drive every element of patient care for osteopathic physicians. Osteopathic physicians are motivated to identify and treat the source of an issue for proper healing. By understanding the intricate relationship that disease has with the human body, an appropriate intervention can be chosen to return the system to normal rather than merely masking the side effects produced by the disease (Table 23.5).

Osteopathic physicians are dedicated to providing a holistic approach to patient care, therefore it is imperative that they include the health of the intestinal microbiome as a contributing factor in the prevention and treatment of clinical diseases. Individualized medical treatment approaches should include the intestinal microbiome, and when appropriate the local microbiome, as factors in the algorithm of care. Clinically-driven technologic advances will

TABLE 23.5

Tenets of Osteopathic Medicine

1. The body is a unit; the person is a unit of body, mind, and spirit.
2. The body is capable of self-regulation, self-healing, and health maintenance.
3. Structure and function are reciprocally interrelated.
4. Rational treatment is based upon an understanding of the basic principles of body unity, self-regulation, and the interrelationship of structure and function.

Osteopathic physicians adhere to the tenets of their profession, recognizing the importance of body, mind, and spirit in the health of the individual. Microorganisms and their participation in overall health are vital to the body's ability to heal itself.

continue to unveil the intricate communication between microorganisms and the host which can be employed to promote health and prevent disease for current and future generations.

ACKNOWLEDGMENTS

The authors would like to thank Ms. Sarah Quinlan for her assistance. Additionally, the authors and editors of this chapter would like to acknowledge the scholarly contributions of Drs. Robert Orenstein, Mihai Covasa, and Vishwanath Venketaraman for prior editions of this chapter.

REFERENCES

1. Wilkins LJ, Monga M, Miller AW. Defining dysbiosis for a cluster of chronic diseases. *Sci Rep.* 2019;9:12918.
2. Fan Y, Pedersen O. Gut microbiota in human metabolic health and disease. *Nat Rev Microbiol.* 2021;19(1):55–71.
3. Polak K, Bergler-Czop B, Szczepanek M, Wojciechowska K, Frątczak A, Kiss N. Psoriasis and gut microbiome—current state of the art. *Int J Mol Sci.* 2021;22(9):4529.
4. Mahmud MR, Akter S, Tamanna SK, et al. Impact of gut microbiome on skin health: gut-skin axis observed through the lenses of therapeutics and skin diseases. *Gut Microbes.* 2022;14(1):e2096995.
5. De Filippis F, Paparo L, Nocerino R, et al. Specific gut microbiome signatures and the associated pro-inflammatory functions are linked to pediatric allergy and acquisition of immune tolerance. *Nat Commun.* 2021;12:5958.
6. Hu W, Lu W, Li L, et al. Both living and dead *Faecalibacterium prausnitzii* alleviate house dust mite-induced allergic asthma through the modulation of gut microbiota and short-chain fatty acid production. *J Sci Food Agric.* 2021;101(13):5563–5573.
7. Chiu CY, Chan YL, Tsai MH, et al. Cross-talk between airway and gut microbiome links to IgE responses to house dust mites in childhood airway allergies. *Sci Rep.* 2020;10:13449.
8. Horta-Baas G, Romero-Figueroa M DS, Montiel-Jarquin AJ, Pizano-Zárate ML, García-Mena J, Ramírez-Durán N. Intestinal dysbiosis and rheumatoid arthritis: a link between gut microbiota and the pathogenesis of rheumatoid arthritis. *J Immunol Res.* 2017;2017:4835189.
9. He J, Chu Y, Li J, et al. Intestinal butyrate-metabolizing species contribute to autoantibody production and bone erosion in rheumatoid arthritis. *Sci Adv.* 2022;8(6):eabm1511.
10. Scher JU, Sczesnak A, Longman RS, et al. Expansion of intestinal Prevotella copri correlates with enhanced susceptibility to arthritis. *Elife.* 2013;2:e01202.
11. Cryan JF, Mazmanian SK. Microbiota–brain axis: context and causality. *Science.* 2022;376(6595):938–939.
12. Needham BD, Funabashi M, Adame MD, et al. A gut-derived metabolite alters brain activity and anxiety behaviour in mice. *Nature.* 2022; 602(7898):647–653.
13. Lynch SV, Pedersen O. The human intestinal microbiome in health and disease. *N Engl J Med.* 2016;375(24):2369–2379.
14. Marchesi JR, Ravel J. The vocabulary of microbiome research: a proposal. *Microbiome.* 2015;3:31.
15. Bordenstein SR, Theis KR. Host biology in light of the microbiome: ten principles of holobionts and hologenomes. *PLoS Biol.* 2015; 13(8):e1002226.
16. Zilber-Rosenberg I, Rosenberg E. Role of microorganisms in the evolution of animals and plants: the hologenome theory of evolution. *FEMS Microbiol Rev.* 2008;32:723–735.
17. Lloyd-Price J, Abu-Ali G, Huttenhower C. The healthy human microbiome. *Genome Med.* 2016;8:51.
18. Allaband C, McDonald D, Vazquez-Baeza Y, et al. Microbiome 101: studying, analyzing, and interpreting gut microbiome data for clinicians. *Clin Gastroenterol Hepatol.* 2019;17(2):218–230.
19. Gilbert J, Blaser MJ, Caporaso G, Jansson JK, Lynch SV, Knight R. Current understanding of the human microbiome. *Nat Med.* 2018;24(4): 392–400.
20. Lambring CB, Siraj S, Patel K, Sankpal UT, Mathew S, Basha R. Impact of the microbiome on the immune system. *Crit Rev Immunol.* 2019;39(5):313–328.
21. Berg G, Rybakova D, Fischer D, et al. Microbiome definition re-visited: old concepts and new challenges. *Microbiome.* 2020;8:103.
22. Ley RE, Peterson DA, Gordon JI. Ecological and evolutionary forces shaping microbial diversity in the human intestine. *Cell.* 2006;124:837–848.
23. Lozupone CA, Stombaugh JI, Gordon JI, Jansson JK, Knight R. Diversity, stability and resilience of the human gut microbiota. *Nature.* 2012;489(7415):220–230.
24. David LA, Maurice CF, Carmody RN, et al. Diet rapidly and reproducibly alters the human gut microbiome. *Nature.* 2014;505(7484):559–563.
25. Song SJ, Lauber C, Costello EK, et al. Cohabiting family members share microbiota with one another and with their dogs. *Elife.* 2013;2:e00458.
26. Human Microbiome Project Consortium. Structure, function, and diversity of the healthy human microbiome. *Nature.* 2012;486:207–214.
27. Gonzalez A, Vazquez-Baeza Y, Knight R. SnapShot: the human microbiome. *Cell.* 2014;158(3):690–690.e1.
28. Frank DN, Feazel LM, Bessesen MT, Price CS, Janoff EN, Pace NR. The human nasal microbiota and *Staphylococcus aureus* carriage. *PloS One.* 2010;5(5):e10598.
29. Oh J, Byrd AL, Deming C, et al. Biogeography and individuality shape function in the human skin metagenome. *Nature.* 2014;514(7520):59–64.
30. Zhou Y, Mihindukulasuriya KA, Gao H, et al. Exploration of bacterial community classes in major human habitats. *Genome Biol.* 2014;15:R66.
31. Man WH, de Steenhuijsen Piters WAA, Bogaert D. The microbiota of the respiratory tract: gatekeeper to respiratory health. *Nat Rev Microbiol.* 2017;15:259–270.
32. Chen M, He S, Miles P, et al. Nasal bacterial microbiome differs between healthy controls and those with asthma and allergic rhinitis. *Front Cell Infect Microbiol.* 2022;12:841995.
33. DiBaise JK, Zhang H, Crowell MD, Krajmalnik-Brown R, Decker GA, Rittmann BE. Gut microbiota and its possible relationship with obesity. *Mayo Clin Proc.* 2008;83(4):460–469.
34. Martinez-Guryn K, Leone V, Chang EB. Regional diversity of the gastrointestinal microbiome. *Cell Host Microbe.* 2019;26(3):314–324.
35. Byrd AL, Belkaid Y, Segre JA. The human skin microbiome. *Nat Rev Microbiol.* 2018;16:143–155.
36. Chen C, Song X, Wei W, et al. The microbiota continuum along the female reproductive tract and its relation to uterine-related diseases. *Nat Commun.* 2017;8:875.
37. Neugent ML, Hulyalkar NV, Nguyen VH, Zimmern PE, De Nisco NJ. Advances in understanding the human urinary microbiome and its potential role in urinary tract infection. *mBio.* 2020;11:e00218–e00220.
38. Knight R, Vrbanac A, Taylor BC, et al. Best practices for analysing microbiomes. *Nat Rev Microbiol.* 2018;16 (7);410–422.
39. Beghini F, McIver LJ, Blanco-Míguez A, et al. Integrating taxonomic, functional, and strain-level profiling of diverse microbial communities with bioBakery 3. *eLife.* 2021;10:e65088.
40. Bolyen E, Rideout JR, Dillon MR, et al. Reproducible, interactive, scalable and extensible microbiome data science using QIIME 2. *Nat Biotechnol.* 2019;37(8):852–857.

41. McMurdle PJ, Holmes S. PhyloSeq: an R package for reproducible interactive analysis and graphics of microbiome census data. *PlosOne.* 2013;8(4): e61217.
42. Meslier V, Qjuinquis B, DaSilva K, et al. Benchmarking second and third-generation sequencing platforms for microbial metagenomics. *Sci Data.* 2022;9(1):694.
43. Kim CY, Ma J, Lee I. HiFi metagenomic sequencing enables assembly of accurate and complete genomes from human gut microbiota. *Nat Commun.* 2022;13(1):6367.
44. Eren AM, Esen OC, Quince C, et al. Anvi'o: an advanced analysis and visualization platform for 'omics' data. *PeerJ.* 2015;3:e1319.
45. Meyer F, Bagchi S, Chaterji S, et al. MG-RAST version 4—lessons learned from a decade of low-budget ultra-high-throughput metagenome analysis. *Brief Bioinform.* 2019;20(4):1151–1159.
46. Lagier JC, Dubourg G, Million M, et al. Culturing the human microbiota and culturomics. *Nat Rev Microbiol.* 2018;16:540–550.
47. Long S, Yang Y, Shen C, et al. Metaproteomics characterizes human gut microbiome function in the colorectal cancer. *NPJ Biofilms Microbiomes.* 2020;6(1):14.
48. Zhang X, Li L, Butcher J, Stintzi A, Figeys D. Advancing functional and translational microbiome research using meta-omics approaches. *Microbiome.* 2019;7:154.
49. Zhang X, Ning Z, Mayne J, et al. MetaPro-IQ: a universal metaproteomic approach to studying human and mouse gut microbiota. *Microbiome.* 2016;4:31.
50. Heyer R, Schallert K, Zoun R, Becher B, Saake G, Benndorf D. Challenges and perspectives of metaproteomic data analysis. *J Biotechnol.* 2017;261:24–36.
51. Starr AE, Deeke Sa, Li L, et al. Proteomic and metaproteomic approaches to understand host-microbe interactions. *Anal Chem.* 2018;90:88–109.
52. Tian Y, Zhang L, Wang Y, Tang H. Age-related topographical metabolic signatures for the rat gastrointestinal contents. *J Proteome Res.* 2012; 11:1397–1411.
53. Chassaing B, Compher C, Bonhomme B, et al. Randomized controlled-feeding study of dietary emulsifier carboxymethylcellulose reveals detrimental impacts on the gut microbiota and metabolome. *Gastroenterology.* 2022;162(3):743–756.
54. Melnik AV, da Silva RR, Hyde ER, et al. Coupling targeted and untargeted mass spectrometry for metabolome-micobiome-wide association studies of human fecal samples. *Anal Chem.* 2017;89:7549–7559.
55. Escobar-Zapeda A, Godoy-Lozano EE, Raggi L, et al. Analysis of sequencing strategies and tools for taxonomic annotation: defining standards for progressive metagenomics. *Sci Rep.* 2018;8:12034.
56. Liu Y, Wang Y, Ni Y, et al. Gut microbiome fermentation determines the efficacy of exercise for diabetes prevention. *Cell Metab.* 2020;31: 77–91.
57. McCoubrey LE, Thomaidou S, Elbedawi M, Gaisford S, Orlu M, Basit AW. Machine learning predicts drug metabolism and bioaccumulation by intestinal microbiota. *Pharmaceutics.* 2021;13:2001.
58. Cammarota G, Ianiro G, Ahern A, et al. Gut microbiome, big data and machine learning to promote precision medicine for cancer. *Nat Rev Gastroenterol Hepatol.* 2020;17(10):635–648.
59. Unal M, Bostanci E, Ozkul C, Acici K, Asuroglu T, Guzel MS. Crohn's disease prediction using sequence based machine learning analysis of human microbiome. *Diagnostics.* 2023;13(17):2835.
60. Dominguez-Bello MG, Good-Vitorino F, Knight R, Blaser MJ. Role of the microbiome in human development. *Gut.* 2019;1108–1114.
61. Yatsunenko T, Rey FE, Manary MJ, et al. Human gut microbiome viewed across age and geography. *Nature.* 2012;486:222–228.
62. Tun HM, Bridgeman SL, Chari R, et al. Roles of birth mode and infant gut microbiota in intergenerational transmission of overweight and obesity from mother to offspring. *JAMA Pediatr.* 2018;172(4):368–377.
63. Backhed F, Roswall J, Peng Y, et al. Dynamics and stabilization of the human gut microbiome during the first year of life. *Cell Host & Microbe.* 2015;17:690–703.
64. Combellick JL, Shin H, Shin D, et al. Differences in the fecal microbiota of neonates born at home or in the hospital. *Sci Rep.* 2018;8:15660.
65. Perez-Muñoz ME, Arrieta MC, Ramer-Tait AE, Walter J. A critical assessment of the "sterile womb" and "in utero colonization" hypotheses: implications for research on the pioneer infant microbiome. *Microbiome.* 2017;5:48.
66. Borghi E, Massa V, Severgnini M, et al. Antenatal microbial colonization of mammalian gut. *Reprod Sci.* 2019;26(8):1045–1053.
67. Nagpal R, Tsuji H, Takahaski T, et al. Sensitive quantitative analysis of the meconium bacterial microbiota in healthy term infants born vaginally or by cesarean section. *Front Microbiol.* 2016;7:1997.
68. Hansen R, Scott KP, Khan S, et al. First-pass meconium samples from healthy term vaginally-delivered neonates: an analysis of the microbiota. *PLoS One.* 2015;10:e0133320.
69. Liu CJ, Liang X, Niu ZY, et al. Is the delivery mode a critical factor for the microbial communities in the meconium? *EBioMedicine.* 2019;49: 354–363.
70. Dominguez-Bello MG, Costello EK, Contreras M, et al. Delivery mode shapes the acquisitions and structure of the initial microbiota across multiple body habitats in newborns. *Proc Natl Acad Sci U S A.* 2010;107(26):11971–11975.
71. Dos Santos SJ, Pakzad A, Albert AYK, et al. Maternal vaginal microbiome composition does not affect development of the infant gut microbiome early in life. *Front Cell Infect Microbiol.* 2023;13:1144254.
72. Asnicar F, Manara S, Zolfo M, et al. Studying vertical microbiome transmission from mothers to infants by strain-level metagenomic profiling. *mSystems.* 2017;2(1):e00164–16.
73. Martley M, Woolcott CG, Langley JM, Brown MM, Ashley-Martin J, Kuhle S. Birth by caesarean section and otitis media in childhood: a retrospective cohort study. *Sci Rep.* 2020;10:5219.
74. Kikuchi J, Ranjit A, Jiang W, Witkop C, Hamlin L, Koehlmoos TP. Early childhood outcomes among infants born by vaginal birth after cesarean and repeat cesarean delivery in the military health system. *Mil Med.* 2021; 186:e1124–e1128.
75. Korvel-Hanquist A, Koch A, Lous J, Olsen SF, Homøe P. Risk of childhood otitis media with focus on potentially modifiable factors: a Danish follow-up cohort study. *Int J Pediatr Otorhinolaryngol.* 2018;106:1–9.
76. Auger N, Soullane S, Luu TM, Lee GE, Wei SQ, Quach C. Association of cesarean delivery with childhood hospitalization for infections before 13 years of age. *J Pediatr.* 2021;231:178–184.
77. Dominguez-Bello MG, De Jesus-Laboy KM, Shen N, et al. Partial restoration of the microbiota of cesarean-born infants via vaginal microbial transfer. *Nat Med.* 2016;22(3):250–253.
78. Liu Y, Li HT, Zhou SJ, et al. Effects of vaginal seeding on gut microbiota, body mass index, and allergy risks in infants born through cesarean delivery: a randomized clinical trial. *Am J Obstet Gynecol MFM.* 2023; 5(1):100793.
79. Ronan V, Yeasin R, Claud EC. Childhood development and the microbiome: the intestinal microbiota in maintenance of health and development of disease during childhood development. *Gastroenterology.* 2021; 160(2):495–506.
80. Walker WA. The importance of appropriate initial bacterial colonization of the intestine in newborn, child and adult health. *Pediatr Res.* 2017;82(3):387–395.
81. Ballard O, Morrow AL. Human milk composition: nutrients and bioactive factors. *Pediatr Clin North Am.* 2013;60(1):49–74.
82. Jost T, Lacroix C, Braegger C, Chassard C. Impact of human milk bacteria and oligosaccharides on neonatal gut microbiota establishment and gut health. *Nutr Rev.* 2015;73(7):426–437.
83. Notarbartolo V, Giuffrè M, Montante C, Corsello G, Carta M. Composition of human breast milk microbiota and is role in children's health. *Pediatr Gastroenterol Hepatol Nutr.* 2022;25(3):194–210.
84. Garcia-Ricobaraza M, García-Santos JA, Escudero-Marin M, Diéguez E, Cerdó T, Campoy C. Short- and long-term implications of human milk microbiota on maternal and child health. *Int J Mol Sci.* 2021;22:11866.
85. Stinson LF, Ma J, Lai CT, Rea A, Perrella SL, Geddes DT. Milk microbiome transplantation: recolonizing donor milk with mother's own milk microbiota. *Appl Microbiol Biotechnol.* 2024;108:74.
86. Zwierz A, Domagalski K, Masna K, Walentowicz P, Burduk P. Impact of breastfeeding duration on adenoid hypertrophy, snoring and acute otitis media: a case-control study in preschool children. *J Clin Med.* 2023;12:7683.
87. Bowatte G, Tham R, Allen KJ, et al. Breastfeeding and childhood acute otitis media: a systematic review and meta-analysis. *Acta Paediatr.* 2015;104:85–95.

88. Al-Nawaiseh FK, Al-Jaghbir MT, Al-Assaf MS, Al-Nawaiseh HK, Alzoubi MM. Breastfeeding initiation and duration and acute otitis media among children less than two years of age in Jordan: results from a case-control study. *BMC Pediatr.* 2022;22:370.
89. Kørvel-Hanquist A, Kock A, Lous J, Olsen SF, Homøe P. Risk of childhood otitis media with focus on potentially modifiable factors: a Danish follow-up cohort study. *Int J Pediatr Otorhinolaryngol.* 2018;106:1–9.
90. Turroni F, Milani C, Duranti S, et al. Bifidobacteria and the infant gut: an example of co-evolution and natural selection. *Cell Mol Life Sci.* 2018;75:103–118.
91. Zivkovic AM, German JG, Lebrilla CB, Mills DA. Human milk glycobiome and its impact on the infant gastrointestinal microbiota. *Proc Natl Acad Sci U S A.* 2011;108(Suppl 1):4653–4658.
92. Pacheco AR, Barile D, Underwood MA, Mills DA. The impact of the milk glycobiome on the neonate gut microbiota. *Annu Rev Anim Biosci.* 2015;3:419–445.
93. Planer JD, Peng Y, Kau AL, et al. Development of the gut microbiota and mucosal IgA responses in twins and gnotobiotic mice. *Nature.* 2016;534:263–266.
94. Cong X, Xu W, Janton S, et al. Gut microbiome developmental patterns in early life of preterm infants: impacts of feeding and gender. *PloS One.* 2016;11:e0152751.
95. Wernroth ML, Peura S, Hedman AM, et al. Development of gut microbiota during the first 2 years of life. *Sci Reports.* 2022;12:9080.
96. De Muinck EJ, Trosvik P. Individuality and convergence of the infant gut microbiota during the first year of life. *Nat Commun.* 2018;9:2022.
97. Kawamoto S, Maruya M, Kato LM, et al. Foxp3(+) T cells regulate immunoglobulin A selection and facilitate diversification of bacterial species responsible for immune homeostasis. *Immunity.* 2014;41: 152–65.
98. Robak OH, Heimesaat MM, Kruglov AA, et al. Antibiotic treatment-induced secondary IgA deficiency enhances susceptibility to *Pseudomonas aeruginosa* pneumonia. *J Clin Invest.* 2018;128:3535–3545.
99. Nikawa T, Odahara K, Koizumi H, et al. Vitamin A prevents the decline in immunoglobulin A and Th2 cytokine levels in small intestinal mucosa of protein-malnourished mice. *J Nutr.* 1999;129:934–941.
100. Wu W, Sun M, Chen F, et al. Microbiota metabolite short-chain fatty acid acetate promotes intestinal IgA response to microbiota which is mediated by GPR43. *Mucosal Immunol.* 2017;10:946–956.
101. Kim MH, Kang SG, Park JH, Yanagisawa M, Kim CH. Short-chain fatty acids activate GPR41 and GPR43 on intestinal epithelial cells to promote inflammatory responses in mice. *Gastroenterology.* 2013;145:396–406.e10.
102. Yeaman MR, Yount NY. Mechanisms of antimicrobial peptide action and resistance. *Pharmacol Rev.* 2003;55:27–55.
103. Cullen T, Schofield W, Barry N, et al. Gut microbiota. Antimicrobial peptide resistance mediates resilience of prominent gut commensals during inflammation. *Science.* 2015;347:170–175.
104. Datta A., Ghosh A., Airoldi C, et al. Antimicrobial peptides: insights into membrane permeabilization, lipopolysaccharide fragmentation and application in plant disease control. *Sci Rep.* 2015;5:11951.
105. Wehkamp J, Harder J, Weichenthal M, et al. Inducible and constitutive β-defensins are differentially expressed in Crohn's Disease and ulcerative colitis. *Inflamm Bowel Dis.* 2003;9(4):215–223.
106. Nancey S, Bienvenu J, Coffin B, Andre F, Descos L, Flourié B. Butyrate strongly inhibits *in vitro* stimulated release of cytokines in blood. *Dig Dis Sci.* 2002;47:921–928.
107. Cavaglieri CR, Nishiyama A, Fernandes LC, Curi R, Miles EA, Calder PC. Differential effects of short-chain fatty acids on proliferation and production of pro- and anti-inflammatory cytokines by cultured lymphocytes. *Life Sci.* 2003;73:1683–1690.
108. Smith PM, Howitt MR, Panikov N, et al. The microbial metabolites, short-chain fatty acids, regulate colonic Treg cell homeostasis. *Science.* 2013;341:569–573.
109. Russo P, López P, Capozzi V, et al. Beta-glucans improve growth, viability and colonization of probiotic microorganisms. *Int J Mol Sci.* 2012; 13:6026–6039.
110. Miyamoto J, Watanabe K, Taira S, et al. Barley β-glucan improves metabolic condition via short-chain fatty acids produced by gut microbial fermentation in high fat diet fed mice. *PLoS One.* 2018;13:e0196579.
111. Lee C, Verma R, Byun S, et al. Structural specificities of cell surface β-glucan polysaccharides determine commensal yeast mediated immunomodulatory activities. *Nat Commun.* 2021;12:3611.
112. Kumpitsch C, Koskinen K, Schöpf V, Moissl-Eichinger C. The micobiome of the upper respiratory tract in health and disease. *BMC Biology.* 2019;17:87.
113. Proctor DM, Relman DA. The landscape ecology and microbiota of the human nose, mouth, and throat. *Cell Host Microbe.* 2017;21:421–432.
114. Costello EK, Lauber CL, Hamady M, Fierer N, Gordon JI, Knight R. Bacterial community variation in human body habitats across space and time. *Science.* 2009;326:1694–1697.
115. Mika M, Mack I, Korten I, et al. Dynamics of the nasal microbiota in infancy: a prospective cohort study. *J Allergy Clin Immunol.* 2015;135: 905–912.e11.
116. Toto-Ascuy D, Cárdenas JP, Zorondo-Rodriguez F, et al. Microbiota profile of the nasal cavity according to lifestyles in healthy adults in Santiago, Chile. *Microorganisms.* 2023;11:1635.
117. Basis CM, Tang AL, Young VB, Pynnonen MA. The nasal cavity microbiota of healthy adults. *Microbiome.* 2014;2:27.
118. Liu CM, Price LB, Hungate BA, et al. *Staphylococcus aureus* and the ecology of the nasal microbiome. *Sci Adv.* 2015;1:e1400216.
119. Camarinha-Silva A, Wos-Oxley ML, Jáuregui R, Becker K, Pieper DH. Validating T-RFLP as a sensitive and high-throughput approach to assess bacterial diversity patterns in the human anterior nares. *FEMS Microbiol Ecol.* 2012;79:98–108.
120. Wos-Oxley ML, Plumeier I, Von Eiff C, et al. A poke into the diversity and associations within human anterior nare microbial communities. *ISME J.* 2010;4:839–851.
121. Elgamal Z, Singh P, Geraghty P. The upper airway microbiota, environmental exposures, inflammation and disease. *Medicina (Kaunas).* 2021;57: 823.
122. Bomar L, Brugger SD, Yost BH, Davies SS, Lemon KP. *Corynebacterium accolens* releases antipneumococcal free fatty acids from human nostril and skin surface triacylglycerols. *MBio.* 206;7(1):e01725–15.
123. Yan M, Pamp SJ, Fukuyama J, et al. Nasal microenvironments and interspecific interactions influence nasal microbiota complexity and *S. aureus* carriage. *Cell Host Microbe.* 2013;14:631–640.
124. Lysenko ES, Ratner AJ, Nelson AL, Weiser JN. The role of innate immune responses in the outcome of interspecies competition for colonization of mucosal surfaces. *PloS Pathog.* 2005;1:e1.
125. Celedón JC, Milton DK, Ramsey CD, et al. Exposure to dust mite allergen and endotoxin in early life and asthma and atopy in childhood. *J Allergy Clin Immunol.* 2007;120:144–149.
126. Kim YS, Kim NH, Seong SY, Kim KR, Lee GB, Kim KS. Prevalence and risk factors of chronic rhinosinusitis in Korea. *Am J Rhinol Allergy.* 2011;25(3):117–121.
127. Schwitzguébel AJP, Jandus P, Lacroix JS, Seebach JD, Harr T. Immunoglobulin deficiency in patients with chronic rhinosinusitis: systematic review of the literature and meta-analysis. *J Allergy Clin Immunol.* 2015;136:1523–1531.
128. Petalas K, Goudakos J, Konstantinou GN. Targeting epithelium dysfunction and impaired nasal biofilms to treat immunological, functional, and structural abnormalities of chronic rhinosinusitis. *Int J Mol Sci.* 2023;24:12379.
129. Sedaghat AR. Chronic rhinosinusitis. *Am Fam Physician.* 2017;96(8): 500–506.
130. Loperfido A, Cavaliere C, Begvarfaj E, et al. The impact of antibiotics and steroids on the nasal microbiome in patients with chronic rhinosinusitis: a systematic review according to PICO criteria. *J Pers Med.* 2023;13:1583.
131. Gan W, Zhang H, Yang F, Liu S, Liu F, Meng J. The influence of nasal microbiome diversity and inflammatory patterns on the prognosis of nasal polyps. *Sci Rep.* 2021;11:6364.
132. Lee E, Lo J, Tran J, et al. Osteopathic manipulative treatment for sinusitis relief: a pilot study. *OFP.* 2022;14(2):10–14.
133. Dewhirst FE, Chen T, Izard J, et al. The human oral microbiome. *J Bacteriol.* 2010;192:5002–5017.
134. Human Microbiome Project Consortium. Structure, function and diversity of the healthy human microbiome. *Nature.* 2012;486:207–214.

135. Zhang Y, Wang X, Li H, Ni C, Du Z, Yan F. Human oral microbiota and its modulation for oral health. *Biomed Pharmacother.* 2018;99: 883–893.
136. Zarco MF, Vess TJ, Ginsburg GS. The oral microbiome in health and disease and the potential impact on personalized dental medicine. *Oral Dis.* 2012;18:109–120.
137. Welch JLM, Rossetti BJ, Rieken CW, Dewhirst FE, Borisy GG. Biogeography of a human oral microbiome at the micron scale. *Proc Natl Acad Sci U S A.* 2016;113:E791–E800.
138. Caselli E, Fabbri C, D'Accolti M, et al. Defining the oral microbiome by whole-genome sequencing and resistome analysis: the complexity of the healthy picture. *BMC Microbiol.* 2020;20:120.
139. Wilbert SA, Welch JLM, Borisy GG. Spatial ecology of the human tongue dorsum microbiome. *Cell Rep.* 2020;30:4003–4015.
140. Bowen WK, Burne RA, We H, Koo H. Oral biofilms: pathogens, matrix, and polymicrobial interactions in microenvironments. *Trends Microbiol.* 2018;26(3):229–242.
141. Graves DT, Corrêa JD, Silva TA. The oral microbiota is modified by systemic diseases. *J Dent Res.* 2019;98(2):148–156.
142. Voorhis A, Miranda-Sanchez F, Dewhirst FE, et al. Expanded human oral microbiome database V3.1. Accessed August 29, 2023.www.homd.org.
143. Eren AM, Borisy GG, Huse SE, Mark Welch JL. Oligotyping analysis of the human oral microbiome. *Proc Natl Acad Sci U S A.* 2014;111(28): E2875–E2884.
144. Lazarevic V, Whiteson K, Hernandez D, François P, Schrenzel J. Study of inter- and intra-individual variation in the salivary microbiota. *BMC Genomics.* 2010;11:523.
145. Bik EM, Long CD, Armitage GC, et al. Bacterial diversity in the oral cavity of ten healthy individuals. *ISME J.* 2010;4(8):962–974.
146. Aas JA, Pastor BJ, Stokes LN, Olsen I, Dewhirst FE. Defining the normal bacterial flora of the oral cavity. *J Clin Microbiol.* 2005;43(11): 5721–5732.
147. Valm AM. The structure of dental plaque microbial communities in the transition from health to dental caries and periodontal disease. *J Mol Biol.* 2019;431(16):2957–2969.
148. Ghannoum MA, Jurevic RJ, Mukherjee PK, et al. Characterization of the oral fungal microbiome (mycobiome) in healthy individuals. *PloS Pathog.* 2010;6(1):e1000713.
149. Shrivastava A, Patel VK, Tang Y, Yost SC, Dewhirst FE, Berg HC. Cargo transport shapes the spatial organization of a microbial community. *Proc Natl Acad Sci U S A.* 2018;115 (34):8633–8638.
150. Abusleme L, Dupuy AK, Dutzan N, et al. The subgingival microbiome in health and periodontitis and its relationship with community biomass and inflammation. *ISME J.* 2013;7:1016–1025.
151. Sanz M, Beighton D, Curtis MA, et al. Role of microbial biofilms in the maintenance of oral health and in the development of dental caries and periodontal diseases. Consensus report of group 1 of the Joint EFP/ ORCA workshop on the boundaries between caries and periodontal disease. *J Clin Periodontol.* 2017;44(Suppl 18):S5–S11.
152. Marcy Y, Ouverney C, Bik EM, et al. Dissecting biological "dark matter" with single-cell genetic analysis of rare and uncultivated TM7 microbes from the human mouth. *Proc Natl Acad Sci U S A.* 2007;104 (29): 11889–11894.
153. Hajishengallis G. Periodontitis: from microbial immune subversion to systemic inflammation. *Nat Rev Immunol.* 2015;15:30–44.
154. Socransky SS, Haffajee AD, Cugini MA, Smith C, Kent RL Jr. Microbial complexes in subgingival plaque. *J Clin Periodotol.* 1998;25:134–144.
155. Maekawa T, Krauss JL, Abe T, et al. *Porphyromonas gingivalis* manipulates complement and TLR signaling to uncouple bacterial clearance from inflammation and promote dysbiosis. *Cell Host Microbe.* 2014;15:768–778.
156. Lamont RJ, Koo H, Hajishengallis G. The oral microbiota: dynamic communities and host interactions. *Nat Rev Microbiol.* 2018;16(12): 745–659.
157. Griffen AL, Beall CJ, Campbell JH, et al. Distinct and complex bacterial profiles in human periodontitis and health revealed by 16s pyrosequencing. *ISME J.* 2012;6:1176–1185.
158. Shang L, Deng D, Buskermolen JK, et al. Multi-species oral biofilm promotes reconstructed human gingiva epithelial barrier function. *Sci Rep.* 2018;8(1):16061.
159. Tanner ACR, Kressirer CA, Rothmiller S, Johansson I, Chalmers NI. The caries microbiome: implications for reversing dysbiosis. *Adv Dent Res.* 2018;29(1):78–85.
160. Liu Y, Daniel SG, Kim H-E, et al. Addition of cariogenic pathogens to complex oral microflora drives significant changes in biofilm compositions and functionalities. *Microbiome.* 2023;11:123.
161. Xiao C, Ran S, Huang Z, et al. Bacterial diversity and community structure of supragingival plaques in adults with dental health or caries revealed by 16s pyrosequencing. *Front Microbiol.* 2016;7:1145.
162. Notarbartolo V, Giuffrè M, Montante C, Corsello G, Carta M. Composition of human breast milk microbiota and its role in children's health. *Pediatr Gastroenterol Hepatol Nutr.* 2022;25(3):194–210.
163. Arishi RA, Lai CT, Geddes DT, Stinson LF. Impact of breastfeeding and other early-life factors on the development of the oral microbiome. *Front Microbiol.* 2023;14:1236601.
164. World Health Organization. Breastfeeding. Accessed March 24, 2024. https://www.who.int/health-topics/breastfeeding#tab=tab_1
165. Kharouba J, Mansour S, Ratson T, Naishlos S, Weissman G, Blumer S. Knowledge of breastfeeding mothers regarding caries prevention in toddlers. *Children.* 2023;10:136.
166. Tham R, Bowatte G, Dharmage SC, et al. Breastfeeding and the risk of dental caries: a systematic review and meta-analysis. *Acta Paediatr.* 2015;104(467):62–84.
167. Khan SY, Schroth RJ, de Jesus VC, et al. A systematic review of caries risk in children <6 years of age. *Int J Paediatr Dent.* 2023;00:1–22.
168. Akpan A, Morgan R. Oral candidiasis. *Postgrad Med J.* 2002;78(922): 455–459.
169. Montelongo-Jauregui D, Lopez-Ribot JL. Candida interactions with the oral bacterial microbiota. *J Fungi (Basel).* 2018;4:122.
170. Vila T, Sultan AS, Montelongo-Jauregui D, Jabra-Rizk MA. Oral candidiasis: a disease of opportunity. *J Fungi (Basel).* 2020;6(1):15.
171. Brzezińska-Zając A, Sycińska-Dziarnowska M, Spagnuolo G, Szyszka-Sommerfeld L, Woźniak K. *Candida* species in children undergoing orthodontic treatment with removable appliances: A pilot study. *Int J Environ Res Public Health.* 2023;20:4824.
172. Shenoy A, Gottlieb A. Probiotics for oral and vulvovaginal candidiasis: a review. *Dermatol Ther.* 2019;32:312970.
173. Fokam J, Nka AD, Semengue NJ, et al. Characterization of oral candidiasis according to antiretroviral treatment status, immunological and virological profiles amount HIV infected patients in two health facilities in Yaounde-Cameroon: a cross-sectional and analytical study. *Pan Afr Med J.* 2023;44:33
174. Mohammadi F, Charkhchian M, Mirzadeh M. Phenotypic and genotypic characterization of virulence markers and antifungal susceptibility of oral Candida species from diabetic and non-diabetic hemodialysis patients. *BMC Oral Health.* 2023;23:261.
175. Akram Z, Al-Kheraif AA, Kellesarian SV, Vohra F, Javed F. Comparison of oral *Candida* carriage in waterpipe smokers, cigarette smokers, and non-smokers. *J Oral Sci.* 2018;60(1):115–120.
176. Hellstein JW, Marek CL. Candidiasis: red and white manifestations in the oral cavity. *Head Neck Pathol.* 2019;13(1):25–32.
177. Lewis M, Williams D. Diagnosis and management of oral candidosis. *Br Dent J.* 2017;223 (9), 675–681.
178. Irfan M, Delgado RZR, Frias-Lopez J. The oral microbiome and cancer. *Front Immunol.* 2020;11:591088.
179. Kapila YL. Oral health's inextricable connection to systemic health: special populations bring to bear multimodal relationships and factors connecting periodontal disease to systemic diseases and conditions. *Periodontol 2000.* 2021;87:11–16.
180. Dominy SS, Lynch C, Ermini F, et al. *Phophyromonas gingivalis* in Alzheimer's disease brains: evidence for disease causation and treatments with small-molecule inhibitors. *Sci Adv.* 2019;5:eaau3333.
181. Ryder MI, Xenoudi P. Alzheimer disease and the periodontal patient: new insights, connections, and therapies. *Periodontol 2000.* 2021;87:32–42.
182. Pattatoni C, Watzenboeck ML, Schneidegger S, et al. Early-life formation of the microbial and immunological environment of the human airways. *Cell Host Microbe.* 2018;24(6):857–865.e4.
183. Marsland BJ, Trompette A, Gollwitzer ES. The gut–lung axis in respiratory disease. *Ann Am Thorac Soc.* 2015;12(Suppl 2):S150–S156.

184. Dang AT, Marsland BJ. Microbes, metabolites, and the gut-lung axis. *Mucosal Immunol.* 2019;12(4):843–850.
185. Morris A, Beck JM, Schloss PD, et al; Lung HIV Microbiome Project. Comparison of the respiratory microbiome in healthy nonsmokers and smokers. *Am J Respir Crit Care Med.* 2013;187(10):1067–1075.
186. Remien K, Woo MJ, Vilella RC. Osteopathic manipulative treatment: lymphatic procedures. [Updated 2024 January 29]. In: *StatPearls [Internet]*. StatPearls Publishing; 2024. https://www.ncbi.nlm.nih.gov/books/NBK559051
187. Mogayzel PJ, Naureckas ET, Robinson KA, et al; Pulmonary Clinical Practice Guidelines Committee. Cystic fibrosis pulmonary guidelines chronic medications for maintenance of lung health. *Am J Respir Crit Care Med.* 2013;187(7):680–689.
188. van Dorst JM, Tam RY, Ooi CY. What do we know about the microbiome in cystic fibrosis? Is there a role for probiotics and prebiotics? *Nutrients.* 2022;14(3):480.
189. Fouhy, F, Ronan, NJ, O'Sullivan, O, et al. A pilot study demonstrating the altered gut microbiota functionality in stable adults with cystic fibrosis. *Sci Rep.* 2017;7:6685.
190. Di Nardo, G, Oliva, S, Menichella, A, et al. *Lactobacillus reuteri* ATCC55730 in cystic fibrosis. *J Pediatr Gastroenterol Nutr.* 2014;58(1):81–86.
191. von Mutius E, Vercelli D. Farm living: effects on childhood asthma and allergy. *Nat Rev Immunol.* 2010;10:861–868.
192. Ridler J, Braun-Fahrländer C, Eder W, et al. Exposure to farming in early life and development of asthma and allergy: a cross-sectional survey. *Lancet.* 2001;358:1129–1133.
193. Stein MM, Hrusch CL, Gozdz J, et al. Innate immunity and asthma risk in Amish and Hutterite farm children. *N Engl J Med.* 2016;375:411–421.
194. Biasucci G, Rubini M, Riboni S, Morelli L, Bessi E, Retetangos C. Mode of delivery affects the bacterial community in the newborn gut. *Early Hum Dev.* 2010;86:13–15.
195. Sirilun S, Takahashi H, Boonyaritichaikij S, et al. Impact of maternal Bifidobacteria and the mode of delivery on Bifidobacterium microbiota in infants. *Benef Microbes.* 2015;6:767–774.
196. Jakobsson HE, Abrahamsson TR, Jenmalm MC, et al. Decreased gut microbiota diversity, delayed Bacteroidetes colonisation and reduced Th1 responses in infants delivered by caesarean section. *Gut.* 2014;63:559–66.
197. Ozdemir O. Various effects of different probiotic strains in allergic disorders: an update from laboratory and clinical data. *Clin Exp Immunol.* 2010;160:295–304.
198. Lynch NR, Medouze L, DiPrisco-Fuenmayor MC, Verde O, López RI, Malavé C. Incidence of atopic disease in a tropical environment: partial independence from intestinal helminthiasis. *J Allergy Clin Immunol.* 1984;73:229–233.
199. Yazdanbakhsh M, Kremsner PG, van Ree R. Allergy, parasites, and the hygiene hypothesis. *Science.* 2002;296:490–494.
200. Masters S, Barrett-Connor E. Parasites and asthma-predictive or protective? *Epidemiologic Rev.* 1985;7:49–58.
201. Beasley R. Worldwide variation in prevalence of symptoms of asthma, allergic rhinoconjunctivitis, and atopic eczema: ISAAC. *Lancet.* 1998;351(9111):1225–1232.
202. Bäckhed F, Ley RE, Sonnenburg JL, Peterson DA, Gordon JI. Host-bacterial mutualism in the human intestine. *Science.* 2005;307:1915–1920.
203. Jumpstart Consortium Human Microbiome Project Data Generation Working Group. Evaluation of 16S rDNA-based community profiling for human microbiome research. *PLoS One.* 2012;7:e39315.
204. Tropini C, Earle KA, Huang KC, Sonnenburg JL. The gut microbiome: connecting spatial organization to function. *Cell Host Microbe.* 2017;21(4):433–442.
205. Vasapolli R, Schütte K, Schulz C, et al. Analysis of transcriptionally active bacteria throughout the gastrointestinal tract of healthy individuals. *Gastroenterol.* 2019;157:1081–1092.
206. Ruan W, Engevik MA, Spinler JK, Versalovic J. Healthy human gastrointestinal microbiome: composition and function after a decade of exploration. *Dig Dis Sci.* 2020;65:695–705.
207. Berry D, Stecher B, Schintlmeister A, et al. Host-compound foraging by intestinal microbiota revealed by single-cell stable isotope probing. *Proc Natl Acad Sci U S A.* 2013;110:4720–4725.
208. Albenberg L, Esipova TV, Judge CP, et al. Correlation between intraluminal oxygen gradient and radial partitioning of intestinal microbiota. *Gastroenterol.* 2014;147:1055–1063.
209. Shetty SA, Hugenholtz F, Lahti L, Smidt H, de Vos WM. Intestinal microbiome landscaping: insight in community assemblage and implications for microbial modulation strategies. *FEMS Microbiol Rev.* 2017;41:182–199.
210. Gu S, Chen D, Zhang JN, et al. Bacterial community mapping of the mouse gastrointestinal tract. *PLoS One.* 2013;8(10):e74957.
211. Sundin OH, Mendoza-Ladd A, Zeng M, et al. The human jejunum has an endogenous microbiota that differs from those in the oral cavity and colon. *BMC Microbiol.* 2017;17:160.
212. Seedorf H, Griffin NW, Ridaura VK, et al. Bacteria from diverse habitats colonize and compete in the mouse gut. *Cell.* 2014;159:253–266.
213. Fusco W, Lorenzo MB, Cintoni M, et al. Short-chain fatty-acid–producing bacteria: key components of the human gut microbiota. *Nutrients.* 2023;15:2211.
214. Peng L, Li ZR, Green RS, Holzman IR, Lin J. Butyrate enhances the intestinal barrier by facilitating tight junction assembly via activation of AMP-activated protein kinase in Caco-2 cell monolayers. *J Nutr.* 2009;139:1619–1625.
215. Said HM. Recent advances in transport of water-soluble vitamins in organs of the digestive system: a focus on the colon and the pancreas. *Am J Physiol Gastrointest Liver Physiol.* 2013;305(9):G601–G610.
216. Magnúsdóttir S, Ravcheev D, de Crécy-Lagard V, Thiele I. Systematic genome assessment of B-vitamin biosynthesis suggests co-operation among gut microbes. *Front Genet.* 2015;6:148.
217. Cryan JF, O'Riordan KJ, Cowan CSM, et al. The microbiota-gut-brain axis. *Physiol Rev.* 2019;99:1877–2013.
218. Sarkar A, Lehto SM, Harty S, Dinan TG, Cryan JF, Burnet PWJ. Psychobiotics and the manipulation of bacteria-gut-brain signals. *Trends Neurosci.* 2016;39(11):763–781.
219. Barrio C, Arias-Sanchez A, Martín-Monzón I. The gut microbiota-brain axis, psychobiotics and its influence on brain and behavior: a systematic review. *Psychoneuroendocrinology.* 2022;137:105640.
220. Baxter NT, Schmidt AW, Venkataraman A, Kim KS, Waldron C, Schmidt TM. Dynamics of human gut microbiota and short-chain fatty acids in response to dietary interventions with three fermentable fibers. *mBio.* 2019;10:e02566–18.
221. Vendrik KEW, Ooijevaar RE, DeJong PRC, et al. Fecal microbiota transplantation in neurological disorders. *Front Cell Infect Microbiol.* 2020;10:98.
222. Moussaoui N, Jacobs JP, Larauche M, et al. Chronic early-life stress in rat pups alters basal corticosterone, intestinal permeability, and fecal microbiota at weaning: influence of sex. *J Neurogastroenterol Motil.* 2017;23(1):135–143.
223. Kiecolt-Glaser JK, Wilson SJ, Bailey ML, et al. Marital distress, depression, and a leaky gut: translocation of bacterial endotoxin as a pathway to inflammation. *Psychoneuroendocrinology.* 2018;98:52–60.
224. Cryan JF, Dinan TG. Mind-altering microorganisms: the impact of the gut microbiota on brain and behaviour. *Nat Rev.* 2012;13:701–712.
225. Van Hemert S, Breedveld AC, Rovers JM, et al. Migraine associated with gastrointestinal disorders: review of the literature and clinical implications. *Front Neurol.* 2014;5:241.
226. Pascale A, Marchesi N, Govoni S, Barbieri A. Targeting the microbiota in pharmacology of psychiatric disorders. *Pharmacol Res.* 2020;157:104856.
227. Strandwitz P. Neurotransmitter modulation by the gut microbiota. *Brain Res.* 2018;1693(pt B):128–133.
228. Yano JM, Yu K, Donaldson GP, et al. Indigenous bacteria from the gut microbiota regulate host serotonin biosynthesis. *Cell.* 2015;161:264–276.
229. Fukumoto S, Tatewaki M, Yamada T, et al. Short-chain fatty acids stimulate colonic transit via intraluminal 5-HT release in rats. *Am J Physiol Regul Integr Comp Physiol.* 2003;284(5):R1269–R1276.
230. Dinan TG, Stilling RM, Stanton C, Cryan JF. Collective unconscious: how gut microbes shape human behavior. *J Psychiatr Res.* 2015;63:1–9.
231. Agus A, Planchais J, Sokol H. Gut microbiota regulation of tryptophan metabolism in health and disease. *Cell Host Microbe.* 2018;23(6):716–724.

232. Pokusaeva K, Johnson C, Luk B, et al. GABA-producing *Bifiobacterium dentium* modulates visceral sensitivity in the intestine. *Neurogastroenerol Motil.* 2017;29:e12904.
233. Barrett E, Ross RP, O'Toole PW, Fitzgerald GF, Stanton C. γ-Aminobutyric acid production by culturable bacteria from the human intestine. *J Appl Microbiol.* 2012;113:411–417.
234. Janik R, Thomason LAM, Stanisz AM, Forsythe P, Bienenstock J, Stanisz GJ. Magnetic resonance spectroscopy reveals oral *Lactobacillus* promotion of increases in brain GABA, N-acetyl aspartate and glutamate. *Neuroimage.* 2016;125:988–995.
235. Tette RM, Kwofie SK, Wilson MD. Therapeutic anti-depressant potential of microbial GABA produced by *Lactobacillus rhamnosus* strains for GABAergic signaling restoration and inhibition of addiction-induced HPA axis hyperactivity. *Curr Issues Mol Biol.* 2022;44:1434–1451.
236. Altaib H, Kozakai T, Badr Y, et al. Cell factory for γ-aminobutryic acid (GABA) production using *Bifidobacterium adolescentis. Microb Cell Fact.* 2022;21:33.
237. Bravo JA, Forsythe P, Chew MV, et al. Ingestion of Lactobacillus strain regulates emotional behavior and central GABA receptor expression in a mouse via the vagus nerve. *Proc Natl Acad Sci U S A.* 2011;108(38):16050–16055.
238. Matsumoto M, Kibe R, Ooga T, et al. Cerebral low-molecular metabolites influenced by intestinal microbiota: a pilot study. *Front Syst Neurosci.* 2013;7:9.
239. Boonstra E, de Kleijn R, Colzato LS, Alkemade A, Forstmann BU, Nieuwenhuis S. Neurotransmitters as food supplements: the effects of GABA on brain and behavior. *Front Psychol.* 2015;6:1520.
240. Hamamah S, Aghazarian A, Nazaryan A, Hajnal A, Covasa M. Role of microbiota-gut-brain axis in regulating dopaminergic signaling. *Biomedicines.* 2022;10(2):436.
241. Rehman MU, Ghazanfar S, Haq RU, et al. Probiotics (*Bacillus clausii* and *Lactobacillus fermentum* NMCC-14) ameliorate stress behavior in mice by increasing monoamine levels and mRNA expression of dopamine receptors (D1 and D2) and synaptophysin. *Front Pharmacol.* 2022;13:915595.
242. Asano Y, Hiramoto T, Nishino R, et al. Critical role of gut microbiota in the production of biologically active, free catecholamines in the gut lumen of mice. *Am J Physiol Gastrointest Liver Physiol.* 2012;303:G1288–G1295
243. Braniste V, Al-Asmakh M, Kowal C, et al. The gut microbiota influences blood-brain-barrier permeability in mice. *Sci Transl Med.* 2014; 6(263):263ra158.
244. Azpiroz F, Dubray C, Bernalier-Donadille A, et al. Effects of scFOS on the composition of fecal microbiota and anxiety in patients with irritable bowel syndrome: a randomized, double-blind, placebo-controlled study. *Neurogastroenterol Motil.* 2017;29:e12911.
245. Wallace CJK, Milev T. The effects of probiotics on depressive symptoms in humans: a systematic review. *Ann Gen Psychiatry.* 2017;16:14.
246. Rudzki L, Ostrowska L, Pawlak D, et al. Probiotic *Lactobacillus plantarum 299v* decreases kynurenine concentration and improves cognitive functions in patients with major depression: a double-blind, randomized, placebo-controlled study. *Psychoneuroendocrinology.* 2019;100:213–222.
247. Ridlon JM, Kang DJ, Hylemon PB, Bajaj JS. Bile acids and the gut microbiome. *Curr Opin Gastroenterol.* 2014;30(3):332–338.
248. Guzior DV, Quinn RA. Review: microbial transformations of human bile acids. *Microbiome.* 2021;9:140.
249. Heinken A, Ravcheev DA, Baldini F, Heirendt L, Fleming RMT, Thiele I. Systematic assessment of secondary bile acid metabolism in gut microbes reveals distinct metabolic capabilities in inflammatory bowel disease. *Microbiome.* 2019;7:75.
250. McElhanon BO, McCracken C, Karpen S, Sharp WG. Gastrointestinal symptoms in autism spectrum disorder: a meta-analysis. *Pediatrics.* 2014;133:872–883.
251. Buie T, Fuchs GR III, Furuta GT, et al. Recommendations for evaluation and treatment of common gastrointestinal problems in children with ASDs. *Pediatrics.* 2010;125(suppl 1):S19–S29.
252. Rodakis J. An n=1 case report of a child with autism improving on antibiotics and a father's quest to understand what it may mean. *Microb Ecol Health Dis.* 2015;26:26382.
253. Bundgaard-Nielsen C, LauritsenMB, Knudsen JK, et al. Children and adolescents with attention deficit hyperactivity disorder and autism spectrum disorder share distinct microbiota compositions. *Gut Microbes.* 2023;15(1):2211923.
254. Grimaldi R, Gibson GR, Vulevic J, et al. A prebiotic intervention study in children with autism spectrum disorders (ASDs). *Microbiome.* 2018;6:133.
255. deMagistris L, Familiari V, Pasotto A, et al. Alterations of the intestinal barrier in patients with autism spectrum disorder and their first-degree relatives. *J Pediatr Gastroenterol Nutr.* 2010;51(4):418–424.
256. Adams JB, Johansen LJ, Powell LD, Quig D, Rubin RA. Gastrointestinal flora and gastrointestinal status in children with autism-comparisons to typical children and correlation with autism severity. *BMC Gastroenterol.* 2011;11:22.
257. Sun H, You Z, Jia L, Wang F. Autism spectrum disorder is associated with gut microbiota disorder in children. *BMC Pediatr.* 2019;19:516.
258. Needham BD, Adame MD, Serena G, et al. Plasma and fecal metabolite profiles in autism spectrum disorder. *Bio Psychiatry.* 2021;89(5):451–461.
259. Altieri L, Neri C, Sacco R, et al. Urinary *p*-cresol is elevated in small children with severe autism spectrum disorder. *Biomarkers.* 2011;16(3):252–260.
260. DeAngelis M, Piccolo M, Vannini L, et al. Fecal microbiota and metabolome of children with autism and pervasive developmental disorder not otherwise specified. *PloS One.* 2013;8(10):e76993.
261. Saito Y, Sato T, Nomoto K, Tsuji H. Identification of phenol- and p-cresol-producing intestinal bacteria by using media supplemented with tyrosine and its metabolites. *FEMS Microbiol Ecol.* 2018;94:fiy125.
262. Zheng Y, Bek MK, Prince NZ, et al. The role of bacterial-derived aromatic amino acids metabolites relevant in autism spectrum disorders: a comprehensive review. *Front Neurosci.* 2021;15:738220.
263. Lobzhanidze G, Japaridze N, Lordkipanidze T, Rzayev F, MacFabe D, Zhvania M. Behavioural and brain ultrastructural changes following the systemic administration of propionic acid in adolescent male rats. Further development of a rodent model of autism. *Intl J Dev Neurosci.* 2020;80(2):139–156.
264. Slattery J, MacFabe DF, Kahler SG, Frye RE. Enteric ecosystem disruption in autism spectrum disorder: can the microbiota and macrobiota be restored? *Curr Pham Des.* 2016;22:6107–6121.
265. Kwak MJ, Kim SH, Kim HH, et al. Psychobiotics and fecal microbial transplantation for autism and attention-deficit/hyperactivity disorder: microbiome modulation and therapeutic mechanisms. *Front Cell Infect Microbiol.* 2023;13:1238005.
266. Mancini JD, Yao S, Martinez LR, Shakil H, Li TS. Gut microbiome changes with osteopathic treatment of constipation in Parkinson's disease: a pilot study. *Neurology.* 2021;13(2):19–33.
267. Tansey MG, Wallings RL, Houser MC, Herrick MK, Keating CE, Joers V. Inflammation and immune dysfunction in Parkinson disease. *Nat Rev Immunol.* 2022;22(11):657–673.
268. Savica R, Carlin JM, Grossardt BR, et al. Medical records documentation of constipation preceding Parkinson disease: a case-control study. *Neurology.* 2009;73:1752–1758.
269. McComick D. Managing costs and care for chronic idiopathic constipation. *Am J Manag Care.* 2019;25:S63–S69.
270. Scheperjans F, Aho V, Pereira PAB, et al. Gut microbiota are related to Parkinson's disease and clinical phenotype. *Mov Disord.* 2015;30: 350–358.
271. Romano S, Savva GM, Bedarf JR, Charles IG, Hildebrand F, Narbad A. Meta-analysis of the Parkinson's disease gut microbiome suggests alterations linked to intestinal inflammation. *NPJ Parkinsons Dis.* 2021;7:27.
272. Aho VTE, Pereira PAB, Voutilainen S, et al. Gut microbiota in Parkinson's disease: temporal stability and relations to disease progression. *EBioMedicine.* 2019;44:691–707.
273. Almeida KA, de Queiroz Andrade E, Burns G, et al, The microbiota in eosinophilic esophagitis: a systematic review. *J Gastroenterol Hepatol.* 2022;37:1673–1684.
274. Furuta GT, Fillon SA, Williamson KM, et al. Mucosal microbiota associated with eosinophilic esophagitis and eosinophilic gastritis. *J Pediatr Gastroenterol Nutr.* 2023;76(3):347–354.
275. Catassi C, Verdu EF, Bai JC, Lionetti E. Coeliac disease. *Lancet.* 2022;399:2413–2426.
276. Stsepetova J, Simre K, Tagoma A, et al. Maternal breast milk microbiota and immune markers in relation to subsequent development of celiac disease in offspring. *Sci Rep.* 2022;12:6607.

277. Constante M, Libertucci J, Galipeau HJ, et al. Biogeographic variation and functional pathways of the gut microbiota in celiac disease. *Gastroenterology.* 2022;163:1351–1363.
278. Galipeau HJ, McCarville JI, Huebener S, et al. Intestinal microbiota modulates gluten-induced immunopathology in humanized mice. *Am J Pathol.* 2015;185(11):2969–2982.
279. Nadal I, Donant E, Ribes-Koninckx C, Calabuig M, Sanz Y. Imbalance in the composition of the duodenal microbiota of children with coeliac disease. *J Med Microbiol.* 2007;56(Pt 12):1669–1674. Erratum in: *J Med Microbiol.* 2008;57(Pt 3):401. Donant, Esther [corrected to Donat, Ester].
280. Collado MC, Donat E, Ribes-Koninckx C, Calabuig M, Sanz Y. Imbalances in faecal and duodenal Bifidobacterium species composition in active and non-active coeliac disease. *BMC Microbiol.* 2008;8:232
281. De Palma G, Nadal I, Medina M, et al. Intestinal dysbiosis and reduced immunoglobulin-coated bacteria associated with coeliac disease in children. *BMC Microbiol.* 2010;10:63.
282. Nieuwenhuizen WF, Pieters RH, Knippels LM, Jansen MC, Koppelman SJ. Is *Candida albicans* a trigger in the onset of coeliac disease? *Lancet.* 2003;361(9375):2152–2154.
283. De Palma G, Cinova J, Stepankova R, Tuckova L, Sanz Y. Pivotal advance: Bifidobacteria and gram-negative bacteria differentially influence immune responses in the proinflammatory milieu of celiac disease. *J Leukoc Biol.* 2010;87(5):765–778.
284. de Almeida NEC, Esteves FG, Dos Santos-Pinto JRA, et al. Digestion of intact gluten proteins by Bifidobacterium species: reduction of cytotoxicity and proinflammatory responses. *J Agric Food Chem.* 2020;68(15): 4485–4492.
285. Devkota S, Wang Y, Musch MW, et al. Dietary-fat-induced taurocholic acid promotes pathobiont expansion and colitis in Il10$^{-/-}$ mice. *Nature.* 2012;487(7405):104–108.
286. Nishida A, Inoue R, Inatomi O, Bamba S, Naito Y, Andoh A. Gut microbiota in the pathogenesis of inflammatory bowel disease. *Clin J Gastroenterol.* 2018;11(1):1–10.
287. Caparrós E, Wiest R, Scharl M, et al. Dysbiotic microbiota interactions in Crohn's disease. *Gut Microbes.* 2021;13(1):1949096.
288. Sokol H, Leducq V, Aschard H, et al. Fungal microbiota dysbiosis in IBD. *Gut.* 2017;66(6):1039–1048.
289. Li XV, Leonardi I, Putzel GG, et al. Immune regulation by fungal strain diversity in inflammatory bowel disease. *Nature.* 2022;603(7902):672–678. Erratum in: *Nature.* 2022;608(7922):E21.
290. Kedia S, Virmani S, Vuyyuru SK, et al. Faecal microbiota transplantation with anti-inflammatory diet (FMT-AID) followed by anti-inflammatory diet alone is effective in inducing and maintaining remission over 1 year in mild to moderate ulcerative colitis: a randomised controlled trial. *Gut.* 2022;71(12):2401–2413.
291. Costello SP, Hughes PA, Waters O, et al. Effect of fecal microbiota transplantation on 8-week remission in patients with ulcerative colitis: a randomized clinical trial. *JAMA.* 2019;321(2):156–164.
292. El Hage Chehade N, Ghoneim S, Shah S, et al. Efficacy of fecal microbiota transplantation in the treatment of active ulcerative colitis: a systematic review and meta-analysis of double-blind randomized controlled trials. *Inflamm Bowel Dis.* 2023;29(5):808–817.
293. Zhou S, Cui Y, Zhang Y, Zhao T, Cong J. Fecal microbiota transplantation for induction of remission in Crohn's disease: a systematic review and meta-analysis. *Int J Colorectal Dis.* 2023;38(1):62.
294. Xiong J, Liao XS, Yin T, Liu XC, Bao L, Li LQ. Alterations of the gut microbiota and short chain fatty acids in necrotizing enterocolitis and food protein-induced allergic protocolitis infants: a prospective cohort study. *Front Cell Infect Microbiol.* 2022;12:1030588.
295. Xia J, Claud EC. Gut microbiome-brain axis as an explanation for the risk of poor neurodevelopment outcome in preterm infants with necrotizing enterocolitis. *Microorganisms.* 2023;11:1035.
296. Nino DF, Sodhi CP, Hackam DJ. Necrotizing enterocolitis: new insights into pathogenesis and mechanisms. *Nat Rev Gastroenterol Hepatol.* 2016;13:590–600.
297. Neu J, Walker WA. Necrotizing enterocolitis. *N Engl J Med.* 2011;364:255–264.
298. Mai V, Young CM, Ukhanova M, et al. Fecal microbiota in premature infants prior to necrotizing enterocolitis. *PLoS ONE.* 2011;6:e20647.
299. Wang Y, Hoenig, JD, Malin KJ, et al. 16S rRNA gene-based analysis of fecal microbiota from preterm infants with and without necrotizing enterocolitis. *ISME J.* 2009;3:944–954.
300. Zhou Y, Shan G, Sodergren E, Weinstock G, Walker WA, Gregory KE. Longitudinal analysis of the premature infant intestinal microbiome prior to necrotizing enterocolitis: a case-control study. *PLoS ONE.* 2015;10:e0118632.
301. Bin-Nun A, Bromiker R, Wilschanski M, et al. Oral probiotics prevent necrotizing enterocolitis in very low birth weight neonates. *J Pediatr.* 2005;147:192–196.
302. Hoyos AB. Reduced incidence of necrotizing enterocolitis associated with enteral administration of *Lactobacillus acidophilus* and *Bifidobacterium infantis* to neonates in an intensive care unit. *Int J Infect Dis.* 1999;3: 197–202.
303. Lin H-C, Hsu C-H, Chen H-L, et al. Oral probiotics prevent necrotizing enterocolitis in very low birth weight preterm infants: a multicenter, randomized, controlled trial. *Pediatrics.* 2008;122:693–700.
304. Lin H-C, Su B-H, Chen A-C, et al. Oral probiotics reduce the incidence and severity of necrotizing enterocolitis in very low birth weight infants. *Pediatrics.* 2005;115:1–4.
305. Gopalakrishna KP, Macadangdang, BR, Rogers MB, et al. Maternal IgA protects against the development of necrotizing enterocolitis in preterm infants. *Nat Med.* 2019;25:1110–1115.
306. Shiou SR, Yu Y, Chen S, et al. Erythropoietin protects intestinal epithelial barrier function and lowers the incidence of experimental neonatal necrotizing enterocolitis. *J Biol Chem.* 2011;286:12123–12132.
307. Meinzen-Derr J, Poindexter B, Wrage L, Morrow AL, Stoll B, Donovan EF. Role of human milk in extremely low birth weight infants' risk of necrotizing enterocolitis or death. *J Perinatol.* 2009;29:57–62.
308. Lawson MAE, O'Neill IJ, Kujawska M, et al. Breast milk-derived human milk oligosaccharides promote Bifidobacterium interactions within a single ecosystem. *ISME J.* 2020;14:635–648.
309. Liou AP, Paziuk M, Luevano JM Jr, Machineni S, Turnbaugh PJ, Kaplan LM. Conserved shifts in the gut microbiota due to gastric bypass reduce host weight and adiposity. *Sci Transl Med.* 2013;5(178):178ra41.
310. Ley RE, Bäckhed F, Turnbaugh P, Lozupone CA, Knight RD, Gordon JI. Obesity alters gut microbial ecology. *Proc Natl Acad Sci U S A.* 2005; 102(31):11070–11075.
311. Turnbaugh PJ, Hamady M, Yatsunenko T, et al. A core gut microbiome in obese and lean twins. *Nature.* 2009;457:480–484.
312. Kaplan RC, Wang Z, Usyk M, et al. Gut microbiome composition in the Hispanic Community Health Study/Study of Latinos is shaped by geographic relocation, environmental factors, and obesity. *Genome Biol.* 2019;20:219.
313. Leone V, Gibbons SM, Martinez K, et al. Effects of diurnal variation of gut microbes and high-fat feeding on host circadian clock function and metabolism. *Cell Host Microbe.* 2015;17:681–689.
314. Martinez-Guryn K, Hubert N, Frazier K, et al. Small intestine microbiota regulate host digestive and absorptive adaptive responses to dietary lipids. *Cell Host Microbe.* 2018;23:458–469.e5.
315. Turnbaugh PJ, Bäckhed F, Fulton L, Gordon JI. Diet-induced obesity is linked to marked but reversible alterations in the mouse distal gut microbiome. *Cell Host Microbe.* 2008;3:213–223.
316. Xu Z, Jiang W. Huang W, Lin Y, Chan FKL, Ng SC. Gut microbiota in patients with obesity and metabolic disorders-a systematic review. *Genes Nutr.* 2022;17:2.
317. Poteres E, Hubert N, Poludasu S, et al. Selective regional alteration of the gut microbiota by diet and antibiotics. *Front Physiol.* 2020;11:797.
318. Alang N, Kelly CR. Weight gain after fecal microbiota transplant. *Open Forum Infect Dis.* 2015;2(1):ofv004.
319. Vrieze A, Van Nood E, Holleman F, et al. Transfer of intestinal microbiota from lean donors increases insulin sensitivity in individuals with metabolic syndrome. *Gastroenterology.* 2012;143:913–6.e7.
320. Turnbaugh P, Ley R, Mahowald M, Magrini V, Mardis ER, Gordon JI. An obesity-associated gut microbiome with increased capacity for energy harvest. *Nature.* 2006;444(7122):1027–1031.
321. Van den Abbeele P, Belzer C, Goossens M, et al. Butyrate-producing *Clostridium* cluster XIVa species specifically colonize mucins in an *in vitro* gut model. *ISME J.* 2013;7:949–961.

322. Ríos-Covián D, Ruas-Madiedo P, Margolles A, Gueimonde M, de Los Reyes-Gavilán CG, Salazar N. Intestinal short chain fatty acids and their link with diet and human health. *Front Microbiol.* 2016;7:185.
323. Liu KH, Owens JA, Saeedi B, et al. Microbial metabolite delta-valerobetaine is a diet-dependent obesogen. *Nat Metab.* 2021;3(12):1694–1705.
324. Depommier C, Everard A, Druart C, et al. Supplementation with *Akkermansia muciniphila* in overweight and obese human volunteers: a proof-of-concept exploratory study. *Nat Med.* 2019;25(7):1096–1103.
325. Rabot S, Membrez M, Gerard P, et al. Germ-free C57BL /6J mice are resistant to high-fat-diet-induced insulin resistance and have altered cholesterol metabolism. *FASEB J.* 2010;24(12):4948–4959.
326. Hooper LV, Wong MH, Thelin A, Hansson L, Falk PG, Gordon JI. Molecular analysis of commensal host-microbial relationships in the intestine. *Science.* 2001;291(5005):881–884.
327. Semova I, Carten JD, Stombaugh J, et al. Microbiota regulate intestinal absorption and metabolism of fatty acids in the zebrafish. *Cell Host Microbe.* 2012;12(3):277–288.
328. Kuang Z, Wang Y, Li Y, et al. The intestinal microbiota programs diurnal rhythms in host metabolism through histone deacetylase 3. *Science.* 2019;365(6460):1428–1434.
329. Wang Y, Kuang Z, Yu X, Ruhn KA, Kubo M, Hooper LV. The intestinal microbiota regulates body composition through NFIL3 and the circadian clock. *Science.* 2017;357(6354):912–916.
330. Bäckhed F, Ding H, Wang T, et al. The gut microbiota as an environmental factor that regulates fat storage. *Proc Natl Acad Sci U S A.* 2004; 101:15718–15723.
331. Mohammad S, Thiemermann C. Role of metabolic endotoxemia in systemic inflammation and potential interventions. *Front Immunol.* 2021;11:594150.
332. Lassenius MI, Pietiläinen KH, Kaartinen K, et al. Bacterial endotoxin activity in human serum is associated with dyslipidemia, insulin resistance, obesity, and chronic inflammation. *Diabetes Care.* 2011;34(8):1809–1815.
333. Trikha SRJ, Lee DM, Ecton KE, et al. Transplantation of an obesity-associated human gut microbiota to mice induces vascular dysfunction and glucose intolerance. *Gut Microbes.* 2021;13(1):1940791.
334. Ruuskanen MO, Åberg F, Männistö V, et al. Links between gut microbiome composition and fatty liver disease in a large population sample. *Gut Microbes.* 2021;13:1–22.
335. Hoyles L, Fernandez-Real JM, Federici M, et al. Molecular phenomics and metagenomics of hepatic steatosis in non-diabetic obese women. *Nat Med.* 2018;24:1070–1080.
336. Sharifnia T, Antoun J, Verriere TGC, et al. Hepatic TLR4 signaling in obese NAFLD. *Am J Physiol Gastrointest Liver Physiol.* 2015;309:G270–G278.
337. Hsu CL, Schnabl, B. The gut–liver axis and gut microbiota in health and liver disease. *Nat Rev Microbiol.* 2023;21(11):719–733.
338. Oh TG, Kim SM, Caussy C, et al. A universal gut-microbiome–derived signature predicts cirrhosis. *Cell Metab.* 2020;32(5):878–888.e6.
339. Aron-Wisnewsky J, Vigliotti C, Witjes J, et al. Gut microbiota and human NAFLD: disentangling microbial signatures from metabolic disorders. *Nat Rev Gastroenterol Hepatol.* 2020;17(5):279–297.
340. Fei N, Miyoshi S, Hermanson JB, et al. Imbalanced gut microbiota predicts and drives the progression of nonalcoholic fatty liver disease and nonalcoholic steatohepatitis in a fast-food diet mouse model. *bioRxiv.* 2023: 2023.01.09.523249.
341. Le Roy T, Llopis M, Lepage P, et al. Intestinal microbiota determines development of non-alcoholic fatty liver disease in mice. *Gut.* 2013; 62:1787–1794.
342. Zhang X, Coker OO, Chu ES, et al. Dietary cholesterol drives fatty liver-associated liver cancer by modulating gut microbiota and metabolites. *Gut.* 2021;70:761–774.
343. Xue L, Deng Z, Luo W, He X, Chen Y. Effect of fecal microbiota transplantation on non-alcoholic fatty liver disease: a randomized clinical trial. *Front Cell Infect Microbiol.* 2022;12:759306.
344. Craven L, Rahman A, Parvathy N, et al. Allogenic fecal microbiota transplantation in patients with nonalcoholic fatty liver disease improves abnormal small intestinal permeability: a randomized control trial. *Am J Gastroenterol.* 2020;115(7):1055–1065.
345. Osborn LJ, Schultz K, Massey W, et al. A gut microbial metabolite of dietary polyphenols reverses obesity-driven hepatic steatosis. *Proc Natl Acad Sci U S A.* 2022;119(48):e2202934119.
346. Sharpton SR, Maraj B, Harding-Theobald E, Vittinghoff E, Terrault NA. Gut microbiome–targeted therapies in nonalcoholic fatty liver disease: a systematic review, meta-analysis, and meta-regression. *Am J Clin Nutr.* 2019;110(1):139–149.
347. Smith MI, Yatsunenko T, Manary MJ, et al. Gut microbiomes of Malawian twin pairs discordant for Kwashiorkor. *Science.* 2013;339(6119): 548–54.
348. Subramanian S, Huq S, Yatsunenko T, et al. Persistent gut microbiota immaturity in malnourished Bangladeshi children. *Nature.* 2014;510: 417–421.
349. Reyes A, Blanton LV, Cao S, et al. Gut DNA viromes of Malawian twins discordant for severe acute malnutrition. *Proc Natl Acad Sci U S A.* 2015;112(38):11941–11946.
350. Blanton LV, Charbonneau MR, Salih T, et al. Gut bacteria that prevent growth impairments transmitted by microbiota from malnourished children. *Science.* 2016;351(6275):10.1126/science.aad3311 aad3311.
351. Hibberd MC, Wu M, Rodionov DA, et al. The effects of micronutrient deficiencies on bacterial species from the human gut microbiota. *Sci Transl Med.* 2017;9(390):eaal4069.
352. Gehrig JL, Venkatesh S, Chang HW, et al. Effects of microbiota-directed foods in gnotobiotic animals and undernourished children. *Science.* 2019;365(6449):eaau4732.
353. Chen RY, Mostafa I, Hibberd MC, et al. A microbiota-directed food intervention for undernourished children. *N Engl J Med.* 2021;384(16): 1517–1528.
354. Tang WHW, Wang Z, Levison BS, et al. Intestinal microbial metabolism of phosphatidylcholine and cardiovascular risk. *N Engl J Med.* 2013;368(17):1575–1584.
355. Brown JM, Hazen SL. The gut microbial endocrine organ: bacterially derived signals driving cardiometabolic diseases. *Annu Rev Med.* 2015; 66:343–359.
356. Koeth RA, Wang Z, Levison BS, et al. Intestinal microbiota metabolism of L-carnitine, a nutrient in red meat, promotes atherosclerosis. *Nat Med.* 2013;19(5):576–585.
357. Robinson WH, Lepus CM, Wang Q, et al. Low-grade inflammation as a key mediator of the pathogenesis of osteoarthritis. *Nat Rev Rheumatol.* 2016;12(10):580–592.
358. Wang Q, Rozelle AL, Lepus CM, et al. Identification of a central role for complement in osteoarthritis. *Nat Med.* 2011;17(12):1674–1679.
359. Longo UG, Lalli A, Bandini B, et al. Role of the gut microbiota in osteoarthritis, rheumatoid arthritis, and spondylarthritis: an update on the gut-joint axis. *Int J Mol Sci.* 2024;25:3242.
360. Marchese L, Contartese D, Giavaresi G, Di Sarno L, Salamanna F. The complex interplay between the gut microbiome and osteoarthritis: a systematic review on potential correlations and therapeutic approaches. *Int J Mol Sci.* 2024;25:143.
361. Favazzo LJ, Hendesi H, Villani DA, et al. The gut microbiome-joint connection: implications in osteoarthritis. *Curr Opin Rheumatol.* 2020; 32(1):92–101.
362. Chen C, Zhang Y, Yao X, et al. Characterizations of the gut bacteriome, mycobiome, and virome in patients with osteoarthritis. *Microbiol Spectr.* 2023;11(1):e0171122.
363. Zhao Y, Chen B, Li S, et al. Detection and characterization of bacterial nucleic acids in culture-negative synovial tissue and fluid samples from rheumatoid arthritis or osteoarthritis patients. *Sci Rep.* 2018; 8:14305.
364. Jespers V, Menten J, Smet H, et al. Quantification of bacterial species of the vaginal microbiome in different groups of women, using nucleic acid amplification tests. *BMC Microbiol.* 2012;12:83.
365. Ravel J, Gajer P, Abdo Z, et al. Vaginal microbiome of reproductive-age women. *Proc Natl Acad Sci U S A.* 2011;108(Suppl 1):4680–4687.
366. Mirmonsef P, Modur S, Burgad D, et al. An exploratory comparison of vaginal glycogen and *Lactobacillus* levels in pre- and post-menopausal women. *Menopause.* 2015;22(7):702–709.
367. Stoyancheva G, Marzotto M, Dellaglio F, Torriani S. Bacteriocin production and gene sequencing analysis from vaginal Lactobacillus strains. *Arch Microbiol.* 2014;196:645–653.
368. Gajer P, Brotman RM, Bai G, et al. Temporal dynamics of the human vaginal microbiota. *Sci Trans Med.* 2012;4(132):132ra52.

369. Romero R, Hassan SS, Gajer P, et al. The composition and stability of the vaginal microbiota of normal pregnant women is different from that of non-pregnant women. *Microbiome.* 2014;2:4.
370. Kwon MS, Lee HK. Host and microbiome interplay shapes the vaginal microenvironment. *Front Immunol.* 2022;13:919728.
371. Barrientos-Durán A, Fuentes-López A, de Salazar A, Plaza-Díaz J, García F. Reviewing the composition of vaginal microbiota: inclusion of nutrition and probiotic factors in the maintenance of eubiosis. *Nutrients.* 2020;12:419.
372. Brotman RM, He X, Gajer P, et al. Association between cigarette smoking and the vaginal microbiota: a pilot study. *BMC Infect Dis.* 2014;14:471.
373. Lehtoranta L, Ala-Jaakkola R, Laitila A, Maukonen J. Healthy vaginal microbiota and influence of probiotics across the female life span. *Front Microbiol.* 2022;13:819958.
374. Fredricks DN, Fiedler TL, Marrazzo JM. Molecular identification of bacteria associated with bacterial vaginosis. *N Engl J Med.* 2005;353:1899–1911.
375. Aagaard K, Riehle K, Ma J, et al. A metagenomic approach to characterization of the vaginal microbiome signature in pregnancy. *PloS One.* 2012;7(6):e36466.
376. Serrano MG, Parikh HI, Brooks JP, et al. Racioethnic diversity in the dynamics of the vaginal microbiome during pregnancy. *Nat Med.* 2019;25(6):1001–1011.
377. Freitas AC, Bocking A, Hill JE. Increased richness and diversity of the vaginal microbiota and spontaneous preterm birth. *Microbiome.* 2018;6:117.
378. Allsworth JE, Peipert JF. Severity of bacterial vaginosis and risk of sexually transmitted infection. *Am J Obstet Gynecol.* 2011;205(2):113.e1–113.e6.
379. Nieves-Ramírez ME, Partida-Rodríguez O, Moran P, et al. Cervical squamous intraepithelial lesions are associated with differences in the vaginal microbiota of Mexican women. *Microbiol Spectr.* 2021;9(2):e00143–21.
380. Zeng M, Xin L, Jiao X, et al. Roles of vaginal flora in human papillomavirus infection, virus persistence and clearance. *Front Cell Infect Microbiol.* 2023;12:1036869.
381. Oakley BB, Fiedler TL, Marrazzo JM, Fredricks DN. Diversity of human vaginal bacterial communities and associations with clinically defined bacterial vaginosis. *Appl Environ Microbiol.* 2008;74(15):4898–4909.
382. American College of Obstetrics and Gynecology. Vaginitis in nonpregnant patients: ACOG practice bulletin, number 215. *Obstet Gynecol.* 2020;135:e1–e17.
383. Chen X, Lu Y, Chen T, Li R. The female vaginal microbiome in health and bacterial vaginosis. *Front Cell Infect Microbiol.* 2021;11:631972.
384. Koumans EH, Sternberg M, Bruce C, et al. The prevalence of bacterial vaginosis in the United States, 2001–2004;associations with symptoms, sexual behaviors, and reproductive health. *Sex Transm Dis.* 2007;34(11):864–869.
385. Fethers KA, Fairley CK, Morton A, et al. Early sexual experiences and risk factors for bacterial vaginosis. *J Infect Dis.* 2009;200:1662–1670.
386. Allsworth JE, Peipert JF. Severity of bacterial vaginosis and the risk of sexually transmitted infection. *Am J Obstet Gynecol.* 2011;203(2):113.e1–113.e6.
387. Ignacio MAO MA, Buesso TS, Morales JAP, Silva MC, da Silva MG, Duarte MTC. Factors associated with bacterial vaginosis in women with homosexual, bisexual and heterosexual practices. *Braz J Infect Dis.* 2023;27(3):102760.
388. Hesham H, Mitchell AJ, Bergerat A, Hung K, Mitchell CM. Impact of vaginal douching products on vaginal *Lactobacillus*, *Escherichia coli*, and epithelial immune responses. *Sci Rep.* 2021;11:23069.
389. Nelson TM, Borgogna JC, Michalek RD, et al. Cigarette smoking is associated with an altered vaginal tract metabolomic profile. *Sci Rep.* 2018;8:852.
390. Esber A, Miguel RDV, Cherpes TL, Klebanoff MA, Gallo MF, Turner AN. Risk of bacterial vaginosis among women with herpes simplex virus type 2 infection: a systematic review and meta-analysis. *J Infect Dis.* 2015;212:8–17.
391. Hellberg D, Nilsson S, Mårdh PA. Bacterial vaginosis and smoking. *Int J STD AIDS.* 2000;11(9):603–606.
392. Ravel J, Moreno I, Simón C. Bacterial vaginosis and its association with infertility, endometritis, and pelvic inflammatory disease. *Am J Obstet Gynecol.* 2021;224(3):251–257.
393. Taylor BD, Darville T, Haggerty CL. Does bacterial vaginosis cause pelvic inflammatory disease? *Sex Transm Dis.* 2013;40(2):117–122.
394. Leitich H, Kiss H. Asymptomatic bacterial vaginosis and intermediate flora as risk factors for adverse pregnancy outcome. *Best Pract Res Clin Obstet Gynaecol.* 2007;21(3):375–390.
395. Abbe C, Mitchell CM. Bacterial vaginosis: a review of approaches to treatment and prevention. *Front Reprod Health.* 2023;5:1100029.
396. Sobel R, Sobel JD. Metronidazole for the treatment of vaginal infections. *Expert Opin Pharmacother.* 2015;16(7):1109–1115.
397. Fethers KA, Fairley CK, Hocking JS, Gurrin LC, Bradshaw CS. Sexual risk factors and bacterial vaginosis: a systematic review and meta-analysis. *Clin Infect Dis.* 2008;47(11):1426–1435.
398. Li C, Wang T, Li Y, et al. Probiotics for the treatment of women with bacterial vaginosis: a systematic review and meta-analysis of randomized clinical trials. *Eur J Pharmacol.* 2019;864:172660.
399. Lopez-Moreno A, Aguilera M. Vaginal probiotics for reproductive health and related dysbiosis: systematic review and meta-analysis. *J Clin Med.* 2021;10:1461.
400. Wolfe AJ, Toh E, Shibata N, et al. Evidence of uncultivated bacteria in the adult female bladder. *J Clin Microbiol.* 2012;50:1376–1383.
401. Nelson DE, Van Der Pol B, Dong Q, et al. Characteristic male urine microbiomes associate with asymptomatic sexually transmitted infection. *PLoS One.* 2010;5(11):e14116.
402. Kenneally C, Murphy CP, Sleator RD, Culligan EP. The urinary microbiome and biological therapeutics: novel therapies for urinary tract infections. *Microbiol Res.* 2022;259:127010.
403. Antunes-Lopes T, Vale L, Coelho AM, et al; EAU Young Academic Urologists (YAU) Functional Urology Working Group. The role of urinary microbiota in lower urinary tract dysfunction: a systematic review. *Eur Urol Focus.* 2020;6:361–369.
404. Foxman B. Urinary tract infection syndromes: occurrence, recurrence, bacteriology, risk factors, and disease burden. *Infect Dis Clin N Am.* 2014; 28:1–13.
405. Karstens L, Asquith M, Davin S, et al. Does the urinary microbiome play a role in urgency urinary incontinence and its severity? *Front Cell Infect Microbiol.* 2016;6:78.
406. Siddiqui NY, Ma L, Brubaker L, et al. Updating urinary microbiome analyses to enhance biologic interpretation. *Front Cell Infect Microbiol.* 2022;12:789439.
407. Karstens L, Asquith M, Caruso V, et al. Community profiling of the urinary microbiota: methodological considerations for low microbial biomass biological samples. *Nat Rev Urol.* 2018;15(12):735–749.
408. Stamm WE, Norrby SR. Urinary tract infections: disease panorama and challenges. *J Infect Dis.* 2001;183(Suppl 1):S1–S4.
409. Schappert SM, Rechsteiner EA. Ambulatory medical care utilization estimates for 2007. *Vital Health Stat.* 2011;13:1–38.
410. Long B, Koyfman A. The emergency department diagnosis and management of urinary tract infection. *Emerg Med Clinc N Am.* 2018;36:685–710.
411. Flores-Mireles AL, Walker JN, Caparon M, Hultgren SJ. Urinary tract infections: epidemiology, mechanisms of infection and treatment options. *Nat Rev Microbiol.* 2015;13(5):269–284.
412. Chu CM, Lowder JL. Diagnosis and treatment of urinary tract infections across age groups. *Am J Obstet Gynecol.* 2018;219(1); 40–51.
413. Mancuso G, Midiri A, Gerace E, Marra M, Zummo S, Biondo C. Urinary tract infections: the current scenario and future prospects. *Pathogens.* 2023;12:623.
414. Klein RD, Hultgren SJ. Urinary tract infections: microbial pathogenesis, host-pathogen interactions and new treatment strategies. *Nat Rev Microbiol.* 2020;18(4):211–226.
415. Schreiber HL, Conover MS, Chou WC, et al. Bacterial virulence phenotypes of *Escherichia coli* and host susceptibility determine risk for urinary tract infections. *Sci Transl Med.* 2017;9(382):eaaf1283.
416. Mulvey MA, Lopez-Boado YS, Wilson CL. Induction and evasion of host defenses by type 1-piliated uropathogenic *Escherichia coli. Science.* 1998;282:1494–1497.
417. Mulvey MA, Schilling JD, Hultgren SJ. Establishment of a persistent *Escherichia coli* reservoir during the acute phase of bladder infection. *Infect Immun.* 2001;69(7):4572–4579.
418. Gajdács M, Ábrók M, Lázár A, Burián K. Increasing relevance of Gram-positive cocci in urinary tract infections: a 10-year analysis of their prevalence and resistance trends. *Sci Rep.* 2020;10:17658.

419. Stapleton AE. Urinary tract infection pathogenesis: host factors. *Infect Dis Clin N Am.* 2014;28:149–159.
420. Morand A, Cornu F, Dufour JC, Tsimaratos M, Lagier JC, Raoult D. Human bacterial repertoire of the urinary tract: a potential paradigm shift. *J Clin Microbiol.* 2019;57(3):e00675–18.
421. Grice EA, Kong HH, Conlan S, et al. Topographical and temporal diversity of the human skin microbiome. *Science.* 2009;324(5931):1190–1192.
422. Findley K, Oh J, Yang J, et al. Topographic diversity of fungal and bacterial communities in human skin. *Nature.* 2013;498(7454):367–370.
423. Oh J, Conlan S, Polley EC, Segre JA, Kong HH. Shifts in human skin and nares microbiota of healthy children and adults. *Genome Med.* 2012;4(10):77.
424. Kalliomäki M, Salminen S, Arvilommi H, Kero P, Koskinen P, Isolauri E. Probiotics in primary prevention of atopic disease: a randomised placebo-controlled trial. *Lancet.* 2001;357(9262):1076–1079.
425. Totté JEE, Feltz WT, Hennekam M, van Belkum A, van Zuuren EJ, Pasmans SGMA. Prevalence and odds of *Staphylococcus aureus* carriage in atopic dermatitis: a systematic review and meta-analysis. *Br J Dermatol.* 2016;175:687–695.
426. Cau L, Williams MR, Butcher AM, et al. *Staphylococcus epidermidis* protease EcpA can be a deleterious component of the skin microbiome in atopic dermatitis. *J Allergy Clin Immunol.* 2020;147:955–966.e16.
427. Umborowati MA, Damayanti D, Anggraeni S, et al. The role of probiotics in the treatment of adult atopic dermatitis: a meta-analysis of randomized controlled trials. *J Heal Popul Nutr.* 2022;41:37.
428. Iemoli E, Trabattoni D, Parisotto S, Borgonovo L, Toscano M, Rizzardini G, et al. Probiotics reduce gut microbial translocation and improve adult atopic dermatitis. *J Clin Gastroenterol.* 2012;46(Suppl):S33–S40.
429. Buhaş MC, Gavrilaş LI, Candrea R, et al. Gut microbiota in psoriasis. *Nutrients.* 2022;14:2970.
430. Quan C, Chen X-Y, Li X, et al. Psoriatic lesions are characterized by higher bacterial load and imbalance between Cutibacterium and Corynebacterium. *J Am Acad Dermatol.* 2020;82:955–961.
431. Groeger D, O'Mahony L, Murphy EF, et al. *Bifidobacterium infantis* 35624 modulates host inflammatory processes beyond the gut. *Gut Microbes.* 2013;4:325–339.
432. Moludi J, Khedmatgozar H, Saiedi S, Razmi H, Alizadeh M, Ebrahimi B. Probiotic supplementation improves clinical outcomes and quality of life indicators in patients with plaque psoriasis: a randomized double-blind clinical trial. *Clin Nutr ESPEN.* 2021;46:33–39.
433. Valentini V, Silvestri V, Marraffa F, et al. Gut microbiome profile in psoriatic patients treated and untreated with biologic therapy. *J Dermatol.* 2021;48:786–793.
434. Hill C, Guarner F, Reid G. et al. Expert consensus document. The International Scientific Association for Probiotics and Prebiotics consensus statement on the scope and appropriate use of the term probiotic. *Nat Rev Gastroenterol Hepatol.* 2014;11:506–514.
435. Sanders ME, Merenstein DJ, Ouwehand AC, et al. Probiotic use in at-risk populations. *J Am Pharm Assoc (2003).* 2016;56:680–686.
436. Jenickova E, Aronsson CA, Bergo AM, Cinek O, Havlik J, Agardh D. Effects of *Lactiplantibacillus plantarum* and *Lacticaseibacillus paracasei* supplementation on the faecal metabolome in children with coeliac disease autoimmunity: a randomised, double-blinded placebo-controlled clinical trial. *Front Nutr.* 2023;10:1183963.
437. Gibson G, Hutkins R, Sanders M, et al. Expert consensus document: The International Scientific Association for Probiotics and Prebiotics (ISAPP) consensus statement on the definition and scope of prebiotics. *Nat Rev Gastroenterol Hepatol.* 2017;14:491–502.
438. Swanson KS, Gibson GR, Hutkins R, et al. The International Scientific Association for Probiotics and Prebiotics (ISAPP) consensus statement on the definition and scope of synbiotics. *Nat Rev Gastroenterol Hepatol.* 2020;17(11):687–701.
439. Salminen S, Collado MC, Endo A, et al. The International Scientific Association of Probiotics and Prebiotics (ISAPP) consensus statement on the definition and scope of postbiotics. *Nat Rev Gastroenterol Hepatol.* 2021;18:649–667.
440. Marco ML, Sanders ME, Gänzle M, et al. The International Scientific Association for Probiotics and Prebiotics (ISAPP) consensus statement on fermented foods. *Nat Rev Gastroenterol Hepatol.* 2021;18(3):196–208.
441. Arnett DK, Blumenthal RS, Albert MA, et al. 2019 ACC/AHA guideline on the primary prevention of cardiovascular disease: executive summary: a report of the American College of Cardiology/American Heart Association Task Force on Clinical Practice Guidelines. *Circulation.* 2019;140(11):e563–e595.
442. Colberg SR, Sigal RJ, Yardley JE, et al. Physical activity/exercise and diabetes: a position statement of the American Diabetes Association. *Diabetes Care.* 2016;39(11):2065.
443. Nelson AE, Allen KD, Golightly YM, Goode AP, Jordan JM. A systematic review of recommendations and guidelines for the management of osteoarthritis: the chronic osteoarthritis management initiative of the US bone and joint initiative. *Semin Arthritis Rheum.* 2014;43(6):701–712.
444. Boytar AN, Skinner TL, Wallen RE, Jenkins DG, Dekker Nitert M. The effect of exercise prescription on the human gut microbiota and comparison between clinical and apparently healthy populations: a systematic review. *Nutrients.* 2023;15:1534.
445. Cerdá B, Pérez M, Pérez-Santiago JD, Tornero-Aguilera JF, González-Soltero R, Larrosa M. Gut microbiota modification: another piece in the puzzle of the benefits of physical exercise in health? *Front Physiol.* 2016;7:51.
446. Grosicki GJ, Langan SP, Bagley JR, et al. Gut check: unveiling the influence of acute exercise on the gut microbiota. *Exp Physiol.* 2023;108(12):1466–1480.
447. Tabone M, Bressa C, García-Merino JA, et al. The effect of acute moderate-intensity exercise on the serum and fecal metabolomes and the gut microbiota of cross-country endurance athletes. *Sci Rep.* 2021;11(1):3558.
448. Domínguez-Balmaseda D, García-Pérez-de-Sevilla G. The relationship between the gut microbiota and exercise: a narrative review. *Hygiene.* 2022;2(4):152–162.
449. Sales KM, Reimer RA. Unlocking a novel determinant of athletic performance: the role of the gut microbiota, short-chain fatty acids, and "biotics" in exercise. *J Sport Health Sci.* 2023;12(1):36–44.
450. Evans CC, LePard KJ, Kwak JW, et al. Exercise prevents weight gain and alters the gut microbiota in a mouse model of high fat diet-induced obesity. *PloS One.* 2014;9(3):e92193.
451. Allen JM, Mailing LJ, Niemiro GM, et al. Exercise alters gut microbiota composition and function in lean and obese humans. *Med Sci Sports Exerc.* 2018;50(4):747–757.
452. Silva JS, Seguro CS, Naves MMV. Gut microbiota and physical exercise in obesity and diabetes–a systematic review. *Nutr Metab Cardiovasc Dis.* 2022;32(4):863–877.
453. Uchida M, Fujie S, Yano H, Iemitsu M. Aerobic exercise training-induced alteration of gut microbiota composition affects endurance capacity. *J Physiol.* 2023;601(12):2329–2344.
454. De Souza PB, de Araujo Borba L, Castro de Jesus L, Valverde AP, Gil-Mohapel J, Rodrigues ALS. Major depressive disorder and gut microbiota: role of physical exercise. *Int J Mol Sci.* 2023;24(23):16870.
455. Ge X, Cheng L, Liu Y, Wu Z, Zhang X. Regulation of the gut microbiota by diet and exercise: improvements in cognition and emotion. *Future Foods.* 2023;8:100256.
456. Lu H, Wang S, Tian M, et al. Exercise preconditioning ameliorates cognitive impairment in mice with ischemic stroke by alleviating inflammation and modulating gut microbiota. *Mediators Inflamm.* 2022;2022:2124230.
457. Watanabe C, Oyanagi E, Aoki T, et al. Antidepressant properties of voluntary exercise mediated by gut microbiota. *Biosci Biotechnol Biochem.* 2023;87(11):1407–1419.
458. Zhu Y, Zhu J, Song G. The impact of aerobic exercise training on cognitive function and gut microbiota in methamphetamine-dependent individuals in the community. *Physiol Behav.* 2023;270:114302.
459. Mach N, Fuster-Botella D. Endurance exercise and gut microbiota: a review. *J Sport Health Sci.* 2017;6(2):179–197.
460. Mohr AE, Jäger R, Carpenter KC, et al. The athletic gut microbiota. *J Int Soc Sports Nutr.* 2020;17(1):24.
461. Jang LG, Choi G, Kim SW, Kim BY, Lee S, Park H. The combination of sport and sport-specific diet is associated with characteristics of gut microbiota: an observational study. *J Int Soc Sports Nutr.* 2019;6(1):21.
462. Dubourg G, Lagier JC, Robert C, et al. Culturomics and pyrosequencing evidence of the reduction in gut microbiota diversity in patients with broad-spectrum antibiotics. *Int J Antimicrob Agents.* 2014;44(2):117–124.

463. Blaser M. Antibiotic overuse: stop the killing of beneficial bacteria. *Nature.* 2011;476:393–394.
464. Patangia DV, Ryan CA, Dempsey E, Paul Ross R, Stanton C. Impact of antibiotics on the human microbiome and consequences for host health. *Microbiologyopen.* 2022;11:e1260.
465. Guh AY, Kutty PK. *Clostridioides difficile* infection. *Ann Intern Med.* 2018;169(7):ITC49–ITC64.
466. Johnson S, Samore MH, Farrow KA, et al. Epidemics of diarrhea caused by a clindamycin-resistant strain of *Clostridium difficile* in four hospitals. *N Engl J Med.* 1999;341:1645–51.
467. National Institute for Health and Care Excellence. *Clostridium difficile* infection: risk of broad spectrum antibiotics. *NICE.* 2015. www.nice.org.uk/guidance/esmpb1
468. Bakken JS, Borody T, Brandt LJ, et al; Fecal Microbiota Transplantation Workgroup. Treating *Clostridium difficile* infection with fecal microbiota transplantation. *Clin Gastroenterol Hepatol.* 2011;9(12):1044–1049.
469. Bibbo S, Settanni CR, Porcari S, et al. Fecal microbiota transplantation: screening and selection to choose the optimal donor. *J Clin Med.* 2020;9:1757.
470. Eiseman B, Silen W, Bascom GS, Kauvar AJ. Fecal enema as an adjunct in the treatment of pseudomembranous enterocolitis. *Surgery.* 1958;44:854–859.
471. Zhang F, Luo W, Shi Y, Fan Z, Ji G. Should we standardize the 1,700-year-old fecal microbiota transplantation? *Am J Gastroenterol.* 2012;107(11):1755;author reply p.1755–1756.
472. Brandt LJ, Aroniadis OC. An overview of fecal microbiota transplantation: techniques, indications, and outcomes. *Gastrointest Endosc.* 2013;78(2):240–249.
473. Vaughn BP, Fischer M, Kelly C, et al. Effectiveness and safety of colonic capsule fecal microbiota transplantation for recurrent *Clostridioides difficile* infection. *Clin Gastroentrol Hepatol.* 2023;21:1330–1337.
474. Nicco C, Paule A, Konturek P, Edeas M. From donor to patient: collection, preparation and cryopreservation of fecal samples for fecal microbiota transplantation. *Diseases.* 2020;8(2):9.
475. https://www.rebyota.com/rebyota-support-resources/?scroll_id=faqs. Accessed November 3, 2024.
476. Kahn SA, Vachon A, Rodriquez D, et al. Patient perceptions of fecal microbiota transplantation for ulcerative colitis. *Inflamm Bowel Dis.* 2013;19(7):1506–1513.
477. Cheng YW, Phelps E, Nemes S, et al. Fecal microbiota transplant decreases mortality in patients with refractory severe or fulminant *Clostridioides difficile* infection. *Clin Gastroenterol Hepatol.* 2020;18(10):2234–2243.
478. Nicholson MR, Mitchell PD, Alexander E, et al. Efficacy of fecal microbiota transplantation for *Clostridium difficile* infection in children. *Clin Gastroenterol Hepatol.* 2020;18(3):612–619.
479. Davidovics ZH, Michail S, Nicholson MR, et al; FMT Special Interest Group of the North American Society of Pediatric Gastroenterology Hepatology, Nutrition, the European Society for Pediatric Gastroenterology Hepatology, Nutrition. Fecal microbiota transplantation for recurrent *Clostridium difficile* infection and other conditions in children: a joint position paper from the North American Society for Pediatric Gastroenterology, Hepatology, and Nutrition and the European Society for Pediatric Gastroenterology, Hepatology, and Nutrition. *J Ped Gastroenterol Nutr.* 2019;68(1):130–143.
480. Romano KA, Nemet I, Prasad Saha P, et al. Gut microbiota-generated phenylacetylglutamine and heart failure. *Circ Heart Fail.* 2023;16(1):e009972.
481. Magill SS, O'Leary E, Janelle SJ, et al; Emerging Infections Program Hospital Prevalence Survey Team. Changes in prevalence of health care-associated infections in U.S. hospitals. *N Engl J Med.* 2018;379(18):1732–1744.
482. Quraishi MN, Widlak M, Bhala N, et al. Systematic review with meta-analysis: the efficacy of faecal microbiota transplantation for the treatment of recurrent and refractory *Clostridium difficile* infection. *Aliment Pharmacol Ther.* 2017;46(5):479–493.
483. Rossen NG, MacDonald JK, de Vries EM, et al. Fecal microbiota transplantation as novel therapy in gastroenterology: a systematic review. *World J Gastroenterol.* 2015;21(17):5359–5371.

24 Environmental Issues

NATALIE A. NEVINS

KEY CONCEPTS

- Environmental health is the field of science that studies how the environment influences human health and disease.
- Health is a product of one's polygenetic inheritance and the environment that interacts with it.
- An environmental health history should be included in every new patient evaluation and is a key component to obtaining an accurate picture of the patient's complete health status.
- When a patient presents with signs and symptoms of disease that do not respond to therapeutic interventions, the clinician should go back to the patient's history and make sure to perform a complete environmental history.

INTRODUCTION

The environment can be broken down into the natural world such as air, water, and earth, and the man-made world such as homes, buildings related to work, pollution, and chemicals.

- The environment includes buildings, foods, clothes, weather, infectious agents, man-made and natural materials, and even socioeconomic status.
- Humans have an intimate relationship with the environment. There is no separation from the air, food, and water used to sustain life and the environment from which they came.
- As an osteopathic physician, it is vitally important to remember these aspects when evaluating patients. An environmental history is a key component to obtaining an accurate picture of the patient's complete health status.

THE INTERACTION OF GENETICS AND ENVIRONMENT

Some liken the role of genetics in overall health as a loaded gun, and the environment as the actual trigger. Patients often ask themselves the "Why me?" question. How is it possible for one person to smoke excessively for years and never develop lung cancer, and another individual who doesn't have a smoking history to develop lung cancer? Current research suggests that most diseases (especially chronic complex disorders) are caused by interactions between an individual's genome, epigenome, microbiome, and their environment.[1] Quantifying a person's exposure experience from conception to death with the related biologic response is referred to as the exposome.[2] Environmental exposures such as pollution, man-made chemicals, nanomaterials, naturally occurring gases and radiation, and infectious agents interacting with our genetics may be setting us up for disease.[2] The developmental stage or age of an individual related to the timing of an environmental exposure also critically influences the level of gene–environment interaction.[1] The latest studies suggest that harmful exposures early in life may increase the risk for disease later in life, and a variety of diseases and conditions that are believed to result partly from intrauterine or childhood exposure include obesity, insulin resistance, type 2 diabetes, asthma, behavioral disorders, reproductive disorders, neurodegenerative disorders, and some cancers.[3]

The Centers for Disease Control and Prevention (CDC) state that 1 in 6 children in the United States has a developmental disability. Childhood exposure to environmental contaminants can negatively affect developing nervous systems.[4]

- A study in 2022 evaluated the association of polychlorinated biphenyl (PCB) and polybrominated diphenyl ether (PBDE) serum concentrations on executive functioning in adolescents.[5]
  - The study found that "higher blood serum concentrations were associated with poorer cognitive flexibility as measured on the Intradimensional/Extradimensional Set-Shifting (ID/ED) task."
  - "Higher serum total PCB concentrations were also associated with more errors on the Delayed Matching to Sample (DMS) task ($\beta = 1.15$, 95% CL: 1.00, 1.31, $p < 0.05$)."
  - "These findings suggest that exposure to PCBs or PBDEs during adolescence may be associated with impaired cognitive flexibility and that adolescent PCB exposure may be associated with visual recognition memory deficits."
- PCBs were banned in the 1970s. They are classified as persistent organic pollutants which have long half-lives that bioaccumulate in mammals.[5]
  - They were used in many everyday items such as wood flooring, adhesives, and paints to name just a few.
  - Many homes and buildings that were built with the use of PCB-contaminated items continue to be a health threat, especially to those patients of lower socioeconomic status.
  - Exposure to PCBs and PBDEs today is common through diet. Those who eat sport-caught fish from contaminated waters tend to have an elevated chemical burden.
- Per- and Polyfluoroalkyl Substances (PFAS) are man-made chemicals manufactured since the 1940s for industrial and consumer products such as nonstick cookware, cosmetics, and stain-resistant fabrics.[6]
  - PFAS can migrate to soil, water, and air, and generally do not break down, thus are persistent in the environment, and can build up in people and animals with repeated exposure.

If physicians do not ask patients about their living and working environment, they will miss important epidemiologic information that will help to diagnosis, treat, and, more importantly, prevent disease.

TABLE 24.1

Examples of Environmental Health Factors

Natural World	Air	Water	Soil	Chemical	Biologic	Social
	Dust	Microbes Arsenic (well water)	Arsenic	Nitrogen	Mold	Pollen
	Radon gas	Mercury	Tetanus toxin	Salts Uranium	Fungi	
Man-Made World	**Structures Home and Work**	**Schools Land**	**Land/Sea Farms Waste Management**	**Factories Pollution**	**Community Buildings Chemicals**	**Transportation Roads**
	Organophosphates	Latex	Asbestos	Epoxy resins	Cigarette smoke	Carbon monoxide
	Lead paint	Noise	Pesticides	Ozone		
	Pharmaceuticals		PCBs and PBDEs	PCBs and PBDEs		
	PCBs and PBDEs					
	Air quality	Air quality		Air quality	Air quality	

PCBs, polychlorinated biphenyls; PBDE, polybrominated diphenyl ethers.

Environment as the Trigger for Disease Development

Several common environmental factors can impact health,[6–9] as shown in Table 24.1.

Examples of work-related environmental diseases include the following:

- Asbestosis/pleural plaques
- Carpal tunnel syndrome
- Hearing loss
- Musculoskeletal pain
- Pneumoconiosis (lung diseases from dust, e.g., silicosis, black lung)
- Vibrational trauma

Examples of environmental diseases related to chemical/biologic/radiation sources include the following:

- Allergies
- Asthma
- Birth defects
- Cancer
- Dermatitis
- Emphysema
- Fertility problems
- Kidney/liver disease
- Lead/mercury poisoning
- Nervous system disorders
- Neurodevelopmental disorders
- Vision problems
- Waterborne diseases

PATIENT HISTORY

Assessing the social history of a patient must also include an environmental history, both occupational and nonoccupational information.

- Clearly ask about ALL previous work history, and do not forget to ask about prior or current military exposures.
  - Prior and current military service members may or may not have exposure histories they are aware of. They may already be on a military exposure registry that is being tracked.
- Keep in mind that chemicals leave residue behind, even outdoors.
- Children and pets crawl on floors and play outside, and young children place almost everything in their mouths.
- Close contact with pets could contaminate indoor living spaces.
- Most patients are not aware of what kinds of chemicals are in their home-cleaning products or pesticides, or the chemicals used where they work.
  - All employers are mandated by the government to maintain a Material Safety Data Sheet (MSDS) that is accessible to all employees giving a complete list of all chemicals used in the workplace.
  - Patients should be encouraged to maintain a file with a copy of the MSDS from all their jobs.[8]

Occupational and Nonoccupational Environmental Health History

Box 24.1 provides a sample of some of the key questions to ask patients. It is not intended to be a comprehensive list of all possible questions. The general history should include asking open-ended questions. See Chapter 27 for examples of questions to ask during history taking. An environmental history should be focused on the details; be a detective.

Box 24.2 provides an example of how environmental toxins affect health.

Box 24.3 provides resources for further information.

PATIENT EDUCATION: EASY STEPS TO PERSONAL ENVIRONMENTAL HEALTH

A physician not only diagnoses and treats medical problems but also educates patients on how to prevent health problems in the first place. Below are some important tips to help educate patients on how to maintain personal environmental health.

1. Read labels on house and garden chemicals. Cross contamination is common and can lead to accidental self-poisonings. Patients should carefully follow instructions on the handling of chemicals especially around children and pets. Use gloves,

BOX 24.1 Key Questions in an Environmental Health History

- Is the problem acute or chronic?
- Are the symptoms worse when at home or work?
- Are you currently, or have you ever served in the military? If yes, when, and are you aware of any environmental exposures? Are you already on any military or VA exposure registries?
- What chemicals are used in and outside the home (e.g., pesticides, paints, solvents, glue, cleaners, etc.)?
- Do any of the chemicals have a warning label (such as "Do not use around small children or pets")?
- Is the home near any manufacturing companies? If so, what kind?
- Does a family member work around chemicals? If so, what are the chemicals?
- Are any of the household pets sick?
- Does anyone else in the home or neighborhood have the same symptoms?
- Is there peeling paint around the home or in the neighborhood? Are there abandoned buildings accessible to the children?
- Is there new construction in or around the home?
- Are medications and chemicals out of reach of children?
- Has there been any recent water leakage in the home? Is there black mold growing on walls?
- What protective equipment is used when handling chemicals in and outside the home? Are these chemicals used around pets or children's toys?
- Have there been visitors to the home from another country? Has there been travel outside the country?
- Has the home been tested for carbon monoxide or radon gas?
- Does anyone smoke in or around the home?
- Do you use well water?
- Is the patient eating a strict vegan diet?

Focused Occupational History Questions

- Type of work: current and past 10 years
- Chemical or radiologic exposures
- If there are chemicals in the workplace, does the patient have a copy of the MSDS?
- If working with or around chemicals, what protective gear does the patient use?
- If working with or around chemicals, does the patient shower at work and change clothes before going home?
- Does the patient work in manufacturing? If so, what kind?
- Does the patient work outside? If so, in what capacity?
- Is any machinery used (e.g., heavy, loud, grinding, vibrational, etc.)?
- If working with or around machinery, what kind of protective equipment is used?
- Does the patient work with animals? If so, what kind?

BOX 24.2 Case Vignette: Environmental Illness

Mary is a 40-year-old health care worker who is in good health with a medical history of only reactive airway disease (RAD). She reports to the clinic with chief complaints of new-onset shortness of breath, nonproductive cough, and wheezing that started 3 weeks ago. She denies any other symptoms. She states that she has not had a flare-up of her RAD for over 5 years. Her RAD is known to be triggered by dust mites, mold, and dog dander. She admits to trying allergy medication and an albuterol inhaler without significant improvement in her symptoms. The patient reports that she moved into a new house 3 weeks ago, that is, a new construction home. It has been professionally cleaned three times, but her symptoms seem to be getting worse. She reports that she has attempted to "dust proof" her new house (hardwood floors, no drapes, dust mite covers on her pillows and mattress, air purifier in her bedroom). She has a cat that does not go outside.

Physical examination reveals normal vital signs. The head examination revealed dark circles (allergic shiners) under each eye. Nasal and throat examination revealed boggy and pale nasal mucosa with clear drainage and cobble stoning of the posterior pharynx. On pulmonary evaluation, the patient had both inspiratory and expiratory wheezing. The remainder of the physical examination was normal.

Investigation of the patient's new home revealed an access panel in her bedroom closet that connected to the room for the washer and dryer. When the panel was removed, black mold (*Stachybotrys*) was found covering all of the inner drywall in the access space. A professional mold removal company was hired to eradicate the mold. The patient's symptoms completely resolved after the space was cleaned.

masks, and eye protection when recommended. When possible, use nontoxic, biodegradable products in and around the home.

2. Turn down the volume. Noise pollution is real and can cause permanent hearing damage. Use ear plugs when working with loud equipment and when attending loud concerts.[9]
3. Use a carbon monoxide detector at home. Carbon monoxide can leak from faulty heaters and is produced from the exhaust of cars. Detectors are inexpensive and easy to install.
4. Know the hazards of the job and its site. All businesses are required to have an MSDS file of the known chemicals used on a job site. Encourage patients to ask their employer for a copy of this information to include with their chart.
5. Immediately deal with any water leakage in the home. Look for any signs of mold (commonly found in wet areas around washing machines, windows, and bathrooms). Remove all mold from the home.[10]
6. Keep chemicals and medications out of reach of children. Use childproof locks on all accessible cabinets that contain household cleaners/chemicals.
7. Don't smoke/don't allow others to smoke around you. There are over 4,000 known chemicals in tobacco smoke, and it is a known carcinogen.
8. Allergy sufferers and asthmatics should consider using an air purifier in their homes. Use dust mite covers on pillows and bedding. Avoid being outside, and exercising outside when air pollution levels are rated as "high"; this is especially important for young children with asthma.[10–12]
9. Wash hands! Many diseases such as COVID, the common cold, flu, and diarrheal diseases are passed passively by people touching bacteria- or virus-laden objects and then introducing

BOX 24.3 Resources Box

There are many resources to assist the practicing clinician with understanding the impact of environmental issues on health.

- Child-Specific Exposure Factors Handbook (Final Report) 2008. **EPA/600/R-06/096 F | September 2008 |** https://cfpub.epa.gov/si/si_public_record_report.cfm?Lab=NCEA&dirEntryId=199243
- **Child-Specific Exposure Scenarios Examples:** Outlines scenarios for various child-specific exposure pathways and to demonstrate how data from the *Exposure Factors Handbook* (U.S. EPA, 2011a) may be applied for estimating dose. **EPA 600/R-14/217 F | September 2014.|** https://cfpub.epa.gov/ncea/risk/recordisplay.cfm?deid = 262211
- 2011 edition of the Exposure Factors Handbook, Chapter 1: This report highlights the 2011 edition of the Exposure Factors Handbook, summarizing the latest findings. https://www.epa.gov/expobox/about-exposure-factors-handbook
- Advisories and technical Resources for Fish and Shellfish Consumption. https://www.epa.gov/fish-tech

Other useful sites are as follows:

- The National Center for Environmental Assessment (NCEA). https://www.epa.gov/archive/epa/aboutepa/about-national-center-environmental-assessment-ncea.html
- The National Institute for Occupational Safety and Health (NIOSH). www.cdc.gov/niosh/
- National Institute of Environmental Health Sciences (NIEHS). www.niehs.nih.gov/
- CDC's **National Center for Environmental Health (NCEH).** https://www.cdc.gov/nceh/

those pathogens into their own system, or contaminating venues affecting many people, such as a food buffet. Handwashing after using the bathroom or changing an infant's diaper is common knowledge, but reminding patients can be helpful. Alcohol-based hand sanitizers and plain soap and water will kill many of these pathogens.

10. Be careful with the use of pesticides around and in the home. Extreme caution should be used when applying insect repellents to children. They should never be applied over open wounds or directly to the face or hands. Use the smallest amount possible, and never under clothing.
11. Use sun block. Apply according to instructions and repeat the application if remaining outdoors for an extended period or after getting wet. Even waterproof sunscreens need to be reapplied after prolonged time in the water. Use age-appropriate sun block.
12. Eat a healthy balanced diet with plenty of fresh fruits and vegetables that are free of pesticides—wash or peel the skin if unsure. (See Chapters 21 and 22 for more details on nutrition and diet.) If a patient is eating a strict vegan diet, supplements may be needed to get all the basic nutrients required, especially for young children. Vegetable protein can be less bioavailable than animal protein sources. The average adult should be getting approximately 0.8 g of protein per day per kilogram of weight, and the protein sources used should be able to provide all the essential amino acids needed. (See Chapter 22 for further information.)
13. Use caution when visiting the beach. It can pose serious health threats to the young, old, and those with a compromised immune system from contaminated water. Patients should always pay attention to signs for beach closures due to pollution and bacterial contamination.[13]
14. Grow plants. Plants have been shown to help reduce toxins in the environment, and they make and release oxygen into the air.

SUMMARY

Every individual on this planet is impacted by the environment. Sometimes that impact moves one toward health and sometimes toward illness. A complete patient history, considering the potential environmental impact, along with a thorough physical examination will provide the information necessary to come up with a functional differential diagnosis. Every patient encounter is an opportunity to counsel patients on how to improve their quality of life. Always include "patient education" on environmental issues; it will go a long way toward helping patients have the happy healthy life they deserve.

REFERENCES

1. Olden K, Freudenberg N, Dowd J, Shields AE. Discovering how environmental exposures alter genes and could lead to new treatments for chronic illnesses. *Health Aff (Millwood).* 2011;30(5):833–841.
2. Vermeulen R, Schymanski EL, Barabási A-L, Miller GW. The exposome and health: where chemistry meets biology. *Science.* 2020;367(6476):392–396.
3. National Institute of Environmental Health and Research. *Developmental origins of health and disease.* Accessed February 5, 2023. https://www.niehs.nih.gov/research/supported/health/developmental/index.cfm
4. Centers for Disease Control and Prevention. Accessed April 8, 2023. https://ephtracking.cdc.gov/assets/images/content/DevDis_final.jpg
5. Sprowles JLN, Monaikul S, Aguiar A, et al. Associations of concurrent PCB and PBDE serum concentrations with executive functioning in adolescents. *Neurotoxicol Teratol.* 2022;92:107092.
6. Agency for Toxic Substances and Disease Registry. *What are PFAS?* Accessed April 8, 2023. https://www.atsdr.cdc.gov/pfas/health-effects/overview.html
7. Rather IA, Koh WY, Paek WK, Lim J. The sources of chemical contaminants in food and their health implications. *Front Pharmacol.* 2017;8:830.
8. USGS. *Most arsenic presumed to be from naturally occurring sources.* Accessed April 8, 2023. https://www.usgs.gov/news/national-news-release/study-estimates-about-21-million-people-using-wells-high-arsenic
9. Nussbaumer-Streit B, Mayr V, Dobrescu AI, et al. Household interventions for secondary prevention of domestic lead exposure in children. *Cochrane Database Syst Rev.* 2020;10(10):CD006047.
10. EPA. *A brief guide to mold, moisture and your home.* Accessed April 8, 2023. https://www.epa.gov/mold/brief-guide-mold-moisture-and-your-home
11. Zuiani C, Custovic A. Update on house dust mite allergen avoidance measures for asthma. *Curr Allergy Asthma Rep.* 2020;20(9):50.
12. Furlong MA, Alexander GE, Klimentidis YC, Raichlen DA. Association of air pollution and physical activity with brain volumes. *Neurology.* 2021;98(4):e416–e426.
13. Landrigan PJ, Stegeman JJ, Fleming LE, et al. Human health and ocean pollution. *Ann Glob Health.* 2020;86(1):151.

PART TWO

The Patient Encounter

25 Medical Professionalism and the Physician–Patient Relationship

REGINA K. FLEMING ▪ KENDI L. HENSEL ▪ REBECCA E. GIUSTI

KEY CONCEPTS

- A critical task for osteopathic physicians is the formation of professional identity.
- Professionalism is the behavioral manifestation of a professional identity, and it is foundational for many tasks of a physician, such as communication, working with a team, and creating a positive physician–patient relationship.
- One study identified four categories of professional behavior—engagement, integrity, respect, and self-awareness.
- Emotional intelligence is often described as being comprised of self-awareness, self-management, social awareness, and relationship management. While emotional intelligence may not be extensively taught in medical school curriculum, it can be learned and refined. Physicians with high emotional intelligence often have more fulfilled and enriched lives enabling them to be better team players and leaders.

At the end of every word, action, and deed is a patient.
—Paula Crone, DO, Provost, Western COMP and COMP-NW

INTRODUCTION

Formation of a professional identity is a critical task in the development of an osteopathic physician. It involves learning, both from mentors as well as from academic sources, to better incorporate important concepts and behaviors. Professional identity manifests in professional behavior, which affects many aspects of medical practice, including interacting with the medical team, fostering the physician–patient relationship, and engaging in personal growth and wellness. Professionalism is intentional and is a skill that physicians commit to developing over their lifetime.

PROFESSIONAL IDENTITY AND PROFESSIONALISM

In addition to the cognitive tasks of medicine—building a knowledge base, developing technical and psychomotor skills, and learning the logistics of medical practice—another critical task is the formation of a professional identity. Professional identity has many definitions. One is simply the way of being and relating in professional contexts.[1–3] Professional identity will likely evolve and continue to form over a physician's lifetime. Professional identity formation is a recently studied process. Very little could be found in the literature until around 2000. Since then, many authors have tried to define professional identity, dissect out its components, and propose the best way to aid learners to develop one.

During a lifetime, individuals take on roles related to their developmental stage and activities. For example, individuals begin in the role of a child, move through adolescence and teen roles, and become associated with activities such as sports, music, or employment. Individuals have roles in peer groups, such as leader or follower. Each role has behavioral expectations, along with the traditions of the role and the institution the role is a part of, such as a sports team, band, or employer's company. For osteopathic medical students, entry into osteopathic medical school endows the role of a "legitimate peripheral participant"[4] into medical society. The institution of medical society has long-standing traditions of "the way things are done" along with acceptable and nonacceptable behaviors. Learning these behaviors and consistently demonstrating them, is critical for an individual to develop professional identity and to be accepted as a member of a medical society, with its norms, values, and roles.[3] The practice of medicine is an institution that requires collaboration and teamwork built on trust and respect, which are best cultivated through professionalism.

As members of a minority profession, osteopathic medical students and osteopathic physicians may have a larger responsibility for professional conduct. As much of the US population is not clear on the difference between an MD and DO, it is more important for osteopathic students and physicians to be able to describe their professional identity without comparisons to other professions, as well as to describe how DOs are distinctive and contribute uniquely to medical society.

During medical education, the development of professional identity can be both implicitly and explicitly influenced. Implicit teaching involves modeling by preceptors, senior learners, and others. Explicit teaching involves clear direction and action to develop a learner's knowledge attitude, judgment, and skills.[5]

Due to the evolution and dynamic nature of societal norms, defining professionalism has posed a challenge. One systematic review evaluated published literature for examples of unprofessional behavior. The authors found 205 different descriptions of unprofessional behavior, which were coded into 30 descriptors, which were grouped into 4 themes: failure to engage, dishonest behavior, disrespectful behavior, and poor self-awareness.[5] By defining and classifying what professionalism is not, this study helped to define four components of professionalism: engagement, integrity, respect, and self-awareness.[5] These components are crucial not only during medical training, but also throughout a physician's life. Other related components, such as poor initiative, irresponsibility, and diminished capacity for self-improvement have been shown to relate to future unprofessional behaviors as

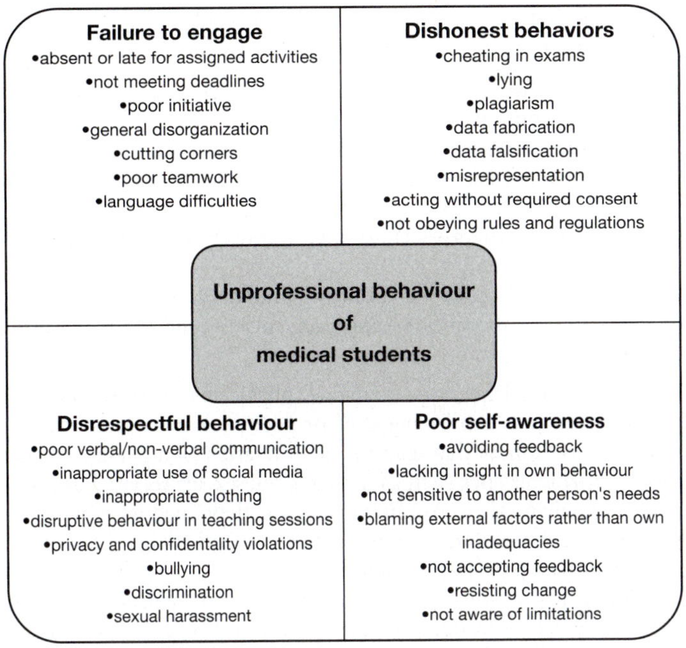

Figure 25.1. Four themes including 30 descriptors for unprofessional behaviors of medical students. (Reprinted from Mak-van der Vossen M, van Mook W, van der Burgt S, et al. Descriptors for unprofessional behaviours of medical students: a systematic review and categorisation. *BMC Med Educ.* 2017;17(1):164. http://creativecommons.org/licenses/by/4.0/)

physicians.[6,7] The remainder of this chapter will use this framework to discuss components of professionalism and examples of unprofessional conduct (Fig. 25.1).

ENGAGEMENT

Engagement in professionalism has many definitions, but most simply it is the focused alignment of personal resources with a meaningful purpose outside of oneself.[8] Engaged professionalism is the application of values and knowledge in the service of work that benefits society.[8]

Failure to engage can be loosely defined as "insufficiently handling one's tasks."[5] Broad examples of lack of engagement include poor reliability and responsibility, lack of conscientiousness, poor initiative and motivation, and seeking a minimally acceptable level of performance.[5] One specific example of poor engagement is poor timeliness.

> ***"Early is on time, on time is late and late is unacceptable!"***
>
> **—Eric Jerome Dickey**

Timeliness is critical in the health care industry. Being on time is a way to show respect for patients, colleagues, and oneself. While everyone may run late at some point, the professional response is to contact the person they are inconveniencing or the clinic (determined by the circumstances of the situation) and notify them as soon as possible. This demonstrates not only ownership and responsibility for the tardiness, but consideration for others.

For a physician, timeliness is more than simply showing up on time. It is also completing charts and other paperwork in a timely manner. While the Centers for Medicare & Medicaid Services do not provide a specific period, some Medicare fiscal intermediaries have defined a reasonable time frame to complete the medical record as 24 to 48 hours.[9] Timely documentation helps provide the physician and other health team members the most accurate information regarding a patient which will lead to better care for the patient.[9]

Another aspect of engagement is to truly understand and respect what it means to be an osteopathic physician. When caring for patients, it is no longer about the physician, the physician's preferences, or what the physician has going on at that moment. It is about the person in front of them, the patient, and how they can best serve that patient with all of their knowledge, skill, and abilities. This is interwoven with life-long learning, a willingness to engage daily at the task at hand, humility, and respect. It is important to remember that it is a privilege to care for others and to have their trust. Patients come to physicians because they need assistance. Oftentimes, for the patient, it can be a scary experience; they find themselves in a vulnerable position—not understanding the seriousness of the situation and experiencing a loss of control over the situation. Physicians should put the patient at ease, support them in their vulnerability, and provide appropriate and timely care.

INTEGRITY

Integrity has been referred to as the "bedrock virtue, defined as a commitment to practice medicine in accord with the standard of intellectual and moral excellence."[10] Integrity includes honesty, keeping one's word, and accountability, which are critical factors for maintaining the public's trust in the profession, as well as maintaining trust with patients, colleagues, and team members.[11] Behaviors that demonstrate a lack of integrity are dishonest behaviors, such as cheating, lying, plagiarism, and not obeying rules and regulations.[5]

One specific behavior that demonstrates integrity is the obtaining of informed consent. Informed consent is a process that involves providing understandable information to a person so they can make an informed decision about whether or not to participate in a procedure or research study. Presenting the information requires honest, clear, and effective communication skills by the physician. The physician must ensure that the information is presented at a level that the patient or participant can understand. The physician must demonstrate trustworthiness, along with patience, to answer any questions, while allowing the patient or participant time to process the information accurately. The procedure or research must be explained objectively, covering the procedure, risks, benefits, and alternative options so the patient or participant understands what to expect, including the possibility of less-than-ideal outcomes. Opportunity for questions must be given, along with communication from the patient or participant that signifies their understanding. Ultimately, it is the patient or participant who makes the decision to proceed or not, and the physician should respect their autonomy and not use position or power to influence their decision. In addition, the physician should support the patient in their decision and should have no vested interest in the outcome. Having an informed consent discussion with a patient or participant may take time, but it is necessary in maintaining an ethical practice; it benefits the physician–patient relationship.[12]

As osteopathic physicians, obtaining informed consent before performing examinations or osteopathic manipulative treatment (OMT) on patients is critical to maintaining trust and demonstrating professionalism in the physician–patient relationship. Examinations and OMT can involve touching sensitive areas, and informing patients respectfully about why touch is necessary is crucial for patients to understand and give consent. If patients seem uncomfortable, physicians can offer to have a chaperone present. When examining or treating children with their parents present, parental consent must be obtained, along with the child's assent, if possible. A good practice is to position the patient and the parent so that the parent is able to observe all actions of the physician. By taking these actions, the physician exhibits honesty, trustworthiness, and respect, all components of integrity.

RESPECT

In the society of medicine, respect means acknowledging and valuing the autonomy, diversity, culture, and preferences of others, or simply, showing consideration for another person's interests and well-being.[13] A respectful patient–physician relationship can directly affect patient outcomes as well as patient satisfaction,[14] and patient suffering may be reduced when providers demonstrate respect for patients.[15]

Disrespectful behavior, on the other hand, has a negative effect on others. Unprofessional behavior that is disrespectful varies widely in severity.[5] Examples are poor communication, either verbal, nonverbal (body language), or electronic (email or social media); ignoring emails or other forms of contact; privacy or confidentiality violations, such as discussing patient issues on social media. More serious examples of disrespect are cultural insensitivity, discrimination, sexual harassment, and bullying.[5] These kinds of behaviors can have a significant impact on all involved persons, including patients and their families, staff, team members, and other students.

Much of communication in the 21st century is asynchronous, meaning there is a delay between when a message is sent and when it is received and interpreted. Examples are email, text messaging, file sharing, and instant messaging. One manifestation of respect and professionalism is prompt attention to asynchronous communication. Habitually failing to respond or excessive delays in response can be interpreted as disorganization, disengagement, or disrespect. Dr. Grant, an organizational psychologist states, "Ignoring email is an act of incivility."[16] Responding in a timely manner shows that one is conscientious, organized, dependable, and hardworking.[16] Not answering messages in a timely manner can strain relationships with patients, colleagues, and others. However, oftentimes physicians are directly involved in patient care and responding to emails may be distracting and could potentially lead to medical errors. In those situations, physicians may find an automatic message system that notifies patients of when to expect a reply to inquiries helpful. An example may be an electronic message that states "Dr. X" is rounding on patients from 7 AM to 12 noon. They will be responding to your inquiry early this afternoon. If this is an emergency, please contact Dr. X's assistant at _." Ensuring that the medical or office staff are also aware of the physician's schedule and times to review electronic inquiries or messages is helpful in communicating to patients. If a patient calls the office with an inquiry that is nonemergent, the front desk person may respond, "Dr. X is generally in surgery Mondays from 6 AM–12 noon. They return to the office around 1:30 PM, and I will let them know you called and relay the message. You may expect a response from Dr. X later this afternoon. If there is an emergency, and this is not possible, I will call you and let you know." This allows the patient to know that Dr. X is providing care to others, but they are important as well, and their question will be answered.

> **"We will all profit from a more diverse, inclusive society, understanding, accommodating, even celebrating our differences, while pulling together for the common good."**
>
> **—Ruth Bader Ginsburg**

One aspect of demonstrating respect for others is being inclusive. As physicians are commonly placed in leadership roles, it is important that they strive to be inclusive leaders. Six traits that demonstrate respect and distinguish inclusive leaders include:

1. Visible commitment—authentic, challenges status quo, and accepts accountability
2. Humility—admits mistakes and creates space for participation
3. Awareness of bias—works to build awareness of personal blind spots
4. Curiosity of others—has an open mindset and actively listens without judgment
5. Cultural intelligence—is attentive and adapts as necessary.
6. Effective collaboration—empowers others and provides psychological safety[17]

As inclusive leaders in medicine, physicians need to consider bias. Implicit bias can be negative or positive associations outside conscious awareness that lead to the evaluation of a person on the basis of characteristics such as race, gender, sex, attire, etc. For physicians to deliver respectful impartial care, they need to be wary of any negative evaluation they make that is linked to membership of a group or to a particular characteristic.[18]

Physician's attire in the workplace is an example of how appearance can both demonstrate respect and be a source of bias. Defining how to dress professionally can be challenging, given regional differences, as well as differences in perception by the patient population the physician serves. For example, some pediatricians prefer to not wear a white coat when visiting with young children. In contrast, older patients in hospital settings preferred more formal attire with white coats.[19]

A study done in Hawaii showed that the majority of participants approved of physicians wearing scrubs and blue jeans and 52% preferred physicians to not wear a white coat.[20] Petrilli et al. performed a literature review looking at the role of physician attire on patient perceptions and of the studies that surveyed patients following a clinical encounter only 25% reported that attire influenced patient perceptions of their physician.[21] Conversely, clear preferences regarding physician attire were reported in 89% of the studies where patients received written descriptions or pictures of physician attire without a corresponding clinical interaction with a physician.[21] This suggests that the physician–patient encounter plays a significant role in the patient's perception of their physician. When there is no encounter the patients are more likely to fall back on their own implicit bias regarding what they believe a physician should look like.

While patient perception is one factor and may play a significant role in the physician–patient relationship, physicians must also consider the perception of their colleagues, administrators, etc. Dressing too casually can give an impression of lack of respect for the situation or patient.

However, not all aspects of the ideal professional dress for physicians may be founded in bias or be situationally driven. For instance, keeping fingernails clean and short for proper hand hygiene would be an appropriate standard for ideal dress. This is based on studies that have found less bacterial transmission from health care workers to patients when fingernails were short. When fingernails were longer than 2 mm, there was an increased carriage rate of *Staphylococcus aureus* and an increased number of microbes and number of microbe species.[22–24] Therefore, based on current evidence, physicians should keep their fingernails clean and short.

SELF-AWARENESS

The fourth component of professional behavior is self-awareness. Self-awareness is the ability to be aware of one's own thoughts, feeling, and actions, and the ability to perceive and understand what makes up a person as an individual, including personality, values, and beliefs. Poor self-awareness is simply defined as inappropriately handling one's own performance.[5] Examples include avoiding feedback, the inability to accept or incorporate feedback, having defensive behavior towards criticism, lacking insight into their behavior, blaming external factors, and failing to accept responsibility for actions. In addition, poor self-awareness can mean a person is not aware of their limitations and may act beyond their level of competence or not respect professional boundaries.

> ***"If your emotional abilities aren't in hand, if you don't have self-awareness, if you are not able to manage your distressing emotions, if you can't have empathy and have effective relationships, then no matter how smart you are, you are not going to get very far."***
>
> **—Daniel Goleman, PhD**

Self-awareness depends heavily on accurate self-assessment. Through reflection, a person may be honest about their own strengths and weaknesses, be clear about their own goals, and be comfortable with who they are as an individual.[25] The ability to perform an honest and accurate self-assessment is an important skill which enables self-improvement.

Certain types of mindfulness can help a person increase their self-awareness. Mindfulness is a type of meditation where the focus is on being intensely aware of what is sensed and felt in the moment without judgment.[26] Practicing mindfulness allows physicians to pause, pay attention to which thoughts and emotions they are experiencing, and process them calmly so that they do not become controlled by them.[25,27,28]

Self-awareness is a key component of emotional intelligence. Medicine can be a highly complex, emotionally demanding environment. The ability to manage oneself and one's relationships is a skill that osteopathic medical students, residents, and physicians must strive to master as they form their professional identity. Increasing one's emotional intelligence will enhance the well-being and professional performance of osteopathic medical students, residents, and physicians.

While there are several models of emotional intelligence published, three common domains other than self-awareness are self-management, social awareness, and relationship management.[27,29–32] Much of osteopathic medical school focuses on building medical knowledge, but many do not address specific leadership or emotional intelligence training, even though physicians are typically expected to either be leaders of a team or display strong leadership skills in medical settings. It is sometimes assumed that since physicians are intelligent and possess vast medical knowledge that this should translate to knowing how to manage a team effectively and be skilled leaders. While there is no correlation between high medical knowledge and high emotional intelligence, the good news is that emotional intelligence, like medical knowledge, can be learned and honed. Once the individual is aware of the four components, they can actively work to enrich their emotional intelligence which will better their own lives and allow them to improve their team player and leadership skills.

SELF-MANAGEMENT

Self-management is the ability to control disruptive impulses and moods, the propensity to suspend judgment, and the ability to think before acting. It involves the application of self-control, trustworthiness, adaptability, achievement orientation, and initiative.[30]

Self-control in this context is the ability to cope with negative or disruptive feelings and not allow them to "hijack" the situation. It is the ability to self-direct and behave professionally in situations where the other party may be behaving in a nonprofessional manner. Reacting impulsively to a situation may result in many negative emotions that can worsen the encounter. It is possible to condition the mind to let go of these negative thoughts through continuous training in mindfulness. Mindful people are more able to quickly notice and reflect on the negative emotions, and thus more likely to choose an appropriate response in these heated situations.[25] As such, self-control is crucial for maintaining professionalism in the workplace.

SOCIAL AWARENESS

Social awareness involves the application of empathy and altruism in medicine. Empathy is the ability to experience and understand what others feel.[25] Several studies have demonstrated that physician empathy was associated with long-term patient satisfaction and better health outcomes.[33–36] Empathy has also been found to positively correlate with clinical competence in medical students.[37]

A study published in 2019 compared patient perceptions of their physician's interpersonal manner, empathy, and communication style. Patients reported more favorable perceptions of DOs on interpersonal manner and empathy compared to MDs.[38] It is theorized that the incorporation of osteopathic philosophy in osteopathic medical education may make it a more humanistic approach, allowing for osteopathic physicians to demonstrate greater empathy in patient care.

Altruism is the unselfish concern for the welfare of others. Altruism results in behavior that supersedes self-interest without any expectation of reward and in some cases may involve a risk or cost to oneself.[39,40] Many physicians would claim that they were motivated to become doctors, in part, because of altruism—what is often referred to as a "calling" to help others.

RELATIONSHIP MANAGEMENT

Relationship management is the ability to relate to others and build relationships and rapport. Teamwork is an essential element of health care delivery. At the heart of a physician–patient relationship is professionalism and clear communication. Effective teams communicate well among themselves and with the patient, delivering a better outcome, safer experience, and a higher level of service at a more efficient cost.[41]

Another important aspect of relationship management is conflict management. Conflict is a disagreement among individuals. Conflict management seeks to resolve the disagreement with a positive outcome that is at a minimum beneficial to the group as a whole.[42] One model for conflict management includes the following:

1. Set rules for respectful communication
2. Ask all to set aside preconceived opinions of each other
3. Ask all to practice active listening without interruption
4. Ask each party to state the problem
5. Ask each party what they think the solution should be
6. Discuss each solution and the pros and cons of all proposed solutions[42]

Following these steps in managing conflict allows each party to speak and be heard. Conflict is not necessarily bad; if managed properly it can promote team building, critical thinking, and new ideas.[42]

So far, this chapter has outlined and described components of professional and unprofessional behavior, and reviewed the importance of the formation of a professional identity. These last two sections will cover work-life harmony as an expression of the four components of professionalism as it relates to a physician's nonprofessional lives, and humility, as a foundational component of service in the medical profession.

FINDING WORK-LIFE HARMONY IN MEDICINE

> ***"Thousands of candles can be lighted from a single candle and the life of the candle will not be shortened. Happiness never decreases by being shared."***
>
> **—Buddha**

A manifestation of these four components of professionalism—engagement, integrity, respect, and self-awareness—is self-care and finding work-life harmony. Engagement, for example, as previously defined as "focused alignment of personal resources with a meaningful purpose"[8] can be thought of as committed attention to self-care. Integrity, as "commitment to excellence" can be applied to self-care as keeping promises to oneself, such as taking a break at the end of a long project, or ending a workday at a certain time. Respect, defined as appreciating the value in others, is easily applied to self-respect, and appreciating one's own strengths and qualities. Finally, self-awareness is also part of self-care, as physicians need to be aware of their own risk of burnout and take steps to address it.

Too often, the demands a physician may place on themselves trying to be the ideal physician, along with their altruistic character may wear them down. A common phrase being used in society today is "work-life balance." However, for many physicians, work is their passion; it is their calling. Because of their altruistic character, work is not in opposition to life. It is part of their life. "Work-life harmony" is a more correct term as physicians' work and life should not be at odds with each other. Instead, they should be interwoven with each other.

One way for a physician to achieve "work-life harmony" is to discuss and agree to reasonable expectations with not only their employers but with their friends and family. With work, this is often manifested by having an employment contract. However, physicians may fail to manage expectations with their loved ones, which can create stress and tension in their lives. Some ideas to try:

1. Not taking work home. When arriving at home focus on loved ones and their day. Learn to leave work at work.
2. Returning home from work by an agreed upon time to the best of their ability.
3. Make plans with friends and family when there is availability and keep to those plans. There is always more work to be done, but unless it is an absolute emergency, avoid cancelling plans. It is important to spend quality time with friends and family. Just as being professional is intentional so too is maintaining relationships with others.

A physician should spend time with those that support them and care for them as it is important for their mental and emotional health. Having a strong network of friends, whether at work or outside of work, is important for happiness. Being happy in general will help bring harmony to life. Some ways to help increase the ability to be happy are:

1. Express gratitude for all of the good things in life.
2. Spend time focusing on one's health.
   a. Exercise
   b. Eat healthy, nutritious food
   c. Get adequate sleep
   d. Manage stress
3. Reduce negative thoughts, and instead practice positive affirmations.
   a. Reduce judgment of oneself and others. Focus on the good not the bad.
   b. Forgive oneself and others for mistakes. Show grace.
4. Start a new hobby.
5. Choose to be happy.
   a. Kindly smile. Even when one doesn't feel like it.
6. Spend meaningful time with supportive family and friends.[43,44]

Another way to achieve "work-life harmony" is to learn to set boundaries by saying "No." Many physicians have altruistic characters, thus it is often difficult for them to say "no." They want to help and be there for others. However, before physicians say "yes," they need to pause and evaluate where they are in their own life. Do they have time to take on another project? Do they have the infrastructure and support in place to take on another project? How much of a demand will this truly place on them? If a physician is already feeling overwhelmed and overburdened then they need to say "no." Saying "no" does not imply they do not care, nor does it imply that they do not believe it to be a worthwhile project. It simply means that the physician needs to not overextend themselves to the detriment of their own physical or mental health or to the detriment of their relationships.

Another aspect of the concept of "work-life harmony" is resilience, the ability to withstand or recover quickly from difficult conditions. Oftentimes, it can be mentally, physically, and emotionally taxing to be a physician. Physicians may lose patients to disease and trauma, despite their best efforts. Sometimes they need to inform their patients of a terminal illness, knowing what this signifies, not only for the patient, but for their whole family. It is important that physicians recognize that resilience is essential to their functioning to serve others. Therefore, to the best of their ability, physicians should ensure that they develop and maintain resilience so that they can best care for their patients and avoid their own burn out.

If a physician finds themselves feeling overwhelmed or overburdened, then it may mean they need to recharge or boost their resilience. It may also mean that they need to evaluate their life and see what needs to change. Physicians cannot continue to give and give if they do not take care of themselves first or soon there will be nothing of themselves left to give. To be at their best for others, they first need to take care of themselves. Interestingly, ways to recharge and ways to be happy can be very similar. The best way to recharge is different for everyone, but some ideas to try:

1. Take a break
   a. Get up for a few minutes and walk outside for a few breathes of fresh air to clear the mind.
   b. If possible, take a trip. The change of scenery may help.
2. Focus on one's health
   a. Exercise and stretch
   b. Eat healthy, nutritious food
   c. Get adequate sleep
3. Manage stress
   a. Meditation
   b. Breathing exercises
   c. Treat oneself to something enjoyable
4. Connect with one's support group (family and friends)[45,46]

HUMILITY IN MEDICINE

> ***"Humility is the solid foundation of all virtues."***
>
> **—Confucius**

Humility is defined as "freedom from pride or arrogance: the quality or state of being humble."[47] Humility is important for developing clinical expertise and providing better patient care. A humble physician is aware of and appreciates the limitations to their abilities and knowledge. These limitations and knowledge gaps fuel the intrinsic motivation to seek further education; thus, leading to lifelong learners in an ever-changing profession.[48,49]

Furthermore, several studies have looked at physician humility from the perspective of the patient. Physicians that are generally perceived to be humbler are rated by patients as communicating more effectively, and patients report having greater patient satisfaction, trust, and self-reported health.[50,51] According to patients, the physician behaviors that contribute to their perception of humility are friendliness and approachability, patient focus, respect for the patient, and knowledge and admission of their own limitations.[52] In fact, physicians using an abrasive tone of voice or nonverbally signaling dominance and authority, which would be the opposite of humility, are associated with an increased likelihood of malpractice claims and litigation.[53]

Humility is also important for effective teamwork. It is necessary to build a good working relationship with all members of the health care team. If an individual is arrogant or abrasive, or communicates poorly, they may create a dysfunctional team and have a negative impact on patient care.[54]

Professionalism and humility are intentional behavior choices; thus, incorporating humble behaviors into daily practice can aid in being a humble physician. Consider the following simple actions:

1. Practice active listening and refrain from interrupting.
2. Express gratitude by saying "thank you" and "please."
3. Acknowledge others' presence by smiling and saying "Hello" or "Good morning/afternoon."
4. Ask for help when it is needed.
5. Admit when an error is made and apologize. Don't blame someone else.
6. Admit to knowledge gaps.
7. Treat everyone with respect.
8. Give credit where credit is due. Do not take credit for someone else's work.

SUMMARY

Professionalism is intentional just as is taking care of oneself and others is intentional. To be their best professional selves, to have the best patient–physician relationships, physicians need to engage in their own version of "work-life harmony." It will be different for everyone, and it may evolve over time or vary depending on what is occurring at that moment in time.

Professionalism is the cornerstone of the physician–patient relationship. Professionalism is intentional and is a skill that physicians commit to developing over their lifetime. There are many aspects of professionalism, and all are important for establishing and maintaining a healthy, successful physician–patient relationship.

Both the institution of medical education and the institution of medical practice bear responsibility for defining the components of professionalism and professional identity. Implicit and explicit guidance is needed to assist learners in professional identity formation. This process is dynamic, iterative, and longitudinal; ultimately, it is up to the learner to determine who they wish to become.

REFERENCES

1. Chandratilake M, McAleer S, Gibson J. Cultural similarities and differences in medical professionalism: a multi-region study. *Med Educ.* 2012;46(3):257–266.
2. Wynia MK, Papadakis MA, Sullivan WM, Hafferty FW. More than a list of values and desired behaviors: a foundational understanding of medical professionalism. *Acad Med.* 2014;89(5):712–714.
3. Goldie J. The formation of professional identity in medical students: considerations for educators. *Med Teach.* 2012;34(9):e641–e648.
4. Lave J, Wenger E. *Situated learning.* Cambridge University Press; 1991.
5. Mak-van der Vossen M, van Mook W, van der Burgt S, et al. Descriptors for unprofessional behaviours of medical students: a systematic review and categorization. *BMC Med Educ.* 2017;17(1):164.
6. Ainsworth MA, Szauter KM. Medical student professionalism: are we measuring the right behaviours? A comparison of professional lapses by students and physicians. *Acad Med.* 2006;81(10, Suppl):S83–S86.
7. Papadakis MA, Teherani A, Banach MA, et al. Disciplinary action by medical boards and prior behavior in medical school. *N Eng J Med.* 2005; 353(25):2673–2682.
8. Mueller MK. *Communication from the Inside Out: Strategies for the Engaged Professional.* F. A. Davis Company; 2010, Chapter 2.
9. Constantine D. Medical record documentation: time is of the essence. *CAPsules.* 2022:1–2. Accessed January 23, 2023. https://www.capphysicians.com/articles/medical-record-documentation-time-essence
10. Coverdale JH, Roberts LW, Balon R, et al. Professional integrity and the role of medical students in professional self-regulation. *Acad Psychiatry.* 2016;40(3):525–529.
11. Levinson W, Ginsburg S, Hafferty F, Lucey C. *Understanding Medical Professionalism.* McGraw-Hill Education; 2014, Chapter 5.
12. Anderson OA, Wearne IM. Informed consent for elective surgery–what is best practice? *J R Soc Med.* 2007;100(2):97–100.
13. https://ccaps.umn.edu/story/10-ways-show-professionalism-health-care-field#:~:text=In%20the%20health%20care%20profession,informed%20decisions%20about%20their%20care. Accessed June 4, 2024.
14. Otani K, Herrmann PA, Kurz, RS. Improving patient satisfaction in hospital care settings. *Health Serv Manage Res.* 2011;24(4):163–169.
15. ANA Position statement: The ethical responsibility to manage pain and the suffering it causes. *Online J Issues Nurs.* 2018;24(1).
16. Grant A. *No, You Can't Ignore Email. It's Rude.* The New York Times; 2019. Accessed November 25, 2022. https://www.nytimes.com/2019/02/15/opinion/sunday/email-etiquette.html
17. Bourke J, Titus A. Why inclusive leaders are good for organizations and how to become one. *Harv Bus Rev.* 2019. Accessed January 17, 2023. https://hbr.org/2019/03/why-inclusive-leaders-are-good-for-organizations-and-how-to-become-one
18. FitzGerald C, Hurst S. Implicit bias in healthcare professionals: a systematic review. *BMC Med Ethics.* 2017;18(1):19.
19. Petrilli CM, Saint S, Jennings JJ, et al. Understanding patient preference for physician attire: a cross-sectional observational study of 10 academic medical centres in the USA. *BMJ Open.* 2018;8(5):e021239. Published 2018 May 29.
20. Reddy R. Slippers and a white coat? (Hawai'i physician attire study). *Hawaii Med J.* 2009;68(11):284–285.
21. Petrilli CM, Mack M, Petrilli JJ, Hickner A, Saint S, Chopra V. Understanding the role of physician attire on patient perceptions: a systematic review of the literature–targeting attire to improve likelihood of rapport (TAILOR) investigators. *BMJ Open.* 2015;5(1):e006578. Published online January 19, 2015.
22. Moolenaar RL, Crutcher JM, San Joaquin VH, et al. A prolonged outbreak of Pseudomonas aeruginosa in a neonatal intensive care unit: did staff fingernails play a role in disease transmission? *Infect Control Hosp Epidemiol.* 2000;21(2):80–85.
23. Fagernes M, Lingaas E. Factors interfering with the microflora on hands: a regression analysis of samples from 465 healthcare workers. *J Adv Nurs.* 2011;67(2):297–307.
24. Rupp ME, Fitzgerald T, Puumala S, et al. Prospective, controlled, crossover trial of alcohol-based hand gel in critical care units. *Infect Control Hosp Epidemiol.* 2008;29(1):8–15.

25. Tan CM, Goleman D, Kabat-Zinn J. *Search Inside Yourself: The Unexpected Path to Achieving Success, Happiness (And World Peace).* HarperOne; 2012:268.
26. Kabat-Zinn J. *Wherever You Go, There You Are: Mindfulness Meditation in Everyday Life.* Hyperion; 2005:280.
27. Uchino R, Yanagawa F, Weigand B, et al. Focus on emotional intelligence in medical education: from problem awareness to system-based solutions. *Int J Acad Med.* 2015;1(1):9–20.
28. Brefczynski-Lewis JA, Lutz A, Schaefer HS, Levinson DB, Davidson RJ. Neural correlates of attentional expertise in long-term meditation practitioners. *Proc Natl Acad Sci USA.* 2007;104(27):11483–11488.
29. Salovey P, Mayer JD. Emotional intelligence. *Imagin Congn Pers.* 1990; 9:185–211.
30. Goleman D. *Emotional Intelligence.* Bantam Books; 1995:352.
31. Bar-On R. The Bar-On Emotional Quotient Inventory (EQ-i): rationale, description and summary of psychometric properties. In: Geher G, ed. *Measuring Emotional Intelligence: Common Ground and Controversy.* Nova Science Publishers; 2004:115–145.
32. Petrides KV, Furnham A. Trait emotional intelligence: psychometric investigation with reference to established trait taxonomies. *Eur J Pers.* 2001; 15:425–448.
33. Kim SS, Kaplowitz S, Johnston MV. The effects of physician empathy on patient satisfaction and compliance. *Eval Health Prof.* 2004;27(3):237–251.
34. Hojat M, Louis DZ, Markham FW, Wender R, Rabinowitz C, Gonnella JS. Physicians' empathy and clinical outcomes for diabetic patients. *Acad Med.* 2011;86(3):359–364.
35. Del Canale S, Louis DZ, Maio V, et al. The relationship between physician empathy and disease complications: an empirical study of primary care physicians and their diabetic patients in Parma, Italy. *Acad Med.* 2012;87(9):1243–1249.
36. Weng HC, Hung CM, Liu YT, et al. Associations between emotional intelligence and doctor burnout, job satisfaction and patient satisfaction. *Med Educ.* 2011;45(8):835–842.
37. Hojat M, Gonnella JS, Mangione S, et al. Empathy in medical students as related to academic performance, clinical competence and gender. *Med Educ.* 2002;36(6):522–527.
38. Licciardone JC, Schmitt ME, Aryal S. Empathy in medicine osteopathic and allopathic physician interpersonal manner, empathy, and communication style and clinical status of their patients: a pain registry–based study. *J Am Osteopath Assoc.* 2019:119(8):499–510.
39. Feldman MD. Altruism and medical practice. *J Gen Intern Med.* 2017; 32(7):719–720.
40. Chestnut DH. On the road to professionalism. *Anesthesiology.* 2017;126(5): 780–786.
41. Trastek VF, Hamilton NW, Niles EE. Leadership models in health care—a case for servant leadership. *Mayo Clin Proc.* 2014;89(3):374–381.
42. Ronquillo Y, Ellis VL, Toney-Butler TJ. Conflict management. In: *StatPearls.* NCBI Bookshelf version. StatPearls Publishing; 2022. Accessed January 17, 2023. https://www.ncbi.nlm.nih.gov/books/NBK470432/
43. Pietrangelo A. *How to Be Happy: 27 Habits to Add to Your Routine.* Healthline; 2019. Updated March 10, 2023. Accessed May 16, 2023. https://www.healthline.com/health/how-to-be-happy
44. Psychological and Counseling Services. *Positive Psychology Strategies for Increased Happiness.* University of New Hampshire; Updated 2023. Accessed May 16, 2023. https://www.unh.edu/pacs/positive-psychology-strategies-increased-happiness
45. Cirino E. *Recharge Your Personal Battery with These Activities.* Healthline; 2018. Accessed May 16, 2023. https://www.healthline.com/health/how-to-recharge
46. Shumake K. *How to Recharge: Tips from a Stanford Wellness Coach.* Stanford News; 2021. Accessed May 16, 2023. https://news.stanford.edu/2021/06/30/recharge-tips-stanford-wellness-coach/
47. Humility. In: *Merriam-Webster.com Dictionary.* Merriam-Webster; 2023. Accessed May 8, 2023. https://www.merriam-webster.com/dictionary/humility
48. Wadhwa A, Mahant S. Humility in medical practice: a qualitative study of peer-nominated excellent clinicians. *BMC Med Educ.* 2022;22(1):88.
49. Krumrei-Mancuso EJ, Haggard MC, LaBouff JP, Rowatt WC. Links between intellectual humility and acquiring knowledge. *J Posit Psychol.* 2020;15(2):155–170.
50. Huynh HP, Dicke-Bohmann A. Humble doctors, healthy patients? Exploring the relationships between clinician humility and patient satisfaction, trust, and health status. *Patient Educ Couns.* 2020;103(1):173–179.
51. Ruberton PM, Huynh HP, Miller TA, Kruse E, Chancellor J, Lyubomirsky S. The relationship between physician humility, physician-patient communication, and patient health. *Patient Educ Couns.* 2016;99(7):1138–1145.
52. Huynh HP, Dicke-Bohmann A, Nelson C. What do humble doctors do? A conceptualization of clinician humility from the patient's perspective. *Patient Educ Couns.* 2021;104(12):3066–3071.
53. Ambady N, Laplante D, Nguyen T, Rosenthal R, Chaumeton N, Levinson W. Surgeons' tone of voice: a clue to malpractice history. *Surgery.* 2002;132(1):5–9.
54. Berger AS. Arrogance among physicians. *Acad Med.* 2002;77(2):145–147.

26 The Five Models of Osteopathic Patient Care

RYAN A. SEALS

KEY CONCEPTS

- The five models of osteopathic patient care represent an anatomical and a physiologic approach to the patient.
- It was developed by the Educational Council on Osteopathic Principles (ECOP) of the American Association of Colleges of Osteopathic Medicine (AACOM) and approved by the Council of Deans in 1987.
- It uses a health-oriented, patient-centered approach based on the philosophy and principles of osteopathic medicine as expounded by its founder A. T. Still, DO.
- The five-model concept can be used as an aid to understand differential diagnoses of possible underlying pathophysiology for any given symptom or chief complaint, as well as to assist the physician in organizing the assessment and management plan.

INTRODUCTION AND BACKGROUND

This chapter will expand and apply the basic ideas of osteopathic philosophy as a patient-centered and health-oriented approach by introducing the Five Models of Osteopathic Patient Care. Recall that the fourth principle of osteopathic medicine states "rational treatment is based upon an understanding of the basic principles of body unity, self-regulation, and the interrelationship of structure and function."[1] In order to best understand the *unity* of the body, it is helpful to break down the different components into the individual *structures* and *functions*.

Anatomy is the study of the *structure* of organisms while physiology is the study of their *functions*[2,3]; these sciences provide foundational understanding of the human body and osteopathic medicine. Some physiology texts (e.g., Vander) have described 10 basic coordinated body functions, namely:

1. Control of posture and body movement
2. Respiration
3. Circulation
4. Regulation of water and electrolyte balance
5. Digestion and absorption of nutrients and elimination of wastes
6. Metabolism and energy balance
7. Protective mechanisms
8. The sensory system
9. Reproduction
10. Consciousness and behavior

Using this framework, the Educational Council on Osteopathic Principles (ECOP) of the American Association of Colleges of Osteopathic Medicine (AACOM) worked to develop osteopathic medical curriculum consistent with anatomy, physiology, and osteopathic philosophy. This group combined these concepts into the five basic body functions that became the five models of osteopathic care that "articulate how an osteopathic practitioner seeks to influence a patient's physiological processes."[1] The five models are (Table 26.1):

- Biomechanical–Structural
- Respiratory–Circulatory
- Neurologic
- Metabolic–Energetic
- Behavioral–Biopsychosocial

The original focus of the five models was to help guide treatment approaches; however, the concepts are equally valid from a diagnostic perspective. The five models provide different lenses and perspectives to address the multifaceted nature of the patient. By organizing the various anatomical and physiologic functions in this way, one can mitigate the temptation to become too focused on one aspect of health, dysfunction, or disease. After considering the five different models, one must reintegrate the diagnosis and treatment into a holistic picture of the entire body inclusive of mind, body, spirit, and the surrounding environment.

THE FIVE MODELS OF OSTEOPATHIC PATIENT CARE

Biomechanical–Structural Model

The biomechanical model views the patient from a structural and mechanical perspective and is foundational to the osteopathic philosophy. The focus is on the muscles, fascia, bones, tendons, and ligaments. These are the primary structures involved in the posture and movement of the body and play an integral role in osteopathic practice. Many of the somatic dysfunctions we identify are the result of joint restrictions and altered muscle tone. Irvin Korr, PhD referred to the musculoskeletal system as the "primary machinery of life" and Dr. Still named his original science "osteopathy" because one should start with the bones when investigating the underlying pathology.[4,5]

When applying the biomechanical model to diagnosis, an osteopathic physician can observe a patient's posture in standing, seated, and supine positions to assess symmetry, tissue mobility, muscle tension, and other tissue changes. After identifying areas of somatic dysfunction, osteopathic manipulative techniques such as high-velocity low-amplitude (HVLA), muscle energy, balanced ligamentous tension, ligamentous articular strain, myofascial release, and others aim to improve the structure and function of the musculoskeletal system by restoring ligamentous balance and normalizing muscle tone.

The goal in this model is to restore an ideal balance between skeletal, myofascial, and neurologic components that allows the body to have the greatest adaptive potential to stressors. For example, in a case of low back pain (LBP) a goal would be to optimize the posture around proper arches of the foot, a level sacral base, and

TABLE 26.1

Osteopathic Five Models in the Context of the Three Domains of a Philosophy of Medicine

Model	Anatomical Structures	Associated Body Regions	Physiologic Functions
Biomechanical–Structural	Postural muscles, spine, and extremities	Muscles and joints of the spine, back, and extremities	Posture and motion
Respiratory–Circulatory	Heart, lungs, blood and lymphatic vessels, thoracic inlet, costal cage, thoracic and pelvic diaphragms	Thoracic cage and diaphragm	Movement of body fluids and critical gas exchange
Neurologic	Head (including brain and organs of special sense), spinal cord, autonomic nervous system, peripheral nerves	Cranium and spine	Control, communication, and coordination of voluntary and involuntary actions of the body; information gathering and processing
Metabolic–Energetic	Internal organs and endocrine glands	Abdominopelvic cavity	Digestion, cellular and organ functions such as assimilation of nutrients, excretion of wastes, metabolic processes, tissue repair, protection from infection, and reproduction
Behavioral–Biopsychosocial	Brain (mind and consciousness)	N/A	Psychological and social activities, behaviors, habits, values, attitudes, and beliefs

vertical alignment of the ankles, legs, and spine. Research investigating the relationship between postural asymmetry and musculoskeletal pain does not support a cause-and-effect relationship,[6] but this does not rule out the value of evaluating and treating posture and biomechanics. Optimizing posture can be an important component of evaluation and treatment, but it is only one facet that must be considered for a particular patient.

This example illustrates why it is so important not to become reductionistic in the application of the five models. Static posture is one component involved in adapting to life's stressors, but it does not give a full picture of the function of the musculoskeletal system. The osteopathic approach incorporates the musculoskeletal system and how it interacts with the rest of the body. Posture alone cannot be fully isolated from the neurologic model because of the complex relationships between afferent inputs (proprioceptive, nociceptive, and interoceptive) and efferent outputs controlling myofascial tone.[7] Additionally, postural alterations in the bones, joints, ligaments, tendons, muscles, and fascia can impede vascular, lymphatic, and neurologic structures. These impediments can then affect the associated physiologic processes and homeostatic capacity of the body.

RESPIRATORY–CIRCULATORY MODEL

The respiratory–circulatory model focuses on critical gas exchange and the movement of the fluids of the body. The body fluids serve to maintain optimum function of the cells by transporting nutrients to the tissues and removing waste products. The adult body is about 50% to 70% fluid with two-thirds being intracellular (i.e., located inside individual cells) and one-third extracellular. The extracellular fluids contain the nutrients and ions needed to maintain the life of cells and are in constant motion throughout the body. In the respiratory–circulatory model, we should specifically consider the following types of extracellular fluid: arterial, venous, lymphatic, interstitial, and cerebrospinal.[8,9] Dr. Still emphasized role of proper fluid circulation in maintaining health with his quote: "The rule of the artery and vein is universal in all living beings."[10]

Respiration is the process by which an organism supplies its cells and tissues with oxygen and removes the carbon dioxide formed during energy production.[11] Respiration can occur at the cellular level via the diffusion of gases across cell membranes or at the level of the lungs where gas is exchanged with the external environment. Pulmonary respiration has traditionally been the focus of the respiratory–circulatory model, but the same principles apply to fluid and gas exchange at the cellular level.

The thoracic cage and diaphragm are the primary anatomical focus areas in this model because of their relationship to the lungs. The thoracic cage contains over 150 articulations and with normal breathing involves over 3 million combined joint movements daily.[12] The diaphragm moves inferiorly during inhalation to create negative intrathoracic pressure. This pressure change allows air to fill the lungs and pulls venous and lymphatic fluids into the thorax to facilitate their return to the heart. The diaphragm descends about 1 cm with normal respiration, but up to 4.7 cm with deep respiration.[13] Consider how restrictions in either the diaphragm and/or thoracic cage impact these pressure changes and the subsequent fluid movement. Similarly, restrictions of the pelvic diaphragm, thoracic inlet, and other fascial structures can also impede fluid movements in the body and should be considered in the diagnostic and treatment process.

The respiratory–circulatory screen of Zink assesses the mechanics of breathing, areas of passive fluid congestion, and fascial preferences at important transition zones and is a valuable diagnostic approach in this model. Osteopathic manipulation can be applied to the thoracic cage, structures of the fascial transition zones (e.g., the diaphragm), and areas of tissue congestion. Somatic dysfunction in structures of the thoracic inlet should always be identified and treated first given the importance of removing impediments to the terminal lymphatic drainage to the thoracic duct and right lymphatic duct. Fluid techniques and lymphatic pumps belong in this osteopathic model of treatment as well. Chapman's reflexes are considered neurolymphatic reflex points related to specific organs and would be considered in both the neurologic and respiratory–circulatory model.

To conclude this section, we will consider how the other four models influence respiration and circulation in the body. Biomechanical–structural alterations influence the movement of the diaphragm and rib cage; therefore, somatic dysfunction in these structures can influence ventilation and fluid movements. For example, scoliosis can impact exercise capacity and even heart and lung function if it becomes severe enough.[14] The nervous system, and thus the neurologic model, influences respiratory rate, vascular tone, and other factors related to ventilation and fluid exchange. The metabolic–energetic model overlaps via the relationship between inflammation, infection, nutrition, and metabolism on fluid and gas exchange in the cells. The inflammation associated with pneumonia, for example, can create pain and discomfort that makes breathing more difficult. The infectious consolidation in the lungs also limits gas exchange by interrupting the normal function of the alveoli in the area. Finally, behaviors such as smoking, and exposure inhaled toxins influence lung function and makes one more susceptible to a variety of maladies.

NEUROLOGIC MODEL

The neurologic model seeks to understand the influence of the autonomic nervous system, nociception, proprioception, and other functions of the nervous system on health and disease. The nervous system receives and processes sensory input and controls a variety of conscious and unconscious functions of the body. This section will highlight nociception, viscerosomatic reflexes, facilitation/sensitization, and the autonomic nervous system because of their importance to osteopathic theory and practice.

Patients often present to a physician's office with a complaint of pain. Pain is defined as "an unpleasant sensory and emotional experience associated with actual or potential tissue damage or described in terms of such damage."[15] Nociceptors are specific nerve fibers that carry information about harmful chemical, mechanical, or thermal stimuli to the central nervous system.[16] To properly evaluate pain, the osteopathic physician needs to understand the local and systemic conditions that result in nociceptive signaling and the complex neurologic circuitry involved in pain perception.

For acute pain, there is a relatively clear connection between an injury or disease and the appearance of pain. Chronic pain, however, involves more adaptive changes in the spinal cord and brain that makes diagnosis and management more complex. In chronic pain, the central nervous system becomes sensitized and interprets nonnociceptive signals as painful.[16] The term "facilitation" is similar to sensitization and describes a region of the spinal cord that is more reactive to afferent signals than normal.[1] Somatic dysfunction can both contribute to and be the result of spinal cord facilitation. One example of facilitation is the tissue texture changes related to viscerosomatic reflexes. Viscerosomatic reflexes occur when afferent input from a viscera causes a tissue response in a somatic structure of the related spinal segment. For example, gall bladder dysfunction can lead to pain and muscle hypertonicity of the ipsilateral posterior shoulder due to involvement of the phrenic nerve (from C3 to C5).

As we have seen previously, the neurologic model also overlaps with all the other models. The posture and movements of the biomechanical model are under tight control by the nervous system through proprioception and motor control. The autonomic nervous system is involved in heart rate, respiratory rate, vascular tone, and other components essential to the respiratory–circulatory model. The autonomic nervous system overlaps with the metabolic–energetic model by controlling peristalsis and blood flow to the digestive system and influencing inflammation on a cellular level. Finally, as we will see in the behavioral model section, emotional stress impacts the brain and sympathetic nervous system through the hypothalamic-pituitary-adrenal (HPA) axis.

METABOLIC–ENERGETIC (NUTRITIONAL) MODEL

The metabolic–energetic model focuses on nutrient absorption, energy conservation and expenditure, and the related immune, endocrine, and organ functions. The immune system creates an inflammatory response to protect the body and promote tissue repair in the short term, but chronic inflammation can contribute to a variety of diseases.[17] Reproduction is included in this model because of the hormonal and energy signals necessary for reproduction to occur.

From a diagnostic perspective, one should evaluate the patient's subjective energetic state by investigating symptoms such as fatigue and tolerance of various levels of exertion. Assessing the patient's nutritional status based on body composition (e.g., BMI, waist circumference) and metabolic parameters (e.g., insulin, lipid panes, glucose) are important to evaluate metabolic fitness. Palpatory findings such as the amplitude of the CRI can give indications of the body's overall energy status, while tissue texture findings can be identified that correlate with inflammation and autoimmune conditions.

Inflammatory diseases of the gastrointestinal tract are prototypical for the metabolic–energetic model. For example, celiac disease is caused by an inflammatory response to dietary gluten that causes structural changes to the small intestine villi and interrupts nutrient absorption. The impact of these changes can be muscle wasting, electrolyte imbalance, lethargy, and a variety of micronutrient deficiencies.[18] This condition illustrates the inflammatory, nutritional, and metabolic aspects of this model.

Treatments in this model focus on balancing the body's energy expenditure and enhancing immune, endocrine, and organ function. Many medications fall into the metabolic–energetic model, especially those addressing inflammation, glucose, insulin, and lipids. Osteopathic manipulation to the abdominopelvic viscera is included in this model, while lymphatic pumps and other fluid techniques can influence inflammation and nutrient exchange on the cellular level. Lymphatic and fluid approaches are typically considered in the respiratory–circulatory model but overlap with the metabolic–energetic model when influencing inflammation and metabolism. A patient's biomechanics and posture can influence the efficiency of movements and the overall allostatic load, thus connecting with the biomechanical model. Nutritional interventions and limiting environmental toxins involve habit changes related to the behavioral model.

BEHAVIORAL (BIOPSYCHOSOCIAL) MODEL

The behavioral model is also called the biopsychosocial model because it recognizes that a patient's health encompasses mental, emotional, and spiritual influences along with one's habits and behaviors. The term biopsychosocial model was coined in 1977 by George Engel,[19] but Dr. Still outlined a similar concept within

Osteopathy when he described the interconnectedness of the body, mind, and spirit.[20] Osteopathic physicians are encouraged to look beyond the symptoms, diseases, and somatic dysfunctions to other factors in the patient's life that help disease recovery and prevention.[4]

The behavioral model's impact on health and disease is supported by an abundance of evidence. It is well established that chronic stress impacts the HPA axis, can increase inflammation, and contribute to a variety of diseases.[21] Depression, anxiety, and emotional distress are often the best predictors of disability, mortality, and healthcare costs in patients with chronic pain. Conversely, positive affect, optimism, and strong social support are associated with less pain and dysfunction in these individuals.[22]

In patients with acute and chronic LBP, being nonemployed and demonstrating catastrophizing behaviors are strong predictors for disability; fear of pain is significantly associated with disability in chronic LBP.[23] Individuals with past traumas have up to a threefold increase in risk of developing chronic, widespread pain conditions such as fibromyalgia, irritable bowel syndrome, temporomandibular joint disorders, and chronic pelvic pain.[22] Even though these are associations and not causations, these examples provide strong support for addressing the patient's trauma history, emotional state, and social support. If we fail to consider these vital elements, we are not truly addressing the entire burden of disease.

The behavioral model also addresses lifestyle factors such as substance use, physical activity, and food choices. More than two-thirds of chronic diseases can be attributed to modifiable risk factors such as alcohol consumption, body mass index (BMI), cigarette smoking, unhealthy diet, and physical inactivity.[24] Behavior changes are essential for directly impacting disease pathogenesis and improving prognosis. As an example, exercise leads to extensive benefits against disease by decreasing cardiovascular risk factors, decreasing osteoporotic fractures, improving pain and physical function, decreasing fall risk, improving cognitive function, improving mood, and improving all-cause mortality.[25] The benefits of smoking cessation (or avoidance) and maintaining a healthy body weight cannot be overemphasized.

The patient's home and/or work environment, ergonomics, repetitive activities, and toxin exposure are all part of the behavioral model of osteopathic medicine. Family relationships, social support, hobbies, spiritual traditions, and community engagement are also considered in this model. Osteopathic physicians utilize a patient-centered approach to compassionately address the mind and spirit. The quality of the physician–patient relationship is an important aspect of the care process. Physicians perceived as being trustworthy, friendly, and supportive have higher levels of patient satisfaction.[26]

The osteopathic approach addresses the psychological, social, cultural, behavioral, and spiritual elements within the plan of care. Cognitive behavioral therapy (CBT), biofeedback, meditation, and group therapy are treatment approaches in this model. Finally, OMT can be employed through the lens of the behavioral model. OMT may indirectly impact stress by decreasing hypersympathicotonia, normalizing heart rate variability, and modulating blood flow to the prefrontal brain regions. Additionally, there is mechanistic support for OMT influencing this model by impacting stress hormones, vagal tone, and central mediators of nociception.[9] The behavioral–biopsychosocial model is an essential part of our osteopathic distinctiveness because it addresses the nonphysical components of disease. Furthermore, this model promotes a partnership with the patient to address habits, attitudes, and beliefs that improve health and well-being.

APPLYING THE FIVE MODELS IN ASSESSMENT AND TREATMENT

To better understand how these models relate to patient care, the following case presentations will illustrate how to incorporate the five models during the history, examination, diagnosis, and treatment. One of A. T. Still's students, Arthur Hildreth, DO, recorded Dr. Still's thought process during a patient encounter:

> When a patient comes to me for examination and begins to talk to me about symptoms…while listening, I am seeing in my mind's eye the combinations of systems which go to make up the whole of that body structure. I am concentrating on her story, trying to determine through the description given to me the structural alterations, which have occurred to produce the symptoms described. I am seeing first the bony framework and the joints, which hold it together as one system, the foundation upon which all other structures in the human body are built. I am seeing, especially, the positions of those bony parts and their relationships, one with the other. Then I see the ligaments…the muscles…the nervous system in all its relationships, in every function of the body…controlling the functions of the internal organs, the circulation of body fluids, and nutrition of the various body parts…I further see the arterial system….the venous system…the lymphatic system (and their functions)…and last but not least I see the glandular system of the body and wonder how it brings about its effect in each particular case.[27]

Notice how he uses an anatomical–physiologic approach, thinking about how the structures and their functions relate to the patient's symptoms and how he considers the structural, neurologic, circulatory, and metabolic effects first singularly and then as interrelated components.

The Five Models framework helps organize and apply the unique osteopathic approach to the history, physical exam, assessment, and treatment plan. Table 26.2 organizes common patient presentations and their differential diagnoses using the Five Models. It is useful to consider all the models to avoid being overly reductionist, but each individual patient or disease condition may warrant more emphasis on certain models.

CASE PRESENTATIONS

PARESTHESIA

Originally submitted by: Edwin Amirianfar (DO 2019), WUHS-COMP.

Chief Complaint

"I am having neck pain and numbness/tingling in my fingers."

History of the Present Illness

A 54-year-old female patient presents to the clinic with bilateral neck pain. The pain began 5 years ago and is described as tightness and stiffness in nature. She has a history of a motor vehicle collision 25 years ago in which she sustained a "whiplash" injury. The patient admits to pain radiating to her left hand associated with numbness and tingling in her fingers and thumb. Neck flexion makes the pain worse, but nothing seems to alleviate the pain. Pain is rated 5/10 in intensity and described as intermittent, worse at nighttime, and occasionally awakens her from sleep. The patient has tried chiropractic, yoga, and pain medications with no lasting relief. She denies history of head or neck trauma since the collision. She has not had an MRI or CT scan performed for this complaint.

TABLE 26.2

Differential Diagnoses Organized by Symptom Using the Five Models

Symptom/Models	Structural	Respiratory–Circulatory	Neurological	Metabolic	Behavioral
Head pain	Somatic dysfunction,[a] congenital deformities, fracture, herniated cervical disk, ocular muscle strain, trauma, temporomandibular joint disorder	Arteriovenous malformation, cerebral aneurysm, Chiari malformation, glaucoma, hydrocephalus, epidural, subdural, or subarachnoid hemorrhages, pseudotumor cerebri	Peripheral and/or central sensitization/facilitated spinal cord segment, fibromyalgia, hemicrania continua, migraine, occipital neuralgia, tension-type headache	Arthritis, bacterial endocarditis, cancer, dental abscess, gum or tooth infection, herpes zoster, iritis, retropharyngeal abscess, meningitis, pharyngitis, sinusitis, vasculitis, THoVoFIS	ADOI, caffeine withdrawal, alcohol abuse (hangover)
Neck pain	Somatic dysfunction,[a] congenital malformations, cervical spinal stenosis with myopathy, fracture, herniated cervical disk, spondylosis, spondylolysis, spondylolisthesis, temporomandibular joint disorder, torticollis	Carotidynia, dissecting carotid aneurysm, vertebral artery dissection or rupture	Peripheral and/or central sensitization/facilitated spinal cord segment, fibromyalgia, spinal cord injury	Arthritis, bacterial endocarditis, cancer, epiglottitis, herpes zoster, peritonsillar or dental abscess, pharyngitis, thyroiditis, lumphadenitis, THoVoFIS	ADOI
Low back pain	Somatic dysfunction,[a] congenital malformations, degenerative or ruptured disk, fracture, lumbar spinal stenosis with myopathy, spondylosis, spondylolysis, spondylolisthesis, short leg syndrome, trauma	Dissecting aortic aneurysm, epidural venous anomaly, ischemic claudication	Peripheral and/or central sensitization/facilitated spinal cord segment, fibromyalgia, multiple sclerosis, hemiplegia	Arthritis, bacterial endocarditis, cancer (primary or metastasis), cholecystitis, diskitis, endometriosis, herpes zoster, inflammatory bowel disease, nephritis, osteomyelitis, osteoporosis, Paget disease, pancreatitis, penetrating ulcer, prostatitis, spinal or paraspinal abscess, ureteral colic from stone, urinary tract infection, THoVoFIS	Compensable injury, Seeking disability or narcotics, somatoform or delusional disorder, ADOI, drug abuse
Chest pain	Somatic dysfunction,[a] fracture, cervical or thoracic spondylosis	Angina, dissecting thoracic aorta aneurysm, myocardial infarction, pleural effusion, pneumothorax, primary pulmonary hypertension, pulmonary embolus	Peripheral and/or central sensitization/facilitated spinal cord segment, fibromyalgia	Bronchitis, bacterial endocarditis, cardiomyopathy, cancer, cholecystitis, costochondritis, esophagitis, esophageal rupture or spasm, gastritis, gastric ulcer, herpes zoster, hiatal hernia, liver or subdiaphragmatic abscess, mastitis, pericarditis, pneumonitis, pleural effusion, pleurisy, pneumonia, THoVoFIS	ADOI, tobacco abuse

(*continued*)

TABLE 26.2 (Continued)

Differential Diagnoses Organized by Symptom Using the Five Models

Symptom/Models	Structural	Respiratory–Circulatory	Neurological	Metabolic	Behavioral
Dyspnea	Somatic dysfunction,[a] diaphragm or intercostal muscle rupture, foreign body in trachea or bronchi, thoracic spine or rib cage fracture	Anemia, congestive heart failure, COPD, ischemic heart disease, pericardial tamponade, pulmonary edema, pleural effusion, pneumothorax, primary pulmonary hypertension, pulmonary emboli, valvular heart disease	Cardiac arrhythmia, peripheral and/or central sensitization/ facilitated spinal cord segment	Asthma, bacterial endocarditis, bronchitis, cancer, granulomatosis with polyangiitis, laryngeal edema, pericarditis, pneumonitis, pneumoconiosis, pleurisy, pleural effusion, pneumonia, sarcoidosis, systemic lupus erythematosus, THoVoFIS	ADOI
Abdominal pain	Somatic dysfunction,[a] abdominal muscle strain or tear, adhesions, bowel obstruction, intussusception, lower costal cage fracture or dislocation, paraspinal muscle spasms	Acute mesenteric ischemia, aortic aneurysm, splenic rupture, ascites, intra-abdominal hemorrhage, leukemia, myocardial infarction, sickle cell anemia	Peripheral and/or central sensitization/facilitated spinal cord segment, fibromyalgia, abdominal migraine	Adrenal insufficiency, appendicitis, bacterial endocarditis, cancer, cholecystitis, colitis, diabetic ketoacidosis, diverticulitis, duodenal ulcer, ectopic pregnancy, enteritis, gastritis, hepatitis, ovarian torsion, pancreatitis, pelvic inflammatory disease, peritonitis, renal colic, tuboovarian abscess, THoVoFIS	ADOI, opiate withdrawal, alcohol abuse, "functional abdominal pain"
Pelvic pain	Somatic dysfunction,[a] adhesions, congenital deformities, fracture, muscle or ligament rupture, muscle spasms, trauma	Blood clots, ischemia, varicose veins	Peripheral and/or central sensitization/facilitated spinal cord segment, fibromyalgia	Arthritis, cancer, cystitis, dysmenorrhea, ectopic pregnancy, endometriosis, ovarian torsion, pelvic inflammatory disease, pregnancy, labor and parturition, abruptio placenta, prostatitis, urinary tract infection, THoVoFIS	ADOI, sexually transmitted disease
Shoulder pain	Somatic dysfunction,[a] adhesive capsulitis, congenital deformities, dislocation, fracture, impingement, muscle, capsule or ligament tear, tendonosis	Avascular necrosis, hemarthrosis, ischemia, thoracic outlet syndrome	Peripheral and/or central sensitization/facilitated spinal cord segment, brachial, axillary or subscapular nerve palsy, cervical radiculopathy, diabetes mellitus, fibromyalgia, hemiplegia, multiple sclerosis, referred pain from thoracic or abdominal organic disease	Arthritis, cancer, bursitis, sprain, bacterial endocarditis, septic joint, tendonitis, THoVoFIS	ADOI
Elbow pain	Somatic dysfunction,[a] cervical disk disease, cervical spondylosis, congenital deformities, thoracic outlet syndrome	Hemiplegia from cerebral vascular accident, ischemia	Fibromyalgia, multiple sclerosis, amyloidosis, brachial plexopathy, cervical radiculopathy, complex regional pain syndrome, hemiplegia, neuropathy	Arthritis, bacterial endocarditis, bursitis, cancer, epicondylitis, septic joint, sprain, tenosynovitis, tendonitis, THoVoFIS	ADOI

Wrist pain	Somatic dysfunction,[a] cervical disk disease, cervical spondylosis, congenital deformities, pronator teres syndrome, thoracic outlet syndrome	Compartment syndrome, hemiplegia from cerebral vascular accident, ischemia, Reynaud syndrome	Amyloidosis, carpal tunnel syndrome, fibromyalgia, hemiplegia, multiple sclerosis, brachial plexopathy, neuropathy, complex regional pain syndrome, syringomyelia	Acromegaly, arthritis, bacterial endocarditis, cancer, diabetic neuropathy, hypothyroidism, leprosy, Lyme disease, pregnancy, renal failure on dialysis, sprain, tenosynovitis, THoVoFIS	ADOI
Hip pain	Somatic dysfunction,[a] congenital deformities, degenerative joint disease, dislocation, fracture	Avascular necrosis, hemarthrosis, ischemia	Peripheral and/or central sensitization/facilitated spinal cord segment, fibromyalgia, hemiplegia, lumbar radiculopathy, meralgia paresthetica, multiple sclerosis, amyloidosis, neuropathy, complex regional pain syndrome, syringomyelia	Arthritis, bacterial endocarditis, bursitis, cancer, Lyme disease, septic joint, sprain, tendonitis, THoVoFIS	ADOI
Knee pain	Somatic dysfunction, congenital deformities, meniscal or ligament tear, patellofemoral syndrome, degenerative joint disease	Avascular necrosis, hemarthrosis, ischemia	Peripheral and/or central sensitization/facilitated spinal cord segment, fibromyalgia, hemiplegia, multiple sclerosis, amyloidosis, neuropathy, complex regional pain syndrome, syringomyelia	Arthritis, bacterial endocarditis, bursitis, cancer, septic joint, sprain, tendonitis, THoVoFIS	ADOI
Ankle pain	Somatic dysfunction, congenital deformities, degenerative joint disease, fracture, muscle or ligament tear	Avascular necrosis, hemarthrosis, ischemia	Peripheral and/or central sensitization/facilitated spinal cord segment, fibromyalgia, hemiplegia, multiple sclerosis, amyloidosis, neuropathy, complex regional pain syndrome, syringomyelia	Arthritis, bacterial endocarditis, bursitis, cancer, septic joint, sprain, tendonitis, THoVoFIS	ADOI

THoVoFIS acronym for Tuberculosis, Hepatitis, other Viral or Fungal Infections, Syphilis. ADOI acronym for Anxiety, Depression, Overuse Injury (i.e., work or sports).
[a]See parts three and four of this book for more details on evaluating each of these body regions.

Allergies

No known drug allergies.

Medications

Omeprazole, 40 mg, daily; baclofen, 10 mg, daily; oxycodone, 5 mg, as needed for severe pain; tylenol as needed for HA.

Past Medical History

Gastroesophageal reflux disease, neck pain.

Past Surgical History

Left Hallux Valgus repair in 2014.

Family Medical History

Parents alive in their late 70s and healthy. Three siblings alive and well. No family history of neurologic problems or depression.

Social History

Happily married for 30 years with three adult children, works as a legal secretary, has moderate stress, never smoked tobacco, and denies alcohol or drug use.

REVIEW OF SYSTEMS

General

Denies appetite changes, weight changes, fevers, chills, night sweats.

HEENT

Denies sore throat, sinus congestion, and changes in vision, smell, hearing, or taste.

Cardiovascular

Denies chest pain, shortness of breath.

Respiratory

Denies cough, dyspnea, and phlegm.

Gastrointestinal

Denies abdominal pain, nausea, vomiting, diarrhea, constipation, changes in bowel control.

Genitourinary

Denies dysuria, recurrent urinary tract infections, or issues with bladder control.

Gynecologic

She is G3P3, perimenopausal, last menses 3 months ago. Last pap, pelvic, breast, and mammogram exams were normal 3 months ago. She does experience hot flashes. She is not taking hormone replacement therapy.

Endocrine

Denies polydipsia, polyphagia, polyuria, heat or cold intolerance.

Dermatologic

Denies rashes, itching.

Neurologic

Denies weakness, back or leg pains, seizures, stroke, paralysis.

Psychiatric

Denies depression, crying spells, emotional lability, sleep disturbance, anxiety, and hallucinations.

DIFFERENTIAL DIAGNOSIS

At this point, the physician considers the five models and makes another assessment of potential diagnoses prior to the physical examination. For example, the following cannot yet be ruled out by the history alone:

Biomechanical

Somatic dysfunction; congenital malformations; cervical spinal stenosis with myopathy; herniated cervical disk; spondylosis; spondylolysis; spondylolisthesis; upper cross syndrome; torticollis.

Neurologic

Peripheral and/or central sensitization/facilitated spinal cord segment; fibromyalgia; cervical radiculopathy; carpal tunnel syndrome; thoracic outlet syndrome; brachial plexopathy; median neuropathy.

Respiratory–Circulatory

Stroke; cerebral or spinal cord ischemia.

Metabolic

Arthritis; cancer; infection.

Biopsychosocial

Overuse injury; drug seeking; malingering; secondary gain; stress.

PHYSICAL EXAMINATION

Vitals

Blood Pressure: 97/61, pulse: 65 beats per minute, respirations: 12 per minute, temperature: 97 °F, weight: 115 lb, height: 5′4″.

General

Well-developed, well-nourished, well-hydrated female in no apparent distress.

HEENT

No pharyngeal erythema, exudates, no lymphadenopathy, thyromegaly. Pupils equal, round, reactive to light, no auditory deficits, nares clear.

Heart

Rate and rhythm regular, no murmurs.

Lungs

Clear to auscultation bilaterally.

Abdomen

Soft, nontender, no hepatosplenomegaly, negative Murphy sign, no rebound tenderness.

Gynecologic

Deferred per patient request.

Extremities

No cyanosis, clubbing, edema.

Skin

Dry, no rashes, ecchymosis, lesions.

Neurologic

Biceps, triceps, and brachioradialis reflexes +2/4 bilaterally; Negative Spurling test for radiculopathy bilaterally; Negative Tinel and Phalen signs at the left wrist. Positive Adson test on the left.

OSTEOPATHIC STRUCTURAL EXAM

Cervical

Active range of motion diminished in left side bending and rotation. Paraspinal muscle tension on the left is tender to palpation. Occipital–atlantal joint is extended, side bent left, and rotated right; atlantoaxial joint is rotated left; C4 is extended, side bent, and rotated left. Anterior, medial, and posterior scalene muscles are hypertonic on the left side.

Thoracic

Flattened kyphotic curvature; T1 extended, rotated, and side bent left; T2–T5 neutral, rotated left, and side bent right.

Rib Cage

Left first rib has inhalation somatic dysfunction.

Upper Extremity

Left pectoralis minor muscle hypertonicity and tenderness; left posterior radial head; left wrist flexion dysfunction; restricted left transverse carpal ligament.

Lumbar

Right paraspinal muscle hypertonicity.

Pelvis, Sacrum, Lower Extremities, Head, and Abdominal Regions

No significant findings.

Assessment

Based on the history and osteopathic physical examination, the most likely diagnosis is thoracic outlet syndrome caused by compression of the neurovascular bundle as it passes between one or more of the following structures (see Figure 26.1):

- The anterior and middle scalene muscles
- The first rib and clavicle
- The pectoralis minor muscle and rib cage

If there is higher suspicion cervical spinal stenosis with myopathy, herniated cervical disk, spondylosis, spondylolysis, or spondylolisthesis would need to be further assessed by CT and MRI studies.

PLAN

The goals of treatment are to alleviate symptoms caused by the compression of the neurovascular structures exiting the thoracic outlet. Each of the Five Models plays a role in the treatment approach for this patient.

BIOMECHANICAL

The patient was treated with OMT to improve the somatic dysfunctions of the upper thoracic spine, scalene, and pectoralis muscles. OMT helped restore normal muscle tone and posture. Stretches were prescribed to help restore a more optimum posture.

RESPIRATORY–CIRCULATORY

By addressing the above somatic dysfunctions, the respiratory–circulatory model was influenced by removing restrictions to blood flow and restoring rib cage motion.

NEUROLOGIC

By addressing the above somatic dysfunctions, the neurologic model was influenced by removing restrictions to the nerve structures exiting the thoracic outlet region.

METABOLIC–ENERGETIC

Consider NSAIDs to address any inflammation contributing to neck pain and plan to discontinue oxycodone.

BEHAVIORAL

The patient was instructed on proper ergonomics at work to minimize the muscle imbalances that led to the clinical condition. A plan was developed with the patient to incorporate home stretching into her daily routine.

FOLLOW-UP

The patient received OMT once weekly for 6 weeks which reduced the hypertonicity of the scalene and pectoralis muscles;

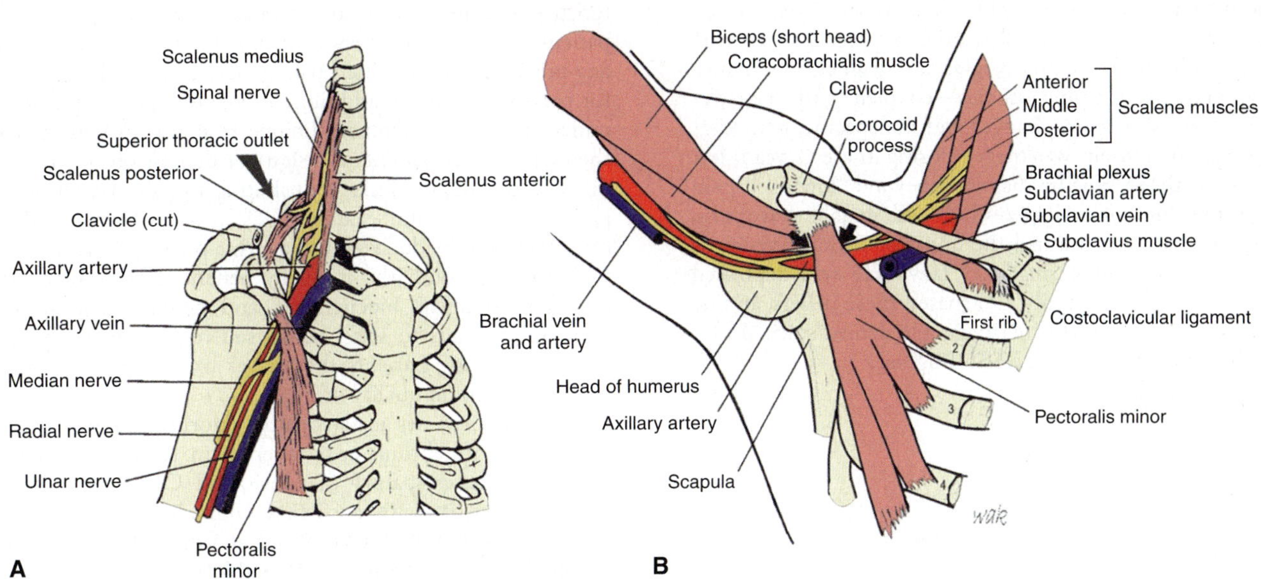

Figure 26.1. Thoracic Outlet Syndrome. A. Normal anatomy of right shoulder. **B.** Compression of neurovascular structures upon right shoulder abduction. (Illustration modified by William A. Kuchera, DO, FAAO, used with permission.)

the left first rib was repositioned and had normal physiologic motion during respiration; the thoracic spine mobility improved; the involved muscles of the left upper extremity were relaxed; the patient's pain, stiffness, and tension were relieved as motion and function were restored to the cervical spine and musculature of the neck and left upper extremity. The patient was instructed on proper ergonomic positions at work and home, stretching of the hypertonic muscles on a daily basis, postural education, and decreased dependency on medications. Sleep improved as did her confidence in her body to heal itself when obstructions to health were removed. The paresthesia was gone by the fourth visit and remained quiescent at successive follow-up visits.

ADULT WITH CHRONIC PAIN AND DEPRESSION

Originally submitted by Michael Kuchera, DO and John Jerome, PhD.

CHIEF COMPLAINT

"I have had chronic back pain for 3 years."

HISTORY OF PRESENT ILLNESS

Chuck, a 45-year-old farmhand, was seen in the clinic with a complaint of back pain. The pain first occurred while the patient carried a small bale of hay in front of his body. He had stepped in an unseen pothole, stumbled, and fell. The next day, he noticed severe back pain, which persisted as recurring episodes for several months. Between and during episodes, he achieved only partial relief with ibuprofen (800 mg/d). Physical therapy reportedly aggravated his pain. His discomfort, present on his right side, was described as deep, nagging, and constant, with periods of acute exacerbation into the right hip, groin, and down the back of the leg to just above the knee. Full symptoms would occur with prolonged walking or standing and would persist for several weeks. The patient was unable to lift more than 25 lb (11 kg) without aggravating his symptoms. His back took several hours to fully relax after lying down.

The patient visited several physicians over a 3-year period prompted by three to four substantial recurrences per year. Negative results from electromyographic, magnetic resonance imaging, and radiographic studies—coupled with negative results from tests of reflex changes and nonspecific, nonradicular patterns of muscle weakness—during these 3 years left the patient with no specific diagnosis beyond "low back pain with recurrent lumbosacral sprain." He was unable to work on the farm and said that he had the impression that physicians believed he was "malingering," or "lazy." He was depressed because he thought his family also shared these beliefs, and he became concerned about his marriage. He denied suicidal ideations. He denied smoking or illicit drug use.

Past Medical History

None.

Medications

Ibuprofen prn.

Past Surgical History

None.

Review of Systems

Noncontributory to chief complaint.

PHYSICAL EXAMINATION

General

Slim statured, appeared his stated age.

Neurologic

Negative straight leg raise, symmetric deep tendon reflexes at patella and Achilles, negative Babinksi.

Musculoskeletal

Negative Lloyd kidney tap test, Trendelenburg test of the right leg was equivocal, mild scoliosis curve and unlevel iliac crests noted (suggestive for short leg syndrome).

OSTEOPATHIC STRUCTURAL EXAM

Lumbar Spine

Reduced lumbar lordosis, tenderness noted over the right iliolumbar ligament.

Pelvis

Left iliacus tenderpoint, right superior innominate shear.

Sacrum

Tenderness noted over right sacroiliac ligament, right piriformis tenderpoint.

Rib Cage

Diaphragm inhalation dysfunction.

Assessment

See Table 26.2 for considerations of possible diagnoses using the five-model approach in a patient with LBP. The patient was informed that this constellation of somatic dysfunction could cause chronic LBP that often responded favorably to OMT.

CHRONIC LOW BACK PAIN

Persistent nonmalignant pain is not a single entity. It has many different causes and manifestations, each with varied characteristics and names. In an osteopathic approach, a complete patient history and physical examination are used to reveal any previously unidentified pain generator or underlying cause for persistent pain. In addition, osteopathic physicians need to understand the individual's unique response to pain and will therefore screen patients for signs of depression or other significant nonsomatic links contributing to pain. Based on such patient histories and examinations, osteopathic practitioners can develop individualized osteopathic prescriptions to address their findings, with the mutually beneficial goals of decreasing biomechanical, biochemical, and psychological stressors, removing barriers to self-healing, self-regulating mechanisms, and empowering patients themselves to reduce the impact of persistent pain on quality of life.

Table 26.3 shows an osteopathic algorithm for management of patients with chronic or recurrent pain. An OMM approach that integrates palpatory diagnosis and OMT provides balance for patients with persistent nonmalignant pain seeking both state-of-the-art interventions and individualized patient-centered care. The various osteopathic models offer strategies both to decrease pain and to enhance physiologic function.

TABLE 26.3

Osteopathic Algorithm for Management of Patients with Chronic or Recurrent Pain

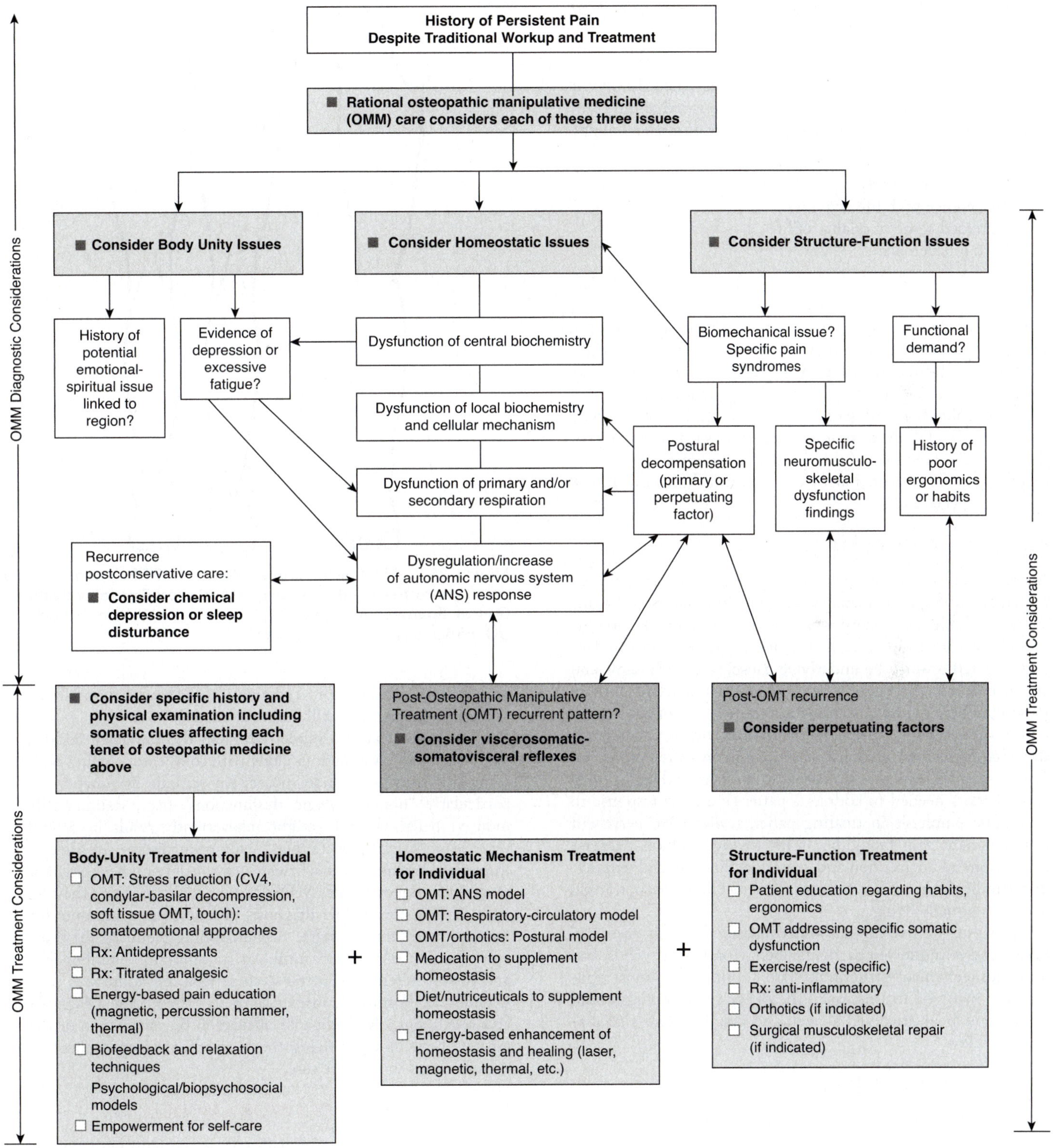

In this fashion, the osteopathic perspective offers two major recognized advantages: an expanded differential of potentially treatable etiologies and an individualized, patient-centered pain prescription based on the application of osteopathic principles.

DEPRESSION

Chuck's depression appears more situational (i.e., dysthymic disorder) and secondary to his pain as there is irritability, sadness, lack of interest in enjoyed activities, fear of movement and reinjury by heavy farm work. He has:

Reduction in activity
Interference with life activities
Decreased sense of quality of life
Work interference

PLAN

OMT provided to the patient consisted of applying the springing, direct method muscle energy technique to the right innominate shear, counterstrain to the iliacus and piriformis tender points, and indirect balanced ligamentous tension to the thoracolumbar and sacral regions. Fascial patterns were treated with HVLA techniques aimed toward symmetry of the transition junctions of the spine, and abdominal and pelvic diaphragms were treated with indirect and direct myofascial release, respectively.

DISCUSSION OF PLAN

In addition to providing appropriate strategies for management of pain, an osteopathic management algorithm (such as the one shown in Table 26.3 incorporates the five common osteopathic models of care to identify and address a variety of host factors directed toward the underlying cause, secondary signs and symptoms, and the tangible and persistent impact of both in patients. These models also provide a framework for the patient education needed to foster compliance built on an understanding of complex interrelationships among many different factors. Each osteopathic prescription seeks to discover and incorporate those factors needed to address a patient's unique response to pain. The emphasis in treating patients who have persistent nonmalignant pain should be on improving function, decreasing peripheral nociception and central facilitation, and empowering individuals to move forward in resuming their normal activities of daily living.

Each of the five models was considered in this case history and two models in particular, behavioral–biopsychosocial and biomechanical–structural, were found to be most specifically involved in this case. The other three models could easily have been involved as well and are therefore also discussed below.

BIOMECHANICAL MODEL

In the biomechanical–structural model, OMT is applied primarily to remove somatic dysfunctions and their objective manifestations of tenderness, asymmetry, ROM alteration, and tissue texture change. That said, identifying and addressing the "key lesions" (or primary somatic dysfunctions) becomes the goal of the model. For example, postural imbalance and compensatory somatic dysfunction above the innominate shear was a real, albeit secondary, consequence in Chuck's case. Obviously, without specific palpatory examination for sacral, innominate, and pubic shears, they will be overlooked.

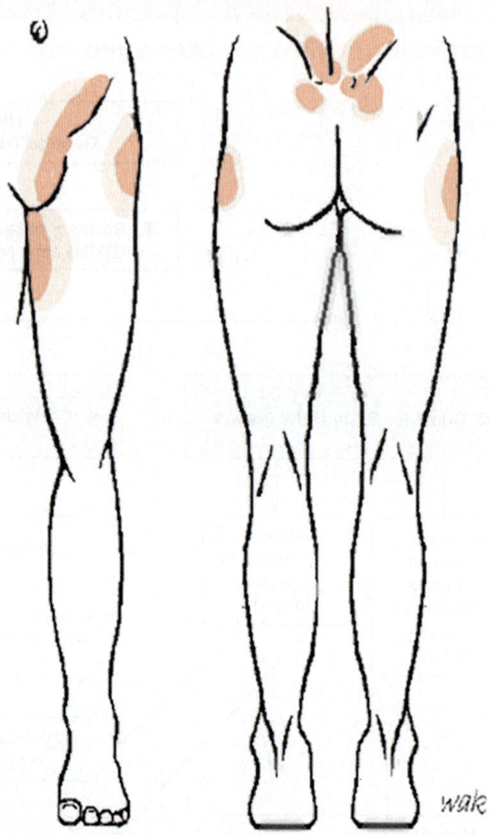

Figure 26.2. Myofascial Trigger Points (MFTrPs) and referred pain syndromes from lumbosacral and sacroiliac joint dysfunction or ligamentous sprains. (Illustration by William A. Kuchera, DO, FAAO, used with permission.)

The biomechanical model can help the physician address the key somatic dysfunctions along with compensatory sites with somatic dysfunction. Undiagnosed, key somatic dysfunctions—particularly "nonphysiologic dysfunctions" (e.g., traumatically induced pelvic shears)—might inadvertently result in several years of persistent pain (either locally or at distant sites linked through compensatory mechanisms) or the development of latent myofascial trigger points (MFTrPs) that recur whenever they are stressed (Fig. 26.2). The diagnosis of "short leg syndrome" (or more properly that of sacral base unleveling requiring lift therapy) should be reserved until—at a minimum—lumbopelvic and lower extremity somatic dysfunctions are addressed. (See Chapter 92 Postural Considerations in Osteopathic Diagnosis and Treatment.) Reduction or alleviation of pain is one of the greatest benefits of applying the biomechanical model, as was demonstrated in Chuck's case.

RESPIRATORY–CIRCULATORY MODEL

Note that mentally or emotionally stressed patients with chronic pain often breathe more shallowly and rapidly. As pain and stress are relieved, often the patient will sigh deeply and switch their respiration over to a slower, deeper, and more effective respiration. This, in turn, helps to maintain that pain reduction. To this end, the respiratory–circulatory model has been applied by osteopathic physicians in managing chronic pain patients.

Maximizing the mobility of the thoracic and pelvic diaphragms, and the thoracic inlet structures, enhances venous and lymphatic drainage. Patients with chronic lumbosacral spine and pelvic somatic dysfunction typically have dysfunctional diaphragmatic motion as well. Thus, addressing the thoracolumbar junction as well as the lumbosacral junction and the associated muscular diaphragms will improve respiratory efficiency. Maximizing the respiratory system to act as a suction pump to reduce local pain is accomplished not only through mechanical intervention by the osteopathic physician using OMT and postural strategies.

NEUROLOGIC MODEL

Pelvic shears often disrupt muscle balance both related to their pelvic attachments and to the body's compensation for these disruptive somatic dysfunctions. Piriformis hypertonicity is common with innominate shears because of its sacral attachments. Such piriformis dysfunction can manifest with posterior pelvis and thigh pain, rarely moving below the knee, secondary to MFTrPs or mechanical pressure upon—or even entrapment of—a portion of the sciatic nerve. Counterstrain or even procaine injection of the piriformis muscle may provide temporary relief from the referred pain, but it will likely recur until the pelvic shear is corrected.

METABOLIC–ENERGETIC MODEL

The HPA axis is affected by the chronic pain state. This system serves as a bridge between the neurologic and the metabolic–energetic models. The resultant increases in cortisol influence interleukin and other components of the immune system and may impact overall health.

BEHAVIORAL MODEL

The behavioral model of chronic pain emphasizes pain as a multidimensional (i.e., mind, body, and spirit) phenomenon expressed as interactions among somatosensory inputs, cognitive and behavioral processes, emotions, and various adaptive/maladaptive coping strategies. Chronic pain is punctuated by high incidence, high relapse, and low rate of recovery. Osteopathic physicians treating chronic back pain often encounter returning symptoms. Patients like Chuck who have had pain for 3 years are particularly frustrating to healthcare providers trying to identify pain generators, somatic dysfunction, and a return to optimal function and health.

In Chuck's case, loss of job, probable financial instability, and the family and physician questioning his intent create tremendous chronic stress affecting immune, neurologic, endocrine, and musculoskeletal systems. Couple this with shame or guilt for not being able to work and not living up to family expectations, perhaps anger for not being believed, and the sheer burden of persistent nociception, and it is clear that secondary losses outweigh any value added by pain. Given any chance of hope, Chuck, like most chronic pain patients, will strive to regain health and function. The art of managing the doctor–patient relationship is essential to success in this case.

Negative attitudes and beliefs by the family physician toward Chuck can greatly expand fear of pain and avoidance of movement and activity. Osteopathic practitioners know that motion is the basic function of life. There is strong evidence in the treatment of chronic back pain that staying active, continuing normal activities, and returning to work as soon as possible leads to faster recovery and lowers rates of disability.

FOLLOW-UP

Post-OMT iliac crest heights and flexion measurements were normal. The patient left with instructions to drink lots of fluid, switch to acetaminophen as needed, avoid jumping or lifting until his next visit, and return in 1 week for follow-up examination.

At the 1-week follow-up, the patient noted that both his acute and nagging pains had been relieved for nearly 4 days, but mild nagging pain had since recurred. A recurrence of innominate shear (~40% of original) and piriformis muscle dysfunction were also noted and retreated with OMT. Two weeks later, the patient returned with no symptoms and no recurrence of pain. He was instructed to make an appointment for 1 month later, but to cancel the appointment if he remained symptom-free. He phoned 1 month later, reporting that he was without pain and able to function normally at home.

CONCLUSION

The Five Models of Osteopathic Care is a useful paradigm to organize health information and apply the osteopathic philosophy and its principles to patient care. It leads to a patient-centered, health-oriented approach that is thorough and effective. This approach is not the whole of how osteopathic physicians think, but merely the unique aspect that may serve to differentiate the osteopathic approach from other approaches used by health care professionals. It is also the foundational perspective that has enabled osteopathic physicians to stand out in their communities as offering exceptional, personal, and comprehensive care to satisfied patients for over 125 years.

ACKNOWLEDGMENTS

The author and editors of this chapter would like to acknowledge the scholarly contributions of Drs. Michael Seffinger, Edwin Amirianfar, Michael L. Kuchera, and John Jerome for prior editions of this chapter.

REFERENCES

1. Giusti R, ed. *Glossary of Osteopathic Terminology*. 3rd ed. American Association of Colleges of Osteopathic Medicine; 2017.
2. Anatomy. 2011. Merriam-Webster.com. Accessed May 8, 2011. from https://www.merriam-webster.com/dictionary/anatomy
3. Physiology. 2011. Merriam-Webster.com. Accessed May 8, 2011. from https://www.merriam-webster.com/dictionary/physiology
4. Korr IM. An explication of osteopathic principles. In: Ward RC, ed. *Foundations of Osteopathic Medicine*. 2nd ed. Lippincott Williams and Wilkins; 2002:12–17.
5. Still AT. *Autobiography of Andrew T. Still. Revised ed.* The Author; 1908.
6. Chaitow L. Is postural-structural-biomechanical model within manual therapies viable?: a JBMT debate. *J Bodyw Mov Ther*. 2011;15(2):130–152.
7. Hruby RJ. Pathophysiologic models and the selection of osteopathic manipulative techniques. *J Osteopath Med*. 1992;6(4):25–30.
8. Hall JE. *Guyton and Hall Textbook of Medical Physiology*. 14th ed. Saunders Elsevier; 2021. Chapter 1.
9. Hruby RJ. *The Five Osteopathic Models: Rationale, Application, Integration.* Handspring Publishing; 2015:245–246.
10. Still AT. *Philosophy of Osteopathy*. The Author: 1899. Reprinted, Academy of Applied Osteopathy, Carmel, CA; 1946.

11. Respiration. 2011. Merriam-Webster.com. Accessed May 8, 2011. https://www.merriam-webster.com/dictionary/respiration
12. Barral JP. *The Thorax.* Eastland Press; 1991.
13. Boussages A, Gole Y, Blanc P. Diaphragmatic motion studied by mode ultrasonography: methods reproducibility and normal values. *Chest.* 2009; 135(2):391–400.
14. Koumbourlis AC. Scoliosis and the respiratory system. *Paediatric Respiratory Reviews.* 2006;7(2):152–160.
15. Raja SN, Carr DB, Cohen M, et al. The revised International Association for the Study of Pain definition of pain: concepts, challenges, and compromises. *Pain.* 2020;161(9):1976–1982.
16. Sandkuhler J. Spinal cord plasticity and pain. In: McMahon SB, Koltzenburg M, Tracey I, Turk D. *Wall & Melzack's Textbook of Pain.* 6th ed. Elsevier; 2013:94–110.
17. Furman, D, Campisi, J, Verdin, E, et al. Chronic inflammation in the etiology of disease across the life span. *Nat Med.* 2019;25:1822–1832.
18. Catassi C, Verdu EF, Bai JC, Lionetti E. Coeliac disease. *Lancet.* 2022; 399(10344):2413–2426.
19. Engel GL. The need for a new medical model: a challenge for biomedicine. *Science.* 1977;196(4286):129–136.
20. Still AT. *Philosophy and Mechanical Principles of Osteopathy.* Originally copyrighted by the author in 1892; then Hudson-Kimberly Pub. Co. in 1902; Republished and distributed by Osteopathic Enterprise, Inc.; 1986.
21. Vissoci Reiche EM, Vargas Nunes SO, Morimoto HK. Stress, depression, the immune system, and cancer. *Lancet Oncol.* 2004;5(10):617–625.
22. Meints SM, Edwards RR. Evaluating psychosocial contributions to chronic pain outcomes. *Prog Neuropsychopharmacol Biol Psychiatry.* 2018; 87(B):168–182.
23. Grotle M, Foster NE, Dunn KM, Croft P. Are prognostic indicators for poor outcome different for acute and chronic low back pain consulters in primary care? *Pain.* 2010;151(3):790–797.
24. Ng R, Sutradhar R, Yao Z, Wodchis WP, Rosella LC. Smoking, drinking, diet and physical activity-modifiable lifestyle risk factors and their associations with age to first chronic disease. *Int J Epidemiol.* 2020;49(1): 113–130.
25. Galloza J, Castillo B, Micheo W. Benefits of exercise in the older population. *Phys Med Rehabil Clin N Am.* 2017;28(4):659–669.
26. Chipidza FE, Wallwork RS, Stern TA. Impact of the doctor-patient relationship. *Prim Care Companion CNS Disord.* 2015;17(5):10.4088/ PCC.15f01840.
27. Hildreth AG. *The Lengthening Shadow of Dr. Andrew Taylor Still.* Privately published. 1942; Republished and distributed by Osteopathic Enterprise, Inc.; 1986:181–183.

27 Osteopathic History and Physical Exam

JANICE U. BLUMER ▪ REBECCA E. GIUSTI

KEY CONCEPTS

- The osteopathic history and physical exam are crucial steps in understanding how structure and function relate to illness in a patient.
- A thorough osteopathic history and physical examination generally leads to an accurate diagnosis, is cost effective, time efficient, and increases patient safety and satisfaction.
- This chapter discusses using four distinct stages and four patient positions to optimize physical diagnosis and information gathered with the least amount of effort exerted by both patient and physician.
- Patient rapport is established in the process of completing an osteopathic history and physical exam.
- The elements of the osteopathic history and physical examination and its underlying thought process are key to osteopathic distinctiveness and the osteopathic profession.
- Motivational interviewing allows the patient and physician to partner together to determine and execute realistic goals with respect to the patient's health and wellness.
- The osteopathic physical and structural examination includes components of the osteopathic screening and regional examinations and the osteopathic segmental examination.
- The osteopathic history and physical exam are critical to guiding the physician to areas of somatic dysfunction which may be addressed with osteopathic manipulative treatment (OMT) as part of a comprehensive care plan.
- During the conclusion of the encounter, clear communication between physician and patient allows the patient to understand the tentative diagnosis and the next steps in the health care process.

INTRODUCTION

The taking of the patient's history and the performance of a physical exam have been a foundation for medical diagnosis for centuries. As technology, imaging, and laboratory diagnosis continue to advance, physical exam skills in medical education have been deemphasized. In a 2020 study, residents cited "being too busy" and lack of feedback by faculty as the most significant barriers to performing the physical exam. It was felt that "faculty demonstration at the bedside was the most effective teaching method."[1] In a study at Johns Hopkins University, only 12% of an intern's time was spent in patient care, and nearly two-thirds of residents' time was spent on administrative duties, such as electronic medical records (EMRs).[2] One study performed at a community hospital estimated physicians spend 4 to 6 hours of their workday documenting and reviewing EMRs.[3] Given the increase in documentation demands, history and physical exam skills are competing for the clinician's time. However, history-taking and physical exam skills remain critical to medical education and optimal patient care. Osteopathic physicians incorporate a thorough history-taking and physical exam skillset that includes a distinctive osteopathic structural evaluation during patient encounters. The evaluation of structure and function and the understanding that the two are reciprocally interrelated assist in the discovery of what is contributing to or causing the health or disease state of the patient. This chapter focuses on a comprehensive osteopathic-oriented patient history and osteopathic structural exam, along with surface anatomical findings to accurately diagnose both somatic dysfunction and systemic disease.

During the 2019 SARS-CoV COVID-19 pandemic, many physicians transitioned to a virtual format for patient encounters to prevent transmission of the virus. While there is a place for a virtual physical examination, this chapter will not address virtual physical examination formats, but rather in-person format for physical examination skills.[4]

History and physical exam skills are a mainstay of education in both osteopathic and allopathic medical schools. In the first moments with the patient, much information can be gleaned. Visual, auditory, and tactile information can help focus the physical examination.

It is estimated that 88% of all diagnoses are made at the end of a brief history and some portion of a physical exam. The accuracy of the diagnosis dropped to 56% with history alone.[5] Inaccuracy in the physical exam may lead to unnecessary exposure to contrast, radiation, and/or delay in diagnosis.[6] In addition, excellent history and physical exam skills are essential in building rapport with the patient.[7] Osteopathic physicians have been educated to view the patient through the framework of the osteopathic tenets and models of care and are well-trained in palpation which enhances the osteopathic history and physical exam.

Osteopathic physicians emphasize the somatic components of physical examination for the purpose of determining somatic dysfunction in the context of systemic, visceral, or local disease processes. As such, they assess for tissue texture changes, asymmetry, tenderness, and variations of temperature to an area including the presence of viscerosomatic, viscerovisceral, somatosomatic, or somatovisceral reflexes and Chapman reflex points. These findings ultimately help ascertain an accurate diagnosis, leading to effective treatment for the patient to restore or maintain health. It also benefits the patient by deterring unnecessary costs or delays in diagnosis.

THE THERAPEUTIC RELATIONSHIP

Building a therapeutic relationship with the patient is an essential part of any history and physical exam. It is a mutually beneficial

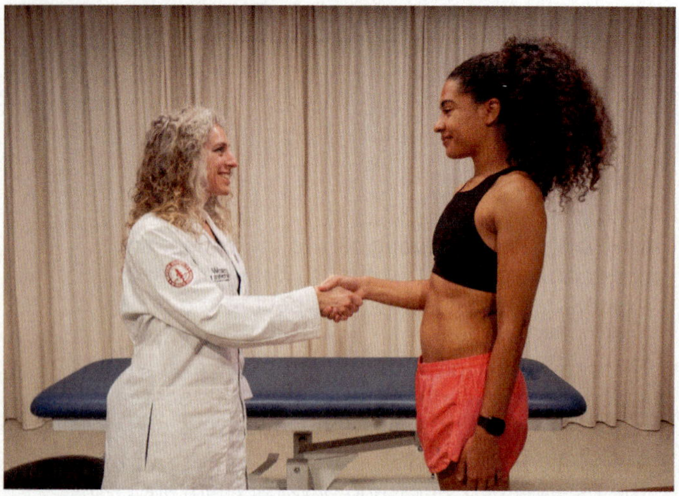

Figure 27.1. Greeting the patient at the onset of the encounter. (Photo courtesy of Western University of Health Sciences, Pomona, CA, with permission.)

relationship that improves both physician and patient satisfaction and assists in achieving the health care goals of the patient.[8]

Common interviewing skills used to build a therapeutic relationship with the patient are active listening, guided questioning, open-ended questions, and patient reassurance, validation, and empowerment. This collaborative style of interaction with the patient is commonly called *motivational interviewing*, a term employed to help the patient partner in their care.[9]

PART I—BEGINNING THE HISTORY AND PHYSICAL EXAM (FIG. 27.1)

Subjective Information from the Patient

- Chief complaint (CC)
- History of present illness (HPI)
- Current medications and allergies
- Past medical history
- Birth and development history (pediatrics)
- Immunizations
- Trauma history
- Past surgical history
- Family history
- Social and personal history
- Social determinants of health
- Review of systems (ROS)[10]

The subjective section includes documentation of the complaint in the patient's own words, medication (including over-the-counter), supplements, and allergy assessment. In addition, screening for the patient's use of illicit substances, tobacco, and alcohol, as well as the patient's social determinants of health, is essential. Examples of social determinants of health are food insecurity, unemployment, or unstable housing.[11]

Below is a scenario that will help elucidate the steps involved in the osteopathic history and physical examination.

CHIEF COMPLAINT

This is the main presenting complaint as stated in the patient's own words. This is often recorded by the medical assistant but may also be documented by the physician in the medical record. Sometimes the true CC is not what the patient describes to the staff but is elicited by the physician during the history. An open-ended question that elicits the CC might be "What is the reason for your visit today?"

HISTORY OF PRESENT ILLNESS

- Associated symptoms of the CC
- Duration and timing of CC
- Assessment of the impact the CC has on the patient
- Disruptions in daily activity of the patient due to the CC

In this section, it is best to utilize open-ended questions to allow the patient to relate the CC in their own words. It is best not to "bundle" questions but to ask simple questions the patient can answer one at a time. An example of "bundling" a question is "Does anything make it better or worse?," which may confuse the patient.

When conducting the HPI, utilizing the acronym, OPQRST may be helpful especially if the patient is experiencing pain.

O-onset
P-palliation/provoking factors
Q-quality or nature of pain
R-radiation
S-severity or situation
T-timing[10]

A scenario is found below which may serve as an example of asking open-ended questions designed to elicit the nature of the problem. Note that questions are bundled here for spacing purposes but should be asked individually so as not to overwhelm the patient.

Scenario: Elizabeth Sorrenti, DO is examining Ms. Johnson, a 26-year-old woman for the first time.

A. Doctor	B. Patient	C. Osteopathic Considerations
"How can I help you today?" "Tell me about this problem you are having." "When did the problem begin?" "Where on your body do you feel this problem?"	"Doctor I am having headaches that began when a box fell off a shelf and hit me on the top of my head." "I feel it mostly on the top of my head, but sometimes the neck as well."	Could the patient's headaches be biomechanical in nature, or related to the injury? Try to clearly define what the patient means, especially with vague terms such as "fatigue."
"Can you tell me about its characteristics, such as its quality, radiation, or severity?" "What are the precipitating factors?" "How frequently are they occurring?" "How long do they last?"	"They are dull and throbbing in nature and seem to come on after a day at work. I am getting them about every other day and they usually last 4–6 hours."	The quality of the headache leads to a better understanding of the origin of the headache. Dull and throbbing pain is often related to tension headaches.

"Does anything make them better? Worse?" "Are you getting any other symptoms along with it?" "Do you know when they are going to happen?"	"The only thing that makes them better is sleep and time, and I am getting nausea with them. Lights seem too bright when I have them. I do not know when they are coming."	Associated symptoms such as nausea and vomiting may help to differentiate tension headaches from migraine headaches. It also helps to orient treatment to areas potentially involved, such as the suboccipital triangle.
"Have you ever had any other headaches before?" "Have you ever had any other head traumas before?" (See below for trauma questions in general)	"Yes, when ....." or "No." "Yes, when......." or "No."	If there is clear correlation between injury and headaches, often the injury creates somatic dysfunction leading to the headache.

Other questions to ask in the HPI are as follows:

- How does the CC affect activities of daily living (ADLs) (e.g., getting dressed, eating, doing housework, using the toilet)?
- How does the CC affect the patient's ability to work?
- In patients who were injured, what was the patient doing at the time of the injury, and the mechanism of injury?
- In addition to timing and duration, trending/progression should be noted (i.e., has the patient had prior episodes? Are the symptoms getting worse/better, more frequent/less frequent)?

Are there symptoms of visceral disease related to the CC, for example, are there visual, hearing, smell, or taste changes, auras, dizziness, weakness, fatigue, nausea, vomiting, chest pain, and shortness of breath? Negative answers become "pertinent negatives" to the history, meaning the negative reply rules out or makes highly unlikely to be present, conditions that typically have those symptoms associated with them. See the section "Review of Systems" below.

MEDICAL HISTORY

Inquire about the date of diagnosis of any medical condition. Immunization history, significant childhood illnesses, and trauma history are usually included in this section. Example questions and answers are listed in the table.

A. Doctor	B. Patient	C. Osteopathic Considerations
"Can you tell me your past medical history?" "What conditions are you being treated for?" "Do you have any history of hospitalizations and when?" "Are you taking medications for anything?"	"I was hospitalized for asthma as a kid but am otherwise healthy and take no medications."	Past medical history gives clues to the patient's overall wellbeing. There may be comorbid conditions in the patient's diagnosis. Note names of hospitals for access to medical records.
"Tell me about your monthly menstrual cycles, when did they begin, how heavy are they, and how many days apart? "Do you have children? How many and how were they delivered? Any complications?" "Any history of sexually transmitted diseases?" "What form of contraception do you use?" "When was your last Pap and mammogram?"	"My cycles are regular and last 4 days, not heavy." "They started at 14 years old." "I have only one child, vaginal delivery at 39 weeks (about 9 months), no complications." "I have never had an STD." "I use oral birth control pills." "I had a Pap smear a year ago, but never a mammogram."	In head injury, menstrual cycles may change or stop entirely, and it is a clue to the impact of the head injury. Headaches that begin after a delivery may be due to the epidural anesthesia and a leak in the cerebrospinal fluid or may be due to sacral somatic dysfunction resulting from delivery positioning.

TIP—Many practices use a health screening and information form to gather a history from patients in a timely fashion.

SURGICAL HISTORY

Inquire about date of surgery, indication, if it was emergent or elective, location, and outcome (any complications).

Below is a sample interaction in the surgical section:

A. Doctor	B. Patient	C. Osteopathic Considerations
"Can you list any surgeries you have had, including in childhood and dental procedures? Have you had any organs removed? Were there any prolonged hospitalizations?" "Have you undergone any cosmetic surgeries including breast implants?" "Have you ever been under anesthesia? How did you react?"	"I had my wisdom teeth out and my appendix when I was a kid, and I was out in a day." "No cosmetic surgeries." "Yes, for both wisdom teeth and appendectomy and I had no problems."	Adhesions after surgery may interfere with blood supply or proper physiology in that region. Be sure to ask if they have had any problems since the surgery. Many patients forget to mention cosmetic or elective surgeries. Anesthesia reactions are important to document in the chart for future surgeries.

TRAUMA HISTORY

From an osteopathic standpoint, the onset of a traumatic event and its sequelae are essential in understanding how the patient's structure and function may have changed leading up to present symptoms and signs. Thus, spend adequate time obtaining the details of any fall, accident, and injury from birth onward as this knowledge can help to discern the cause of the current illness. Traumas to the body are cumulative and often have long-lasting effects, as each one has the potential to set off a series of compensatory changes until symptoms become so intolerant to lead the patient to the doctor for alleviation or palliation. Trauma usually affects all five models of osteopathic care.

A. Doctor	B. Patient	C. Osteopathic Considerations
"Can you tell me if you have had any accidents, fractures, falls, or major injuries?"	"I was rear-ended in a car accident about 4 years ago and told I had a whiplash injury. I broke my leg skiing as a child."	Motor vehicle accidents, like all traumas, can set the stage for somatic dysfunction throughout the body. Structural damage can lead to impediment of the respiratory/circulatory and metabolic systems which is detrimental to the body's self-healing capabilities. From the neurologic standpoint, trauma is related to pain which may affect the patient's ADLs, relationships, and ability to work, thus impacting the biopsychosocial model.

FAMILY MEDICAL HISTORY

Inquire about the age at diagnosis. If parents, siblings, or grandparents are deceased, inquire about the cause of death and age. This is important so early screening can be initiated for the patient as needed.

A. Doctor	B. Patient	C. Osteopathic Considerations
"Help me to understand your family's medical history by including conditions or diseases your family has experienced. Let us start with your grandparents, then parents, siblings, and your own children. Does anyone have a condition like what you are experiencing today?" "Does anyone have diseases that could run in the family, such as heart disease, diabetes, cancer?"	"My grandparents died in old age on both sides, my mother has diabetes II, but father is healthy. I have one brother who also has headaches but relates them to stress. My kids are healthy."	Osteopathic education focuses on prevention of disease when possible. A family history of diabetes is an opportunity to educate and inform with the goal of prevention.

TIP—Some patients may not be familiar with a family member or side of a family's medical history (for example in some cases of divorce or death) or they may be adopted. Using the question, "*Can* you tell me about your family's medical history?" gives space for the patient to relate their family's medical history to the best of their knowledge.

IMMUNIZATIONS AND CHILDHOOD ILLNESSES

This includes screening for diseases such as mumps, rubella, rubeola, and varicella and helps to guide the need for immunizations and informed decision making. Some childhood illnesses may have long-term sequelae, such as chicken pox and future herpes zoster infections.

A. Doctor	B. Patient	C. Osteopathic Considerations
"Can you tell me if you have had the regular childhood immunizations, tetanus-diphtheria, pertussis, polio, *Haemophilus influenza* type B, varicella, human papillomavirus (HPV), measles, mumps, rubella (MMR), and hepatitis?"	"Yes, I am up to date on all of those vaccines."	In establishing care for a new patient, this information is critical to document, especially in the presence of abnormal vital signs, such as elevated temperature. While the patient's CC is a headache, it is important to recall that recent immunizations are relevant to the metabolic model of osteopathic care by potentially causing fever.
"Have you had any diseases in childhood such as scarlet fever, rheumatic fever, mumps, or polio?"	"No."	
"Have you had a tetanus booster in the last 5–10 years?"	"Yes, when I stepped on a nail last year."	Childhood diseases can be associated with somatic dysfunction from scar tissue or disease processes.
"What about influenza or pneumonia vaccine?"	"Not yet."	Travel is an important diagnostic clue for patients with fever of unknown origin.
"Any travel immunization such as malaria vaccine?"	"No, I have only traveled to Mexico."	

CHILDHOOD DEVELOPMENT

In both children and adults, particularly those with chronic problems, a birth and developmental history may provide insight into the anatomical and physiologic development and supply clues to persistent problems in structure and function and all aspects of health.

A. Doctor	B. Patient	C. Osteopathic Considerations
"Tell me about your growth and development as a child. When did you first sit, creep, crawl, walk, talk? What was your birth history like? Did you have any trouble in school?"	"I did everything at the usual times, I do not know much about my birth history, I was slow to read but was never 'held back' in school."	From a biopsychosocial and neurologic standpoint, birth trauma may be associated with growth and developmental delays as well as learning disabilities. For pediatric patients, the Denver Developmental Screening Exam is a useful tool to assess childhood development.

TIP—Adverse Childhood Experiences (ACEs) screening

Screening for ACEs and childhood trauma involves asking a patient about exposures to emotional stresses known to impact their health during childhood. High scores are associated with higher all-cause mortality. Adequate social support allows patients to be more resilient to support health and wellness. Appropriate questions can help the physician to understand the patient's resources.[12,13]

DIET HISTORY

Much can be learned about a patient by asking about diet, including sugary drinks and caffeine intake. Gaining a diet history opens a conversation about healthy food balance, food choices, personal habits, diabetes, and obesity. It may also lead to valuable information about possible food insecurity.

A. Doctor	B. Patient	C. Osteopathic Considerations
"Can you describe what you eat on a typical day?"	"I eat 3 meals a day, light breakfast, lunch, and dinner."	AT Still emphasized the importance of good nutrition to the health of the patient.[7] Appropriate food and hydration are key building blocks to the body's make-up. From a biopsychosocial perspective, body image is a concern for many patients. Additionally, is the patient under- or overnourished? Is this truly due to biopsychosocial factors related to personal habits (overeating, undereating) or is it due to a metabolic condition?
"Can you tell me how much sugar, salt, fat, and caffeine you have in a day?"	"I avoid sugar snacks but like a flavored coffee daily, I don't salt my food, I don't like fried foods."	
"Who does the cooking in your family?"	"I do the cooking on the weekends for the week."	
"How many servings of fruit, vegetables, and dairy do you get in a day?"	"I usually get one vegetable serving with lunch and dinner and snack on fruit."	
"Are you happy with your weight currently?"	"I am happy with my current weight."	
"How many times do you consume fast food a week?"	"I do use food coupons in order to help pay for groceries."	
"Do you ever worry about paying for groceries?"		

TIP—Having patients keep a dietary log for several days, including all snacks and beverages, can help gain valuable insight into a patient's eating habits.

PERSONAL/SOCIAL HISTORY

Include inquiries about relationships; occupation; personal health habits, such as sleep, diet, and exercise; tobacco use including vaping; recreational drug use, and alcohol use. If the patient denies tobacco use, inquire if the patient has ever used tobacco. Tobacco use history should include amount, frequency, and duration. Alcohol and recreational drug use history should also include amount, frequency, and last time used. This section of the history should include the patient's living situation, sexual history, and stressors. Personal safety considerations such as access to firearms, the use of safety belts when in the car, and helmets when riding bicycles or motorcycles should also be documented here.

A. Doctor	B. Patient	C. Osteopathic Considerations
"Can you tell me if you are single, married, divorced, or widowed? What is your preferred sexual orientation?"	"I am married to a man, heterosexual."	Understanding personal and social history can help to identify barriers to healing, such as unemployment, unhealthy habits, or toxic relationships as well as identify areas that may promote well-being; strong social support system, job satisfaction. AT Still discusses "The Triune Man" or the unity of body, mind, and spirit as all are important in healing.[14]
"Are you sexually active? Do you have concerns you want to discuss?"	"Yes. No concerns to discuss."	
"What does your husband do? Is he supportive?"	My husband is currently unemployed. He is as supportive as he can be.	
"Do you have financial or other stressful situations that may impact your health that you would like to discuss?"	My husband being unemployed is very stressful.	
"Do you have children and if so, how old?"	"I have a daughter who is 4."	
"What is your living situation?"	"I live with my husband and child in a house."	
"Do you smoke or chew tobacco products or vape?"	"My religion prohibits smoking, but I do vape occasionally."	

"Do you drink alcohol? If so, how many drinks per day?	"I drink only occasionally on weekends and usual a beer or two."	
"Do you use recreational drugs?"	"No drugs."	
"Do you affiliate with a religion? Any medical preferences associated with your belief?"	"I am Jehovah's Witness, no medical abortion or assisted suicide and no blood products."	Knowing a patient's religious background can be an important consideration and should be documented in the medical record.
"Do you wear seat belts?"	"Yes, always."	
"Do you have a gun in the house? Is it in a locked cabinet?"	"Yes, for protection, it is locked in the safe."	Gun safety should be assessed for prevention of accidental death.
"Are there times at home when you feel unsafe? Why?"	"I live in a rough neighborhood, that's why the gun."	
"What is your social support system?"	"My husband and daughter, my mother and brother."	
"Are there any stressors in your life right now? "	"Money is always tight since my husband lost his job."	
"Do you have an advanced directive?"	"No—I don't know what that is."	
"What is your level of education? Occupation?"	"I finished one year of community college and work as a bank teller."	Knowing a patient's educational background may help direct care and appropriate communication.

TIP—From the perspective of the biopsychosocial model, adequate social and spiritual support systems enable patients to be more resilient and knowledge of these helps the physician to understand the patient's resources.[12]

PART II—REVIEW OF SYSTEMS

The ROS is a complete survey of the patient's experienced symptoms generally within the last year. The ROS is typically related to the CC in the routine office visit. In the context of a full physical exam, the ROS will include every system in the body. A thorough ROS may uncover problems the patient was unaware of, or systemic connections to the current complaint. Experienced physicians often do the ROS while performing the physical exam of the area. However, this approach is not recommended for physicians in training.[10]

Questioning should be open-ended and general in the beginning, with more specific questioning occurring around the area of concern. When executed effectively, the ROS can be performed in a timely matter which will reduce costs and potential missed diagnoses.[6,15]

Continuing the encounter between Dr. Sorrenti and Ms. Johnson, below is one approach to eliciting the ROS.

A. Doctor	B. Patient	C. Osteopathic Considerations
General—"Within the last year have you had any weight change, appetite change, weakness or fatigue, fevers, chills or night sweats, or changes in your mood?"	"I have lost 5 pounds but attribute that to stress from my husband losing his job. I do feel tired but no more than usual."	Excessive weight gain or loss may indicate systemic disease or be truly related to biopsychosocial aspects. Identifying onset, insidious or acute, can be helpful in classifying cause.
Head, Eyes, Ears, Nose, and Throat/ Mouth—"Can you tell me if you have experienced any problems or changes with vision, hearing, swallowing, or breathing through your nose? Tell me more about your headaches when they come."	"I have not had problems with vision, hearing, or breathing but the headaches have been bad. Light hurts when I have one, and I do not like noise either. They throb and are on the right side usually."	Changes in vision or the visual field may indicate a tumor as origin of the headache. Light intolerance is usually associated with migraine headache. Sinusitis, cysts, esophageal masses or disorders, brain tumors, ischemia, or aneurysms can alter neurologic functions as well as cause pain. Cervicogenic headache is a common cause of tension-type headache. Neck tumors and enlarged lymph nodes noted by the patient may indicate a metastatic cancer or infectious component, and thyroid enlargement may indicate a hyperthyroid or hypothyroid condition.
Respiratory—"Do you ever find it difficult to breathe or feel short of breath? Do you have any problems with seasonal allergies or allergies to pets? Do you cough or wheeze? Any blood or mucus with the cough?"	"I had asthma as a kid, but "outgrew" it. I also cannot be around cats. I do not wheeze currently and am not coughing."	Identifying barriers to self-healing capabilities is critical. Molds, animal dander, chemicals such as cleaning products, perfumes, air fresheners, and cockroach and/or mouse allergens can trigger asthma exacerbations. Children in daycare often bring home upper respiratory illnesses to the rest of the family, so ensuring proper immune function such as adequate sleep, nutrition, and hand washing are essential. Report of hemoptysis warrants further questioning.

A. Doctor	B. Patient	C. Osteopathic Considerations
Cardiovascular—"Are you experiencing any chest pain, skipped heart beats, irregular heartbeats, swelling, or discoloration of your limbs? How many stairs can you climb without being short of breath?" "Do you have any hemorrhoids or varicose veins?"	"I have not had any chest pain. I haven't been able to exercise as much and notice I get short of breath after going up 3 flights of stairs. I do not notice swelling or change in color. No varicose veins but I have a small hemorrhoid after my pregnancy."	As related to the respiratory/circulatory and metabolic models, AT Still stated "The rule of the artery must be absolute, universal and unobstructed, or disease will be the result."[7] Appropriate vascular supply provides oxygenation and nutrition. If it is lacking, it is imperative to identify the obstruction to flow and how it is impacting the patient's health and then provide rational treatment. Additionally, the proper functioning of the thoracoabdominal and pelvic diaphragms maintain pressure gradients that support adequate lymphatic and vascular drainage. The presence of hemorrhoids and varicose veins may indicate suboptimal functioning of this hydraulic system.
Endocrine/Metabolic—"With regards to your weight loss, how rapidly did you lose weight? Do you have to urinate frequently? Are you excessively hungry or thirsty? Any fevers, night sweats, hair loss, or brittle nails? What about salt cravings? Is your hat or glove size getting bigger?"	"I lost weight over the past year, mostly due to stress. No, I do not notice any of the other symptoms."	Homeostasis is the key feature of this system. For example, the endocrine system is responsible for producing hormones that control metabolism and the hypothalamic–pituitary–adrenal axis in neuroendocrine response to stress. What and where are disruptions in the patient's ability to maintain homeostasis?
Musculoskeletal—"Have you noticed any swelling, redness, and/or pain in your joints, back, or neck? Do you notice your muscles are unusually sore? Have you noticed any weakness or numbness in any area?" "What distance (quantify if possible) can you walk without pain?"	"My fingers go numb at night, and I need to shake them out. No, I do not notice swelling or joint pain, but I do notice my neck is very tight, sometimes I cannot turn it to back the car up."	The musculoskeletal system is key to understanding where somatic dysfunction lies within the patient. This knowledge may guide the structural component of the exam. If movement or positions modulate symptoms (relieve them or worsen them), there is often underlying somatic dysfunction. Foot and other lower extremity issues may limit a patient's ability to walk, stand, and exercise. Inquire about footwear, orthotics, heel lifts (height and recent changes), and walking devices or assists.

A. Doctor	B. Patient	C. Osteopathic Considerations
Neurologic—"Can you tell me more about when the headaches occur? Where are they located and what are the associated symptoms? Do you wake up with headaches? Are they all over or in a specific location? Does it affect your vision or hearing?" "Do you feel your speech is impacted by your headaches?" "Tell me about the frequency and intensity of these headaches as well as modifying factors." "Tell me about your hand numbness. Which fingers go numb or is it your entire hand? How long does it stay numb? Does it affect movement? Do you have trouble moving your legs ever?" Other general questions in this section may pertain to dizziness, vertigo, loss of balance, difficulty walking, muscle weakness, paralysis, loss of sensation or numbness, tingling, confusion, problems with memory or concentration, difficulty speaking, tremors, or seizure history.	"I don't wake with the headaches but often have them when I go to bed. There is no rhyme or reason for when they occur, but I am getting one about 3 times a week. I notice my neck is often tight and sore with the headaches. My first three fingers go numb when I sleep, and I can usually shake it out to make it go away. I don't notice any numbness anywhere else or weakness in my legs."	With neurologic concerns, it is helpful to categorize the condition as focal or systemic, and central or peripheral when possible. To elucidate the pathophysiology of the complaint, obtain details of what happened prior to the onset of symptoms, for example, trauma, injury, and biopsychosocial stress. As per the third tenet, the musculoskeletal and neurologic systems are interrelated, as a tight muscle can cause a neurologic condition, and neurologic dysfunction can affect muscles. Further questioning about the patient's sleep position and repetitive motions may help determine the cause of the patient's carpal tunnel symptoms.

Gastrointestinal—"Tell me about your bowel function, how often do you have a bowel movement? Is it loose or firm? Any changes in your bowel habits lately? Any blood or discharge from your rectum? How about indigestion or upper or lower abdominal pain? Are you able to eat a variety of foods or are there some foods that you cannot eat?" "Have you ever had an ulcer?" "Have you ever had a colonoscopy and/or endoscopy? If so, why?" "Do you notice bleeding from your hemorrhoids or any blood in your stools? How about "black tarry" stools?" "Do you notice any vomiting or yellowing of your skin and eyes?"	"I am regular daily in my bowel habits, firm to very firm at times. I avoid milk products because they cause flatulence. I do get indigestion with fried foods and try to avoid those. No, there are no foods that I cannot eat or am allergic to." "No." "No, none of that." "No, I have not."	Gastrointestinal health can give clues to the patient's fiber intake and hydration status. Hard stools may indicate a lack of water or fiber in the diet. Linking symptoms to a specific food may indicate an underlying food sensitivity or allergy. Affirmative responses in this section may prompt the physician to check for the presence of viscerosomatic reflexes or Chapman reflexes on the structural exam.[16] If a patient notices "black tarry" stools, it may be a sign of upper gastrointestinal tract bleeding. Jaundice is a sign of hepatitis and may present as yellowing of the skin.
Female Reproductive—"Tell me about your menses? Age when it started? Are your periods regular, heavy, or light? How far apart? Tell me about your pregnancy and delivery. Do you have any pain or discomfort in your pelvis? Any current discharge from your vaginal area?" "Do you have any breast lumps, pain, or tenderness? What about discharge?" Inquire about date of last menstrual period, birth control method, and consistency of use if not already asked in past medical history (PMHX). May also include questions regarding intermenstrual bleeding and dysmenorrhea, number of pregnancies, deliveries, and abortions (spontaneous or induced). If postmenopausal, inquire about age at onset and postmenopausal symptoms or postmenopausal bleeding. Inquire about any genital sores, itching, masses, and prior sexually transmitted infection/HIV exposure (or risk) and treatment.	"I had regular periods until my first child, now they are not, usually every 6 weeks. They are heavy when they occur. I do have an odor but no discharge in my vaginal area. I had diabetes during pregnancy, but otherwise, it was a normal pregnancy and delivery." "No."	A patient's menstrual history can give clues to conditions such as polycystic ovary syndrome. Pregnancy history may provide clues for the patient's future health. Many patients with gestational diabetes go on to develop diabetes type II. Pain and discomfort in the pelvis may indicate somatic dysfunction or local disease. Somatic dysfunction of the lumbar, pelvic, and sacral regions may contribute to neurologic dysfunction, restriction of the pelvic diaphragm, and impaired vascular and lymphatic flow which may compromise the viscera of the region and contribute to pathology.
Male Reproductive—"Have you noticed difficulty with urination, hesitancy of urination, or decreased flow? Any masses in your scrotum? Any discharge from your penis?" Any changes in erection or ejaculation? What about pain or swelling in your groin?" Inquire about testicular/scrotal pain, masses, or swelling, or any history of prostate problems or interrupted stream, genital sores, itching, masses, and prior sexually transmitted infection/HIV exposure (or risk) and treatment.	(Not applicable as patient is female.)	In men, frequent urination and nocturia often indicate an enlarged prostate. Somatic dysfunction of the lumbar, pelvic, and sacral regions may contribute to neurologic dysfunction, restriction of the pelvic diaphragm, and impaired vascular and lymphatic flow which may compromise the viscera of the region and contribute to pathology.
Urologic—"Do you find you urinate frequently or lose urine on occasion? Does it hurt to urinate? Any blood in the urine? Do you ever have trouble making it to the bathroom on time? Have you had any sharp back pain in the flank recently? Have you ever had kidney stones? Have you ever had a urinary tract infection?"	"No, none of those things."	When asking about the urologic system it is helpful to break it into regions, kidney, ureter, bladder, and urethra to determine the etiology of the issue. Problems in this area may prompt evaluation of thoracoabdominal diaphragm motion, as this may affect kidneys, the linea alba due to its attachment to the bladder and for the presence of viscerosomatic reflexes and Chapman points.

Psychiatric—"Have you experienced any sadness, hopelessness, or helplessness recently? Do you feel a sense of impending doom? Have you had a sense of panic or rapid heart rate for no reason? How is your sleep? Have you had extended periods of time where you feel you do not need sleep, overspend, or do things out of the ordinary for you?" "Do you feel nervous or moody?"	"I do not sleep well at night and I have been feeling overwhelmed since I am the only one working, but not sad. No, I do not have any sense of panic and I am always on top of my budget."	As the person is a unit of body, mind, and spirit, the psychiatric component is critical. Psychiatric conditions may be difficult to diagnose if they are not asked about. Family history may provide clues to hereditary conditions that may affect the patient such as schizophrenia or bipolar disorder. Screen for suicidal thoughts if there is any hopelessness, helplessness, or sadness. Biopsychosocial stressors may cause reactive depression. Any trauma, emotional or physical can cause physiologic dysfunction.
Dermatologic—"Have you seen any changes in color or texture of moles or freckles, bleeding of skin, rashes, itching or dryness? Any change in your hair or nails?"	"I get dry skin on occasion but have no other rashes. No, my hair and nails are fine."	Skin conditions often are the first signs of underlying disease but can be primary skin disorders as well.
Hemopoietic—"Any unusual bleeding, swelling, or easy bruising? Have you had any unexplained swelling of lymph nodes? What about frequent infections?" Ask about a history of anemia or history of prior blood transfusions.	"I have some bumps on my neck but had a cold recently. No bleeding."	The lymphatic system can be addressed with osteopathic manipulation. Drainage of lymph fluid can be assisted through lymphatic techniques.

TIP—Remember to screen for biopsychosocial factors, such as depression and anxiety comorbidities. There are many screening tools to help with this, such as the PHQ-9 scale.[17] In geriatric or impaired patients, a "Mini-Mental Status Exam" may be helpful.

TIP—If positives are found in the ROS, delve deeper into the "what, where, when, and how often" questions to understand the problem further.

In summary, a thorough review of each system will help to focus the physical examination and guide the diagnosis for the patient. It provides an accurate timeline of what symptoms occurred first and how these symptoms might be interrelated. In a time-pressed office visit, this critical step is often abbreviated. That can lead to prolongation of diagnosis as well as unnecessary testing. Take the time upfront to do a thorough ROS for the benefit of the patient.

PART III—THE OSTEOPATHIC PHYSICAL EXAMINATION

The osteopathic physical examination should maximize the information gathered toward the goal of eliciting a diagnosis, of both somatic dysfunction as well as disease process, while minimizing the physical effort and change in position of the patient. Completing all portions of the examination in one position (e.g., with the patient standing) before moving to the next position establishes a flow and sequence for the physician, ensuring that no steps are skipped and conserving energy for both the patient and the physician. The osteopathic structural exam, the evaluation, and diagnosis of somatic dysfunction are woven seamlessly into what may be thought of as the traditional physical examination steps, providing another dimension and level of comprehension to patient care. The exam is performed through the lens of the five models of osteopathic patient care, guiding the physician toward relating the biomechanical–structural, respiratory–circulatory, neurologic, metabolic–energetic, and behavioral–psychosocial aspects of the patient's condition. These concepts will be further delineated in this section.

The osteopathic structural examination and evaluation and diagnosis of somatic dysfunction can be incorporated into the traditional physical examination in many ways. Sally Sutton DO, FAAO described a method of examining the patient by anatomic positioning which incorporates physical examination with the osteopathic structural examination.[18] The patient is examined in the order of standing (including gait), seated, supine, and prone positions.

When an abnormal finding is detected, experienced clinicians recommend evaluating the finding in more than one position to assess its stability and relation to gravity; this is especially applicable to cardiovascular, respiratory, neurologic, and musculoskeletal problems. When a problem is found in one organ, the entire system should be evaluated, for example, any vascular, dermatologic, neurologic, or musculoskeletal problem found in one region of the body requires an assessment of the entire system throughout the body. It is important to develop a system and flow for each of the following components and perform the exam in a similar manner each time so that no element is missed.

Once the examination is completed, diagnoses are made or conjectured, further tests as needed are ordered, and a management plan is designed, which may include OMT for addressing somatic dysfunction.

While every physician will eventually develop their own "style," this model guides the learner in a method that accomplishes history and physical examination, physical diagnosis, and osteopathic structural diagnosis.

Logistics of Patient Evaluations

In the primary care setting, attention to the scheduling of the patient is critical to the physician's productivity and ability to accurately diagnose and treat the patient.

- Office staff record patient information in order to schedule the appointment as a new patient visit or a follow-up return visit. Each office varies, but in general, a new patient exam visit may be 45 minutes to 1 hour, and a follow-up appointment is usually 15 to 30 minutes.

- If a procedure is performed in addition to a physical evaluation, additional time may be allotted.
- Time-saving measures include having the "back office" medical assistant or nurse gather information in the rooming process, including CC, vital signs, medications, allergies, social history, past medical history, accident, and surgical history. Intake forms may also be used to maximize time available with the patient. This varies based on the physician's level of comfort.
- Most often patient intake forms are reviewed prior to the physician entering the room, so the physician can begin with focused CC history and physical examination soon after greeting the patient.
- Review chart notes prior to a return visit. Review or arrange for transfer of previous records, if any, for a new patient.
- Dictation or utilizing a medical scribe can expedite the charting and documentation process.
- Most clinics and hospital systems utilize a form of EMR and have a computer in the exam room. It can be time efficient to document and type while seeing the patient as long as it does not interfere with good patient rapport.
- Accurate documentation is the key to reimbursement by insurance companies. Ensure to accurately document services performed.

VITAL SIGNS

In most offices, vital signs are performed by the medical assistant who is also responsible for leading the patient into the examination room. Common vital signs include heart and respiratory rates, blood pressure, temperature, weight, and height (first visit in adults; in children, height is checked at each visit). Some clinics routinely assess pulse oximetry and calculate the BMI. In addition, the visual analog or verbal pain scale (0 to 10) assessment can be used.

Sequence of Physical Exam

POSITION 1—*WITH THE PATIENT STANDING*

(Height and weight are usually assessed in Position 1 or during intake.)

Gait Assessment—Much can be learned by watching the patient as they move from the waiting area to the exam room. Is the patient ambulatory, or do they require assistive devices to walk? Is the gait steady or shuffling? Is there a limp? In addition, much can be learned about posture in the first few minutes. Does the patient have a stooped posture possibly indicating kyphosis? Iliac crest heights can be observed and give clues to whether the patient has a short leg.

The "Timed Up and Go" (TUG) test is a helpful tool to assess if a patient is struggling with mobility and thus at risk for falls. The TUG test is a timed measurement of how long it takes for a patient to get up out of a chair with arms, walk 3 meters, turn around to walk back and sit down.[19] Taking longer than 12 seconds[20] to complete the task indicates that the patient is at an increased risk of falls; as the time to complete the TUG test increases further, patients may require greater assistance to perform daily tasks[21] (Fig. 27.2).

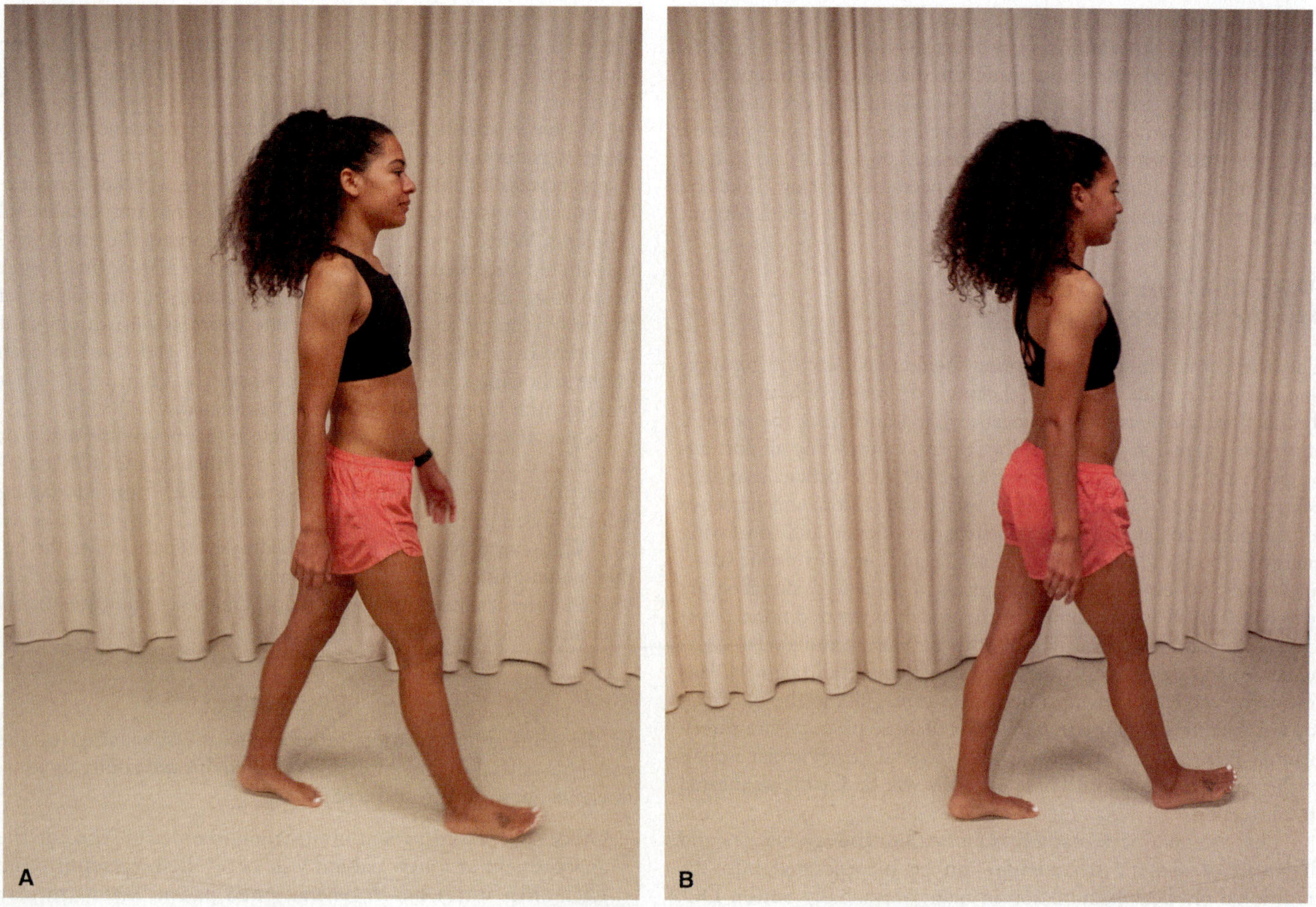

Figure 27.2. A, B. Gait assessment. It should include observation of stride length, heel strike, toe off, symmetry of arm swing, cadence, and smoothness of weight transfer. (Photo courtesy of Western University of Health Sciences, Pomona, CA, with permission.)

A. Doctor Can Assess the Following:

Gait—Observe the following in the anterior, lateral, and posterior views.

Observe stride length, cadence, and arm swing. Is there a limp or antalgic gait? Does the patient shuffle when they walk? Is the patient bent forward? Observe heel strike and toe off for symmetry and smoothness. Does the patient walk fluidly? How is their postural balance? Do they show signs of pain? Is the patient using an assistive device such as a crutch, cane, or walker?

B. Osteopathic Considerations

Gait is often affected in both the neurologic and the musculoskeletal models of the five models of osteopathic care. Observing and investigating gait abnormalities is helpful in pinpointing whether they stem from the brain, or spinal column as in neurologic model (stroke or Parkinson disease), or peripheral musculoskeletal or joint injury, trauma, or somatic dysfunction as in the structural model. Osteoarthritis of the knee can cause a limp for example, which can lead to somatic dysfunction of the pelvis and lower back. Restriction of the psoas muscle may cause the patient to be flexed forward. Asymmetry of arm swing may be observed post-CVA, but more commonly it is due to postural accommodations and somatic dysfunction and may respond to OMT.

TIP—If the doctor does not see the patient walk into the room, have the patient arise and walk in the hallway as an alternative. Sometimes it is helpful to observe their gait with both shoes on and barefoot.

A. Doctor Can Assess the Following:

General—Patient Stationary

Posterior view: Observe levels of earlobes, shoulders, scapulae inferior angles, iliac crest heights, and posterior superior iliac spines (PSIS) (Fig. 27.3) and observe for any obvious lateral spinal curves that may indicate scoliosis. Perform the passive hip shift test to screen for spinal, pelvic, and/or lower extremity somatic dysfunction (Fig. 27.4). Pronation or supination of the feet may be observed. Rib angles can be assessed for tenderness and position.

B. Osteopathic Considerations

Unlevel iliac crest heights may be a sign of a short leg or a pelvic somatic dysfunction. In this case, a ***shim*** should be used under the heel of the lower iliac crest.

Tissue texture abnormalities, asymmetry of anatomical landmarks, restriction of motion, and tenderness (TART) can be assessed in the standing position to gain input from postural loading.

Asymmetry of the head, neck, and shoulders may indicate underlying somatic dysfunction or scoliosis. Head tilt may be associated with ocular or visual issues.

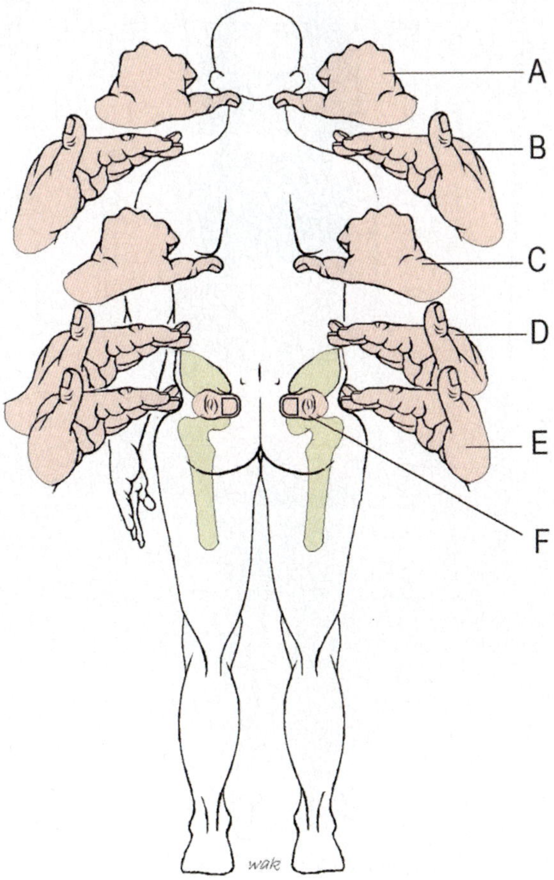

Figure 27.3. Patient standing, physician evaluates levels of (**A**) earlobes, (**B**) shoulders, (**C**) scapulae, (**D**) iliac crest heights, (**E**) greater trochanters, and (**F**) posterior superior iliac spines (PSIS). (Illustration courtesy of William A. Kuchera, DO, FAAO, with permission.)

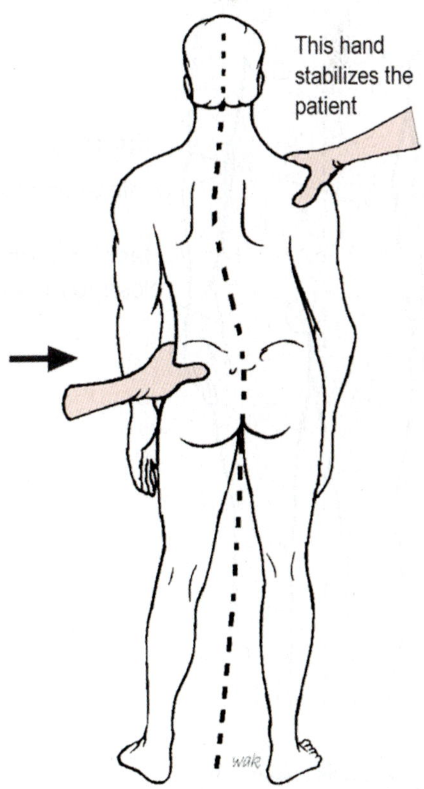

Figure 27.4. Hip shift test to assess for lumbopelvic somatic dysfunctions, including short leg syndrome and scoliosis. (Illustration courtesy of William A. Kuchera, DO, FAAO, with permission.)

Anterior view: Observe for eye levels, levels of earlobes, facial symmetry, tilt of head, shoulder levels, and symmetry of the space between the arms and torso (Fig. 27.5). Observe costal cage contour, and sternal region for any deformities (pectus excavatum or carinatum). Observe for evidence of a barrel chest. Observe the patient in the anatomical position (Fig. 27.6) to evaluate upper extremities at the patient's sides for elbow abduction or adduction as well as elbow carrying angle (Fig. 27.7A); for the lower extremities, observe the Q-angle of the knee for genu valgum or varum (Fig. 27.7B), the lower legs and ankles for swelling or varicosities, the arches of the feet for pes planus or cavus, supination or pronation and the toes for cyanosis.

The Quick test assesses gross upper extremity and glenohumeral mobility. A "squat" test assesses gross hip, knee, and ankle mobility and function.

Certain orthopedic tests, such as the Thessaly test are performed in the standing position.

Body type and weight distribution can also be noted.

Sternal deformities may indicate underlying conditions and may impair functioning of the cardiopulmonary systems. A barrel chest may be a normal variant but may also indicate underlying pathology such as chronic obstructive pulmonary disease (COPD) or cystic fibrosis.

Excessive carrying angle may lead to elbow instability, especially in the pediatric population.

Carrying angle of the arm will be more pronounced in female patients but should measure between 5 and 15 degrees. The Q-angle should be about 10–12 degrees.

Osteopathic assessment of the feet and knees is important in the evaluation of low back pain. If there is pes planus of the feet or collapse of the arch, the resulting kinetic chain can be experienced as low back pain. The etiology of genu varum and valgum should be determined as it can alter mechanics of the body and cause abnormal wear of joints.

Pes cavus and planus may be normal variants, although pes cavus can be associated with certain neurologic condition. Pronation or supination of the foot warrants further evaluation to determine if orthotics or exercises are needed or if they are due to other issues; for example, short leg, scoliosis, etc.

A positive Quick test indicates a restriction of the upper extremity complex while a positive squat test indicates dysfunction of the lower extremity complex. A positive Thessaly test may indicate a torn meniscus.

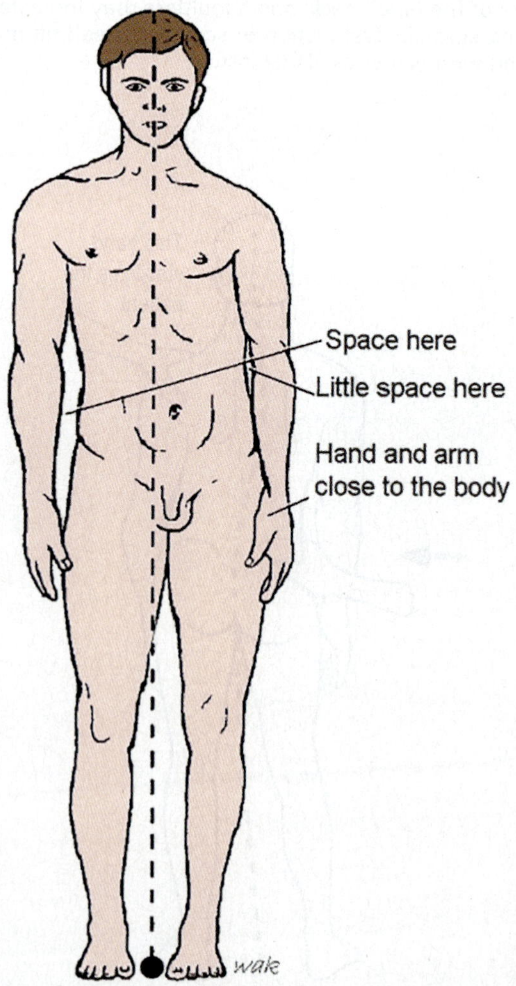

Figure 27.5. Anterior view with patient standing. Notice asymmetrical space between arm and trunk, indicative of spinal lateral curvatures (scoliosis). (Illustration courtesy of William A. Kuchera, DO, FAAO, with permission.)

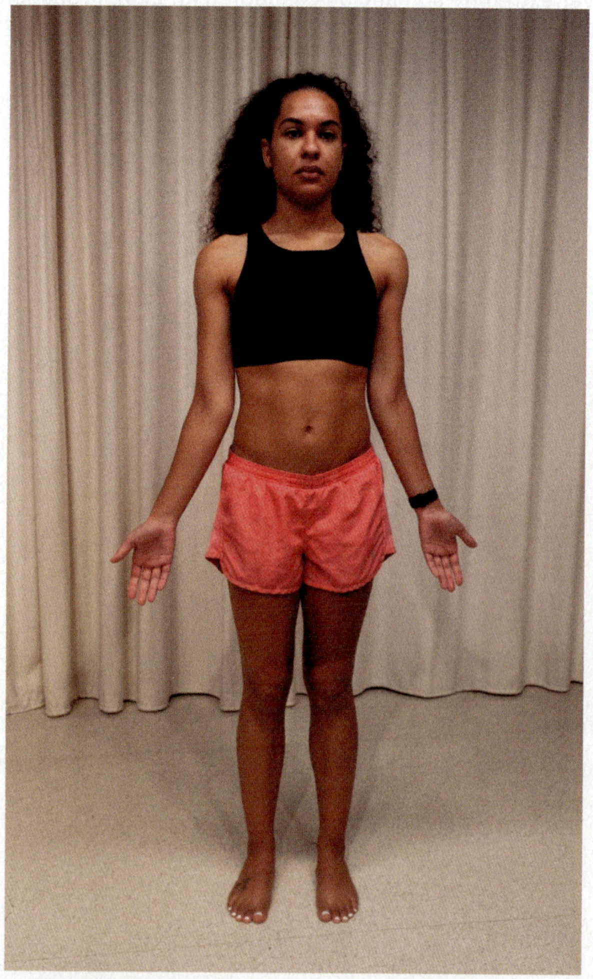

Figure 27.6. Observe the patient in the anatomical position for carrying angle of the elbow, presence of genu varum or valgum and pes cavus or planus, and pronation or supination of feet. (Photo courtesy of Western University of Health Sciences, Pomona, CA, with permission.)

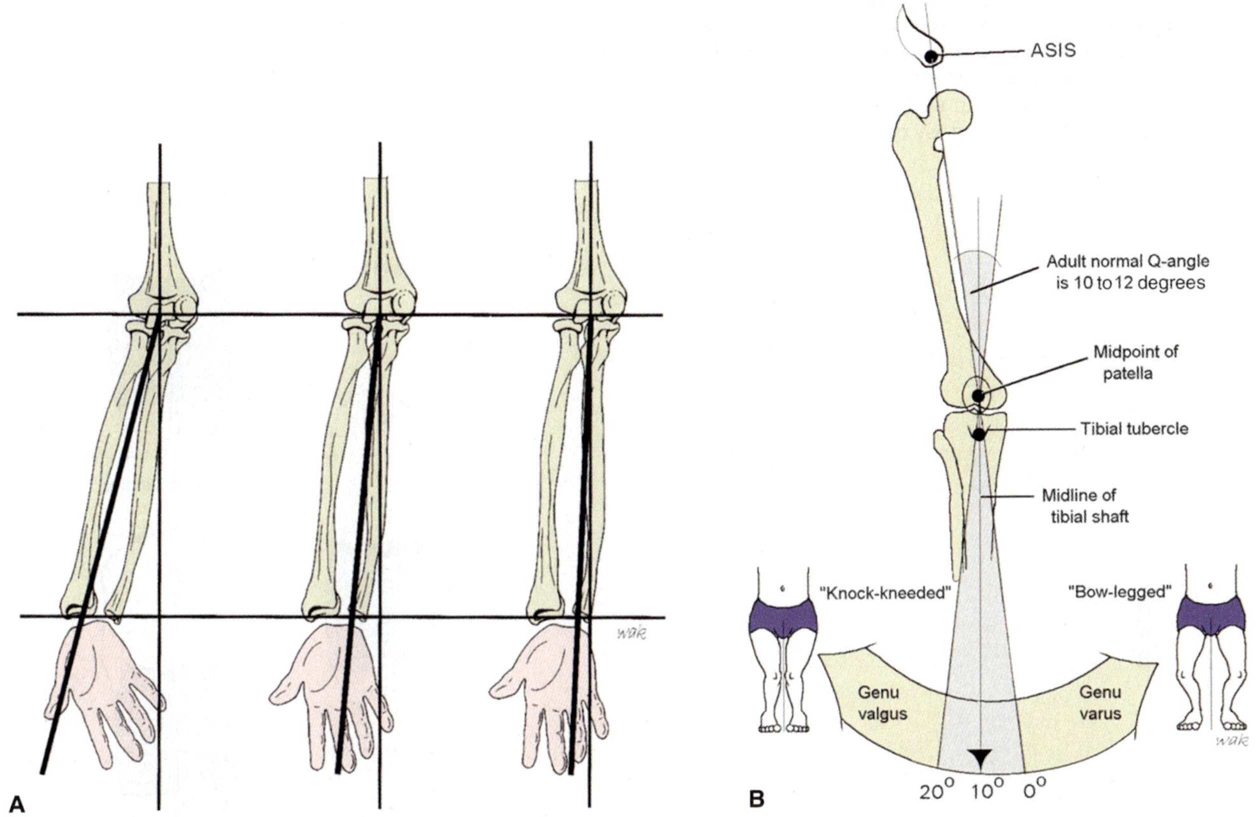

Figure 27.7. **A.** Carrying angle of the right elbow. Left is excessive, right is diminished, and middle is within normal range. **B.** Q-angle of the right knee. (Illustration courtesy of William A. Kuchera, DO, FAAO, with permission.)

Standing Flexion Test—Physician places their thumbs on the inferior slopes of the posterior superior iliac spines (PSIS) and asks the patient to bend forward slowly without bending the knees as if to touch the toes (Fig. 27.8).

In ***iliosacral somatic dysfunction*** one PSIS will move further in an anterior superior direction in comparison to the other. This indicates the side of dysfunction.

While the patient is flexing forward the examiner may also look for a ***rib hump*** which may indicate functional or anatomical scoliosis (Fig. 27.9). If a rib hump is noted, then lateral side bending in the forward position will determine if the scoliotic curve is functional, that is, tight musculature or anatomical, that is, related to a short leg or altered spinal anatomy (Fig. 27.10).

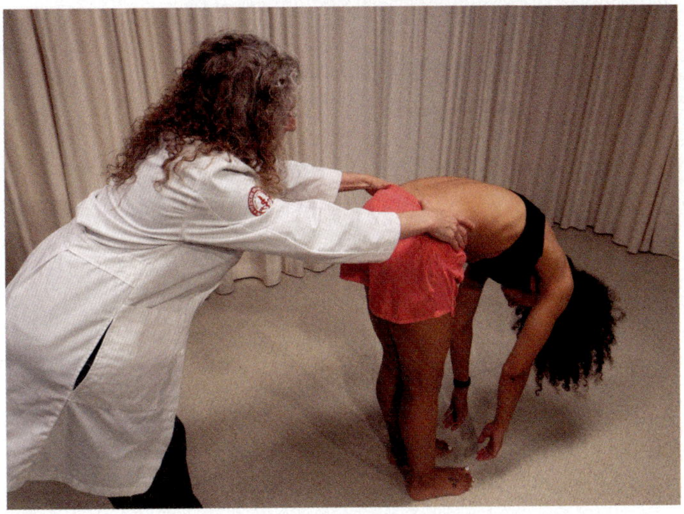

Figure 27.8. **Performance of the standing flexion test.** (Photo courtesy of Western University of Health Sciences, Pomona, CA, with permission.)

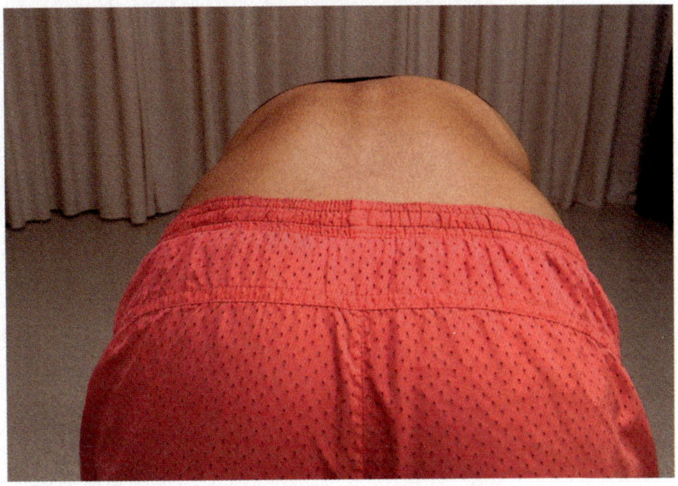

Figure 27.9. **Presence of right rib hump noted during performance of standing flexion test.** May indicate functional or anatomical scoliosis. (Photo courtesy of Western University of Health Sciences, Pomona, CA, with permission.)

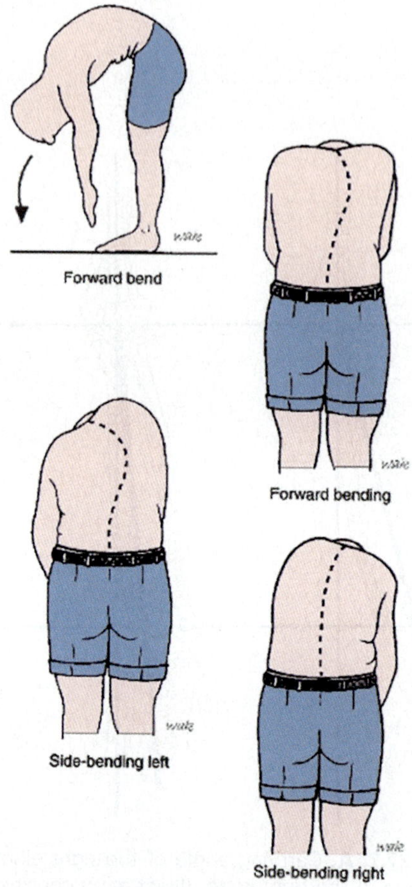

Figure 27.10. Forward bending test for scoliosis: patient bends forward with knees extended and then side bends left and then right while physician observes posteriorly for accentuation or improvement of the spinal curve. Functional curves improve or resolve with side bending, whereas anatomical curves do not. (Illustration courtesy of William A. Kuchera, DO, FAAO, with permission.)

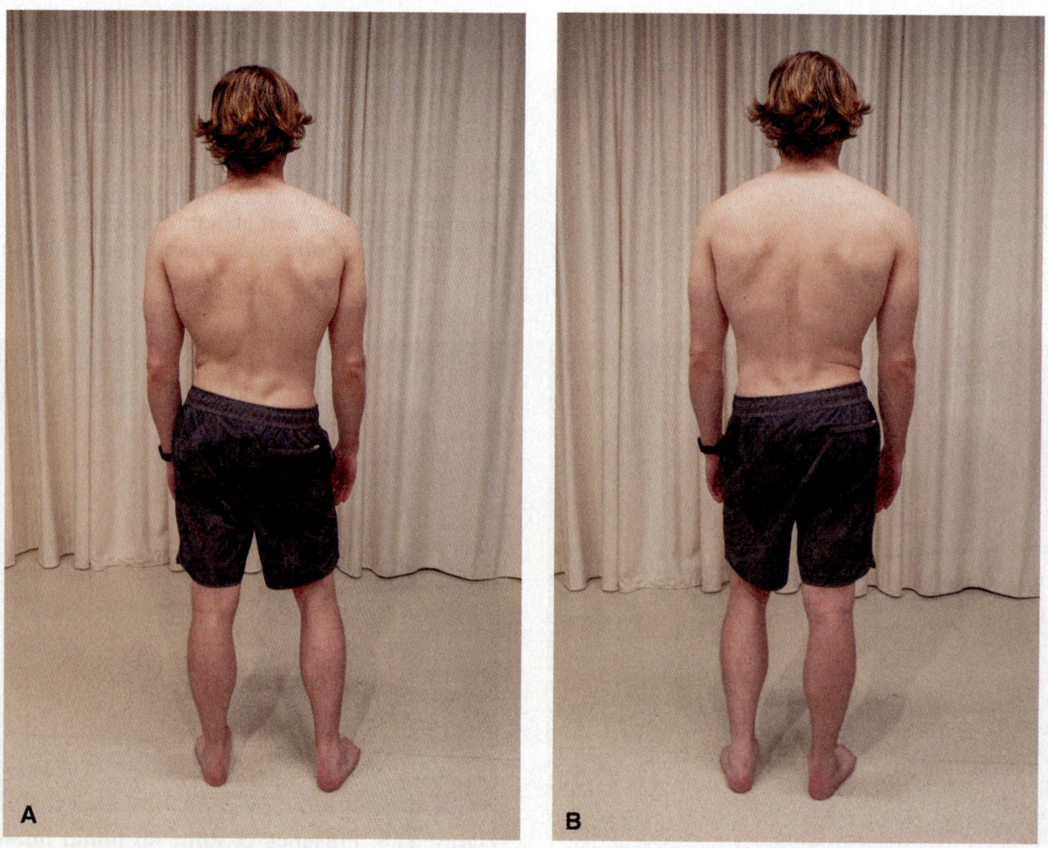

Figure 27.11. A and **B.** (**A**) reflects a negative hip drop test. As the patient bends the right knee, the lumbar spine side bends to the left to accommodate for the unleveling of the sacral base. (**B**) reflects a positive hip drop test which would be described as a positive left hip drop test. As the patient bends the left knee, the lumbar spine remains straight and does not side bend to the right to compensate for the unleveling of the sacral base.

Hip Drop Test—The hip drop test can be performed in a standing position to assess for somatic dysfunction of the lumbar region. While the patient is standing, feet shoulder-width apart, the examiner asks the patient to bend one knee while keeping the other knee straight and both feet on the ground (Fig. 27.11A,B).	A positive test indicates somatic dysfunction of the lumbosacral region. As the patient bends the right knee, left-side bending of the lumbar spine should occur to compensate for the unleveling of the sacral base and the opposite should occur with bending the left knee. This compensatory side bending of the lumbar spine should be equal on both sides. If rotoscoliosis is present, there will be impaired side bending on the side of the convexity. In addition, skin folds will be lower on the side of the convexity.
Posterior Paraspinal Palpation—Palpate the paraspinal skin and muscles to assess for tissue texture abnormalities and tenderness from the suboccipital region to the lumbosacral junction (Fig. 27.12). Consider the biomechanics of the transition areas of the spine as they demonstrate unique structural characteristics (Fig. 27.13). Most somatic dysfunctions involve these areas. In the scoliotic spine, these junctional areas demonstrate altered biomechanics, and new stress points are created at the transitions of the lateral curves.	Tissue texture abnormalities, asymmetry of anatomical landmarks, restriction of motion, and tenderness (TART) are assessed by palpation with the patient standing, seated, supine, and prone. TART changes can be assessed in the standing position to gain input from postural loading (Fig. 27.12).
Lateral View—Observe anteroposterior spinal curvatures (lordosis and kyphosis) in the sagittal plane. Gravitational line can be observed from the anterior aspect of the lateral malleolus to the greater trochanter of the femur, to the acromion process at the shoulder, and to the external auditory meatus.	Excessive or diminished lordotic or kyphotic curves may be normal variants or may indicate areas of somatic dysfunction, compensation, or weakness. The gravitational line is important to assess the patient's overall posture and effects of trauma or somatic dysfunction. In a head-forward posture, the patient leads with their head. This may be from sitting, studying in forward bent posture, or from neck somatic dysfunction.

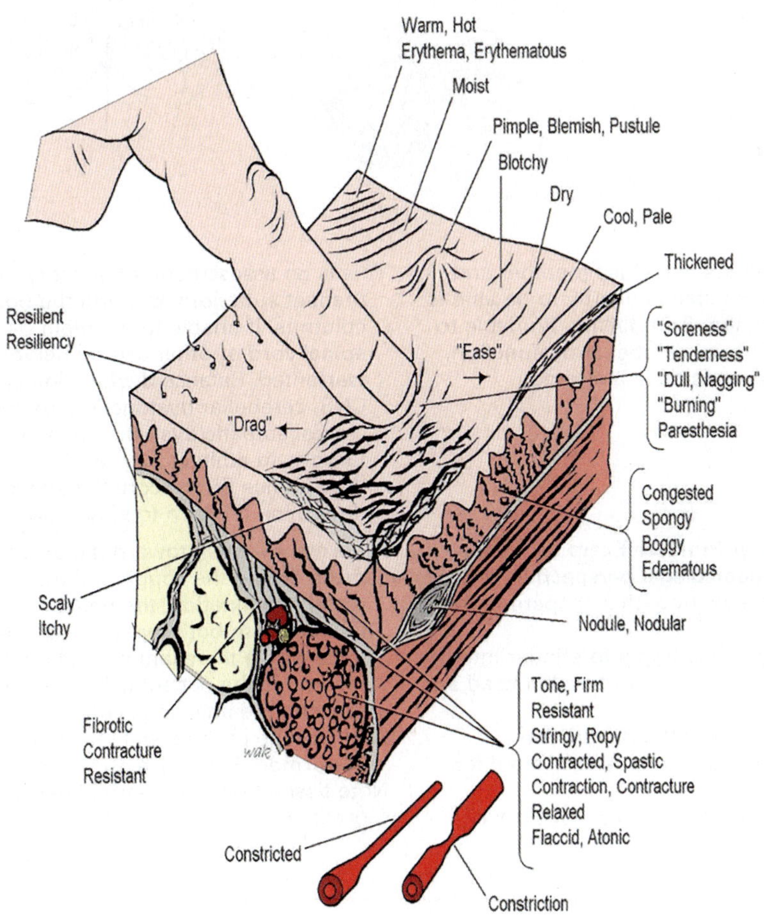

Figure 27.12. Palpation of the skin layers to assess autonomic function, which determines tissue texture. (Illustration courtesy of William A. Kuchera, DO, FAAO, with permission.)

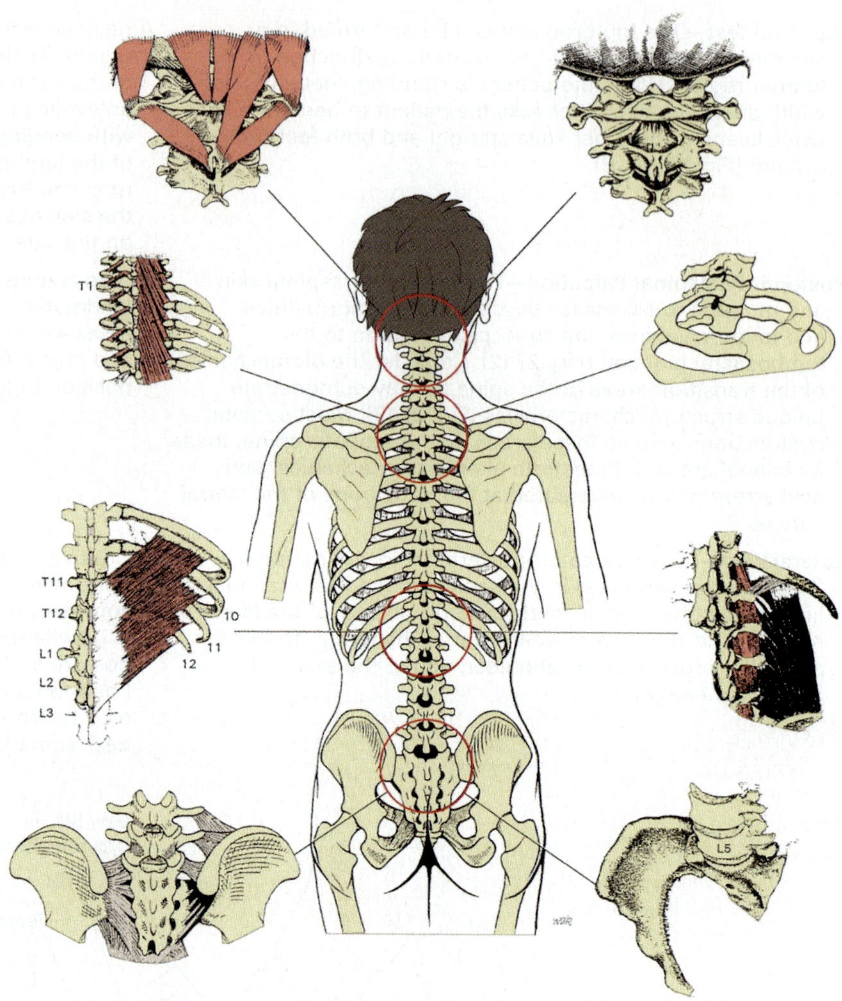

Figure 27.13. Transition areas of the spine have distinctly unique biomechanical characteristics and are subject to somatic dysfunction and compensatory changes. (Illustration courtesy of William A. Kuchera, DO, FAAO, with permission.)

Romberg Sign—The patient stands feet close together and closes their eyes. The physician stands nearby to be able to catch the patient or prevent them from falling. If unable to maintain balance other testing for cerebellar dysfunction, peripheral neuropathy, or concussion is indicated.	This is an assessment for sensory information ascending from the feet superiorly through the posterior sensory spinal columns. If unable to maintain balance, additional testing for spinal cord or other central nervous system (CNS) disease is warranted. Balance dysfunction can be from many sources: CNS, cerebellar dysfunction, peripheral nervous system, cranial somatic dysfunction, age, concussions, trauma, or tumors. In athletes who are prone to concussions in sports, the Balance Error Score System is a useful test to help determine if return to play is advisable.
Evaluation for Hernia and Rectal/Prostate Exam for Males—If clinically indicated, from a medicolegal perspective, it is best to perform this portion of the exam with a chaperone (MA) present. Examine for inguinal hernias by inserting a forefinger into the patient's inguinal canal and asking him to turn his head and cough. Perform rectal examination to assess the rectum for hemorrhoids, masses, and/or anal tears. Assess stool for occult blood with hemoccult slide. Assess the prostate for enlargement, masses, asymmetry, consistency, and tenderness. Penile discharge can be cultured if infection is a possibility.	A hernia will push toward the examiner's finger as a bulging mass during the cough and may recede again afterward. For rectal examination, the patient is standing up and leaning forward with both forearms resting on the examination table, while the examiner places a gloved forefinger into the rectum as the patient is instructed to push the finger out, thus relaxing the anal sphincter. A full sweep of the distal rectal vault (360 degrees) should be performed. For males, the prostate should also be palpated. Note tissue texture abnormalities and/or enlargement of the prostate.

POSITION 2—WITH THE PATIENT SEATED ON EXAM TABLE OR CHAIR (FIG. 27.14)

As indicated earlier, vital signs are usually taken in this position for accuracy; temperature, blood pressure, pulse, respiratory rate, pulse oximetry if indicated, as well as a patient assessment of pain prior to the beginning of the encounter.

The general appearance of the patient, such as their clothing (disheveled or unkempt or well put together), overall appearance (pale, diaphoretic or unwell, or winded from walking), nutritional status (gaunt, obese, overweight), and emotional state (anxious or depressed) can also be noted at this time.

After assessing the patient in the standing position, the following may be assessed in the seated position: (However, note that certain elements such as observation of general appearance and evaluation of the patient's skin may also done in other positions.) As a general note, seated posture is an indicator of motor tone of the patient. Poor motor control may cause the patient to slump when seated.

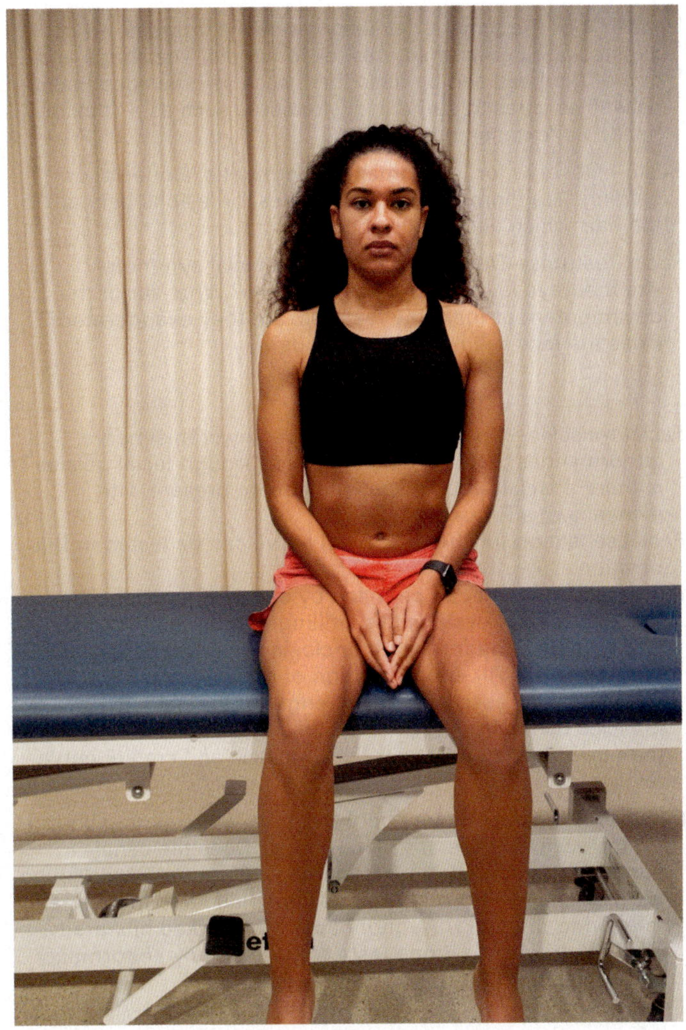

Figure 27.14. The next part of the exam may be conducted with the patient seated on the exam table or a chair. (Photo courtesy of Western University of Health Sciences, Pomona, CA, with permission.)

A. Doctor Can Assess the Following:	B. Osteopathic Considerations
General appearance—Is the patient well nourished, over or underweight? Is there evidence of muscle wasting? What is their emotional state? What is their attitude? Does the patient have an appropriate level of consciousness? Does the thought process seem coherent and intellectual process appropriate?	What the patient does not say is often as important as what they do say. The way someone presents themselves can be indicative of their mental state. The biopsychosocial issues impacting the patient may not be the chief complaint but often interfere with health. Note if the patient maintains eye contact, if they have a "flat affect," or if they appear fearful. All are clues to underlying mental health concerns. Inability to find the right words or memory issues can be a sign of early dementia. Consider evaluating for depression if the patient appears to have a flat affect or admits to depression.
Skin—The physician observes and palpates for the presence of dryness, oiliness, scaliness, hyperhidrosis, tenderness, petechial, rashes, eruptions, dermatitis, temperature, texture, and tenderness. In addition, suspicious moles can be evaluated, and the physician can check hair and nails for signs of systemic disease.	Evaluation of the skin can provide important clues related to TART (*temperature, tissue texture change, asymmetry, restriction in motion, and tenderness*) and therefore, somatic dysfunction. Areas of chronic somatic dysfunction may present with cool, dry skin, whereas acute somatic dysfunction may present with increased moisture, heat, and edema or "bogginess." Hair and nail abnormalities can indicate chronic disease states, such as hypothyroidism or chronic renal disease.

Head—Does the patient have any swellings, masses, exostoses, ridging of sutures, or fontanels? The shape and size of the head can be described, such as brachiocephalic, as well as clues to somatic dysfunction, such as a "flexion head," or "extension head."	Differences in the shape and configuration of the head and position and shape of the eyes and ears may be related to somatic dysfunction from birth or trauma.[22]
Scalp—Observe for inflammation, dermatitis, alopecia, or balding. Are there any moles, freckles, or lesions beneath the hair which need to be checked?	The presence of excessive flaking of skin (commonly called dandruff) may be associated with underlying conditions such as eczema and seborrheic dermatitis.
Facial features—Does the patient have facial symmetry? Are their eye levels and ear levels even? What about the development of the bony features, are they exaggerated? Does the face seem myxedematous?	Unlevel eyes and ears may be evidence of cranial or cervical somatic dysfunction. Epicanthal folds may be present in patients with Down syndrome or maybe a normal finding in certain ethnicities. From the neurologic model, evaluating facial symmetry assesses CNVII. Myxedema is a sign of systemic disease and hypothyroidism.
Facial muscles—Does the patient have any cranial nerve abnormalities that can be diagnosed through facial palsies? Is there a facial droop? Does the patient present with evidence of a TIA or CVA? Facial sensation for the trigeminal nerve can be tested in this position. Further assessment can be made by asking the patient to make facial expressions like smiling, puffing out the cheeks, and wrinkling the forehead, or closing the eyelids against resistance (CNVII). Motor portion of cranial nerve V can be checked by assessing the strength of the patient's jaw muscles by having the patient clench their teeth or move their jaw. See Table 27.1 for facial muscle and cranial nerve testing chart.	Evaluation of the cranial nerves is a critical component of the neurologic model of osteopathic care. This evaluation may provide information on compression or irritation of cranial nerves and their foramina with respect to cranial somatic dysfunction. Many of the ocular muscles attach to the tendinous ring of the sphenoid. If it is malpositioned, this may place abnormal tension on those muscles causing ocular dysfunction. Bell's palsy is a condition in which the facial nerve is affected and causes a facial and eyelid droop. Compression of the stylomastoid foramen or that region may also place tension on CNVII as it exits the skull resulting in CNVII dysfunction. Abnormal tension on muscles of mastication and ligaments of the jaw may affect chewing and eating and cause uneven wear of teeth.
Ears—Can the patient hear spoken voice, watch ticking sound? Do the auricles have any skin lesions? Does the canal appear patent and tympanic membrane normal? What is the position of the ears on the horizontal plane and the pinna in relation to the head? Auditory acuity is checked bilaterally. The Weber and the Rinne tests are done if any abnormality is detected with further testing as needed.	From a structural model, ear position may indicate somatic dysfunction of the temporal bones. Dysfunction of temporal bones may be related to Meniere's disease, tinnitus, or chronic ear infections. It is important to check one ear relative to the other. Checking for hearing acuity helps assess cranial nerve VIII. This neurologic component may contribute to the biopsychosocial model as patients who cannot hear well sometimes feel isolated and will not participate in social events.
Eyes—Examine the patient's orbits for size variation. Is there any ptosis, inflammation, or discharge of the eyelid? What is the shape and size of the pupils and are they equally reactive to light? Do the eyes track properly or is amblyopia present? What is the color of the sclera and conjunctiva? Is there any pterygium? Check visual acuity with a Snellen Chart (may also be available in a pocket version) and check for colorblindness. What does the lens look like? Does the patient wear glasses or contacts? Look for bilateral red reflex and perform a fundoscopic examination looking at optic disks, blood vessels, macula, and fovea. Are the funduscopic exam, optic nerve pressure, and blood vessels normal? Check extraocular muscles by having the patient follow physician's finger movement with both eyes. Check all four quadrants of the visual fields. Check eye pressure (presence of glaucoma) if indicated, usually after age 39.	Eye conditions often reflect other neurologic conditions such as tumors or progressive degeneration in conditions such as multiple sclerosis. Vision decline may be due to cataracts, the aging process, or can reflect complications from diabetes. Cranial nerve II is assessed by checking for visual acuity, visual fields, and the funduscopic examination. Abnormalities of the fundoscopic exam may indicate systemic diseases such as diabetes or hypertension. When checking visual acuity, the eyes should be checked together as well as individually. Indicate whether the values reported were while wearing glasses (corrected vision). Extraocular movement assesses the integrity of cranial nerves III, IV, and VI. Abnormal motion may indicate presence of somatic dysfunction, either of the cranium or as a compensation for other somatic dysfunction of the body.

TIP—Cerumen can obstruct the tympanic membrane. If present, an ear lavage may be performed in order to visualize the tympanic membrane and canal. Discourage the use of cotton swabs for patients as cotton swabs may further impact the cerumen in the ear canal.

TABLE 27.1

Evaluation of Facial Muscles

Instructions to Patient	Muscles Involved	Cranial Nerve Involved
Close eyes tightly	Orbicularis oculi	VII
Raise eyebrows	Occipitofrontalis	VII
Draw eyebrows medially and downward	Corrugator supercilii	VII
Lift upper eyelids and look upward	Levator palpebrae superioris	III
Look up and to the right	Obliquus oculi inferior, right Rectus oculi superior, left	IV III
Look down and to the left	Obliquus oculi superior, left Rectus oculi inferior, right	IV III
Look to the right	Rectus oculi lateralis, right Rectus oculi medialis, left	VI III
Look to the left	Rectus oculi lateralis, left Rectus oculi medialis, right	VI III
Lift lateral borders of nostrils	Procerus	VII
Flare nostrils	Dilator naris posterior, anterior	VII
Compress nostrils	Nasalis	VII
Approximate and compress lips	Orbicularis oris	VII
Protrude upper lip	Levator labii superioris	VII
Lift upper border of lip on one side without raising lateral angle of mouth	Levator anguli oris	VII
Smile	Zygomaticus major	VII
Grimace	Risorius	VII
Approximate lips and blow	Buccinator	VII
Protrude lower lip (pout)	Depressor labii inferioris	VII
Draw corners of mouth down strongly	Depressor anguli oris, platysma	VII
Draw tip of chin upward	Mentalis	VII
Close jaw tightly	Temporalis, masseter, pterygoideus medialis	V
Move mandible laterally, forward, and to the right	Pterygoideus lateralis, medialis, left	V
Move mandible laterally, forward, and to the left	Pterygoideus lateralis, medialis, right	V
Depress mandible	Digastricus, suprahyoid muscle	V, VII, C1

Adapted from Sutton S. An osteopathic method of history taking and physical examination: part 1. *J Am Osteopath Assoc.* 1978;77:780–788.

Nose—Examine the patient for external lesions on the nares; then use the otoscope to view the nasal mucosa, septum, and turbinates for abnormalities. Ask the patient to breathe with one nostril closed and then the other to assess ventilation. Palpate or percuss the maxillary and the frontal sinus regions bilaterally looking for tenderness.

Optional: Cranial nerve I can be assessed by blocking one nostril at a time and having the patient identify a familiar smell with the open nostril.

Congestion or sinusitis may be an indication for lymphatic techniques, such as facial effleurage which reduces congestion of superficial soft tissues and enhances drainage of the face. This technique is useful if the patient is having difficulty with ventilation or sinus infection.[23]

Mouth—Assess the external mouth for abnormalities; then use a light source to look internally for lesions on and under the tongue, of the buccal mucosa and gums, and on the posterior hard or soft palate. Examine the gums and under the tongue for evidence of jaundice. Use the otoscope to visualize the posterior oropharynx and tonsillar pillars, using a tongue depressor if needed to lower the tongue, which often impedes visualization. Have the patient say "Ah," and watch the palate and uvula elevate, assessing for symmetry. Check the gag reflex by touching the posterior aspect of the tongue or pharyngeal wall with the tongue depressor. Ask the patient to stick out their tongue and move it from side to side and notice any asymmetry.

Examine the teeth for state of repair, missing or broken teeth, caries, evidence of bruxism, and occlusion. Examine the temporomandibular joint while the patient is opening the mouth for deviation of the chin and crepitus of the joint.

The gingiva reflects the overall health of the patient. Does the gingiva bleed easily? Is there hyperplasia or gingival recession? Do they look friable or inflamed? The lips and tongue may provide evidence of hydration status. Cranial nerves IX and X are assessed when the patient says "Ah" and the palate and uvula remain midline; deviation is abnormal. Cranial nerve XII can be assessed by the active movement of the protruded tongue. Abnormalities here, especially in newborns and infants, may indicate condylar compression. Cranial dysfunction may be associated with abnormalities of cranial nerves. The temporomandibular joint is usually assessed with this region. It may be painful in the presence of malocclusion, missing teeth, or bite problems. Temporomandibular joint disorder (TMD) may be related to multiple areas of somatic dysfunction including cranial, cervical, pelvic and sacral.

Neck—Check to see that the trachea is midline. Assess cranial nerve XI by having the patient shrug both shoulders against resistance. Examine the anterior neck for thyroid enlargement and lymphadenopathy and auscultate for bruits of the carotid arteries. Examine the neck and head posture. Examine active and passive cervical range and quality of motion (Fig. 27.15). For passive range of motion, palpate facet and spinous process motion, and note any abnormalities in ranges of motion and tissue tension.

While the somatic dysfunction diagnosis of the cervical spine is often performed in the supine position, the facet joint mechanics are easier to feel in the seated position. With one hand on the head and the other on the C2–7 region, test flexion, extension, side bending, and rotation. Assess for normal joint mechanics and abnormal palpatory findings such as crepitus. Cervical lordosis can be assessed and may be decreased, increased, or normal.

Thorax—The chest wall should be inspected anteriorly and posteriorly for any abnormalities, in both appearance and movement. If chest pain is reported, the area should be palpated for tenderness, deformities, or tissue changes. For respiratory complaints, the patient should be assessed for signs of respiratory distress such as accessory muscle use or intercostal retractions. The lung examination involves inspection, palpation for rib movement and chest expansion, and percussion and auscultation of the anterior, posterior, and lateral aspects of the chest bilaterally in a stepwise manner looking for any abnormal breath sounds. When warranted, the lung examination also involves checking for tactile fremitus and transmitted voice sounds such as egophony, bronchophony, or whisper pectoriloquy. The patient should have a thorough cardiac examination to assess for arrhythmias, murmurs, extra heart sounds, point of maximal impulse, and heart rate (Fig. 27.16).

Percuss the thoracolumbar junction costovertebral angle region (Lloyd test for kidney disease). If indicated, assess the breasts for symmetry and any abnormalities.

When clinically indicated, from a medicolegal perspective, it is best to perform this portion of the exam with a chaperone (MA) present.

From a metabolic consideration, thoracic kyphosis may indicate bone degeneration from age or medications, or it may be an inherited condition. Thoracic kyphosis from aging is often from osteoporosis and may prompt appropriate evaluation of bone density.

As the physician palpates the paraspinal tissues, the structural and neurologic models must be considered. Tissue texture and temperature changes may indicate somatic dysfunction and the presence of viscerosomatic reflexes (generally from T1–L2). These reflexes may signify underlying conditions that may confirm a suspected diagnosis or elicit further investigation.[24] The sympathetic chain ganglia are found in the posterior thorax and can be irritated by somatic dysfunction of the thoracic vertebral joints; certain osteopathic techniques are designed to affect autonomic nervous system activity by taking advantage of the costotransverse joint articulation's proximity to the posterior sympathetic chain. An example of this is called *rib raising*.[23]

Chapman reflexes may also be found midway between the transverse processes and spinous processes and be associated with underlying visceral dysfunction.

Lower thoracic costovertebral angle tenderness upon percussion may indicate a kidney stone or disease. In the seated female patient, for a general physical or when there is a problem with the breasts, during breast inspection, the patient is asked to do certain maneuvers to bring out abnormalities. These include raising the arms above the head, pressing the hands against the hips, and leaning forward.

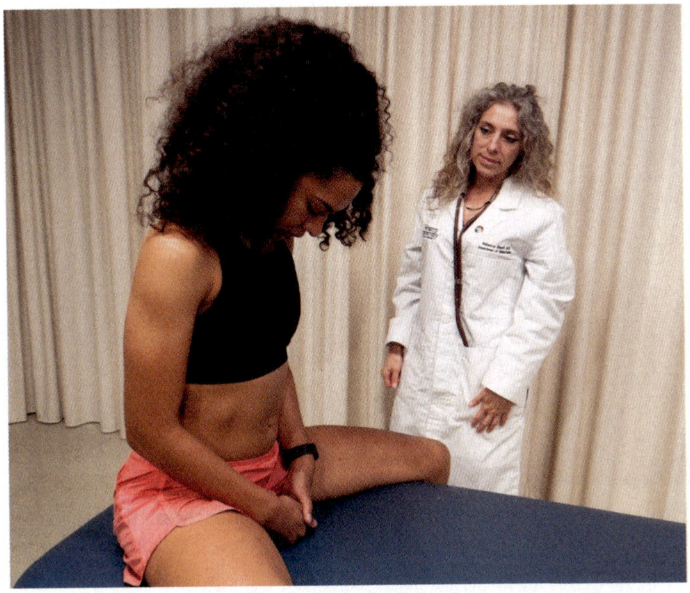

Figure 27.15. Active range of motion of the cervical, thoracic, and lumbar regions may be performed in the seated position. Here, the physician evaluates the patient's active range of motion of cervical flexion. (Photo courtesy of Western University of Health Sciences, Pomona, CA, with permission.)

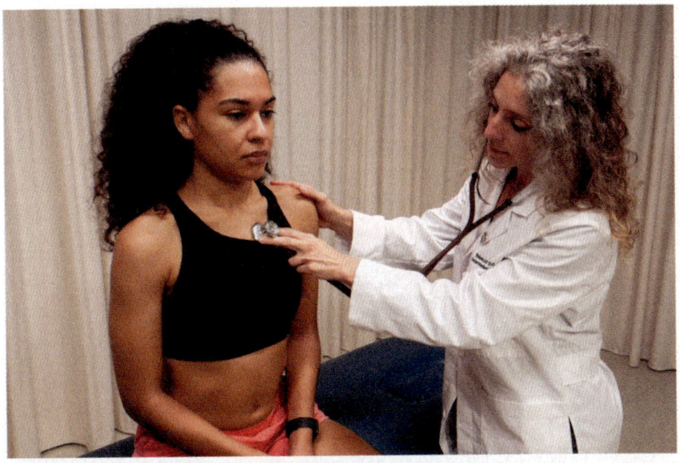

Figure 27.16. The physician can conduct a thorough heart and lung examination to assess for arrhythmias, murmurs, point of maximal impulse, pulse rate, abnormal breath sounds, and the presence of egophony and pectoriloquy in the seated position. (Photo courtesy of Western University of Health Sciences, Pomona, CA, with permission.)

A. Doctor Can Assess the Following:	B. Osteopathic Considerations
Spine—In the seated position, the mechanics of the lower extremity have been removed which may alter any compensatory changes of the spine. Lateral spinal curvatures in the neutral seated position may be compared to the standing view for apices, convexities, and number of segments involved. Also, observe for excessive or diminished thoracic kyphosis and lumbar and cervical lordosis. Assessment of active and passive vertebral flexion, extension, side bending, and rotation both regionally and segmentally in cervical, thoracic, and lumbar regions may be done. In the seated position, the degrees of trunk flexion can be visualized. Thoracic and lumbar spinous process rotation in a neutral position can be observed. Lumbar lordosis can be observed while performing the seated flexion test and may be fixed, reversed, or changed minimally with forward bending.	When assessing the patient in this position, it is important that the patient's feet are on the floor and they are sitting up straight. Determine regional as well as segmental levels of somatic dysfunction. Deviation of spinous processes may indicate somatic dysfunction; the spinous process is rotated opposite the position of the body of the vertebra. If control of the patient's body is an issue when assessing passive range of motion due to operator-patient size discrepancy, the physician may ask the patient to sit on a lower stool, which will offer more stability and ease of the maneuvers of flexion, extension, rotation, and side bending. The trunk is often used as a lever to examine facet joint mechanics, active range of motion, and quality of motion of the lower thoracic spine and the lumbar spine. The head is used as a lever to assess active and passive range of motion of the upper thoracic spine (Fig. 27.17). Some conditions, such as Cushing syndrome, cause a prominence of fat in the upper thoracic region called a *buffalo hump*.[10]
Seated Flexion Test—With the patient seated on a low stool, feet and knees shoulder width apart, and feet on the floor, the examiner places their thumbs on the inferior slope of the posterior inferior iliac spine. The patient then bends forward and may put their flexed elbows between their knees. Anterior superior excursion of the PSIS is compared to the opposite side.	This test is for *sacroiliac somatic dysfunction*. The side of maximum excursion is considered the dysfunctional or restricted side and is called a positive test. This indicates that the motion of the sacrum on the ilium has been affected. Figure 27.18 shows an example of a slightly modified seated flexion test in that the patient's arms are not between the knees, thus not limiting potential side bending of the trunk that can affect the test results or interpretation.

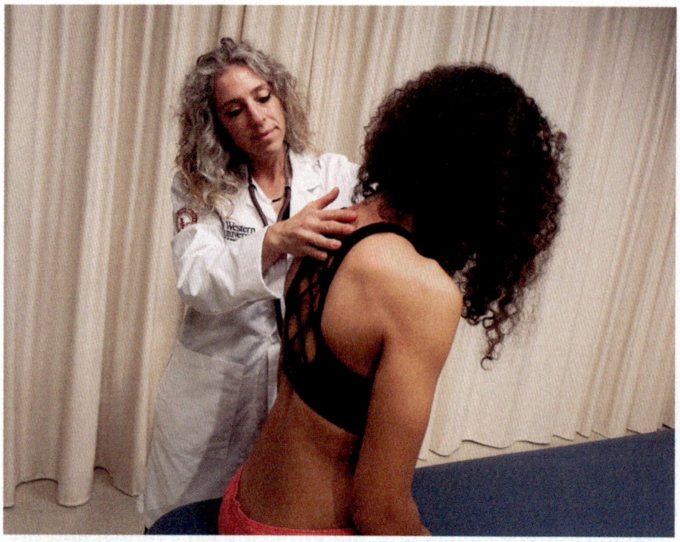

Figure 27.17. Assessment of passive range of motion or quality of motion of the upper thoracic spine with the patient in the seated position. (Photo courtesy of Western University of Health Sciences, Pomona, CA, with permission.)

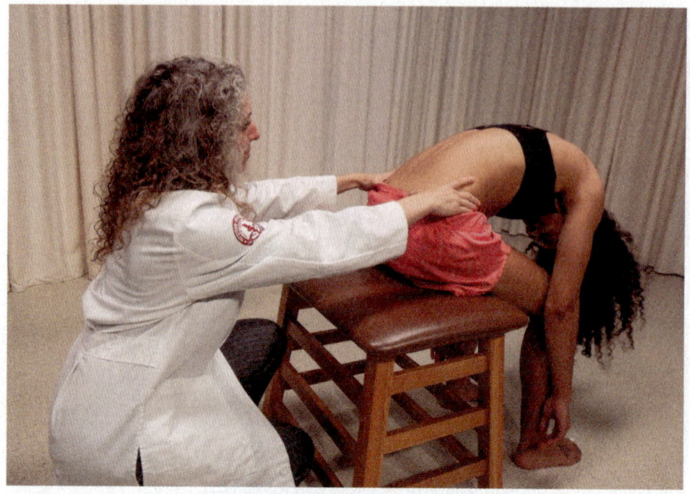

Figure 27.18. Performance of seated flexion test. (Photo courtesy of Western University of Health Sciences, Pomona, CA, with permission.)

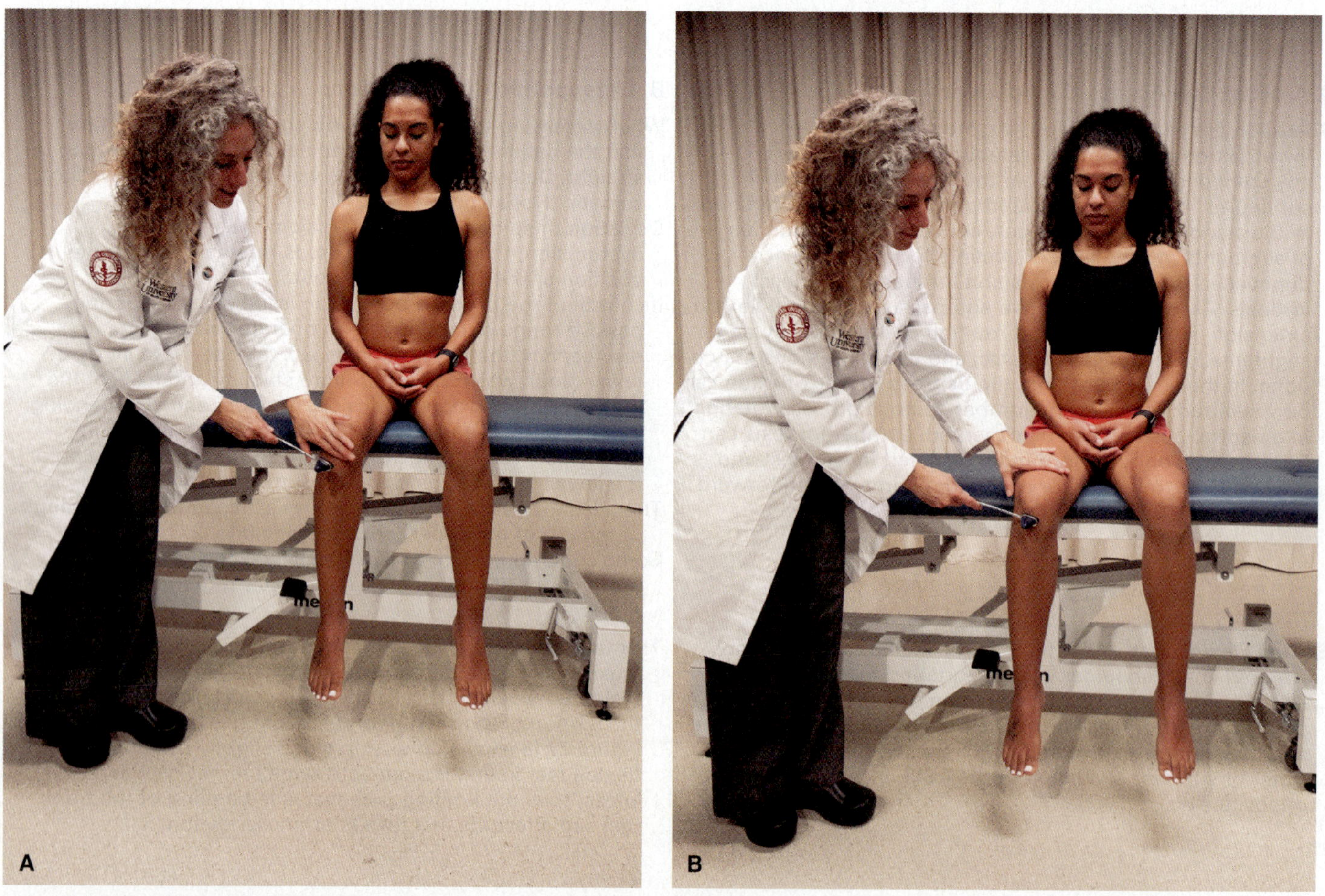

Figure 27.19. Assessing the patellar reflex. A. If there is difficulty eliciting any deep tendon reflex, it may be beneficial to palpate for the tendon first. **B.** Then elicit the reflex with the reflex hammer. (Photo courtesy of Western University of Health Sciences, Pomona, CA, with permission.)

Lower Extremities—Observe how the patient sits. Are the knees extended? Are they unable to flex the knee past a certain angle? Observe for scars that may indicate surgery or joint replacement. Can the patient bend forward at the waist indicating adequate hip mobility?

Knee examination assesses for patellar tracking and crepitus with flexion and extension as well as fibular head motion. Assess the knees for swelling, erythema, edema, and ballottement (also can be performed with patient supine; see below). Assess sensation by dermatomes and motor strength of the muscles. Check the patellar (Fig. 27.19A,B) and Achilles tendon reflexes (deep tendon reflexes or tendon stretch reflexes). Perform muscle strength testing for the quadriceps, biceps femoris, and gastrocnemius muscles. Examine the feet for hammer toes, calluses, and bunions. Vascular assessment (dorsalis pedis and/or posterior tibialis pulses) and sensory examination using a monofilament are especially important for patients with diabetes. Vibration testing is important in diabetes using a tuning fork on the distal interphalangeal joint of the great toe.

This evaluation truly encompasses all five osteopathic models as the lower extremity is responsible for locomotion and thus interfacing with the ground reactive force (GRF). Overall, GRF increases during ambulation and the vertical component of the GRF can be three to five times the body weight during running.[25] Inappropriate posture, conditions such as cervical and lumbar stenosis,[26–28] altered mechanics of the ground striking pattern, altered joint kinematics due to injury or trauma,[29] systemic factors such as peripheral arterial disease,[30,31] and neurologic deficits such as the diabetic foot[25] can increase GRF. This can cause overall increased energy expenditure, pain during ambulation, and/or increased and abnormal impact to joints and the axial spine risking and perpetuating further damage.[32]

Upper Extremity—Examination of the upper extremities should include inspection of the skin, nails, pulses, and all joints, range, and quality of motion, glenohumeral joint static position, protracted and retracted, and static and active position of the clavicle and scapulae. Assess sensation by dermatomes, the deep tendon reflexes of the biceps, triceps, and brachioradialis tendons, and the Tinel test may be performed to assess nerve entrapment in the carpal tunnel at the wrist. Perform muscle strength testing of the rotator cuff muscles, the deltoid, biceps\triceps, wrist flexors/extensors, and intrinsic hand muscles as well as special tests such as Adson test to evaluate for thoracic outlet syndrome (TOS). Fingernails should be inspected for clubbing, koilonychia, pitting, cyanosis, or splinter hemorrhages. Hand temperature should be assessed along with radial pulses.

The upper extremity complex is intricate, dynamic, and wide-reaching and must be evaluated and treated as an integrated system. Sensory testing for the cervical and upper thoracic dermatomes provides information about the cervical disk integrity or nerve entrapment syndromes.

Seventeen muscles attach to the scapula and compromise of their mechanics, vascular, lymphatic, and neurologic supply can lead to a wide range of dysfunction. Thoracic outlet syndrome may affect the upper extremity by compression of the brachial plexus and subclavian artery. Osteopathic evaluation and treatment are well-suited to elucidate contributory factors to dysfunction of the upper extremity and restore them to proper physiologic function.

Dr. Still was known for stating "The rule of the artery must be absolute, universal and unobstructed or disease will be the result.[7]" He pointed out to his students that when circulatory flow was obstructed to the distal parts of the body, changes in the hands or feet were evident. Nail clubbing in chronic obstructive pulmonary disease (COPD) demonstrates when lack of oxygen occurs chronically, changes to the underlying structure can ensue. Raynaud disease is another example of impairment from altered circulation. Hand temperature may be abnormal in Raynaud disease or circulatory decline. OMT can maximize the arterial flow, thereby decreasing the impact on the distal site.

From a biopsychosocial aspect, the upper extremity is prone to repetitive overuse injuries either from daily habits or from work-related activities. This strain pattern may be evident from the structural exam or may be elucidated through the history. Once the inciting activity is identified, the physician may be able to work with the patient on how to modify those activities.

TIP—Some physicians prefer to do the entire musculoskeletal examination and neurologic examination as separate examinations, rather than incorporate into each position as in this approach. Either approach is fine but may entail the patient moving around more than necessary. Often the chief complaint focuses the examination on a particular system, or if the physician notices an abnormality during the examination, the entire system related to that abnormality is usually thoroughly investigated to determine the cause. The neurologic examination, for example, may entail a head-to-toe assessment such as gait and coordination (cerebellar examinations such as rapid alternating movements and finger-to-nose examination or heel-to-shin); Romberg and pronator drift tests; mental status check to determine if the patient is alert, oriented to person, place, time, and situation; assessment of each cranial nerve; assessment for sensation, deep tendon reflexes, and muscle strength of the upper and lower extremities bilaterally; and Babinski reflex. Likewise, the entire surface of the skin can be examined with the patient standing, looking for jaundice, rashes, lesions, masses, or abnormal-appearing skin changes.

POSITION 3—WITH THE PATIENT SUPINE ON EXAM TABLE

A. Doctor Can Assess the Following:	B. Osteopathic Considerations
Head—Palpate the cranium using the vault hold (Fig. 27.20) to assess for symmetry, motion, compliance, and amplitude of CRI. Note the presence of any SBS strain patterns. **Cervical spine**—Passive range of motion in side bending, flexion, extension, and rotation. **Occipitoatlantal (OA) Joint**—Passively assess by laterally translating the occiput with hands posterior to the occipitomastoid suture and comparing it with the opposite side. **Atlantoaxial (AA) Joint**—The physician stands at the head of the table and flexes the cervical spine maximally. Rotation is compared on the left and right, and side of ease is noted as the somatic dysfunction of the AA.	Presence of somatic dysfunction in the cranial region can have a profound effect on the CNS, cranial nerve function, and conditions such as anxiety and depression. Due to the reciprocal tension membrane, somatic dysfunction of the cranium can have implications throughout the spine and even beyond its attachment at S2. Ensure that the neck is fully relaxed before trying to accurately diagnose cervical joint mechanics. The *sternocleidomastoid muscle* is often contracted if the patient is not relaxed. OA joint motion is similar to Fryette Type I mechanics in that it side bends and rotates in opposite directions, but unlike the thoracic and lumbar spine, it maintains this relationship whether it is flexed, extended, or in neutral position. AA joint motion is purely rotational. The detection of and resolution of somatic dysfunction of the cervical region may positively affect the following: • From the neurologic model of care: pain generated by structural problems, vagal nerve function at the cranial base and upper cervical complex, proper function of the thoracoabdominal diaphragm with optimization of the phrenic nerve at C3–5, and herniated disks or areas of nerve root compression. • With regards to the respiratory/circulatory model: glymphatic system drainage of the head to the deep cervical lymph nodes and blood flow to the brain and organs such as the thyroid via the vertebral and the internal and external carotid arteries.
Typical Cervical Segments C2–C7—In this region, lateral translation of the articular pillars is generally used to arrive at the diagnosis. With physician's fingers on the articular pillars, laterally translate the segment while the neck is neutral, then flexed and extended. Compare sides to confirm if there is more ease of translation while the cervical spine is flexed or extended to arrive at the somatic dysfunction diagnosis.	Typical cervical vertebral joint mechanics are often described as "Fryette Type II-like," because side bending and rotation occur on the same side and in flexed or extended positions. Exceptions to this rule are found with extreme compression injuries of the cervical spine.[33] Please see above for further osteopathic considerations of the typical cervical region.
Breast and Axillae If clinically indicated, from a medicolegal perspective, it is best to perform this portion of the exam with a chaperone such as a Medical Assistant (MA) present. The physician looks for asymmetry, scars, dimpling, edema, inflammation, and gross evidence of masses, areas of tenderness, and nipple discharge. Palpate the axillary and supraclavicular regions for lymphadenopathy or tender lymph nodes. The breasts are examined one at a time, with the ipsilateral arm above the patient's head.	Breast examination may be done in the context of a full physical examination and with patient permission.

TIP—For women who are still menstruating, it is helpful to know chronologically where they are during their menstrual cycle, as they may experience tenderness during the breast exam depending on where they are with the cycle.

Figure 27.20. Vault hold hand placement used to assess cranial contour and motion with patient supine. (Illustration courtesy of William A. Kuchera, DO, FAAO, with permission.)

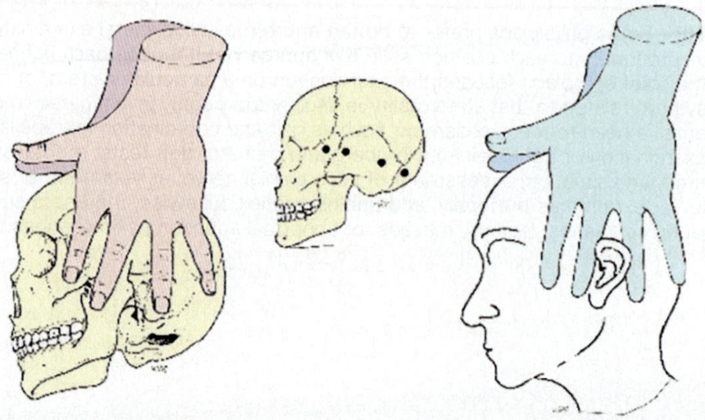

A. Doctor Can Assess the Following:	B. Osteopathic Considerations
Heart—Supine evaluation of the heart should be performed with the head of the bed elevated 15 to 30 degrees. Left lateral auscultation may also be indicated. Point of maximal impulse may also be evaluated in this position. If jugular venous distention (JVD) evaluation is indicated, it would be done with head of the bed elevated 30–45 degrees and the patient's head turned to the left.	Jugular venous distention (JVD) indicates increased central venous pressure, or the pressure of the right atrium. The external jugular vein will be seen as distended or bulging if the patient has elevation of the central venous pressure in conditions such as congestive heart failure. If JVD is present, the jugular venous pulse should be measured in relationship to the sternal angle. Signs of heart failure must be thoroughly evaluated as this is a multisystem process and has neurohormonal implications.[34] Osteopathic care is an important adjuvant treatment for heart failure.[35]
Thoracic Cage—Rib motion abnormalities are best examined in the supine position. In this position, the physician can evaluate first rib motion, pump handle motion, mixed, and bucket handle motion with active inhalation and comparison with the opposite side (Fig. 27.21). The motion of the floating ribs is best palpated in the prone position. The sternum and costochondral cartilages may also be examined in this position for tenderness or pectus excavatum or carinatum. The thoracic cage can be evaluated for symmetry from left to right.	Rib motion abnormalities can be seen with respiratory complaints or from injury to the region. Asymmetry in the thoracic cage may indicate scoliosis or developmental abnormality and should be investigated further. Improvement of rib motion with OMT may positively affect the thoracoabdominal diaphragm and its ability to maintain appropriate pressure gradients for adequate vascular and lymphatic flow.

TIP—Before initiating the exam of the thoracic cage it is recommended to explain to the patient the nature of the exam. Clear communication with the patient is especially important when examining regions such as the breast area. Communicate to the patient what is being done and why it is being done and inform the patient that they are in control and can ask the physician to stop this portion of the exam if they feel uncomfortable.

When performing the thoracic cage and rib motion evaluation on a woman, she may place her hands over her breasts for comfort and also be asked to move the breast tissue medially and/or inferiorly during different parts of the exam in order to allow the physician to accurately assess rib motion.

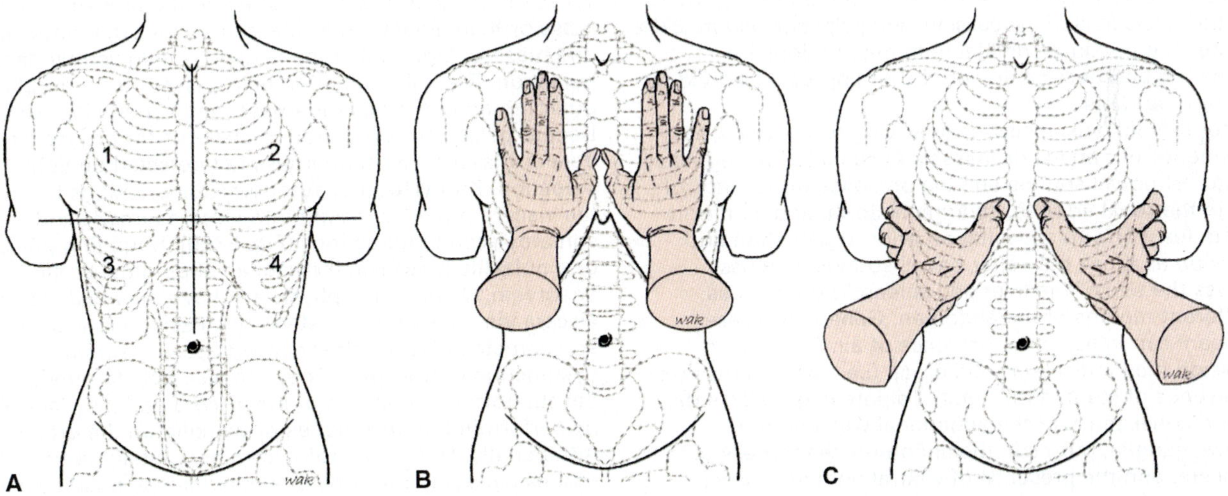

Figure 27.21. Hand placement for supine assessment of costal cage contour and active motion. A. Costal cage divided into four quadrants. **B.** Hand placement for pump handle type rib motion assessment. **C.** Hand placement for bucket handle type rib motion. (Illustration courtesy of William A. Kuchera, DO, FAAO, with permission.)

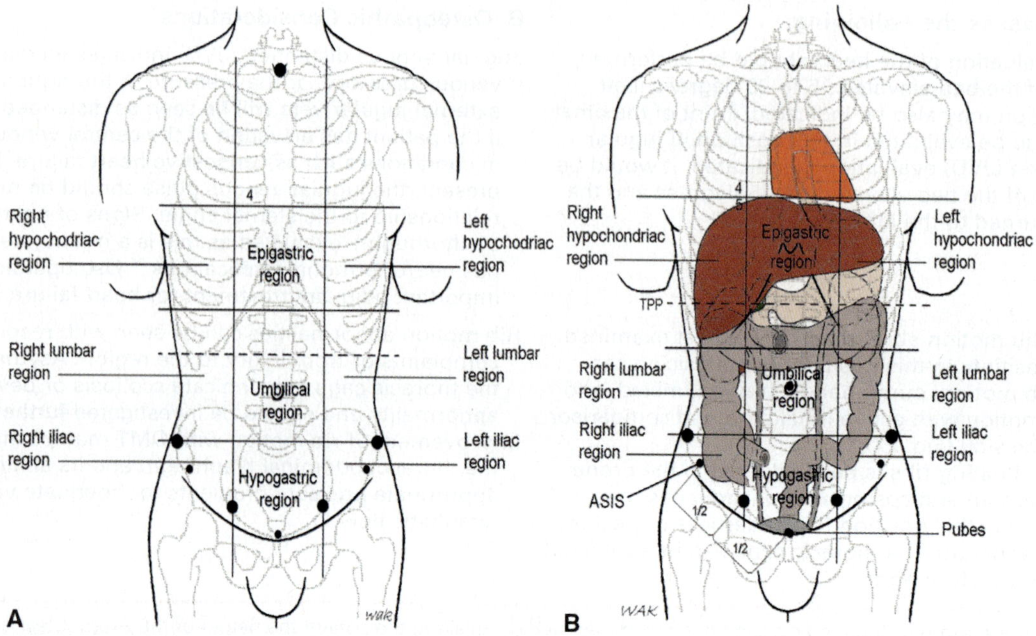

Figure 27.22. Supine assessment of abdomen. A. Division of the abdomen into nine quadrants. **B.** Boney and organ relationships underlying the nine quadrants. Spleen, gallbladder, small intestines, and pancreas not shown. ASIS, anterior superior iliac spine; TPP, trans pyloric plane. (Illustration courtesy of William A. Kuchera, DO, FAAO, with permission.)

A. Doctor Can Assess the Following:

Abdomen—The abdomen is examined in the following order: inspection, auscultation, percussion, and palpation. Figure 27.22 illustrates the abdomen divided into nine regions for examination and documentation. Other approaches divide it into four quadrants.

Inspect for skin lesions, incisions or scars, swelling or striae, and evidence of hernias or masses. Auscultate for frequency and pitch of bowel sounds and the presence or absence of bruits in the renal arteries, abdominal aorta, and common iliac arteries. Perform auscultation prior to palpation and percussion as those may alter bowel sounds. Percuss to assess the size of the liver and spleen. Then percuss the different regions of the abdomen. General increase in tympani can indicate the presence of air. Dullness to percussion may indicate a solid organ (i.e., liver), a mass, or the presence of stool in the colon. Palpate (Fig. 27.23)—the tone and consistency of the abdominal wall and the collateral ganglia, pulses in the abdomen, tenderness of the viscera, and the presence of ventral hernias. Assess compliance of the root of the mesentery and the colonic flexures. If a hernia is suspected, have the patient attempt to sit up to increase abdominal pressure and elucidate further. Dermatomal testing may also be performed during this time (Fig. 27.24). Consider autonomic innervations as the supine patient is being examined (Fig. 27.25). Abdominal organs may be assessed for mobility and motility.

Special tests are performed as needed. These special tests include palpation for tenderness at McBurney point and Rosving, psoas, and obturator signs for appendicitis, the presence of rebound tenderness for peritoneal inflammation, and Murphy sign for gallbladder disease or cholecystitis.

B. Osteopathic Considerations

Percussion helps assess organ size and the presence of a mass or fluid. Palpation also assesses for organomegaly and masses. Light palpation is usually followed by deeper palpation. The light palpation helps assess for muscular guarding and rigidity, tenderness, and superficial masses. Deeper palpation is required to evaluate for organomegaly, deeper masses, and tenderness not detected on light palpation. Knowledge of autonomic innervations to the viscera provides insight into viscerosomatic and somatovisceral interactions (Fig. 27.25). Bounding pulsations or a pulsatile mass can indicate an abdominal aortic aneurysm. Osteopathic physicians have the ability to affect viscera via the somatic system, decreasing viscerosomatic and somatovisceral reflexes by addressing somatic dysfunction of the spine. They are also able to directly address the supporting structures of the viscera and the viscera itself by performing lift techniques or working on the organ directly. Additionally, from a neurologic standpoint, inhibition of the tissues overlying the collateral ganglia may positively affect the organs they innervate.

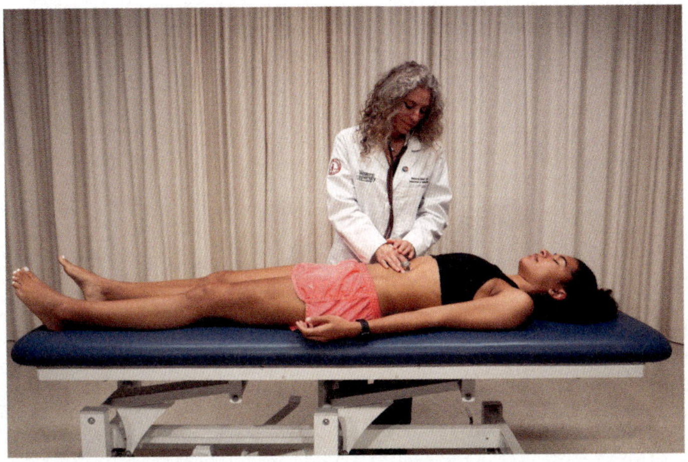

Figure 27.23. Palpation of the abdomen. (Photo courtesy of Western University of Health Sciences, Pomona, CA, with permission.)

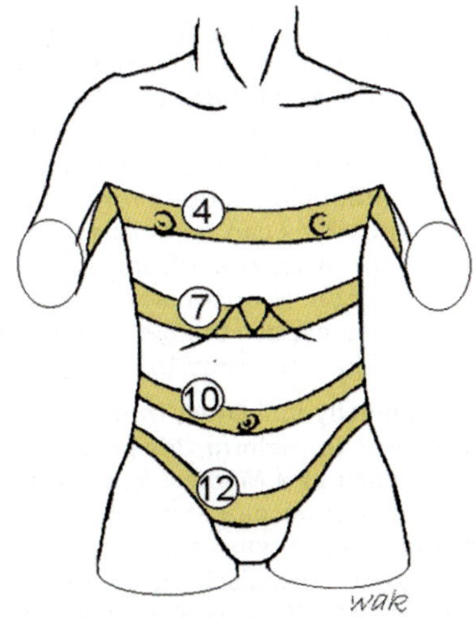

Figure 27.24. Dermatomes on the anterior torso. (Illustration courtesy of William A. Kuchera, DO, FAAO, with permission.)

Pelvis Landmarks—Ask the patient to perform a hip flop by having the patient bend their knees and lift their hips while stabilizing their ankles. Then draw the legs out along the treatment table. This may assist with relaxing the abdominal musculature and provide more accurate assessment of pelvic landmarks. Assess the levels of the inferior aspect of the medial malleoli. Anterior superior iliac spine levels and relation to a midline structure are assessed and compared from side to side. Keep in mind the side of the positive standing flexion test as this will indicate the dysfunctional side. It is helpful to list the findings on the dysfunctional side to generate the appropriate diagnosis. Pubic tubercle levels are also assessed to determine somatic dysfunction of the pelvis (Fig. 27.26).

Anterior and posterior innominate rotations, innominate and pubic shears, and innominate inflares and outflares can all be determined using pelvic landmarks as a guide. The pelvic diaphragm is an important structure to evaluate in concerns of the pelvis in both male and female patients. Evaluation and treatment of pelvic somatic dysfunction can be performed in the supine, prone, and lateral recumbent positions.[36]

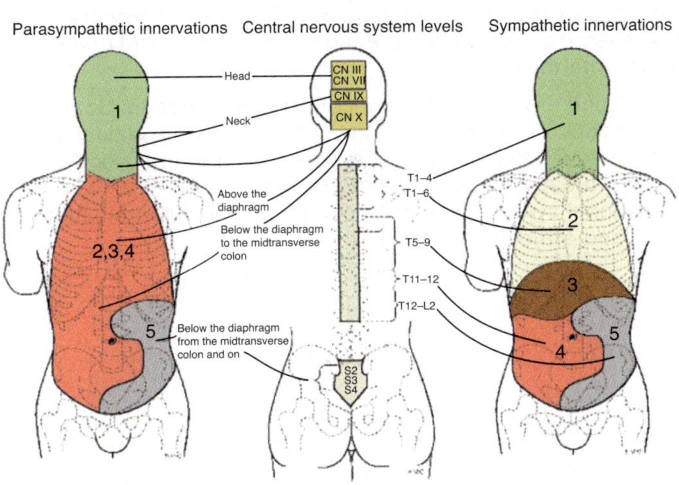

Figure 27.25. Autonomic innervation patterns to consider while examining the patient's head, neck, chest, and abdominal regions. (Illustration courtesy of William A. Kuchera, DO, FAAO, with permission.)

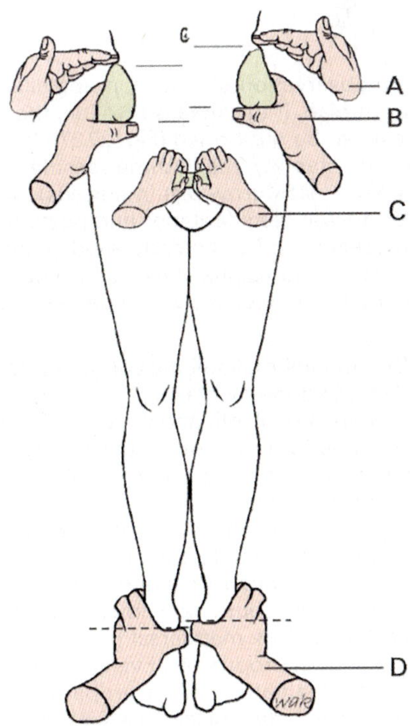

Figure 27.26. Supine assessment of symmetry (levels) of (A) iliac crests, (B) anterior superior iliac spines (ASIS), (C) pubic symphysis, and (D) medial malleoli. The patient's left innominate, left pubic tubercle, and left leg are superior to the right counterparts. (Illustration courtesy of William A. Kuchera, DO, FAAO, with permission.)

Male pelvis—If clinically indicated, from a medicolegal perspective, it is best to perform this portion of the exam with a chaperone such as a Medical Assistant (MA) present. Evaluate the scrotum for lesions, incisions, scars, and masses. Seminal vesicle and varicocele evaluation is also performed. Transillumination is done for hydrocele and masses. Cremasteric reflex can be evaluated here. The penis is examined for discharge, ulcers, rashes, condyloma, carcinoma, and infection. In uncircumcised males, the foreskin is retracted to expose the glans. After the glans is inspected, the foreskin is returned to the original position.	If the penis foreskin cannot be retracted or does not return to the original position, suspect phimosis.
Female pelvis—If clinically indicated, from a medicolegal perspective, it is best to perform this portion of the exam with a chaperone such as a Medical Assistant (MA) present. In lithotomy position, a gynecologic examination can be performed, first looking at skin, labia, and external rectum for rashes, lesions, masses, discharge, cysts, or secretions. Then, using a speculum, the cervix and vagina can be evaluated and Papanicolaou smear or cultures obtained. Rectum–lithotomy position is used to examine the rectum: check for rectocele, cystocele, or hemorrhoids. Assess stool for occult blood using a hemoccult slide.	Structural and physical examination of the obstetric patient may require modification of patient position as many women in the third trimester are uncomfortable laying supine.[36]

A. Doctor Can Assess the Following:	B. Osteopathic Considerations
Hips—Degrees of motion in abduction, adduction, flexion, and internal and external rotation (knee at 90 degrees) can be measured bilaterally. The Thomas test can be performed to assess for iliopsoas restriction and the straight leg raise test for hamstring restriction or sciatic nerve stretch. Other tests include the FABER test (flexion, abduction, and external rotation) for hip dysfunction and the Ober test for iliotibial band tightness.	Short leg will cause the pelvis to shift toward the long leg side in a standing position; this should clue the examiner to evaluate for a short leg in the supine position.[37] A restricted psoas may cause the patient to be flexed forward altering posture. Adequate hip mobility and strength are critical to proper ambulation and joint mechanics of the trunk and lower extremity. Muscle imbalance of the hip complex, injury such as a labral tear, or conditions such as osteoarthritis may cause pain and alter joint kinematics. Careful evaluation of the hip can elicit the underlying cause of pain or dysfunction of the region and depending on the condition, OMT may correct or improve it.
Knees—General observation of patella, prepatellar, and suprapatellar bursae. If the knee is swollen, the ballottement and bulge test can be performed (Fig. 27.27). In concerns for intra-articular stability, the Lachman test (anterior cruciate ligament), McMurray test (meniscus), and anterior and posterior drawer tests (anterior and posterior cruciate ligaments, respectively) can be performed bilaterally for comparison. Varus and valgus stress tests (lateral and medial collateral ligaments, respectively) can be performed as well (Fig. 27.28).	Varus and valgus deformity of the lower extremity causes increased wear on the knees, and osteoarthritis can result. If a patient experiences knee pain, it is important to evaluate the feet for pes planus or cavus and supination and pronation. Often the source of the knee pain begins at the feet.[38] If the exam indicates a meniscal or collateral ligament injury, conservative treatment including OMT may help resolve the issue or minimize pain negating the need for surgery. However, if a surgical intervention is warranted, OMT can assist with the recovery.
Ankle/Foot—The medial malleoli are compared for short leg assessment. This is done by placing thumbs on the inferior slopes of the medial malleoli, and the examiner determines if one is more superior to the other, which may indicate a short leg on that side. The ankle joint is palpated as well as the distal end of the fibular for joint integrity. If the ankle is swollen or injured, the anterior drawer test of the ankle may be performed to evaluate anterior talofibular ligament integrity. Evaluate the foot for conditions that may alter gait or cause pain such as subungual hematomas, bunions, or hammer toes. Palpate the metatarsal bones to ensure that they are positioned appropriately. Evaluate sensation using a monofilament if the patient has neuropathy or diabetes. Check and compare pedal pulses. Check for clubbing, cyanosis, edema, and capillary refill.	The foot and ankle complex are critical to locomotion. Somatic dysfunction of the area may be addressed with a wide variety of techniques to restore joint mechanics, optimize vascular flow, and decrease energy expenditure. Tarsal tunnel syndrome may be corrected with a combination of OMT and orthotics.[39]

TIP—With extremity issues, it may be helpful to evaluate the joint above and below the painful joint/area for somatic dysfunction, although the source of the issue may be even more wide-reaching. Pain may be a secondary effect rather than primary to the joint itself.

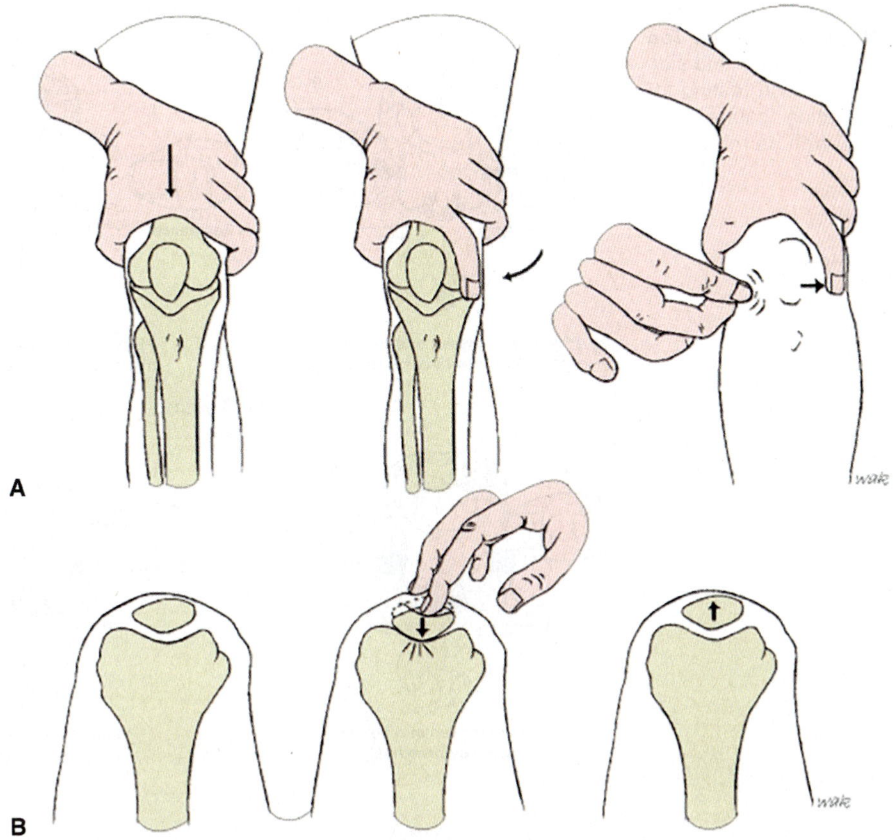

Figure 27.27. Hand placement to assess knee effusion. A. The ballottement test of the right knee of a patient. **B.** The bulge test also assesses for effusion. (Illustration courtesy of William A. Kuchera, DO, FAAO, with permission.)

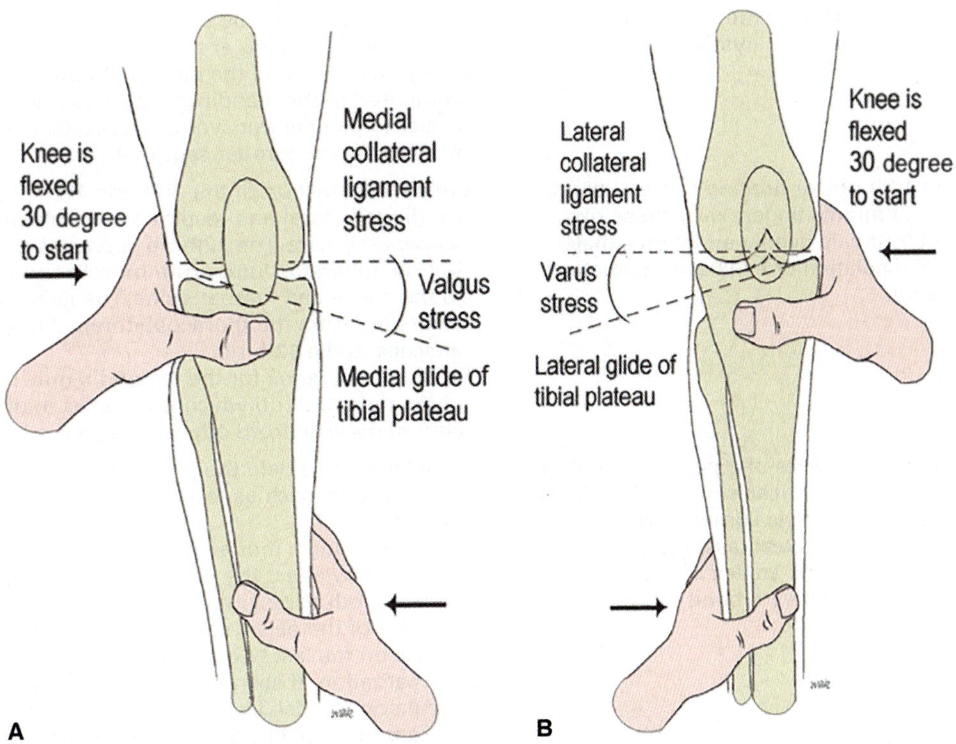

Figure 27.28. Hand placements to assess the integrity of lateral and medial collateral ligaments of a patient's right knee. A. Valgus stress test to assess medial collateral ligament integrity. **B.** Varus stress test to assess lateral collateral ligament integrity. (Illustration courtesy of William A. Kuchera, DO, FAAO, with permission.)

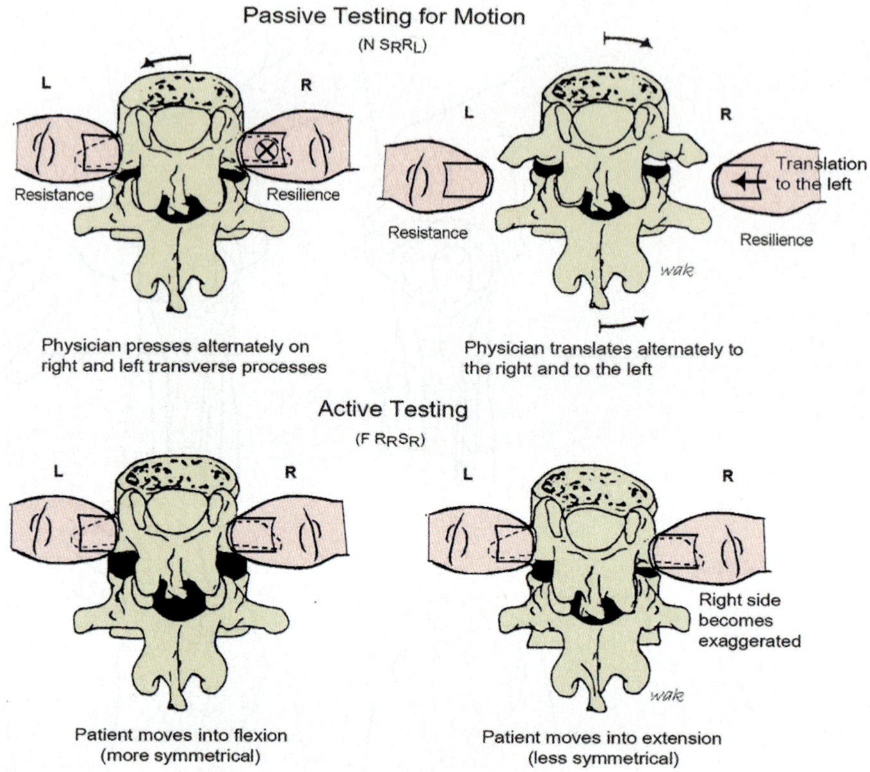

Figure 27.29. Thumb placement for vertebral joint assessment with patient prone. Top shows passive motion testing for rotation and side bending. **Bottom** shows active motion testing for flexion and extension. (Illustration courtesy of William A. Kuchera, DO, FAAO, with permission.)

POSITION 4—WITH THE PATIENT PRONE

A. Doctor Can Assess the Following:	B. Osteopathic Considerations
Spine—The skin can be palpated for hyperhidrosis or dryness. Posterior transverse processes can be palpated in this position to diagnose rotation of the thoracic and lumbar spine (Fig. 27.29). Paravertebral asymmetry in a prone position can help determine somatic dysfunction.	Skin qualities such as dryness or excessive moisture, as well as temperature (cool or hot), provide information about the acuity and timing of an injury to a region. Many patients do not see their backs; be sure to evaluate suspicious moles or rashes while looking at the spine. In the prone position, the paraspinal muscles are relaxed as compared to the standing and seated positions and it may be easier to palpate transverse processes to determine rotation of thoracic and lumbar segments.
Rib Cage—The 11th and 12th ribs or floating ribs are examined by placing the index and middle fingers over these ribs and asking the patient to inhale deeply and then exhale. Determine if structural inhalation or exhalation somatic dysfunctions are present.	Somatic dysfunction of the 11th and 12th ribs has implications for the structural and respiratory/circulatory models of osteopathic care. The 12th rib serves as an attachment site for the quadratus lumborum muscle and therefore is related to the pelvis and lumbar spine. The lateral arcuate ligament extending from the thoracoabdominal diaphragm also attaches to the 12th rib. The Chapman reflex for the appendix may be found at the tip of the right 12th rib which may assist in differentiating lower abdominal pain from other etiologies.
Pelvic and sacral landmarks—In cases of a positive standing flexion test, the posterior superior iliac spines (PSIS) levels are assessed to determine the pelvic somatic dysfunction. In cases of a positive seated flexion test, assess for the depth of the sacral sulcus, inferior lateral angles of the sacrum, rotation of L5 (if applicable), backward bend (Sphinx), and lumbosacral spring test (Fig. 27.30).	Sacral landmarks help the physician diagnose sacral somatic dysfunctions, such as torsions, flexions, or extensions of the sacrum. From a neurologic model of care, somatic dysfunction of the sacrum may affect the pelvic splanchnic nerves, S2–S4, which provide both parasympathetic and motor innervation to muscles of the pelvic cavity and floor. The levator ani muscle inserts on the last two segments of the sacrum, therefore normalization of sacral mechanics may affect the respiratory/circulatory model. In addition, somatic dysfunction of the sacrum may affect cranial mechanics due to the reciprocal tension membrane and the dura mater attachment to S2.

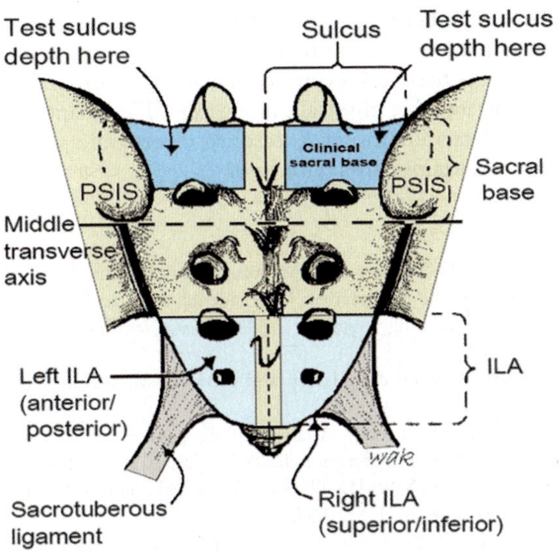

Figure 27.30. Sacral landmarks for thumb placement to assess sacral motion with patient prone. (Illustration courtesy of William A. Kuchera, DO, FAAO, with permission.)

A. Doctor Can Assess the Following:	B. Osteopathic Considerations
Hips—Hip extension can be performed in the prone position by stabilizing the pelvis with one hand and lifting the thigh just above the knee. Internal and external rotation of the hip can also be measured in this position by placing the knees together and flexed to 90 degrees and allowing them to fall out laterally (internal rotation) or medially (external rotation). Dermatomes of L4–S3 can be assessed and the musculature of the posterior pelvis and hip may be palpated for tissue texture changes and tenderness.	Restriction of hip extension may indicate a contracted iliopsoas which has implications on lumbar, pelvic, and gait mechanics. As a strong external rotator of the thigh, hypertonicity of the piriformis may contribute to pelvic and sacral somatic dysfunction, piriformis syndrome, and also be a source of sciatic pain. OMT may resolve or improve somatic dysfunction of structures contributing to hip dysfunction, restriction, or pain.
Knees—The popliteal fossa can be evaluated for fascial restrictions, evidence of deep vein thrombosis (DVT), and cysts. Degrees of flexion at the knee in the prone position should be measured.	Fascial restriction of the popliteal fossa may impede lymphatic drainage from the distal lower extremity. A Baker cyst is a fluid-filled cyst that bulges behind the knee in the popliteal fossa and may result from trauma, osteoarthritis, or torn cartilage. A history of trauma involving the lower extremity may prompt clinical index of suspicion of DVT. Evaluation of the region by ultrasound should be incorporated or follow the physical exam to confirm the diagnosis.
Feet—The Achilles tendons, calcaneus, and plantar fascia are palpated for the presence of tenderness. Assess motion of the tarsal bones, metatarsal bones, phalangeal joints, and interphalangeal joints. Inspect for calluses, deformities, and foot ulcerations.	Inferior displacement of tarsal bones may be treated in this position with a maneuver known as the *Hiss whip*, a high-velocity low-amplitude technique.

Alternative Structural Screening Options Helpful in Clinical Practice

The "10-Step exam"

Screening Exam—The "10-Step exam" is an alternative option for experienced physicians to incorporate into their practice once they have mastered the above. These 10 distinct osteopathic structural evaluation elements may prompt the physician to further examine that region for somatic dysfunction contributing to the patient's CC. The steps are listed as follows:

1. Gait, posture, and iliac crest heights from anterior, lateral, and posterior views
   - □ Determines gait abnormalities, postural abnormalities such as kyphoscoliosis, and possible asymmetries relating to a short leg or cranial base or pelvic dysfunction.
2. Standing flexion test
   - □ Determines the presence and lateralization of iliosacral dysfunction.
3. Lateral flexion test, aka "hip drop" test
   - □ Determines the presence and lateralization of iliolumbar/lumbosacral dysfunction.
4. Seated flexion test
   - □ Determines the presence and lateralization of sacroiliac dysfunction.
5. Seated trunk rotation
   - □ Determines range of motion abnormalities in rotation of the thoracic and lumbar spine.
6. Seated lateral flexion (Side bending)
   - □ Determines range of motion abnormalities in side bending of the thoracic and lumbar spine.
7. Seated cervical testing
   - □ Determines range of motion abnormalities and quality of motion of the cervical spine.
8. Supine rib testing of three regions (pump, bucket, and caliper rib regions)
   - □ Determines rib inhalation or exhalation abnormalities.

9. Supine upper extremity testing
    - □ Determines range of motion abnormalities of the glenohumeral joint.
10. Supine and prone lower extremity testing
    - □ Determines range of motion abnormalities in the hip, knee, and ankle.[40]

For a clinician with limited time, this 10-step osteopathic screening exam can be performed in a matter of minutes leading to a diagnosis of somatic dysfunction in a timely manner without excess movement for patient or physician. Appropriate OMT could then be rendered to the area that would be most beneficial to the patient.

PART IV—CONCLUDING THE ENCOUNTER

Assessment and Plan

When the physician is done gathering data during the patient encounter, the last steps to the office visit include developing a differential diagnosis, formulating an assessment and treatment plan, and communicating with the patient what the next steps will be. In many instances, this includes *motivational interviewing*, or a style of communication that allows intrinsic motivation of the patient to achieve better health outcomes. It is patient-centered and goal-oriented. The plan should include clear steps for both the patient and the physician that may include further testing, bloodwork, imaging, medications, and/or lifestyle changes.

If the assessment includes the presence of somatic dysfunction, then osteopathic manipulation should be offered when appropriate as a part of the plan and with the patient's informed consent (discuss risks, benefits, alternatives, and possible treatment reactions such as mild soreness or fatigue). Many osteopathic techniques can be administered within minutes which provide patients with immediate relief. OMT may also remove primary obstructions to the patient's self-healing and regulating mechanism, so they often note improvement in symptoms in the days following the treatment. It is ideal to provide OMT at the same-day appointment if possible, but reevaluation and treatment can occur at a future date.

Physicians must use clinical judgment, patient history, and experience to know which portions of the exam need to be included during the encounter, or if a complete exam is required.

To finalize the encounter, most physicians will discuss when to return, review the next steps for the patient, and provide take-home information if appropriate. Clear communication is important to ensure patient compliance, especially if there are new medications, dietary recommendations, or exercises being prescribed. Some physicians use the "teach back" method to ensure the patient understands what they need to do next, by asking the patient to repeat their portion of the plan. Ask the patient if they have any questions or clarifications before concluding the encounter. Many electronic record-keeping systems have "meaningful use" documentation that the patient must take upon discharge from the clinic.

SUMMARY

This chapter is meant to be an all-inclusive and comprehensive review of a complete osteopathic history and physical and screening structural exam, highlighting how each region should be approached and evaluated from an osteopathic lens and perspective. It is an example of how experienced osteopathic physicians include structure and function in their exams for the purpose of gaining useful information about somatic dysfunction in relation to the patient's CC. This osteopathic history and physical examination will help to establish rapport with patients and is a part of the distinctive osteopathic approach to patient care. With practice and time, the osteopathic thought process becomes second nature and is incorporated naturally into the osteopathic physical examination. This chapter is the first step in understanding how a seasoned osteopathic physician can perform this examination with ease.

REFERENCES

1. Ragsdale J, Habashy C, Warrier S. Developing physical exam skills in residency: comparing the perspectives of residents and faculty about values, barriers, and teaching methods. *J Med Educ Curric Dev*. 2020: 7:2382120520972675.
2. Shultz MA, Doty M. Why the history and physical examination still matter. *JAAPA*. 2016;29(3):41–45.
3. Verma G, Ivanov A, Benn F, et al. Analyses of electronic health records utilization in a large community hospital. *PLoS One*. 2020;15(7):e0233004.
4. Ansary AM, Martinez JN, Scott JD. The virtual physical exam in the 21st century. *J Telemed Telecare*. 2021;27(6):382–392.
5. Jauhar S. The demise of the physical exam. *N Engl J Med*. 2006:354(6): 548–551.
6. Verghese A, Charlton B, Kassirer JP, Ramsey M, Ioannidis JPA. Inadequacies of physical exam as a cause of medical errors and adverse events: a collection of vignettes. *Am J Med*. 2015;128(12):1322–1334.e3.
7. Still AT. *The Autobiography of Andrew T. Still*. Self; 1908.
8. Seffinger MA, Hruby RJ, Kuchera WA. *Evidenced-Based Manual Medicine: A Problem Oriented Approach*. Saunders Elsevier; 2007.
9. Frost H, Campbell P, Maxwell M, et al. Effectiveness of motivational interviewing on adult behaviour change in health and social care settings: a systematic review of reviews. *PLoS One*. 2018;13(10):e0204890.
10. Bickley L, Szilagyi G, Hoffman R. *Bates' Guide to Physical Examination and History Taking*. 13th ed. Wolters Kluwer; 2021.
11. Owens MR, Brito-Silva F, Kirkland T, et al. Prevalence and social determinants of food insecurity among college students during the COVID-19 pandemic. *Nutrients*. 2020;12(9):2515.
12. Gertis AKS, Schwerdtfeger AR. When rumination counts: perceived social support and heart rate variability in daily life. *Psychophysiology*. 2016;53(7):1034–1043.
13. Hunt TKA, Slack KS, Berger LM. Adverse childhood experiences and behavioral problems in middle childhood. *Child Abuse Negl*. 2017;67: 391–402.
14. Still AT. *The Philosophy and Mechanical Principles of Osteopathy*. Hudson-Kimberly Publishing Co; 1892.
15. Chi J, Artandi M, Kugler J, et al. The five-minute moment. *Am J Med*. 2016;129(8):792–795.
16. Chapman F. *An Endocrine Interpretation of Chapman's Reflexes*. 5th ed. American Academy of Osteopathy; 1937.
17. Ma S, Yang J, Yang B, et al. The patient health questionnaire-9 vs. the Hamilton rating scale for depression in assessing major depressive disorder. *Front Psychiatry*. 2021;12:747139.
18. Sutton SE. An osteopathic method of history taking and physical examination part 1. *J Am Osteopath Assoc*. 1978;77(10):780–788.
19. Beauchet O, Fantino B, Allali G, Muir SW, Montero-Odasso M, Annweiler C. Timed up and go test and risk of falls in older adults: a systematic review. *J Nutr Health Aging*. 2011;15(10):933–938.
20. https://www.cdc.gov/steadi/media/pdfs/steadi-assessment-tug-508.pdf. Accessed November 28, 2024.
21. Podsiadlo D, Richardson S. The timed "Up & Go": a test of basic functional mobility for frail elderly persons. *J Am Geriatr Soc*. 1991;39(2): 142–148.
22. Hruby RJ. *Craniosacral Osteopathic Technique: A Manual*. 2nd ed. The Institute for Osteopathic Studies; 1996.
23. Nelson KE, Glonek T. *Somatic Dysfunction in Osteopathic Family Medicine*. Lippincott Williams & Wilkins; 2007.
24. Johnston WL, Friedman HD. *Functional Methods: A Manual for Palpatory Skill Development in Osteopathic Examination and Manipulation of Motor Function*. American Academy of Osteopathy; 2006.
25. Nilsson J, Thorstensson A. Ground reaction forces at different speeds of human walking and running. *Acta Physiol Scand*. 1989;136(2):217–227.

26. Natarajan P, Fonseka RD, Kim S, Betteridge C, Maharaj M, Mobbs RJ. Analysing gait patterns in degenerative lumbar spine diseases: a literature review. *J Spine Surg*. 2022;8(1):139–148.
27. Haddas R, Ju KL, Patel S, Belanger TA, Arakal RG. Altered ground reaction forces in adult cervical spondylotic myelopathy compared to controls. *J Spine*. 2017;17(10):S44
28. Haddas R, Ju KL. Gait alteration in cervical spondylotic myelopathy elucidated by ground reaction forces. *Spine (Phila Pa 1976)*. 2019;44(1):25–31.
29. Lanier AS, Knarr BA, Stergiou N, Snyder-Mackler L, Buchanan TS. ACL injury and reconstruction affect control of ground reaction forces produced during a novel task that simulates cutting movements. *J Orthop Res*. 2020;38(8):1746–1752.
30. McGrath D, Judkins TN, Pipinos II, Johanning JM, Myers SA. Peripheral arterial disease affects the frequency response of ground reaction forces during walking. *Clin Biomech (Bristol, Avon)*. 2012;27(10):1058–1063.
31. Rahman H, Anderson CP, Pipinos II, et al. Muscle forces and power are significantly reduced during walking in patients with peripheral artery disease. *J Biomech*. 2022;135:111024.
32. Farahpour N, Jafarnezhad A, Damavandi M, Bakhtiari A, Allard P. Gait ground reaction force characteristics of low back pain patients with pronated foot and able-bodied individuals with and without foot pronation. *J Biomech*. 2016;49(9):1705–1710.
33. Fryette HH, Strachan WF. *Principles of Osteopathic Technic*. Vol. 2. Academy of Applied Osteopathy; 1954.
34. Hartupee J, Mann DL. Neurohormonal activation in heart failure with reduced ejection fraction. *Nat Rev Cardiol*. 2017;14(1):30–38.
35. Nelson KE, Glonek T. *Somatic Dysfunction in Osteopathic Family Medicine*. Lippincott Williams & Wilkins; 2007:279–289.
36. Nelson KE, Glonek T. *Somatic Dysfunction in Osteopathic Family Medicine*. Lippincott Williams & Wilkins; 2007:110.
37. Nelson KE, Glonek T. *Somatic Dysfunction in Osteopathic Family Medicine*. Lippincott Williams & Wilkins; 2007:418–421.
38. Speece CA, Crow WT, Simmons SL. *Ligamentous Articular Strain. Osteopathic Manipulative Techniques for the Body*. Eastland Press; 2001.
39. Kokubo R, Kim K, Isu T, et al. The impact of tarsal tunnel syndrome to cold sensation in the pedal extremities. *World Neurosurg*. 2016;92:249–254.
40. Moran PS, Pruzzo NA, Mitchell FL Jr, ed. *An Evaluation and Treatment Manual of Osteopathic Manipulative Procedure*. 2nd ed. The Postural-Structural Model: Volume I. The Institute for Continuing Education In Osteopathic Principles; 1973.

28 An Osteopathic Approach to Case-Based Learning

NATALIE A. NEVINS

KEY CONCEPTS

- With a foundation in osteopathic philosophy, use a systematic approach to gather information from the patient, complete the physical examination, and formulate an assessment and treatment plan for the patient.
- An algorithmic approach will help the student to begin to "think" like an osteopathic physician.

THE OSTEOPATHIC ALGORITHM FOR CASE-BASED LEARNING

Chief Complaint

A short description of why the appointment was made in the patient's own words.

Subjective History/History of Present Illness

Allow the patient to give a primary summary of the chief complaint. Then, use additional open- and closed-ended questions to create a complete picture of the patient's problem.

Review pertinent past medical, surgical, family, and social history.

- A complete social history is vital. Historical jobs and military service are often overlooked. Without this information, key environmental exposures may be missed.

Review any pertinent injury history and environmental exposures.

- Patients often forget historical injuries, especially concussions, and may downplay environmental exposures. Directed questions such as "have you ever hit your head," rather than just asking about a history of concussion may help the patient recall pertinent information.

Review all current medications and allergies.
Review of Systems:

Decide if questions need to be asked regarding all systems or focus on systems pertinent to the subjective patient information and the reason for the visit.

Considering all above information and using the five models of osteopathic patient care as a guide, list the top potential differential diagnoses based on the history, first impressions, and knowledge of potential diagnoses, including those that are most probable or most common, as well as probable but not likely. Even the most unlikely diagnoses must be kept in the back of the physician's mind at this point until ruled out completely or at least considered so improbable that it would be considered only after all other diagnoses have failed to explain the history and subsequent physical findings.

1. Biomechanical–Structural
2. Respiratory–Circulatory
3. Neurologic
4. Metabolic–Energetic
5. Behavioral–Biopsychosocial

See Chapter 26, Table 26.2 for examples of using the five models to help develop differential diagnoses of many common chief complaints.

Objective Findings

Consider if a complete physical examination or focused examination is required based on the information above.

If a focused examination is most appropriate, ensure that all pertinent areas are examined and in the most logical order.

Ensure the musculoskeletal/osteopathic structural exam (MSK/OSC) is completed for all pertinent areas.

Document diagnostic palpation (TART) findings in each region: tissue texture changes, temperature variations, asymmetrical anatomical landmarks, restriction of joint motion, and tenderness. Assess the following:

- Gait
- Head
- Cervical
- Thoracic
- Lumbar
- Pelvic/IS joint
- Sacral/SI joint
- LE
- UE
- Costal cage
- Abdomen

Based on the physical exam and objective findings, adjust the top (most likely) differential diagnoses.

Laboratory/Testing

Are laboratory tests required to confirm or assist in determining the diagnosis?

If yes, which labs need to be reviewed or ordered?

Imaging

Are imaging/radiologic studies required to confirm or assist in determining the diagnosis?

If yes, which studies need to be reviewed or ordered?

Assessment

Based on all the gathered information, *what is the final diagnosis*? Which of the five models (or more than one) does the final diagnosis best nest under?

1. Biomechanical–Structural
2. Respiratory–Circulatory
3. Neurologic
4. Metabolic–Energetic
5. Behavioral–Biopsychosocial

Plan

Based on the final diagnosis, what *treatment plan* is recommended?

1. Biomechanical–Structural
2. Respiratory–Circulatory
3. Neurologic
4. Metabolic–Energetic
5. Behavioral–Biopsychosocial

Use the five models to write up a plan, and ensure to cover each of the following as appropriate:

1. Osteopathic manipulation
   - □ Ideally, broken down into the five models being addressed by which techniques are most appropriate for the somatic dysfunction, and what types of techniques are most appropriate for the patient.
   - □ Patients that are acutely ill, or in severe pain may need shorter duration and more indirect techniques. Always consider what is best for the patient, not what your preferred manipulation techniques may be.
2. Medication/supplements
   - □ Metabolic model
3. Referral to a medical specialist
   - □ Metabolic model, to address the disease with medication
   - □ Biopsychosocial model, to develop medical team support
   - □ Respiratory–circulatory model if this addresses vascular and/or breathing issues
4. Referral to surgical specialist
   - □ Structural–biomechanical model
   - □ Biopsychosocial model
5. Diet counseling and education by you or a nutritionist
   - □ Metabolic model
6. Referral to psychiatry/psychotherapy
   - □ Biopsychosocial model
7. Counseling and education: Home exercise program, workstation ergonomics, relaxation techniques, etc.
   - □ Biopsychosocial model
8. How often should the patient follow up in clinic
   - □ Biopsychosocial model

STUDENT CASE EXAMPLES

Patient One

Chief Complaint

"My head has been hurting."

Subjective History/History of Present Illness

An 8-year-old boy presents with multiple complaints:

1. He has been having a headache since this morning. The headache is at the top of his head and in the frontal region. It has been constant since this morning. He says it's a dull achy type of pain. No visual, auditory changes, no weakness, nausea, or vomiting. The patient's mother denies he has had fever, chills, fatigue, or joint achiness. History of concussion 8 months ago.
2. He has also had nonradiating right middle thigh pain for the past 2 days. The pain is an aching pain that has been occurring intermittently. It typically lasts 3 to 4 minutes and has started occurring since he has been skateboarding more. The patient denied trauma or redness to the area.

Note: Patient has been doing well with occupational therapy (OT) and has started reading again (eye therapy/vision therapy). Patient's diet has also improved (previously malnourished).

Past medical history (PMHx): Pediatric autoimmune neuropsychiatric disorders associated with streptococcal infections (PANDAS) diagnosed 1 year ago, Lyme disease diagnosed 2 years ago, obsessive compulsive disorder (OCD), attention deficit hyperactivity disorder (ADHD), sensory integration disorder.

Past surgical history (PSH): None

Trauma Hx: Blunt head trauma in bicycle accident, had a concussion, recovered, 8 months ago.

Immunization: Up-to-date

Medications: (All prescriptions, homeopathic, over-the-counter [OTC], herbal remedies) folic acid, Tox-Ease (supplement), Paragard, glutathione, Chlorella, Nystatin, Bar1 (for Borrelia), BB2 (for Bartonella).

Allergies: Wheat, dairy, walnuts, food dye, pesticides, nitrates in meat (patient gets hives, hyper and OCD-like behavior); red dye → rash; Benadryl → hyperactivity

Family History (FHx)

- Father: Skin cancer on face with lymph involvement
- Maternal grandfather: Bipolar disorder

Risk factors

- No TB exposure
- No tobacco exposure
- No lead exposure

Social history (Soc Hx): Parents are requesting a referral to OT. He used to see an OT for arm–neck–eye for sensory integration disorder and OCD but is taking a break from it because he was getting frustrated, as he was adjusting to a new school. He participates in baseball 2 to 3 times/wk. He stopped vision therapy and wants to restart after baseball season ends. Using magnet therapy. One year ago he saw a Lyme specialist for hematotoxicity. The mother states on a follow-up appointment the Dr. found a "tape worm" in his duodenum, which passed through his stool this past week. He did not tolerate mebendazole, as his mother states that the medication was "too harsh" on his body.

Review of Systems (ROS): Denies chills, ear pain, runny nose, cough, fatigue, myalgias, arthralgias, wheezes, shortness of breath, chest pain, and palpitations.

Admits to changes in appetite (eating more).

Biopsychosocial: denies tuberculosis, hepatitis, other viral or fungal infections, syphilis (THoVoFIS); ADOI, anxiety, depression, overuse injury (i.e., work or sports).

Objective Findings

Vital Signs

Ht: 55 in.; Wt: 57.1 lb; HR: 79; Temp 98.3; RR: 18; BP: 99/62

Physical Examination

General: Well-developed and well-nourished (WDWN) 8-year-old male. Active, pleasant, and cooperative

Psychiatric: Alert and oriented, normal range of facial expressions, mood stable, speech not pressured

Skin: No rashes or lesions

Preliminary Differential Diagnoses (from Table 26.2)

	Biomechanical–Structural	Respiratory–Circulatory	Neurologic	Metabolic–Energetic	Behavioral–BPS
Head pain	Somatic dysfunction[a], congenital deformities, fracture, herniated cervical disk, ocular muscle strain, trauma, temporomandibular joint disorder	Arteriovenous malformation, cerebral aneurysm, Chiari malformation, glaucoma, hydrocephalus, epidural, subdural, or subarachnoid hemorrhages, pseudotumor cerebri	Peripheral and/or central sensitization/facilitated spinal cord segment, fibromyalgia, hemicrania continua, migraine, occipital neuralgia, tension-type headache	Arthritis, bacterial endocarditis, cancer, dental abscess, gum or tooth infection, herpes zoster, iritis, retropharyngeal abscess, meningitis, pharyngitis, sinusitis, vasculitis, THoVoFIS	ADOI, caffeine withdrawal, alcohol abuse (hangover)
Hip or thigh pain	Somatic dysfunction, congenital deformities, degenerative joint disease, dislocation, fracture	Avascular necrosis, hemarthrosis, ischemia	Peripheral and/or central sensitization/facilitated spinal cord segment, fibromyalgia, hemiplegia, lumbar radiculopathy, meralgia paresthetica, multiple sclerosis, amyloidosis, neuropathy, complex regional pain syndrome, syringomyelia	Arthritis, bacterial endocarditis, bursitis, cancer, Lyme disease, septic joint, sprain, tendonitis, THoVoFIS	ADOI

THoVoFIS, tuberculosis, hepatitis, other viral or fungal infections, syphilis; ADOI, anxiety, depression, overuse injury (i.e., work or sports).

Ext: No cyanosis or edema

HEENT: Nasal turbinates swollen, pale, white mucous discharge bilaterally, no sinus pressure tenderness, tympanic membranes intact without erythema or bulging, pharynx hyperemic, tonsils without exudates or hypertrophy, no lymphadenopathy at jugulodigastric node, but shotty nodes palpable in the posterior auricular region

Heart: Regular rate and rhythm (RRR), normal S1/S2, systolic flow murmur

Lungs: Chest wall symmetric, clear to auscultation bilaterally (CTAB), no wheezing or crackles

Abdomen: Normal bowel sounds (BS) × 4, abdomen was soft, no hepatomegaly or splenomegaly noted

Neuro: Normal rhythmic gait, muscular strength (MS) 5/5 in upper and lower extremities bilaterally (B/L), sensation intact in upper and lower extremities B/L. No tics visible today

Musculoskeletal/Osteopathic Structural Examination (MSK/OSE):

- Gait: See Neuro above
- Head: Sphenobasilar symphysis (SBS) compression, dural tension noted, rotated clockwise
- Cervical: Atlantoaxial (AA) rotated right RR
- Thoracic: T2FRLSL, T10-12NRRSL
- Lumbar: L1FRLSL, L3FRRSR
- Sacral: Left unilateral sacral flexion
- Pelvis: Rotated left, left pelvic inflare. Left posterior rotated innominate. Right lower pole restriction. Left upper pole restriction
- Lower extremities: Limited B/L internal rotation, less so on the left. Left leg shorter
- Upper extremities: Full range of motion (ROM)
- Rib region: Left 1st rib inhalation somatic dysfunction (ISD), right 2nd rib exhalation somatic dysfunction (ESD), left 3rd rib ISD, right 4th rib ISD
- Abdomen: Soft, nontender, no counterstrain or Chapman reflex tender points

Labs:

Intestinal Microbial Overgrowth		
Arabinose	**67 (H)**	Reference range: ≤50
HPHPA	**661 (H)**	Reference range: ≤220

Neurotransmitter Metabolites		
Phenylalanine and tyrosine metabolites		
Homovanillic *(dopamine)*	12	Ref: 0.49–13
Vanillylmandelic *(NE, EPI)*	1.7	Ref: 0.72–6.4
HVA/VMA ratio	**6.8 H**	**Ref: 0.23–2.8**
Tryptophan metabolites		
5-Hydroxyindoleacetic *(serotonin)*	0.32	Ref: ≤11
Quinolinic	4.0	Ref: 0.48–8.8
Quinolinic/5-HIAA ratio	**13 H**	**Ref: ≤2.5**

Lyme IgM Western Blot
IGeneX IGM result: Positive
CDC/NYS result: Negative

HPHPA, 3-(3-hydroxyphenyl)-3-hydroxypropionic acid; HVA, homovanillic; VMA, vanillylmandelic; 5-HIAA, 5-hydroxyindoleacetic; CDC, Center for Disease Control; NYS, New York State.

Imaging

None provided for review

Assessment

1. Biomechanical–Structural
   a. Somatic dysfunction: head, cervical, thoracic, lumbar, lower extremity, costal cage regions

2. Respiratory–Circulatory:
   a. Systolic heart murmur
   b. Upper respiratory infection (URI)
3. Neurologic
   a. Tourette syndrome
   b. PANDA/pediatric acute-onset neuropsychiatric syndrome (PANS)
   c. Sensory integration disorder
   d. S/P biomagnetism therapy
4. Metabolic–Energetic
   a. Irritable bowel syndrome (IBS)
   b. Celiac disease
   c. Lactose intolerance
   d. Malnutrition
   e. Lyme disease
5. Behavioral–Biopsychosocial
   a. OCD
   b. Anxiety
   c. PANDAS
   d. ADHD

Plan

1. Biomechanical–Structural
   a. Muscle energy (costal cage, thoracic, pelvic, sacral, and lower extremity regions)
   b. Still technique (lower pole right SI joint, upper pole left SI joint)
   c. HVLA (lumbar region)
   d. Myofascial release (lower extremity region)
   e. Soft tissue (cervical spine region)
2. Respiratory–Circulatory
   a. Lymphatic drainage techniques
   b. Articulatory (rib articulatory)
   c. Osteopathic cranial manipulative medicine (OCMM) (SBS decompression)
3. Neurologic
   a. OCMM (SBS decompression)
   b. Cognitive behavioral therapy
   c. Selective serotonin reuptake inhibitor (SSRI)
4. Metabolic–Energetic
   a. Nutritional and dietary support
5. Behavioral–Biopsychosocial
   a. Cognitive behavioral therapy
   b. Antidepressant medication management
   c. OT
   d. Patient education: review proper way to partake in safe skateboarding and exercising using helmet and protective gear.
      - No further labs or radiologic studies are needed at this time.
      - OMT consent by patient and parent obtained prior to treatment.
      - Follow-up (F/U) in 4 weeks

Case presentation by Diane Padre, DO originally submitted while OMS-III, College of Osteopathic Medicine of the Pacific, Western University of Health Sciences

Patient Two

Chief Complaint

"My leg is swollen; I was struck from behind by a truck."

Subjective History/History of Present Illness

A 52-year-old male who presented to the emergency department (ED) 6 months ago following a motor vehicle collision whereby he was struck from behind by a truck while walking alongside a highway. Injuries sustained at the time include the following from referral note:

- Comminuted fractures of the distal shaft of the right tibia and fibula with lateral displacement and angulation
- Comminuted mildly displaced fractures of the head of the right fibula
- Posterior hip dislocation
- Closed acetabular fracture
- Lower lumbar transverse process fractures

The patient was treated at that time with the following:

- Intramedullary nail of the right open tibia fracture
- Irrigation and debridement of the right hip
- Skin grafting over right lower extremity open wound
- Nonadherent periwound graft
- Arrangement for continuing outpatient wound care

Two months ago, the patient had the following complications:

- Admitted for postoperative infection of right lower extremity RLE pinning
- Inpatient treatment preferred due to concerns of noncompliance with treatment plan and patient unreliability
- Discharged to skilled nursing facility (SNF) 3 weeks later
- Medically stable but mobilizing slowly

Currently, the patient was admitted for the following:

- Readmitted for scheduled free tissue transfer to right lower extremity
- Preoperative examination revealed right leg edema and erythema consistent with worsening infection of pinning and cellulitis
- Orthopedics wanted to remove pinning as the nidus of infection but were concerned about bone stability

Past Medical History (PMHx)

- Methicillin-resistant *Staphylococcus aureus*–positive (MRSA [+] culture of right leg)
- Recurrent depression
- Anxiety
- Post-traumatic stress disorder (PTSD) following motor vehicle accident (MVA) and leg injury
- Full dentures
- Microcytic anemia
- IBS
- Diverticulitis
- Lumbago

Past Surgical History (PSHx)

- Closed reduction of right acetabular fracture
- External fixation of tibia with irrigation and debridement (I&D) and wound-vac placement
- Bilateral shoulder surgery
- Left inguinal hernia repair

Family History (FHx)

- Chronic back pain (Mother)
- Crohn disease (Mother)
- Atrial fibrillation (Father)
- Diabetes (Brother)

Social History (SocHx)

- Divorced 8 years ago, living with girlfriend, notable social stress

- Daily smoker using a pipe for 20 years
- Does not drink alcohol (last drink 6 months ago)
- Previous history of methamphetamine use (last used 6 months ago)
- Medical marijuana
- Tried cocaine decades ago
- Self-employed as a carpenter

Allergies

- No known allergies

Medications

- Clindamycin 450 mg oral tid
- Olanzapine 10 mg po qd
- Morphine 30 mg po bid
- Lovenox 40 mg sub-q qd
- Ascorbic acid 500 mg po qd
- Ferrous sulfate 325 mg po bid
- Omeprazole 20 mg po qd

Review of Systems

No fevers, chills, night sweats, nausea, vomiting, diarrhea, constipation, hematochezia, hematemesis, abdominal pain, chest pain, shortness of breath, lymphadenopathy.

Preliminary Differential Diagnoses

The patient was referred to the NMM/OMM clinic to assess for somatic dysfunction and provide OMT as indicated as part of the management plan. The patient has known diagnoses, and OMT is requested to help restore motion and reduce edema. Thus, the osteopathic medical student modified the algorithm and listed the problems to be addressed by OMT and application of osteopathic principles using the five models as a guide.

STRUCTURAL–BIOMECHANICAL: Right leg deformities and foreign objects; assess for somatic dysfunction

RESPIRATORY–CIRCULATORY: Edema, erythema in RLE; assess obstruction to lymphatic drainage

METABOLIC: Inflammation and infection from open wound, fractures, and foreign bodies; identify factors inhibiting natural healing.

NEUROLOGIC: Mental health problems may be interfering with healing/compliance; assess for evidence of somatic dysfunction that may interfere with autonomic nerve activity, peripheral nerve entrapments, facilitated spinal cord segments, tender points, or trigger points.

BIOPSYCHOSOCIAL: PTSD, anxiety, depression, decreased mobility, activities of daily living challenges due to medical problems, social stress, drug dependency/abuse history; research and address these issues with the patient as they may be preventing healing.

Objective Findings

Focused physical examination done as complete physical was performed by the referring physician.

Osteopathic Structural Examination *(positive findings listed only)*

Upper extremity: Left clavicle superior, tender left supraclavicular fossa

Thoracic and lumbar spine: T10–L2 NRRSL

Sacrum: R/R forward sacral torsion

Pelvis: Right innominate anterior rotation

Lower extremity: Right leg inflammation and lymphedema, externally rotated right femur, internally rotated right tibia

Laboratory/Testing

None provided for review

Imaging

No images or reports provided; reviewed referral note for findings

Assessment

1. Structural–Biomechanical
   a. Somatic dysfunction of upper and lower extremities, thoracic, lumbar, sacral, and pelvic regions
   b. Compound/comminuted fractures due to high-velocity impact
2. Respiratory–Circulatory
   a. Lymphatics

See Chapter 14 Anatomy and Physiology of the Lymphatic System for further information.

3. Neurologic
   a. Somatic dysfunction in the T10–L2 region may cause irritation or facilitation that can alter sympathetic activity and affect blood flow to the extremities
4. Metabolic
   a. Nicotine[1]
      i. Delayed fracture and wound healing
   b. Cannabis[2]
      i. Cannabis users have a higher risk for delayed bone-healing
      ii. Demonstrate lower bone mineral density
   c. Methamphetamine[3]
      i. Users have a threefold increase in reoperation after 1 year
      ii. Reoperation resulting from major complications such as: deep wound infections, failure of fixation, and hematoma
   d. Alcohol[4]
      i. Decreased fracture callus formation
      ii. Slower fracture healing
5. Biopsychosocial
   a. Unstable behavior
      i. Multiple reports on record of unreliability
      ii. Noncompliance complicates recovery
   b. PTSD
      i. Flashbacks
      ii. Fear of reinjury
   c. Depression
      i. Preexisting
      ii. Uncertain root diagnosis
   d. Amount of activity
      i. Patient frustration with limitations
      ii. Fears of immobility

Plan

1. Structural–Biomechanical
   a. Osteopathic manipulation of areas of somatic dysfunction to improve motion
   b. Shoulder girdle/clavicle
      i. Free tissue around left thoracic outlet/supraclavicular fossa
      ii. Release myofascial restrictions
   c. Lower extremity areas of restriction
      i. Fibular head
      ii. Interosseous membrane

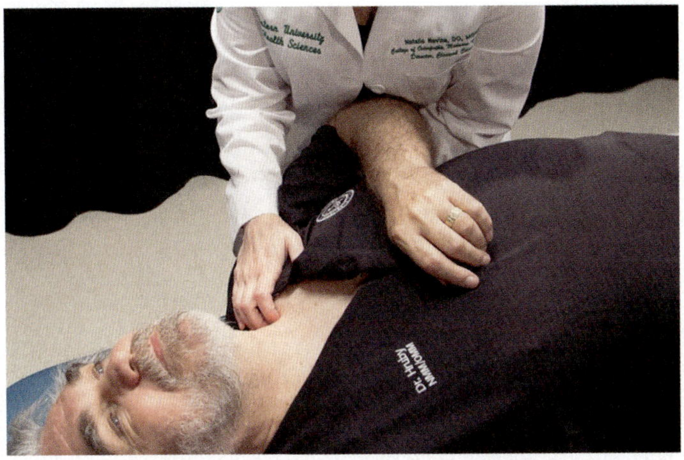

Figure 28.1. Myofascial release OMT for the left thoracic outlet, supraclavicular space, where left lymphatic duct drains into the left subclavian vein, as first procedure for lymphatic drainage of edema from the lower extremities. (Photo courtesy of Western University of Health Sciences, Pomona, CA, with permission.)

2. Respiratory–Circulatory
   a. Treat sacrum somatic dysfunction to release tension that could be affecting pelvic diaphragm functions
   b. Lymphatic technique
      i. Free up fascia around lymphatic channels in sequence from proximal (left supraclavicular space, diaphragms, and thigh) to distal (leg and foot) (Fig. 28.1)
      ii. Goal of alleviating lymphedema of lower extremity
         1. Kneading soft tissues and myofascial traction twist for extremities
         2. Manually mobilize lymph
      iii. See Chapter 50 Lymphatic Drainage Procedures for more information
3. Metabolic
   a. Reduce or eliminate nicotine, alcohol, marijuana, and sugar intake
   b. Improve nutritional intake, appointment with nutritionist
4. Neurologic
   a. Treat somatic dysfunctions to release tension that could be affecting sympathetic ganglia functions
   b. Refer the patient to mental health resources
5. Biopsychosocial
   a. Arrange appropriate discharge to SNF to help with patient care and compliance
   b. Behavioral therapy, hypnosis, or other cognitive behavioral therapy to help patient to discontinue use of nicotine, marijuana, methamphetamines, and alcohol and address PTSD, anxiety, and depression.
   c. Healthy diet education/nutritional counseling.
      - No further labs or radiologic studies are needed at this time.
      - OMT consent by patient and parent obtained prior to treatment.
      - Follow-up (F/U) in 2 weeks

Case submitted by Matthew Albright, DO originally submitted while OMS-III at College of Osteopathic Medicine of the Pacific-Northwest, Lebanon, Oregon.

ACKNOWLEDGMENTS

The author and editors of this chapter would like to acknowledge the scholarly contributions of Drs. Scott Helf, Diane Padre, and Matthew Albright for prior editions of this chapter.

REFERENCES

1. Smith DH, McTague MF, Weaver MJ, Smith JT. Durability of smoking cessation for elective lower extremity orthopaedic surgery. *J Am Acad Orthop Surg*. 2019;27(16):613–620.
2. Heath DM, Koslosky EJ, Bartush KC, Hogue GD. Marijuana in orthopaedics: effects on bone health, wound-healing, surgical complications, and pain management. *JBJS Rev*. 2022;10(2):10.2106/JBJS.RVW.21.00184.
3. Zusman NL, Woelber E, McKibben NS, et al. Methamphetamines and acetabular reoperation rates: poor outcomes from the front lines. *J Orthop Trauma*. 2021;35(12):e491–e495.
4. Natoli RM, Yu H, Meislin MC, et al. Alcohol exposure decreases osteopontin expression during fracture healing and osteopontin-mediated mesenchymal stem cell migration in vitro. *J Orthop Surg Res*. 2018;13(1):101.

PART THREE

The Somatic Component

29

Palpatory Examination Skills and Exercises for Developing the Sense of Touch

WALTER C. EHRENFEUCHTER ▪ REBECCA E. GIUSTI

KEY CONCEPTS

- No known device has yet been developed that exceeds the tactile sensitivity of the human hand.
- Palpation can be developed through various exercises.
- The physician never stops learning and acquiring new experiences.
- Developing a high level of palpatory skill is an ongoing process that requires patience and practice.

INTRODUCTION

Palpation remains central to being a physician. Palpation is used during the physical examination to determine the presence of masses, the size and shape of organs, the point maximal impulse of the heart, tactile fremitus of the lungs, to evaluate lymph nodes, and to assess pulses, just to name a few.[1] For the osteopathic physician, palpation provides even more information on the health of the tissues and the presence of somatic dysfunction. The osteopathic palpatory examination is used to scan all body regions with abnormalities, as identified from the screening exam. Therefore, findings of asymmetry, spinal curve abnormalities, and alterations of body posture, combined with range of motion testing, guide the physician to the location(s) of abnormality/somatic dysfunction for performing layer-by-layer palpation. When more than one area of abnormality is identified, typically the region of greatest motion loss is evaluated first, since it is most likely the location of the area of greatest restriction, or what is sometimes referred to as the key somatic dysfunction.

Strong palpation skills enable the osteopathic physician to both accurately diagnose somatic dysfunction and perform effective osteopathic manipulative treatment (OMT).

The good news regarding palpation for those on their osteopathic journey is this:

> "…but the fundamental information comes from the sense of touch. This is not of necessity a special sense of touch, **but an ordinary one developed to a high degree**."[2]

This means that an osteopathic physician, much like a musician or an athlete who practices their drills and refines their skills, can develop, hone, and improve their palpation skills.

DEFINITION

The *Glossary of Osteopathic Terminology* defines palpation as "the application of variable manual pressure to the surface of the body for the purpose of determining the shape, size, consistency, position, inherent motility, and health of the tissues beneath."[3] Another definition is "The light placement of the hands or fingers on the patient's body to discover abnormal changes of the soft tissues, bones, organs, and skin itself."[4] No device has yet been developed that comes close to mimicking, let alone exceeding the tactile sensitivity of the human hand.

KEY TERMS RELATED TO PALPATION

Those studying osteopathic medicine should be familiar with the terms below in order to better appreciate the following discussion on palpation and exercises designed to enhance palpatory skills.

Receptive field: An area within which a stimulus can excite a cell or alter the firing of the neuron associated with it. Large receptive fields are found on the back which enable the cell to detect changes over a vast area but with less precision. The finger pads have smaller receptive fields which gives them a higher degree of discriminatory sensitivity.[5]

Two-point discrimination: The ability to discriminate the detailed features of a stimulus. If the skin is touched at two separate points within a single receptive field in the brain, the subject will not perceive those two points. However, if the two points span more than a single field, the subject will be able to distinguish those two points. The smaller more densely clustered the receptive field, the higher the resolution and thus ability to distinguish separate stimuli at short distances apart.[6] Meissner and Merkel corpuscles both have small receptive fields and are located mainly in the finger pads. Therefore, the finger pads have a much better discriminatory tactile sense than the back of the hand where those structures are sparser.[7]

Threshold: The least amount of energy or force that causes a measurable response. When palpating, vary the amount of pressure used to sense the nature of the layers of the anatomy beneath the skin surface. The threshold of each of the receptors in the hands differs.[8]

Adaptation: When a continuous sensory stimulus is first applied, the receptors respond at a very high impulse rate initially, then progressively less rapidly until finally many of them no longer respond at all. So, altering the amount of pressure used during palpation also allows the sensory receptors to recover from adaptation.[9]

Stereognosis: The ability to recognize the three-dimensional shape of an object solely based on the sense of touch. The center of the palms are uniquely constructed to assess stereognosis and are used to assess three-dimensional structures, such as elbows, ischial tuberosities, and the size of an enlarged uterus.[10]

Fulcrum: A structure that serves as a point of support or something that supplies capability for action. It is usually established by the physician's elbow of the palpating hand being supported by a firm structure. This tends to relieve any tension in the hand and finger pads themselves and allows for a full palpatory experience[11] as the physician is free from extraneous interference and can remain relaxed and comfortable.[1]

End-feel: Perceived quality of motion as an anatomic or physiologic restrictive barrier is approached.[3] Joints have normal ranges of motion. Normal end-feels can be soft due to soft tissue approximation, firm, due to capsular or ligamentous stretching, or hard, usually when a bone meets another bone. A pathologic end-feel can be firm and resistant due to scar tissue or shortened connective tissue, soft but still resistant (almost a "rubbery" feel) due to increased muscle tone or edema, or what is described as an "empty" end-feel.

Bind: Relative palpable resistance to motion of an articulation or tissue.[3]

Ease: Relative palpable freedom of motion, compliance, or resilience of an articulation or tissue.[3]

Compression: Force applied perpendicularly to the skin surface.[3]

Shear: Force applied parallel to the skin surface. Sometimes deep palpation requires both compression and shear to explore the underlying structures.[12]

Skin drag: The estimation of resistance experienced when the pads of the fingers are lightly applied to the skin and then moved or "dragged" over the surface. The physician should note if there is an increase in skin drag secondary to excessive perspiration, oiliness of the skin, or edema; or if there is a decrease secondary to excessive dryness, atrophy of the skin or the underlying structures.[13]

Trophic changes: This is a change resulting from the interruption of a nerve supply. While trophic changes can have a variety of presentations, they may manifest as areas of "scaliness," absence of hair, or feel unusually smooth.[14]

Red reflex: The erythematous biochemical reaction (reactive hyperemia) of the skin in an area that has been stimulated mechanically by friction. The reflex is greater in degree and duration in an area of acute somatic dysfunction as compared to an area of chronic somatic dysfunction. It is a reflection of the segmentally related sympathicotonia commonly observed in the paraspinal area.[3]

INTRODUCTION TO LAYER-BY-LAYER PALPATION

When performing palpation in a given region of the body, it is best to apply a layer-by-layer approach. This consists of:

- Observation
- Temperature
- Skin topography and texture
- Superficial fascia
- Muscle
- Tendons
- Ligaments
- Bone

Palpation always includes noting any areas of tenderness elicited by palpation, and the amount of pressure needed to reach the various layers. Light surface palpation requires only a few grams of pressure. Deep bony palpation requires about 1,500 g of pressure or about 3.33 pounds.[15–17]

Consent

Prior to palpating a patient, the osteopathic physician should describe where and what they will be palpating and gain permission from the patient to do so. If consent is initially obtained, it is generally best practice to ask for consent again if the physician needs to palpate a new area that is considered to be more sensitive such as the chest and pelvic regions.

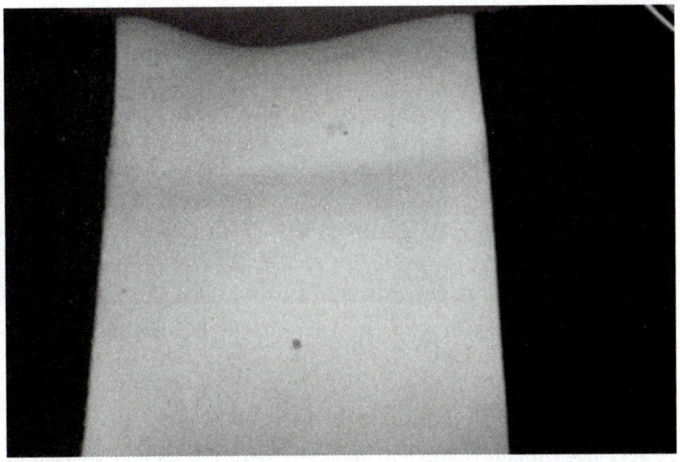

Figure 29.1. Observation.

Observation

Visual observation of the skin surface must precede any palpatory examination (Fig. 29.1).

Observe the skin's color and any adnexal alterations such as the presence of:

- Pustules
- Dryness or scaliness
- Folliculitis
- Pigmentary changes
- Scars

The spinal segments or body surface associated with any findings are noted for further review during the examination. These may reflect local sympathetic nervous system changes and trophic changes[14] that are segmentally associated with somatic dysfunction.

Temperature

The use of skin temperature differences in diagnosis dates to Hippocrates' time. He searched for hot spots, by having an assistant smear the patient with a thin layer of mud. Areas that dried first were warmer than those that required more time.[18]

- Today, skin temperature may be evaluated with the volar aspect of the wrist, or the dorsal surface of the hypothenar eminence of the hand.
- The wrists or hands are placed a few centimeters above the area to be tested. Both hands simultaneously evaluate the paraspinal areas bilaterally, searching for areas of thermal asymmetry (Fig. 29.2).
- Some physicians best perceive variations in skin temperature using the dorsum of the hand, especially the dorsum of the middle phalanges of fingers two, three, and four. Others prefer using the palmar surface. Physicians should test both methods to determine which is more personally effective.
- Heat radiation may be palpated in many other areas of the body (e.g., the abdomen or extremities).
- If a temperature difference is unable to be discerned while off the skin surface, then very light contact may be made with area to be examined.[19]
- The hands are then lifted off, not dragged along the surface, and replaced gently on the next levels to be examined.

The spinal segments or body regions of abnormality are noted. Changes in temperature reflect a change in local blood flow that may be due to inflammation or to the changes in sympathetic tone associated with segmental somatic dysfunction.

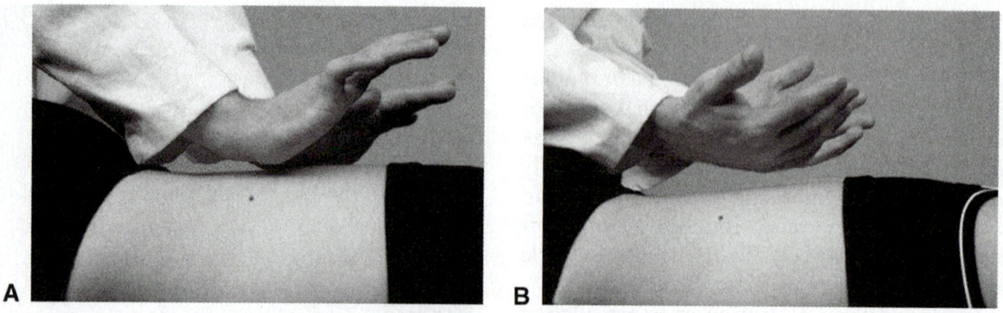

Figure 29.2. A, B. Temperature assessment.

Skin Topography and Texture

A very light touch is applied, generally with the palmar surface of the fingertips. This pressure will permit the finger pads to glide smoothly over the skin surface without excessive friction.

The skin is evaluated for:

- Sweat gland activity
- Greasiness (sebaceous gland activity)
- Thickening
- Roughness

Again, note the spinal segments or body regions of abnormality. Gently press the fingers into the skin surface to evaluate for changes in skin turgor and tension, which may reflect a change in local sympathetic nervous system activity associated with segmental somatic dysfunction. Using the same contact, the physician may run their finger pads over a region of skin or using the index finger and middle finger of one hand, run these finger pads down the paraspinal muscles of the back to assess for any sensation of "drag." This suggests a resistance to the easy passage of the finger pad over the skin and may represent an area of greater moisture or turgor.[13]

ERYTHEMA FRICTION RUB

To perform the erythema friction rub, the pads of the physician's second and third fingers are placed paraspinally, and in two or three quick strokes drawn superiorly to inferiorly down the spine (Fig. 29.3).

The normal tissue response is initial blanching of the skin surface, followed by reddening or darkening of the skin, which is known as the red reflex, followed by a slow fading back to the original skin color. This is described by Cox et al.[20] as the following: "Red reflex" (RR); Cutaneous stimulation was applied digitally in both paraspinal areas simultaneously by twice briskly stroking the skin in a caudad direction. Patients were divided arbitrarily into three groups. (a) grade 1: erythema of the paraspinal tissues lasting less than 15 seconds after cutaneous stimulation. (b) grade 2: erythema persisting 15–30 seconds after stimulation. (c) grade 3: erythema persisting longer than 30 seconds after stimulation."

Note any abnormal deviation by the tissues, which may be indicative of a viscerosomatic reflex, areas of vasoconstriction (rapidly fading color), or a facilitated segment. This may be evidenced by the skin remaining pale, remaining red or darker in color, or becoming red or darker in color initially instead of pale as compared to the surrounding tissue.[20,21]

The spinal levels and laterality of the abnormal findings should also be noted.

It is important to note that the erythema friction rub, while still possible, may be more difficult to interpret in patients with darker skin tones. This reflex may also be variable depending on the sensitivity of the skin.

Superficial Fascia

Make a broader contact with the skin's surface, by pressing gently with the palm of the hand to engage the fascia. The necessary amount of pressure typically causes slight reddening of the physician's nail beds (Fig. 29.4).

To elicit motion tensions, as well as directions of ease and bind in the superficial fascia, the physician gently moves the hands:

- Superior and inferior (if performed on the paraspinal muscles, this correlates with flexion and extension)

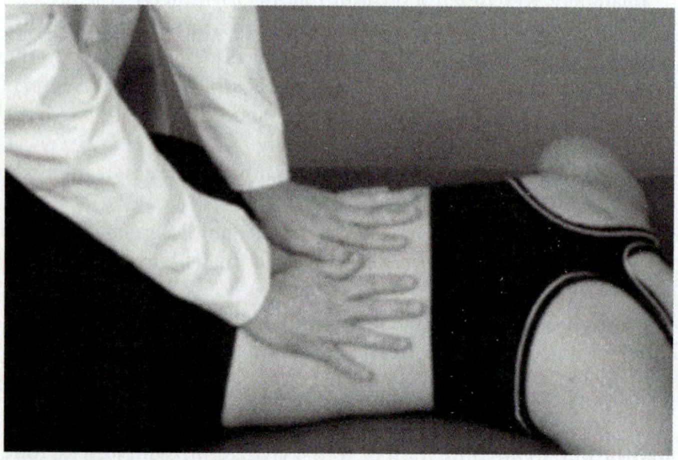

Figure 29.3. Palpating fascia.

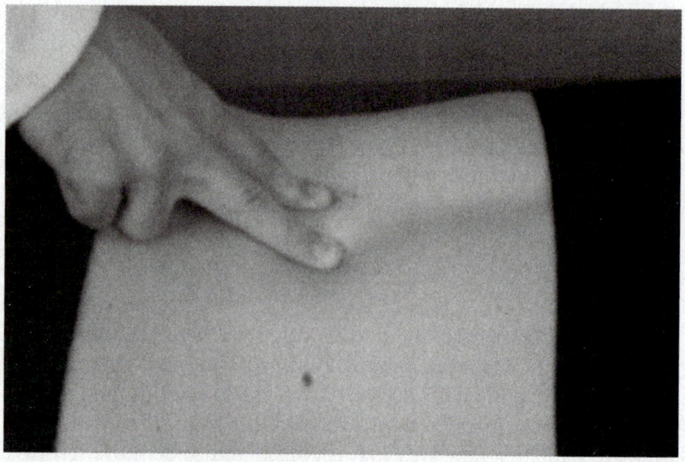

Figure 29.4. Palpating muscle.

- Side to side or right and left (if performed on the paraspinal muscles, this correlates with rotation)
- Clockwise and counterclockwise (if performed on the paraspinal muscles, this correlates with side bending)

Gradually applying more pressure allows for the evaluation of deeper layers of fascia, such as the muscular investing fascia. Note the segmental levels or body regions associated with the fascias' asymmetric bind, and the depth of penetration necessary to elicit that alteration. Likewise, note any areas of tenderness.

Muscle

Deeper palpation may be used to palpate the muscle just inferior to the investing layer of fascia.

- The amount of pressure varies from patient to patient, depending on the thickness of the subcutaneous fat layers.
- The thicker the layer of subcutaneous fat, the more difficult it can be to palpate changes in the deeper tissues.
- Typically, the pads of the fingers are aligned perpendicular to the direction of the muscle fibers, pressed firmly into the muscle, and then rolled across the fiber bundles (Fig. 29.5).
- Sufficient pressure is typically necessary to blanch the physician's nail beds.
- An irritable muscle may twitch in response to this "plucking" of the muscle.

The muscle is evaluated for:

- Turgor
- Tension
- Thickness
- Shape
- Irritability
- Other terms that are used to describe the changes felt in abnormal musculature include ropiness, stringiness, fibrotic, and dense. More examples are found in Table 29.1.

Note the segmental location of any of these changes and the character of the muscle tissue at that location. While muscle hypertonicity may extend for a number of levels (e.g., T4–9 left paraspinal), also note the level of peak muscular change in the paravertebral muscles (e.g., T6 left paravertebral muscles). In addition, note the location of any tenderness elicited or trigger points discovered.

Tendons

Although tendons are not readily palpable in the paraspinal tissues, they should be traced in the periphery to their bony attachments and their continuity with the muscle. Take note of any:

- Fibrous thickening
- Change in elasticity
- Tenderness

Tenderness of a tendinous attachment to bone may be due to an enthesopathy, a change in the fibrillar structure of the tendon due to injury.

Ligaments

Palpation should include the following:

- Presence or absence of the ligament (absence indicating a traumatic rupture or congenital absence)
- Tension in the ligament (normal, excessive, or lax)
- Elicited tenderness

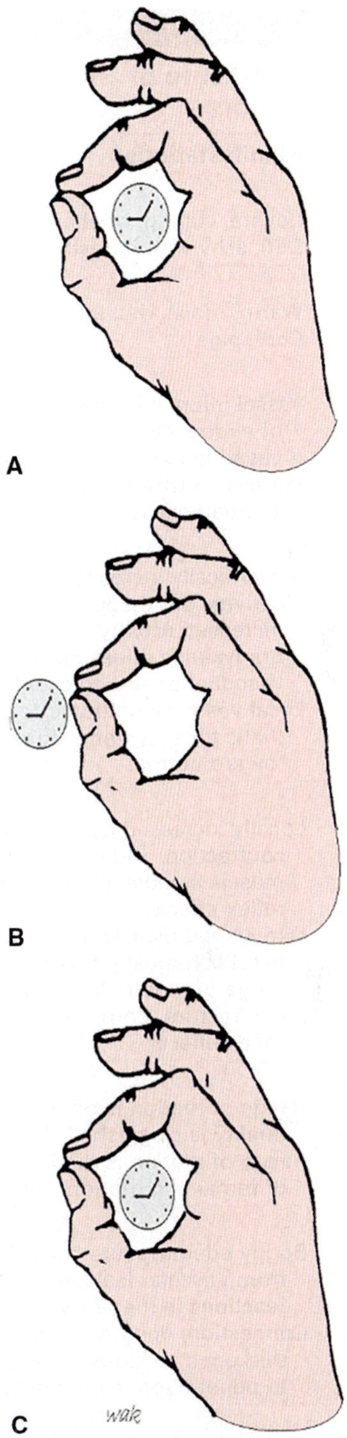

A

B

C

Figure 29.5. Right eye dominance. A. Both eyes are open. **B.** Right eye closed; left eye open. **C.** Left eye closed; right eye open. (Modified from Kuchera WA, Kuchera ML, eds. Palpation of soft tissue. In: *Osteopathic Principles in Practice*. 2nd ed. Greyden Press; 1994:23, 112. Reprinted with permission from Michael L. Kuchera, DO, FAAO.)

Bone

Deeper pressure allows for palpation of the bony structures beneath the musculature. The bone is evaluated for normal:

- Contour
- Tenderness
- Motion

TABLE 29.1

Palpatory Signs of Acute or Chronic Somatic Dysfunction

Signs	Manifestations
Pain	
Acute	Severe, cutting, or sharp
Chronic	Dull, achy with paresthesias
Skin Changes	
Acute	Warm, moist, red, inflamed
Chronic	Cool, pale
Vasculature	
Acute	Vessel injury with resultant release of endogenous peptides, chemical vasodilation, inflammation, and edema
Chronic	Vessels constricted due to increased sympathetic tone
Sympathetic Activity	
Acute	Systemically increased sympathetic activity, but the local effect of this increased activity is overpowered by bradykinins released, so there is local vasodilation due to chemical effect
Chronic	Local vasoconstriction due to hypersympathetic tone; systemic tone has returned toward normal
Musculature	
Acute	Locally increased muscle tonus, muscle contraction, and spasm mediated via the muscle spindle. Minimal somatosomatic reflex effects
Chronic	Diminished muscle tone, ropiness, flaccidity, mushy feeling. Limited range of motion likely due to fascial contracture. Common somatosomatic reflex effects[9]
Mobility	
Acute	Range of motion is often normal, but the quality is sluggish
Chronic	Range of motion is diminished, but quality of remaining motion is normal
Soft Tissues	
Acute	Boggy edema, acute congestion, fluids from vascular leakage, and chemical reactions in the tissues
Chronic	Congestion, doughy, stringy, fibrotic, thickened, exhibits increased resistance to penetration, contracted, contractured
Adnexa	
Acute	Moist skin, no trophic changes
Chronic	Scaly, dry skin, pimples, folliculitis, altered pigmentation (trophic changes)
Visceral	
Acute	Minimal somatovisceral reflex effects
Chronic	Common somatovisceral reflex effects[10]

Chaitow L. *Palpation and Assessment Skills: Assessment through Touch.* 3rd ed. Churchill Livingstone Elsevier; 2010:44.

PALPATION

Steps of palpation[1]:

The steps of palpation are commonly referred to as detection or reception, transmission, and interpretation with amplification being described by some texts as an additional step in this process.[22]

- *Reception/Detection:* This is a matter of being aware of the possible findings in the region being palpated and practicing techniques required to expose these possibilities. This step serves to discover the nature of the object being palpated. It is here that the proprioceptors and mechanoreceptors of the hand receive stimulation from the tissues that they are interfacing with. This step may be difficult for a beginning student as many have depended mostly on sight and have not developed the sense of touch to its full capacity. Osteopathic physicians need to develop a profound sense of touch as most palpation depends on that which cannot be visualized. The fingers become the eyes and are trained to detect subtle change in the tissues being palpated. This step requires localized concentration on a specific task and the ability to shut out extraneous information. It demands focus and directed concentration on the palpatory input from the hands and elimination of other distracters.
- *Amplification or magnification:* It refers to a localized concentration on a specific task and the ability to shut out extraneous information. It demands focus and directed concentration on the palpatory input from the hands and elimination of other distractors.
- *Transmission:* The information gathered by the sense of touch is relayed through the peripheral and central nervous system to the brain.
- *Interpretation:* This step is the ability to translate palpatory observations into meaningful knowledge about anatomic, physiologic, or pathologic states. This requires proficient knowledge of anatomy, physiology, and pathologic states. As the osteopathic physician continues to practice palpating both physiologic normal and abnormal states their ability to accurately interpret the information and therefore precisely diagnose will be greatly accentuated. This can be termed "thinking fingers."

Fine palpation is used unconsciously on a daily basis, in activities such as picking coins out of a pocket or purse by touch. Dimes, nickels, pennies, and quarters are readily differentiated based on the known characteristics of each coin.

There is no substitute for experience. Inexperienced examiners have been able to palpate motions as small as 1 mm in excursion, while experienced examiners have been shown to palpate motion as small as 0.0846 mm (3/100″). A study was conducted to explore the ability of the human hands to perceive expansion in a manner similar to palpating respiratory motion of the rib cage, or expansion of the skull with the cranial rhythmic impulse. The average examiner was able to palpate motion of just 148 μm. Two-thirds of the subjects were able to palpate motion of 50 to 200 μm, and one-third of the subjects palpated motions of 50 μm or less, which is 5/100 of a millimeter.[23]

In defining somatic dysfunction, three elements are typically used; asymmetry, range of motion changes, and tissue texture abnormalities,[24] while a fourth, tenderness is also utilized.

The regional or scanning examination, applied to abnormal areas previously discovered through screening, provides further information on asymmetry, tenderness, range of motion changes, and tissue texture changes associated with the somatic dysfunction. It also provides an opportunity for segmental localization.

The results of the palpatory examination will then be examined on a level-by-level basis. Table 29.1 outlines the changes expected in the presence of either acute or chronic somatic dysfunction.

This allows the physician to ascertain whether a somatic dysfunction is new (acute), old (chronic), or perhaps a combination of the two (acute exacerbation of a chronic condition). Correct identification is crucial for choosing the appropriate manipulative techniques in treatment.

KEY CONCEPTS FOR ACCURATE PALPATION

- Utilize the thumb and/or the first two finger pads, rather than the fingertips for palpation due to smaller receptive fields, greatest number of kinesthetic nerve endings, and enhanced two-point discrimination[5,7]
- Utilize the palm to palpate more three-dimensional structures such as organs during an abdominal exam due to the palm's ability to detect stereognosis.[10]
- When palpating, utilize a fulcrum in order to eliminate extraneous sensory stimuli and fully concentrate on what is being palpated.[1,19]
- Maintain both joint flexibility and strength of the upper extremity, especially the elbows, wrists, and fingers.
- This can be accomplished by:
  - □ Using a finger exerciser
  - □ Squeezing a ball
  - □ Playing a musical instrument that requires fingering
- Because the hands are an important, sensitive diagnostic instrument for the physician, they should be carefully protected and cared for. Attempt to avoid callous formation on the palmar surface of the hands and fingers. Keep fingernails short and clean.[1] If fingernails are long, they may cause pain and/or injury to the patient. Furthermore, the physician may have to angle the palpating hand causing strain or injury to the physician's upper extremity in an effort to avoid hurting the patient.
- Maintain "relaxed and soft" hands and fingers when palpating. Tension or intense pressure on the proprioceptors and mechanoreceptors may detract from their ability to feel or perceive accurately.[25]
- Light touch is considered the most useful and easily applied modality by many experienced physicians. Very light touch, or light touch, involves passively laying the hands on the skin, or moving the hands lightly over it.
- This can be used to determine the skin's:
  - □ Temperature
  - □ Texture
  - □ Moistness
  - □ Oiliness
  - □ Resistance
  - □ Tone

Elasticity

- Firmer pressure communicates with deeper cutaneous layers and fascial sheaths. It allows for the exploration of tone and mobility of superficial muscles. Further increasing pressure and compression will convey the relationships between deeper muscle, fascia, and bony structures. Note that firm pressure should still be applied with a relaxed hand, by using the physicians' body weight to sink into the tissues. If pressure is applied too firmly or without consideration to the tissues, there may be a "defensive retraction of the palpated tissues, tensing superficial musculature, making assessment difficult or its interpretation invalid."[25] Also, as stated above, applying too firm of a pressure may lessen the sensitivity of the palpating structure.[25]
- When palpating, attempt to use adjectives to describe what is being felt. Oftentimes, comparing and contrasting is most beneficial and builds a virtual library and context of palpation. Comparative descriptors include: superficial/deep, pliable/rigid, warm/cold, moist/dry, relaxed/tense, hypertonic/hypotonic, painful/pain-free, resistant/compliant.[26] Familiarity with osteopathic terminology permits the description of palpatory findings in consistent terms.
- Effective palpation cannot be learned by observation or merely by watching another physician perform it. It must be experienced and performed on as many patients as possible to begin to understand the variations of how normal and abnormal tissues may feel and distinguish between them.[19]
- Experiencing a variety of palpation skills can also bring about a greater understanding of the different types of palpation. For some physicians, experiencing the palpation of a skilled practitioner may actually assist them in improving their own manner of palpation, having now "felt how it is supposed to feel."

PALPATORY EXERCISES

Exercise 1: Palpating Inanimate Objects[27]

PURPOSE

- To perceive slight tactile differences in tissue texture and motion through exercises on inanimate objects, which sharpens tactile concentration and attention
- To practice three of the steps related to the process of palpation in a mindful manner[1]:
  1. Detection/reception
  2. Internal amplification or magnification
  3. Analysis and interpretation

As the following exercises are performed remember that concentration is essential. The physician may close their eyes to eliminate extraneous stimuli (amplification) and pay attention to the kinesthetic sensation received through the fingers.

PROCEDURE

1. Put a mixture of coins in a pocket or purse. By touch, distinguish between heads and tails, and between pennies, dimes, nickels, and quarters. Identify date lines on the coins.
2. Locate a hair, string, or thread that has been placed under a sheet of paper. Attempt to estimate its length. Palpate for its ends and palpate its contour. Determine if it is resting in a curved or straight position. Add sheets of paper until the hair can no longer be palpated.
3. An instructor may place some everyday items made out of different materials in a paper bag such as a metal item (i.e. paperclip), a plastic item, a shell, a piece of wood, something made from clay, a rubber eraser, etc. Without looking into the bag, the student may then palpate one item at a time, describing it and attempting to determine what it is and what it is made out of before removing it from the bag to see if they are correct. Special care may be taken to ascertain if organic materials have a different feel from nonorganic materials.
4. Palpate several types of human bones. Identify the bones and their component parts, envisioning the tissue that normally surrounds them.
5. Palpate a human bone and a solid plastic imitation of the same bone. Identify the characteristics of the human bone that distinguish it from the replica.

These exercises greatly assist with the final step in the process of palpation. While the above exercises tune the physician into greater awareness of their palpatory findings and utilize the information they receive to interpret if an object is organic or nonorganic or to actually determine what it is, this will translate to live human beings into a determination of meaningful anatomic, physiologic, or pathologic states.

Dr. Frymann states the following regarding palpation:

> "The interpretation of analysis of the observations made by palpation is the key which makes the study of the structure and function of the tissues meaningful. Nevertheless, it is like the first visit to a foreign country. Numerous strange and unfamiliar sights are seen, but without some knowledge of the language with which to ask questions or a guide to interpret these observations in the life and history of the country they have little meaning for us. The third step in our study then, is to be able to translate palpatory observations into meaningful anatomic, physiologic, or pathologic states. Past, present, and future osteopathic research must be called upon if an accurate translation of findings is to be made."[19]

Exercise 2: Determining the Dominant Hand

Many physicians have a dominant hand that they prefer to palpate or motion test with, which may be different from their dominant writing hand.

PURPOSE

To determine the dominant hand: It is believed that the dominant hand is unconsciously placed on top when the hands are clasped together. The dominant hand may be stronger than the other and therefore may unwittingly apply more pressure into the structure being palpated. It may need to be calibrated in order to palpate more lightly and intelligently. Awareness of the dominant hand will also allow the physician to practice applying equal pressure over equivalent structures, in order to develop accurate interpretation of dominant and nondominant proprioceptive feedback from each hand.

POSITION

Standing or sitting.

PROCEDURE

Without consciously thinking about it, clasp the hands together in front of the body, with one hand on top of the other.

RESULTS

The top hand will most likely be the dominant hand.

Exercise 3: Determining the Dominant Eye

PURPOSE

To determine the dominant eye: Palpation and palpatory results are thought to be more accurate when the dominant eye is directly over the area being palpated. It is also clinically relevant for comparing two landmarks for symmetry. For example, if the physician is comparing the inferior aspect of the anterior superior iliac spine (ASIS), the dominant eye should be placed midway between the two structures to determine if they are level or if one is superior to the other.[1]

POSITION

Standing or sitting, with a distant clock or object to look at.

PROCEDURE

1. Look at the distant object with both eyes open (Fig. 29.5).
2. Fully extend the dominant arm, and make a circle with the thumb and index finger, enclosing the distant object. Or, extend both arms and form a small circle with the thumb and index finger of each hand, ensuring that the distant object is in the center of the circle.[1]
3. Close one eye, open it, and then close the other eye.

RESULT

The dominant eye will continue to see the encircled object while the other eye is closed, whereas the encircled object will have moved when viewed solely by the nondominant eye.[2]

Exercise 4: Palpating Through a "Colloid" Glove to Mimic Live Tissue

PURPOSE

Colloid suspensions or non-Newtonian fluids can be easily made with cornstarch and water and placed in a surgical glove that is then tied off or a plastic sealable bag.[28] Palpation of the colloid fluid may assist the physician with the speed of palpation and how to better interact with live tissue that exhibits viscoelastic properties.

POSITION

The physician is seated comfortably resting the elbow of the palpating hand on the table with access to the colloid glove.

PROCEDURE

1. Quickly "jab" at the colloid glove and observe the effects. The colloid suspension will typically harden when encountered with a quick sharp force. This mimics live viscoelastic tissue which defensively retracts tissues when this type of force is applied.
2. Now, allow the palpating digits to slowly "sink" into the colloid suspension. Observe the effects. With this method of palpation, the water in the colloid suspension has time to move out of the way and the physician can palpate down to the layer of the table. The physician should remove the palpating digits at the same speed back up to the surface of the glove.

This exercise may help physicians better appreciate George Webster, D.O.'s following statement and assist in a thoughtful transition to palpation of a living being:

> "Each tissue is composed of cells and each cell is a living thing. Living things prefer persuasion to force; consideration to trauma, intelligence to ill-expended energy. It is better to work with the tissues rather than at the tissues. Nature has her regards and also her penalties for the manner in which lesions are treated. As osteopathic physicians, our highest duty is to cooperate with nature."[29]

Exercise 5: Layer Palpation

PURPOSE

To perceive various layers and structures of the body, by palpating tissues on the physician's own body and varying the amount of pressure applied.

POSITION

Seated comfortably beside a table, with the nondominant arm resting on the table.

PROCEDURE

1. Close the eyes and relax. Concentrate all attention through the palpating fingers of the dominant hand.
2. Lightly palpate the dorsum of the nondominant hand using the fingers of the dominant hand. Scarcely touching the surface, feel the contour of the hand.
3. Assess temperature with the dorsal and then the palmar aspects of the palpating fingers, to determine which is more sensitive to temperature.

4. Using very light touch, palpate and describe the skin's texture, moisture, and thickness.
5. Gently pinch the skin on the back of the hand. Elevate and release it.
   a. How long did it take for the skin to resume its normal configuration?
6. Evaluate skin drag on both the palm and dorsum of the hand. Skin drag is an estimate of the amount of resistance experienced when the pads of the fingers are lightly applied and moved (dragged) over the skin surface.
   a. On which aspect of the hand do the palpating fingers move most easily? Why?
   b. Describe any increase in skin drag that may be due to excessive dryness, slight perspiration, or edema.
   c. Describe any decrease in drag that may be the result of excessive perspiration, oiliness, or atrophy.
7. Locate the veins and note their size and texture. Make a fist several times to engorge the veins, and then describe the differences observed.
8. Locate the radial artery, and describe how it differs from a vein.
9. Increase the contact between the palpating fingers and the skin of the hand, in order to create a shearing stress in the subcutaneous tissues. Shearing in this context refers to the movement of tissues between layers. Note that with this palpation, shearing can progress only so far before the palpating fingers slide on the skin.
   a. Describe how it feels to shear across the hand in various directions.
   b. Does the skin move equally and easily in all directions?
10. Palpate the extensor tendon of the ring finger. Place two fingers along the length of the tendon, flex the ring finger, and palpate the sense of the linear movement along the tendon.
11. Palpate the tendon of the biceps at the elbow.
   a. How does it feel? It should be ropelike, smooth, and firm.
12. Place the thumb and index finger of the palpating hand on either side of the midphalangeal articulation of a finger on the opposite hand. Note the quality and range of various elements during flexion and extension. Now lighten the touch while performing the same movements. Notice how little contact is needed to distinguish flexion and extension.
13. Place the palpating fingers on the anterior surface of the proximal third of the other forearm. Apply slightly more pressure than that applied to the skin to palpate the muscles used to flex the fingers. Maintain palpatory contact during flexion of the middle finger.
   a. Describe the feel of these flexor muscles and fascia during the maneuver.

Exercise 6: Palpating a Partner's Forearm

PURPOSE

To determine the characteristics of different structures in the forearm of another person.

Important Notes

When examining a patient, explain the procedure in general terms throughout the process. This is especially important if significant tenderness might be elicited during deep palpation. Take the necessary time, moving gently and deliberately. It is common to apply too much pressure at first, in an attempt to feel the tissue. Avoid poking, prodding, tickling, or "stirring" (performing a circular motion) the tissue. These actions can cause reflex irritation.[10]

Louisa Burns, a noted early osteopathic researcher, made the following suggestions for developing palpatory skills[30]:

- Palpate the objects with the lightest possible touch, scarcely touching the surface.
- Be aware of surface elevations and temperature differences.
- Palpate the surface using slightly more contact.
- Try to ascertain the qualities or characteristics of the object's substance.
- Describe perceptions as accurately as possible.

Mitchell[31] calls palpation a two-way communication system, in which the patient's tissues react to the presence of the physician's hand. While this is more likely to be easily experienced by physicians who have practiced palpation for a long period of time, it is a skill that can be developed with practice and dedication.

POSITION

Seated comfortably, facing a partner.

Partner is seated facing the physician from across a narrow table.

PROCEDURE

1. Grasp the partner's left forearm with the nondominant hand.
2. Lightly place the palm and fingers of the dominant hand over the dorsal forearm of the partner, just distal to the elbow. Close the eyes, relax, and concentrate attention through the palmar surface of the fingers.
3. Without moving the hand, try to perceive and describe skin temperature, texture, thickness, and moisture.
4. Compare the dorsal and palmar aspects of the forearm, and describe the differences.
   a. Which aspect is smoother? Thicker? Warmer? Drier?
5. With a slightly firmer touch, concentrate on the second layer, the subcutaneous fascia. Gently move the skin of the forearm longitudinally and horizontally.
   a. How thick is it?
   b. How loose?
   c. Many of the tissue texture changes associated with somatic dysfunction are within this layer.
6. Gently and slowly increase the depth of touch until the deep fascial layer, which is forming a sheath around the underlying structures, is palpated.
   a. Is it smooth? Continuous? Firm?
7. While palpating the deep fascial layer, slowly move the hand horizontally across the partner's forearm to identify areas of thickening, which form the fascial compartments between bundles of muscles. Identifying the enveloping layers of deep fascia is often helpful in separating one muscle from another. Use this technique to work with even deeper structures.
8. While palpating through the deep fascia, concentrate on the underlying muscle.
   a. Is it soft and compliant?
   b. How is its elasticity?
      Pay attention to individual muscle fibers and the directions in which they run.
9. The partner slowly opens and closes the hand. Note the quality and range of movement created by the contracting and relaxing muscle.
   a. Describe the difference.
      Palpate the forearm muscles as the hand is clenched. This simulates the feel of the most common tissue texture abnormality at the level of muscle, or in areas of somatic dysfunction.

10. Still palpating at the level of muscle, move the hand slowly distally down the partner's forearm until the musculotendinous junction is felt. This is an area or region where the muscle is vulnerable to injury.
11. Move past the musculotendinous junction toward the wrist. Note the transition from muscle to musculotendinous junction, then to the smooth, round, firm feel of tendons.
12. Follow the tendons distally until a structure, that is binding them at the wrist, is felt. These are the transverse carpal ligament (flexor retinaculum) and palmar carpal ligament (a thickening of the deeper anterolateral fascia). Note fiber direction, thickness, and firmness.
    a. How does it feel in comparison with the tendon? Compare the palpatory sensation over this area with that over the more superficially located tendons.
13. Place the index finger over the proximal radiohumeral joint at the dimple of the partner's elbow. Place the thumb opposite the index finger, on the ventral side over the lateral side of the humeroulnar attachments. This allows for the palpation of the head of the radius.
    a. Describe the characteristics.
    b. Compare the feel of this living bone with a plastic model or with the memory of a cadaver bone.
14. Move the thumb and index finger proximally until they fall into the joint space, thus locating it. The joint capsule should not be palpable, since those that are palpable signal pathologic changes.

Palpatory skill involves more than a mechanism for finely tuned sensory perception. Even more essential is the ability to focus on the mass of information perceived, pay close attention to those qualities associated with tissue texture abnormalities, and bypass many other palpatory clues not relevant at the time. These skills may be enhanced by palpating a hair through several sheets of paper.

Exercise 7: Palpatory Sensitivity

PURPOSE

To determine and improve sensory awareness.

POSITION

Sit comfortably in front of a table, with a notebook or several sheets of paper and objects of various thicknesses, including a human hair.

PROCEDURE

1. Starting with the thickest object, place the objects, one at a time, under a sheet of paper and see if their edges and dimensions can be palpated.
2. Then add pages until the objects' dimensions can no longer be palpated.
    a. How many pages were between the fingers and each object before it could no longer be palpated?
    b. Can the human hair be palpated through a single page?

Palpatory sensitivity requires a process of developing mental filters. Consider an analogy in music, where the orchestra conductor focuses on the violins. The conductor is aware of the entire orchestra's melody but diverts attention to a specific portion of the perceived sound. The brain cannot process everything at once. Likewise, it is easier and faster to detect areas of significant tissue texture abnormalities by focusing on only one portion at a time.

In a comparison of student musculoskeletal examinations with those of experienced examiners, Kappler et al.[32] observed that experienced examiners recorded fewer findings than student examiners, but the experienced examiner's findings were more significant. This demonstrates a filtering process that unconsciously rejects insignificant findings from the palpatory data. In contrast, the student has not yet developed this filtering process, is unable to reduce the data to manageable portions, and thus may start off overwhelmed by the mass of information until they gain more palpatory experience.

MOTION PERCEPTION

If any motion is present, describe the sensations transmitted through the fingers. Also, estimate the weight of the objects, the amount of pressure needed to move them, and the resistance or force exerted against the applied pressure.

The perception of motion is an important component in the palpation of living tissue. Three types of motion in the body may be described as:

1. Passive motion: motion the physician induces on the patient
2. Active motion: deliberate, conscious muscular activity that the patient performs
3. Inherent motion[2]: activity unconsciously generated within the body, such as respiratory motion or peristalsis

Inherent motion is postulated to occur in several ways:

- Biochemically, at the cellular or subcellular level
- As part of multiple electrical patterns
- As a combination of a number of circulatory and electrical patterns
- As some periodic patterns are not yet understood

Experts agree that tissue movement as minute as 1 mm^2 can be perceived. Therefore, inherent motion may be palpated with practice and patience.

Successive layers of tissue can be distinguished by varying the amount of pressure applied. In palpating superficial tissue, use the lightest possible effective touch. To palpate successively deeper layers, apply only as much additional pressure as necessary. As a general rule, palpate to the depth of the tissue or structure to be examined, that is, down to but not through them. The use of various depths of touch differs from physician to physician, usually depending on their chosen model of diagnosis and treatment.

Exercise 8: Palpating Spinal Motion and Paravertebral Tissues

PURPOSE

To learn how to palpate living tissue in the classroom, with an instructor available to demonstrate and interpret as needed.

To palpate the thoracic and lumbar spinal areas, testing for and finding any regions with relative resistance of the vertebrae and their spinous processes when passive flexion is introduced.

POSITION

Physician stands behind the partner, who's seated on the table.

PROCEDURE

1. Using the fingers of both hands, palpate for temperature differences along the paravertebral thoracic and lumbar spine. Use either the palmar or dorsal surface of the fingers, depending on which is more sensitive for the physician.
2. Using both hands simultaneously, stroke the back from C7 to L5. Which areas are warmer? Try to find a segment within the thoracic area that is either warmer or cooler than another segment.

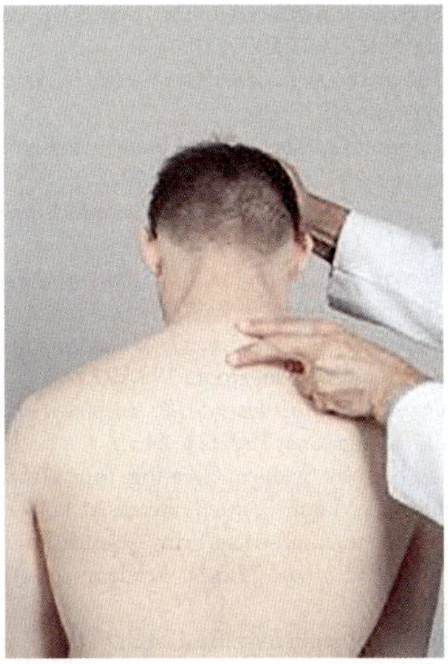

Figure 29.6. Palpating upper thoracic flexion–extension. (Reprinted with permission from Nicholas AS, Nicholas EA. *Atlas of Osteopathic Techniques*. 3rd ed. Wolters Kluwer; 2016:44.)

Compare left with right sides, and superior with inferior. Stroking of this type is useful in identifying changes in contour, as well as in identifying areas of edema and increased tissue tension.

3. Palpate for moisture differences, noting stickiness, dryness, wetness, waxiness, and slipperiness. The physician places the pads of the first three fingers of the dominant hand between the spinous processes of T1 and T2, T2 and T3, and T3 and T4. Remember to use the pads of the fingers. Place the other hand on the top of the partner's head.
4. Locate the spinous processes and interspinous ligaments. Note how they feel. Compare differences between the feel of the bone and the feel of the ligament.
5. Passively flex the partner's head and neck while sensing for increasing tension of the interspinous ligaments. Note: one spinous process may move more easily than another (Fig. 29.6).
6. Proceeding from T2 to L5, lightly compress the paravertebral soft tissues. Then, use deeper pressure, but less pressure than that required to palpate bone. In some areas, tissues compress more easily than in others, where there is more resistance. Significant resistance indicates an area of tissue texture abnormality,[3] which bears further investigation.
7. Lightly palpate the skin and subcutaneous tissue over the resistant site. This helps to identify the outer limits of tissue texture involved.

DEVELOPING ADVANCED SKILLS IN PALPATION OF TISSUE TEXTURE ABNORMALITY

Advanced palpatory skills require practice and experience. This text defines and describes what the tissues feel like. Nonetheless, words are inadequate to illustrate the perceived sensation imprinted in the brain. This sensation must be experienced. It is vital to compare an area of abnormal tissue with an adjacent area without the abnormality. Experiences that involve such COMPARISON are far more valuable than palpating an abstract area.

A skilled osteopathic physician has developed a store of information in the brain regarding what tissues feel like, and especially of the tissue texture changes in somatic dysfunction. When palpating an area, the physician is able to compare the current sensation with the mental store of information. At times, this may be difficult to put into words. The osteopathic physician may palpate a resistance to the tissues that is more indicative of that related to a somatic dysfunction based on the hundreds of patients they have palpated. At other times, they may palpate a paraspinal level that has a strange almost "rubbery" end feel. In the past, when this sensation was palpated, it correlated to a malignant or metastatic process. This palpatory finding, when linked to the patient's history, may prompt further clinical evaluation. This critical information store can only be gained by experience and the continued development and enhancement of palpatory skills.

Once the physician has developed this advanced skill, it is never lost.

SUMMARY

This chapter provides a method for obtaining the practical skills in developing the art of palpation. Many additional exercises to improve and enhance palpation exist. Initially, palpation is practiced on a partner in the skills laboratory. During clinical clerkships, additional experience is gained from examining actual patients. Ultimately, palpatory experience is gained from examination of the physician's own patients. The physician never stops learning and gaining new experiences.

Developing a high level of palpatory skill is an ongoing process that requires patience and practice.

As the osteopathic journey continues, these words from Dr. Sutherland may resonate:

> "The admonition, 'Touch Not', was not written for the osteopathic physician....Let him touch....But first instruct him how to feel. His professional task to a great degree is a finger task-that of locating etiological factors beneath as well as throughout all bodily tissues, being as problematic as is the 'searching for a needle in a haystack' and requiring fingers with brain cells in their tips. Fingers capable of feeling, thinking, seeing...The finger-feel, the finger-thought, and the finger-sight are the only way to read the diagnostic message. His fingers should be like detectives, skillful in the art of locating things hidden. The mere tracing by fingers up and down, here and there, is not 'getting in touch' with things hidden; the 'hit and miss' not being the proper osteopathic application of tactile sense. His fingers should pause, here and there, pressing in deeply to the deeper things that concern. Sojourning in a city for a day or two affords more opportunity for an acquaintance with the populace than merely driving through. So it is with the sense of touch. The fingers should tarry, resting firmly, yet gently, yet deeply on articulations, on ligaments, on muscles, here and there, and thus form an acquaintance with the 'populace' in the 'burg'. The populace of the spinalburg is inclined to inform and will tell the fingers many important things."[33]

REFERENCES

1. DeStefano LA. *Greenman's Principles of Manual Medicine*. 5th ed. Wolters Kluwer; 2017:12–13.
2. Van Allen P, Stinson J. The development of palpation. *J Am Osteopath Assoc*. 1941;40(5):207, 208.
3. Educational Council on Osteopathic Principles. Glossary of osteopathic terminology. American Association of Colleges of Osteopathic Medicine. 2017 (see appendix in this volume).
4. DiGiovanna EL, Schiowitz S, Dowling DJ. *An Osteopathic Approach to Diagnosis and Treatment*. 3rd ed. Williams & Wilkins; 2005.
5. Deflorio D, Di Luca M, Wing AM. Skin and mechanoreceptor contribution to tactile input for perception: a review of simulation models. *Front Hum Neurosci*. 2022;16:862344.
6. Bickley L, Szilagyi PG. *Bates' Guide to Physical Examination and History-Taking*. 9th ed. Lippincott Williams & Wilkins; 2007.

7. Fleming MS, Luo W. The anatomy, function, and development of mammalian Aβ low-threshold mechanoreceptors. *Front Biol (Beijing).* 2013; 8(4):10.1007/s11515-013-1271-1.
8. Shepherd GM. *Biology of Sensory Systems.* 2nd ed. Wiley-Blackwell; 2009.
9. Adibi M, Lampl I. Sensory adaptation in the whisker-mediated tactile system: physiology, theory, and function. *Front Neurosci.* 2021;15:770011.
10. Kuchera WA, Kuchera ML. *Osteopathic Principles in Practice.* 2nd ed. Greyden Press; 1994;23:112.
11. Chaitow L. *Palpation and Assessment Skills: Assessment and Diagnosis through Touch.* Churchill Livingstone; 1997:125–126.
12. Nakazawa N, Ikeura R, Inooka H. Characteristics of human fingertips in the shearing direction. *Biol Cybern.* 2000;82(3):207–214.
13. Chaitow L. *Palpation Skills- Assessment and Diagnosis Through Touch.* Churchill Livingstone; 1997:43–44.
14. Chaitow L. *Palpation and Assessment Skills: Assessment and Diagnosis Through Touch.* Churchill Livingstone; 1997:147–149.
15. Patterson MM, Shamus E, Carter K. Determination of pressures used in osteopathic palpatory diagnosis. *J Am Osteopath Assoc.* 2003;103(8):382.
16. Patterson MM, Shamus E, Carter K. Determination of pressures used in osteopathic manipulative treatments. *J Am Osteopath Assoc.* 2003;103(8):381.
17. Valibo AB, Johansson RS. Properties of cutaneous mechanoreceptors in the human hand related to touch sensation. *Hum Neurobiol.* 1984;3(1):3–14.
18. Bronzino JD, ed. Medical devices and systems. *The Historical Development of Thermometry and Thermal Imaging in Medicine.* 1st ed. CRC Press; 2006.
19. Frymann VM. *Palpation Part I: Its Study in the Workshop. AAO 1963 Yearbook.* The Academy of Applied Osteopath in affiliation with the American Osteopathic Association; 16–19.
20. Cox JM, Gorbis S, Dick LM, Rogers JC, Rogers FJ. Palpable musculoskeletal findings in coronary artery disease: results of a double-blind study. *J Am Osteopath Assoc.* 1983:82(11):832–836.
21. Chaitow L. *Palpation Skills-Assessment and Diagnosis Through Touch.* Churchill Livingstone; 1997:107–110.
22. Chaitow L. *Palpation Skills-Assessment and Diagnosis Through Touch.* Churchill Livingstone; 1997: 20.
23. Kasparian H, Signoret G, Kasparian J. Quantification of motion palpation. *J Am Osteopath Assoc.* 2015;115(10):604–610.
24. DeStefano LA. *Greenman's Principles of Manual Medicine.* 5th ed. Wolters Kluwer; 2017:41.
25. Chaitow L. *Palpation and Assessment Skills: Assessment and Diagnosis through Touch.* Churchill Livingstone; 1997:61.
26. Chaitow L. *Palpation and Assessment Skills: Assessment and Diagnosis Through Touch.* Churchill Livingstone; 1997:21.
27. Chaitow L. *Palpation and Assessment Skills: Assessment and Diagnosis Through Touch.* Churchill Livingstone; 1997:22–24.
28. Science Buddies. Starchy Science: Creating Your Own Colloid. Scientific American. Published March 7, 2023. Accessed January 5, 2024. https://www.scientificamerican.com/article/bring-science-home-colloids/
29. Webster GV. *The Feel of the Tissues.* Academy of Applied Osteopathy Yearbook; 1947:33.
30. Burns L. Palpation and pathology. Beal MC, *Exec. Ed. AAO 1994 Yearbook.* American Academy of Osteopathy; 1994:230–234.
31. Mitchell FL Jr. The training and measurement of sensory literacy in relation to osteopathic structural and palpatory diagnosis. *J Am Osteopath Assoc.* 1976;75(10):874–884.
32. Kappler RE, Larson NJ, Kelso AF. A comparison of osteopathic findings on hospitalized patients obtained by trained student examiners and experienced osteopathic physicians. *J Am Osteopath Assoc.* 1971;70(10): 1091–1092.
33. Sutherland AS, Wales AL, eds. *Contributions of Thought.* 2nd ed. Published by Sutherland Cranial teaching Foundation. 1998:201.

30 Osteopathic Structural Examination

WALTER C. EHRENFEUCHTER ▪ REBECCA E. GIUSTI ▪ RAYMOND J. HRUBY

KEY CONCEPTS

- The osteopathic structural exam is comprised of three parts; screening, regional, and segmental to assess for and identify somatic dysfunction.
- The screening osteopathic structural examination is a comprehensive assessment of gait and posture, symmetry of anatomical landmarks, skin and soft tissue contours, and dynamic regional motion characteristics.
- The screening osteopathic structural examination assesses for the presence of any somatic dysfunction and/or musculoskeletal problems.
- If there is evidence of somatic dysfunction, the regional component helps to locate the problem within a particular area. This is accomplished by palpating the identified and related area(s) from the screening portion for tissue texture changes, temperature changes, tenderness and asymmetry, and a quality of motion or passive range-of-motion assessment.
- The ability to accurately locate anatomical landmarks is mandatory for initiating motion challenges related to the structural exam.

INTRODUCTION

The osteopathic structural examination is performed to determine the presence of clinically significant somatic dysfunction in a given patient. This examination can be performed independently or as part of a focused or complete history and physical examination. The examination consists of three components: (1) the screening component; (2) the regional component; and (3) the segmental component. The screening portion of the examination is used to determine whether somatic dysfunction(s) may be present and in which body region(s). One may think of this portion of the osteopathic structural exam as asking the question: "Is there a structural problem present?" This part of the examination typically consists of visual observation of the musculoskeletal system, palpation of static landmarks to assess for symmetry, and the use of active and sometimes passive range-of-motion maneuvers to assess for restricted motion of joints or tissues.

Once the physician has used the screening portion to determine whether any region(s) of the body may need further evaluation for the presence of somatic dysfunction, they then perform the regional and segmental evaluations of the affected area(s). The regional portion is comprised of two parts; assessment of tissue texture changes including differences in temperature and tenderness, and passive range of motion to assess the quality of joint and/or tissue motion to localize the problem more specifically. This part of the examination may be thought of as asking the question "Where is the structural problem?" The segmental portion then defines and describes the specific joint or tissue restriction that was localized using the regional examination. This part of the examination may be thought of as asking the question: "What is the problem?" The components of the exam may almost be thought of as a funnel leading the osteopathic physician to a specific diagnosis to which a rational treatment may now be applied.

The bulk of this chapter will focus on the screening and regional portions of the osteopathic structural examination.

SCREENING PORTION OF THE OSTEOPATHIC STRUCTURAL EXAMINATION

The screening portion of the osteopathic structural examination is designed to rapidly locate the most significant somatic dysfunctions in the body and to simultaneously find larger structural abnormalities that may be responsible for these dysfunctions.

The screening portion of the osteopathic structural exam consists of two components:

1. A static postural examination
2. A dynamic part, which includes regional range-of-motion testing and gait observation

The structural osteopathic screening examination identifies gross asymmetries of structural landmarks and range-of-motion abnormalities, thus addressing two of the four physical exam findings that support the diagnosis of somatic dysfunction as described in the acronym T.A.R.T. This acronym stands for **T**issue texture abnormalities, **A**symmetry of anatomical landmarks, **R**estriction of range of motion and **T**enderness.[1] The other two components, tissue texture abnormalities and tenderness, are generally assessed during the regional palpatory component of the exam. The presence of any one of these four components is necessary for the regional diagnosis of somatic dysfunction.[1]

OBSERVATION—GAIT

Anterior View

If possible, the physician should observe the patient's natural gait when the patient is being escorted to the examination room. Otherwise, the patient should be observed walking the length of the examination room or hallway several times. This allows for evaluation of the patient's customary walking speed, stride length, and step rate, all of which are a result of the patient's own amalgamation of joint mobility and mechanics, muscular strength,

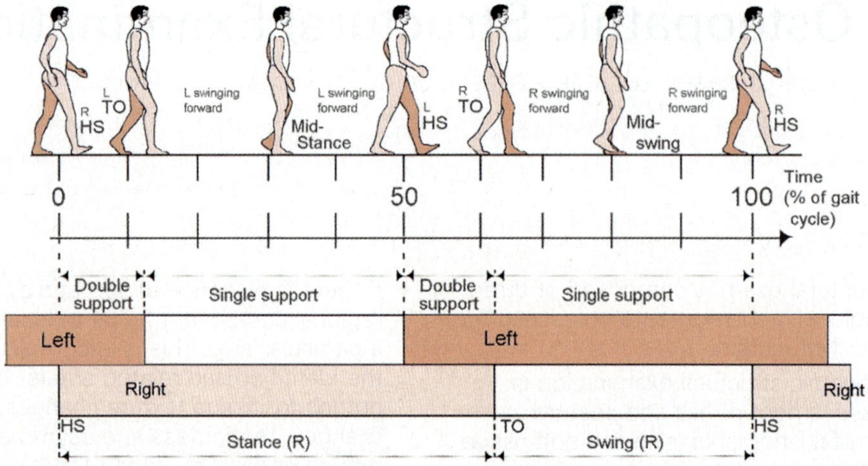

Figure 30.1. Gait cycle. HS, Heal Strike; L, Left; R, Right. (With permission William A. Kuchera, D.O., F.A.A.O.)

posture, neural control, and energy. The following vocabulary and definitions are used to describe the gait cycle:

- **Stride length:** the distance between the sequential points of the initial contact by the same foot.
- **Cadence:** step rate per minute. It is typically faster in women (117 steps per minute) compared to men (111 steps per minute), generally to compensate for a shorter stride length.[2]
- **Arm swing:** the motion of the upper extremity as it correlates to the ipsilateral lower extremity during ambulation. Normally the shoulder should flex as the ipsilateral hip extends providing a counterforce to minimize the rotatory displacement of the body during locomotion.[2]
- **Out-toeing** or excess external rotation: greater-than-normal external rotation for a particular phase of the gait cycle.[2]
- **In-toeing** or excess internal rotation: greater-than-normal internal rotation for a particular phase.[2]
- **Supination:** the excessive outward rolling motion (inversion) of the foot or ankle during walking or running.
- **Pronation:** the excessive inward rolling motion (eversion) of the foot or ankle during walking or running.
- **Stance phase:** the entire period where the limb is in contact with the ground during ambulation. It is further divided into four parts: initial contact; loading response; midstance; and terminal stance.[3]
- **Swing phase:** the period of time when the foot comes off the ground during ambulation. It is further divided into four parts: pre-swing; initial swing; mid swing; and terminal swing.[3]

Observe for the following:

- Length of stride
- Cadence
- Arm swing
- Out-toeing or in-toeing
- Supination or pronation
- Heel strike
- Toe off
- Pelvic tilt
- Disruption in weight transfer (limping)

Recognize that there are essentially two components to the gait, as depicted in Figure 30.1:

1. Stance phase
2. Swing phase

Assess for the following:

- Are both smooth and unencumbered?
- Is the weight transferred in a smooth manner from heel strike to toe off?
- Do the toes point inward or outward?
- Is there excessive pronation or supination of the feet?
- Is there internal or external rotation of either leg?

The observation of gait during the osteopathic screening portion of the structural examination is meant to assess the functional performance of the gait rather than the pathologic entities looked for during a more typical musculoskeletal or neurologic examination (e.g., shuffling-type gait seen in patients with Parkinson disease). Any abnormalities noted during gait observation may indicate the presence of certain systemic or degenerative diseases, or somatic dysfunction, especially in the thoracic, lumbar, sacral, pelvic, or upper or lower extremity regions. Assess the patient's gait from the anterior, lateral (Fig. 30.2A,B) and posterior views.

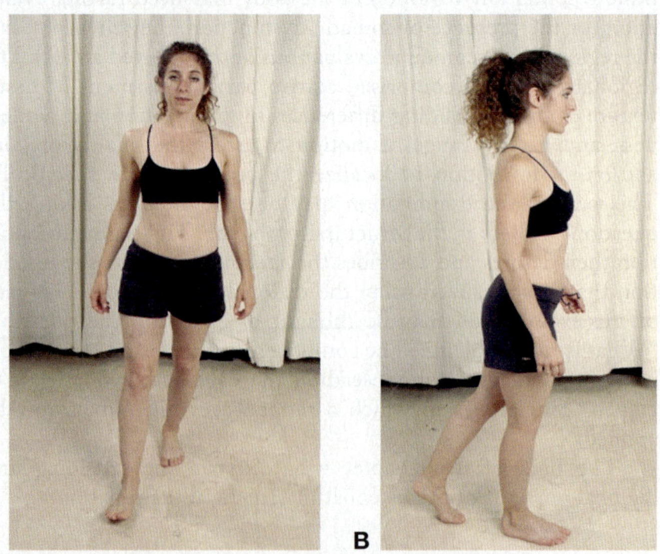

A B

Figure 30.2. A. Gait—Anterior view. (Photo courtesy of Western University of Health Sciences, Pomona, CA, with permission.) **B.** Gait—Lateral view. (Photo courtesy of Western University of Health Sciences, Pomona, CA, with permission.)

- *Asymmetry of arm swing, supination,* or *pronation* and *alteration in stride length and cadence* may indicate muscular imbalances and/or somatic dysfunction of the aforementioned regions.
- *Out-toeing* may indicate an external rotation contracture that may have developed due to a surgery of the lower extremity, tightness of the iliotibial (IT) band, or tightness or overactivity of the gluteus maximus, and when accompanied by abduction during the swing phase, may be an indication of a long leg compared to the other.[2]
- *In-toeing* may be the result of overactivity of the internal rotators of the hip such as the semimembranosus, semitendinosus, adductors, femoral anteversion, and/or weak quadriceps.[2]

OBSERVATION—STATIC POSTURAL EXAMINATION

Please see Table 30.1 for an overview of the elements that comprise both the static postural examination and screening range-of-motion testing. Note that skin should be assessed in all views.

Posterior View—Patient Standing

The patient is undressed enough for the overall configuration of the body to be observed, without being obscured by clothing. This also allows the patient to be examined for evidence of other disease conditions.

TABLE 30.1

Overview of Screening Exam—Static Postural Examination and Screening Range-of-Motion Tests

Posterior View	Anterior View	Lateral View
Feet and arches	Feet	Knees
Achilles tendons	Knees	Thighs
Knees	Thighs	Pelvis
Thighs	Pelvis	Curvatures of spine
Gluteal region	Abdomen	Shoulders
Iliac crests	Rib cage	Head alignment
PSIS	Shoulder	Gravitational line
Thoracic/lumbar spine	Overhead upper extremity quick test	Squat test
Paravertebral musculature	Cervical	
Arm position and length	Head	
Slope of shoulder	Facial asymmetry	
Rib angles	TMJ assessment	
Cervical spine		
Head		
Hip drop test		
Standing flexion test		
Pelvic side shift test		
Seated flexion test		

SKIN

The skin should be observed for such characteristics as erythema, pallor, pigmentation and/or scars, tattoos, lesions, masses, implanted devices, and any observable evidence of excessive moisture or dryness.

The skin may provide clues to the patient and any underlying conditions. Scarring may be the result of trauma or surgical intervention and may be associated with motion restriction of the musculoskeletal structures in the region of the scar. Excessive moisture or dryness may be associated with increased or decreased sympathetic nervous system activity in the noted body region which may lead to discovery of facilitated segments on further evaluation. Different forms of skin cancer may be observed. Masses such as lipomas, goiters, or foreign-body placements such as pacemakers and continuous glucose monitors (CGMs) may be noted and provide clues to the patient's medical history.

BODY SYMMETRY

The second portion of the structural examination involves an assessment of body symmetry, to determine the presence of any abnormal asymmetries in the patient. Some minor asymmetry is present in virtually all human beings. Figure 30.3 shows symmetry assessment of the posterior landmarks on the body. Those commonly used in the osteopathic screening structural examination are discussed below.

Feet and Arches

Alterations in the normal posture and positioning of the foot may be the result of somatic dysfunction within the structure of the foot itself, or injury or instability of the foot's stabilizing ligaments. Such alterations may have profound effects on the patient's posture and gait, and may result in compensatory somatic dysfunctions elsewhere, such as in the lower extremities, pelvis, or lumbar region. Likewise, somatic dysfunction or conditions from above may contribute to altered foot position.

The foot is observed for the following: the height of the longitudinal arches of the foot, the existence of pes planus or pes cavus, and excessive pronation or supination. The height of the arches should be evaluated for relative symmetry. This is more important than whether or not one or both are diminished.

Unilateral arch collapse with valgus hindfoot can occur to compensate for an anatomically longer leg on the ipsilateral side, and for pelvic dysfunctions that create a functionally long leg on the ipsilateral side (anterior rotation of the innominate, inferior innominate shear, etc.).

- Observe the height of the arches on each foot.
  - ☐ Their relative symmetry is more important than whether or not one or both are flat.
  - ☐ Is there excessive pronation or supination of the feet?
  - ☐ Observe the longitudinal arches of the feet. Is the curvature of the arch excessive (pes cavus) or markedly reduced (pes planus)? (Fig. 30.4)
- **Pes planus:** (flat foot) is a deformity of the foot where the medial longitudinal arch is abnormally flattened or lost. It can occur in about 20% of the adult population. Most patients are asymptomatic and do not require treatment, but it may also be associated with congenital fusion of the midfoot and hindfoot or connective tissue disorders. It may be helpful to ask the patient to lift their foot to observe if an arch is present or not.
- **Pes cavus:** a descriptive term for a foot deformity with an abnormally high medial longitudinal arch. While it may be a normal variant, it may also be seen in neuromuscular conditions such as

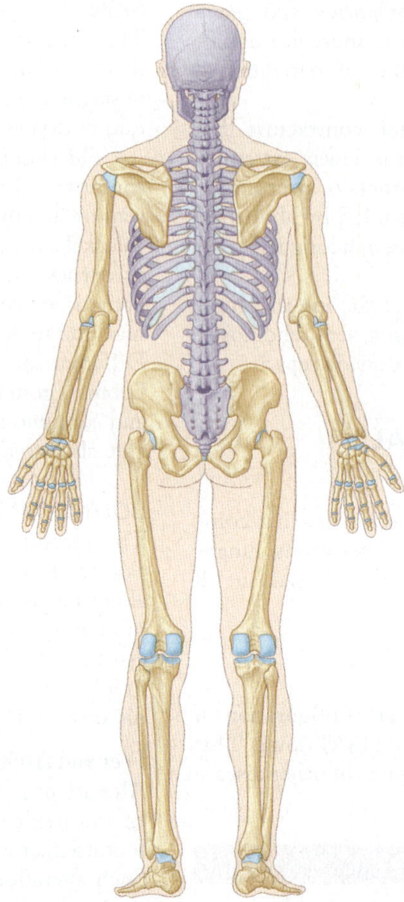

Figure 30.3. Examination for symmetry of posterior landmarks of the body. (Reprinted with permission from Moore KL, Agur AMR, Dalley AF II. *Essential Clinical Anatomy*. 5th ed. Wolters Kluwer Health; 2015.)

Charcot–Marie–Tooth disease, spinal anomalies, and conditions causing spastic paralysis.

- **Supination:** a patient may have a normal medial longitudinal arch but upon standing may demonstrate inversion of the forefoot and a medial arch elevation.
- **Pronation:** the patient may have a normal medial longitudinal arch but upon standing may demonstrate an eversion of the hindfoot and a depressed medial arch.

Achilles Tendons

- Observe the medial and lateral surfaces of the tendon (Figs. 30.5 and 30.6).
  - The curve of the tendon should be symmetric.
  - Flattening of the normal curve on the medial side of the Achilles tendon indicates the likely presence of a valgus hindfoot deformity. The valgus hindfoot accompanies longitudinal arch collapse in the foot.

LEGS

- Observe the size and symmetry of the gastrocnemius and soleus muscles. If asymmetric, determine if one is larger or smaller than the other. Surgery of the spine or the lower extremity itself may result in asymmetry of the legs. Conditions such as edema or venous insufficiency may contribute to a larger calf, while muscle atrophy due to chronic entrapment of the S1 or S2 nerve roots, or even of the sciatic nerve itself may result in a smaller calf.

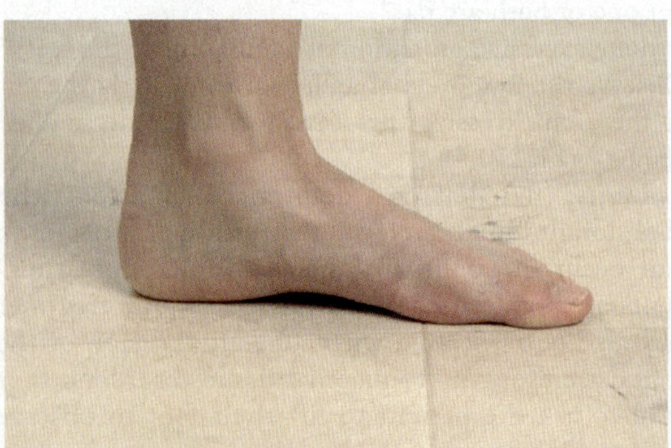

Figure 30.4. Foot arch evaluation. Medial view allows observation of the longitudinal arch. (Photo courtesy of Western University of Health Sciences, Pomona, CA, with permission.)

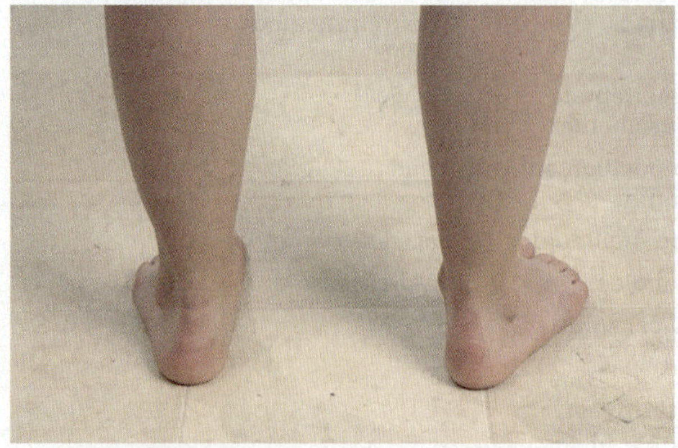

Figure 30.5. Achilles tendon evaluation. Posterior view (evaluator standing) provides a view of the foot in relation to the calf. (Photo courtesy of Western University of Health Sciences, Pomona, CA, with permission.)

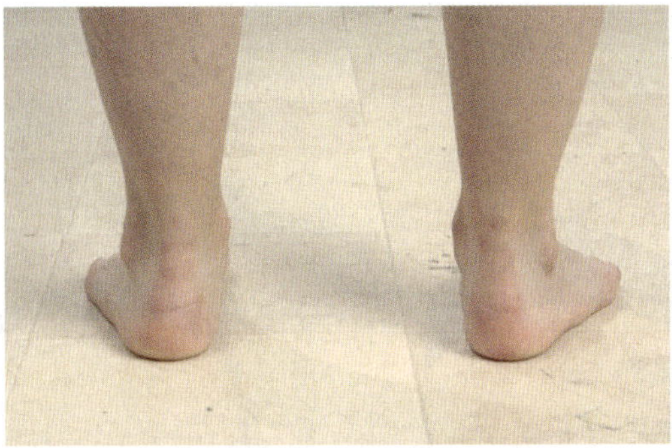

Figure 30.6. Achilles tendon evaluation. Posterior view (physician squatting) can offer a better view for evaluation of the Achilles tendons, pes planus, and pes cavus. Notice the relative straightening of the medial border of the right Achilles tendon. (Photo courtesy of Western University of Health Sciences, Pomona, CA, with permission.)

KNEES

- Observe the popliteal creases.
  - If they are found to be unlevel in the presence of normal ankles and feet, this may indicate the presence of a shortened tibia and fibula on one side.
- Observe the shape of the popliteal fossa.
  - A flattened popliteal fossa or the presence of genu recurvatum, suggests hyperextension of the knee and possibly the presence of laxity of the posterior cruciate ligament.
  - If unilateral, this may represent a compensatory change for an anatomic or functional long leg on the ipsilateral side.

THIGHS

- Observe the posterior thigh muscle mass.
  - Unilaterally enlarged muscle mass may be due to:
    - Venous insufficiency
    - Thrombosis
    - An underlying tumor[1]
  - Unilaterally decreased muscle mass may indicate a chronic entrapment of the:
    - L5, S1, or S2 nerve roots
    - Sciatic nerve's tibial division

GLUTEAL REGION

- The gluteal folds should be symmetric; asymmetry may indicate a leg-length inequality.
- The greater trochanters should be palpated and assessed for levelness to check for leg-length inequality.
- The gluteal muscle mass should be assessed for asymmetry.
  - Enlargement may indicate the presence of a tumor (lipoma being the most common).
  - Atrophy may indicate chronic entrapment of the S1 nerve root, or entrapment of the superior and inferior gluteal nerves in the greater sciatic foramen due to hypertrophy of the piriformis muscle.

ILIAC CRESTS

- Assess the iliac crests for symmetric height over their lateral aspect (Fig. 30.7).

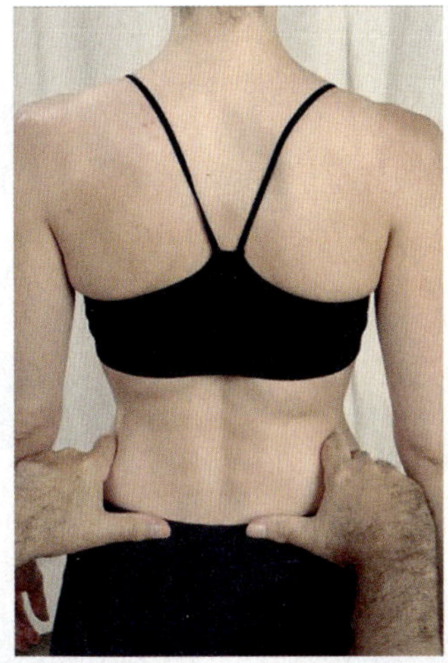

Figure 30.7. Posterior view of iliac crest level assessment. (Photo courtesy of Western University of Health Sciences, Pomona, CA, with permission.)

- Asymmetry may indicate the presence of a short hemipelvis, *coxa vera* or *coxa valga*, or a leg-length discrepancy (i.e., a shortened lower extremity due to normal anatomic variation or due to other causes such as surgery).

POSTERIOR SUPERIOR ILIAC SPINES

- Assess for symmetric localization relative to vertical displacement and anterior–posterior displacement.
  - The patient stands erect with the feet a shoulder width apart.
  - The physician stands or kneels behind the patient, with eyes at the level of the patient's posterior superior iliac spines (PSISs).
  - The physician's thumbs are placed on the inferior slope of the PSISs (Fig. 30.8).
  - Using the dominant eye along the patient's midline, assess level of the PSISs.
- Asymmetric PSISs may be caused by:
  - An anatomic or functional leg-length inequality
  - A short hemipelvis
  - Innominate somatic dysfunction
- An inferior PSIS may result from a posteriorly rotated innominate or an inferior innominate shear.
- A superior PSIS may result from an anteriorly rotated innominate or a superior innominate shear.
- A posterior displacement of the PSIS may indicate the presence of a posteriorly rotated innominate or an anteriorly displaced and anteriorly rotated innominate on the contralateral side.

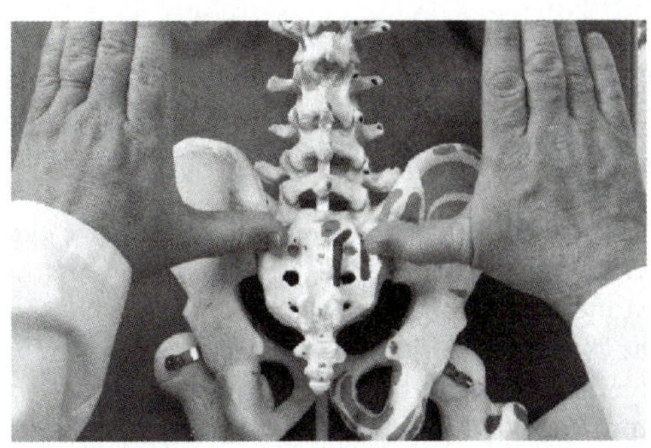

Figure 30.8. Posterior view demonstrating placement of physician's thumbs for assessing levelness of the posterior superior iliac spines on a skeleton model. (Photo courtesy of Western University of Health Sciences, Pomona, CA, with permission.)

[1]Clinical Note: One of the authors (WE) examined a patient who presented with low back pain and asymptomatic enlargement of one thigh. Further examination, imaging, and surgery ultimately resulted in the removal of a football-sized liposarcoma from the patient's thigh.

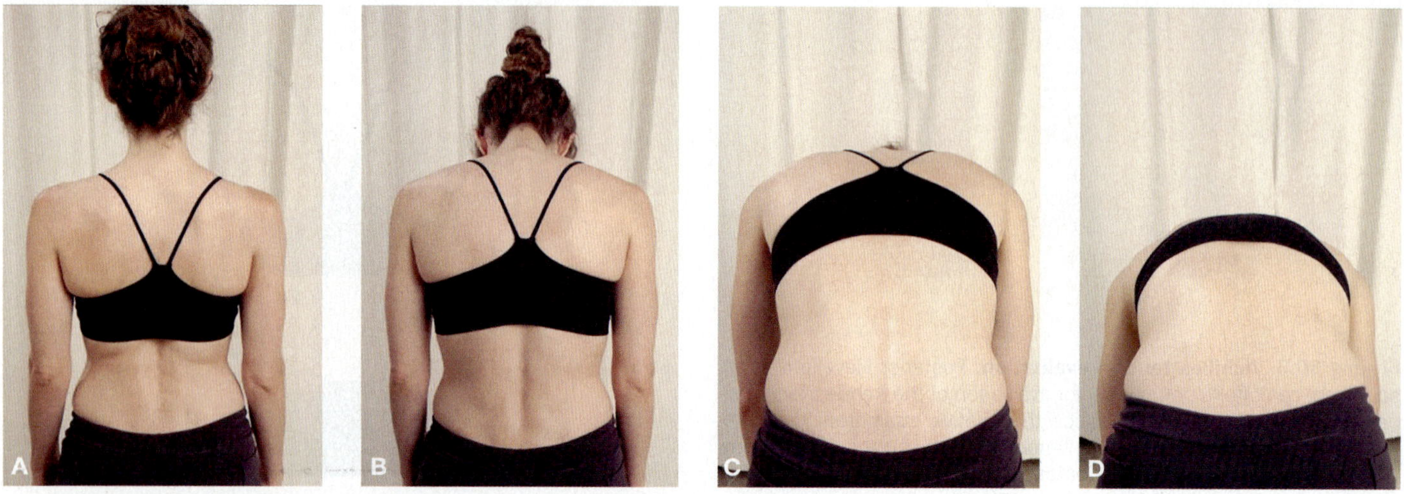

Figure 30.9. A. Posterior view, checking for curvature in the spine. (Photo courtesy of Western University of Health Sciences, Pomona, CA, with permission.) **B.** Posterior view, patient standing and bent forward at the cervical spine level with chin to chest to assess for scoliosis in the upper thoracic and cervical regions. (Photo courtesy of Western University of Health Sciences, Pomona, CA, with permission.) **C.** Partial forward bent position while standing to assess for scoliotic curves in the thoracic and lumbar spinal regions. (Photo courtesy of Western University of Health Sciences, Pomona, CA, with permission.) **D.** Full forward bent position while standing to assess for scoliosis in the thoracic and lumbar spinal regions. (Photo courtesy of Western University of Health Sciences, Pomona, CA, with permission.)

- Posterior rotation or superior shear of the innominate is a common compensatory mechanism for an anatomic long leg.

THORACIC AND LUMBAR SPINE

- The spinous processes should all be in a vertical straight line. Deviations from this may indicate various underlying conditions.
- Scoliosis
- Scoliosis is the most common cause of a lateral curvature of the spine. There are different forms of scoliosis. There is true anatomic scoliosis which is usually called "idiopathic" (its etiology is undetermined), or it may be due to congenital anomalies, trauma, degenerative bone or muscle diseases. These represent a true actual curvature of the spine and are usually noted by a rib hump during forward flexion. Functional scoliosis may be due to repetitive postures or positions, or it may be secondary to somatic dysfunction, either in the spinal regions or in the pelvis or lower extremities. Scoliosis and/or a rib hump that reduces or disappears when the patient sidebends indicates more of a functional type of scoliosis and may be more amenable to treatment with osteopathic manipulative treatment (OMT), bracing, stretching, and other exercises, or lift therapy.
- Mild scoliosis may be produced by segmental or group somatic dysfunction.
- The direction of the curve gives a general indication of the sidebending component of the segmental dysfunctions.
  - If the curve is due to a group Fryette type I dysfunction, all segments generally exhibit sidebending and rotation in opposite directions.
  - If the curve is generated from a single Fryette type II dysfunction, the dysfunction will generate compensatory Fryette type I mechanics in the adjacent regions of the spine.
    - The type II dysfunction may be located at the inferior or superior aspect of the curve, or in the middle.
  - The presence of a thoracic scoliosis can indicate:
    - Primary thoracic curvature
    - Secondary thoracic curvature compensating for a primary lumbar curve or a secondary lumbar curve from unleveling of the sacral base due to a short leg
    - Secondary thoracic curvature compensating for an unleveling of the cranial base which may be due to:
      - Cervical spine abnormalities (e.g., Klippel–Feil syndrome)
      - Head tilt due to asymmetric cervical muscle tone (torticollis)
      - Somatic dysfunction of the cranial base
- Large side-to-side deviations indicate the presence of a scoliosis (Fig. 30.9A–D).

In the presence of a leg-length inequality, the sacral base will be unlevel and will be lower on the side of the short leg.[4] The convexity of the lumbar scoliotic curve will be on the same side of the inferior sacral base and short leg. Determining whether the scoliosis is due to leg-length inequality or to a separate condition may necessitate radiographic imaging (Fig. 30.10).

To assess for scoliosis, the osteopathic physician stands behind the patient who is instructed to stand with their feet a comfortable distance apart.

The patient is instructed to bend the head toward their chest and then continue to bend forward slowly through the thoracic and lumbar spine as though trying to touch the floor with their fingers. As the patient is flexing forward the physician should attempt to closely observe the spine and the paravertebral musculature and note the following items:

- Whether there is normal or restricted flexion motion in the patient's spine. This can be assessed by noting how close to the floor the patient's fingertips are.
- Whether the spine is aligned in the midline or whether any lateral curvature (scoliosis) is noted, and if so, whether it is noted in the cervical, thoracic, or lumbar regions, whether it is convex to the left or right, and where the apex of each curve is located.
- Whether there is any rib hump present.
- If there are any lateral curves and/or rib hump present, the physician asks the patient, while forward bent to that level, to sidebend their trunk left and right. The physician notes whether there is any change in the spinal curves or rib hump with the sidebending motion. It is important that the physician observes the full flexion of the spine to observe any lateral curves and/or

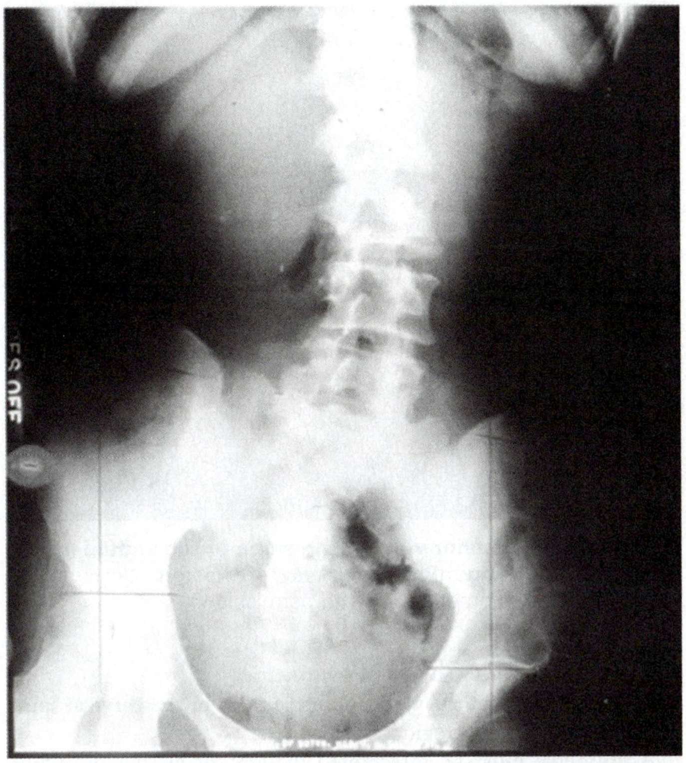

Figure 30.10. Anterior view of radiograph demonstrating left convex lumbar scoliosis due to 2-inch sacral base unleveling from an anatomic short left leg. (Original photograph, Walter C. Ehrenfeuchter, D.O., F.A.A.O., with permission.)

rib humps that may be present before asking the patient to forward bend to the levels of greatest curvature and perform the sidebending.

Further Observations of the Spine and its Curvatures:

- Excessive prominence of a spinous process may indicate the presence of an angular kyphosis, which can be the result of a congenital anomaly of the vertebral body, or of a possible compression fracture.
  - ☐ Flattening of the kyphotic thoracic curve can be due to:
    - Extended segmental dysfunctions
- Exaggeration of the kyphotic thoracic curve can be due to:
  - ☐ Flexed segmental dysfunctions
  - ☐ Scheuermann disease
  - ☐ Spondyloarthropathies
- Diffuse idiopathic skeletal hyperostosis (DISH), which occurs more frequently in patients with type II diabetes mellitus
- Exaggeration of the lumbar lordotic curve can be due to:
  - ☐ Extended segmental dysfunction
  - ☐ Flexed or anteriorly rotated sacrum or pelvis
- Flattening of the lumbar lordotic curve can be due to:
  - ☐ Flexed segmental dysfunction
  - ☐ Extended or posteriorly rotated sacrum or pelvis
  - ☐ Muscle spasm
  - ☐ Ankylosing spondylitis
- Observe the lumbosacral junction for the presence of skin anomalies.
- These include:
  - ☐ A hairy patch
  - ☐ Pigmented nevus
  - ☐ Port-wine stain
  - ☐ Pilonidal sinus
  - ☐ Pilonidal cyst
  - ☐ Lipoma
- The presence of a skin lesion has strong correlation with the presence of an underlying congenital bony abnormality, including many forms of occult spinal dysraphism.

PARAVERTEBRAL MUSCLES

- Observe for symmetry.
  - ☐ Prominence of the paravertebral muscle mass can indicate:
    - Vertebral rotation to the ipsilateral side
    - Hypertrophy or hypertonicity of the larger muscle mass
    - Tumor or abscess in the musculature (though uncommon)

LATERAL BODY LINE

- The lateral body line is the silhouette of the contour of the sides of the trunk, below the rib cage.
- They are especially useful in obese patients, where the condition of the lumbar vertebrae and the paravertebral muscles is harder to assess.
  - ☐ For example, flattening of the left lateral body line, and exaggeration of the curvature of the right lateral body line suggest the presence of a scoliosis in the lumbar region convex to the left. In more obese patients, the presence of skin folds and their depth and/or number could provide similar information. For example, the left lateral body line could exhibit two skin folds, and the right lateral body line three skin folds, indicating the presence of the same sidebending curve.

SCAPULAR LANDMARKS

- The relative positions of the scapulae are under numerous muscular and postural influences. The most important landmarks are the:
  - ☐ Acromion process
  - ☐ Inferior angle
  - ☐ Spine of the scapula
  - ☐ Medial scapular border
- A line across the shoulders should be perpendicular to the spinal column, regardless of the spinal column's activity in the upper thoracic region.
- Assess the level of the inferior angles of the scapulae (Fig. 30.11A,B).
- If the spinal column is vertical, the shoulders should be symmetrically horizontal.
- If a scoliosis sidebends the spinal column to the right in this region, the right scapular landmarks will be more inferior than those of the left.
- Normally, the medial scapular border is approximately 2 to 3 inches from the spinous processes and should be roughly parallel to the spine, regardless of the spine's configuration at this level.
- Forward carriage of one shoulder will result in the medial scapular border being farther from the spinous processes than normal.
- Rotation of the scapula due to shoulder muscle imbalances will result in a loss of the parallel relationship between the spine and the medial border of the scapula.
- A vertically straight spine with unlevel scapulae indicates a problem with the shoulder girdle.
- Typically, the spine of the scapula is even with the spinous process of T3.
- Generally, the inferior angle of the scapula is even with the spinous process of T7 (transverse processes of T8).

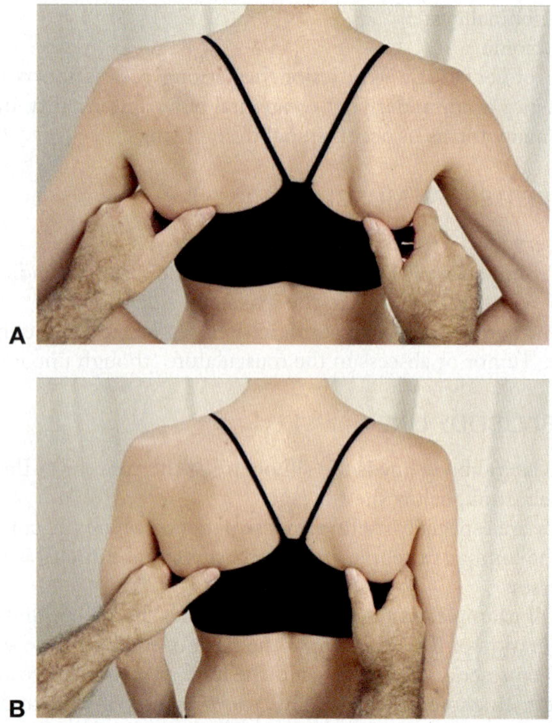

Figure 30.11. **A.** Patient's hands placed on lumbar spine to aid physician in locating the inferior angles of the scapulae. (Photo courtesy of Western University of Health Sciences, Pomona, CA, with permission.) **B.** Palpation for scapulae levels with patient standing at ease. (Photo courtesy of Western University of Health Sciences, Pomona, CA, with permission.)

- A scapula positioned more superiorly than normal, *scapula alta*, implies the presence of hypertonic or contractured musculature involving the shoulder elevators:
  - Upper trapezius muscles
  - Rhomboids
  - Levator scapulae

  Note: A scapula that is sufficiently high and present from birth represents a congenital Sprengel deformity.
- On the other hand, a scapula positioned more inferiorly than normal, *scapula infra*, may represent weakness of the shoulder elevators instead of hypertonicity of the shoulder depressor muscles such as the latissimus dorsi, lower trapezius, and lower serratus anterior.

ARM POSITION AND LENGTH

- Viewing the arms' position in relation to the trunk can provide further insight into dysfunctions of the shoulder girdle musculature, by revealing rotations of the entire extremity.
- The distance of the arms from the torso also elucidates the possibility of scoliosis decompensation or pelvic side shift.
- Observe the length of the arms from acromion to fingertip.
  - A patient may present with a short arm in the same manner as they present with a short leg, giving the false impression of spinal or shoulder dysfunction or deformity.
  - This asymmetry may be significant for work and sports involving the upper extremities.

SLOPE OF THE SHOULDER

- Observe the region where the slope of the shoulder meets the neck (Fig. 30.12).

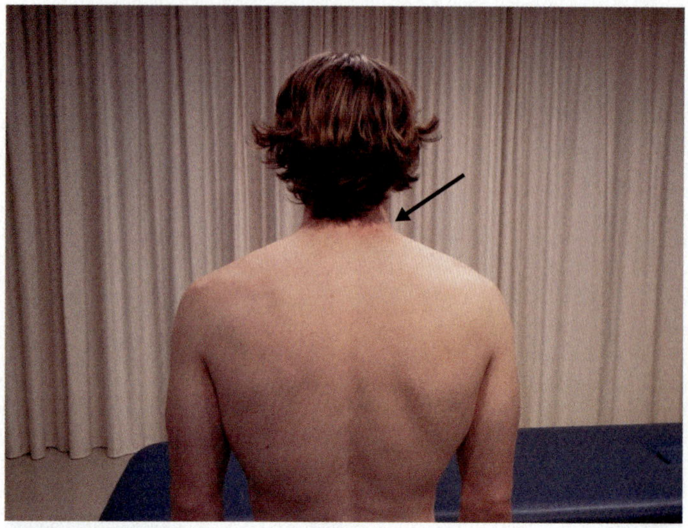

Figure 30.12. **Posterior view of the slope of the shoulder indicated by the *arrow*.** (Photo courtesy of Western University of Health Sciences, Pomona, CA, with permission.)

- These two surfaces should be symmetric.
- They should meet the vertical muscle mass of the cervical spine in the mid-cervical region.
- Asymmetry must be interpreted in light of all the preceding data regarding scapular position.
  - A fold of skin that attaches to the neck at a location higher than the mid-cervical region constitutes as a web neck or pterygium colli. It may even attach as high as the mastoid process. This condition is associated with congenital disorders such as Klippel–Feil syndrome or Turner syndrome.

RIB ANGLES

- Observe for symmetry.
- Instruct the patient to grasp opposite shoulders, crossing the arms in front of the chest, to move the scapulae laterally, and expose the rib angles (Fig. 30.13).
- Assess the rib angles for symmetry and tenderness by palpating the ribs with the palms and finger pads bilaterally.
- Any abnormalities found indicate the need to further examine the rib cage for segmental somatic dysfunction.

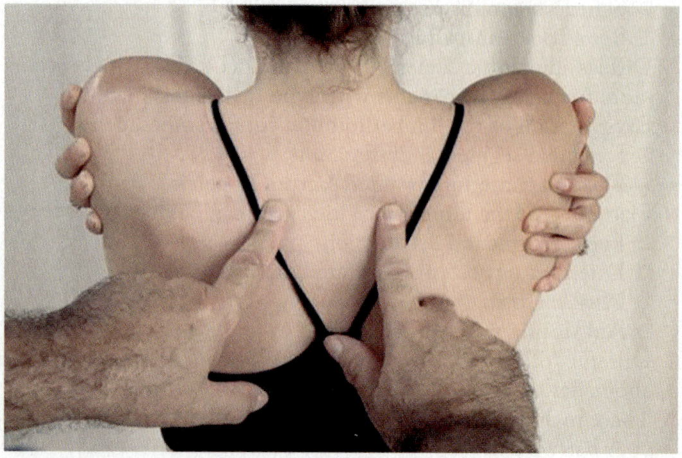

Figure 30.13. **Rib cage contour.** Assessing rib cage symmetry by visual inspection and by palpation. (Photo courtesy of Western University of Health Sciences, Pomona, CA, with permission.)

- Asymmetrical rib cage contours may arise from scoliosis, healed rib fractures or dislocations, metastatic cancer lesions, or bony cysts.
- Tenderness upon palpation may indicate somatic dysfunction or underlying pathology that may require imaging for a definitive diagnosis.

CERVICAL SPINE

- The cervical spinous processes should be vertically oriented.
  - Slight deviations from the ideal position are normal since the mid-cervical spinous processes are bifid, and it is not unusual for one fid to be longer than the other. This in turn gives the false impression that a cervical vertebra is out of alignment with the rest of the neck.
- The paravertebral muscle masses should be symmetric.
- Prominence of muscle mass unilaterally may indicate the presence of:
  - Unilateral facet dislocation with overriding
  - Enlarged facet joints due to arthritic changes
  - Local muscle hypertonicity
  - Hematoma within the musculature

HEAD

- The head should sit level on top of the cervical spine.
- A tilt of the head on the cervical spine may indicate:
  - Asymmetric suboccipital muscle tone
  - Hypertonicity or spasm of one of the larger muscles that attach to the cranium (torticollis).
  - The sidebending component of an occipitoatlantal somatic dysfunction may be a compensatory mechanism for diplopia.
- The mastoid processes should be level and the inion positioned in the midline.
  - Asymmetry of the mastoid processes, in the presence of a symmetrically positioned head upon the neck, suggests the possibility of cranial somatic dysfunction with involvement of the temporal bones.
- Likewise, observe the position of the pinnae of the ears.
  - Asymmetry would again suggest the presence of cranial somatic dysfunction involving the temporal bones in the presence of a symmetrically positioned head upon the neck.

Posterior View—Patient Seated

- Examine the same landmarks of the torso, shoulders, neck, and head with the patient seated.
  - Any changes from what was observed in the erect posture indicate a strong influence from the lower extremities. This is often associated with asymmetry or dysfunction of the hip girdle musculature (especially the psoas muscle) but can also be the result of aberrations anywhere in the lower extremity.

These problems would need to be identified and addressed before any clear conclusions can be made regarding the presence of somatic dysfunction in the pelvis and above.

Anterior View—Patient Standing (Fig. 30.14)

Some structural and postural abnormalities of the body are more obvious when viewed anteriorly.

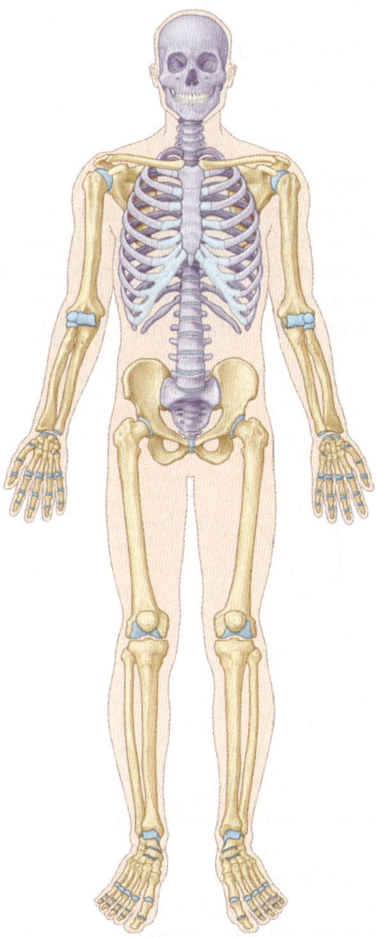

Figure 30.14. Examination for symmetry of anterior landmarks of the body. (Reprinted with permission from Moore KL, Agur AMR, Dalley AF II. *Essential Clinical Anatomy*. 5th ed. Wolters Kluwer Health; 2015.)

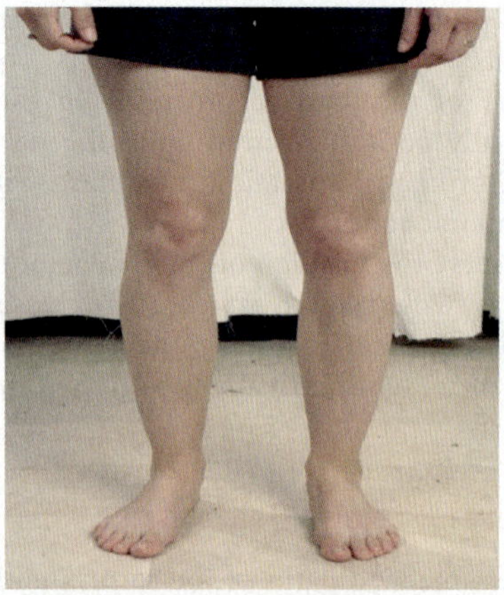

Figure 30.15. Anterior view allows observation of the knees, foot, and ankle in relation to the lower leg. (Photo courtesy of Western University of Health Sciences, Pomona, CA, with permission.)

FEET

- Observe for symmetry (Fig. 30.15).
- Apparent in-toeing ("pigeon toed") and out-toeing ("duck footed") positions of the feet may be due to normal variants, asymmetric muscle tensions or conditions such as:
  - Metatarsus adductus
  - Lower leg abnormalities like tibial torsion
  - Femoral abnormalities such as anteversion or retroversion of the femoral neck
- The following may also influence the position of the entire lower extremity:
  - A shortened piriformis muscle (out-toeing)
  - A shortened iliopsoas muscle (in-toeing)
  - Somatic dysfunction of the pelvis
    - Posterior innominate rotation and innominate outflare are generally associated with external rotation of the lower extremity.
    - Anterior innominate rotation and innominate inflare are generally associated with internal rotation of the lower extremity.

KNEES

- Observe for symmetry (Fig. 30.15).
- Observe any medial or lateral deviation of the legs at the knees (genu valgus ["knock-kneed"] or genu varus ["bow-legged"] or genu recurvatum [hyperextensibility] Fig. 30.16). These can all be normal physiologic variants of the anatomy. However, they may also be due to pathologic causes.[2]
  - Typically, these are congenital or developmental deformities, although they can also occur with advanced unilateral compartment arthritis of the knee.
  - The presence of a unilateral varus or valgus deformity may shorten the ipsilateral leg and affect the structures above.
  - If bilateral, asymmetry may indicate a worsening of the condition, again, as a result of an anatomic or functional long leg.
  - Genu varum is physiologic in infants up to about the time when they learn to walk.
  - Genu valgum may also be the result of ipsilateral abductor weakness and/or ipsilateral trunk lean.[2]
  - Pathologic causes of genu varum and valgum can include genetic disorders, trauma, obesity, rickets, and Blount disease, among others.
  - Genu recurvatum may be due to trauma or certain illnesses such as polio, and may signal weakness or paralysis of the hamstring and/or quadratus femoris muscle(s).
  - While genu varum, valgum, and recurvatum may be normal variants, they may also be the source of pain or weakness and may need to be addressed with proper footwear or appropriate strengthening exercises or stretches. These variants can predispose a patient to degenerative joint disease in the knees and can have profound effects on the patient's posture and gait. They may also be the source of compensatory somatic dysfunctions elsewhere, such as in the lower extremities, pelvis, or lumbar region.
- Observe the tibial tuberosities for prominence, as this may represent a case of Osgood–Schlatter disease.
- Observe the height of the patellas relative to the tibial tuberosities.
  - Search for the presence of *patella alta* (high-riding patella) or *patella baja* (low-riding patella).

THIGHS

- Observe the symmetry of the thigh muscle mass.
- Enlargement of the musculature may be due to normal variants such as a dominant leg, especially in athletes. Pathologic causes may be the presence of a tumor or edema. Atrophy may be due to surgery, history of immobilization of the extremity (such as wearing a cast), or entrapment of the femoral nerve or L2, L3, L4 nerve roots.

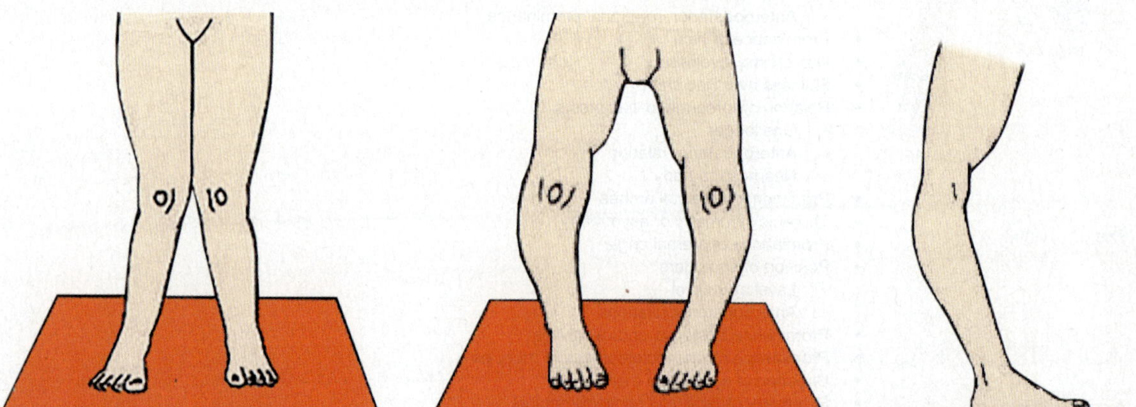

Figure 30.16. Deformities of the knees—Anterior View. From left to right: *genu valgum, genu varum, genu recurvatum.* (From Department of Neuromusculoskeletal Medicine/Osteopathic Manipulative Medicine at Western University of Health Sciences, College of Osteopathic Medicine of the Pacific. *Osteopathic Principles and Practice: Osteopathic Manipulative Treatment.* 1st ed. Western University of Health Sciences; 2015–2016, with permission.)

PELVIS

- Observe the position of the anterior superior iliac spines (ASIS) and pubic bones.
  - They should reside in the same anterior coronal plane.
  - If not, this may indicate either an anterior or a posterior pelvic tilt that could be causing changes in the lumbar lordotic curve (anterior tilt—increased lordosis; posterior tilt—flattening of lordosis).
    - Changes in the lumbar curve can force changes in the tilt of the pelvis.
    - Pelvic tilt is also under the influence of the hip girdle musculature.
      - Anterior tilt may be caused by hypertonic or contractured iliopsoas muscles.
      - Posterior tilt by hypertonic or contractured hamstrings. Leg-length discrepancy may also contribute to an anterior or posterior tilt of the pelvis.
  - Pelvic rotation about a vertical axis is also readily viewed from the anterior aspect, with shifting of the ASIS anteriorly or posteriorly in response to positioning of the entire pelvis.
- Observe the pelvis for evidence of pelvic side shift.
  - This can again be associated with either anatomic or functional leg-length inequality.
  - Side shift will increase the prominence of the greater trochanter on the side to which the pelvis has shifted and will increase the tension in the IT band.
  - The symmetry of the ASIS may also be altered by the presence of virtually any of the innominate dysfunctions.

ABDOMEN

- The prominence of the abdomen is often dependent on the shape of the lumbar lordosis.
  - A flattened lordosis may flatten the abdomen.
  - An increased lordosis will generally make the abdomen appear more protuberant.
- Protuberance of the lower abdomen is common:
  - In the presence of an increased kyphosis
  - From flattening of the diaphragm due to respiratory conditions such as emphysema or asthma
- If the spinal curves are normal and no respiratory condition exists, the protuberant abdomen may provide evidence of visceroptosis, and the patient should be evaluated accordingly.
- Normally, there is about three or four fingerbreadths of space between the superior aspect of the iliac crest and the lower costal margin.
  - This can be decreased by the presence of scoliosis.
  - In severe or decompensated scoliosis, one side of the costal cage can essentially be sitting on top of the iliac crest. This may adversely impact the underlying viscera.

RIB CAGE

Observe rib cage contours for symmetry in relationship to the abdomen (Fig. 30.17).

- Asymmetrical costal margins can occur from many factors including scoliosis, congenital or acquired rib cage deformities, diaphragmatic asymmetries, rickets, and internal organ pathologies or surgeries.
- Observe the costal cartilages for any deformity or swelling.
  - A common abnormality is an outflaring of the lower rib cage.
  - A visible or palpable ridge at one or more costochondral joints can indicate the presence of a "separated rib."

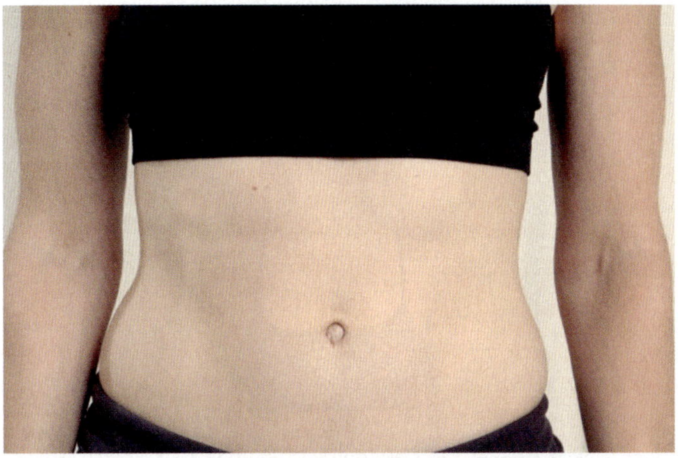

Figure 30.17. Evaluation of abdomen and rib cage contours. (Photo courtesy of Western University of Health Sciences, Pomona, CA, with permission.)

  - When deformity is present at the time of injury, the articulation will often heal with a slight anteroposterior deformity.
    - This is not amenable to correction after the injury has already healed.
  - Swelling of one or more costal cartilages (typically the second or the third) can be due to a viral infection and may indicate the likelihood of Tietze syndrome.[5,6]
    - This must be differentiated from the more common costochondritis, which does not cause swelling of the cartilage, only tenderness.
- Note the prominence of the xiphoid process.
  - It is not uncommon for the xiphoid to become more prominent with age.
  - Prominence can also be increased with clothing pressure or from sleeping prone. Consequentially, the xiphoid becomes tender to touch, and the patient presents with "midepigastric pain" with the unnecessary resultant workup. Palpation of the xiphoid will reproduce the patient's pain and render a diagnosis of xiphalgia.
- Observe the patient for any deformities of the sternum.
  - *Pectus excavatum* (funnel breast) is the most common (Fig. 30.18).
  - *Pectus carinatum* (pigeon breast) is less common.

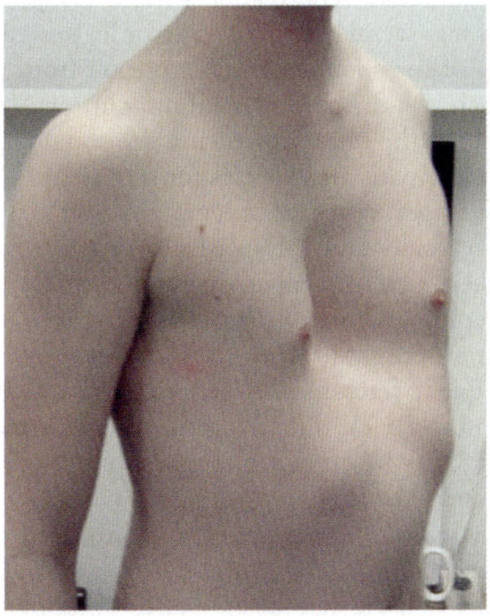

Figure 30.18. Pectus excavatum. (Original photograph, Walter C. Ehrenfeuchter, D.O., F.A.A.O., with permission.)

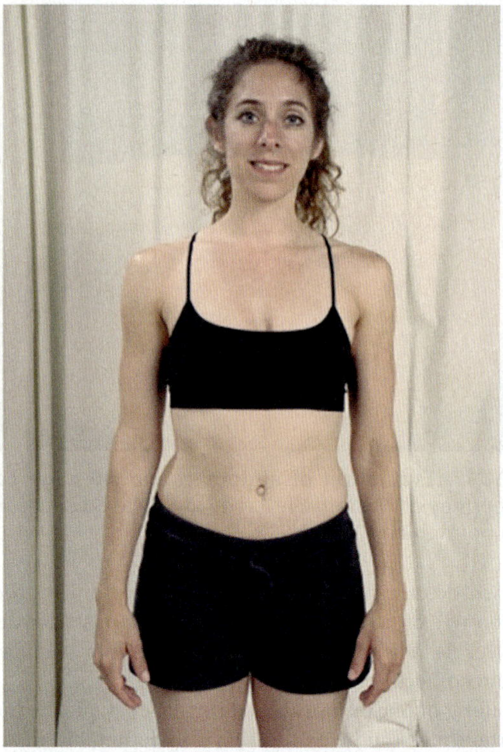

Figure 30.19. Evaluation of the shoulder levels. (Photo courtesy of Western University of Health Sciences, Pomona, CA, with permission.)

- Any deformity of the sternum should prompt an examination for occult congenital heart defects.
  - Though it is not a 100% correlation, heart defects are more common in patients with sternal abnormalities than in the general population.[7,8]

SHOULDERS

- Observe for symmetry (Fig. 30.19).
- Stand facing the patient. Observe if the shoulder levels appear to be level on a horizontal plane. The physician may also observe the arms hanging by the patient's side. Do they appear symmetrical or does one seem to be closer to the body? Is there any excessive internal or external rotation of the upper extremity? If the shoulder levels are not level this could indicate a cervical somatic dysfunction, scoliosis, or a more distant somatic dysfunction such as sacral base unleveling or leg-length discrepancy.
- Asymmetry of the shoulder may also result from trauma to the shoulder such as a dislocation, a rotator cuff or AC injury, or an injury to one of the nerves supplying the shoulder.
- Observe and palpate the clavicles for symmetry.
  - It is rare to see a case of congenital absence of the clavicles such as in cleidocranial dysplasia.
  - A clavicle can be misshapen due to:
    - Congenital anomaly
    - Fracture during birth
    - Subsequent fracture at a later date. Figure 30.20 shows a deformed clavicle due to old fracture with malunion.
  - The length of the clavicle from sternum to acromion determines in part the shoulder's position.
  - The clavicle is the upper extremity's only bony connection to the axial skeleton.
    - A shortened clavicle often causes anterior shoulder carriage, pulling the scapula farther away from the spinal column than its mate on the uninjured side.

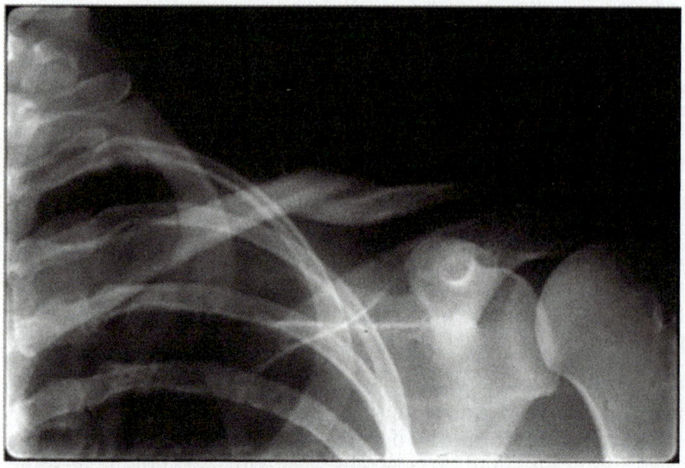

Figure 30.20. Deformed clavicle due to old fracture with malunion. (Original photograph, Walter C. Ehrenfeuchter, D.O., F.A.A.O., with permission.)

CERVICAL REGION

- Observe the patient for prominence of the sternocleidomastoid muscles and scalene muscles.
  - These commonly injured muscles can be shortened by:
    - Hypertonicity
    - Contracture
    - Hematoma
  - Neck and head carriage are altered by unequal tone or length of these muscles.[9]
  - Tracheal deviation, neck masses, or thyromegaly can be easily observed from this view as well.

HEAD

- Observe the alignment of the head atop the neck. Observe whether the patient's head is in a vertical position, or whether there is rotation or sidebending in relation to the midline.
  - Rotation and/or sidebending of the head may indicate somatic dysfunction of the cervical or upper thoracic regions or may be compensatory to spinal scoliosis or somatic dysfunctions in the lower thoracic, lumbar or pelvic regions, or leg-length discrepancy.
  - Some dysfunctions in this region will be more obvious from an anterior rather than posterior view.
- Observe the position of the symphysis menti relative to the midline of the body and to the midline of the face.
- Observe the jaw for symmetry relative to the rest of the head.
  - Asymmetry of the jaw can also be generated by somatic dysfunction of the temporal bones.
  - Lateral deviation of the jaw can signify a shortened portion of the mandible, with resultant:
    - Dental abnormalities
    - Potential for temporomandibular dysfunction syndrome and pain
    - Often, the presence of cranial somatic dysfunctions can be determined visually, prior to palpating the motion of the head.

Facial Asymmetry (Fig. 30.21)

- Assess the face for symmetry. Observe the overall shape of the face; is it round or oval, narrow or elongated? The shape and contour of the face may provide preliminary information regarding such influences as heredity, trauma, or cranial somatic dysfunction. Are there any observable asymmetries? Asymmetry

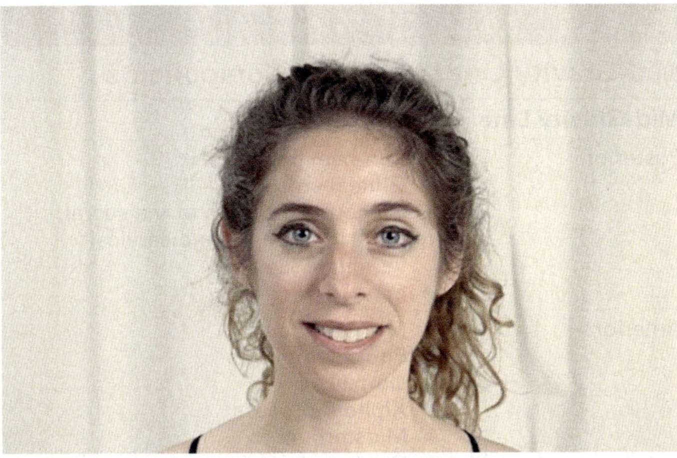

Figure 30.21. Patient position for observation of facial asymmetry. (Photo courtesy of Western University of Health Sciences, Pomona, CA, with permission.)

from side to side may indicate the presence of cranial somatic dysfunction, especially of the cranial base. Obvious drooping of one side of the face may indicate more serious pathologies such as those listed above or neurologic dysfunction of the cranial nerves or brain.

- Observe the midline of the face; is there symmetry from side to side?
- Are there asymmetries in the forehead skin creases or the nasolabial skin creases?
- Are the eyes the same shape?
- Is there any obvious drooping of one side of the face, eye, cheek, or mouth that could be the result of brain or cranial nerve disease or dysfunction?
- Difference in the size of the orbits may indicate cranial somatic dysfunction.
- Facial asymmetry can occur due to:
  - □ Congenital malformation of the skull
  - □ Birth trauma to the sphenobasilar synchondrosis
  - □ Acquired sphenobasilar somatic dysfunction as a result of head trauma or dental work
  - □ Facial bone somatic dysfunction resulting from trauma to the face

Observe the eye levels from side to side on a horizontal plane. The physician can evaluate the orbital sizes by placing a thumb at the most inferolateral corner of each orbit, and then visually estimate the distance of each thumb to the glabella. Inequality of these distances from side to side may indicate cranial somatic dysfunction.

- Also note the overall shape and symmetry of the orbits as facial asymmetry may be most evident in the shape of the orbits.
- Asymmetry of the actual orbits may indicate hereditary influences, the effect of trauma, or cranial somatic dysfunction.
- If the eyes are not level in the horizontal plane, this may indicate a postural compensation for somatic dysfunction in the cervical region, scoliosis in other spinal regions, or more distant somatic dysfunctions such as sacral base unleveling or leg-length discrepancy.

Observe the ear levels from side to side on a horizontal plane. Imagine a horizontal line drawn from the bottom of one ear lobe to the bottom of the other ear lobe.

- If the ears are not level in the horizontal plane, this may indicate a postural compensation for somatic dysfunction in the cervical region, scoliosis in other spinal regions, or more distant somatic dysfunctions such as sacral base unleveling or leg-length discrepancy.

Temporomandibular Joint

- Instruct the patient to open and close the jaw several times.
- Observe for any deviation on opening or closing, or any limitation in opening the jaw.

Deviation of the mandible on opening or closing, or any observed limitation of jaw opening, requires further evaluation. If dysfunction of the temporomandibular joint (TMJ) is suspected, the physician should perform an active range-of-motion test as part of the screening exam as described below in the "Range-of-Motion Testing."

Lateral View—Patient Standing (Fig. 30.22)

KNEES

- The genu recurvatum or flexion contracture of the knee may be most easily observed laterally. Again, symmetry can be more important than the mere presence of deformities.

THIGHS

- The lateral thigh surface should be smooth. The presence of a deep groove, running from the greater trochanter of the femur to the knee, suggests shortening and contracture of the IT band.

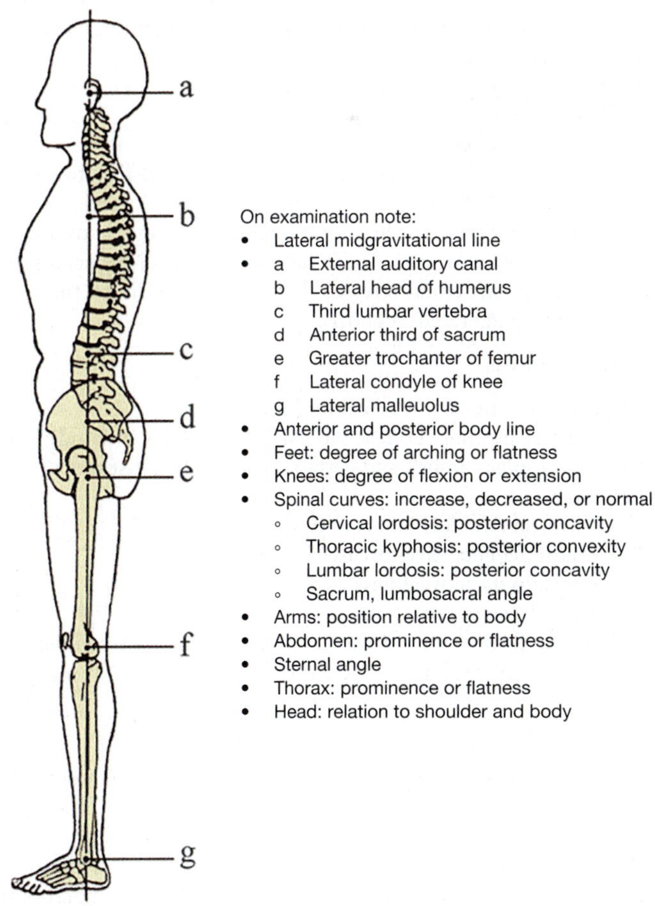

Figure 30.22. Lateral view of normal posture with midgravitational line. (Reprinted with permission from Nicholas AS, Nicholas EA. *Atlas of Osteopathic Techniques*. 3rd ed. Wolters Kluwer; 2016.)

PELVIS

- Anterior or posterior pelvic tilt is readily seen from the lateral aspect.

SPINAL CURVATURE AND GRAVITATIONAL LINE

The patient is standing. The physician stands to either side of the patient so as to have a posterolateral view, in order to gain the best sense of appreciation for the curves of the spine. Observe the spinal curves in the **lumbar, thoracic, and cervical** regions.

Lumbar Lordosis

- Observe for a normal lumbar lordotic curve.
- **Lordosis** is a curve in the spine in a sagittal plane with the convexity anterior. Some lordosis is normally present in the lumbar and cervical regions of the spine. Loss of the normal lumbar lordosis may be due to paravertebral muscle spasm, certain diseases such as ankylosing spondylitis, or somatic dysfunction in the lumbar, pelvic, or lower extremity regions.
- Excessive lumbar lordosis can occur in certain situations such as:
  - Pregnancy
  - Obesity
  - Certain diseases of the vertebrae
  - Certain spinal muscle diseases
  - Fixed flexion deformity of the hip
  - Anterior abdominal wall muscle weakness

Thoracic Kyphosis

- Observe for a normal thoracic kyphotic curve.
- **Kyphosis** is a curvature in the spine in the sagittal plane with the convexity posterior. If present, it is most commonly seen in the thoracic spine.
- Exaggerated kyphosis can result from:
  - Poor posture
  - Muscle imbalance
  - Certain bone diseases, such as osteoporosis and Paget disease
  - Certain medications, such as long-term steroid usage.
- Somatic dysfunction in the thoracic region, or somatic dysfunctions in other areas, such as the lumbar spine and pelvis, might also result in structural stresses that can contribute to the formation of exaggerated kyphosis.

Cervical Lordosis

- Observe for a normal cervical lordotic curve.
- Loss of the normal cervical lordosis can be seen in conditions such as whiplash injury and certain degenerative diseases of the vertebrae.
- Excessive cervical lordosis can occur with:
  - Certain degenerative diseases of the vertebrae
  - Cervical muscle weakness
  - Postural decompensations
  - Somatic dysfunction of the cervical spine, or as a compensatory mechanism for somatic dysfunction in other body regions.

SHOULDERS

- Assess for presence of anterior shoulder carriage or posterior carriage (posterior carriage has been referred to as a "military-type" posture).
- Anterior shoulder carriage with the scapula shifting superiorly and laterally will cause the acromion process to impinge upon the supraspinatus tendon. This can result in:
  - Subacromial bursitis
  - Rotator cuff tendonitis
  - Frozen shoulder (fibrous adhesive capsulitis)
  - Partial or total rupture of the supraspinatus portion of the rotator cuff

TABLE 30.2

Mid-Gravity Lines and Their Components

Mid-Gravity Line	Components
Posterior	• Mid-heel point • Gluteal crease • Spinous processes of the sacral, lumbar, thoracic, and cervical vertebrae • Inion
Anterior	• Mid-heel point • Pubic symphysis • Umbilicus • Xiphoid process • Midsternum • Episternal notch • Symphysis menti • Glabella
Lateral	• Lateral malleolus • Patella • Greater trochanter of the femur • Sacral promontory • Mid-body of L3 • Greater tuberosity of the humerus • Odontoid process of C2 • External auditory meatus

HEAD ALIGNMENT

Note the position of the head relative to the rest of the trunk.

Mid-Gravity Lines

- Components of the posterior mid-gravity, anterior mid-gravity, and lateral mid-gravity lines are shown in Table 30.2.

POSTERIOR MID-GRAVITY LINE

Instruct the patient to stand with their feet together. The medial line where the heels approximate each other is referred to as the "mid-heel point."

- The posterior mid-gravity line begins at a mid-heel point and passes directly through the:
  - Gluteal cleft
  - Spinous processes of the sacral, lumbar, thoracic and cervical vertebrae
  - Inion
- Assessment of body symmetry about this line makes readily apparent any:
  - Pelvic side shift
  - Minor scoliotic curves
  - Head tilt
- If the line is reversed and started instead at the inion, passing down through the spine, then other information can be gathered.
- In the presence of a scoliosis, no matter how severe, if it is a compensated curve, this plumb line will fall through the spinous process of S1.
- If decompensated, the plumb line will fall laterally to one side or the other.
- If the body as a whole has compensated for a decompensated or traumatic spinal curve, even when the plumb line does not fall mid-sacrum, it may still fall normally at the mid-heel point.

- If the body is unable to compensate for any deformity above the feet, the plumb line will fall off of the mid-heel point to one side or the other.
- Posturing, which relieves or minimizes pain in any part of the body, can also shift this plumb line off of the mid-heel point.

ANTERIOR MID-GRAVITY LINE

- The anterior mid-gravity line originates at the mid-heel point, and passes upward through the:
  - Pubic symphysis
  - Umbilicus
  - Xiphoid process
  - Midsternum
  - Suprasternal notch
  - Symphysis menti
  - Glabella
- Again, some truncal asymmetries and deformities are most visible from an anterior perspective, especially those involving the rib cage, jaw, and face.
- A plumb line hung from the glabella can be used similar to the way a plumb line from the inion is used.

LATERAL MID-GRAVITY LINE

- The normal lateral mid-gravity line (see Fig. 30.22) passes:
  - Just anterior to the lateral malleolus
  - Just posterior to the patella
  - Through the:
    - Greater trochanter of the femur
    - Sacral promontory
    - Midbody of L3
    - Greater tuberosity of the humerus
    - Odontoid process of C2
    - External auditory meatus
- However, the following landmarks; just anterior to the lateral malleolus, the greater trochanter, the acromion process, and the external auditory meatus may be the most easily visible and readily used to assess the lateral gravitational line in a clinical setting.
- Shifts in posture due to trauma, muscle imbalance, or repetitive poor ergonomics may cause deviations in the gravitational line.
- An extreme abnormality of this weight bearing occurs when all of the gravitational line landmarks are anterior to the lateral malleolus.
  - The patient may appear to be on the verge of falling forward and are often contracting every posterior truncal muscle they have to fight this gravitational tendency.
  - Often, such patients have had their sense of normal posture disrupted by some trauma and have come to accept this distorted posture as correct.
  - In addition to OMT, these patients will frequently require postural reeducation.
- The alignment of the lateral malleolus and greater trochanter, but not the knee may indicate the presence of knee flexion contracture or genu recurvatum.
- An increased lumbar lordosis may carry the points of L3 and the sacral promontory anteriorly, but leave all the other gravitational landmark points aligned. This is often due to:
  - A bilaterally flexed sacrum
  - Other anterior sacral dysfunctions
  - An extended dysfunction of the one or more of the lower lumbar vertebrae
  - Weak lower abdominal musculature
- In increased lumbar lordosis, sometimes referred to as "sway back" posture, typically the lateral malleolus and acromion or greater tuberosity of the humerus are aligned but all other gravitational landmarks are anterior to this line.
  - This posture is common during pregnancy due to the body accommodating for the growth of the fetus. However, post-delivery, this posture may persist and then become fixed. To avoid this fixation, abdominal strengthening exercises, OMT, and postural reeducation may be employed to restore normal physiologic posture.
- Increased thoracic kyphosis tends to shift all gravitational landmark points below the shoulder posterior to the weight-bearing line, except for the malleolar reference point.
  - Often, the head is carried anterior to the line for balance.
  - To a lesser degree, this is the same posture assumed by students while studying in a seated position.
- Anterior shift of the external auditory meatus may result in "forward head carriage" which places more stress on the suboccipital and posterior cervical musculature. This can lead to altered proprioceptive input of the musculature to the central nervous system which may ultimately lead to symptoms of dizziness, pain, lightheadedness, and headaches.[9]
  - Relearning to sit upright can correct this shift.
  - This can be assisted by raising the reading materials and propping them on something akin to a music stand.
    - These devices are commercially available.
    - Artists and draftsmen have long used tilt-top tables that relieve strain from the neck and shoulders and facilitate the upright seated position.
- Some physicians prefer to reference the lateral mid-gravity line to the external auditory meatus, rather than to the lateral malleolus. This changes the relative position of the landmarks for all conditions listed above but does not change the diagnoses.[10–12]

SCREENING RANGE-OF-MOTION TESTING

Head Region—Patient Seated or Standing

THE TEMPOROMANDIBULAR JOINT

The physician stands in front of the patient and places the pads of the index fingers on the sides of the patient's head, just anterior to the external auditory meatus (Figs. 30.23 and 30.24).

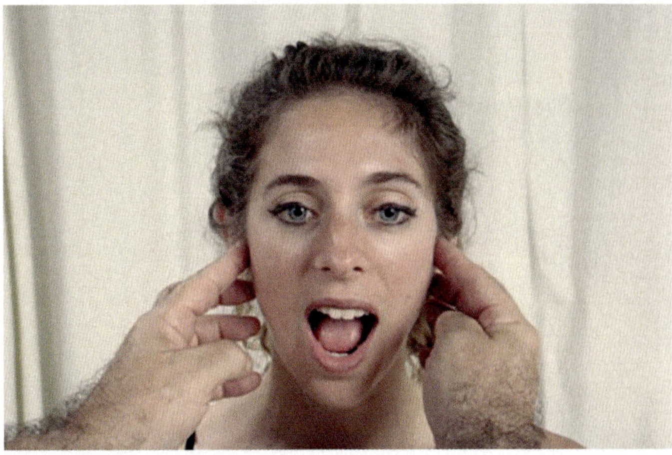

Figure 30.23. Palpation and observation of mandibular motion—anterior view. (Photo courtesy of Western University of Health Sciences, Pomona, CA, with permission.)

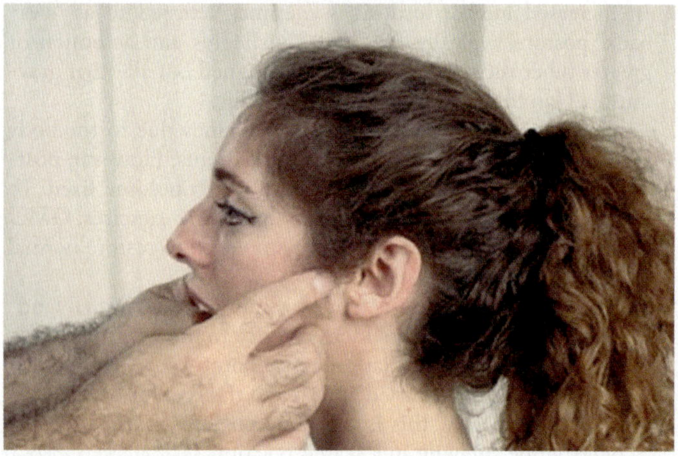

Figure 30.24. Palpation and observation of mandibular motion—lateral view. (Photo courtesy of Western University of Health Sciences, Pomona, CA, with permission.)

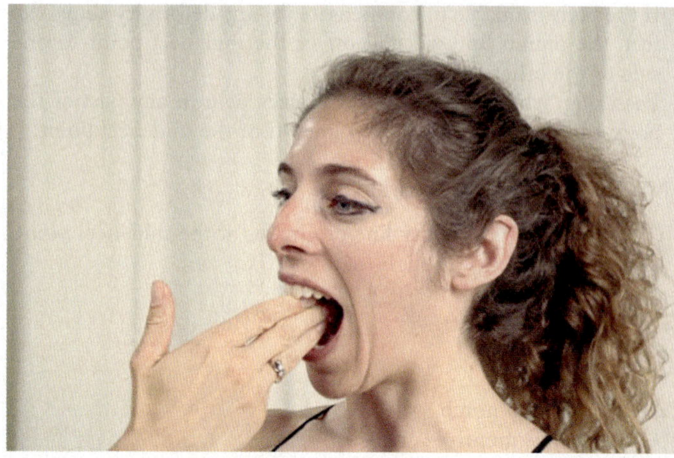

Figure 30.26. Clinical estimate of degree of jaw opening present. (Photo courtesy of Western University of Health Sciences, Pomona, CA, with permission.)

(Alternatively, the physician may stand behind the patient and place the pads of the index or little fingers into the external auditory meatus on each side of the patient's head, with the pads of the little fingers facing anteriorly, and the palmar surfaces pressing lightly anteriorly to contact the head of the mandible as it articulates with the temporomandibular fossa) (Fig. 30.25).

Physician asks the patient to slowly open and close the jaw several times and notes the following:

- Jaw opening: The normal range of jaw opening is around 40 to 50 mm. Alternatively, the physician can observe if the patient is able to fit three fingerbreadths between the front teeth (incisors), after opening the mouth as wide as possible (Fig. 30.26).
- Chin deviation: Note whether the chin deviates to one side or the other, either during opening or after having opened the jaw as far as comfortable.
- Crepitus and/or joint sounds: Note whether there is any crepitus (a peculiar crackling, crinkly, or grating feeling or sound under the skin, around the lungs, or in the joints), popping, clicking, or other joint sounds. In addition to being heard, crepitus, popping, or clicking of the TMJ may also be palpated.

Limitation in jaw opening, or deviation of the chin to one side on jaw opening, can be indicative of underlying TMJ dysfunction.

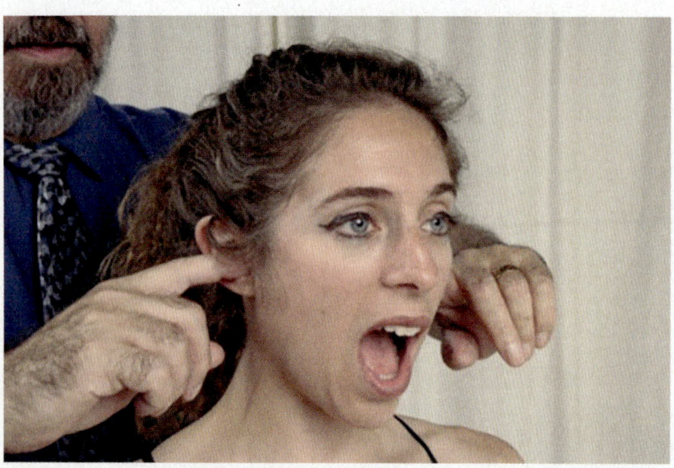

Figure 30.25. Palpation and observation of mandibular motion—alternative method. (Photo courtesy of Western University of Health Sciences, Pomona, CA, with permission.)

This may also indicate the possibility of related cranial or cervical somatic dysfunction. The presence of crepitus may be a sign of TMJ dysfunction and indicate cartilage wear in the joint space.

Upper Extremities Region—Patient Standing

OVERHEAD UPPER EXTREMITY QUICK TEST

This is a screening test for possible somatic dysfunction of the upper extremities. This is typically observed from the anterior vantage point.

- The patient can be standing or seated.
- The patient actively fully abducts both arms in the coronal plane over the head, first with the palms together and again with dorsal surfaces of the hands together (Fig. 30.27A and B).

The test is ***negative*** if the patient, with their head and neck in the neutral position, can raise the arms fully overhead, with the

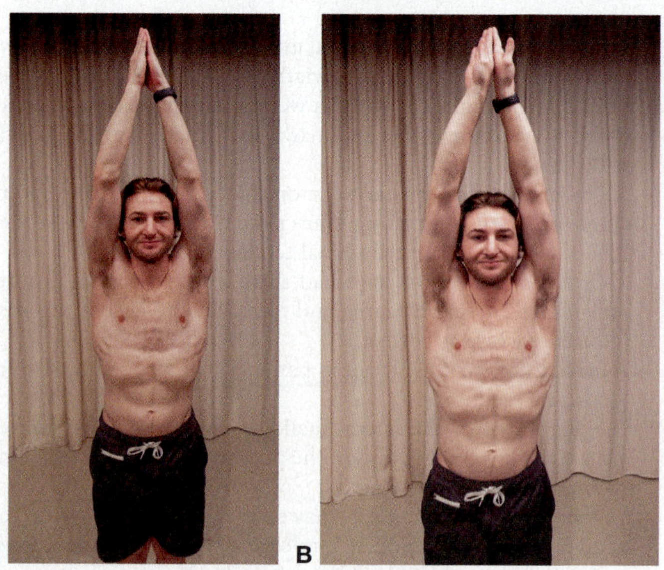

A B

Figure 30.27. A. Negative overhead upper extremity Quick test: arms abducted, palmar surfaces of hands together. (Photo courtesy of Western University of Health Sciences, Pomona, CA, with permission.) **B.** Negative overhead upper extremity Quick test: arms abducted, dorsal surfaces of hands together. (Photo courtesy of Western University of Health Sciences, Pomona, CA, with permission.)

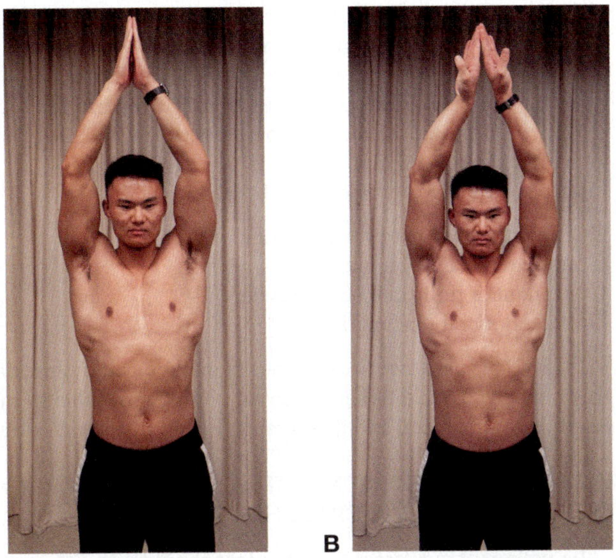

A B

Figure 30.28. **A.** Positive overhead upper extremity Quick test: arms abducted, palmar surfaces of hands together. (Photo courtesy of Western University of Health Sciences, Pomona, CA, with permission.) **B.** Positive overhead upper extremity Quick test: arms abducted, dorsal surfaces of hands together. (Photo courtesy of Western University of Health Sciences, Pomona, CA, with permission.)

medial surfaces of the upper arms touching the ears, the elbows fully extended, the forearms fully pronated, and the backs of the hands together over the head. When the test is repeated, the patient should be able to accomplish the same position with the forearms fully supinated and the palms together over the head. If the patient can do this, then somatic dysfunction of the joints of the shoulders, elbows, radioulnar regions, and wrists are not as likely to be present.

The test is ***positive*** if the patient is unable to bring the medial surfaces of the upper arms against their ears, the elbows and/or wrists cannot be fully extended, and/or the backs of the hands or palms of the hands cannot be placed together over the head. This indicates possible upper extremity somatic dysfunction and means that the joints and tissues of the upper extremity need to be more specifically examined for motion restriction and the presence of somatic dysfunction (Fig. 30.28A and B).

Somatic dysfunction of the upper extremity may also occur due to restricted motion of the acromioclavicular joint, sternoclavicular joint, clavicle, scapulae, upper ribs, upper thoracic region, and the large muscle groups of the shoulder. If the patient is having specific hand, wrist, or elbow pain or dysfunction, further evaluation to those areas should be done.

Lower Extremities Region—Patient Standing

SQUAT TEST

This test requires normal lower extremity muscle strength and bilateral mobility of the hips, knees, feet, and ankles. If the patient cannot perform this test, then further structural evaluation of the joints and tissues of the lower extremities is indicated (Fig. 30.29). A positive test would include the patient's heels lifting off of the floor in order to accomplish this maneuver and/or the patient being unable to bend the knees past 90 degrees.

- The patient is standing.
- The physician stands so as to have a posterolateral view of the patient.

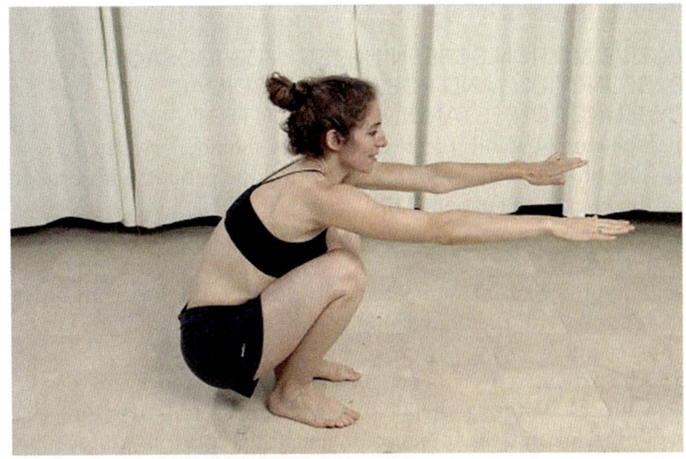

Figure 30.29. **Squat test.** Active range-of-motion screening test for lower extremities. Negative test is when the knees can fully flex with the heels flat on the ground as depicted. (Photo courtesy of Western University of Health Sciences, Pomona, CA, with permission.)

- The patient is instructed to raise their arms 90 degrees, as though reaching toward the wall in front of them.
- The patient squats down as far as possible, maintaining the feet flat on the floor, and then returns to the standing position.

The Hip Drop Test

The hip drop test is performed to screen for sidebending/passive range of motion in the lumbar region. It is interpreted as passive motion since the lumbar spine spontaneously responds to an artificially produced sacral base declination:

- The standing patient flexes one knee, allowing the pelvis to drop on that side of the body (Fig. 30.30A and B). A positive test is indicated by the inability of the lumbar spine to sidebend and is named for the side of the flexed knee (Fig. 30.30B indicates a positive left hip drop test.).
- From a posterior vantage point, the physician observes for symmetry of range and quality of motion. Many lower extremity conditions can interfere with this test, such as inflexible knees, a hypertonic IT band and/or the inability to dorsiflex the ankle.

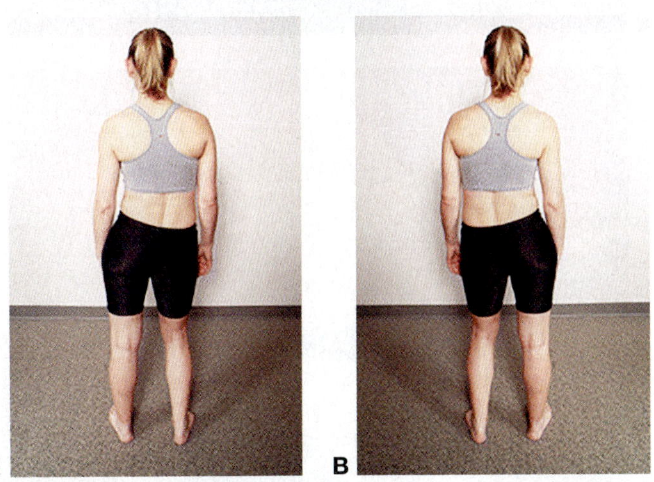

A B

Figure 30.30. **A** and **B.** Hip drop test to assess for lumbar spine sidebending range of motion. **A.** Right hip drop assesses for compensatory left lumbar sidebending. **B.** Left hip drop assesses for compensatory right lumbar sidebending. (Reprinted with permission from Nicholas AS, Nicholas EA. *Atlas of Osteopathic Techniques*. 3rd ed. Wolters Kluwer; 2016.)

Pelvic Region Screening

ACTIVE MOTION SCREENING TEST FOR ILIOSACRAL DYSFUNCTION (AND POSSIBLY SACROILIAC DYSFUNCTION): STANDING FLEXION TEST

1. The patient stands erect with the feet shoulder-width apart.
2. The physician stands or kneels behind the patient, with eyes at the level of the patient's PSISs (Fig. 30.31A).
3. The physician's thumbs are placed on the inferior slope of the PSISs.
4. The physician maintains a firm contact on the PSISs in order to move with the bony landmarks, and not shift due to skin or fascial drag.
5. The patient actively bends forward, trying to touch the toes.
   Clinical Note: If the iliac crest heights, and therefore the PSISs, are unlevel, it is recommended that prior to performing a standing flexion test, a shim be placed under the heel of the foot on the side of the inferior iliac crest in order to make the iliac crests and PSISs level. This is done to avoid false-positive or false-negative results from this test or difficulties in trying to perform and interpret the test.[13,14]
6. The test is positive when asymmetry of the PSIS's excursions occurs during and/or at the end of active forward bending. The side of a positive test is the one where the thumb on the PSIS moves at least one thumb breadth more superiorly and anteriorly at the end range of motion as compared to the other side, indicating the side of likely iliosacral dysfunction (Fig. 30.31B).

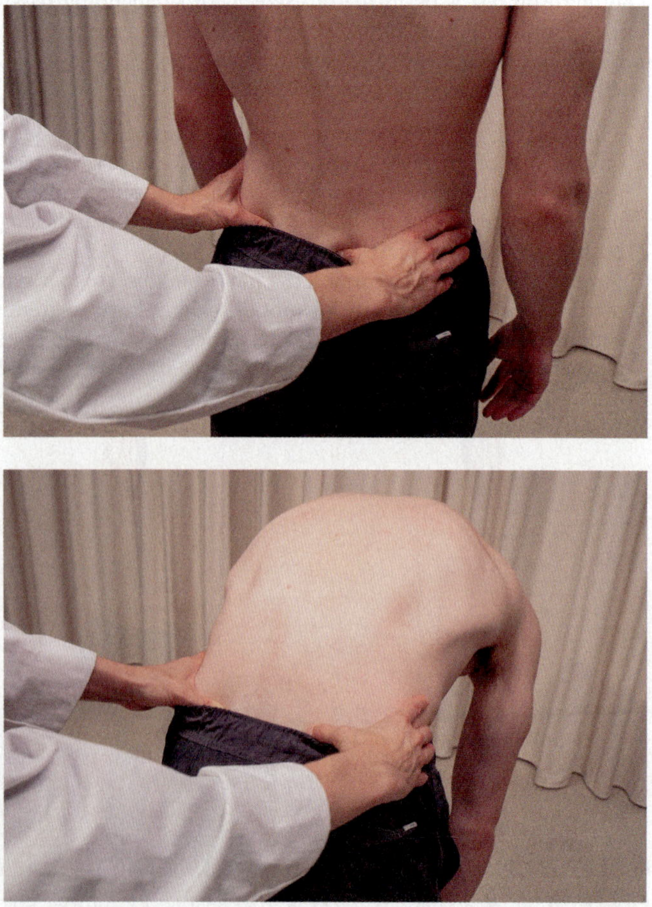

A

B

Figure 30.31. **A.** Palpating the PSISs for the standing flexion test. (Photo courtesy of Western University of Health Sciences, Pomona, CA, with permission.) **B.** Positive right standing flexion test. (Photo courtesy of Western University of Health Sciences, Pomona, CA, with permission.)

- ☐ Normally, the sacrum moves anteriorly and superiorly along with the lumbar spine during forward bending, and the innominates maintain relative stability and levelness. If one of the iliosacral joints is not functioning properly, the sacrum and innominate move together anteriorly/superiorly along with the lumbar spine.

A false-positive test can be created by a:

- Leg-length discrepancy >½ inch
- Contralateral tight hamstring
- Contralateral tight iliopsoas muscle
- Unilateral sacral dysfunction

If this test is negative, the presence of an iliosacral dysfunction is highly unlikely. An additional screen for short leg or other dysfunctions of the lumbosacral and iliosacral regions is the pelvic side shift.

PASSIVE MOTION SCREENING TEST FOR ILIOSACRAL DYSFUNCTION: PELVIC SIDE SHIFT TEST

1. The patient stands erect with the feet shoulder-width apart.
2. The physician stands behind the patient.
3. The physician places one hand on the patient's iliac crest and the other on the opposite deltoid/shoulder area.
4. The physician gently pushes the iliac crest/pelvis laterally (translates) to the opposite side, utilizing the hand on the patient's deltoid/shoulder to stabilize the thoracic spinal segments. The ease and amount of motion is noted.
5. The physician switches hand positions and introduces motion to the opposite direction comparing the two.
6. A positive pelvic side shift reveals freer translation to the side of the side shift and is named for that direction. The sacrum (base of support) is positioned on the side of the freer motion and may indicate a possible long leg to the side of, and/or a tight psoas muscle to the opposite side of the pelvic side shift.

Sacral Region—Patient Seated

ACTIVE MOTION SCREENING TEST FOR UNILATERAL SACRAL DYSFUNCTION: SEATED FLEXION TEST

1. The patient is seated on a low stool or on the side of a treatment table, with feet touching the floor.
2. The physician stands or kneels behind the patient, with eyes at the level of the patient's PSISs.
3. The physician's thumbs are positioned on the inferior slopes of the PSISs.

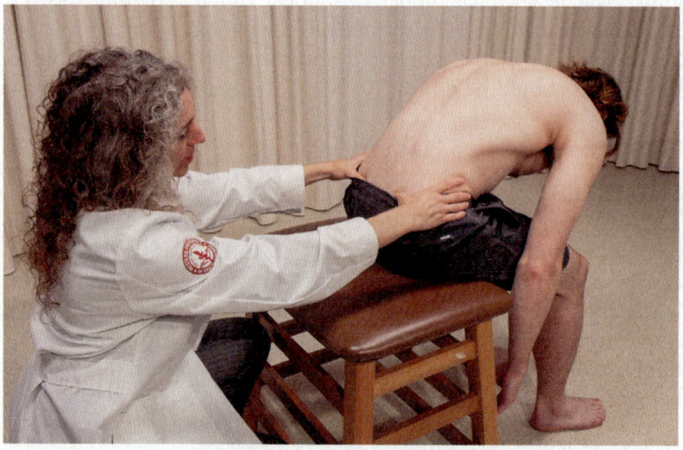

Figure 30.32. **Positive right seated flexion test.** (Photo courtesy of Western University of Health Sciences, Pomona, CA, with permission.)

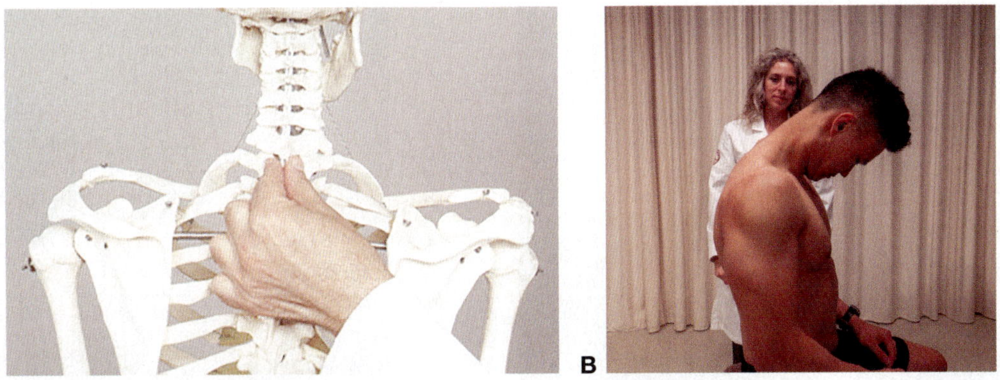

A B

Figure 30.33. **A.** Using a skeleton model, physician demonstrates hand placement so thumb and forefinger pads palpate between the spinous processes of C7 and T1 in order to assess cervical flexion–extension ranges of motion. (Reprinted with permission from Nicholas AS, Nicholas EA. *Atlas of Osteopathic Techniques.* 3rd ed. Wolters Kluwer; 2016.) **B.** Cervical active range-of-motion assessment—flexion. Physician stands at side of patient and may palpate C7–T1 or observe the motion. (Photo courtesy of Western University of Health Sciences, Pomona, CA, with permission.)

4. The patient bends forward as far as possible (Fig. 30.32).
5. A positive test is one where the PSIS moves more superiorly by at least one thumb breadth at the end of the range of motion as compared to the other side. Potential dysfunctions here include anterior and posterior torsions, and unilateral flexed and extended sacrum.[13]

At this point in the osteopathic structural examination, the osteopathic physician has assessed static landmarks for asymmetry with observation and where needed, palpation. Key regions have also been assessed grossly with active range of motion to determine if these regions warrant further evaluation.

ACTIVE RANGE-OF-MOTION TESTING

The next component of the screening portion of the exam is the active range-of-motion exam of the axial spine. The patient will be instructed to actively flex, extend, sidebend and rotate the cervical, thoracic, and lumbar spine. Note the following when performing this segment of the exam:

1. Any region with diminished range of motion is abnormal.
2. Any region with increased range of motion is abnormal and may be compensating for an adjacent area that is hypomobile.
3. For the paired motions of sidebending and rotation, any left-to-right asymmetry is abnormal, even if the overall range of motion is normal.

Cervical Region

The patient may be standing or seated on a fixed-legged stool with foot support or straddling the examination table.

- To localize the cervical spine motion in flexion, extension, sidebending, and rotation the physician should observe the motion from the occiput to T1. Active motion testing can be localized to the region by palpating just below the region and telling the patient when to stop, that is, when the next region, in this case, the thoracic region at T1, begins to move. To facilitate this, the physician may monitor the T1 vertebra. For flexion, the physician stands to one side of the patient and asks the patient to try to touch their chin to the chest. The patient then returns to the neutral position (Fig. 30.33A and B).
- For extension, the patient is asked to tilt their head backward as far as is comfortably possible and look toward the ceiling (Fig. 30.34).
- For sidebending the physician stands behind or in front of the patient and asks the patient to try to touch their left ear to the left shoulder, return to neutral, and then try to touch their right ear to the right shoulder (Fig. 30.35A). For these motions, the physician is observing individual segmental articulation versus vertebral units moving as a group.
- To observe rotation, the physician stands posterior to the patient (Fig. 30.35B), and then asks the patient to turn their head as far as is comfortably possible to the left, return to neutral, and then turn the head in the same manner toward the right The physician may also monitor at the C7–T1 junction while observing the active range of motion of sidebending and rotation from the posterior vantage point to ensure that range of motion is limited to that specific region (Fig. 30.35C).

Active range-of-motion values vary greatly depending on the manner in which it is measured and the age of the patient.

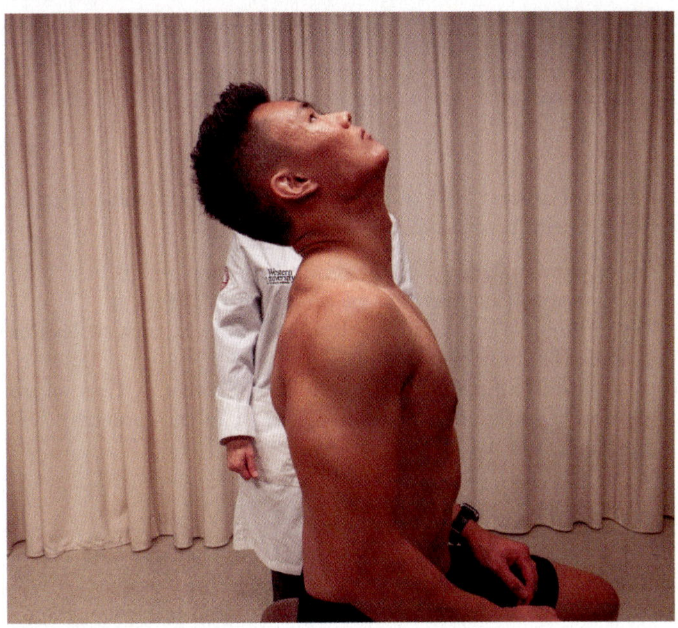

Figure 30.34. Cervical active range-of-motion assessment—extension. Physician stands at side of patient and may palpate C7–T1 or observe the motion. (Photo courtesy of Western University of Health Sciences, Pomona, CA, with permission.)

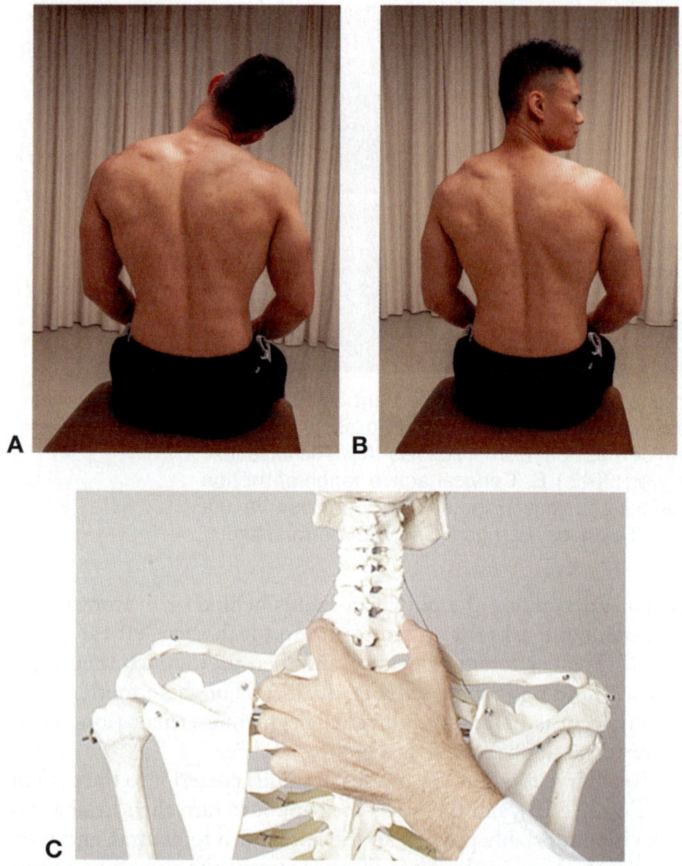

Figure 30.35. A. Cervical active range-of-motion assessment—sidebending. Physician stands at side of patient and may palpate C7-T1 or observe the motion. (Photo courtesy of Western University of Health Sciences, Pomona, CA, with permission.) **B.** Cervical active range-of-motion assessment—rotation. Physician stands at side of patient and may palpate C7–T1 or observe the motion. (Photo courtesy of Western University of Health Sciences, Pomona, CA, with permission.) **C.** Using a skeleton model, physician demonstrates hand placement so thumb and forefinger pads palpate over the intertransverse spaces bilaterally between C7 and T1 in order to assess cervical side bending and rotation ranges of motion. (Reprinted with permission from Nicholas AS, Nicholas EA. *Atlas of Osteopathic Techniques*. 3rd ed. Wolters Kluwer; 2016.)

Loss of around 50% of rotation in the cervical spine may be associated with several types of dysfunctions:

- Since approximately 50% of cervical rotation occurs at C1 on C2, a dysfunction may thus be present at this level.
- Hypertonic spasm of a long restrictor muscle, such as levator scapulae or sternocleidomastoid
- A group dysfunction of all joints from C2 to C7. Less severe motion losses are typically due to one or more segmental dysfunctions from C2 to C7.

Thoracic Region

The patient may be standing or seated comfortably on the examination table or stool.

To localize the upper thoracic spine motion in flexion, extension, sidebending, and rotation the physician should observe the motion from T1 to T4. To facilitate this, the physician may monitor the T4 vertebra until motion is palpated there for each range of motion tested.

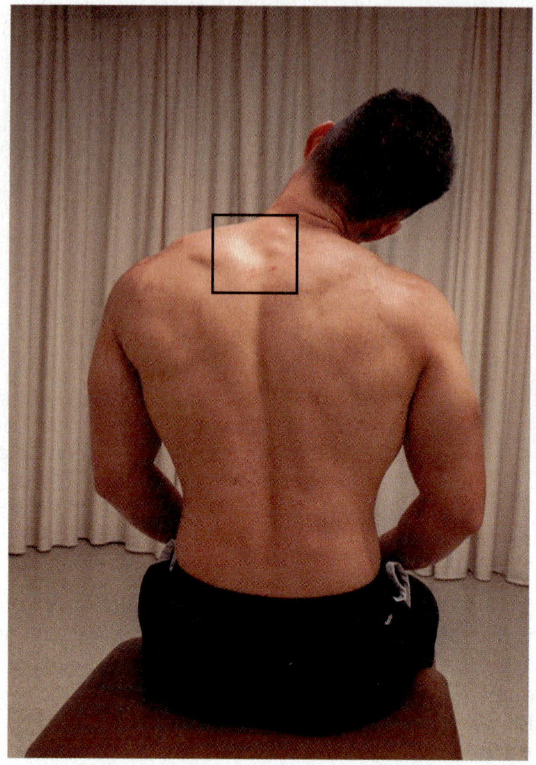

Figure 30.36. Observation of active range of motion of T1–T4. Note that the physician is observing the motion of the area in the box.

- For flexion, the physician stands to one side of the patient and asks the patient to try to touch their chin to the chest. The patient then returns to the neutral position.
- For extension, the patient is asked to tilt their head backward as far as is comfortably possible and look toward the ceiling.
- For sidebending the physician stands behind the patient and asks the patient to try to touch their left ear to the left shoulder, return to neutral, and then try to touch their right ear to the right shoulder. For flexion, extension, and sidebending, the physician is observing the region for individual segmental articulation versus vertebral units moving as a group.
- To observe rotation, the physician stands behind the patient and then asks the patient to turn their head as far as is comfortably possible to the left, then return to neutral, and then turn the head in the same manner toward the right. These active ranges of motion will look very similar to Figures 30.33B, 30.34, and 30.35A and B except that the observational focus will be on the motion of T1–T4. See Figure 30.36.

To localize the lower thoracic spine motion in flexion, extension, sidebending, and rotation the physician should observe the motion from T5 to T12. To facilitate this, the physician may monitor the T12 vertebra. For flexion and extension, the physician observes the motion from a lateral vantage point.

- The patient is asked to bend their head forward slowly and continue the forward bending until the physician notes motion at the T12 vertebra (Fig. 30.37). The patient then returns to the neutral position.
- To observe extension, the patient is asked to raise their chin and look toward the ceiling, and to continue this motion into the thoracic spine (instructions such as "push your belly forward" or "allow your back to arch" may be helpful to the patient) until the physician notes motion at the T12 vertebra (Fig. 30.38).

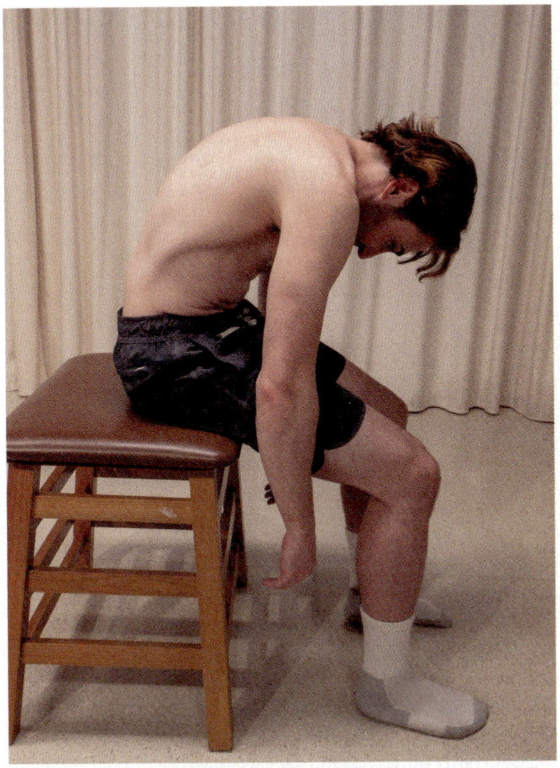

Figure 30.37. Observation of active range of motion of the lower thoracic spine (T5–T12) in flexion. (Photo courtesy of Western University of Health Sciences, Pomona, CA, with permission.)

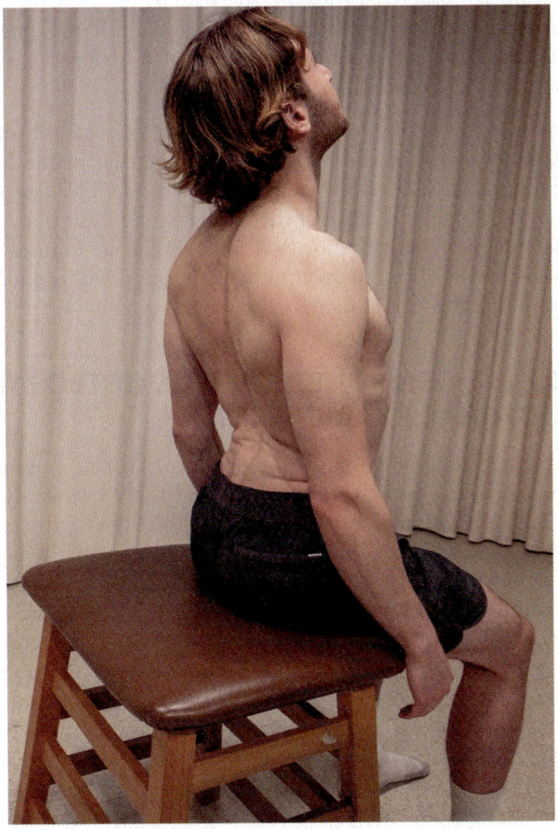

Figure 30.38. Observation of active range of motion of the lower thoracic spine (T5-T12) in extension. (Photo courtesy of Western University of Health Sciences, Pomona, CA, with permission.)

For these motions, the examiner notes the degree of movement, the smoothness of the motion, and whether there is any deviation of the thoracic and/or lumbar spine to the left or right. Generally, there are about 50 degrees of flexion[15] and about 10 degrees of extension in the thoracic spine.

To observe sidebending, the physician stands behind the patient and asks the patient to sit erect with their arms at their sides and their fingertips pointing toward the floor.

- The patient is then instructed to sidebend to one side by slowly moving their hand toward the floor. The patient sidebends without moving into flexion or extension and continues this motion until the physician observes or palpates motion at the T12 vertebra.

The degree of movement and the smoothness of the motion can be compared from side to side. The normal amount of combined sidebending motion in the thoracic spine is about 30 degrees to each side.

For flexion, extension, and sidebending, the physician is observing the region for individual segmental articulation versus vertebral units moving as a group (Fig. 30.39A and B).

- Rotation is observed by asking the patient to cross their arms in front and turn the trunk to one side until the physician notes motion at the T12 vertebra. This process is then repeated to the other side.

Again, observe the amount and smoothness of the motion from side to side. The normal amount of rotation in the thoracic spine varies greatly depending on the study and the region of the thoracic spine examined, but a general range is 30 to 55[15] degrees to each side (Fig. 30.40A and B).

Lumbar Region

To localize the lumbar spine motion in flexion, extension, sidebending, and rotation the physician should observe the motion from T12 to lumbosacral junction. To facilitate this, the physician may monitor the lumbosacral junction.

- For flexion, the physician stands to one side of the patient ensuring a lateral view of the lumbar spine and asks the patient to bend their head forward slowly and continue the forward bending until the physician notes motion at the lumbosacral junction. If seated, the patient's hips should not lift off the stool. The patient then returns to the neutral position.
- To observe extension, the patient is asked to raise their chin and look toward the ceiling, and to continue this motion into the lumbar spine until the physician notes motion at the lumbosacral junction.

The examiner notes the degree of movement, the smoothness of the motion, and whether there is any deviation of the lumbar and/or lumbar spine to the left or right during both lumbar flexion and extension.

There are generally about 40 to 50[16] degrees of flexion and about 20 to 25[16] degrees of extension in the lumbar spine.

- To observe sidebending, the physician stands behind the patient and asks the patient to sit erect with their arms at the sides and their fingertips pointing toward the floor.
- The patient is then instructed to sidebend to one side by slowly moving their hand down their lateral thigh toward the floor. The patient sidebends without moving into flexion or extension.

The degree of movement and the smoothness of the motion can be compared from side to side. The normal amount of

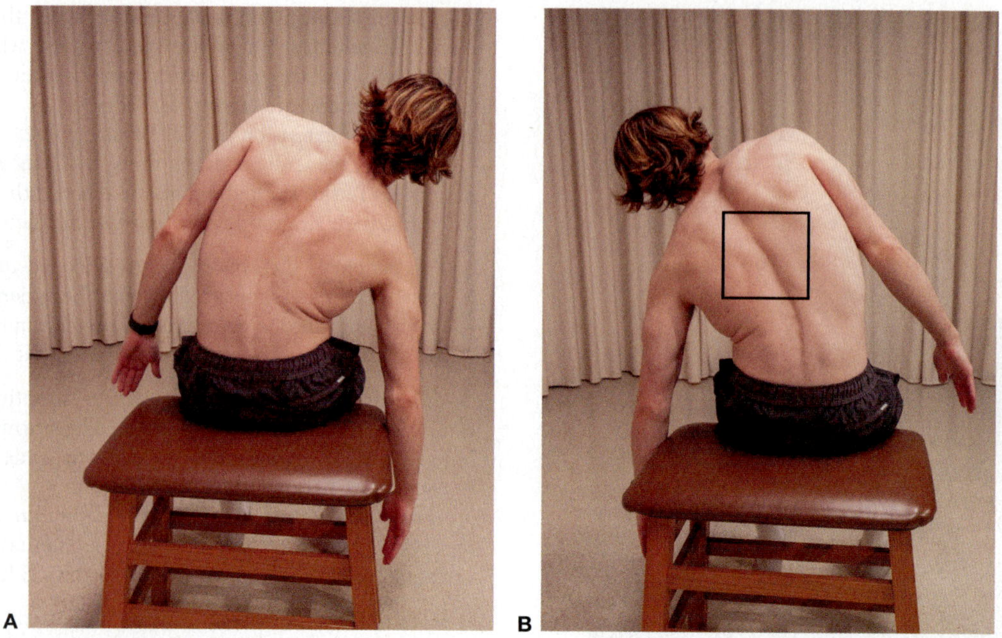

Figure 30.39. A. Observation of active range of motion of the lower thoracic spine (T5–T12) in right sidebending. Note the arc or curve made by the lumbar spine through the lower thoracic spine as it appears that each segment is able to articulate individually into right sidebending. Contrast this with Figure 30.39B where there is a flattening of this curve with respect to left sidebending. (Photo courtesy of Western University of Health Sciences, Pomona, CA, with permission.) **B.** Observation of active range of motion of the lower thoracic spine (T5–T12) in left sidebending. Note the flattening of the curve of the lower thoracic spine (indicated by the box) where it appears that these segments are moving more as a group as compared to right sidebending. (Photo courtesy of Western University of Health Sciences, Pomona, CA, with permission.)

combined sidebending motion in the lumbar spine is about 30 to 45[16] degrees to each side. Note where the sidebending occurs. There should be an "arc" of motion during sidebending. Restriction may cause a "hinge" at a certain level or a straight line instead of a rounded arc.

- For flexion, extension, and sidebending, the physician observes individual segmental articulation versus vertebral units moving as a group.

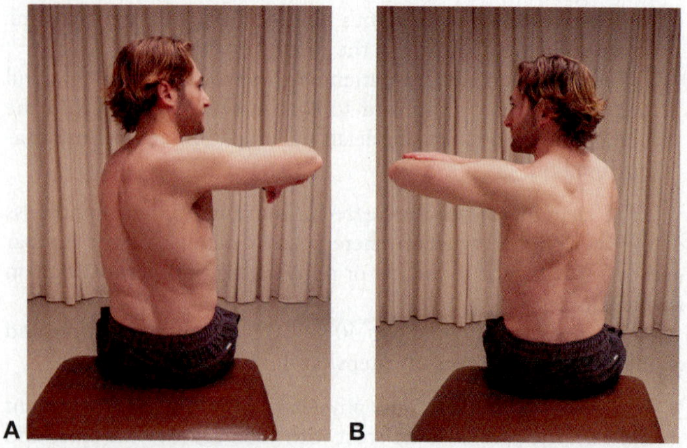

Figure 30.40. A. Observation of active range of motion of the lower thoracic spine (T5–T12) in right rotation. (Photo courtesy of Western University of Health Sciences, Pomona, CA, with permission.) **B.** Observation of active range of motion of the lower thoracic spine (T5–T12) in left rotation. Note that left rotation is diminished as compared to right rotation. (Photo courtesy of Western University of Health Sciences, Pomona, CA, with permission.)

- Rotation is observed by asking the patient to cross their arms in front and turn the trunk to one side until the physician notes motion at the lumbosacral junction. This process is then repeated to the other side.

Again, observe the amount and smoothness of the motion from side to side. The normal amount of rotation in the lumbar spine ranges from 12[17] to 33[16] degrees to each side. The assessment of the active range of motion of the lumbar spine in flexion, extension, sidebending, and rotation will look similar to Figures 30.37 to 30.40A and B with the exception that motion will occur to the level of the lumbosacral junction.

REGIONAL COMPONENT OF THE OSTEOPATHIC STRUCTURAL EXAMINATION

The screening component of the osteopathic structural examination asks the question, "Is there a problem?" The above examination for asymmetry and assessment for general restriction of range of motion may reveal findings that indicate the presence of somatic dysfunction. The next question is "Where is the problem?" It is important to assess the body or variations in temperature, tissue texture abnormalities, and tenderness. This may lead the physician to a particular region or regions to assess for quality range of motion. For example, if a positive hip drop test was noted along with restriction of active range of motion of the lumbar region, it is now important to palpate along the axial spine for tissue texture abnormalities, tenderness, and paravertebral fullness to determine if the findings are due to an issue with the lumbar spine itself or another region. If the lumbar spine is felt to be the source of the problem, this region may now be assessed for quality of motion to determine where within the lumbar region the source of the issue may be.

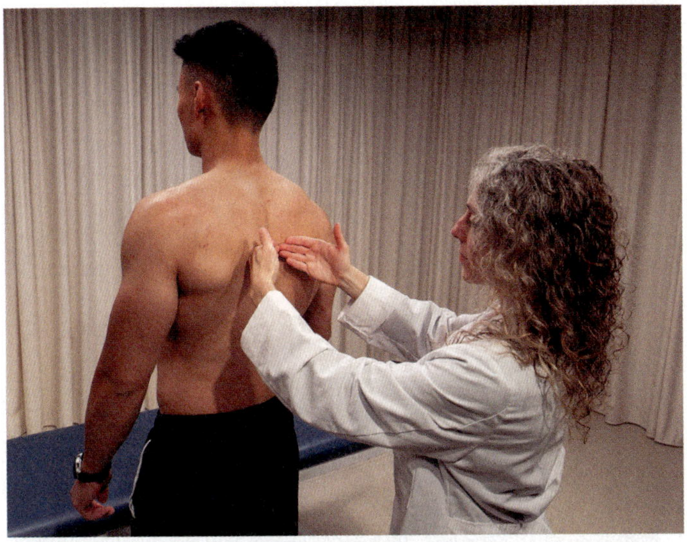

Figure 30.41. One method of assessing temperature during the regional portion of the osteopathic structural exam. (Photo courtesy of Western University of Health Sciences, Pomona, CA, with permission.)

Palpation for temperature variations, tissue texture abnormalities, and tenderness:

- This portion of the osteopathic screening exam can be accomplished in different ways.

One method may be the following:

Temperature Assessment:

- With the patient seated or standing, the physician stands behind the patient.
- The physician brings the dorsum of their hands close to the patient's skin of the T5–T6 region until the warmth is detected.
- Maintaining the same distance away from the surface of the patient's skin, the physician will then slowly move their hands superiorly to the cervical region, then inferiorly to the lumbosacral region, and then laterally on either side of the spine assessing for variations in temperature.

An area of increased warmth may indicate a sign of increased metabolism such as trauma (fracture) and/or infection (osteomyelitis, pneumonia) (Fig. 30.41).

Assessment for Tissue Texture Change and Tenderness:

- With the patient seated or standing, the physician may stand slightly behind the patient.
- The physician stabilizes the patient's right shoulder with their right hand and uses the left hand to palpate the right paraspinal cervical musculature starting at the suboccipital region.
- At the cervicothoracic junction, the physician continues to use the left hand to palpate the left paraspinal musculature and tissues all the way to the lumbosacral region.
- The physician then assesses the opposite side in a similar manner.

The physician is assessing the tissues for the following: hypotonicity, hypertonicity, atrophy, hypertrophy, ropiness, bogginess, dryness, excessive moisture and noting the spinal levels at which these occur. At the same time, the physician may ask if any of these areas are tender upon palpation or ask the patient to report tenderness as they palpate (Fig. 30.42A–C).

Quality of Motion Testing:

If any areas of the spine are found to be the source of the problem, they can now be assessed with passive motion to determine

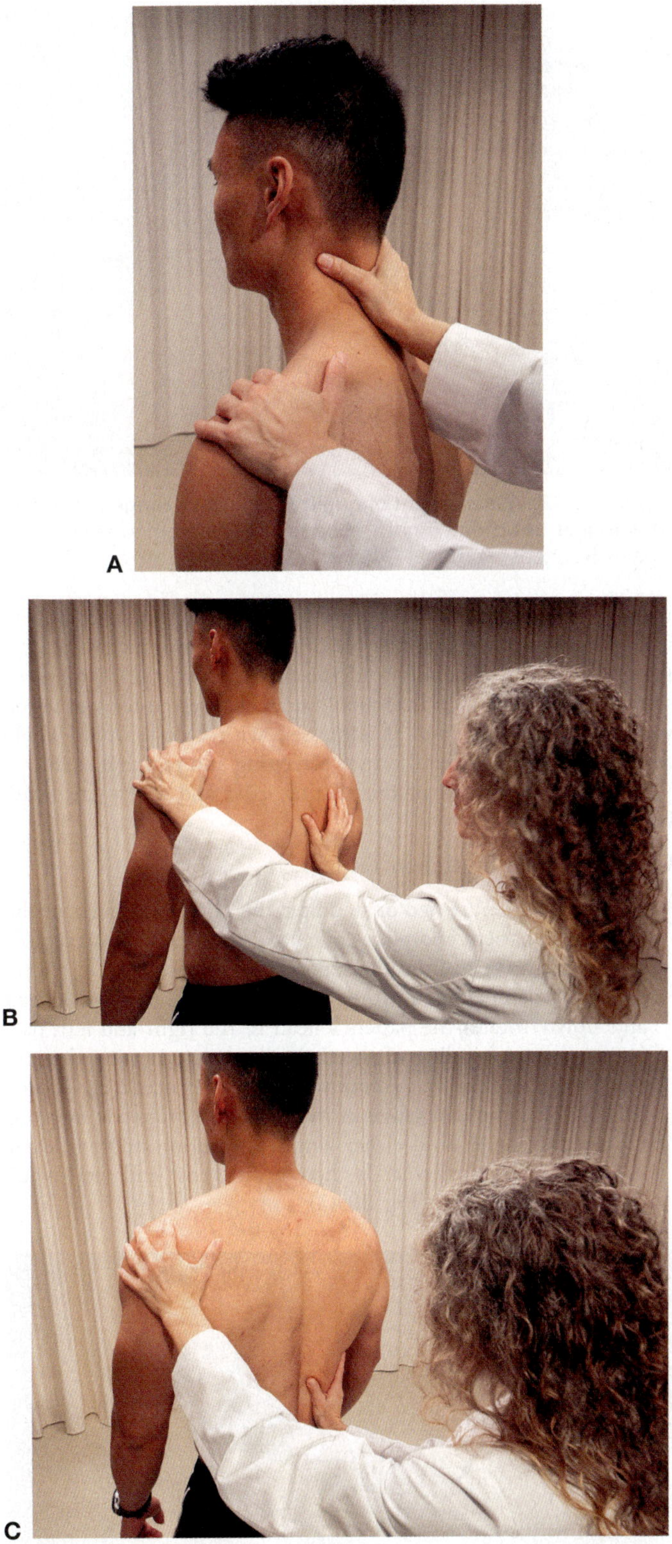

Figure 30.42. A, B, and C: These figures demonstrate the palpatory component of the regional exam in which the physician assesses for tissue texture changes and tenderness. A. The physician begins the palpation of the tissues at the suboccipital region and then continues down the length of the spine to the lumbosacral region as shown in Figures 30.42B and C. (Photo courtesy of Western University of Health Sciences, Pomona, CA, with permission.)

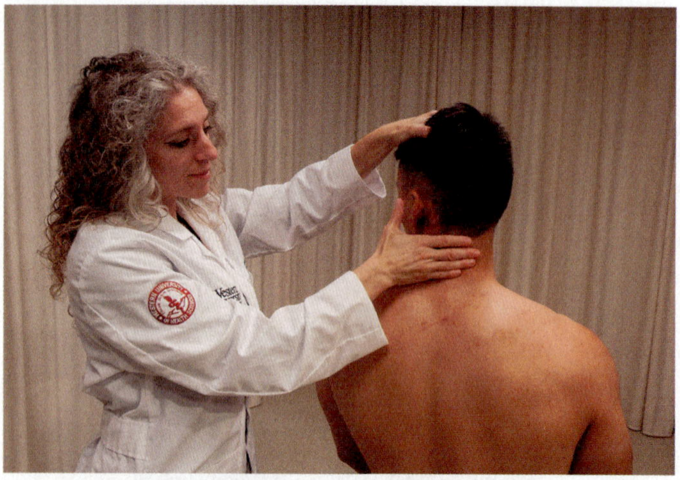

Figure 30.43. Assessment of quality or passive range of motion of cervical rotation. (Photo courtesy of Western University of Health Sciences, Pomona, CA, with permission.)

if the segments are moving individually or as a group and if there is any binding of the musculature or ligamentous structures of the region. This will generally lead the physician to the segment or segments of that region that should now be assessed for segmental somatic dysfunction, and if addressed with OMT, would likely resolve the findings found on the screening and regional exam.

Different methods of this testing exist and a few are listed below.

Cervical Quality of Motion Testing:

- With the patient seated or standing, the physician stands at the side of the patient and places one hand over the cervical region, attempting to span from the suboccipital region to T1.
- The physician places the other hand on top of the patient's head and slowly rotates the patient's head to the right and left, palpating for any binding of the tissues and determining the end feel. Is the motion free, smooth with binding occurring appropriately near the end range of motion in a symmetric fashion? Or do the tissues bind either within the region or from levels superior or inferior to it? Is there a different "end feel" when comparing the sides? (Fig. 30.43)

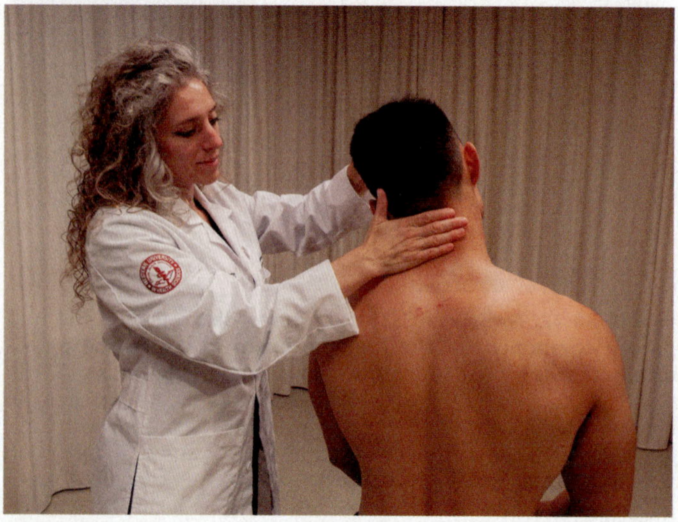

Figure 30.44. Assessment of quality or passive range of motion of cervical sidebending. (Photo courtesy of Western University of Health Sciences, Pomona, CA, with permission.)

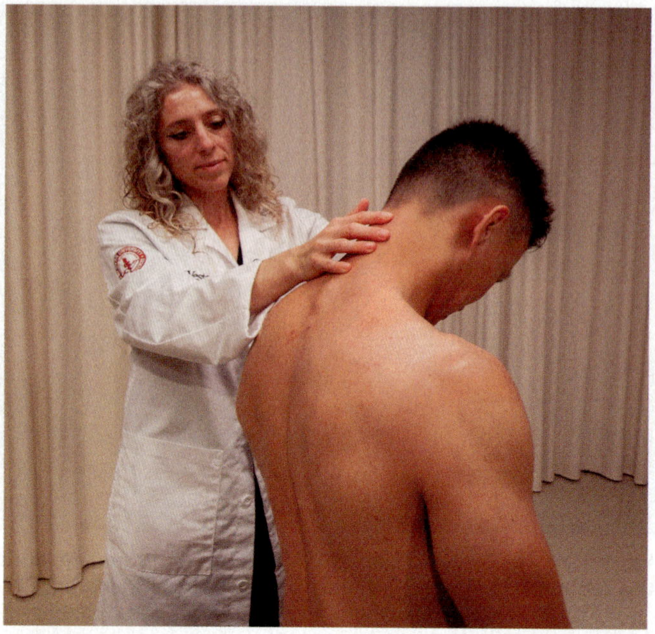

A

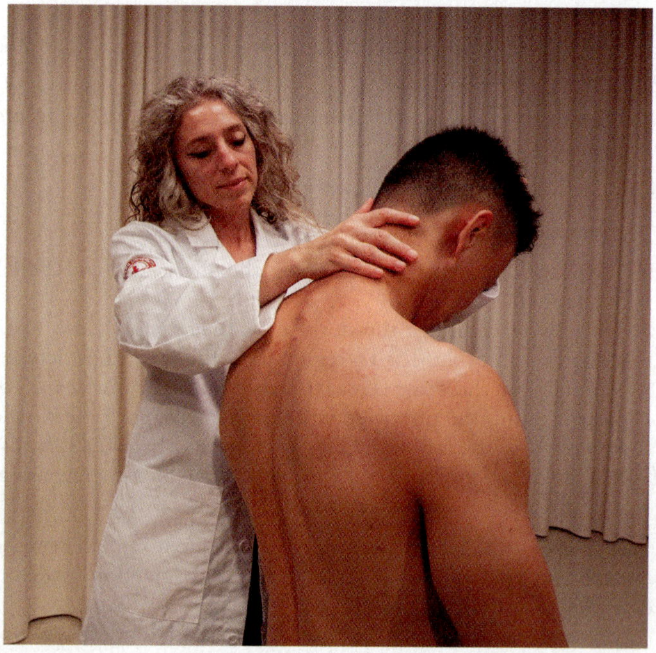

B

Figure 30.45. A and B: Figures A and B demonstrate assessment of quality or passive range of motion of flexion of the cervical spine. A depicts the physician attempting to assess the individual vertebrae while **B** depicts a broader contact over the cervical spine. (Photo courtesy of Western University of Health Sciences, Pomona, CA, with permission.)

- The same is repeated with the physician moving the patient into passive sidebending to the right and left and then into flexion and extension (Fig. 30.44). With flexion and extension, the physician may also choose to place their finger pads on individual spinous processes to determine if the spinous processes are gapping during flexion and approximating during extension appropriately (Figs. 30.45A and B and 30.46).

Thoracic Quality of Motion Testing:

- Passive motion testing of the upper versus the lower thoracic spine can be used to isolate areas that are perhaps related to

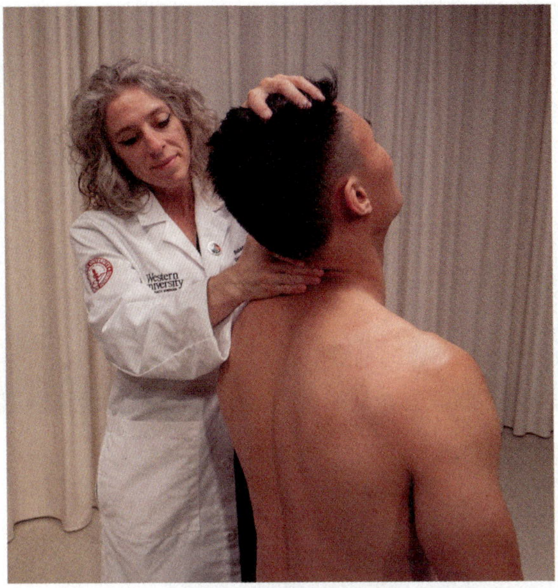

Figure 30.46. Assessment of quality or passive range of motion of the cervical extension. (Photo courtesy of Western University of Health Sciences, Pomona, CA, with permission.)

head and shoulder mechanics versus shoulder or low back and pelvis mechanics, respectively.

Upper Thoracic Region:

- The steps above for assessing the cervical region are repeated except that the physician is now palpating the region from T1 to about T4. The physician uses the head and neck as a lever by placing one hand on the patient's head and induces passive rotation, sidebending and flexion, and extension, palpating for the same qualities as listed above (Fig. 30.47A–D).

Lower Thoracic Region:

The steps above are repeated except that the physician is now monitoring the region from about T5–T12 with one hand.

- The physician now utilizes the trunk as a lever by placing the other arm across the patient's chest, contacting the patient's opposite shoulder and their axilla over the patient's ipsilateral shoulder. The physician's elbow should be in the region of the patient's sternum and the patient is instructed to hold onto the physician's arm or elbow with their hands.
- The physician maintains the patient over their center of gravity throughout the assessment to allow as much relaxation of the musculature as possible.

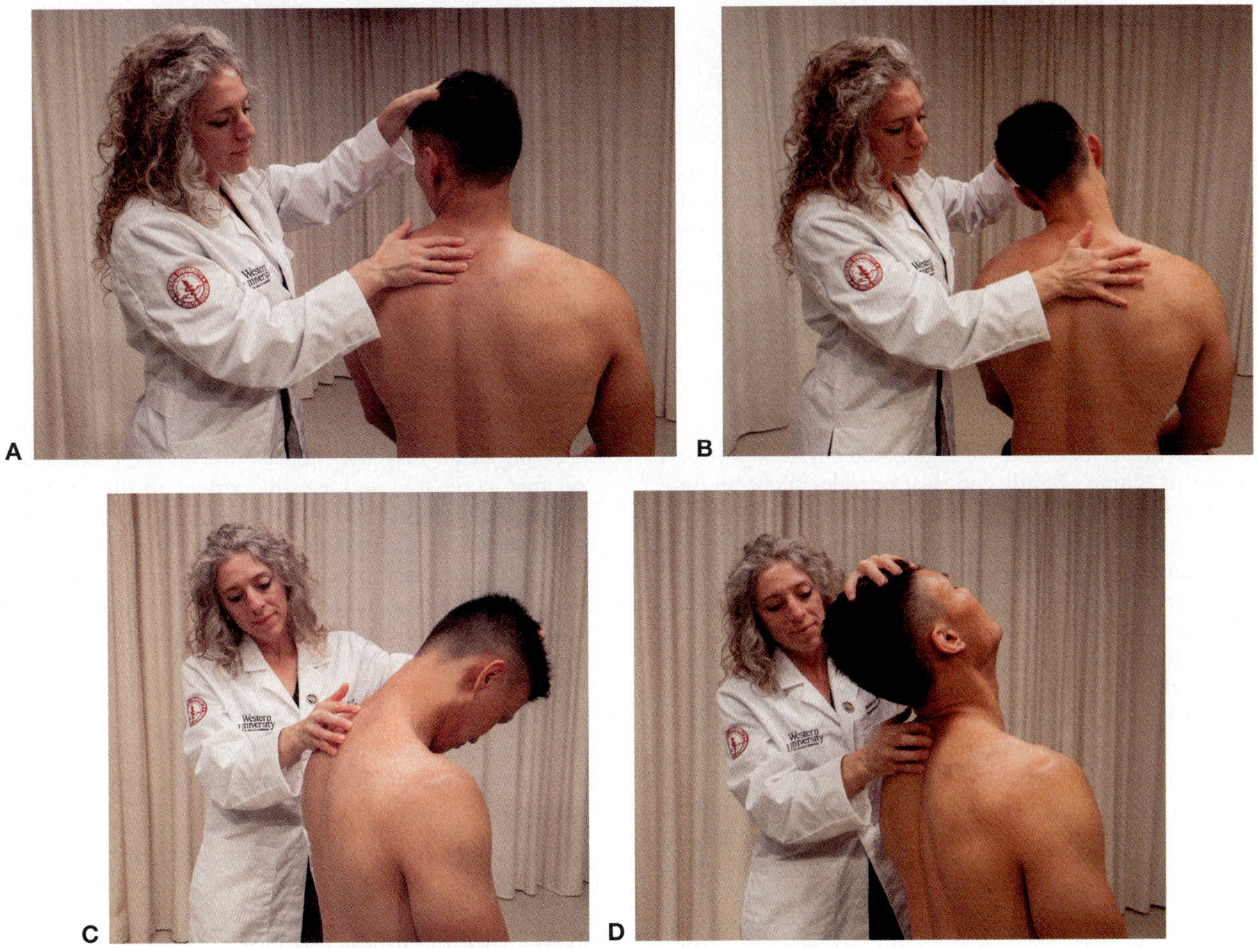

Figure 30.47. A. Assessment of quality or passive range of motion of upper thoracic rotation. (Photos courtesy of Western University of Health Sciences, Pomona, CA, with permission.) **B.** Assessment of quality or passive range of motion of upper thoracic sidebending. Note, that the physician may use finger pads on individual vertebrae or use a broader contact during the assessment as depicted here. (Photos courtesy of Western University of Health Sciences, Pomona, CA, with permission.) **C.** Assessment of quality or passive range of motion of upper thoracic flexion. (Photos courtesy of Western University of Health Sciences, Pomona, CA, with permission.) **D.** Assessment of quality or passive range of motion of upper thoracic extension. (Photos courtesy of Western University of Health Sciences, Pomona, CA, with permission.)

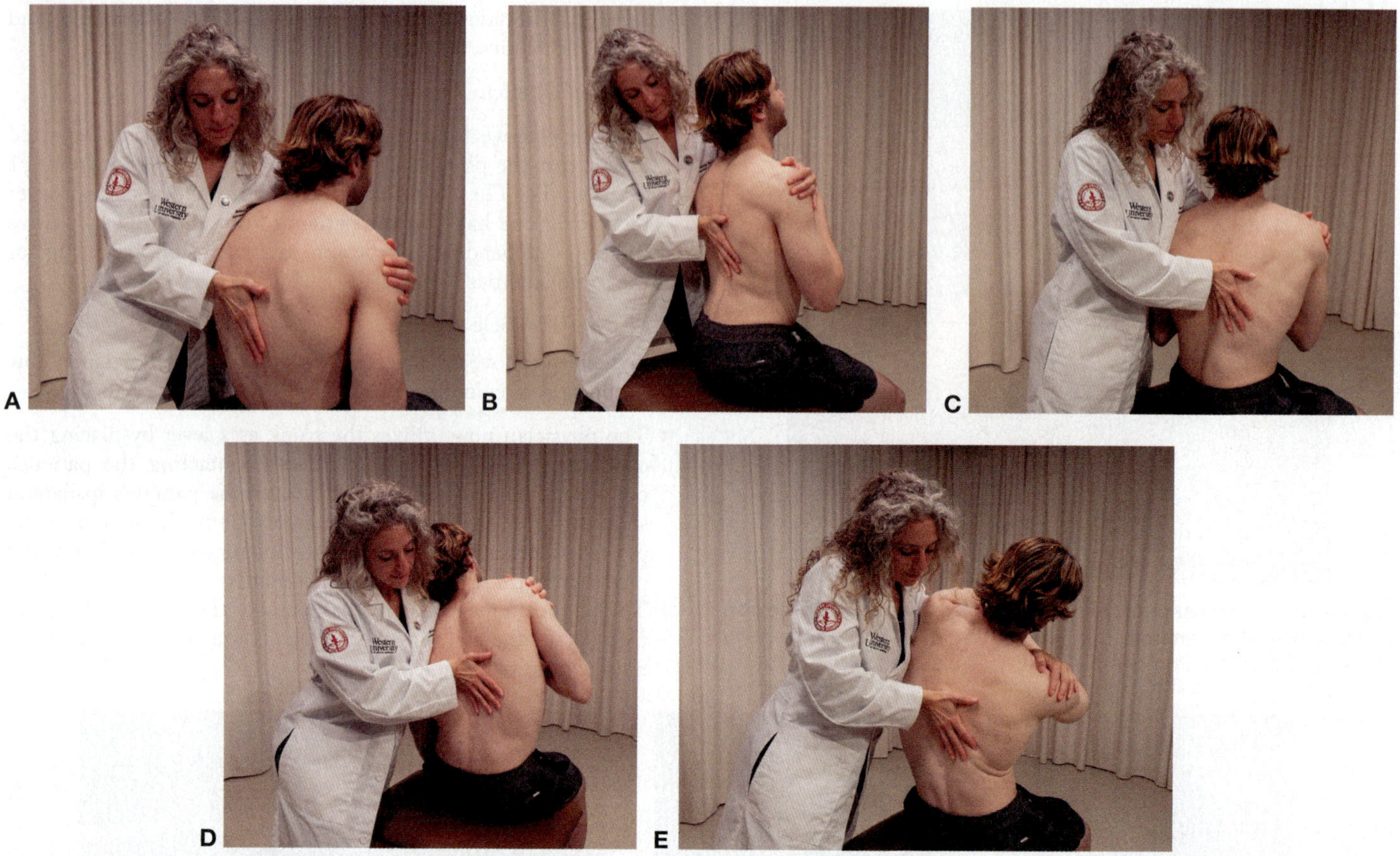

Figure 30.48. **A.** Assessment of quality or passive range of motion of lower thoracic flexion. (Photo courtesy of Western University of Health Sciences, Pomona, CA, with permission.) **B.** Assessment of quality or passive range of motion of lower thoracic extension. (Photo courtesy of Western University of Health Sciences, Pomona, CA, with permission.) **C.** Assessment of quality or passive range of motion of lower thoracic rotation. (Photo courtesy of Western University of Health Sciences, Pomona, CA, with permission.) **D.** Assessment of quality or passive range of motion of lower thoracic left sidebending. (Photo courtesy of Western University of Health Sciences, Pomona, CA, with permission.) **E.** Assessment of quality or passive range of motion of lower thoracic right sidebending. (Photo courtesy of Western University of Health Sciences, Pomona, CA, with permission.)

- Therefore, to induce flexion to the region, the physician instructs the patient to "slump" slightly and then provides slight pressure through the elbow to induce further flexion through the whole region taking care not to induce hip flexion. The physician should strive to maintain proper ergonomics by maintaining a straight spine and performing a lunge to induce flexion (Fig. 30.48A).
- To induce extension, the physician may instruct the patient to sit slightly forward toward their pubic bones. The physician then lunges the opposite way, pressing slightly anteriorly on the region of T5 to T12 to move the patient into extension but maintaining them over their center of gravity (Fig. 30.48B).
- The patient is returned to neutral.
- For rotation, the physician passively rotates the patient toward them keeping the patient over their center of gravity and, if seated, ensuring that the patient's hips remain on the exam table and do not lift.
- The physician then goes to the other side of the patient and repeats the process. To maintain control and fully support the patient through the exam, the physician maintains close contact with the patient and always rotates the patient toward them. This will also help avoid injury to the physician (Fig. 30.48C).
- To induce sidebending, the physician induces inferior and oblique pressure through their axilla into the thoracic region (Fig. 30.48D).
- The physician may then repeat this on the other side or stay on that same side and ask the patient to lift their arms and fold them on top of the other. The physician then brings their shoulder under the patient's axilla and brings their arm across the patient's chest to contact the patient's opposite shoulder. The physician induces inferior and oblique pressure now toward the physician to induce sidebending in the opposite direction (Fig. 30.48E).

Lumbar Quality of Motion Testing:

- The same procedure is repeated as described in the lower thoracic region except that the physician is now monitoring the region from about L1–L5.

Other methods of passive motion testing of the thoracic spine include:

PASSIVE SIDEBENDING T1 TO T4

1. The patient is seated on the side of the table.
2. The physician stands behind the patient, on the side to be tested.
3. The physician palpates the transverse processes of T4.
4. The physician's first metacarpal–phalangeal joint is placed over the patient's first rib at the base of the neck.

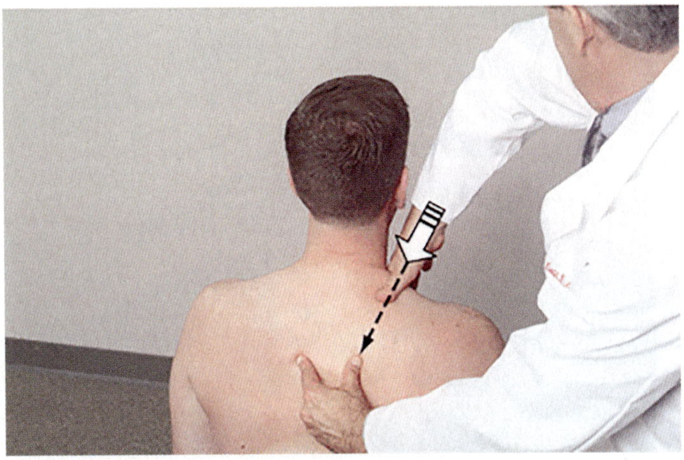

Figure 30.49. Thoracic vertebrae 1 to 4 passive side bending—right range and quality of motion assessment, exerting a springing force from the patient's ipsilateral first rib directed at the patient's T4 spinous process. (Reprinted with permission from Nicholas AS, Nicholas EA. *Atlas of Osteopathic Techniques*. 3rd ed. Wolters Kluwer; 2016.)

5. The physician's elbow is held high above the shoulder, to deliver a springing force toward the spinous process of T4 (Fig. 30.49). This produces passive sidebending of T1–T4.
6. Steps 1 to 3 are repeated on the opposite side.

PASSIVE SIDEBENDING T5 TO T8

1. The patient is seated on the side of the table.
2. The physician stands behind the patient, on the side to be tested.
3. The physician palpates over the transverse processes of T8.
4. The physician's first metacarpal–phalangeal joint is placed over the midpoint of the patient's shoulder.
5. The physician's elbow is held high above the shoulder, to deliver a springing force toward the spinous process of T8 (Fig. 30.50). This produces passive sidebending of the thoracic spine from T5 to T8.
6. Steps 1 through 4 are repeated on the opposite side.

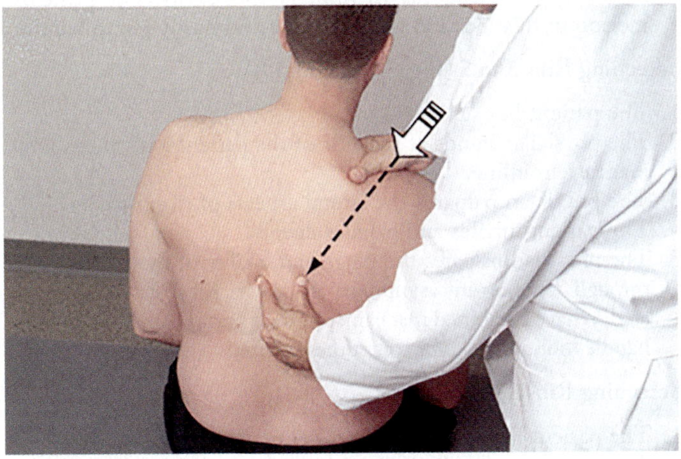

Figure 30.50. Thoracic vertebrae 5 to 8 passive side bending—right range and quality of motion assessment, using a springing force directed at the patient's T8 spinous process from the midpoint of the patient's ipsilateral shoulder. (Reprinted with permission from Nicholas AS, Nicholas EA. *Atlas of Osteopathic Techniques*. 3rd ed. Wolters Kluwer; 2016.)

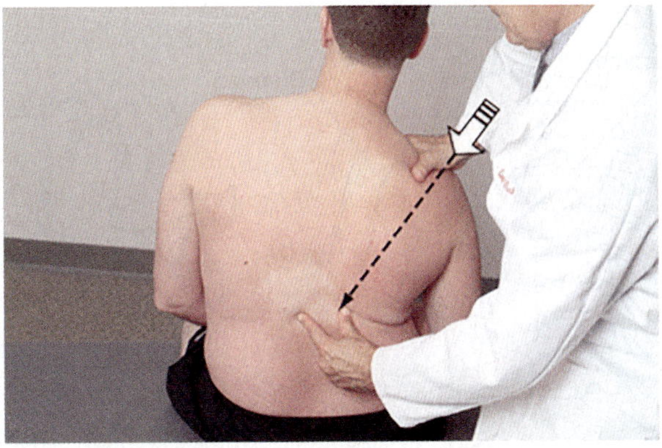

Figure 30.51. Thoracic vertebrae T9–12 passive side bending—right range and quality of motion assessment, using a springing force directed at the patient's T12 spinous process from the patient's ipsilateral acromioclavicular joint. (Reprinted with permission from Nicholas AS, Nicholas EA. *Atlas of Osteopathic Techniques*. 3rd ed. Wolters Kluwer; 2016.)

PASSIVE SIDEBENDING T9 TO T12

1. The patient is seated on the side of the table.
2. The physician stands behind the patient, on the side to be tested.
3. The physician palpates over the transverse processes of T12.
4. The physician's first metacarpal–phalangeal joint is placed over the acromioclavicular joint.
5. The physician's elbow is held high above the shoulder, to deliver a force toward the spinous process of T12 (Fig. 30.51). This produces passive sidebending from T9 to T12.
6. Steps 1 through 3 are repeated on the opposite side.

PASSIVE ROTATION T9 TO T12

1. The patient is seated on the side of the table, with the arms crossed and holding onto the shoulders.
2. The physician stands behind the patient, on the side to be tested.
3. The physician palpates over the transverse processes of T12.
4. The physician grasps the patient's contralateral arm and then rotates both of the patient's arms farther in the same direction. This is the passive range of motion (Fig. 30.52).
5. Steps 1 to 4 are repeated on the opposite side.

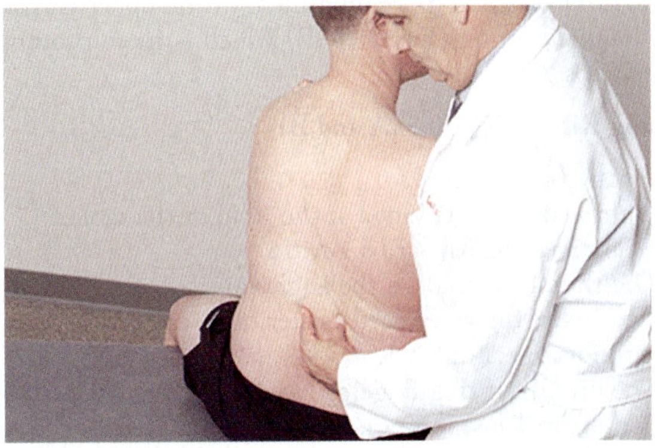

Figure 30.52. T9–12 rotation passive range and quality of motion assessment. (Reprinted with permission from Nicholas AS, Nicholas EA. *Atlas of Osteopathic Techniques*. 3rd ed. Wolters Kluwer; 2016.)

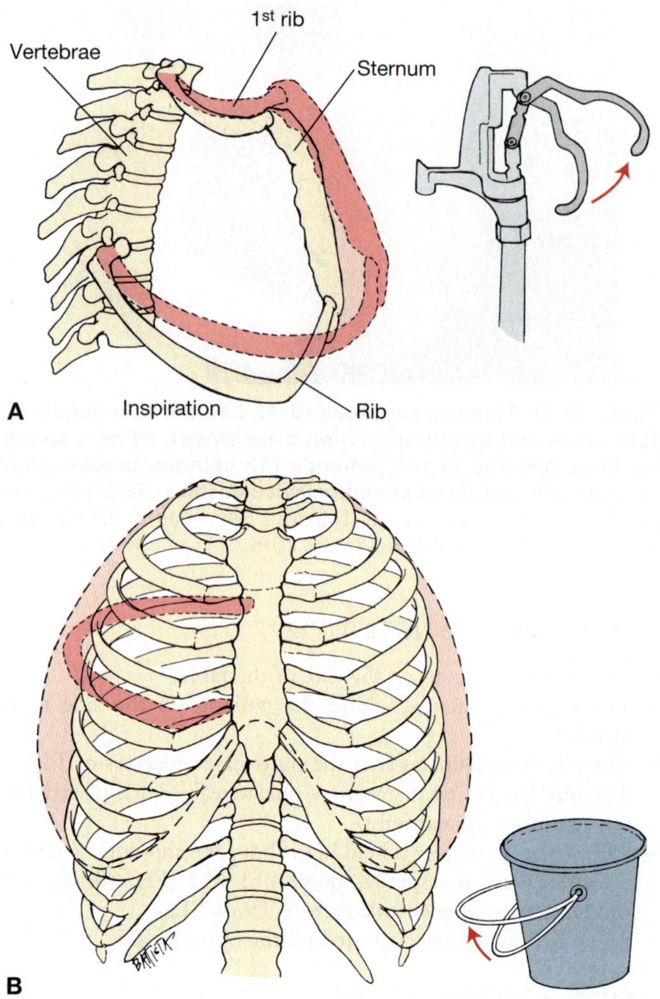

Figure 30.53. **A.** Rib pump handle motion. (From Clay JH, Pounds DM. Basic Clinical Massage Therapy: Integrating Anatomy and Treatment. Lippincott Williams & Wilkins; 2003, with permission.) **B.** Rib bucket handle motion. (Reprinted with permission from Clay JH, Pounds DM. *Basic Clinical Massage Therapy: Integrating Anatomy and Treatment.* Lippincott Williams & Wilkins; 2003.)

Assessment of Costal Cage Motion:

If the costal cage was thought to be the source of the problem during the screening exam (i.e., asymmetry and/or tenderness of the rib angles upon palpation), the costal cage may be assessed for motion. This involves palpating for pump handle motion (Fig. 30.53A) which is more prominent in the upper ribs, and for bucket handle motion (Fig. 30.53B) which is more prominent in the lower ribs.

Screening Rib 1 (Fig. 30.54A and B)

1. The patient lies supine.
2. The physician is positioned at the head of the table.
3. The physician palpates ribs 1 with:
   a. The thumbs placed on the angles of rib 1.
   b. The index fingers placed posterior to the clavicle, over the anterior aspect of rib 1.
   c. The middle or ring fingers placed at the costochondral junction of rib 1 just inferior to the clavicular heads.
4. The patient inhales and exhales deeply.
5. The physician palpates the range and quality of motion of the first rib, noting any asymmetry that may exist. The principal motion in this location is designated as pump handle.

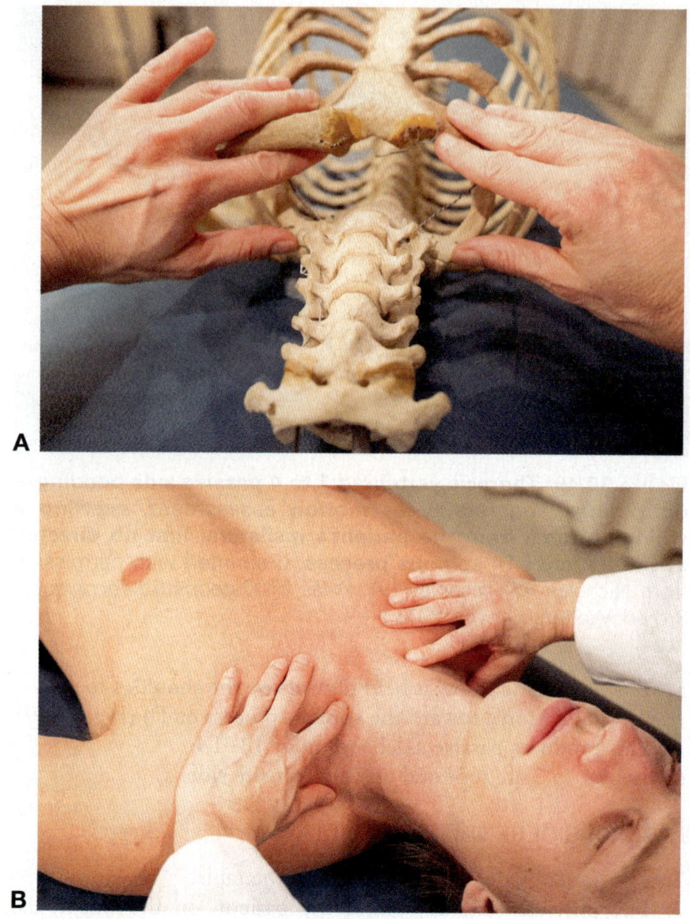

Figure 30.54. A and B Skeleton model to show assessment of rib 1 and then on patient. (Photos courtesy of Western University of Health Sciences, Pomona, CA, with permission.)

Screening Ribs 2 to 4 (Fig. 30.55A and B)

1. The patient lies supine.
2. The physician stands at the head of the table.
3. The physician palpates over the anterolateral aspect of ribs 2 to 4.
4. The patient inhales and exhales deeply.
5. The physician palpates the range and quality of motion of ribs 2 through 4 noting any asymmetry that exists. The principal motion in this location is described as primarily pump handle.

Screening Ribs 5 to 7 (Fig. 30.56A and B)

1. The patient lies supine.
2. The physician stands at the side of the patient with their dominant eye midline.
3. The physician palpates the lateral aspects of ribs 5 to 7.
4. The patient inhales and exhales deeply.
5. The physician palpates the range and quality of motion of ribs 5 through 7, noting any asymmetry that exists. Ribs 5 to 7 are considered to have combined mechanics of both pump handle and bucket handle motion, which is sometimes referred to as "mixed motion".

Screening Ribs 8 to 10

1. The patient lies supine.
2. The physician stands at the side of the patient with dominant eye midline.
3. The physician palpates the lateral aspects of ribs 8 to 10.
4. The patient inhales and exhales deeply.
5. The physician palpates the range and quality of motion of ribs 8 to 10, noting any asymmetry that exists (Fig. 30.57A and B)

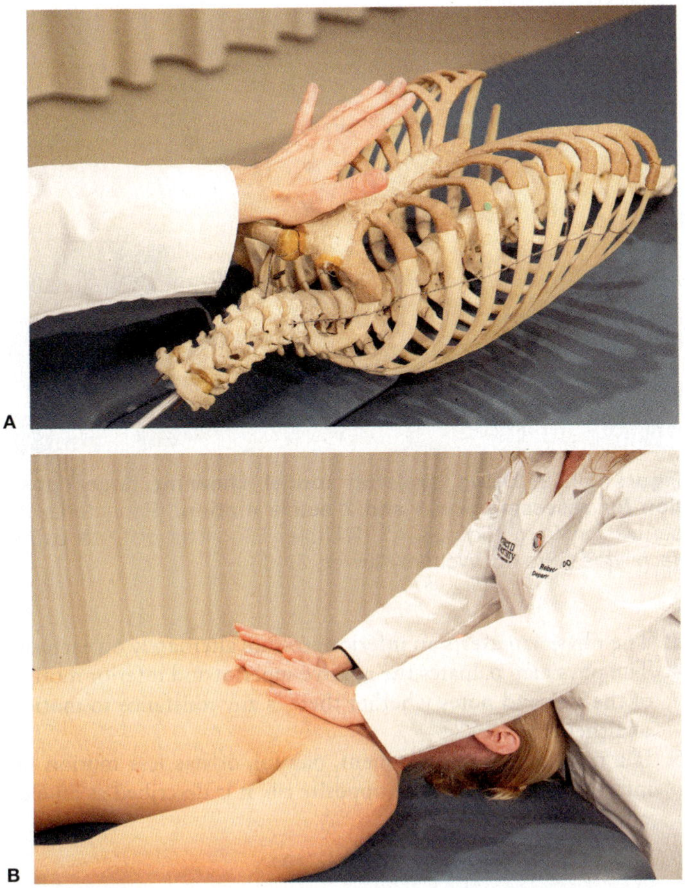

Figure 30.55. **A.** Using skeleton model to demonstrate hand placement over the anterior aspect of ribs 2 to 4 to evaluate active motion. (Photo courtesy of Western University of Health Sciences, Pomona, CA, with permission.) **B.** The physician palpates over the anterior aspect of ribs 2 to 4 while patient inhales and exhales to assess symmetry, range, and quality of motion. (Photo courtesy of Western University of Health Sciences, Pomona, CA, with permission.)

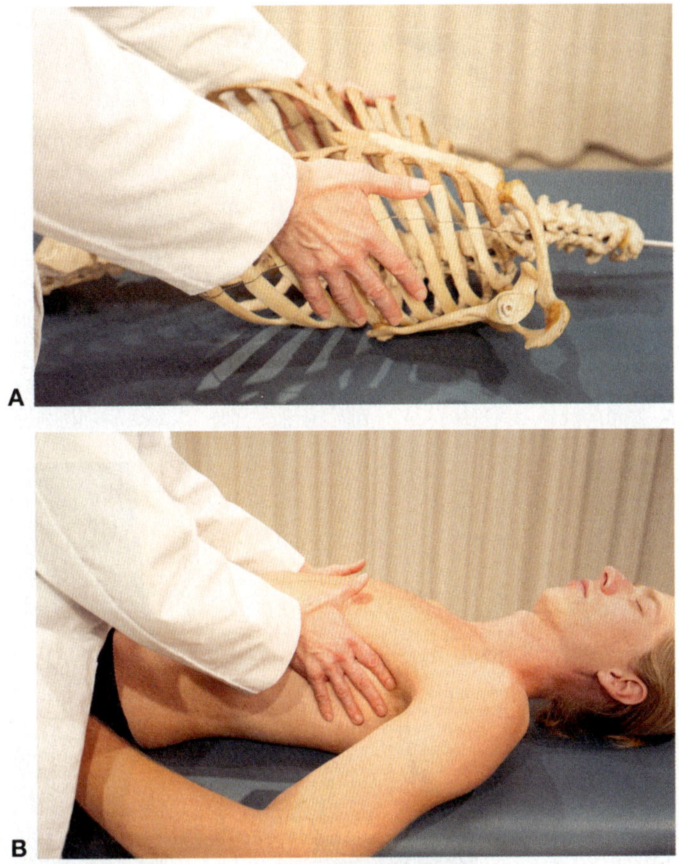

Figure 30.56. **A.** Using skeletal model to demonstrate hand placement on the lateral aspects of ribs 5 to 7 to assess active motion. (Photo courtesy of Western University of Health Sciences, Pomona, CA, with permission.) **B.** The physician palpates the lateral aspects of ribs 5 to 7 while patient inhales and exhales to assess symmetry, range, and quality of motion. (Photo courtesy of Western University of Health Sciences, Pomona, CA, with permission.)

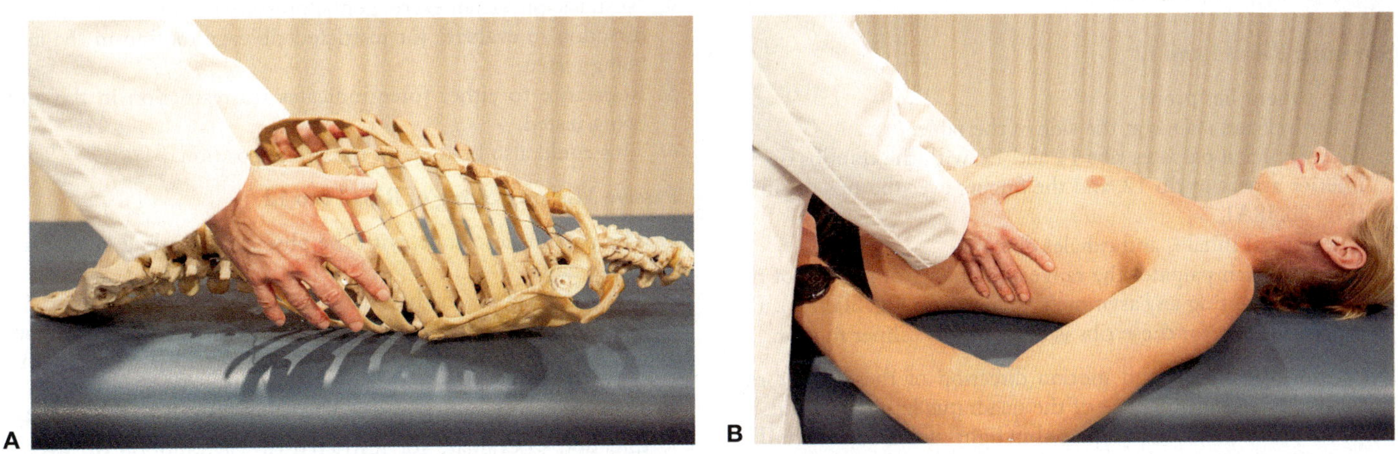

Figure 30.57. **A.** Using skeletal model to demonstrate hand placement on the lateral aspects of ribs 8 to 10 to assess active motion. (Photo courtesy of Western University of Health Sciences, Pomona, CA, with permission.) **B**. The physician palpates the lateral aspects of ribs 8 to 10 while patient inhales and exhales to assess symmetry, range, and quality of motion. (Photo courtesy of Western University of Health Sciences, Pomona, CA, with permission.)

A

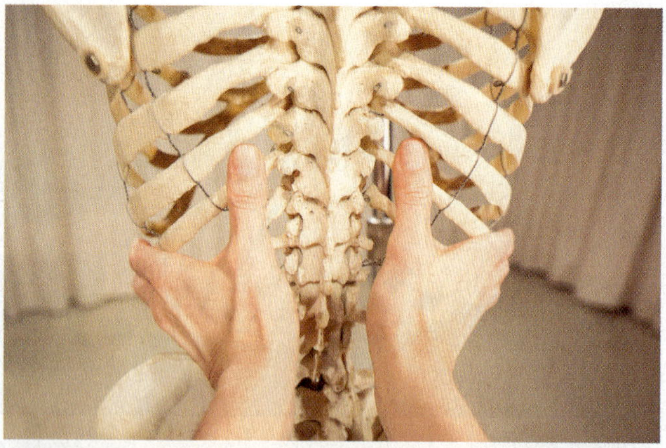

B

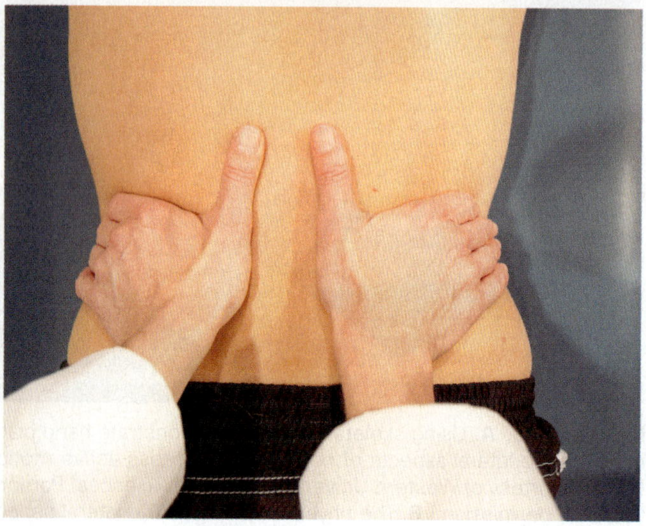

Figure 30.58. A. Using skeletal model to demonstrate hand placement for evaluation of active motion of ribs 11 and 12. (Photo courtesy of Western University of Health Sciences, Pomona, CA, with permission.) **B.** The physician palpates ribs 11 and 12 while patient inhales and exhales to assess symmetry, range, and quality of motion. (Photo courtesy of Western University of Health Sciences, Pomona, CA, with permission.)

Screening Ribs 11 and 12

1. The patient lies prone.
2. The physician stands at the side of the table.
3. The physician palpates ribs 11 and 12, with the thumbs on the inferior aspect of rib 12, and the fingers over the tips of rib 11 (Fig. 30.58A).
4. The patient inhales and exhales deeply.
5. The physician palpates the range and quality of motion of ribs 11 and 12, noting any asymmetry that exists (Fig. 30.58B). The typical motion for these ribs is described as caliper motion.

Restriction of motion and motion direction of these lower ribs is under the strong influence of the quadratus lumborum muscle. Any restriction must be interpreted in light of this influence. The passive range of motion or quality of motion of the ribs may be assessed as follows:

Passive Motion Testing of Rib 1

1. The patient is seated or supine.
2. The physician palpates each 1st rib at the posterolateral shaft and immediately lateral to the costotransverse articulation (Fig. 30.59).

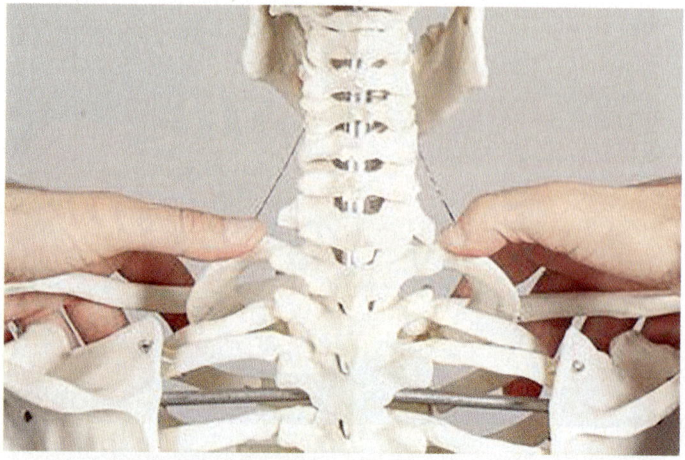

Figure 30.59. Using skeleton model showing finger position for assessing ribs 1 and 2 active motion. (Reprinted with permission from Nicholas AS, Nicholas EA. *Atlas of Osteopathic Techniques*. 3rd ed. Wolters Kluwer; 2016.)

3. The physician exerts an inferior pressure alternately on each rib.
4. The physician palpates the relative superior and inferior motion of the ribs and notes whether there is any resistance to motion of either rib.
5. If a rib feels more prominent, painful, or has less motion on inferior pressure than the opposite rib, it is described as an elevated rib dysfunction.

Passive Motion Testing of Ribs 2 to 10

1. The patient lies supine, with the physician standing at the side of the table.
2. The physician places their hands bilaterally over the anterolateral aspects of the ribs[2–10] to be evaluated. The hand placement should be between the midclavicular and midaxillary lines bilaterally.
3. The physician then exerts gentle pressure in an anterior-posterior direction to evaluate for restricted rib cage motion in the area being tested.
4. Next, the physician exerts gentle pressure in a lateral-to-medial direction to evaluate for restricted rib cage motion in the area being tested.
5. Resistance to either force indicates rib restriction in the area being tested.
6. This could also be done in the prone position.

Passive Motion Testing of Ribs 11 to 12

1. The patient lies prone, with the physician standing at the side of the table.
2. The physician places their hands bilaterally over ribs 11 and 12.
3. The physician then exerts gentle pressure in an anterior-posterior direction to evaluate for restricted rib cage motion in the area of ribs 11 and 12.
4. Next, the physician exerts gentle pressure in a lateral-to-medial direction to evaluate for restricted rib cage motion of ribs 11 and 12.
5. Resistance to either force indicates rib restriction in this rib cage region.

Assessment of Sacrum:

A positive seated flexion test in the presence of a positive or negative standing flexion indicates a sacroiliac dysfunction. Passive motion testing of the sacrum may be accomplished as follows.

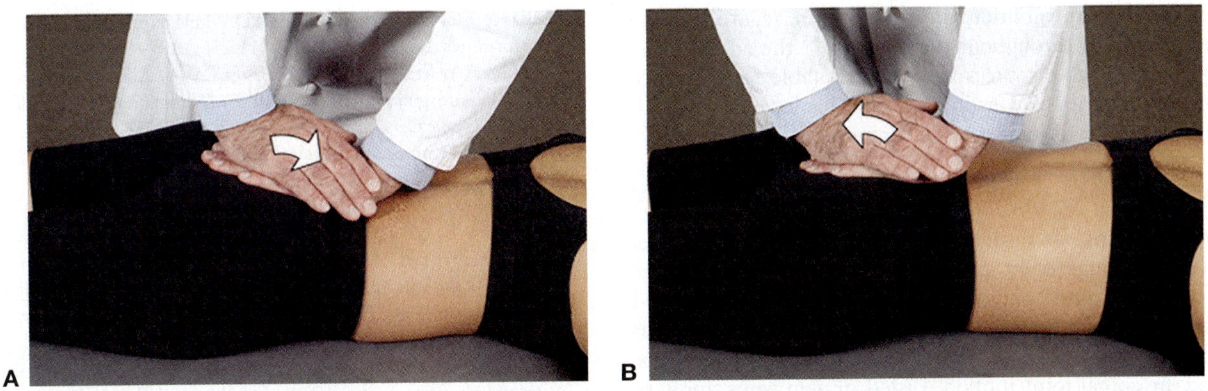

Figure 30.60. **A.** Sacral rock—passive flexion of the sacrum. (From Nicholas AS, Nicholas EA. *Atlas of Osteopathic Technique*. 3rd ed. Lippincott Williams & Wilkins; 2015, with permission.) **B.** Sacral rock—passive extension of the sacrum. (Reprinted with permission from Nicholas AS, Nicholas EA. *Atlas of Osteopathic Techniques*. 3rd ed. Wolters Kluwer; 2016.)

Sacral Region—Patient Prone

SACRAL SPINE PASSIVE MOTION

Screening Test for Bilateral Sacral Dysfunction: Sacral Rock Test

1. The patient lies prone.
2. The physician stands at the side of the patient, at the level of the patient's pelvis.
3. The physician places one hand on the sacrum, with the heel of the hand on the sacral base, and the fingers pointing toward the coccyx.
4. The physician's other hand reinforces the first hand, with the thumb and the index finger creating a space for the wrist of the superior hand.
5. The physician presses straight down into the sacrum so that any body movement is imparted to the sacrum.
6. The physician rocks the sacrum through flexion (Fig. 30.60A) and extension (Fig. 30.60B). Bilateral sacral dysfunction feels exceptionally rigid and decreased compliance may palpated with sacral flexion, extension, or both.[18]

In ambulatory practice, examining the patient first in the standing, then seated, and finally, the supine and prone positions is a common and efficient method often used for the ease of the patient. Screening the active range of motion of the upper extremity, lower extremity, lumbar, and pelvis is easily accomplished within the standing portion of the structural exam. With the patient seated, the head, cervical, thoracic, lumbar, and sacral regions may be assessed from superior to inferior. With the patient supine, assess costal cage motion. Lastly, with the patient prone, assess motion of the 11th and 12th ribs. Passive sacral motion tests can also be done while the patient is in the prone position. In actual clinical practice, tests may be done in a different order, depending on the location, condition of the patient, and physician preference. When communicating with the patient, it is important to convey to them what is about to be done and why. It is recommended that the physician communicate what region is about to be palpated and ensure that they have permission to palpate. When moving to a potentially sensitive region, such as the chest or pelvis, it is recommended that the physician again ask for consent to palpate and communicate the area they will be palpating and why. When asking the patient to perform the active range of tests, language such as "move," "bend," "turn," or "breathe in and out" may be better understood and easier for a patient to follow than technical terms, such as flex, extend, and rotate.

TABLE 30.3

Common Structures Responsible for Motion Loss and Conditions Whose Symptoms are Exacerbated by Spinal Range of Motion

Structure	Motion	Condition
Cervical Spine	Flexion	Disk herniation Hypertonic posterior muscles
	Extension	Facet joint disease Hypertonic anterior muscles
	Sidebending	Hypertonic trapezius Levator scapulae muscles
	Rotation	Hypertonic splenius capitis, splenius cervicis, and sternocleidomastoid muscles
Thoracic Spine	Flexion	Hypertonic paraspinal Posterior shoulder girdle muscles Disk herniation
	Extension	Facet joint disease
	Sidebending	Hypertonic intercostal Serratus anterior muscles
	Rotation	Hypertonic abdominal oblique muscles
Lumbar Spine	Flexion	Disk herniation Hypertonic lumbar paravertebral muscles Lumbosacral ligaments
	Extension	Spondylolisthesis Facet syndrome Spinal stenosis Psoas spasm
	Sidebending	Hypertonic lateral abdominal wall muscles IT band syndrome
	Rotation	Hypertonic abdominal oblique muscles Iliolumbar ligaments Piriformis syndrome[16]

Note: As there are variations in the literature regarding normal ranges of motion throughout the body,[13,19–25] the editors have compiled several reliable sources to develop a table for reference throughout this volume: see Chapter 8 Biomechanics Boxes 8.1-8.7 for the normal ranges of joint motion throughout the body.

Symptom Exacerbation or Remission

Aside from screening for dysfunctional regions or joints, another important goal of range-of-motion testing is the provocation, exacerbation, or remission of patient symptoms, which serves to aid in the diagnosis of the underlying condition. Table 30.3 includes a partial list of structures that would be affected, and conditions exacerbated, by spinal joint motion. Listed muscle pains apply to both injury and muscle hypertonicity or spasm.

CONCLUSION

In summary, the screening and regional components of the structural osteopathic examination provide regional data as to asymmetry and range-of-motion changes. Following the screening and regional portion of the exam, the segmental component determines the definitive diagnosis of the joints or soft tissues that are at the root of the somatic dysfunction. The components and flow of the osteopathic structural exam embody one quote by A.T. Still: "We know that if we ever know the whole, we must first know the parts."[26]

REFERENCES

1. Educational Council on Osteopathic Principles. *Glossary of Osteopathic Terminology*. American Association of Colleges of Osteopathic Medicine; 2017.
2. Perry JM, Burnfield M. *Gait Analysis: Normal and Pathological Function*. 2nd ed. Slack Incorporated; 2010.
3. The Pathokinesiology Service and the Physical Therapy Department of Rancho Los Amigos National Rehabilitation Center. *Observational Gait Analysis Handbook*. Los Amigos Research and Education Institute, Inc. Rancho Los Amigos National Rehabilitation Center; 2001.
4. Kappler RE. Postural balance and motion patterns. In: Peterson B, ed. *Postural Balance and Imbalance*. American Academy of Osteopathy; 1983:6–12.
5. Gregory PL, Biswas AC, Batt ME. Musculoskeletal problems of the chest wall in athletes. *Sports Med*. 2002;32(4):235–250.
6. Rokicki W, Rokicki M, Rydel M. What do we know about Tietze's syndrome? *Kardiochir Torakochirurgia Pol*. 2018;15(3):180–182.
7. Blanco FC, Elliott ST, Sandler AD. Management of congenital chest wall deformities. *Semin Plast Surg*. 2011;25(1):107–116.
8. Fokin AA, Steuerwald NM, Ahrens WA, Allen KE. Anatomical, histologic, and genetic characteristics of congenital chest wall deformities. *Semin Thorac Cardiovasc Surg*. 2009;21(1):44–57.
9. Sung Y-H. Suboccipital muscles, forward head posture, and cervicogenic dizziness. *Medicina (Kaunas)*. 2022;58(12):1791.
10. Cathie AG. The applied anatomy of some postural changes (1945). In: Peterson B, ed. *Postural Balance and Imbalance*. American Academy of Osteopathy; 1983:44–46.
11. Cathie AG. Soft tissue changes that may follow postural defects (1949). In: Peterson B, ed. *Postural Balance and Imbalance*. American Academy of Osteopathy; 1983:47–49.
12. Cathie AG. The influence of the lower extremities upon the structural integrity of the body (1950). In: Peterson B, ed. *Postural Balance and Imbalance*. American Academy of Osteopathy; 1983:50–53.
13. Mitchell FL, Mitchell PKG. *The Muscle Energy Manual-Volume One*. MET Press; 1995:100–110.
14. Marquez AP, Yim M, Zelimkhanian B, et al. Does using a shim improve the diagnostic reliability of the standing flexion test? A pilot study. *AAOJ*. 2016;26(3):21–25.
15. Johnson KD, Kim K-M, Yu B-K, Saliba SA, Grindstaff TL. Reliability of thoracic spine rotation range-of-motion measurements in healthy adults. *J Athl Train*. 2012;47(1):52–60.
16. Ng JK, Kippers V, Richardson CA, Parnianpour M. Range of motion and lordosis of the lumbar spine: reliability of measurement and normative values. *Spine (Phila Pa 1976)*. 2001;26(1):53–60.
17. Greene WB, Heckman JD. *The Clinical Measurement of Joint Motion*. American Academy of Orthopaedic Surgeons; 1994:71.
18. Nicholas AS, Nicholas EA. *Atlas of Osteopathic Techniques*. 4th ed. Wolters Kluwer; 2023:16–28.
19. Moll JM, Wright V. Normal range of spinal mobility. An objective clinical study. *Ann Rheum Dis*. 1971;30:381–386.
20. Macrae IF, Wright V. Measurement of back movement. *Ann Rheum Dis*. 1969;28:584–589.
21. Mitchell FL Jr, Moran PS, Pruzzo NA. *A General Osteopathic Postural/Structural Screening Examination: The Ten Step Screening Examination*. 1st ed. Mitchell, Moran & Pruzzo Associates; 1985.
22. Cathie AG. *Regional Ranges of Passive Spinal Motion*. 1974 Year Book of the American Academy of Osteopathy; 1974:68–72.
23. https://ama-guides.ama-assn.org/
24. DeStefano, LA. *Greenman's Principles of Manual Medicine*. 5th ed. Wolters Kluwer; 2017:21–35.
25. Simons DG, Janet G, et al. *Myofascial Pain and Dysfunction: The Trigger Point Manual*. 2nd ed. Lippincott Williams & Wilkins; 1999.
26. Still AT. *The Philosophy and Mechanical Principles of Osteopathy*. Hudson-Kimberly Publishing Co.; 1902:29.

31 Osteopathic Segmental Examination

WALTER C. EHRENFEUCHTER ▪ REBECCA E. GIUSTI ▪ RAYMOND J. HRUBY

KEY CONCEPTS

- The characteristics of vertebral unit position and motion are essential for an accurate understanding of segmental definition.
- Accurate segmental definition enhances recognition of somatic dysfunctions responsible for symptomatology or disordered physiology.
- Osteopathic manipulative treatment corrects somatic dysfunctions that maintain symptomatology or disordered physiology.
- The goal of osteopathic diagnosis and treatment is to improve the patient's overall body physiology.

INTRODUCTION

Segmental definition serves as the final component of the osteopathic structural examination. The spinal levels examined are discovered through the screening (asymmetry, motion restriction) and regional (layer palpation assessing for tissue texture change and tenderness) components of the structural exam. In the absence of such findings, significant somatic dysfunction is unlikely to exist at that segment, and segmental definition is unnecessary.

CORE CONCEPTS FOR SEGMENTAL EVALUATION

The Vertebral Unit

The vertebral unit is defined as two adjacent vertebrae with their associated intervertebral disk, arthrodial, ligamentous, muscular, vascular, neural, and lymphatic elements (Fig. 31.1).

Conventionally, the motion of a single vertebra is referred to as that segment's vertebral unit. For example, the motion of L3 is in fact referring to the motion of L3 in reference to L4.

Potential Segmental Motions

Using a Cartesian coordinate system, the position or motion of any vertebra can be described in space as a combination of rotation

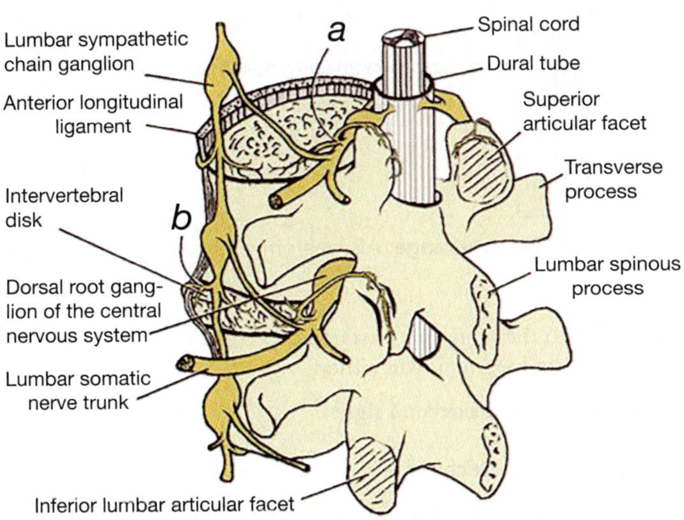

Figure 31.1. The vertebral unit.

about, and translation along any of the three axes. This system is clinically cumbersome, though useful for biomechanical research purposes. For simplicity, the movements of the individual vertebrae are broken into three components:

1. Flexion or extension
2. Rotation
3. Sidebending (Table 31.1)

When referencing the position or motion of a vertebra, the position of a point on the superior end plate at the most anterior aspect of that end plate is used (Fig. 31.2).

Conventionally, the diagnosis of a segmental dysfunction may be described in one of two ways:

1. The vertebra's position relative to the vertebra below
2. The vertebra's directions of motion restriction, relative to the vertebra below

For example:

- Positional diagnosis: L5 flexed, sidebent right, and rotated right
- Motion restriction diagnosis: L5 restricted in extension, left sidebending, and left rotation

The examples above describe the same segment, from two different points of view.

- In positional language: words end in "-ed" and "-ent," as in flexed, extended, rotated, and sidebent.
- When diagnosing somatic dysfunction, the positional diagnosis is determined and named for the vertebra's direction of freest motion, that is, the direction of ease.

TABLE 31.1

Vertebral Movements

Movement	Definition
Rotation	Movement in a transverse plane about a vertical axis
Sidebending	Movement in a coronal plane about an anterior–posterior axis
Flexion	Anterior movement in a sagittal plane about a transverse axis
Extension	Posterior movement in a sagittal plane about a transverse axis

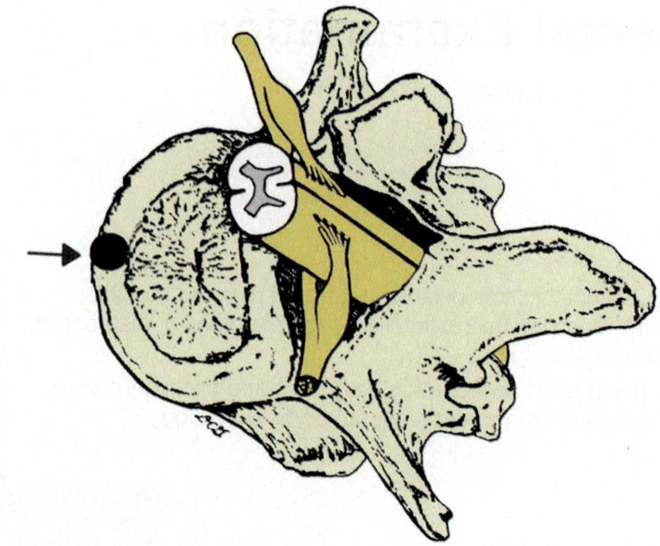

Figure 31.2. Point of reference for vertebral motion.

- In motion restriction language: words end in "-ing" and "-ion," as in flexion, extension, rotation, and sidebending.

PHYSIOLOGIC LAWS OF SPINAL MOTION: FRYETTE'S PRINCIPLES

Fryette's principles regarding the physiologic laws of spinal motion include the following:

I. In the neutral range, sidebending and rotation are coupled in opposite directions.
II. In sufficient flexion or extension, sidebending and rotation are coupled in the same direction.[1]
III. Initiating movement of a vertebral segment in any plane of motion will modify the movement of that segment in other planes of motion.

Fryette's first and second principles apply to thoracic and lumbar motion only. Sidebending and rotation are considered coupled motions (i.e., they occur together). They were described by Harrison H. Fryette, DO, in 1918. All of his observations regarding vertebral mechanics were made using palpation only, without the benefit of x-rays. The third principle was described by C.R. Nelson, DO, in 1948.

Neutral Is a Range

Neutral in spinal mechanics is not a single point, but rather a range in which the weight of the trunk is borne onto the vertebral bodies and disks, and the facets are "idling"[2] (Fig. 31.3).

In this range, Fryette's first principle applies. That is, when one or the other is introduced, sidebending and rotation will be coupled in opposite direction. The motion segment will either:

- Sidebend right and rotate left
- Sidebend left and rotate right

This is referred to as type I mechanics (Fig. 31.4).

A dysfunctional segment held in this position is referred to as a type I dysfunction.

Nonneutral Mechanics

In the thoracic and lumbar spine, when sufficient flexion or extension occurs beyond the neutral range, sidebending and rotation will be coupled to the same side as stated by Fryette's second principle. The nonneutral segment will either:

- Rotate right and sidebend right
- OR
- Rotate left and sidebend left

This is referred to as type II mechanics (Fig. 31.5).

A dysfunctional segment held in this position is referred to as a type II dysfunction.

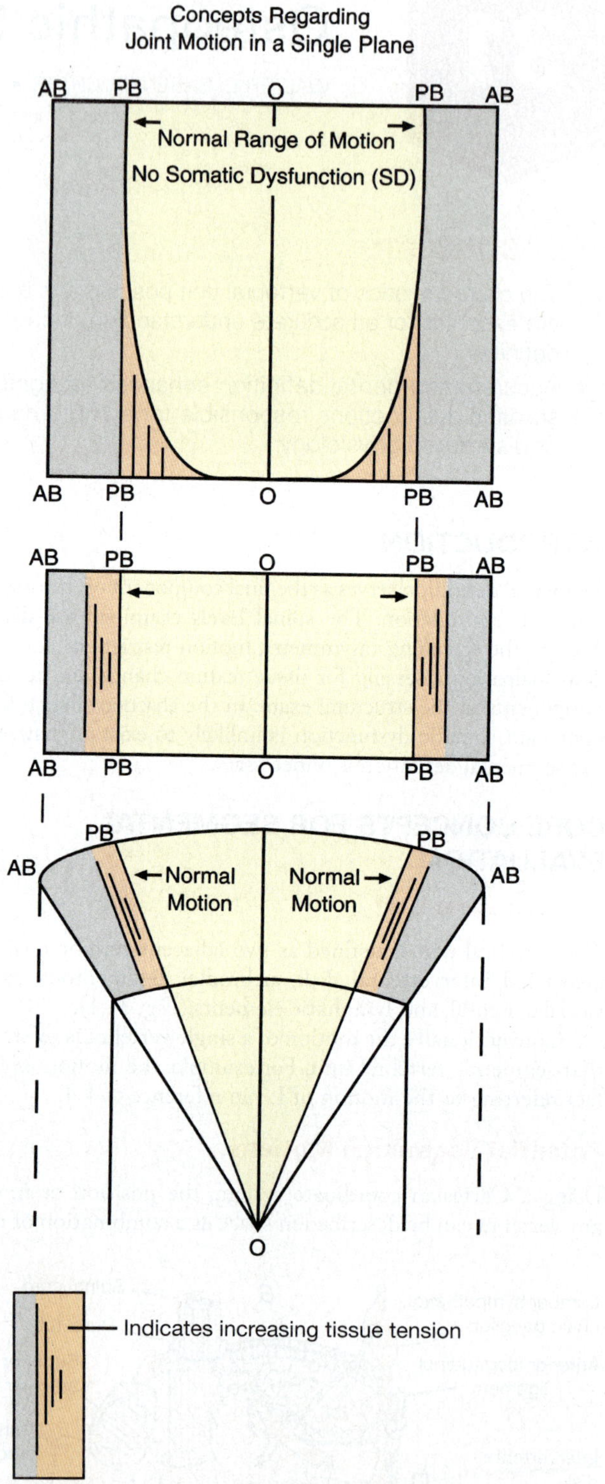

Figure 31.3. Neutral range. AB, anatomic barrier; PB, physiologic barrier.

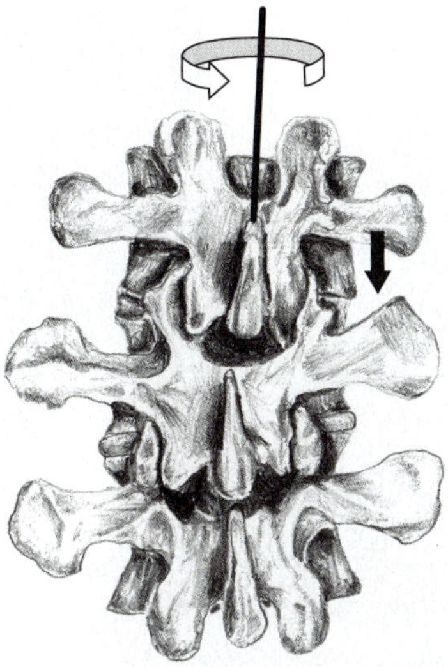

Figure 31.4. **Fryette type I mechanics.** (Courtesy of Adam Ehrenfeuchter, San Francisco, CA.)

SIGNIFICANCE OF THE THIRD LAW OF SPINAL MOTION

The third principle or Nelson's law suggests that if motion is restricted in any one direction (e.g., rotation), then motion will also be restricted in sidebending and flexion/extension. Likewise, if motion is improved in any one direction (e.g., flexion/extension), its rotation and sidebending will also improve.

Since longhand descriptions of vertebral position are cumbersome, clinical shorthand abbreviations and notations are listed in Box 31.1.

Characteristics of Type I Dysfunctions

Type I dysfunctions tend to occur in groups,[2] such as T1–T7 NR_RS_L. This constitutes typical scoliosis mechanics but does not preclude their singular occurrence, like T5 NR_RS_L. Groups of type I dysfunctions generally compensate for a single type II dysfunction that is typically present at the apex of the group dysfunction, or at either end of it.

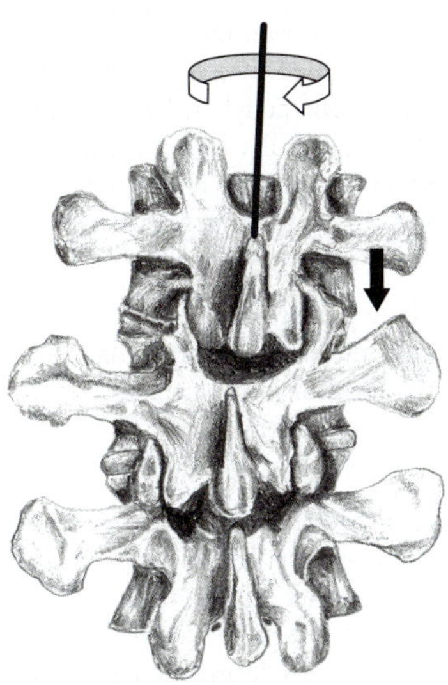

Figure 31.5. **Fryette type II mechanics.** (Courtesy of Adam Ehrenfeuchter, San Francisco, CA.)

BOX 31.1 Shorthand Abbreviations and Notations for Segmental Dysfunctions

Abbreviations
- N—Neutral
- F—Flexed
- E—Extended
- L—Left
- R—Rotated
- R—Right
- S—Sidebent

Notations

Type I dysfunction:
- L5 neutral, rotated left, sidebent right
- Or L5 NRLSR
- Or L5 RLSR

Type II dysfunction:
- L5 flexed, rotated right, sidebent right
- Or L5 FRRSR
- Or L5 FRSR

Characteristics of Type II Dysfunctions

Type II dysfunctions tend to occur singularly. Two type II dysfunctions may exist adjacent to each other,[3] but more than that is rare. In addition to trauma or altered postural mechanics, extended type II dysfunctions may represent segmental muscle contraction resulting from a viscerosomatic reflex prompting further evaluation through history and/or physical for visceral disease and dysfunction.

Classic Spinal Mechanics

Classic Fryette mechanics is typically exhibited by the thoracic and lumbar vertebrae. The motion pattern in these regions is determined by patterns of force generated by the disks, ligaments, and musculature.

- Motion patterns in the cervical spine are largely determined by the shape of the facet and uncovertebral joints, which are independent of the disks, ligaments, and musculature.
- Motion in the cervical region is often described in terms of Fryette-"like" mechanics, since unlike Fryette mechanics, it is independent of sagittal plane position.
- The occiput on C-1 always exhibits type I–like mechanics in that sidebending and rotation are always coupled to opposite sides, regardless of whether the occiput is flexed, extended, or neutral.[4]
- C1 on C2, the atlantoaxial (AA) joint is considered to be almost purely rotational. Even though considerable (20 degrees) sagittal plane motion is possible, dysfunctions are typically discovered only in the rotational component of C-1 motion.[5]
- C2–C6 always exhibit type II–like mechanics in that sidebending and rotation are always coupled to the same side, regardless of whether these segments are flexed, extended, or neutral.[6]
- C7 has inferior facet joints that are more thoracic in configuration and thus tend to follow classical Fryette mechanics.[1,7]

Exceptions to the Laws of Spinal Mechanics

- Single-plane dysfunctions are quite possible and involve restriction of motion on both facet joints. For example, T10 flexed or L5 extended.

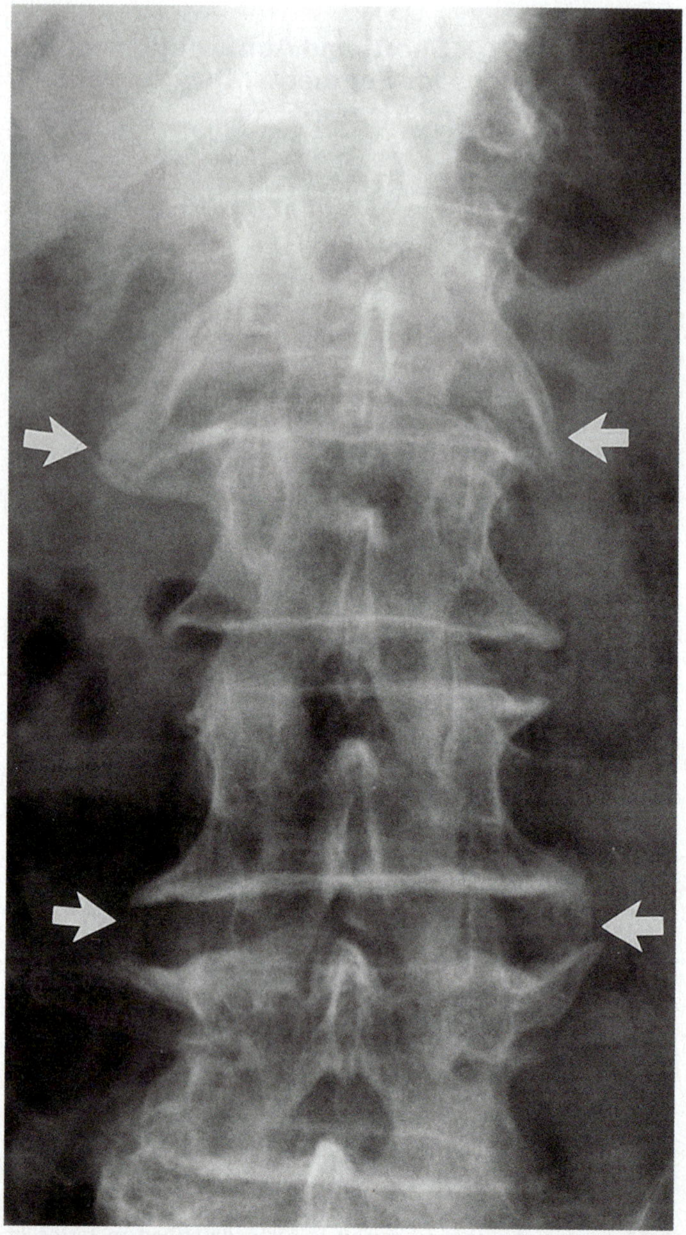

Figure 31.6. Detailed view of lumbar vertebral column showing large osteophytes.

- Similarly, compressive dysfunctions are possible and also involve restriction of motion of both facet joints. For example, occiput compressed on C1.
- Trauma to the supporting ligaments and/or disks can generate segmental instability in any direction. These dysfunctions are caused by external traumatic forces, not by exaggerated physiologic motion of the spine.
- Advanced degenerative disk disease and degenerative facet joint disease also lead to segmental instability in any direction, along with neural entrapment due to a phenomenon called dynamic lateral stenosis. Figure 31.6 shows a detailed view of lumbar vertebral column showing large osteophytes.
- Congenital anomalies of the vertebrae or facet joints will also alter motion characteristics of those segments. Facet tropism, a turning of the facet joints from their usual orientation, can dramatically alter the motion characteristics of a segment, present with bony asymmetry, and thus congenital asymmetric vertebral motion. Figure 31.7 shows a transitional lumbosacral segment causing atypical lumbosacral mechanics.

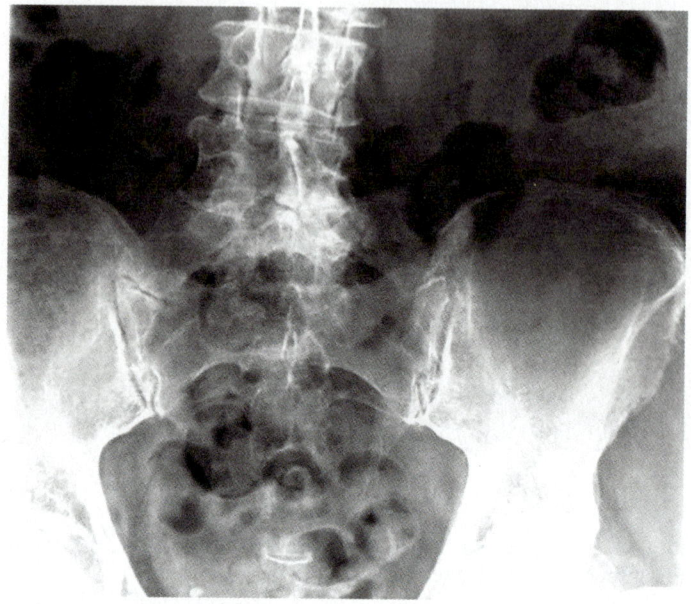

Figure 31.7. Transitional lumbosacral segment causing atypical lumbosacral mechanics. (Photograph courtesy of Walter C. Ehrenfeuchter, DO, FAAO.)

CATEGORIZING SOMATIC DYSFUNCTION

Somatic dysfunction can be categorized by the tissue or structure most responsible for the motion restriction at that segment.[8] Most dysfunctions result from a combination of types, but it is helpful for the purpose of technique selection to determine the underlying cause for segmental restriction.

Types of somatic dysfunction include:

- Arthrodial restriction
- Muscular restriction
- Fascial and ligamentous restriction
- Edema-causing restriction

Arthrodial Restriction

The articular restriction is maintained by the facet joint structure itself. It is often accompanied by a reflex muscle guarding response that will not relax until the articular "lock" is released. These dysfunctions can be quite painful when acquired by acute injury, but patients often derive instantaneous relief when properly treated.

Articular restrictions may be generated by:

- Acute trauma
- Sustained muscle hypertonicity
- Repetitive motion injuries (microtrauma)
- Cartilage degeneration of joint surfaces[9]
- Fascial or ligamentous contracture
- Poor posture

They are maintained by a combination of thin layer adherence and muscle guarding response. If the dysfunction becomes chronic, it will lead to fascial contracture and desiccation of the facet joint.

Thin layer adherence is a process where two congruent surfaces adhere together by a typically lubricating substance, when the said substance is spread thinly enough. For thin layer adherence to occur, both congruent surfaces and a lubricating substance must be present.

In a congruent joint, all joint surfaces are in complete contact with each other in the anatomic position. The spinal facet joints are congruent joints.

Synovial fluid, when present in normal amounts, is an exceptionally effective lubricant that makes joint surfaces approximately 10 times more slippery than ice on ice. It is also very viscous due to its high molar mass of hyaluronan[10] and possesses a high surface tension. Therefore, if there are congruent facet surfaces with both the viscous synovial fluid and a force that compresses the facet surfaces together, a thin layer adherence and an articular dysfunction will likely result.

In the acute, traumatically induced articular dysfunction, where does the synovial fluid go? Some is squeezed out of the joint space and distends the capsule, serving as one source of pain. Over time, the synovial fluid is also absorbed into the surface of the cartilage and removed from the capsule and surrounding tissues by the lymphatics.

Muscular Restriction

One very common cause of asymmetric and restricted segmental motion is the attached musculature. A detailed analysis on the influence of every muscle attached to the axial skeleton is beyond the scope of this book. However, some broad generalizations may be made.

- Short restrictor muscles generally only cross one vertebral segment, or one joint in the peripheral skeleton. When hypertonic, they will only alter the positional and motion characteristics of a single vertebral segment.
- Long restrictor muscles cross more than one vertebral segment on more than one joint in the peripheral skeleton. When hypertonic, they will alter the positional and motion characteristics of groups of vertebrae.

DEEP SEGMENTAL SPINAL MUSCLES

They are short restrictors that run only a segment or two adjacent to the spinal column and rib cage. These muscles include the following:

- Rotatores brevis
- Levator costorum brevis
- Interspinalis
- Lateral intertransverse
- Rectus capitis posterior minor

These muscles are completely involuntary in their action. For instance, it is not possible to consciously contract only the lateral intertransverse muscle in order to sidebend L4 on L5.

They also balance the spinal column in response to larger movements of the trunk and long restrictor muscles. More importantly, the deep segmental spinal muscles respond rapidly and in predictable patterns to facilitation of spinal cord segmental influences. They are believed to produce and maintain the extended Fryette type II dysfunctions in response to viscerosomatic and somatosomatic reflexes observed in some clinical practices. However, little is known about their complex function as a group in truncal posturing and locomotion.

INTERMEDIATE SPINAL MUSCLES

They are long restrictors that run parallel to the spinal column and cross anywhere from two to eight or more segments. These muscles include the following:

- Multifidus
- Semispinalis
- Longissimus
- Iliocostalis
- Quadratus lumborum
- Psoas major

The intermediate spinal muscles are voluntary, motor muscles that move the trunk with volitional thought. They also function unconsciously in large truncal movements, such as those necessary to maintain balance and propulsion in the gait cycle. When hypertonic, they produce sidebending of the spinal column and group curves usually composed of vertebrae engaged in Fryette type I mechanics.

SUPERFICIAL BACK MUSCLES

They are attached to the spinal column or ribs and are thus incidentally involved in spinal motion. They are actually used to brace or move the extremities. These muscles include the following:

- Trapezius
- Latissimus dorsi
- Rhomboideus major and minor
- Serratus anterior
- Pectoralis minor

When hypertonic, they influence both the motion of an extremity and spinal motion. For example, a hypertonic rhomboid minor muscle would draw the scapula medially and superiorly. If the scapula is anchored by its other attached musculature, its attachment to the spinous processes of C7 and T1 would rotate these vertebrae away from the side of the hypertonic rhomboid (remember the reference point for vertebral rotation is the anterior aspect of the vertebra).

When these muscles go into a true spasm, they produce significant pain and grossly distort the normal curves of the spine and body posture. They can also produce a host of body-wide adaptational responses.

Fascial and Ligamentous Restriction

Ligaments of the spine can shorten due to fibrosis resulting from trauma, or to inflammatory diseases of the spine. The ligaments that shorten or lose elasticity the most will determine the directions that a vertebral segment can and cannot move.

Likewise, the fascial envelope in which the contractile elements of the muscles reside can shorten from a host of causes (congenital, developmental, disuse, injury, inflammatory diseases of muscle). Again, when shortened, they produce patterns of restriction identical to those that would occur if the same muscle was hypertonic. However, even with the musculature's contractile elements relaxed, its more static investing fascia will remain shortened.

Edema-Causing Restriction

The presence of fluid in the interstices of any body region will create motion restriction. This is partially due to the presence of pain from fascial stretching and compartmental distention and partially to the mechanical presence of the fluid itself, which distends fascial compartments and stretches tissues. Consequentially, some of the "slack" is taken out of the fascia or joint capsules themselves. While no set pattern of dysfunction has been ascribed to segmental or regional edema, the osteopathic profession has long acknowledged its importance.

END FEEL

End feel encompasses how the tissue feels at the end of range-of-motion testing for large joint motions, or for segmental motion testing. This concept has significant implications for the osteopathic physician. The quality of the end feel is used to determine the most likely etiology of the motion restriction (articular, muscular, fascial, edema). This palpatory information guides the physician in selecting the most appropriate manipulative technique to address that particular region or dysfunction.

Each etiologic agent of somatic dysfunction produces one distinct end feel. Edema produces a mushy or fluid-filled sponge kind of end feel. Muscle hypertonicity has a stretchy or rubbery end feel. Articular dysfunctions have a more solid end feel, with palpated loss of elasticity usually in the muscles associated with the articular restrictions. Ligamentous and fascial restrictions often have a very hard, abrupt end feel with near total loss of tissue elasticity.

It is not uncommon for a patient to exhibit several types of restrictions in a single dysfunction, especially if the dysfunction is chronic.

- For instance, a muscle energy technique can be initially applied to a segmental dysfunction. On retesting, the contractile elements of the muscle could have relaxed, and the segment may now exhibit a more fascial restriction type of end feel, calling for a direct myofascial release technique to now be applied.
- Another example would be in applying indirect myofascial release or lymphatic approaches where edema is present. With the new-found absence of edema, the end feel can subsequently reveal an articular restriction, calling for an articulatory or high-velocity, low-amplitude thrust technique.

An osteopathic manipulative technique may be applied perfectly but would still be unsuccessful if applied for the wrong tissue etiology of the restriction. Likewise, a technique may also fail to work due to a misinterpretation of the end feel by the inexperienced physician, rather than to poor application of a given technique.

PRIMARY AND SECONDARY SOMATIC DYSFUNCTIONS

A primary dysfunction is one that is caused by a trauma, or repetitive microtrauma. It initiates a variety of symptoms and events such as:

- Local pain
- Somatosensory referred pain
- Local muscle guarding responses
- Initiation of somatosomatic and somatovisceral reflexes
- Creation of secondary somatic dysfunctions[11]

Secondary somatic dysfunction can arise secondary to a variety of other conditions. The following list is not exhaustive but contains many of the more common causes:

- Local diseases of the spine such as degenerative disk disease or facet joint osteoarthritis
- Mechanical effects of larger deformities such as kyphosis or scoliosis
- Compensatory for primary or other secondary somatic dysfunctions
- Viscerosomatic reflex–generated dysfunctions
- Somatosomatic reflex–generated dysfunctions[11]

THE KEY SOMATIC DYSFUNCTION

The key somatic dysfunction is the somatic dysfunction that causes and maintains an entire pattern of dysfunction, including secondary somatic dysfunctions. It frequently represents, on a percentage basis, the *most* restricted structure in a patient's body. A great deal of time and effort is often expended searching for this key dysfunction, since its correction may result in the greatest improvement in the patient's overall physiology.[11]

SPECIFIC ELEMENTS OF THE SEGMENTAL EXAMINATION

One of the distinctive features of osteopathic medicine is the incorporation of the structural exam or evaluation which may be performed alone or incorporated into the physical exam to assess for the presence of somatic dysfunction. With respect to the patient's symptoms, somatic dysfunction may be the actual cause, it may be a contributing factor, or it may be a reflection of an underlying process (e.g., viscerosomatic reflex).

The structural exam consists of three components: (1) the screening component; (2) the regional component; and (3) the segmental component. The screening portion of the examination is used to determine whether somatic dysfunction(s) may be present and in which body region(s). One may think of this portion of the osteopathic structural exam as asking the question: "Is there a structural problem present?"

Once the physician has used the screening portion to determine whether any region(s) of the body need further evaluation for the presence of somatic dysfunction, they then perform the regional and segmental evaluations to the affected area(s). The regional portion is comprised of two parts; assessment of abnormal tissue texture changes, and passive range of motion to assess the quality of joint and/or tissue motion and to localize the problem more specifically. This part of the examination may be thought of as asking the question "Where is the structural problem?" The segmental portion then defines and describes the specific joint or tissue restriction that was localized using the regional examination. This part of the examination may be thought of as asking the question: "What is the problem?" The components of the exam may almost be thought of as a funnel leading the osteopathic physician to a specific diagnosis to which a rational treatment may now be applied.

FINDINGS RELATED TO THE SEGMENTAL EXAM

The following represents specific segmental findings or somatic dysfunction related to the different regions of the body. For further information on the anatomy of each region and how to perform the actual segmental exam of each, please see the "Functional Anatomy and Segmental Exam" chapters of each region.

HEAD REGION

In general, the cranium may be palpated for evidence of the following:

- Unusually increased or decreased angulation of bones
- Abnormal approximation or separation of sutures
- Decreased resiliency of the bones
- Painful areas

Somatic dysfunction of the cranium may include:

- Sphenobasilar synchondrosis (SBS) strain patterns or dysfunction including:
  - ☐ Torsions (right or left)
  - ☐ Sidebending rotation (right or left)
  - ☐ Vertical (superior or inferior)
  - ☐ Lateral (right or left)

- SBS compression often manifests as absence of cranial flexion and extension
  - □ Sutural or joint restrictions
  - □ Membranous articular strains
  - □ Ligamentous strains including petrosphenoid, sphemomandibular, stylomandibular and stylohyoid ligaments
  - □ Intraosseous strains
  - □ Cranial rhythmic impulse (CRI)

The CRI is palpated for:

- Rate (cycles per minute)
- Rhythm (symmetrical, asymmetrical)
- Amplitude (large, small)
- Vitality (a general assessment of the energy level of the CRI)

CERVICAL REGION

Segmental examination of the cervical spine should be divided into two regions for diagnosis. The atypical cervical vertebral segments include the OA and AA joints. The typical cervical segments include the C2 through C7 segments.

- Atypical Cervical Vertebral Segments:
  - □ OA (neutral, extended, flexed, sidebending and rotation occur in opposite directions)
  - □ AA (AA rotated left [AARL], AA rotated right [AARR])
- Typical Cervical Vertebral Segments
  - □ C2–C7 (extended or flexed with sidebending and rotation occurring in the same direction. There is ongoing discussion on whether neutral somatic dysfunction exists within the typical cervical spine.)

THORACIC REGION

The upper thoracic and lower thoracic regions differ with respect to the mechanical levers used for their assessment. The head and neck are utilized to assess the upper thoracic region and the trunk is utilized to assess the lower thoracic region.

- Upper thoracic (typically T1–T4): exhibits Type I (neutral, sidebending and rotation occurring in opposite directions) or Type II mechanics (flexed or extended with sidebending and rotation occurring in the same direction)
- Lower thoracic (typically T5–T12): exhibits Type I (neutral, sidebending and rotation occurring in opposite directions) or Type II mechanics (flexed or extended with sidebending and rotation occurring in the same direction)

RIB CAGE

Somatic dysfunction of the ribs may be related to dysfunction of the thoracic region. In the presence of rib somatic dysfunction, it is generally advised to assess the thoracic region for dysfunction and address those first. The rib region may be then be reevaluated to determine if rib dysfunction remains. Dysfunction of the ribs is designated as either structural or respiratory. Specific structural dysfunction include the following:

- Superior subluxation of the first rib
- Anterior or posterior subluxations
- External rib torsions
- Anteroposterior compression
- Lateral compressions
- Laterally flexed ribs

Respiratory rib somatic dysfunction is classified as either inhalation or exhalation and may involve either a single rib or a group of ribs.

- **Inhalation somatic dysfunction** signifies a rib or group of ribs that move more easily and through a greater range of motion during inhalation and are restricted in motion during exhalation as relative to a comparable rib or group of ribs on the contralateral side.
- **Exhalation somatic dysfunction** signifies a rib or group of ribs that move more easily and through a greater range of motion during exhalation and are restricted in motion during inhalation as relative to a comparable rib or group of ribs on the contralateral side.
- **Key rib:** Groups of ribs held in an inhalation and exhalation somatic dysfunction are generally maintained by a "key rib." The key rib of an inhalation somatic dysfunction is usually located toward the inferior aspect or bottom of the group of ribs, maintaining the ribs superior to it in an inhaled position. The key rib of an exhalation somatic dysfunction is usually located toward the superior aspect or top of the group of ribs, maintaining the ribs inferior to it in an exhaled position. The acronym, BITE (**B**ottom-**I**nhalation somatic dysfunction; **T**op-**E**xhalation somatic dysfunction)[12] may be a useful tool for recalling assessment of the key rib.

Other somatic dysfunction of the rib cage includes sternal compression and dysfunction of the various joints of the sternum. These may result from seat belt injuries and surgeries involving the costal cage such as coronary bypass surgery.

Lumbar Region

The lumbar region is an important crossroads between the pelvis and the thoracic cage and is also the site of the crura insertion (L1–L3) of the thoracoabdominal diaphragm.

- Lumbar somatic dysfunction may exhibit Type I (neutral, sidebending and rotation occurring in opposite directions) or Type II mechanics (flexed or extended with sidebending and rotation occurring in the same direction)

Pelvis Region (Iliosacral)

The pelvis is a complex and multifaceted region that includes the innominates and the sacrum. The diagnoses of the pelvis and sacrum have been separated here but clinically, should always be considered as a functional unit.

A positive standing flexion test often indicates the presence of an iliosacral somatic dysfunction. The seated flexion test may also be positive. Landmarks used to determine iliosacral somatic dysfunction include ASIS levels and their distance from a midline structure, pubic tubercle levels, and PSIS levels.

Iliosacral somatic dysfunctions include the following:

- Innominate rotations, anterior and posterior
- Innominate subluxations (shears), superior and inferior
- Innominate flares (inflares and outflares)
- Pubic shears (subluxations), superior and inferior

Related somatic dysfunctions include:

- Unequal hamstring length
- Unequal iliopsoas length

Please see Tables 31.2 and 31.3 for a summary of iliosacral and pubic dysfunctions and their structural findings.

TABLE 31.2

Iliosacral Somatic Dysfunctions

Side of Positive Standing Flexion Test	Anterior Superior Iliac Spine (ASIS)	Posterior Superior Iliac Spine (PSIS)	Diagnosis
Right	Inferior right	Superior right	Anterior rotation right
	Superior right	Inferior right	Posterior rotation right
	Superior right	Superior right	Superior shear right
	Inferior right	Inferior right	Inferior shear right
	Medial right	Lateral right	Inflare right
	Lateral right	Medial right	Outflare right
Left	Inferior left	Superior left	Anterior rotation left
	Superior left	Inferior left	Posterior rotation left
	Superior left	Superior left	Superior shear left
	Inferior left	Inferior left	Inferior shear left
	Lateral left	Medial left	Outflare left
	Medial left	Lateral left	Inflare left

TABLE 31.3

Pubic Symphysis Somatic Dysfunction

Side of Positive Standing Flexion Test	Pubic Tubercle Height	Diagnosis
Right	Superior	Superior right
	Inferior	Inferior right
Left	Superior	Superior left
	Inferior	Inferior left

Sacral Region (Sacroiliac)

Three systems of nomenclature currently used to define sacropelvic mechanics are those described by

1. Mitchell (muscle energy)
2. Chicago Model (Strachan)
3. Van Buskirk (Still technique)

A positive seated flexion test and oftentimes a positive standing flexion test indicate sacral somatic dysfunction. The degree of asymmetry between the following anatomical landmarks is of interest here:

1. Sacral sulcus
2. Inferior lateral angles (ILAs) of the sacrum
3. Position of L5 relative to S1

Confirmatory tests include:

- The backward bend or Sphinx test: change in sacral sulcus depth or ILA levels with backward bending test of the lumbar spine (increased symmetry or asymmetry)
- Lumbosacral spring test: amount of stiffness palpable in the lumbosacral area during a lumbosacral spring test (increased stiffness is described as a positive test while decreased stiffness or compliance indicates a negative test)

The most common and standard diagnoses of SI somatic dysfunction include (but are not limited to) the following:

- Sacrum anterior[13]
- Sacrum posterior[13]
- Anterior/forward torsions (rotation of the sacrum on the same oblique axis):
  - ☐ Left rotation on left oblique axis
  - ☐ Right rotation on right oblique axis
- Posterior/backward torsions (rotation of the sacrum on the opposite oblique axis):
  - ☐ Right rotation on left oblique axis
  - ☐ Left rotation on right oblique axis
- Bilateral sacral flexion
- Bilateral sacral extension
- Unilateral sacral flexion (sacral shear)
- Unilateral sacral extension (sacral shear)

Please see Table 31.4 for a summary of the Mitchell and Chicago sacroiliac somatic dysfunctions and their structural findings.

Please see Table 31.5 for a summary of sacral diagnoses using the Still model.

Upper Extremity

Somatic dysfunction in the extremities was conventionally named according to the direction of motion preference. However, documenting the restriction of certain joints has become increasingly more common. Chapter 91 Osteopathic Approach to Diagnosing and Treating Somatic Dysfunction in the Extremities has several tables that list the commonly used nomenclature for various extremity joint somatic dysfunctions and are referred to in this section.

THE SHOULDER AND PECTORAL GIRDLE

THE GLENOHUMERAL JOINT

Somatic dysfunction of the glenohumeral joint occurs in the minor motions of the joint. Restrictions of translatory motions in many directions may occur due to the ball-and-socket nature of the glenohumeral joint. Some authors call this "joint play," "translation," or "glide." These gliding dysfunctions of the shoulder joint are active

TABLE 31.4

Summary of the Mitchell and Chicago Sacroiliac Somatic Dysfunctions and Their Structural Findings

Test/Findings	Forward Sacral Torsions (L on L)	Backward Sacral Torsions (R on L)	Bilateral Sacral Flexion	Bilateral Sacral Extension	Unilateral Sacral Flexion (Right Shear)	Unilateral Sacral Extension (Right Shear)	Chicago Anterior Sacrum (Right)	Chicago Posterior Sacrum (Right)
(+) Seated flexion test	Right	Right	Neither (negative)	Neither (negative)	Right	Right	Right	Right
Sacral base (sacral sulcus)	Deep/anterior on right Shallow/posterior on left	Shallow/posterior on right Deep/anterior on left	Deep/anterior on both sides	Shallow/posterior on both sides	Deep/anterior on right Shallow/posterior on left	Deep/anterior on left Shallow/posterior on right	Deep/anterior on right Shallow/posterior on left	Deep/anterior on left Shallow/posterior on right
Inferior lateral angle (ILA) position	Posterior and inferior on left	Posterior and inferior on right	Posterior and inferior on both sides	Anterior and superior on both sides	Posterior and inferior on right	Anterior and superior on right	Posterior and inferior on left	Posterior and inferior on right
Tissue texture change	N/A	N/A	N/A	N/A	N/A	N/A	Right sulcus	Right lower pole of SI joint
Passive sacral motion testing	N/A	N/A	N/A	N/A	N/A	N/A	Freedom about left oblique axis	Freedom about right oblique axis
Lumbar lateral curve	Convex right	Convex left	None	None	Convex right	Convex left	N/A	N/A
Lumbar lordosis (spring test)	Increased (negative spring test)	Reduced (positive spring test)	Increased or normal (negative spring test)	Reduced (positive spring test)	Increased or normal (negative spring test)	Reduced (positive spring test)	N/A	N/A
Supine medial malleolus (leg length)	Short left	Short right	Symmetrical	Symmetrical	Short left	Short right	Short right	Short left
L5	Neutral and rotated right	Flexed or extended and rotated left	Neutral, nonneutral or normal	Neutral, nonneutral or normal	Neutral and rotated right	Neutral and rotated left	N/A	N/A
Sphinx test	Negative (decreased asymmetry/ findings improved)	Positive (increased asymmetry/ findings worsen)	N/A	N/A	Negative (decreased asymmetry/ findings improved)	Positive (increased asymmetry/ findings worsen)	N/A	N/A
Innominate rotation	N/A	N/A	N/A	N/A	N/A	N/A	Right posterior ilium	Right anterior ilium
Muscle reactivity/ tension	N/A	N/A	N/A	N/A	N/A	N/A	Right gluteus medius	Right piriformis

SI, sacroiliac.

TABLE 31.5

Summary of Sacral Diagnoses Using the Still Model

Diagnosis	Characteristics
Diagonal right	Positive right seated flexion test
	Positive left ILA test
Diagonal left	Positive left seated flexion test
	Positive right ILA test
Unilateral right	Positive right seated flexion test
	Positive right ILA test
Unilateral left	Positive left seated flexion test
	Positive left ILA test

or passive exaggerations of its cardinal movements. The humeral head tends to glide more anteriorly during extension and external rotation, posteriorly during flexion up to 90 degrees and internal rotation, superiorly with adduction, and inferiorly with abduction and flexion from 90 to 180 degrees.[14] These gliding restrictions may be evaluated with each plane of motion and treated using principles of muscle energy technique or articulatory techniques.

STERNOCLAVICULAR JOINT

Please see *Table 91.1 Sternoclavicular Joint (SCJ) Somatic Dysfunction* for a summary of SCJ somatic dysfunction and its nomenclature.

THE ACROMIOCLAVICULAR JOINT

Please see *Table 91.2 Acromioclavicular Joint Somatic Dysfunction* for a summary of acromioclavicular joint somatic dysfunction and its nomenclature.

THE SCAPULOTHORACIC REGION

The scapulothoracic joint is a physiologic joint as there are no boney articulations between the scapula and the posterior thorax. However, the 17 muscles attaching to the scapula and those acting on the pectoral girdle allow for significant scapular mobility on the thoracic wall.

Scapular position and motion on the thoracic wall, independent of glenohumeral motion is dependent on several of the muscles attaching the scapula to the spine and ribs as well as influences from gravity and the inferior sternocostal head of the pectoralis major[15]:

1. Elevation
2. Depression
3. Protraction (Abduction)
4. Retraction (Adduction)
5. Upward rotation (Lateral rotation of inferior angle)
6. Downward rotation (Medial rotation of inferior angle)

The Elbow

The elbow joint consists of three joints within one joint capsule

1. The humero-ulnar joint (ulnohumeral joint) (Table 91.4)
2. The humero-radial joint (radiohumeral joint) (Table 91.5)
3. The proximal radio-ulnar joint

The elbow joint may be evaluated for restriction in abduction and adduction, flexion and extension, and pronation and supination. The radial head is also assessed for somatic dysfunction.

The motion and the nomenclature for somatic dysfunction of these joints are described in *Table 91.4 The Ulnohumeral (Elbow) Joint Somatic Dysfunction* and *Table 91.5 Radial Head Somatic Dysfunction (Combined Humeroradial and Proximal Radioulnar Joint Motion)*.

THE WRIST AND HAND

WRIST (RADIOCARPAL) JOINT

The wrist (radiocarpal) joint is an ellipsoid synovial joint formed by the concave distal end of the radius, three convex proximal carpal bones (the scaphoid, lunate, and triquetral bones), and an articular disk. The articular disk separates the cavity of the distal radio-ulnar joint from the cavity of the wrist joint.[11] The wrist joint moves around A/P and transverse axes, allowing for the movements of flexion, extension, abduction (radial deviation), and adduction (ulnar deviation). Somatic dysfunction is not related to the gross motions of the wrist but instead to dysfunction of the small gliding motions of the proximal carpal bones on the radius as the wrist is moved. The carpals can move slightly anteriorly, posteriorly, medially, or laterally.

Somatic dysfunction of the wrist was conventionally named according to the direction of motion preference. However, documenting the restriction has become increasingly more common. The motions include:

- Dorsiflexion
- Palmar flexion
- Ulnar deviation pronated
- Radial deviation pronated
- Ulnar deviation supinated
- Radial deviation supinated

For further information on motion and somatic dysfunction nomenclature see

- *Table 91.6 The Radiocarpal (Wrist) Joint Somatic Dysfunction*
- *Chapter 91 Box 91.1 Intercarpal Joint Diagnostic Findings*[16]

CARPOMETACARPAL (CMC) AND INTERMETACARPAL (IM) JOINTS

The carpometacarpal (CMC) and intermetacarpal (IM) joints are all classified as plane synovial joints, except the CMC of the thumb, which is a saddle joint. The medial four CMC joints and each of their three IM joints share a common joint cavity. Their gliding motion is primarily anterior and posterior; however, each digit's quantity of motion differs.

METACARPOPHALANGEAL (MP) AND INTERPHALANGEAL (IP) JOINTS

The metacarpal–phalangeal (MP) joints are condyloid joints permitting flexion–extension and adduction–abduction, while the interphalangeal (IP) joints of the hand are gliding joints that permit gross flexion and extension. The MP and IP joints may develop somatic dysfunction in any one of a combination of six minor gliding motions that cannot be initiated directly by muscle action:

- Anteroposterior glide
- Mediolateral glide
- Internal–external rotational glide

The Lower Extremity

Like the Upper Extremity section, descriptions of the specific examinations for the various joints of the lower extremities are described in Chapter 91 Osteopathic Approach to Diagnosing and Treating

Somatic Dysfunction in the Extremities. That chapter includes several tables that list the commonly used nomenclature for various extremity joint somatic dysfunctions and are referred to in this section.

THE FEMOROACETABULAR JOINT

The hip (femoroacetabular) joint forms the connection between the lower extremity and the pelvis. The stable multiaxial ball-and-socket synovial joint allows for weight bearing and motion in flexion, extension, abduction, adduction, internal (medial) rotation, external (lateral) rotation, and circumduction. Average ranges of motion of the hip differ when the knee is flexed or extended.

Table 91.7 Hip Joint Somatic Dysfunction for a summary of the femoroacetabular joint motion and the somatic dysfunction nomenclature.

The Knee

The knee is a compound synovial joint consisting of three separate articulations within one joint capsule—the medial and lateral femorotibial articulations and the patellofemoral articulation.[15] The fibula is not considered part of the knee joint. However, dysfunction at the proximal tibiofibular joint, the distal tibiofibular syndesmosis, and the interosseous membrane can also affect knee and ankle mechanics (REF Kingston).

The knee is a compound synovial joint consisting of three separate articulations within one joint capsule—the medial and lateral femorotibial articulations and the patellofemoral articulation.[17] The fibula is not considered part of the knee joint. However, dysfunction at the proximal tibiofibular joint, the distal tibiofibular syndesmosis, and the interosseous membrane can also affect knee and ankle mechanics.[18]

Femorotibial Articulations

The major motions of the knee joint are flexion and extension. Because of the irregular shape of the joint surfaces, these two motions are combined with some minor involuntary glides, rolling, and rotational motions. Minor motions of the tibial plateau at the knee include:

- Anterior and posterior glides
- Medial and lateral glides
- Internal rotation with posterolateral glide
- External rotation with anteromedial glide

See *Table 91.8 Knee (Femorotibial) Joint Somatic Dysfunction* for a summary of the femorotibial joint motion and the somatic dysfunction nomenclature.

Patellofemoral Joint Dysfunction

Patellofemoral joint dysfunction and structural change of the patella may each arise from abnormal patella tracking or pressure on the patella. This is often seen when the Q-angle is excessive. An increased Q-angle is referred to as genu valgum (knock-kneed). A decreased Q-angle is referred to as genu varum (bow-legged).

The Fibular Joints and Proximal Fibular Dysfunction

The fibula lies posterolateral to the tibia and is connected by the proximal tibiofibular joint, the distal tibiofibular syndesmosis, and the interosseous membrane between the two shafts.

There is reciprocal anterior–posterior motion between the distal and proximal ends of the fibula. When the distal fibula moves posteriorly, the proximal fibular head moves anteriorly. This motion can be induced by ankle dorsiflexion and plantarflexion or through translatory motion at either fibular end. Restricted ankle motion warrants examination and treatment of any tibial rotations and tibiofibular syndesmosis tension prior to treating fibular dysfunction.

Fibular head somatic dysfunction is classically named for the preferred position of anterior or posterior glide. It is checked by gliding the fibular head posteriorly (and slightly medial) and anteriorly (and slightly lateral).

See *Table 91.9 The Proximal Tibiofibular Joint/Fibular Head Somatic Dysfunction* for a summary of the fibular head somatic dysfunction nomenclature.

The motion of the fibula is tightly coupled with the rotation of the tibia and pronation/supination of the subtalar joint.

See *Table 91.10 The Distal Tibiofibular Joint/Distal Fibula Somatic Dysfunction* for a summary of the distal fibular somatic dysfunction nomenclature.

The Ankle and Foot

The ankle joint complex is comprised of the kinetic linkage between the lower leg and the foot. It is comprised of the tibiotalar (talocrural), talocalcaneal (subtalar), and transverse-tarsal (talocalcaneonavicular) joints.[19] The talus has no direct muscular attachments, so its movements are determined by muscle actions on the bones above and below it.[19] The combined proper functions of all the lower extremity joints are needed for mobility and balance.[19,20]

The Tibiotalar Joint (Talocrural Joint)

The tibiotalar joint forms the junction between the distal tibia and fibula of the lower leg and the talus. Dorsiflexion and plantarflexion are the primary motions of the talocrural joint, with an oblique axis of rotation that travels through the medial malleolus, the talar head, and the lateral malleolus.[21,22]

See *Table 91.11 Tibiotalar/Talocrural Joint (Ankle) Somatic Dysfunction* for a summary of the tibiotalar somatic dysfunction nomenclature.

The Subtalar Joint

The subtalar joint is comprised of anterior (talocalcaneonavicular) and posterior (talocalcaneal) articulations that are separated by the tarsal canal.[21] The subtalar joint's major motions are inversion and eversion of the ankle and foot, yet it has its own defined distinct pronation and supination.

See *Table 91.12 Subtalar/Talocalcaneal Joint (Ankle) Somatic Dysfunction* for a summary of the talocalcaneal somatic dysfunction nomenclature.

The Transverse Tarsal and Intertarsal Joints

The transverse tarsal joint, or *Chopart's* joint, is the joint between the hindfoot (talus and calcaneus) and the midfoot (navicular and cuboid). It contains the talonavicular, the calcaneocuboid and two small talocalcaneal articulations, which are separate joints that act together as a functional unit, responding to eversion or inversion of the calcaneus.

The navicular, cuboid, and three cuneiform bones (medial, intermediate, and lateral) make up the midfoot. This region acts as a bridge between the hindfoot and the forefoot. The bones of the midfoot form the medial longitudinal, the lateral longitudinal, and the transverse arches. The function of the midfoot is to transmit and attenuate force and allow the foot to accommodate to the variable surface of the ground.[21]

Somatic dysfunction of the tarsal bones (cuboid, navicular, or cuneiforms) is relatively common and is summarized in *Table 91.13 Transverse Tarsal (Talonavicular and Calcaneocuboid) Joint and Intertarsal Joint (Cuneiform Bones) Somatic Dysfunction.*

The Tarsometatarsal, Metatarsophalangeal, and Interphalangeal Joints

The tarsometatarsal (TMT) joint is the articulation between mid and forefoot segments and consists of the medial and lateral columns of the foot.[21] The forefoot is composed of the metatarsals and the phalanges. It may be divided into the medial and lateral forefoot. The joint capsules and the medial collateral, and lateral collateral ligaments provide stability for each of the metatarsophalangeal and IP joints.

Each of these bones may exhibit motion in the following directions:

- Dorsal and plantar glide
- Internal and external rotation (about an anterior–posterior axis)
- Small amounts of medial and lateral glide

In addition to the above, the physician should also examine the regions for the following:

- Myofascial restrictions
- Counterstrain tender points
- Chapman reflexes as is appropriate

SUMMARY

The overall osteopathic structural exam aims to search for:

- Larger deformities that give rise to secondary somatic dysfunctions
- Evidence of musculoskeletal diseases that give rise to somatic dysfunction
- Somatic dysfunctions that may be responsible for the patient's symptomatology or dysfunctional physiology
- The location of the key somatic dysfunction
- The tissue responsible for maintaining the somatic dysfunction

The ultimate goal of the osteopathic physician is to improve the quality of their patients' lives. An important element of this process is accurately identifying somatic dysfunction pertinent to the patient's condition so that it can be addressed with osteopathic manipulative treatment to alleviate the direct source of the patient's condition or remove allostatic load associated with it.

REFERENCES

1. Fryette HH. *Principles of Osteopathic Technic.* Academy of Applied Osteopathy; 1954:22–26.
2. Fryette HH. *Principles of Osteopathic Technic.* Academy of Applied Osteopathy; 1954:19.
3. Kimberly PE. *Outline of Osteopathic Manipulative Procedures (The Kimberly Manual).* Walsworth Publishing Company; 2000:11–12.
4. Fryette HH. *Principles of Osteopathic Technic.* Academy of Applied Osteopathy; 1954:30.
5. Fryette HH. *Principles of Osteopathic Technic.* Academy of Applied Osteopathy; 1954:29–30.
6. Fryette HH. *Principles of Osteopathic Technic.* Academy of Applied Osteopathy; 1954:27–29.
7. Nicholas AS, Nicholas EA. Intersegmental motion testing. In: *Atlas of Osteopathic Techniques.* Lippincott Williams & Wilkins; 2008.
8. Greenman PE. *Principles of Manual Medicine.* 4th ed. Williams & Wilkins; 2011:47.
9. Furmann D, Nečas D, Rebenda D, Čípek P, Vrbka M, Křupka I, Hartl M. The effect of synovial fluid composition, speed and load on frictional behaviour of articular cartilage. *Materials (Basel).* 2020;13(6):1334.
10. Tamer TM. Hyaluronan and synovial joint: function, distribution and healing. *Interdiscip Toxicol.* 2013;6(3):111–125.
11. American Association of Colleges of Osteopathic Medicine. *Glossary of Osteopathic Terminology.* American Association of Colleges of Osteopathic Medicine; 2011:53.
12. Mitchell FL. *The Muscle Energy Manual: Evaluation and Treatment of the Thoracic Spine, Lubar Spine and Rib Cage.* Vol 2. MET Press; 1998:60.
13. Walton WJ. *Osteopathic Diagnosis and Technique, Sacroiliac Diagnosis.* 1st ed. Matthews Book Co.; 1966:187–197. Distributed, Colorado Springs, CO: American Academy of Osteopathy; reprinted, 1970.
14. Kimberly PE, Halma K, Kirksville College of Osteopathic Medicine. *Outline of Osteopathic Manipulative Procedures: The Kimberly Manual 2006.* Updated 2008 ed. Walsworth Publishing Company; 2006, 2008; 235–236.
15. Dalley AF, Agur AMR. *Moore's Clinically Oriented Anatomy.* 9th ed. Wolters Kluwer; 2023;142–295.
16. Kimberly PE, Halma K, Kirksville College of Osteopathic Medicine. *Outline of Osteopathic Manipulative Procedures: The Kimberly Manual 2006.* Updated 2008 ed. Walsworth Publishing Company; 2006, 2008;255.
17. Dalley AF, Agur AMR. *Moore's Clinically Oriented Anatomy.* 9th ed. Wolters Kluwer; 2023:672–838.
18. Kingston, B. *Understanding Joints, A Practical Guide to Their Structure and Function.* Stanley Thornes; 2000:163–182.
19. Brockett CL, Chapman GJ. Biomechanics of the ankle. *Orthop Trauma.* 2016;30(3):232–238.
20. Ombregt L, Bisschop P, J ter Veer H. *A System of Orthopaedic Medicine.* 2nd ed. Elsevier Limited; 2003;1161–1165.
21. Fraser JJ, Feger MA, Hertel J. Midfoot and forefoot involvement in lateral ankle sprains and chronic ankle instability. Part 1: Anatomy and biomechanics. *Int J Sports Phys Ther.* 2016;11(6):992–1005.
22. Scott SH, Winter DA. Talocrural and talocalcaneal joint kinematics and kinetics during the stance phase of walking. *J Biomech.* 1991;24(8):743–752.

Descriptive and Functional Regional Anatomy (Introduction to Chapters 32–41)

KEY CONCEPTS

- Knowledge of anatomy is important for the following:
  - The accurate palpation of musculoskeletal structures
  - The performance of the physical examination
  - The performance of the osteopathic structural examination
  - Anatomy assists in the understanding of orthopedic, neurologic, and musculoskeletal disorders.
- Anatomy also assists the physician with interpreting symptoms and radiologic images.

INTRODUCTION

Anatomy is arguably the foundation of all aspects of clinical practice. Osteopathic physicians rely on their anatomical knowledge for the following:

- Performing physical examinations (including osteopathic structural examinations)
- Formulating differential diagnoses
- Communicating clinical findings to patients and colleagues

Andrew Taylor Still taught that anatomical discord engenders physiologic discord. One of the objectives of osteopathic medicine is to prevent and cure disease. Disease manifests itself as disordered function. The presence of disordered function is recognized through knowledge of healthy function. However, healthy function cannot be understood without knowledge of normal structure, which is learned through the study of anatomy.

32 Head Region

KURT P. HEINKING ▪ REBECCA E. GIUSTI

KEY CONCEPTS

- Osteopathic manipulative treatment can improve functional outcomes in patients with conditions such as concussion, sinus, eye, and ear disorders.
- Identifying the drainage patterns of the paranasal sinuses, the lymphatic channels, and the venous system assists the physician in identifying possible points of connective tissue blockage.
- Identifying the parasympathetic and sympathetic innervation of the head and neck, as well as the consequences of autonomic nerve dysfunction, can guide the physician in treatment.
- Evaluation of osteopathic cranial motion and consideration of dural continuity are essential to addressing and treating the head and its related regions.
- Somatic dysfunction plays a significant role in a number of clinical conditions that affect the head, suboccipital regions, and ultimately the entire body.

INTRODUCTION

Osteopathic manipulative treatment (OMT) to the head region is based on anatomy and physiologic function of the neurologic, vascular, muscular, articular, and lymphatic systems. Physicians must be as comfortable diagnosing and treating somatic dysfunctions occurring in the head and face region, as with those occurring in other regions of the body.

Treatment of such dysfunctions is thought to

- Diminish tissue congestion
- Improve sinus drainage
- Resolve motion restrictions
- Normalize autonomic tone
- Decrease pain

OMT may be used as a primary treatment, or as an adjunct to pharmacologic agents, hot or cold compresses, gargles, dental appliances, corrective lenses, hearing aids, creams or ointments, shampoos, eye- or eardrops, massage, acupuncture, or other treatments.

Structural exam and diagnosis of this region may be integrated with the traditional evaluation performed for the head, eyes, ears, nose, and throat (HEENT). Many studies have shown that the diagnosis of cranial somatic dysfunction and the use of OMT improves patient outcome in a variety of conditions.

DEFINITION

The head region is defined as any of the topographical divisions of the cranium in relation to the bones of the cranial vault, including the following:

- Frontal region
- Parietal region
- Occipital region
- Temporal region[1]

The uppermost part of the human body, which contains the brain, eyes, ears, nose, and mouth. This anatomical region is crucial for housing essential sensory organs and the control center for the nervous system.[1]

DESCRIPTIVE AND FUNCTIONAL ANATOMY

Skeletal Structures

THE ADULT SKULL

The adult skull is composed of 29 bones (Figs. 32.1 to 32.3), which are summarized in Table 32.1.

From an osteopathic cranial perspective, these bones can be divided into midline and paired bones. See Chapter 53 for a detailed description of cranial motion mechanics and terminology. In normal physiologic motion, the following should occur:

- During osteopathic cranial flexion, the midline bones (sphenoid, occiput, ethmoid, and vomer) move into flexion around their respective transverse axes.
- The paired bones externally rotate during osteopathic cranial flexion.
- During cranial extension, the reverse occurs.[2]

THE INFANT SKULL

The infant skull is divisible into two parts:

1. The neurocranium (vault and base) that surrounds and protects the brain and consists of eight bones
2. The facial skeleton or viscerocranium (face) that consists of 13 bones

The neurocranium (vault and base) can be divided into two parts:

1. The vault or calvaria, from a membranous origin
2. The base, from a cartilaginous origin[3]

The bones of the vault are separated by membranous spaces, the sutures. The fontanelles are present at the angles of the parietal bones, and at the junctions between several sutures of the calvarial bones. There are six fontanelles: two are medial and unpaired (the anterior or bregmatic, posterior or lambdatic) and four are lateral and paired (the sphenoid and mastoid), two on either side.[3]

At birth, the skull is quite large in proportion to the other parts of the skeleton. The neurocranium (vault and base) is, in turn, much larger than the viscerocranium (face). There is a significant

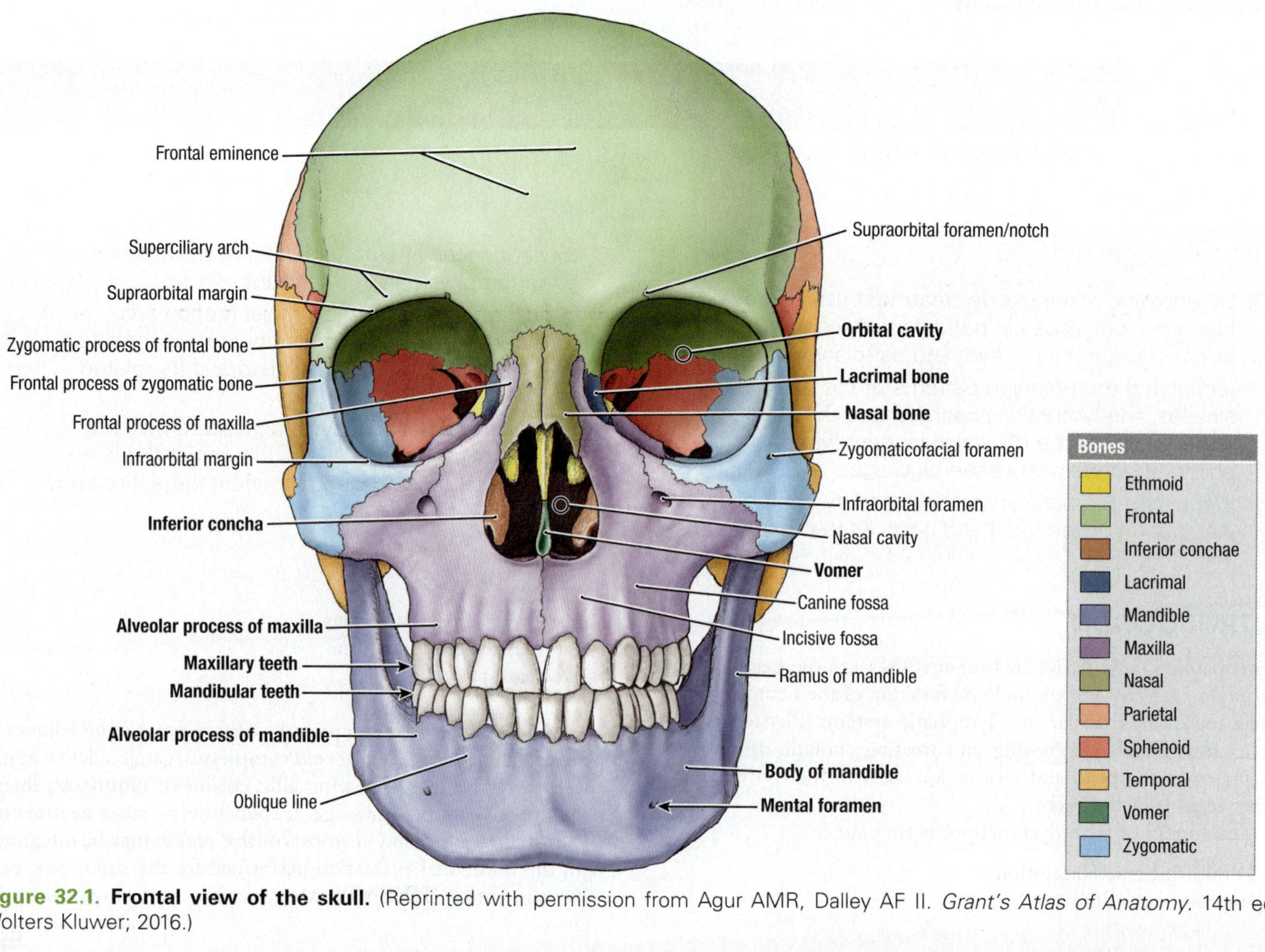

Figure 32.1. Frontal view of the skull. (Reprinted with permission from Agur AMR, Dalley AF II. *Grant's Atlas of Anatomy*. 14th ed. Wolters Kluwer; 2016.)

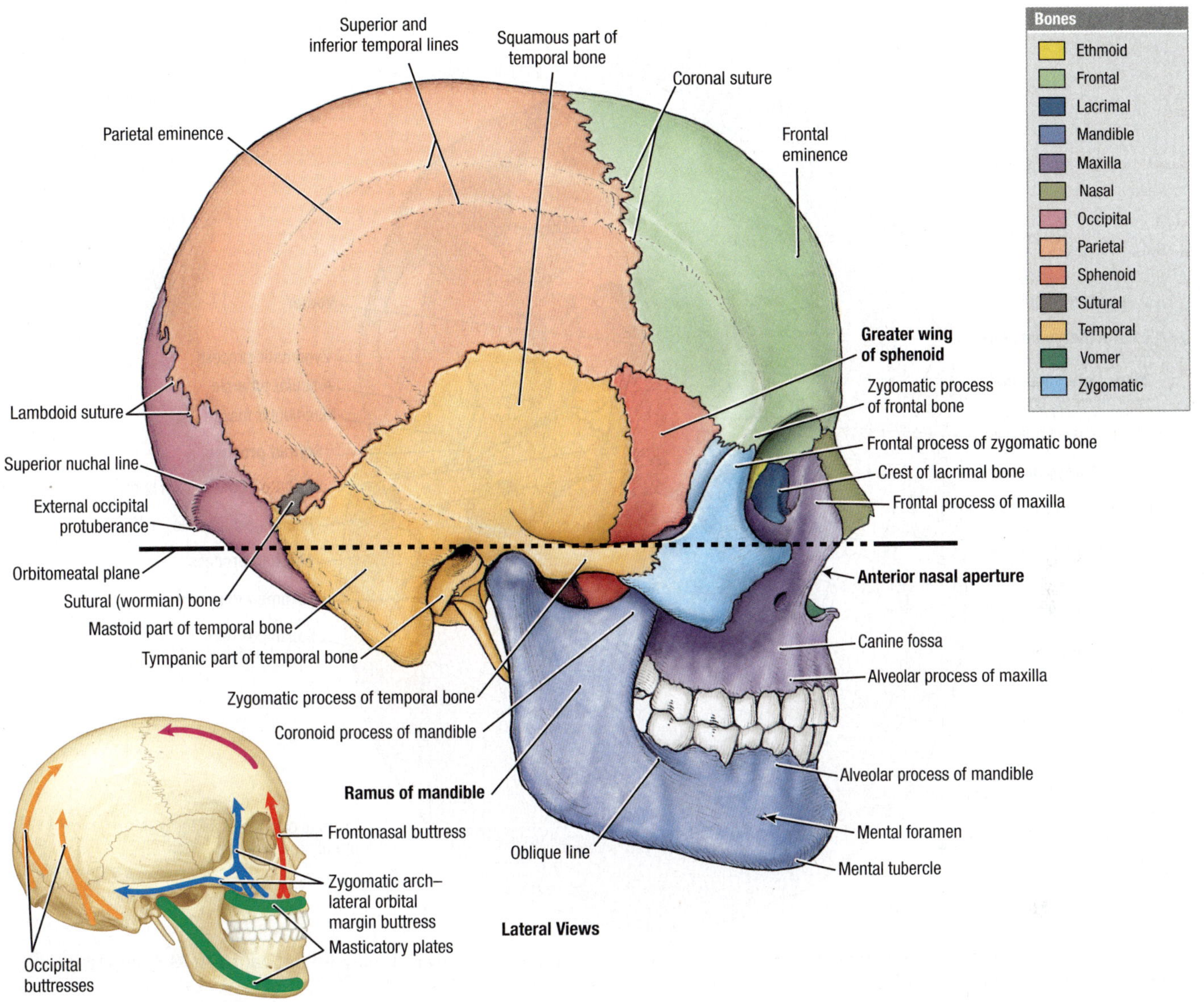

Figure 32.2. Lateral view of the skull. (Reprinted with permission from Agur AMR, Dalley AF II. *Grant's Atlas of Anatomy*. 14th ed. Wolters Kluwer; 2016.)

difference in the growth rate of the neurocranium as compared to that of the viscerocranium. The neurocranium grows quickly from birth to about the 7th year. At about 5 years of age, although brain growth is almost complete, the face has grown to only half of its adult size.[3] The bones of the orbital cavity—the frontal, lacrimal, palatine, zygomatic, ethmoid, maxilla, and sphenoid—develop in membrane and are very reactive to trauma and growth.

Most individual bones of the skull arise from multiple centers of ossification.

- The cartilaginous portion of the occipital bone is not fused at birth. Instead, it is derived from five primary centers of ossification.
- The sphenoid bone is a more complex structure with multiple centers of ossification that unite to result in the three units.
- The occiput, sphenoid, and temporal bones demonstrate both endochondral and intramembranous types of ossification.
- When developed, the ossification centers form the bones of the calvaria. They are as follows:
  - □ The frontal bones
  - □ The parietals
  - □ The squamous portions of the temporal bones
  - □ The upper portion of the occipital (supraoccipital) squama[3]

The sutures separating these bones are as follows:

- The sagittal suture between the parietal bones
- The metopic suture between the frontal bones
- The paired coronal sutures between the two frontal and two parietal bones
- The paired lambdoidal sutures between the supraoccipital and parietal bones
- The squamous sutures between the parietal, temporal, and sphenoid bones

At birth, ossification is not yet complete for most of the bones, which still consist of several component parts. For example, consider the occiput, sphenoid, and temporals.

- At birth, the occiput consists of four portions: the basiocciput, two "exocciputs," and the squama. The different articulations of the cranial base are named synchondroses. By definition, synchondroses are cartilaginous joints in which two bones are united by fibrocartilage.

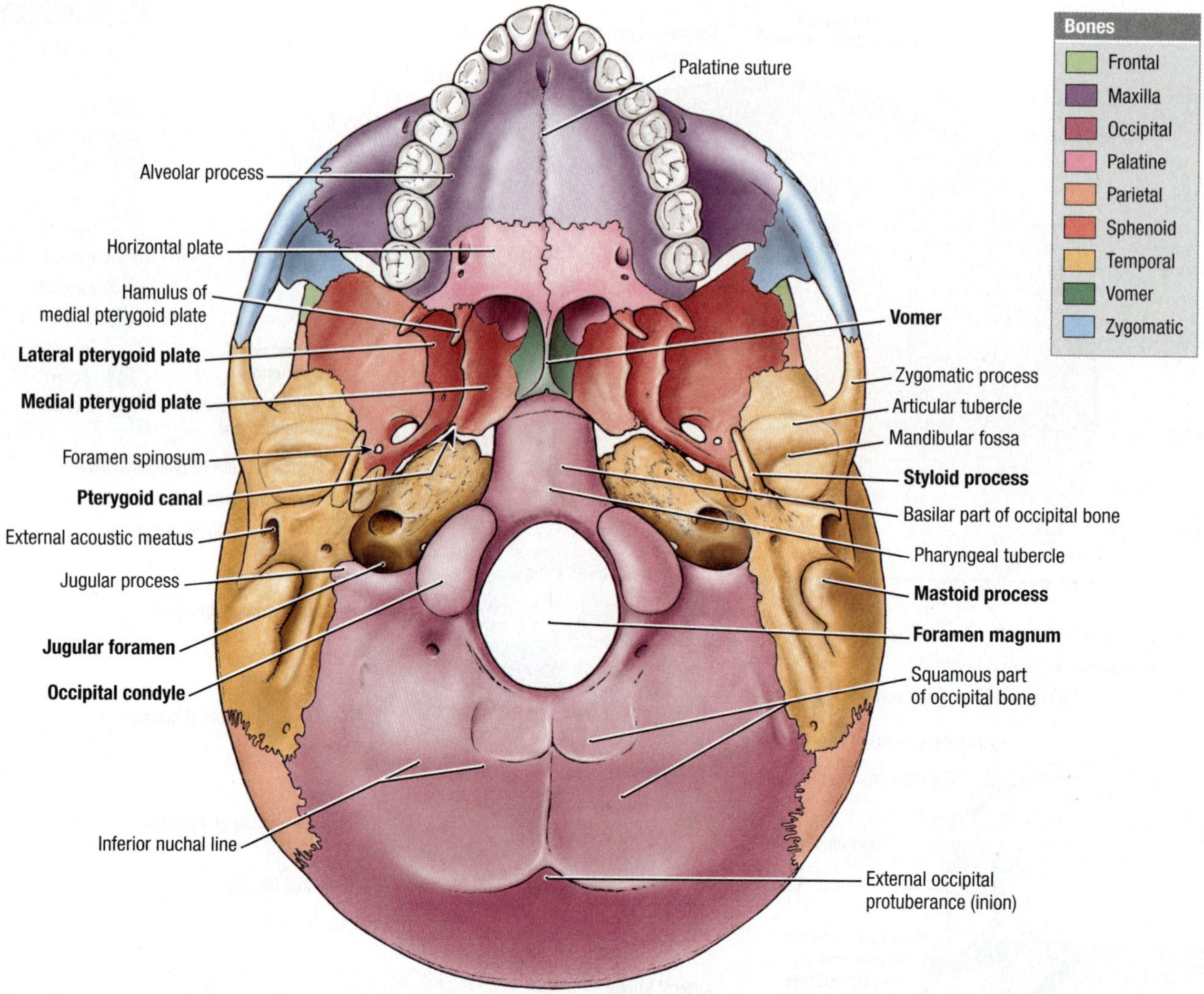

Figure 32.3. Inferior view of the skull. (Reprinted with permission from Agur AMR, Dalley AF II. *Grant's Atlas of Anatomy.* 14th ed. Wolters Kluwer; 2016.)

- At birth, the sphenoid presents essentially as three main parts: a central part that is the body and the lesser wings, and two lateral parts, each consisting of a greater wing and the associated pterygoid process.
- At birth, the temporal bones each consist of four parts: the squamous, petrous and tympanic portions, and the styloid process.

TABLE 32.1

Bones of the Adult Skull

Cranial Group (8)	Facial Group (14)	Miscellaneous (7)
Occiput	Vomer	Paired sets of three middle ear ossicles
Sphenoid	Mandible	Hyoid bone
Ethmoid	Paired maxillae	
Frontal	Paired palatines	
Paired temporals	Paired zygomae	
Paired parietals	Paired lacrimals Paired nasals Paired inferior conchae	

The petrous portion is cartilaginous in origin. The squamous and tympanic portions are membranous in origin.[3]

During delivery and expulsion of the fetus, the occiput is positioned under the pubic symphysis around which extension of the craniocervical junction takes place. The superior and the inferior parts of the occipital squama may be stressed with resultant cranial somatic dysfunction.

THE PARANASAL SINUSES

The paranasal sinuses are air-filled extensions of the nasal cavity into the following cranial bones:

- Frontal
- Ethmoid
- Sphenoid
- Maxillae

The paranasal sinuses are small at birth and develop at different rates between individuals. Frontal and sphenoidal sinuses are absent at birth, although a few ethmoid cells and small maxillary sinuses are present. The maxillary and sphenoidal sinuses develop first, at about the 4th month of gestation. This is followed by development of the frontal and ethmoidal sinus in the 6th month. The ethmoidal air cells reach mature size at 12 to 13 years of age.

The maxillary sinuses assume their pyramidal shape between 5 and 8 years, reaching full size by age 15. The sphenoidal sinuses become pneumatized, at about 5 years.[3]

The sinuses are lined with mucous membranes and connect via openings within the nasal cavities. All of the paranasal sinuses drain directly or indirectly into the nasal cavity. The balance of parasympathetic and sympathetic tone determines the nature of the mucosal secretions.

Parasympathetic fibers from cranial nerve (CN) VII synapse in the sphenopalatine ganglion and promote thin, watery, saliva-like secretions. Sympathetic fibers from T1 to T4 synapse in the cervical ganglia and promote thick, sticky secretions. Sinus headache referral patterns are predictable because branches of the trigeminal nerve innervate the sinuses.

Frontal Sinuses

- The frontal sinuses drain into the middle meatus.
- The innervation arises from the supraorbital nerves.[4]

Ethmoid Sinuses

- The anterior and middle ethmoid cells drain into the middle meatus.
- The posterior ethmoid cells drain into the superior meatus.
- The innervation arises from the anterior and posterior ethmoidal nerves (sensory supply), and from the orbital branches of the pterygopalatine ganglion (parasympathetic secretomotor fibers).[4]

Sphenoid Sinuses

- These drain into the sphenoethmoidal recess in close approximation to the cavernous sinuses.
- The innervation arises from the posterior ethmoidal nerves (sensory) and orbital branches of the pterygopalatine ganglion (secretomotor fibers).[4]
- Infections of the sphenoid sinus are especially dangerous because of its close association with the pituitary, brainstem, cavernous sinus, and CNs. Sphenoidal sinusitis is usually severely disabling and associated with severe, deep head pain.

Maxillary Sinuses

- The largest of the paranasal sinuses drain into the middle meatus.
- The innervation is derived from the infraorbital and the anterior, middle, and posterior superior alveolar nerves.[4]
- Sinus dysfunction (acute and chronic sinusitis and chronic postnasal drip) may result from dysfunction in the cranium.
- The physician should focus on improving the general health of the mucous membranes by the following:
  - □ Correcting ventilation and circulation
  - □ Restoring autonomic balance
  - □ Eliminating stagnant secretions by removing mechanical hindrances[2]
- Associated dysfunction in the upper thoracic spine, cervical spine, and sacrum should also be treated.

THE TEETH

When considering the effect of the dentition on somatic dysfunction of the head, face, and jaw, the physician must understand the basics of dental anatomy and malocclusion.

There are two sets of teeth that develop in a lifetime:

1. The primary teeth (also called the baby, milk, or deciduous teeth)
   - □ Most infants are born with no visible teeth as the teeth are forming inside the gums.
   - □ Children have 20 primary teeth that form approximately during age 6 months to 1 year.
   - □ Primary teeth fall out and are replaced by 32 permanent teeth approximately during age 6 to 14 years. They are replaced by the permanent teeth by about age 13.
2. The permanent teeth (also called the adult or secondary teeth)
   - □ Adults have 32 permanent teeth.
   - □ Wisdom teeth (also called the third molars) are molars that usually erupt from the ages of 17 to 21.

When examining teeth:

- The crown is the part of the tooth seen on the surface of the gum. It is made up of the enamel, dentine, and pulp.
- The front incisor teeth have a straight edge and are used for cutting.
- The canine or "eye teeth" are the pointed long teeth between the incisor and the premolar teeth.
- Premolar teeth (bicuspids) have two cusps.
- Molar teeth each have four or more cusps.

The enamel is the white hard covering over the crown of the tooth.

- It is the hardest material in the body and does not have a nerve or blood supply.
- Chipping or damage to enamel only will not be painful.
- Enamel cannot heal or repair itself as bone or dentine can.

Dentine is an off white colored hard material that makes up the bulk of the tooth.

- Dentine can heal itself.
- It can also register pain.
- The tooth becomes sensitive to temperature changes and feels painful when the dentine is exposed.

The pulp is composed of the nerves and blood vessels of the tooth.

- When the pulp is exposed to infection, by decay or injury, it will die and cause severe pain. An abscess will also develop on the root.
- The roots are embedded in the tooth socket in the mandible, covered by cementum, and held in place by the periodontal ligament.
- The periodontal ligament attaches the roots to the alveolar surface of the mandible. It has both a nerve and a blood supply. The ligament provides an elastic cushion between the tooth and the bone. It also makes the slight movement of a tooth possible.

Teeth are not rigidly joined to bone. There is flexibility. Teeth change their position based on stresses and occlusion patterns. Occlusion refers to the alignment of teeth and the way they fit together. Ideally, the points of the molars fit the grooves of the opposing molar, and all teeth are aligned, straight, and spaced evenly.

Malocclusion is the most common reason for orthodontist referrals. Very few people have perfect occlusion, or bite. By treating moderate or severe malocclusion, the teeth are easier to clean, and have less risk for decay and periodontal diseases. Some malocclusions have a hereditary component, but others can be acquired from habits, bruxism, and strains of the sphenobasilar synchondrosis (SBS). When hereditary, malocclusion may be due to disproportionate upper and lower jaw sizes, or from disproportionate tooth size resulting in an overcrowding of teeth. During infancy and childhood, personal habits can greatly affect the shape of the jaws, such as:

- Thumb sucking
- Tongue thrusting
- Pacifier use beyond the age of three
- Prolonged use of a bottle

In adults, malocclusion can also be attributed to the improper fit of dental fillings, crowns, appliances, retainers, or braces.

The position of the teeth and jaw affects motion of the cranial mechanism. Receiving cranial treatment will change bite patterns and jaw position. Braces and retainers can decrease the palpable motion of the primary respiratory mechanism, causing headaches, jaw pain, and many other complaints. Therefore, osteopathic physicians must work closely with dentists to achieve the best functional outcome for their patients.

THE MANDIBLE

The mandible develops from membranous ossification[3] and forms the lower jaw. It is not part of the neurocranium, nor is it part of the viscerocranium. The mandible has a horizontal body convex anteriorly, and two rami ascending posteriorly. Union of its two halves forms the symphysis menti, which is prominent inferiorly as that of the mental protuberance. The upper, alveolar part of the mandible contains the teeth, below which a mental foramen is visible. The angle of the mandible is the meeting point between its inferior margin, and the posterior margin of the vertical mandibular ramus. The superior part of the ramus extends upward to form a coronoid process and a condylar process. The head of the condylar process articulates with the mandibular fossa of the temporal bone to form the temporomandibular joint (TMJ).

THE TEMPOROMANDIBULAR JOINT

The TMJ is formed by the head of the mandible and the mandibular fossa of the temporal bone. A fibrocartilaginous articular disk separates these structures. The stylomandibular ligament connects the angle of the mandible to the styloid process of the temporal bone. The sphenomandibular ligament then connects the lingula (medial aspect) of the mandible to the spine of the sphenoid. The lateral pterygoid muscle arises from the sphenoid bone and attaches to the articular disk. This muscle draws the articular disk anteriorly when the mouth is opened.

MUSCULATURE

It is important to be familiar with the muscles of the head and face, and of those that attach from the spine to the head. This will help the physician to accurately palpate and identify tender points, fascial tension, and tightness of the various muscles. Understanding their innervation and action is also crucial, especially in the study of plastic surgery, neurosurgery, or otolaryngology.

SUPPORTIVE TISSUES

The dura mater lines the skull. It produces folds, or intracranial membranes, that act as partitions between and support for the cerebral hemispheres and cerebellum (Fig. 32.4).[2]

These structures form the reciprocal tension membrane and are integrally involved in osteopathic cranial motion. The dura lining the skull extends through the cranial sutures and becomes continuous with the periosteal covering of the skull. The falx cerebelli extends inferiorly from the straight sinus and firmly attaches to the foramen magnum. It then attaches to the bodies of the second and the third cervical vertebrae and extends downward as a tube that ultimately attaches to the second sacral segment (Fig. 32.5).

The dura becomes continuous with the extracranial fascia at various foramina in the base of the skull and continues outward as sheaths (perineurium) surrounding various cranial and spinal nerves. Extracranial and intracranial dural continuity is one mechanism in which dysfunction of the periphery can be referred to the head.[2]

Neural Structures

CRANIAL NERVES

Knowledge of CN anatomy and function is important in treating patients with a variety of disorders referable to the head, eyes, ears, nose, and throat. CNs can become:

- Inflamed
- Infected

Figure 32.4. Dural reflections within the skull.

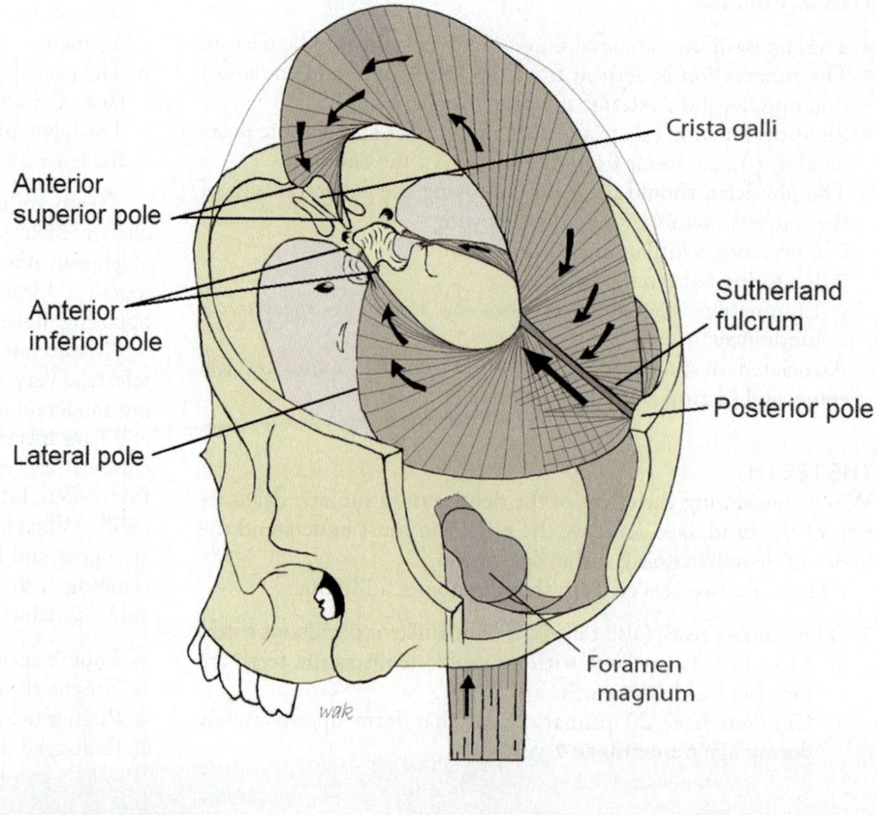

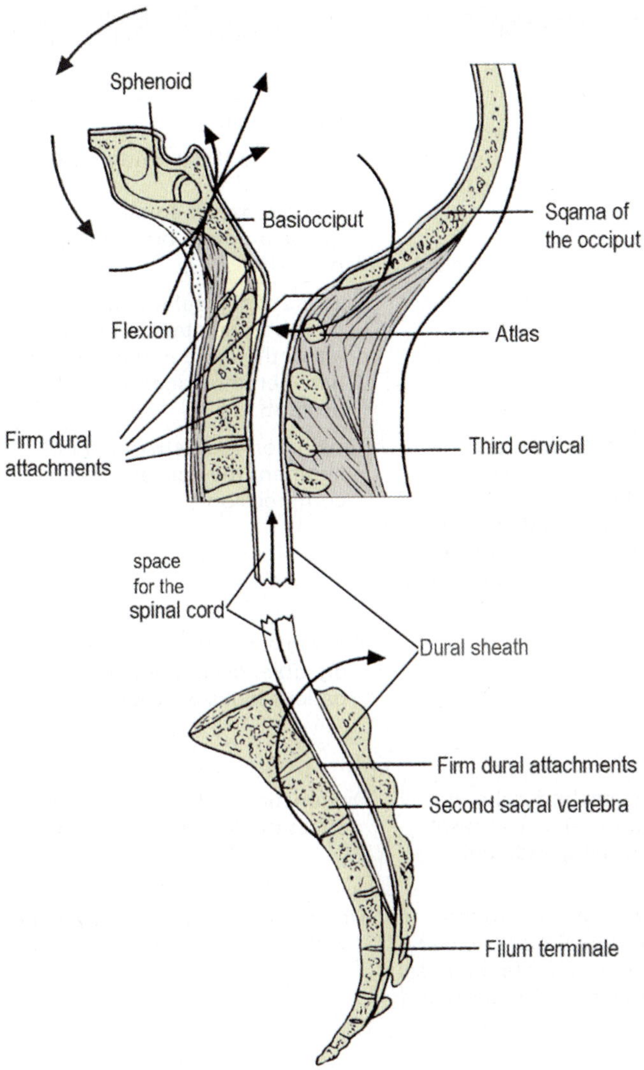

Figure 32.5. Dural continuity of the skull, cervical vertebrae, and sacrum. (Adapted with permission from Magoun HI Sr. *Osteopathy in the Cranial Field*. 3rd ed. The Journal Printing Company; 1976:39. Figure 20.)

- Entrapped
- Traumatized

Cranial strains/dysfunction of the SBS can affect their function as well. Table 32.2 highlights important aspects of the CNs.

PARASYMPATHETIC INNERVATION

- Parasympathetic nerve fibers to the pupil are supplied by CN III (oculomotor nerve) (Fig. 32.6).
  - They innervate the ciliary muscle and cause constriction of the pupil.
  - Parasympathetic activity shortens the focal length of the lens and is associated with visual disturbance.
- Parasympathetic fibers to the lacrimal gland and nasopharyngeal mucosa originate in CN VII (facial nerve).
  - They synapse in the sphenopalatine ganglion (Fig. 32.7).
  - The postganglionic fibers travel in the maxillary branch of CN V to the lacrimal gland.
  - Parasympathetic hyperactivity resulting from sphenoid, maxilla, and palatine dysfunction results in excessive tear production and profuse, clear, thin secretions from the mucosa of the nasopharynx and sinuses.
- Parasympathetic nerves to the thyroid gland arise from the superior and inferior laryngeal nerves, a branch of the main vagus nerve (CN X).[5]

SYMPATHETIC INNERVATION

The structures of the head and neck obtain their sympathetic innervation from cell bodies located at spinal cord levels T1–T4 (Fig. 32.8).

Preganglionic and postganglionic fibers synapse in the upper thoracic region and/or cervical sympathetic ganglia. Sympathetic fibers to the head generally form sympathetic plexi that follow the course of the arterial supply.[5] The superior, middle, and inferior cervical paraspinal ganglia lie in the fasciae of the cervical region at levels C2, C6, and C7, respectively. Upper thoracic, upper rib, and cervical somatic dysfunction can increase sympathetic tone to the structures of the head.

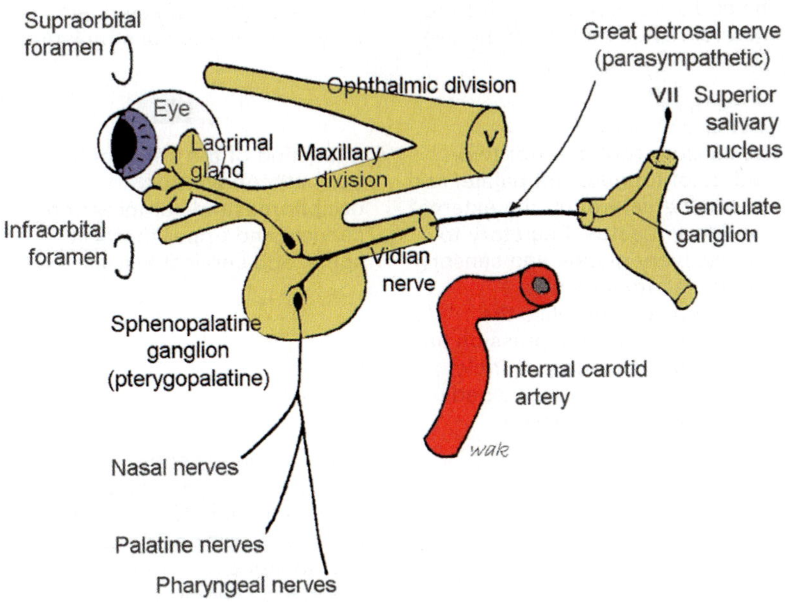

Figure 32.6. Parasympathetic nerves to orbital and nasal areas. (From Kuchera ML, Kuchera WA. *Osteopathic Considerations in Systemic Dysfunction*. 2nd ed. Greyden Press; 1994. Reprinted with permission from Michael L. Kuchera, DO, FAAO.)

TABLE 32.2

Cranial Nerves

Cranial Nerve	Anatomic Location	Innervation	Dysfunction
I. Olfactory	Foramina of the cribriform plate of the ethmoid bone		Crosses the lesser wing of the sphenoid[2] Altered sense of smell Impression of an odor that does not exist[5]
II. Optic	Optic canal (in the lesser wing of the sphenoid)		Lesions of the sphenoid or membranous tension may affect the optic nerve anywhere between the sphenoid and occiput[2]
III. Oculomotor	Midbrain, lateral wall of cavernous sinus, top of the petrosphenoidal ligament, superior orbital fissure	Levator palpebrae extraocular muscles of the eye (except the superior oblique and lateral rectus). Parasympathetic fibers supply the smooth muscle in the sphincter pupillae and ciliary muscles[6]	Tension on the petrosphenoid ligament may cause compression
IV. Trochlear	Passes through the petrosphenoidal ligament and enters the orbit via the superior orbital fissure		The most common symptom, diplopia, occurs when the patient looks downward
V. Trigeminal			
V1. Ophthalmic branch	Passes through the lateral wall of the cavernous sinus Enters the orbit through the superior orbital fissure	Upper eyelid, scalp, forehead, eyeball, ethmoid sinus, nasal cavity, lacrimal gland, and conjunctiva	Dysfunction of temporal bone may affect the function of this nerve
V2. Maxillary branch	Courses through: inferior portion of cavernous sinus, middle cranial fossa, foramen rotundum, pterygopalatine fossa, infratemporal fossa, inferior orbital fissure	Supplies sensory fibers to the dura, maxillary sinus, maxillary premolar and molar teeth, nasal septum, lower eyelid, nose, and upper lip	Tic douloureux may be associated with dysfunction of this nerve
V3. Mandibular branch	Exits the middle cranial fossa via the foramen ovale	It contains both motor and sensory fibers. Supplies the teeth, gingiva, skin of the temporal region, the ear, lower face, muscles of mastication, floor of the oral cavity, and tongue	Trigeminal neuralgia affecting this division. Sensory information from structures innervated by the trigeminal nerve (sinuses) may be perceived as headache
VI. Abducens	Courses underneath the petrosphenoid ligament, through the cavernous sinus, enters the orbit via the superior orbital fissure[6]	The abducens nerve supplies the lateral rectus muscle of the eye	Nerve most often affected and may result in medial strabismus
VII: Facial	Arises from the pons, enters the internal acoustic meatus of the temporal bone, joins the facial canal, and exits the skull via the stylomastoid foramen[6]	The sensory root anterior two-thirds of tongue, soft palate, and a small area around the external auditory meatus. Secretory to the salivary glands and sensory to the lacrimal glands. The motor root supplies the muscles of facial expression and muscles of the scalp, auricle, buccinator, platysma, stapedius, stylohyoid, and digastric	Dysfunction of the sphenoid, occiput (condylar or occipitomastoid compression) cervical and upper thoracic spine, and cervical fascia[2]
VIII. Auditory	Both divisions arise in a groove between the pons and medulla and course through the internal acoustic meatus with the facial nerve[6]		Lesions of the sphenoid, occiput, and temporals may affect the functioning of this nerve, producing vertigo or hearing dysfunctions[2]

TABLE 32.2 (Continued)

Cranial Nerves

Cranial Nerve	Anatomic Location	Innervation	Dysfunction
IX. Glossopharyngeal	It arises from the medulla and leaves the skull through the jugular foramen[6]	Stylopharyngeus muscle Secretomotor to the parotid gland Sensory to the pharynx, tonsils, and posterior portion of the tongue	Dysfunctions affecting the jugular foramen (temporal, occiput, occipitomastoid suture, or cervical fascia) may interfere with normal function of this nerve[2]
X. Vagus	It arises from the medulla and exits the skull via the jugular foramen[6]	Head, neck, thorax, abdomen, half of colon	Referred pain and parasympathetic reflexes headache, nausea, bradyarrhythmia cough
XI. Accessory	It arises from both the cervical spinal cord and the medulla and exits the skull through the jugular foramen	Sternocleidomastoid and trapezius muscles; it also supplies muscles in the pharynx and palate	Dysfunctions affecting the jugular foramen, sternocleidomastoid dysfunction
XII. Hypoglossal	It arises from the medulla and exits the skull via the foramen magnum. It courses through the hypoglossal canal in the occipital bone[6]	The hypoglossal nerve is the motor nerve of the tongue	Dysfunction of the condylar parts of the occipital bone may affect functioning of this nerve,[2] suckling disorders in infants, dysphagia, dysarthria, and swallowing difficulties in adults

Visceral afferent nerves stimulated by organ dysfunction usually follow the same fascial pathways as the efferent sympathetic fibers of innervation. Excessive afferent input from head and neck structures is a factor in the production of facilitation in upper thoracic cord segments. Facilitation of cord segments is associated with excessive sympathetic outflow from the affected regions of the cord (T1–T4 to head and neck). Hypersympathetic stimulation to associated viscera, over time, produces physiologic changes in the viscera and in the somatic tissues innervated by the involved cord segments.[5] Relevant palpatory changes mediated by viscerosomatic reflexes from HEENT structures can therefore be found in T1–T4 paraspinal tissues, and in predictable anterior Chapman points on the anterior chest wall above the second rib.

Palpatory changes in the upper thoracic and cervical paraspinal tissues can therefore suggest structural or functional involvement of the head and neck structures, innervated by sympathetic fibers.

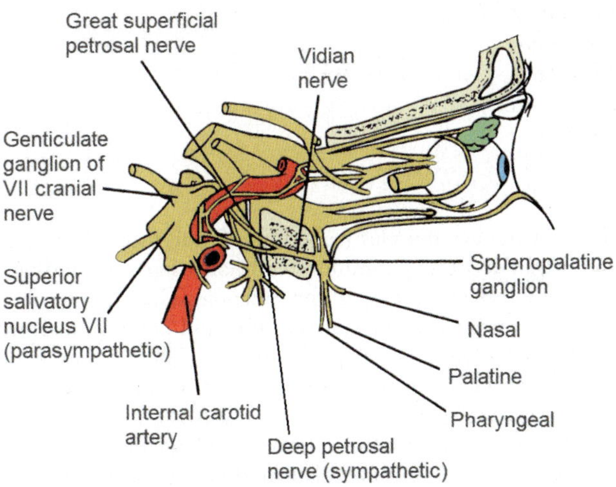

Figure 32.7. Sphenopalatine ganglion. (Modified from Kuchera ML, Kuchera WA. *Osteopathic Considerations in Systemic Dysfunction.* 2nd ed. Greyden Press; 1994. Reprinted with permission from Michael L. Kuchera, DO, FAAO.)

- Conditions such as Horner syndrome (constricted pupil, ptosis, and facial anhidrosis on the affected side) indicate significant structural involvement or blockage of the sympathetic nervous system.
- Increased sympathetic tone also leads to functional photophobia, unsteadiness, and tinnitus.
- Hyperesthesia of the pharyngeal tissues causes patients to cough and expectorate in an attempt to rid themselves of an imaginary foreign body in the throat.[5]

Increased sympathetic activity alters the normal physiologic responses that the tissues can provide.

- Vasoconstriction results in decreased nutrient supply to, as well as reduced lymphatic and venous drainage from, target organs and tissues. The body's ability to mount an immune response and obtain effective concentrations of medications is reduced in such areas of vasoconstriction and tissue congestion.[5]
- Prolonged sympathetic stimulation changes the composition of the cells of the respiratory epithelium. This results in nasal and pharyngeal secretions that are thick and sticky, thereby reducing effective cleaning and clearing by the pseudostratified ciliated epithelium of the mucosa. Epithelial hyperplasia is present, with
  - Relative increase in the activity and number of goblet cells
  - Constriction of arterioles
  - Decreased vascular and lymphatic drainage of the tissues
  - Mechanical difficulty in moving the mucus
- Sympathetic stimulation also produces vasoconstriction and inhibits secretion, leading to dryness of the nasopharyngeal mucosa. Dryness and cracking of the mucosa break down the normal mucosal defenses, thereby permitting secondary bacterial infection.[5]
- Dilation of the pupil (mydriasis) also occurs with increased sympathetic activity to the eye. This elevates intraocular pressures in patients with narrow angle glaucoma. Prolonged upper thoracic and cervical dysfunctions have been associated with the development of cloudiness of the lens.[5]
- The Barre–Lieou syndrome (vertigo, ataxia, vasodilation, and eye pain) results from hypersympathetic activity and proprioceptive dysfunction that often follows whiplash injuries.

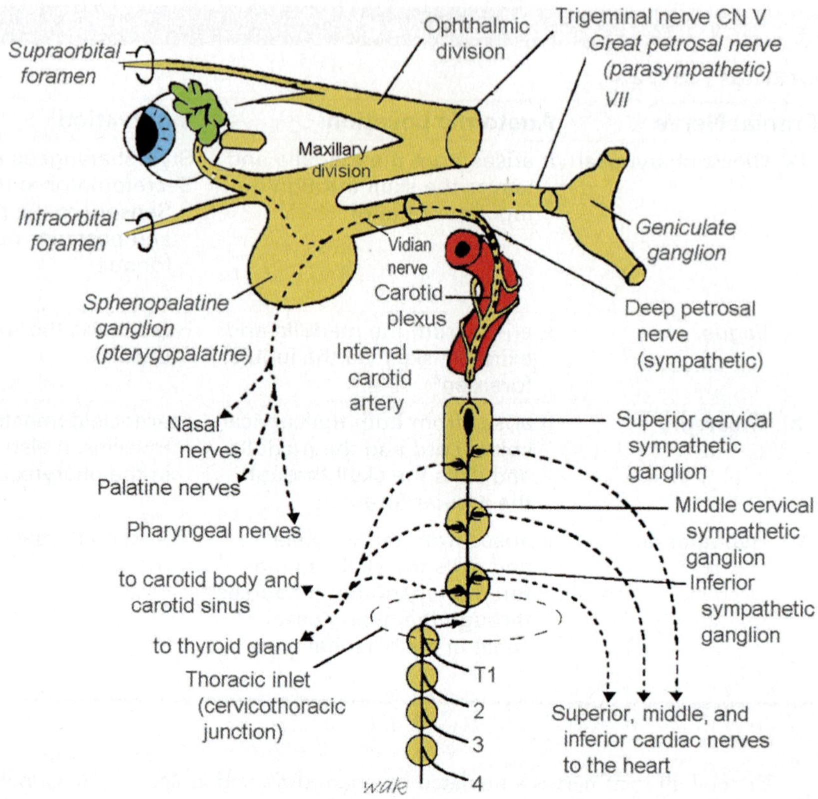

Figure 32.8. Sympathetic nerves to the head. (Modified from Kuchera ML, Kuchera WA. *Osteopathic Considerations in Systemic Dysfunction*. 2nd ed. Greyden Press; 1994. Reprinted with permission from Michael L. Kuchera, DO, FAAO.)

- The sympathetic nervous system innervates blood vessels that supply the thyroid, as well as the cells that produce thyroid secretions. Thus, increased sympathetic stimulation may alter thyroid gland secretion.[5]

DORSAL RAMI OF THE UPPER CERVICAL NERVES

Familiarity with the anatomy of the cervical nerves' dorsal rami is important for understanding how somatic dysfunction at C2 and C3 may be related to tension headaches and "occipital neuritis." The greater and lesser occipital nerves have been implicated in the production of tension headaches, so this is a region commonly treated by OMT. These branches of the dorsal rami of the upper cervical segments pierce through the fascia just below the superior nuchal line. Tension in this fascia has been hypothesized to cause compression and irritation of the greater occipital nerve.

The greater occipital nerve is the medial branch of the dorsal ramus of the second cervical nerve. It ascends between the muscles of the suboccipital triangle and the semispinalis capitis. This nerve pierces the semispinalis capitis and the trapezius near their attachments to the occipital bone and ascends on the back of the scalp with the occipital artery. The greater occipital nerve supplies the skin of the occipital part of the scalp, lateral to the median line, and as far superiorly as the vertex of the skull. Its lateral branches communicate with those of the lesser occipital nerve. The greater occipital nerve gives off muscular branches to semispinalis capitis joins with occipitalis tertius, the cutaneous branch of the third cervical nerve. The occipitalis tertius then supplies the skin of the upper part of the back of the neck, near the median line, and the skin of the scalp over the external occipital protuberance.

The cutaneous branches of the cervical plexus are:

- The lesser occipital
- The great auricular
- The transverse cervical
- The supraclavicular nerves

The lesser occipital nerve (C2, sometimes also C3) ascends in the neck along the posterior border of the sternocleidomastoid muscle. It pierces the superficial layer of cervical fascia near the insertion of the muscle and divides into branches. These supply the skin and subcutaneous tissue of the scalp behind and above the ear, and of the upper portion of the cranial surface of the ear. The great auricular nerve (C2, C3) arises in the posterior triangle at the lateral border of the sternocleidomastoid muscle. It travels below the lesser occipital nerve and crosses obliquely in a course toward the ear and the angle of the mandible.

Sensory Organs

EYE

Each orbit is composed of seven bones[2]:

1. Frontal
2. Sphenoid
3. Maxilla
4. Zygomatic
5. Palatine
6. Ethmoid
7. Lacrimal

Four of the eye muscles (superior, inferior, medial, and lateral rectus) originate from a common tendinous ring surrounding the optic canal in the lesser wing of the sphenoid. The superior oblique muscle arises from the body of the sphenoid bone, superomedial to the common tendinous ring. The inferior oblique muscle originates on the maxilla in the floor of the orbit. All are involved in eye movements (Fig. 32.9).[6]

Dysfunction of the frontal, sphenoid, and maxillae may produce muscle imbalance of the eye.[2] Restrictions of the orbital bones, through fascial connections, contribute to venous stasis in head structures.[2] A lateral stain pattern, maintained by unilateral condylar compression, is often associated with strabismus. A vertical

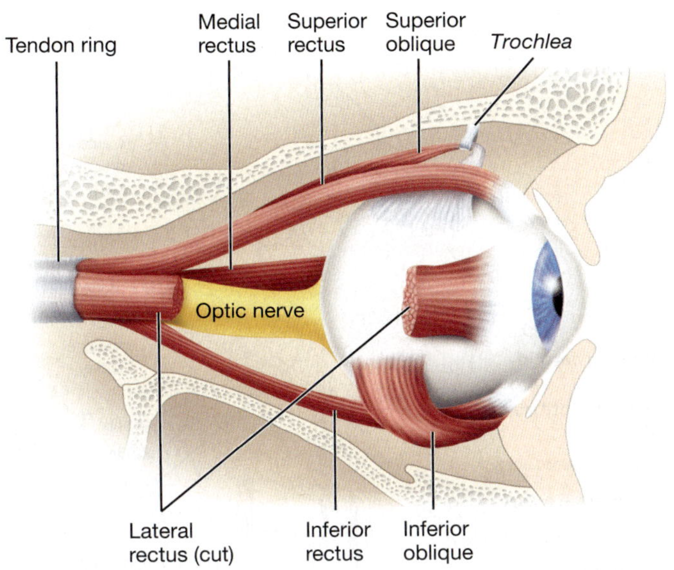

Figure 32.9. External eye muscles (right eye). The extraocular eye muscles originate on the bones (not shown) or the tendon ring of the eye orbit and insert into the sclera. (Reprinted with permission from McConnell TH, Hull KL. Human Form, *Human Function: Essentials of Anatomy & Physiology*. Wolters Kluwer Health/Lippincott Williams & Wilkins; 2011.)

strain pattern, maintained by bilateral condylar compression, is often associated with either myopia or hyperopia. Dysfunction of the occipital bone can obstruct the jugular foramen, leading to backward venous pressure in the orbit. These factors may contribute to such conditions as[2]:

- Amblyopia
- Astigmatism
- Diplopia
- Hyperopia
- Myopia
- Strabismus

The patient receives clinical benefit from the removal of cranial somatic dysfunction. Gentle eye mobilization using indirect techniques may also decrease ocular tension resulting from glaucoma.

EAR

The ear serves two major functions:

1. Maintenance of equilibrium
2. Hearing[6]

Most of the structures of the ear reside within the petrous portion of the temporal bone. Hence, dysfunction of the temporal bone can be a factor in impaired hearing, and asynchrony of temporal bone motion can be associated with vertigo (Fig. 32.10).

The eustachian tube connects the middle ear to the nasopharynx.[6] It functions to equalize middle ear pressure with atmospheric pressure. Fixed internal rotation of the temporal bone, typically secondary to occipitomastoid or sphenosquamous compression, maintains partial or complete closure of the eustachian tube. This is associated with two effects: perception of high-pitched noises and impaired drainage from the middle ear, thereby producing a media for recurrent ear infections. Fixed external rotation maintains patency of the eustachian tube and is associated with the perception of a roar or low-pitched noises.[1] Eustachian tube dysfunction is the most common precursor of otitis media. In addition, it is often responsive to treatment of somatic dysfunction affecting the

- Cranium
- Cervical and thoracic spine
- Medial pterygoid muscle
- Cervical fasciae
- Sacrum

THROAT

Impaired arterial supply to, and/or decreased venous and lymphatic drainage from the throat predisposes this region to infection. Patients with pharyngitis and tonsillitis often present with one or more of the following dysfunctions:

- Sacrum
- Upper thoracic and cervical spine
- Hyoid bone

Vasculature

ARTERIAL STRUCTURES

- The face and scalp are supplied by branches of the external carotid artery (primarily the facial artery).[6]
- The internal structures of the head are primarily supplied by the internal carotid and vertebral arteries (Fig. 32.11).

INTERNAL CAROTID ARTERIES

The internal carotid artery passes through the carotid canal in the petrous portion of the temporal bone. It supplies the anterior portions of the cerebrum.[6] Cranial dysfunction of the articulations between the temporal bones, occiput, and sphenoid can alter the normal function of these arteries.[6] This can produce symptoms including weakness and altered sensation on the opposite side of the body.

EXTERNAL CAROTID ARTERIES

The external carotid artery travels from the upper border of the thyroid cartilage to the neck of the mandible. Here, it divides into

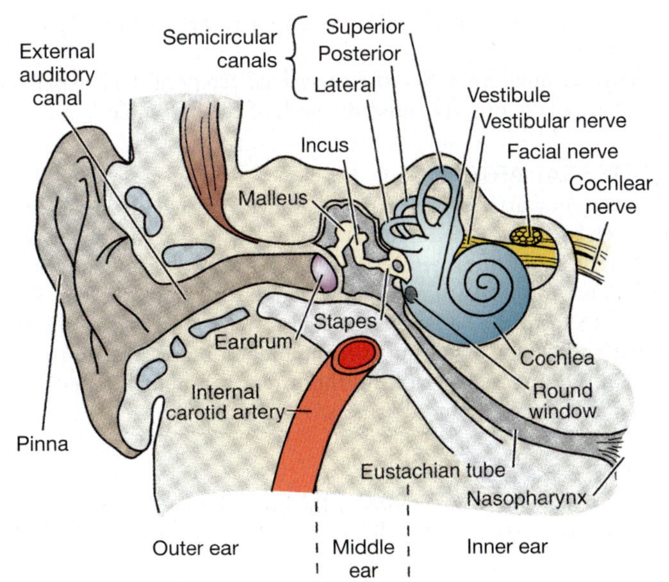

Figure 32.10. Basic structure of the human ear. Each ear consists of three basic parts: the external, middle, and inner ear. The structures of the middle and inner ear are encased in the temporal bone of the skull. The external and middle portions of the ear transmit airborne sound waves to the fluid-filled inner ear, amplifying sound waves in the process. (Reprinted with permission from Rhoades RA, Bell DR. *Medical Physiology: Principles for Clinical Medicine*. 4th ed. Wolters Kluwer Health/Lippincott Williams & Wilkins; 2013.)

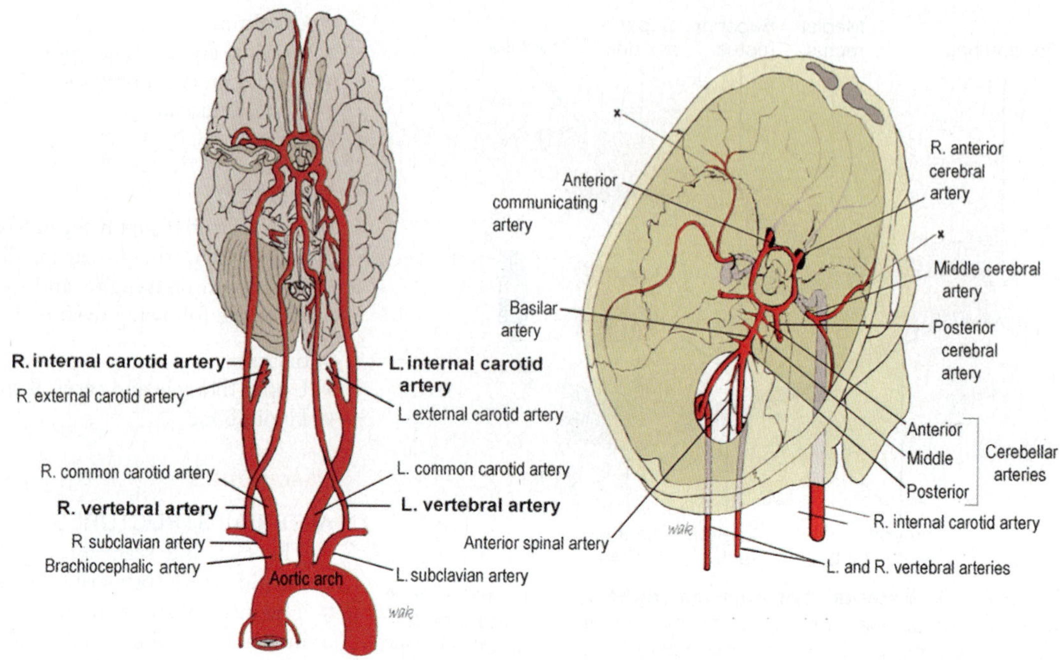

Figure 32.11. Arterial supply to the brain.

the superficial temporal and maxillary arteries. The artery is relatively superficial in the carotid triangle, where it is covered by the superficial layer of cervical fascia and overlapped by the anterior border of the sternocleidomastoid muscle. Leaving the carotid triangle, the artery is crossed by the posterior belly of the digastric and the stylohyoid muscles. It thus separates these muscles from the stylopharyngeus muscle. The facial nerve crosses both vessels.

The external carotid artery has eight branches.

- Four arise in the carotid triangle: the superior thyroid, the lingual, and the facial arteries.
- Two posterior branches, the occipital and posterior auricular arteries, arise at the level of the posterior belly of the digastric muscle.
- Two terminal branches, the superficial temporal and maxillary arteries, take origin behind the neck of the mandible.[7]

VERTEBRAL ARTERIES

The vertebral arteries arise from the subclavian arteries and ascend through the transverse foramina of C6–C3. At C2, they make several right angle turns before piercing the dura to angle anteriorly and enter the skull through the foramen magnum.[6] Here, they merge to form the basilar artery. The vertebral arteries supply the visual area of the cerebrum (occipital lobe), brainstem, and cerebellum. Dysfunctions affecting this artery can be associated with visual abnormalities and dizziness.[6]

CIRCLE OF WILLIS

The vascular interconnections of the brain, known as the cerebral arterial circle (circle of Willis), serve to equalize the blood supply to the various parts of the brain under conditions of fluctuating pressure through the major vessels. This anatomic design is unique and is crucial whenever a major source vessel becomes thrombosed or has to be ligated. The vertebral arteries join to form the basilar artery. The basilar artery splits into the two posterior cerebral arteries. The anterior and posterior communicating arteries indirectly connect the internal carotid arteries of the two sides and the basilar system, so that an arterial circle is formed at the base of the brain.[7] The terminal vessels in and on the brain anastomose, but the larger arteries do not, except in this arterial circle. Effects from an occlusion of one vertebral artery may be dampened by these vascular interconnections.

VENOUS STRUCTURES (FIG. 32.12)

Venous blood flows peripherally via superficial cerebral veins, and centrally via the deep cerebral veins into the venous sinuses, which lie between the outer endosteal and the inner meningeal layer of the dura. The cerebral veins are thin walled and have no valves. There are numerous venous connections between cerebral veins and dural sinuses, as well as among venous systems of the meninges, skull, scalp, and nasal sinuses. This anatomic arrangement not only allows the spread of infection but also allows cranial techniques to affect the venous drainage of the cerebral vessels.

- The venous drainage of the brain begins with the superior and inferior sagittal sinuses, as they drain into the transverse then sigmoid sinuses, and finally into the internal jugular vein.
- The ophthalmic veins from the orbit drain backward to the cavernous sinus, or forward to the facial vein.
- The cavernous sinus drains to the pterygoid plexus of veins, through the superior petrosal sinus, to the transverse sinus, and through the inferior petrosal sinus to the internal jugular vein.
- The veins of the scalp drain through veins that accompany the arteries, or through emissary veins, which connect the venous plexus of the scalp with the dural venous sinuses.
- The maxillary and superficial temporal veins form the retromandibular vein behind the angle of the mandible. The retromandibular vein communicates with the external jugular vein and the internal jugular vein.
- The facial vein drains into the internal jugular vein.
- The internal jugular vein lies in the carotid sheath. As it passes down the neck, it receives the superior and middle thyroid veins.
- The external jugular vein lies subcutaneous on the sternocleidomastoid muscle. It joins the subclavian vein.
- The internal jugular vein and the subclavian vein form the brachiocephalic veins on the right and left.

With the patient in the supine position, approximately 85% of the venous drainage from the head occurs via the internal jugular

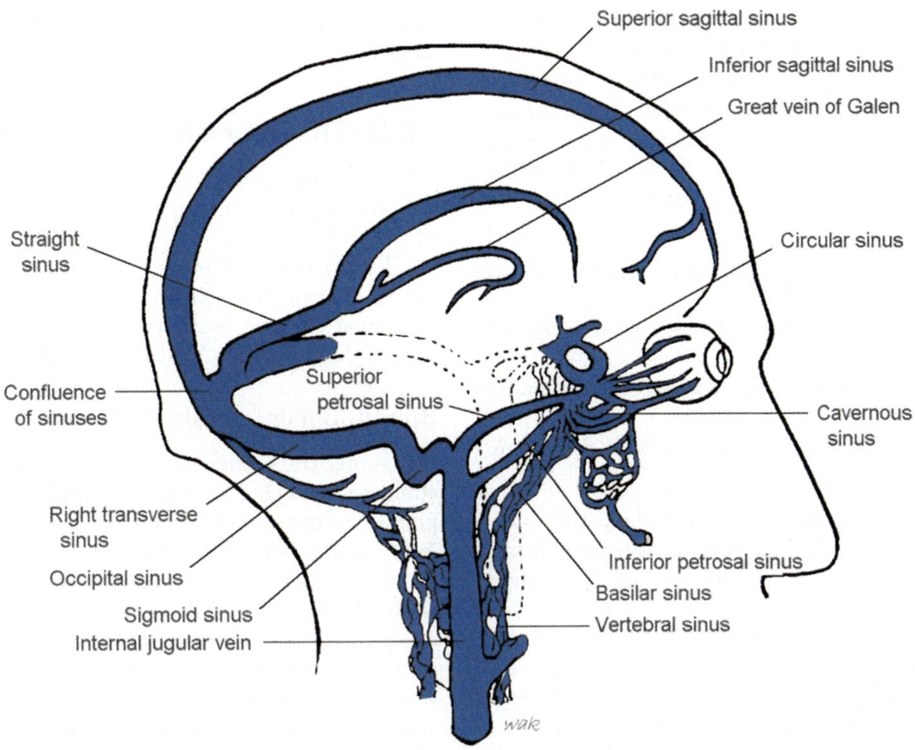

Figure 32.12. Venous drainage of the head. (Adapted with permission from Magoun HI Sr. *Osteopathy in the Cranial Field.* 3rd ed. The Journal Printing Company; 1976:21. Figure 12.)

veins. These veins pass through the jugular foramen, formed by both the occiput and the temporal bones, and are located along the occipitomastoid suture. CNs IX to XI course along with the internal jugular vein, and also exit through the jugular foramen, which is located between the occiput and the temporal bones. Suboccipital tension of this area is thought to cause fascial obstruction to flow and venous congestion. Specifically, an occipitomastoid compression can compromise venous flow through the jugular foramen, leading to congestion of the large valveless venous sinuses within the head. Sacral, upper thoracic, cervical, and associated regional connective tissue dysfunction can also contribute to congestion and impaired venous flow from the head.[5]

LYMPHATIC STRUCTURES

Understanding the lymphatic drainage patterns assists the physician in localizing pathologic conditions in the head (Fig. 32.13).

- Lymphatic vessels in the forehead and anterior part of the face drain into the submandibular lymph nodes.
- Lymph vessels from the lateral face and eyelids drain inferiorly toward the parotid lymph nodes and ultimately into the deep cervical lymph nodes.[6]

The superficial lymph nodes of the head include the submandibular, occipital, retroauricular, and superficial parotid lymph nodes.

The presence of lymphatics in human dura mater had been described by an Italian anatomist, Mascagni in 1787 in "Vasorum lymphaticorum corporis humani historia et ichnographia." However, the study could not be reproduced at that time and this observation faded from view for centuries. Therefore, until recently, it was thought that a lymphatic system for the brain and spinal cord did not exist. However, the recent "rediscovery" of the glymphatic system (or glymphatic clearance pathway) has revised this thinking.

Interestingly, over half a century prior to this "rediscovery," W.G. Sutherland, DO, stated that such a system did exist. "Such alternating membranous tension and relaxation probably aid in the regulation of venous blood, lymph and cerebrospinal fluids along the longitudinal sinus channels (superior sagittal sinus)."[8] In studies done by Absinta and Albayram[9,10] "dural lymphatics are seen running parallel to the dural venous sinuses, especially the superior sagittal and straight sinuses, and alongside branches of the middle meningeal artery." In addition, dorsal meningeal lymphatic vessels were apparent around almost all dural venous–parasagittal structures and were continuous with fluid channels from the skull base to the deep cervical lymph nodes.

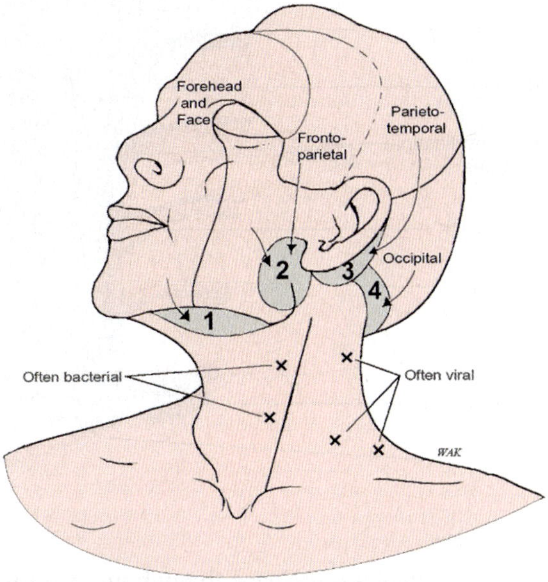

Figure 32.13. Lymphatic drainage of the head.

The glymphatic pathway consists of a para-arterial route for cerebrospinal fluid (CSF) to enter the brain parenchyma. It is connected with a clearance mechanism for the removal of interstitial fluid (ISF) and extracellular solutes from the interstitial compartments of the brain and spinal cord. The exchange of these solutes between the CSF and the ISF is thought to be driven by arterial pulsation and regulated during sleep by the expansion and contraction of brain extracellular space.[11,12]

- Lymph from the occipital region of the scalp drains into the occipital lymph nodes.
- The temporoparietal region drains into the retroauricular lymph nodes.
- The frontoparietal region drains into the superficial parotid lymph nodes.
- Lymph from the superficial lymph nodes eventually drains into the cervical lymph nodes.

The deep cervical lymph nodes are located along the internal jugular vein. Lymph from the deep cervical structures passes through the jugular trunk into the left (thoracic duct) and right lymphatic trunks (Fig. 32.14).[6]

All drainage from the head passes through the neck, cervical fasciae, and thoracic inlet to return to general circulation. Dysfunction in any of these structures can hinder the pathways and lead to lymphatic congestion. Increased sympathetic stimulation constricts the smooth muscle of the larger lymphatic vessels of the head and neck (associated with upper thoracic and cervical dysfunction), leading to decreased lymphatic drainage.[5]

SOMATIC DYSFUNCTION OF THE CRANIUM

There is a multitude of cranial somatic dysfunction that can occur and just like any other region, somatic dysfunction of other regions of the body and their resolution can impact cranial dysfunction.

The following is an overview of possible cranial somatic dysfunction, some of which may overlap. For an in-depth discussion of cranial somatic dysfunction, please refer to the Osteopathic Cranial Manipulative Medicine (OCMM) Chapter 53.

Sphenobasilar Strain Patterns

Dr. Sutherland's extensive work led to a model of sphenobasilar strain patterns that are often identified in clinical practice.[13] The premise of the model is that there exists a residual histologic flexibility at the SBS, even after the sphenoid and occiput are said to be fused according to standard osteologic descriptions.[14] This allows degrees of movement of that region that may represent normal physiology, such as cranial flexion and extension. However, it may be altered by factors such as the mechanics of birth, trauma, sutural restrictions, muscular, membranous or ligamentous imbalance, or somatic dysfunction distal to the cranial region. These SBS strain patterns consist of torsions and side-bending rotations,

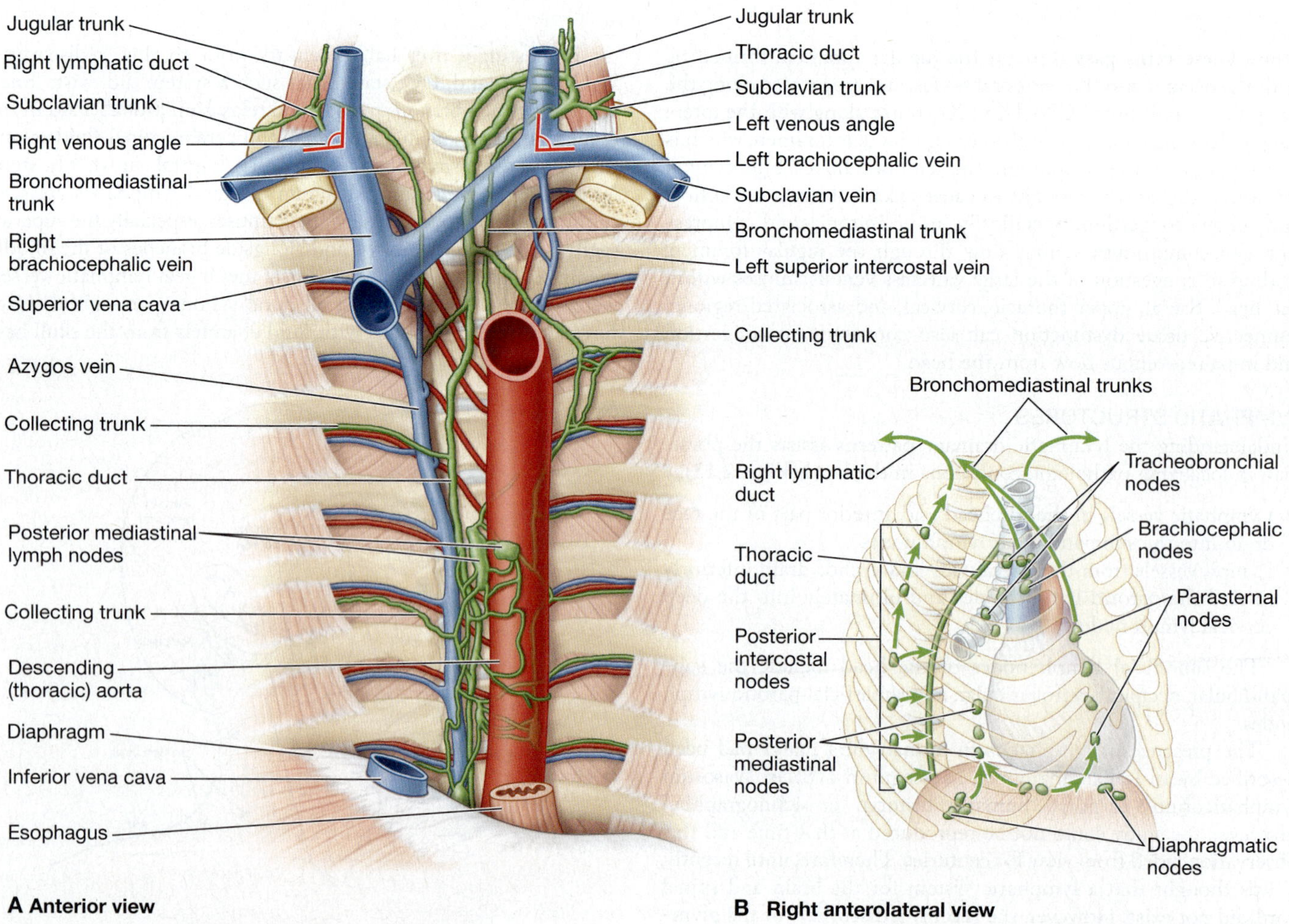

Figure 32.14. Lymphatic drainage through the thoracic inlet. (Reprinted with permission from Moore KL, Dalley AF II, Agur AMR. *Clinically Oriented Anatomy*. 8th ed. Wolters Kluwer; 2018.)

which are considered more physiologic in nature, and vertical and lateral SBS strain patterns, which are considered to be nonphysiologic. Compression of the SBS may also occur in which there is an absence of cranial flexion and extension.

Sutural/Joint Restrictions

The cranium is rich with various forms of sutures; serrate (sagittal), squamous (overlapping such as parietosquamous), squamoserrate (coronal or lambdoidal), harmonic (lacrimoethmoidal), gomphosis (peg and socket such as the great wings of the sphenoid), irregular (frontosphenoidal or parietomastoid), and schindylesis (plate and fissure such as vomeroid). Cranial joints include syndesmosis, a ligamentous union such as petrosphenoid and synchondrosis, a cartilaginous union such as the sphenobasilar joint as described above. These sutures and joints can become compressed or exhibit restrictions that can cause cranial somatic dysfunction.[15]

Membranous Articular Strains

The inside of the cranium is covered in dura mater which has two layers, the periosteal layer which adheres to the inner skull and the meningeal layer. Duplications or folds of the meningeal layer form the sickle-shaped falx cerebri and falx cerebelli between the hemispheres and form the double sickle-shaped transverse fold, the tentorium cerebelli, between the cerebrum and the cerebellum. The falx and the tentorium cerebelli join along the straight sinus, which is also called the Sutherland fulcrum. The diaphragm sellae is a horizontal fold of the meningeal layer of dura mater covering the sella turcica with a central foramen for the stalk of the pituitary. The meningeal layer envelopes the spinal cord tube, blending with the periosteum of foramen magnum, attaching to C2 and C3 and continuing down to its attachment site at the posterior aspect of S2. Disturbed membranous tension balance or membranous strain can limit or prevent articular freedom in one or more directions.

In addition, the periosteal layer provides a tubular sheath for the CNs as they exit their respective foramina. Therefore, tension on the dura, via articular dysfunction and/or altered membranous tension, can affect CN function, especially as they pass through their foramen.

Ligamentous Strains

Several ligamentous structures exist within the cranium including the petrosphenoid, sphemomandibular, stylomandibular, and stylohyoid ligaments. Restriction or abnormal tension of these ligaments may contribute to cranial somatic dysfunction resulting in clinical conditions such as esotropia and temporomandibular joint disorder (TMD).

Intraosseous Strains

Intraosseous strains can occur when a time-dependent load is applied to bone.[16] This may occur in utero, depending on fetal positioning, and with birth trauma, whether with regular delivery or instrument induced. It may also occur in craniums that have not yet ossified with repetitive or frequent positioning (e.g., infants placed on their backs), or trauma.

EVALUATION OF THE CRANIUM

During the screening portion of the osteopathic structural examination, the osteopathic physician assesses the patient's gait and overall structure. Facial asymmetry and abnormality noted on active motion testing of the TMJ are among some elements that may indicate the presence of cranial somatic dysfunction.

Segmental Structural Examination

If a cranial somatic dysfunction is suspected further evaluation is warranted.

PALPATION

If cranial somatic dysfunction is suspected, the general contours of the cranium may be palpated for evidence of:

- Unusually increased or decreased angulation of bones
- Abnormal approximation or separation of sutures
- Decreased resiliency of the bones
- Painful areas

Individual cranial bones can be examined in this manner. The physician may additionally wish to take photographs of the patient at this time, especially when tracking the progress of a newborn or a pediatric patient with plagiocephaly. These can be valuable for pre- and posttreatment comparisons and used as part of the medicolegal record of the patient's treatment.

The physician may then palpate the cranium for the presence of flexion and extension, any SBS strain patterns, and the cranial rhythmic impulse.

Palpation of the Cranium

1. The physician sits at the head of the table.
2. The patient is supine.
3. The physician contacts the patient's head using the vault hold; index fingers on the greater wings of the sphenoid, third fingers just anterior to the external auditory meatus on the temporal bone, ring fingers on the mastoid processes of the temporal bone, and fifth finger on the lateral angles of the occiput.
4. Using this contact, the physician may palpate the cranial rhythmic impulse (CRI) for:
   - □ Rate (cycles per minute)
   - □ Rhythm (regular vs. irregular)
   - □ Amplitude (large, small)
   - □ Vitality (a general assessment of the energy level of the CRI)
5. The physician should also palpate for the presence of motion. The absence of flexion and extension may indicate an SBS compression. If motion is present, the physician may assess for the following:
   - □ Signs of appropriate flexion and extension
   - □ Evidence of SBS strain patterns (e.g., torsion, side-bending rotation, vertical and lateral)
   - □ Any areas of restriction
   - □ It is recommended to evaluate these items before proceeding with any motion testing.

Other procedures used to determine the presence of specific somatic dysfunction(s) of the head include the following:

- Temporal drawer test
- Parietal lift test
- Frontal lift test
- Cranial base and quadrant evaluation
- Evaluation of sacral motion (which may elucidate dysfunction of the cranium)
- Evaluation of the TMJ
- Palpation of medial and lateral pterygoid muscles

The details of these procedures are given below. See also Chapter 53 Osteopathic Cranial Manipulative Medicine, for further details on evaluation of the head region or cranium.

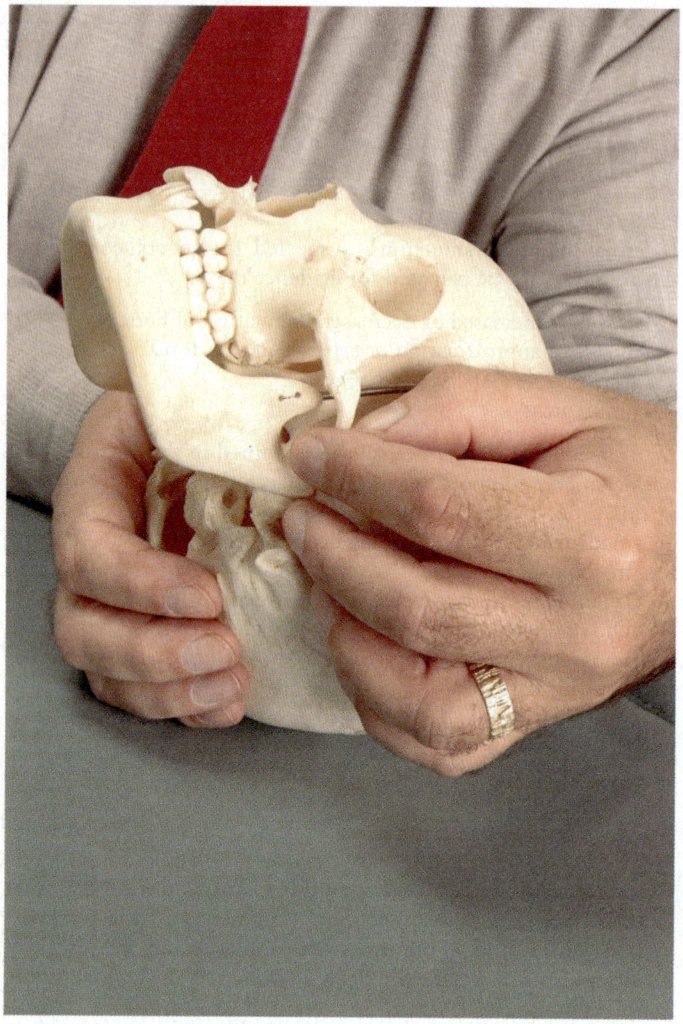

Figure 32.15. The "five-finger" hold for the temporal bone—shown for the left temporal bone. (Reprinted with permission from Hruby RJ. *Exploring Osteopathy in the Cranial Field.* Author; 2013.)

Temporal Drawer Test

1. The physician sits at the head of the table.
2. The patient lies supine.
3. The physician assumes a "five-finger hold" (Fig. 32.15) on each temporal bone (zygomatic arch between thumb and index finger, third finger in external ear canal, fourth and fifth fingers on mastoid portion of the temporal bone).
4. The physician gently applies traction on both temporal bones simultaneously, in order to lift the temporal bones superiorly (i.e., toward the top of the patient's head). The physician then gently releases the traction.
5. The physician notes whether the motion in the temporal bones is normal, springing ("joint play"), or if it is restricted on one or both sides.
6. Lack of normal spring-like motion of one or both temporal bones indicates possible somatic dysfunction of the temporal bone(s) and/or somatic dysfunction at the base of the cranium.

Parietal Lift Test (Fig. 32.16)

1. The physician sits at the head of the table.
2. The patient lies supine.

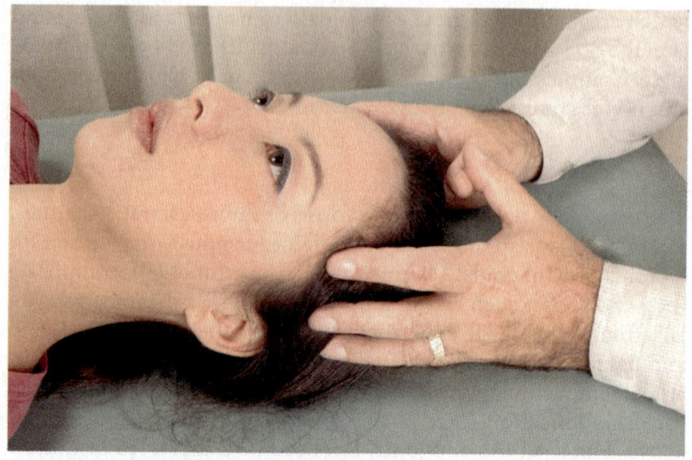

Figure 32.16. Hand position for the parietal lift test. (Reprinted with permission from Hruby RJ. *Exploring Osteopathy in the Cranial Field.* Author; 2013.)

3. The physician rests their forearms on the table and places the finger tips on the inferior border of the two parietals, just superior to the parietosquamous suture.
4. The physician's thumbs are crossed above, but not in contact with the sagittal suture.
5. The physician firmly presses one thumb against another (i.e., one thumb presses superiorly as the other resists this motion by pressing inferiorly).
   - Thus, the fingers will approximate and induce internal rotation of the inferior border of the parietal bones.
6. At the same time, the physician lifts both hands in a superior direction (toward the physician), noting whether there is any restriction in the expected "joint play" motion of the parietal bones.
7. The physician gently releases contact on the parietal bones.
8. Palpation of tissue texture abnormality, asymmetry, restriction of motion, and tenderness (TART) changes in the tissues of the parietal region, or of resistance in the "joint play" motion of the parietal bones, suggests possible somatic dysfunction in this area of the cranial vault.

Frontal Lift Test (Fig. 32.17)

1. The physician sits at the head of the table.
2. The patient lies supine.

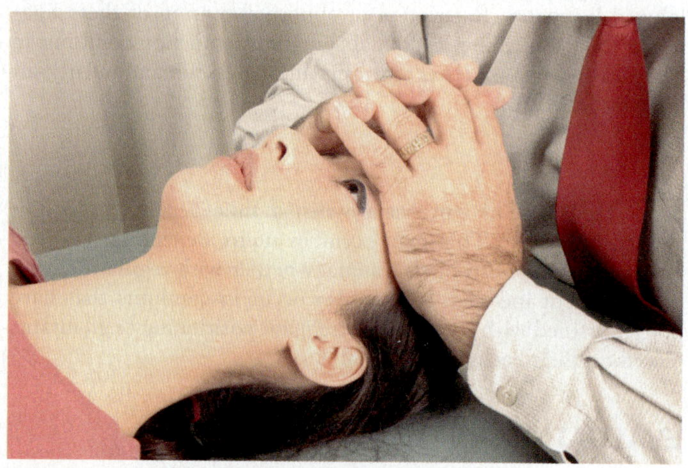

Figure 32.17. Hand position for the frontal lift test. (Reprinted with permission from Hruby RJ. *Exploring Osteopathy in the Cranial Field.* Author; 2013.)

3. The physician rests their elbows on the table, with the hypothenar eminences of the hands placed on the lateral angles of the patient's frontal bones. The fingers of the physician are interlaced over, but not in contact with, the patient's forehead.
4. The physician draws the fingers of one hand from the fingers of the other, yet at the same time, grips the fingers of the one hand with the other (action of the lumbrical muscles).
   - This way, the hypothenar eminences exert an influence of internal rotation on the lateral angles of the frontal bones.
5. The physician coordinates this action with a lifting of the frontal bone anteriorly (toward the ceiling), noting whether there is any restriction in the expected "joint play" motion of the frontal bones.
6. The physician gently releases the hands from the patient's forehead.
7. Palpation of TART changes in the tissues of the frontal region, or of resistance in the "joint play" motion of the frontal bones, indicates possible somatic dysfunction in this area of the cranial vault.

Cranial Base and Quadrant Evaluation

1. The physician sits at the head of the table.
2. The patient lies supine.
3. The physician assumes a vault hold on the patient's head (Fig. 32.18) in which the index fingers of each hand rest on the greater wings of the sphenoid, the middle fingers rest just anterior to the external auditory meatus on the temporal bone (thereby enabling evaluation of the two anterior quadrants), the ring fingers contact the mastoid process of the temporal bones and the fifth fingers rest on the lateral angles of the occiput (thereby enabling evaluation of the two posterior quadrants).
4. The head can be visualized (from a superior viewpoint) as divided into four quadrants, two anterior and two posterior (Fig. 32.19).
5. The physician then notes:
   - Whether there is symmetry or asymmetry of motion at the points of contact on the greater wings of the sphenoid and the angles of the occiput.
   - Whether, in general, there is one quadrant of the head that has less motion compared to the other three quadrants.
6. Using this procedure, the physician can determine if motion restriction is present at the cranial base, and/or in any of the anterior or posterior quadrants of the cranium.
   - This information allows the physician to then examine any restricted quadrant for specific suture restrictions, that is, perform a segmental examination of the region.

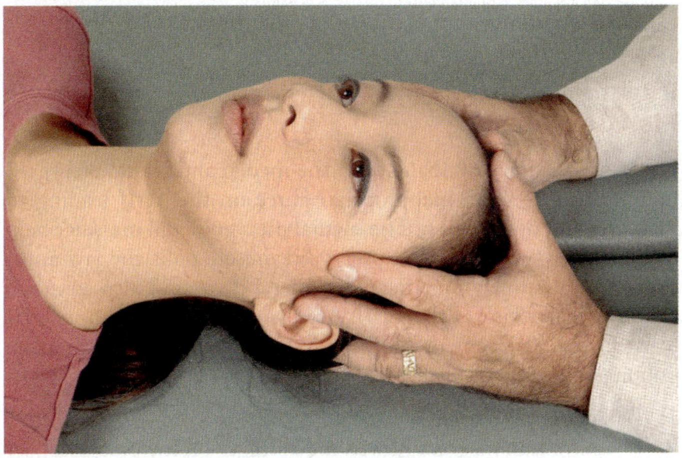

Figure 32.18. The vault hold. (Reprinted with permission from Hruby RJ. *Exploring Osteopathy in the Cranial Field.* Author; 2013.)

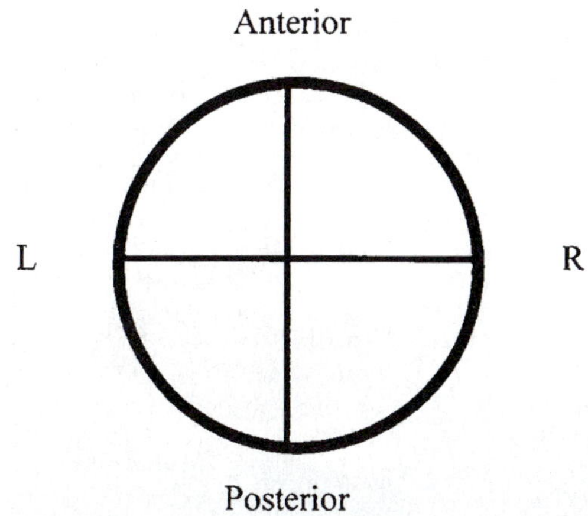

Figure 32.19. The four quadrants of the head—superior view. (Reprinted with permission from Hruby RJ. *Exploring Osteopathy in the Cranial Field.* Author; 2013.)

SACRAL MOTION EVALUATION

Due to the nature of the reciprocal tension membrane and the dural attachments to the posterior aspect of S2, it is often helpful to assess sacral flexion and extension to provide additional information on where restriction may exist within the system.

1. The physician sits by the side of the supine patient looking toward the patient.
2. The physician asks the patient to bend their contralateral knee and lift their hips slightly off the table.
3. Using the hand closest to the patient, the physician contacts the sacrum so that the thumb and fifth digit are on the SI joints with the rest of the finger pads spread across the sacral base and the heel of the hand or the thenar and hypothenar eminences are near the apex of the sacrum and the coccyx (Fig. 32.20A,B). To ensure that the physician's hand is placed at the midline of the sacrum, the physician's arm will be between the patient's thighs.
4. The patient may then be instructed to lower their hips and allow their legs to extend fully on the table in a relaxed manner.
5. The physician ensures that their elbow and forearm of the hand contacting the sacrum are resting on the table, providing a fulcrum. To achieve proper ergonomics, the physician may ask the patient to move closer to the physician so that the physician's elbow is placed on the table at about a right angle, minimizing stress to the physician's shoulder and neck. There should be a straight line from the physician's elbow to the finger pads contacting the sacral base, without deviation of the elbow or wrist.
6. Once both physician and patient positioning are optimized, sacral motion is evaluated.
7. When the physician concludes their assessment, they may ask the patient to flex the contralateral knee once again and lift their hips, enabling the physician to remove their hand from the sacrum.

EVALUATION OF THE TEMPOROMANDIBULAR JOINT

In the screening portion of the exam, the physician observes the patient opening and closing their jaw to note the amount of opening and any chin deviation. The physician may also palpate the TMJ as the patient opens and closes their mouth to assess for crepitus, popping, and clicking. Limitation of motion, chin deviation, and joint sounds may indicate that the TMJ should be further

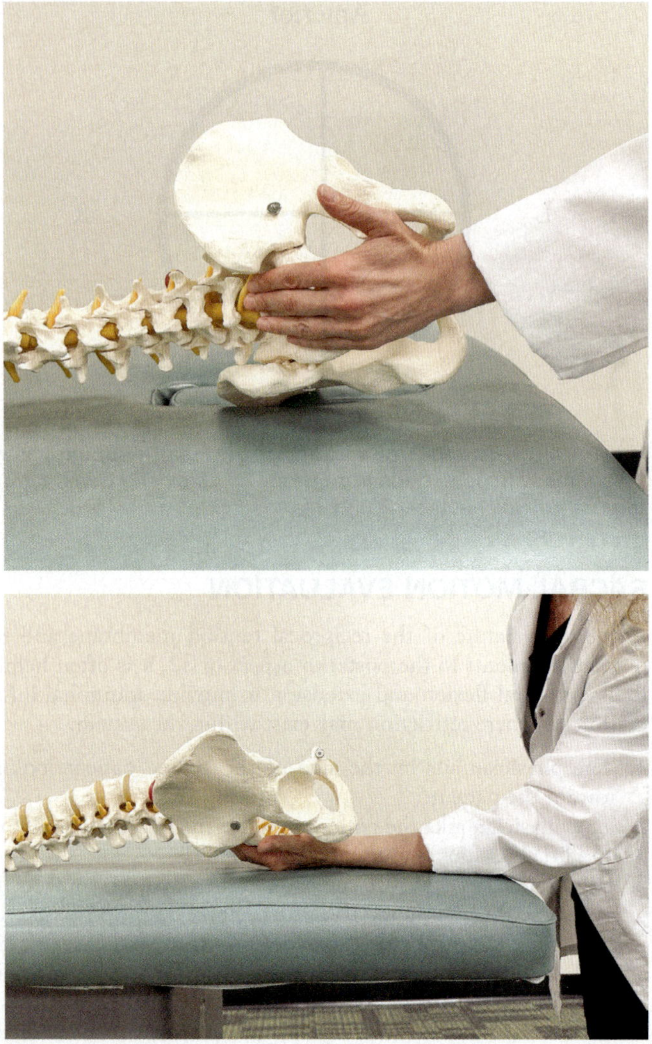

A

B

Figure 32.20. A, B: Sacral motion evaluation hand placement. (Photos courtesy of Western University of Health Sciences, Pomona, CA, with permission.)

evaluated for somatic dysfunction. Further evaluation may involve the following:

- Palpation of the muscles of mastication such as the temporalis and masseter for tenderness or tissue texture changes
- Assessment of deviation of midincisural lines at rest (the patient may passively open lips to view), with the teeth edge to edge and then with the jaw protruded
- Assessment of the sphenomandibular ligament, stylomandibular ligament, and the joint capsule

Assessment of the Sphenomandibular Ligament

1. The patient is supine.
2. The physician stands at the side of the table opposite the side to be evaluated.
3. The physician places the superior (cephalad) hand over the patient's forehead monitoring the grater wings of the sphenoid with the thumb and index or middle finger.
4. With a gloved inferior (caudad) hand, the physician places their thumb on the occlusal surface of the last lower molar of the side being evaluated and wraps the rest of the fingers around the ramus and body of the mandible.
5. The physician exerts slight pressure on the mandible with the gloved thumb to move the mandible inferiorly. If restriction of the sphenomandibular ligament exists, the greater wing of the sphenoid will move superiorly (toward cranial extension) which will be palpated or sensed with the monitoring hand indicating that it may be addressed with balanced ligamentous tension or another modality of OMT.

Assessment of the Stylomandibular Ligament

1. The patient is supine.
2. The physician stands at the side of the table opposite the side to be evaluated.
3. With the superior (cephalad) hand, the physician contacts the temporal bone by placing the middle finger in the external auditory meatus, the index finger and thumb grasping the zygomatic arch, and the fourth and fifth finger contacting the mastoid process.
4. The physician places the inferior (caudad) gloved thumb onto the occlusal surface of the last lower molar on the side of the mouth being evaluated and wraps the rest of the fingers around the angle of the mandible.
5. The physician applies gentle traction to the mandible by drawing it in an inferior, lateral, and anterior direction to assess the compliance of the stylomandibular ligament. Decreased compliance and/ or restriction may indicate the need for treatment with balanced ligamentous tension or another modality of OMT.

Assessment of the TMJ Capsule

1. The patient is supine.
2. The physician stands at the side of the table opposite the side to be evaluated.
3. With the superior (cephalad) hand, the physician contacts the temporal bone by placing the middle finger in the external auditory meatus, the index finger and thumb grasping the zygomatic arch, and the fourth and fifth finger contacting the mastoid process.
4. The physician places the inferior (caudad) gloved thumb onto the occlusal surface of the last lower molar on the side of the mouth being evaluated and wraps the rest of the fingers around the angle of the mandible.
5. The physician attempts to decompress the TMJ by placing slight anteroinferior pressure on the mandible. If the mandible does not move easily, it may indicate an area of restriction around the glenoid fossa which may be amenable to gentle compression of the head of the mandible into the glenoid fossa until spontaneous decompression occurs or another modality of OMT.

Palpation of the Medial and Lateral Pterygoid Muscles

Excessive tension or imbalance of the medial and lateral pterygoid muscles can exert an inappropriate force on the TMJ leading to irritation and dysfunction. The medial pterygoid and masseter help to close the jaw. The lateral pterygoid muscle pulls the jaw anteriorly to initiate jaw opening. The lateral pterygoid also connects to the articular disk of the TMJ. Abnormal tension can contribute to anterior displacement of the TMJ which may result in pain, popping, clicking, or restriction of motion.[17]

1. The patient is supine.
2. The physician inserts a gloved index finger on the medial aspect of the mandible in the region of the angle of the mandible to palpate the lower insertion of the medical pterygoid muscle.

The physician assesses the muscle for excessive tenderness, tissue congestion or hypertonicity which may be amenable to treatment with gentle steady pressure or inhibition.

3. To palpate the lateral pterygoid muscle, insert the gloved little finger along the lateral aspect of the upper teeth on the side to be palpated. Slide the finger along the outside of the upper teeth to a point just beyond the last molar.
4. The physician gently presses laterally and feels for the bony aspect of the coronoid process of the mandible.
5. The physician may instruct the patient to open and close the jaw slightly to better palpate the coronoid process. Asking the patient to shift the jaw slightly toward the side to be examined will create more space between the coronoid process and the teeth allowing the physician to move the palpating finger further posteriorly and medially.
6. Instructing the patient to open the jaw slightly will contract the muscle, allowing the physician to confirm the correct location of the lateral pterygoid.
7. The physician assesses the muscle for excessive tenderness, tissue congestion, or hypertonicity which may be amenable to treatment with gentle steady pressure or inhibition.[17]

In addition to the above assessments, the physician may also examine for the presence of counterstrain tender points.

REFERENCES

1. Stedman TL. Stedman's Medical Dictionary. 28th ed. Lippincott Williams & Wilkins; 2006. Accessed September 26, 2024. https://www.wolterskluwer.com/en/solutions/lippincott-medicine/medical-education/stedmansonline-medical-dictionary.
2. Magoun HI. *Osteopathy in the Cranial Field.* 3rd ed. The Journal Printing Co.; 1976.
3. Sergueef N. *Cranial Osteopathy for Infants, Children, and Adolescents.* Churchill Livingston, Elsevier; 2007:23–35, 45–47, 301.
4. Sandring S, ed. *Gray's Anatomy.* 39th ed. Elsevier Churchill Livingstone; 2005.
5. Kuchera ML, Kuchera WA. *Osteopathic Considerations in HEENT Disorders.* Greyden Press; 2012.
6. Moore KL, Dalley AF II, Agur AMR. *Clinically Oriented Anatomy.* 7th ed. Lippincott Williams & Wilkins; 2014.
7. Woodburne RT. *Essentials of Human Anatomy.* 7th ed. Oxford University Press; 1983:147–148, 160–161, 283–284.
8. *Contributions of Thought: the Collected Writings of William Garner Sutherland, D.O.* 2nd ed. The Sutherland Cranial Teaching Foundation, Inc.; 1998:95.
9. Absinta, M, Ha SK, Nair G, et al. Human and nonhuman primate meninges harbor lymphatic vessels that can be visualized noninvasively by MRI. *eLife.* 2017;6:e29738.
10. Albayram M, Smith G, Tufan F, et al. Non-invasive MRI imaging of human brain lymphatic networks with connections to cervical lymph nodes. *Nat Commun.* 2022;13(1):203.
11. Iliff JJ, Lee H, Yu M, et al. Brain-wide pathway for waste clearance captured by contrast-enhanced MRI. *J Clin Invest.* 2013;123(3):1299–1309.
12. Iliff JJ, Wang M, Liao Y, et al. A paravascular pathway facilitates CSF flow through the brain parenchyma and the clearance of interstitial solutes, including amyloid β. *Sci Transl Med.* 2012;4(147):147ra11.
13. Capobianco JD, Shemon S. Taxonomy of the lateral strain patterns at the sphenobasilar synchondrosis for osteopathic cranial manipulative medicine. *J Am Osteopath Assoc.* 2020;120(1):25–29.
14. Pritchard JJ, Scott JH, Girgis FG. The structure and development of cranial and facial sutures. *J Anat.* 1956;90(1):73–86.
15. Magoun HI, ed. *Osteopathy in the Cranial Field.* 1st Edition, 1951. Second printing, SCTF; 1997.
16. Hong J. Intraosseous pressure and strain generated potential of cylindrical bone samples in the drained uniaxial condition for various loading rates. *J Mater Sci Mater Med.* 2008:19(7):2589–2594.
17. Hruby RJ. *Exploring Osteopathy in the Cranial Field.* Published by the author; 2013:109.

33 Cervical Region

KRISTIN PUTNAM

KEY CONCEPTS

- Describe the anatomy relevant to the cervical regional and segmental examinations.
- List the components of the cervical regional and segmental examinations.
- Describe the purpose of performing the cervical regional and segmental examinations.
- Correctly perform each component of the cervical regional and segmental examinations.
- Correctly diagnose cervical somatic dysfunction.

INTRODUCTION

Neck pain represents a common complaint of patients and per the Global Burden of Disease, Injuries and Risk Factor Study (GBD) is reported to be a major cause of disability that will likely increase in future years.[1,2] Dysfunction of the cervical spine may be related to various mechanical, systemic, and traumatic factors that can contribute and/or stem from a myriad of clinical scenarios; head and neck infections, trauma, somatic stress, and aberrant posture, sleep disturbance, overuse syndromes, breathing abnormalities, orthopedic or rheumatologic conditions. A comprehensive knowledge of cervical regional anatomy is critical for accurate diagnosis and management of this area. A thorough understanding of the region and its intimate connections allows the physician to know when further work-up such as imaging, lab work, or other diagnostic testing is warranted and makes the physician less likely to miss a serious condition such as cervical spine fracture, instability, or neurovascular compromise.

The cervical region is a pathway between the head and the thorax with significant neural, vascular, and musculoskeletal communication. Injury, pathology, or dysfunction may interfere with these vital communications.

This chapter will provide an overview of cervical spine anatomy, biomechanics, dysfunction, and common conditions that would necessitate osteopathic diagnosis and/or manipulative treatment of cervical somatic dysfunction.

FUNCTIONAL ANATOMY

Proficiency in regional and segmental examinations and accurate diagnosis of somatic dysfunction in the cervical spine requires an understanding of the functional anatomy of the cervical region. The pertinent anatomy of the cervical spine, including bony structures, joints and articulations, intervertebral disks, ligaments, fascial structures, musculature, neurologic structures, and vascular structures are reviewed in this section.

DEFINITION

The cervical region encompasses the various anatomic regions of the neck, including the following:

- Anterior region
- Lateral region
- Posterior cervical region
- Region over the sternocleidomastoid muscle[3]

MUSCULOSKELETAL

Bony Structures

The cervical spine consists of seven vertebrae with eight vertebral segments (Fig. 33.1). A vertebral segment refers to two adjacent vertebrae and their associated arthrodial, ligamentous, muscular, vascular, neural, and lymphatic elements. A vertebral segment is named for the superior vertebra contributing to the unit, for example, C3 refers to C3 on C4 and the joint space between them (C3–C4). Additionally, a vertebra's motion is described relative to the position of the segment below. For example, if C3 is described as flexed, it is flexed relative to C4.

The atlas (C1) and the axis (C2) are atypical vertebrae and their articulations with the occiput and axis respectively are considered atypical cervical segments. The remaining cervical vertebral articulations are considered typical cervical segments. There are six typical cervical segments extending from the C2–C3 articulations through the C7–T1 articulations.

The first cervical vertebra, or atlas, consists of an anterior and posterior arch, joining to form the heavy lateral masses that bear the superior and inferior articular surfaces. The superior facets articulate with the occiput forming the occipitoatlantal (OA) joint, and the inferior facets articulate with the axis forming the atlantoaxial (AA) joint. The atlas has a facet for articulation with the odontoid process or dens of the axis on its internal surface, as well as an anterior tubercle for muscular attachments. The posterior arch is longer and bears a small posterior tubercle in place of a spinous process. The transverse processes of the atlas, called lateral masses, are modified and palpable. Each transverse process has a transverse foramen for the vertebral artery. The vertebral arteries traverse through the foramina of C6 through the atlas and pierce the tectorial membrane to enter the foramen magnum.

The second cervical vertebra, or axis, is identified by the projection of the odontoid process, or dens, which develops from the embryologic body of the first vertebra. The dens articulates with the inner anterior surface of the ring-like atlas and acts as a pivot point about which the atlas rotates. The posterior surface of the dens has a facet that accommodates the synovial bursa that separates it from the transverse band of the cruciate ligament. The axis does not form a neural foramen for spinal roots. Its transverse processes are the only ones in the cervical spine that are not grooved to allow exit of a nerve root.[4] The spinous process of the axis is larger, palpable, and prominent on x-ray. The spinous process of C2 can serve as an important landmark to orient an osteopathic physician to begin their diagnosis of the typical cervical segments.

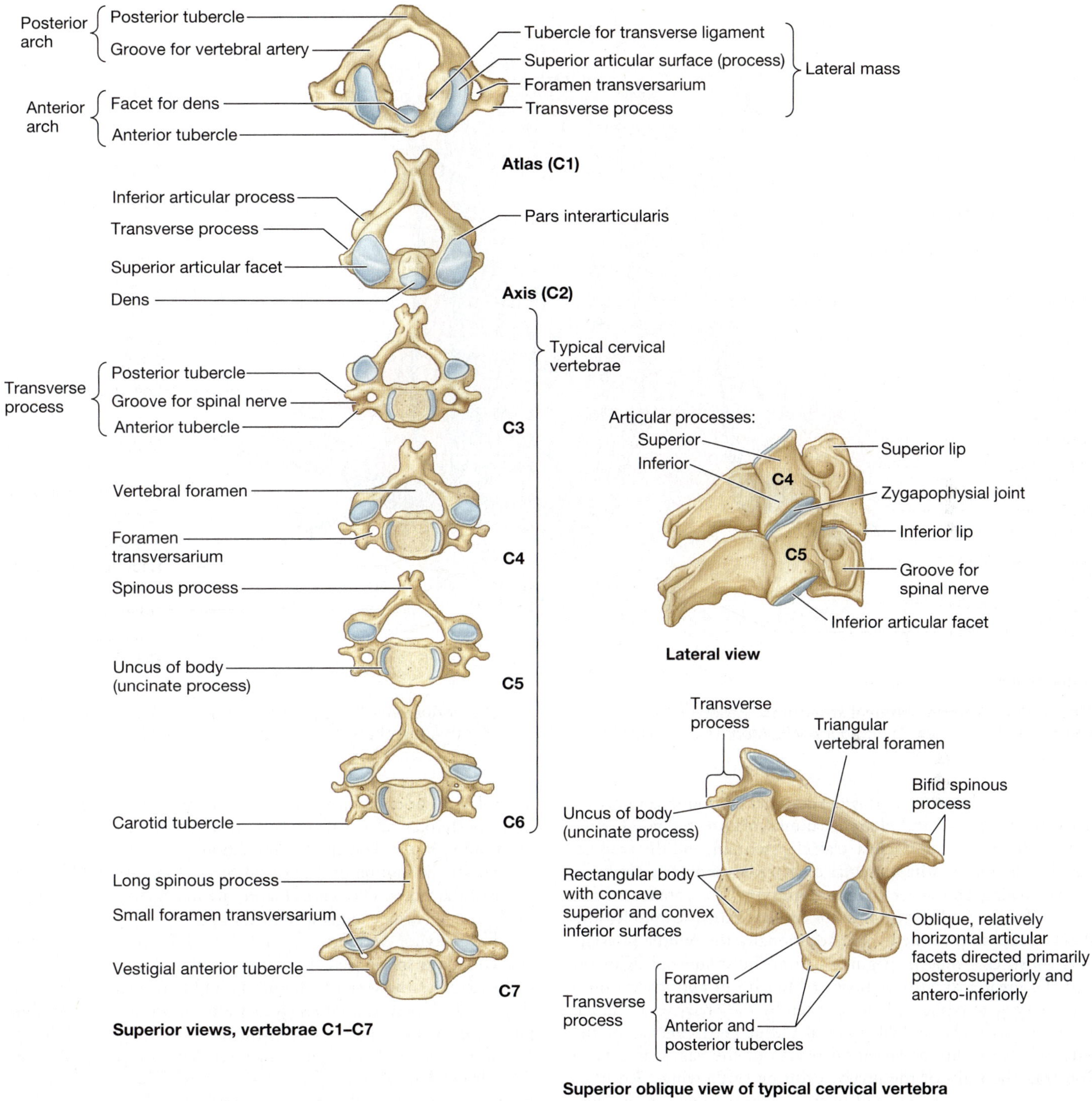

Figure 33.1. Cervical vertebrae and their articulations. (Reprinted with permission from Dalley AF II, Agur AMR. *Moore's Clinically Oriented Anatomy*. 9th ed. Wolters Kluwer; 2023. Figure 9.2A,B,D.)

The cervical transverse processes are unique and different from the transverse processes of the thoracic and lumbar spine. The typical cervical transverse processes contain a gutter that runs obliquely from anterior to posterior, through which the spinal nerves traverse. These nerves exit the spine through the neural foramina, which are largest at the C2–C3 level, and decrease in size progressively to the C6–C7 level. Flexion of the cervical spine increases the vertical diameter of the neural foramen, whereas extension decreases it. The anterior portion of the cervical transverse process is developmentally a rib, whereas the posterior portion is a true transverse process.[4] These portions fuse, but between them persists the transverse foramen, which allows for the passage of the vertebral artery and vein from C1 to C6. Although this provides protection for the vertebral artery, it also creates the possibility of trauma to the artery from bony insult. The transverse processes of the C7 vertebra contain a small foramen that allows passage of the vertebral vein, but not the vertebral artery. C7 is also called "vertebra prominens" as the spinous process is long and easily palpable.[5]

The hyoid bone is contained in the anterior cervical region (Fig. 33.2). The hyoid bone develops from the embryologic second and third pharyngeal arches. Through its ligamentous and

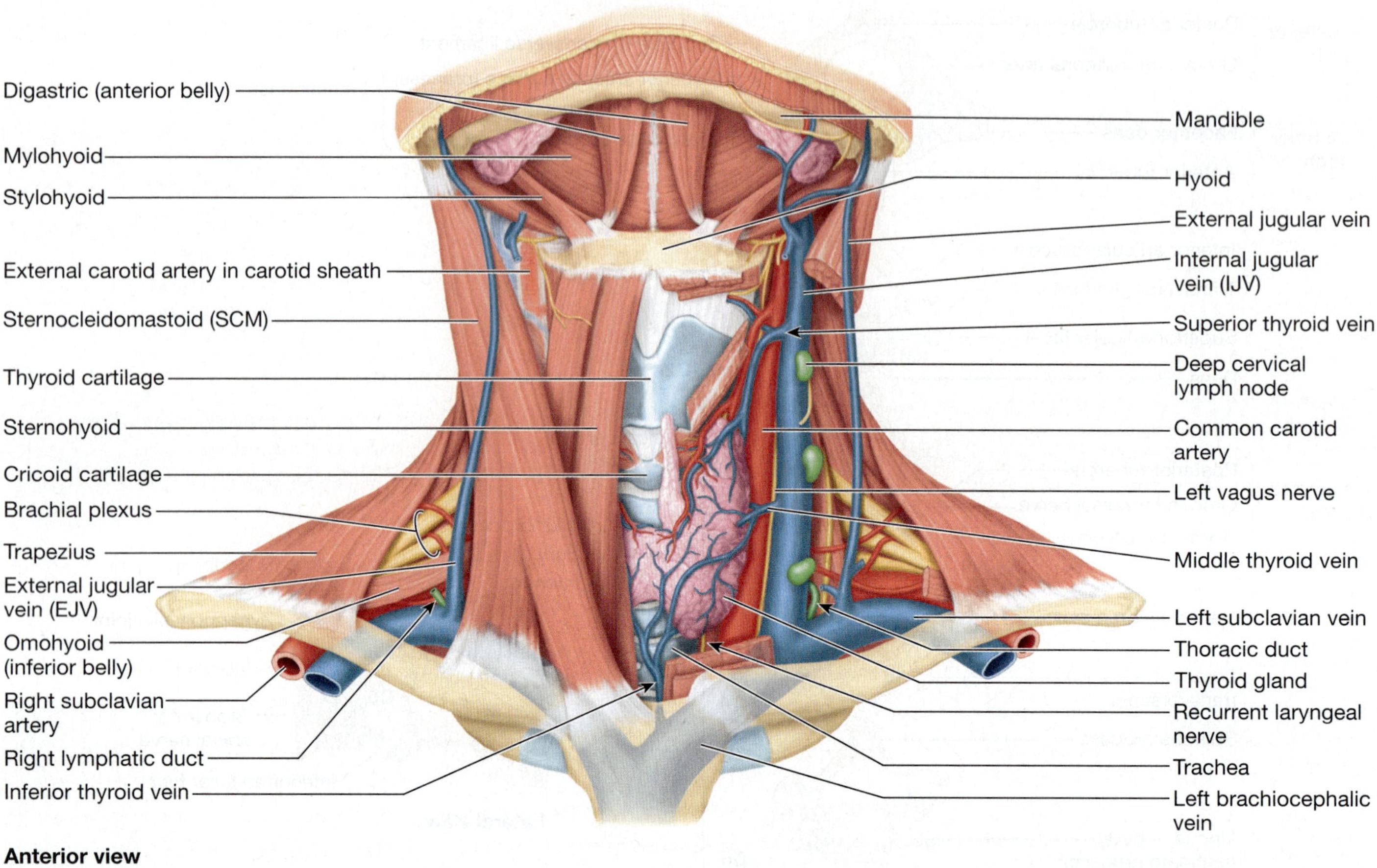

Figure 33.2. Anterior cervical structures. (Based on Gest TR. *Lippincott® Atlas of Anatomy*. 2nd ed. Wolters Kluwer; 2020. Reprinted with permission from Dalley AF II, Agur AMR. *Moore's Clinically Oriented Anatomy*. 9th ed. Wolters Kluwer; 2023. Figure 9.1.)

muscular attachments, it provides a direct anatomic connection between the glossal and pharyngeal musculature, temporal bone, larynx, thyroid gland, trachea, clavicle, sternum, and the scapula. The hyoid bone and its muscular connections provide a vital role in swallowing and speech while preserving the patency of the airway. Table 33.1 lists the anterior cervical extrinsic muscles and their relationship to the hyoid. Additionally, the middle pharyngeal constrictor muscle originates from the stylohyoid ligament and the greater and lesser horns of the hyoid and inserts onto the pharyngeal raphe. It is innervated by the pharyngeal branch of the vagus nerve and pharyngeal plexus and branches of the external and recurrent laryngeal nerves of the vagus. It acts to constrict the walls of the pharynx during swallowing.[6] An inferior and posterior positioned hyoid has been shown to be correlated with upper airway obstruction, such as in obstructive sleep apnea.[7] The hyoid is an important anatomic structure responsible for maintaining the functional integrity and postural support of the cervical region and contributes to a bony and myofascial ring around the upper cervical region (Table 33.1). The hyoid should be assessed in any patient with dysfunction involving the cervical or cranial regions.

Joints/Articulations

The facet joints, or zygapophyseal joints, of the cervical spine are enclosed in a fibrous capsule that is lax to allow movement in multiple planes. The smooth mass of bone between the superior and inferior articular facets of the cervical vertebrae from C2 to C7 is called the articular pillar. Due to the relatively small and anterolateral orientation of the cervical transverse processes, the broad posterolateral articular pillars are used to determine vertebral positioning in the segmental examination.

Rotational motion of the typical cervical segments follows the plane of the facets. The cervical facets are in a plane oriented superiorly at a 45-degree angle toward the eye.

The cervical vertebrae from C2 to C7 are saddle shaped and contain a specialized set of small synovial joints on the lateral surface of the vertebral bodies in addition to the facet joints (Fig. 33.1). These specialized joints are known as uncovertebral joints (or uncinate joints) of Luschka, which provide stability to the cervical spine. They contain menisci that protect articular surfaces from damage during cervical motion. These menisci may become entrapped in the joint and cause cervical dysfunction. The uncinate processes also act as a barrier to lateral disk herniations in the cervical region. Most lateral disk herniations in the cervical spine occur at the C7–T1 level where the uncinate processes are rudimentary or absent.[8,9]

The combination of the orientation of the zygapophyseal joints and the uncovertebral joints in the typical cervical spine results in coupled rotation and side bending to the same side during sagittal flexion or extension.[8]

Landmarks

There are important anatomical landmarks that help one to identify both the location of cervical vertebral levels and sites for procedures such as cricothyroidotomy and tracheostomy. However, these landmarks may be altered due to patient position (erect or

TABLE 33.1

Muscles of Anterior Cervical Region and Hyoid (Extrinsic Muscles of Larynx)

Muscle	Origin	Insertion	Innervation	Main Action(s)
Suprahyoid Muscles				
Mylohyoid	Mylohyoid line of mandible	Mylohyoid raphe and body of hyoid	Nerve to mylohyoid, a branch of inferior alveolar nerve (from mandibular nerve, CN V_3)	Elevates hyoid, floor of mouth, and tongue during swallowing and speaking
Geniohyoid	Inferior mental spine of mandible	Body of hyoid	C1 via hypoglossal nerve (CN XII) and nerve to geniohyoid	Pulls hyoid anterosuperiorly; shortens floor of mouth; widens pharynx
Stylohyoid	Styloid process of temporal bone		Stylohyoid (preparotid) branch of facial nerve (CN VII)	Elevates and retracts hyoid, thus elongating floor of mouth
Digastric	*Anterior belly:* digastric fossa of mandible *Posterior belly:* mastoid notch of temporal bone	Intermediate tendon to body and greater horn of hyoid	Nerve to mylohyoid, a branch of inferior alveolar nerve Digastric (preparotid) branch of facial nerve (CN VII)	Working with infrahyoid muscles, depresses mandible against resistance; elevates and steadies hyoid during swallowing and speaking
Infrahyoid Muscles				
Sternohyoid	Manubrium of sternum and medial end of clavicle	Body of hyoid	C1–C3 by a branch of ansa cervicalis	Depresses hyoid after elevation during swallowing
Omohyoid	Superior border of scapula near suprascapular notch	Inferior border of hyoid		Depresses, retracts, and steadies hyoid
Sternothyroid	Posterior surface of manubrium of sternum	Oblique line of thyroid cartilage	C2 and C3 by a branch of ansa cervicalis	Depresses hyoid and larynx
Thyrohyoid	Oblique line of thyroid cartilage	Inferior border of body and greater horn of hyoid	C1 via hypoglossal nerve (CN XII) and nerve to thyrohyoid	Depresses hyoid and elevates larynx

Modified with permission from Dalley AF II, Agur AMR. *Moore's Clinically Oriented Anatomy.* 9th ed. Wolters Kluwer; 2023. Table 9.3.

supine) and the body habitus of the patient. The hyoid is typically located at the level of C3.[10] The thyroid cartilage is the largest of the cartilages of the larynx. Its superior border is typically located at the level of the C4 vertebra[11] and it spans C4–C5. The cricoid cartilage is inferior to the thyroid cartilage and typically spans the level of C6–C7.[12,13] Both the trachea and esophagus begin at about the level of C6. The common carotid artery bifurcates at the level of C4.[10]

Intervertebral Disks

Each cervical intervertebral disk is situated between the cartilaginous endplates of two consecutive typical cervical vertebrae. There are no disks found at the OA or AA joints. Each intervertebral disk is composed of a gelatinous nucleus pulposus surrounded by a laminated, fibrous annulus fibrosus. Cervical disks are thicker anteriorly than posteriorly and are responsible for the normal cervical lordotic curve.[14] Positions of the cervical spine affect intradiskal pressure (IDP). Pressure is least in the supine position and greatest during extension of the cervical spine.[4] Each intervertebral disk is composed of a gelatinous nucleus pulposus surrounded by a laminated, fibrous annulus fibrosus. Successive layers of the annulus fibrosus slant in alternate directions, so that they cross each other at different angles depending on the IDP of the nucleus pulposus. At birth, the disk has a high water content (88%), which mechanically allows it to absorb a significant amount of stress. However, with age, the percentage of water decreases, and the ratio of proteoglycans changes. After 50 years of age, the nucleus pulposus becomes a fibrocartilaginous mass with characteristics similar to those of the outer zone of the annulus fibrosis. Positions of the cervical spine, disease processes, and surgical procedures can affect IDP.[15,16] For example, anterior cervical diskectomy and fusion (ACDF) will drastically reduce the amount of IDP at the fused segments, however IDP has been shown to increase at the vertically adjacent segments. This increase in IDP has been postulated to contribute to the increased likelihood of adjacent segment degeneration seen post-ACDF.[16]

Ligaments

The anterior and posterior longitudinal ligaments (PLLs) run along both sides of the spinal column and give support to the bony structures and the natural cervical lordosis. They also help to contain the intervertebral disks. The anterior longitudinal ligament is a broad, strong ligament on the anterior aspect of the vertebral bodies, extending from the atlas to the sacrum. Its superior attachment is to the anterior arch of the atlas and the anterior OA membrane. The PLL lies on the posterior surface of the bodies of the vertebrae from the axis to the sacrum. This ligament is wider in the upper cervical spine and narrower in the lower cervical spine. Its lateral expansions over the disks are thin, weak, and represent a vulnerable area for disk herniation as compared to its strong central band. Lateral disk herniations are more likely at the lower cervical

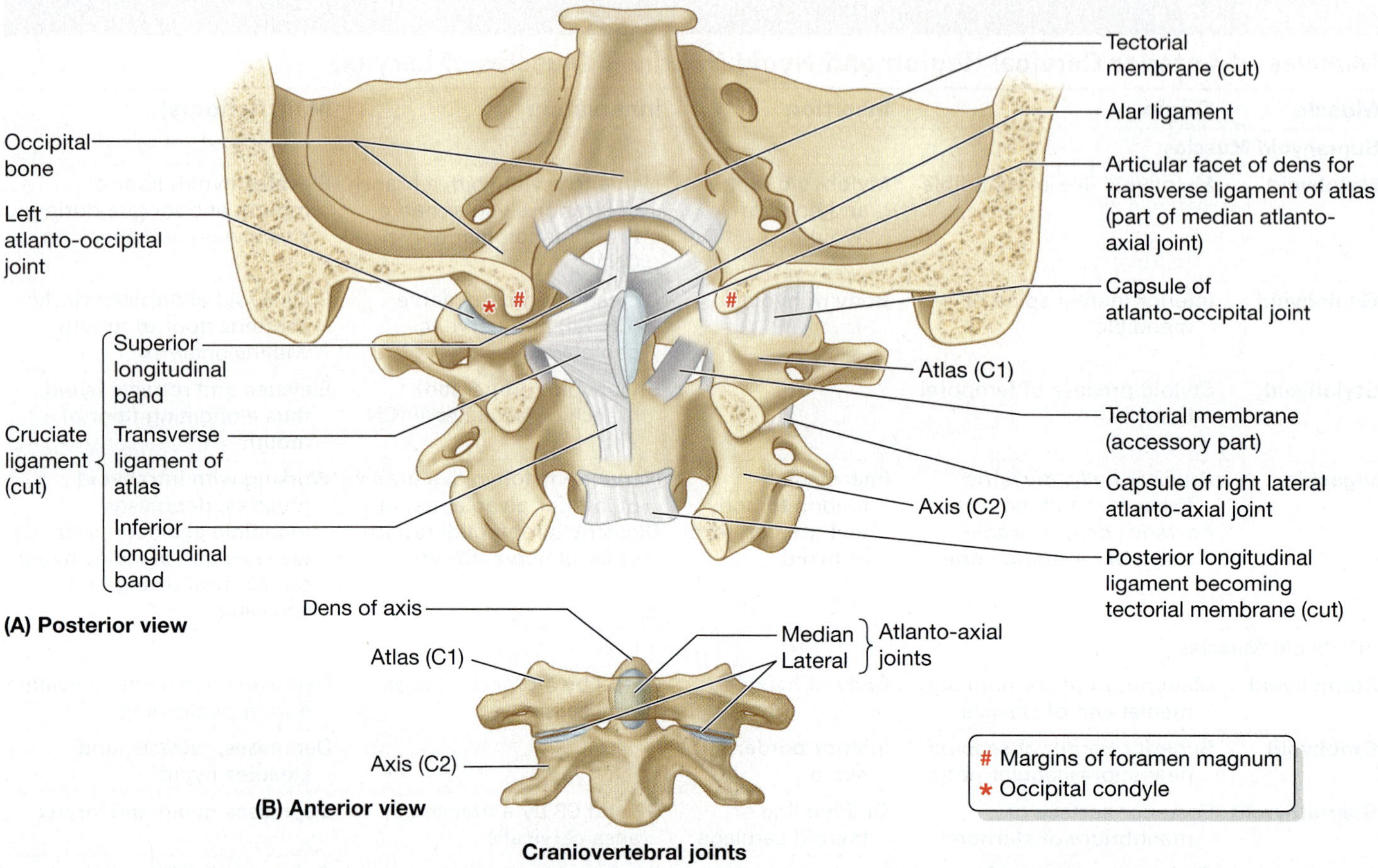

Figure 33.3. Ligaments of the upper cervical articulations. (Reprinted with permission from Dalley AF II, Agur AMR. *Moore's Clinically Oriented Anatomy*. 9th ed. Wolters Kluwer; 2023. Figure 2.23.)

levels due to the decreased height of the uncinate processes combined with the weak lateral expansions of the PLL. At the base of the skull, the tectorial membrane (occipitoaxial ligament) is a continuation of the PLL and lies immediately behind the body of the axis. The tectorial membrane connects the posterior aspect of the dens and vertebral bodies of C2 and C3 to the clivus of the cranial base.

The atypical cervical segments have a series of specific ligaments that help govern the stability and motion of the OA and AA joints (Fig. 33.3). The transverse ligament of the atlas is a broad, strong, triangular ligament arching across the ring of the atlas and anchored firmly on each side to a tubercle on the medial surface of both lateral masses of the atlas. It has two fascicles layered in a crosswise fashion, which gives it a cruciate configuration. The transverse ligament portion of the cruciate ligament complex supports the atlas in rotating about the dens. The anterior surface of the spinal cord lies immediately posterior to the transverse ligament. Rupture (or laxity, which may occur in conditions such as rheumatoid arthritis) of this ligament creates the possibility of the dens contacting the spinal cord, causing catastrophic neurologic damage.[17] The alar ligaments are short, strong bundles of fibrous tissue that extend superolateral in an oblique orientation from both sides of the superior portion of the odontoid process of the axis and attach to the medial aspect of the occipital condyles. They are often referred to as the "check" ligaments.

The typical cervical vertebrae, C2–C7, have a similar ligamentous configuration to the thoracic and lumbar regions of the axial spine. The supraspinous and interspinous ligaments, found between adjacent spinous processes, attach each spinal vertebra to one another. The highly elastic ligamentum flavum connects the ventral portions of vertically adjacent laminae. There are two ligamentum flavum at each spinal level, separated by a small posteromedial cleft.

Fascial Structures

The three fascial layers of the cervical spine are superficial, intermediate, and deep (Fig. 33.4).

The superficial fascia exists as a single sheet over the anterior and posterior cervical triangles. It surrounds subcutaneous fat, the platysma muscle, the external jugular vein, and cutaneous sensory nerves.

The intermediate fascia layer consists of the alar fascia. The alar fascia spreads behind the esophagus and surrounds the carotid sheath.

The deep layer of fascia has superficial (investing), anterior (pretracheal), and posterior (prevertebral) layers. The investing layer of the deep fascia extends from the trapezius muscle over the posterior triangle and then splits to enclose the sternocleidomastoid (SCM) muscle. The pretracheal layer of the deep cervical fascia encloses the strap muscles and extends laterally to the scapula. The prevertebral fascia covers the muscles surrounding the vertebral column, scalene muscles, longus colli muscle, and the anterior longitudinal ligament of the vertebral column.

Fascia from the cervical spine follows a "tube within tube" structure and continues into the mediastinum to blend with the pericardium and great vessels.

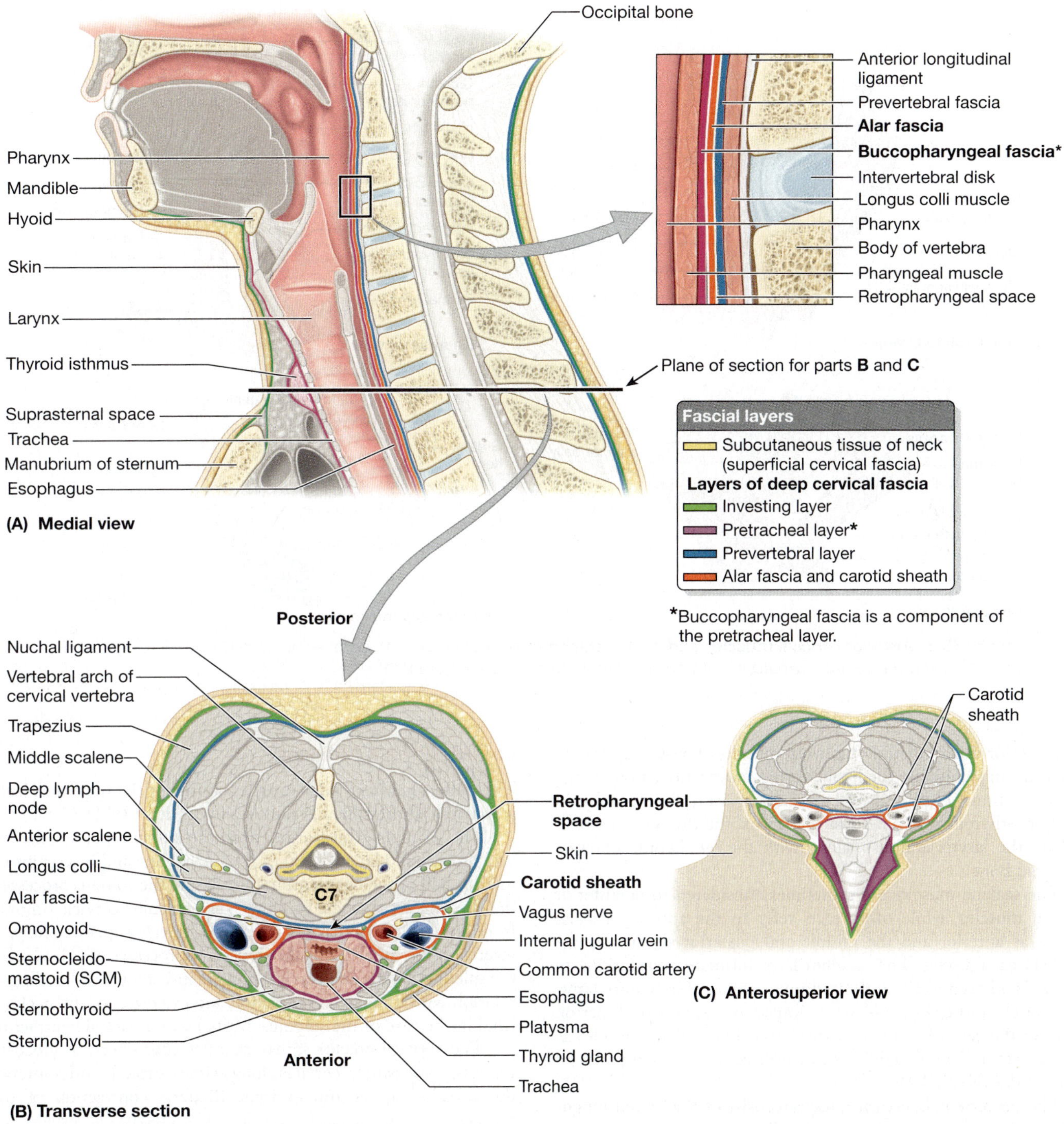

Figure 33.4. Fascial layers of the neck. (Based on Gest TR. *Lippincott® Atlas of Anatomy.* 2nd ed. Wolters Kluwer; 2020. Reprinted with permission from Dalley AF II, Agur AMR. *Moore's Clinically Oriented Anatomy.* 9th ed. Wolters Kluwer; 2023. Figure 9.4A.)

Musculature

The neck muscles may be categorized as anterior, lateral, and posterior neck.

Anterior Neck Muscles

Anteriorly, many muscles travel from the mandible to the hyoid, sternum, and clavicle (Figs. 33.5 and 33.6). The anterolateral cervical muscles function to flex and rotate the head and neck as well as provide protection and support for the visceral structures in the anterior neck. The anterior cervical muscles include the platysma, SCM, suprahyoid, infrahyoid, scalene, and prevertebral cervical muscles.

The anterior superficial neck muscles include the platysma and SCM muscles. Their actions and innervations are found in Table 33.2.

The suprahyoid muscles attach the hyoid bone to the mandible, tongue, and temporal bone. These muscles are void of muscle spindles and are capable of reversing origin and insertion to facilitate effective swallowing. These muscles also help to provide upper cervical postural stability.[7]

The suprahyoid muscles consist of those found in Table 33.3.

The infrahyoid "strap muscles" attach to the hyoid, thyroid cartilage, and sternum. They traverse medial to the SCM (except for

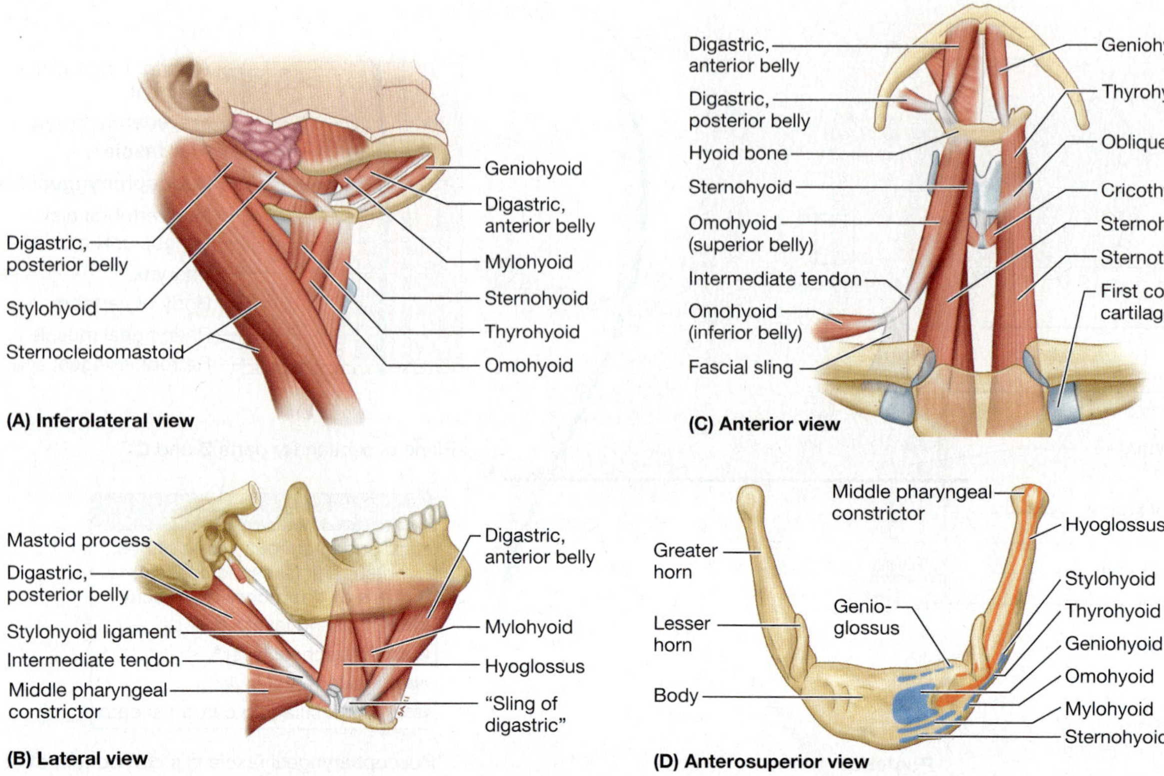

Figure 33.5. Anterior cervical muscles and hyoid attachments. (Reprinted with permission from Dalley AF II, Agur AMR. *Moore's Clinically Oriented Anatomy*. 9th ed. Wolters Kluwer; 2023. Figure 9.19.)

the posterior aspect of the omohyoid muscle). These muscles are important in stabilizing the hyoid during mastication, swallowing, and respiration.[2] The infrahyoid muscles consist of the sternohyoid and sternothyroid which depress the larynx, the thyrohyoid which elevates the larynx and also, along with the omohyoid depresses the hyoid bone.

The scalene muscles are sometimes considered to be anterior cervical muscles, while other texts refer to the anterior scalene muscle as anterior and the middle and posterior scalene as lateral cervical muscles. The scalenes have intimate connections to the first and second rib and oftentimes osteopathic manipulative treatment to those ribs will have an impact on somatic dysfunction found in the cervical spine and vice versa. The scalene muscles as a group act as lateral stabilizers, as well as accessory muscles of respiration (Table 33.4).

The prevertebral cervical muscles consist of the paired longus colli and longus capitis. The longus colli muscles extend from C1 to T3, spanning the lateral portions of the vertebral bodies, and attaching at the anterior tubercles of the lateral masses of C3–C6. Bilateral contraction flexes the neck. Unilateral contraction provides contralateral rotation and ipsilateral side bending. The longus capitis muscles arise on the anterior tubercles of C3–C6 and extend superiorly to the basiocciput. They act to flex the neck with bilateral contraction and provide ipsilateral rotation with unilateral contraction.

Lateral Neck Muscles

The lateral neck muscles consist of the rectus capitis anterior which flexes the head at the OA joint and the rectus capitis lateralis which provides ipsilateral lateral head flexion at the OA joint. The longus colli and capitis are oftentimes considered to be lateral muscles.

Posterior Neck Muscles

The more superficial back muscles consist of the trapezius, levator scapulae, and the splenius capitis and cervicis (Table 33.5).

The splenius capitis arises from the lateral aspect of the mastoid process and lateral third of the nuchal line and inserts into the inferior half of the ligamentum nuchae and the spinous processes of the superior six thoracic vertebrae. The splenius cervicis originates from the spinous processes of T3–T6, travels superolaterally, and inserts on the tubercles of the transverse processes of C1–C3. Both the splenius capitis and cervicis provide ipsilateral side bending and rotation with unilateral contraction and extension of the neck (and head in the case of the splenius capitis) with bilateral contraction.[6]

The cervical erector spinae muscles consist of the iliocostalis cervicis, longissimus cervicis, longissimus capitis, and sometimes the spinalis capitis and cervicis. Bilateral contraction of these muscles provides cervical extension. The iliocostalis cervicis is the most lateral and originates on the posterior tubercles of C4–C6 and inserts on the posterior rib angles of ribs 3 to 6. It sidebends the neck with unilateral contraction. The longissimus capitis arises from the transverse processes of C4 and/or C5 and inserts at the posterior edge of the mastoid process. Unilateral contraction induces ipsilateral side bending and rotation. The longissimus cervicis originates from the transverse processes of C2–C6 and inserts into the transverse processes of T1–T4 or T5. Unilateral contraction provides ipsilateral side bending. When present, the spinalis capitis, which consists of fibers of the semispinalis muscle, originates from the midline of the occiput and inserts on the spinous processes of C7 and T1. Likewise, the spinalis cervicis, when present originates from the spinous processes of the axis, C3 and C4, and may insert on the inferior aspect of the ligamentum nuchae, and spinous processes of C7, T1, and T2.[18,19]

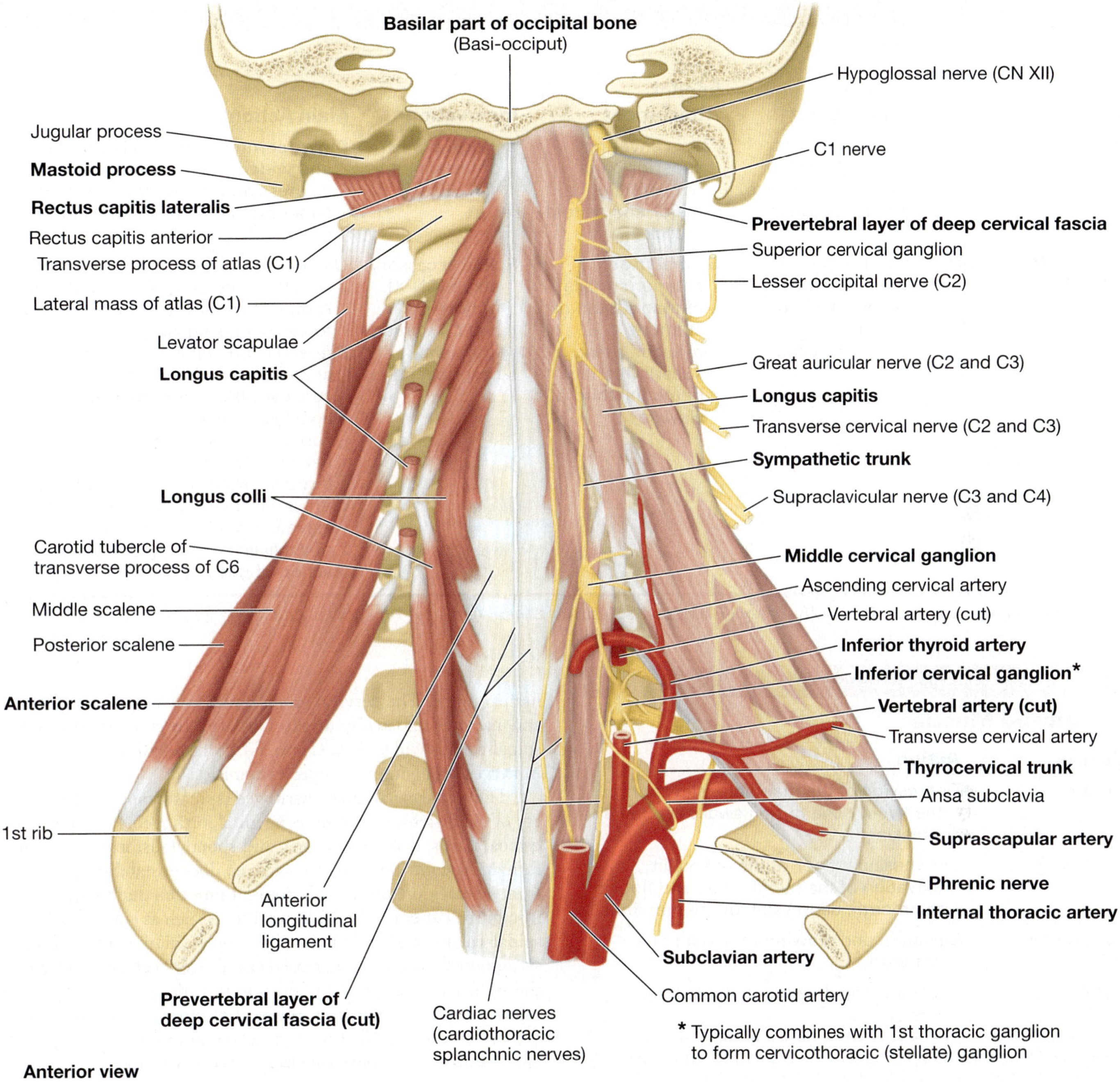

Figure 33.6. Cervical prevertebral region. (Reprinted with permission from Dalley AF II, Agur AMR. *Moore's Clinically Oriented Anatomy*. 9th ed. Wolters Kluwer; 2023. Figure 9.25B.)

The transversospinales muscles consist of the semispinalis capitis and cervicis which provide extension of the head, cervical and thoracic spine with bilateral contraction and ipsilateral side bending and contralateral rotation of the head, cervical and thoracic spine with unilateral contraction. Also included in this group are the rotatores cervicis which extend the spine with bilateral contraction and induce ipsilateral side bending with unilateral contraction, the interspinales which accomplish extension of the cervical spine and the intertransversarii which assist in both side bending and stabilization of the spine.

The suboccipital muscles lie deep to the semispinalis capitis muscle and consist of the rectus capitis posterior major and minor and the obliquus capitis superior and inferior (Fig. 33.7). They all provide extension of the head at the AA joint with bilateral contraction and ipsilateral head rotation at the AA joint with unilateral contraction. In addition to their motor function, these muscles are integral in the proprioception of the positioning of the head on the cervical spine. The connective tissue between the rectus capitis posterior major and minor and the obliquus capitis inferior muscles and the cervical spinal dura mater forms a myodural bridge. Disruption or irritation of this myodural bridge has been implicated in the etiology of cervicogenic headache.[20–22]

NEUROLOGIC

In adults, the spinal cord extends from the medulla in the brain, through the cervical and thoracic spine, to the L2 level of the

TABLE 33.2

Superficial Cervical Muscles

Muscle	Superior Attachment	Inferior Attachment	Innervation	Main Action(s)
Platysma	Inferior border of mandible, skin, and subcutaneous tissues of lower face	Fascia covering superior parts of pectoralis major and deltoid muscles	Cervical branch of facial nerve (CN VII)	Draws corners of mouth inferiorly and widens it as in expressions of sadness and fright; draws skin of neck superiorly when teeth are clenched, indicating tension
Sternocleidomastoid (SCM)	Lateral surface of mastoid process of temporal bone and lateral half of superior nuchal line	*Sternal head:* anterior surface of manubrium of sternum *Clavicular head:* superior surface of medial third of clavicle	Spinal accessory nerve (CN XI, motor); C3 and C4 nerves (pain and proprioception)	*Unilateral contraction:* tilts head to same side (i.e., laterally flexes neck) and rotates it so face is turned superiorly toward opposite side *Bilateral contraction:* (1) extends neck at atlanto-occipital joints, (2) flexes cervical vertebrae so that chin approaches manubrium, or (3) extends superior cervical vertebrae while flexing inferior vertebrae, so chin is thrust forward with head kept level With cervical vertebrae fixed, may elevate manubrium and medial ends of clavicles, assisting pump-handle action of deep respiration

Reprinted with permission from Agur AMR, Dalley AF II. *Moore's Essential Clinical Anatomy.* 7th ed. Wolters Kluwer; 2024:600. Table 9.1.

TABLE 33.3

Suprahyoid Muscles

Muscle	Action
Digastric	Depression of the mandible, elevation of the hyoid bone during swallowing and speaking
Mylohyoid	The muscular floor of the oral cavity, elevation of the hyoid bone, and floor of the mouth, depression of the mandible
Geniohyoid	Elevation and drawing of hyoid bone anteriorly
Stylohyoid	Elevation and drawing of hyoid bone posteriorly

Modified with permission from Dalley AF II, Agur AMR. *Moore's Clinically Oriented Anatomy.* 9th ed. Wolters Kluwer; 2023. Table 9.3.

lumbar spine. The cervical spinal canal is widest at the AA level and narrows maximally at the C6 level. In contrast, the cervical spinal cord is wider from C3 to T2, corresponding to the increase in nerves supplying the upper extremities.

The spinal canal can be narrowed (spinal stenosis) due to a variety of conditions, including congenital, orthopedic disease such as osteoarthritis, disk protrusions, and spondylolisthesis. Osteophyte formation contributes to stenosis, as does instability with excess front-to-back or side-to-side translation often due to ligamentous instability. Patients who have conditions such as congenitally small spinal canals, disk herniations, Arnold–Chiari malformation, or syringomyelia are all at increased risk for cervical cord injury, given the right circumstances. In addition to canal stenosis, spinal cord injuries can also occur from physical traumatic events or ischemic damage to the cord due to vascular compromise. Cord injury due to any etiology can have catastrophic consequences.

TABLE 33.4

Scalene Muscles

Muscle	Superior Attachment	Inferior Attachment	Innervation	Main Action(s)
Anterior scalene	Transverse processes of C3–C6 vertebrae	1st rib	Cervical spinal nerves C4–C6	Flexes neck laterally; elevates 1st rib during forced inspiration
Middle scalene	Posterior tubercles of transverse processes of C5–C7 vertebrae	Superior surface of 1st rib; posterior to groove for subclavian artery	Anterior rami of cervical spinal nerves	Flexes neck laterally; elevates 1st rib during forced inspiration
Posterior scalene	Posterior tubercles of transverse processes of C5–C7 vertebrae	External border of 2nd rib	Anterior rami of cervical spinal nerves C7 and C8	Flexes neck laterally; elevates 2nd rib during forced inspiration

Modified with permission from Dalley AF II, Agur AMR. *Moore's Clinically Oriented Anatomy.* 9th ed. Wolters Kluwer; 2023. Table 9.4.

TABLE 33.5

Trapezius and Levator Scapulae Innervations and Actions

Muscle	Superior Attachment	Inferior Attachment	Innervation	Main Action(s)
Trapezius	Medial third of superior nuchal line, external occipital protuberance, nuchal ligament, spinous processes of C7–T12 vertebrae	Lateral third of clavicle, acromion, and spine of scapula	Spinal accessory nerve (CN XI; motor); C3 and C4 nerves (pain and proprioception)	Elevates, retracts, and rotates scapulae superiorly *Descending (superior) fibers:* elevate scapulae/shoulders; maintain level of shoulders against gravity or resistance *Transverse (middle) fibers:* retract scapulae *Ascending (inferior) fibers:* depress scapulae/shoulders *Descending and ascending fibers together:* rotate spinous process of scapulae superiorly With shoulders fixed, *bilateral contraction* extends neck; *unilateral contraction* produces lateral flexion to same side
Levator scapulae	Posterior tubercles of transverse processes C2–C6 vertebrae	Superior part of medial border of scapula	Dorsal scapular nerve C5 and cervical spinal nerves C3 and C4	Downward rotation of scapula and tilts its glenoid cavity inferiorly by rotating scapula

Modified with permission from Dalley AF II, Agur AMR. *Moore's Clinically Oriented Anatomy.* 9th ed. Wolters Kluwer; 2023. Tables 9.2 and 9.4.

Cervical Spinal Nerves

The cervical spinal cord gives rise to the cervical plexus (Fig. 33.8) and the brachial plexus.

Because the brachial plexus innervates the upper extremity, nerve root impingement at the cervical intervertebral foramen produces neck pain and upper extremity neurologic symptoms. Impingement of the nerve roots commonly occurs from disk protrusion or osteophyte encroachment. The mixed spinal nerve contains motor fibers, sensory axons of the dorsal root ganglia, and preganglionic fibers from the autonomic nervous system.

There are eight cervical nerve roots. In contrast with the nerves in the thoracic and lumbar spine, the nerves in the cervical spine take the name of the pedicle above which they exit. For

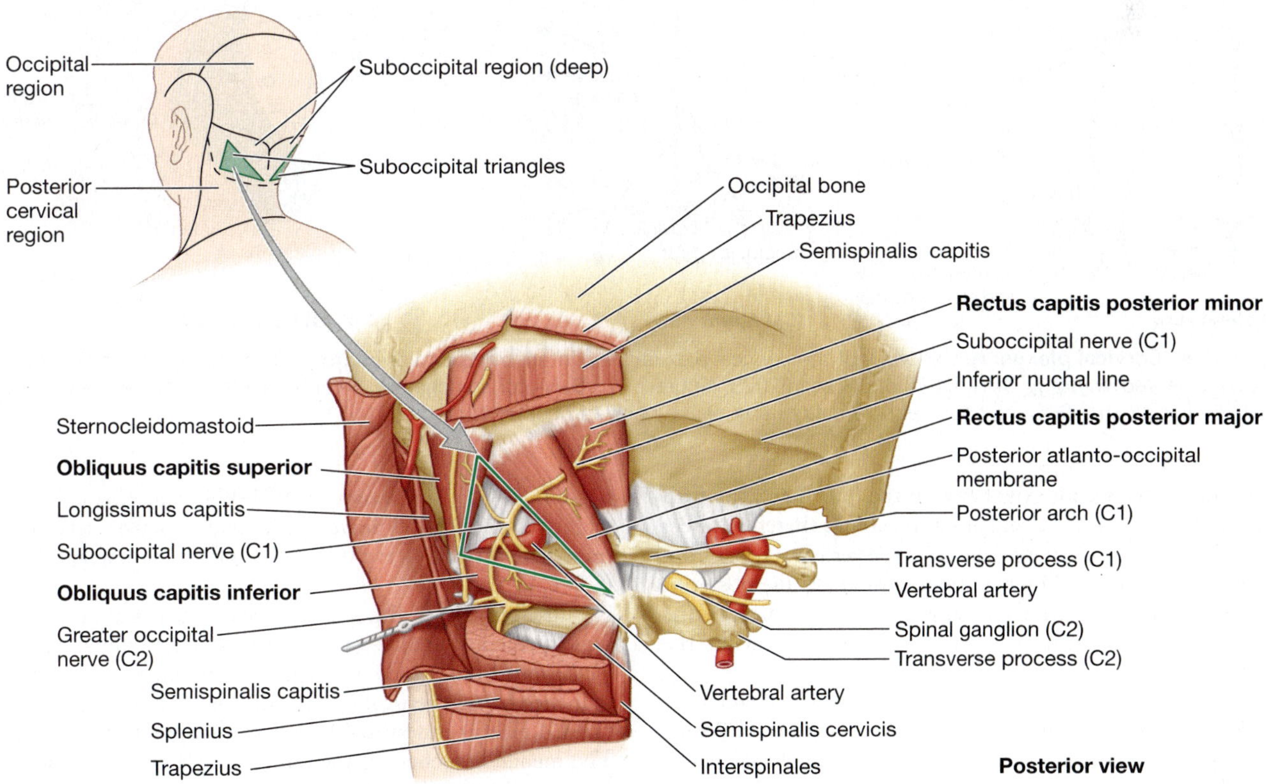

Figure 33.7. Suboccipital region. (Reprinted with permission from Dalley AF II, Agur AMR. *Moore's Clinically Oriented Anatomy.* 9th ed. Wolters Kluwer; 2023. Figure 9.14.)

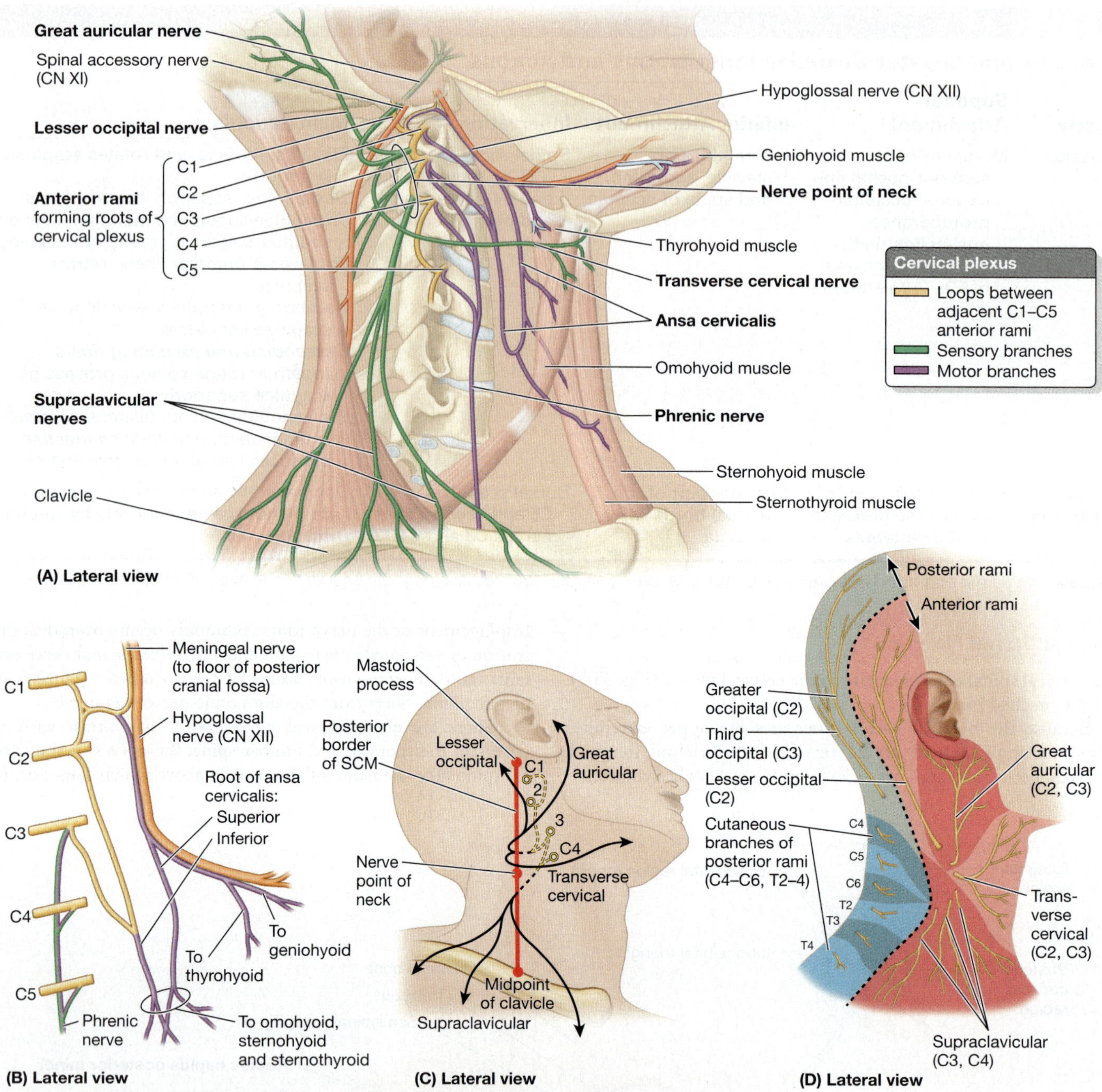

Figure 33.8. Cervical plexus. A. Overview of the cervical plexus. (Reprinted with permission from Dalley AF II, Agur AMR. *Moore's Clinically Oriented Anatomy*. 9th ed. Wolters Kluwer; 2023. Figure 2.42.) **B.** Motor branches of the cervical plexus. **C.** Sensory branches of the cervical plexus. **D.** Cutaneous sensory distribution of the neck and posterior cranium.

example, the C5 nerve root exits between the fourth and the fifth cervical vertebra. A C4–C5 disk herniation would therefore affect the C5 nerve root. The C1 nerve root exits the vertebral canal from an orifice in the posterior OA membrane just above the posterior arch of the atlas and posterior medially to the lateral mass of the atlas. The C8 nerve root exits between the seventh cervical and the first thoracic vertebrae.

Many of the cervical nerve roots have specialized anatomy (Fig. 33.8). The C1 ventral primary ramus unites with the C2 ventral primary ramus to contribute fibers to the hypoglossal nerve. The dorsal primary ramus of C1 enters the suboccipital triangle, supplying the muscles of this region, but has no cutaneous sensory branches. The cervical plexus provides innervation to the phrenic nerve (C3–C5), ansa cervicalis (C1–C3), and cutaneous branches of the lesser occipital nerve (C2), great auricular nerve (C2–C3), transverse cervical nerve (C2–C3), and the supraclavicular nerves (C3–C4).

Of clinical note, the spinal nerve dorsal ramus provides a small sensory medial branch to the cervical facet joints. The cervical facet joints from the C3–C7 segments are innervated by the medial branches of two vertically adjacent dorsal rami. For example, the C3–C4 facet is innervated by the medial branches of C3 and C4. The medial branches are the target of radiofrequency ablation for facet-mediated pain.[23] The C2–C3 facets differ in that they are innervated solely by the third occipital nerve, which is the superficial medial branch of C3. The OA and AA do not have medial branch innervation of their facet articulations. The C1 ventral ramus provides innervation to the OA joint. The C2 ventral ramus and C1–C3 sinuvertebral nerves innervate the AA joint.[24]

Cervical Sympathetic Nerves

The cervical sympathetic system consists of preganglionic and postganglionic autonomic fibers, as well as three cervical sympathetic ganglia. The preganglionic fibers originate in the intermediolateral gray column of the T1–T5 spinal cord segments. In addition to efferent fibers, small, nociceptive afferents (C fibers) travel with sympathetic fibers and synapse in the upper thoracic cord as well. Nociceptive input from the cervical spine produces palpable musculoskeletal changes in the upper thoracic spine and ribs and also increases sympathetic activity from this area.[25,26]

There are three cervical sympathetic ganglia (Fig. 33.6). The superior cervical ganglion, the largest ganglion, is located at the C2–C3 level. It contributes sympathetic fibers to the carotid plexus, orbital structures, sweat glands of the face, pharyngeal plexus where it joins the vagus and hypoglossal nerves, C1–C4 spinal nerves, and the cardiac plexus. The middle cervical ganglion, the smallest ganglion, is located at the C6 level. It contributes sympathetic fibers to the esophagus, pharynx, larynx, trachea, C5–C6 spinal nerves, and the cardiac plexus. The inferior cervical ganglion is located between the transverse process of C7 and the first rib. The first thoracic and inferior cervical ganglia fuse to form the stellate ganglion which contributes sympathetic fibers to the subclavian and vertebral arteries, C7–T1 spinal nerves, and the cardiac plexus.

Sinuvertebral Nerve

The sinuvertebral nerves at each cervical vertebral level arise from the ventral ramus distal to the dorsal root ganglion. This small branch recurs into the intervertebral foramen to reach the vertebral canal. The terminal branches supply the PLL, periosteum on the posterior aspect of the vertebral body, outer layers of the intervertebral disks, and the anterior surface of the spinal dura. The cervical sinuvertebral nerves supply the level of entry and the disk above.

Irritation of the small caliber primary afferent fibers in the sinuvertebral nerve can refer pain several segments up or down the spinal cord, as well as to the contralateral side of the body. The sinuvertebral nerve does not supply skeletal muscle or skin. The sinuvertebral nerve contains only sensory and sympathetic fibers and is sensitive to stretch and ischemia. Overactivation of the C1–C3 sinuvertebral nerves has been implicated in the etiology of cervicogenic headache.[27]

Vagus Nerve

The vagus nerve originates from the medulla oblongata and exits the skulls via the jugular foramen. A superior ganglia of the vagus nerve is found within the jugular foramen and an inferior ganglia is found after the nerve exits the foramen.[28,29] The cell bodies of the vagus nerve originating from the nucleus ambiguous have efferent special visceral (ESV) nerve fibers that help mediate swallowing and phonation. Those from the dorsal motor nucleus of the vagus nerve are efferent general visceral (EGV) and provide involuntary muscle control of organs it innervates (cardiac, pulmonary, esophageal) and innervates glands throughout the gastrointestinal tract. The superior ganglion provides afferent general somatic innervation to the external ear and tympanic membrane and the inferior ganglion provides afferent visceral fibers to the carotid and aortic bodies as well as taste sensation to the pharynx, relaying all of this information to the nucleus tractus solitarius.[28–31]

The vagus nerve continues by traveling inferiorly within the posterior portion of the carotid sheath where it is located posterior and lateral to the internal and common carotid arteries, and medial to the internal jugular vein. The right vagus nerve passes anterior to the first part of the subclavian artery and posterior to the brachiocephalic vein and sternoclavicular joint to descend into the thoracic cavity by traveling to the right of the trachea, and posterior to the hilum on the right. It then moves medially to form the esophageal plexus with the left vagus nerve. The left vagus nerve travels between the left common carotid artery and left subclavian arteries and posterior to the sternoclavicular joint to enter the thorax.[6] It then travels posterior to the phrenic nerve and left lung before traveling medially to join the right vagus to form the esophageal plexus.[28,30,31]

The four branches of the vagus nerve within the neck are the:

- pharyngeal branches: arising from the inferior ganglion of CN X they contain both sensory and motor fibers. These fibers form the pharyngeal plexus–branches of which innervate the pharyngeal and palate muscles (except the tensor palatine muscle) and also supplies the innervation to the intercarotid plexus which mediates information from the carotid body.[30,32]
- superior laryngeal nerve: travels between the external and internal carotid arteries before dividing into internal and external branches near the level of the hyoid. The internal laryngeal nerve goes through the thyrohyoid membrane entering the larynx. The external portion travels distally with the superior thyroid vessels and supplies the cricothyroid muscle, whereas the internal branch supplies the mucosa superior to the glottis, recurrent laryngeal nerve, and the superior cardiac nerve.[32]
- recurrent laryngeal: The right recurrent laryngeal nerve's fibers branch from the vagus nerve inferior to the right subclavian artery at about the T1–T2 level and then travel superiorly to enter the larynx between the cricopharyngeus muscle and the esophagus. The left recurrent laryngeal nerve loops inferior to the aortic arch distal to the ligamentum arteriosus at about the T4–T5 level.[6] After looping, the recurrent laryngeal nerves track superiorly to the posteromedial aspect of the thyroid gland where they ascend in the tracehoesophageal groove, supplying both trachea and esophagus and all the intrinsic muscles of the larynx except the cricothyroid (supplied by the laryngeal nerve).[6,30]
- superior cardiac nerve: while the vagus nerve is within the carotid sheath, it gives off the superior cardiac nerve which provides postganglionic sympathetic innervation to the heart.[31,33]

Additionally, the vagus nerve gives off:

- anterior and posterior bronchial branches in which the anterior branches form the anterior pulmonary plexus and the posterior branches form the posterior pulmonary plexus.[30,32]
- anterior (left vagus) and posterior (right vagus) esophageal branches to form the esophageal plexus.[30,32]
- gastric branches that supply the stomach. The celiac branches are mainly derived from the right vagus nerve and supply the pancreas, kidneys, adrenals, and small intestine.[28,30,31,34]

Somatic dysfunction of the cranium, especially that which affects the jugular foramen, and somatic dysfunction of the upper cervical complex where the vagus nerve courses may cause irritation or dysfunction of the vagus nerve.

Phrenic Nerve

The phrenic nerves originate from C4 but also receive contributions from C3 and C5 nerves. The phrenic nerves contain motor,

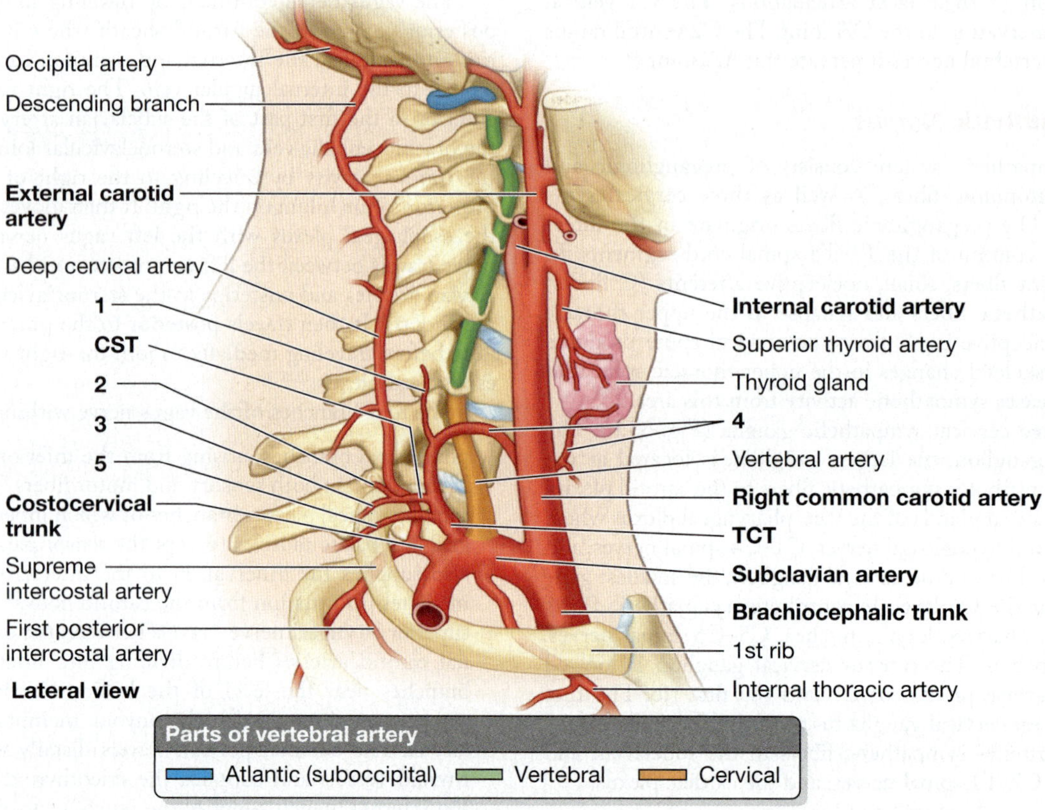

Figure 33.9. Arteries of the neck. 1, Ascending cervical artery; 2, Superficial cervical/transverse cervical artery; 3, Suprascapular artery; 4, Inferior thyroid artery; 5, Dorsal scapular artery; CST, Cervicodorsal trunk; SA, Subclavian artery; TCT, Thyrocervical trunk. (Reprinted with permission from Dalley AF II, Agur AMR. *Moore's Clinically Oriented Anatomy*. 9th ed. Wolters Kluwer; 2023. Figure 9.26C.)

sensory, and sympathetic nerve fibers and provide the sole motor supply to the diaphragm and sensation to its central region.

VASCULATURE

Arterial

The carotid, vertebral, and subclavian arteries supply the head and neck with arterial blood (Fig. 33.9). The carotid arteries lie anterior to the cervical vertebra. The carotid pulse may be palpated for diagnostic purposes. Avoid pressure over the carotid arteries while palpating the cervical spine.

The vertebral artery is the major source of blood supply for the cervical spine and the cervical portion of the spinal cord. The vertebral arteries typically originate off the subclavian artery on the right and aorta on the left and travel through the intervertebral foramen (Fig. 33.9). They then enter the cranium through the foramen magnum. The vertebral arteries join after passing through the foramen magnum to form the basilar artery. Just before joining, one or both vertebral arteries give off a branch that joins with the branch from the other side and descends in the ventral medial fissure on the anterior aspect of the spinal cord as the anterior spinal artery.

The vertebral artery can become occluded by thrombosis, dissection, or mechanical insult which may be precipitated by injury to the artery as it passes through the intervertebral foramina and over the atlas. Signs and symptoms of vertebral artery insufficiency can be remembered through the mnemonic "5D's And 3N's": dizziness, drop attacks, diplopia, dysarthria, dysphagia, ataxia of gait, nausea, numbness, and nystagmus.[35] If there is clinical suspicion of vertebral artery compromise by the history and physical findings, then high-velocity low-amplitude (HVLA) manipulation of the cervical spine should not be attempted and further investigation of the integrity of the vertebral artery should be performed. Extension and rotation have been found to be the position most likely to occlude the vertebral artery.[14] In a patient without suspicion of vertebral artery insufficiency, evidence implicating cervical manipulations as the primary cause of vertebral artery compromise is conflicting, especially because even normal neck movements have been associated with spontaneous dissections.[35] Caution and clinical judgment should be used in all patients where extension and rotation are used as part of cervical treatment positioning.

Vascular and neurologic compromise often occur simultaneously due to the close anatomic relationship of these structures. For example, thoracic outlet syndrome (TOS) is a condition arising from compression of the vascular and neural components of the brachial plexus in the thoracic outlet. Compression in TOS can occur between the anterior and middle scalene, between the clavicle and first rib, or between the pectoralis minor muscle and the costal cage. Venous return from the upper extremity is not as impacted by scalene compression, as the subclavian vein passes in front of the anterior scalene muscle.

Provocative tests used to differentiate the site of compression in TOS can be used to identify timing, severity, and location of symptoms, however, they lack specificity and reliability.[14,36] Generally, shoulder abduction and external rotation worsen the symptoms of TOS. Symptoms such as paresthesia or hand weakness typically affect the ulnar side of the hand after an inciting activity or position.

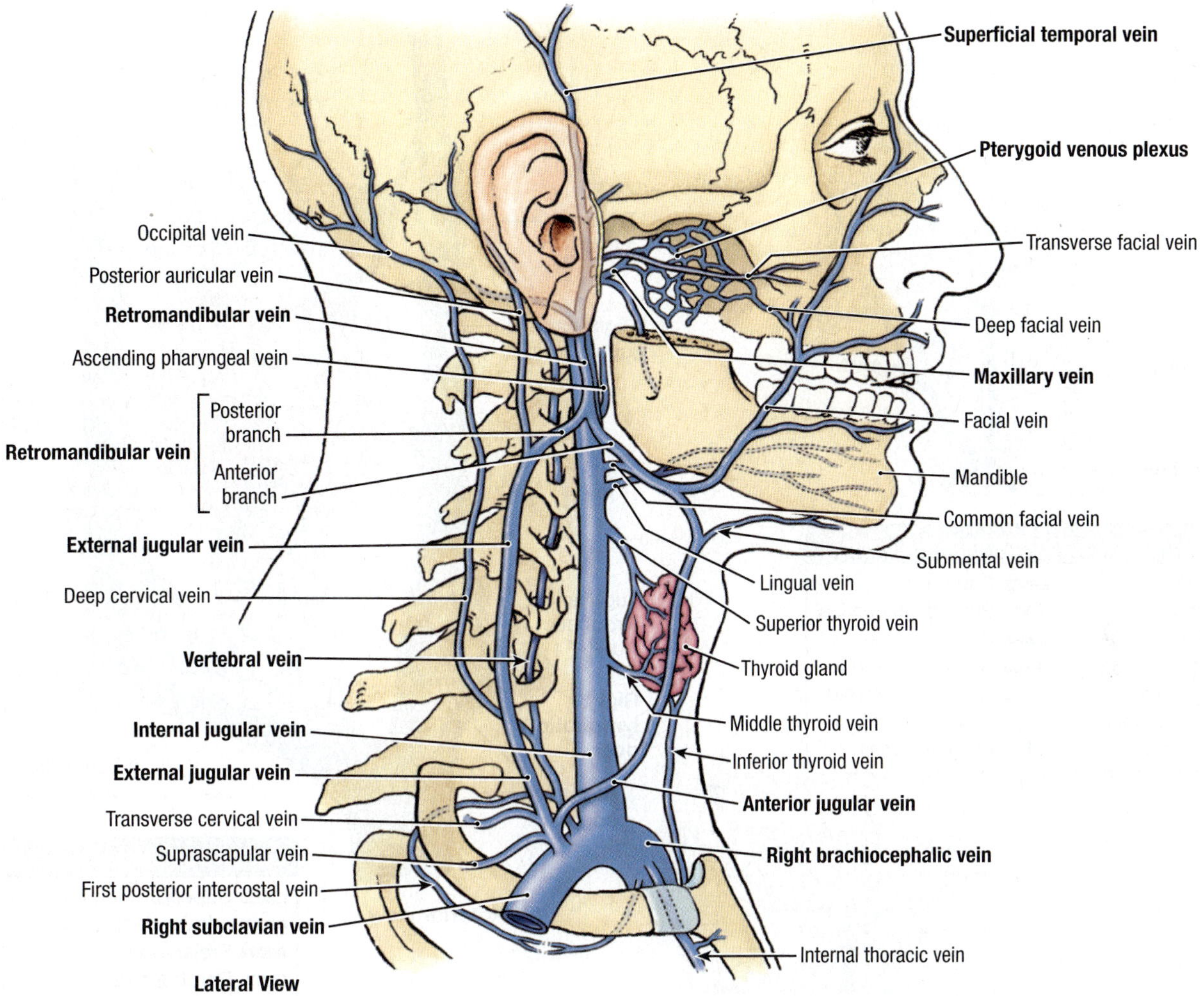

Figure 33.10. Venous drainage and lymphatic structures of the neck. (Reprinted with permission from Kupinski AM. Vascular anatomy. In: Kupinski AM, ed. *The Vascular System*. 3rd ed. Wolters Kluwer; 2023:44. Figure 4-9.)

Symptoms often resolve within minutes of cessation of the inciting activity or position. Occasionally, distal pulses are absent or decreased, and digital cyanosis can be present. Somatic dysfunction of the upper thoracic spine and ribs often contributes to the compression of the neurovascular structures in this syndrome.

Venous

The venous system of the cervical spine drains into the brachiocephalic veins via the internal and external jugular veins (Fig. 33.10). Disorders such as heart failure may cause visible jugular venous distension. The spinal venous system includes a valveless complex of venous plexi and veins that allow for retrograde flow and that form a continuous connection between the pelvis and the dural sinuses.

Lymphatics

The cervical region has many superficial and deep lymph nodes (Fig. 33.11). Superficial nodes penetrate the investing fascia to connect with the deeper channels that return lymph to the vascular compartment of the thorax. The thoracic inlet and thoracic ducts should be free of any restrictions before applying fascial or lymphatic techniques to the cervical region to improve lymphatic drainage. The glymphatic system of the cranium drains into the deep cervical lymph nodes.

VISCERA

The cervical region provides the passageway for multiple visceral organs between the head and the thoracic cavity, including the pharynx, larynx, trachea, esophagus, thyroid gland, and parathyroid glands. The cervical region also provides passage of vital neurologic, arterial, and venous structures. Dysfunction of these organs and structures can contribute to cervical spine dysfunction and should be addressed clinically.

STRUCTURAL EXAMINATION

As a quick recap of the screening examination, asymmetry and restriction of active range of motion of the region(s) may indicate that further evaluation is warranted with the regional portion of the structural exam which includes palpatory assessment and passive range of motion/quality of motion assessment.

During the palpatory evaluation of the paraspinal tissues, evidence of acute or chronic somatic dysfunction, viscerosomatic or somatovisceral reflexes, infectious processes, and even trauma may be found with the assessment of temperature changes (excessive warmth or coolness), tissue texture changes such as bogginess, thickness, ropiness, stringiness, firmness, and excessive moisture or dryness, patient tenderness to palpation and asymmetry on palpation. The suboccipital region contains muscles that are more lateral

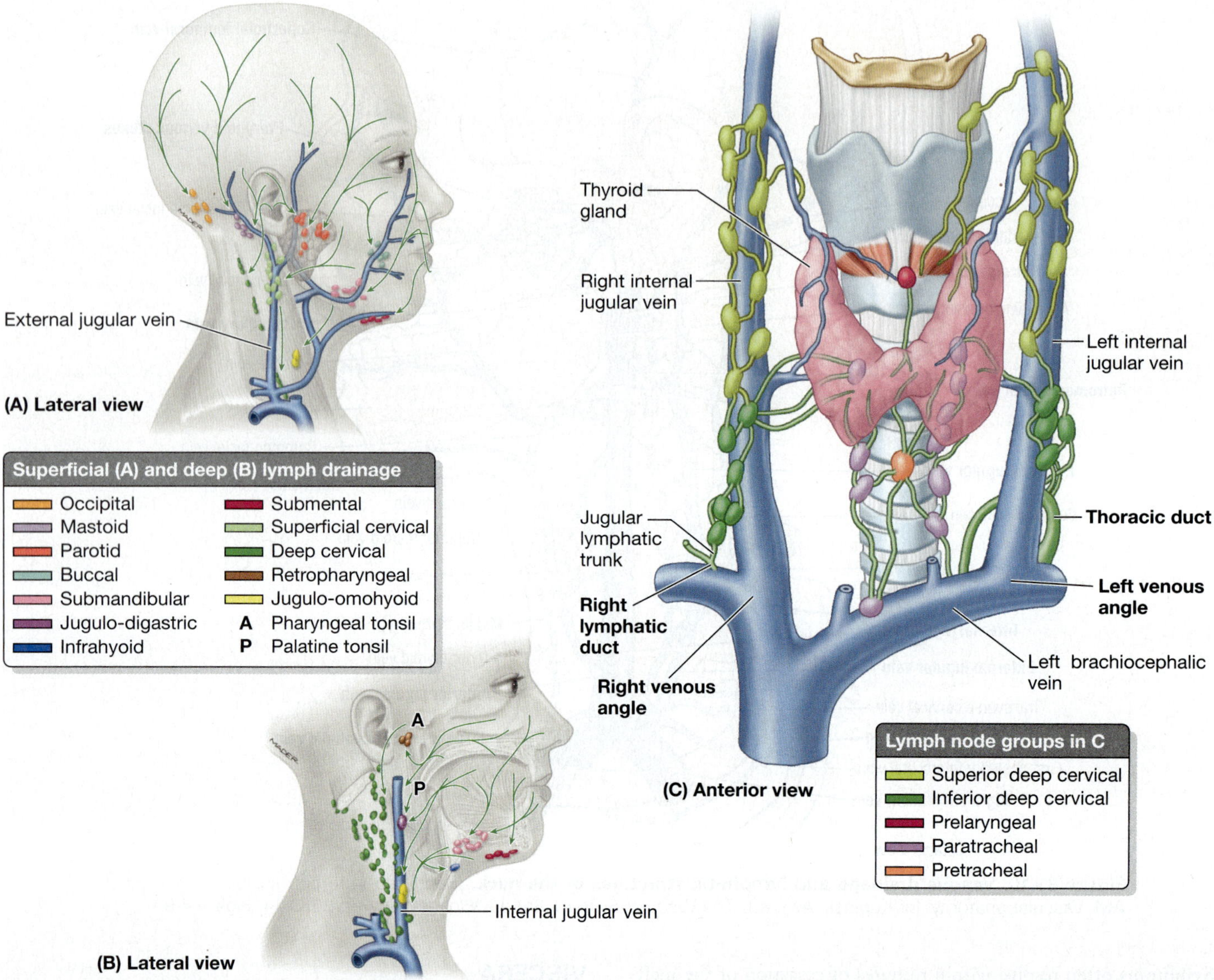

Figure 33.11. Lymphatic drainage of head and neck. A. Superficial lymphatic drainage. **B.** Deep lymphatic drainage. **C.** Lymph nodes, lymphatic trunks, and thoracic duct. (Reprinted with permission from Dalley AF II, Agur AMR. *Moore's Clinically Oriented Anatomy*. 9th ed. Wolters Kluwer; 2023. Figure 9.51.)

than the mid- and lower cervical region, so accurate paraspinal palpation involves more lateral finger placement.

Additionally, the hyoid may be palpated and assessed for any asymmetry, restricted range of motion, or tenderness by contacting the lateral greater horns and translating the hyoid left and right. The suprahyoid and infrahyoid musculature should also be palpated for muscle tension, asymmetry, and tissue texture abnormality.

The regional examination is continued with the evaluation of passive range of motion or quality of motion.

Abnormal findings here will lead the osteopathic physician to a further refinement of the differential diagnosis and provide indication for the segmental exam.

SEGMENTAL EXAMINATION COMPONENTS

Segmental Diagnosis

- Atypical cervical vertebral segments:
  - □ OA
  - □ AA
- Typical cervical vertebral segments
  - □ C2–C7

SEGMENTAL EXAMINATION

The experienced clinician tests those segments in which the screening and regional examinations suggest evidence of somatic dysfunction. Segmental examination of the cervical spine should be divided into two regions for diagnosis. The atypical cervical vertebral segments include the OA and AA joints. The typical cervical segments include the C2 through C7 segments.

Atypical Cervical Vertebral Segments

The suboccipital area is anatomically complex. C1 and C2 are considered a common neurologic segment and act as a functional vertebral unit.[37] Therefore, dysfunction of the suboccipital region potentially involves three joints: the OA, AA, and C2 vertebral segment. Positive palpatory findings in the suboccipital region require individual assessment of each of these three joints. Chronic

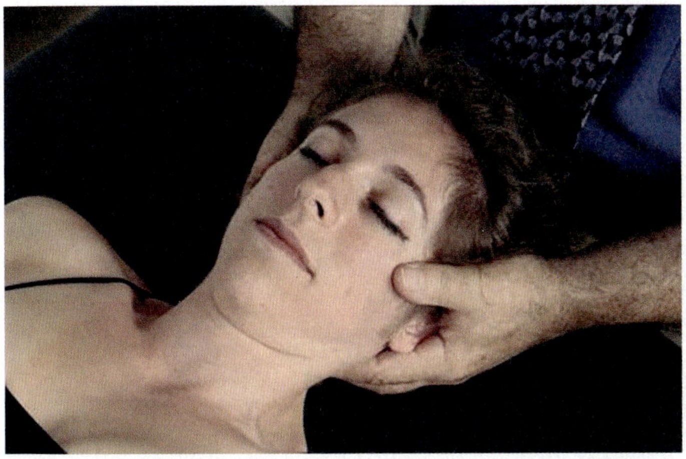

Figure 33.12. Initial positioning for assessment of the OA joint. (Photo courtesy of Western University of Health Sciences, Pomona, CA, with permission.)

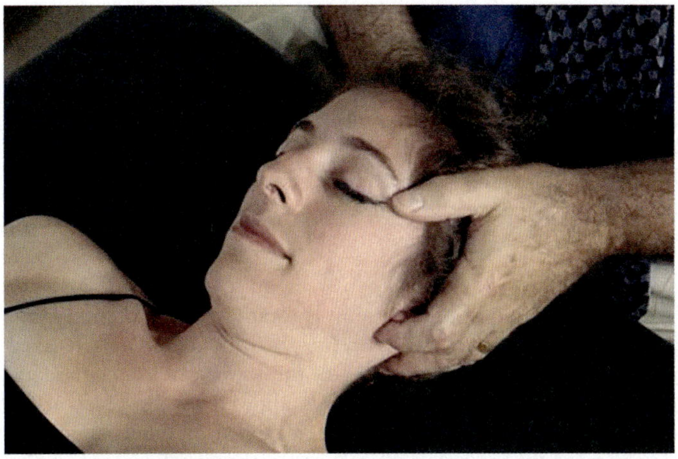

Figure 33.13. Assessment of the OA joint in flexion. (Photo courtesy of Western University of Health Sciences, Pomona, CA, with permission.)

dysfunction or dysfunction refractory to appropriate manipulative treatment in this region can be indicative of a cranial etiology.

Occipitoatlantal Joint (OA or C0–C1)

The major motions at the OA joint are flexion and extension.[38] The OA provides the majority of flexion and extension of the upper cervical complex. There is approximately 20 to 25 degrees of sagittal motion induced at the OA. Side bending and rotation are considered minor motions and are coupled in opposite directions. This contralateral coupling is a function of the orientation of the occipital condyles and the articular surfaces on the atlas. The convex occipital condyles converge anteriorly and diverge posteriorly. The lateral portions of the concave articulations on the atlas are more cephalad than the medial portions. The bilateral condyles glide anteriorly in extension and posteriorly in flexion relative to the atlas. If one condyle glides anteriorly while the other glides posteriorly, the occiput rotates and sidebends in opposite directions relative to the atlas. Although considered a minor motion of the joint, this asymmetric gliding motion is involved in occipital joint restriction.

One method of diagnosing the OA joint is via lateral translation in which the physician performs the following:

1. The physician sits or stands at the head of the table.
2. The patient lies supine.
3. The physician grasps the base of the patient's head with both hands oftentimes placing the finger pads of the index and middle fingers over the occipital articulation (Fig. 33.12).
4. Assess the OA joint first in the neutral position, then in the flexed and extended positions by doing the following:
   a. In the neutral position, perform left side bending at the OA joint by translating the base of the skull to the right, and then right side bending by translating the base of the skull to the left. Evaluate for range and quality of motion and a sense of freedom and restriction during the translatory maneuvers. Determine if the translatory motion is easier when moving from left to right or from right to left.
   b. Glide the occipital condyles posteriorly on C1 to provide slight flexion of the OA joint and repeat the same translatory motion (Fig. 33.13). Perform the same lateral translatory assessment with the head in slight extension by gliding the occipital condyles anteriorly on the atlas (Fig. 33.14). Ensure that all motion testing is localized to the OA joint region.

Interpretation: If the lateral translation is easier (has more freedom) going from left to right, the occiput is sidebent left. If the motion is easier (has more freedom) going from right to left, the occiput is sidebent right. One can infer that the occiput is rotated to the side opposite the side bending due to the biomechanics of the OA joint.

For example, with greater ease of motion noted in:

- Extension and right side bending, the diagnosis is ESRRL. The physician would state that the OA joint is extended, sidebent right, and rotated left. In this example, the right occipital condyle prefers to glide anteriorly on the atlas with restriction in posterior glide. The left occipital condyle exhibits freedom of motion in anterior and posterior glide. This same diagnosis is sometimes referred to as a right anterior occipital condyle.
- Neutral (more restriction in both flexion and extension) and left side bending, the diagnosis is NSLRR. The physician would state that the OA joint is neutral, sidebent left, and rotated right.
- Flexion and left side bending, the diagnosis is FSLRR. The physician would state that the OA joint is flexed, sidebent left, and rotated right. In this example, the left occipital condyle prefers to glide posteriorly on the atlas with restriction in anterior glide. The right occipital condyle exhibits freedom of motion in

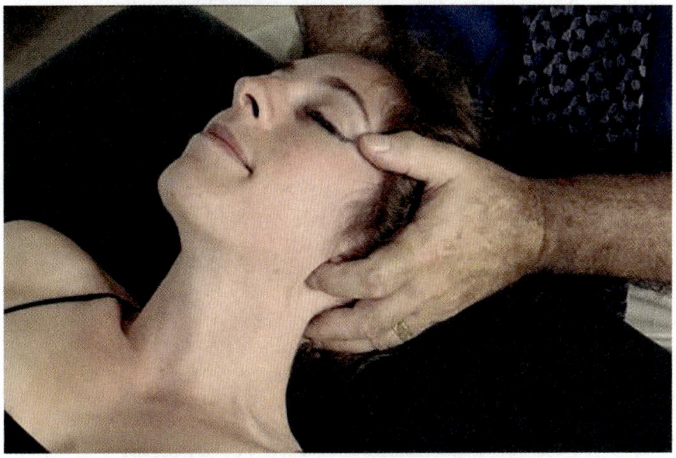

Figure 33.14. Assessment of the OA joint in extension. (Photo courtesy of Western University of Health Sciences, Pomona, CA, with permission.)

anterior and posterior glide. This same diagnosis is sometimes referred to as a left posterior occipital condyle.

As seen in the examples above, some osteopathic physicians describe an anterior or posterior occiput, or an extended or flexed condyle, to describe the dysfunction found at the OA. Discussion of these dysfunctions is beyond the scope of this chapter but can be diagnosed and treated clinically.

Altantoaxial Joint (C1–C2)

The major motion of the AA joint is rotation.[39] AA rotation averages 45 to 50 degrees, which represents about half of the axial rotation in the cervical region, with the lower cervical spine contributing the remainder. Rotation is allowed by the pivot articulation between the odontoid process (dens) of the axis and the ring formed by the anterior arch and transverse ligament of the atlas. Side bending is not a significant component of AA motion as the atlas moves inferiorly bilaterally during rotation, maintaining a horizontal orientation. Flexion and extension at the AA are limited by the tectorial membrane's connection between the cranial base and the dens. However, there is a small degree of sagittal motion of the anterior arch of the atlas on the odontoid process of the axis.

To perform the diagnostic segmental test of the AA joint, the physician performs the following[40]:

1. The physician stands at the head of the table.
2. The patient lies supine.
3. The physician flexes the patient's head **markedly** to provide physiologic locking of C2–C7, thereby reducing rotation from the lower vertebrae (Fig. 33.15). (This will provide a more localized and accurate diagnosis of the atlas in relation to the axis.)
4. The physician passively rotate patient's head to the motion barrier on each side maintaining the flexion throughout the procedure.
5. The physician compares the quantity and quality of the rotational motion to the right (Fig. 33.16) and to the left (Fig. 33.17).

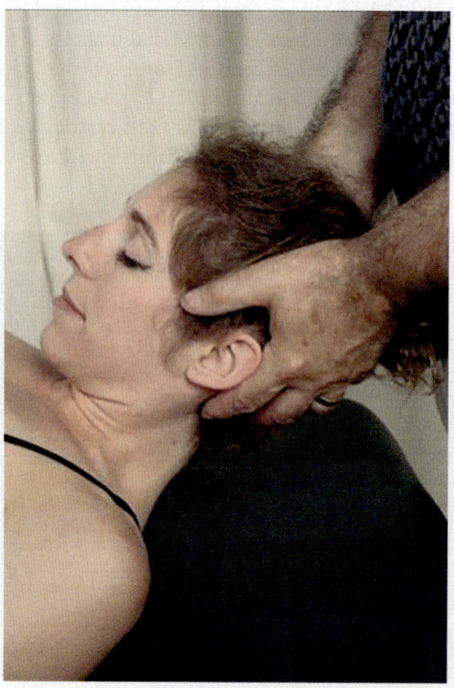

Figure 33.15. Initial positioning for assessment of the AA joint. (Photo courtesy of Western University of Health Sciences, Pomona, CA, with permission.)

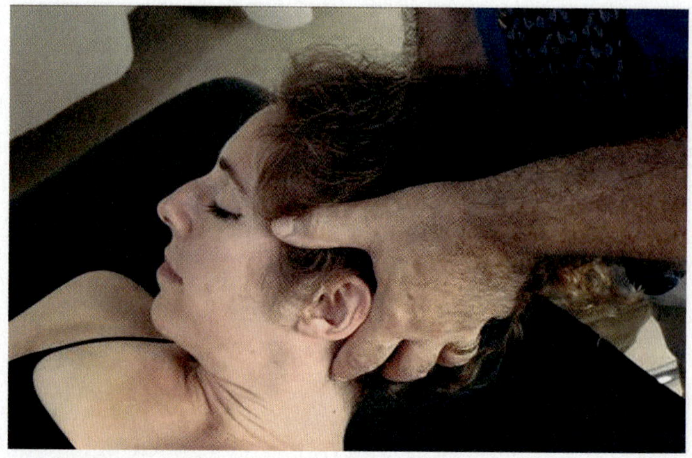

Figure 33.16. Assessment of the AA joint, rotation to the right. (Photo courtesy of Western University of Health Sciences, Pomona, CA, with permission.)

The physician may find that the AA rotates smoothly and within normal range to each side or that it rotates more easily in one direction than the other. The side to which the AA rotates more easily is the side to which it is rotated and is described as rotated left or rotated right (e.g., AA RL or RR).

Typical Cervical Vertebral Joints (C2–C7)

Motion of the typical cervical segments (C2 through C7) involves sagittal flexion or extension with coupled rotation and side bending to the same side due to the orientation of the cervical facet joints and the uncovertebral joints on the vertebral bodies.[8]

The diagnostic motion testing of the typical cervical vertebral segments involves testing lateral translation and rotation while inducing sagittal flexion or extension.

To diagnose the typical cervicals using lateral translation, the physician stands or sits at the head of the supine patient[41]:

1. The physician supports the patient's head with their hands while palpating the lateral aspect of the articular pillars of each vertebral segment. The physician provides localized side bending by inducing lateral translation from right to left and from left to right to each individual segment in the neutral position

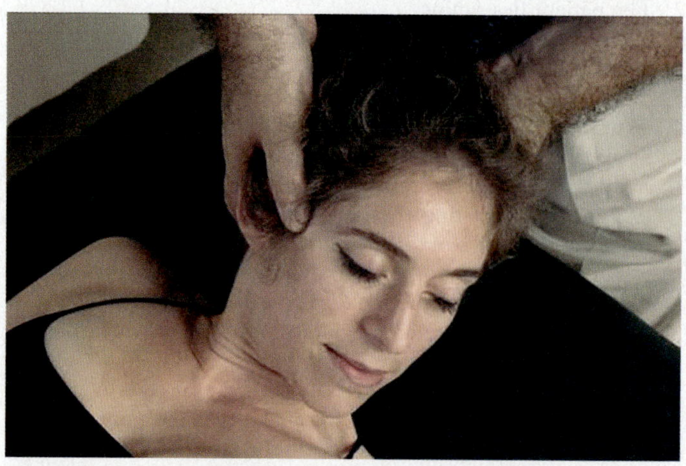

Figure 33.17. Assessment of the AA joint, rotation to the left. (Photo courtesy of Western University of Health Sciences, Pomona, CA, with permission.)

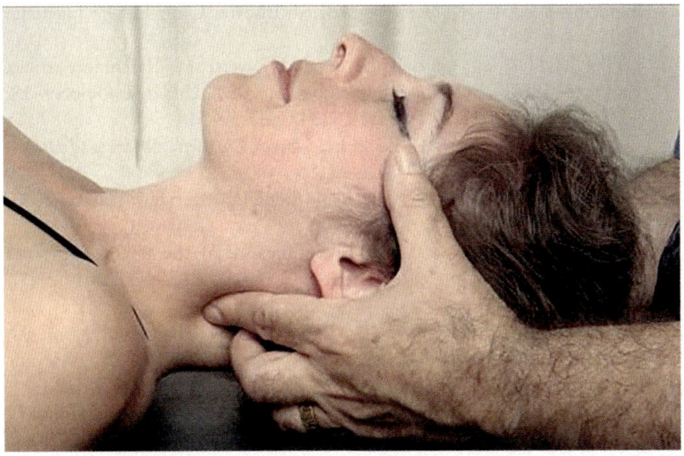

Figure 33.18. Assessment of a typical cervical vertebra in neutral. (Photo courtesy of Western University of Health Sciences, Pomona, CA, with permission.)

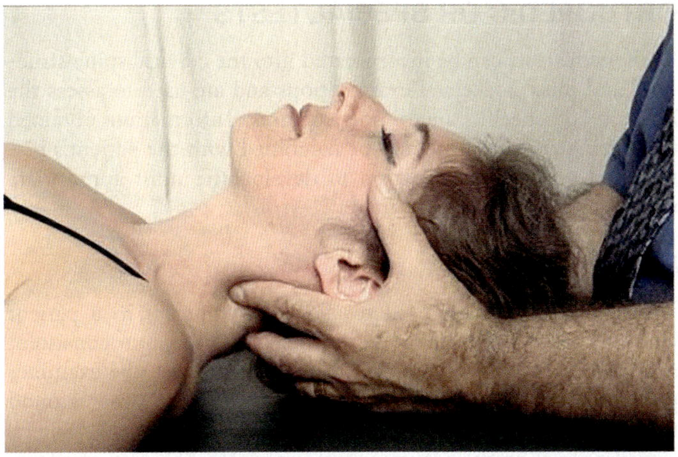

Figure 33.20. Translation of a typical cervical vertebra in extension. (Photo courtesy of Western University of Health Sciences, Pomona, CA, with permission.)

to identify any TART changes including restriction and freedom of motion (Fig. 33.18).

2. The physician then tests each restricted segment found in neutral in the flexed and extended positions by:
   a. Inducing localized side bending to the segment by testing right and left lateral translation with the segment flexed to that level (Fig. 33.19). This is repeated with the segment extended to the level in question (Fig. 33.20). For example, if the segment in question is C4, flexion and extension should be produced until they are palpated at the C4–C5 joint space before assessing the translation of the segment.

The physician may infer the rotational component using the knowledge of the specific anatomy of the cervical facet and uncovertebral joints, and the understanding that the typical cervical vertebrae will sidebend and rotate to the same side in neutral, flexion, or extension.

The segmental diagnosis is recorded using the position of ease format. Somatic dysfunction would be recorded as C7 FRLSL, C7 ERLSL, C7 FRRSR, or C7 ERRSR. For example, if C7 has ease of translation from right to left but is restricted in translation from left to right and these findings become more pronounced in flexion but improve (less resistance with translation from left to right) with extension, the physician would state that C7 is extended, rotated right, and sidebent right and this somatic dysfunction would be written as C7 ERRSR.

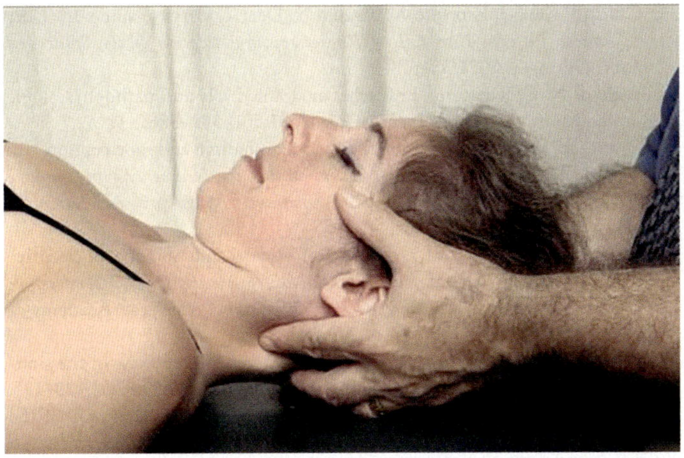

Figure 33.19. Translation of a typical cervical vertebra in flexion. (Photo courtesy of Western University of Health Sciences, Pomona, CA, with permission.)

Additionally, a segmental diagnosis may be obtained of the typical cervical spine by utilizing rotation instead of lateral translation. This is accomplished with the physician standing or sitting at the head of the table, contacting the posterior aspect of the articular pillars and inducing segmental rotation by lifting the articular pillar anteriorly on the right to rotate the segment to the left, then lifting the articular pillar anteriorly on the left to rotate the segment to the right of the supine patient. The physician should localize the force to one segment and follow the plane of the facets with the segment flexed and then extended. To follow the plane of the facets, the physician's force is directed superiorly at an angle toward the patient's eye, rather than in a horizontal plane. Restriction of right rotation in the extended position with freedom of right rotation in flexion, and freedom of left rotation in both flexion and extension suggests the typical cervical segment is flexed, rotated left, sidebent left.

It is generally easier to feel the side bending or translatory ease and/or restriction than the rotational component but both methods have been included here for sake of completeness.

Additional Segmental Evaluation

Additional components of the HEENT exam can be performed as clinically warranted.

In addition to the joint motion restrictions described above, the physician should also evaluate for the presence of other possible somatic dysfunction manifestations such as myofascial restrictions and counterstrain tender point.

CONCLUSION

Appropriate diagnosis and treatment of the cervical spine requires a thorough understanding of the functional anatomy of the cervical region. Rational treatment of the cervical region requires accurate diagnoses and sound clinical reasoning. Osteopathic manipulative medicine should be integrated throughout the treatment plan of patients with a variety of conditions including, but certainly not limited to neck pain, cervicogenic headache, TOS, cervical radiculopathy, torticollis, swallowing or speech difficulties, and other HEENT conditions. Due to the cervical region's anatomic connections, improving motion and tissue restrictions of the cervical region will influence other regions of the body, particularly the cranium, upper extremity, upper thorax, and ribcage.

ORTHOPEDIC OR SPECIAL TESTS

Orthopedic tests can be incorporated into the cervical spine structural and musculoskeletal examinations and are used to assess the integrity of specific anatomic structures. Information obtained from using these tests should be combined with the patient's history and physical examination to develop the most appropriate treatment plan for the patient.

Distraction Test

The distraction test is used to alleviate symptoms in a patient who presents with a history and physical examination consistent with radicular pain. To perform the distraction test, the examiner places one hand under the patient's chin and the other around the occiput. Axial traction is then applied to the cervical spine by slowly distracting the patient's head superiorly. This test is considered positive if pain is decreased or relieved when the head is tractioned, indicating the pressure on nerve roots has been relieved.[14]

Spurling Maneuver (Foraminal Compression Test)

Spurling Maneuver is utilized to test for nerve root compression or irritation. This maneuver is designed to provoke the patient's symptoms. The test is performed in three stages, each of which is more provocative. If symptoms are produced, the test is considered positive, and the physician does not proceed to the next stage. The first stage involves axial compression with the head in neutral. The second stage places the head in extension and then adds axial compression. The third stage places the head sidebent away from the affected side and then toward the affected side and adds axial compression. Dermatomal pain down the arm in the distribution of the compressed or irritated nerve root is considered a positive test. While sensitivity of the Spurling test is variable, the specificity is greater than 90%, thus it is clinically useful in confirming the absence of cervical radiculopathy when negative.[14]

Static Vertebral Artery Test (VAT)

The static VAT has been used to rule out vertebral artery insufficiency prior to manipulative procedures that can place the vertebral artery under stretch, such as cervical HVLA. Coupled extension and rotation have been found to be the position most likely to occlude the vertebral artery.[14] To perform the static VAT, place the supine patient's head in full neck and head extension, ipsilateral rotation, and side bending. An alternative positioning is to simulate the mobilization or manipulation position. Hold this position for at least 10 to 30 seconds unless the patient starts to exhibit symptoms of vertebral artery insufficiency. Signs and symptoms of vertebral artery insufficiency can be remembered by the mnemonic "5D's And 3N's."[35] If signs or symptoms are induced this is a positive test, cervical manipulations should be discontinued and further workup of the integrity of the vertebral artery should be obtained.

REFERENCES

1. GBD 2021 Neck Pain Collaborators. Global, regional, and national burden of neck pain, 1990–2020, and projections to 2050: a systematic analysis of the Global Burden of Disease Study 2021. *Lancet Rheumatol.* 2024;6(3):e142–e155.
2. Kazeminasab S, Nejadghaderi SA, Amiri P, et al. Neck pain: global epidemiology, trends and risk factors. *BMC Musculoskelet Discord.* 2022; 23(1):26.
3. Dalley AF, Agur AMR, Moore KL. *Moore's Clinically Oriented Anatomy.* 9th ed. Table 9.1. Wolters Kluwer; 2023.
4. Sandring S, ed. *Gray's Anatomy.* 39th ed. Elsevier Churchill-Livingstone; 2005.
5. Luijkx T, Hacking C, Bell D, et al. C7 vertebra. Reference article, Radiopaedia.org. Published September 6, 2014. Updated October 18, 2022. Accessed April 29, 2024. 10.53347/rID-30851
6. Dalley AF II, Agur AMR. Back. In: *Moore's Clinically Oriented Anatomy.* 9th ed. Wolters Kluwer; 2023.
7. Auvenshine RC, Pettit NJ. The hyoid bone: an overview. *Cranio.* 2020; 38(1):6–14.
8. Hartman J. Anatomy and clinical significance of the uncinate process and uncovertebral joint: a comprehensive review. *Clin Anat.* 2014;27(3): 431–440.
9. Raveendranath V, Kavitha T, Umamageswari A. Morphometry of the uncinate process, vertebral body, and lamina of the C3–7 vertebrae relevant to cervical spine surgery. *Neurospine.* 2019;16(4):748–755.
10. Edney G, Awal W, Plant L, et al. Vertebral levels (anatomical landmarks). Reference article, Radiopaedia.org. Published January 4, 2018. Updated October 14, 2023. Accessed April 29, 2024. 10.53347/rID-57629
11. Spencer T, Hacking C, Yu Y, et al. Thyroid cartilage. Reference article, Radiopaedia.org. Published April 21, 2016. Updated February 21, 2024. Accessed April 29, 2024. 10.53347/rID-44430
12. Siribumrungwong K, Sinchai C, Tangtrakulwanich B, Chaiyamongkol W. Reliability and accuracy of palpable anterior neck landmarks for the identification of cervical spinal levels. *Asian Spine J.* 2018;12(1):80–84.
13. Bilkey W. Manual medicine approach to the cervical spine and whiplash injury. *Phys Med Rehabil Clin North Am.* 1996;7:749–759.
14. Magee D, Manske R. *Orthopedic Physical Assessment.* 7th ed. Elsevier; 2021.
15. Wu LP, Huang YQ, Zhou WH, et al. Influence of cervical spine position, turning time, and cervical segment on cadaver intradiscal pressure during cervical spinal manipulative therapy. *J Manipulative Physiol Ther.* 2012; 35(6):428–436.
16. Ansaripour H, Ferguson SJ, Flohr M. In vitro biomechanics of the cervical spine: a systematic review. *J Biomech Eng.* 2022;144(10):100801.
17. Shin JJ, Kim KR, Shin J, et al. Surgical versus conservative management for treating unstable atlas fractures: a multicenter study. *Neurospine.* 2022;19(4):1013–1025.
18. Yee J, Mellam Y, Hacking C, et al. Erector spinae group. Reference article, Radiopaedia.org. Published May 20, 2016. Updated March 6, 2023. Accessed April 29, 2024. 10.53347/rID-45291
19. Ocran E. Deep back muscles. Kenhub.com. Updated October 30, 2023. Accessed April 30, 2024. https://www.kenhub.com/en/library/anatomy/intrinsic-back-muscles
20. Enix D, Scali F, Pontell M. The cervical myodural bridge, a review of literature and clinical implications. *J Can Chiropr Assoc.* 2014;58(2):184–192.
21. Zheng N, Chung B, Li YL, et al. The myodural bridge complex defined as a new functional structure. *Surg Radiol Anat.* 2020;42:143–153.
22. Kitamura K, Cho KH, Yamamoto M, et al. Suboccipital myodural bridges revisited: application to cervicogenic headaches. *Clin Anat.* 2019; 32(7):914–928.
23. Ghosh P, Shah J, Esposito M, Azeem N, Deer T. Cervical spine. In: Deer T, Azeem N, eds. *Essentials of Radiofrequency Ablation of the Spine and Joints.* Springer; 2021:55–67.
24. Bogduk N. Cervicogenic headache: anatomic basis and pathophysiologic mechanisms. *Curr Pain Headache Rep.* 2001;5(4):382–386.
25. Payan D. Peripheral neuropeptides, inflammation and nociception. In: Willard F, Patterson M, eds. *Nociception and the Neuroendocrine-Immune Connection, 1992 International Symposium.* American Academy of Osteopathy; 1992:3446.
26. deGroat W. Spinal cord processing of visceral and somatic nociceptive input. In: Willard F, Patterson M, eds. *Nociception and the Neuroendocrine-Immune Connection, 1992 International Symposium.* American Academy of Osteopathy; 1992:4773.
27. Shayota B, Wong T, Fru D, David G. A comprehensive review of the sinuvertebral nerve with clinical applications. *Anat Cell Bio.* 2019;52(2):128–133.
28. Berthoud HR, Neuhuber WL. Functional and chemical anatomy of the afferent vagal system. *Auton Neurosci.* 2000;85(1–3):1–17.
29. Freitas CAF, Santos LRMD, Santos AN, Amaral Neto ABD, Brandão LG. Anatomical study of jugular foramen in the neck. *Braz J Otorhinolaryngol.* 2020;86(1):44–48.

30. Erman AB, Kejner AE, Hogikyan ND, Feldman EL. Disorders of cranial nerves IX and X. *Semin Neurol.* 2009;29(1):85–92.
31. Yuan H, Silberstein SD. Vagus nerve and vagus nerve stimulation, a comprehensive review: part II. *Headache.* 2016;56(2):259–266.
32. Hammer N, Glätzner J, Feja C, et al. Human vagus nerve branching in the cervical region. *PLoS One.* 2015;10(2):e0118006.
33. Ter Horst GJ, Hautvast RW, De Jongste MJ, Korf J. Neuroanatomy of cardiac activity-regulating circuitry: a transneuronal retrograde viral labelling study in the rat. *Eur J Neurosci.* 1996;8(10):2029–2041.
34. Wiley RG, Oeltmann TN. Anatomically selective peripheral nerve ablation using intraneural ricin injection. *J Neurosci Methods.* 1986;17(1):43–53.
35. Dutton M. *Dutton's Orthopaedic Examination, Evaluation, and Intervention.* 6th ed. McGraw Hill; 2023.
36. Hixson K, Horris H, McLeod T, Bacon C. The diagnostic accuracy of clinical diagnostic tests for thoracic outlet syndrome. *J Sport Rehabil.* 2017;26(5):459–465.
37. Cisler T, ed. *Are We on the Path? The Collected Works of Robert C. Fulford, DO, FCA.* The Osteopathic Cranial Academy; 2003.
38. DeStefano LA. *Greenman's Principles of Manual Medicine.* 5th ed. Wolters Kluwer; 2017:53.
39. DeStefano LA. *Greenman's Principles of Manual Medicine.* 5th ed. Wolters Kluwer; 2017:54.
40. DeStefano LA. *Greenman's Principles of Manual Medicine.* 5th ed. Wolters Kluwer; 2017:188.
41. DeStefano LA. *Greenman's Principles of Manual Medicine.* 5th ed. Wolters Kluwer; 2017:185–187.

34 Thoracic Region

RAYMOND J. HRUBY ▪ REBECCA E. GIUSTI

KEY CONCEPTS

- Importance of the thoracic spinal region for normal function
- Descriptive and functional anatomy of the thoracic spine
- Clinical aspects of thoracic structures and functional interrelationships, including the costal cage
- The impact of somatic dysfunction in the thoracic region
- Diagnosis of somatic dysfunction in the thoracic region
- Performance of the segmental exam to the thoracic region

INTRODUCTION

Because the heart and lungs are contained in the thorax, this region's unique significance in life has long been recognized. The inability to draw breath or the perception of pain in the thorax often constitutes real or imagined life-threatening problems. Since much of the regulatory outflow of the sympathetic nervous system originates in the thoracic spinal cord, disturbances in the muscles and joints of the thoracic region may mimic life-threatening problems. Injury to thoracic vertebrae can also cause long-term sequelae for health and survival. The complexities of the thoracic region, and the vital importance of its organ systems, underscore the necessity for the osteopathic physician to understand its many functions, to be able to accurately diagnose this region, including evaluation for somatic dysfunction and apply potential treatment approaches.

DEFINITION

The thoracic region is bounded by the cervical region above, and by the lumbar region below. In diagnosis and treatment, it cannot be considered as separate from the other body regions, since such dysfunction is always interdependent.[1]

This section focuses on the thoracic vertebrae and its associated structures and functions. See Chapter 35 for information on the rib cage structures and functions.

DESCRIPTIVE AND FUNCTIONAL ANATOMY

Skeletal Structures

The thoracic spinal region includes 12 thoracic spinal vertebrae and their associated bony structures (Fig. 34.1).

Although the scapula overlies the posterior portion of the rib cage, it is connected to the sternum through the clavicle and is often involved in thoracic injuries and pain syndromes. Therefore, this structure is more properly considered a part of the upper extremity (see Chapter 39). This section will focus on the thoracic spine itself. For more detailed information on the rib cage region, see Chapter 35.

White and Panjabi[2] divide the thoracic spine into three anatomical regions:

1. Upper (T1–T4)
2. Middle (T4–T8)
3. Lower (T8–L1)

It is also helpful to divide the thoracic and upper lumbar spine into four functional divisions that roughly correspond to the thoracolumbar outflow of the sympathetic system:

1. T1–T4: Sympathetics to head and neck, with T1–T6 to the heart and lungs
2. T5–T9: All upper abdominal viscera: stomach, duodenum, liver, gallbladder, pancreas, and spleen
3. T10–T11: Remainder of the small intestines, kidneys, ureters, gonads, and right colon
4. T12–L2: Left colon and pelvic organs

This functional division is often very useful to the physician because visceral, afferent neurons tend to follow the same pathway as the sympathetic outflow. Visceral disturbances usually cause increased musculoskeletal tension in the somatic structures innervated from the corresponding spinal level, through the viscerosomatic reflexes (see Chapter 43). Manipulative treatment at that spinal level is used to reduce somatic afferent input from the associated facilitated segments, which in turn reduces somatosympathetic activity to the affected viscus.[3]

Generally, the thoracic spine has a mildly kyphotic, forward-bending curve that varies from person to person. In osteoporotic or older patients, the angle of this curve can become more acute. This causes biomechanical problems and necessitates compensatory adaptation in other regions of the spine, as well as in general posture. Individual thoracic vertebrae are parts of a continuum with the cervical and lumbar vertebrae. Size increases from cervical to lumbar to account for increased weight bearing. The spinous processes of the thoracic vertebrae are particularly large and easily palpated, pointing increasingly inferior from T1 through T9, and back to an almost anteroposterior orientation from T10 to T12.

Thoracic vertebral facet joints are plane-type synovial joints. The interarticular surfaces of these joints are smooth, shiny, and compact bone covered with hyaline cartilage. They are surrounded by a thin, loose articular capsule lined with synovial membrane. The facet joints guide and limit gross, segmental, and coupled movements.

- The superior facets of each thoracic vertebra are slightly convex and face posteriorly, somewhat superiorly, and laterally. Their angle of declination averages 60 degrees relative to the transverse plane, and 20 degrees relative to the coronal plane.
- This contrasts with the cervical and lumbar regions, where the superior facets face posteriorly, superiorly, and slightly medially.
- In the lower portion of the thoracic spine, the superior facet surface begins to face more posteriorly than laterally. At T12, it

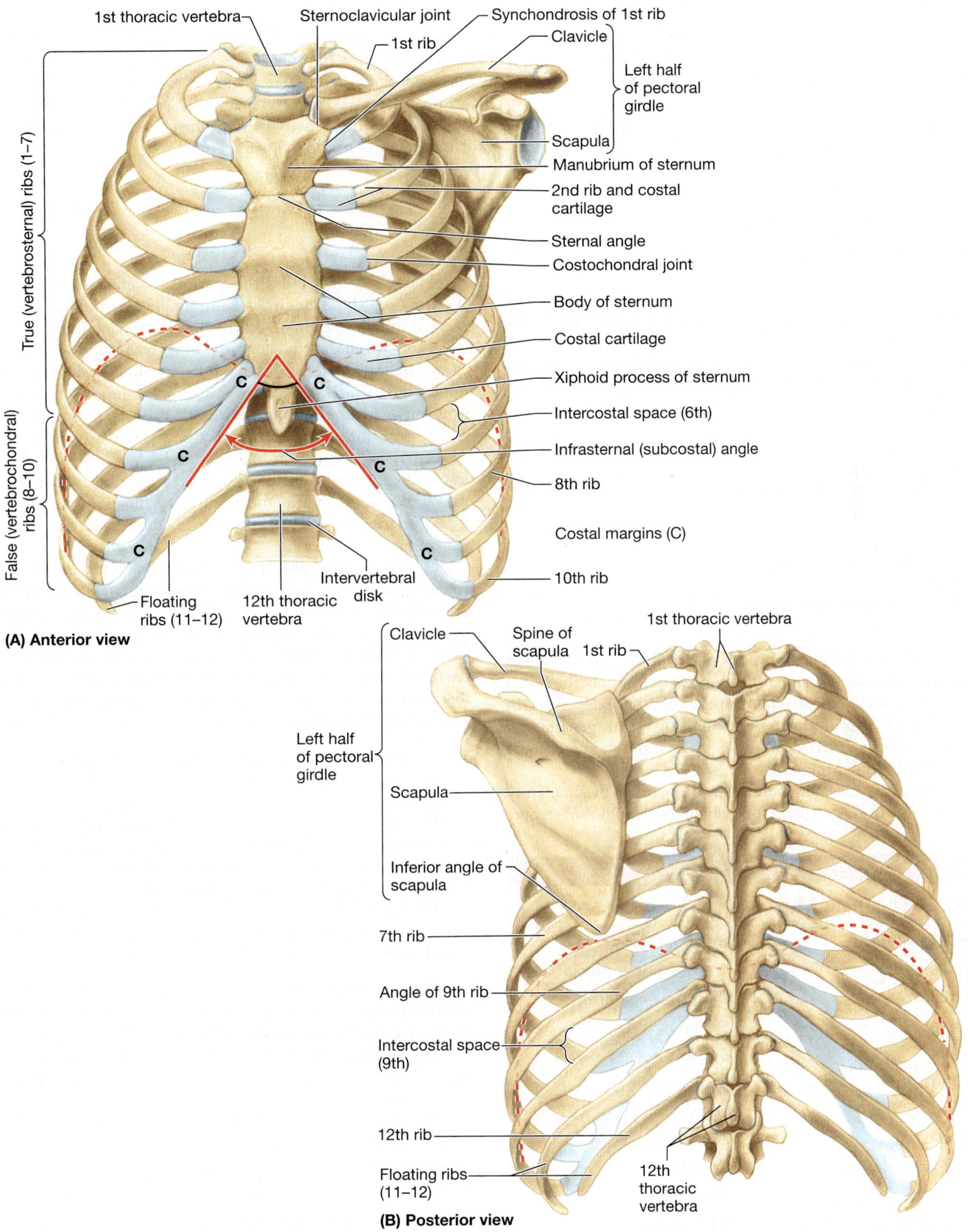

Figure 34.1. A and B. Thoracic skeleton. The osteocartilaginous thoracic cage includes the sternum, 12 pairs of ribs and costal cartilages, and 12 thoracic vertebrae and intervertebral disks. The clavicles and scapulae form the pectoral (shoulder) girdle, one side of which is included here to demonstrate the relationship between the thoracic (axial) and upper limb (appendicular) skeletons. The *red dotted lines* indicate the position of the diaphragm, which separates the thoracic and abdominal cavities.

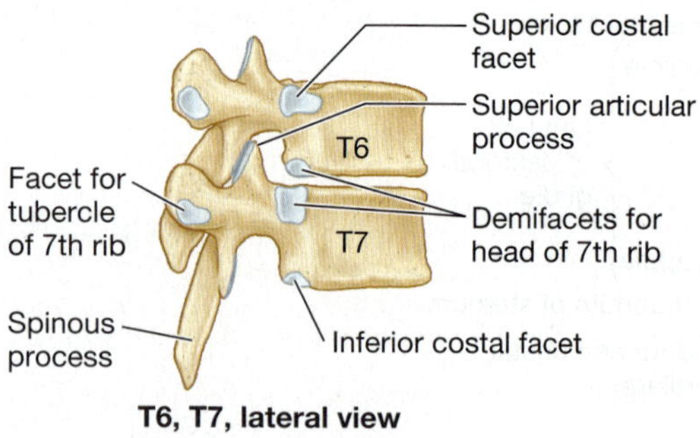

Figure 34.2. Thoracic vertebral anatomy.

may even face medially, as part of a functional transition to the lumbar spine.

- The inferior facet of each thoracic vertebra faces in the opposite direction from the superior and has a slightly concave surface (Fig. 34.2).

Musculature

The muscles of the thoracic spinal area are involved in the following:

1. Posture
2. Head and neck control
3. Locomotion
4. Stabilization of the extremities
5. Visceral function

Table 34.1 lists the major muscles of the thoracic area. Altered tone in these muscles can affect the function of not only the bones to which the muscles are attached but also of other body areas. In addition, increased or decreased tone may alter both general and microcirculation in a myriad of ways, such as through homeostatic regulation and cellular immunity.

As with all muscles, the thoracic muscles are fed by circulatory elements, in addition to physiologically active trophic substances delivered directly by nerves.[4] There is also evidence that the sympathetic nerve supply to striated and smooth muscles alters muscle tone and contractile forces. Therefore, attention to the palpatory cues associated with altered muscle tone implies the presence of many differential diagnostic factors discussed throughout this text.

Much of the activity of the thoracic cage is controlled by the larger muscles of the following:

- Head
- Neck
- Shoulder girdle
- Thorax

These help to stabilize the cervical and cranial areas, as well as the arms and shoulder girdle. For example, the splenius capitis and cervicis muscles originate on the lower cranial and upper cervical areas and attach distally along the middle thoracic spine. In some cases, this can be as low as T6–T8. Vertebral dysfunction in the upper thoracic areas can affect the action of these muscles, causing problems with motion outside the thoracic area in the head and neck. More inferiorly, the internal and external oblique muscles are generally viewed as trunk rotators, but they also attach to the lower ribs along with the diaphragm. Altered tone in these muscles can alter diaphragmatic and respiratory function and vice versa. These relationships are readily identified by those experienced in palpations.

Of special note with respect to this chapter are the erector spinae groups (Fig. 34.3), which extend and sidebend the vertebral column, and allow for smooth flexion by gradually decreasing resistance to forward bending. The erector spinae group consisting of the spinalis (most medial), longissimus, and iliocostalis (most lateral) all arise from a broad tendon from the posterior part of the iliac crest, posterior aspect of the sacrum, sacroiliac ligaments, sacral and inferior lumbar spinous processes and supraspinous ligament.

- The spinalis fibers (thoracic, cervicis, capitis) course superiorly and attach to the spinous processes of the upper thoracic region and the cranium.
- The longissimus fibers (thoracis, cervicis, capitis) run superiorly to attach to the ribs between the tubercles and angles, to the transverse processes of the thoracic and cervical regions and to the mastoid process of the temporal bone.
- The iliocostalis fibers (lumborum, thoracis, cervicis) course superiorly to the angles of the lower ribs and cervical transverse processes.

Osteopathic physicians can access the transverse processes of the thoracic segments for diagnostic and therapeutic purposes via the fascial cleft between the longissimus and iliocostalis muscles.[5,6]

These muscles are often involved in group or multiple movement dysfunction and are vulnerable to insult with unplanned movements or trauma.

The deep layer of the intrinsic back muscles of the thoracic region includes the transversospinales, semispinalis, mutifidus, and rotatores. They are more involved in the maintenance of a single vertebral unit somatic dysfunction or Type II somatic dysfunctions.[5]

- The transversospinales attach to the transverse processes and the spinous process of the superior vertebrae and provide extension.[5]
- The semispinalis fibers (thoracis, cervicis, capitis) arise from the transverse processes of C4–T12, course superomedially to span 4–6 segments before inserting on the occipital bone and spinous processes of the thoracic and cervical regions. They extend the head and thoracic regions of the vertebral column and rotate them contralaterally.[5]

TABLE 34.1

Regional Thoracic Muscles

Pectoralis Major	Subcostals
Pectoralis minor	Transversus thoracis
Teres major	Levatores costarum
Teres minor	Splenius
Trapezius	Spinalis
Latissimus dorsi	Semispinalis
Levator scapulae	Longissimus
Rhomboid	Iliocostalis
Quadratus lumborum	Rotatores
Serratus anterior	Multifidus
Serratus posterior (superior/ inferior)	Interspinales
Intercostals	Intertransversarii
External intercostals	Diaphragm
Internal intercostals	Obliquus capitis inferior
Innermost intercostals	Subclavius

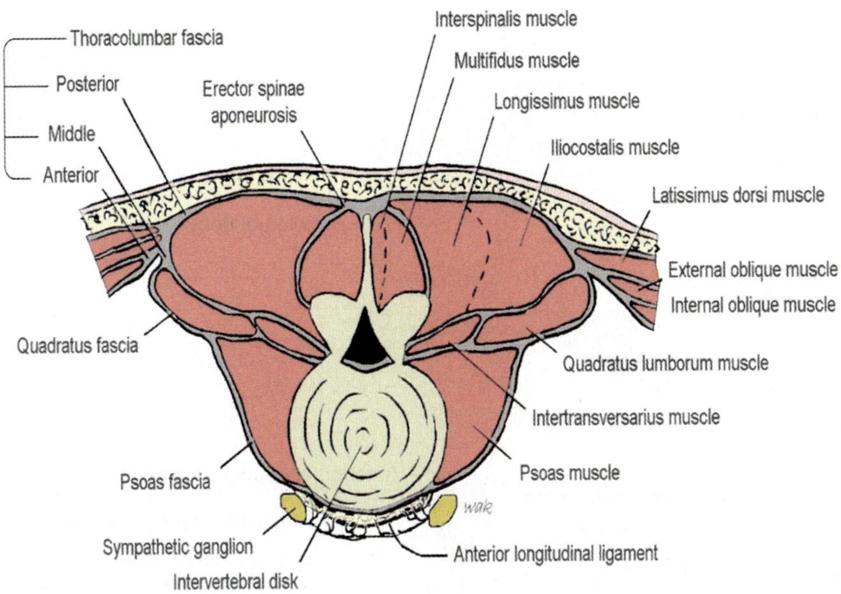

Figure 34.3. Erector spinae muscle and surrounding structures.

- The multifidus are most developed in the lumbar region. They arise from the posterior sacrum, posterior superior iliac spine, aponeurosis of the erector spinae, sacroiliac ligaments, mammillary processes of the lumbar vertebrae, transverse processes of T1–T3 and the articular processes of C4–C7 and course superomedially to insert on the spinous processes 2–4 segments superior to the origin.[5]
- The rotatores brevis and longus are best developed in the thoracic region. They arise from the transverse processes of the vertebrae. The rotatores brevis attach to the lamina and transverse process or spinous process of the vertebra one level superior while the longus usually inserts two levels superior to the origin. They stabilize the vertebrae and assist with local extension and rotation, as well as likely act as proprioceptors.[5]

Muscles are also described as polyarticular or monoarticular. Because the monoarticular rotatores are positioned at an oblique angle from origin to insertion, they have a strong vertical component to their contraction, making them extenders as well as rotators.[7]

These small muscles are richly innervated with muscle spindles, which provide proprioception. In fact, one of their primary tasks is to signal position and speed of motion of the vertebral column. (This task makes them important in the maintenance of posture and in directing movement.) The deep back muscles are also very vulnerable to sudden stretch and unplanned movement, which appears to alter the sensory input to the spinal cord and brain, with the resultant development of altered motion and pain typical of vertebral somatic dysfunction.[8–10]

The minor deep layer of muscles includes the interspinales and intertransversarii which are both more developed in the cervical and lumbar regions. However, the levatores costarum insert on the rib between the tubercle and angle and attach to the tips of the transverse processes of C7 and T1–T11 vertebrae. They function in respiration by elevating ribs and assist with lateral flexion of the spine.[5]

Supportive Tissues

Connective tissue unites and surrounds all other tissues. It is found:

- Between the cells of organs
- As tendons of muscles
- As ligaments joining skeletal parts

Of special importance to the osteopathic physician are the fasciae of the body. These connective tissues surround virtually all organs, muscles, and vessels.[2,11] The fascial elements, the pericardium and pleura even surround the heart and lungs, respectively. Fascia is a fibrous tissue that is effectively wound around the invested organs at various angles.

Trauma, chemical alterations of the bathing fluids (immune changes), and other pathologic agents alter the angles of the fascial bands and change cross-linkages between the bands, causing altered tensions of the fasciae throughout the body. An increase in tension in the fascial sheets leads to the following:

- Altered interstitial fluid (lymph) flows
- Decreased blood flow
- Decreased efficiency of organ function

Normalization of the fascial tensions returns the body to more efficient function, and thereby the body expends less energy. Osteopathic manipulative techniques, including direct and indirect myofascial release, help restore this normal physiologic state. The thoracic fasciae are often involved in dysfunction due to thoracic trauma.

The thoracic vertebrae are separated by disks, as are the cervical and lumbar vertebrae.[2] The disks act as shock absorbers and permit flexibility between the vertebrae. Each disk is composed of an outer annulus fibrosus and an inner nucleus pulposus.

- The inner nucleus pulposus resembles a gel at the center of the disk and acts like a semifluid hydrophilic ball bearing that becomes less hydrated and broader under sustained compression.
- The annulus fibrosus is composed of concentric lamellae of fibrocartilage, running at right angles to the fibers of adjacent layers. Its structural arrangement is more vulnerable to tears posteriorly, where the lamellae are thinner and less numerous.

Ligaments of the thoracic region may be categorized as an intersegmental system which includes the anterior and posterior longitudinal ligaments, and the supraspinal ligaments and an intrasegmental system which includes the ligament flavum, the interspinous and intertransverse ligaments. Other ligaments of the region are involved in the costovertebral and costotransverse joints. The costovertebral ligaments include the intra-articular ligament of the head of the rib and the radiate ligament, which extends from the joint capsule and fans out from the anterior margin of the head

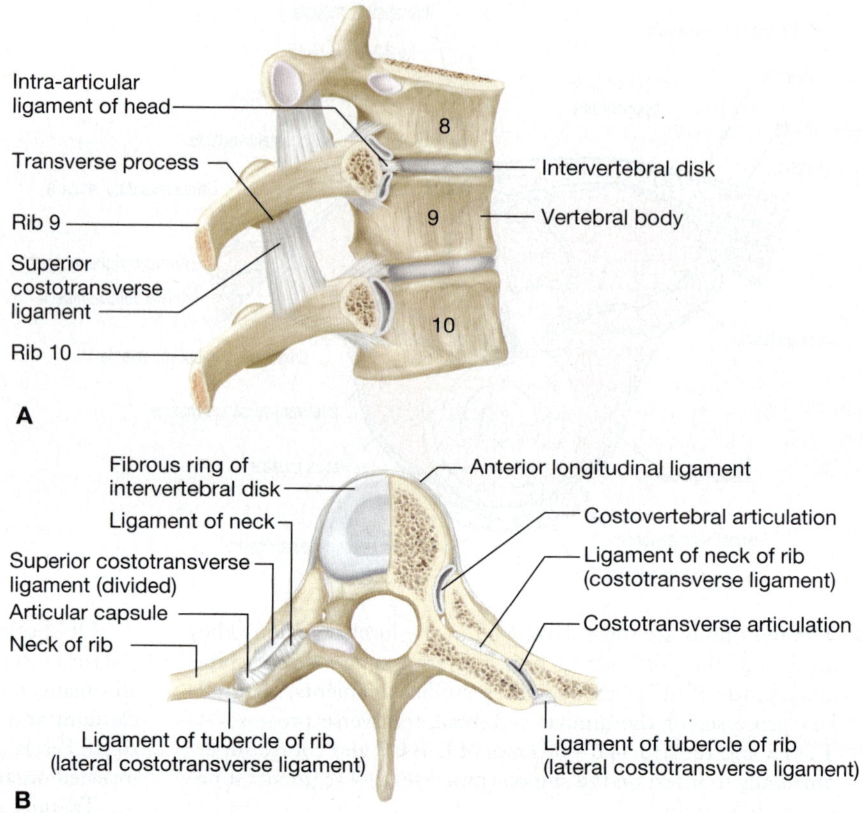

Figure 34.4. Ligaments of the vertebral column. **A.** Lateral view. **B.** Superior view.

of the rib to the sides of the bodies of the two vertebrae and the disk between them.[5] The costotransverse joints are reinforced in strength and limited in motion by a costotransverse ligament which runs from the neck of the rib to the transverse process, a lateral costotransverse ligament, and a superior costotransverse ligament.[5]

The restricted motion of the thoracic spine due to the attachments of the rib cage and the fairly broad posterior longitudinal ligament make ruptured thoracic disks relatively uncommon. On the other hand, diskopathy from trauma, aging, and degenerative disease is relatively common in the thoracic area (Fig. 34.4).

Neural Structures

The neural connections of the thoracic area are of vital importance to all body functions. In the thoracic region, not only do the usual connections to the musculoskeletal system exit the spinal cord but it is also where a large part of the sympathetic nervous system originates (Fig. 34.5).

Knowledge of the relationships between the thoracic nerves, as well as their relationships to the bony landmarks, is vital to understanding the associated neurologic problems in this region.

The spinal cord, which runs from the brainstem to about the level of L3, is a continuous structure with no segmentation. During embryologic development, the spinal nerve bundles are gathered into spinal nerve roots that course between the encircling bones, through the intervertebral foramina. This imposes what appears to be a dermatomal segmentation effect. However, the function of the spinal cord is not inherently segmented.[2]

The spinal nerves exit through the intervertebral foramina, which identifies their vertebral level. Each spinal nerve is numbered for the level at which it exits, except in the cervical region, as there are eight cervical nerve roots and seven cervical vertebra. Spinal nerve C1 exits above the atlas, and the eighth root exits below C7. All other roots exit below their corresponding vertebrae.[2,11]

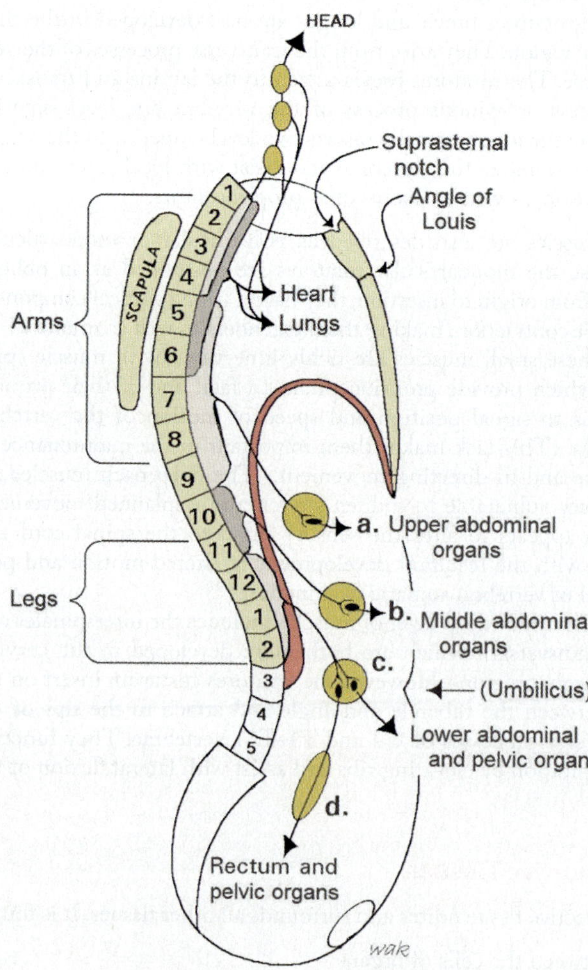

Figure 34.5. Sympathetic nervous system relationships in the thoracic and abdominal regions.

- Because the intervertebral foramen is a bounded space, and the nerve roots share that space with other tissues, the roots are especially vulnerable to pressure from herniated nucleus pulposus and even edema.
- Somatic dysfunction in a thoracic area may cause local edema and tissue tightening, which can exert pressure on the nerve root. Importantly, it can alter blood and fluid flows to and from the nerve sheaths.
- Such pressure may alter neural conductivity in the affected roots. The lack of proper blood and fluid flow to the sheaths can irritate the nociceptors of the sheath, causing pain along the nerve distribution.[12]

Local disturbances may often be relieved with proper manipulative treatment designed to restore motion and fluid flow to the region. As stated previously, radiculopathy is somewhat rare in the thoracic region, even though diskopathy is less rare. These problems in the thoracic area are not easy to diagnose due to overlapping dermatome, and the lack of readily testable deep tendon reflexes.

The abdominal diaphragm receives its motor innervation through the phrenic nerves coming from C3–C5.

Perhaps more importantly, sensory nerves of the diaphragm innervate the following:

- Mediastinal pleura
- Fibrous pericardium
- Parietal layer of the serous pericardium[2]

This relationship helps explain the common palpatory findings of cervical tension and somatic dysfunction associated with pericardial or diaphragmatic irritation, mediated via the viscerosomatic reflexes (see Chapter 43). Manipulative treatment of the involved cervical segments is designed to ameliorate thoracic and diaphragmatic dysfunction through somatovisceral reflex pathways.

Parasympathetic innervation to the thoracic viscera and many of the abdominal viscera is via the vagus nerve (cranial nerve X).[2] Treatment of conditions related to the thoracic viscera must include assessment and treatment of cranial and cervical areas to normalize vagal function.

The majority of sympathetic system outflow originates in the thoracic region.[2] The distribution of the sympathetic system to almost every tissue and area of the body renders it a crucial system for all body functions (see Fig. 34.5). Evidence is also demonstrating that the sympathetic system is vital in regulating immune function.[13] Thus, its importance for all body functions suggests that disturbances within the thoracic vertebra, and their associated musculature that affect the function of the sympathetic system, can have widespread consequences. Identification and treatment of somatic dysfunction in the thoracic region is especially important in addressing conditions ranging from infectious processes to functional abnormalities.

Visceral Considerations

Visceral dysfunction that alters input to the spinal cord not only increases the sympathetic outflow back to the visceral areas through viscerovisceral reflex pathways but it also often alters somatic outflow in unexpected patterns. Understanding this phenomenon provides insight on how to treat many painful and/or functional problems. Due to the overlap of visceral afferents onto spinal pathways that also receive somatic afferents, the sensory experience of visceral irritation is often one of referred pain to a somatic structure, with concomitant increased somatic muscle tone. One of the most common patterns is shoulder pain and muscle tension associated with acute myocardial infarction. The nociceptive input from the compromised myocardium is experienced as shoulder or chest pain. Often, a vicious circle of increased somatic involvement results, as increased somatic activity also increases sympathetic outflow to the heart, further exacerbating the pathologic process.

Although it is not the only course of treatment, treating the somatic component of the process can be beneficial.

- Recognizing the visceral origin of referred pain patterns can save the physician much time and missed diagnoses.
- Likewise, knowledge of the appropriate osteopathic treatment for addressing the involved somatic structures is also helpful.
- Understanding the somatic areas likely to show effects of underlying visceral pathologic conditions through viscerosomatic reflexes[2] serves as another important diagnostic and treatment tool.

Vascular Structures

The arterial blood supply to the thoracic viscera is largely obtained from branches of the descending thoracic aorta. These include the following:

- Pericardial arteries
- Bronchial arteries
- Mediastinal arteries
- Phrenic arteries
- Posterior intercostal arteries
- Subcostal arteries

The venous drainage of the thoracic visceral structures is accomplished by way of a corresponding system of veins that parallel the arteries. Several other structures that participate in the venous drainage of the thoracic regional viscera are the following:

- Superior vena cava
- A short section of the inferior vena cava
- The azygos and hemiazygos system of veins

The thoracic portion of the spinal cord derives its arterial blood supply from three longitudinal structures: a single anterior and two posterior spinal arteries. In addition, the posterior intercostal arteries make contributions to the longitudinal arterial system.[2,11]

The arterial supply of the thoracic vertebrae and musculature is derived from branches of the posterior intercostal arteries (Fig. 34.6).

- Each posterior intercostal artery gives rise to a spinal branch, which provides arterial blood to its corresponding spinal vertebra, along with the spinal cord and meninges at that vertebral level.
- The spinal branch then further divides into medial and lateral musculocutaneous branches.
  - □ The medial branch provides arterial blood to the spinalis and longissimus thoracis muscles, and a corresponding area of skin.
  - □ The lateral branch provides arterial blood for the longissimus thoracis and iliocostalis muscles, the medial aspects of the latissimus dorsi and trapezius muscles, and a corresponding area of skin.

There is a corresponding network of veins that provide for venous drainage of the thoracic spinal region (Fig. 34.7). These include the following:

- Anterior and posterior internal plexus of vertebral veins
- Anterior and posterior external plexus of vertebral veins
- Basivertebral and intervertebral veins[2,5,11]

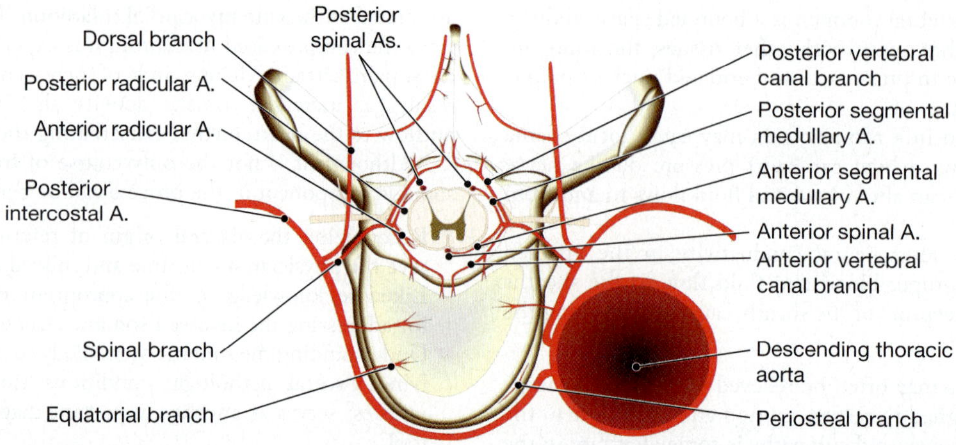

Figure 34.6. Distribution of spinal branches from the posterior intercostal artery (transverse section).

Lymphatics

As blood moves through the capillaries, fluid filters into the interstitial tissues. The return of interstitial fluid through the lymphatic system is necessary for health and proper function and is even more important in the diseased state.

There are two main divisions to the human lymphatic system. Lymph from the lower extremities, abdomen, pelvis, left upper extremity, left hemithorax, left upper lobe of the lung, and left side of head drain into the left lymphatic system and therefore into the thoracic duct. Lymph from the right upper extremity, right hemithorax, left lower lobe and right lung, liver, most of the heart, tracheobronchial lymph nodes, and right side of head empty into the right lymphatic system and ultimately into the right lymphatic duct[13,14] (Fig. 34.8).

The thoracic duct develops from outgrowths of the jugular lymphatic sacs and the cisterna chyli. While there are wide variations in the final anatomic structure of the main ductal system, the thoracic duct generally originates in the abdomen at the cisterna chyli, which is located around the level of the second lumbar vertebra. The thoracic duct extends into the thorax through the aortic hiatus of the thoracoabdominal diaphragm into the right posterior mediastinum before crossing to the left at the level of the fifth or sixth thoracic vertebra, ascends posteriorly to the aortic arch and into the posterior neck to the junction of the subclavian and internal jugular veins.[13] Other common variations include a double system rising from the cisterna or a multiple ductal pattern at the level of the diaphragm. Within the chest, a profuse collateral system originates from intercostal spaces, the posterior mediastinum, and visceral lymphatics which communicate with the main duct via collecting trunks. The wall of the thoracic duct has three layers: the intima, media, and adventitia. The media is comprised of connective tissue and smooth muscle which is capable of contracting regularly with enough force to propel lymph superiorly toward the jugular venous junction at a rate of 50 to 200 mL/hr.[13,15] The thoracic duct contains valves that may be unicuspid, bicuspid or tricuspid, but are usually bicuspid. At the junction of the lymphatic and venous system, a bicuspid valve prevents venous backflow into the lymphatic

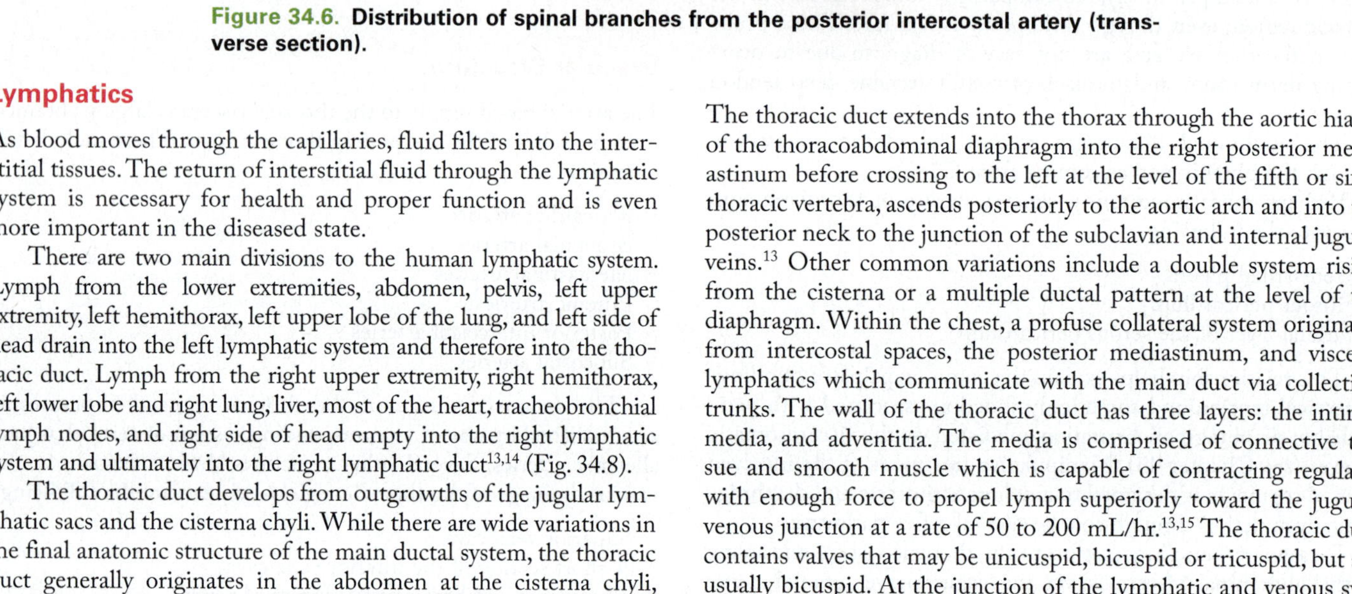

Figure 34.7. Venous drainage of vertebral column. A. Pattern of drainage. The venous drainage parallels the arterial supply and enters the external and internal vertebral venous plexuses. There is also anterolateral drainage from the external aspects of the vertebrae into segmental veins. **B.** Nature of veins. The dense plexus of thin-walled vessels within the vertebral canal, the internal vertebral venous plexuses, consists of valveless anastomoses between anterior and posterior longitudinal venous sinuses. (Reprinted with permission from Dalley AF II, Agur AMR. *Moore's Clinically Oriented Anatomy*. 9th ed. Wolters Kluwer; 2023. Figure 2.30.)

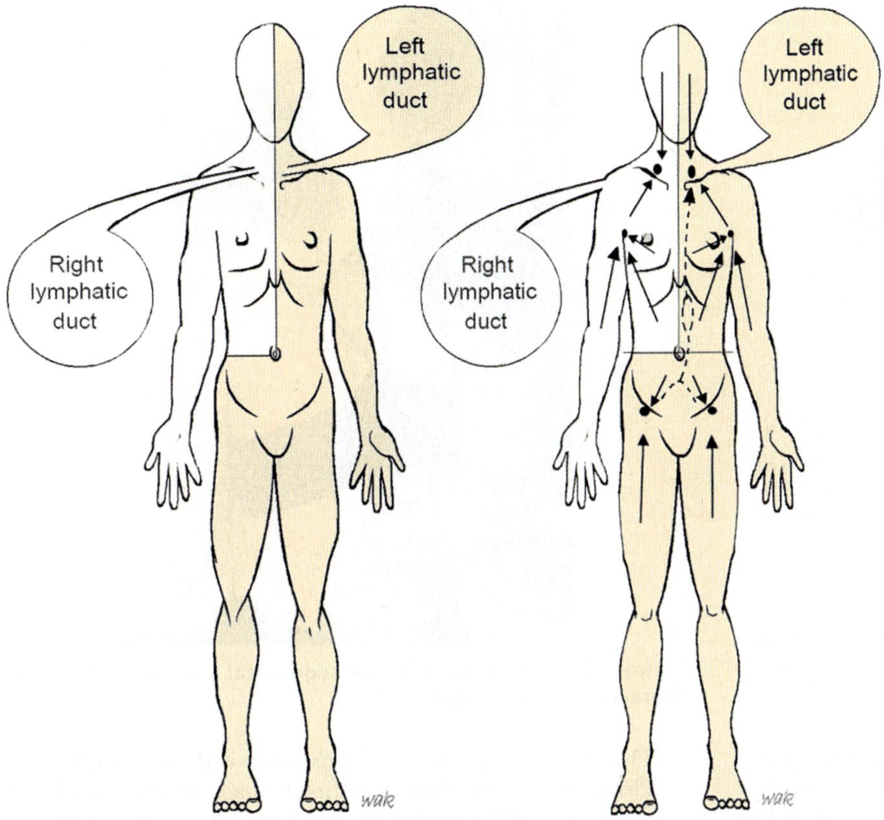

Figure 34.8. Lymphatic drainage of the body.

system.[15] The right lymphatic duct ascends in the right posterior mediastinum and enters the junction of the right subclavian and internal jugular veins.[2,5,11,14]

In approximately 20% of the population, three trunks join to form the right lymphatic duct:

1. The right jugular
2. The right subclavian
3. The right transverse cervical

The remainder of the population varies in the way the three trunks empty into the jugulosubclavian junction in the anterior neck.

STRUCTURAL EXAMINATION

For the screening and regional examination of the thoracic region the reader is referred to Chapter 30.

As a quick recap of the screening examination, asymmetry and restriction of active range of motion of the region(s) may indicate that further evaluation is warranted with the regional portion of the structural exam which includes palpatory assessment and passive range of motion/quality of motion assessment.

During the palpatory evaluation of the paraspinal tissues, evidence of acute or chronic somatic dysfunction, viscerosomatic or somatovisceral reflexes, infectious processes and even trauma may be found with the assessment of temperature changes (excessive warmth or coolness), tissue texture changes such as bogginess, thickness, ropiness, stringiness, firmness and excessive moisture or dryness, patient tenderness to palpation and asymmetry on palpation.

The regional examination is continued with the evaluation of passive range of motion or quality of motion.

Abnormal findings here will lead the osteopathic physician to a further refinement of "what is the problem" or the segmental exam. As with the passive and active range of motion testing, the segmental examination of the upper thoracic and lower thoracic regions differs with respect to the mechanics of the head and neck utilized to assess the upper thoracic region and the trunk utilized to assess the lower thoracic region.

SEGMENTAL EXAM

1. The physician stands behind the patient with the dominant eye over the patient's midline.
2. Patient sits on a fixed stool or straddles one end of the table, facing the other end. The patient may also sit on the side of the table with feet supported.
3. Patient's spine is in the neutral position.
4. Physician chooses the area with the greatest tissue texture changes as assessed during the screening and regional examinations, then locates the most posterior transverse process within the vertebral segments being examined.

To assess T1–T4—Method 1:

1. The physician places one hand on the patient's head and uses the patient's head and cervical spine as a lever to induce flexion/extension, sidebending, and rotation in the upper thoracic spine.
2. Physician uses the thumb and index finger of the other hand to monitor motion of thoracic vertebrae (see Fig. 34.9). Physician contacts the segment with the most posterior transverse process by placing the thumb and index finger on the lateral aspects of the patient's transverse processes.
3. Physician assesses the amount and quality of sidebending, rotation, and flexion/extension, of the individual vertebra.

To assess T1–T4—Method 2:

1. The physician places their thumbs on the transverse processes of the segment being examined. The posterior transverse process may be cross-referenced by applying anterior pressure

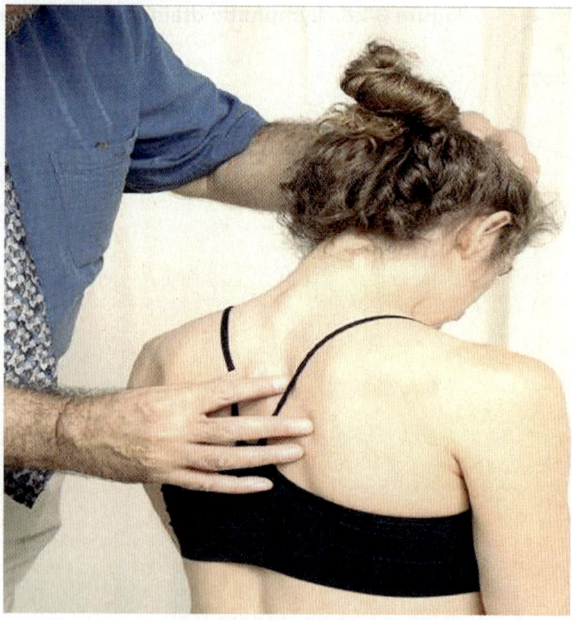

Figure 34.9. Hand position for segmental evaluation of upper thoracic vertebrae—Method 1.

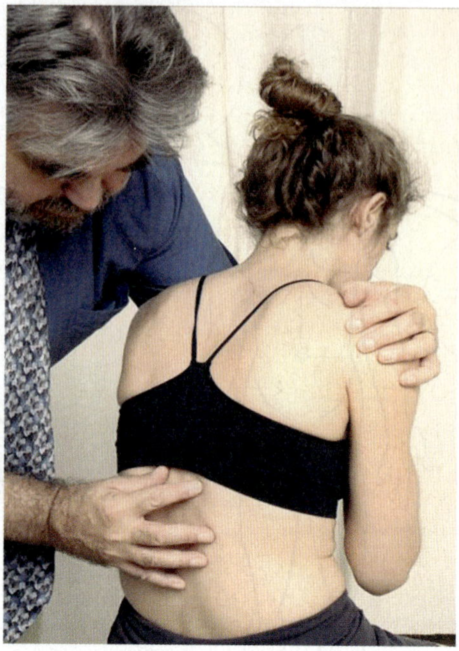

Figure 34.11. Hand position for segmental evaluation of lower thoracic vertebra—Method 1.

to one transverse process and then the other. The posterior transverse process will generally resist anterior spring or pressure as compared to the other side (i.e., T2 is found to have a right posterior transverse process. This resists anterior spring or pressure, but the left transverse process has compliance to anterior spring or pressure as the segment is rotated right).

2. To assess for flexion and extension, maintain the thumbs in this position. Instruct the patient to flex their neck until motion is felt just through the level of the segment being examined (i.e., if T2 is being examined, to the T2–T3 joint space). Assess rotation as described above and note if the posterior transverse process still feels posterior or if it feels more symmetrical as compared to the other side.
3. Then instruct the patient to return to neutral and then extend their neck until motion is felt to the appropriate level. Assess for rotation in the same manner[16–18] (Fig. 34.10A–C).

To assess T5–T12—Method 1:

1. The physician reaches across the patient's chest with one arm and grasps the patient's opposite shoulder.
2. The patient grasps the physician's elbow with both hands.
3. Physician uses the thumb and index finger of the other hand to monitor motion of thoracic vertebrae. Physician contacts the segment with the most posterior transverse process by placing the thumb and index finger on the lateral aspects of the patient's transverse processes (see Fig. 34.11).
4. Physician assesses the amount and quality of sidebending, rotation, and flexion/extension, of the individual vertebrae.
   - The side of the more prominent transverse process, or of greater resistance to motion from posterior pressure, is the side to which the vertebra is rotated.

To assess T5–T12—Method 2[19]:

1. The physician places their thumbs on the transverse processes of the segment being examined. The posterior transverse process may be cross-referenced by applying anterior pressure to one transverse process and then the other. The posterior transverse process will generally resist anterior spring or pressure as compared to the other side.
2. To assess for flexion and extension, maintain the thumbs in this position. Instruct the patient to slump or flex their neck and

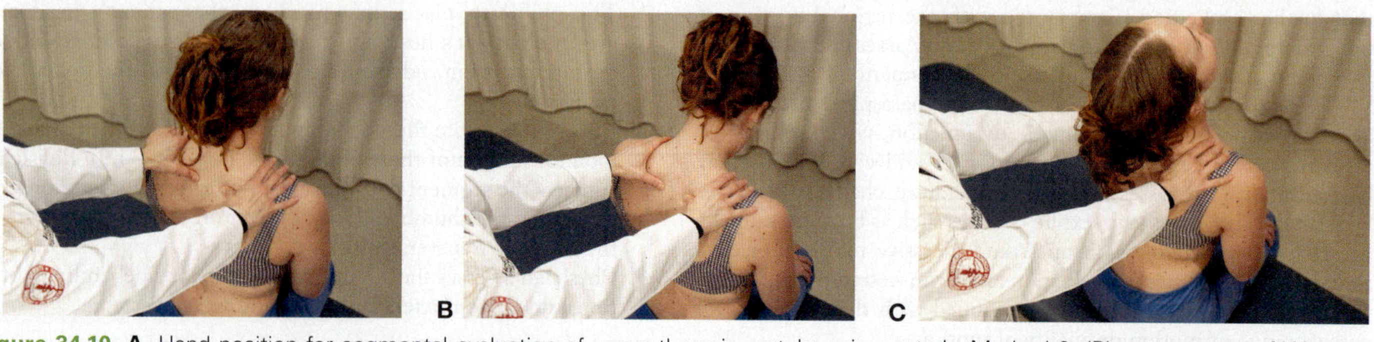

A B C

Figure 34.10. **A.** Hand position for segmental evaluation of upper thoracic vertebrae in neutral—Method 2. (Photo courtesy of Western University of Health Sciences, Pomona, CA, with permission.) **B.** Hand position for segmental evaluation of upper thoracic vertebrae in flexion—Method 2. (Photo courtesy of Western University of Health Sciences, Pomona, CA, with permission.) **C.** Hand position for segmental evaluation of upper thoracic vertebrae in extension—Method 2. (Photo courtesy of Western University of Health Sciences, Pomona, CA, with permission.)

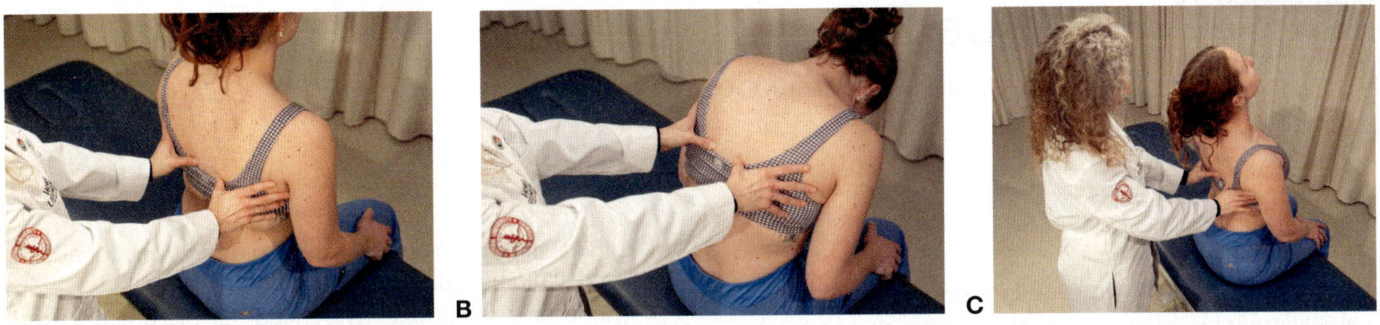

A B C

Figure 34.12. A. Hand position for segmental evaluation of lower thoracic vertebrae in neutral—Method 2. (Photo courtesy of Western University of Health Sciences, Pomona, CA, with permission.) **B.** Hand position for segmental evaluation of lower thoracic vertebrae in flexion—Method 2. (Photo courtesy of Western University of Health Sciences, Pomona, CA, with permission.) **C.** Hand position for segmental evaluation of lower thoracic vertebrae in extension—Method 2. (Photo courtesy of Western University of Health Sciences, Pomona, CA, with permission.)

trunk until motion is felt just through the level of the segment being examined (i.e., if T7 is being examined, to the T7–T8 joint space). Assess rotation as described above and note if the posterior transverse process still feels posterior or if it feels more symmetrical as compared to the other side.

3. Then instruct the patient to return to neutral and then extend their trunk (push their abdomen anteriorly) until motion is felt to the appropriate level. Assess for a posterior transverse process in the same manner (Fig. 34.12A–C).

The following types of somatic dysfunction diagnoses are possible:

1. If the transverse processes are most symmetrical with the patient in extension, then the vertebra is described as extended, sidebent, and rotated to the same side, for example, T7 ER_RS_R.
2. If the transverse processes are most symmetrical with the patient in flexion, then the vertebra is described as flexed and will be sidebent and rotated to the same side, for example, T7 FR_RS_R.[20]
3. If the transverse processes are most symmetrical with the patient in the neutral position, then the vertebra is described as neutral and based on Fryette's first principle of spinal joint mechanics, will be sidebent and rotated to opposite sides, for example, T7 NR_RS_L. This result also indicates that there is a group dysfunction present, and all vertebrae in this region where TART changes were found would be described in the same fashion, for example, T5–T9 NR_RS_L. T7 would be the apex of this group curve, since it demonstrated the most posterior transverse process or the greatest amount of restricted motion within this group of vertebrae.

In addition to diagnosing the thoracic vertebrae in the above fashion, the physician should also evaluate the thoracic spinal region for the following:

1. Myofascial restrictions. The reader is referred to Chapter 52 for more information about the evaluation of myofascial restrictions.
2. Counterstrain tender points. Chapter 47 elaborates on evaluation for counterstrain points.
3. Chapman reflex points. Chapters 43 and 58 provides further details regarding the evaluation of Chapman reflex points.

SUMMARY

An in-depth knowledge of thoracic regional anatomy, along with the skilled use of osteopathic palpatory diagnosis, can help to inform the successful practice of osteopathic medicine. Such a combination of knowledge and skills can lead to more efficient and accurate patient diagnoses, and more rational and effective treatment decisions.

REFERENCES

1. Schuenke M, Schulte E, Schumacher U, Johnson N, eds. *Thieme Atlas of Anatomy: General Anatomy and Musculoskeletal System*. 3rd ed. Georg Thieme Verlag; 2020.
2. Galbusera F, Wilke H-J, eds. *Biomechanics of the Spine*. Elsevier; 2018.
3. Patterson MM, Howell JN, eds. *The Central Connection: Somatovisceral/Viscerosomatic Interaction*. American Academy of Osteopathy; 1992.
4. Korr IM. The spinal cord as an organizer of disease processes. IV. Axonal transport and neurotrophic function in relation to somatic dysfunction. *J Am Osteopath Assoc*. 1981;80(7):451–459.
5. Dalley AF, Agur AMR. *Moore's Clinically Oriented Anatomy*. 9th ed. Lippincott, Williams & Wilkins; 2022.
6. Mitchell, FL. *The Muscle Energy Manual: Evaluation and Treatment of the Thoracic Spine, Lumbar Spine and Rib Cage*. Vol. 2. MET Press; 1998:114.
7. Mitchell, FL. *The Muscle Energy Manual: Evaluation and Treatment of the Thraocic Spine, Lumbar Spine and Rib Cage*. Vol. 2. MET Press; 1998:18–19.
8. Korr IM. Proprioceptors and somatic dysfunction. *J Am Osteopath Assoc*. 1975;74(7):638–650.
9. Patterson MM, Steinmetz JE. Long-lasting alterations of spinal reflexes: a basis for somatic dysfunction. *Man Med*. 1986;2:38–42.
10. Van Buskirk RL. Nociceptive reflexes and the somatic dysfunction: a model. *J Am Osteopath Assoc*. 1990;90(9):792–804.
11. Standring S, ed. *Gray's Anatomy*. 42nd ed. Elsevier Churchill Livingston; 2021.
12. Budgell B, Sato A. Somatoautonomic reflex regulation of sciatic nerve blood flow. *J Neuromusculoskel Syst*. 1994;2:170–177.
13. Puligandla P, Laberge JM. Infections and Diseases of the Lungs, Pleura, and Mediastinum. In: Holcomb G, Murphy J, Ostlie D, eds. *Ashcraft's Pediatric Surgery*. Elsevier; 2006.
14. Ferguson MK. Thoracic Duct. In: *Thoracic Surgery Atlas*. 2nd ed. Elsevier; 2024:71.
15. Woodcock T. Fluid physiology part 1: Volume and distribution of water and its major solutes between plasma, the interstitium and intracellular fluid. In: Malbrain ML, Wong A, Nasa P, Ghosh S, eds. *Rational Use of Intravenous Fluids in Critically Ill Patients*. Springer; 2024:47–74.
16. Nelson KE, Glonek T. *Somatic Dysfunction in Osteopathic Family Medicine*. Lippincott Williams & Wilkins; 2007:21.
17. Mitchell, FL. *The Muscle Energy Manual: Evaluation and Treatment of the Thoracic Spine, Lumbar Spine and Rib Cage*. Vol. 2. MET Press; 1998: 114–115.
18. DeStefano LA. *Greenman's Principles of Manual Medicine*. 5th ed. Wolters Kluwer; 2017:215–216.
19. DeStefano LA. *Greenman's Principles of Manual Medicine*. 5th ed. Wolters Kluwer; 2017:2167.
20. Mitchell, FL. *The Muscle Energy Manual: Evaluation and Treatment of the Throacic Spine, Lumbar Spine and Rib Cage*. Vol. 2. MET Press; 1998:115.

35

Rib Cage

RAYMOND J. HRUBY ▪ REBECCA E. GIUSTI

KEY CONCEPTS

- Importance of the rib cage for normal function
- Relationship of the rib cage with the thoracic vertebrae
- Important structures and functions of the rib cage
- Clinical relevance of the rib cage
- Descriptive and functional anatomy of the costal cage
- Clinical aspects of costal structures and functional interrelationships, including the thoracic spine
- The impact of somatic dysfunction of the costal cage
- Identification and diagnosis of somatic dysfunction of the costal cage; both structural respiratory
- Performance of the segmental exam to the costal cage
- Define inhalation and exhalation somatic dysfunctions
- Define and identify the key rib

INTRODUCTION

Respiration is a process involving the participation of several systems of the body, none the least of which is the musculoskeletal system. As Cathie[1] noted, "Respiratory activity requires motion in a greater number of articulations and with a greater frequency than any other musculoskeletal function." This includes not only the intervertebral joints of the thoracic spine but also the costovertebral and costotransverse joints at the posterior aspects of the ribs. In addition to the articular motion, optimal respiration also requires a degree of elasticity of the ribs and costal cartilages. The biomechanical architecture among the vertebrae and ribs may be thought of as a complex system of levers. Anything that alters the normal movement of this system of levers may impair respiration.

DEFINITION

The rib cage is the bony enclosing wall of the chest. It is a structure formed by the thoracic vertebrae, the ribs, the sternum, and the costal cartilages.[2,3]

Figure 35.1. Bones of the thorax, anterior view.

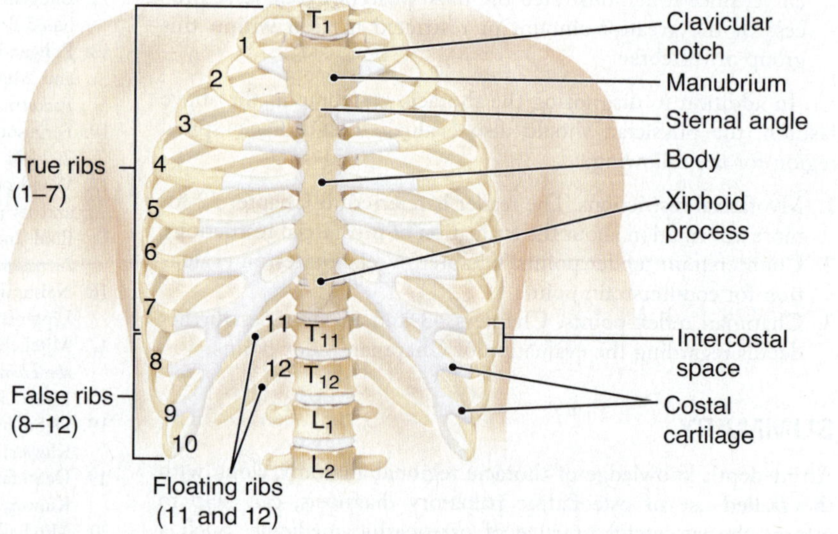

DESCRIPTIVE AND FUNCTIONAL ANATOMY

Skeletal Structures (See Fig. 35.1)

The 12 sets of ribs correspond with the 12 thoracic vertebrae. All ribs are composed of a bony segment and a costal cartilage. Each rib has a cup-shaped depression in its bony segment where the costal cartilage fits into the costochondral joint, and where the periosteum of the rib joins the perichondrium of the rib cartilage. The rib heads join with the thoracic vertebrae at the costovertebral articulations. The heads of ribs 2 through 9 articulate with a demifacet on the vertebra above and below. For example, rib 2 articulates by demifacets with T1 and T2. The heads of ribs 1 and 10 to 12 articulate with unifacets on their corresponding vertebrae. The transverse processes of vertebrae T1–T10 also have synovial costotransverse joints with the tubercle of the corresponding rib.[2,3]

Ribs 1, 2, 11, and 12 are called atypical ribs (see Fig. 35.1)

- Rib 1 is the flattest, shortest, broadest, strongest, and most curved. The subclavian artery and the cervical plexus are vulnerable to muscular compression where they pass over the first

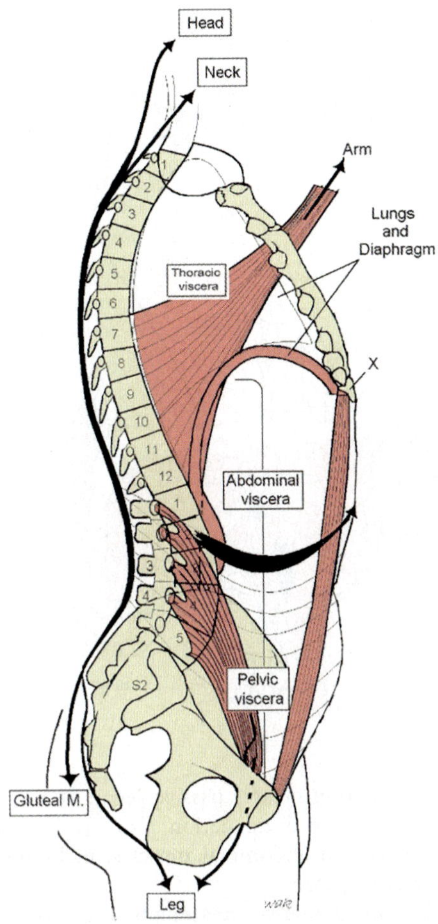

Figure 35.2. The thoracic region and its relationships.

rib between the tubercles and attachments of the anterior and the middle scalene muscles. The subclavian vein may also be compressed between the first rib and the clavicle.

- Rib 2 is considered anatomically atypical because of its tuberosity that attaches to the proximal portion of the serratus anterior muscle.
- Ribs 11 and 12 are anatomically atypical because they do not have tubercles, do not attach to the sternum or other costal cartilages, and have tapered ends. These two ribs are also called floating or vertebral ribs.
- Rib 10 is sometimes considered atypical because of its single articulation between the rib head and T10.[2,3]

The anatomy of the thoracic region and its relationships is shown in Figure 35.2.

Anatomically typical ribs (3–9, and in most respects 10) have heads, necks, tubercles, angles, and shafts that connect directly or via chondral masses to the sternum.

- Rib 1 and ribs 2 to 7 connect directly with the sternum by their own individual cartilaginous synovial joints (rib 1 with a stable synchondrosis); therefore, they are often called the true ribs.
- Ribs 8 to 10 merge into a single cartilaginous mass that attaches to the sternum; therefore, these are called vertebral chondral ribs.
- Ribs 11 and 12 do not connect with the sternum and are hence called floating ribs. Because ribs 8 to 12 do not connect directly to the sternum, they are often called false ribs (see Fig. 35.1).

The costovertebral joints between the heads of the ribs and the vertebral bodies allow gliding or sliding costal motions. The costotransverse joints at the tubercle of the typical ribs, with the facets at the tip of the transverse processes of their own vertebra, a synovial membrane, and a thin articular capsule, allow gliding and slight rotational motions. When these motions are restricted, respiratory movements are commonly impeded.

The sternum has three parts (see Fig. 35.1):

1. Head or manubrium
2. Body or gladiolus
3. Tail or xiphoid process

The superior portion of the manubrium cradles the clavicles at the sternoclavicular joints, forming the sternal notch or jugular notch, which is a landmark for several anterior thoracic strain/counterstrain tender points. The sternal notch lies almost directly anterior to the T2 vertebral body. The manubrium joins the sternal body via a fibrocartilaginous symphysis, or secondary cartilaginous joint, called the *sternal angle*. This joint lies anterior to the fourth thoracic vertebra. Because the second rib attaches to the manubrium and sternal body with a synovial joint, the sternal angle is an anterior landmark for counting the ribs. The xiphisternal joint is located anterior to the ninth thoracic vertebra. It is also a hyaline cartilage symphysis that fuses into a synostosis in the fifth decade.[3]

Musculature

The muscles of the thoracic area are involved in the following:

1. Actions of the ribs and vertebrae
2. Head and neck control
3. Breathing

For specific information regarding individual muscles of the rib cage, see Table 34.1 in Chapter 34. The muscles involved in respiration are discussed in greater detail below in the "Rib Motion" section. As with all muscles, the rib cage muscles are fed not only by circulatory elements but also by physiologically active trophic substances delivered directly by nerves themselves.[2] In addition, there is evidence that the sympathetic nerve supply to striated and smooth muscles alters muscle tone and contractile forces. Attention to the palpatory cues associated with altered muscle tone, therefore, implies the presence of many differential diagnostic factors that are discussed throughout this text.

The abdominal diaphragm is the primary muscle of respiration (Fig. 35.3).

It forms the floor of the thorax and attaches to the xiphoid process, the internal surface of the inferior six ribs, and its crura attach to the upper two (left) or three (right) lumbar vertebrae and their intervertebral disks. Its fibers converge into a common central tendon that has no bony attachment. When the diaphragm contracts with inhalation, it descends into the abdomen; when it relaxes during exhalation, it moves upward into the thorax. This piston-like motion produces pressure gradients between the thoracic and abdominal cavities and is important for both efficient respiration and circulation. Because there are one-way valves in the larger lymphatic vessels, the pressure gradients also enhance the movement of lymph and venous blood toward the heart. When the dome of the diaphragm is flattened because of asymmetric load and/or tonus, respiration and lymphatic drainage from anywhere in the body becomes less efficient.[2]

Three apertures occur in the diaphragm:

1. One for the vena cava at about the level of T8
2. One for the esophageal hiatus at T10
3. One for the aorta at the level of T12 (Fig. 35.4)

Diaphragmatic muscle fibers are arranged so that upon contraction during inspiration, the vena cava opening dilates, permitting

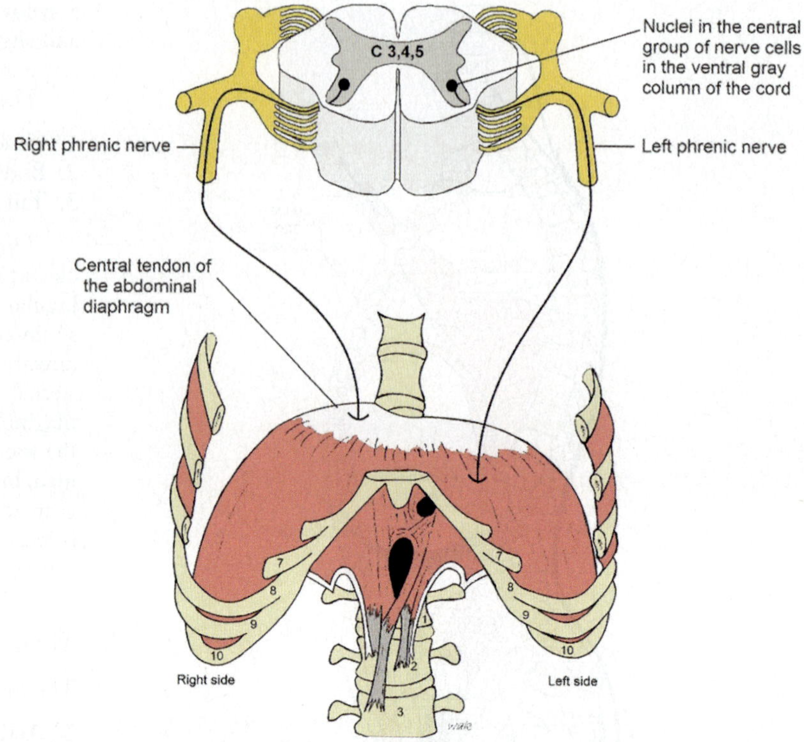

Figure 35.3. Phrenic nerve innervation to the thoracoabdominal diaphragm.

more venous blood to pass from the abdomen to the thorax. At the same time, the esophageal hiatus constricts to prevent gastric contents from rising in the esophagus. Its contraction has no influence on the aortic hiatus, which lies posterior to the diaphragm and does not truly pierce the diaphragm.

The diaphragm does most of the work of breathing under normal conditions and during moderately forced inspiration. With increased respiratory demands, accessory muscles of respiration become involved to move the ribs even more. The scalene muscles, attached to the upper two ribs, assist inhalation. Hypertonicity or hypotonicity of segmental intercostal muscles alters rib behavior, making breathing less efficient. Actual spasm in these muscles can result in pain at rest or especially with each deep breath or cough. Quiet exhalation creates passive recoil of the lung as the diaphragm relaxes. Forced exhalation also involves the inferior internal intercostal and abdominal muscles, including the trunk rotators and erector spinae.

Osteopathic manipulative treatments can often restore or partially rehabilitate altered diaphragmatic function. Treatments designed to resolve somatic dysfunction of the attachment sites of the diaphragm such as the lower costal cage, lumbar spine, and even the thoracoabdominal muscle itself may improve diaphragmatic excursion. This, in turn, helps improve breathing mechanics and assists in venous blood return and lymphatic flow. This approach can be especially helpful for individuals with asthma, respiratory infections, loss of general lung compliance, and associated disorders.

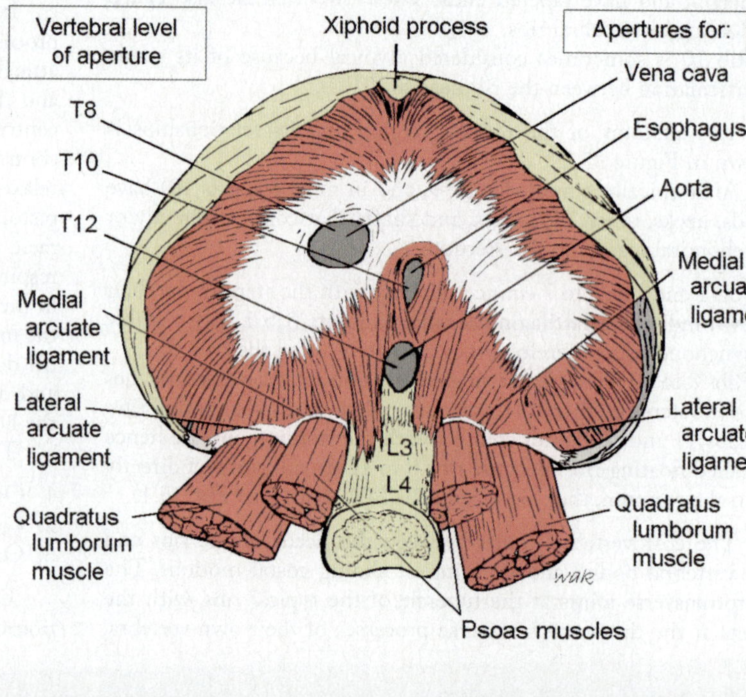

Figure 35.4. Apertures of the thoracoabdominal diaphragm.

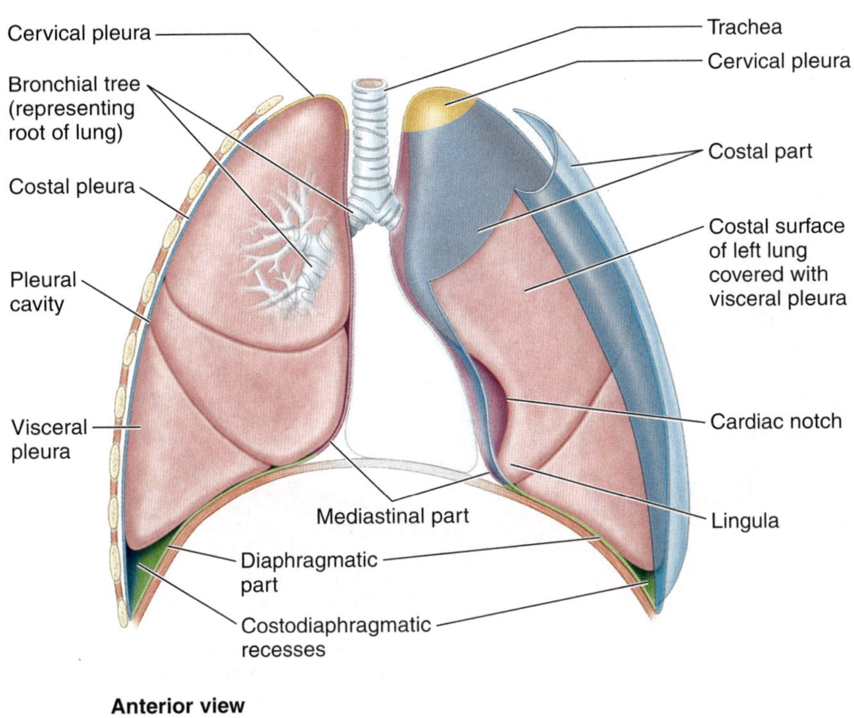

Figure 35.5. Supportive structures of the costal region-fascia and pleura.

Supportive Tissues (Fig. 35.5)

Like all other muscles of the body, the muscles of the thoracic cage are invested with fascia. The internal thoracic wall is covered by a parietal layer of fascia called the endothoracic fascia. This deep fascia invests the internal intercostal, subcostal, and transversus thoracis muscles.[3] This fascia blends with the periosteum of the ribs and sternum and with the perichondral tissue of the costal cartilages. The endothoracic fascia also covers the superior surface of the diaphragm, thus becoming the superior diaphragmatic fascia. The endothoracic fascia is also continuous with the prevertebral layer of the cervical fascia and with the scalene fascia (also called Sibson fascia), where it attaches along the inner border of the first rib. Behind the sternum, it is also continuous with the fascia of the infrahyoid muscles. This parietal thoracic fascia proceeds through the openings of the diaphragm to become continuous with the transversalis fascia of the abdomen. In addition, there are specialized fascial elements that comprise the pericardium, pleura, and mediastinum.[2]

Neural Structures

A detailed description of the nerve supply to the thoracic area is given in Chapter 34. The ventral rami of the first 11 thoracic nerves are called *intercostal* nerves.[4] They are located between the ribs (see Figs. 35.6 and 35.7), although the 12th thoracic nerve lies below the last rib and is thus called the *subcostal nerve*. Each of these nerves is connected to the sympathetic chain ganglia via the *white and gray rami communicantes*. The intercostal nerves provide innervation chiefly to the thoracic and abdominal walls. The first six nerves provide innervation to the thoracic wall, with the first two nerves also providing fibers to the upper extremity. The lower five nerves are distributed to the thoracic and abdominal walls, and the subcostal nerve innervates the abdominal wall and the skin of the gluteal area.

The thoracoabdominal diaphragm receives its motor innervation through the phrenic nerves coming from C3 to C5 (see Fig. 35.3).

Perhaps more importantly, sensory nerves of the diaphragm innervate the following:

- Mediastinal pleura
- Fibrous pericardium
- Parietal layer of the serous pericardium[3]

This relationship helps explain the very common palpatory findings of cervical tension and somatic dysfunction associated with pericardial or diaphragmatic irritation that are mediated via viscerosomatic reflexes (see Chapter 13). Manipulative treatment of the involved cervical segments is designed to ameliorate thoracic and diaphragmatic dysfunction through somatovisceral reflex pathways.

Vasculature

The arterial blood supply to the walls of the thoracic cage comes from three main sources: the axillary and subclavian arteries, and the aorta (Fig. 35.8).

1. The axillary artery provides its contribution to the arterial blood supply of the thoracic cage walls by way of two of its branches: the superior thoracic and lateral thoracic arteries.
2. The subclavian artery gives rise to the internal thoracic artery, which in turn provides arterial blood to the thoracic cage from the following branches: anterior intercostal, perforating, and musculophrenic arteries. It also gives rise to the superior intercostal artery.
3. The aorta gives rise to the posterior intercostal arteries. The superior intercostal artery branches into the first and second intercostal arteries and then anastomoses with the third intercostal artery.[2–4]

The venous drainage of the thoracic walls is accomplished by way of several venous structures (Fig. 35.9).

These include the following:

- Internal thoracic veins
- Anterior, posterior, and superior intercostal veins
- Azygos and hemiazygos veins[2–4]

The intercostal veins accompany the intercostal arteries and nerves and occupy the most superior aspect of the costal grooves. There are 11 posterior intercostal veins and 1 subcostal vein on

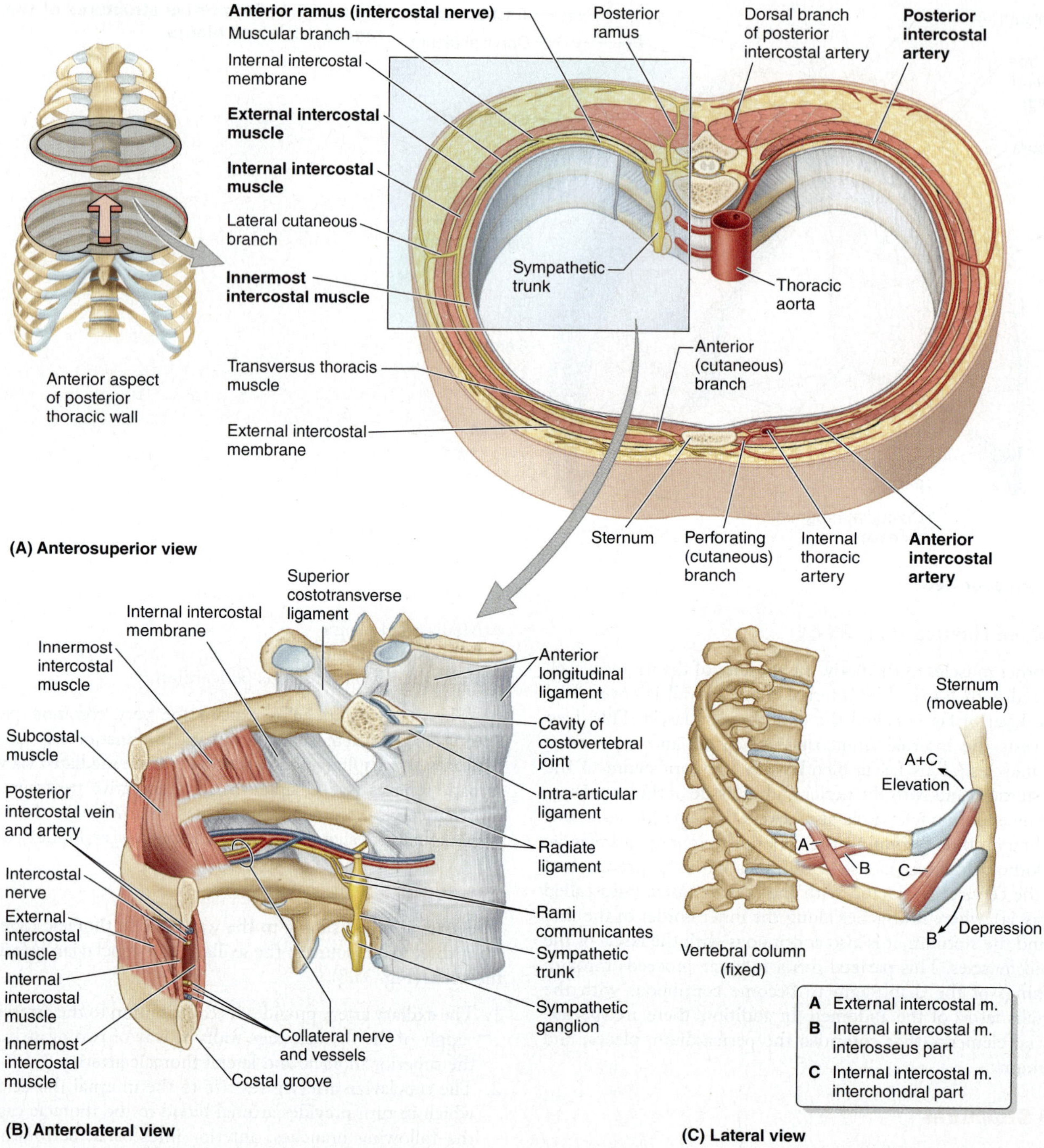

Figure 35.6. Contents of an intercostal space. (Reprinted with permission from Dalley AF II, Agur AMR. *Moore's Clinically Oriented Anatomy*. 9th ed. Wolters Kluwer; 2023. Figure 4.15.)

each side. The posterior intercostal veins anastomose with the anterior intercostal veins which are tributaries of the internal thoracic veins. As the posterior intercostal veins approximate the vertebral column, they receive a posterior branch, which accompanies the posterior ramus of the spinal nerve of that level, and an intervertebral vein draining the vertebral venous plexuses associated with the vertebral column. Most posterior intercostal veins (4–11) end in the azygos/hemi-azygos venous system, which conveys venous blood to the superior vena cava (SVC). The posterior intercostal veins of the first intercostal space usually enter directly into the right and left brachiocephalic veins. The posterior intercostal veins of the second, third and occasionally fourth intercostal spaces unite to form a trunk, the superior intercostal vein.[4]

Lymphatic Structures

In general, the superficial lymph vessels of the thoracic wall ramify subcutaneously and converge on the axillary nodes.[2,5] The lymph nodes from the deeper tissues of the thoracic wall drain into three groups of nodes (Fig. 35.10):

1. The parasternal (internal thoracic) lymph nodes. These are four or five pairs of nodes located at the anterior ends of the intercostal spaces.
2. The intercostal lymph nodes, located in the posterior parts of the intercostal spaces in relation to the heads and necks of the ribs.
3. The diaphragmatic (phrenic) lymph nodes, located on the thoracic surface of the diaphragm.

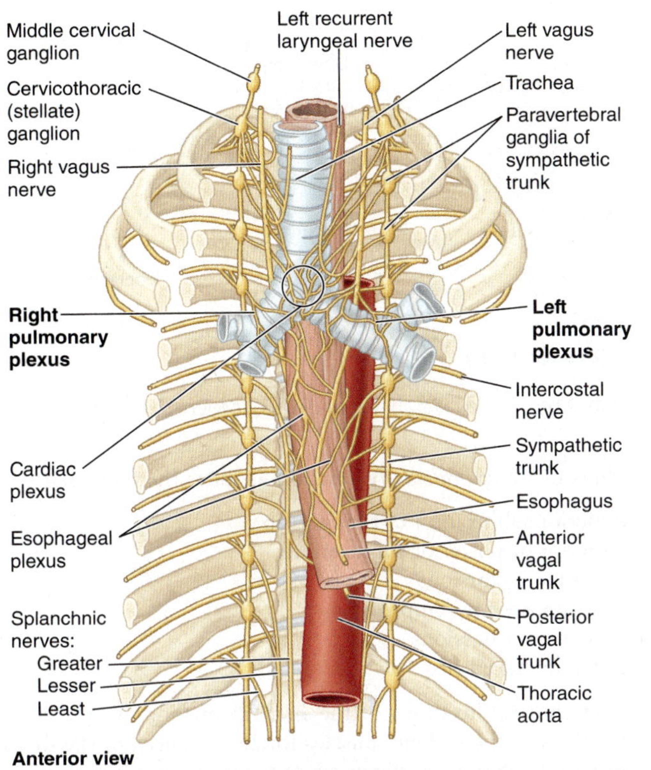

Figure 35.7. Nerves of lungs and visceral pleura. (Reprinted with permission from Dalley AF II, Agur AMR. *Moore's Clinically Oriented Anatomy*. 9th ed. Wolters Kluwer; 2023. Figure 4.40.)

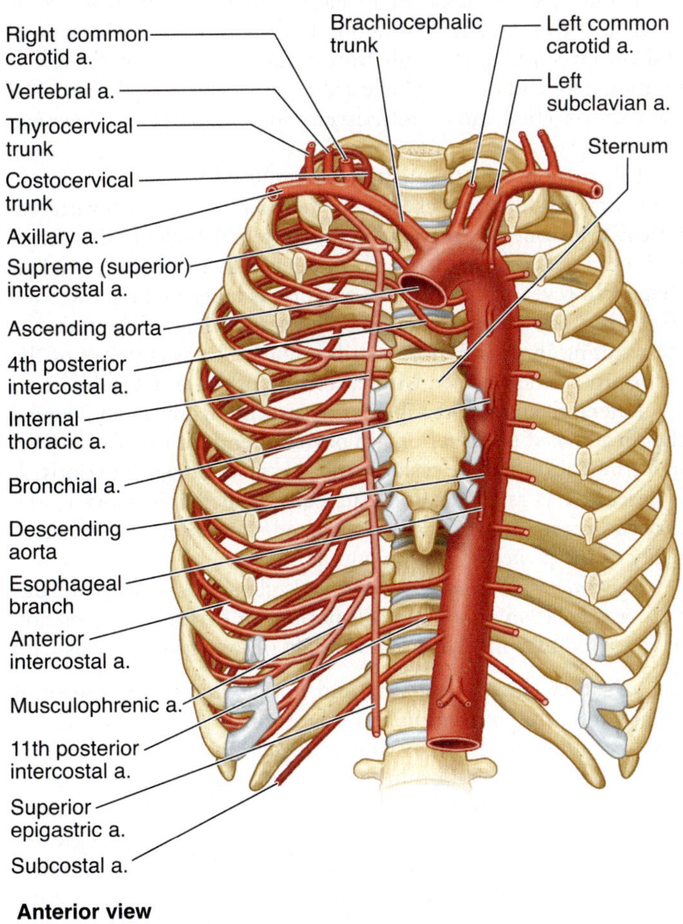

Figure 35.8. Arterial supply to the costal region.

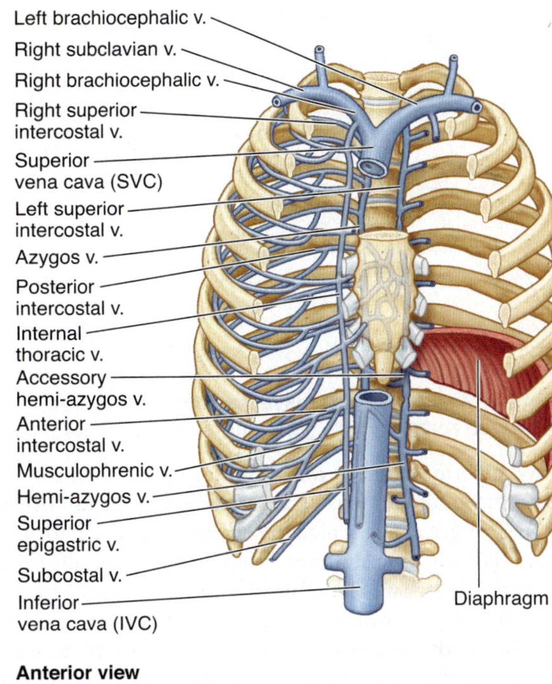

Figure 35.9. Venous drainage of the costal region.

Rib Motion

Rib motion is multifactorial and can be extremely nuanced. Ribs move with complex combinations of pump handle, bucket handle and/or caliper motion. However, ribs 2 to 4 display predominantly pump handle motion; ribs 8 to 10 display predominantly bucket handle motion, ribs 11 to 12 more caliper type motion and ribs 5 to 7 display a mix of pump and bucket handle motion.[6]

- Pump handle motion: During inhalation, there is an increase in the anterior-posterior diameter as the anterior aspect of these

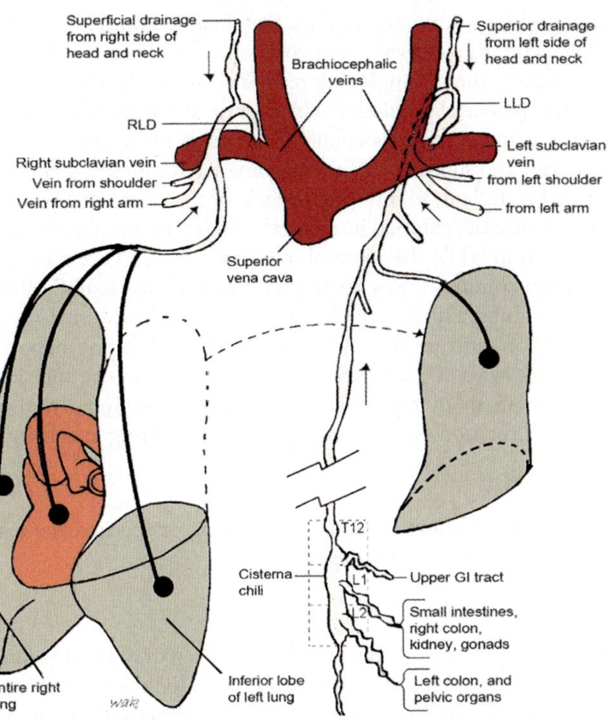

Figure 35.10. Lymphatic drainage of the costal region.

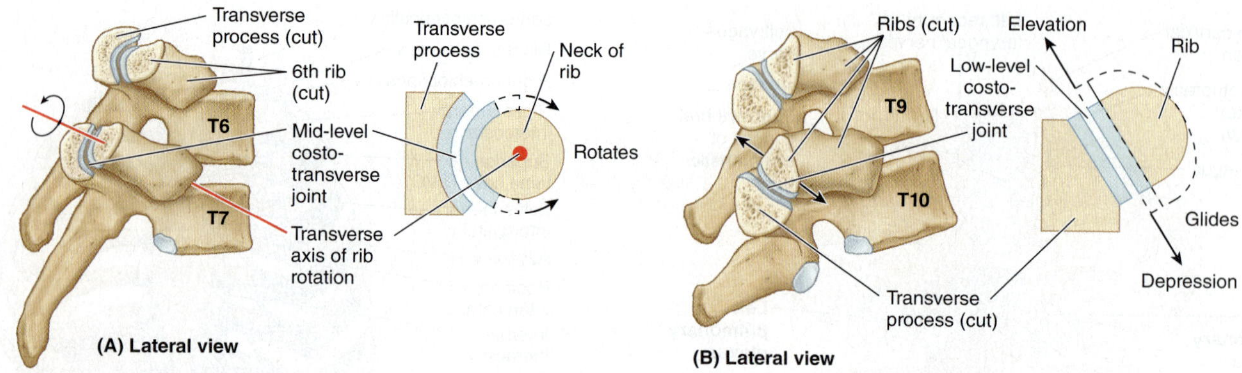

Figure 35.11. Costotransverse joints. (Reprinted with permission from Dalley AF II, Agur AMR. *Moore's Clinically Oriented Anatomy*. 9th ed. Wolters Kluwer; 2023. Figure 4.9.)

ribs move superiorly due to the respiratory axis of the rib about the costovertebral and costotransverse facets being oriented almost in a direct coronal plane. Additionally, ribs 2 to 4 tend to rise and fall with the sternum, lifted by the pectoralis minor.[6]

- Bucket handle motion: The transverse processes of about T7 to T10 are angled posteriorly towards the sagittal plane as compared to the upper thoracics. Therefore, the costotransverse articulation is posterior shifting the respiratory axes of the lower ribs closer to the sagittal plane. During inhalation, the anterior and posterior ends of the ribs are relatively fixed as the anterior aspect and the body of the rib "swing" superiorly and laterally, increasing the transverse diameter of the chest wall. During exhalation, the motion is medial and inferior.[6]
- Caliper motion: This type of motion is primarily exhibited by ribs 11 and 12 as there are no costotransverse articulations posteriorly and no anterior articulations. They move posterior and lateral during inhalation and anterior and medial during exhalation (Figs. 35.11 and 35.12).[7]
- Muscles involved in respiration: The thoracoabdominal diaphragm is the primary muscle of respiration. The secondary muscles of inhalation include the scalenes (ribs 1and 2), pectoralis minor (ribs 3–5), pectoralis major (pump handle components of ribs 2–8), serratus anterior (bucket handle components of ribs 2–9) and the external intercostal muscles. Posteriorly, during inhalation, the rib angles are restrained somewhat by the actions of the iliocostalis muscles which draw the rib angles inferiorly causing the anterior portions of the same rib to move relatively anterior and superior.[8] While ongoing EMG studies demonstrate that it is difficult to interpret the role of the intercostal muscles, it seems that the external intercostal muscles are most active during inspiration while the internal intercostal muscles are most active during expiration.[4] Respiratory motion also causes subtle changes to the limbs. During inhalation, there is slight external rotation, abduction, and flexion of the extremities while the opposite is observed with exhalation. An external rotation of the anterior tissues occurs in an inferior spiral direction during inhalation while internal rotation occurs in a superior spiral during exhalation.[8]

Structural Exam

For the screening and regional examination of the rib cage region, the reader is referred to Chapter 30.

Segmental Exam

When the history and the screening and regional portions of the examination indicate rib cage dysfunction, look for more specific signs of somatic dysfunction of the ribs. Motion dysfunction of the ribs is designated as either structural or respiratory.

Specific *structural rib dysfunction* includes the following[9]:

- Superior subluxation of the first rib
- Anterior or posterior subluxations
- External rib torsions
- Anteroposterior compression
- Lateral compressions
- Laterally flexed ribs

Superior subluxations of the first rib may occur by a sudden contraction of the scalene muscles forcing the neck of the first rib from its articulation on the anterior-facing facet of the transverse process of T1. It may then become lodged in a superior and slightly posterior position at the superior aspect of the transverse process. This positioning may persist even with relaxation of the scalenes.[10]

While ribs are designed to have a good deal of pliability in order to withstand anteroposterior and lateral forces, subluxations and compressions may result from trauma such as sports-related injuries, falls, and motor vehicle accidents in which the integrity of the costovertebral and costotransverse joint capsules and ligamentous articulations are compromised.[11]

Rib torsions are frequently the result of a Type II thoracic segmental dysfunction caused by tension of the costovertebral articulations due to rotation of the vertebral body. If the vertebral rotation is corrected, the rib will generally recoil to its original shape. However, if the vertebral rotation is longstanding, the bone of the rib may undergo microscopic restructuring of the trabeculae resulting in an intraosseous rib lesion and a persistence of the deformity of the rib even with correction of the vertebra.[9]

Lateral flexion is described as occurring mainly at rib 2 where the rib acts as if the anterior and posterior ends of the rib are fixed in a true bucket handle fashion and the rib is drawn superiorly. It is described as resulting from an acute sidebending injury to the cervicothoracic junction with associated shortening and hypertonicity of the posterior scalene muscle.[11]

Respiratory rib somatic dysfunction is classified as either inhalation or exhalation restriction (of motion) or dysfunction (position of ease) and may involve either a single rib or a group of ribs.

- Evaluation entails observing and noting restriction or ease of motion during inhalation and exhalation.
- Conventionally, the term *somatic dysfunction* is used to describe the phase of respiration in which a rib or group of ribs moves most easily; for example, *inhalation somatic dysfunction* signifies a rib or group of ribs that moves smoothly and through a greater range or distance than a comparable rib or ribs on the contralateral or ipsilateral side during inhalation and exhibit restriction during exhalation as compared to the contralateral side. The position of ease is termed *inhaled position*.

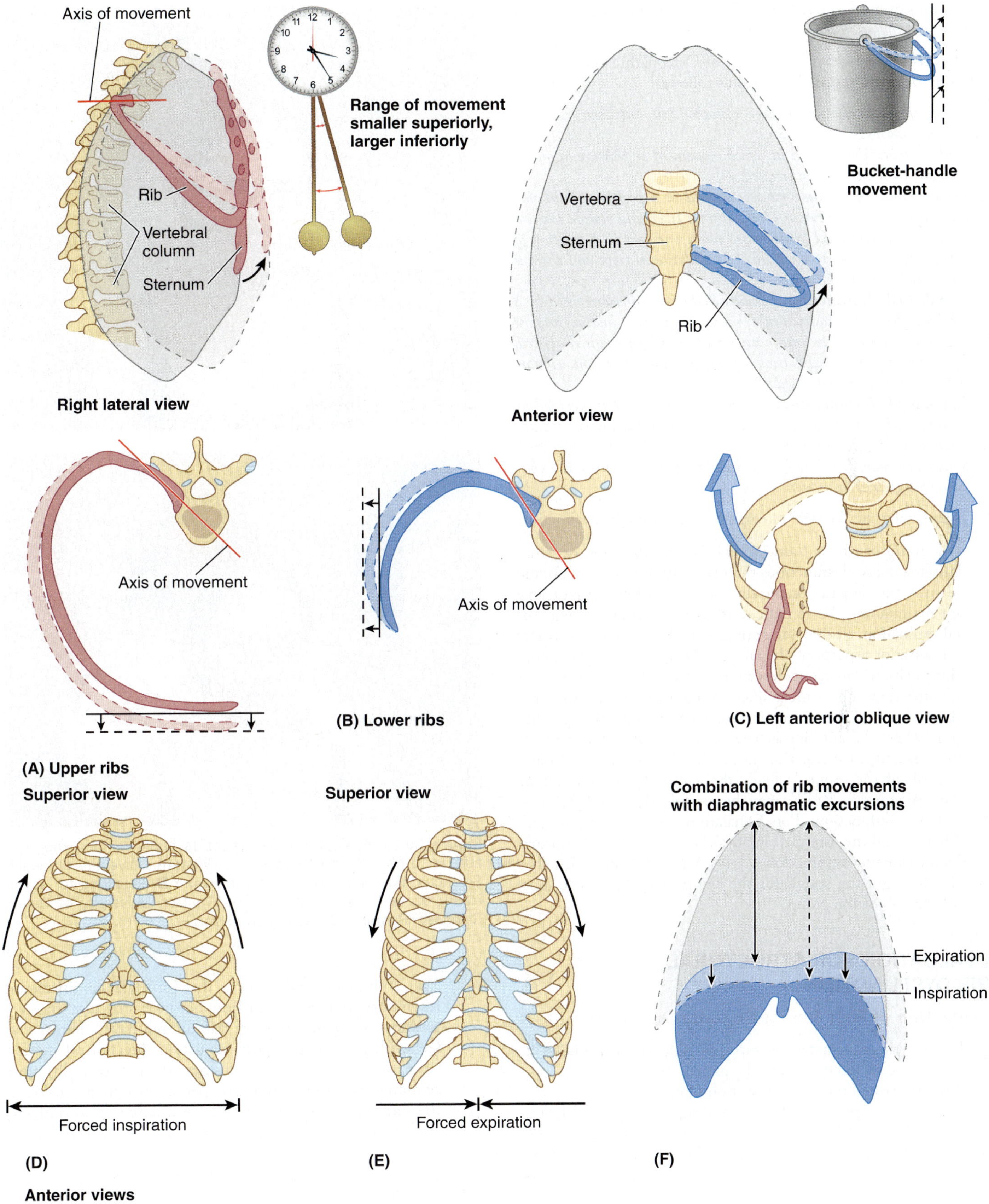

Figure 35.12. Movements of thoracic wall. (Reprinted with permission from Dalley AF II, Agur AMR. *Moore's Clinically Oriented Anatomy*. 9th ed. Wolters Kluwer; 2023. Figure 4.10.)

- In terms of motion restriction, that rib or group of ribs is noted to have *exhalation motion restriction.*

In accordance with the Glossary of Osteopathic Terminology, **rib somatic dysfunction** is defined as follows[12]:

- *A somatic dysfunction of rib cage, costochondral, costovertebral, sternal, and sternochondral regions;*
- *And a somatic dysfunction in which movement or position of one or several ribs is altered or disrupted.*
- *For example, an elevated rib is one held in a position of inhalation such that motion toward inhalation is freer, and motion toward exhalation is restricted. A depressed rib is one held in a position of exhalation such that motion toward exhalation is freer and there is a restriction in inhalation.*
- **Exhaled rib dysfunction.** *Somatic dysfunction characterized by a rib being held in a position of exhalation such that motion toward exhalation is more free and motion toward inhalation is restricted. Synonyms: caught in exhalation, exhalation rib dysfunction, inhalation rib restriction, depressed rib.*
- **Inhaled rib dysfunction.** *A somatic dysfunction characterized by a rib being held in a position of inhalation such that motion toward inhalation is freer and motion toward exhalation is restricted. Synonyms: caught in inhalation, inhalation rib dysfunction, exhalation rib restriction, elevated rib.*

Identifying the "key rib" of respiratory rib somatic dysfunction:

If a group of ribs is found to exhibit an inhalation or exhalation somatic dysfunction, the osteopathic physician should identify the "key rib" or the rib that is most likely responsible for maintaining the somatic dysfunction during the segmental evaluation. For an inhalation somatic dysfunction, where the anterior aspects of the ribs are held in a relatively superior position and resist descending in exhalation, an inferior rib in the group is most likely responsible for maintaining the somatic dysfunction. In an exhalation somatic dysfunction, where the anterior aspects of the ribs are held relatively inferior and resist superior motion during inhalation, a superior rib of the group is likely the cause of the dysfunction. The mnemonic BITE may be useful: **B**ottom-**I**nhalation somatic dysfunction; **T**op-**E**xhalation somatic dysfunction.[13] Therefore, if the osteopathic physician has identified an inhalation somatic dysfunction of ribs 5 to 7 on the right, they should begin the search for the key rib with rib 7, the most inferior rib of the group.

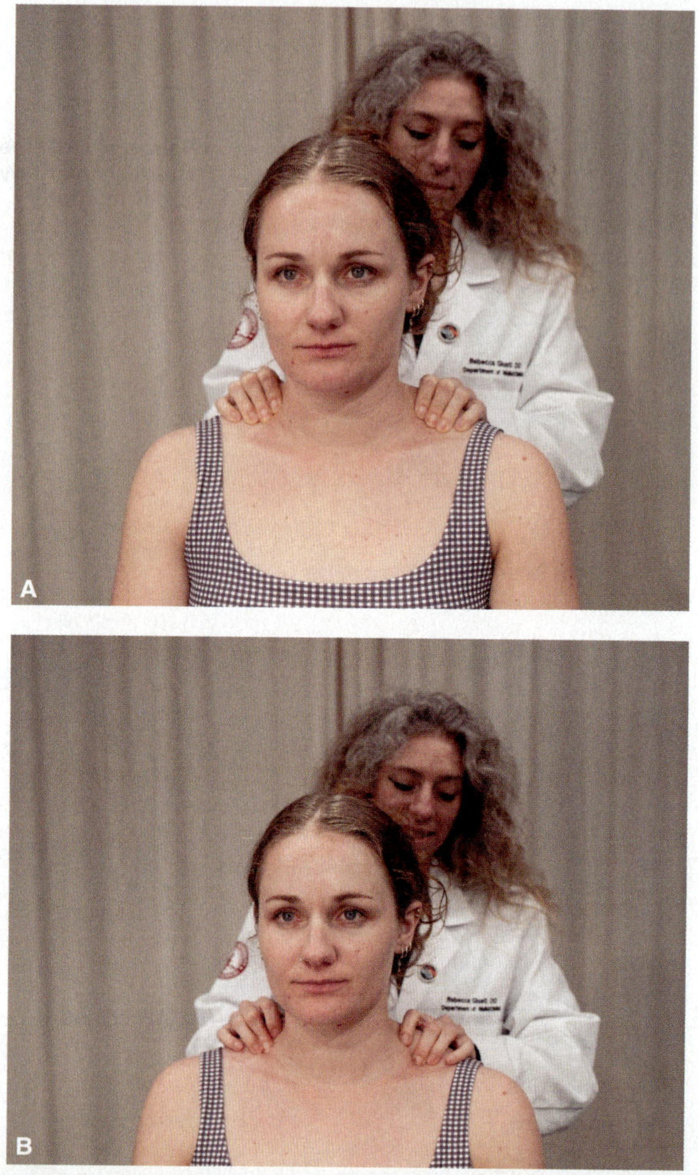

Figure 35.13. A. Drawing the trapezius superiorly for improved access to rib 1. (Photo courtesy of Western University of Health Sciences, Pomona, CA, with permission.) **B.** Palpating for asymmetry of rib 1. (Photo courtesy of Western University of Health Sciences, Pomona, CA, with permission.)

EVALUATION FOR STRUCTURAL RIB DYSFUNCTION

Evaluation of First Rib for Superior Subluxation

1. The first rib is evaluated for superior subluxation as follows[14]: The physician stands behind the patient.
2. Patient is seated on the examination table.
3. The physician grasps the anterior and superior aspect of the trapezius muscle on both sides and retracts the tissues posteriorly.
4. The long fingers of the physician are directed inferiorly to make bilateral contact with the posterior shafts of the patient's first ribs.
   - □ A positive finding is unleveling of the first ribs.
5. The patient is instructed to inhale and exhale deeply.
   - □ The inability of one or the other first rib to descend into the exhalation position confirms the diagnosis of superior subluxation of that rib.
   - □ This is the same evaluation as that for a first rib inhalation respiratory somatic dysfunction; however, structural rib subluxations are generally more painful and have a harder end feel with springing toward exhalation direction of motion since the joint is in effect dislocated. It is typically more symptomatic and has more compensatory muscle tension in the surrounding musculature that is attempting to compensate for the dysfunctional first rib joint (Fig. 35.13A,B).

Evaluation of Ribs 2 to 10 for Structural Rib Restrictions

Evaluate for structural rib restrictions in this region as follows[15]:

1. The patient is seated on the examination table.
2. The physician first stands behind the patient and assesses the posterior contour of the rib cage by palpating over the area of

the rib angles. The physician assesses whether one rib angle is more or less prominent than another.

3. The physician then assesses whether there is a normal posterior convexity with the inferior border of each rib, as being more easily palpated than the superior border.
4. The posterior rib cage is assessed for muscle hypertonicity and tenderness.
5. The width of the intercostal spaces is evaluated for symmetry, intercostal muscle hypertonicity, and tenderness. Each intercostal space should be symmetrical with the one on the opposite side and with the ones immediately above and below it.
6. The physician stands in front of the patient and examines the anterior contour of the rib cage. They then palpate the costochondral junctions to assess the rib contours and intercostal spaces in a manner like that described in step 5 above.
7. The physician then similarly evaluates the lateral rib cage, palpating in the midaxillary line.

The diagnostic criteria for structural rib dysfunction are described as follows[16]:

1. Anterior subluxation
   a. Posteriorly, the rib angle is less prominent.
   b. Anteriorly, the rib shaft is more prominent.
   c. There is associated tenderness and muscle hypertonicity.
2. Posterior subluxation
   a. Posteriorly, the rib angle is more prominent.
   b. Anteriorly, the rib angle is less prominent.
   c. There is associated tenderness and muscle hypertonicity.
3. External rib torsion
   a. The superior border of the involved rib is more prominent.
   b. The inferior border of the involved rib is less prominent.
   c. There is a wider intercostal space above and a narrower intercostal space below the involved rib, with associated muscle hypertonicity and tenderness.
4. Anteroposterior rib compression
   a. There is less prominence of the involved rib both anteriorly and posteriorly.
   b. There is increased prominence of the involved rib in the midaxillary line.
   c. The intercostal space above and below the involved rib reveals tenderness and increased muscle tension.
5. Lateral rib compression
   a. There is more prominence of the involved rib in the anterior and posterior rib cage.
   b. There is less prominence of the involved rib in the midaxillary line.
   c. The intercostal space above and below the involved rib reveals tenderness and increased muscle tension.
6. Laterally flexed rib
   a. There is prominence of the involved rib in the midaxillary line.
   b. There is a narrow intercostal space above and a wider intercostal space below the involved rib.
   c. There is marked tenderness, usually in the intercostal space above the involved rib.
   d. This restriction is most commonly seen in the second rib.

Evaluation of the First Rib for Respiratory Rib Somatic Dysfunction

The first rib is evaluated for respiratory somatic dysfunction as follows:

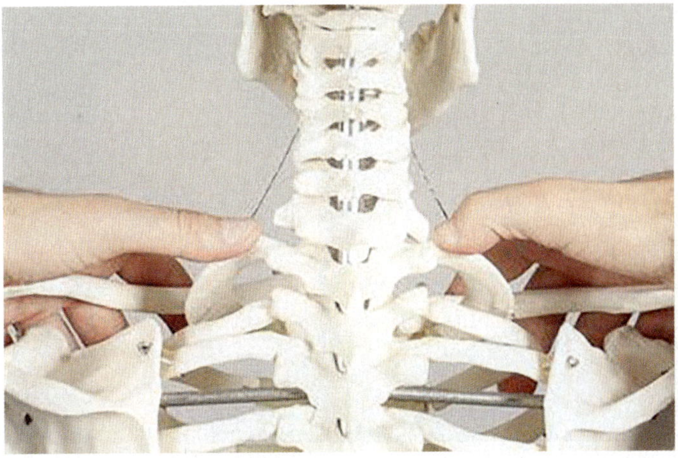

Figure 35.14. Contacting the posterior shafts of the first rib.

1. The patient is seated or supine on the examination table.
2. The physician stands behind the patient if the patient is seated or sits at the head of the table if the patient is supine.
3. The physician uses the thumbs to make bilateral contact with the posterolateral shafts of the patient's first ribs, immediately lateral to the costotransverse articulation (Fig. 35.14).
4. The patient is instructed to inhale and exhale deeply.
   - ☐ The inability of one or the other first rib to descend into the exhalation position indicates *exhalation restriction* and is diagnosed as an *inhalation somatic dysfunction* or *inhaled rib*.
   - ☐ The inability of one or the other first rib to ascend into the inhalation position indicates *inhalation restriction* or an *exhalation (exhaled rib) somatic dysfunction* of that rib.

Evaluation of Ribs 2 to 10 for Respiratory Rib Somatic Dysfunctions (Figs. 35.15 to 35.17)

During regional exam of the costal cage, asymmetry of motion in any of the rib cage areas indicates the presence of respiratory rib dysfunction in that region. Respiratory rib dysfunction has either inhalation or exhalation somatic dysfunction, which is usually maintained by one rib within a group of ribs. This rib is referred to as the key rib and must be identified and treated to remove the group restriction.

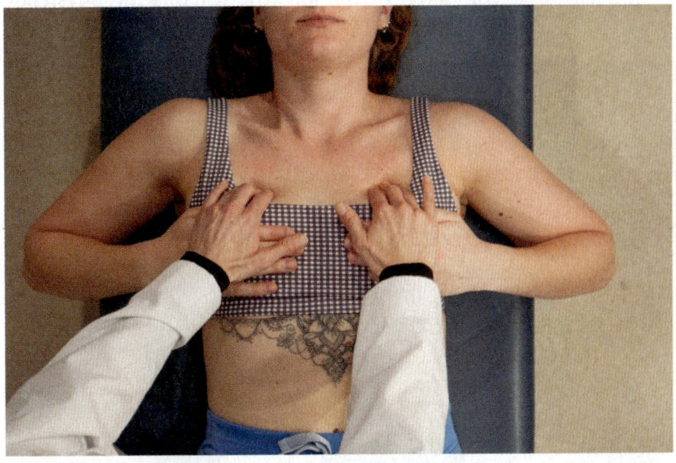

Figure 35.15. Assessing for key rib dysfunction of the pump handle ribs, in this example rib 4. Note that the physician may instruct the patient to cover any sensitive areas of anatomy if needed. (Photo courtesy of Western University of Health Sciences, Pomona, CA, with permission.)

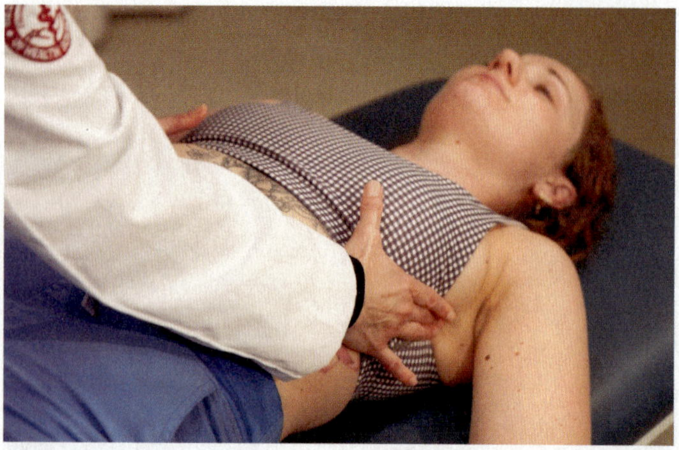

Figure 35.16. Assessing for key rib dysfunction of the mixed ribs, in this example rib 7. (Photo courtesy of Western University of Health Sciences, Pomona, CA, with permission.)

To identify the key rib within a group of ribs, the osteopathic physician may utilize the BITE mnemonic and evaluate the most superior pair of ribs of a group with exhalation somatic dysfunction and the most inferior pair of ribs of a group with an inhalation somatic dysfunction. These ribs may be examined individually by performing the following[17]:

1. Place a finger or finger pads on each pair of ribs to be examined, the parasternal area for pump handle ribs, and the midaxillary line for bucket handle ribs.
2. For each placement, ask the patient to inhale and exhale and note for asymmetry or symmetry of motion.
3. Palpate successive pairs of ribs within the group until symmetry of motion on respiration is noted. If the physician needs to assess ribs in a sensitive area, such as near the nipple, they may instruct the patient to place their hands over the sensitive region so that the physician can work around this area and not cause the patient discomfort.
4. If an inhalation somatic dysfunction was noted on the right ribs 5 to 7, the osteopathic physician should contact the most inferior pair of ribs (using the BITE mnemonic), ribs 7 bilaterally as described above. The patient is instructed to inhale and exhale. If the right rib 7 does not descend well during exhalation as compared to the left, the osteopathic physician should then assess ribs 8. If symmetric motion is noted at ribs 8 during inhalation and exhalation, right rib 7 is the key rib maintaining the somatic dysfunction. If ribs 8 continued to exhibit asymmetrical motion, the osteopathic physician should evaluate ribs 9.
5. If an exhalation somatic dysfunction was noted on the right ribs 5 to 7, the physician should begin the evaluation with the most superior pair of ribs, ribs 5. If the right rib 5 is restricted in rising superiorly during inhalation as compared to the left, the physician should then assess ribs 4. If they move symmetrically during inhalation and exhalation, then the right rib 5 is the key rib, maintaining the group exhalation somatic dysfunction.

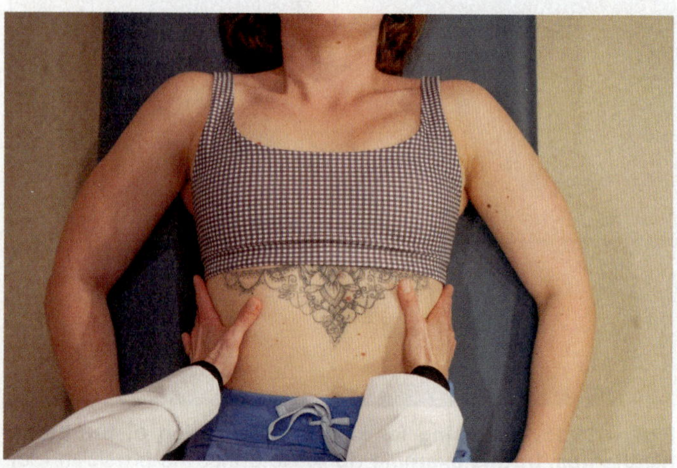

Figure 35.17. Assessing for key rib dysfunction of the bucket handle ribs, in this example rib 9. (Photo courtesy of Western University of Health Sciences, Pomona, CA, with permission.)

In summary, inhalation somatic dysfunctions (restricted in descending during exhalation) involve a rib or group of ribs that stop moving first during exhalation. The key rib is generally the most inferior rib of the group. Exhalation somatic dysfunctions involve ribs that are restricted in ascending during inhalation. The key rib is generally the most superior rib in the group.

Evaluation of Ribs 11 and 12 (Fig. 35.18)

Ribs 11 and 12 have no anterior cartilaginous attachment and therefore exhibit a caliper type of motion by moving posteriorly and laterally with inhalation, and anteriorly and medially during exhalation.

Assessment for respiratory dysfunction of ribs 11 and 12 is as follows:

1. The patient lies prone on the examination table.
2. The physician stands at the side of the patient, with the dominant eye over the patient's midline.
3. The physician's hands are placed over the 11th and 12th ribs, contacting the rib shafts with the thumbs and thenar eminences.
   a. Ask the patient to inhale and exhale fully; note any asymmetry of motion in the ribs.

      If either of the ribs do not move posteriorly with inhalation, an inhalation restriction or exhalation somatic dysfunction is present.

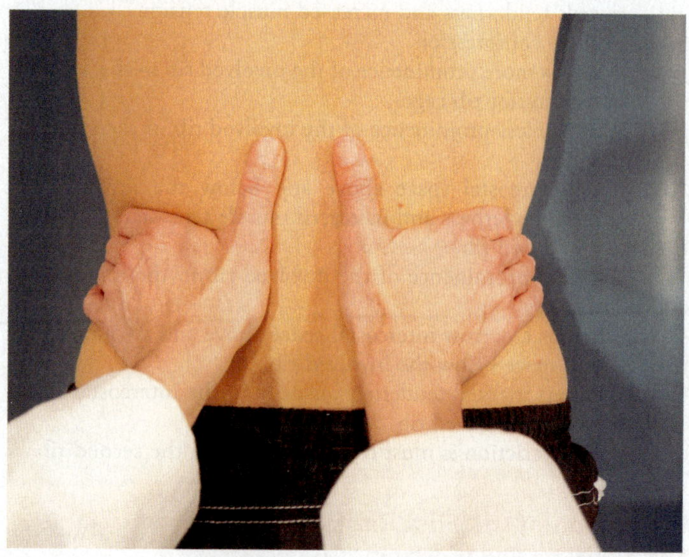

Figure 35.18. Assessing ribs 11 and 12 for key rib dysfunction. (Photo courtesy of Western University of Health Sciences, Pomona, CA, with permission.)

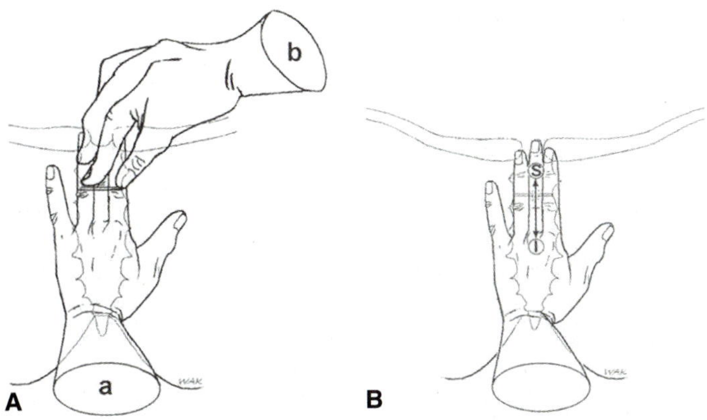

Figure 35.19. Osteopathic Segmental Exam. Evaluation of the sternum.

b. Conversely, if the ribs do not move anteriorly with exhalation, an exhalation restriction or inhalation somatic dysfunction is present.

Sternum Evaluation

Compression and decompression of the sternum can be a valuable diagnostic test, especially when there has been a history of trauma or surgery. Two common examples are sternocostal problems associated with seat belt injuries in motor vehicle accidents, and mechanical chest wall problems secondary to coronary artery bypass surgery.

Sternal Compression

Testing the sternum *involves* gentle compression and release with particular attention to respiratory, mechanical, and pain-related responses arising both locally and from distant points.

To test the motion of the sternum:

1. Place one hand longitudinally on the manubrium and the body of the sternum, and the fingers of the other hand on top of the first hand (Fig. 35.19A).
2. Compress slightly, noting any indication that the tissue moves more easily in one or more directions as the patient goes through the respiratory cycle.
3. Place one hand longitudinally on the manubrium and the body of the sternum, and apply a superior and inferior gliding motion, noting whether motion is restricted in one direction or the other (Fig. 35.19B).

Sternal Segmental Examination

The sternum may also be examined segmentally as follows:

1. The manubrium may be tested by placing the thumbs first on the upper and lower portions of the manubrium in the midline (Fig. 35.20), then on the anterolateral aspects of the middle portion of the manubrium, and finally on the upper and lower opposite corners of the manubrium. Motion of the manubrium can be tested around transverse, longitudinal, and oblique axes, respectively.
2. A similar approach may be used to test the motion of the body of the sternum (Fig. 35.21).
3. Perform a motion test at the xiphisternal joint using one thenar eminence on the sternum and a single finger (or the thumb and a finger) on the inferior border of the xiphoid. Maintain slight pressure on the sternum while depressing and then lifting the xiphoid with slight anterosuperior pressure. Note any tendency for the tissues to move toward a position of ease.

In addition to the above evaluations, the physician should also examine the rib cage for the following:

1. Myofascial restrictions. See Chapter 52 for more information on the evaluation of myofascial tissues for somatic dysfunction.
2. Counterstrain tender points. See Chapter 47 for more information on counterstrain diagnosis and treatment.

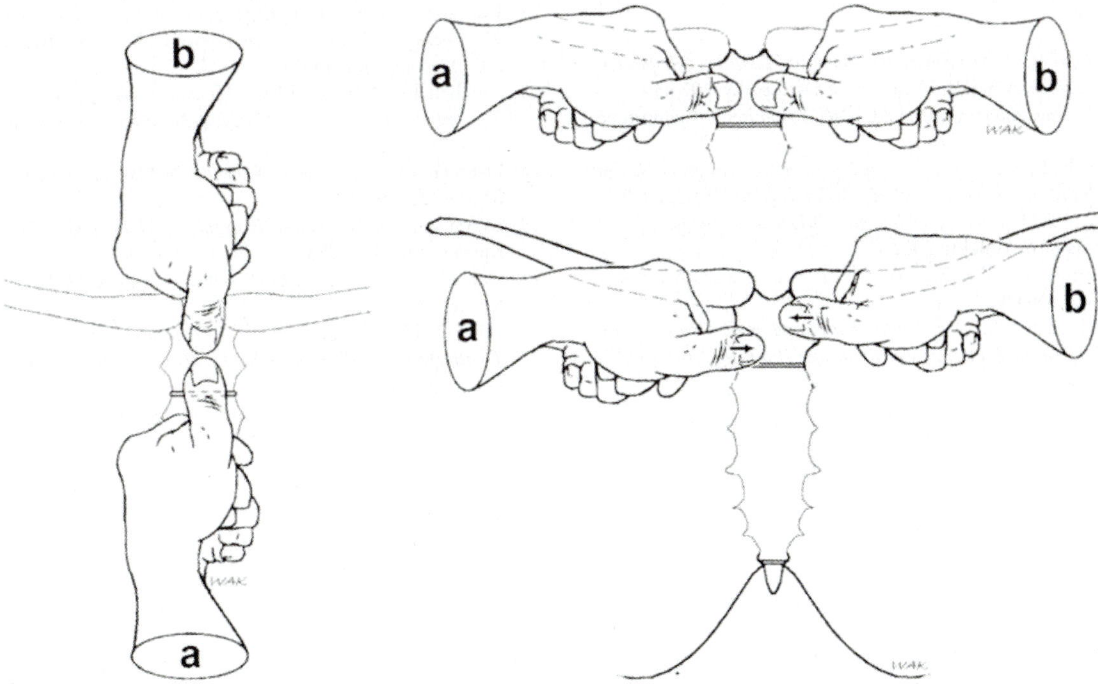

Figure 35.20. Segmental evaluation of the manubrium of the sternum.

Figure 35.21. Segmental evaluation of the manubrium of the sternum.

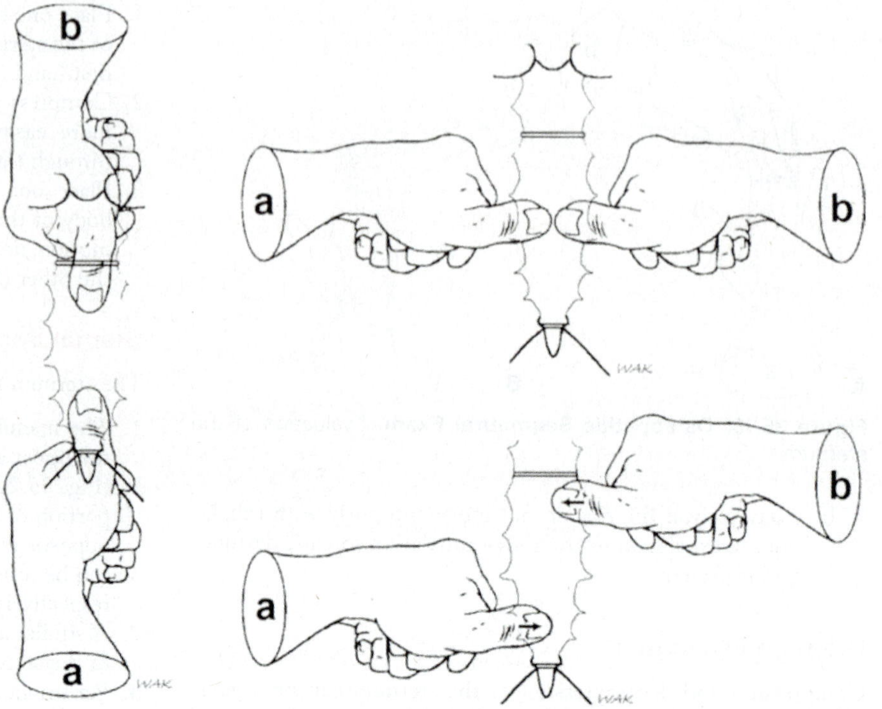

3. Chapman reflexes. See Chapter 58 for further details regarding Chapman reflexes.

SUMMARY

An in-depth knowledge of the anatomy of the rib cage region, along with the skilled use of osteopathic palpatory diagnosis, can help to inform the successful practice of osteopathic medicine. Such a combination of knowledge and skills can lead to more efficient and accurate patient diagnoses, and more rational and effective treatment decisions.

REFERENCES

1. Cathie AH. *Physiological Motions of the Spine as Related to Respiratory Activity. AAO Yearbook*. American Academy of Osteopathy; 1974:59.
2. Standring S, ed. *Gray's Anatomy*. 42nd ed. Elsevier Churchill Livingstone; 2021.
3. Schunke M, Schulte E, Schumacher U, eds. *Thieme Atlas of Anatomy: General Anatomy and Musculoskeletal System*. 3rd ed. Georg Thieme Verlag; 2020.
4. Dalley AF, Agur AMR. *Moore's Clinically Oriented Anatomy*. 9th ed. Lippincott, Williams & Wilkins; 2022.
5. Hruby RJ, Martinez ES. The lymphatic system: an osteopathic review. *Cureus*. 2021;13(7):e16448.
6. Mitchell FL, Mitchell PKG. *The Muscle Energy Manual: Evolution and Treatment of the Thoracic Spine, Lumbar Spine and Rib Cage*. Vol. 2. MET Press; 1998:50–51.
7. DeStefano LA. *Greenman's Principles of Manual Medicine*. 5th ed. Wolters Kluwer; 2017:249–250.
8. Mitchell FL, Mitchell PKG. *The Muscle Energy Manual: Evolution and Treatment of the Thoracic Spine, Lumbar Spine and Rib Cage*. Vol. 2. MET Press; 1998:52.
9. Mitchell FL, Mitchell PKG. *The Muscle Energy Manual: Evolution and Treatment of the Thoracic Spine, Lumbar Spine and Rib Cage*. Vol. 2. MET Press; 1998:133–141.
10. Mitchell FL, Mitchell PKG. *The Muscle Energy Manual: Evolution and Treatment of the Thoracic Spine, Lumbar Spine and Rib Cage*. Vol. 2. MET Press; 1998:87.
11. DeStefano LA. *Greenman's Principles of Manual Medicine*. 5th ed. Wolters Kluwer; 2017:257.
12. Educational Council on Osteopathic Principles. *Glossary of Osteopathic Terminology*. American Association of Colleges of Osteopathic Medicine; 2017 (see appendix in this volume).
13. Mitchell FL, Mitchell PKG. *The Muscle Energy Manual: Evolution and Treatment of the Thoracic Spine, Lumbar Spine and Rib Cage*. Vol. 2. MET Press; 1998:60.
14. DeStefano LA. *Greenman's Principles of Manual Medicine*. 5th ed. Wolters Kluwer; 2017:253.
15. DeStefano LA. *Greenman's Principles of Manual Medicine*. 5th ed. Wolters Kluwer; 2017:251–253.
16. DeStefano LA. *Greenman's Principles of Manual Medicine*. 5th ed. Wolters Kluwer; 2017:257–258.
17. Mitchell FL, Mitchell PKG. *The Muscle Energy Manual: Evolution and Treatment of the Thoracic Spine, Lumbar Spine and Rib Cage*. Vol. 2. MET Press; 1998:61–63.

36 Lumbar Region

KAREN T. SNIDER ▪ ADRIAN L. WOOLLEY

KEY CONCEPTS

- Descriptive and functional anatomy of the lumbar spine
- Clinical aspects of lumbar structure and function interrelationships
- The impact of somatic dysfunction in the lumbar region
- Screening and diagnosis of somatic dysfunction in the lumbar region

INTRODUCTION

Common patient complaints that require evaluation of the lumbar region include, but are not limited to, the following:

- Gastrointestinal complaints
- Urogenital complaints
- Numbness in the lower extremities
- Pain in the abdomen, lower back, pelvis, or lower extremities

In the presence of any of these symptoms, and as part of an integrated physical examination, the lumbar region should be examined for somatic dysfunctions that may be contributing to the patient's complaint. If potentially contributing somatic dysfunctions are found, osteopathic manipulative treatment (OMT) may be used as part of a comprehensive treatment plan that includes other interventions, such as medications, lifestyle interventions, and stretches or exercises. This chapter highlights the anatomical basis for applying osteopathic principles and practices (OPP), including OMT, to the evaluation and management of conditions involving the lumbar region.

DEFINITION

The lumbar region comprises the five vertebrae at the distal end of the spinal column between the twelfth thoracic vertebra (T12) and the first sacral vertebra (S1). It also includes the supporting ligaments and myofascial structures between the twelfth ribs and the iliac crests.

DESCRIPTIVE AND FUNCTIONAL ANATOMY

Skeletal Structures

The lumbar spine normally consists of five vertebrae arranged in a lordotic curve just above the pelvis. The five lumbar vertebrae are the largest individual vertebral segments in the spinal column and serve the functional need of carrying the weight of the upper half of the body without supporting bony elements, such as ribs. The regional anatomy allows for more gross range of motion than that permitted in the adjacent thoracic cage and pelvic region. However, greater range of motion with less bony support makes the lumbar region more prone to injury, thus resulting in low back pain as one of the most common musculoskeletal complaints globally.[1]

The functional relationship between each individual vertebra and its surrounding structures is contingent on proper anatomy that, when disturbed by disease states or trauma, can lead to somatic dysfunctions which may impact the rest of the body. The location of a patient's symptoms does not necessarily indicate the location of the etiology of the patient's complaint. Consistent with the osteopathic tenet of body unity, dysfunction throughout the body can impact, or be impacted by, dysfunctions in the lumbar region.

VERTEBRAL BODIES (FIG. 36.1)

The lumbar vertebrae can be distinguished from the other spinal vertebrae by the absence of costal facets, which are present in the thoracic vertebrae, and by the absence of transverse foramina, which are present in the cervical vertebrae. The lumbar vertebral body is wider transversely and deeper anteroposteriorly than any other vertebra.[2] This large, cross-sectional area—and its longitudinal and vertical trabecular arrangement—increases its strength and stability. Lumbar vertebrae are capable of sustaining the heavy, functional, longitudinal loads that are typically placed on them. However, the compressive strength tends to decrease with age.[3] The vertebral bodies can also act as accessory organs for hematopoiesis in patients with impaired erythropoiesis like thalassemia major.[4]

Lumbosacral transitional vertebrae are congenital anomalies affecting the transition between L5 and S1 (Fig. 36.2). Types of transitional vertebrae include lumbarization, which occurs when S1 does not fuse properly with S2 and can appear as a sixth lumbar vertebra, and sacralization, which occurs when L5 fuses to S1 to become part of the sacrum, leaving only four functional lumbar vertebrae. These anomalies can affect the anatomy and function of the vertebral body, the transverse processes, the facet joints, and the intervertebral disks.[5] Further, these anomalies can present as a complete fusion, incomplete fusion, or as a unilateral anomaly that is only fused on one side.[5] The altered anatomy is associated with altered function and can lead to local degenerative changes. Symptoms originating from these anomalies will typically occur at the level above a complete fusion or at the contralateral facet when there is unilateral fusion.[5] Because transitional vertebrae affect the apparent number of vertebrae in the lumbar region, identifying the presence of these anomalies is important for proper localization when interventional procedures or surgery are being considered.[5]

INTERVERTEBRAL DISKS (FIG. 36.3)

An intervertebral disk is located between each lumbar vertebra. Combined, the intervertebral disks account for 20% to 25% of the length of the vertebral column, but in the lumbar spine, they account for approximately 35% of the length of the region.[6,7] Intervertebral disks are commonly named according to adjacent superior and inferior vertebrae. For example, the intervertebral disk between L2 and L3 is referred to as the L2/L3 disk.[6]

Lumbar disks are large and built to tolerate and dissipate heavy loads. They consist of water, collagen, proteoglycans, and glycoproteins.

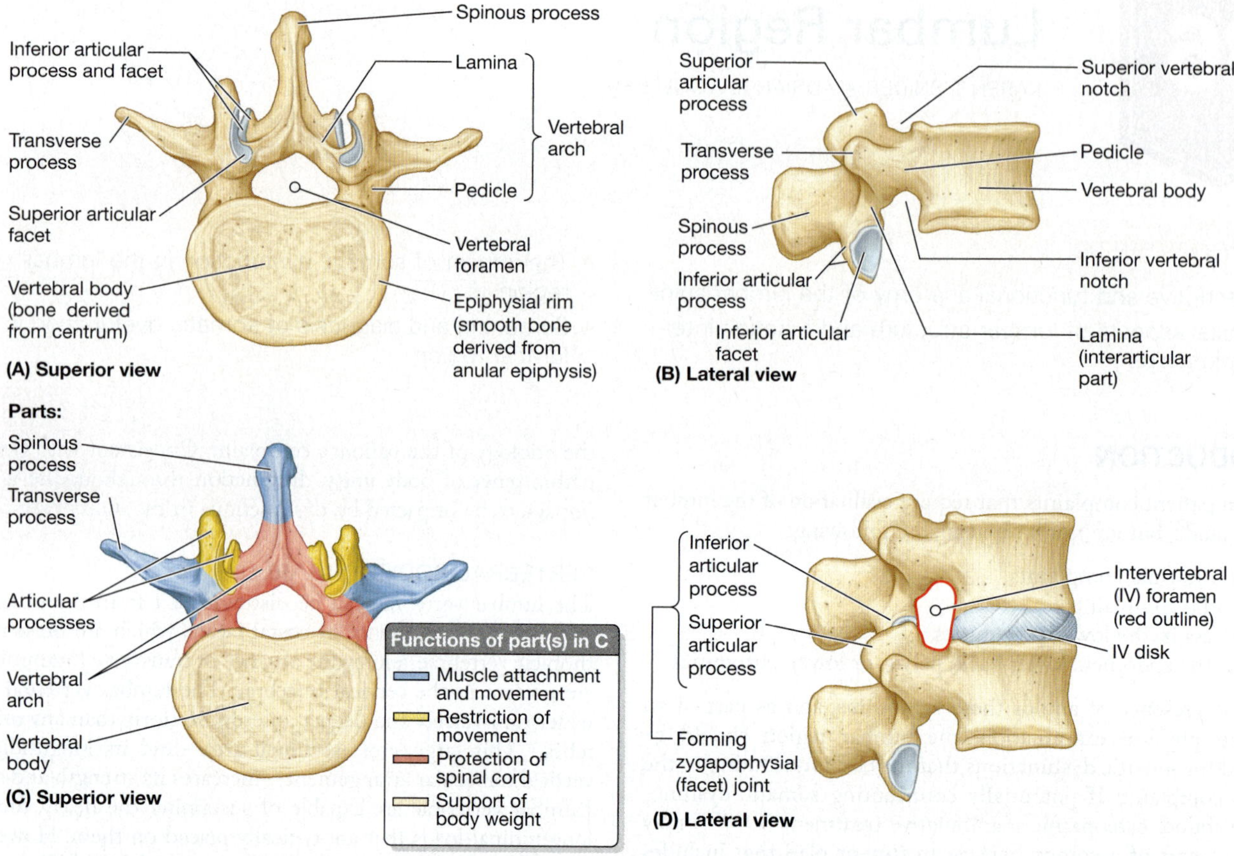

Figure 36.1. **Typical lumbar vertebra as represented by the L2 vertebra. A, B.** Bony features. **C.** Functional components. **D.** Formation of intervertebral foramen between the vertebral unit. (Reprinted with permission from Agur AMR, Dalley AF II. *Moore's Essential Clinical Anatomy*. 7th ed. Wolters Kluwer; 2024:49. Figure 2.2.)

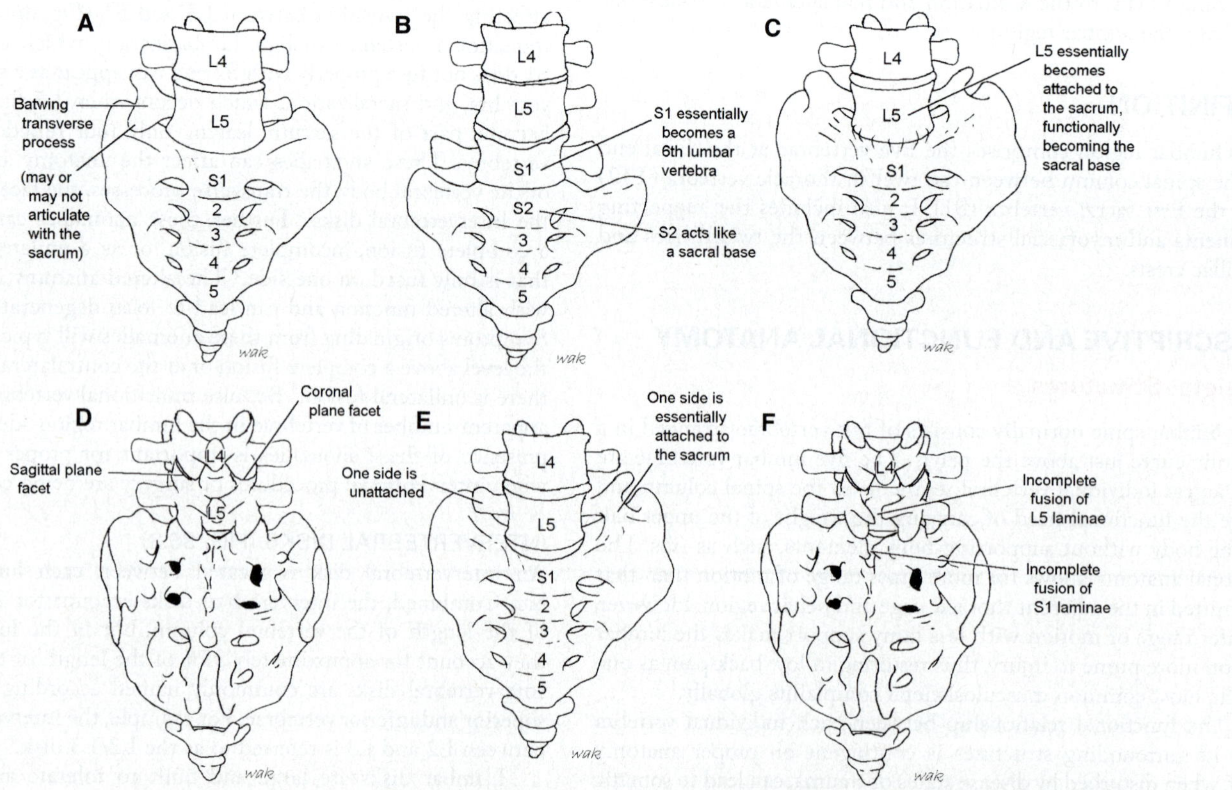

Figure 36.2. **Lumbar transitional vertebrae and common lumbosacral abnormalities. A.** Batwing transverse process of L5. **B.** Lumbarization of S1. **C.** Sacralization of L5. **D.** Facet asymmetry (zygapophyseal facet tropism) of L4. **E.** Partial sacralization of L5. **F.** Spina bifida occulta of L5 and S1. (Courtesy of William Kuchera, DO, FAAO.)

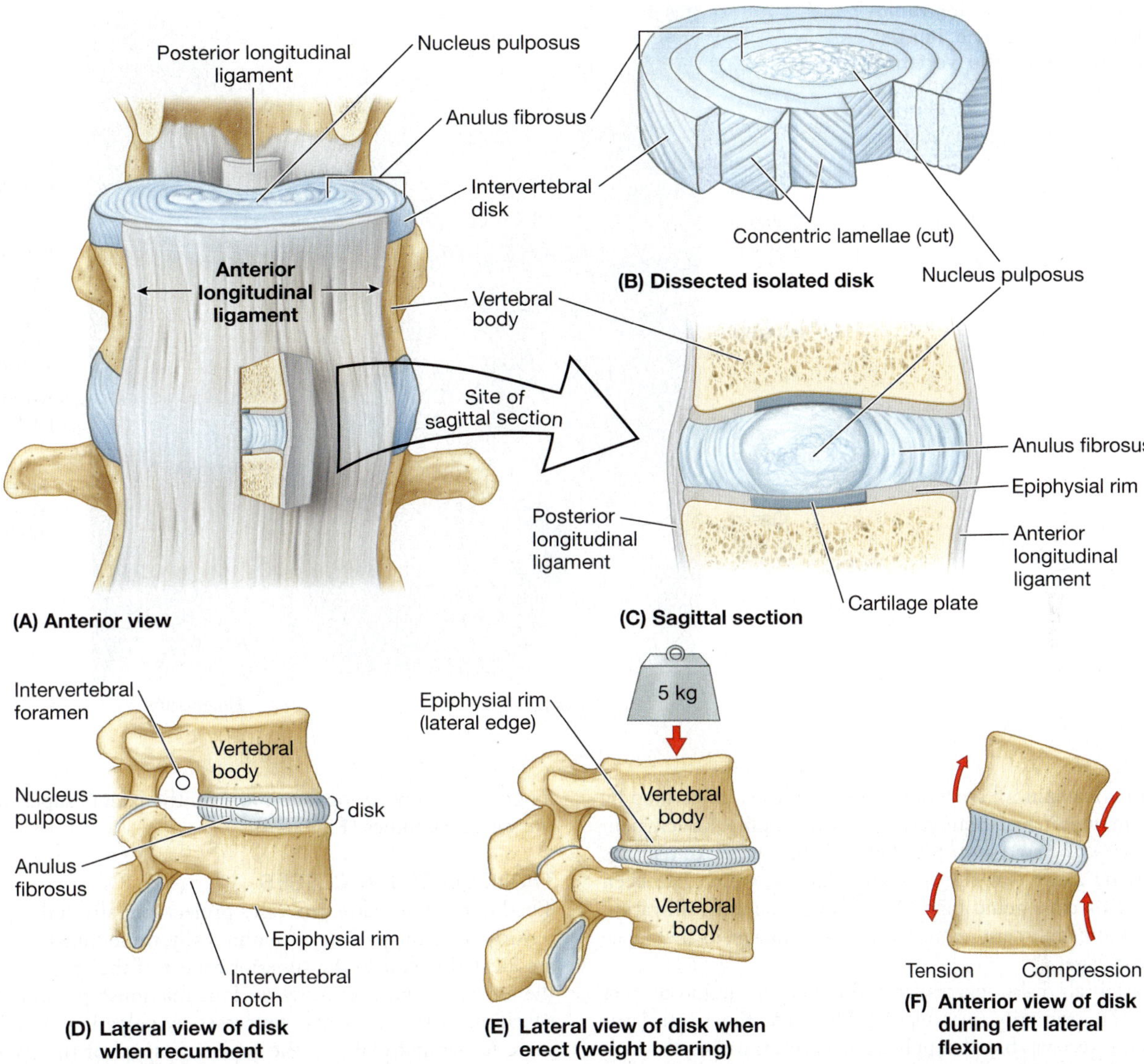

Figure 36.3. Structure of the intervertebral disk. A. Anterior view. **B.** Dissected isolated disk. **C.** Sagittal section. **D.** Non–weight-bearing. **E, F.** Intervertebral disk during loading and movement. (Reprinted with permission from Agur AMR, Dalley AF II. *Moore's Essential Clinical Anatomy.* 7th ed. Wolters Kluwer; 2024:60. Figure 2.8.)

Each disk is joined superiorly and inferiorly to the adjacent cartilaginous endplates of the vertebral body endplates and joined anteriorly and posteriorly to the respective longitudinal ligaments.[8] The center of the disk contains a gelatinous nucleus pulposus surrounded by layers of the annulus fibrosus. The annulus is composed of 70% water, bound in collagenous fibers that provide high tensile strength.[8] Smaller amounts of hydrophilic proteoglycans, such as chondroitin, and glycoproteins, such as elastin, are also present and provide resilience to compression.[8] These annulus fibers are arranged in concentric lamellae oriented at a diagonal angle of greater than 60 degrees.[6,8] Each layer alternates obliquely as it encircles and contains the nucleus pulposus.[6,8] These alternating layers of lamellae allow for a small amount of intersegmental rotation while providing strong structural support.[6] In the lumbar spine, the annulus of a lumbar disk is thicker anteriorly than posteriorly, which contributes to the lordosis.[6] Even though the annular fibers are strong, herniations are most likely to occur posteriorly where the annulus fibers are thinner; 95% of nucleus pulposus protrusions occur at the L4–L5 or L5–S1 levels.[6]

The nucleus pulposus is composed of approximately 80% water, randomly distributed proteoglycans and collagen, and small amounts of glycoproteins.[8] This composition allows the nucleus pulposus to be elastic and deform under stress, while also remaining resilient and able to resist compression.[8] During postural weight bearing, the nucleus absorbs and redistributes the load radially to the annulus and vertically to the endplates, thus acting as a shock absorber.[8,9] When a vertical load is applied to the disk, the annulus and the nucleus are compressed and lose water.[9] Throughout the day, sustained vertical loading can result in 20% to 25% of the water being lost from the disks.[9] In the supine position, when the pressure is released, fluid will move back into the disk, resulting in a diurnal change in the disk height.[9] As part of the aging process, the large hydrophilic macromolecules in the annulus and nucleus pulposus break down into smaller molecules that bind and retain less water under compressive loads, which contributes to age-related degenerative changes, such as loss of disk height.[8] This loss of height of the disks combined with a decrease in height of the vertebral body contributes to the loss of overall body height seen with aging.[3]

In the normal disk, only the outer one-third of the annulus is innervated, and the nucleus pulposus receives no innervation.[10] Anteriorly, the annulus receives sensory innervation from the ventral rami of the adjacent spinal nerves, and the gray rami communicates from

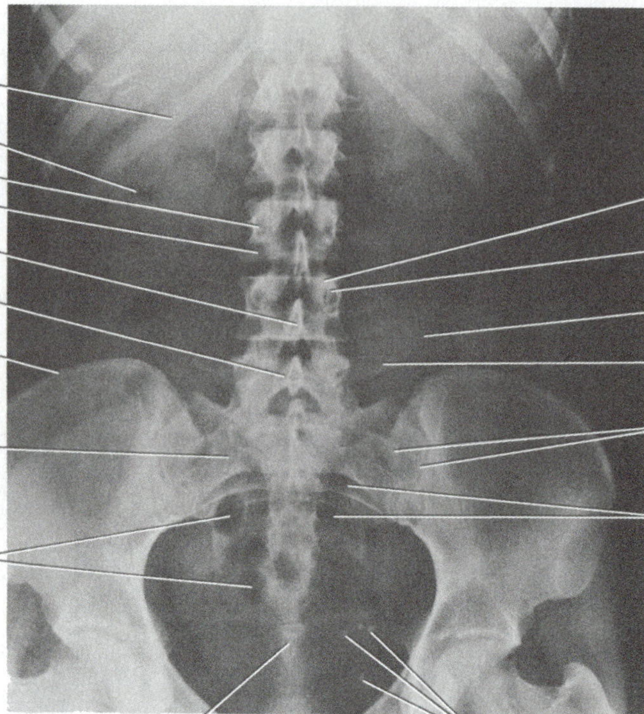

Figure 36.4. Anteroposterior radiograph of the lower thoracic, lumbar, and sacral regions of the vertebral column. (Reprinted with permission from Wineski LE. *Snell's Clinical Anatomy by Regions.* 10th ed. Wolters Kluwer; 2019:79. Figure 2.31.)

the sympathetic chain.[8,10] Posteriorly, the annulus is innervated by the recurrent meningeal branches of ventral rami.[8,10] Back pain symptoms are associated with a higher incidence of nerve endings infiltrating the inner two-thirds of the annulus, which has been correlated with diskogenic pain.[8,10] Although neural infiltration tends to be more abundant in areas with disk damage, its incidence increases with age.[8,10]

Intervertebral disks, particularly the nucleus pulposus, are thought to be primarily avascular.[8,11] However, the outer layer of the annulus receives blood supply from vessels traveling through the surrounding longitudinal ligaments.[11] Although this blood supply is robust early in life, it typically decreases with age. Disk degeneration and injury, such as disk protrusions, extrusions, and sequestrations, are associated with vascular invasion into the inner layers of the annulus.[11] The nucleus has been shown to be avascular throughout its lifespan, and its nutrition is primarily obtained through passive diffusion from the endplates or through the annulus.[11] Altered nutrient delivery to the disk is associated with aging and disk degeneration.[11]

PEDICLES

Pedicles connect the vertebral body to the posterior elements, including the lamina, the facet joints, and the transverse and spinous processes. The pedicles of each vertebral unit form the superior and inferior borders of the intervertebral foramen. The exiting nerve roots contact the superior border along the pedicles of the superior vertebra of the unit.[12] The medial aspects of the pedicles form the lateral recess of the spinal canal and contact the dural sac in the upper lumbar region and nerve roots in the lower lumbar region.[12] The lateral aspect of the lumbar pedicles is in contact with the psoas muscle.[12] In the lumbar region, pedicles project from the upper third of the posterior vertebral body. This position provides space for the nerve root to exit even in the presence of a herniation of the intervertebral disk at the same vertebral unit. On an anteroposterior (AP) radiograph, the pedicles appear as two longitudinal rows of opaque ovals on the lateral, superior third of the vertebral bodies (Fig. 36.4).

TRANSVERSE PROCESSES

The lumbar transverse processes project laterally and slightly posteriorly from the pedicles. Anatomically, these transverse processes are located lateral to the superior aspect of the spinous process of the associated lumbar vertebra. This relationship allows for identification of the transverse processes by palpating laterally in the same horizontal plane to the superior aspect of the spinous processes (Fig. 36.1). The transverse processes of the lumbar spine are the attachment site for a large number of muscles, including the psoas anteriorly and the iliocostalis, longissimus, multifidi, and lumbar aponeurosis posteriorly[13] (see Lumbar Musculature). Somatic dysfunctions, such as hypertonicity of these muscular structures, can present as asymmetry of the transverse processes, which can impact the postural balance.[13,14]

SUPERIOR AND INFERIOR ARTICULAR PROCESSES AND FACET JOINTS

The articular processes of the lumbar vertebra project from the pedicles inferiorly and superiorly and articulate with the adjacent vertebrae at the cartilage-covered facets of the zygapophyseal or facet joints[15] (Fig. 36.1). The facets at the end of the inferior articular process face laterally, while the facets at the end of the superior articular process face medially.[15] In the lumbar region, the synovial facet joints are at the level of the base of the spinous processes.[15] The facet joints are vertical and gradually change from a sagittal orientation at T12/L1 and to coronal orientation at L5/S1.[15] Congenital lumbosacral anomalies of facet orientation are fairly common (Figs. 36.2D and 36.5) and can affect the function of the lumbar region.[16] Facet tropism, which is asymmetry of the sagittal orientation between the left and right facet joints, results in asymmetrical loading forces on the facets during lumbar movement.[16] The presence of facet tropism is associated with an

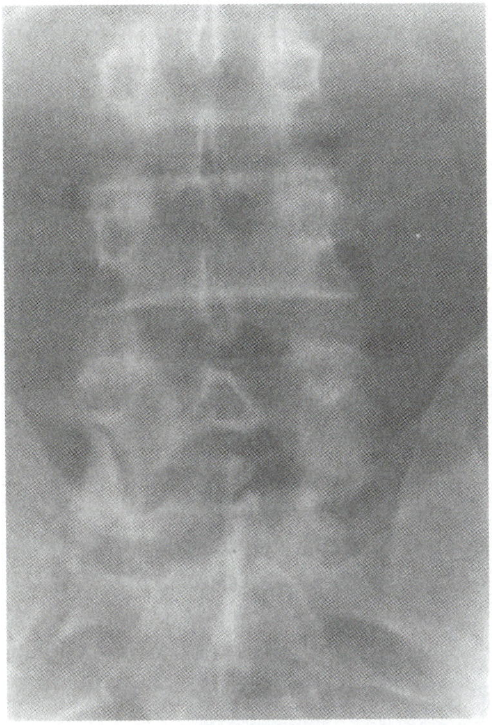

Figure 36.5. Facet tropism of L5–S1. Note asymmetry of the sagittal orientation between the left and right L5–S1 facet joints. (Reprinted with permission from Anrig CA, Plaugher G. *Pediatric Chiropractic*. 2nd ed. Wolters Kluwer Health/Lippincott Williams & Wilkins; 2013. Figure 4-11.)

increased incidence of low back pain and pathologic changes in the vertebral disk, most notably at the L4–L5 level.[16,17] However, some controversy exists about whether this is a congenital deformity or caused by progressive remodeling of the joint secondary to degenerative changes.[18]

Lumbar facet joints have long been considered a source of low back pain and are often targeted for interventional pain management procedures, such as facet nerve ablations.[19] The facet joint is richly innervated by branches from the medial divisions of the dorsal rami above and below the joint; however, the majority of the innervation is thought to be from efferent sympathetic fibers rather than sensory.[20] The lumbar facet joints contain both nociceptive and proprioceptive innervation.[21] Pain from the facet joints may be referred to the lower extremity but not typically below the knee.[19]

LAMINAE

The laminae connect the pedicles to the spinous process of the vertebra. The laminae project medially and inferiorly and connect at the posterior midline to form the spinous process. In some people, the laminae will not completely close or fuse in the midline during development, causing a spina bifida deformity.[7] The most serious form of spina bifida occurs when the neural tube fails to close and the spinal membranes protrude, with or without cord tissue, forming a meningocele or meningomyelocele, respectively. Spina bifida occulta occurs when the posterior elements of the spine do not close completely, but there is no impact on the spinal cord or meninges. This anomaly, which is present in up to 10% of the population, most commonly occurs at L5/S1 and is often undetected until an imaging study of the lumbar spine reveals its presence.[22,23] Most patients are asymptomatic, but spina bifida occulta is associated with instability at the base of the lumbar spine and an increased incidence of spondylolysis.[24] Spondylolysis is a pars defect characterized by a fracture of the pars interarticularis, which is associated with back pain. Without the support of the posterior elements, the vertebra can slip anteriorly or posteriorly resulting in a spondylolisthesis[24,25] (Fig. 36.6) or a retrolisthesis.

SPINOUS PROCESSES

Clinically, the spinous process of a lumbar vertebra is located at about the same horizontal plane as its associated transverse processes. Lumbar spinous processes are distinguished from the other vertebra by their palpable thick, quadrangular, distal ends (Fig. 36.1). The transition between the fingertip-shaped thoracic spinous processes and the much larger lumbar spinous processes can be used to identify L1. The third spinous process tends to be the largest, and the fifth spinous process is the smallest.[26] The height of the spinous processes increases with age and contributes to the reduced extension range of motion and anterior disk space narrowing seen with age-related degenerative changes.[3]

The superior root of the lumbar spinous processes is in the same horizontal plane as the transverse processes. The intercristal line between the iliac crests, also known as Tuffier line, most often intersects the L4 body or its inferior endplate in men and the L5 body or superior endplate in women. However, because of this variability, using only the intercristal line as the sole landmark for palpatory identification of lumbar segmental level is insufficient.[27] When attempting to identify the different levels of the lumbar spine, a clinician may use this landmark as an initial starting point and cross-reference with the insertion of the 12th rib on T12.

Palpation of a shelf or step-off may indicate a spondylolisthesis with a pars defect, thus suggesting instability that needs additional evaluation (Fig. 36.6). Lateral radiographs with flexion and extension views can be used to determine whether instability is present with motion. Anterior or posterior translation of the affected vertebra of more than 3 mm between flexion and extension positions indicates that significant instability is present.[28,29]

SPINAL CANAL

The spinal canal, also known as the vertebral canal, is the anatomic space bordered by the posterior margin of a vertebral body, the medial pedicles, and the posterior laminae. It contains the dural tube, spinal cord, and origins of the spinal nerves down to approximately the L1–L2 or L2–L3 level, where the spinal cord terminates as the conus medullaris. Extending distally from the conus medullaris is the cauda equina, which consists of the L2–S5 spinal nerve roots and the filum terminale, an extension of pia mater, which terminates at the periosteum of the dorsal aspect of the coccyx.[30]

INTERVERTEBRAL FORAMINA (FIG. 36.1)

Intervertebral foramina are located bilaterally and are bordered anteriorly by the two adjacent vertebral bodies and the intervertebral disk between them. The superior and inferior borders are formed by the pedicles of the adjacent vertebrae. The posterior aspect of the foramina is bordered by the facet joint and the inferior articular process of the superior adjacent vertebra and the articular process of the inferior adjacent vertebra. In addition to arterial, venous, and lymphatic vessels, a spinal nerve passes through each foramen. A recurrent meningeal nerve also branches off the spinal nerve lateral to the opening and travels back through the foramen to innervate the ligaments and dura in the spinal canal.[6] The foramina also contains several ligaments that stabilize the nerve roots. These nerves occupy approximately one-third of the lumbar foraminal area,[31] thus providing space for the nerve to move and not become compressed. During flexion, the pedicles move superiorly as the facet surfaces glide away from one another, and the size of the intervertebral foramen increases. During extension, the

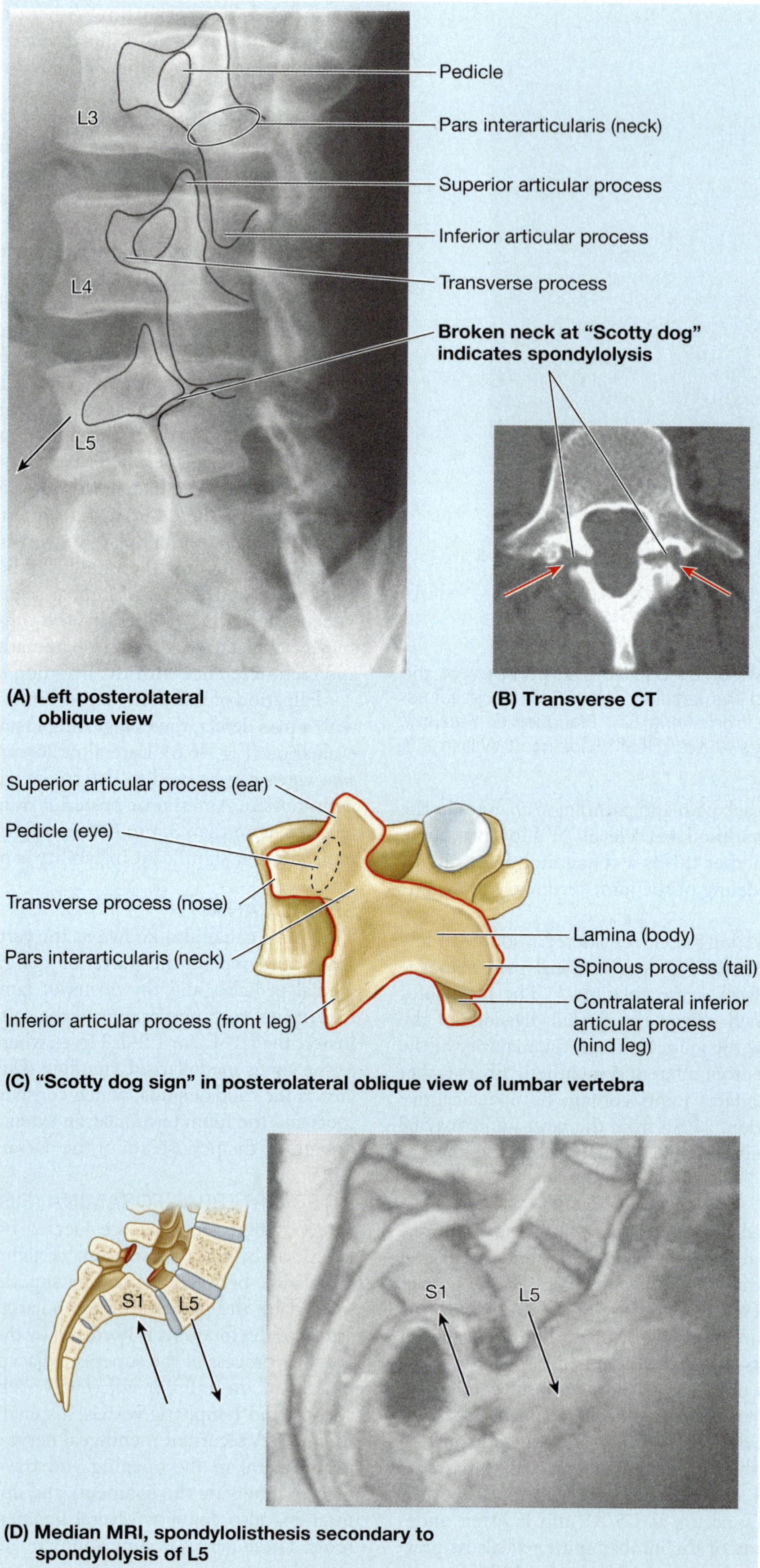

Figure 36.6. Spondylolysis and spondylolisthesis. (Reprinted with permission from Moore KL, Dalley AF II, Agur AMR. *Clinically Oriented Anatomy*. 7th ed. Wolters Kluwer Health/Lippincott Williams & Wilkins; 2014:479. Figure B4.16.)

pedicles move inferiorly as the facets glide toward one another and the foramen is reduced in size. Reduction of the foramen size can also result from the following:

- Arthritis, osteophytes, or hypertrophy of the facets
- Hypertrophy of the posterior longitudinal ligament
- Disk widening, displacement, or extrusion
- Tissue congestion or edema
- Inflammation
- Perineural edema

Removal or reduction of the compressive effect produced by any of these factors may allow a symptomatic patient with complaints of back pain, radiculopathy, or paresthesia to become asymptomatic, thus leading to a better quality of life.

Supportive Tissues

MUSCULATURE

The lumbar musculature stabilizes the spine and provides dynamic motion. The muscles—through their origins, insertions, and actions—directly link the lumbar spine with the adjacent body regions. Their fascial sheaths are connected to the fascia of adjacent structures. The combined effect is a myofascial continuity of the lumbar region with the rest of the body.[32,33] For example, the psoas muscle originates at the lumbar transverse processes and intervertebral disks and inserts at the lesser trochanter of the femur. The psoas muscle fibers descend from the lumbar region, cross the sacral and pelvic regions, and join with the iliacus muscle before inserting in the lower extremity region.[34] Its enveloping fascia blends with the muscle at its bony attachments, but it also blends with the fascia of the neighboring muscles, such as the quadratus lumborum and iliacus, which in turn blend with the fascia of their neighboring structures.[35] Somatic dysfunction, such as localized muscular hypertonicity, can directly impact the function of each body region associated with that muscle's origins, insertions, and actions, but it can also indirectly affect other body regions through the myofascial continuity.[32,33]

The muscles relating to the lumbar region can be thought of as being located anterior or posterior to the spine (Fig. 36.7).

Anterior Muscles

1. Psoas major (and psoas minor when present)[35]
2. Iliacus and iliopsoas musculotendinous unit[36]
3. Abdominal muscles (rectus abdominis, external and internal obliques, and transversus abdominis)

Posterior Muscles

The posterior muscles can be classified as superficial, intermediate, or deep.

Superficial Muscles

1. Latissimus dorsi

Intermediate Muscles

1. Serratus posterior inferior
2. Erector spinae
   a. Iliocostalis
   b. Longissimus
   c. Spinalis

Deep Muscles

1. Transversospinales
   a. Semispinalis
   b. Rotatores
   c. Multifidus
2. Segmental
   a. Interspinales
   b. Intertransversarii
3. Quadratus lumborum

Table 36.1 lists the muscles of the lumbar spine and includes information about their origins, insertions, actions, and innervations.[37–40] Impaired or altered function of the musculature can cause, or be caused by, vertebral articular somatic dysfunction. In addition, muscle dysfunction may be compensatory to dysfunction in other areas of the body, so examination should also include surrounding body regions, including the shoulder girdle and the thoracic, pelvic, sacral, and lower extremity regions.

LIGAMENTS (FIG. 36.8)

The ligaments of the lumbar spine provide structural support to the bony framework, limit range of motion, and provide protection to the spinal canal and its neural elements. Most ligaments are continuous from the cervical to the thoracic and to the lumbosacral regions. Some ligaments cross over into the pelvis and play a key role in the self-bracing mechanism of the pelvis, which functions to maintain the integrity of the low back and pelvis during the transfer of energy from the spine to the lower extremities.[41] Ligaments, such as the iliolumbar ligament, also provide attachment sites for muscles. Nociceptive innervation of the longitudinal and spinous ligaments is primarily through the recurrent meningeal nerves and the gray rami communicantes from the sympathetic chain. Because of this structural continuity from the occiput and sacrum, these longitudinal ligaments are integral to the craniosacral mechanism and the concept of body unity. As a result, dysfunction throughout the body can impact or be impacted by dysfunction in the lumbar region.

In addition, the lumbar spine with its intimate connections to the thoracoabdominal diaphragm, may have a significant impact on the pressure gradients of the thorax and abdomen and on respiration. The crura of the diaphragm are musculotendinous bands that arise from the anterior longitudinal ligament, the anterior surfaces of the bodies of the three superior lumbar vertebrae, and their disks. The right crus arises from the first three or four lumbar vertebrae and ascends to the left of the spine forming the esophageal hiatus.[42] The vagus nerve also passes through the esophageal hiatus. The left crus arises from the first two or three lumbar vertebrae. The crura are united by the median arcuate ligament, which forms a fibrous arch (the aortic hiatus) over the anterior aspect of the aorta. The azygous vein and the thoracic duct also pass posterior to the diaphragm through the aortic hiatus.[42,43] The crura then ascend to the central tendon of the thoracoabdominal diaphragm. The corresponding crus of the median arcuate ligament then continues laterally as a thickening of fascia becoming the medial arcuate ligament (also called medial lumbocostal arch and internal arcuate ligament). The medial arcuate ligament attaches to the side of the body of the first or second lumbar vertebrae, crosses over the anterior aspect of the psoas major, and inserts into the anterior aspect of the transverse processes of L1 and sometimes L2.[42] From this insertion point, it continues as the lateral arcuate ligament (external arcuate ligament) which typically runs from the anterior aspect of the L1 transverse process to the tip and lower margin of the 12th rib, forming an arch over the quadratus lumborum muscle.[43] The sympathetic trunks enter the abdomen by piercing the crura of the diaphragm or by passing posterior to the medial arcuate ligament.[44]

Ligamentum Flavum

The ligamentum flavum, which is also known as the yellow ligament, extends from each pedicle to the lamina and makes up the

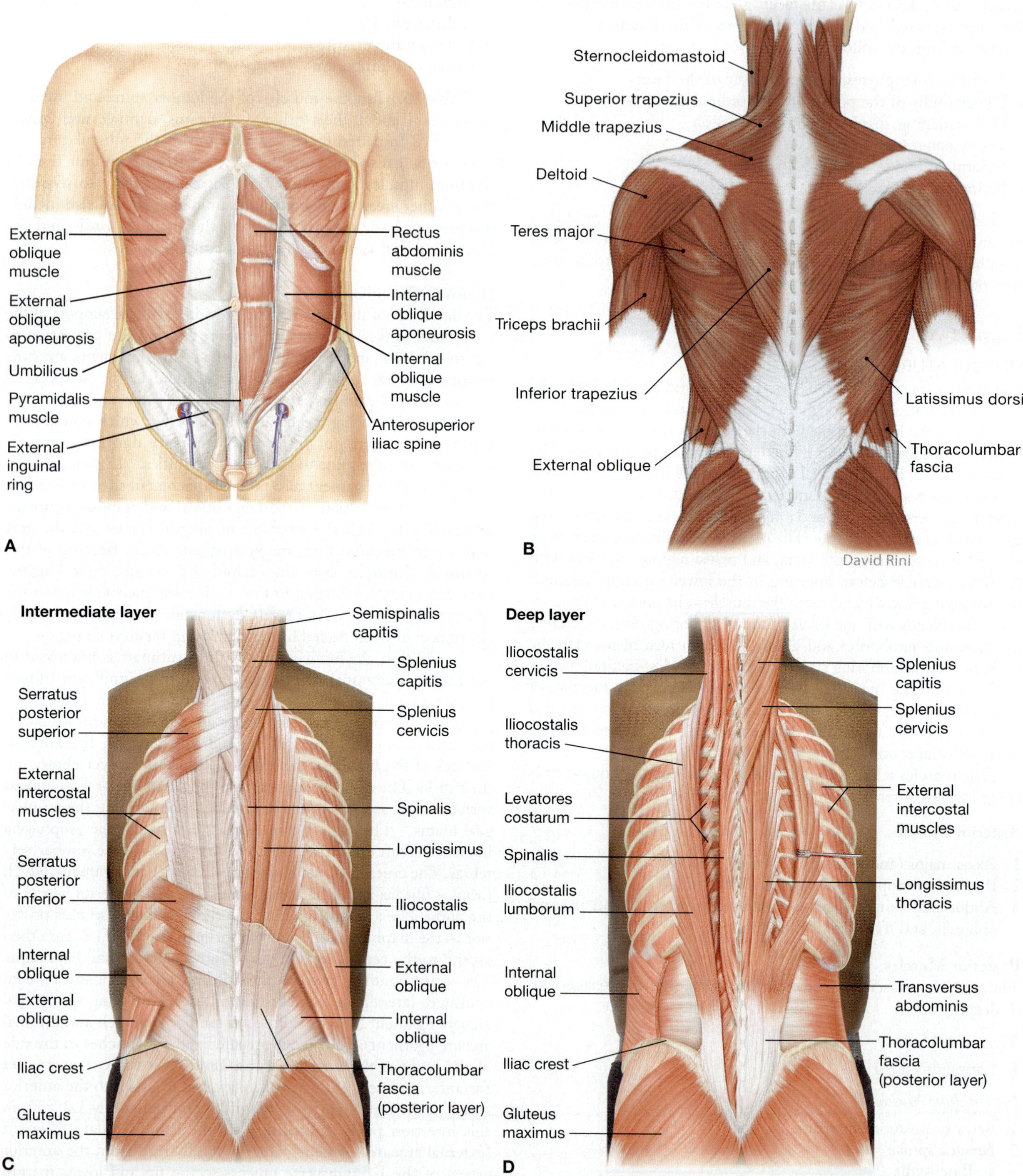

Figure 36.7. Anterior and posterior lumbar musculature. A. Anterior. **B.** Superficial posterior. **C.** Intermediate posterior. **D.** Deep posterior. (**A,** Reprinted with permission from Scott DJ, Rondon LA. Anatomy and pathophysiology of hernias. In: Jones DB, ed. *Master Techniques in Surgery: Hernia*. Wolters Kluwer Health/Lippincott Williams & Wilkins; 2013:3. Figure 1.2. **B,** Reprinted with permission from Werner R. *Scheumann's the Balanced Body: A Guide to the Integrated Deep Tissue Therapy System*. 4th ed. Wolters Kluwer; 2018:93. Figure 6-21B. **C, D,** Reprinted with permission from Nicholas AS, Nicholas EA. *Atlas of Osteopathic Techniques*. 4th ed. Wolters Kluwer; 2023:33. Figures 4.9 and 4.10.)

TABLE 36.1

Muscles of the Lumbar Region Origin, Insertion, Action, and Innervation—Includes Closely Related Thoracic and Abdominal Musculature That Influence the Lumbar Spine[36–39]

Muscles	Origin	Insertion	Action	Innervation
Psoas	Vertebral bodies, transverse processes, and intervertebral disks of T12 and L1–L5 (when present, psoas minor originates at T12–L1)	Lesser trochanter of the femur (when present, psoas minor inserts on medial innominate at pectineal line)	Flexion and external rotation of the hip	Anterior rami of L1–L3
Iliacus	Iliac fossa, anterior sacroiliac and iliolumbar ligaments, and superolateral surface of sacrum	Lesser trochanter of the femur	Flexion and external rotation of hip	Femoral nerve (L2–L4)
Rectus abdominis	Pubic symphysis, pubic crest, and pubic tubercle	Costal cartilage of ribs 5–7 and xiphoid process	Flexion of trunk Maintains abdominal wall tension which provides spine and pelvic stability	Ventral rami of T7–T12
Internal oblique	Lateral inguinal ligament, iliac crest, and thoracolumbar fascia	Inferior border of ribs 10–12, linea alba, xiphoid process, pubic symphysis, pubic crest, and pectineal line	Flexion of trunk when contracting bilaterally Flexion with ipsilateral rotation of trunk when contracting unilaterally Assists in maintaining intra-abdominal pressure Assists in forceful expiration by depressing the lower ribs	Ventral rami of T7–T12 and L1
External oblique	External surfaces of ribs 5–12	Anterolateral iliac crest, linea alba, xiphoid process, pubic symphysis, and pubic tubercle	Flexion of trunk when contracting bilaterally Flexion with contralateral rotation of trunk when contracting unilaterally Assists in maintaining intra-abdominal pressure Assists in forceful expiration by depressing lower ribs	Ventral rami of T7–T12
Transversus abdominis	Costal margin of ribs 7–12, lateral inguinal ligament, iliac crest, and thoracolumbar fascia	Linea alba, xiphoid process, and pubic symphysis	Maintains abdominal wall tension which provides spine and pelvic stability	Ventral rami of T7–T12 and L1
Latissimus dorsi	Spinous processes of T7–T12, ribs 10–12, thoracolumbar fascia, and iliac crest	Intertubercular sulcus of humerus	Extension, adduction, and medial rotation of humerus	Thoracodorsal nerve (C6–C8)
Serratus posterior inferior	Spinous processes of T11–L3	Inferior border of ribs 9–12	Depress ribs 9–12	Ventral rami of T9–T12
Iliocostalis thoracis/lumborum (lateral erector spinae)	Rib angles of ribs 7–12, transverse processes of T10–L4, sacrum, iliac crest, and thoracolumbar fascia	Rib angles of ribs 1–6 and transverse processes of C7, rib angles of ribs 6–12	Extension of vertebral column or control speed of spinal flexion when contracting bilaterally Side bending when contracting unilaterally	Dorsal rami of spinal nerves
Longissimus thoracis et lumborum (intermediate erector spinae)	Transverse processes of L1–L5, sacrum, iliac crest, and erector spinae aponeurosis	Transverse processes of T1–T12 and rib angles of ribs 3–12	Extension of vertebral column or control speed of spinal flexion when contracting bilaterally Side bending when contracting unilaterally	Dorsal rami of spinal nerves
Spinalis thoracis (medial erector spinae)	Spinous processes of T10–L2	Spinous processes of T1–T8	Extension of vertebral column or control speed of spinal flexion when contracting bilaterally Side bending when contracting unilaterally	Dorsal rami of spinal nerves

(*continued*)

TABLE 36.1 (*Continued*)

Muscles of the Lumbar Region Origin, Insertion, Action, and Innervation—Includes Closely Related Thoracic and Abdominal Musculature That Influence the Lumbar Spine[36–39]

Muscles	Origin	Insertion	Action	Innervation
Semispinalis thoracis dorsi	Transverse processes of T6–T10	Spinous processes of C7–C8 and T1–T4	Extension of vertebral column when contracting bilaterally Contralateral rotation and ipsilateral side bending when contracting unilaterally	Dorsal rami of spinal nerves
Rotatores thoracis/ lumborum	Transverse processes of T1–T12 and L1–L5	Spinous processes of adjacent and two vertebral levels superior to origin	Extension and rotation of vertebral column	Dorsal rami of spinal nerves
Multifidus	Sacrum, erector spinae aponeurosis, posterior superior iliac spine, posterolateral articular processes of L1–L5, transverse processes of T1–T12, and articular processes of C3–C7	Spinous processes of 2–4 vertebra levels superior to origin	Stabilizes vertebrae in local movements of vertebral column Contracting bilaterally will extend the spine Contracting unilaterally will side bend and ipsilaterally rotate spine	Dorsal rami of spinal nerves
Interspinales	Spinous processes of C1–L5	Spinous processes of adjacent vertebral level superior to origin	Stabilizes adjoining vertebrae during spinal movement	Dorsal rami of spinal nerves
Intertransversarii	Transverse processes of C2–L5	Transverse processes of adjacent vertebrae superior to origin	Stabilizes adjoining vertebrae during spinal movement	Dorsal rami of spinal nerves
Quadratus lumborum	Transverse processes of L5, iliac crest, and iliolumbar ligament	Transverse processes of L1–L4 and inferior border of rib 12	Lumbar extension when contracting bilaterally Lumbar side bending when contracting unilaterally	Ventral rami of T12 and L1–L4

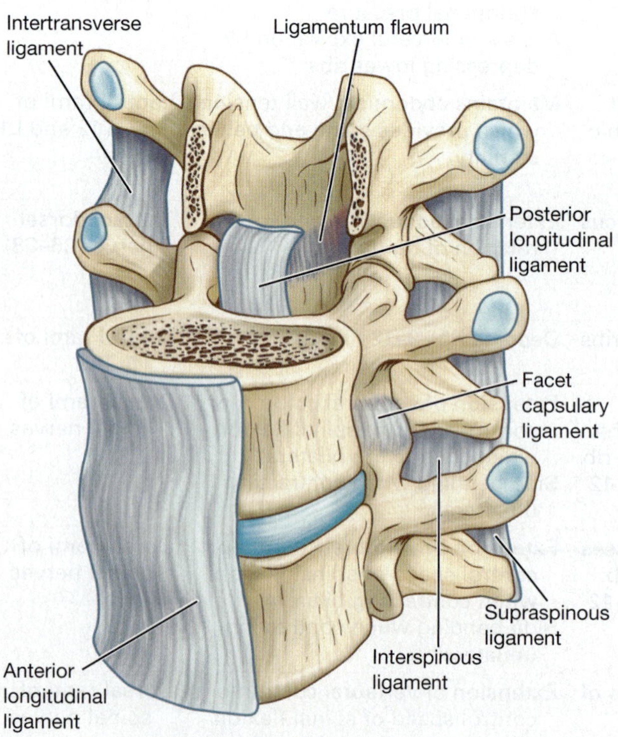

Figure 36.8. Ligaments of the lumbar spine. (Reprinted with permission from Anderson MK. *Foundations of Athletic Training: Prevention, Assessment, and Management.* 6th ed. Wolters Kluwer; 2017:783. Figure 22.2.)

posterolateral boundary of the neural foramen. It extends vertically to connect the posterior elements of each vertebra. This ligament is the most elastic in the spine; it has the highest elastin-to-collagen ratio and an average thickness of 6 mm in the lumbar area, which is thicker than any other region in the spine.[6,45] This high elasticity aids in straightening the spine after flexing.[6] Thickening and calcification of this ligament can cause foraminal narrowing, spinal stenosis, and nerve root compression.[6]

Interspinous Ligament

The interspinous ligaments are thin membranes located between each spinous process. These ligaments join with the ligamentum flava anteriorly and the supraspinatus ligament posteriorly.[6] The fibers run obliquely in a medial to lateral direction from the superior aspect of one spinous process to the spinous process above. These ligaments limit the forward bending of the spine by restricting separation of the spinous processes. In conjunction with the supraspinous ligaments, the interspinous ligaments help maintain the sagittal stability of spinal segments.[46] Pathology such as chondrification and ossification of this and other ligaments is present in ankylosing spondylitis and limits the flexion–extension motion of the spine.[47]

Supraspinous Ligament

The strong fibrous supraspinous ligament is a continuum of the ligamentum nuchae that attaches to the external occipital protuberance and continues to the spinous process of C7. From there, the supraspinous ligament courses the length of the spine connecting the posterior tips of the spinous processes from C7 to the sacrum.[6] In the lumbar region, the structure is thicker and broader and is intimately blended with the surrounding thoracolumbar fascia. This structure also serves as the attachment site for the erector spinae muscles.[6] In conjunction with the interspinous ligament, the supraspinous ligament assists in preventing hyperflexion of the lumbar spine. Injury to this ligament can lead to Baastrup disease, also known as "kissing spines syndrome," which is characterized by close approximation and hyperostosis of the spinous processes and by low back pain.[46] Degeneration of this ligament can contribute to spinal stenosis and spondylolisthesis.[46]

Anterior Longitudinal Ligament

The anterior longitudinal ligament continuously connects the anterior vertebral bodies from the basilar part of the occipital bone to the anterior sacrum, where it blends into the ligamentous encapsulation of the sacrum and ends at the first coccygeal vertebra.[45] The longitudinal fibers are strongly adherent to the intervertebral disks, the margins of the adjacent vertebral bodies, and the hyaline cartilage end plates.[48] The crura of the diaphragm are attached to the anterior longitudinal ligament in the lumbar region.[42] As previously described, the right crus attaches to the upper 3 to 4 lumbar vertebrae, and the left crus attaches to the upper 2 to 3 vertebrae.[42] In the lumbar spine, the anterior longitudinal ligament is wider and thicker than the posterior longitudinal ligament and limits the extension of the lumbar spine.[6]

Posterior Longitudinal Ligament

The posterior longitudinal ligament continuously connects the posterior vertebral bodies from the endocranial surface of the basiocciput to the sacrum and first coccygeal vertebra.[45] Like the anterior longitudinal ligament, the posterior ligament also attaches to the intervertebral disks, the margins of the adjacent vertebral bodies, and the hyaline cartilage end plates.[48] The posterior longitudinal ligament is broad and of uniform width throughout the cervical and upper thoracic regions. In the lower thoracic and lumbar region, the ligament becomes scalloped as it narrows over the vertebral bodies and widens over each intervertebral disks.[48] The posterior longitudinal ligament is separated from the lumbar vertebral bodies by a venous plexus, but it is strongly adherent to the annulus of the disks.[45] The widening of the ligament over the disks prevents or redirects disk herniations away from the spinal cord and accounts for the greater incidence of posteromedial disk herniations in the lumbar region.[6,45] Hyperflexion injuries, such as that seen with whiplash, can injure the posterior longitudinal ligament as well as the other posterior ligaments.[45]

Iliolumbar Ligament

The iliolumbar ligament connects the transverse processes of L4 and L5 to the iliac crest and to the anterior sacroiliac joint.[45,48] This ligament also integrates into the attachment of the quadratus lumborum muscle. In children, the iliolumbar ligament contains muscle fibers that are gradually replaced with ligamentous fibers during the next three or four decades.[48] The major function of the ligament is to stabilize the lumbosacral junction, and it can be strained during lumbar flexion from acute injuries or chronically poor posture.[49] When irritated, this ligament refers pain to the ipsilateral groin, sacroiliac joint, and lateral thigh.[50] Patients with iliolumbar ligament syndrome will present with pain and tenderness at the iliolumbar insertion at the medial iliac crest and have the characteristic referral pattern as described above.[51,52]

THORACOLUMBAR FASCIA (FIG. 36.9)

The thoracolumbar fascia, which is also known as the fascia profundis or thoracolumbar aponeurosis, is a composite of aponeurotic tissue and fascia that continuously connects with the paraspinal fascia of the thoracic and cervical regions, thereby connecting the cranial base to the sacrum.[48] This fascia is also continuous with the anterior abdominal wall and its musculature. A number of the trunk and extremity muscles insert into this connective tissue plane and assist with modulating tension, the maintenance of static and dynamic posture, facilitate the work of breathing, and contribute to lumbopelvic stability.[3,48]

There are three layers of the thoracolumbar fascia in the lumbar region. Anteriorly, this fascia lies between the psoas and quadratus lumborum muscles and is attached to the lumbar transverse processes, the iliolumbar ligament, and the iliac crest.[48] The middle layer is also attached to the transverse processes and to the intertransverse ligaments, the lower border of the 12th rib, and the lumbocostal ligament.[48] The posterior layer is attached to the spinous processes of the lumbar and sacral vertebrae and to the supraspinous ligaments.[48] The posterior and middle layers fuse to form the lateral margin of the erector spinae and combine with the anterior layer to form the lateral margin of the quadratus lumborum muscle and the aponeurotic origin of the transversus abdominis.[48] Because of the continuity of the thoracolumbar fascia with the muscles throughout the back, pelvis, and abdomen, this fascia is affected by the muscle's actions, especially the large muscles like the latissimus dorsi, gluteus maximus, and hamstrings.[48] Since this continuity also includes attachments to the vertebrae, somatic dysfunction affecting muscles or vertebrae can place asymmetric tension on this three-dimensional fascial structure, impacting the tensegrity of the musculoskeletal system.

The thoracolumbar fascia is innervated by a high density of sympathetic fibers that include nociceptors and mechanoreceptors capable of proprioception.[53] Dysfunction of the thoracolumbar fascia can contribute to low back pain symptoms through microinjuries that irritate nociceptors, impaired proprioceptive signaling, and regional segmental facilitation.[53] The interaction between the fascia and the sympathetic nervous system has been proposed as one of the mechanisms that explain why some patients with low back pain report increased pain severity when under psychological stress.[53]

Viscera

MESENTERIES

Approximately 30 feet of small intestines and portions of the ascending and descending colon are located anterior to the lumbar region. The abdominal mesenteries are formed by reflections of the parietal peritoneum from the posterior abdominal wall. These mesenteries carry arteries and efferent autonomic nerve fibers to the viscera. They also carry veins, lymphatic vessels, and visceral afferent nerves away from the viscera. Therefore, somatic dysfunction of the myofascial tissues of the lumbar region has the potential to functionally influence the local environment of the abdominal viscera.

Neural Structures

The neural structures of the lumbar region provide an important link between the region and the rest of the body. The spinal cord and nerve roots are covered by the three layers of the meninges—spinal dura mater, arachnoid mater, and pia mater—that support and protect the nerves and surround them with cerebrospinal fluid. These tissues, especially the dense dura mater, form the "core link" of the reciprocal tension membrane that transmits biomechanical forces throughout the body through the link between the cranium and the sacrum and coccyx.[54] In addition, the sensory innervation of the lumbar structures provides proprioceptive and nociceptive information that can affect the biomechanical and autonomic nervous functions of other body regions.

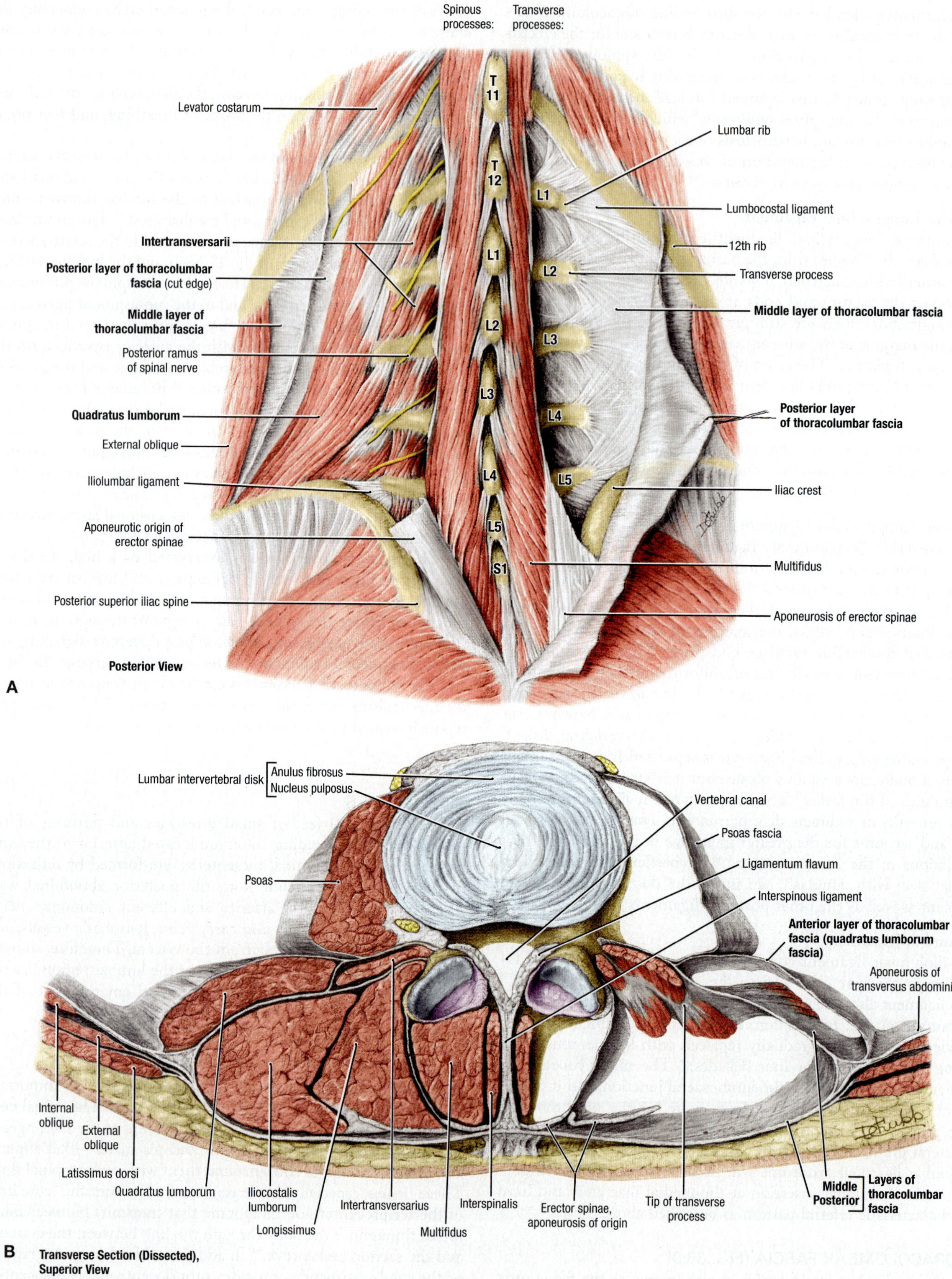

Figure 36.9. Thoracolumbar fascia. A. Posterior view. **B.** Transverse section. (Reprinted with permission from Agur AMR, Dalley AF II. *Grant's Atlas of Anatomy*. 15th ed. Wolters Kluwer; 2021. Figures 1.31 and 1.32.)

SPINAL CORD (FIG. 36.10)

In the adult lumbar spine, the spinal cord usually terminates at the level of the L1–L2 vertebrae at the conus medullaris. The remaining lumbar, sacral, and coccygeal spinal nerve roots diverge at the conus medullaris and continue as a loose bundle of individual nerve roots known as the cauda equina. A connective tissue filament known as the filum terminale descends from the apex of the conus medullaris to attach to the first coccygeal vertebra.[55] The upper portion of the filum terminale, known as the filum terminale internum, is comprised of extensions of the dural and arachnoid meninges and descends to the caudal border of S2.[56] The lower portion, known as the filum terminale externum, is continuous with the spinal pia mater and descends to attach to the posterior periosteum first coccygeal vertebra.[56]

In the lumbar region, the spinal canal has a triangular configuration that decreases in its AP dimension as it progresses from L1 to L5. A variety of conditions can narrow the lumbar spinal canal or intervertebral foramen, causing central canal or neuroforaminal stenosis, and lead to impingement or compression of the spinal cord, nerve roots, or exiting spinal nerves. Examples of these conditions include the following:

- Hypertrophy of the ligaments bordering the spinal canal
- Arthritides, exostoses, and osteophytes
- Tumors, cysts, and vascular lesions
- Intervertebral disk protrusions, extrusions, and sequestrations
- Spinal trauma

In the upper lumbar region, compression of the conus medullaris can cause conus medullaris syndrome, which is characterized by symmetric saddle anesthesia and lower extremity motor deficit with atonic bladder dysfunction. Compression at the level of the cauda equina can cause cauda equina syndrome, which is characterized by asymmetric saddle anesthesia and lower extremity motor deficit with atonic bladder dysfunction and a flaccid anal sphincter. Both syndromes are medical emergencies that require

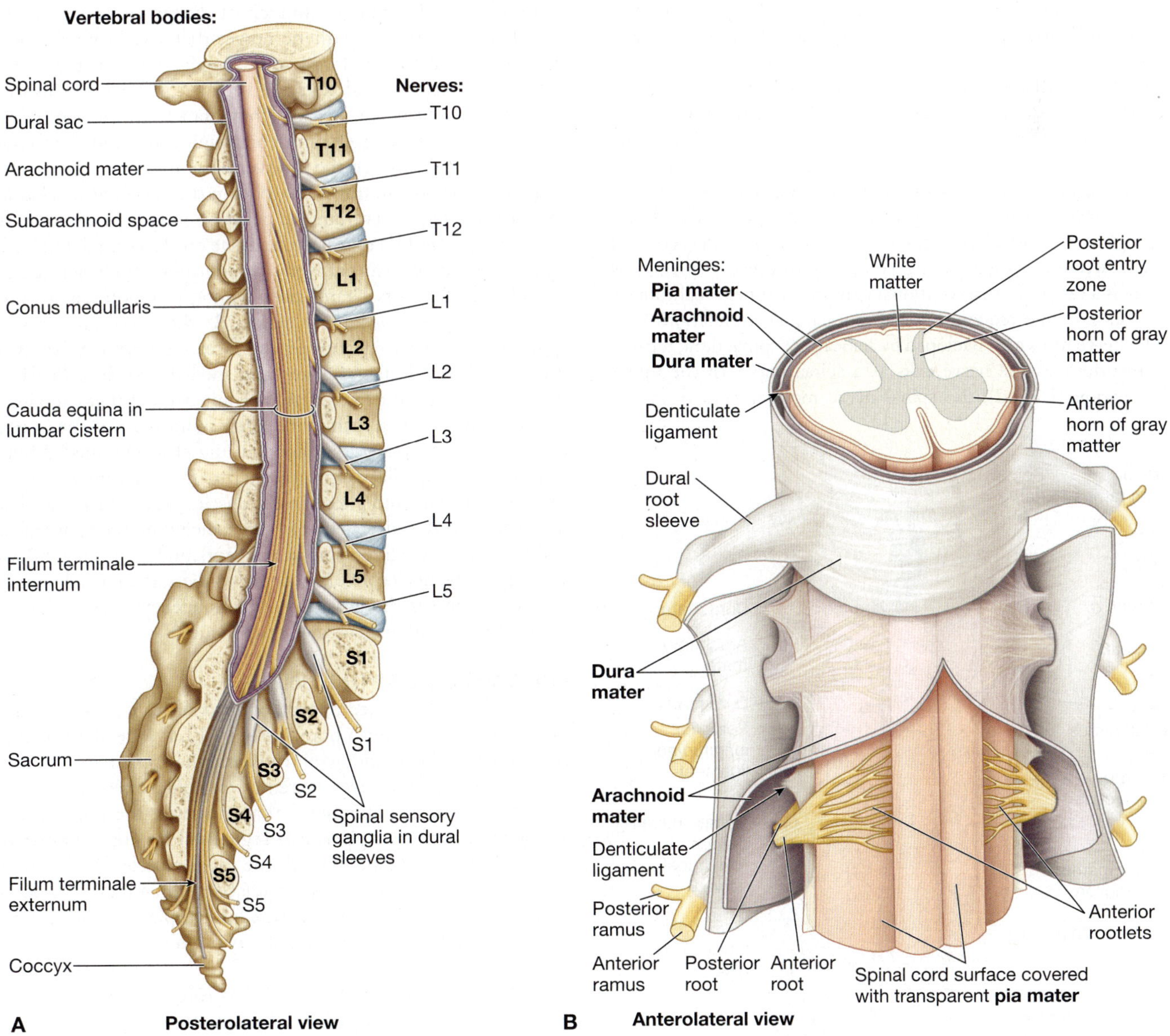

Figure 36.10. Spinal cord and spinal meninges. A. Posterolateral view of the spinal cord showing the relationships of the spinal cord, conus medullaris, filum terminale internum, and filum terminale externum to the lumbar and sacral regions. **B.** Anterolateral view of the spinal cord showing reflection of meninges. (**A** reprinted with permission from Dalley AF II, Agur AMR. *Moore's Clinically Oriented Anatomy*. 9th ed. Wolters Kluwer; 2023. Figure 2.46. **B** reprinted with permission from Dalley AF II, Agur AMR. *Moore's Clinically Oriented Anatomy*. 9th ed. Wolters Kluwer; 2023. Figure 1.31.)

emergent surgical decompression to avoid potential irreversible nerve ischemia and damage.[56]

Tethered cord syndrome occurs when the filum terminale is unusually short and restricts motion of the spinal cord. In children, this syndrome is often congenital and associated with other anomalies. In adults, impingement of the filum terminale in the spinal canal can cause tethering and may occur at either the upper internum or lower externum portions of the structure. This condition is characterized by low back or perianal pain symptoms with sensory symptoms, muscular weakness of the lower extremities, and bowel or bladder dysfunction. On imaging, this condition will often appear as a low positioning of the conus medullaris, suggesting caudal traction on the spinal cord.[55,56] In the presence of progressively deteriorating symptoms, this syndrome can be treated with surgical detethering.[57]

SPINAL NERVE ROOTS AND SPINAL NERVES (FIG. 36.11)

At each vertebral level, a pair of mixed sensory and motor spinal nerves exits through the intervertebral foramina. Within the spinal canal, the root of these spinal nerves is composed of a pair of ventral (anterior) and dorsal (posterior) nerve roots, which in turn are each composed of six to eight individual rootlets in a vertical row that exit the spinal cord and unite to form a single root before then joining together to form a spinal nerve root. The ventral spinal nerve roots contain efferent motor somatic and, at L1 and L2, preganglionic efferent sympathetic nerve fibers. The dorsal spinal nerve roots carry afferent sensory somatic and visceral fibers and form a ganglion just proximal to joining with the ventral root.[56] The dorsal root ganglion is most commonly located within the intervertebral foramen. Because this ganglion is composed of sensory fibers, this structure is a target for interventional pain management techniques, such as pulsed radiofrequency dorsal root ganglia stimulation.[58]

The nerve roots are enveloped by a sheath of spinal dura, termed the epineurium, as the nerve exits as a spinal nerve. In the upper lumbar region (L1–L2), the spinal nerve roots emerge from the

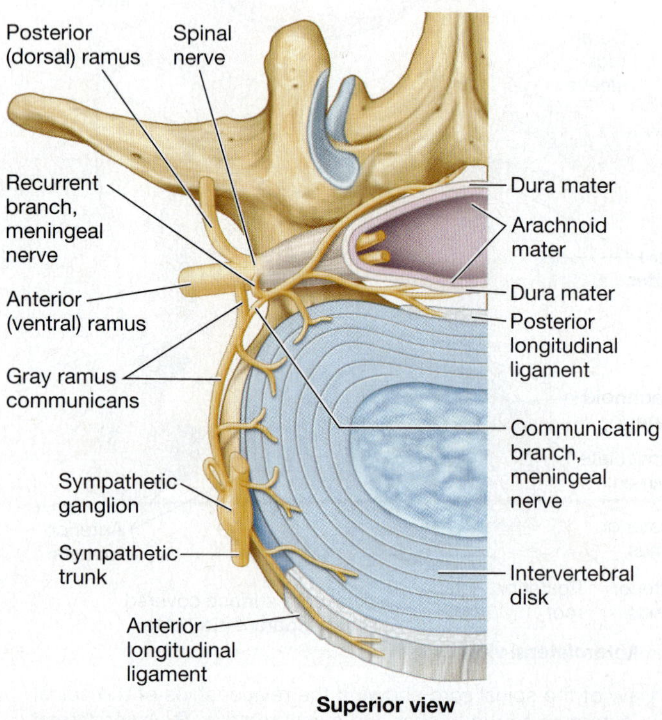

Figure 36.11. Spinal nerve roots and nerves. (Reprinted with permission from Agur AMR, Dalley AF II. *Moore's Essential Clinical Anatomy*. 7th ed. Wolters Kluwer; 2024:66. Figure 2.16.)

spinal cord at least two vertebral segments superior to the exiting foramina.[56] The remaining lumbar and sacral nerve roots exit the spinal cord at the conus medullaris and descend as the cauda equina before exiting at their respective intervertebral foramina. In the vertebral canal, the nerve roots travel laterally and inferiorly to the pedicle of the same numbered vertebra and then cross over the surface of the corresponding intervertebral disk as exiting spinal nerves.

After exiting the foramina, the spinal nerves branch into ventral and dorsal rami, both of which carry sensory and motor fibers. In the lumbar region, the larger ventral rami branch into a small recurrent meningeal nerve and the peripheral lumbar nerves, which join into either the lumbar plexus (L1–L4) or the sacral plexus (L4–L5). The peripheral lumbar nerves carry sensory and motor fibers to the anterolateral trunk and lower extremities, including the muscles along the anterior spine.[56] At L1 and L2, the ventral rami also contribute white rami communicantes that travel to the sympathetic ganglia.[2] The recurrent meningeal nerves are known by several names, including the sinuvertebral nerve, recurrent nerve of Luschka, and meningeal branch of the spinal nerve,[59] and are mixed sensory and sympathetic nerves that arise from the ventral rami just distal to the dorsal root ganglia. These nerves contain both proprioceptive and nociceptive fibers.[59] They are also considered recurrent nerves because they branch off the ventral rami, join the sympathetic grey rami communicantes, and then reenter the spinal canal through the intervertebral foramen. The recurrent meningeal nerves can travel up or down the vertebral canal at least two or three segments from the point of entry.[59] In addition, they can cross the midline to innervate tissue on the contralateral side.[60] The variability of their pathways complicates pain localization.

The smaller dorsal rami carry motor, vasomotor, and sensory fibers to the posterior lumbar region. As the dorsal rami leave the spinal nerve, they wrap around the facet joint directly below and divide into lateral, intermediate, and medial branches. The lateral branch innervates the lateral fascial compartment that contains the long postural muscles, such as the longissimus muscle. The intermediate branch innervates the iliocostal muscles. The medial branch innervates the medial fascial compartment that contains muscles like the multifidus and interspinalis muscles. The medial branch also innervates the dorsal skeletal elements, including the vertebral arch and facet joints, the interspinous ligaments, and the ligament flavum. Because of the nociceptive role of these fibers, the medial branch of the dorsal rami is the target for radiofrequency rhizotomies as an interventional pain management technique.[55]

LUMBAR PLEXUS[61] (FIG. 36.12)

The lumbar plexus is composed of the ventral rami of the spinal nerve roots L1–L4 and a branch from T12. It joins the L4 and L5 nerve roots at the lumbosacral trunk and the sacral plexus to innervate the pelvic and lower extremity regions. These nerves carry both sensory and motor fibers that innervate the lumbar, pelvic, and lower extremity regions in a segmental fashion. Lumbar ventral rami of L1–L4 pass through the psoas muscle. Dysfunction of the psoas muscle from spasm or adjacent inflammatory processes, such as diverticulitis, can irritate the lumbar plexus, causing pain or sensory disturbances in the thigh, hip, or gluteal areas.[61]

SYMPATHETIC NERVOUS SYSTEM (FIG. 36.13)

The preganglionic sympathetic nerves arise from the intermediolateral nucleus of the ventral horn of the spinal cord from T1 to L2. In the lumbar region, preganglionic sympathetic fibers exit from the spinal cord at L1 and L2. These fibers accompany the ventral roots of the spinal nerves exiting the intervertebral foreman and then follow the white rami communicantes, where they

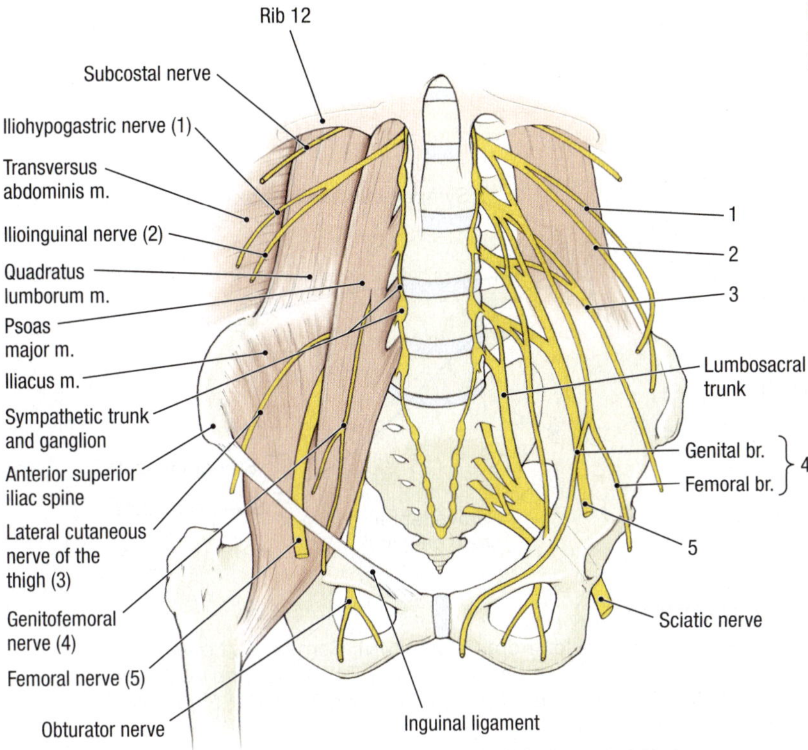

Figure 36.12. Lumbar plexus. (Reprinted with permission from Tank PW. *Grant's Dissector.* 15th ed. Wolters Kluwer Health/Lippincott Williams & Wilkins; 2013:121. Figure 4.47.)

either synapse within the paravertebral chain ganglia and exit as grey rami, or pass through the paravertebral chain ganglia to synapse at the prevertebral collateral ganglia that lie next to the major abdominal arteries arising from the aorta.[61] The fibers that pass through the chain ganglia to synapse at the collateral ganglia are known as lumbar splanchnic nerves and they innervate the viscera and their blood vessels in the lower abdomen and pelvis. The four lumbar splanchnic nerves are named after the four ganglia of the sympathetic chain in the lumbar region. These sympathetic nerves travel anteriorly to synapse within the celiac, inferior mesenteric, and hypogastric plexuses.

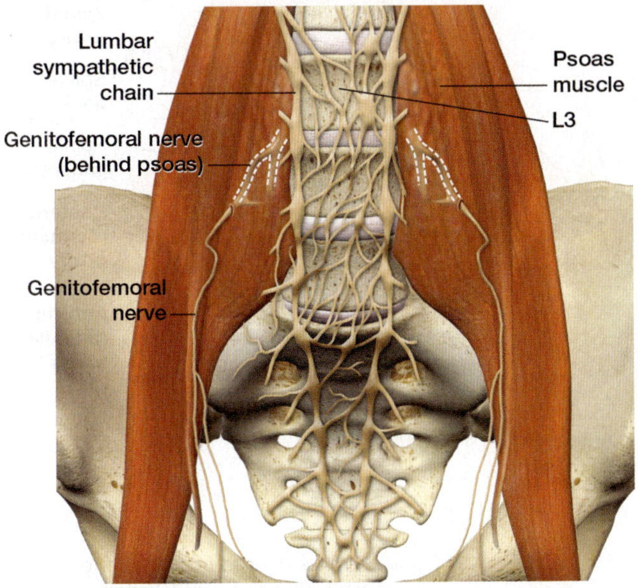

Figure 36.13. Lumbar sympathetic chain. (Reprinted with permission from Hoppenfeld JD. *Fundamentals of Pain Medicine: How to Diagnose and Treat Your Patients.* Wolters Kluwer Health; 2014:181. Figure 24-14.)

The sympathetic fibers that synapse at the paravertebral chain ganglia exit to travel with the peripheral nerves, providing segmental sympathetic innervation to the vasculature, skin, and muscles of the lumbar, pelvic, and lower extremity regions.[61] The paravertebral chain ganglia in the lumbar region run along the medial margin of the psoas major muscle and are anterolateral to the lumbar vertebral bodies.[61] Somatic dysfunctions of the lumbar vertebrae or psoas muscle may directly irritate the sympathetic chain affecting segmentally innervated structures.

SOMATOVISCERAL INFLUENCE OF THE LUMBAR SPINE (FIG. 36.14)

Within the dorsal horn of the spinal cord, afferent stimuli converge from the viscera, somatic structures, and higher centers. This close proximity allows for interactions between somatic and visceral systems and for the development of segmental facilitation or sensitization in the dorsal horn[62] (see Chapter 6). Segmental facilitation can lead to somatovisceral, viscerosomatic, viscero-visceral, and somato-somatic reflex arcs, allowing somatic or visceral dysfunction that is innervated within the lumbar region to affect segmentally innervated structures. As such, a person presenting with somatic symptoms may have a visceral origin to their symptoms. Likewise, OMT can be used to reduce somatic dysfunction and potentially disrupt these reflex arcs, thus impacting somatic and visceral dysfunction of segmentally innervated structures.[62]

Vascular and Lymphatic Structures of the Lumbar Spine

The anatomical relationships between the vascular and lymphatic structures and the bony, articular, ligamentous, and myofascial musculoskeletal structures provide the foundation for the respiratory-circulatory model of osteopathic diagnosis and treatment.[63] The biomechanical function of the regional musculoskeletal structures, in conjunction with the thoracic inlet and the respiratory and pelvic diaphragms, can directly impact vascular

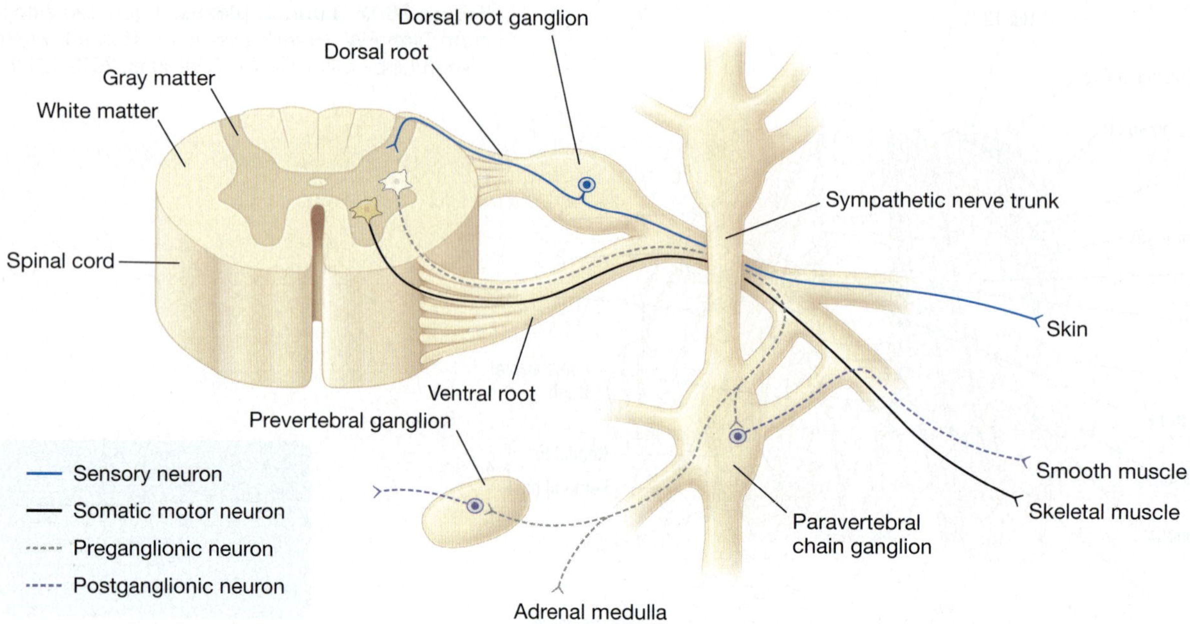

Figure 36.14. Sympathetic nerve fiber tracks. (Reprinted with permission from Galanter JM, Cornes SB, Lowenstein DH. Principles of nervous system physiology and pharmacology. In: Golan DE, Armstrong EJ, Armstrong AW, eds. *Principles of Pharmacology: The Pathophysiologic Basis of Drug Therapy*. 4th ed. Wolters Kluwer; 2017:112. Figure 9-1.)

and lymphatic functions in the lumbar region. With this model, diagnosis should be directed toward identifying somatic dysfunctions of the lumbar and adjacent musculoskeletal structures, including the diaphragms. Then, OMT can be applied to improve musculoskeletal function with the goal of optimizing regional vascular and lymphatic function.[63]

ARTERIAL SUPPLY

The lumbar spine and spinal cord receive most of their arterial blood supply from the anterior and posterior spinal arteries that travel from the head to the conus medullaris and from the four paired lumbar arteries that branch off the dorsal abdominal aorta[64] (Fig. 36.15). The lumbar arteries pass under the psoas tendons

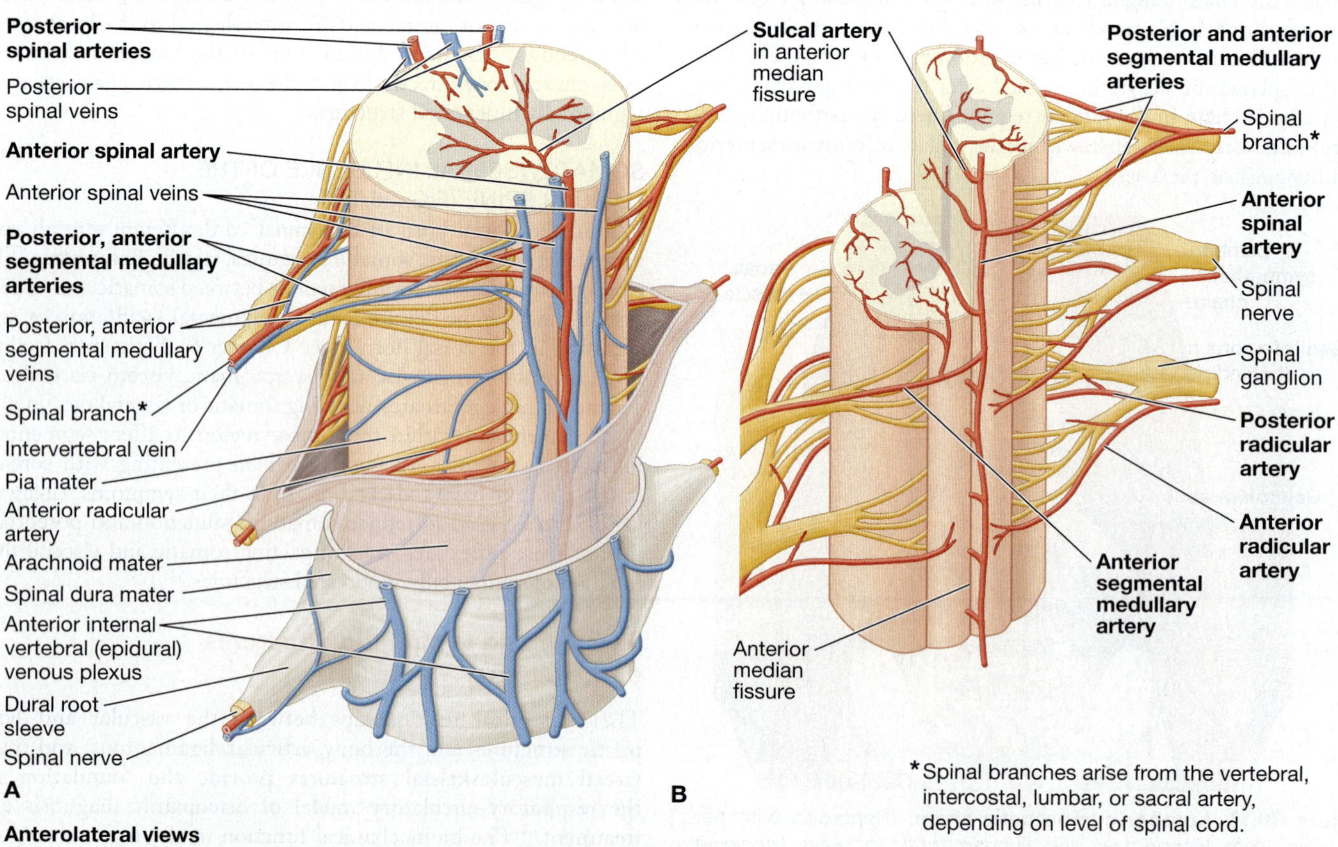

Figure 36.15. Blood supply of the spinal cord. A. Spinal veins. **B.** Spinal arteries. (Reprinted with permission from Dalley AF II, Agur AMR. *Moore's Clinically Oriented Anatomy*. 9th ed. Wolters Kluwer; 2023. Figure 2.53.)

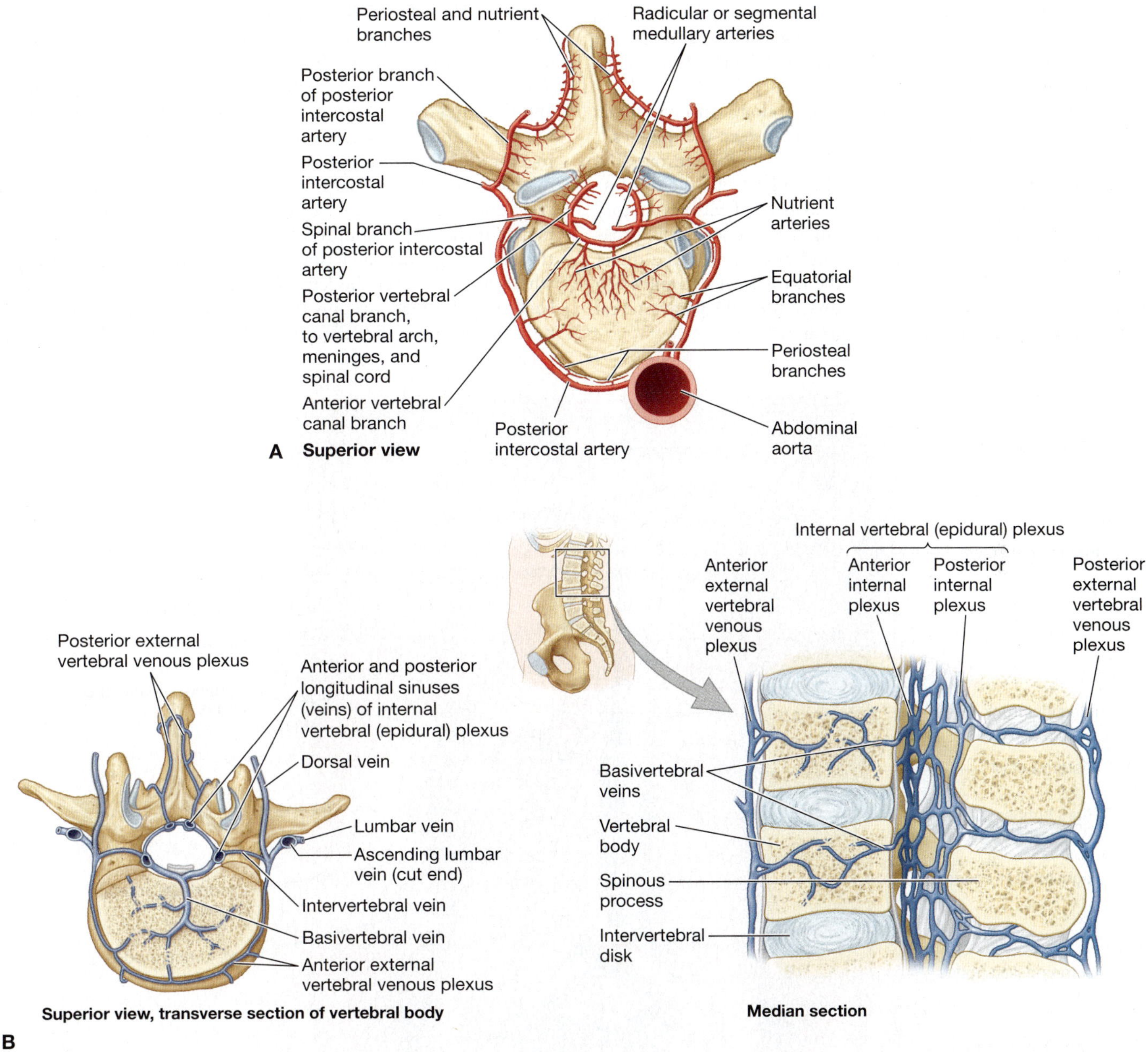

Figure 36.16. Blood supply of the vertebra. A. Arterial supply. **B.** Venous drainage. (Reprinted with permission from Agur AMR, Dalley AF II. *Moore's Essential Clinical Anatomy*. 7th ed. Wolters Kluwer; 2024:66. Figures 2.14 and 2.15.)

and then curve around the vertebrae to supply the vertebral bodies (Fig. 36.16). Dorsal branches pass under the sympathetic chain and branch again to enter the intervertebral foramen, supplying the structures within the canal or travel posteriorly to supply the posterior elements of the vertebrae, myofascial structures of the back, and skin.[48] Although the anatomy may vary, lumbar branches of the iliolumbar arteries or a fifth pair of lumbar arteries may arise from the middle sacral artery to supply the lower lumbar region. Once in the foramen, these arteries branch to supply the structures in the canal and anastomose with the spinal arteries. One segmental branch is generally larger than the others and is the primary source of blood for the inferior two-thirds of the spinal cord.[2] This artery—which is known as the greater anterior segmental medullary artery, the radiculomedullary artery of Adamkiewicz, or the arteria radicularis magna—most commonly arises from the left upper lumbar artery.[2,65] Pathology of the aorta in the abdominal region, such as an aneurysm, or surgical damage to the lumbar arteries can impact the blood supply to the lumbar region and present as back pain due to ischemia of the spine or spinal cord.[66,67]

VENOUS DRAINAGE (SEE FIG. 36.16)

Venous drainage from the spinal cord occurs via the anterior and posterior spinal veins into anterior and posterior internal plexuses of thin-walled valveless veins that also drain bony and ligamentous structures within the vertebral canal. These internal veins communicate with external plexuses on the anterior and posterior sides of the vertebrae that also drain the bony and ligamentous structures outside the vertebral canal.[48] In the lumbar region, this system eventually drains into the inferior vena cava. The profuse, valveless venous plexuses of the spinal cord, vertebrae, and communicating veins are of great clinical importance because they are continuous throughout the spine and with the intracranial venous sinuses. Elevated intra-abdominal pressures, postural alterations, and obstructions can reverse the flow of venous blood and become a factor in the metastasis of primary abdominal and pelvic malignancies to the spine and brain.[48,68]

Venous drainage from the back muscles, along with lymphatic drainage, travels through the fascial spaces between the muscles.[41] This drainage is facilitated by contractions of the surrounding muscles and by the alternating diastolic and systolic blood pressures and the intra-abdominal pressures associated with respiratory and pelvic diaphragms during breathing.[69,70] The anatomic proximity of these vessels to the muscles and fascia provides a direct mechanism by which dysfunction of the myofascial structures can impair local venous and lymphatic drainage from the paravertebral tissues, thereby affecting local tissue textures.[63]

LYMPHATIC STRUCTURES (FIG. 36.17)

Lymphatic drainage from the lumbar vertebral column and associated soft tissues flows to the lateral aortic and retroaortic nodes.[48] These nodes are located in close proximity to the psoas muscles and the crura of the respiratory diaphragm, and they drain into the lumbar lymphatic trunks or the intestinal lymphatic trunk, which together join to form the cisterna chyli.[68] The cisterna chyli is a dilated lymphatic sac that is located anterior to L1–L2.[35] The thoracic duct exits from the cisterna chyli to pass through the aortic hiatus of the diaphragm into the mediastinum. The thoracic duct travels through the mediastinum to the left thoracic inlet region, where it arches over the left subclavian artery before descending back into the mediastinum to empty into the venous circulation near the union of the left internal jugular and subclavian veins.[68]

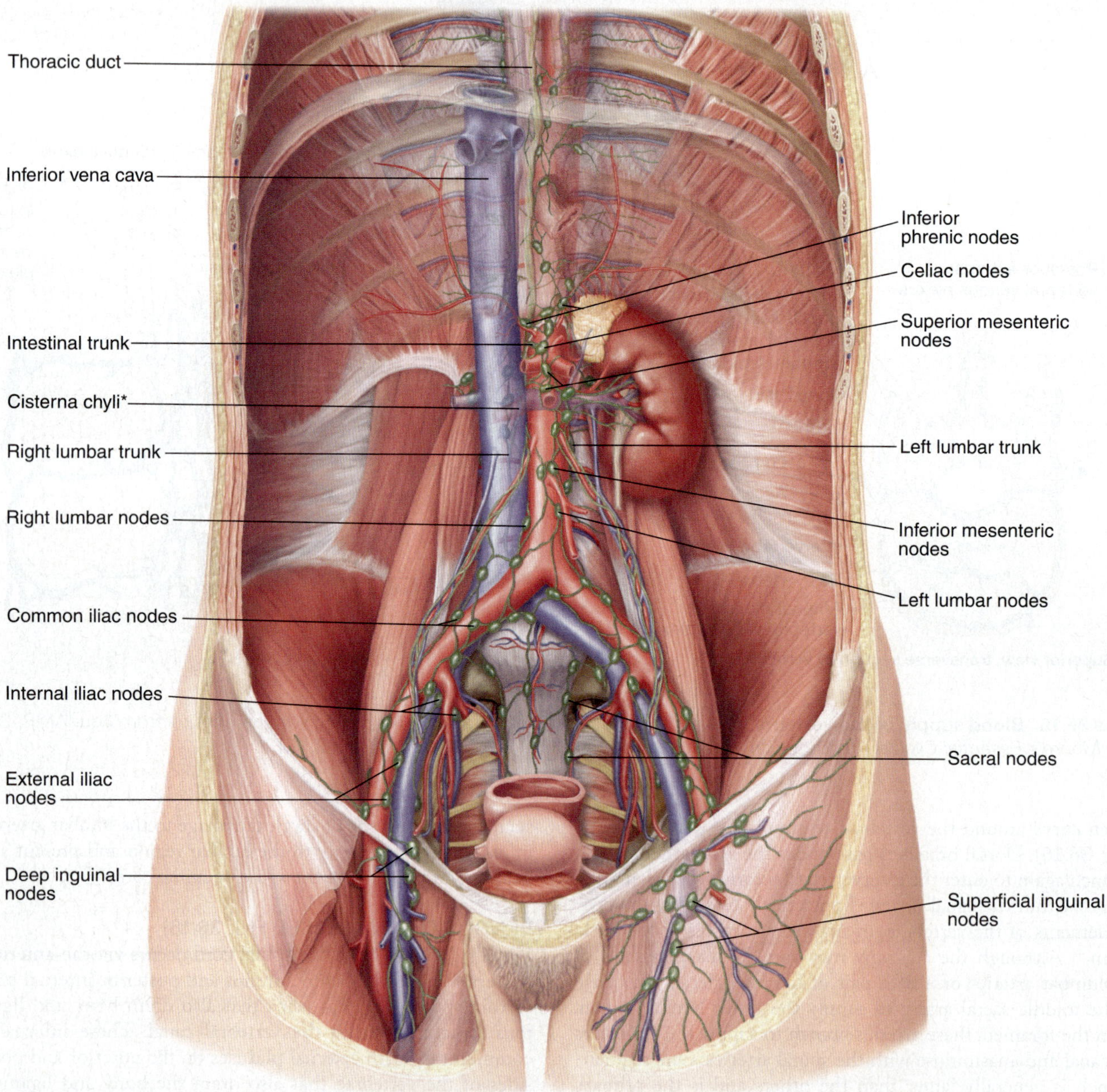

Figure 36.17. Lymphatic drainage of the lumbar spine as illustrated at the left and right lumbar (periaortic) lymph nodes. (Reprinted with permission from Gest TR. *Lippincott® Atlas of Anatomy*. 2nd ed. Wolters Kluwer; 2020:271. Plate 5-39.)

Somatic dysfunction of the upper lumbar region, psoas muscles, thoracic diaphragm, and/or the left thoracic inlet can all potentially impede lymphatic drainage from the lumbar region.

STRUCTURAL EXAMINATION OF THE LUMBAR SPINE

Assessing for somatic dysfunction in the lumbar region involves the screening and regional components of the structural exam to identify potential areas of dysfunction and then focusing the physical examination to identify discrete dysfunctions that are amenable to OMT. Somatic dysfunction in the lumbar spine can be identified by the presence of one or more of the TART physical findings associated with somatic dysfunction. The TART findings include tenderness, asymmetry, restricted range of motion, and tissue texture abnormalities.

Screening for Lumbar Somatic Dysfunction

Screening for somatic dysfunction in the lumbar spine involves a brief assessment for regional asymmetry, restricted range of motion, and tissue texture abnormalities. If findings are indicative of somatic dysfunction, then assess for local myofascial dysfunction, such as tender points, trigger points, or muscular imbalance, and for articular segmental vertebral somatic dysfunction. For additional information (see Chapter 30).

Screening Component of the Structural Exam

The screening component of the structural exam consists of evaluating the patient for asymmetry and restriction of active range of motion.

Screening for Asymmetry

Screening for asymmetry in the lumbar region can be performed through visualization and palpation for asymmetry of anatomic landmarks, such as the spinous processes or the paravertebral muscles overlying the transverse processes. Spinous processes should be midline without deviation to the right or left sides and equidistant apart. Indications of somatic dysfunction include variable distance between the spinous processes and lateral deviation of one or more spinous processes (Fig. 36.18). Visual asymmetry of spinous processes is considered a screen because spinous process deviation can occur as a developmental anomaly without abnormality of the joint structures.[71] Paravertebral muscle asymmetry is common with neutral type I curves, such as those that occur with scoliosis.[72,73] In scoliosis, the paravertebral muscles on the convexity of the curve tend to be larger and stronger than the muscles on the concavity of the curve, which show electrical and histologic changes consistent with muscle degeneration.[74–76]

Active Range of Motion Screen

Instruct the patient to flex, extend, rotate, and side bend their lumbar spine. Note pain or reduced range of motion in any plane. Asymmetric range of motion between right and left rotation and right and left side bending may also indicate segmental vertebral somatic dysfunction. The hip drop test uses active patient motion to screen for passive lumbar side bending that should occur in response to sacral base declination[77,78] (Fig. 36.19). This test is

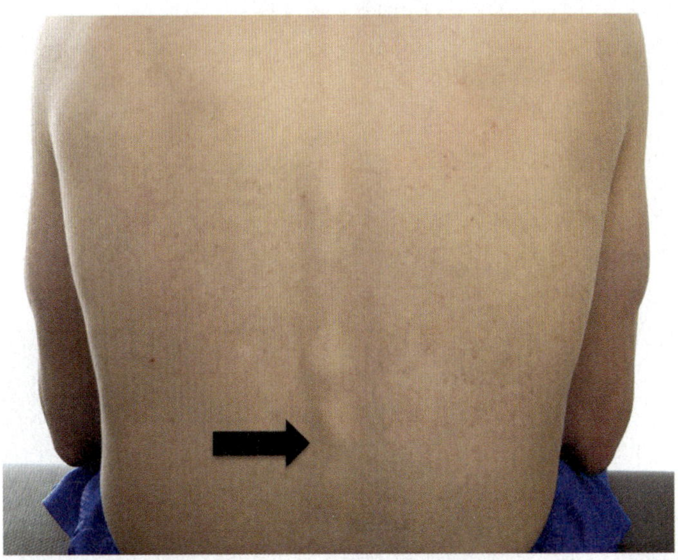

Figure 36.18. Deviation of a lumbar spinous process to the right indicative of segmental vertebral somatic dysfunction. (Used with permission from A.T. Still University's Kirksville College of Osteopathic Medicine.)

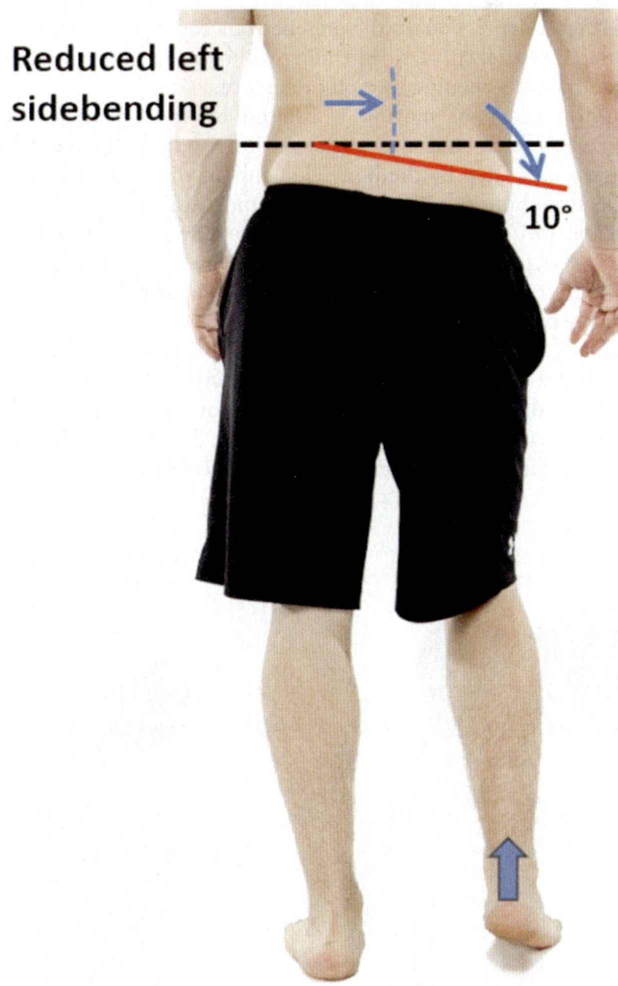

Figure 36.19. Hip drop test is performed by having the standing patient bend one knee while keeping their ipsilateral foot in contact with the floor. Compare both sides. The positive side is named for the side with reduced contralateral lumbar side bending and is accompanied by reduced ipsilateral iliac crest depression. (Used with permission from Western University of Health Sciences, Pomona, CA.)

TABLE 36.2

Average Active Range of Motion Values for the Lumbar Spine[78]

Lumbar Motion	Average Active Range of Motion (Degrees)
Flexion	40–60
Extension	20–35
Side bending[a]	15–20
Rotation[a]	3–18

[a]Side-bending and rotation ranges of motion represent global range of motion that is inclusive of both right and left ranges of motion.

Adapted from Magee DJ, Manske RC. Lumbar spine. In: *Orthopedic Physical Assessment*. 7th ed. Elsevier; 2021:627–723.

performed by having the standing patient bend one knee while keeping their ipsilateral foot in contact with the floor. The hip should "drop" on the side of the bent knee. This maneuver should induce compensatory lumbar side bending to the opposite side in response to the sacral base declination that occurs with ipsilateral iliac crest depression. In the presence of a somatic dysfunction with a large neutral curve, side bending will be reduced on the side opposite the side-bending motion preference.

Flexion range of motion is limited by the ligaments of the vertebral arch and the posterior longitudinal ligament.[79] Extension is limited by the bony elements of the vertebral arch and the stretching of the anterior longitudinal ligament.[79] Side bending is limited by lateral ligaments and the vertebral articular facets.[79] Rotation is also limited by the facets.[79] Right and left side bending and rotation may be unequal in the presence of facet tropism due to anatomical asymmetry of the orientation of the facets.[16] Published regional range of motion values for the lumbar spine vary in the literature depending on the measurement method. In addition, the range of motion of the lumbar spine can vary from person to person and it decreases with age. Average values for active lumbar range of motion are presented in Table 36.2.

Regional Component of Structural Exam

The regional or scanning component of the structural exam consists of palpating for tissue texture abnormalities, tenderness, temperature changes, and asymmetry and evaluating the patient's passive range of motion or quality of motion for the areas identified as being the likely source of somatic dysfunction.

ASSESS FOR TISSUE TEXTURE ABNORMALITIES

Assess for tissue texture abnormalities by palpating the lumbar paravertebral myofascial tissues for localized areas of temperature variation and for tissue texture variation, including boggy, tight, ropy, or fibrotic tissue. Acute somatic dysfunction can present as warm or boggy tissue texture. Chronic somatic dysfunction may present as cool or tight, ropy, or fibrotic tissue.

PASSIVE RANGE OF MOTION EVALUATION (FIG. 36.20)

In addition to the passive range of motion testing described in Chapter 30 The Osteopathic Structural Examination, passive range of motion of the lumbar region can be performed by inducing regional lumbar motion in one or more planes and noting localized areas of asymmetrical motion or excess motion restriction.

Rotational Motion Evaluation

1. With the patient seated, supine, prone, or lateral recumbent, apply a rotational springing force to multiple transverse processes on one side to induce rotation to the opposite side. Note resistance to anterior motion.
2. Repeat rotational motion evaluation to the transverse processes on the opposite side.
   - □ The evaluation is positive if one or more transverse processes resist the anterior springing force when compared with the opposite transverse processes at the same vertebral levels.

Side-Bending Motion Evaluation

1. With the patient seated and the lumbar spine in neutral, apply a side-bending springing force through the shoulder to induce ipsilateral lumbar side bending.
2. Palpate the lumbar transverse processes on either the ipsilateral or contralateral side to the side bending. Note posterior motion

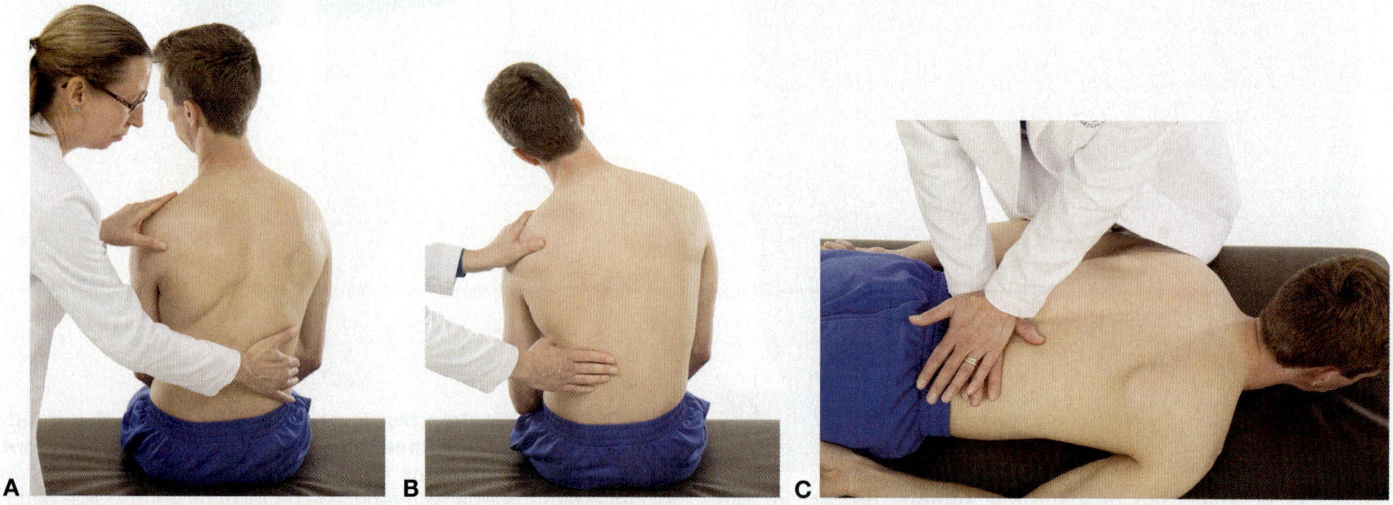

Figure 36.20. Passive range of motion evaluation. A. Rotational motion evaluation assessing for resistance to anterior motion of transverse processes. **B.** Side-bending motion evaluation monitoring for ipsilateral transverse process motion. **C.** Sagittal motion evaluation using prone posteroanterior springing. (Used with permission from A.T. Still University's Kirksville College of Osteopathic Medicine.)

of the transverse processes. With the lumbar spine in the neutral position, type I side-bending motion should result in transverse process rotation to the side opposite the side bending.

3. Repeat side-bending motion evaluation on the opposite side.
   - □ The evaluation is positive if the transverse processes do not become prominent on the opposite side of the side bending or remain posterior on the same side as the side bending.

Sagittal Motion Evaluation

1. With the patient seated, supine, prone, or lateral recumbent, apply anterior pressure on one or more lumbar spinous processes and note either excess resistance to anterior motion or excessive springiness characterized by a localized decrease in resistance to anterior motion.
2. Repeat posteroanterior springing evaluation on all lumbar spinous processes.
   - □ The evaluation is positive if there is localized excess resistance to anterior motion, which suggests flexed dysfunction, or there is excessive springiness, which suggests extended dysfunction.

Diagnosing Lumbar Somatic Dysfunction

Somatic dysfunction in the lumbar spine primarily presents as impaired or altered motion of the myofascial structures or the articular elements of the lumbar vertebra, or segmental somatic dysfunction. However, dysfunction can also manifest as impaired or altered functioning in regional neural, vascular, or lymphatic structures. Lumbar somatic dysfunction may be primary in nature or secondary to compensation from dysfunction in other body regions.

Myofascial Somatic Dysfunction in the Lumbar Region

Muscular somatic dysfunction can be identified by hypertonicity of individual muscles or tenderness. Muscular hypertonicity may manifest as texture abnormalities, such as tight, ropy, or fibrotic myofascial tissue; restricted range of motion characterized by muscle shortening with reduced active and passive range of motion; or tenderness that may present as tender points and trigger points that refer pain. Muscular hypertonicity may occur when a muscle imbalance, such as lower crossed syndrome, is present. With this condition, hypertonic postural muscles are associated with hypotonic phasic muscles. The resulting muscle imbalance can impact the postural stability and function of the body below the diaphragm.[80] In the case of the lower crossed syndrome, physical examination will reveal a tight quadratus lumborum in the lumbar region and tight iliopsoas, piriformis, hamstrings, rectus femoris, gastrocnemius, and soleus muscles. The abdominal oblique muscles, rectus abdominis, glutei muscles, vastus muscles, tibialis anterior, and peroneus muscles will also be functionally weak.[80–83]

Myofascial somatic dysfunction can also present as fascial tension, trigger points[84] (Fig. 36.21), or tender points at the attachment sites of muscles and ligaments. Lumbar tender points, commonly treated with counterstrain osteopathic manipulative

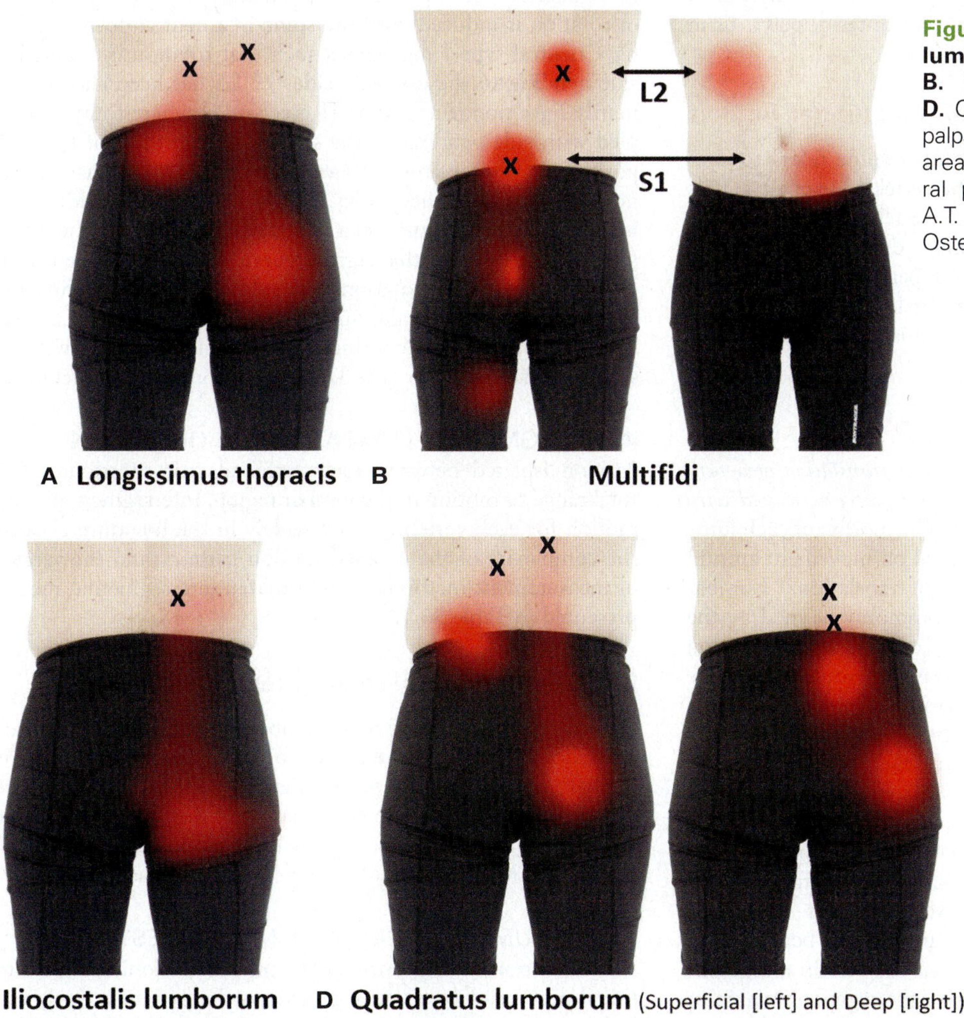

Figure 36.21. Trigger points found in the lumbar region. A. Longissimus thoracis. **B.** Multifidi. **C.** Iliocostalis lumborum. **D.** Quadratus lumborum. "X" indicates the palpable location of the trigger point. The area shaded in *red* indicates the pain referral pattern. (Used with permission from A.T. Still University's Kirksville College of Osteopathic Medicine.)

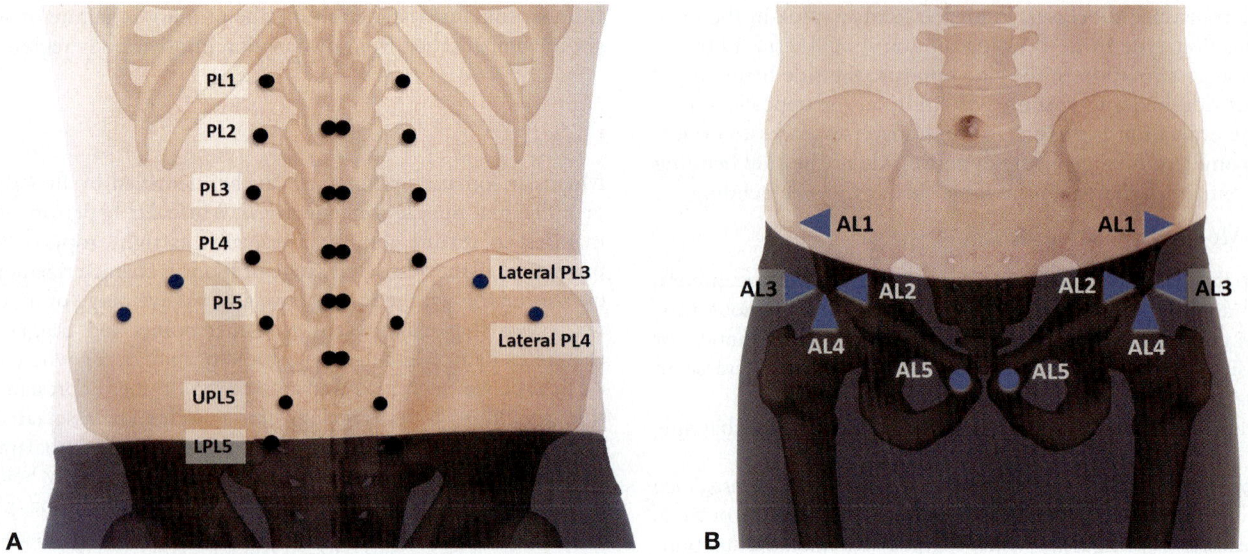

Figure 36.22. Lumbar counterstrain tender points. A. Posterior lumbar tender points, including those on the transverse processes and inferolateral spinous processes. Additional posterior lumbar tender points include lateral posterior L3 (PL3), lateral posterior L4 (PL4), upper pole L5 (UPL5), and lower pole L5 (LPL5). **B.** Anterior lumbar tender points along the pelvic brim. *Arrows* indicate direction of palpatory pressure to assess the points. (Used with permission from Snider KT, Glover JC. *Atlas of Common Counterstrain Tender Points.* A.T. Still University; 2014.)

technique (see Chapter 47), are often found on the vertebrae at the posterolateral aspects of the transverse processes and at the midline and inferolateral aspects of the spinous processes[85–87] (Fig. 36.22). Tender points that are thought to reflect somatic dysfunction in the lumbar spine can also be found along the anterior pelvic brim and in the posterior pelvis[85–87] (Fig. 36.22).

Articular Somatic Dysfunction of the Lumbar Region

Articular somatic dysfunction in the lumbar spine refers to dysfunction that occurs at joints between the vertebral segments. This somatic dysfunction may occur as a single vertebral unit or a group of segments. By convention, when a somatic dysfunction occurs at a single vertebral unit, it is named for the superior of the two vertebral segments. Diagnosis of articular vertebral somatic dysfunction is made when segmental motion restriction is present and named for the motion preference.

Intersegmental Lumbar Vertebral Motion

Coupled motion is defined as *the rotation or translation of a vertebral body about or along one axis that is consistently associated with rotation or translation about a second axis.*[88] The motion of each lumbar vertebra has 6 degrees of freedom based on movement around three axes of rotation and along three axes of translation.[90] Lumbar segmental somatic dysfunction is most commonly defined by the triplanar rotational preference around the x, y, and z axes. Flexion and extension motions are sagittal rotations that occur around the transverse x-axis, axial rotation occurs around the vertical y-axis, and side-bending (lateral flexion) rotation occurs around the AP z-axis. These three types of rotation are each accompanied by translatory motion along their respective axis. For example, flexion and extension (anterior or posterior rotation about the x-axis) are coupled with translation along the z-axis. In side bending, there is rotation around the AP z-axis, translation along the horizontal x-axis as well as rotation around the vertical y-axis. The z-axis and x-axis directions depend on the direction of side bending, but the y-axis direction varies as it depends on the vertebral segment involved. In side bending to the right, the right zygapophysial joint "closes" and the left zygapophysial joint "opens."[90] Rotation of a vertebra is described as rotation around the y-axis with the translatory motion being dependent on the involved vertebral segment. It is generally a component of side bending.[90] When side bending or rotation is induced with the spine in a neutral position, L1–L4 have neutral type I mechanics such that rotation is coupled with side bending to the opposite side.[89,91] L5 has been shown to primarily have nonneutral type II mechanics, where rotation is coupled with side bending to the same side regardless of the sagittal position.[89,91] Some studies have found that L4 also has primarily nonneutral type II mechanics.[89,91] When rotation or side bending is induced with the spine in a flexed or extended position, the vertebra at the apex of the sagittal curve will have nonneutral type II mechanics, where rotation is coupled with side bending to the same side.[92] When evaluating the lumbar spine from an articular standpoint, an osteopathic physician may find no evidence of somatic dysfunction or type I or type II somatic dysfunctions.

INTERSEGMENTAL LUMBAR RANGE OF MOTION

Motion isolated between each vertebral unit contributes to the total range of motion in the lumbar region. Intersegmental range of motion for each vertebra varies widely in the literature because of the complexity of the coupled motion patterns and the variability of measurement methods.[93,94] Estimated intersegmental motion is presented in Table 36.3.[48,95]

Lumbar Segmental Motion Testing

Segmental motion testing of the lumbar spine is used to assess motion restriction and motion preference for each plane of motion of each lumbar vertebra. Motion testing may be performed using active or passive motion testing or a combination of the two testing methods. The segmental findings for each plane of motion are combined for a triplanar vertebral segment somatic dysfunction diagnosis.

ACTIVE LUMBAR SEGMENTAL MOTION TESTING

Active motion testing involves the physician monitoring for rotational motion of vertebral segments as the patient actively moves

TABLE 36.3

Estimated Lumbar Intersegmental Range of Motion[44,89]

	Lumbar Intersegmental Range of Motion			
Vertebral Level	Flexion (Degrees)	Extension (Degrees)	Side Bending[a] (Degrees)	Rotation[a] (Degrees)
L1–L2	8	5	3–8	<3
L2–L3	10	<5	3–9	<3
L3–L4	12	<5	5–10	<3
L4–L5	13	<5	5–7	<3
L5–S1	9	5	2–3	<3

[a]Side-bending and rotation ranges of motion represent global range of motion that is inclusive of both right and left ranges of motion.

through lumbar flexion and extension. Vertebral rotation and side bending should not occur with normal active lumbar flexion and extension.[89] This method can be used to assess vertebral segments that were identified during the screening and regional component of the structural exam as areas with tissue texture abnormalities, asymmetry, or motion restriction. Active motion testing is most commonly performed with the patient seated.

Active Motion Testing Assessment (Fig. 36.23)

1. With the patient's lumbar spine in a neutral position, palpate the lumbar transverse processes bilaterally of the suspected dysfunctional vertebra and note asymmetry. The transverse processes can be found approximately two finger widths away from the associated spinous process. A unilateral posterior prominence of a transverse process will typically be present on the side of rotation preference.
2. Instruct the patient to flex and then extend. Note the change in asymmetry between the left and right transverse processes.
3. Repeat the procedure on the vertebra above and below the suspected area of dysfunction to determine the extent of the dysfunction and to confirm findings.

Interpretation (Table 36.4)

- Rotational motion preference
  - □ Posterior prominence of the right transverse process is consistent with a right rotation preference. Diagnose as rotated right.
  - □ Posterior prominence of the left transverse process is consistent with a left rotation preference. Diagnose as rotated left.
- Sagittal motion preference
  - □ A preference for flexion motion will demonstrate increased asymmetry between the right and left transverse processes when the dysfunctional vertebra is extended and decreased asymmetry when flexed. Diagnose as flexed (Fig. 36.24).
  - □ A preference for extension motion will demonstrate increased asymmetry between the right and left transverse processes when the dysfunctional vertebra is flexed and decreased asymmetry when extended. Diagnose as extended.
  - □ A preference for neutral motion will demonstrate minimal to no change in asymmetry of the transverse processes in neutral, flexion, and extension. In addition, neutral type I dysfunctions will typically occur as a group of vertebrae demonstrating the same asymmetrical motion pattern. Diagnose as neutral.

A

B

C

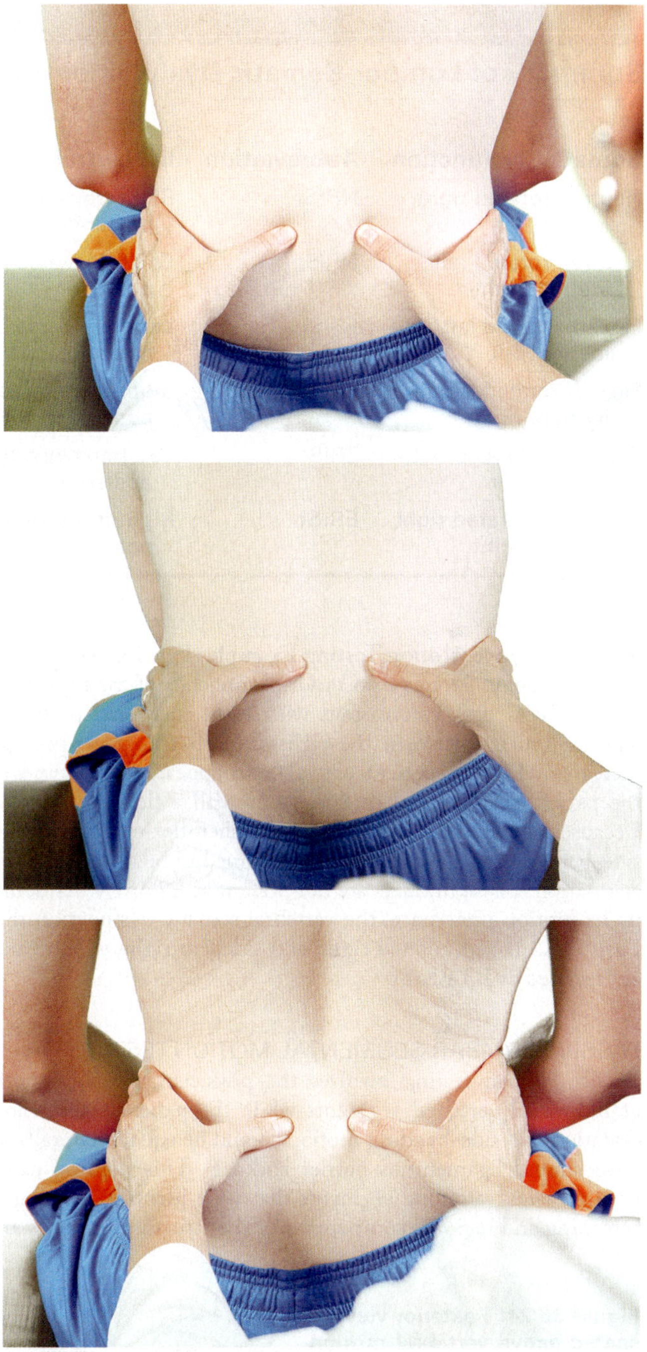

Figure 36.23. Seated active motion testing for lumbar rotational preference. With the lumbar spine in (**A**) neutral, palpate the lumbar transverse processes bilaterally and note asymmetry. Monitor transverse processes for change in asymmetry in (**B**) flexion and (**C**) extension. (Used with permission from A.T. Still University's Kirksville College of Osteopathic Medicine.)

- Side-bending motion preference
  - □ Side bending is not assessed using the active motion testing.
  - □ Side-bending motion is assumed to be to the same side as the rotation preference if there is a flexion or extension preference.
  - □ Side-bending motion is assumed to be to the opposite side as the rotation preference if there is a preference for neutral motion.

TABLE 36.4

Summary of Lumbar Somatic Dysfunction Findings Using Active Motion Testing

		Transverse Process Findings		
Somatic Dysfunction	**Abbreviation**	**In Neutral**	**In Flexion**	**In Extension**
Neutral, rotated right, sidebent left	NRrSl	Right transverse process posterior	Right transverse process posterior	Right transverse process posterior
Neutral, rotated left, sidebent right	NRlSr	Left transverse process posterior	Left transverse process posterior	Left transverse process posterior
Flexed, rotated left, sidebent left	FRlSl	Left transverse process posterior	No asymmetry	Left posterior transverse process more prominent
Flexed, rotated right, sidebent right	FRrSr	Right transverse process posterior	No asymmetry	Right posterior transverse process more prominent
Extended, rotated left, sidebent left	ERlSl	Left transverse process posterior	Left posterior transverse process more prominent	No asymmetry
Extended, rotated right, sidebent right	ERrSr	Right transverse process posterior	Right posterior transverse process more prominent	No asymmetry

Triplanar Active Motion Testing Example (Fig. 36.24)

A patient demonstrates a posterior prominence of the right transverse process of L3 consistent with right rotational preference. The asymmetry between the right and left transverse processes increases when the patient extends and appears to resolve when the patient flexes, which is consistent with a flexion preference. Because the findings improve with either flexion or extension, side-bending motion preference is assumed to be to the same side as rotation. These findings are not present at L2 or L4. As defined by its motion preference, the vertebral somatic dysfunction diagnosis is L3 flexed, rotated right, and sidebent right, which can be abbreviated as L3 FRrSr.

PASSIVE LUMBAR SEGMENTAL MOTION TESTING

Passive motion testing involves the physician inducing motion at individual vertebral segments while the patient stays relaxed. Rotation and side-bending motion should be equal bilaterally and have similar ligamentous barrier end feel. This method can be used to assess vertebral segments that were identified during the screening and regional components of the structural exam as areas with tissue texture abnormalities, asymmetry, or motion restriction. Passive motion testing can be performed with patient seated, supine, lateral recumbent, or prone.

Passive Rotational Motion Assessment (Fig. 36.25)

1. With the patient's lumbar spine in a neutral position, palpate the posterior aspect of the transverse processes bilaterally of the suspected dysfunctional vertebra and note asymmetry. The transverse processes can be found approximately two finger widths away from the associated spinous process. A unilateral posterior prominence of a transverse process will typically be present on the side of rotation preference.
2. Apply alternating anterior pressure to the posterior aspect of each transverse process to assess for passive rotational motion restriction to the opposite side. Note asymmetry of resistance to the anterior motion.
   a. Apply anterior pressure to the right transverse process to induce left vertebral rotation.
   b. Apply anterior pressure to the left transverse process to induce right vertebral rotation.

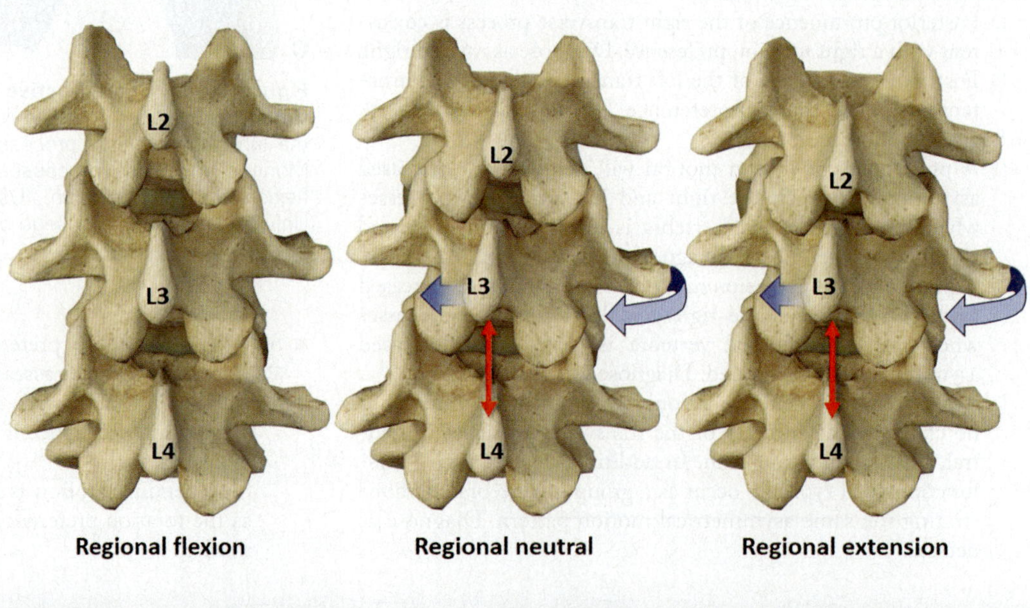

Figure 36.24. Posterior view of seated active vertebral motion assessment of L3. L3 is flexed, rotated right, and sidebent right in (**A**) flexion, (**B**) neutral, and (**C**) extension demonstrating posterior prominence of the right transverse process, deviation of the spinous process to the left, and increased space between the spinous processes of L3 and L4 in regional neutral and extension. (Used with permission from A.T. Still University's Kirksville College of Osteopathic Medicine.)

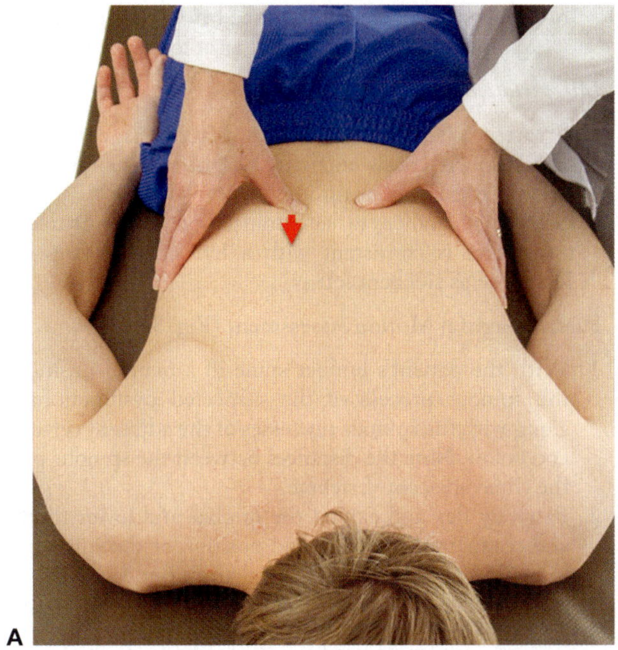

Figure 36.25. Prone passive motion testing for lumbar rotational preference. A. Apply posteroanterior pressure to the right transverse process to induce left vertebral rotation. **B.** Apply posteroanterior pressure to the left transverse process to induce right vertebral rotation. (Used with permission from A.T. Still University's Kirksville College of Osteopathic Medicine.)

Interpretation

- The posterior transverse process will typically demonstrate greater resistance to anterior pressure than the side that is not posteriorly prominent.
- The presence of a posterior right transverse process with greater resistance to anterior pressure is consistent with a right rotational preference. Diagnose as rotated right.
- The presence of a posterior left transverse process with greater resistance to anterior pressure is consistent with a left rotational preference. Diagnose as rotated left.

Passive Side-Bending Motion Assessment (Fig. 36.26)

1. With the patient's lumbar spine in a neutral position, palpate the suspected dysfunctional vertebra at the level of the inferior facet joints by palpating slightly inferior and medial to the transverse processes bilaterally.
2. Apply alternating medial translatory pressure to each side to induce passive side bending on each side. Note asymmetry of the resistance to the translatory motion.
   a. Apply a left translatory force by pushing medially from right to left at the level of the right facet to induce right side bending.

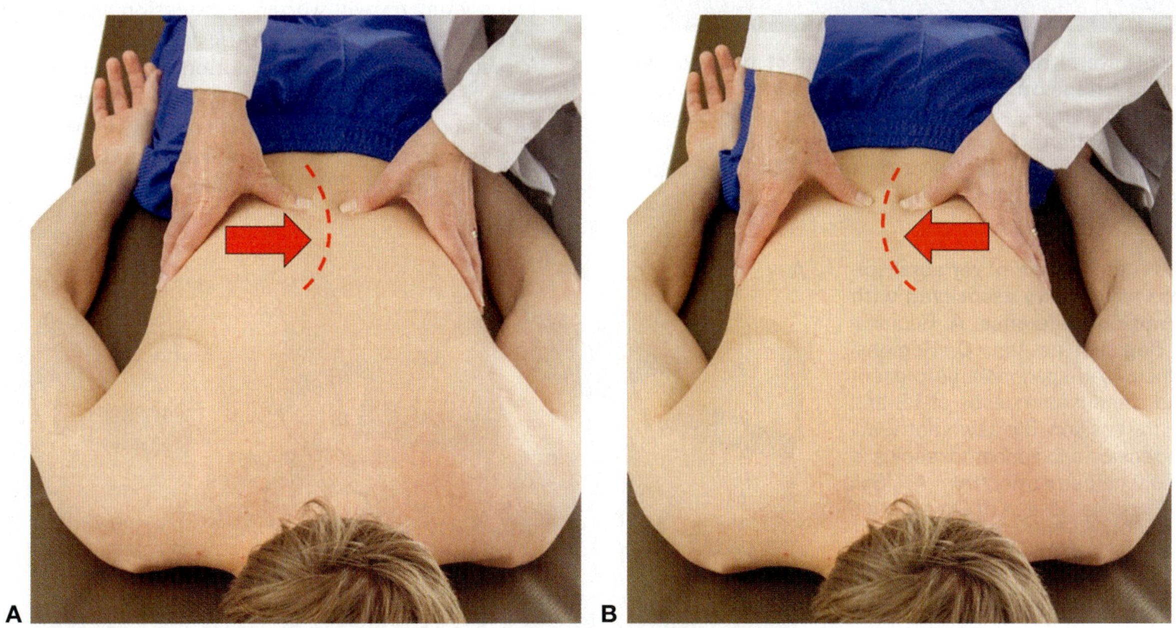

Figure 36.26. Prone passive motion testing for lumbar side-bending preference. A. Apply a left translatory force by pushing medially at the level of the right facet to induce right side bending. **B.** Apply a right translatory force by pushing medially at the level of the left facet to induce left side bending. (Used with permission from A.T. Still University's Kirksville College of Osteopathic Medicine.)

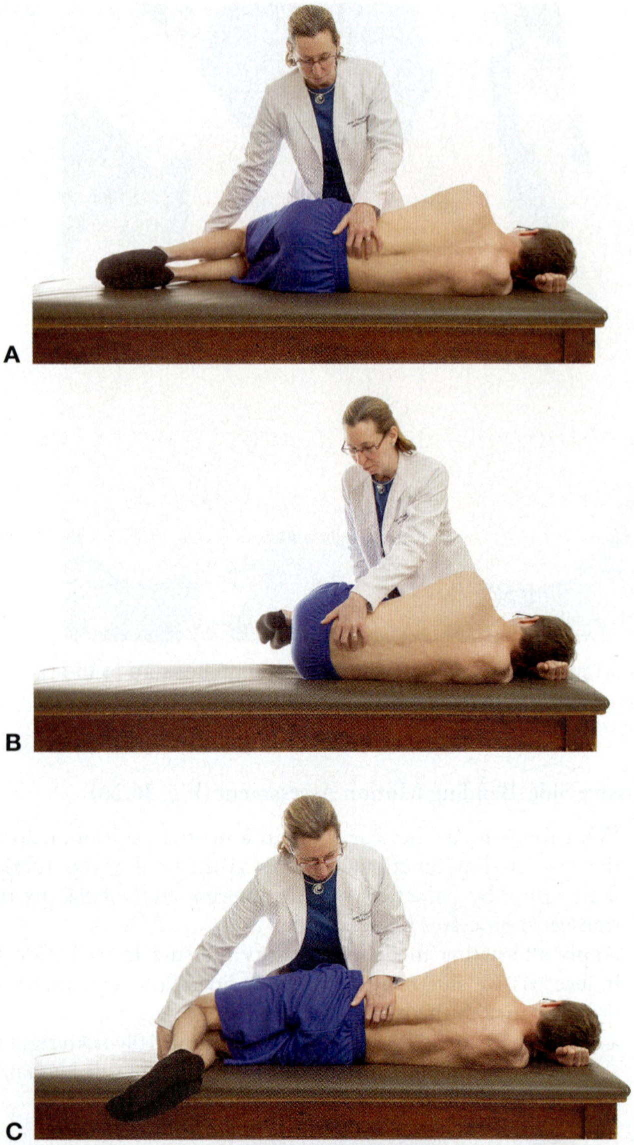

Figure 36.27. Lateral recumbent assessment of passive lumbar flexion and extension. Monitor lumbar spinous process asymmetry and motion of three adjacent vertebrae as the lumbar spine is passively moved from (**A**) neutral into (**B**) flexion and then into (**C**) extension. (Used with permission from A.T. Still University's Kirksville College of Osteopathic Medicine.)

b. Apply a right translatory force by pushing medially from left to right at the level of the left facet to induce left side bending.

Interpretation

- Greater resistance to right translation as compared to left translation is consistent with a right side-bending preference. Diagnose as sidebent right.
- Greater resistance to left translation as compared to right translation is consistent with a left-side–bending preference. Diagnose as sidebent left.

Passive Sagittal Motion Assessment (Fig. 36.27)

1. With the patient's lumbar spine in a neutral position, palpate the spinous process of the suspected dysfunctional vertebra along with the spinous processes of the adjacent vertebrae above and below. Note the distances between the spinous processes of the three adjacent vertebrae.
2. Passively flex and extend the lumbar and lower thoracic spine and compare the motion and position of the spinous processes in neutral and then when flexed and extended.
   a. With the lumbar spine in the neutral position, the spinous processes should be equidistant apart.
   b. With the lumbar spine in flexion, the spinous processes should separate equally until maximal flexion is reached.
   c. With the lumbar spine in extension, the spinous processes should approximate equally until maximal extension is reached.
3. If needed, repeat the procedure on the three vertebrae above and below the suspected area of dysfunction to determine the extent of the dysfunction and to confirm findings.

Note: This procedure can be modified for use as an active sagittal motion assessment by monitoring for changes in spinous process asymmetry while the patient actively flexes and extends.

Interpretation

- A preference for flexion motion will demonstrate increased space between the spinous process of the affected vertebra and the spinous process of the vertebra below in the neutral position. The asymmetry will worsen in extension and appear to resolve in flexion (Fig. 36.28). Diagnose as flexed.
- A preference for extension motion will demonstrate decreased space between the spinous process of the affected vertebra and the spinous process of the vertebra below in the neutral position. The asymmetry will worsen in flexion and appear to resolve in extension (Fig. 36.29). Diagnose as extended.

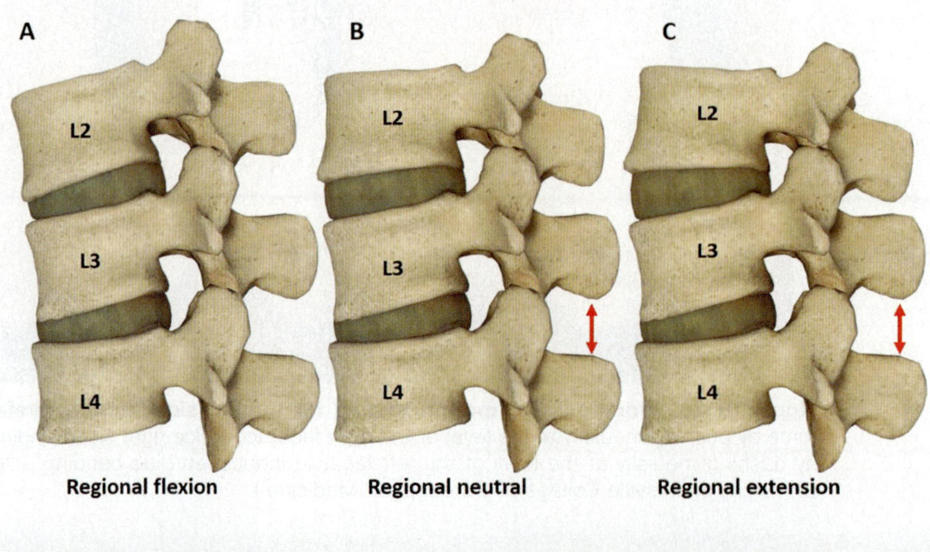

Figure 36.28. Lateral view of vertebral spinous process asymmetry associated with L3 flexion motion preference. A. Regional flexion. **B.** Regional neutral. **C.** Regional extension. Increased space will be present between the spinous processes of L3 and L4 in the neutral position. The asymmetry will worsen in extension and appear to resolve in flexion. (Used with permission from A.T. Still University's Kirksville College of Osteopathic Medicine.)

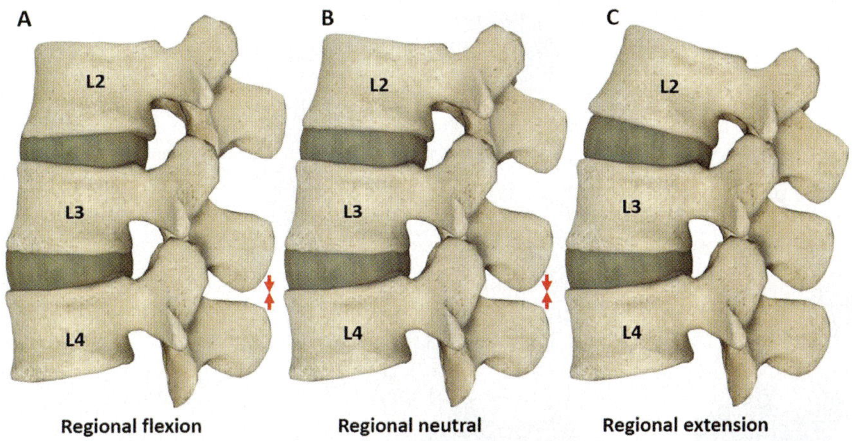

Figure 36.29. Lateral view of vertebral spinous process asymmetry associated with L3 extension motion preference. A. Flexion. **B.** Neutral. **C.** Extension. Decreased space will be present between the spinous processes of L3 and L4 in the neutral position. The asymmetry will worsen in flexion and appear to resolve in extension. (Used with permission from A.T. Still University's Kirksville College of Osteopathic Medicine.)

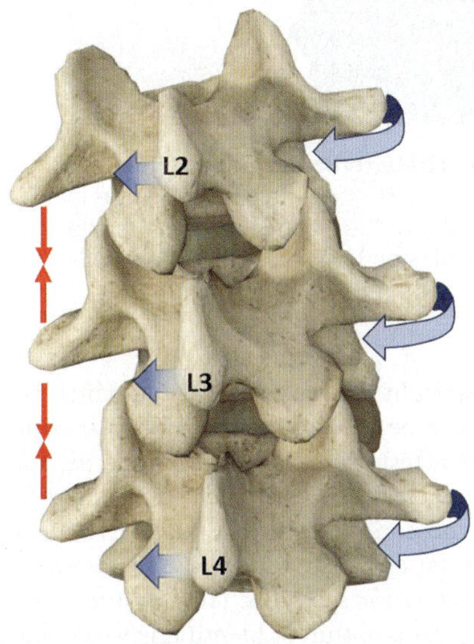

Figure 36.30. L2–L4 Neutral, rotated right, and sidebent left. Demonstrating deviation of the spinous processes to the left, posterior prominence of the right transverse processes, and decreased vertical distance between the left transverse processes. (Used with permission from A.T. Still University's Kirksville College of Osteopathic Medicine.)

- A preference for neutral type 1 motion will demonstrate equidistant spinous processes in neutral, flexion, and extension. Diagnose as neutral.

Triplanar Passive Motion Testing Example (Fig. 36.30)

A patient demonstrates a posterior prominence of the right transverse process of L3. The right transverse process of L3 resists anterior pressure to a greater degree than the left transverse process which is consistent with a right rotational preference at L3. At the level of the L3 inferior facets, there is less resistance to translation from left to right than from right to left, which is consistent with a left-side–bending preference. The spinous processes of L2–L4 are equidistant apart when the lumbar spine is in neutral and remain equidistant in both flexion and extension. The rotation and side-bending findings are also present at L2 and L4. As defined by its motion preference, the triplanar vertebral somatic dysfunction diagnosis is L2–L4 neutral, rotated right, and sidebent left, which can be abbreviated as L2–L4 NRrSl.

Comprehensive Lumbar Evaluation

A comprehensive approach to evaluation of the lumbar region involves assessment for somatic dysfunction and identification of dysfunction that may need additional evaluation for structural

TABLE 36.5

Lumbar Nerve Root Assessment in the Lower Extremity[91]

Nerve Root	Deep Tendon Reflex	Movement Assessment	Innervated Muscle or Muscle Group	Sensory Dermatome
L1	None	Hip flexion	Psoas	Back, groin, and lateral hip
L2	None	Hip adduction	Psoas, hip adductors	Back, anterior thigh
L3	Patellar (variable)	Knee extension	Iliopsoas; quadriceps; adductor brevis, longus, and magnus	Anteromedial thigh
L4	Patellar	Ankle dorsiflexion	Quadriceps; tibialis anterior; adductor brevis, longus, and magnus; hip abductors	Lateral or anterior thigh, medial leg and knee
L5	Medial hamstring (variable)	Great toe dorsiflexion (cannot walk on heels)	Extensor hallucis longus and brevis, gluteus, fibularis longus and brevis, hip abductors	Posterolateral thigh, anterolateral leg, middorsal foot
S1	Achilles	Ankle plantar flexion (cannot walk on toes) and knee flexion	Hamstrings, gastrocnemius, soleus, peroneus longus and brevis, flexor hallucis longus, flexor digitorum longus and brevis	Posterior thigh and calf, lateral and plantar foot

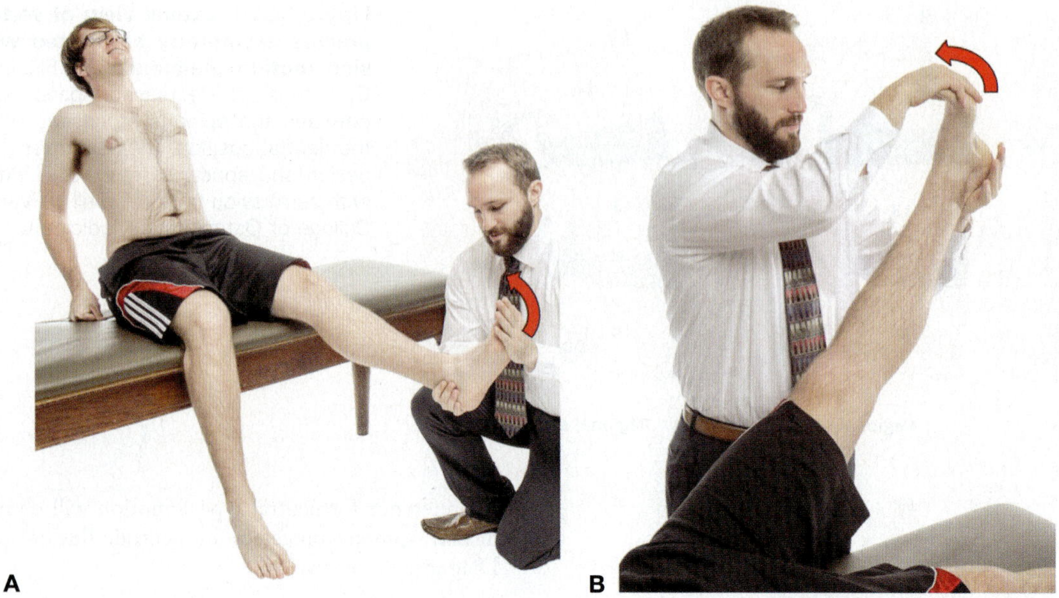

Figure 36.31. Straight leg raise (SLR) test is used to recreate or exacerbate radicular pain. A. Seated. **B.** Supine. The SLR test is performed by passively flexing the patient's hip while maintaining the knee in full extension. If pain occurs, slowly lower the leg until the pain resolves and then apply ipsilateral ankle dorsiflexion. A positive test is reproducible radicular pain. (Used with permission from A.T. Still University's Kirksville College of Osteopathic Medicine.)

pathology, such as nerve root compression, or areas that need specific therapeutic interventions, such as core strengthening. Evaluation should include lower extremity muscle strength testing, deep tendon reflex assessment, and sensory testing[96] (Table 36.5).

Special tests should also be included to further localize functional and structural dysfunction. The choice of special tests is based on symptoms and the tests can be used to identify the origin of pain symptoms. The following tests are just a few of the many options. The straight leg raise (SLR) test, which is also known as Lasègue sign, can be used to identify radicular pain[97] (Fig. 36.31). The crossed SLR test is considered more specific for radiculopathy because it can recreate or exacerbate the patient's radicular pain when flexing the contralateral leg.[97] FABER (flexion, abduction, and external rotation) test, which is also known as Patrick test, can be used to test for sacroiliac joint dysfunction[98] (Fig. 36.32). Trendelenburg test is useful for identifying weak gluteal muscles[81,98]

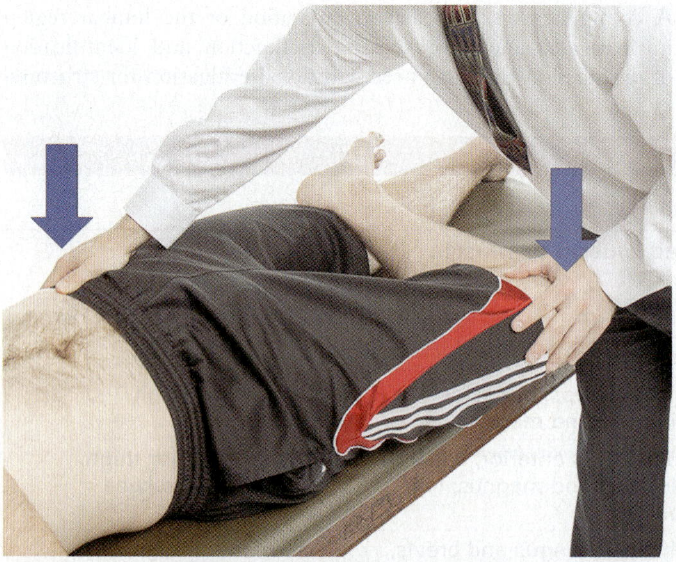

Figure 36.32. FABER (Patrick) test for sacroiliac dysfunction. The test is performed with the ipsilateral knee flexed and the hip flexed, abducted, and externally rotated (FABER) and placed in a "figure-4" position. While stabilizing the opposite hip, apply posterior pressure to the ipsilateral knee. The test is considered positive if pain occurs in the ipsilateral sacroiliac joint. (Used with permission from A.T. Still University's Kirksville College of Osteopathic Medicine.)

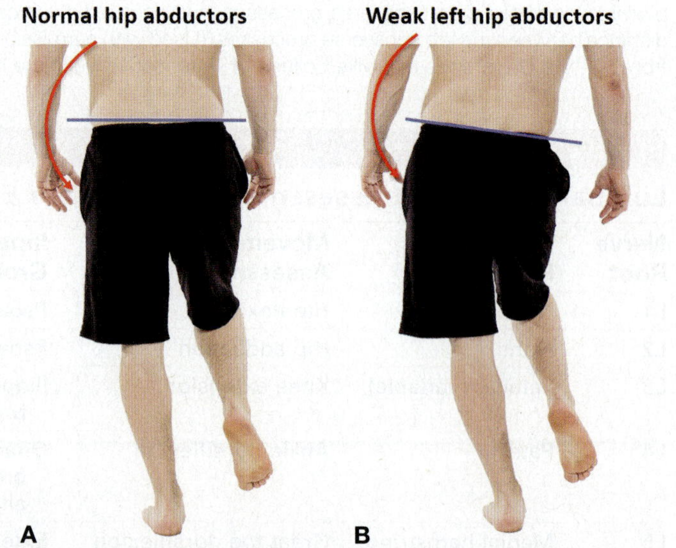

Figure 36.33. Trendelenburg test is performed by having the patient stand unassisted on one leg while observing their iliac crests. A. In the presence of normal hip abductors, the iliac crests should stay level. **B.** Inferior depression of the iliac crest on the non–weight-bearing side indicates weak abductors on the weight-bearing side. (Used with permission from A.T. Still University's Kirksville College of Osteopathic Medicine.)

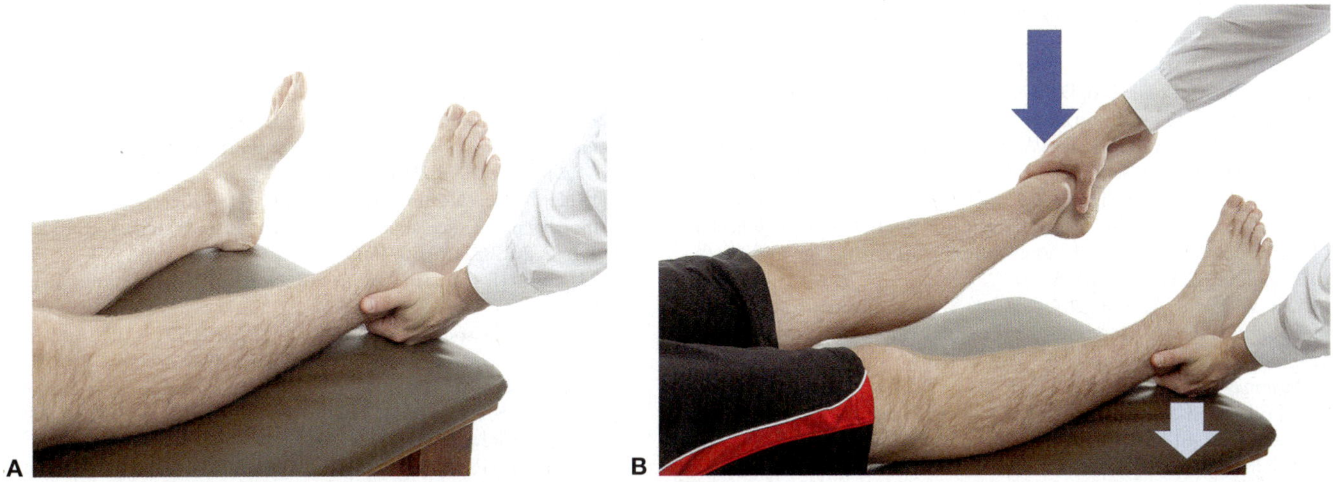

Figure 36.34. Hoover test is performed with the patient supine. A. Place one hand under the heel to be assessed. **B.** Instruct the patient to lift their contralateral leg against physician resistance while monitoring for involuntary downward pressure of the ipsilateral heel. Lack of downward heel pressure is positive for either ipsilateral paresis or poor patient cooperation, which may occur with malingering. (Used with permission from A.T. Still University's Kirksville College of Osteopathic Medicine.)

(Fig. 36.33). The Hoover test can be used to identify malingering[81,97] (Fig. 36.34) (see Chapter 84).

SUMMARY

Identification and treatment of somatic dysfunction in the lumbar region is part of the comprehensive management of regional symptoms, such as low back pain. People with low back pain have been shown to have altered lumbar spinal mechanics when compared to people without low back pain.[99] In addition, people with chronic low back pain have been shown to have more severe lumbar somatic dysfunction, including increased severity of tissue texture abnormalities, motion restriction, and tenderness.[100,101] Somatic dysfunction is the clinical indication for OMT,[102] and OMT has been shown to reduce pain and improve function in people with low back pain.[103] As a result, the American Osteopathic Association recommends that OMT be integrated into the care of patients with low back pain.[104] But, through the interconnectedness of the lumbar region with the rest of the body via myofascial, ligamentous, neural, vascular, and lymphatic structures, treatment of lumbar somatic dysfunction can also impact symptoms throughout the body.

REFERENCES

1. Chen S, Chen M, Wu X, et al. Global, regional and national burden of low back pain 1990–2019: a systematic analysis of the Global Burden of Disease Study 2019. *J Orthop Translat.* 2022;32:49–58.
2. Moore KL, Dalley AF II, Agur AMR. *Clinically Oriented Anatomy.* 8th ed. Wolters Kluwer; 2018.
3. Sénégas J, Bouloussa H, Liguoro D, Yoshida G, Vital JM. Morphologic and functional evolution of the aging spine. In: Vital JM, Cawley DT, eds. *Spinal Anatomy: Modern Concepts.* Springer Nature; 2020:75–112.
4. Suresh SC, Raju B, Jumah F, Nanda A. Lumbosacral extradural extramedullary hematopoiesis in thalassemia major causing spinal canal stenosis. *Surg Neurol Int.* 2020;11:331.
5. Konin GP, Walz DM. Lumbosacral transitional vertebrae: classification, imaging findings, and clinical relevance. *AJNR Am J Neuroradiol.* 2010;31(10):1778–1786.
6. Dalley AF II, Agur AMR. Back. In: *Moore's Clinically Oriented Anatomy.* 9th ed. Wolters Kluwer; 2023:71–141.
7. Dimeglio A, Bonnel F, Canavese F. The growing spine. In: Vital JM, Cawley DT, eds. *Spinal Anatomy: Modern Concepts.* Springer Nature; 2020:25–52.
8. Chen S, Fu P, Wu H, Pei M. Meniscus, articular cartilage and nucleus pulposus: a comparative review of cartilage-like tissues in anatomy, development and function. *Cell Tissue Res.* 2017;370(1):53–70.
9. Chan SC, Ferguson SJ, Gantenbein-Ritter B. The effects of dynamic loading on the intervertebral disc. *Eur Spine J.* 2011;20(11):1796–1812.
10. Groh AMR, Fournier DE, Battié MC, Séguin CA. Innervation of the human intervertebral disc: a scoping review. *Pain Med.* 2021;22(6):1281–1304.
11. Fournier DE, Kiser PK, Shoemaker JK, Battie MC, Séguin CA. Vascularization of the human intervertebral disc: a scoping review. *JOR Spine.* 2020;3(4):e1123.
12. Obeid I, Vital JM. Surgical anatomy of the vertebral pedicle. In: Vital JM, Cawley DT, eds. *Spinal Anatomy: Modern Concepts.* Springer Nature; 2020:153–160.
13. Vital JM. The normal and pathological spinal muscle. In: Vital JM, Cawley DT, eds. *Spinal Anatomy: Modern Concepts.* Springer Nature; 2020:251–272.
14. DeStefano LA. Lumbar spine technique. In: *Greenman's Principles of Manual Medicine.* 5th ed. Wolters Kluwer; 2017:288–313.
15. Louis C, Louis R. Anatomy of the thoraco-lumbar facet joint. In: Vital JM, Cawley DT, eds. *Spinal Anatomy: Modern Concepts.* Springer Nature; 2020:217–228.
16. Alonso F, Kirkpatrick CM, Jeong W, et al. Lumbar facet tropism: a comprehensive review. *World Neurosurg.* 2017;102:91–96.
17. Ko S, Chae S, Choi W, Kim JY, Kwon J, Doh J. The prevalence of facet tropism and its correlation with low back pain in selected community-based populations. *Clin Orthop Surg.* 2019;11(2):176–182.
18. Samartzis D, Cheung JP, Rajasekaran S, et al. Is lumbar facet joint tropism developmental or secondary to degeneration? An international, large-scale multicenter study by the AOSpine Asia Pacific Research Collaboration Consortium. *Scoliosis Spinal Disord.* 2016;11:9.
19. Varlotta GP, Lefkowitz TR, Schweitzer M, et al. The lumbar facet joint: a review of current knowledge. Part II: diagnosis and management. *Skeletal Radiol.* 2011;40(2):149–157.
20. Lavignolle B. Spinal nerves (innervation of the spine). In: Vital JM, Cawley DT, eds. *Spinal Anatomy: Modern Concepts.* Springer Nature; 2020:391–402.
21. McLain RF, Pickar JG. Mechanoreceptor endings in human thoracic and lumbar facet joints. *Spine (Phila Pa 1976).* 1998;23(2):168–173.
22. Gregerson DM. Clinical consequences of spina bifida occulta. *J Manipulative Physiol Ther.* 1997;20(8):546–550.
23. Illeez OG, Ulger FEB, Aktas I. The effect of transitional vertebrae and spina bifida occulta on disc herniation, disc degeneration, and end-plate changes in pediatric patients with low back pain. *Acta Orthop Belg.* 2022;88(2):275–283.

24. Morimoto M, Sugiura K, Higashino K, et al. Association of spinal anomalies with spondylolysis and spina bifida occulta. *Eur Spine J.* 2022;31(4):858–864.
25. Sedney CL, McConda DB, Daffner SD. Natural history of spondylolysis and spondylolisthesis. *Semin Spine Surg.* 2014;26(4):214–218.
26. Aylott CE, Puna R, Robertson PA, Walker C. Spinous process morphology: the effect of ageing through adulthood on spinous process size and relationship to sagittal alignment. *Eur Spine J.* 2012;21(5):1007–1012.
27. Snider KT, Kribs JW, Snider EJ, Degenhardt BF, Bukowski A, Johnson JC. Reliability of Tuffier's line as an anatomic landmark. *Spine (Phila Pa 1976).* 2008;33(6):E161–E165.
28. Chan V, Marro A, Rempel J, Nataraj A. Determination of dynamic instability in lumbar spondylolisthesis using flexion and extension standing radiographs versus neutral standing radiograph and supine MRI. *J Neurosurg Spine.* 2019;31(2):229–235.
29. Oh JY, Liang S, Louange D, Rahmat R, Hee HT, Kumar VP. Paradoxical motion in L5-S1 adult spondylolytic spondylolisthesis. *Eur Spine J.* 2012; 21(2):262–267.
30. Sakka L. Anatomy of the spinal meninges. In: Vital JM, Cawley DT, eds. *Spinal Anatomy: Modern Concepts*. Springer Nature; 2020:403–420.
31. Vital JM. The spinal canal. In: Vital JM, Cawley DT, eds. *Spinal Anatomy: Modern Concepts*. Springer Nature; 2020:345–362.
32. Ajimsha MS, Shenoy PD, Gampawar N. Role of fascial connectivity in musculoskeletal dysfunctions: a narrative review. *J Bodyw Mov Ther.* 2020;24(4):423–431.
33. Bordoni B, Zanier E. Clinical and symptomatological reflections: the fascial system. *J Multidiscip Healthc.* 2014;7:401–411.
34. Neumann DA. Pelvic girdle, hip, gluteal region and thigh. In: Standring S, ed. *Gray's Anatomy: The Anatomical Basis of Clinical Practice*. 42nd ed. Elsevier; 2021:1352–1394.
35. Tubbs RS. Posterior abdominal wall and retroperitoneum. In: Standring S, ed. *Gray's Anatomy: The Anatomical Basis of Clinical Practice*. 42nd ed. Elsevier; 2021:1137–1149.
36. Dalley AF, Agur AMR, Moore KL. *Moore's Clinically Oriented Anatomy*. 9th ed. Wolters Kluwer; 2023.
37. Drake RL, Vogl AW, Mitchell AWM. Back. In: Drake RL, Vogl AW, Mitchell AWM, ed. *Gray's Anatomy for Students*. 4th ed. Elsevier; 2020: 49–122.
38. Drake RL, Vogl AW, Mitchell AWM. Abdomen. In: Drake RL, Vogl AW, Mitchell AWM, ed. *Gray's Anatomy for Students*. 4th ed. Elsevier; 2020: 249–412.
39. Drake RL, Vogl AW, Mitchell AWM. Lower limb. In: Drake RL, Vogl AW, Mitchell AWM, ed. *Gray's Anatomy for Students*. 4th ed. Elsevier; 2020:525–670.
40. Drake RL, Vogl AW, Mitchell AWM. Upper limb. In: Drake RL, Vogl AW, Mitchell AWM, ed. *Gray's Anatomy for Students*. 4th ed. Elsevier; 2020:671–821.
41. Bonnel F, Dimeglio A. Vertebral column: muscles, aponeurosis, and fascia. In: Vital JM, Cawley DT, eds. *Spinal Anatomy: Modern Concepts*. Springer Nature; 2020:279–320.
42. Dalley AF II, Agur AMR. Abdomen. In: *Moore's Clinically Oriented Anatomy*. 9th ed. Wolters Kluwer; 2023:410–558.
43. Tubbs RS. Abdomen and pelvis: overview and surface anatomy. In: Standring S, ed. *Gray's Anatomy: The Anatomical Basis of Clinical Practice*. 42nd ed. Elsevier; 2021:1107–1121.
44. Gardner ED, Bunge RP. Chapter 2 – Gross anatomy of the peripheral nervous system. In: Dyck PJ, Thomas PK, eds. *Peripheral Neuropathy*. 4th ed. W.B. Saunders; 2005:11–33.
45. Vital JM. The spinal ligaments. In: Vital JM, Cawley DT, eds. *Spinal Anatomy: Modern Concepts*. Springer Nature; 2020:229–242.
46. Hatgis J, Granville M, Jacobson RE. Baastrup's disease, interspinal bursitis, and dorsal epidural cysts: radiologic evaluation and impact on treatment options. *Cureus.* 2017;9(7):e1449.
47. Yu T, Zhang J, Zhu W, et al. Chondrogenesis mediates progression of ankylosing spondylitis through heterotopic ossification. *Bone Res.* 2021;9:19.
48. Baron E, Tunstall R. Back. In: Standring S, ed. *Gray's Anatomy: The Anatomical Basis of Clinical Practice*. 42nd ed. Elsevier; 2021:814–855.
49. Ashby K, Yilmaz E, Mathkour M, et al. Ligaments stabilizing the sacrum and sacroiliac joint: a comprehensive review. *Neurosurg Rev.* 2022;45(1):357–364.
50. Tortland PD. Evaluation and treatment of low back pain in athletes. *J Am Osteopath Assoc.* 1997;97(11 suppl):S13–S14.
51. Peeters L. The iliolumber ligaments: a literature study. *AAO J.* 2011; 21(2):23–29.
52. Rucco V, Basadonna PT, Gasparini D. Anatomy of the iliolumbar ligament: a review of its anatomy and a magnetic resonance study. *Am J Phys Med Rehabil.* 1996;75(6):451–455.
53. Willard FH, Vleeming A, Schuenke MD, Danneels L, Schleip R. The thoracolumbar fascia: anatomy, function and clinical considerations. *J Anat.* 2012;221(6):507–536.
54. Magoun HI. *Osteopathy in the Cranial Field*. 2nd ed. Journal Publishing Company; 1966.
55. Guérin J. The spinal cord. In: Vital JM, Cawley DT, eds. *Spinal Anatomy: Modern Concepts*. Springer Nature; 2020:363–390.
56. Baron E, Solanki G. Spinal cord and spinal nerves: gross anatomy. In: Standring S, ed. *Gray's Anatomy: The Anatomical Basis of Clinical Practice*. 42nd ed. Elsevier; 2021:856–868.
57. O'Connor KP, Smitherman AD, Milton CK, et al. Surgical treatment of tethered cord syndrome in adults: a systematic review and meta-analysis. *World Neurosurg.* 2020;137:e221–e241.
58. Vuka I, Došenović S, Marciuš T, et al. Efficacy and safety of pulsed radiofrequency as a method of dorsal root ganglia stimulation for treatment of non-neuropathic pain: a systematic review. *BMC Anesthesiol.* 2020;20:105.
59. Shayota B, Wong TL, Fru D, et al. A comprehensive review of the sinuvertebral nerve with clinical applications. *Anat Cell Biol.* 2019;52(2):128–133.
60. Breemer MC, Malessy MJA, Notenboom RGE. Origin, branching pattern, foraminal and intraspinal distribution of the human lumbar sinuvertebral nerves. *Spine J.* 2022;22(3):472–482.
61. Standring S. The anatomy of the peripheral nervous system. In: Standring S, ed. *Gray's Anatomy: The Anatomical Basis of Clinical Practice*. 42nd ed. Elsevier; 2021:e11–e55.
62. Beal MC. Viscerosomatic reflexes: a review. *J Am Osteopath Assoc.* 1985; 85(12):786–801.
63. Zink JG. Respiratory and circulatory care: the conceptual model. *AAO J.* 2012;22(1):86–90.
64. Liguoro D, Barreau X. Spinal vascularization. In: Vital JM, Cawley DT, eds. *Spinal Anatomy: Modern Concepts*. Springer Nature; 2020:427–446.
65. Biglioli P, Roberto M, Cannata A, et al. Upper and lower spinal cord blood supply: the continuity of the anterior spinal artery and the relevance of the lumbar arteries. *J Thorac Cardiovasc Surg.* 2004;127(4):1188–1192.
66. Johnson SM, Shah LM. Imaging of acute low back pain. *Radiol Clin North Am.* 2019;57(2):397–413.
67. Roman PEF, Grewal AS, Taylor BS, Grigore AM. Advances in spinal cord protection from perioperative ischemic injury. *Adv Anesth.* 2014; 32(1):205–235.
68. Standring S. The anatomy of the vascular and lymphatic systems. In: Standring S, ed. *Gray's Anatomy: The Anatomical Basis of Clinical Practice*. 42nd ed. Elsevier; 2021:e56–e129.
69. van Schoor A. Respiratory diaphragm and phrenic nerves. In: Standring S, ed. *Gray's Anatomy: The Anatomical Basis of Clinical Practice*. 42nd ed. Elsevier; 2021:1038–1046.
70. Ward JPT. Smooth muscle and the cardiovascular and lymphatic systems. In: Standring S, ed. *Gray's Anatomy: The Anatomical Basis of Clinical Practice*. 42nd ed. Elsevier; 2021:127–144.
71. Van Schaik JP, Verbiest H, Van Schaik FD. Isolated spinous process deviation: a pitfall in the interpretation of AP radiographs of the lumbar spine. *Spine (Phila Pa 1976).* 1989;14(9):970–976.
72. Ng PTT, Claus A, Izatt MT, Pivonka P, Tucker K. Is spinal neuromuscular function asymmetrical in adolescents with idiopathic scoliosis compared to those without scoliosis? A narrative review of surface EMG studies. *J Electromyogr Kinesiol.* 2022;63:102640.
73. Shahidi B, Yoo A, Farnsworth C, Newton PO, Ward SR. Paraspinal muscle morphology and composition in adolescent idiopathic scoliosis: a histological analysis. *JOR Spine.* 2021;4(3):e1169.
74. Reuber M, Schultz A, McNeill T, Spencer D. Trunk muscle myoelectric activities in idiopathic scoliosis. *Spine (Phila Pa 1976).* 1983;8(5):447–456.
75. Shafaq N, Suzuki A, Matsumura A, et al. Asymmetric degeneration of paravertebral muscles in patients with degenerative lumbar scoliosis. *Spine (Phila Pa 1976).* 2012;37(16):1398–1406.

76. Xie H, Liu J, He Y, et al. Surface electromyography study on asymmetry in paravertebral muscle degeneration in patients with degenerative lumbar scoliosis. *Sci Rep.* 2022;12(1):18675.
77. DiGiovanna EL, Amen CJ, Burns DK. *An Osteopathic Approach to Diagnosis and Treatment.* 4th ed. Wolters Kluwer; 2021.
78. Sutton SE. An osteopathic method of history taking and physical examination: part 2. *J Am Osteopath Assoc.* 1978;77(11):845–858.
79. Kapandji AI. *The Physiology of the Joints: The Spinal Column, Pelvic Girdle and Head.* Vol 3. 7th ed. Handspring Publishing; 2019.
80. Frank C, Liebenson C, Veverková M. Evaluation of muscular imbalance. In: Liebenson C, ed. *Rehabilitation of the Spine: A Patient-Centered Approach.* 3rd ed. Wolters Kluwer; 2020:339–359.
81. Magee DJ, Manske RC. Lumbar spine. In: *Orthopedic Physical Assessment.* 7th ed. Elsevier; 2021:627–723.
82. Magee DJ, Manske RC. Assessment of posture. In: *Orthopedic Physical Assessment.* 7th ed. Elsevier; 2021:627–723.
83. Puagprakong P, Kanjanasilanont A, Sornkaew K, Brady WS. The effects of lower crossed syndrome on upper body posture during sitting in female office workers. *Muscles Ligaments Tendons J.* 2022;12(4):621–627.
84. Donnelly JM, ed. *Travell, Simons & Simons' Myofascial Pain and Dysfunction: The Trigger Point Manual.* 3rd ed. Wolters Kluwer; 2019.
85. Jones LH. *Strain and Counterstrain.* American Academy of Osteopathy; 1981.
86. Jones LH. *Jones Strain-Counterstrain.* JonesStrain-Counterstrain, Inc.; 1995.
87. Snider KT, Glover JC. *Atlas of Common Counterstrain Tender Points.* A.T. Still University; 2014.
88. White AA III, Panjabi MM. *Clinical Biomechanics of the Spine.* 2nd ed. Lippincott Williams & Wilkins; 1990:646.
89. Harrison DE, Harrison DD, Troyanovich SJ. Three-dimensional spinal coupling mechanics: part I. A review of the literature. *J Manipulative Physiol Ther.* 1998;21(2):101–113.
90. DeStefano LA. *Greenman's principles of Manual Medicine*, 5th ed. Wolters Kluwer; 2017:49–50.
91. Cook C. Coupling behavior of the lumbar spine: a literature review. *J Man Manip Ther.* 2003;11(3):137–145.
92. Fryette HH. *Principles of Osteopathic Technic.* Academy of Applied Osteopathy; 1954:22–26.
93. Lee R. Measurement of movements of the lumbar spine. *Physiother Theory Pract.* 2002;18(4):159–164.
94. Zhang C, Mannen EM, Sis HL, et al. Moment-rotation behavior of intervertebral joints in flexion-extension, lateral bending, and axial rotation at all levels of the human spine: a structured review and meta-regression analysis. *J Biomech.* 2020;100:109579.
95. White AA III, Panjabi MM. The basic kinematics of the human spine. A review of past and current knowledge. *Spine (Phila Pa 1976).* 1978;3(1):12–20.
96. Apaydin N, Woodley SJ. Pelvic girdle and lower limb: overview and surface anatomy. In: Standring S, ed. *Gray's Anatomy: The Anatomical Basis of Clinical Practice.* 42nd ed. Elsevier; 2021:1333–1351.
97. De Luigi AJ, Fitzpatrick KF. Physical examination in radiculopathy. *Phys Med Rehabil Clin N Am.* 2011;22(1):7–40.
98. Magee DJ, Manske RC. Hip. In: *Orthopedic Physical Assessment.* 7th ed. Elsevier; 2022:765–868.
99. Saito H, Watanabe Y, Kutsuna T, et al. Spinal movement variability associated with low back pain: a scoping review. *PLoS One.* 2021;16(5):e0252141.
100. Snider KT, Johnson JC, Degenhardt BF, Snider EJ. Low back pain, somatic dysfunction, and segmental bone mineral density T-score variation in the lumbar spine. *J Am Osteopath Assoc.* 2011;111(2):89–96.
101. Snider KT, Johnson JC, Degenhardt BF, Snider EJ, Burton DC. Association of low back pain, somatic dysfunction, and lumbar bone mineral density: reproducibility of findings. *J Am Osteopath Assoc.* 2014;114(5):356–367.
102. Snider KT, Jorgensen DJ. Billing and coding for osteopathic manipulative treatment. *J Am Osteopath Assoc.* 2009;109(8):409–413.
103. Franke H, Franke JD, Fryer G. Osteopathic manipulative treatment for nonspecific low back pain: a systematic review and meta-analysis. *BMC Musculoskelet Disord.* 2014;15:286.
104. Task Force on the Low Back Pain Clinical Practice Guidelines. American Osteopathic Association guidelines for osteopathic manipulative treatment (OMT) for patients with low back pain. *J Am Osteopath Assoc.* 2016; 116(8):536–549.

37 Pelvis

KURT P. HEINKING ▪ MIHO YOSHIDA ▪ REBECCA E. GIUSTI

KEY CONCEPTS

- Osteopathic manipulative treatment of the pelvic girdle is dependent on applying functional anatomical knowledge of the region.
- Knowledge of the anatomy, biomechanics, and physiologic motion of the innominates, pubic bones, and sacroiliac joints (SIJs) is essential to understanding the somatic dysfunction of this region.
- Physical examination is integrated with palpatory diagnosis and motion testing of the pelvic region.
- Diagnosis of somatic dysfunction in the pelvic region.
- Performance of the segmental exam to the pelvic region.
- Knowledge of pelvic anatomy is necessary for the diagnosis and evaluation of viscerosomatic and somatovisceral reflexes in this region.

INTRODUCTION

Accurate and efficient diagnosis of the pelvic girdle is of great importance to practitioners of manual medicine. The pelvis holds a central role in coupling the mechanical forces of the lower extremities with the axial skeleton above. It is also the foundation for body support and locomotion. Alterations and restrictions of motions in the pelvic girdle may have a profound effect on the following:

- Vertebral function
- Thoracoabdominal diaphragm
- Pelvic diaphragm
- The craniosacral mechanism
- Lower extremities

Somatic dysfunction of the pelvic girdle may be causative, contributory, or diagnostic for a wide range of patient complaints. Such complaints may be somatic, visceral, or emotional in nature. Common patient complaints that require evaluation of the sacrum and pelvis include but are not limited to the following:

- Abdominal pain
- Pelvic pain
- Gynecologic disorders
- Lower back pain (including during pregnancy)
- Urinary tract problems
- Lower gastrointestinal issues
- Neuralgia of the lower extremities

In each of these situations, the patient's sacrum and pelvis should be evaluated and if appropriate, treated with osteopathic manipulation. In addition to a focused physical exam, an osteopathic evaluation for somatic dysfunction of the cranium and lumbar spine is integrated with sacral–pelvic diagnoses. If somatic dysfunction is found and related to the patient's condition, osteopathic manipulative treatment (OMT) may be utilized in the treatment plan along with other applicable therapies. The role of manual medicine in the management of the pelvic girdle is to restore function and optimize coordination between the arthrodial, neural, vascular, lymphatic, and connective tissue elements.

DEFINITION

The pelvis (plural pelves or pelvises) is either the lower part of the trunk,[1] between the abdomen and the thighs (also referred to as the pelvic region of the trunk), or the skeleton embedded in it (also referred to as the bony pelvis, or pelvic skeleton).[2]

The pelvic region of the trunk includes the following[1]:

- Bony pelvis
- Pelvic cavity (the space enclosed by the bony pelvis)
- Pelvic floor
- Perineum

The pelvic skeleton is formed posteriorly, by the sacrum and the coccyx, and anteriorly and laterally, by a pair of hip bones or the innominates. The innominates connect the spine with the lower limbs. They are attached to the sacrum posteriorly, connected to each other anteriorly, and joined with the two femurs at the acetabular joints. The gap enclosed by the bony pelvis, called the pelvic cavity, is the section of the body inferior to the abdomen containing the reproductive organs and the rectum.

The pelvis consists of three bones and three joints forming an open ring shape. The false pelvis is a part of the lower abdomen and is walled laterally by ilia. The true pelvis is located inferior and posterior to the abdomen. It begins at the level of the sacral promontory, arcuate line, pectinate line, and pubic bones and ends with the inferior fascia of the pelvic diaphragm.

DESCRIPTIVE AND FUNCTIONAL ANATOMY

Skeletal Structures (Fig. 37.1)

THE ILIA

Functionally, each innominate can be viewed as a lower extremity bone; and the sacrum, as a component part of the vertebral axis. The innominates are composed of three bones joined together at the acetabular notch; the ischium, ilium, and pubis.

- The innominate is formed from a single cartilaginous model where the ischium, ilium, and pubis are the primary ossification centers before birth.
- Epiphyseal centers form in the cartilaginous iliac crest, anterior superior iliac spine (ASIS), and ischial tuberosities (at puberty) and eventually fuse in the late teens or early 20s.
- The only remnants of the original cartilaginous model are the bilateral SIJs.[3]

The acetabulum occupies the lateral aspect of the ilium and articulates with the head of the femur to create the hip joint. The

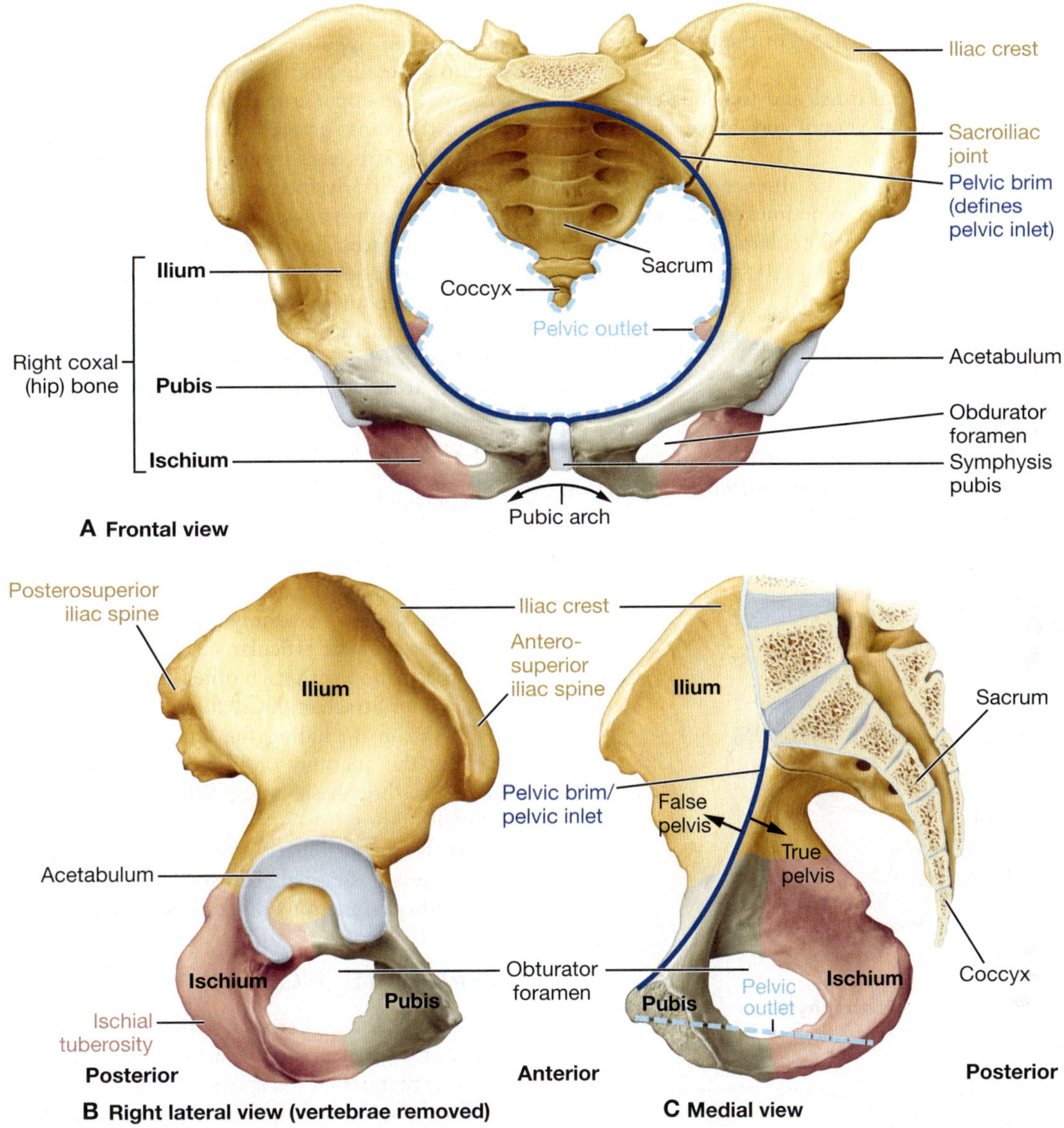

Figure 37.1. Bones of the pelvic girdle. The pelvic girdle consists of two coxae fused together. Each coxa consists of one ilium, one ischium, and one pubic bone fused together. **A.** Frontal view. **B.** Right lateral view. **C.** Medial view. (Reprinted with permission from McConnell TH, Hull KL. *Human Form, Human Function: Essentials of Anatomy & Physiology*. Wolters Kluwer Health/Lippincott Williams & Wilkins; 2011.)

two innominate bones are joined anteriorly by the pubic symphysis, and superiorly with the sacrum via the bilateral SIJs. Male and female skeletons can be notably distinguished by the pelvic girdles. The differences are related to the heavier build and larger muscles of most men leading to a thick and heavy structure and narrow and deep lesser pelvis and the adaptation of the pelvis in women for parturition, developing a thin and light structure and wide, shallow lesser pelvis.[1]

SPINAL ARTICULATIONS

The three joints of the pelvis include the symphysis pubis and the two SIJs. The sacrum is attached to the lumbar vertebra by a lumbosacral disk, two lumbosacral synovial joints, and ligaments. The superior articular processes of the sacrum are concave and generally face posteromedially. They articulate with the inferior articular processes of the fifth lumbar vertebrae. Anomalous development commonly results in asymmetric lumbosacral facets (facet tropism), and less commonly in incomplete separation and differentiation of the fifth lumbar vertebrae (sacralization). When the transverse processes of the fifth lumbar vertebra are atypically large, pseudoarthrosis may occur with the sacrum or ilia (ilium).

THE PUBIC BONES AND PUBIC SYMPHYSIS

The pubic symphysis is a fibrocartilaginous joint that has motion determined by its anatomic shape, ligaments, and muscular attachments. The pubic rami are also subject to a wide range of muscular forces which can produce somatic dysfunction.

THE SACRUM AND COCCYX

The sacrum is shaped like an inverted triangle with the superior aspect being the base, and the inferior aspect being the apex.

- The most anterior and superior portion of the first sacral vertebral body is called the sacral promontory.
- The anterior (pelvic) surface is smooth and concave, and the dorsal surface is rough and convex with palpable spinous tubercles.
- The medial row of tubercles is formed by fusion of the sacral articular processes.

- The lateral row is formed by the fusion of sacral transverse processes and inferiorly ends in a curve of the bone called the inferolateral angle.
- The sacrum contains the sacral canal and four bilateral sacral foramina for the passage of the ventral and dorsal rami of the first four sacral spinal nerves.
- The sacral hiatus is formed from the absence of the laminae and spinous process the fifth (and sometimes fourth) sacral vertebra. It is at this location that sacral epidural nerve blocks are performed.

The coccyx attaches to the sacral apex via the sacrococcygeal joint. The ganglion impar (where the right and left sympathetic chains join) rests on the anterior surface of the coccyx.

THE PELVIC ARTICULATIONS

The SIJs have been described as L or C shaped and are contoured with a shorter upper arm and longer lower arm, with the junction occurring approximately at S2 (Fig. 37.2).

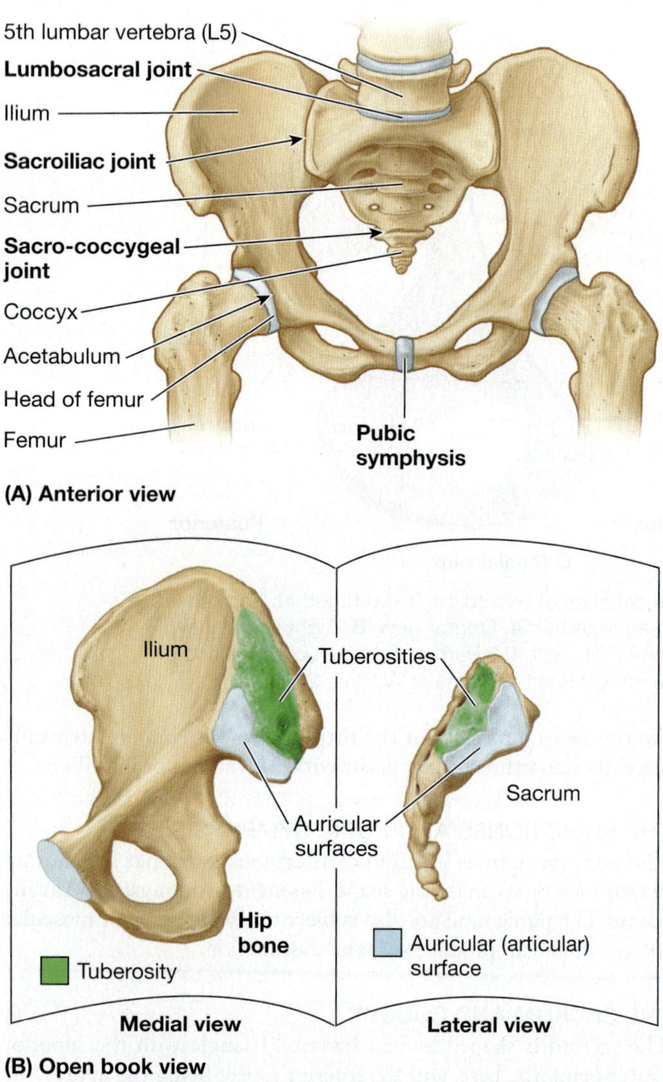

Figure 37.2. Joints of the pelvic girdle. A. Overview. The sacroiliac joints unite the axial and inferior appendicular skeletons. The lumbosacral and sacrococcygeal joints are joints of the axial skeleton directly related to the pelvic girdle. **B.** Open book view of articulating surfaces of sacroiliac joint. (Reprinted with permission from Dalley AF II, Agur AMR. *Moore's Clinically Oriented Anatomy*. 9th ed. Wolters Kluwer; 2023. Figure 6.4.)

The articular surfaces are subject to a great deal of variation, including on opposite sides of the same bone.[4] The apex of the sacrum generally points anteriorly. The SI articulation is typically convex at the upper arm and concave at the lower arm. The longer arm of the joint surface is directed posteriorly and inferiorly, and the shorter arm faces posteriorly and cranially; therefore, the SIJs converge inferiorly and posteriorly. It is a diarthrodial joint because it contains both synovial fluid and matching articular surfaces. The articular surfaces, however, are different from those in any other joint in the body. It is in this joint alone that hyaline articular cartilage faces and moves against fibrocartilage. On the sacral side, this hyaline cartilage is usually 1 to 3 mm in depth. The ilial side is composed of fibrocartilage.[3] The sacrum decreases in width from superior to inferior and it is wedged between the two ilia. The predominant direction of fibers of the SI ligaments is such that they prevent excessive separation of the innominates and inferior gliding of the sacrum.[4]

The lumbosacral facets are predominantly coronal with the surface of the inferior lumbar facet slanting posteriorly. The sacral sulcus is a palpable groove just medial to the PSIS.

Much variation exists between anatomic description and an individual patient's anatomy. Weisl's work[5] demonstrates the varying contours of the articular surfaces of the sacrum and the ilia at their articulation with each other. In extensive study of sacral anatomy, Frazier Strachan, DO,[4] found significant anatomic variations of the sacrum including the amount of curvature present. After studying the anatomy of numerous sacrums, he concluded that there were three basic types, differentiated by the dorsal and ventral width ratios.

Anatomic asymmetry affects the sacrum's stability as well as the way it is positioned against the ilia. This also affects the types of somatic dysfunction and applicable treatment.[4]

LIGAMENTS (FIG. 37.3)

The bilateral sacrotuberous ligaments run from the inferior medial border of the sacrum and insert on the ischial tuberosities and the posterior margins of the sciatic notches.

The bilateral sacrospinous ligaments lie anterior to the sacrotuberous ligaments and attach to the ischial spines, dividing this space into the greater and lesser sciatic foramen. The sacrospinous and sacrotuberous ligaments restrain the anterior movement of the sacrum within the pelvic bones. The long head of the biceps femoris, piriformis, and gluteus maximus muscles often have direct attachments to the sacrotuberous ligament. It has been shown that the muscles interacting with the sacrotuberous ligament have a role in SIJ mobility and stability.[6] Detailed dissections of anatomic material by Vleeming et al.[7] noted that the gluteus maximus fascia was connected to the sacrotuberous ligament in all sections. In most dissections, a portion of the long head of the biceps femoris tendon is in continuity with the sacrotuberous ligament, traversing the ischium.

In the weight-bearing position, force is transmitted through the bodies of the lumbar vertebrae to the superior end of the sacrum, and the sacral base tends to be pushed anteriorly and inferiorly due to the weight being anterior to the axis of the SIJs. The downward effects of gravity, combined with environmental and genetic factors, can stress the tensile strength of these ligaments. Unbalanced ligamentous stresses can contribute to lumbosacral imbalance, chronic back pain, and joint degeneration.

Lumbosacral instability may cause irritation of the iliolumbar ligament resulting in tenderness upon palpation at its attachment at the posterior iliac crest and the transverse processes of L4–L5.

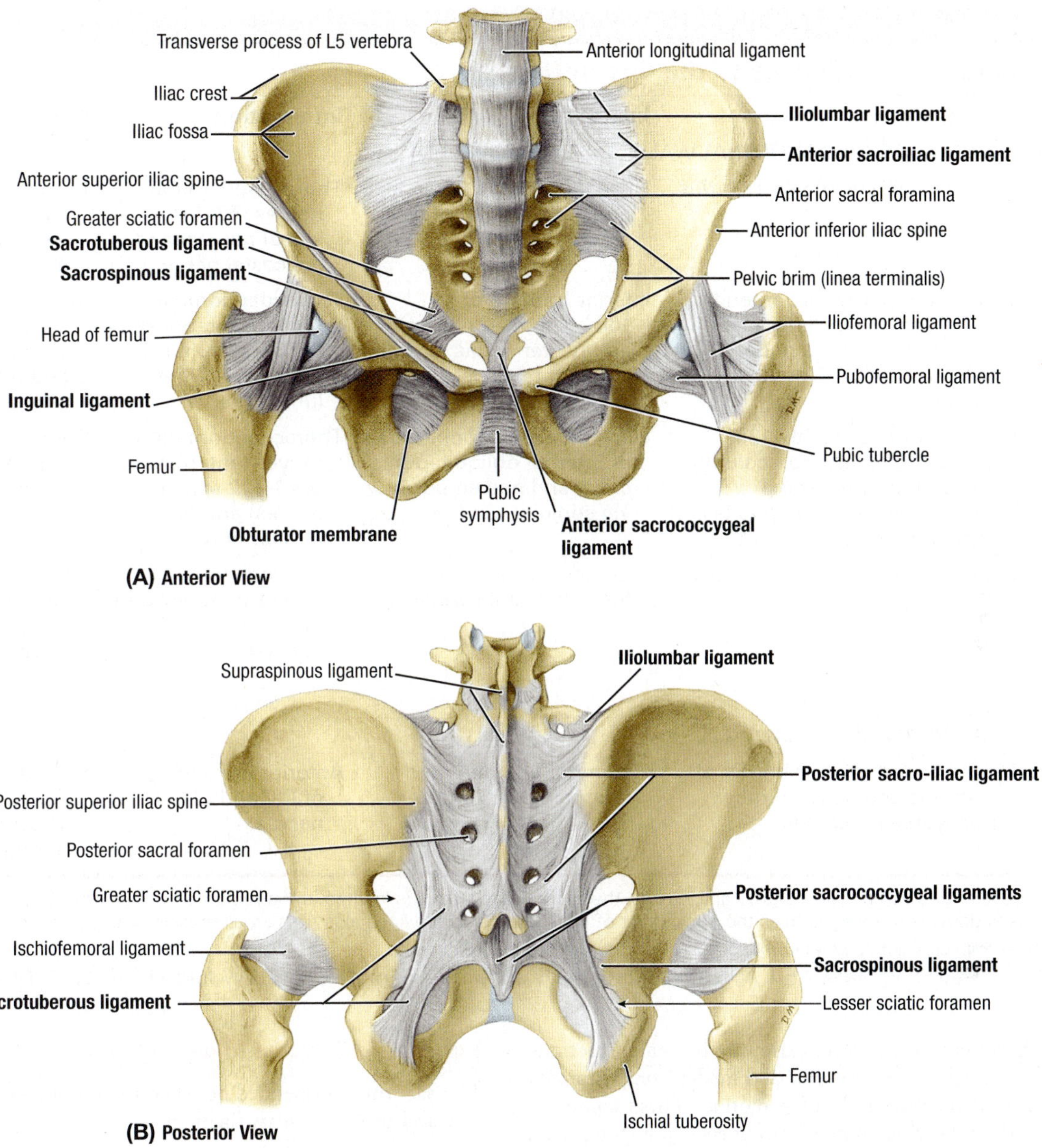

Figure 37.3. Ligaments of the pelvic girdle. The sacrotuberous and sacrospinous ligaments convert the greater and lesser sciatic notches into foramina. (Reprinted with permission from Agur AMR, Dalley AF II. *Grant's Atlas of Anatomy*. 15th ed. Wolters Kluwer; 2021. Figure 1.20A-B.)

Pain may be referred to the groin via the ilioinguinal nerve, mimicking the pain felt in an inguinal hernia. Palpatory diagnosis should therefore always include these ligamentous attachments.

Musculature

Muscles acting on or through the pelvis can be classified as

1. Primary (intrinsic muscles of the pelvic diaphragm)
2. Secondary (muscles considered to have partial attachment to the true pelvis)

Primary muscles and connective tissue intrinsic to the pelvic girdle include the pelvic and urogenital diaphragms. The pelvic diaphragm consists of the levator ani and coccygeus muscles, which form a basin, supporting the pelvic viscera and closing the pelvic outlet. The levator ani group includes the pubococcygeus, puborectalis, and iliococcygeus muscles. The urogenital diaphragm spans the area between the ischiopubic rami and is formed by the deep transverse perineal and sphincter urethra muscles and their fasciae. The pelvic diaphragm slants inferiorly from the lateral wall to the midline perineal structures, while the urogenital diaphragm is relatively level. This creates a small potential finger-like space (ischiorectal fossa) on either side superior to the urogenital diaphragm and inferior to the pelvic diaphragm, which may provide an anterior avenue for the spread of perineal infections. The pelvic floor muscles work in a synergistic way with the abdominal diaphragm to increase intra-abdominal pressure. They also provide support during defecation, inhibit bladder activity, and assist in providing lumbosacral pelvic support.[8]

Respiration may also be affected by pelvic dysfunction due to the relationship of the secondary muscles that connect the pelvis to the costal cage including the rectus abdominis, transverse abdominis, internal and external oblique, and the quadratus lumborum (Table 37.1).

TABLE 37.1

Muscular Relationship of Pelvis to the Costal Cage

Muscle	Origin	Insertion	Innervation	Main Action[a]
MUSCLES OF ANTEROLATERAL ABDOMINAL WALL				
External oblique	External surfaces of 5th–12th ribs	Linea alba, pubic tubercle, and anterior half of iliac crest	Thoracoabdominal nerves (T7–T11 spinal nerves) and subcostal nerve	Compresses and supports abdominal viscera[b] and flexes and rotates trunk
Internal oblique	Thoracolumbar fascia, anterior two-thirds of iliac crest, and connective tissue deep to lateral, third of inguinal ligament	Inferior borders of 10th–12th ribs, linea alba, and pecten pubis via conjoint tendon	Thoracoabdominal nerves (anterior rami of T6–T12 spinal nerves) and first lumbar nerve	Compresses and supports abdominal viscera[b] and flexes and rotates trunk
Transversus abdominis	Internal surfaces of 7th–12th costal cartilages, thoracolumbar fascia, iliac crest, and connective tissue deep to lateral third of inguinal ligament	Linea alba with aponeurosis of internal oblique, pubic crest, and pecten pubis via conjoint tendon	Thoracoabdominal nerves (anterior rami of T6–T12 spinal nerves) and first lumbar nerve	Compresses and supports abdominal viscera[b]
Rectus abdominis	Pubic symphysis and pubic crest	Xiphoid process and 5th–7th costal cartilages	Thoracoabdominal nerves (anterior rami of T6–T12 spinal nerves)	Flexes trunk (lumbar vertebrae) and compresses abdominal viscera[b]; stabilizes and controls tilt of pelvis (antilordosis)
MUSCLES OF POSTERIOR ABDOMINAL WALL				
Quadratus lumborum	Medial half of inferior border of 12th ribs and tips of lumbar transverse processes	Iliolumbar ligament and internal lip of iliac crest	Anterior branches of T12 and L1–L4 nerves	Extends and laterally flexes vertebral column; fixes 12th rib during inspiration

[a]Approximately 80% of people have an insignificant muscle, the *pyramidalis*, which is located in the rectus sheath anterior to the most inferior part of the rectus abdominis. It extends from the pubic crest of the hip bone to the linea alba. This small muscle draws down on the linea alba.

[b]In so doing, these muscles act as antagonists of the diaphragm to produce expiration.

Reprinted with permission from Dalley AF II, Agur AMR. *Moore's Clinically Oriented Anatomy*. 9th ed. Wolters Kluwer; 2023. Tables 5.2 and 5.13.

Each compartment of the lower extremity has unique actions on the sacrum and pelvis. The anterior and medial compartments of the thigh can affect iliac and pubic motion. These compartments contain the following muscles: pectineus, adductor group, gracilis, rectus femoris, sartorius, obturator externus, and iliopsoas (Table 37.2).

The muscles of the "lateral compartment" of the leg include only the tensor fascia lata muscle and the iliotibial band. The deep fascia of the thigh (fascia lata) is continuous with the superficial thoracolumbar fascia of the thorax and splits to form the compartments of the lower extremity.

The extensors, abductors, and external rotators of the thigh include gluteus maximus, minimus, and medius, piriformis, obturator internus, and superior and inferior gemelli (Table 37.3).

Dysfunction of muscles or fascia of the posterior compartment or gluteal region can affect the function of the pelvic girdle. The fascia covering the posterior aspect of the piriformis muscle and the biceps femoris have been found to be continuous with the posterior SI ligament. The implication of these findings is that physical activity and diagnostic tests, such as the straight leg raise, stress the SIJ due to this configuration. Inflammation of the SIJ could affect the piriformis muscle and biceps femoris through resultant reactive muscle spasm (Table 37.4).

Collectively, the muscles of the gluteal region, the quadratus femoris, and the iliopsoas constitute the rotator cuff of the hip (Fig. 37.4).

Supportive Tissues (Figs. 37.5 and 37.6)

The sacrum is suspended between the innominate bones by three true and three accessory ligaments.

- The true pelvic ligaments form a direct bone-to-bone connection and include the following:
  - ☐ Anterior SI ligaments
  - ☐ Interosseous SI ligaments
  - ☐ Posterior SI ligaments
- The accessory pelvic ligaments include the following:
  - ☐ Sacrotuberous ligaments
  - ☐ Sacrospinous ligaments
  - ☐ Iliolumbar ligaments
  - ☐ Inguinal ligaments

The iliolumbar ligaments attach from the anterior surface of the posterior iliac crest, and the anterior surface of the sacral base to the transverse processes of L4 and L5. The lower fibers blend in with the anterior SI ligament, thus integrating SI mechanics with the lumbar spine.

The anterior SI ligaments are flat bands, while the posterior ligaments are thicker with multiple layers. The long dorsal SI ligament, which connects the PSIS to the lateral aspect of the third and fourth sacral segments, has a close anatomic relationship with the erector spinae muscles, posterior layer of the thoracolumbar fascia, and a specific part of the sacrotuberous ligament.[7] Another

TABLE 37.2

Musculature of the Anterior and Medial Compartments of the Thigh That May Affect Iliac and Pubic Motion

Muscle	Proximal Attachment[a]	Distal Attachment	Innervation[b]	Main Action(s)
MUSCLES OF ANTERIOR THIGH ACTING AT HIP JOINT				
Pectineus	Superior ramus of pubis	Pectineal line of femur, just inferior to lesser trochanter	Femoral nerve (**L2,** L3); may receive a branch from obturator nerve	Adducts and slightly flexes hip joint; assists with lateral rotation
Iliopsoas				
Psoas major	Sides of T12–L5 vertebrae and disks between them; transverse processes of all lumbar vertebrae	Lesser trochanter of femur	Anterior rami of lumbar nerves (**L1, L2,** L3)	
Psoas minor	Sides of T12–L1 vertebrae and intervertebral disks	Pectineal line and iliopubic eminence via iliopectineal arch	Anterior rami of lumbar nerves (LI, L2)	Act conjointly in flexion and lateral rotation of hip joint and in stabilizing this joint when standing[c]
Iliacus	Iliac crest, iliac fossa, ala of sacrum, and anterior sacroiliac ligaments	Tendon of psoas major, lesser trochanter, and femur distal to it	Femoral nerve (**L2,** L3)	Act conjointly in flexion and lateral rotation of hip joint and in stabilizing this joint when standing[c]
Sartorius	Anterior superior iliac spine and superior part of notch inferior to it	Superior part of medial surface of tibia (as part of pes anserinus)	Femoral nerve (L2, L3)	Flexes, abducts, and lateral rotates hip joint; flexes knee joint (medially rotates leg when knee joint is flexed)[d]
Muscle[e]	**Proximal Attachment**	**Distal Attachment**	**Innervation**	**Main Action**
MUSCLES OF MEDIAL THIGH				
Adductor langus	Body of pubis inferior to pubic crest	Middle third of linea aspera of femur	Obturator nerve and branch of anterior division (L2, **L3,** L4)	Adducts hip joint
Adductor brevis	Body and inferior ramus of pubis	Pectineal line and proximal part of linea aspera of femur	Obturator nerve and branch of anterior division (L2, **L3,** L4)	Adducts hip joint and, to some extent, flexes it
Adductor magnus	Adductor part: inferior ramus of pubis and ramus of ischium Hamstring part: ischial tuberosity	Adductor part: gluteal tuberosity, linea aspera, and medial supracondylar line Hamstring part: adductor tubercle of femur	Adductor part: obturator nerve (L2, **L3, L4**) and branches of posterior division Hamstring part: tibial part of sciatic nerve (**L4**)	Adducts hip joint Adductor part: flexes hip joint Hamstring part: extends hip joint
Gracilis	Body and inferior ramus of pubis	Superior part of medial surface of tibia (as part of pes anserinus)	Obturator nerve (**L2,** L3)	Adducts hip joint; flexes knee joint, medially rotating it when flexed
Obturator externus	Margins of obturator foramen and obturator membrane	Trochanteric fossa of femur	Obturator nerve (L3, **L4**)	Laterally rotates hip joint; stabilizes hip joint

[a]The Latin word *insertio* means *attachment*. The terms insertion and origin (L. *origo*) have not been used here (or elsewhere) since they change with function.

[b]The spinal cord segmental innervation is indicated (e.g., "LI, L2, L3" means that the nerves supplying the psoas major are derived from the first three lumbar segments of the spinal cord). Numbers in boldface (**LI, L2**) indicate the main segmental innervation. Damage to one or more of the listed spinal cord segments, or to the motor nerve roots arising from them, results in paralysis of the muscles concerned.

[c]The psoas major is also a postural muscle that helps control the deviation of the trunk and is active during standing.

[d]The four actions of the sartorius (L. *sartor*, tailor) produce the once common cross-legged sitting position used by tailors, hence the name.

[e]Collectively, the four of five muscles listed are the adductors of the thigh, but their actions are more complex (e.g., they act as flexors of the hip joint during flexion of the knee joint and are active during walking).

TABLE 37.3

Muscles of Gluteal Region: Extensors, Abductors and Rotators of the Thigh

Muscle	Proximal Attachment	Distal Attachment	Innervation[b]	Main Action
MUSCLES OF GLUTEAL REGION: EXTENSORS, ABDUCTORS AND ROTATORS OF THIGH[a]				
Gluteus maximus	Ilium posterior to posterior gluteal line; dorsal surface of sacrum and coccyx; sacrotuberous ligament	Most fibers end in iliotibial tract, which inserts into lateral condyle of tibia; some fibers insert on gluteal tuberosity.	Inferior gluteal nerve (L5, **SI**, **S2**)	Extends hip joint (especially from flexed position) and assists in lateral rotation; fixes hip joint and assists in rising from sitting position
Gluteus medius	External surface of ilium between anterior and posterior gluteal lines	Lateral surface of greater trochanter of femur	Superior gluteal nerve (**L5**, S1)	Abduct and medially rotate hip joint; keep pelvis level when ipsilateral limb is weight bearing and advance opposite (unsupported) side during its swing phase.
Gluteus minimus	External surface of ilium between anterior and inferior gluteal lines	Anterior surface of greater trochanter of femur	Superior gluteal nerve (**L5**, S1)	Abduct and medially rotate hip joint; keep pelvis level when ipsilateral limb is weight bearing and advance opposite (unsupported) side during its swing phase.
Tensor fasciae latae	Anterior superior iliac spine; anterior part of iliac crest	Iliotibial tract, which attaches to lateral condyle of tibia	Superior gluteal nerve (**L5**, S1)	Abduct and medially rotate hip joint; keep pelvis level when ipsilateral limb is weight bearing and advance opposite (unsupported) side during its swing phase.
Piriformis	Anterior surface of sacrum; sacrotuberous ligament	Superior border of greater trochanter of femur	Branches of anterior rami of **S1** and S2	Laterally rotate extended hip joint and abduct hip joint when flexed; stabilize hip joint
Obturator internus	Pelvic surface of obturator membrane and surrounding bones	Medial surface of greater trochanter (trochanteric fossa) of femur[c]	Nerve to obturator internus (L5, **S1**)	Laterally rotate extended hip joint and abduct hip joint when flexed; stabilize hip joint
Superior and inferior gemelli	Superior: ischial spine Inferior: ischial tuberosity	Medial surface of greater trochanter (trochanteric fossa) of femur[c]	Superior gemellus: same nerve supply as obturator internus Inferior gemellus: same nerve supply as quadratus femoris	Laterally rotate extended hip joint and abduct hip joint when flexed; stabilize hip joint
Quadratus femoris	Lateral border of ischial tuberosity	Quadrate tubercle on intertrochanteric crest of femur and area inferior to it	Nerve to quadratus femoris (L5, S1)	Laterally rotates hip joint[d]; stabilizes hip joint

[a]Collectively, the muscles are listed as abductors and rotators of the hip joint but their actions are more complex.

[b]The spinal cord segmental innervation is indicated (e.g., "S1, S2" means that the nerves supplying the piriformis are derived from the first two sacral segments of the spinal cord). Numbers in boldface (**S1**) indicate the main segmental innervation. Damage to one or more of the listed spinal cord segments, or to the motor nerve roots arising from them, results in paralysis of the muscles concerned.

[c]The gemelli muscles blend with and share the tendon of the obturator intern us as it attaches to the greater trochanter of the femur, collectively forming the triceps coxae.

[d]There are six lateral rotators of the thigh: piriformis, obturator internus, superior and inferior gemelli, quadratus femoris, and obturator externus. These muscles also stabilize the hip joint.

Reprinted with permission from Dalley AF II, Agur AMR. *Moore's Clinically Oriented Anatomy*. 9th ed. Wolters Kluwer; 2023. Table 7.6.

significant relationship of the long dorsal SI ligament is that this ligament becomes stretched when the sacrum is rotated in a posterior manner relative to the ilium.[7] Thus, in situations where there is a decrease in lumbar lordosis, such as in the early stages of pregnancy or in aging, this ligament may be stretched via backward torsions or unilateral/bilateral sacral extensions.

According to anatomic dissections by Vleeming et al.,[7] in all specimens, traction on the posterior layer of the thoracolumbar lumbar fascia transmits force to the contralateral side, specifically into the fascia of the gluteus maximus. The relationship of the contralateral latissimus dorsi to the involved gluteus maximus could affect the stability of the SIJs due to the connecting fascia. Stability of the SI region is achieved by a combination of ligamentous and dynamic muscular functions crossing the SIJs.[8]

- Anatomic studies have shown that gluteus maximus tendon fibers blend with the posterior sacroiliac ligaments and overlie the lower half of the SIJ.

TABLE 37.4

Muscles of Posterior Thigh: Extensors of Hip and Flexors of Knee

Muscle[a]	Proximal Attachment	Distal Attachment	Innervation[b]	Main Action[c]
MUSCLES OF POSTERIOR THIGH: EXTENSORS OF HIP AND FLEXORS OF KNEE				
Semitendinosus	Ischial tuberosity	Superior part of media surface of tibia (as part of pes anserinus)	Tibial division of sciatic nerve part of tibia (**L5, S1**, S2)	Extend hip joint; flex knee joint and medially rotate it when flexed. When hip and knee joints are flexed (as when sitting), these muscles can extend trunk at hip joint (to rise).
Semimembranosus	Ischial tuberosity	Posterior part of medial condyle of tibia. Reflected attachment forms oblique popliteal ligament (to lateral femoral condyle).	Tibial division of sciatic nerve part of tibia (**L5, S1**, S2)	Extend hip joint; flex knee joint and medially rotate it when flexed. When hip and knee joints are flexed (as when sitting), these muscles can extend trunk at hip joint (to rise).
Biceps femoris	Long head: ischial tuberosity Short head: linea aspera and lateral supracondylar line of femur	Lateral side of head of fibula. Tendon is split at this site by fibular collateral ligament of knee.	Long head: tibial division of sciatic nerve (L5, **S1**, S2) Short head: common fibular division of sciatic nerve (L5, **S1**, S2)	Flexes knee joint and laterally rotates it when flexed; long head extends hip joint (e.g., accelerating mass during first step of gait and when rising from sitting position).

[a]Collectively, these three muscles are known as hamstrings.

[b]The spinal cord segmental innervation is indicated (e.g., "L5, SI, S2" means that the nerves supplying the semitendinosus are derived from the fifth lumbar segment and first two sacral segments of the spinal cord). Numbers in boldface (**L5, S1**) indicate the main segmental innervation. Damage to one or more of the listed spinal cord segments or to the motor nerve roots arising from them results in paralysis of the muscles concerned.

[c]Collectively, the muscles are listed as extensors of the hip joint and flexors of the knee joint but their actions are more complex.

Reprinted with permission from Dalley AF II, Agur AMR. *Moore's Clinically Oriented Anatomy*. 9th ed. Wolters Kluwer; 2023. Table 7.7.

- The tendons of the erector spinae run inferiorly from the paraspinal areas to attach to the posterior surface of the sacrum directly, through the perimysial membranes of the multifidus muscles.
- The multifidus muscle takes its origin from the median sacral crest and runs laterally to attach to the medial PSIS.[9]

Integrated Function

There is an integrated function between the muscles of the gluteal region, the abdominal diaphragm, and the muscles of the pelvic and urogenital diaphragms. The pelvic diaphragm consists of the levator ani and coccygeus muscles, which form a basin and work synchronously with the abdominal diaphragm. This synchronous movement with the abdominal diaphragm preserves interstitial fluid homeostasis in the true pelvic region. A properly functioning pelvic diaphragm is necessary for the efficient movement of lymphatic fluids away from the pelvis and perineal tissues. Somatic dysfunction of the symphysis pubis or disturbed ilioilial mechanics (asymmetry of the relationship between the two innominates) can place asymmetric tensions on the pelvic and urogenital diaphragms. These tensions may result in the following:

- Tension myalgia or pain of the pelvic floor
- Levator ani syndrome

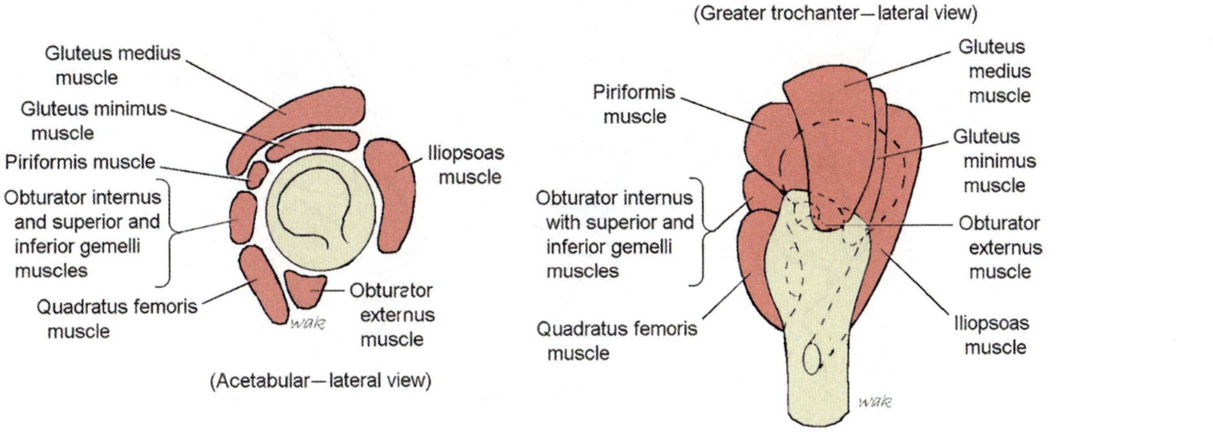

Figure 37.4. Rotator cuff muscles of the right hip. (Modified from Kuchera WA, Kuchera ML. *Osteopathic Principles in Practice*. 2nd ed. Greyden Press; 1994. Reprinted with permission from Michael L. Kuchera, DO, FAAO.)

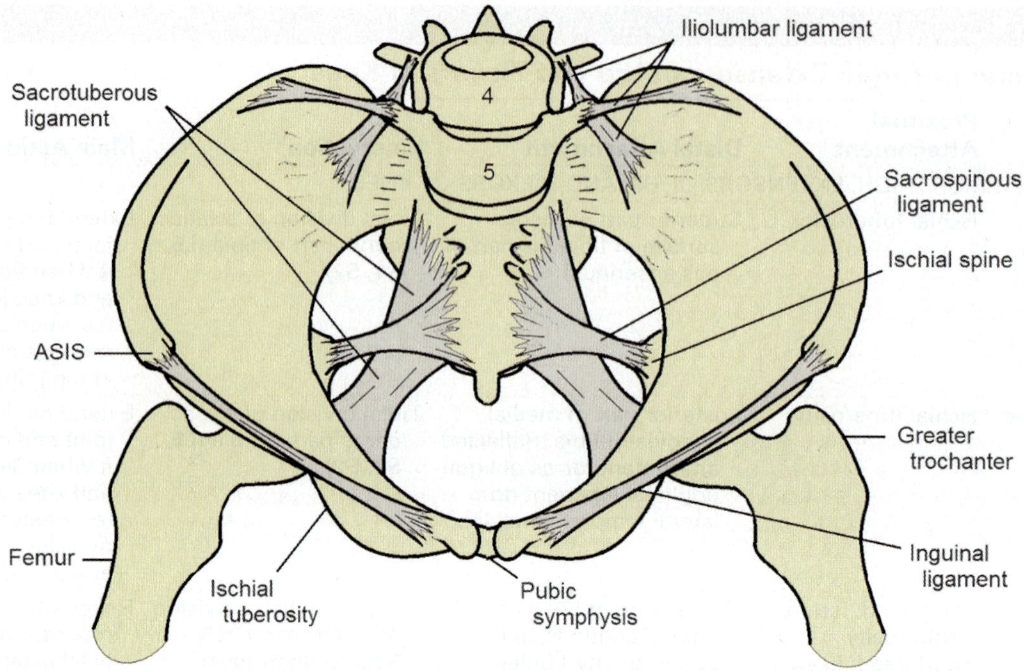

Figure 37.5. Ligaments of the pelvis—anterior view. (Modified from Kuchera WA, Kuchera ML. *Osteopathic Principles in Practice*. 2nd ed. Greyden Press; 1994. Reprinted with permission from Michael L. Kuchera, DO, FAAO.)

- Low back pain
- Dyspareunia
- Painful defecation with associated constipation[10]

Somatic dysfunction of this region may cause hypertonicity and tenderness of the gluteal muscles. Tension on the pubovesicular and puboprostatic fascia from innominate dysfunction (especially pubic shears and compressions) may produce urinary tract symptoms such as burning, frequency, fullness, and a weak stream. Such tensions on the inguinal ligament from disturbed ilioilial mechanics can affect the lateral femoral cutaneous nerve, resulting in anterior thigh pain.

Dysfunction of any of the abdominal muscles or their fasciae may disrupt respiratory excursion, compromising the intra-abdominal pressure changes that promote lymphatic and venous return. The thoracolumbar and lumbosacral fasciae contribute to the origin of the internal abdominal oblique and the transverse abdominis muscles. Fascial restrictions in these areas can restrict both thoracolumbar and sacral motion. The inner membranous

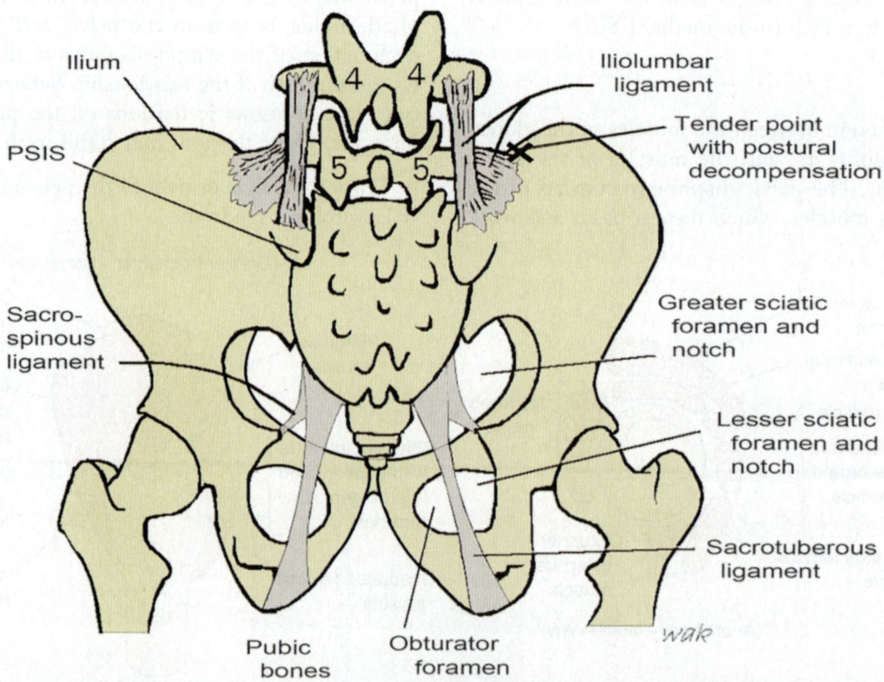

Figure 37.6. Ligaments of the pelvis—posterior view. (Modified from Kuchera WA, Kuchera ML. *Osteopathic Principles in Practice*. 2nd ed. Greyden Press; 1994. Reprinted with permission from Michael L. Kuchera, DO, FAAO.)

layer of the superficial thoracolumbar fascia (Scarpa) attaches to the iliac crest and pubic symphysis. It is continuous with the following:

- Fascia of the thigh inferior to the inguinal ligament (fascia lata)
- Posterior perineal membrane
- Tunica dartos scrota

Fascial restrictions along its course may affect the thigh, perineum, or abdomen, as fluid collections can traverse along these planes.

Dysfunction of the rectus femoris, the iliacus, or the ipsilateral adductor group may cause an anterior rotation of the innominate and inferior shear at the pubic bones.

- Adductor dysfunction may be related to reflex changes at the ipsilateral iliolumbar ligament, while a pubic shear may affect the pelvic and urogenital diaphragms.
- Gait may be affected by lumbosacral somatic dysfunction, affecting the superior gluteal nerve (L4–L5, S1) and the gluteus medius and minimus.
- Piriformis hypertonicity related to sacral somatic dysfunction may produce sciatica.
- Hamstring tension may cause a posterior rotation of the innominate and affect pelvic mechanics.
- Pregnant patients are prone to pelvic somatic dysfunction due to the influence of hormonal and structural changes. There are many biomechanical causes such as a shift in the center of gravity, increased lumbar lordosis, and anterior rotation of the pelvis (see Chapters 81 and 82, for osteopathic considerations in obstetrics and gynecology).

Neural Structures

The lumbar plexus lies between the anterior and posterior masses of the psoas major, anterior to the transverse processes of the lumbar vertebrae (see Chapter 36). The plexus is formed by the contributions of the ventral rami from T12 to L4, with only partial contributions from T12. The lumbar plexus gives motor supply to muscles in the abdomen and thigh, which act on the pelvic girdle and supplies sensation to the thigh, buttocks, lower abdomen, and pubic area.

The sacrum contains sacral foramina for passage of the sacral nerve roots, which exit anteriorly and posteriorly. The innervation of the SIJ and its ligaments is derived exclusively from the dorsal branches of the sacral spinal nerves. The joint capsule contains complex encapsulated and unencapsulated nerve endings capable of providing proprioceptive and pressure information. The numerous thick myelinated axons in the nerve branches to the SIJ ligaments indicate the presence of special encapsulated mechanoreceptors and nociceptors.[3,7]

- The posterior innervation to the SIJs is from the posterior primary rami of L4 through S3.[3]
- The anterior innervation arises from branches of the anterior primary rami from L2 to S2.
- The posterior and anterior rami are variable, and this may account for the inconsistent pain referral pattern seen with SIJ syndrome.[11]

Since the sacroiliac joints have a wide distribution of innervation, it is possible that pain referred from this region will not be associated with any motor, reflex, or sensory deficit on physical examination.

The lumbosacral trunk (ventral rami of L4 and L5) comprised of the first three sacral ventral rami, and a portion of the fourth, form the sacral plexus. The ventral rami divide into anterior and posterior branches. The anterior branch forms anterior nerves that innervate the flexors and adductors; the posterior branch forms posterior nerves that innervate the extensors and abductors.

The sacral plexus has motor and sensory innervations in the pelvis and lower extremities and also contains parasympathetic fibers (S2, S3, and S4) for innervation of the left colon and pelvic organs (Fig. 37.7).

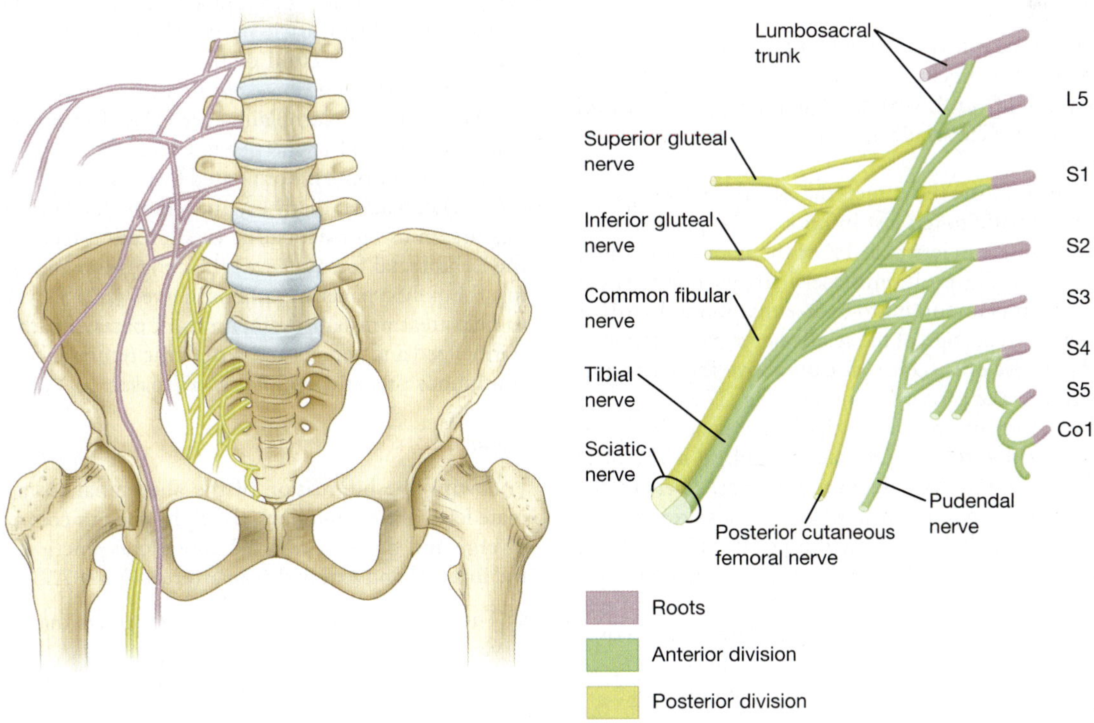

Figure 37.7. Sacral plexus. The sacral plexus is formed by the segmental nerves L4 through S5. This plexus innervates the lower leg, ankle, and foot via the tibial and common peroneal nerves. (Reprinted with permission from Anderson MK. *Foundations of Athletic Training: Prevention, Assessment, and Management*. 6th ed. Wolters Kluwer; 2017.)

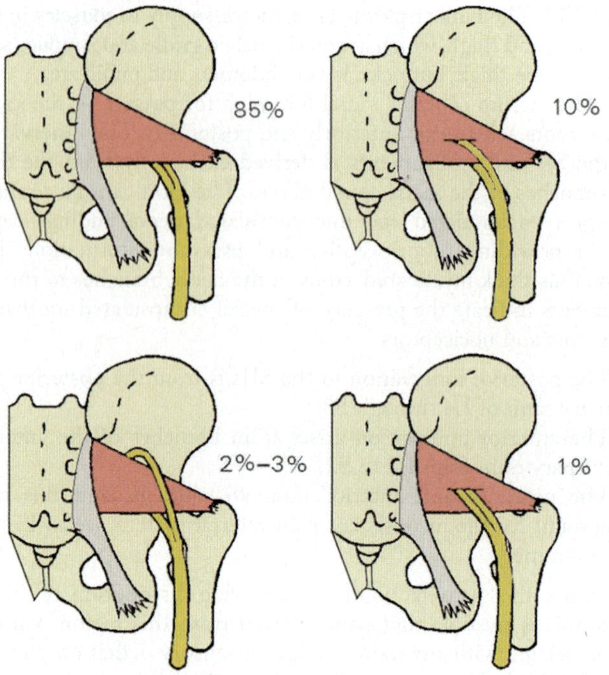

Figure 37.8. Relationship of the sciatic nerve to piriformis. **A.** Inferior to piriformis. The sciatic nerve usually emerges from the greater sciatic foramen inferior to the piriformis. **B.** Common fibular division piercing piriformis. In 12.2% of 640 limbs studied by Dr. JCB Grant, the sciatic nerve divided before exiting the greater sciatic foramen; the common fibular division (*yellow*) passed through the piriformis. **C.** Common fibular division superior to piriformis. In 0.5% of cases, the common fibular division passed superior to the muscle, where it is especially vulnerable to injury during intragluteal injections. (Reprinted with permission from Dalley AF II, Agur AMR. *Moore's Clinically Oriented Anatomy*. 9th ed. Wolters Kluwer; 2023. Figure 7.46.)

The sciatic nerve is a muscular branch of the lumbar and sacral plexi and is composed of fibers from the ventral rami of L4–S3. Pathology at the L4–L5 or L5–S1 level is usually the cause of nerve root compression. The sciatic nerve is closely associated with the piriformis muscle.

Eighty-five percent of the time, the sciatic nerve passes through the greater sciatic notch just inferior to the piriformis; it passes through the muscle in less than 1% of the population. Since injections are sometimes given in myofascial trigger points when the muscle is spastic, it is important to realize that more than 10% of the time, the peroneal portion of the sciatic nerve passes through the muscle. In 2% to 3% of instances, it exits above the piriformis and passes posterior to the piriformis muscle (Fig. 37.8).[12]

Piriformis hypertonicity can cause sciatica. Evidence indicates that this may not be due to pressure, but instead, to a chemical reaction that irritates the peroneal (common fibular) fibers of the sciatic nerve and thus the referred pain down the posterior thigh.

The coccygeal plexus is located on the pelvic surface of the coccygeus muscle and is formed by the coccygeal nerve with contributions from S4 to S5. This plexus gives rise to the anococcygeal nerve that pierces the coccygeus and anococcygeal ligament to supply the skin between the tip of the coccyx and the anus.

The autonomic nerves of the pelvis include the following:

1. Sacral sympathetic trunks
2. Parasympathetic nerves of the pelvic splanchnic nerves
3. Hypogastric plexuses
4. Peri-arterial plexuses

The right and left sacral sympathetic trunks are extensions of the lumbar sympathetic chain ganglia and are located on the ventral surface of the sacrum medial to the sacral foramina. They contain four or five ganglia that eventually fuse over the coccyx, to form the single ganglion impar. The sacral sympathetic trunks have gray rami communicantes that follow the sacral and coccygeal nerves for innervation of blood vessels and sweat glands in the body wall and extremities. Because the sacral and coccygeal nerves do not have white rami, visceral afferent impulses returning from sites of sympathetic innervation by the sacrum and coccyx refer viscerosomatic symptoms to the thoracolumbar region of the body. Examples include anterior lower thoracic or sacral exostoses and anterior disk protrusions or ruptures. Contractions of the uterus refer pain to the thoracolumbar region, as the visceral afferent nerves travel to this level from the uterine body.

The sacral splanchnic nerves come off the chain and contribute to the formation of the inferior hypogastric plexus. The pelvic splanchnic nerves arise directly off the ventral rami of S2–S4 and supply parasympathetic innervation to the left colon and inferior hypogastric plexus for pelvic viscera. Visceral afferent nerves following parasympathetic nerve pathways produce viscerosomatic symptoms over the sacrum. An example is sacral pain and pressure from uterine contractions. The inferior hypogastric plexus contains both sympathetic and parasympathetic fibers; it gives rise to subplexuses referred to as the pelvic plexuses associated with the following:

- Lateral aspects of the rectum
- Inferolateral surfaces of the bladder
- Prostate and seminal glands
- Cervix of the uterus
- Lateral fornices of the vagina

Somatic dysfunction of the lumbar spine may affect the lumbar plexus and produce symptoms in both the pelvis and lower extremity. Dysfunction of the quadratus lumborum may produce symptoms similar to a groin pull or hernia, by irritating the ilioinguinal and iliohypogastric nerves (L1) as they pass just anterior to this muscle. Dysfunction of the piriformis, or sacrum, can affect the sciatic nerve and cause signs and symptoms of sciatica.

Many visceral complaints are related to an imbalance in the autonomic control of the pelvic viscera. For example, when irritable bowel syndrome is dominated by parasympathetic hyperactivity (headache, nausea, diarrhea, and cramps), relaxation of the pelvic diaphragm using osteopathic manipulation techniques directed to the ischiorectal fossa relieves the congestion and pain by influencing the pelvic parasympathetic nerves (S2, S3, S4). Additionally, to help treat primary dysmenorrhea, parasympathetic tone can be normalized and venous and lymphatic return encouraged with firm continuous pressure over the sacral base.

Vasculature

Following the bifurcation of the abdominal aorta at the approximate level of the umbilicus, the right and left common iliac arteries diverge and descend to the lumbosacral junction and divide into the internal and external iliac arteries (Fig. 37.9).

- The internal iliac arteries have two trunks that supply the pelvic viscera, perineum, and gluteal region.
- The proximal anterior trunk supplies the urinary bladder, uterus, vagina, and rectum.
- Distally, the anterior division of the internal iliac artery branches into the internal pudendal artery, supplying the genitalia and perineum and the inferior gluteal artery, which supplies the pelvic diaphragm, sciatic nerve and muscles of the gluteal region.

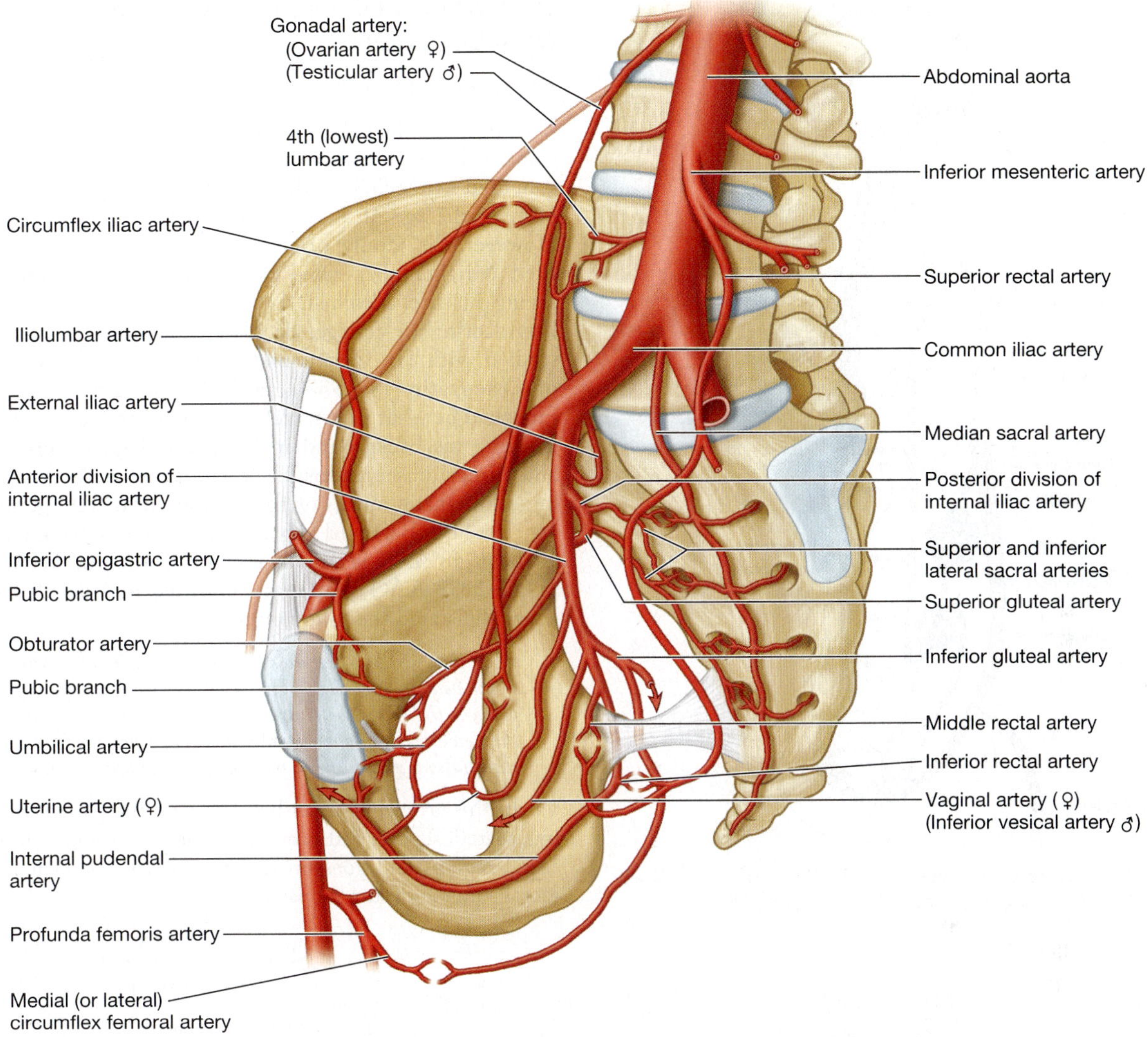

Figure 37.9. Arteries and arterial anastomoses in the pelvis. (Reprinted with permission from Dalley AF II, Agur AMR. *Moore's Clinically Oriented Anatomy*. 9th ed. Wolters Kluwer; 2023. Figure 6.16.)

- The posterior trunk contains the iliolumbar, lateral sacral, and superior gluteal arteries, which collectively supply the intrinsic muscles of the pelvis, the sacrum, and the superior gluteal region.

Veins of the pelvic girdle form venous plexi, which encircle the pelvic organs and the sacrum, and generally follow the arterial distribution. The rectal venous plexus communicates with the portal system via the superior rectal vein, which is valveless (Fig. 37.10).

Lymphatic Structures (Fig. 37.11)

Lymphatic drainage from the pelvic girdle generally follows the corresponding arteries. Lymphatic flow from the lower extremities and pelvic viscera (apart from the gut) passes through the pelvic girdle, ultimately terminating in the lateral aortic groups. Organs and tissues drained by these groups include the following:

- Testes
- Ovaries
- Fallopian tubes
- Uterus
- Kidneys
- Ureters
- Posterior abdominal, pelvic, and perineal walls

Lymph from the remaining viscera (bladder) and gluteal region passes initially to regional nodes along the internal iliac arteries. The external genitalia drain to the inguinal nodes, and then deeper into the external iliac and the intermediary lumbar groups.[13]

Lymphatic drainage of the rectum and anal canal is unique in that, above the pectinate line, lymph follows a deep course to the internal iliac nodes and preaortic nodes. Below the pectinate line, the lymph drains superficially to the inguinal nodes. As lymph flows through a number of intermediary groups in the lumbar region, then to the cisterna chyli and thoracic duct, the diameter of the thoracic duct and lymphatic channels is under sympathetic control similar to the blood vessels. Hypersympathetic activity can reduce lymphatic flow capacity.

Accumulation of pelvic lymph may occur in the preaortic, lateral aortic, or retroaortic lymph node groups. Peripherally compromised lymphatic drainage has been linked to the pathogenesis of atherosclerosis, and to the development of hypertension.[14] Correction of pelvic girdle dysfunction and piriformis tension may allow improved lymphatic and venous return, blood flow, and ambulation for a patient whose activities of daily living are compromised by a preexisting atherosclerotic cardiovascular condition.

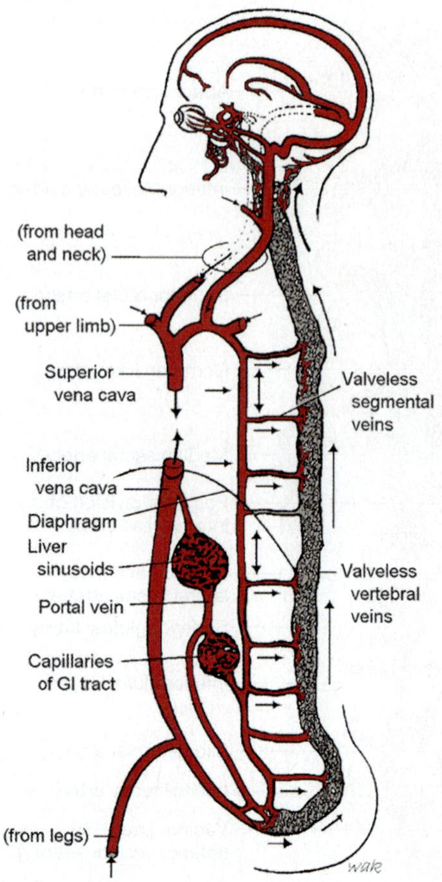

Figure 37.10. **Overview of Venous System of the Body.** (Illustration by W. A. Kuchera, adapted from G. Zink, DO.)

DIAGNOSIS OF PELVIC SOMATIC DYSFUNCTION

Historical Perspective

The model of the pelvis that is commonly taught and its possible somatic dysfunctions are derived from Fred Mitchell, Sr, DO. His son, Fred Mitchell, Jr. suffered third degree burns over 50% of his body at the age of 5. In 1934, this was considered to be fatal. However, the family physician, Charles Owens, DO, reversed Fred Mitchell, Jr.'s renal failure by using Chapman reflexes, saving his life. Mitchell, Sr., who had majored in Mechanical Engineering in college, decided to become an osteopath. He studied with Dr. Owens and enrolled in the Chicago College of Osteopathy in 1937, graduating in 1941.[15] He remained intrigued by what Owens referred to as the "balanced pelvis" and utilizing his background in Mechanical Engineering, anatomy, and clinical observations, he set about researching and developing a kinematic model of this region, ultimately publishing two articles; "The Balanced Pelvis in Relation to Chapman's Reflexes" in the 1948 AAO yearbook and the "Structural Pelvic Function" in the 1958 AAO Yearbook (reprinted in 1965).[15] In his 1958 article he stated the following:

> *The pelvic girdle is the cross-roads of the body, the architectural center of the body, the meeting place of the locomotive apparatus, the resting place of the torso, the temple of the reproductive organs, the abode of the new life's development, the site of the two principal departments of elimination, and, last but not least, a place upon which to sit.*[16]

In this article, he describes assessing the patient in the standing, seated, supine, and prone positions to evaluate the pelvic and sacral regions and goes on to describe several related pelvic and sacral somatic dysfunctions:

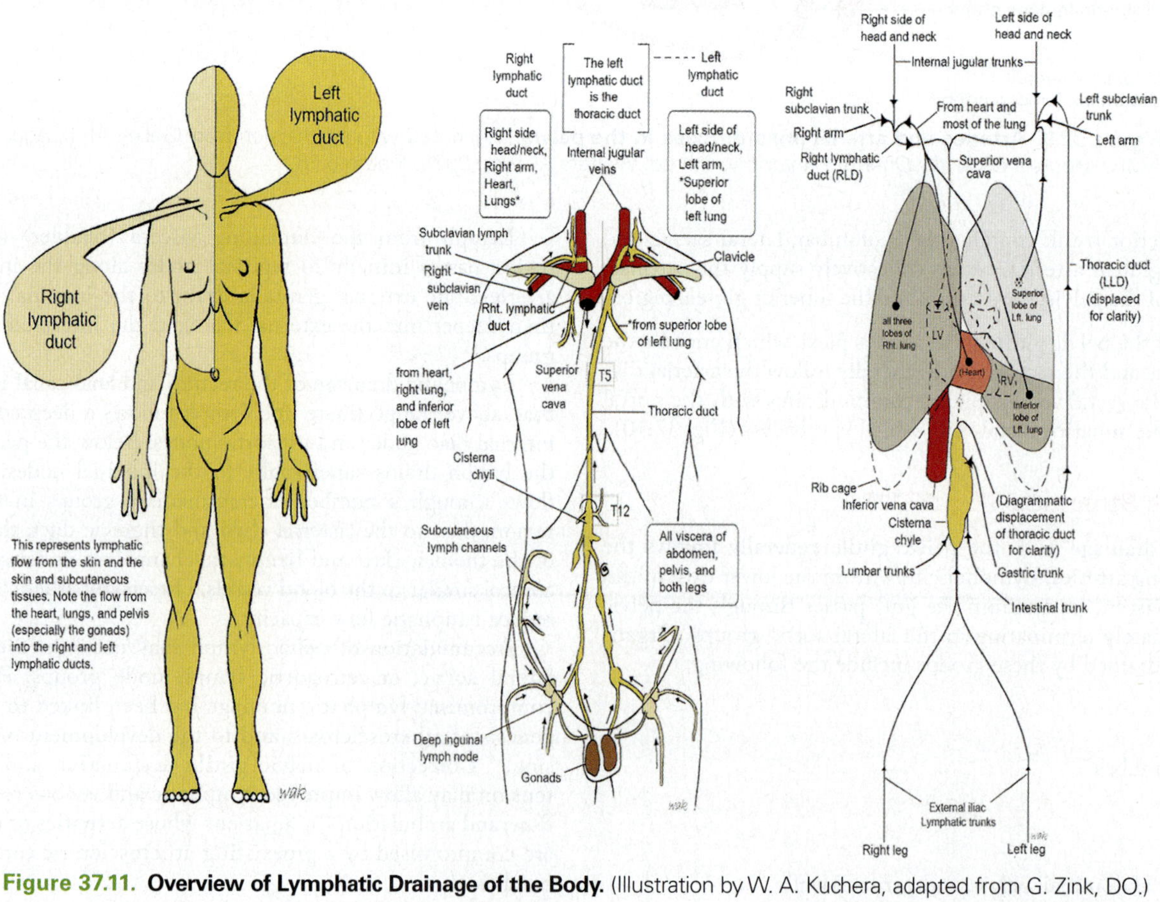

Figure 37.11. **Overview of Lymphatic Drainage of the Body.** (Illustration by W. A. Kuchera, adapted from G. Zink, DO.)

1. *Ilium in extension (Posterior innominate left) Patient supine—check anterior landmarks. The anterior superior spine has moved superiorly and posteriorly on the left. The pubic tubercle shows no measurable change. The medial malleolus moves superiorly or cephalad on the left*
2. *Ilium in flexion on right (Anterior innominate right). Patient supine. The anterior superior spine has moved anteriorly and inferiorly on right. The pubic tubercle shows no measurable change. The medial malleolus is caudal on right. Patient prone. The posterior superior spine is anterior and superior on the right. The sulcus is shallow on right. The inferior lateral angle shows no change. The medial malleolus is caudal on right.*
3. *Out-flare innominate on right. (Can occur only with convex articular surface of sacrum). May have flexion or extension as an associated component. Use finding in 1 and 2 to determine. Patient supine. Anterior superior spine moves laterally and to the right in relation to the sagittal cardinal plane and its fellow. Pubic tubercle shows no measurable change other than stress. Medial malleoli show no change unless complicated by anterior or posterior innominate, which frequently is the case. Patient prone. Posterior superior spine on right approximates sagittal cardinal plane. Sulcus is narrowed on right. Inferior lateral angle shows no change. Medial malleoli show no change.*
4. *In-flare innominate on left. (Occurs only with convex sacral articulation). Patient supine. Anterior superior spine on left moves medially and approximates sagittal cardinal plane. Sulcus is wider, ligament tense. Inferior lateral angle shows no change. Medial malleolus shows no change.*
5. *Up-slip innominate. (Not physiologic but for completeness, is included.) Produced by extreme force when weight is caught on one leg with the body in the upright position. The arc-like movement of the innominate is not accomplished. There is a shearing, cephalic movement of the innominate in the sagittal plane, producing a relaxed sacro-tuberous ligament. There is a short leg on the same side. Both anterior superior spine and posterior superior spine superior on same side.*[17]

He also describes "lesions of the pubic symphysis." The pubic tubercles are assessed to see if they are inferior or superior and the inguinal ligament is palpated for tenderness or tension. Somatic dysfunction of the sacrum, torsional or hinge-like locking as a result of bilateral sacral flexion, may be determined by springing the symphysis with the heel of the hand.[17]

Biomechanical Considerations

The pelvic girdle holds a central role in coupling the mechanical forces from the lower extremities to the axial skeleton. The two primary functions of the SIJ are to dissipate the load of the upper trunk to the lower extremities and to facilitate childbearing by ligamentous relaxation during pregnancy. Somatic dysfunction of the pelvis occurs when there are motion preferences during an activity that do not return to a physiologic state once the activity is completed. The joint now remains in an abnormal resting position. While the innominates and the sacrum are intrinsically linked, this chapter will be primarily focused on pelvic somatic dysfunctions.

INNOMINATES

The innominates can be functionally considered as part of the lower extremity. The innominates rotate anteriorly and posteriorly about the inferior transverse axis of the sacrum. The innominates may also be considered to rotate posturally around an axis passing through the greater trochanters of the femur. Reynolds[18] demonstrated that there were multiple varying instantaneous axes of rotation of the ilium about the sacrum when the thigh was used to introduce motion at the SIJ.

If the clinician considers the ilium functionally, each lower extremity, including the attached innominate, is likely to shear superiorly or inferiorly as well as have rotation around a horizontal/transverse axis. Innominate motion can be induced by hip motion as during gait, or by muscular forces from below or above.

- When the innominate rotates anteriorly, it glides in the direction of the short arm of the "L" and posteriorly along the longer length of the "L."
- When the innominate rotates posteriorly, it glides in the direction of the longer length of the "L" and superiorly up the short length of the "L".[19]
- According to Fryette,[20] it is thought that the sacrum follows the motion of the ilia, but to a lesser degree.

PURPOSE OF STANDING AND SEATED FLEXION TESTS

Flexion tests are used to determine whether there is movement restriction of an iliosacral/sacroiliac joint on one side for screening and lateralization purposes.[21] The standing and seated flexion tests have been used clinically to distinguish if an iliosacral or sacroiliac somatic dysfunction is predominant. Mitchell, Sr. stated that the physician places their "thumbs on the posterior superior spines of the patient ensuring that their feet are about 4 inches apart and then asks the patient to bend forward with their arms hanging freely. If the sacrum is free to move, the posterior superior spines will maintain their positional relationship to each other. However, if the sacrum or ilium is locked, the ilium will be picked up and carried forward and up, indicating the restriction to postural movement, a point in differentiating the lesioned side."[22]

He then described the seated flexion test: "Place thumbs over the posterior superior spines and have the patient bend forward. Note if posterior superior spines do not move, allowing sacrum to freely extend, or if it is locked, thus carrying the fixed ilium (posterior superior spine) superiorly. If the fixation is on the same side sitting as determined when the patient was standing, you know on which side the lesion is, and you are now ready to make the final diagnosis with the patient lying."[22]

INTERPRETATION OF FLEXION TESTS

Based on Mitchell, Jr.'s description, it has been classically taught that if there is greater excursion (superior and anterior movement of the PSIS) with the standing flexion test as compared to the seated flexion test, an iliosacral somatic dysfunction may be the predominant dysfunction. If the seated flexion test exhibits greater excursion, a sacroiliac dysfunction may be the predominant dysfunction. A positive flexion test necessitates an evaluation of iliosacral and sacroiliac landmarks to make a definitive diagnosis.[23] Generally, the more positive flexion test determines the primary somatic dysfunction, which should be treated first. The pelvis can then be reevaluated to determine if the secondary dysfunction is still present. If so, that dysfunction is treated and then reevaluated.

If the amount of unilateral excursion is the same for both the standing and seated flexion tests, this likely represents a "carryover factor" or a combination of iliosacral and sacroiliac dysfunction on the same side. Evaluation of all pelvic landmarks will resolve the question.

Generally, if a restriction exists, it manifests as positive on the same side for both the standing and seated flexion tests. However, restrictions may be present on both sides and be slightly different in nature. Thus, it is possible for a patient to have a positive left standing flexion test and a right positive seated flexion test, indicating a left iliosacral somatic dysfunction and a right sacroiliac somatic dysfunction.

It is also possible to have a negative standing flexion test and positive seated flexion which may be more indicative of a sacroiliac dysfunction while a positive standing flexion test and a negative seated flexion test are more indicative of an iliosacral dysfunction.

If both the standing and seated flexion tests are negative, this may indicate an absence of somatic dysfunction or a bilateral dysfunction.[23]

Theorized Biomechanics

When there is a dysfunction of the sacroiliac or iliosacral joint, the sacrum and ilium will become compressed together. In the standing flexion test, the sacrum will flex or nutate with L5. The ilia rotate about their acetabular axis. However, if an ilia is "stuck to" or compressed to the sacrum, that ilia will continue to travel with the sacrum while the other side will have ceased moving at the end of its normal range of motion. In the seated flexion test, the innominates are resting on the seat and therefore braced by the femurs. If the sacrum is "stuck to" an ilia, once again, that ilia will be pulled forward by the sacrum as compared to the other side resulting in a side of greater excursion of the PSIS or the positive side.[21] While these different attributes of the standing and seated flexion exist, they are slight.

Additionally, the standing flexion test is highly sensitive to restrictors influencing the pelvis from the lower extremity while these influences are removed in the seated position and results in greater sensitivity to restrictors from the sacroiliac joints and trunk.[24]

It is also assumed that the physician has ruled out and/or treated conditions that might give a false-positive standing flexion test such as:

- Hamstring, quadratus lumborum, or iliopsoas tightness
- Anatomical short leg

Unequal Hamstring Length or Tension

Unequal hamstring length or tension can be considered either a pelvic or a lower extremity somatic dysfunction because the hamstrings are attached to both the pelvis, and the lower extremity.

- If the hamstrings are of unequal length or tone, standing flexion test results may be either falsely positive or negative. Therefore, it is imperative to treat the hamstrings and retest.
  - □ If the standing flexion test and pelvic landmark positions normalize, the dysfunctional hamstrings were the problem.
  - □ Otherwise, treat as indicated by the second diagnosis.

Unequal Psoas Length

Unequal psoas length or tension may be suspected when pelvic side shift is present, when the upper lumbar lordotic curve is flattened, or when seated or prone evaluation suggests upper lumbar flexed somatic dysfunction.

1. To test the ability of the psoas muscle to lengthen, place the patient in a prone position. Stand at the side of the table facing the patient at the level of the patient's thigh.
2. Stabilize the ipsilateral pelvis with the closest hand to the pelvis.
3. Grasp the thigh just above the knee with the other hand that is closest to the patient's knee and extend the hip until the ASISs begin to rise off the table. Repeat this test on the other side.
4. Note the ease ("end feel") and degrees (quality and quantity) of hip extension on both sides.
5. Compare the two sides.
6. Note that on the tighter side, the leg feels heavier, as well as its range and quality of motion are diminished.

ILIOSACRAL SOMATIC DYSFUNCTIONS

Iliosacral somatic dysfunctions include the following:

- Innominate rotations, anterior and posterior
- Innominate subluxations (shears), superior and inferior
- Innominate flares (inflares and outflares)
- Pubic shears (subluxations), superior and inferior
- Unequal hamstring length
- Unequal iliopsoas length

Anterior Innominate Rotation

This may be found when the dysfunctional side has the following positional characteristics:

- Entire innominate appears to be rotated in a direction anterior to the other hip bone or innominate
- ASIS is more inferior (caudad)
- PSIS is more superior (cephalad)

Subjective complaints may include ipsilateral hamstring tightness and spasm and sciatica (secondary to piriformis dysfunction). Assess for the following palpatory findings:

- Positive standing flexion test on the involved side
- Tissue texture changes at the ipsilateral ILA of the sacrum
- Iliolumbar ligament tenderness
- Generally positive ASIS compression test on the involved side (Fig. 37.12)
- Motion characteristics should indicate freedom of anterior rotation, about an inferior transverse axis, on supine motion testing, and resistance to posterior rotation.

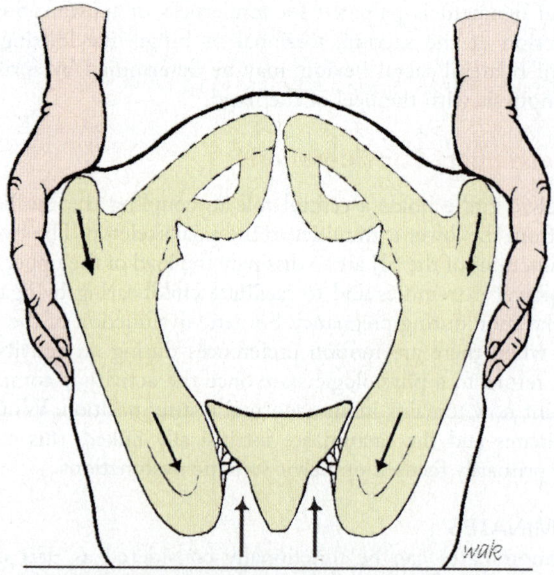

Figure 37.12. ASIS compression test. A positive test is restricted motion and/or pain elicited at either or both SI joints. (Modified by William A. Kuchera, DO, FAAO, from Kuchera WA, Kuchera ML. *Osteopathic Principles in Practice.* 2nd ed. Greyden Press; 1994. Reprinted with permission from Michael L. Kuchera, DO, FAAO.)

Posterior Innominate Rotation

This may be found when the dysfunctional side has the following positional characteristics:

- Entire innominate appears to be rotated in a direction posterior to the other hip bone or innominate.
- ASIS is more superior (cephalad).
- PSIS is more inferior (caudad).

Subjective complaints may include inguinal/groin pain (secondary to rectus femoris dysfunction) and/or medial knee pain (secondary to sartorius dysfunction).

Assess for the following palpatory findings:

- Positive standing flexion test on the involved side
- Inguinal ligament tenderness
- Tissue texture change at the ipsilateral sacral sulcus
- Generally positive ASIS compression test on the involved side (Fig. 37.12)
- Motion characteristics include freedom of posterior rotation about an inferior transverse axis on supine motion testing and resistance to anterior rotation.

Superior Innominate Shear (Subluxation)

This was originally described by Fryette (1914) but is defined by Mitchell, Jr. as "essentially a vertical shear between the sacrum and ilium which shortens the distance between the sacrotuberous ligament and its ischial tuberosity attachment."[25] Mitchell, Sr. states that it is nonphysiologic and is generally produced "by extreme force when weight is caught on one leg with the body in the upright position. The arc-like movement of the innominate is not accomplished. There is a shearing, cephalic movement of the innominate in the sagittal plane, producing a relaxed sacrotuberous ligament."[17]

This may be found when the dysfunctional side has the following characteristics:

- Positive standing flexion test on the involved side.
- ASIS is more superior (cephalad).
- PSIS is more superior (cephalad).
- Pubic ramus may be more superior (cephalad).
- Generally positive ASIS compression test on the involved side (Fig. 37.12).
- *Note:* There can also be rotation of the contralateral innominate as compensation for the shear, or the two innominates may appear to be sheared with one hip bone subluxed more superiorly to the other.

Subjective complaints may include pelvic pain. Assess for the following palpatory findings:

- Tissue texture changes at the ipsilateral SIJ and ipsilateral pubic bones.
- Passive motion testing shows freedom of superior translation of the affected innominate.

Inferior Innominate Shear (Subluxation)

As a historical note, this somatic dysfunction was not described by Mitchell, Sr. Mitchell, Jr. states that "downslipped innominate lesions have been reported despite the obvious curative effects of gravity, but it is rare enough to have eluded the author."[26]

This may be found when the dysfunctional side has the following characteristics:

- ASIS is more inferior (caudad).
- PSIS is more inferior (caudad).
- Pubic ramus may be more inferior.
- Positive ASIS compression test on the involved side (Fig. 37.12).
- Positive standing flexion test on the involved side.

The two innominates appear to be sheared so that the one ilium is subluxed inferiorly to the other. This condition is rare, and walking tends to reduce it. Subjective complaints may include pelvic pain. Assess for the following palpatory findings:

- Tissue texture changes at the ipsilateral SIJ and ipsilateral pubic bones.
- Passive motion tests show freedom of inferior translation of the affected innominate.

Innominate Flares

This condition is a positional change of an innominate in which the ASIS is medial or lateral to its usual position. This may be thought of as rotation of an innominate in relation to a vertical axis.

- If the ASIS is more lateral on the dysfunctional side, the patient has an innominate outflare.
- If the ASIS is more medial on the dysfunctional side, the patient has an innominate inflare.
- According to Mitchell. Jr., DO, until innominate rotations are treated, medial and lateral displacement of the ASIS may not be a valid indicator or an inflared or outflared innominate.
  - Clinically, an inflared innominate results in the ipsilateral pubic crest being slightly posterior compared to the other side while an outflared innominate results in the ipsilateral pubic crest being slightly anterior.
- Subjective complaints may include pelvic or SI pain.
- Assess for the following palpatory findings:
  - Greater laxity in the muscles on the side that is more lateral and more tautness on the side that is more medial.
  - Passive motion tests show freedom of motion medially for inflare and laterally for outflare dysfunctions.

Table 37.5 provides a description of possible iliosacral somatic dysfunction.

PUBIC BONE MOTION

Pubic bone motion is complex. The pubic bones are thought to correspond to ilial motion by rotating anteriorly and posteriorly about a transverse axis.

Dysfunction of the pubic symphysis is common and often overlooked. Muscle imbalances between the abdominal muscles and the adductor muscles may be responsible for the presence and persistence of this somatic dysfunction. Pubic symphysis shears have also been attributed to standing for long periods of time with the body weight mostly on one leg. These somatic dysfunctions may produce symptoms that mimic those of cystitis (pain and/or a burning sensation on urination).

Note that pubic symphysis somatic dysfunction is named for the side of the positive standing flexion test. For example, if the standing flexion test is positive on the left, and the pubic tubercle is more superior on the left (possibly along with tenderness and tension in the inguinal ligament on the left), this is a SUPERIOR pubic symphysis shear or a superior pubic tubercle on the left, NOT an inferior pubic symphysis shear on the right. The diagnostic criteria for pubic symphysis shears are summarized in Table 37.6.

- With anterior rotation of the ilium, the ipsilateral pubic bone is commonly found to be inferior.
- With posterior rotation of the ilium, the ipsilateral pubic bone is commonly found to be superior.

TABLE 37.5

Iliosacral Somatic Dysfunctions

Diagnosis	Characteristics
Anterior rotation right	Positive right standing flexion test Inferior right ASIS Superior right PSIS
Anterior rotation left	Positive left standing flexion test Inferior left ASIS Superior left PSIS
Posterior rotation right	Positive right standing flexion test Superior right ASIS Inferior right PSIS
Posterior rotation left	Positive left standing flexion test Superior left ASIS Inferior left PSIS
Outflare right	Positive right standing flexion test Lateral right ASIS Medial right PSIS
Outflare left	Positive left standing flexion test Lateral left ASIS Medial left PSIS
Inflare right	Positive right standing flexion test Medial right ASIS Lateral right PSIS
Inflare left	Positive left standing flexion test Medial left ASIS Lateral left PSIS
Superior shear (upslip) right	Positive right standing flexion test Superior right ASIS Superior right PSIS
Superior shear (upslip) left	Positive left standing flexion test Superior left ASIS Superior left PSIS
Inferior shear (down slip) right	Positive right standing flexion test Inferior right ASIS Inferior right PSIS
Inferior shear (down slip) left	Positive left standing flexion test Inferior left ASIS Inferior left PSIS

ASIS, anterior superior iliac spine; PSIS, posterior superior iliac spine.

TABLE 37.6

Pubic Symphysis Dysfunctions

Diagnosis	Characteristics
Superior right	Positive right standing flexion test Superior right pubic tubercle Tense, tender right inguinal ligament
Superior left	Positive left standing flexion test Superior left pubic tubercle Tense, tender left inguinal ligament
Inferior right	Positive right standing flexion test Inferior right pubic tubercle Tense, tender right inguinal ligament
Inferior left	Positive left standing flexion test Inferior left pubic tubercle Tense, tender left inguinal ligament

- However, the pubic bones may also be sheared (subluxed) superiorly or inferiorly along with the rest of the respective innominate.
- Pubic somatic dysfunctions usually occur when iliac movement is maximal.
- Strachan came to these conclusions in his SI research in the 1930s.[27]
- Anterior and posterior pubic shears can also occur, as well as a "gapped" pubic symphysis. These are rare and usually result from a significant traumatic event.

PALPATION OF PELVIC ANATOMIC LANDMARKS

Iliosacral Landmarks

Iliosacral (innominate) somatic dysfunctions are most commonly characterized by the combination of a positive standing flexion test and a negative seated flexion test or a positive standing and seated flexion test with the greater excursion found on the standing flexion test. Any asymmetry between certain anatomical landmarks will help to determine the exact type of somatic dysfunction present. These anatomical landmarks consist of the following:

1. Pubic tubercles
2. Anterior superior iliac spines (ASIS)
3. Posterior superior iliac spines (PSIS)
4. Medial malleoli

EXAMINING THE ILIOSACRAL ANATOMICAL LANDMARKS

The Hip Flop Maneuver or Patient Alignment[28] (Figs. 37.13 and 37.14) and Assessment of Medial Malleoli Levels

The hip flop maneuver or patient alignment is performed as follows:

1. The patient lies supine with legs fully extended.
2. The physician stands at the foot of the table.
3. The patient is asked to flex the knees and place the feet flat on the table surface.
4. The physician grasps the patient's feet by placing the hands over the dorsal aspects of the patient's feet.
5. The patient's feet are maintained in this position for the remainder of this maneuver.
6. Physician asks the patient to raise the hips slightly off the table, then drop the hips onto the table.

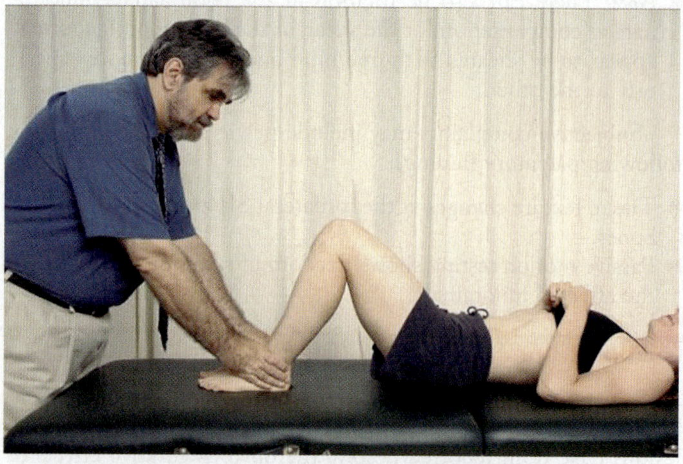

Figure 37.13. Patient positioning prior to hip flop. (From Department of Neuromusculoskeletal Medicine/Osteopathic Manipulative Medicine at Western University of Health Sciences, College of Osteopathic Medicine of the Pacific. *Osteopathic Principles and Practice: Osteopathic Manipulative Treatment.* 3rd ed. Western University of Health Sciences; 2021–2022, with permission.)

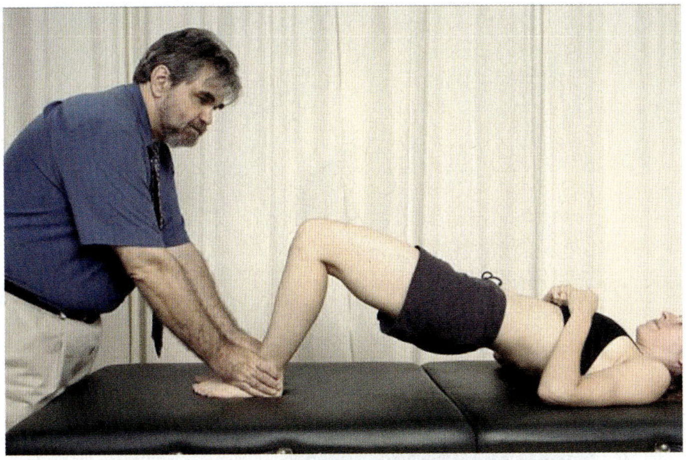

Figure 37.14. Patient performing hip flop. (From Department of Neuromusculoskeletal Medicine/Osteopathic Manipulative Medicine at Western University of Health Sciences, College of Osteopathic Medicine of the Pacific. *Osteopathic Principles and Practice: Osteopathic Manipulative Treatment.* 3rd ed. Western University of Health Sciences; 2021–2022, with permission.)

7. The physician then passively extends the patient's legs until they are fully extended on the table.
8. The physician internally rotates the patient's hips by springing the toes medially in order to relax the external rotators.
9. The physician places the thumbs on the inferior aspects of the patient's medial malleoli while applying a mild traction force on the patient's feet. Physician compares the height of the thumbs to each other.
   - □ An unequal height of the thumbs may be an indication of unequal leg lengths, iliosacral, or other somatic dysfunction.

The purpose of this maneuver is to make sure the patient is aligned on the examination table, so that the postural muscles are as relaxed as possible. This should be a comfortable position for the patient. The hip flop maneuver must be performed prior to any other structural evaluation of the pelvis or lower extremities, such as palpating pelvic landmarks or estimating leg lengths of which assessment of medial malleoli levels may be one component.

THE PUBIC TUBERCLES (FIG. 37.15A–E)

The pubic tubercles are evaluated as follows:

1. The patient lies supine on the examination table.
2. The physician stands at the side of the table with the dominant eye over the patient's midline.
3. The physician places the palm of one hand on the patient's abdomen at the umbilicus. The physician moves the hand inferiorly until the heel of the hand meets the superior aspect of the patient's pubic symphysis.
4. The physician places the pads of the index fingers on the superior aspect of the patient's pubic symphysis in the midline.
5. The physician moves the index fingers laterally until the superior aspects of the pubic tubercles are palpated.

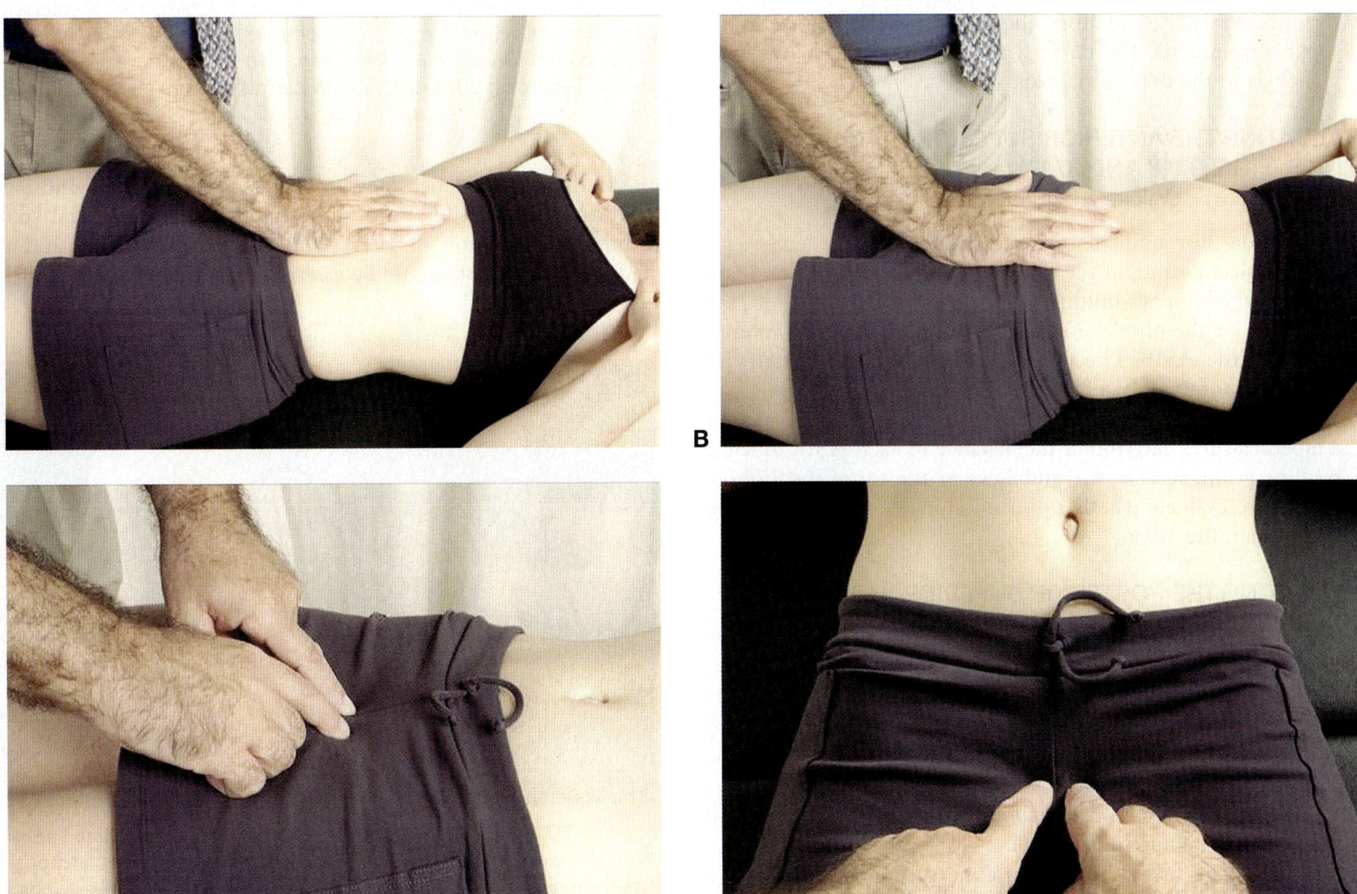

A B C D

Figure 37.15. A–E. The pubic symphysis. A. Initial physician hand placement at umbilicus applying slight posterior pressure. **B.** Thenar and hypothenar eminences contacting the pubic symphysis. **C.** Lateral view of physician's index fingers palpating the medial portion of the pubic symphysis. **D.** Anterior view of index fingers on the medial aspect of the patient's pubic symphysis. *(continued)*

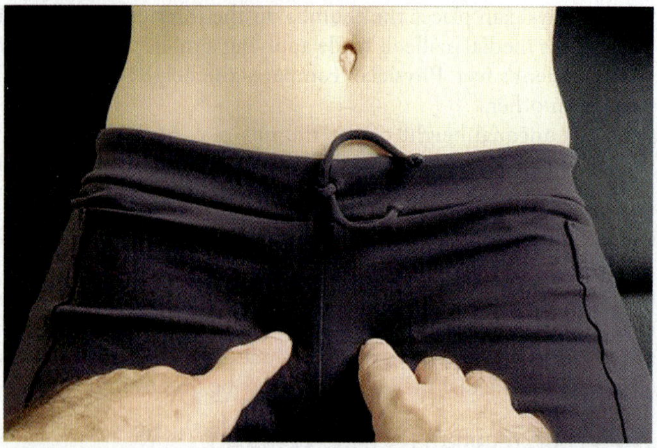

E

Figure 37.15. *(Continued)* **E.** Anterior view of index fingers at the superior aspect of the pubic tubercles. (From Department of Neuromusculoskeletal Medicine/Osteopathic Manipulative Medicine at Western University of Health Sciences, College of Osteopathic Medicine of the Pacific. *Osteopathic Principles and Practice: Osteopathic Manipulative Treatment.* 3rd ed. Western University of Health Sciences; 2021–2022, with permission.)

- □ A positive finding occurs when one pubic tubercle is more superior or inferior than the other.
- □ Tenderness may also be noted at the medial attachment of the inguinal ligament on the side of the positive standing flexion test.
- □ Note that a pubic tubercle may also be anterior or posterior compared to the other side due to the compliance of the pubic symphysis. The pubic symphysis itself may be widened such as in the case of diastasis.

EVALUATING THE ANTERIOR SUPERIOR ILIAC SPINES (FIGS. 37.16 AND 37.17)

The ASIS may be evaluated as follows:

1. The patient lies supine on the examination table.
2. The physician stands at the side of the table with the dominant eye over the patient's midline.
3. The pads of the physician's thumbs are placed on the inferior slopes of the ASIS. The physician observes for symmetry or asymmetry of the ASIS in the horizontal plane.
4. The physician (using the hand or a measuring device such as a tape measure) determines the distance of each ASIS to some midline point, such as the umbilicus or the tip of the xiphoid process, to evaluate whether one innominate is more medial or lateral than the other.

EVALUATING THE POSTERIOR SUPERIOR ILIAC SPINES (FIGS. 37.18 AND 37.19)

The PSIS may be evaluated as follows:

1. The patient lies prone on the examination table.
2. The physician stands at the side of the table with the dominant eye over the patient's midline.
3. The physician's thumbs are placed on the inferior slopes of the PSISs. The physician observes for symmetry or asymmetry of the PSIS in the horizontal plane.
4. The physician (using the hand or a measuring device such as a tape measure) determines the distance of each PSIS from some midline point, such as the spinous process of L5, to evaluate whether one innominate is more medial or lateral than the other.

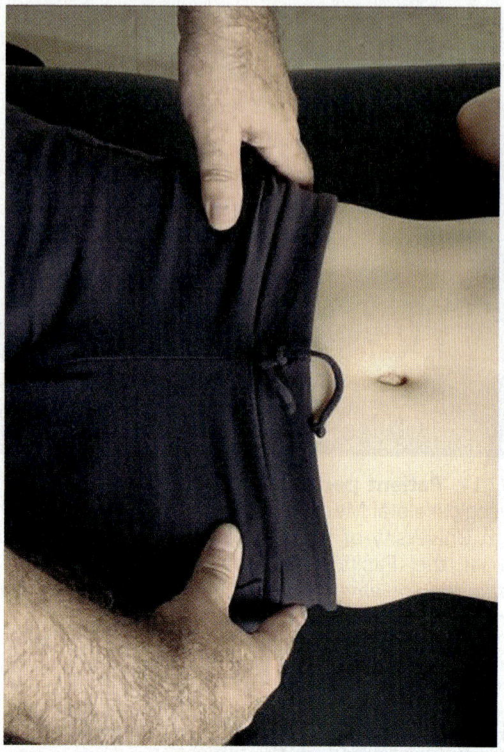

Figure 37.16. Evaluating the anterior superior iliac spines. Superior view of ASIS level assessment. (From Department of Neuromusculoskeletal Medicine/Osteopathic Manipulative Medicine at Western University of Health Sciences, College of Osteopathic Medicine of the Pacific. *Osteopathic Principles and Practice: Osteopathic Manipulative Treatment.* 3rd ed. Western University of Health Sciences; 2021–2022, with permission.)

If there is evidence of sacroiliac dysfunction, the landmarks relating to sacral somatic dysfunction, rotation L5, sacral sulcus depths, the position of ILAs, lumbosacral spring test, and the backward bend test should be assessed (Please see Chapter 38). In

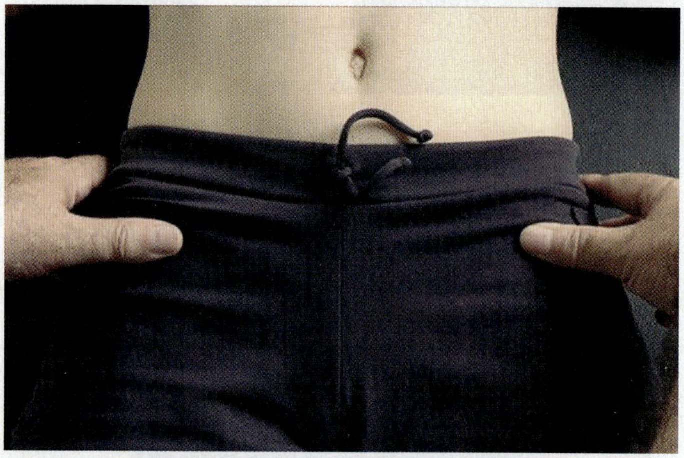

Figure 37.17. Evaluating the anterior superior iliac spines. Anterior view of ASIS level assessment. (From Department of Neuromusculoskeletal Medicine/Osteopathic Manipulative Medicine at Western University of Health Sciences, College of Osteopathic Medicine of the Pacific. *Osteopathic Principles and Practice: Osteopathic Manipulative Treatment.* 3rd ed. Western University of Health Sciences; 2021–2022, with permission.)

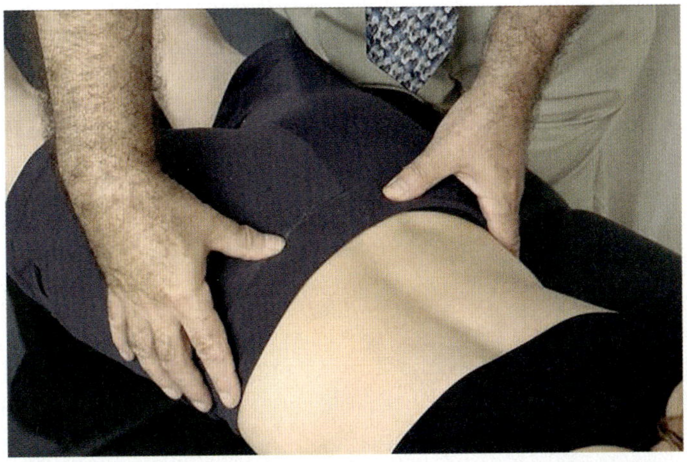

Figure 37.18. Evaluating the posterior superior iliac spines. Lateral oblique view of thumb placement for PSIS evaluation. (From Department of Neuromusculoskeletal Medicine/Osteopathic Manipulative Medicine at Western University of Health Sciences, College of Osteopathic Medicine of the Pacific. *Osteopathic Principles and Practice: Osteopathic Manipulative Treatment.* 1st ed. Western University of Health Sciences; 2021–2022, with permission.)

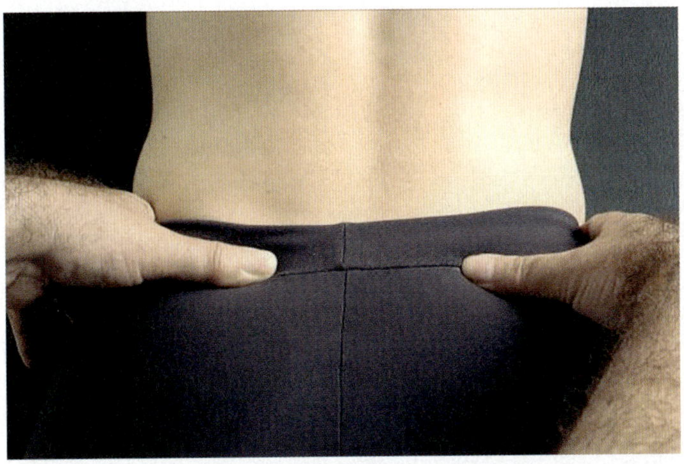

Figure 37.19. Evaluating the posterior superior iliac spines. Posterior view of thumb placement for evaluation of PSISs. (From Department of Neuromusculoskeletal Medicine/Osteopathic Manipulative Medicine at Western University of Health Sciences, College of Osteopathic Medicine of the Pacific. *Osteopathic Principles and Practice: Osteopathic Manipulative Treatment.* 3rd ed. Western University of Health Sciences; 2021–2022, with permission.)

addition to the above evaluations, the physician should also examine the pelvis region for the following:

- Myofascial restrictions. See Chapter 52 for more information about evaluation of myofascial structures.
- Counterstrain tender points. See Chapter 47 for more information about counterstrain.
- Chapman reflexes. See Chapter 58 for more information about Chapman reflexes.

SUMMARY

The pelvis is a complicated and intricate region. When Owens, DO saved his son's life with the application of Chapman reflex points, Mitchell, Sr. was motivated to become an osteopathic physician and to create a model of this region in order to elucidate how to restore and maintain balance to the pelvis. From the structural osteopathic model of care, this chapter endeavored to provide the osteopathic physician with resources to evaluate the pelvis with respect to iliosacral somatic dysfunction. Structural balance may optimize the functioning of the pelvic diaphragm, thoracoabdominal pressure gradients, and lymphatic and vascular flow and thereby positively impact the respiratory/ circulatory model. It may reduce impingement on the different nerve plexi of the region decreasing pain and restoring autonomic imbalance of the viscera of the region. It may also optimize compensation for short leg, scoliosis, or somatic dysfunction thereby affecting related energy expenditure and positively influencing the metabolic model. An in-depth knowledge of how to evaluate for and diagnose somatic dysfunction of this region enables osteopathic physicians to provide distinctive and individualized care to their patients for a wide range of conditions that affect the pelvis and its related structures.

REFERENCES

1. Agur AMR, Dalley AF. *Moore's Clinically Oriented Anatomy.* 9th ed. Wolters Kluwer; 2022.
2. Standring S, Editor-in-Chief. *Grays Anatomy.* 39th ed. Elsevier Churchill Livingston; 2005:1357.
3. Bernard TN. The role of the sacroiliac joints in low back pain: basic aspects of pathophysiology and management. In: Vleeming A, ed. *Movement, Stability and Lumbopelvic Pain.* Churchill Livingstone; 1997:73–86.
4. Strachan WF. Applied anatomy of the pelvis and perineum. *J Am Osteopath Assoc.* 1939;38(8):57–58.
5. Weisl H. The articular surfaces of the sacro-iliac joint and their relationship to the movements of the sacrum. *Acta Anat.* 1954;22:1–14.
6. Novoseltsev SV, Vcherashny DB. Biomechanical disorders in the patients with lumbar discal hernias and their osteopathic correction. *AAOJ.* 2010;20(1):11–15.
7. Vleeming A, Snijders CJ, Stoeckart R, et al. The role of the sacroiliac joints in coupling between spine, pelvis, legs and arms. In: Vleeming A, ed. *Movement, Stability and Lumbopelvic Pain.* Churchill Livingstone; 1997:53–71.
8. Dutton M. The sacroiliac joint. In: *Orthopedic Examination, Evaluation, Intervention.* McGraw-Hill; 2004.
9. VanBuskirk RL. *The Still Technique Manual.* 2nd ed. American Academy of Osteopathy; 2006.
10. Thiele GH. Coccygodynia: cause and treatment. *Dis Colon Rectum.* 1963; 6:422–436.
11. Mooney V. Sacroiliac joint dysfunction. In: Vleeming A, ed. *Movement, Stability and Lumbopelvic Pain.* Churchill Livingstone; 1997:37–43.
12. Beaton LE, Anson BJ. The sciatic nerve and the piriformis muscle: their interrelationship a possible cause of coccygodynia. *J Bone Joint Surg (Br).* 1938;20:686–688.
13. Chikly B. *Silent Waves: Theory and Practice of Lymph Drainage Therapy.* IHH Publishing; 2002.
14. Korr IM. Sustained sympathicotonia as a factor in disease. *The Collected Papers of Irvin M. Korr.* American Academy of Osteopathy; 1979:77–89.
15. Mitchell FL. *The Muscle Energy Manual, Volume Three: Evaluation and Treatment of the Pelvis and Sacrum.* MET Press; 1999:xvi–xvii.
16. Mitchell FLS. *Structural pelvic function.* Academy of Applied Osteopathy Yearbook; 1965:178.
17. Mitchell FLS. *Structural pelvic function.* Academy of Applied Osteopathy Yearbook; 1965:190–191.
18. Reynolds HM. Three dimensional kinematics in the pelvic girdle. *J Am Osteopath Assoc.* 1980;80:277–280.
19. Dutton M. The sacroiliac joint. In: *Orthopedic Examination, Evaluation, Intervention.* McGraw-Hill; 2004: Chapter 27.
20. Fryette HH. *Principles of Osteopathic Technique.* Academy of Applied Osteopathy; 1954.
21. Mitchell FL. *The Muscle Energy Manual, Volume Three: Evaluation and Treatment of the Pelvis and Sacrum.* MET Press; 1999:76, 83.
22. Mitchell FLS. *Structural pelvic function.* Academy of Applied Osteopathy Yearbook; 1965:189.

23. Mitchell FL. *The Muscle Energy Manual, Volume Three: Evaluation and Treatment of the Pelvis and Sacrum*. MET Press; 1999:89.
24. DeStefano LA. *Greenman's Principles of Manual Medicine*, 5th ed. Wolters Kluwer; 2017:319.
25. Mitchell FL. *The Muscle Energy Manual, Volume Three: Evaluation and Treatment of the Pelvis and Sacrum*. MET Press; 1999:56.
26. Mitchell FL. *The Muscle Energy Manual, Volume Three: Evaluation and Treatment of the Pelvis and Sacrum*. MET Press; 1999:57.
27. Strachan WF, Beckwith CG, Larson NJ, et al. A study of the mechanics of the sacroiliac joint. *JAOA*. 1938;37(12):575–578.
28. Mitchell FL. *The Muscle Energy Manual, Volume Three: Evaluation and Treatment of the Pelvis and Sacrum*. MET Press; 1999:95–96.

38

Functional Anatomy and Diagnosis of the Sacrum

KENDI L. HENSEL ▪ LISA A. DESTEFANO ▪ KURT P. HEINKING

KEY CONCEPTS

- Descriptive and functional anatomy of the sacrum and sacroiliac (SI) joints
- Biomechanics of the sacrum and sacroiliac joints
- Identification and diagnosis of somatic dysfunction of the sacrum based on the three models of sacral dysfunction
- Clinical implications of sacral dysfunction
- Clinical aspects of sacroiliac structures and functional interrelationships
- Performance of the segmental exam to the sacroiliac region

INTRODUCTION

The sacroiliac (SI) joint, its mechanics, and its interplay with the rest of the body are incredibly nuanced. Dysfunction of this complex can lead to a host of acute and chronic issues including back and pelvic pain. Both normal and abnormal sacral mechanics can be challenging to learn but a comprehensive understanding of this complexity and the ability to apply that understanding to clinical scenarios is vital for thorough osteopathic treatment and patient care.

> "It [the sacrum] is the seat of the transverse center of gravity, the keystone of the pelvis, the foundation of the spine. It is closely associated with our greatest abilities and disabilities, with our greatest romances and tragedies, our greatest pleasures and pains."
> —Fryette,[1] p. 68.

SACRAL ANATOMY

Skeletal

The sacrum is formed by five fused elements of the sacral vertebrae, which fuse in the midsecond to the early third decade of life and articulate superiorly with the last lumbar vertebra and inferiorly with the coccyx.[2,3] In clinical practice, it is critical to consider the sacrum as a component of the vertebral axis.[1]

The SI joints, formed at the lateral margins of sacral segments S1, S2, and S3, are diarthrodial joints with a joint space, a capsule that secretes synovial fluid, and articular cartilage.[4] They are unique because the cartilage on the concave sacral surface is thick hyaline cartilage, while the cartilage on the convex ilial surface is thin fibrocartilage.[2,5] Abundantly innervated with mechanoreceptors, proprioceptors, and nociceptors, this joint has intricate neural-reflexive qualities.[6,7] The joints are L-shaped in contour with a shorter upper arm and a longer lower arm[3] (Fig. 38.1).

The joint contour usually has a depression on the sacral surface at approximately S2 and a congruent prominence on the ilial surface.[8–10] The SI joints are relatively flat but not smooth, with irregular ridges and depressions. Like most relatively flat articular surfaces, they need specific adaptation to resist shear forces, especially with rotation or translation. Given the location of the sacrum and its crucial role in supporting the spine, the lack of resistance to shear forces can be problematic.[11,12]

Since the time of Hippocrates, motion of the SI joint has been postulated. Over the past 200 years, many authors have described significant anatomic asymmetry of the sacrum and the SI joints between individuals and in the same individual.[2] In the osteopathic profession, these concepts were popularized in the early 20th century, when Harrison Fryette, DO described his observational studies of the sacrum and SI joints to the osteopathic profession. Fryette described three types of anatomic asymmetries of the sacrum (A, B, C) and three anatomic asymmetries of the SI joints (D, E, F). The difference between these types is primarily related to the varying widths of the dorsal transverse sacral segments. In general, however, the sacrum is wider superiorly than inferiorly and broader anteriorly than posteriorly. This "keystone-shape" configuration is necessary for the sacrum to wedge between the ilia and reduce its susceptibility to shear.[11,13]

The sacrum also requires complex continuous muscular and ligamentous tensile forces to protect it from vulnerability and yet allow it to function within the pelvis as a stable platform critical for the transferal of force from the pelvis to and from the lumbar spine and legs, often referred to as "form and force closure."[4,14–19]

Landmarks

The primary palpatory landmarks on the sacrum include the sacral base, apex, sulcus, and inferior lateral angles (ILAs). The sacral base is the most superior aspect of the sacrum, just below L5. The

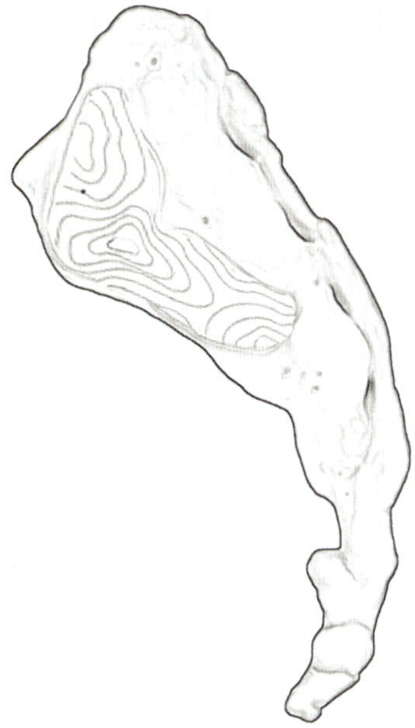

Figure 38.1. SI joint.

Figure 38.2. **Ligaments of the pelvis—anterior view.**

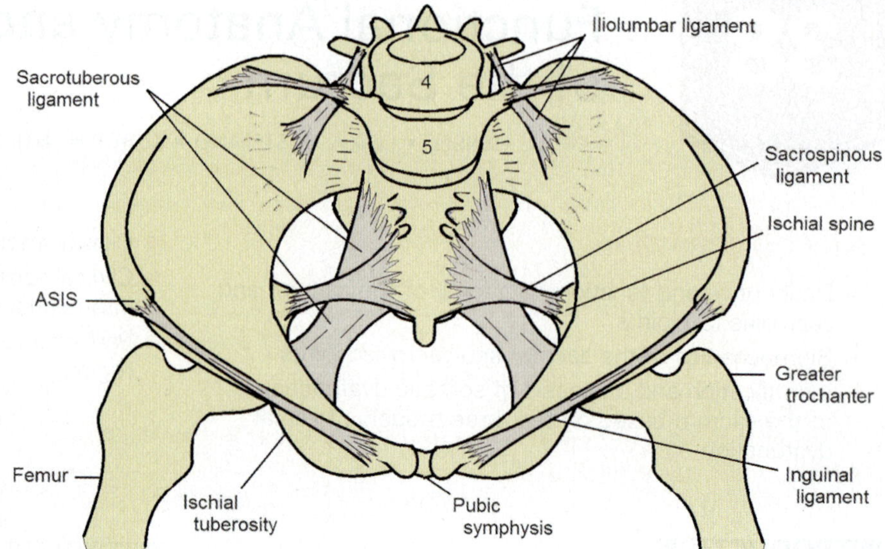

sacral sulcus is the drop-off medially from the posterior superior iliac spine (PSIS) to the sacrum. The easiest way to palpate these is to find the iliac crests bilaterally with the 2nd digits' MCP joints, then drop the thumbs; they will fall into the area of the PSIS at approximately the level of S2. With the pads of the thumbs on the PSIS, roll the tips of the thumbs medially so that the tip of the thumb sinks into either side of the sulcus, just medial to the PSIS. The sulcus is assessed by the comparative depth of the left and right sides (Figs. 38.2 and 38.3).

The sacral apex is the inferior aspect of the sacrum and is roughly triangular, with the coccyx descending from the midline. The ILAs are the inferior edges of the sacrum just to each side of the coccyx. Assessment of the ILAs is to compare their inferior/superior and their posterior/anterior positions related to each other.

Muscle and Fascial Structures

In addition to the psoas major, the iliacus, piriformis muscle, gluteus medius, sartorius, and thigh adductors all contribute to somatic dysfunction in the sacral–pelvic region. The iliacus muscle lies in the fossa of the ilium and has been clinically thought to contribute to a recurrent anterior ilium somatic dysfunction. The iliacus muscle joins the psoas major to form the iliopsoas muscle passing through the groin and inserting on the lesser trochanter of the femur.

The piriformis muscle is flat, oblique, and pyramid-shaped. The piriformis muscle arises from ventrolateral surface of the S2–S4 sacral vertebrae, gluteal surface of the ilium, and SI joint capsule, and from the anterior sacrospinous ligament and the pelvic portion of the sacrotuberous ligament.[20,21] It runs laterally through the greater sciatic foramen, becomes tendinous, and inserts into the piriformis fossa at the medial aspect of the greater trochanter of the femur.[20] Also coursing through the foramen and emerging along the inferior border of the piriformis muscle are the inferior gluteal nerve and artery, the posterior cutaneous nerve of the thigh, and the pudendal nerve.[21] The piriformis muscle receives innervation from nerve branches coming off L5, S1, and S2. The sciatic nerve has genetic variations that may predispose it to compression by the piriformis muscle. There are six categories of anatomic variations of the relationship between the piriformis muscle and sciatic nerve, originally reported in 1938 by Beaton and Anson.[20] In >80% of the population, the sciatic nerve courses deep to and exits inferiorly to the piriformis muscle belly/tendon (see Fig. 38.4).

Figure 38.3. **Ligaments of the pelvis—posterior view.**

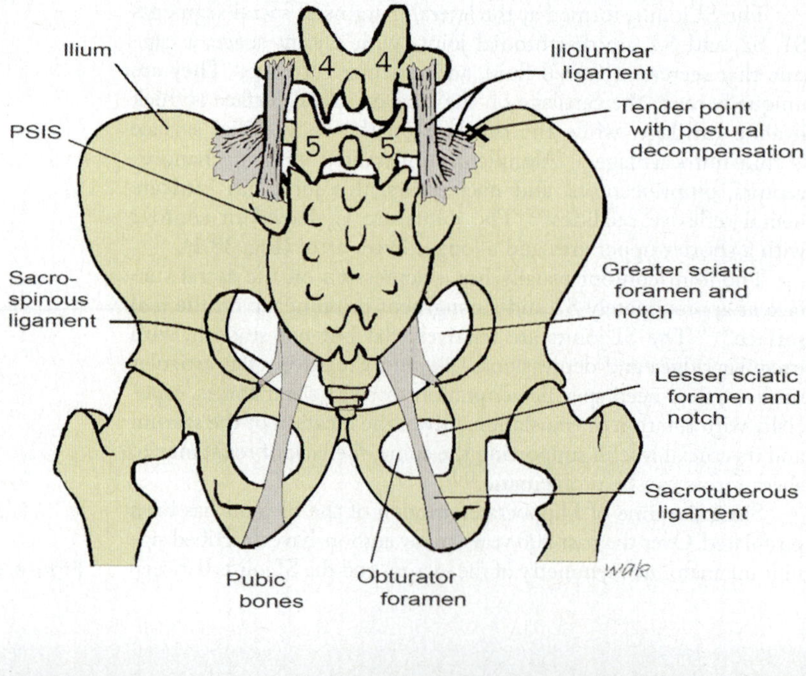

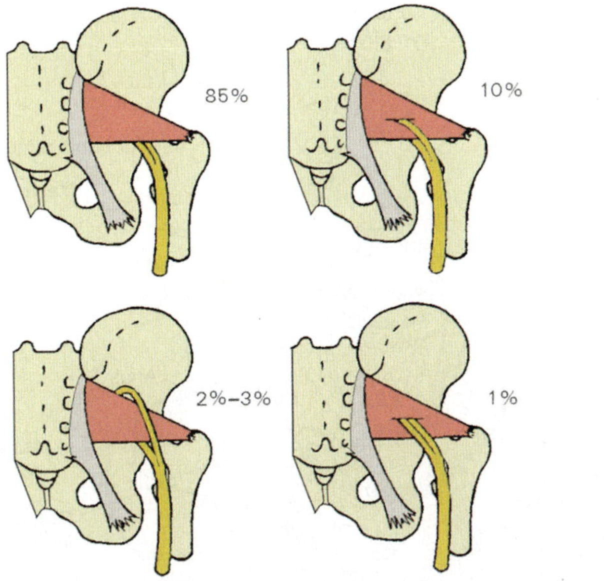

Figure 38.4. Position of the sciatic nerve in relation to the piriformis muscle. (Adapted with permission from Beaton LE, Anson BJ. The sciatic nerve and the piriformis muscle: their interrelation a possible cause of coccygodynia. *J Bone Joint Surg Am.* 1938;20(3):686–688. Copyright © 1938 by The Journal of Bone and Joint Surgery, Incorporated.)

The piriformis muscle has a unique relationship to the sciatic nerve. The sciatic nerve typically passes beneath the piriformis muscle. However, anatomic variation exists. The possible anatomical relationships between the sciatic nerve and the piriformis muscle include the following[20]: (a) Sciatic nerve passes below the piriformis muscle; (b) Divided nerve passes through and below the muscle; (c) A divided nerve passes above and below the muscle; (d) Undivided nerve passes through the piriformis; (e) Divided nerve passes through and above the muscle; or (f) Smaller accessory piriformis with its own separate tendon and sciatic nerve passes through the piriformis (Fig. 38.4). Sciatic nerve irritation due to piriformis spasm typically causes posterior thigh pain that stops at the knee.

When the patient is standing or the hip is extended, the muscle acts primarily as an external rotator, but when the hip is in flexion, the piriformis muscle restricts posterior translation of the femoral head and acts like a hip abductor.[20] If the hip is flexed greater than 90 degrees the piriformis acts as an internal rotator.[22] The abduction role is important during walking to shift the body's weight to the other side. The piriformis also tilts the pelvis slightly posterior and lateral.[23] Under normal function, the sciatic nerve can stretch and glide to accommodate the strain or compression associated with joint movement.[20]

The gluteus medius is a stabilizer of the pelvis, especially during gait. Weakness and tenderness of this muscle have been seen clinically within ipsilateral anterior sacrum dysfunction. It has a referral pattern that can closely mimic that of the piriformis. The muscle is vital in maintaining the coupling of forces between the sacrum and pelvis to the lumbar spine during ambulation, jogging, and other postural movements. When the muscle is dysfunctional, the opposite hip will drop during one leg standing posture (Trendelenburg test).

The sartorius muscle originates on the anterior inferior iliac spine and inserts on the medial aspect of the proximal tibia. When the muscle contracts, it moves the hip into the figure-4 position. A posteriorly rotated innominate dysfunction may create medial knee pain through the tension of the sartorius muscle.

The pelvic floor muscles are depicted in the following Figures 38.5 and 38.6.

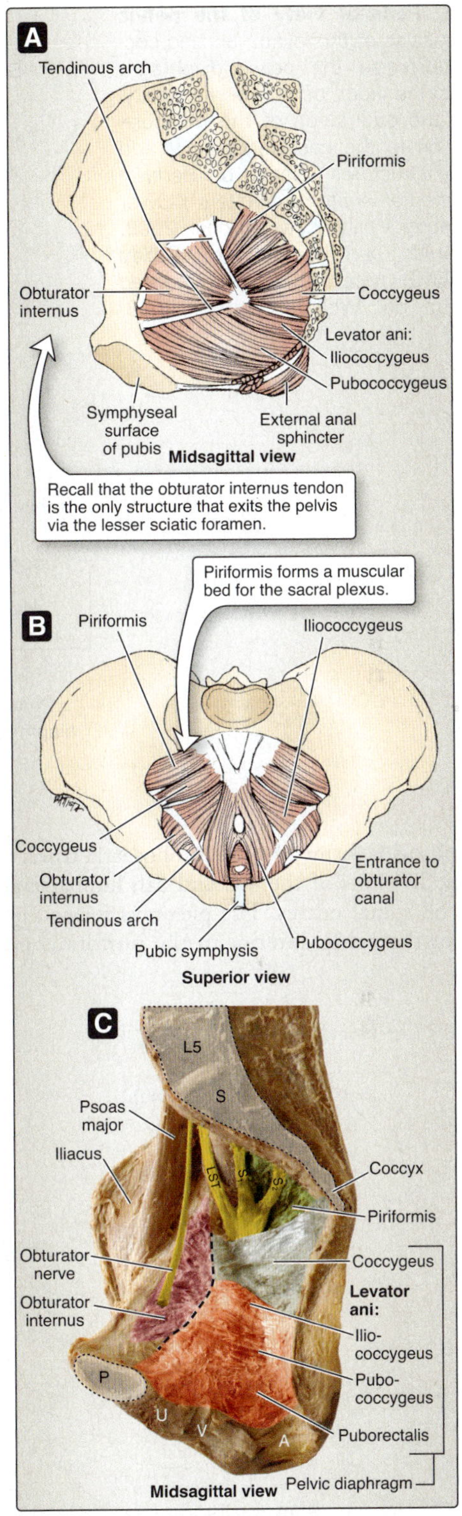

Figure 38.5. Floor and walls of pelvis. (**A**) Midsagittal view of the pelvic floor muscles: The pelvic muscular wall includes the piriformis and obturator internus. (**B**) Superior view of the pelvic floor muscles: The pelvic floor is formed by the pelvic diaphragm, encircled by and suspended in part from the pubic symphysis and pubic bones anteriorly, the ilia laterally, and the sacrum and coccyx posteriorly. (**C**) Midsagittal view of the pelvic floor muscles: Cadaveric specimen with pelvic viscera and vasculature removed. (Based on *Stedman's Medical Dictionary*. 28th ed. Lippincott Williams & Wilkins; 2006 (artist: Neil O. Hardy, Westport, CT). Reprinted with permission from Dalley AF II, Agur AMR. *Moore's Clinically Oriented Anatomy*. 9th ed. Wolters Kluwer; 2023. Figure B6.9.)

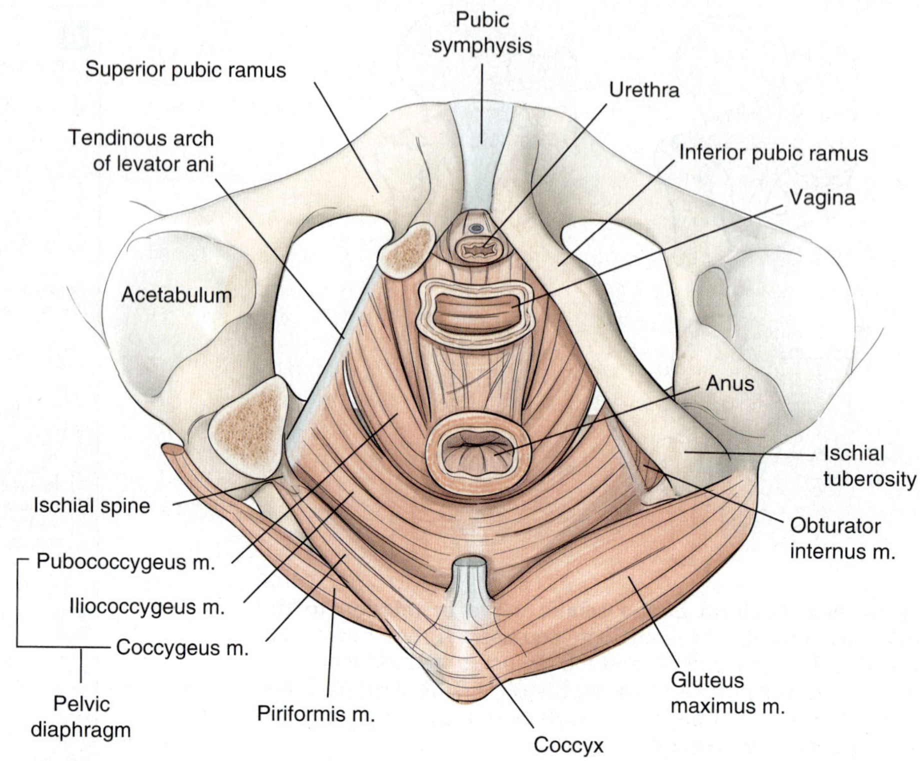

Figure 38.6. Perineal view of the pelvic floor. The muscles of the levator ani and coccygeus compromise the pelvic diaphragm which forms the floor of the pelvic cavity. Depicted is the orientation of the musculature in relation to the coccyx, ischium, and genitourinary structures. (Based on Hartwig WC. *Fundamental Anatomy.* Wolters Kluwer Health/Lippincott Williams & Wilkins; 2008. Reprinted with permission from Dalley AF II, Agur AMR. *Moore's Clinically Oriented Anatomy.* 9th ed. Wolters Kluwer; 2023. Figure B6.10.)

Neurologic Structures

The sacral plexus is formed by the lumbosacral trunk from anterior primary divisions of the 4th and 5th lumbar and 1st, 2nd, and 3rd sacral spinal nerves. The plexus is formed on the posterior wall of the pelvis anterior to the piriformis muscle. The lumbosacral trunk, from the 4th and 5th lumbar spinal nerves, belongs to both the lumbar and sacral plexuses, and passes directly anterior to the SI joint. As such, somatic dysfunction of L4, L5, or the sacrum can lead to sciatic nerve complaints (p. 24)[24,25] (Fig. 38.7).

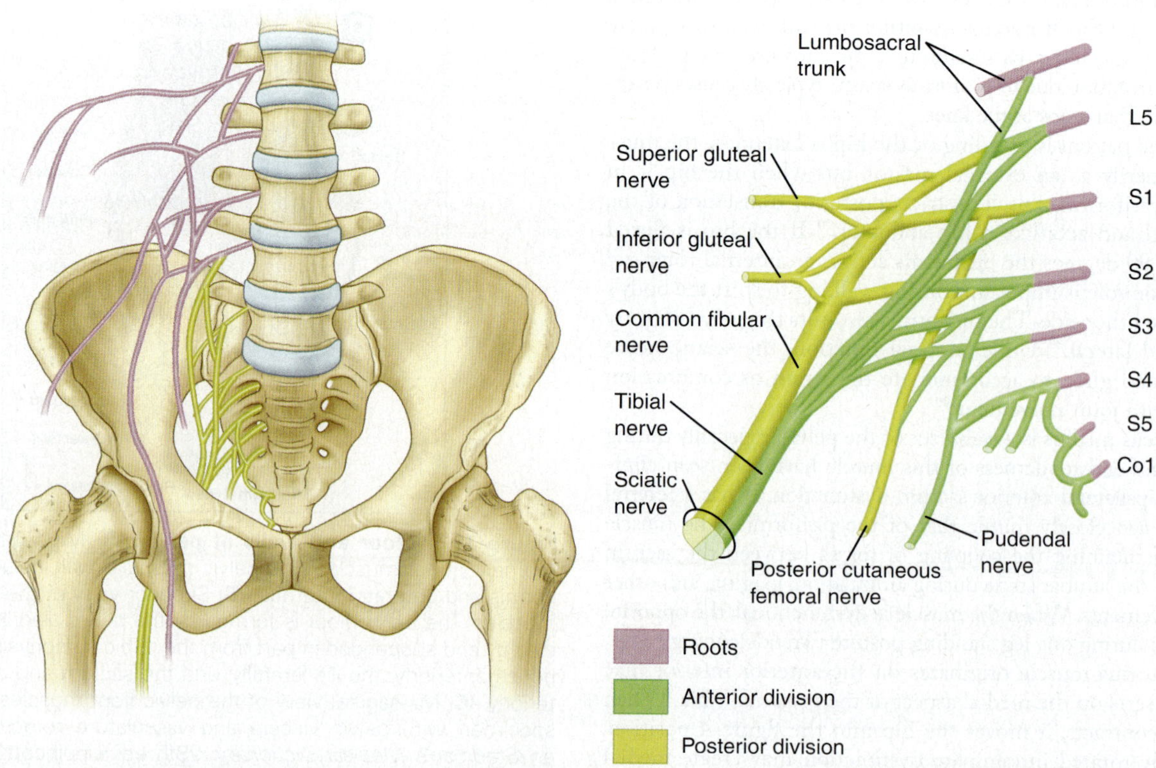

Figure 38.7. Sacral plexus. The sacral plexus is formed by the segmental nerves L4 through S5. This plexus innervates the lower leg, ankle, and foot via the tibial and common peroneal nerves. (Reprinted with permission from Anderson MK. *Foundations of Athletic Training: Prevention, Assessment, and Management.* 6th ed. Wolters Kluwer; 2017.)

The fibers forming the sacral plexus gradually come together as they pass inferiorly through the pelvis until they converge into a flat cord-like structure that passes through the greater sciatic foramen to emerge as the sciatic nerve. This nerve should be referred to as a "trunk" rather than a nerve because it is comprised of two main nerves, the common peroneal and anterior tibial (p. 24).[24,25]

The contribution to the autonomic nervous system found here is unique in its arrangement and shall be discussed as "sacral outflow" below in the section on the autonomic nervous system.

The Sacral Plexus

Nerve	Segmental Origin	Distribution
Superior gluteal nerve	L4, L5, S1	Muscular: Gluteus minimus, gluteus medius, and tensor fasciae latae muscles
Inferior gluteal nerve	S1, S2, S3	Muscular: Gluteus maximus muscle
Quadratus femoris and gemellus inferior nerve	L4, L5, S1	Muscular: Gemellus inferior and quadratus femoris muscles
Nerve to obturator internus and gemellus superior nerve	L5, S1, S2	Muscular: Obturator internus and gemellus superior muscles
Posterior femoral cutaneous nerve	S1, S2, S3	Cutaneous: Inferior portion of the buttock, the posterior thigh to the mid portion of the leg, the upper medial thigh, the scrotum (male), and the labium majus (female)
Nerve to piriformis muscle	S1, S2	Muscular: Piriformis muscle
Pudendal nerve	S2, S3, S4	All muscles of the perineum and the overlying skin
Sciatic: Tibial nerve, through its branches, the medical and lateral plantar nerves	L4, L5, S1, S2, S3, S4	Muscular: Gastrocnemius, plantaris, soleus, tibialis posterior, abductor hallucis, flexor digitorum longus, flexor digitorum brevis, flexor hallucis longus, flexor hallucis brevis, Interossei muscles, lumbrical muscles (1st lumbrical S2, S3, S4) and all of the muscles of the sole of the foot Cutaneous: Through (a) the sural nerve to the lower third of the posterior aspect of the calf and the lateral aspect of the foot to the 5th toe, and (b) the medial plantar nerve to the sole of the foot and the webs of toes Articular: Hip joint (from the common sciatic trunk), tibiofibular joint, knee joint, and ankle joint
Sciatic: Common peroneal nerve through its branches, the musculocutaneous and anterior tibial nerves	L4, L5, S1, S2	Muscular: Peroneus longus and brevis muscles, tibialis anterior, exterior hallucis longus exterior digitorum longus, peroneus tertius. Cutaneous: Through the musculocutaneous nerve to the lateral aspect of the ankle and the dorsum of all toes except the lateral side of 5th toe. Articular: Ankle joint

The nerves of the pelvis and lower limbs originate from sympathetic, parasympathetic, and somatic nerves. Somatic innervation for the pelvis arises from nerve roots S2 through S4. Somatic nerves of the pelvis supply purely motor, purely sensory, or both motor and sensory information. Afferent fibers carry sensory information, while efferent fibers carry motor. The autonomic nerves of the pelvis include the sympathetic component (which comes from roots T12 through L2) and the parasympathetic component (from roots S2 through S4). The sympathetic component reaches the pelvis through the superior hypogastric plexus. These nerves are known as sacral splanchnic nerves. The parasympathetic components are referred to as pelvic splanchnic nerves. Their anatomy and function will be described in Chapter 6 Autonomic Nervous System. Nerve roots L2 through L4 and L4 through S3 supply all the motor and some sensory information for the lower limbs.[26] Generally, nerves with motor information supply all muscles within a given compartment. The cutaneous sensation is in a dermatomal distribution.

The 4th and 5th lumbar spinal nerves arise from the lumbosacral trunk. The lumbosacral trunk joins the 1st through 4th sacral nerves as they exit the sacrum to form the sacral plexus. The sacral plexus runs down on the posterior pelvic wall anterior to the piriformis muscle. The sacral plexus is comprised of the following nerves: The sciatic nerve, the pudendal nerve, the superior and inferior gluteal nerves, the nerve to the quadratus femoris and obturator internus muscles, the nerve to the piriformis muscle, the posterior femoral cutaneous nerve, some cutaneous perforating nerves, and pelvic splanchnic nerves providing parasympathetic innervation to the pelvic viscera.[27]

Some other important nerves of the pelvic region and their clinical significance are listed below:

- The superior and inferior gluteal nerves supply motor information to the gluteal muscles and the tensor fascia latae.
- The lateral femoral cutaneous nerve provides sensation to the anterior and lateral aspects of the thigh through an anterior and posterior branch.
- The femoral nerve, artery, and vein are in the femoral triangle. The femoral nerve supplies the anterior compartments and a few medial compartment muscles with motor information. The femoral nerve also supplies the anterior and medial aspects of the thigh with cutaneous sensation. It continues as the saphenous nerve to provide cutaneous sensation to the lower extremity.
- The obturator nerve sends motor information to the medial compartment of the thigh through posterior and anterior branches.
- The genitofemoral nerve is composed of two separate branches: the genital branch and the femoral branch. The genital branch runs within the spermatic cord and supplies motor information to the scrotum, specifically the cremasteric muscle. The femoral branch supplies cutaneous sensation to the inner aspect of the upper thigh.
- The ilioinguinal nerve travels through the inguinal canal outside of the spermatic cord, providing sensation to the scrotum, labia, and the upper anterior-medial thigh.

Somatic dysfunction of the ilium, pubic bones, and hip can affect any of these nerves due to muscular attachments and fascial relationships. Many lower extremity symptoms can be produced by somatic dysfunction of the lumbar spine, sacrum, and pelvis.

- The 4th and 5th sacral spinal nerves and the coccygeal nerves form the coccygeal plexus of nerve fibers. This plexus supplies the coccygeus and levator ani muscles and the sacrococcygeal joint.

Vasculature

The median sacral artery is a small posterior branch of the abdominal aorta arising from the aorta above its bifurcation. It descends in the midline, anterior to the fourth and fifth lumbar vertebrae, the sacrum, and the coccyx. There are anastomoses with the rectum, lumbar branches of the iliolumbar artery, and lateral sacral arteries (Fig. 38.8).

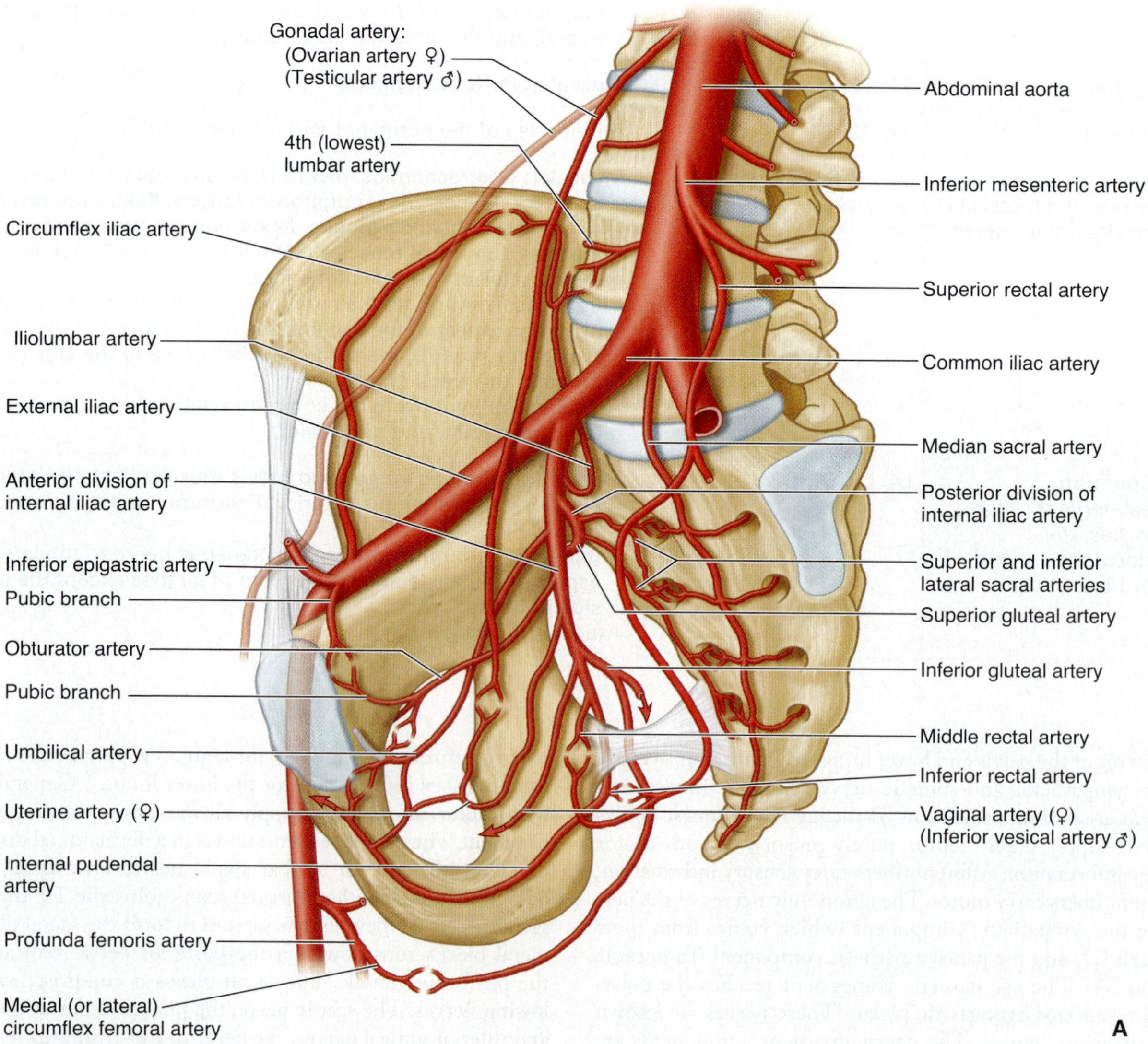

Figure 38.8. **A.** Arteries of the pelvis. (Reprinted with permission from Moore KL, Dalley AF II, Agur AMR. *Clinically Oriented Anatomy*. 8th ed. Wolters Kluwer; 2018.)

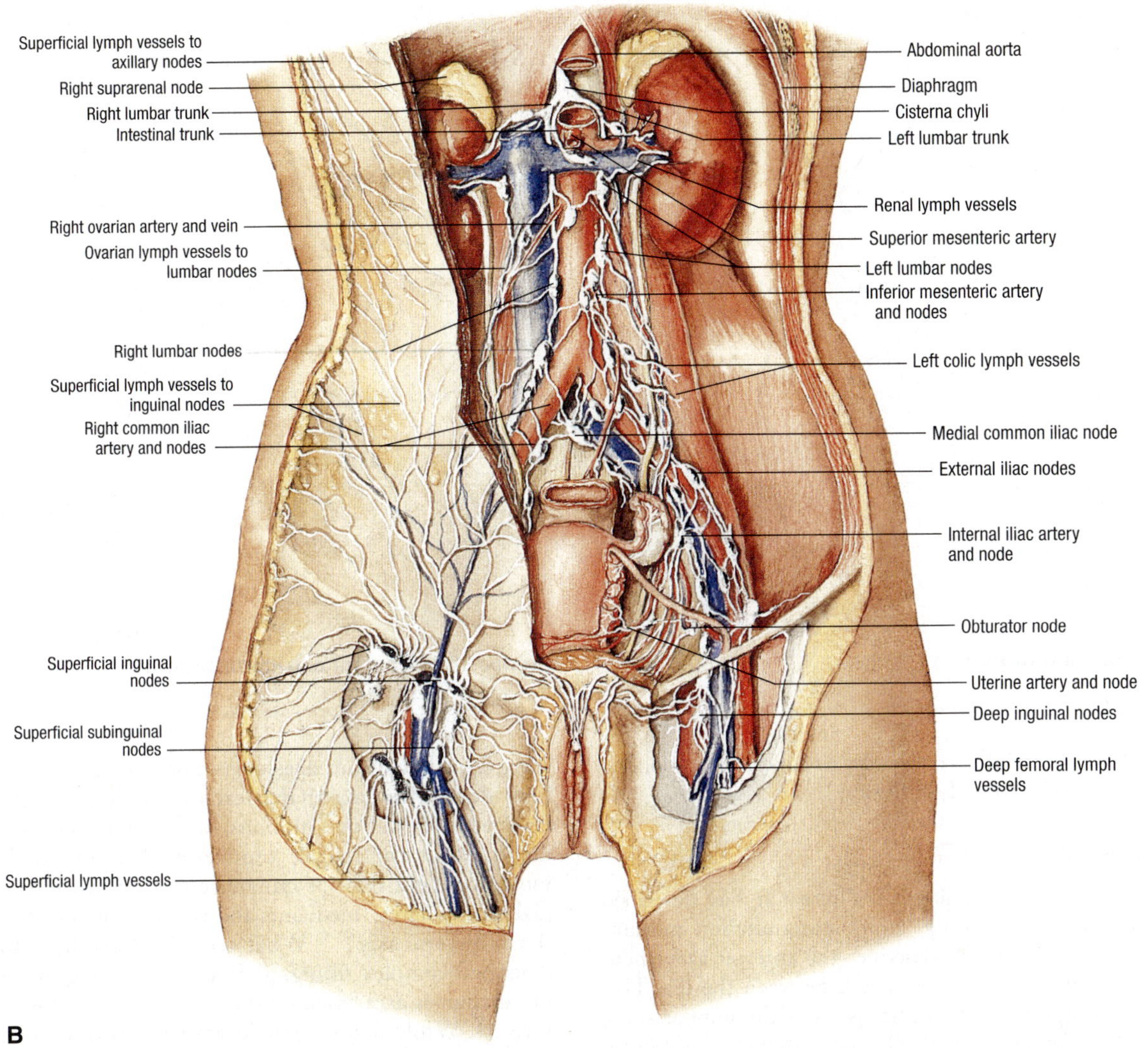

Figure 38.8. (*Continued*) **B.** Pelvic lymph nodes. (Reprinted with permission from Halperin EC, Wazer DE, Perez CA, Brady LW. *Perez & Brady's Principles and Practice of Radiation Oncology*. 7th ed. Wolters Kluwer; 2019.)

The lymphatic drainage of the sacrum includes four main groups of lymph nodes. These include the sacral nodes, internal iliac nodes, external iliac nodes, and common iliac nodes. They are generally named by the arteries with which they are associated. Most lymph nodes drain into the common iliac nodes, and the common iliac nodes drain into the lumbar nodes.

Sacral lymph nodes: Within the pelvis, at the concavity of the sacrum, lies the sacral group of lymph nodes. They receive lymphatic vessels, which course along the median sacral blood vessels. Specifically, they receive lymph from the posteroinferior pelvic viscera and drain either to the internal or common iliac group of lymph nodes.

Tension of the piriformis muscle, the pelvic floor/pelvic basin muscles, and their fascial attachments can limit lymphatic drainage into the pelvic region. Somatic dysfunction of the SI joint, ilium, and pubic bones can all affect the tension and function of the pelvic floor.

FUNCTIONAL BIOMECHANICS

Normal Sacral Biomechanics

The sacrum is unique in the body in that it has three joints—the lumbosacral joint at L5–S1 and the two SI joints connecting with the innominates. Understanding and describing this three-joint arrangement and its complex biomechanics can be difficult. Although sacral motion between the ilia is limited to about 2 to 4 degrees, the composite function of the three independently moving joints allows for a wide variation in possible motions.[28–35] In this manner, the sacrum functions as the body's differential system in distributing forces to and from the spine and legs.[36,37] When describing any sacral motion, it is essential to specify which of these three joints is being discussed and to which joint component(s) the sacral motion is being compared.

L5–S1 (Lumbosacral) Flexion and Extension

Describing lumbosacral motion is complicated because, at times, it is appropriate to refer to the sacrum as part of the spine. At other times the sacrum is described independently of spinal motion in relation to the SI joint or ilia.[38] One must be careful to refer to the joint, not the involved structures. Reference should be made to the lumbosacral joint in flexion/extension, not the sacrum.[1] Doing so, changes from a global reference frame (lumbosacral joint) to a local reference frame (sacrum) and can confuse learners. For example, when the lumbosacral joint flexes, both L5 and S1 flex. Looking at each structure, however, L5 moves anteriorly relative to the sacrum, while S1 moves posteriorly relative to L5. Osteopathic

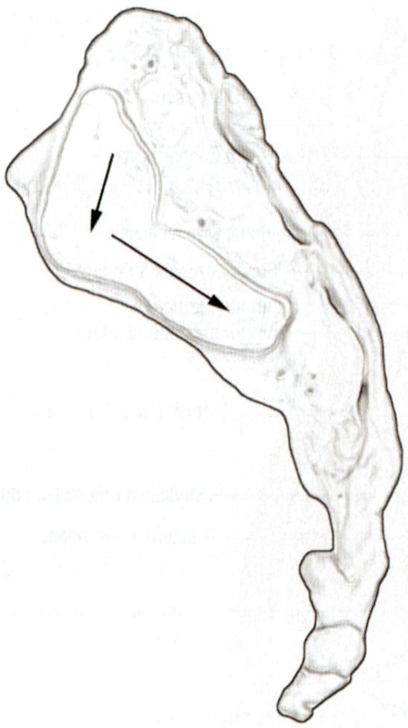

Figure 38.9. Sacral nutation.

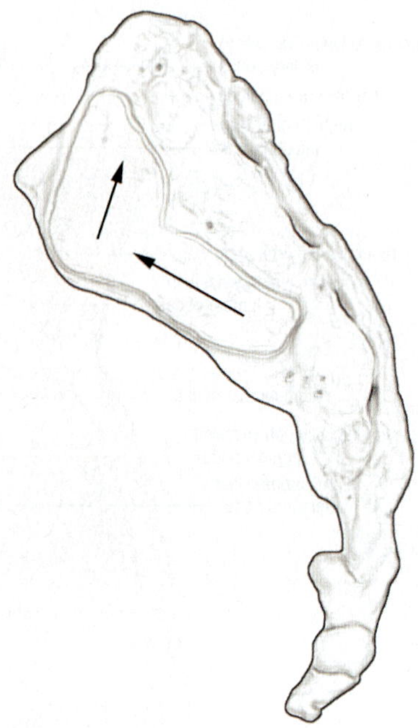

Figure 38.10. Sacral counternutation.

nomenclature describes a joint's motion by its superior component, and thus, this motion is called L–S flexion.

Sacral Motion About the Transverse Axes

Ample biomechanical and radiographic research has described sacral nutation (anterior nodding) and counternutation motions relative to the ilia.[39–42] Nutation describes the anterior movement of the sacral base around a transverse axis between the ilia. This motion of the sacrum occurs with extension of the lumbar spine and lumbosacral joint (Fig. 38.9). During nutation, the sacrum glides in a curving motion anteriorly along the short arm of its articulation and inferiorly along the long arm of its articulation.[43] Nutation allows for sacral stability, as it generates medial compression of the ilia onto the sacrum, wedging it between the ilia, known as form closure.[11,44]

Counternutation describes the posterior movement of the sacral base around a transverse axis between the ilia. Counternutation occurs with flexion of the lumbar spine and lumbosacral joint (Fig. 38.10). During counternutation, the sacrum glides superiorly along the long arm of its articulation and posteriorly along the short arm of its articulation.[43] Counternutation makes the sacrum vulnerable to shearing by "unlocking" it from its protective ilial compression or form closure.[11]

The sacrum acts like any other spinal segment in its motion around a transverse axis. The transverse axis around this anteroposterior nutation appears to be related to the junction of the upper and lower limbs of the SI joint around S2.[2,29,33,40,45–49] This axis is the middle transverse axis in Fred Mitchell Sr. DO's terminology.[37] It is important to remember that SI motion is more of an arc of motion along both arms of the joint and less of a wheel-like rotation around this axis.[40] Due to the L-shape of the SI articulation, nutation and counternutation include a component of inferior and superior translatory movement, respectively.

The osteopathic profession utilizes three *hypothetical* transverse axes of the sacrum as an educational construct to describe sacral motion patterns seen clinically. Research in sacral kinematics has shown that fixed axes for sacral motion do not occur and that variable instantaneous axes of motion can occur even in the same individual.[3] It is taught that each of the three transverse axes is engaged with various motions; with spinal motion, the sacrum moves about the middle transverse axis; with walking, the ilia move about the inferior transverse axis; and with osteopathic cranial manipulative medicine, the sacrum rotates about the superior transverse axis.[50–52] What occurs is most likely the previously described complex tilting, gliding, and shifting of the sacrum on instantaneous axes based on the form and force closure of the joint surfaces. While this is the educational construct used to describe sacral motions, no evidence currently exists for the coexistence of multiple simultaneous sacral axes[53] (Fig. 38.11).

When considering anatomic flexion or extension of the spine, the sacrum follows along, acting as the lower segment of the vertebral unit. Motion is described as occurring about the middle transverse axis (S2). The terms flexion and extension of the sacrum in relation to the relatively fixed ilium are generally used.[2,37]

When considering osteopathic cranial manipulative medicine, the superior transverse axis is described and taught due to the attachment point of the dura (S2). The cranial flexion phase provides a cephalad pull on the dura, causing the sacrum to rotate posteriorly in relation to the ilia. This movement is considered cranial flexion, although it can be confused with biomechanical extension, as the motions of the sacrum appear the same to the learner.[50,51]

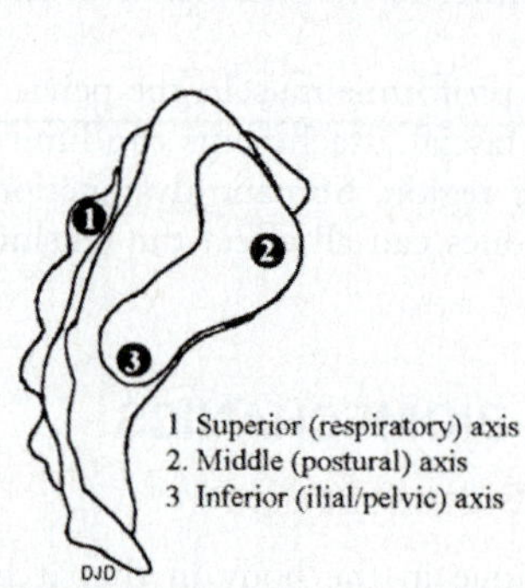

Figure 38.11. Sacral transverse axes—lateral view.

Sacral Motion about the Oblique Axes

In contrast to the relatively simple transverse axes, sacral motion during the gait cycle is a complex polyaxial motion termed axial rotation. In this model, the sacrum is viewed as the last five segments of the vertebral axis. The axial rotation of the sacrum is likely a derivative of the relative position of side bending and coupled rotation in the lumbar spine. This sacral motion has been described as "torsion" to describe the coupling of side bending and rotation to opposite sides.[1,37,43]

The reason for the coupled motion lies in the unusual structure of the SI joints. SI joints are flat, L-shaped synovial joints with irregular elevations and depressions. The apex of the L-shape points anteriorly with the upper, short-arm of the L-angled cephalad and posteriorly at approximately 45 degrees relative to the sacrum's longitudinal axis. The lower, long-arm of the L, is angled caudad and posteriorly at also approximately 45 degrees.[8]

Since the motion of the sacral base between the joint surfaces must track along this short arm, any anterior motion of the sacral base relative to the ilium (nutation) requires that the ipsilateral side of the sacrum glides inferiorly along its long arm. Conversely, any posterior motion of the sacral base relative to the ilium (counternutation) requires that the sacrum glides superiorly.[43] Thus, for left rotation of the sacrum in a neutral lumbosacral joint position, the right side of the sacrum glides anteriorly and, therefore, inferiorly (into nutation), and simultaneously the left side of the sacrum moves posteriorly and, therefore, superiorly (into counternutation), within a neutral range of motion. This motion causes the right-side bending coupling with the left rotation position of the sacrum. Keep in mind that this sacral side bending is not the same single-axis motion observed in the spine but a motion involving multiple axes and occurring functionally.

Described as "torsional," this polyaxially coupled, complex movement occurs around an "oblique axis," which by convention is named for its superior pole. The left oblique axis runs from the short upper arm of the left SI joint to the lower long arm of the right SI joint. The right oblique axis runs from the short upper arm of the right SI joint to the lower long arm of the left SI joint.[37] Although the biomechanics of the torsional movements of the sacrum are derived from a combination of lumbopelvic and SI motion and fascial tension, the hypothetical left and right oblique axes are useful for descriptive purposes. In other words, the sacral motion (including all the combined related motions) defines the axis, as it is hypothetical, not that the axis is an anatomical structure that allows the motion (Fig. 38.12).

STRUCTURAL EXAM

Assessment for somatic dysfunction of the sacrum includes standing and seated flexion tests, landmark assessment, backward bend (sphinx), and lumbosacral spring tests, among other assessments. Further details of this exam can be found in Chapter 30 Osteopathic Structural Examination and Chapter 31 Osteopathic Segmental Examination.

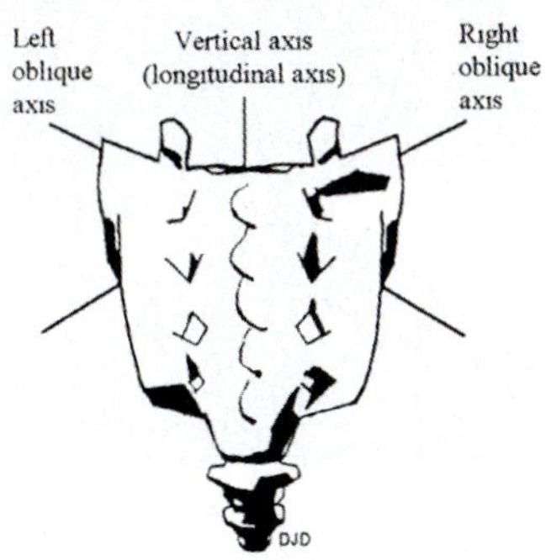

Figure 38.12. **Axes of sacral motion—posterior view.**

In addition, there are some key physical exam findings of gait and posture assessment that may indicate lumbosacral and/or SI somatic dysfunction and include the following:

- One foot turns outward or inward.
- One hip hikes superiorly.
- Weight is distributed unequally, causing the patient to lean to one side or limp.
- Positive standing or seated flexion test and/or positive pelvic side shift test.
- Unlevel iliac crests as well as greater trochanters.
  - An ipsilateral inferior greater trochanter, inferior iliac crest, and deep sacral sulcus, with a pelvic side shift away from this side, may be indicative of a leg length inequality.
- This situation will unlevel the sacral base and affect pelvic stability.
- A group curve in the thoracic or lumbar region. This finding generally correlates with sacral base unleveling and is commonly seen with forward sacral torsions.
- A reversal of the thoracic and lumbar A–P curves.
  - A flattened upper lumbar spine and an increased lumbar lordosis of the lower segments generally correlate with bilateral iliopsoas tension.
- If the entire lumbar spine is flattened, the sacral base may be held in extension (counternutation).
- An increase in the lumbar lordosis.
- This can be due to the sacrum being bilaterally flexed, almost parallel to the ground.
  - In this situation, L5 frequently is unstable and may develop disk protrusions or other pathologic changes.
- A positive Trendelenburg test indicates gluteus medius weakness in lumbosacral and sacroiliac joint (SIJ) somatic dysfunctions.

DIAGNOSIS OF SOMATIC DYSFUNCTION

Screening Component of Structural Exam: Flexion Tests

> Evidence of an SI somatic dysfunction may be found during the screening and regional components of the structural exam with a positive seated flexion test and oftentimes a positive standing flexion test. Based on Mitchell Jr.'s description, it has been classically taught that if there is greater excursion (superior and anterior movement of the PSIS) with the standing flexion test as compared to the seated flexion test, an iliosacral somatic dysfunction may be the predominant dysfunction. If the seated flexion test exhibits greater excursion, an SI dysfunction may be the predominant dysfunction. A positive flexion test necessitates an evaluation of iliosacral and SI landmarks to make a definitive diagnosis.[66] The side of the greatest excursion indicates the side of dysfunction. It is also possible to have a negative standing flexion test and positive seated flexion which may be more indicative of an SI dysfunction while a positive standing flexion test and negative seated flexion test are more indicative of an iliosacral dysfunction.

If the amount of unilateral excursion is the same for both the standing and seated flexion tests, this could represent a combination of iliosacral and SI dysfunction on the same side. Evaluation of all pelvic landmarks will resolve the question.

If both the standing and seated flexion tests are negative, this may indicate an absence of somatic dysfunction or a bilateral dysfunction.[66]

Palpation of Sacral Anatomical Landmarks and Performance of Confirmatory Tests for Sacroiliac Somatic Dysfunction

After screening with the flexion tests, a more focused exam of the lumbar and sacral regions is appropriate. Any lumbar rotation which is not compensating for the SI dysfunction should be corrected.[124] Normal lumbar compensation to SI dysfunction is in neutral, with side-bending and rotation in opposite directions, with the rotation in the direction of the deeper sacral sulcus.[124]

Lumbar spine quality of motion or passive motion testing for somatic dysfunction should be assessed. The presence of a positive seated flexion test or a history that suggests a possible bilateral sacral flexion or extension with an equivocal seated flexion test should elicit an assessment of asymmetry between the following anatomical landmarks and performance of the following tests:

1. Sacral sulcus depth/position of the sacral base
2. ILAs of the sacrum
3. Position of L5 relative to S1

Confirmatory tests include:

- The backward bending or Sphinx test: change in sacral sulcus depth or ILA levels with backward bending test of the lumbar spine (increased symmetry or asymmetry)
- Lumbosacral spring test or spring test: amount of stiffness palpable in the lumbosacral area during a lumbosacral spring test (increased stiffness is described as a positive test while decreased stiffness or compliance indicates a negative test)

Palpation of sacral sulcus (Fig. 38.13):

The sacral sulcus may be evaluated as follows (Fig. 38.14):

1. The patient lies prone on the examination table.
2. The physician stands at the side of the table with the dominant eye over the patient's midline.
3. The pads of the physician's thumbs are placed on the most posterior aspects of the PSISs. The thumbs are curled medially, approximately 30 degrees inferiorly, and then anteriorly until contact is made with the sacral base. The physician assesses the depth of each side of the sacral sulcus. The depth of a sulcus is considered to be the distance from the peak of a PSIS to the bottom of the patient's adjacent sulcus.[124]

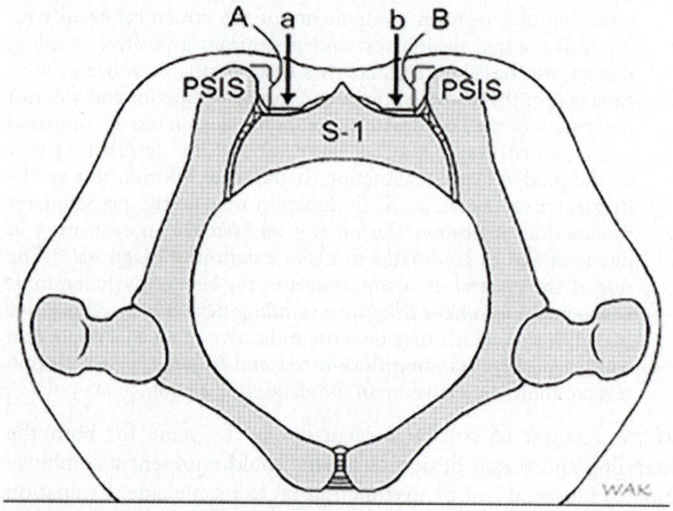

Figure 38.13. Cross-section of pelvis. Differential static landmarks for determining sacral sulcus depth (*A* and *B*) *versus sacral base anterior or posterior (a and b).* (Illustration courtesy of William A. Kuchera, DO, FAAO, with permission.)

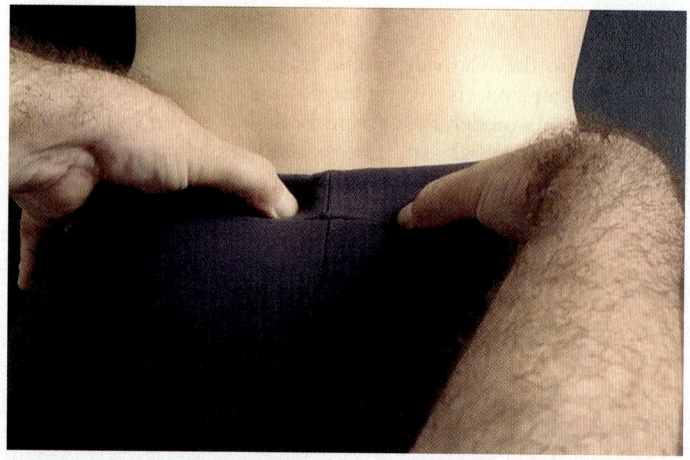

Figure 38.14. Hand placement for evaluation of sacral sulcus depth. (Photo courtesy of Western University of Health Sciences, Pomona, CA, with permission.)

Palpation of the ILAs of the sacrum (Fig. 38.15).

The ILAs may be evaluated by examining both the posterior and inferior aspects as follows:

1. The patient lies prone on the examination table.
2. The physician stands at the side of the table with the dominant eye over the patient's midline.
3. The physician palpates the sacral hiatus at the inferior end of the sacrum.
4. The pads of the physician's thumbs are placed in the midline at the sacral hiatus. The thumbs are moved laterally about ¾″ on each side at equal distances until the posterior aspects of the ILAs are contacted. Physician assesses the posterior ILAs for levelness relative to the coronal plane (anterior/posterior).
5. The physician's thumbs are then rolled onto the inferior aspects of the ILAs to determine if one is inferior compared to the other. The ILA is the most inferior aspect of the sacrum, where the bone tapers medially, and further inferior palpation will drop off the edge onto soft tissue laterally or coccyx in the midline.
6. Alternatively, the physician may place the heel of the hand closest to the patient on the sacral base and palpate inferiorly until a "drop off" is palpated. The "drop off" is generally at the level of the ILAs. The physician lifts the thenar eminence so that the

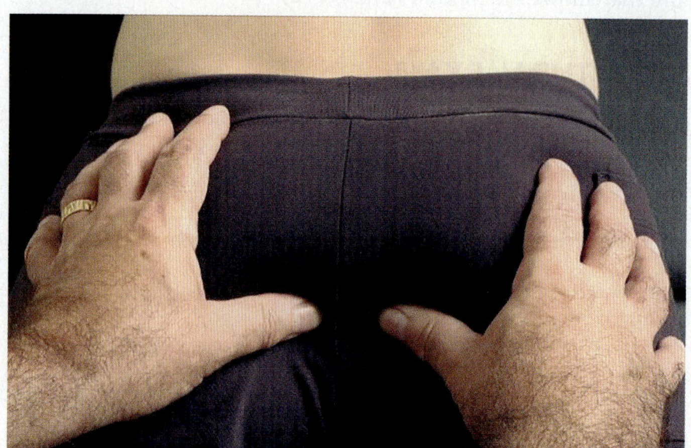

Figure 38.15. Hand placement for evaluation of inferior aspect of ILAs. (Photo courtesy of Western University of Health Sciences, Pomona, CA, with permission.)

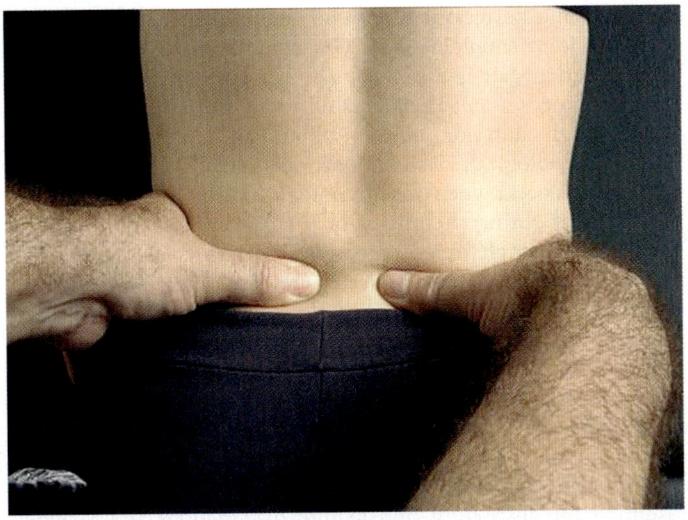

Figure 38.16. Evaluation of L5 position by assessing posterior rotation of the transverse process of L5. (Photo courtesy of Western University of Health Sciences, Pomona, CA, with permission.)

hypothenar eminence rests on the midline of the sacrum and palpates the posterior aspect of the ILA with the other hand. Then the physician uses the hand that was used to palpate for the "drop off" to contact the opposite posterior aspect of the ILAs.

7. The physician determines whether one ILA is more posterior and/or inferior than the other.

Position of L5:

The position of L5 may be evaluated as follows (Fig. 38.16):

1. The patient lies prone on the examination table.
2. The physician stands beside the table close to the patient and places the hands on the superior aspects of both iliac crests of the patient using this as a landmark to identify the spinous process of L4 with their thumbs, recognizing that the iliac crests are generally at the same level as the spinous process of L4.
3. Once the spinous process of L4 is located, the physician moves the thumbs inferiorly to one vertebra to the spinous process of L5 and then places thumbs over the lamina of L5 (as the transverse processes may be difficult to palpate)[125] to evaluate the position of the vertebra.
4. The physician assesses the rotational and side bending position of the L5.

Performance of confirmatory tests:

Backward bend/Sphinx test (Fig. 38.17)

The backward bending test is performed as follows:

1. The patient lies prone on the examination table.
2. The physician stands at the side of the table with the dominant eye over the patient's midline.
3. The pads of the physician's thumbs are placed in the sacral sulcus bilaterally.
4. The patient is asked to rise up on the elbows, thus assuming a position of trunk extension.
5. The physician assesses the depth of each side of the sacral sulcus in the coronal plane.
6. The physician compares the depth of each side of the sacral sulcus in this position with the depth noted with the patient in the prone neutral position.
7. This test may also be applied in a similar fashion to the ILAs. The physician's thumbs are placed on the inferior or posterior aspects of the ILAs. Physician notes any change in ILA position from the neutral prone position to the trunk extension position.

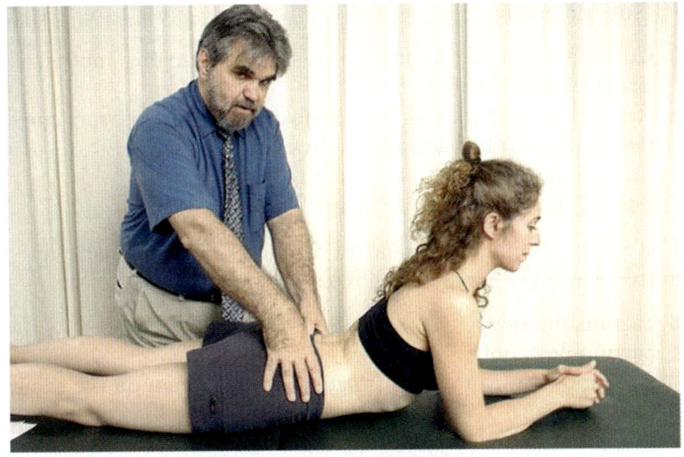

Figure 38.17. The backward bending test/Sphinx test. (Photo courtesy of Western University of Health Sciences, Pomona, CA, with permission.)

Interpretation: The physician is assessing for the landmarks to become more symmetrical, asymmetrical or there may be no change.

Lumbosacral spring or spring test (Fig. 38.18):

The lumbosacral spring test is performed as follows:

1. The patient lies prone on the examination table.
2. The physician stands at the side of the table, with the dominant eye over the patient's midline.
3. The physician places the palm of one hand over the midline of the lumbar region, with the thenar eminence of the hand over the lumbosacral junction (L5 and base of sacrum), and the fingers extending superiorly over the spinous processes and paravertebral tissues.
4. The physician provides a short quick push in an anterior direction with the heel of the hand causing lumbar extension and sacral nutation and evaluates for compliance ("springiness") or resistance of the lumbar spine.

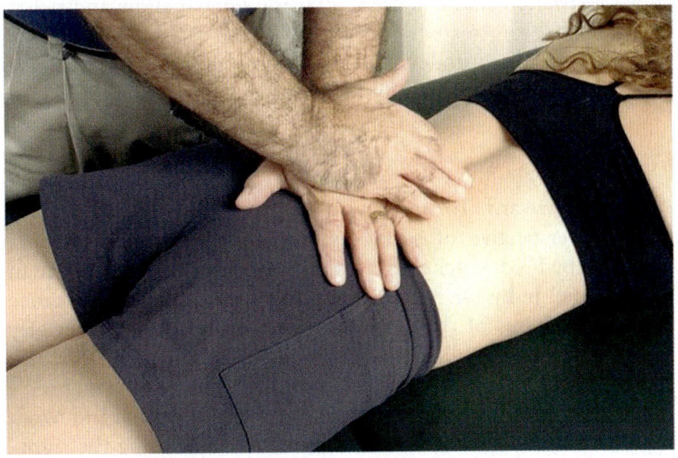

Figure 38.18. The lumbosacral spring test. (Photo courtesy of Western University of Health Sciences, Pomona, CA, with permission.)

Interpretation:

- Compliance of the lumbar spine to this springing motion is described as a negative test.
- Resistance (stiffness) of the lumbar spine to this springing motion is described as a positive test.

Types of Sacral Dysfunctions

The most common and standard diagnoses of SIJ somatic dysfunction include (but are not limited to) the following:

- Sacrum anterior[125]
- Sacrum posterior[125]
- Anterior/forward torsions (rotation of the sacrum on the same oblique axis):
  - □ Left rotation on a left oblique axis
  - □ Right rotation on a right oblique axis
- Posterior/backward torsions (rotation of the sacrum on the opposite oblique axis):
  - □ Right rotation on a left oblique axis
  - □ Left rotation on a right oblique axis
- Bilateral sacral flexion
- Bilateral sacral extension
- Unilateral sacral flexion (sacral shear)
- Unilateral sacral extension (sacral shear)

See this textbook's Glossary of Osteopathic Terminology for illustrations of these dysfunctions.

In the osteopathic profession, several models of SI dysfunction have been described. Three systems of nomenclature currently used to define sacropelvic mechanics are those described by

1. Mitchell (muscle energy)
2. Chicago Model (Strachan)
3. Van Buskirk (Still technique)

The Chicago model is described in Walton's text, *Osteopathic Diagnosis and Technique, Sacroiliac Diagnosis.*[125] Both the Chicago and Mitchell models describe similar events but from differing points of reference. Both systems are based on the physiologic motion of the sacrum, pelvis, and lumbar spine. However, the Chicago model does not describe or identify what the Mitchell system refers to as backward sacral torsions, just as the Mitchell system has no equivalent for Strachan posterior sacrum.

The Still (Van Buskirk) model looks at the sacrum in a unique way (Van Buskirk). It looks at sacral dysfunction as more of a myofascial restriction that is present after the lumbar spine and pelvis have already been treated. The student of the osteopathic medical profession needs to understand these three approaches to engage with SI and pelvic somatic dysfunctions.

Mitchell Model of Sacral Dysfunction

Anterior (Forward) Torsion Dysfunction

The perspective of sacral motion during the gait cycle as described by Fred Mitchell Sr., DO, is more highly referenced than Dr. Mitchell Jr. by Dr. Mitchell Sr. model, during both the stance and swing phases of the gait cycle, the sacrum rotates anteriorly around alternating oblique axes. When the left leg is in the stance phase, it induces a left-on-left torsional sacral movement.[36,57] Alternately, when the right leg is in the stance phase, it induces a right-on-right torsional sacral movement.[36,57–63] During the right-on-right torsional movement, the left sacral base nutates, moving anteriorly and inferiorly along the neutral plane of the L-shaped track of the SI joint; the right sacral base counternutates or moves superiorly and posteriorly along the neutral plane L-shaped track of the SI joint simultaneously. Understanding the normal sacral motion during gait is essential to fully appreciate the impact of sacral dysfunction on gait and stability.[64]

Although anterior motion about an alternating oblique axis is physiological, dysfunctions can occur. Most commonly, dysfunctions occur when one physiologic SI joint position becomes predominant during the phases of the gait cycle[62,65] (Fig. 38.19). A common example of a dysfunctional pattern would be when an individual has a leg length discrepancy and short leg/pelvic tilt syndrome. During the walking cycle, an individual with a short right leg will spend more time in the left stance phase and have more left-on-left SI predominance, according to the Mitchell Sr. gait cycle model.[66] This predominance of motion can become dysfunctional, as evidenced by limitations in the motion of the SI joint during motion testing and static landmark symmetry. The following description of anterior torsion sacral landmarks is described assuming the absence of non-neutral dysfunctions at L5, which can influence lumbosacral mechanics (Fig. 38.19).

There are two types of forward torsions:

1. Left rotation on a left oblique axis (left on left)
2. Right rotation about the right oblique axis (right on right)

Example of a left-on-left forward torsion due to a short right leg.

1. Patient standing:
   a. In the absence of intrinsic L5 dysfunction, L5 can compensate for the sacral asymmetry. The lumbar spine will appear to be rotated right and side-bent left in neutral mechanics. L5 may have intrinsic dysfunction (non-neutral mechanics) that makes it appear to be noncompensatory relative to the sacrum.
   b. The sacral base is rotated to the left.
   c. The iliac crest is lower on the right.
2. Patient seated:
   a. Right seated flexion test positive.
   b. The sacral base becomes asymmetric when the patient forward bends.
   c. L5 follows the sacrum to the left in forward bending.
3. Patient prone:
   a. Spring test negative.
   b. The lumbar spine is rotated to the right and side-bent left; neutral mechanics rotated opposite the sacral dysfunction. L5 follows the sacrum into symmetry in backward bending.
   c. The sacrum is rotated to the left at the base (deep right sacral sulcus), and the left ILA is posterior and inferior compared to the right (more posterior than inferior).
   d. Sacral landmarks become more symmetrical in the backward bending test/Sphinx test.

POSTERIOR (BACKWARD) TORSION DYSFUNCTION

Posterior (backward) torsional movement of the sacrum generally occurs when the lumbar spine is flexed and side bent or rotated to one side. This maneuver results in non-neutral behavior of the lumbar spine with side bending and rotation coupled to the same side. The sacrum between the ilia responds with a backward or posterior torsional movement opposite the side of lumbar rotation, which can occur around a right or left oblique axis.[61,65]

With the lumbar spine in flexion (non-neutral lumbar mechanics), the sacrum is positioned superiorly and posteriorly (counternutated) bilaterally as both sides track along the L-shaped SI joint. Introducing a left lumbar side-bending (coupled with left rotation) causes the sacrum to compensate by rotating to the right.[61,65]

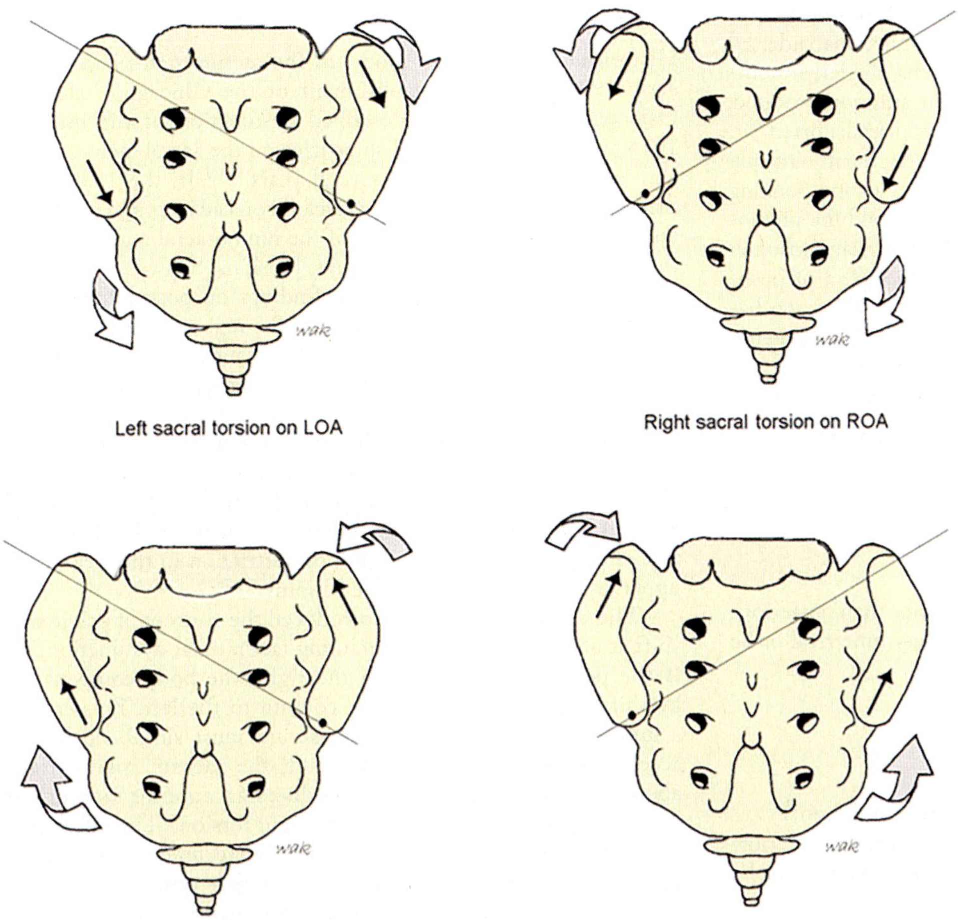

Left sacral torsion on LOA

Right sacral torsion on ROA

Right sacral torsion on LOA

Left sacral torsion on ROA

Figure 38.19. Lumbosacral torsion mechanics as described by Mitchell. Above two drawings are forward sacral torsions; below two are backward sacral torsions. Note that axes of motion are through the superior pole of the sacroiliac joint and inferior pole of the contralateral sacroiliac joint. LOA, left oblique axis; ROA, right oblique axis; L, lumbar; S, side bent; R, rotated; R, right; L, left. (Courtesy of William A. Kuchera, DO, FAAO, with permission.)

Because of the constraints placed upon both SI joints, the sacrum can only accomplish this if the right side counternutates more (glide superiorly and posteriorly along the L-shaped joint surface). The left side responds by limited nutation anteriorly and inferiorly along the L-shaped track. As the left sacral base moves anteriorly and inferiorly, the sacrum essentially side bends to the left and rotates to the right, producing a left oblique axis.[61,65] Counternutation of the right base, beyond its physiologic range of motion, can lock and cause a posterior sacral torsion. So, flexion, left-side bending, and left rotation of the lumbar spine take the sacrum into a posterior torsion to the right on a left oblique axis (right-on-left).[61,65]

In the posterior torsional movement, the anatomical constraints placed upon both SI joints commonly cause one side of the sacral base to accommodate more rotational torque and move beyond neutral into posterior nutation, thereby becoming dysfunctional.[18,61,65] These posterior torsional movements are considered hypomobile nonphysiologic SI mechanics as they are not part of the normal gait cycle. The following description of posterior torsion sacral landmarks is described assuming the absence of non-neutral dysfunctions at L5, which can influence lumbosacral mechanics.

There are two types of backward sacral torsions:

1. Right rotation on a left oblique axis (right on left)
2. Left rotation on a right oblique axis (left on right)

Example of a left-on-right backward torsion.

1. Patient standing:
   a. In the absence of intrinsic L5 dysfunction, L5 can compensate for the sacral asymmetry and will appear to be rotated right and side-bent left in neutral mechanics. L5 may have intrinsic dysfunction (non-neutral mechanics) that makes it appear to be noncompensatory relative to the sacrum.
   b. The sacral base is rotated to the left.
   c. The iliac crests are level.
2. Patient seated:
   a. The left seated flexion test is positive.
   b. The sacral base becomes symmetric when the patient forward bends.
   c. L5 follows the sacrum in forward bending.
3. Patient prone:
   a. The spring test positive.
   b. L5 is rotated to the right (non-neutral mechanics rotated opposite the sacral dysfunction) but then rotates to the left in backward bending as it follows the sacrum.
   c. The sacrum is rotated to the left at the base (deep right sacral sulcus) and the left ILA is posterior and inferior as compared to the right (more posterior than inferior).
   d. Backward bending test/Sphinx test becomes more asymmetrical.

UNILATERAL SACRAL DYSFUNCTION (SACRAL SHEAR)

A unilateral sacral dysfunction is a somatic dysfunction that results from a restriction within the upper and lower arm of the sacrum on one side relative to its respective ilium, leaving the other SI joint nondysfunctional. Diagnostic palpation of the sacrum reveals a deep sulcus on the same side of a posterior ILA. A deep sacral sulcus and posterior ILA on the right define a right unilateral sacral flexion or a left unilateral sacral extension. Seated flexion and/or spring tests are necessary to determine the dysfunctional side.[61,65] With either of the abovementioned dysfunctions, the left innominate appears posteriorly rotated and the right anteriorly rotated, and the shape and motion of the whole pelvis appear distorted.[61,65]

The SI joints have irregular and completely congruent joint surfaces; for every bump on the joints' surface, there is a corresponding hollow on the facing joint surface. Thus, carried beyond the physiologic range of motion, a bump on one side of the joint may encounter a bump on the facing side of the joint, having the effect of pushing the two bony surfaces apart and creating a joint locking mechanism.[13,18,65,67] This puts increased tension on the supporting ligaments.

The two types of unilateral sacral dysfunctions include:

- Unilateral sacral flexion–more common on the left
- Unilateral sacral extension–more common on the right

Left unilateral sacral flexion

- Positive left seated flexion test.
- The spring test is negative.
- The sacral sulcus deep on the left.
- The left ILA is posterior/inferior (more inferior than posterior).
- Backward bending/Sphinx test may remain asymmetrical or be unaffected.

Right unilateral extension

- Positive right seated flexion test
- The spring test is positive
- The sacral sulcus is deep on the left (shallow on the right)
- The left ILA is posterior/inferior (more inferior than posterior)
- Backward bending/Sphinx test may remain asymmetrical or be unaffected

Bilateral sacral nutation and counternutation dysfunctions

Both SI joints can move into nutation (flexion) or counternutation (extension) beyond the physiologic boundaries and become dysfunctional. Bilateral nutational dysfunctions are less likely to occur and are not commonly diagnosed because of this SI position's physiologic appearance. Bilateral counternutational dysfunctions of the sacrum must be considered as they cause considerable clinical instability of the pelvis.[61,65]

The mechanisms of these bilateral counternutation dysfunction vary and could include dorsal lithotomy birth mechanics and repetitive forward bending. Subjectively, the patient complains of low back pain that becomes worse when bending backward.

Bilateral sacral extension

- The seated flexion test is equivocal when bilateral and hard to rely on. Be suspicious when the PSIS elevates soon after the patient bends forward.
- The sacral sulcus is shallow bilaterally.
- There is a decreased lumbar curve.
- There is a positive lumbar spring test.

Sacrum resists posterior-to-anterior pressure at the base but yields to posterior-to-anterior pressure on the apex

Bilateral sacral flexion

- The seated flexion test is equivocal when bilateral and hard to rely on. Be suspicious when the PSIS elevates soon after the patient bends forward.
- The sacral sulcus is bilaterally deep.
- There is increased lumbar curve.
- There is a negative lumbar spring test.
- Sacrum resists posterior-to-anterior pressure at the apex but yields to posterior-to- anterior pressure on the base (Table 38.1).

Chicago Model of Sacral Dysfunctions

Historically, the Chicago model of the sacrum dates back to the early 1900s with the establishment of the Chicago College of Osteopathy. HH Fryette described dysfunction of the ilium in 1914 and continued to publish articles on the sacral–pelvic region and iliopsoas over the next several years.[68–70] In the 1930s, WF Strachan performed anatomical research on cadavers and published results regarding the mechanics of the lumbosacral region.[71] With the advancement of postural x-rays, Hoskins, Schwab, and Beilke (Chicago faculty) published their findings on postural factors in relationship to somatic dysfunction of the region.[72,73] The research by Strachan and publications by other Chicago faculty describe sacral dysfunction influenced by the lumbar spine and named in relation to the ilium.[71,74,75] From this initial research, x-ray studies, and clinical practice, the faculty of Chicago delineated two primary sacral dysfunctions, the anterior sacrum, and the posterior sacrum, defined by either the upper or lower arm of the L-shaped SI joint, respectively. Each dysfunction is identified by tissue texture changes, tenderness, and motion restriction in the area of the upper arm and lower arm of the SI joints.[71,76]

The Chicago Model also introduced the concept of pelvic side shift as an etiology and a maintaining factor of SI dysfunction.[77,78] If the pelvis is side shifted to the right, the body compensates by shifting the lumbar vertebral column to the left. This creates a lumbar curve convex left. The sacrum must side bend left to accommodate the curve. As a result, the sacrum rotates right about a right oblique axis; this produces an anterior sacrum left or a posterior sacrum right (right on right torsion). The differentiator is the side with the tissue texture change, tenderness, and the positive seated flexion test. Pelvic side shift is typically the result of long-restrictor muscle influence, dominantly from the psoas (left in this case) and or from postural imbalance due to a short leg (left in this case).[77,79]

Mitchell described sacral restrictions about an oblique axis as two-joint, two-arm composite asymmetries relative to L5. Interestingly, HH Fryette did describe compensation of an SI lesion (due to short leg syndrome) at L5 based upon an anatomic variation of the facets.[69] The Chicago model does not have an equivalent dysfunction to the backward torsion of the Mitchell model, and the Mitchell model does not explicitly describe a lower arm SI dysfunction. The Chicago model does recognize bilateral sacral flexion (nutation) and extension (counternutation) dysfunctions.[54]

The Chicago Model also recognizes sacral movement around an oblique axis as in an anterior/forward torsion. However, the description of the dysfunction relates to the ipsilateral ilium rather than its position relative to L5. The Chicago model only defines two SI dysfunctions occurring about a theoretical oblique axis. These dysfunctions are named in reference to the ipsilateral ilium, and the corresponding ilium is named opposite the sacrum (anterior sacrum = posterior ilium).

The specific dysfunction, diagnosed by tissue texture abnormality, tenderness, passive motion testing, and the seated flexion test, becomes the focus of treatment.[80,81] Treatment methodologies (direct action techniques) initially described by HH Fryette were expanded and published by Walton.[1,54,69,70] Many of these technique methods are still part of contemporary teachings.[80,81]

ANTERIOR SACRUM

An anterior sacrum is a positional term describing a somatic dysfunction in which the sacral base rotates forward, and side bends to the side opposite the rotation. An anterior sacrum (e.g., anterior sacrum left) has the following characteristics:

TABLE 38.1

Summary of the Examination Findings for Somatic Dysfunctions of the SIJ in the Mitchell and Chicago (Strachan) Models

Mitchell and Chicago Models: Sacral Diagnoses Summary

Test/Findings	Forward Sacral Torsions (L on L)	Backward Sacral Torsions (R on L)	Bilateral Sacral Flexion	Bilateral Sacral Extension	Unilateral Sacral Flexion (Right Shear)	Unilateral Sacral Extension (Right Shear)	Chicago Anterior Sacrum (Right)	Chicago Posterior Sacrum (Right)
(+) Seated flexion test	Right	Right	Neither (negative)	Neither (negative)	Right	Right	Right	Right (possibly left)
Sacral base (sacral sulcus)	Deep/anterior on right Shallow/posterior on left	Shallow/posterior on right Deep/anterior on left	Deep/anterior on both sides	Shallow/ posterior on both sides	Deep/anterior on right Shallow/posterior on left	Deep/anterior on left Shallow/posterior on right	Deep/anterior on right Shallow/posterior on left	Deep/anterior on left Shallow/posterior on right
Inferiro lateral angle (ILA) position	Posterior and inferior on left	Posterior and inferior on right	Posterior and inferior on both sides	Anterior and superior on both sides	Posterior and inferior on right	Anterior and superior on right	Posterior and inferior on left	Posterior and inferior on right
Tissue texture change	N/A	N/A	N/A	N/A	N/A	N/A	Right sulcus	Right lower pole of SI joint
Passive sacral motion testing	N/A	N/A	N/A	N/A	N/A	N/A	Freedom of left rotation about the left oblique axis	Freedom of right rotation about right oblique axis
Lumbar lateral curve	Convex right	Convex left	None	None	Convex right	Convex left	N/A	N/A
Lumbar lordosis (spring test)	Increased (negative spring test)	Reduced (positive spring test)	Increased or normal (negative spring test)	Reduced (positive spring test)	Increased or normal (negative spring test)	Reduced (positive spring test)	+/– Lumbar lateral curve, convex right	+/– Lumbar lateral curve, convex left
Supine medial malleolus (leg length)	Short left	Short right	Symmetrical	Symmetrical	Short left	Short right	N/A	N/A
L5	Neutral and rotated right	Flexed or extended and rotated left	Neutral, non-neutral, or normal	Neutral, non-neutral, or normal	Neutral and rotated right	Neutral and rotated left	N/A	N/A
Sphinx test	Negative (decreased asymmetry/ findings improved)	Positive (increased asymmetry/ findings worsen)	N/A	N/A	Negative (decreased asymmetry/ findings improved)	Positive (increased asymmetry/ findings worsen)	N/A	N/A
Innominate rotation	N/A	N/A	N/A	N/A	N/A	N/A	Right posterior ilium	Right anterior ilium
Muscle reactivity/ tension	N/A	N/A	N/A	N/A	N/A	N/A	Right gluteus medius	Right piriformis

SI, sacroiliac.

- Deep sulcus left (right ILA posterior)
- Tissue texture abnormality and tenderness in the deep sulcus
- Right rotated about a right oblique axis, left side bent
- Positive seated flexion test left
- When pressure is applied to the right ILA, the left sacral base will not move posteriorly (This passive motion test would involve the right oblique axis.)

Clinical pearls include the following:

- The upper limb of the SIJ has restricted motion, and the dysfunction is named for the side with the deep sacral sulcus and tissue texture change, as well as on which forward rotation occurs.
- The conceptual model is that an anterior sacrum is a dysfunction in the upper pole (upper part of the "L"-shaped articulation).
- Because the sacrum is side bent left, the left SI is the "compressed side." The left sacral base will be lower (inferior) in the standing position.
- Gluteus medius hypertonicity and tenderness are commonly found on the side of the anterior sacrum.
- An anterior sacrum is probably one type of Mitchell's forward torsion. For example:

  Anterior sacrum left describes a condition in which the sacrum is rotated right and side bent to the left, the directions of ease of motion (This could also be considered right rotation about a right oblique axis.).

  There is a restriction of left rotation and right side bending.

  The sacral sulcus is deep on the left, with tenderness and tissue texture abnormality in the left sulcus.

  When downward pressure is applied over the right ILA, attempting to rotate the sacrum about the right oblique axis, the left superior portion of the sacrum resists moving posteriorly toward the ilium.

- The anterior sacrum is an "oblique axis dysfunction." Therefore, it is one form of forward torsion with motion restriction, tissue texture abnormality, and tenderness associated with the deep sulcus side.

POSTERIOR SACRUM

A posterior sacrum (e.g., posterior sacrum right) has the following characteristics:

- Right ILA posterior (deep sulcus left)
- Tissue texture abnormality and tenderness at the right inferior pole (lowest part of the SI joint)
- Right rotated, left side bent
- Positive seated flexion test on the right (usually)

Clinical pearls include the following:

- The patient experiences discomfort at the inferior arm of the right SIJ and possibly sciatic pain.
- There is a pelvic side shift to the side of dysfunction, spinal asymmetry, and postural imbalance.
- The seated flexion test may be positive on either side of a posterior sacrum dysfunction.
- There is ipsilateral piriformis tension, and the ipsilateral ILA is posterior and inferior.
- There may be contralateral psoas tension, and there is generally a contralateral short leg.
- As in the example above:
  - □ A posterior sacrum right has rotated right about the right oblique axis, and side bent left. Rotation left, and side bending right are restricted.
  - □ A posterior sacrum involves the restriction of motion at the lower limb of the SI articulation.
  - □ Tissue texture abnormality and tenderness are located over the inferior portion of the dysfunctional SIJ; in this example, the tenderness is on the right.
- A posterior sacrum is probably a form of forward torsion in which the major joint motion restriction is on the side opposite the deep sulcus. A confirmatory passive motion test for lower pole (lower limb of the L) restriction (e.g., posterior sacrum right) is to contact the inferior borders of the sacrum with both thumbs and apply a cephalad/anterior force, attempting to glide the sacrum in the direction of the lower limb of the joint. Restriction is felt on the posterior sacral side.
- Although there are similarities between the posterior sacrum and the forward torsion, there is no true Mitchell equivalent to Chicago posterior sacrum. A posterior sacrum should not be confused with a backward torsion, a posterior or counternutation of the sacral base, or a unilateral extension of the sacrum.
- A confirmatory motion test for lower pole (lower limb of the L) restriction (e.g., posterior sacrum right) is to contact the inferior borders of the sacrum with both thumbs and apply a cephalad/anterior force.

PATIENT LYING PRONE

Physician applies pressure on the inferior surface of the sacrum in a superior and anterior direction, trying to glide the sacrum superiorly along the lower limb of the "C"-shaped articulation. It is met with resistance.

The ILA is inferior and resists moving superiorly.

- The conceptual model is that of a lower pole SI restriction.
- From a side-bending perspective, the posterior sacrum is on the "stretch side" of the SI problem.
- The piriformis muscle may become tender and hypertonic on the side of a posterior sacrum dysfunction. It may also become tight or irritable on the side of the pelvic side shift. This is due to the origin and insertion being separated. Manipulative treatment of the posterior sacrum dysfunction will often improve the tension of the piriformis muscle, improving hip internal rotation.

The Still Model of Sacral Dysfunction

Another essential concept is the emergence of SI disturbances that remain after treatment of the lumbar spine and pelvis somatic dysfunctions, which may be due to ligamentous and fascial tissues in contrast to a bony positional change of the sacrum and the ilium. The Still model demonstrates that after treatment of lumbar and innominate somatic dysfunctions, only two types of sacral dysfunctions seem to remain; a "diagonal" dysfunction or a "unilateral" dysfunction.

Both of these sacral dysfunctions behave as if the sacrum was fixated at two of four restriction points, one superior and one inferior on each side[55]:

- The two superior restrictive axis points are on the sacral base just medial to the PSISs of the ilia and inferior to L5.
- The two inferior restrictive axis points are in the area of the origins of the sacrotuberous ligaments on the ILAs of the sacrum.

Dr. Richard Van Buskirk proposes a clinically useful model for diagnosing sacral dysfunction in "The Still Technique Manual."[55] Based on active patient movement, it is simple and quick. The patient evaluation includes performing two seated flexion tests. The first is a modified seated flexion test with the physician's thumbs over the sacral sulcus instead of the PSIS. The second is the same assessment but performed with the physician's thumbs over the ILAs of the sacrum. The pattern of movement of the physician's thumbs determines the diagnosis.

Test 1: Monitoring sacral sulcus:

A restriction in one of the two superior axis points is identified during a seated flexion test in which the sensing fingers are firmly placed on the sacral sulcus.

- If there is a restriction, the sacral sulcus will move superiorly during the patient's flexion at the waist. *Note:* The seated flexion test, as done by Van Buskirk, differs from the Mitchell model seated flexion test.
- The tips of the sensing fingers are placed over the SI joint just medial to the PSIS at the sacral base or sulcus level.
- A positive test is indicated when the patient bends forward, and the sensing finger travels superior in relation to the other side.

TEST 2: MONITORING ILAS

The second test is the position of the ILA, with the patient seated.

- A restriction in one of the inferior axis points can be identified by the tightness of the tissues to any form of direct motion testing, tightness of the sacrotuberous ligament, and the inferior and/or posterior position of one of the ILAs in relation to the other.
- It is considered positive if one ILA is posterior and does not move anteriorly, if the sacrotuberous ligament is tight on that side, or if the ILA is more inferior.
- The positive side is that of restriction.

Diagonal sacrum (Still technique model):

A positive seated flexion test on one side and a positive ILA test on the other are diagnostic of a *diagonal sacrum.*

- Van Buskirk describes that there will be a corresponding single-segment lumbar neutral dysfunction whenever a diagonal SI dysfunction is found.
- This neutral lumbar dysfunction commonly will be found at L5.

Unilateral sacrum (Still technique model):

If the positive seated flexion test and the positive lateral angle test (ILA) are on the same side, the diagnosis is a *unilateral sacrum.*

Dr. Van Buskirk also describes a supine technique for each dysfunction in his manual.[55]

To review sacral diagnoses using the Still model, refer to Table 38.2.

The sacral diagnosis will be named for the pattern of free axis points (i.e., whether they are diagonal to each other or on the same side) and the free direction of rotation of the sacral base. These dysfunctions are effectively treated with a Still technique (see Chapter 56 for further information).

Innominate function and dysfunction involve shifts in iliosacral motion among the three described axes. Van Buskirk finds that most of the motion is across the superior and inferior axes, with little or no motion in the middle axis.[55] The Still model uses the following five tests to evaluate the ilia:

1. PSIS position
2. ASIS position
3. Pelvic translation or ASIS compression test
4. ASIS tender point
5. Standing flexion test

No single test or even pair of tests predicts the nature of the iliosacral somatic dysfunction. Van Buskirk finds that innominate somatic dysfunctions act as if the normal axis of motion at the middle pole of the SIJ has been transferred to the other axes.

- The anterior innominate dysfunction, characterized by PSIS superior and ASIS inferior on the affected side, acts as if there were a restriction at the inferior pole of the SIJ. Attempts to move the innominates seem to isolate the inferior SI pole rather than the normal middle pole.
- The posterior innominate dysfunction, characterized by PSIS inferior and ASIS superior on the affected side, acts as if there were a restriction at the superior pole of the SIJ.

The Still model also recognizes up-slipped and down-slipped innominates. Down-slipped innominates are rare in clinical practice and are usually created by a traumatic pull to the leg. However, VanBuskirk proposes that that the "upslipped" or superior sheared innominate is not sheared at the SI joint as described. Rather the innominate is sidebent with the iliac crest closer to the midline. Similarly, a "downslipped" or inferiorly sheared innominate is sidebent with the iliac crest tilted away from the midline. The physical findings will be the same as in the originally described upslipped and downslipped models. Likewise, both of these dysfunctions occur far more commonly than would be expected if the problem was traumatic vertical shearing.

Listed below, Van Buskirk relates how up-slipped or superior innominates can occur:

- Asymmetrical weight bearing on one leg for a prolonged time
- Upward or superior shear on the side of the shoe lift
- The longer leg may develop an upward pelvic shear
- Trendelenburg gait (hip drop during the swing phase from a weak contralateral gluteus medius muscle) can cause an up-slipped innominate on the side of the weak muscle

No single treatment using the Still technique has been found that resolves the up-slipped or superior innominate completely. According to Van Buskirk, complete success only requires treating the two commonly restricted poles (superior and inferior) and the middle pole. When treatments focused on each of the three poles are performed during the same session, the dysfunction seems fully released and does not reoccur as readily. A newer Still Technique treatment simply uses the supine leg beginning in an abducted position (thereby replicating and relaxing a superior sidebent or "upslipped" innominate) and then carrying the leg across the midline with an appropriately vectored force. The superior sidebent innominate is most restricted at the S1 site in the SI joint. The inferior sidebent innominate (downslipped) is just the opposite and has its restriction at S3.[56]

TABLE 38.2

Sacral Diagnoses Using the Still Model

Diagnosis	Characteristics
Diagonal right	Positive right seated flexion test Positive left ILA test
Diagonal left	Positive left seated flexion test Positive right ILA test
Unilateral right	Positive right seated flexion test Positive right ILA test
Unilateral left	Positive left seated flexion test Positive left ILA test

PUBIC BONES

Regarding the pubic bones, Van Buskirk states that pubic ramus evaluation is a poor test for iliosacral dysfunction. Per Van Buskirk, treating the innominate dysfunction with the Still technique model often reduces pubic ramus dysfunctions which is why he evaluates and treats the innominate dysfunctions first. Clinically, Van Buskirk will evaluate and treat the external abdominal oblique and the ilioinguinal ligament when there is a pubic dysfunction. When diagnosing these muscles and the pubic bones, evaluation includes palpating for tender points on the ASIS and lateral pubic bones.

- The dysfunction will involve the external abdominal oblique if a tender point is present at both sites.
- If the tender point includes only the insertion on the lateral pubic bones, the ilioinguinal ligament is involved.
- The pubic dysfunction is treated before the external abdominal oblique and/or the ilioinguinal ligament.

PSOAS

With psoas dysfunction, leg extension will be markedly restricted, and the foot will tend to be everted. The leg extension is evaluated with the ilium stabilized. Another finding related to psoas dysfunction is a referred tender point found on the anterolateral aspect of the thigh, just inferior and about 1 cm medial to the inferior ASIS.[55] Van Buskirk finds this tender point routinely when there is a psoas restriction.

ANTERIORLY OR POSTERIORLY TRANSLATED SACRUM (STILL TECHNIQUE MODEL)

These are rare and are difficult to diagnose as there is no asymmetry between bilateral sacral sulcus depths or seated flexion test results. Passive motion tests discern freer motion in the direction of the dysfunction. For example, passive anterior translatory motion is easier in an anteriorly translated sacrum.

Table 38.3 summarizes commonly used osteopathic structural examination tests to differentiate the above SI diagnoses.

TABLE 38.3

Commonly Used Osteopathic SI Tests

Osteopathic SI Tests	Characteristics
Standing flexion test	PSIS moves superiorly indicates SIJ dysfunction
Seated flexion test	PSIS moves superiorly indicates SIJ dysfunction
Pelvic side shift	Pelvis shifts off to one side indicates contralateral psoas, lumbar, sacral, pelvis, or short leg somatic dysfunction
Hip drop	Hip drop (patient flexes one knee while standing) fails to produce lumbar spine convexity on ipsilateral side of the inferior innominate indicates lumbar dysfunction
Backward bending test	Prone, prop up alters sulcus depth Asymmetry of sulcus depth increases
Spring test	Prone, anterior springing of L5 Poor spring = positive test
Iliac compression test	Supine, posterior/lateral compression Poor motion = positive test
Posterior sacrum confirmatory test	Prone, superior glide of sacral lower pole Restricted superior glide = positive test
Kappler seated translation test	Seated, palpate sacral sulcus for motion as the lumbar spine is translated toward the sulcus. Restricted motion = positive test

Clinical Implications of Sacral Dysfunctions

SI dysfunction is described in this chapter using the most consistent criteria of all three of the above systems. No matter which model is used, to integrate the following information into the clinical arena, the physician must consider three questions:

1. Is the sacrum restricted or demonstrating dysfunction?
2. Why is the sacrum restricted?
3. What needs to be done to correct the dysfunction for the patient?

Recurring episodes of low back pain can be extremely frustrating to the patient and the clinician. When faced with this situation, it is critical to document the dysfunctional pattern(s) of the thoracolumbar, lumbosacral, and pelvis and establish an appropriate home exercise program.[82] Regarding the pelvis, one of the goals of appropriate osteopathic treatment is to restore the motion of the sacrum during the gait cycle, which includes restoration of anterior motion around oscillating oblique axes.

The literature is consistent in determining that SI joint dysfunctions can cause back pain.[61,64,83,84] However, the exact mechanism or cause is often unknown.[85,86] The etiology of the pain is reportedly due to loss of form and force closure of the sacrum and alterations in the kinematic chain leading to cumulative microtrauma.[57,87–91]

However, in attempts to diagnose SI joint dysfunction, interrater reliability among all clinicians in the sacrum position relative to ilia has been poor,[86,92–94] and clear evidence of functional improvement with manipulation to the SI joints is limited.[95–98] Therefore, anatomical and functional information is used to educate osteopathic students to address somatic dysfunction of the pelvis.

POSTERIOR SACRAL TORSIONS

Loss of nutation of the sacrum is the primary cause of pain and dysfunction for two reasons: loss of form and loss of force closure. According to Vleeming, "Form closure refers to a stable situation with closely fitting joint surfaces, in which no extra forces are necessary to maintain the state of the system."[14] Force closure refers to compression generated by muscles and ligaments that accommodate the specific pelvic loading situation.[14]

As discussed above, the sacrum is wider superiorly than it is inferiorly and broader anteriorly than posteriorly. This "keystone-shape" configuration is necessary for the sacrum to wedge anteriorly between the ilia.[99] The SI joints are relatively flat, and like most flat articular surfaces, they cannot resist shear forces.[12] Given the location of the sacrum, the lack of resistance to shear forces can be problematic. The shape of the sacrum and its ability to anteriorly nutate between the ilia seems to protect it from shear. However, the sacrum requires sophisticated continuous muscular and ligamentous tensile forces to protect it from vulnerability and allow optimal function.[11,16,57,100]

Force closure of the sacrum begins in the lower extremity just after heel strike, with the force-couple of the peroneus longus and biceps femoris into the sacrotuberous ligament and across the ipsilateral SI joint. During the single support phase, the biceps femoris' downward pull is replaced by the myofascial force-couple between the gluteus maximus ipsilaterally and the latissimus dorsi contralaterally through the thoracolumbar fascia.[11,88,100,101] This stabilizing force closure of the sacrum is a longitudinal muscle-tendon–fascial sling, in which the timing of the muscle firing is critical. Delay in firing any of the synergistic muscles results in altered motor strategies, dysfunctional load transfer through the pelvis, and decreased force closure.[101–107] The exact mechanism responsible for the delay in muscle firing is unknown. However, pain, joint position, or dysfunction may play a role.[104,105,108–110]

Studies in the knee show that specific muscle responses during joint movement are reflexive and originate from proprioceptors in the corresponding capsule of the joint.[108,111] Termed arthrokinetic reflex, its responses are sensitive to position and movement and are part of the same reflex, which employs reciprocal innervation and function to coordinate the movement of the joint.[112,113]

When considering sacral stability, the relationship between joint mechanics and related muscle activity is essential. If the joint is dysfunctional and does not move freely, the lack of motion is reflected as a signal loss. It causes a delay in coordinated muscle contraction, termed arthrogenic inhibition. This inhibition primarily affects the joint stabilizer muscles, which for the sacrum, would include the gluteal muscle group. Poorly timed reflexive contraction of the gluteals subsequently diminishes the force closure capacity of the SI joint.[101,114,115]

The most common inciting posture for posterior torsion is bending forward at the waist while twisting. When bending forward and to the right, the lumbar spine is forward bent, right rotated, and right side bent. Concurrently, the sacrum moves into left rotation around a right oblique axis. Because of the destabilizing nature of this counternutated position,[19] the sacrum can remain locked in this position.[61,65] If the fifth lumbar remains in a dysfunctional flexed side bent and rotated right position (consistent with the bending and twisting posture), with the sacrum preferring left rotation along the right axis, it exposes the L5–S1 intervertebral disk to a great deal of torque.[65,116] The lumbar spine is thus at risk for annular tears of the intervertebral disk and joint dysfunction of the zygapophyseal joints.[61,65,117] If, in this case, the patient has pre-existing non-neutral dysfunctions at thoracolumbar segments consistent with psoas innervation, they may also be at risk for acute iliopsoas muscle facilitation or spasms.[65]

ANTERIOR SACRAL TORSIONS

While anterior torsions in and of themselves do not seem to cause failed back syndrome, the short leg/pelvic tilt syndrome has been clinically observed to be a component.[118] It would be prudent to correct the leg length discrepancy if suspected based on anatomical landmark levels and combined with a recurrent anterior innominate on and lumbar convexity toward the side of the short lower extremity.[119]

A unilateral chronically tight piriformis is not unusual in runners or those who speed walk for exercise.[65] The syndrome is typically due to the need of the piriformis muscle to decelerate the ipsilateral hip during overpronation or uncontrolled pronation.[65] The piriformis attaches proximally onto the anterior surface of the sacrum and functions as a hip external rotator and abductor. When facilitated, it pulls the ipsilateral sacral base forward and can contribute to recurrent anterior sacral torsions.[120] In addition to treating the sacral dysfunction and stretching the hip external rotators, treatment consists of limiting the overpronation or uncontrolled pronation.[65]

UNILATERAL SACRAL DYSFUNCTIONS

Patients with recurrent unilateral sacral dysfunctions present with chronic, disabling back pain with minimal radiation to the lower extremity below the buttocks. They find it difficult to stand for any period because the back pain progressively increases while standing without being mobile; hence the term "cocktail party syndrome."[61,65] It is significant in patients who must stand for long periods. The pain is lessened by walking activities or by sitting. People who suffer from this problem are frequently one-legged standers who do not bear weight symmetrically on their lower extremities resulting in chronic postural imbalance.[65]

Clinically, unilateral flexed (nutated) is far more common on the left than right.[118] Patients presenting out of the pattern, that is, a right sacral flexion (nutation) or left sacral extension (counternutation), are more likely present in patients following pelvic fractures or major pelvic trauma. In the "cocktail party syndrome," the structural diagnostic findings usually consist of the problem on the left side with the left pubis superior, a left unilateral flexion, left innominate posterior, and an ERS left type-II lumbar somatic dysfunction at L5.[61] They frequently present with tight erector spinae muscles, weak pelvic stabilizers, and weak abdominals from a muscle imbalance perspective.[65]

Treatment of these patients is challenging and frustrating because recurrent exacerbations are frequent. Self-treatment is necessary for this population and should begin with de-rotating the innominate and self-mobilizing the sacrum. They may require appropriate OMT for the dysfunctions described and a lifelong exercise program to maintain pelvic, trunk, and abdominal muscle control. The patient must maintain a balanced standing posture and refrain from a one-legged stance or sitting with one foot under the pelvis.[65]

THE CHICAGO MODEL ANTERIOR OR POSTERIOR SACRUM DYSFUNCTIONS

The Chicago Model anterior sacrum and posterior sacrum clinical implications are similar to the anterior torsions. Somatic dysfunction of L5 may or may not be involved in either dysfunction; however, pelvic side shift usually plays a role. Pelvic side shift moves more freely away from the anterior sacrum side and the short leg or hypertonic psoas. Pelvic side shift may be a factor in maintaining the anterior sacrum and corresponding ipsilateral gluteus muscle dysfunction.[69,78,79] It is common to have a "chronic" anterior sacrum on the side of an anatomic short leg, as this corresponds to the low ipsilateral sacral base. Depending on the compensatory factors and duration, the anterior sacrum can occur on the other side.[77–79] The characteristic findings accompanying an anterior sacrum are a flexed Type II dysfunction in the upper lumbar spine, an ipsilateral tight iliopsoas, L5 extended, and an anterior sacrum dysfunction.[77,80,81] Many times, the ipsilateral gluteus muscle is tender and weak. Patients usually present with mechanical lower back pain but may also have many different presentations. These are generally amenable to OMT and respond well to restoration of the core abdominal musculature and correction of postural imbalance.

The seated flexion test may be positive on either side in a posterior sacrum, so its use is not as reliable in this dysfunction. Tenderness and tissue texture changes are located over the lower pole of the dysfunctional SI joint. In addition, many times, palpating the piriformis muscle on the dysfunctional side reveals tenderness and muscle tension.[54,76,80,81] The ipsilateral PSIS may be superior, and the ipsilateral ASIS is usually inferior to the other side. Somatic dysfunction of L5 may or may not be involved in the posterior sacrum dysfunction. However, pelvic side shift usually plays a role. The pelvic side shift moves more freely toward the posterior sacrum side and away from the short leg or hypertonic psoas.[77,78] Pelvic side shift may be a factor in maintaining the posterior sacrum and corresponding ipsilateral piriformis muscle dysfunction. Many times, the ipsilateral piriformis muscle is tender and tight. In this situation, there is a separation between the origin and insertion of the piriformis, which may cause muscle irritability and resultant sciatica.[77,121] Patients usually present with mechanical lower back pain and ipsilateral sciatica that does not go below the knee (piriformis syndrome). Treatment of postural imbalances, core strengthening, and pelvic side shift elimination are vital components for long-term patient improvement.[77,78]

GLOBAL STATEMENT ON TREATMENT

Treating the lumbosacral region is crucial in improving the patient's gait and mobility, posture, spinal stabilization, and visceral function. Frequent reevaluation throughout the treatment process guides the clinician. Many clinicians begin their treatment in the pelvis to obtain a stable and level base of support that functions smoothly during gait. Another common approach is improving non-neutral segmental dysfunctions in the lumbar spine, iliopsoas tension, innominate/pubic position, and motion before diagnosing sacral dysfunction. Somatic dysfunction in the lumbopelvic region comprises articular, myofascial, reflex, and dural components. Therefore, multiple osteopathic diagnostic and treatment models are equally efficacious in improving the function of this region.

FINAL THOUGHTS

The Sacrum and the Walking Cycle

In the normal walking cycle, each side of the sacral base moves anteriorly in an oscillating fashion around alternating oblique axes. In other words, nutation on one side, return to neutral, then nutation on the opposite side, and then a return to neutral. How the axis is formed and when during the gait cycle it occurs was first described to the osteopathic community by Fred Mitchell Sr. in 1948 and again in 1958.[29,37] His son, Fred Mitchell Jr., DO, has disputed his father's premise[46,66]; therefore, this chapter describes both versions. Both models assume symmetric leg lengths and normal, nondysfunctional mechanics.

FRED MITCHELL SR., DO

The stability of the trunk and pelvis is critical for walking, which begins when the heel contacts the ground to prepare for toe-off and stability during a single-leg stance. The ground exerts the ground reaction force on the body in contact with it.

Right heel strike engages the tibialis anterior and peroneus longus muscles, which attach to the fibular head. Shortly after heel strike, these myofascial forces are continuous along the biceps femoris to the ischial tuberosity. From there, the fascia continues superiorly, stabilizing the right sacroiliac joint, and allowing the left sacral base to move forward with the advancing left leg. During bipedal support, before lifting the left leg, the pelvis is rotated to the left. The left innominate is rotated anteriorly, and the right innominate posteriorly. The trunk is rotated to the right. In this stance, there is a high torsional load at the thoracolumbar junction. The lumbar spine is neutral, rotated left, and side bent right (convex left) as left toe-off begins (left swing phase and right stance phase), the ground reaction force, superincumbent weight, and adaptive response from the lumbar spine brace the right upper pole of the sacrum. This fascial stability allows the lumbar spine to unload and move the lumbar convexity from left to right as the left leg is carried forward. The fascial bracing of the right SI joint also produces a right oblique axis. The sacrum is then carried forward with the advancing left leg into right rotation upon this right oblique axis. So, from left toe-off through right stance phase gait, the sacrum moves into right rotation about a right oblique axis (right-on-right). Relative to the sacrum, the lumbar spine simultaneously rotates to the left, and the side bends to the right.[43,123]

After left heel strike, as left stance phase gait begins, the sacral base on the right begins to move anteriorly as it is carried forward by the advancing right ilia. As the sacrum begins to rotate to the left, its coupled motion is side bending to the right. The oblique sacral axis, generated from this polyaxial movement, is left. So, during the left stance phase, the sacrum moves into left rotation about a left oblique axis (left-on-left). Relative to the sacrum, the lumbar spine concurrently rotates to the right, and side bends to the left.[37,66]

FRED MITCHELL JR., DO

There are considerable differences between the descriptions of sacral motion during gait between father and son. Fred Mitchell Jr. agrees that right heel strike allows ground reaction fascial support from the foot to the pelvis. The divergence in opinion is the effect of the fascial support on the sacrum's axis of motion. Dr. Mitchell Sr. states that right heel strike engages fascial support to stabilize the right upper pole of the sacrum, creating a right oblique axis.[37] Dr. Mitchell Jr. believes the fascial support from the lower extremity results in fascial tension following the piriformis path, thus stabilizing the inferior pole of the right SI joint, creating a left oblique axis.[66]

Fred Mitchell Jr. contends that the sacrum faces forward during bipedal support before left toe-off.[122] The left innominate is anteriorly rotated, and the right innominate is posteriorly rotated. He then states that at initial left leg swing phase, the left anterior innominate rotation facilitates left quadratus lumborum contraction, first concentrically and then eccentrically, causing left side bending of the lumbar spine, which concurrently pushes the sacrum into left rotation around a left oblique axis. To simplify, Dr. Mitchell Jr. describes that during the initial left leg swing phase, the fascial and muscular pull from the lumbar spine carries the sacrum into left rotation around a left oblique axis. So, from left toe-off through right midstance, the right sacrum is carried forward with the stance leg into left rotation about a left oblique axis (left-on-left).

Despite differences in opinions, both Drs. Mitchell agree that the sacrum is carried forward around an alternating oblique axis during the gait cycle. Because the nutational component of this normal walking movement is anterior in direction, left torsion on the left oblique axis (left-on-left) and right torsion on the right oblique axis (right-on-right) describe anterior torsional movements. The nutational movement in normal walking is anterior on one side, returns to neutral, anterior to the opposite side, and returns to neutral. The counternutational movement does not appear past neutral in the normal walking cycle because of the sacroiliac joint motion.

Although described decades ago, current literature searches contain no published studies demonstrating proof of either Mitchell model. Detection and analysis of sacral motion during gait are challenging to study, partially due to the density of tissue lying between the sacrum and the skin placement of motion detection sensors.

Since much of the musculoskeletal system activity involves the walking cycle, maintenance of normal left-on-left and right-on-right sacral movements is an important therapeutic objective. Since walking occurs with the vertebral column in an erect, neutral (neither flexed nor extended) position, the anterior torsional sacral movements are called neutral mechanics. During walking, the thoracolumbar spine side bends left and rotates right, and then side bends right and rotates left with each step. This neutral movement of the vertebral column requires normal segmental mobility.[123]

As the sacrum side bends right and rotates left, L5 side bends left and rotates right, reflecting inversions of the same lumbosacral joint movement. Each vertebra above L5 should appropriately respond as part of the adaptive neutral curve. A vertebra with a non-neutral dysfunction, particularly in the lower lumbar spine, results in a "nonadaptive" vertebral response to the sacrum.

The difference in opinion in describing sacral motion is difficult to rectify. Studies on the influence of fascial tension on sacral motion are nonexistent, and studying sacral mechanics is very technically complex. The reviewed literature was limited to English-only publications, and the small number of pertinent texts is a testament to the relative lack of scientific data underlying our understanding of sacral mechanics. As such, we are left with the option of basing our teaching and clinical practice on anatomical principles, as AT Still did.

ACKNOWLEDGMENTS

The authors and editors of this chapter would like to acknowledge the scholarly contributions of the ECOP Sacral White Paper Subcommittee 2016 to 2019: Walter C. Ehrenfeuchter, DO; Heather Ferrill DO, MEdL; Stacey Pierce-Talsma, DO, MS; and members of ECOP 2020 to 2022.

REFERENCES

1. Fryette HH. *Principles of Osteopathic Technic.* Academy of Applied Osteopathy; 1954:246.
2. Vleeming A, Schuenke MD, Masi AT, Carreiro JE, Danneels L, Willard FH. The sacroiliac joint: an overview of its anatomy, function and potential clinical implications. *J Anat.* 2012;221(6):537–567.
3. Beal MC. The sacroiliac problem: review of anatomy, mechanics, and diagnosis. *J Am Osteopath Assoc.* 1982;81(10):667–679.
4. Brooke R. The sacro-iliac joint. *J Anat.* 1924;58(Pt 4):299–305.
5. Poilliot AJ, Zwirner J, Doyle T, Hammer N. A systematic review of the normal sacroiliac joint anatomy and adjacent tissues for pain physicians. *Pain Physician.* 2019;22(4):E247–E274.
6. Fortin JD, Kissling RO, O'Connor BL, Vilensky JA. Sacroiliac joint innervation and pain. *Am J Orthop (Belle Mead NJ).* 1999;28(12):687–690.
7. Indahl A, Holm S. Chapter 7: the sacroiliac joint: sensory-motor control and pain. In: Vleeming A, Mooney V, Stoeckart R. *Movement, Stability and Lumbopelvic Pain: Integration of Research and Therapy.* 2nd ed. Churchill Livingstone; 2007:103–111.
8. Kapandji IA. *The Physiology of the Joints: The trunk and the vertebral column.* 2nd ed. Vol. 3. Churchill Livingstone; 1974.
9. Vleeming A, Stoeckart R, Volkers AC, Snijders CJ. Relation between form and function in the sacroiliac joint. Part I: clinical anatomical aspects. *Spine (Phila Pa 1976).* 1990;15(2):130–132.
10. Wilder DG, Pope MH, Frymoyer JW. The functional topography of the sacroiliac joint. *Spine (Phila Pa 1976).* 1980;5(6):575–579.
11. Vleeming A, Stoeckart R. Chapter 8: the role of the pelvic girdle in coupling the spine and the legs: a clinical–anatomical perspective on pelvic stability. In: Vleeming A, Mooney V, Stoeckart R, eds. *Movement, Stability and Lumbopelvic Pain: Integration of Research and Therapy.* 2nd ed. Churchill Livingstone; 2007:113–137.
12. Snijders CJ, Vleeming A, Stoeckart R. Transfer of lumbosacral load to iliac bones and legs Part 1: biomechanics of self-bracing of the sacroiliac joints and its significance for treatment and exercise. *Clin Biomech (Bristol, Avon).* 1993;8(6):285–294.
13. Harrison DE, Harrison DD, Troyanovich SJ. The sacroiliac joint: a review of anatomy and biomechanics with clinical implications. *J Manipulative Physiol Ther.* 1997;20(9):607–617.
14. Vleeming A, Schuenke M. Form and force closure of the sacroiliac joints. *PM R.* 2019;11(Suppl 1):S24–S31.
15. Vleeming A, Van Wingerden JP, Dijkstra PF, Stoeckart R, Snijders CJ, Stijnen T. Mobility in the sacroiliac joints in the elderly: a kinematic and radiological study. *Clin Biomech (Bristol, Avon).* 1992;7(3):170–176.
16. Pardehshenas H, Maroufi N, Sanjari MA, Parnianpour M, Levin SM. Lumbopelvic muscle activation patterns in three stances under graded loading conditions: proposing a tensegrity model for load transfer through the sacroiliac joints. *J Bodyw Mov Ther.* 2014;18(4):633–642.
17. Walker JM. The sacroiliac joint: a critical review. *Phys Ther.* 1992; 72(12):903–916.
18. Grieve EF. Mechanical dysfunction of the sacro-iliac joint. *Int Rehabil Med.* 1983;5(1):46–52.
19. Snijders CJ, Vleeming A, Stoeckart R. Transfer of lumbosacral load to iliac bones and legs Part 2: loading of the sacroiliac joints when lifting in a stooped posture. *Clin Biomech (Bristol, Avon).* 1993;8(6):295–301.
20. Carro LP, Hernando MF, Cerezal L, Navarro IS, Fernandez AA, Castillo AO. Deep gluteal space problems: piriformis syndrome, ischiofemoral impingement and sciatic nerve release. *Muscles Ligaments Tendons J.* 2016;6(3):384–396.
21. Burdett PH. *Piriformis Syndrome, MRI Web Clinic.* Radsource LLC; 2010.
22. Delp SL, Hess WE, Hungerford DS, Jones LC. Variation of rotation moment arms with hip flexion. *J Biomech.* 1999;32(5):493–501.
23. Kendall FP, McCreary EK, Provance PG. In: Piriformis muscle and its relationship to Sciatic Pain. *Muscle Testing and Function.* 4th ed. 1993; Lippincott, Williams and Wilkins. p. 365.
24. Heinking K. Chapter 28f. Pelvis. In: Seffinger M. (2018). *Foundations of Osteopathic Medicine* (4th ed.). Lippincott Williams and Wilkins.
25. Walton W. *Textbook of Osteopathic Diagnosis and Technique Procedures.* 2nd ed. Published by the author; 1972.
26. Glenesk NL, Lopez PP. *StatPearls [Internet].* StatPearls Publishing; 2022. Anatomy, Bony Pelvis and Lower Limb: Thigh Nerves.
27. Spence KT, Forro SD. Anatomy, bony pelvis and lower limb: nerves. [Updated 2022 Jul 25]. In: *StatPearls [Internet].* StatPearls Publishing; 2023. https://www.ncbi.nlm.nih.gov/books/NBK532304/
28. Bogduk N. The anatomical basis for spinal pain syndromes. *J Manipulative Physiol Ther.* 1995;18(9):603–605.
29. Sturesson B, Selvik G, Uden A. Movements of the sacroiliac joints. A roentgen stereophotogrammetric analysis. *Spine (Phila Pa 1976).* 1989; 14(2):162–165.
30. Joukar A, Kiapour A, Elgafy H, Erbulut DU, Agarwal AK, Goel VK. Biomechanics of the sacroiliac joint: surgical treatments. *Int J Spine Surg.* 2020;14(3):355–367.
31. Hammer N, Scholze M, Kibsgard T, et al. Physiological in vitro sacroiliac joint motion: a study on three-dimensional posterior pelvic ring kinematics. *J Anat.* 2019;234(3):346–358.
32. Kissling RO, Jacob HA. The mobility of the sacroiliac joint in healthy subjects. *Bull Hosp Jt Dis.* 1996;54(3):158–164.
33. Jacob HA, Kissling RO. The mobility of the sacroiliac joints in healthy volunteers between 20 and 50 years of age. *Clin Biomech (Bristol, Avon).* 1995;10(7):352–361.
34. Zheng N, Watson LG, Yong-Hing K. Biomechanical modelling of the human sacroiliac joint. *Med Biol Eng Comput.* 1997;35(2):77–82.
35. Rebello da Veiga T, Custodio da Silva A, Gomes da Silva RT, Carvalho SL, Orsini M, Silva JG. Intra-observer reliability in three-dimensional kinematic analysis of sacroiliac joint mobility. *J Phys Ther Sci.* 2015; 27(4):1001–1004.
36. Alderink GJ. The sacroiliac joint: review of anatomy, mechanics, and function. *J Orthop Sports Phys Ther.* 1991;13(2):71–84.
37. Mitchell FL. Structural pelvic function. *The AAO J.* 2012;22(1):63–84.
38. Strachan WF, Beckwith CG, Larson NJ, Grant JH. A study of the mechanics of the sacroiliac joint. *J Am Osteopath Assoc.* 1938;37:576–578.
39. Giusti R, ed. *Glossary of Osteopathic Terminology.* 3rd ed. American Association of Colleges of Osteopathic Medicine; 2017.
40. Weisl H. The movements of the sacroiliac joint. *Acta Anat (Basel).* 1955; 23(1):80–91.

41. Frigerio NA, Stowe RR, Howe JW. Movement of the sacroiliac joint. *Clin Orthop Relat Res.* 1974;(100):370–377.
42. Grieve E. Lumbo-pelvic rhythm and mechanical dysfunction of the sacroiliac joint. *Physiotherapy.* 1981;67(6):171–173.
43. DeStefano LA. *Greenman's Principles of Manual Medicine.* 5th ed. Lippincott Williams and Wilkins; 2016:522.
44. Barker PJ, Hapuarachchi KS, Ross JA, Sambaiew E, Ranger TA, Briggs CA. Anatomy and biomechanics of gluteus maximus and the thoracolumbar fascia at the sacroiliac joint. *Clin Anat.* 2014;27(2):234–240.
45. Goldthwait JE. Osgood RB. A consideration of the pelvic articulations from an anatomical, pathological and clinical standpoint. *Boston Med Surg J.* 1905;152(21):593–601.
46. Pitkin H, Pheasant AB. Sacrathrogenetic telalgia: II. A study of sacral mobility. *J Bone Joint Surg.* 1936;18(2):365–374.
47. Colachis SC Jr., Worden RE, Bechtol CO, Strohm BR. Movement of the sacroiliac joint in the adult male: a preliminary report. *Arch Phys Med Rehabil.* 1963;44:490–498.
48. Egund N, Olsson TH, Schmid H, Selvik G. Movements in the sacroiliac joints demonstrated with roentgen stereophotogrammetry. *Acta Radiol Diagn (Stockh).* 1978;19(5):833–846.
49. Brunner C, Kissling R, Jacob HA. The effects of morphology and histopathologic findings on the mobility of the sacroiliac joint. *Spine (Phila Pa 1976).* 1991;16(9):1111–1117.
50. Sutherland WG. *Contributions of Thought: The Collected Writings of William Garner Sutherland, DO.* 2nd ed. Rudra Press; 1998:364.
51. Magoun HI. *Osteopathy in the Cranial Field.* 3rd ed. The Journal Printing Company; 1976:367.
52. Mitchell FL, Jr., Pruzzo NA. Investigation of voluntary and primary respiratory mechanisms. *J Am Osteopath Assoc.* 1971;70(10):1109–1113.
53. Nelson KE. The Sacrum; a bone of contention. *AAOJ.* 1997;(Winter 1997):17–24.
54. Walton WW. *Osteopathic Diagnosis and Technique.* Chicago College of Osteopathic Medicine; 1966.
55. VanBuskirk RL. *The Still Technique Manual.* American Academy of Osteopathy; 2000:87.
56. Goldman SI, Van Buskirk RL. Rethinking superior and inferior sacroiliac shear: a new approach to diagnosis and treatment. *AAOJ.* 2018;28(1): 21–28.
57. Greenman P. Clinical aspects of sacroiliac function in walking. In: Paterson JK BL, ed. *Back Pain.* SpringerLink; 1990.
58. Kuchera DF, Kuchera WA, Kuchera ML. *Osteopathic Principles in Practice.* Greyden Press; 1994.
59. Richard R. *Osteopathic Lesions of the Sacrum: Physio-pathology and Correction Techniques.* Thorsons; 1986.
60. DiGiovanna EL, Schiowitz S, Dowling DJ. *An Osteopathic Approach to Diagnosis and Treatment.* Lippincott Williams & Wilkins; 2005.
61. Isaacs ER, Bookhout MR, Bourdillon JF. *Bourdillon's Spinal Manipulation.* Butterworth-Heinemann; 2002.
62. Chila AG, Association AO. *Foundations of Osteopathic Medicine.* Wolters Kluwer Health/Lippincott Williams & Wilkins; 2010.
63. Brolinson PG, Kozar AJ, Cibor G. Sacroiliac joint dysfunction in athletes. *Curr Sports Med Rep.* 2003;2(1):47–56.
64. DonTigny RL. Anterior dysfunction of the sacroiliac joint as a major factor in the etiology of idiopathic low back pain syndrome. *Phys Ther.* 1990;70(4):250–265; discussion 262–265.
65. DeStefano L. *Greenman's Principles of Manual Medicine.* 5th ed. Wolters Kluwer; 2017.
66. Mitchell FL MP. *The Muscle Energy Manual: Evaluation and Treatment of the Pelvis and Sacrum.* Vol 3. MET Press; 1999:89.
67. Dreyfuss P, Dryer S, Griffin J, Hoffman J, Walsh N. Positive sacroiliac screening tests in asymptomatic adults. *Spine.* 1994;19(10):1138–1143.
68. Fryette HH. Four innominate lesions, their cause, diagnosis and treatment. *J Am Osteopath Assoc.* 1914;105–111.
69. Fryette HH. Some reasons why sacroiliac lesions recur. *J Am Osteopath Assoc.* 1936;36(3):119–121.
70. Fryette HH. The psoas muscle. *J Am Osteopath Assoc.* 1937;36(10): 441–444.
71. Strachan WF. Applied anatomy of the pelvis and perineum. *J Am Osteopath Assoc.* 1939;38(8):57–58.
72. Hoskins ER. The development of posture and its importance: No3. Short leg. *J Am Osteopath Assoc.* 1934;34(September):125–126.
73. Beilke MC. Roentgenological spinal analysis and the technic for taking standing x-ray plates. *J Am Osteopath Assoc.* 1936;35(May):414–418.
74. Beckwith CG. Pelvic mechanics. *J Am Osteopath Assoc.* 1944;43(12): 102–105.
75. Strachan WF, Beckwith CG, Larson NJ, Grant JH. A study of the mechanics of the sacroiliac joint. *J Am Osteopath Assoc.* 1938;37(12):576–578.
76. Walton WJ. Palpatory diagnosis of the osteopathic lesion. *J Am Osteopath Assoc.* 1971;70(August):1295–1309.
77. Kappler RE. Role of psoas mechanism in low-back complaints. *J Am Osteopath Assoc.* 1973;72(8):794–801.
78. Kappler RE. Postural balance and motion patterns. *J Am Osteopath Assoc.* 1982;81(9):598–606.
79. Beilke MC. Simple mechanics of the sacrolumbar group. *J Am Osteopath Assoc.* 1939;39(3):165–167.
80. Heinking KP, Kappler RE. Pelvis and sacrum. In: Chila AG, ed. *Foundations of Osteopathic Medicine.* 3rd ed. Lippincott Williams & Wilkins; 2011:575–601.
81. Seffinger M. *Foundations of Osteopathic Medicine: Philosophy, Science, Clinical Applications, and Research.* Wolters Kluwer; 2018.
82. Prather H, Bonnette M, Hunt D. Nonoperative treatment options for patients with sacroiliac joint pain. *Int J Spine Surg.* 2020;14(Suppl 1):35–40.
83. Booth J, Morris S. The sacroiliac joint–victim or culprit. *Best Pract Res Clin Rheumatol.* 2019;33(1):88–101.
84. Cusi MF. Paradigm for assessment and treatment of SIJ mechanical dysfunction. *J Bodyw Mov Ther.* 2010;14(2):152–61.
85. Cohen SP, Chen Y, Neufeld NJ. Sacroiliac joint pain: a comprehensive review of epidemiology, diagnosis and treatment. *Expert Rev Neurother.* 2013;13(1):99–116.
86. Palsson TS, Gibson W, Darlow B, et al. Changing the narrative in diagnosis and management of pain in the sacroiliac joint area. *Phys Ther.* 2019;99(11):1511–1519.
87. Voorn R. Case report: can sacroiliac joint dysfunction cause chronic Achilles tendinitis? *J Orthop Sports Phys Ther.* 1998;27(6):436–443.
88. van Wingerden JP, Vleeming A, Snijders CJ, Stoeckart R. A functional-anatomical approach to the spine-pelvis mechanism: interaction between the biceps femoris muscle and the sacrotuberous ligament. *Eur Spine J.* 1993;2(3):140–144.
89. Feeney DF, Capobianco RA, Montgomery JR, Morreale J, Grabowski AM, Enoka RM. Individuals with sacroiliac joint dysfunction display asymmetrical gait and a depressed synergy between muscles providing sacroiliac joint force closure when walking. *J Electromyogr Kinesiol.* 2018;43:95–103.
90. Hodges PW, Cholewicki J, Popovich JM Jr, et al. Building a collaborative model of sacroiliac joint dysfunction and pelvic girdle pain to understand the diverse perspectives of experts. *PM R.* 2019;11(Suppl 1):S11–S23.
91. Capobianco RA, Feeney DF, Jeffers JR, et al. Patients with sacroiliac joint dysfunction exhibit altered movement strategies when performing a sit-to-stand task. *Spine J.* 2018;18(8):1434–1440.
92. Nejati P, Sartaj E, Imani F, Moeineddin R, Nejati L, Safavi M. Accuracy of the diagnostic tests of sacroiliac joint dysfunction. *J Chiropr Med.* 2020;19(1):28–37.
93. Consorti G, Basile F, Pugliese L, Petracca M. Interrater reliability of osteopathic sacral palpatory diagnostic tests among osteopathy students. *J Am Osteopath Assoc.* 2018;118(10):637–644.
94. Kmita A, Lucas NP. Reliability of physical examination to assess asymmetry of anatomical landmarks indicative of pelvic somatic dysfunction in subjects with and without low back pain. *Int J Osteopath Med.* 2008;11(1):16–25.
95. Kamali F, Zamanlou M, Ghanbari A, Alipour A, Bervis S. Comparison of manipulation and stabilization exercises in patients with sacroiliac joint dysfunction patients: a randomized clinical trial. *J Bodyw Mov Ther.* 2019;23(1):177–182.
96. Nejati P, Safarcherati A, Karimi F. Effectiveness of exercise therapy and manipulation on sacroiliac joint dysfunction: a randomized controlled trial. *Pain Physician.* 2019;22(1):53–61.
97. Wojtowicz S, Sajko I, Hadamus A, Mosiolek A, Bialoszewski D. Effect of sacroiliac joint manipulation on selected gait parameters in healthy subjects. *Ortop Traumatol Rehabil.* 2017;19(4):323–331.

98. Cattley P, Winyard J, Trevaskis J, Eaton S. Validity and reliability of clinical tests for the sacroiliac joint. A review of literature. *Australas Chiropr Osteopathy*. 2002;10(2):73–80.
99. Zlomislic V, Garfin SR. Anatomy and biomechanics of the sacroiliac joint. *Techniques in Orthopaedics*. 2019;34(2):70–75.
100. van Wingerden JP, Vleeming A, Buyruk HM, Raissadat K. Stabilization of the sacroiliac joint in vivo: verification of muscular contribution to force closure of the pelvis. *Eur Spine J*. 2004;13(3):199–205.
101. Lee D. Instability of the sacroiliac joint and the consequences to gait. *J Man Manip Ther*. 2013:4(1):22–29.
102. Cibulka MT, Rose SJ, Delitto A, Sinacore DR. Hamstring muscle strain treated by mobilizing the sacroiliac joint. *Phys Ther*. 1986;66(8):1220–1223.
103. Cibulka MT. Sacroiliac joint dysfunction as a reason for the development of acetabular retroversion: a new theory. *Phyiother Theory Pract*. 2014;30(4):249–253.
104. Cibulka MT, Morr B, Wedel J, et al. Changes in pelvic tilt during three different reciprocal stance positions in patients with sacroiliac joint regional pain. *Int J Sports Phys Ther*. 2019;14(6):967–977.
105. Hungerford B, Gilleard W, Hodges P. Evidence of altered lumbopelvic muscle recruitment in the presence of sacroiliac joint pain. *Spine*. 2003;28(14):1593–1600.
106. Kato K, Otoshi K-I, Tominaga R, et al. The prevalence and clinical characteristics of sacroiliac joint dysfunction in adolescent baseball players. *J Orthop Sci*. 2022;27(2):335–341.
107. Bashir MS, Noor R, Hadian MR, Olyaei G. Pattern of changes in latissimus dorsi, gluteus maximus, internal oblique and transverse abdominus muscle thickness among individuals with sacroiliac joint dysfunction. *Pak J Med Sci*. 2019;35(3):818–823.
108. Indahl A, Kaigle A, Reikeras O, Holm S. Sacroiliac joint involvement in activation of the porcine spinal and gluteal musculature. *J Spinal Disord*. 1999;12(4):325–330.
109. Holm S, Indahl A, Solomonow M. Sensorimotor control of the spine. *J Electromyogr Kinesiol*. 2002;12(3):219–234.
110. Arab AM, Nourbakhsh MR, Mohammadifar A. The relationship between hamstring length and gluteal muscle strength in individuals with sacroiliac joint dysfunction. *J Man Manip Ther*. 2011;19(1):5–10.
111. Cohen LA, Cohen ML. Arthrokinetic reflex of the knee. *Am J Physiol*. 1956;184(2):433–437.
112. Panayi S. The need for lumbar-pelvic assessment in the resolution of chronic hamstring strain. *J Bodyw Mov Ther*. 2010;14(3):294–298.
113. Bullock-Saxton JE, Janda V, Bullock MI. Reflex activation of gluteal muscles in walking. An approach to restoration of muscle function for patients with low-back pain. *Spine*. 1993;18(6):704–708.
114. Hossain M, Nokes LDM. A model of dynamic sacro-iliac joint instability from malrecruitment of gluteus maximus and biceps femoris muscles resulting in low back pain. *Med Hypotheses*. 2005;65(2):278–281.
115. Added MAN, de Freitas DG, Kasawara KT, Martin RL, Fukuda TY. Strengthening the gluteus maximus in subjects with sacroiliac dysfunction. *Int J Sports Phys Ther*. 2018;13(1):114–120.
116. Keklicek H, Demirel A, Kirdi E, Yalcin A, Ulger O. P 139 – Investigating the effects of sacroiliac joint dysfunction on gait in individuals with lumbar herniation nucleus pulposus. *Gait Posture*. 2018;65(Suppl 1): 467–467.
117. Madani SP, Dadian M, Firouznia K, Alalawi S. Sacroiliac joint dysfunction in patients with herniated lumbar disc: a cross-sectional study. *J Back Musculoskelet Rehabil*. 2013;26(3):273–278.
118. Greenman P. Sacroiliac dysfunction in the failed low back pain syndrome. In: Vleeming A, Mooney V, Snijders C, Dorman T, eds. *Proceedings from the First Interdisciplinary World Congress on Low Back Pain and Its Relation to the Sacroiliac Joint*. San Diego, California; 1992:329–352.
119. Ayanniyi O, Raji FS, Adegoke BOA. Prevalence of asymptomatic sacroiliac joint dysfunction and its association with leg length discrepancies in male students in selected junior secondary schools in Ibadan. *Afr J Med Med Sci*. 2008;37(1):37–42.
120. Boyajian-O'Neill LA, McClain RL, Coleman MK, Thomas PP. Diagnosis and management of piriformis syndrome: an osteopathic approach. *J Am Osteopath Assoc*. 2008;108(11):657–664.
121. TePoorten BA. The piriformis muscle. *J Am Osteopath Assoc*. 1969;69(2): 150–160.
122. Mitchell FL, Jr. Evaluation and treatment of the pelvis and sacrum. *The Muscle Energy Manual*. Vol 3. MET Press; 1999:175.
123. Greenman PE. Chapter 19: Clinical aspects of the sacroiliac joint in walking. In: Vleeming A, ed. *Movement, Stability and Low Back Pain: The Essential Role of the Pelvis*. Churchill Livingstone; 1997:235–242.
124. Institute for Continuing Education in Osteopathic Principles, Moran PS, Pruzzo NA, Mitchell FL. *An Evaluation & Treatment Manual of Osteopathic Manipulative Procedure*. The Institute for Continuing Education in Osteopathic Principles; 1973.
125. Bourdillon JF. *Spinal Manipulation*. 2nd ed. Heinemann Medical Books Ltd.; Appleton-Century-Crofts; 1973.

39 Upper Extremity

KRISTA LUND ▪ KURT P. HEINKING ▪ SHELDON C. YAO ▪ MICHAEL L. KUCHERA

KEY CONCEPTS

- Familiarity with functional anatomy of the upper extremities is required for its accurate assessment and manipulative treatment procedures.
- Knowledge of muscle anatomy, actions, and innervations is necessary for addressing extremity complaints.
- Sympathetic stimulation from thoracic dysfunction can cause symptoms in the upper extremities.
- Peripheral nerves of the upper extremity can become entrapped by muscular, fascial, or ligamentous tension.
- Fascial restrictions can impede venous and lymphatic drainage of the upper extremities.

INTRODUCTION

The upper extremities are vital to performing the activities of daily living (ADLs). Coordination and mobility of the upper extremity joints is paramount for precise and fluid movement. Even minor injuries may produce disabilities that significantly affect overall function. Effective diagnosis and treatment necessitate a thorough understanding of the structure and function within this region.

DEFINITION

The upper extremity can be divided into four major segments[1]:

- Shoulder
- Arm
- Forearm
- Hand

The upper extremity is also referred to as the upper limb.[1]

DESCRIPTIVE AND FUNCTIONAL ANATOMY

Skeletal, Arthrodial, and Ligamentous Structures

The aspects of the upper limb skeletal structures are depicted in Figure 39.1. Notice the palpable bony structures, which are important landmarks for the osteopathic screening and segmental examination.

Functionally the upper extremity can be divided based on mobility of the joints:

- Shoulder
  - ☐ Acromioclavicular joint (ACJ)
  - ☐ Sternoclavicular joint (SCJ)
  - ☐ Glenohumeral joint (GHJ)
  - ☐ Scapulothoracic joint
- Elbow
  - ☐ Ulnohumeral joint
  - ☐ Radiohumeral joint
  - ☐ Radioulnar joint
- Forearm
  - ☐ Radioulnar interosseous membrane
- Wrist
  - ☐ Radiocarpal joint
  - ☐ Distal radioulnar joint
  - ☐ Ulnocarpal joint
- Hand
  - ☐ Intercarpal joints
  - ☐ Carpometacarpal joints
  - ☐ Metacarpal phalangeal joints
  - ☐ Interphalangeal joints

THE SHOULDER

The shoulder (or pectoral girdle) consists of three bones, the clavicle, scapula, and humerus. These bones articulate at the glenohumeral (GH or shoulder joint), sternoclavicular (SC), and acromioclavicular (AC) joints. The clavicle forms a strut that holds the scapula and GHJ away from the thorax, so it can move freely.[1]

The Acromioclavicular Joint (ACJ)

The ACJ is formed by the articulation of the lateral end of the clavicle with the acromion process of the scapula. The joint is a planar synovial joint, with a crescent-shaped rudimentary incomplete meniscus.[2] The acromion has a variable shape and slope that forms the roof of the coracoacromial arch.[3] The coracoacromial ligament attaches from the outer portion of the coracoid process to the undersurface of the acromion and makes up the anterior portion of the coracoacromial arch.[1,3] Under the coracoacromial arch are the subacromial bursa and rotator cuff tendons. Extrinsic or outlet impingement of the rotator cuff occurs in this region. The ACJ depends on its ligamentous attachments for stability: the acromioclavicular and coracoclavicular ligaments. The strongest ligament between the clavicle and scapula is the coracoclavicular ligament. It has two portions:

- The conoid portion that prevents anterior rotation of the distal clavicle.
- The trapezoid portion that resists posterior rotation of the distal clavicle.

Although it is functionally a planar joint, the AC joint acts like a ball and socket joint, providing anterior/posterior, superior/inferior, and rotational motion of the clavicle relative to the acromion. A small yet important amount of clavicular motion occurs with shoulder movement. However, the amount of motion occurring is

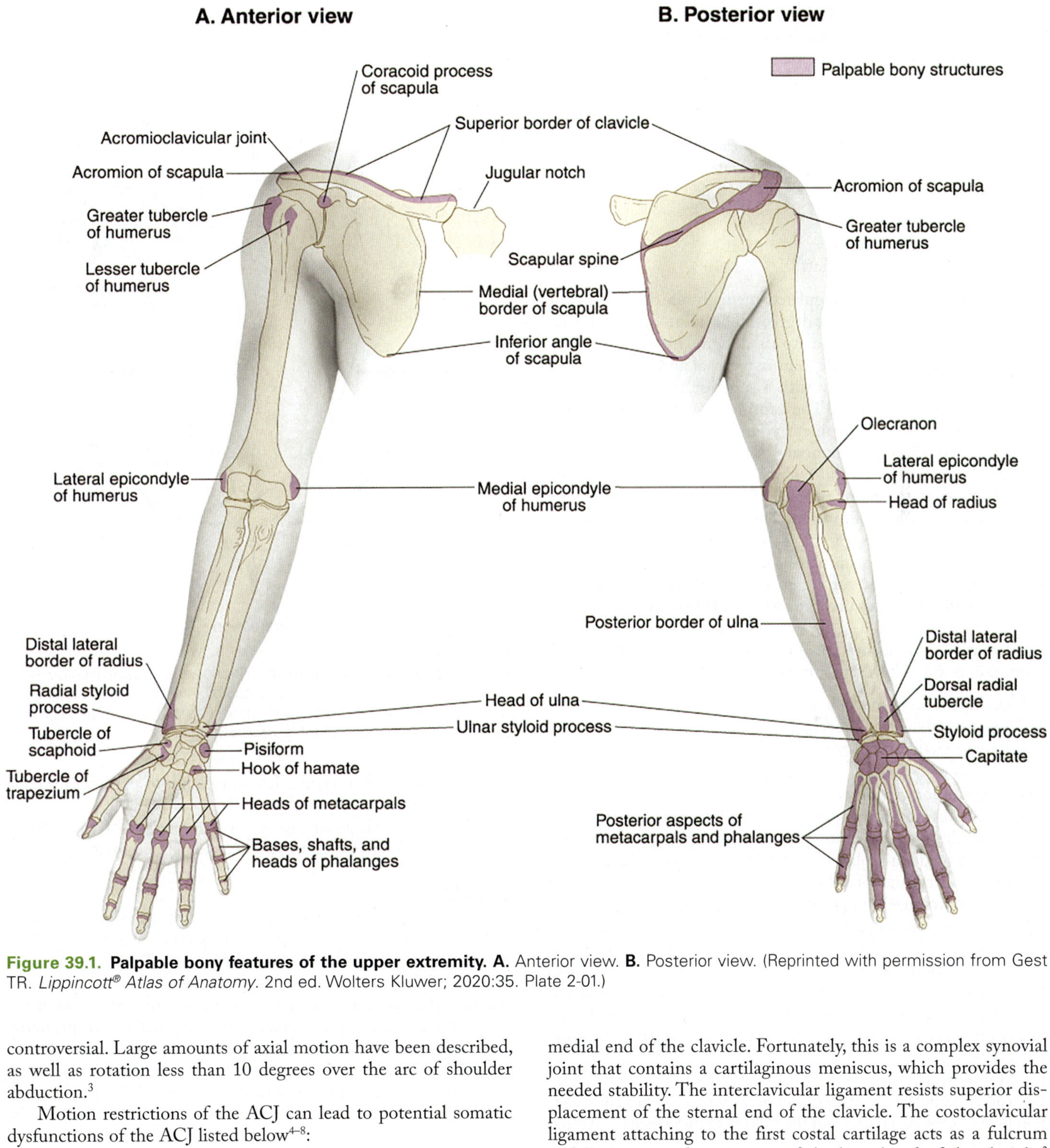

Figure 39.1. Palpable bony features of the upper extremity. A. Anterior view. **B.** Posterior view. (Reprinted with permission from Gest TR. *Lippincott® Atlas of Anatomy*. 2nd ed. Wolters Kluwer; 2020:35. Plate 2-01.)

controversial. Large amounts of axial motion have been described, as well as rotation less than 10 degrees over the arc of shoulder abduction.[3]

Motion restrictions of the ACJ can lead to potential somatic dysfunctions of the ACJ listed below[4–8]:

- Abduction/adduction movement
- Superior/inferior movement
- Anterior/posterior rotation movement
- Internal/external rotation movement

The Sternoclavicular Joint

The SCJ is formed by the articulation of the medial end of the clavicle with the manubrium of the sternum. It has a saddle-shaped articular surface. The clavicular notch on the sternum is shallow and small compared to the articular surface of the medial end of the clavicle. Fortunately, this is a complex synovial joint that contains a cartilaginous meniscus, which provides the needed stability. The interclavicular ligament resists superior displacement of the sternal end of the clavicle. The costoclavicular ligament attaching to the first costal cartilage acts as a fulcrum and limits upward movement of the lateral end of the clavicle.[2] As the clavicle abducts, this ligament helps produce a downward glide to its sternal end. The subclavius muscle depresses and pulls the medial end of the first rib forward as the lateral end of the clavicle is elevated. Potential SCJ somatic dysfunctions can occur in the following motions[5–8]:

- Abduction/abduction movement
- Superior/inferior movement
- Anterior/posterior rotation movement

The Glenohumeral Joint (GHJ)

The GHJ is formed by the articulation of the head of the humerus with the glenoid fossa of the scapula.

The humeral head is large, smooth, slightly elliptical, and covered in articular cartilage.

The glenoid is small, concave, and has a cartilaginous lip (labrum) that helps locate the humeral head into the glenoid.

The proximal humerus has four separate anatomic parts:

- The articular surface
- The lesser tuberosity
- The greater tuberosity
- The diaphyseal humeral shaft[3]

The humeral head is angulated medially 45 degrees to the long axis and retroverted 30 degrees. The joint has significant mobility but lacks stability due to its design. It undergoes spinning, sliding, and rolling. The joint is synovial and is enclosed by a strong ligamentous capsule with a superior, middle, and inferior GH ligament complex. The capsule is weak anteriorly and inferiorly (inferior GH ligament complex), allowing for instability or dislocation to commonly occur in that direction. The posterior capsule is often tight which causes anterior translation and elevation of the humeral head. This can lead to secondary impingement of the rotator cuff.[3] The fibrocartilaginous labrum surrounds the periphery of the glenoid. The labrum acts as an attachment site for the capsular ligamentous structures and acts as a cup to increase the surface area of the glenoid. It also provides a negative intracapsular pressure that helps to center or capture the humeral head.

Potential somatic dysfunction of the GHJ can occur with restriction of the following joint motions[4,5]:

- Flexion/extension movement
- Abduction/abduction movement
- Internal/external rotation movement

The Scapulothoracic Joint

The scapulothoracic joint is a functional joint formed by the articulation of the scapula's anterior surface with the posterior thorax. It is a pseudo articulation, not being a true joint, however its motion is paramount for GH motion. Movement of the scapula on the thoracic cage is required for full shoulder motion. During GH abduction, the motion at the scapulothoracic junction allows the scapula to elevate and protract at a 2:1 ratio to motion at the GHJ (scapulohumeral rhythm). For every 3 degrees of abduction, approximately 2 degrees occurs at the GHJ and 1 degree at the physiologic scapulothoracic joint. So, at 180 degrees of abduction, 120 degrees occurs at the GHJ and 60 degrees occurs at the scapulothoracic joint.[1]

Motion restrictions due to muscular imbalance or restrictions can lead to scapular motion restrictions. Potential somatic dysfunction of the scapula can occur in the following movements depicted in Figure 39.2[4–6]:

- Superior/inferior movement
  - Also called elevation and depression
  - Elevation may have an associated anterior tilt component
- Medial/lateral movement
  - This may also be called adduction and abduction or retraction and protraction
  - Retraction has a posteromedial glide toward midline while protraction has an anterolateral glide due to the rib cage contour
- Internal/external rotation

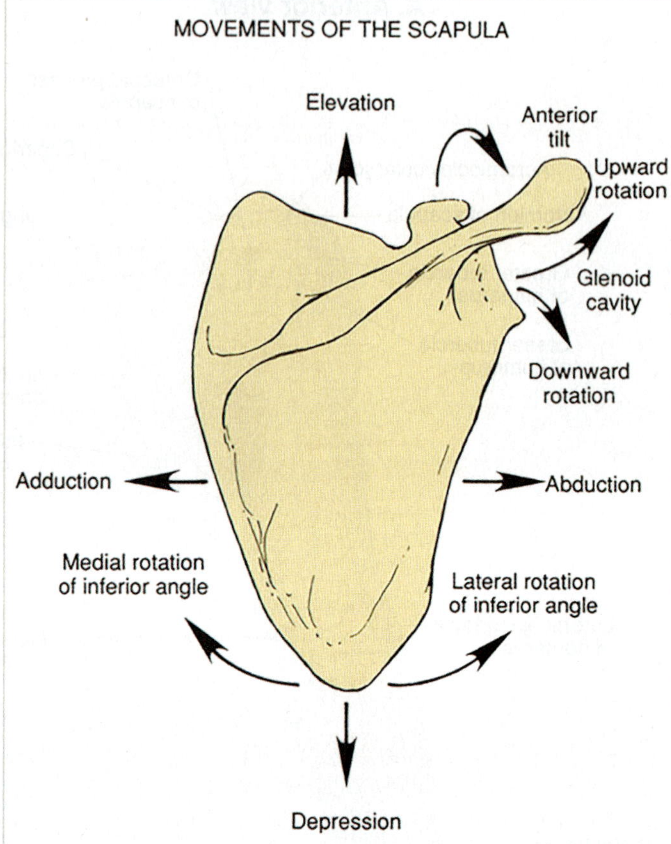

Figure 39.2. Scapular motion. (Reprinted with permission from Conroy VM, Murray B, Alexopulos QT, McCreary JB. *Kendall's Muscles: Testing and Function with Posture and Pain*. 6th ed. Wolters Kluwer; 2024:251. Figure 6-47.)

  - Internal rotation creates lateral rotation of the inferior angle and upward rotation of the glenoid cavity
  - External rotation creates a medial rotation of the inferior angle and downward rotation of the glenoid cavity

THE ELBOW

The elbow joint is the articulation of the humerus with the ulna and radius of the forearm. There are three synovial joints: the ulnohumeral, radiohumeral, and radioulnar joint, all within one joint capsule.[1] All three joints participate in elbow function; however flexion, extension, abduction, and adduction primarily occur at the ulnohumeral joint while pronation and supination are primarily a combined radiohumeral and proximal radioulnar joint movement. The ligamentous capsule is thicker on the medial and lateral aspects than on the anterior and posterior aspects. Muscles such as the biceps brachii and triceps serve as joint stabilizers in the anterior and posterior directions.

The trochlear notch of the ulna is closely fitted to the trochlea of the humerus. The surfaces are lined with articular cartilage and fit together in a spiraled fashion. This positions the hands away from the body (carrying angle) when the elbows are extended and positions the hands near the head when the elbows are flexed. The motion occurs without requiring any rotation of the humerus at the shoulder. The minor motions such as abduction (with medial ulnar glide) and abduction (with lateral glide) are permitted by the relative looseness of the trochlea's fit in the trochlear notch, and by the presence of articular cartilage.[2] Abduction of the ulna with medial glide at the elbow coincides with an increased

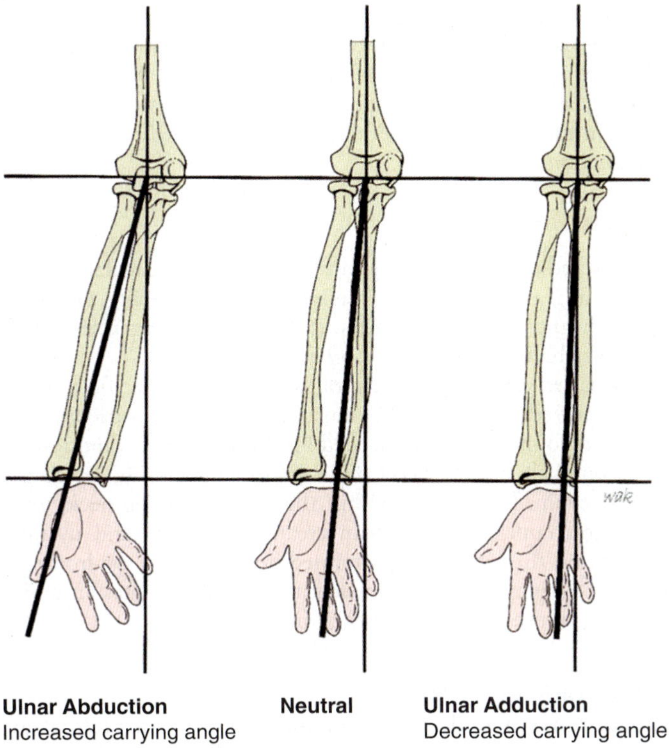

Figure 39.3. Ulnar abduction and adduction. (Illustration by William. A. Kuchera, DO, FAAO, with permission.)

carrying angle, while conversely adduction with lateral glide occurs in patients with a decreased carrying angle (Fig. 39.3). Potential somatic dysfunctions of the ulnohumeral joint include flexion/extension movements and abduction/abduction movements.

Besides flexion and extension, the forearm can rotate around its longitudinal axis to position the hand. When evaluating supination and pronation, the elbow joint should be flexed 90 degrees. In supination, the ulna and radius are parallel at the proximal and distal radioulnar joints and the hand faces palm up. In pronation, the ulna and radius cross and the palm faces down. Due to anatomical structure, there is coupled motion of the radial head with pronation and supination. Posterior glide of the radial head occurs with pronation of the forearm and anterior glide is coupled with supination[3,4,6] (Fig. 39.4). Somatic dysfunction is evaluated by assessing for tissue texture change or tenderness within the forearm and at the radial head, noting any asymmetry to the quality and range of forearm pronation/supination, and any restriction within the radial head's posterior/anterior glide. Restriction of the interosseous membrane between the ulna and radius in the forearm can also affect forearm motion.[8] Nomenclature for the somatic dysfunctions can vary and is further described in Table 91.5 Radial Head Somatic Dysfunction (Combined Humeroradial and Proximal Radioulnar Joint Motion). When naming for the position of ease, pronation dysfunctions are associated with a posterior radial head. Supination dysfunctions are associated with an anterior radial head.

THE WRIST

The wrist joint is formed by the junction of the ulna, radius, and the carpal bones. The joint is considered an ellipsoidal synovial

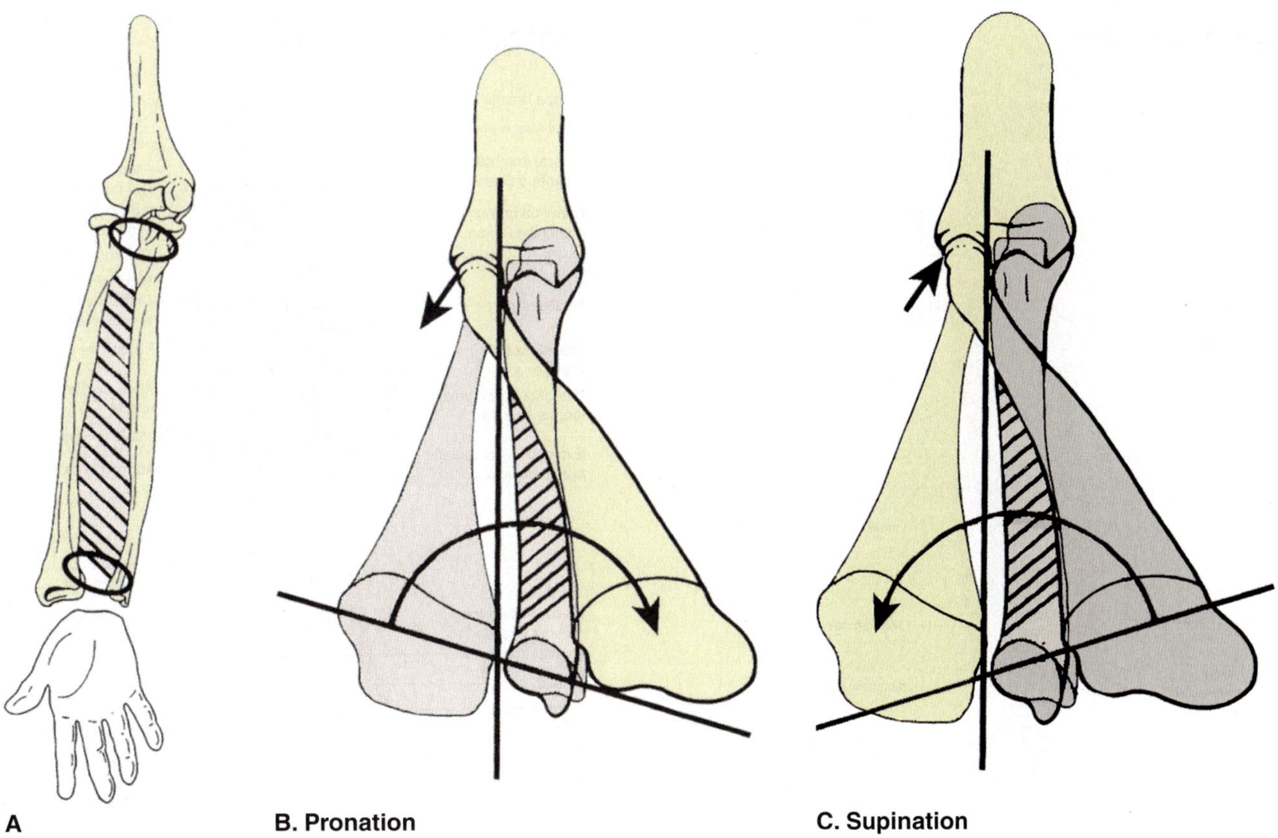

Figure 39.4. Forearm pronation and supination. A. Reciprocal motion occurs at the proximal and distal radioulnar joints during pronation and supination. **B.** During pronation, as the distal radius moves anteriorly, the proximal radial head glides posteriorly. **C.** During supination, as the distal radius moves posteriorly, the proximal radial head glides anteriorly. (Illustration by William A. Kuchera, DO, FAAO, with permission.)

articulation. The true wrist joint is the radiocarpal joint, formed by the distal end of the radius and three proximal carpal bones:

- Scaphoid
- Lunate
- Triquetral

The convexity of these bones fits into the concavity of the radius and articular disk. The disk separates the distal radioulnar joint from the wrist joint cavity and attaches the ulna to the radius. The capsular ligaments are sufficiently loose to allow some minor movements of the carpal bones.[2]

Somatic dysfunction of the wrist joint includes dysfunctions that occur in the major motions of the wrist: flexion/extension and abduction/abduction movements.[5–7] Abduction of the wrist is also named radial deviation and adduction is also named ulnar deviation. Naming is in reference to the anatomic position with the forearm supinated. Flexion and adduction of the wrist typically possesses more range compared to extension and abduction.

THE HAND

In the hand, the scaphoid, lunate, and the triquetral articulate with the greater and lesser multangular bones (aka trapezium and trapezoid), the capitate and hamate forming the intercarpal joint or midcarpal joint. The first carpometacarpal articulation is cavoconvex and is classified as a saddle-shaped joint. The second to fifth carpometacarpal joints are gliding joints. The metacarpal phalangeal joints allow for flexion, extension, abduction, and adduction, as well as a slight amount of rotation; all accompanied by associated minor glides of one bone on the other for the joint involved. Each joint is surrounded by a joint capsule and a synovial membrane. The interphalangeal joints of the hand are commonly referred to as the proximal interphalangeal (PIP) joints, and as the distal interphalangeal (DIP) joints, respectively. Somatic dysfunction of the joints in the hand can be defined by the positional freedom of the dysfunctional joint.[5–7]

Musculature

Understanding the location and function of the musculature when performing a physical exam is essential for developing the differential diagnosis and osteopathic treatment plan, regardless of the patient's chief complaint (Fig. 39.5).

Muscles generally act in groups to produce specific motions. Synchronized action of the muscles influencing various upper extremity joint motion are needed for normal range of motion and to accomplish specific tasks. This sequencing can be viewed as a kinetic chain. Imbalances within the muscles of the neck, upper back, and upper extremity can create restrictions and dysfunction within the kinetic chain termed upper crossed syndrome.[9] A detailed assessment of the upper extremity necessitates an understanding of these groups and their innervations.[2]

SHOULDER MOTION

Efficient and smooth motion of the shoulder and pectoral girdle requires synchronized motion of the SC, AC, GH, and scapulothoracic joints. Table 39.1 identifies the muscles and nerves influencing GH (shoulder) motion, through the actions of both scapulothoracic and GH joint motion.[1,2]

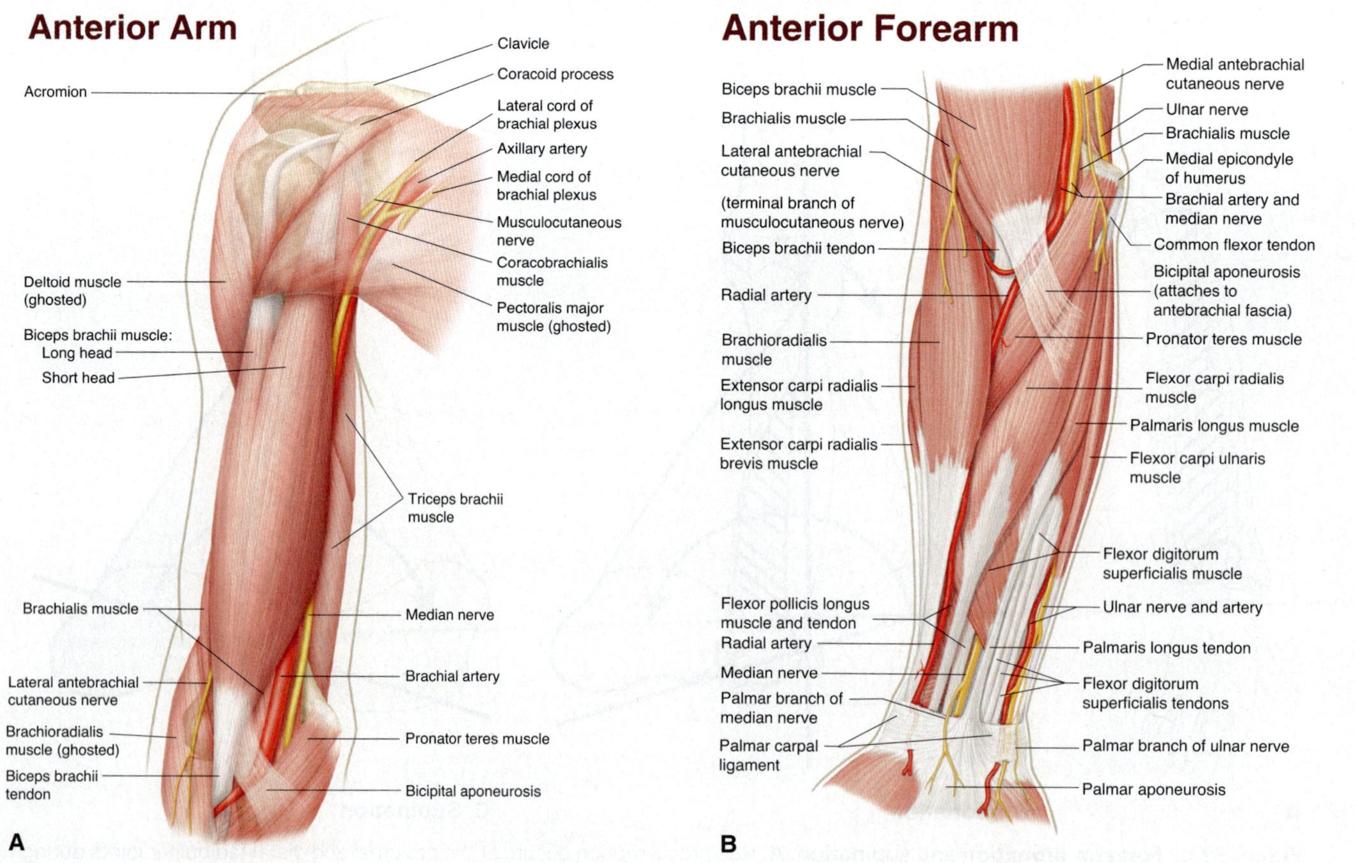

Figure 39.5. Upper limb—location of muscles and surface landmarks. A–C. Anterior view. **D, E.** Posterior view. (Courtesy of ACC Charts, Wolters Kluwer, 2022.)

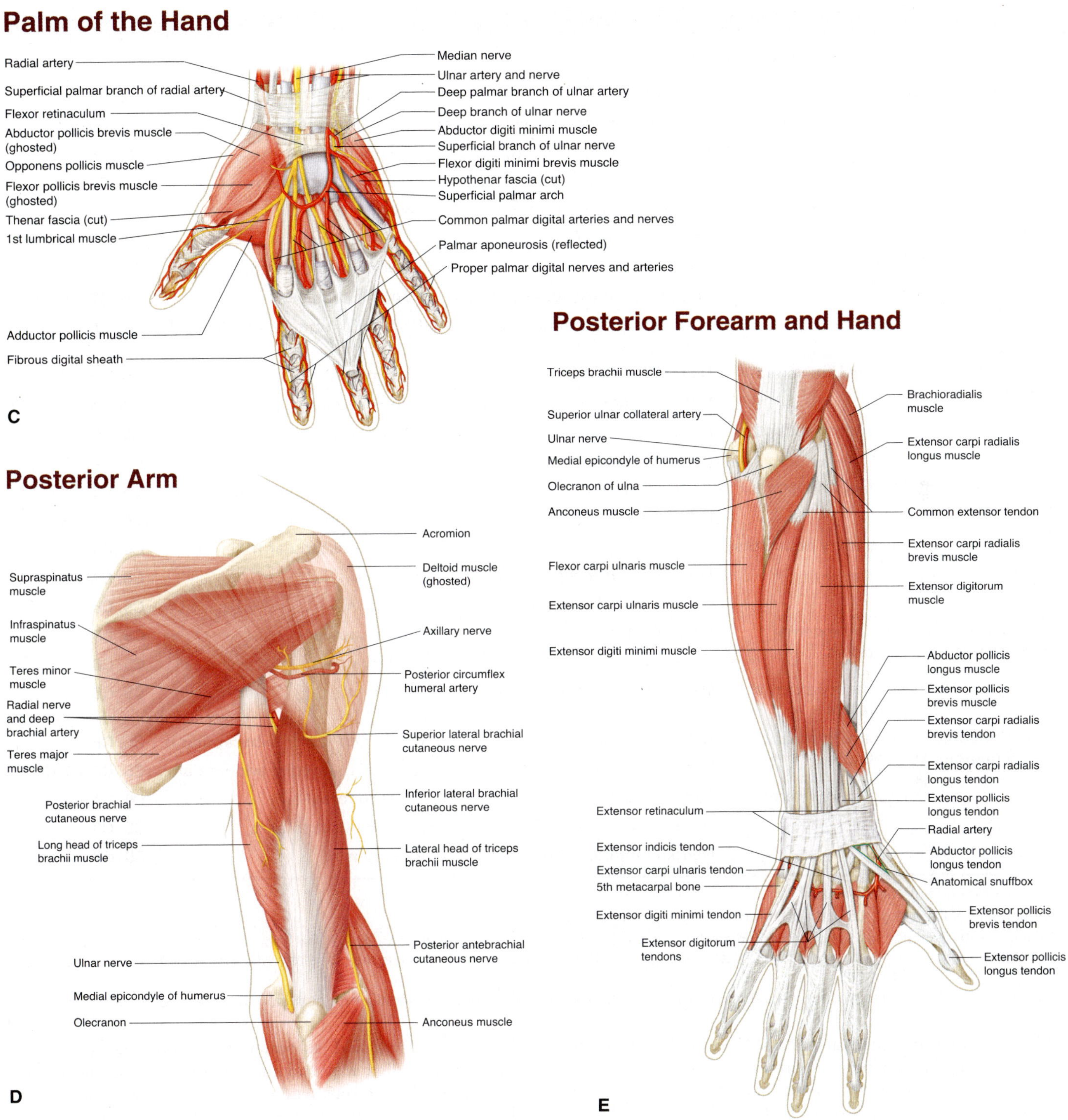

Figure 39.5. *(Continued)*

The rotator cuff muscles are critical to maintaining stability of the GHJ. Their primary function is to hold the humeral head in the glenoid cavity of the scapula during all movements of the GH (shoulder) joint.[1] They also provide precision movements and propulsion in throwing or swinging motions. The cuff is formed by the insertion of the following muscles onto the humerus:

- Confluent tendon of the supraspinatus (greater tuberosity)
- Infraspinatus (greater tuberosity)
- Teres minor (greater tuberosity)
- Subscapularis (lesser tuberosity)

The supraspinatus initiates the first 15 degrees of abduction and then assists the deltoid through the entire arc of abduction. The supraspinatus muscle passes under the coracoacromial arch and subacromial bursa. Inflammation in this area and the shape of the acromion can lead to impingement of the cuff between the humeral head and undersurface of the acromion.[1]

The teres minor and infraspinatus depress, extend, and externally rotate the humerus. The infraspinatus is more active with the arm at the side, and the teres minor with the shoulder elevated 90 degrees, respectively.

TABLE 39.1

Muscles and Nerves Affecting Shoulder Motion[1,2]

Shoulder Motion and Range[a]		Muscle	Innervation	Root[b]
Flexion 0–180 degrees	Primary flexors	Pectoralis major (clavicular head)	Pectoral n. (medial and lateral)	C5, **C6**
		Deltoid (anterior portion)	Axillary n.	**C5**, C6
	Secondary flexors	Coracobrachialis	Musculocutaneous n.	C5, **C6**, C7
Extension 0–60 degrees	Primary extensors	Deltoid (posterior portion)	Axillary n.	**C5**, C6
	Secondary extensors	Latissimus dorsi	Thoracodorsal n.	**C6**, **C7**, C8
		Teres major	Lower subscapular n.	C5, **C6**
		Long head of triceps brachii	Radial n.	C6, **C7**, **C8**
		Pectoralis major (sternocostal head)	Pectoral n. (medial and lateral)	C5, **C6**
Abduction[c] 0–80 degrees	Primary abductors	Deltoid (midportion)	Axillary n.	**C5**, C6
		Supraspinatus	Suprascapular n.	C4, **C5**, C6
	Secondary abductors	Deltoid (anterior, posterior)	Axillary n.	**C5**, C6
		Serratus anterior	Long thoracic n.	C5, **C6**, **C7**
Adduction[c] 0–75 degrees	Primary adductors	Pectoralis major	Pectoral n. (medial and lateral)	C5, **C6**, **C7**, **C8**, T1
		Latissimus dorsi	Thoracodorsal n.	**C6**, **C7**, C8
	Secondary adductors	Teres major	Lower subscapular n.	C5, **C6**
		Long head of triceps brachii	Radial n.	C6, **C7**, **C8**
		Deltoid (anterior portion)	Axillary n.	**C5**, C6
External Rotation[d] 0–90 degrees	Primary external rotators	Infraspinatus	Suprascapular n.	**C5**, C6
		Teres minor	Axillary n.	**C5**, C6
	Secondary external rotators	Deltoid (posterior portion)	Axillary n.	**C5**, C6
Internal rotation[d] 0–100 degrees	Primary internal rotators	Subscapularis	Upper and lower subscapular n.	C5, **C6**, C7
		Pectoralis major	Pectoral n. (medial and lateral)	C5, **C6**, **C7**, **C8**, T1
	Secondary internal rotators	Latissimus dorsi	Thoracodorsal n.	**C6**, **C7**, C8
		Teres major	Lower subscapular n.	C5, **C6**
		Deltoid (anterior portion)	Axillary n.	**C5**, C6

[a]Degrees of motion are approximate.[2]

[b]Numbers in boldface (e.g., **C5**) indicate the main segmental innervation.

[c]Abduction and adduction ranges documented are for vertical ab-/adduction in the coronal plane. Horizontal abduction of 0–45 degrees and horizontal adduction (sometimes called horizontal flexion) of 0–130 degrees occur in the transverse plane after the arm is vertically abducted in the coronal plane to 90 degrees.

[d]Shoulder internal/external rotation range of motion is with the elbow flexed to 90 degrees and the arm abducted to 90 degrees (to the horizontal).

The subscapularis internally rotates, flexes, and depresses the humeral head. The tendinous insertion is continuous with the anterior capsule, which helps to limit anterior instability. The subscapularis is currently considered a GHJ stabilizer. Because of the subscapularis' angle of insertion (70 degrees from the glenoid), it acts as a fulcrum, applying a compressive force to stabilize the humeral head in the glenoid as the supraspinatus and deltoid abduct the humerus.

During throwing and eccentric activity, the subscapularis and infraspinatus are the two most important stabilizing forces of the shoulder.[3]

The long head of the biceps is intimately associated with the rotator cuff and has been considered as its "fifth tendon."[3] The long head of the biceps originates from the supraglenoid tubercle.[1] Thus, the biceps tendon is intra-articular yet extra synovial and passes deep to the "rotator interval," a space between the supraspinatus and subscapularis tendon insertions. The coracohumeral ligament and the superior GH ligament complex surround the biceps tendon and act as a pulley as it enters the intertubercular groove. The long head of the biceps tendon then travels in the intertubercular sulcus, which has a variable shape and slope. This allows the tendon to translate back and forth, which causes degenerative changes within it. The bicep's function is controversial, as some believe that it is a humeral head depressor, while others consider it a passive player in most shoulder motions.[3]

The short head of biceps brachii muscle originates via a short flat tendinous aponeurosis on the apex of the coracoid process of scapula. This origin site is anterosuperior to the coracobrachialis muscle's origin site.[10] The muscle bellies of the long and short heads of biceps brachii converge to a single biceps brachii tendon, which inserts onto the radial tuberosity. This tendon has a flat tendinous aponeurosis, which attaches to the antebrachial fascia.[10]

The pectoralis minor is frequently tight and tender in patients with shoulder complaints. The pectoralis minor originates from the margins of the third to fifth ribs near the costochondral junction. The fibers run upward and laterally to insert into the medial border and superior surface of the coracoid process of the scapula.[11] It is crucial in the stabilization of the scapula by pulling it downward and anteriorly against the thoracic wall.[11] Shortening of pectoralis minor causes protraction of the shoulder which can contribute to shoulder impingement and neurovascular compression, causing thoracic outlet syndrome (TOS).[12] Trigger points in pectoralis minor refer pain to the front of the shoulder, down the inside of the arm, and to the elbow, forearm, palm of the hand, and fingers.[13]

The teres major muscle is not a muscle of the rotator cuff. It is sometimes used as a donor muscle in shoulder surgeries. The teres major acts in synergy with the latissimus dorsi muscle, to cause humeral extension internal rotation and abduction.[14]

SCAPULAR MOTION

Seventeen muscles attach to the scapula. The position of the scapula is primarily controlled by the tension in the rhomboids, trapezius, serratus anterior, pectoralis minor, and levator scapulae,[1] however, asymmetric muscle imbalance of any of the attachments can affect the overall scapular glide and impact motion throughout the shoulder and pectoral girdle.

1. Supraspinatus
2. Infraspinatus
3. Teres major
4. Teres minor
5. Trapezius
6. Deltoid
7. Triceps (long head)
8. Subscapularis
9. Serratus anterior
10. Rhomboid major
11. Rhomboid minor
12. Levator scapula
13. Omohyoid (inferior belly)
14. Biceps brachii (long and short head)
15. Coracobrachialis
16. Pectoralis minor
17. Latissimus dorsi

The levator scapulae and trapezius provide postural support, while the middle trapezius and rhomboids retract the scapula, and serratus anterior protracts it. When contracting with the upper trapezius, these muscles will cause scapular upward rotation and elevation.[3] The position and motion of the scapula controls the GHJ. Somatic dysfunction of a single rib, or a group of ribs, will affect the smooth gliding motion of the scapula over the posterior rib cage. In conditions such as scoliosis, abnormal position of the ribs will affect the positional alignment of the scapula bringing it into a more protracted and elevated position on the convex side of the scoliotic curve. The function of the muscles and motion of the shoulder on the convex side of the spinal curve will be different than that on the concave side. The rotator cuff muscles attach the humeral head to the scapula. If the scapular position is abnormal, these muscles are required to function differently, based on their length/tension relationships. The various motions and innervations of the scapula are listed in Table 39.2[1,2]:

ELBOW MOTION

The elbow moves in flexion and extension, pronation and supination, and minor abduction and adduction. Seventeen muscles cross the elbow and extend to the forearm and hand and have potential to affect elbow movement.[1] The muscles of flexion and extension are listed in Table 39.3.

WRIST MOTION

Wrist movement is primarily due to the "carpi" muscles as listed in Table 39.4.

Supportive Tissues

The deep fascia of the arm can be divided into the following:

- Brachial fascia, which joins superiorly with the pectoral and axillary fascia, has medial and lateral septa that functionally divide the arm into anterior and posterior musculofascial compartments.
- Antebrachial fascia, which surrounds the forearm, joins with the brachial and deep fascia of the hand.
- An interosseous membrane separates the forearm into anterior and posterior musculofascial compartments.
- Distally, the fascia forms the palmar carpal ligament, which is continuous with the flexor retinaculum.
- The deep fascia of the hand forms the palmar aponeurosis.
- The flexor retinaculum, or transverse carpal ligament, forms the carpal tunnel.[15]

Neural Structures

CERVICAL NERVE ROOTS

Nerve roots C5–C8 and T1 form the brachial plexus (Fig. 39.6). These nerve roots pass through the intervertebral foramen of the cervical vertebrae, and between the anterior and middle scalene muscles.[15]

The roots unite to form successive trunks, divisions, cords, and branches. The nerve trunks extend from the scalene triangle (formed by the anterior and middle scalenes and the clavicle) to the clavicle. Nerve divisions extend from a position posterior to the clavicle, to the axilla. Nerve cords found in the axilla divide into branches that innervate various structures in the upper extremity. The neurovascular bundle of the arm contains the following:

- Subclavian artery
- Subclavian vein
- Brachial plexus
- Sympathetic nerve plexus

THE THORACIC OUTLET

The thoracic outlet is an anatomic region that contains three important structures: the subclavian artery and vein and the brachial plexus. The subclavian artery passes between the anterior scalene and middle muscles, and over the first rib through the interscalene triangle. The subclavian vein follows a similar course but does not pass through the interscalene triangle. It courses just medial and anterior to the anterior scalene muscle.[16] The brachial plexus travels similarly to the subclavian artery. These three structures pass under the clavicle through the costoclavicular space, between the clavicle and first rib. The costoclavicular space is a triangular area bordered anteriorly by the medial portion of the clavicle and underlying subclavian muscle, its tendon, and costocoracoid ligament.[16] It is bordered posteromedially by the first rib and the insertion of both anterior and middle

TABLE 39.2

Muscles and Nerves Influencing Scapulothoracic Motion[1]

Motion Type and Range of Movement/Displacement		Muscle	Innervation	Root
Elevation 10–12 cm	Primary	Trapezius, descending part	Spinal accessory n.	CN XI
		Levator scapulae	Dorsal scapular n.	C3, C4, **C5**
	Secondary	Rhomboids major and minor	Dorsal scapular n.	C4, **C5**
Depression	Primary	Gravity		
	Secondary	Pectoralis major, inferior sternocostal head	Pectoral n. (medial and lateral)	C5, **C6**, **C7**, **C8**, T1
		Latissimus dorsi	Thoracodorsal n.	**C6**, **C7**, C8
		Trapezius, lower/ascending part	spinal accessory (CNXI), sensory ventral rami	CN XI and C3,4
		Serratus anterior, inferior part	Long thoracic n.	C5–C7
		Pectoralis minor	Medial pectoral n.	C8, T1
Protraction 40–45 degrees, 15 cm	Primary	Serratus anterior	Long thoracic n.	C5–C7
	Secondary	Pectoralis major	Pectoral n. (medial and lateral)	C5, **C6**, **C7**, **C8**, T1
		Pectoralis minor	Medial pectoral n.	C8, T1
Retraction	Primary	Trapezius muscle (middle portion)	Spinal accessory (CNXI), sensory ventral rami C3, 4	CN XI and C3, 4
	Secondary	Rhomboid major and minor	Dorsal scapular n.	C4, **C5**
		Latissimus dorsi	Thoracodorsal n.	**C6**, **C7**, C8
Lateral (upward) Rotation 60 degrees (10–12 cm at inferior angle; 5–6 cm at superior angle)	Primary	Trapezius, descending part	Spinal accessory n.	CN XI
		Serratus anterior	Long thoracic n.	C5–C7
	Secondary	Trapezius, lower/ascending part	Spinal accessory (CNXI), sensory ventral rami	CN XI and C3, C4
Medial (downward) Rotation	Primary	Latissimus dorsi	Thoracodorsal n.	**C6**, **C7**, C8
	Secondary	Levator scapulae	Dorsal scapular n.	C3, C4, **C5**
		Rhomboids major and minor	Dorsal scapular n.	C4, **C5**
		Pectoralis minor	Medial pectoral n.	C8, T1
		Pectoralis major, inferior sternocostal head	Pectoral n. (medial and lateral)	C5, **C6**, **C7**, **C8**, T1
		Gravity		

TABLE 39.3

Muscles and Nerves of the Elbow Joint[1]

Motion		Muscle	Innervation	Root
Flexors	Primary	Brachialis	Musculocutaneous n.	C5, C6
		Biceps brachii	Musculocutaneous n.	C5, C6
	Secondary	Brachioradialis	Radial n.	C5, **C6**, C7
		Pronator teres	Median n.	C6, **C7**
Extensor	Primary	Triceps brachii (especially the medial head)	Radial n.	C5, **C6**, C7
	Secondary	Anconeus	Radial n.	C7, C8, T1
Supinators	Primary	Biceps brachii	Musculocutaneous n.	C5, C6
		Supinator	Radial n. (deep branch)	**C7**, C8
	Secondary	Brachioradialis	Radial n.	C5, **C6**, C7
Pronators	Primary	Pronator teres	Median n.	C6, **C7**
		Pronator quadratus	Median n. (ant. interosseous branch)	**C8**, T1

TABLE 39.4

Muscles and Nerves of the Wrist[1]

Motion	Muscle	Innervation	Root
Flexors	Flexor carpi radialis	Median n.	C6, **C7**
	Flexor carpi ulnaris	Ulnar n.	C7, **C8**
	Palmaris longus	Median n.	C7, C8
Extensors	Extensor carpi radialis longus	Radial n.	C6, C7
	Extensor carpi radialis brevis	Radial n. (deep branch)	**C7**, C8
	Extensor carpi ulnaris	Radial n. (deep branch)	**C7**, C8
Abductors (Radial deviation)	Abductor pollicis longus	Posterior interosseous n. (from deep branch of radial n.)	C7, **C8**
	Flexor carpi radialis	Median n.	C6, **C7**
	Extensor carpi radialis longus	Radial n.	C6, C7
	Extensor carpi radialis brevis	Radial n. (deep branch)	**C7**, C8
Adductors (Ulnar deviation)	Flexor carpi ulnaris	Ulnar n.	C7, **C8**
	Extensor carpi ulnaris	Radial n. (deep branch)	**C7**, C8

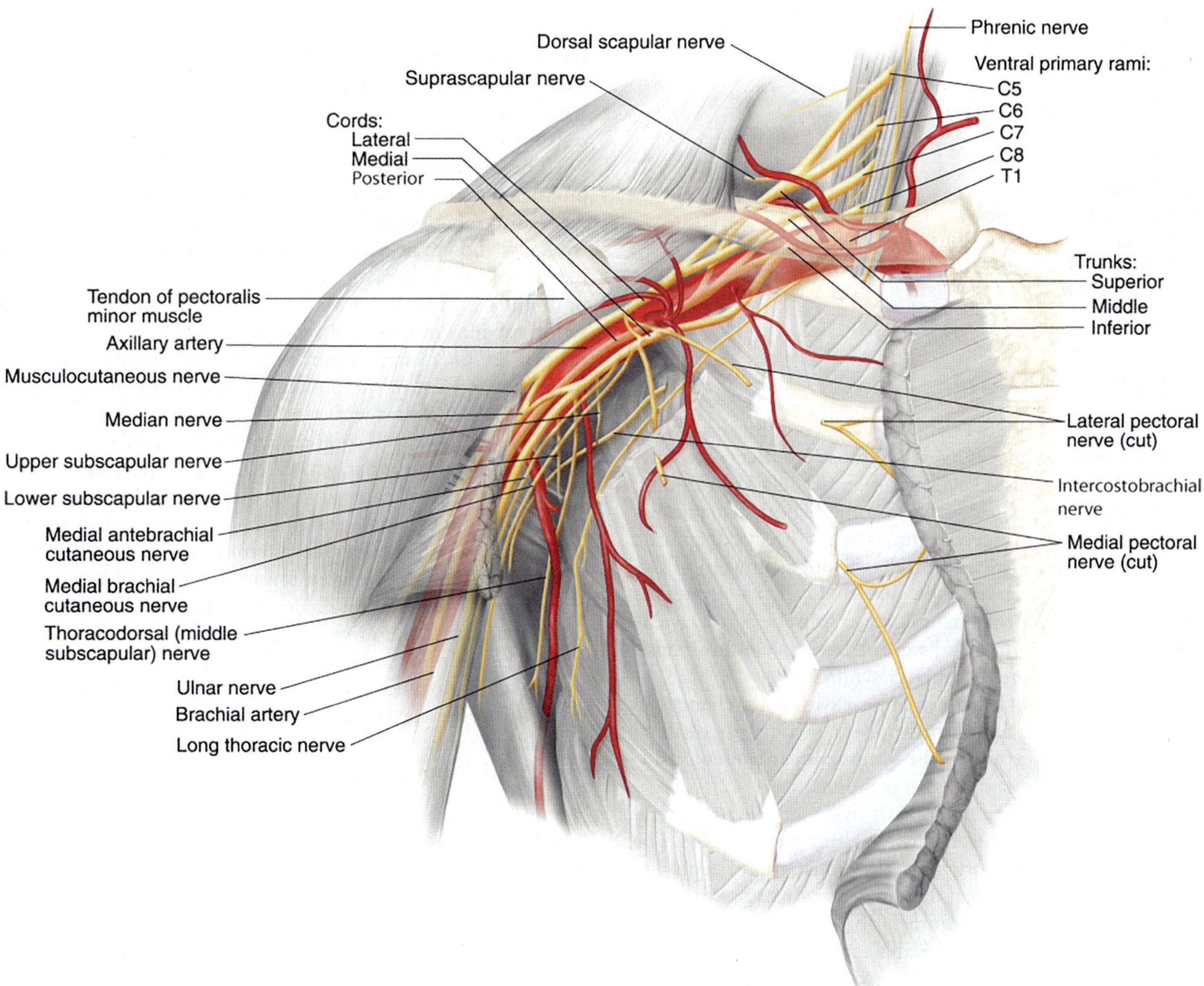

Figure 39.6. Brachial plexus and nerves of the axilla. (Reprinted with permission from Gest TR. *Lippincott® Atlas of Anatomy.* 2nd ed. Wolters Kluwer; 2020:47. Plate 2-13.)

scalene muscles. From here, the three anatomic structures travel below the pectoralis minor muscle through the subpectoral minor space.[16]

Thoracic outlet syndrome (TOS) is a group of conditions in which compression can occur to nerves of the brachial plexus, the subclavian artery, or vein. Nonspecific symptoms occur such as numbness, tingling, and weakness in the upper extremities.[17] The history and physical exam will help determine if the condition is neurologic, arterial, or venous and suggest the site in which the compression is occurring. However, the physical exam tests do not have a high sensitivity or specificity. Narrowing classically occurs in three different regions listed below:

- Interscalene space or triangle
  - Between the anterior and middle scalene muscle
  - Adson test suggests arterial compression
- Costoclavicular space
  - Between the clavicle and first rib
  - Military brace (Eden test)
- Subpectoral minor space:
  - Underneath the pectoralis minor
  - During the hyperabduction test, the neurovascular structures may be compressed by the taut pectoralis minor muscle
  - If neurogenic, it is also called pectoralis minor syndrome[17]
  - Subpectoral minor space compression is less frequently encountered than interscalene or costoclavicular space compression[16]

Multiple etiologies of TOS include:

- Cervical ribs
- Fibrous bands
- Clavicular fracture/deformity
- Tumors/space occupying lesions
- Muscle deficiency, causing the shoulder to depress
- Athletic overuse
- Trauma
- DVT
- Somatic dysfunction

Several variants of TOS exist; however, compression of the brachial plexus (neurogenic TOS) is the most prevalent, accounting for over 90% of all cases.[17] Gilliatt–Sumner hand is a finding in which the abductor pollicis brevis and the hypothenar muscles become atrophied due to nerve compression.[17] Electrodiagnostic studies are a classic diagnostic tool for diagnosing neurogenic TOS.

Venous thoracic outlet may be due to DVT and produces vague symptoms and a normal neurologic exam. The costoclavicular ligament plays an important role in subclavian vein thrombosis (effort thrombosis) or Paget Schroetter syndrome.[16]

The arterial variant of TOS can appear with color changes in the upper extremity and diminished pulses.[17,18] Due to collateral blood flow in the upper extremity, the symptoms can present insidiously and only appear in certain arm positions.

OMT for associated regional somatic dysfunction and postural correction is a common approach in osteopathic management. The way the patient sleeps is important, as they must avoid sleeping in overhead arm positions. Physical therapy is a mainstay as first-line treatment for patients suffering from TOS. For many patients, the cause of the condition is muscular imbalance.

See Chapter 91 Osteopathic Approach to Diagnosing and Treating Somatic Dysfunction in the Extremities—section Common Shoulder Conditions and the Osteopathic Approach—for further detailed explanation about TOS and the osteopathic approach.

PERIPHERAL NERVES OF THE UPPER EXTREMITY

Cutaneous innervation to the upper extremity is supplied by nerves from all five terminal branches and the medial cord of the brachial plexus. However, the three main peripheral nerves of the upper extremity are the following:

- Median nerve
- Ulnar nerve
- Radial nerve

It is crucial to understand the innervation of each, as well as their site(s) of potential compression (Fig. 39.7).

The Median Nerve

The median nerve arises from the lateral (C6, C7) and medial (C8, T1) cords of the brachial plexus and provides motor innervation to the anterior forearm and hand and sensory innervation to the palmer surface of the radial 3½ digits of the hand. The median nerve can be compressed at several locations in the arm, particularly around the elbow and forearm.

The most proximal level of compression of the median nerve may produce pronator syndrome: a compression of the median nerve as it passes through the pronator teres muscle, the bicipital aponeurosis, or under the ligament of Struthers.[1]

Pronator syndrome is associated with pain in the proximal volar forearm, as well as sensory signs and symptoms in the radial 3½ digits of the hand. This syndrome may affect the function of the median nerve–innervated muscles in the C6 and C7 distribution and symptoms typically mimic C6 and C7 radiculopathy. Symptoms are generally aggravated by flexion of the elbow against resistance.[1]

The median nerve has a motor branch known as the anterior interosseous nerve. In anterior interosseous syndrome, there are no sensory abnormalities. Motor abnormalities are manifested as weakness and are referred to muscles innervated by this nerve—the flexor pollicis longus, pronator quadratus, and flexor digitorum profundus of the index finger. Therefore, anterior interosseous syndrome may mimic a C8 radiculopathy. This results in difficulty making an "O.K." sign or pinching objects between the thumb and index finger. Pain in the proximal forearm is typically aggravated by exercise and abates with rest.[1]

The next region of compression for the median nerve is at the carpal tunnel of the wrist, which results in carpal tunnel syndrome.

Typical sensory symptoms of carpal tunnel syndrome include night pain, paresthesias, and numbness in the radial 3½ digits of the hand. Symptoms may be referred proximally from the hand toward the forearm, and even toward the elbow. They may also be reproduced or elicited by Phalen maneuver or Tinel sign. Thenar muscle weakness and atrophy represent advanced disease. Sensory symptoms may mimic C6 and C7 radiculopathy, but no C6 or C7 muscle demonstrates abnormalities since they are all innervated proximal to the carpal canal. Thenar motor weakness may mimic T1 radiculopathy due to abnormalities of the opponens pollicis and the abductor pollicis brevis. However, other T1-innervated muscles are normal.[1]

The Ulnar Nerve

The ulnar nerve arises from the medial cord of the brachial plexus (C7, C8, and T1) and provides motor innervation to two muscles in the anterior forearm (the flexor carpi ulnaris and the ulnar half of the flexor digitorum profundus) and most of the intrinsic muscles of the hand. Sensory innervation is to the ulnar 1½ digits of the hand.[1]

The ulnar nerve can become entrapped at the elbow, resulting in cubital tunnel syndrome.[1] The cubital tunnel is a narrow space

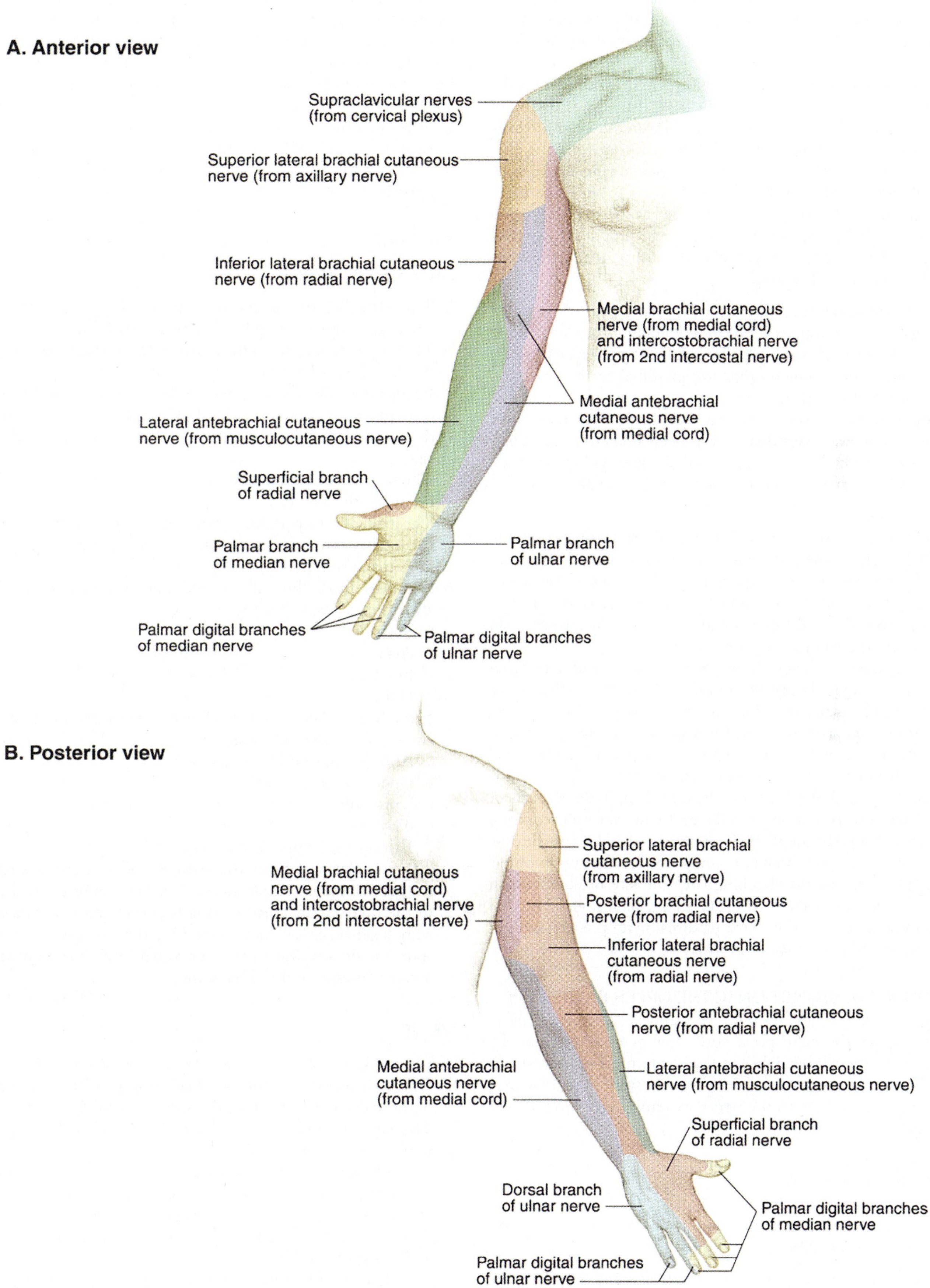

Figure 39.7. Cutaneous innervation of the upper limb. A. Anterior view. **B.** Posterior view. (Reprinted with permission from Gest TR. *Lippincott® Atlas of Anatomy*. 2nd ed. Wolters Kluwer; 2020:87. Plate 2-53.)

formed by the medial epicondyle of the humerus and the olecranon process of the ulna. Cubital tunnel syndrome can result from trauma, repetitive elbow flexion, prolonged pressure on the elbow, and overuse.

The most typical symptom of cubital tunnel syndrome is aching pain on the medial aspect of the elbow, although radiation of the pain and paresthesia may migrate distally on the ulnar forearm, and into the ulnar 1½ digits of the hand. Symptoms may be elicited by percussion of the nerve behind the medial epicondyle, or by acute, prolonged flexion of the elbow.[1]

The ulnar nerve may also be compressed at the wrist in Guyon canal, which usually affects both its superficial and deep branches. The superficial branch is essentially all sensory, while the deep branch is essentially all motor.

- Sensory symptoms are referred to the volar aspect of the ulnar 1½ fingers. The dorsal aspect of these digits remains unaffected because that area of skin is supplied by the dorsal sensory branch of the ulnar nerve, which originates proximal to the wrist and does not traverse Guyon canal.
- Motor symptoms, weakness, and atrophy are referable only to those muscles innervated by the deep branch of the ulnar nerve—the hypothenar, interossei, and abductor pollicis muscles.
- This syndrome may mimic T1 and C8 radiculopathy.[1]

The Radial Nerve

The radial is the largest branch of the plexus, arising from the terminal branch of the posterior cord and receiving fibers from C5–T1. It provides motor innervation to all muscles of the posterior compartments of the arm and forearm and sensory innervation of the posterior and inferolateral arm, posterior forearm, and the dorsum of the hand's radial four digits.[1]

The radial nerve divides into the deep motor and superficial sensory branches just lateral to the brachialis in the cubital fossa. The deep branch penetrates the supinator muscle and emerges in the posterior compartment of the forearm as the posterior interosseous nerve. The deep branch can become compressed in the radial tunnel, resulting in posterior interosseous syndrome.[1] This condition is characterized by pain along the dorsal and radial aspects of the proximal forearm, often exacerbated by movements requiring pronation and supination of the forearm or resisted elbow flexion. Because only the motor branch is compressed, sensory symptoms are rare. However, localized aching over the site of compression may be present and elicited with full elbow extension. The most common site of compression is the proximal margin of the supinator muscle, called the arcade of Frohse.[19]

AUTONOMIC DYSFUNCTION TO THE UPPER EXTREMITY

The sympathetic innervation to the upper extremities arises from the upper thoracic spinal cord. The sympathetic ganglia lie anterior to the rib head, in the fascia common to both structures.[1] Dysfunction in the upper thoracic spine and ribs may affect sympathetic tone to the upper extremity and produce the following:

- Altered motion
- Nerve dysfunction
- Vasoconstriction
- Lymphatic and venous congestion
- Sudomotor dysfunction

Nociceptive afferents from the cervical spine travel in the sympathetic chain and synapse in the intermediolateral cell columns of the upper thoracic (T2–T7) cord. This produces an irritable focus in the spinal cord, resulting in facilitation and sympathetic hyperactivity.[20] Increased sympathetic tone is often accompanied by palpatory findings in the upper thoracic and rib area, with increased sensitivity to painful stimulus. These musculoskeletal findings may be primary somatic dysfunctions in the area, reflex from the cervical spine, or viscerosomatic facilitations. Hypersympathetic tone can cause vasoconstriction, preventing arterial blood from reaching the structures of the arm and reducing the amount of lymphatic fluid returning from the arm via the lymphatic vessels.[21]

Vasculature

ARTERIES (FIG. 39.8)

- The left subclavian artery arises from the posterior part of the aortic arch and passes posterior to the left SCJ.
- The right subclavian artery arises from the brachiocephalic trunk.[15] The subclavian arteries pass over the top of the first rib between the anterior and middle scalene muscles. This is an area of compression in TOS. Consider an elevated first rib dysfunction and or dysfunction of the clavicle narrowing this space.
- The subclavian artery becomes the axillary artery at the lateral border of the first rib.
- The axillary artery passes posterior to the pectoralis minor muscle and becomes the brachial artery at the inferior border of the teres major muscle.
- Branches from the axillary and brachial arteries supply the structures of the following:
  - Shoulder
  - Arm
  - Forearm
  - Hand
- Somatic dysfunction of the following structures may affect arterial supply to the following:
  - Anterior and middle scalenes
  - Upper thoracic vertebrae
  - Upper ribs
  - Clavicles
  - Fascia of the upper extremity
- The vascular supply of the rotator cuff has been extensively studied. There is a "critical zone" of anastomotic blood supply to the rotator cuff muscles. It is hypothesized that rotator cuff tears begin in this critical zone. One such area is in the supraspinatus tendon immediately proximal to its insertion into the greater tuberosity of the humerus.[3]

VEINS

- The axillary vein lies on the medial side of the axillary artery. The vein receives tributaries that correspond to the branches of the axillary artery, and venae comitantes of the brachial artery. The axillary vein ends at the lateral border of the first rib, where it becomes the subclavian vein.[6]
- The subclavian vein passes over the first rib anterior to the anterior scalene muscle.[15] The vein then unites with the internal jugular vein to become the brachiocephalic vein.[15]
- The left brachiocephalic vein passes posterior to the left SCJ and crosses the midline.
- The right brachiocephalic vein passes posterior to the right SCJ. The vein then joins the left brachiocephalic vein to form the superior vena cava.[15]

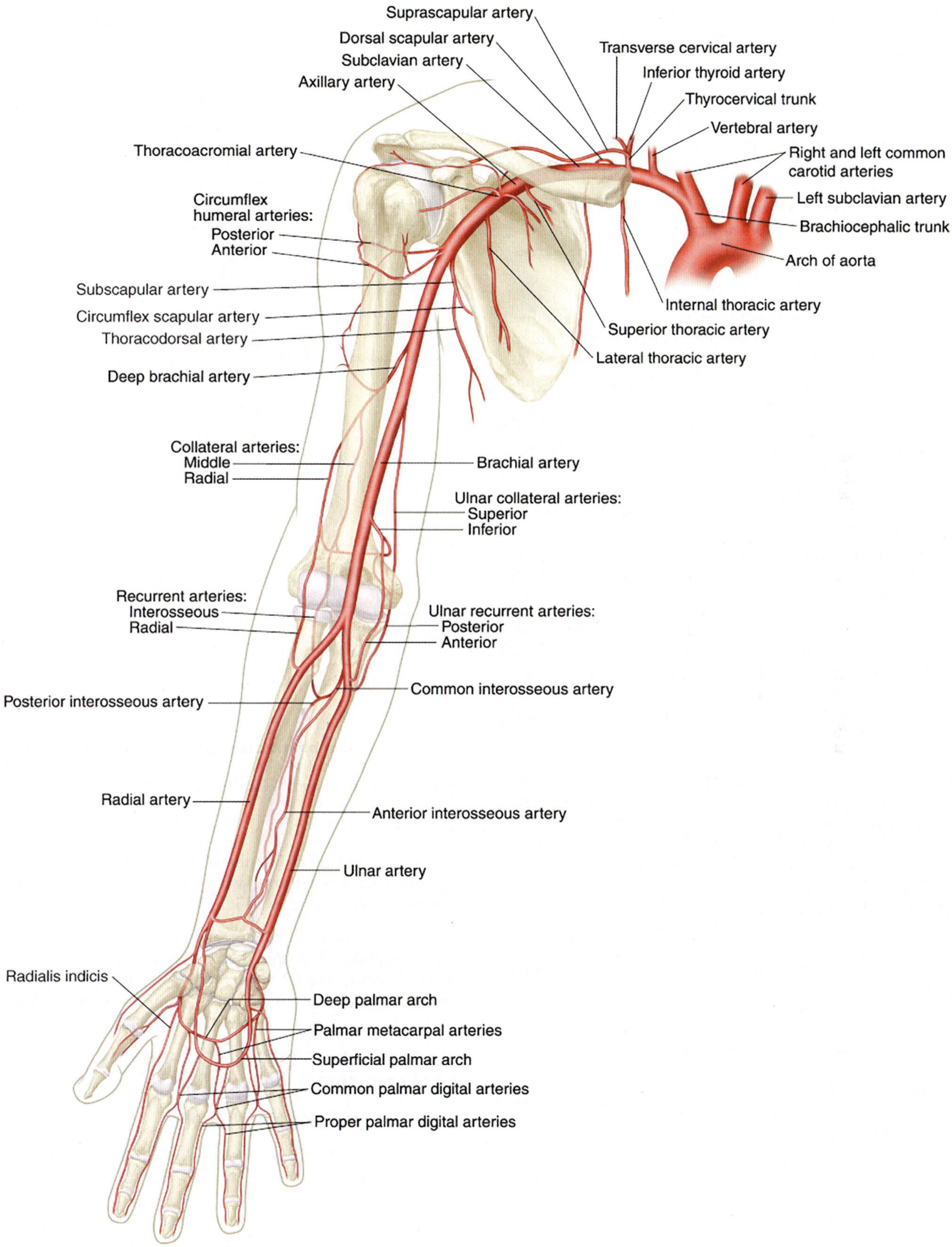

Figure 39.8. Arterial of the upper limb. (Reprinted with permission from Gest TR. *Lippincott® Atlas of Anatomy*. 2nd ed. Wolters Kluwer; 2020:80. Plate 2-46.)

- Dysfunction in the following may impair venous return:
  - □ Upper thoracic vertebrae (causing increased sympathetic tone to the upper extremities)
  - □ Upper ribs
  - □ Clavicles
  - □ Fascia of the upper extremities
- Because the subclavian vein passes anterior to the scalene muscles, scalene tension does not create venous distention of the upper extremity.
- A thrombosis in the subclavian vein can cause swelling in the breast and upper extremity due to venous obstruction.[22]

Lymphatic Structures

The final terminal drainage sites, the left and right lymphatic ducts, drain into the subclavian veins near the junction with the internal jugular veins (Fig. 39.9). In a small percentage of people, the duct drains into the internal jugular vein.[1] The subclavian vein courses just medial and anterior to the anterior scalene muscle[16] and passes under the clavicle through the costoclavicular space, between the clavicle and first rib. Therefore, tension within the pectoral girdle and somatic dysfunction of the clavicle may restrict the associated lymphatic drainage that terminates on that side.

The major lymph nodes of the upper extremities are found in the connective tissue of the axilla. They are arranged in five groups, four of which lie inferior to the pectoralis minor tendon[1] (Fig. 39.10). These groups of axillary lymph nodes are pectoral, humeral, subscapular, central, and apical.

- The pectoral (anterior) axillary lymph nodes receive lymph mainly from the anterior thoracic wall and breast. The efferent vessels from these nodes pass from here to the central and apical groups.
- The humoral (lateral) axillary lymph nodes lie along the lateral wall of the axilla. This group receives lymph from most of the upper limbs. The efferent vessels from these nodes pass from here to the central and apical groups.
- The subscapular (posterior) lymph nodes are located along the posterior aspect of the thoracic wall and scapular region. Efferent vessels pass from here to the central group.
- The central axillary lymph nodes are situated deep into the pectoralis minor, near the base of the axilla. This group receives lymph from the anterior, lateral, and posterior groups. Efferent vessels from the central nodes pass lymph to the apical group.
- The apical axillary lymph nodes are situated in the apex of the axilla. This group receives lymph from the central lymph nodes. The efferent vessels from this group unite to form the subclavian lymphatic trunk.

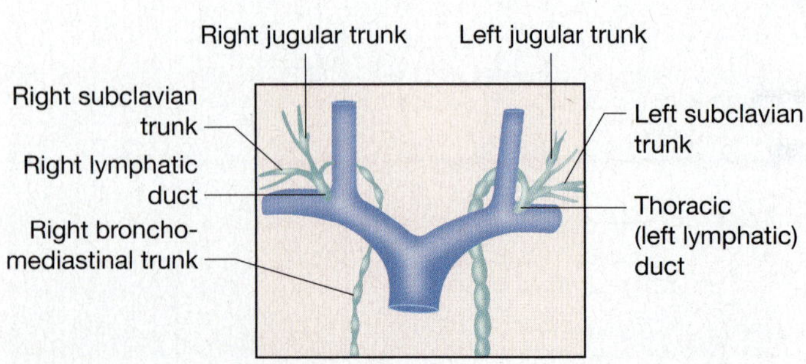

Figure 39.9. Terminal lymphatic drainage sites—the left and right lymphatic ducts. (Reprinted with permission from Tanner JM. Structure and function of the cardiovascular system. In: Norris TL, ed. *Porth's Pathophysiology: Concepts of Altered Health States.* 10th ed. Wolters Kluwer; 2019:709. Figure 25.21.)

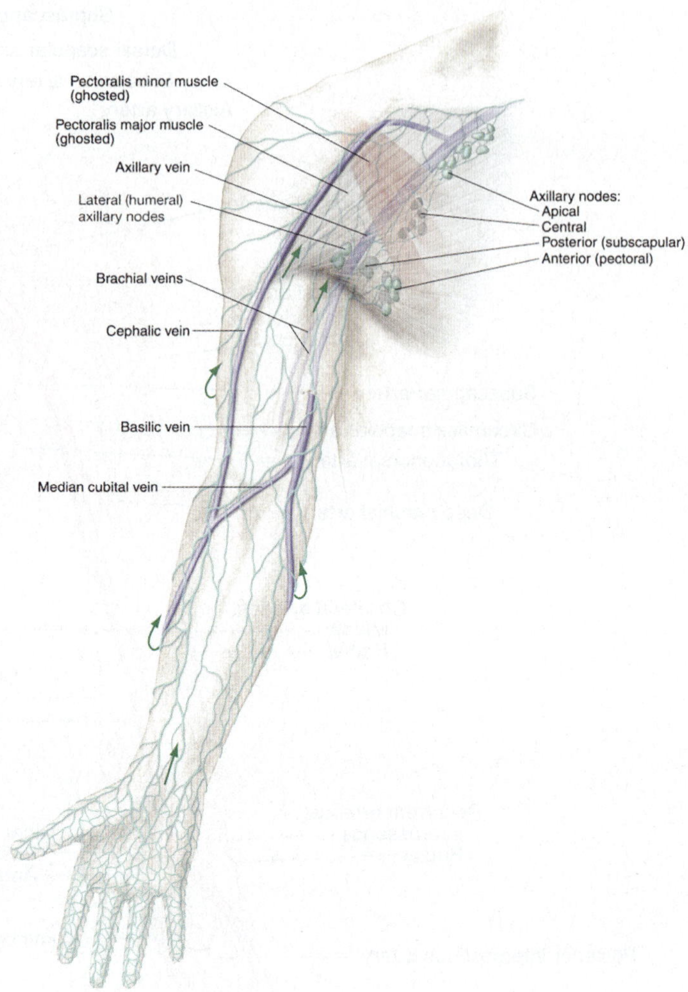

Figure 39.10. Lymphatic drainage of the upper limb. (Reprinted with permission from Gest TR. *Lippincott® Atlas of Anatomy.* 2nd ed. Wolters Kluwer; 2020:89. Plate 2-55.)

- The right subclavian lymphatic trunk drains into the right lymphatic duct. The left subclavian lymphatic trunk drains into the thoracic duct[1] (see above Fig. 39.9).

Somatic dysfunction affecting the venous system may also affect lymphatic drainage, thereby producing congestion in the upper extremity. Fascial restriction of the thoracic inlet and pectoral fascia can also cause lymphatic stasis of the upper extremity.

DIAGNOSIS OF UPPER EXTREMITY SOMATIC DYSFUNCTION

SCREENING EXAMINATION

Please refer to Chapter 30 Osteopathic Structural Examination to understand how the upper extremity exam is integrated into the entire patient evaluation.

Initially, assess for any acute fractures, neurologic injuries, significant soft tissue injuries, wounds, and medical conditions associated with the patient presentation. A detailed history and a problem-focused physical are required to rule out the most significant issues first. Once accomplished, it is equally important to perform a structural examination and directly visualize landmarks and asymmetries.

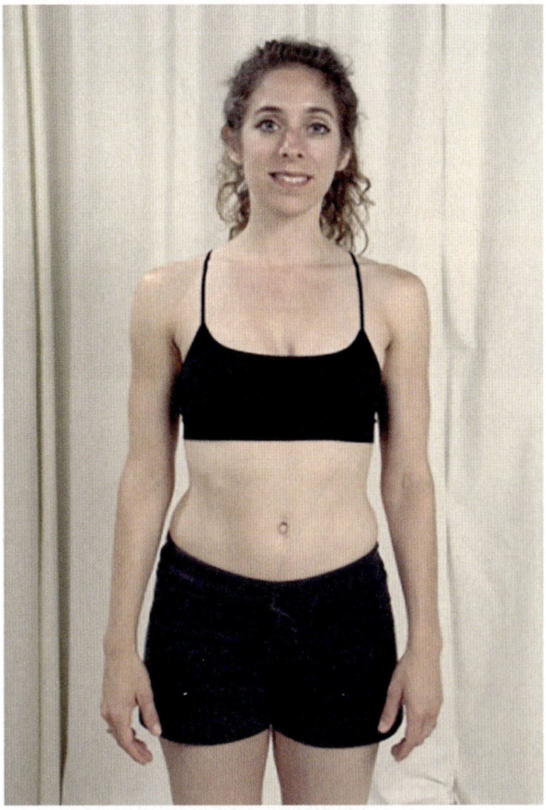

Figure 39.11. Observing shoulder symmetry. (Photo courtesy of Western University of Health Sciences, Pomona, CA, with permission.)

Shoulders

- Observe for symmetry of position and level (Fig. 39.11).
- Observe if the shoulders appear to be level on a horizontal plane from the anterior view and from the posterior view.
  - If the shoulders are not level this could indicate a cervical somatic dysfunction, spinal scoliosis, or a more distant somatic dysfunction such as sacral base unleveling or leg-length discrepancy.
  - Asymmetry of the shoulder may also result from trauma to the shoulder such as a dislocation, or a rotator cuff or AC injury, or an injury to one of the nerves supplying the shoulder.
  - It is not uncommon for the shoulder to be lower on the side of the patient's handedness.
- Assess for presence of anterior shoulder carriage (protraction) or posterior carriage (retraction), also known as a "military-type" posture.
  - This is best observed from the lateral view but is also seen in the anterior and posterior views.
  - Anterior shoulder carriage with the scapula shifting superiorly and laterally can cause the acromion process to impinge upon the supraspinatus tendon. This can result in:
    - Subacromial bursitis
    - Rotator cuff tendonitis
    - Frozen shoulder (fibrous adhesive capsulitis)
    - Partial or total rupture of the supraspinatus portion of the rotator cuff

SLOPE OF THE SHOULDER

- Observe the region where the slope of the shoulder meets the neck (Fig. 39.12) from the anterior and posterior views.
  - These two surfaces should be symmetric and meet the vertical muscle mass of the cervical spine in the midcervical region.

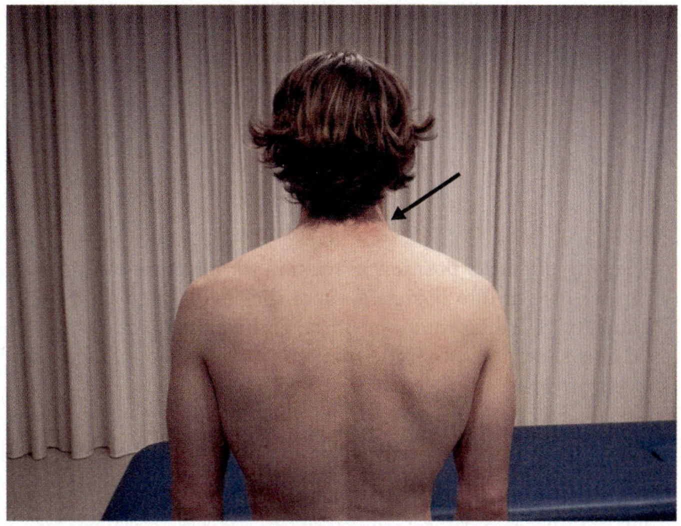

Figure 39.12. Observing slope of the shoulder. (Photo courtesy of Western University of Health Sciences, Pomona, CA, with permission.)

  - Asymmetry may indicate cervicothoracic scoliosis
  - Asymmetry must be interpreted with consideration of the scapular position.
    - A fold of skin that attaches to the neck at a location higher than the midcervical region constitutes a web neck, or pterygium colli. It may even attach as high as the mastoid process. This condition is associated with congenital disorders such as Klippel–Feil syndrome or Turner syndrome.

Clavicles

- Observe and palpate the clavicles for symmetry.
  - It is rare to see a case of congenital absence of the clavicles such as in cleidocranial dysplasia.
  - A clavicle can be misshapen due to:
    - Congenital anomaly
    - Fracture during birth
    - Subsequent fracture later typically shows a deformed clavicle due to old fracture with malunion (Fig. 39.13).
  - The length of the clavicle from sternum to acromion determines in part the shoulder's position.

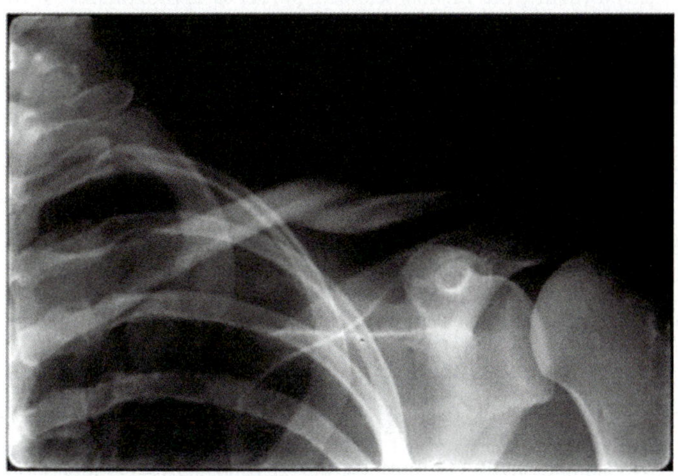

Figure 39.13. Observing the clavicles. (Courtesy of Western University of Health Sciences, Pomona, CA, with permission.)

- ☐ The clavicle is the upper extremity's only bony connection to the axial skeleton.
  - A shortened clavicle often causes anterior shoulder carriage (shoulder protraction), pulling the scapula farther away from the spinal column than it is on the contralateral side.

Arm Position and Length

- Viewing the arms' position in relation to the trunk can provide further insight into dysfunctions of the shoulder girdle musculature, by revealing rotations of the entire extremity.
  - ☐ This should be observed from the anterior, lateral, and posterior views.
- The distance of the arms from the torso also elucidates the possibility of scoliosis, postural decompensation, or pelvic side shift.
- Observe the symmetry of carrying angle of the arms.
- Observe the length of the arms from acromion to fingertip.
  - ☐ A patient may present with a short arm, in the same manner they present with a short leg, giving the false impression of spinal or shoulder dysfunction or deformity.
  - ☐ This asymmetry becomes significant for work and sports involving the upper extremities.

Scapular Landmarks

- The relative positions of the scapulae are under numerous muscular and postural influences. The most important scapular landmarks are the:
  - ☐ Acromion process
  - ☐ Spine of the scapula (T3 spinous process level)
  - ☐ Inferior angle of the scapula (T7 spinous process level)
  - ☐ Medial scapular border
- If the spinal column is vertical, the scapular landmarks (along with the shoulder level) should be symmetrically horizontal.
- Asymmetry to scapular position and motion may be due to in imbalance of the scapular musculature (scapular dyskinesia) or an injury to the long thoracic or spinal accessory nerve (scapular winging).
- Assess the level of the inferior angles of the scapula (Fig. 39.14).
  - ☐ If a scoliosis side bends the spinal column to the right, in this region the right scapular landmarks will be more inferior than those of the left.
- Assess the medial borders and spine of the scapula.
  - ☐ Normally, the medial scapular border is approximately 2 to 3 inches from the spinous processes and should roughly be parallel to the spine, regardless of the spine's configuration at this level.
  - ☐ Forward carriage of one shoulder will result in the medial scapular border being farther from the spinous processes than normal.
  - ☐ Rotation of the scapula due to shoulder muscle imbalances will result in a loss of the parallel relationship between the spine and the medial border of the scapula.
    - Medial rotation may be due to weakness of the serratus anterior muscle or from long thoracic nerve dysfunction (scapular winging).
    - Lateral scapular rotation may be due to weakness in the trapezius muscle or spinal accessory nerve (CN XI) dysfunction.
- A scapula positioned more superiorly than normal, *scapula alta*, implies the presence of hypertonic or contractures of the musculature involving the shoulder elevators:

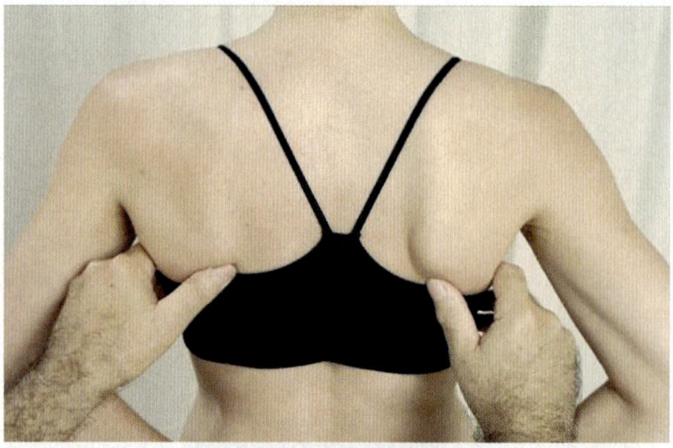

A

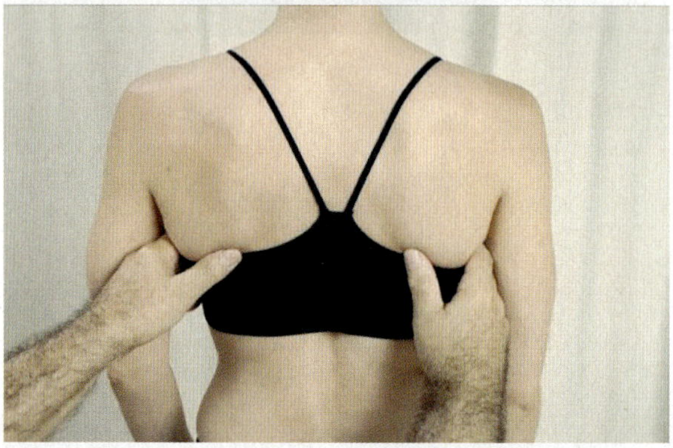

B

Figure 39.14. Assessing the level of the inferior angles of the scapula. A. Patient's hands placed on lumbar spine to aid physician in locating the inferior angles of the scapulae. **B.** Palpation for scapulae levels with patient standing at ease. (Photo courtesy of Western University of Health Sciences, Pomona, CA, with permission.)

  - ☐ Upper trapezius muscles
  - ☐ The rhomboids
  - ☐ Levator scapulae

  Note: A scapula that is sufficiently high and present from birth represents a congenital Sprengel deformity.
- A scapula positioned more inferiorly than normal, *scapula infra*, may represent weakness of the shoulder elevators instead of hypertonicity of the shoulder depressor muscles:
  - ☐ Latissimus dorsi
  - ☐ Lower trapezius
  - ☐ Lower serratus anterior
- If the patient complains of shoulder pain or if scapular asymmetry is observed during screening, further evaluation of scapular position and motion should include observing symmetry during active shoulder ROM and passive translation of the scapula in each of the three planes of motion.[9]

Upper Extremity Screening, Neurologic, and Orthopedic Tests

The *Overhead Upper Extremity Quick Test* is a screening test for possible somatic dysfunction of the upper extremities. Other upper extremity joint–specific neurologic and orthopedic tests would be performed after observing, palpating, and assessing the range of motion for a given region.

OVERHEAD UPPER EXTREMITY QUICK TEST

This is a screening test for possible somatic dysfunction of the upper extremities. This is typically observed from the anterior vantage point. The patient may be standing or seated.

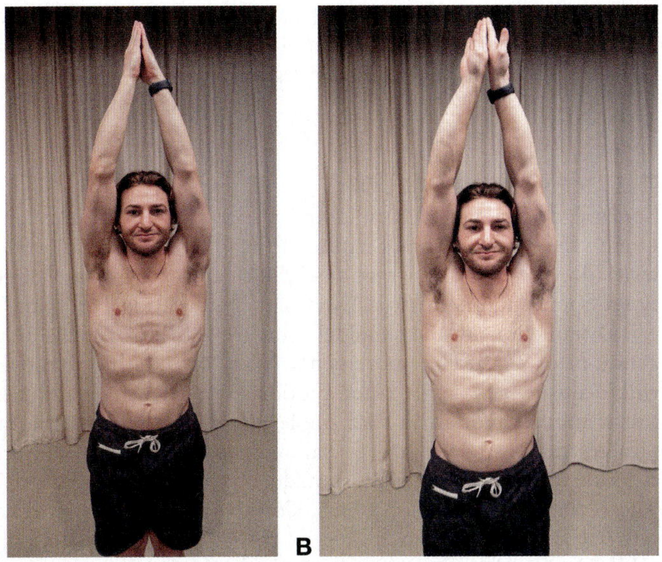

A B

Figure 39.15. Negative Overhead Upper Extremity Quick Test. **A.** Palms together. **B.** Dorsal surfaces of hands together. (Photo courtesy of Western University of Health Sciences, Pomona, CA, with permission.)

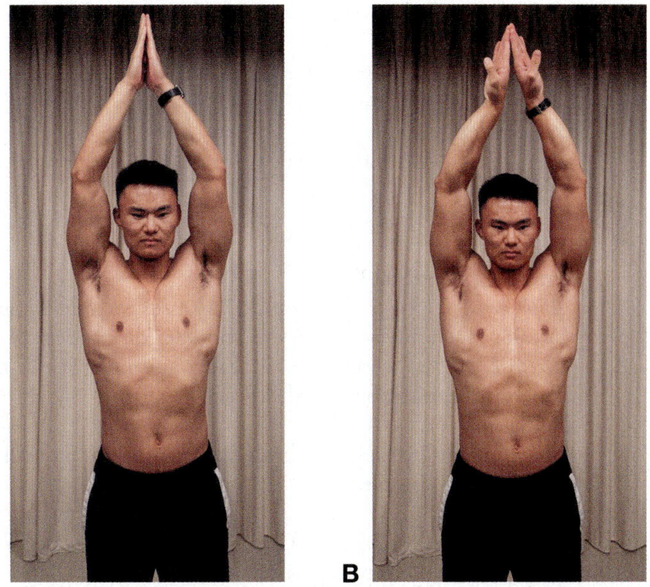

A B

Figure 39.16. Positive Overhead Upper Extremity Quick Test. **A.** Palms together. **B.** Dorsal surfaces of hands together. (Photo courtesy of Western University of Health Sciences, Pomona, CA, with permission.)

The patient actively fully abducts both arms in the coronal plane over the head, first with the palms together and again with dorsal surfaces of the hands together (Fig. 39.15).

The test is ***negative*** if the patient, with their head and neck in the neutral position, can raise the arms fully overhead, with the medial surfaces of the upper arms touching the ears, the elbows fully extended, the forearms fully pronated, and the backs of the hands together over the head. When the test is repeated, the patient should be able to accomplish the same position with the forearms fully supinated and the palms together over the head. If the patient can do this, then somatic dysfunction of the joints of the shoulders, elbows, radioulnar regions, and wrists are not as likely to be present.

The test is ***positive*** if the patient is unable to bring the medial surfaces of the upper arms against their ears, the elbows and/or wrists cannot be fully extended, and/or the backs of the hands or palms of the hands cannot be placed together over the head. This indicates a possible orthopedic condition and/or upper extremity somatic dysfunction. The joints and tissues of the upper extremity need to be more specifically examined to determine a diagnosis (Fig. 39.16).

Keep in mind that somatic dysfunction of the upper extremity can occur because of restricted motion in the ACJ, SCJ, clavicle, scapulae, upper ribs, upper thoracic region, and the large muscle groups of the shoulder. Also, if the patient has specific hand, wrist, or elbow pain or dysfunction, further evaluation to those areas should be done.

NEUROVASCULAR TESTS FOR THE UPPER EXTREMITY[23,24]

- *Cervical Nerve Root Compression Test* (Spurling sign, test, or maneuver) assesses for nerve root compression syndromes, cervical radiculopathy.
  - Extension, sidebending, and axial compression of the cervical spine toward the side being tested can narrow the intervertebral foramina. A positive test produces symptoms of nerve root compression such as pain, numbness, and tingling that radiate down the arm.
  - Conversely, applying manual traction (distraction) to the cervical region usually offers relief
- *Adson Test* assesses for neurovascular compression in the thoracic outlet.
  - The patient is instructed to side bend head away from affected side. Then the shoulder on affected side is abducted and extended (horizontal abduction) while monitoring the radial pulse.
  - A decrease in radial pulse indicates likely vascular compression in the thoracic outlet region. Reproduced radicular symptoms in the upper extremity indicates likely neurologic compression in the thoracic outlet region.
- *Roos Test* assesses for neurovascular compression in the thoracic outlet.
- *Allen Test* and *Modified Allen Test* determine if the radial and ulnar arteries are supplying the hand to their full capacity.
- *Tinel sign of the elbow* assesses for ulnar nerve entrapment at the cubital tunnel.
- *Tinel sign of the wrist* assesses for median nerve entrapment at the transverse carpal ligament.
- *Hoffmann sign* is an involuntary flexion of the DIP joints of the patient's thumb and little finger may be indicative of an upper motor neuron lesion and corticospinal pathway dysfunction.

Many of the above tests are described in Chapter 73 Osteopathic Considerations in Neurology.

ORTHOPEDIC TESTS FOR THE UPPER EXTREMITY[23,24]

- Shoulder:
  - ACJ
    - *Horizontal Adduction Stress Test (Cross Arm Adduction/Scarf Sign)* assesses for ACJ sprain or inflammation.
    - *Hawkins–Kennedy Test* assesses for shoulder impingement.
      - Involved structures include supraspinatus tendon, the long head of the biceps, and/or the ACJ.
  - Rotator Cuff
    - *Neer Impingement Test* assesses for impingement and irritation of the supraspinatus muscle.

  - *Empty Can Sign (Jobe Test)* assesses for a tear of the supraspinatus muscle.
  - *Drop Arm Test** assess for rotator cuff tears (especially in the supraspinatus muscle).
- □ Bicep Tendon
  - *Speeds Test* assesses for a tear or irritation of the long head of the biceps.
  - *Yergason Test** assesses for biceps pathology and SLAP lesions.
- □ Labral/Ligament Stability
  - *Apprehension Sign* of the shoulder* assesses for anterior and inferior instability secondary to shoulder dislocations.
  - *Biceps Load Test** assesses for stability and integrity of the superior glenoid labrum (SLAP tear).
- □ Range of motion
  - *Apley Scratch Test** assesses for decreased range of motion of the shoulder complex

- Elbow
  - □ *Resisted wrist extension test (Cozen Sign/Tennis Elbow Test)* assesses for lateral epicondylitis.
  - □ *Tinel sign of the elbow* assesses for ulnar nerve entrapment at the cubital tunnel.
- Wrist
  - □ *Allen Test** assesses radial and ulnar artery supply to the hand.
  - □ *Tinel Sign* of the carpal tunnel, *Phalen Test,* and *Reverse Phalen Test* all assess for median nerve entrapment at the wrist/carpal tunnel syndrome.
  - □ *Finklestein Test*[25] assesses for radial styloid (first compartment) tenosynovitis also known as De Quervain tenosynovitis.

The above orthopedic tests marked with * are described fully Chapter 84 Osteopathic Considerations in Orthopedics section Specific Orthopedic Tests (Organized by Chief Complaint).

JOINT-SPECIFIC EXAMINATION

When evaluating a complaint of a specific area of the upper extremity, it is important to compare that region bilaterally as well as inspect and palpate the joint above and below the area of concern. Please refer to Chapter 31 Osteopathic Segmental Examination to understand how specific components of the upper extremity exam are integrated into the entire patient evaluation.

Please refer to Chapter 91 Osteopathic Approach to Diagnosing and Treating Somatic Dysfunction in the Extremities for detailed descriptions of joint motion and tables identifying various joint somatic dysfunction nomenclature.

Function of the upper extremity is essential in performing ADLs. Minor injury and somatic dysfunction can have profound effects on these. It is very important to palpate for acute and chronic tissue texture changes and determine restrictions of motion and tenderness of various tissues. TART findings are commonly seen with orthopedic injuries, both traumatic and overuse. For patients with upper extremity symptomology, diagnose any segmental and group axial articular dysfunctions, especially in the thoracic and cervical regions. Evaluate the soft tissues of the anterior chest wall, the periscapular muscles, the trapezius, rhomboids, and scalene and the rotator cuff muscles. The latissimus dorsi is frequently involved and often forgotten. Remember how broad of an anatomic origin it has. Pay equal attention to palpating for articular dysfunctions, local tender points, and myofascial tissue tightness or looseness.

In addition to the articular and muscular joint motion asymmetry described below, the physician should also evaluate for the presence of other possible somatic dysfunction manifestations, such as myofascial restrictions (see Chapter 52), counterstrain tender points (see Chapter 47), and Chapman reflex points (see Chapter 58) within the applicable regions.

The Shoulder and Pectoral Girdle

THE GLENOHUMERAL JOINT

Somatic dysfunction occurs in the minor motions of the joint. Due to the ball-and-socket nature of the GHJ, this would include restrictions of translatory motions, which can occur in many directions. Some authors call this "joint play," "translation," or "glide."

Dysfunctions of the shoulder joint are active or passive exaggerations of its cardinal movements. Many osteopathic physicians will evaluate each single-plane motion (i.e., extension) and treat restrictions of motion in that single plane. In addition to articular restrictions, there are fascial restrictions that can traverse the shoulder joint and limit shoulder motion (see Chapter 52). Jones strain–counterstrain points, along with Simons and Travel myofascial tender points, occur in the muscles controlling the GHJ. Dysfunctions elsewhere in the body can produce symptoms referable to the shoulder joint. For example, an ACJ dysfunction can cause deltoid muscle tension, just as a sacroiliac dysfunction can cause latissimus dorsi tightening. Both situations will produce shoulder pain. Greenman states that the primary motion loss involves abduction and external rotation.[6] The humeral head moves superiorly and inferiorly on the glenoid during abduction. Loss of this ability is significant in shoulder function.

THE STERNOCLAVICULAR JOINT

Potential SCJ somatic dysfunctions can occur in the following motions:

- Abduction/abduction movement
- Superior/inferior movement
- Anterior/posterior rotation movement

Please see Table 91.1 Sternoclavicular Joint (SCJ) Somatic Dysfunction for a summary of SCJ somatic dysfunction and its nomenclature.

Evaluation for Restriction in Superior/Inferior Glide of SCJ

1. Patient sits (Fig. 39.17) or lies supine (Fig. 39.18) with arms at the sides.
2. Physician stands at the side of the table.
3. The pads of the physician's index fingers are used to palpate the superior aspect of the medial ends of the patient's clavicles.
4. Patient is asked to raise the shoulders toward the ears (shoulder shrug) bilaterally.
5. Physician notes the movement of the medial ends of the clavicles.
   - □ Normally, the medial ends of the clavicles move inferiorly as the shoulders move superiorly.
   - □ If one clavicle fails to move inferiorly as compared to the opposite clavicle, then SC somatic dysfunction is present in the affected clavicle.

Evaluation for Restriction in Anterior/Posterior Glide of SCJ

1. Patient sits (Fig. 39.19) or lies supine (Fig. 39.20) with arms at the sides.
2. Physician stands at the side of the table.
3. The pads of the physician's index fingers are used to palpate the anterior aspect of the medial ends of the patient's clavicles.
4. Patient is asked to extend the arms by reaching toward the ceiling (bench press maneuver).

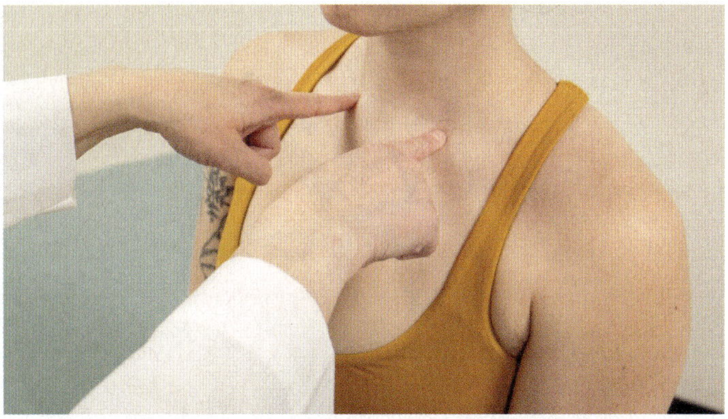

Figure 39.17. Seated evaluation of superior/inferior glide of medial clavicle. (Photo courtesy of Western University of Health Sciences, Pomona, CA, with permission.)

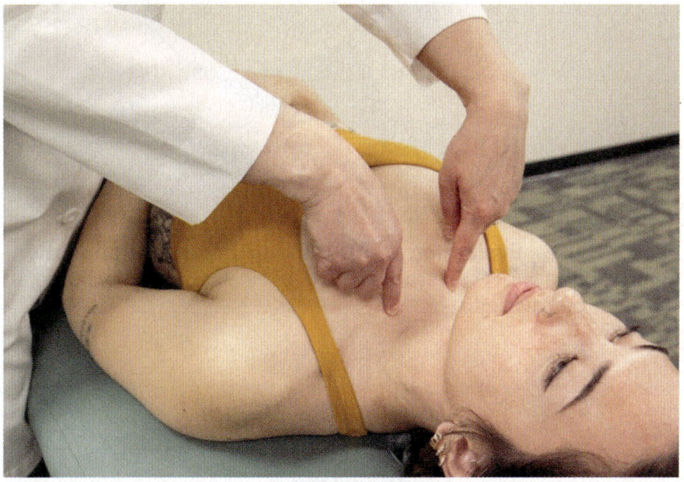

Figure 39.18. Supine evaluation of superior/inferior glide of medial clavicle. (Photo courtesy of Western University of Health Sciences, Pomona, CA, with permission.)

5. Physician notes the movement of the medial ends of the clavicles.
   a. Normally, the medial ends of the clavicles move posteriorly as the lateral ends of the clavicles move anteriorly.
   b. If one clavicle fails to move posteriorly as compared to the opposite clavicle, then SC somatic dysfunction is present in the affected clavicle.

THE ACROMIOCLAVICULAR JOINT

When evaluating the ACJ for each of the planes of motion described below, the physician should place one finger on the acromion and another on the distal clavicle to monitor for motion (rotation) of the clavicle compared to the acromion. Please see Table 91.2 Acromioclavicular Joint Somatic Dysfunction for a summary of ACJ somatic dysfunction and its nomenclature.

Evaluation for Restriction in Adduction and Abduction

1. Patient is seated.
2. The physician stands behind the patient.

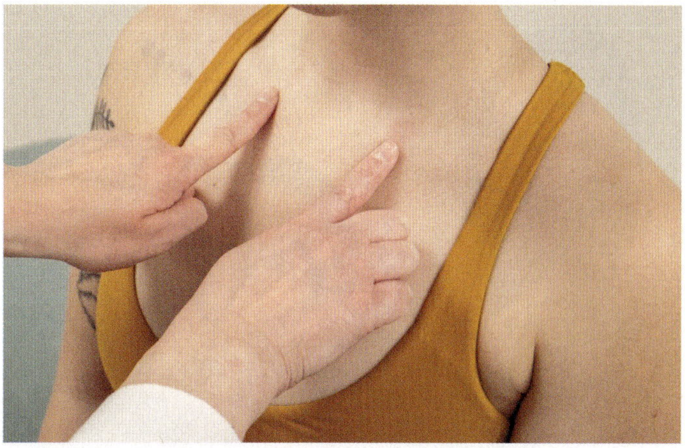

Figure 39.19. Seated evaluation of anterior/posterior glide of medial clavicle. (Photo courtesy of Western University of Health Sciences, Pomona, CA, with permission.)

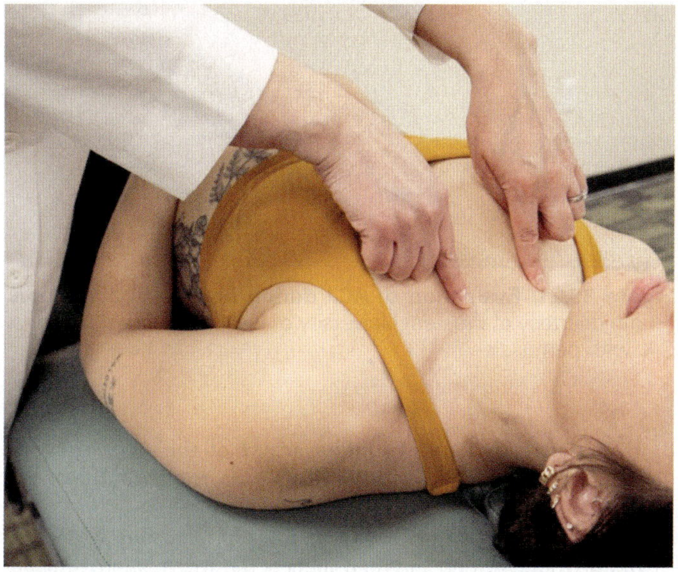

Figure 39.20. Supine evaluation of anterior/posterior glide of medial clavicle. (Photo courtesy of Western University of Health Sciences, Pomona, CA, with permission.)

3. Physician palpates the superior aspect of the ACJ with one hand while grasping the patient's forearm with the other hand.
4. Physician introduces adduction and external rotation of the patient's forearm while monitoring for a gapping motion at the ACJ (Fig. 39.21).
5. Comparison is made with the opposite ACJ.
   - Absence of the gapping motion indicates the presence of somatic dysfunction of the ACJ.
6. Physician then introduces abduction and internal rotation of the patient's arm while monitoring for a gapping motion at the ACJ (Fig. 39.22).
7. Comparison is made with the opposite ACJ.
   - Absence of the gapping motion indicates the presence of somatic dysfunction of the ACJ.

Evaluation for Restriction in Internal and External Rotation

1. Patient is seated.
2. Physician stands behind the patient.

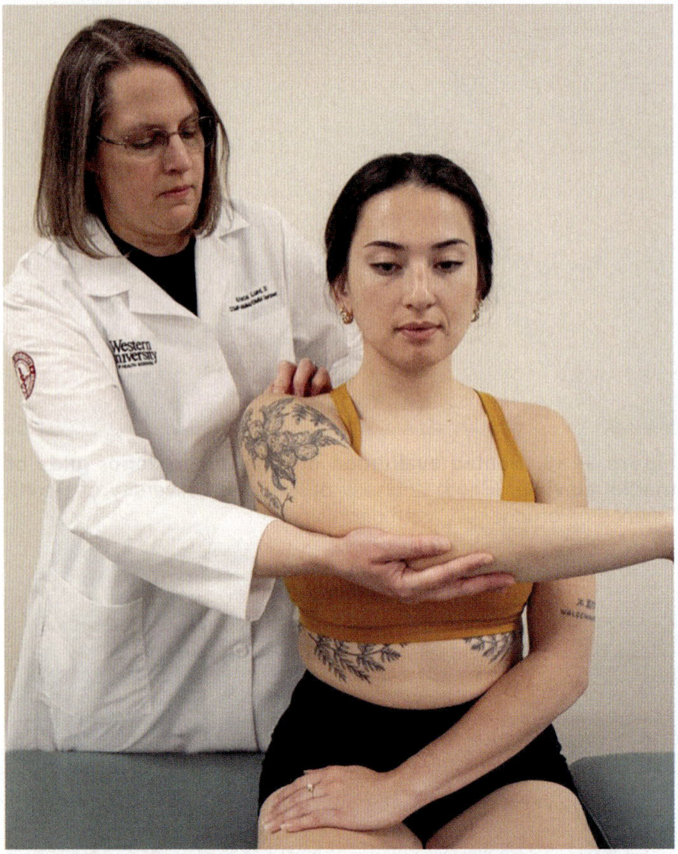

Figure 39.21. Evaluation of ACJ during horizontal adduction. (Photo courtesy of Western University of Health Sciences, Pomona, CA, with permission.)

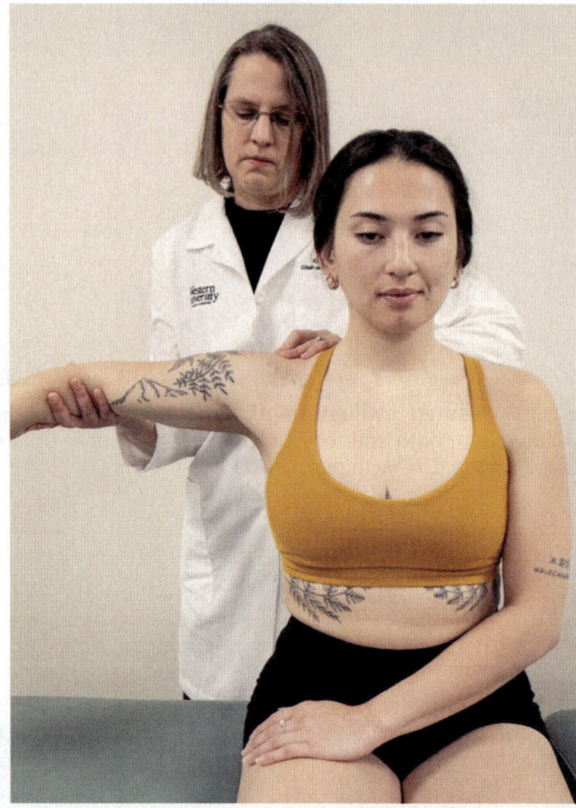

Figure 39.22. Evaluation of ACJ during horizontal abduction. (Photo courtesy of Western University of Health Sciences, Pomona, CA, with permission.)

3. Physician palpates the superior aspect of the ACJ with one hand while grasping the patient's forearm with the other hand.
4. Physician places the patient's arm into approximately 30 degrees of horizontal flexion and then abducts the arm to approximately 90 degrees.
5. Physician then introduces internal (Fig. 39.23) and external rotation (Fig. 39.24) of the patient's arm while monitoring for motion at the ACJ.
6. Comparison is made with the opposite ACJ.
   - Absence of motion at either ACJ indicates the presence of somatic dysfunction of the ACJ.

Evaluation for Restriction in Flexion and Extension

1. Patient is seated.
2. Physician stands behind the patient.
3. Physician palpates the superior aspect of the ACJ with one hand while grasping the patient's forearm with the other hand.
   - Note: This may also be performed with the patient's elbow flexed and slightly abducted. Physician would grasp the patient's arm under the elbow.
4. Physician then introduces flexion (Fig. 39.25) and extension (Fig. 39.26) of the patient's arm while monitoring for motion at the ACJ.
5. Comparison is made with the opposite ACJ.
   - Absence of motion at either ACJ indicates the presence of somatic dysfunction of the ACJ.

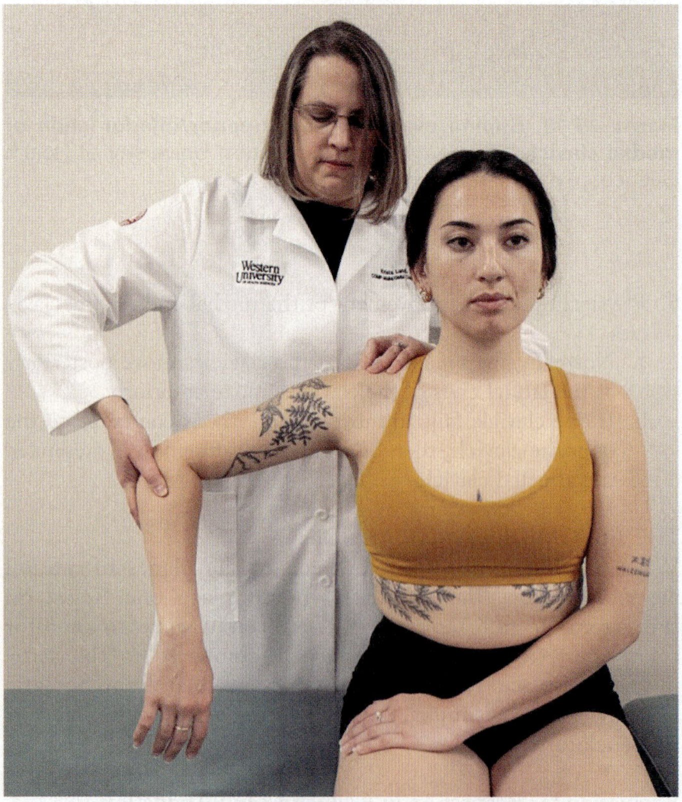

Figure 39.23. Evaluation of ACJ during internal rotation. (Photo courtesy of Western University of Health Sciences, Pomona, CA, with permission.)

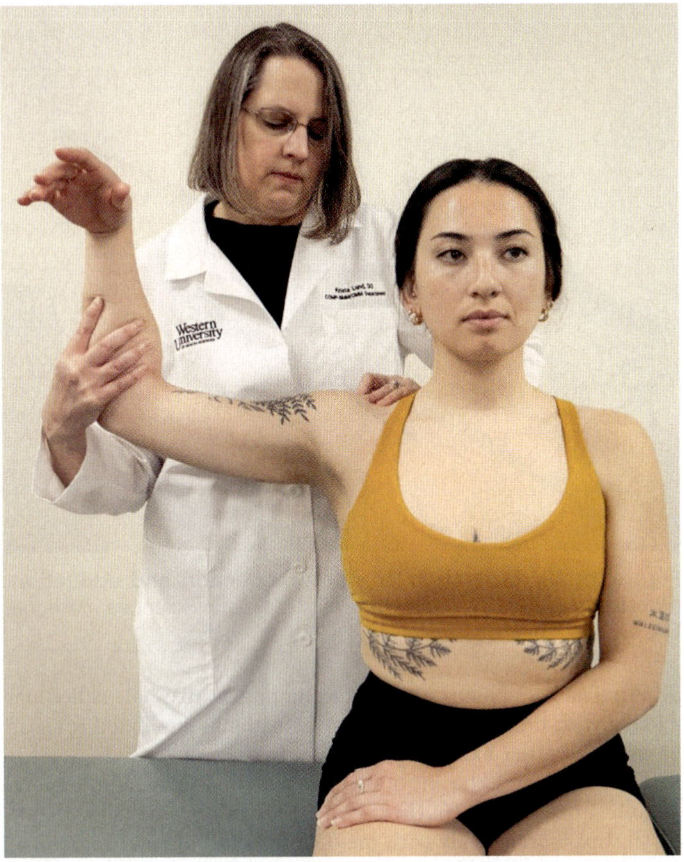

Figure 39.24. **Evaluation of ACJ during external rotation.** (Photo courtesy of Western University of Health Sciences, Pomona, CA, with permission.)

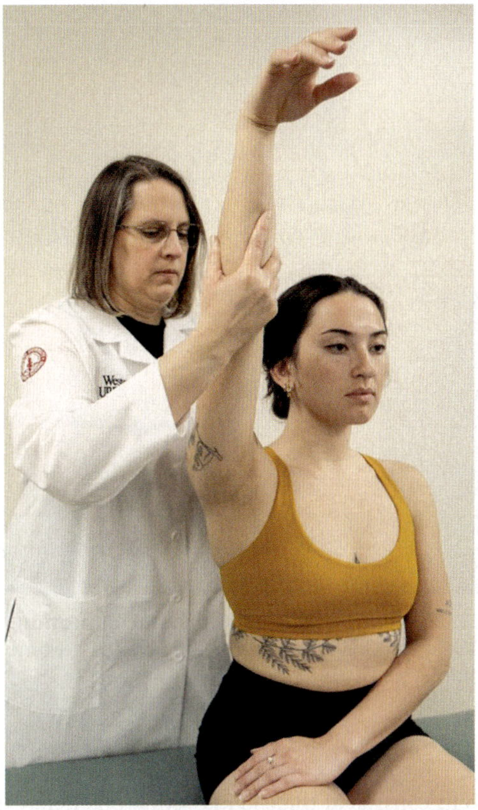

Figure 39.25. **Evaluation of ACJ during flexion.** (Photo courtesy of Western University of Health Sciences, Pomona, CA, with permission.)

THE SCAPULOTHORACIC REGION

Scapular position and motion on the thoracic wall, independent of GH motion is dependent on several of the muscles attaching the scapula to the spine and ribs as well as influences from gravity and the inferior sternocostal head of the pectoralis major[1,7]:

1. Elevation
2. Depression
3. Protraction
4. Retraction
5. Internal rotation (Lateral rotation of inferior angle)
6. External rotation (Medial rotation of inferior angle)

Evaluation for Restriction in Scapulothoracic Motion

1. Patient lies on the table in the lateral recumbent position.
2. Physician stands at the side of the table facing the patient.
3. Physician grasps the patient's scapula with both hands (Fig. 39.27).
4. Physician tests the following scapular motions:
   - □ Superior and inferior glide
   - □ Medial and lateral glide
   - □ Rotation (clockwise and counterclockwise)
5. Patient then lies on the opposite side. Steps 3 to 4 are repeated, and comparison of the motions of the two scapulae is made.
   - □ Restriction in any of the motions tested is indicative of somatic dysfunction in the scapular region.

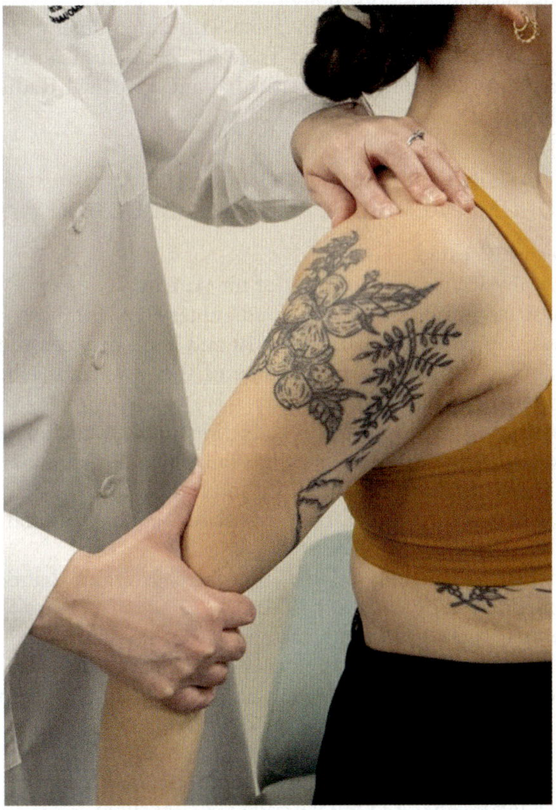

Figure 39.26. **Evaluation of ACJ during extension.** (Photo courtesy of Western University of Health Sciences, Pomona, CA, with permission.)

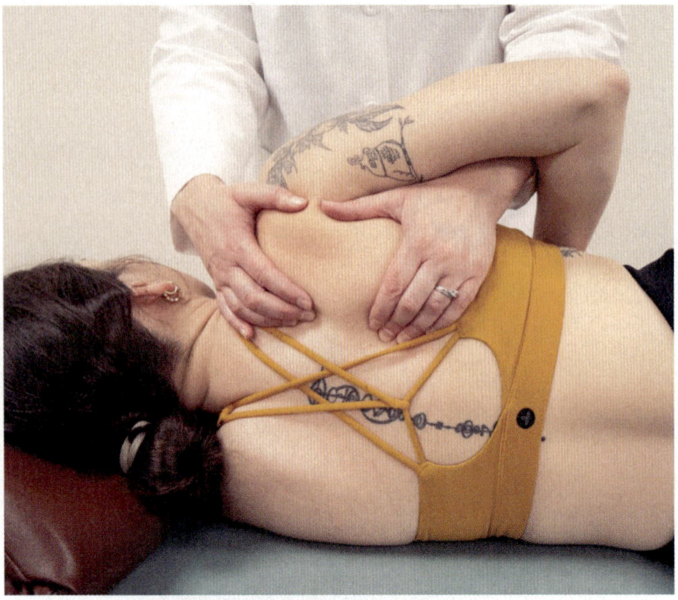

Figure 39.27. Evaluation of scapulothoracic motion. (Photo courtesy of Western University of Health Sciences, Pomona, CA, with permission.)

The Elbow

The elbow joint consists of three joints within one joint capsule:

1. The humero-ulnar joint (ulnohumeral joint)
2. The humero-radial joint (radiohumeral joint)
3. The proximal radio-ulnar joint

The motion and the nomenclature for somatic dysfunction of these joints are described in Table 91.4 Ulnohumeral (Elbow) Joint Somatic Dysfunction and Table 91.5 Radial Head Somatic Dysfunction (Combined Humeroradial and Proximal Radioulnar Joint Motion).

EVALUATION FOR RESTRICTION IN ELBOW (ULNOHUMERAL) ABDUCTION AND ADDUCTION

1. Patient is seated.
2. The physician stands in front of the patient.
3. Physician grasps the proximal radioulnar area with both hands.
4. Physician places the patient's wrist and hand between the physician's trunk and the medial side of the physician's elbow, to support it (Fig. 39.28).
5. Physician introduces ulnar abduction and adduction (elbow goes laterally and hand goes medially) of the radioulnar joint by translating the joint medially and laterally.
   - □ Ulnar abduction: Elbow translates medially, hand goes laterally
   - □ Ulnar adduction: Elbow translates laterally, hand goes medially
6. Comparison is made with the opposite radioulnar joint.
   - □ Restriction of adduction or abduction indicates the presence of somatic dysfunction of the ulnohumeral radioulnar joint.

EVALUATION FOR RESTRICTION IN ELBOW (ULNOHUMERAL) FLEXION AND EXTENSION

1. Patient is seated.
2. Physician stands in front of the patient.

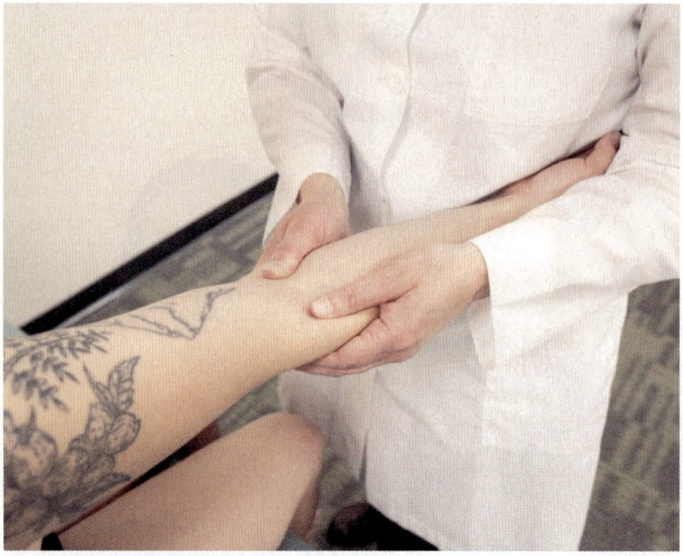

Figure 39.28. Evaluation of elbow abduction and adduction. (Photo courtesy of Western University of Health Sciences, Pomona, CA, with permission.)

3. Physician stabilizes the distal humerus/proximal radioulnar area with one hand and grasps the patient's supinated forearm with the other hand.
4. Physician tests the motion of the ulnohumeral radiohumeral joint from full flexion (Fig. 39.29) to full extension (Fig. 39.30).
5. Comparison is made with the opposite ulnohumeral/radioulnar joint.
   - □ Restriction of flexion or extension indicates the presence of somatic dysfunction of the ulnohumeral/radioulnar joint.

EVALUATION OF FOREARM PRONATION AND SUPINATION AND RADIAL HEAD MOTION

1. Patient is seated with arms in neutral position (no humoral flexion or extension) and elbow flexed to 90 degrees.
2. Physician stands in front of the patient.

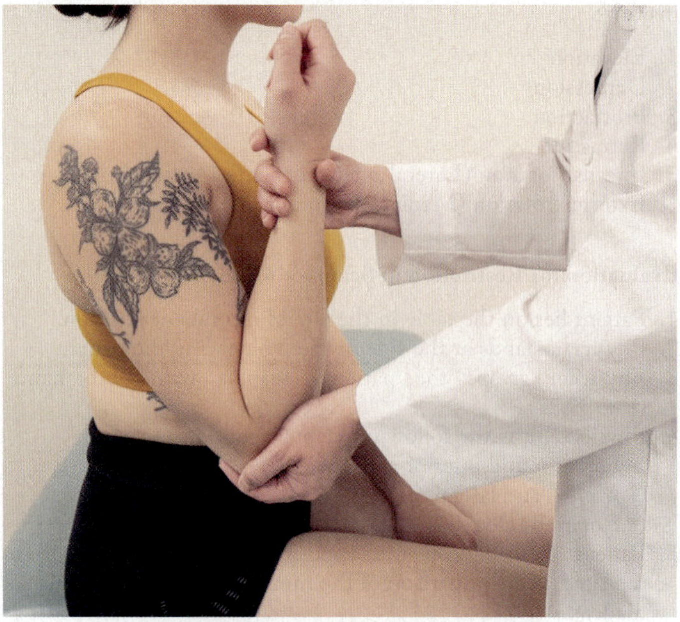

Figure 39.29. Evaluation of elbow flexion. (Photo courtesy of Western University of Health Sciences, Pomona, CA, with permission.)

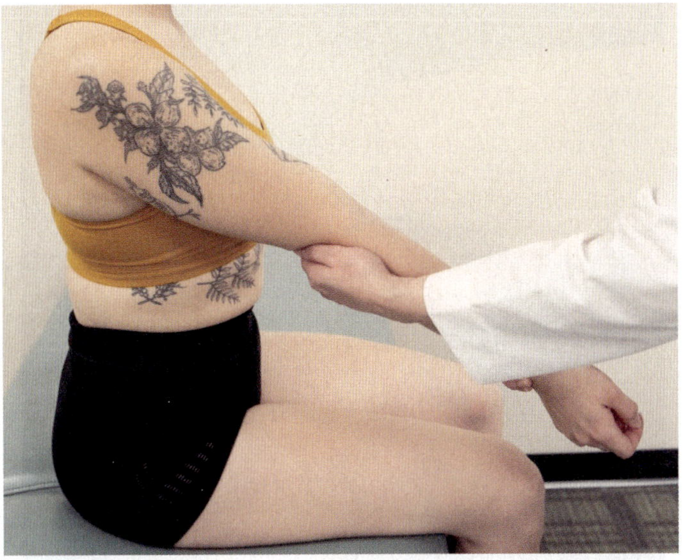

Figure 39.30. Evaluation of elbow extension. (Photo courtesy of Western University of Health Sciences, Pomona, CA, with permission.)

3. Physician stabilizes the proximal radial head with one hand and grasps the patient's distal forearm with the other hand, placing it in a neutral position with the patient's thumb in a vertical position, pointed superiorly.
   - □ Note: Radial head motion is a combination of humeroradial and proximal radioulnar joint motion.
4. Physician introduces pronation and supination (Fig. 39.31), noting any restriction of that motion, and noting any restriction of the anterolateral–posteromedial motion of the radial head.
   - □ Restriction of forearm pronation or supination in the absence of other radial head findings like tissue texture change, tenderness or palpable anterolateral–posteromedial motion of the radial head indicates the presence of other musculoskeletal or myofascial somatic dysfunction within the elbow, forearm, and/or wrist.
   - □ Restriction of anterolateral–posteromedial motion of the radial head, tenderness or tissue texture change at the radial head indicates articular radial head somatic dysfunction. Table 91.5 Radial Head Somatic Dysfunction (Combined Humeroradial and Proximal Radioulnar Joint Motion)

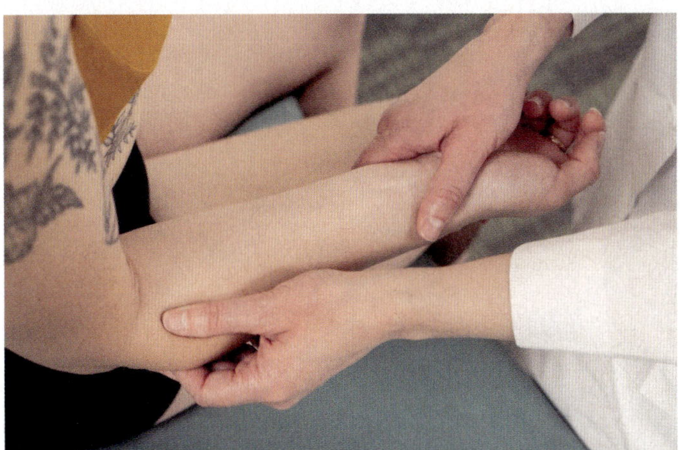

Figure 39.31. Evaluation of forearm pronation and supination and radial head motion. (Photo courtesy of Western University of Health Sciences, Pomona, CA, with permission.)

The Wrist and Hand

The wrist joint moves around A/P and transverse axes, allowing for the movements of flexion, extension, abduction (radial deviation), and adduction (ulnar deviation). Somatic dysfunction is not related to the gross motions of the wrist but instead to dysfunction of the small gliding motions of the proximal carpal bones on the radius as the wrist is moved. The carpals can move slightly anteriorly, posteriorly, medially, or laterally. Somatic dysfunction of the wrist was conventionally named according to the direction of motion preference. However, documenting the restriction has become increasingly more common.

For further information on motion and somatic dysfunction nomenclature see:

- Table 91.6 Radiocarpal (Wrist) Joint Somatic Dysfunction
- Box 91.1 Intercarpal Joint Diagnostic Findings[8]

EVALUATION OF RESTRICTION OF THE WRIST REGION

1. Patient is seated.
2. Physician stands in front of the patient.
3. Patient's arms are at the sides, with the elbows flexed to 90 degrees.
4. Physician tests the following motions in each of the patient's wrists by stabilizing the patient's wrist:
   - □ Dorsiflexion (extension) (Fig. 39.32)
   - □ Palmar flexion (flexion) (Fig. 39.33)
   - □ Ulnar deviation (adduction) pronated
   - □ Radial deviation (abduction) pronated
   - □ Ulnar deviation (adduction) supinated (Fig. 39.34)
   - □ Radial deviation (abduction) supinated (Fig. 39.35)
     - **Note:** Ulnar and radial deviation restrictions may differ when the forearm is positioned in pronation or supination due to reciprocal motion of ulnohumeral and radiocarpal joints. Restriction of wrist flexion and extension does not significantly differ with forearm supination or pronation. Always compare findings bilaterally.
   - □ Any restrictions of these motions noted may indicate the presence of somatic dysfunction of the wrist region.
5. Physician may then repeat motion testing for any specific radiocarpal or intercarpal joint by contacting the specific carpal

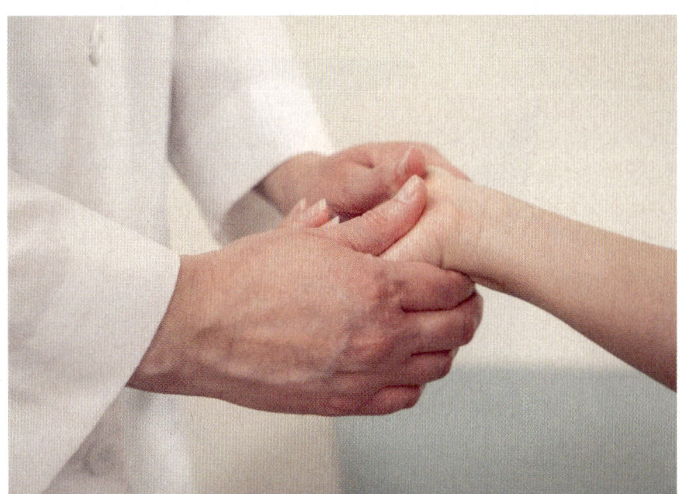

Figure 39.32. Evaluation of wrist extension with forearm supinated. (Photo courtesy of Western University of Health Sciences, Pomona, CA, with permission.)

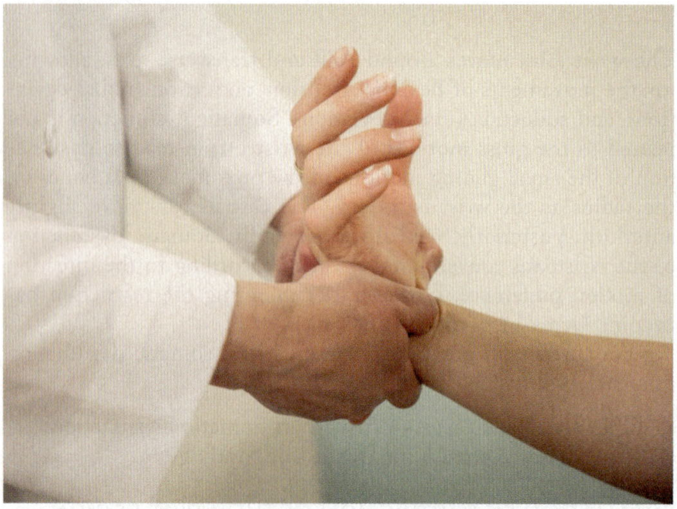

Figure 39.33. Evaluation of wrist flexion with forearm supinated. (Photo courtesy of Western University of Health Sciences, Pomona, CA, with permission.)

bone, stabilizing the proximal area, and inducing the following gliding motions on that carpal bone:

- □ Extension with anterior glide
- □ Flexion with posterior glide
- □ Adduction with lateral glide
- □ Abduction with medial glide
  - Any restrictions of these motions noted may indicate the presence of somatic dysfunction of a specific carpal bone in relation to the surrounding bones.

EVALUATION FOR RESTRICTION OF THE METACARPALS AND PHALANGES

1. Patient is seated.
2. Physician stands in front of the patient.
3. Patient's arms are at the sides, with the elbows flexed to 90 degrees.
4. Physician tests the following metacarpal and phalangeal motions by stabilizing the proximal bone and moving the distal bone upon it in each hand:
   - □ Anterior and posterior glide (Figs. 39.36 and 39.37)

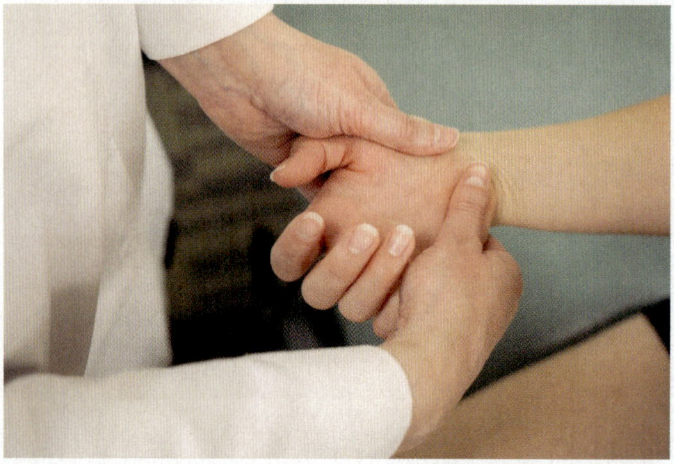

Figure 39.34. Evaluation of wrist ulnar deviation with forearm supinated. (Photo courtesy of Western University of Health Sciences, Pomona, CA, with permission.)

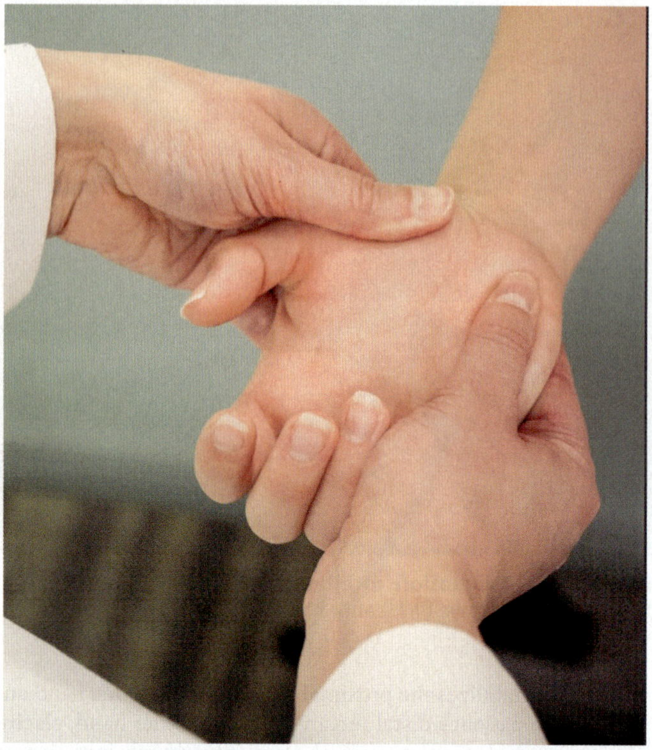

Figure 39.35. Evaluation of wrist radial deviation with forearm supinated. (Photo courtesy of Western University of Health Sciences, Pomona, CA, with permission.)

   - □ Medial and lateral glide
   - □ External and internal rotation
     - Any restrictions of these motions noted may indicate the presence of somatic dysfunction of the associated structure.

In addition to the above joint motion restrictions, the physician should also examine the upper extremity for the following:

- Myofascial restrictions. See Chapter 36 for more information about evaluation of myofascial structures.
- Counterstrain tender points. See Chapter 37 for more information about counterstrain.

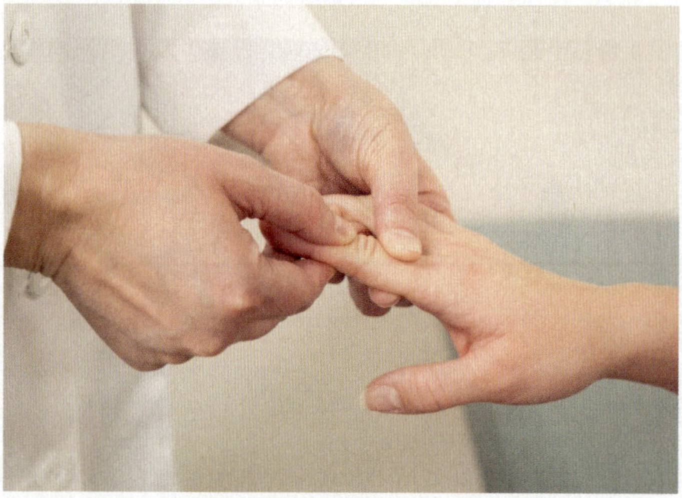

Figure 39.36. Evaluation of phalangeal (PIP) anterior glide (extension). (Photo courtesy of Western University of Health Sciences, Pomona, CA, with permission.)

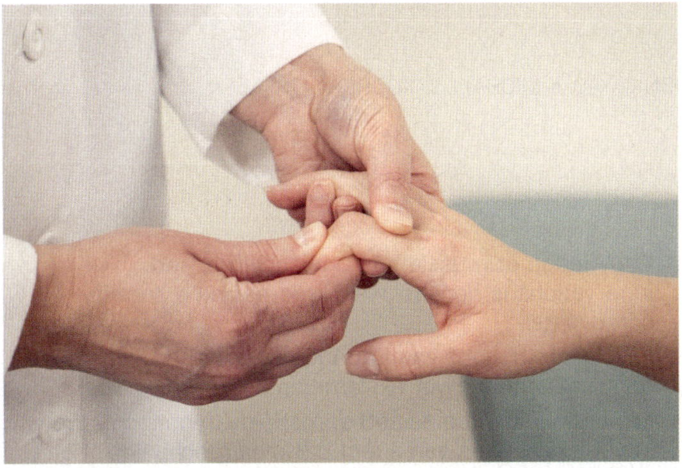

Figure 39.37. **Evaluation of phalangeal (PIP) posterior glide (flexion).** (Photo courtesy of Western University of Health Sciences, Pomona, CA, with permission.)

- Chapman reflexes. See Chapter 40 for more information about Chapman reflexes.

SUMMARY

Osteopathic diagnosis and treatment of upper extremity conditions has its foundation in the knowledge and application of functional anatomy. Applying structure and function relationships between various systems and regions in the patient provides a much more thorough understanding and specific treatment plan. Local and distant areas of somatic dysfunction may be involved in patients with upper extremity symptoms. Consider the upper extremity on a systems basis looking at the articular, myofascial, muscular, vascular/lymphatic, and ligamentous aspects. Try to synthesize your history, physical and palpatory findings, and orthopedic tests into a differential diagnosis prior to ordering diagnostic studies. The five models of osteopathic medicine can assist in developing the differential as well as an osteopathic treatment plan.

REFERENCES

1. Dalley AF II, Agur AMR. *Moore's Clinically Oriented Anatomy*. 9th ed. Wolters Kluwer; 2023:142–295.
2. Hoppenfeld S. *Physical Examination of the Spine and Extremities*. Appleton & Lange; 1976.
3. Strachan F. Part IV appendicular technic. In: Fryette H, ed. *Principles of Osteopathic Technic*. Academy of Applied Osteopathy; 1954:134–199.
4. Seffinger MA; American Osteopathic Association. *Foundations of Osteopathic Medicine: Philosophy Science Clinical Applications and Research*. 4th ed. Wolters Kluwer; 2018:598–602.
5. DiGiovanna EL, Amen CJ, Burns DK. *An Osteopathic Approach to Diagnosis and Treatment*. 4th ed. Wolters Kluwer; 2021:359–396.
6. DeStefano LA. *Greenman's Principles of Manual Medicine*. 5th ed. Wolters Kluwer; 2017:375–418.
7. Nicholas AS, Nicholas EA. *Atlas of Osteopathic Techniques*. 4th ed. Wolters Kluwer Health/Lippincott Williams & Wilkins; 2022:347–364.
8. Kimberly PE, Halma K; Kirksville College of Osteopathic Medicine. *Outline of Osteopathic Manipulative Procedures: The Kimberly Manual 2006*. Updated 2008 ed. Walsworth Publishing Company; 2008:231–265.
9. Chang MC, Choo YJ, Hong K, Boudier-Revéret M, Yang S. Treatment of upper crossed syndrome: a narrative systematic review. *Healthcare (Basel)*. 2023;11(16):2328.
10. Crichton JCI, Funk L. The anatomy of the short head of biceps—not a tendon. *Int J Shoulder Surg*. 2009;3(4):75–79.
11. Baig MA, Bordoni B. Anatomy, shoulder and upper limb, pectoral muscles. [Updated August 28, 2023]. In: *StatPearls [Internet]*. StatPearls Publishing; 2024. https://www.ncbi.nlm.nih.gov/books/NBK545241/
12. Castelein B, Cagnie B, Parlevliet T, Cools A. Serratus anterior or pectoralis minor: which muscle has the upper hand during protraction exercises? *Man Ther*. 2016:22:158–164.
13. Travell JG, Simons DG. *Myofascial Pain and Dysfunction: The Trigger Point Manual*. Williams & Wilkins; 1983.
14. Syros A, Rizzo MG. Anatomy, shoulder and upper limb, teres major muscle. [Updated April 7, 2023]. In: *StatPearls [Internet]*. StatPearls Publishing; 2024. https://www.ncbi.nlm.nih.gov/books/NBK580487/
15. Kuchera WA, Kuchera ML. *Osteopathic Principles in Practice*. 2nd rev ed. Greyden Press; 1994.
16. Atasoy E. Thoracic outlet syndrome: anatomy. *Hand Clin*. 2004;20(1):7–14, v.
17. Kaplan J, Kanwal A. Thoracic outlet syndrome. [Updated April 10, 2023]. In: *StatPearls [Internet]*. StatPearls Publishing; 2024. https://www.ncbi.nlm.nih.gov/books/NBK557450/
18. Grunebach H, Arnold MW, Lum YW. Thoracic outlet syndrome. *Vasc Med*. 2015;20(5):493–495.
19. Benes M, Kachlik D, Kunc V, Kunc V. The arcade of Frohse: a systematic review and meta-analysis. *Surg Radiol Anat*. 2021;43(5):703–711.
20. Dey S, Guthmiller KB, Varacallo M. Complex regional pain syndrome. [Updated August 7, 2023]. In: *StatPearls [Internet]*. StatPearls Publishing; 2024. https://www.ncbi.nlm.nih.gov/books/NBK430719/
21. Nelson KE, Glonek T. *Somatic Dysfunction in Osteopathic Family Practice*. 2nd ed. Wolters Kluwer Health; 2015:13.
22. Chikly B. *Silent Waves: Theory and Practice of Lymph Drainage Therapy*. IHH Publishing; 2002.
23. Bickley L. *Bates' Guide to Physical Examination and History Taking*. 13th ed. Wolters Kluwer; 2021.
24. Ombregt L, Bisschop P, J ter Veer H. *A System of Orthopaedic Medicine*. 2nd ed. Elsevier Limited; 2003.
25. Wu F, Rajpura A, Sandher D. Finkelstein's test is superior to Eichhoff's test in the investigation of de Quervain's disease. *J Hand Microsurg*. 2018; 10(2):116–118.

40 Lower Extremity

KRISTA LUND ▪ KURT P. HEINKING ▪ SHELDON C. YAO ▪ MICHAEL L. KUCHERA

KEY CONCEPTS

- Familiarity with functional anatomy of the lower extremities is required for its accurate assessment and manipulative treatment procedures.
- The lower extremities supply the final common platform for postural alignment.
- The lower extremities provide support and locomotion through strong bones and powerful muscles.
- Knowledge of muscle anatomy, actions, and innervations is necessary for addressing extremity complaints.
- Fascial restrictions can impede venous and lymphatic drainage of the lower extremities.
- Structural pathologies and somatic dysfunction in the lower extremities can affect basic biomechanics of gait and have local, postural, and systemic implications.

INTRODUCTION

The structure and function of the lower extremities allow them to play several significant roles.

- They contribute to balance and to the body's postural strategies.
- They support and facilitate locomotion.
- They house the muscular "pumps" involved in locomotion, making them a major contributor in the return of venous and lymphatic fluids back to the central vascular system.
- Their condition is a key factor in designing exercise protocols important for a person's general health.

Understanding the complexity of the lower extremity anatomic relationships and their functions leads to a better discernment of the roles the lower extremities play. For example, in each foot alone, there are

- 126 muscles and ligaments
- 33 joints
- 26 articulating bones (plus two sesamoid bones under the first metatarsophalangeal joint)

Due to their many roles, structural pathologies and somatic dysfunction in the lower extremities have local, postural, *and* systemic implications. Effective diagnosis and treatment necessitate a thorough understanding of the structure and function within this region.

DEFINITION

The lower extremity includes the following regions[1]:

- Gluteal region—buttocks and hip
- Femoral region—thigh
- Knee region
- Leg region—connecting knee to ankle
- Ankle (talocrural) region
- Foot region

The lower extremity is also referred to as the lower limb.[1]

DESCRIPTIVE AND FUNCTIONAL ANATOMY

Skeletal, Arthrodial, and Ligamentous Structures

The aspects of the upper limb skeletal structures are depicted in Figure 40.1. Notice the palpable bony structures, which are important landmarks for the osteopathic screening and segmental examination.

The joints are covered in articular cartilage. The majority are synovial joints consisting of a capsule and synovial membrane. However, the distal tibiofibular joint is a fibrous syndesmosis with an interosseous membrane. Each of these joints is stabilized by ligaments, which limit joint motions and are a part of the normal end feel sensed when palpating joint motion.

HIP JOINT (FEMOROACETABULAR ARTICULATION)

The hip joint, or *coxa*, is a term used to indicate the articulation of the femoral head with the acetabular socket of the innominate (pelvic) bone. The acetabulum is the junction of the ilium, ischium, and pubic bones. Throughout this chapter, *hip* will be used interchangeably with the structural and functional elements associated with the femoroacetabular joint. The hip is a ball-and-socket synovial joint with a socket deeper than that of the glenoid fossa of the shoulder. The hip demonstrates the characteristic stability of this type of joint while allowing for mobility.

The *iliofemoral ligament* on the anterior aspect of the hip joint is the strongest ligament in the body. Because it is shaped like the letter Y, it is also called the Y ligament of Bigelow. This ligament tenses with full hip extension and helps to maintain ideal standing posture (military at-ease position) with minimal muscle activity. On the posterior side, the *ischiofemoral ligament* attaches to the ischial portion of the acetabular rim and wraps over the posterior and superior part of the hip joint where it attaches just medially to the base of the greater trochanter of the femur. This important anatomic configuration tends to screw the femoral head into the acetabulum with extension, which prevents hyperextension. Normal extension is typically limited to less than 35 degrees.[2] Functional hip ligaments are illustrated in Figure 40.2.

Restrictions of the hip joint movement can lead to potential somatic dysfunctions of the hip in the following directions[3–5]:

- Flexion/extension
- Abduction/adduction
- Internal/external rotation

It is important to note that the degree of flexion and extension possible at the hip joint depends on the position of the knee. If the knee is flexed, relaxing the hamstrings, the hip joint can be further flexed than when the knee is extended.

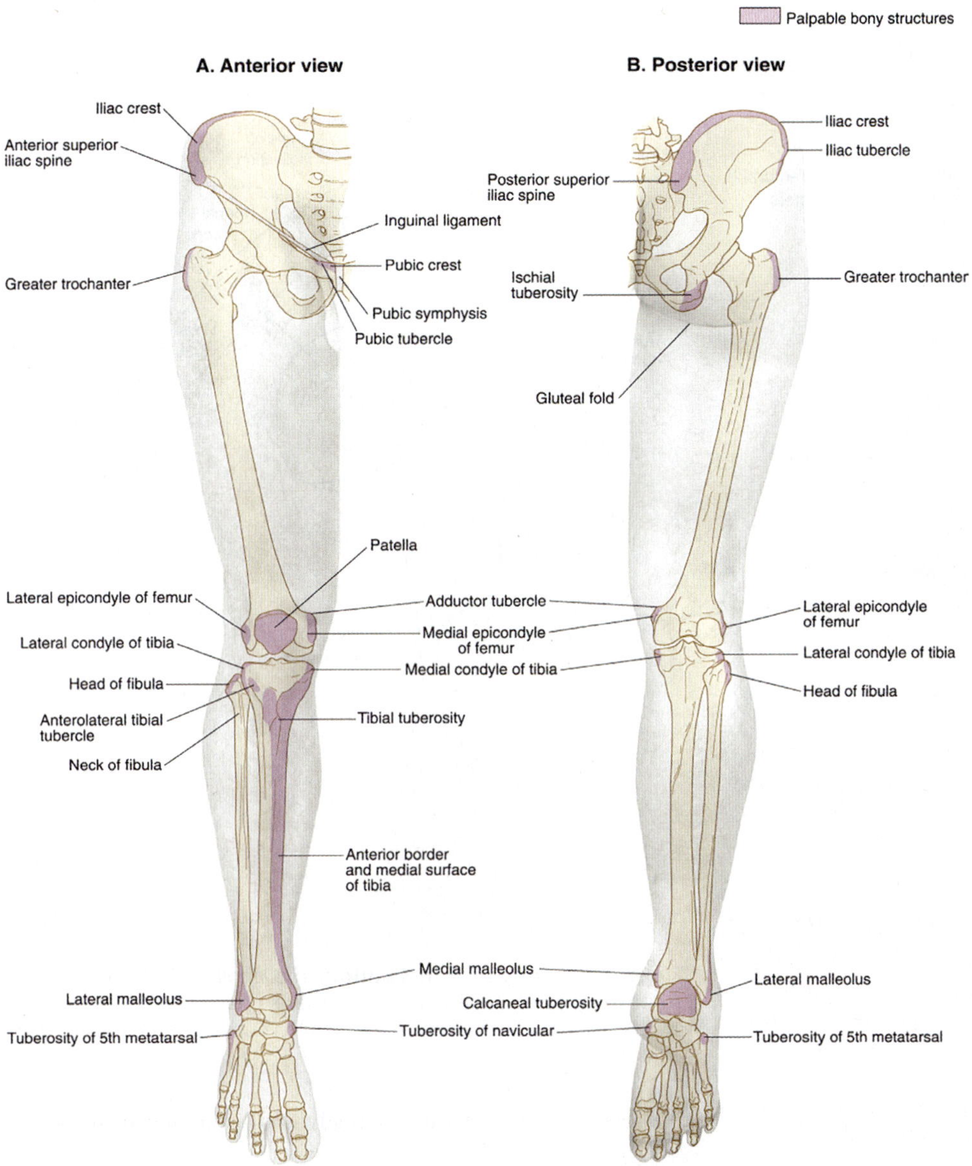

Figure 40.1. Palpable bony features of the upper extremity. (Reprinted with permission from Gest TR. *Lippincott® Atlas of Anatomy*. 2nd ed. Wolters Kluwer; 2020:35. Plate 2-01.)

FEMUR

The femur is the longest and heaviest bone in the body, attaining a length about one-fourth the height of an adult.[1] Therefore, a forensic pathologist or archaeologist can estimate an individual's height based on the femur alone.

The angle formed by the intersection of the long axis of the femoral neck and the femoral shaft is termed the *angle of inclination*.

- This angle varies with age, sex, and development of the femur.
- It normally measures 120 to 135 degrees in adults.
- If the angle is greater than 135 degrees, the condition is referred to as *coxa valga*, and if less than 120 degrees, then as *coxa vara*, respectively (Fig. 40.3).[6]
- The femoral shaft is twisted so that the condyles of the distal femur are in a transverse plane, even though the femoral neck angles forward 12 to 15 degrees; this is called the *angle of anteversion*.

Angle deviation at the femur can contribute to postural and gait disturbances and is an important factor in hip replacements. (See Chapter 84 Osteopathic Considerations in Orthopedics.)

KNEE JOINT

The knee, *genu*, is a compound synovial joint consisting of three separate articulations within one joint capsule:

- The medial femorotibial articulation
- The lateral femorotibial articulation
- The patellofemoral articulation

The knee is primarily a hinge joint, allowing for flexion (0 to 135 degrees) and extension (0 to 15 degrees). However, the hinge movements are combined with minor gliding, rolling, and rotational motions. Internal and external rotation of the knee ranges from 0 to 10 degrees.

Femorotibial Articulations

Evaluation of the bony features of the femorotibial articular surfaces is essential to understanding the mechanics of the knee. Stability and motion of the joint depend on the strength and actions of the surrounding muscles, tendons, ligaments, and menisci (Fig. 40.4).

The medial condyle of the tibia has a longer contact point and is more concave than the articular surface of the lateral condyle. It also has a slightly more oblique orientation than the lateral condyle. This ensures that the tibia rotates during flexion and extension.

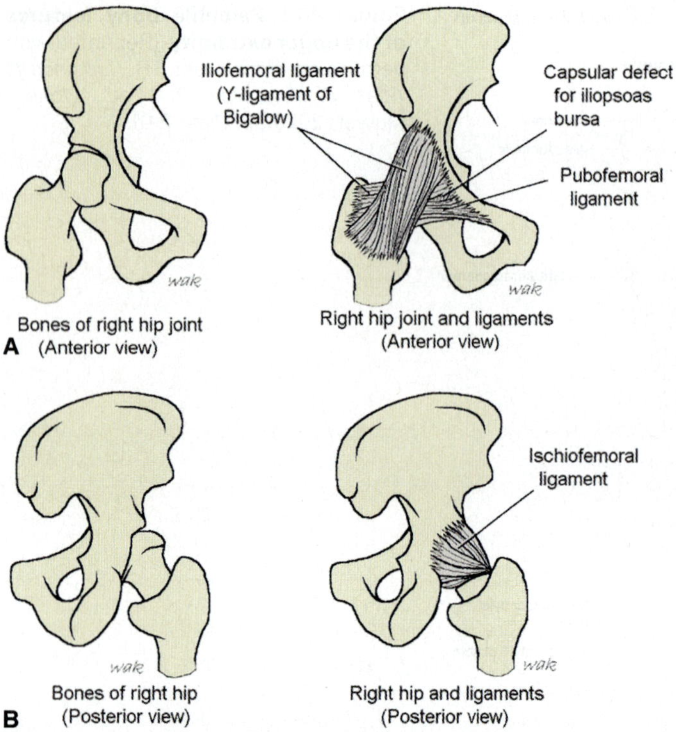

Figure 40.2. Functional hip ligaments. A. Anterior view of the right hip joint, the iliofemoral ligament (Y ligament of Bigelow) and the pubofemoral ligament. **B.** Posterior view of the right hip joint and the ischiofemoral ligament. (Illustration by William A. Kuchera, DO, FAAO, with permission.)

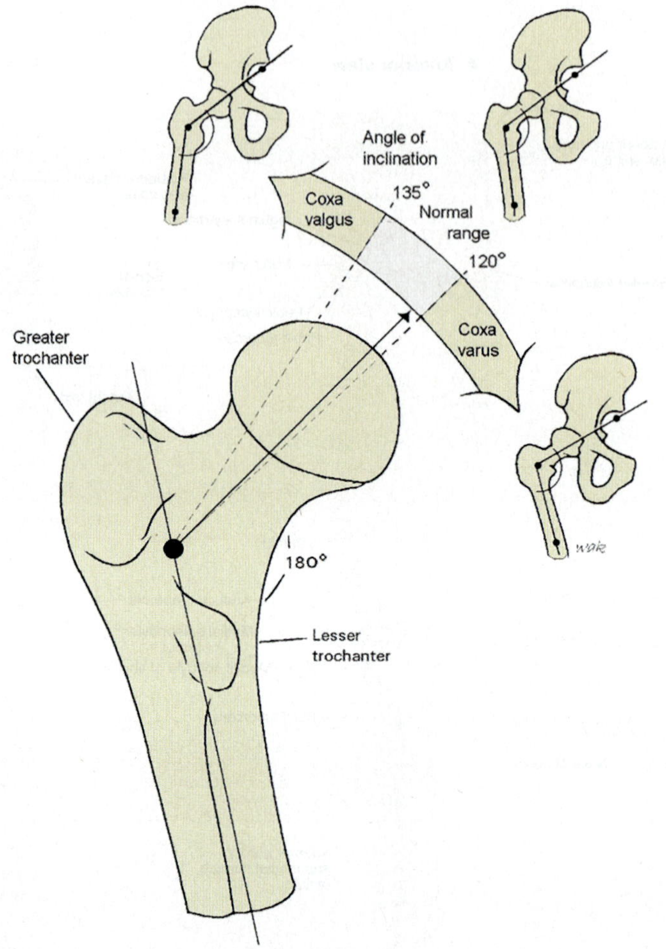

Figure 40.3. Angle of inclination. The angle of inclination measures less than 120 degrees in *coxa vara*; greater than 135 degrees in *coxa valga*. (Illustration by William A. Kuchera, DO, FAAO, with permission.)

Lateral and medial collateral ligaments (LCLs and MCLs) of the knee, adapted to limit lateral glide of the tibia with adduction and medial glide of the tibia with abduction, stabilize the joint. The lateral (fibular) collateral ligament does not attach to the lateral semilunar cartilage (*lateral meniscus*), while the medial (tibial) collateral ligament does attach to the medial semilunar cartilage (*medial meniscus*) (see Fig. 40.4). This anatomic arrangement makes the medial meniscus more susceptible to the following:

- Tears
- Displacement, especially from a blow to the knee that comes through the knee, from the lateral to the medial side
- Twisting injuries of the knee

The cruciate ligaments run between the tibia and the femur and are named according to their tibial attachments.

- The posterior cruciate ligament (PCL) attaches to the posterior part of the tibia and prevents excessive posterior glide of the tibia at the knee joint.
- The anterior cruciate ligament (ACL) attaches to the anterior part of the tibia and prevents excessive anterior glide of the tibia.

As the knee fully extends, or "locks", the condylar shape and orientation as well as the tightening of the cruciate and collateral ligaments will, cause external rotation of the tibia, or an internal rotation of the femur, depending on which bone is held stationary. This motion has been called the "screw home effect" of the knee. The contraction of the popliteus muscle unlocks the knee during knee flexion. When seated there is tibial motion on the femur and when standing the femur moves on the tibia, as seen in Figure 40.5.

This combined rotation which accompanies flexion/extension should not be confused with the active additional rotatory movements that are an important part of normal knee function. When the knee is flexed, it can internally and externally rotate about 10 degrees.[5]

Normal knee function depends on appropriate gliding of the femorotibial articulations:

- Posterolateral glide of the tibia is associated with tibial internal rotation.
- Anteromedial glide of the tibia is associated with tibial external rotation.
- Lateral glide is associated with tibial adduction.
- Medial glide is associated with tibial abduction.
- The tibia may also glide anteriorly or posteriorly on the femur.

Potential somatic dysfunctions of the tibial glide cause restrictions in mobility.

Patellofemoral Articulation

The patella is a sesamoid bone in the tendon of the quadriceps femoris muscle group. The patellofemoral articulation is between the patella and the anterior condyles of the femur. Tension of the quadriceps muscles, the quadriceps tendon, and the patellar tendon maintain the joint's stability in knee flexion and extension. Any muscle imbalance or structural changes to the movement of the patella on the femur can result in inflammation, pain, and motion restrictions. Assessment of the quality of motion and evaluation for tender points of both the quadricep muscles and the patellar bone can assist in diagnosis and treatment of patellofemoral joint dysfunctions.[4,5]

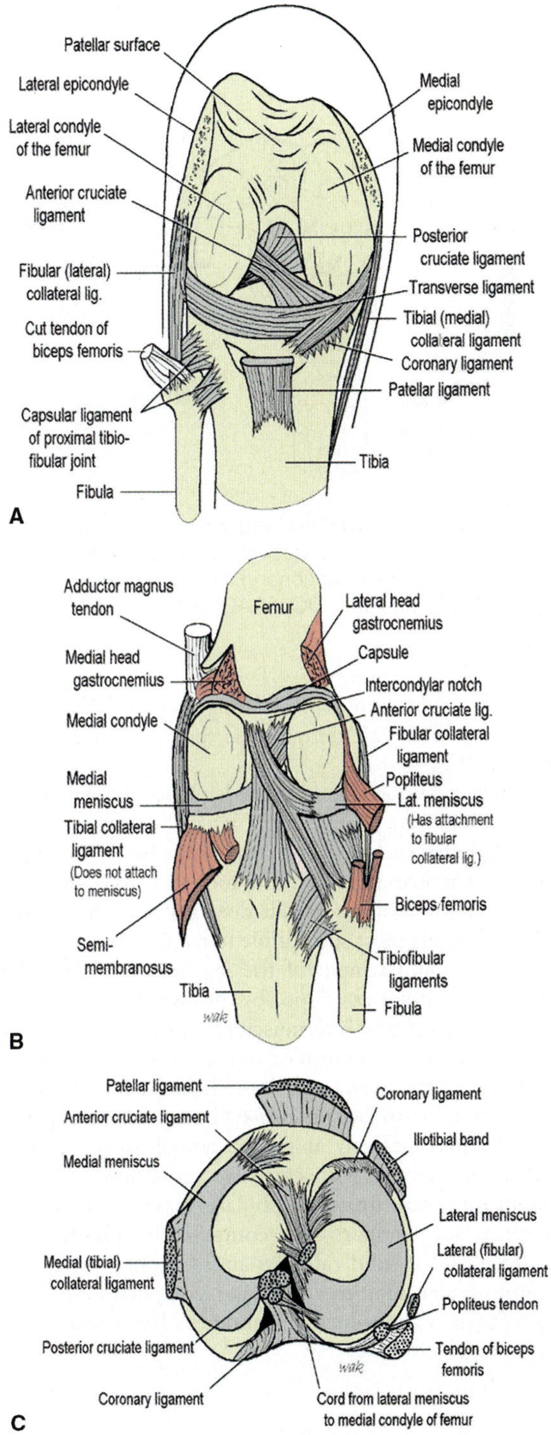

Figure 40.4. Knee joint. A. Anterior view. **B**. Posterior view. **C**. Relationship of collateral ligaments to knee cartilage (anterior view). (Illustration by William A. Kuchera, DO, FAAO, with permission.)

Q Angle and the Patella

The angle formed by the intersection of the functional longitudinal axis of the femur and the tibial longitudinal axis is clinically referred to as the *Q (or Quadriceps) angle*. It may be calculated by measuring the degree of force between the quadriceps muscle group and the tendon of the patella in the extended knee.[7] Although clinically it is more often estimated by drawing a line from the anterior superior iliac spine (ASIS) to the middle of the patella and extrapolating a second (vertical) line passing through the middle of the patella and tibial tuberosity.[1] The Q-angle typically averages 14 degrees for men and 17 degrees for women, due to the wider female pelvis.[7] An increased Q angle, around 20 degrees or higher is referred to as genu valgum (knock-kneed.) A decreased Q angle around 10 degrees or less is referred to as genu varum (bow-legged) (Fig. 40.6).

Biomechanically, coxa varus increases the Q angle, as does a pronated foot, and both enhance the possibility of genu valgus. An excessive Q angle also interferes with smooth movement of the patella in the femoral groove, leading to increased biomechanical stress during repetitive knee activities.[8] Patellofemoral joint dysfunction and structural change may arise from the abnormal tracking and pressure on the patella.

LEG REGION

The leg region includes the tibia and fibula. The tibia transmits the body's weight and articulates with the femur superiorly and the talus inferiorly. The fibula is not considered part of the knee joint. However, dysfunction can affect knee mechanics.[9] The fibula primarily functions as an attachment site for nine muscles and has a role in ankle stability.[1] It lies posterolateral to the tibia and is connected by the proximal synovial tibiofibular joint, the interosseous membrane, and the distal tibiofibular syndesmosis. The syndesmosis consists of three parts—the anterior tibiofibular ligament, the posterior tibiofibular ligament, and the interosseous tibiofibular ligament, which continues superiorly with the interosseous membrane. The membranous fibers span the two shafts, running inferiorly from the tibia to the fibula. This allows slight superior motion of the fibula but resists the downward pull placed on the fibula by eight of the nine muscles attaching to it.[1]

Movement at the superior tibiofibular joint is impossible without movement at the inferior tibiofibular syndesmosis.[1] The angulation of the tibiofibular articulations and tensions from the attached ligaments and muscles create a reciprocal anterior–posterior motion between the proximal and distal ends of the fibula.

During dorsiflexion and pronation of the foot, ligamentous attachments glide the distal tibiofibular joint posteriorly and allow the fibula to move superior and laterally to accommodate the increased width of the talus. Through reciprocal motion, the fibular head glides anteriorly, superiorly, and laterally. Plantarflexion and supination will induce the opposite inferior and medial fibular motion with anterior motion of the distal fibula and posterior motion of the fibular head. Similar anterior–posterior motion of the distal and proximal fibula may be induced with rotation of the tibia and ankle. External rotation of the tibia and ankle carry the distal fibula posteriorly and glide the proximal fibular head anteriorly. The opposite occurs with internal rotation of the tibia and ankle (Fig. 40.7).

Somatic dysfunctions of the superior tibiofibular joint are named by motion preference of anterior or posterior glide at the proximal aspect of the fibula (the fibular head).[3–5,10] Somatic dysfunctions of the inferior tibiofibular joint are named by motion preference of anterior or posterior glide at the distal aspect of the fibula (the lateral malleolus). Fibular somatic dysfunction, as well as tibial somatic dysfunctions, and restrictions within the interosseous membrane[6] can all affect muscle tension and lower extremity biomechanics, especially at the ankle joint.

Fascial Compartments in the Leg

The lower leg is divided into four fascial compartments:

- Anterior compartment
- Lateral compartment
- Two posterior compartments—deep and superficial

The muscles of each compartment share common functions and innervations.[1] Clinically, a compartment syndrome can arise

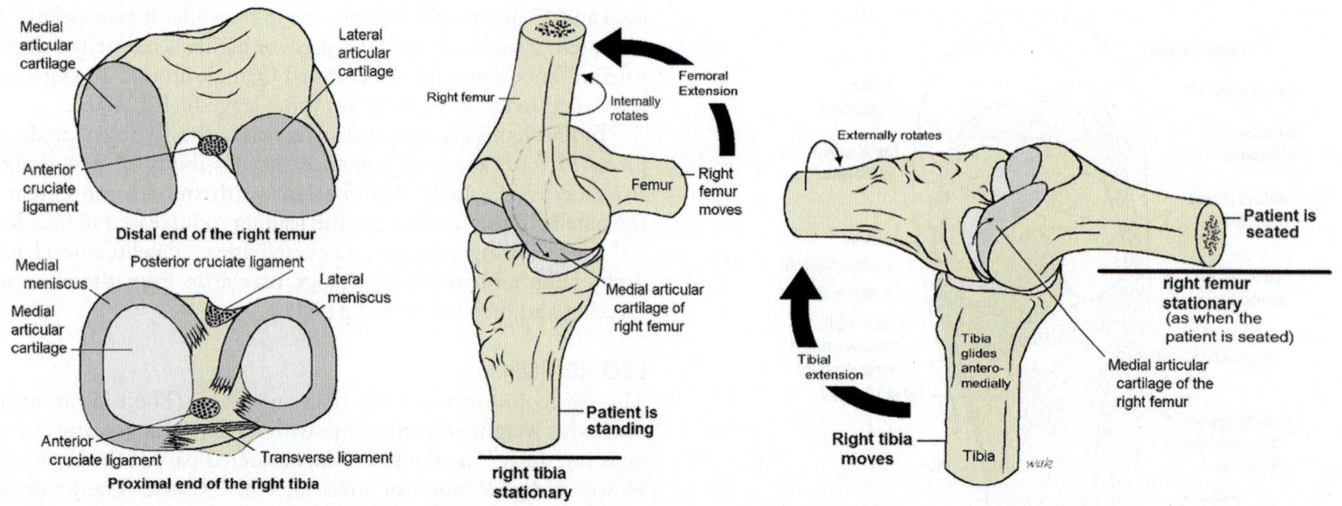

Figure 40.5. Structure–function relationship of the medial condyle of the femorotibial joint. The longer medial condyle influences knee joint function. In knee extension, the medial, but not the lateral, femoral condyle will continue to track posteriorly, resulting in internal rotation of the femur (if the tibia is stationary) or external rotation of the tibia (if the femur is held stationary). The condylar glide occurring with external rotation of the tibia is called the anteromedial glide. (Illustration by William A. Kuchera, DO, FAAO, with permission.)

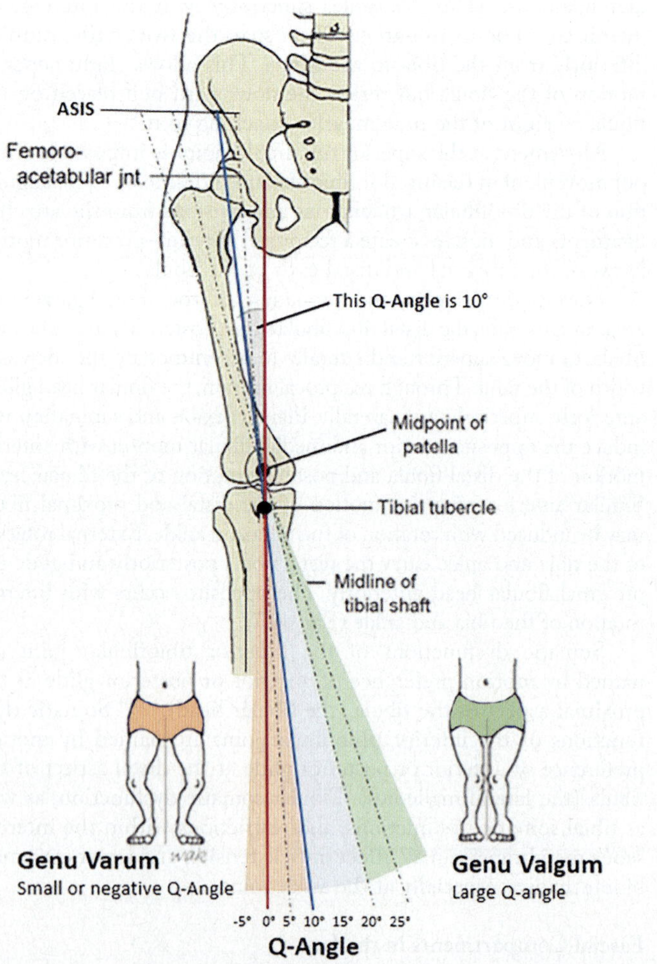

Figure 40.6. Q-Angle of the right knee. The Q-Angle is estimated by drawing a line from the anterior superior iliac spine (ASIS) to the middle of the patella (blue line) and extrapolating a second (vertical) line passing through the middle of the patella and tibial tuberosity (red line). A person with wider hips will have a larger Q-angle and a person with narrow hips will have a smaller Q-angle. (Illustration courtesy of William A. Kuchera, DO, FAAO, with permission.)

from trauma or vigorous overuse, leading to a rise in intracompartmental pressure. This can compromise the circulation within that compartment (Fig. 40.8).

The anterior compartment of the leg is located anterior to the interosseous membrane, between the lateral surface of the shaft of the tibia and medial surface of the shaft of the fibula. It contains the dorsiflexor or extensor muscles of the foot and ankle and is covered anteriorly by relatively nonexpansile deep fascia of the leg and skin. This confined area is most susceptible to compartment syndromes.[1]

The lateral compartment of the leg is located lateral to the shaft of the fibula and is enveloped by the deep fascia of the leg and skin between the anterior intermuscular septum of the leg and the posterior intermuscular septum of the leg. It contains two evertor muscles (the fibularis brevis and fibularis longus) and the superficial fibular nerve.[1] Pain from increased lateral intracompartmental pressure is located diffusely along the lateral aspect of the lower leg. It recurs in runners with excessive pronation of the foot or might result from rupture of the fibularis longus muscle.

The posterior compartment contains the plantarflexion or flexor muscles and is subdivided by an intracompartmental transverse intermuscular septum.[1] Posterior compartment syndromes typically refer pain anteromedially and are often bilateral and difficult to manage conservatively.

ANKLE

Anatomically, the talocrural (tibiotalar) joint is often considered the "ankle joint" while the talocalcaneal (subtalar) and talocalcaneonavicular (transverse-tarsal) are considered part of the "foot joint."[1] However, the talus has no direct muscular attachments, so its movements are determined by the muscle actions on the bones above and below it.[1,3] The ankle joint complex is comprised of the kinetic linkage between the lower leg and the foot.[11] The combined function of these joints is needed for mobility and balance.[11,12]

The key movements of the ankle joint complex are

- Dorsiflexion/plantarflexion: ankle and foot move in the sagittal plane about a transverse axis, toes pointing upward and downward
- Abduction/adduction: ankle moves in the transverse plane about a vertical axis through the tibia, rotating the foot to point toes medial (toe-in) or lateral (toe-out)

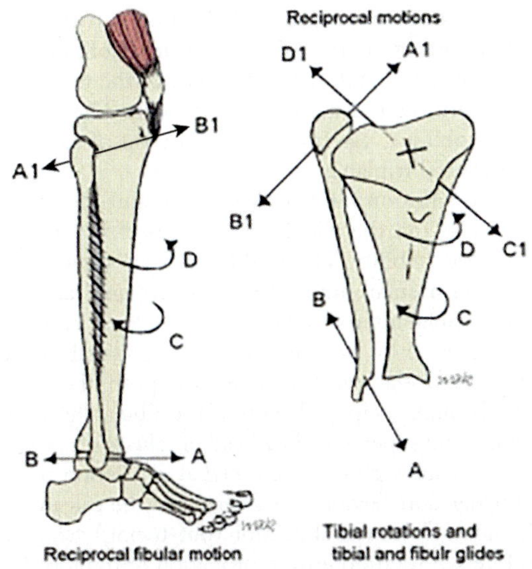

Figure 40.7. Reciprocal fibular motions. Inducing external rotation of the tibia and ankle (C) moves the distal fibula posteriorly (B) and is reciprocally associated with the fibular head moving anteriorly (B1). The opposite is true (A, A1) when inducing internal rotation (D) of the lower leg. (Illustration by William A. Kuchera, DO, FAAO, with permission.)

- Inversion/eversion: ankle and foot in the frontal (coronal) plane about an anterior–posterior (long) axis through the ankle and foot, rotating the sole of the foot to face in or face out (Fig. 40.9).

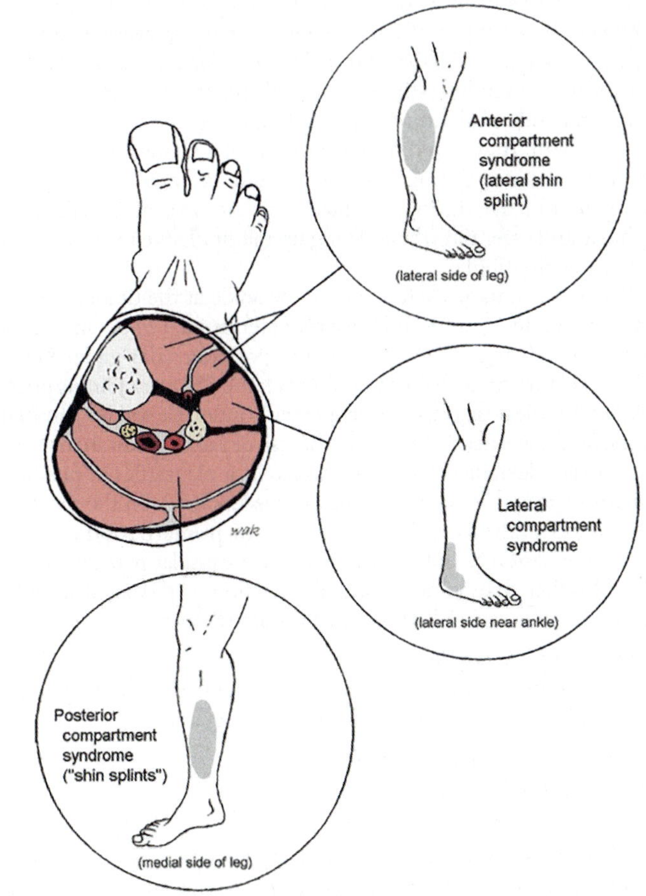

Figure 40.8. Fascial compartments of the lower extremity. (Illustration by William A. Kuchera, DO, FAAO, with permission.)

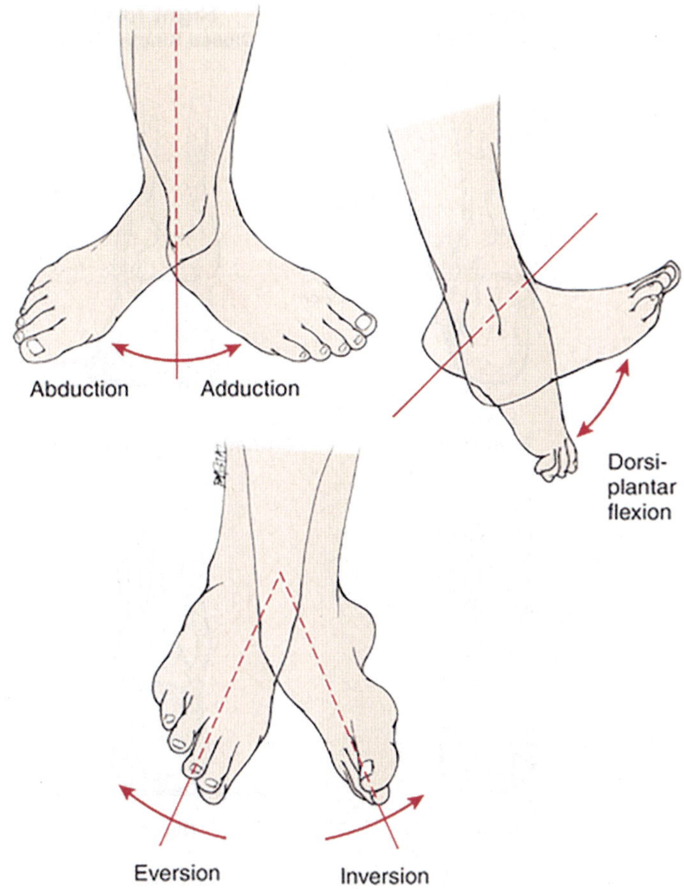

Figure 40.9. Motions of the ankle joint complex. Dorsiflexion/plantarflexion occurs about a transverse axis moving the foot and ankle in the sagittal plane; abduction and adduction occur about a vertical (long) axis through the tibia moving the foot and ankle in the transverse plane; eversion and inversion occur about anterior posterior axis through the ankle and foot rotating in the frontal (coronal) plane.

A combination of these motions across the tibiotalar and subtalar joints create supination and pronation in the foot (Fig. 40.10).[11,13]

1. The talocrural (tibiotalar) joint primarily allows dorsiflexion and plantarflexion of the ankle.
   a. Talocrural dorsiflexion has associated components of talar eversion and adduction (tibial internal rotation).
   b. Talocrural plantarflexion has associated components of talar inversion and abduction (tibial external rotation).
2. The subtalar (talocalcaneal) joint allows hindfoot pronation (hindfoot valgus) coupled with tibial internal rotation and hindfoot supination (hindfoot varus) coupled with tibial external rotation.
   a. Subtalar pronation is a combination of calcaneal eversion (tilting outward), dorsiflexion, and abduction (out-toeing)
   b. Subtalar supination is a combination of calcaneal inversion (tilting inward), plantarflexion, and adduction (in-toeing)
3. The transverse tarsal joint is considered part of the same functional unit as the subtalar joint, sharing a common axis of motion contributing to pronation and supination of the foot.

Motions of the foot-ankle complex, their joints, ligaments, and muscular attachments can have different compensation and deformability when weight bearing. Reciprocal rotations of multiple joints of the ankle and foot occur in response to force

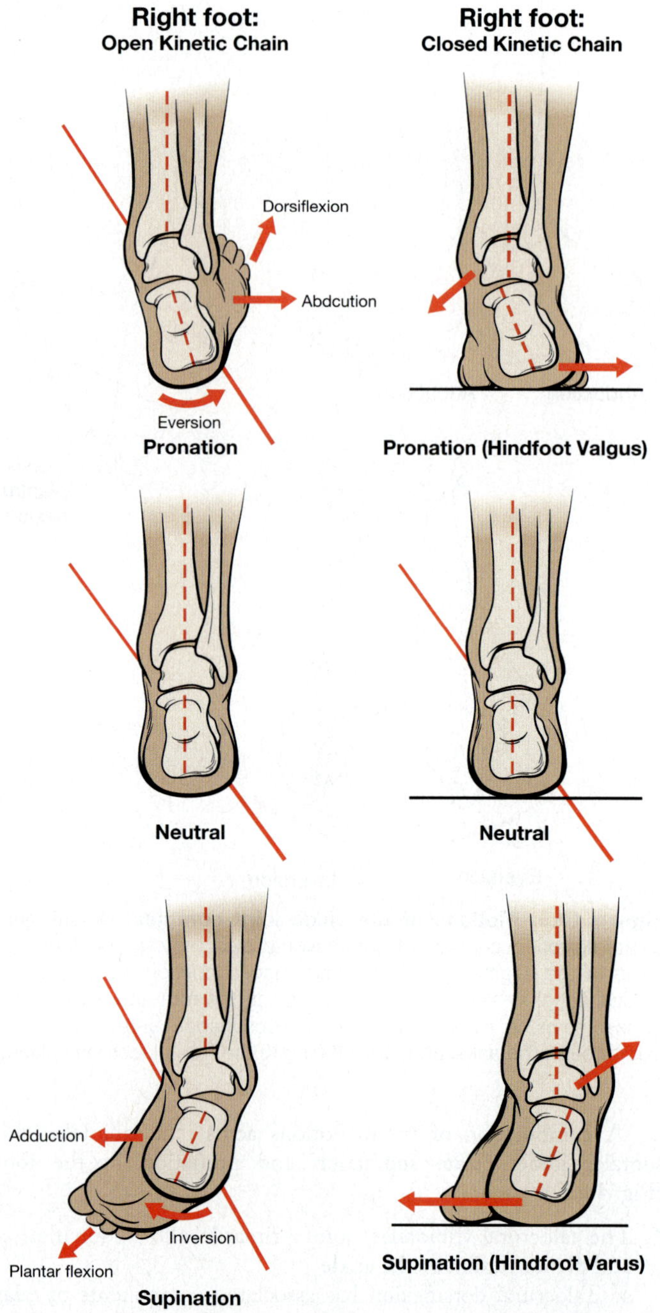

Figure 40.10. Pronation and supination of the right foot. In an open kinetic chain, with the foot off the ground, the foot and ankle move on a fixed tibia at the talocrural and subtalar joints. Pronation is produced by eversion, abduction, and dorsiflexion. Supination is produced by inversion, abduction, and plantarflexion. In a closed kinetic chain, with the foot on the ground, most of the pronation and supination are produced by the weight of the body acting on the talus. In this weight-bearing position, the tibia moves on the talus (talocrural) and the talus moves on the fixed calcaneus (subtalar) to produce pronation and supination. (Reprinted with permission from Hamill J, Knutzen K, Derrick TR. *Biomechanical Basis of Human Movement*. 5th ed. Wolters Kluwer; 2022:250. Figure 6-34.)

distributions to maintain balance.[11,13] See Chapter 92 Postural Considerations in Osteopathic Diagnosis and Treatment.

Tibiotalar/Talocrural Joint

The tibiotalar (or talocrural joint) is a synovial joint located within the talo-tibiofibular complex, between the *malleolar mortise* (formed by the inferior surface of the tibia, the two malleoli, and the inferior transverse part of the posterior tibiofibular ligament) and the trochlea of the talus. The trochlea of the talus is structurally wider anteriorly and narrower posteriorly. The tibiotalar axis of rotation is oblique, passing through the tip of each malleolus, creating associated triplanar motions.

During dorsiflexion the trochlea of the talus glides posteriorly into the mortise and the wider anterior aspect fits more securely, increasing ankle stability. The slightly oblique orientation of the axis also allows a small amount of talar eversion and adduction which leads to tibial internal rotation and calcaneal eversion (tilting outward). The width of trochlea will push the distal fibula slightly posterolateral and the everted ankle will push the distal fibula superiorly. Through reciprocal motion the fibular head will move anterolaterally and superiorly. The head of talus glides slightly inferior and base of talus glides anteromedial in relation to calcaneus, allowing further dorsiflexion and eversion of the calcaneus in relation to the talus. Calcaneal abduction (out-toeing), talar adduction, and tibial internal rotation lead to pronation of the foot.[11,13,14]

During plantarflexion, the trochlea of the talus glides anteriorly within the mortise placing the less stable, narrower posterior portion of the talus within the ankle mortise. Small amounts of talar inversion and abduction lead to tibial external rotation and calcaneal inversion (tilting inward). The distal fibula will be pulled anteriorly and inferiorly leading to a posteromedial and inferior position of the fibular head. The head of talus glides slightly superiorly and base of talus glides posterolaterally in relation to calcaneus. This allows for further calcaneal plantarflexion, inversion, and adduction (in-toeing) leading to supination of the foot.[11,13,14]

The gross ranges of motion (ROM) for the ankle vary significantly between individuals due to geographical and cultural differences in activities of daily living but tend to average around 15 degrees for dorsiflexion and 45 degrees for plantarflexion.[11,15] Axis position may be estimated by placing the fingertips at the most distal ends of the malleoli and visualizing the transverse axis between them. Associated minor motions of a posterior talar glide within the mortise during dorsiflexion and an anterior talar glide within the mortise during plantarflexion are helpful in palpatory diagnosis and essential when setting up manipulative techniques of the talus or the fibula.

Recurrent somatic dysfunction of the ankle at the tibiotalar joint commonly prefers plantarflexion with anterior talar glide and has a resistant barrier to full dorsiflexion and posterior talar glide. Acute ankle sprains are more likely to occur when the tibiotalar joint is plantarflexed. Studies suggest that people with inflexible ankles (limited dorsiflexion) have nearly five times the risk of ankle sprain than those with average flexibility.[16] This is because in a plantarflexed position the narrow posterior portion of the talus is less stable in the mortise. This clinical finding can be associated with plantarflexion somatic dysfunction patterns. Note that the tibiotalar capsular pattern seen in arthritis, rather than joint somatic dysfunction, is restricted in both directions and is especially resistant to plantarflexion.

Ligaments of the Ankle

Three separate ligaments stabilize the lateral side of the ankle (Fig. 40.11). From anterior to posterior, these are:

1. Anterior talofibular ligament
2. Calcaneofibular ligament
3. Posterior talofibular ligament

When functioning properly these ligaments stabilize the ankle during inversion. However, they are prone to inversion/supination sprains, especially during exaggerated plantarflexion when the less stable, narrow, posterior aspect of the talus is in the mortise.[11]

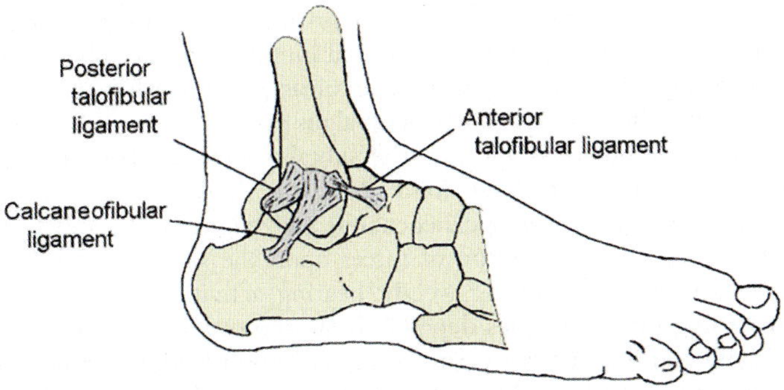

Figure 40.11. Ligaments stabilizing the lateral ankle. (Illustration by William A. Kuchera, DO, FAAO, with permission.)

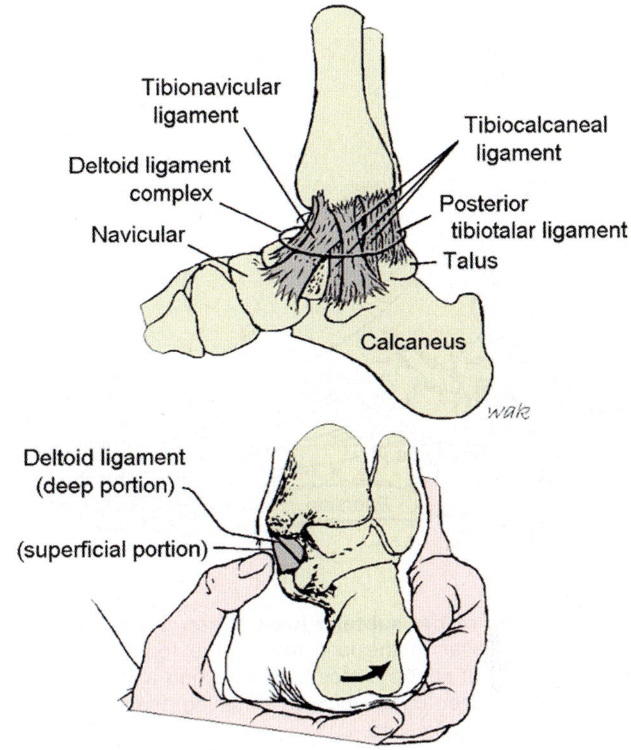

Figure 40.12. The deltoid ligament. (Illustration by William A. Kuchera, DO, FAAO, with permission.)

The medial side of the ankle is stabilized by the strong medial ligament of the ankle (deltoid ligament) and attaches proximally to the medial malleolus. The distal aspect fans out, attaching to the talus, calcaneus, and navicular bones (Fig. 40.12). It stabilizes the ankle joint during eversion and prevents subluxation of the joint.[1]

FOOT

The anatomy of the foot can be classified into three main sections: the hindfoot, midfoot, and forefoot, each comprising distinct bones and structures (Fig. 40.13).[1]

- Hindfoot: the talus, the calcaneus, and the subtalar joint
- Midfoot: the navicular, cuboid, and three cuneiform bones (medial, intermediate, and lateral)
- Forefoot: the metatarsals, phalanges, and two sesamoid bones

Subtalar Joint

The subtalar joint is a synovial joint comprised of anterior (talocalcaneonavicular) and posterior (talocalcaneal) articulations that are separated by the tarsal canal[13] and stabilized by the strong medial, lateral, posterior, and interosseous talocalcaneal ligaments.[1] The subtalar joint's axis of rotation is oriented from anterior-superomedial to posterior-inferolateral. The oblique declining axis transects all three cardinal planes (Fig. 40.14).[1,13] It is often described as a "mitered hinge" because its triplanar orientation allows for the coupling of tibial rotation and rearfoot supination and pronation.[11,13]

The declination of the subtalar oblique axis is more horizontal in people with flat feet which allows for greater foot motion. Those with a more vertical axis have a more rigid, pes cavus foot. Supination and pronation and, as complex triplanar motions of the foot are accompanied by calcaneus inversion or eversion, ankle plantarflexion or dorsiflexion, and forefoot adduction or abduction (see Figs. 40.9 and 40.10).

Subtalar Supination[11,13,17]:

- Plantarflexion of the ankle joint complex—a summation of the talocrural and subtalar joints pointing toes downward.[18]
  - Talar plantarflexion: the trochlea of talus glides anteriorly within the mortise
  - Calcaneal plantarflexion: head of talus glides superiorly on the anterior aspect of calcaneus
- Inversion of the calcaneus—the base of the calcaneus tilts inward (inverts), faces towards midline of the body (sole of foot arches and tilts inward)
  - Talus also inverts compared to tibia but to a lesser degree
  - Base of talus glides posterolaterally over the calcaneus (talus abducts and tibia externally rotates)

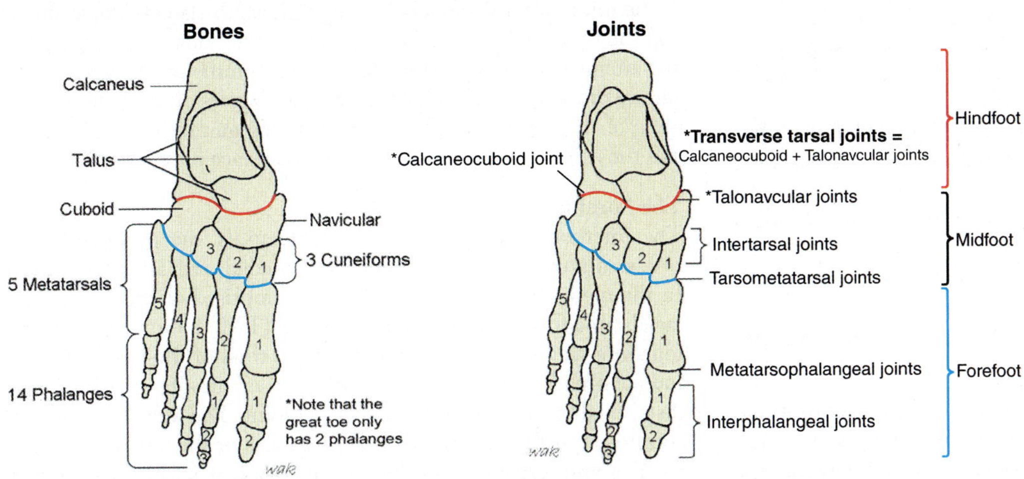

Figure 40.13. The bones and joints of the right foot. (Illustration by William A. Kuchera, DO, FAAO, with permission.)

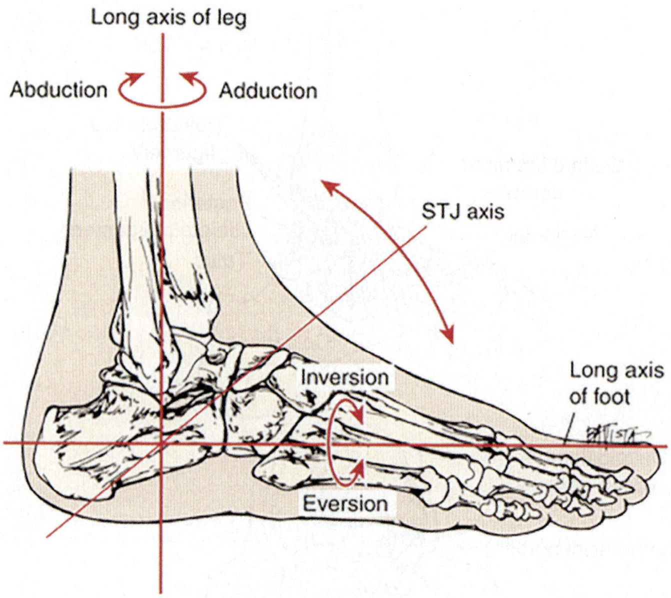

Figure 40.14. Axes of the subtalar joint. When the axis of the subtalar joint lies closer to the long axis of the foot, motion at the subtalar joint (STJ) consists mostly of inversion and eversion. When the axis lies closer to the long axis of the leg, the abduction–adduction component increases.

  - Inversion is primarily produced by the tibialis anterior, tibialis posterior, extensor hallucis longus, flexor hallucis longus, and flexor digitorum longus muscles.
  - The average range of motion for subtalar inversion is about 30 degrees
- Adduction of the forefoot—the forefoot moves towards midline of the body (toes pointing medially).
  - Calcaneus and tarsals adduct as base of talus glides posterolaterally over the calcaneus

Subtalar Pronation[11,13,17]:

- Dorsiflexion of the ankle joint complex—a summation of the talocrural and subtalar joints approximating the foot and shin (toes pointing upward).[18]
  - Talar dorsiflexion: the trochlea of talus glides anteriorly within the mortise
  - Calcaneal dorsiflexion: head of talus glides inferiorly on the anterior aspect of calcaneus)
- Eversion of the calcaneus—the base of the calcaneus tilts outward (everts), faces away from midline of the body (sole of foot flattens or tilts outward)
  - Talus also everts compared to tibia but to a lesser degree
  - Base of talus glides anteromedially over the calcaneus (talus adducts and tibia internally rotates)
  - Eversion is primarily produced by the fibularis longus, fibularis brevis, and fibularis tertius muscles with assistance from the toe extensor muscles.
  - The average range of motion for subtalar eversion is about 18 degrees during gait.
- Abduction of the forefoot—the forefoot moves away from midline of the body (toes pointing laterally).
  - Calcaneus and tarsals abduct as base of talus glides anteromedially over the calcaneus

Clinically, these mechanics are palpable talocalcaneal motions. The mechanics may also be visualized from the posterior view of a standing patient when they are asked to turn the trunk and pelvis to the right. The right leg (talo-tibiofibular complex) will externally rotate while the left leg will internally rotate. The right calcaneus will invert into a subtalar varus position while the left calcaneus will evert into a subtalar valgus position.[14]

In addition to its motion, the subtalar joint has been called the main shock-absorber joint[6,19] of the lower extremity. In coordination with the calcaneocuboid and talonavicular joints, it determines the distribution of forces upon the skeleton and soft tissues of the foot during weight-bearing activities. The shock-absorbing function varies depending on impact level of a person's activity and their body weight. A higher impact load, like running or jumping, can result in greater injury and pathologic changes.

Running is one of the most widespread activities during which overuse injuries of the lower extremity occur. Many biomechanical risk factors for such injuries stem from the hindfoot.[20] Examples of overuse injuries that commonly occur during running include the following:

- Stress fractures
- Medial tibial stress syndrome (shin splints)
- Chondromalacia patellae
- Plantar fasciitis
- Achilles tendinitis

Normal subtalar joint function is critical to normal foot and lower extremity functions[11]; and should be a major focus of physical examination and assessment for sports medicine physicians.

Transverse Tarsal Joint

The transverse tarsal joint, or *Chopart* joint, is the joint between the hindfoot (talus and calcaneus) and the midfoot (navicular and cuboid). It contains the talonavicular, the calcaneocuboid, and two small talocalcaneal articulations, which are separate joints that act together as a functional unit. Because the unit responds to eversion or inversion of the calcaneus, it exerts its greatest influence during the stance phase of the walking cycle (Fig. 40.15). When amputating a foot, the surgeon follows the articulations of the Chopart joint.[12]

Between the intertarsal joints and the subtalar joint is a groove called the *sinus tarsi*. Attached along this groove is the very strong interosseous talocalcaneal ligament that provides stability for the subtalar and intertarsal joints. Following injury or overuse, an inflammatory sinus tarsi syndrome may occur, leading to medial or lateral heel pain on weight bearing. A conservative biomechanical approach is typically successful in addressing this condition.[21]

The Midfoot

The midfoot contains five tarsal bones: the navicular, cuboid, and three cuneiform bones (medial, intermediate, and lateral). This region acts as a bridge between the hindfoot and the forefoot. The bones of the midfoot form the medial longitudinal, the lateral longitudinal, and the transverse arches. The function of the midfoot is to transmit and attenuate force and allow the foot to accommodate to the variable surface of the ground.[13] There are various degrees of mechanical coupling of the forefoot to the hindfoot during gait (midtarsal locking) and the control of dorsiflexion during the stance phase.[13]

The Forefoot

The forefoot is composed of the metatarsals, the phalanges and, two sesamoid bones. It contains the medial and lateral forefoot. In the medial forefoot, the first ray is comprised of the first metatarsal, cuneiform, and the tarsometatarsal (TMT) joint. The first ray functions as a pillar and forms the distal truss of the medial longitudinal arch.[13,22] The hallux is comprised of the first proximal and distal phalanx and the interphalangeal joint. The lateral forefoot is comprised of the metatarsals and phalanges of the lateral four digits. The joint capsules and the medial collateral, and LCLs provide

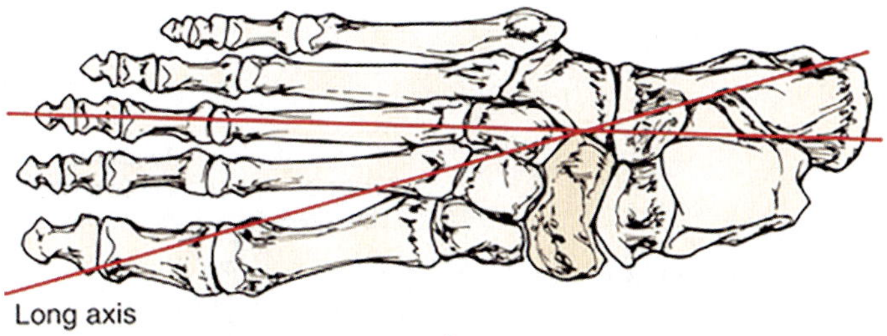

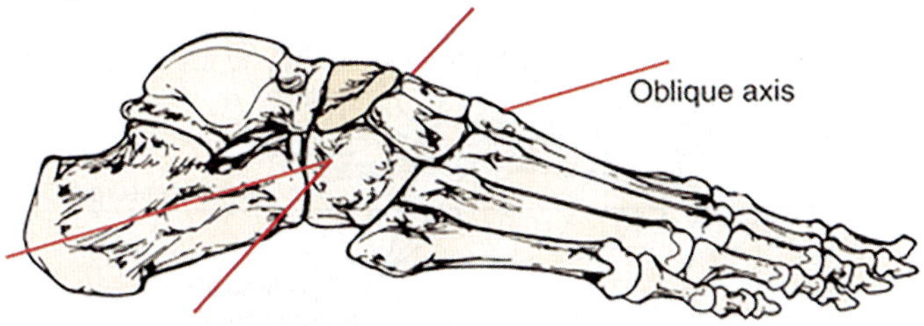

Figure 40.15. Axes of the transverse tarsal joint. Motion about the theoretical long axis of the transverse tarsal joint contributes to more eversion and inversion of the foot, while motion about the theoretical oblique axis of the transverse tarsal joint contributes mostly to dorsiflexion and plantarflexion of the foot.

stability for each of the metatarsophalangeal and interphalangeal joints. These joints play a crucial role in propulsion and toe-off.

The medial and lateral sesamoid bones (sesamoid of the 1st metatarsal) are embedded in the flexor hallucis brevis tendon. The flexor hallucis longus tendon runs between them. These bones elevate the first metatarsal, absorbing pressure and protecting the flexor hallucis longus tendon during terminal stance and toe-off phase of gait. The sesamoids of the 1st metatarsal and the head of the 2nd metatarsal make up the ball of the foot. They share the body's weight and pressure laterally with the 3rd, 4th and 5th metatarsal heads as necessary for balance and comfort.[1]

Functional Arches of the Foot

The three main functional arches of the foot are the medial longitudinal arch, the lateral longitudinal arch, and the transverse arch. Together they act as a unit spreading the weight in all directions.[1] They are formed and maintained by both passive and dynamic supports from the following:

- Interlocking articular facets of the bones
- Interosseous ligaments
- Plantar aponeurosis and ligaments
- Long tendons extending into the foot
- Intrinsic muscles of the foot
- Shoes of proper width (transverse arch) and insole (longitudinal arches)

A so-called metatarsal arch is not a functional arch; it refers to the heads of the five metatarsals. Restrictions or altered relationships here are usually secondary to dysfunction of the other foot arches.[3]

Longitudinal Arches

The longitudinal arch is divided into medial and lateral components.

- The bony medial longitudinal arch consists of the calcaneus, talus, navicular, the three cuneiforms, and the first three metatarsals.
- The bony lateral longitudinal arch is the calcaneus, the cuboid, and the 4th and 5th metatarsals.

The lateral longitudinal arch is typically flatter than the medial component and it usually rests on the ground while standing. The alignment of the lateral and medial longitudinal axes of the midtarsal joint is influenced by subtalar pronation and supination. During pronation, the axes become more parallel which permits them to be more flexible and to adapt to different surfaces. During supination nonparallel alignment of the midtarsal axes permits the foot to become rigid, supporting the body's weight and providing a rigid lever for propulsion.

Transverse Arch

The transverse arch is composed of the cuboid, the navicular, the three cuneiforms, and the proximal ends of the metatarsals. The shape and alignment of the united bones are especially important for this arch.

Supporting Structures for the Arches of the Foot[1]

Dynamic support for the arches of the foot includes the intrinsic muscles of the foot and the long tendons of the foot. The transverse arch also receives stirrup-like support from a major inverter (tibialis posterior) and evertor (fibularis longus).[1]

The fibrous tissues that passively bowstring the longitudinal arch (superficial to deep) are (Fig. 40.16):

1. The *plantar aponeurosis,* which extends from the calcaneus to the phalanges and encompasses the sesamoid bones under the great toe.
2. The *long plantar ligament,* which runs from the calcaneus to the lateral three metatarsals.
   - □ It forms a tunnel for the passage of the fibularis longus muscle, as that tendon passes under the foot to the first cuneiform and first metatarsal.
3. The *plantar calcaneocuboid (short plantar) ligament*, which lies medial to the lateral longitudinal arch and is attached between the calcaneus and the proximal end of the cuboid.
4. The *plantar calcaneonavicular (spring) ligament* (not pictured in Fig. 40.16), strengthens the medial longitudinal arch and runs from the sustentaculum tali of the calcaneus to the navicular.
   - □ It assists in transferring weight from the talus to the navicular bone, which is essential for effective load distribution across the foot during standing and walking.

Musculature

Proper functioning of the lower limbs depends upon the integrity of their joints, muscles, nerves, and vascular supply. Actions of individual muscles are often described as if they are acting in isolation. However, the totality of somatic structures should be viewed as a "kinetic chain." A kinetic chain is described as a sequencing of individual body segments and joints functioning in a predictable movement pattern to accomplish a task.[23] The lower limbs provide energy-efficient bipedal gait and a base of support for the body.

Imbalance of concentric and eccentric lower extremity and postural muscles can lead to disruption of the kinetic chain in a condition called lower cross syndrome (LCS) (Fig. 40.17).[24] If left unidentified and untreated, the muscle imbalance and any associated somatic dysfunction may lead to altered muscle-firing patterns resulting in overload to connective tissues (capsular laxity and instability, labral tears) or the joint itself (osteoarthritis, etc.).

The muscles of the lower extremity (Fig. 40.18) can be grouped as follows[3]:

1. Hip and thigh
   a. Flexors
   b. Extensors
   c. Abductors
   d. Adductors
   e. External rotators
   f. Internal rotators

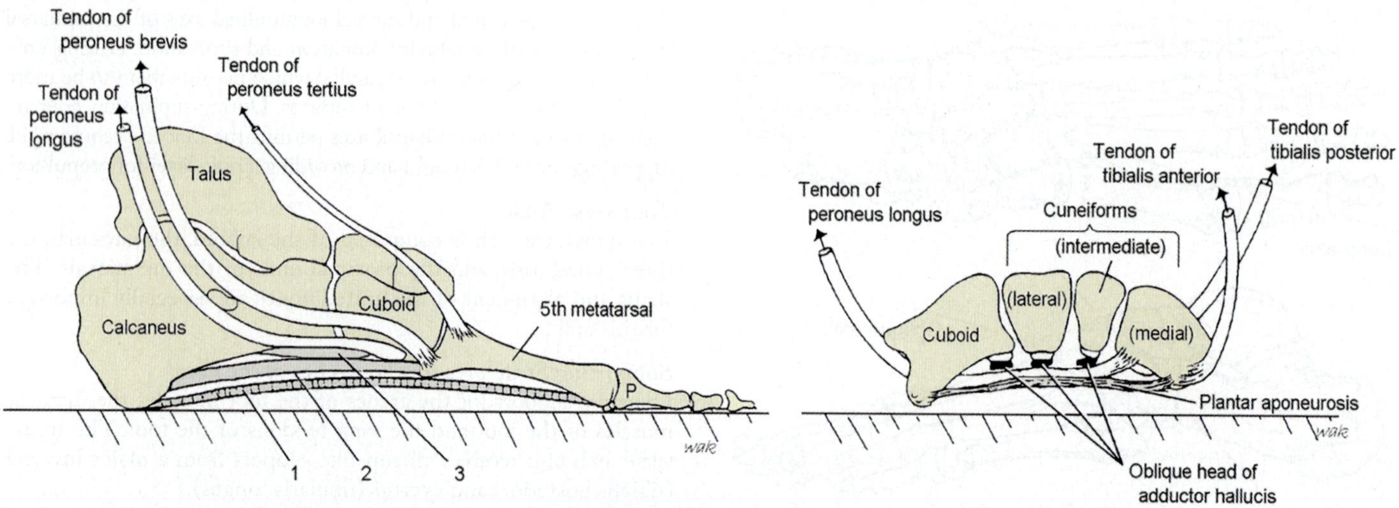

Figure 40.16. Plantar tendons and ligaments supporting the arches of the foot. 1. Plantar aponeurosis. 2. Long plantar ligament. 3. Plantar calcaneocuboid (short plantar) ligament. (Illustration by William A. Kuchera, DO, FAAO, with permission.)

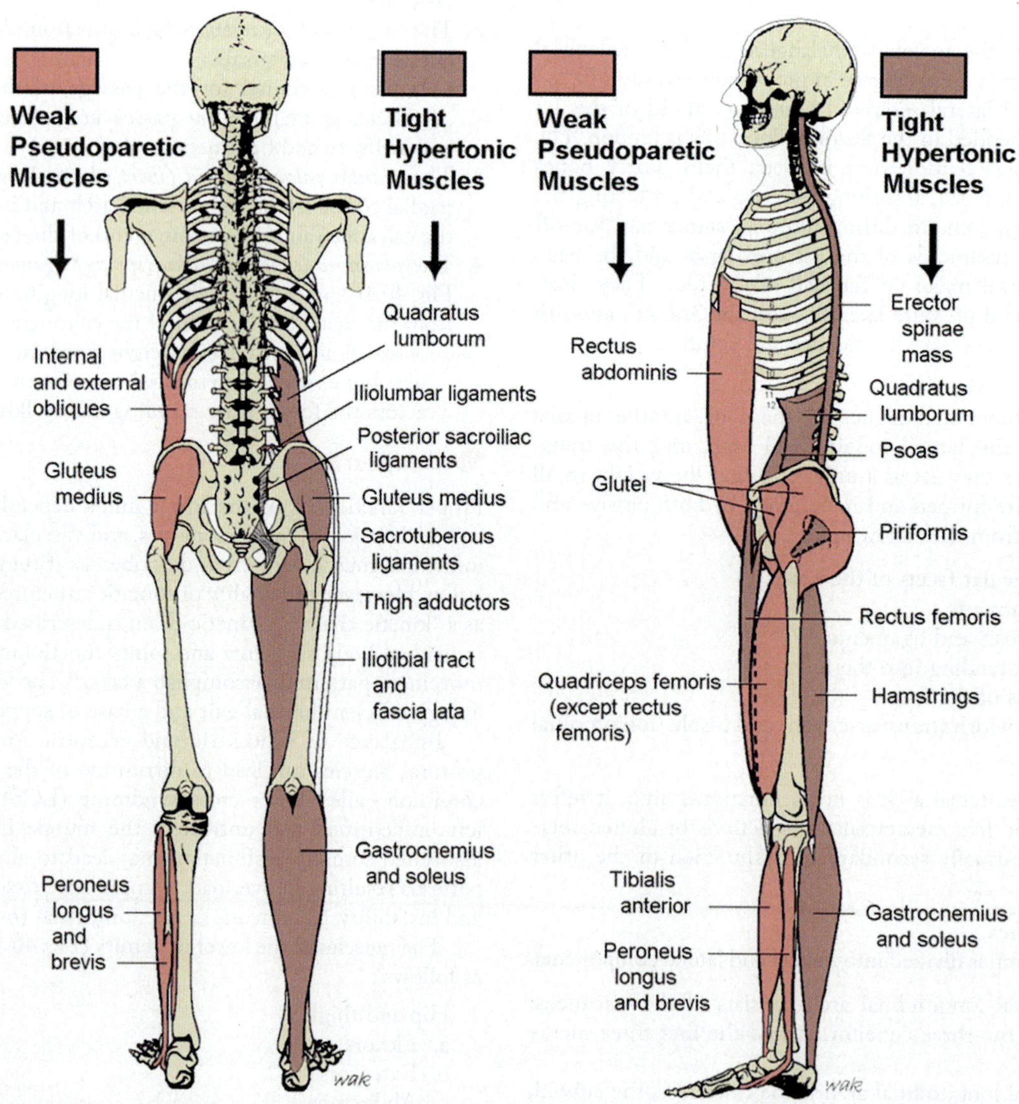

Figure 40.17. Postural pattern of tight (postural) and weak (postural antagonist) muscles. (Illustration by William A. Kuchera, DO, FAAO, with permission.)

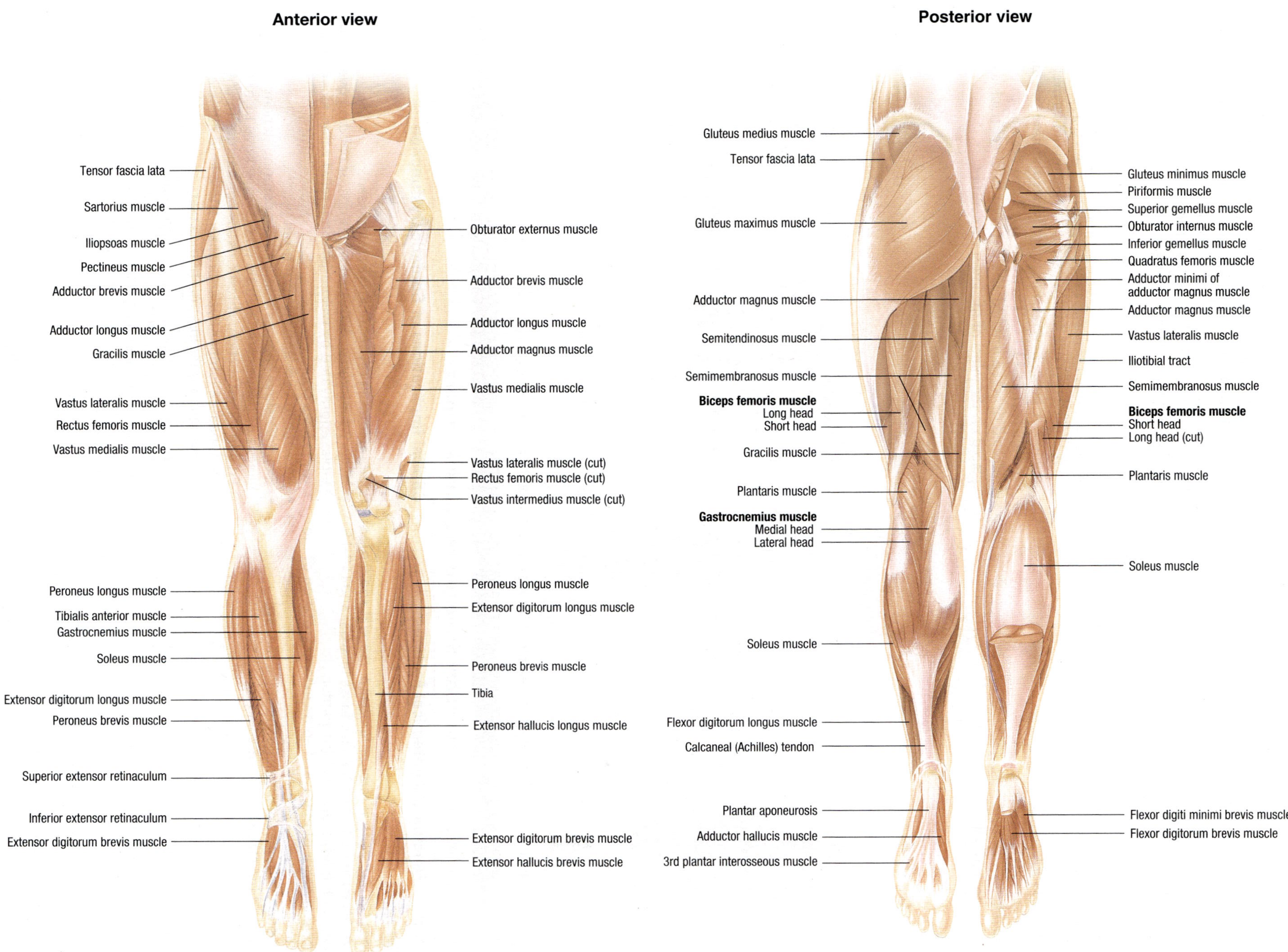

Figure 40.18. Lower limb muscles. (Reprinted with permission from Springhouse. *ACC Atlas of Human Anatomy*. Lippincott Williams & Wilkins; 2001.)

2. Knee
   a. Flexors
   b. Extensors
   c. External rotator
   d. Internal rotators
3. Ankle and foot
   a. Dorsiflexors
   b. Plantar flexors
4. Foot
   a. Supinators
   b. Pronators
5. Foot and/or toe
   a. Flexors
   b. Extensors
6. Intrinsic foot muscles

The specific muscles in each of the above groups are listed in Tables 40.1 to 40.3, along with information about their clinical implications of somatic dysfunctions. Postural and phasic designation of each muscle is also listed. Postural muscles tend to become hypertonic when stressed while phasic muscles tend to be inhibited or pseudo-paretic when stressed.

Bursae

Bursae are small, synovial tissue-lined structures that help different tissues glide over one another, such as a tendon sliding over another tendon or bone. Several bursae are located around the hip, knee, and ankle (Fig. 40.19). They may swell and become painful when infected or when irritated as a response to direct trauma or stress placed on the joints of the lower extremities.

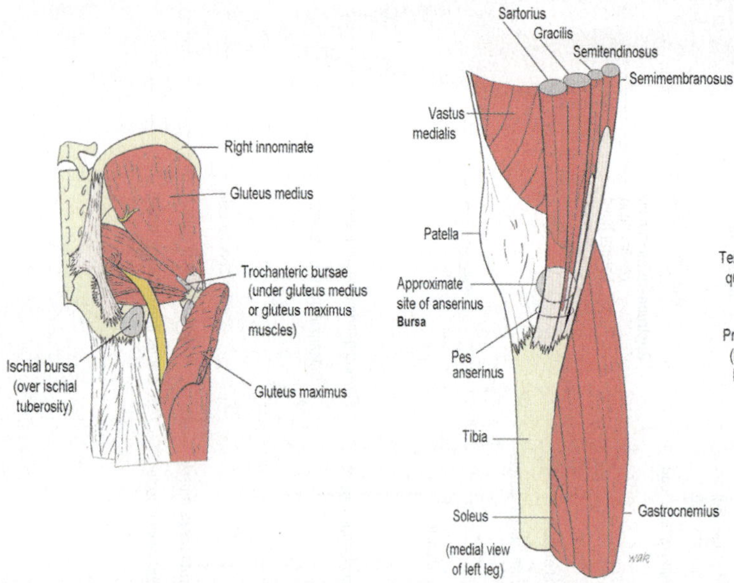

Figure 40.19. Bursae of the lower extremity. (Illustration by William A. Kuchera, DO, FAAO, with permission.)

TABLE 40.1

Hip Joint Myofascial Dysfunction: Structure and Clinical Impact

Structure → Functional Anatomical Features[1]	Clinical Implications of Somatic Dysfunction
Hip Flexors	
Iliopsoas (*L1–L4; ventral rami of lumbar n. (psoas) and femoral nerve (iliacus)*)—attaches the iliac fossa (iliacus) and T12–L5 (psoas) to the femoral lesser trochanter • Strongest flexor of thigh; and some external rotation of the hip joint • Activation with feet planted: Bends spine forward • Spine and hip stabilizer when standing	Postural muscle (hypertonic when stressed) • History/symptoms: Activated by sit-ups or bending over a low table; aggravated by weight-bearing; relief when recumbent with knees bent • Referral: To back and anterior groin • Exam: Positive Thomas test; psoas posturing; tender over iliacus or psoas counterstrain points; may have L1 or L2 Fryette II dysfunction; chronic psoas contracture might demonstrate lumbar hyperlordosis and a loud audible pop (psoas tendon) during the Thomas test
Tensor fasciae latae (*L5–S1; superior gluteal n.*) • Hip flexor (attachment on anterior iliac crest and ASIS), mild hip abductor, and internal rotator • Knee flexion and lateral rotation (via the iliotibial band when knee is flexed) • Stabilizes hip and knee when knee is extended • TFL tightens the iliotibial band to increase power of hip flexors and it steadies the trunk on the thigh	Postural muscle (hypertonic when stressed) • History/symptoms: perpetuated by sitting or excessive use; stiff hips, pain extending hips or running • Referral: from hip joint down toward knee along the outer/lateral thigh
Other contributors to hip flexion: **sartorius; the thigh adductors;** and **rectus femoris** (only when knee extended)	Sartorius is the "tailor muscle." It flexes, abducts, and externally rotates the hip.

TABLE 40.1 (Continued)

Hip Joint Myofascial Dysfunction: Structure and Clinical Impact

Structure → Functional Anatomical Features[1]	Clinical Implications of Somatic Dysfunction
HIP Extensors	
Gluteus maximus (*L5–S2; inferior gluteal n*) • Most powerful extensor of thigh and assists in hip external rotation • Location/size unique; provides anatomic basis for upright posture; type I (slow twitch) muscle fibers suited for continuous postural use	Phasic muscle (inhibited when stressed) • History/symptoms: Restlessness; sit or walk uphill = pain • Referral: To buttock • Exam: Antalgic gait
Hamstrings (*L5–S2; sciatic nerve*) • Hip extension (accelerating step of gait and rising from seated position) • Restrains hip flexion produced by body weight during stance phase of gait • See knee flexion below for individual actions of **semitendinosus, semimembranosus, and long head of the biceps femoris**	Postural muscle (hypertonic when stressed) • History/symptoms: Perpetuated by chair pressure under thighs; pain sitting and walking; disturbs sleep • Referral: To posterior thigh • Exam: Decreased hip flexion with straight leg raising test
Adductor magnus—hamstring portion (*L4; tibial part of sciatic n.*)—attaches from ischial tuberosity to adductor tubercle of femur • "Hamstring part" adducts and extends hip joint	Postural muscle (hypertonic when stressed) • Referral: To inner thigh
HIP Abductors	
Gluteus medius and Gluteus minimus (*L4–S1; superior gluteal innervation*) • Abductor and internal rotators of the hip • Stabilizes/levels pelvis during single limb stance and prevents contralateral nonstance innominate from falling inferiorly (negative Trendelenburg test)	Phasic muscles (inhibited when stressed) • History/symptoms: TrPs aggravated by walking, slouching in chair, or lying on back • Referral: G. medius to posterior iliac crest, sacroiliac joint, sacrum, and minor to buttock • Referral: G. minimus to buttock, lateral, and posterior thigh; mistaken for L5 or S1 radiculopathy (but may coexist) • Exam: Positive Trendelenburg test = weakness in hip abductors; antalgic Trendelenburg gait = "abductor lurch"

Piriformis (*S1–S2; branches of anterior rami innervation*)
• Activation can either externally or internally rotate the hip depending on the orientation of the femur. This paradoxical motion is due to the muscle's insertion on the superior apex of the greater trochanter.
  ○ When the femur is positioned within a range from full hip extension to about 70-degree hip flexion the piriformis externally rotates the femur.
  ○ Once the femur flexes past about 70 degrees the piriformis will internally rotate the femur.[25]
• Hip abduction when the femur is in flexion
	Postural muscle (hypertonic when stressed)
	• History/symptoms: perpetuated by sacroiliac somatic dysfunction (especially sacral shear) or irritation (sitting on billfold); might have fallen/missed step; Due to the anatomic location, piriformis spasm may entrap entire or fibular portion of sciatic nerve; may see footdrop
	• Referral: To pelvic floor; sciatica to knee if entrapped sciatic n.
	• Associated with pelvic floor dysfunction, dyspareunia, prostatodynia

Hip abductors to lesser extent: **Sartorius, Tensor fascia latae, gluteus maximus, iliopsoas,** and **obturator internus** (only when thigh is flexed)	
HIP Adductors	
Pectineus (*L2–L3; femoral ± obturator n*) • Adduction, slight flexion of the hip • Assists with external rotation of the hip	Postural muscle (hypertonic when stressed) • Referral: As deep-seated groin ache • Designed for power, not speed
Adductor magnus—adductor portion (*L2–L4; obturator n.*)—attaches from inferior ramus of pubis and ramus of ischium to the gluteal tuberosity, linea aspera, and medial supracondylar line of the femur • "Adductor part" adducts and flexes hip joint • Early in swing phase, muscles pull limb toward midline	Postural muscle (hypertonic when stressed) • Referral: To inner thigh
Adductor longus and brevis (*L2–L4; obturator n.*) • Adducts hip and to some extent brevis flexes it • Early in swing phase, muscles pull limb toward midline	Postural muscle (hypertonic when stressed) • Referral: To inguinal ligament, inner thigh, and upper medial knee

(*continued*)

TABLE 40.1 (*Continued*)

Hip Joint Myofascial Dysfunction: Structure and Clinical Impact

Structure → Functional Anatomical Features[1]	Clinical Implications of Somatic Dysfunction
Gracilis (*L2–L3; obturator n.*) • Gracilis is the second longest muscle in the body crossing hip and knee • Adducts hip joint; flexes knee joint and internally rotates tibia when knee is flexed.	Phasic muscles (inhibited when stressed) • Pain from gracilis is described as a hot stinging, superficial pain in the medial thigh; it may be relieved by walking
HIP External Rotators	
Piriformis (*S1–S2*) • External rotation when the femur is extended, neutral, or flexed less than about 70 degrees. See hip abductors, above.	See hip abductors above
Obturator externus (*L3–L4; obturator n*) • Externally rotates the hip; stabilizes the hip joint actions **Obturator internus, Superior and Inferior Gemelli** (*L5–S1*) (*n to obt. internus innervates superior gemellus. N to quadratus femoris innervates inferior gemellus*) • When the thigh is extended, causes external rotation at hip (when flexed, causes abduction) **Quadratus femoris** (*L5–S1; n to quadratus femoris*) • Externally rotates the hip; stabilizes the hip joint actions	Phasic muscles (inhibited when stressed) • History/symptoms: Responsible for pelvic floor symptoms (fullness in rectum) • Referral: To anococcygeal region (some to posterior thigh)
Gluteus maximus, Iliopsoas, pectineus and sartorius • Externally rotate the hip as secondary muscle actions	See hip extension for glut max, hip flexion for Iliopsoas, and knee extension for sartorius
HIP Internal Rotators	
Primary hip internal rotators: **Gluteus medius and gluteus minimus** (L4–S1)	See hip abductors above
Secondary hip internal rotators: **Tensor fascia latae** and **Piriformis** (only when thigh is flexed).[25]	See hip flexor for Tensor fascial latae information and hip abductors for Piriformis information above

TABLE 40.2

Knee Joint Myofascial Dysfunction: Structure and Clinical Impact

Structure → Functional Anatomical Features[1]	Clinical Implications of Somatic Dysfunction
Knee Flexors	
Biceps femoris (*L5–S2; sciatic n.; long head = tibial portion; short head = fibular portion*); attachment—both muscle heads plus the lateral collateral ligament establish a tripartite anchor on the fibular head • Long head crosses the hip (ischial tuberosity attachment) and knee for hip extension and knee flexion • Short head only crosses the knee (posterior femur attachment) and is active in knee flexion for toe clearance during walking • Active contraction also induces some external rotation of the knee	Postural muscle (hypertonic when stressed) • History/symptoms: Perpetuated by chair pressure under thighs; pain sitting and walking; disturbs sleep, often wakes patient at night • Referral: Distal from TrPs in the posterior thigh to the back of the knee or to the region of the fibular head • Exam: Decreased hip flexion with straight leg raising test (knees extended) and/or difficulty bending to touch toes without bending knees
Semimembranosus and **semitendinosus** (*L5–S2; sciatic n. tibial portion*) • Hip extensors and knee flexors • Hamstrings are not consistently active for all knee flexion during walking (passive gravitational knee flexion occurs more commonly with hip flexion) • Active contraction also induces some internal rotation of the tibia	Postural muscle (hypertonic when stressed) • History/symptoms: Aggravated by walking, often causing limp; TrPs often misdiagnosed as "sciatica" or "osteoarthritis of the knee" or "growing pains"; TrPs remaining postop often cause of "postlaminectomy syndrome" • Referral: Proximally to lower buttock • Exam: Tightness in the hamstrings is associated with secondary inhibition and laxity of the gluteal muscles
Sartorius (*L2–L3; femoral n.*) • Sartorius is the longest muscle in the body crossing both hip and knee • Flexes, abducts, and externally rotates the hip • Flexes the knee and internally rotates the tibia when the knee is flexed	Phasic muscles (inhibited when stressed) • Pain from the sartorius in the anterior thigh is superficial and described as tingling or sharp; may exhibit symptoms of meralgia paresthetica (entrapment of lateral femoral cutaneous nerve)

TABLE 40.2 (*Continued*)

Knee Joint Myofascial Dysfunction: Structure and Clinical Impact

Structure → Functional Anatomical Features[1]	Clinical Implications of Somatic Dysfunction
Popliteus (*L4–S1; Tibial n.*) • During swing phase of gait: Internally rotates tibia on femur. • During stance phase: externally rotates femur on Tibia. • Weakly flexes knee joint and unlocks it from full extension by rotating the femur 5 degrees.	See knee internal rotators below.
Gracilis (*L2–L3; obturator n.*) • Gracilis is the second longest muscle in the body crossing hip and knee • Adducts hip joint; flexes knee joint and internally rotates tibia when knee is flexed.	Phasic muscles (inhibited when stressed) Pain from gracilis is described as a hot stinging, superficial pain in the medial thigh; it may be relieved by walking
Knee Extensors	
Quadriceps (*L2–L4; femoral n.*); attachments—all four tendons unite into patellar tendon with patella; anchored to tibial tuberosity by patellar ligament • **Rectus femoris** crosses both hip and knee joints (proximal attachment to anterior inferior iliac spine [AIIS]); knee extension and assist with hip flexion and stabilization • The **vastus lateralis, medialis, and intermedius** only cross the knee joint, extending the knee • *Q-angle* or quadriceps angle is the angle of intersection for a line from ASIS to mid patella and a second (vertical) line from mid patella to tibial tuberosity	Rectus femoris is a postural muscle (hypertonic when stressed); the three vasti are phasic muscles (inhibited when stressed) • History/symptoms: Thigh and knee pain and weakness of knee extension especially going up stairs may interrupt sleep. TrPs in v. medialis cause "buckling knee" and may cause patient to fall; TrPs in v. lateralis may restrict motion of the patella; pain with walking; TrPs in v. intermedius create difficulty straightening knee after prolonged sitting • Referral: Anterior knee pain is referred from v. medialis and rectus femoris; posterior knee pain and pain anywhere along the lateral thigh to the iliac crest referred from v. lateralis • Exam: Include Q-angle and patellar grind tests; imbalance in quadriceps with one another or with the hamstrings predispose to chondromalacia patellae (as does an increased Q-angle); direct trauma to the quadriceps should be observed for myositis ossificans
Knee External Rotator	
Biceps femoris (*L5–S2; sciatic n.*) • Primarily knee flexor but also externally rotates knee	See description with Knee Flexors above
Knee Internal Rotators	
Popliteus (*L4–S1; tibial n.*) • Unlocks knee at the start of weight bearing by externally rotating the femur on the fixed tibia; internally rotates tibia when femur is fixed • Prevents posterior glide of tibia relative to femur while crouching	• History/symptoms: Aggravated by braking forward motions during twists (e.g., skiing), high heels by excessive foot pronation, and by training on uneven ground • Referral: Pain behind the knee when crouching, walking downstairs, or running downhill • Exam: Mimics symptoms of Baker cyst but no associated swelling in the region
Semimembranosus, semitendinosus, sartorius, and **gracilis** also internally rotate the knee when it is flexed.	See descriptions above in Knee Flexors for first three muscles and see Hip adductor for gracilis.

TABLE 40.3

Ankle–Foot Joints Myofascial Dysfunction: Structure and Clinical Impact

Structure → Functional Anatomical Features[1]	Clinical Implications of Somatic Dysfunction
Ankle Dorsiflexors	
Tibialis anterior (*L4–L5; deep fibular n.*) • Dorsiflexes the talocrural joint • Inverts the subtalar joint • Supinates foot at the talocalcaneal and transverse tarsal joints • An anterior compartment muscle	Phasic muscle (inhibited when stressed) • History/symptoms: Might complain of tripping over carpets, dragging foot, or "foot slap." Weakness in muscle may be caused by L5 radiculopathy, fibular mononeuropathy, the habit of crossing the legs at the knee, or posterior fibular head somatic dysfunction • Referral: Pain and tenderness referred into great toe and anteromedial ankle • Exam: Weakness leads to varying degrees of footdrop (rule out other causes)

(*continued*)

TABLE 40.3 (*Continued*)

Ankle–Foot Joints Myofascial Dysfunction: Structure and Clinical Impact

Structure → Functional Anatomical Features[1]	Clinical Implications of Somatic Dysfunction
Fibularis (Peroneus) tertius (*L5–S1; deep fibular n.*); attachment—tendon passes in front of lateral malleolus to insert on proximal 5th metatarsal • Weakly dorsiflexes the talocrural joint • Everts the subtalar joint (balancing inversion of tibialis anterior muscle) • Pronates the foot • An anterior compartment muscle	Phasic muscle (inhibited when stressed) • History/symptoms: Weakness in ankle dorsiflexion predisposing to ankle instability and repeat sprains; might be mistaken for ankle arthritis. Weakness in muscle might be caused by L5 radiculopathy, fibular mononeuropathy, the habit of crossing the legs at the knee, posterior fibular head somatic dysfunction, or prolonged immobilization (as in an ankle cast) • Referral: Anterolateral ankle and sometimes to lateral heel • Exam: Failure to identify and treat TrPs post ankle sprain can prolong rehabilitation process. Weakness in ankle dorsiflexion predisposing to ankle instability and repeat sprains
Extensor digitorum longus (*L4–S1; deep fibular n.*) • Dorsiflexes ankle • Dorsiflexes (extends) the lateral four digits • Helps prevent posterior postural sway • An anterior compartment muscle	Postural muscle (hypertonic when stressed) • History/symptoms: Dysfunction often results in foot slap after heel strike • Referral: Dorsum of foot and ankle • Exam: TrPs might entrap deep fibular nerve fibers; muscle imbalance → formation of hammer toes
The **Extensor Hallucis Longus**, although mostly a great toe extender, also weakly dorsiflexes the ankle	See below under Foot and/or Toe Extensors
Ankle Plantar Flexors	
Gastrocnemius (*L5–S2; posterior tibial n.*); shares Achilles tendon attachment to calcaneus • Plantarflexes ankle joint when knee joint is extended • Raises heel during waking • Flexes knee joint • *The gastrocnemius–soleus complex is referred to as* ***triceps surae*** *and constitutes a close functional unit* • A superficial posterior compartment muscle	Postural muscle (hypertonic when stressed) • History/symptoms: Often nocturnal leg cramps; "tennis leg" (partial tearing of gastrocnemius) with a sudden intense calf pain, as if kicked, followed by swelling and local tenderness • Referral: Upper posterior calf and/or to instep • Exam: Failure to recognize "tennis leg" might lead to a posterior compartment syndrome
Soleus (*S1–S2; tibial n.*); shares Achilles attachment to calcaneus • Plantarflexes ankle joint independent of knee position • Stabilizes ankle joint • Pumps venous and lymphatic fluid from lower extremity (e.g., fainting with military attention position) • *Gastrocnemius–soleus complex constitutes close functional unit* • A superficial posterior compartment muscle	Postural muscle (hypertonic when stressed) • History/symptoms: Pain severe walking up hill or stairs; may cause growing pains in children • Referral: Heel pain with TrPs in this muscle and/or may refer proximally to sacroiliac joint or even temporomandibular joint • Exam: May restrict dorsiflexion at ankle; soleus TrPs easily mistaken for Baker cyst, thrombophlebitis, and/or Achilles tendinitis
Fibularis (Peroneus) longus and brevis (*L5–S2; superficial fibular n.*) attachments—**f. longus** attaches to fibular head and to upper 2/3 of lateral fibula, crosses behind the lateral malleolus over the cuboid, and divides to attach to the 1st cuneiform and the base of the 1st metatarsal; **f. brevis** travels with **f. longus** but inserts on the lateral aspect of the 5th metatarsal • Plantarflexes the ankle • Pronate the foot and evert the subtalar joint • Lateral compartment muscles	Phasic muscles (inhibited when stressed) • History/symptoms: TrPs initiated by inversion twisting of ankle or prolonged immobilization in ankle cast; predispose to weak ankles and recurrent sprains; pain easily mistaken for arthritis in ankle; numbness often noted in web of great toe • Referral: Lateral malleolus and some of lateral leg • Exam: May have deep fibular nerve entrapment with some footdrop; f. longus and brevis aggravated by Morton foot structure; TrPs in p. longus can entrap the common fibular nerve and weaken both anterior and lateral compartment muscles
Tibialis posterior (*L4, L5; tibial n.*) • Plantarflexes the ankle • Inverts the foot • Maintains medial longitudinal arch • Deep posterior compartment muscles	Postural muscle (hypertonic when stressed) • History/symptoms: Symptoms mimic plantar fasciitis and acquired flatfoot • Referral: posterior calf and heel, plantar surface of heel, foot, and toes. • Exam: May have weak deep posterior compartment muscles, foot drop, degenerative changes to the tendon, and loss of medial longitudinal arch support, acquired pes planus

TABLE 40.3 (Continued)

Ankle–Foot Joints Myofascial Dysfunction: Structure and Clinical Impact

Structure → Functional Anatomical Features[1]	Clinical Implications of Somatic Dysfunction
Foot Supinators	
Tibialis anterior (*L5–S1; deep fibular n.*) • Supinates foot at talocalcaneal and transverse tarsal joints • Also dorsiflexes at the talocrural joint	See above Ankle dorsiflexors
Tibialis posterior (*L4, L5; tibial n.*)	See above Ankle plantar flexors
Foot Pronators	
Fibularis (Peroneal) (*L5–S1; deep fibular n.*); • All three pronate the foot (eversion and abduction) • F. tertius also dorsiflexes the ankle joint • F. longus and F. brevis also plantarflex the ankle joint • Anterior (tertius) and Lateral (longus and brevis) compartment muscles	Phasic muscles (inhibited when stressed) • History/symptoms: May be mistaken for ankle arthritis. Weakness in muscle may be caused by L5 radiculopathy, fibular mononeuropathy, the habit of crossing the legs at the knee, posterior fibular head somatic dysfunction, or prolonged immobilization (as in an ankle cast) • Referral: Lateral ankle and foot; sometimes to lateral heel • Exam: Failure to identify and treat TrPs post ankle sprain can prolong rehabilitation process.
Foot and/or Toe Flexors	
Flexor digitorum longus (*S2–S3; tibial n.*) • Flexes lateral four digits and plantarflexes ankle • Supports longitudinal arches of foot • Deep posterior compartment muscle	• History/symptoms: TrP perpetuation by Morton foot, running on uneven ground, or barefoot in the sand; pain worse with walking • Referral: Sole of foot
Flexor hallucis longus (*S2–S3; tibial n.*) • Flexes great toe and weakly plantarflexes ankle • Supports medial longitudinal arch of foot • Deep posterior compartment muscles	• History/symptoms: TrP perpetuation by Morton foot, running on uneven ground or barefoot in the sand • Referral: Plantar surface of great toe and first metatarsal head
Also **intrinsic foot muscles**	• History/symptoms: Intolerably sore feet, limited walking range, limp
Foot and/or Toe Extensors	
Extensor digitorum longus (*L4–S1; deep fibular n.*) • Dorsiflexes the lateral four digits and the ankle • Anterior compartment muscle	See above under Ankle Dorsiflexors
Extensor hallucis longus (*L4–S1; deep fibular n.*) • Dorsiflexes the great toe • Weakly dorsiflexes the ankle • Anterior compartment muscle	• Dysfunction makes foot less adaptable to the ground while walking • History/symptoms: TrPs may be perpetuated by L4–L5 radiculopathy; often created following anterior compartment syndrome, prolonged jogging, or dorsiflexed ankle position during sleep • Referral: Dorsum of foot at the base of the great toe
Also **intrinsic foot muscles**	• History/symptoms: Intolerably sore feet, limited walking range, limp

Bursitis is inflammation of a bursa. There is typically palpable swelling that can be defined and is sensitive to deep pressure.

Neural Structures

Because many neurologic symptoms and functional deficits in the lower extremities are related to the lumbar nerve roots, a solid foundation of lumbar neuroanatomy is important. This includes understanding the sensory, motor, and reflex changes that can occur, and conditions that warrant emergent intervention.

Motor and sensory innervation to the lower extremities arise from the lumbar plexus and sacral plexus (Fig. 40.20)[1]:

- The lumbar plexus (L2–L4) gives rise to the femoral and obturator nerves.
  - □ The femoral nerve conveys fibers to the hip flexors and knee extensors, along with multiple anterior cutaneous nerves of the thigh, the anteromedial leg, and medial aspect of the ankle and foot.
  - □ The obturator nerve conveys fibers to the hip adductors and a variable area of skin on the medial thigh, above the knee.
- The sacral plexus (L4–S3) gives rise to the sciatic nerve which descends in the posterior compartment of the thigh and further separates into the tibial and common fibular nerve components proximal to the knee.
  - □ The tibial nerve supplies the posterior compartment of the leg and the muscles of the foot.
  - □ The deep fibular (peroneal) nerve supplies the anterior compartment of the leg with sensation to the webbing between the first and second toes.
  - □ The superficial fibular (peroneal) nerve supplies the lateral compartment of the leg as well as the skin on the anterolateral side of the leg, and the dorsum of the foot.

Muscle innervations for the hips, knees, ankles, and feet are summarized in Tables 40.1 to 40.3. Pathologic or biomechanical entrapment of a nerve root, plexus, or peripheral nerve can leave weakness or myofascial trigger points (MTrP) in the muscles distal

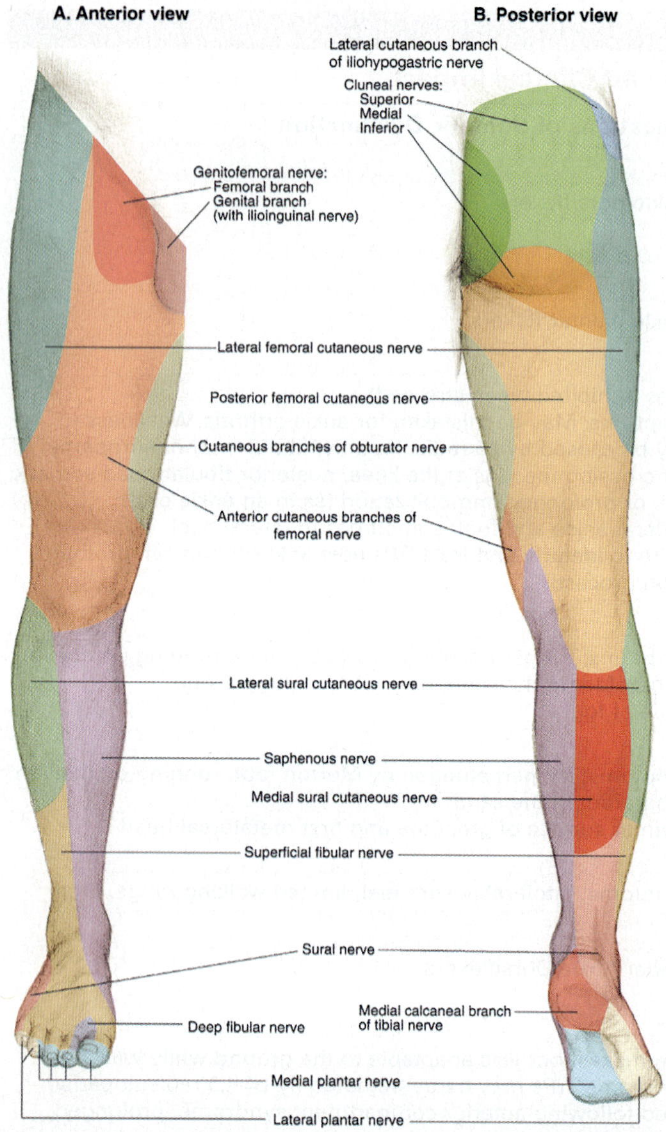

Figure 40.20. Cutaneous innervation of the lower limb. (Reprinted with permission from Gest TR. *Lippincott® Atlas of Anatomy*. 2nd ed. Wolters Kluwer; 2020:167. Plate 3-69.)

to that site in the neural pattern associated with the involved structure.

Pain descriptions and pattern distributions can extend beyond dysesthesia or anesthesia associated with a nerve root or dermatomal pattern. Other lower extremity patterns of pain occur in sclerotomal and myotomal distributions. Sclerotomal pain arises from ligaments, tendons, disks, periosteum, and apophyseal joints. Sclerotomal pain is typically described as deep, ill-defined, dull aching, and diffuse.[26] A myotome is defined as a group of muscles that are innervated by the ventral root of a single spinal nerve and are the motor equivalent of dermatomes.[27]

Often, the pain quality and patterns are mixed. For example, pain patterns referred from the facet joints of the lumbar spine (sclerotomal structures) overlap MTrP pain (Fig. 40.21) that arises from the somatic dysfunction in following muscles (myotomal structures)[28]:

- Multifidi
- Quadratus lumborum
- Glutei
- Piriformis
- Obturator internus

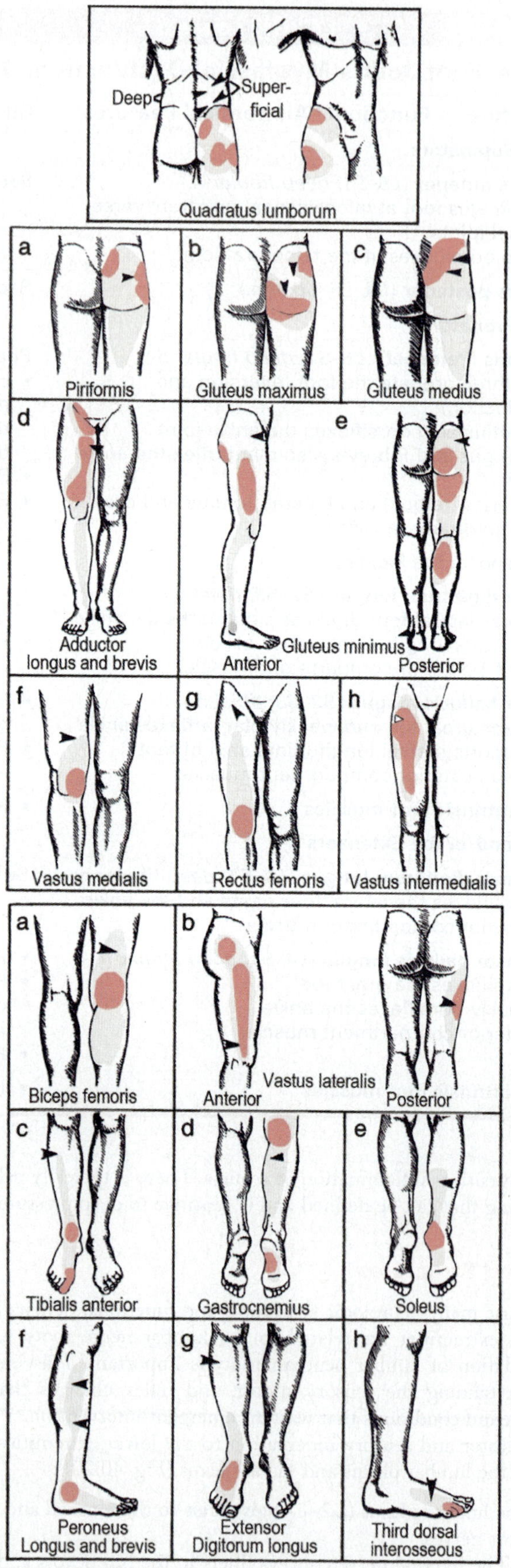

Figure 40.21. Travell MTrP patterns in the lower extremity. (Reprinted with permission from Travell JG, Simons DG. *Myofascial Pain and Dysfunction: The Trigger Point Manual. The Lower Extremities*. Vol 2. Williams & Wilkins; 1992:429–459.)

Sclerotomal (bony/ligamentous) distribution has also been mapped out, but it is often overlooked, and patients might dismiss it as lower extremity arthritic pain. There can also be confusion due to the overlap of joint and spinal level distributions. For example, different aspects of the knee and the hip joints share the L3 and L4 sclerotomes. Additionally, a vulnerable site for entrapment or trauma exists as the common fibular nerve passes behind the fibular head.

In general, referred pain is reproducible; therefore, diagnosis can be enhanced by stimulating the postulated pain generator to cause the pain symptom and by anesthetizing (or deactivating) that structure to see if the pain is eliminated. An understanding of the patterns associated with each referral improves patient diagnosis and treatment design. Failure to appreciate nondermatomal patterns may lead a practitioner to ineffectively treat symptoms rather than causes or to incorrectly consider a patient with legitimate symptoms a malingerer.

Circulatory Structures

ARTERIES

Arterial supply to the lower extremities begins with the internal and external branches of the common iliac arteries.

The internal iliac artery primarily supplies the pelvic viscera and pelvic girdle musculature—including the gluteal region, iliac fossa, and the most proximal part of the medial thigh.[1] The inferior margin of the acetabulum is incomplete, forming an acetabular notch through which the hip joint receives its blood vessels. These vessels could easily be disrupted by a femoral neck fracture, which creates the possibility of delayed healing or nonunion; somatic dysfunction rarely causes problems with these large vessels.

The external iliac artery becomes the femoral artery, which is the major vessel supplying the lower extremities.[1] It is easily located in the femoral triangle, bounded by the sartorius and adductor muscles, and the inguinal ligament. The mnemonic NAVEL (***N***erve, ***A***rtery, ***V***ein, ***E***mpty space, ***L***ymphatics) provides a reminder of the order, from lateral to medial, of the structures in the femoral triangle (Fig. 40.22).

The arterial pulse in the femoral triangle helps to establish the distal pulses, including the popliteal pulse, the posterior tibial pulse, and the dorsalis pedis pulse within their palpatory landmarks of the lower limb (Fig. 40.23). Acute loss of pulses in the lower extremity is a contraindication to the use of osteopathic manipulative treatment (OMT).

Treatment of lower thoracic and lumbar somatic dysfunction is postulated to improve blood delivery to the lower extremities by reducing hypersympathetic activity. Cell bodies for the sympathetic nerve supply to the lower extremities' vasculature are found at the levels of T10-L2. This is important for the nutritional status of the tissues. It would also benefit the delivery of medications, such as nonsteroidal anti-inflammatory drugs to target tissues in the lower extremities where pharmacologic effectiveness is proportionate to tissue or synovial concentration of the drug.

As an example, the vascular supply to the menisci in the knees (especially the central section) and to synovial joint tissues in general is very poor. Generally, nutrition to the joints depends on good blood flow to the region, and subsequent bidirectional exchange of nutrients and metabolic waste products via the synovial fluids.[29]

VENOUS AND LYMPHATIC STRUCTURES

The lower limb has both superficial and deep venous and lymphatic vessels, which typically travel alongside each other. There are also perforating veins that pierce the deep fascia to shunt blood from the superficial veins to the deep veins.

The superficial veins typically course through the subcutaneous tissue. Superficial lymphatic vessels converge and travel along the saphenous veins (Fig. 40.24). The great saphenous vein passes anterior to the medial malleolus and ascends approximately one hand's breadth posterior to the patella traveling toward the inguinal region where it drains into the femoral vein. The lymphatics accompanying the great saphenous vein end in the vertical group of superficial inguinal lymph nodes, which then primarily drain into the external iliac lymph nodes.[1]

Superficial lymphatic vessels of the lateral foot and posterolateral leg accompany the small saphenous vein posteriorly and enter the popliteal lymph nodes in the popliteal fossa, where they join with the deep lymphatics of the leg. From there, the lymph continues to ascend the femoral vessels and drain into the deep inguinal lymph nodes and then passes to the external and common iliac lymph nodes and enters the lumbar lymphatic trunks.[1]

The popliteal vein is formed by the union of the anterior and posterior tibial veins. These deep veins, along with the deep veins of the thigh and the deep lymphatics are internal to the deep fascia and usually course along the arteries.[1] They are clinically significant as a common site for venous thrombosis formation, which can cause life-threatening pulmonary embolus.

The femoral vein is a continuation of the popliteal vein after it passes proximal to the adductor hiatus. Within the femoral triangle, it receives the deep vein of the thigh and the great saphenous vein and then becomes the external iliac vein as it passes proximal to the inguinal ligament.

Ideally, venous and lymphatic return are improved by addressing myofascial restriction and by using lymphatic drainage techniques, especially in the setting of lower extremity lymphedema.

DIAGNOSIS OF LOWER EXTREMITY SOMATIC DYSFUNCTION

The structure and function of the lower extremities allow them to play significant roles in the body's balance, posture, and locomotion as well as venous and lymphatic fluid return to the central vascular system. The lower extremities are vital to successful participation in most occupations and recreational activities. Screening the lower extremities is an essential part of a total body screening examination, regardless of the chief complaint. Chapter 30 Osteopathic Structural Examination provides a full description of the static postural examination and the dynamic screening components, including regional range of motion testing and gait observation. This section will focus more on screening and regional examination for lower extremity dysfunction.

Dysfunction in the lower extremities can be a significant source of debility for patients. When evaluating a patient, begin with pertinent screening tests and progress to more specific regional examination and special tests. Always compare both sides as well as the joint above and below the affected area. OMT and therapeutic exercises are generally useful in treating lower extremity complaints due to somatic dysfunction.

SCREENING EXAMINATION

Observation—Gait

The physical examination of the lower extremity begins when the patient walks into the clinic. It is important for the osteopathic physician to observe the patient's gait, station, and body habitus. Observation of gait during the osteopathic screening portion of the structural examination is intended to assess the functional

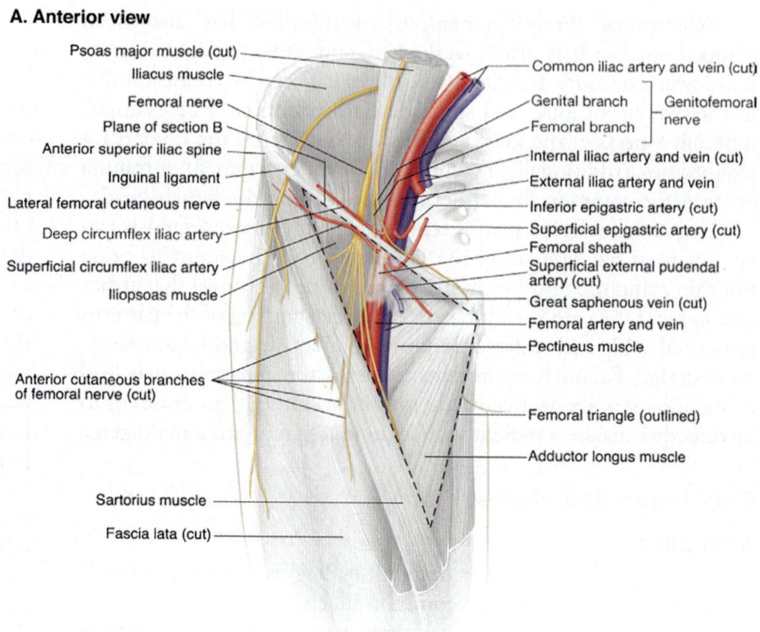

Figure 40.22. Femoral triangle. (Reprinted with permission from Gest TR. *Lippincott® Atlas of Anatomy*. 2nd ed. Wolters Kluwer; 2020:116. Plate 3-18.)

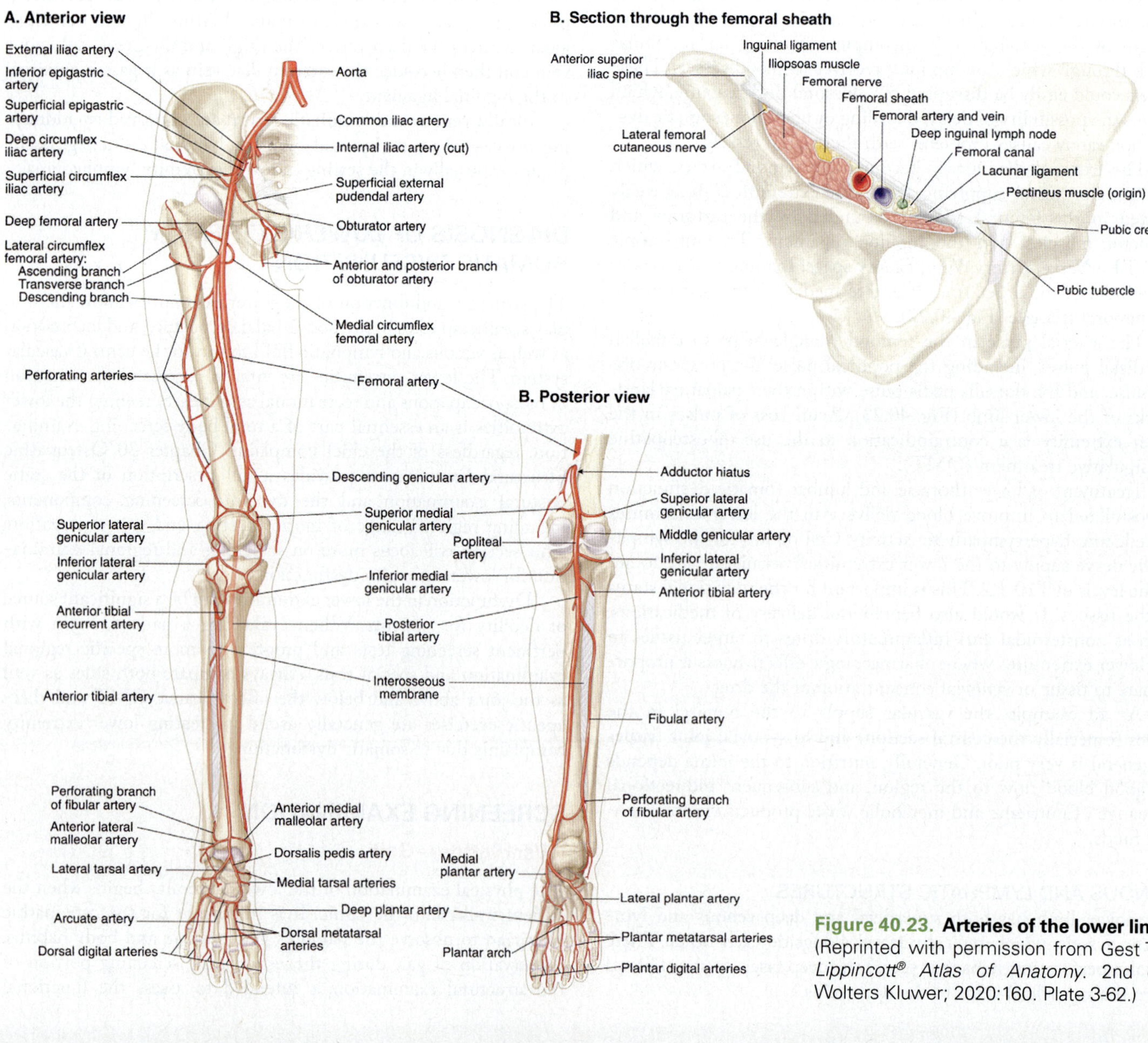

Figure 40.23. Arteries of the lower limb. (Reprinted with permission from Gest TR. *Lippincott® Atlas of Anatomy*. 2nd ed. Wolters Kluwer; 2020:160. Plate 3-62.)

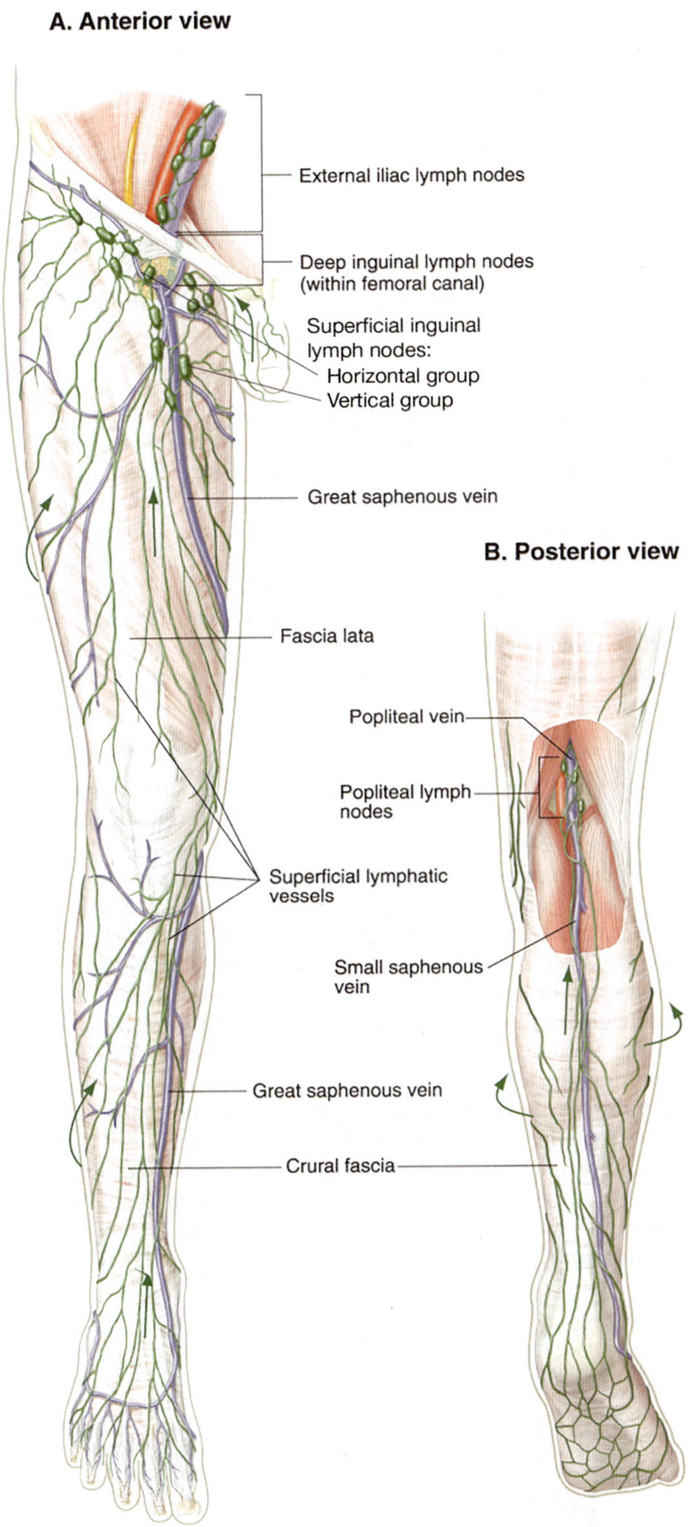

Figure 40.24. Superficial veins and lymphatics of the lower limb. (Reprinted with permission from Gest TR. *Lippincott® Atlas of Anatomy*. 2nd ed. Wolters Kluwer; 2020:169. Plate 3-71.)

performance of gait regardless of presence or absence of musculoskeletal or neurologic pathology. Watching the patient walk without shoes, viewing them from an anterior position and a posterior position gives useful information to the clinician. It is also important to note the patient's shoe wear and balance.

Assess for the following:

- Stride length
- Cadence
- Arm swing
- Out-toeing or in-toeing
- Supination or pronation
- Heel strike
- Toe off
- Pelvic tilt
- Balance
- Disruption in weight transfer (limping)

See Chapter 30 Osteopathic Structural Examination for definitions of each of these components of gait observation. Restriction or asymmetry in any of these components can either be caused by lower extremity somatic dysfunction or can produce and maintain lower extremity somatic dysfunction. As these various aspects of the gate cycle are visualized, recall the biomechanical motions of the innominates and sacrum that are expected to occur during the different phases of gait. (For further detail than what was described earlier in this chapter, see Chapter 38 Functional Anatomy and Diagnosis of the Sacrum—section: "The Sacrum and the Walking Cycle.") For health and wellbeing, there needs to be unencumbered movement of the lower extremities and pelvis, coupled through the axial spine to the upper extremities and the rest of the body.

Common observations include asymmetry of arm swing, a declination of the pelvis during mid-stance (Trendelenburg gait), and in-toeing or out-toeing. Although there are orthopedic causes for the following, some of the more common somatic dysfunctions that correspond to these findings include:

- Asymmetry of arm swing
  - ☐ Myofascial tension and tender points of the pectoral girdle
  - ☐ Thoracic scoliosis or group curve somatic dysfunction
  - ☐ Somatic dysfunction of the shoulders, clavicles, and scapula
- Declination of the pelvis during mid-stance
  - ☐ Weak gluteus medius causes a contralateral pelvic declination during gait
- In-toeing
  - ☐ Weak hip abductors
  - ☐ Tight hip adductors
  - ☐ High arch
- Out-toeing
  - ☐ Weak hip adductors
  - ☐ Tight hip abductors
  - ☐ Collapsed arch

Observation—Static Postural Examination

Observing the standing patient from the anterior, lateral, and posterior views will allow the clinician to notice skin abnormalities and any asymmetries of tissue, muscular, and bony alignment. Ideally, the patient is uncovered enough for the overall configuration of the body to be observed, without being obscured by clothing.

Although the generalized static posture examination should include the full head-to-toe inspection, as described in Chapter 30, this chapter will focus on specific observations within the lower extremities. Additionally, some elements of static observation commonly include simultaneous palpation to confirm asymmetries.

SKIN

The skin should be observed for such characteristics as erythema, moisture, pallor, pigmentation and/or scars, tattoos, lesions, masses, implanted devices, muscle atrophy, hair loss, deformity, and edema.

The skin may provide clues to any underlying patient conditions. Scarring may be the result of trauma or surgical intervention and may be associated with motion restriction of the musculoskeletal structures in the region of the scar. Excessive moisture or dryness (as well as edema) may be associated with increased or decreased sympathetic nervous system activity in the noted body region which may lead to discovery of facilitated segments on further evaluation. Different forms of skin cancer may be observed.

BODY SYMMETRY

Some minor asymmetry is present in virtually everyone. The standing structural exam can be applied before and after treatment to determine clinical effects of treatments. See Chapter 30 Osteopathic Structural Examination for the list of all commonly used landmarks throughout the body observed during the osteopathic screening structural examination. It is useful to determine asymmetry in the sagittal and coronal planes while the patient is standing on a level floor. Some of the key standing landmarks for lower extremity evaluation include:

- Iliac crest
- Posterior superior iliac spine (PSIS)
- Sacral sulcus
- Greater trochanter
- Popliteal creases
- Fibular head
- Lateral malleolus
- Arches of the feet

Pelvic and Hip Landmarks

Iliac crest heights, PSIS levels, sacral sulcus depth, and greater trochanter levels relate to one another when interpreting asymmetric anatomic landmark findings during the structural examination. It is important for the clinician to utilize the same part of the anatomic structure during each assessment. If the patient has a low iliac crest, low PSIS, low greater trochanter, and deep sacral sulcus all on the ipsilateral side, an anatomic short leg may be present. Another common finding with short leg syndrome is a lumbar group curvature or scoliosis. Over time the lumbar spine compensates for the sacral base declination with convexity toward the short leg side. Asymmetry of these landmarks may also be due to functional causes such as myofascial tension, spasms of the iliopsoas, quadratus lumborum, and erector spinae muscles or somatic dysfunction of the lumbar spine, sacrum, and pelvis. Therefore, it is important to repeat these landmark assessments following OMT or other treatments.

Gluteal Region

The gluteal folds should be symmetric. Asymmetry may indicate a leg-length inequality. The gluteal muscle mass should be assessed for asymmetry and atrophy. Atrophy may indicate disuse or neurologic impairment such as chronic entrapment of the S1 nerve root, or entrapment of the superior and inferior gluteal nerves in the greater sciatic foramen due to hypertrophy of the piriformis muscle.

Thighs

Observe thigh muscle mass from anterior, posterior, and lateral views. Unilaterally enlarged muscle mass may be due to hypertrophy on one side or atrophy on the opposite side. Enlargement of the musculature may be due to normal variants such as a dominant leg, especially in athletes. Pathologic enlargement may occur with venous insufficiency, thrombosis, tumor, edema, or hematoma. Unilateral decreased muscle mass or atrophy can occur with chronic entrapment of the associated lumbar nerve roots. The lateral thigh surface should be smooth. The presence of a deep groove, running from the greater trochanter of the femur to the knee may suggest shortening and contracture of the iliotibial band.

Knees

Observe the knees' positions and look for any asymmetry, bony deformity, swelling, bruising, and/or scars from trauma, surgeries, or other procedures.

From an anterior view note the Q-angle. A patient with an increased Q-angle, *genu valgum*, appears knock-kneed. While a patient with a decreased Q-angle, *genu varum*, appears bow-legged (Fig. 40.25). Observe the tibial tuberosities for prominence, as this may represent a case of Osgood-Schlatter disease. Also, observe the height of the patella relative to the tibial tuberosities. Search for the presence of *patella alta* (high-riding patella) or *patella baja* (low-riding patella).

Observe the shape of the popliteal fossa posteriorly or laterally. A bulging popliteal fossa may be indicative of a Baker cyst and internal derangement. A flattened popliteal fossa suggests the presence of *genu recurvatum* (hyperextension of the knee). If unilateral, this may represent a compensatory change for an anatomic or functional long leg on the ipsilateral side.

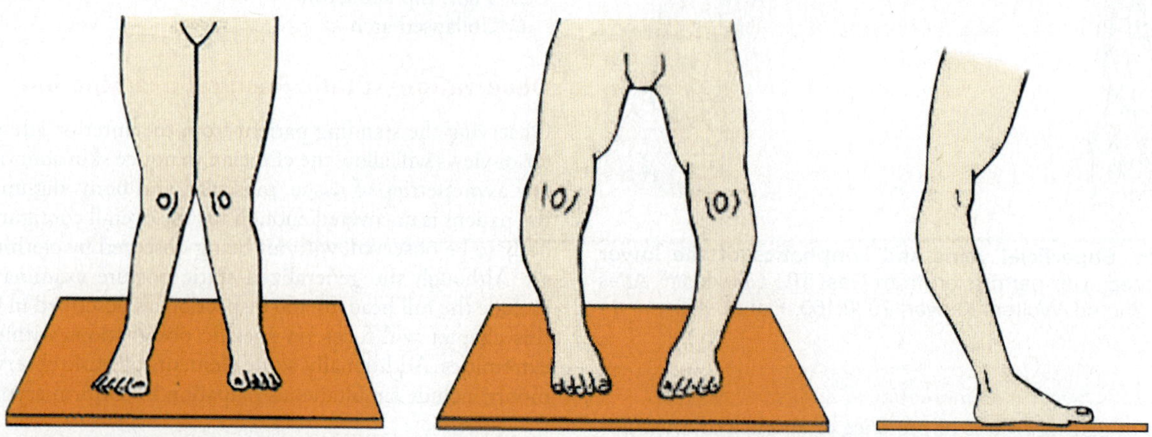

Figure 40.25. Deformities of the knees—anterior and lateral view. From left to right: *genu valgum, genu varum, genu recurvatum*. (From Department of Neuromusculoskeletal Medicine/Osteopathic Manipulative Medicine at Western University of Health Sciences, College of Osteopathic Medicine of the Pacific. *Osteopathic Principles and Practice: Osteopathic Manipulative Treatment.* 1st ed. Western University of Health Sciences; 2015–2016, with permission.)

Note if the knees appear flexed or hyperextended. A flexed knee (restricted extension) may be related to muscle imbalance like tight hamstrings or could be from internal derangement including bony, capsular, or ligamentous deformity, or effusion. Genu recurvatum can be a normal physiologic variant, a congenital misalignment, or may be related to somatic dysfunction, injury, or pathologic conditions like hypermobility. Some causes include trauma to an extended knee, instability of the ligaments and joint capsule, connective tissue disorders, irregular alignment of the femur and tibia, leg length discrepancy, and certain diseases that lead to muscle imbalance like cerebral palsy, multiple sclerosis, and muscular dystrophy.

Although palpating the major bony landmarks of the knee is typically more of a focused segmental examination, it may be done during the screening examination when identifying the landmarks. The major bony landmarks including the medial and lateral joint lines, femoral condyles, tibial plateaus, tibial tuberosity, pes anserine region, Gerdy tubercle (insertion of the IT band), margins of the patella, infrapatellar tendon, MCLs and LCLs, and the hamstring tendon insertions.

Lower Leg

Observe the color, size, and symmetry of the calves in the standing and seated position. If one side appears smaller, measure each at the same location with a tape measure. Look for skin changes from conditions that may contribute to a larger calf such as cellulitis, peripheral edema, compartment syndrome, or deep venous thrombosis. Varicose veins and spider veins are common and can become painful. In athletes or laborers, an overdevelopment of one calf may occur due to repetitive overuse. Muscle atrophy due to chronic entrapment of the S1 or S2 nerve roots, or of the sciatic nerve itself may result in a smaller calf. Patients who have had veins harvested from their legs, vascular surgery, or orthopedic surgery of the limb or spine can all have asymmetry of the legs.

Ankles

Evaluate the ankles for scars, edema, hypertrophy, deformity, and discoloration. Include the Achilles tendons in the assessment. View the ankles posteriorly and look for evidence of hindfoot varus or valgus deformity. This will affect the smooth contour of the Achilles tendon. Hindfoot valgus occurs with a collapsed arch and overpronation. Hindfoot varus occurs with high arches and supination. Chronic edema and lipomatous changes can occur around the lateral or medial aspect of the ankle.

Feet and Arches

The clinician should inspect the overall structure of the patient's foot, noting any deformities, calluses, and the height of the longitudinal arches of the foot, evaluating for the existence of pes planus or pes cavus, and excessive pronation or supination. It is also helpful to compare the patient's gait and structural foot findings to the patient's shoes and insoles.

- Pes planus (flat foot): a deformity of the foot where the medial longitudinal arch is abnormally flattened or lost. It can be helpful to ask the patient to lift their foot to observe if the flattened arch is fixed or flexible. About 20% to 40% of the population has some degree of pes planus.[30] Most patients are asymptomatic and do not require treatment, but it may also be associated with congenital fusion of the midfoot and hindfoot or connective tissue disorders.
- Pes cavus: a foot morphology with an abnormally high longitudinal arch that does not flatten with weight bearing. While it may be a normal variant, it may also be seen in neuromuscular conditions such as Charcot-Marie-Tooth disease, spinal anomalies, and conditions causing spastic paralysis.
- Supination: a patient may have a normal medial longitudinal arch when the foot is elevated but upon weight bearing may demonstrate inversion of the forefoot and elevated medial arch. When ambulating most of the weight is transferred to the lateral edge of the foot.
- Pronation: the patient may have a normal medial longitudinal arch when the foot is elevated but upon weight bearing may demonstrate an eversion of the hindfoot and a depressed medial arch. Patients who overpronate may have more visible toes when viewed posteriorly. Their shoes will often wear out the medial heel.

Collapsed arches are common and may be related to somatic dysfunction (dropped navicular, cuboid, or cuneiforms). Recall passive support for the arches of the foot include the ligaments and plantar aponeurosis. Dynamic support includes the intrinsic muscles of the foot and the long tendons of the foot.[1] Tensions or weakness within any of those supporting structures may lead to somatic dysfunction of the tarsal bones.

As the body's weight is transferred anteriorly the foot pronates and everts. A flat foot is frequently associated with overpronation (foot eversion). This will place excessive stress on the ligaments of the medial ankle and may lead to pain in this area. Overpronation may also be associated with shin splints. A high arch is frequently associated with excessive supination (foot inversion). This will place excessive strain on the ligaments of the lateral ankle and may lead to lateral foot pain.

The height of the arches should also be evaluated for relative symmetry. Unilateral arch collapse with valgus hindfoot can occur to compensate for an anatomically longer leg on the ipsilateral side, and for pelvic dysfunctions that create a functionally long leg on the ipsilateral side (anterior rotation of the innominate, inferior innominate shear, etc.).

Structural foot deformities and issues with the toes and metatarsals are common and can be related to dysfunction elsewhere. Although, some patients have a genetic predisposition to having a longer 2nd toe (Morton foot); hammer toes, calluses, and bunions can develop or worsen in any patient due to poor foot and lower extremity mechanics, and improper shoes.

Alterations in the normal posture and positioning of the foot may be the result of somatic dysfunction within the structure of the foot itself, or from injury or instability of the foot's stabilizing ligaments. Such alterations may have profound effects on the patient's posture and gait, and may result in compensatory somatic dysfunctions elsewhere, such as in the lower extremities, pelvis, or lumbar region. Likewise, somatic dysfunction, medical conditions, overuse, and obesity can contribute to altered foot mechanics and dysfunction.

Lower Extremity Functional Screening, Neurologic, and Orthopedic Tests

THE SQUAT TEST

The squat test is a quick way to assess the full lower extremities and assists with determining if there is presence of lower extremity somatic dysfunction. This screening test is useful when a patient's chief complaint is related to another region of the body but dysfunction in the lower extremity could be contributing to that complaint.

The squat test requires normal lower extremity muscle strength and bilateral mobility of the hips, knees, feet, and ankles. If the patient cannot perform this test, then further structural evaluation of the joints and tissues of the lower extremities is indicated (Fig. 40.26).

- The physician stands so they have a posterolateral view of the standing patient.

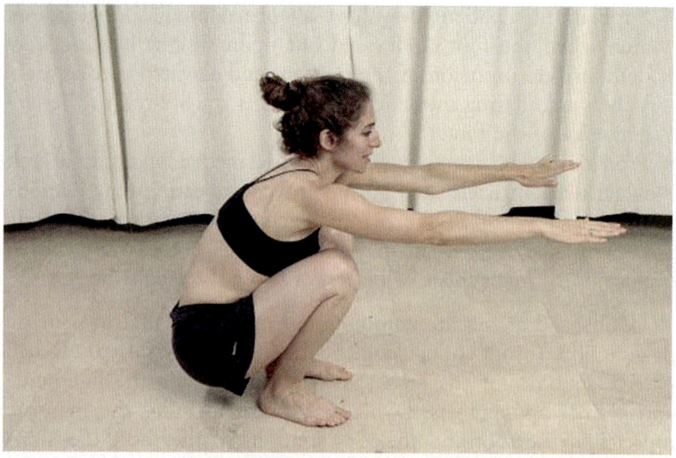

Figure 40.26. Squat test. Active range of motion screening test for lower extremities. A negative test is when the knees can fully flex with the heels flat on the ground as depicted. (From Department of Neuromusculoskeletal Medicine/Osteopathic Manipulative Medicine at Western University of Health Sciences, College of Osteopathic Medicine of the Pacific. *Osteopathic Principles and Practice: Osteopathic Manipulative Treatment.* 1st ed. Western University of Health Sciences; 2015–2016, with permission.)

- The patient is instructed to raise their arms 90 degrees, as though reaching toward the wall in front.
- The patient squats down as far as possible, maintaining the feet flat on the floor, and then returns to the standing position.

A negative test is when the knees can fully flex with the heels flat on the ground.

A positive test would include the patient's heels lifting off the floor to accomplish this maneuver and/or the patient being unable to bend the knees past 90 degrees.

ORTHOPEDIC AND NEUROVASCULAR TESTS FOR THE LOWER EXTREMITY

Other lower extremity joint-specific orthopedic tests are generally performed after observing, palpating, and assessing the range of motion for a given region. Many of the orthopedic and neurologic tests for the lower extremity are listed here. The orthopedic tests marked with * are described fully in Chapter 84 Osteopathic Considerations in Orthopedics—section: "Specific Orthopedic Tests (Organized by Chief Complaint"). There are also brief descriptions of a few of the neurologic tests in Chapter 73 Osteopathic Considerations in Neurology.

- Low back, sacroiliac, and/or hip pathology tests
  - □ Trendelenburg sign
    - Assesses hip abductor (gluteus medius) muscle strength
  - □ *Straight-leg raising (SLR) test (Lasègue test)
    - Assesses for radiculopathy and/or hamstring muscle tension
  - □ Log roll
    - Assesses for hip pathology
    - With the patient supine and leg straight on the table, the entire leg is internally and externally rotated. Restriction of internal rotation is sensitive for capsular lesions of the hip, including osteoarthritis.
  - □ FABER (Patrick) test
    - Assesses for hip or sacroiliac pathology
    - The acronym FABER describes the motion of the femur at the hip joint performed during this orthopedic screening test—***F***lexion, ***Ab***duction, and ***E***xternal ***R***otation
    - With the patient supine, the hip and knee are passively flexed. Then the femur is abducted and externally rotated. This should result in a "figure 4" position, with the ankle crossed on the opposite distal thigh. The evaluator then stabilizes the opposite ASIS and applies further abduction and external rotation of the femur by applying a gentle downward force on the medial knee or distal thigh (Fig. 40.27).
    - There are some osteopathic sources that also include "extension" as a third plane of motion when the femoral abduction and external rotation are applied toward the table[4,5,31] however this aspect of motion is not typically included in orthopedic and physical therapy texts.[32,33]
  - □ FADIR test
    - Assesses for hip pathology (femoroacetabular impingement)
    - The acronym FADIR describes the motion of the femur at the hip joint performed during this orthopedic screening test—***F***lexion, ***Ad***duction, and ***I***nternal ***R***otation.
    - With the patient supine, the hip and knee are passively flexed. Then the femur is adducted and internally rotated, monitoring for restriction or pain in the anterolateral hip (Fig. 40.28).
  - □ *Ober test
    - Assesses for iliotibial band tightness due to tensor fascia latae (TFL) muscle hypertonicity

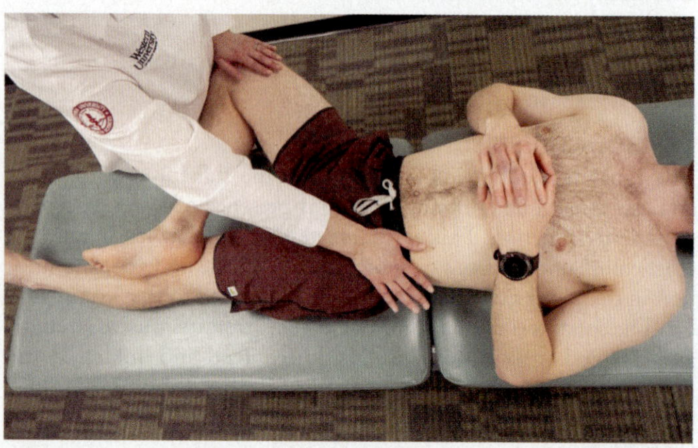

Figure 40.27. FABER test. Flexion, abduction, external rotation. (Photo courtesy of Western University of Health Sciences, Pomona, CA, with permission.)

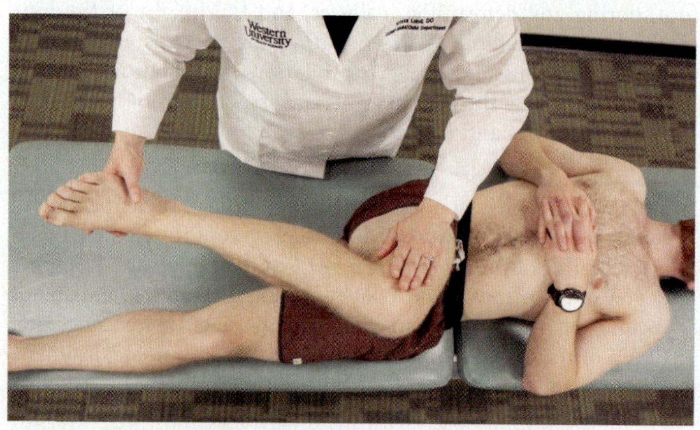

Figure 40.28. FADIR test. Flexion, adduction, internal rotation. (Photo courtesy of Western University of Health Sciences, Pomona, CA, with permission.)

- □ *Psoas (Thomas) test
  - Assesses for psoas tension (hip flexion contracture)
- □ *Prone knee bending (Nachlas or Ely test)
  - Assesses for muscle tension of the rectus femoris, femoral nerve irritation, upper lumbar disk herniation, sacroiliac or hip pathology.

■ Knee–ligament/cartilage integrity tests

- □ *Anterior and posterior drawer test of the knee
  - Assesses for integrity of the ACL and PCL (knee flexed 90 degrees)
- □ *Lachman test
  - Assesses for integrity of the ACL (knee flexed 20 to 30 degrees)
- □ *Varus and valgus
  - Assesses for integrity of the LCLs and MCLs, respectively
- □ Apley distraction
  - Assesses integrity of the collateral ligaments of the knee in the prone position with the knee flexed to 90 degrees
- □ Apley compression
  - Assesses integrity of the medial and lateral menisci of the knee in the prone position with the knee flexed to 90 degrees
- □ *McMurray (medial and lateral meniscus) test
  - Assesses for medial, lateral, or posterior meniscus injuries. In these tests, start with the patient's knee fully flexed while the patient is supine.
- □ *Thessaly test
  - Assesses for meniscal tears with the patient in the standing position

■ Knee—patellar provocation tests

- □ Patellar grind (clarke's test)
  - Assesses for patellofemoral joint pathology
  - With the patient supine and the knee extended, the examiner places pressure on the superior pole of the patella while the patient contracts the quadriceps muscle. The presence of pain or grinding sensations during this maneuver is considered a positive sign, indicating potential patellofemoral joint pathology.
- □ *Patellar apprehension/subluxation
  - Assesses for patella or patellar tendon injury or dislocation
  - With the patient supine and the knee extended, the evaluator translates the patella laterally. Observe for pain, apprehension, and/or subluxation of the patella.
- □ Patellar bulge sign and patellar ballottement tests (Fig. 40.29)
  - The patellar bulge sign is used to assess for <u>small</u> effusions. With the patient's knee in full extension, begin by stroking upward along the medial surface of the patella to force the fluid to the lateral side. Then compress the lateral side and observe for any fluid bulging on the medial side.
  - The patellar ballottement test is used to confirm the presence of a <u>large</u> effusion. With the patient's knee in full extension, the evaluator compresses the suprapatellar patch distally to force the fluid below the patella. The patella will appear to float when compressed into the trochlear groove and rebound when it is released.

■ Leg, ankle, and foot tests

- □ Squeeze test
  - Assesses integrity of the interosseous membrane of the leg
  - Assesses for high ankle sprain
- □ Thompson test
  - Assesses for ruptured Achilles tendon
- □ *Anterior drawer test of the ankle
  - Evaluates the integrety of the anterior talofibular ligament
- □ Posterior drawer test of the ankle
  - Evaluates the integrity of the posterior talofibular ligament
- □ Talar tilt
  - Evaluates the integrity of the calcaneofibular ligament with inversion and the integrity of the deltoid ligament with eversion
- □ Metatarsal compression/squeeze (Morton test)
  - Assesses for an intermetatarsal (Morton) neuroma

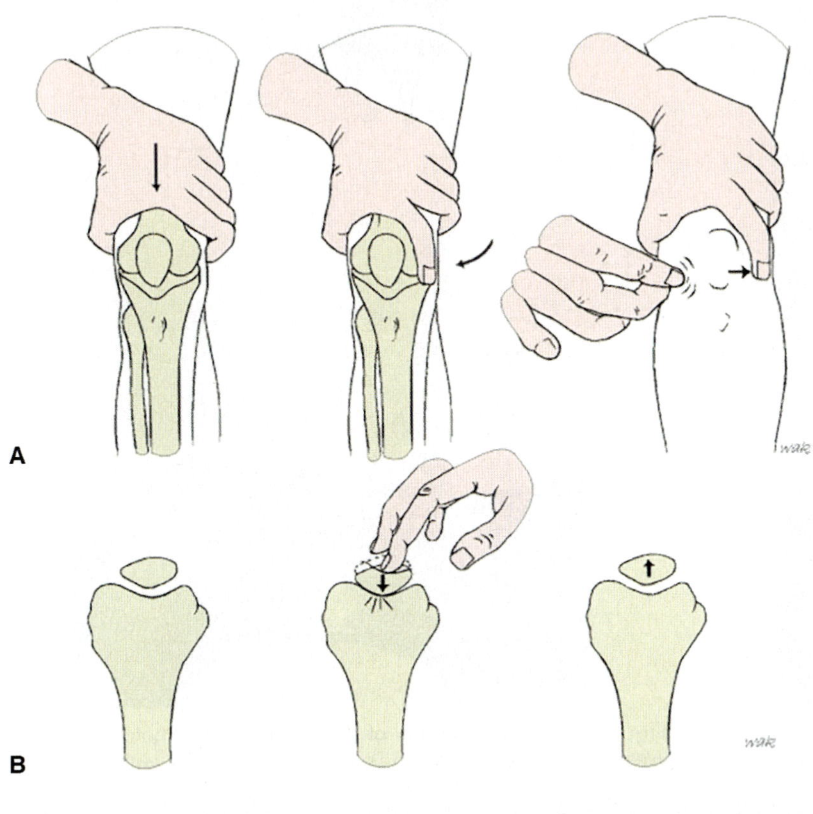

Figure 40.29. Assessing knee effusion. A. Bulge sign. **B.** Ballottement test. (Illustration by William A. Kuchera, DO, FAAO, with permission.)

- ☐ Tinel sign of the tarsal tunnel
  - Assesses for irritation of the posterior tibial nerve

JOINT SPECIFIC EXAMINATION

This section describes the evaluation of muscle and/or articular tensions affecting specific joint ROM. Please refer to Chapter 31 Osteopathic Segmental Examination for further explanation of how specific components of the lower extremity exam are integrated into the entire patient evaluation. Chapter 91 Osteopathic Approach to Diagnosing and Treating Somatic Dysfunction in the Extremities also has tables describing joint motion and varying articular somatic dysfunction nomenclature for each of the extremity joint regions. The specific tables are identified for each joint region.

In addition to the articular and muscular joint motion asymmetry described below, the physician should also evaluate for the presence of myofascial restrictions, tissue texture changes, and tenderness within the applicable regions.

The Hip Joint

The major motions of the hip are flexion-extension, abduction-adduction, and internal-external rotation. The physician should evaluate these motions actively and passively along with evaluating strength, sensation, tissue tension, and tender points. Restrictions in motion may be related to imbalance of hip and thigh musculature, loss of femoroacetabular joint play, capsular restriction, or other hip joint pathology. Some examples of hip pathology include osteoarthritis, labral tears, capsulitis, femoroacetabular impingement, and iliopectineal bursitis.

The minor motions of the femoroacetabular joint are anterior and posterior glide. The head of the femur will glide anteriorly with external rotation of the hip and will glide posteriorly with internal rotation of the hip. Somatic dysfunctions of the hip may involve any of the major motions and can also include dysfunction in minor gliding motions or joint play motions.

See *Table 91.7 Hip Somatic Dysfunction* for a summary of the femoroacetabular joint motion and the somatic dysfunction nomenclature.

EVALUATION FOR RESTRICTION OF HIP ABDUCTION

1. Patient lies supine on the examination table.
2. Physician stands at the end of the table.
3. Physician grasps the leg to be examined at the ankle, lifts it slightly, and abducts the leg, noting the range and quality of the motion (Fig. 40.30)
4. Step 3 is repeated with the patient's opposite leg.
5. Physician compares the range and quality of abduction of the involved leg with that of the opposite leg.
   - ☐ Asymmetric range of motion can indicate restricted adductor muscles, other femoroacetabular somatic dysfunction, or hip pathology.
   - ☐ Tight adductors may include the pectineus, gracilis, and the adductor magnus, longus, and brevis.

EVALUATION FOR RESTRICTION OF HIP ADDUCTION

1. Patient lies supine on the examination table.
2. Physician stands at the end of the table.
3. Physician grasps the leg to be examined at the ankle, lifts it slightly, and adducts it in front of the opposite leg, noting the range and quality of the motion (Fig. 40.31).
4. Step 3 is repeated with the patient's opposite leg.

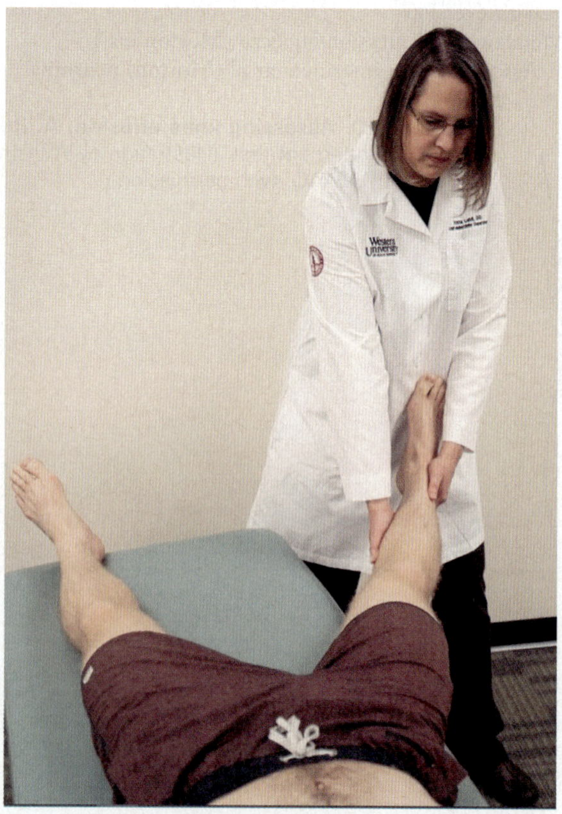

Figure 40.30. Evaluation of hip abduction. (Photo courtesy of Western University of Health Sciences, Pomona, CA, with permission.)

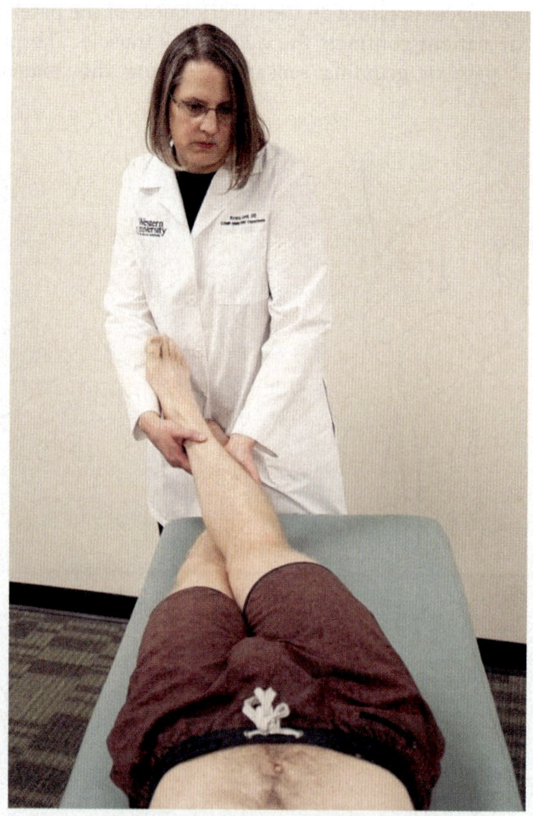

Figure 40.31. Evaluation of hip adduction. (Photo courtesy of Western University of Health Sciences, Pomona, CA, with permission.)

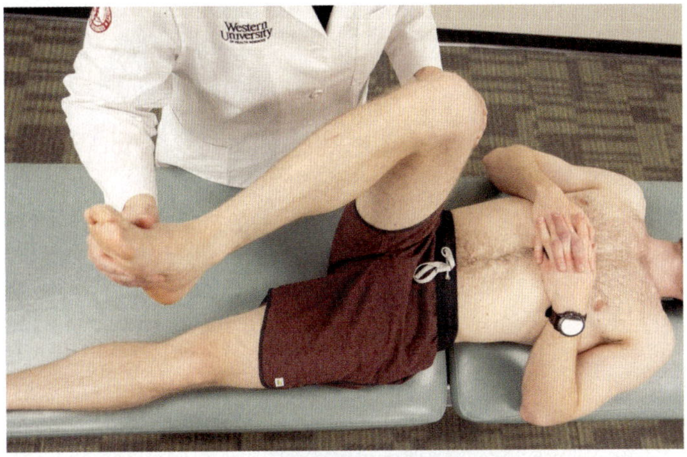

Figure 40.32. Evaluation of hip external rotation. (Photo courtesy of Western University of Health Sciences, Pomona, CA, with permission.)

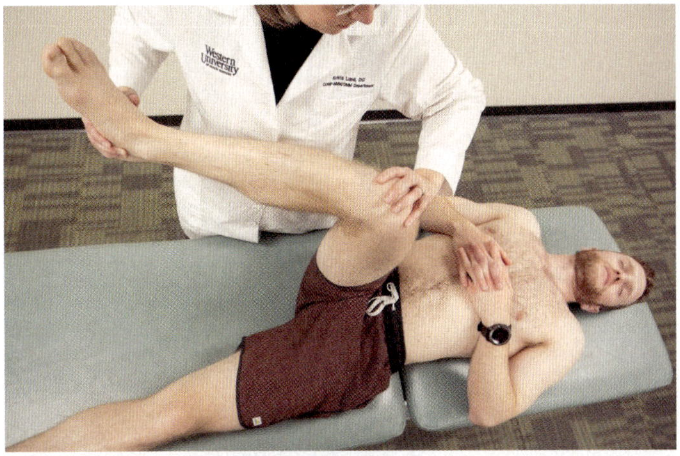

Figure 40.33. Evaluation of hip internal rotation. (Photo courtesy of Western University of Health Sciences, Pomona, CA, with permission.)

5. Physician compares the range and quality of adduction of the involved leg with that of the opposite leg.
   - Asymmetric range of motion can indicate restricted abductor muscles, other femoroacetabular somatic dysfunction, or hip pathology.
   - Tight abductors may include the gluteus medius, gluteus minimus, piriformis, and to a lesser extent sartorius, TFL, gluteus maximus, iliopsoas. (Recall obturator internus is only a hip abductor when the hip is flexed)

EVALUATION FOR RESTRICTION OF HIP EXTERNAL (FIG. 40.32) AND INTERNAL ROTATION (FIG. 40.33)

1. Patient lies supine on the examination table.
2. Physician stands at the side of the extremity to be tested.
3. Physician grasps the leg to be tested and flexes the hip and the knee, each to 90 degrees.
4. Physician then externally rotates the femur by moving the foot and ankle medially, noting the range and quality of motion.
5. Physician then internally rotates the femur by moving the foot and ankle laterally, noting the range and quality of motion.
6. Steps 2 to 5 are repeated with the patient's opposite leg.
7. Physician compares the quality and range of external rotation of the involved leg with that of the opposite leg.
   - Asymmetric range of motion can indicate restricted external or internal rotator muscles, other femoroacetabular somatic dysfunction, or hip pathology.
   - Articular somatic dysfunction of the femoroacetabular joint can restrict the head of the femur from gliding anteriorly with external rotation of the hip or from gliding posteriorly with internal rotation of the hip.
   - Tight internal rotators will restrict external rotation. The internal rotators include the gluteus medius and gluteus minimus and to a lesser extent the TFL.
   - Tight external rotators will restrict internal rotation. The external rotators include obturator externus, obturator internus, superior and inferior gemelli, quadratus femoris, and to a lesser extent gluteus maximus, iliopsoas, pectineus, and sartorius.
   - The piriformis, although typically classified as an external rotator, may function as an internal rotator, when the hip is flexed to 90 degrees.[25]

To evaluate all six primary external rotator muscles (the piriformis, obturator externus and internus, superior and inferior gemelli, and quadratus femoris) the patient should lie prone, with the thigh remaining flat on the table and the knee flexed to 90 degrees. External rotation of the hip can be induced by allowing the foot to fall medially. Internal rotation of the hip may be induced by allowing the foot to fall laterally. Range of motion and strength evaluation for both internal and external rotation as well as treatment with muscle energy, articulatory technique, or stretching of the hip rotators may all be performed in the prone position.

EVALUATION FOR RESTRICTION OF HIP FLEXION

Straight leg raising at the hip is limited by the hamstring muscles (semitendinosus, semimembranosus, and biceps femoris) which cross the hip and knee joints. When the knee is bent, hamstring influence is removed, and the thigh can be flexed almost to the torso.[1] Assessing hip flexion with the knee straight (Fig. 40.34) and then with the knee bent (Fig. 40.35) can assist with differentiating tight hamstrings from other hip somatic dysfunction and/or pathology.

1. Patient lies supine on the examination table.
2. Physician stands to the side of the extremity to be tested.
3. Physician grasps the ankle of the leg to be tested with one hand (ipsilateral side).
4. The physician's other hand is placed on the patient's contralateral ASIS to monitor for motion.
5. Physician lifts the involved leg, introducing hip flexion with the knee extended until motion is noted at the contralateral ASIS. The range and quality of the motion that is limited by hamstrings muscles are noted (Fig. 40.34).
6. The physician's monitoring hand is then moved to the patient's ipsilateral PSIS.
7. Physician then lifts the involved leg, introducing hip flexion with the knee flexed until motion is noted at the ipsilateral PSIS. The range and quality of the motion is noted (Fig. 40.35).
8. Steps 2 to 7 are repeated with the patient's opposite leg.
9. Physician compares the quality and range of hip flexion for both legs for both straight leg raise and hip flexion with knee bent.
   - Asymmetric range of motion of straight leg raise but not of hip flexion with knee flexed indicates restricted hamstring muscle tension. Recall straight leg raise can also be limited by lumbar pathology and radicular pain.

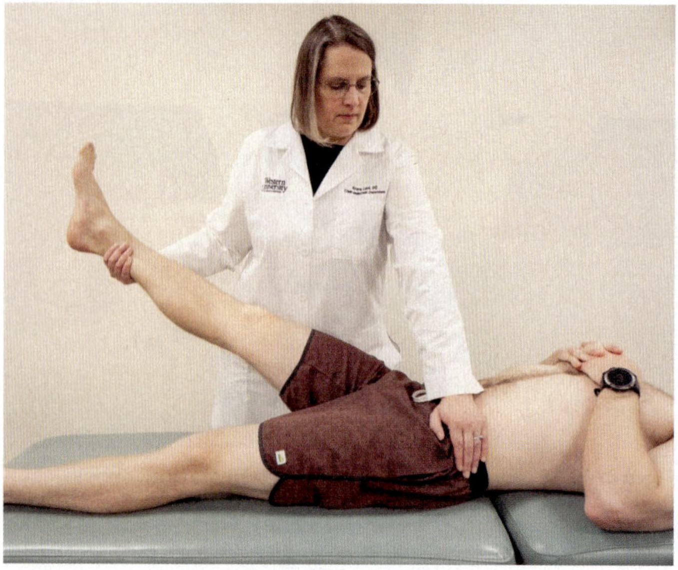

Figure 40.34. Evaluation of hip flexion/straight leg raise. (Photo courtesy of Western University of Health Sciences, Pomona, CA, with permission.)

- □ Asymmetric hip flexion range of motion with knee bent can indicate restricted gluteus maximus or adductor magnus, other femoroacetabular somatic dysfunction, or hip pathology.

EVALUATION FOR RESTRICTION OF HIP EXTENSION (FIG. 40.36)

1. Patient lies supine, with their pelvis at the end of the examination table, so that the femur can hang over the edge of the table/extension at the femoroacetabular joint.
2. Physician stands at the end of the examination table, facing the patient.
3. Patient flexes both hips and knees, bringing the knees close to the chest.
4. Patient grasps one knee and holds the leg close to the chest, while the physician passively extends the leg to be tested (Fig. 40.36).
5. The range and quality of the leg motion is noted.
6. Steps 3 to 5 are repeated with the opposite leg.
7. Physician compares the range and quality of hip extension of the involved leg with that of the opposite leg.
   - □ Asymmetric range or quality can indicate restricted hip flexor muscles, other femoroacetabular somatic dysfunction, or hip pathology.
   - □ Tight hip flexors may include the iliopsoas, tensor fasciae latae, and to a lesser extent the sartorius and the thigh adductors. (The rectus femoris can also flex the hip when the knee is extended but is better evaluated as a knee extensor.)
   - □ Notice this patient setup is identical to the orthopedic Psoas (Thomas) test.

The Knee

The major motions of the knee joint are flexion and extension. Because of the irregular shape of the joint surfaces, these two motions are combined with some minor involuntary glides, rolling, and rotational motions of the medial and lateral femorotibial articulations. Minor motions of the tibial plateau at the knee include:

- Anterior and posterior glides
- Medial and lateral glides

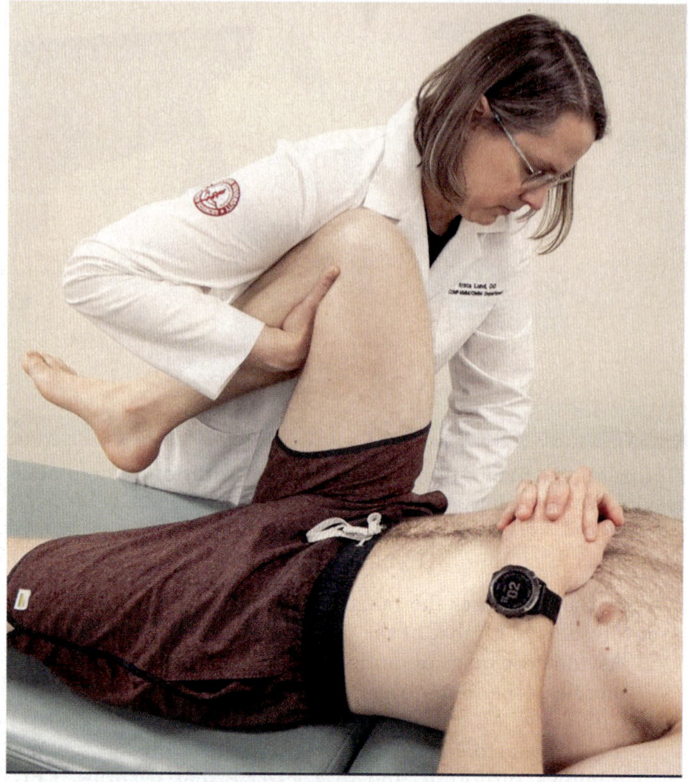

Figure 40.35. Evaluation of hip flexion with knee bent. (Photo courtesy of Western University of Health Sciences, Pomona, CA, with permission.)

- Internal rotation with posterolateral glide
- External rotation with anteromedial glide

Excessive tension in the muscles, fascia, and joint capsule can alter the minor motions of the knee and have an adverse effect on overall function.

See *Table 91.8 Knee (Femorotibial) Joint Somatic Dysfunction* for a summary of the femorotibial joint motion and the somatic dysfunction nomenclature.

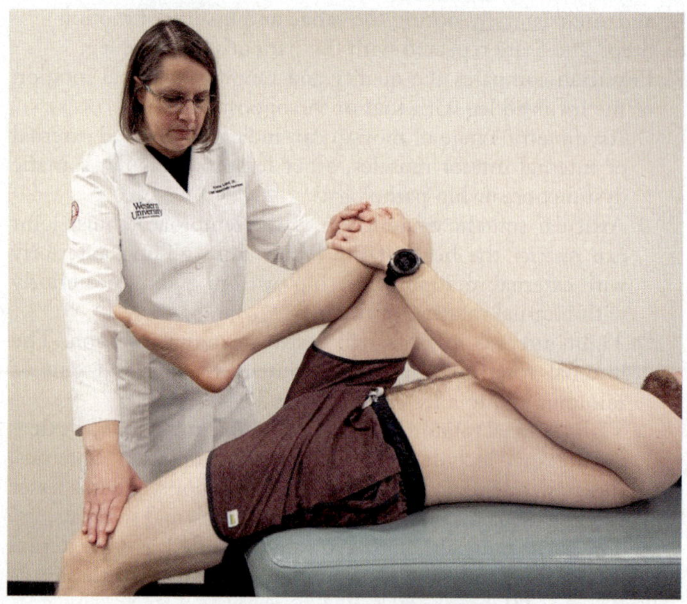

Figure 40.36. Evaluation of hip extension/psoas (modified Thomas) test. (Photo courtesy of Western University of Health Sciences, Pomona, CA, with permission.)

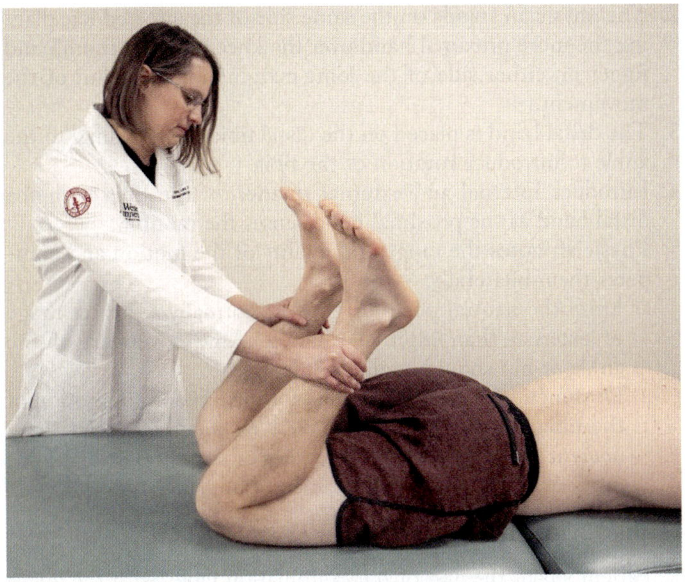

Figure 40.37. **Evaluation of knee flexion.** (Photo courtesy of Western University of Health Sciences, Pomona, CA, with permission.)

EVALUATION FOR RESTRICTION OF KNEE FLEXION

1. Patient lies prone on the examination table.
2. Physician stands to the side of the patient's legs, facing the patient.
3. Physician grasps patient's ankles and passively flexes both knees. Physician notes the range and quality of the motion and compares them bilaterally (Fig. 40.37).
   - Asymmetric range or quality can indicate restricted knee extensor muscles, other femoroacetabular somatic dysfunction, or hip pathology.
   - Tight knee extensors may include any of the quadricep muscles—rectus femoris, vastus lateralis, vastus medialis, and vastus intermedius.
   - Note: if the patient is unable to lie prone, evaluation can be done unilaterally with the patient lying in the lateral recumbent position. Evaluate right knee flexion while the patient is lying on their left side and evaluate left knee flexion while the patient is lying on their right side.

EVALUATION FOR RESTRICTION OF KNEE EXTENSION

Observe if the knees appear flexed or hyperextended. A flexed knee (restricted extension) may be related to muscle imbalance like tight hamstrings or could be from internal derangement including bony, capsular, or ligamentous deformity, or effusion. Genu recurvatum (hyperextended knee) can be a normal physiologic variant, a congenital misalignment, or may be related to somatic dysfunction, injury, or pathologic conditions.

Knee extension is passively assessed with the patient supine, flexing the hip with the knee straight because the hamstrings extend the hip and flex the knee (see Fig. 40.34). Also, palpate these muscles for tension. Restriction of these muscles will often have a significant effect on the pelvis and knee.

EVALUATION OF TIBIAL ABDUCTION AND ADDUCTION

Abduction and adduction of the tibia are passive motions of the knee that typically cannot be voluntarily created by the patient. Examining these motions with valgus and varus stress testing provides information about somatic dysfunction and the stability of the collateral ligaments. Restriction of glide in one direction suggests somatic dysfunction; laxity in one direction suggests ligamentous sprain or tear.

- Valgus stress testing of the knee at 30 degrees of flexion (Fig. 40.38A) induces abduction of the tibia and medial glide of the tibial plateau. Laxity suggests instability of the MCL.
- Varus stress testing at 30 degrees of flexion (Fig. 40.38B) induces adduction of the tibia and lateral glide of the tibial plateau. Laxity suggests instability of the LCL.

EVALUATION OF TIBIAL ROTATION

Tibial rotation is a natural part of the biomechanics of gait. The irregular shape of the femorotibial joint surface creates simultaneous minor gliding motions:

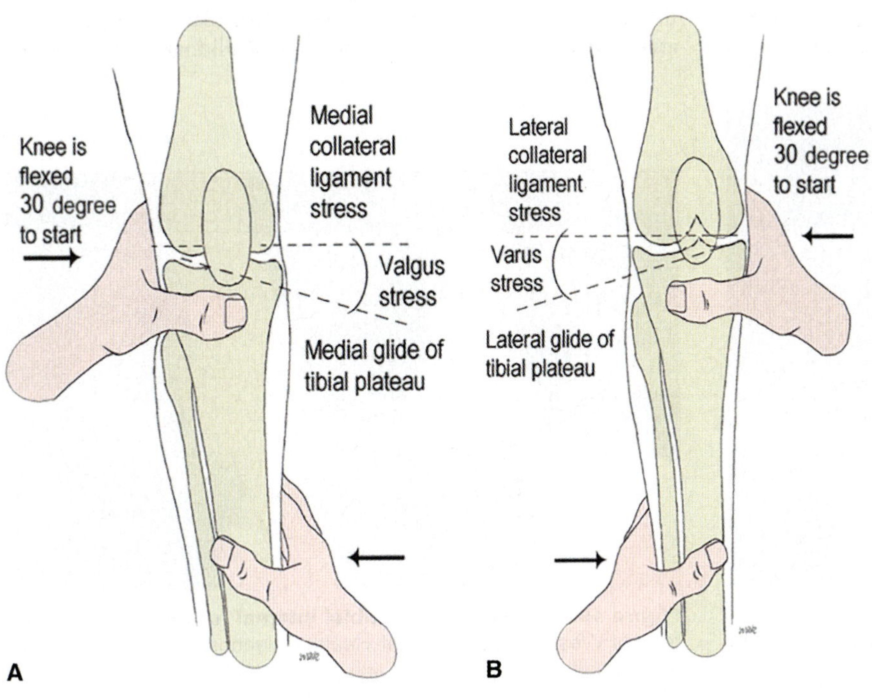

Figure 40.38. **Hand placements to assess the integrity of lateral and medial collateral ligaments of a patient's right knee. A.** Valgus stress test to assess MCL and medial glide of the tibia. **B.** Varus stress test to assess LCL and lateral glide of the tibia. (Illustration by William A. Kuchera, DO, FAAO, with permission.)

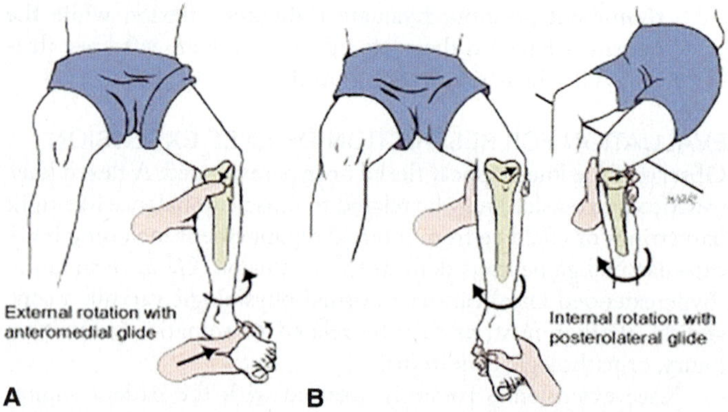

Figure 40.39. Physical examination of minor tibial glides. **A.** Palpate for anteromedial tibial glide with external rotation. **B.** Palpate for posterolateral tibial glide with internal rotation of the knee. (Illustration by William A. Kuchera, DO, FAAO, with permission.)

- Posterolateral glide of the tibia on the femur with tibial internal rotation
- Anteromedial glide of tibia on the femur with tibial external rotation

Testing of minor motions of the joint and ligament assessment should be performed with the knee in variable degrees of flexion because complete extension of the knee creates a bony lock or "screw home" effect.

Evaluation of the minor articular gliding motion during tibial rotation is best performed unilaterally (as shown in Method 1) and comparing both sides. The normal knee should be tested first to determine the pattern and assist with recognizing minor restrictions in the affected knee.

Bilateral motion testing (as shown in Method 2) provides a more generalized assessment of the muscular, fascial, and interosseous tensions that influence tibial rotation.

Method 1: Evaluating Tibial Glide on the Femur—Rotational Somatic Dysfunction

Evaluation may be performed in the seated position as shown in Figure 40.39 or in a supine position:

1. The patient is supine, with the knee slightly flexed over a pad 3 to 4 inches thick, and the heel of the foot resting on the table.
2. The physician stands on the same side of the affected leg, placing the more proximal hand over the knee with the thumb and finger on either side of the joint margins for palpation of the movement.
3. The distal hand is placed on the distal tibia just proximal to the ankle to introduce rotation of the tibia.
4. Introduce internal and external rotation of the tibia with the distal hand as the proximal hand senses the motion.
5. Physician notes the range and quality of the motion and compares them bilaterally.
   - □ From the neutral position, there is normally a greater range of external than internal rotation. Any movement of the ankle or hip should be disregarded.
   - □ Dysfunction is typically named for the freedom of motion of the tibia on femur. See *Table 91.8 Knee (Femorotibial) Joint Somatic Dysfunction* for a summary of the femorotibial joint motion and the somatic dysfunction nomenclature.

Method 2: Evaluating Generalized Tibial Rotation

1. Patient sits at the end of the examination table, with the lower legs dangling over the table edge.
2. Physician sits in front of the patient.
3. Physician grasps the patient's feet, dorsiflexes the ankles, and <u>externally</u> rotates the lower extremities, noting the range and quality of the motion (Fig. 40.40).
4. While maintaining the dorsiflexion, the physician then <u>internally</u> rotates the lower extremities, noting the range and quality of the motion (Fig. 40.41).
5. Physician compares the range and quality of external and internal rotation of each leg.
   - □ Less range of motion in one leg as compared to the opposite leg may indicate a restriction related to muscular, fascial, and/or interosseous tensions that influence tibial rotation.

The Fibular Joints and Proximal Fibular Dysfunction

There is reciprocal anterior–posterior motion between the distal and proximal ends of the fibula. This motion can be induced by ankle dorsiflexion and plantarflexion or through translatory motion at either fibular end. Motion is affected by tension of the interosseous membrane as well as muscular and ligamentous attachments. Dysfunction of the normal gliding motion of the

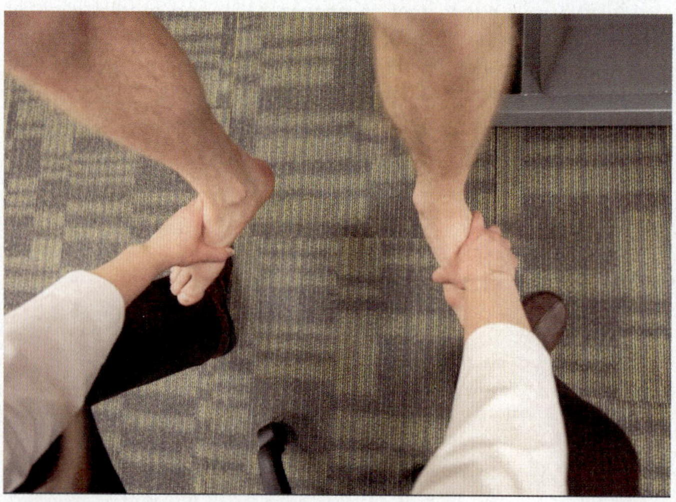

Figure 40.40. Evaluation of tibial external rotation. (Photo courtesy of Western University of Health Sciences, Pomona, CA, with permission.)

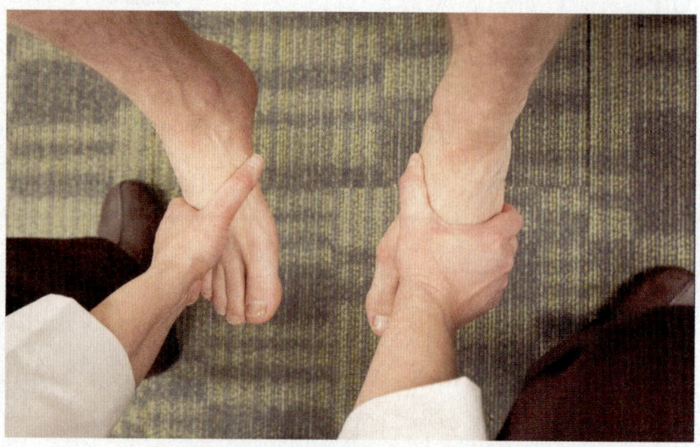

Figure 40.41. Evaluation of tibial internal rotation. (Photo courtesy of Western University of Health Sciences, Pomona, CA, with permission.)

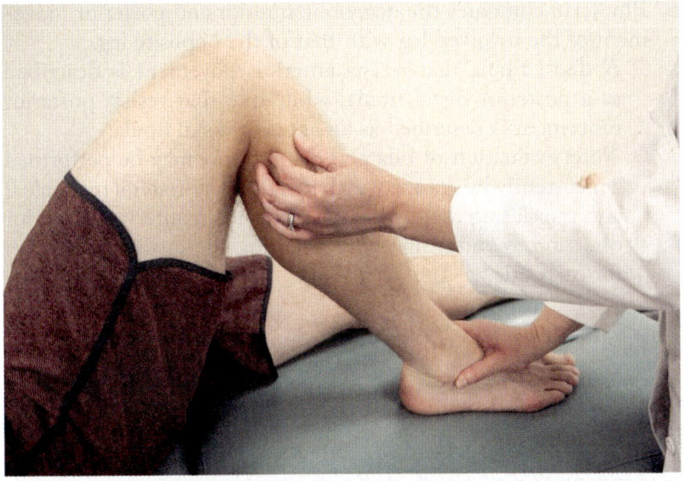

Figure 40.42. Evaluation of fibular head translation motion. Induce anterior and posterior gliding motion at the fibular head and compare bilaterally. (Photo courtesy of Western University of Health Sciences, Pomona, CA, with permission.)

fibular head can produce unusual mechanical strain at the knee (acting via the biceps femoris and the LCL) or at the ankle. This will, in turn, alter knee and ankle motion and may be a source of pain.

Fibular head somatic dysfunction is classically named for the preferred position of anterior or posterior glide.

EVALUATING FIBULAR HEAD MOTION

See *Table 91.9 The Proximal Tibiofibular Joint/Fibular Head Somatic Dysfunction* for a summary of the fibular head somatic dysfunction nomenclature.

Evaluation of fibular head motion may be performed with the patient seated or supine. Motion can be induced through translatory motion at the fibular head (Fig. 40.42) or through long lever induction of ankle dorsiflexion and plantarflexion (Fig. 40.43).

Evaluation of Fibular Head with Anterior–Posterior Translation Motion (Short Lever):

1. Patient lies supine on the examination table, with the hip and knee flexed, and the foot flat on the table surface.
2. Physician stands at the end of the table, facing the patient.
3. Physician grasps the proximal fibular head, with their thumb placed on the anterior part of the fibular head, and the fingers on the posterior aspects (Fig. 40.42).
   - □ Physician must take care not to cause undue pressure on the fibular nerve, which lies directly posterior to this structure.
4. Physicians opposite hand stabilizes the foot and can monitor for fascial tensions or palpable reciprocal motion of the distal fibula.
5. Physician passively moves the proximal fibular head anteriorly and posteriorly in the plane of the joint, noting the range and quality of the movement, as well as any tissue texture changes or tenderness.
6. Steps 1 to 5 are repeated with the opposite leg.
7. Physician compares the quality and range of anterior and posterior movement of the radial head with that of the opposite leg.
   - □ A proximal fibular head that resists anterior movement is described as a posterior fibular head, while one that resists posterior movement is described as an anterior fibular head.
   - □ Note: evaluation of bilateral distal fibula may be performed concurrently by grasping each lateral malleolus and translating them simultaneously in an anterior–posterior direction, monitoring and comparing the quality of motion for each side.

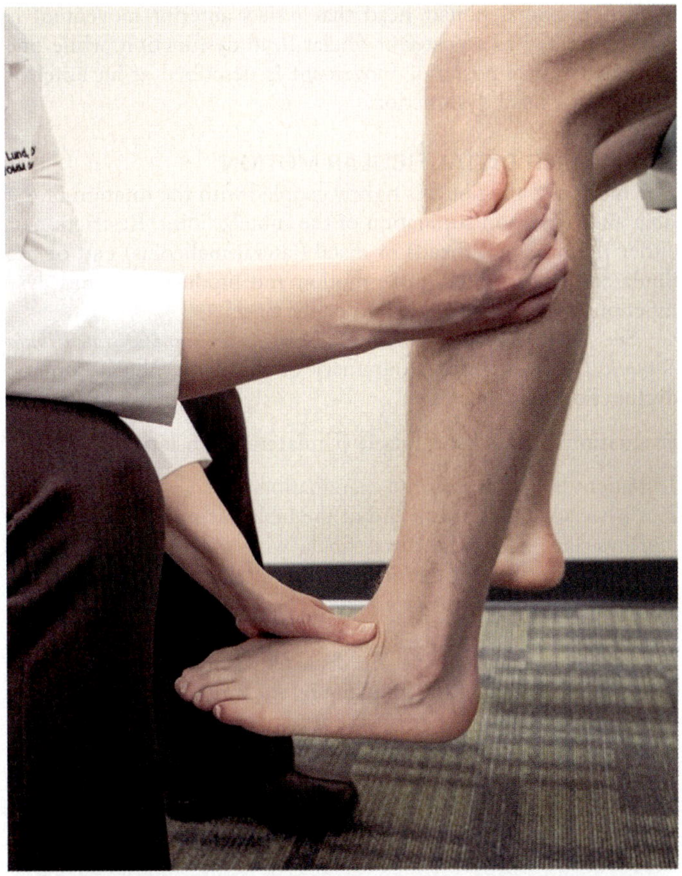

Figure 40.43. Evaluation of fibular head motion using foot as long lever. Inducing dorsiflexion should cause anterolateral glide of the fibular head. Conversely, plantarflexion should induce posteromedial glide of the fibular head. (Photo courtesy of Western University of Health Sciences, Pomona, CA, with permission.)

Evaluation of Fibular Head Motion Using Foot as Long Lever:

1. Patient sits at the end of the examination table, with the lower legs dangling over the table edge.
2. Physician sits in front of the patient.
3. Physician grasps the proximal fibular head with their lateral hand, so the thumb is placed on the anterior part of the fibular head, and the fingers on the posterior aspects.
   - □ Physician must take care not to cause undue pressure on the fibular nerve, which lies directly posterior to this structure.
4. Physician grasps the foot with their medial hand and places it in a neutral position (Fig. 40.43).
5. Physician induces dorsiflexion and plantarflexion of the ankle, noting range and quality of both the ankle motion and the anterolateral–posteromedial motion of the fibular head.
   - □ During dorsiflexion, the fibular head should glide anteriorly and slightly lateral.
   - □ During plantarflexion, the fibular head should glide posterior and slightly medial.
   - □ There may also be tissue texture changes or tenderness at the fibular head.
6. Steps 3 to 5 are repeated with the opposite leg.
7. Physician compares the range and quality of anterior and posterior movement bilaterally.

- □ A proximal fibular head that resists anterior movement is described as a posterior fibular head dysfunction, while one that resists posterior movement is described as an anterior fibular head dysfunction.

EVALUATING DISTAL FIBULAR MOTION

The motion of the fibula is tightly coupled with the rotation of the tibia and pronation/supination of the subtalar joint. Restriction at either the proximal (head) or distal (lateral malleolus) end of the fibula can alter normal ankle motion and produce pain and dysfunction in either the ankle and/or the knee.

See *Table 91.10 The Distal Tibiofibular Joint/Distal Fibula Somatic Dysfunction* for a summary of the distal fibular somatic dysfunction nomenclature.

Evaluation of the Distal Fibula (Unilateral Translation)

1. Patient lies supine on the examination table.
2. Physician stands at the end of the table, facing the patient.
3. Physician grasps the distal fibula with the thumb placed on the anterior part of the distal fibula (lateral malleolus), and the fingers on the posterior aspects. The other hand stabilizes the calcaneus (Fig. 40.44).
4. Physician passively moves the distal fibula anteriorly and posteriorly in the plane of the joint, noting the range and quality of the movement, as well as any tissue texture changes or tenderness.
5. Steps 1 to 5 are repeated with the opposite leg.

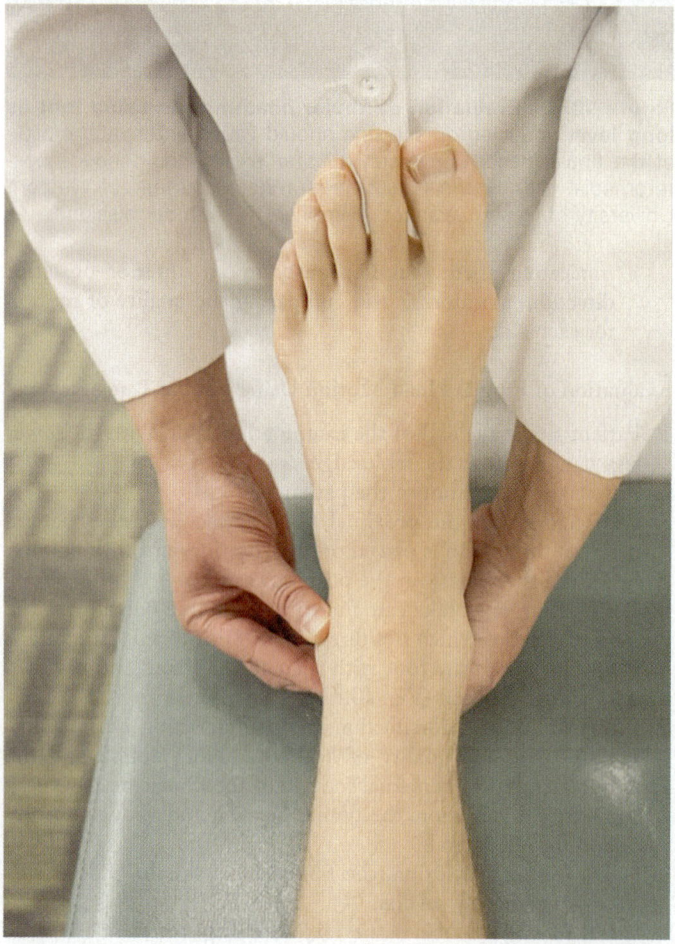

Figure 40.44. Evaluation of the distal fibular motion. Induce anterior and posterior gliding motion and compare bilaterally. (Photo courtesy of Western University of Health Sciences, Pomona, CA, with permission.)

6. Physician compares the degree of anterior and posterior movement of the involved leg with that of the opposite leg.
   - □ A distal fibula that resists anterior movement is described as a posterior distal fibula, while one that resists posterior movement is described as an anterior distal fibula.
   - □ Note: evaluation of bilateral distal fibula may be performed concurrently by grasping each distal fibular (lateral malleolus) and translating them simultaneously in an anterior–posterior direction, monitoring and comparing the quality of motion for each side.

The Ankle and Foot

The ankle joint complex is comprised of the kinetic linkage between the lower leg and the foot. The combined proper functions of all the lower extremity joints are needed for mobility and balance.

THE TIBIOTALAR JOINT (TALOCRURAL JOINT)

During dorsiflexion, the talus glides posteriorly within the mortise. During plantarflexion, the talus glides anteriorly making the head of the talus more palpable.

Evaluation of Tibiotalar Joint Motion:

1. Patient is seated on the examination table, with the feet dangling.
2. Physician sits facing the patient.
3. Physician grasps the patient's feet. The physician's thumbs monitor just distal to the tibia to palpate talar motion, and the palms encircle the plantar surface of the foot to induce motion (Fig. 40.45).
   - □ Note: this may also be performed unilaterally with the patient's legs extended on the table, one hand supporting the calcaneus, and the other monitoring talar motion.

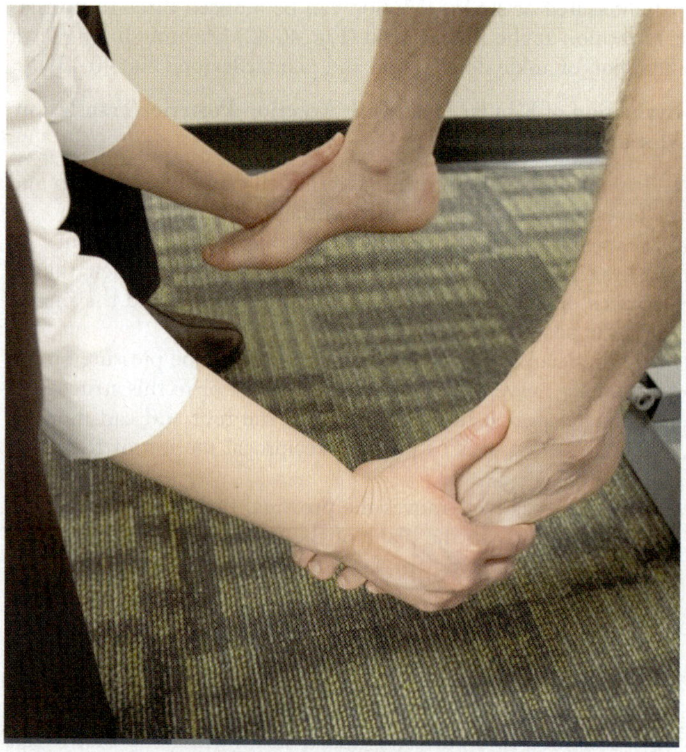

Figure 40.45. Evaluation of tibiotalar motion. (Photo courtesy of Western University of Health Sciences, Pomona, CA, with permission.)

4. Physician dorsiflexes and plantarflexes both the patient's feet, noting the range and quality of movement of the feet and the ability of the talus to glide anteriorly and posteriorly under the tibia.
   - □ A tibiotalar joint that resists ankle dorsiflexion and posterior glide of the talus into the mortise (or resists plantarflexion and anterior glide of the talus) within the mortise likely has somatic dysfunction which is typically named for the position of ease.
   - □ See *Table 91.11 Tibiotalar/Talocrural Joint (Ankle) Somatic Dysfunction* for a summary of the options of nomenclature for tibiotalar somatic dysfunction.

THE SUBTALAR JOINT

The subtalar joint's major motions are inversion and eversion of the ankle and foot, yet it has its own defined distinct pronation and supination.

See *Table 91.12 Subtalar/Talocalcaneal Joint (Ankle) Somatic Dysfunction* for a summary of the talocalcaneal joint motion and somatic dysfunction nomenclature.

Evaluation of Subtalar Joint Motion:

1. Patient lies supine on the examination table.
2. Physician stands at the end of the table, facing the patient.
3. Physician grasps the ankle to be examined with one hand, stabilizing the talus with the web of the thumb and index finger, and stabilizing the medial and lateral malleoli with the distal aspects of the thumb and fingers.
   - □ Depending on which hand the physician uses, this may be done by placing the palm over the distal leg (Fig. 40.46) or with the palm over the dorsum of the foot. Either position is acceptable to stabilize the talocrural joint.
4. Physician grasps the calcaneus with their opposite hand.
5. With the patient's ankle maintained at a 90-degree angle and stabilized, the physician moves the calcaneus medially into inversion and laterally into eversion noting the range and quality of the motion.
   - □ As the calcaneus inverts the talus will glide posterolateral on the calcaneus.
   - □ As the calcaneus everts the talus will glide anteromedial on the calcaneus.
6. Steps 3 to 5 are repeated for the opposite foot, and the motion of the involved calcaneus is compared with that of the noninvolved one.
   - □ A calcaneus that resists inversion and posterolateral glide of the talus is typically named for the position of ease: *eversion of the calcaneus with anteromedial glide of the talus.* The opposite restriction would place the subtalar joint in an *inversion of the calcaneus with posterolateral glide of the talus* somatic dysfunction.

THE TRANSVERSE TARSAL AND INTERTARSAL JOINTS

The talus, cuboid, and calcaneus make up the functional unit of the transverse tarsal joint (Fig. 40.47A). The tarsals respond to eversion or inversion of the calcaneus. Somatic dysfunction of the tarsal bones (cuboid, navicular, or cuneiforms) typically occurs in response to subtalar supination or pronation causing a medial or lateral shift of the transverse tarsals. Medial shift tends to affect the navicular and lateral shift tends to affect the cuboid.

- Cuboid somatic dysfunction involves the edge nearest the middle of the foot. This edge glides toward the plantar surface of the foot and rotates laterally around its AP axis (everting or flattening the transverse arch) (Fig. 40.47C).
- Navicular somatic dysfunction involves the edge nearest the middle of the foot gliding toward the plantar surface and rotating medially around its AP axis (inverting or flattening the transverse arch) (Fig. 40.47C).
- Cuneiform somatic dysfunction usually manifests from one of the cuneiforms gliding in the plantar direction (downward). Primary somatic dysfunction of the cuneiform bones is rare, although secondary restrictions following navicular or cuboid somatic dysfunction are common.[34] The second cuneiform is most commonly involved.[6,35]

Nomenclature is summarized in *Table 91.13 Transverse Tarsal (Talonavicular and Calcaneocuboid) Joint and Intertarsal Joint (Cuneiform Bones) Somatic Dysfunction.*

Evaluation of *Talonavicular* Joint Motion:

1. Patient lies supine on the examination table.
2. Physician stands at the end of the table, facing the patient.
3. Physician grasps the foot to be examined, placing one hand over the dorsal aspect of the foot and ankle to stabilize the talus.

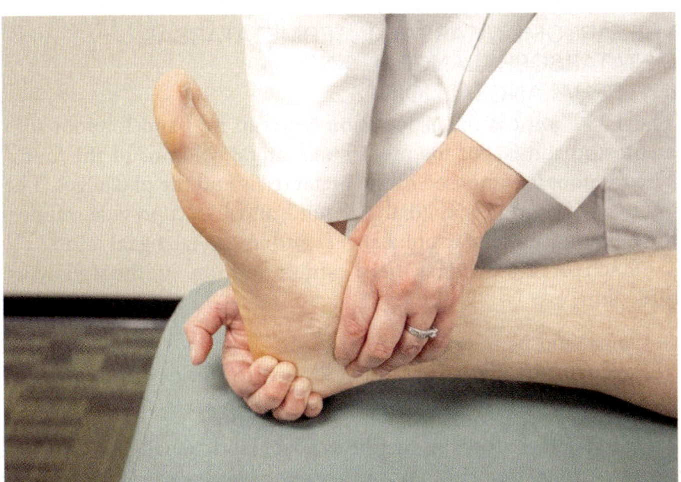

Figure 40.46. Evaluation of the subtalar joint. (Photo courtesy of Western University of Health Sciences, Pomona, CA, with permission.)

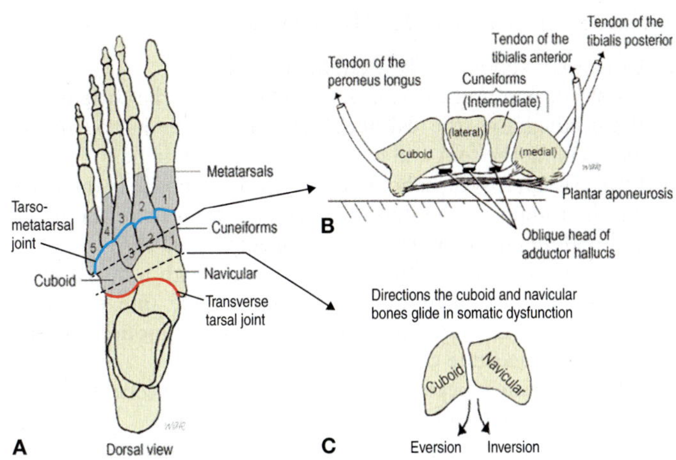

Figure 40.47. Navicular, cuboid, and cuneiform somatic dysfunction; relation to supports of the transverse arch of the foot. **A.** Foot skeletal anatomy. **B.** Muscle tendons forming the transverse arch of the foot. **C.** Cuboid and navicular somatic dysfunction. (Illustration by William A. Kuchera, DO, FAAO, with permission.)

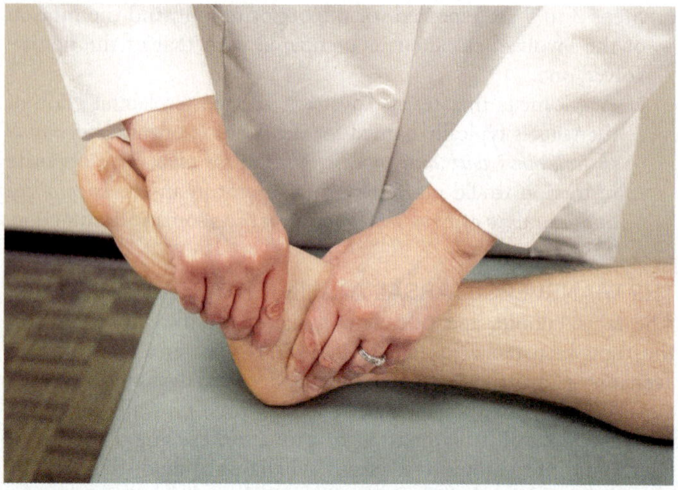

Figure 40.48. Evaluation of the talonavicular joint. (Photo courtesy of Western University of Health Sciences, Pomona, CA, with permission.)

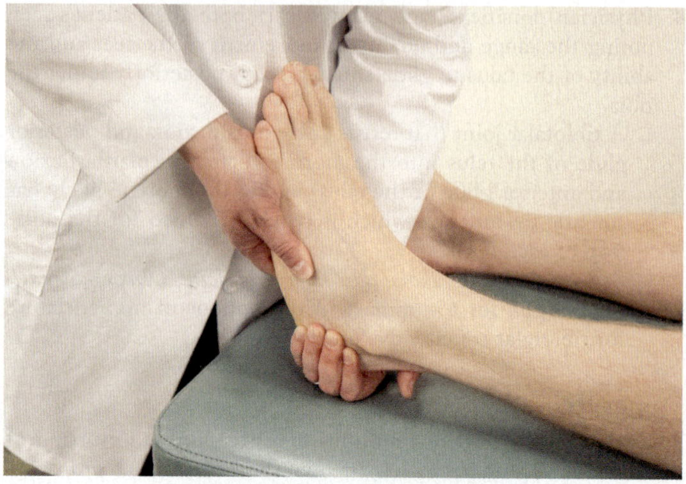

Figure 40.49. Evaluation of the calcaneocuboid joint. (Photo courtesy of Western University of Health Sciences, Pomona, CA, with permission.)

4. Physician grasps the navicular bone with the opposite hand, placing the thumb on the dorsal aspect, and the pads of the index and middle fingers on the ventral aspect.
   - □ If grasping the navicular is too tender for the patient, the physician can monitor navicular motion with their index finger while stabilizing the cuneiforms and metatarsals with their hand on the dorsum of the foot (Fig. 40.48).
5. Physician then moves the navicular bone through a dorsal glide into eversion/pronation and a plantar glide into inversion/supination, noting the range and quality of the motion.
6. Steps 3 to 5 are repeated with the opposite talonavicular joint.
   - □ The navicular typically has an everted (pronated) position to maintain the transverse and medial longitudinal arches. Somatic dysfunction occurs when there is restriction of the dorsal glide, the navicular is more palpable inferiorly, and/or there is tenderness over the plantar aspect. This is sometimes referred to as a dropped navicular or inverted navicular.
   - □ See *Table 91.13 Transverse Tarsal (Talonavicular and Calcaneocuboid) Joint and Intertarsal Joint (Cuneiform Bones) Somatic Dysfunction* for the variations of nomenclature of this positioning.

Evaluation of *Calcaneocuboid* Joint Motion:

1. Patient lies supine on the examination table.
2. Physician stands at the end of the table, facing the patient.
3. Physician grasps the calcaneus of the foot to be examined, maintaining the foot and ankle at a 90-degree angle.
4. Physician grasps the cuboid bone with the opposite hand, placing the thumb on the dorsal aspect, and the pads of the index and middle fingers on the ventral aspect (Fig. 40.49).
5. Physician then moves the cuboid bone through a dorsal glide into inversion/supination and a plantar glide into eversion/pronation, noting the range and quality of the motion, as well as any tissue texture change or tenderness.
6. Steps 3 to 5 are repeated with the opposite calcaneocuboid joint noting the range and quality of the motion,
   - □ A cuboid typically has an inverted (supinated) position to maintain the transverse and lateral longitudinal arches. Somatic dysfunction occurs when there is restriction of the dorsal glide, the cuboid is more palpable inferiorly, and/or there is tenderness over the plantar aspect. This is sometimes referred to as a dropped cuboid or everted cuboid.
   - □ See *Table 91.13 Transverse Tarsal (Talonavicular and Calcaneocuboid) Joint and Intertarsal Joint (Cuneiform Bones) Somatic Dysfunction* for the variations of nomenclature of this positioning

Evaluation of the *Cuneiform Bones*:

1. Patient lies supine on the examination table.
2. Physician stands at the end of the table, facing the patient.
3. Physician grasps the cuneiform bone to be tested and stabilizes the one next (Fig. 40.50) to it by placing the thumbs on the dorsal surfaces of the two bones, and the fingers of both hands on the plantar surfaces. Physician then moves each cuneiform bone in a dorsal and plantar direction while stabilizing the bone next to it.
4. Note the quality and range of motion, any palpable bony prominence on the plantar surface, tenderness, or other tissue texture change.
5. Repeat steps 3 and 4 for each of the three cuneiforms, bilaterally.
6. Compare the motion of the cuneiform bones of the involved foot to that of the opposite foot.
   - □ A cuneiform bone that resists dorsal motion is described as being inferior in position or "dropped." (Again, see Table 91.13 for variations of somatic dysfunction nomenclature.)

THE TARSOMETATARSAL, INTERMETATARSAL, METATARSOPHALANGEAL, AND INTERPHALANGEAL JOINTS

The TMT joint is the articulation between mid and forefoot segments and consists of the medial and lateral columns of the foot.[13] The forefoot is composed of the metatarsals and the phalanges. The joint capsules and the medial collateral, and LCLs provide stability for each of the metatarsophalangeal and interphalangeal joints.

Each of these bones may exhibit motion in the following directions:

- Dorsal and plantar glide
- Internal and external rotation (about an anterior–posterior axis)
- Small amounts of medial and lateral glide

Each of these motions may be evaluated individually for *the TMT and intermetatarsal* (Fig. 40.51), *metatarsophalangeal* (Fig. 40.52A and B), *and interphalangeal* (Fig. 40.53) *joints* as follows:

1. Patient lies supine on the examination table.
2. Physician stands at the end of the table, facing the patient.

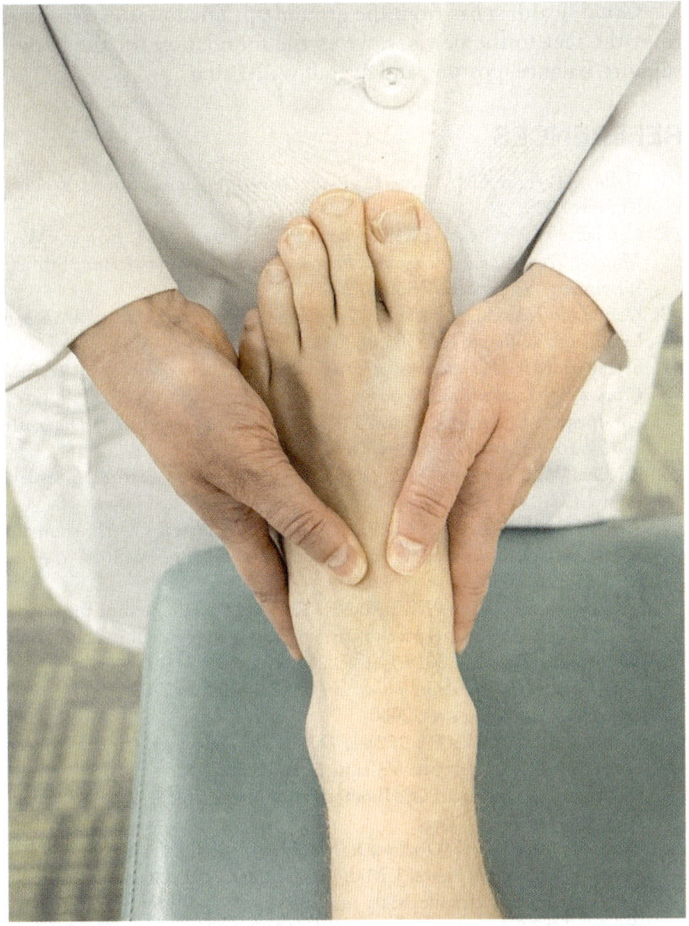

Figure 40.50. Evaluation of the cuneiform bones. (Photo courtesy of Western University of Health Sciences, Pomona, CA, with permission.)

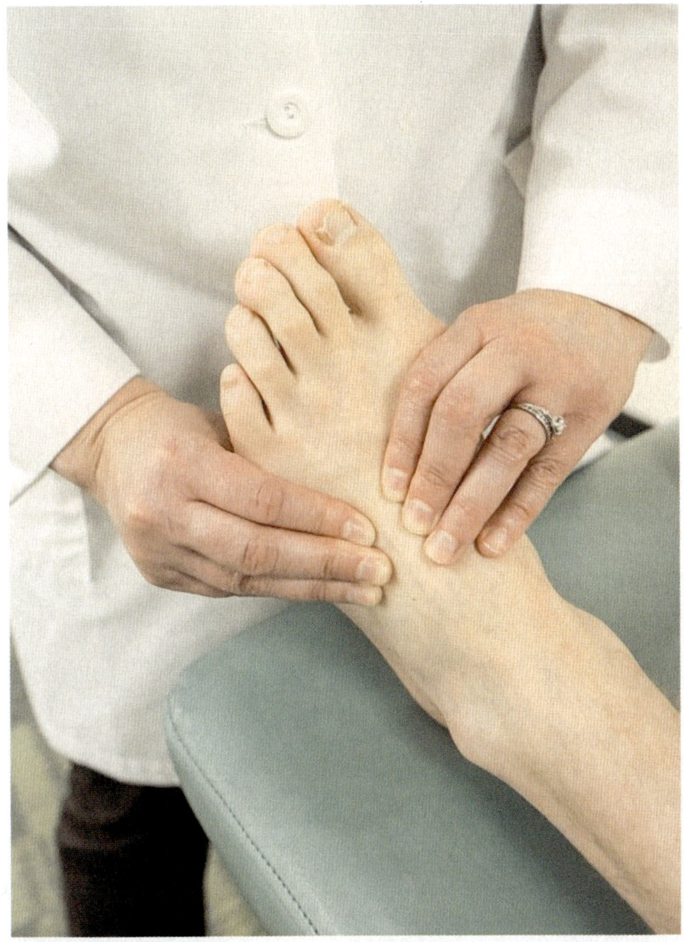

Figure 40.51. Evaluation of the tarsometatarsal and intermetatarsal joints. For evaluation of tarsometatarsal motion stabilize the proximal tarsal bones while moving the metatarsal bone. For evaluation of intermetatarsal joint motion stabilize one metatarsal and motion test the metatarsal next to it. (Photo courtesy of Western University of Health Sciences, Pomona, CA, with permission.)

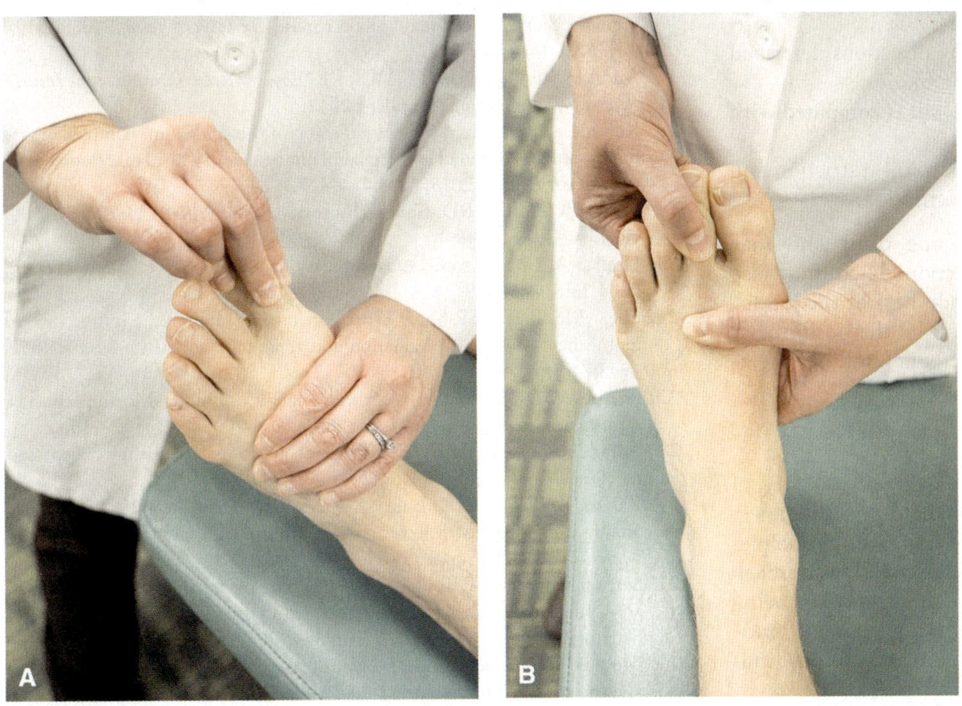

Figure 40.52. Evaluation of the metatarsophalangeal joints. A. Proximal stabilizing thumb is on plantar surface. **B.** Proximal stabilizing thumb is on dorsal surface. (**A, B:** Photo courtesy of Western University of Health Sciences, Pomona, CA, with permission.)

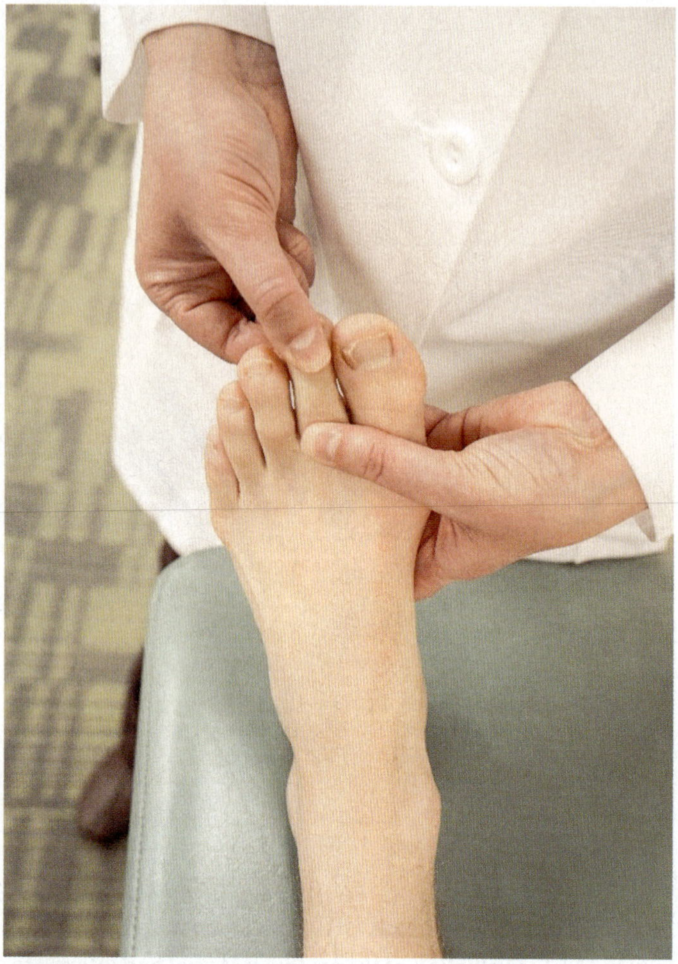

Figure 40.53. Evaluation of the interphalangeal joints. (Photo courtesy of Western University of Health Sciences, Pomona, CA, with permission.)

3. Physician grasps the bone being tested and stabilizes the bones proximal to it (or to the side in the case of intermetatarsal motion.)
4. Physician moves the bone passively in the directions described above, noting the range and quality of the motion.
5. The motion of the bones in the involved foot is compared with that of the opposite foot.
6. Physician notes the specific bone(s) that exhibit restriction and in which direction(s) there was motion restriction.

Restrictions can occur in more than one plane and may involve compression or, less commonly, traction. There may also be associated tissue texture changes and tenderness of the joint.[36] Somatic dysfunction nomenclature may describe the positions of ease or define the restrictions of the specific bone motion in relation to its surrounding bones/joint.

SUMMARY

A thorough understanding of the functional anatomy of the lower extremities, coupled with a grounding in osteopathic principles and practice, establishes a foundation for the osteopathic approach to patients presenting with conditions that are affecting or being affected by dysfunction in the lower extremities. Accurately identifying somatic dysfunction pertinent to presenting conditions leads to a better osteopathic management plan.

Good health starts from the ground up. The lower extremities, from the feet to the pelvis, serve as the foundation for the body's support, balance, posture, and overall well-being.

REFERENCES

1. Dalley AF, Agur AM. *Moore's Clinically Oriented Anatomy*. 9th ed. Wolters Kluwer; 2023.
2. Kendall FP, McCreary EK, Provance PG, Rodgers MM, Romani WA. *Muscles: Testing and Testing and Function with Posture and Pain*. 5th ed. Lippincott Williams & Wilkins; 2005.
3. DeStefano LA. Chapter 19. In: *Greenman's Principles of Manual Medicine*. Lippincott Williams & Wilkins; 2011.
4. Seffinger MA. *Foundations of Osteopathic Medicine: Philosophy, Science, Clinical Applications, and Research*. 4th ed. Wolters Kluwer; 2018.
5. DiGiovanna E, Amen C, Burns DK. *An Osteopathic Approach to Diagnosis and Treatment*. 4th ed. Wolters Kluwer; 2021.
6. Kuchera WA, Kuchera ML. *Osteopathic Principles in Practice*. Greyden Press LLC; 1994.
7. Sharma R, Vaibhav V, Meshram R, Singh B, Khorwal G. A systematic review on quadriceps angle in relation to knee abnormalities. *Cureus*. 2023;15(1):e34355.
8. Khasawneh RR, Allouh MZ, Abu-El-Rub E. Measurement of the quadriceps (Q) angle with respect to various body parameters in young Arab population. *PLoS One*. 2019;14(6):e0218387.
9. Kingston B. *Understanding Joints: A Practical Guide to Their Structure and Function*. Nelson Thornes; 2000.
10. Nicholas AS, Nicholas EA. *Atlas of Osteopathic Techniques*. 4th ed. Wolters Kluwer Health/Lippincott Williams & Wilkins; 2022.
11. Brockett CL, Chapman GJ. Biomechanics of the ankle. *Orthop Trauma*. 2016;30(3):232–238.
12. Ombregt L. *A System of Orthopaedic Medicine*. Churchill Livingstone; 2003.
13. Fraser JJ, Feger MA, Hertel J. Midfoot and forefoot involvement in lateral ankle sprains and chronic ankle instability. Part 1: anatomy and biomechanics. *Int J Sports Phys Ther*. 2016;11(6):992–1005.
14. Ghanem I, Massaad A, Assi A, et al. Understanding the foot's functional anatomy in physiological and pathological conditions: the calcaneopedal unit concept. *J Child Orthop*. 2019;13(2):134–146.
15. Roaas A, Andersson GB. Normal range of motion of the hip, knee and ankle joints in male subjects, 30–40 years of age. *Acta Orthop Scand*. 1982; 53(2):205–208.
16. de Noronha M, Refshauge KM, Herbert RD, Kilbreath SL, Hertel J. Do voluntary strength, proprioception, range of motion, or postural sway predict occurrence of lateral ankle sprain? *Br J Sports Med*. 2006;40(10): 824–828; discussion 828.
17. Andrews JR, Harrelson GL, Wilk KE. *Physical Rehabilitation of the Injured Athlete, 4th Ed*. 4th ed. Saunders; 2012.
18. Koo S, Lee KM, Cha YJ. Plantar-flexion of the ankle joint complex in terminal stance is initiated by subtalar plantar-flexion: a bi-planar fluoroscopy study. *Gait Posture*. 2015;42(4):424–429.
19. Nack JD, Phillips RD. Shock absorption. *Clin Podiatr Med Surg*. 1990; 7(2):391–397.
20. Hreljac A. Impact and overuse injuries in runners. *Med Sci Sports Exerc*. 2004;36(5):845–849.
21. Shear MS, Baitch SP, Shear DB. Sinus tarsi syndrome: the importance of biomechanically-based evaluation and treatment. *Arch Phys Med Rehabil*. 1993;74(7):777–781.
22. Glasoe WM, Coughlin MJ. A critical analysis of Dudley Morton's concept of disordered foot function. *J Foot Ankle Surg*. 2006;45(3):147–155.
23. Karandikar N, Vargas OOO. Kinetic chains: a review of the concept and its clinical applications. *PM R*. 2011;3(8):739–745.
24. Zahari Z, Naga DNA, Bukry SA. Motor control on gait performance among individuals with lower crossed syndrome: a scoping review. *Med J Malaysia*. 2024;79(Suppl 1):168–175.
25. Michel F, Decavel P, Toussirot E, et al. The piriformis muscle syndrome: an exploration of anatomical context, pathophysiological hypotheses and diagnostic criteria. *Ann Phys Rehabil Med*. 2013;56(4):300–311.
26. Meyr AJ, Diprimio R. Lower-extremity sclerotomes: clinical applications and the modified mayo block. *J Am Podiatr Med Assoc*. 2009;99(3):232–235.

27. Harrow-Mortelliti M, Reddy V, Jimsheleishvili G. Physiology, Spinal Cord. In: *StatPearls*. StatPearls Publishing; 2023. Accessed May 22, 2024. http://www.ncbi.nlm.nih.gov/books/NBK544267/
28. Travell JG, Simons DG. *Myofascial Pain and Dysfunction: The Trigger Point Manual: The Lower Extremities*. Vol. 2. Williams & Wilkins; 1992.
29. Pasiński M, Zabrzyńska M, Adamczyk M, et al. A current insight into human knee menisci. *Transl Res Anat*. 2023;32:100259.
30. Raj MA, Tafti D, Kiel J. Pes Planus. In: *StatPearls*. StatPearls Publishing; 2023. Accessed May 13, 2024. http://www.ncbi.nlm.nih.gov/books/NBK430802/
31. Krabak BJ, Jarmain SJ, Prather H. Chapter 8: physical examination of the hip. In: Malanga GA, Nadler SF, eds. *Musculoskeletal Physical Examination (Fourth Edition)*. Hanley & Belfus; 2006:251–278.
32. American Academy of Orthopaedic Surgeons. *AAOS Essentials of Musculoskeletal Care*. 6th edition. Jones & Bartlett Learning; 2021.
33. Lotke PA, Abboud JA, Ende J. *Lippincott's Primary Care Orthopaedics*. 2nd ed. Lippincott Williams & Wilkins; 2013.
34. Fryette H, Styrachan WF. *Principles of Osteopathic Technic*. Academy of Applied Osteopathy; 1954.
35. Kimberly PE, Halma K. Chapter 12. In: *Outline of Osteopathic Manipulative Procedures: The Kimberly Manual 2006*. Walsworth Publishing Company; 2008:269–311.
36. Kimberly PE. *Outline of Osteopathic Manipulative Procedures: The Kimberly Manual 2006*. Walsworth Publishing Company; 2008.

41

Abdominal Region

RAYMOND J. HRUBY

KEY CONCEPTS

- The abdomen is the region of the trunk below the thoracic diaphragm. It consists of the abdomen proper and the lesser pelvis.
- Evaluation of the abdominal region from an osteopathic perspective dates back to the time of A. T. Still, DO. Evidence to support Still's concepts and clinical applications continues to grow.
- Knowledge of abdominal anatomy is critical to understanding the somatic and visceral interchanges resulting in viscerosomatic and somatovisceral reflexes in the region.
- An osteopathic regional exam of the abdominal area will be discussed as well as a brief summary of the segmental exam.

INTRODUCTION

Osteopathic manipulative treatment (OMT) can be used within a complete treatment approach to abdominal visceral problems. Such techniques have been part of osteopathic practice dating back to the founder of osteopathic medicine, Dr. Andrew Taylor Still. One early description of abdominal visceral treatment by Still is his first case of "flux," or dysentery, in a 4-year-old boy. He describes his examination of the child, noting that the back was hot, while the abdomen was cold to the touch. In his writing, Dr. Still stated:

> I began at the base of the brain, and thought by pressures and rubbings I could push some of the hot to the cold places, and in so doing I found rigid and loose places on the muscles and ligaments of the whole spine, while the lumbar was in a very congested condition. I worked for a few minutes on that philosophy, and told the mother to report next day, and if I could do anything more for her boy I would cheerfully do so. She came early next morning with the news that her child was well.[1]

Still described having treated many other similar cases with a high degree of success. His knowledge of the structure–function relationships involved in abdominal conditions was extensive enough to warrant an entire chapter, in one of his books.[2]

Osteopathic physicians, since the time of Still, continue to promote the use of OMT directed toward the abdominal viscera.

- Hazzard described the protocol for abdominal examination, along with treatment approaches for various abdominal visceral diseases.[3]
- Conrad[4] also devoted a section of his book to diseases of the abdomen. He described and illustrated specific manual techniques for diseases of the stomach, intestines, liver, kidneys, and spleen.
- In a rather extensive treatise on the abdomen, McConnell[5] discussed the osteopathic approach from the ventral plane of the body, as well as "ventral technique."
- Tender points, termed "gangliform contractions" by Frank Chapman, DO, became known as "Chapman reflexes."
- The only noted reference text on this topic was published by Owens.[6]

In later years, other osteopathic researchers published studies on the use of OMT for abdominal conditions.

- Hermann[7] demonstrated that applying OMT prior to abdominal surgery greatly reduced the incidence of postoperative ileus. He also showed that OMT could be successfully used to treat the incidence of postoperative ileus.
- Radjieski et al.[8] concluded that OMT could significantly reduce the length of hospital stay in patients with acute pancreatitis.

Researchers in other health care professions have also reported the clinical relationship between the soma and the viscera.

- Pikalov and Kharin[9] found that using spinal manipulative techniques, as part of the treatment plan for duodenal ulcer disease, resulted in pain relief and clinical remission that was much faster than with conventional medical treatment alone.
- Travell and Simons[10] noted that abdominal myofascial trigger points may produce visceral symptoms such as diarrhea, vomiting, belching, food intolerance, and infantile colic.
- Barral has published extensively on the use of manual techniques for treatment of the abdominal viscera.[11,12]
- Other authors in this area include Finet[13] and Lossing, who has contributed to several editions of this textbook in addition to providing numerous courses through the American Academy of Osteopathy on the visceral and whole body approach.

Thus, it becomes apparent that the optimum treatment of abdominal visceral conditions requires an understanding of its underlying structure–function relationships, and of its involved segmental viscerosomatic reflex phenomena. Knowledge of osteopathic philosophy and principles, as well as of usage of OMT as part of a complete treatment approach to abdominal disease, is one of the most unique characteristics of the osteopathic physician.

DEFINITION

The abdomen may be simply defined as the region of the trunk below the thoracic diaphragm, which consists of two parts:

- An upper part, the *abdomen proper*
- A lower part, the *lesser pelvis*[14] (Fig. 41.1)

These areas are continuous at the plane of the inlet of the lesser pelvis. This inlet is bounded by the following:

- Sacral promontory
- Arcuate lines of the innominate bones
- Pubic crests
- Upper border of the symphysis pubis

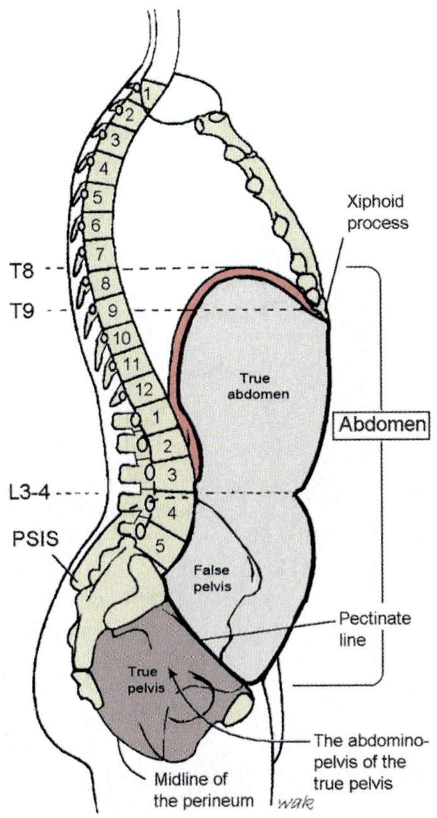

Figure 41.1. Boundaries and skeletal elements of the abdomen. (Illustration by William A. Kuchera, DO, FAAO, with permission.)

The *abdomen proper* is bounded *superiorly* by the thoracolumbar diaphragm. *Inferiorly*, it becomes continuous with the pelvis or, as some anatomists describe it, the abdominopelvic portion of the abdominal cavity,[15] by way of the superior aperture of the lesser or true pelvis.

Anteriorly, the abdomen is bounded by the abdominal muscles, which include the following:

1. Rectus abdominis
2. Pyramidales
3. External obliques
4. Internal obliques
5. Transversus abdominis

Posteriorly, the abdomen is bounded by the following:

1. Lower thoracic and the lumbar vertebrae
2. Crura of the diaphragm
3. Psoas muscles
4. Quadratus lumborum muscles
5. Posterior parts of the iliac bones

The *lesser pelvis*, or abdominopelvic portion of the abdomen, is shaped like an inverted cone. Its *anterolateral* boundary consists of those parts of the hip bones below the arcuate lines, the pubic crests, and the obturator internus muscles. Its *superior* and dorsal boundary includes the following:

- Sacrum
- Coccyx
- Piriformis and coccygeus muscles

Its *inferior* boundary includes the following:

- Levator ani muscles
- Fascial coverings (which together form the pelvic diaphragm)

The abdominal structures of interest in this chapter are the following:

- Stomach
- Small intestine
- Large intestine
- Liver
- Gallbladder
- Spleen
- Pancreas
- Kidney
- Parts of the ureters
- Suprarenal or adrenal glands
- Numerous blood and lymph vessels
- Lymph nodes
- Nerves

DESCRIPTIVE AND FUNCTIONAL ANATOMY

Skeletal Structures

The skeletal elements of the abdomen (see Fig. 41.1) are the following:

- Lumbar vertebrae
- Sacrum
- Coccyx
- Innominate bones

Muscular Structures

The muscles of the abdominal region may be divided into anterolateral and posterior groups.

The anterolateral group includes the following muscles:

1. Rectus abdominis
2. Pyramidalis
3. External oblique
4. Internal oblique
5. Transversus abdominis

The posterior group consists of the following:

1. Quadratus lumborum
2. Psoas major
3. Psoas minor
4. Erector spinae
5. Iliacus[14]

Note that somatic dysfunctions of these posterior muscles may mimic the pain of certain abdominal disorders or may be painful because of viscerosomatic reflex activity associated with abdominal problems. The thoracoabdominal diaphragm, while not usually considered part of the abdominal wall, should nevertheless be considered when evaluating the abdomen for somatic dysfunction.

Supportive Structures

The muscles of the abdominal region have associated fascial sheaths. The deep fascial layers have names associated with the various abdominal regions. Table 41.1 shows these fascial layers and their associated regions.

The *peritoneum* is a large serous membrane that consists of two layers:

1. The *parietal* layer, which lines the abdominal wall
2. The *visceral* layer, which is reflected over the abdominal viscera

TABLE 41.1

Abdominal Regions and Their Associated Deep Fascial Layers

Region	Fascial Layer
Internal surface of the transversus abdominis	Transversalis fascia
Inferior surface of thoracolumbar diaphragm	Diaphragmatic fascia
Psoas and iliac areas	Iliac fascia
Anterior surface of the quadratus lumborum muscles	Anterior layer of the thoracolumbar fascia
Muscles of the pelvis	Pelvis fascia

The parietal peritoneum angles from the posterior wall of the abdomen to form very defined mesenteric connections to the abdominal viscera.

- These mesenteries carry the sympathetic and parasympathetic fibers and arteries to the viscera.
- They also carry visceral afferent fibers, veins, and lymphatic vessels away from the viscera.
- The visceral peritoneum is sensitive to stretch.

It produces visceral pain only when the distention of the viscus exceeds the length of the visceral peritoneum, on the outside of the mesentery. The root of the mesentery for approximately 30 feet of small intestines is only about 6 inches long. It is located on the posterior wall of the abdominal cavity, posterior to a point about 1 inch to the left of and 1 inch superior to the umbilicus (Fig. 41.2).

The root of the mesentery runs inferolaterally to a second point just anterior to the right sacroiliac joint.[14] Mental visualization of these mesenteries allows the physician to determine the origin of palpable masses more accurately, and of auscultated abnormal sounds. It is also crucial in performing visceral manipulation to free fascial pathways and to improve visceral function.

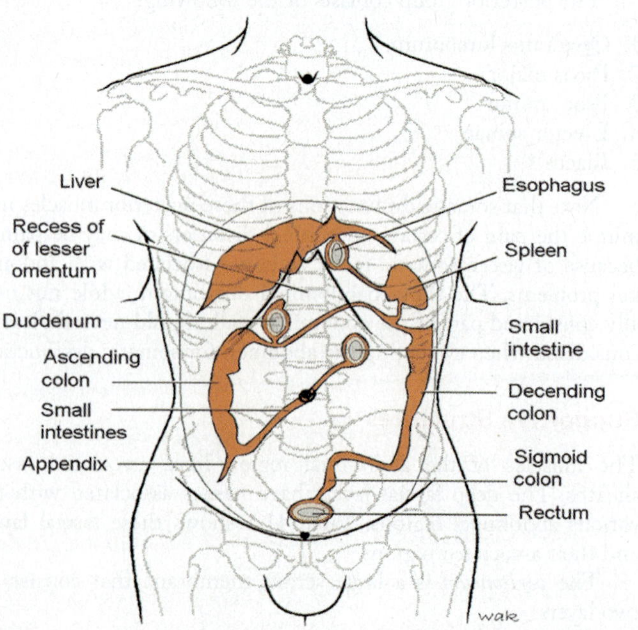

Figure 41.2. Roots of the abdominal mesenteries. (Illustration by William A. Kuchera, DO, FAAO, with permission.)

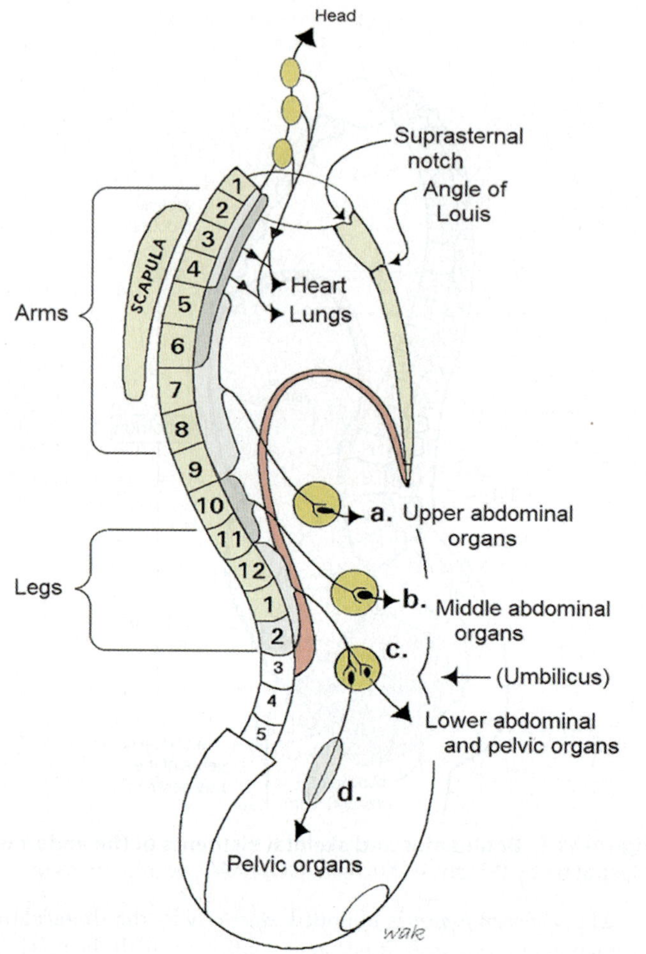

Figure 41.3. Primary sympathetic (efferent) nerves of the body. (Illustration by William A. Kuchera, DO, FAAO, with permission.)

Neurologic Structures

Primary sympathetic fibers for innervation of all organs below the diaphragm, except the descending colon and pelvic organs, pass from the intermediolateral cells in the thoracic spinal cord through the thoracoabdominal diaphragm. In the abdomen, these primary fibers enter the collateral ganglia, where they synapse (Fig. 41.3). These ganglia are the following:

1. Celiac
2. Superior mesenteric
3. Inferior mesenteric

Secondary or postganglionic fibers continue on to innervate specific groups of organs in the abdomen and pelvis. Parasympathetic innervation is supplied from the craniosacral outflow. All abdominal organs down to the midtransverse colon are supplied by the vagus nerve (cranial nerve X); the rest of the abdominal organs and all of the pelvic viscera receive their parasympathetic innervation from the pelvic splanchnic nerves (S2–S4).

Visceral afferent impulses travel back to the cord using the same course as that used by the sympathetic efferent nerves to the organ (Fig. 41.4).

This pain tends to be:

- Vague and gnawing
- Deep
- Poorly localized
- Midabdominal

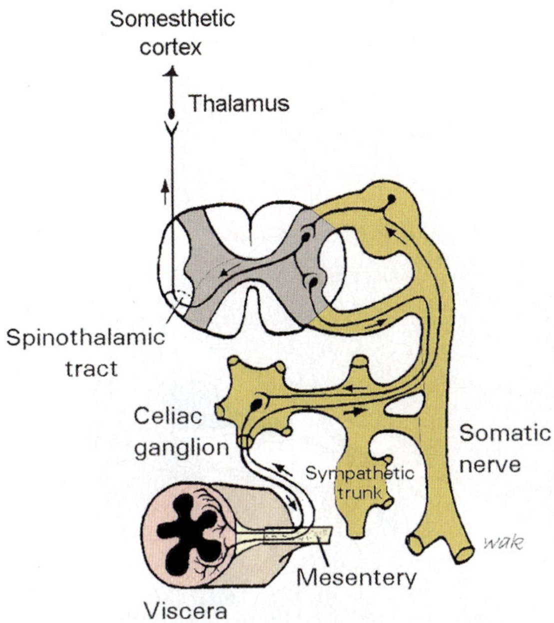

Figure 41.4. Neurologic pathway of visceral pain (afferent fibers). (Illustration by William A. Kuchera, DO, FAAO, with permission.)

Visceral afferent fibers from the root of the mesentery report to the somatic cord segment of that organ's sympathetic innervations.[14] This type of sensory input produces the paraspinal tissue changes that help the physician locate the viscus that is most likely dysfunctional. The tissue changes (TART) are as follows:

1. *T*enderness
2. *A*symmetry
3. *R*ange-of-motion differences
4. *T*issue texture changes

The pain and tissue texture changes are primarily localized at the paraspinal level, which is consistent with the organ's sympathetic innervation (Figs. 41.5 and 41.6).

Somatic pain may also be caused by what is known as the percutaneous reflex of Morley. This pain is usually located directly over the inflamed organ and is produced by direct contiguous irritation of the parietal peritoneum and the abdominal wall (Fig. 41.7).

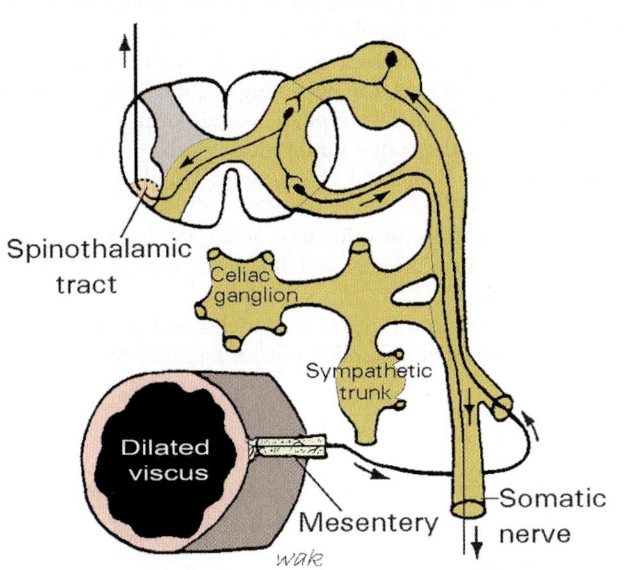

Figure 41.5. Neurologic pathway of viscerosomatic pain. (Illustration by William A. Kuchera, DO, FAAO, with permission.)

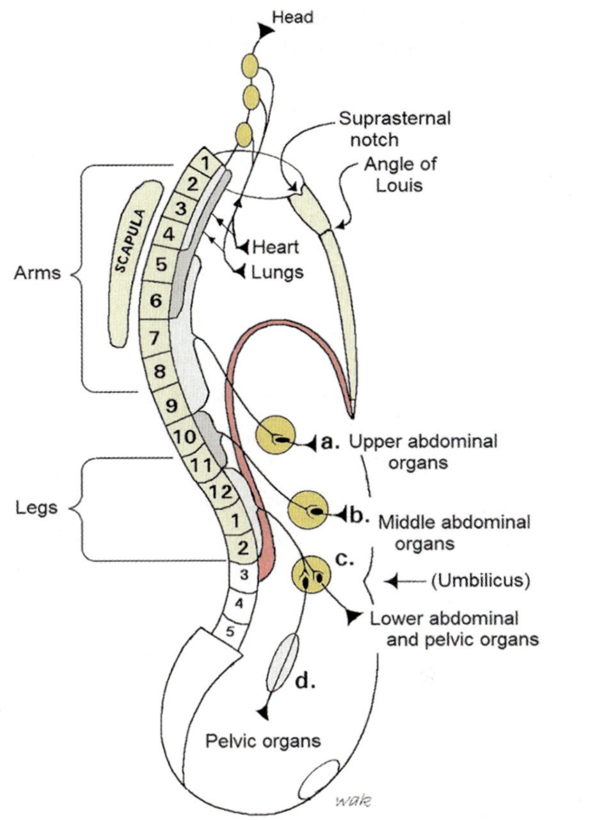

Figure 41.6. Visceral afferent fibers. (Illustration by William A. Kuchera, DO, FAAO, with permission.)

It is responsible for rebound tenderness and abdominal guarding associated with more severe abdominal pain.

Vascular Structures

ARTERIES

The thoracic aorta lies along the anterior and left anterolateral side of the thoracic vertebrae.

- It enters the abdominal cavity through the aortic hiatus in the abdominal diaphragm, at the level anterior to the 12th thoracic vertebra.

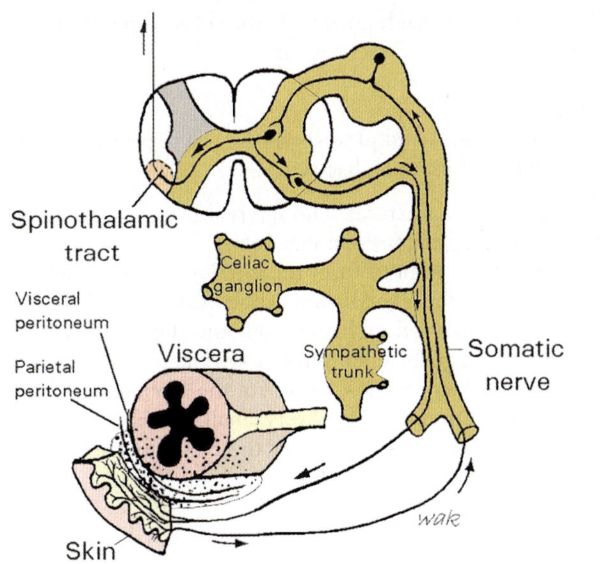

Figure 41.7. Neurologic pathway of pain from the percutaneous reflex of Morley. (Illustration by William A. Kuchera, DO, FAAO, with permission.)

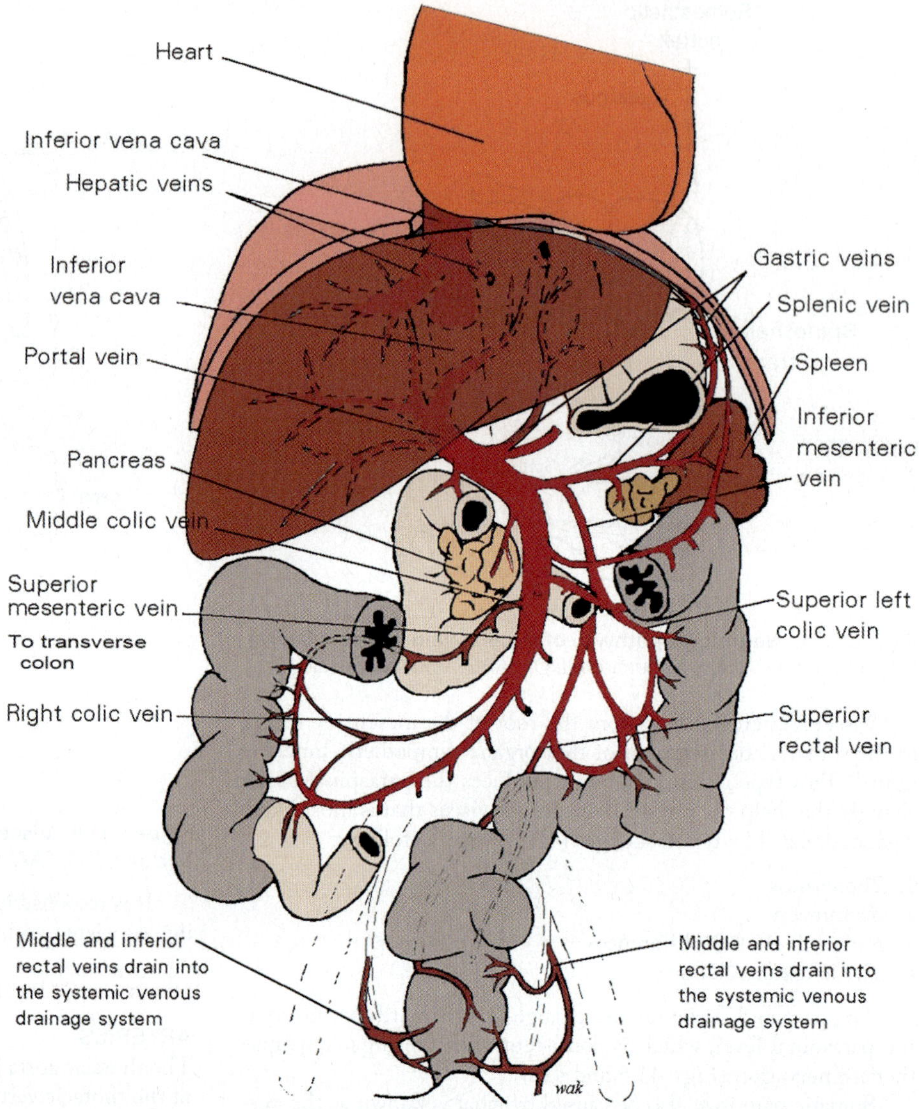

Figure 41.8. Venous drainage: portal venous drainage for the abdominal viscera. (Illustration by William A. Kuchera, DO, FAAO, with permission.)

- Here, it becomes the abdominal aorta.
- Its main abdominal branches are the celiac, superior mesenteric, renal, and inferior mesenteric arteries.[14]

VEINS

Various small veins and plexuses in the pelvis eventually flow into the external and internal iliac veins.

- The two pairs of external and internal iliac veins unite to form the left and right common iliac veins.
- These in turn unite to form the inferior vena cava, which conveys blood to the right atrium of the heart (Fig. 41.8).
- The veins that collect blood from the digestive tract, spleen, pancreas, and gallbladder join to form the portal vein.
- The portal vein carries blood to the liver, where this vein branches out into a series of very small vessels called sinusoids.
- From here, hepatic veins convey the blood to the inferior vena cava.[14]

Lymphatic Structures

The left lymphatic duct (the thoracic duct) drains interstitial fluids from the lower extremities, the pelvic and abdominal viscera, the left arm, and the left side of the head (Fig. 41.9).

- It begins as the *cisterna chyli*, a 2-inch, yellowish, cylindrical structure that lies just to the left of the thoracolumbar junction, at about the level of the first lumbar vertebra.
- It receives lymphatic vessels that drain interstitial fluids from all the abdominal organs, the pelvic organs, the lower extremities, and all of the superficial lymphatic vessels located below a horizontal plane of the body running through the umbilicus.
- The superficial lymphatic vessels drain lymph into superficial inguinal nodes.
- Lymph then travels into the deep nodes, the deep trunks along the common iliac arteries and the aorta, and finally into the cisterna chyli.
- Note that lymph from the ovary, testicles, and prostate does not drain into the inguinal nodes, but instead into the deep pelvic nodes.[16]

Visceral Structures

The major visceral structures in the abdomen are the following (Fig. 41.10):

- Adrenal glands
- Colon
- Gallbladder

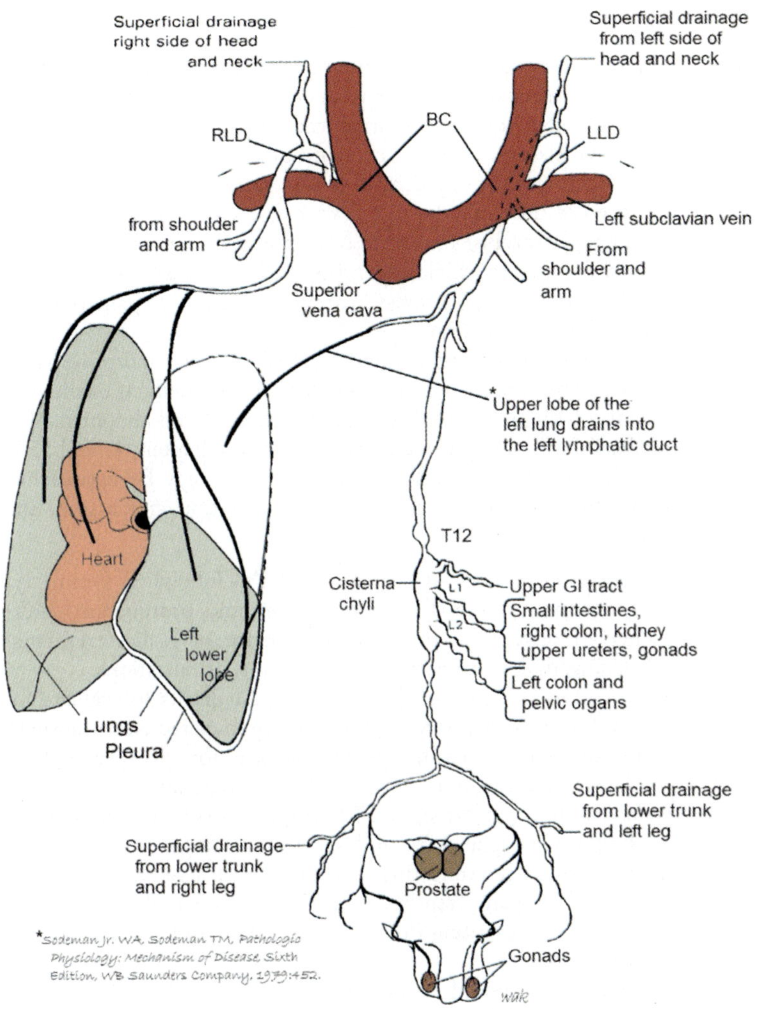

Figure 41.9. Lymphatic drainage pathways for the abdominal viscera. (Illustration by William A. Kuchera, DO, FAAO, with permission.)

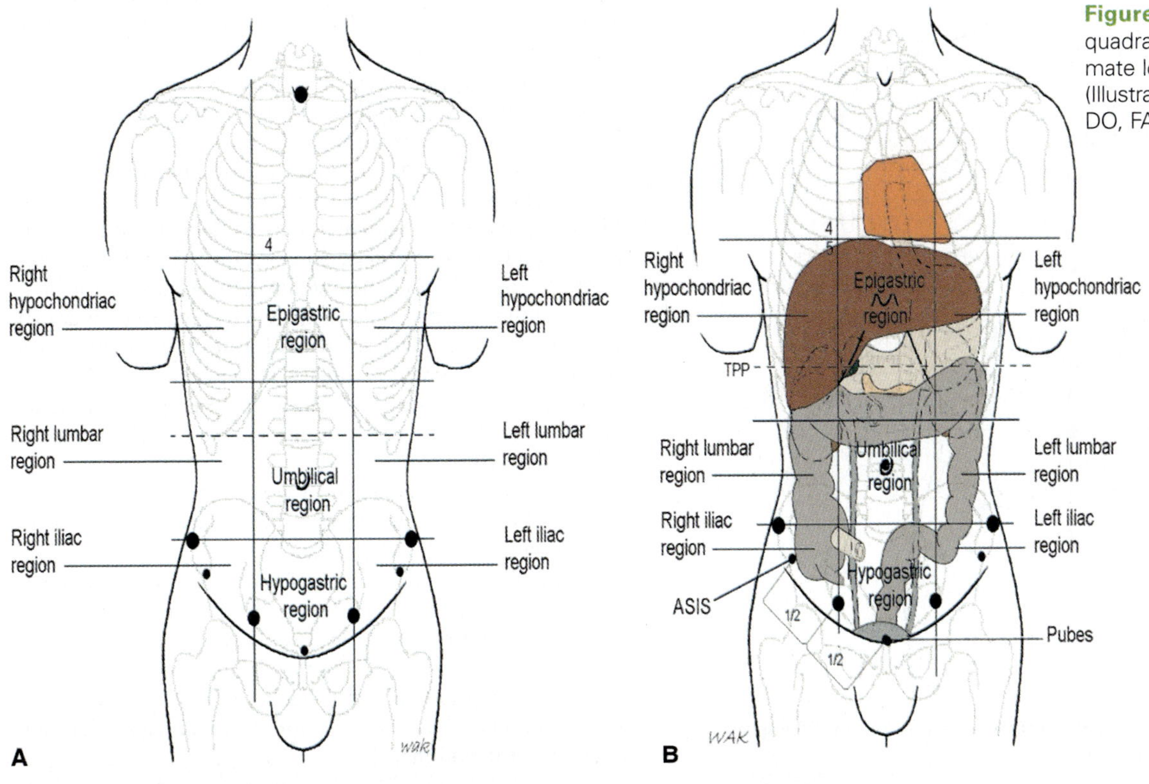

Figure 41.10. A. The nine-quadrant abdomen. **B.** Approximate location of visceral organs. (Illustration by William A. Kuchera, DO, FAAO, with permission.)

- Kidneys
- Large intestine
- Liver
- Pancreas
- Small intestine
- Spleen
- Stomach
- Urinary bladder

Topographic Anatomy

There are certain surface landmarks of the abdomen that are palpable,[17] which include the following:

- Anterior superior iliac spines
- Costal margins
- Iliac crests
- Inguinal ligaments
- Ischial tuberosities
- Pubic arches, crests, symphysis, and tubercles
- Umbilicus
- Xiphisternal joint
- Xiphoid process

For purposes of locating abdominal structures and describing abnormalities, the abdomen is conventionally divided into four quadrants (Fig. 41.11).

Another method divides the abdomen into nine sections (see Fig. 41.10).

Either method may be used, although the division into quadrants is most common.

Structural Exam

For the screening examination of the abdominal region, the reader is referred to Chapter 30.

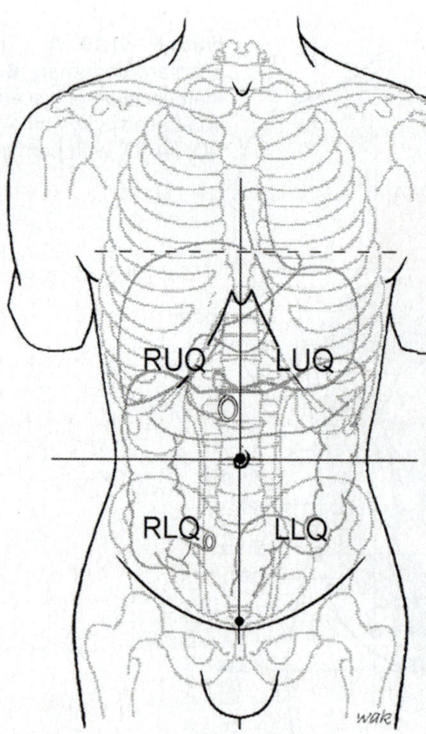

Figure 41.11. The four-quadrant abdomen. (Illustration by William A. Kuchera, DO, FAAO, with permission.)

Regional Exam

The palpatory component of the regional exam consists of assessing the paraspinal region for temperature, tissue texture changes, tenders, and asymmetry. During the palpatory evaluation of the paraspinal tissues, evidence of acute or chronic somatic dysfunction, viscerosomatic or somatovisceral reflexes, infectious processes, and even trauma may be found with the assessment of temperature changes (excessive warmth or coolness), tissue texture changes such as bogginess, thickness, ropiness, stringiness, firmness, and excessive moisture or dryness, patient tenderness to palpation and asymmetry on palpation.

Findings of facilitated segments, viscerosomatic and/or somatovisceral reflexes may assist the physician with refinement of the next portion of the assessment, the examination of the abdomen. (For further information, the reader is directed to Chapters 42 and 55.)

The abdomen should be undraped and may be approached in the following order: inspection, auscultation, percussion, and palpation:

- Inspection consists of evaluation of the following: symmetry/asymmetry, contour (flat, rounded, scaphoid, protuberant), presence of distension, presence or absence of rashes/erythema/bruising/moles/scars/striae, dilated veins, or pulsations.
- Auscultation is performed in all four quadrants to evaluate for bowel sounds (hypoactive, normoactive, hyperactive, or absent). Auscultation is performed to evaluate for the presence or absence of aortic, renal, and iliac bruits bilaterally.
- Percussion is performed in all four quadrants by rapidly striking a finger lying against the abdomen with a finger from the other hand, usually the third finger on each hand. The physician notes areas of tympany (representing gas and is a hollow sound) or dullness (representing fluid, mass, or organ and is a dull sound).
- Palpation:
  - Palpation should be performed across the entire abdomen, covering all four quadrants as well as the epigastric, periumbilical, and suprapubic regions. First, palpate with light palpation and proceed to deeper palpation throughout these locations. The patient should be instructed to report any tenderness upon palpation.
  - The osteopathic physician should note any areas of tenderness, guarding, or rigidity and assess for the presence or absence of masses or organomegaly.
  - The physician should assess for thoracoabdominal diaphragm motion and excursion.
  - A listening test of the abdomen may be done as the physician compresses through the skin, adipose, superficial fascia, muscle, transversalis fascia, peritoneum with the dominant hand at the midline of the abdomen, fingers pointing superiorly. At each layer, the physician should note if there is a tissue pull in a certain direction, and if so, where is the center of the tension. By palpating in this manner, the physician identifies the area of dysfunction that should likely be assessed and treated first.
  - The linea alba may be tested for compliance by gently compressing through the tissue layers from just inferior to the xiphoid process to the umbilicus.
  - The regions of the collateral ganglia may be assessed for compliance or restriction by grouping the finger pads together and compressing through the tissue layers at the area of the celiac ganglion (just inferior to the xiphoid process), superior mesenteric ganglion (midway between the xiphoid process and the umbilicus) and the inferior mesenteric ganglion (just superior to the umbilicus).

TABLE 41.2

Common Chapman's Reflexes and Points Related to the Abdominal Region

Stomach acidity (Left)—5th intercostal space, midclavicular line to the sternum.
Liver (Right)—5th and 6th intercostal spaces, from the midclavicular line to the sternum.
Gallbladder (Right)—6th intercostal space, midclavicular line to the sternum.
Pancreas (Right)—7th intercostal space, close to the approximation of the costal cartilages.
Appendix (Right)—tip of the 12th rib
Small intestine (Bilateral)—8th, 9th, and 10th intercostal spaces near the costal cartilage (e.g., enteritis).
Left colon—A band 1 to 2 inches wide on the anterolateral aspect of the left femur, from 1 inch above the patella to the greater trochanter (left distal femur = left half of transverse colon, left midfemur = descending colon, left proximal femur = sigmoid colon).
Right colon—same instructions as for left colon (right distal femur = right half of transverse colon; right midfemur = ascending colon; right proximal femur = cecum)

- □ Assess the viscoelasticity of the root of the mesentery and the cecal and sigmoid suspensory ligaments by drawing them at an angle perpendicular to their mesenteric attachments.
- □ The physician may assess for appropriate Chapman's reflexes if there is a clinical index of suspicion of a particular disease process. Please see Table 41.2 for Chapman's points related to conditions of the abdominal region.

Segmental Exam

A more directed type of palpation can be used for somatic dysfunctions related to visceral dysfunction. Such directed palpation would include diagnosing segmentally related spinal somatic dysfunction and assessing for the presence of counterstrain tender points. Based on the findings of the regional abdominal exam, the mobility and motility of various abdominal organs and/or structures may be assessed using palpation methods associated with visceral osteopathic techniques (see Chapter 42).

Special Assessments Related to the Abdominal Exam

Osteopathic medicine encompasses comprehensive diagnosis and treatment of the patient. Additional assessments of the abdomen may be done to narrow the patient's differential, including:

- McBurney point: located one-third of the distance between the right ASIS and the umbilicus (about 2 inches from the ASIS). The physician palpates this point. Tenderness may indicate appendicitis.
- Psoas sign: the physician places their hand just superior to the patient's right knee and asks the patient to raise that thigh against the resistance provided. Tenderness may indicate appendicitis. Alternatively, the physician can extend the right leg at the hip (can be performed with the patient lying on the left side) and ask the patient if there is any tenderness.
- Obturator sign: the physician flexes the patient's right thigh at the hip with the knee flexed and then internally rotates the right lower extremity at the hip. Tenderness with this maneuver may indicate appendicitis.
- Rovsing sign: the physician presses deeply in the left lower quadrant (LLQ) and then quickly withdraws the palpating hand. The physician asks about the presence of pain and location of pain (if present). Tenderness in the right lower quadrant (RLQ) during LLQ pressure indicates a positive Rovsing sign, suggestive of acute appendicitis.
- Murphy sign: the physician palpates the right upper quadrant (RUQ) near the costal margin and, while observing respiration, instructs the patient to inhale deeply. Abrupt halt in inspiration is a positive Murphy sign and may indicate cholecystitis.
- Rebound tenderness: the physician presses deeply into abdominal regions and quickly withdraws the palpating hand. The physician asks the patient which hurts more, when pressure is applied or when pressure is removed. A positive finding is more pain on release of pressure and is suggestive of peritonitis.[18]

SUMMARY

An in-depth knowledge of abdominal region anatomy, along with the skilled use of osteopathic palpatory diagnosis, can help to inform the successful practice of osteopathic medicine. Such a combination of knowledge and skills can lead to more efficient and accurate patient diagnoses, and more rational and effective treatment decisions.

REFERENCES

1. Still AT. *Autobiography of A.T. Still*. Published by the author; 1897.
2. Still AT. *The Philosophy and Mechanical Principles of Osteopathy*. Hudson-Kimberly Publishing Company; 1902.
3. Hazzard C. *The Practice and Applied Therapeutics of Osteopathy*. The Journal Printing Company; 1901.
4. Conrad CF. *A Manual of Osteopathy*. 4th ed. The University Book Company; 1919.
5. McConnell CP. *Ventral Technique*. The American Academy of Osteopathy, Yearbook; 1951.
6. Owens C. *An Endocrine Interpretation of Chapman's Reflexes*. Reprinted by the American Academy of Osteopathy; 1932.
7. Hermann E. *The DO*. 1965;6(2):163–164.
8. Radjieski JM, Lumley MA, Cantieri MS. Effect of osteopathic manipulative treatment on length of stay for pancreatitis: a randomized pilot study. *J Am Osteopath Assoc*. 1998;98:264–272.
9. Pikalov AA, Kharin VV. Use of spinal manipulative therapy in the treatment of duodenal ulcer: a pilot study. *J Manipulative Physiol Ther*. 1994; 17:310–313.
10. Donnelly JM, Editor-in-Chief. *Travell, Simons & Simon's Myofascial Pain and Dysfunction: The Trigger Point Manual*. 3rd ed. Wolters Kluwer; 2019.
11. Barral JP, Mercier P. *Visceral Manipulation*. Rev. ed. Eastland Press; 2006.
12. Barral JP. *Visceral Manipulation II*. Rev. ed. Eastland Press; 2007.
13. Finet G, Wiallame C. *Treating Visceral Dysfunction*. Stillness Press; 2000.
14. Standring S, ed. *Gray's Anatomy*. 42nd ed. Elsevier Churchill Livingstone; 2021.
15. Anderson DM, ed. *Mosby's Dictionary of Medicine, Nursing & Health Professions*. 11th ed. Elsevier; 2022.
16. Hruby RJ, Martinez ES. The lymphatic system: an osteopathic review. *Cureus*. 2021;13(7):e16448.
17. Suneja M, Szot F, LeBlond RF, Brown DD. *DeGowin's Diagnostic Examination*. 11th ed. McGraw Hill; 2020.
18. Bickley LS, Szilagyi PG, Hoffman RM, Soriano RP. Abdomen. In: *Bates' Guide to Physical Examination and History Taking*. 13th ed. Wolters Kluwer; 2021:613–676. Accessed May 14, 2024. https://meded.lwwhealthlibrary.com/book.aspx?bookid=2964

42 Internal Organ Assessment for Visceral Motion Dysfunction

KENNETH LOSSING ▪ REBECCA E. GIUSTI

KEY CONCEPTS

- Viscera (internal organs) have inherent motility, that seem to follow electrochemical principles, and mobility that follow mechanical principles.
- Assessment of viscera for impaired or altered mobility and motility requires a detailed knowledge of anatomy and physiology.
- Abnormal motion tests and changes in distensibility and/or viscoelasticity of visceral attachments support the diagnosis of visceral dysfunction.
- Visceral dysfunctions are determined based on the principles of diagnosis, palpation, and assessment specific to each organ.

DEFINITION

A visceral dysfunction is impaired or altered mobility or motility of the visceral system and related fascial, neurological, vascular, skeletal, and lymphatic elements.[1]

Visceral dysfunctions may be associated with:

- Local symptoms (e.g., gastroesophageal reflux disease or stress incontinence)
- Distant symptoms (shoulder pain from gallbladder disease)
- Presymptomatic strain patterns

HISTORY

Dr. A.T. Still pioneered osteopathic diagnosis of the viscera.[2] A little-known fact is that Dr. Still palpated temperature changes when looking for the dysfunctional areas. Hildreth[3] states that he often observed Dr. Still running his hand along the patient's spine, throat, thorax, abdomen, and pelvis, looking for areas of heat or variation in temperature.

Since the time of Hippocrates, there have been clinical associations between problem areas of the body and increased output of heat within that area. Hippocrates is said to have put wet mud on a person, to see where it dried first, in an attempt to localize the problem. What has been less clear is why there are so many small temperature variations in a person's body. Clinical research using temperature recording devices over the past 10 years has concluded that somatic and visceral dysfunctions (functional problems) project heat imbalances, which are generally warmer, but sometimes cooler, relative to the surrounding area. For example, often in ankle sprains, the area of the injured ligament is warmer.

Two of Dr. Still's earliest students, Carl McConnell[4] and Elmer Barber,[5] attempted to record the visceral techniques as they were taught by Dr. Still through books and scientific journal articles. Apart from his legacy in osteopathy of the cranial field, William G. Sutherland, DO, was also a student of Dr. Still, and published on the principles of visceral diagnosis:

> "When you want to observe the abdominal viscera that may be in ptosis, with the patient supine gently place one hand over or just below the area of interest. This hand is passive; it does nothing. Then place your other hand over it. You use the upper hand for gentle lifts and observation. That gentle application will tell you a great deal about where you are so that you can feel what the tissues can reveal. The lower hand can be permitted to sink into the tissues below, but the upper hand does the lifting in cooperation with the exhalation excursion of the diaphragm.[6]"

Several other osteopathic physicians added to this body of knowledge; Gaddis,[7] Teal,[8] Smith,[9] Woodall,[10] Hoover,[11–13] Young,[14,15] Hazzard,[16] Riggs,[17] Murray,[18] and Goetz.[19] As is the case with all clinical sciences, with time, improved imaging techniques and clinical experience, the knowledge base increased.

The 1982 book, *Traite d'osteopathie Viscerale* by Jacques Weischenck, described the normal exchange of pressure in the abdomen, visceral dysfunction chains, normal and dysfunctional axis of motion of the organs during respiration, palpatory diagnosis, and manipulative treatment for all of the abdominal viscera.[20]

The biggest driving force for the dissemination of visceral technique has been Jean-Pierre Barral.[21–26] He generated the concepts of:

- "General and local listening" of the tissues
- Manual thermal diagnosis
- Visceral emotional connections
- Visceral motility

Additionally, authors and educators including Bensky,[27] Lossing,[28] Davidson,[29] and Blackman[30] have added to the accumulating evidence and teaching of visceral motion and manipulative techniques.

Research on the motions of the viscera has exploded onto the scene with the advent of MRI-guided and CT-guided radiotherapy for cancer treatment, as well as with other interventions reliant on detailed comprehension of respiratory organ motion. Visceral motion is being explored in both normal patients and patients with different medical conditions. The implications of maintaining normal physiologic visceral motion by the application of osteopathic manipulative techniques may have a profound effect on restoration of normal physiologic processes, supportive care, and perhaps even in disease prevention.

MECHANICAL PRINCIPLES OF VISCERA

Visceral ligaments or attachments are viscoelastic and therefore are subject to tensile and compressive forces, which are always in relationship with each other. Buckminster Fuller[31] coined the term tensegrity to describe architectural buildings/structures invented in 1948 by Kenneth Snelson. Tension occurs when something is stretched. Integrity is a state of wholeness. So, tensegrity is the balancing of tensile and compressive forces in a whole structure. When these forces are balanced and relatively evenly distributed, the structure as a whole is stronger and is able to withstand more stress. When the forces are unequally distributed, weakness and strain result. In the human body, bones are subjected to compressive forces, the connective tissues distribute tension, but the viscera interact with both of these forces. Besides the static forces generated in architecture of buildings, the human frame also has the constantly changing forces of:

- Respiration
- Circulation
- Physical movement
- Gravity
- Digestion
- Other factors

Visceral and somatic dysfunctions cause an imbalance in the distribution of tension and compressive forces, weakening the whole structure.

While structural problems (like tumors) are relatively easy to document on standard medical tests, functional problems (like sustained abnormal mechanical tension) are less easy to document but are palpable. Sustained abnormal mechanical tension in the tissues:

- Adversely affects the exchange of fluids and nutrition
- Overstimulates the nervous system leading to facilitation
- Decreases the exchange of pressures
- Taxes the homeostatic mechanisms of the body

Conversely, treating the sustained abnormal mechanical tension improves:

- Neurologic exchange
- Homeostatic mechanisms
- Exchange of fluids, nutrition, and pressures

In the case of viscera, the main tissue addressed is the attachments (ligaments, peritoneum, pleura, and mediastinum).

Osteopathic principles include the concept that one part of the body may affect another part and indeed have a global effect on the body as a whole. The osteopathic profession's neurologic model describes:

- Somatosomatic reflexes
- Somatovisceral reflexes
- Viscerosomatic reflexes
- Viscerovisceral reflexes[32]

Visceral diagnosis follows Dr. Still's adage that "life is motion." About 100 years ago, Carl McConnell, DO, said that "[t]he viscera ride in the tide of respiration."[4] Research in recent years appears to confirm these statements. Respiration-induced motions of the abdominal visceral are well documented.[33–35]

- With each inhalation, the rib cage raises, while the respiratory diaphragm, thoracic inlet, pelvic floor, and all of the viscera descend.
- Visceral motion is permitted in part by the viscoelasticity of the visceral ligaments.
- During respiration, the diaphragm and abdominal organs move inferior/superior (more so laterally than near the midline), and anterior/posterior, as measured by MRI.[36]

An osteopathic perspective is that abnormal mechanical tension in these structures decreases their respiratory motion and adversely affects their function. Preliminary work has been done measuring the respiratory movements of the abdominal organs in symptom-free and symptom-present states, showing normal and abnormal axes of motion.[37] The viscera are found to move and to have potential restrictions in the same three planes of motion described for all joints and sutures.

Along with the mechanical displacement of these structures, there is a corresponding change in the exchange of fluids. Arteries, veins, and lymphatic vessels travel through many of the visceral attachments and are sensitive to dysfunctional forces.

MECHANISMS OF RESPIRATION

To adequately assess and treat the viscera, it is critical to understand the respiratory mechanics of the body, along with its implications and interrelatedness to the anatomical structures and viscera of the thorax, abdomen, and pelvis. These respiratory motions are much larger and more important than was previously understood.

In quiet respiration, the thoracoabdominal diaphragm moves about 1.5 cm in a superior and inferior direction. The chest circumference changes to 1.2 cm when erect, and 0.7 cm when supine. With deep respiration, the diaphragm moves from 7 to 13 cm in a superior and inferior direction, and the chest circumference changes between 5 and 11 cm. Wade found that with deep respiration in a full vital capacity breath, one-quarter of the ventilation was due to chest expansion, and three-quarters was due to diaphragm displacement.[38] Based on Gierada's work, the thoracoabdominal diaphragm exhibits the most motion at the domes and its posterior aspects.[36]

The inferior wall of the heart moves an average of 1.5 cm with normal tide respiration as measured by MRI. Not only do the viscera move with respiration, but arterial and venous circulation are also affected by respiratory motion.[21] Blood flow in the descending aorta and superior vena cava increases during inspiration due to decreased intrathoracic pressure. Likewise, blood flow to these vessels decreases during exhalation.

In the abdomen, blood flow in the portal vein is greatest during exhalation, and lowest during inhalation, due to increased positive pressure. Pulsatility or cardia intercycle variability differentiates between the minimum and maximum values during a cycle. In healthy subjects, cardiac pulsititiy of portal venous flow is usually minimal, with larger flow variations seen with respiration. The average flow rate of the portal vein is about 970 mL/min, with the respiration varying the flow to an average of 539 mL/min, and cardiac cycle varying to an average of 296 mL/min. In other words, over half of portal vein blood flow is respiration dependent.

Diaphragmatic, abdominal, thoracic, and pelvic viscera motions have been measured by various forms of radiology (such as fluoroscopy, MRI, CT, and ultrasound), for their normal range of motion.[39] The viscera and the thoracoabdominal diaphragm have been found to move in three dimensions

1. Inferior-superior
2. Lateral
3. Anterior–posterior

With the establishment of normal motion, technology can now identify perturbed motion. Typically, in a dysfunction, either by medical diagnosis or by motion testing, the visceral organs are found to have decreased respiratory motion.[40,41] In addition to their normal physiologic motion with respiration, the viscera must also be able to slide relative to the neighboring organs. This ability is reduced in the presence of tumors, adhesions, and visceral dysfunctions diagnosed with MRI,[42] ultrasound, and motion testing palpation.

DYNAMIC INTERPLAY

What occurs during normal respiration has just been described. To further explore the global implications of dysfunction from an osteopathic perspective, examine for a moment the complex interplay during respiration and pulmonary ventilation.

The movement of air into and out of the lungs depends on a few basic factors:

- The pressure and volume inverse relationship (as volume increases, the pressure decreases)
- The volume itself, which is dependent on the movement of the diaphragm and ribs
- The internal and external air pressure
- The compliance of the lungs

As the ribcage expands during inhalation:

- The anterior ribcage moves superiorly (pump handle rib motion)
- The lateral ribcage moves laterally (bucket handle rib motion)
- The respiratory diaphragm descends

The excursion of the diaphragm during normal volume respiration is 1.5 to 4 cm, as measured by CT scan,[36] but can go as far as 7 cm. At the same time venous blood flow in the superior vena cava increases, and blood flow in the portal vein decreases. Simultaneously, the pericardium swings around the attachments for the great vessels, with its inferior border moving 1.5 cm medial and inferior.[43] The thoracic contents are stretched mechanically, so that the tension increases in the pericardium, pulmonary ligaments, and lung parenchyma, as the negative pressure inside the lungs becomes more negative,[22,24,25] and the negative pleural pressure becomes more negative. The negative pleural pressure keeps the visceral and parietal pleura in contact, which also increases the mechanical tension to the lung parenchyma. Normal tidal volume is about 500 mL of air.

The thoracic contents expand and the diaphragm contracts, causing a compression of the abdominal contents. The splenic flexure of the colon descends an average of 1.43 cm and the sigmoid colon descends about 0.25 cm.

The lymphatic system of the lungs has many roles; immune response, disease resistance, and fluid drainage. The lymphatic system may become congested due to infection, inflammation, inhalation allergies, and mechanical tension of the surrounding tissues.

If the fluid drainage is impaired, the mechanical tension increases, leading to less compliance in the lungs.

During rest and exercise, the tidal volume changes, not only depending on demand but also depending on the functional capacity of the overall structure. For instance, it is evident that if a rib is dysfunctional, its normal physiologic movement will be perturbed, and the thorax will not be able to expand as well. Less intrathoracic volume translates into less air inhaled and exhaled. What may not be as immediately evident is the fact that the compliance of the lungs can be impaired by mechanical factors, which also reduce tidal volume. A visceral dysfunction of a lung will reflect itself in reduced compliance.

Stretch receptors of the lungs connect via the vagus nerve to the ventral respiratory group of the medulla. Visceral afferent receptors send information to the spine, and also to the brain. They are chemosensitive, mechanosensitive, and thermosensitive.

The sensory system can be overstimulated, leading to a decreased threshold required for stimulation.

- Osteopathic literature has called this facilitation, which is very similar to the current medical terminology of peripheral and central sensitization.
- Whatever the mechanism, and whatever the current terms, the functional result is an associated mechanical tension.
- In the case of the sympathetics to the lung, the upper thoracic spine between T1 and T6 and its associated costal region will demonstrate an area of restriction.
- The parasympathetics to the lung can likewise be irritated.
- Cranial dysfunction near the jugular foramen can compress the vagus nerve, and there is reason to think that the parasympathetic nerves may also become facilitated.

To summarize, a visceral dysfunction of the lungs and airways may have related:

- Spinal and rib dysfunctions
- Cranial dysfunctions
- Neurologic dysfunctions
- Lymphatic or other fluid dysfunctions
- Temperature imbalances

Traditional osteopathic thought has always promoted the idea that the intelligent physician would find the most primary dysfunction, address it, and then allow the body to do the rest. The art of this practice is to determine the most efficient treatment order, and the most effective treatment that the body can tolerate. When the viscera presents as the primary dysfunction, it should be addressed first, perhaps using the diagnostic procedure presented in this chapter.

PRINCIPLES OF DIAGNOSIS

Osteopathic examination of the abdomen, thorax, and pelvis extends the normal medical exam of percussion, auscultation, and palpation, to include the following:

- Tissue pull (listening)
- Motion testing structures (organs, attachments)
- Palpation of fluid (arterial and lymphatic)
- Density changes

Palpatory diagnosis should be performed both globally (to find the total body pattern) and locally. Appropriate medical tests should be ordered when indicated. Similar to cranial and musculoskeletal structures, each organ can be evaluated for motion.

There are different aspects/models of dysfunction for evaluation, each equally valid, which are presented as follows:

- Fascial model—tested with motion testing and fascial pull ("listening" technique).
- Fluid model—arterial and venous blood, interstitial fluids, and lymphatics can be tested with palpation, Doppler ultrasound, or perfusion studies as necessary.
- Inherent motions model—tested with palpation/sensing (described as motility by Sutherland).
- Mechanical model—evaluation of associated musculoskeletal structures (rib cage, attachments through the posterior peritoneum to the anterior longitudinal ligament and spine, etc.) and associated cranial structures (e.g., the esophagus attaches to the temporal bones, occiput, and sphenoid by the pharyngeal constrictor muscles).
- Metabolic model—evaluation of Chapman reflexes.

- Neurologic model—tested with palpation and motion testing, or EMG, and taking into consideration the sympathetic and parasympathetic connections (viscerosomatic and somatovisceral reflexes).
- Respiratory model—excursion of tissue with respiration can be tested with palpation (described as mobility by Sutherland), fluoroscopy, or real-time MRI.

Temperature changes/energy/emotions—tested with palpation, or thermography.

As with all osteopathic diagnosis, the general area of the body with the primary or greatest dysfunction needs to be identified. One diagnostic technique termed "general listening" uses a fascial continuity model (see Chapter 52). Bones, muscles, blood vessels, and viscera are seen as tissues encased in a three-dimensional covering, the fascia. The fascia is tighter in an area of abnormal mechanical tension and pulls into that location.

- With the patient's body in the standing anatomical position, the physician's hand is placed on the top of the patient's head, to feel for which direction the fascia is pulling.
- In general:
  - An anterior pull results from a visceral restriction, anterior rib, or sternal restriction.
  - A posterior pull indicates a spinal or dural dysfunction.
  - A lateral pull indicates an issue in the extremities, or paired bilateral viscera.

Once the general area has been determined, specific localization of the restriction can be found using palpation of tissue pull in the local area, called "local listening" or "listening." At that point, a thorough knowledge of anatomy becomes paramount.

- In the case of suspected visceral restrictions, the specific organ is palpated and evaluated for motion during respiration and is named for the direction of motion ease.
- Next, motion testing is performed to evaluate the distensibility of all the attachments. Inherent motion (similar, but distinctly different from the cranial rhythmic impulse) may also be evaluated by palpating the viscera with a hand on the longitudinal axis.
- Palpation of the specific spinal segments of sympathetic innervation will reveal any tissue texture changes.[32]
- Areas of parasympathetic innervation, and other mechanically associated structures, are also examined for tissue texture changes.

A simple test may then be performed to identify which of the structures is the most primary, by palpating two related structures.

- Gently press on one of the structures to inhibit it and assess if the other responds immediately with decreased fascial tension. If this occurs, the structure is selected as the one to treat.
- This test may be used to determine whether the problem is viscerosomatic, somatovisceral, or viscerovisceral.

ILLUSTRATIVE TECHNIQUES

Palpatory Tests

"LISTENING" TEST OF THE ABDOMEN

This is a layer palpation designed to help identify the most problematic region and/or organ. The physician slowly compresses through the abdominal wall, noting the different layers:

- Skin
- Adipose
- Superficial fascia
- Muscle
- Transversalis fascia
- Peritoneum

Layer palpation utilizes Newton's third law which is: for every action, there is a reaction.

- Each layer has a different texture and will press back against the physician's hand.
- A dysfunction will generally pull connective tissues and surrounding structures (nerves, vasculature, etc.) toward it.
- At each layer, the physician should note if there is a tissue pull in a certain direction, and if so, determine the center of the tension.
- By palpating in this manner, the physician identifies the area of dysfunction that should likely be assessed and treated first.

The palpation is performed as follows:

1. The dominant hand is placed on the midline of the abdomen, with the fingers pointing superiorly, and the palms inferiorly (Fig. 42.1A,B).
2. Palpate through the abdominal wall to the "potential space" or the peritoneal cavity, before reaching the intraperitoneal viscera.
3. Palpate for a sense of tissue pull. If one is identified, move the dominant hand to that area in order to localize it.

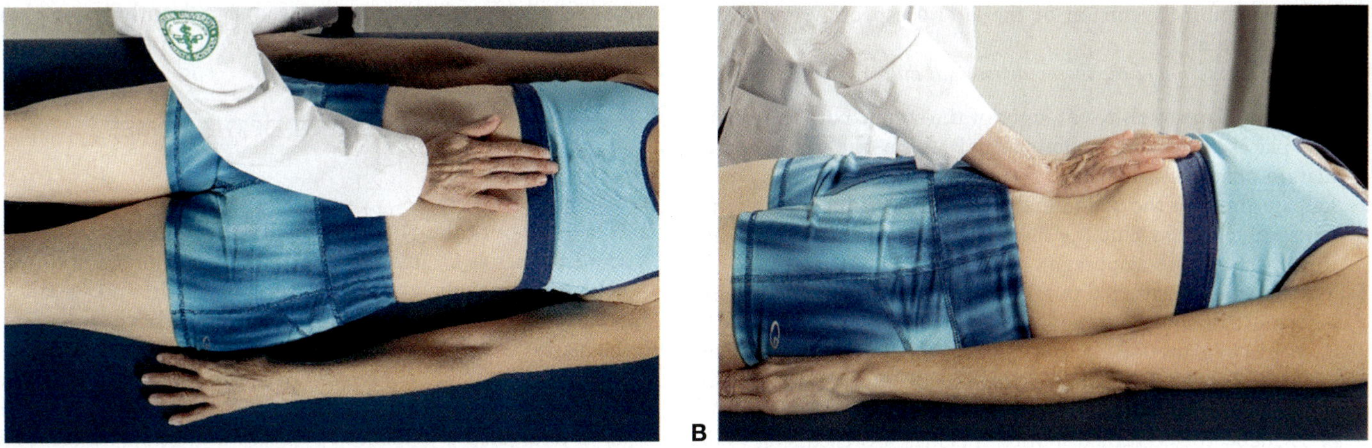

A B

Figure 42.1. "Listening test" to the upper abdomen. A. Anterior view. **B.** Lateral view. (Courtesy of Western University of Health Sciences, College of Osteopathic Medicine of the Pacific, with permission.)

4. Pay attention to the depth of the pull, and identify if it is superficial, middle, or deep (retroperitoneal).
5. The same process can be repeated in the mid- and lower abdomen as well.

Motion Testing

Motion testing involves palpating the organ in question and then checking its ability to be moved in an inferior–superior, medial–lateral, and anterior–posterior directions. The "end feel" of the motion should also be noted. In motion testing of a nondysfunctional organ, the distensibility will be within the physiologic normal parameters. A dysfunctional organ will have restrictions upon motion testing, and a harder than normal end feel.

Lymphatic Palpation

The lymphatic system has been found to contract not only in the thoracic duct but also between the valves, the lymphatic collectors, trunks, and ducts.[21,37] The channels expand and contract to propel the lymph toward the heart. The rhythmic contractions occur at a rate of 5 to 8 per minute at rest but may increase with exercise and direct stimulation. It is possible to palpate these contractions. Sites to experience this palpation include the following:

- The terminal areas of lymphatic drainage near the medial ends of the clavicles
- On the surface of an organ
- Near any lymphatic nodes

The physician palpates lightly into the fluid system and identifies the rhythmic contractions. The direction of the fluid motion and the strength of the contraction should be assessed. Less than optimal lymphatic flow will be found in any area of mechanical tension.

The Thoracoabdominal Diaphragm

Thoracoabdominal diaphragmatic motion has been studied with CT, MRI, fluoroscopy, and ultrasound. There is a displacement of about 1.7 cm on shallow breathing and a displacement of 13 cm on deep breathing. In 1995, Gierada et al. [36] used fast gradient-recalled MRI, on supine patients with maximal respiration. The study demonstrated that absolute excursion of the domes of the diaphragm was 4.4 cm on the right and 4.2 cm on the left. Excursion increased from the anterior portion of the diaphragm to the middle and was greatest at the posterior portion. Excursion of the lateral aspects was greater than the middle.

To test the motion of the thoracoabdominal diaphragm (Fig. 42.2):

1. The physician stands to the right of the supine patient's pelvis and places the thumbs approximately 2 cm below the costal margin bilaterally, about 4 to 5 cm from the midline.
2. Palpate through the abdominal wall until the abdominal contents are felt, then slide the thumbs slightly superior to engage the tension of the diaphragm.
3. The patient is instructed to take a deep inhalation, followed by a deep exhalation.
   a. With free motion, both sides of the diaphragm descend about 2 to 4 cm with inhalation. The diaphragm will ascend during exhalation with a similar amplitude.
   b. Evidence of perturbed motion includes less excursion than 2 to 4 cm, lack of descent, or superior displacement with inhalation.

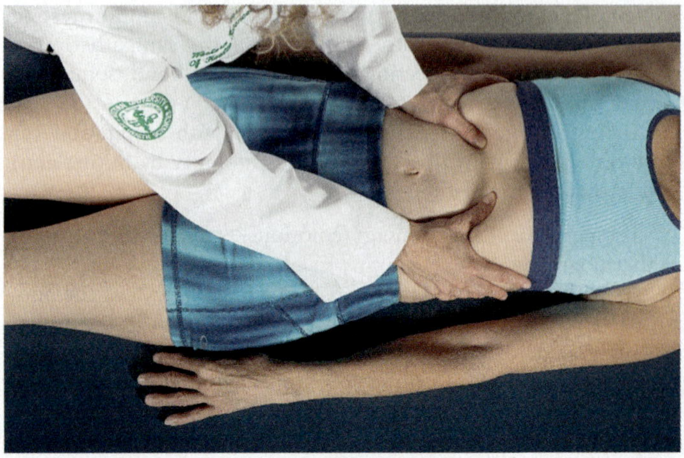

Figure 42.2. Testing thoracoabdominal diaphragm excursion. (Courtesy of Rebecca E. Giusti, DO, Western University of Health Sciences, College of Osteopathic Medicine of the Pacific, with permission.)

The Lungs and Associated Structures

During inhalation, the thoracoabdominal diaphragm descends. The costodiaphragmatic recess opens, the anterior ribs rise superiorly, and the pericardium descends, which increases tension on the pulmonary ligaments, vessels, and lung parenchyma. Dysfunction or tension of the costal cage, pleura, pericardium, and lung can therefore contribute to a decrease in respiratory volume.

The parietal pleura of the thorax is attached to the:

- Thoracoabdominal diaphragm
- Mediastinum
- Visceral pleura
- Ribcage

As the anterior upper ribs rise superiorly during a deep inhalation, the pleural domes are pulled inferiorly by the thoracoabdominal diaphragm.

The lungs have been found to move with respiration in three dimensions and were measured in over 11 different studies, mostly with resting respiration. Only one study[44] assessed lung motion with deep vital capacity breathing. Several studies have shown that the lower lung is displaced about 5 cm inferiorly/superiorly, with less motion in the medial/lateral and anterior/posterior planes, and even less motion in the upper lungs. Studies have also shown that areas of a lung with a tumor showed significantly less mobility and have also been found to have paradoxical motion, compared to what is expected.[45]

PALPATION AND ASSESSMENT OF THE DOMES OF THE LUNGS (FIG. 42.3)

1. The patient is supine.
2. The thumbs of the physician are placed on the patient's pleural dome, which is located posterior to the clavicle, lateral to spine, and anterior to the posterior portion of the first rib.
3. The patient is instructed to take a deep breath while the physician assesses for motion of the pleural domes.
   a. In normal physiologic motion, both domes should move inferiorly with inhalation.
   b. Dysfunction is evidenced by a lack of motion, or worse still, paradoxical motion where the pleural dome or domes move superiorly during inhalation.

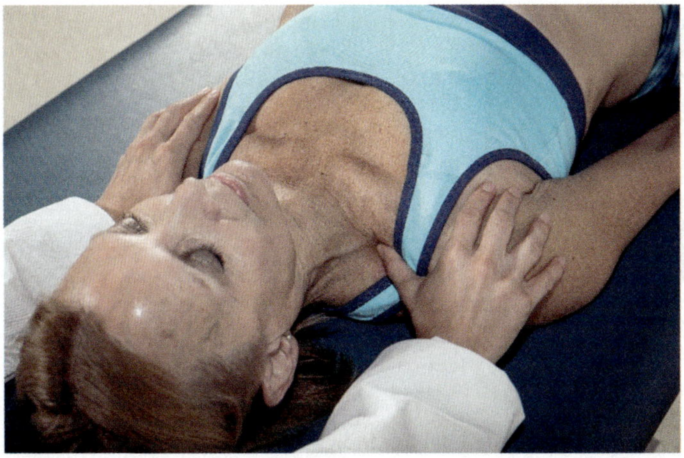

Figure 42.3. **Pleural dome testing.** (Courtesy of Rebecca E. Giusti, DO, Western University of Health Sciences, College of Osteopathic Medicine of the Pacific, with permission.)

PALPATION AND ASSESSMENT OF THE LUNGS

Before motion testing the lungs, perform a local "listening" test by placing the dominant hand over the sternum and identifying if there is a side of increased tension and reduced motion (Fig. 42.4).

Next, check the thoracoabdominal diaphragm's ability to appropriately descend during a deep inhalation (see Fig. 42.2), to confirm that it correlates with the side of tension found with the "listening" test. Once the side of greatest tension and least amount of motion is determined, the lung itself may be tested as follows:

1. The patient is in a lateral recumbent position on the unaffected side (Fig. 42.5).
2. The physician stands behind the patient and performs a layer palpation through the skin, ribcage, pleura, and then to the actual lung tissue.
3. Once the lung tissue has been contacted, the physician performs a "listening" test. A medial pull may indicate a dysfunction of the hilum, interpulmonary ligament of mediastinum.
4. The physician then motion tests the lung by assessing its superior/inferior motion and medial and lateral rotation.
5. In addition, the physician compresses the lung and then appreciates its return or recoil to assess its viscoelasticity.

The lung's ability to distend laterally may be compromised by tension of the interpulmonary ligament, and/or tension of the pulmonary vasculature. To test the ability of the lung to distend laterally:

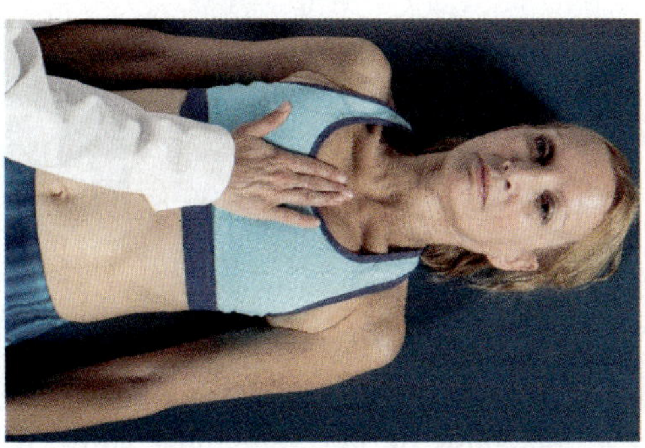

Figure 42.4. **"Listening" test of the midthorax.** (Courtesy of Rebecca E. Giusti, DO, Western University of Health Sciences, College of Osteopathic Medicine of the Pacific, with permission.)

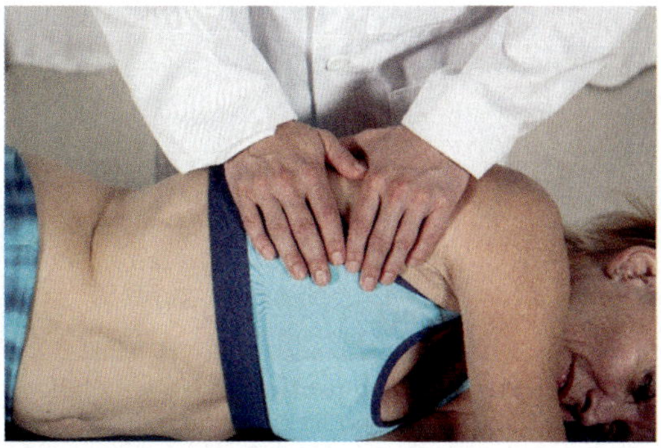

Figure 42.5. **Testing the lung.** (Courtesy of Rebecca E. Giusti, DO, Western University of Health Sciences, College of Osteopathic Medicine of the Pacific, with permission.)

1. The physician stands behind the lateral recumbent patient.
2. The physician places one forearm anteriorly along the patient's sternum, with the other arm placed posteriorly along the patient's costovertebral junction.
3. The physician compresses the patient's costal cage through the forearms to catch the lung and then lifts it laterally, away from the patient's midline (Fig. 42.6A–C).

PALPATION AND ASSESSMENT OF THE BRONCHI AND TRACHEA (FIG. 42.7)

1. The patient is supine.
2. The physician stands near the patient's head.
3. The physician palpates the trachea with one hand, tractioning it superiorly, while palpating about 2 cm lateral to the midline on each second intercostal space, until a slight tug is felt.
   a. Normal distensibility is about 2 cm. If the distensibility is less than that, there may be lymphatic congestion in the airways, or mechanical tension in the trachea and/or airways.

Pericardium

During inhalation, the great vessels act as a fulcrum above the heart for the pericardium to swing on. The inferior pericardium moves inferior and medially by at least 1.5 cm during a tidal respiration.[21] Using fast gradient MRI, Wang found that during tidal respiration, the inferior margin of the heart moves 1.81 cm inferior during inhalation, while the anterior margin moved 0.24 cm anterior. The coronary arteries had less motion.[46] Forced breathing has not been measured. Another study done by Shechter[47] used coronary angiography to demonstrate that during tidal respiration, the heart translates inferiorly, rotates superiorly and posteriorly, and translates anteriorly. Additionally, there is a decrease in the left ventricular stroke volume, and an increase in left ventricular end systolic volume, as well as an increase in right ventricular stroke volume. Respiration also seemed to change the shape of the heart during diastole.[46]

PALPATION AND ASSESSMENT OF THE PERICARDIUM

1. The patient is supine with the knees flexed.
2. The physician uses one hand as the palpating hand on the sternum, between the sternal angle and xiphoid. The palm of the hand should be near the xiphoid, a little to the left of the sternum, with the fingers pointing to the manubrium.
3. The physician's other hand is placed over the palpating hand to apply pressure.

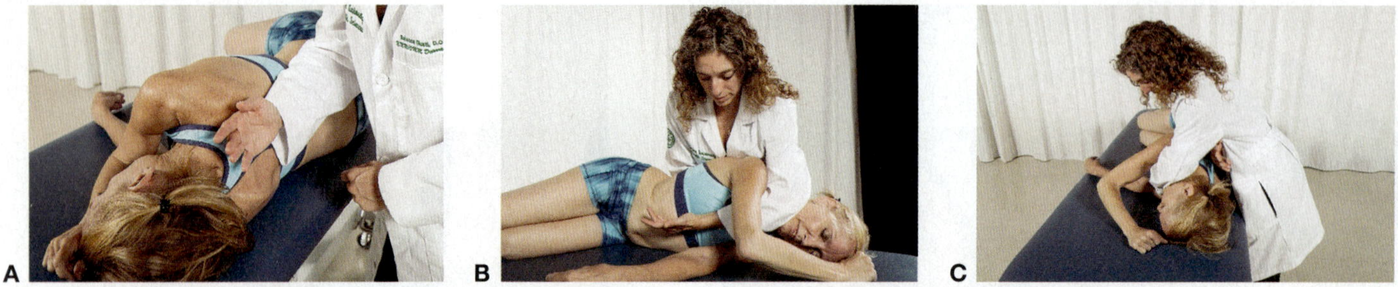

Figure 42.6. Testing lateral lung motion. A. Place inferior forearm along costovertebral junction. **B.** Place superior forearm along patient's sternum. **C.** "Catch" between the forearms and lift laterally. (Courtesy of Rebecca E. Giusti, DO, Western University of Health Sciences, College of Osteopathic Medicine of the Pacific, with permission.)

4. The physician compresses sagittally through the first osteocartilagious barrier.
5. The second barrier is met once the heart beat is palpated.
6. At this point, the physician adds a slight compression before motion testing the area of the pericardium in a superior and inferior direction, translating it to the right and left, and assessing the rotation of the inferior pericardium around the axis of the superior pericardium.

Aorta

The aorta pierces the crus of the diaphragm at the level of T11 and then extends inferiorly to its bifurcation at the level of L4 to L5. All of the abdominal and pelvic viscera receive their arterial blood from it. Mechanical stress in the walls of the arteries can affect arterial blood flow.

PALPATION AND ASSESSMENT OF THE AORTA (FIG. 42.8A,B)

In this palpation, the physician's goal is to contact the walls of the aorta superiorly and inferiorly.

1. The physician stands to the right of the supine patient, with a clear field of the patient's abdomen.
2. The physician's thumbs are used to palpate just to the right of the xiphoid–umbilical line, and the fingers to palpate to the left of this line.
3. The physician palpates deeply until the aortic pulse is found.
4. To precisely locate the walls of the aorta, the physician softly palpates laterally with the thumbs until the aortic pulse is no longer appreciated, which indicates that the aorta is no longer being palpated.
5. The physician then palpates incrementally medially until the tunica externa of the aortic wall is palpated. The aortic pulse will be felt through the walls. This is repeated with the fingers to ensure appropriate contact with the opposite walls of the aorta.
6. A "listening" test is now performed at the aorta to assess for dysfunction.
7. The aorta may then be motion tested to the right and left.
8. Last, the physician attempts to gently elongate or stretch the aorta, assessing its viscoelasticity.

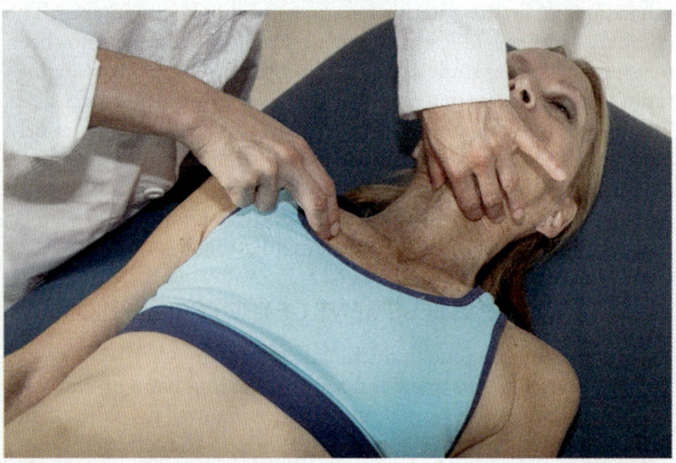

Figure 42.7. Palpating the bronchi and trachea. (Courtesy of Rebecca E. Giusti, DO, Western University of Health Sciences, College of Osteopathic Medicine of the Pacific, with permission.)

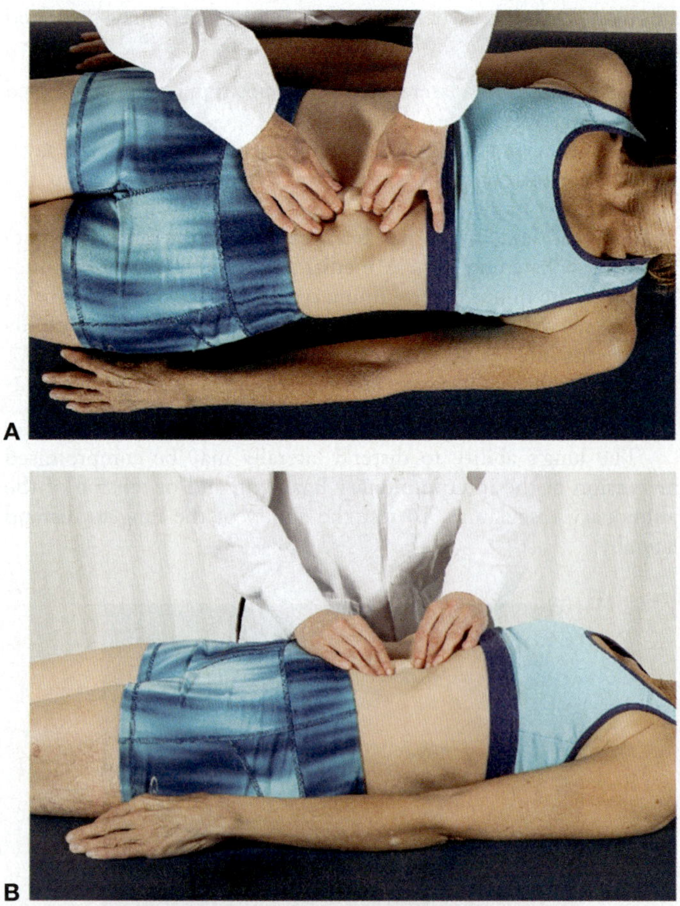

Figure 42.8. Palpation of the abdominal aorta. A. Anterior view. **B.** Lateral view. (Courtesy of Rebecca E. Giusti, DO, Western University of Health Sciences, College of Osteopathic Medicine of the Pacific, with permission.)

Celiac Trunk, Plexus, Ganglion, and Lymph Nodes

At the height of the superior border of L1, just anterior to the aorta, is the:

- Celiac trunk (which branches into the common hepatic, left gastric and splenic arteries)
- Celiac plexus and ganglion (supplying the esophagus, stomach, liver gallbladder, adrenal glands, duodenum, pancreas, and spleen)
- Celiac lymph nodes that drain the same organs as above

The paraaortic lymph nodes have been found to move during respiration less than the respiratory diaphragm, as measured by 4D CT, cranial/superior 0.45 to 0.86 cm, left/right 0.06 to 0.28 cm, and anterior/posterior 0.57 cm.[48] Palpation of the celiac trunk, celiac plexus, and celiac nodes should precede any treatment of the viscera that they supply.

PALPATION AND ASSESSMENT OF THE CELIAC TRUNK, PLEXUS, GANGLION, AND LYMPH NODES (FIG. 42.9A,B)

1. The physician stands to the right of the supine patient and uses the left hand to palpate posteriorly to identify the spinous process of L1. The spinous process of L1 is larger than that of T12.
2. The physician uses the right hand to palpate anteriorly at the same height near the midline.
3. Using layer palpation, the physician palpates through the abdominal wall, superficial abdomen, middle abdomen, and deep abdomen until the aortic pulse is felt.
4. Slightly soften the fingers and palpate to the right until the pulse is lost, then return toward the midline to find the left wall of the aorta. The same procedure is repeated to identify the right wall of the aorta.
5. Once both lateral walls of the aorta have been identified, the physician palpates in the mid aorta, lightening the fingers until the size of the pulse becomes smaller. At this level, the lighter pulse in the midaorta is the celiac trunk.

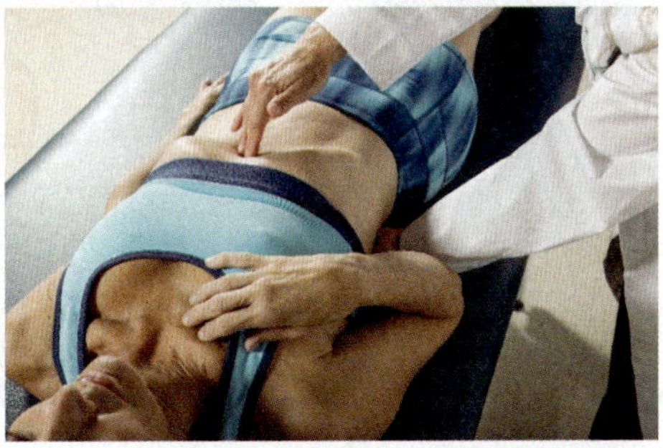

A

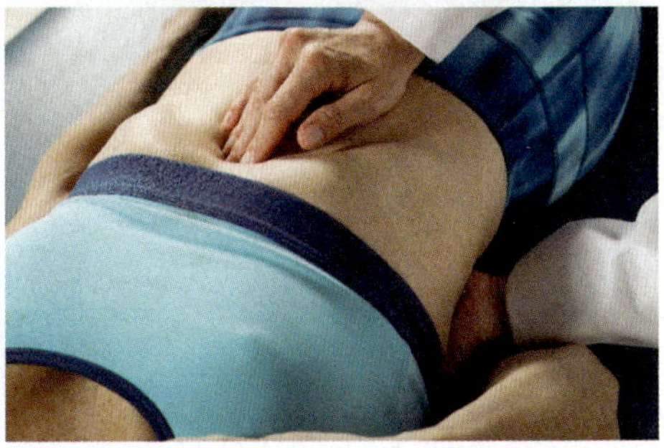

B

Figure 42.9. A. Identification of the celiac ganglion, trunk, and nodes. **B.** Palpation of the celiac ganglion, trunk, and nodes. (Courtesy of Rebecca E. Giusti, DO, Western University of Health Sciences, College of Osteopathic Medicine of the Pacific, with permission.)

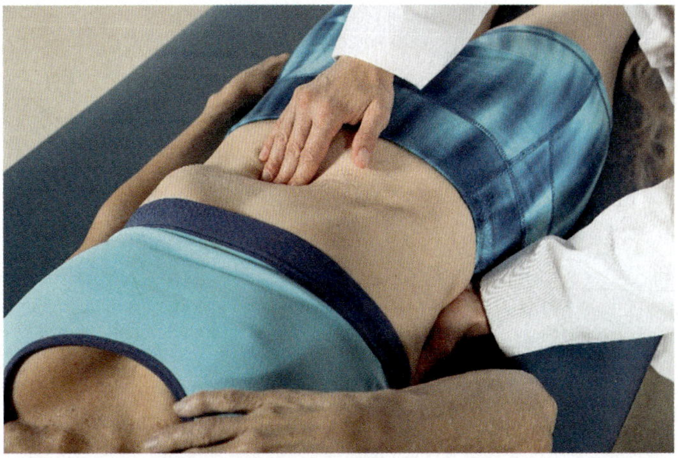

Figure 42.10. Palpation of the superior mesenteric artery, ganglion, and nodes. (Courtesy of Rebecca E. Giusti, DO, Western University of Health Sciences, College of Osteopathic Medicine of the Pacific, with permission.)

6. The physician appreciates the strength of the pulse and also palpates the lymphatic rhythm in this location. Does it seem to be strong or weak? The celiac ganglion is slightly superior to celiac trunk.
7. Assess the celiac ganglion with "listening," to determine if there is a pull in a particular direction and palpates for a feeling of congestion.
8. A motion test is then performed in a superior/inferior direction, and then to the right and left.

Superior Mesenteric Artery, Ganglion, and Lymph Nodes

The superior mesenteric artery branches off of the aorta about 1 cm inferior to the celiac trunk, at the level of the L1–L2 disk or the superior border of L2 vertebral body. It is accompanied by the superior mesenteric ganglion and superior mesenteric lymph nodes. These all supply the small intestine, as well as the large intestine from the cecum to about the first two-thirds of the transverse colon.

PALPATION AND ASSESSMENT OF THE SUPERIOR MESENTERIC ARTERY, GANGLION, AND NODES (FIG. 42.10)

The palpation is the same as that described above for the celiac trunk and ganglion but is instead performed at the level of the superior aspect of the L2 vertebral body.

Inferior Mesenteric Artery Ganglion and Lymph Nodes

The inferior mesenteric artery branches off the aorta at the level of L3, slightly to the left of midline. Surrounding it are the inferior mesenteric ganglion and inferior mesenteric lymph nodes. These supply the distal third of the transverse colon through the descending colon.

PALPATION AND ASSESSMENT OF THE INFERIOR MESENTERIC ARTERY GANGLION AND LYMPH NODES

The palpation is the same as that described for the celiac and superior mesenteric trunks but is instead performed slightly more inferiorly at the level of L3.

Liver

The liver has been studied by MRI, ultrasound, and nuclear imaging. Using CT and ultrasound, Suramo[40] found the liver to move

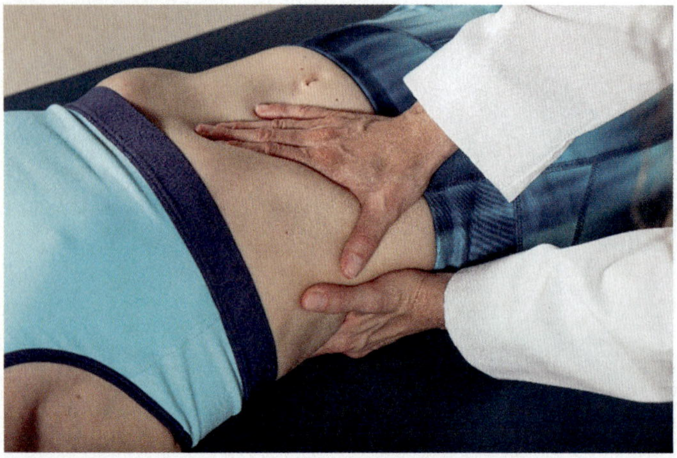

Figure 42.11. Palpation and assessment of the liver. (Courtesy of Rebecca E. Giusti, DO, Western University of Health Sciences, College of Osteopathic Medicine of the Pacific, with permission.)

in the superior/inferior direction at an average of 5.5 cm (3 to 8 cm range) with maximal inhalation, and at an average of 2.5 cm (1 to 4 cm range) with normal respiration. The liver has also been found to move in the medial/lateral and anterior/posterior planes.[41] Finet and Williame found an average of 2.31 cm inferior displacement with tidal inhalation, as measured by ultrasound.[37]

PALPATION AND ASSESSMENT OF THE LIVER (FIG. 42.11)

1. The physician stands at the right side of the supine patient.
2. The physician's right hand is placed just inferior to the costal margin, near the midline, to access the inferior part of the liver.
3. The liver should first be assessed for its consistency. A cirrhotic liver is palpably firmer than a normal one.[49]
4. The physician's left hand is then placed posteriorly against the patient's right lower ribcage. The physician compresses the two hands together to "catch" the liver.
5. The liver is then motion tested inferiorly and superiorly as a screening test.
6. If the liver is unable to move well either superiorly or inferiorly, it should then be motion tested to the left and right, and also in rotation in an anterior and posterior direction.
7. If dysfunction is found, the area of the celiac trunk should be palpated to assess for strength of arterial pulse, nerve congestion, and lymphatic movement.

Pancreas

Using ultrasound, Suramo[40] showed the pancreas to move an average of 4.3 cm with deep breathing (3 to 8 cm range), and an average of 2 cm with shallow breathing (1 to 3 cm range). The pancreatic duct diameter increases with inhalation. The pancreas seems to move relative to the superior mesenteric artery. On full inspiration, it is inferior to the origin of the superior mesenteric artery, and at full exhalation, it is found partly superior to that origin. The tail of the pancreas is more mobile than the body, in some cases displacing 8.8 cm. The pancreas has been found to move not only with respiration but also with changes in posture.[50] Kivisaari et al. [51] studied pancreatic motion in patients with a normal pancreas, chronic pancreatitis, and pancreatic head cancer. They found the following:

1. The head displacement averaged
   - □ 3.2 cm (normal pancreas)
   - □ 3.2 cm (chronic pancreatitis)
   - □ 2.2 cm (pancreatic head cancer)
2. The body displacement averaged
   - □ 3.0 cm (normal pancreas)
   - □ 2.9 cm (chronic pancreatitis)
   - □ 2.5 cm (pancreatic head cancer)
3. The tail displacement averaged
   - □ 4.1 cm (normal pancreas)
   - □ 3.2 cm (chronic pancreatitis)
   - □ 1.4 cm (pancreatic head cancer)

This demonstrates a tendency for larger reductions in motion with more significant medical problems.

PALPATION AND ASSESSMENT OF THE PANCREAS (FIG. 42.12A,B)

1. The physician stands to the right of the supine patient and places the right hand on the abdomen with the hypothenar eminence 2 in superior and 2 in to the right of the patient's umbilicus, with the fingertips pointing to the area of the spleen.
2. The physician compresses slowly through the abdominal wall, performing layer palpation, into the peritoneum, and eventually reaching all the way to the pancreas. The pancreas has a slightly softer consistency.
3. At this point, a screening exam should be performed by motion testing the pancreas superiorly, then back to neutral, and then inferiorly.
4. "Normal" distensibility should be around 4 cm. If the motion is less, the physician should check the translation to the left and to the right.
5. The physician should also check the "listening," by very slightly softening the palpating hand.
6. The area of the celiac trunk should also be assessed for the strength of the arterial pulse, tension in the ganglion, and lymphatic movement.

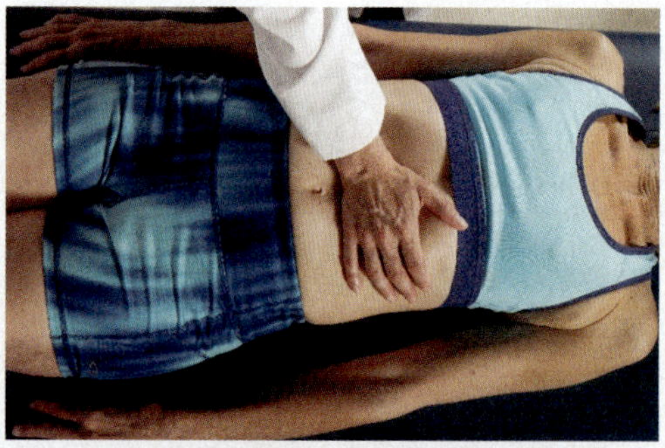

A

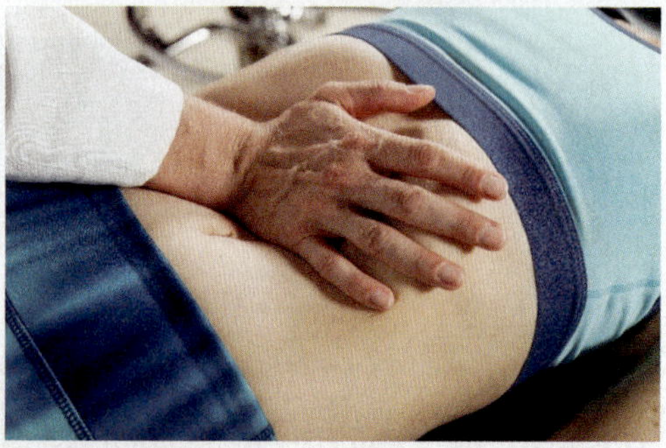

B

Figure 42.12. Palpation of the pancreas. A. Anterior view. **B.** Oblique view. (Courtesy of Rebecca E. Giusti, DO, Western University of Health Sciences, College of Osteopathic Medicine of the Pacific, with permission.)

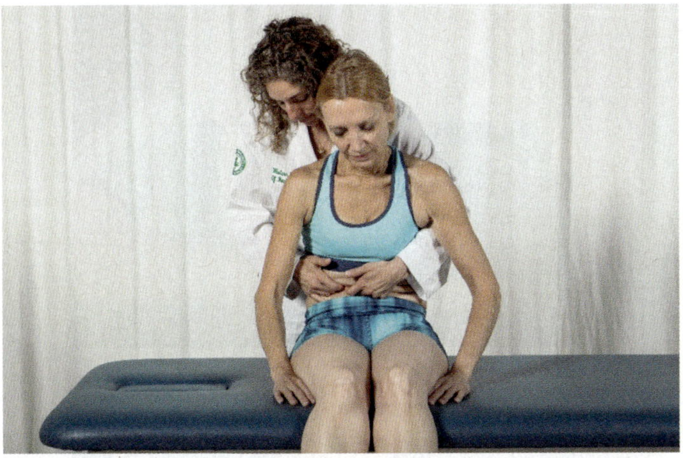

Figure 42.13. Palpation of the gallbladder. (Courtesy of Rebecca E. Giusti, DO, Western University of Health Sciences, College of Osteopathic Medicine of the Pacific, with permission.)

Gall Bladder and Sphincter of Oddi

The gallbladder's motion has not been studied radiographically. As it is firmly attached to the liver, it should move a similar amount.

PALPATION AND ASSESSMENT OF THE GALLBLADDER AND SPHINCTER OF ODDI (FIG. 42.13A,B)

1. The physician stands behind the seated patient and reaches around the patient, contacting the costal margins.
2. At about the midnipple line on the right, the physician palpates the lower edge of the liver and then palpates just inferior to that point.
3. Palpating more posteriorly toward the backside of the liver, the physician attempts to palpate the medial and lateral borders of the gallbladder.
4. The gallbladder's consistency is assessed and then motion tested to the left and to the right.
5. The patient is then asked to lie supine.
6. The sphincter of Oddi is located about 2 cm superior and to the right of the umbilicus. The physician uses a flat soft hand to perform a layer palpation through the abdominal wall and contents to the duodenum, and finally to the sphincter of Oddi.
7. A "listening" test is performed, and the area is motion tested inferior/superior, and then medially and laterally.

Stomach

During inhalation, the gastric fundus moves from superior to inferior an average of 2.9 cm, posterior to anterior 2 cm. It shifts to the right 0.6 cm, and tends to incline to the left. During inhalation, the body of the stomach descends 0.8 cm, advances anteriorly 0.95 cm, and shifts to the left or right.[39]

PALPATION AND ASSESSMENT OF THE STOMACH (FIG. 42.14)

1. The physician stands to the right of the supine patient and places the right hand under the patient's left costal margin, superior to the umbilicus.
2. The left hand of the physician is placed over the right to add the compressive force.
3. The physician palpates through the abdominal wall using layer palpation to arrive at the abdominal contents.
4. The stomach should first be tested for consistency. A normal stomach has a soft consistency. An irritated stomach, for instance, in gastroesophageal reflux, will feel much "harder."

A

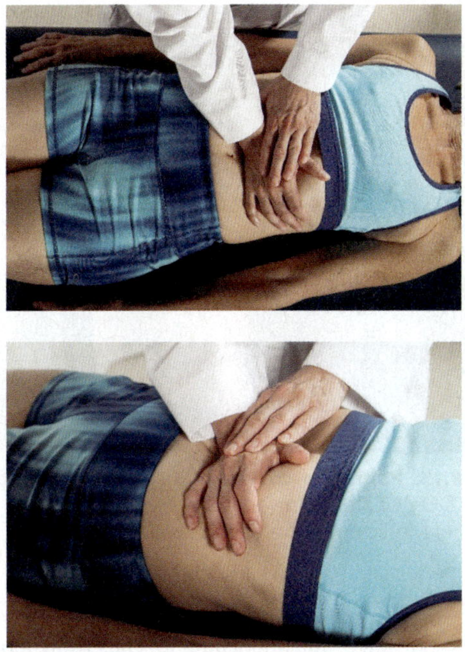

B

Figure 42.14. Palpation of the stomach. A. Anterior view. **B.** Oblique view. (Courtesy of Rebecca E. Giusti, DO, Western University of Health Sciences, College of Osteopathic Medicine of the Pacific, with permission.)

5. The stomach should have nearly 4 cm of superior/inferior motion. If the motion is less, it should be assessed with left-to-right translation and a "listening" test.
6. The gastroesophageal junction is tested by drawing the stomach inferiorly and to the left toward the left anterior superior iliac spine (ASIS), along the axis of the esophagus where it pierces the diaphragm and then continues to the stomach.

The Pylorus

The pylorus is between the antrum of the stomach and the first section of the duodenum. It is normally in a closed position. However, when the stomach contents are ready to be transferred to the duodenum, the pyloric sphincter relaxes, allowing the contents to be transferred. The pyloric sphincter then closes once again. Normal physiologic sphincter tone, along with proper contraction and relaxation, is imperative to the coordination and dynamics of the digestive tract.

PALPATION AND ASSESSMENT OF THE PYLORUS (FIG. 42.15A,B)

1. The pylorus is palpated about four to five fingers superior to the umbilicus, to the right of the midline.
2. Its fibers are normally slightly more firm than the surrounding area. The palpatory quality may resemble an almond.
3. The pylorus is assessed with "listening," superior and inferior displacement, medial and lateral distensibility, and rotation clockwise and counterclockwise.

The Small Intestine

The small intestine consists of the duodenum, jejunum, and ileum. It extends from the pylorus to the ileocecal valve. It is normally about 5 m long in an adult but may be as short as 3 or as long as 7 m. The jejunum and ileum are attached to the peritoneum by the root of the mesentery.

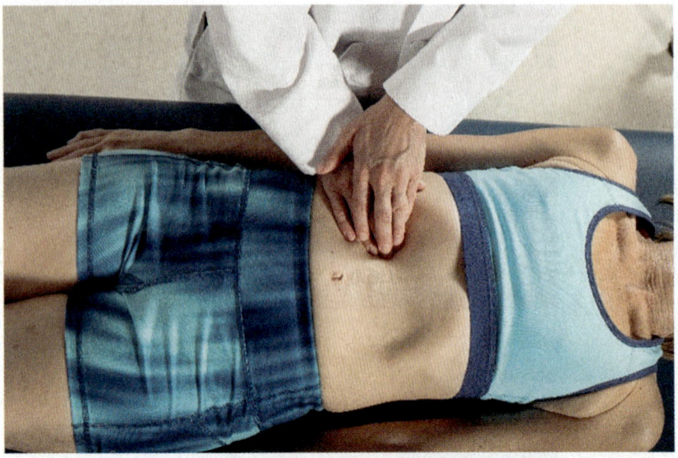

Figure 42.15. Palpation of the pylorus. (Courtesy of Rebecca E. Giusti, DO, Western University of Health Sciences, College of Osteopathic Medicine of the Pacific, with permission.)

Duodenum

- The first portion of the duodenum ascends from about the level of T12 to the posterior surface of the liver. It is intraperitoneal and very flexible. This portion connects to the portal vein, proper hepatic artery, and common bile duct through the lesser omentum.
- The second section of the duodenum descends anterior to the spine, connecting with the right perirenal fascia, the transverse mesocolon, and the pancreatic head down to a level of about L3.
- The third section crosses the midline and has attachments to the root of the mesentery, and right psoas muscle, left psoas muscle, and the inferior duodenal fold.
- The fourth section ascends to the duodenal–jejunal junction, which also opens and closes like a sphincter, with connections to the muscle or ligament of Treitz.

During tidal inhalation, the duodenum globally descends about 0.55 cm, closes on itself, advances anteriorly about 0.66 cm, and shifts to the left.[37]

PALPATION AND ASSESSMENT OF THE DUODENUM (FIG. 42.16A,B)

1. The physician stands to the right of the supine patient and places the right hand with the base of the palm at the level of the umbilicus, and the fingers pointed toward the patient's head to contact the abdomen.
2. Using layer palpation, the physician palpates through the abdominal wall, through the superficial abdomen, to the deep abdomen.
3. The physician's hand is soft and relaxed, as a tense hand can be uncomfortable for the patient.
4. The physician performs a "listening" test to assess for tissue pull or tension.
5. The physician then translates the duodenum superiorly, inferiorly, to the left, and to the right, noting distance and end feel.

The Duodenal–Jejunal Junction

The duodenal–jejunal junction acts like a sphincter, opening when required to pass the duodenal contents into the jejunum. This ability can be compromised due to abnormal tension in the root of the sigmoid, root of the mesentery, or muscle/ligament of Treitz.

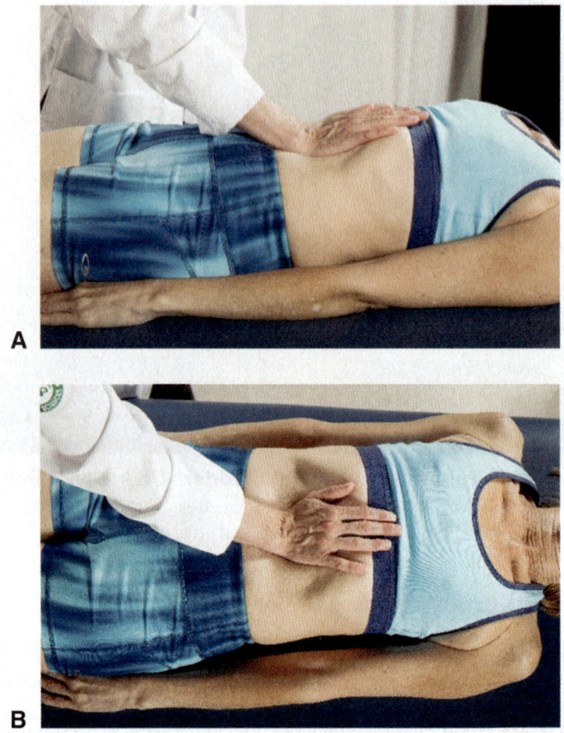

Figure 42.16. Palpation of the duodenum. A. Lateral view. **B.** Anterior view. (Courtesy of Rebecca E. Giusti, DO, Western University of Health Sciences, College of Osteopathic Medicine of the Pacific, with permission.)

PALPATION AND ASSESSMENT OF THE DUODENAL–JEJUNAL JUNCTION

1. The physician stands to the right of the supine patient and then locates the region two-finger width superior to the umbilicus, and two-finger width lateral to the midline.
2. At this location, a layer palpation is performed through the abdominal wall, the superficial abdomen, to the deep abdomen.
3. A "listening" test is performed to assess for a direction of tissue pull.
4. A motion test is then performed to the right, left, superiorly, and inferiorly, noting distance and end feel.

Jejunum and Ileum

The root of the mesentery contains the superior mesenteric artery and vein, superior mesenteric nerves, and the lymphatic vessels of the jejunum and ileum. Any increase in tension of the root can potentially have an adverse effect on those structures.

The jejunum descends 0.3 cm, shifts to the right or the left, and spreads out to the left. The ileum descends and spreads to the right.[20] Globally, during inhalation, the jejunum and ileum descend, advance anteriorly in the sagittal plane, and spread laterally in the frontal plane.

PALPATION AND ASSESSMENT OF THE JEJUNUM AND ILEUM

The specific loops of the jejunum and ileum are virtually impossible to distinguish by palpation. It is possible to check the distensibility of the root of the mesentery area (Fig. 42.17) and to specifically palpate the area of the peritoneum's reflections.

In a small intestine that is functioning well and not congested, the region of the mesentery's root will be more clearly delineated than that of a congested small intestine (as may be found

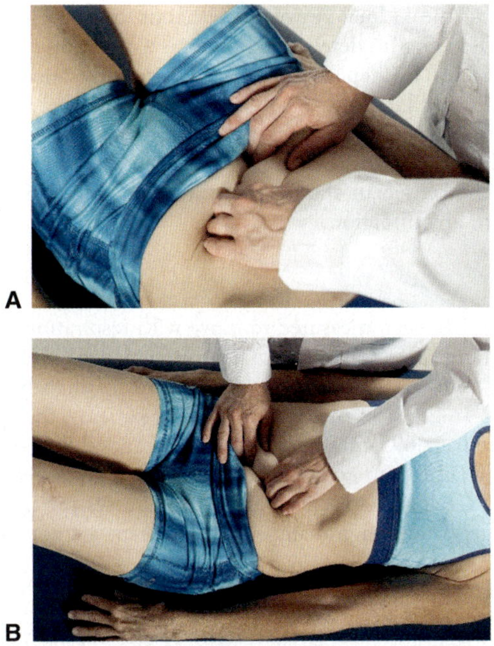

Figure 42.17. Palpation of the root of the mesentery. A. Right superior oblique view. **B.** Anterior view. (Courtesy of Rebecca E. Giusti, DO, Western University of Health Sciences, College of Osteopathic Medicine of the Pacific, with permission.)

in patients with food sensitivities). The root of the mesentery is palpated with the thumbs superior to the region, and the fingers inferior to it. This can be performed either in a supine position or in the left lateral recumbent position.

1. The physician gently palpates through the small intestine until the root is clearly appreciated. The area of the root is then motion tested.
2. The superior root is drawn inferiorly, and the inferior portion is drawn superiorly.
3. The lateral portion should be drawn inferiorly, and the medial portion superiorly before reversing this. Simultaneously, compliance and end feel are also assessed.
   a. In cases of food sensitivities, small intestinal bacteria overgrowth, adhesions, and small bowel obstructions, there is generally less compliance with the above motion testing.

Ileocecal Valve

The ileocecal valve is found on a line from the umbilicus to the ASIS. If this line is divided into thirds, the ileocecal valve is generally located about two-thirds of the distance from medial (umbilicus) to lateral (ASIS). The valve opens to allow the contents of the small intestine to move into the large intestine and then closes to prevent reflux. Tension in any of the structures attaching to it or in the region, such as the appendix, ovaries, iliacus, and psoas muscles, can affect proper functioning of the ileocecal valve.

PALPATION AND ASSESSMENT OF THE ILEOCECAL VALVE

1. The physician stands to the right of the supine patient, finds the location of the ileocecal valve, and performs a layer palpation to the level of the valve.
2. The physician then performs a "listening" test to identify the direction of any abnormal tension.
3. A motion test is then performed in a superior/inferior, medial/lateral, clockwise, and counterclockwise direction.

Large Intestine

The large intestine is about 1.5 m long. It is thickest at the cecum and narrows at the level of the midrectum. The superior mesenteric artery and inferior mesenteric artery provide the arterial supply to the colon. The ascending colon, descending colon, and rectum are considered to be retroperitoneal structures, while the cecum, appendix, transverse, and sigmoid are intraperitoneal structures. Retroperitoneal structures were thought to be "fixed." However, radiographic evidence demonstrates mobility of these areas. With inhalation, the following has been found[37]:

- Cecum: descends 0.42 cm, advances 0.54 cm, inclines posteriorly and to the right.
- Ascending: descends 0.38 cm, advances 0.62 cm, shifts either to the right or the left.
- Right flexure: descends 1.18 cm, advances 0.86 cm, shifts to the left 0.29 cm, inclines to the left.
- Right transverse: descends 0.89 cm, advances 0.85 cm, inclines, and shifts to the left.
- Left transverse: descends 0.73 cm, advances 1.05 cm, shifts and inclines to the left.
- Left flexure: descends 1.43 cm, advances 1.63 cm, shifts either to the right or the left.
- Descending: descends 0.72 cm, advances 0.85 cm, shifts to the left, and inclines to the right and anteriorly.
- Iliac: descends 0.25 cm, advances 0.27 cm, inclines to the left.
- Sigmoid: descends 0.13 cm, inclines to the left and anteriorly.
- Rectum: very small motion detected, but seems to shift inferiorly and to the right, and to incline to the left and posteriorly.
- Global: rotation clockwise, descends, advances, and inclines anteriorly.

PALPATION AND ASSESSMENT OF THE LARGE INTESTINE (FIG. 42.18A,B)

Screening tests of the large intestine involve motion testing of each region of the intestine in a superior and inferior direction. If significant restriction of motion is found, that area is further tested with medial/lateral motion and with rotation. Lack of mobility in the area of the cecum tends to be associated with diarrhea. Lack of mobility in the area of the sigmoid tends to be associated with constipation.

Kidneys

The kidneys are quite mobile and slide within the perirenal fat encased in the perirenal fascia. Of all the organs, renal respiratory motion has been the best studied.

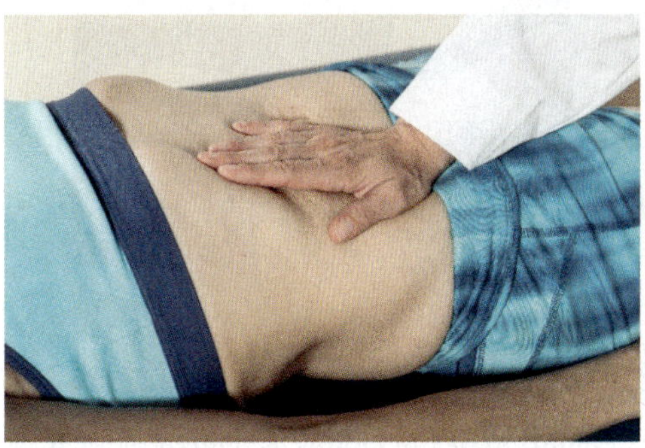

Figure 42.18. Palpation of the large intestine. (Courtesy of Rebecca E. Giusti, DO, Western University of Health Sciences, College of Osteopathic Medicine of the Pacific, with permission.)

- Using ultrasound, Suramo et al. found renal displacement with normal breathing to average 1.9 cm (1 to 4 cm range) with tidal respiration, and 4 cm (2 to 7 cm range) with deep respiration.[40]
- Ultrasound imaging has demonstrated displacement of the kidneys with tidal breathing: the right kidney averaging 1.89 cm, and the left kidney 1.29 cm in the superior/inferior direction. Both kidneys move from posterior to anterior by 0.85 cm, and in 70% of cases have a slight posterior inclination at the end of inhalation.[37]
- In the first study of its kind,[52] ultrasound measurements were taken of normal and restricted kidney motion, as diagnosed by palpation. Normal kidneys moved about 4.4 to 5.9 cm with deep inhalation. Restricted kidneys were found to move about 1 cm less than the normal kidneys. The kidneys with restricted motion, as found by palpation and confirmed by ultrasound, were then treated. Postmanipulative treatment restored motion to the restricted kidneys. Kidneys can also drop inferiorly in ptosis, which can be fixed medially, posteriorly, superiorly, laterally, and have restricted internal or external rotation. Ultrasound often shows adhesions in the area where restricted motion is found.

PALPATION AND ASSESSMENT OF THE KIDNEYS (FIG. 42.19)

1. Physician stands at the ipsilateral side of the supine patient of the kidney to be palpated.
2. One hand is used to palpate Grynfelt space posteriorly, lateral to the spine, inferior to the 12th ribs, and superior to the iliac crest.
3. Physician palpates through the latissimus dorsi muscle to identify the posterior border of the kidney and then places the other hand anteriorly over the patient's abdomen at the level of the umbilicus.
4. With the anterior hand, the physician attempts to separate the colon from the psoas muscle, gradually sinking deeper until the anterior aspect of the kidney is palpated. Thus, the physician "catches" the kidney between the hands and checks the tissue with "listening" to determine if there is a direction of tissue pull.
5. The kidney is then motion tested anteriorly and posteriorly, medially and laterally, and superiorly and inferiorly.
6. If there is no hard end feel, and the motion tests demonstrate compliance in all directions, the kidney is likely free of dysfunction. The physician should be aware that kidney fixations can occur in any direction.

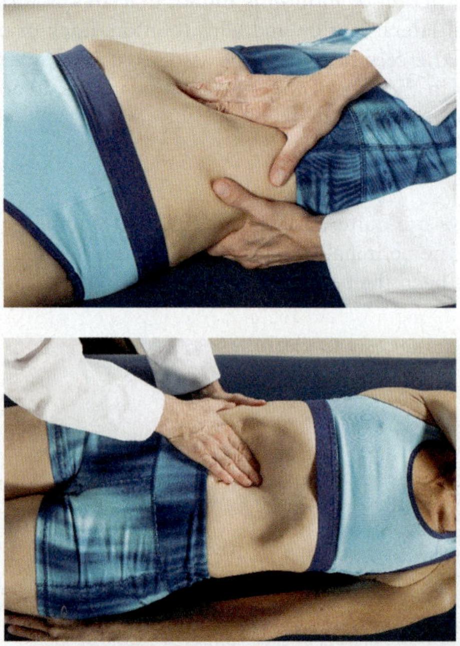

A

B

Figure 42.19. Palpation of the kidney. A. Lateral view. **B.** Anterior view. (Courtesy of Rebecca E. Giusti, DO, Western University of Health Sciences, College of Osteopathic Medicine of the Pacific, with permission.)

Spleen

The spleen has been measured to move with respiration by 4D CT 1.06 cm craniosuperiorly, 0.12 cm left to right, and 0.11 cm anterior/posterior.[48] Studies with ultrasound have shown a slightly larger displacement. In 29 cases of nonsymptomatic patients, the spleen was found to move 1.695 cm superior to inferior, and in 70% of the cases, there was a shift from posterior to anterior of about 0.39 cm.[37] The finding of a palpable spleen on an exam increases the possibility of splenomegaly,[53] although many enlarged spleens are not palpable.

PALPATION AND ASSESSMENT OF THE SPLEEN

1. The physician stands to the right of the supine patient and slides the right hand posteriorly under the patient to contact the left lower ribcage, spanning the left ribs 8 to 12.
2. The physician then places the left hand anteriorly, just inferior to the costal margin on the left.
3. The physician's hands are compressed together to "catch" the spleen.
4. Normally, unless the spleen is enlarged, it cannot be palpated readily.
5. A "listening" test is performed while maintaining the compression between the hands.
6. The physician then motion tests the spleen superiorly and inferiorly.

Adrenal Glands

The adrenal glands rest superior to the kidneys, inside the perirenal fascia. They have not been studied radiographically for motion. Clinical experience shows that they move with the motion of the respiratory diaphragm. However, in cases of dysfunction, the region of the adrenals is palpably tighter and typically has less distensibility. This has been found clinically in patients suffering from anxiety.

PALPATION AND ASSESSMENT OF THE ADRENAL GLANDS

1. The physician stands to the right of the patient's pelvis and slides the left hand under the patient to locate T12.
2. The physician's right hand is placed anteriorly at the level of T12 and is used to palpate into the abdomen to locate the pulse of the celiac trunk.
3. The fingers on the patient's abdomen are then moved slightly to the right and superior to perform a "listening" test.
4. The physician performs a motion test in a superior–lateral direction.
5. The same procedure is repeated for the patient's left adrenal gland. The lymphatic rhythm and flow may also be palpated in this region.

Greater Omentum

The greater omentum is suspended from the transverse colon and can be pulled to regions of infection where it may be tethered to that local tissue. This may occur in instances of appendicitis or pelvic infection.

PALPATION AND ASSESSMENT OF THE GREATER OMENTUM

1. The physician stands to the right of the patient and places the right hand inferior to the umbilicus, with the fingers pointed superiorly.
2. They then perform a layer palpation through the abdominal wall to the intraperitoneal contents.
3. A "listening" test should be performed, along with motion testing in an inferior and superior direction, and then to the left and right.

The Pelvis

Osteopathic theory has long held that the pelvic floor moves inferiorly during inhalation. This has recently been verified by real-time dynamic MRI.[54] In asymptomatic patients, the pelvic floor was found to displace inferiorly an average of 0.48 cm in quiet breathing, 0.5 cm in forceful breathing, and 0.74 cm with coughing.

Pelvic viscera has been studied for respiratory motion using MRI and ultrasound and compared to the motions of the uterus, ovaries, rectum, and intestines.[55] These viscera have been found to move more than 1 cm relative to each other. This motion is reduced in cases of pelvic adhesions.

PALPATION AND ASSESSMENT OF THE PELVIS REGION: "LISTENING" TEST

Examination of the pelvis begins with a "listening" test (Fig. 42.20) in the midline of the lower abdomen, just superior to the pubic symphysis, in order to identify the side of tension, and to approximate the depth or layer of that tension.

PALPATION AND ASSESSMENT OF THE ISCHIORECTAL FOSSA (FIG. 42.21A,B):

1. The patient is prone.
2. The physician palpates the ischial tuberosities and uses the thumb pads to palpate the region just medial to the ischial tuberosities. The thumb pads will be posterior to the sacrum, and lateral to the rectum, contacting the levator ani musculature.
   a. The levator ani should descend with inhalation and ascend with exhalation.

A

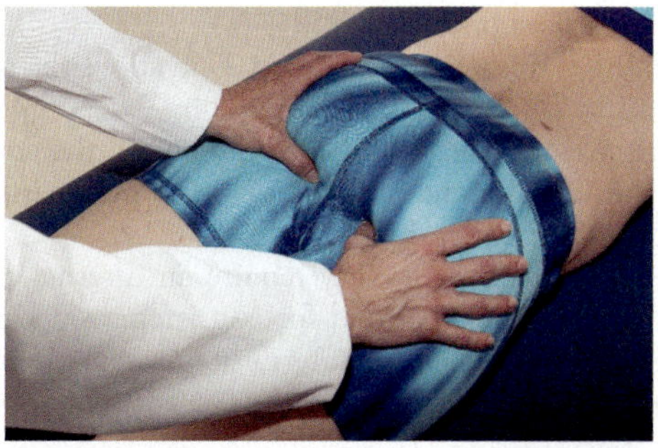

B

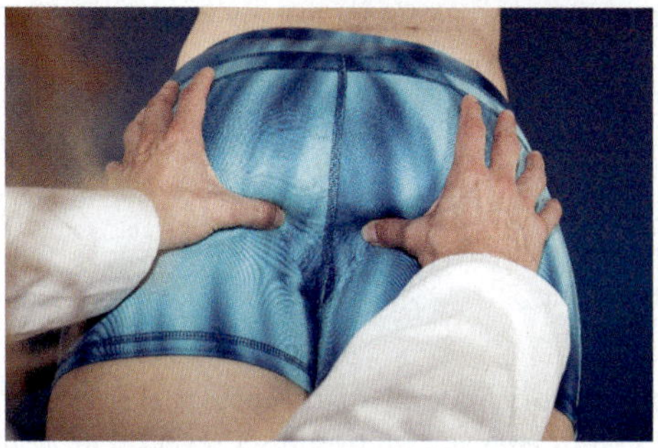

Figure 42.21. Assessment of pelvic diaphragm at ischiorectal fossa. A. Right superior oblique view. **B.** Posterior view. (Courtesy of Rebecca E. Giusti, DO, Western University of Health Sciences, College of Osteopathic Medicine of the Pacific, with permission.)

PALPATION AND ASSESSMENT OF THE BLADDER (FIG. 42.22)

1. The pubovesical ligaments of the bladder can be tested by palpating the top of the bladder on either side of the pubic symphysis, about 1 to 2 cm lateral to the symphysis.
2. The physician presses inferiorly and medially, palpating for distensibility, and then checking the other side.
3. In cases of stress incontinence, the bladder may also be checked internally. Pay attention to the urethra, sphincter area, general distensibility superiorly, and the wall of the detrusor muscle.

PALPATION AND ASSESSMENT OF THE CERVIX

1. The mobility of the cervix should be checked in cases of low back pain, infertility, and pelvic pain.

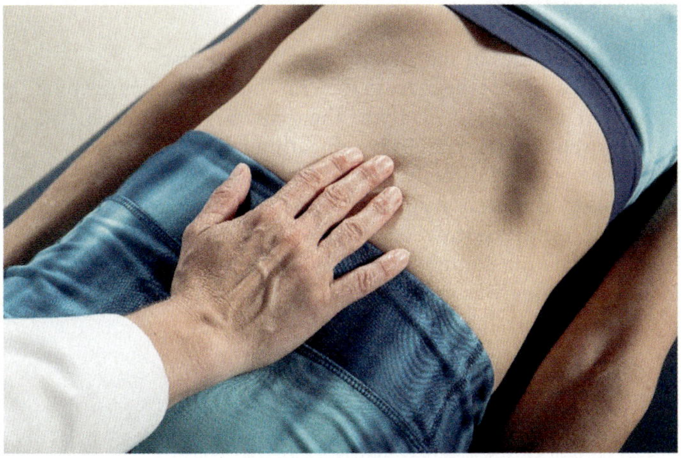

Figure 42.20. Listening test of the pelvis. (Courtesy of Rebecca E. Giusti, DO, Western University of Health Sciences, College of Osteopathic Medicine of the Pacific, with permission.)

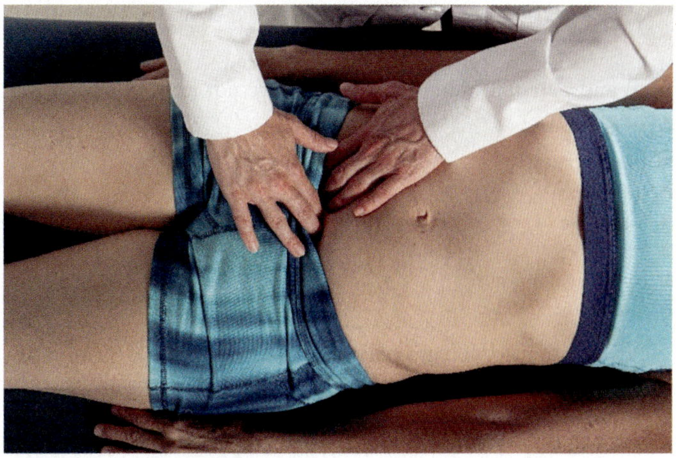

Figure 42.22. Testing the bladder. (Courtesy of Rebecca E. Giusti, DO, Western University of Health Sciences, College of Osteopathic Medicine of the Pacific, with permission.)

2. The patient is supine.
3. A listening test is performed about 2 cm above the pubis, on the middle line.
4. The physician uses layer palpation to obtain the correct depth.
5. After checking for the presence of tissue pull, perform motion testing to the right and left.
6. More complicated cases may require an internal examination, where the cervix is palpated for consistency, motion tested to the right and left, and also anteriorly to assess the distensibility of the uterosacral ligaments.

PALPATION AND ASSESSMENT OF THE PROSTATE

Check the prostate for:

- Size
- Presence of sulcus
- Nodules or areas of enlargement
- Consistency
- Motion testing
- Tissue pull

The respiratory motion of the prostate is small,[56] averaging about 0.05 cm. However, motion tests reveal that a slightly larger motion is possible in anterior/posterior, superior/inferior, and left/right directions. Palpation can be done externally, or internally, which is far more accurate.

Externally

1. The patient is supine or lateral recumbent.
2. The physician identifies the suprapubic region, either to the right or left of the middle line, and palpates deeply. While it is not possible to directly palpate the prostate in this fashion, the region's ability to distend and its available motion in the right and left planes can be assessed.

Internally

1. The physician palpates the size of the prostate, the presence or absence of a sulcus, and notes whether there are any hard nodules. If a nodule is present, the patient should be referred to urology for possible biopsy.
2. In the absence of nodules, the physician tests the prostate by bringing the left side to the right, the right side to the left, lifting the whole prostate superiorly, and by checking its distensibility.[57]

Rectum

Anal and perianal lesions include, but are not limited to, the following:

- Hemorrhoids
- Fissures
- Verrucae
- Herpes
- Syphilitic chancre
- Carcinoma

In addition to doing a perianal exam and internal rectal exam for these where indicated, motion testing of the rectal area can provide information about normal distensibility or loss of it. In a noncongested rectum, there should be a distensibility of about 1 cm. In a congested rectum, or in one with dysfunction of the pelvic floor musculature, the area of the rectum will not distend superiorly.

PALPATION AND ASSESSMENT OF THE RECTUM

1. The patient is supine.
2. The physician places the palpating hand just superior to the pubic symphysis. In males, palpation should occur about 1 cm above the symphysis; in females, about 4 cm above. The height in females will vary depending on the position of the uterus: anteflexed, normal position, or retroflexed.
3. Palpate posteriorly until the walls of the rectum are felt.
4. The physician palpates for a sense of tissue pull and then motion tests the region superiorly and inferiorly, to the left and to the right.

Related Palpatory Diagnostic Methods

Frank Chapman and Charles Owens first described Chapman reflex points. These are viscerosomatic reflex points on the anterior and posterior body that appear to correlate to different organs and regions of the body. See Chapter 58 for further information.

Strain/counterstrain tender points often correlate well with visceral problems in the corresponding area of sympathetic innervation. For example, in cases of gastroesophageal reflux, there is usually an anterior T5 or T6 tender point. See Chapter 47 for further information.

CASE STUDY

A 78-year-old woman presented to the office with a history of bronchitis for the last week. She continued to cough and feel sick in spite of medical therapy.

PHYSICAL EXAMINATION

Vital signs were normal. Pulmonary exam revealed diffuse rhonchi. Structural exam revealed restriction of ribs 1 and 2 on the left, and rib 12 bilaterally. The left occipitomastoid suture was restricted. Decreased compliance of the lungs, increased tension in the trachea and bronchus, and congested lymphatics of the lungs, airways, and thoracic cage were noted.

DIAGNOSIS

1. Acute bronchitis
2. Somatic dysfunction—thoracic, rib, cranial regions

TREATMENT PLAN

- The lymphatics of the airways were treated first.
- The ribs were then treated with balanced ligamentous tension technique. By then, the thoracic compliance had improved and the patient was breathing more easily.
- The lungs were directly treated last, as it was now possible to more accurately palpate their compliance. Compression and decompression were used, which resulted in markedly improved lung compliance, and again improved respiration.
- The coughing was reduced significantly within an hour.

REFERENCES

1. Giusti R, Ex. ed. *Glossary of Osteopathic Terminology*. 3rd ed. American Association of Colleges of Osteopathic Medicine; 2017.
2. Still AT. *Research and Practice of Osteopathy*. Andrew Taylor Still; 1911.

3. Hildreth A. *The Lengthening Shadow of Andrew Taylor Still.* Simpson Printing; 1942.
4. McConnell CP. *Selected Writings of Carl Philip McConnell.* Squirrel's Tail Press; 1994.
5. Barber E. *Osteopathy Complete.* Press of Hudson-Kimberly publishing Company; 1898.
6. Sutherland WG. *Teachings in the Science of Osteopathy.* Rudra Press; 1990.
7. Gaddis CJ. Bedside technique. *J Am Osteopath Assoc.* 1922;21:691.
8. Teal CC. Palpation of the colon with special reference to the cecum. *J Am Osteopath Assoc.* 1922;21:492.
9. Smith RK. Mechanical principles of the human body. *J Am Osteopath Assoc.* 1912;12:210.
10. Woodall PH. *Intra-Pelvic Technic.* Williams Publishing Co., 1926.
11. Hoover HV. A consideration of an osteopathic lesion of the whole liver and its effects on hepatic dysfunction. In: Northup TL, ed. *AAO Yearbook.* American Academy of Osteopathy; 1948:135–140.
12. Hoover HV. Liver and gall bladder technique. In: Northup TL, ed. *AAO Yearbook.* American Academy of Osteopathy; 1947:137–139.
13. Hoover HV. Technique for removing still lesion usually found in gall bladder disease. In: Page LE, ed. *AAO Yearbook.* American Academy of Osteopathy; 1950:80–83.
14. Young MD. Head's law and its relation to the treatment of the viscera. Osteopathic Profession. August, 1946. Reprinted in Northup TL, ed. *AAO Yearbook.* American Academy of Osteopathy; 1947:65–69.
15. Young MD. Illustration of visceral technique. In: Northup TL, ed. *AAO Yearbook.* Academy of Applied Osteopathy, now called American Academy of Osteopathy; 1948.
16. Hazzard C. The Practice and Applied Therapeutics of Osteopathy. 1905.
17. Riggs W. A Manual of Osteopathic Manipulations and Treatment. 1901.
18. Murray C. Practice of Osteopathy: Its Practical Application to the Various Diseases of the Human Body. 6th ed. 1925. Accessed September 7, 2018. http://www.mcmillinmedia.com/eamt/files/murray/murcont.htm
19. Goetz E. A Manual of Osteopathy. 2nd ed. 1909. Accessed September 7, 2018. http://www.mcmillinmedia.com/eamt/files/goetz/goecont.htm
20. Weischenck J. *Traire D'Osteopathis Viscerale.* Malione; 1982.
21. Barral J, Mercier P. *Viscera Manipulation.* Eastland Press; 1988.
22. Barral J. *Visceral Manipulation II.* Eastland Press; 1989.
23. Barral J. *Urogenital Manipulation.* Eastland Press; 1993.
24. Barral J. *The Thorax.* Eastland Press; 1991.
25. Barral J. *Manual Thermal Diagnosis.* Eastland Press; 1996.
26. Barral JP, Croibier A. *Trauma an Osteopathic Approach.* Eastland Press; 1999.
27. Bensky D. Asthma treated by visceral manipulation. *AAOJ.* 1995;5(1): 15–17.
28. Lossing KJ. *An Osteopathic Approach to Gastroesophageal Reflux Disease (residency thesis).* Ohio University; 1997.
29. Davidson SM. *Vitalize the viscera.* Seminar; 1992.
30. Blackman E. *Posterior Midline.* 2001.
31. Baldwin J. *Bucky Works: Buckminster Fuller's Ideas for Today.* John Wiley and Sons; 1996.
32. The Central Connection: Somatovisceral/Viscerosomatic Interaction. Paper presented at the American Association of Osteopathy 1989 International Symposium.
33. Moerland M, van den Bergh AC, Bhagwandien R, et al. The influence of respiration induced motion of the kidneys on the accuracy of radiotherapy treatment planning, a magnetic resonance imaging study. *Radiother Oncol.* 1994;30(2):150–154.
34. Davies S, Hill AL, Holmes RB, Halliwell M, Jackson PC. Ultrasound quantitation of respiratory organ motion in the upper abdomen. *Br J Radiol.* 1994;67(803):1096–1102.
35. Korin HW, Ehman RL, Riederer SJ, Felmlee JP, Grimm RC. Respiratory kinematics of the upper abdominal organs: a quantitative study. *Magn Reson Med.* 1992;23(1):172–178.
36. Gierada D, Curtin JJ, Erickson SJ, Prost RW, Strandt JA, Goodman LR. Diaphragmatic motion: fast gradient-recalled-echo MRI imaging in healthy subjects. *Radiology.* 1995;194:879–884.
37. Finet G, Williame C. *Treating Visceral Dysfunction.* Stillness Press; 2000.
38. Wade OL. Movements of the thoracic cage and diaphragm in respiration. *J Physiol.* 1954;124:193–212.
39. Barral JP, Crobier A. *Visceral Vascular Manipulations.* Elsevier; 2011.
40. Suramo J, Paivansalo M, Myllyla V. Craniocaudal movement of the liver, pancreas and kidneys in respiration. *Acta Radiol Diagn (Stockh).* 1984;25:129–131.
41. Clifford MA, Banovac F, Levy E, Cleary K. Assessment of hepatic motion secondary to respiration for computer assisted intervention. *Comput Aided Surg.* 2002;7:291–299.
42. Lienemann A, Sprenger D, Steitz HO, Korell M, Reiser M. Detection and mapping of intraabdominal adhesions by using functional cine MR imaging: preliminary results. *Radiology.* 2000;217(2):421–425.
43. Fredrickson JO. *J Radiol.* 1995;195:169–175.
44. Bieder J, Hintze C, Fabel M, Dinkel J. Magnetic resonance imaging and computed tomography of respiratory mechanics. *Magn Reson Imaging.* 2010;32:1388–1397.
45. Kauczor HU, Plathow C. Imaging tumor motion for radiotherapy planning using MRI. *Cancer Imaging.* 2006;6:S140–S144.
46. Wang Y, Riederer SJ, Ehman RL. Respiratory motion of the heart: kinematics and the implications for the spatial resolution in coronary imaging. *Magn Reson Med.* 1995;33(5):713–719.
47. Shechter G, Ozturk C, Resar JR, McVeigh ER. Respiratory motion of the heart from free breathing coronary angiograms. *IEEE Trans Med Imaging.* 2004;23(8):1046–1056.
48. Main X, Liu M, Li Q, Cai L, Zhang L, Hu Y. Analysis of abdominal organ motion using four-dimensional CT. *Chin J Cancer.* 2009;28(9):989–993.
49. Gierada D. Physical examination of the liver, is it still worth it? *Am J Gastroenterol.* 1995;90(9):1428–1432.
50. Bhasin D, Rana S, Chandail V. The pancreas and respiration: oblivious to the obvious. *JOP.* 2006;7(6):578–583.
51. Kivisaari L, Makela M, Aaimaa M. Pancreatic mobility: an important factor in pancreatic computed tomography. *J Comput Assist Tomogr.* 1982;6:854–856.
52. Heller R. Motion characteristics of kidneys with visceral somatic dysfunction. Sonographic pilot study before and after osteopathic manipulative treatment. *Man Med.* 2013;51:317–324.
53. McGee S. *Evidence-Based Physical Diagnosis.* 3rd ed. Elsevier; 2012.
54. Talasz H, Kremser C, Kofler M, Kalchschmid E, Lechleitner M, Rudisch A. Phase-locked parallel movement of diaphragm and pelvic floor during breathing and coughing-a dynamic MRI investigation in healthy females. *Int Urogynecol J.* 2011;22:61–68.
55. Katayama M, Masui T, Kobayashi S, et al. Using multiphase and multislice MR imaging with kinematic display. *AJR Am J Roentgenol.* 2001;177:107–110.
56. Lin Y, Liu T, Yang X, Wang Y, Khan MK. Respiratory-induced prostate motion using wavelet decomposition of the real-time electromagnetic tracking signal. *Int J Radiat Oncol Biol Phys.* 2013:87(2):370–374.
57. Barral JP. *Manual Therapy for the Prostate.* North Atlantic Books; 2010.

43 Clinical Assessment: Viscerosomatic, Somatosomatic, Somatovisceral Reflexes; Counterstrain Points, Myofascial Trigger Points, and Chapman Reflexes

SHARON GUSTOWSKI ▪ MICHAEL L. KUCHERA ▪ HUGH M. ETTLINGER ▪ MICHAEL A. SEFFINGER

KEY CONCEPTS

- The osteopathic structural examination includes palpatory assessment of the musculoskeletal tissues to identify areas of tissue texture abnormalities, restricted motion, asymmetries, and tenderness (TART).
- The TART exam identifies somatic dysfunction. Somatic dysfunction may be due to direct tissue injury or related to an underlying pathologic process.
- Information gathered from a structural exam is synthesized with information from the history, physical examination, and imaging and/or laboratory tests, to formulate a diagnosis and treatment plan.
- Tenderness is a subjective experience of the patient upon palpation and may indicate the cause of the patient's problem or a manifestation of an underlying visceral or somatic condition.
- Tissue texture abnormalities are objective findings upon palpation and may indicate the cause of a patient's problem or be a manifestation of an underlying visceral or somatic condition.
- Exam findings of tenderness and/or tissue texture changes can indicate the presence of a viscerosomatic, somatosomatic, or somatovisceral reflex. These reflexes can be utilized for generating a diagnosis and treatment plan.
- Chapman reflex points (CRPs) are tender, palpable nodular soft tissue masses found near the body surface and are an autonomic and lymphatic response to internal organ dysfunction or pathology and therefore a viscerosomatic reflex.
- Counterstrain (CS) points are a type of somatosomatic reflex, or manifestation of somatic dysfunction in a proximal or distant body structure, such as a joint.
- Trigger points (TrPs) are discrete areas of soft tissue tenderness that typically radiate pain in fairly predictable patterns upon palpation. They often indicate local muscle dysfunction but also can be classified as viscerosomatic or somatosomatic reflexes.
- Somatic dysfunction in any form can manifest as tissue texture abnormalities and tenderness. Multiple palpatory diagnostic models exist and can be used in clinical practice for enhancing diagnosis and designing a comprehensive treatment plan that includes OMT.

INTRODUCTION

An integral component of an osteopathic structural exam is a palpatory assessment for tenderness and tissue texture abnormalities which are two of four criteria required to diagnose somatic dysfunction. Distinguishing somatic dysfunction as primary or due to one of the following reflexes: viscerosomatic, somatovisceral, and somatosomatic, can be challenging. Palpatory assessment should begin after history gathering as a component of a physical exam and can be performed at any time and throughout the physical exam.

- Consent should always be obtained prior to performing a physical exam.
- Clear explanation should be given to the patient as to why, where, and what to expect during the examination.
- Patients should be made aware that some areas may be tender with palpation and to state when tenderness occurs.
- The physical exam should include examination of all relevant body systems as tenderness and tissue texture changes alone are not sufficient for making a diagnosis beyond somatic dysfunction. Often patients have comorbidities. Physical exam findings that are normal may ensure there isn't underlying pathology beyond somatic dysfunction.
- Palpatory exam findings can be used in the formulation of a differential diagnosis, to recommend additional exams or diagnostic testing and/or can be confirmatory in generating a diagnosis.
- Palpatory exam findings can also be used as an indicator of treatment effectiveness.
- Often, tenderness and tissue texture abnormalities are found within the same tissues. However, tissues with texture abnormalities are generally tender, but not always. Although less likely, tissues with tenderness may not exhibit tissue texture abnormalities.

This chapter builds on the basic science foundations presented in Chapter 3 (Anatomy), on the nervous system structure and function (Chapters 6, 9, 11, 13, 74), Chapter 12 (Inflammation), and relevant osteopathic manipulative technique chapters. Reviewing those chapters first before reading this chapter will facilitate comprehension and contextualize the applications in clinical practice.

TENDERNESS—EVALUATION AND CLASSIFICATION

Tenderness is defined as "discomfort or pain elicited by an osteopathic practitioner through palpation and a state of heightened sensitivity to touch or pressure"[1] reported by the patient upon palpation during a physical exam. Tenderness is the most reproducible of all manual diagnostic exams.[2] However, tenderness as an isolated finding does not always indicate the origin or cause of the pathologic process or indicate that somatic dysfunction alone caused the tenderness. This is because the sensation of pain is a multifactorial phenomenon that includes a subjective evaluation by the patient (see Chapter 11 Nociception and Pain and Chapter 74 Chronic Pain Management). Therefore, the finding of tenderness must be evaluated in the context of the entire patient encounter, including the patient's history, all physical exam findings, and diagnostic test results when available.

Contextualizing the exam finding of tenderness or absence of tenderness helps formulate a diagnosis, including indications for diagnostic imaging and/or laboratory tests. Therefore, it is important to understand some common types and causes of tenderness.

Tenderness can be due to any of the following:

- Major injuries, such as: fractures, dislocations, strains, sprains, muscle/tendon/ligament tears, bruises, cuts, burns, etc.
- Systemic pathologic processes such as: myositis, myofascial pain syndrome, inflammatory arthropathies (e.g., rheumatoid arthritis, ankylosing spondylitis), fibromyalgia, chronic regional pain syndrome.
- Musculoskeletal conditions such as: costochondritis, peripheral nerve entrapments (e.g., carpal tunnel syndrome [CTS], tarsal tunnel syndrome), enthesopathies (e.g., biceps tendonitis) bursitis (e.g., trochanteric, pes anserine) plantar fasciitis, compartment syndrome.
- Somatic dysfunction, which includes tenderness as a component. Tenderness associated with somatic dysfunction can be discrete or generalized.
  - Discrete areas of tenderness include counterstrain (CS) points and Chapman reflex points (CRPs).
  - Generalized tenderness can include somatic dysfunction in joints, musculature (individual muscles or groups of muscles), and/or fascia.
  - Myofascial trigger points (TrPs), are discrete areas of tenderness and usually related to somatic dysfunction. The TrP model was developed independently from somatic dysfunction theories but there is significant overlap with TrPs and somatic dysfunction.
- Visceral diseases, such as: cholecystitis, angina, pneumonia, gastroesophageal reflux disease, dysmenorrhea, etc.
  - Tenderness due to visceral diseases can be classified as a viscerosomatic reflex which is a neurologically mediated somatic dysfunction, or directly related to organ dysfunction (stretch or rupture), such as when an appendix ruptures and the abdominal wall becomes rigid and tender.
  - Viscerosomatic reflexes can be discrete, such as CS points, CRPs, or manifest as generalized tenderness in soft tissues that is associated with articular, muscular, or fascial somatic dysfunction.

TISSUE TEXTURE ABNORMALITIES—EVALUATION AND CLASSIFICATION

Tissue texture abnormalities are palpable changes in soft tissues, including skin, fascia, and musculature. They can be classified as acute, chronic, or acute overlying chronic.

Acute changes are often distinguishable from chronic changes. Acute changes elicit an acute inflammatory response which includes local vasodilation, release of inflammatory mediators, and numerous chemical and molecular signaling for healing. Patients report pain in the tissues and tenderness with palpation. The skin is warm, moist, mildly edematous (boggy), and the musculature is congested (see Chapter 29, Table 29.1).

Chronic changes involve more complex adaptive responses involving the neuroendocrine and immune systems and include diminished localized blood flow. The tissues are described by the patient as itchy, tingling/numb, and on exam the skin is dry and cool. The tissues exhibit contraction, fibrosis, and tenderness with palpation (see Chapter 29, Table 29.1).

Similar to tenderness, tissue texture abnormalities can be due to any of the following:

- Major injuries, such as: fractures, dislocations, strains, sprains, muscle/tendon/ligament tears, bruises, cuts, burns, etc.
- Systemic pathologic processes such as: spasticity poststroke, flaccidity postspinal cord lesion, multiple sclerosis, etc.
- Musculoskeletal conditions such as: postural abnormalities (e.g., Scoliosis, kyphosis) sprains, strains, etc.
- Somatic dysfunction. Tissue texture abnormalities associated with somatic dysfunction can be discrete or generalized and may or may not be tender.
- Visceral diseases, such as: cholecystitis, angina, pneumonia, gastroesophageal reflux disease, dysmenorrhea, etc.
  - Tissue texture abnormalities due to visceral diseases can be classified as a viscerosomatic reflex or a neurologically mediated somatic dysfunction or directly related to organ dysfunction (stretch or rupture), such as when an appendix ruptures and the abdominal wall becomes rigid and tender.
  - Tissue texture changes associated with viscerosomatic reflexes are often nondiscrete and span multiple vertebral and costal levels.

VISCEROSOMATIC REFLEXES—GENERALIZED AND CHAPMAN REFLEXES

A viscerosomatic reflex is a "localized visceral stimuli producing patterns of reflex response in segmentally related somatic structures."[1] A viscerosomatic reflex is manifested as TART changes in the somatic system reflexively generated from a visceral disorder or disease. The palpable changes due to a viscerosomatic reflex occurs in the segmentally related spinal levels of internal organs based on visceral efferent nerve fibers, which are more anatomically consistent than the variable and divergent visceral afferent fibers. See Table 6.1 in Chapter 6 for a list of spinal levels.

- The palpable changes can be generalized tissue texture changes and/or tenderness in the paraspinal or intercostal musculature and often also associated with articular somatic dysfunction.
- The changes can also be discrete tenderness and tissue texture abnormalities of a CRP.
- Often, both CRPs and generalized paraspinal tissue texture abnormalities are present. CRPs are "a group of palpable points occurring in predictable locations on (or near) the anterior and posterior surfaces of the body that are considered to be reflections of visceral dysfunction or disease."[1]
- CRPs are often nodular or gangliform in consistency, located just beneath the skin, are tender, and do not radiate pain upon palpation. Refer to Chapter 58 for more detail.

When the patient's history or other exam findings indicate the possibility of visceral disease, palpatory examination for somatic dysfunction in both the segmentally related spinal level(s) and CRP should be performed. Used in this context, the finding of a CRP and/or paraspinal tissue texture changes can add further evidence for a diagnosis of visceral disease.

Regardless of the manifestation of the viscerosomatic reflex as generalized or discrete, the neurologic mechanisms are similar. Visceral afferents are stimulated by inflammation or expansion of an organ, and the cause can be inflammatory or stretching of the capsule of an organ without inflammation.

- Examples of inflammation in an organ, its capsule, or surrounding fascia:
  - Appendicitis, colitis, pancreatitis, cholecystitis, gastritis, hepatitis, pericarditis, esophagitis, pneumonitis, pneumonia, nephritis, appendicitis, endocarditis, coronary artery disease, reactive airway disease
- Examples of stretching of an organ's capsule:
  - Hepatomegaly, splenomegaly, cardiomyopathy, tumors, or cysts

Visceral afferents can initiate long or short reflexes. With minor irritation or stretch of visceral receptors, initial afferent information might be conveyed just to an associated collateral ganglion (short reflex) and this is referred to as a visceral reflex. With more substantial afferent stimuli, a long reflex may be added to the short reflex. In the long reflex, the visceral afferent information reaches the central nervous system where the efferent response can be generated; when this response affects somatic tissues, it is referred to as a viscerosomatic reflex. Viscerosomatic reflex findings typically create TART changes including the following:

- CRPs, located on the anterior and/or posterior aspects of the body
- Sympathetically mediated tissue texture changes in muscles, often the paraspinals, sharing a common facilitated segment (Fig. 43.1)

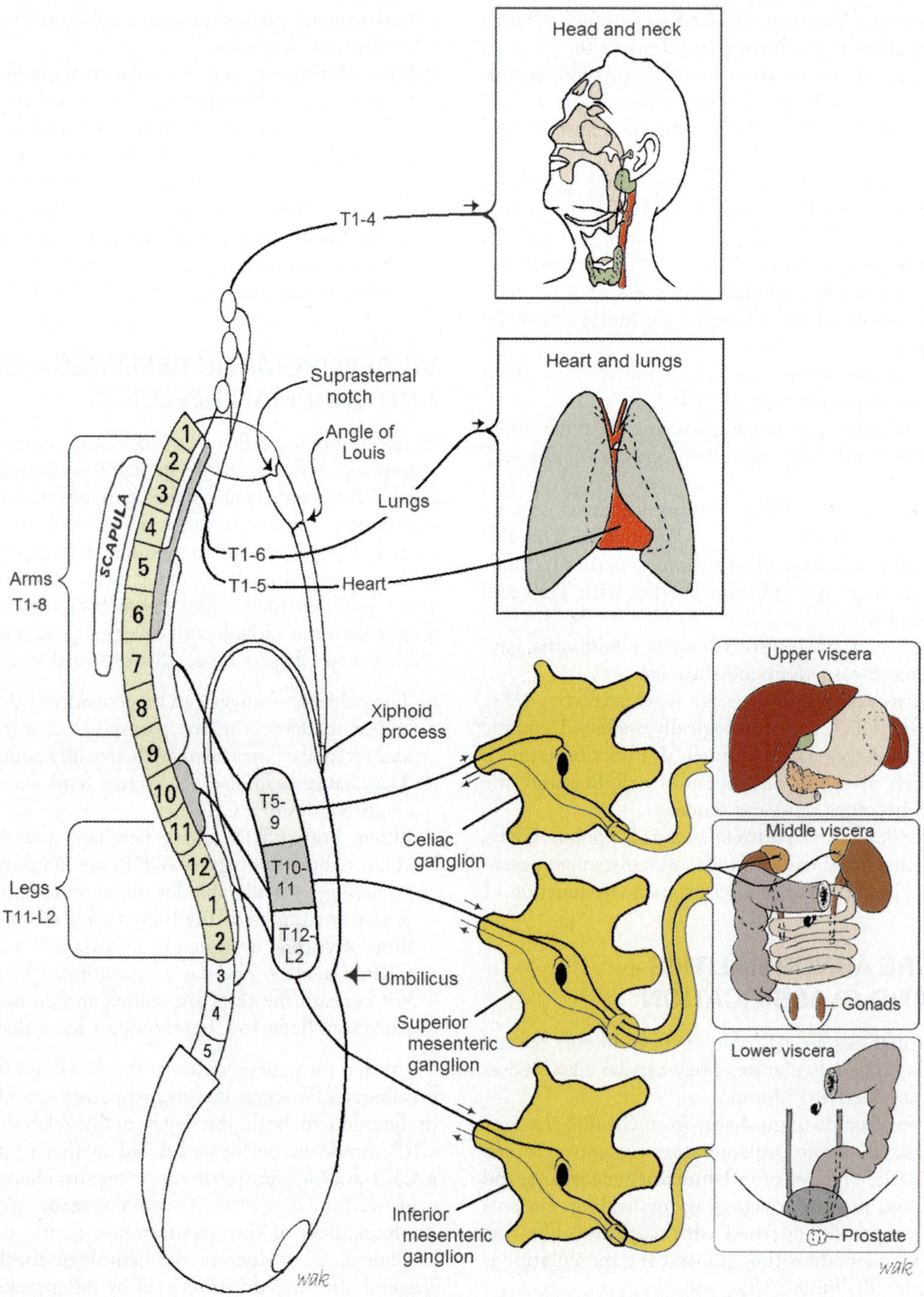

Figure 43.1. General scheme of sympathetic innervations to the organs. (Illustration courtesy of William A. Kuchera, DO, FAAO, with permission.)

In the long reflex, the visceral afferent nociceptive information that travels from the organ to the spinal dorsal root, dorsal horn, and interneurons typically elicits an excitatory signal from the spinal cord interneurons on which they synapse. The interneurons stimulate both autonomic motor and somatic, alpha motor neurons originating from the same segmental level. The autonomic nerves innervate not only the viscera but also the blood vessels and sweat glands of the body wall of the segmental level, producing palpable tissue texture changes in the paraspinal region of the segments involved. The somatic motor neurons activate the skeletal muscles, producing tonic muscular contraction and splinting of the muscles in the referral area. These changes in the paraspinal, intercostal, and other neurologically related musculature can be palpated. The palpable findings in the referred area either in the paraspinal tissues or anteriorly are a type of viscerosomatic reflex.

Reflex somatic dysfunction provides important clues to the presence of acute and/or chronic disease. The information gathered is combined with the rest of the physical examination to reach a working differential diagnosis. In order to most accurately interpret structural findings as they relate to the systemic diseases they reflect, reflex somatic dysfunction must be differentiated from postural, traumatic, and other purely somatic causes of somatic dysfunction.[3] There are unique qualities of viscerosomatic reflexes, which are related to the known pathophysiology of the reflex and the unique tissue changes they create. Reflexes may not be evident in a patient with a malignant tumor if the tumor is not causing irritation, pressure, stretch, or inflammation.

Stimulation of segmental autonomic efferent nerves produces changes in blood supply and sweat gland activity at the body surface, in addition to visceral motor changes. Korr et al. measured the cutaneous changes produced by segmental facilitation via alterations in skin resistance (sweat) and temperature (blood flow).[4] These changes are palpable as increased temperature and sweat (moisture and/or skin drag) in the paraspinal tissues and are excellent and reliable indicators of segmental facilitation at that level of the spinal cord. In a study of the palpatory findings in patients with acute myocardial infarction, Nicholas and colleagues found increased temperature as the second most common tissue finding.[5]

Short visceral reflexes initially produce vague, midline, gnawing deep pain (see Chapter 41, Fig. 41.4). As they progress to long viscerally initiated reflexes, they involve neuromuscular changes in the segmentally related tissues; this reflex effect on muscle tone is important, as it identifies their spinal segmental level, suggests the involvement of a facilitated segment (central sensitization) and distinguishes them at a paraspinal level (see Chapter 41, Figs. 41.5 and 41.6).

- In his work with Korr, Denslow describes "doughy, boggy" paraspinal myofascial tissues at the levels of spinal segmental facilitation.[6]
- Patriquin describes a "fusiform soft tissue change in the paraspinal muscles" occurring over several segments which "tails out on the ends."[7] He continues to say, "The multifidus and rotatores are the best place in the spinal region to palpate for changes of viscerosomatic origin."[7]
- Beal, in his studies of cardiac and pulmonary patients, found a supine compression test to be the most accurate indicator of reflex dysfunction.[8,9] Beal's description of the response to the compression test is at the level of joint motion but is considered secondary to deep muscle splinting.
- Nicholas et al., most often found "firmness" in the upper thoracic paraspinal muscles in patients with acute myocardial infarction.[5] Osseous/articular motion changes also occur, but these findings are most likely secondary to the altered muscle tone produced by the acute viscerosomatic reflex processes.
- William Johnston, DO, describes a "linkage" of thoracic vertebral and rib motion that he considers indicative of a viscerosomatic reflex.[10] This linkage of articular motion finding is considered to be secondary to an altered neuromuscular response to a motion challenge.
- The movement restriction, found at a joint involved in this reflex process, is soft, with a springy feel, which, when palpated, suggests the viscerosomatic reflex.
- Regions of reflex somatic dysfunction also show unusual resistance to manipulative treatment, especially high velocity/low amplitude, when directed toward primary joint somatic dysfunction.
- Somatic dysfunction that rapidly recurs after successful manipulative treatment also suggests viscerosomatic origin or accentuation.
- When visceral inflammation involves the parietal peritoneum, the patient's discomfort becomes localized over the viscera involved and brings in palpable somatic dysfunction related to their innervation; this is referred to as the peritoneo-cutaneous reflex[11] (see Chapter 41, Fig. 41.7). Palpable tissue texture change and acute pain is found directly over the organ and segmentally at the innervation level of the peritoneum or pleura.

Acute segmental facilitation creates a variety of palpable tissue changes that may be used to identify the presence of an underlying disease process.

- The skills required to consistently identify reflexes develop with time and experience. For the practitioner learning to recognize the unique tissue changes of viscerosomatic reflexes, it is helpful to evaluate reflex patterns in patients with clearly identified, acute disease processes. In this way the physician develops the skills required to recognize reflexes and to identify their unique qualities.
- Some generalizations by experienced physicians include the following:
  - The most superficial clues, temperature and skin drag or moisture, are among the most useful and are easy to identify in the seated position.
  - Viscerosomatic reflexes in the spine exhibit motion restriction *without* a firm, stiff end point.

Studies examining the relationship between palpatory findings and visceral disease include the following:

- Snider et al. describe significant positive associations between various gastrointestinal diseases and specific spinal level TART changes, CRPs, and tenderness.[12]
- Licciardone et al. found that patients with type 2 diabetes mellitus had tissue texture abnormalities in the right side of the T11–L2 spinal levels.[13]
- Washington et al. identified that hospitalized patients with pneumonia had CRPs.[14]

If a reflex persists as part of a chronic condition, the tissues, including the joints, become stiff and the qualities palpated become different. Beal states,

"The chronic phase of reflex activity is ... characterized by trophic changes in the skin, increased thickening of the skin and subcutaneous tissues and localized muscle contraction. The muscles are hard and tense and may be hypersensitive to palpation."[15]

The chronic muscle spasm ultimately stiffens the joints, giving the articular motion restriction a more firm, definite end feel that is much closer to a typical postural or somatic problem. When someone with a chronic problem has an acute exacerbation, a

TABLE 43.1

Segmental Facilitation

Type	Characteristics
Acute	Increased temperature (a local chemical physiologic reaction), increased moisture and/or skin drag. Prolonged red reflex Boggy, fusiform muscular changes Articular motion restrictions *without* a firm, stiff end point
Chronic	Thickened skin and subcutaneous tissues. Rapid fading red reflex Localized muscle contraction (increased muscular tone) Muscles are hard, tense, and hypersensitive to palpation Stiff joints with articular motion restrictions that are firm with more definite end feel
Acute on chronic	Warm, moist, and boggy superimposed on deeper hard, stiff tissues

warm, moist, boggy tissue reaction will be superimposed on the deeper hard, stiff tissues, leading to a separate tissue diagnosis that may be called "an acute on a chronic problem." This finding may clarify the history of a current problem where the patient may be unaware of previous episodes of the problem (Table 43.1).

SOMATOSOMATIC REFLEXES—COUNTERSTRAIN POINTS

- A CS point is defined as, "a discrete area of tissue texture abnormality which often exhibits tenderness and responds to a positional release technique."[1]
- Typically, CS points are assessed in the region in which somatic dysfunction is diagnosed with palpation at defined, specific, point locations. See Chapter 47 for detailed discussion, point locations, and treatment procedures.
- CS points are a type of somatosomatic reflex in that they are often associated with joint or muscular dysfunctions in the region in which they are found. However, as yet, no randomized clinical trials have assessed whether alleviation of either the related joint somatic dysfunction or the CS point will alleviate the other.
- In clinical practice, it is prudent to assess and treat both joint dysfunctions and any associated tender points as components of central and peripheral sensitization, or facilitation.
- CS points associated with visceral dysfunction are being investigated by clinicians, but no clinical trials have as yet been published.

MYOFASCIAL TRIGGER POINTS—VISCEROSOMATIC, SOMATOSOMATIC AND PRIMARY MUSCULOSKELETAL

Travell and Simons[16,17] developed the most widely recognized myofascial point system used in diagnosis and treatment. Diagrammatic summaries of TrP maps affecting different regions are shown in Figure 43.2. When a patient complains of pain in a particular region, consider examining these or related points.

- A myofascial TrP is a specific form of impaired or altered myofascial function with distinctive clinical and pathophysiologic characteristics; these characteristics are extremely well documented in the literature.[18] A TrP is defined as "a hyperirritable spot in skeletal muscle that is associated with a hypersensitive palpable nodule in a taut band. The spot is painful on compression and can give rise to characteristic referred pain, referred tenderness, motor dysfunction, and autonomic phenomena."[16] In short, a TrP is a specific form of somatic dysfunction.

TrPs can be viewed as a particular subset of somatic dysfunction. They represent impaired or altered function of the myofascial system and its related neural, lymphatic, and circulatory elements. Several TrPs have been linked to viscerosomatic and somatovisceral reflexes; others are known to entrap circulatory and/or neural structures. Many have autonomic sequelae, and most involve pain and/or musculoskeletal dysfunction. All require careful and skilled palpation for diagnosis and an understanding of the underlying anatomy and physiology for successful treatment.

As a form of somatic dysfunction, TrPs respond to an osteopathic approach that integrates manual techniques, behavioral modification, and nutritional factors that reestablishes the homeostatic relationship between the musculoskeletal system and the central nervous system.

TrP Classification and Evaluation

Diagnosis of myofascial TrPs is based on distinctive palpatory findings (local spot, palpable band, and twitch response); muscle testing (strength and range of motion); distribution of the pain pattern; and the patient's history. TrPs are locally very tender. They are palpated as small nodular or spindle-shaped thickenings within a taut band of tissue.

The activation of a TrP is usually associated with some degree of mechanical abuse of the muscle. This may be associated with:

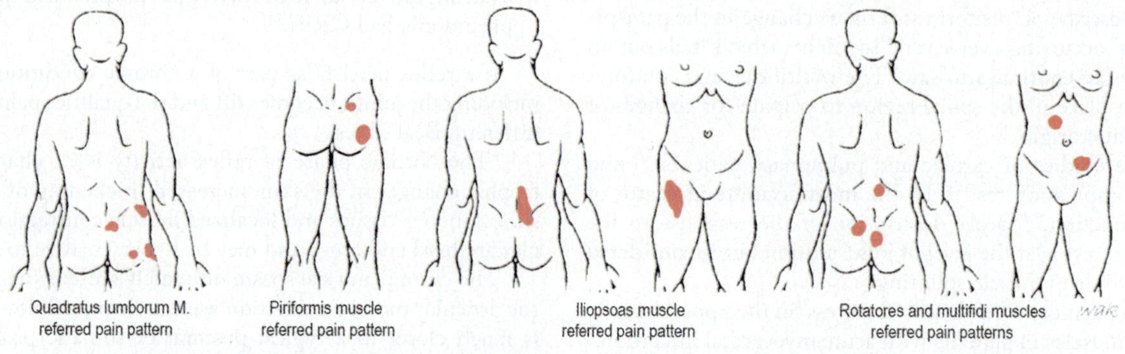

Figure 43.2. Myofascial trigger points. (Illustration courtesy of William A. Kuchera, DO, FAAO, with permission.)

- Muscle overload (acute, sustained, and/or repetitive)
- Myofascial postural stress
- Leaving a muscle in a prolonged shortened position (especially if the muscle is then contracted while in the shortened position)
- Muscle chilling
    - TrPs are classically classified as "active" or "latent" depending on whether or not pain is referred with palpation in the characteristic distribution empirically mapped for each point.
        - Active points refer pain at rest, with muscular activity, or with palpation.
        - Latent points often restrict motion or cause stiffness without causing referred pain; potentially becoming active only with a precipitating cause. Unless a skilled palpatory examination is conducted, latent points are often overlooked, and the true cause of dysfunction may be misdiagnosed.
    - All muscles in which a TrP is suspected should be examined. Muscles to examine are identified using the patient's history of the onset of the complaint.
    - TrPs are palpated by applying pressure with the fingertip across the long axis of the muscle and the patient responds with a generalized "jump sign" along with a "local twitch" of the taut band of musculature. The two findings are not synonymous.
        - The jump sign is a patient response to pain characterized by wincing or a voluntary withdrawal response.
        - The local twitch response is a transient contraction of the taut band of fibers where the TrP is located. The local twitch response is clinically significant because it is usually absent in the fibromyalgia syndrome but present in myofascial pain syndromes due to TrPs.[16]
    - Precise localization of the TrP is required for accurate diagnosis and treatment. Depending on the muscle examined, use either flat palpation or palpation with a pincer-type grip (Fig. 43.3).
        - In large, flat muscles like the quadratus lumborum, fingertips can be drawn across the muscle perpendicular to its fibers.
        - Some muscles, like the trapezius or those in the axillary folds, are better palpated with a pincer grip.
        - The most appropriate palpation for a TrP is that which permits pressure to be applied perpendicular to the long axis of the muscle suspected of harboring the point. Palpatory findings in the area of a TrP include an alteration of cutaneous temperature and humidity. There is a small nodular or spindle-shaped thickening of the tissues, representing the myofascial point itself. There may be localized goose flesh or trophic changes at the site. A summary of these palpatory findings is proposed in Table 43.2.
    - The joints that the muscles with TrPs attach to may exhibit restricted ranges of motion in the direction of stretch, and the muscles are painful with either active or passive stretching. Patchy weakness during muscle testing may result from a conscious or unconscious desire to avoid pain. If present, attention to the precise pain patterns is extremely important in the diagnosis, because the empirically mapped patterns for each given muscle are fairly consistent among patients (see Fig. 43.2).[16,17]

Current recommended diagnostic criteria are summarized in Table 43.2.

Laboratory, imaging, and neuroelectrodiagnostic tests are not diagnostic for primary myofascial TrPs or for most other forms of somatic dysfunction. They may prove useful, however, in identifying factors that perpetuate TrPs or in ruling out a variety of clinical conditions from which secondary myofascial TrPs may arise. For example, in the presence of nerve compression sufficient to alter axoplasmic flow and create peripheral electromyographic changes, an increased number of active TrPs will be found in the affected muscles.[19]

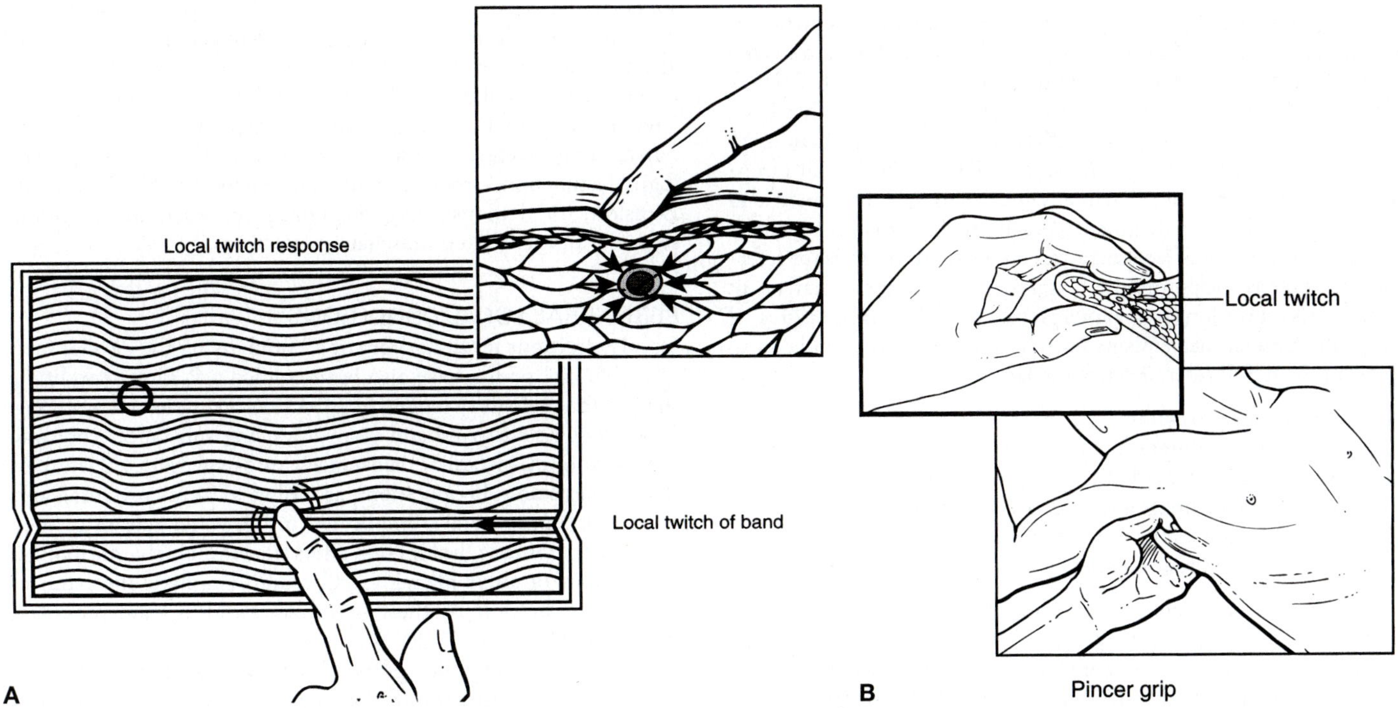

Figure 43.3. Palpation for myofascial trigger points. A. Draw fingertips across large, flat muscles, (**B**) use pincer grip for muscles like trapezius or those in axillary folds. (Reprinted with permission from Travell JG, Simons DG. *Myofascial Pain and Dysfunction: The Trigger Point Manual. The Upper Extremities.* Vol 1. Williams & Wilkins; 1983:60, 61, 398.)

TABLE 43.2

Criteria and Comparative Reliability for Trigger Point Diagnosis

A. Recommended criteria for identifying a latent trigger point or an active trigger point

Essential criteria

1. Taut band palpable (if muscle accessible)
2. Exquisite spot tenderness of a nodule in a taut band
3. Patient's recognition of current pain complaint by pressure on the tender nodule (identifies an active trigger point)
4. Painful limit to full stretch range of motion

Confirmatory observations

1. Visual or tactile identification of local twitch response
2. Imaging of a local twitch response induced by needle penetration of tender nodule
3. Pain or altered sensation (in the distribution expected from a trigger point in that muscle) on compression of tender nodule
4. Electromyographic demonstration of spontaneous electrical activity characteristic of active loci in the tender nodule of a taut band

B. Comparative reliability of diagnostic examinations for trigger points, estimate of the relative difficulty performing the examinations, and estimated relative diagnostic value of each examination by itself, regardless of other findings

Presence of	No. of studies	Mean kappa	Difficulty	Diagnostic value alone
Spot tenderness	3	0.70	+	+[a]
Pain recognition	3	0.59	++	+++
Palpable band	3	0.54	+++	++[a]
Referred pain	4	0.47	+++	+
Twitch response	3	0.23	++++	++++

[a]The combined presence of these two will likely have a high diagnostic value for sufficiently skilled examiners.

Reprinted with permission from Simons DG, Travell JG, Simons LS. *Travell and Simons' Myofascial Pain and Dysfunction: The Trigger Point Manual. Upper Half of Body.* Vol 1. 2nd ed. Williams & Wilkins; 1999. Tables 2.4A and 2.4B.

Referred Pain Mechanisms and Causation

Regardless of the exact mechanism or mechanisms proposed, afferent information to the central nervous system from peripheral somatic and visceral structures figures prominently in the proposed origin of all myofascial points. In the Travell system, overuse of somatic structures, especially chilled muscle and joint dysfunction, is often implicated.[16,18] Although primary visceral dysfunction related to facilitated segments is more frequently associated with CRPs,[20] Travell and Simons also noted the association of segmentally related visceral dysfunction in TrP initiation and/or perpetuation.[16,18] Proponents of CRPs,[20] CS points,[3] and Travell TrPs[16,18] all recognize the importance of segmentally related somatic dysfunction in the interpretation and treatment of each myofascial point system.

Unless physicians recognize and understand the basis for referral phenomena, inappropriate diagnosis and treatment may result from mislocalization or misinterpretations of the true origins of the pain. Several mechanisms have been historically postulated to play a role in TrP referral phenomena[20]:

1. Convergence projection
2. Convergence facilitation
3. Activity of the sympathetic nervous system
4. Convergence or image projection at the supraspinal level
5. Peripheral axon branching from certain dorsal root ganglion cells to two different muscles

Most of the central mechanisms applied to understanding TrPs suggest that pain referral may result from nociceptive information being misdirected in the spinal cord to reach somatotopically inappropriate dorsal horn neurons. The first and fifth mechanisms relate to the structure of the nervous system, although the others relate to functional factors. (Further discussion of referred pain may be found in Chapter 11 Nociception and Pain.)

CENTRAL NERVOUS SYSTEM

The central integration of afferent data with generalized, predictable modification of efferent responses is a neurologic model used to explain causation and maintenance of somatic dysfunction (including TrPs), referred pain, and several reflexes between the soma, the viscera, and the sympathetic systems.[18,21] This view is consistent with Korr's observations[22] that the spine can be viewed as an "organizer" of disease and dysfunctional processes and may harbor a segmentally related "neurologic lens" for a wide variety of stressors (Fig. 43.4). In fact, Mense and Simons credit Korr as "an outstanding osteopathic pioneer in the establishment of physiologic dysfunction associated with articular dysfunction" and, with Denslow, for demonstrating the linkage between the facilitated segment and its related muscular connections.[18]

PERIPHERAL LOCAL CONDITIONS

Local conditions resulting from or accompanying the development of myofascial points have also been studied.[18,23] These conditions suggest that palpatory tenderness and TrPs are increased by endogenous tissue-sensitizing and pain-producing substances (bradykinins, serotonin, histamine, substance P, prostaglandin E2, etc.).[18,23] Branching axon subpopulations, as well as local microtrauma and/or macrotrauma, are also implicated in the wider release of these substances. Somatic dysfunction alters the local biochemical milieu and impairs or alters neural, vascular, and lymphatic mechanisms, preventing removal of these sensitizing and/or pain-producing substances.[24,25]

Physiologically, one proposal known as the "Integrated Concept of TrP Formation"[18] has suggested that a local metabolic (energy) crisis arises in the presence of impaired circulation, a factor that leads to tissue texture abnormalities that aid in finding the myofascial point by palpation.

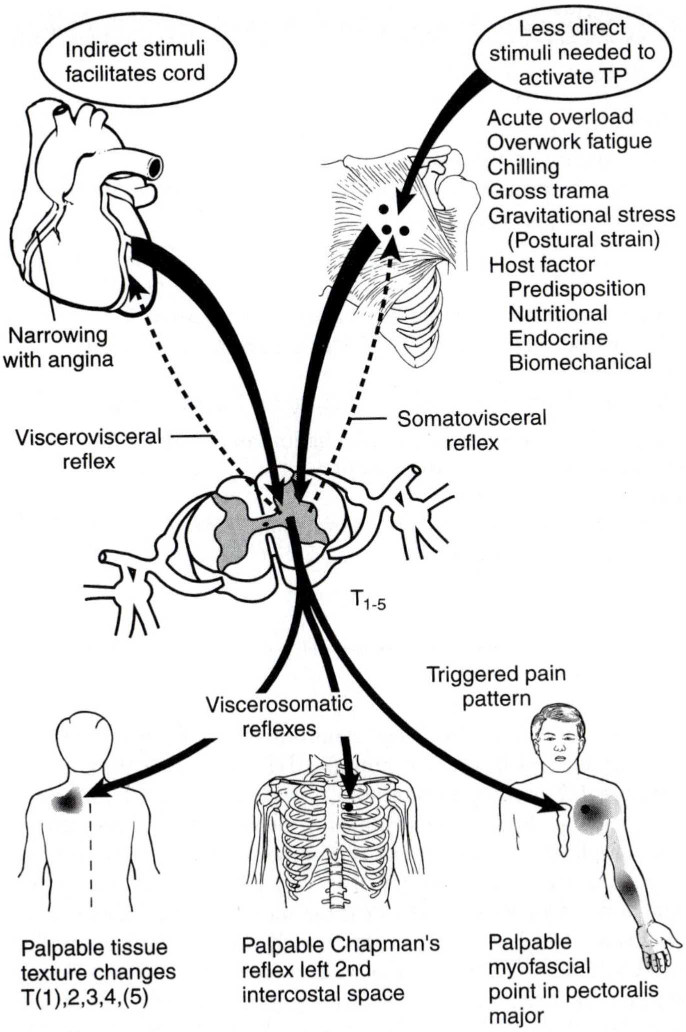

Figure 43.4. The spinal cord as an organizer of disease processes. (Illustration courtesy of William A. Kuchera, DO, FAAO, with permission.)

Trigger Points Affecting Regional Somatic Functions

TrPs typically result in weakness and/or dysfunction of the muscle harboring them.[16,18] Overuse in the myotatic unit because of this primary myofascial point may cause secondary associated myofascial points, resulting in further weakness and reduced function. If the point is latent,[16] it may be clinically silent unless it is palpated directly or the muscle harboring it is functionally stressed. If the point is active,[16] it weakens and prevents full lengthening of the muscle. It may produce referred pain and/or autonomic phenomena in a predictable trigger or reference zone. These zones are characteristic for each muscle and have been empirically mapped and documented (Fig. 43.2).[17,18,23] Altered somatic function that has been noted includes the following[17,18]:

- Disturbed proprioceptor and motor coordination
- Temporomandibular joint dysfunction
- Depressed deep tendon reflexes
- Muscular stiffness and weakness
- Diminished ranges of motion

The patient often complains of these symptoms, as well as dysesthesia, paresthesia, and pain. The pain is described as steady, deep, and achy in nature. Symptoms are often aggravated by[16,18]:

- Overuse or prolonged repetitive use of the muscle
- Chilling
- Psychogenic stress
- Viral infection
- Prolonged shortening of the muscle
- Pressure over the TrP
- Chronic pain may lead to secondary depression, sleep disturbance, and chronic pain behavior

Diminished range of motion (ROM) caused by myofascial TrPs should be differentiated from structural limitations of the joints, such as occur in osteoarthritis, and functional arthrodial limitations, such as occur in other forms of somatic dysfunction. In particular, Travell myofascial points should be distinguished from fibromyalgia syndrome and other rheumatologic disorders.[16,26,27] Appropriate recognition and treatment of TrPs have provided dramatic restoration of function in numerous patients previously misdiagnosed with these other conditions.

As a component element of somatic dysfunction, myofascial TrPs must sometimes be specifically addressed to allow complete resolution of the joint dysfunction.[16,28] Conversely, because articular dysfunction may lead to the creation of muscle dysfunction,[18] it may be necessary to correct the articular component such as in treatment of a sacral shear prior to treating a piriformis TrP. Clinically, this is often the case in recurrent exhalation somatic dysfunction of rib 12 related to quadratus lumborum TrPs. The presence of TrPs must be considered when the usual treatment for shoulder dysfunction fails to respond fully to manipulative techniques, such as the seven stages of Spencer (see Chapter 57). Table 43.3 delineates the TrPs associated with Spencer technique.

Many clinical diagnoses have associated myofascial TrPs in which the dysfunctional trigger zone overlaps with the structural symptoms profile. Although a cause-and-effect relationship has not been demonstrated, treatment of those myofascial elements contributes significantly to patient management and symptom reduction. This point is very well illustrated by two common clinical diagnoses: lateral epicondylitis and carpal tunnel syndrome (CTS).

- In lateral epicondylitis, or tennis elbow syndrome, TrPs in the supinator, wrist, and finger extensor muscles, anconeus, and triceps are all capable of referring symptoms to the lateral epicondyle.[16,21] Conversely, all become significantly stressed with the altered biomechanics adopted in a true inflammatory process of the lateral epicondyle.

TABLE 43.3

Limitations of Shoulder Range of Motion (ROM)

Motion Restriction[a]	Myofascial Point Found
Flexion	Triceps
Abduction	Subscapularis Infraspinatus Supraspinatus Teres major (levator scapulae)
Internal rotation	Teres minor Infraspinatus
External rotation	Subscapularis Pectoralis minor

[a]Stage of Spencer with restricted motion. Note: The majority of muscles are rotator cuff muscles.

TABLE 43.4

Common Clinical Conditions Linked to Somatic Dysfunction or TrPs

Region	CONDITION/DISORDER: Dysfunctional Muscle(s)
HEENT	TMJ: masseter, medial pterygoid, lateral pterygoid, digastric, temporalis HEADACHE BEHIND EYE with ANS SYMPTOMS: sternocleidomastoid (sternal head or counterstrain point AC8) EUSTACHIAN TUBE DYSFUNCTION/OTITIS MEDIA: medial pterygoid SINUSITIS: lateral pterygoid (especially)
Upper extremity	FROZEN SHOULDER: especially subscapularis LATERAL EPICONDYLITIS (TENNIS ELBOW): supinator, wrist/finger extensors, anconeus, triceps MEDIAL EPICONDYLITIS (GOLFER'S ELBOW) AND CARPAL TUNNEL SYNDROME: pronator teres, wrist/finger flexors, thenar muscles THORACIC INLET/ENTRAPMENTS: scalenes, pectoralis minor, combination of shoulder internal rotators
Torso	UPPER CROSSED SYNDROME: hypertonic upper trapezius, levator scap, sternocleidomastoid, pectoralis major with inhibited/weak deep cervical flexors, lower trapezius and serratus anterior CHEST PAIN IN ANGINA PATTERN: pectoralis major LOWER CROSSED SYNDROME: hypertonic iliopsoas, quadratus lumborum, piriformis, hamstrings, gastroc/soleus with inhibited/weak abdominals, glutei, vasti, tibialis ant/peroneus
Pelvis	RECURRENT SACROILIAC DYSFUNCTION: glutei (force closure) PELVIC FLOOR PAIN AND DYSFUNCTION: levator ani

- In CTS, TrPs are found in the pronator teres, and wrist, finger, and thumb flexors.[16] Here also, triggered referral zones from the myofascial points overlap with the wrist pain, finger and thumb paresthesias, grip weakness, and referred forearm pain perception common to patients with CTS. Forearm muscles also become significantly stressed with the altered extremity mechanics adopted by patients with CTS.
- Failure to address TrPs results in failure to help a significant number of these patients. For example, in CTS, osteopathic treatment protocols that specifically address treatment of these myofascial structures in addition to traditional conservative care have been more effective than wrist splints and medication alone.[29]
- Table 43.4 summarizes some examples of frequently encountered clinical conditions linked to common sites for somatic dysfunction or TrPs. These conditions often benefit from osteopathic consideration, palpation and, if dysfunction is found, treatment of the muscle involved.[16–18,30,31]

Trigger Points and Posture

TrPs may result from and/or contribute to postural disorders.[18,32–34] Patterns of recurrent TrPs in various combinations should alert the clinician to an underlying postural disorder. Likewise, all patients with postural disorders should be evaluated for patterns of TrPs to address in the postural treatment regimen.

Patients with postural decompensation have a higher propensity to develop patterns of recurrent somatic dysfunction, TrPs, facilitated segments, and related visceral dysfunction[35] (also see Chapter 92 Postural Considerations in Osteopathic Diagnosis and Treatment). Whether the muscles become hypertonic or weak is fairly predictable from a postural perspective with the tonic, postural muscles, which usually cross two or more joints having palpable tightness and reactivity while postural antagonists may demonstrate weakened during strength testing.[18] For these reasons, numerous clinicians cite postural disorders as one of the primary precipitating and/or perpetuating factors of myofascial TrPs, even stating that "postural training should be one of the first parts, if not the first part of the treatment program."[17]

The so-called "short leg syndrome" (see Chapter 92) has been implicated in causing multiple TrPs, including those in the paraspinal,[16] sternocleidomastoid,[16] and quadratus lumborum[17] muscles. Quadratus lumborum and iliopsoas TrPs have already been implicated as an extremely common primary cause of myogenic low back pain and are often aggravated by sacroiliac dysfunction.[18] Conversely, TrPs in these muscles are capable of producing a false short leg syndrome as well as perpetuating sacroiliac dysfunctions.[17,18] This situation is likely to result in compensatory postural charges, recurrent somatic dysfunction, and TrPs in local and distant areas. Failure to consider the influence of muscular imbalance and TrPs may lead to lift therapy being incorrectly or inappropriately instituted.

Autonomic Effects of Travell Myofascial Points

Clinically, autonomic effects of myofascial dysfunction are common.[16,26] Travell's term "referred autonomic phenomena"[16] refers to the vasoconstriction (blanching), coldness, sweating, pilomotor response, ptosis, and/or hypersecretion that are caused by activity of a TrP in a region separate from the TrP. The phenomena usually appear in the same area as the pain referral for that TrP.[16]

Travell and Simons,[16] and Korr[22] have postulated an organizing role for the spinal cord by relating somatic and visceral inputs to palpatory and symptomatic findings in both systems (Fig. 43.4). Afferent input to the spinal cord may facilitate the segment at the spinal level it enters. Efferent consequences include sympathetic changes to somatic and visceral tissues at the same spinal level, and palpable somatic dysfunction, including tissue texture changes. A series of reflexes and referred symptoms result.

Trigger zones for each muscle have been mapped by Travell and Simons.[16,17] Viscerosomatic reflexes have been documented by Chapman (see Chapter 58). The autonomic effects produced in both somatic and visceral systems should be recognized in the patient and elicited in the history. Furthermore, the associated tissue texture changes should be actively sought throughout the physical examination to enhance the differential diagnosis process.

Clinical symptoms attributed to the autonomic sequelae of myofascial dysfunction include the following[16–18]:

- Diarrhea and dysmenorrhea due to autonomic control changes in the activity of smooth muscle
- Diminished gastric motility and aggravation of duodenal ulcer activity
- Vasoconstriction with headache
- Dermatographism
- Proprioceptive disturbances and dizziness
- Excessive secretion from the maxillary sinus
- Localized sweating
- Cardiac arrhythmias
- Gooseflesh
- Ptosis, excessive lacrimation, conjunctival reddening

Trigger Points Associated with Viscerosomatic and Somatovisceral Reflexes

When considering the interaction between somatic and visceral systems, recognizing somatovisceral and viscerosomatic reflexes is important for arriving at a differential diagnosis. TrPs in the pectoralis major muscle provide an example of each phenomenon. They illustrate the clinical concern that should be raised by the discovery of this important somatic clue. Pectoralis TrPs may result in cardiac rhythm dysfunction, a demonstrable somatovisceral reflex. Supraventricular tachyarrhythmias have been documented to arise from TrPs located in the right pectoralis major muscle (at the level of the fifth intercostal space), midway between the sternal margin and the nipple line (Fig. 43.5).[16] (Pectoralis TrPs are also common in patients with slumped posture and rounded shoulders.) Treatment of the somatovisceral reflex involves both removing the TrP and correcting the underlying postural problem if present. Correction of this somatic dysfunction results in immediate return of normal cardiac function.[16]

Pectoralis major TrPs occur as a viscerosomatic reflex in the majority of patients with cardiac disease.[16] They arise as a consequence of coronary artery insufficiency and, unless treated, often persist replicating the pain even after the original cardiac insult

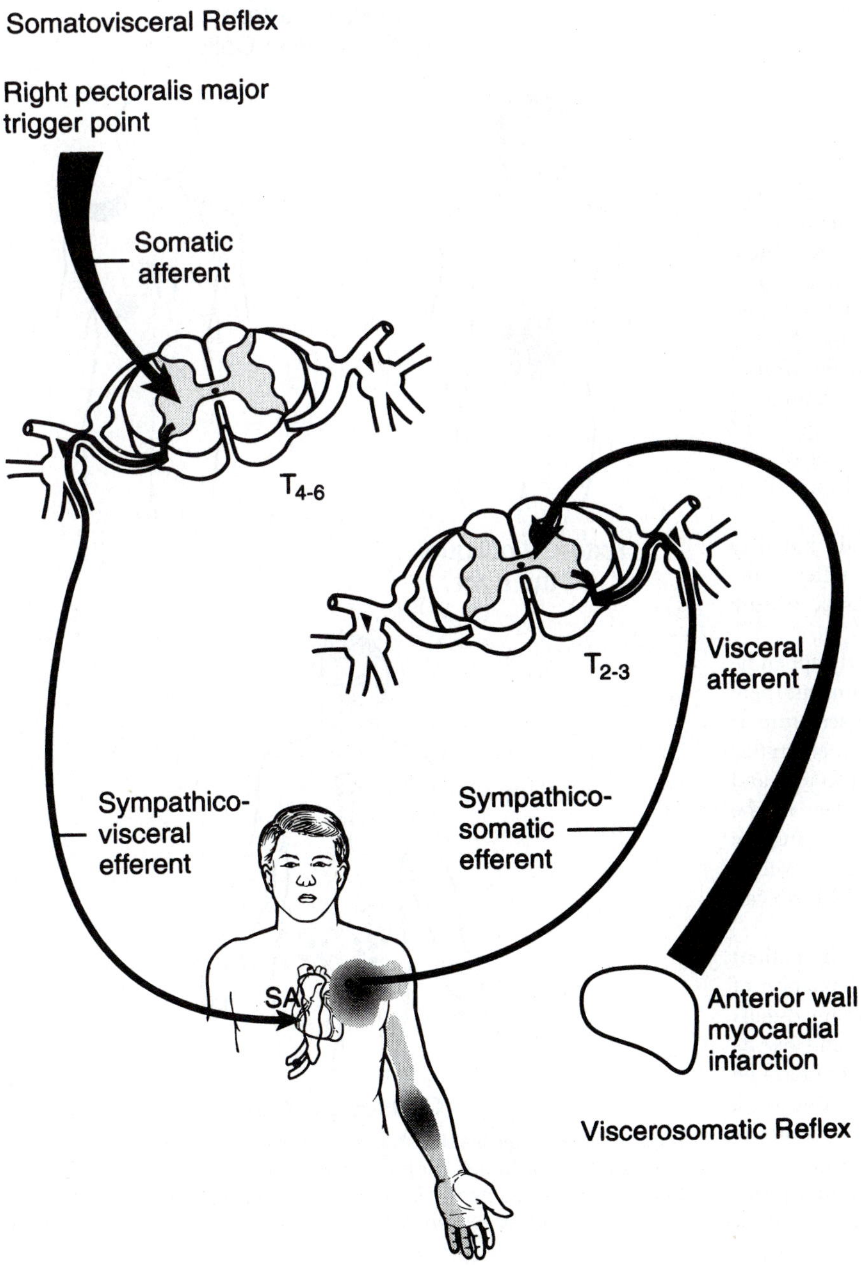

Figure 43.5. Pectoralis trigger points and associated reflexes. *SA*, sinoatrial node of the heart. (Illustration courtesy of William A. Kuchera, DO, FAAO, with permission.)

resolves.[18] This example of a viscerosomatic reflex has a significant prevalence as demonstrated by one study of 72 patients. Chest muscle TrPs were reported in 61% of patients with cardiac disease.[16] Treatment of these TrPs is an important factor in reducing reflex coronary artery spasm,[16] but reduction of chest pain in this particular situation may inadvertently present an associated clinical dilemma. Symptomatic relief provided by treatment of somatic findings does not eliminate the need clinically to assess and treat a specific underlying primary visceral cause.

In the case of somatic findings resulting from viscerosomatic reflexes, healing of the primary visceral component does not mean that the secondary somatic dysfunction will spontaneously resolve. Pectoralis major TrPs originating in this manner have been shown to be self-perpetuating and a source of referred chest/arm pain even after recovery from or successful treatment for the initial visceral event.[16] Precipitated by cold or overuse of the pectoralis muscles, these somatically referred symptoms may unfortunately promote unnecessary emotional distress and disability in a cardiac patient until identified and removed. Similar myofascial points occur in patients with a variety of visceral disorders, including duodenal ulcer[16] (Fig. 43.6) and postcholecystectomy syndrome.[20]

Differentiating Viscerosomatic Reflexes from Referred Pain

Not only are spinal pathways for somatic and visceral afferent input often shared, but the ascending pathways to the brain are also shared; there are also significant neural interconnections between the cranial nerves. Such interconnectivity and central overlap help explain why visceral nociceptive information is perceived as a generalized somatic pain. In addition, there is less visceral input than somatic as the viscera are less densely innervated, meaning that the individual is more likely to interpret the input in a somatic context. Another important aspect of the viscerosomatic interrelationship is that some of these visceral sensory receptors in the spinal cord extend for several spinal segments and give off a number of collaterals. This is the cause of the nonspecific nature and sometimes wide somatic distribution of referred visceral pain.

Referred pain is a sensation perceived by the brain but may not have palpable somatic findings. A viscerosomatic reflex manifest palpable finding, including tenderness and/or tissue texture changes.

For example, in the case of a patient with acute early appendicitis, the patient may experience vague periumbilical pain, but there will not be palpable changes in the abdominal wall musculature or related ganglion and/or spinal level because a viscerosomatic reflex has not yet developed. With increased severity of the infection and inflammation, palpable findings may eventually manifest in the periumbilical area as tension over the involved collateral ganglion site and also in the paraspinal muscles of the lower thoracic vertebral levels. In addition, a CRP on the tip of the right 12th rib can manifest as a viscerosomatic reflex.

For another example, a patient with cholecystitis, the patient may feel referred pain in the right shoulder due to stimulation of the thoracoabdominal diaphragm muscle from the inflamed gallbladder. This activates afferents via the phrenic nerve and results in a sensation in the C3–C5 dermatome in the right shoulder. The shoulder tissues will be without palpable findings. In contrast, a viscerosomatic reflex would manifest in the paraspinal muscles between around the T6 and T9 vertebral levels on the right.

In both patient examples above, the inflamed organ may progress in severity to the point where it irritates or otherwise elicits

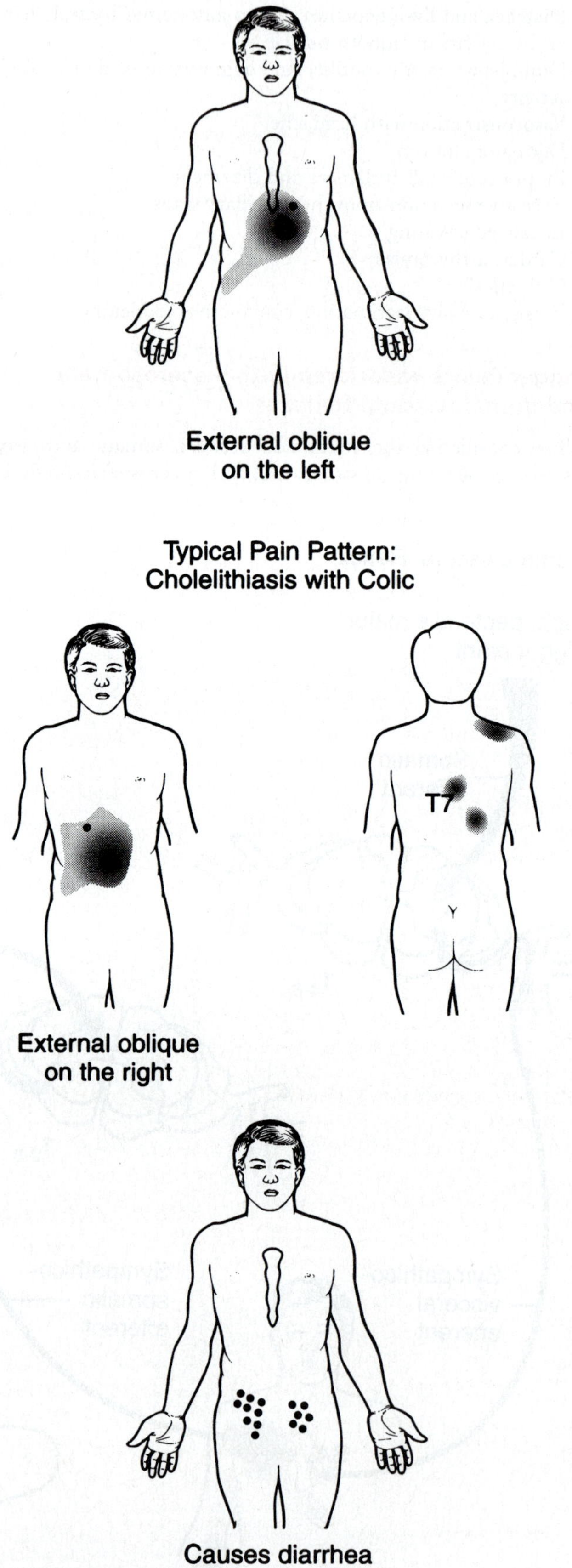

Figure 43.6. Myofascial trigger points associated with viscerosomatic reflexes. (Reprinted with permission from Travell JG, Simons DG. *Myofascial Pain and Dysfunction: The Trigger Point Manual. The Upper Extremities.* Vol 1. Williams & Wilkins; 1983:662.)

local guarding of the surrounding musculature. While the pathway is not truly a viscerosomatic reflex, this pattern change, too, provides a palpable somatic clue that may help the clinician understand the underlying visceral disturbance.

- In appendicitis, the right lower quadrant muscles (i.e., external oblique muscle) contract when anterior to posterior pressure is applied to the peritoneum overlying the appendix, forcing it to contact adjacent structures. This is called "guarding." It may also directly irritate the right psoas muscle lying posterior to it.
- In cholecystitis, when the clinician presses superiorly under the right costal margin forcing the inflamed gallbladder to be pressed by the force of the diaphragm descending upon it during inhalation, the diaphragm reflexively ceases from further contraction and inhalation is arrested. This is known as Murphy sign.

Differentiating Viscerosomatic from Somatosomatic Reflexes

A somatosomatic reflex is defined as, "localized somatic stimuli producing patterns of reflex response in segmentally related somatic structures."[1] Since viscerosomatic reflexes are identified in part by their similarity to somatic muscular strains, the question may be asked: how does one tell the difference between the two? Over time, the practitioner must learn to differentiate changes caused by visceral dysfunction and those that are related to mechanical somatic dysfunction. In addition, the patient's history should be considered.

Since an inflamed or diseased organ theoretically stimulates afferent nerve fibers continuously, there is a constant barrage of input into the spinal cord at the associated spinal segment, as well as to the brain. Somatosomatic reflexes on the other hand are most commonly postural or movement related. Since visceral afferent input is constant, and divergent, it is most likely that more than one spinal cord segment will be involved, thus generating a larger receptive field for this afferent input. The spinal cord efferent output will therefore entail a wider range of paraspinal muscles, usually at least two segments, but possibly three to five segments. So, the first assessment is to determine if the somatic findings of a thoracic vertebral segment are focused at only one segment, or are the findings really several segments in a row? A viscerosomatic reflex typically affects more than one spinal cord segment[10,15] and is often rotated and sidebent to the side of the organ.[3,20]

Also, as previously mentioned concerning TART objective findings, often a predominance of sympathetically mediated tissue texture changes characterizes a viscerosomatic reflex, while the quality and pattern of motion restriction is more prevalent in somatosomatic reflexes. Another characteristic of viscerosomatic reflexes is the extension of paraspinal soft tissue findings laterally into the rib intercostal soft tissues at the same level of the primary or central dysfunctional segment. There are compensatory changes above and below, and reciprocal changes on opposite sides of the spine in both somatovisceral and viscerosomatic reflexes. However, the similarity of findings of paraspinal soft tissues alongside a dysfunctional central vertebra and its ipsilateral associated intercostal soft tissues distinguishes the viscerosomatic reflex; this phenomenon is called "linkage."[1,10]

Finally, an important differentiating factor lies in the pattern of somatic clues that are uncovered.[3,20] The finding of a singular somatic dysfunction regardless of its TART characteristics, local spinal distribution, or even relationship to visceral symptomatology is not adequate to properly differentiate a viscerosomatic from a somatosomatic reflex or even from a localized somatic process. Such a differential requires seeking a potentially related pattern of palpatory clues including possibly related collateral ganglia, thoracolumbar or craniosacral dysfunction, CRPs, and responses of the tissues adjacent to the dysfunction.

SOMATOVISCERAL REFLEXES

A somatovisceral reflex, aka somatoautonomic reflex, is defined as, "localized somatic stimuli producing patterns of reflex response in segmentally related visceral structures."[1] Identifying somatic dysfunctions is the primary goal of the osteopathic structural examination; interpreting this diagnosis in relation to the history, physical findings, ancillary tests, and other diagnoses is the distinctive advantage of applying osteopathic principles and practices. It is possible that any somatic dysfunction can be a source of somatic stimuli that produces a reflex response to segmentally related visceral structures. More globally, as discussed elsewhere, somatic sources of stimuli can generate total body reflex responses via the autonomic, peripheral, and central nervous systems, and the endocrine and immune systems as well.

Somatovisceral reflexes can be identified during the osteopathic structural examination if exaggeration, accentuation, or provocation of the TART findings alters autonomic/visceral functions. For example, if a dysfunctional second rib is positioned for performance of a direct osteopathic technique and this stimulus causes the patient's heart to beat faster, or irregularly, but is reversed when the rib dysfunction is corrected and normal motion and function is restored, then that would be considered a somatovisceral reflex phenomenon. Somatovisceral reflexes should be considered in the differential diagnosis of patients with visceral symptoms in the absence of organ pathology or disease.[20] In treatment regimens, somatovisceral reflexes are commonly used, as is discussed in Chapter 78 Osteopathic Considerations and Approaches in the Acutely Ill or Hospitalized Patient.

VISCEROVISCERAL REFLEXES

A viscerovisceral reflex could be defined as, "localized visceral stimuli producing patterns of reflex response in segmentally related visceral structures"; however, most of the literature on this topic is from animal studies, and the preferred term is autonomic reflex (see Chapter 6 Autonomic Nervous System and Chapter 11 Nociception and Pain). Chapter 42 Internal Organ Assessment for Visceral Motion Dysfunction also provides more detail on this topic. Viscerovisceral reflexes are assessed during the osteopathic structural examination most commonly in terms of peripheral blood flow abnormalities and/or sweat gland activity, which alters skin turgor and surface friction; together, both alter palpatory sense of skin temperature variations (see Chapters 29 and 31 for further information on the palpatory examination). Alterations of vital signs (e.g., heart rate, respiratory rate, blood pressure, and temperature) are linked via autonomic reflexes.

Discerning between somatovisceral and viscerovisceral reflexes can be challenging. However, if a thorough osteopathic structural examination does not find somatic dysfunction or somatic sources of nociceptive stimuli, then a visceral cause of abnormal autonomic/visceral reflex activity is more likely. It is also possible to have both somatovisceral and viscerovisceral reflex phenomenon occurring simultaneously. This makes it imperative to perform a thorough history and physical examination, combined with appropriate ancillary laboratory and radiologic tests, in order to accurately interpret palpatory findings.

BOX 43.1 Types of Tenderness

- A trauma patient with altered consciousness in which pain provocative maneuvers are performed to assess brain and spinal cord integrity and functionality.
- A middle-aged male who has severe chest pain may have musculoskeletal chest wall pain. Reproducible chest wall pain upon examining with digital palpation in subjects with known or suspected stable angina pectoris has been shown to substantially differentiate cardiac from musculoskeletal origin and be predictive of normal myocardial scintigraphy,[2] meaning that if the pain is reproducible upon digital pressure of the pectoralis muscles alone, then it is not likely to be related to angina.
- Symmetric peripheral small joint tenderness coupled with swelling often indicates arthritis.
- Symmetric non–joint-related soft tissue tenderness both above and below the level of the diaphragm, including the extremities, coupled with irritable bowel disorder, depression, and sleep irregularities, is associated with fibromyalgia syndrome and is thought to be due to central or peripheral sensitization phenomenon and failure of the descending antinociceptive system (see Chapter 11 Nociception and Pain for further details).
- Palpable abnormal findings in the musculoskeletal system that are compensatory or responsive to distal somatic dysfunctions signify somatosomatic reflexes.

Often, the experienced physician will recognize characteristics or patterns that discern one type of tenderness from another. Examples shown in Clinical Correlations Box 43.1.

There is a tremendous amount and variety of information available to the osteopathic physician provided through the evaluation for the presence of segmental reflexes. Although practice will obviously improve the accuracy of the examination, each of the authors' decades of experience doing structural examinations in the acute care setting has demonstrated that the great majority of cases present with significant, obvious reflex patterns, which are easily recognized.

1. *The presence or absence of an acute process* (perhaps the most fundamental difference). Although this information alone should not determine workup and treatment, it can be a factor in how aggressively a patient should be worked up, especially with a somewhat vague complaint. The presence of an acute reflex indicates an underlying acute process. For example, in a patient with right lower quadrant abdominal pain, appendicitis, a ruptured ovarian cyst, or Crohn disease will all produce an acute reflex pattern. Simple cramping or mild gastroenteritis may not.
2. *Identification of visceral disease in the presence of an acute paraspinal reflex finding.* There are some diseases that may be differentiated by localization of reflexes and some that may not. For example, the heart is innervated by levels T1–T5, whereas the stomach is innervated by levels T5–T9. Although there is anatomic variation within these levels, it is usually clear if substernal pain has its origin in the heart or the stomach. On the other hand, the gallbladder and the duodenum are both innervated via the right side of the celiac ganglion, and cholecystitis and nonperforated duodenal ulcer could produce a similar, if not identical reflex pattern. Although many sources identify unique sympathetic innervation levels for each visceral organ, clinically there are four important groupings which are easy to remember and practical for use (see Chapter 6, Table 6.1 and Fig. 43.7).

   Parasympathetic nerve innervations of the organs can be divided into three general regions (Fig. 43.8). Palpable viscerosomatic findings related to vagal afferents are found in the upper cervical area, especially around the C1 and C2 paraspinal musculature.[15]

   Grouping the viscera by general level makes reflex phenomena easy to remember and, therefore, more clinically useful. When utilizing reflexes clinically, however, the following limitations must be considered. It is not easy to clinically differentiate between different viscera within a given segmental level alone if their innervation comes from the same side. For example, it is difficult to distinguish appendicitis from a right-sided ovarian cyst; however, appendicitis can be differentiated from cholecystitis or a left-sided ovarian cyst. Nevertheless, it is a good idea to have some way of recalling the basic autonomic innervation to the viscera of the body.
3. *Assessing degree of disease by degree of reflex facilitation.* This is an intriguing thought, but one fraught with potential pitfalls. Different individuals have different reactivity within their nociceptive nervous systems and will therefore present with varying degrees of reflex facilitation with the same degree of inflammatory process and/or disease. One particular example from clinical practice would be the patient with diabetic neuropathy, which affects small caliber peripheral nerves. These patients often have blunted reflexes that are more difficult to identify and interpret. Once a baseline level or pattern of dysfunction is established, and compared to other clinical indicators of disease severity, it may be possible to follow the progress of the disease by changes in the intensity of the reflex, although this has not been studied. However, it is not uncommon to find whether a reflex has changed or disappeared, indicating a change in the patient's clinical status before other indicators have changed.
4. *Differentiating acute versus chronic processes.* This can be important in several ways. First, it may allow the identification of a long-standing process in the face of an acute presentation (i.e., the "acute on chronic" tissue changes). Surprisingly, patients do not always recall past episodes of a problem. The examiner can also identify if a known chronic problem is, in fact, the cause of a present complaint. A chronic reflex pattern, without an acute overlay in that region, makes it unlikely that the chronic organ or system is the source of the acute disease process. This might be useful in the evaluation of chest pain in a patient with a history of ischemia or myocardial infarction, who will in most cases demonstrate chronic findings with or without an acute process superimposed (see Table 43.1).
5. *Assessing the impact and involvement of the lymphatic system.* Optimal venous and lymphatic drainage depends on unobstructed myofascial pathways through which these circulatory vessels pass, and on respiratory–circulatory mechanisms efficiently creating pressure differentials. Zink[36,37] stated the relevance of this perspective to the osteopathic clinician. Travell and Simons have also documented the effect of certain myofascial points in creating lymphatic dysfunction and have reported improvement of congestive sequelae by removing this type of somatic dysfunction.

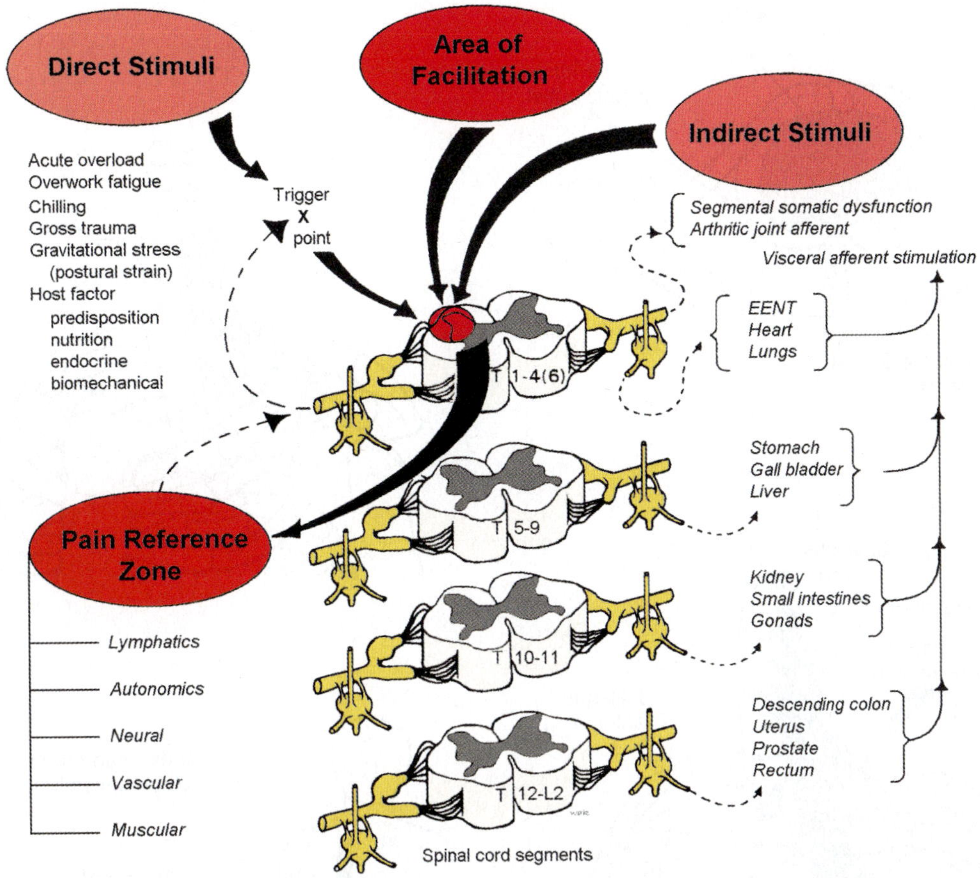

Figure 43.7. Trigger point causing further stimulation of facilitated spinal cord segment along with other pain and visceral afferents. The spinal cord can be viewed as a neurologic lens for a variety of stressors that initiate somatic and/or visceral symptoms. (Illustration courtesy of William A. Kuchera, DO, FAAO, with permission.)

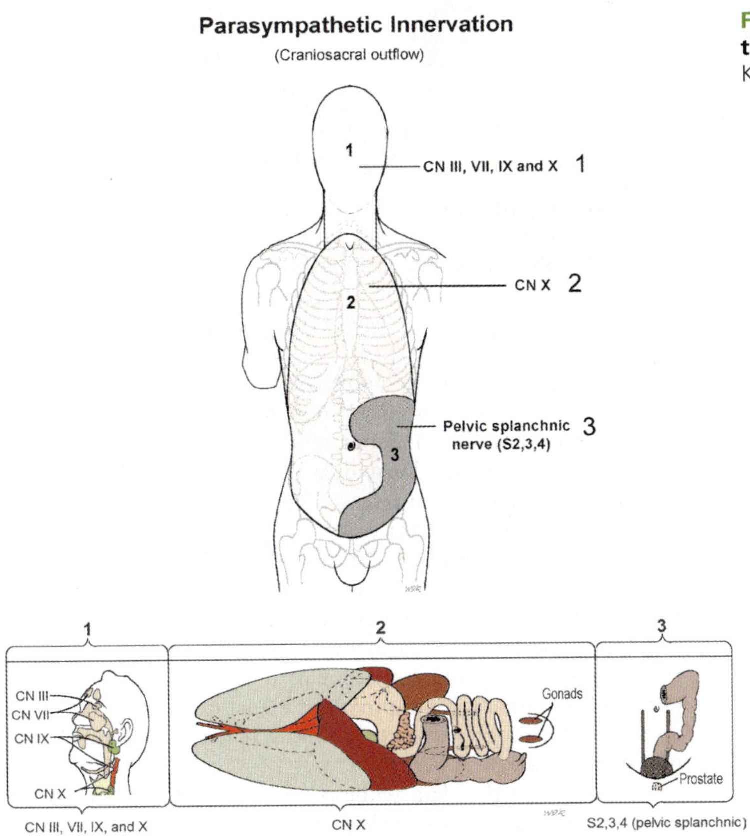

Figure 43.8. Parasympathetic innervation divided into three general areas. (Illustration courtesy of William A. Kuchera, DO, FAAO, with permission.)

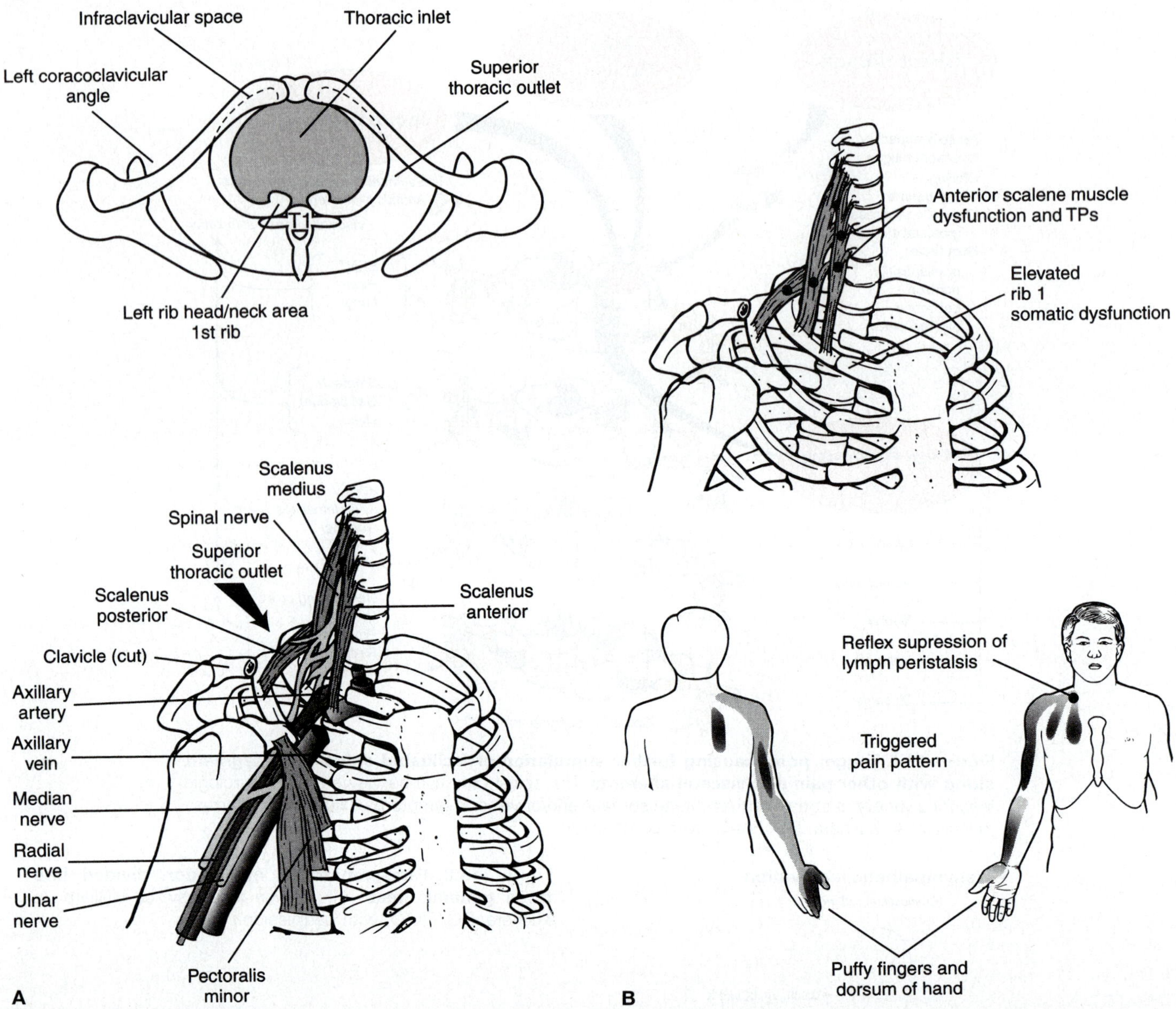

Figure 43.9. **A.** Entrapment of vascular and lymphatic structures in the thoracic inlet, (**B**) anterior scalene muscle referred pain and lymphatic/venous congestion in affected extremity. (Reprinted with permission from Travell JG, Simons DG. *Myofascial Pain and Dysfunction: The Trigger Point Manual. The Upper Extremities.* Vol 1. Williams & Wilkins; 1983:345, 356; **A**, top illustration by William A. Kuchera, DO, FAAO, with permission.)

The subclavian lymphatic trunk and the subclavian vein are particularly susceptible to muscular compression caused by TrPs in the anterior scalene muscles (Fig. 43.9A). This compression is further aggravated by elevation of the first rib, which may result from a variety of dysfunctional phenomena, including TrPs in the anterior or middle scalene muscles. Scalene TrP activity has been implicated in reflex suppression of lymphatic duct peristaltic contractions in the affected extremity (Fig. 43.9B).[16]

Palpation of the posterior and anterior axillary folds for evidence of myofascial dysfunction is clinically important in assessing the degree of lymphatic dysfunction affecting the upper extremities and/or breasts. The posterior axillary fold is the location of palpable myofascial points in the subscapularis, teres major, and latissimus dorsi muscles. It is also the site of terminal lymphatic drainage dysfunction for the upper extremities (Fig. 43.10A). Zink[38] discusses diagnosis and treatment of this region to relieve lymphatic congestion in the upper extremity. Those findings closely parallel the palpatory and clinical findings described independently by Travell and Simons, using myofascial points located in the posterior axillary fold.[16] Figure 43.10B shows that points higher in the posterior axillary fold correlate predominantly with shoulder referral, although lower points refer distally. Zink and Travell both report that treatment of myofascial dysfunction in this area results in reduction of swelling, joint dysfunction, and dysesthesia (Fig. 43.11). Likewise, appropriate treatment of anterior axillary fold dysfunction results in reduction of breast tenderness and congestive changes attributed to entrapment of breast lymphatics traveling around and through the pectoralis muscle toward the subclavicular lymph nodes.[16]

To interpret the data gathered from palpation, osteopathic practitioners need a clear understanding of the neurologic levels

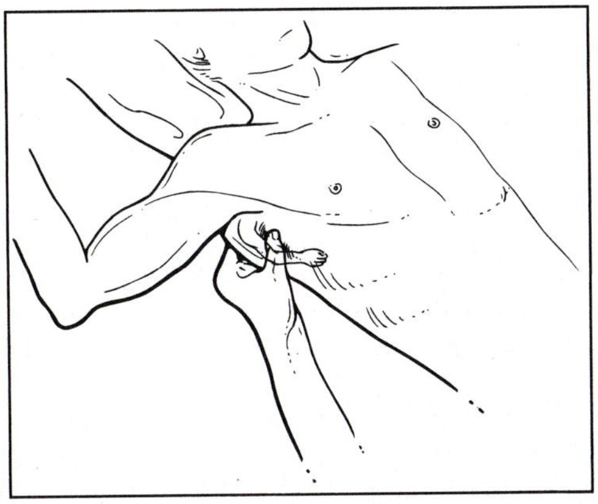

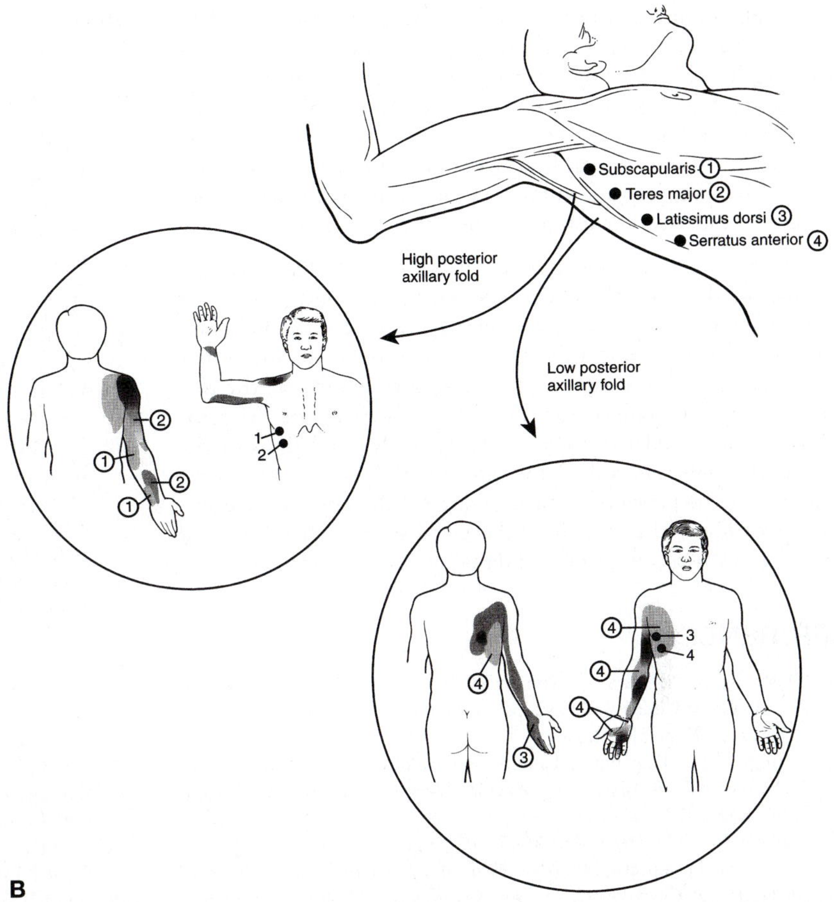

Figure 43.10. A. Zink's posterior axillary fold technique, (**B**) location and overlapping patterns of Travell and Simons' trigger points located in the posterior axillary fold. (*1*), subscapularis; (*2*), teres major; (*3*), latissimus dorsi; (*4*), serratus anterior. Overlapping patterns between (*1*) and (*2*) and between (*3*) and (*4*) are shown in black. (Reprinted with permission from Travell JG, Simons DG. *Myofascial Pain and Dysfunction: The Trigger Point Manual. The Upper Extremities.* Vol 1. Williams & Wilkins; 1983:398.)

involved and/or the organ systems involved in the disease process. Interpreting the severity of a given visceral condition may benefit from understanding pattern progression resulting from the pathophysiologic process that stimulates local and adjacent receptors. For example:

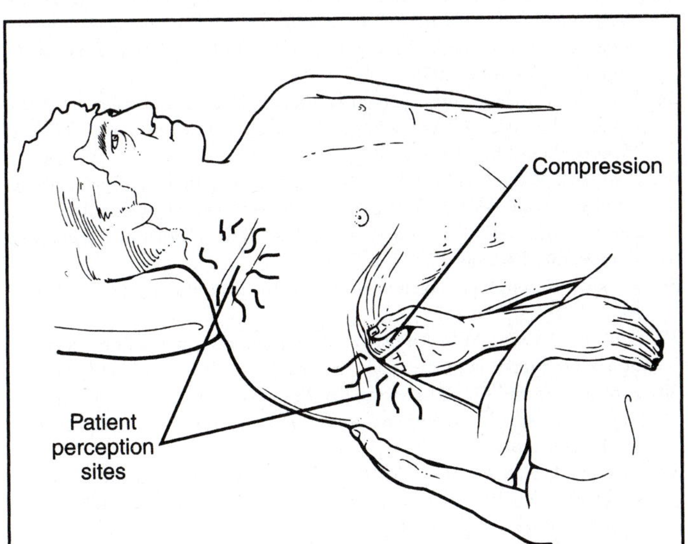

Figure 43.11. Compression of the posterior axillary fold at the palpatory site of each thickened tender point. (Reprinted with permission from Travell JG, Simons DG. *Myofascial Pain and Dysfunction: The Trigger Point Manual. The Upper Extremities.* Vol 1. Williams & Wilkins; 1983:418.)

- Dilated cardiomyopathy is neither infectious nor inflammatory and most often not painful since the heart dilates over an extended period of time. The palpable paraspinal findings from a viscerosomatic reflex would be less acute and intense compared to the findings from an inflammatory and/or infectious condition.
- Coronary artery disease is an inflammatory condition that produces distinguishable palpatory findings in the thoracic paraspinal tissues, pectoralis major muscle, and cervical spine.[18,39,40]
- Pneumonia is both an infectious and inflammatory condition that generates pain and creates viscerosomatic and viscerovisceral reflexes. Pneumonia is accompanied by:
  - □ Somatic clues related to visceral receptors that sense nociceptive elements from the visceral tissues, relay that information to spinal cord in the upper thoracic region, and reflexively create tissue texture changes and/or CRPs that may be palpated in the upper thoracic cage.[14] This is accompanied by sympathetic physiologic responses to multiple tissues sharing the underlying spinal segmental facilitation.
  - □ Somatic clues related to visceral receptors that sense alveolar distension, relay their information via vagal afferents leading to central facilitation of the brainstem, and produce a number of parasympathetic and phrenic mediated physiologic responses. Somatic clues to this may be palpated in the craniocervical junctional region.[8,15]
  - □ Local reduction in rib excursion. This somatic phenomenon may extend *beyond* a typical viscerosomatic reflex, since the dysfunction levels in lower lobe pneumonia that involve the lower ribs are outside the levels of the sympathetic innervation of the lung. In such a case, it is more likely that they are produced through the parietal pleura, which carries a

local, intercostal innervation. These reflex changes are likely involved in pleuritic chest pain (see Chapter 41, Fig. 41.7), which often accompanies pneumonia, and are very useful in locating and making the diagnosis of pulmonary consolidation.

- For each visceral system, similar examples can be cited that involve the discovery and interpretation of somatic clues as they relate to the organ involved and the severity of condition.[20]

Although this chapter puts emphasis on palpable structural findings in the musculoskeletal system, the physician must not disregard visceral conditions and just assess and treat the soma. Therefore, be aware that a life-threatening visceral condition may be at the root of the symptoms and signs assessed during the history and physical examination. The safety of looking for a viscerosomatic reflex is relative to the stability of the vital signs of the patient. It is only safe and appropriate to spend the time and effort to assess for the presence of these reflexes if the physician's attention is not diverted to the musculoskeletal system when it should instead be focused on unstable internal organ conditions.

REFERENCES

1. Giusti R, ed. *Glossary of Osteopathic Terminology*. 3rd ed. American Association of Colleges of Osteopathic Medicine. Education Council on Osteopathic Principles; 2017.
2. Seffinger MA. Palpation reliability and validity. In: Chaitow L, eds. *Palpation and Assessment in Manual Therapy*. 4th ed. Handspring Publishing; 2017.
3. Kuchera ML. Counterstrain: differential diagnosis of myofascial points, an integrated perspective. In: Myer HM, ed. *Compendium Edition: Clinical Application of Counterstrain*. Tucson Osteopathic Medical Foundation; 2012:15–28.
4. Korr IM, Wright HM, Thomas PE. Effects of experimental myofascial insults on cutaneous patterns of sympathetic activity in man. *Acta Neuroveg (Wien)*. 1962;23(22):329–355.
5. Nicholas AS, DeBias DA, Ehrenfeuchter W, et al. A somatic component to myocardial infarction. *Br Med J (Clin Res Ed)*. 1985;291(6487):13–17.
6. Denslow JS, Korr IM, Krems AD. Quantitative studies of chronic facilitation in human motoneuron pools. *Am J Physiol*. 1947;150(2):229–238.
7. Patriquin DA. Viscerosomatic reflexes. In: Patterson MM, Howell JN, eds. *The Central Connection: Somatovisceral and Viscerosomatic Interaction*. University Classics, Ltd; 1992.
8. Beal MC, Morlock JW. Somatic dysfunction associated with pulmonary disease. *J Am Osteopath Assoc*. 1984;82(4):179–183.
9. Beal MC. Palpatory testing for somatic dysfunction in patients with cardiovascular disease. *J Am Osteopath Assoc*. 1983;82(11):822–831.
10. Johnston WL. Segmental definition: III. Definitive basis for distinguishing somatic findings of visceral reflex origin. *J Am Osteopath Assoc*. 1988;88(3):347–353.
11. Morley J. Visceral pain. *Br Med J*. 1937;2(4016):1270–1273.
12. Snider KT, Schneider RP, Snider EJ, et al. Correlation of somatic dysfunction with gastrointestinal endoscopic findings: an observational study. *J Am Osteopath Assoc*. 2016;116(6):358–369.
13. Licciardone JC, Fulda KG, Stoll ST, Gamber RG, Cage AC. A case-control study of osteopathic palpatory findings in type 2 diabetes mellitus. *Osteopath Med Prim Care*. 2007;1:6.
14. Washington K, Mosiello R, Venditto M, et al. Presence of Chapman reflex points in hospitalized patients with pneumonia. *J Am Osteopath Assoc*. 2003;103(10):479–483.
15. Beal MC. Viscerosomatic reflexes: a review. *J Am Osteopath Assoc*. 1985;85(12):786–801.
16. Simons DG, Travell JG, Simons LS. *Travell and Simons' Myofascial Pain and Dysfunction: The Trigger Point Manual. Volume I: Upper Half of Body*. 2nd ed. Williams & Wilkins; 1999.
17. Travell JG, Simons DG. *Myofascial Pain and Dysfunction: The Trigger Point Manual. Volume II. The Lower Extremities*. Williams & Wilkins; 1992:547.
18. Mense S, Simons DG, Russell IJ. *Muscle Pain: Understanding Its Nature, Diagnosis, and Treatment*. Lippincott Williams & Wilkins; 2001.
19. Wu C-M, Chen H-H, Hong C-Z. Inactivation of myofascial trigger points associated with lumbar radiculopathy: surgery versus physical therapy. *Arch Phys Med Rehabil*. 1997;78:1022–1055. https://doi.org/10.1016/S0003-9993(97)90071-X
20. Kuchera ML, Kuchera WA. *Osteopathic Considerations in Systemic Dysfunction*. 2nd ed. rev. Greyden Press; 1994:200–201.
21. Van Buskirk RL. Nociceptive reflexes and somatic dysfunction: a model. *J Am Osteopath Assoc*. 1990;90(9):792–809.
22. Korr IM. The spinal cord as organizer of disease processes. In: Peterson B, ed. *The Collected Papers of Irvin M. Korr*. American Academy of Osteopathy; 1979:207–221.
23. Simons DG. *Myofascial Pain Syndrome Due to Trigger Points. International Rehabilitation Medicine Association Monograph Series Number 1*. Rademaker Printing; 1987.
24. Hubbard DR, Berkoff GM. Myofascial trigger points show spontaneous needle EMG activity. *Spine*. 1993;18(13):1803–1807.
25. Gilliar WG, Kuchera ML, Giulianetti DA. Neurologic basis of manual medicine. *Phys Med Rehabil Clin N Am*. 1996;7(4):693–714.
26. Bennett RM. Myofascial pain syndrome and the fibromyalgia syndrome: a comparative analysis. *J Man Med*. 1991;6:34–45.
27. Fernández-de-Las-Peñas C, Arendt-Nielsen L. Myofascial pain and fibromyalgia: two different but overlapping disorders. *Pain Manag*. 2016;6(4):401–408.
28. Lewit K. *Manipulative Therapy in Rehabilitation of the Locomotor System*. 2nd ed. Butterworth-Heinemann; 1991.
29. Strait B, Kuchera ML. Osteopathic manipulation for patients with confirmed mild, modest, and moderate carpal tunnel syndrome. *J Am Osteopath Assoc*. 1994;94(8):673.
30. Meyers HL. *Compendium Edition: Clinical Application of Counterstrain*. Osteopathic Press; Tucson Osteopathic Medical Foundation; 2012.
31. Teachey WS. Otolaryngic myofascial pain syndromes. *Curr Pain Headache Rep*. 2004;8(6):457–462.
32. Kuchera ML. Gravitational stress, musculoligamentous strain and postural alignment. *Spine State Art Rev*. 1995;9(2):463–490.
33. Kuchera ML. Gravitational strain pathophysiology, Parts I and II. In: Vleeming A, ed. *Low Back Pain: The Integrated Function of the Lumbar Spine and Sacroiliac Joints*. Proceedings of the 2nd Interdisciplinary World Congress, November 1995.
34. Janda V. Muscles, central nervous motor regulation, and back problems. In: Korr IM, ed. *The Neurobiologic Mechanisms in Manipulative Therapy*. Plenum Publishing; 1978:27–41.
35. Korr IM, Wright HM, Chace JA. Cutaneous patterns of sympathetic activity in clinical abnormalities of the musculoskeletal system (1964). In: Peterson B, ed. *The Collected Papers of I. M. Korr*. American Academy of Osteopathy; 1979:66–72.
36. Zink JG. Respiratory and circulatory care: the conceptual model. *Osteopath Ann*. 1977;5(3):108–112.
37. Zink JG, Lawson WB. An osteopathic structural examination and functional interpretation of the soma. *Osteopath Ann*. 1979;7(12):433–440.
38. Zink JG, Fetchik WD, Lawson WB. The posterior axillary folds: a gateway for osteopathic treatment of the upper extremities. *Osteopath Ann*. 1981;9(3):81–88.
39. Cox JM, Gorbis S, Dick LM, Rogers JC, Rogers FJ. Palpable musculoskeletal findings in coronary artery disease: results of a double-blind study. *J Am Osteopath Assoc*. 1983;82(11):832–836.
40. Beal MC, Kleiber GE. Somatic dysfunction as a predictor of coronary artery disease. *J Am Osteopath Assoc*. 1985;85(5):302–307.

44 Osteopathic Manipulative Treatment (OMT) as Part of the Patient's Treatment Plan

RAYMOND J. HRUBY

KEY CONCEPTS

- Determining when and how to use osteopathic manipulative treatment (OMT).
- Creating a rational treatment plan that includes the use of OMT.
- Important considerations for the use of OMT.

INTRODUCTION

The ultimate development of a patient treatment plan typically starts with some combination of the following activities:

- Gathering a detailed patient history
- Performing a careful and precise physical examination, including an osteopathic structural examination
- Obtaining other information as needed, by way of laboratory testing, imaging, other diagnostic procedures, or further consultations

Once all pertinent information is received and a diagnosis is established, an individual treatment plan can be formulated for the patient. Depending on the specific diagnosis, the plan may include interventions such as medication, surgery, nutritional approaches, counseling, and patient education, to name a few. These interventions are prescribed to optimize the patient's rapid return to health in a manner that is also efficient, safe, and cost-effective.

The presence of clinically relevant somatic dysfunction, amenable to the use of OMT, requires certain additional considerations. As with any other component of the patient's treatment plan, the use of OMT must also be precise, and rationally formulated to assist in the patient's return quickly, safely, and effectively to health and wellness.

COMPONENTS OF A TREATMENT PLAN THAT INCLUDES OMT

A treatment plan that includes the use of OMT must consider certain components in order to provide for the most appropriate, effective, and efficient treatment of the patient's condition. These components are:

Method

This refers to the specific OMT modality or combination of modalities to be utilized (e.g., muscle energy technique, osteopathic cranial manipulative medicine, and articulatory technique). For more information about OMT modalities see Sections VIII and IX.

OMT is indicated for the treatment of somatic dysfunction. Many types, or modalities, of OMT are available, and the choice of which is/are used in each situation can be based on any number of considerations. These include:

- The expected goals of the treatment, which may involve the desire to achieve any of the following:
  - □ Changes in circulation, such as to improve movement of body fluids, or to provide a tonic effect for the body
  - □ Modification of neurologic reflexes (e.g., viscerosomatic or somatovisceral)
  - □ A maintenance OMT program for chronic conditions[1,2]
- The Five Models of Osteopathic Care. These conceptual models assist the osteopathic physician in determining the nature of the patient's pathophysiologic processes, formulating a diagnosis, and in the case of somatic dysfunction, selecting the most appropriate type(s) of OMT. These models are:
  - □ Biomechanical
  - □ Neurologic
  - □ Respiratory/Circulatory
  - □ Metabolic
  - □ Biopsychosocial

For more detailed information on the five models of osteopathic medicine and their clinical usage, the reader is referred to Chapter 26.

- Tissue End-feel. This is the sensation imparted to the examiner's hands at the end point of the available range of motion, which varies according to the limiting structure or tissue.[3] Knowledge of the different types of end-feel allows the physician to determine which structures and/or tissues are involved in each somatic dysfunction, and in turn, to select for the appropriate OMT modalities to address these tissues and/or structures.[4,5] For more information on end-feel, see Chapter 30.
- Direct versus Indirect Approach. The presence of somatic dysfunction implies the presence of a restrictive barrier in the tissues and/or structures involved, preventing normal physiologic motion in that area. The physician may choose to utilize OMT modalities that approach the restrictive barrier directly or indirectly.
  a. When direct methods are used, the restrictive barrier is engaged, and a final activating force is applied to correct the somatic dysfunction.
  b. With indirect methods, the restrictive barrier is disengaged, and the dysfunctional body part is moved away from the restrictive barrier, until tissue tension is equal in one or all planes and directions. The dysfunctional tissues are guided along the path of least resistance until free movement is achieved.[6]

ACTIVATING FORCES

Activating forces are additional maneuvers or energy introduced that causes a given OMT maneuver to produce its effect. These forces can be further classified as extrinsic or intrinsic. DeStefano[2] listed the extrinsic and intrinsic activating forces as follows:

1. Extrinsic activating forces are those that are applied externally and directly to the patient.
   a. Operator effort, such as guiding, springing, and thrust
   b. Adjunctive, such as straps, pads, and traction
   c. Gravity, activated with a combination of the patient's body weight and the patient's positioning
2. Intrinsic activating forces are those that arise from within the patient and are used to help achieve the therapeutic effect.
   a. Inherent force, or nature's tendency toward balance and homeostasis
   b. Respiratory force
      i. Inhalation, which straightens the spinal curves and externally rotates the extremities
      ii. Exhalation, which enhances the spinal curves and internally rotates the extremities
   c. Muscle force of the patient
      i. Muscle cooperation
      ii. Muscle energy, especially isometrics
   d. Reflex activity
      i. Eye movements
      ii. Muscle activation

OTHER FACTORS THAT INFLUENCE THE CHOICE OF METHODS AND ACTIVATING FORCES

1. Patient condition
   a. Acute versus chronic.
      i. Acute conditions are frequently more painful and physiologically stressing to the patient, and thus may require shorter, more frequent treatment sessions, along with the use of more passive and/or indirect OMT techniques.
      ii. Chronic conditions may require longer treatment sessions, less frequent visits, and more active and/or direct technique approaches, along with patient cooperation.[7]
   b. Complicating factors (comorbidities). These issues affect the use of certain types of OMT modalities and activating forces.
      i. For example, a patient with advanced osteoporosis may not be a candidate for more forceful or direct types of OMT.
      ii. Likewise, a patient with acute congestive heart failure may not be able to exert themselves with extrinsic activating forces.
   c. Hospital versus ambulatory setting. Expert consensus within the osteopathic profession states that techniques may need to be modified depending on the treatment setting. (For more information on this topic, see Chapter 78 Osteopathic Considerations and Approaches in the Acutely Ill & Hospitalized Patient.)
      i. Acutely ill, hospitalized patients respond better to shorter, more frequent treatments, often using passive and indirect approaches.
      ii. Patients in the ambulatory setting often respond well to more active and direct approaches, with less frequent treatment intervals.
   d. Contraindications. The physician must be aware of the contraindications to various OMT modalities and avoid any situation that would endanger the patient. In addition, there are certain conditions that call for special precautions, and are listed by DeStefano[2] as:
      i. The vertebral artery in the cervical spine.
      ii. Primary joint disease, such as rheumatoid arthritis.
      iii. Metabolic bone disease, such as osteoporosis.
      iv. Primary or metastatic malignant bone disease.
      v. Genetic disorders, such as Down syndrome, particularly in the cervical spine.
      vi. Hypermobility in the involved segments. Hypermobile areas should not be treated with OMT; rather, the physician should look for *hypomobility* elsewhere.
   e. Patient preference. Patients having had prior OMT treatments may prefer certain modalities. Typically, this preference can be honored, unless the physician has a clear reason for the use of other modalities. However, other modalities should not be performed without the patient's full knowledge and consent.

DOSAGE

The dosage, or amount, of OMT refers to the time spent during a treatment session, and the amount of patient energy required to accomplish the treatment. This will vary from one patient to another, and from one treatment session to another. Only general guidelines for treatment dosage can be given, as this is often dictated by a combination of the patient's response to treatment and the physician's skill and experience. Kimberly[1] described appropriate OMT dosage as:

1. Enough to effect a physiologic response
2. Not enough to overwhelm the patient

Many of the factors that affect the choice of OMT modalities and activating forces (see above) also affect the treatment dosage.

FREQUENCY

The frequency of OMT is also largely dictated by the patient's condition and the physician's skill and experience. The correct and optimum frequency of treatment requires that the patient be evaluated at each visit with the physician. Evaluation of the patient's functional improvement, as reported by the patient and/or observed by the physician, along with objective findings on the osteopathic structural examination, are noted at each patient visit. These factors, along with any other pertinent information are used to determine whether the frequency of OMT needs to be adjusted. A few general guidelines for OMT frequency are:

1. Each treatment should build on the effects achieved from previous treatments.
2. Infrequent treatments may result in the physician repeating the same techniques for the same somatic dysfunctions, without achieving long-term effects.
3. Giving treatments too frequently may not allow the patient sufficient time to benefit from each treatment.[1]

Many of the factors that affect the choice of OMT modalities and activating forces (see above) also affect treatment frequency.

DURATION

How long OMT should be continued for a given patient situation is also a matter of clinical judgment. The same considerations given above for dosage and frequency or OMT also apply to the determination of duration of OMT treatment. Some general guidelines for treatment duration are:

1. For acute conditions, the aim of OMT treatment is to continue until normal function is restored, or until the condition is returned to baseline or plateaus.
2. If unable to effect continued improvement, the physician should reassess the patient's condition and adjust the management plan.
3. For chronic conditions, the duration of treatment is determined by the nature of the patient's condition, needs, and response.

Following these principles, the physician can create a specific and appropriate plan for the use of OMT in any given patient situation. The plan will also be safe, effective, and helpful to the patient in returning to, and maximizing health and wellness.

SUMMARY

The decision to use OMT in the overall treatment plan for a patient requires the consideration of multiple factors and must be rationally derived based on the application of fundamental osteopathic principles. Each patient must be considered individually, and must be re-evaluated at each physician–patient encounter in order to correctly, rationally, and optimally apply OMT in the context of the patient's overall treatment plan.

REFERENCES

1. Kimberly PE. Formulating a prescription for osteopathic manipulative treatment. *J Am Osteopath Assoc.* 1980;79(8):506–513.
2. DeStefano LA, ed. *Greenman's Principles of Manual Medicine.* 5th ed. Lippincott Williams & Wilkinson; 2016.
3. Anderson DM, ed. *Mosby's Dictionary of Medicine, Nursing & Health Professions.* 11th ed. Elsevier; 2022.
4. Hruby RJ. Somatic dysfunction: a principled approach to diagnosis and the selection of OMT modalities. *AAOJ.* 2016;26(1):7–16.
5. Hruby RJ. Pathophysiologic models and the selection of osteopathic manipulative techniques. *J Osteop Med.* 1992;6(4):25–30.
6. Giusti RE, ed. *Glossary of Osteopathic Terminology.* American Association of Colleges of Osteopathic Medicine; 2017.
7. Seffinger MA, Hruby RJ. *Evidence-Based Manual Medicine: A Problem-Oriented Approach.* Saunders Elsevier; 2007:62.

45 Osteopathic Neuromusculoskeletal Medicine

BRIAN LOVELESS ▪ MINDY A. CHILMAN MCCOMB ▪ REBECCA E. GIUSTI

KEY CONCEPTS

- The development of the earned postdoctoral designation conferred by the American Academy of Osteopathy, FAAO (Fellow of the American Academy of Osteopathy) generated the evolution of the American Osteopathic Association (AOA) certification in neuromusculoskeletal medicine and osteopathic manipulative medicine (NMM/OMM).
- The specialty of Osteopathic Neuromusculoskeletal Medicine (ONMM) was created by the Accreditation Council for Graduate Medical Education (ACGME) in 2014.
- There is a unique role of the ONMM specialist in clinical practice and academic medicine.
- The development of the hospital-based OMM consultation and treatment service was unique to the osteopathic profession.
- The osteopathic examination, structural diagnosis, and treatment of acutely ill hospitalized patients employ the procedures introduced in other chapters in this volume and may be employed at the specialty practice level by the ONMM specialist as well as other osteopathic physicians.
- The four osteopathic tenets and the five osteopathic models of care provide a scaffolding by which the ONMM specialist interfaces with every patient.

INTRODUCTION

Every osteopathic physician is educated in osteopathic principles and practices (OPP) and osteopathic manipulative treatment (OMT), which are incorporated into the everyday practice of osteopathic medicine. Like other areas of medicine, a need has developed over time for experts in the field. This has led to the development of a primary certification in neuromusculoskeletal medicine and osteopathic manipulative medicine (NMM/OMM) through the American Osteopathic Board of Neuromusculoskeletal Medicine (AOBNMM). The single accreditation system under the Accreditation Council for Graduate Medical Education (ACGME) led to the establishment of the Osteopathic Neuromusculoskeletal Medicine (ONMM) specialty. Specialists are responsible for further expanding the osteopathic concepts and methods. They contribute to the profession through teaching, writing, and specialized clinical practice.

HISTORY OF THE DEVELOPMENT OF THE FAAO AND THE ONMM SPECIALTY

In 1958, representatives from the Academy of Applied Osteopathy (AAO, now called the American Academy of Osteopathy) and the AOA formed a committee to establish the fellowship program of the AAO (FAAO). The intent of the program was to recognize doctors of osteopathy (DOs) with special expertise in manipulation and to encourage other DOs to improve their skills. In 1959, the following paragraph appeared in the directory of the AAO:

> A proposal was presented to the Board of Governors of the Academy, and to a special committee of the Advisory Board for Osteopathic Specialists for the formation of a new certifying board called the American Osteopathic Board of Manipulative Arts and Sciences. The proposal was made by a group of osteopathic physicians headed by Dr. T.F. Schooley, Phoenix, Arizona. Proposals for certification in the field of manipulative therapy have been studied for several years with no success in reaching agreement relative to the propriety and value of such a program. Those favoring such a step contend that there must be established a means of recognizing and accrediting the members of the profession who have developed a high degree of knowledge and skill in the field, and whose practices are based principally upon the structural approach. Those opposed to certification in the field contend that the manipulative application of osteopathic principles is basic to every osteopathic physician's approach to the problems presented by his patients, and certification of this basic and fundamental aspect of osteopathy would be improper and would limit the profession. All who have studied the matter agree that a means must be established for recognizing ability in the field.[1]

In 1960, the committee presented detailed recommendations for the duties of the Board on Fellowship, which was adopted by the Academy's Board of Governors and the AOA's Board of Trustees. The FAAO process required certain prerequisites, a 5,000-word written thesis, as well as oral, written, and practical examinations. Therefore, it was established as an "earned" fellowship.

In 1971, a joint committee of representatives from the AAO and the AOA discussed the necessary steps for converting the FAAO process to a certification in OMM. The AOA Board approved the resolution in 1977. This created the American Osteopathic Board on Fellowship in the American Academy of Osteopathy (AOBFAAO), a committee directly responsible to the Board of Trustees, and was given the role of establishing residency programs in OMM.

In 1989, to align with similar processes in other AOA specialty colleges, the AOA requested the separation of the processes for OMM certification and conferring of the FAAO. Consequentially, the FAAO became adjudicated by a Committee on Fellowship within the AAO. Becoming an FAAO continues to be a prestigious achievement in which the osteopathic physician has this title conferred on them after a 2-year process in which they demonstrate their mastery of application of the osteopathic principles and philosophy and present a thesis.[2] Those interested in applying for this fellowship can find the requirements at the American Academy of Osteopathy's website.

A new certifying board was formulated and named the American Osteopathic Board of Special Proficiency in Osteopathic Manipulative Medicine (AOBSPOMM), which was also directly responsible to the AOA Board of Trustees. In 1999, the

AOBSPOMM was renamed the "American Osteopathic Board of Neuromusculoskeletal Medicine" (AOBNMM). Osteopathic physicians who successfully pass this board's examination are certified in NMM and OMM.

In 2014, the AOA, the American Association of Colleges of Osteopathic Medicine (AACOM), and the ACGME jointly established a single accreditation system for graduate medical education. As part of the agreement, the ACGME formed a new position, the Senior Vice President of Osteopathic Accreditation, and a new Residency Review Committee, thus recognizing ONMM as a specialty within the broader medical community.[3]

ONMM is a medical specialty certified by the AOBNMM. Physicians who are certified through the predecessor examination are also recognized by the AOBNMM. To sit for the ONMM boards, a physician must have completed a residency in ONMM. Historically, there have been three ways to complete this residency training:

1. A 2-year residency in ONMM.
2. A 1-year (Plus-1) residency after completing another primary residency certified by the AOA.
3. Completing a combined residency such as in Family Medicine and ONMM or Internal Medicine and ONMM. These programs required completion of all basic standards in each specialty and are generally 4 years long.

Under the ACGME there are the following options:

1. ONMM1 Level of Entry: This is a 36-month training program. https://www.acgme.org/globalassets/pfassets/programrequirements/275_osteopathicneuromusculoskeletalmedicine_2023.pdf. Accessed November 7, 2024.
2. ONMM2 Level of Entry: To be eligible for entry into the program at the ONMM2 level, residents must have successfully completed, prior to appointment, a broad-based clinical year (postgraduate year 1 [PGY-1] or internship year). They then complete a 2-year ONMM residency. https://www.acgme.org/globalassets/pfassets/programrequirements/275_osteopathicneuromusculoskeletalmedicine_2023.pdf. Accessed November 7, 2024.
3. ONMM3 Level of Entry: Residents accepted at the ONMM3 level must have completed a residency program and have met other eligibility criteria prior to entry. The length of the educational program for a resident entering at the ONMM3 level is 12 months. https://www.acgme.org/globalassets/pdfs/faq/275_osteopathic_neuromusculoskeletal_medicine_faqs.pdf. Accessed November 7, 2024.

All osteopathic physicians are trained in OPP as well as OMT. They are trained to evaluate and treat all patients through this distinctive lens and may use OMT wherever indicated. ONMM residency programs further educate physicians in the diagnosis, prevention, treatment, and rehabilitation of neuromusculoskeletal conditions at the level of a specialist.[3] It is a primary residency focused on the neuromusculoskeletal system's comprehensive relationship to other organ systems and its dynamic function of locomotion. The discipline is osteopathic, and patient centered, accounting for the structure and function interrelation of the body, its unity, and its inherent ability to self-maintain and self-heal.

OVERVIEW OF ONMM SPECIALTY

ONMM specialists must demonstrate specialized knowledge of the basic and clinical sciences, clinical evaluation, and management of disorders of the neuromusculoskeletal system and its related visceral and somatic structures. They must also be able to identify the indications, risks, and benefits of manipulative medicine in the treatment of patients with neuromusculoskeletal disorders.

ONMM specialists may focus their practice primarily on hospital patients (inpatient), clinic patients (outpatient), academic medicine (teaching at a College of Osteopathic Medicine), medical administration (directing an ONMM residency program), or a combination of any of the former.

The ONMM specialist's approach to patient evaluation and treatment differs based on the setting (inpatient or outpatient) and on the acuity of the patient:

- Hospital setting:
  - Patient population unique considerations:
    - Generally, patients are more acute.
    - Consultation is generally based upon the interplay of the musculoskeletal system with the patient's disease process, visceral dysfunctions that are amenable to OMT, secondary musculoskeletal pain related to other medical problems, and/or severe debilitating musculoskeletal pain.
    - Patients have limited mobility secondary to their illness and medical equipment/interventions.
      - Modified structural evaluation should be completed as part of a complete physical examination.
      - Regional TART evaluation may supplant segmental diagnosis for regions where a segmental diagnosis may be difficult or inappropriate to obtain.
    - The treatment may be shorter in duration (5 to 15 minutes) depending on the severity of illness. In addition, indirect techniques may be more appropriate for hospitalized patients than direct techniques, but clinical judgment should always be utilized. For example, rib raising and suboccipital release are generally considered to be direct techniques but may be indicated for a hospitalized patient to optimize their function.
  - Unique treatment considerations:
    - The treatment plan implements a five-model approach with the focus on primary functions (respiration, lymphatic flow, autonomic balance, pain reduction).
    - Basic techniques (thoracic inlet/outlet release, lymphatic drainage, thoracic diaphragm release, suboccipital release, SI decompression, paraspinal inhibition/release, rib raising) may be the focus of the OMT utilized during the clinical encounter.
    - OMT delivery positional considerations:
      - Techniques are usually performed with the patient supine, or laterally recumbent, and seated or prone techniques are often modified.
      - Techniques may need additional modifications based on a patient's clinical presentation and limitations.
      - OMT techniques are often modified to work safely around hospital equipment (hospital bed, ventilators, IVs, invasive lines).
    - Requires interprofessional work as a consultant/specialist with the primary medical providers (e.g., internists, family medicine, ob/gyn, or pediatricians) or other subspecialists (e.g., cardiologists, intensivists, neonatologists, or pulmonologists).
      - May order additional diagnostic tests, prescribe or recommend changes to medications and participate in treatment.
      - May function as a primary care provider if dual board certified in a primary care specialty.
    - Treatment is covered by Medicare and many health insurance plans.

- Outpatient clinical setting:
  - Patient population unique considerations:
    - Patient chief complaints are predominantly primary and secondary musculoskeletal pain, but occasionally patients present with primary systemic disease complaints.
  - Unique treatment considerations:
    - Treatment positions may vary greatly depending on the individual patient's mobility.
      - Regional and segmental evaluations are generally included in the structural evaluation.
      - In addition to the osteopathic structural exam, a complete or focused physical examination is done within the context of the chief complaint and patient presentation.
    - Longer treatment duration of 30 to 60 minutes is generally well tolerated by patients.
    - The treatment plan implements a five-model approach. Direct and indirect techniques may be utilized.
    - The visit and treatment plan often have a broad focus that considers lifestyle modifications influencing the patient's complaints and general patient well-being, including exercise and nutrition education. (see Chapter 21 Lifestyle Medicine—Osteopathic Perspectives for further information and discussion)
    - Patients may be referred from other healthcare providers or may self-refer.
    - ONMM specialists are not considered a primary care provider unless dually board certified in a primary care specialty.
    - Treatment may be covered by insurance and depends on the individual patient plan and physician negotiation with the health plans. Some ONMM specialists choose to maintain cash-only reimbursement policies.

THE DEVELOPMENT OF THE HOSPITAL-BASED ONMM CONSULTATION AND TREATMENT SERVICE

As osteopathic hospitals were developed in the early years of the profession, OMT was essential to the treatment of hospitalized patients. However, the emergence of specialties and subspecialties within the profession resulted in increased patient loads, time constraints, and overall demands of specialty practices. As a result, it became more difficult for DOs to provide regular OMT to their hospitalized patients. Those with more extensive training in OMT were called on to provide consultation and treatment and were viewed as specialists in OMM.

This practice gained impetus and expanded with the development of a unique program at the Waterville Osteopathic Hospital in Maine, in 1973. The hospital hired a director of osteopathic medicine and a full-time osteopathic physician to provide consultation and treatment service in OMT and OPP. Its first director was Edward G. Stiles, DO, whose successful leadership inspired other osteopathic hospitals to provide similar services. In addition, Dr. Stiles did much to establish the role of the OMM specialist in such a setting. He described the duties of the director of osteopathic medicine as follows:

1. The director is to provide clinical consultation services for referred patients and to properly document the osteopathic diagnosis and treatment utilized.
2. The director is to be an educator and to increase the staff's expertise and awareness of the applications and indications for osteopathic care. Creating a service of osteopathic medicine in a hospital setting provides tremendous educational potential. The following educational tools can be utilized:
   a. Consultation reports
   b. Courses in technique and principles
   c. Committee reports on utilization of osteopathic manipulation
   d. Departmental educational meetings
   e. Staff educational meetings

   Each of these tools provides an opportunity to increase the awareness of the staff of the implications, applications, and indications for utilization of osteopathic care in a hospital environment. This naturally increases the awareness of the staff as to the types of patients who should be referred to this service and offers a challenge to staff members to improve their own levels of expertise in the delivery of healthcare.
3. The director of osteopathic medicine is to fill a public relations role for the hospital.[4]

Dr. Stiles also made note of the research potential afforded by a hospital-based service of this nature. The emergence of residency programs in NMM/OMM throughout the country continued this tradition in many teaching hospitals.

Most hospitals require that physicians serving as consultants complete a credentialing process and be granted privileges in their area of specialty. This credentialing also applies to specialists in ONMM.

THE ONMM SPECIALIST IN THE HOSPITAL/ INPATIENT SETTING

History Taking and Data Gathering

An open-ended approach to obtaining the patient's chief complaint and history is like other medical practices, except that the ONMM specialist tends to highlight the data that affect or may be affected by the neuromusculoskeletal system. If the patient is unable to give the history due to cognitive impairment, age (i.e., neonate, pediatric patient), intubation, or other causes, a family member may be asked to provide the history.

The history for the neuromusculoskeletal evaluation includes the typical intake done when admitting patients or following them in the hospital; history of present illness, medical and surgical history, allergies (environmental, medical, and food), medications and supplements, family and social history, and review of systems.

An ONMM specialist additionally may inquire and place emphasis on the following during the intake:

- Episodes of loss of consciousness
- Previous injuries, history motor vehicle accidents, falls, fractures
- Any trauma, but especially that of the head
- Presence of known short leg
- Known structural abnormalities such as scoliosis and plagiocephaly
- Exercise level and activities
- Sports and repetitive motion activities
- Hobbies (sedentary and active)
- Social living and working environment
- Chronic pain syndromes
- Chronic organic diseases, especially those which have neuromusculoskeletal components or effects
- Medications and/or supplements that affect the neuromusculoskeletal system
- Previous experience with OMT and response to it
- Previous experience with other manual medicine modalities

- Previous other manipulative interventions (physical therapy, chiropractic, massage therapy, and other body workers), as well as alternative medical interventions (acupuncture, Reiki, and other types of healers)

The physician's intake of the above assists in the:

- Identifying the musculoskeletal areas containing the primary somatic dysfunction
- Identifying secondary somatic dysfunction(s) produced by biomechanical responses (somatosomatic, nociceptively mediated response, or muscle imbalance) and/or somatovisceral or viscerosomatic reflexes
- Selecting the most appropriate OMT techniques

PHYSICAL EXAMINATION

Preferably, prior to performing the physical examination, the ONMM specialist would review the patient's chart and the patient's original imaging studies. This is crucial, since imaging reports often focus upon orthopedic and neurologic findings and may not mention the bony and fascial abnormalities amenable to OMT or other interventions that the ONMM specialist may recommend. The ONMM specialist integrates the osteopathic palpatory and structural examination into the patient encounter. The history and chief complaint may indicate areas of the body that should be investigated more thoroughly. When evaluating the patient, the ONMM specialist is expected to follow the institution's protocol on personal protective equipment (PPE).

Structural Exam Components of the Physical Exam of the Hospitalized Patient

The structural component of the physical examination may focus on the respiratory/circulatory, and neurologic models of osteopathic care.[5,6] This may involve:

- Assessment of the major diaphragms of the body, as well as their bony and fascial attachments as restrictions of these structures may impede normal vascular and lymphatic flow.
- Assessment of proper rib motion due to the relationship both with the respiratory/circulatory model and the reflexes mediated by the sympathetic nervous system (SNS) via the chain ganglia, lying anterior to the rib heads.
- Evaluation of the paraspinal myofascial elements of the suboccipital, thoracolumbar, and sacral regions due to their involvement with autonomic reflexes that manifest in those areas.

Physical examination of the patient during an ONMM consult usually includes body systems related to the patient's underlying medical condition (i.e., HEENT, cardiovascular, lungs, abdomen, and neurologic). A pertinent osteopathic structural exam is incorporated into the patient's overall physical examination. Examples of regions and findings that may be entered into the hospital electronic medical record (EMR) are as follows:

Cranial region
- Overall motion—rate, quality, amplitude
- Sutural restrictions
- SBS strain pattern
- SBS compression

Cervical region
- TART level(s)
- OA diagnosis
- AA diagnosis
- C2–C7 segmental diagnosis

Thoracic inlet
- Supraclavicular fossa
- Clavicular mobility

Thoracic diaphragm (supine)

Thoracic region
- TART level(s)
- Segmental rotational diagnosis

Lumbar region
- TART level(s)
- Segmental rotational diagnosis

Rib region
- Rib angles
- TART levels
- Rib regional motion examination (supine)

Pelvis region
- SI joint TART
- Passive motion testing (vertical axis)
- ASIS levels

Performance of the Hospital Structural Exam Component

If the patient is ambulatory, the examination is not significantly different from an outpatient structural evaluation. However, in many cases within the hospital setting, an acutely ill patient may be evaluated in the supine position.

A suggested examination is as follows:

1. Observe the patient for their overall status which may include alertness and orientation, hydration, and nutritional state (i.e., presence of cachexia), and any distress.
2. Begin with bilateral compression of the anterior superior iliac spines (ASISs), the ASIS compression test.
   a. This indicates restrictions in iliosacral mobility that may interfere with sacral and pubic motion, and pelvic diaphragm tension (Fig. 45.1).
3. Evaluate the sacral and lumbar regions from the patient's side. Generally, the patient is lying on an absorbent pad over a draw sheet and a fitted mattress sheet.

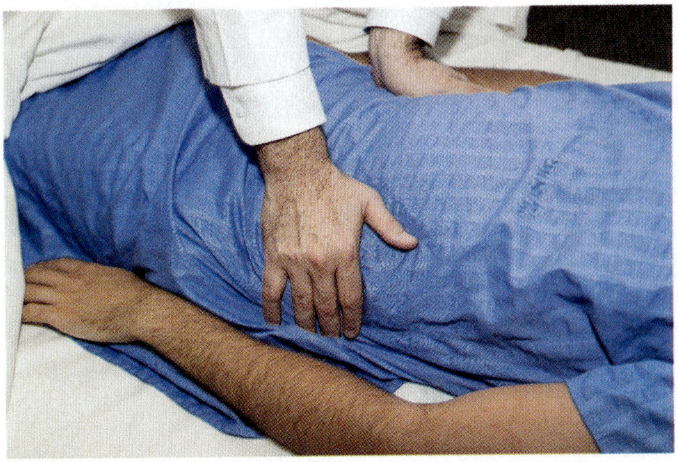

Figure 45.1. Anterior superior iliac spine compression test. (Photo courtesy of Western University of Health Sciences, with permission.)

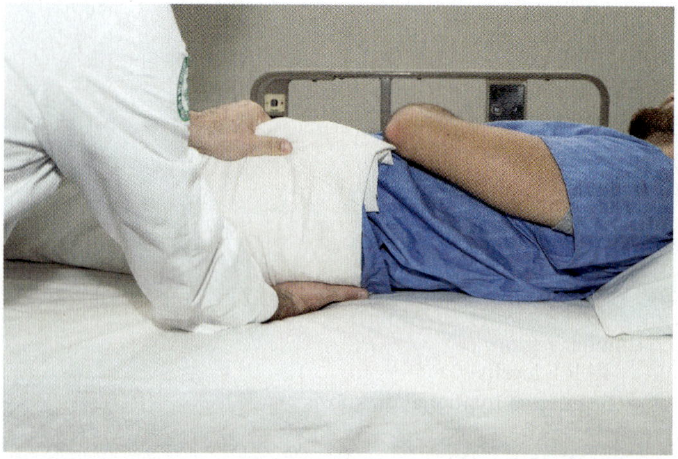

Figure 45.2. Draw sheet sling for posterior palpation and treatment of the patient. (Photo courtesy of Western University of Health Sciences, with permission.)

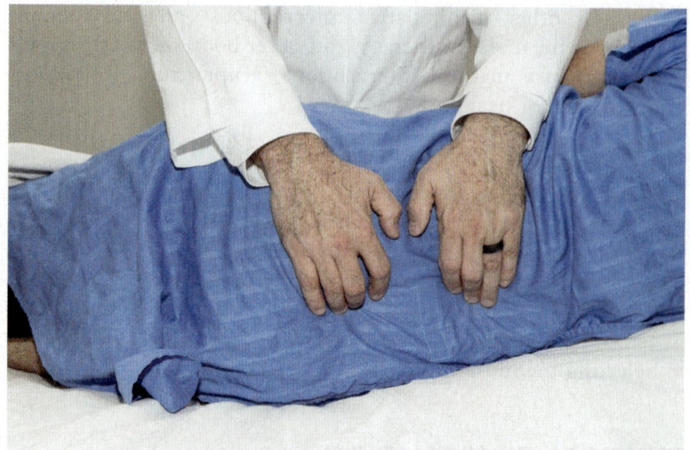

Figure 45.4. Sacral palpation. (Photo courtesy of Western University of Health Sciences, with permission.)

a. The sacral and lumbar regions are easily approached by slipping the hands under the patient, palms up, between the two sheets. This is made easier by loosening the draw sheet from under the mattress and rolling it up parallel to the patient on either side of the bed (Fig. 45.2).

b. This rolled-up draw sheet serves as a sling with which the patient can be gently lifted and rolled away, enabling the physician to place a hand under the pelvic or lumbar regions without requiring any effort by the patient (Fig. 45.3).

c. Although this treatment procedure requires palpating and treating through the thickness of the absorbent pad and draw sheet, it becomes easier with practice. This approach also protects the patient's modesty and minimizes the physician's contact with any bodily fluids that may be present.

4. Place the hands side by side so that the finger pads of one hand contact the ipsilateral sacral base and the finger pads of the other contact the inferolateral angle of the sacrum. Assess for tissue texture changes and tenderness at this SI joint. Then exert alternate pressure in an anterior direction with the finger pads, ascertaining the ability of the sacrum to "rock" on its L-shaped articulation about its biomechanical transverse axis (Fig. 45.4).

   a. To assess the lumbar spine, place one or both hands under the patient's ipsilateral lumbar paraspinal region and press anteriorly to assess the tissue texture changes and motion restrictions of the lumbar spine.[7] Evidence of viscerosomatic reflexes may be discerned by layer palpation.[7]

   b. Then note ease of rotatory motion by applying a springing anterior pressure to the transverse processes. Repeat the same procedure on the patient's opposite side. As a note, both sides may be evaluated at the same time with the physician contacting the paraspinal regions of the lumbar spine and applying alternating pressure to each level of the paraspinal tissues and transverse processes in a methodical fashion. With the patient relaxed as much as possible, estimate the amount of lumbar lordosis as it may contribute to dysfunction of the thoracoabdominal diaphragm via the crural attachments.

5. If the patient is not in the immediate postoperative period after abdominal or pelvic surgery, palpate the abdomen for visceral dysfunction.

   a. The thoracoabdominal diaphragm may be assessed for restrictions by placing one hand under the patient at the T10–L2 area posteriorly, and the other hand anteriorly, just inferior to the xiphoid process.

   b. One hand gently twists the underlying fascia clockwise, while the other hand twists counterclockwise; then, reverse the direction of testing (Fig. 45.5).

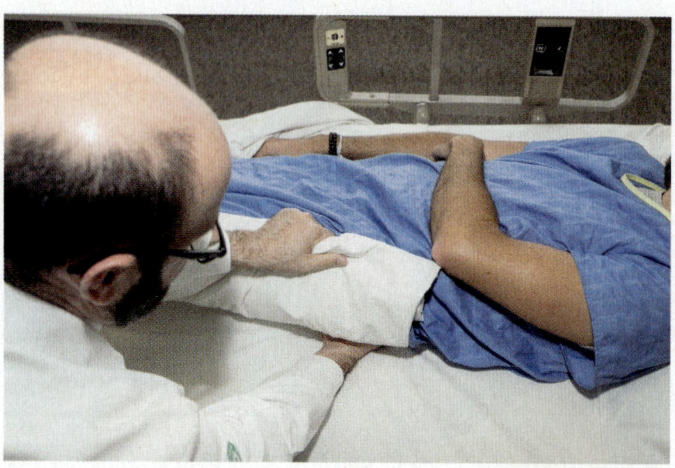

Figure 45.3. Place hands between the draw sheet and the mattress to contact lumbar areas. (Photo courtesy of Western University of Health Sciences, with permission.)

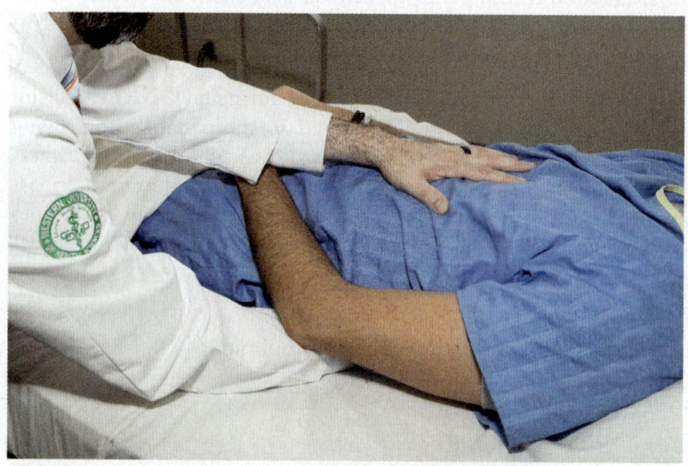

Figure 45.5. Assessing the thoracoabdominal diaphragm. (Photo courtesy of Western University of Health Sciences, with permission.)

c. The thoracoabdominal diaphragm dysfunction is named according to the direction of preferred fascial movement sensed by the abdominal hand.

6. Assess the excursion of the lower and upper ribs by instructing the patient to inhale and exhale deeply.
   a. To assess motion of the lower ribs, contact the costal cage at the midaxillary line avoiding the chondral cartilage.
   b. To assess motion of the upper ribs place hands over the ribs lateral to the sternum at the midclavicular line.
   c. If the patient has a chest tube in place or is on a ventilator, follow the motion present by lightly resting hands on the rib cage. Gently rest the palpating hand on the sternum and follow its motion, noting any fascial pulls and any costosternal articular restrictions.
   d. Note the symmetry of the thoracic cage and any tension of the accessory muscles of respiration.
7. A screen of the anterior Chapman reflexes[8] may be considered while assessing the thorax and abdomen.
8. Depending on the patient's presentation, a screen of the Jones tender points[9] in the cervical, thoracic, and abdominal regions may also be considered (see Chapter 43 for further details on these procedures).
9. Adjust the bed to place the patient in the low Fowler position (approximately 15 degrees of head elevation), elevating the mattress until it is even with the top of the headboard (Fig. 45.6). Move to the head of the bed. The patient's pillow may be removed depending on their comfort.
   a. This positioning allows treatment with minimal stooping and without requiring removal of the headboard. However, the headboard may be removed to ensure proper ergonomics for the physician.
   b. If the Fowler position is contraindicated, the entire bed may be elevated.
   c. The bed may need to be pushed away from the wall to permit access to the head of the bed.
   d. Be careful not to disturb peripheral and central lines, suction tubing, urinary catheters, and other medical equipment.
   e. Follow this same procedure in the intensive care unit. If the patient is on a ventilator, treat them in the position dictated by the life support systems.
   f. From the head of the bed, place a hand on each side of the patient's head, with the palms facing upward. Glide the hands between the draw sheet and the bed or between the bedsheet and the mattress, down to the T12–L2 area of the patient's back (Figs. 45.6 and 45.7). With elbows leaning on the head of the bed for support, contact the transverse processes with the finger pads. Press anteriorly with the finger pads of both hands, first assessing for tissue texture changes, fascial restrictions, and tenderness. Next, alternate anterior pressure with the finger pads of one hand followed by the other to assess the rotatory motion of the vertebral segments.

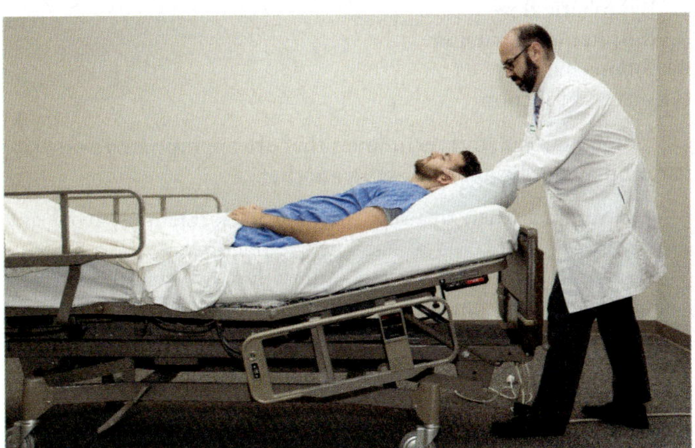

Figure 45.6. The low Fowler position. (Photo courtesy of Western University of Health Sciences, with permission.)

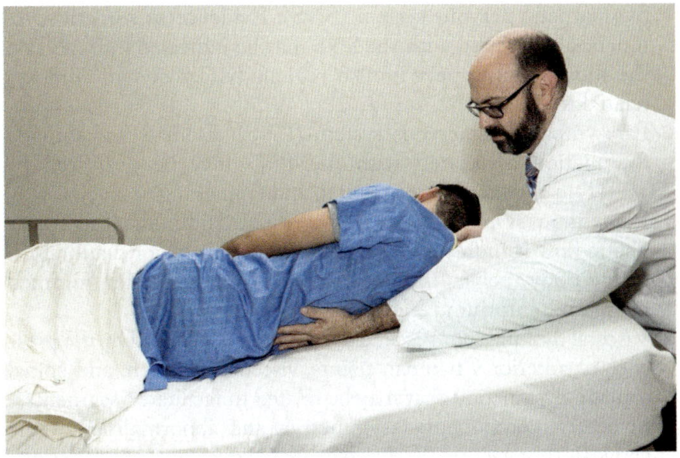

Figure 45.7. Demonstration of hand position for palpation of posterior thoracic area. (Photo courtesy of Western University of Health Sciences, with permission.)

   g. Move the finger pads up stepwise and repeat the process until the entire thoracic spine has been evaluated. Using areas of thoracic segmental dysfunction or the information gathered on the rib motion screening exam earlier, consider further evaluation of rib somatic dysfunction by moving the finger pads of one hand laterally to palpate the rib head and costotransverse joint of the affected rib and the finger pads of the other hand anteriorly to the costochondral junction of the same rib. Apply gentle anterior pressure with the finger pads on the posterior aspect to assess for compliance.
10. Evaluate the thoracic inlet for fascial restrictions (see Chapter 52).
    a. If the patient has any central venous lines, the hand on that side must be placed more laterally, near the acromioclavicular joint. The presence of these lines may actually be an indication for evaluation and treatment of this region and does not represent a contraindication.
11. Evaluate the cervical region for the presence of somatic dysfunction.
12. The suboccipital region may be assessed for tissue texture changes, tenderness, and condylar compression. A segmental diagnosis may be obtained for the occipitoatlantal (OA) and atlantoaxial (AA) joints (see Fig. 45.6).
13. The soft tissues of the cervical region are assessed, and segmental motion is evaluated by translating the articular pillars in an alternating fashion. This process is repeated for the entire cervical region.
14. To assess the cranium for somatic dysfunction, the bed may be in the low Fowler position with the physician resting their elbows on the head of the bed for support. The cranium can be evaluated using the vault hold (see Chapter 53) or any other cranial hand contact the physician deems appropriate.

The above assessment has considered evaluation of the following:

- Sympathetic nervous system (SNS): Evidence of somatic dysfunction associated with the SNS may be indicated by TART in the thoracic and upper lumbar regions (viscerosomatic reflexes related to the SNS).
- Parasympathetic nervous system (PNS): Evidence of somatic dysfunction associated with the PNS may be indicated by TART in the sacral, suboccipital, and cranial regions.
- Lymphatic system: Evidence of dysfunction affecting lymphatic flow is indicated by assessing the four major diaphragms of the body (pelvic, thoracoabdominal, thoracic inlet, foramen magnum–tentorium cerebelli) and rib motion.
- Visceral dysfunction: Visceral dysfunction is reflected by the presence of anterior Chapman points, visceral palpation, and spinal somatic dysfunction that may be related to facilitated segments.
- Structural component: Asymmetries and abnormalities of the cervical, thoracic, rib, and pelvic areas affect optimal functioning of the biomechanical, neurologic, and respiratory-circulatory models of care.

TREATMENT OF THE HOSPITALIZED PATIENT

General Considerations

The ONMM specialist must weigh the risks and benefits of different OMT techniques in designing a unique plan for each hospitalized patient. Several studies on hospitalized patients including those with pneumonia and pancreatitis, have demonstrated efficacy in utilizing OMT. Findings include decreased length of hospital stay, reduced amount of medication needed and decreased morbidity.[10–16]

The overall goal is to promote homeostasis and the body's innate ability to self-heal. Each intervention requires energy input from the patient, to incorporate the bodily changes induced by the manipulation. Therefore, treatment for the very ill may be directed toward only those dysfunctions that impede the homeostatic processes. Long-standing or unrelated problems are often left for outpatient care. For example, it might not be necessary to address a short leg and mild functional scoliosis during a hospitalization for pneumonia, unless they are a contributing factor to impaired homeostasis during the acute illness. Experts in hospital-based OMT agree that the acutely ill patient may only tolerate short periods of treatment at a time, so manipulative efforts should focus on body regions that require immediate attention[7] (see Chapter 78 Osteopathic Considerations and Approaches in the Acutely Ill or Hospitalized Patient).

Differences in TART findings are helpful for following the patient's medical progress. Changes at a given level may represent viscerosomatic reflexes and may indicate possible early organ dysfunction. Likewise, improvement of TART findings that are thought to be related to a viscerosomatic reflex may indicate improved organ function. One notable exception occurs when treating the severely ill patient, whose vital resources or immune system has been exhausted or overwhelmed. These patients will fail to show the expected tissue texture changes at the site of organ dysfunction. Therefore, the presence of new tissue texture change in areas appropriate for the patient's illness can be a favorable sign.

When formulating a manipulative prescription[17] for an inpatient osteopathic treatment, determine the appropriate frequency and duration of treatment based on the patient's condition. In general, for very ill patients, it is better to provide frequent treatments of short durations utilizing techniques easily tolerated by the patient. The patient is usually treated once daily, although some literature suggests more frequent applications.[18–21] As the patient improves, the interval between treatments and treatment duration may be lengthened, if needed. The patient may also be able to tolerate the use of more direct techniques. Treat only those areas most likely to impair the recovery process, considering both lymphatic flow and autonomic balance. Psychiatric inpatients and those in drug and alcohol inpatient treatment programs may require a different schedule and are discussed separately.

If the patient is unfamiliar with OMT the ONMM specialist will briefly explain the philosophy and purpose of OMT and obtain informed consent for the OMT procedure.

- Simple language is key, such as "There are nerves from your spine that go to both the back muscles and the organs inside. When an internal organ is sick, a reflex is created that causes your back muscles to get tense. By treating your back, the reflex is calmed so that the organs can heal faster."
- Another example may be "When you have pneumonia (or congestive heart failure, etc.), the fluids in your body pool in your lungs, making you sicker. Your ribs don't move normally, making it more difficult to get rid of this fluid. The osteopathic treatment will help your ribs work more normally and help pump the fluids out of your lungs."

Though generally not used to describe OMT, one coauthor (BL) has found that most patients understand the concept of "therapy," which is thus a useful term for describing treatment. Further explanation may be provided if the patient expresses an interest in learning more about this type of treatment.

Treatment Protocol

The ONMM specialist must decide:

- Which areas most impair the patient's homeostatic balance
- Which techniques are best suited for the patient
- How much treatment the patient is likely to tolerate

In other words, a unique manipulative prescription is created, tailored to the patient's needs and findings. A general rule of thumb is to select at least one or two principal areas for treatment that are most relevant to the patient's recovery. Additional areas may be added, depending on the patient's response. This prevents important areas from being missed and the patient from being overtreated.

The ONMM specialist considers a treatment plan incorporating the five models of osteopathic care, with emphasis on any or all the following:

1. Autonomic nervous system function
2. Lymphatic flow
3. Respiratory excursion
4. Biomechanics
5. Visceral function

Some manipulative techniques that are appropriate in one situation may not be appropriate in another.

- For example, when treating a patient with fractures, avoid any positioning that could destabilize the fracture site.
- A patient in the intensive care unit with a myocardial infarction generally should not receive techniques using isometric patient contractions.

The decision of where and why to treat the patient resides with the physician and is part of the medical decision-making process.

Although the use of "protocols" is generally inconsistent with the osteopathic approach to patient care (which involves selecting the appropriate treatment for a patient based on the somatic

TABLE 45.1

Protocol for Treatment of Patients after Surgery or Trauma[a]

Type of Patient	Area	Technique
Postsurgical/trauma patient* Thoracic (i.e., thoracotomy, rib fracture, chest drainage tube, etc.)		
Sympathetic	T1–T5	PI, CS, DA
Parasympathetic	OA, cranium	Suboccipital ST, cranial,[b] CS, DA
Lymphatic	TI, abd. diaphragm	MR, RR, DA (no vigorous lymphatic pumps)
Other	Viscera	Visceral[c]
Abdominal surgery (cholecystectomy, bowel resection, etc.)		
Sympathetic	T1–T5 T5–T9 T10–L2	PI (to decrease respiratory complications), RR, CS, DA PI (if upper GI surgery), RR, CS, DA PI (to decrease ileus), RR, CS, DA
Parasympathetic	OA, cranium Sacrum	Suboccipital ST, cranial,[b] CS, DA Sacral rocking, CS, DA
Lymphatic	T1–T12 Thoracic inlet, abd. diaphragm	RR, CS, DA MR, DA
Other	Viscera	Visceral[c]
Medical patient (i.e., MI, pneumonia, peritonitis, etc.)		
Sympathetic	T1-T5	PI, CS, DA
Parasympathetic	OA, cranium	Suboccipital ST, cranial,[b] CS, DA
Lymphatic	T1–T12 Thoracic inlet, abd. diaphragm	RR MR lymphatic pump, DA
Other	a. Respiratory muscles, rib; b. abdomen	a. ST, MR, CS, DA; b. ST mesenteric release (to decrease sluggish bowel function), visceral[c]
Newborn infant feeding disorder/colic	Suboccipital area	ST, condylar decompression (to improve sucking and swallowing), reduce irritability[b]

PI, paraspinal inhibition; CS, counterstrain; DA, direct action (muscle energy, articular, etc.); ST, soft tissue; TI, thoracic inlet; abd. diaphragm, abdominal diaphragm; MR, myofascial release; RR, rib raising.

[a]This table is organized to encourage a thoughtful approach to treatment. It is time-efficient and does not miss treatment of critical areas. The protocol is organized under the headings of Sympathetic, Parasympathetic, Lymphatic, and Other for each area. The physician is encouraged to pick one or two techniques for each of the three functions to be assisted with OMT, yielding 3–6 techniques for each treatment encounter.

[b]For recommendations of appropriate cranial techniques indicated for patients with various medical illnesses, refer to *Osteopathy in the Cranial Field,*[22] *Craniosacral Therapy,*[27] or other texts on cranial technique.

[c]For recommendations of appropriate visceral techniques, see Barral JP, Mercier P. *Visceral Manipulation.* Eastland Press; 1988.

dysfunction(s) found), a review of the literature demonstrates how to formulate a treatment plan. The above examination protocol evaluates the neurologic, respiratory–circulatory, and biomechanical models of the patient, with a focus on the "transition areas" of transverse restrictors of fluid flow, that is, the diaphragms, and TART changes in the regions related to autonomic activity. A consistent approach to treatment can be derived from an analysis of these findings from the screening examination, coupled with a knowledge of the pathophysiology of the presenting complaint. Table 45.1 demonstrates different conditions the ONMM specialist may encounter in the hospital setting and what treatments may be considered.

Special Considerations

PATIENTS UNDERGOING DRUG AND ALCOHOL DETOXIFICATION AND REHABILITATION

During acute drug or alcohol detoxification, OMT may not be well tolerated. After the completion of detoxification, OMT may be useful in aiding the recovery process. Most patients undergoing drug or alcohol treatment have a long history of trauma and/or abuse. OMT should thus address the lasting effects of that trauma on both the musculoskeletal and emotional systems. Biopsychosocial considerations should also be addressed. Any medical or surgical conditions are treated according to the guidelines described earlier.

OMT in the inpatient psychiatric or drug/alcohol treatment setting is generally more effective than when used in the outpatient setting. Presumably, the intensive setting, where nutrition, medication, exercise, peer support, situation control, and counseling are structured into the patient's existence, increases the recovery rate holistically, in terms of the body, mind, and spirit.

PATIENTS IN THE INTENSIVE CARE UNIT AND/OR ON A VENTILATOR

Request assistance when moving a patient in the bed, or when changing the bed position, in order to prevent destabilizing any medical lines or tubes. Patients on ventilators can and should be treated with OMT. Depending on the patient's condition, consider using techniques that may alter the respiratory rate such as the pedal pump or classic lymphatic pump with caution.

PATIENTS IN ISOLATION

If the patient has been placed in some form of isolation, follow the required PPE protocol. While palpatory examination and OMT performed with gloves is not ideal, it is still assisting in optimizing the patient's health. Depending on the situation, even in the absence of isolation protocol, appropriate PPE should be donned to minimize risk of infection to the physician. In addition, during evaluation and treatment, both the physician and the patient should be positioned in a manner that reduces the physician's risk for infection.

PEDIATRIC PATIENTS

Newborns may require treatment in the nursery for cranial entrapment neuropathies, that have resulted in colic and feeding disorders.[22]

Evaluation of hospitalized pediatric patients is similar to what is listed above for adults. Treatment of pediatric patients for medical illnesses (such as pneumonia) and postoperative OMT for infants may focus on the following techniques:

- Articular
- Balanced ligamentous tension
- Balanced membranous tension
- Myofascial release

One treatment for children described by Max Gutensohn, DO (Personal communication—RJH), enables the physician to simultaneously articulate vertebral levels and encourage lymphatic flow while seemingly playing a game with the child. This is especially helpful in assisting recovery from respiratory disease.

1. The child is held in the air with the physician's hands encircling the child's chest, under the axillae.
2. The child's legs are then gently swung in a circle, thereby mobilizing the area just distal to the physician's hands on the torso.
3. To articulate other areas, hold the child higher or lower on the torso.

Gentle rib raising and spinal articulatory procedures in the lateral recumbent, supine, or seated positions are also well tolerated.

PATIENTS IN THE POSTOPERATIVE PHASE

There are numerous considerations for patients in the postoperative phase. Utilize caution when applying techniques near the postoperative site or site of injury. Vigorous techniques that could destabilize these areas should be avoided. Monitor for atelectasis which may be addressed with various forms of lymphatic pumps, rib raising or other appropriate techniques. Paraspinal inhibition may be useful in postoperative ileus.

INPATIENT PSYCHIATRY SETTING

The first osteopathic tenet states that the person is a unit of body, mind, and spirit. This supports the concept of treating a patient who has a mental health illness with OMT. If the psychiatric patient is hospitalized for a medical or surgical condition, the condition should be treated following the guidelines described earlier. Patients hospitalized for a mental health illness warrant an osteopathic structural evaluation and manipulative treatment, if indicated.

Older literature established dysautonomia as a significant factor in psychiatric disease, based in part on clinical observations at the Still-Hildreth Osteopathic Sanatorium. Dunn[23] discusses the association of autonomic dysfunction with psychiatric disease and supports this association with data from 1,000 patients who were diagnosed with schizophrenia. More than 50 of these patients demonstrated palpable somatic dysfunction at C2 and T4–T6 paravertebral regions of the spine. Per Alvares et al., "combined findings confirm substantial reductions in heart rate variability (HRV) across psychiatric disorders, and these effects remained significant even in medication-free individuals. Reductions in HRV may therefore represent a significant mechanism contributing to elevated cardiovascular risk in individuals with psychiatric disorders. The negative impact of specific medications on HRV suggests increased risk for cardiovascular disease in these groups, highlighting a need for treatment providers to consider modifiable cardiovascular risk factors to attenuate this risk." Evidence from pilot studies demonstrates that OMT affects HRV. While more research is needed, OMT may affect the ANS either with the utilization of Osteopathic Cranial Manipulative Medicine (OCMM) or by decreasing somatic load to regions exhibiting viscerosomatic reflexes, reducing the cardiovascular risk in this patient population.[24]

In addition to affecting autonomic reflexes, OMT may be beneficial to certain patients with mental health illness as patients may find it to be calming and soothing, and that the physician is engaging with them in a therapeutic manner.[25,26] Older studies indicate that while OMT provided within 24 hours of an electroconvulsive shock treatment (ECT) event does not appear to be productive, it has been observed to be effective when provided on the day after treatment.[27] In 2,288 examinations, Woods[28] demonstrated an altered rate of the cranial rhythmic impulse in patients with various psychiatric diseases, as compared with controls. Therefore, evaluation and treatment of the cranial and sacral regions should be highly considered in this patient population.[27]

Osteopathic physicians with experience in treating patients in an inpatient psychiatric setting report finding that the cranial base is "locked up" or the presence of sphenobasilar synchondrosis compression on structural exam. Treatment modalities included OCMM and emotional release techniques among others. The main goal of treatment was to free any restrictions of the cranium and any other areas of greatest restriction. They reported success in treating patients diagnosed with schizophrenia, manic depression, and multiple diagnoses (Personal communication K. Lossing, DO and B. Nourani, DO March 2024). One physician reported that he was the physician on duty at a state inpatient psychiatry ward one weekend a month. After treating several patients, he reported that they and others began to look forward to his visits and would request OMT when he was on duty. He emphasizes that one of the most important aspects of care is to treat and talk to each individual as a human being. As a healthcare provider in an institutional-like setting, it is critical to uphold each person's dignity and treat them according to the first osteopathic tenet; that they are a unique unit of body, mind and spirit, deserving of high-quality comprehensive osteopathic healthcare that includes OMT (Personal communication K. Lossing, DO March 2024).

While OMT is indicated for many patients with mental health illness, it may be contraindicated in some situations or diagnoses.

- A patient with paranoid schizophrenia may interpret a hands-on treatment modality as threatening and may not tolerate it well.
- Touch may be misinterpreted by patients with difficulty in differentiating fantasy from reality.
- For those with a history of abuse, manipulation may be seen as a sexual advance or assault.
- The physician may decide against providing OMT due to concerns of personal safety.

- It is generally advised not to utilize OMT as treatment when addressing patients with borderline personality disorder due to the intense and unstable relationships that often accompany this disorder (Personal communication K. Lossing, DO March 2024).

Some studies have been conducted in an out-patient setting to determine the effects of OMT on anxiety and depression including anxiety and depression related to chronic pain. While further research is needed, these studies indicate that OMT may reduce cortisol levels, pain, anxiety, mental health dysfunction and result in improvement in social-psychological self-assessments and self-care.[29–31]

As with all patients, the benefits of OMT for those with mental health illness must be weighed against its potential adverse outcomes. Most patients in inpatient settings tolerate and respond to the treatment extremely well (Personal communication K. Lossing March 2024).

Documenting the ONMM Consult

After evaluating and treating a patient, the ONMM consultation should be documented as follows:

1. Date and time of consult.
2. Name of the attending physician and reason for consult request.
3. History and a statement that the history was obtained from the patient or other, such as family member.
4. Physical and structural examination findings: include the position(s) in which the patient was examined, for example, sitting, supine, and lateral recumbent and location of TART findings.
5. Labs, diagnostic tests, imaging reviewed.
6. Procedure Note: include date and time of procedure, indication for treatment, duration of procedure, discussion of risks, benefits and alternatives, counseling of potential side effects and aftercare, informed consent, regions treated, what techniques were used, how well patient tolerated the procedure, subjective and objective improvements, and what complications, if any, arose. Use standard nomenclature as defined in the *Glossary of Osteopathic Terminology* (see "Glossary").
7. Assessment: List the medical diagnoses, including identified somatic dysfunction diagnoses. Include those diagnoses that are directly related to the somatic dysfunction, the disease process, and the viscerosomatic and somatovisceral reflexes.
8. Treatment Plan: This includes the manipulative prescription if OMT is indicated, recommendations for imaging, and if appropriate, lifestyle modifications, exercise prescription, nutrition recommendations/counseling. Recommendations for further evaluation and/or specialties, for example, OT, PT, respiratory therapists, medical specialties, etc., may be included here. Direct discussion with other consultants and/or the primary team regarding recommendations often results in more timely and comprehensive care and management of the patient and should be documented. Follow-up recommendations should be included in the treatment plan. Note that a specialist's participation in continued follow-up care is at the discretion of the attending physician; however the ONMM specialist may document their recommendation to "follow as indicated by examination findings and response to treatment" or "no continued ONMM follow-up necessary in the hospital setting."
9. An expression of thanks to the requesting physician for the consultation and allowing for the participation in the care of this patient.

FOLLOW-UP EVALUATION AND TREATMENT

1. Begin the follow-up examination with a review of any new imaging, followed by a review of the medical record since the last evaluation.
2. Take an interval history.
3. Perform the physical and osteopathic structural examination following the protocol described above, noting any changes in response to the previous treatment or in the disease process.
4. The areas to be treated may change with each evaluation and are determined by the interval history and physical and structural examination findings. The tolerance for a longer treatment may increase as the patient improves. Less frequent treatment may be needed as the patient's overall health improves.

THE ONMM SPECIALIST IN THE OUTPATIENT/AMBULATORY SETTING

A distinctive element of a visit to an ONMM specialist is the lens through which the specialist views the patient with regard to the OPP. The patient is typically viewed through the four osteopathic tenets; the person is a unit of body, mind, and spirit, the body has self-healing and regulating capabilities, structure and function are interrelated and that rational treatment is based on the above.

Patients may be referred to an ONMM specialist by their primary care physician or other specialties or may self-refer. This is a critical point to understand, as this may be the patient's first encounter with any physician. The ONMM specialist may be the first physician to evaluate a patient's chief complaint. Conversely, ONMM specialists may also see a patient who has seen multiple healthcare providers in various healthcare settings or patients who feel that they have exhausted all avenues of medicine and view the ONMM specialist as a "last resort."

Therefore, it is imperative that the ONMM specialist conducts a comprehensive history and physical. They will often start with a "clean slate" and gather the history, perform their evaluation and execute their treatment plan within the context of the osteopathic philosophy and four tenets. The ONMM specialist will often evaluate and treat the patient utilizing the five osteopathic models of care; biomechanical, respiratory-circulatory, metabolic-energetic, neurologic, and biopsychosocial as a framework.

Osteopathic History and Data Gathering

The ONMM specialist obtains the chief complaint and a detailed history within the context of the osteopathic tenets. This should include the history of present illness, medical and surgical history, allergies (environmental, medical and food), medications and supplements, family and social history and review of systems. The ONMM specialist generally focuses on those elements that interfere with the unity of the body–mind–spirit relationship, disturb the normal homeostatic processes and self-healing mechanisms of the body, and alter the dynamic interplay of structure and function.

Therefore, the ONMM specialist may place particular emphasis on the following while gathering the patient's history:

- Birth history
- Childhood illnesses
- Vaccination history
- Dental history including orthodontia, appliances, dental surgeries and procedures, etc.
- Hospitalizations and reason for hospitalization
- History of abuse including physical, sexual, emotional, verbal, mental, etc.

- Episodes of loss of consciousness
- Previous injuries, motor vehicle accidents, trauma, falls, fractures, etc.
- Presence of known short leg
- Known structural abnormalities such as scoliosis and plagiocephaly
- Exercise level and activities
- Sports and repetitive motion activities
- Hobbies (sedentary and active)
- Social, living and work environments
- Chronic pain syndromes
- Chronic organic diseases, especially those which have neuromusculoskeletal components or effects
- Medications and/or supplements that affect the neuromusculoskeletal system
- Previous experience with OMT and response to it
- Previous experience with other manual medicine modalities
- Previous other manipulative interventions (physical therapy, chiropractic, massage therapy, and other body workers), as well as alternative medical interventions (acupuncture, Reiki, and other types of healers)

The ONMM specialist may review notes from other healthcare providers and any available diagnostic data (lab results, original imaging, electromyography, and nerve conduction studies, etc.) before proceeding with the physical exam. This additional information may help in guiding portions of the physical and structural examination, especially in complex patient cases. Depending on the patient, this information may be summarized in the patient's history or included below in the objective findings.

Physical Examination

The ONMM specialist integrates the osteopathic palpatory and structural examination into the overall physical examination of the patient. This should include general observation of the patient's condition, a detailed neurologic and musculoskeletal exam and examination of other body systems relevant to the patient's chief complaint and general overall health.

The screening portion of the osteopathic structural exam will identify regions of the body warranting further osteopathic evaluation and is followed by a regional and then a segmental exam. The patient is typically examined in at least two positions (standing, seated, supine, prone, lateral recumbent). Changes in palpatory findings with changes in the patient's position can provide clues to primary and secondary somatic dysfunctions and where the specialist may need to focus their treatment for that particular visit.

TREATMENT PLAN

The history and physical examination allow the ONMM specialist to generate a differential diagnosis and determine whether OMT is indicated at the time of the office visit, whether further workup is needed prior to considering OMT, or whether OMT is not indicated. If OMT is indicated, consent for treatment is obtained. The ONMM specialist will then select the most appropriate osteopathic techniques to address areas of somatic dysfunction, taking into consideration the four osteopathic tenets and incorporating the five models of osteopathic care.

Further development of the treatment plan generally includes shared decision making with the patient on how to continue to optimize the patient's health through appropriate nutrition and exercise, lifestyle modifications and improved ergonomics at home and at work. The ONMM specialist may recommend other specialties or interventions including dentistry, PT, OT, mental health therapists or other medical specialties such as cardiology, GI, neurology, pain management, orthopedics, etc. Imaging, diagnostic tests and lab work may also be ordered.

Potential side effects of the treatment should be reviewed with the patient. The expected short- and long-term goals of treatment should also be discussed with the patient. Some patients with acute issues may necessitate one to a few visits before their symptoms completely resolve and then return only when another issue arises. In the presence of chronic conditions some patients may require more regular evaluation and treatment. Follow-up is generally on a case-by-case basis. As with any other medical visit, emergency department protocol or guidance should be provided in the case of symptoms worsening or if there is an adverse event.

As with all medical encounters, the documentation of the office visit and the billing and coding for the visit should be completed in an accurate and timely fashion.

CONCLUSION

The ONMM specialist is a valuable addition to the osteopathic profession. The role of the ONMM specialist is to provide clinical expertise upon request and to expand the ever-evolving osteopathic concept. The ONMM specialist plays a crucial role in the development and application of OPP, especially in the areas of education, research, and service.

ACKNOWLEDGMENTS

The authors and editors of this chapter would like to acknowledge the scholarly contributions of Drs. Ray Hruby, Karen Steele, and Natalie Nevins.

REFERENCES

1. Eggleston A. *President's Report. Academy of Applied Osteopathy Directory.* American Academy of Osteopathy; 1959.
2. Academy of Osteopathy. AAO Fellowship Program. Accessed February 27, 2024. https://www.academyofosteopathy.org/aao-fellowship-program
3. ACGME Program Requirements for Osteopathic Neuromusculoskeletal Medicine (ONMM). 2022. Accessed February 27, 2024. https://www.acgme.org/globalassets/pfassets/programrequirements/275_onmm_2022
4. Stiles EG. Osteopathic manipulation in a hospital environment. *J Am Osteopath Assoc.* 1976;76(4):243–258.
5. Hruby RJ. Pathophysiologic models: aids to the selection of manipulative techniques. *J Am Osteopath Assoc.* 1991;1(3):8–10. Accessed November 6, 2024. https://www.academyofosteopathy.org/assets/aaoj/AAOJ_Fall1991.pdf
6. Zink JG. Respiratory and circulatory care: the conceptual model. *Osteopath Ann.* 1977;5(3):10. Accessed November 6, 2024. https://archive.org/details/sim_osteopathic-annals_1977_5_index/page/50/mode/2up
7. Larson NJ. Summary of site and occurrence of paraspinal soft tissue changes of patients in the intensive care unit. *J Am Osteopath Assoc.* 1976; 75(9):840–842.
8. Owens C. *An Endocrine Interpretation of Chapman's Reflexes by the interpreter.* American Academy of Osteopathy; 1963.
9. Jones LH. *Strain Counterstrain.* American Academy of Osteopathy; 1981.
10. Radjieski JM, Lumley MA, Cantieri MS. Effect of osteopathic manipulative treatment of length of stay for pancreatitis: a randomized pilot study. *J Am Osteopath Assoc.* 1998;98(5):264–272.
11. Noll D, Shores JH, Gamber RG, Herron KM, Swift J Jr. Benefits of osteopathic manipulative treatment for hospitalized elderly patients with pneumonia. *J Am Osteopath Assoc.* 2000;100(12):776–782.

12. Clark RC, McCombs TM. Post operative osteopathic manipulative protocol for delivery by students in an allopathic environment. *AAO J.* 2006: 19–21. Retrieved June 2, 2016.
13. Noll DR, Degenhardt BF, Fossum C, Hensel K. Clinical and research protocol for osteopathic manipulative treatment of elderly patients with pneumonia. *J Am Osteopath Assoc.* 2008;108(9):508–516.
14. Crow WT, Gorodinsky L. Does osteopathic manipulative treatment (OMT) improve outcomes in patients who develop postoperative ileus: a retrospective chart review. *Int J Osteopath Med.* 2009;12(1): 32–37.
15. Baltazar GA, Betler MP, Akella K, Khatri R, Asaro R, Chendrasekhar A. Effect of osteopathic manipulative treatment on incidence of postoperative ileus and hospital length of stay in general surgical patients. *J Am Osteopath Assoc.* 2013;113(3):204–209. Erratum in: *J Am Osteopath Assoc.* 2013;113(4):271.
16. Probst P, Büchler E, Doerr-Harim C, et al. Randomised controlled pilot trial on feasibility, safety and effectiveness of osteopathic manipulative treatment following major abdominal surgery (OMANT pilot trial). *Int J Osteopath Med.* 2016;20:31–40.
17. Kuchera WA, Kuchera ML. *Osteopathic Principles in Practice.* 2nd ed. Greyden Press; 1994:297–302.
18. Herrmann EP. Postoperative adynamic ileus: its prevention and treatment by osteopathic manipulation. *Precepts Pract.* 1965:163–164. Accessed November 6, 2024. https://osteopathic.org/index.php?aam-media=/wp-content/uploads/2019-rome-southeast-bowers-handout-3.pdf
19. Young GS. Post-operative osteopathic manipulation. *Academy of Applied Osteopathy Yearbook.* American Academy of Osteopathy; 1970:77–82.
20. Rumney IC. Osteopathic manipulative treatment of infectious disease. *Osteopath Ann.* 1974:29–33.
21. Noll DR, Degenhardt BF, Morley TF, et al. Efficacy of osteopathic manipulation as an adjunctive treatment for hospitalized patients with pneumonia: a randomized controlled trial. *Osteopath Med Prim Care.* 2010;4:2.
22. Magoun HI. *Osteopathy in the Cranial Field.* 2nd ed. Journal Printing Co.; 1966:234, 263.
23. Dunn FE. Osteopathic concepts in psychiatry. *J Am Osteopath Assoc.* 1950;49(7):354–357.
24. Curi ACC, Maior Alves AS, Silva JG. Cardiac autonomic response after cranial technique of the fourth ventricle (cv4) compression in systemic hypertensive subjects. *J Bodyw Mov Ther.* 2018;22(3):666–672.
25. Ching LM. The Still-Hildreth Sanatorium: a history and chart review. *AAO J.* 2014;24(4):12–25.
26. Bradford SG. Role of osteopathic manipulative therapy in emotional disorders: a physiologic hypothesis. *J Am Osteopath Assoc.* 1965;64: 484–493.
27. Upledger JE, Vredevoogd JD. *Craniosacral Therapy.* Eastland Press; 1983:268.
28. Woods JM, Woods RH. A physical finding related to psychiatric disorders. *J Am Osteopath Assoc.* 1961;60:988–993.
29. Edwards DJ, Toutt C. An evaluation of osteopathic treatment on psychological outcomes with patients suffering from chronic pain: a prospective observational cohort study collected through a health and well-being academy. *Health Psychol Open.* 2018;5(1):2055102918774684.
30. Dixon L, Fotinos K, Sherifi E, et al. Effect of osteopathic manipulative therapy on generalized anxiety disorder. *J Am Osteopath Assoc.* 2020;120(3):133–143.
31. Abraham C, Sloan SNB, Coker C, et al. Osteopathic manipulative treatment as an intervention to reduce stress, anxiety, and depression in first responders: a pilot study. *Mo Med.* 2021;118(5):435–441.

46 Balanced Ligamentous Tension and Ligamentous Articulatory Strain

WILLIAM THOMAS CROW

KEY CONCEPTS

- Balanced ligamentous tension (BLT) and ligamentous articular strain (LAS) are original osteopathic techniques derived from the teachings of A. T. Still, preserved and articulated by his early students through the successive generations.
- In BLT and LAS techniques, emphasis is placed on the role of ligaments in maintaining articular dysfunction.
- The three cardinal principles of BLT and LAS are disengagement of the dysfunctional area (compression/decompression), exaggeration of the dysfunctional pattern (returning to the original position of injury), and balanced tension of ligaments (maintained until release).
- Retracing the path of injury via ligamentous tension and strain is done anatomically and facilitated by respiratory cooperation of the patient.

CASE STUDY

SUBJECTIVE

A 50-year-old man complains of pain in the left hip. It started several weeks ago after climbing six flights of stairs at work. The pain is worse in flexion and going up the stairs. He tolerates going down the stairs easier. The pain radiates from the groin mainly into the left thigh region. However, he is more functional and can bear weight on his left leg. Rest makes it better. It is worse at the end of the day than in the morning. Ibuprofen relieves most of his pain, but it is now causing him some "stomach burn."

OBJECTIVE

Physical exam is normal except as follows:

Neurologic: Less sensitivity to touch noted in the S1–S2 distribution.

Musculoskeletal: Muscle spasm noted in the left adductors. His gait is antalgic.

Osteopathic Structural Exam

Patient was found to have tenderness, asymmetry, restriction of range of motion, and tissue texture changes (TART) in the following areas:

Lumbar spine: Lumbar paraspinal muscles tight bilaterally, L4–L5 extended, rotated left, and sidebent left
Sacrum: Posterior sacrum—left
Pelvis: Inferior pubic symphysis shear, right; tight piriformis, left
Lower extremities: Adductors tight—left

ASSESSMENT

Left hip pain
Muscle spasm
Somatic dysfunction of the lumbar spine, sacrum, pelvis, and lower extremity regions

PLAN

OMT using BLT and LAS to the four regions of somatic dysfunction, tolerated well with no complications. Rest and ice to painful areas, if needed. He is to try acetaminophen as needed for pain and is advised to discontinue ibuprofen use. Increase in oral fluids for 24 to 48 hours. Stretching exercises provided for the lumbar spine, pelvis, and lower extremities.

INTRODUCTION

Balanced ligamentous tension (BLT) and balanced membranous tension (BMT) techniques to treat ligamentous and membranous articular strains, respectively, were concepts of Dr. Andrew Taylor Still, founder of osteopathy. William G. Sutherland, DO, an early student of Still, reinforced these concepts in his teaching. Rebecca Lippincott, DO, and Howard Lippincott, DO, students of Sutherland, wrote the principles and techniques down and subsequently published them as the "Osteopathic Technique of Wm. G. Sutherland" in the 1949 *Year Book of the Academy of Applied Osteopathy*.[1] Anne Wales, DO, another student of Sutherland, from the northeastern region of the United States, used the term "BLT" to describe her treatment style utilizing these principles. Another student of Sutherland, Rollin Becker, DO, from Dallas, Texas, used the term "ligamentous articular strain (LAS)" to describe his treatment style utilizing the same principles. The terms come from the abovementioned article where it states "Osteopathic lesions are strains of the tissues of the body. When they involve joints it is the ligaments that are primarily affected so the term 'ligamentous articular strain' is the one preferred by Dr. Sutherland. The ligaments of a joint are normally on a balanced, reciprocal tension and seldom if ever are they completely relaxed throughout the normal range of movement... Since it is the ligaments that are primarily involved in the maintenance of the lesion it is they, not muscular leverage, that are used as the main agency for reduction....This is the point of balanced tension."[1]

HISTORY

At the time that Dr. Sutherland received his osteopathic training at Kirksville, Dr. Still was still supervising the instruction given at the college. The principles that were taught had to conform exactly to his concept. Dr. Sutherland made good use of every opportunity to learn and understand them and adhered closely in his thinking and practice to Dr. Still's principles throughout his professional career.

"In consequence, the technique, which he presented to us, is a reflection of the clear vision of our founder."[2] Sutherland related the following:

> Dr. Still gave me a lesson one day along with the rest of our class. A member of our class had stepped on a rusty nail. All the appropriate surgical management and cleansing had been used, but it would not heal. It began to look an angry red, so we called in the Old Doctor. He said, 'You damn fools!' and we were. We had not stopped to consider that when the patient stepped on that nail he drew his leg up away from it. The lasting problem was not the nail or the original wound; it was what occurred in the sudden jerk of the patient that caused a membranous strain between the fibula and the tibia.[2]

Sutherland's student H. A. Lippincott, DO, elaborated on this:

> Since it is the ligaments that are primarily involved in the maintenance of the lesion it is they, not muscular leverage, that are used as the main agency for reduction. The articulation is carried in the direction of the lesion position as far as is necessary to cause tension of the weakened elements of the ligamentous structure to be equal to or slight in excess of the tension of those that are not strained. This is the point of balanced tension. Forcing the articulation back and away from the direction of lesion strains the ligaments that are normal and unopposed, and if it is done with thrust or jerks there is a definite possibility of separating fibers of ligaments from their bony attachments. When the tension is properly balanced the respiratory or muscular cooperation of the patient is employed to overcome the resistance of the defense mechanism of the body to the release of the lesion.[1]

Sutherland is best remembered for his application of osteopathic techniques for the cranium and sacrum. (See Chapter 53 Osteopathic Cranial Manipulative Medicine for further information about this approach.) However, it is clear that he had learned Dr. Still's techniques for treating the whole body and was only expounding more on an area that was receiving insufficient attention at that time, that is, the motion of the individual bones in the cranium. This is why Sutherland, later in his life, held that he had just pulled back a veil so that others could see more clearly.

While LAS techniques may not be the only techniques used by Drs. Still and Sutherland, they are the ones that both of them described. For example, Dr. Still wrote:

> Without going into detail further, I will say that all dislocations, partial or complete, can be adjusted by this rule: First loosen the dislocated end from other tissues, then gently bring it back to its original place.[3]

Carl Phillip McConnell, DO, MD, who had been treated by Still and was one of the faculty at the American School of Osteopathy, described Still's treatment technique in his book, *The Practice of Osteopathy*, by writing:

> Disengage the articular points that have become locked. Reduce the dislocation by retracing the path along which the parts were dislocated. One can readily see that a dislocated ball and socket joint could be reduced only by the dislocated bone retracing the path through which it left its socket as the capsular ligament would at once prevent its returning to the socket by any path other than that taken when dislocated. This applies to all dislocations to a greater or lesser extent.[4]

In 1917, Edythe Ashmore, DO, wrote that there were two methods commonly employed by osteopaths in the correction of lesions, the older of which is the traction method and the latter the direct method or thrust.[5] In a footnote, she wrote:

> The term "direct" is preferred for the reason that the imitators of osteopathy have given to the word "thrust" an objectionable meaning of harshness.[5]

As noted previously, the older method is now known as LAS techniques, while the newer methods refer to high-velocity–low-amplitude techniques. Of the former, she wrote:

> Those who employ the traction method secure the relaxation of the tissues about the articulation by what has been termed exaggeration of the lesion, a motion in the direction of the forcible movement which produced the lesion, as if its purpose were to increase the deformity. C. P. McConnell states that this disengages the tissues that are holding the parts in the abnormal position. The exaggeration is held, traction made upon the joint, replacement initiated and then completed by reversal of the forces.[5]

RECIPROCAL TENSION

Sutherland coined the terms "reciprocal tension ligaments" and "reciprocal tension mechanism" to describe the role of ligaments in joints.[2]

- An example of this is the wrist as it moves into flexion displacing the distal row of carpal bones toward the dorsal surface of the arm. During extension, the reverse occurs. Each bone then rotates as the group is moved. The tension of the carpal ligaments remains constant and constantly shifts its balance. This is a key concept in Dr. Sutherland's approach.

The type of motion which may occur at any given articulation is determined by the following three elements:

1. The shape of the joint surfaces
2. The position of the ligaments
3. The forces of the muscles acting upon the joint

Ligaments do not stretch and contract as muscles do; consequently, the tension in a ligament has very little variation.

- The tension distributed throughout the ligaments of any given joint is balanced.
- In normal movements, as the joint changes position, the relationships between the joint's ligaments also change, but the total tension within the ligamentous articular mechanism does not.

The distribution of tension between the ligaments is altered, however, when the joint is affected by injury, inflammation, and/or mechanical forces. This is what happens in somatic dysfunction.

- The distribution and vector of tension within any given ligament will change according to the position of strain in the joint.
- However, the shared tension within the ligamentous articular mechanism of any given joint remains constant as long as the ligament is not damaged.
- While the latter case will most assuredly result in a strain to the balance of the articular ligaments, the ligaments do not need to be disrupted for the balance to be distorted.
- The distortion in balance is a mechanical strain, which may or may not involve an anatomical one.

In any somatic dysfunction, there is always a strain. H. A. Lippincott, DO, describes LAS as follows:

> Osteopathic lesions are strains of the tissues of the body. When they involve joints, it is the ligaments that are primarily affected, so the term 'ligamentous articular strain' is the one preferred by Dr. Sutherland. The ligaments of a joint are normally on a balanced, reciprocal tension and seldom if ever are they completely relaxed throughout the normal range of movement. When the motion is carried beyond that range, the tension is unbalanced and the elements of the ligamentous structure that limit motion in that direction are strained and weakened. The lesion is maintained by the overbalance of the reciprocal tension by the elements that have not been strained. This locks the articular mechanism or prevents its free and normal movement. The unbalanced tension causes the bones to assume a position that nearly reproduces that of the original strain produced than would be the case if the tension were normal, and the weakened part of the ligaments permits motion in the direction of the lesion in excess of normal. The range of movement in the opposite direction is limited by the more firm and unopposed tension of the elements which had not been strained.[1]

FASCIA

Still looked to the fascia for the source of disease.[3] Strains in the fascia not only pull bones out of position and impinge on nerves, vessels, and lymphatics but also impede the flow of the interstitial fluid. At the 1998 Cranial Academy Conference, the osteopathic anatomist Frank Willard, PhD, stated that the fascia should be defined and studied as a system unto itself and not simply as an obscuring material hiding more important tissues.[6] From an embryologic standpoint, the fascia, bone, and all the connective tissues arise from the mesenchyme. See Chapter 7 The Fascial System of the Body for further information.

CONNECTIVE TISSUE

Connective tissue makes up about 16% of the body's weight and stores approximately 25% of the body's total water.

- It forms the biologic building blocks of the skin, muscles, nerve sheaths, tendons, ligaments, fascia, blood vessels, joint capsules, periosteum, aponeuroses, bones, adipose tissue, and cartilage and the framework for the internal organs.[7]
- Connective tissue, with a special emphasis on fascia, has unique deformative characteristics.

CRIMPING

If there are abnormal stresses found in the collagen that makes up the tendons and ligaments, then the tendons and ligaments will be deformed and their basic functions will be affected.

- Tendons attach muscle fibers to bones and transmit muscle forces, and the ligaments check excess motion of the joints and guide joint motion.[8]
- Ligaments have a less consistent parallel arrangement of collagen than tendons.[9]
- There was a loss of water and of glycosaminoglycans in the ground substance, a lubricant found between the collagen fibers, which are the primary connective tissue fibers that compose the fascia.[10,11]
- Pascal's law states that "Pressure applied to a liquid at rest from any point is transmitted equally in all directions."[13] The human body consists of many closed fluid systems like the plastic bags that respond exactly as predicted by Pascal's principle; that is, an increase in the pressure of fluid in one of the plastic bags will distribute its pressure to other portions of the body.

The effects of the hydrodynamic fluctuation of body fluids restore motion and life to "dead spots," or somatic dysfunctions, changing the structure of the tissues.

- Research has shown that changes in the structure of the tissues of the body alter the structure of the cytoskeleton, which in turn can actually alter gene expression and cellular metabolism.[14]
- Therefore, it is reasonable to deduce that by manipulating the tissues of the body, one can bring about significant change on all levels. This concept is echoed in the osteopathic literature.

Every organ in the body exhibits the phenomenon of pulsations or rhythmic action, which is incessantly active, dynamic, and highly mobile, resulting in forward, backward, sideways, and rotational fluid movement.[12] These pulsations appear to be ubiquitous. They propel the extracellular fluids into and across the semipermeable membranes of cells everywhere and deliver nutrients and remove metabolic waste products even from synovial spaces, bursae, and other nonvascular compartments. Every cell membrane of the body is continuously and rhythmically bathed with these essential fluids in a fashion similar to the ebb and flow of the ocean upon the beach. See Chapter 4 Inherent Motion, Rhythms, and Oscillations for further information.

Fluid dynamics, joint physiology, fascia, and vectors of injury may look on the surface to be unrelated but, on a deeper level, are found to be closely connected. Osteopathic physicians are continuously advancing palpatory diagnostic and manual treatment skills and studying the interrelatedness of biomechanics and the health/illness/disease spectrum. With the acquisition of knowledge, skill, and experience, the osteopathic student's perspective changes from a view of the human body as a skeleton, with other tissues hanging on as it were, to a view of the body as a moving, living organism with a skeleton found within it. As a result, attention will move from the bones and joints to the fascia and fluid dynamics. It is important to understand the scientific principles upon which these techniques are based in order to apply them most successfully. If one understands the principles, one can then create one's own techniques.

PROPOSED MECHANISM OF ACTION

As Lippincott so elegantly described, the ligaments of a joint are normally on a balanced, reciprocal tension and seldom if ever are they completely relaxed throughout the normal range of movement. When the motion is carried beyond that range, the tension is unbalanced and the elements of the ligamentous structure that limit motion in that direction are strained and weakened. The lesion is maintained by the overbalance of the reciprocal tension by the elements that have not been strained. This locks the articular mechanism or prevents its free and normal movement. The unbalanced tension causes the bones to assume a position that nearly reproduces that of the original strain produced than would be the case if the tension were normal, and the weakened part of the ligaments permits motion in the direction of the lesion in excess of normal. The range of movement in the opposite direction is limited by the more firm and unopposed tension of the elements which had not been strained.[1]

When an injury occurs, the joint becomes compressed and/or subluxed, altering its normal physiologic position and thereby affecting the state of BLT. The goal of treatment is to restore and maintain balanced tension within the affected ligamentous structures of the joint.[15]

INDICATIONS

BLT and LAS are used to treat somatic dysfunction that include LASs.

CONTRAINDICATIONS

Most of the contraindications are relative and involve the actual site being treated. The osteopathic physician should use clinical judgment at all times but it is best to either avoid or use caution performing these techniques at the site of a fracture, open wound, soft tissue or bony infection, abscess, deep venous thrombosis, aortic aneurysm, recent postoperative site (avoid dehiscence) and in conditions of anticoagulation and disseminated or focal neoplasm.

SAFETY AND EFFICACY

BLT and LAS are generally safe and well-tolerated. There are no known reports of complications arising from these two treatment methods. Side effects similar to post exercise soreness have been observed and are generally self-limiting.

PRINCIPLES OF DIAGNOSIS

Once an area has been localized through a screening exam and palpatory exam, passive motion testing for a region, local tissues or a joint is performed to identify a restrictive barrier and a position of ease. This is often done with small precise movements to allow the physician to assess the tension in the ligaments in all directions of motion.

PRINCIPLES OF CORRECTIVE TECHNIQUE

The first and most important step in treatment is establishing BLT in the articular mechanism so that the body's inherent forces can resolve the strain. The point of BLT exists somewhere between the tension created by the strain and the physiologic normal setting of the joint. When placed in this precise position, where the ligaments have the least amount of strain, the physiologic forces of the body become the activating forces to resolve the somatic dysfunction.[16]

Somatic dysfunction may be regarded as an impediment to the flow of the interstitial fluid.

- The fluid moves around areas of dysfunction like a stream flows around a stone.
- The goal of the treatment is to remove the stone and let the stream flow through unimpeded.
- Take that which is palpated as hard and make it soft.
- When one feels the flow come through the dysfunctional area, the treatment of that area is complete.[17]

Once an area of dysfunction has been located, compress or decompress the joint or fascial plane to disengage the injury so that the displaced bone can be moved. (This is similar to pushing in the clutch on a car to shift gears.)

Then, carry the injured part in the direction of least resistance, which is usually returning it to the position to which it was forced during the original injury.

The steps are as follows:

1. Disengage: Compress or decompress the joint or fascial plane, increasing the pressure or traction until able to move the injured part.
2. Exaggerate: Carry the injured part back to the original position of injury by, for example, rotating, flexing, "sidebending," or "side shifting" until the balance point or still point is found. For example, if the right ankle is slightly inverted, exaggerate the position of the ankle by taking it into a more inverted position, which is how the injury occurred originally.
3. Balance: Maintain the area of dysfunction in the position of injury, that is, the balance point or still point, until a release occurs. The bone will move slightly farther in the direction of exaggeration. When the strain corrects, the physician will palpate a shift or change in tension as the joint moves spontaneously toward physiologic neutral.[18] The cranial rhythmic impulse or tide returns through the tissues that were injured. Once the correction has occurred, the injured ligaments may start their 3-month healing process.

ILLUSTRATIVE TECHNIQUES

BLT of the Axial Spine: Thoracic[19]

Symptoms/diagnosis: Thoracic pain due to somatic dysfunction and/or degenerative processes of the thoracic spine.

1. The patient is supine on the treatment table.
2. The physician sits at the side of the table.
3. The physician slides their hands under the patient, contacting the spinous processes of the affected segment(s) with the finger pads.
4. The physician observes the flexion/extension movement of the vertebrae with inhalation and exhalation through their finger pads and also notes any lateral motion.
5. Using the spinous processes as handles, encourage the spinous processes into flexion or extension with the appropriate phase of breath and apply gentle pressure to encourage right and left rotation to assess freedom of rotation.
6. The physician uses the spinous process to direct the vertebra into a position of balance (flexion or extension, rotation and sidebending) relative to the one inferior to it.
7. The patient may be asked to augment sidebending by dorsiflexing the ipsilateral foot for segments inferior to T6 or by elevating the opposite shoulder or sidebending the head for segments superior to T6. Flexion and extension may be augmented by asking the patient to inhale or exhale.
8. Once the point of balance is established, the position is held through a few respiratory cycles until the point of balance shifts to a physiologic state and there is decreased tension of the affected ligaments.

BLT of the Ribs[19]

Symptoms/diagnosis: Rib pain or altered mechanics and motion due to rib somatic dysfunction.

1. The patient is supine.
2. The physician is seated at the side of the dysfunctional rib.
3. The physician places one hand on the posterior aspect the affected rib. The other hand contacts the transverse or spinous processes of the vertebrae articulating with the rib.
4. The rib is gently tractioned anterolaterally while the physician uses the transverse or spinous processes to establish balance

between the vertebra-rub unit (comprised of the rib and the articulating vertebrae). Postural and respiratory cooperation may be used to find the point of balanced tension.

5. The point of balanced tension is held through a series of the patient's respiratory cycle until a change of tension is palpated.
6. This may also be accomplished with the patient in the seated position. To optimize the point of balanced tension, the patient may be instructed to rotate their body toward the affected side.

BLT of the Upper Extremity: Clavicle[20]

Symptoms/diagnosis: Pain and/or decreased range of motion of the upper extremity, shoulder, and clavicles.

1. The physician assesses the position of the clavicle by comparing the levels of the clavicular heads at the sternoclavicular joints. Address the inferior clavicle first.
2. The patient is seated facing the physician.
3. The costoclavicular ligament is the fulcrum for superior/inferior motion of the clavicle, located about 1-inch lateral to the sternoclavicular joint. In order to utilize this fulcrum to address the clavicle, the physician does the following:
   a. The physician contacts the distal end of the affected clavicle with one hand resting the fingers across the acromioclavicular (AC joint) and the pad of the thumb under the distal clavicle. The other thumb is placed under the proximal end of the clavicle just lateral to the sternoclavicular joint.
   b. The patient is instructed to lean forward onto the physician's thumbs.
   c. The physician applies gentle pressure to the shoulder at the acromial end until a subtle disengagement or "give" is palpated at the AC joint. This may be described as carrying the thumbs slightly laterally, superiorly, and posteriorly.[21] The patient is instructed to move the contralateral shoulder posteriorly to disengage the sternal portion. These two movements are performed to establish a balance in the ligaments of the articulation.
   d. This position is held as the patient performs several respiratory cycles until a "shift" or "glide" of the clavicle is palpated (usually in a lateral and posterior direction).[21]
   e. The patient is instructed to slowly bring the contralateral shoulder back to neutral and to sit up straight.
   f. The physician maintains contact with the clavicle until the patient is seated upright and all weight is removed from the physician's thumb.
   g. The clavicles are reassessed and if needed, the opposite clavicle is addressed.

LAS of the Forearm and Elbow[22]

Symptoms/diagnosis: Pain and/or decreased range of motion of the elbow due to somatic dysfunction of the upper extremity and/or strains of the interosseous membrane between the radius and ulna.

1. The patient may be seated or supine.
2. The physician is positioned slightly in front of and at the side of the affected elbow, facing the patient.
3. Flex the patient's elbow to 90 degrees. The physician then contacts the patient's proximal olecranon process with the thumb and index finger of one hand so that they are located on the edge of the grooves on either side of the olecranon process. The physician uses the other hand to contact the dorsum of the affected hand, palmarflex the wrist, and fully pronate the forearm.
4. The physician compresses the forearm between the two hands, drawing the patient's elbow toward extension.
5. If dysfunction is present, the physician will have the sense of a firm barrier as the elbow is brought into extension.
6. The physician maintains steady balanced pressure against the barrier until the elbow extends and the thumb and index finger slide through the grooves on either side of the olecranon process.
7. This complex is reassessed for any torsional strains of the radial head, lateral or medial deviations of the ulna, pain, and range of motion.

BLT of the Sacroiliac Joint[20]

Symptoms/diagnosis: Low back pain or hip pain due to somatic dysfunction of the pelvis and/or sacrum.

1. The patient is supine.
2. The physician sits at the affected side of the supine patient.
3. The hand furthest from the patient contacts the medial aspect of the affected SI joint while the hand closest to the patient contacts the affected innominate over the ASIS.
4. While monitoring the SI joint posteriorly, apply pressure to the innominate to rotate it anteriorly and posteriorly, assessing the tension of the articular mechanism of the SI joint.
5. The joint is placed in a position of BLT using the innominate to establish neutral. The joint may be further decompressed by applying anterior pressure to the sacrum.
6. Once the point of BLT is established, it is held until the patient's inherent forces correct the strain. Respiration may be used to augment the positioning and release.
7. Reassess the joint for improved motion.

LAS Hip Technique

Symptoms/diagnosis: Hip pain, often due to a force transferred up from the lower extremity or a fall directly on the hip: lower extremity somatic dysfunction.

Procedure (Fig. 46.1 depicts a patient with left hip dysfunction from LAS):

1. The patient is supine on the treatment table.
2. The physician stands facing the patient aside the treatment table as shown in Figure 46.1.

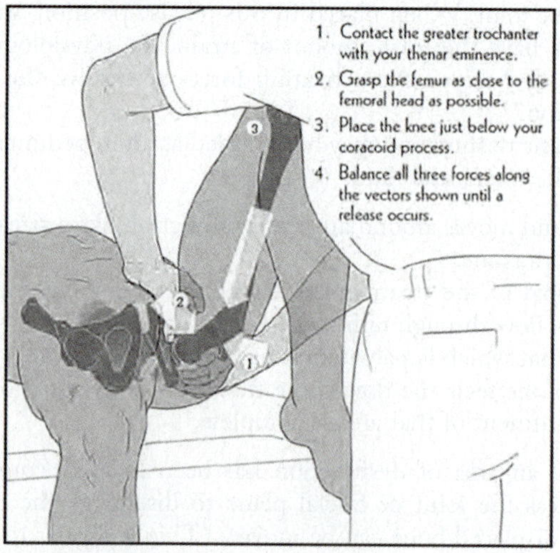

Figure 46.1. LAS technique for the left hip. (Reprinted with permission from Speece CA, Crow WT, Simmons SL. *Ligamentous Articular Strain: Osteopathic Manipulative Techniques for the Body.* Eastland Press; 2009.)

3. The physician rolls the patient's ipsilateral knee, on the affected hip side, medially to raise the symptomatic hip slightly off the table.
4. The physician places the thenar eminence of the hand farthest from the table (right hand depicted in the figure) between the patient's greater trochanter and the table and then places the patient's knee in the depression just below the coracoid process on the side nearest the patient to control the patient's distal femur (at the left shoulder as depicted in the figure).
5. The physician grasps the medial proximal aspect of the patient's femur close to the femoral head with the index, middle finger, and thumb of the other hand (physician's left hand depicted in the figure).
6. The physician uses the shoulder to increase or decrease the flexion at the patient's hip and to slightly internally or externally rotate the femur. The patient's foot is dangling just off the table. The hip is compressed slightly anteriorly and medially with the thenar eminence on the greater trochanter.
7. With the medial hand (left hand in the figure) grasping the femur close to the femoral head, generate pressure posteriorly and laterally with the middle finger, index finger, and thumb.
8. Using the (left) shoulder, locate the direction of balanced tension in the hip by slightly increasing or decreasing the flexion of the femur and slightly internally or externally rotating the femur.
9. Balance the forces at the patient's hip joint from all three contact points.
10. When the release occurs, the connective tissue surrounding the head of the femur will readjust itself, all three vectors of force will "melt," and the femur will move back to its anatomical and functional (physiologic) position.

LAS Treatment for Externally Rotated Legs

Symptoms/diagnosis: Hip pain, often due to a force transferred up from the lower extremity or a fall directly on the hip: pelvis and/or lower extremity somatic dysfunction.

1. Active range of motion is assessed with the patient standing facing the physician and the physician slowly passively moving the patient's foot into internal and external rotation with the patient seated.
2. Restriction of active motion is noted by assessing movement at the pelvis.
3. The treatment is performed with the patient sitting facing the physician.
4. The leg to be treated is crossed so that the ankle rests over the contralateral knee.
5. The physician places one hand upon the medial aspect of the femur near the femoral neck to externally rotate the femur.
6. The other hand grasps the patient's knee.
7. The physician establishes a point of balance between the femoral head and the acetabulum.
8. The patient also places their hands upon their knee.
9. The patient holds the knee down and laterally while rotating the body away from the affected leg and backward.

LAS Treatment for Internally Rotated Legs

Symptoms/diagnosis: Hip pain, often due to a force transferred up from the lower extremity or a fall directly on the hip: pelvis and/or lower extremity somatic dysfunction.

1. In this instance, the physician's handhold is more proximal so that there is less torque at the acetabulum.
2. The physician establishes a point of balance between the femoral head and the acetabulum.
3. The patient draws the knee medially and upward while rotating forward and toward the affected side.

LAS Treatment for the Fibular Head[23]

Symptoms/diagnosis: Posterior and lateral knee pain or unstable ankle due to ankle sprain. Somatic dysfunction of the lower extremity and/or displacement of the fibular head.

1. The patient is supine.
2. The physician is seated facing the table at the level of the affected extremity.
3. The physician flexes the hip and knee of the affected side to about 90 degrees and slightly externally rotates the femur.
4. With the cephalad hand, the physician bends the elbow to 90 degrees and places it on the table. The thumb contacts the posterior superior aspect of the fibular head, pressing it slightly inferiorly toward the foot while the fingers contact the opposite side of the knee.
5. The distal hand inverts the foot and rotates the foot slightly medially which tractions on the distal end of the fibula.
6. Balance the connective tissue surrounding both ends of the fibula and interosseous membrane between the tibia and fibula until a release is palpated. This may be felt as the fibular head gliding inferiorly and anteriorly, sliding back into its socket.
7. Reassess the motion of the fibula.

ACKNOWLEDGMENTS

The author and editors of this chapter would like to acknowledge the scholarly contributions of Drs. Jane Carreiro and Rebecca E. Giusti.

REFERENCES

1. Lippincott HA. *The Osteopathic Technique of Wm. G. Sutherland.* American Academy of Applied Osteopathy; 1949.
2. Sutherland WG. Chapter 14. Clinical experience in the practice of osteopathy. In: Wales AE, ed. *Teachings in the Science of Osteopathy.* Rudra Press; 1990:188.
3. Still AT. *Osteopathy: Research and Practice.* The Journal Printing Company; 1910.
4. McConnell CP. *The Practice of Osteopathy.* The Journal Printing Company; 1906.
5. Ashmore E. *Osteopathic Mechanics.* The Journal Printing Company; 1915.
6. Willard F. *Fascia as an organ system.* Lecture at Cranial Academy Conference; 1995.
7. Ham AW, Gomak DH. *Histology.* JB Lippincott; 1979.
8. Frankel VH, Nordin M. *Basic Biomechanics of the Skeletal System.* Lea and Febiger; 1980.
9. Kennedy JC, Hawkins RJ, Willis RB, Danylchuck KD. Tension studies of human knee ligaments, yield point, ultimate failure and disruption of the cruciate and tibial collateral ligaments. *J Bone Joint Surg Am.* 1976;58(3):350–355.
10. Woo SL, Matthews JV, Akeson WH, Amiel D, Convery FR. Connective tissue response to immobility. *Arthritis Rheum.* 1975;18:257–264.
11. Akeson WH, Amiel D, LaViolette D, Secrist D. The connective tissue response to immobility: an accelerated aging response. *Exp Gerontol.* 1968;3(4):289–301.
12. Evans EB, Eggers G, Butler J, Blumel J. Experimental immobilization and mobilization of rat knee joints. *J Bone Joint Surg.* 1960;42A(5): 737–758.
13. Stedman TL. *Stedman's Medical Dictionary.* 26th ed. Williams & Wilkins; 1995.

14. Chen CS, Ingber DE. Tensegrity and mechanoregulation: from skeleton to cytoskeleton. *Osteoarthritis Cartilage.* 1999;7(1):81–94.
15. Speece CA, Crow WT. *Ligamentous Articular Strain: Osteopathic Manipulative Techniques for the Body.* Eastland Press; 2001:23.
16. Carreiro JE. Chapter 59: Balanced ligamentous tension techniques. Ward RC, ex ed. *Foundations for Osteopathic Medicine.* 2nd ed. Lippincott Williams & Wilkins; 2003:918.
17. Speece CA, Crow WT. *Ligamentous Articular Strain: Osteopathic Manipulative Techniques for the Body.* Eastland Press. 2001:34.
18. Carreiro JE. Chapter 59: Balanced ligamentous tension techniques. Ward RC, ex ed. *Foundations for Osteopathic Medicine.* 2nd ed. Lippincott Williams & Wilkins; 2003:919.
19. Carreiro JE. Chapter 59: Balanced ligamentous tension techniques. Ward RC, ex ed. *Foundations for Osteopathic Medicine.* 2nd ed. Lippincott Williams & Wilkins; 2003:924–925.
20. Carreiro JE. Chapter 59: Balanced ligamentous tension techniques. Ward RC, ex ed. *Foundations for Osteopathic Medicine.* 2nd ed. Lippincott Williams & Wilkins; 2003:926–927.
21. Speece CA, Crow WT. *Ligamentous Articular Strain: Osteopathic Manipulative Techniques for the Body.* Eastland Press; 2001:116.
22. Speece CA, Crow WT. *Ligamentous Articular Strain: Osteopathic Manipulative Techniques for the Body.* Eastland Press; 2001:123.
23. Speece CA, Crow WT. *Ligamentous Articular Strain: Osteopathic Manipulative Techniques for the Body.* Eastland Press; 2001:50.

47 Strain–Counterstrain

JOHN C. GLOVER ▪ PAUL R. RENNIE

KEY CONCEPTS

- This approach was developed from astute clinical observation (Jones), followed by progressive exploration of a line of thought.
- Correlations between symptoms, history and physical examination, structural findings, and associated counterstrain points are necessary to obtain maximum benefit.
- Counterstrain points are most commonly, but not exclusively, found in muscle tissue. Research continues to explore muscle involvement within various body systems.
- Finding the key counterstrain point, typically the most tender point, and not just any counterstrain point that is tender, is critical.
- All anterior and posterior counterstrain points in a key region need to be checked before deciding where to begin treatment.
- Treatment of somatic dysfunction is accomplished by placing the patient's body in a position of maximum comfort.
- To obtain the maximum response to treatment, the physician needs to use a combination of response in the affected tissue in combination with feedback from the patient.

INTRODUCTION

Lawrence H. Jones, DO, FAAO, initially referred to his new treatment approach as *spontaneous release by positioning*,[1] but later changed to *strain–counterstrain*, which he believed was more descriptive of the mechanism of injury and the underlying physiologic mechanism he used to treat somatic dysfunction. Once Jones formalized his teachings, he termed the model strain–counterstrain, which is referred to in this chapter as *counterstrain*, the terminology currently in use by the Glossary of Osteopathic Terminology[2] and by most practitioners.

Similar to the way Jones changed the title of his approach, he also changed the terms used to describe the small discrete areas of tissue texture changes signifying the presence of somatic dysfunction. Initially, Jones referred to these areas as trigger points, after the work of Janet Travell, MD, author of *Myofascial Pain and Dysfunction: The Trigger Point Manual*. However, after a discussion with Travell, Jones believed that the significant tissue changes in his model were different from hers and subsequently referred to his as tender points (see Table 47.1). Later, in the 1995 update of Jones' book, these two words were combined, resulting in the term "tenderpoint."

The authors of this chapter further proposed a new designation for these points, counterstrain points, which has been adopted by the Educational Council on Osteopathic Principles (ECOP). This change is supported by several factors:

1. Tender point and tenderpoint are generic terms that do not communicate their uniqueness or ties to the counterstrain model. Jones constantly added points to his model and encouraged those who used his model to continually look for new points.
2. Importantly, not all tender points are tender. Jones described stoics, patients who had points that did not elicit tenderness when palpated and were identifiable solely by tissue texture changes. Thus, the new term defines an area of tissue texture change, primarily tension, associated with a somatic dysfunction that typically, but not always, produces local tenderness when palpated and resolves with specific patient positioning.

Manipulative treatment models fall into two primary divisions: direct and indirect, based on the initial positioning of the patient relative to the restrictive barrier of the dysfunctional tissues. Counterstrain is an indirect model with initial positioning away from the restrictive barrier. It has a unique advantage over other such models, in that the patient can provide feedback indicating when they are in the correct position for treatment. The model is also highly accessible to physicians with limited palpatory skills and treatment experience. Hence, counterstrain is often taught early in an osteopathic curriculum. With additional clinical experience, the physician will be able to detect subtle tissue changes occurring during evaluation and treatment. In turn, this will guide effective treatment decisions using counterstrain integrated with other diagnostic findings and manipulative models, which will produce long-lasting results. Additionally, by paying attention to the tissue changes under the monitoring hand, the physician will learn to palpate subtle tissue changes required to effectively apply other manipulative treatment models. While counterstrain can be learned early in manual skills development, it can be used effectively either in combination with other treatment models or as the sole treatment model by experienced physicians.

HISTORY

Counterstrain began as an unexpected discovery in 1955. A young, athletic-looking man visited Dr. Jones[3] after having developed a psoitis 2½ months before seeking treatment. This left him in pain and unable to stand erect. The injury was not caused by trauma and had gradually worsened over the 2½ months. Since the onset, the man had received treatment from two chiropractors with no substantial improvement. Jones treated the man several times with high velocity/low amplitude thrust technique over the course of 6 weeks, also with little improvement.

At one visit, the man reported difficulty sleeping due to pain and asked if Dr. Jones could help him find a comfortable sleeping position. After working with the patient for 20 minutes, Jones found this position and then left him in the position to treat another patient. When Jones returned and assisted him to a standing position, to their mutual surprise, the young man stood erect and pain free for the first time in 4 months. Jones was impressed by the results and decided to investigate further.

Jones experimented by treating patients with whole-body positions of comfort. After finding frequent success, he then experimented to shorten the time spent in the treatment position. He also observed discrete tender paravertebral areas prior to treatment, which became pain free after being placed in the position of comfort. Therefore, Jones began positioning only the region of the body where the tissue changes occurred, which reduced the time required in the treatment position. He also experimented with the amount of time required for treatment and concluded that 90 seconds in the position of maximum comfort was optimal. Shorter periods did not always produce lasting relief, and longer periods did not necessarily produce a better response. However, he felt that probably some skilled practitioners in the use of counterstrain would be able to reduce the time further.[1] Jones then began mapping the discrete areas of tenderness and correlating them to specific somatic dysfunctions identified by the traditional structural exam he learned in osteopathic medical school.

Jones could only identify the discrete paravertebral areas of tenderness in about half of his patients. A theory as to why came when Jones was treating a patient for psoitis, who was presumed to have developed a hernia by pulling hard to free a stuck garden hoe. Although Jones found no inguinal hernia, there was a discrete area of tenderness in the pelvis. Jones placed the patient in a position of comfort to treat the psoitis and then palpated the tender area. To their mutual surprise, the tissue was no longer tender. After 90 seconds, Jones slowly returned the patient to a neutral position, palpated the area again, and found no evidence of tenderness.

Based on his experience with the patient injured while gardening, Jones reasoned there were anterior tender points in addition to the posterior tender points, and thus began his search for tender points on the front of the body.[4] This observation is consistent with the osteopathic principle of the body as a unit, whereas the traditional emphasis on spinal function and posterior diagnostic evaluation had eclipsed this connection.

As previously discussed, Jones noted important differences between the trigger points elaborated by Travell[5] and the tender points he had identified.[6] Jones described over 300 specific tender points, and new tender points continue to be found. Through their correspondences, Travell and Jones identified similarities and differences between their points. Table 47.1 provides a comparison of trigger and counterstrain points.

Dr. Jones made two important discoveries:

1. Placing the body in a position of maximum comfort can effectively treat somatic dysfunction.
2. The anterior aspect of the patient must be evaluated, in addition to the posterior, to effectively diagnose and treat somatic dysfunction.

PROPOSED MECHANISMS OF ACTION

Physiologic Basis of Counterstrain

At the time Jones was formulating his ideas about counterstrain, Irwin Korr[7] published an article on proprioceptors and somatic dysfunction. Jones proposed that the gamma system was responsible for the development of an inappropriate proprioceptive reflex associated with somatic dysfunction.[3,6] That is, a sudden "panic" response of the antagonist muscle to the initially strained and painful agonist muscle, set up by a dysfunction of the antagonist muscle due to the rapid muscle lengthening. Consequentially, hypertonic myofascial tissue and restricted motion of the joint are affected by the dysfunctional antagonist muscle. Jones treated the counterstrain point found in the antagonist by shortening the muscle the central nervous system interpreted as strained in countering the original agonist muscle strain. This places the originally strained and painful muscle back into a stretched position and reduces the tension of the antagonist muscle tissues. Since the theory of counterstrain methodology was originally proposed, greater understanding of the involved physiology has been achieved.

TABLE 47.1

Comparison of Trigger Points and Counterstrain Points

Trigger Point	Counterstrain Point
Patient presents with characteristic pain pattern	Typically, no characteristic pain pattern
Located in muscle tissue	Located in muscle, tendons, ligaments, and fascia
Locally tender	Locally tender
Elicits jump sign when pressed	Elicits jump sign when pressed
Elicits a radiating pain pattern when pressed	No radiating pattern when pressed
Present within a taut band of tissue	Taut band not present
Elicits twitch response with snapping palpation	Twitch response not present
Responds to spray, stretch, needling, and often responds to positioning	Responds to specific positioning
Dermographia of skin over point	Dermographia not present

- Muscle spindle reactivity decreases during muscle contraction and increases when the muscle is stretched.[8] Hypoxic conditions can also reduce muscle spindle influence on muscle tension (stretch reflex) and impair central nervous system control on motor coordination and quality of movement.[9]
- The gamma motor fibers attached to the peripheral ends of the intrafusal fiber stretch the central portion of this fiber to increase the sensitivity of the muscle spindle to contract the homonymous muscle (deep tendon reflex).
- Group Ia fibers respond to both static length and dynamic length changes and have impulse activity at all muscle lengths.
- Group II fibers respond only to length changes and are not active when the muscle is relaxed.
- Golgi tendon organ receptors are connected to Group Ib afferents and are arranged in series at the transition zone of the muscle and tendons. They respond to compression and are excited by muscle contraction and muscle stretch to inhibit the homonymous muscle. Counterintuitively, these organs are also very sensitive to stretch, wherein the contraction of a few muscle fibers is sufficient for activation.[10,11]
- The ligament muscular reflex also influences muscle tone. When a ligament is sprained, muscles in which further contractions would increase the strain are inhibited, while those that would reduce the strain are stimulated in order to protect the ligament.[12–16] This ligament muscular reflex[14,17] demonstrates the close relationship

between specific muscles and ligaments to preserve joint integrity and muscle balance. Ligamentous injury produces muscular contraction and/or inhibition that becomes symptomatic.

With regard to tendon injury, one study on the effect of counterstrain treatment for Achilles tendinitis demonstrated that the use of osteopathic manipulative treatment (OMT) produced a 23.1% decrease in the stretch reflex amplitude of the soleus, in subjects with Achilles tendinitis.[18] Similarly, significant responses were measured in the lateral and medial heads of the gastrocnemius in the OMT treatment group. Subjects who received OMT reported various ratings of soreness, stiffness, and swelling during the 1-week period following counterstrain treatment. Mean ratings of soreness and stiffness were significantly reduced between pre- and post-treatment levels at 6 hours and also daily for 7 days following treatment. Subjects also reported significantly reduced swelling on post-treatment days 2 through 6. In another related study, counterstrain was also found to be clinically effective for the treatment of plantar fasciitis.[19]

Furthermore, the understanding of the counterstrain method requires a study of the circulatory and nociceptive processes that are present with somatic dysfunction.[20] It is important to recognize that under normal conditions, sympathetically induced vasoconstriction in the skeletal muscle and viscera restrains vasodilatation in order to maintain arterial perfusion pressure, the exercise pressor reflex.[21] This is designed to maintain vital organ functions while simultaneously reducing extracardiac and respiratory work stress (increased cardiac output).

However, at the same time, adequate arterial pressure within the blood vessels is required to overcome the compression force (and therefore blood vessel flow resistance) of the contracting muscle. Part of the sympathetic effect is attenuated through neural receptors in the muscle and fascial tissues that sense metabolic and mechanical alterations in the tissues. Sustained elevated intramuscular pressure is also a factor in reducing metabolic recovery in the muscles where blood flow is restricted, often due to prolonged static positioning, repetitive motion, or direct compressive forces on the tissues.[20,22–24]

The nociceptive reflex functions in the presence of actual or threatened tissue damage and sets forth a chain of afferent, biochemical, and tissue-altering responses.[9,24–26] Nociceptors are constantly monitoring for potential injury to tissues[27] and do not typically respond to weak locally applied pressure, normal physiologic contractions, and normal joint ranges of motion.[9,28] However, when activated, nociceptors trigger noxious afferent information to the spinal cord and brain via the axonal reflex (widening the receptive field). In addition, nociceptive activation generates tissue edema from increased tissue permeability and vasodilation.

Nociceptors accomplish this through close proximity with the blood vessels and group III and IV muscle afferents. Group III and IV afferents are the primary nociceptive fibers from the skeletal and cardiac muscles.[21,29–31] The receptors connected to the group III afferents predominately report on mechanical deformation in the muscles and fascia, while those connected to the group IV afferents predominately report on metabolic alterations in the same areas. A number of neuropeptides are involved in this process.

ATP activates P2 (purinergic) receptors that elicit the exercise pressor reflex by sensitizing group III mechanoreceptors and stimulating group IV metaboreceptors.[21,32] Injections of ATP and P2X receptor agonist into the rat hind paw have been shown to increase behavioral indexes of pain (hind paw licking, lifting, and flinching).[10,33] However, ATP release from red blood cells and the interstitium contributes to the functional sympatholysis effect by countering norepinephrine, resulting in vasodilatation. ATP has an amazing number of different functions that assist in the myosin-to-actin filament movement necessary for muscle contraction. This contributes to arterial dilation, which increases nutrient and oxygen delivery, and elicits nociceptive information when bound to the P2 receptors.[21]

Bradykinin is a biochemical derived from the plasma protein kallidin. Rather than opening an ion channel, bradykinin activates a G-protein that regulates intracellular metabolic changes leading to sensitization of the nerve ending.[34] In noninflamed tissues, bradykinin elicits this sensitization by acting on B1 receptors. Inflamed tissues sensitize newly synthesized B2 receptors. Such differentiation shows a peripheral neuroplastic change of the nerve ending. Bradykinin is released by noxious stimulation, which is further accentuated under ischemic conditions.

Prostaglandins (predominately PGE_2) are released from the endothelial lining of the blood vessels and other tissue cells. Serotonin (5-HT3) is released from the platelets. Together, PGE_2 and 5-HT3 induce a chain of intracellular sequences that increase the sensitivity of the Na+ channels by activating protein kinase A (PKA).[10,21,34] PGE_2 not only stimulates group IV afferents but also enhances the effect of bradykinin. The ion currents running through this channel protein subsequently sensitize the nerve ending to external stimuli.

Lactic acid activation of ASIC (acid-sensing ion channels), particularly to ASIC3, leads to increased sensation under ischemic conditions.[9,28,31] ASIC3 channels open when pH drops from 7.4 to 7.0, common with ischemic exercise. ATP also enhances the responsiveness of this channel. The ATP augmentation of the current through this channel remains high for minutes after ATP is removed. It is interesting to note that circulatory changes do not always occur instantaneously, which parallels the counterstrain model with regard to the classic 90-second treatment time.

Substance P (SP) releases histamine from mast cells along with calcitonin gene-related peptide (CGRP), which causes vasodilatation and an increase in vascular permeability of the blood vessels around the nerve ending.[21,31,34,35] This results in a shift of blood plasma from the intravascular to the interstitial space, allowing pain-generating biochemicals, released from the blood vessels, to react with the receptors.

Transient receptor potential (TRPV1) can be stimulated by capsaicin, elevated H+ levels, and heat. Elevated acid levels also lower the threshold for heat to activate this receptor. Moreover, stimulation of TRPV1 may be associated with the muscle aches from systemic viral illness.[10,28,34] TRPV4 is a mechanosensitive ion channel sensitive to both weak and strong noxious intensities of local pressure.

Excitation of a nociceptive receptor releases neuropeptides into the interstitial tissues that affect microcirculation and chemistry of the region. In this setting, a nontraumatic noxious mechanical stimulus can elicit a local region of vasodilatation, edema, and further sensitization of nociceptors.[9,20,28,31] Pressing on these tissues elicits a tenderness response and elaborates tissue texture findings characteristic of somatic dysfunction.

The following factors may also contribute to pain and affect muscle activity, resulting in impaired metabolism, circulation, altered proprioceptive control, and the maintenance of sensitivity in the tissues[9,14,17,22,23,36–39]:

- Stimulation of nociceptors, augmented with the accumulation of metabolites
- Myofascial force transmission (intermuscular and extramuscular forces between agonist and synergist muscle fibers during contraction efforts)

- Altered ligament–muscular reflexes
- Intramuscular shear forces (where a low percentage of muscle fibers are activated under low-intensity contraction effort)
- Cinderella motor unit loading (muscle damage from low-intensity tasks)
- Calcium ion accumulation in the muscle fibers and mitochondria
- Sustained increased intramuscular pressure (without adequate metabolic recovery time)
- Reinforced sympathetic activity particularly induced by stressful activities
- Impaired lymphatic drainage and interstitial inflammatory stasis

The location of specific counterstrain points is consistent from one patient to another and can be mapped. These areas of tenderness and/or tissue texture changes can be found in different myofascial structures including tendons, ligaments, fascia, and muscle bellies.[3,35,40–42] Additionally, motor points (the site where the motor nerve pierces the investing fascia and enters the muscle it innervates) are also sites rich with afferent neural fibers. Sensitized neural tissues can also be found in these regions.[20,35,37,43]

Locations of group III and IV muscle afferents and receptors correspond closely with counterstrain point locations. The superficial lamina of the thoracolumbar fascia has CGRP and SP containing free nerve endings, found mainly in the subcutaneous layer and also between the fascia and the surface of the multifidus muscle.[10] Nerve fiber density of the group III and IV afferents in the rat calcaneal tendon peritendineum is several times higher than that in the gastrosoleus muscle.[10,44] Other key locations include the perimysium surrounding larger or smaller bundles of muscle fibers, adventitia of arterioles, venules, lymphatic vessels, and the sheaths of the nerve fiber bundles from the nervi nervorum.[10,45,46] This connection between neural pain fibers in addition to blood and lymphatic vessels demonstrates the interconnections between pain generation and metabolic processing.

To reinforce the importance of the neural and circulatory unity in function, it is vital to recognize that nutrients and oxygen are delivered through sympathetically controlled blood vessels that traverse within blood vessels to reach target organs. When tissue abnormality emerges, blood flow in the skeletal muscle is increased to meet the metabolic demand triggered by changes in the chemical environment. From studies involving dynamic exercise, it has been determined that intravascular release of ATP from red blood cells exerts direct sympatholytic (vasodilator) effects, a functional sympatholysis[32,47] occurring in response to a decrease in erythrocyte and plasma oxygen levels.[32,48] This vasodilatory effect appears to result from ATP inhibition of noradrenaline-mediated vasoconstriction via the P2 receptors and also occurs when nitric oxide is released in the blood vessel.

In the counterstrain model, the patient is placed into a passive position that reduces or ideally eliminates the tenderness at the counterstrain point site. With regard to blood flow, cadaveric studies have shown that when the shoulder was passively abducted, relaxation on the supraspinatus muscle allowed almost complete filling of micropaque in the vessels throughout the tendon to the muscle's point of insertion, so that in the rested position, blood vessel filling is reduced with the tendon being squeezed flatter over the head of the humerus.[49] Additionally, the supraspinatus tendon has a zone of avascularity that also corresponds to where degeneration typically first appears. With the onset of degeneration, an inflammatory response follows with vascular changes of granulation tissue. However, these areas are also the most common locations where spontaneous tendon ruptures occur.

The nociceptive quality of counterstrain point locations relates segmentally and participates with viscerosomatic, somatovisceral, somatosomatic, and viscerovisceral reflex patterns of dysfunction. These reflect the sensory and motor arm of the reflexes. Therefore, an understanding of the spinal level associated with the counterstrain point allows for mapping of the dysfunction. Since the soma may be manifesting a visceral dysfunction, areas of tenderness that cannot be resolved with counterstrain treatment may suggest a visceral-level dysfunction that requires further evaluation. Nonetheless, past visceral dysfunction that has resolved could also manifest with lingering soma-level tenderness that has not resolved with the original visceral dysfunction and may be amenable to counterstrain treatment.

However, patients with heart failure have also demonstrated augmented sympathetic nerve activity, in which studies suggest that it is due to the sensitization of mechanoreceptors, leading to an exaggerated exercise pressor reflex.[21] Studies in rats have shown group III afferents to be responsible for this reflex. If group IV afferents are desensitized or not present, group III afferents will overcompensate and augment the exercise pressor reflex in the heart failure population. Here, the mechanical predominant receptor group III afferents override the metabolic predominant receptor group IV afferents. Is this a permanent structural abnormality, or can manipulative treatment enhance the functional sympatholysis effect?

Another study on the in vitro effects of indirect OMT established a model that simulates repetitive motion strain (RMS) and demonstrated reduction in fibroblast proliferation and a delayed inflammatory response.[50,51] Indirect models of OMT, including those of counterstrain and indirect myofascial release, did not produce such a response. IOMT (indirect OMT) also reversed the inflammatory effects in cells that had been strained repetitively. The IOMT model was performed for 60 seconds, which closely parallels the counterstrain model. Inhibitors of fibroblastic growth, IL-1β and IL-6, were increased in the RMS and 24-hour RMS profiles and were reduced in the 24-hour IOMT and 24-hour RMS+IOMT profiles. These results contribute to the clinical efficacy of indirect osteopathic manipulative medicine techniques. In addition, IL-1β has been shown to increase production of substance P and prostaglandin E_2 in neuronal and glial cells.[52–54] IL-6 is associated with neuropathic pain following nerve injury.[52,55]

Additional studies have indicated the benefits of counterstrain on various conditions. A partial list includes:

- Forearm strength[56]
- Chronic ankle instability[57]
- Length of stay for pancreatitis (via combination OMT treatment involving counterstrain)[58]
- Counterstrain point tenderness in the upper trapezius in patients with mechanical neck pain[59]
- Low back pain and disability[60]
- Complex regional pain syndrome associated with ankle sprain[61]
- Chondromalacia patellae[62]
- Shoulder pain and repetitive strain injury to the supraspinatus muscle[63]
- Piriformis syndrome[64]

INDICATIONS

The use of counterstrain is indicated for any acute or chronic somatic dysfunction with an associated counterstrain point. It is important to remember that while counterstrain points are typically tender when palpated locally, tissue tension can also be identified in some individuals who do not report tenderness. The rationale for deciding to use counterstrain may include better tolerance to indirect models for acute somatic dysfunction, where positioning at the restrictive barrier is less tolerated due to pain or the mechanism of injury. A counterstrain point may be primary in the development of somatic dysfunction or develop secondary to another primary cause, such as a joint restriction or a specific postural pattern. Points can also be found in association with viscerosomatic reflexes. Counterstrain should be considered in any patient who has persistent dysfunction after three treatments with direct manipulative models. Also, consider using counterstrain for a patient who has been treated by another practitioner because most practitioners do not evaluate a patient for counterstrain points. Counterstrain is a good choice for any patient who is hesitant about the forces used in other forms of manipulative treatment, such as those who are frail or find high-velocity, low-amplitude thrust to be uncomfortable. Counterstain may also be used to assess a patient's tolerance to manual treatment. This model is valuable for any somatic dysfunction where a neural reflex is identified or suspected, and a counterstrain point can be identified.

CONTRAINDICATIONS

Absolute contraindications are rare when considering the use of counterstrain (Table 47.2).

These include:

- A patient who does not consent to the procedure.
- The presence of a fracture that would be directly affected by the positioning used for treatment.
- The presence of a torn ligament in the area to be treated, whereby counterstrain positioning would risk further tearing.
- Positioning that exacerbates potentially life-threatening symptomology, in which case the treatment should be stopped immediately.

All other contraindications are relative. While the following situations are considered relative contraindications, it is the magnitude of the problem that is most crucial, which requires sound clinical judgment and the use of common sense to determine if the treatment is warranted. A major consideration is if the positioning would increase pressure on sensitive or diseased tissue. This is especially true of the developing fetus or an osteoporotic bone. The use of counterstrain on a hospitalized patient whose oxygen saturation and EKG are being monitored in real time can provide feedback to more precisely evaluate the immediate effect of the treatment on the patient.

- Children who cannot remain passive during the time required for treatment are not good candidates for counterstrain.
- Patients who cannot voluntarily relax are also poor candidates for counterstrain. Patients need to be instructed on how to properly relax so they do not confuse being still with being relaxed for this method to be most effective.
- Osteoporosis must be evaluated for severity and location. Counterstrain is contraindicated if positioning the patient for treatment poses risk for a fracture, although this is typically uncommon since the treatment position is within a patient's range of motion. Patients with osteoporosis usually benefit from counterstain due to relaxation of the hypertonic spinal muscles that increase pressure on the spine and, in turn, produce pain.
- Counterstrain treatment that is directed at hypertonic muscles exacerbating pain at a fracture site can often relax such muscles, thus decreasing pain and the need for analgesic medications. This decision should be made by an experienced physician.
- Treatment of the cervical spine in patients with vertebral artery disease may be contraindicated when the disease is severe and especially when the treatment position requires marked extension and rotation.
- Patients with Down syndrome must be evaluated for spinal anomalies prior to treatment of the upper cervical spine.
- In addition, gravely ill patients who may not be able to tolerate a severe treatment reaction are not good candidates, although counterstrain has been used very effectively in the hospital setting, including intensive care units.
- Patients with a cardiac event and presenting with minimal symptomatology are also a challenge.
- Those with a classic presentation, displaying all the signs and symptoms, should be immediately transferred to an emergency department for treatment.
- If any neurologic symptoms (dizziness, nystagmus, pain radiation, etc.) develop during the course of treatment, it is prudent to immediately return the patient to a neutral position and evaluate further for the cause of the symptoms.
- Postsurgical cases are also challenging. One of the primary goals of treatment is to maximize function. If positioning would compromise the surgical outcome, treatment is not warranted. This is especially true in thoracic surgery involving a sternotomy and in joint replacements. Counterstrain treatment of these patients can provide many benefits, but the effects on the surgical sites need to be weighed before treatment is initiated.

TABLE 47.2

Contraindications for Counterstrain

Absolute	Relative
Fracture directly affected by positioning	Cardiac event
Ligamentous tear directly affected by positioning	Deep vein thrombosis
Potentially life-threatening symptomatology exacerbation	Development of neurologic symptoms with positioning
Request not to be treated (a medicolegal issue not technique specific)	Gravely ill patient Inability to relax Inability to remain passive during treatment Joint replacement Osteoporosis Pregnancy Rheumatoid arthritis Sternotomy Down syndrome Vertebral artery disease

PALPATION OF COUNTERSTRAIN POINTS

Phases of Development

There are two basic phases in the development of palpatory and treatment skills associated with counterstrain. The first is to identify the various locations where counterstrain points may be found by following the descriptions given in a counterstrain text, pressing on the location, and asking the patient if it is tender (Fig. 47.1A).

Initially, many physicians are unable to identify the tissue texture abnormalities associated with the presence of a counterstrain

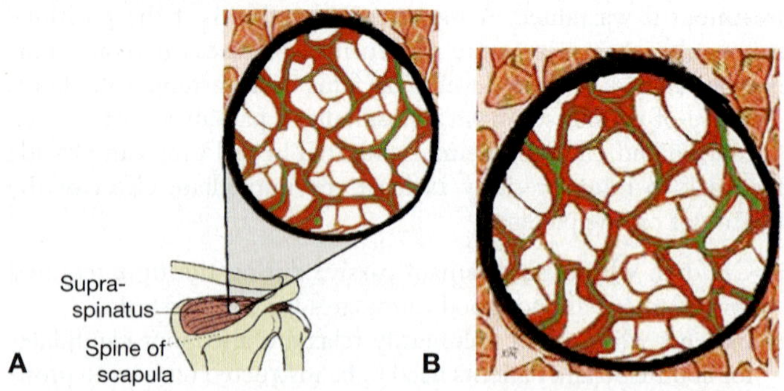

Figure 47.1. Phases of palpatory development. A. Counterstrain point located in the supraspinatus muscle. **B.** Close-up of a theoretical counterstrain point.

point and thus rely on the patient's response to the point being pressed. This method can be used to position the patient. The novice practitioner moves the patient in a direction that should shorten the dysfunctional myofascial tissue (or that reproduces a classic treatment position illustrated in a counterstrain text) and assesses the patient's response to level of tenderness. This method is effective but can be time-consuming while learning to use the model.

A patient who does not perceive tenderness of a counterstrain point, despite the presence of tissue texture changes at the counterstrain point, was referred to by Jones as a *stoic* patient. The physician who relies solely on the patient's response of tenderness at the point for positioning will not be successful with such patients. When tissue texture changes become the key determinant for assessment and positioning, the efficiency and speed of treatment dramatically increase. These tissue texture changes can also be used for patients who have difficulty sensing or quantifying varying degrees of tenderness.

Therefore, the second phase of learning begins when the physician learns to perceive the tissue texture abnormalities characteristic of a counterstrain point (Fig. 47.1B) and palpate how positional changes affect them.

These tissue abnormalities will alert the physician to the presence of a counterstrain point before the patient experiences tenderness and then presses the counterstrain point for tenderness.

POSITION OF COMFORT

The position of comfort used in counterstrain treatment is a very specific three-dimensional position in space, where the tenderness of the counterstrain point disappears or becomes insignificant. Another vital skill for the physician is the ability to palpate changes in the tissue texture abnormality of the counterstrain point during treatment. A change toward the position of maximal comfort will be palpated as decreased tension or softening of the tissue involved with the counterstrain point. This indicates to the physician whether the patient is being moved in the correct direction for treatment. Experience will also allow the physician to correlate the degree of tissue change with the required amount of positional change and with the required amount of time spent in the treatment position.

A clue for the treatment time arises with the palpation of a pulsation, the *therapeutic pulse*, at a counterstrain point location. The frequency of the pulsation is often the same as the cardiac rate and therefore suggests a circulatory relationship. Recall the physiologic mechanisms discussed earlier. Of note is that the pulsation is not present before positioning; it develops after the patient has been moved close to the position of comfort and then disappears after myofascial tissue relaxation. Occasionally, the *therapeutic pulse* does not begin until the patient has been in the treatment position for 20 to 30 seconds. The pulsation phenomenon does not occur with every counterstrain point; however, when palpated, it is correlated with markedly improved treatment response.

SAFETY AND EFFICACY

Counterstrain is a safe and effective OMT model. Adverse events occurring with this technique have rarely, if ever, been reported in published literature. Post-treatment soreness occurs in approximately 30% of patients and usually resolves or reduces within 1 to 2 days, rarely 5 days after treatment. In rare cases, a patient may experience nausea or vomiting after treatment. See the above list of contraindications and relative contraindications. Clinical judgment should always be used in prescribing treatment for any disease condition.

PRINCIPLES OF DIAGNOSIS

Several different diagnostic approaches can be used.

- Taking a good trauma history and observation of a patient's gait and body habitus can aid in locating key counterstrain points.
- If the patient can accurately recount the mechanism of the injury, this can help guide the physician to the counterstrain point. For example, a patient whose injury occurred in a flexed position will typically result in a counterstrain point on the anterior aspect of the body, and the treatment position would approximate the position of injury.
- Observation of the patient's habits provides valuable clues to the location of significant counterstrain points.
- A patient who has difficulty standing upright and is more comfortable in a forward-bent position typically has counterstrain points on the anterior aspect of the body.
- The more forward or backward bent without side bending and rotation, the more likely the counterstrain point will be located close to the midline.
- If the patient is most comfortable with a side bent and/or rotated position, then the counterstrain points are more likely to be located lateral to the midline.
- The pain patterns reported by the patient can be used to identify specific muscle groups that may contain counterstrain points.[41]
- Another method is to perform a neuromusculoskeletal (structural) exam. After segmental diagnosis is made the counterstrain points associated with the dysfunctional segment can be identified.
- If the segment is flexed, rotated, and side bent to the right, there is commonly a counterstrain point on the anterior aspect of the body on the left side. There may also be counterstrain points on the right anterior. Additionally, there could also be counterstrain points to the right or left side on the posterior aspect of the body.
- An additional method is to scan the counterstrain points in the region of the complaint, both anterior and posterior, and also in one body region above and below the area of the complaint. For instance, a thoracic complaint may yield significant counterstrain points in the thoracic, cervical, lumbar, or costal regions, as well as in the upper extremities. It is crucial not to narrow the evaluation only to the site of the presenting complaint.

- Many physicians first scan the patient for counterstrain points to identify the most dysfunctional segment in a region and then perform a multiplane segmental diagnosis. With this information, the physician can decide whether to use a counterstrain or another manipulative model.

See Chapter 43 Clinical Assessment: Viscerosomatic, Somatosomatic, Somatovisceral Reflexes; Counterstrain Points, Myofascial Trigger Points, and Chapman Reflexes for further discussion on the assessment of tenderness during the physical examination.

PRINCIPLES OF TREATMENT

Counterstrain is a very gentle technique that is well tolerated by most patients. The patient is not subjected to any external force other than gentle positioning. Basic counterstrain treatment also does not require force generated from the patient's muscle contractions. It is an indirect technique, with positioning away from restrictive barriers, and is therefore applicable for both acute and chronic problems.

The basic counterstrain procedure involves identifying significant counterstrain points associated with a somatic dysfunction and then positioning the patient to eliminate the tenderness of the point, which results in structural changes following successful treatment. Counterstrain is easy to understand and to apply. However, mastery requires:

- Time to learn the location of counterstrain points.
- Ability to palpate the tissue changes associated with the counterstrain point and dynamic changes that occur over the course of treatment.
- Skill in fine-tuning the treatment position for maximum results.
- The clinical experience to understand the correlations between symptoms, structural findings, and associated counterstrain points.

The basic steps for treating somatic dysfunction with counterstrain after a relevant osteopathic neuromusculoskeletal exam are as follows:

1. Find the most significant/relevant counterstrain point associated with the somatic dysfunction.
2. Establish a tenderness scale with the patient for effective feedback.
3. Continuously monitor the counterstrain point tenderness and tissue texture changes.
4. Place the patient passively in a position that results in the greatest reduction of tenderness and tissue texture changes at the counterstrain point (position of comfort/ease).
    a. Slowly position the patient toward a position of comfort/ease, initially with large movement, while the patient remains passive.
    b. Fine-tune the position through small arcs of movement to below 3, preferably 0, on the tenderness scale, in multiple planes of motion, to find the position of greatest comfort.
5. Maintain this position for 90 seconds while the patient remains passive.
    a. Continuously monitor the counterstrain point for tissue texture changes.
    b. Periodically retest for tenderness (about every 30 seconds).
6. Slowly return the patient passively to the pretreatment position while maintaining contact with the counterstrain point.
7. Re-evaluate for resolution of tenderness and tissue texture abnormalities at the counterstrain point and at the associated TART findings.

Step 1: Find the Most Significant/Relevant Counterstrain Point Associated with the Somatic Dysfunction

Counterstrain points are typically located at tendinous attachments or in the belly of a muscle (Fig. 47.2A–C).

Additional counterstrain points are found in other myofascial tissues (ligaments and fascial sheets) associated with a somatic dysfunction. Counterstrain points are typically exquisitely tender locally, nonradiating, discrete, small, tense, somewhat edematous areas of tissue change smaller than a fingertip. It requires about four times more pressure to elicit tenderness in adjacent healthy tissue than in a significant counterstrain point. A counterstrain point may range in size from a few millimeters to several inches. Palpation of the counterstrain point reveals more tension than the surrounding tissue.

It is essential to identify the most significant counterstrain point associated with a specific somatic dysfunction rather than simply finding a point that is tender. One method to gauge the tenderness and significance of a counterstrain point is to ask the patient if the discomfort is mild, moderate, or severe. Due to the exquisite tenderness of significant counterstrain points, a patient will typically jump, wince, guard, or push the physician's hand away when the counterstrain point is pressed. Patients are often surprised by the amount of tenderness, especially when unaware of the existence of the counterstrain point. In rare cases, a *stoic* patient, as termed by Jones, will not perceive tenderness when a significant counterstrain

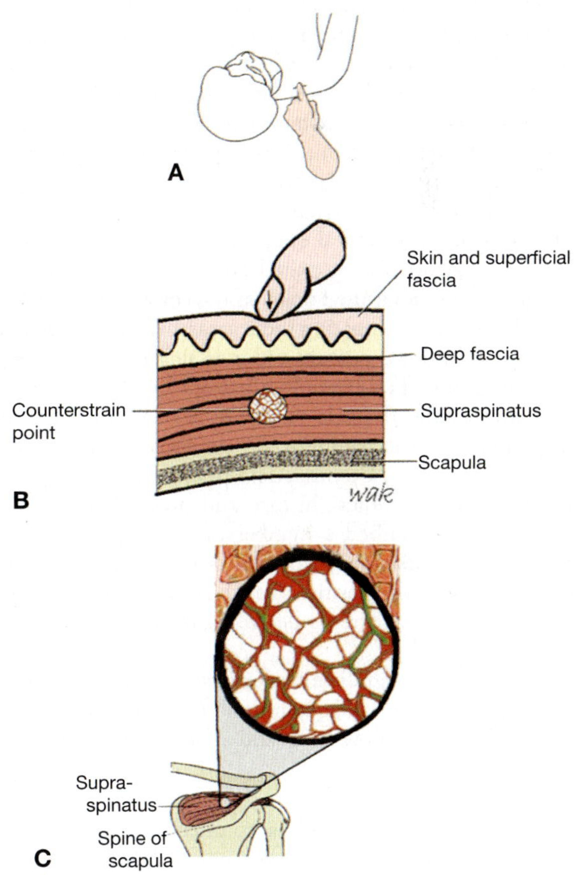

Figure 47.2. Counterstrain treatment: Step 1: Find the most significant/relevant counterstrain point associated with the somatic dysfunction. A. Scanning for tissue texture changes. **B** and **C.** Identification of a significant counterstrain point in the supraspinatus muscle.

point is pressed. Such patients can still be treated with counterstrain by monitoring tissue changes rather than the typically associated tenderness.

A counterstrain point should be palpated with the pad of the physician's finger or thumb. The pads of the fingers are profoundly more sensitive to tactile input and are better at identifying the location of counterstrain points. Avoid using the fingertips, especially if the fingernails are long. Fingertips are less sensitive and can elicit iatrogenic tenderness.

Palpation should be slow and firm but gentle. The pressure used to elicit a counterstrain point is typically a few ounces and not strong enough to elicit tenderness in normal tissue. Jones recommended using the amount of force necessary to blanch tissue under the fingernail of the physician's palpating finger. Note that the pressure required to elicit tenderness increases as the depth of the counterstrain point in the body increases. The vector of pressure is also important. Typically, the tissue of the counterstrain point is pressed 90 degrees to the more rigid underlying tissue, such as bone or cartilage. Do not forget to consider other pathologies capable of producing tenderness unrelated to neuromusculoskeletal counterstrain points, such as a fracture, infection, inflammation, or pathology of visceral origin.

Before beginning to palpate for counterstrain points, ask the patient to identify any points that are tender when pressed. Then, if tender, rate the tenderness as mild, moderate, or severe. The physician can palpate tissue texture changes before the patient experiences tenderness by scanning with light pressure. Verify the presence of a counterstrain point by increasing the contact pressure for a brief second and then asking the patient if the area is tender. The tenderness of a counterstrain point becomes an objective sign when elicited by physical palpation, relating the magnitude of tenderness to the tenderness scale. In contrast, pain is a subjective symptom that the patient may experience without palpation. Jones found that counterstrain points are often located in areas the patient does not report as painful, on the opposite side of the body.

One method for identifying counterstrain points is to perform an osteopathic structural examination, noting any alteration of movement, asymmetry of paired landmarks, or tissue texture abnormalities. Jones identified many of the counterstrain points he originally described by palpating these areas: evaluating the patient for variations from ideal posture and assessing those locations for counterstrain points. For example, a patient presenting with flattening of the normal thoracic curvature is likely to have one or more posterior thoracic counterstrain points associated with the extension in this region. Counterstrain point locations can also be anticipated based on clinical history and presenting complaints. Jones and Myers described a number of such clinical presentations.[3,6,41] The most likely areas of significant counterstrain points can be deduced from the position that the original injury occurred. Many myofascial pain patterns described by Travell may provide further correlations.[41]

A patient with a significant counterstrain point will unconsciously attempt to maintain a comfortable posture to alleviate the functional distress by shortening and relieving tense myofascial tissues.

- Patients tend to bend around a counterstrain point. That is, counterstrain points are often, but not always, located at the focal point of the concavity of the postural adaptation.
- If the patient is forward bent, counterstrain points tend to be anterior.
- If a patient is backward bent, counterstrain points tend to be posterior.
- Jones found that a patient who is side bent to one side usually has a counterstrain point on the opposite side of the spine (L.H. Jones, *personal communication*, 1993).

Counterstrain points are frequently found in areas other than those of reported pain or discomfort. The primary or key strain may induce a secondary or compensatory strain elsewhere, which may be more symptomatic. For example, when the psoas muscle is chronically shortened and irritated, patients seldom complain of abdominal or anterolateral hip pain. Instead, they complain of pain in the lumbosacral or sacroiliac regions, due to the strain and compensation of those regions to the psoas spasm. Counterstrain points may be 180 degrees around the body from the site of the presenting pain. For example, in a patient with pain between the shoulder blades, the counterstrain point is often on the sternum. Counterstrain points are mediated through the nervous system and can result in multiple points from a single somatic dysfunction. Therefore, it is also possible to have both anterior and posterior or right and left counterstrain points associated with the same segmental dysfunction. If multiple counterstrain points are located in a given area, ask the patient which is the most tender and treat that point first. This is the most efficient treatment method since associated but less significant counterstrain points often disappear after successful treatment of the primary counterstrain point.

If the counterstrain point results from a viscerosomatic reflex, tenderness returns within minutes or hours, not days. This requires a thorough review of the patient's medical history, a more careful physical examination, and consideration of all possible causes for the original tenderness (For more information about viscerosomatic reflexes, refer to the discussion of viscerosomatic reflexes in the basic science section of this book, and the article by Beal).[65] This understanding is also important when treating patients in the hospital. (Refer to the article by Schwartz[66] on the treatment of hospitalized patients with counterstrain.)

The physician will first palpate the anatomical location of a counterstrain point as described by Jones and others and then test for the presence of a counterstrain point. As the physician's skill develops, finding tissue texture abnormalities, most typically increased tension, will become evident well before the patient reports any tenderness. The skilled palpating hand will zero in on the area of greatest tissue change and then confirm the identification of a significant counterstrain point by pressing on the tissue to elicit tenderness from the patient. This ability to palpate these tissue changes will also help guide the physician to more accurate positioning as well as in treating stoic patients.

Step 2: Establish a Tenderness Scale with the Patient for Effective Feedback

To facilitate the communication between physician and patient, it is important to establish a means to monitor the level of tenderness of the counterstrain point. Physicians typically use a tenderness scale to enhance verbal feedback from the patient, several of which have been used effectively. The most common is a 0-to-10 scale, with 10 being equal to the level of pretreatment tenderness and 0 being the absence of tenderness (Fig. 47.3A).

The number only represents a relative relationship, not a fixed quantity of tenderness. The quantity of tenderness for a designation of 10 for one counterstrain point may be different from the 10 for another point. Nonetheless, the scale allows the patient to communicate the changes in tenderness in correlation with palpatory changes. The same amount of pressure should be used each time to elicit tenderness of a specific point, although different pressures are

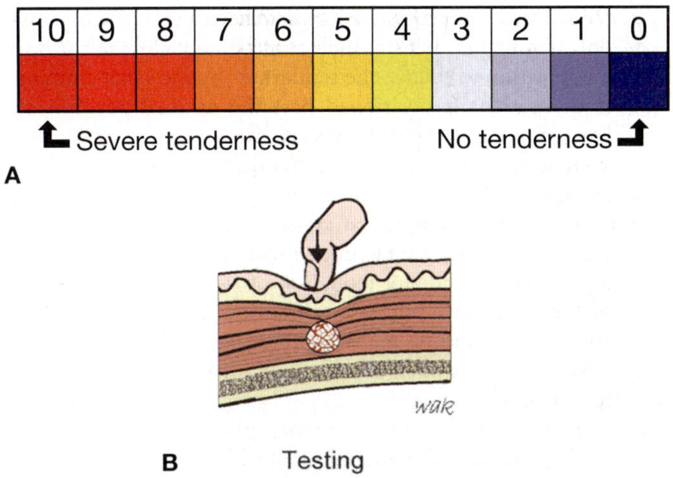

Figure 47.3. Counterstrain treatment: Step 2: Establish a tenderness scale with the patient for effective feedback. A. Ten-point tenderness scale. **B.** Testing tenderness of a counterstrain point.

needed for different counterstrain points because of the different amounts of tissue over each point (Fig. 47.3B).

It should be emphasized to the patient that the applied pressure is not acupressure or a form of massage. It is used for evaluation, not treatment. Firm pressure is provided only to determine the level tenderness. At other times, only light contact is maintained. This feedback provides a means for monitoring the effectiveness of positioning and treatment for both patient and physician. Asking the patient to define a point as mild, moderate, or severe initially, rather than as a number, reduces confusion with the tenderness scale.

Step 3: Continuously Monitor the Counterstrain Point Tenderness and Tissue Texture Changes

Maintaining contact with the counterstrain point throughout treatment is vital for palpating tissue changes occurring at the point and showing the patient that the post-treatment assessment is the exact same point. This helps guide the physician to the optimal treatment position as well as to the end point of treatment. Note that the pressure used to monitor the counterstrain point is less than that used to test for tenderness. Monitoring pressure allows enough force to maintain contact with the myofascial tissues of the counterstrain point without eliciting tenderness (Fig. 47.4A,B).

After a significant counterstrain point is selected for treatment, it is monitored as the physician moves the patient toward the position of comfort described by Jones and others. The myofascial tissues of the counterstrain point will begin to relax as the patient is moved toward the correct treatment position. The patient is first positioned in the classic position described for that specific counterstrain point. The physician then tests for the level of tenderness, with the initial goal of rating as a 3 or less from the initial tenderness. The pressure used to test for the level of tenderness is increased to the firm pressure initially used to test for the presence of a counterstrain point. Jones[6] found it would take about four times this pressure to cause tenderness in healthy tissue. The pressure should be applied as a very short quick push, not a long, slow, and sustained amount of pressure. If the physician moves the patient in the correct direction, the tenderness will decrease. The closer to the optimal position, the less tenderness is present. Once the physician is able to palpate changes in tissue texture, these changes can be used to determine if the patient is positioned correctly. For example, moving the patient toward the optimal position will typically cause the tissues to relax, while moving the patient away from the optimal position will typically cause the tissue tension to increase. With experience, the physician will gather the correlation between tissue changes and the level of tenderness, which will be used to determine the optimal position of comfort more efficiently. Each new position is accompanied by retesting the tenderness of the counterstrain point.

Step 4: Place the Patient in the Position of Maximum Comfort

One of the advantages of counterstrain is that treatment is always performed in a position of comfort or ease, so that discomfort is avoided, and further injury is unlikely to occur (Fig. 47.5A,B).

Counterstrain can be used for patients with a wide variety of medical conditions unless gently moving the patient into the specific treatment position is contraindicated. A word of caution: medical judgment must always be used to determine the appropriateness of any treatment. Every patient needs to be evaluated thoroughly on an individual basis. The only absolute requirement for counterstrain is for the patient to be relaxed while the dysfunctional area of the body is placed into the position of comfort, where it is maintained during treatment.

The optimal position of comfort is a very specific position in space. While the position is similar for the same counterstrain point in different patients, the exact position is unique for each patient and varies with differences in range of motion between various patients. To determine this exact position, the physician uses a combination of palpation and feedback from the patient. Maintaining continuous light contact with the counterstrain point during treatment is crucial for maximum effectiveness and efficiency.

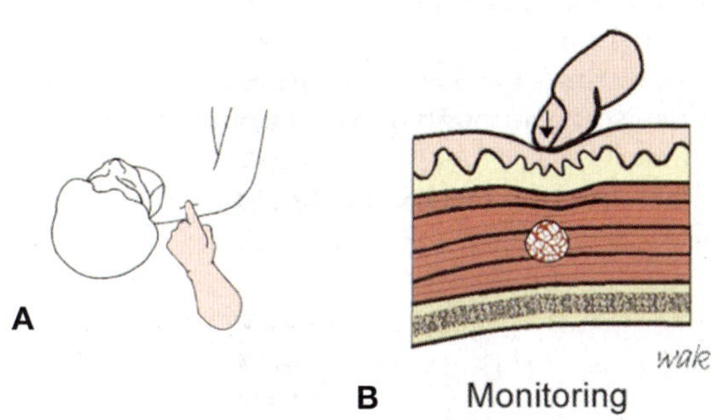

Figure 47.4. Counterstrain treatment: Step 3: Continuously monitor the counterstrain point tenderness and tissue texture changes. A. Monitoring a supraspinatus counterstrain point. **B.** Use of light pressure to monitor a counterstrain point.

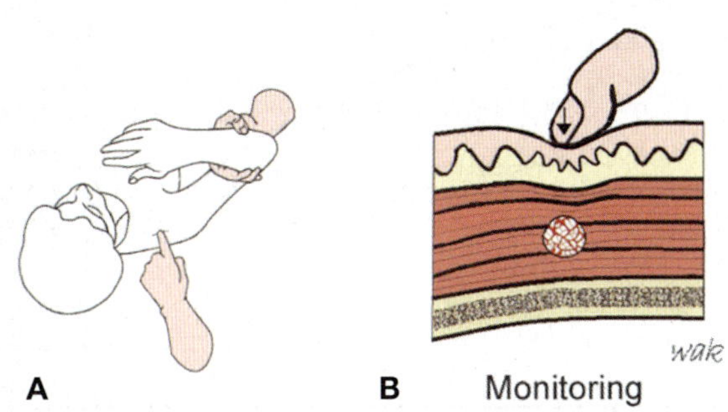

Figure 47.5. Counterstrain treatment: Step 4: Place the patient in the position of maximum comfort. A. Treatment position or position of maximum comfort for the supraspinatus counterstrain point. **B.** Use of light pressure to monitor a counterstrain point.

The first step in positioning is to approximate the expected position. This approximation may be based on previous clinical experience, patient history, or an illustration of the position in a counterstrain textbook. The purpose of the positioning is to reduce the tension of the dysfunctional myofascial structures and to eliminate the reflex maintaining the counterstrain point. As a general rule, the closer the counterstrain points are to the midline, the more flexed or extended the patient's presenting posture, and the more flexion or extension is required for the treatment position. With counterstrain points more lateral to the midline, more side bending and rotation are usually required for treatment. Side bending and/or rotation of the body away from the counterstrain point is the most common position necessary for effective treatment.

A protocol for arriving at this expected position is as follows:

1. Slowly move the patient toward the described or expected position of comfort while monitoring the counterstrain point for tissue relaxation. When marked relaxation of the counterstrain point is palpated, stop moving the patient.
2. Press the counterstrain point and ask for the level of tenderness. If the level is reported as being greater than 3 on the 10-point scale, continue to move the patient in the same direction. Then, as more significant relaxation is palpated or if the patient has been placed in the described position, stop movement and test again.
3. Repeat this process until the level of tenderness is lowered to 3 or less. If the number increases instead, return in the direction just traveled, and retest, since most likely, the patient has been positioned beyond the optimal position. It may be necessary to change direction or add other directions to find the correct position.
   a. Figure 47.6 shows the changes in tenderness as the patient is moved from a neutral starting position to the position of comfort and beyond.
   b. Note the reduction of tenderness to the distance traveled for optimal positioning is not linear.
4. From the beginning of positioning to about halfway to the position of optimal comfort, large movements are typically used, because the reduction in tenderness is small for the distance traveled.
5. As the patient is moved into a position close to the optimal position, fine-tune the position with small movements, monitoring with constant light contact of the counterstrain point and retesting the counterstrain point for reduction of tenderness with each new position. A small change in position at this point markedly reduces tenderness.
   a. For example, movement of 20% toward the optimal position (e.g., several inches) from the neutral starting position may reduce the tenderness by one on the scale, whereas it may only require one-quarter inch of movement close to the optimal position to reduce the tenderness by the same amount.
   b. If the patient is positioned past the optimal position, the level of tenderness will increase.
6. Fine-tune the position until the tenderness has been reduced by at least 70% (3 on the scale) and preferably by 100%. The position of comfort must be at least 70% improved over the initial tenderness or the technique will be ineffective.
   a. Jones recommended a reduction of two-thirds, while other practitioners have suggested three-fourths.
   b. An effort should be made to maximally reduce the tenderness since this will significantly increase the effectiveness of the treatment.
   c. If the patient cannot be easily brought to a position without tenderness, this also provides valuable diagnostic information and suggests another counterstrain point needs to be treated first.
7. A common mistake is the application of constant firm pressure on the counterstrain point throughout the treatment sequence. Instead, once the optimal treatment position has been determined, maintain only light contact with the myofascial tissue of the counterstrain point. There are three important reasons for maintaining contact:
   a. Tissue changes that occur in the counterstrain point can be monitored and can aid in determining the end point of treatment.
   b. The counterstrain point can continue to be fine-tuned while maintaining the optimal position of comfort, because the position may change slightly during treatment.
   c. Both the patient and the practitioner can be confident of the location of the counterstrain point.
      i. The third reason may seem unimportant, but when contact with the counterstrain point is lost, the patient may question whether the same point is being pressed. Also, the practitioner may have difficulty re-establishing contact with the point with enough confidence to allow for an accurate recheck.
8. At times, a pulsation in the counterstrain point may be palpated. This is referred to as the therapeutic pulse. Although its intensity may vary, it is often close to the intensity of the radial pulse. In fact, simultaneously palpating the patient's radial artery with the other hand typically shows it to be synchronous with the therapeutic pulse. Thus, the position of release is postulated to result in a sympatholytic vasodilation of small arterioles in the myofascial tissue.
   a. Occasionally, the therapeutic pulse will be palpated while attempting to determine the position of maximal comfort, enabling the practitioner to establish the position more accurately.
   b. At other times the therapeutic pulse will not be palpated until the treatment position has been maintained for a period of time.

In either case, the therapeutic pulse can be used to enhance treatment.

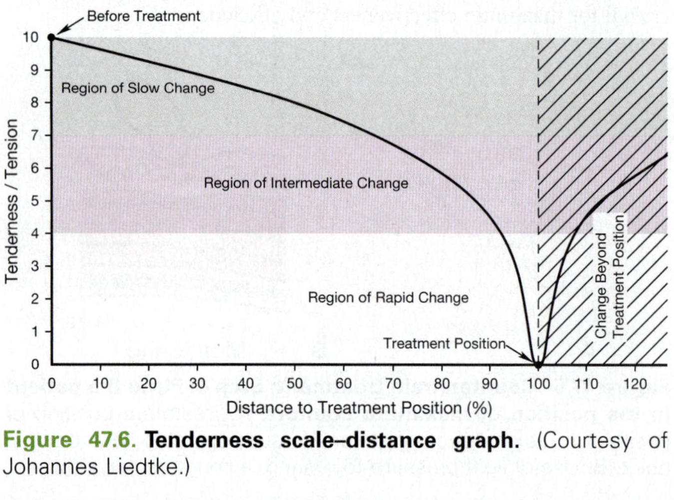

Figure 47.6. Tenderness scale–distance graph. (Courtesy of Johannes Liedtke.)

Step 5: Maintain the Treatment Position for 90 Seconds While the Patient Remains Passive

1. Once the position of comfort has been established, hold the position for 90 seconds (Fig. 47.7A,B).
2. Note that the patient must remain relaxed without contracting the dysfunctional myofascial tissue. The 90 seconds does not

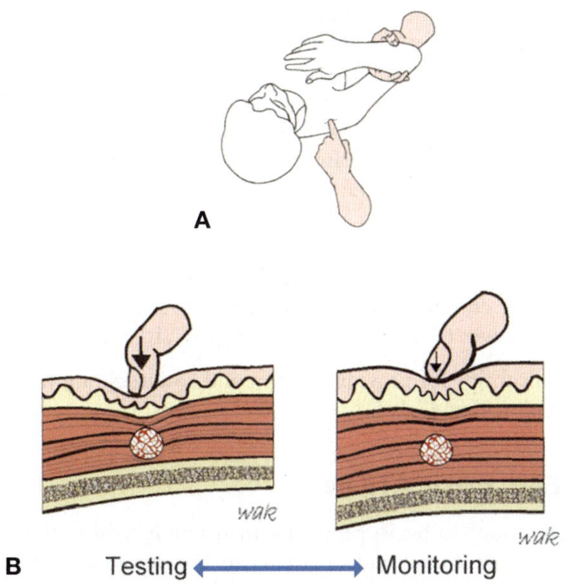

Figure 47.7. Counterstrain treatment: Step 5: Maintain the treatment position for 90 seconds while the patient remains passive. **A.** Supraspinatus treatment position. **B.** Alternating testing and monitoring the counterstrain point while in the treatment position.

begin until the patient is completely relaxed. It may be necessary to remind the patient to stay relaxed several times during the 90 seconds because patients often tend to contract the muscles unconsciously. Such a contraction is indicated by an apparent decrease in the weight of the body part being supported in the treatment position.

a. It is critical that the physician use good body mechanics for positioning. If not, they will not be able to support the patient during the treatment or may cause personal injury.
b. Patients who are not comfortable will not be able to relax for the entire 90 seconds.
c. Likewise, it will be difficult for a physician who is not comfortable to hold the patient in the treatment position for 90 seconds.
d. Trial and error may be required to determine the ideal positions for both patient and physician.
e. Each patient and clinical setting offers different challenges requiring a different setup. This is especially true with pregnant patients, patients with some degree of paralysis, hospitalized patients, and with physician–patient size mismatches. In all cases, good body mechanics are essential.

3. Jones recommended treatment of rib dysfunctions for 120 seconds. Though rib counterstrain points were not different from other counterstrain points, Jones observed that most patients tend to be slightly uncomfortable leaning up against the physician. Therefore, he added an additional 30 seconds for the patient to relax. Once the patient is placed in the position of maximal comfort for the rib counterstrain point, treatment time is the same 90 seconds used for all counterstrain points. This illustrates the importance of the physician being aware of the patient's state of relaxation and comfort at all times and is a common reason why a good response may not be achieved.
4. Feel for tissue changes in the counterstrain point and surrounding tissue. As time in the treatment position increases, the tissue relaxes, and a softening should be palpated. The myofascial tissue around the counterstrain point may begin to move in a seemingly random pattern. This sensation is due to relaxation of the myofascial tissue in different planes.
5. Although treatment time may not always require exactly 90 seconds, it is important to maintain the treatment position for 90 seconds when beginning to learn counterstrain.
   a. The ability to palpate myofascial release patterns enhances counterstrain treatment and can also be applied toward improving palpatory skills for myofascial release techniques and other models where subtle changes need to be palpated.
6. As discussed previously, the therapeutic pulse may be felt. Once the random motion becomes symmetrical or the therapeutic pulse disappears, move the patient back to the starting position.
7. Once a physician can confidently palpate the tissue changes signaling the end of treatment, watching a clock is no longer necessary.

Step 6: Slowly Return the Patient Passively While Maintaining Contact with the Counterstrain Point

1. After maintaining the position of comfort for 90 seconds, the patient is slowly returned to the starting position while monitoring the counterstrain point.
2. Before starting to move, ask the patient to remain passive and not assist by actively moving, otherwise, patients often try to help during the return.
3. If the patient starts to help or move, stop the return and remind the patient to remain passive.
   When the patient has relaxed, start moving again, more slowly.
4. An apparent decrease in the patient's weight while being moved is another indication that the patient is contracting muscles.
5. A common error when learning counterstrain is to move the patient too quickly. A slow return is critical, especially for the first few degrees of motion.
   a. Watch the patient for signs of flinching or other guarding gestures during the return, as this may be an indication they fear pain will occur.
   b. Palpating for muscle contraction could also provide a sign that the patient is being moved too quickly (Fig. 47.8).

Step 7: Re-evaluate for Resolution of Tenderness, Tissue Texture Abnormalities, and Associated TART Findings at the Counterstrain Point

1. Once the patient has been returned to the starting neutral position, re-evaluate the tenderness and tissue texture of the counterstrain point (Fig. 47.9A,B).
2. To consider the treatment successful, no more than 30% (3 on the 10-point scale) of the original tenderness should remain. Ideally, all of the tenderness will have resolved. More than 30% of the tenderness may remain due to several reasons:
   a. The patient may not have been optimally positioned.
   b. The physician may have let the position change during treatment.

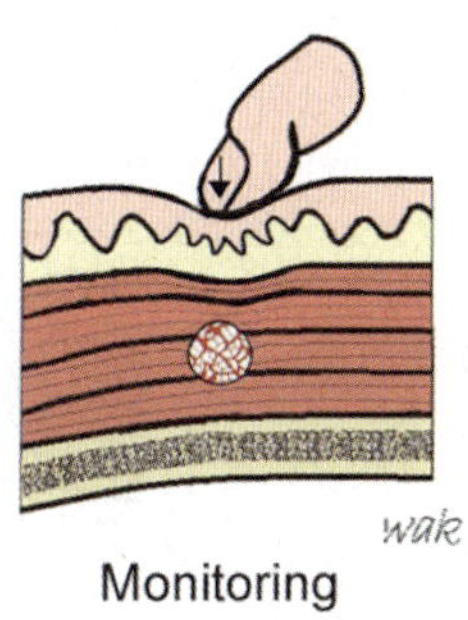

Figure 47.8. Counterstrain treatment: Step 6: Slowly and passively return the patient to the neutral position while maintaining contact with the counterstrain point.

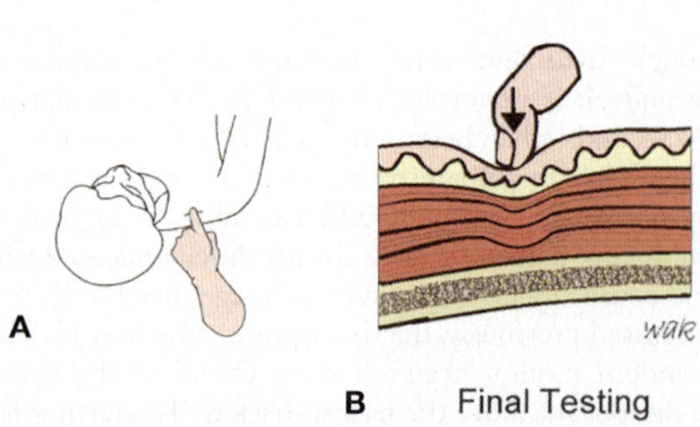

Figure 47.9. Counterstrain treatment: Step 7: Re-evaluate for resolution of tenderness, tissue texture abnormalities, and associated TART findings at the counterstrain point. A. Supraspinatus counterstrain point. **B.** Final testing of counterstrain point after treatment.

   c. The patient may have contracted the muscle being treated.
   d. The physician may have lost contact with the counterstrain point.

   In all cases, repeat the positioning, with particular attention to obtaining and maintaining the optimal position with the patient completely relaxed.

3. Another cause for failure may be that another counterstrain point is the primary problem, and therefore, the most significant point was not treated.
   a. Evaluate the counterstrain points in the area near the counterstrain point just treated and the corresponding area on the opposite side of the body to determine if another, more significant counterstrain point is present.
   b. This is especially relevant if the point treated was part of a sequential line of counterstrain points.
   c. Consider the possibility that the primary counterstrain point is distant from the area evaluated or is on the opposite side of the body from the reported problem.
4. More than one treatment session may be necessary to completely resolve a counterstrain point.
5. Failure to completely resolve the tenderness also does not necessarily indicate an ineffective treatment. Some of the most challenging counterstrain points to treat occur when both anterior and posterior counterstrain points are present at the same level (e.g., AT4 and PT4).
6. Reevaluate the original structural findings to assess the effectiveness of the treatment. Since the goal is to treat a somatic dysfunction and not simply decrease the tenderness of a counterstrain point, the importance of revaluation cannot be overstated.
   a. Motion restrictions, asymmetry, and tissue texture abnormalities should improve or disappear after an effective treatment.
   b. With chronic somatic dysfunction, the tissue changes may be slower to return to normal (Fig. 47.10 and Table 47.3).

Clinical tips for providing strain and counterstrain techniques are found in Box 47.1.

PATIENT EDUCATION

It is important to begin providing instructions before the patient gets off the treatment table. Patients are curious to see if the treatment eliminated the presenting complaint.

1. Warn the patient not to test previously restricted motions and to avoid extremes of motion for several days.
   a. This is especially true if the movement approximates the original position of injury, because it may reproduce the inappropriate reflex just treated.
   b. Active movement that reproduces the position of injury is different from the careful positioning performed by the physician while the patient is passive.
2. The patient should stay well hydrated for several days after treatment. This helps to eliminate the increased products of metabolism that may have been released into circulation after relaxation of the tense myofascial tissue.
   a. Water is recommended over other fluids, which may contain sugar and other dissolved substances.
   b. The patient is especially recommended to avoid consuming alcoholic beverages for about 3 days.

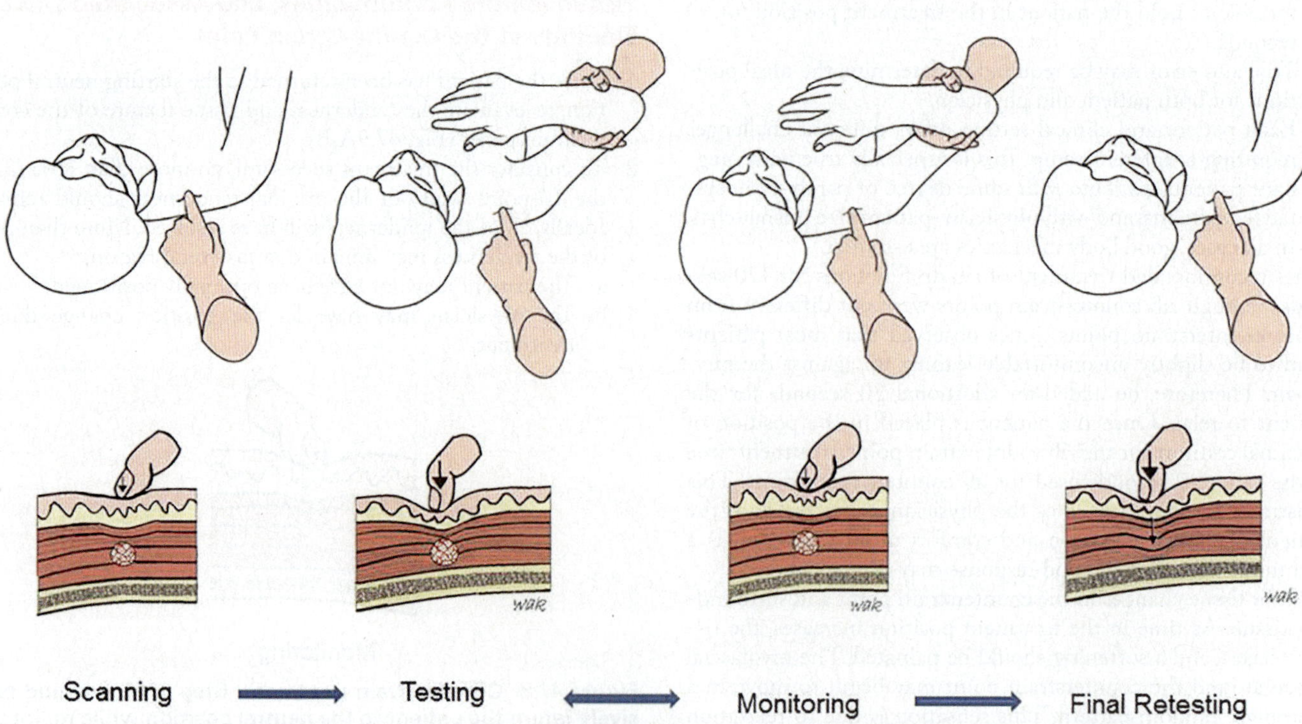

Figure 47.10. Overall process of scanning, testing, monitoring, and final testing of a counterstrain point.

TABLE 47.3

Basic Steps for Treating Somatic Dysfunction with Counterstrain

Step	Procedural Steps	Step Illustrations
1	• Identify the most significant counterstrain point associated with the somatic dysfunction by ○ History ○ Observation ○ Structural exam ○ Scanning appropriate regional counterstrain points. ○ Point is identified by ■ local tenderness ■ tissue tension • When a point is identified, ask the patient if the tenderness is mild, moderate, or severe • Significant points are severe and the worst is treated first	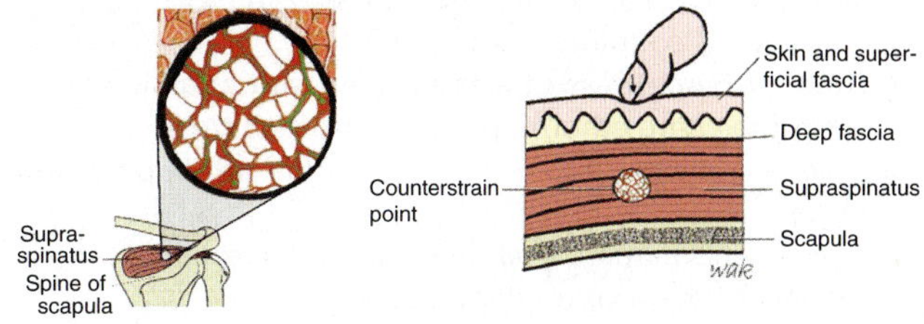
2	• Establish a tenderness scale with the patient for effective feedback of tenderness changes during positioning and treatment with "10" representing the tenderness before treatment and "0" being no tenderness, only pressure	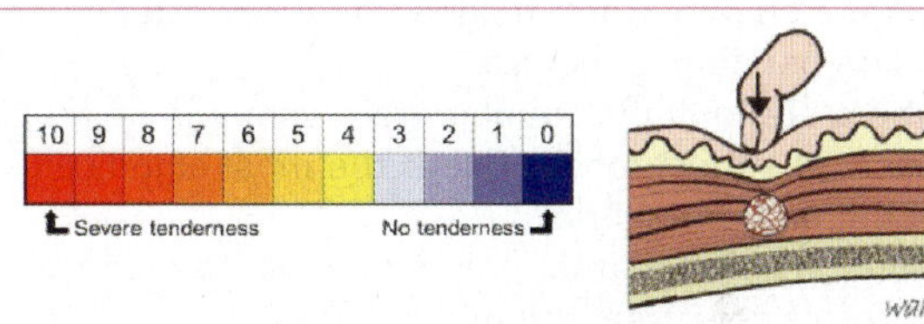
3	• Continuously monitor the counterstrain point tenderness and tissue texture changes with light pressure while adjusting patient position as needed during the procedure • The tissue tension directly correlates with tenderness, so also monitor tension changes • Keep your finger on the counterstrain point throughout the procedure	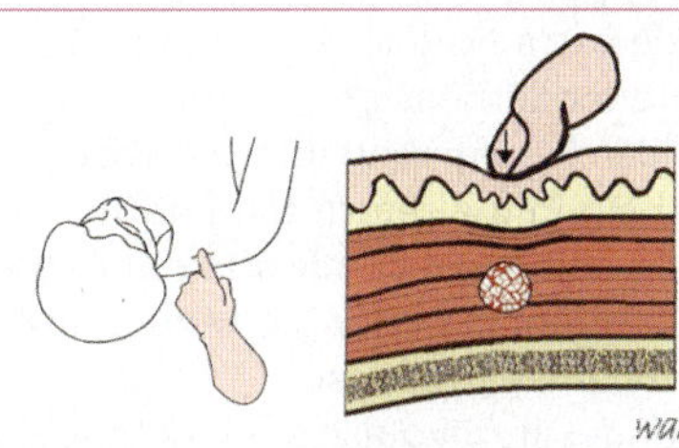
4	• Place the patient in a position to reduce tenderness of the counterstrain point, ideally to "0," but no higher than "3" on a 10-point scale (70% reduction of tenderness) • Initial large motions of the patient toward the treatment position yield small reductions in tenderness/tension, while small motions close to the treatment position produce large changes	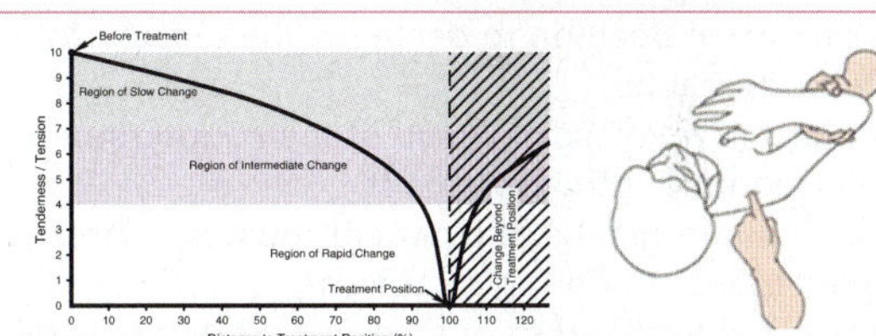
5	• Maintain the position of maximal comfort/minimal tenderness for 90 seconds with the patient passive while continuously monitoring tissue texture with light pressure • Test the tenderness about every 30 seconds with brief added pressure, adjusting patient position to ideally stay at "0"	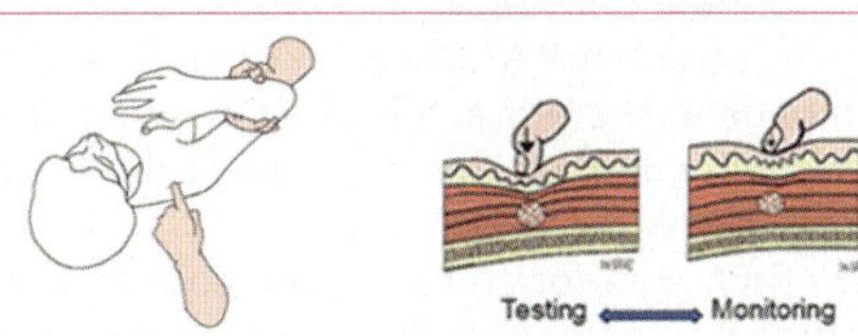
6	• Before beginning the slow return to the pretreatment position, instruct the patient to remain passive during the return • Monitor to feel if patient assists by contracting the muscle being treated during the return • Remember to keep your finger on the counterstrain point throughout procedure	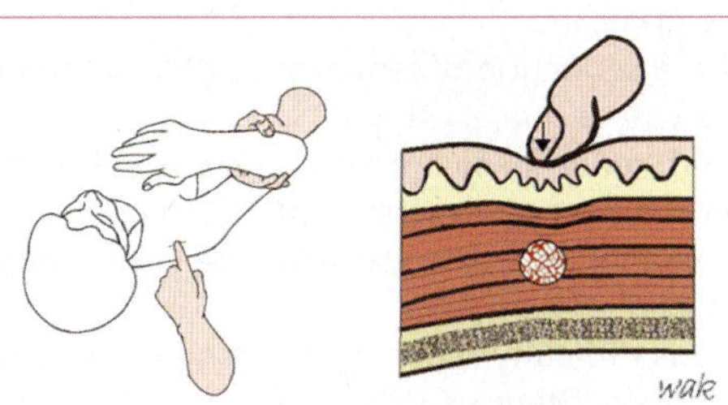
7	• Recheck tenderness level of counterstrain point once patient is back in pretreatment position • Then recheck structural, TART findings, and other regional counterstrain points	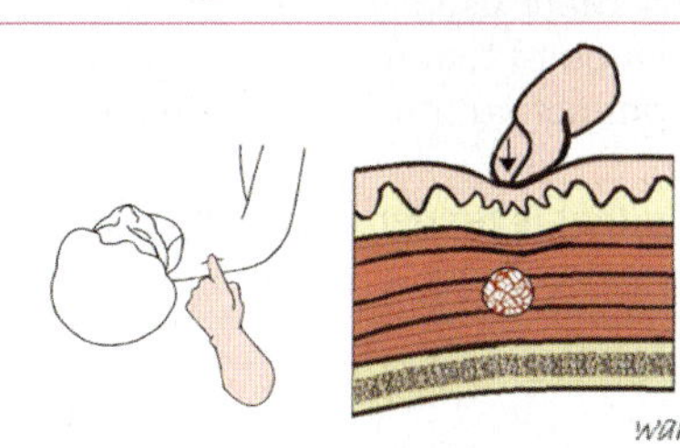

BOX 47.1 Clinical Tips for Using Counterstrain

- A single somatic dysfunction may have more than one associated counterstrain point
- Test for tenderness of a specific counterstrain point with the same amount of pressure each time
- Use less pressure to monitor a counterstrain point than to test it
- Physician's palpatory abilities are more reliable than a patient's report of tenderness
- Anterior points typically require flexion and posterior points typically require extension
- Midline points typically require pure flexion (if anterior) or pure extension (if posterior), whereas the more lateral a point is from midline, the more rotation and/or side bending is required
- If there are multiple counterstrain points in an area, usually the most tender one is the most significant and should be treated first
- If several counterstrain points of equal tenderness occur in a row, treat the middle one first
- Spend a little extra time to fine-tune and completely eliminate the tenderness of a counterstrain point
- The patient can help getting into the position of comfort, but cannot help in the return to neutral
- The optimal position of comfort is obtained when the counterstrain point is no longer tender and the tissue tension is maximally reduced
- Monitor changes in myofascial tension and adjust the treatment position to decrease the tension for maximum results
- Monitor the myofascial tissue of the counterstrain point throughout the treatment
- For maximum results, the patient must be completely relaxed (passive) during treatment
- Recheck the tenderness of a point several times while in the treatment position
- Causative factors and mechanism of injury are unique to each patient. Therefore, the exact position of ease will vary depending on the response of the tissue during positioning
- Scan for both anterior and posterior counterstrain points within a region/functional unit to determine the most significant
- Aim for a reduction of tenderness of less than or equal to 70% with a goal of 100%
- Use both tenderness and tissue texture abnormalities to find the best treatment position
- The presence of a therapeutic pulse indicates good myofascial relaxation
- If there is difficulty reducing the tenderness to zero is experienced, there usually is another more significant counterstrain point that needs to be treated first or the patient is contracting muscles near the counterstrain point
- Every tissue that is tender to palpation is not a counterstrain point

Although counterstrain techniques are well tolerated, a post-treatment reaction may occur. Approximately 30% of patients experience a generalized soreness or a flu-like reaction 1 to 48 hours after treatment. This usually occurs on the morning after treatment, and typically only after the first treatment. The reaction may last for 1 to 5 days, although 1 to 2 days are most common. The cause is unclear but could be related to the washout of the products of metabolism from the dysfunctional myofascial tissue. In any case, the patient should be alerted to the possibility of a post-treatment reaction. Prescribing an analgesic for 1 or 2 days may help reduce discomfort. The possibility of a post-treatment reaction also cautions the use of counterstrain on some gravely ill patients.

Patients generally want to know how often they need to be treated and how long it will take to resolve the complaint. As with all forms of manipulative treatment, there is no single, definitive answer. One treatment may eliminate the somatic dysfunction, although other dysfunctions may require treatment over a more extended period of time. Jones had patients return in 3 to 7 days after the initial treatment, although 1 to 2 weeks may be more practical for many physicians. If the same somatic dysfunctions and associated counterstrain points recur beyond three to four treatments, without any resolution, rethinking the cause and treatment plan are indicated. As the somatic dysfunction resolves, the time between treatments is increased. The end point of treatment depends on the:

- Cause of the problem, especially if work related
- Underlying tissue damage
- Preexisting medical problems
- Response of the patient
- Cooperation by the patient to avoid painful positions
- Skill of the physician

EVOLUTION OF THE COUNTERSTRAIN MODEL

It is not the nature of an osteopathic physician to learn a manipulative model by memorizing a group of techniques and then repeating them over and over. Andrew Still did not write a technique manual. Instead, he emphasized learning anatomy and concepts that can be applied to meet the unique needs of each patient. Therefore, it is no surprise that osteopathic physicians have modified Larry Jones model. Classical counterstrain involves maintaining the position of release for 90 seconds, but this is not always necessary nor the best option. Just as each patient is unique, the time required for treatment is not a constant.

Two critical factors affect the treatment time required:

1. The physician's ability to accurately position the patient.
2. The patient's ability to keep the myofascial tissue being treated completely passive.

The best indicator that a treatment is complete is the palpatory response gained by monitoring the counterstrain point and adjacent tissues. Over the course of treatment, the tissues relax, and the initial random motion of the surrounding myofascial tissue becomes symmetrical and rhythmic. If the myofascial tissues in the region being treated begin to unwind, the physician may choose to change from counterstrain to myofascial release to treat the somatic dysfunction. Counterstrain is classically a positional release model, but it is the physician's experience and decision that determine whether remaining in a relatively static position or moving the dysfunctional tissue offers the best treatment.

Other alternatives may be used to accelerate or enhance the release.

- Instead of treating a single counterstrain point with a position of ease, Ross Pope, DO, FAAO, stacked several regional counterstrain points and treated them all at once in a single position, which greatly increased his efficiency.
- Facilitated Positional Release, developed by Stanley Schiowitz, DO, FAAO, reduces treatment time by adding compression, distraction, or a torque force to the indirect treatment position.
- Richard Van Buskirk, PhD, DO, FAAO, used counterstrain points as he worked on redeveloping the Still technique. He would identify a somatic dysfunction and find an associated counterstrain point, followed by a position to eliminate the tenderness. He then adds a compressive force and brings the joint from its indirect position in a continuous arc, past neutral, and through the restrictive barrier. He also applied distractive and torque forces as in Facilitated Positional Release.
- A number of osteopathic physicians, including Larry Jones, studied Janet Travell myofascial pain syndromes and its associated trigger points. A number of trigger point locations were identical to those of the counterstrain points. Naturally, physicians attempted to treat trigger points with a counterstrain positional release approach and found it to be quite effective.[41,67] Harmon Myers, DO, spent much of his career integrating the two models, produced excellent results, and passed on his knowledge to many physicians who took courses from him.
- Paul Rennie, DO, FAAO, found combining counterstrain with muscle energy and exercise to be another approach that increases treatment efficiency and accelerates patient recovery. In the counterstrain treatment position, the patient contracts the antagonist muscle to the muscle being treated by lengthening the antagonist muscle to further reduce both tenderness of the counterstrain point and tissue texture changes. This contraction is a postisometric relaxation of the antagonist muscle and reciprocal inhibition of the agonist, commonly involved in muscle energy technique. Specific exercises are combined with the treatment of specific counterstrain points to reinforce the balance and reduce reinjury.[40]

Other physicians have also contributed to the evolution of the counterstrain model. These include:

- G. Bradley Klock, DO, FAAO, who modified treatment of the six sacral counterstrain points with a gentle traction of the myofascial tissues over the sacrum. He has also identified 18 specific counterstrain points that correlate with Dr. Zink's common compensatory pattern and emphasized the importance of sequencing the counterstrain points.
- John Glover, DO, FAAO, who brought the cranial rhythmic impulse into the counterstrain point to complete a treatment.
- William Devine, DO, who added traction into the counterstrain point through the myofascial tissue.
- Faculty at the Jones Institute, including Edward Goering, DO, have identified and successfully treated both visceral and lymphatic counterstrain points, thus expanding the model into new areas. These counterstrain points are treated in one-third of the time required for treating a typical counterstrain point, and the results are exciting.
- Other modifications also continue to be developed.

The nomenclature of the counterstrain points is a component of the counterstrain model that is often confusing for novice physicians. Jones identified these points over a number of years and named them in several ways, such as:

- The dysfunctional segment
- A nearby landmark
- An associated diagnostic finding
- Muscle in which the point was located

Jones changed the names of several points between the publication of his two books,[3,6] in most cases, to identify the muscle he felt was associated with the somatic dysfunction. This evolution of the model must continue in order to clearly delineate the anatomical relationships of the counterstrain point and to allow physicians to learn both the names and treatment positions more effectively.

DIAGNOSES AND TREATMENTS BY BODY REGION

The treatment illustrations that follow are intended as an introduction to the counterstrain technique model. An example from each of the 10 codable regions of the body has been chosen to illustrate a variety of treatment options. More in-depth counterstrain reference texts are available for greater coverage of the body regions.[3,6,40,41,67]

The treatment positions presented may be modified according to the needs of the physician and patient. Therefore, knowledge of the three-dimensional position typically used to treat a counterstrain point is helpful in changing the position from that described in a text. Either the physician or patient may prefer a change to seated, supine, or side lying. Certain conditions may also necessitate changing a preferred position of treatment. For example, a pregnant patient in the third trimester may need to be treated in a side lying position. Such adaptations allow for the successful performance of the treatment. An effective treatment position should also be one that reduces the patient's tenderness to zero.

With the introduction of ICD-10, the osteopathic code numbers have changed. The new codes all begin with M99 and have two digits after the decimal point. These range from M99.00 to M99.09 for the same ten regions and follow the same sequence. Each of the 10 regions given below shows the new ICD-10 code, followed by the former ICD-9 code in parentheses and the name of the region. Some of the counterstrain points present a challenge with regard to how they should be recorded.[68] Most of the posterior counterstrain points are located on the structures from which their names were derived, but many of the anterior counterstrain points are not. Therefore, the physician must decide whether to record them in the physical region where they are located or in the functional region related to the somatic dysfunction diagnosis proposed by Jones. The physician needs to be consistent in the charting. This brings up an important point: the rationale for Jones' nomenclature as was taught in his courses is different from that being taught in counterstrain courses today. Thus, this is a source of confusion and frustration for many students learning the counterstrain points for the first time. A thorough review of the nomenclature would benefit students in the future. Nevertheless, more basic science investigation and electromyogram studies of the exact tissue location of counterstrain points are necessary to propose a revised nomenclature.

ILLUSTRATIVE TREATMENT TECHNIQUES

M99.00: Segmental and Somatic Dysfunction of Head Region

Jones described a number of counterstrain points on the head, many of which are associated with cranial dysfunctions. The reader should refer to a counterstrain text for a description of these points. In addition, several of the cervical counterstrain points are located

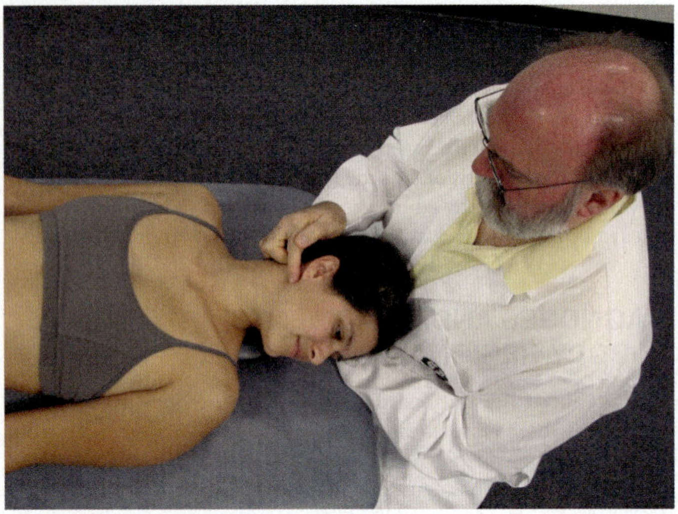

Figure 47.11. **Anterior first cervical (AC1), right.**

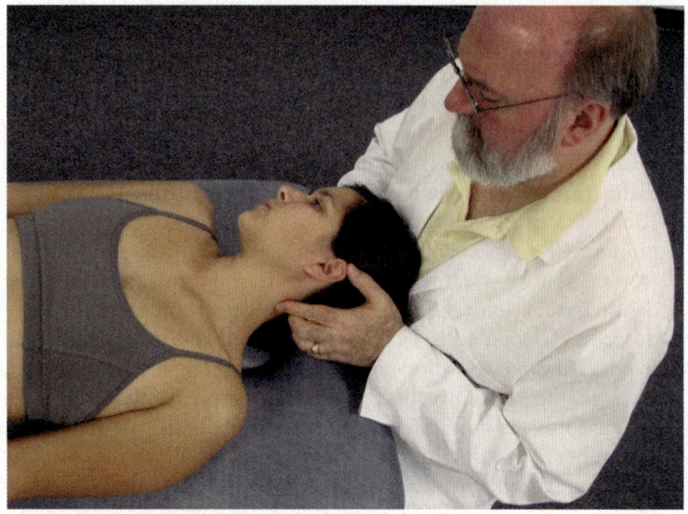

Figure 47.12. **Anterior fourth cervical (AC4), left.**

on the skull, with the two most common being the anterior first cervical and posterior second cervical.

M99.01: Segmental and Somatic Dysfunction of Cervical Region

The cervical spine has several maverick counterstrain points (points where the position of comfort differs from that expected). Anterior counterstrain points are typically located on the most anterolateral aspect of the anterior tubercles of the cervical vertebra. Posterior counterstrain points are found on the occiput, associated with the tip of the spinous processes or lateral to the spinous processes.

ANTERIOR FIRST CERVICAL (AC1)

Counterstrain Point Location
Found on the posterior surface of the ascending ramus of the mandible, approximately 1 cm from the angle of the jaw, pressing anteriorly (Fig. 47.11).

Treatment Position (Patient Supine)
Slight *flexion* of the head and upper neck, *rotation* away from the side of the counterstrain point close to the end range of motion, and slight *side bending* to fine-tune.

ANTERIOR FOURTH CERVICAL (AC4)

Counterstrain Point Locations
Found at the anterior lateral surface of the anterior tubercle of the fourth cervical vertebrae, pressing anterolateral to posteromedial (Fig. 47.12).

Treatment Position (Patient Supine)
Flexion of the head and upper neck to the fourth cervical vertebra (approximately 45 degrees). *Side bend* and *rotate* the head and upper neck away from the side of the counterstrain point.

M99.02: Segmental and Somatic Dysfunction of Thoracic Region

Anterior thoracic spine counterstrain points are located in two major areas:

1. The first group of counterstrain points, AT1-6, is located midline on the sternum. They can be identified by palpating for tense, tender tissue overlying the sternum.
2. The second group is located in the abdominal wall. Most are within the rectus abdominis muscle and can be found an inch or two lateral to midline on the right or left.

Posterior thoracic counterstrain points are found on two parts of each vertebra.

1. One location is associated with the spinous process and is more tender on either the left or right side.
2. The second location is on either transverse process.

The treatment described is given for different spinal levels, but they are not hard and fast requirements. Extension, side bending, and rotation to any level can be introduced either from above or below the segment. The physician's decision is based on the flexibility of the patient, patient comfort, and the relative size of the patient and physician.

POSTERIOR FIFTH THORACIC (PT5)

Counterstrain Point Location
On the inferolateral side of the spinous process of the fifth thoracic vertebra, pressing anteriorly (Fig. 47.13).

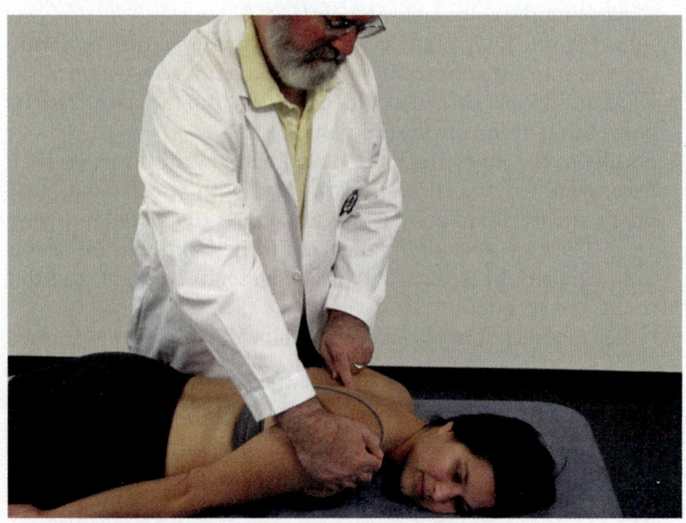

Figure 47.13. **Posterior fifth thoracic (PT5), left.**

Even though the spinous process is a midline structure, there will be more tenderness on one side than on the other. In addition, look for deviation in the spinous process.

Treatment Position (Patient Prone)

Side bend the trunk away from the side of the deviated spinous process by pulling the opposite shoulder in an inferior and posterior direction. This creates extension with rotation and side bending away from the deviated side.

M99.03: Segmental and Somatic Dysfunction of Lumbar Region

- Anterior lumbar spine counterstrain points are mostly located around the rim of the pelvis anteriorly. They can be found in association with the anterior superior iliac spine (ASIS), anterior inferior iliac spine, and anterior surface of the pubic rami.
- Posterior lumbar counterstrain points are found mostly in the same areas as in the thoracic spine, although the counterstrain points found on the tips of the transverse processes need to be approached by pressing anteromedially at about a 45-degree angle.

The naming convention for spinal dysfunction involves describing the dysfunctional segment relative to the segment below it. If motion is introduced from below the dysfunctional segment, the vertebral segment below it moves first, producing a position relative to the dysfunctional segment that can seem confusing. As an example, if the vertebra below the dysfunctional segment is rotated to the right, then the relative position of the dysfunctional segment relative to the vertebra below is described as rotated left. Take note of this when reading the treatment descriptions for this section.

POSTERIOR FIFTH LUMBAR (PL5)

Counterstrain Point Location

On the tip of the spinous process, test the right and left sides of the spinous process to identify the most tender side, by pressing anteriorly (Fig. 47.14).

Treatment Position (Patient Prone)

Extend the trunk on the ipsilateral side of the spinous process by lifting the pelvis in a posterior direction. This creates extension with the needed rotation of the upper vertebrae away from the counterstrain point side.

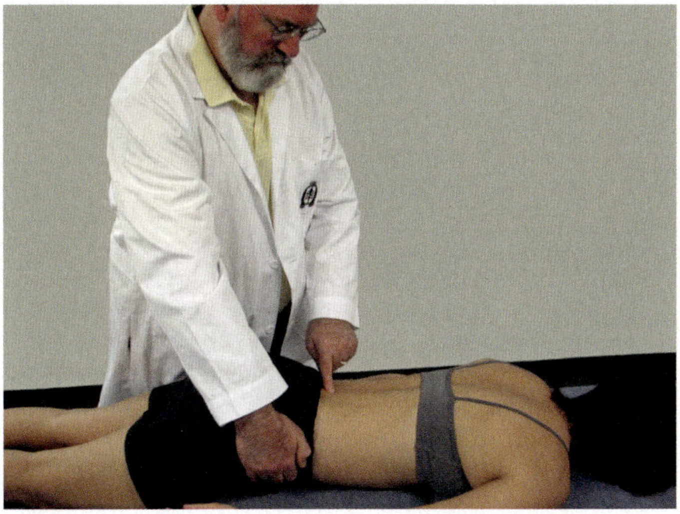

Figure 47.14. Posterior fifth lumbar (PL5), right.

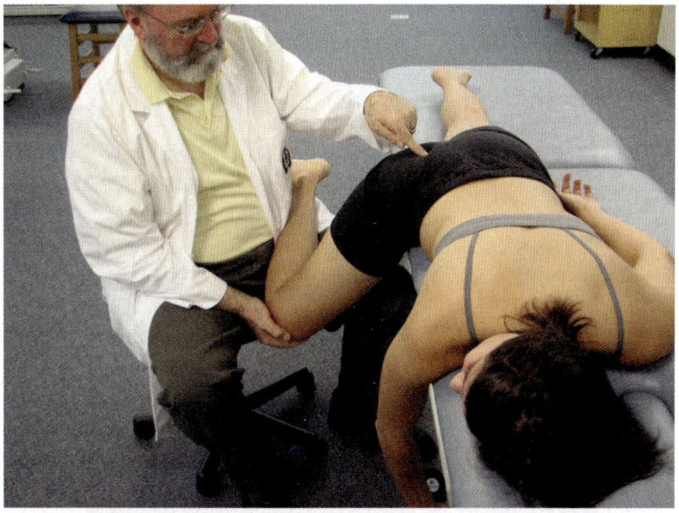

Figure 47.15. Piriformis (PIR), right.

M99.04: Segmental and Somatic Dysfunction of Sacral Region

Several anterior counterstrain points and several posterior counterstrain points are vital for diagnosis and treatment of pelvic somatic dysfunction. The anterior points typically require flexion, with varying amounts of rotation, and side bending, to a lesser degree. Posteriorly, counterstrain points are associated with sacral problems and muscles of the pelvis. Extension is the predominant motion associated with the posterior counterstrain points, although several points also require some degrees of flexion.

PIRIFORMIS (PIR)

Counterstrain Point Location

In the middle of the piriformis muscle, halfway between the greater trochanter and its attachment to the lateral side of the sacrum, pressing posterolateral to anteromedial (Fig. 47.15).

Treatment Position (Patient Prone)

Marked flexion of the ipsilateral hip to about 135 degrees and marked *abduction*. *Lateral rotation* of the hip may also be required, particularly if tenderness is found more lateral on the piriformis muscle.

M99.05: Segmental and Somatic Dysfunction of Pelvic Region

A number of counterstrain points are located on the sacrum and are associated with the musculature of the posterior pelvis. The counterstrain point locations and treatments demonstrate the counterstrain approach to the sacrococcygeal region. Since many counterstrain points are located in the sacrococcygeal region, consulting a text devoted to counterstrain is recommended for further discussion of the points in this region.

ILIACUS (ILA)

Counterstrain Point Location

At the level of the ASIS, one-third of the way toward midline, from the ASIS deep in the abdomen over the iliacus, pressing anterior to posterior (Fig. 47.16).

Treatment Position (Patient Supine)

Marked *flexion* of the hips bilaterally to shorten both of the iliacus muscles. Both hips are *laterally rotated*, with the knees *abducted* from the center of the body.

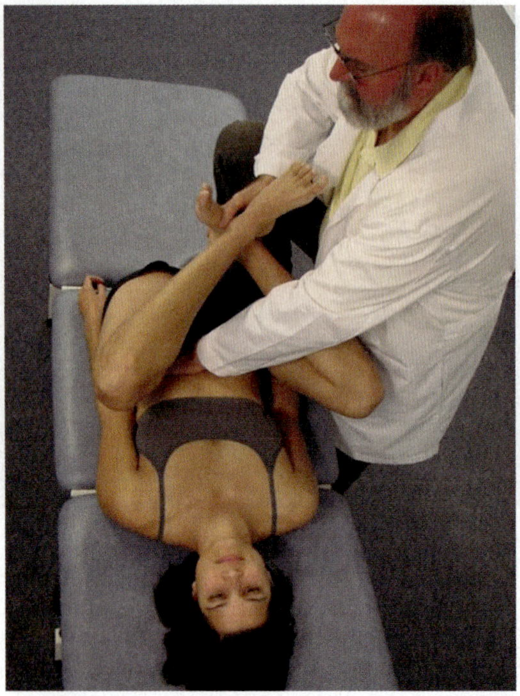

Figure 47.16. **Iliacus (ILA), right.**

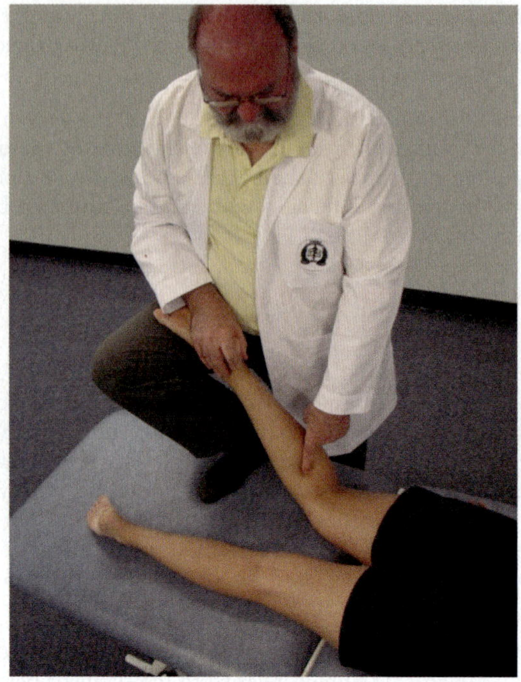

Figure 47.17. **Extension ankle (EXA), left.**

M99.06: Segmental and Somatic Dysfunction of Lower Extremity

The counterstrain point location and treatment demonstrate the counterstrain approach to the lower extremity. Because many counterstrain points are present in the lower extremity, consulting a text devoted to counterstrain is recommended for further discussion of the points associated with this region. Counterstrain points may be found at attachment points for muscles or ligaments, as well as in the belly of a dysfunctional muscle.

EXTENSION ANKLE (EXA)

Counterstrain Point Location
Within the two bellies of the gastrocnemius, just below the lower popliteal margin, pressing posterior to anterior (Fig. 47.17).

Treatment Position (Patient Prone)
Marked *plantar flexion* of the ankle. This is usually accomplished with the patient prone, and the dorsum of the patient's involved foot supported on the physician's thigh. Pressure is applied on the calcaneus to produce plantar flexion.

M99.07: Segmental and Somatic Dysfunction of Upper Extremity

The counterstrain point location and treatment demonstrate the counterstrain approach to the upper extremity. Because many counterstrain points are present in the upper extremity, consulting a text devoted to counterstrain is recommended for further discussion of the points associated with this region. Counterstrain points may be found at attachment points for muscles or ligaments, as well as in the belly of a dysfunctional muscle.

SUPRASPINATUS (SPI)

Counterstrain Point Location
In the middle of the supraspinatus muscle, superior to the spine of the scapula, pressing superiorly to inferiorly (Fig. 47.18).

Treatment Position (Patient Supine)
Flexion and *abduction* to about 45 degrees and *external rotation* of the humerus.

M99.08: Segmental and Somatic Dysfunction of Rib Cage

Jones used the terms "depressed" and "elevated" to refer to the counterstrain points associated with rib somatic dysfunction in order to emphasize the position of maximum comfort with a patient. The current convention involves naming the counterstrain points for their location, anterior or posterior on the body. In the example provided here, both conventions have been combined.

Anterior counterstrain points correspond to Jones' depressed ribs and posterior counterstrain points correspond to Jones' elevated ribs. The anterior rib counterstrain points start just below the medial end of the clavicle, where the first rib attaches to the

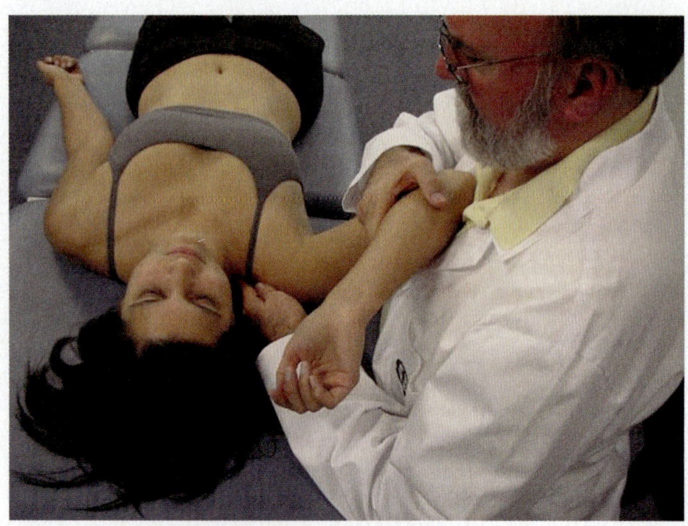

Figure 47.18. **Supraspinatus (SPI), right.**

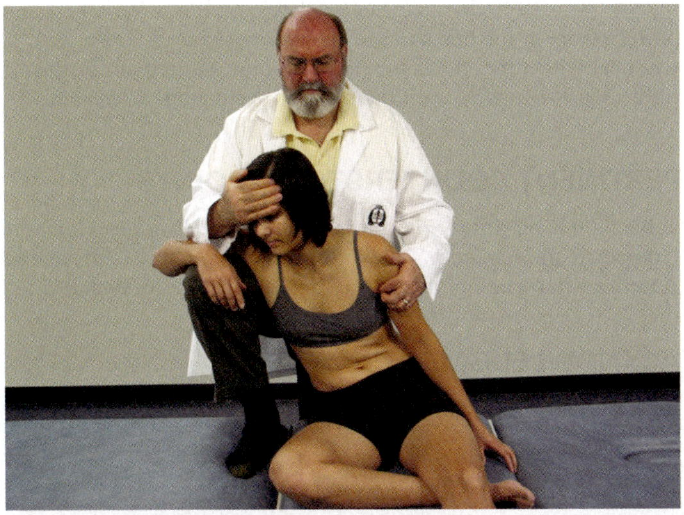

Figure 47.19. Anterior third rib (AR3), left.

sternum and moves laterally in an arc to the anterior axillary line. Most of the anterior rib counterstrain points are located on the ribs, along the anterior axillary line. It is uncommon, but not impossible, to find counterstrain points below the sixth rib. The posterior counterstrain points, with the exception of the first rib, are located on the angle of the ribs.

ANTERIOR (DEPRESSED) THIRD RIB (AR3)

Counterstrain Point Location

On the third rib in the anterior axillary line, pressing from anterolateral to posteromedial (Fig. 47.19).

Treatment Position (Patient Seated)

Depression of the ipsilateral costal cage is elicited by:

- *Side bending* of that side
- *Flexion* of the thoracic cage, head, and neck with elevation of the contralateral shoulder
- Translation away from (side bend toward) the counterstrain point. Fine tune with *rotation* of the body, usually toward the counterstrain point. Side bending can be increased with patient's legs placed on the table opposite the elevated shoulder, which is usually supported on the physician's thigh.

M99.09: Segmental and Somatic Dysfunction of Abdomen and Other Regions

A number of counterstrain points are found in the abdominopelvic region and different practitioners have recorded them in different regions.[68] Jones felt that some were reflexes from spinal dysfunctions, anterior thoracic seven to eleven for example, while others are related to muscle dysfunction, such as the iliacus and psoas points. The counterstrain points in this region may also represent viscerosomatic reflexes.

ANTERIOR EIGHTH THORACIC (AT8)

Counterstrain Point Location

In the medial aspect of the rectus abdominis muscle, halfway between AT7 and AT9 (Fig. 47.20).

Treatment Position (Patient Seated)

Mild *flexion* of the torso with side bending toward the counterstrain point and rotation away.

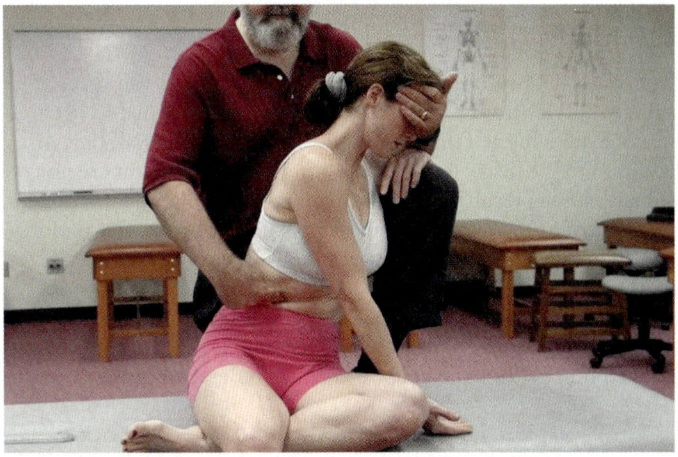

Figure 47.20. Anterior eighth thoracic (AT8), right.

CASE

A 45-year-old male presented to the office with a complaint of nonradiating right-sided low back pain of 2 weeks' duration. He described the pain as alternating between an intense deep pain and an achy pain, which becomes worse when he tries to stand upright. The problem began 2 weeks ago when he spent a day cleaning out his garage. After working most of the day bending and lifting to go through boxes and move them into a storage cabinet, he lifted a very heavy box of books. The patient was bent over at the waist and had barely lifted the box off the ground when he felt a sharp pain in his lower back. He dropped the box and, as a reflex reaction, stood up quickly. The patient went inside to sit down and rest. When trying to stand up from the chair, he experienced a low back spasm and could not stand upright. Over the course of the following 2 weeks, the patient tried hot showers, a heating pad, a topical analgesic cream, and Extra Strength Tylenol, all without much benefit. He denies any change in bladder or bowel function.

PHYSICAL EXAMINATION

- Vital signs were within normal limits (P: 72, R: 14, BP: 118/74, T: 98°F).
- Head, Eyes, Ears, Nose and Throat, cardiovascular, pulmonary, and abdominal exams were also normal.
- Neurologic exam showed normal lower extremity DTRs (2+/4+ bilaterally) and normal sensation in the lower extremities.
- Straight leg raising test was negative.
- Structural exam revealed a discrete area of intense tenderness to palpation. Tissue texture abnormalities were also found at the level of the ASIS, one-third the distance to midline, and deep in the abdomen bilaterally over the right iliopsoas muscle.

DIAGNOSIS

1. Lumbar strain, right greater than left
2. Somatic dysfunction—lumbar spine and pelvis

PLAN

Osteopathic manipulative treatment using counterstrain produced good results and was well tolerated by the patient.

DISCUSSION

The initial injury occurred when the patient used the erector spinae muscles from a stretched position, as the agonist to lift a heavy load. Muscle fatigue from lifting and bending all day, in addition to the heavy load, caused him to strain the right erector spinae muscle, resulting in back pain. When the patient stood up rapidly to move away from the position of pain, the rapid lengthening of the shortened right iliopsoas muscle (antagonist to the erector spinae muscle) reported a strain to the central nervous system before an actual strain occurred. This concluded in a hyper-shortened right iliopsoas muscle and a counter-strain point within the muscle. While the erector spinae was protected from further damage by the mechanical strain and will heal with time, the counterstrain point will remain in the right iliopsoas muscle until the somatic dysfunction is treated.

PERTINENT COUNTERSTRAIN POINTS

Table 47.4 is reprinted with permission from *A Teaching Guide for Osteopathic Manipulative Medicine*, 2nd ed., by the ECOP of the American Association of Colleges of Osteopathic Medicine.

ACKNOWLEDGMENTS

Illustrations by William A. Kuchera.

TABLE 47.4

Pertinent Counterstrain Points

Region Tender Points	General Anatomical Location Palpate in the area of the described tender point to find the point of maximum tenderness and associated tension related to the dysfunction.	General Treatment Position This is in reference to the position of the tender point.
Cervical		
Anterior cervical 2–8	2–6—On the anterolateral aspect of the corresponding anterior tubercle of the transverse process 7—On the clavicular attachment of the SCM 8—At the sternal attachment of the SCM on the medial end of the clavicle	2–6—Flexed, rotated away, side bent away 7—Flexed, rotated away, side bent toward 8—Flexed, rotated away, side bent away
Anterior cervical 1	Mandible—posterior aspect of the ascending ramus of the mandible at the level of the earlobe	Marked rotation away with slight side bending to fine tune
Posterior Cervical		
C1 inion	On the inferior nuchal line lateral to the inion	Marked flexion with fine tuning
C2 (occiput)	On the inferior nuchal line at the attachment of semispinalis capitis	Extended, with fine tuning
C1 (occiput)	On the inferior nuchal line at the splenius capitis (midway between inion and mastoid)	Extended, with fine tuning
2–8 (spinous processes)	2—On the superior aspect of the spinous process 3—At the side or inferolateral aspect of the spinous process of C2 4–8—On the inferior or inferolateral aspect of the tip of the spinous process. PC4 is inferior to the C3 spinous process. Remainder of tender points follows this pattern.	2—Extended, with fine tuning 3—Flexed, side bent away, and rotated away 4–8—Extended, side bent away, and rotated away
Thoracic		
Anterior Thoracic		
1–6 midline	May have some degree of lateralization: AT1—Suprasternal notch AT2—From midpoint of the manubrium to the sternal angle AT3–6—Located on sternum, corresponding to costal level	Primarily flexion with minor rotation and/or side bending
7–12 bilateral	Points are lateral to the midline within the rectus abdominus. Using the area between the tip of the xiphoid and the umbilicus divided into quarters: AT7 is upper ¼ AT8 is ½ of distance AT9 is ¾ below	Shorten the tissues around the tender point, which may involve rotating the torso away or rotating the pelvis toward with flexion and side bending toward the tender point.

TABLE 47.4 (Continued)

Pertinent Counterstrain Points

Region Tender Points	General Anatomical Location Palpate in the area of the described tender point to find the point of maximum tenderness and associated tension related to the dysfunction.	General Treatment Position This is in reference to the position of the tender point.
	Using the area between the umbilicus and the pubic symphysis divided into quarters, AT10 is ¼ below umbilicus slightly more lateral than AT9 AT11 is ½ of distance and slightly more lateral than AT10 AT12 is midaxillary line on the inner iliac crest.	
Anterior Thoracic		
Pectoralis minor	Inferior and medial to the coracoid process at the myotendinous junction or in the muscle belly	Arm adducted diagonally across the chest, tractioned inferomedially
Rhomboids	Along the medial border of the scapula at the attachment of the muscle	Extend and adduct shoulder by positioning arm posteriorly to approximate the medial border of the scapula to the spine
Posterior Thoracic		
1–12 spinous process	On the inferior midline or inferolateral aspect of the tip of the spinous process	Primarily extension with rotation and/or side bending away
1–12 transverse process	At the lateral aspect of the transverse process	Extension, side bending away and rotation toward
Rib		
Anterior rib (depressed) 1–10	1—Inferior to the clavicle on the first chondrosternal articulation 2—Superior aspect of rib 2 in midclavicular line 3–10—On the anterior axillary line on the corresponding rib	1–2—Using the cervical-thoracic spine, flex, side bend and rotate toward the tender point 3–10—Sidebend and rotate toward and flex
Posterior rib (elevated) 1–10	On posterior–superior aspect of rib 1 just lateral to the costotransverse articulation 2–10—On the superior aspect of the corresponding rib angle	Using the cervical-thoracic spine, side bend away, rotate toward, and slightly extend 2–10—Sidebend and rotate away with flexion
Upper Extremity		
Subscapularis	Anterolateral border of the scapula on the subscapularis muscle pressing from an anterior-lateral to posteromedial direction	Shoulder extension and internal rotation
Supraspinatus	In the belly of the supraspinatus muscle	Flexion of shoulder, abduction, with marked external rotation
Levator scapulae	Superior medial border of the scapula at the attachment of the levator scapula	Glide the scapula superiorly and medially to shorten the muscle. May alternatively be treated by marked internal rotation of the shoulder with traction and slight abduction
Long head of biceps, short head of biceps/ coracobrachialis	Long head—Over the tendon of the bicep muscle in the bicipital groove Short head/coracobrachialis—At the inferolateral aspect of the coracoid process	Long head—flexion of elbow, shoulder flexion, abduction, internal rotation Short head/coracobrachialis—flexion of elbow, shoulder flexion, adduction and internal rotation
Radial head-lateral	Anterolateral aspect of the radial head at the attachment of the supinator	Elbow in full extension, forearm in marked supination, and slight valgus force
Medial epicondyle	At the medial epicondyle of the humerus at the common flexor tendon and the attachment of pronator teres	Flexion, marked pronation, and slight adduction of the forearm with slight flexion of the wrist
Dorsal wrist	Surface of any of the proximal 2nd to 5th metacarpals and in the muscles of the extensor carpi radialis and ulnaris	Wrist extension, with slight radial or ulnar deviation

(*continued*)

TABLE 47.4 (Continued)

Pertinent Counterstrain Points

Region Tender Points	General Anatomical Location Palpate in the area of the described tender point to find the point of maximum tenderness and associated tension related to the dysfunction.	General Treatment Position This is in reference to the position of the tender point.
Upper Extremity		
Palmar wrist	Base of any of the proximal 2nd to 5th metacarpals and in the muscles of the flexor carpi radialis and ulnaris	Wrist flexion, with slight radial or ulnar deviation
Abductor policis brevis (first carpometacarpal)	Anterioradial aspect of the base of the first metacarpal bone	Flexion of wrist with abduction of thumb
Lumbar		
Anterior lumbar 1–5	1—Medial aspect of ASIS 2—Medial aspect of AIIS 3—Lateral aspect of the AIIS 4—Inferior aspect of the AIIS 5—On the anterior, superior aspect of the pubic ramus just lateral to the symphysis	1—Flex to spinal level, rotate pelvis toward (achieves relative trunk rotation away) and sidebend toward 2–4—Flex to spinal level, rotate pelvis away (achieves relative trunk rotation toward) and sidebend away 5—Flex to spinal level, rotate pelvis toward (achieves relative trunk rotation away) and sidebend away
Posterior Lumbar 1–5		
1–5 (spinous process)	On the inferior midline or inferolateral aspect of the tip of the spinous process	Extension to spinal level, side bending, and rotation pelvis toward
1–5 (transverse process)	At the lateral aspect of the transverse process	Extension to spinal level, side bending, and rotation pelvis toward
Pelvis		
Anterior		
Iliacus	Starting at 1/3 of the distance from the ASIS to the midline and pressing deep in a posterior-lateral direction toward the iliacus	Marked bilateral flexion and external rotation of the hips with the knees flexed
Psoas	Starting at 2/3 of the distance from the ASIS to the midline and pressing deep in a posterior direction toward the belly of the psoas	Marked bilateral hip flexion with some external rotation of the hips and slight ipsilateral side bending of the lumbar spine
Low ilium	Superior surface of the iliopectineal (iliopubic) eminence associated with the attachment of psoas minor	Marked ipsilateral hip flexion
Inguinal	Medial aspect of the inguinal ligament near the pubic tubercle in association with the attachment of the pectineus	Flexion of thighs with contralateral thigh crossed over the ipsilateral thigh. Ipsilateral lower leg pulled laterally to create slight internal rotation of the hip on the affected side
Posterior		
Piriformis	Midpoint between the lower half of the lateral aspect of the sacrum and ILA and the greater trochanter	Marked flexion of the hip and abduction. Fine tune with external or internal rotation
Upper and lower pole L5	Upper pole-superior medial aspect of PSIS Lower pole-On the ilium just inferior to PSIS pressing superiorly	Upper pole-hip extension with fine tuning in adduction and ER/IR Lower pole-hip flexion to ~90 degrees, adduction, and slight internal rotation
High ilium sacroiliac	2–3 cm lateral to the PSIS pressing medially toward the PSIS	Hip extension with fine tuning in abduction and external rotation
Gluteus medius (posterior lumbar 3 and 4)	Upper outer portion of the gluteus medius at the level of the PSIS PL3—2/3 lateral from PSIS to tensor fasciae latae PL4—Posterior margin of tensor fasciae latae	Hip extension with fine tuning in abduction and external rotation
High ilium flare out (coccygeus)	Lateral aspect of the ILA and/or lateral aspect of the coccyx	Hip extension and adduction

TABLE 47.4 (Continued)

Pertinent Counterstrain Points

Region Tender Points	General Anatomical Location Palpate in the area of the described tender point to find the point of maximum tenderness and associated tension related to the dysfunction.	General Treatment Position This is in reference to the position of the tender point.
Lower Extremity		
Lateral trochanter	Along the iliotibial band distal to the greater trochanter	Moderate abduction of the thigh, slight flexion
Medial meniscus	Medial meniscus-anteromedial aspect of the meniscus on the joint line	Medial meniscus-moderate knee flexion, internal rotation and slight adduction of the tibia
Lateral meniscus/ popliteus	Lateral meniscus-lateral aspect of the meniscus on the joint line	Lateral meniscus-Moderate knee flexion, slight abduction of the tibia. May require some mild internal or external rotation
Navicular	Plantar surface of the navicular bone	Plantar flexion, supination, and inversion
Medial ankle (tibialis anterior)	Medial ankle-inferior to the medial malleolus along the deltoid ligament	Medial ankle-place a fulcrum on the medial aspect of the ankle. Apply an inversion force with slight shear.
Lateral ankle (fibularis or peroneus longus and brevis)	Lateral ankle-inferior and anterior to the lateral malleolus in the sinus tarsi (talocalcaneal sulcus)	Lateral ankle-place a fulcrum on the lateral aspect of the ankle. Apply an eversion force with slight shear.
Flexion calcaneus (quadratus plantae)	Anterior aspect of the calcaneus on the plantar surface of the foot at the attachment of the plantar fascia	Marked flexion of the forefoot approximating the forefoot to the calcaneus
Extension ankle (gastrocnemius)	Within the proximal gastrocnemius muscles distal to the popliteal margin	Marked plantar flexion of the ankle with knee flexion
Biceps femoris (lateral hamstring)	In the posterior thigh lateral to the midline approximately halfway down the shaft of the femur	Flexion of the knee with external rotation and slight abduction of the tibia, and plantar flexion of the ankle by compression on the calcaneus
Semimembranosus (medial hamstring)	In the posterior thigh medial to the midline approximately halfway down the shaft of the femur	Flexion of the knee with internal rotation and slight adduction of the tibia, and plantar flexion of the ankle by compression on the calcaneus

REFERENCES

1. Jones LH. Spontaneous release by positioning. *DO*. 1964;4:109–116.
2. Educational Council on Osteopathic Principles. *Glossary of Osteopathic Terminology*. 3rd ed. American Association of Colleges of Osteopathic Medicine; 2017.
3. Jones LH. *Strain and Counterstrain*. American Academy of Osteopathy; 1981.
4. Jones LH. Missed anterior spinal lesions: a preliminary report. *DO*. 1966;6:75–79.
5. Travell JG, Simons DG. *Myofascial Pain and Dysfunction: The Trigger Point Manual*. Vol. 1. Williams & Wilkins; 1999.
6. Jones LH, Kusunose R, Goering E. *Jones Strain-Counterstrain*. Jones Strain-Counterstrain; 1995.
7. Korr IM. Proprioceptors and somatic dysfunction. *J Am Osteopath Assoc*. 1975;74:638–650.
8. Kandel ER, Schwartz JH, Jessell TM, Siegelbaum SA, Hudspeth AJ. *Principles of Neural Science*. 5th ed. McGraw-Hill Companies, Inc.; 2013:790–801.
9. Mense S, Simons D. *Muscle Pain: Understanding Its Nature, Diagnosis, and Treatment*. Lippincott Williams & Wilkins; 2001.
10. Mense S, Gerwin RD, eds. *Muscle Pain: Understanding the Mechanisms*. Springer-Verlag; 2010:17–48.
11. Crago PE, Houk JC, Rymer WZ. Sampling of total muscle force by tendon organs. *J Neurophysiol*. 1982;47(6):1069–1083.
12. Dyhre-Poulsen P, Krogsgaard MR. Muscular reflexes elicited by electrical stimulation of the anterior cruciate ligament in humans. *J Appl Physiol*. 2000;89:2191–2195.
13. Melnyk M, Faist M, Gothner M, Claes L, Friemert B. Changes in stretch reflex excitability are related to "giving way" symptoms in patients with anterior cruciate ligament rupture. *J Neurophysiol*. 2007;97:474–480.
14. Solomonow M. Ligaments: a source of musculoskeletal disorders. *J Bodyw Mov Ther*. 2009;13:136–154.
15. Solomonow M. Sensory-motor control of ligaments and associated neuromuscular disorders. *J Electromyogr Kinesiol*. 2006;16:549–567.
16. Petrie S, Collins J, Solomonow M, Wink C, Chuinard R. Mechanoreceptors in the palmar wrist ligaments. *J Bone Joint Surg Br*. 1997;79-B:494–496.
17. Krogsgaard MR, Dyhre-Poulsen P, Fischer-Rasmussen T. Cruciate ligament reflexes. *J Electromyogr Kinesiol*. 2002;12:177–182.
18. Howell JN, Cabell KS, Chila AG, Eland DC. Stretch reflex and Hoffman reflex responses to osteopathic manipulative treatment in subjects with Achilles tendinitis. *J Am Osteopath Assoc*. 2006;106(4):537–545.
19. Wynne MM, Burns JM, Eland DC, et al. Effect of counterstrain on stretch reflexes, Hoffmann reflexes, and clinical outcomes in subjects with plantar fasciitis. *J Am Osteopath Assoc*. 2006;106(9):547–556.
20. Rennie PR. Counterstrain tender points as indicators of sustained abnormal metabolism: advancing the counterstrain mechanism of action theory. *AAO J*. 2007:17–23.
21. McCord JL, Kaufman MP. Chapter 12: Reflex autonomic responses evoked by Group III and IV muscle afferents. In: Kruger L, Light AR, eds. *Translational Pain Research: From Mouse to Man*. CRC Press; 2010.
22. Jarvholm U, Palmerud G, Karlsson D, Herberts P, Kadefors R. Intramuscular pressure and electromyography in four shoulder muscles. *J Orthop Res*. 1991;9(4):609–619.

23. Jensen BR, Jorgensen K, Huijing PA, Sjogaard G. Soft tissue architecture and intramuscular pressure in the shoulder region. *Eur J Morphol.* 1995;33(3):205–220.
24. Luckenbill-Edds L, Bechill GB. Nerve compression syndromes as models for research on osteopathic manipulative treatment. *J Am Osteopath Assoc.* 1995;95(5):319–326.
25. Van Buskirk RL. Nociceptive reflexes and the somatic dysfunction: a model. *J Am Osteopath Assoc.* 1990;90(9):792–794, 797–809.
26. Bailey M, Dick L. Nociceptive considerations in treating with counterstrain. *J Am Osteopath Assoc.* 1992;92(3):334, 337–341.
27. Baliki MN, Apkarian AV. Nociception, pain, negative moods and behavior selection. *Neuron.* 2015;87(3):474–491.
28. Kandel ER, Schwartz JH, Jessell TM, Siegelbaum SA, Hudspeth AJ. *Principles of Neural Science.* 5th ed. McGraw-Hill Companies, Inc.; 2013:530–555.
29. Amann M. Significance of group III and IV muscle afferents for the endurance exercising human. *Clin Exp Pharmacol Physiol.* 2012;43:831–835.
30. Amann M, Blain GM, Proctor LT, Sebranek JJ, Pegelow DF, Dempsey JA. Implications of group III and IV muscle afferents for high-intensity endurance exercise performance in humans. *J Physiol.* 2011;589(21):5299–5309.
31. Mense S. Pathophysiologic basis of muscle pain syndromes: an update. *Phys Med Rehabil Clin N Am.* 1997;8(1):23–53.
32. Rosenmeier JB, Hansen J, Gonzalez-Alonso J. Circulating ATP-induced vasodilation overrides sympathetic vasoconstrictor activity in human skeletal muscle. *J Physiol.* 2004;558(Pt 1):351–365.
33. Bland-Ward PA, Humphrey PPA. Acute nociception mediated by hindpaw P2X receptor activation in the rat. *Br J Pharmacol.* 1997;122:365–371.
34. Kandel ER, Schwartz JH, Jessell TM, Siegelbaum SA, Hudspeth AJ. *Principles of Neural Science.* 5th ed. McGraw-Hill Companies, Inc.; 2013:289–306.
35. Kruger L, Silverman JD, Mantyh PW, Sternini C, Brecha NC. Peripheral patterns of calcitonin-gene-related peptide general somatic sensory innervation: cutaneous and deep terminations. *J Comp Neurol.* 1989;280(2):291–302.
36. Visser B, van Dieen JH. Pathophysiology of upper extremity muscle disorders. *J Electromyogr Kinesiol.* 2006;16:1–16.
37. Gunn CC, Milbrandt WE. Tenderness at motor points: an aid in the diagnosis of pain in the shoulder referred from the cervical spine. *J Am Osteopath Assoc.* 1977;77:196–212.
38. Korner L, Parker P, Almstrom C, Herberts P, Kadefors R. Relation between spectral changes of the myoelectric signal and intramuscular pressure of human skeletal muscle. *Eur J Appl Physiol.* 1984;52:202–206.
39. Tuckey B, Srbely J, Rigney G, Vythilingam M, Shah J. Impaired lymphatic drainage and interstitial inflammatory stasis in chronic musculoskeletal and idiopathic pain syndromes: exploring a novel mechanism. *Front Pain Res.* 2021;2:691740.
40. Rennie PR, Glover JC, Carvalho C, Key LS. *Counterstrain and Exercise: An Integrated Approach.* 3rd ed. RennieMatrix; 2012.
41. Myers HL, Devine WH, Fosum C, Glover JC, Kuchera M, Kusunose RS, Van Buskirk RL. *Clinical Application of Counterstrain.* Compendium ed. Osteopathic Press; 2012.
42. Yates HA, Glover JC. *Counterstrain: A Handbook of Osteopathic Technique.* Y Knot Publishers; 1994.
43. Gunn CC, Milbrandt WE. Tenderness at motor points. A diagnostic and prognostic aid for low-back injury. *J Bone Joint Surg Am.* 1976;58(6):815–825.
44. Reinert A, Kaske A, Mense S. Inflammation-induced increase in the density of neuropeptide-immunoreactive nerve endings in rat skeletal muscle. *Exp Brain Res.* 1998;121(2):174–180.
45. Nakamoto T, Matsukawa K. Muscle mechanosensitive receptors close to the myotendinous junction of the Achilles tendon elicit a pressor reflex. *J Appl Physiol.* 2007;102:2112–2120.
46. Von Düring M, Andres KH. Topography and ultrastructure of group III and IV nerve terminals of the cat's gastrocnemius-soleus muscle. In: Zenker W, Neuhuber WL, eds. *The Primary Afferent Neuron: A Surgery of Recent Morpho-Functional Aspects.* Plenum; 1990:35–41.
47. Saltin B, Mortensen SP. Inefficient functional sympatholysis is an overlooked cause of malperfusion in contracting skeletal muscle. *J Physiol.* 2012;590(24):6269–6275.
48. Gonzalez-Alonso J. ATP as a mediator of erythrocyte-dependent regulation of skeletal muscle blood flow and oxygen delivery in humans. *J Physiol.* 2012;590(20):5001–5013.
49. Rathbun J, Macnab I. Microvascular pattern at the rotator cuff. *J Bone Joint Surg Br.* 1970;52:540–553.
50. Meltzer KR, Standley PR. Modeled repetitive motion strain and indirect osteopathic manipulative techniques in regulation of human fibroblast proliferation and interleukin secretion. *J Am Osteopath Assoc.* 2007;107:527–536.
51. Dodd JG, Good MM, Nguyen TL. In vitro biophysical strain model for understanding mechanisms of osteopathic manipulative treatment. *J Am Osteopath Assoc.* 2006;106:157–166.
52. Zhang J-M, An J. Cytokines, inflammation and pain. *Int Anesthesiol Clin.* 2007;45(2):27–37.
53. Jeanjean AP, Moussaoui SM, Maloteaux JM, Laduron PM. Interleukin-1β induces long-term increase of axonally transported opiate receptors and substance P. *Neuroscience.* 1995;68(1):151–157.
54. Schweizer A, Feige U, Fontana A, Müller K, Dinarello CA. Interleukin-1 enhances pain reflexes. Mediation through increased prostaglandin E2 levels. *Agents Actions.* 1988;25(3–4):246–251.
55. DeLeo JA, Yezierski RP. The role of neuroinflammation and neuroimmune activation in persistent pain. *Pain.* 2001;90:1–6.
56. Wong CK, Moskovitz N, Fabillar R. The effect of strain counterstrain (SCS) on forearm strength compared to sham positioning. *Int J Osteopath Med.* 2011;14:86–95.
57. Collins CK, Masaracchio M, Cleland JA. The effectiveness of strain counterstrain in the treatment of patients with chronic ankle instability: a randomized clinical trial. *J Man Manip Ther.* 2014;22(3):119–128.
58. Radjieski JM, Lumley MA, Cantieri MS. Effect of osteopathic manipulative treatment on length of stay for pancreatitis: a randomized pilot study. *J Am Osteopath Assoc.* 1998;98:264–272.
59. Meseguer AA, Fernandez-de-las-Penas C, Navarro-Poza JL, Rodrıguez-Blanco C, Gandia JJB. Immediate effects of the strain/counterstrain technique in local pain evoked by tender points in the upper trapezius muscle. *Clin Chiropract.* 2006;9:112–118.
60. Lewis C, Flynn TW. The use of strain-counterstrain in the treatment of patients with low back pain. *J Man Manip Ther.* 2001;9(2):92–98.
61. Collins CK. Physical therapy management of complex regional pain syndrome I in a 14-year-old patient using strain counterstrain: a case report. *J Man Manip Ther.* 2007;15(1):25–41.
62. Haman JL. An osteopathic approach to treating chondromalacia-patellae with counterstrain manipulation. *Am Acad Osteopath J.* 1994;Spring:26–27.
63. Jacobson EC, Lockwood MD, Hoefner VC Jr, Dickey JL, Kuchera WL. Shoulder pain and repetition strain injury to the supraspinatus muscle: etiology and manipulative treatment. *J Am Osteopath Assoc.* 1989;89(8):1037–1040, 1043–1045.
64. Boyajian-O'Neill LA, McClain RL, Coleman MK, Thomas PP. Diagnosis and management of piriformis syndrome: an osteopathic approach. *J Am Osteopath Assoc.* 2008;108:657–664.
65. Beal MC. Viscerosomatic reflexes: a review. *J Am Osteopath Assoc.* 1985;85(12):786–801.
66. Schwartz HR. The use of counterstrain in an acutely ill in-hospital population. *J Am Osteopath Assoc.* 1986;86(7):433–442.
67. Ravin T, Cantieri M, Pasquarello G. *Principles of Prolotherapy.* American Academy of Manual Medicine; 2008.
68. Snider KT, Johnson JC. Survey of billing and coding for counterstrain tender points. *J Am Osteopath Assoc.* 2012;112(6):356–365.

RECOMMENDED READING

Jones LH, Kusunose R, Goering E. *Jones Strain-Counterstrain.* Jones Strain-Counterstrain; 1995.

Myers HL, Devine WH, Fosum C, Glover JC, Kuchera M, Kusunose RS, Van Buskirk RL. *Clinical Application of Counterstrain.* Compendium ed. Osteopathic Press; 2012.

Nicholas AS, Nicholas EA. *Atlas of Osteopathic Techniques.* 4th ed. Wolters Kluwer; 2022.

Ravin T, Cantieri M, Pasquarello G. *Principles of Prolotherapy.* American Academy of Manual Medicine; 2008.

Rennie PR, Glover JC, Carvalho C, Key LS. *Counterstrain and Exercise: An Integrated Approach.* 3rd ed. RennieMatrix; 2012.

48

Facilitated Positional Release

DENNIS J. DOWLING

KEY CONCEPTS

- Facilitated positional release aims to decrease muscle hypertonicity involved in the maintenance of articular dysfunction.
- The dysfunctional region is initially placed in a relatively neutral position.
- An activating force of compression, traction, or torsion is applied to effect immediate release of tissue tension, articular restriction, or both.
- Subsequent positioning into resistance seeks to affect larger (regional) muscle groups or smaller (intrinsic) deep muscles involved in joint mobility.

DEFINITION

Facilitated positional release (FPR) is defined by the Glossary of Osteopathic Terminology as the following[1]: An osteopathic treatment method in which a dysfunctional body region or structure is addressed with a combination of neutral positioning, application of an activating force (e.g., compression, distraction, or torsion), and placement into position of ease.[2] A technique developed by Stanley Schiowitz, DO, FAAO.

HISTORY

Stanley Schiowitz, DO, FAAO, graduated from the Philadelphia College of Osteopathy in 1944 and operated a solo practice for over 30 years in Brooklyn, New York. He states in his book "FPR and Beyond":

> "To balance my busy practice, to keep up with my studies, to stay involved in my professional organizations and to have time left for my family, I needed to develop a quick and accurate method of administering manipulative techniques. Over time, I began to work out fast and efficient manipulative diagnostic and treatment methods that expended minimal effort. These techniques freed me up to attend to the general practice and manipulative medicine needs of my patients- all during the same visit."[1]

In 1977, Dr. Schiowitz was asked to create the Osteopathic Manipulative Medicine department at the newly opened New York College of Osteopathic Medicine of the New York Institute of Technology.[1] During his tenure, he served as the associate dean and chairman of the Department of Osteopathic Principles and Practices (OPP) at the New York College of Osteopathic Medicine. His clinical practice on campus gave the undergraduate OPP fellows a great opportunity to practice osteopathic manipulation under the supervision of an experienced practitioner. Time after time, they would describe the same experience: Dr. Schiowitz would enter the treatment room after the students had treated a patient. The fellows would describe some finding or restriction that was recalcitrant to treatment. Dr. Schiowitz would then perform some quick maneuver that was unfamiliar to them, and the patient's somatic dysfunction would be improved. Dr. Schiowitz would quickly exit to see other patients. As the fellows exchanged notes on what they observed with his treatments, the group found that they were able to successfully perform them. Whenever possible, Dr. Schiowitz taught the fellows one-on-one or in small groups. It appeared that he had a cohesive approach for treatment that was, as of that time, without a name. The OPP fellows referred to it as "IO," or "instant osteopathy."

Because of his busy practice and time limitations, Dr. Schiowitz sought out and adapted methods of treatment that were rapid, effective, and based on anatomical and physiologic principles. Some of his students have remarked that Dr. Schiowitz had to develop a quick approach to treatment since he couldn't stay in one place for 90 seconds. Dr. Schiowitz admitted that he may have seen some practitioners using some elements or aspects of his approach on very specific diagnoses, but not in a globally designed system. By 1990, Dr. Schiowitz had standardized his treatment approach to the extent that it was published in the JAOA[2] and taught the technique at national meetings. The OPP fellows and some faculty members became his earliest table trainers at some of these sessions.

FPR is primarily an indirect method of treatment. However, Dr. Schiowitz practiced and taught FPR as a mixed treatment of indirect followed by direct techniques. The physician initially attempts to modify the sagittal posture by placing the region of somatic dysfunction into a position between flexion and extension, in order to approach the neutral position as defined by Fryette.[2,3] An activating force of compression, traction, or torsion is then applied to facilitate an immediate release of tissue tension and/or joint motion restriction. The region is then placed into its directions of dysfunction for a few seconds and then repositioned to neutral or, if desired, in the barrier directions, followed by reevaluation. This latter aspect, the positioning into the barriers, brings FPR into greater resemblance with the Still technique.[4] The goals of treatment are to decrease the muscle hypertonicity that maintains somatic dysfunction, whether by affecting larger regional groups or by modifying smaller more intrinsic deep muscles involved in joint mobility.

FPR is easily applied, effective, and time efficient. Often, patients report immediate relief of tension and/or tenderness, as well as restoration of function. Because treatment of specific dysfunctions is accomplished in seconds, repeat application can be attempted, or other methods of treatment can be subsequently applied.

PROPOSED MECHANISM OF ACTION

Korr[5] wrote that the immobility of a lesioned segment was initiated or maintained by an increased gain in gamma motor neuron activity of the muscles of that segment. The gamma motor neurons specifically innervate the intrinsic muscles, the muscle spindle apparatus that acts as sensors for overall muscle tonicity. When a gamma motor neuron stimulates a muscle spindle, such as a nuclear bag fiber, the fiber shortens in length, and the stretch receptor, either annulospiral or flower spray, becomes more sensitive to stretch than it was previously. Even if the overall extrinsic muscle is in a rest position, the lengthening nerve fibers of the muscle spindles may be sending signals back to the spinal cord, which in turn stimulates alpha motor neuron fibers innervating the same muscles. In effect, the muscle may remain in tension even in a so-called neutral position and may worsen with further stretching. Bailey[6] proposed that this high gain set of the muscle spindles result in changes of the soft tissues that are characteristic of somatic dysfunction. Due to these aspects, FPR is an indirect form of osteopathic manipulation in which the patient remains passive throughout treatment.

According to Carew's[7] discussion of the feedback mechanism of the muscle spindle stretch reflex, compressing muscles past their neutral position results in an inverse spindle output. The afferent excitatory input to the spinal cord through the group Ia and II fibers is eliminated. This results in a "quieting" of the gamma motor gain to the spindle, reduction of the stretch stimuli, and resultant elimination of the reflex activation of the alpha motor neuron. The tension and hypertonicity of the extrafusal muscle fibers are also reset.

Specific diagnosis in three planes is required for accurate treatment with FPR. The primary step in the application of FPR is the placement of the region of somatic dysfunction into its neutral position. This unloads the joints and may also affect both proprioceptive and nociceptive elements. The dysfunction can then respond more easily and rapidly to the applied therapeutic position, motion, and force. For the spine, the articular facets are placed into an "idling" position between the flexed and the extended extremes. A facilitating force, typically compression and/or torsion, is applied and maintained throughout the treatment. This tends to unload the facet joints and creates a "loose-packed" position.[8] The force is maintained as, using the triplanar diagnosis, further positioning of the somatic dysfunction is applied into all of the directions of relative freedom. Immediate soft tissue softening and relaxation is usually noted at this point.[8] This position is held for approximately 5 seconds, after which the region is returned to neutral. In practice, Dr. Schiowitz often followed neutral by bringing the dysfunction into the barrier directions and then returning the region again to neutral. The dysfunction is then reassessed. The tension that was noted in the area is most typically eliminated or at least reduced. Joint motion symmetry increases after treatment with the FPR if the etiology or maintenance of the dysfunction is due to muscular hypertonicity. If the asymmetry of joint motion is caused by other factors, such as degenerative changes, congenital malformation, meniscal injury, synovial entrapment, or ligamentous damage, the joint may remain restricted. Other modalities of osteopathic manipulation or repeated treatment with FPR may be necessary to complete treatment of the dysfunction.

INDICATIONS

As with all OMT, somatic dysfunction is an indication for FPR. However, FPR may be more specifically utilized in addressing the muscle fibers involved in somatic dysfunction. The treatment procedures are divided into two categories. The first is directed toward the normalization of palpable tissue texture abnormalities, such as hypertonicity while the other is modified to influence the deep muscles involved in joint mobility. Dr. Schiowitz recommended that if the physician was in doubt, to address the palpable tissue texture changes first and "If motion restriction persists, then a technique designed to normalize the deep muscles involved in the specific joint motion restriction is applied."[2]

SIDE EFFECTS AND CONTRAINDICATIONS

There are few contraindications, and most are relative in nature in the clinical application of FPR. If the patient is not able to tolerate the positioning or experiences discomfort, either alternative positioning of the region or alternative techniques should be used. FPR to the cervical region approximates a Spurling maneuver. If the patient experiences radicular pain, then repositioning or traction may be used. Lumbar techniques may put torsion into the knees or hips that have degenerative changes or prosthetics. Performing lumbar diskogenic treatment as described in this chapter would be contraindicated with a patient who has had a hip replacement, since the external rotation and torque forces may possibly disarticulate the joint. The same can be said for the use of the first rib technique with patients with shoulder pathology. The compression and twisting involved with the treatment may exacerbate conditions associated with new or chronic shoulder dislocations or separations. Any recent history of trauma to any region should raise suspicion of fracture or dislocation. Compression, even the relatively small forces used in FPR, may make a stable fracture unstable. Accurate diagnosis and integration of clinical knowledge should direct the use of any intervention with osteopathic manipulation. Caution should be used in the event of osteoporosis, malignancy, rheumatologic disorders, congenital malformations, stenosis, or other clinical diseases, although these are not absolute contraindications.

Generally, patients experience relief and few side effects when treated with FPR. As with any other treatment, there may be transient fatigue, soreness, or stiffness due primarily to the restoration of circulation to previously dysfunctional tissue and release of muscular waste products. In rare cases, the patient experiences these discomforts on subsequent treatments.

PRINCIPLES OF DIAGNOSIS

The diagnostic methods used to determine somatic dysfunction can vary. The use of FPR does not require special diagnostic tests unique to this modality. However, diagnosis is a prerequisite to treatment. Mennell[9] has described a method of skin rolling. Mitchell et al.[10] have used the coupled vertebral motion as described by Fryette to conduct rotoscoliosis testing, while Johnston[11] incorporates a method of scanning and screening to progressively narrow the findings to specific diagnoses.

Schiowitz utilized a very rapid method of diagnosis that incorporates the introduction of small motions to test all cardinal planes of motion. The appreciated palpatory response indicating relative freedom and resistance results in a specific diagnosis. For superficial muscular diagnosis, the pads of the physician's fingers are placed on the area of dysfunction to determine elements of sensitivity (tenderness), tissue texture changes, asymmetry, and restriction of motion (STAR or TART).[12] This can be accomplished in seconds, after which FPR can be applied. For specific segmental dysfunction, the physician introduces motion in all three planes by alternating forces in opposite directions. In the spine, the pads of the physician's fingers apply anterior force to create rotation, both to the left and to the right. When pressure is placed on the right transverse process, it creates a slight left rotation. Segmental dysfunctions have directions of relative ease and restriction. The direction of restriction demonstrates greater resistance to the applied pressure and allows for less freedom. Lateral motion, or sidebending in the spine, is tested by applying pressure to deviate one transverse process into a more superior direction and the opposite side simultaneously into the inferior direction. Relative ease and restriction to the forces are noted, and the opposite directions are tested. Sagittal planar motions of flexion and extension require observation of the resistance to anterior deviation of one vertebra with the next lower one. The pads of the physician's fingers are pressed anteriorly on the superior surfaces of the upper vertebra's transverse processes for flexion and on the inferior surfaces for extension. The combination of all findings results in a triplanar diagnosis of segmental dysfunction. For the extremities, similar methods are utilized to determine flexion–extension, abduction–adduction, and rotation. The directions of ease will be introduced immediately after placing the joint into neutral and adding the facilitating force. Using a combination of methods can further increase the accuracy of the diagnosis and therefore the treatment.

PRINCIPLES OF TREATMENT

FPR can be used to address superficial tissue texture abnormalities, as well as to influence the deep intrinsic muscles involved in segmental joint mobility. When there is a clear diagnostic differentiation as to which is primarily involved in the somatic dysfunction, the superficial soft tissue changes should be initially treated. If the dysfunction persists after this treatment, FPR should then be directed toward treatment of the deeper muscular component involved in the specific joint motion restriction. FPR is primarily an indirect technique that requires the patient to remain passive. However, particularly in the case of lower thoracic somatic dysfunction, the patient can initially assist with attaining a neutral position as the physician can ask them to "sit up straight" to reduce any thoracic kyphosis present[2] FPR can be adapted to treat the patient in a supine, prone, lateral recumbent, or upright position.

The basic steps of treating somatic dysfunction with FPR after a comprehensive osteopathic neuromusculoskeletal exam are as follows:

The somatic dysfunction is monitored continuously.

1. Place the affected body area in its "neutral" position (i.e., mechanically unloaded) where the anteroposterior curve is flattened.
2. Add a facilitating force (e.g., compression, distraction, torsion or a combination usually of compression and torsion).
3. Maintaining the facilitating force, place the dysfunctional structure into all planes of freedom monitoring for the greatest ease.
4. Hold the position for 3 to 5 seconds.
5. Return to the starting position while maintaining the facilitating force.
6. Release the facilitating force.
7. Re-evaluate the somatic dysfunction.
8. Optional: depending on the region, at the completion of holding the position for 3 to 5 seconds, maintaining the facilitating force, the structure(s) is moved into the restrictive barrier(s) and an oscillatory component may be added if needed.

Tissue Texture Change Treatment

1. The physician places the patient in a relaxed position.
2. The physician monitors the region to be treated.
3. The anteroposterior spinal curve of the treatment area is flattened. The lordoses of the lumbar and cervical regions are slightly flexed, while the thoracic spine is extended. When treating the patient in the supine or prone positions, pillows can be used to attain approximation of the neutral position. This position places that region of the spine into an idling position, which shortens and softens the associated muscle. A palpatory softening is customarily noted immediately.
4. A facilitating force is applied. This may be compression, torsion, or a combination of the two. At times, traction may be used with or without torsion.
5. Physician places the patient (patient's musculature) into its ease of motion. This usually requires approximating the origins and insertions by further compression and/or torsion. Additional softening is often noted.
6. The position is held for 3 to 5 seconds and then all facilitating forces are released.
7. The patient's condition is reevaluated. In some cases, passive stretch can be introduced.

Intervertebral Motion Restriction Treatment

The same basic procedures are used to address intervertebral motion restrictions, with the additional requirement that the physician places the vertebra into a position that allows freedom of motion in all planes. For the cervical spine, the patient can be treated in the seated position but is more frequently treated in the supine position. The thoracic and lumbar regions are typically treated in the seated or prone positions, but the techniques can be adapted for side-lying positions:

1. The dysfunction is monitored continuously.
2. The lordosis or kyphosis is flattened.
3. A facilitating force, either compression, torsion, or a combination, is applied specifically to the monitored dysfunction. Often, regional tension decreases immediately.
4. The directions of the somatic dysfunction are added just to the level of the dysfunction. Further relaxation is noted. The sequencing can be varied depending on the skill and experience of the physician. In fact, motion into all directions can be applied simultaneously rather than in a stepwise fashion. Some clinicians have even found the treatment effective by placing the dysfunction into neutral, applying the directions of relative freedom, and then adding the facilitating force.
5. The position is held for 3 to 5 seconds and then the region is returned to neutral. (Oftentimes, Dr. Schiowitz would maintain the facilitating force as he returned the region to neutral.)
6. The dysfunction is reevaluated. When appropriate, the physician can bring the patient past neutral and into the barrier directions before returning to neutral to reevaluate the somatic dysfunction.

SUMMARY

FPR is an easily administered, nontraumatic, and efficient technique. When it is properly performed, the patient often reports immediate relief of point tenderness and restoration of function. If complete normalization is not achieved, FPR can be repeated, or other methods of treatment can be applied immediately. Since FPR treatments may only last a few minutes, they can be easily incorporated into a busy clinical, nonmanipulative specialist practice. Although primarily axial procedures have been described in this chapter, it is possible to use FPR for other regions of articular and soft tissue dysfunction.

ILLUSTRATIVE TREATMENT TECHNIQUES

Cervical Somatic Dysfunction

SOFT TISSUE TREATMENT

Findings

Posterior cervical muscle hypertonicity (soft tissue texture abnormalities)

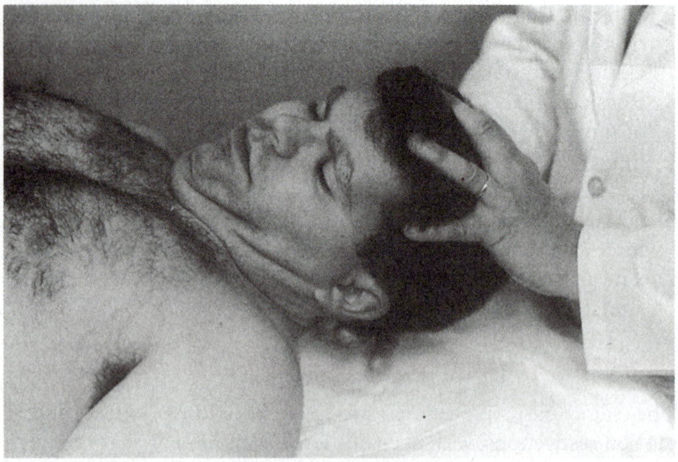

Figure 48.1. **Cervical soft tissue technique.**

Patient Position

Supine, with head beyond the end of the table, resting on a pillow on the physician's lap. Alternatively, the patient could be fully on the table. (Dr. Schiowitz was known to use both methods.) The patient's head off the table enables the physician to better extend the patient's neck if that is required.

Procedure

1. The physician sits at the head of the table (Fig. 48.1).
2. The palm of the physician's hand, which is on the opposite side of the dysfunctional region, cradles the patient's neck. When treating the left side, the right hand is used. The pad of a finger, either the index or another, acts as both the monitoring finger and the fulcrum on the contralateral muscular spasm.
3. The physician's other hand is placed on the top of the patient's head to straighten the patient's cervical lordosis, by slightly bending the neck forward.
4. Using the hand on the top of the patient's head, the physician applies a compressive axial facilitating force to the neck through the patient's head, sufficient enough to be appreciated and to create a relaxation of the tissue noted at the monitored location (usually less than 1 lb).
5. Maintaining the compressive force, extension is introduced to the neck to the level of the monitoring finger. This should cause further relaxation of the tissue being treated.
6. Sidebending and rotation, usually toward the side of the tense tissues, are added to the point that the tissues continue to soften.
7. The position is maintained for 3 to 5 seconds before returning the neck slowly to a neutral position.
8. The tissue being treated is reevaluated. A mild stretch can be applied into the barrier directions while monitoring the tissue tension.

Note: In general, tissues along the posterior aspect of the spine that exhibit tissue texture abnormalities are shortened with extension and ipsilateral sidebending. If tissue changes are found anteriorly, flexion is usually required instead.[2] Some muscles, such as the sternocleidomastoid, have side-bending and rotation components in opposite directions. Knowledge of anatomy is important to determine the direction in which muscles must be placed to achieve their individual shortened positions; this is guided by palpation and tissue response. Careful localization of the component motions of forward/backward bending, sidebending/rotation, and compression to the area of tissue texture change will result in faster and more efficient results.[2]

CERVICAL SEGMENTAL SOMATIC DYSFUNCTION

Findings

C3 ES_LR_L and C7 FS_LR_L

Patient Position

Supine, with head beyond the end of the table, resting on a pillow on the physician's lap. Alternatively, the patient could be fully on the table. (Dr. Schiowitz was known to use both methods.) The patient's head off the table enables the physician to better extend the patient's neck if that is required.

Procedure

1. The physician sits at the head of the table (Fig. 48.2).
2. The palm of the physician's hand cradles the patient's neck. When treating the left side, the right hand is used. The pad of a finger monitors posterior to the left articular pillar of C3.
3. The physician's other hand is placed on the top of the patient's head. This hand then introduces straightening of the patient's cervical lordosis, by slightly flexing the neck down to the level of the monitoring finger on C3, reducing the anteroposterior curve at this level and introducing a neutral positioning to this vertebral unit.
4. The physician's hand on the top of the patient's head now adds a compressive force directed through the head to the neck, until noted at the monitored level.
5. Slight extension is added to the neck through the level of the monitored C3 while maintaining the compression.
6. Introduce a translatory force to the right through the monitoring finger at the level of C3; this effectively adds the relative freedom of motion of the somatic dysfunction by sidebending C3 to the left.
7. Rotate the patient's head and neck to the left only through the level of C3. This places C3 into all three planes of freedom of motion.
8. This position is held for 3 to 5 seconds. The patient's neck is then slowly returned to the neutral position.
9. The C3 motion freedoms and restrictions are reevaluated.

Note: If the diagnosis is **flexed** rather than **extended** (e.g., C7 FS_LR_L), then replace step 5 with adding **flexion** instead of extension through the level of C7. Similarly, if the diagnosis is one of **right** sidebending and **right** rotation, then the appropriate adjustments should be made to engage these relative freedoms.

This procedure can be specifically applied to the occipitoatlantal articulation. The flexion or extension component can be localized by introducing a nodding motion to the skull. Any further flexion or extension of the cervical spine is nonspecific. The

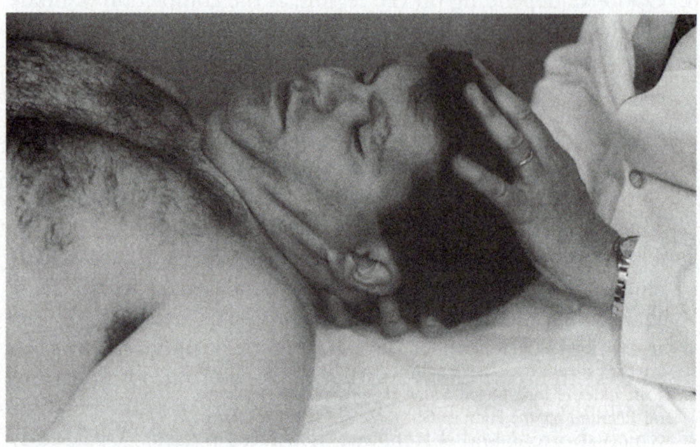

Figure 48.2. **Typical cervical C3 ERS_LR_L technique.**

typical and restrictive motions of the occipitoatlantal joint involve sidebending and rotation in opposite directions.[2] The appropriate directions of relative freedom should be used.

Thoracic Somatic Dysfunction

THORACIC SEGMENTAL SOMATIC DYSFUNCTION

Findings

T6 FS_LR_L

Patient Position

Seated on the end of the table

Procedure

1. The physician stands behind and to the side of the dysfunction to be treated (the T6 FS_LR_L somatic dysfunction). In the case shown, this is to the left of the patient (Fig. 48.3).
2. The physician's index or middle finger of the right hand monitors the left T6 transverse process. The palm of the hand can be used to support the region during the next step.
3. Although FPR is a passive technique, attaining a neutral position in the seated position requires patient cooperation. The patient is asked to sit up as straight as possible and to push the chest forward. This will straighten the thoracic kyphosis and add to the initial neutral component.
4. The physician's left axilla is placed over the patient's left shoulder, as close to the cervicothoracic junction as possible. The physician places their forearm across the patient's chest, grasping the patient's right shoulder with their left hand.
5. The physician adds a downward compressive force through the left axilla onto the patient's left shoulder. This both adds the facilitating force and introduces a localized left sidebending down through to the level of the monitoring finger at T6.
6. Physician adds flexion to the level of T6 by pulling forward on both of the patient's shoulders while maintaining the sidebending.

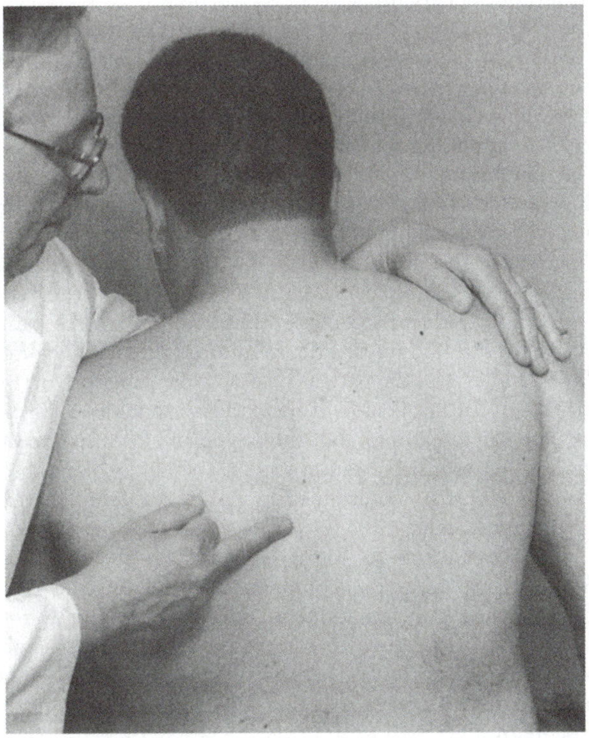

Figure 48.3. **Thoracic spine T6 FS_LR_L technique, seated.**

7. The physician rotates the patient's thoracic spine to the left, down through the level of T6, by pulling the patient's right shoulder forward.
8. This position is held for 3 to 5 seconds. The patient is then slowly returned to a neutral position.
9. The somatic dysfunction is reassessed.

Note: If the diagnosis is **extended** rather than **flexed** (e.g., T6 ES_LR_L), the flexion in step 6 is replaced with adding **extension** through the level of T6. This is accomplished by the physician pushing the patient's shoulders posteriorly. Similarly, if the diagnosis is sidebent and rotated to the **right**, then the appropriate adjustments to the relative freedoms of the somatic dysfunction are made. If the somatic dysfunction is a neutral group curve, then neither flexion nor extension is used. The physician stands at the side of the curve concavity (where the patient is sidebent, e.g., for T5-7N R_RS_L, the physician would stand at the patient's left side), and monitors at the apex of the curve. Adjustments are applied so that the sidebending and rotation are achieved in opposite directions.

ALTERNATIVE THORACIC SEGMENTAL SOMATIC DYSFUNCTION (EXTENSION DYSFUNCTIONS), PRONE

Findings

T6 ES_LR_L

Patient Position

Prone, with arms placed at the sides and pillows beneath the abdomen and head. This creates a flattening of the thoracic kyphosis.

Procedure

1. The physician stands at the side of the table opposite to the somatic dysfunction. For T6 ES_LR_L, the physician stands on the right side of the patient (Fig. 48.4).
2. The physician palpates and monitors the T6 posterior left transverse process with their right hand.
3. The physician's left hand grasps the patient's entire left shoulder, with palm and fingers placed on the superior and lateral portion of the shoulder.
4. The patient's left shoulder is compressed medially toward the spine (this flattens the spine in the anteroposterior plane) and then toward the patient's feet (this compressive force creates left sidebending). The combination of forces creates a force vector that is parallel to the patient's thoracic spine.
5. Some extension of the spine is created through the level of T6 by maintaining traction on the shoulder as the patient's

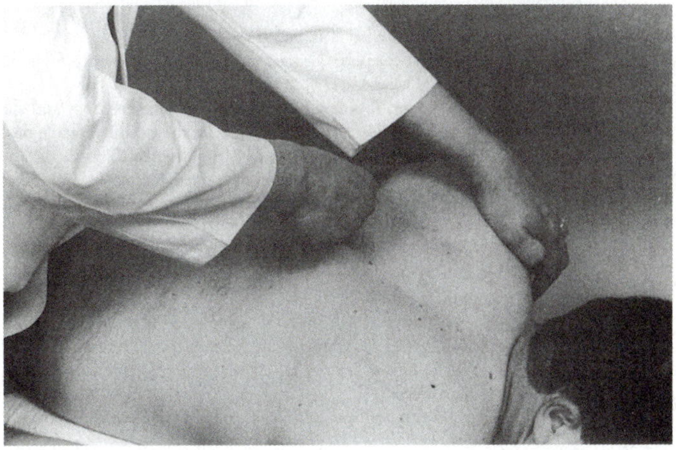

Figure 48.4. **Thoracic spine T6 FS_LR_L technique, prone.**

shoulder is lifted from the table until motion can be palpated at the level of the monitoring fingers.

6. To create greater extension, the physician stands up straighter, pulling the patient's shoulder further posteriorly. This also creates additional left rotation down through the level of T6.
7. This position is held for 3 to 5 seconds. The patient's shoulder and thoracic region are then slowly returned to the neutral position.
8. The T6 somatic dysfunction is then reevaluated.

Note: If the diagnosis is a **flexed** somatic dysfunction, FPR is more easily accomplished with the patient in the seated position as previously described.

Lumbar Somatic Dysfunction

DISKOGENIC PAIN SYNDROME TREATMENT

Findings

Left lumbar disk herniation or bulge with left radiculitis

Position

Prone, close to the left edge of the table, with a sufficient number of pillows beneath the abdomen to cause flattening of the lumbar lordosis

Procedure

1. The physician sits on a rolling stool at the (left) side of the table of the dysfunction, with thighs parallel to the table, at the level of the patient's pelvis, facing the patient's head (Fig. 48.5).
2. The physician monitors the posterior transverse process (left) of the level to be treated (L4–L5) with a finger of the (right) hand that is closer to the patient.
3. The physician's operating (left) hand grasps the patient's (left) knee and flexes the patient's (left) hip and knee on the involved side.
4. The patient's thigh is placed across the physician's anterior thighs. This creates abduction and external rotation. The patient's distal lower extremity is lateral to the physician's thighs, and the physician grasps the patient's (left) ankle.
5. Motion is localized to the involved segment by moving the patient's thigh in a superior direction. This is accomplished by rolling the stool closer to the head of the table.
6. The physician's outer (left) knee is raised by lifting the heel off the floor. The lateral part of the physician's (left) knee is pressed into the popliteal fossa of the patient's (left) knee. The physician's knee is further raised and moved laterally, creating a traction force through the patient's proximal lower extremity that can be modified, until motion is palpated at the monitoring finger. The physician's knee is now at the medial surface of the popliteal fossa of the patient's knee. The medial surface of the physician's knee acts as a fulcrum for the rest of the technique.
7. The physician's operating (left) hand presses the patient's (left) ankle toward the floor until motion is palpated with the monitoring finger. There may be a slight amount of tension noted at the monitored location. Often, the patient will state that the symptoms are reduced while in this position.
8. The position is held for 3 to 5 seconds until there is a sudden release of the somatic dysfunction, and then the patient is slowly returned to the initial position.
9. The lumbar region is reevaluated.

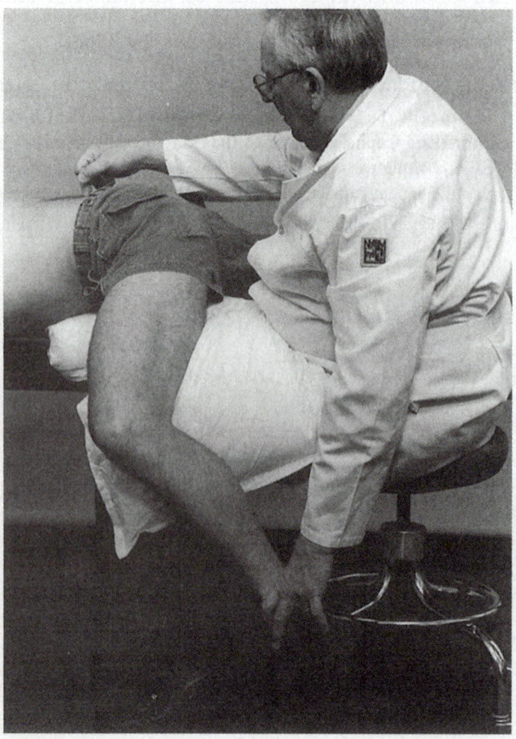

Figure 48.5. Diskogenic pain syndrome treatment.

Rib Somatic Dysfunction

FIRST RIB

Findings

First rib elevated on the left

Patient Position

Supine

Procedure

1. The physician stands at the side of the elevated rib, facing toward the head of the table. In the current example, this is to the left of the patient.
2. The physician places the monitoring finger of the hand that is closer to the patient (left hand for an elevated left first rib) over the posterior portion of the elevated first rib. The finger serves primarily as a monitoring component. The physician's forearm serves as a fulcrum for some of the subsequent steps.
3. The physician's other (right) hand grasps the patient's left elbow. The shoulder is flexed to approximately 90 degrees and abducted slightly (10 to 20 degrees) from the vertical. This should be adjusted until the tissues soften maximally (Fig. 48.6A).
4. Physician introduces a compressive force through the patient's left elbow, directed toward the monitoring finger (Fig. 48.6B).
5. Physician deviates the patient's elbow more superiorly to introduce slight further flexion of the patient's shoulder. This causes the patient's forearm to abut the physician's forearm and introduces some internal rotation into the shoulder. The absolute position should be determined by the relaxation of the monitored rib soft tissue.
6. This position is held for 3 to 5 seconds.
7. While maintaining the compressive force and the internal rotation, the physician adducts and further internally rotates the patient's upper arm. To complete the treatment, the physician circumducts the patient's arm through a curving motion and back into a neutral position alongside the patient's torso (Fig. 48.6C).
8. The first rib is reevaluated.

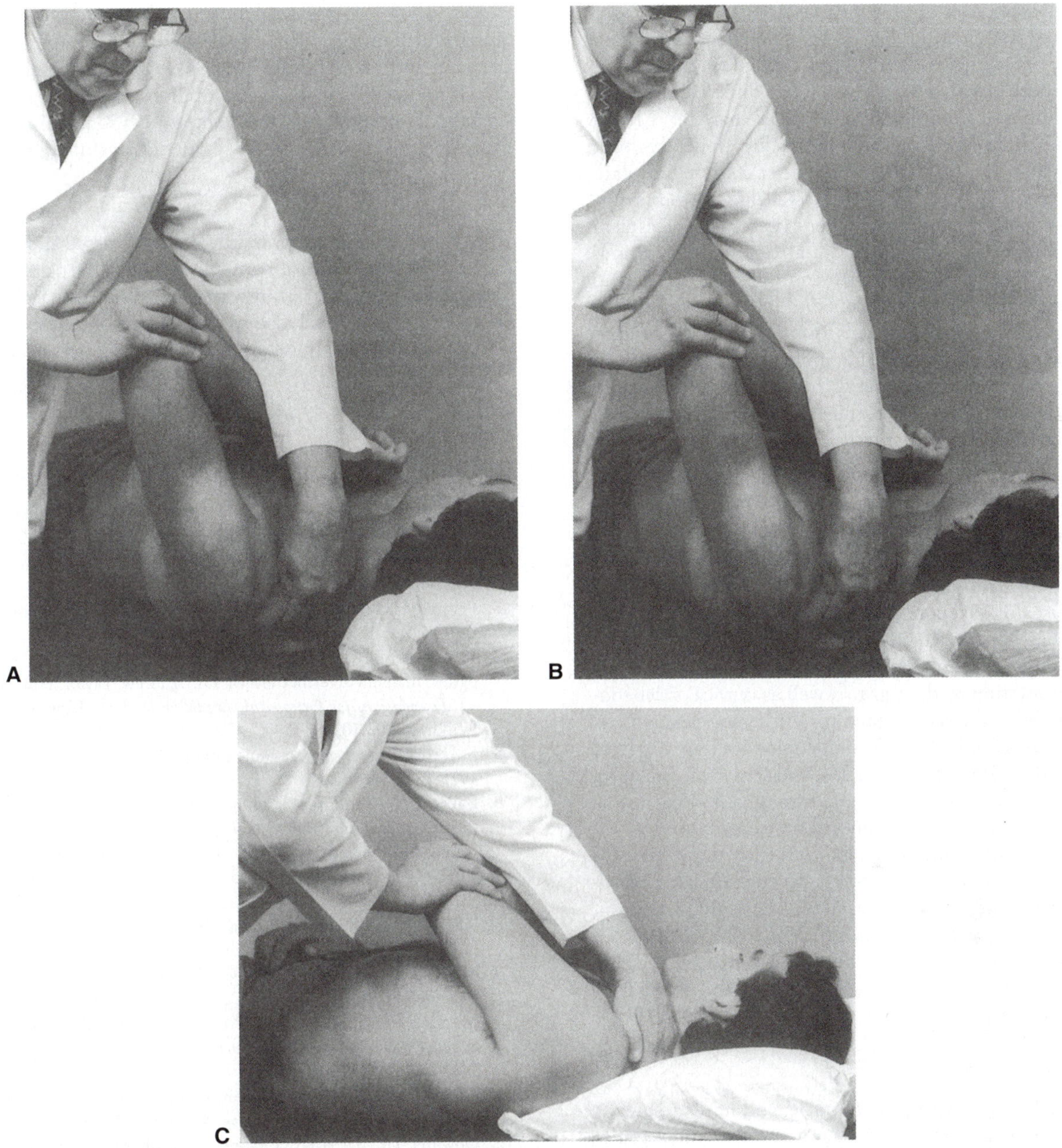

Figure 48.6. Treatment for elevated left first rib. A. Flex and abduct the patient's left arm. **B.** Introduce compression, further flexion, and internal rotation. **C.** Add further internal rotation, adduction, followed by circumduction (not shown).

CASE STUDY

The patient is a 48-year-old woman who presented with several complaints of chronic lower back pain, neck pain, left shoulder pain, and frequent headaches. She described these as originating in her early 20s with no noted precipitating event. The symptoms have been gradually increasing over the years. The most recent symptom to appear has been intermittent radiating pain and tingling from the left lower back to the left buttock and sometimes the left lower leg. The level of pain is 3–4/10 and is worse in the morning after awakening. She describes the headaches as tightness at the back of her head radiating to her temple area. She denies any aura or other symptoms associated with the headaches. She denies any other constitutional symptoms.

She has been seen by several physicians and health practitioners including orthopedists, a neurologist, a rheumatologist, physical therapists, a massage therapist, an acupuncturist, and a nutritionist. The massage therapy helped but was only of short benefit. Radiologic findings included some mild degenerative changes in the cervical and lumbar spinal regions with a paracentral herniated disk on the left at L4–L5. Neurophysiologic tests (EMG/NCS) only demonstrated some involvement of the L5 paraspinal muscles. Blood serology has been negative.

She has no known allergies. She has been prescribed a tricyclic antidepressant, a selective serotonin reuptake inhibitor, gabapentin, various nonsteroidal anti-inflammatories, muscle relaxants, and narcotic analog medications. She discontinued all of the medications either because of side effects or ineffectiveness. She occasionally takes acetaminophen for headaches.

She has been married for 25 years, has three children, and works full time as a librarian. She describes that she is happy and satisfied in her private and professional life. In her free time, she exercises and does volunteer work at her church. She states that both activities often, but not always, help with her symptoms. The patient is up to date with her gynecologic, breast, and physical examinations; is not menopausal. She is monogamous; and utilizes barrier methods for birth control. Her bone density studies have revealed minimal osteopenia. She has never smoked or used recreational drugs, has one to two glasses of wine per week, and has never had surgery. Her only hospitalizations were for her pregnancies, which were all full-term and resulted in spontaneous vaginal deliveries. Family history is essentially negative, with the exception of her father's controlled hypertension.

PHYSICAL EXAMINATION

On physical examination, the patient is a well-nourished, well-developed woman who appears younger than her stated age and is in no apparent distress. Gait and posture are normal. Regional musculoskeletal examination demonstrates full range of motion that appears equal, with the exception of reduced left shoulder flexion/abduction/internal rotation, lumbar side bending, and rotation to the right, as well as cervical sidebending and rotation to the right. Standing and seated flexion tests, straight leg raising, and Spurling compression tests are negative. Motor strength is 5/5, reflexes are 2/4, and sensory is intact for touch/sharp/dull and is symmetrical throughout. The rest of the physical examination is benign and noncontributory.

Specific structural findings include left trapezius spasm, C3 ESLRL, C7 FSLRL, elevated first rib on the left, T6 FSLRL lumbar paravertebral muscle spasm on the right, latissimus dorsi muscle spasm on the left, L3 ESLRL, and L4 FSLRL. A mild flexion pattern with a cranial rhythmic impulse (CRI) of 8 cycles per minute was noted, and the sacrum and pelvis were symmetrical and mobile.

DIAGNOSES

Diagnoses included cervical, rib, thoracic, and lumbar somatic dysfunctions, lumbar herniated disk, and lumbar radiculopathy, along with lumbar and cervical strain and sprain. The shoulder pain and restriction of motion were determined to not be directly related to shoulder restriction or pathology but were secondary to the spasms of the trapezius and latissimus muscles as well as the cervical and rib segmental dysfunctions.

TREATMENT

The patient was treated primarily with soft tissue and FPR techniques. After the first treatment, she described the pain as a 1–2/10 and less frequent. She also reported less frequent headaches. The course of treatment included weekly evaluation and treatment for 3 weeks, then biweekly, followed by monthly intervals.

REFERENCES

1. Schiowitz S, Ellis EP. FPR and beyond facilitated positional release: A quick and accurate manual medicine method. *Decamus LLC.* 2016:3.
2. Schiowitz S. Facilitated positional release. *J Am Osteopath Assoc.* 1990; 901:145–155.
3. Fryette HH. *Principles of Osteopathic Technic.* Academy of Applied Osteopathy; 1980:19.
4. Van Buskirk RL. Treatment of somatic dysfunction with an osteopathic manipulative method of Dr. Andrew Taylor Still. In: Ward RC, ed. *Foundations for Osteopathic Medicine.* 2nd ed. Lippincott Williams & Wilkins; 2003:1094–1114.
5. Korr IM. Proprioceptors and somatic dysfunction. *J Am Osteopath Assoc.* 1975;75:638–650.
6. Bailey HW. Some problems in making osteopathic spinal manipulative therapy appropriate and specific. *J Am Osteopath Assoc.* 1976;75:486–499.
7. Carew TJ. The control of reflex action. In: Kandel ER, Schwartz JH, eds. *Principles of Neural Science.* 2nd ed. Elsevier Science Publishing Co Inc.; 1985:464.
8. Schiowitz S, Ellis EP. FPR and beyond facilitated positional release: a quick and accurate manual medicine method. *Decamus LLC.* 2016:15.
9. Mennell JM. *Back Pain: Diagnosis and Treatment Using Manipulative Techniques.* Little, Brown and Company; 1960:75.
10. Mitchell FL Jr, Moran PS, Pruzzo NA. *An Evaluation and Treatment Manual of Osteopathic Muscle Energy Procedures.* Mitchell, Moran & Pruzzo Assoc; 1979:229–253.
11. Johnston WL. Segmental definition. Part 1: a focal point for diagnosis of somatic dysfunction. *J Am Osteopath Assoc.* 1988;88:99–105.
12. Dowling DJ. S.T.A.R.: a more viable alternative descriptor system of somatic dysfunction. *AAOJ.* 1998;8(2):34–37.

49 High-Velocity Low-Amplitude (HVLA) Thrust

REBECCA E. GIUSTI ▪ RAYMOND J. HRUBY

KEY CONCEPTS

- The high-velocity low-amplitude (HVLA) (thrust) approach is a direct-action osteopathic manipulative treatment (OMT) procedure characterized by positioning a dysfunctional joint against the appropriate restrictive barrier, followed by a rapid and brief corrective thrust to move the joint through the barrier.
- There is a significant amount of research that has investigated the mechanisms underlying the efficacy of HVLA procedures.
- Accurate diagnosis with a distinct endpoint and precise engagement of the barrier are key to successful performance of HVLA (thrust) techniques.

DEFINITION

The Glossary of Osteopathic Terminology defines high-velocity low-amplitude (HVLA) technique as, "An osteopathic method in which the restrictive barrier is engaged in one or more planes of motion and then a rapid, therapeutic force of brief duration traveling a short distance is applied within the anatomic range of motion."[1]

HVLA is a direct method manipulative treatment that uses HVLA activation to passively move a dysfunctional joint through its restrictive barrier. Once the dysfunctional joint is appropriately addressed, improved physiologic motion and a reduction of pain should result. The term direct refers specifically to the positioning of the restricted joint toward the restrictive barrier. After this precise positioning, the final force is a short (low-amplitude), quick (high-velocity) thrust. Although not necessary for a successful result, a cavitation (sometimes described as a "click" or "pop") is often heard at the time the force is applied.

HVLA is not unique to osteopathic physicians. Other healthcare professions, such as chiropractic and physical therapy, may use similar procedures. Oftentimes, this is referred to as "spinal manipulation."

"Spinal manipulative therapy (SMT) is a manual treatment where a vertebral joint is passively moved between the normal range of motion and the limits of its anatomic range, though a universally accepted definition does not seem to exist."[2] This understanding of SMT often involves an HVLA thrust, a technique in which the joints are adjusted rapidly, often accompanied by popping sounds.[3,4]

This is an important note as patients may be confused by the word "manipulation" and assume that all osteopathic manipulative medicine or treatment connotes the performance of a thrust maneuver. Osteopathic physicians must be able to clearly explain how each osteopathic modality or method of treatment is administered along with its benefits and risks to their patients in the context of their patients' somatic dysfunction.

HISTORY

Thrust styles of manipulation have been documented worldwide throughout history.[5] Hippocrates, the "father of medicine," described spinal manipulative techniques as did Galen. European immigrants brought the techniques of the "bone setters" to America.[6] Robert Kappler, DO, MS, FAAO (DIST), has theorized on the development of HVLA as a distinctly osteopathic modality as follows:

> "Thrust technique has been the major type of technique taught in colleges of osteopathic medicine and has been practiced by osteopathic physicians for years. In the 1970s, the osteopathic medical school curricula began to include other types of techniques. Until recently, however, osteopathic manipulation and high-velocity technique were essentially synonymous. Graduates are now exposed to a complete spectrum of direct and indirect techniques; therefore, osteopathic manipulation is no longer synonymous with thrust technique."[7]

It is interesting to speculate why osteopathic manipulative techniques taught in the colleges evolved into the exclusive domain of thrust techniques and then remained as such for many years. This change was likely initiated by faculty and students who assisted with teaching in the early days. Thrust techniques can be taught by describing the nature of the restriction and by providing techniques for treating the dysfunction, both of which can be memorized and practiced.

In contrast, fascial release and indirect techniques require proficiency in assessing motion patterns in the tissues. These release techniques are often difficult to describe because the physician is responding to tactile and proprioceptive input from the hands. Thus, faculty often find these techniques challenging to teach, and students may find them to be abstract. In contrast, thrust techniques may be more easily taught since they can be described in a precise manner. However, the motor coordination necessary to apply them effectively requires extensive practice and experience.

PROPOSED MECHANISM OF ACTION

Current thinking regarding the mechanism of action of HVLA technique is that the sudden stretch or change in the joint alters the afferent activity of the mechanoreceptors, resulting in a neural change at the related spinal cord segment and the release of muscle hypertonicity surrounding the joint. The following paragraphs summarize the current level of knowledge regarding this mechanism and other proposed mechanisms of action of HVLA technique.

Proposed Causes of Joint/Somatic Dysfunction

Based on evidence in published literature, a somatic dysfunction is likely caused by a mechanical overload resulting from cumulative stresses or a single event.

- An inflammatory response gives rise to inflammatory and biomechanical changes that then lead to sensitivity, in addition to reduced function and mobility of the involved region.
- Depending on the nature of the insult and the condition of the patient, the response may remain local or have widespread effects.[8]

Contributing causes of somatic dysfunction appear to be multifactorial. Some evidence cites the following:

- Trapped synovial folds within the facet joints
- Alteration in the periarticular and articular structures of a joint
- Buckling of motion segments that have undergone disproportionate displacement[9]
  - This may result in the misalignment of joint surfaces and a change in the thixotropic property of the synovial fluid, which can make joint surfaces more adhesive or sticky.[10]

The facet joints and surrounding supportive structures are rich in mechanoreceptors capable of detecting motion and tissue distortion with fairly large receptive fields. These include the following:

- Ruffini corpuscles (type I afferents), which respond to mechanical stress
- Pacinian corpuscles (type II afferents), which respond to acceleration of a joint
- Golgi tendon organs (type III afferents), which respond to tensile forces and provide feedback on joint position or muscle tendon tension
- Free nerve endings (type IV afferents), which act as nociceptors and respond to high threshold mechanical stimuli (e.g., intense stretch or strain)

These mechanoreceptors provide proprioceptive feedback and information to the nervous system, which has implications for the following:

- Tonicity of the surrounding musculature
- Perception of pain in a region
- Function of the region

Postulated Effect of HVLA Technique on Restoration of Joint Mobility

- Somatic dysfunction may in part be caused by an increase in fiber cross-link formation resulting in adhesions.[11]
- Articular and periarticular restrictions have been shown to result from joint immobilization.[11]
- In the absence of movement, joint capsule contractures and intra-articular capsular adhesions occur, promoting joint stiffness.
- Fibrofatty joint infiltration and cartilage degeneration may also occur.[12]

Research has demonstrated improved range of motion following HVLA technique applied to various regions of the body.

- Several studies have reported a statistically significant increase in range of motion after HVLA was administered to the cervical spine.[13–15]
- Another study comparing mobilization and HVLA of the metacarpophalangeal (MP) joints showed an increase in range of motion in both treatment groups, but the increase was significantly greater in the group that received HVLA.[16]
- Yet another study showed a significant increase in ankle dorsiflexion after HVLA was administered to the tibiofibular and talocrural joints in subjects with decreased range of motion in ankle dorsiflexion, when compared to the change in subjects who had received stretching exercises.[17]
- Other research studies on HVLA to the ankle have reported no improvements in range of motion. However, such studies were carried out on asymptomatic patients.[18,19]

Postulated Effect of HVLA Technique on Pain Reduction

Several studies have shown that HVLA technique applied to different regions of the body reduces pain in those areas.[20–23]

- González-Iglesias et al. found that patients with mechanical neck pain who received thoracic spine manipulation had greater improvements in pain, cervical range of motion, and disability compared to patients who received a program of electrothermal therapy interventions.[24]

Other researchers have focused on whether greater improvement is achieved with either mobilization (low-velocity, variable-amplitude movements) or manipulation (HVLA thrust).

- Hurwitz et al. concluded that cervical mobilization is as effective as manipulation in reducing neck pain and related disability in chiropractic patients. Moreover, heat and electromagnetic stimulation (EMS) alone, or in conjunction with manipulation or mobilization, were not found to improve clinical outcomes.[25]
- Leaver also did not find cervical manipulation to be superior to mobilization with respect to the number of days taken to recover from an episode of neck pain.[26]
- However, a review by Coronado et al. demonstrated that SMT had an immediate effect on increasing the mechanical pressure pain threshold, which was favorable over other interventions.[27]

Yu et al. showed a significant effect of SMT on increased pressure pain threshold at remote sites from the application of the stimulus, indicating potential central nervous system involvement.[28]

Many neurologic mechanisms have been proposed to explain how HVLA could reduce pain to an area of somatic dysfunction.

- HVLA may activate the descending inhibitory pathways from the dorsal periaqueductal gray area of the midbrain causing not only hypoalgesia to the targeted area but also sympathoexcitation.[29]

Several studies on New Zealand white rabbits have demonstrated that the somatosensory units of the lumbar facet joints may play a role in low back pain.

- The facet joints contain group-III and group-IV mechanosensitive units that may serve as nociceptors and proprioceptors.[30]
  - The 24 discrete mechanosensitive units have been identified in the facet joint, including in:
    - The ligamentum flavum
    - Twelve in the rotatores, intertransversarii, and multifidus muscles and tendons near the insertion into the facet joint
    - Two in the interspinous ligament.
- The lumbar intervertebral disk may be a pain source, but the mechanosensitive units identified in the disk region are sparse and are only sensitive to strong noxious stimuli. Nonetheless, these group III and IV units may become sensitive to mechanical stimuli in an inflamed joint.[31]
- The mechanical thrust from HVLA may either stimulate or quiet non-nociceptive mechanosensitive receptive nerve endings in paraspinal tissues, including the following:
  - Skin
  - Ligaments
  - Muscles
  - Tendons

- Facet joints
- Intervertebral disks

- Thus, the inflow of sensory signals from these structures is altered in a manner that improves physiologic functioning. The mechanoreceptors include the following:
  - Proprioceptors (muscle spindles and Golgi tendon organs)
  - Low- and high-threshold mechanoreceptors
  - High threshold polymodal nociceptors
- Therefore, all groups of sensory neurons, groups Ia, Ib, II, III, and IV fibers, could be positively affected by HVLA.[32]
- A study by Bishop et al. showed that HVLA reduced temporal sensory summation, a short-lasting aspect of the central sensitization system. They theorized that this reduction may decrease the potential for central sensitization and thereby reduce the risk of progression to persistent pain states.[33]
- Herzog, Scheele, and Conway demonstrated that HVLA elicited consistent, measurable, and repeatable electromyography (EMG) responses to the targeted area as well as reflex activation of the upper and lower limbs with spinal and sacroiliac (SI) treatments.
  - The study could not determine whether the origin of the EMG response was from mechanoreceptors in the capsule of the spinal facet joints, pain and cutaneous receptors, skeletal muscle proprioceptors, the muscle spindles, or the Golgi tendon organs.
  - However, the authors proposed that these reflex responses may explain some of the clinical effects of HVLA such as decreased pain and hypertonicity of muscles to the involved region.[34]
- A study by Colloca and Keller showed similar findings in patients with low back pain.
  - In addition, they found that patients with frequent to constant low back pain had more marked surface EMG (sEMG) responses compared to patients with occasional to intermittent low back pain.
  - They also observed neuromuscular reflex responses to HVLA at segments superior and inferior to the targeted segment, likely due to the sensory inputs that ascend or descend as much as three to four spinal levels via interneuronal connections with motor neurons.[35]
- Pickar explores several theories of pain reduction.
  - One of which is the gate theory of Melzack and Wall, which states that non-noxious mechanical stimuli from HVLA input traveling on A fiber neurons can inhibit the response of dorsal horn neurons to nociceptive stimuli from C fibers.
  - HVLA may also modulate pain via the neuroendocrine system.[32]

Postulated Effect of HVLA Technique on Muscle Relaxation

HVLA is believed to relax the periarticular muscles by possibly stimulating joint receptors, causing reflexive relaxation of those structures.[36]

- Herzog found that HVLA caused an EMG response followed by a decrease in hypertonicity of the musculature.[34]
- Shambaugh noted a 25% reduction in paraspinal muscle electrical activity after application of HVLA.[37]

Postulated Effect of HVLA Technique on Improvement of Muscle Strength

A number of studies have reported muscle strength improvement post-HVLA intervention.

- Keller and Colloca demonstrated that low back pain patients who received HVLA showed improved erector spinae strength with spinal extension via EMG, when compared to the responses of the control group.[38]
- A study by Liebler et al. noted a significant increase in isometric muscle strength of the lower trapezius in patients who received Grade-IV mobilization compared to those in the control group who received Grade-I mobilization.[39]
- A study by Suter et al. supported previous research demonstrating that HVLA to SI joint dysfunction in patients with anterior knee pain resulted in a decrease in muscle inhibition and an increase in knee extensor torques and muscle activation.[40]
- Yerys et al. postulated that a loss of hip extension in the geriatric population may arise from neutrally mediated inhibition of the articular mechanoreceptors.
  - They hypothesized that improving mobility of hip extension would remove the inhibitory influence of the arthrokinematic reflex (AKR) on the gluteus maximus muscle, thus improving gait.[41]
  - They found a 14% increase in strength of the gluteus maximus after performing Grade VI-P-A mobilization of the anterior hip capsule.[41]

Postulated Effect of HVLA Technique on Improvement of Joint Nutrition

Articular surfaces are avascular and depend on the flow of unimpeded synovial fluid for nutrition. A joint that is motion restricted due to mechanical or neurophysiologic impairments may have reduced circulation of synovial fluid within its synovium.

- HVLA is thought to reduce these mechanical restrictions or alleviate neurophysiologic factors, thus improving joint motion and synovial fluid circulation within the joint. At this time, no published research has been found addressing this postulation.[36]

Postulated Effect of HVLA Technique on Correction of Positional or Mechanical Faults

Joint surfaces can alter their position relative to each other. In severe cases, this is termed "dislocation" and if this alteration is minimal, it is called "subluxation."[36]

Even minimal alteration to a segment may result in profound changes to its periarticular and articular structures, in addition to its feedback to the central nervous system, which potentially causes pain or dysfunction. Studies provide contradictory information on the "movement" of joints and their correlation to pain. Some sources state that joints change position after HVLA,[42] while others state that these changes, if they do exist, are not apparent on radiography.[36]

Postulated Effect of HVLA Technique on the Elimination of Meniscoid Impingement

- Engel and Bogduk examined 82 cadaveric specimens (age range 22 to 90) and identified three types of intra-articular structures:
  - Adipose tissue pads
  - Fibroadipose meniscoids
  - Connective tissue rims
- However, they concluded that the morphology of the fibroadipose meniscoids was incompatible with the proposed "meniscus entrapment theory," which states that:
  - A meniscus with fibrous apices, when interposed between articular processes, could deform the articular cartilage; this

traps the apex of the meniscus, which in turn would cause capsular strain, resulting in pain and muscle spasm around the affected joint.[43]

- No specific study has been completed on the positioning of meniscoids in a dysfunctional joint, or on the effect of HVLA on that joint.[36] However, research has emerged on synovial folds within the cervical spine,[44,45] their potential role in creating somatic dysfunction, and how HVLA may alleviate such dysfunction.[46]

Postulated Effect of HVLA Technique on Reduction of Spinal Disk Herniation

Mechanical compression of the dorsal root or the dorsal root ganglia may alter both impulse-based neural transmission (action potentials) and non–impulse-based mechanisms (axoplasmic transport).

- As little as 10-mm Hg pressure to the dorsal root reduces nutritional transport to the peripheral axons by 20% to 30%.[32]
- Compression of the dorsal root ganglia also increases endoneurial fluid pressure and causes edema and hemorrhage within the dorsal root ganglia.[47]
- HVLA may alter neural function mechanically or by reducing the inflammatory mediators pervading the dysfunctional joint.

Postulated Effect of HVLA Technique on Mediation of the Central Nervous System

Central facilitation, also referred to as central sensitization, is described as the increased excitability or enhanced responsiveness of dorsal horn neurons to an afferent input.

- This may manifest through increased spontaneous central neural activity, enhanced discharge of central neurons to an afferent input, or a change in the receptive field properties of central neurons.[48]
- Alpha motoneurons may be held in a facilitated state due to increased or aberrant sensory input from segmentally related paraspinal structures.
- Once the central neurons are sensitized, subthreshold mechanical or chemical stimuli may initiate pain. HVLA may remove that subthreshold stimuli[32] and normalize the segment.

Cao et al. reported that HVLA likely affects the muscle spindle apparatus.

- It is most likely stretched after application of HVLA, which results in an increase in resting spindle input to secondary neurons in the spinal cord.
- Normalization of the muscle spindle discharge would feed back to the spinal cord and return muscle functioning to a more physiologic state.
- Other mechanoreceptors within the lumbar spine are likely responsible for sustaining the effects of the HVLA.[42]

Postulated Effect of HVLA Technique on Improved Circulation

Altered circulation may be due to the hypertonicity of the area surrounding the facilitated segment. Due to both neural and biomechanical components, tissue fluid congestion and circulatory stasis may occur perpetuating the cycle of inflammation, pain production, and dysfunction. These effects may either be local or far-reaching.

- A report by Salamon, Zhu, and Stefano, while not specific to HVLA, did demonstrate that OMT-like maneuvers augment blood flow and vasodilation by increasing the concentration of nitric oxide (NO) within the blood and vasculature.
- They proposed that this may be a mechanism of action of OMT and recommended further studies in this realm.[49]

Postulated Effect of HVLA Technique on the Autonomic Nervous System

It would appear that HVLA and manual therapy in general would have an effect on the autonomic nervous system based on its organization.

- Non-noxious paraspinal sensory input inhibits sympathetic outflow, whereas noxious input has an excitatory effect.[32]

However, studies are still limited on exactly how HVLA can affect those reflexes and end-organ function.[20,32]

- Sato and Swenson applied a non-noxious mechanical stimulus to the thoracic and lumbar regions of rats, which reflexively decreased the level of renal and adrenal sympathetic nerve activity by 25% to 40%, thereby inhibiting sympathetic nerve activity for a short duration.[50]
- Budgell and Hirano found that in healthy young adults, when compared to sham, cervical manipulation indicated a possible shift in the balance of autonomic control of the heart toward the parasympathetic nervous system.[51]
- Budgell and Polus reported that thoracic HVLA influenced the autonomic output influencing heart rate variability.[52]

Postulated Effect of HVLA Technique on the Immune System

It appears that HVLA may also have an effect on the immune system.

- Brennan et al. found that spinal manipulation primed polymorphonuclear leukocytes (PMNs) and enhanced the respiratory burst of these white blood cells to a particulate challenge.
- The spinal manipulation also primed the PMNs for enhanced production of cytokines.[53,54]

INDICATIONS, CONTRAINDICATIONS, AND USES

Indications

- Articular somatic dysfunction
- Joint motion restriction with a firm articular barrier

HVLA can be used in the following situations:

- When a somatic dysfunction is determined to be an actual joint motion restriction (such as facet locking), not an exclusive restriction of the soft tissues
- In the face of joint fixation
- To disrupt connective tissue adhesions
- To treat chronic dysfunction resistant to other treatment modalities
- To modify reflexes
- As a maintenance treatment in irreversible situations
- Hypomobile joints
- Restoration of bony alignment
- Meniscoid entrapment
- Pain modulation
- Reprogramming of the CNS
- Displaced disk fragment
- Reflex relaxation of affected muscles

Contraindications[55]

Absolute (regionally or segmentally specific)

- Upper cervical
  - Rheumatoid arthritis
  - Down syndrome
  - Achondroplastic dwarfism
  - Chiari malformation
- Fracture/dislocation/spinal or joint instability
- Ankylosis/spondylosis with fusion
- Surgical fusion
- Klippel–Feil syndrome
- Vertebrobasilar insufficiency
- Inflammatory joint disease
- Joint infection
- Bony malignancy
- Patient refusal

Note: Patient refusal is a medicolegal issue for all manual procedures and is not specific to HVLA.

Relative (regionally or segmentally specific)

- Acute herniated nucleus pulposus
- Acute radiculopathy
- Acute whiplash/severe muscle spasm/strain/sprain
- Osteopenia/osteoporosis
- Spondylolisthesis
- Metabolic bone disease
- Hypermobility syndromes

SAFETY AND EFFICACY

Similar to everything else in medicine, there are potential side effects, complications, and adverse events with manipulative procedures.

- Manipulation remains as possibly one of the safest procedures in medicine, but like all modalities, it must be used properly.
- This requires taking a complete history, doing a thorough physical examination, and selecting the appropriate OMT modalities to fit the clinical context.

Compared to the incidence of adverse effects (including death) associated with pharmaceuticals, manipulative treatment is an extremely safe and therapeutic modality when performed by a knowledgeable and skilled practitioner.

- Reported complications from manipulation range from about 1:400,000 to 1:1,000,000 depending on the author cited.[56,57]
- Kuchera et al., citing data from the Swiss Manual Medical Society in 1981, noted that out of 1,408 reported manipulative "complications," 1,255 (about 89%) were associated with cervical manipulative procedures.[56] Most of the complications in this series were described as "minor vertigo," while a loss of, or alteration in, consciousness occurred in a minority of individuals.
- Vick et al. examined the reports of adverse sequelae from manipulation from 1925 to 1993 and noted a total of 185 cases of "major" complications from spinal "manipulation."
  - These complications ranged from strokes, cardiac arrest, disk herniation, and bone fracture to vascular complications.
  - Interestingly, about 20% of the complications were either "spontaneous" or occurred at the hands of an unskilled operator.
  - Spontaneous or accidental events were from self-turning of the head or injuries that occurred while painting a ceiling (presumptively looking up with the neck extended eliciting vertebrobasilar artery compromise), sustained in a fall, or during exercise.[58]
- Other authors estimate the risk of cerebrovascular accident (stroke, presumably from carotid or vertebrobasilar arterial dissection) to be 1 to 3 per million manipulations.[59]
- For all serious adverse effects, the estimated incidence is 5 to 10 per 10 million manipulations.[60]
- Haldeman et al. concluded, based on a retrospective review, that cerebrovascular accidents occurring after spinal manipulation appear to be *unpredictable* and should be considered an inherent, idiosyncratic, and *rare* complication of spinal manipulative treatment.[61]
- The results of a study by Cagnie et al.[62] indicated that reactions to spinal manipulation may be relatively common but are *benign* in nature and short in duration.
- A study by Haneline et al.[63] was conducted to determine the relationship between manipulative therapy (as administered by chiropractors) and internal carotid artery dissection (a splitting of the layers or "tunics" of the vascular wall resulting in impaired circulation).
  - Utilizing a MEDLINE literature search from 1966 through 2000, many confounding factors such as connective tissue aberrations, native arteriopathy, and concomitant infection were noted. This obfuscated any obvious etiologic relationship between HVLA manipulation and the provocation of arterial dissection.
  - Thirteen cases of internal carotid arterial dissection related to chiropractic manipulative therapy were identified.
  - Most internal carotid artery dissections appeared to occur spontaneously (e.g., not related to spinal manipulative treatment).
  - Indeed, Selim et al.[64] remarked that *spontaneous* dissection of the carotid artery is a *relatively common disorder.* It is believed that most dissections are spontaneous, possibly related to activities that cause a sudden stretch of the pharyngeal portion of the carotid artery.

Most complications of the cervical spine occur with maneuvers employing coupled cervical extension and rotation. Of the two components, the cervical rotation appeared to be the more important aspect in eliciting adverse outcomes.

It must be stressed, however, that the overall incidence of adverse outcomes remains very low. As chiropractors perform the majority of cervical HVLA in the United States, there is more data available from this profession. Specifically, data suggests that a chiropractor will be aware of an arterial dissection occurring following cervical manipulation only once in 8.06 million office visits with only 1 in 48 chiropractors experiencing such an event in their entire careers.[65] If cervical manipulative procedures were inherently dangerous, the incidence of obvious adverse outcomes would have been widely reported in medical literature. Thus, in the hands of competent practitioners, after a thorough evaluation has been performed, and inclusion criteria have been met, manipulation can prove very efficacious where other techniques may not suffice.

The American Academy of Osteopathy created a white paper on the use of HVLA technique on the cervical spine. The American Osteopathic Association's House of Delegates passed a resolution in July of 2004 to accept this document as their official position on the teaching and use of HVLA technique. This was reaffirmed in 2017 and again in 2024.[66]

PRECAUTIONS

- In general, adverse effects of HVLA technique can be avoided by following certain principles.

- In particular, a thorough history and physical examination are essential for uncovering possible diseases or conditions that would contraindicate the use of HVLA.
  - In addition, when addressing the cervical spine, ***avoid hyperextension and excessive rotation*** when positioning the patient and performing any HVLA maneuver.

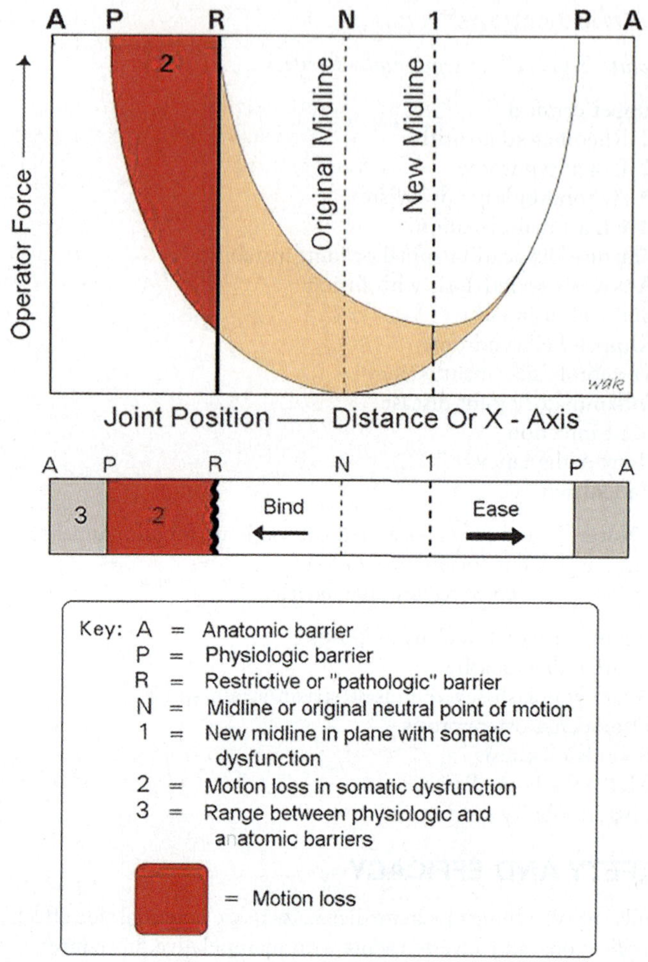

Figure 49.1. Somatic dysfunction quantity and quality of joint motion. (From Kappler RE, Jones JM III. Thrust (high velocity/low-amplitude) techniques. In: Ward RC, ed. *Foundations for Osteopathic Medicine.* 2nd ed. Lippincott Williams & Wilkins; 2003:852–880.)

PRINCIPLES OF DIAGNOSIS

It cannot be stated strongly enough that the key to properly performing thrust manipulation with the greatest efficacy and the least side effects is the ability to diagnose accurately and to only use HVLA technique when the diagnosis warrants it.

The variety of etiologic elements is reflected in the wide variety of both somatic dysfunction diagnoses and treatment options. A methodology is thus essential for differentiating among these disparate diagnostic possibilities and for selecting the optimal treatment modality.

- Manipulation is much more efficacious when the modality chosen is correctly matched to the type of somatic dysfunction present.

When examining an area for somatic dysfunction, identify changes from the norm by using the acronym TART:

- Are there palpable tissue texture changes (T)?
- Is there visually observable asymmetry (A)?
- Is there a restriction of motion (R)?
- Does the palpatory exam elicit tenderness (T)?

BARRIER MECHANICS

To understand the type of somatic dysfunction that is amenable to HVLA manipulation, an understanding of the Barrier Concept is essential.

- The Barrier Concept refers to the movement capabilities of a joint during normal and restricted motion.
- These movement capabilities are evaluated during the palpatory exam for both quantity and quality of motion.
  - *Quantity of motion* refers to the amount of movement from the joint's midline, or neutral point of motion, to a motion barrier; it is determined by the amount of movement from the neutral point.
  - The neutral point of motion is the position of a nondysfunctional joint at rest, with equal myofascial forces pulling it in all directions (Fig. 49.1).
- When a healthy joint is actively moved during normal activity, the end of motion occurs at the *physiologic* barrier.
- When the range of motion of a joint is tested passively during a physical examination, the end of the furthest motion is the *anatomic* barrier.
  - Motion beyond the anatomic barrier implies disruption of osseous or ligamentous structures of that joint.
  - Both the anatomic and the physiologic barriers are present in healthy joints without any dysfunction.
- A third barrier, the *restrictive* or *pathologic barrier*, is found when a joint has motion loss due to somatic dysfunction.
  - The quantity of motion required to arrive at the restrictive barrier is less than the amount required to reach the physiologic barrier.
  - This shifts the midline of joint motion away from the restrictive barrier.
  - The palpatory experience of a restrictive barrier sense occurs when the examining physician feels the decreased joint range of motion in at least one direction, or the joint moves better in one direction than in the other.
- One of the goals of manipulative treatment is to aid a return to normal, unrestricted motion.

The *quality of motion* refers to the palpatory sense of how smoothly a joint can be moved through its range of motion.

- A resistance or hesitance through motion implies some type of dysfunction of the joint.
- End feel is a term describing the quality of motion palpated when a joint is brought passively to its final barrier of motion.
  - End feel can be a function of both the focal tissue turgor at the region of the somatic dysfunction and the tethering actions of the muscle and fascia, which are being stretched.
  - The end feel is typically nebulous or rubbery with reflex-related somatic dysfunctions.
  - It is typically firm and distinct, with mechanical-type arthrodial dysfunctions.
- The quantity and quality of motion, along with the end feel, allow the physician to determine the restriction of motion component of the diagnostic TART mnemonic mentioned earlier.
  - TART defines somatic dysfunction.
  - The component(s) of TART that predominate for a given dysfunction can help guide the physician to the appropriate manipulative treatment(s).

HVLA or thrust manipulation is ideal for addressing a somatic dysfunction with distinct barrier mechanics involving a palpable loss of motion at a restrictive barrier and a firm end feel. HVLA is designed to resolve motion loss, regain normal quantity and quality of motion, and restore normal barriers. In weighing the importance of the TART components in a somatic dysfunction to be treated with HVLA, it would look like this: **TART**. Similarly weighed, the TART for counterstrain diagnosis might look like: **T**ART. Thus, it becomes apparent how the parameters of a somatic dysfunction can guide the physician to the most appropriate treatment modality.

PRINCIPLES OF TREATMENT

To understand why HVLA works in an area of somatic dysfunction, the reason for *why* the dysfunctional segment has restriction of motion must first be understood.

- A somatic dysfunction exhibiting barrier mechanics is *not* "subluxed," "out of place," "out of joint," or "dislocated." Like a door that will not fully close, it is inhibited from completing its full normal motion.
- Some external or internal force or factor may have caused local segmental irritation sufficient to create focal edema and swelling in a small discrete area.[67]
  - □ This in turn causes a tightening of the fascial structures, myofascial component, and capsular components of a specific arthrodial joint.
  - □ The articular distortion results in reflex hypertonicity of the musculature crossing the given joint.
  - □ Thus, there is a resultant decrease in the range of motion around that area.
  - □ This is discussed in the osteopathic and scientific literature on proprioceptors and somatic dysfunction.[68–73]

As previously discussed, restoring motion to the articulation is theorized to result in the restoration of normal proprioceptive input from the joint and reflex relaxation of muscles surrounding the joint.

- There are special considerations when treatment is applied to a vertebral joint as opposed to an appendicular joint.
- The "typical" vertebral joints (C2–L5) are assessed in the three cardinal planes of motion.
- Restrictions are classically found in:
  1. Side bending
  2. Rotation
  3. Flexion/extension
- The thrust treatment, however, is along a summed vector of findings.
  - □ The unique motion patterns found in the SI, atlantoaxial (AA), and occipitoatlantal (OA) joints are addressed in Chapter 8 Biomechanics, Chapter 33 Cervical Region, and Chapter 38 Functional Anatomy and Diagnosis of the Sacrum.
  - □ The HVLA treatments for SI and OA joint dysfunctions also tend to be along a summed vector.
  - □ AA dysfunctions are diagnosed and treated in a rotational manner along a vertical axis.

The entire gamut of appendicular motion patterns does not lend itself to treatment generalizations, but a few trends do predominate.

- Many appendicular joints have a predominant major joint motion as well as lesser minor joint motions.
- The patient typically presents with loss of, and pain with, the major joint motion.
  - □ This is frequently the result of a restricted minor joint motion.
  - □ Treatment is focused along a single vector of the minor joint motion loss.

The audible "pop" or "snap" frequently heard with the thrust is a subject of great debate.[74] If present, it may be the harbinger of a successful treatment or merely incidental, resulting from treatment forces spilling over to a joint above or below the targeted dysfunction. Similarly, a lack of audible articulation does not mean a technique was unsuccessful. Treatment should always be followed with thorough reassessment which can demonstrate resolution or persistence of somatic dysfunction.

TECHNIQUE METHODOLOGY

The HVLA approach involves the following:

- Initial positioning
- Engagement and stacking of barriers
- Accumulation of forces
- Final corrective thrust

Initial Positioning

- Initial positioning refers to the positions of both the patient and the physician.
- The physician assumes a relaxed and balanced position. This frees up the cortex, allowing attention to the diagnostic input from the fingers and hands as the technique is continually fine-tuned during its application.
  - □ If the physician's own proprioceptors are firing due to imbalance from an awkward stance, or from straining to hold up more weight than the physician's strength allows, it will be difficult to focus on the treatment at hand.
  - □ A patient will feel imbalance or lack of confidence on the part of a treating physician, and in response, will tense the muscles in anticipation of a fall or drop.
- Position the patient comfortably at the start of the treatment.
  - □ This allows the patient to relax.
  - □ In turn, this decreases the tonicity of the longer muscles overlying the dysfunction and the tensile forces or "pull" from muscles above and below the dysfunction.
- When performing a treatment using HVLA, focus the vector forces as precisely as possible, and use only the minimum force necessary. The more variables that can be eliminated from the manipulative equation, the more likely that a successful solution will be obtained.

Engagement and Stacking of Barriers

Engage barriers in side bending, rotation, and flexion/extension. The physician "stacks" these individual components to address each barrier of the somatic dysfunction, similar to the method used with muscle energy or myofascial release techniques.

- Maintain each previously engaged barrier as the next barrier is engaged, and the forces accumulate.
- With experience, this summation of vector forces, along with the arrival at a single summed vector, becomes very fast and efficient.
- Experienced physicians are able to sense how the tissues respond to the force being applied and make subtle alterations in the direction of force to effectively engage the barrier in all planes.

- If the setup is painful to the patient or the physician, the procedure should be stopped immediately.
  - Move the patient back to the neutral position and reassess.
  - The technique setup may be incorrect, or the patient may have a type of somatic dysfunction not amenable to HVLA. In that case, another modality may be used or further evaluation is warranted.
  - Correction may simply require first treating some overlying soft tissue dysfunction and then retrying the HVLA.

Accumulation of Forces

- The basis of most HVLA treatments is addressing the dysfunctional relationship between two bones.
- To treat them, the physician generally holds one bone still and moves the other bone in the direction of the restriction.
- The discomfort, if any, that a patient experiences during HVLA, occurs at the moment when all of the forces are stacked against the restrictive barrier.
- This is a natural conclusion to correct stacking, as mentioned above.
- A novice frequently runs into trouble at this stage, by losing concentration and relaxing the forces on the segment. If this occurs, do not continue with the thrust.

FINAL CORRECTIVE THRUST

- HVLA thrust techniques use a short, rapid thrust, hence the term high velocity low amplitude.
- Once the barrier is engaged, the final force is applied quickly from that position.
  - The proper application has been described as a tack hammer blow, which is sudden and short, but not forceful.
  - The term *impulse* applied to HVLA technique recognizes that the force is a sudden acceleration and deceleration.
  - Do not back off before delivering the corrective thrust.
  - The final force is often applied during exhalation. The exhalation phase of respiration is the relaxation phase.
  - If intuition suggests against the thrust, then don't. The physician's intuition is probably based on proprioceptive feedback indicating that some part of the treatment is not balanced properly.

Some thrust techniques are not executed at high velocity, and others have a larger or variable amplitude of motion during the articulation. Consider an experience where the patient undergoes treatment for a joint restriction and, as the physician is positioning the patient and localizing the forces, the restriction is released with a "pop" or "click." Occasionally, a joint may instead be manipulated with carefully and slowly applied forces. Again, experience is beneficial in applying the proper force. Although HVLA is described as thrust technique, the actual speed and force may be modified to fit the patient's needs.

DOSAGE

- In most circumstances, treating the same segment more than once a week using thrust technique is discouraged.[75]
- When treating hospitalized patients on a daily basis, Larson (N.J. Larson, *personal communication*, 1967, 1978) would vary the technique, so as to not repeat the same technique on a given area.
- If the same somatic dysfunction keeps recurring, the physician must assess and address the underlying cause.

ILLUSTRATIVE TREATMENT TECHNIQUES

HVLA Techniques for Somatic Dysfunctions in the Cervical Region

Occipitoatlantal Joint

Possible Objective Findings (and their corresponding restriction objective findings)

OA: FS_RR_L (restriction toward ES_LR_R); FS_LR_R (restriction toward ES_RR_L)

OA: ES_RR_L (restriction toward FS_LR_R); ES_LR_R (restriction toward FS_RR_L)

Note: *Some physicians diagnose and treat neutral OA somatic dysfunctions as well.*

Example

OA FS_RR_L (restriction toward ES_LR_R)

Treatment Position

Patient: Supine
Physician: Standing at the head of the table

Procedure

- After diagnosis and soft tissue preparation, using the right palm or forearm, the physician cups the patient's chin, supporting the patient's head at the right zygomatic process
- Place the left index MP joint on the patient's bony calvarium, and with the left thumb contacting the patient's left zygomatic process (Caution: Avoid the mastoid portion of the temporal bone.) (Fig. 49.2).
- Add mild extension with the left MP joint by pressing the MP joint slightly anteriorly, ensuring that the extension is localized and limited to the OA joint (Caution: Avoid typical cervical spine extension past neutral.).
- Minimally rotate the patient's head to the right with the right hand, engaging the rotational barrier of the OA joint. Ensure that the patient's head is well-supported on the physician's right forearm for maximum control of both the patient and the procedure.
- The physician engages the side bending barrier of the patient's OA joint by translating inferior with the left MP joint and slightly superior with the right hand (inducing left side bending at OA).
- The patient is instructed to inhale and exhale fully. As they exhale, the physician approaches the restriction barriers (extension, left

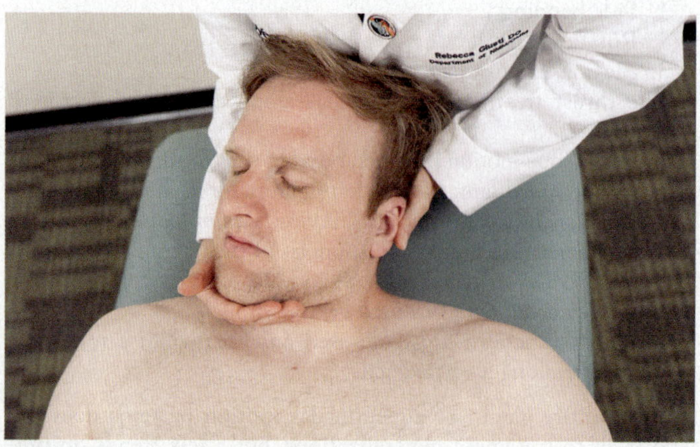

Figure 49.2. Initial positioning for O-A FS_RR_L. (Photo courtesy of Department of Neuromusculoskeletal Medicine/Osteopathic Manipulative Medicine at Western University of Health Sciences, Pomona, CA, with permission.)

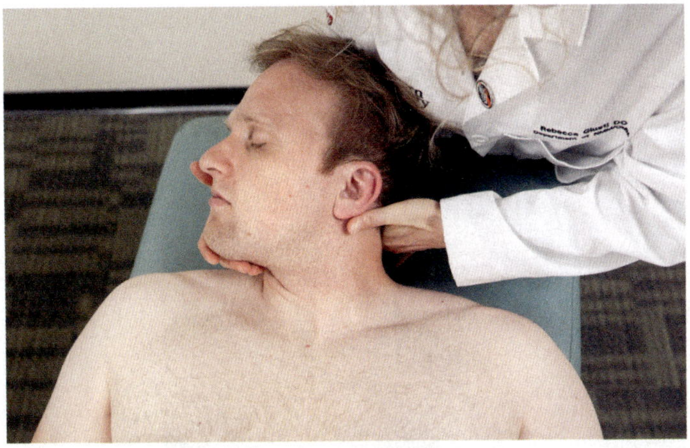

Figure 49.3. O-A FS_RR_L. Thrust toward patient's right eye. (Photo courtesy of Department of Neuromusculoskeletal Medicine/Osteopathic Manipulative Medicine at Western University of Health Sciences, Pomona, CA, with permission.)

side bending, right rotation) until they reach the end point of free motion at the patient's OA joint.

- At the end of exhalation, the physician applies an HVLA thrust through the restrictive barrier by translating through the left MP joint, directing the force toward the patient's right eye (Fig. 49.3).
- Retest: The physician uses the same method to reassess as was used to find the initial somatic dysfunction.

Atlantoaxial Joint—Rotation Only

Possible Objective Findings (and their corresponding restriction objective findings)

AA: R_L (restriction toward R_R); R_R (restriction toward R_L)

Example

AA R_R (restriction toward left atlantoaxial rotation)

Treatment Position

Patient: Supine
Physician: Standing to the right of the patient, at the head of the table

Procedure

- After diagnosis and soft tissue preparation, the physician slightly flexes the patient's head and neck. (**Note:** *Some physicians flex the neck to 45 degrees.*)
- Using the left palm or forearm, the physician cups the patient's chin, supporting the patient's head at the left zygomatic process
- Supporting the patient's head on the left forearm, rotate the patient's head to the left with the left hand, toward the AA joint's restrictive barrier.
- Then, place the right index MP joint on the soft tissue of the patient's AA joint with the right thumb contacting the lateral aspect of the patient's face on the right zygomatic process (avoid the mastoid process) (Fig. 49.4).
- The patient inhales and exhales fully. As the patient exhales, rotate the patient to the end point of free motion into the restrictive barrier at the patient's AA joint. At the end of exhalation, the physician applies an HVLA left rotational thrust through the restrictive barrier, using the right index finger MP joint as a fulcrum (Fig. 49.5).
- Retest: The physician uses the same method to reassess as was used to find the initial somatic dysfunction.

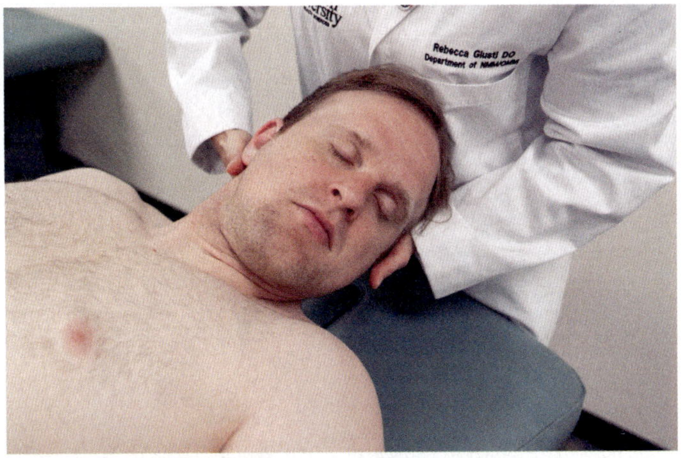

Figure 49.4. AA R_R—performing the set-up for HVLA to the AA joint. (Photo courtesy of Department of Neuromusculoskeletal Medicine/Osteopathic Manipulative Medicine at Western University of Health Sciences, Pomona, CA, with permission.)

Typical Cervical Vertebrae (C2–C7)—Type II Rotational Focus

Possible Objective Findings (and their corresponding restriction objective findings)

C2–C7: FR_RS_R (restriction toward ER_LS_L); FR_LS_L (restriction toward ER_RS_R)
C2–C7: ER_RS_R (restriction toward FR_LS_L); ER_LS_L (restriction toward FR_RS_R)

Example

C3 FR_RS_R (restriction toward ER_LS_L)

Treatment Position

Patient: Supine
Physician: Standing to the right of the patient, at the head of the table

Procedure

- After diagnosis and soft tissue preparation, the physician localizes the dysfunctional segment by contacting the articular pillars with the index finger or middle finger pads. The physician induces mild

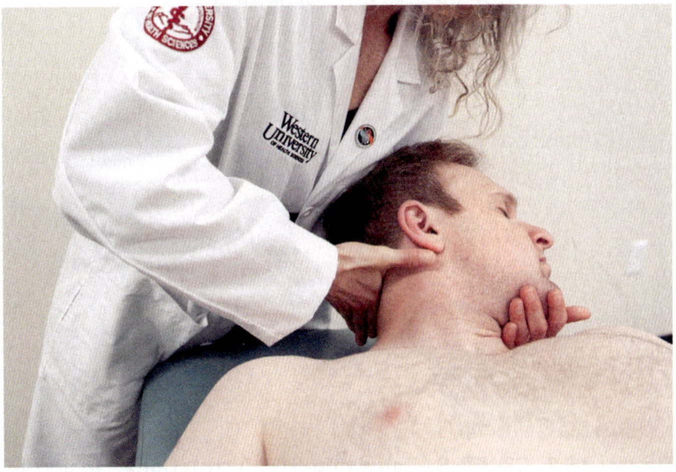

Figure 49.5. AA R_R—rotational thrust to the AA joint. (Photo courtesy of Department of Neuromusculoskeletal Medicine/Osteopathic Manipulative Medicine at Western University of Health Sciences, Pomona, CA, with permission.)

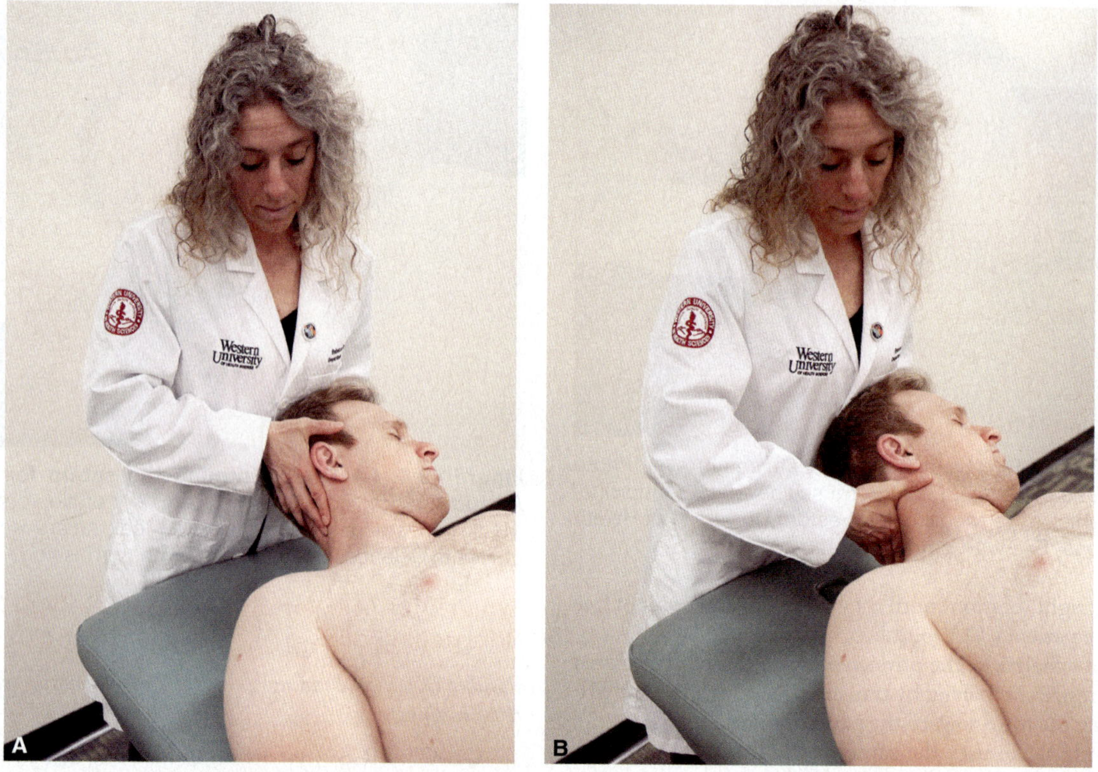

Figure 49.6. **A** and **B. C3 FR_RS_R—A.** Initial positioning: After diagnosis and soft tissue preparation, the physician localizes the dysfunctional segment by contacting the articular pillars with the index finger or middle finger pads. The physician induces mild flexion to the cervical spine and then rotates the patient's head slightly to the left to better visualize the right articular pillar. **B.** The physician places the right index MP joint against the posterolateral aspect of the patient's right C3 articular pillar with the right palm supporting the patient's neck and occiput. (Photo courtesy of Department of Neuromusculoskeletal Medicine/Osteopathic Manipulative Medicine at Western University of Health Sciences, Pomona, CA, with permission.)

flexion to the cervical spine and then rotates the patient's head slightly to the left to better visualize the right articular pillar. The physician places the right index MP joint against the posterolateral aspect of the patient's right C3 articular pillar with the right palm supporting the patient's neck and occiput (Fig. 49.6A,B).

- Maintaining this contact, the physician localizes flexion to the C3–C4 joint space, using the right palm to support the patient's neck and occiput to induce flexion to that level.

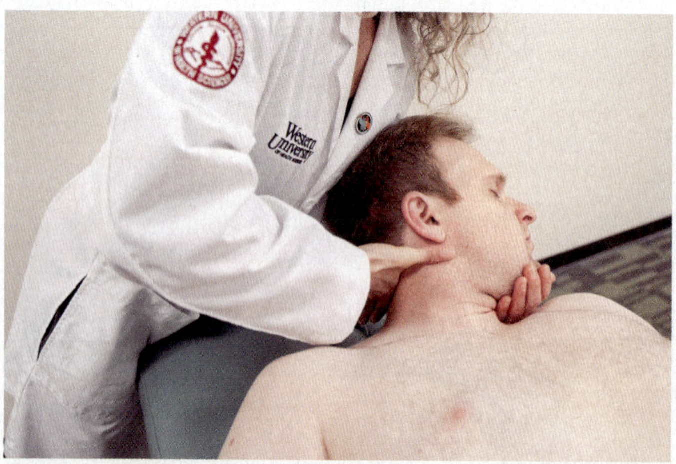

Figure 49.7. **C3 FR_RS_R—applying HVLA rotational focus to typical cervical region.** (Photo courtesy of Department of Neuromusculoskeletal Medicine/Osteopathic Manipulative Medicine at Western University of Health Sciences, Pomona, CA, with permission.)

- Using the right palm to stabilize the patient's occiput, the physician gently cups the patient's chin with the left hand and then rotates the patient's head to the left into the restrictive barrier while supporting the patient's head with the left palm or forearm.
- The physician's right MP joint induces right side bending at the patient's C3–C4 joint, into the position of ease. The right side bending may be augmented by the physician lifting the left forearm (patient's head) toward the ceiling.
- The physician applies a small amount of anterior translation of the patient's C3 vertebra with the right MP joint fulcrum engaging the extension barrier of the somatic dysfunction.
- The physician adjusts flexion, extension, and rotation as needed to confront the restrictive barrier of the joint.
- The patient is instructed to inhale and exhale fully. During exhalation, the physician will further approximate the barrier in all planes of motion until the "lock out" position is engaged. At the end of exhalation, the physician applies an HVLA left rotational thrust using the right index MP joint as a fulcrum, directing the force toward the patient's opposite eye (Fig. 49.7).
- Retest: The physician uses the same method to reassess as was used to find the initial somatic dysfunction.

Typical Cervical Vertebrae (C2–C7)—Type II Side Bending Focus

Possible Objective Findings (and their corresponding restriction objective findings)

C2–C7: FR_RS_R (restriction toward ER_LS_L); FR_LS_L (restriction toward ER_RS_R)

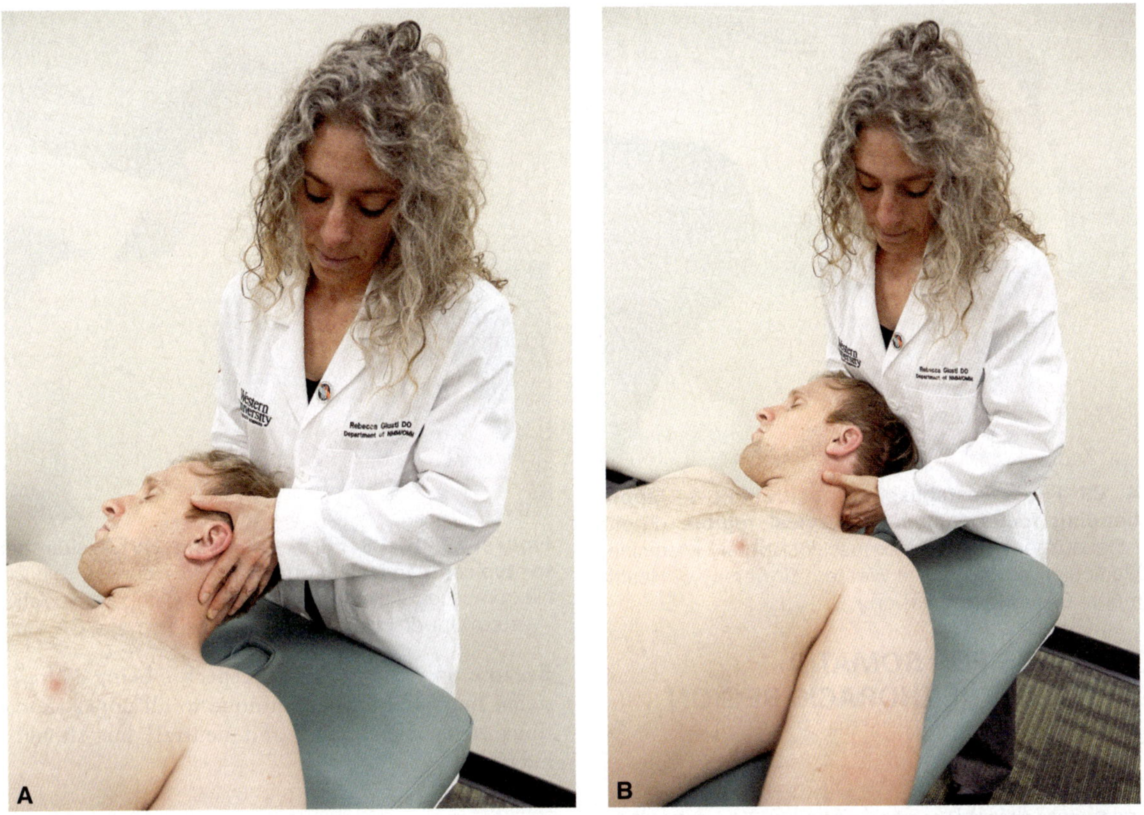

Figure 49.8. **A** and **B. C3 FR_RS_R. A.** Initial positioning: After diagnosis and soft tissue preparation, the physician localizes the dysfunctional segment by contacting the articular pillars with the index finger or middle finger pads. The physician induces mild flexion to the cervical spine and then rotates the patient's head slightly to the right to better visualize the left articular pillar. **B.** The physician places the left index MP joint against the posterolateral aspect of the patient's left C3 articular pillar with the left palm supporting the patient's neck and occiput. (Photo courtesy of Department of Neuromusculoskeletal Medicine/Osteopathic Manipulative Medicine at Western University of Health Sciences, Pomona, CA, with permission.)

C2–C7: ER_RS_R (restriction toward FR_LS_L); ER_LS_L (restriction toward FR_RS_R)

Example

C3 FR_RS_R (restriction toward ER_LS_L)

Treatment Position

Patient: Supine
Physician: Standing to the right of the patient, at the head of the table

Procedure

- After diagnosis and soft tissue preparation, the physician localizes the dysfunctional segment by contacting the articular pillars with the index finger or middle finger pads. The physician induces mild flexion to the cervical spine and then rotates the patient's head slightly to the right to better visualize the left articular pillar. The physician places the left index MP joint against the posterolateral aspect of the patient's left C3 articular pillar with the left palm supporting the patient's neck and occiput (Fig. 49.8A,B).
- Maintaining this contact, the physician localizes flexion to the C3–C4 joint space, using the left palm to support the patient's neck and occiput to induce flexion to that level.
- Using the left palm to stabilize the patient's occiput, the physician gently cups the patient's chin with the right hand and then rotates the patient's head to the right into the position of ease while supporting the patient's head with the right palm or forearm (Fig. 49.9A).
- The physician's left MP joint further induces left side bending at the patient's C3–C4 joint, into the restrictive barrier. The left side bending may be augmented by the physician lifting the right forearm (patient's head) toward the ceiling.
- The physician applies a small amount of anterior translation of the patient's C3 vertebra with the left MP joint fulcrum engaging the extension barrier of the somatic dysfunction.
- The physician adjusts flexion, extension, side bending as needed to confront the restrictive barrier of the joint.
- The patient is instructed to inhale and exhale fully. During exhalation, the physician will further approximate the barrier in all planes of motion until the "lock out" position is engaged. At the end of exhalation, the physician applies an HVLA left-to-right translational thrust using the left index MP joint as a fulcrum, directing the force toward the patient's opposite shoulder (Fig. 49.9B).
- Retest: The physician uses the same method to reassess as was used to find the initial somatic dysfunction.

When utilizing the side bending focus to address C2–C7 from superior to inferior, the physician should gradually alter the angle of the thrust in order to match the changing angle of the facets. This change in direction will form an approximate arc from the tip of the opposite shoulder ending just medial to the opposite nipple. For example, the direction of the thrust at C6–C7 is aimed more in the direction of the opposite nipple.

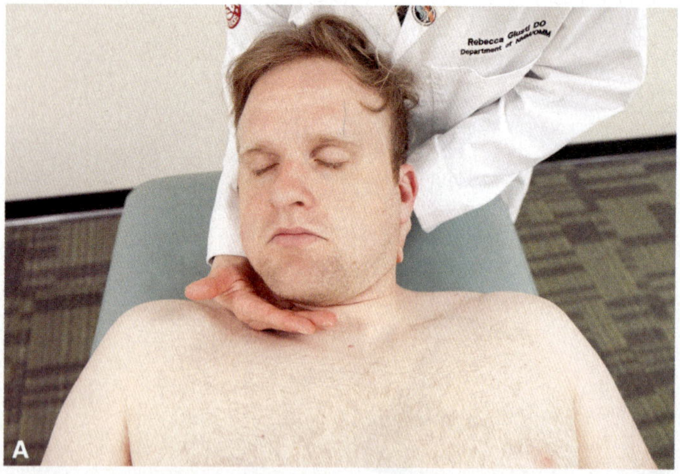

Figure 49.9A. C3 FR_RS_R—establishing positioning to apply HVLA side bending focus to typical cervical region. (Photo courtesy of Department of Neuromusculoskeletal Medicine/Osteopathic Manipulative Medicine at Western University of Health Sciences, Pomona, CA, with permission.)

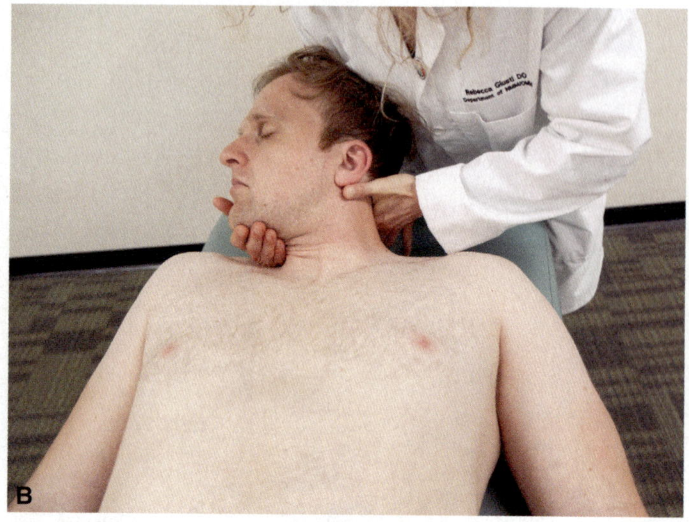

Figure 49.9B. C3 FR_RS_R—applying HVLA side bending focus to typical cervical region. (Photo courtesy of Department of Neuromusculoskeletal Medicine/Osteopathic Manipulative Medicine at Western University of Health Sciences, Pomona, CA, with permission.)

HVLA TECHNIQUES FOR SOMATIC DYSFUNCTIONS IN THE THORACIC REGION

Upper Thoracic Prone Cross-Hand Technique (T1–T4): Type I and Type II[76]

(Note: Some texts state that this method of treatment can be done from T1–T5.)

Possible Objective Findings (and their corresponding restriction objective findings):

T1–T4: FR_RS_R (restriction toward ER_LS_L); FR_LS_L (restriction toward ER_RS_R)
ER_RS_R (restriction toward FR_LS_L); ER_LS_L (restriction toward FR_RS_R)
NS_RR_L (restriction toward NS_LR_R); NS_LR_R (restriction toward NS_RR_L)

(Note: Utilization of prone cross-hand technique is generally recommended for neutral and flexed somatic dysfunction. Because only the rotational aspect is being addressed, the physician may apply this technique to all upper thoracic dysfunctions [flexed, extended, and neutral] but should use clinical judgment.)

Example

T2 FR_LS_L (restriction toward ER_RS_R)

Treatment Position

Patient: Prone with chin resting on the treatment table
Physician: Standing at the head of the table to the side of the patient's posterior transverse process (left in this example)

Procedure

- After diagnosis and soft tissue preparation, grasp the patient's head with both hands and passively sidebend the patient's head and neck toward the restrictive barrier (to the patient's right) localizing at the T2–T3 joint space (Fig. 49.10A).

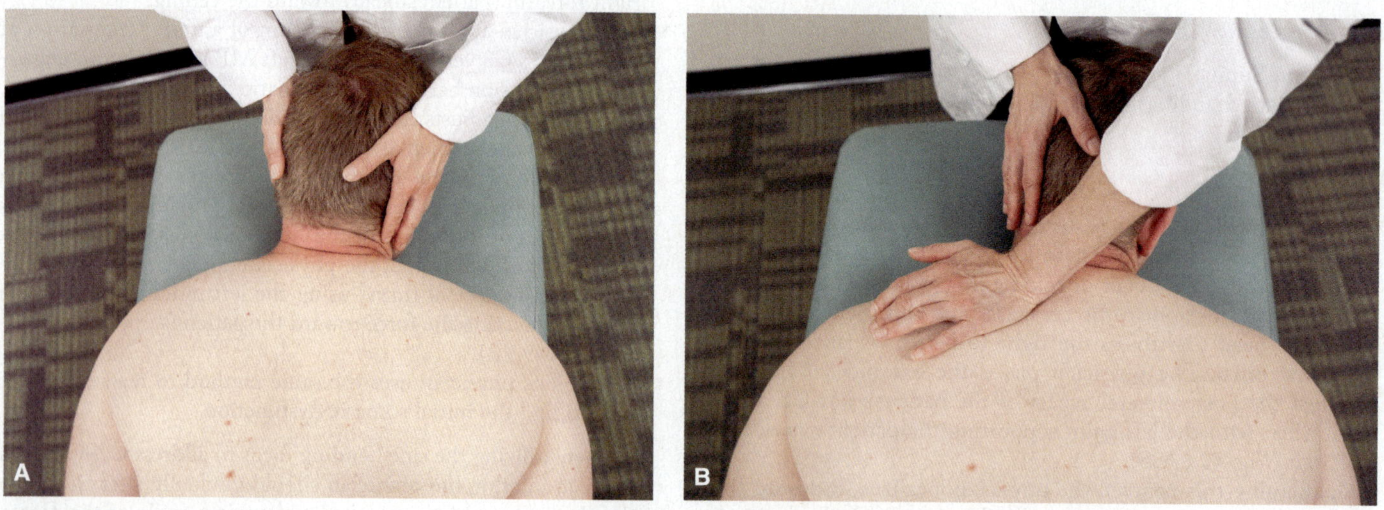

Figure 49.10. A and **B. T2 FS_LR_L A**. After diagnosis and soft tissue preparation, grasp the patient's head with both hands and passively sidebend the patient's head and neck toward the restrictive barrier (to the patient's right) localizing at the T2–T3 joint space. **B.** The physician's right hand contacts the patient's left occipital region; the left hypothenar or thenar eminence is placed over the patient's posterior (*left*) transverse process of T2. (Photo courtesy of Department of Neuromusculoskeletal Medicine/Osteopathic Manipulative Medicine at Western University of Health Sciences, Pomona, CA, with permission.)

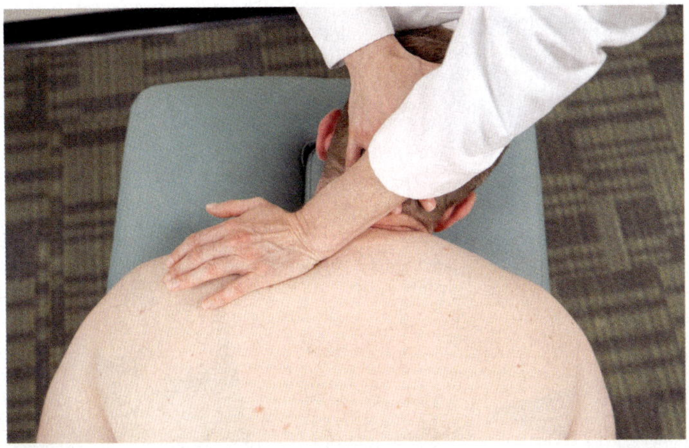

Figure 49.11. T2 FS_LR_L. Applying upper thoracic cross-hand HVLA. (Photo courtesy of Department of Neuromusculoskeletal Medicine/Osteopathic Manipulative Medicine at Western University of Health Sciences, Pomona, CA, with permission.)

- The physician's right hand contacts the patient's left occipital region; the left hypothenar or thenar eminence is placed over the patient's posterior (left) transverse process of T2 (Fig. 49.10B).
- The patient's head, cervical spine, and T1 vertebra are rotated to the left by gently pushing the patient's left occipital region away from the physician; resulting in ligamentous locking (the segments superior are "locked" in left rotation) to further localize forces at T2.
- The patient is instructed to inhale and exhale fully. During exhalation, the physician takes up the slack in the tension between the two hands by using opposing forces.
- At the end of exhalation, the physician applies an HVLA thrust through the left hypothenar or thenar eminence in a posteroanterior and inferior direction, thus inducing a small amount of right rotation at T2 (Fig. 49.11), while simultaneously, the physician's right hand stabilizes the patient's head by inducing a slight opposing (left) rotation/right side bending force.
- Retest: The physician uses the same method to reassess as was used to find the initial somatic dysfunction.

Note: A dysfunctional rib 1 may also be treated in a similar manner. For a dysfunctional left rib 1, the set-up for HVLA would be the same as above, but the physician would contact the posterior aspect of the dysfunctional rib 1 with their left hypothenar or left pisiform and induce a thrust in an oblique fashion (slightly anterior, inferior and lateral) in accordance with its costovertebral and costotransverse joints.

Supine Thoracic Multiple Planes (T3–T12): Type I

Possible Objective Findings (and their corresponding restriction objective findings):

T3–T12: NS_RR_L (restriction toward NS_LR_R); NS_LR_R (restriction toward NS_RR_L)

Example

T5–T9 NS_RR_L (restriction toward NS_LR_R), apex at T7

Treatment Position

Patient: Supine
Physician: Standing at the side of the patient opposite the patient's posterior transverse process (the patient's right)

Procedure

- After diagnosis and soft tissue preparation, the patient crosses their arms over the chest, with the left arm superior to the right arm. The elbows are aligned midline, with the hands grasping the shoulders firmly (Fig. 49.12).

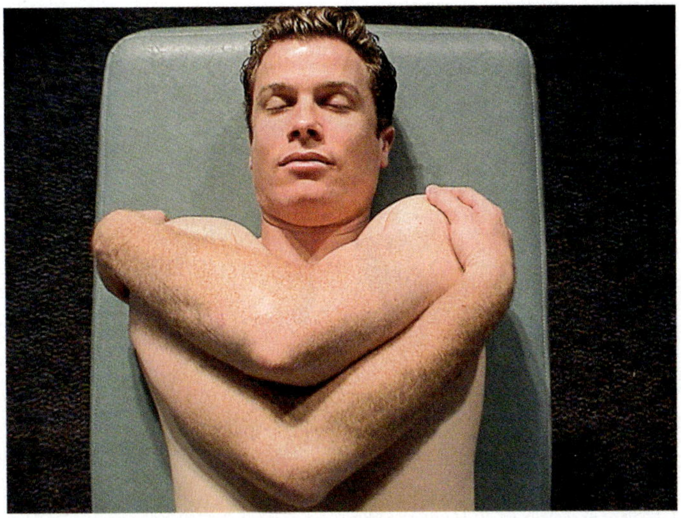

Figure 49.12. T5–T9 NS_RR_L—initial position. (Photo courtesy of Department of Neuromusculoskeletal Medicine/Osteopathic Manipulative Medicine at Western University of Health Sciences, Pomona, CA, with permission.)

- The physician's left hand is placed on the patient's left shoulder and is used to rotate the patient toward the physician.
- The physician reaches across the patient with the right hand and places the thenar eminence on the patient's posterior transverse process at T7 with the palm cradling the spinous processes.
- The physician's right hand may be flat or in a fist with the second, third, fourth, and fifth fingers flexed.
- The physician rolls the patient supine onto the right thenar eminence, which acts as a fulcrum.
- The patient's elbows are placed in the physician's epigastrium. The physician localizes a force over the fulcrum by adjusting their body weight through the patient's elbows, which act as a lever.
- The physician supports the patient's head, neck, and spine with the left hand/arm as flexion and left side bending is induced through T7 to the dysfunctional joint space (T7–T8).
- The patient inhales and exhales fully. During exhalation, the physician increases localization by applying their body weight through the patient's elbows.
- At the end of exhalation, the physician applies an HVLA thrust by dropping their body weight through the patient's thorax toward the floor (Fig. 49.13).
- The thrust forces the upper vertebra of the dysfunctional joint (T7) into right rotation relative to the lower vertebra (T8).
- Retest: The physician uses the same method to reassess as was used to find the initial somatic dysfunction.

Note: For a type II (i.e., flexed or extended) somatic dysfunction in the thoracic region, the procedure is similar as long as the physician localizes the dysfunctional joint toward its restrictive motion barriers. For an extended somatic dysfunction, the physician provides a thrust at a 45-degree vector toward the patient's head instead of a perpendicular vector toward the table.

Prone Cross-Hand Thoracic Technique (T5–T10): Type II (Flexed)[77]

Possible Objective Findings (and their corresponding restriction objective findings):

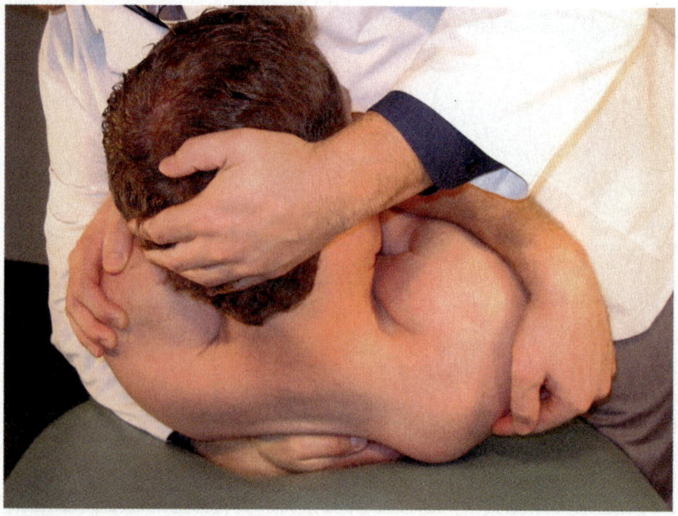

Figure 49.13. T5–T9 NS_RR_L—applying the thrust force. (Photo courtesy of Department of Neuromusculoskeletal Medicine/Osteopathic Manipulative Medicine at Western University of Health Sciences, Pomona, CA, with permission.)

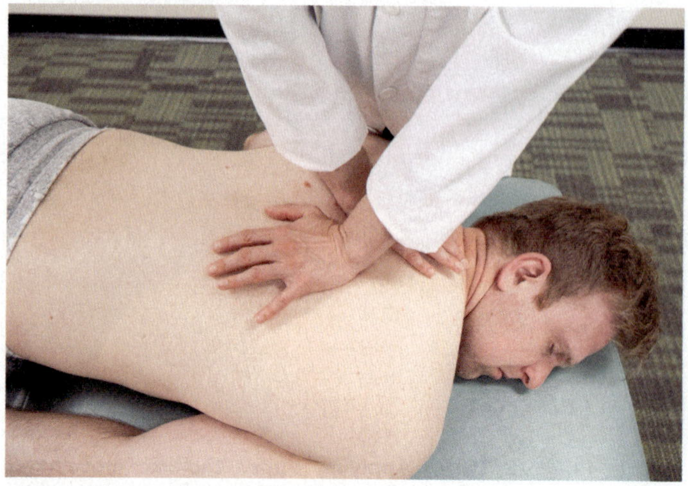

Figure 49.15. Prone cross-hand thoracic technique, T6 FR_LS_L—hand position prior to thrust. (Photo courtesy of Department of Neuromusculoskeletal Medicine/Osteopathic Manipulative Medicine at Western University of Health Sciences, Pomona, CA, with permission.)

T5–T12: FR_RS_R (restriction toward ER_LS_L); FR_LS_L (restriction toward ER_RS_R)

Example

T6 FR_LS_L (restriction toward ER_RS_R)

Treatment Position

Patient: Prone, with arms lying by their sides

Physician: Standing at the side of the patient's posterior transverse process (on the left)

Procedure

- The patient's head is turned away from the physician to assist rotation to the restricted side (right).
- The physician contacts the inferior aspect of the patient's posterior (left) transverse process (T6) with the right hypothenar eminence and the fingers pointing toward the patient's head (Fig. 49.14).
- The thenar eminence of the physician's left hand contacts the superficial tissues over the patient's opposite (right) transverse process on the same vertebra (T6), with the fingers pointing toward the patient's feet.

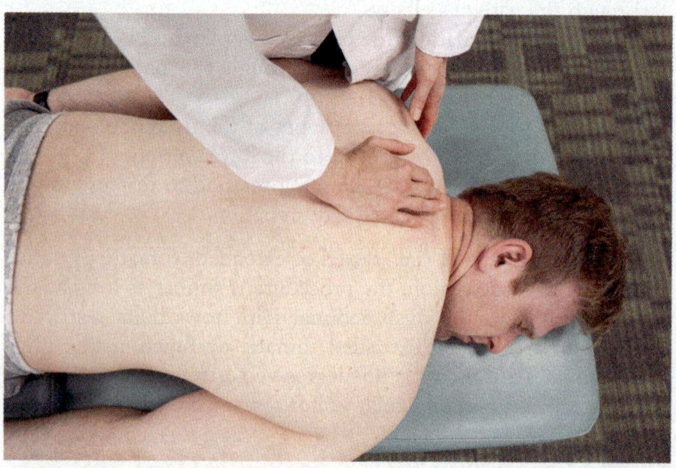

Figure 49.14. Prone cross-hand thoracic technique, T6 FR_LS_L—initial position. (Photo courtesy of Department of Neuromusculoskeletal Medicine/Osteopathic Manipulative Medicine at Western University of Health Sciences, Pomona, CA, with permission.)

- The physician localizes forces under both hands by applying an anterior–superior pressure over the patient's posterior (left) transverse process with the right hand and an anterior–inferior pressure over the patient's opposite (right) transverse process with the left hand (Fig. 49.15).
- Rotation of the vertebra to the restricted side (right) is induced by an anterior force, thereby inducing mobilization. Right side bending is produced by the longitudinal vectors (the superior and inferior pressure described above). The physician induces a translatory force to the region by moving both hands toward themself, thereby decreasing the dysfunctional side bending.
- The patient inhales and exhales fully. During exhalation, the physician increases localization through the hands with both elbows held rigid in extension. At the end of exhalation, the physician applies an HVLA thrust by using a momentary drop of their body weight to transmit the force through the wrists and elbows.
- Retest: The physician uses the same method to reassess as was used to find the initial somatic dysfunction.

Note: Only neutral type I and flexed type II somatic dysfunctions are treated by using prone cross-hand thoracic HVLA from T5–T12. The technique should not be used to address extended somatic dysfunctions in this region.

HVLA TECHNIQUES FOR SOMATIC DYSFUNCTIONS IN THE RIB REGION

Rib Inhalation Somatic Dysfunction (Ribs 2 to 10)

Possible Objective Findings (and its corresponding motion restriction):

Ribs 2 to 10: R/L rib(s) move(s) easier in inhalation than exhalation (the rib resists exhalation; exhalation restriction)

Example

Left rib 5 inhalation somatic dysfunction (left rib 5 resists exhalation)

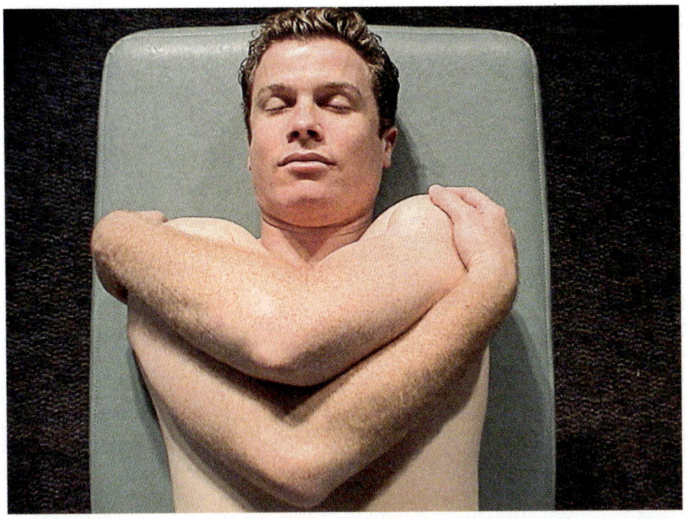

Figure 49.16. Left rib 5 inhalation somatic dysfunction—initial position. (Photo courtesy of Department of Neuromusculoskeletal Medicine/Osteopathic Manipulative Medicine at Western University of Health Sciences, Pomona, CA, with permission.)

Treatment Position

Patient: Supine
Physician: Standing at the patient's right side (opposite side of the dysfunctional rib)

Procedure

- After diagnosis and soft tissue preparation, the patient is instructed to cross their arms over the chest with the left arm superior to the right arm. The patient's elbows are aligned midline, with the hands grasping the shoulders firmly (Fig. 49.16).
- The physician's left hand is placed on the patient's left shoulder and is used to rotate the patient.
- The physician reaches across the patient with the right hand and places the thenar eminence on the inferior border of the patient's left 5th rib at the rib angle, applying a superior traction to the rib angle (Fig. 49.17).

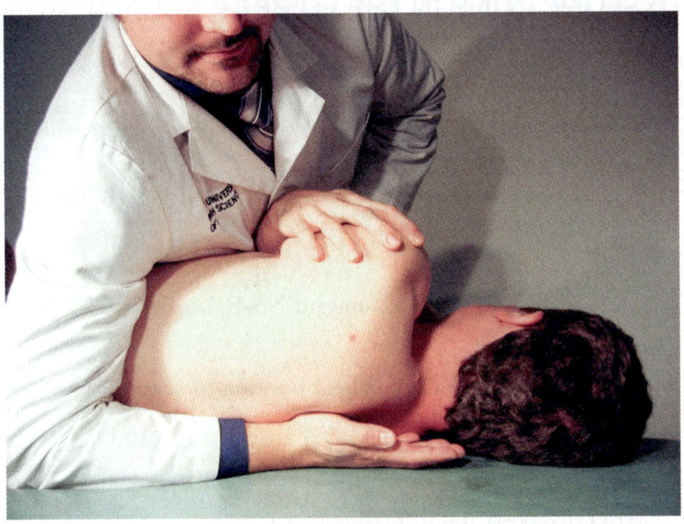

Figure 49.17. Placing the thenar eminence on the inferior border of the rib, at the rib angle. (Photo courtesy of Department of Neuromusculoskeletal Medicine/Osteopathic Manipulative Medicine at Western University of Health Sciences, Pomona, CA, with permission.)

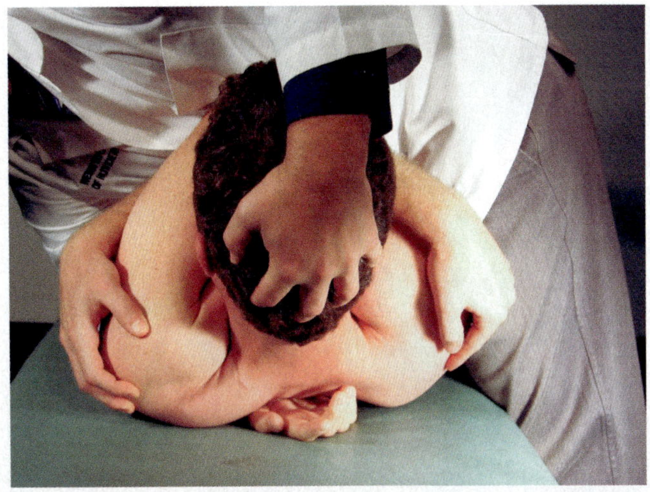

Figure 49.18. Rib thrust—inhalation somatic dysfunction. (Photo courtesy of Department of Neuromusculoskeletal Medicine/Osteopathic Manipulative Medicine at Western University of Health Sciences, Pomona, CA, with permission.)

- The physician rolls the patient supine, beyond midline, onto the right thenar eminence, which acts as a fulcrum.
- The patient's elbows are placed in the physician's epigastrium. The physician localizes a force to the patient's dysfunctional left 5th rib by adjusting their body weight through the patient's elbows, which act as a lever.
- The physician supports the patient's head, neck, and spine with the left hand/arm as flexion is induced until motion is felt at the left 5th rib.
- The patient inhales and exhales fully, and the physician follows the restricted motion to the barrier with the force of the physician's body weight.
- At the end of exhalation, the physician directs an HVLA thrust through the patient's elbows to the involved rib by abruptly dropping their body weight to the localized somatic dysfunction (Fig. 49.18).
- Retest: The physician uses the same method to reassess as was used to find the initial somatic dysfunction

Note: To address an exhalation somatic dysfunction, the physician contacts the superior aspect of the key rib angle and provides inferior traction with their thenar eminence.

Seated HVLA First Rib—Elevated[78]

HOW TO DIAGNOSE

The physician contacts the posterior shafts of the patient's first ribs. This can be done with the patient seated or supine. A positive finding is unleveling of the first ribs. The patient is instructed to inhale and exhale deeply. The inability of one or the other first rib to descend into the exhalation position confirms the diagnosis of superior subluxation of that rib. This is the same evaluation as that for a first rib inhalation respiratory somatic dysfunction; however, structural rib subluxations are more painful and have increased resistance to springing as compared to the other side. The patient may complain of tenderness upon palpation of the affected rib. Tenderness may be noted over the costotransverse articulation palpated anterior to the trapezius muscle. There may be a sense of deep anterior cervical muscle hypertonicity, as well as relatively restricted cervical side bending away from this dysfunctional 1st rib.

Possible Objective Findings (and its corresponding restriction objective findings)

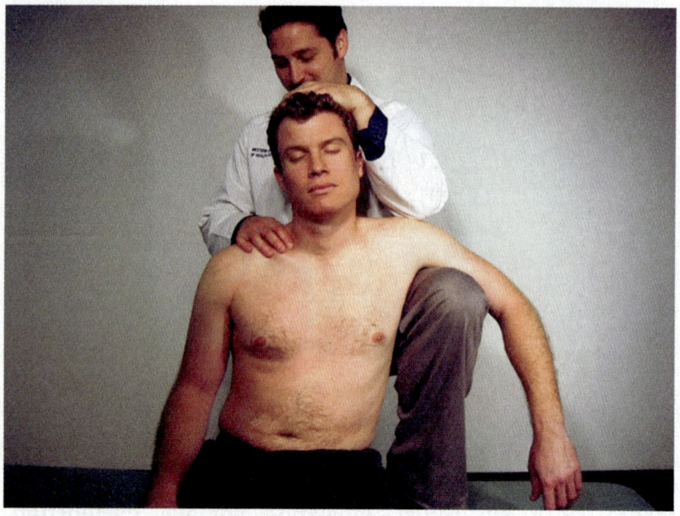

Figure 49.19. Elevated 1st rib—initial positioning. (Photo courtesy of Department of Neuromusculoskeletal Medicine/Osteopathic Manipulative Medicine at Western University of Health Sciences, Pomona, CA, with permission.)

R/L 1st rib: Superior elevated or subluxed (the L/R 1st rib resists depression and exhalation)

Example

Right 1st rib: Superiorly elevated (the right 1st rib resists depression and exhalation)

Treatment Position

Patient: Seated
Physician: Standing behind the patient

Procedure

- After diagnosis and soft tissue preparation, the physician's left foot is placed beside the patient's left side so the knee is in the patient's axilla OPPOSITE the superior 1st rib (Fig. 49.19).
- The physician places the right index MP joint against the patient's superior 1st rib head. The physician's wrist is straight to slightly dorsiflexed so there is a straight line from the MP joint through the wrist to the elbow. The physician's elbow is flexed (Fig. 49.20).

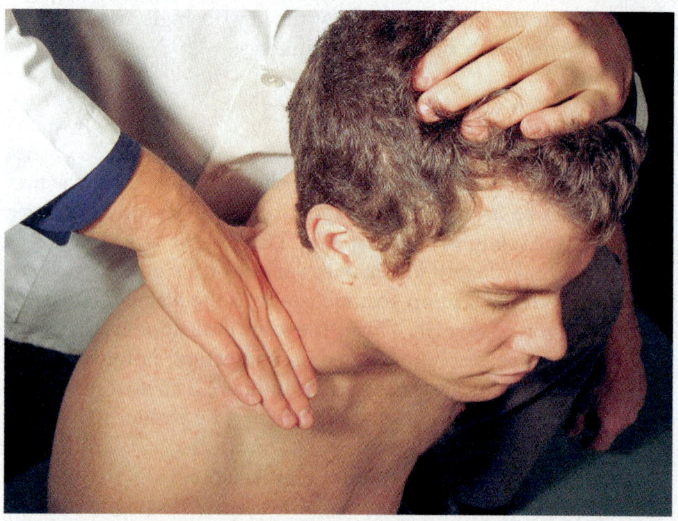

Figure 49.20. Elevated 1st rib—contact on the rib head. (Photo courtesy of Department of Neuromusculoskeletal Medicine/Osteopathic Manipulative Medicine at Western University of Health Sciences, Pomona, CA, with permission.)

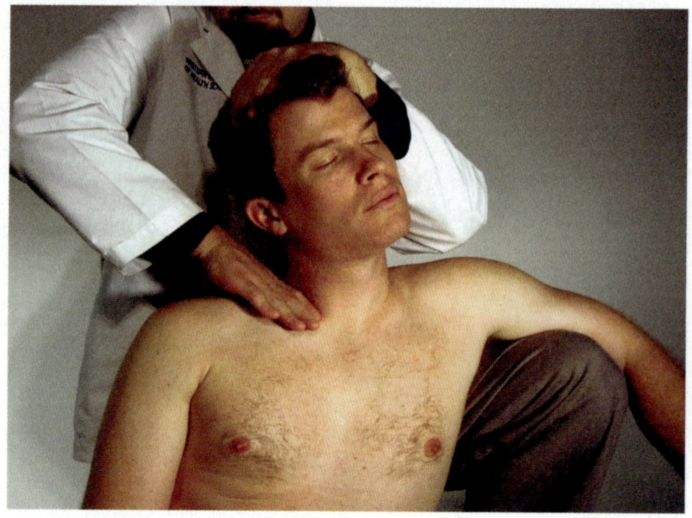

Figure 49.21. Elevated 1st rib thrust. (Photo courtesy of Department of Neuromusculoskeletal Medicine/Osteopathic Manipulative Medicine at Western University of Health Sciences, Pomona, CA, with permission.)

- The physician contacts the top of the patient's head with the left hand and sidebends the head and neck to the right. The physician then slowly rotates the patient's head and neck away from the patient's superior 1st rib (to the left), while maintaining right side bending in order to localize and engage the restrictive barrier.
- The physician instructs the patient to inhale and exhale fully. As the patient exhales, the physician further localizes the restrictive barriers to achieve a "locked out" position. At the end of exhalation, the physician applies a corrective HVLA thrust with the right index MP joint against the patient's superior 1st rib. The force is at an angle across the patient's body and toward the opposite costal margin (midclavicular line) (Fig. 49.21).
- Retest: The physician uses the same method to reassess as was used to find the initial somatic dysfunction.

HVLA TECHNIQUES FOR SOMATIC DYSFUNCTIONS IN THE LUMBAR REGION

Lumbar Technique (L1–L5)—Type I Neutral (Group) Somatic Dysfunction[79]

Possible Objective Findings (and their corresponding restriction objective findings)

L1–L5: NS_RR_L (restriction toward NS_LR_R); NS_LR_R (restriction toward NS_RR_L)

Example

L2–L4 NS_LR_R (restriction toward NS_RR_L), apex at L3

Treatment Position

Patient: Right lateral recumbent position (posterior transverse process toward the table)
Physician: Standing in front of the patient

Procedure

After diagnosis and soft tissue preparation:

- The fingers of the physician's left hand are used to monitor the patient's L3–L4 joint space.
- The physician flexes the patient's knees with the right hand until motion is felt at the patient's L3–L4 joint space (Fig. 49.22).

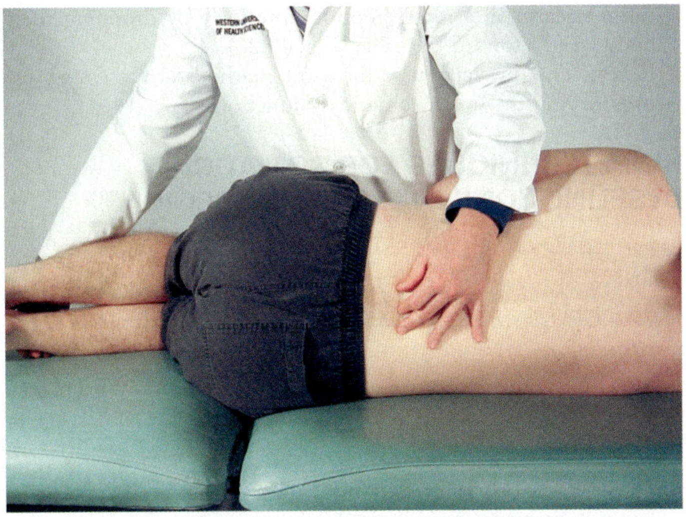

Figure 49.22. L2–L4 NS_LR_R—initial positioning. (Photo courtesy of Department of Neuromusculoskeletal Medicine/Osteopathic Manipulative Medicine at Western University of Health Sciences, Pomona, CA, with permission.)

- The patient straightens the right leg while the physician maintains flexion of the L3–L4 joint space.
- The physician places the patient's left foot into the popliteal fossa of the patient's right leg (Fig. 49.23).
- The physician changes hands so the right hand is palpating the patient's L3–L4 joint space.
- The physician's left hand grasps the patient's right arm and pulls it anteriorly and laterally to induce left truncal rotation to the level of L3, and inferiorly to induce right side bending of L3 on L4 (Fig. 49.24).
- The patient interlocks their fingers and places them across the chest or side.
- The physician slips their left hand beneath the patient's left arm and contacts the patient's left anterior axilla (pectoral area) with the left forearm to maintain left rotation, while the physician's left hand palpates the patient's spinous process of L3.
- The physician's right forearm is placed on the patient's left gluteal region across the SI area, with the right hand palpating the patient's spinous process of L4, to assist right rotation of L4 relative to L3 using the patient's pelvis as a lever.

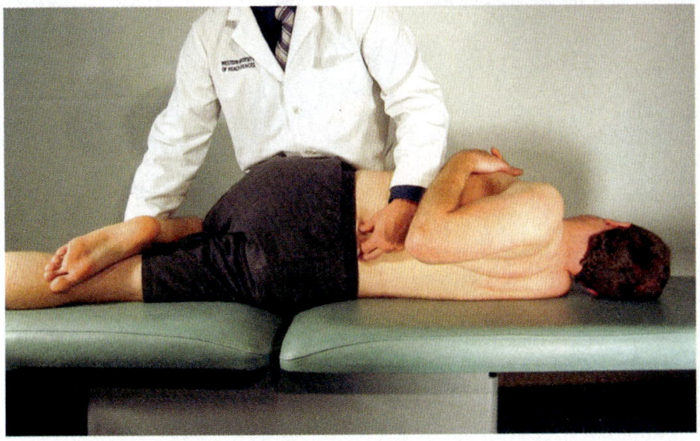

Figure 49.23. L2–L4 NS_LR_R—left foot in right popliteal fossa. (Photo courtesy of Department of Neuromusculoskeletal Medicine/Osteopathic Manipulative Medicine at Western University of Health Sciences, Pomona, CA, with permission.)

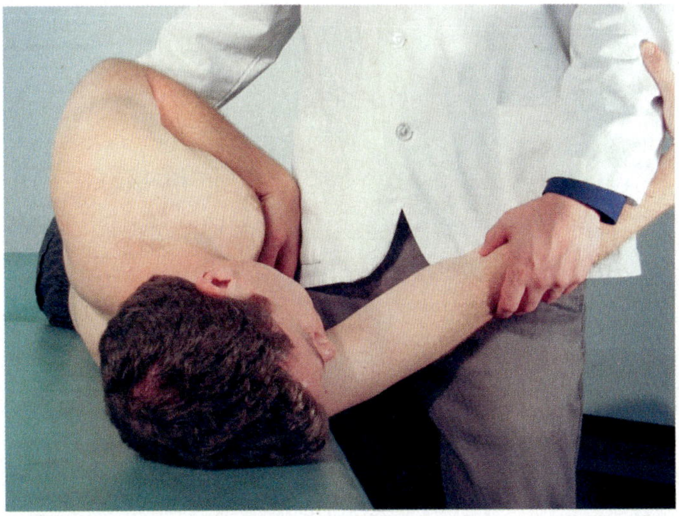

Figure 49.24. L2–L4 NS_LR_R—inducing left rotation and right side bending. (Photo courtesy of Department of Neuromusculoskeletal Medicine/Osteopathic Manipulative Medicine at Western University of Health Sciences, Pomona, CA, with permission.)

- While maintaining slight flexion, left rotation, and right side bending localization of L3 on L4, the patient is rolled as a unit toward the physician as the patient inhales. This serves to bring the dysfunctional facet joint perpendicular to the table which is theorized to facilitate the corrective thrust.
  - □ The patient exhales fully, while the physician induces left truncal rotation by increasing posterior pressure against the patient's left axilla and anterior pressure to the gluteal region to further localize the barrier.
- At the end of exhalation, the physician applies an HVLA thrust through the right forearm in a rotary motion anteriorly by dropping their body weight toward the table.
- Retest: The physician uses the same method to reassess as was used to find the initial somatic dysfunction.

Lumbar Roll (L1–L5)—Type II Flexed Somatic Dysfunction

Possible Objective Findings (and their corresponding restriction objective findings)

L1–L5: FR_RS_R (restriction toward ER_LS_L); FR_LS_L (restriction toward ER_RS_R)

Example

L3 FR_RS_R (restriction toward ER_LS_L)

Treatment Position

Patient: Right lateral recumbent (posterior transverse process toward the table)
Physician: Standing in front of the patient

Procedure

- After diagnosis and soft tissue preparation, the fingers of the physician's left hand are used to monitor the patient's L3–L4 joint space.
- The physician's right hand is used to flex the patient's left hip and knee and to place the patient's left foot in the popliteal fossa of the patient's right leg. The physician extends the patient's right leg until motion is palpated at the L3–L4 joint space (Fig. 49.25).
- The physician changes hands so the right hand is palpating the L3–L4 joint space.

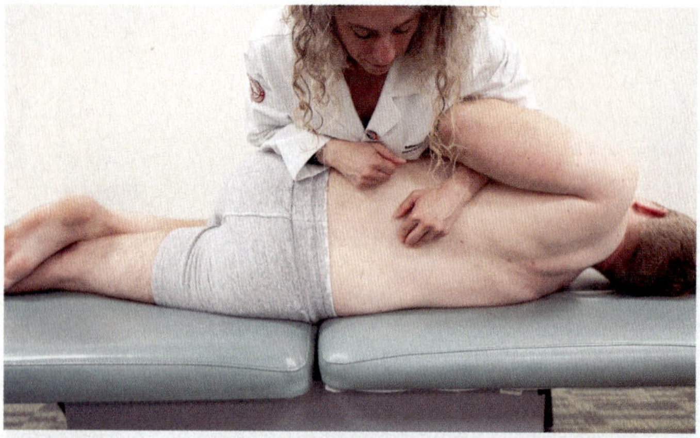

Figure 49.25. L3 FR_RS_R—positioning of patient for HVLA technique. (Photo courtesy of Department of Neuromusculoskeletal Medicine/Osteopathic Manipulative Medicine at Western University of Health Sciences, Pomona, CA, with permission.)

- The physician's left hand grasps the patient's right arm and pulls it anteriorly and laterally to induce left trunk rotation to the level of patient's L3, and superiorly to induce left side bending of L3 on L4.
- The patient interlocks their fingers and places them across the chest or side.
- The physician slips their left hand beneath the patient's left arm and contacts the patient's left anterior axilla (pectoral area) with the left forearm to maintain left rotation and the left hand palpates the patient's spinous process of L3.
- The physician places the right forearm on the patient's left gluteal region across the SI area, and the right hand palpates the patient's spinous process of L4, to assist right rotation of L4 relative to L3 using the patient's pelvis as a lever.
- While maintaining extension, left rotation, and left side bending localization of L3 on L4, the patient is rolled as a unit toward the physician while the patient inhales. This serves to bring the dysfunctional facet joint perpendicular to the table which is theorized to facilitate the corrective thrust.
- The patient exhales fully, while the physician induces left truncal rotation by increasing posterior pressure against the patient's left axilla and anterior pressure to the gluteal region to further localize the barrier.
- At the end of exhalation, once the physiologic barrier has been reached, the physician applies an HVLA thrust through the right forearm in a rotary motion anteriorly by dropping their body weight toward the table (Fig. 49.26).
- Retest: The physician uses the same method to reassess as was used to find the initial somatic dysfunction.

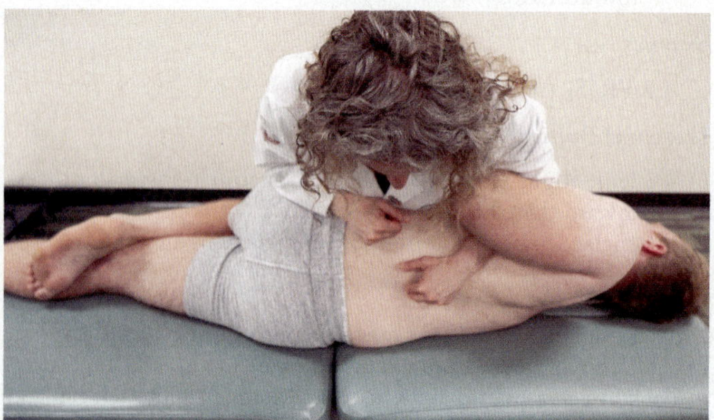

Figure 49.26. L3 FR_RS_R—applying the HVLA thrust force. (Photo courtesy of Department of Neuromusculoskeletal Medicine/Osteopathic Manipulative Medicine at Western University of Health Sciences, Pomona, CA, with permission.)

HVLA TECHNIQUES FOR SOMATIC DYSFUNCTIONS IN THE PELVIC REGION[80]

Iliosacral Dysfunctions: Anteriorly Rotated Innominate

Possible Objective Findings (and their corresponding restriction objective findings):

R/L/bilateral anterior innominate(s) (restriction toward posterior rotation of the innominate)

Example:

Right anteriorly rotated innominate (right innominate restriction toward posterior rotation)

Treatment Position

Patient: Left lateral recumbent
Physician: Standing in front of the patient

Procedure

After diagnosis and soft tissue preparation:

- The physician monitors the lumbosacral junction with the fingers of the left hand.
- Keeping the patient's spine in the neutral position, the physician rotates the patient's trunk to the right to induce right rotation and pulls the patient's left arm in an inferior direction to induce left side bending down to and including the lumbosacral junction (Fig. 49.27).
- The physician now uses the fingers of the right hand to monitor the patient's lumbosacral junction.
- The physician places the patient's right foot in the patient's left popliteal space (Fig. 49.28).
- The physician stabilizes the patient's trunk with the right forearm and uses the fingers of the right hand to monitor motion at the patient's right SI joint.
- The physician places the left forearm on the patient's right ischial tuberosity (below the axis of rotation of the right innominate).

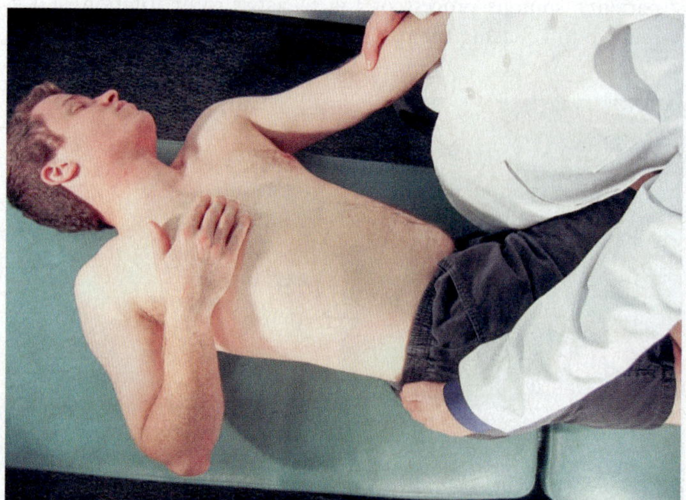

Figure 49.27. Anteriorly rotated innominate—initial position. (Photo courtesy of Department of Neuromusculoskeletal Medicine/Osteopathic Manipulative Medicine at Western University of Health Sciences, Pomona, CA, with permission.)

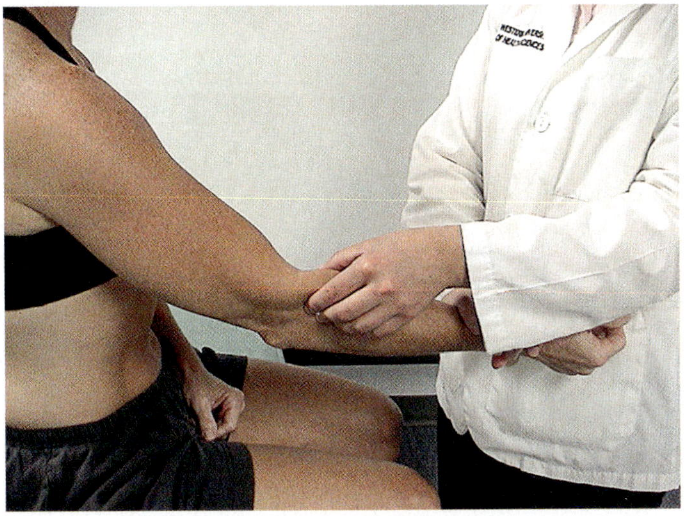

Figure 49.34. Posterior radial head technique—initial position. (Photo courtesy of Department of Neuromusculoskeletal Medicine/Osteopathic Manipulative Medicine at Western University of Health Sciences, Pomona, CA, with permission.)

Treatment Position

Patient: Seated on the table
Physician: Standing in front of the patient

Procedure

- The physician grasps the patient's right proximal forearm with the left thumb contacting the anterior aspect of the patient's right radial head (Fig. 49.36).
- The physician uses the right hand to pronate and flex the patient's right forearm while using their left thumb to engage the radial head posteriorly into the restrictive barrier.
- The patient is instructed to inhale and as they exhale, the physician further engages the restrictive barrier with increased elbow flexion. At the end of exhalation, the physician applies a slight HVLA thrust by applying a short posterior thrust to the anterior radial head (Fig. 49.37).
- Retest: The physician should use the same method to recheck as was used in the initial assessment of the restriction.

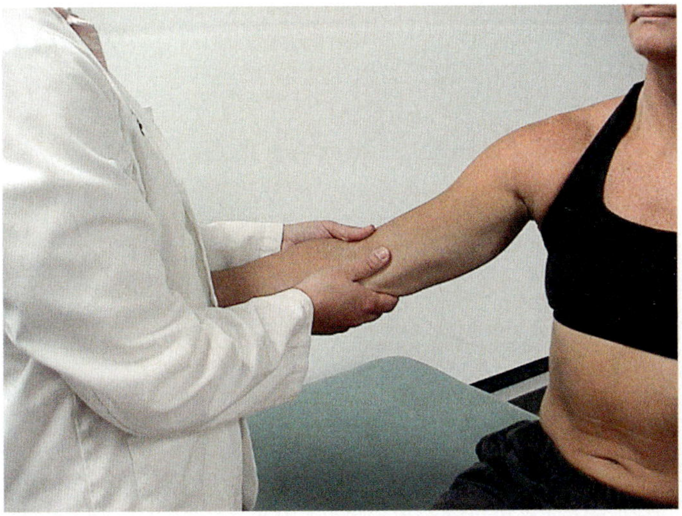

Figure 49.35. Posterior radial head technique—applying the thrust force. (Photo courtesy of Department of Neuromusculoskeletal Medicine/Osteopathic Manipulative Medicine at Western University of Health Sciences, Pomona, CA, with permission.)

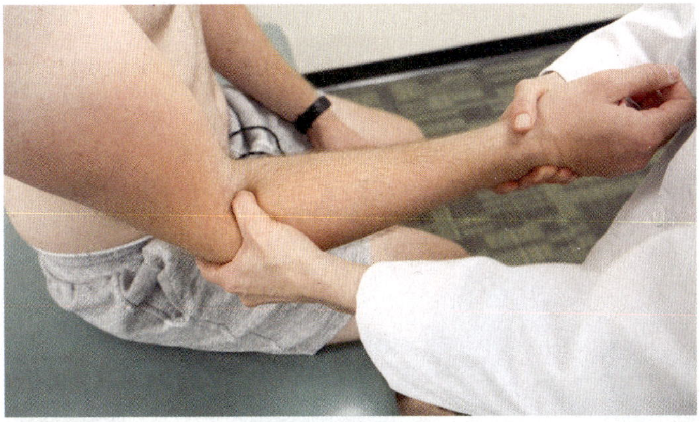

Figure 49.36. Anterior radial head contact. (Photo courtesy of Western University of Health Sciences, Pomona, CA, with permission.)

HVLA TECHNIQUES FOR SOMATIC DYSFUNCTIONS OF THE LOWER EXTREMITIES

Posterior Fibular Head

Possible Objective Findings (and their corresponding restriction objective findings)

R/L/bilateral posterior fibular head(s) (restriction in anterior glide of the fibular head)

Example

Right posterior fibular head (right fibular head restriction in anterior glide)

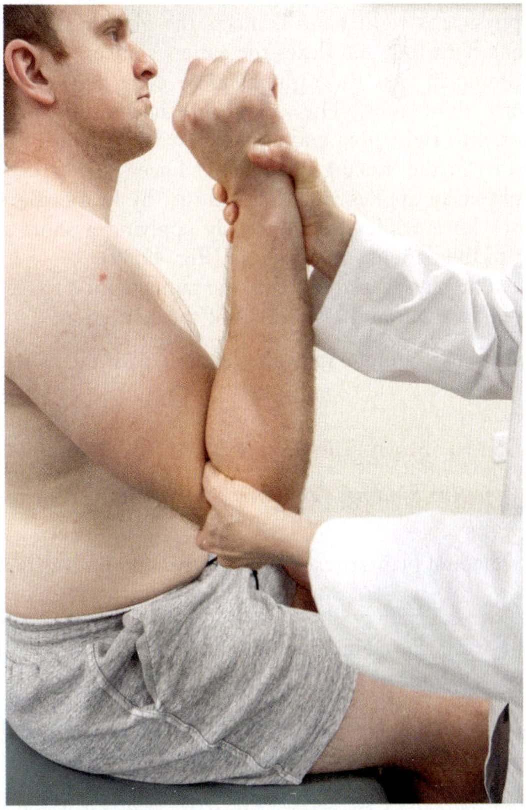

Figure 49.37. Anterior radial head technique—applying the thrust force. (Photo courtesy of Department of Neuromusculoskeletal Medicine/Osteopathic Manipulative Medicine at Western University of Health Sciences, Pomona, CA, with permission.)

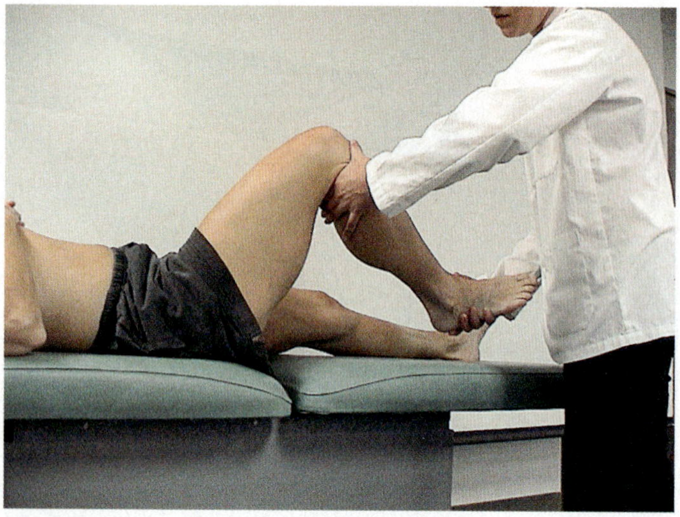

Figure 49.38. Posterior fibular head technique—initial position. (Photo courtesy of Department of Neuromusculoskeletal Medicine/Osteopathic Manipulative Medicine at Western University of Health Sciences, Pomona, CA, with permission.)

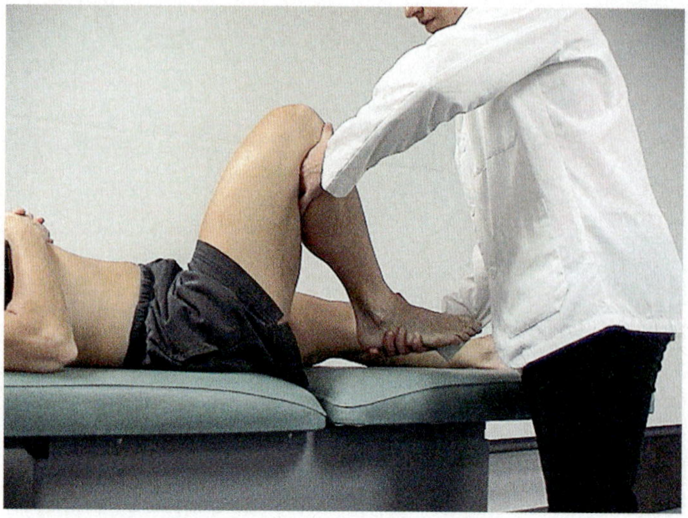

Figure 49.39. Posterior fibular head technique—applying the thrust force. (Photo courtesy of Department of Neuromusculoskeletal Medicine/Osteopathic Manipulative Medicine at Western University of Health Sciences, Pomona, CA, with permission.)

Treatment Position

Patient: Supine
Physician: Standing on the same side of the table as the leg being treated

Procedure

- The physician places the left hand gently across the patient's right popliteal fossa with the 1st metacarpal–phalangeal joint in contact with the patient's posterior fibular head.
- The physician's right hand contacts the plantar surface of the patient's right foot and flexes the patient's knee.
- The physician uses the right hand to evert and dorsiflex the patient's right foot. The physician then externally rotates the patient's right tibia and approaches the patient's restrictive barrier by further flexing the patient's knee (Fig. 49.38).
- The physician applies an HVLA thrust by further flexing the patient's knee while simultaneously applying a short anterior thrust to the patient's fibular head (Fig. 49.39).
- Retest: The physician should use the same method to recheck as was used in the initial assessment of the restriction.

Note: This technique may also be done with the patient lying prone.

Ankle Dysfunction- Talus Plantarflexed

Possible Objective Findings (and their corresponding restriction objective findings)

R/L/bilateral plantarflexed talus (restriction in dorsiflexion)

Example

Right plantarflexed talus (right talus restriction in dorsiflexion)

Treatment Position

Patient: Supine
Physician: Standing at the foot of table

Procedure

- The physician interlocks their fingers and places them on the anterosuperior surface of the patient's right talus with both thumbs contacting the plantar surface of the foot.
- The physician dorsiflexes the patient's ankle to the restrictive barrier.
- The physician applies an HVLA thrust inferiorly on the patient's talus while further dorsiflexing the ankle to free the talus from the crura (Fig. 49.40).
- Retest: The physician should use the same method to recheck as was used in the initial assessment of the restriction.

Foot/Tarsal Displacement—Cuboid Displacement

Note: In a "dropped" arch, the cuboid is frequently everted in which the plantar surface is turned laterally.

Possible Objective Findings (and their corresponding restriction objective findings):

R/L/bilaterally inverted cuboid(s) (restriction in eversion of cuboid bone)

R/L/bilaterally everted cuboid(s) (restriction in inversion of cuboid bone)

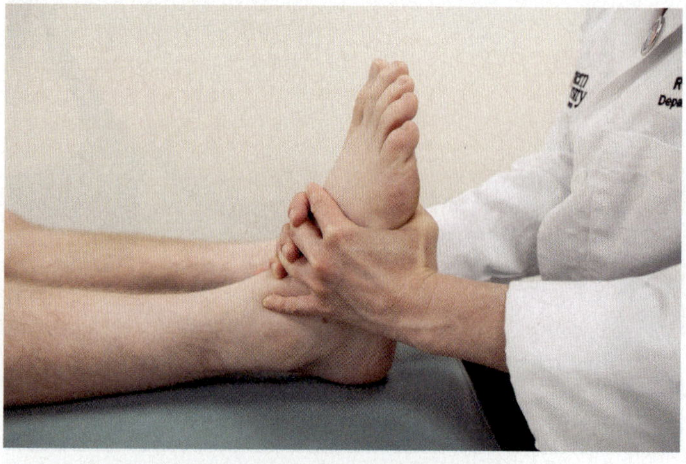

Figure 49.40. Talus plantar flexed. (Photo courtesy of Department of Neuromusculoskeletal Medicine/Osteopathic Manipulative Medicine at Western University of Health Sciences, Pomona, CA, with permission.)

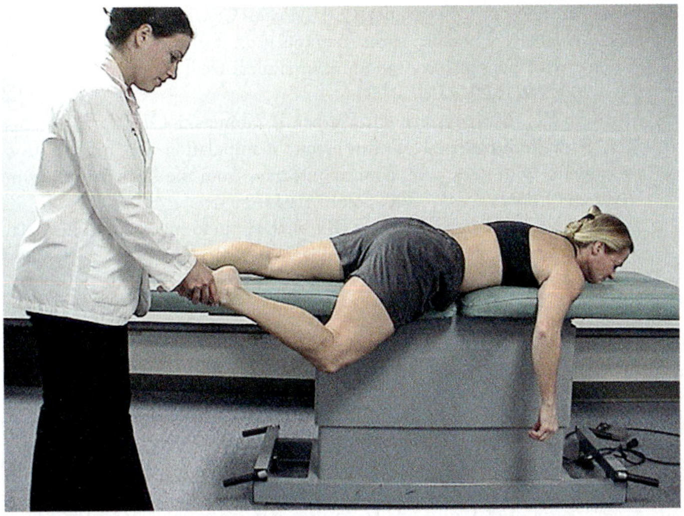

Figure 49.41. Cuboid technique—initial position. (Photo courtesy of Department of Neuromusculoskeletal Medicine/Osteopathic Manipulative Medicine at Western University of Health Sciences, Pomona, CA, with permission.)

Example

Right cuboid displacement—Everted (i.e., eversion of right cuboid bone, resists inversion, the medial aspect of the plantar surface of the cuboid is displaced inferiorly and laterally)

Treatment Position

Patient: Prone, with the right (dysfunctional) foot off the side of the table.

Physician: Standing at the foot of the table to the patient's dysfunctional (right) side.

Procedure

- The physician grasps the patient's right forefoot with both hands while the thumbs are placed on the plantar surface of the cuboid to be treated (Fig. 49.41).
- The physician plantar flexes the patient's right foot and engages the restrictive barrier at the cuboid (Fig. 49.42).

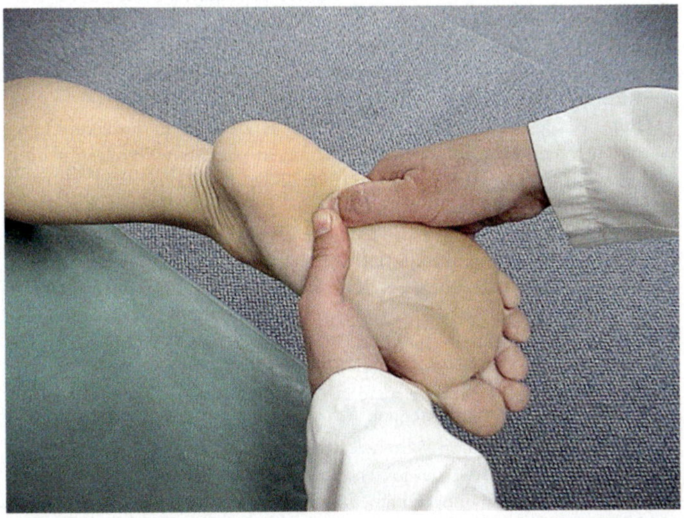

Figure 49.42. Cuboid technique—engaging the restrictive barrier. (Photo courtesy of Department of Neuromusculoskeletal Medicine/Osteopathic Manipulative Medicine at Western University of Health Sciences, Pomona, CA, with permission.)

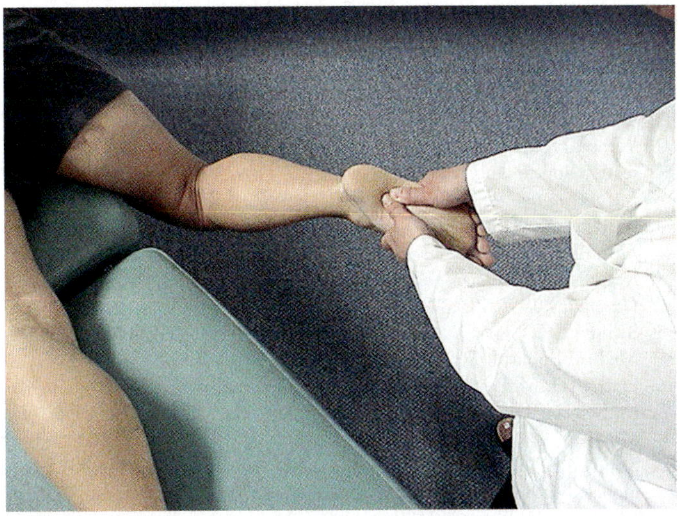

Figure 49.43. Cuboid technique—applying the thrust force. (Photo courtesy of Department of Neuromusculoskeletal Medicine/Osteopathic Manipulative Medicine at Western University of Health Sciences, Pomona, CA, with permission.)

- When the barrier is engaged in plantar flexion, the physician applies an HVLA thrust through the thumbs, toward the floor and laterally, while the foot is plantar flexed (Fig. 49.43).
- Retest: The physician should use the same method to recheck as was used in the initial assessment of the restriction.

Note: If the longitudinal arch of the foot is flattened, the cuboid will often be everted, the cuneiforms will be depressed or displaced inferiorly and the navicular will be inverted (the lateral aspect of the plantar surface of the navicular will be displaced inferiorly and medially). To correct the cuneiforms, the set-up for HVLA is the same as above but the thrust is applied straight down toward the floor to the affected cuneiform. To correct the inverted navicular, the set-up is the same, but the physician contacts the plantar surface of the navicular and applies a thrust toward the floor and medially.

CASE STUDY

DJ is a 27-year-old woman who presented with right-hand numbness for 1-month duration. She started a new job as a cashier about 2 months ago. She stated that at first, her entire right hand started to "fall asleep" occasionally while working at her cash register. At the time of her visit, the numbness occurred within 5 minutes of working and was relieved with rest. She had also noted right-sided upper back pain over the past month. There was no history of injury or previous numbness. There was no past medical or surgical history. She tried ibuprofen and a wrist splint without improvement.

Physical examination revealed normal vital signs, normal cardiac, and pulmonary exams. Neuromusculoskeletal exam revealed normal motor strength, reflexes, and sensation in the right upper extremity. Tinel and Phalen tests were negative. Acute tissue texture changes and tenderness were noted over the transverse process area of T3 right. Motion changes were noted at T3 consistent with somatic dysfunction at T3 extended side bent and rotated right with a distinct barrier found with attempts to flex, side bend, and rotate T3 to the left. The presence of distinct barrier mechanics indicates that this type of somatic dysfunction would be amenable to HVLA treatment.

REFERENCES

1. Giusti R, ex ed. *Educational Council on Osteopathic Principles. Glossary of Osteopathic Terminology.* 3rd ed. American Association of Colleges of Osteopathic Medicine; 2017:36.
2. Vernon H, Mrozek J. A revised definition of manipulation [published correction appears in J Manipulative Physiol Ther. 2005 Jul–Aug;28(6):460]. *J Manipulative Physiol Ther.* 2005;28(1):68–72.
3. Brodeur R. The audible release associated with joint manipulation. *J Manipulative Physiol Ther.* 1995;18(3):155–164.
4. Reggars JW. The manipulative crack. Frequency analysis. *Australas Chiropr Osteopathy.* 1996;5(2):39–44.
5. Schiotz EH, Cyriax J. *Manipulation Past and Present.* William Heinemann Medical Books, Ltd.; 1975.
6. Harris JD, McPartland JM. Historical perspectives of manual medicine. In: Stanton DF, Mein EA, eds. *Phys Med Rehabil Clin N Am.* 1996;7(4): 679–692.
7. Kappler RE, Jones JM III. Thrust (high velocity/low amplitude) techniques. In: Ward RC, ex. ed. *Foundations of Osteopathic Medicine.* 2nd ed. Lippincott Williams & Wilkins; 2003:854.
8. Triano JJ. Biomechanics of spinal manipulative therapy. *Spine J.* 2001; 1(2):121–130.
9. Shekelle PG. Spine update: spinal manipulation. *Spine (Phila Pa 1976).* 1994;19(7):858–861.
10. DeStefano LA. *Mobilization With And Without Impulse Technique. In: Greenman's Principles of Manual Medicine.* 5th ed. Wolters Kluwer; 2017: 109.
11. Edmond S. *Joint Mobilization/Manipulation: Extremity and Spinal Techniques.* 2nd ed. Mosby Elsevier; 2006:6.
12. Triano JJ. The mechanics of spinal manipulation. *Clinical Biomechanics of Spinal Manipulation.* Churchill Livingstone; 2000:113.
13. Cassidy JD, Lopes AA, Yong-Hing K. The immediate effect of manipulation vs mobilization on pain and range of motion in the cervical spine: a randomized controlled trial. *J Manipulative Physiol Ther.* 1992;15(9): 570–575.
14. Nansel DD, Peneff A, Quintoriano J. Effectiveness of upper vs lower cervical adjustments with respect to amelioration of passive rotational vs lateral-flexion end-range asymmetries in otherwise asymptomatic subjects. *J Manipulative Physiol Ther.* 1992;15(2):99–105.
15. Whittingham W, Nilsson N. Active range of motion of the cervical spine increases after spinal manipulation (toggle recoil). *J Manipulative Physiol Ther.* 2001;24(9):552–555.
16. Mierau D, Cassidy JD, Bowen V, Dupuis P, Noftall F. Manipulation and mobilization of the third metacarpophalangeal joint: a quantitative radiographic and range of motion study. *Man Med.* 1988;3:135–140.
17. Dananberg HJ, Shearstone J, Guiliano M. Manipulation method for the treatment of ankle equines. *J Am Podiatr Med Assoc.* 2000;90(8):385–389.
18. Nield S, Davis K, Latimer J, Maher C, Adams R. The effect of manipulation on range of movement at the ankle joint. *Scand J Rehabil Med.* 1993;25(4):161–166.
19. Fryer GA, Mudge JM, McLaughlin PA. The effect of talocrural joint manipulation on range of motion at the ankle. *J Manipulative Physiol Ther.* 2002;25(6):384–390.
20. Bialosky JE, Bishop MD, Price DD, Robinson ME, George SZ. The mechanisms of manual therapy in the treatment of musculoskeletal pain: a comprehensive model. *Man Ther.* 2009;14(5):531–538.
21. Cleland JA, Glynn P, Whitman JM, Eberhart SL, MacDonald C, Childs JD. Short-term effects of thrust versus nonthrust mobilization/manipulation directed at the thoracic spine in patients with neck pain: a randomized clinical trial. *Phys Ther.* 2007;87(4):431–440.
22. Ruiz-Sáez M, Fernández-de-las-Peñas C, Blanco CR, Martínez-Segura R, García-León R. Changes in pressure pain sensitivity in latent myofascial trigger points in the upper trapezius muscle after a cervical spine manipulation in pain-free subjects. *J Manipulative Physiol Ther.* 2007;30(8): 578–583.
23. Puentedura EJ, Cleland JA, Landers MR, Mintken PE, Louw A, Fernández-de-Las-Peñas C. Development of a clinical prediction rule to identify patients with neck pain likely to benefit from thrust joint manipulation to the cervical spine. *J Orthop Sports Phys Ther.* 2012;42(7):577–592.
24. González-Iglesias J, Fernández-de-las-Peñas C, Cleland JA, Gutiérrez-Vega Mdel R. Thoracic spine manipulation for the management of patients with neck pain: a randomized clinical trial. *J Orthop Sports Phys Ther.* 2009;39(1):20–27.
25. Hurwitz EL, Morgenstern H, Harber P, Kominski GF, Yu F, Adams AH. A randomized trial of chiropractic manipulation and mobilization for patients with neck pain: clinical outcomes from the UCLA neck-pain study. *Am J Public Health.* 2002;92(10):1634–1641.
26. Leaver AM, Maher CG, Herbert RD, et al. A randomized controlled trial comparing manipulation with mobilization for recent onset neck pain. *Arch Phys Med Rehabil.* 2010;91(9):1313–1318.
27. Coronado RA, Gay CW, Bialosky JE, Carnaby GD, Bishop MD, George SZ. Changes in pain sensitivity following spinal manipulation: a systematic review and meta-analysis. *J Electromyogr Kinesiol.* 2012;22(5): 752–767.
28. Yu X, Wang X, Zhang J, Wang Y. Changes in pressure pain thresholds and Basal electromyographic activity after instrument-assisted spinal manipulative therapy in asymptomatic participants: a randomized, controlled trial. *J Manipulative Physiol Ther.* 2012;35(6):437–445.
29. Sterling M, Jull G, Wright A. Cervical mobilisation: concurrent effects on pain, sympathetic nervous system activity and motor activity. *Man Ther.* 2001;6(2):72–81.
30. Yamashita T, Cavanaugh JM, El-Bohy AA, Getchell TV, King AI. Mechanosensitive afferent units in the lumbar facet joint. *J Bone Joint Surg Am.* 1990;72(6):865–870.
31. Yamashita T, Minaki Y, Oota I, Yokogushi K, Ishii S. Mechanosensitive afferent units in the lumbar intervertebral disc and adjacent muscle. *Spine (Phila Pa 1976).* 1993;18(15):2252–2256.
32. Pickar JG. Neurophysiological effects of spinal manipulation. *Spine J.* 2002;2(5):357–371.
33. Bishop MD, Beneciuk JM, George SZ. Immediate reduction in temporal sensory summation after thoracic spinal manipulation. *Spine J.* 2011;11(5):440–446.
34. Herzog W, Scheele D, Conway PJ. Electromyographic responses of back and limb muscles associated with spinal manipulative therapy. *Spine (Phila Pa 1976).* 1999;24(2):146–153.
35. Colloca CJ, Keller TS. Electromyographic reflex responses to mechanical force, manually assisted spinal manipulative therapy. *Spine (Phila Pa 1976).* 2001;26(10):1117–1124.
36. Edmond S. *Joint Mobilization/Manipulation: Extremity and Spinal Techniques.* 2nd ed. Mosby Elsevier; 2006:9.
37. Shambaugh P. Changes in electrical activity in muscles resulting from chiropractic adjustment: a pilot study. *J Manipulative Physiol Ther.* 1987; 10(6):300–304.
38. Keller TS, Colloca CJ. Mechanical force spinal manipulation increases trunk muscle strength assessed by electromyography: a comparative clinical trial. *J Manipulative Physiol Ther.* 2000;23(9):585–595.
39. Liebler EJ, Tufano-Coors L, Douris P, et al. The effect of thoracic spine mobilization on lower trapezius strength testing. *J Man Manipulative Ther.* 2001;9(4):207–212.
40. Suter E, McMorland G, Herzog W, Bray R. Decrease in quadriceps inhibition after sacroiliac joint manipulation in patients with anterior knee pain. *J Manipulative Physiol Ther.* 1999;22(3):149–153.
41. Yerys S, Makofsky H, Byrd C, Pennachio J, Cinkay J. Effect of mobilization of the anterior hip capsule on the gluteus maximus strength. *J Man Manipulative Ther.* 2002;10(4):218–224.
42. Cao DY, Reed WR, Long CR, Kawchuk GN, Pickar JG. Effects of thrust amplitude and duration of high-velocity, low-amplitude spinal manipulation on lumbar muscle spindle responses to vertebral position and movement. *J Manipulative Physiol Ther.* 2013;36(2):68–77.
43. Engel R, Bogduk N. The menisci of the lumbar zygapophyseal joints. *J Anat.* 1982;135(Pt 4):795–809.
44. Webb AI, Rassoulian H, Mitchell BS. Morphometry of the synovial folds of the lateral atlanto-axial joints: the anatomical basis for understanding their potential role in neck pain. *Surg Radiol Anat.* 2012;34(2):115–124.
45. Inami S, Kaneoka K, Hayashi K, Ochiai N. Types of synovial fold in the cervical facet joint. *J Orthop Sci.* 2000;5(5):475–480.
46. Webb AL, Collins P, Rassoulian H, Mitchell BS. Synovial folds—a pain in the neck? *Man Ther.* 2011;16(2):118–124.

47. Rydevik BL, Myers RR, Powell HC. Pressure increase in the dorsal root ganglion following mechanical compression. Closed compartment syndrome in nerve roots. *Spine (Phila Pa 1976)*. 1989;14(6):574–576.
48. Cook AJ, Woolf CJ, Wall PD, McMahon SB. Dynamic receptive field plasticity in rat spinal cord dorsal horn following C-primary afferent input. *Nature*. 1987;325(7000):151–153.
49. Salamon E, Zhu W, Stefano GB. Nitric oxide as a possible mechanism for understanding the therapeutic effects of osteopathic manipulative medicine (Review). *Int J Mol Med*. 2004;14(3):443–449.
50. Sato A, Swenson RS. Sympathetic nervous system response to mechanical stress of the spinal column in rats. *J Manipulative Physiol Ther*. 1984;7(3):141–147.
51. Budgell B, Hirano F. Innocuous mechanical stimulation of the neck and alterations in heart-rate variability in healthy young adults. *Auton Neurosci*. 2001;91(1-2):96–99.
52. Budgell B, Polus B. The effects of thoracic manipulation on heart rate variability: a controlled crossover trial. *J Manipulative Physiol Ther*. 2006; 29(8):603–610.
53. Brennan PC, Kokjohn K, Kaltlinger CJ, et al. Enhanced phagocytic cell respiratory burst induced by spinal manipulation: potential role of substance P. *J Manipulative Physiol Ther*. 1991;14(7):399–408.
54. Brennan PC, Triano JJ, McGregor M, Kokjohn K, Hondras MA, Brennan DC. Enhanced neutrophil respiratory burst as a biological marker for manipulation forces: duration of the effect and association with substance P and tumor necrosis factor. *J Manipulative Physiol Ther*. 1992;15(2): 83–89.
55. Hensel K. *A Teaching Guide for Osteopathic Manipulative Medicine*. American Association of Colleges of Osteopathic Medicine; 2015:43.
56. Kuchera ML, DiGiovanna EL, Greenman PE. Efficacy and complications. In: Ward RC, ed. *Foundations of Osteopathic Medicine*. 2nd ed. Lippincott Williams & Wilkins; 2003:1147–1148.
57. Klougart N, Leboeuf-Yde C, Rasmussen LR. Safety in chiropractic practice, Part I; The occurrence of cerebrovascular accidents after manipulation to the neck in Denmark from 1978-1988. *J Manipulative Physiol Ther*. 1996;19(6):371–377.
58. Vick DA, McKay C, Zengerle CR. The safety of manipulative treatment: review of the literature from 1925 to 1993. *J Am Osteopath Assoc*. 1996;96(2):113–115.
59. Dabbs V, Lauretti WJ. A risk assessment of cervical manipulation versus NSAIDS for the treatment of neck pain. *J Manipulative Physiol Ther*. 1995;18:530–536.
60. Hurwitz EL, Aker PD, Adams AH, Meeker WC, Shekelle PG. Manipulation and mobilization of the cervical spine. A systematic review of the literature. *Spine (Phila Pa 1976)*. 1996;21(15):1746–1760.
61. Haldeman S, Kohlbeck FJ, McGregor M. Unpredictability of cerebrovascular ischemia associated with cervical spine manipulation therapy: a review of sixty-four cases after cervical spine manipulation. *Spine (Phila Pa 1976)*. 2002;27(1):49–55.
62. Cagnie B, Vinck E, Beernaert A, Cambier D. How common are side effects of spinal manipulation and can these side effects be predicted? *Man Ther*. 2004;9(3):151–156.
63. Haneline MT, Croft AC, Frishberg BM. Association of internal carotid artery dissection and chiropractic manipulation. *Neurologist*. 2003;9(1):35–44.
64. Selim M, Caplan LR. Carotid artery dissection. *Curr Treat Options Cardiovasc Med*. 2004;6(3):249–253.
65. Haldeman S, Carey P, Townsend M, Papadopoulos C. Arterial dissections following cervical manipulation: the chiropractic experience. *CMAJ*. 2001;165(7):905–906.
66. American Osteopathic Association. *Osteopathic Manipulative Treatment (OMT) of the Cervical Spine: Policy Statement*. Accessed December 23, 2024. https://osteopathic.org/index.php?aam-media=/wp-content/uploads/policies/Policy_H322-A-24-Osteopathic-Manpulative-Treatment-of-the-Cervical-Spine-H324-A19.pdf
67. Denslow JS. Pathophysiologic evidence for the osteopathic lesion: the known, unknown, and controversial. *J Am Osteopath Assoc*. 1975;75(4):415–421.
68. Hargrove-Wilson. Symposium: manipulative treatment. *Med J Aust*. 1967;24:274–280.
69. Kappler R. Role of psoas mechanism in low back pain. *J Am Osteopath Assoc*. 1973;72:784–801.
70. Korr IM. *The Collected Papers of Irwin Korr*. American Academy of Osteopathy; 1979.
71. Korr IM. Proprioceptors and somatic dysfunction. *J Am Osteopath Assoc*. 1975;74:638–650.
72. Patterson M. A theoretical neurophysiologic mechanism for facilitated segment. *J Am Osteopath Assoc*. 1978;77(5):399.
73. Patterson M. A model mechanism for spinal segmental facilitation. *J Am Osteopath Assoc*. 1976;1:62–72.
74. Van Buskirk R. Nociceptive reflexes and the somatic dysfunction: a model. *J Am Osteopath Assoc*. 1990;9:792–809.
75. Kimberly PE. Formulating a prescription of osteopathic manipulative treatment. In: Beal MC, ed. *The Principles of Palpatory Diagnosis and Manipulative Technique*. American Academy of Osteopathy; 1992:146–152.
76. DeStefano LA. *Greenman's Principles of Manual Medicine*. 5th ed. Wolters Kluwer; 2017:229–230.
77. DeStefano LA. *Greenman's Principles of Manual Medicine*. 5th ed. Wolters Kluwer; 2017:231.
78. DeStefano LA. *Greenman's Principles of Manual Medicine*. 5th ed. Wolters Kluwer; 2017:283.
79. DeStefano LA. *Greenman's Principles of Manual Medicine*. 5th ed. Wolters Kluwer; 2017:303.
80. DeStefano LA. *Greenman's Principles of Manual Medicine*. 5th ed. Wolters Kluwer; 2017:372.
81. DeStefano LA. *Greenman's Principles of Manual Medicine*. 5th ed. Wolters Kluwer; 2017:373.
82. DeStefano LA. *Greenman's Principles of Manual Medicine*. 5th ed. Wolters Kluwer; 2017:401.

50 Lymphatic Drainage Procedures

TURNER SLICHO ▪ MICHAEL L. KUCHERA

KEY CONCEPTS

- The lymphatic system plays a major role in numerous homeostatic mechanisms of the body.
- The lymphatic system is particularly vulnerable to fascial dysfunctions, especially in the region of the superior thoracic inlet.
- Draining the lymphatic system begins with consideration of terminal areas.
- The benefit-to-risk ratio for lymphatic techniques is quite favorable. No known significant complications resulting from osteopathic lymphatic treatment have been reported to date. Clinical judgment, however, should always be applied when prescribing treatment for a patient in any disease state.

DEFINITION AND BACKGROUND

Lymphatic techniques are defined as "a diverse group of techniques designed to remove impediments to lymphatic circulation and to promote and augment the flow of interstitial fluid and lymph."[1] As the lymphatic and venous vasculature have similar embryologic origins and anatomical features (such as one-way valves), many of the lymphatic strategies using these techniques may be expected to enhance venous return.[2]

The lymphatic system plays a major role in numerous homeostatic mechanisms of the body:

- Transports fats to the blood from digestive processes
- Facilitates immune function
- Is a vital component of the overall circulatory system of the body
- Assists the body in removing interstitial tissue fluid and plasma proteins that accumulate as a result of tissue metabolism, inflammation, infection, trauma, or somatic or systemic dysfunctions
- Regulates edema

For these reasons, a coordinated, systematic approach known as the "respiratory–circulatory model" of osteopathic care, and numerous lymphatic treatment techniques have been incorporated clinically by osteopathic professionals treating patients with various conditions, such as edema and infection. This model is illustrative of the third osteopathic tenet, "structure and function are interrelated" and demonstrates an approach commonly employed by osteopathic practitioners in their objective and subjective interpretation of the physical findings that lead to rational diagnoses and treatment. It also codifies a systemic osteopathic approach to deliver treatment that specifically and effectively accomplishes lymphaticovenous homeostatic goals; it may even provide useful respiratory–circulatory strategies aimed toward enhancing intrinsic, host-maintained health levels. In order to systematically set clinical goals applying the "respiratory–circulatory model," osteopathic physicians incorporate a number of important principles that influence both the choice of OMT techniques and the sequence of their application.

HYDRODYNAMICS OF LYMPH TRANSPORT

See Chapter 14 Anatomy and Physiology of the Lymphatic System for a comprehensive discussion regarding lymphatic structures and functions.

In humans, 8 to 12 L of fluid and protein per day are returned to the vascular system from the extravascular compartments by way of the lymphatic system.[3] Without this return of fluid, metabolic waste products would congest the extracellular matrix, ultimately influencing the ability for proper physiologic functioning of the underlying tissue. Under steady states, most interstitial fluid pressures are either near atmospheric or subatmospheric pressure, however, pressure measured in early lymphatic collecting vessels are on average slightly positive.[4] This pressure gradient does not favor fluid entering the lymphatic system. Cyclical changes in both interstitial fluid pressure and lymphatic system pressure must therefore occur to produce a pressure gradient that favors the formation of lymph.[4] This is done through a combination of extrinsic (passive) and intrinsic (active) forces acting on the lymphatic system and surrounding tissues.

The endothelium of the initial lymphatics is unique in that they have valves not only across their lumen but also in-between adjacent lymphatic endothelial cells.[4] These endothelial cells are also tethered to the tissues they invest by anchoring filaments and other connective tissue proteins. Initial lymphatics consist of pure endothelial channels without perivascular cells and smooth muscle cells.[4] Changes in pressure gradients across these valves cause them to open and close. When either the intrinsic lymphatic contraction or the extrinsic tissue deformation enters a phase of relaxation or decompression, the initial lymphatic structures are "pulled open" because of the transmission of stored tissue energy through the anchoring filaments to the initial lymphatic wall, creating a situation where pressure gradients favor lymph formation.[4] As the initial lymphatics fill and the intraluminal pressure increases, the resulting pressure gradient causes the valves to close to prevent backflow of the fluid into the surrounding tissue.

Extrinsic forces such as skeletal muscle contraction, heart contraction, gastrointestinal muscle contraction, and intrinsic contraction lymphatic system are activities known to be important to this process of cyclical tissue deformation.[4] The introduction of manual forces during manipulative technique application can act on these structures in a similar fashion. The analogy of repeatedly wringing out a sponge under a running faucet provides a good visual of the process of fluid entering the initial lymphatics during the creation of lymph.

INTRINSIC MOVEMENT OF FLUID THROUGH THE LYMPHATIC SYSTEM

The vessels of the lymphatic system are lined with smooth muscle which is nonstriated and shares biochemical and functional characteristics with both vascular and cardiac muscle.[3] Lymphatic vessels resemble arterioles in that they develop a basal tone and exhibit myogenic constriction to pressure elevation.[3] Coordinated contractions move lymphatic fluid along the vessels through functional units called lymphangions, which is defined as a length of the vessel between the half-moon shaped valves found within the lumen. Proper movement of fluid requires synchronous contractions of the muscles from one lymphangion to the next, along with properly functioning valves to prevent backflow.

The muscles undergo synchronous contractions along the length of the vessel similar to that of the cardiac pumping cycle, with the lymphangion going through a contraction (systole) phase and a relaxation (diastole) phase. During the systole phase, intraluminal pressure rises to overcome outflow pressure, causing the downstream valve to open and lymphatic fluid to be ejected into the next lymphangion. The lymphatic muscle cell then relaxes, causing the outflow valve to close and the inflow valve to open to allow filling. These functional lymphangion units work to overcome the hydrostatic pressure gradient that exists, largely due to gravity, from foot to head. In the average height, upright human, there is a potential hydrostatic pressure gradient of −150 cm H_2O from the feet to the great veins of the neck, with the peripheral lymphatic structures having a lower hydrostatic pressure than the final outflow tracts (thoracic duct and right lymphatic duct).[4] The presence of valves and nodal structures throughout the lymphatic system helps to reduce this gradient, however, lymph does not normally "drain" passively as it is commonly described. Energy must be imparted to the lymph fluid in some fashion in order to transport it along the lymphatic network.[4]

The influences on lymphatic flow are similar to that of the cardiac cycle: lymphatic preload, afterload, spontaneous contraction rate, contractility, and neural influences. Osteopathic technique can affect various aspects of these influences. Given the thin-walled structure of lymphatic vessels, they are prone to distortion via tensegrity issues found with somatic dysfunction in the body. Fascial distortions can affect preload and afterload, with distortions affecting the ability of fluid to move through the lumen of vessels, as well as the extrinsic pumping mechanism in the early lymphatic tissues previously described. A variety of techniques can be utilized by the practitioner depending on the type and location of the dysfunction found.

While research is still ongoing regarding neural influences of the autonomic nervous system and lymphatic flow, recent evidence shows that the lymphatic system is widely innervated with sympathetic nerve fibers, particularly in the nodal structures.[5] Discrete nerves were observed in relation to T cells and non-T cell-rich areas such as the hilar and capsular connective tissue, suggesting neural influences over immune response as well.[5] Patients in one study suffering from unilateral peripheral edema related to complex regional pain syndrome had marked improvement after sympathectomy, suggesting that peripheral lymph flow was under control of the autonomic nervous system.[6] In addition to approaching the lymphatic system from a hydrodynamic, fluid-flow approach, the astute osteopathic practitioner must also evaluate and treat somatic dysfunction in anatomic areas associated with sympathetic innervation to affected tissue to ensure that the autonomic nervous system has the optimal ability for self-regulation.

HISTORY

Systematic

The lymphatic system, which is integral to the understanding of health and disease, was first accurately described as a system by Olaf Rudbeck (Sweden) in 1653.[7] From its onset, the osteopathic profession embraced the importance of the lymphatic system and attempted to document its role in health. Dr. AT Still emphasized that diagnosis of the fascia and treatment of the lymphatic system were vital for maintaining health and treating disease going as far as to recommend that "…the fascia is the place to look for the cause of disease and the place to consult and begin the action of remedies in all diseases."[8] In 1898, the American School of Osteopathy faculty in Kirksville used skiagraphy (an early form of x-ray) to research the distribution of the vascular and lymphatic systems, reinforcing Still's emphasis on the lymphatic system.[9]

Later, one of Still's students, Frederic Millard, DO, researched the structure and functions of the lymphatic system and published *Applied Anatomy of the Lymphatics* in 1922.[10] Millard, the first DO to specifically describe physical examination of fluid and lymphatic status,[11,12] based aspects of his surgical versus nonsurgical recommendations on the state in which he found the lymph nodes. He noted that:

- The lymph vessels were "pliable and readily compressed."
- "For every congested tissue, there is a corresponding lymph disturbance."
- "Attempts to clear the lymph stream before clearing the edema in the clavicular regions is to overtax the general lymph stream and cause profound reactions."[10]

In addition, Millard also described a series of "lymphatic drainage" techniques,[10,13,14] while admonishing the osteopathic practitioner to "never work over an enlarged or indurated lymph node" and to instead "free the efferents and the lymph will drain".[10]

J. Gordon Zink, DO, FAAO, acknowledging the work of Millard as his major inspiration, expanded the approach by popularizing the concept that "respiration and circulation are unifiable functions"[15] and that, for homeostasis, external respiration determines internal respiration. Zink's influence and teaching led to the profession's general adoption of the "respiratory–circulatory" model, and acceptance of technique sequences designed to enhance cellular-level health (internal respiration) by maximizing external respiration. In his extensive teaching of the respiratory–circulatory model, Zink placed special emphasis on the:

- Fascial restrictions (particularly at anatomic transitional zones) that limited venous and lymphatic return.
- Value of creating pressure differentials in the body cavities for effective venous–lymphatic flow.
- Central importance of coordinated optimal diaphragmatic functions for the thoraco-abdominopelvic to maintain lymphatic homeostasis.[15–17]
- Optimization of venous return to enhance lymphatic return.

While the idea that respiration affected venous return was known at this time, it was only quantified and confirmed with Doppler studies in the 1980s.[18]

Specific lymphatic treatments outside the osteopathic profession were first defined and described by Emil Vodder, a French PhD in the 1930s, and consisted largely of manual lymph drainage.[19] Based upon manual therapies for draining lymphedema, the Vodder method was developed further in Europe during the 1960s and applied to the treatment of lymphedema patients, as a part of Complex Decongestive Therapy. Schools teaching the Vodder technique to therapists and physicians opened in the 1970s, around the same time that Zink was popularizing a codified approach for osteopathic physicians to enhance the lymphatics.

Zink, and subsequently Bruno Chikly, MD, described diagnostic sites for identification of regional lymphatic dysfunction (sites of "terminal lymphatic drainage")[15,20] and integrated concepts from osteopathic cranial manipulative medicine (OCMM). In addition, Zink specifically linked "primary and secondary respiration" via what he termed the "craniosternosacral mechanism."[21]

Osteopathic Lymphatic Technique

Still preferred that his students create techniques to accomplish their clinical goals, that is, to perform techniques based upon their knowledge of anatomy rather than to memorize a maneuver ("I am not here to teach a bunch of parrots," he wrote).[22] Probably for this reason, the lymphatic techniques used by Still, as early as the 1870s, were not described by his students until later.[23] Nonetheless, some specific osteopathic lymphatic techniques, involving a few minutes of local manual pumping to reduce swelling in and around organs (such as the pressure-sensitive liver), were described in the profession's literature as early as 1898.[24]

Like that over the liver, rhythmic manual pumping over the spleen (a secondary lymphoid organ) was described and researched very early in the profession, and continues to be used today. Clement A. Whiting, DO, studied the effects of using splenic pump on immune function in 1910[25] as did MA Lane, DO in 1920,[26] in addition to Yale Castlio, DO and Louise Ferris-Smith, DO in the 1930s.[27,28] Modern research, investigating lymphatic pump techniques on enhancing immune function, began again in earnest with the work of Measel[29,30] in the 1980s and continues with funding from both the osteopathic profession and the NIH. The work of Lisa Hodge, PhD and associates at the Osteopathic Research Center (ORC) located at the University of North Texas Health Science Center—Texas College of Osteopathic Medicine has contributed greatly to both an understanding of the osteopathic lymphatic pump technique and its physiologic role.[31–33] Further research has focused on the physiologic effects of osteopathic manipulation as it applies to immune function and fluid movement.[14]

Osteopathic techniques expanded to the use of muscle pumps and respiratory pumps, each improving normal homeostatic mechanisms to move fluids in the vascular–lymphatic system.

- C. Earl Miller, DO in 1926 first described and then researched the effects of the classic thoracic lymphatic pump along with other lymphatic approaches (Fig. 50.1A).[34,35]
- TJ Ruddy, MD, DO, developed a muscle pump system termed "rapid rhythmic resistive duction" for treating lymphatic congestion in multiple areas (especially the head and neck).[36] Ruddy's system was the precursor to the later development of muscle energy techniques (Fig. 50.1B).
- William Galbreath, DO, in 1929, described the Galbreath technique, a method for mobilizing lymphatic fluid in the mandibular region and for draining accumulated fluid from the middle ear (Fig. 50.1C).[37,38]

Another student of Dr. AT Still, and a contemporary of Millard, William Garner Sutherland, DO, also focused on fluid diagnosis and treatment. Best known for his contributions to OCMM, Sutherland emphasized Webster's definition of "fluctuation" as "the movement of a fluid within a natural or artificial cavity and observed by palpation or percussion." The techniques he described and taught within the profession were simple and effective. Sutherland noted, "(with) the method I described of facilitating the movement of lymph and controlling the Tide by bringing the fluctuation to the short rhythmic period, you have the interchange of all the fluids of the body."[39]

The lymphatics were postulated by osteopathic physicians to play a diagnostic and therapeutic role in visceral function. For example, in the 1930s, Frank Chapman, DO, another student of Still, elucidated a series of so-called neurolymphatic reflexes believed to correspond to visceral structures. These Chapman reflexes (see "Chapman Reflexes" in Chapter 58) may be associated with viscerosomatic reflexes in distribution with the sympathetic nervous system.

The lymphatic system is also an avid area of research outside the osteopathic community, with funded NIH projects exploring topics such as the coupling of the lymphatic/glymphatic system in central nervous system (CNS) fluid homeostasis, cardiac lymphatics, inflammatory lymphatic signaling in stroke, and pulmonary lymphatics in inflammation and disease.[40] Properly employed lymphatic techniques offer a wide potential range of effects to a variety of disease states, with the end goal of helping the body find a state of health through better homeostatic regulation of fluid exchange within tissue. Sutherland offered the most cogent insight, as true now as it was then: "(t)he science of Osteopathy is simple. You realize you are a mechanic of the fluids of the body as well as of the skeletal system."[39]

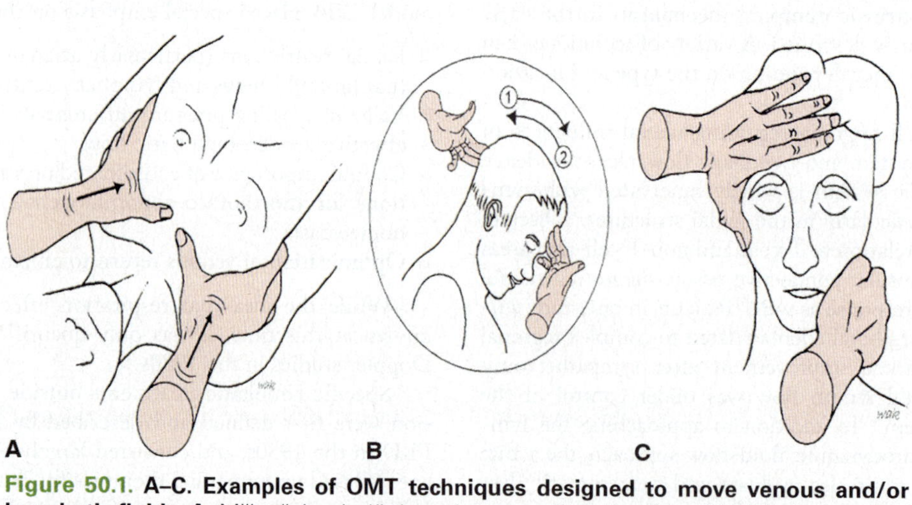

Figure 50.1. A–C. Examples of OMT techniques designed to move venous and/or lymphatic fluids. A. Miller "classical" thoracic pump. (See also Fig. 50.27.) **B.** Ruddy rapid resistive duction muscle pump. **C.** Galbreath mandibular drainage technique. (Illustration courtesy of William A. Kuchera, DO, FAAO, with permission.)

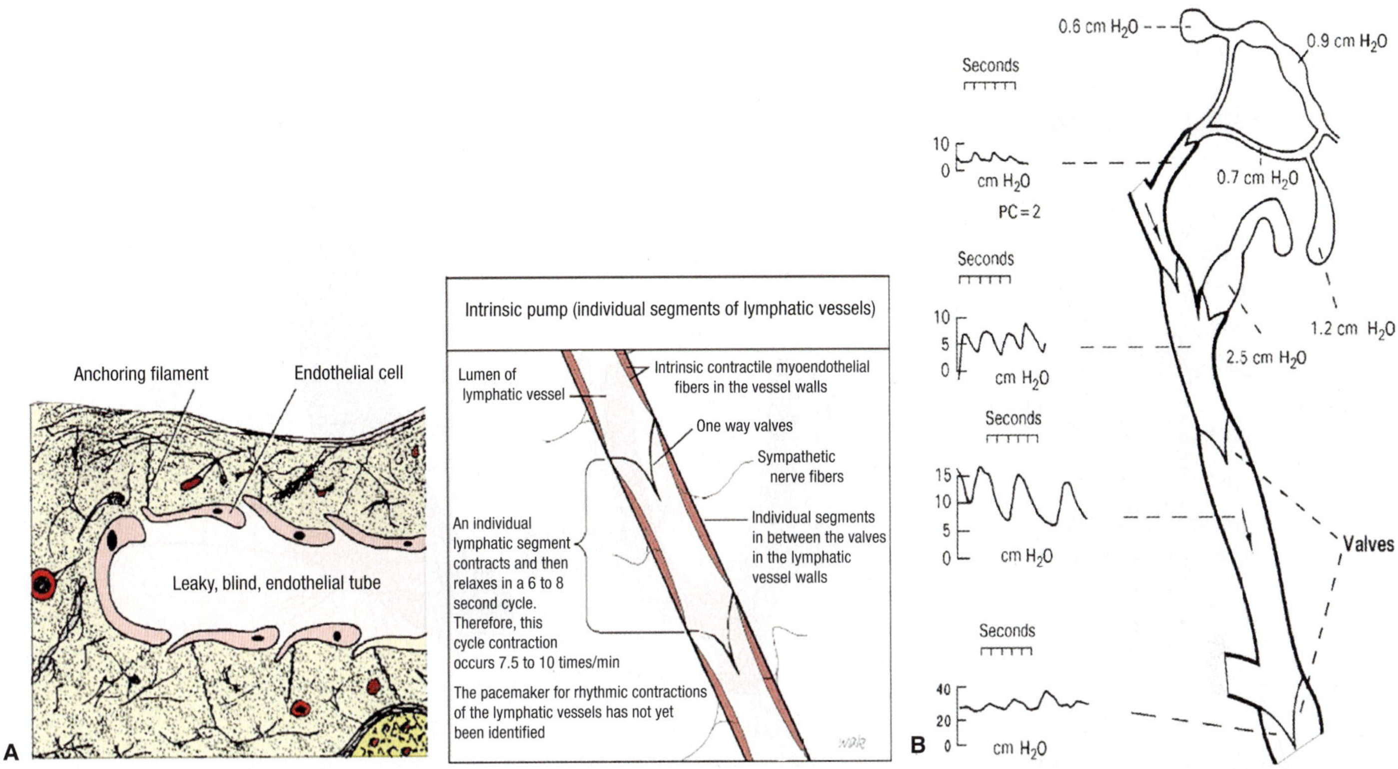

Figure 50.2. **A** and **B.** Lymph propulsion results from extrinsic and intrinsic forces pumping the lymph from blind endings (**A**) to lymphatic capillaries to larger collecting vessels (**B**) made up of a series of lymphangions which also have sympathetic innervation. The lymphangion is the functional unit that is located between semilunar unidirectional valves; they act like "primitive hearts" with intrinsic pacemaker contractions. Smooth muscle cell numbers increase from distal to proximal along the lymphatic route. (Illustration courtesy of William A. Kuchera, DO, FAAO, with permission.)

PROPOSED MECHANISM OF ACTION

To improve treatment outcomes, different strategies might be selected to enhance homeostatic mechanisms specifically linked to the different phases of lymphatic function (see Figs. 50.2 to 50.4).[41]

For example:

- Any OMT technique that improves *local tissue motion* should enhance the *lymph formation phase*, consequently reducing edema and improving cellular level nutrition. While tensegrity principles suggest that this can be indirectly accomplished with almost any technique that removes somatic dysfunction throughout the body, the most effective choice should be specific local manual techniques that include oscillatory movement, various manual techniques focused upon the soft (myofascial) tissues, or any addition of a host of energy-transmitting physical therapy modalities (such as pulsed ultrasound or Fulford percussion hammer) that could increase local tissue motion.
- Application of other types of ancillary modalities such as rest, ice, compression, and elevation during acute edematous states should be properly timed to limit local swelling (to prevent it from overwhelming the local homeostatic mechanisms and allowing entry into the blind end lymphatic capillaries) and otherwise remove impediments to the lymph *formation phase*.
- Several osteopathic manipulative treatments affect lymphatic channels as they travel between fascial layers and throughout body regions. Any treatment that reduces myofascial restriction can theoretically improve lymphatic flow by optimizing the *vascular phase* and thereby increase the efficacy of intrinsic lymphatic pumps. Myofascial release (MFR), balanced ligamentous tension (BLT), and ligamentous articular strain techniques seem suited for removing such local and regional fascial obstructions.
- Also, numerous OMT modalities employ direct external forces that act as extrinsic pumps mobilizing lymphatic fluid in the *vascular phase*. Some of these modalities or methods improve the lymph flow by applying external pressure (soft tissue effleurage, massage, petrissage, etc.), whereas others remove somatic dysfunction that generally restricts fluid or employ directed muscle energy OMT to speed propulsion using muscle pumps. This latter mechanism is especially effective in the periphery when combined with ruddy rapid resistive duction OMT, where isometric contraction–relaxation rates may be two to three times the normal heart pulsation (see Fig. 50.1B). Significant increases in lymphatic flow rates in the thoracic duct[42,43] have been measured as well, using both the muscle pumps involved in exercise and the passive pressure changes of various lymphatic pump OMT techniques (Fig. 50.5E).
- Osteopathic treatment that seeks to enhance the efficacy of respiratory mechanisms (primary and secondary) in order to maximize venous and lymphatic return, during either the vascular or the terminal phase, typically focuses upon improving diaphragm or chest cage functions. (See as an example: thoracic diaphragm release technique, Fig. 50.5D).
- Such respiratory approaches to circulation function largely through amplifying rhythmic pressure changes between compartments, as well as through the Bernoulli principle shown in Figure 50.3. Addressing the abdominal diaphragm with osteopathic manipulative treatment has been shown with ultrasound to significantly increase the mobility of the diaphragm with a single treatment.[44]

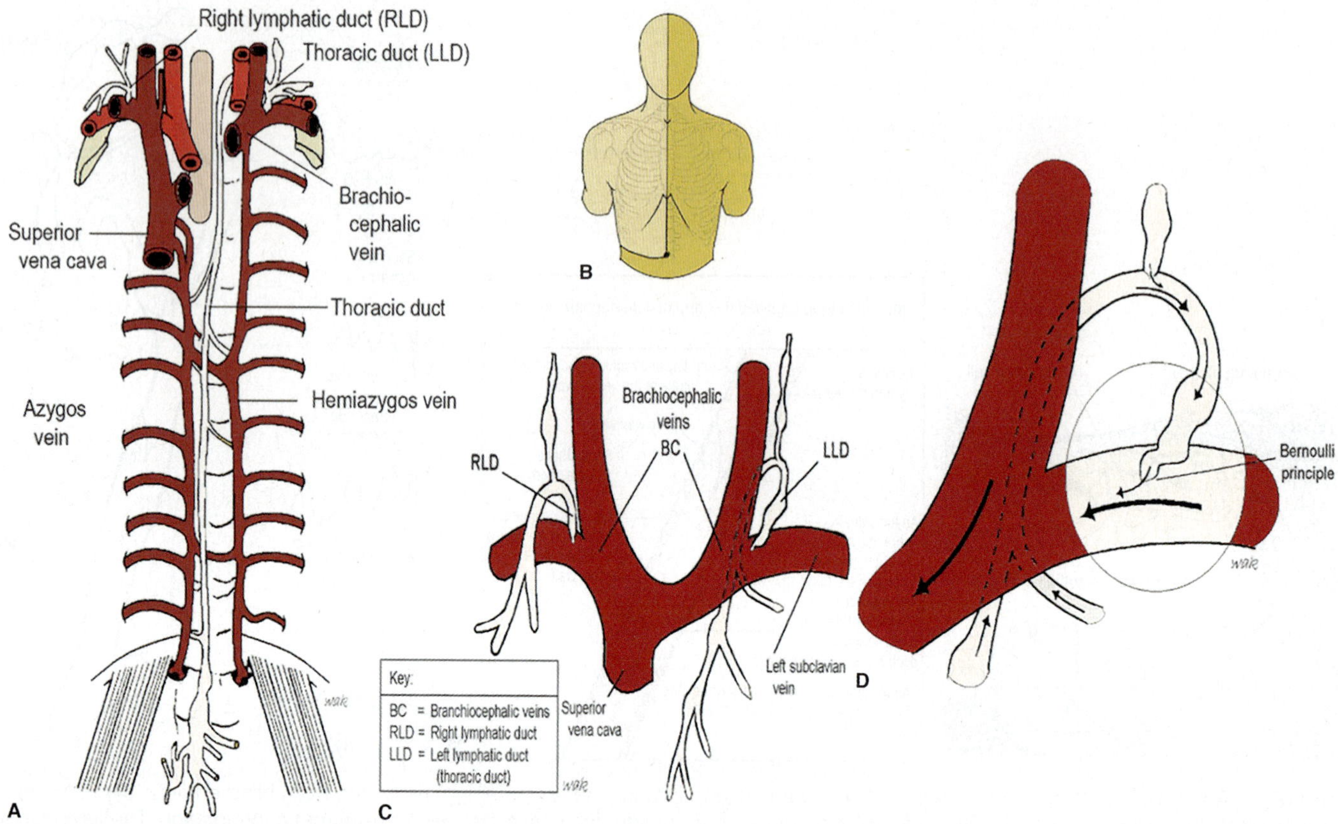

Figure 50.3. A–D. Terminal drainage phase: lymphatic ducts, drainage regions, and Venturi effect (Bernoulli principle) noting that increased venous return to the heart augments lymphatic return as well. (Illustration courtesy of William A. Kuchera, DO, FAAO, with permission.)

- Lymphatic pump manipulative techniques are also used over the spleen, liver, chest cage, abdominal wall, or from the feet. The direct motion against the tissues could affect the formation phase; the systemic and rhythmic pumping could affect the vascular phase; and the additional pressure changes in intra-abdominal and intrathoracic cavities could affect the terminal phase. (See as examples: splenic pump and Dalrymple pedal pump, respectively.)

Other mechanisms of action for OMT have been postulated and are worthy of exploration. For example, the role of endothelial nitric oxide synthetase (eNOS) is of particular interest due to the lymphatic pump mechanics. Nitric oxide (NO) is not only produced in the walls of blood vessels but also in the luminal wall of lymphatic vessels.[45] NO causes dilation of the contractile lymphatic vessels, similar to vasodilation in the cardiovascular system.

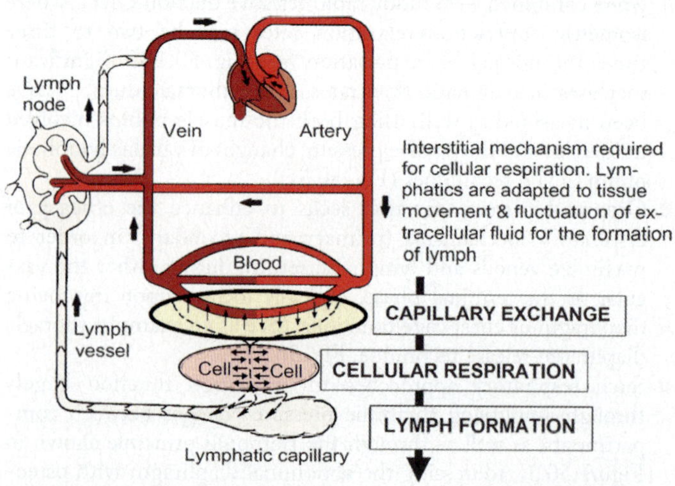

Figure 50.4. Formation phase involved in cellular respiration lymph formation. (Illustration courtesy of William A. Kuchera, DO, FAAO, with permission.)

Research analyzing ejection fraction and lymphatic output of individual contractions of the intrinsic lymphatic pump has confirmed that eNOS in lymphatic endothelial cells is required for robust lymphatic contractions under physiologic conditions and may be dynamically modulated by fluid shear stress on the lymphatic endothelium in a cyclical manner.[46] Flow of fluid through the vessels (increased shear stress) causes upregulation of eNOS, which results in increased in NO production by endothelial cells leading to vasodilation, inhibiting contraction of the lymphangion to allow for fluid to be received by the downstream functional unit. As this lymphangion unit fills and the next downstream valve opens due to hydrostatic pressure, fluid moves to the next lymphangion, reducing concentration of NO in the upstream unit (favoring vessel constriction), and shear stress causing eNOS-mediated NO production in the downstream lymphangion (favoring vessel dilation). This process repeats itself in a rhythmical fashion until the fluid reaches its terminal drainage into the vascular system.

In the inflammatory state, this dynamic modulation of eNOS has been shown to be overridden by inducible nitric oxide synthase (iNOS) producing myeloid cells infiltrating the surrounding tissue, creating a constant increased concentration of NO within the local tissue environment.[46] This overwhelms the subtle flow-dependent NO production from eNOS, preventing contraction and effectively inhibiting the intrinsic pumping motion of the lymphatic system.[46]

As previously mentioned, thoracic and abdominal pump techniques have been shown to increase lymphatic flow at the thoracic duct.[42] The intermittent movement associated with the Dalrymple pedal lymphatic pump also has the potential to increase shear stress (fluid flow) on the lymphatic endothelium

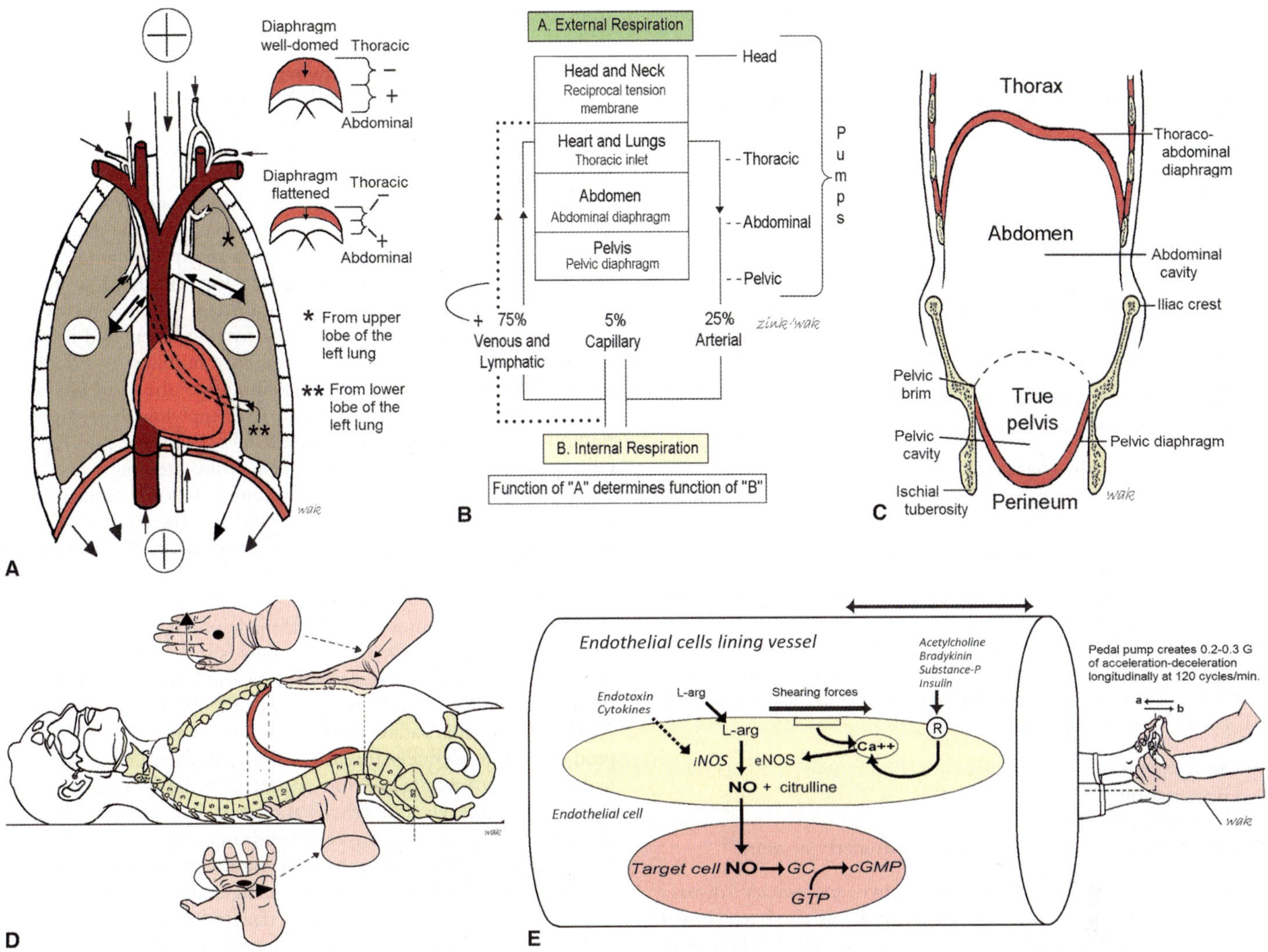

Figure 50.5. A–E. Maximizing Venous-Lymphatic Return: A–B. Pressure differentials between chest and abdominopelvic cavities, the Venturi effect (Bernoulli principle), and the relationship between internal and external respiration are fundamental to understanding respiratory physiology and lymphatic treatment strategies. **C.** Compartmentalization with an active thoracolumbar diaphragm and a passive pelvic diaphragm acting in synchrony creates an effective "ThoracoAbdominoPelvic (TAP)" pump. **D.** Hand placement for indirect myofascial diaphragmatic release OMT; treatment maximizes pressure changes created by the TAP pump. **E.** Upregulation of endothelial nitric oxide (NO) is a postulated mechanism for some of the actions of lymphatic pedal (Dalrymple) pump OMT; immune cell mobilization has also been demonstrated.

(Fig. 50.5E). Arguably, these rhythmical fluctuations artificially increase eNOS-mediated production of NO during the active treatment of tissue, resulting in vasodilation throughout the system to promote fluid movement, particularly in the proximal portions of the system. Research on isolated rat lymphatic tissue showed that fluid shear forces due to flow gradients caused a loss of basal tonic contraction strength, reductions in the contraction frequency, amplitude of the phasic lymphatic contractions, ejection fraction, and fractional pump flow.[4] This inhibition was even greater in the thoracic duct in comparison to the mesenteric lymph.[4] As stagnant fluid begins to move through the system, constant NO concentrations resulting from iNOS mediated release decrease, and the flow-dependent eNOS regulation of the intrinsic lymphatic pump mechanism are allowed to resume. As more is elucidated on the mechanisms of action for various OMT techniques, additional strategies may be found for the existing techniques and for fine-tuning the frequency and duration of their application.

For many decades, it has been known that scarring or thickening of tissues might occur after trauma if only water is resorbed, and interstitial proteins remain; poorly rehabilitated ankle sprains with thickening of the Achilles tendon is one such example. Efficient lymphatic drainage might effectively prevent this problem by facilitating removal of proteins in edematous states. Furthermore, prevention of the production of or removal of inflammatory cytokines and the subsequent resolution of the pain and sequelae associated with an inflammatory process depend on enhancing physiologic homeostasis.[47–49]

A wide range of lymphatic drainage techniques have been shown to be effective in reducing pain, edema, and tissue turgor secondary to numerous traumatically induced inflammatory processes. Furthermore, evidence is growing for the use of manual techniques and exercise to enhance immune function.[2,50,51] Osteopathically delivered lymphatic techniques as opposed to lymphatic techniques delivered by a therapist may have farther reaching outcomes in that they are delivered in the context of the needs and knowledge of the specific patient and their (patho)physiology.[52] Regardless of the professional degree of the health care practitioner, a growing number of techniques have each been documented to accomplish particular physiologic responses, ranging from:

- Massage (including effleurage and petrissage)[53] to indirect OMT (such as counterstrain)[54,55]
- Mechanical tissue movement (such as vibration)[56]
- Exercise strategies targeting extremities, chest wall, and/or the cardiovascular system
- Elevation to allow the effect of gravity to improve lymphatic drainage
- Various stroking or compressive lymphatic drainage manual methods with alternating pressures from those of Vodder to those of the massage therapists including effleurage
- Counterstrain (and other indirect OMT) techniques to block production of inflammatory cytokines and apoptosis postrepetitive motion (*in vitro*) and to prevent postexercise muscle soreness after repetitive eccentric arm-curls (in vivo)

The osteopathic respiratory–circulatory model also generally depends on the role of OMT to improve:

1. Compliance of the chest wall
2. Diaphragmatic excursion (both mechanical and neurologic targets)
3. General efficacy of the respiratory process

Although the logic is convincing, less extensive evidence has been published concerning the application. Nonetheless, such evidence includes that while restriction of chest wall excursion limits forced expiratory vital capacity and forced expiratory volume in 1 second,[57] treatment of chest wall somatic dysfunction with OMT has been shown to increase:

- Chest expansion
- O_2 saturation
- Total lung capacity
- Vital capacity as much as incentive spirometry or more[58–60]

In patients with chronic obstructive pulmonary disease (COPD), manual treatment of the chest wall has also been shown to increase respiratory efficacy (including so-called "chest wall gymnastics").[58,61–63]

In the last few decades, significant documentation has been made with respect to immune function and the lymphatic model in part due to the current emphasis in the osteopathic profession's research funding. The production of lymphocytes is noted to increase greatly as lymph passes through the nodes. Research indicates that T-lymphocytes remain approximately 30 minutes in the blood circulation, about 5 to 6 hours in the spleen, and 20 hours in the lymphatic vascular system.[20]

In the early 1980s, Measel[29] tested immune response in healthy individuals using the classic thoracic (Miller) pump technique. He found a greater immune response to several subserotypes of pneumococcal polysaccharide in the treatment group relative to the control group. Since that study, several other research teams have explored immune function in response to different lymphatic pumps in isolation. For example, one study[64] found that of 39 healthy subjects provided with the hepatitis B vaccine, those who were also treated with lymphatic and splenic pump techniques, three times weekly for 2 weeks, experienced a faster rise in antibody titers when compared to the control group. By 13 weeks, 50% of OMT-treated subjects versus only 16% of controls achieved protective antibody titers. At all points in time after 6 weeks, antihepatitis titers in the treatment group were higher than in the control. However, by the end of the study period, both groups had similar numbers of individuals with protective antibody titers. In a different study that used splenic pump alone on nursing home residents, the researchers failed to show improved influenza vaccine antibody titers after the use of splenic pump but did document a reduction in antibiotic use during the influenza season.[65]

Recent research studies conducted at the ORC, located at the University of North Texas Health Sciences Center—Texas College of Osteopathic Medicine (UNTHSC-TCOM), clearly support the claim that lymphatic pump OMT techniques (thoracic or abdominal) are capable of enhancing both lymphatic flow and leukocyte flux. Innovative protocols employing dogs with surgically cannulated thoracic ducts were designed to answer the question of "how much lymph could a lymph pump pump if a lymph pump could pump lymph?"[66] The model (see Fig. 50.5A) allowed the researchers to directly measure an approximate threefold increase in thoracic duct lymph flow, as well as a five- to seven-fold increase in the number of active immune cells per milliliter of lymph in response to the lymphatic pumps, similar to the increases seen in exercise. They also demonstrated that applying the lymphatic pump in dogs repetitively at intervals of two hours could repeatedly enhance their thoracic duct flow, leukocyte count and flux, and other measures important in immune function.[31] Additionally, researchers at the ORC have been studying the impact of lymphatic pump in reducing morbidity and mortality in a rat model infected with highly pathogenic pneumonia-causing bacteria and in another with lung carcinomas.

Using a human model at the Philadelphia College of Osteopathic Medicine (PCOM), researchers showed the Dalrymple pump to significantly increase serum NO, at levels consistent with those expected from eNOS release[67] (see Fig. 50.5E). Furthermore, NO levels from this passive intervention were consistent with those produced by moderately intense exercise. Researchers at this site had previously investigated the impact of pedal lymphatic pump OMT on NO levels and other parameters in subjects with conditions ranging from fibromyalgia syndrome to Parkinson disease. Preliminary studies performed collaboratively by these PCOM and UNTHSC-TCOM researchers using real-time NO probes in dogs have shown this biomarker to rise and fall in venous blood and thoracic duct lymph with each respiration and to increase with the application of a lymphatic pump maneuver. There is also demand for research centered around the respiratory–circulatory model, ranging from the reduction of postmastectomy lymphedema[68,69] to strategies for the reduction of mortality risk in any future influenza pandemic.[70–73]

INDICATIONS

General indications for use of lymphatic treatment techniques within the framework of the respiratory–circulatory model include (see also Refs. 74 and 75):

- Acute somatic dysfunction
- Sprains and strains
- Edema, tissue congestion, or lymphatic/venous stasis
- Pregnancy
- Infection
- Inflammation
- Pathologies with significant venous and/or lymphatic congestion
- Most systemic or organ-specific diseases/disorders

CONTRAINDICATIONS

Clinical judgment must be used in employing lymphatic techniques, with particular attention to the patient's diagnosis, clinical condition, and medical therapy. These factors influence choice of the appropriate technique, dose, duration, and frequency of treatment (see also).[74]

1. Absolute
   a. Lack of patient consent and/or cooperation—as with any medical procedure
   b. Anuresis if not on dialysis, due to potential risk of pulmonary edema
   c. Necrotizing fasciitis (in area involved)
2. Relative
   a. Inability of patient with congestive heart failure (CHF) to tolerate excessive preload
   b. COPD (thoracic pump with activation) due to increased residual volume posttreatment
   c. Acute asthma exacerbation (thoracic pump) due to risk of increasing reflexive bronchospasm
   d. Unstable cardiac conditions
   e. Most authorities support judicious use of OMT in cancer patients. Treatment over metastatic sites or involved nodes is contraindicated while exercise and osteopathic lymphatic treatments that increase lymphatic flow have not been demonstrated to increase cancer risk. (See Chapter 76 Osteopathic Considerations in Oncology for further discussion.)
   f. Study of lymphatic treatment in the animal model has shown some benefit in pulmonary infectious disease and pulmonary neoplasm.
   g. Osseous fracture or crushed tissue (in area involved)
   h. Bacterial infections with risk of dissemination
   i. Chronic infections with risk of reactivation (e.g., abscess, chronic osteomyelitis)
   j. Diseased organ (i.e., treating thyroid in the presence of hyperthyroidism, splenomegaly as in infectious mononucleosis)
   k. Pregnancy (uterus/deep abdominal work)
   l. Circulatory disorders (venous obstructions, embolism, hemorrhage)
   m. Untreated coagulopathies or patients on anticoagulants (modify technique to be less vigorous)
   n. Acutely herniated nucleus pulposus (modify pumping techniques to be less vigorous)

SAFETY AND EFFICACY

Clinically, the benefit-to-risk ratio for lymphatic techniques is quite favorable. No known significant complications have resulted from osteopathic lymphatic treatment to date, and multiple published studies have documented the efficacy of various treatments. Nonetheless, clinical judgment should always be used when prescribing treatment for a patient in any disease state. For example, since the pediatric population generally exhibits highly effective immune function, be sure to warn caregivers that a lymphatic treatment approach may transiently increase their child's fever; this being a normal response to the pyrogens produced in fighting infection. Treatment of the fever may or may not be necessary depending on its level and duration.

Of special note is the safety of returning fluids back into an already fluid-overloaded condition, like that found in a patient with CHF. In such a state, the thoracic duct may be dilated 16 times its normal size; subsequent leakage can cause ascites and congestive backflow can compromise other organs (e.g., pulmonary edema or hepatomegaly). However, in a study of severe CHF patients where death was imminent, a surgical shunt created between the thoracic duct and venous system resulted in stabilization (fluid–electrolyte improvement) within 24 hours.[75] This has been cited to suggest that the much slower homeostatic lymphatic fluid return may not overload the system, even in severe CHF.[76]

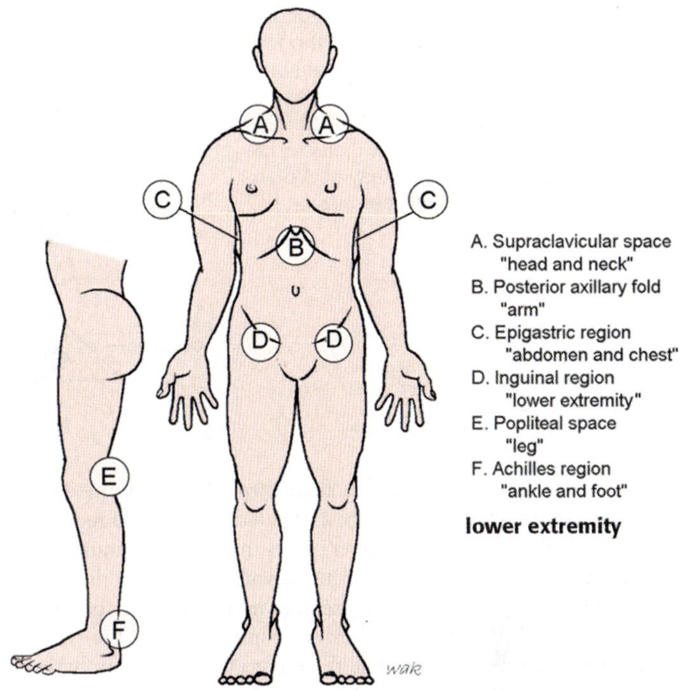

Figure 50.6. Palpation sites for terminal lymphatic drainage dysfunction from body regions. (Illustration courtesy of William A. Kuchera, DO, FAAO, with permission.)

PRINCIPLES OF DIAGNOSIS

The use of the respiratory–circulatory model in a coordinated systematic manner, including indicated lymphatic techniques may be of benefit to many patients in the context of their unique parameters:

1. Indications/benefit-to-risk ratio: Obtain a thorough history and physical examination to determine if the patient's given pathologic condition has a significant lymphatic component. This is helpful in deciding the degree of emphasis on the respiratory–circulatory model and the use of lymphatic techniques. Palpable tension, tenderness, or full, boggy tissue texture changes in the regional terminal lymphatic drainage sites are particularly useful in determining if regional tissue congestion exists (see Fig. 50.6). The initial history and examination should also for potential absolute and relative contraindications to the use of lymphatic techniques.
   - ☐ Swelling
   - ☐ Organ dysfunction and disease
   - ☐ Shortness of breath
   - ☐ Areas of swelling or puffiness
   - ☐ Tissue trauma
   - ☐ Infection
2. Central myofascial pathways: Palpate anatomical transition zones and consider the fascial compensated or uncompensated patterns described by Zink (Fig. 50.7) to identify common fascial restrictions such as torsion or rotational patterns, which may cause restriction of lymphatic flow.

   Restriction in any direction or pattern indicates dysfunction; however, a pattern of fascial motion restrictions that does not alternate in direction for adjacent regions is considered to be "uncompensated" or "traumatic," often seems associated with congestive symptoms, and is an indication for treatment under this model. Even compensated patterns of fascial somatic dysfunction may cause symptoms. This is especially true in patients restricted to bed rest, where the peripheral muscular pumps normally activated by walking fail to simultaneously alter the relationships between

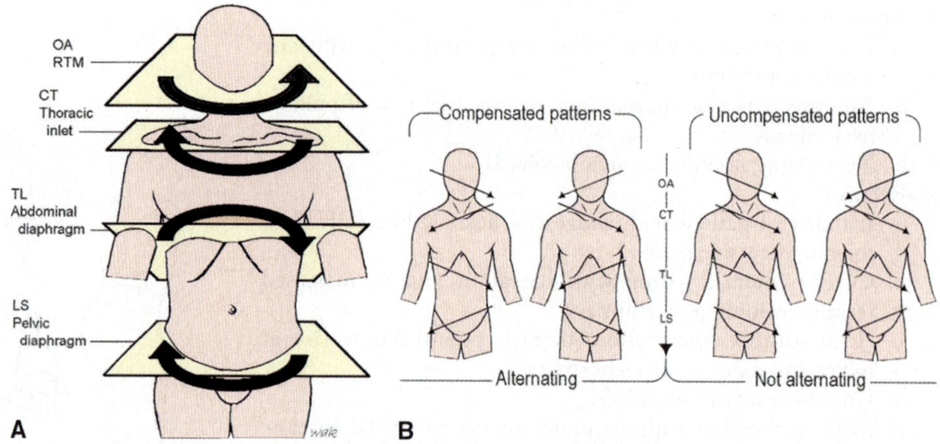

Figure 50.7. A and B. Regional diagnosis and transitional zone relationship to the four major transverse diaphragms (compensated and uncompensated fascial pattern examples). A, occipitoatlantal; RTM, reciprocal tension membranes; CT, cervicothoracic; LS, lumbosacral. (Illustration courtesy of William A. Kuchera, DO, FAAO, with permission.)

adjacent regions to permit free fluid flow. Other key myofascial somatic dysfunctions that can be associated with general reduction in lymphatic flow include trigger points in the scalene muscles.

3. Fluid pumps: Observe and palpate muscular and fascial diaphragmatic function, including thoracic inlet restrictions, for conditions that may limit lymphatic flow. In the supine position, the motion of respiration should extend all the way to the pubic symphysis in a patient who is breathing passively and in a non–self-conscious manner; failure to do so could indicate a need for improvement of thoracic diaphragm function. Likewise, palpate the pelvic diaphragm, which should normally move synchronously with the abdominothoracic diaphragm, and exhibit equal tension to the medial wall of both ischiorectal fossae. A poorly functioning abdominothoracic diaphragm that does not respond to redoming OMT or to treatment of the inferior thoracic outlet may warrant diagnosis and treatment of any C3–C5 (phrenic) somatic dysfunction. Attempts to "redome" the pelvic floor with OMT generally follow treatment of any bony articular pelvic somatic dysfunctions. Diaphragmatic motion and contraction of the pelvic floor musculature (PFM) correlate with breathing and proper contraction of the diaphragms can optimize breathing. Therefore, physicians may consider adding PFM strengthening exercises to the treatment protocol, especially with respiratory rehabilitation programs.[77]
4. Spinal Involvement: After treatment of the central pathways and diaphragms, the patient should experience a uniform sensation of warmth down to the sacrum when the physician places a hand high on the abdomen, below the costal arch, and uses firm pressure downward toward the table and cephalad, as if to "raise" or "re-dome" the diaphragm. This maneuver stops the action of the diaphragm while costal breathing is made to take over, as well as creating a positive pressure in the abdomen. This effectively causes a back-flushing of blood in the superior and inferior vena cava and ultimately the venous drainage of the entire CNS—Zink "Warmth Provocative test"[78] (Fig. 50.8).

   A spinal area perceived to be warmer than others may be interpreted as a site of somatic dysfunction requiring treatment to maximize fluid return. Other key somatic dysfunctions interfering with the respiratory–circulatory model would include:
   - ☐ Dysfunctions of the thoracic, rib, and sternum that restrict motion of the chest cage (secondary respiration) and cranial base.
   - ☐ Attention should be paid to the spinal levels corresponding to sympathetic innervation of the anatomic areas of lymphatic-related somatic dysfunction.
   - ☐ C2 somatic dysfunction.
   - ☐ C3 to C5 should be assessed for any somatic dysfunction that may contribute to suboptimal firing of the phrenic nerve.
   - ☐ Sacral somatic dysfunctions which may contribute to the inhibition of the primary respiratory mechanism.
5. Peripheral/Regional pathways: Evaluate sites of terminal lymphatic drainage associated with early regional lymphatic congestion (see Fig. 50.6). Congestion in the terminal lymphatic drainage sites may indicate the need for comprehensive treatment using the respiratory–circulatory model. Palpate other regional and local tissues to evaluate for the presence of congestion and excess fluid in the interstitial tissues. This helps to identify the region that might benefit from local fluid techniques which is typically the last step in this model's protocol.

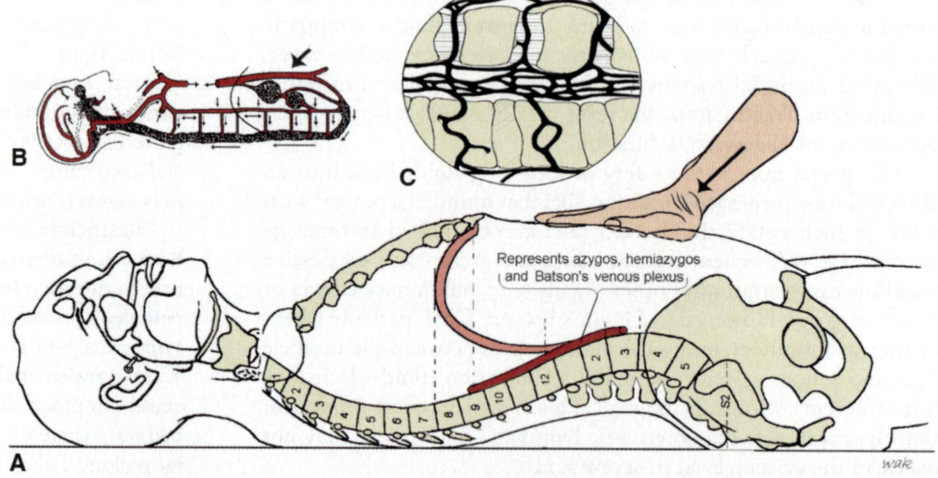

Figure 50.8. A–C. Zink "Warmth Provocative" test for a significant somatic dysfunction using the respiratory–circulatory model may be performed after first treating transition zones. (Illustration courtesy of William A. Kuchera, DO, FAAO, with permission.)

CASE STUDY

This case and its discussion at the end of the chapter were chosen to illustrate the rationale and manual components associated with applying the respiratory–circulatory model. The ultimate result of the OMT portion of the patient's care in this regard included:

- Reduction of upper extremity edema
- Resolution of the signs and symptoms of carpal tunnel syndrome (CTS)
- Increased function in both arms and several other systems

INITIAL CASE PRESENTATION

After 14 years at the same job without complaint, a 32-year-old woman who works as a transcriptionist presented with 6-week progressive numbness and tingling in her right (dominant) hand (Fig. 50.9).

Awakening her nearly every night, the distribution of her dysesthesia included her thumb and the next 2½ digits. For the last month, the patient had difficulty opening jars and has nearly dropped objects. Now early in the second trimester of her first pregnancy, she has taken no medications or nutritional supplements other than a prenatal vitamin.

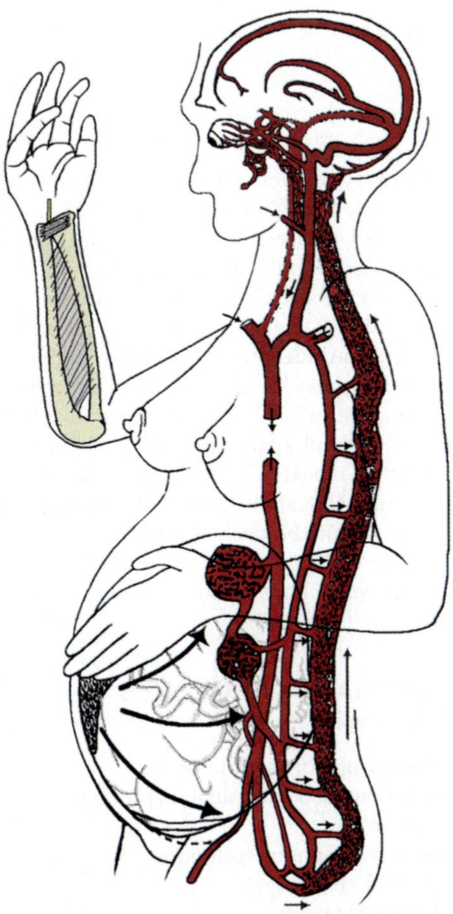

Figure 50.9. Case Study: Pregnant medical transcriptionist with finger swelling and tingling. (Illustration courtesy of William A. Kuchera, DO, FAAO, with permission.)

The distribution of the numbness and weakness coupled with an almost pathognomonic night-waking symptom is classic for CTS, a median entrapment neuropathy at the wrist. The five osteopathic models of care and approach may be used as a framework to approach this patient and her condition.

- Biomechanical risk factors (e.g., overuse on the computer, square wrists, forearm somatic dysfunction including trigger points, etc.)
- Neurologic risk factors (e.g., double crush conditions including cervical radiculopathy or dysfunction, scalene entrapment, etc.)
- Metabolic: hormonal risk factors (e.g., hypothyroidism, diabetes, etc.)
- Respiratory/circulatory: fluid overload/edema due to pregnancy
- Biopsychosocial: how is this affecting her work, relations with employer, etc.

PHYSICAL EXAMINATION

The patient's right thenar eminence appeared smaller than that on the left and manifested reduced grip strength; all fingers on the right hand were puffy. On the right, positive neurologic tests included Phalen (at 20 seconds) and Tinel (just distal to the wrist's flexor crease). There were no other historical or physical findings to indicate thyroid disorder, cervical radiculopathy, diabetes, vascular disease, or other significant health issues.

The common compensatory pattern of Zink was violated by her superior thoracic inlet that preferred rotation and sidebending to the left. The right supraclavicular region and posterior axillary fold exhibit fullness and are tender on palpation; in the supine position, her shallow, rapid breaths were observed to extend only halfway down to the umbilicus. Spinal palpatory revealed only grade I severity and Fryette type I somatic dysfunctions; no Chapman points or collateral ganglion findings were identified. The patient had a right posterior radial head somatic dysfunction. Active myofascial trigger points (MTrPs) were palpated in the right pronator teres and in several forearm and finger flexor muscles.

EMG consisting of nerve conduction studies (NCS) with needle examination confirmed moderate severity of median entrapment neuropathy at the wrist, with positive sensory and motor NCS, but no fibrillation potentials in the thenar eminence; it also ruled out a concomitant cervical radiculopathy. The presence of both sensory and motor problems suggested that this condition was probably at least moderate in severity and that treatment was warranted. The EMG confirmed this, but without fibrillation potentials, indicating that conservative management was possible. The EMG also ruled out a cervical radiculopathy as might coexist in a low, but significant percentage of cases, and could itself predispose that extremity to MTrPs.

Coupled with several ruled-out risk factors, her pregnancy (including edema, signs of terminal lymphatic drainage dysfunction, poorly effective respiration, and multiple somatic dysfunctions impeding both optimal fluid return and optimal biomechanical efficiency) suggested that the optimal first conservative step might be a combination of applying the respiratory–circulatory model in conjunction with a biomechanical approach.

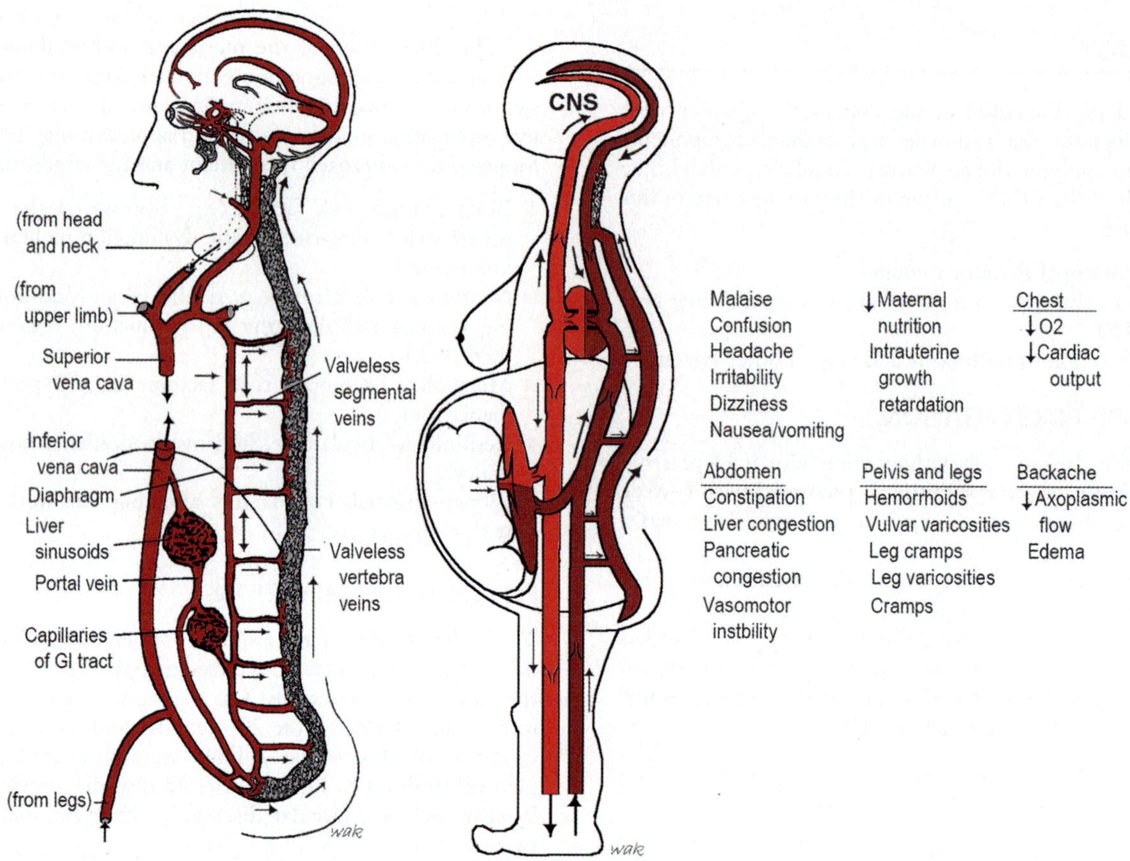

Figure 50.10. Congestive phase of pregnancy. (Illustration courtesy of William A. Kuchera, DO, FAAO, with permission.)

OVERVIEW OF APPROACH WITH OMT

While the findings in this particular case confirmed the manifestation of a neurologic pathology, they also suggested that the majority of the dysfunctional components (and perhaps the structural changes themselves) were related to overwhelming the patient's underlying myofascial and fluid homeostatic mechanisms (Fig. 50.10).

It was therefore determined that this case would best be primarily addressed by applying the respiratory–circulatory model and by emphasizing education and exercises derived from the biomechanical model.

The primary goals selected for this patient included correcting somatic dysfunction to:

1. Remove pathway impediments to fluid return.
2. Maximize the use of respiratory and muscle pumps to augment that return.

It was felt that additional goals were needed to empower the patient through education, in order to reduce ergonomic stress and maintain appropriate fluid flow with certain exercises. The resultant homeostatic improvement in her ability to manage systemic fluid changes (seen in pregnancy) simultaneously with local edema (that may have resulted from overuse and trigger points associated with her job) eliminated her CTS symptoms and, in this case, modified several of the pathogenic causes of median entrapment so that her self-healing mechanisms could take over.

Care in this case consisted of OMT at each of her remaining prenatal visits (employing from those techniques listed later only as needed to accomplish the clinical goals of the respiratory–circulatory model) and asking her to take a short rest with forearm–wrist stretches every few hours. This simple regimen successfully resolved her symptoms after the second visit, even as she continued to work. After vaginal delivery and 1 month of maternity leave, the patient returned to work. Her thenar eminence on the right returned to normal, and she had no further hand symptoms. With clinical improvement, she refused to repeat the EMG and remained empowered with her prior education concerning wise ergonomics, self-stretch exercises for the neck and forearm, and breathing exercises. She now seeks OMT occasionally "when she feels overly stressed at work" but is ultimately responsible for her own health.

SPECIFIC LYMPHATIC TECHNIQUES USED IN THIS CASE

1. Thoracic inlet lymphatic technique
2. Doming of the thoracoabdominal diaphragm
3. Pectoral traction
4. Upper extremity lymphatic technique
5. Anterior cervical effleurage
6. Thoracic lymphatic pump

The patient was also given specific self-stretch exercises.[79,80]

PRINCIPLES OF TREATMENT

Treatment protocols using this model are typically designed to:

1. Remove impediments to lymphatic flow.
2. Enhance mechanisms involved in respiratory–circulatory homeostasis.
3. Extrinsically augment the flow of lymph and other immune system elements.
4. Further mobilize lymphatic fluids from local or regional tissues that would benefit from decongestion.

Theoretically, all manipulative treatments can influence the lymphatic system through change in:

- Muscle tone
- Myofascial pathways
- Neural reflexes
- Autonomic tone
- Effects of respiration

Certain osteopathic techniques, however, have been long identified as "lymphatic techniques" because of their efficiency and efficacy.

- Some of these techniques are postulated to remove somatic dysfunctions that interfere with various motions needed for lymph formation or lymph flow.
- Others remove key somatic dysfunctions that impede flow between or through somatic structures.
- Others seem to augment homeostatic mechanisms important in respiration and circulation.

The logical order of techniques used in the respiratory–circulatory model may be summarized by the following series of statements:

1. First, ensure that the lymphatic channels, especially the terminal channels, are free of obstruction and functioning properly in order to permit appropriate fluid movement,
2. Ensure that the thoraco-abdominopelvic pump is functioning optimally.
3. Accomplish clinical goals with respect to the involved target tissues.

With this simple mechanical sequence in mind, the order of integrating choices from the varying broad categories of "lymphatic treatment" techniques proceeds roughly as follows:

1. Open myofascial pathways at transition areas of the body.
2. Maximize normal diaphragmatic motions.
3. Increase pressure differentials or transmit motion to pump or otherwise augment fluid flow beyond normal levels.
4. Mobilize targeted tissue fluids into the lymphaticovenous system.

ILLUSTRATIVE TECHNIQUES

Consistent with the logical sequencing recommendations above, several illustrative techniques used to implement respiratory-circulatory model clinical goals follow. By virtue of the anatomy addressed, some OMT techniques may be used to accomplish more than clinical goal or even address more than one osteopathic model of care. For instance, some thoracoabdominal redoming techniques may both optimize fascial pathways between those two compartments as well as maximize diaphragmatic motion. Likewise, some treatments addressing the anatomic structures making up the superior thoracic inlet (a common first step in implementing the respiratory-circulatory model) not only opens the final common fascial diaphragm for lymphatic fluid to return to the central vascular system but may also address somatic dysfunction of T1–4 (important in the neurologic-autonomic model in HEENT and patients who suffer from cardiopulmonary conditions).

It is important to emphasize that the lymphatic system is one continuous system. Restriction of fluid movement through one area of this system can cause a shunting effect of fluid flow in other parts of the system creating or augmenting unwanted congestion and reduced fluid exchange in tissue, that is, myofascial restriction of the right thoracic duct will indirectly affect fluid flow through the left thoracic duct. Therefore, significant somatic dysfunction affecting anatomical areas that may not be in direct relationship to the target area of treatment should also be addressed and treated to optimize physiologic functioning.

Superior Thoracic Inlet (Sibson Fascia) Lymphatic Drainage Technique—Left Side

Clinical Goal: remove obstruction to terminal lymphatic drainage

Treatment Position

Patient: supine
Physician: sitting on the left side of the patient, facing the patient's head
Possible diagnosis: left-sided supraclavicular myofascial resistance with terminal lymphatic congestion

Procedure

1. The physician abducts the patient's arm to 90 degrees and externally rotates the arm with the elbow flexed to 90 degrees. The physician's knee supports the patient's elbow. The physician's right hand supports the patient's wrist, while the left hand is placed on the superior aspect of the supraclavicular fossa (Fig. 50.11).
2. The physician applies an inferior–anterior pressure to the patient's clavicle while moving the patient's arm in an arc, from external rotation to internal rotation (Fig. 50.12).
3. The physician maintains anterior pressure with the fingers on the posterior aspect of the clavicle, while arcing the patient's arm back into external rotation (Fig. 50.13).
4. Steps 2 and 3 are repeated with the fingers of the physician wrapping further around the posterior aspect of the clavicle, as the fascia of that region begins to relax.
5. This motion is repeated until a sense of fascial release and decongestion of the thoracic inlet is palpated.

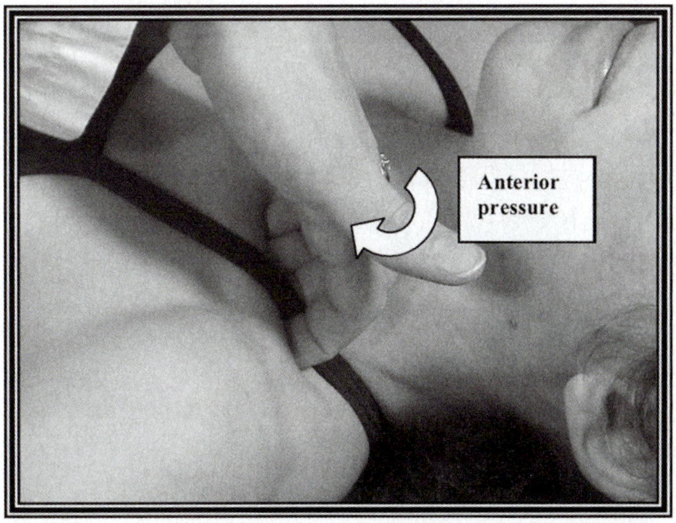

Figure 50.11. Lymphatic drainage of the thoracic inlet—finger position behind the clavicle over Sibson fascia. (Photo courtesy of Western University of Health Sciences, College of Osteopathic Medicine of the Pacific, Department of NMM/OMM, with permission.)

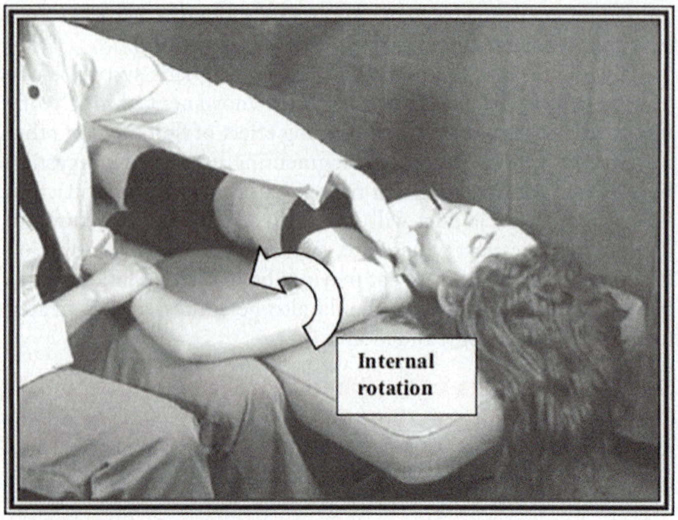

Figure 50.12. Lymphatic drainage of the thoracic inlet—internal rotation of the arm. (Photo courtesy of Western University of Health Sciences, College of Osteopathic Medicine of the Pacific, Department of NMM/OMM, with permission.)

6. This same procedure is typically repeated for the right thoracic inlet, as this is considered a bilateral technique.
7. Retest: Physician retests using the same method as was used in the initial assessment. For example: increased compliance of the previously restricted inlets with less supraclavicular terminal lymphatic congestion.

Note #1: *This same procedure is typically repeated for the right thoracic inlet, as this is considered a bilateral technique.*

Note #2: *Consider also treating the scalene muscles to optimize outcomes. The scalene fascia is continuous with Sibson fascia.*

Bilateral Superior Thoracic Inlet–Indirect Regional "Opening" (BLT & MFR)

Clinical goal(s): Optimize transverse thoracic inlet diaphragm to enhance lymphaticovenous drainage; remove regional somatic dysfunction. This technique may also address the neurologic-autonomic model as the correction of the thoracic inlet may address dysfunction of structures associated with T1–4 and thus may normalize T1–4 sympathetic activity or decrease associated segmental facilitation. Ribs 1 to 2, the manubrium and attached myofascial structures including Sibson fascia may also be positively affected.

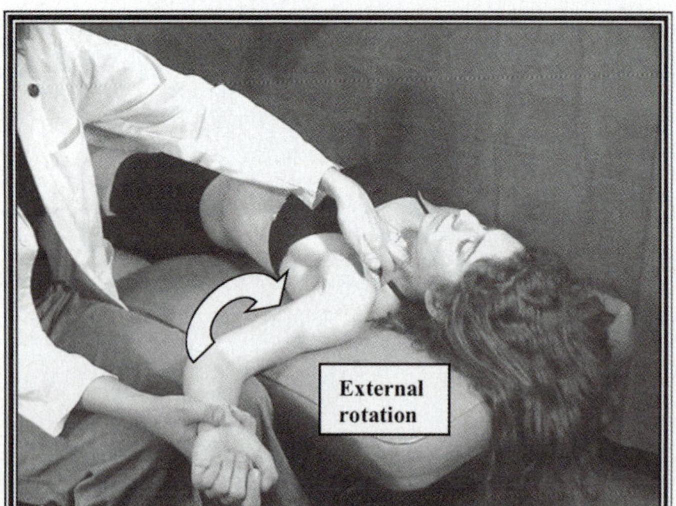

Figure 50.13. Lymphatic drainage of the superior thoracic inlet—external rotation of the arm. (Photo courtesy of Western University of Health Sciences, College of Osteopathic Medicine of the Pacific, Department of NMM/OMM, with permission.)

Treatment Position

Patient: supine (or seated)
Physician: sitting at head of table/bed (or standing behind the patient)
Possible diagnosis: thoracic inlet sidebent and rotated left

Procedure

1. The physician places their hands over the thoracic inlet with fingers spread over the anterior thorax (below the clavicle but at or above rib 2) and thumbs over the upper thoracic transverse processes posteriorly.
2. Regional myofascial motion preference is assessed in all three cardinal planes.
3. Using both hands simultaneously (like hands on a car's steering wheel), the physician carries the superior thoracic inlet region as a unit, stacking all directions of freedom to a 3-D point of ligamentous balance (left rotation, left sidebending and slight flexion or extension) (Fig. 50.14).
4. Often additional balance is obtained by adding a slight compressive force from the thumb on the concave side toward the opposite nipple seeking to release first rib head tension.
5. The physician tests both respiratory phases and may add an activating force by instructing the patient to hold their breath (if they can) "for as long as possible" in the phase that provides the best ligamentous balance as they make continuous minor adjustments in all three planes as the release takes place. (The release generally occurs in the directions of ease.)
6. This is continued until the tissues begin to return to the neutral position or until maximum tissue response has been obtained.
7. Retest using same procedure as in Step 1.

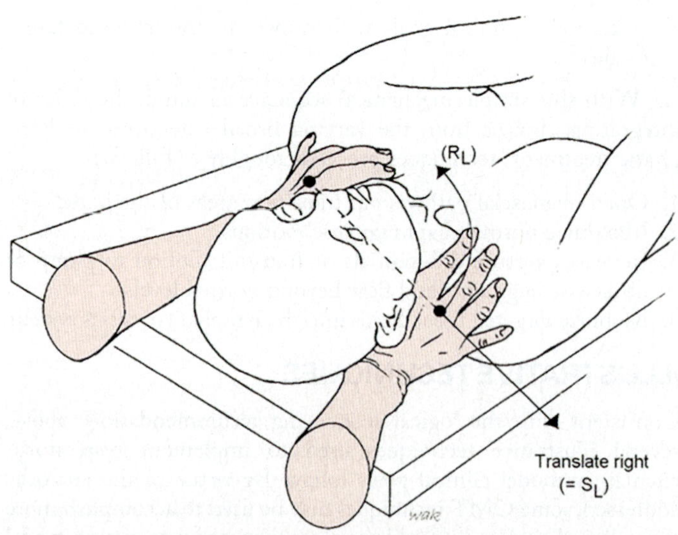

Figure 50.14. Bilateral Superior Thoracic Inlet–Indirect Regional "Opening" (BLT & MFR) that is sidebent and rotated left. Translate superior thoracic inlet region to the right to create sidebending left and rotate the region to the left—both into the position of ease The physician may add slight flexion or extension into the position of ease. (Modified from Kuchera ML, Kuchera WA. *Osteopathic Considerations in HEENT Disorders: Head, Eyes, Ears, Nose, Throat.* Greyden Press; 2012. Reprinted with permission from Michael L. Kuchera, DO, FAAO.)

Note: This technique can be modified from an indirect BLT to an indirect MFR simply by shifting attention from a ligamentous multiarticular balance to balancing the more superficial myofascial layers.

Note: This technique can also be performed as a direct technique as follows:

Steps 1 and 2 are the same.

Then translate both hands simultaneously to the left and compress through the web-trapezius contact to sidebend the superior thoracic inlet to the right (stop at the edge of the myofascial barrier). Add rotation to the right by turning both hands simultaneously (like turning a steering wheel) to rotate the entire T1–4 and first two ribs to the myofascial barrier. Finally, add a small amount of inlet flexion or extension as needed to maximize the restrictive barrier in the sagittal plane. (See Fig. 50.14 as set-up steps 1 and 2 are the same as in that technique.)

Maintain the tension at the edges of the myofascial barriers and follow the "creep" phenomenon until a complete release is achieved.

Recheck the motion characteristics of the superior thoracic inlet to ensure that all planes of motion are equally free.

Anterior Cervical Effleurage

Clinical Goal(s): Targeting local lymphatic drainage of head and neck structures. (It has been noted clinically that the first sign of sternocleidomastoid (SCM) dysfunction seems to be edematous change in the fascial sheathe around that muscle.)

Treatment Position

Patient: supine
Physician: sitting at the head of the patient

Procedure

NOTE: DO NOT put pressure on the carotid bodies causing a vasovagal response.

1. Physician rotates the patient's head away from the side being treated. The patient's head is slightly flexed manually or with a pillow for comfort and to facilitate lymphatic drainage.
2. The physician's thumb pad is placed on the anterior margin of the SCM muscle in the inferior portion of the patient's neck (Fig. 50.15).

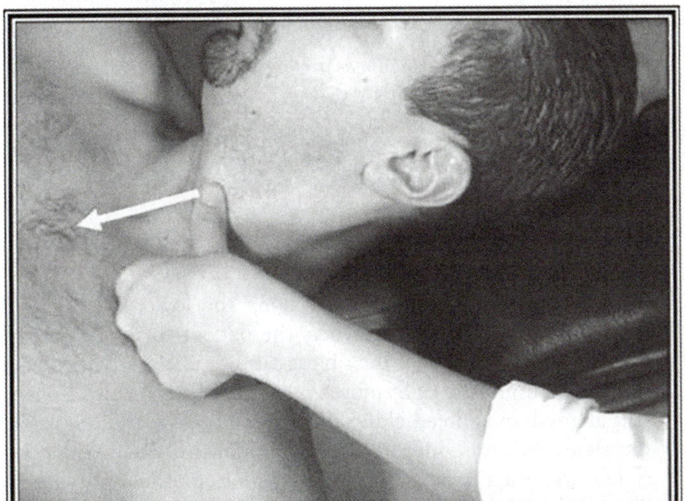

Figure 50.15. Anterior cervical effleurage—fingers on inferior aspect of sternocleidomastoid muscle. (Photo courtesy of Western University of Health Sciences, College of Osteopathic Medicine of the Pacific, Department of NMM/OMM, with permission.)

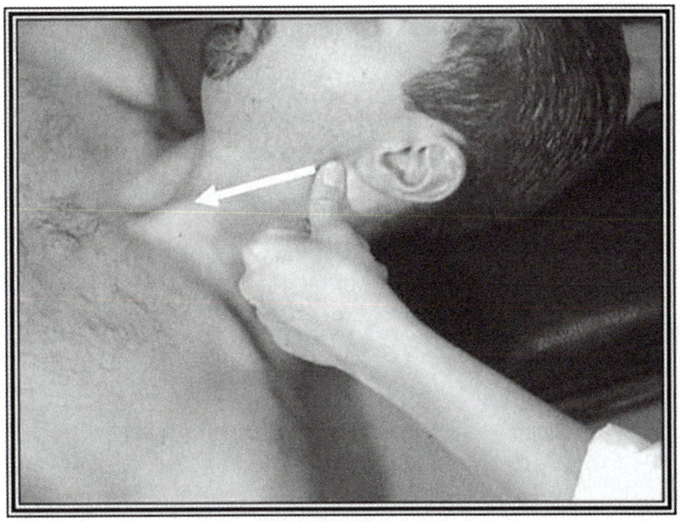

Figure 50.16. Anterior cervical effleurage—fingers at superior aspect of sternocleidomastoid muscle. (Photo courtesy of Western University of Health Sciences, College of Osteopathic Medicine of the Pacific, Department of NMM/OMM, with permission.)

3. Physician applies slow, steady strokes along the inferior part of SCM margin toward the clavicle several times.
4. Physician replaces the thumb in the middle portion of the patient's neck and repeats the stroking to the clavicle.
5. This is then repeated from the mastoid tip in the superior section (Fig. 50.16).
6. Physician repeats the entire process inferiorly to superiorly until congestion is reduced and the tissues move freely.
7. Retest: Physician will retest by assessing the area for increased tissue warmth, increased tissue compliance, and flexibility. The patient may also report a sense of drainage.

Supine Direct Doming of Diaphragm

Clinical goal(s): Optimize lymphaticovenous pathway between abdominal and thoracic compartment. Maximize thoracoabdominal diaphragmatic pump function.

Treatment Position

Patient: supine (optimally with knees bent to soften abdomen)
Physician: standing at the patient's side, facing the patient's head

Procedure

1. The fingers of both the physician's hands are placed on the anterolateral aspect of the inferior border of the ribs, with the thumbs placed medial to the costal margins, directly inferior to the xiphoid process of the sternum (Fig. 50.17).
2. The patient inhales deeply and then exhales fully. As the patient exhales, the physician's thumbs are gently pressed posteriorly toward the table and slightly superiorly, following the motion of the diaphragm.
3. The physician holds this endpoint as the patient inhales again. (The thumbs may sense resistance to respiration.)
4. As the patient exhales again, the physician presses in further, posteriorly toward the table, continuing to monitor the superior movement of the diaphragm.
5. This process is continued through several respiratory cycles until the diaphragm domes easily at the end of exhalation.
6. Retest: Physician attempts to sense decreased resistance under the thumbs to all phases of respiration.

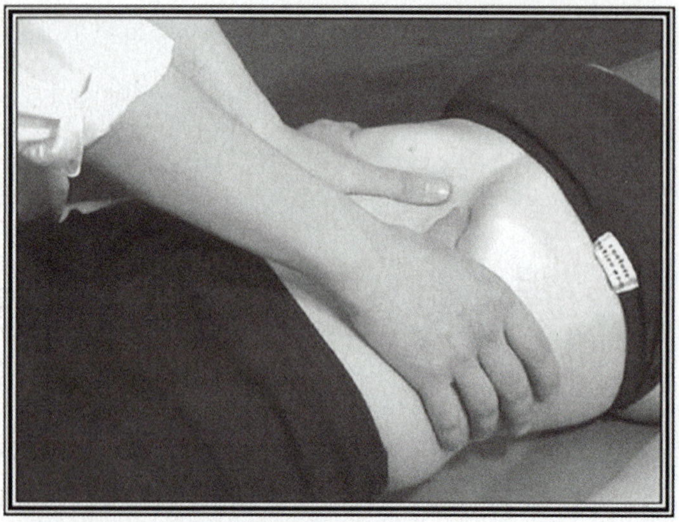

Figure 50.17. **Supine doming of the abdominal diaphragm.** (Photo courtesy of Western University of Health Sciences, College of Osteopathic Medicine of the Pacific, Department of NMM/OMM, with permission.)

Supine Indirect Myofascial Release (MFR) of Thoracoabdominal Diaphragm/Thoracoabdominal Diaphragm "Redoming" Myofascial Release

Clinical goal(s): Optimize lymphaticovenous pathways between the abdominal and thoracic compartments. Maximize thoracoabdominal diaphragmatic pump function. (Also, this may address thoracolumbar somatic dysfunction as well as vagophrenic connections related to the neurologic-autonomic model).

Treatment Position

Patient: supine, preferably with knees bent to relax the abdominal musculature

Physician: standing at the patient's side, facing the patient's head

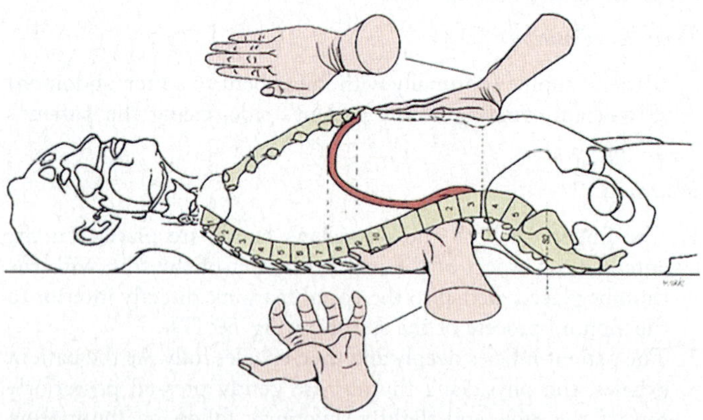

Figure 50.18. **Supine indirect myofascial release (MFR) of thoracoabdominal diaphragm/thoracoabdominal diaphragm "redoming" myofascial release.** A–P hand positions for performing MFR technique to redome this diaphragm. Both hands are coordinated in all three planes to focus on the myofascial diaphragmatic attachments. Imbalance between sides of the diaphragm will pull through the crura resulting in an additional alternate clockwise or counterclockwise hand preference which can be followed. (Modified from Kuchera ML, Kuchera WA. *Osteopathic Considerations in HEENT Disorders: Head, Eyes, Ears, Nose, Throat.* Greyden Press; 2012. Reprinted with permission from Michael L. Kuchera, DO, FAAO.)

Procedure (see Fig. 50.18)

1. The physician bridges L1–3 vertebrae (posterior diaphragm attachment) contacting erector spinae masses with thenar eminence ipsilaterally and digits 2 to 4 contralaterally.
2. The physician's hand nearest the patient compresses the subxiphoid region down to deep fascia lining anterior abdominal wall.
3. Both physician's hands move as unit away from restrictions to create balanced regional sidebending and rotation.
4. Both the physician's hands move reciprocally clockwise-counterclockwise to achieve indirect MFR balance of diaphragm.
5. The physician follows indirect MFR until both hands appreciate the release.
6. Recheck balance. (Ensure that passive breathing extends to pubic level).

Direct MFR of Inferior Thoracic Outlet/Direct Method, MFR Activation to Treat Thoracolumbar Region

Clinical goal(s): Release somatic dysfunction of regional thoracolumbar junction; maximize thoracoabdominal diaphragmatic function; enhance respiratory-circulatory model goals; optimize pressure-sensitive spleen with goal of enhancing immune function by optimization of diaphragmatic pumping.

Treatment Position

Patient: supine

Physician: standing on either side of the patient at approximately the level of the greater trochanter of the femur

Potential diagnosis: regional inferior thoracic outlet $S_L R_L$ (sidebending left and rotation left)

Procedure

1. With fingers aligned and spread along the lower rib cage on both sides, translate the entire inferior thoracic outlet to the left (sidebending it right) and then rotate the entire region to the right—each direction to the myofascial barrier (Fig. 50.19).
2. Maintain tension as the "creep" phenomenon occurs and follow in all planes as the regional tissues release fully moving through all barriers.
3. Recheck motion characteristics and note whether supine passive breathing extends to the pubic symphysis.

Note: *This technique can also be performed as an indirect technique.*

Another variation of this can be accomplished as described below:

Redoming of the Thoracoabdominal Diaphragm: Direct MFR with Respiratory Cooperation for Thoracoabdominal Diaphragm (Lateral Approach)

1. With fingers aligned and spread along the lower rib cage on both sides, the physician instructs the patient to inhale deeply to ascertain which side of the rib cage moves anteriorly the most (in this example, the right moves more anteriorly). With fingers still aligned and spread along the lower rib cage, the physician translates the entire inferior thoracic outlet to the left (sidebent right) and then rotates the entire region to the right—each direction to the myofascial barrier. (Refer back to Fig. 50.19.) Perfect balance may also require fine-tuning in the sagittal plane.
2. The physician instructs the patient to inhale and concentrates on diaphragmatic excursion under each hand; when the left side stops moving, the physician adds additional compression

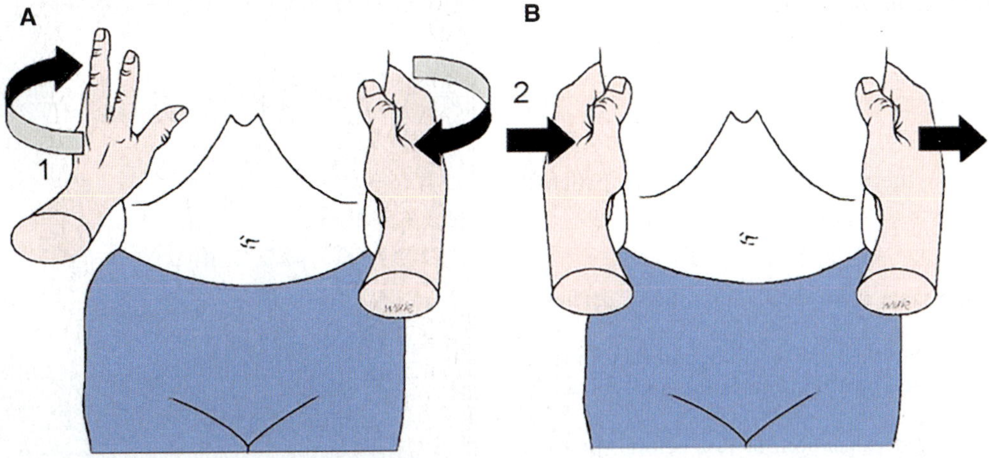

Figure 50.19. Direct method, MFR activation to treat a thoracolumbar region that is sidebent and rotated to the left. A. Using both hands simultaneously, rotate the lower chest cage and thoracolumbar region to the feather-edge of the myofascial rotational barrier. **B.** Using both hands simultaneously and maintaining the rotational component achieved in part A, translate this same region to "stack" the combined tension to the direct barrier. Adjust both A & B to maintain the barrier until the release is complete. (Modified from Kuchera ML, Kuchera WA. *Osteopathic Considerations in HEENT Disorders: Head, Eyes, Ears, Nose, Throat.* Greyden Press; 2012. Reprinted with permission from Michael L. Kuchera, DO, FAAO.)

to limit the right side from moving more than the left. (This is to "encourage" the non-functional side to work). During exhalation the physician follows the chest cage's release, maintaining tension at its barrier in all planes as the "creep" phenomenon occurs.

3. The physician asks the patient to repeat inhalation concentrating on the diaphragmatic element (again restricting the side of the "functioning diaphragm" to balance its motion with the side with less activity) and again follow the MFR of the chest cage during exhalation (in all three planes) as the regional tissues release fully moving through all barriers.
4. This is continued until the less functional side of the diaphragm is sensed to dramatically increase its excursion to match the functional side.
5. Recheck motion characteristics and note whether supine passive breathing extends to the pubic symphysis.

Supine or Lateral Recumbent *Direct* Pelvic Diaphragm Release (Ischiorectal Fossa Technique)

See "Pelvic Diaphragm Release" technique description in Chapter 78 Osteopathic Considerations and Approaches in the Acutely Ill or Hospitalized Patient; the hand position is depicted in Figure 50.20.

Supine *Indirect* Pelvic Diaphragm Release

Exhaled position (Exhalation) of the pelvic diaphragm (the pelvic diaphragm appears to be held superiorly and does not descend fully in response to active thoracoabdominal diaphragm inhalation)

Treatment Position

Patient: supine
Physician: standing at the patient's side, facing the patient's head

Procedure

1. Using rigid, straightened fingers of one of the physician's hands follow along the posteromedial aspect of the ischial tuberosity to monitor the pelvic floor in the ischiorectal fossa (Fig. 50.20).
   The physician's other hand is placed just below the costal margin on the same side to monitor movement of the thoracic diaphragm.
2. The patient inhales deeply, then exhales fully, and holds the breath until *forced* to inhale.
3. At the moment of forced inhalation, or just before, the diaphragm will descend.
4. The physician rechecks pelvic diaphragmatic motion during the next breathing cycle.
5. If the somatic dysfunction is not felt to be completely resolved, repeat steps 2 through 4 until both the thoracic and pelvic diaphragms are in phase. (Both descend and ascend simultaneously with good amplitude during the appropriate respiratory phase.)
6. Retest: The physician evaluates bilaterally to ensure that both sides are moving freely equally and without restriction.

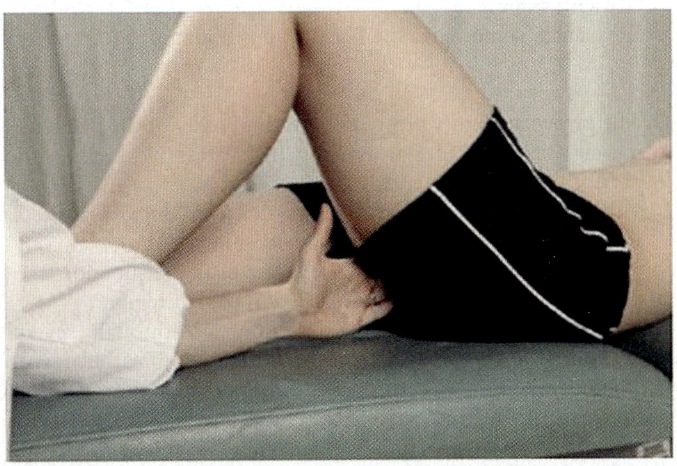

Figure 50.20. Supine direct or indirect pelvic diaphragm treatment technique. See Figure 78.2 for precise diagrammatic location. (Photo courtesy of Western University of Health Sciences, College of Osteopathic Medicine of the Pacific, Department of NMM/OMM, with permission.)

Inhaled Position (*Inhalation*) of the Pelvic Diaphragm (the pelvic diaphragm is inferior in inhalation position and does not ascend during exhalation)

Treatment Position

Patient: supine
Physician: standing at the patient's side, facing the patient's head

Procedure

1. Steps 1, 4 to 6 are the same as for exhalation somatic dysfunction above.
2. The patient inhales deeply, then exhales fully, and then inhales fully. The patient holds the breath in inhalation until forced to exhale.
3. At the moment of forced exhalation, or just before, the diaphragm will ascend.
4. This may also be addressed in a direct manner; as the patient exhales, the physician may apply gentle superior pressure to the pelvic diaphragm and maintain this pressure as the patient inhales. This may be repeated three to five times until improved motion of the pelvic diaphragm is noted.

Pectoral Traction

Pectoral traction may influence lymph flow by means of influencing the pectoralis minor muscle. By exerting a superior traction on the pectoralis minor, the range of motion of the upper rib cage is augmented during inhalation, thereby increasing the negative pressure in the thorax and the intrathoracic volume of the chest. It is estimated that a 1 cm increase in the diameter of the chest increases air intake by 200 to 400 cc. This is a useful technique that can be used for patients with osteoporosis, postsurgical patients, and, with relative caution, on patients in the ICU with multiple intravenous lines in place.

Clinical goal(s): Similar to a lymphatic pump, this technique may help to enhance pressure differentials between the thoracic and other compartments to augment lymphatic flow without the use of significant pressures or motion forces.

Note: Best performed after opening fascial pathways particularly, at the superior thoracic inlet.

Treatment Position

Patient: supine
Physician: standing at the head of the patient

Procedure

1. The physician gently grasps the inferior border of the pectoralis muscles of each anterior axilla, taking care not to gouge the patient with the fingertips.
2. With arms fully extended, the physician produces a bilateral superior traction by leaning backward (Fig. 50.21).
3. The physician may feel that one side resists the superior traction. This may be noted as a restriction of that region.
4. The physician maintains bilateral traction through several respiratory cycles, instructing the patient to breathe deeply. The combination of traction and respiratory motion will help to release any restriction of the pectoralis muscle/anterior axilla region. (During exhalation, the physician may follow the tissues inferiorly and add slight compression into the passive chest cage motion; reinitiate pectoral traction with the inhalation traction cycle. If there is asymmetrical pectoral tension, seek to balance it by adding slightly more tension on the restricted side during inhalation to release dysfunction.)

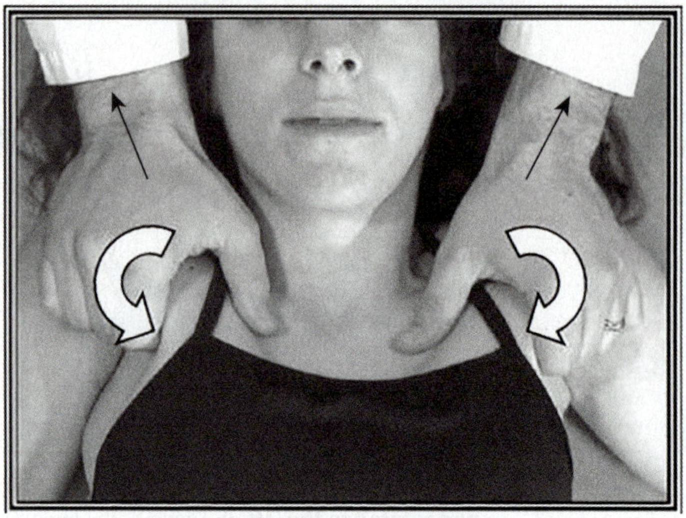

Figure 50.21. Pectoral traction technique. (Photo courtesy of Western University of Health Sciences, College of Osteopathic Medicine of the Pacific, Department of NMM/OMM, with permission.)

5. The superior traction is continued until the myofascial restrictions are reduced or eliminated or for approximately 2 minutes.
6. The physician then gently releases the tissue.
7. Retest: The physician may retest by again administering superior traction into the anterior axilla region, noting equal compliance of both regions.

Lymphatic Drainage of the Upper Extremities

Clinical goal(s): targeting local lymphatic drainage of upper extremity structures.

Treatment Position

Patient: supine
Physician: standing to the affected side of the patient

Procedure

1. The patient's arm is held in the physician's axilla (e.g., if right arm, stand on the right and hold the patient's right arm in the left axilla).
2. The physician grasps the patient's upper arm close to the shoulder. The physician's two hands are placed on either side of the limb, applying a rotatory motion with compression directing fluid toward the axillary region (Fig. 50.22).
3. The physician repeats this motion from proximal to distal until the patient's elbow is reached. The physician then returns to the proximal upper extremity and repeats this entire proximal to distal process of lymphatic drainage an additional three to four times or until adequate drainage has been achieved.
4. The physician then moves to the forearm. The physician's thumbs are placed on the ventral surface between the flexor and extensor muscle masses, with the fingers around the patient's other side.
5. The physician gently squeezes the muscle masses simultaneously toward the patient's axilla before relaxing the compression (Fig. 50.23).

This "milking"-type action is continued from proximal (near distal elbow) to distal (wrist) three to four times or more, depending on the patient's response, in order to reduce edema. Note that while proximal areas are addressed before distal ones, each region being addressed is ALWAYS compressed from

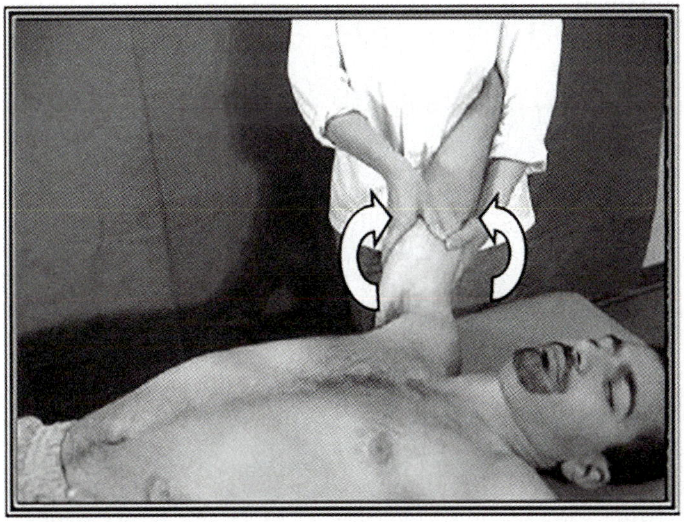

Figure 50.22. Lymphatic drainage of the proximal portion of the upper extremity. (Photo courtesy of Western University of Health Sciences, College of Osteopathic Medicine of the Pacific, Department of NMM/OMM, with permission.)

distal to proximal to accommodate fluid motion through the one-way valves toward the heart.

6. Retest: Physician may retest by palpating the upper extremity for decreased edema and increased compliance. See also alternative OMT of "Lateral fluctuation of the forearm" in Chapter 78.

Lymphatic Drainage of the Lower Extremities

Clinical goal(s): targeting local lymphatic drainage of lower extremity structures.

Treatment Position

Patient: supine
Physician: sitting on the table, facing the patient

Procedure

1. The patient's affected leg is balanced on the physician's shoulder.

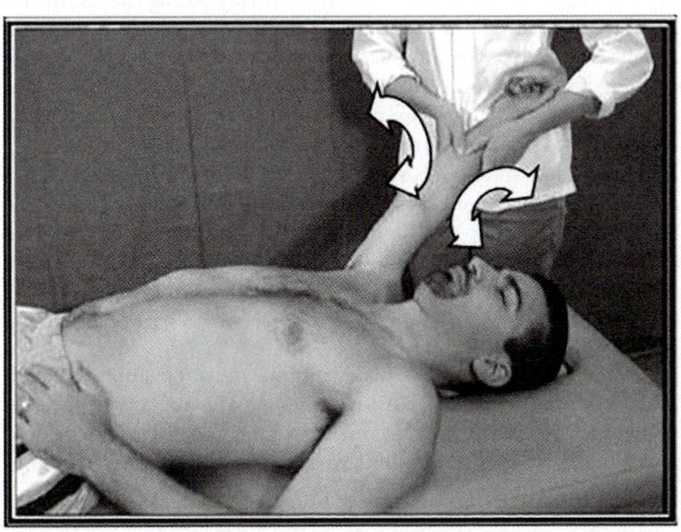

Figure 50.23. Lymphatic drainage of the distal portion of the upper extremity. (Photo courtesy of Western University of Health Sciences, College of Osteopathic Medicine of the Pacific, Department of NMM/OMM, with permission.)

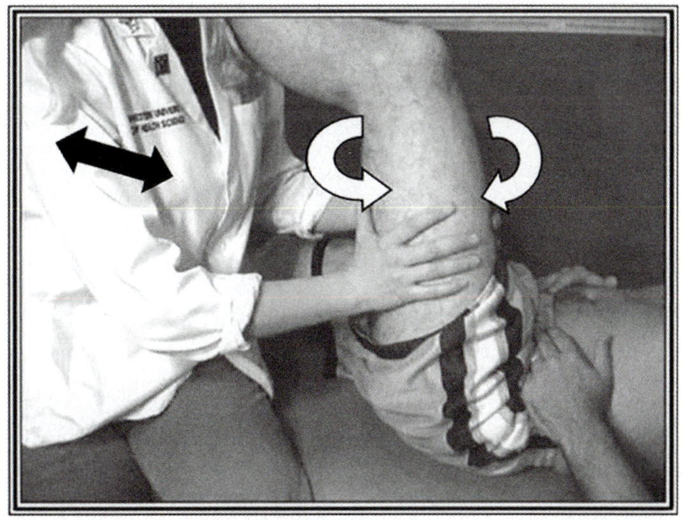

Figure 50.24. Lymphatic drainage of the proximal femoral region. (Photo courtesy of Western University of Health Sciences, College of Osteopathic Medicine of the Pacific, Department of NMM/OMM, with permission.)

2. Physician flexes the patient's hip and knee both to right angles so that the patient's thigh is perpendicular and the lower leg is parallel to the table.
3. Starting at the proximal end of the thigh, the physician places the palmer surface of both hands on opposing sides of the leg and then performs a rotatory motion with compression toward the pelvis and the inguinal region. This motion is repeated several times (Fig. 50.24).
4. As tissue change takes place, the physician moves distally down the thigh toward the knee, one hand's width at a time, performing the same action as described in step 2 (Fig. 50.25).
5. This sequence may be performed multiple times in order to effectively reduce edema.
6. When the tissues have softened and there is less congestion in the tissues, the physician moves distal to the knee joint.
7. The physician's two hands are placed on either side of the patient's lower leg, with the thumbs pressing deeply between

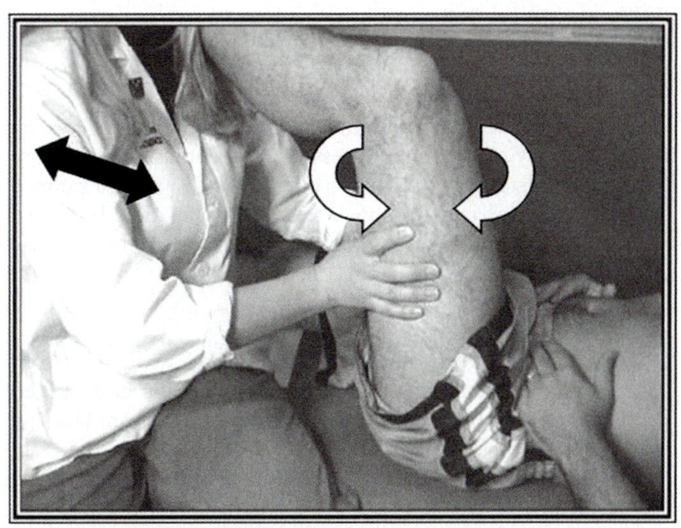

Figure 50.25. Lymphatic drainage of the femoral region—progressively addressing more distal regions, enabling fluids to move distal-to-proximal. (Photo courtesy of Western University of Health Sciences, College of Osteopathic Medicine of the Pacific, Department of NMM/OMM, with permission.)

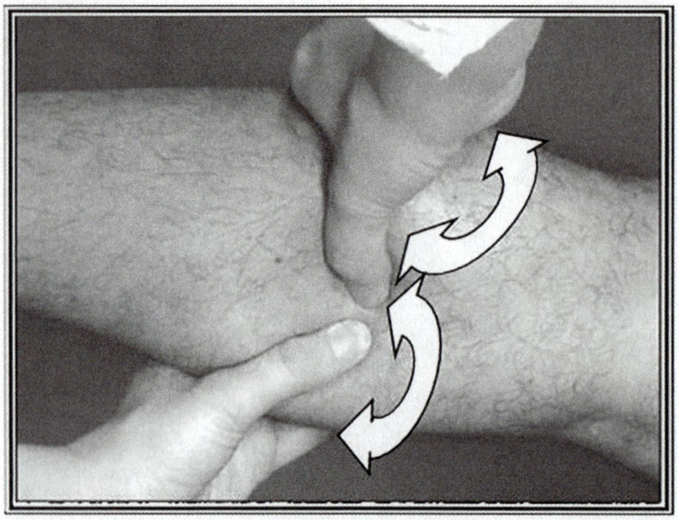

Figure 50.26. Lymphatic drainage of the distal lower extremity—starting at gastrocnemius muscle heads, just distal to the knee joint. (Photo courtesy of Western University of Health Sciences, College of Osteopathic Medicine of the Pacific, Department of NMM/OMM, with permission.)

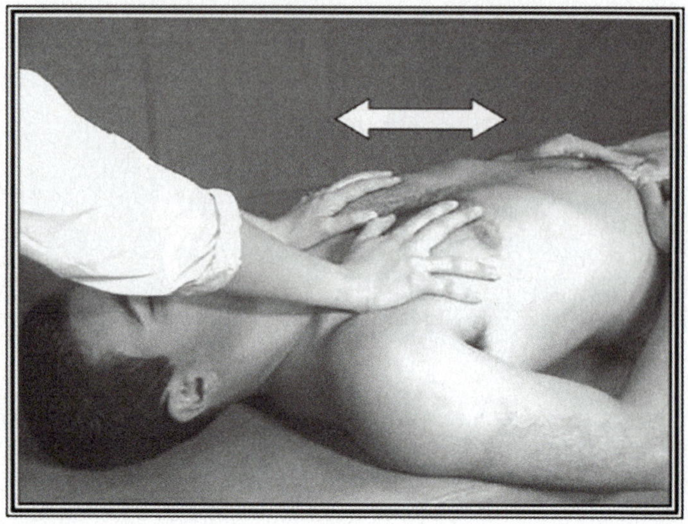

Figure 50.27. Classical thoracic pump technique. (Photo courtesy of Western University of Health Sciences, College of Osteopathic Medicine of the Pacific, Department of NMM/OMM, with permission.)

the two gastrocnemius heads close to the popliteal fossa (Fig. 50.26).

8. The physician's thumbs and fingers are squeezed together rhythmically several times performing a "milking" action to this region encouraging fluid from distal to proximal.
9. During each squeezing motion, the physician rocks forward, using body weight to flex the patient's knee and hip, further encouraging fluid drainage from distal to proximal. The physician then moves their hand placement further distally toward the ankle and repeats this procedure until the entire appropriate distal extremity has been addressed.
10. This may be performed for up to 5 minutes to effectively reduce edema, depending on the patient's response, moving from distal to proximal.
11. Retest: The physician may retest this region by assessing for increased warmth and decreased edema.

See also "Lateral fluctuation at the knee" in Chapter 78.

Classical Miller Thoracic Pump Technique

Clinical Goal(s): Enhance respiratory-circulatory model goals via enhancing body compartment pressure differentials. Is utilized to enhance mobilization of pulmonary secretions, introduce pulmonary toilet, and enhance immune titers post vaccination. Indicated in infection, fever, pneumonia, productive cough, and lymphaticovenous congestion.[80]

Treatment Position

Patient: supine with mouth open breathing (without gum or any foreign body that might be aspirated) and head turned right or left (to avoid the patient's expired air from blowing into the physician's face)

Physician: standing at the head of table with hands broadly spread out over the patient's sternum or upper chest wall with the thenar eminence of each hand just distal to the respective clavicle, avoiding the breast tissue. Female patients may be instructed to cover their breasts with their hands to assist the physician in avoiding direct contact with a potentially sensitive region (Fig. 50.27)

Procedure

1. To initiate the treatment, the physician follows the direction of motion with slightly exaggerated compression into the passive chest wall range of motion during the exhalation phase. Then, throughout the underlying periodicity of the patient's breathing cycle, the physician maintains a rhythmic compression-decompression (pumping action) at a faster rate to add extra cycles of pressure change; during the patient's exhalation cycles, the physician adds even more compression to begin to add recoil from the passive motion range. The motion is generated through a slight extension/flexion of the physician's elbows, with forearm, wrist, and hand acting as a fixed lever. The oscillatory force of the motion should come from the physician's whole body.
2. The rate of the pumping should be approximately 110 to 120 times/min and with a force adequate to comfortably add to the passive range of motion available in the patient's chest cage.
3. The patient is instructed to breathe normally during this treatment.
4. The physician continues the oscillatory pumping until an increased sense of soft tissue compliance is palpated and decreased tissue congestion is attained. Alternatively, if the goal is fluid movement through periodic pressure change, then, the technique should be performed for approximately 2 minutes.
5. Retest: As stated in Step 4 the physician may palpate an increased soft tissue compliance and decreased tissue congestion. Objectively, the physician may note an increase in the patient's oxygen saturation as measured by an apparatus such as a pulse oximeter. The patient may also subjectively comment that breathing is easier and that a fuller breath may be obtained.

Note: A variation of this technique may be applied called **"thoracic pump with activation"**. This may be applied to patients with conditions such as atelectasis and lung congestion to create a pressure differential to mobilize fluid. The setup for the procedure is the same as above.

1. Instruct the patient to breathe in fully through the mouth and during the exhalation phase add an oscillatory pumping motion increasing compression into the passive range of motion at about 120 cycles per minute.

2. As the patient inhales, the physician maintains compression to the chest wall, providing moderate resistance to inhalation, and then resumes the oscillatory pumping during exhalation. Further compression is added with each cycle for about two to three cycles of breathing.
3. At the start of inhalation on the third or fourth cycle, the physician may either resist open mouth inhalation momentarily but then rapidly release compression or instruct the patient to hold their breath out in exhalation and then take a sudden deep inhalation. During this sudden inhalation, the physician removes their hands and thus the pressure to the chest wall. This three to four cycle series may be repeated two to five times (depending on the patient) ending with the largest pressure change.

Note: *Avoid the thoracic pump with activation in patients with COPD or those with emphysematous changes where the sudden inhalation might inadvertently rupture a bleb.*

The thoracic duct siphon technique described by Sutherland is described in Chapter 78.

Abdominal Pump

Clinical goal(s): To enhance pressure differentials between the abdominal and thoracic compartments; also to enhance immune function

Treatment Position

Patient: supine (knees may be flexed)
Physician: standing at the patient's side

Procedure

1. Both of the physician's palms are placed on the patient's abdomen, with the fingers pointing to the patient's head and the thumbs side by side. For small patients, or for greater control, the physician's two hands can be placed on top of one another (Fig. 50.28).
2. Both of the physician's arms should be extended, with the elbows locked.
3. The physician then pumps in a superior and inferior direction in a rhythmic manner. The pumping motion is similar to that of the pedal or thoracic pump. The rate should be approximately 20 to 30 times/minute but varies according to the patient's needs and response to treatment. Often this technique is performed for about 2 minutes to mobilize immune cells and/or move fluid.
4. Retest: The retest for this technique is difficult to assess at the time of treatment. The patient may report decreased edema to an affected area and/or improvement in symptoms noted prior to treatment. In a patient with an infection, a warning that their temperature may transiently rise shortly afterward due to pyrogen activity from enhanced immune function may be warranted. Abdominal lift and cisterna chyli techniques are additional abdominal lymphatic techniques that assist in drainage of the abdominopelvic viscera.

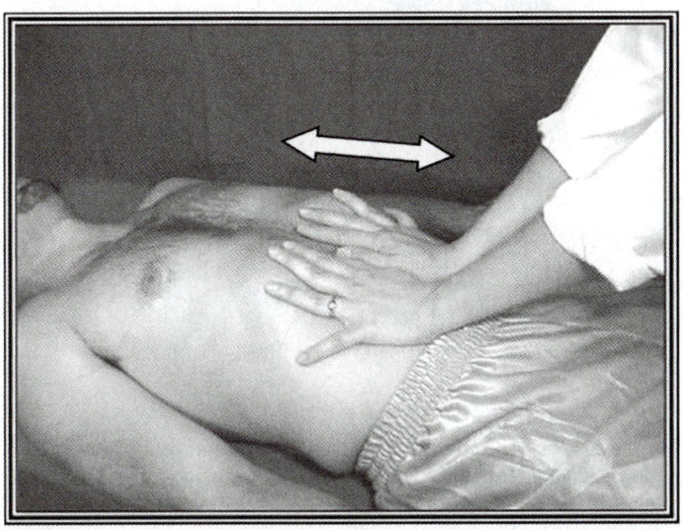

Figure 50.28. Abdominal lymphatic pump. (Photo courtesy of Western University of Health Sciences, College of Osteopathic Medicine of the Pacific, Department of NMM/OMM, with permission.)

Splenic Pump (Including Pediatric Variation)

Clinical goal: enhance immune function

Treatment Position

Patient: supine
Physician: seated or standing on patient's left side

Procedure

1. The physician places one hand under the lower posterior rib cage at approximately rib 10 to stabilize chest wall and the other thenar-hypothenar hand anteriorly, over the splenic site (Fig.50.29A).
   Pediatric variation: *Replace the anterolateral hand with the operator's forearm such that the palm of the hand is facing downward (see Fig. 50.29B).*
2. Being mindful that the spleen is a pressure-sensitive organ, the physician creates periodic compression at a rate of 20 to 60 compressions per minute from the anterior site toward the posterior stabilizing site by both moving into the passive range of motion of the chest wall and recognizing the bucket-bale motion of the overlying ribs when doing so. *(In the pediatric variation "waving" the hand at the wrist, or pretending to bounce a ball, transmits an appropriate amount of pressure through the physician's forearm into the pediatric chest cage.)*
3. This may be continued for 1 to 2 minutes or until a softening of the involved tissues is noted.
4. In pediatric cases, warn the parents that the child's fever may initially rise before falling. This is likely due to an increased release of immune-fighting cells from the spleen causing an increase in resultant pyrogens.

Note: *This technique is often contraindicated in individuals with hepatosplenomegaly, as may occur in conditions such as infectious mononucleosis, hemolytic anemia, and cirrhosis.*

Pedal (Dalrymple) Lymphatic Pump Clinical Goal(s): To Enhance Pressure Differentials between the Abdominal and Thoracic Compartments; also to Enhance Immune Function

Treatment Position

Patient: supine
Physician: standing at the feet of the patient

Procedure

1. The physician dorsiflexes the patient's ankles and contacts the balls of the feet to initial tension. Maintaining the ankle dorsiflexion, the physician introduces a superior oscillatory rhythmic force that may further dorsiflex the patient's feet. The umbilicus may be used as a landmark to appreciate a wave of motion.[81]

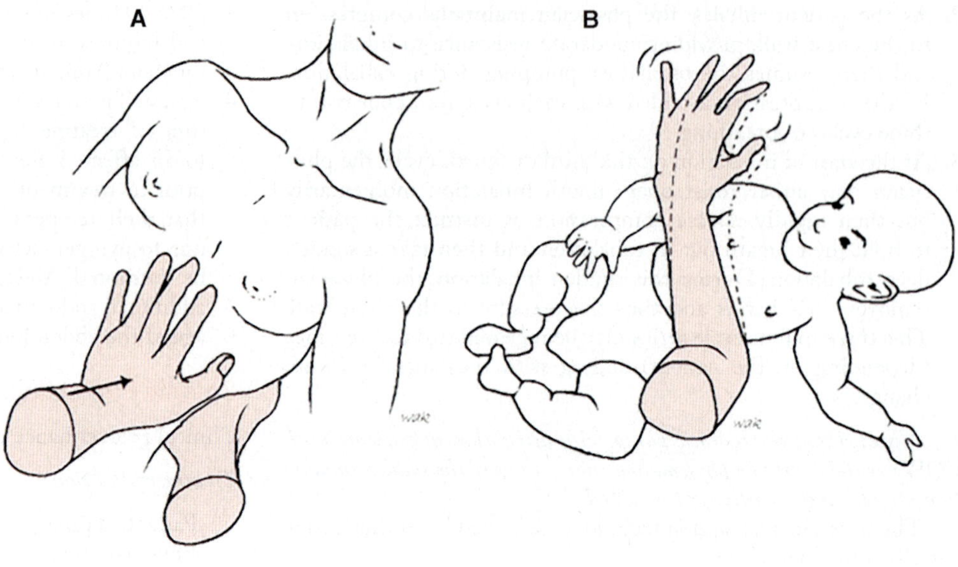

Figure 50.29. Splenic pumps over the rib cage. (**A**) Classic splenic pump and (**B**) splenic pump for treating an infant where the "waving of the hand" interests the infant and yet allows the physician's forearm to provide mild splenic compression. An alternative splenic pump can be applied through the left upper abdominal quadrant. (Modified from Kuchera ML, Kuchera WA. *Osteopathic Considerations in HEENT Disorders: Head, Eyes, Ears, Nose, Throat.* Greyden Press; 2012. Reprinted with permission from Michael L. Kuchera, DO, FAAO.)

2. As the rebound wave returns to the feet, the feet are allowed to return toward neutral but just back to the initial dorsiflexion tension. The rhythmic dorsiflexion force is reapplied at a rate of 110 to 130 cycles per minute as needed to have the abdominal contents push or "slosh" against the thoracoabdominal diaphragm, thereby creating an oscillatory pump[81] (Fig. 50.30).
3. Retest: The pump is typically performed for about 2 minutes; over time, the physician should evaluate the affected area for any decrease in edema or tissue congestion.

Auricular Drainage

Clinical goal(s): lymphatic drainage related to the ears such as otitis externa and otitis media

Treatment Position

Patient: supine or seated

Physician: adjacent to the patient approaching from the front to allow webs between 3rd and 4th digits bilaterally to glide cephala from the earlobe with the 3rd and 4th digits on either side of each ear. This handhold places the bulk of the anterior surface of fingers two to five over the soft tissues on either side of the ears. (This is a superficial OMT technique and does not address temporal bone motion.)

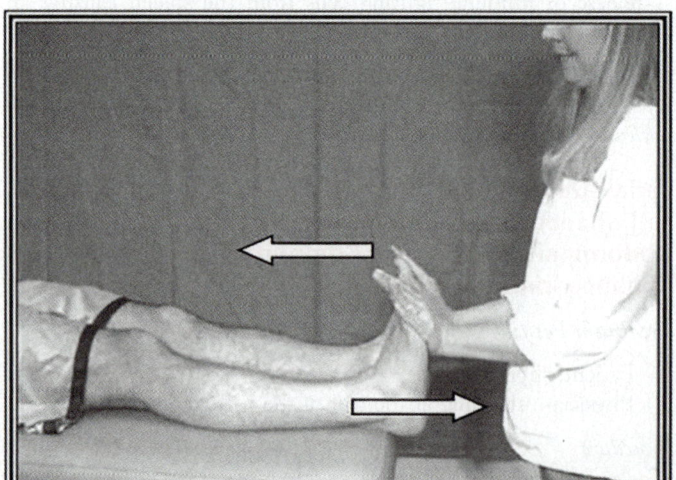

Figure 50.30. Pedal (Dalrymple) lymphatic pump. (Photo courtesy of Western University of Health Sciences, College of Osteopathic Medicine of the Pacific, Department of NMM/OMM, with permission.)

1. Applying a light pressure over the contracted soft tissues, the physician provides an alternating clockwise and counterclockwise rotation of each ear and adjacent tissues of the scalp. This is continued for 1 to 2 minutes (Fig. 50.31).
2. Reassess in the same manner as diagnosed.

Mandibular Drainage and Opening the Eustachian Tube (Galbreath)

Clinical goal(s): Enhance the lymphatic drainage around the pterygoid plexus; remove myofascial dysfunction, MTrPs, and/or stretch the medial pterygoid (MP) muscle; establish conditions to permit the eustachian tube (ET) to open and function properly. The technique is especially useful in the treatment of otitis media or barometric dysacusia[81]; useful in the prevention of otitis media; and has been found to be clinically useful in treatment of TMD if

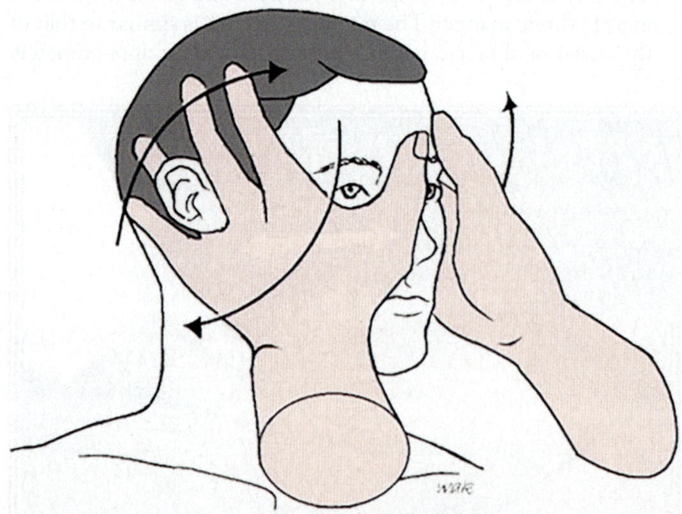

Figure 50.31. Auricular myofascial drainage technique. Alternating clockwise/counterclockwise motions encourage lymphatic drainage from the region of soft tissues and structures around the ear. (Modified from Kuchera ML, Kuchera WA. *Osteopathic Considerations in HEENT Disorders: Head, Eyes, Ears, Nose, Throat.* Greyden Press; 2012. Reprinted with permission from Michael L. Kuchera, DO, FAAO.)

asymmetrical jaw opening motion disappears when the tongue is placed on the hard palate.

Treatment Position

Patient: supine; head turned slightly away from the side to be treated

Physician: one hand stabilizes the head during the technique; the other hand contacts the jaw with the 4th and 5th digits curled behind and along the ascending ramus of the mandible and the hypothenar eminence near the tip of the chin

Procedure

1. The physician asks the patient to relax their jaw as the physician applies a slight inferior traction to the jaw. The physician may request that the patient translate their lower jaw away from their hand. The physician palpates the feeling of the vector involved in that motion in order to duplicate it.
2. The physician applies a slow, rhythmic inferior and lateral translatory motion to carry the inferior jaw to its first myofascial barrier and then allows it to return. This is repeated over a course of 30 to 90 seconds with each cycle lasting 3 to 5 seconds. A short MFR period could be applied at the apex of each cycle. The patient may assist with the treatment motion during the first few cycles to allow them to relax and feel at ease with the procedure.
3. Once completed, this procedure is repeated on the other side.

Note: This technique alternately compresses and releases the pterygoid plexus of veins and lymphatics on one side and stretches the MP muscle on the other. The vessels constitute the primary drainage path for the middle ear and ET; the MP muscle must be pushed aside by the tensor veli palatini to open the ET so this technique is designed to remove MP hypertonicity or triggerpoints.

ACKNOWLEDGMENTS

The authors and editors of this chapter would like to acknowledge the scholarly contributions of Dr. Elaine Wallace for prior editions of this chapter.

REFERENCES

1. Educational Council on Osteopathic Principles (ECOP). *Glossary of Osteopathic Terminology*. American Association of Colleges of Osteopathic Medicine (AACOM); 2011:24.
2. Mortimer PS, Pearson IC. Lymphatic function in severe chronic venous insufficiency. *Phlebolymphology*. 2004;44:253–257.
3. Scallan JP, Zawieja SD, Castorena-Gonzalez JA, Davis MJ. Lymphatic pumping: mechanics, mechanisms and malfunction. *J Physiol*. 2016;594(20): 5749–5768.
4. Zawieja DC. Contractile physiology of lymphatics. *Lymphat Res Biol*. 2009;7(2):87–96.
5. Cleypool CGJ, Mackaaij C, Bruinenberg DL, Schurink B, Bleys RLAW. Sympathetic nerve distribution in human lymph nodes. *J Anat*. 2021;239(2):282–289.
6. Howarth D, Burstal R, Hayes C, Lan L, Lantry G. Autonomic regulation of lymphatic flow in the lower extremity demonstrated on lymphoscintigraphy in patients with reflex sympathetic dystrophy. *Clin Nucl Med*. 1999;24(6):383–387.
7. Chikly B. Who discovered the lymphatic system [published correction appears in Lymphology 1998 Jun;31(2):92]. *Lymphology*. 1997;30(4):186–193.
8. Still AT. The lymphatics. In: *Philosophy of Osteopathy*. A.T. Still; 1899: 105–106.
9. Smith W. Skiagraphy and the circulation. *J Osteopath*. 1899:3:356–378.
10. Millard FP. *Applied Anatomy of the Lymphatics*. Journal Printing Company; 1922.
11. Millard FP. New method of diagnosing various diseases by palpating lymphatic glands. *J Am Osteopath Assoc*. 1920;19:405–408.
12. Millard FP. A lymphatic examination. *J Osteopath*. 1922;29:78–81.
13. Goode GW, Millard FP. Manipulative lymphatic therapy. In: *Selected Papers from the Section of Manipulative Therapeutics*. Vol. 2. American Academy of Osteopathy; 1940:11–14.
14. Millard FP. Lymphatics: prevention of complications of diseases sought through clearance of stasis. *Osteopath Prof*. 1945;13(3):20–23, 56.
15. Zink JG. Respiratory and circulatory care: the conceptual model. *Osteopath Ann*. 1977;5(3):108–112.
16. Zink JG, Lawson WB. The role of pectoral traction in the treatment of lymphatic flow disturbances. *Osteopath Ann*. 1978;6(11):493–496.
17. Zink JG, Fetchik WD, Lawson WE. The posterior axillary folds: a gateway for osteopathic treatment of the upper extremities. *Osteopath Ann*. 1981;9(3):114–117.
18. Smith HJ, Grøttum P, Simonsen S. Ultrasonic assessment of abdominal venous return: I. Effect of cardiac action and respiration on mean velocity pattern, cross-sectional area and flow in the inferior vena cava and portal vein. *Acta Radiol Diagn (Stockh)*. 1985;26(5):581–588.
19. Vodder E. *Le Drainage Lymphatique, Une Nouvelle Méthode Thérapeutique*. Santé Pour Tous; 1936.
20. Chikly B. *Silent Waves: Theory and Practice of Lymph Drainage Therapy: [With Applications for Lymphedema, Chronic Pain and Inflammation]*. 2nd ed. International Health & Healing Publishing; 2011.
21. Zink JG. The osteopathic holistic approach to homeostasis: 1969 Academy Lecture. *1970 Yearbook of the Academy of Applied Osteopathy*. Academy of Applied Osteopathy; 1970:1–5.
22. Still AT. H.H. Gravett Papers. In: Trowbridge C, ed. *Andrew Taylor Still, 1828–1917*. Thomas Jefferson University Press (NMSU); 1991:156.
23. Chikly BJ. Manual techniques addressing the lymphatic system: origins and development. *J Am Osteopath Assoc*. 2005;105(10):457–464.
24. Barber ED. Diseases of the lymphatic system. In: *Osteopathy Complete*. Hudson-Kimberly Publishing Co.; 1898:131–146.
25. Whiting CA. Investigations of the phagocytic index (reprint). 1916. *1955 Yearbook of the Academy of Applied Osteopathy*. Academy of Applied Osteopathy; 1955:107–109.
26. Lane MA. On increasing the antibody content of the serum by manipulation of the spleen. *J Osteopath*. 1920;27:361–364.
27. Castilio Y, Ferris-Swift L. Effects of splenic stimulation in normal individuals on the actual and differential blood cell count, and the opsonic index (reprint). 1932. *1955 Yearbook of the Academy of Applied Osteopathy*. Academy of Applied Osteopathy; 1955:111–120.
28. Castilio Y, Ferris-Swift L. The effect of direct splenic stimulation on the cells and the antibody content of the blood stream in acute infectious diseases (reprint). 1934. *1955 Yearbook of the Academy of Applied Osteopathy*. Academy of Applied Osteopathy; 1955:121–138.
29. Measel JW Jr. The effect of the lymphatic pump on the immune response: I. Preliminary studies on the antibody response to pneumococcal polysaccharide assayed by bacterial agglutination and passive hemagglutination. *J Am Osteopath Assoc*. 1982;82(1):28–31.
30. Measel JW, Kafity AA. The effect of the lymphatic pump on the B and T cells in peripheral blood (abstract). *J Am Osteopath Assoc*. 1986;86(9):608.
31. Schander A, Padro D, King HH, Downey HF, Hodge LM. Lymphatic pump treatment repeatedly enhances the lymphatic and immune systems. *Lymphat Res Biol*. 2013;11(4):219–226.
32. Huff JB, Schander A, Downey HF, Hodge LM. Lymphatic pump treatment augments lymphatic flux of lymphocytes in rats. *Lymphat Res Biol*. 2010;8(4):183–187.
33. Hodge LM, Bearden MK, Schander A, et al. Lymphatic pump treatment mobilizes leukocytes from the gut associated lymphoid tissue into lymph. *Lymphat Res Biol*. 2010;8(2):103–110.
34. Miller CE. The lymphatic pump, its application to acute infections. *J Am Osteopath Assoc*. 1926;25:443–445.
35. Miller CE. Osteopathic principles and thoracic pump therapeutics proved by scientific research. *J Am Osteopath Assoc*. 1927;26:910–914.
36. Ruddy TJ. Osteopathic manipulation in eye, ear, nose, and throat disease. In: Barnes MW, ed. *1962 Year Book of Selected Osteopathic Papers*. 1962;133–140.
37. Galbreath WO. Acute otitis media: including its postural and manipulative treatment. *J Am Osteopath Assoc*. 1929;28:377–379.

38. Pratt-Harrington D. Galbreath technique: a manipulative treatment for otitis media revisited. *J Am Osteopath Assoc.* 2000;100(10):635–639.
39. Sutherland WG. *Teachings in the Science of Osteopathy.* Sutherland Cranial Teaching Foundation Inc.; 1990:13.
40. U.S. Department of Health and Human Services. *Reporter - Active Projects.* National Institutes of Health. August 8, 2023. Accessed July 1, 2024. https://reporter.nih.gov/
41. Kuchera ML, Kuchera WA. *Osteopathic Considerations in Head, Eyes, Ears, Nose Throat (HEENT) Disorders.* Greyden Press LLC; 2011:191–213.
42. Knott EM, Tune JD, Stoll ST, Downey HF. Increased lymphatic flow in the thoracic duct during manipulative intervention. *J Am Osteopath Assoc.* 2005;105(10):447–456.
43. Hodge LM, King HH, Williams AG Jr, et al. Abdominal lymphatic pump treatment increases leukocyte count and flux in thoracic duct lymph. *Lymphat Res Biol.* 2007;5(2):127–133.
44. Mancini D, Cesari M, Lunghi C, Benigni AM, Antonelli Incalzi R, Scarlata S. Ultrasound evaluation of diaphragmatic mobility and contractility after osteopathic manipulative techniques in healthy volunteers: a prospective, randomized, double-blinded clinical trial. *J Manipulative Physiol Ther.* 2019;42(1):47–54.
45. Leak LV, Cadet JL, Griffin CP, Richardson K. Nitric oxide production by lymphatic endothelial cells in vitro. *Biochem Biophys Res Commun.* 1995;217(1):96–105.
46. Schmid-Schönbein GW. Nitric oxide (NO) side of lymphatic flow and immune surveillance. *Proc Natl Acad Sci U S A.* 2012;109(1):3–4.
47. Didem K, Ufuk YS, Serdar S, Zümre A. The comparison of two different physiotherapy methods in treatment of lymphedema after breast surgery. *Breast Cancer Res Treat.* 2005;93(1):49–54.
48. Földi E, Földi M, Clodius L. The lymphedema chaos: a lancet. *Ann Plast Surg.* 1989;22(6):505–515.
49. Zein-Hammoud M, Standley PR. Modeled osteopathic manipulative treatments: a review of their in vitro effects on fibroblast tissue preparations. *J Am Osteopath Assoc.* 2015;115(8):490–502.
50. da Silveira MP, Fagundes KKS, Bizuti MR, Starck E, Rossi RC, Silva DTR. Physical exercise as a tool to help the immune system against COVID-19: an integrative review of the current literature. *Clin Exp Med.* 2021;21(1):15–28.
51. Walkowski S, Singh M, Puertas J, Pate M, Goodrum K, Benencia F. Osteopathic manipulative therapy induces early plasma cytokine release and mobilization of a population of blood dendritic cells. *PLoS One.* 2014;9(3):e90132.
52. Remien K, Woo MJ, Vilella RC. Osteopathic manipulative treatment: lymphatic procedures. In: *StatPearls.* StatPearls Publishing; 2024.
53. Zainuddin Z, Newton M, Sacco P, Nosaka K. Effects of massage on delayed-onset muscle soreness, swelling, and recovery of muscle function. *J Athl Train.* 2005;40(3):174–180.
54. Dodd JG, Good MM, Nguyen TL, Grigg AI, Batia LM, Standley PR. In vitro biophysical strain model for understanding mechanisms of osteopathic manipulative treatment. *J Am Osteopath Assoc.* 2006;106(3):157–166.
55. Meltzer KR, Standley PR. Modeled repetitive motion strain and indirect osteopathic manipulative techniques in regulation of human fibroblast proliferation and interleukin secretion. *J Am Osteopath Assoc.* 2007; 107(12):527–536.
56. Leduc A, Lievens P, Dewald J. The influence of multidirectional vibrations on wound healing and on regeneration of blood- and lymph vessels. *Lymphology.* 1981;14(4):179–185.
57. Cline CC, Coast JR, Arnall DA. A chest wall restrictor to study effects on pulmonary function and exercise. 1. Development and validation. *Respiration.* 1999;66(2):182–187.
58. Howell RK, Allen TW, Kappler RE. The influence of osteopathic manipulative therapy in the management of patients with chronic obstructive lung disease. *J Am Osteopath Assoc.* 1975;74(8):757–760.
59. Sleszynski SL, Kelso AF. Comparison of thoracic manipulation with incentive spirometry in preventing postoperative atelectasis. *J Am Osteopath Assoc.* 1993;93(8):834–845.
60. Pratt-Harrington D, Neptune-Ceran R. The effect of OMT in the post-abdominal surgery patient. *Acad Appl Osteopath J.* 1995;9:9–13.
61. Kakizaki F, Shibuya M, Yamazaki T, et al. Preliminary report on the effects of respiratory muscle stretch gymnastics on chest wall mobility in patients with COPD. *Respir Care.* 1999;44(4):409–414.
62. Minoguchi H, Shibuya M, Miyagawa T, et al. Cross-over comparison between respiratory muscle stretch gymnastics and inspiratory muscle training. *Intern Med.* 2002;41(10):805–812.
63. Shanmugananth E, Chandramouli E, Nambi SG, Parthasarathy S. Effect of respiratory muscle stretch gymnastics on chest expansion and peak expiratory flow rate among sawmill workers. *Asian J Pharm Res Health Care.* 2022;14(4):220–223.
64. Jackson KM, Steele TF, Dugan EP, Kukulka G, Blue W, Roberts A. Effect of lymphatic and splenic pump techniques on the antibody response to hepatitis B vaccine: a pilot study. *J Am Osteopath Assoc.* 1998;98(3):155–160.
65. Noll DR, Degenhardt BF, Stuart MK, Werden S, McGovern RJ, Johnson JC. The effect of osteopathic manipulative treatment on immune response to the influenza vaccine in nursing homes residents: a pilot study. *Altern Ther Health Med.* 2004;10(4):74–76.
66. Gevitz N. Center or periphery? The future of osteopathic principles and practices. *J Am Osteopath Assoc.* 2006;106(3):121–129.
67. Overberger R, Hoyt JA, Daghigh F, et al. Comparing changes in serum nitric oxide levels and heart rate after osteopathic manipulative treatment (OMT) using the Dalrymple pedal pump to changes measured after active exercise. *J Am Osteopath Assoc.* 2009;109(1):41–42.
68. Ota KS. Postmastectomy lymphedema: a call for osteopathic medical research. *J Am Osteopath Assoc.* 2006;106(3):110–111.
69. Opipari MI, Perrotta AL, Essig-Beatty DR. Oncology. In: Ward RC, ed. *Foundations of Osteopathic Medicine.* 2nd ed. Lippincott Williams & Wilkins; 2003:473–474.
70. Patterson MM. The coming influenza pandemic: lessons from the past for the future [published correction appears in J Am Osteopath Assoc. 2006 Jan;106(1):3]. *J Am Osteopath Assoc.* 2005;105(11):498–500.
71. D'Alonzo GE Jr. Influenza epidemic or pandemic? Time to roll up sleeves, vaccinate patients, and hone osteopathic manipulative skills. *J Am Osteopath Assoc.* 2004;104(9):370–371.
72. Hruby RJ, Hoffman KN. Avian influenza: an osteopathic component to treatment. *Osteopath Med Prim Care.* 2007;1:10.
73. Martinez E, Redding D. Osteopathic response to the COVID-19 pandemic. *J Am Osteopath Assoc.* 2020.
74. Hensel K, ex. ed. *A Teaching Guide for Osteopathic Manipulative Medicine.* American Association of Colleges of Osteopathic Medicine; 2015:55–56.
75. Dumont AE, Clauss RH, Reed GE, Tice DA. Lymph drainage in patients with congestive heart failure. Comparison with findings in hepatic cirrhosis. *N Engl J Med.* 1963;269:949–952.
76. Kuchera ML, Kuchera WA. *Osteopathic Considerations in Systemic Function.* Greyden Press; 1994:53–78.
77. Park H, Han D. The effect of the correlation between the contraction of the pelvic floor muscles and diaphragmatic motion during breathing. *J Phys Ther Sci.* 2015;27(7):2113–2115.
78. Zink JG. Applications of the osteopathic holistic approach to homeostasis. *Am Acad Osteo Yearb.* 1973;37–47:42.
79. Sucher BM. Myofascial release of carpal tunnel syndrome. *J Am Osteopath Assoc.* 1993;93(1):92–94, 100–101.
80. Nicholas AS, Nicholas EA. *Atlas of Osteopathic Techniques.* Wolters Kluwer Health/Lippincott Williams & Wilkins; 2008:504–507.
81. Kuchera ML, Irwin J, Myers NE, Ferencz V, Nelson J. Documenting and comparing frequencies and forces used to perform lymphatic pump OMT manually and with use of a machine. *JAOA* 2011;111(8):489–490.

51 Muscle Energy

WALTER C. EHRENFEUCHTER ▪ REBECCA E. GIUSTI

KEY CONCEPTS

- Muscle energy is a direct osteopathic treatment method in which a patient, on request, actively uses their muscles from a controlled position and in a specific direction against a distinct counterforce.
- While postisometric relaxation is a widely used principle of muscle energy technique, other physiologic principles may be used alone or in combination to address somatic dysfunction including joint mobilization using muscle force, respiratory assist, oculocephalogyric reflex, reciprocal inhibition, crossed extensor reflex, isokinetic strengthening, isolytic lengthening, muscle force to move one region of the body to achieve motion in another region and multiple mini isotonic contractions.
- The versatility of this modality allows for its combination with any of the other osteopathic manipulative techniques, in total patient management.

DEFINITION

- Muscle energy is a direct osteopathic treatment method in which a patient, on request, actively uses their muscles from a controlled position and in a specific direction against a distinct counterforce. These techniques involve the patient's active cooperation to:
  - □ Contract a muscle or muscles.
  - □ Inhale or exhale
  - □ Move one bone of a joint in a specific direction relative to the adjacent bone.

For these reasons, muscle energy cannot be used if the patient is in a coma, uncooperative, or unresponsive.[1]

HISTORY

Muscle energy is a system of osteopathic approach to patient-specific diagnosis and treatment with roots extending back to Andrew Taylor Still. Dr. Still did not record the way he treated. Instead, he preferred that his students have a thorough understanding of anatomy and physiology, determine the root of the patient's problem through history and diagnostic palpation and then apply osteopathic principles and philosophy as rational treatment.

As the osteopathic profession sought to increase the efficiency of teaching manipulative treatments, certain individuals made key contributions. Fred Mitchell, Sr. developed a plan of patient-specific diagnosis and treatment he termed muscle energy, because of its reliance on active patient effort through a muscular restrictive barrier. Mitchell[2] credited Kettler as the first to focus attention on the importance of the vast amount of tissue involved between joints, muscle, and fascia, and the changes they undergo in the lesioning process. Kettler also emphasized that without establishing bilateral myofascial harmony, the lesion pattern will not be obliterated and will return again and again.

Some sources allege that muscle energy techniques (METs) are an outgrowth of the resistive duction method developed by T. J. Ruddy.[3] In the Ruddy approach, the patient is instructed to move quickly, often at a rate of 60 excursions per minute (or that equal to the patient's pulse rate), while the physician offers resistance to this active movement. The purpose for the patient's quick and repetitive muscle contraction was twofold:

1. To increase blood (and other tissue fluid) movements to remove metabolic waste products from the cells and circulate oxygen.
2. To tone inactive muscles that may be weak.

Mitchell (personal communication, 1970–1974) expanded Ruddy's concept of the unyielding counterforce as a treatment strategy to functionally reverse the origin and insertion of the muscle(s).

Mitchell and Kettler were likely unaware of the proprioceptive neuromuscular facilitation (PNF) techniques developed by Kabat, Knott, and Voss at the Kabat-Kaiser Institute during the late 1940s. These techniques were not widely known. PNF uses skills to reeducate muscle for several reasons[4]:

1. "To gain inhibition in muscles which may be in a protective spasm."
2. "To improve range (of motion) at an intervertebral level"

Mitchell first published his description of the model in 1948, in the Academy of Applied Osteopathy Yearbook, in "The Balanced Pelvis in Relation to Chapman Reflexes" which did not include all the diagnostic pelvic landmarks and tests and only referenced high-velocity, low-amplitude (HVLA) as a treatment modality. In his 1958 publication "Structural Pelvic Function," he expanded his understanding to include all the diagnostic pelvic landmarks and tests and the treatments described were METs.

- He described one method of correction in which the physician provided the extrinsic activating force as a guide to the patient's intrinsic respiratory and muscular cooperation.
- He wrote about the direct method treatments of soft tissues (with attention to fasciae) using Neidner fascial release prior to articular correction.
- He argued that muscular energy technique, with its many ramifications, is a useful tool in preparation of the soft tissues. Ligamentous stretching may also be of use before articular correction is attempted.[2]

12 years after his last publication, Mitchell Sr. taught his MET diagnostic and treatment approach for the whole body to numerous physicians through tutorials. He held his first 6-day tutorial in Fort Dodge, IA, in 1970, which was attended by osteopathic physicians John Goodridge, Philip Greenman, Rolland Miller, Devota Nowland, Edward Stiles, and Sara (Sally) Sutton. Several

5-day tutorials were subsequently given across the country and internationally. In 1972, Mitchell examination and treatment procedures were videotaped at Michigan State University's College of Osteopathic Medicine, as part of an initiative to introduce MET into the curriculum.

After Mitchell Sr.'s death in 1974, the American Academy of Osteopathy organized a committee of physicians who had taken a Mitchell Sr. tutorial, to develop a manual for a 5-day course to familiarize others with Mitchell Sr.'s work, chaired by Sally Sutton with members: Fred Mitchell Jr., Philip Greenman Jr., Edward Stiles, Paul Kimberly, Steve Blood, and Lauren Rex. Drs. Greenman, Stiles, Sutton, and Mitchell Jr. also began teaching courses nationally and internationally over the ensuing 4 decades. Initially, the five earlier established osteopathic colleges began to integrate muscle energy procedures into their curricula. Additional tutorials were conducted from 1977 to 1981, for faculty at the newly established colleges of osteopathic medicine.

Lewit and Simons[5] stated that postisometric relaxation was pioneered by Mitchell Sr., and clearly described by F. L. Mitchell Jr., as a mobilization technique that applies gentle force to improve "articulation," thereby restoring previously restricted movement. Later authors believed that Mitchell muscle energy approach accomplished this more quickly than did the PNF techniques. Because Mitchell work was not recorded in indexed allopathic literature, Travell and Simons[6] credited the concept of applying postisometric relaxation in the treatment of myofascial pain to Lewis, who first presented the idea in a North American journal in 1984.

In 1979, Mitchell Jr. et al.[7] published the manual currently in use as reference by most osteopathic medical colleges. In 1999, Mitchell, Jr. published an exhaustive text on the muscle energy approach.[8] His muscle energy diagnostic and treatment procedures are a standard component of the osteopathic manipulative medicine curriculum today and are also used by many physical therapists. Unfortunately, a lot of the patient-specific finetuning and treatment concepts that Mitchell, Sr. taught in the tutorials was never published.

DEFINITIONS RELATED TO MUSCLE ENERGY TECHNIQUE

The definitions of the terms listed below are critical for a thorough comprehension of METs and their proposed mechanisms of action:

1. *Contraction*: Shortening and/or development of tension in a muscle.
2. *Contracted muscle*: The physiologic response to a neuromuscular excitation that may be characterized by histologic change in which noncontractile tissue is substituted for muscle tissue which prevents the muscle from reaching its normal relaxed length.
3. *Contracture*: A condition of fixed high resistance to passive stretch of a muscle, resulting from fibrosis of the tissues supporting the muscles or the joints, or from disorders of the muscle fibers.
4. *Concentric contraction*: Contraction of a muscle resulting in the approximation of the origin and insertion.
5. *Eccentric contraction*: The muscle tension allows the origin and insertion to separate, in effect to lengthen.
6. *Isometric contraction*: The distance between the origin and the insertion of the muscle is maintained at a constant length. The involved joint or limb does not move. For example, if a patient provides a force against a physician, the physician responds with equal force; therefore there is a change in the tension of the muscle but no approximation of the muscle origin and insertion.
7. *Isolytic contraction*: A form of eccentric contraction in which the patient's voluntary concentric muscle contraction is overpowered by a stronger counterforce applied by the physician. Thus, the affected muscle is lengthened. As the muscle contracts, it is forced to elongate. This is most commonly used for the treatment of fibrotic or chronically shortened myofascial tissues or to disrupt adhesions.
8. *Isokinetic contraction*: A concentric contraction against resistance in which the angular change of joint motion is at the same rate. The counterforce is less than the patient force.
9. *Isotonic contraction*: A technique that involves voluntary muscular contraction by the patient against a steady but *yielding* counterforce of the physician (the involved joint angle will increase or decrease), allowing the contracted muscle to maintain its tone through the range of motion.
10. *Sherrington Law*: (a) Every posterior spinal nerve root supplies a specific region of the skin, although fibers from adjacent spinal segments may invade such a region. (b) When a muscle receives a nerve impulse to contract, its antagonist receives, simultaneously, an impulse to relax.
11. *Golgi tendon organ*: A spindle-shaped end organ within a tendon that provides information about muscle tension. It becomes relatively stretched during muscular contraction where the overall length of the muscle does not change. When a critical amount of tension occurs, its increased activity provides a reflex relaxation of the muscle as a whole.
12. *Monoarticular Muscles*: Also referred to as short restrictors, considered key in maintaining Type II segmental dysfunctions.
13. *Polyarticular Muscles*: Also referred to as long restrictors, considered key in maintaining Type I group dysfunctions.

OVERVIEW OF MUSCLE ENERGY AND PROPOSED MECHANISM OF ACTION

Overview

METs are often considered to be direct (engaging the restrictive barrier[s]) and active (the patient contributes a corrective force).[9] In distinguishing MET from other techniques, Mitchell, Jr., discussed the indication and diagnostic criteria for MET. He described vertebral articular mobilization as the primary application of MET. He regarded muscle spasm and tightness, when they occur, as neurologic consequences of postural and locomotor adaptation to articular dysfunction, usually located elsewhere in the body.[10]

He stated that MET is occasionally used to:

- Lengthen tight or short muscles
- Strengthen weak muscles
- Remove peripheral edema
- Reduce articular subluxations
- Stretch deep fascia[10]

The criteria for diagnosing articular restriction are based on motion restriction as determined by assessing changes in the static positions of bony landmarks before and after movement.

Research continues to evolve which may provide a more comprehensive picture of the clinical effectiveness of this technique.[10]

What is emerging is that muscles are not isolated but embedded in a three-dimensional connective tissue network that links them to adjacent muscles and other nonmuscular structures in the body. Therefore, changes in length, activation level, or disruption of the connective tissue of neighboring muscles, can affect how muscles interact and produce force on the skeleton.[11]

The "motor unit" or the "muscle" has long been considered the quantal element in the control of movement, but it now seems that there is a strong interaction between muscle fibers and intramuscular connective tissue, and between muscles and fasciae, suggesting that the muscles can no longer be considered the only elements that organize movement. In addition, innervation and vascularization of muscle is strongly connected with intramuscular connective tissue.[12]

With these emerging findings, the clinical effectiveness and sometimes wide-reaching effects of muscle energy may be further elucidated.

Proposed Mechanism of Action

The following physiologic principles of MET have been described:

1. Postisometric relaxation
2. Joint mobilization using muscle force
3. Respiratory assistance
4. Oculocephalogyric reflex
5. Reciprocal inhibition
6. Crossed extensor reflex
7. Isokinetic strengthening
8. Isolytic lengthening
9. Using muscle force to move one region of the body to achieve movement of another bone or region
10. Multiple mini isotonic contractions (personal communication, Mitchell, Sr.)

The following section describes the goals, physiologic basis, and contraction force for each of these principles. Each treatment section then describes the role of each principle in the treatment of somatic dysfunction.

1. **Postisometric Relaxation**
   Goal
   Muscle relaxation
   Physiologic Basis
   Mitchell Jr.[13] postulated that immediately after an isometric contraction, the neuromuscular apparatus is in a refractory state during which passive stretching may be performed without encountering strong myotatic reflex opposition. The physician only needs to resist the contraction, and then take up the slack in the muscles during the relaxed refractory period. With muscle contraction, there may also be increased tension on the Golgi organ proprioceptors in the tendons; this inhibits the active muscle's contraction.
   Force of Contraction
   Sustained gentle pressure (minimum amount of pressure to produce the maximal effect.)
2. **Joint Mobilization Using Muscle Force**
   Goal
   Restoration of joint motion in an articular dysfunction.
   Physiologic Basis
   Distortion of articular relationships and motion loss results in a reflex hypertonicity of the musculature crossing the dysfunctional joint, similar to thrust (HVLA) technique. This increase in muscle tone tends to compress the joint surfaces, and results in thinning of the intervening layer of synovial fluid and adherence of the joint surfaces. Restoration of motion to the articulation results in a gapping or reseating of the distorted joint relations with reflex relaxation of the previously hypertonic musculature.
   Force of Contraction
   Maximal muscle contraction that can be comfortably resisted by the physician
3. **Respiratory Assistance**
   Goal
   To improve body physiology with the patient's voluntary respiratory motion.
   Physiologic Basis
   The muscular forces involved in these techniques are generated by the simple act of breathing. This may involve the use of the respiratory muscles themselves, or of the motion transmitted to the spine, pelvis, and extremities in response to ventilation motions. A fulcrum is usually applied against which the respiratory forces can work.
   Force of Contraction
   Exaggerated respiratory motion
4. **Oculocephalogyric Reflex**
   Goal
   To affect reflex muscle contractions using eye motion.
   Physiologic Basis
   Functional muscle groups are contracted in response to the patient's voluntary eye motion, which reflexively affect the cervical and truncal musculature as the body attempts to follow the lead provided by the motion. This approach can be used to produce very gentle postisometric relaxation or reciprocal inhibition.
   Force of Contraction
   Exceptionally gentle
   Contraindications
   - □ Fracture, dislocation, or moderate to severe segmental instability in the cervical spine.
   - □ Evocation of neurologic symptoms or signs on rotation of the neck.
   - □ Recent eye surgery or trauma
5. **Reciprocal Inhibition**
   Goal
   To lengthen a muscle shortened by cramp or acute spasm.
   Physiologic Basis
   Initiating a gentle contraction in the spastic muscle's ANTAGONIST muscle results in a reflex relaxation of the spastic muscle and its agonistic group.
   Force of Contraction
   Very gentle (think ounces, not pounds of pressure)
6. **Crossed Extensor Reflex**
   Goal
   To treat muscles located in the extremities, in an area so severely injured (e.g., fractures or burns) that it is not directly manipulable or accessible.
   Physiologic Basis
   This technique makes use of the learned cross pattern locomotion reflex engram in the central nervous system. When the flexor muscle in one extremity is contracted voluntarily, the flexor muscle in the contralateral extremity relaxes, and the extensor contracts.
   Force of Contraction
   Very gentle (think ounces, not pounds of pressure)
7. **Isokinetic Strengthening**
   Goal
   To reestablish normal tone and strength in a muscle weakened by reflex hypertonicity of the opposing muscle group.
   Physiologic Basis
   Where asymmetry of range of motion exists, there is also the potential for asymmetry in muscle strength. If there is

shortening of an antagonist muscle, attend to that first. Jull and Janda[14] believe that the length of the agonists spontaneously increases if the shortened or hypertonic fibers are lengthened first. Further restoration of strength can then be accomplished through an isokinetic contraction, in which length change occurs at a constant velocity. Typically, concentric contractions are used, where the muscle is permitted to shorten, but at a controlled, slow rate.

Force of Contraction

Sustained gentle pressure

8. **Isolytic Lengthening**

   Goal

   To lengthen a muscle shortened by contracture and fibrosis.

   Physiologic Basis

   The vibration used in this technique is postulated to have some effect on the myotatic units, in addition to its mechanical and circulatory effects.[15]

   Force of Contraction

   Maximal contraction that can be comfortably resisted by the physician.

9. **Using Muscle Force to move one region of the body to achieve movement of another bone or region**

   Goal

   To treat somatic dysfunction.

   Physiologic Basis

   For some dysfunctions, especially those involving the pelvis, it is often more effective to move one body structure by moving another body structure adjacent to it. Muscular force is used to move the first structure, and the body's response to that force is then transmitted to another region of the body.

   Force of Contraction

   Sustained gentle pressure

10. **Multiple mini isotonic contractions**

    Goal

    To treat somatic dysfunction.

    Physiologic Basis

    When employing isotonic procedures, the classic law of reciprocal innervation and inhibition must be considered. When an agonist muscle contracts and shortens, there is reciprocal inhibition of the antagonist muscle causing the antagonist to relax and lengthen so that smooth motion directed by the agonist can occur.[16]

    For example, for a thoracic ERS_L, the patient's muscular contraction to the left will inhibit the left short restrictors (likely the Golgi system), enabling the left facet pair to open. Simultaneously the left long muscle mobilizers micro-shorten. The isometric contraction becomes a mini-isotonic contraction and enables the vertebra to flex, sidebend, and rotate right.

    Force of Contraction

    Minimum amount of force for maximal beneficial effect

INDICATIONS

Presence of somatic dysfunction in the absence of contraindications.

CONTRAINDICATIONS

- Postisometric relaxation and joint mobilization using muscle force type techniques are contraindicated for:
  - Acutely injured or painful muscles. These would be better addressed using a reciprocal inhibition technique.
  - A patient with low vitality, whose condition can be further compromised with active muscle exertion.
  - For instance, a postsurgical patient or a patient in an intensive care unit immediately following a myocardial infarction.
  - These patients could still be treated with techniques requiring the use of respiratory assistance, oculocephalogyric reflex, reciprocal inhibition, or the crossed extensor reflex, as these techniques are exceptionally gentle.
- Oculocephalogyric reflex techniques are contraindicated for:
  - Anyone who has undergone recent eye surgery or has recently sustained trauma to the eye.
- METs are contraindicated for:
  - Any individual unable or unwilling to follow the physician's verbal directions.
- At the site of treatment:
  - Infection, hematoma, tear in the muscle involved
  - Fracture, avulsion, or dislocation of involved joint
  - Severe osteoporosis that is unable to tolerate sustained or resisted muscle contraction
  - Metastatic disease of bone or soft tissue
  - Rheumatologic/inflammatory conditions or congenital spinal abnormalities, for example, causing instability of the cervical spine
- Relative contraindications at site of treatment include:
  - Undiagnosed joint swelling of involved joint
  - Positioning that compromises vasculature
  - Open wounds

COMPLICATIONS

- Minor complications such as posttreatment muscle or joint soreness tend to be self-limiting and resolve within 24 to 36 hours without additional treatment. This soreness is likely due to the metabolic process of muscular contraction which results in the release of carbon dioxide, lactic acid, and other metabolic waste products that need to be transported and metabolized.[16]
- Complications are minimized with judicious application of the appropriate type of MET.
- Use of inappropriately excessive force has been reported to result in tendon avulsion from bone (in an 85-year-old man) and rib fracture (in a patient with osteoporosis).
- Inappropriate application of oculocephalogyric reflex with cervical range-of-motion METs resulted in anterior chamber intraocular hemorrhage in a single patient postcataract removal and lens implant surgery (author's personal experience).

SAFETY AND EFFICACY

METs have inherent safety due to the patient's intrinsic application of corrective force. Too vigorous a contraction on the part of the patient can render the technique less effective, and result in posttreatment soreness or muscle spasm. Therefore, it is imperative that the osteopathic physician correctly instructs the patient on how much force to generate when performing the treatment.

PRINCIPLES OF DIAGNOSIS

The physician should make an accurate diagnosis prior to initiating any treatment sequence. Although a diagnosis of somatic dysfunction from the muscle energy perspective has some unique elements, they are well described in the chapters on the osteopathic structural exam and the functional anatomy and segmental examination of the body regions. The reader is referred to those chapters (Chapters 30 to 40) for further information on appropriate diagnostic techniques.

PRINCIPLES OF TREATMENT

Muscle energy may be applied to various somatic dysfunctions including two types of muscle restrictions that affect vertebral articular mobilization:

- Monoarticular muscles
  - Also referred to as short restrictors, considered to be instrumental in maintaining type II segmental dysfunctions
- Polyarticular muscles
  - Also referred to as long restrictors, considered to be involved in the maintenance of type II groups dysfunctions

Based on an accurate diagnosis, a muscle energy procedure follows these principles:

1. The physician positions the body part to be treated as follows:
   - At the position of initial resistance—It is important that only the "feather edge" of the restrictive barrier is engaged for maximal efficacy of these techniques. The "feather edge" is the point where the restrictive barrier is just beginning to be engaged, or where the tissue tension is just palpable.
   - With finetuning—Using small movements in every direction such that any movement is localized at the "feather edge" of the restrictive articular barrier (facet, joint).
2. The physician helps the patient obtain an effective *direction* of movement for the limb, trunk, or head, then instructs the patient on the appropriate *intensity* and *duration* of the muscle contraction. The force should be the minimum amount of pressure to produce the maximal beneficial effect.
3. The physician directs the patient to contract the appropriate muscle(s) or muscle group.
4. The physician provides an unyielding counterforce in opposition to and equal to the patient's muscle contraction and maintains forces until an appropriate patient contraction is perceived at the critical articulation or area.
   - This generally requires 3 to 5 seconds, but the duration may vary with the size of the muscle being treated.
5. The patient is directed to relax the area being treated by gently ceasing the contraction, while the physician simultaneously matches the decrease in patient force. It is important to maintain the new positioning against the remaining part of the restrictive barrier.
   - The physician's proprioceptors are used to sense tissue relaxation as the patient relaxes.
   - This usually takes 1 to 2 seconds (postrelaxation phase).
6. The physician takes up the slack permitted by the procedure (e.g., moving the joint toward the remaining part of the restrictive barrier in all three planes in the case of an isometric muscle energy procedure). The slack is formed by the decreased tension in the tight muscle, allowing for it to be passively lengthened. The physician notes increased range of motion.
7. Steps 1 to 6 are generally repeated 3 to 5 times until the best possible increase in motion is obtained. The quality of response often peaks at the third excursion, with diminishing return thereafter. (However, 3 to 5 times is the standard, especially when first learning to correctly apply the technique.)
8. The physician reevaluates the original dysfunction.

Positive treatment outcomes depend on:

- Accurate diagnosis
- Sufficient localization
- Appropriate levels of force

Negative outcomes are most often caused by:

- Inaccurate diagnosis
- Improperly localized forces
- Forces that are too strong

DIAGNOSIS

An inaccurate diagnosis may lead to inappropriate treatment and prevent the desired improvement in the patient's condition. Even with an accurate segmental diagnosis, complicating factors and the patient's entire clinical picture must be considered. Treatment may not improve due to a more primary somatic dysfunction elsewhere in the body. For example, a careful diagnosis may indicate that side-bending is restricted at a segment superior to the one identified for treatment; this then interferes with the localization required, and the superior segment may need to be treated before the inferior segment.

LOCALIZATION

The localization of force is more important than the intensity of force. Localization depends on the physician's palpatory perception of movement (or resistance to movement) at or about a specific articulation. Such perception enables the physician to make subtle assessments about a dysfunction, and to create variations of suggested treatment procedures.

Monitoring the localization of forces and confining the direction of force by the diagnosed muscle group to the level of somatic dysfunction are important to achieve desired results. Imprecise localization, such as motion introduced into an articulation that is a segment or two below the dysfunctional one, decreases the probability of success as the forces have been directed to the wrong segment and facet pair and therefore the wrong corresponding muscles.

AMOUNT OF FORCE

Using excessive force is a commonly made mistake in applying MET. This is not a wrestling match between the patient and physician. Excessive force recruits other muscles to assist with stabilizing the body part being treated, which may completely negate the intent of the technique. Excessive forces used on older patients can result in tendon avulsion from bone. The force required is just enough to restore harmonious motion to the restricted region.

ASYMMETRICAL MUSCLE STRENGTH

Where asymmetrical range of motion occurs, consider and test for possible asymmetrical strength. Some ranges of motion may be asymmetrical due to weakness of a group of muscles, rather than to the shortness of the antagonist group. If asymmetry of muscle strength is present, employ a method to increase the strength of the weak muscle group.

Progressive resistance exercises are used to strengthen weakened muscle groups. If weakness and shortness occur in different muscle groups, but on the same side, attend to the shortness first. According to Jull and Janda,[14] the agonists spontaneously increase their strength if shortened, or if hypertonic fibers are lengthened.

ILLUSTRATIVE TREATMENT TECHNIQUES

M99.00 Craniocervical Somatic Dysfunction

Example

DIAGNOSIS
Acute cervical sprain and strain (Whiplash)

POSITION
Occiput is flexed on C1

RESTRICTION
Occiput is restricted in extension on C1

TYPE OF MUSCLE ENERGY
Postisometric relaxation

TREATMENT POSITION
Patient: Supine
Physician: Seated at the head of the table

PROCEDURE

1. One of the physician's hands is placed beneath the occiput, with the fingers in contact with the suboccipital musculature.
2. The index and middle fingers of the physician's other hand are placed on top of the patient's chin (Figs. 51.1 and 51.2).
3. The patient is instructed to very gently tilt the head backward, so that the chin lifts against the physician's fingers.
   - The physician should be able to palpate the contraction of the suboccipital muscles with the hand beneath the occiput.
4. This contraction is maintained for a full 3 to 5 seconds.
5. The patient is instructed to relax, while the physician simultaneously ceases the applied counterforce. Wait 2 seconds for the tissues to relax.
6. The physician's fingers shift from the front of the patient's chin, to just below the chin.
7. The physician lifts the chin superiorly, while simultaneously pressing inferiorly with the hand beneath the occiput until the new restrictive barrier is engaged.
8. The fingers of the physician are then shifted once again to the anterior surface of the chin.
9. Steps 3 to 8 are repeated 3 to 5 times.
10. Success of the technique is determined by retesting occipitoatlantal segmental motion.

M99.01 Cervical Somatic Dysfunction

Example 1

DIAGNOSIS
Cervical segmental somatic dysfunction: C5FRSR

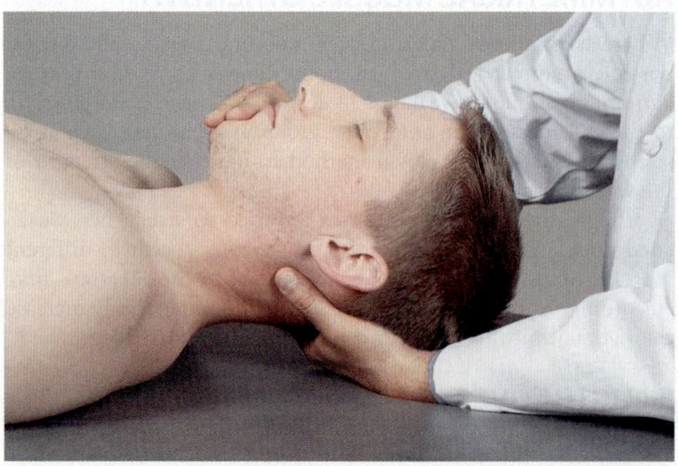

Figure 51.1. Occipitoatlantal (C0–C1) dysfunction example. C0 ES_LR_R—Postisometric relaxation. (Reprinted from Nicholas AS, Nicholas EA. *Atlas of Osteopathic Technique*. Lippincott Williams & Wilkins; 2008:238, with permission.)

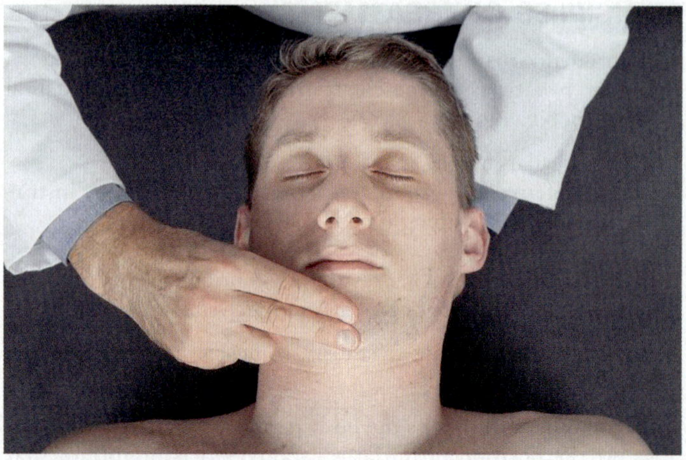

Figure 51.2. Occipitoatlantal (C0–C1) dysfunction example. C0 ES_LR_R—Postisometric relaxation. (Reprinted from Nicholas AS, Nicholas EA. *Atlas of Osteopathic Technique*. Lippincott Williams & Wilkins; 2008:238, with permission.)

POSITION
C5FRSR; C5 is flexed, rotated right, and sidebent right

RESTRICTION
C5 Restricted in extension, left rotation and left sidebending

TYPE OF MUSCLE ENERGY
Postisometric relaxation

TREATMENT POSITION
Patient: Supine
Physician: Seated at the corner of the head of the table

PROCEDURE (FIG. 51.3)

1. The physician's two hands cradle the head and neck, with the index fingers palpating the articular pillar of C5 and the middle finger palpating C6, enabling the physician to monitor and control the entire joint complex.
2. Lift the head anteriorly until the cervical spine is straightened.
3. With the patient completely relaxed, extend the head posteriorly until the feather edge of the restrictive extension barrier is felt at the C5–C6 joint space.

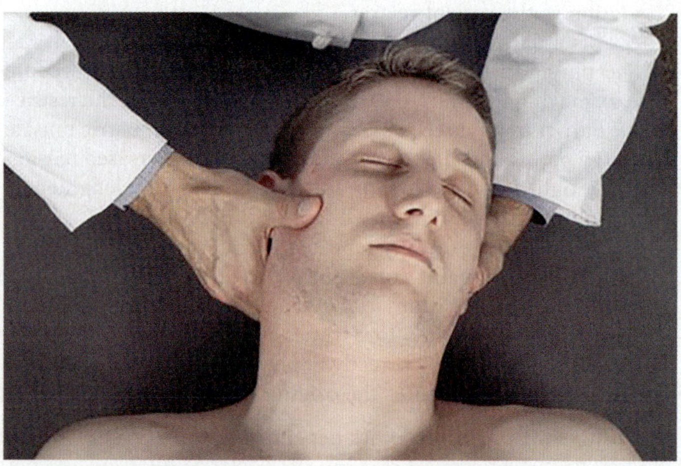

Figure 51.3. Treatment for cervical segmental dysfunction, C2–C6. (Reprinted from Nicholas AS, Nicholas EA. *Atlas of Osteopathic Technique*. Lippincott Williams & Wilkins; 2008:243, with permission.)

4. Maintaining the extension barrier, induce left sidebending by passively translating C5 from left to right until resistance to segmental motion is palpated. As the neck is sidebent, simultaneous left rotation may be added to localize the restrictive barriers or it may be added after. As sidebending and rotation are compound movements in the cervical spine, generally only a small amount of rotation is needed. However, a translation from left to right until resistance is palpated may provide localized sidebending to the joint space.
5. Once the pathologic barrier is localized in three planes with localized extension, left sidebending and left rotation, instruct the patient to either flex (i.e., "look toward your chin") or sidebend ("gently push your head toward your right shoulder").
6. The patient maintains the contraction for 3 to 5 seconds against the physician's unyielding counterforce.
7. The patient is then asked to relax completely.
8. Wait 2 seconds for the tissues to relax, then relocalize C5 until the new restrictive barrier is engaged.
9. Steps 5 to 8 are repeated 3 to 5 times or until a release of the desired motion is palpated.
10. Success of the technique is determined by retesting segmental motion at the C5–C6 level.

Example 2

DIAGNOSIS
Restriction of regional cervical rotation

POSITION
Cervical region rotated left

RESTRICTION
Cervical region restricted in right rotation

TYPE OF MUSCLE ENERGY
Oculocephalogyric reflex

CONTRAINDICATIONS

- Fracture, dislocation, or moderate-to-severe segmental instability in the cervical spine.
- Evocation of neurologic symptoms or signs on rotation of the neck.

TREATMENT POSITION
Patient: Supine
Physician: Seated at the head of the table

PROCEDURE

1. Rotate the patient's head and neck to the right, to the feather edge of the regional motion barrier.
2. Instruct the patient to "look as far left as possible."
3. This position is held for a full 3 to 5 seconds.
4. Direct the patient to "look straight ahead again and relax."
5. Wait 2 seconds for the tissues to relax, and then rotate the head and neck further to the right, engaging the new regional restrictive barrier.
6. Steps 2 to 5 are repeated 3 to 5 times.
7. Success of the technique is determined by reassessing cervical regional rotation.

Example 3

DIAGNOSIS

- Torticollis due to acute sternocleidomastoid muscle spasm
- Acute left sternocleidomastoid spasm

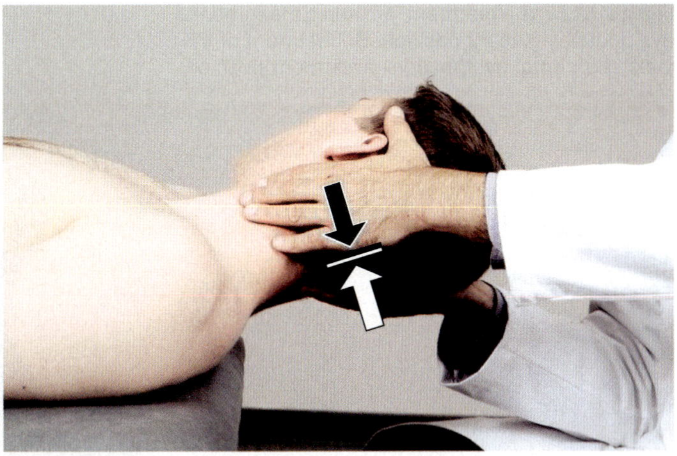

Figure 51.4. Left sternocleidomastoid spasm (acute torticollis); reciprocal inhibition. (Reprinted from Nicholas AS, Nicholas EA. *Atlas of Osteopathic Technique*. Lippincott Williams & Wilkins; 2008:234, with permission.)

TYPE OF MUSCLE ENERGY
Reciprocal inhibition

CONTRAINDICATIONS

- Fracture, dislocation, or moderate-to-severe segmental instability in the cervical spine.
- Evocation of neurologic symptoms or signs on rotation of the neck.

TREATMENT POSITION
Patient: Supine with the head positioned off the end of the table
Physician: Seated at the head of the table, supporting the patient's head

PROCEDURE (FIG. 51.4)

1. The patient's head is flexed approximately 45 degrees, then rotated so that the hypertonic sternocleidomastoid muscle is positioned superiorly.
2. Lower the patient's head straight toward the floor, until the restrictive barrier produced by this hypertonic muscle is engaged.
3. The physician instructs the patient to very gently extend the head (*black arrow*, Fig. 51.4) while the physician applies an equal counterforce (*white arrow*). Or, the physician may also tap the patient's right mastoid process and instruct the patient to "think about pushing down against my finger."
4. The patient is instructed to relax. After 2 seconds of relaxation, the head is again lowered toward the floor until the new restrictive barrier is engaged.
5. Steps 3 to 5 are repeated 3 to 5 times.
6. Success of the technique is determined by palpating the involved sternocleidomastoid muscle for reduction in tone, and by observing the patient's head in the erect posture for improved body carriage.

M99.02 Lower Thoracic Somatic Dysfunction (T5–T12)

Example 1

DIAGNOSIS
Thoracic segmental somatic dysfunction

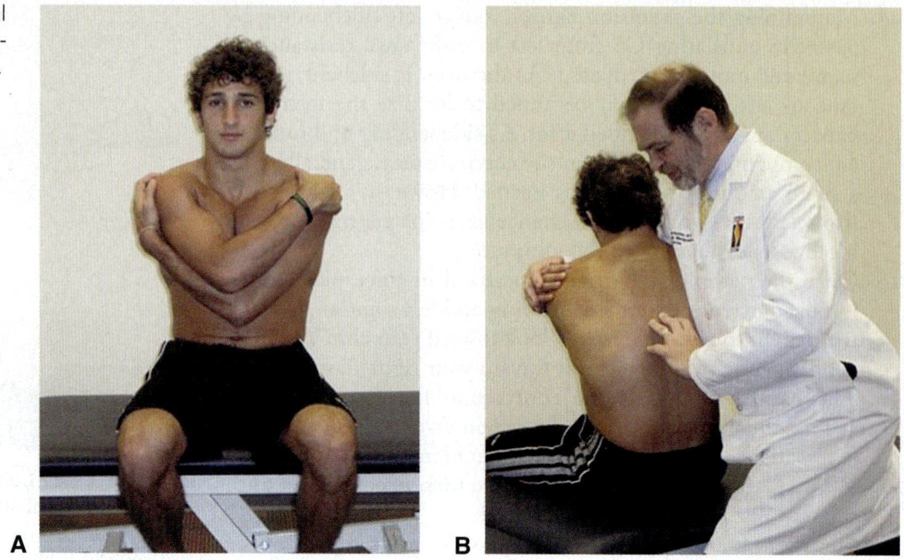

Figure 51.5. **A.** Treatment of thoracic segmental dysfunction—patient position. **B.** Treatment of thoracic segmental dysfunction—treatment position.

POSITION
T8ERSR; T8 is extended, rotated, and sidebent left

RESTRICTION
T8 is restricted in flexion, rotation, and sidebending right

TYPE OF MUSCLE ENERGY
Postisometric relaxation

TREATMENT POSITION
Patient: Seated on the side of the treatment table, grasping the shoulders with arms crossed
Physician: Standing behind the patient, on the side opposite of the direction of rotation

PROCEDURE (FIG. 51.5)

1. The finger pads of the physician's right hand are placed between the facet pair of T8 and T9.
2. Instruct the patient to slowly bend forward, until a slight separation of these spinous processes is palpated.
3. The physician maintains this flexion at the T8–T9 joint space and places the right axilla over the top of the patient's right shoulder. The physician's right hand reaches across the front of the patient, to grasp the patient's left shoulder.
4. The physician adds a compressive force through the patient's right shoulder to the T8–T9 joint space until a sidebending motion is palpated at the T8 level.
5. The physician may add a small degree of right rotation into the restrictive barrier but it is minimal as sidebending and rotation are coupled motions in the thoracic spine.
6. The physician instructs the patient to "pull the left shoulder down toward the floor."
7. This contraction is held for a full 3 to 5 seconds.
8. The patient is directed to relax, while the physician simultaneously ceasing the applied counterforce.
9. The patient is then further localized into the new restrictive barrier with small degrees of flexion, sidebending right, and rotation right.
10. Steps 5 to 9 are repeated 3 to 5 times.
11. Success of the technique is determined by retesting segmental motion at the T8 level.

Example 2

DIAGNOSIS
Thoracic segmental somatic dysfunction

POSITION
T5–T9 NRRSL; T5–T9 are neutral, rotated right, and sidebent left

RESTRICTION
T5–T9 are restricted in left rotation, and right sidebending

TYPE OF MUSCLE ENERGY
Postisometric relaxation

TREATMENT POSITION
Patient: Seated on the side of the treatment table with the left hand behind their neck and the right hand on their left elbow. (The position would be reversed for a dysfunction with the opposite rotational components.) (Fig. 51.6A)
Physician: Standing behind the patient, at the side opposite of the direction of rotation.

PROCEDURE (FIG. 51.6A–C)

1. The physician contacts the patient's spine by placing their right index finger pad between the spinous processes of T6 and T7; middle finger pad between the spinous processes of T7 and T8 and ring finger pad between the spinous processes of T8 and T9. Localization of the forces will be directed toward the middle or apex of the group dysfunction, in this case, T7 (Fig. 51.6B). Alternatively, the physician may also contact the transverse processes of T7 with their thumb and index or middle finger pad (Fig. 51.6C).
2. The physician places their left arm under the patient's left axilla and then contacts the patient's opposite shoulder with the left hand (Fig. 51.6A).
3. The physician induces mild flexion through the patient's spine until slight gapping is palpated between the spinous processes of T7 and T8.
4. The physician then rotates and sidebends into the restrictive barrier. This is accomplished by rotating the patient's trunk to

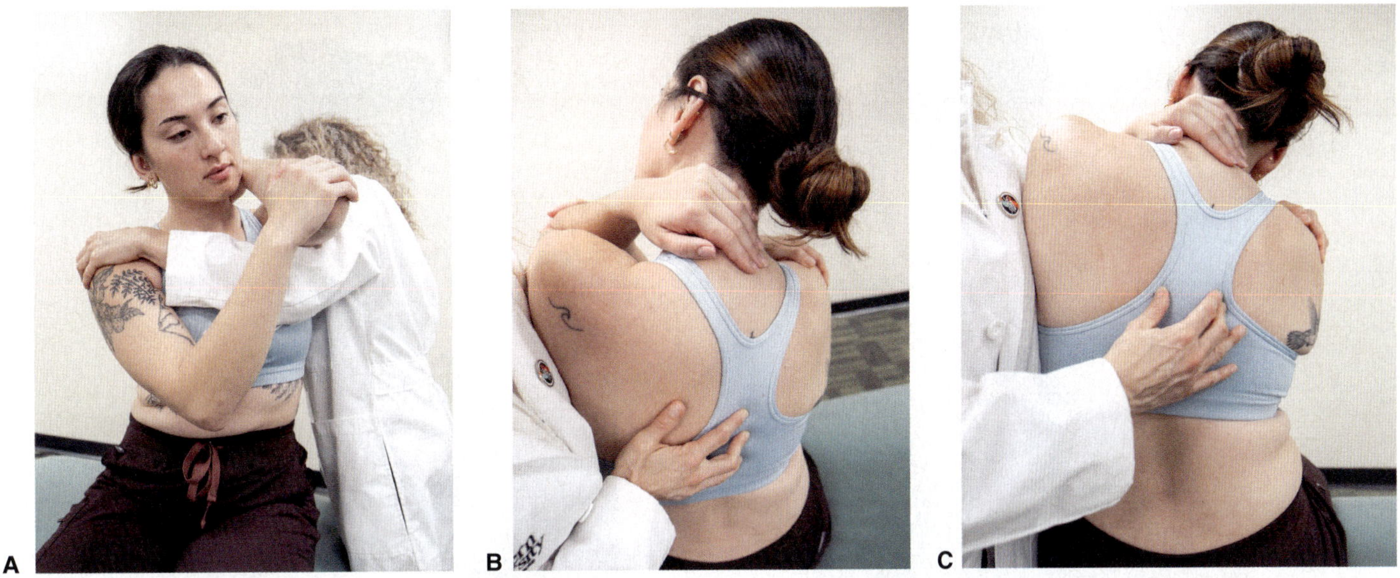

Figure 51.6. A–C. Treatment setup for T5–9 NRRSL. A. Anterior view- patient seated on the side of the treatment table with the left hand behind their neck and the right hand on their left elbow. B. The physician contacts the patient's spine by placing their right index finger pad between the spinous processes of T6 and T7; middle finger pad between the spinous processes of T7 and T8 and ring finger pad between the spinous processes of T8 and T9. C. The physician may also contact the transverse processes of T7 with their thumb and index or middle finger pad. (Photo courtesy of Western University of Health Sciences, Pomona, CA, with permission.)

the left to the T7–T8 joint space. The physician induces right sidebending by compressing the patient's right shoulder inferiorly and translating the patient's body slightly medially to the T7–T8 joint space until the edge of the restrictive barrier is palpated.

5. Once the patient is positioned into the initial restrictive barrier, the physician instructs the patient to attempt to "turn your shoulders to the right matching my force" or to "rotate your right shoulder backward and up toward the ceiling matching my force."
6. The patient is instructed to maintain this contraction for 3 to 5 seconds against the physician's unyielding counterforce.
7. The patient is then directed to relax while the physician simultaneously ceases the applied counterforce.
8. The physician waits for about 2 seconds (postisometric phase) before engaging the new restrictive barrier by adding further left rotation and right sidebending localized to the T7–T8 joint space. The motions here are generally quite small.
9. Steps 5 to 8 are repeated 3 to 5 times or until the somatic dysfunction appears to be maximally improved.
10. Success of the technique is determined by reassessing restored segmental motion of the T5–T9 region.

M99.02 Upper Thoracic Somatic Dysfunction (T1–T4)

Example 3

DIAGNOSIS

Thoracic segmental somatic dysfunction

POSITION

T4ERSL; T4 is extended, rotated, and sidebent left

RESTRICTION

T4 is restricted in flexion, rotation, and sidebending right

TYPE OF MUSCLE ENERGY

Postisometric relaxation

TREATMENT POSITION

Patient: Seated on the side of the treatment table

Physician: Standing behind the patient, on the side opposite of the direction of rotation

PROCEDURE (FIG. 51.7A AND B)

1. The physician palpates the somatic dysfunction by contacting the T4–T5 joint space (Fig. 51.7A) or by contacting the transverse processes of T4 with left thumb and index or middle finger (Fig. 51.7B). This is considered to be the "monitoring hand" for the duration of the procedure. The physician contacts the patient's left parietal bone with the palmar surface of their right hand (the "positioning" hand).
2. The physician utilizes their right hand to induce flexion, right rotation and right sidebending to the T4–T5 joint space until the edge of the restrictive barrier is palpated.
3. The physician instructs the patient to "extend your head while turning it and sidebending it to the left matching my force" or "lift your head up into my hand matching my force."
4. The patient is instructed to maintain this contraction for 3 to 5 seconds against the physician's unyielding counterforce.
5. The patient is then directed to relax while the physician simultaneously ceasing the applied counterforce.
6. The physician waits for about 2 seconds (postisometric phase) before engaging the new restrictive barrier by adding further flexion, right rotation and right sidebending localized to the T4–T5 joint space. The motions here are generally quite small.
7. Steps 3 to 6 are repeated 3 to 5 times or until the somatic dysfunction appears to be maximally improved.
8. Success of the technique is determined by reassessing restored segmental motion between T4 and T5.

*Note: For a flexed upper thoracic somatic dysfunction, extension may be induced to the affected joint space by instructing the patient to "straighten up" and/or by inducing anterior translation to the affected segment with the "monitoring" hand. Care should be taken to avoid inducing hyperextension of the cervical spine in order to engage the restrictive barrier of the upper thoracic segments.

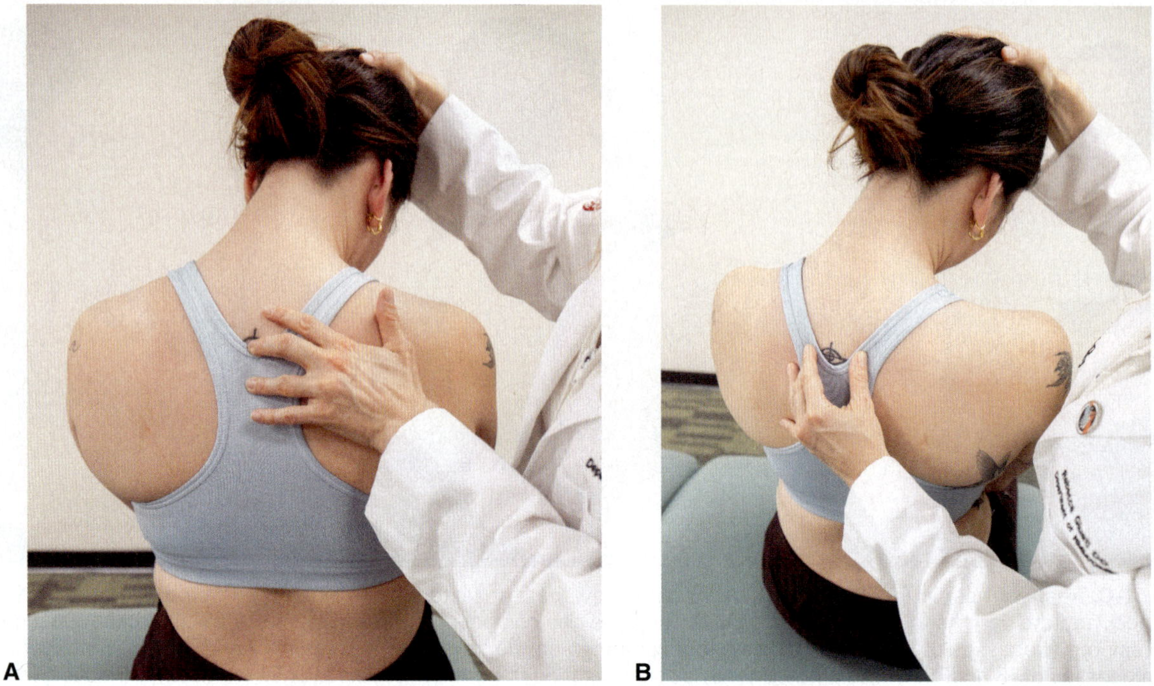

Figure 51.7. A and B. Treatment for T4ERLSL. **A.** The physician may palpate the somatic dysfunction by contacting the T4–T5 joint space. **B.** The physician may also contact the transverse processes of T4 with left thumb and index or middle finger. This is considered to be the "monitoring hand" for the duration of the procedure. The physician contacts the patient's left parietal bone with the palmar surface of their right hand (the "positioning" hand). (Photo courtesy of Western University of Health Sciences, Pomona, CA, with permission.)

M99.03 Lumbar Somatic Dysfunction

Example

While segmental lumbar somatic dysfunction may be addressed in the seated position, the lateral recumbent position oftentimes allows for the forces of gravity to be more effectively controlled and utilized. The positioning of the patient with the upper torso rotating opposite the dysfunctional segment and the regions below rotating toward the same side creates an effective torque on the spinal column and allows for the contrarotational forces to be localized at the dysfunctional segment.

DIAGNOSIS

Lumbar segmental somatic dysfunction[17]

POSITION

L5FRRSR; L5 (a type II dysfunction) is flexed, rotated right, and sidebent right.

RESTRICTION

L5 is restricted in extension, left rotation, and left sidebending.

TYPE OF MUSCLE ENERGY

Postisometric relaxation

TREATMENT POSITION

Patient: Right lateral recumbent (most posterior transverse process on table). The hips and knees are flexed.

Physician: Standing facing the patient.

PROCEDURE (FIG. 51.8)

1. Palpate the interspinous space between L5 and S1 with the superior hand.
2. Passively flex and extend the lumbar spine, by flexing and extending the hips until the dysfunctional segment is positioned in neutral, relative to flexion and extension.
3. Instruct the patient to straighten the bottom leg and place the top foot into the popliteal fossa of the bottom leg.
4. Induce mild extension to the level of L5 by pressing the patient's right thigh slightly posteriorly until motion is felt at that level.
5. The physician then monitors the segment with the inferior hand while the superior hand guides the patient's left shoulder posteriorly until resistance is palpated at the L5 segment.
6. Palpating the L5–S1 interspinous space with the inferior hand, the physician instructs the patient to "push the shoulder gently

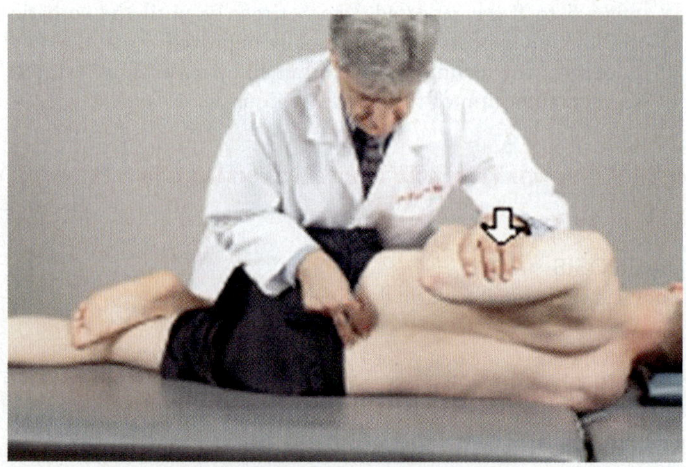

Figure 51.8. Treatment for lumbar type II segmental dysfunction, lateral recumbent position. (Reprinted from Nicholas AS, Nicholas EA. *Atlas of Osteopathic Technique*. Lippincott Williams & Wilkins; 2008:278, with permission.)

forward meeting my force." The isometric contraction is held for 3 to 5 seconds.

7. After 2 seconds of relaxation, the physician carries the shoulder posteriorly until the edge of the new restrictive barrier is met at L5 (as indicated by the white arrow in Fig. 51.8).
   - Repeat each sequence of contraction/relaxation/repositioning 3 to 5 times, or until further segmental motion is being gained.
8. The physician rotates the patient's left hip anteriorly, until resistance is palpated at the segment to be treated.
9. The patient is instructed to "pull the hip gently backward." This isometric contraction is held for a full 3 to 5 seconds.
10. After 2 seconds of relaxation, the physician carries the hip anteriorly until a new restrictive barrier is met, addressing the joint space of L5–S1.
    - Repeat each sequence of contraction/relaxation/repositioning 3 to 5 times, or until further segmental motion is being gained.
    - If coordinated enough, the patient may contract muscles at both the hip and shoulder simultaneously.
11. Additionally, the sidebending component can be addressed by utilizing the patient's lower extremity. In this type II example, once the rotational component of the somatic dysfunction is addressed, the physician continues to monitor the L5–S1 joint space with the superior hand and flexes the patient's knees and hips to 90 degrees and then lifts the ankles toward the ceiling inducing left sidebending until the feather edge of the restrictive barrier is palpated.[18,19]
12. The physician instructs the patient to press the ankles down toward the floor into the restrictive barrier for 3 to 5 seconds against the physician's unyielding counterforce.
13. The patient is then instructed to relax for 2 to 3 seconds.
14. The physician further localizes the segment into the restrictive barrier.
15. Repeat each sequence of contraction/relaxation/repositioning 3 to 5 times, or until further segmental motion is being gained.
16. Success of the technique is determined by reevaluating segmental motion at the dysfunctional lumbar segment.

M99.04 Sacral Somatic Dysfunction

The diagnosis of sacral dysfunction requires the following information:

- Seated flexion test (determines the presence of sacroiliac dysfunction and the side of the dysfunction, i.e., side of greatest excursion)
  - Laterality of the dysfunctional sacral iliac joint. The other SI joint is functional.
- Relative position of the sacral base. Which sacral base is anterior?
- Relative depths of the sacral sulcus. What are the sacral sulcus depths?
- The sacral sulcus on the side of the dysfunction is designated as either deep or shallow. The other may appear relatively shallow or deep but is actually the functional side.
- Relative position of the ILAs. Which ILA is posterior and inferior?
- The ILAs are designated as posterior/inferior or anterior/superior.
- L5 rotation
- Leg lengths
- Lumbosacral spring test
- Backward bend test (Sphinx test)

Example 1

DIAGNOSIS

- A left-on-left sacral torsion (L/L sacral torsion)
- Sacral dysfunction—anterior or forward torsion

POSITION

The sacrum is rotating anteriorly to the left over a left oblique axis.

RESTRICTION

Posterior rotation about the left oblique axis is restricted. The oblique axes are not free to alternate during the gait cycle.

TYPE OF MUSCLE ENERGY

Complex: The technique's mechanism of action is still being debated, but it is likely due to a combination of multiple muscles simultaneously going through postisometric relaxation and mechanisms described above.

TREATMENT POSITION

Patient: Left lateral modified Sims' position (lying on the side of the axis), chest toward the table, right arm hanging off the table and left arm either hanging off the table or placed behind the patient on the table

Physician: Standing at the side of the table, facing the patient

PROCEDURE (FIG. 51.9A AND B)

1. While monitoring the lumbosacral region with the superior hand, the physician uses their other hand to flex the patient's hips and knees to 90 degrees.
2. The physician stands facing the patient with their own hip, knee, and ankle slightly flexed. The physician places the patient's knees on their anterior thigh in order to have control of the patient's hips without utilizing their hands. This also aids in further derotating the L5 segment (Fig. 51.9A).
3. To achieve an optimal position of L5 in a neutral "loose-packed" position, the physician monitors the lumbosacral region with the right hand while utilizing their hips against the patient's knees to slightly flex and extend the patient's spine. Once the optimal mid-neutral position of L5 is achieved, the physician stabilizes the patient in this position.
4. To address the rotated right L5 segment, the physician instructs the patient to inhale fully and as they exhale, to reach for the floor with the right hand, bringing the chest and right shoulder closer to the table. This is repeated 3 to 5 times. A muscle energy component may be added to this step where the physician now monitors L5 with the left hand and contacts the patient's posterior right shoulder. As the patient inhales, they may push the shoulder posteriorly against the physicians' unyielding counterforce for 3 to 5 seconds. As they exhale, they are instructed to reach for the floor with their right hand and the physician may gently encourage this motion with slight posterior–anterior pressure to the right shoulder during exhalation. This may be repeated 3 to 5 times.
5. To address the sacral component of the torsion, the physician switches the monitoring hand so that the superior or right hand monitors the lumbosacral junction. Maintaining the left truncal rotation, the physician lowers the patient's feet and ankles toward the floor, just as far as the patient's anatomy of the hip permits (producing external rotation of the top or right thigh and internal rotation of the left) or until motion is palpated just inferior to the PSIS at the sacral base (Fig. 51.9B).

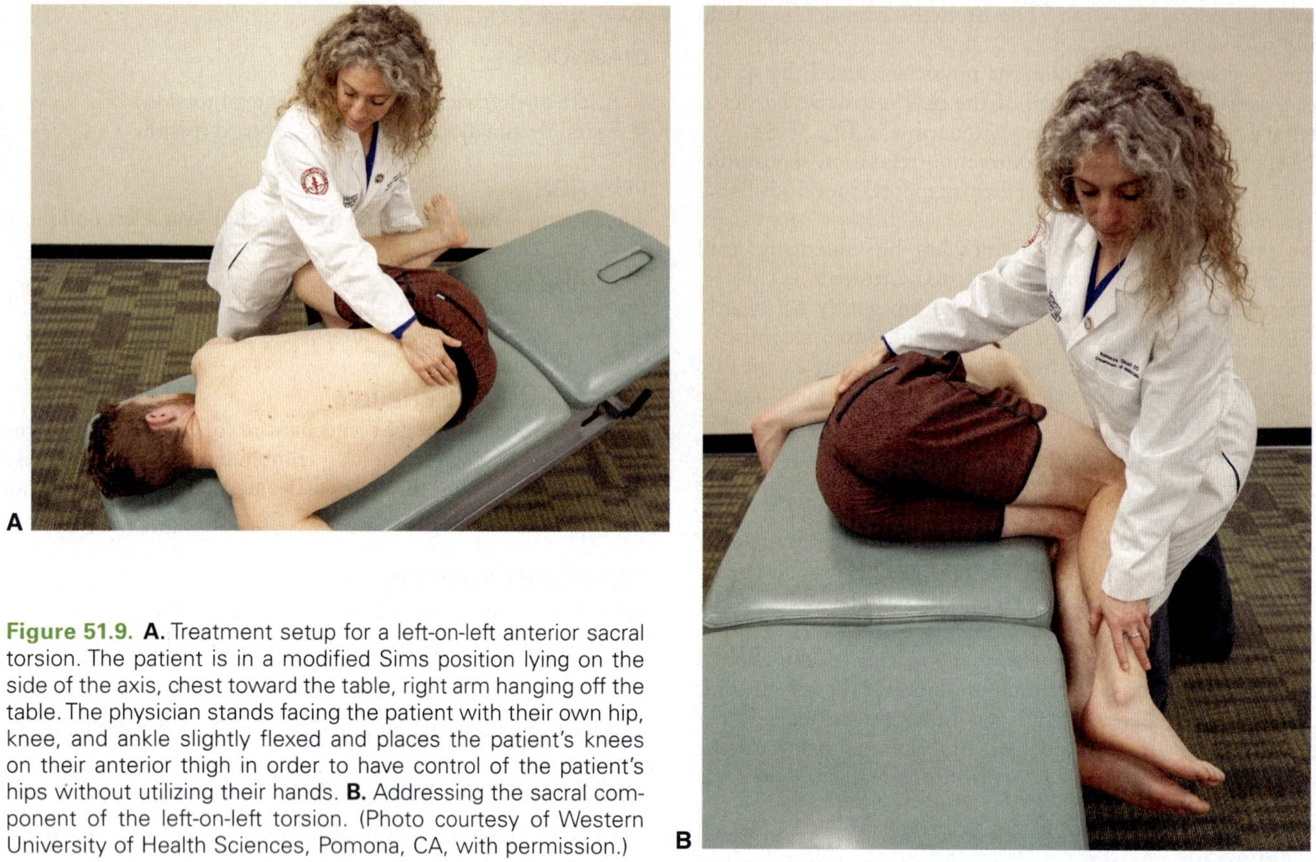

Figure 51.9. **A.** Treatment setup for a left-on-left anterior sacral torsion. The patient is in a modified Sims position lying on the side of the axis, chest toward the table, right arm hanging off the table. The physician stands facing the patient with their own hip, knee, and ankle slightly flexed and places the patient's knees on their anterior thigh in order to have control of the patient's hips without utilizing their hands. **B.** Addressing the sacral component of the left-on-left torsion. (Photo courtesy of Western University of Health Sciences, Pomona, CA, with permission.)

6. The physician instructs the patient to lift the ankles up toward the ceiling for 3 to 5 seconds against the physician's unyielding counterforce.
7. The physician directs the patient to relax, while simultaneously ceasing the applied counterforce.
8. The physician waits 2 seconds for the tissues to relax, then engages the feather's edge of the new restrictive barrier by gently pressing the patient's ankles toward the floor.
9. Steps 6 to 8 are repeated 3 to 5 times.[20]
10. Success of the technique is determined by rechecking the above landmarks and SI motion.

*Note: For improved control of the patient's lower extremity, the entire above procedure may be done with the osteopathic physician sitting on the table at the patient's right side and resting the patient's thighs on the physician's left thigh. Some physicians choose to switch to this option to address the sacral component of the torsion at step 5 (Fig. 51.10A and B).[20]

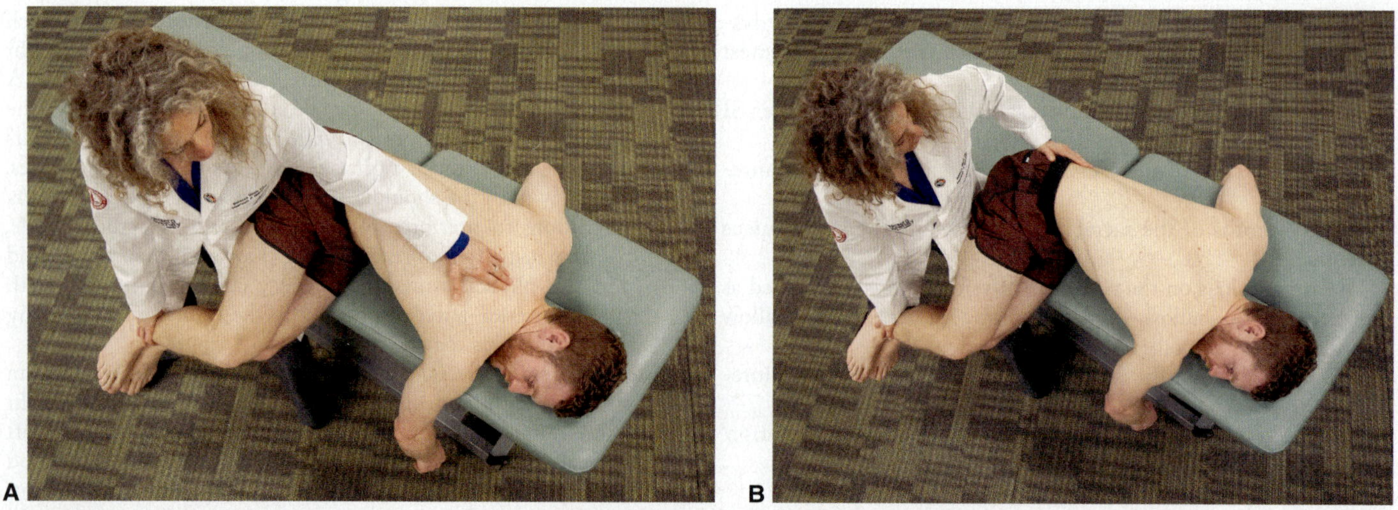

Figure 51.10. **A and B.** Treatment setup for a left-on-left anterior sacral torsion with the physician seated. **A.** Addressing the lumbar rotational component of the left-on-left sacral torsion. **B.** Addressing the sacral component of the left-on-left sacral torsion. (Photo courtesy of Western University of Health Sciences, Pomona, CA, with permission.)

Example 2

DIAGNOSIS

- A left on right sacral torsion (Lon R sacral torsion)
- Sacral dysfunction—posterior or backward torsion

POSITION

The sacrum is rotating posteriorly to the left about a right oblique axis.

RESTRICTION

Anterior rotation about the right oblique axis is restricted. The oblique axes of the sacrum are not free to alternate during the gait cycle.

TYPE OF MUSCLE ENERGY

Complex: the technique's mechanism of action is still being debated, but it is likely due to a combination of joint mobilization using muscle force and postisometric relaxation.

TREATMENT POSITION

Patient: Right lateral recumbent position (lying on the side of the axis)
Physician: Standing at the side of the table, facing the patient

PROCEDURE

1. The physician instructs the patient to lie on their right side with the hips/pelvis as close to the front edge of the table as possible. This will assist in maintaining lumbosacral extension in the final aspects of the procedure. Both knees may be slightly flexed and the patient's top lower extremity (left) is positioned over the bottom leg so that the left foot rests on the table anterior to the bottom foot.
2. The physician then palpates the lumbosacral junction with the superior or left hand while the right hand guides the patient's bottom (right) lower extremity posteriorly, inducing hyperextension of the hips until motion is felt at the lumbosacral junction. Ensure that this extension is maintained throughout the rest of the procedure.
3. The physician monitors the lumbosacral junction with the superior hand and stabilizes the pelvis with the inferior hand by resting the forearm on the posterolateral aspect of the patient's hip. This will prevent the pelvis from rolling while truncal rotation is accomplished.
4. Maintaining the stability of the pelvis, the physician instructs the patient to inhale and exhale and after they exhale to allow the left shoulder to rotate posteriorly in order to de-rotate L5. This is repeated 3 to 5 times. If the patient is able, they are instructed to grasp the back edge of the table with their left hand. More flexible patients may be instructed to grasp the back edge of the table and then move their hand down toward their feet as they continue the series of respirations. Other patients may lack the flexibility to grasp the back edge of the table, and therefore may allow the left arm to hang behind them with shoulder abduction which will still allow for the desired lumbar rotation (Fig. 51.11A).
5. Maintaining the truncal rotation and the pelvic alignment, the physician monitors the lumbosacral junction with the superior hand and using the inferior hand, extends the patient's top (left) knee without inducing any other motion (i.e., further hip flexion). The physician then contacts the patient's top ankle or knee in order to resist hip abduction.
6. The patient is instructed to raise their knee toward the ceiling for 3 to 5 seconds against the physician's unyielding counterforce (Fig. 51.11B)
7. The physician directs the patient to relax, while simultaneously ceasing the applied counterforce.
8. The physician waits 2 seconds for the tissues to relax, before engaging the new restrictive barrier by lowering the patient's top lower extremity toward the floor.
9. Steps 6 to 8 are repeated 3 to 5 times.
10. Success of the technique is determined by rechecking the above landmarks and SI motion.[20]

Example 3

DIAGNOSIS

Bilaterally extended sacrum

POSITION

Bilaterally extended sacrum

RESTRICTION

Sacrum restricted in flexion at both sacroiliac joints

TYPE OF MUSCLE ENERGY

Respiratory assistance

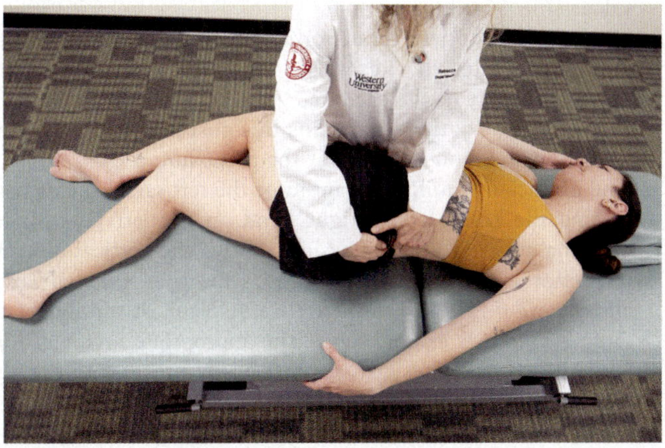

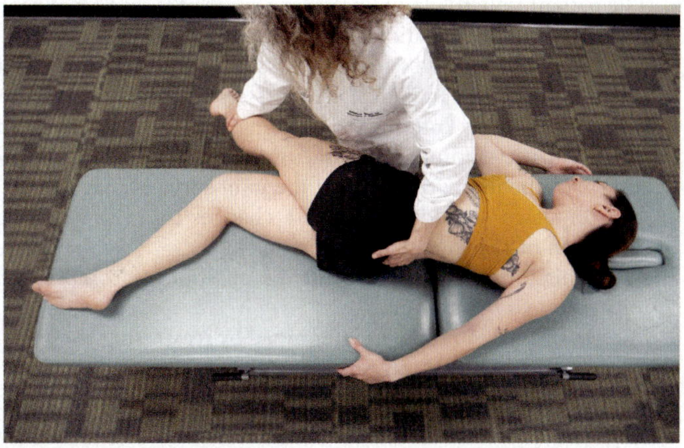

Figure 51.11. A. Treatment setup for a left-on-right posterior sacral torsion. If possible, after inducing truncal rotation to address the lumbar component of the L/R torsion, the patient grasps hold of the back edge of the table. **B.** Treatment of the sacral component of an L/R backward torsion where the patient is instructed to lift their top knee toward the ceiling against the physician's unyielding counterforce. (Photo courtesy of Western University of Health Sciences, Pomona, CA, with permission.)

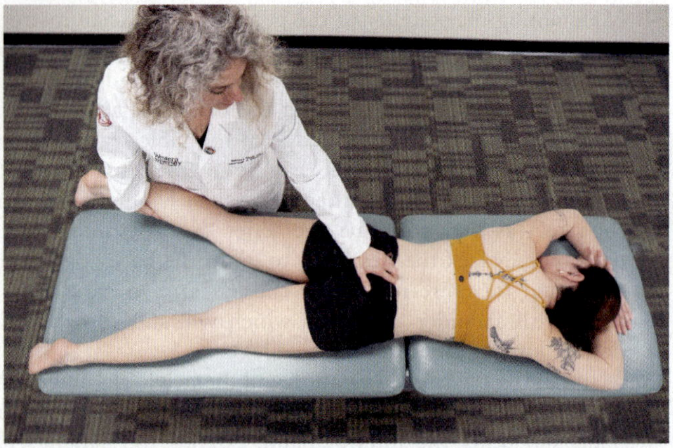

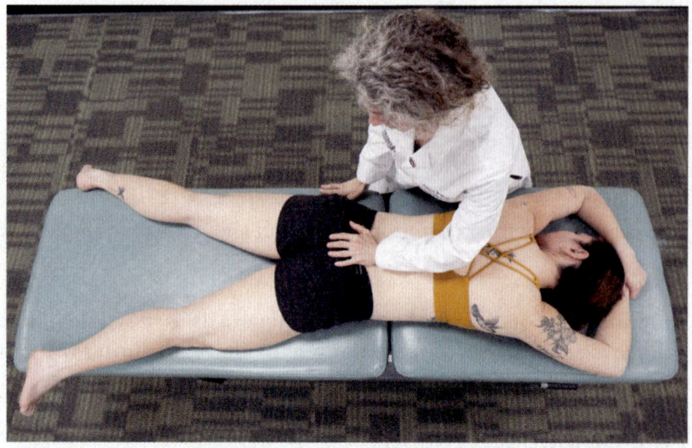

Figure 51.12. **A.** Treatment setup for a bilaterally extended sacrum. The physician uses the finger pads to monitor the sacroiliac joint at the sacral sulcus while using the other hand to adduct the ipsilateral lower extremity until motion is palpated at the sacroiliac joint. **B.** Treatment of a bilaterally extended sacrum. The physician contacts the sacral base with the heel, fingers contacting ILAs to monitor, maintaining pressure as the patient inhales and applying a compressive force anteriorly to the base of the sacrum as the patient exhales. (Photo courtesy of Western University of Health Sciences, Pomona, CA, with permission.)

TREATMENT POSITION

Patient: Prone on the treatment table
Physician: Standing at the side of the treatment table

PROCEDURE

1. The physician uses the finger pads to monitor the sacroiliac joint at the sacral sulcus while using the other hand to adduct the ipsilateral lower extremity until motion is palpated at the sacroiliac joint (Fig. 51.12A)
2. The physician then externally rotates that leg to provide a slight gapping of the sacroiliac joint anteriorly and a loose-packed position at that joint.
3. The process is repeated for the contralateral side.
4. The physician contacts the sacral base with the heel of the hand closest to the patient, fingers pointing inferiorly and if possible contacting ILAs to monitor motion.
5. The physician applies a compressive force anteriorly to the base of the sacrum with the thenar and hypothenar eminences. Alter the direction of the force (medial–lateral and superior–inferior) slightly from straight vertical (posterior to anterior) to find the freest plane of motion at the sacroiliac joint (Fig. 51.12B)
6. The patient is instructed to perform a series of three to five deep inhalations and exhalations. As the patient inhales, the physician maintains the pressure at the sacral base. As the patient exhales, the physician actively compresses the sacral base anteriorly and slightly inferiorly depending on the freest plane of motion of the sacrum. As the sacrum slides along the articular surface of the ilium, the bevel of the joint surfaces may change. The physician should follow these changes to assist with the resolution of the somatic dysfunction.[20]
7. After this series of breaths with the appropriate compressive force, reassess the sacrum.
8. Success of the technique is determined by reassessing the sacral anatomical landmarks, tests, and position.

Example 4

DIAGNOSIS

- Unilateral flexed sacrum—left
- Sacral dysfunction—unilateral flexed sacrum

POSITION

Unilateral flexed sacrum—left

RESTRICTION

Left sacroiliac joint restricted in extension

TYPE OF MUSCLE ENERGY

Respiratory assistance

TREATMENT POSITION

Patient: Prone with head turned either direction for patient comfort
Physician: Standing at the side of the patient, at the side of dysfunction

PROCEDURE

1. The physician monitors the sacral sulcus of the side of dysfunction with their left hand while passively abducting the patient's left lower extremity to loose pack the sacroiliac joint. This is achieved when slight superior compression and inferior traction to the left leg result in palpable motion at the ipsilateral sacral sulcus (Fig. 51.13A).
2. Once the appropriate abduction is achieved, the physician then internally rotates the left thigh in order to slightly gap the posterior aspect of the sacroiliac joint which will enable sacral extension. The patient maintains this position of internal rotation and abduction throughout the procedure.
3. The physician continues to monitor the left sacral sulcus while placing the heel of their right hand on the left ILA, fingers pointing superiorly. The physician varies the vertical direction (posterior–anterior) of pressure to the ILA (medial–lateral and superior–inferior) until the freest plane of motion of the sacroiliac joint is located. Once the appropriate vector of force is identified, the physician applies steady pressure to the ILA along that vector (Fig. 51.13B-C).
4. The patient is then instructed to inhale fully. As they exhale, the physician sustains the anterior pressure to the ILA to prevent the sacral base from flexing or nutating. (As a note, Fred Mitchell, Jr, DO, describes instructing the patient to perform "step breathing" where the patient inhales deeply and holds it

A

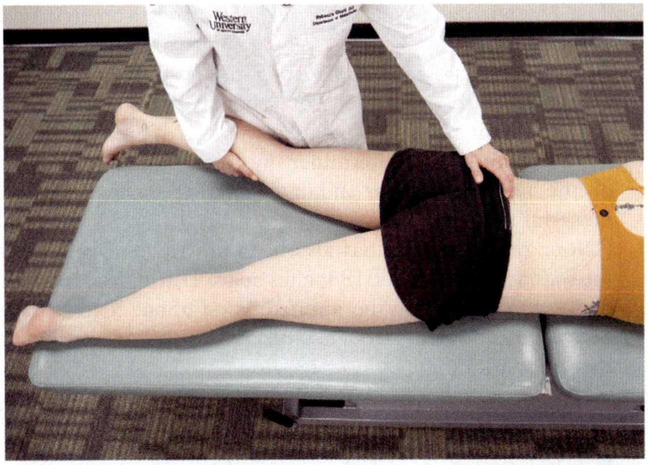

B

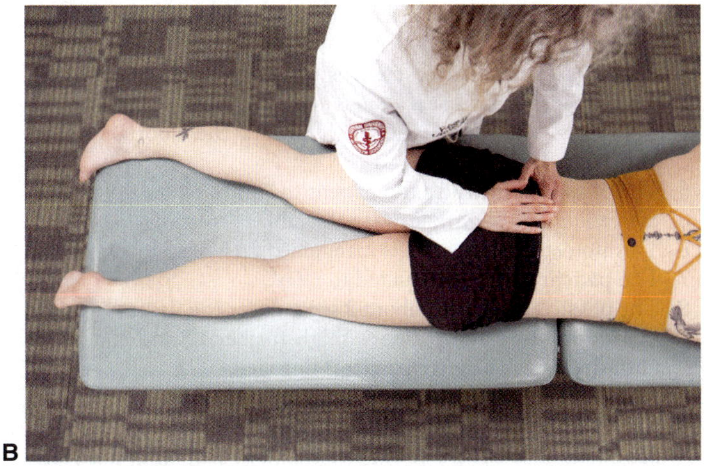

C

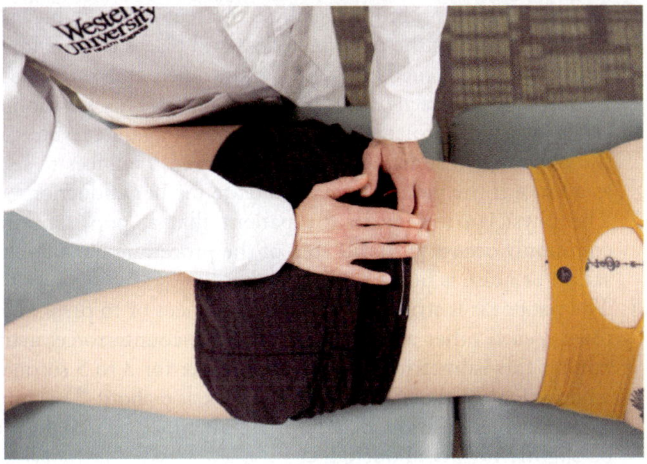

Figure 51.13. A–C. Treatment of a left unilateral sacral flexion. **A.** Treatment set-up for a left unilateral sacral flexion. The physician monitors the sacral sulcus of the side of dysfunction while passively abducting the patient's left lower extremity to loose pack the sacroiliac joint. This is achieved when slight superior compression and inferior traction on the left leg result in palpable motion at the ipsilateral sacral sulcus. **B.** Treatment position for a left unilateral sacral flexion. **C.** Close-up of physician's hand position for treatment of a left unilateral sacral flexion; monitoring left sacral sulcus with heel of other hand applying anterior pressure to left ILA. (Photo courtesy of Western University of Health Sciences, Pomona, CA, with permission.)

and attempts to take in more air before fully exhaling while the physician sustains the anterior pressure, preventing the sacral base from moving anteriorly.[20])

5. Steps 3 to 4 are repeated 3 to 5 times. After each repetition, the physician assesses their pressure to ensure they are still engaging the freest plane of motion of the sacroiliac joint. As the sacrum slides anteriorly along the auricular surface of the ilium, the beveling of the joint surface may be altered and the physician continuously monitors with the pressure hand on the ILA and at the sacral sulcus to avoid any compression of the bony surfaces.[20]
6. Success of the technique is determined by reassessing for improved symmetry of the sacral landmarks, tests, motion and resolution of the seated forward bending test.[20]

M99.05 PELVIC SOMATIC DYSFUNCTION

Example 1

DIAGNOSIS

Superior pubic bone somatic dysfunction

POSITION

Pubic bone on side of dysfunction is displaced superiorly

RESTRICTION

Pubic bone on side of dysfunction resists inferior movement

TYPE OF MUSCLE ENERGY

Joint mobilization using muscle force

TREATMENT POSITION

Patient: Supine, lying near the edge of the table

Physician: Standing at the side of the table, at the side of dysfunction

PROCEDURE (FIG. 51.14)

1. Abduct the patient's ipsilateral thigh, so that the leg and thigh can hang off the side of the table.

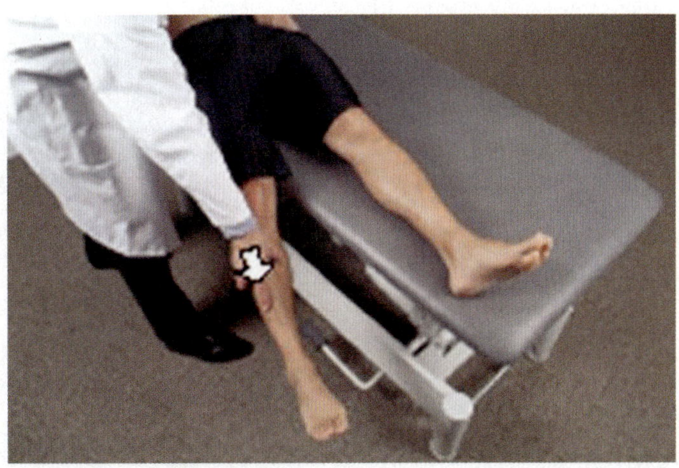

Figure 51.14. Right superior pubic shear dysfunction: muscle contraction mobilized articulation. (Reprinted from Nicholas AS, Nicholas EA. *Atlas of Osteopathic Technique*. Lippincott Williams & Wilkins; 2008:289, with permission.)

2. The physician's superior hand is placed on the contralateral ASIS, to stabilize the patient.
3. The physician's inferior hand is placed just proximal to the patient's ipsilateral knee.
4. The physician presses the thigh toward the floor until the restrictive barrier is engaged.
5. The physician instructs the patient to "lift the knee up toward the ceiling and slightly toward the table."
6. This isometric contraction is maintained for a full 3 to 5 seconds.
7. The patient is then instructed to relax.
8. The physician waits for about 2 seconds for the tissues to relax, then repositions the patient's thigh further toward the floor, until the new restrictive barrier is engaged.
9. Steps 5 to 8 are repeated 3 to 5 times.
10. Effectiveness of the technique is determined by reexamining the position of the pubic tubercles, and by palpating passively induced iliosacral motion.

Example 2

DIAGNOSIS

Normal physiologic pubic symphysis motion is restricted (superior or inferior pubic subluxation, or gapped/abducted or compressed/adducted pubic symphysis)

TYPE OF MUSCLE ENERGY

Joint mobilization with muscle force
Patient: Supine
Physician: Standing at the side of the table

PROCEDURE (SEE FIG. 51.15A AND B)

Part 1: Superior or inferior pubic subluxations and/or gapped/abducted pubic symphysis[21]

1. The physician flexes the patient's knees to about 90 degrees and hips to about 45 degrees with the patient's feet resting flat on the table.
2. The physician holds the patient's knees together with both hands and then instructs the patient to abduct their legs against the physician's unyielding counterforce for 3 to 5 seconds with an instruction such as, "Matching my force, try to press your knees apart."
3. After this isometric contraction is held for 3 to 5 seconds, the patient is instructed to relax.
4. The physician allows about 2 seconds of postisometric relaxation.
5. Steps 2 to 4 are repeated 3 to 5 times. If the patient was diagnosed with a "gapped" or "abducted" pubic symphysis, the treatment may be concluded here and the effectiveness of the technique is determined by reexamining the position of the pubic tubercles, and by palpating passively induced iliosacral motion.
   (*Note: this technique has also been described as being initiated with the feet about 18 inches apart. During the relaxation phase, the knees may be approximated about 3 to 4 inches before repeating the sequence of contraction, relaxation, and then repositioning.[22])

Part 2: Superior or inferior pubic subluxations and/or compressed/adducted pubic symphysis[21]

6. For the next step in this treatment, the patient maintains the flexion of the hips and knees with the feet on the table. The physician abducts the patient's knees and places their palm on the contralateral medial aspect of the knee and their elbow at the medial aspect of the ipsilateral knee. This positioning serves as a brace for the patient to adduct against. Note that the physician's fist could be placed between the knees to serve as a brace if the patient cannot tolerate further abduction.
7. The physician may warn the patient that a "pop" sensation commonly occurs with this step of the procedure but this sensation or noise is benign.
8. The patient is instructed to adduct the knees or to press knees toward each other against the physician's counterforce, maintaining this isometric contraction together for 3 to 5 seconds.
9. The patient is then instructed to relax for about 2 seconds. The patient's position may be maintained, or the knees may be slightly further abducted.
10. Steps 8 to 9 are repeated 3 to 5 times.
11. The effectiveness of the technique is determined by reexamining the position of the pubic tubercles, and by palpating passively induced iliosacral motion.

(*Note: in personal communication with Melicien A. Tettambel, DO, FAAO, instructing the patient to perform a slight posterior pelvic tilt [instructions to patient: bring tailbone slightly toward your umbilicus] during the isometric contractions of the procedure assists in localizing the forces to the pubic symphysis. She felt that this improved efficacy of the procedure for her ob/gyn patients.

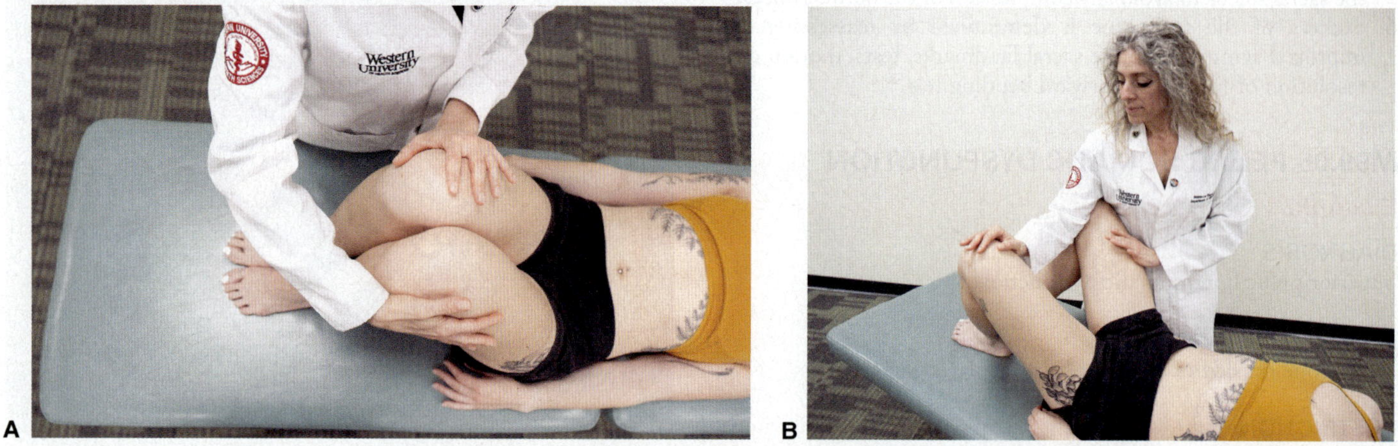

Figure 51.15. A and B. Treatment set-up for Normal physiologic pubic symphysis motion is restricted (superior or inferior pubic subluxation, or gapped/abducted or compressed/ adducted pubic symphysis). **A.** Part 1—for superior or inferior pubic subluxations and/or gapped/adducted pubic symphysis. **B.** Part 2—for superior or inferior pubic subluxations and/or compressed/abducted pubic symphysis. (Photo courtesy of Western University of Health Sciences, Pomona, CA, with permission.)

[Tettambel, M. Personal communication during instruction at COMP, Western University (2009–2012)].)

Example 3

DIAGNOSIS
Acute right hamstring strain with spasm

TYPE OF MUSCLE ENERGY
Crossed extensor reflex

TREATMENT POSITION
Patient: Supine
Physician: Standing at the side of the table, at the side of acute spasm

PROCEDURE (FIG. 51.16)

1. The physician flexes the patient's right hip until initial resistance is palpated while keeping the knee in extension.
2. If range of motion permits, the leg may be placed atop the physician's shoulder.
3. The physician's hands are placed on top of the patient's thigh to maintain the knee in extension throughout the technique.
4. The physician instructs the patient to "very gently push the left knee down against the table."
5. This contraction is held for a full 3 to 5 seconds.
6. The physician directs the patient to relax.
7. The physician waits for 2 seconds for the tissues to relax, then further flexes the right hip until the new restrictive barrier is engaged.
8. Steps 4 to 7 are repeated 3 to 5 times, or until no additional motion can be gained.
9. Effectiveness of the technique is assessed by retesting right hip range of motion in flexion, with the knee extended.

Example 4

DIAGNOSIS
Hamstring shortening resulting in reflex quadriceps weakness

TYPE OF MUSCLE ENERGY
Isokinetic strengthening

TREATMENT POSITION
Patient: Prone
Physician: Standing at the side of the table, at the side of the weakened quadriceps

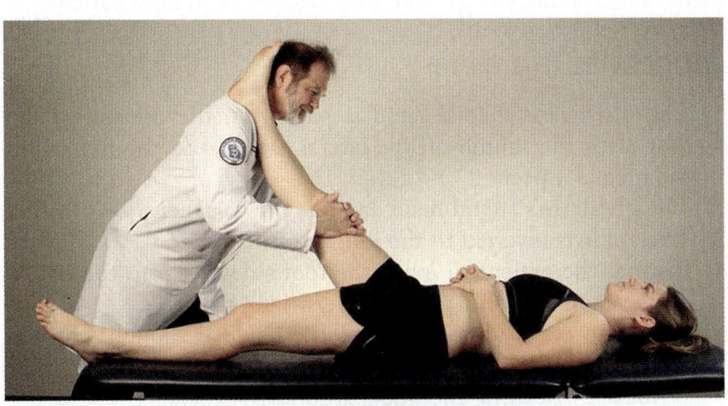

Figure 51.16. **Treatment of hypertonic hamstring muscle.**

PROCEDURE

1. Flex the patient's right knee until the motion barrier for the quadriceps is reached. Restrain the leg just proximal to the ankle.
2. Instruct the patient to "gently push the leg against the physician's hand."
3. While the patient is pushing, slowly allow the knee to extend through the middle of its normal range of motion. This typically requires 3 to 5 seconds.
4. Instruct the patient to stop pushing.
5. Steps 1 to 4 are repeated 3 to 5 times.
6. Success of the technique is determined by retesting quadriceps strength.

Example 5

DIAGNOSIS
Hamstring contracture

TYPE OF MUSCLE ENERGY
Isolytic lengthening

TREATMENT POSITION
Patient: Supine
Physician: Standing at the side of the table, on the side of the contractured hamstring

PROCEDURE

1. Flex the patient's hip to the initial resistance while keeping the knee in extension.
2. The patient's leg is then placed atop the physician's shoulder.
3. One hand of the physician's hands is placed on the thigh, just proximal to the knee. The physician's other is placed just proximal to the ankle, posterior to the Achilles tendon.
4. Instruct the patient to "push the knee down toward the table as hard as possible."
5. While the patient is pushing, create an oscillatory motion with both hands. This repeatedly stretches the muscle at a rate of about 4 times per second (4 Hz).
6. This combined forceful contraction and vibratory stretching is continued for 3 to 5 seconds.
7. Instruct the patient to relax and stop the oscillatory motion.
8. Wait 2 seconds for the tissues to relax, and then further flex the hip to the new restrictive barrier.
9. Steps 4 to 8 are repeated 3 to 5 times.
10. Success of the technique is determined by retesting hip range of motion in flexion, with the knee extended.

Example 6

DIAGNOSIS
Innominate dysfunction—anterior rotation/ anteriorly rotated innominate

POSITION
Innominate rotated anteriorly

RESTRICTION
Innominate restricted in posterior rotation[23]

TYPE OF MUSCLE ENERGY
Can use multiple mechanisms

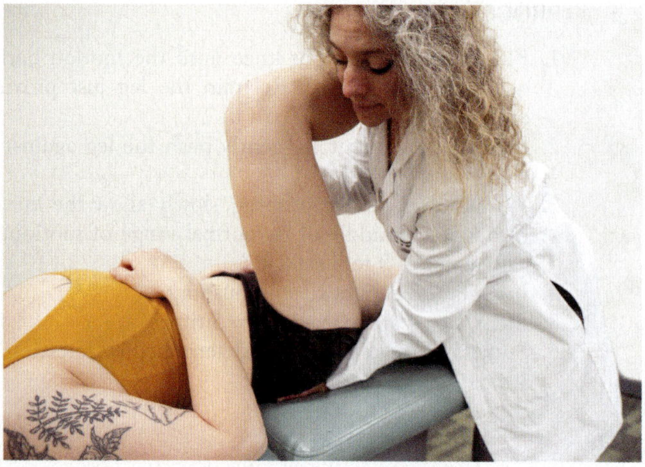

A

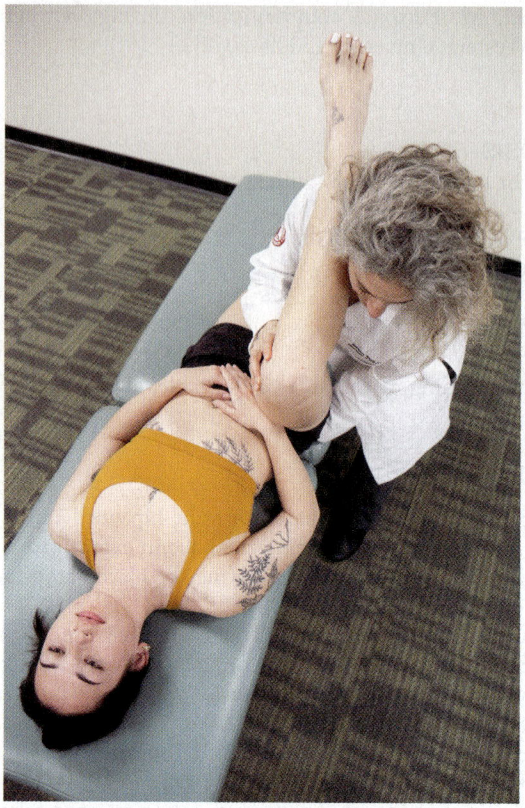

B

Figure 51.17. A. Treatment set-up for a right anteriorly rotated innominate. With the superior hand, the physician may palpate the sacral sulcus with the 4th finger in order to detect iliosacral motion while curling the 2nd and 3rd fingers around the adjacent PSIS in order to encourage de-rotation of the pelvis. Using the inferior hand, the physician contacts the affected lower extremity just superior to the popliteal fossa, flexing the knee to 90 degrees and then flexing and slightly abducting the affected hip to engage the first restrictive barrier within the freest plane of innominate rotation. **B.** Overhead view of treatment of right anteriorly rotated innominate. (Photo courtesy of Western University of Health Sciences, Pomona, CA, with permission.)

TREATMENT POSITION

Patient: Can be done prone, lateral, or supine. For this example, the patient is lying supine. Prone positioning adds advantage of sacral stabilization with physician's forearm. Lateral positioning may be beneficial for patients who experience difficulty lying supine or prone, such as term pregnant patients.

Physician: At the side of dysfunction, facing patient

PROCEDURE (FIG. 51.17A AND B)

1. With the superior hand, the physician may palpate the sacral sulcus with the 4th finger in order to detect iliosacral motion while curling the 2nd and 3rd fingers around the adjacent PSIS in order to encourage de-rotation of the pelvis.
2. Using the inferior hand, the physician contacts the affected lower extremity just superior to the popliteal fossa, flexing the knee to 90 degrees and then flexing and slightly abducting the affected hip to engage the first restrictive barrier within the freest plane of innominate rotation. (The physician should cease this motion before the ilium moves the sacrum.) (Fig. 51.17A)
3. Maintaining this position, the physician instructs the patient extend their hip against the physician's unyielding counterforce for 3 to 5 seconds.
4. The patient is directed to relax, while the physician simultaneously ceases the applied counterforce.
5. The physician waits 2 seconds for the tissues to relax and then repositions the innominate into further posterior rotation by further flexing with finetuning of abduction or adduction of the hip until the next restrictive barrier is engaged. The physician may also assist with de-rotation of the hip by applying slight inferior and anterior pressure on the PSIS.
6. Steps 3 to 5 are repeated 3 to 5 times, or until an improvement of the innominate dysfunction is palpated.
7. Effectiveness of the technique is assessed by reassessing iliosacral motion.

M99.06 LOWER EXTREMITY SOMATIC DYSFUNCTION

Example

DIAGNOSIS

Proximal Fibula Posterior

POSITION

The proximal fibula is posterior

RESTRICTION

The proximal fibula is restricted in anterior glide

TYPE OF MUSCLE ENERGY

Joint mobilization using muscle force

TREATMENT POSITION

Patient: Supine, with hip flexed 45 degrees, and knee flexed 90 degrees

Physician: Standing at the foot of the table, facing the patient

PROCEDURE (FIG. 51.18)

1. The physician's medial hand is placed on the dorsum of the foot, with the thumb on the lateral aspect, and the fingers on the medial aspect.
2. The physician's lateral hand anchors the calcaneus.
3. The ankle is inverted to the initial resistance.
4. Instruct the patient to "push the foot sideways into the physician's thumbs, and up into the physician's hand."
   a. This eversion/dorsiflexion of the ankle is thought to contract the extensor digitorum longus and the tibialis anterior muscles, drawing the fibula anteriorly.
5. This contraction is held for a full 3 to 5 seconds.

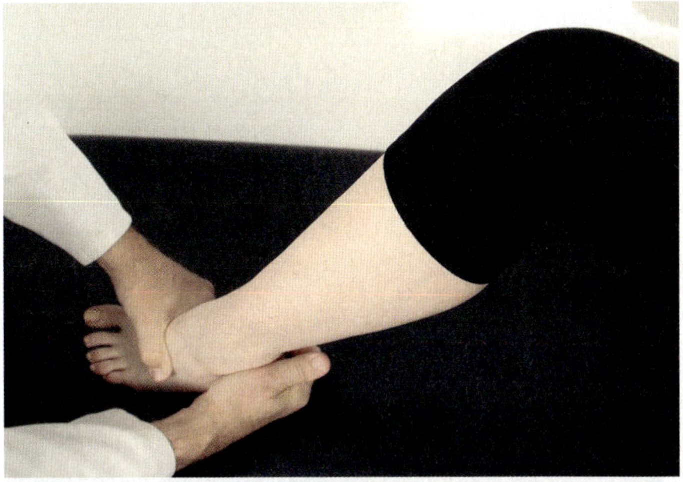

Figure 51.18. **Treatment of posterior proximal fibula.**

6. The patient is directed to relax, while the physician simultaneously ceases the applied counterforce.
7. The physician waits 2 seconds for the tissues to relax, and then further inverts the foot until a new restrictive barrier is met.
8. Steps 4 to 7 are repeated 3 to 5 times or until no additional motion can be gained.
9. Effectiveness of the technique is determined by retesting motion at the proximal tibiofibular articulation.

M99.07 UPPER EXTREMITY SOMATIC DYSFUNCTION

Example

DIAGNOSIS
Hypertonicity of the rhomboid causing medial scapular displacement

POSITION
Scapula medially displaced

RESTRICTION
Scapula resists lateral displacement

TYPE OF MUSCLE ENERGY
Postisometric relaxation

TREATMENT POSITION
Patient: Seated on the side of the table
Physician: Standing behind the patient and to the left

PROCEDURE (FIG. 51.19A AND B)

1. The physician reaches in front of the patient with the left hand and grasps the patient's right forearm.
2. The patient's right arm is drawn across the front of the body, from right to left, and inferiorly in a direction paralleling the direction of the fibers of the rhomboid major and minor.
3. The physician's right hand is placed to the left of the spine, providing a counterforce to truncal rotation.
4. The patient is instructed to "pull the right elbow toward the right," while the physician provides an unyielding counterforce.
5. This contraction is maintained for 3 to 5 seconds.
6. The patient is then instructed to relax.
7. After a second or two of relaxation, the physician increases tension on the rhomboid musculature by drawing the patient's right arm further across the front of the patient's body, until the new restrictive barrier is engaged.
8. Steps 4 to 6 are repeated 3 to 5 times.
9. Success of the technique is determined by palpating the rhomboid musculature and retesting scapular motion.

M99.08 COASTAL SOMATIC DYSFUNCTION

In general, costal somatic dysfunction is divided into two groups:

- Ribs held in inhalation (inhaled ribs)
- To identify the key rib that may be maintaining the group dysfunction, begin assessment at the most inferior rib of the group. Once the key rib is determined, direct treatment to that key rib.
- Ribs held in exhalation (exhaled ribs)
- To identify the key rib that may be maintaining the group dysfunction, begin assessment at the most superior rib of the group. Once the key rib is determined, direct treatment to that key rib.

Example 1

DIAGNOSIS
Rib dysfunction—left ribs 1–3 held in inhalation. The left rib 3 has been identified as the key rib. (The following technique can be performed on ribs that generally exhibit pump handle mechanics, ribs 1–5 with the key rib usually being the most inferior of the group.)

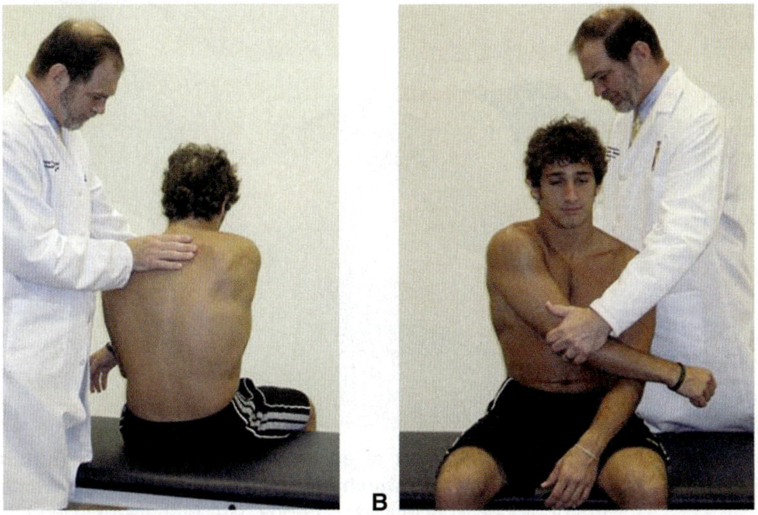

A B

Figure 51.19. **A.** Treatment of hypertonic rhomboid, posterior view. **B.** Treatment of hypertonic rhomboid, anterior view.

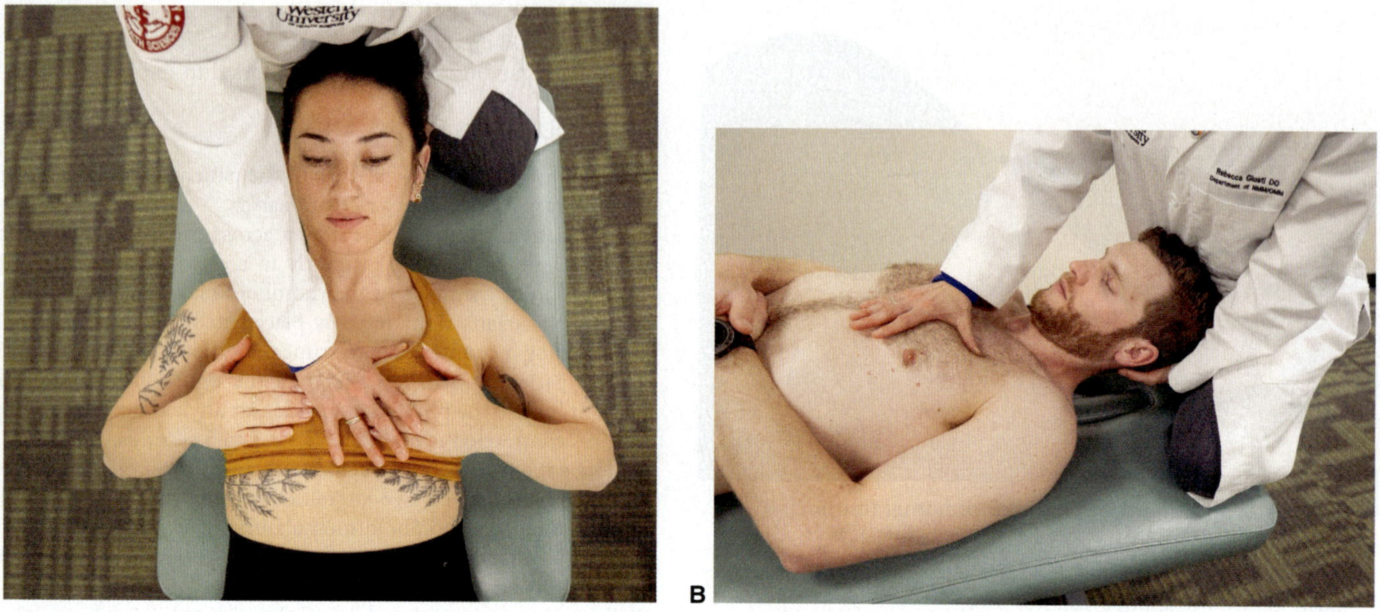

A B

Figure 51.20. A and B. Treatment set-up for an inhalation somatic dysfunction of rib 3 (pump handle mechanics) on two different patients. (Photo courtesy of Western University of Health Sciences, Pomona, CA, with permission.)

POSITION

Inhaled rib; a rib moves fully in inhalation; a rib is held in inhalation.

RESTRICTION

Restriction of exhalation; rib stops early in exhalation; extent and duration of exhalation movement are decreased.

TYPE OF MUSCLE ENERGY

Uses multiple mechanisms including respiratory assistance

TREATMENT POSITION

Patient: Supine. Please note that the patient may place their hands over the midline of the chest as this may be a sensitive area. Please see Figure 51.20.

Physician: Standing at the head of the table

PROCEDURE (FIG. 51.21)

1. The physician contacts the patient's head and neck with the same hand and forearm (right) as the affected rib and induces mild flexion and sidebending toward the affected rib. This localizes the rib into the "exhaled" position. Ensure that the flexion and sidebending are limited to the key rib and do not continue to the rib just inferior to it.
2. The physician then places the opposite thenar eminence and thumb on the anterior superior aspect of the key rib (left rib 3) using slight medial and lateral traction to free the costosternal joint. The physician's two hands work in concert to loose pack the joints (costosternal, costovertebral, and costotransverse) of the affected rib.
3. The physician then flexes the patient's head and neck until the anterior aspect of the key rib glides inferiorly toward the edge of the first restrictive barrier (just before motion is felt at the rib just inferior to it). The monitoring hand takes up slack in the inferior direction but does not transmit excessive force on the rib.
4. The physician then instructs the patient to inhale and exhale.
5. As the patient inhales, the physician resists superior motion of the key rib with the monitoring hand. During exhalation, the physician exaggerates the pump handle motion.
6. At the end of exhalation, the physician relocalizes the key rib into the restrictive barriers with further flexion, sidebending, and any other joint play needed.
7. Steps 3 and 6 are repeated 3 to 5 times until optimal motion of the key rib has been achieved.
8. Success of the technique is determined by reassessing for improved motion of the dysfunctional rib.[24]

Example 2

DIAGNOSIS

Rib dysfunction—Right ribs 1 and 2 held in exhalation, key rib is right rib 1

POSITION

Exhaled rib; the rib moves fully in exhalation; the rib is held in exhalation

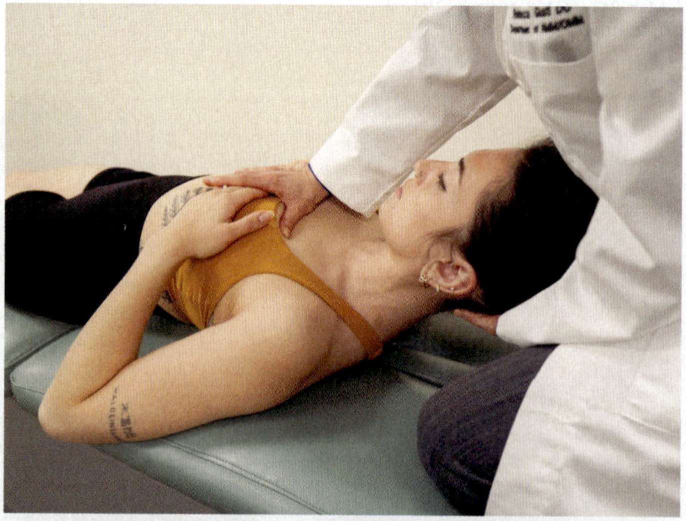

Figure 51.21. Treatment of an inhalation somatic dysfunction of rib 3 (pump handle mechanics). (Photo courtesy of Western University of Health Sciences, Pomona, CA, with permission.)

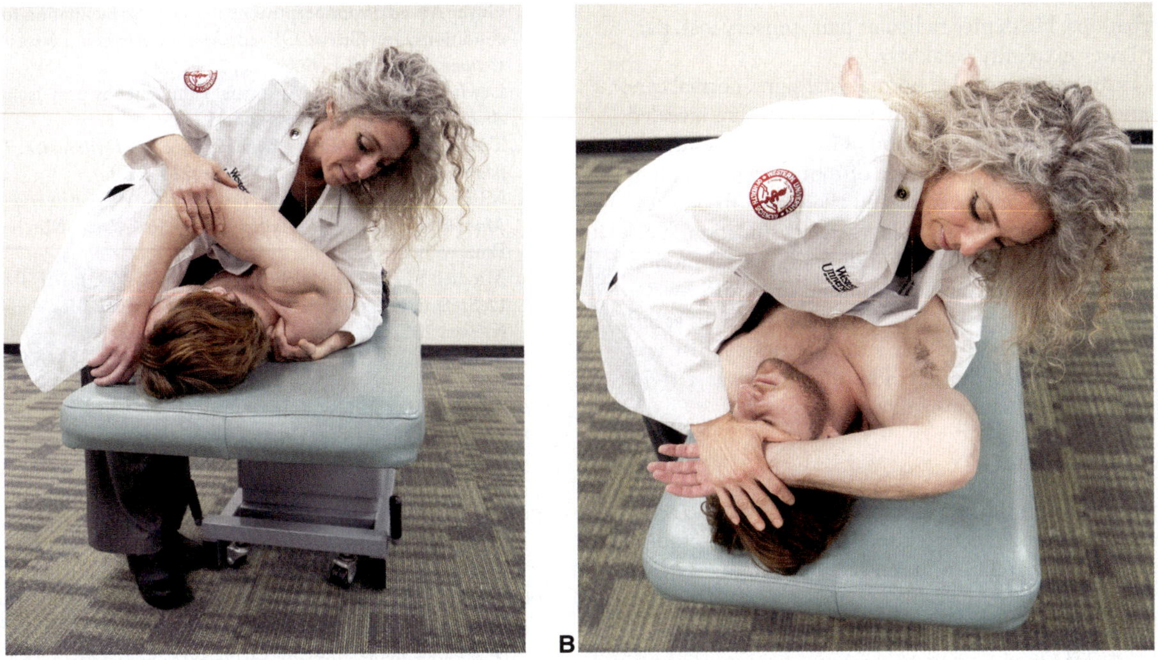

A B

Figure 51.22. **A.** Treatment setup for an exhalation somatic dysfunction of rib 1. **B.** Treatment of an exhalation somatic dysfunction of rib 1. (Photo courtesy of Western University of Health Sciences, Pomona, CA, with permission.)

RESTRICTION

Restriction of inhalation; rib stops early in inhalation; extent and duration of inhalation motion are decreased

TYPE OF MUSCLE ENERGY

Uses multiple mechanisms, including joint mobilization using muscle force

TREATMENT POSITION

Patient: Supine

Physician: Standing at the side of the patient, opposite the side of the dysfunctional rib one.

PROCEDURE

1. The patient lies on the table as close to the physician as possible.
2. The physician rolls the patient toward them and contacts the superior posterior aspect of the shaft of right rib 1 with their left hand, applying tension in an anterior, lateral, and inferior direction (Fig. 51.22A).
3. The physician rolls the patient back to a supine position, allowing the patient's shoulders to rest flat on the table. The patient is instructed to rotate their head contralaterally about 30 degrees (away from the dysfunctional rib). The patient's arm on the side of the dysfunction is placed over the forehead with the dorsum of the hand resting against the patient's forehead with the physician's hand lightly contacting it.
4. The patient is asked to maintain this positioning while contracting their head up against their arm or hand for 3 to 5 seconds against the physician's unyielding counterforce while holding their breath in the inhalation phase. This may be accomplished with the instruction, "Take a deep breath in and hold it while pushing your head toward the ceiling, matching my force." This contraction activates the anterior and middle scalene muscles which may serve to draw the anterior aspect of the rib 1 superiorly and the posterior aspect inferiorly (Fig. 51.22B).
5. The patient is directed to relax the contraction while the physician maintains the tension on rib 1.
6. After about 2 seconds of the relaxation phase, the physician increases the disengagement of the rib by drawing the rib slightly inferiorly, anteriorly, and laterally, further gapping the costovertebral joint.
7. After this repositioning into the new restrictive barrier, steps 4 to 6 are repeated 3 to 5 times.
8. Success of the technique is determined by reassessing for improved motion of the dysfunctional rib.[25]

CASE STUDY

A.J., a 54-year-old man presented with a recent onset of lower back pain. The pain began while he was attempting to push a heavy automobile (Fig. 51.23).

The worst pain is located in the region of the lumbosacral junction, and spreads across the top of the right iliac crest and into the right groin. The pain is worse with truncal flexion and improves with truncal extension. It is a constant dull ache with

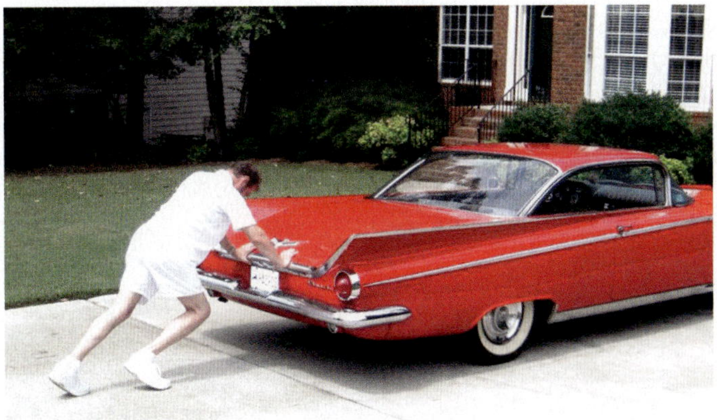

Figure 51.23. **See case study.**

sharp exacerbations. He denies radicular pain, sensory loss, paresthesias, or lower extremity weakness.

Physical examination revealed normal vital signs, normal cardiac and pulmonary exams. Neuromusculoskeletal exam revealed normal motor, reflexes, and sensation. Gross motion testing revealed mildly restricted lumbar range of motion. The standing flexion test was positive on the right and the seated flexion test was negative, suggesting a possible iliosacral dysfunction. This was confirmed by palpating passively induced iliosacral motion and discovering loss of right iliosacral motion. The PSIS on the right was more superior than was on the left and the right sacral sulcus was shallow compared to the left. The right ASIS was more inferior compared to the left. The diagnosis was a right anteriorly rotated innominate somatic dysfunction.

MECHANISM OF INJURY

Excessive contraction of the rectus femoris muscle on the right against an unyielding resistance resulted in the anterior rotation of the innominate bone, relative to the sacrum.

TREATMENT

The appropriate MET was applied to treat the right anterior innominate somatic dysfunction. Reassessment revealed restoration of symmetric passively induced iliosacral motion, and a normal standing flexion test. Additionally, the patient reported immediate substantial pain relief.

REFERENCES

1. Goodridge JP. Muscle energy technique: definition, explanation, methods of procedures. *J Am Osteopath Assoc*. 1981;81:249–254.
2. Mitchell FL Sr, ed. Structural pelvic function. In: Barnes MW, ed. *Yearbook of the Academy of Applied Osteopathy*. American Academy of Osteopathy; 1958:79.
3. Ruddy TJ, ed. Osteopathic rhythmic resistive duction therapy. In: Barnes MW, ed. *Yearbook of the Academy of Applied Osteopathy*. American Academy of Osteopathy; 1961:58.
4. Guyer AF, ed. Proprioceptive neuromuscular facilitation for vertebral joint conditions. In: Grieve GP, ed. *Modern Manual Therapy of the Vertebral Column*. Churchill Livingstone; 1986:626.
5. Lewit K, Simons DG. Myofascial pain: relief by post-isometric relaxation. *Arch Phys Med Rehabil*. 1984;65:453–456.
6. Travell JG, Simons DG. *Myofascial Pain and Dysfunction: The Trigger Point Manual*, Vol. 2. Williams & Wilkins; 1992:10.
7. Mitchell FL Jr, Moran PS, Pruzzo NA. *An Evaluation and Treatment Manual of Osteopathic Muscle Energy Procedures*. Mitchell, Moran, and Pruzzo; 1979.
8. Mitchell FL Jr. *The Muscle Energy Manual*. Vol. 1. MET Press; 1999.
9. DeStefano LA. *Greenman's Principles of Manual Medicine*. 5th ed. Wolters Kluwer. 2017:97.
10. Mitchell FL Jr. *The Muscle Energy Manual*. Vol. 3. MET Press; 2001:xxvi.
11. Finni T, de Brito Fontana H, Maas H. Force transmission and interactions between synergistic muscles. *J Biomech*. 2023 May;152:111575.
12. Stecco A, Giordani F, Fede C, Pirri C, De Caro R, Stecco C. From Muscle to the Myofascial Unit: Current Evidence and Future Perspectives. *Int J Mol Sci*. 2023 Feb 24;24(5):4527.
13. Mitchell FL Jr, Moran PS, Pruzzo NA. *An Evaluation and Treatment Manual of Osteopathic Manipulative Procedure*. 2nd ed. Institute for Continuing Education in Osteopathic Principles, Inc.; 1973:325.
14. Jull GA, Janda V, eds. Muscles and motor control in low back pain; assessment and management. In: Twomaey LT, Taylor JR, eds. *Physical Therapy for the Low Back*. Churchill Livingstone; 1987:272.
15. Mitchell FL Jr. *The Muscle Energy Manual*. Vol. 1. MET Press; 1999:14.
16. DeStefano LA. *Greenman's Principles of Manual Medicine*. 5th ed. Wolters Kluwer. 2017:99.
17. Mitchell FL Jr. *The Muscle Energy Manual*. Vol. 3. MET Press; 2001:201.
18. Mitchell FL Jr. *The Muscle Energy Manual*. Vol. 3. MET Press; 2001: 201–203.
19. Seffinger MA, Hruby RJ. *Evidence-Based Manual Medicine: A Problem-Oriented Approach*. Saunders Elsevier; 2007:107–108.
20. Mitchell FL Jr. *The Muscle Energy Manual*. Vol. 3. MET Press; 2001: 129–141.
21. Mitchell FL Jr. *The Muscle Energy Manual*. Vol. 3. MET Press; 2001:106.
22. Nicholas A, Nicholas E. *Atlas of Osteopathic Techniques*, 4th ed. Wolters Kluwer. Philadelphia. 2023: 318–319.
23. Mitchell FL Jr. *The Muscle Energy Manual*. Vol. 3. MET Press; 2001:146.
24. Mitchell FL Jr. *The Muscle Energy Manual*. Vol. 2. MET Press; 1998: 71–75.
25. Mitchell FL Jr. *The Muscle Energy Manual*. Vol. 2. MET Press; 1998: 66–69.

52 Myofascial Release

JUDITH A. O'CONNELL

KEY CONCEPTS

- This approach emphasizes appreciation and recruitment of the innate and inherent motion of the myofascial structures.
- Patterns of motion and ease are identified across proximal and distal structures, diaphragms, compartments, viscera, and organ systems.
- This family of techniques includes myofascial release (MFR), integrated neuromusculoskeletal release (INR), fascial–ligamentous release, and bioelectric fascial activation and release (BFAR).
- Respiratory assistance, fulcrums, body positions, neuroreflexive activities, oscillations, passive progressive motions, and muscular contractions may aid in the progression of MFR.

DEFINITIONS

MFR is a system of diagnosis and treatment first described by Andrew Taylor Still and his early students, which engages continual palpatory feedback to achieve release of somatic dysfunction involving myofascial tissues. It can be applied as a *direct, indirect, or combined approach.*

- In a direct technique, a restrictive barrier is identified in the myofascial tissues, then engaged with a loaded, constant, directional force until the tissue releases and motion is restored.
- In an indirect technique, the dysfunctional myofascial tissues are loaded and then guided toward the position of greatest ease. The tissues are held at this point of least resistance until free movement of all tissues is achieved.
- In a combined approach, dysfunctional myofascial tissues are engaged in directions of restriction and ease concurrently or sequentially, allowing the MFR to occur through the interactive application of both direct and indirect methods.
- Fascial or myofascial unwinding. An osteopathic treatment method in which the dysfunctional fascial tissues are engaged in a dynamic continuous process in response to palpatory feedback of ease and/or bind.

HISTORY

"As this philosophy (osteopathy) has chosen the fascia as a foundation on which to stand, we hope the reader will chain his patience for a few minutes on the subject of the fascia, and its relation to vitality. It stands before the philosopher as one of, if not the deepest living problem ever brought before the mind of man."[1]

Still

As Dr. Still was developing the science of osteopathy, he spent a great deal of time writing and pondering the importance of fascia in health and disease. Dr. Still did not write detailed instructions on how to perform a treatment. Instead, in *Research and Practice*, he provided a rationale for applying osteopathic principles and integrating osteopathic manipulative treatments (OMTs) into the medical management of diseases. Even though he did not leave a technique manual, and the profession has only one short video of him performing a treatment, Dr. Still's emphasis on the fascia affected the development of early osteopathic methods, which serve as the foundation for this class of techniques today. Dr. Still directed his students and colleagues to hunt in the fascia as "*[t]he ground in which all causes of death do the destruction of Life*,"[1] and many did.

Pioneers in early osteopathic thought and education[2,3] continued to develop methods for diagnosing and treating the fascia by applying the principles of osteopathy: the body is a unit with the innate ability to heal, where structure and function are reciprocally interrelated.

Sutherland, Becker, Fulford

Osteopathic luminaries such as Sutherland, Kaufman, Snyder, Cathie, Cole, Smoot, Zink, Becker (Alan and Rollin), and Fulford all expanded our understanding of fascia and laid the foundation for a renaissance of technique development, beyond a joint-centric model of manipulation.

Within this resurgence of interest in the myofascia, Sutherland's teachings on the treatment of the membranes and ligaments, along with Fulford's percussion vibrator techniques, were incorporated into osteopathic education (see Chapter 53 Osteopathic Cranial Manipulative Medicine and Chapter 59 Fulford Percussion for more details). Harakal and Becker taught the importance of enlisting the aid of the *physician within* a patient to harness self-healing properties in all osteopathic treatments.[4] Fulford challenged the osteopathic physician to engage a patient's life force with proper intention and attention to achieve positive results.[5] An increased interest emerged in the innate motions of connective tissues, in the vibratory changes across tissues, in the bioenergy discussions of Sutherland, Becker, and Fulford, and the fluid properties of palpation and treatment. This shift in focus from joint-based models to the evolving connective tissue models thus fueled a renaissance of osteopathic thought and the expansion of osteopathic technique.

Peckham, Ward, Chila

In the 1980s, Peckham, Chila, and Ward began discussing how to standardize the techniques being developed as MFR (personal communication with Anthony Chila, DO, 2007). Two models emerged from their conversations: the *biomechanical model* of Ward and the *big bandage of fascial continuum model* of Chila.

- The *biomechanical model* (Ward) emphasizes the muscular–fascial relationship. It developed the techniques known as MFR and integrated INR. As the basis for diagnosis and treatment, these techniques emphasize:

TABLE 52.1

Models of MFR Techniques

Models of MFR	Techniques	Tissue Focus	Emphasizes
Biomechanical model	MFR, integrated INR	Muscular–fascial relationships	Mechanics, anatomic relationships, tight/loose concepts, tethering, and interdependent neural relationships
Fascial continuum of the big bandage model	Fascial–ligamentous release, fascial release	Fascia	Fascial continuum, treat proximal to distal, fulcrum with leverage, torsion and traction, respiratory assistance, and reflexive neurologic reset
Bioenergetic model	Bioelectric fascial activation and release, fascial release, MFR	Fascia, holographic interface in homeostasis	Bioresponsive electrical potentials, diaphragms, longitudinal cables and tubes, fascial interface in homeostasis, holographic diagnosing and treating

  - Mechanics
  - Anatomic relationships
  - Tight and loose relationships
  - Tethering and interdependent neural influences
- The *fascial continuum model of the big bandage* (Chila) emphasizes the fascia. It developed into fascial release and fascial–ligamentous release. These techniques treat proximal to distal using:
  - The integrity of the fascial continuum
  - A fulcrum with leverage
  - Torsion and traction
  - Respiratory assistance
  - Reflexive neurologic reset

Ward and Chila began teaching their respective models, both of which influenced the next generation of osteopathic techniques.

O'Connell

During the 1980s, O'Connell was influenced by the osteopathic teachings of Still, Kappler, Larson, Chila, Ward, Harakal, Sutherland, Fulford, Alan, and Rollin Becker. In the 1990s, she explored bioenergetic research in other disciplines and integrated these concepts into diagnosing and treating the fascia. From this emerged the *bioenergetic model*, which emphasizes:

- The bioresponsive electric potentials of the fascia
- The primary and compensatory patterns of dysfunction
- The fascial continuity of diaphragms with longitudinal cables and tubes
- The fascial interface of internal extracellular fluid (ECF) and external (biomechanical) environmental factors on homeostasis

BFAR is a treatment process of intention, attention, and activation of the bioenergetic fascia with holographic palpation, diagnosis, and treatment. O'Connell's approach allows the totality of the human being to be accessed through a single hand placement, or portal of entry.[6] Using the fascia as a portal of entry provides information regarding the whole person, as the fascia connects all structures of the body.

These models are summarized in Table 52.1.

EMBRYOLOGIC, ANATOMIC, AND PHYSIOLOGIC PROPERTIES OF FASCIA

Embryology

Embryologic development of the mesodermal germ layer gives rise to connective tissues and muscles. The largest mesodermal derivative is connective tissue, which encompasses blood, cartilage, bone, and connective tissue proper. Histologically, these tissues are distinguished by the proportions of fiber, cells, and extracellular matrix into six types:

1. Areolar
2. White fibrous
3. Yellow elastic
4. Mucous
5. Retiform
6. Basement membrane

The principal cell types are:

- Fibroblasts
- Fat cells
- Fixed macrophages
- Mast cells
- Plasma cells
- Leukocytes

The extracellular matrix contains:

- Collagenous, elastic, and reticular fibers
- Mucopolysaccharides
- Proteoglycans
- And molecules of:
  - Elastin
  - Mucin
  - Reticulin
  - Chondroitin sulfate
  - Keratin sulfate
  - Heparin
  - Chondroitin acid
  - Hyaluronic acid[7]
  - Collagen

Collagen is a major component of connective tissue proper, and more specifically, of white fibrous tissue. Fascia, the largest component of white fibrous tissue, contains linear sheets of collagen found in superficial, deep, and subserous layers (see Fig. 52.1 and Chapter 7 The Fascial System of the Body for more details).

A special property of connective tissue cells is *embryologic plasticity*.[8] This allows differentiated connective tissue cells, when properly stimulated, to dedifferentiate to a polypotential root cell, and then redifferentiate into another type of connective tissue cell. Histologically, some traumatized tendons or muscle tissues have islands of cartilage or bone exemplifying this process. Experiments by Becker et al.[8] documented that disruption in the collagen of the periosteum creates a bioelectric current, which affects the *charge*

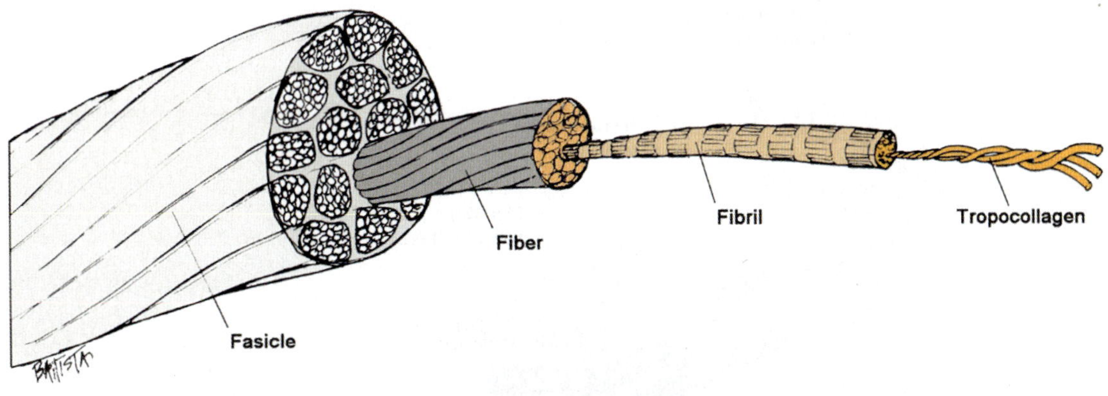

Figure 52.1. **Mobility of collagen is demonstrated in its structure.**

of the cell membrane of fibroblasts. This triggers their *embryologic plasticity* as part of the healing process in fractures. The resultant changes in the DNA and RNA allow for the cell to dedifferentiate into a primitive polypotential root cell, which then redifferentiates into the types of cells needed during the healing process. This illustrates the embryologic plasticity of connective tissues. In the face of traumatic biomechanical stress, connective tissue responds by changing its cell type to meet the demands on the tissue. The process is initiated by bioelectric changes at the tissue, cell, and nuclear levels.

The extracellular matrix of connective tissue contributes to homeostasis through:

- Diffusion
- Absorption
- Secretion
- Diffusion gradients
- Modification of absorbed substances
- Metabolism and catabolism
- Excretion of metabolic end products and waste[8]

All cells contribute to this ECF by interfacing with nerve endings, hormones, and vascular and lymphatic structures. This organization allows for coordination of the internal (metabolic, cellular, and organ systems) components of homeostasis, within the structure of connective tissues.

Anatomy

MUSCLES

There are three types of muscles: smooth, cardiac, and skeletal. They are all related embryologically to connective tissue, the vascular system, cranial nerves (CNs), as well as to the autonomic and peripheral nervous systems through *migratory segmental differentiation*. Skeletal muscle fibers develop from the mesodermal myotomes and regional mesenchyme. They then migrate in a sea of connective tissue, in response to lines of stress in the developing embryo. Skeletal muscle myofibrils extend along these lines in a linear fashion and become bundled as fascicles by the perimysium. Between the fascicles exists the endomysium, which contains the nerves, blood, and lymph vessels. It also acts as lubricant and cushion. Fascicles are bundled by the epimysium and by the tendons that connect muscles to the developing skeleton. This creates a compact integration of multiple systems, residing within a connective tissue container (Fig. 52.2).

Earlier authors like Cathie[9] and Becker[10] suggested that fasciae move independently. A 1987 soft tissue dissection performed by Frank George, D.O., in the anatomy laboratories of Michigan State University demonstrated that fascia and muscle are anatomically inseparable. His findings suggest that complex muscle activities acting on bones, ligaments, and tendons associate with joints as well as the fasciae.

FASCIA

Fascia is associated with all organs, tissues, cells, and structures. Clinically, it is possible to conceptualize such wrapping as being a *big bandage* of the body. Such an analogy is implied in osteopathic literature, where the idea that the body retains form, even if everything except the connective tissue framework is removed, is discussed. The superficial and deep layers of fascia are found everywhere in the body as complete ensheathments. The subserous layer lies in the innermost, deep layer of all body cavities. Of the three layers of fascia, the deep layer is the most complex since it is composed of two layers with intervening septa. Fascia lines, divides separates, and supports the internal organs, great vessels, muscles, bones and joints, and lymphatics. Even the meninges are a form of fascia and have multiple attachments inside the skull, in the spinal canal, along the traversing nerve roots, and onto the sacrum (see Chapter 7 The Fascial System of the Body). This fascial continuum is the one anatomic structure of the body that links the osteopathic principles of the interrelationship of structure and function.

Guimberteau and Armstrong provide a visual tour of living fascia which highlights the structure and expanse of fascia allowing the viewer a unique understanding of fascia and the human condition.[11]

Physiology

PRINCIPLES OF FASCIA

Collagen, fibrin, and reticulin are the connective tissues that act as the body's reactor to motion and stress. They are coupled with the skeletal muscle, and their interaction produces *irritability, contractility, relaxation, distensibility, and elasticity* (Table 52.2).[12]

- *Irritability* is the ability of the muscle fiber to react to stimulation.
- *Contractility* is the ability to actively create tension between its origin and insertion. The opposing passive state is *relaxation*.
- *Distensibility* is the ability of the associated connective tissue to be stretched or deformed by an outside force. If the force does not exceed the tensile strength of the connective tissue, the muscle will not be injured.
- *Elasticity* is the ability of the connective tissue to return to its original resting shape when forces are removed.[12]

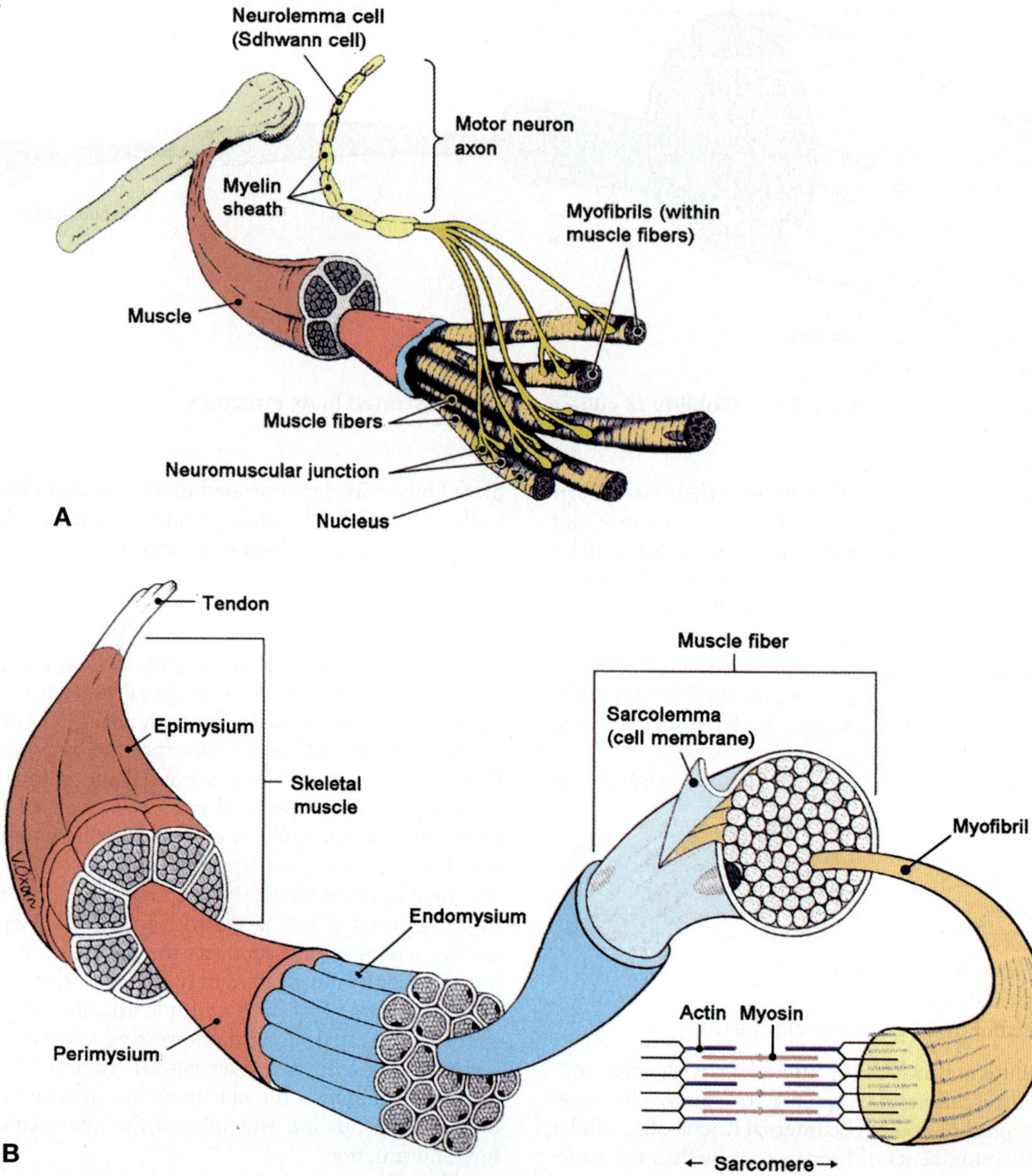

Figure 52.2. A, B. Muscle fiber structure.

TABLE 52.2

Physical Properties of Muscle

Properties	Description
Irritability	Ability of the muscle fiber to react to stimulation
Contractility	Ability to actively create tension between its origin and insertion
Relaxation	Ability to reduce tension between its origin and insertion
Distensibility	Ability of the associated connective tissue to be stretched or deformed by an outside force, and if the force does not exceed the tensile strength of the connective tissue, the muscle will not be injured
Elasticity	Ability of the connective tissue to return to its original resting shape when forces are removed

Other force effects in connective tissue of importance are *plastic deformation, elastic deformation, viscosity, stress, strain, and creep* (Table 52.3).

- In plastic deformation, a stressed, formed, or molded tissue *preserves* its new shape.
- In elastic deformation, a stressed, formed, or molded tissue *recovers* its original shape.
- *Viscosity* is the capability of a solid to continually yield under stress, with a measurable rate of deformation.
- *Stress* is the effect of a force normalized over an area.
- *Strain* is a change in shape as a result of stress.
- *Creep* is the continued deformation of a viscoelastic material under constant load over time (Fig. 52.3).

Hysteresis, or *stress–strain*, is defined as a connective tissue response to loading and unloading. Restoration of the tissue's final length occurs at a rate, and to an extent less than during deformation (loading). This represents energy loss in the connective tissue (Fig. 52.4).[13]

TABLE 52.3

Force Effects in Connective Tissue

Force Effects	Description
Plastic deformation	A stressed, formed, or molded tissue *preserves* its new shape
Elastic deformation	A stressed, formed, or molded tissue *recovers* its original shape
Viscosity	Capability of a solid to continually yield under stress with a measurable rate of deformation
Stress	The effect of a force normalized over an area
Strain	A change in shape as a result of stress
Creep	The continued deformation of a viscoelastic material under constant load over time
Hysteresis or stress–strain	A connective tissue response to loading and unloading where the restoration of the final length of the tissue occurs at a rate and to an extent less than during deformation (loading) representing energy loss in the connective tissue

Generally, the body's connective tissues are under some degree of load and extension (expansion). The increase and subsequent reversal of extension produces a degree of tissue response, less than that of the relatively unloaded state. This phenomenon is referred to as *hysteresis*. It implies the occurrence of some flow and dissipation of energy throughout the loaded tissue. Hysteresis occurs less with successive cycles of extension, indicating stabilization of response.[13]

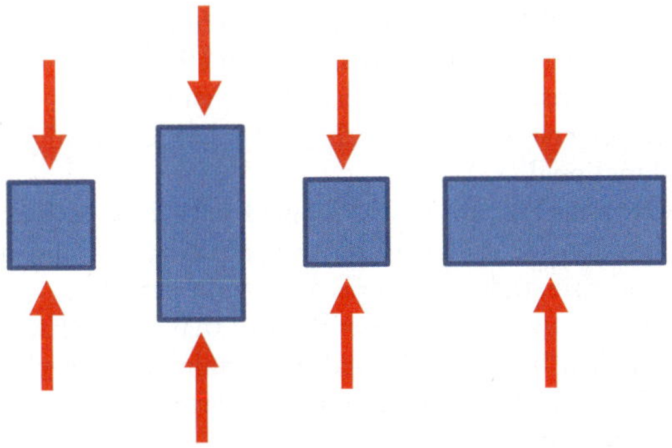

Figure 52.3. Deformation under load.

PHYSIOLOGIC LAWS

It is now clear that the physical properties of fascia and muscles explain how physical laws of adaptability apply to MFR techniques.

- *Hooke law*[14] states that stress applied to stretch or compress a body is proportional to the strain, or the change in length produced, so long as the limit of elasticity of the body is not exceeded.
  - □ Palpatory diagnosis and treatment is the systematic application of directed mechanical pressures and motions while monitoring the tissue response.

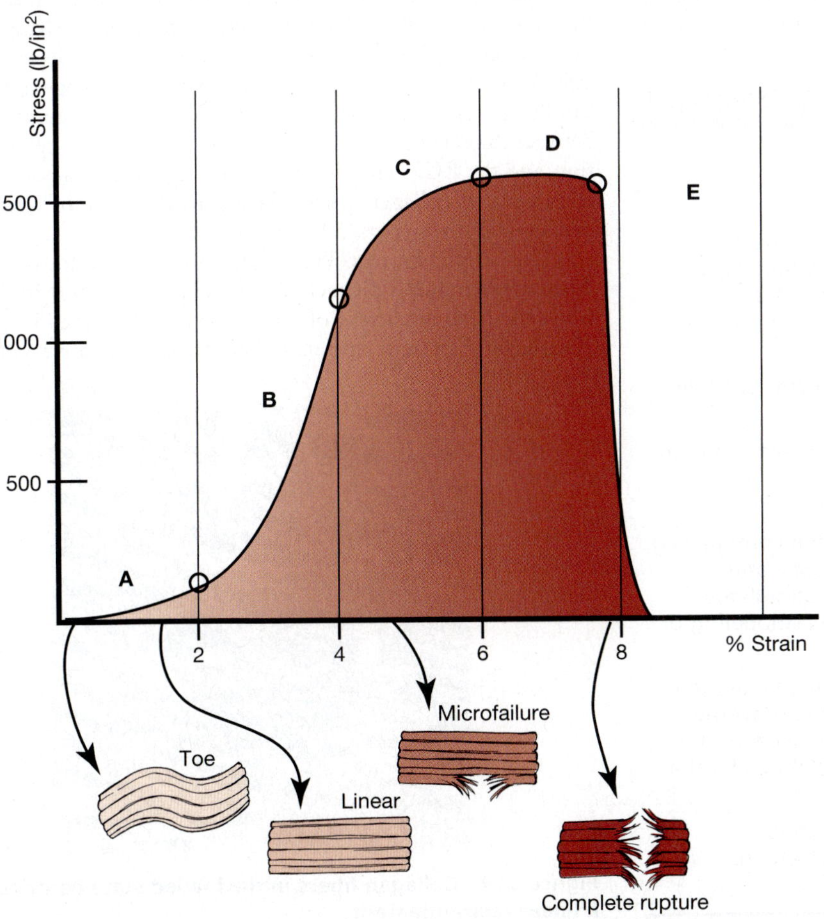

Figure 52.4. The stress–strain curve.

- Perceived alterations in motions, symmetry, tissue texture, and tenderness define somatic dysfunction.[15]
- The response in intact fascia to mechanical stress is predictable, detectable, and treatable with MFR techniques when dysfunctional.
- These physical properties, coupled with Hooke law, are the foundation for the characteristic palpatory findings of barriers and ease, tight and loose, and strain patterns.

■ *Wolff law of bone transformation*[14] states that every change in the function of a bone is followed by certain definite changes in internal architecture and external conformation, in accordance with mathematical laws.

- Function dictate's structure. Every change in the form and function of a bone is followed by certain changes in its internal architecture and secondary alterations in its external conformation.
- Structure also dictates function. Multiple studies examined the application of this law.

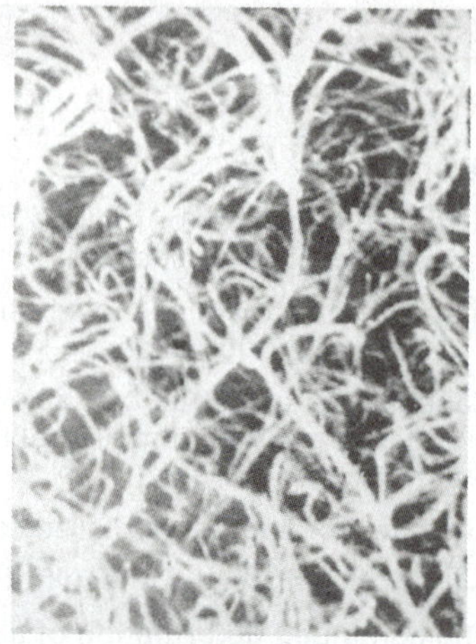

Figure 52.5. Collagen fibers in the unloaded state demonstrating a multidirectional arrangement.

PIEZOELECTRICITY

In the 1950s, Yasuda and Fukada and Bassett and Becker demonstrated that bone is *piezoelectric*. Piezoelectricity is a current produced by a substance that transforms mechanical stress into electrical energy. Piezoelectric substances act as transducers and are able to discharge electrical current when physically stressed. When placed in an electric current, they vibrate at a frequency dependent upon their crystal lattice structure. Further studies identified *collagen* as the piezoelectric substance in bone.[16] *Fascia is a collagen-rich connective tissue with piezoelectric properties* (see Table 52.4).

Piezoelectricity is important in the maintenance of bone, as well as the response of bone to stress. Studies investigating Wolff law noted that a bioelectric gradient is formed in bone in response to stress. The electronegative charge in the compressed bone stimulates osteoblasts, and the electropositive bone stimulates osteoclasts that direct the remodeling of the bone. This concept was further clarified when Becker and Bachman[16] discovered that when mechanically stressed, collagen in bone produces a biphasic signal that is negative with stress (load) and positive with release (unload). This stress-release signal is rectified to a direct current at the junction between the apatite and collagen in the bone. *The strength of this signal indicates the amount of stress, and the changes in polarity identify the direction of the stress.* This signal triggers osteocyte activity, allowing for the bone to remodel and adapt to the mechanical stress.

Collagen is the source of stress-related electrical potentials due to its piezoelectric nature as a transducer. Collagen communicates the presence, location, direction, and strength of mechanical stress by producing a biphasic electric current. This bioelectric current affects the charge-sensitive cells that move and change in response. Studies demonstrate that collagen is the ultimate communicator between biomechanical events, bioelectric changes, cellular function, and the ECF. The electronegative signal also causes the linear alignment of collagen perpendicular to the lines of compressive mechanical stress (Figs. 52.5 and 52.6).

This alignment of collagen becomes the base for ossification. Also, stress-induced piezoelectric potentials are short in duration, while the healing current of bone growth is sustained in duration. The healing current stimulates electrically sensitive connective

TABLE 52.4

Piezoelectric Properties of Collagen

Properties	Description
Transducer	Able to discharge electrical current when physically stressed and when placed in an electric current, vibrate at a frequency dependent upon its crystal lattice structure
Biphasic signal	Negative with stress (load) and positive with release (unload)
Stress-related signal	Strength of this signal indicates the amount of stress, and the polarity changes identify the direction of the stress
Stimulates osteocytes	Electronegative charge in the compressed bone stimulates osteoblasts, and the electropositive bone stimulates osteoclasts directing the remodeling of the bone
Stimulates and directs the migration of electrically sensitive cells	Releases chemotactic factors, creating a gradient and activating the movement of necessary connective tissue cells facilitate the clearing of debris and the repair of injured tissues
Activates cells	Stimulates electrically sensitive connective tissue cells which are embryologically plastic

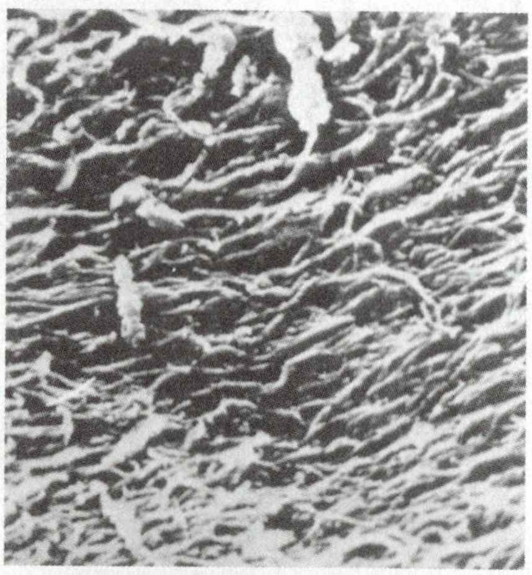

Figure 52.6. Collagen fibers in the loaded state demonstrating a linear rearrangement.

tissue cells that are embryologically plastic and allows the bone to respond to growth or stress appropriately.

The cells of connective tissue are mobile, allowing for the migration of cells to meet the needs of the organism. This ameboid motion is exemplified by the fibroblasts, macrophages, and white blood cells. It is triggered by positive or negative chemotaxis, or in response to a bioelectric potential gradient that directs the cells into and out of the area of need. This movement allows tissues to respond to changes in their environment, both internal and external, by releasing chemotactic factors. This activates the movement of connective tissue cells, facilitates the clearing of debris, and participates in the repair of injured tissues. Disruption and distortion of the fascia trigger a repair process directed at correcting damage and strengthening tissues.

In addition to cellular movement directed by bioelectric potentials and the alignment of collagen, other research highlights the importance of fascia in maintaining general proprioception. Since proprioception is ultimately controlled by interdependent neural and muscular elements, after joint and muscle spindle activity is accounted for, 75% of remaining proprioception occurs in the fascial sheaths.[17] Such responses were demonstrated in the 1960s by Earl[18] and Wilson,[19] in their work with muscles under stretch.

In Dr. Still's words: "I know no part of the body that equals the fascia as a hunting ground … By its actions we live and by its failure we die."[1]

PROPOSED MECHANISM OF ACTION

The continuity of fascia throughout the body, along with structural–functional interrelationships, makes it possible to discuss the proposed mechanism of MFR technique in relationship to the biomechanical attributes of fascia. MFR techniques harness the power of collagen through diagnosing and treating the fascia, the largest collagen pool in the body.

MFR techniques address somatic dysfunction by normalizing motion, relieving edema, reestablishing symmetry, relieving pain, aiding circulatory and lymphatic function, normalizing neuroreflexive activity, supporting visceral function, restoring bioenergetic balance, and supporting homeostatic function. Fascia supports and stabilizes, which helps to maintain postural balance and assists with the production and control of motion. Therefore, MFR techniques are proposed to improve stabilization, balance, and motion of the related tissues biomechanically and neurologically. Consider a patient challenged with chronic pain who may seek a position where the pain lessens or is relieved. This infers that positional relief of pain allows a decrease in some critical level of facilitation in the nervous system. Fascial release techniques are designed to reduce afferent input to the cord either directly or through central brain influences. Muscle proprioceptors and the gamma motor system are affected with reduced excitation of the muscle spindles, and the resumption of normal length and motion.[20]

Palpation introduces compressive and distraction forces into fascial tissue, which responds in predictable patterns of motion, produced by adaptations to the mechanical stress. Alterations in normal patterns and ranges of motion are diagnostic parameters. Abnormal patterns of motion are recognized as restrictions to motion and ease of motion. The asymmetric motion and position of components of the musculoskeletal system are also readily identified through palpation. Adaptive responses in the ECF and surrounding structures to stress-generated electrical potentials produce acute and chronic tissue textures, as well as areas of stiffness, looseness, tenderness, asymmetry, edema, and pain. Further rationales for the mechanism of OMT in releasing dysfunction are found in the works of Korr,[21] Becker,[22] and Patterson.[23]

Tensegrity Systems

Tensegrity systems are another way of looking at the responsiveness of the fascia. As discussed by Edward Stiles, D.O., a tensegrity structure consists of multiple nontouching rods (compression struts) and a continuous connecting system (tension system) embedding or islanding the compression struts. He references Donald Ingber's, M.D., Ph.D., research:

- The bones of the body are compression struts, and the continuous tension system is a tensegrity structure composed of the myofascial and ligamentous tissues of the body.
- These integrated multilevel hierarchical systems exhibit balanced tension, and system-wide adaptation when a force is introduced anywhere in the structure.
- This force can influence any part of the system, from the macro to the micro and vice versa, and can be distributed throughout the system in a nonlinear manner.
- Distortions altering cellular shape and function affect differentiation and specialization, biochemical activity, and genetic expression of the affected cells.

Stiles stresses the importance of these concepts in applying OMT for the removal of somatic dysfunction and in enabling patients to realize their optimal health potential by restoring their tensegrity potential.[24] Further discussion of the importance of tensegrity within the myofascial network is provided by Hohenschurz-Schmidt demonstrating its importance in understanding the body's response in health and disease.[25]

FASCIA, HOMEOSTASIS, ALLOSTASIS, AND ALLOSTATIC LOAD

Homeostasis

Homeostasis involves a complex series of events and interfaces between all systems and the internal and external environment. Homeostasis is both a state of equilibrium and the process by which this balance is maintained. It is a dynamic, ever-adapting, and changing series of events that respond to internal and external environmental changes (Table 52.5). Homeostasis includes

TABLE 52.5

Components of Homeostasis

Components	Description
Internal environment is the ECF	Complex activities coordinating hormones, nerve impulses, gases, nutrients, ions, and electrical potentials by diffusion, gradients, absorption, secretion, modification of substances, excretion, metabolism, and catabolism
External environment is the aggregate of complex events outside of our body that affect us	Adaptation to external stressors and accommodates active manipulation of the environment with posture, movement, coordination, strength, balance, and awareness coordinating cognitive, neural, muscular, skeletal, and vascular structures
Confluence of all organs and systems	Dynamic, ever-adapting, and changing series of events responding to internal and external environmental changes

the interface and interaction among the physical, emotional, mental, and spiritual bodies within an individual. Insights into these connections can be found in many sources outside medical literature. One helpful guide in understanding and interpreting the connections between thought patterns and disease is *Heal Yourself* by Louise Hay. The author has been supporting patients with cancer, AIDS, and other life-altering diseases.

The challenge of homeostasis is to recognize that all events, external and internal, communicate needs for adaptation throughout the organism, and direct responses that are both internal and external. Nothing is isolated.[26]

Allostasis

Allostasis refers to the process that maintains homeostasis with the recognition that control may change with the environment (see Chapter 18 Stress Management). The primary mediators of allostasis include the HPA axis, autonomic nervous system (sympathetic and parasympathetic), and pro- and anti-inflammatory cytokines. Allostatic systems allow the organism to respond to its physical state and to cope with stressors in its environment. Allostatic load and overload refer to the cumulative result of an allostatic state.

McEwen at the Rockefeller Institute postulated that the shift from homeostasis to the disease state is related to the system's response to traumatic, psychological, emotional, physiologic, and/or environmental stress. The body under any source of stress enters a state of allostasis, where epinephrine and cortisol are released. If this state becomes long term, an allostatic load ensues with physiologic consequences, such as elevated blood pressure, heart rate, and risk of cardiovascular disease. Increased cortisol levels can suppress the immune system, affect organ function, alter metabolism, and contribute to depression.

Allostatic Load

The allostatic load may become somaticized and expressed as somatic dysfunction with *body language significance*,[24] which may help in identifying the nonsomatic cause of chronic, recurrent dysfunction in light of appropriate treatment. This is demonstrated when the body acts out its underlying stress condition.

- A patient with chronic emotional stress may have low back pain.
- Mental and emotional feelings of "shouldering" a heavy burden may cause shoulder pain.
- Refusal to change behaviors leads to a stiff neck.

As previously discussed, fascia responds to biomechanical stress, through its collagen fibers, by producing micro electrical potential changes. The changes are communicated through electrical changes in the ECF to cellular, neural, vascular, and lymphatic components. These stress-generated potentials are predictable and precise, whether traumatic or intentional.

In systemic disease, alterations in ECF and electrical potentials cause changes in the biomechanical integrity of the fascia. Areas of acute and chronic congestion, swelling, laxity, stiffness, and pain are produced. Palpatory findings are utilized by skilled physicians to identify the disease-produced somatic dysfunction. Integrating an understanding of the patterns of viscerosomatic and somatovisceral relationships adds a deeper diagnostic and therapeutic dimension to the palpatory exam.[26]

Neuroreflexive coordination is essential to homeostasis Autonomic, sympathetic tone especially affects not only pain perceptions but also the balance of neurovascular exchange that affects edema and effusions. This in turn affects motion and tissue function. Proprioception, integrated with the special senses of sight, hearing, and touch, is essential to balance, posture, and gait.

Disease occurs when one or more system(s) fail to maintain their role in homeostasis. It begins as a clinically undetectable change in ECF and progresses until clinically detectable signs and symptoms appear, making the diagnosis apparent.[26] The goal of the physician is to detect the disease and institute appropriate treatment as early as possible. This limits the amount of damage to the systems and organs and enhances the body's innate healing capabilities. Learning to diagnose and treat with MFR techniques is a clinical advantage, since no disease escapes notice in the fascia, and no cure occurs without its assistance.

INDICATIONS

MFR is used to treat somatic dysfunction involving myofascial tissues or other connective tissues.[27]

The goal is to alleviate the visceral and somatic components of somatic dysfunction in the connective tissues of the body, with a focus on fascia, muscles, and related structures (neuroreflexive, circulatory, lymphatic, respiratory, bioenergetic, systemic, holographic, and homeostatic). In systemic disease, MFR techniques address structural imbalances and somatic dysfunction indicative of and pursuant to changes in homeostasis, thus aiding in the normalization of function in all systems.

CONTRAINDICATIONS

1. **Absolute**
   a. Absence of somatic dysfunction
   b. Lack of patient consent or cooperation
2. **Relative**
   a. Extreme caution should be exercised in patients with:
      i. Fractures
      ii. Open wounds
      iii. Soft tissue or bony infections
      iv. Abscesses
      v. Deep venous thrombosis (threat of embolism)
      vi. Anticoagulation
      vii. Disseminated or focal neoplasm
      viii. Recent postoperative conditions over the site of proposed treatment (wound dehiscence)
      ix. Aortic aneurysm

COMPLICATIONS

A word of caution: overly aggressive interventions are counterproductive. Care should be taken to ensure that any treatment respects the limits of dysfunctional and injured tissues. Exceeding these limits creates a traumatic event. Somatic dysfunction resulting from iatrogenic trauma, layered on already dysfunctional or traumatized tissue, is the most difficult dysfunction to treat.[26]

Patients commonly experience a temporary worsening of discomfort following the first treatment or two. This possibility should be communicated to the patient. The phenomenon is similar to postexercise muscle soreness. Older age groups and general deconditioning are common contributors to the problem. Those with autoimmune, inflammatory, and rheumatologic disorders such as lupus erythematosus and fibromyalgia can experience repeated flare-ups.

SAFETY AND EFFICACY

Direct and indirect MFR are very safe. The efficacy of MFR has been demonstrated in the treatment of carpal tunnel syndrome. MFR for other conditions has not been specifically studied but is believed to be comparable to counterstrain or muscle energy. While theoretically possible, there are no known reports of complications arising from MFR.[27]

The safe introduction of motion depends upon multiple factors: integrity of the tissues (open wounds, fractures, recent surgery), the amount of traumatized tissue (thermal injury, contusions, crushing), concomitant diseases (deep vein thrombosis, disseminated or local neoplasms, aortic aneurysm, uncontrolled diabetes), internal injuries (ruptured viscera or vascular structures), surgical interventions, infections, cooperation of the patient, and the skill of the physician.[27]

TYPES OF MFR

As previously described in the definition of MFR, this technique can be applied in a direct, indirect, or combined approach.

In a direct technique, a restrictive barrier is identified in the myofascial tissues, then engaged with a loaded, constant, directional force until the tissue releases and motion is restored.

In an indirect technique, the dysfunctional myofascial tissues are loaded and then guided toward the position of greatest ease. The tissues are held at this point of least resistance until free movement of all tissues is achieved.

In a combined approach, dysfunctional myofascial tissues are engaged in directions of restriction and ease concurrently or sequentially, allowing the MFR to occur through the interactive application of both direct and indirect methods.

This family of techniques include *MFR, INR, fascial–ligamentous release, and BFAR*. Related techniques (facilitated positional release, functional release, counterstrain, balanced ligamentous and membranous tension, progressive inhibition of neuromuscular structures, soft tissue, articulatory, Still method, osteopathic cranial manipulative medicine, Fulford percussion vibrator, and visceral) are discussed in Section VIII and IX of this book.

Soft tissue techniques are related techniques that are *not* in the family of MFR techniques discussed in this chapter. They treat the soft tissues of the body with inhibitory pressure, stretching and kneading, petrissage and skin rolling, deep friction, tapotement, and effleurage.

Clinical Approach

In choosing the most appropriate approach, it is important to recall that fascia is ubiquitous connective tissue that enrobes the body in a *big bandage*.[6] It contributes to form and function and is accessible by manipulative techniques to alleviate somatic dysfunction.

Muscular relationships to the fascia contribute to the shifting tightness and looseness identified through range of motion changes, and through palpation as direct and indirect barriers.

Appreciation and recruitment of the *innate and inherent motion* of the myofascial structures allow for the identification and treatment of patterns of motion and ease, across proximal and distal structures, diaphragms, compartments, viscera, and organ systems.

The *bioresponsive electrical potentials of the fascia*[6] produce palpable changes in fascial motion and ease, which are related to the status of the internal environment of homeostasis, and the biomechanical response to the external environment. This aids in the diagnosis and treatment of visceral as well as musculoskeletal disorders and diseases.

Evaluating the patient in multiple positions (standing, seated, prone, supine) and activities (walking, standing, squatting, changing positions, bending, work positions) adds another dimension to fascial diagnosis and treatment. Dysfunctions in these areas are important contributors to chronic recurring somatic and visceral dysfunctions. Identification of such patterns and their neuromyofascial components allows the physician the opportunity to affect and extinguish self-perpetuating cycles. Once this is accomplished, repatterning the neuromyofascia into a more physiologic response is appropriate.

The following clinical aids may assist in the implementation of MFR[13,28]:

- Respiratory assistance
- Fulcrums
- Body position
- Patient cooperation
- Sequential guiding by the physician
- Using neuroreflexive activities
- Oscillation
- Passive progressive guiding
- Using muscular contractions and relaxation

SPECIAL CONSIDERATIONS IN DIAGNOSIS AND TREATMENT

Passive range of motion testing for a region, local tissues, or a joint is performed to identify a restrictive barrier and a position of ease. The skilled physician is able to identify altered fascial patterns from any source, internal or external, as somatic dysfunction. Once identified, the pattern, location, and type of somatic dysfunction assist in the diagnosis of visceral and somatic disease. The disease is then treated with the appropriate application of MFR technique, and/or combination of osteopathic techniques with standard medical/surgical care. Monitoring changes, immediate and distant (over time), in the form and function of fascial structures, indicates the status of diseases and their response to all treatment endeavors.

Developing Subtle Palpatory Skills

DR. STILL

"For many years, immersed in extensive study of normal and abnormal positions of the human anatomy, Still had formed in his mind a perpetual image of every articulation in the framework of the human body. Before William Roentgen's discovery of the x-ray machine, visualization, good observation skills, a delicate sense of touch—and that perpetual image—were the only tools Still had to assist him in detecting the abnormal from the normal. He also claimed to see an aura around all of his patients—vibrations emanating from the body—giving him additional clues about his patient's conditions. The Old Doctor, skeptical of the new instrument (x-ray machine), stated to some students, "The x-ray by tremendously increasing the vibrations enables us to see under the surface what our eyes will not discover. Why can't we train our minds to do that?"[29] (see Box 52.1).

WARD

Inherent tissue motions are palpably evident, asymmetrically patterned, neuroreflexive activities in the soft tissues. They constantly move, often at variable rates. Palpation that focuses on these motions identifies patterns of shifting asymmetric tightness and looseness. Asymmetrical end-feels are commonly referred to as direct and indirect barriers. As a rule, inherent movements are

BOX 52.1 Common Causes of Tethering[30]

- The spine, with altered coupled vertebral motions from any source
- Altered soft tissue mechanics (remembering that all tissues and their inherent motions are intrinsically asymmetric)
- The synovial joints and their influences on joint play
- Asymmetric neural inputs arising from:
- Multiple levels of the central nervous system, including CN, brainstem, midbrain, thalamus, and cortex; limbic system and reticular activating system; primary spinal cord; peripheral nervous system at any level
- Viscerosomatic reflexes, somatovisceral reflexes, and somatosomatic reflexes
- Neurohumoral activities of all kinds
- Lowered reflex thresholds from sites of disease, injury, and degeneration
- Biobehavioral and sociocultural factors, environmental stressors
- Treat the effects of disrupted hierarchical balance of patterns of dysfunction by first relieving the iatrogenic effects and then reconstruct and treat the layered dysfunctional patterns in the body.

easier in some directions, less so in others. Myofascially, shifting tightness and looseness identifies unevenly distributed direct and indirect barriers. Many are independent of joint mechanics. Others are tightly linked to joint mechanisms.[13]

During treatments with MFR techniques, there is a link between the intrinsic body movements of both the patient and the physician at some level. How this occurs is unknown, but it is likely that both conscious and subconscious brain-mediated factors are at play. Skilled palpation in the fascia enables the physician to sense anatomic and mechanical detail, much like how a blind person senses the environment.[13]

CHILA

MFR techniques require refinement of palpatory skills to appreciate subtleties of stress patterns and motion characteristics. Technique application engages and assists the patient's own potency, rather than the use of blind external force that overpowers the patient's innate assistance. The physician uses palpation to sense or listen to the effects of the biokinetic energies and forces, while allowing the biodynamic intrinsic force to manifest.[20] These corrective forces engage the identified resistance to motion and direct it to a point of simultaneous balance and decreased tension. This allows the intrinsic force of the tissues to correct the imbalance. The focus is on the quality of movement, particularly on initiation of motion. The correct gauging of force and velocity provides infinite variation in the delivery of technique. Control minimizes force. An effective physician should be able to vary the applications of force over time during a single manipulative treatment. Appropriate use of a fulcrum and leverage can refine the physician's diagnostic touch and treatment effectiveness.

Visualization and synthesis of messages received through the fingers are the basis for clinical behavior. Conceptualization of anatomic–physiologic dysfunction peculiar to a given patient is the key to maximizing manipulative responses. The sustained effective response following treatment is contingent on selective and controlled variation of force from an appropriate fulcrum. When these conditions are met, inherent neuroregulatory mechanisms, acting in accordance with the capacity of the patient, will facilitate the resolution of dysfunction.[20]

O'CONNELL

Fascia can be viewed as an "intelligent tissue," functioning as the interface between internal and external events. It also plays a key role in homeostasis. As discussed previously, embryologic plasticity gives connective tissue the unique ability to respond with cellular adaptations that meet the changing needs of the organism.[6] Through the use of "thinking fingers" (Sutherland), intelligent palpation interfaces with the fascia in a clinical dialogue, giving access to:

- Peripheral and central structures
- Viscera and soma
- The biologic and bioenergetic bodies

The body, mind, and spirit are all available to the skilled physician as the whole of the human condition. They are recorded and assessable in the holographic fascia. As physicians improve their palpatory skills, they gain the awareness that from any portal of entry into the fascia, the whole of the patient's condition (body, mind, and spirit) is available for diagnosis and treatment. Once this skill level is achieved, the physician can identify the primary dysfunction rapidly from contact at any site on the body. Within the holographic fascia, the primary dysfunction is not limited to connective tissue structures and may be anywhere in the body, mind, and spirit continuum. Focused intention to assist in healing, and attention to the homeostatic fascial holographic interface, allows for the activation of far-reaching releases and healing dynamics.

This level of skill has been described by many master osteopaths and healers as a "knowing" sensation, and also as viewing an image or movie like projection that flashes into a stilled mind. The power and potency of techniques at this level demands that the physician maintain an attitude of humility, respect, suspended expectations, and compassion.[6] It is within the patient that the capacity to heal resides.

Dr. Still: "Don't believe for one second that this was the limit of his vision. According to many who studied with him and others who have spent years studying his works it was his hope that the experience of living, dynamic anatomy would awaken dormant centers of perception in the student. Gradually, over a period of years of focused attention, conscious intention of purpose and deep non-judgmental concentration on the experience of life as manifested in the patient, the physician would evolve to a higher level of interaction with the dynamic mechanism of the patient. He would evolve into an osteopath."[30]

PRINCIPLES OF TREATMENT

As described by Ward, the key to clinical success is the systematic development and application of the MAN acronym—Mechanics, Anatomic relationships, and interdependent Neural influences with:

- Tethering
- Tight–loose relationships
- Three-dimensional patterns (Ward)
- Harnessing a fulcrum, balanced points of tension
- Expanding releases of dysfunction over time within the connective tissue continuum (Chila)

- Monitoring for and continuously responding to fascial unwinding.
- Utilizing the holographic fascial structure of tubes, diaphragms, and longitudinal cables
- Identifying primary somatic and visceral dysfunctions with their related patterns of activating releases in the bioenergetic fascial continuum, supporting homeostasis (O'Connell)

Treatment is enhanced when the physician addresses the patient with proper intention (humility and respect for the patient's process), attention (mindfulness of the patient's needs), appropriate application of technique, and activation of releases (supporting the healing process) (Chila, Ward, and O'Connell).

The treatment process for MFR may be summarized as follows[27]:

1. Indirect MFR:
   a. Physician moves patient into the position of ease for all planes, following any tissue release or fascial unwinding until completed. If needed to enhance tissue release, the following may be employed:
      i. Regional compression, distraction, or torsion
      ii. Tissue inhibition or traction
      iii. Respiratory cooperation in the phase that encourages tissue tension
      iv. Eye, tongue, jaw, head, or limb movements
2. Direct MFR:
   a. Physician moves patient into restriction for all planes, applying steady force until tissue release or fascial unwinding is completed.
   b. If needed to enhance tissue release, the following may be employed:
      i. Respiratory cooperation in the phase that encourages tissue tension
      ii. Tissue inhibition
      iii. Oscillation
      iv. Eye, tongue, jaw, head, or limb movements
3. Combined MFR:
   a. In a combined approach, dysfunctional myofascial tissues are engaged in directions of restriction and ease concurrently or sequentially, allowing the MFR to occur through the interactive application of both direct and indirect methods. Enhancing maneuvers as described above may be employed as needed to achieve maximal release.
   b. Indirect, direct, or combined MFR may be employed dynamically depending upon the nature and extent of the diagnosis, in addition to the patient's physical condition, tolerance, and initial response to treatment.

Activating Forces

Activating forces used in MFR techniques are as follows[6,13]:

- *Inherent (intrinsic) force* uses the body's natural tendency to seek homeostasis. Inherent force is the rhythmic activity in all tissues, which works to improve the hydrodynamic and bioenergetic factors around restricted tissues and articulations.
- *Respiratory force (cooperation/assist)* may be used in four ways:
  1. While using a direct or indirect position, *full cycle respiratory effort* is applied as a fascial and/or articulatory activating force.
  2. Once positioned, a *particular phase of respiration* enhances the position of the area being treated.
  3. *Breath holding* for the maximum time that a patient can tolerate causes air hunger and triggers a generalized relaxation of soft tissues.
  4. *Coughing or sniffing on command* produces a respiratory impulse to assist in the release of restrictions.
- *Patient cooperation*: The patient is requested to move in specific directions in various planes of an articulation, to aid in mobilizing an area of restriction.
- *Physician-guided force*: After engaging a barrier or point of ease, the physician sequentially guides the tissue or joint through various positions, following a shifting pattern of easy motion, until the path of dysfunction is retraced and released.
- *Springing/vibration*: Placing the hands or percussion hammer on a dysfunction and applying variable degrees of pressure and/or frequency of force causing springing or vibration in the structure, activates release of the tissues.

GENERAL PRINCIPLES OF THE TECHNIQUES

Fascial–Ligamentous Release—Chila

Fascial–ligamentous release is a dynamic and expansile form of MFR that emphasizes the "cybernetic loop" between the physician and patient. The diagnosis and treatment occur simultaneously by using a selective, controlled reciprocal variation of force and appropriate leverage. This is coupled with inherent neuroregulatory mechanics, to impact the resolution of dysfunction within the capacity of the patient. This form of MFR helps explain the interactive nature of MFR, and the importance of continuously monitoring the involved tissues for response and interpreting and adapting treatment based upon tissue feedback.

Key elements of this dynamic process are as follows:

- Application of force is variable.
- Utilization of time is variable.
- Visualization and synthesis are mandatory.
- Conceptualization is paramount.
- Tolerance and response are individual.
- Inherent capacity is the standard for health or disease.
- Dynamic interchange: Patient allows physician to enter bodily territorial space.
- Physician is a facilitator and observer.
- Patient's life story is available through examination and evaluation of body tissues.
- Energy flows from thought.[20]

In conjunction with these elements, the patient provides breath assistance and/or muscular assistance in the corrective procedure. The physician seeks to establish a fulcrum within their body that matches or balances the fulcrum within the patient's body. This facilitates a continuum of reflex release from the patient. Once local and regional dysfunctions have been addressed with an appropriate fulcrum, expanding leverage is achieved through torsion and traction applied to the extremities to facilitate the release and restore balance. It is the ongoing analysis of dysfunction within this connective tissue continuum that makes possible the integration of multiple manipulative approaches, through variable applications of force.

The establishment of an appropriate fulcrum facilitates diagnostic touch. Under examination, the hands and fingers of the physician are placed on the tissues, with the idea that the fingers can mold themselves to the patient's body. A slight compression at the fulcrum points initiates the pattern and the principles of fulcrum are applied variably, depending on the complaints of the patient. *This process is not time-consuming*. Harnessing internal patient mechanisms are used and only contacted to sense them speaking for themselves. The point(s) of contact is(are) listening posts. Let the tissues tell the story; be quiet and listen. Biokinetic (dysfunctional) energies or forces are always at work in all physiologic and pathologic processes. The biodynamic (healing) intrinsic force within manifests with the appropriate use of diagnostic touch.

Special consideration of respiratory and circulatory function is essential in diagnosis and treatment. Compromised respiratory and circulatory effectiveness results from generalized fascial–ligamentous tension throughout the body. Therefore, the character of respiration provides information about such tension. Observe the following four factors about respiration:

1. Type of respiration: diaphragmatic, costal, or mixed
2. Abdominal wall motion: visible to the level of the umbilicus; visible to the level of the symphysis pubes
3. Rate: slow, rapid; documented before and after treatment
4. Duration of cycle: inspiration and expiration equal, inspiration shorter in duration than expiration, inspiration longer in duration than expiration, dilation of the nares during respiration

The body's connective tissues are generally under a certain amount of load and extension (expansion). As previously discussed, connective tissues under sustained load will extend (expand) in response to the load. In biomechanical terms, this continued extension is referred to as creep. An imposed constant load will result in relaxation, as the extension remains constant. In either situation, the tissue displays less subsequent resistance to extension than in the original state. Patterns of previous mechanical events affect the tissue's response to load and extension. Physician-applied extension effects tend to revert to their pre-extension responses, whether functional or dysfunctional, if the neuroreflexive processes are not altered. This observation is useful in appreciating recurrence of dysfunctional complaints and patterns. The timed release of tissues associated with the fascial–ligamentous release model considers these factors as sequential. Expanding progression of releases allows the patient to tolerate central nervous system modulation by the lowering of afferent inputs. Significant reduction or elimination of sensitization is proportional to the patient's capacity to appropriately respond. This view is attuned to the idea that conditioning the central nervous system over time may be the vehicle for the retention as well as the reduction of dysfunctional states. The physician's role is that of a facilitator. With appropriate facilitation, the physician observes the capacity for change, while the patient expands the power of the change. Success of this interchange depends on the patient's motivation.

Integrated INR—Ward

The ability to identify tethering effects that persistently create and maintain pathologic asymmetries is essential. Tightness suggests tethering, while looseness suggests joint and/or soft tissue laxity with/without neural inhibition. Sometimes, tethering relates directly to changes in coupled vertebral motions and altered joint play, which alters the motion segment. It is vital to know the difference between neutral and nonneutral vertebral mechanics. Common contributors to tethering include both local soft tissue and neuroreflexive and neurocirculatory changes, such as viscerosomatic reflex changes. Tethering arises from many sources, as shown in Box 52.1.

Painful sensations are common at loose sites, particularly in chronic cases. Typically, there is little muscle spasm or tightening. Under these conditions, associated muscles are commonly weak and inhibited. Some physicians refer to these sites as hypermobile, implying that ligamentous laxity and joint instability are the fundamental problems. An alternative idea concludes that loose, painful muscles are weak and inhibited over large, often ill-defined areas, including vertebral mechanics.

From a clinical perspective, whole-body effects are the rule rather than the exception. Loosened sites are often vulnerable to injury under relatively trivial circumstances. Repeated ankle and lumbosacral sprains, as well as neck and shoulder problems arising from altered lumbopelvic and lower limb mechanics, are common examples. The tight–loose concept can be quickly appreciated by the exercise given in Box 52.2.

Tightness of any kind suggests tethering and direct barriers. It also implies the presence of direct barriers and "bind." Some are of bony origin, but many are not. Whether these tethers and areas of bind should be removed requires careful assessment.

Acute muscle spasm is a form of tethering that is almost always self-limited. Another form generally relates to tight muscles, which are not always sources of pain and altered function. Stressful lifestyles and personality issues are common in this group. True spasticity, or centrally mediated neural tethering, arises from upper motor neuron pathologies. Common examples include cerebral palsy, central spinal stenosis, strokes, and the effects of head injuries.

BOX 52.2 Tight–Loose Concept Exercise

A simple laboratory exercise readily demonstrates the tight–loose concept. With the patient lying supine, the operator grasps the patient's wrists. By slowly raising the upper limb toward full overhead extension, one gets a sense of shifting three-dimensional tightness or looseness that begins at the wrists and eventually involves the whole of the patient's body. By carefully attending to both the quality and the amplitude of these passively induced operator forces, clearly defined mechanically asymmetric sites of tightness and looseness become apparent.

As each limb is moved separately and together, tight–loose relationships vary considerably, and their end-feels are different. Some are abrupt, almost like hitting a wall. Others are soft, like either falling into or fluffing a pillow. Importantly, these asymmetric shifts rarely follow classic anatomic patterns. With practice, variable tensions and loads are readily sensed from the hands and wrists distally into the lumbodorsal fascia and pelvis.

BOX 52.3 Concepts for Peeling an Onion of Dysfunctional Patterns

- Always treat the *primary pattern of dysfunction*
- Space out treatments to allow the system to rebalance.
- Acute patterns are always considered primary.
- Identify and treat the next primary pattern of dysfunction and continue this process as the layered patterns of dysfunction emerge, allowing recuperation time between treatments.
- Release activated primordial patterns very carefully as the changes in the body will be monumental, with both wondrous and devastating effects possible.

Scar tissue implies the presence of passive mechanical tethering that may actually stabilize an otherwise unstable site. Scar tissue changes a tissue's ability to respond and move in normal planes and produces a new focus of motion patterning. Acute localized muscle tension and tethering generally imply peripheral neural involvement. A history of direct trauma is common to this group.

Looseness generally occurs in association with indirect barriers, neural inhibition, and painful sites. Since inhibition often accompanies neural injury and Wallerian degeneration, pain reports and muscle weaknesses are a common theme with this group.

Three-dimensional vertical, horizontal, and wraparound patterns are the rule and can be identified with practice. Determining three-dimensionally related areas of tightness and looseness is key.

Tightness and looseness should be evaluated from a patterned three-dimensional context that includes the following:

- Skeletal and soft tissue configurations
- Upper and lower motor neuron influences
- Effects of mechanical modeling and remodeling of bones, joints, and soft tissues
- Effects of general skeletal factors
- Injury history
- Effects of repetitive daily activities
- Psychoemotional states
- Limiting psychosocial and socioeconomic factors

Locating direct and indirect barriers is a useful method for understanding tightness, looseness, and tethering effects. The general goal is to release tightness and to restore three-dimensional patterned functional symmetry without aggravating hypermobility. An experienced physician can efficiently *treat the whole body in a reasonably short time*, by sequentially applying forces against direct and indirect barriers.

Integrated neuromuscular and MFR approaches and treatments are used to diagnose and modify altered reflex and mechanical patterns anywhere in the body. Applying this form of treatment depends on the physician's ability to palpate and interactively respond to shifting reflexes and mechanical changes as they occur. Vital to this process is also the recognition of active and passive elements that influence both local and general myofascial patterns, and skeletal patterns. The key to clinical success is the systematic development and application of the MAN acronym—Mechanics, Anatomic relationships, and interdependent Neural influences.

Bioelectric Fascial Activation and Release—O'Connell

MFR techniques apply compression and distraction forces into the affected fascia, directed toward or away from a barrier of motion. Once the barrier or point of ease is engaged, the fascia responds with a decrease in resistance, and motion resumes. The fascia responds rapidly to the light forces applied by all MFR techniques. As previously discussed, this rapid response is the result of the multiple properties of myofascial tissue within the fascial continuum:

- Irritability
- Distensibility
- Contractility
- Relaxation
- Plasticity
- Elasticity
- Viscosity
- Stress
- Strain
- Creep
- Hysteresis
- Piezoelectric responses
- Neuroreflexive activity

During the technique, the fascia releases its restrictions in stages and leads the physician through a pattern of motion. Depending on the physician's skill, releases occur in two dimensions, three dimensions, or holographically. This pattern of motion is often complex, traversing any direction or plane, structure or region, organ, or system, within the body–mind–spirit continuum.

From the view of the bioenergetic model, the fascia's response is directed and mediated by microelectrical potential changes. Internal or external trauma and dysfunction leaves a pattern of bioelectric potential changes in the fascia that record the direction, strength, and location as somatic dysfunction (see mechanisms mentioned earlier). The application of the diagnostic and corrective forces also produces bioelectric potentials. This activation of bioenergetic tissues opens a diagnostic dialogue within the fascial continuum. Physician-induced patterns interact with the dysfunctional pattern differently than the normal tissue. This discernable difference unmasks the dysfunctional pattern as it leads the physician along its path to the primary dysfunction. With practice, the dysfunctional pattern becomes rapidly obvious, the primary dysfunction becomes evident, and releases begin almost immediately.

The MFR technique of activating a bioenergetic response and following its patterns of release, both diagnostically and therapeutically, is BFAR. BFAR builds on the principles of integrated INR/MFR and fascial–ligamentous release within the family of MFR techniques.

The foundation of BFAR is that the fascia is a holographic system with a structural continuum of tubes, diaphragms, and longitudinal cables that contain the record of all events, internal and external, biologic and bioenergetic, in any person. This design is like a transportation system with many connections, lines, and stations, allowing the rider to enter at any point and travel throughout the entire system. With the understanding of fascia as a readily accessible portal of entry, the physician has the opportunity to engage in a meaningful and far-reaching diagnostic dialogue with the patient. As dysfunction occurs (from any cause), its effects are transported throughout the whole organism via this continuum, interfacing with homeostatic mechanisms, from the bioenergetic to the systemic to the intracellular. To optimize this dialogue, the physician needs to have the appropriate intention to:

- Assist the innate healing properties of the patient to alleviate or eliminate the effects of disease processes.
- Restore the patient's ability to resume command of the clinical situation (Chila).
- Attend to the type, structure, and pattern of dysfunction diagnostically and therapeutically (Ward).
- Activate the holographic homeostatic response throughout the patient to facilitate the release of dysfunction and restore health (O'Connell).

In BFAR, the physician is a partner in this process where the patient's mechanisms are in control. Healing, therefore, is an internal dynamic of the patient and is not imposed by the well-meaning endeavors of the physician.

Considering the concepts of holographic fascia and tensegrity, diaphragms are especially good portals of entry to the fascia, because they occur at important anatomical crossroads where curves change, cavities change, and passage points for major circulatory and lymphatic vessels and organs occur. Diaphragms are muscular and fascial structures that give shape and form to the tubular structure of the body. They also counter the physical effects of gravity, entropy, and enthalpy while preserving the body's ability to function and perform in space.

- The central diaphragms are the tentorium, thoracic inlet/outlet, respiratory diaphragm, and pelvic diaphragm.
- Secondary diaphragms occur in the extremities, at the palmer and plantar fascia.

Myofascial structures act as longitudinal cables connecting all diaphragms, allowing for coordination of motion throughout the system.

The portal of entry to the fascia is chosen based on the patient's history, testing, and imaging results, consults, exams, and provisional diagnosis coupled with knowledge of anatomy and mechanics. This may lead to a very specific structure such as an organ, tendon, or muscle. Active diagnostic palpation may also be needed for further delineation. In the latter case, diagnostic palpation begins with the diaphragm closest to the suspected region, or the diaphragm the physician is most conformable palpating. In all cases, test tightness, looseness, local tissue quality, and range of motion induce motion using compression, distraction, or the full deep respiration cycle. Note the different patterns of interaction between the normal (predictable) and the dysfunctional (unpredictable) tissue responses. With practice, the dysfunctional pattern, whether a barrier or point of ease, becomes rapidly obvious, making the primary dysfunction evident, so releases begin almost immediately. The primary dysfunction may be proximal or distal in any organ or system and be biologic and/or bioenergetics.

- In using BFAR, no more than three deep respiratory cycles are needed to activate the release in a progressive fashion.
- With each respiratory cycle, motion in the tissue begins as a release occurs, and a new endpoint of motion manifests.
- Each successive deep respiratory cycle continues this process until the release is complete.
- The physician then returns to the original portal of entry and reassesses for symmetry and resolution of that pattern of dysfunction.

TRAUMA HISTORY AND PATTERNS

Special dysfunctional patterns resulting from the effects of trauma and ensuing trauma patterns warrant further discussion prior to the discussion on specific techniques. Trauma and alterations in the ECF precipitate a cascade of events mediated by bioelectric potential changes in the collagen-laden fascia. These events have local and distant effects that ultimately affect homeostasis. All musculoskeletal, medical, surgical, rehabilitative, and manipulative treatments engage these properties, whether passively or actively.

Disruption and distortion of the fascia trigger a repair and strengthening process mediated by the release of chemotactic factors, which then activates the congregation and proliferation of fibroblasts.

- Fibroblasts first coat the injured area with a fibrin matrix.
- Collagen is then deposited in a linear fashion in the tissue, along lines of mechanical tension.[24]
- Mechanical tension creates bioelectric current changes that guide the orientation of the fibrin and collagen.
- Healing therefore considers the function of the injured tissue as it repairs its structure.

If neurologic integrity is compromised or the tissue is immobilized, then dense connective tissue is formed. Without the lines of tension and motion, edema and disruptions in circulation as well as lymphatic drainage also cause fibrin and collagen to be deposited in a thick and haphazard scar. These thickened areas impede the normal function of the linear sheets of fascia, causing stiffness, changes in range of motion, pain, and further edema.[6] This process increases the tissue scarring in a vicious self-perpetuating cycle. Chronic alterations in fascial integrity impede the normal function of the ECF, resulting in consequences to the health of the whole organism.

Movement is essential to the appropriate, functional repair of fascia.

The following healing concepts apply to all connective tissues when injured:

- Linear fibrin and collagen are deposited in response to tension in the tissue and are directed by bioelectric potential changes.
- Immobilization causes collagen and fibrin to be condensed and haphazard.
- Motion improves circulation, exchange of lymphatic fluids and metabolites, and encourages the normal distribution of fibrin and collagen.
- It is essential that motion, whether passive or active, be introduced into traumatized tissue as soon as possible.
- Appropriate application of OMT will help to restore normal function in traumatized tissue.

Tensegrity concepts help to explain relationships between trauma and chronic pain.[15] As previously discussed, the body can be viewed as a tensegrity system where trauma affects the whole system, and adaptations occur as the body rebalances. As the trauma is distributed, the most intense area of adaptation is not always at the site of trauma. This site of the pain complaint is secondary, resulting from adaptation to the original site of trauma and its related dysfunction pattern. Therefore, evaluation of the whole patient is necessary to identify the site and pattern of the traumatic event, not just the site of pain. Treating the cause of the pain, rather than the pain itself (the adaptive effect), is more efficient and will yield better results.[31]

A good trauma history is essential to understanding the patient's condition and complaints.[15] Table 52.6 outlines the components of a trauma history, which helps to identify areas and patterns of related dysfunctions and the patient's state of health.

The treatment plan for the dysfunctional and/or traumatized patient incorporates these concepts. Osteopathic management of such patients addresses the trauma and its effects with OMT, in combination with medical, surgical, rehabilitative, and alternative interventions. Treating somatic dysfunction enhances healing and homeostasis in all levels of the body, mind, and spirit. "To find health should be the object of the doctor. Anyone can find disease."[1]

LAYERED DYSFUNCTIONAL PATTERNS ("PEELING THE ONION")

After releasing the primary dysfunction pattern, a new primary pattern of dysfunction is often evident upon reassessment. Throughout life, the body is exposed to many traumatic and stressful events that produce a distinct primary dysfunction pattern. In the same way that the primary dysfunction is defined as the most dysfunctional segment within a pattern of dysfunction, the *primary pattern of dysfunction* is defined as the most dysfunctional of the layered patterns of dysfunction. As this pattern resolves, the next most dysfunctional pattern becomes the primary (52.3).

The process is much like peeling an onion.[6] This onion layer effect continues until all dysfunctional patterns are resolved. A word of caution: After the release of a primary dysfunction

TABLE 52.6

Components of a Trauma History

Components	Description
Chronology of trauma	When, where, and what happened during the trauma
Events surrounding the time of the trauma	Circumstances, state of health, state of mind, age, life changes, etc.
Progression of the trauma-related symptoms	Radiation or migration of pain or symptoms, development of other symptoms, etc.
Mechanism of trauma	Motor vehicle accident, birth trauma, fall, surgery, etc.
Direction and motion of trauma	As detailed as possible, e.g., pivoting left on right foot when tackled on the outside of the right knee
Type of trauma	Blunt, sharp or cutting force, compression, traction, active motion against resistance, repetitive, etc.
Original signs and symptoms	Bruising, pain, swelling, asymmetry, fractures, motion changes, organ symptoms, etc.
Changes in signs and symptoms	Progressing, developing or continuing pain, functional changes, neurologic, mental, or emotional symptoms, improving symptoms, etc.
Types and responses to treatments	Surgery, medication list, physical therapy, supplements, alternative care, etc.
Pretrauma diseases and changes since the trauma	Any changes in types of disease and response to treatment
Post-trauma diseases	New conditions and response to treatment
Previous trauma	List any residuals still present at time of present trauma
Subsequent trauma	Relationship to the presenting trauma, e.g., repetitive work injuries, falls due to unstable joints, etc.
Disabilities related to the presenting trauma	Achieved or applied for, e.g., social security, personal injury, worker's compensation, private disability
Disabilities *not* related to the trauma	Achieved or applied for, e.g., social security, personal injury, worker's compensation, private disability

pattern, the body needs time to respond and adjust. If the physician immediately begins the release of other emerging patterns of dysfunction, the system tends to decompensate. To avoid this, the next emerging primary dysfunction pattern should be addressed in another treatment session.

Another important consideration is when a pattern of dysfunction is associated with an acute condition, such as, but not limited to pneumonia, a cardiac event, or uncontrolled diabetes. These acute patterns are always considered primary and should be addressed first.

A new traumatic event can occasionally exacerbate an old pattern and makes it primary. For instance, heading a soccer ball exacerbates the birth primary dysfunction pattern. In adults, these very early chronic patterns are closest to the core of the onion. All other patterns and dysfunctions are then layered on top of it. The physician must be very careful in releasing these activated primordial patterns, because although changes in the body will be monumental, both wondrous and devastating effects are possible.

Interaction between multiple traumas can also result in an accumulated trauma vector (resulting force vector). This resulting force vector is created by a reaction with existing vectors and does not follow the physical force pattern of the most recent, or past trauma vectors. Care must be taken in their release since changes will also occur in the reactive old trauma patterns. Gradual releases and close follow-up are necessary to safely harness the body's innate ability to heal and find balance.

Be patient: disorderly and aggressive treatments disrupt the hierarchal balance of dysfunction patterns and result in systemic chaos. In these patients, it is significantly challenging to first relieve the iatrogenic effects and then to reconstruct and treat the layered dysfunctional patterns in the body. The tissue knows the needs of the system. The prudent physician honors this and applies the process of release in peeling the onion of dysfunctional patterns accordingly (Box 52.3).

ILLUSTRATIVE TREATMENT TECHNIQUES

Techniques are divided according to body regions of somatic dysfunction. Ward's, Chila's, and O'Connell's techniques are described separately.

TECHNIQUES BY WARD

Head and Cervical Region

CRANIOCERVICAL SPINE

This process is shown in Figure 52.7.

Objective

The goal is to establish three-dimensional movement symmetry in the cervical spine from basiocciput to upper thoracic influences. Particular emphasis is placed on restoration of adequate sidebending and rotation, both generally and in relation to single-segment mobility. This technique is usually more effective after the release of lower cervical, cervicothoracic junction, and upper thoracic, and upper limb factors.

Note: To protect the vertebral arteries, take particular caution to avoid simultaneous sidebending and extension maneuvers. While important for all age groups, most injuries occur under the age of 35 years.

Patient

Supine.

Procedure

1. Patient lies supine with heels on the table, arms comfortably at the sides. This basically ensures that unusual mechanical stresses transmitted through the Achilles tendons and ankles will be neutralized.
   a. For patients with significant kyphosis, it is helpful to use a large pillow to minimize cervical and thoracolumbar problems.
2. Physician sits at the patient's head.

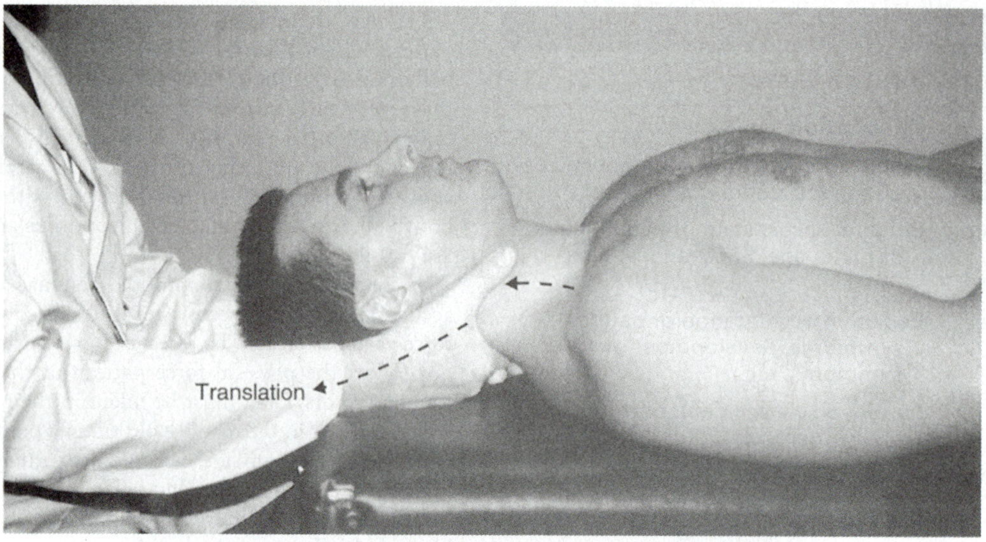

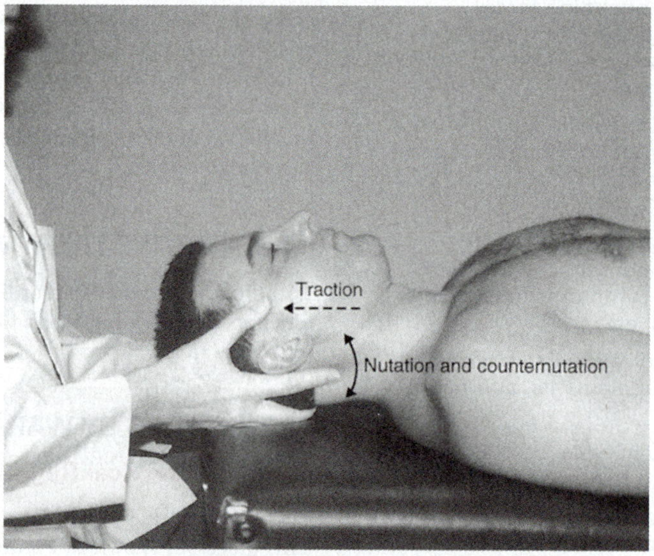

Figure 52.7. A, B. Craniocervical technique.

3. Two hand positions, among many possibilities, are particularly useful:
   a. One hand overlapping the other—this permits carefully controlled and focused, twist, traction, and sidebending maneuvers. The maneuvers are used both separately and with patient cooperation.
   b. By grasping the basiocciput with the palms of each hand, the fingers of the physician are left free to sort out both superficial and deep mechanisms.
4. From either hand position, traction, turning, and sidebending maneuvers assess myofascial and joint-related tightness and looseness.
   a. Pay particular attention to tightness, remembering that loose joints with surrounding inhibited muscle groups are common sources of pain and disability. However, in more acute situations, loose joints are usually associated with tight muscles as they work to protect and stabilize the system. The opposite findings are also common, such as tight joints with accompanying inhibition of overlying muscles.
   b. Facet joints are often tight on one side, and loose on the other. Side-to-side motion testing with only a little rotation will determine which facets are failing to effectively open or close.
   c. The procedure's focus is to carefully, but persistently, apply well-focused stress against tight sites with and without patient assistance.
   d. INR CN and upper limb activities such as finger tapping, and hand rolling are commonly helpful. They also save the physician time.
5. Linking subtle translatory maneuvers (e.g., combinations of distraction and extension with flexion, extension, sidebending, and rotation) is usually helpful. In particular:
   a. Release deep upper cervical muscles by combining CN activities with occipitoatlantal nutation and counternutation.
   b. Remember that SCM, trapezius (CN XI), and scalene mechanics are easily accessible primary neck stabilizers often asymmetric in relation to each other. For example, the left SCM mechanism is typically tighter than the right from origin to insertion.
   c. Commonly, the underlying scalene system is looser (i.e., tightness and looseness occur among ipsilateral layers as well as from side to side, front to back, and circumferentially).
6. In the process:
   a. Atlantoaxial joints and surrounding attachments are carefully rotated against tightness.

A 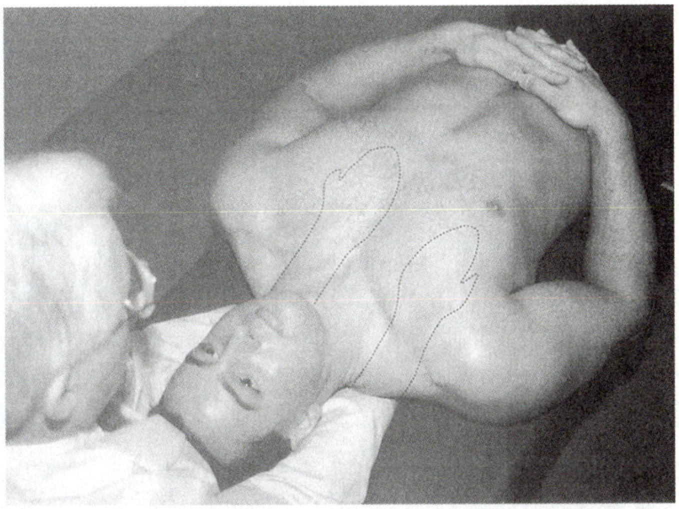 B 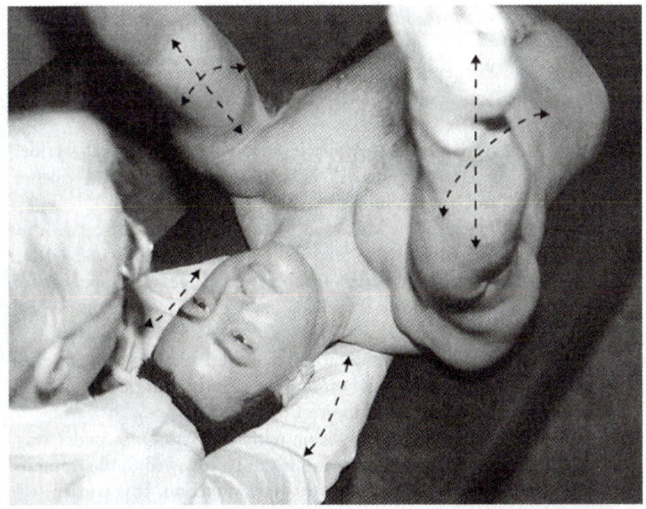

Figure 52.8. A, B. Thoracic and rib technique.

b. Middle and lower cervical attachments and coupled joint movements are stressed using translatory movements with combinations of sidebending, flexion, and extension that avoid excessive rotation (Remember the vertebral arteries!).

7. Treatment is complete when symmetric movements are restored to facet joints and surrounding soft tissues, within the patient's ability to adapt.

Thoracic Region and Ribs

THORACIC CAGE, SPINE, DIAPHRAGM, AND LOWER COSTAL CAGE

This process is shown in Figure 52.8.

Objective

The goal is to three-dimensionally balance scapulothoracic, thoracic spine, and costodiaphragmatic relationships.

Patient

Supine.

Procedure

1. Patient lies supine with heels on the table, arms comfortably at the sides. This basically ensures that unusual mechanical stresses transmitted through the Achilles tendons and ankles will be neutralized.
   a. For patients with significant kyphosis, it is helpful to use a large pillow to minimize cervical and thoracolumbar problems.
2. Physician sits at the head of the table.
3. Physician reaches under the patient, with elbows resting on the table and hands placed firmly against inferior costothoracic attachments on either side of the thoracic spine.
   a. Be sure to maintain whole hand contact across and along the erector spinae as well as around the costal cage.
4. Both positional and movement-related tight–loose asymmetries will become apparent.
5. Focus on the following:
   a. Diaphragmatic asymmetries become apparent as the patient slowly but deeply inhales and exhales.
   b. Upper limb asymmetries that occur as the patient actively moves the upper limbs in a variety of directions.
   c. Repeat the procedure by passively moving each arm and shoulder, with one hand remaining behind the patient.
   d. Thoracolumbar junction asymmetries are assessed with the patient moving the lower limbs in a variety of directions. Focuses on the proximal iliopsoas as well as the response of more distal, lumbopelvic relationships to active patient movements.
6. As inherent tissue movements become apparent, gently, but firmly, lift the thoracolumbar attachments anteriorly and laterally.
   a. Shifting sites of tightness and looseness are balanced against each other until inherent movements become quietly symmetric.
   b. Sometimes, considerable traction and twist are needed to release asymmetrically tight areas.
7. As tightness releases, varieties of release-enhancing activities are helpful. Examples are:
   a. Three-dimensional upper and lower limb movements.
   b. Breath holding at neutral, during moderate and deep inhalation, and then during moderate and deep exhalation, which can be combined with three-dimensional upper and lower limb movements.
8. Treatment is complete when thoracocostal movements are as functionally symmetric as can be expected.

Lumbar Region

THORACOLUMBAR RELEASE

This process is shown in Figure 52.9.

Objective

The goal is to balance the thoracolumbar junction three dimensionally in relation to lumbopelvic, thoracocostal, and diaphragmatic mechanics.

Review

Review cervical, trapezius, shoulder girdle, and costal cage anatomy for their three-dimensional perspectives and functional relationships to the area.

Patient

Prone.

Procedure

1. Patient's feet are off the end of the table to minimize lower limb stresses in relation to the pelvis and low back.
2. Initially, the patient's head is turned to the most comfortable side. Holding the head exclusively in the midline, as many

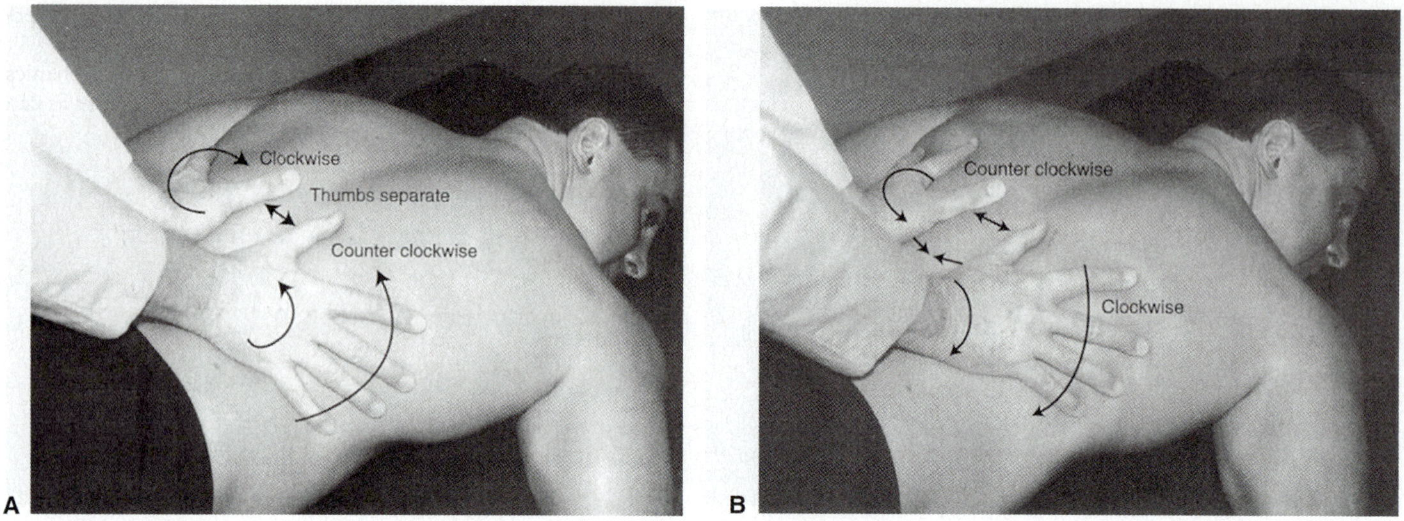

Figure 52.9. Lumbar technique. A. Physician stands beside patient's hip, with head to side. **B.** Head right.

physicians wish to do, often obscures tight–loose effects at the thoracolumbar junction.

3. Patient's hands and arms are comfortably placed either over the sides of the table or on the table beside the hips and thighs.
4. Physician stands beside the patient's hip, facing the patient.
5. The physician's hands are placed at the thoracolumbar junction, covering the posteroinferior rib, trunk rotator, and diaphragmatic sites.
6. The physician's hands are placed widely open, with the thumbs pointed superior along either side of the spinous processes, while the remainder of each hand spreads over the posteroinferior costodiaphragmatic and upper lumbar areas.
7. Identify superficial and deep tightness and looseness patterns three dimensionally.
8. Firmly separate the thumbs across the midline as the left hand creates clockwise and the right hand creates counterclockwise traction. The hands should not slide on the skin.
9. As the skin is stretched between the thumbs, it will initially blanch. As compression, traction, and twist are maintained, tissues begin to relax both reflexively and mechanically in accordance with principles discussed earlier in this chapter.
   a. After initial blanching, the site of major soft tissue tension commonly becomes reddened and warmer, in a process known as the blush phenomenon.
10. Typical releases occur in three dimensions with sustained traction and twist, either singly or in multiples. The latter often creates a wormlike sensation under the palpating hands.
    a. As multiple releases continue, the unwinding phenomena often occur, as shifting patterns of tightness and looseness alter three-dimensional relationships.
    b. With practice, the physician learns to feel deeply into the areas surrounding facet joints.
    c. Symmetric segmental movements to passive three-dimensional stressing suggest that the procedure is complete.
    d. Treatment is complete when repetitive stressing of selected sites no longer creates release activity.

Sacrum

FOCUSED PRONE SACRAL BASE RELEASE: TWO-HANDED TECHNIQUE

This process is shown in Figure 52.10.

Objective

The goal is to three-dimensionally balance the sacral base in relation to L4–L5 mechanics, the iliolumbar ligament, and positional innominate asymmetries.

Review

Review lumbopelvic anatomy, L4–L5 mechanics in relation to the sacrum and pelvis, iliolumbar ligament, and innominate, hip rotator, and pelvic diaphragm relationships, including distal iliopsoas and piriformis muscle influences.

Patient

Prone.

Procedure

1. Patient's feet are off the end of the table to minimize lower limb stresses in relation to the pelvis and low back.
2. Patient's head should be turned to the most comfortable side.

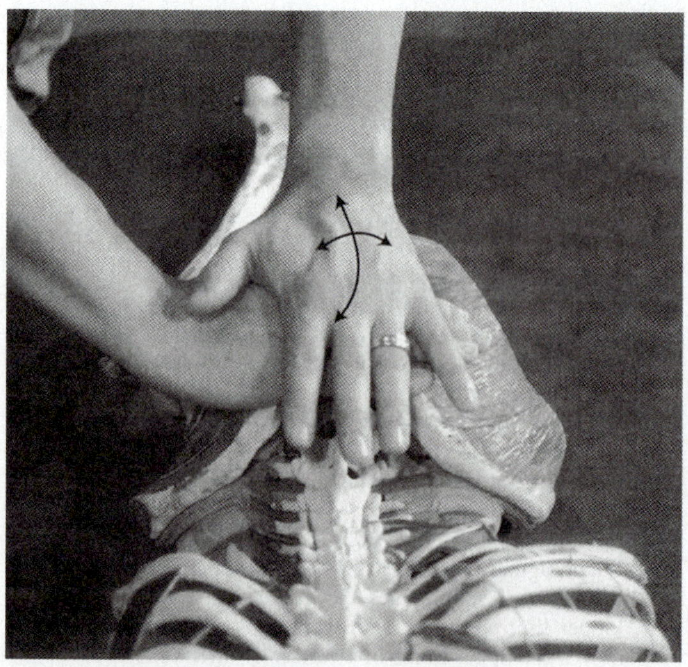

Figure 52.10. Sacral technique. Using a rocking notion, induce lumbosacral joint distraction.

3. Patient's hands and arms are comfortably placed either over the sides of the table or on the table beside the hips and thighs.
4. Physician who is right-handed stands at the patient's left shoulder, facing inferior.
5. Physician places one hand either horizontally or transverse to the sacrum, contacting the posterior superior iliac spines and medial gluteus maximus attachments bilaterally.
6. Physician's other hand is placed over the bottom hand along the long axis of the sacrum between the two innominates, with the index finger overlying one SI joint in an inferior lateral angle. The ring finger covers the other SI joint. In this hand placement, the longer finger naturally falls over the sacral spine and sacral hiatus.
7. Evaluate patterns of tightness and looseness by rocking the sacrum in multiple planes:
   a. Proximally and distally, by distracting the sacrum and lumbar spine at the sacral base, along the long axis of the spine
   b. Circumferentially, by transversely translating each hand across the pelvis in opposite directions.
8. Using a rocking nutation–counternutation gapping motion, induce lumbosacral joint distraction. Create the motion by moving the distal hand inferiorly, as well as up and over the natural curve of the sacrum.
   a. Some sacrums are in a straight-line relationship with the spine.
   b. Others can be acutely angled, with the plane of the sacral base virtually perpendicular to the flow of the physician-imposed forces.
9. Both light- and heavy-handed force can be used, depending on the physician's skill. A key to success is the ability to monitor, induce, and enhance both inherent tissue and craniosacral activities.
10. As both static and dynamic loading is applied, inherent tissue movement–related tightness and looseness usually becomes apparent.
    a. Static forces load the system against direct and indirect barriers without superimposing oscillating movements.
    b. Dynamic forces load the system with subtle physician-induced forces that:
    c. Follow along behind inherent tissue and craniosacral movements
    d. Systematically seek out three-dimensional shifts of direct and indirect barriers as releases occur
11. Success is more apt to occur when special attention is given to the sacral base in relation to L4–L5 mechanics, iliolumbar ligament anomalies, degenerative changes, and nonneutral vertebral mechanics.
12. Treatment is complete when L5 and sacral base mechanics and their associated inherent motions are as symmetric as can reasonably be expected.

Pelvis

PUBIC SYMPHYSIS RELEASE

This process is shown in Figure 52.11.

Objective

The goal is to restore symmetry to the pubic symphysis.

Review

Review the functional three-dimensional relationships among the proximal thigh adductors, anterior and posterior innominates and their asymmetries, as well as changes involving the rectus sheath and transverses abdominis muscles, where they attach to the pubic symphysis.

Patient

Supine.

Procedure

1. Patient lies supine with heels on the table and arms comfortably at the sides or on the abdomen.
   a. Short-armed patients should keep their arms on the table to avoid stressing shoulder and thoracolumbar systems. This ensures that unusual mechanical stresses transmitted through the Achilles tendons and ankles will be neutralized.
   b. For patients with significant kyphosis, use a large pillow to minimize cervical and thoracolumbar problems.
2. Physician sits or stands facing the patient, beside the patient's right thigh, near the knee.
3. First, assess for symphyseal shear and positional asymmetry. Some physicians prefer visual analysis, while others prefer a combination of palpation and vision.
   a. Tightness and looseness in the rectus sheath often identify the most problematic site. Tightness can be on the inferior or superior side.
   b. Though there are usually strong correlations with innominate positioning, the physician must be aware of the exceptions.
4. Place the thenar eminences on either side of the symphysis pubis, with the thumbs pointed superiorly and anteriorly. Proximal adductor and iliacus tendon attachments should be palpably evident under the thenar muscles.

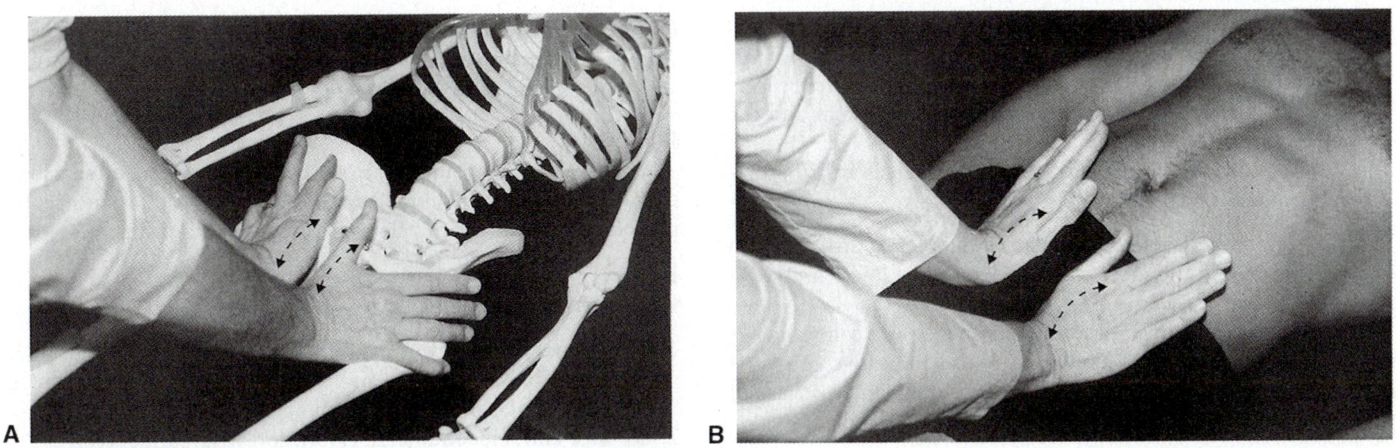

Figure 52.11. Pelvic technique. A. Symphysis release. **B.** Thenar eminences are placed on either side of symphysis pubis, thumbs pointed superiorly and anteriorly.

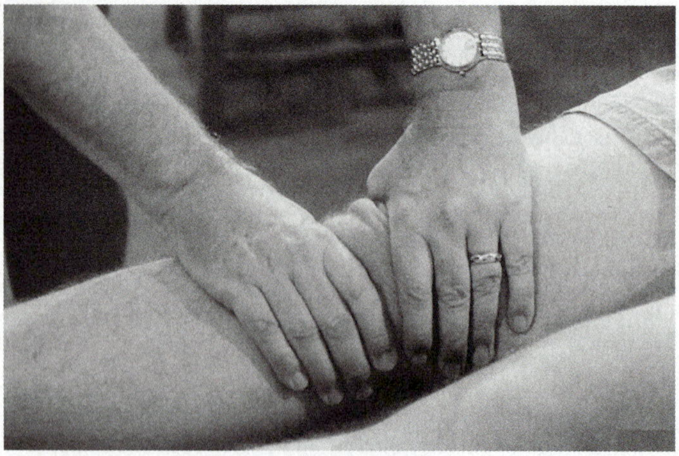

Figure 52.12. Lower extremity technique.

5. Induce firm, slow forces that either exaggerate (indirect barriers) or decrease (direct barriers) symphysis asymmetry.
   a. Direct rocking back and forth, similar to an articular maneuver, is often effective.
   b. Hold against the barriers until releases occur.
   c. Mild oscillations usually become evident as the rectus fasciae, bony pelvis, pelvic diaphragm, trunk rotators, and thigh adductors become more symmetric.

Lower Extremity

LOWER LIMB

This process is shown in Figure 52.12.

Objective

The goal is to release each lower limb from lumbopelvic and hip rotator attachments to the foot and ankle.

Review

Review the following:

1. Functional neurology of the lower limb, including pelvic girdle, low back, trunk rotators, lumbodorsal fascia, latissimus dorsi, and scapulocostal stabilizers.
   a. Understand them in relation to the low back, brachial plexus influences through shoulder girdle structures, and diaphragmatic–phrenic influences.
   b. Remember that the limbs are precisely represented in cerebellopontine functions as well as in multiple areas of the homunculus and precentral gyrus.
2. Functional neuromuscular anatomy of the foot, ankle, knee, and their myofascial elements.
3. Functional neuromuscular anatomy of the hips and upper leg.
4. Circulatory anatomy of both the lumbopelvic system and the lower limbs.
5. The effects of common medical problems, such as arthritis, diabetes, trauma, and surgery.

Note 1: Smoking-related circulatory problems, arthritis, and diabetes are among the most common sources of lower limb dysfunctions.

Note 2: Proprioceptive instability on one leg is a common signal of unilateral muscle weakness. It is also indicative of neural inhibition anywhere from the lower back to the plantar surface of the ipsilateral foot. Pain is a common presenting complaint.

Patient

Supine.

Procedure

1. Patient's heels are on the table with knees extended to minimize lower limb stresses. Patient's head and neck should be comfortable with minimal stress on the spine and pelvis.
   Note: Remember to check for leg-length inequalities and altered hip mechanics both prone and supine. It is common to find differences between supine, prone, and seated positions. Pelvic obliquities are common when these inconsistencies occur.
2. Patient's hands and arms are comfortably placed either on the abdomen or at the sides.
3. Physician sits or stands beside the patient.
4. Grasp distal femur and distal patellar/proximal tibial attachments.
5. Using firm, passive, circumferential movements, assess each fully extended knee for three-dimensional tightness and looseness.
   a. Particular care is taken in assessing medial hamstring and lateral hamstring/iliotibial band/proximal fibular head tight–loose relationships.
   Note: Myofascially, this is a fairly ambiguous area to assess and treat, so one must subjectively rely on tight–loose end feels. Both lumbopelvic and foot–ankle mechanics significantly influence the system.
6. Assess hip function in the same way, with the leg in full extension, followed by varieties of flexion, internal and external rotation, abduction, and adduction.
7. Passively twist the knee in opposite directions (axial twist), with the hand and fingers in firm contact with areas of maximum tightness. Usually, maximum tightness is found in two places:
   a. Laterally around distal iliotibial band attachments and proximal fibular head.
   b. Medially and posteriorly near and around distal hamstring attachments.
8. It is common to find asymptomatic lateral knee/fibular head problems (tightness) in response to medial complaints where the knee is generally more mobile.
   a. Also common to this group are distal tensor fasciae latae problems in conjunction with ipsilateral gluteus medius weakness. A positive standing Trendelenburg test is the most common signal of gluteus medius weakening.
   b. Remember that proximal SI joint and sacrotuberous–sacrospinous ligamentous factors are also common sources of distal difficulties, and vice versa.

Upper Extremity

UPPER LIMB AND SHOULDER

Rotator Cuff and Partially Frozen Shoulder Dysfunctions

This process is shown in Figure 52.13.

Objective

The goal of this treatment is to balance in three dimensions: cervical, shoulder, scapulocostal, anterior chest wall, rotator cuff–glenohumeral, upper arm, elbow, wrist, and hand influences.

Review

Review the following:

1. Functional neurology of the neck in relation to the upper limb, including brachial plexus and cervical autonomic elements, as well as CN sensory and motor functions.
2. Rotator cuff, glenohumeral, elbow, and wrist influences.
3. Craniocervical spine relationships with particular reference to large and small muscle influences from the basiocciput to the

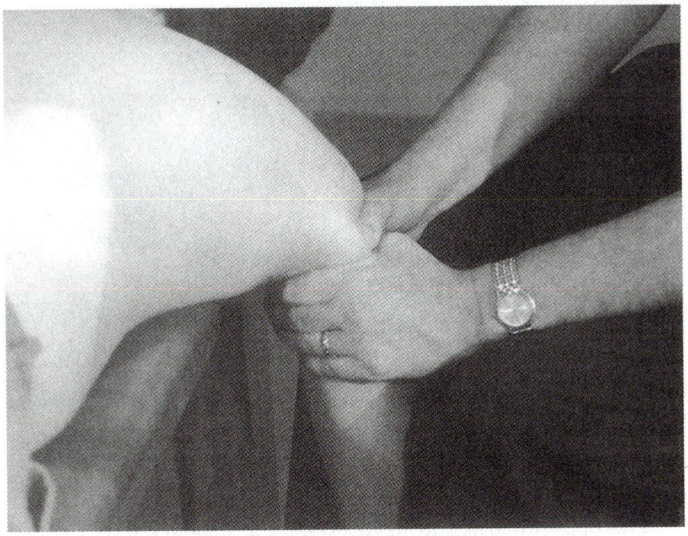

Figure 52.13. **Upper extremity technique.**

upper thoracics, along with related scapulothoracic and scapulocostal influences.

Patient

Prone.

Procedure

1. Patient lies prone with the affected arm and shoulder off the table. Most of the time, this position is used to deal directly with compromised shoulder and scapulocostal mechanics (see also "Spencer Techniques").
   a. Direct myofascial stressing occurs across and around the rotator cuff
      i. Acromioclavicular joint
      ii. Distal glenohumeral attachments
      iii. Inferior subscapularis
      iv. Latissimus dorsi
      v. Infraspinatus
      vi. Teres major and minor attachments
2. Patient's feet are off the end of the table to minimize lower limb stresses in relation to the pelvis and lower limb.
3. Patient's head turned to the most comfortable side. Note the effect of head turning on tightness and looseness across the shoulder in question.
   a. Proximal and superior cervical attachments are often compromised and need to be released along with the shoulder. *Note*: Keeping the head in the midline not only readily neutralizes craniocervical asymmetries but also reduces the chance that significant tight–loose asymmetries go undetected.
4. Patient's hands and arms are comfortably placed either over the sides of the table or on the table beside the hips and thighs. If hands are over the sides of the table, note any asymmetric scapulocostal effects.
5. Physician sits on a rolling stool that allows movement in response to shifting sites of tightness and looseness.
6. Patient's affected arm is held between the physician's knees. Physician uses the rolling stool to guide movements as specific stressing against tight barriers occurs.
7. Initially, place both hands firmly around the glenohumeral attachments immediately lateral to the acromioclavicular joint. The fingers of one hand firmly contact pectoralis major attachments anteriorly, while the other hand contacts teres/infraspinatus attachments posteriorly.
8. Assess tightness and looseness by three-dimensionally stressing the system using distraction, compression, twist, and shear.
9. The process begins with direct and firm stressing against tightness. For example, approximately 5 to 15 lb. of load is common before initial releases begin.
10. Pay particular attention to posterior and inferior glenohumeral restrictions close to the scapula.
11. Long-term problems usually require firmly held movements that assertively stretch the area without interfering with neurocirculatory functions.
12. A well-organized home exercise and/or physical therapy program is usually needed to maintain improvement.
13. Side-lying techniques using a similar approach are also helpful.

TECHNIQUES BY CHILA

Head and Suboccipital Region

CRANIUM

Treatment procedures for the cranium are shown in Figure 52.14.

Occipitoatlantal Articulation

1. One hand contacts the posterior tubercle of the atlas.
2. The other hand contacts the vertex of the patient's head. The fulcrum is established by the placement of the elbow on the tabletop.

Basilar Axes of the Skull

1. Patient's head rests on the interlaced or overlapped fingers of the physician.
2. Thumbs extend above the ears toward the forepart of the patient's head. The fulcrum is established by the placement of the elbows on the tabletop.

Cervical Region, Thoracic Region, and Rib Cage

Place one hand beneath the rib cage, with the fingertips just beyond the spinous processes of the associated thoracic vertebrae (Fig. 52.15).

Place the other hand on the anterior ends of the ribs. The fulcrum is established by the elbow on the knee.

LOWER THORAX

1. Place both hands beneath the patient at the level of the 12th thoracic segment (T12) (Fig. 52.16).

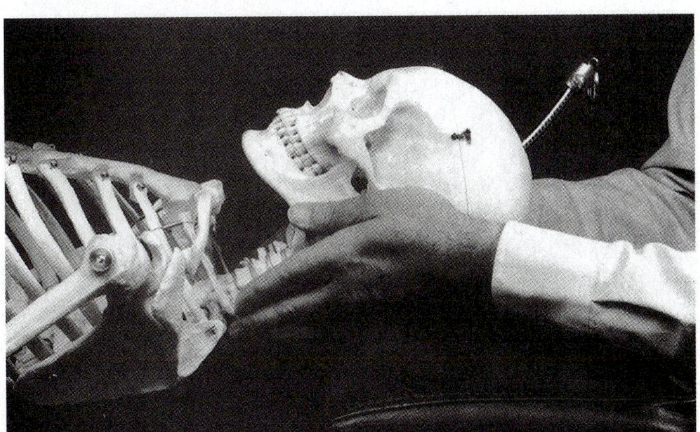

Figure 52.14. **Head and suboccipital technique.**

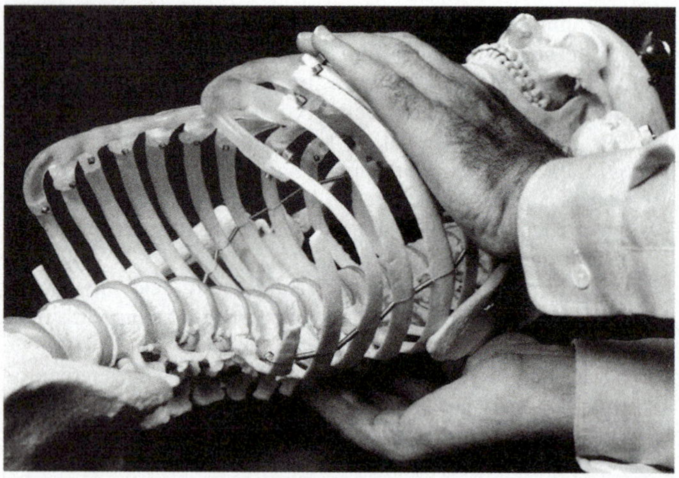

Figure 52.15. **Rib cage technique.**

This area corresponds to the level of the insertion of the trapezium muscles bilaterally. The fulcrum is established bilaterally by the elbows resting on the tabletop.

UPPER THORAX

1. The patient's head rests on a pillow.
2. One hand and arm contact the upper thoracic spinous processes, with the fingers spread slightly to contact the ribs on each side (Fig. 52.17).
3. Place the opposite hand on the sternum. The fulcrum is established by the elbow on the tabletop, beneath the patient's head.

CERVICAL AREA

1. Both hands bridge the entire cervical area from the base of the skull to the upper thorax (Fig. 52.18).

The fulcrum is established bilaterally by the elbows and forearms resting on the tabletop.

Lumbar Region

Patient's knees are flexed, with the feet placed flat on the table. Lateralization of the feet, with inversion of the toes, helps to stabilize the pelvis.

UPPER LUMBAR, PSOAS MUSCLE

1. Place one hand under the upper lumbar area (Fig. 52.19).

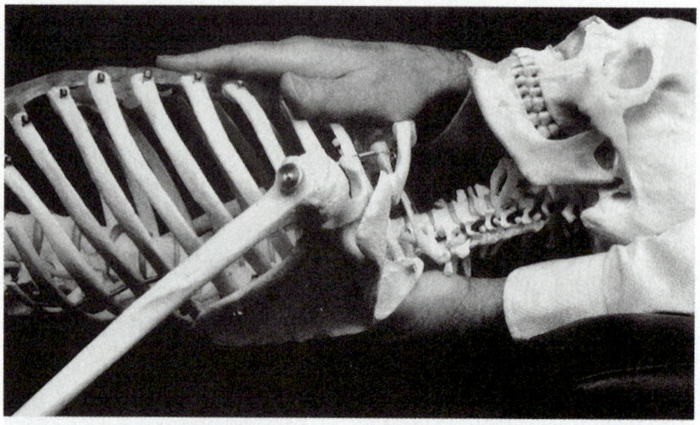

Figure 52.17. **Upper thoracic technique.**

2. The opposite arm and hand bridge the patient's flexed knees. The fulcrum is established by the physician's elbow on the patient's knee (upper lumbar area).

Sacrum and Pelvis

Patient's knees are flexed, with the feet placed flat on the table. Lateralization of the feet, with inversion of the toes, helps to stabilize the pelvis.

SACRUM AND PELVIS

1. Mold the patient's sacrum with one hand.
2. Place the fingertips of this hand at the level of the spinous process of the fifth lumbar segment (L5). The opposite arm and hand bridge the anterior superior iliac spine (ASIS) on each side of the pelvis (Fig. 52.20).
3. The fulcrum is established by the elbow, which is leaning on the treatment table.

SACRUM, ILIOSACRUM, LOWER LUMBAR

1. Mold with the patient's sacrum with one hand (Fig. 52.21).
2. Place the opposite hand under the iliosacral articulation. The fingertips of this hand contact the spinous process of the lower lumbar segments (L3, L4, L5). Both elbows establish the fulcrum: one leaning on the treatment table (sacrum), the other leaning on the physician's knee (iliosacrum; lower lumbar).

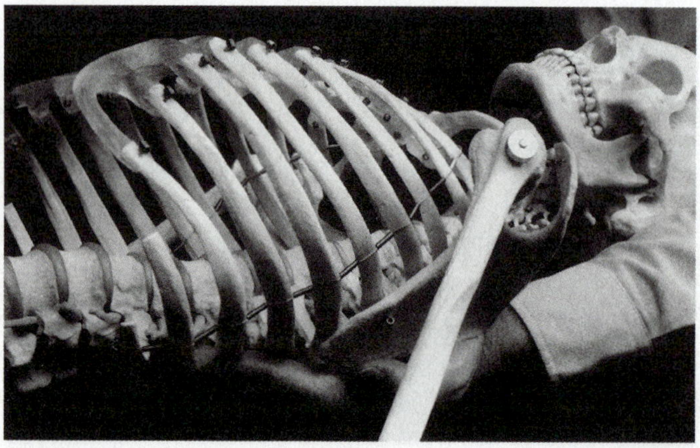

Figure 52.16. **Lower thoracic technique.**

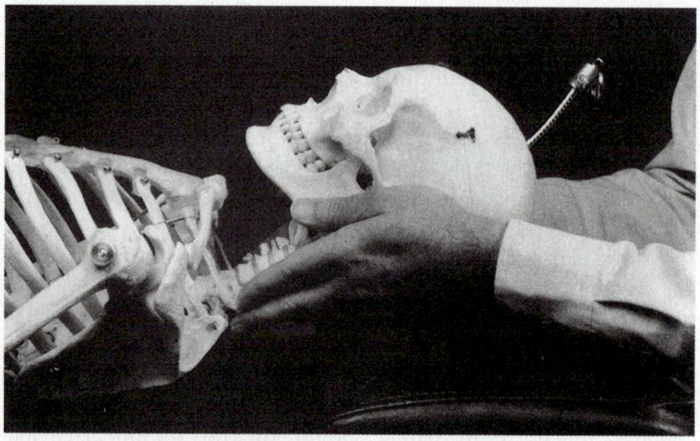

Figure 52.18. **Cervical technique.**

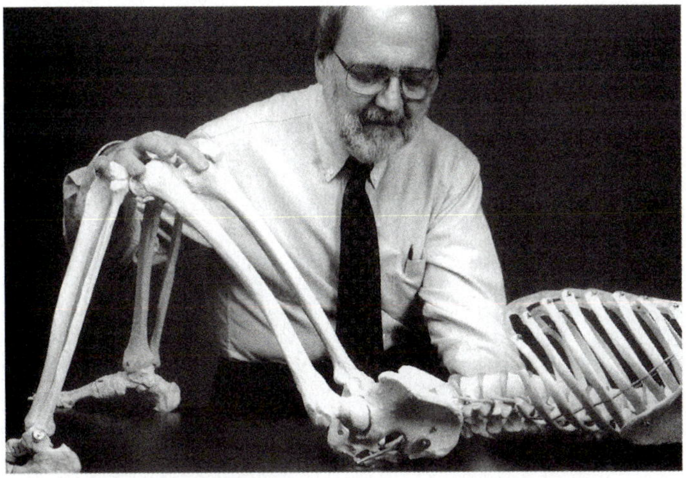

Figure 52.19. **Upper lumbar, psoas muscle technique.**

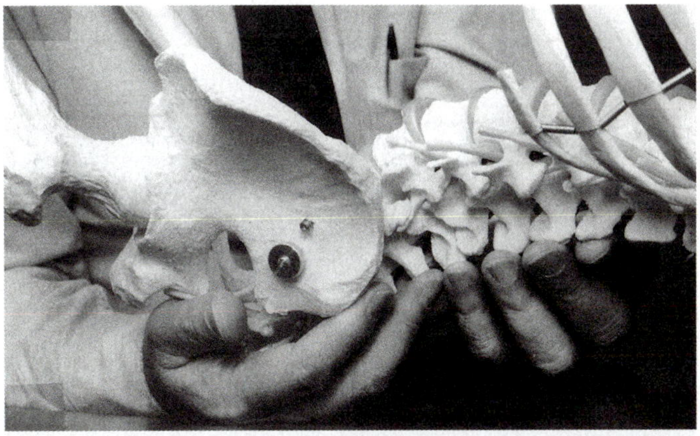

Figure 52.21. **Sacrum, iliosacrum, lower lumbar technique.**

Lower Extremity

LOWER EXTREMITY

1. Selectively employ torsion (rotation) and traction in two phases to release muscular, fascial, ligamentous, and articular dysfunction. The fulcrum is established by the elbows of the physician's arms in supporting the motions of the patient's foot, lower leg, and knee.

ABDUCTION PHASE (LOWER LEG)

1. Invert the plantar surface of the foot (Fig. 52.22).
2. Introduce torsion between the ankle and the knee.
3. Advance the effect of torsion by slowly moving the knee across the lower abdomen, resulting in progressive abduction of the lower leg.
   a. The torsion will be felt in the lateral malleolar area, the medial compartmental area of the knee, the tensor fascia lata area, and the trochanter area.
   b. Upon completion of this phase, gradually extend the lower extremity and slowly return it to the tabletop.

ADDUCTION PHASE (LOWER LEG)

1. Evert the plantar surface of the foot (Fig. 52.23).
2. Introduce torsion between the ankle and the knee.
3. Steadily advance the effect of torsion by slowly moving the knee away from the lower abdomen, resulting in progressive adduction of the lower leg.
   a. The torsion will be felt in the medial malleolar area, the lateral compartmental area of the knee, the medial thigh area, and the inguinal area.
   b. Upon completion of this phase, gradually extend the lower extremity and slowly return it to the tabletop.

FOOT

1. Note tenderness to palpation in the plantar myofascial tissues. Give particular attention to such findings along the medial longitudinal arch. The contour of the foot can be analogized to the spinal complex:
   Tender points can be analogized to the ipsilateral spinal level, including paraspinal tissues.
   a. The calcaneus represents the sacrum.
   b. The tarsal bones represent the lumbar region.
   c. The tarsometatarsal area represents the thoracolumbar junction.
   d. The metatarsal area represents the thoracic region.
   e. The metatarsophalangeal area represents the cervicothoracic junction.
   f. The phalangeal area represents the cervical region.

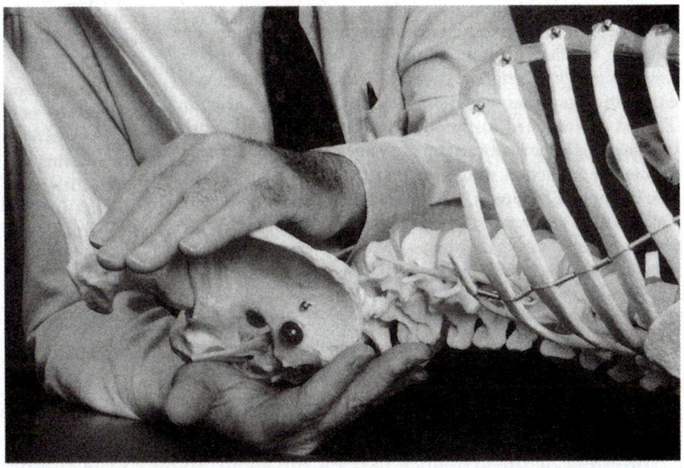

Figure 52.20. **Sacrum and pelvis technique (bridging ASISs).**

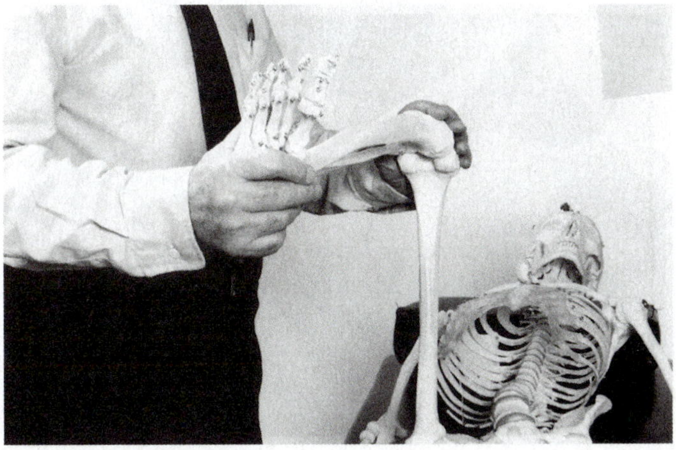

Figure 52.22. **Lower extremity technique, abduction phase.**

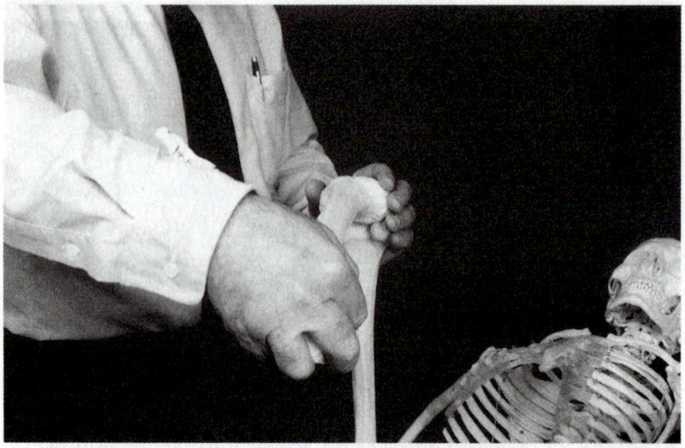

Figure 52.23. Lower extremity technique, adduction phase.

2. Treatment is by increased plantar flexion of the foot to the point of greatest tenderness (Fig. 52.24).
3. Perform articulatory release of the small joints of the toes in sequence, from the great toe to the small toe.

Upper Extremity

UPPER EXTREMITY SCAPULOFASCIAL RELEASE

1. Explore ease and resistance to motion in several planes: superior, inferior, medially, laterally, clockwise, and counterclockwise (Fig. 52.25).
2. Both hands are used to grasp the scapula completely, both medially and laterally.

AXILLARY RELEASE

1. Apply manual decongestion of the posterior axillary tissues and the pectoral tissues.

EXPANSION OF THE INFERIOR THORACIC APERTURE

1. Support the patient's elbow region with one hand, and the patient's wrist region with the other hand. For this and all subsequent procedures, the fulcrum is established by the elbows of the physician's body in support of the motions of the patient's upper extremity.

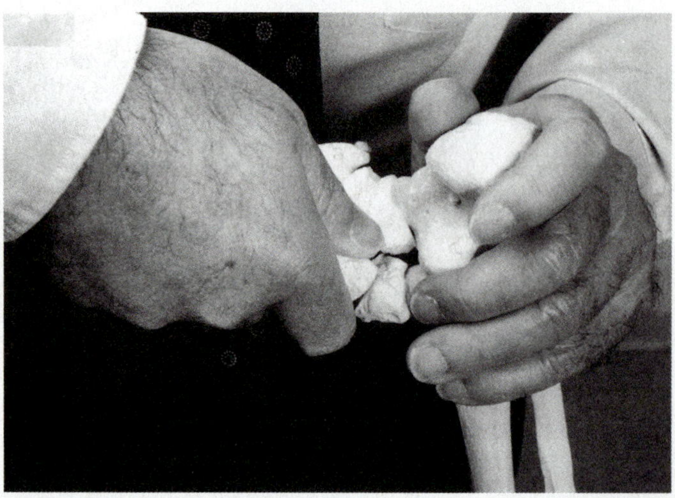

Figure 52.24. Foot technique.

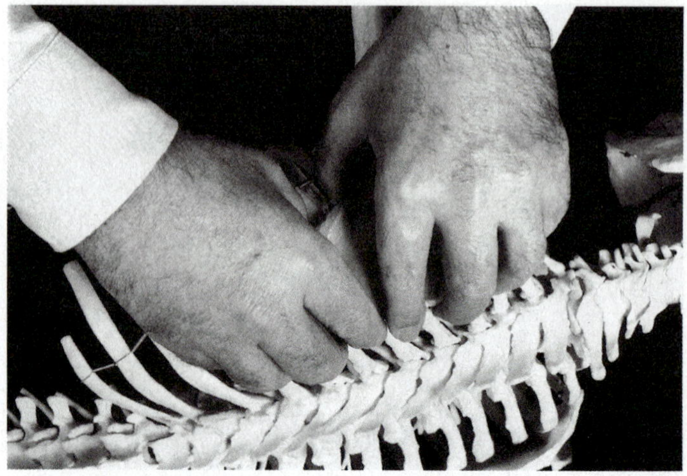

Figure 52.25. Upper extremity technique, scapulofascial release.

2. Bring the extended upper extremity of the patient closer to the side of the body.
3. Sustain supination as the upper extremity is carried toward the posterior thorax, facilitating release of the thoracolumbar junction.
4. Sustain pronation as the upper extremity is carried toward the xiphoid process, facilitating musculofascial release along the costal margin. The cumulative effect of these forces contributes to ligamentous articular release of the elbow region.

EXPANSION OF THE SUPERIOR THORACIC APERTURE

1. Grasp the deep webbing between the index finger and thumb of the patient's extended upper extremity.
2. Sustain alternation between supination and pronation. This facilitates the release of congestion in this area and contributes to the release of the cervicothoracic junction.

CLAVICULAR AND GLENOHUMERAL RELEASE

1. Place the extended upper extremity in a neutral position, with respect to the side of the body, and abduct to the point where a continuum exists between the upper extremity and the position of the clavicle.
2. Sustain pronation as the upper extremity is carried toward the manubrial region. This facilitates the release of the manubrial area, and the sternoclavicular articulation.
3. Sustain supination as the upper extremity is carried toward the posterior thorax. This facilitates the release of the acromioclavicular articulation, and the glenohumeral area (Fig. 52.26).

RADIOULNAR, WRIST, HAND, AND FINGERS RELEASE

1. Sustain alternation between supination and pronation. This facilitates the release of fascial–ligamentous tension along the course of the interosseous membrane to the flexor retinaculum.
2. Alternate flexion and extension of the wrist. This addition facilitates the release of articular dysfunctions of the carpal bones (Fig. 52.27).
3. Fascial–ligamentous release of the palmar area precedes articulatory release of the small joints of the fingers and thumb. The progress of the sequence is from the small finger to the thumb (Fig. 52.28).

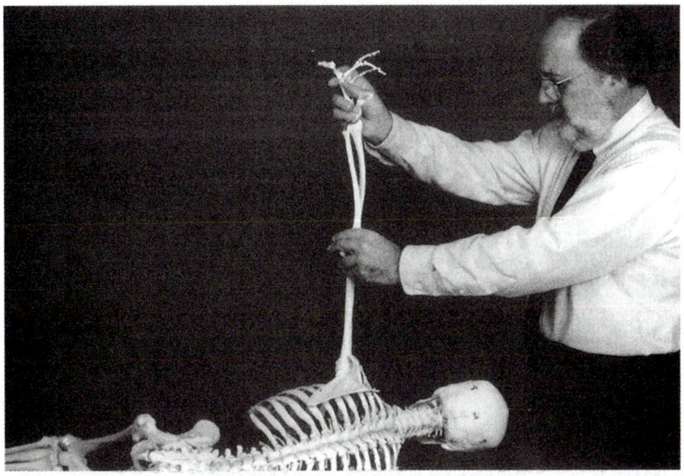

Figure 52.26. **Upper extremity radioulnar release.**

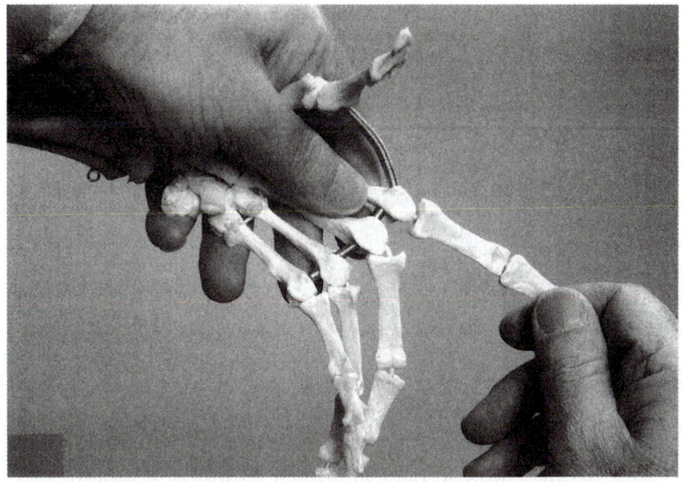

Figure 52.28. **Upper extremity hand and fingers technique.**

TECHNIQUES BY O'CONNELL

Head and Cervical Region

HEAD/CERVICAL

Release across diaphragms (tentorium cerebelli to thoracic inlet) of a trauma pattern into the neck (birth trauma, personal injury, or MVA) (Fig. 52.29).

1. Patient lies supine. Physician sits at the head of the treatment table.
2. Physician's hands are placed on the patient's head, with:
   The palms of the physician's hands are then laid lightly on the patient's head, with the thumbs on the patient's parietals. This allows the physician's hands to capture the tentorium, while allowing contact with the suboccipital fascia.
   a. The index fingers above the zygomatic process
   b. The middle finger below the process
   c. The ring fingers behind and contacting the pinnae, taking care not to overlay the mastoidal suture.
   d. The little finger on the occipital squama
3. Sense the motion of the tentorium and note the asymmetries in motion between temporalis and occiput. Then focus on the motion of the posterior external fascial planes of the head into the neck, while continuing to monitor the tentorium.
4. Introduce a compressive or distractive force into the tissues. A pattern of motion, which travels between the tentorium and the thoracic inlet, will become evident.
   a. Follow this pattern along its ease or oppose the pattern and engage its motion barrier.
   b. Since the fascia is a continuum, the trauma pattern will follow a distinct path and move across multiple structures, organs, and regions as the fascia responds intelligently to the physician-induced forces. This resulting pattern of motion reflects the traumatic strain pattern in the tissues and reproduces the positions of trauma.
5. Choose a direct or an indirect approach and follow the pattern along its responsive moving barrier or its point of ease as the pattern releases. Three deep respiratory cycles facilitate the pattern release through continuous repositioning.
6. Return the patient to neutral and retest as above, taking note as to whether the pattern is extinguished.
7. Trauma patterns are not limited to normal physiologic motion patterns and may be confusing to the physician. But with practice, they can aid in diagnosis and treatment.

Thoracic Region, Upper Extremity, and Ribs

THORACIC/RIBS/STERNUM/CLAVICLE/UPPER EXTREMITY

This approach allows for anatomical access to all structures that converge at this diaphragm, and to the longitudinal connections

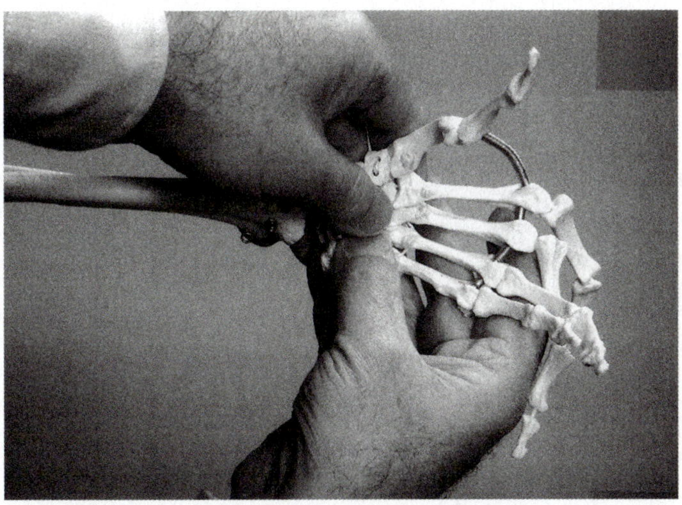

Figure 52.27. **Upper extremity wrist technique.**

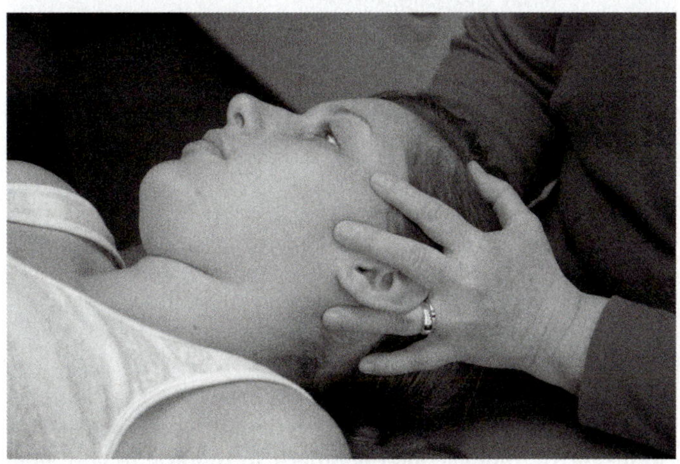

Figure 52.29. **Head and neck technique.**

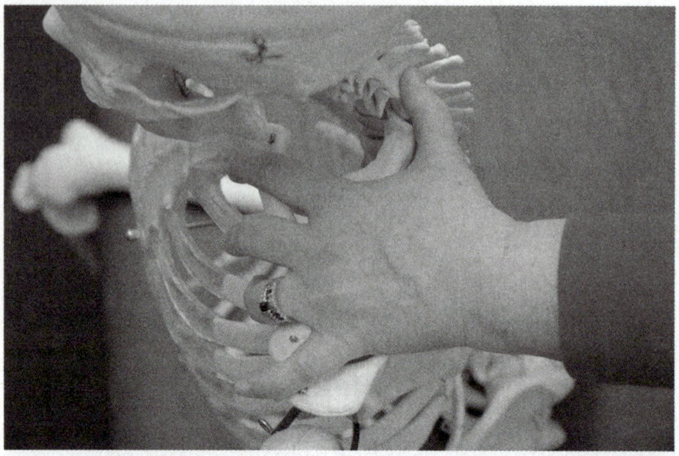

Figure 52.30. Thoracic inlet approach to thoracic region, ribs, and upper extremity, skeletal view.

between diaphragms. It is excellent for experiencing a holographic release (Figs. 52.30 and 52.31).

When accessed, the motions that interface in the region are usually more complex, and of grosser levels. This phenomenon, sensed by the physician and the patient, is referred to as "the dance." Importantly, this approach allows the physician to travel the fascial continuum both diagnostically and therapeutically.

1. Patient sits on the table. Physician stands directly behind the patient. Patient is slightly lower than the physician, so that the physician's hands are placed on the patient's thoracic inlet in a comfortable position.
2. The handhold is designed to capture the whole thoracic inlet with contacts on the bony anchors to the inlet.
   a. The physician's hands are placed on top of the patient's shoulders, with the thumbs pointing posteriorly, and the tips pointing toward the spinous processes of C7 and T1. The third and fourth fingers overly the clavicle, with tips of the fingers contacting the first and second ribs anteriorly.
   b. Place the second finger along the shaft of the clavicle, pointing toward the sternoclavicular joint.
   c. Place the fifth finger laterally toward the acromioclavicular joint. In this position, relax the hands so that the palms overly and contact the tops of the patient's shoulders.
3. Assess the motion patterns in both hands simultaneously, remembering that motion may occur in different planes and directions.

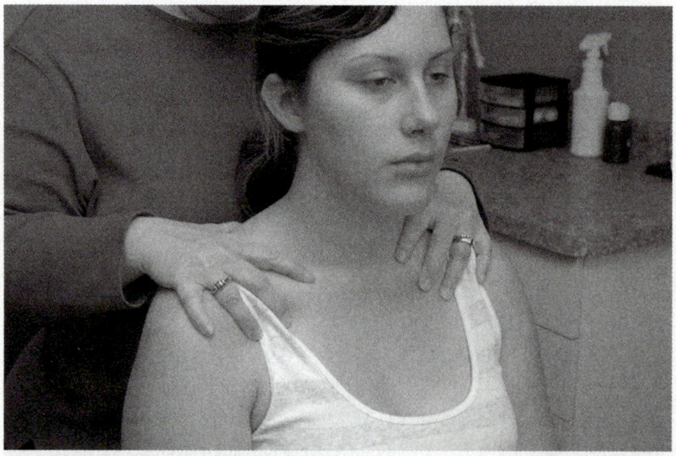

Figure 52.31. Thoracic inlet approach to thoracic region, ribs, and upper extremity.

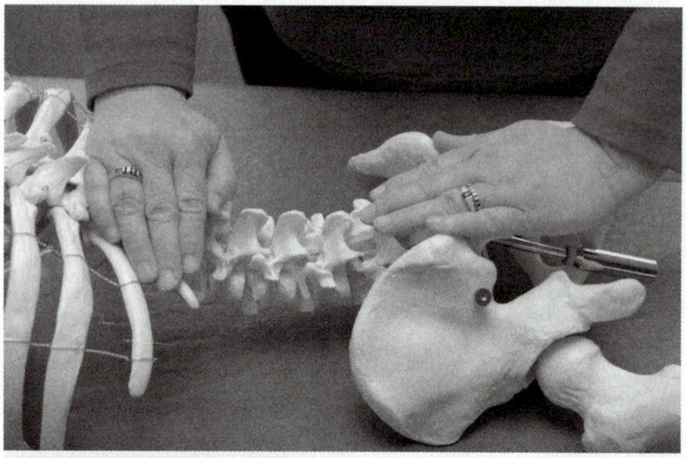

Figure 52.32. Iliopsoas release, skeletal view.

   a. With a respiratory cycle, identify the patterns of motion and choose a direct or indirect approach.
   b. With three deep respiratory cycles, follow the shifting release pattern with both hands. The physician's epigastrium stabilizes the patient's torso, dancing with the patient's release and not limiting the motion.
4. Return the patient to neutral and reevaluate the pattern's resolution.

Lumbar Region

LUMBAR: ILIOPSOAS RELEASE

Lifting injury, short leg accommodation. (Figs. 52.32 and 52.33).

1. Patient lays prone on the table. Physician stands at the side of the patient.
   a. Physician places the hand that is closest to the patient's head perpendicular to the long line of the spine, with the spinous processes of T11–L1 in the midline of the palm.
   b. The physician's hand is laid down, with fingers on the contralateral side of the spine, and the thenar and hypothenar eminences on the ipsilateral side of the spine. This allows for the capture of the posterior fascial attachments of the respiratory diaphragm, and the posterior longitudinal fascial planes of the lumbar spine/torso.
2. Physician's other hand is placed parallel to the long line of the spine, with the palm of the hand at the sacral base. The fingers

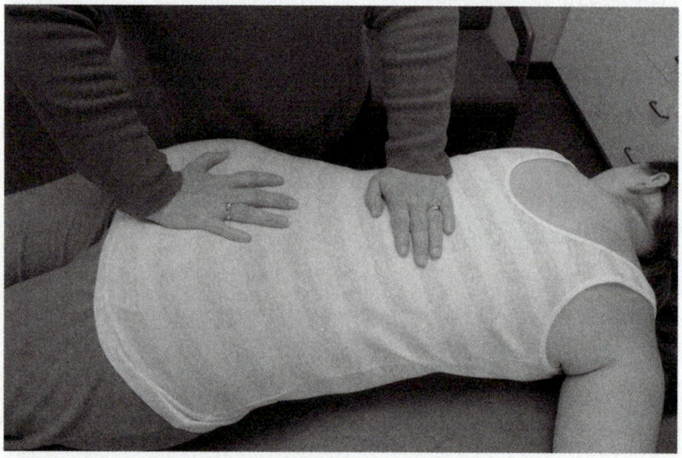

Figure 52.33. Iliopsoas release.

extend superiorly, with its spread capturing the lumbopelvic spine and fascia.

3. The motion in this region is more tubular in character, and as the release occurs, both of the physician's hands will be moving in different directions.
   a. Motion is assessed with a respiratory cycle between the physician's sensing hands, or with palpatory listening to the innate fascial motion.
   b. Identify areas of restriction and ease between these listening posts and choose a direct or indirect approach.
4. Augment the motion with three respiratory cycles and follow the shifting pattern as it releases.
5. Return the patient to neutral and reevaluate the motion.

Sacrum and Pelvis

SACRUM/PELVIS

Sacral sling release in three dimensions (fall, pregnancy pain, post-delivery pain) (Figs. 52.25 and 52.34).

1. Patient lays supine. Physician stands or sits next to the patient, facing the patient's pelvis.
2. Place one hand under the patient's pelvis, perpendicular to the long line of the spine, with the spinous processes in midpalm, the fingertips across to the contralateral SI joint, the thenar/hypothenar eminences on the ipsilateral SI joint. Then relax the hand.
3. With the other hand, reach across the ilia, grasping the contralateral anterior ilia with the fingertips, and contacting the ipsilateral ilia with the forearm or elbow.
4. With the upper arm and hand, compress the ilia toward midline, disengaging the sacrum posteriorly, which now floats in the lumbosacral fascia.
5. With a deep breath, set the fascia in motion.
   a. Identify positions of ease and barriers to motion of the sacrum within the fascia.
   b. Become aware of the relationship between the posterior fascia and the anterior fascia, then of the motion into the pelvic floor and the fascial loop up into the rectus, transversalis, internal and external oblique fascia.
   c. Now become aware of the bony pelvis within this fascial container.
   d. With a deep breath, enter into this system using the sacrum as a guide.
   e. Go through three respiratory cycles, following the three-dimensional release of the structures as direct, indirect, or combined.

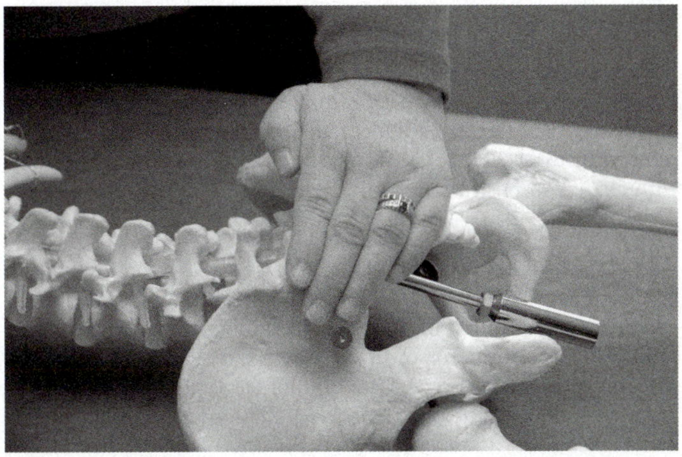

Figure 52.34. Sacrum and pelvis technique, skeletal view.

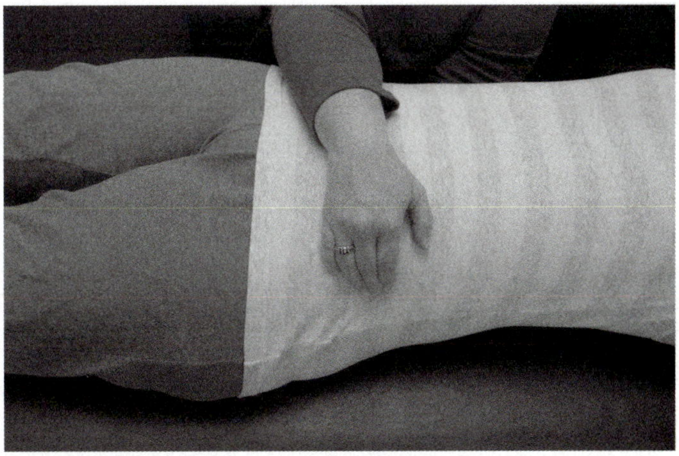

Figure 52.35. Sacrum and pelvis technique.

6. Return the patient to neutral and reassess motion for resolution of the dysfunctions (Fig. 52.35).

Lower Extremity

LOWER EXTREMITY

Tubular release of knee using heel-to-hip approach (twist of knee trauma with a stable knee) (Fig. 52.36).

1. Patient lays supine. Physician stands at the foot of the table.
2. The palm of the physician's outside hand grasps the patient's heel, gripping the patient's calcaneous between the hypothenar eminence, with fingers keeping the patient's leg on the table. Physician's other hand is placed on the dorsum of the patient's foot, with the thumb wrapped under the patient's arch.
3. Place the ankle in neutral position and maintain this throughout the release. Begin the release in segments, from the distal to proximal extremity, allowing a gradual accumulative release below and above the injured joint.
4. With the above handhold, lean back, placing a traction force into the patient's ankle to the calf. Follow the stress pattern in the tissue by positioning the patient's leg, taking care to make small arc motion adjustments.
   a. Continue the release with increased traction to the tibial plateau, allowing for positional pattern adjustments.
   b. Repeat this process while gradually increasing traction.
   c. Follow the pattern to the lower femur, mid femur, then end at the hip.

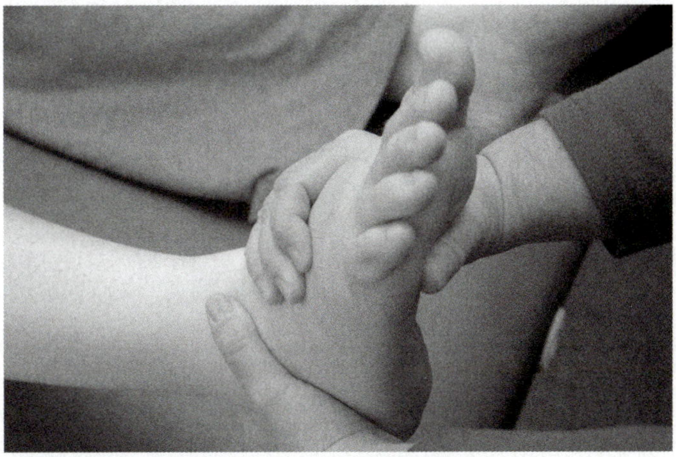

Figure 52.36. Lower extremity technique.

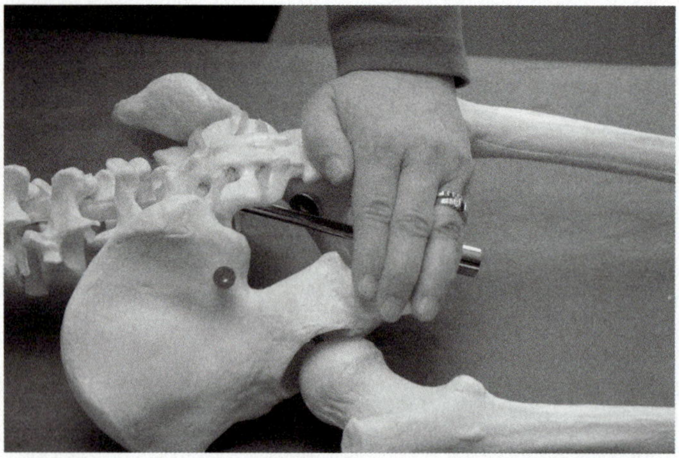

Figure 52.37. **Abdomen and viscera technique, skeletal view.**

5. Hold this position. Patient takes three deep breaths and follows the shifting pattern throughout. Return the limb to neutral and reevaluate motion, pain, and edema of the knee.

Abdomen/Other

ABDOMEN/OTHER

The prostate releases through the pelvic floor. Pelvic floor fascial motion is important to the proper placement and function of the prostate, which sits on top of the diaphragm. Congestion is encouraged by a lack of tone and motion in this diaphragm (Figs. 52.37 and 52.38).

1. Patient lays supine on the table. Physician sits next to the side of the pelvis.
2. The physician's hand that is closest to the patient's head is placed perpendicular to the long line of the spine, with the patient's coccyx in the palm of the hand, contacting the ischial tuberosities contralaterally with the fingers, and capturing the posterior pelvic diaphragm ipsilaterally with the hypothenar eminence.
3. Place the other hand parallel to and in contact with the edge of the fifth digit on the pubic symphysis. Lay the hand down flat, contacting the lower abdominal wall fascia.
4. Be aware of the fascial motion loop between the anterior and posterior fascial planes as they converge in the pelvic diaphragm.
   a. Notice the motion and tension in the tissues while traveling that loop.

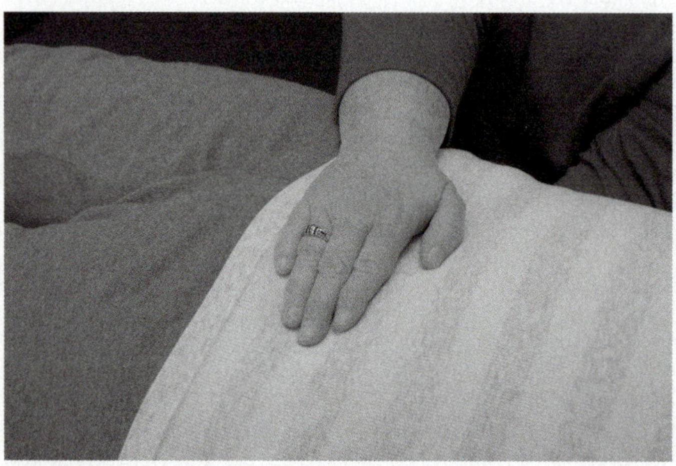

Figure 52.38. **Abdomen and viscera technique.**

   b. Allow a three-dimensional motion to occur between the sensing hands.
5. Sense the placement of the prostate (bladder, vagina, uterus, or rectum), as well as the tension or ease in the fascia surrounding them.
6. Identify the pattern of motion ease and restriction. Choose a direct or an indirect approach.
   a. With three respiratory cycles, follow the shifting pattern as it releases.
   b. Maintain awareness of the viscera while both hands move in response to the tissue tension changes, occurring as the release progresses with the three deep respiratory cycles.
   c. Remember that these motions may take on different directions and traverse multiple viscera. They are diagnostic as well as therapeutic.
7. At the end of the release, return the patient to neutral and reassess the motion pattern.

CASE STUDIES

CASE 1: BIOMECHANICAL MODEL OF WARD

J.M. is a 49-year-old man who has been suffering from right sciatica for 3 months, after beginning a cardiac fitness program. He describes the pain as an ache from his right buttock to posterior thigh, but not below the knee. He notices it while walking and standing. The pain decreases with rest or sitting. He denies any numbness or tingling in his legs, or any weakness with activities. He has noticed that he is wearing out the sole on his left shoe and has had to replace them more frequently. He denies any recent trauma. Ibuprofen helps the pain temporarily.

The rest of his review of systems is noncontributory. Past medical history is negative for neuromusculoskeletal issues other than the present chief complaint and is positive for elevated blood pressure. Family history, both maternal and paternal, is positive for hypertension. Medications are occasional ibuprofen for sciatica.

Physical Exam

BP: 130/72; pulse: 70 regular; resp: 12 regularly, and in moderate distress.

Gait

Antalgic with limp right. Pain in right sacroiliac (SI) joint with full weight bearing on right leg, and reproduction of sciatica right.

Postural Exam

Posterior view: right iliac crest low, right PSIS low with lateral curve changes. Convex right lumbar and left thoracic with downward tilt of right shoulder. The greater trochanter is low right with externally rotated right hip. Pain in right SI joint with change in position seated to standing.

Palpatory Exam

Pain on palpation of the right piriformis with reproduction of chief complaint of sciatica. Tenderness and tightness of left quadratus lumborum and right thoracolumbar fascia, with torsion to the left of the torso, on the pelvis. Contralateral pattern palpated through the rectus abdominis fascia. Inhibited right hamstrings with tight right quadriceps femoris and right piriformis.

Neurologic Exam

No signs of peripheral or central compromise and is otherwise normal.

Vascular Exam

Normal.

Diagnosis

- Postural imbalance with short right leg
- Sciatica
- Somatic dysfunction of thoracic, lumbar, sacrum, pelvis, and lower extremity

Treatment

- Myofascial release (MFR) to the thoracic, lumbar, sacrum, pelvis, and lower extremity
- Postural x-rays
- Consider heel lift after review of x-rays
- Home exercise program

CASE 2: "THE BIG BANDAGE" MODEL OF CHILA

P.R. is a 46-year-old woman who presents with pain in the right shoulder, neck, and upper back after gardening during the weekend. She spent a day weeding and planting in her gardens and went to bed stiff. She woke up this morning in pain, with poor motion of her neck and right shoulder without radiation of pain or numbness. She denies any other recent traumas. She did have a similar problem last spring when she began to garden again and was helped by osteopathic manipulative treatments (OMTs).

Review of systems is positive for ovarian cysts and is otherwise noncontributory.

Past medical and family histories are unchanged from last year.

Tests

X-rays of the cervical spine a year ago demonstrated mild degenerative changes at the facets and disks at C5–C6.

Medications

Ibuprofen 200 mg, two pills every 6 hours since yesterday, with relief of stiffness but not pain. Aleve 1 to 2 q12 prn prior to her periods, and at midcycle for ovarian pain.

Physical Exam

BP: 120/80; pulse: 76 in acute moderate distress.

Neurologic Exam

Normal reflexes and sensation of upper extremities; strength intact with pain, with endpoints of exertion.

Peripheral Vascular Exam

Pulses normal with good capillary refill and no edema of all extremities.

Musculoskeletal Exam

Range of motion of right shoulder limited in abduction with pain, and otherwise both shoulders normal; cervical spine spasms with rotation of head and neck greater than 20 degrees left, otherwise motion intact; thoracic spine limited by pain in all planes of motion with spasms.

Diagnosis

- Sprain/strain right shoulder
- Sprain/strain cervical spine
- Sprain/strain thoracic spine
- Somatic dysfunction of the cervical, thoracic spine, and right upper extremity

Treatment

- MFR
- Stretches
- Continue ibuprofen

CASE 3: BIOENERGETIC MODEL OF O'CONNELL

E.G. is a 3-week-old female infant brought in by her parents for problems with sucking, torticollis, and the inability to move her right arm. She is the product of an uncomplicated term pregnancy that was augmented with synthetic oxytocin for failure to progress, due to being in an occiput posterior position. Labor lasted 22 hours, and she was delivered without further assistance. She weighed 8 lb. 2 oz and had APGARS of 7 and 9. Mom states that E.G. had problems latching on from the start and cried a lot, keeping her from nursing at the breast or with bottles of expressed milk. They noticed that she did not move her right arm like her left and that her head was always turned left and tilted onto her right shoulder. The pediatrician reassured them that this would resolve on its own. Since it did not, they have brought her to seek osteopathic manipulative treatments at the advice of their lactation consultant.

The rest of the review of systems shows steady weight gain in the 25th percentile, no reflux, and is otherwise noncontributory.

Family history is negative for similar conditions. Both parents are healthy and are 22 years old.

Physical Exam

Pulse 140 regular, respirations nonlabored, distressed with certain positions, nursing, and changing clothes.

Neurologic Exam

Inability to actively, grossly move right shoulder. Movement of elbow, wrist, and grip is maintained but weak on the right with the left normal. Torticollis with head turned left and upward gaze, and inability to actively rotate right. Suck is disorganized with posterior tongue position and inability to maintain suction on digit, nipple, or breast with aerophagia and discomfort. The rest of her neurologic exam is appropriate for age.

Musculoskeletal Exam

Torticollis rotated left, with spasm of right sternocleidomastoid (SCM) muscle resulting in pain with passive motion of head and neck right past midline. Group curve cervical spine has the most significant loss of motion at C5 and C1-occiput. Ribs 1 to 2 elevated right with depression of the acromioclavicular joint with a click with motion. The position of ease is head rotated left with upward tilt and right shoulder internally rotated. Cranial motion demonstrates a compression of the mastoidal suture and occipital condyle on the right. T1–T3 are extended, and any attempt at flexion in this region is painful.

The rest of the physical exam is normal and appropriate for age.

Diagnoses

- Erb palsy
- Torticollis, spasmodic
- CN trauma of birth (3 to 5)
- Feeding problems of the newborn
- Somatic dysfunction of head, cervical, thoracic, ribs, and upper extremity right

Treatment

- MFR
- Set up for physical therapy
- Discussed positional support when feeding
- Continue with lactation consultant to support breast feeding

REFERENCES

1. Still AT. *Philosophy of Osteopathy*. American Academy of Osteopathy; 1899:162.
2. Page LE. The role of the fasciae in the maintenance of structural integrity. In: *The American Academy of Osteopathy Yearbook*. American Academy of Osteopathy; 1952:70.
3. Snyder GE. Fasciae—applied anatomy and physiology. In: *The American Academy of Osteopathy Yearbook*. American Academy of Osteopathy; 1956:65.
4. Personal Attendance. *Sutherland Cranial Teaching Foundation*. Introductory Course; 1981.
5. Fulford RC. *Touch of Life*. Pocket; 1997.
6. O'Connell J. *Bioelectric Fascial Activation and Release, The Physician's Guide to Hunting with Dr. Still*. American Academy of Osteopathy; 2000.
7. Gray H. *Anatomy, Descriptive and Surgical 1901 Edition*. Running Press; 1974:1086–1092.
8. Patten BM. *Human Embryology*. 3rd ed. McGraw-Hill Inc.; 1968:59.
9. Cathie AG. The fascia of the body in relation to function and manipulative therapy. In: *The American Academy of Osteopathy Yearbook*. American Academy of Osteopathy; 1974:81–87.
10. Becker RF. The meaning of fascia and fascial continuity. *Osteopath Ann*. 1975:3:8–32.
11. Guimberteau J, Armstrong C. *Architecture of Human Living Fascia*. Handspring Publishing; 2015.
12. Gowitzke BA, Milner M. *Scientific Basis of Human Movement*. 3rd ed. William & Wilkins; 1998:143–145.
13. Ward RC. Integrated neuromusculoskeletal release and myofascial release. In: Ward RC, ed. *Foundations for Osteopathic Medicine*. 2nd ed. Lippincott Williams & Wilkins; 2003:931–932.
14. Stedman TL, Stedman's Medical Dictionary Staff. *Stedman's Medical Dictionary*. 23rd ed. Burns & McEachern; 1976.
15. Kottke FJ, Stillwell GK, Lehman JF. *Krusen's Handbook of Physical Medicine and Rehabilitation*. 3rd ed. W.B. Saunders Company; 1971:391.
16. Becker RO, Seldon G. *The Body Electric*. Quill; 1985:152–155.
17. Bonica JJ. *The Management of Pain*. 2nd ed. Lea and Febiger; 1990:66.
18. Earl E. The dual sensory role of muscles spindles. *Phys Ther J*. 1965;45:4.
19. Wilson VJ. Inhibition in the central nervous system. *Sci Am*. 1966;5: 102–108.
20. Chila AG. *Connective Tissue Continuity: Membranous and Ligamentous Articular Dysfunction*. Ohio University College of Osteopathic Medicine; 2006:48.
21. Korr IM. The spinal cord as organizer of disease processes—some preliminary perspectives. *J Am Osteopath Assoc*. 1976;76:35–45.
22. Becker RF. The gamma system and its relation to the development and maintenance of muscle tone. *J Am Osteopath Assoc*. 1975;75:170–187.
23. Patterson MM. A model mechanism for spinal segmental facilitation. *J Am Osteopath Assoc*. 1976;76:62–72.
24. Stiles E. Stylized osteopathic seminars. Stiles DO on Web.
25. Hohenschurz-Schmidt DJ. Tensegrity in the context of the myofascial network: it's relevance to osteopathic practice. In: Liem T, Tozzi P, Chila A, eds. *Fascia in the Osteopathic Field*. Handspring Publishing; 2017.
26. O'Connell J. Bioelectric responsiveness of fascia: a model for understanding the effects of manipulation. In: *Techniques in Orthopaedics*. Vol. 18(1). Lippincott Williams & Wilkins, Inc.; 2003:67–73.
27. Hensel K. *A Teaching Guide for Osteopathic Manipulative Medicine*. American Association of Colleges of Osteopathic Medicine; 2015:85.
28. Kimberly PE. *Outline of Osteopathic Manipulative Procedures, The Kimberly Manual*. Walsworth Publishing Company; 2006:30–31.
29. Trowbridge C. *Andrew Taylor Still, 1828–1917*. The Thomas Jefferson University Press; 1991:176.
30. Still AT. *Osteopathy: Research and Practice*. Published by the Author; 1910:19–20.
31. O'Connell JA. The Bioenergetic Model of Fascia as Related to Trauma. In: Liem T, Tozzi P, Chila A, eds. *Fascia in the Osteopathic Field*. Handspring Publishing; 2017.

53 Osteopathic Cranial Manipulative Medicine

HOLLIS H. KING

KEY CONCEPTS

- Osteopathic cranial manipulative medicine (OCMM) delineates an anatomically based understanding of range and vector of motion, along with physiologic dynamics of cranial bones and intracranial structures.
- The primary respiratory mechanism (PRM) is a functional unit based on the accommodative actions of cranial articular surfaces.
- The traditional model of OCMM includes five phenomena: the inherent rhythmic motion of the brain and spinal cord, fluctuation of cerebrospinal fluid, mobility of intracranial and intraspinal membranes, articular mobility of cranial bones, and involuntary mobility of sacrum between ilia.
- Evidence-based research supports the OCMM PRM phenomena underlying the palpatory experience of osteopathic practitioners who utilize OCMM in medical practice. Clinical research has demonstrated benefit of OCMM in a number of medical conditions and disorders, especially in pediatrics and the neurosciences.

DEFINITION

Osteopathic cranial manipulative medicine (OCMM), previously called osteopathy in the cranial field (OCF), is a system of diagnosis and treatment by an osteopathic physician using the primary respiratory mechanism (PRM) and balanced membranous tension. It refers to the system of diagnosis and treatment first described by William G. Sutherland, DO.[1]

HISTORY

William G. Sutherland, DO, DSc (Hon) (1873–1954), was an early student of Dr. A.T. Still. Sutherland graduated from the American School of Osteopathy in Kirksville, Missouri, in 1899. While he was a student, Sutherland observed a mounted disarticulated skull. The sphenoid and the squamous portions of the temporal bones caught his attention. Sutherland stated:

> "As I stood looking and thinking in the channel of Dr. Still's philosophy, my attention was called to the beveled articular surfaces of the sphenoid bone. Suddenly there came a thought; I call it a guiding thought—beveled like the gills of a fish, indicating articular mobility for a respiratory mechanism.[2] (pp. 12–13)"

He dismissed the thought but it kept returning, as if goading him to study the details of the various articulations of the skull.

Sutherland was an original thinker, and his application of Still's philosophy is recognized as "one of the most innovative ideas to be advanced by a member of the osteopathic profession.[3] (p. 40)" Anatomy books at that time stated that the sutures of the cranium were immovable. This, however, did not deter Sutherland. He was determined to understand why the articular surfaces have such a unique design and persevered until he understood that the design was accommodative to the function of the central nervous system (CNS), cerebrospinal fluid (CSF), and dural membranes, all of which function as a unit. He named this functional unit the *primary respiratory mechanism* (PRM).

Sutherland established his practice in Minnesota and devoted 30 years to study, to perform original research on himself, and to observe his patients, before he began to share his discovery with his colleagues. The remarkable results that Sutherland obtained with patients aroused the interest of other physicians. They prevailed upon him to teach them his method of treatment. He agreed to do so and began classes at his home. The classes and the interest grew, slowly but steadily, because those who were able to learn the concept and apply this method of osteopathic diagnosis and treatment had similar results of relieving patients of pain and distressful conditions when other forms of treatment failed to help.

DEVELOPMENT OF THE CRANIAL CONCEPT

As more physicians studied and practiced Sutherland's method of osteopathic treatment, they formed an organization, the Osteopathic Cranial Association, for the purpose of joining together to promote further study, support research, and publish literature to help educate physicians and laypersons. This membership organization later changed its name to the Osteopathic Cranial Academy and became a component society of the American Academy of Osteopathic Medicine.

Another, though little known, pioneer of the cranial concept was Charlotte Winger Weaver, DO (1884–1964), a 1912 graduate of the American School of Osteopathy. Dr. Weaver was reintroduced to the osteopathic profession by Margaret A. Sorrel, DO, in the 1998 Sutherland Memorial Lecture. Dr. Weaver considered the cranial bones as modified vertebrae possessing articular surfaces and taught her concepts through the Doctor Weaver Foundation established in 1927. Dr. Weaver performed many dissections of skulls and dural membranous structures and had a special interest in the relationship between lesions of the basicranium and neuropsychiatric disorders. She taught that the basicranium could be distorted by birth trauma. Apparently, Dr. Sutherland knew Dr. Weaver, but they performed their research of the cranium from two different, and thus independent, perspectives.[4]

In 1953, Dr. Sutherland, together with Drs. Chester Handy and Harold I. Magoun, Sr., established the Sutherland Cranial Teaching Foundation, Inc., for the purpose of continuing the teaching of the cranial concept. Dr. Sutherland had established that an accurate diagnosis and successful treatment required sensitive and proficient palpation that could not be learned from a book; expert instructors using hands-on teaching and repeated verification were needed.

Dr. Sutherland's contributions have supplied knowledge that clarifies and expands on the science of osteopathy. Prior to

Dr. Sutherland's work, the body was treated as if the head was incapable of having somatic dysfunction.

OCMM is osteopathy of the entire person because the inherent force that manifests from within the head region functions throughout the body. Therefore, this form of diagnosis and treatment affects the body as a whole rather than being limited to the cranium. Furthermore, the position of the head atop the vertebral column affects the postural balance of the entire neuromusculoskeletal system. For example, if the cranial bone structures have been brought into a state of imbalance through trauma, the cranium will cause compensatory changes throughout the neuromusculoskeletal system in order to keep the equilibrium apparatus efficient in its function.

PROGRESSION AND INTEGRATION OF OCMM IN MEDICAL EDUCATION AND CLINICAL PRACTICE

The teaching and practice of OCMM were continued after Sutherland's death by the Sutherland Cranial Teaching Foundation (SCTF) and The Cranial Academy. In the past 70 years of the teaching and practice of OCMM, there emerged a number of leaders who have preserved and advanced Sutherland's cranial concept through their teachings sponsored by these organizations.

- H.I. Magoun, DO, wrote *Osteopathy in the Cranial Field*,[5] a text that for many years has been a primary reference for those studying OCMM.
- Howard Lippincott, DO, and his wife Rebecca Lippincott, DO, taught with Sutherland for several years and published the first work on ligamentous articular strain based on Sutherland's teaching.[6,7]
- Rollin E. Becker, DO, succeeded Lippincott, DO, as President of the SCTF and was considered the leading teacher of OCMM for many years. His writings are also a primary reference for those studying OCMM.[8,9]
- Robert C. Fulford, DO, was a contemporary of Becker who also studied with Sutherland; his writings elaborate on many cranial principles and elucidate many of the more subtle aspects of OCMM.[10–12]
- Anne L. Wales, DO, along with her husband Chester Handy, DO, taught OCMM with Dr. Sutherland. She also brought many of Sutherland's recorded lectures into print.[13]
- Beryl E. Arbuckle, DO, was a pediatrician and researcher who, as part of her research on OCMM, attended hundreds of autopsies at the Hospital of Philadelphia College of Osteopathic Medicine. These autopsies involved gross or microscopic study of the skull. Dr. Arbuckle was noted for her application of OCMM on special needs children, particularly those with cerebral palsy.[14]
- Viola M. Frymann, DO, FAAO, was also a student of Sutherland and championed OCMM with children.[15] She has been instrumental in the teaching of and research on OCMM internationally, as well as in the United States.[16–18]
- Edna M. Lay, DO, FAAO, has also been a leader in the teaching of OCMM and in working with children. Her writings have shaped the form of this very chapter in previous editions.[19]

The insights and techniques derived from Dr. Sutherland's expansion of basic osteopathic principles are increasingly integrated into osteopathic teaching and clinical care.[20–22] *The International Classification of Disease, Ninth Revision* (*ICD-9-CM*), delineated coding for somatic dysfunction of the cranium, which was continued in the ICD-10; and *Current Procedural Terminology* provides coding for osteopathic manipulative treatment (OMT) of the head. In recent years, the American Osteopathic Association (AOA) has received numerous research grant proposals from both clinicians and basic scientists to study the mechanisms and/or efficacy of this approach; the AOA has funded several of these projects.[23–26]

Instruction in OCMM has been a part of standard training in the departments of osteopathic principles, practice, and manipulative medicine in all osteopathic medical schools. Concepts and terminology pertaining to OCMM have been developed and defined by the Educational Council on Osteopathic Principles of the American Association of Colleges of Osteopathic Medicine. They have been published in the Glossary of Osteopathic Medical Terminology, which is updated regularly and easily accessible online.[27]

The AOA has approved the *Basic Standards for Residency Training in Neuromusculoskeletal Medicine and Osteopathic Manipulative Treatment*. OCMM is one of the OMT models within these basic standards. The AOA is the federally recognized body charged with approval of certifying boards within the osteopathic medical profession. The AOA has chartered the American Osteopathic Board of Neuromusculoskeletal Medicine. This certifying board administers written, oral, and practical examinations that include items relating to OCMM. Questions pertaining to principles of OCMM appear on the written portions of the Comprehensive Osteopathic Medical License Examination (COMLEX-USA) administered by the National Board of Osteopathic Medical Examiners, and COMLEX-USA results are accepted for medical licensure in all 50 of the United States. These same standards, including for OCMM, are maintained by the Accreditation Council of Graduation Medical Education's Residency Review Committee for Osteopathic Neuromusculoskeletal Medicine of the United States.

PROPOSED MECHANISM OF ACTION

Primary Respiratory Mechanism (PRM)

Central to Sutherland's cranial concept is his integration of anatomic structure and physiologic processes into the PRM model. All five components of this model have garnered sufficient research verification over the last four decades to mitigate any criticism regarding lack of scientific proof.

Primary refers to first in importance and precedes thoracic respiration in importance. Dr. Sutherland posited that physiologic centers, located in the floor of the fourth ventricle (which regulate pulmonary respiration, circulation, digestion, and elimination and depend on the function of the CNS) were primary in the maintenance of life.[5]

- Respiratory refers to the exchange of gases and other metabolites at the cellular level.
- Mechanism implies an integrated machine, each part in working relationship with every other part.

The PRM is described as having five anatomic–physiologic components, also often referred to as the five phenomena of OCMM. These five components or phenomena are described in the following sections and include:

1. The inherent rhythmic motion of the brain and spinal cord
2. Fluctuation of CSF
3. Mobility of intracranial and intraspinal membranes
4. Articular mobility of cranial bones
5. Involuntary mobility of sacrum between ilia

1. *The inherent rhythmic motion of the brain and spinal cord*

The inherent motion of the CNS is a subtle, slow, pulse-wave–like movement. It is described as having a biphasic cycle, which may have a rhythmic nature. The entire CNS shortens and thickens during one phase and lengthens and thins during the other.[5] In words still relevant today, Lassek described the brain as being "vibrantly alive...incessantly active...dynamic...highly mobile, able to move forward, backward, sideward, circumduct and to rotate." He further stated, "[t]he normal, human brain is a wondrous, enormously complex, master organ which can be only made by nature. There are probably approximately twenty billion neurons in the CNS of man and it runs on a mere 25 W of electrical power.[5] (p. 23)" As the cerebral hemispheres develop in fetal life, they grow, lengthen, and curl or coil within the developing cranium in the shape of a pair of ram's horns. Specific motion characteristics of cranial palpation are attributed to this configuration of brain structures.

Since the publication of Magoun's text, the delineation of embryologic development principles by Jealous,[28] based in large measure on the work of Blechschmidt,[29,30] has increased the understanding of Sutherland's formulation of the PRM. These writings also enhanced the detailed application of OCMM in clinical practice, through the appreciation of the anatomic positional changes of human structures, as they develop from embryonic to adult human configuration and location.

2. *Fluctuation of cerebrospinal fluid*

The CSF is formed by the choroid plexuses and circulates through the ventricles, over and around the surface of the brain and spinal cord, through the subarachnoid spaces and cisternae, and is reabsorbed in the arachnoid villi. Thus, the CSF is inside and outside of the CNS, bathing, protecting, and nourishing it. Fluctuation is defined as a wavelike motion of fluid in a natural or artificial cavity of the body observed by palpation or percussion.[31] From the perspective of Sutherland's concept of the PRM, as the CNS shortens and lengthens in a biphasic rhythmic motion, the ventricles of the brain change shape slightly and the fluid moves concurrently. Furthermore, the combined motility of the CNS and the fluctuation of CSF manifest as a hydrodynamic activity as well as a bioelectric interchange throughout the body. Stated simply, this combined activity of the CNS and CSF functions both as a pump and as a bioelectric generator. Recording of the bioelectric flow in fascia and connective tissue is in the piezoelectric range.[32]

3. *Mobility of intracranial and intraspinal membranes*

The meninges surround, support, and protect the CNS. The dura mater, the outermost of the three meningeal coverings, is composed of two layers of tough fibrous tissue within the cranial vault.

- The outer layer of dura mater lines the cranial cavity, forming a periosteal covering for the inner aspect of the bones and extends through the sutures of the skull to become continuous with the periosteum on the outer surface of the skull.
- The inner layer of dura mater covers the brain and spinal cord and has reduplications named the falx cerebri and the tentorium cerebelli. These sickle-shaped structures arise from a common origin along the straight sinus and invest the various bones of the cranium. The two layers of dura mater are blended or fused in certain areas and are separated in other areas, forming the intradural venous sinuses

  The dura mater extends down the spinal canal with firm attachment around the foramen magnum and in the spinal canal of the sacrum at the level of the second sacral segment. There are also occasional attachments at C2 and C3 and the lower lumbar. The falx cerebri arises from the straight sinus, attaching to the occiput, parietals, frontals, and the crista galli of the ethmoid. The two halves of the tentorium cerebelli arise or originate at the straight sinus and attach to the occiput, temporals, and sphenoid bone.

The spinal and cranial dura with its reduplications respond to the inherent motion of the CNS and fluctuation of CSF and move through the biphasic cycle, influencing the bones of the cranium and the sacrum. Sutherland named this functional anatomic unit, consisting of the dura mater within the cranium and spinal canal, the reciprocal tension membrane (RTM).[5] It has also been referred to as the "core link"[5] because of the potential to transmit biomechanical forces due to this connection of the cranium to the sacrum. Influences such as trauma and postural strains that affect one part of the mechanism have been clinically observed to affect other parts of the body via this "core link."

4. *Articular mobility of cranial bones*

The most dramatic and debated phenomenon of the PRM has been the articular mobility of the cranial bones. Careful study of the design of the various articulations of the cranium, face, and the RTM, as well as its influence on the motion of the bones, led Sutherland to an appreciation of the mechanical design of this anatomy and their relationship to the inherent motility of the CNS and CSF. At birth, the cranial bones are smooth-edged osseous plates with membrane and/or cartilage between them. With normal growth and motion of intracranial structures, the edges of the cranial bone plates develop and join together with sutures (joints) between them. These sutures allow for a minimal amount of motion while still providing protection for the brain.

5. *Involuntary mobility of sacrum between ilia*

The cranial dura is continuous with the spinal dura; the spinal dura extends through the vertebral canal into the sacral canal, attaching at the level of some cervical and lumbar segments and the second sacral segment. Careful study of the design of the articular surfaces reveals that the sacrum may move on one or several postural axes in relation to the ilia (pelvic bones). In addition to these voluntary or postural movements, the sacrum also responds to the:

- Inherent mobility of the CNS
- Fluctuation of the CSF
- Pull of the intracranial and intraspinal membranes with an involuntary movement that can be observed by palpation in the living body

This slight rocking motion occurs around a transverse axis (called the respiratory axis). Normally, the involuntary motion of the sacrum is synchronous with the involuntary motion of the occiput, each bone being influenced by the rhythmic pull of the spinal and cranial dura mater.

Appreciation of the five phenomena of the PRM in theoretical and practical terms requires an integration of the anatomic and physiologic factors substantiated by empirical research. Experience-derived applications are discussed below. It may help to visualize this physiologic unit of function with all five components moving slightly but steadily in the living body from before birth until death. Becker[33] (p. 57) summarizes its influence on the total body economy as follows:

> "Health requires that the PRM have the capacity to be an involuntary, rhythmic, automatic, shifting suspension mechanism for the intricate, integrated, dynamic interrelationships of its five elements. It is intimately related to the rest of the body through its

fascial connections from the base of the skull through the cervical, thoracic, abdominal, pelvic, and appendicular areas of the body physiology. Since all of the involuntary and voluntary systems of the body, including the musculoskeletal system, are found in fascial envelopes, they, too, are subjected to the 10 to 14 cycle-per-minute rhythm of the craniosacral mechanism in addition to their own rhythms of involuntary and voluntary activity. The involuntary mobility of the craniosacral mechanism moves all the tissues of the body minutely into rhythmic flexion of the midline structures with external rotation of the bilateral structures and, in the opposite cycle, extension of the midline structures with internal rotation of the bilateral structures 10 to 14 times/min throughout life."

MECHANISMS OF PHYSIOLOGIC MOTION

The overall shape of the skull is that of a relative sphere with its inferior surface indented. The sphenoid and occiput meet to create this indentation, which is slightly convex on its superior surface. These two midline bones form the key articulation of cranial bone motion at the sphenobasilar synchondrosis (SBS) (or synostosis) in the base of the skull. This remains a modified cartilaginous union up to the age of 20 years and, thereafter, will have the resiliency of cancellous bone.[34]

The overall motion of the cranium is similar to the motion of the chest during respiration, but the two do not occur simultaneously. Thoracic respiration occurs 12 to 16 cycles/min in adults and up to 44 cycles/min in newborns;[35] the most frequently encountered motion of the PRM normally occurs 10 to 14 cycles/min.[5]

The terminology used to describe the directions of motion of the various bones is similar to that of the motions of the spine and extremities. Midline bones (the sphenoid, occiput, ethmoid, vomer, and sacrum) move through a flexion phase and an extension phase around a transverse axis, while paired bones move through external and internal rotation. They are moved through this biphasic cycle in response to the pull or influence of the dural membranes, which are influenced by the coiling and uncoiling of the CNS and the fluctuation of the CSF. This motion, initiated from within the living body, is referred to as inherent motion or involuntary motion.

With flexion of the SBS, there is slight increase in the convexity of the superior surface of the joint. At the same time, the area where the coronal and sagittal sutures join, called bregma, descends. Palpation in the flexion portion of the biphasic cycle senses that the head widens slightly in its transverse diameter and shortens slightly in its anteroposterior (AP) diameter as the paired bones move toward external rotation. With extension of the midline bones, the head narrows and lengthens slightly as the bregma ascends, and all paired bones move toward internal rotation.

During the biphasic cycle, the osseous cranium changes shape slightly and allows some intracranial fluid volume change. The research of Heisey and Adams[36] and Moskalenko and Kravchenko[37] suggests that there is enough cranial bone compliance and "sutural stretch" to allow as much as a 15-mL intracranial fluid volume change.

During flexion, the sacrum is influenced by the spinal dura and core link and moves posterosuperiorly at its base while the apex moves anteriorly toward the pubic bones. During extension, the base moves anteriorly and the apex moves posteriorly. This motion occurs around a transverse axis in the area of the second sacral segment posterior to the sacral canal and is called the respiratory axis of the sacrum. The other axes of sacral motion are postural axes (Fig. 53.1).

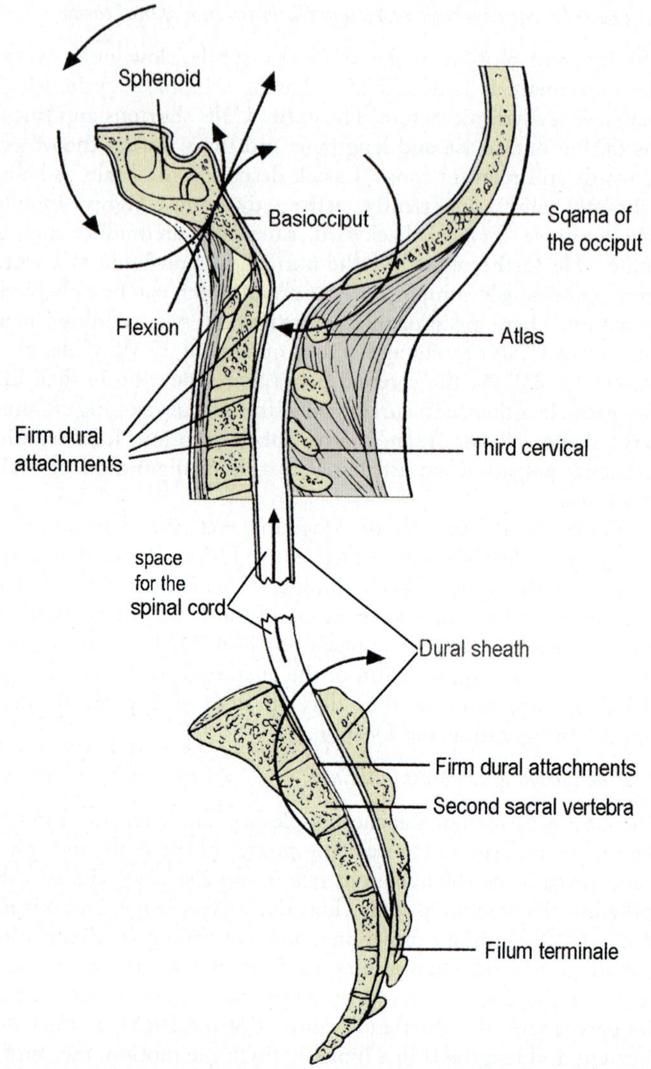

Figure 53.1. Craniosacral mechanism with *arrows* indicating direction of motion during flexion phase of physiologic motion. (From Magoun HI. *Osteopathy in the Cranial Field.* 2nd ed. Journal Publishing Company; 1966, with permission from The Osteopathic Cranial Academy, Indianapolis, IN, https://cranialacademy.org.)

RESEARCH SUPPORTIVE OF THE PRIMARY RESPIRATORY MECHANISM

The Inherent Rhythmic Motion of the Brain and Spinal Cord

As stated above, all five of the phenomena have sufficient evidence-based research supporting their validity to the point where they are no longer controversial. Much of the support for this phenomenon of the PRM derives from research done in basic science and medical laboratories outside the osteopathic profession. Movement of the CNS anatomy is a well-established medical and anatomic function. Representative of this line of research is the work of Greitz et al.[38] who, utilizing magnetic resonance imaging (MRI) technology, demonstrated brain tissue movement is characterized by an inferior, medial, and posteriorly directed movement of the basal ganglia and an inferior and anterior movement of the pons during cardiac systole. The resultant movement vectors created a "funnel-shaped" appearance to the brain resulting in a "piston-like" remolding of the brain. The authors felt that this "piston-like" action of the brain during cardiac systole was the driving force responsible for compression of the ventricular system and thus the driving force for the intraventricular flow of cerebral spinal fluid.

Poncelet et al.[39] using echo-planar MRI, were able to demonstrate pulsatile motion of brain parenchyma. Brain motion in Poncelet's study appeared to consist of a single displacement during systole and a slow return to baseline configuration during diastole. This displacement includes a descent of midbrain and brainstem toward foramen magnum with velocities ≤2 mm/s and medial compression of thalami onto the third ventricle with a velocity of ≤1.5 mm/s.

Feinberg and Mark[40] postulated that the pulsatile nature of CSF flow and brain motion was driven by the force of expansion of the choroid plexus. In their study, which involved observations of pulsatile brain motion via MRI, ejection of CSF into the ventricles occurred simultaneously with reversal of CSF flow in the basal cisterns. These observations suggest that the pumping force for CSF circulation may be a vascularly driven mechanism. They reported the velocity of anterior cortex and corpus callosum movement is 0.4 ± 0.25 mm/s and motion velocity of the basal ganglia and foramen of Monro is 0.63 ± 0.5 mm/s.

These dimensions of motion of cranial and spinal CNS structures suggest that the intracranial structures may not move as far or as fast as spinal cord structures, but these structures do all manifest motion of a precise measurable nature. This motion appears to be related to the vascular dynamics of the circulatory system and the cardiac cycle. This element of the PRM is not controversial as such motion has been well studied and established.

Yet to be fully delineated is whether or not there exists any biomechanical impetus to the palpable characteristics of the PRM by cellular and intracellular activity, motility, as well as mobility possibly associated with a primary respiration process.

Fluctuation of Cerebrospinal Fluid

Movement of the CSF in a fluctuant flow pattern, through the ventricles of the brain and within the subarachnoid space around the brain and spinal cord, is also a well-established phenomenon. In fact, much of research that demonstrated the motion of the brain and spinal cord, also identified features of the CSF fluctuant flow.

Summarizing over a century of research DuBolay et al.[41] (p. 497) stated, "The majority of workers throughout these seven decades have become convinced that the 'cardiac' CSF pressure rise measured in the ventricles, at the cisterna magna and in the lumbar theca, is caused by the rhythmic arterial input of blood to the cranial cavity." DuBolay further states, "Most authors, e.g., Becher,[42] had envisaged the arterial inflow to the head as causing an expansion of the brain and of the vessels within the basal cisterns. O'Connell[43] suggested that the brain's expansion, by compressing the third ventricle, might constitute a CSF pump."

As will be discussed below is the anatomic connection between CSF flow and the lymphatic system, a long-held hypothesis in OCMM practice, which appears to have been established. Research by Walter et al.[44] showed that India ink particles injected into rat subarachnoid space were found distributed around the olfactory nerves and within the lymphatic vessels. The authors commented, "This anatomical communication, thus, allows the CNS to connect with the lymphatic system. The presence of the route may play an important role in the movement of antigens from the subarachnoid space to the extracranial lymphatic vessels, resulting in inducement of an immune response of the CNS"[44] (p. 388). The continuum between the glymphatic and lymphatic systems has been delineated further establishing the CSF and lymphatic flow relationship.[45]

Mobility of Intracranial and Intraspinal Membranes

The existence of the dura mater membrane around the brain and spinal cord is well documented and utilized in anatomic research and medical practice. Every medical student and anatomist who has dissected the central nervous has seen this membrane. Every physician who has done a lumbar puncture (or spinal tap) has felt the "pop" as the needle penetrates the dura in the procedure to obtain a sample of CSF. Those who practice OCMM utilize this anatomy to treat cranial and cervical malalignment from the sacrum, or sacral malalignment from the base of the skull. These types of treatment are believed to be possible because of the hypothesized direct connection between the cranium and sacrum in the form of the dural membrane.

Representative of the pertinent research is based on MRI imagery of in vivo kinematic analysis of head and neck position in extension and flexion positions, Zhu et al.[46] reported relative displacements of brain with respect to skull as the head position changes. The displacements were on the order of 1 to 2 mm when the head changed positions voluntarily. According to the authors, "...these displacements over the normal range of head/neck flexion suggest free interfascial conditions between brain and skull[46] (p. 813)."

Kostopoulos and Keramidas[47] utilized a novel approach to anatomic research on a male cadaver that had been embalmed for 6 months. The brain tissue was removed through two cut windows, leaving the intracranial dural membranes intact. A piezoelectric element attached to the falx cerebri was used to measure the motion which was recorded by an oscilloscope. Application of the frontal lift cranial treatment maneuver then produced a 1.44-mm elongation of the falx cerebri and a parietal lift maneuver produced a 1.08-mm elongation. Even on embalmed tissue, application of the sphenobasilar compression maneuver produced a 0.33-mm movement, and the sphenobasilar decompression maneuver a +0.28-mm movement of the falx cerebri. The Kostopoulos and Keramidas data suggest that, for cranial structures, there is an identifiable association between cranial maneuvers applied to the cranium and the movement of cranial dural membranes.

In the treatment of head and neck pain, one of the more clinically useful applications of the fascia continuity of the body is the myofascial-dural bridge between the rectus capitus posterior minor muscle/fascia and the dura mater of the cervical spine.[48] This is also described in Gray Anatomy[49] (p. 813).

Articular Mobility of Cranial Bones

Recent research on cranial bone mobility,[50] plus prior research discussed below, and lack of concerted criticism of the phenomenon of cranial bone motion for over a decade justifies confidence in the validity of the Sutherland proposed five phenomena of the PRM.[5]

While the preponderance of the evidence demonstrates cranial bone motion, the nature of the cranial sutures regarding the nature of fusion, if it occurs, is fusion the whole depth of the boney suture or just partial? Clinical experience suggests that there is palpable motion in seemingly "fused" sutures. "Obliteration of sutures and synostosis of adjoining bones, *if it happens at all* (italics added), occurs usually after all growth has ceased. In great apes, synostosis of all sutures occurs immediately after growth has ceased, but in man and most laboratory animals sutures may never completely close and become obliterated. These differences have been attributed to the differences in the degree of development of the masticatory apparatus"[51] (p. 81). Anatomic formations support the likelihood of motion in cranial sutures which are constructed in a way that allows for motion beyond simple bony compliance (Fig. 53.2).

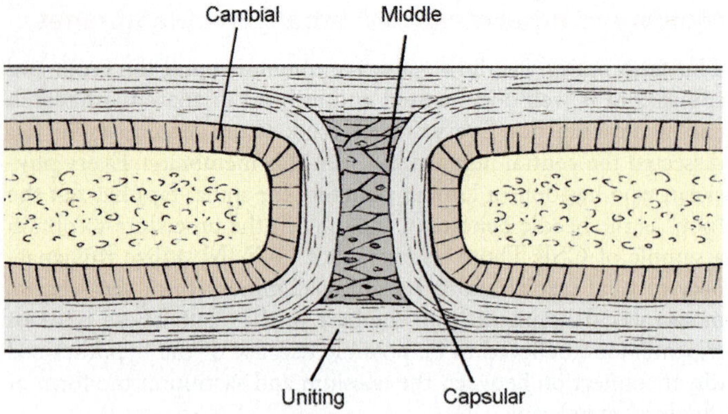

Figure 53.2. Histology of cranial sutures. (From Magoun HI. *Osteopathy in the Cranial Field.* 2nd ed. Journal Publishing Company; 1966, with permission from The Osteopathic Cranial Academy, Indianapolis, IN, https://cranialacademy.org.)

Research by Sabini and Elkowitz[52] provided pictorial and systematic review of 36 human cadaver skulls ranging in age from 56 to 101 years, all well above the age when bone growth is complete. Only 26 of the skulls showed 100% obliteration of the coronal suture, 31 of the skulls had unobliterated lambdoidal sutures, and 24 of the skulls had unobliterated sagittal sutures. The lambdoidal suture was the least fused on a majority of the skulls, and the attachment of musculature on the occipital bone was cited as the probable cause of maintaining sutural patency (nonfusion). Similar to Pritchard et al.,[51] Sabini and Elkowitz speculated that the chewing motion contributes to muscular tension on the bones, maintaining some degree of sutural patency. The endocranial (inner) surface of the skull was not evaluated, so that no estimate of through-and-through fusion of each suture could be made. However, the finding of a significant amount of sutural patency certainly brings into question the idea that all cranial sutures are fused and therefore cannot move.

Research involving assessment of human cranial bone motion has been performed by neurologists, space physiologists, osteopathic medical profession physicians, and basic scientists. In work later cited by NASA scientists, Frymann[53] developed a noninvasive apparatus for mechanically measuring the changes in cranial diameter. Cranial motion was recorded simultaneously with thoracic respiration. On the basis of her extensive recordings on one human subject, Frymann concluded that a rhythmic pattern of cranial bone mobility exists and moves at a rate that is different than that of thoracic respiration.

RUSSIAN AND UNITED STATES SPACE RESEARCH RELATED TO CRANIAL BONE MOTION

One of the most thoroughgoing areas of research, which involved assessment of cranial bone motion, has been that carried out by the Russian Cosmonaut and U.S. Astronaut programs. The concerns that led to this research revolved around the nature of human response to prolonged weightlessness in space. Without gravity, would the human circulation and CNS function normally? While assessing intracranial fluid dynamics, various types of radiographic and ultrasound equipment have been used to measure intracranial volume and cranial bone dimensions. Significant changes in these dimensions have been observed.

Yuri Moskalenko, PhD,[54,55] first published research on cats in space that described "third order waves" similar to that described above in glial cells. After being introduced to OCMM by Viola Frymann, DO, Moskalenko and associates carried out several studies that substantiated cranial bone motion. One utilizing NMR tomograms showed cranial bone motion between 380 μm and 1 mm, and intracranial fluid volume increased by 12 to 15 mL, with a rhythmicity of 6 to 14 cycles/min.[51] This work was followed by a study utilizing bioimpedance measures and transcranial ultrasound Doppler echography to demonstrate slow oscillations of the cranial bones at 0.08 to 0.2 Hz.[56] Moskalenko demonstrated that these oscillations, "...were of intracranial origin and were related to the mechanisms of regulation of the blood supply to and oxygen consumption by cerebral tissue, as well as with the dynamics of CSF circulation.[56] (p. 171)." From this work, Moskalenko and Frymann have formulated a theory that explains the physiology of the PRM.[57]

In the mid-1990s, NASA was also concerned about intracranial fluid volume changes in astronauts in space. NASA carried out research and developed an ultrasound device, pulse phase–locked loop (PPLL), with sensitivity to 0.1 μm, to more precisely assess intracranial anatomy and physiology.[58] This NASA team at the Ames Research Center carried out a series of studies.[59–61]

On two fresh cadavera (<24 hours postmortem), female 83 and male 93, intracranial pressure (ICP) pulsations were generated manually by infusing saline into the intracranial ventricular system at a rate of 1 cycle/s (1 Hz).[59] In this study, an increase in ICP of 15 mL Hg caused a skull expansion of 0.029 mm, and this was interpreted by the authors as similar to that found by Heisey and Adams,[36] and Frymann.[53]

In another study, seven healthy volunteers fitted with the PPLL ultrasound device were placed in 60-degree, 30-degree head-up tilt, supine, and 10-degree head-down tilt positions. The average path length from forehead to occipital bone increased 1.038 ± 0.207 mm at 10-degree head-down tilt relative to 90-degrees upright, "...in other words, when intracranial pressure increases, arterial pulsation produces a higher amplitude ICP pulsation. Increased amplitude of ICP pulsations will be manifested by larger fluctuations in distance across the skull.[61] (p. 3)"

Summarizing their work, the NASA research team stated:

> "Although the skull is often assumed to be a rigid container with a constant volume, many researchers have demonstrated that the skull moves on the order of a few micrometers in association with changes in intracranial pressure[60] (p. 66). In their last publication in this series, they state,...analysis of covariance revealed that there was a significant effect of tilt angle on amplitude of cranial diameter pulsation ($P < 0.001$)....As a result, amplitudes of cranial distance pulsation increased as the angle of tilt decreased. The observed changes in cranial diameter pulsation are considered to be statistically significant[61] (p. 883)."

OSTEOPATHIC RESEARCH ON CRANIAL BONE MOTION

Research comparing palpatory assessment of cranial bone motion with simultaneous assessment by laser Doppler flowmetry technology has been performed. Striking correlations have been found between cranial palpation reports and the technologically measured physiologic motion phenomena identified by the laser Doppler flowmetry. Nelson et al.[62–65] posit that it is the Traube–Hering–Meyer oscillations that they have identified. Based on laser Doppler flowmetry electronically recorded on humans, the authors described oscillations that occur about 4 to 6 cycles/min. In their studies, these oscillations have been shown to correlate with the phases of cranial bone motion as reported by osteopathic cranial practitioners. These investigators proposed that Traube–Hering–Meyer oscillations comprise all or account for most of the cranial bone motion palpated by cranial practitioners. Having instrumented recordings of physiologic activity correlated to the palpatory experience of OCMM practitioners constitutes support for the concepts of the PRM and cranial bone motion.

Another approach to examining cranial bone motion was carried out by Crow et al.[66,67] This group utilized MRI imagery of eight slices each, through the same calvarial plane on the heads of 20 healthy subjects. ImageJ[68] analysis from the National Institutes of Health showed that there were significant differences ($P < .003$) between the means for the largest and smallest cranial bone dimensions for area. The mean difference was 122.69 mm^2 for the area analyzed on the outer table of the cranial bones. The significant differences in this intracranial dimension would be possible only if cranial bones were capable of motion. The authors suggested the intracranial area change may be related to intracranial fluid volume changes.

In the most definitive research to date, Rasmussen and Meulengratch[50] measured temporal bone motion with state-of-the art servo-activator technology which measured motion on the temporal bones bilaterally between 20 and 500 μm while measurements of heart rate and respiratory rate were made simultaneously on 50 healthy subjects. "The mean arterial pulsing on the head was 56.65 cpm (44.00 to 78.28), mean respiratory cpm on the head was 14.34 cpm (9.63 to 20.65), and the mean for the third rhythm was 6.16 cpm (4.25 to 7.07)[50] (p. 26)." As previously stated, it appears that cranial bone motion indeed occurs.

While the evidence for cranial bone motion is definitive, the nature of the motion has more questions to be answered. Commentary that holds to the "cranial bones are fused" perspective is particularly critical of the sphenobasilar junction mobility model.[69] In response, Cook,[70] an OCMM practitioner with a background in engineering and computational fluid mechanics, presents a plausible model based on cranial bone compliance and flexibility that would explain the palpatory experience of OCMM practitioners based on the interaction of all the cranial bones.

Involuntary Mobility of Sacrum between Ilia

Movement of the sacrum in its position between the ilia is an anatomical fact. It would not be possible for humans to walk or run if the iliosacral joints did not allow motion. Though hard to imagine, scientists had believed for centuries that the pelvis was a solid array of bone, with no independent motion of the sacrum.

The biomechanical dimensions of iliosacral joint motion were delineated by Weisl in the mid-1950s.[66,71] Elaboration on iliosacral motion characteristics was accomplished by Kissling,[72] who directed subjects to perform flexion and extension movements of the spine as well as one-legged stance to induce sacroiliac (SI) motion. The range of motion (ROM) observed was 0.2 to 1.6 mm, with an average of 0.7 mm for males and 0.9 mm for females. Other research describes a number of different axes of sacral motion, a concept already well integrated into OMT training programs, with motion noted to be in the range of 1 to 3 mm.[73]

The nature of sacral motion from the perspective of the PRM hinges on the source of the impetus for the sacral motion. There is evidence to support the contention of *involuntary active motion* of the sacrum between the ilia. Mitchell and Pruzzo[74–76] demonstrated a horizontal axis for sacral motion located anterior to the second sacral segment. Movement around this axis was measured at 0.9 to 4.7 mm at the sacral apex, and the impetus for this motion was simply breathing, which associated sacral motion with the normal respiratory excursion.[74] While this research establishes normal respiratory motion as one impetus for sacral motion, other research describes the sacral motion induced by the PRM as separate and distinct from motion caused by respiratory excursion.[53]

OCMM Research Status

Evidence-based research publications appear to support the vast majority of the PRM phenomena and the palpatory experience of osteopathic practitioners who utilize OCMM in medical practice. Advances in imaging technology, cerebral blood flow analysis, and genetic analysis have enabled exploration of the effects of OCMM on humans and animals with state-of-the-art outcome measures that add to the list of clinical benefits attributed to OCMM and suggest mechanisms of action for these procedures. In the review of literature in this chapter, it has not been possible to discuss the design of the studies cited. It is acknowledged that some of researches cited in this chapter are relatively small studies and some are pilot studies. The more recently published research cited and described are more robust in size and quality. The reader who is not familiar with this body of scientific literature is advised to access the original publication(s) for more in-depth information and analysis.

Clinical Research: History

The second edition of Osteopathy in the Cranial Field contains references of research demonstrating the effects of OCMM.[5]

The first reported research was by Dr. Sutherland on himself. "Ingenious mechanisms were contrived to alter his cranial contours in such a way as to approximate the different types he observed among his patients. Through years of tireless experimentation, best described in his biography,[77] he saw and felt significant changes in the mechanics and physiology of his own head....He was able to produce and correct traumatic lesions"[5] (p. 313). Woods and Woods[78] studying psychiatric patients at the Still-Hildreth Osteopathic Hospital in Macon, Missouri reported "In 2,288 examination involving 102 patients the average number of cranial impulses per minute was 6.7, while in a control group of 62 normal subjects, the average was 12.47 per minute"[5] (p. 315). Of historical note, this is the first description of the use of the term "cranial rhythmic impulse (CRI)," a phrase never used by Sutherland himself.

Clinical Research: Conditions and Physiologic Functions Affected by OCMM

OTITIS MEDIA

The location of the eustachian tube within the temporal bone and the possible derangement of the temporal bone during a difficult labor and delivery comprise the anatomy and life circumstances described as the likely basis for the application of OCMM to the treatment of otitis media. The clinical success reported by OCMM clinicians has been validated by positive results in several studies and has become one of the most frequently cited applications of OMT in pediatric cases.[79–83] These studies showed improvement in health as measured by fewer placements of ear tubes, improved tympanography assessment, reduced middle ear effusion, and generally reduced need for antibiotics in children suffering from recurrent ear infections (otitis media).

PREGNANCY, LABOR, AND DELIVERY

The prenatal application of OMT has been a staple of the osteopathic medical profession since its inception.[84] The earliest study cited does not list OCMM as part of the OMT, but to give context, all other citations in this section included OCMM in the treatment protocol. As early as 1911, studies on hundreds of women who received prenatal OMT were published, demonstrating benefits such as shorter durations of labor and fewer reported complications.[85] In one of the largest studies (N = 321 patients), statistical significance was found for fewer preterm deliveries and fewer cases of meconium-stained amniotic fluid in women who received prenatal OMT.[86]

A promising pilot study that awaits a larger follow-up was performed by Gitlin and Wolf on women who were overdue to deliver and had not yet perceived uterine contractions.[87] Eight women were treated using only the OCMM CV4 technique. Two were eliminated due to disruption during post-treatment monitoring, while the other six all began uterine contractions within 34 minutes with an average of 17.5 minutes. The theory underlying the use of the CV4 is that this maneuver "helps nature take its course." Subsequent to publication of this study, there was concern that a CV4 would induce labor before it occurred naturally. However, it was pointed out that all the women in this study were "overdue" and the OCMM only facilitated a normal gestational phase. In fact, utilizing the CV4 in a prenatal OMT protocol, Hensel et al.[88] found reduced pain and improved functional abilities compared to the control group. A follow-up article showed no premature induction of labor because of the use of the CV4.[89]

PEDIATRIC APPLICATIONS

The effects of difficult labor and delivery involve many possible suboptimal outcomes which may be beneficially treated with OCMM. Frymann[90] evaluated the cranial bone mechanics of 1,250 newborns and found that 76% had identifiable malalignment in the form of cranial bone strain patterns. Corroborating the high percentage of cranial dysmorphology was the work of Stellwagen et al.[91] which found that 73% of newborns had cranial asymmetry. The concern raised by these findings is whether or not deviations from the genetically intended configuration of the infant's head will lead to physical and cognitive dysfunctions as the body grows and matures.

Frymann attributed almost all of the problems encountered in pediatric practice to cranial bone distortions,[92](pp. 86–93) with exception of genetic-related problems such as Down syndrome. She published research presenting data indicating benefit of OCMM in the treatment of children with learning problems,[93] neurologic deficits,[94] and seizure disorders.[95]

Inspired by Frymann's work, research was conducted in Russia by Lassovetskaia[96] on children with language and learning problems. In this study, 96 children undergoing neuropsychological tutoring in a large school program due to delayed academic performance were selected and compared to the performance of the rest of the children, before and after receiving OCMM for 6 to 12 weeks. The children who received the OCMM were significantly higher in virtually all categories of academic performance compared to the comparable population of children who did not receive OCMM.

As with all OMT, OCMM is described as an effective means to correct anatomic malalignment and restore optimal physiologic function by improving the anatomic structures associated with those functions. For example, in the treatment of colic, the commonly found impingement of the tenth cranial nerve (which coordinates the peristaltic wave action of the gastrointestinal tract) as it passes through the jugular foramen, caused by compression of the nerve during the birth process, between the occipital and temporal (mastoid area) bones, can be relieved by OCMM to decompress the occipito-mastoid suture and relieve the obstructed flow of vagal nerve supply to abdominal viscera. A pilot study found that the OCMM applied to infants with colic did significantly reduce the symptoms of colic.[97]

In an impressive series of studies, inspired by Dr. Frymann's work, conducted in Italian Neonatal Intensive Care Units (NICU), the effects of OCMM on premature infants were examined. In the first study, the number of gastrointestinal symptoms and the length of stay (LOS) were reduced compared to the control group.[98,99] A follow-up randomized controlled trial showed that the sooner the OCMM was applied, the greater were the reductions in LOS.[100] A multicenter random controlled study showed that premature infants who received the OCMM compared to a control group not only had significantly reduced LOS but also had a significant cost savings of 1,586 € per child.[101] A meta-analysis of this series of studies showed significant benefit for OCMM applied in the NICU.[102] The NICU research has continued and results showed the premature infants receiving OCMM had significantly greater weight gain than controls.[103] Also shown was that OCMM lowered heart rate and increased saturation of peripheral oxygen (SpO_2)[104] all beneficial outcomes for premature infants in a NICU.

Also inspired by Dr. Frymann, another promising area of research on the effects of OCMM for children with nonsynostotic plagiocephaly, also referred to as positional plagiocephaly (PD). Pastor-Pons et al.[105] compared infants who received conventional care with infants who received conventional care plus manipulation which included OCMM and found the group that received the OCMM was significantly improved on the anthropometric measure of cranial vault asymmetry index (CVAI). A case series study by Lessard et al.[106] also showed significant improvement in CVAI in children diagnosed with PD who would otherwise have had helmet therapy. A retrospective chart review study also found significant improvement in cranial bone symmetry using OCMM in infants with PD.[107]

DENTAL APPLICATIONS

Because teeth, considered to be part of the skeletal system in part because they move within their sockets, are housed in cranial bones, application of OCMM for treatment of dental conditions can and has been used successfully in practice. In a series of articles, Magoun[108–110] provided case studies and specific technique for OCMM treatment of individuals whose cranial malalignment involves dentition. Edna Lay carried this work on dental applications forward and described more case studies utilizing OCMM with an emphasis on temporomandibular joint (TMJ) dysfunction.[111] With the publication of these articles, many dentists have been attracted to study and even apply OCMM in their practice. There is even a special membership section within The Cranial Academy for dentists.

Empirical research was performed by Baker,[112] who evidenced measurable changes in the dental arch of a patient receiving OCMM. Serially measured models of maxillary teeth over 6 months showed overall lateral dimensional changes between permanent second molars of 0.0276 of an inch. It is common in the practice of orthodontics today to move the maxillary arch at least this far, and even more, up to 2 mm by dental appliances. However, in the case reported by Baker, the changes were brought about by OCMM alone.

It is worth noting that musculoskeletal deformities, specifically scoliosis and pronounced kyphosis dorsalis (Scheuermann disease), have now been associated with malocclusion.[113] This finding substantiates emphasis on early childhood treatment and prevention championed by practitioners of OCMM.

CONCUSSIONS AND MILD TRAUMATIC BRAIN INJURY

A number of studies have found some degree of benefit for patients with concussions and mild traumatic brain injury (mTBI). In active duty military populations Davis et al.[114] and Wetzler et al.[115] demonstrated that the incorporation of OCMM in their treatment protocol resulted in reduced pain and increased memory function.

Post-concussion syndrome (PCS) is estimated to occur in 10% of high school athletes who sustain a concussion, and estimates for other age groups range from 5% to 30%.[116]

Patel and Sabini[117] collaborated with a neuropsychologist who treated PCS and applied one session of OCMM to 9 of the patients, and 5 of 7 who returned for follow-up reported improvement on the Post-Concussion Symptom Scale scores as well no treatment reactions or adverse events were reported.[117] Yao et al.[118] studied 30 student athletes who were diagnosed with concussion. Sixteen received OMM with an emphasis on OCMM and 14 received concussion education. "The OMM intervention group had a significant decrease in symptom number (P = .002) and symptom severity (P = .001) compared with the concussion education group[118] (p. 607)." On this same group of patients Mazzeo et al.[119] found that the OMM group was significantly able to sleep better as measured by the Sport Concussion Assessment Tool 5th edition (SCAT5). Alexander et al. studied 15 patients recruited from a university concussion clinic and found that 12 sessions of OCMM significantly reduced migraine symptoms as measured by the Migraine Intensity Disability Assessment Scale (MIDAS).[120]

OCMM has been used in the inpatient setting as well. McCallister et al.[121] report two case studies of severe TBI in which OMT/OCMM was utilized early in the acute phase and after medical interventions had been carried out. There was improvement in the reduction of somatic dysfunction in both cases, and no adverse events were reported. Kashyap et al.[122] reported the treatment of 11 severe TBI at a level two trauma center. A standard 51-minute OMT protocol was applied up to three times per patient. All patients meeting the inclusion criteria had an extra ventricular drain (EVD) placed based on clinical presentation and need. EVDs remained open during OMT to allow continued CSF drainage, except for brief periodic closures during treatment to measure accurate ICP values. There was a mean *decrease* in the optical nerve sheath diameter (ONSD) of 0.62 mm from 6.24 mm to 5.62 mm (P = .0001). The mean *increase* in neurologic pupil index (NPi) was 0.18 (P = .01). The mean *decrease* in ICP was 3.33 mm Hg (P = .0001). There was a significant *decrease* in CSF output after treatment (P = .0001). All of these outcomes were beneficial, and no adverse events were reported. It was further noted that OMT is routinely applied to all patients on the neurosurgery service.

CEREBRAL BLOOD FLOW EFFECTS FOLLOWING OCMM

A commonly applied OCMM technique called the "venous sinus technique" has been reported by many who practice OCMM to be successful in the relief of headache and sinus congestion symptoms. A study by Huard[123] suggests that the efficacy of this technique may be in the restoration of optimal intracranial vascular flow. Huard applied the venous sinus technique to 39 subjects, with 39 others receiving light touch only, and another group of 39 subjects receiving no touch at all. The outcome measure was a radiology procedure called the encephalogram, which utilizes ultrasound technology to record blood flow. Huard's results showed that subjects who received the OCMM venous sinus technique had demonstrably improved blood flow in the area of the cranial base.

Advances in technology that can demonstrate the vascular and cerebral flow dynamics changes in response to OCMM have resulted in findings that are both clinically useful and supportive of an understanding of mechanisms of action for OCMM. Roberts et al.[124] utilized Doppler ultrasound to assess blood flow in the middle cerebral artery (MCA), internal carotid artery (ICA), and vertebral artery (VA) before and after the application of occipital–atlantal distraction (OAD) compared to sham touch. End diastolic velocity (EDV) increased after OAD in the MCA, ICA, and VA (all $P < .001$); no change occurred after sham touch (all $P > .05$).

EDV was greater for all post-treatment timepoints after OAD in the MCA, ICA, and VA than sham touch (all $P < .001$). Changes in peak systolic velocity (PSV) in the ICA and VA did not depend on treatment intervention ($P > .06$). Vardy et al.[125] utilized innovative MRI, computerized tomography, and positron emission tomography to measure intracranial vascular and CSF changes in normal subjects and compared with PD patients. "Parkinson patients utilized their right brain hemisphere in contrast to neurologically normal ageing subjects (left hemisphere was dominant) pre- and post all cognitive and orthostatic tests, P = .0039. The left brain hemisphere is normally associated with analytical reasoning, mathematical calculations and logic, and all neurologically normal subjects. In contrast, all PD subjects used their right brain hemispheres for solving the arithmetic cognitive tests.[125] (p. 1)"

One of the new technologies employed in OCMM research is use of arterial spin labeling (ASL). ASL involves the utilization of an endogenous tracer, thus avoiding the risks associated with exogenous radioactive ones. ASL uses magnetically labeled arterial blood water and changes in decay as a measure of cerebral blood perfusion. ASL is specific to intravascular changes and can provide absolute quantification of perfusion values. First used by Tamburella et al.[126] who compared one session of OMT, utilizing OCMM, with one session of placebo intervention on healthy subjects, found that only in the OMT subjects were there any changes in cranial blood perfusion dynamics. Perfusion decreased in cluster comprising the left cingulate cortex and the superior parietal lobule, it increased in the right posterior cingulate cortex.[126]

In patients with chronic low back pain (LBP) randomized to OMT, which included OCMM, or sham groups who each received four intervention sessions, Cerritelli et al.[127] found that the OMT group showed decreased baseline regional cerebral blood flow (rCBF), using ASL, within several regions considered the pain matrix (areas reflecting the experience of pain) compared to sham. These areas were the left posterior insula, left anterior cingulate cortex, and left thalamus. Areas also with decreased rCBF were in sensory regions: left superior parietal lobe, middle frontal lobe, and left cuneus. Conversely, rCBF was increased in the OMT group compared to the sham group in right anterior insula, bilateral striatum, left posterior cingulate cortex, right prefrontal cortex, left cerebellum, and right ventroposterior lateral thalamus, all suggesting an autonomic nervous system (ANS) response to reduced pain. OMT showed a statistically significant negative correlation between baseline High-frequency heart rate variability (HRV) changes and rCBF after the last OMT in left posterior insula and bilateral lentiform nucleus. These findings suggest that OMT can play a significant role in regulating brain–heart interaction mechanisms. The authors concluded, "We interpret the accompanying decrease of CBF in pain-related areas as reflecting the positive influence of osteopathic treatment on heart rate variability and pain perception on LBP patients' physiologic state, hypothesizing a potential OMT effect on central mechanisms of endogenous pain modulation.[127] (p. 10)"

AUTONOMIC NERVOUS SYSTEM EFFECTS

In addition to the Cerritelli et al.[127] study which showed ANS effects, there are a number of studies utilizing OCMM which also demonstrated ANS effects. Cutler et al.[128] showed statistically significant effects of application of the CV4 on sleep latency and reduction of sympathetic nerve activity. In a controlled environment, healthy subjects who received the CV4 treatment went to sleep faster than subjects who received only a light touch control protocol or no touch at all. Sympathetic nerve activity, measured at the peroneal nerve in the popliteal fossa using standard microneurographic technique, was also significantly reduced in the CV4 group compared to control or no-treat groups.

Evidence of the impact of OCMM on ANS physiologic function was demonstrated by the statistically significant improvement in heart rate variability of healthy subjects. In this study, Giles et al.[129] applied soft tissue manipulation to the cervical spine with emphasis on the occipitoatlantal decompression maneuver, a frequently used OCMM technique. In a crossover, subjects as own control, design with N = 24, heart rate variability was best in subjects who received OCMM, when compared to those in the sham- and time-controlled conditions. Using a similar design, Henley et al.[130] also found alterations in heart rate variability as a result of OMT that utilized several OCMM maneuvers. Also using the suboccipital decompression OCMM, Purdy et al.[131] found blood flow to the fingers to be increased.

ANS enhancement of increased HRV was found.[132–136] utilizing OCMM that emphasized or only utilized the compression of the fourth ventricle (CV4) procedure. However, citing the references in this section and articles which used other than OCMM-related procedures it was concluded by Roura et al.,[137] "Research suggests that manual therapy (MT) can produce both a PNS and an SNS short-term effect depending on the ANS measurement method. Skin conductance and heart rate variability are the most frequent autonomic measures to assess ANS. Based on all current evidence; it is difficult to conclude whether the findings on the autonomic effects produce any clinically relevant results in these studies.[137] (p. 28)" Nevertheless, my clinical practice experience and reports of colleagues utilizing OCMM, application OCMM does in fact appear to have clinically beneficial effects mediated by the ANS, and the empirical evidence is mounting as well.

THE SPECIAL CASE OF THE CV4

The best known of the OCMM procedures is the CV4, sometimes referred to by teachers of OCMM as the "osteopathic aspirin" because of the wide variety of clinically reported effects. Besides being the intervention in Cutler et al.[128] study which showed reduction in sleep latency and SNS muscle activity and increase in sleep duration, the use of the CV4 has been the only intervention in other studies. Hanten et al.[138] studied the effect of the CV4 in the treatment of tension-type headaches and reported significant improvement compared to controls. Maina et al.[139] reported data showing increased Alpha Band activity as assessed by qualitative EEG. Shi et al.[140] reported reduced cerebral tissue oxygenation ($S_{CT}O_2$) in the prefrontal lobes, which the authors suggest could be helpful in conditions in which cerebral blood flow is excessive, such as migraine headaches. Gerdner et al.[141] used the CV4 in a population of nursing home patients with dementia and found significant reductions in verbal and aggressive behavior. In a group of six pregnant women more than a week past their due date for delivery, the sole application of the CV4 brought about uterine contractions in less than an hour.[87] This study was cited as a reason to avoid the use of the CV4 in pregnant women until Hensel et al.,[88] reported above, proved otherwise.

The use of the CV4 has not always produced significant results. Both Milnes and Moran[142] and Cardoso-Ribeiro et al.[143] did not find any significant changes in ANS measures after application of the CV4. Nevertheless, the preponderance of the evidence and clinical experience support the expectation of ANS effects from application of the CV4.

EVIDENCE OF BENEFITS IN EQUILIBRIUM, SINUS, INNER EAR, AND IMMUNE SYSTEM FUNCTIONS AND CONDITIONS

Two studies showed benefit to vestibular functions as a result of OCMM treatment. Lopez et al.[144] found significantly improved balance in healthy elders compared to a control group as measured by pressure plate technology. Fraix et al.[145] showed significant reduction in symptoms of dizziness from before to after application of OCMM utilizing the NeuroCom advanced technology equipment. Alexander et al.[146] treated 19 patients with sensory motor tinnitus, 10 responded to treatment, and 9 did not. Eighty percent of the treatment-responsive patients reported lessening of tinnitus with musculoskeletal activity (head turning, cervical flexion, cervical side bending, chewing) whereas none of the unresponsive patients reported this ($P = .0007$). Patients who responded did so after an average of 3.25 treatments and were treated an average total of 5.89 times. Sixty percent of the treatment-responsive group rated their tinnitus volume severity on a scale of 0 to 10 with 10 being the loudest volume. Tinnitus severity ranged from 4 to 10 prior to treatment and 0 to 2 following treatment showing an average reduction of 76.9%. Saggio et al.[147] applied OMT with an emphasis on OCMM on medical students at test times assuming this was a high-stress time and reported significant results for an increase in secretory immunoglobulin A (sIgA) in these high-stress students. Two studies showed benefit in the treatment of sinusitis using OCMM.[148,149]

EVIDENCE OF BENEFITS IN NEURODEGENERATIVE CONDITIONS

A study conducted in Israel evaluated the impact of cranial manipulation on urinary tract function and quality of life in 28 outpatients with multiple sclerosis (MS).[150] Results showed statistically significant reductions in postvoiding residual volume, urinary frequency, urinary urgency, and improvement in quality of life. The authors suggest that the OCMM has impact on parasympathetic centers in the lower brain stem and sacral spinal cord may be the likely mechanism of action.[150] Cordano et al.[1,151] reported on a population of 22 MS patients. Twelve received OCMM compared with 10 MS patients in a control group, and statistically significant improvements in fatigue and depression were found 1 week after the final session ($P = .002$ and $P < .001$, respectively).

In a study of 41 PD patients compared with 43 controls, some received OMT, others received OMT+OCMM. The only significant finding was that with PD patients hip ROM was improved if OCMM was provided in their treatment.[152] King et al. studied 90 PD patients in a 3-armed prospective clinical trial comparing OMT which heavily emphasized OCMM with a sham group and standard care only. The OMT group improved in sleep quality, had reduced perceived stress, and reduced anxiety; none of the gait measures were significant.[153]

With application of the CV4 on transgenic rats bred with Alzheimer disease (AD), Tobey et al.[154] showed that the treated rats were able to complete a maze while untreated rats could not. The biomarker for AD, amyloid-β, was significantly reduced in the treated rats, and there was an increase in the amount of neurotransmitter molecules in the treated rats. Also in this group of OCMM-treated rats, transcriptome analysis revealed that OCMM significantly affected the expression of 36 genes in the neuronal pathway (false discovery rate [FDR] < 0.004.), the top five neuronal genes with largest-fold change were part of the cholinergic neurotransmission mechanism, which is known to affect cognitive function.[155,156]

The presumed mechanism of action for the effects of the CV4 is an increase in the flow of CSF in brain and spinal cord.

If this can be demonstrated empirically, then this simple procedure of the CV4 has much to offer in the neurosciences and helps explain the physiologic function of the glymphatic system which may significantly clear the waste product of cellular metabolism in the brain such as amyloid-β found in Alzheimer, tau protein found in dementia, and the phosphorylated LRRK2 biomarker in PD. Hitscherich et al.[45] extensively reviewed the characteristics of glymphatic system from the perspective of the osteopathic manipulative medicine, and suggest that OCMM could affect the glymphatic–lymphatic system.

Clinical Research—Summary

OCMM clinical research compares favorably with the amount of clinical research conducted on the other commonly used OMT modalities. From a technical perspective, the application of OCMM takes longer than other OMT modalities and is often not applied due to time restraints. Critics of OCMM cite lack of clinical evidence on its benefits thereof and question its risk–benefit ratio. However, there has been only one report of an adverse event from the application of OCMM, and the "stacking" procedure used in that study has been modified and is rarely used today.[157] Nevertheless, improvement reported in the reviewed clinical articles on OCMM is certainly suggestive, if not compelling, evidence of benefit for OCMM.

The succeeding sections will elucidate the classic OCMM concepts taught in osteopathic medical schools and osteopathic training programs worldwide.

INDICATIONS

OCMM is used to treat somatic dysfunction.[158] (p. 102)

Examples of clinical presentations that commonly have relevant somatic dysfunction include but are not limited to:

1. Bell palsy[159]
2. Cranial neuropathy-nerve entrapment*
3. Colic[97]
4. Headache[160]
5. Orofacial pain*
6. Otitis media[79–83]
7. Sinusitis[148,149]
8. TMJ dysfunction and malocclusion[108–110]
9. Vertigo[144,145]
10. Feeding difficulties[161]
11. Plagiocephaly[105–107]
12. Torticollis[106]
13. Trigeminal neuralgia*
14. Tinnitus[146]

*clinical experience

CONTRAINDICATIONS

As with any medical procedure, there are conditions in which the physician must proceed with caution in the application of OCMM procedures. In the case of the application of OCMM procedures, there are a number of relative contraindications based on the training and experience of the physician. The greatest concerns are in conditions of:

a. Acute intracranial bleeding
b. Skull fracture
c. Acute cerebrovascular accident

In these conditions, always in an inpatient setting, the standard of practice in OCMM is to respond to an osteopathic consultation request by the surgeon or treating physician after the patient is initially evaluated, treated, and medically determined to be in a stable condition.

Similar relative considerations are applicable in cases of:

a. Coagulopathies
b. Space-occupying lesions in cranium
c. Increased ICP

This statement was developed by consensus group of the organizations that teach courses on OCMM; The Osteopathic Cranial Academy, The SCTF, Osteopathy's Promise to Children, and the American Academy of Osteopathy.

SAFETY AND EFFICACY

OCMM, when appropriately applied, is very safe and effective for many conditions as noted above.[159, p103] In all of the research reported in this chapter, no adverse effects of OCMM have been reported with the exception of Greenman and McPartland[157] and as noted above the "stacking" procedure used in that study has been modified since publication of that study.

PRINCIPLES OF DIAGNOSIS

The diagnosis of a pathologic condition or malfunction of the PRM is based on history, observation, and palpation. Palpation by a well-trained and sensitive physician is the most reliable source of information.

Palpation of the Primary Respiratory Mechanism

The inherent motion of the cranium is not visible, but it is palpable. This motion is perceived as a subtle, soft, slight movement of fluid (CSF) and semifluid (CNS) inside an osseous case. The first attempt at this palpatory exercise may not reveal anything or the subject's thoracic respiration, transmitted through the neck to the head, may be felt. If the breathing is a distraction, ask the patient to hold the breath for a moment. If the rhythmic motion in the patient's head can still be sensed, then the inherent motion is coming from within the cranium. The ability to distinguish between these different motions is attained with palpatory experience.

Follow these steps to palpate this rhythmic motion:

1. Position the patient supine, with the head 8 to 10 inches from the head of the table.
2. Sit comfortably at the head of the table with the forearms resting on the table and the hands placed on the sides of the patient's head. The patient is asked to move up or down on the table to comfortably accommodate the physician's relaxed posture.
3. Contact the patient's head lightly, allowing the fingers and part of the palms to gently conform to the curvature of the head. (It is essential that the palmar surface of all the fingers, but not the thumbs, contact the head because the nerve endings that sense the subtle cranial motion are proprioceptors located in tendons and around joints. The numerous tactile sensors in the finger pads are not as receptive to this motion. Even though a gentle and light contact is essential, it is not a fingertip contact.)
4. Allow the mind to become quiet and direct attention to the space between the hands, allowing what is sensed by the proprioceptors to be perceived by the brain. Continue to stay

relaxed; do not try to feel something. If the patient's head has fairly normal motion, a slow, rhythmic swelling or widening may be felt, followed by a receding or narrowing. This constitutes one cycle of inherent motion. This cycle is usually steadily repeated. The motion is so mild and subtle that it may actually feel as if the head is breathing.

Subtle motion is easier for some physicians to palpate than for others. Some find this difficult to sense because they try too hard. Their intensity is so set, their effort so strong, that they block their own sensorium. It is essential to be relaxed, physically, mentally, and emotionally. The physician's attitude should be similar to one who is trying to hear a minor sound—complete attention is given to listening.

Keep the hand contact light. Pressure by the hands will suppress the inherent motion and/or distract the sensors (proprioceptors) in the hands. If excessive hand pressure is continued, the patient may get a headache.

If perceiving the motion in one patient proves difficult, try other patients. The cyclic characteristics of the motion and its amplitude (strength or power) usually vary from one individual to another. The biphasic cycle of motion of the PRM most often encountered occurs 10 to 14 times/min, although it can occur at somewhat faster or slower rates. When observing the rate, allow one full minute and count the number of cycles (one flexion phase plus one extension phase equals one complete cycle).

Evaluating the amplitude, or quality rather than rate, of the PRM in patients who have clinical problems requires experience but has been found to be statistically possible.[162,163] This may also reveal the most useful clinical data about the patient. After palpating 5 or 10 individuals, it is possible to determine that the strength or vitality of the rhythm is stronger in one or two individuals, fair or medium in some, and weak or poor in others. Experience with palpation has shown that the rate and amplitude of the PRM, when considered in addition to clinical knowledge of the patient's history and symptoms, becomes an additional diagnostic indication of their state of health and is helpful in determining a prognosis.

There are many scenarios in which the rate and quality of the PRM may be increased slightly:

- Following vigorous physical exercise
- With systemic fevers
- Following effective OMT of the craniosacral mechanism

The rate and quality of the PRM may be decreased in the following situations:

- Stress (mental, emotional, and physical)
- Chronic fatigue
- Chronic infections
- Mental depression and other psychiatric conditions[78]
- Chronic poisoning
- Other debilitating conditions

The cyclic, biphasic motion originating within the PRM is most evident to palpation in the head region but is palpable in every part of the body. The impulse moves longitudinally through the body and extremities, with midline structures moving through flexion/extension and paired structures moving through external/internal rotation. Its presence or absence and its deviation from normal direction are useful diagnostic signs.

The body is subject to stresses and strains from before birth until death. Pressures and forces affect the developing fetus, the neonate during birth, and the individual through childhood, adolescence, and adulthood. These forces cause minor to major distortions of the cranium that result in strains of the SBS. With induced strain, the efficiency of the PRM is compromised, which may have minor to major effects on the individual's health.

Strains

As mentioned previously, Dr. Sutherland spent a great deal of time researching the cranium and its motion on himself and others. His extensive work led to a model of sphenobasilar strain patterns that are often identified in clinical practice.[164] In order to understand a discussion of strain patterns, it is necessary to know some terminology and to recall some basic principles of anatomy. The portion of the occiput that is at the base of the skull and is part of the SBS is called the basiocciput. Likewise, the part of the sphenoid that lies at the base of the skull and is part of the SBS is the basisphenoid. When the motion of these bones is discussed, oftentimes, the motion is named for what is occurring at, the basisphenoid. The major articulation of concern in the following discussion of strain patterns is composed of the anterior portion of one bone (the occiput) and the posterior portion of another bone (the sphenoid). Thus, when motion occurs in the same direction in the two bones, the two bones appear to move in opposite directions at the SBS. Keeping these principles in mind will help in understanding the following discussion of strain patterns.

As mentioned above under "Mechanisms of Physiologic Motion," the midline bones (the sphenoid, occiput, ethmoid, vomer, and sacrum) move through a flexion phase and an extension phase around a transverse axis, while paired bones move through external and internal rotation. The sphenoid moves about a transverse axis that runs through the body of the sphenoid to the region of the sphenosquamous pivot. The occiput moves about a transverse axis that lies just superior to the jugular processes. In normal physiologic cranial flexion, the greater wings of the sphenoid and the lateral angles of the occiput will move slightly inferiorly and the basisphenoid will move slightly superiorly. In normal physiologic cranial extension, the basisphenoid moves slightly inferiorly and the greater wings of the sphenoid and lateral angles of the occiput move slightly superiorly.

If the osteopathic physician is palpating normal physiologic cranial flexion and extension of a supine patient using the vault hold (index fingers on greater wings of the sphenoid, middle fingers anterior to the external auditory meatus, ring fingers on mastoid process of temporal bone and fifth digits on lateral angles of occiput), it may feel as if the physician's index fingers (on the greater wings of the sphenoid) and the fifth digits (on the lateral angles of the occiput) move inferiorly during flexion as the cranium seems to widen, and superiorly during extension as the cranium seems to narrow. Alterations to normal physiologic motion may result in the following strain patterns or conditions.

TORSION

Torsion occurs around an AP axis of the skull that extends from nasion, through the symphysis, to opisthion (Fig. 53.3A).

The sphenoid and related structures of the anterior cranium rotate in one direction about this axis; the occiput and related structures of the posterior cranium rotate in the opposite direction, producing a twist or torsion at the SBS. This strain is named for the side of the more superior wing of the sphenoid, right torsion (RT), or left torsion (LT). Therefore, if the osteopathic physician is palpating a pure RT pattern via the vault hold on a supine patient, they would feel that the right index finger and left fifth finger move superiorly as the left index finger and right fifth finger move inferiorly. The opposite would be true for a LT. Torsions are considered to be physiologic strain patterns as the sphenoid and

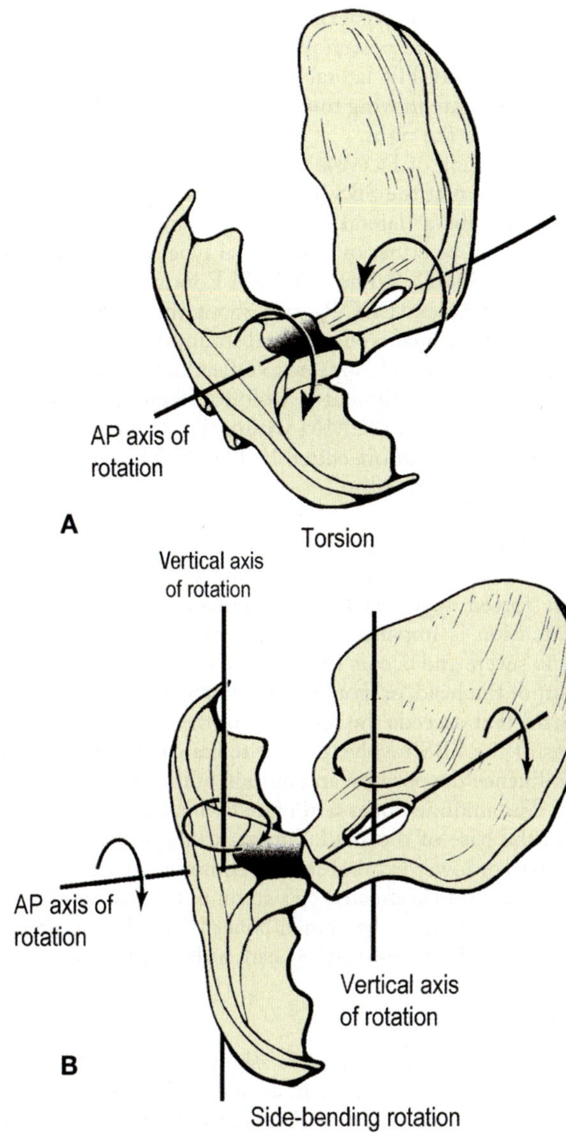

Figure 53.3. Schematic patterns of sphenobasilar junction. In torsion and SBR, sphenoid and occiput rotate in opposite directions about axes indicated. **A.** Torsion with great wing high on the right. Occiput is lower on the side of high great wing. **B.** SBR with convexity to the left. Both great wings of sphenoid and occiput are lower on the side of convexity. (Reprinted with permission from Sutherland WG, Wales AL. *Teachings in the Science of Osteopathy*. Sutherland Cranial Teaching Foundation; 1990.)

occiput are moving in opposite directions relative to each other, as long as their presence does not interfere with the flexion–extension motion of the mechanism.

SIDE BENDING/ROTATION

Side bending/rotation (SBR) at the SBS occurs around an AP axis and around two parallel vertical axes. The AP axis is the same as the axis around which torsions occur. The vertical axes are through the body of the sphenoid and through the foramen magnum, perpendicular to the physiologic transverse axes and the AP axis (Fig. 53.3B).

This is a compound movement similar to physiologic motion in the spine when rotation and side bending are concomitant movements. Because the sphenobasilar symphysis' superior surface is slightly convex as the two bones side bend away from each other (around the two parallel vertical axes), both bones rotate inferiorly on the convex side (around the AP axis) and superiorly on the concave side. This strain pattern is named for the side of the convexity, SBR right (SBR$_R$) or SBR left (SBR$_L$). If the osteopathic physician is palpating a pure right side-bending rotation pattern, they would palpate a fullness of the right side of the cranium as the right index finger and fifth finger move inferiorly and as the left side of the cranium seems to narrow. The opposite would be palpated for a left side-bending rotation pattern. These four strain patterns (RT, LT, SBR$_R$, and SBR$_L$) are common and are considered physiologic if their presence does not interfere with the flexion–extension motion of the mechanism.

EXTREME OR EXAGGERATED FLEXION WITH DECREASED EXTENSION

Extreme or exaggerated flexion with decreased extension of the SBS is considered a strain pattern. Conversely, marked or exaggerated extension with decreased flexion is considered a strain pattern. Normally, the PRM moves through the flexion and extension phases equally and fully.

VERTICAL STRAINS

Vertical strains or displacement occur at the SBS and can be superimposed on the above strains. Vertical strain at the SBS is present when the sphenoid and the occiput rotate in the same direction around their own transverse axes (Fig. 53.4A).

This creates a superior or inferior strain at the SBS and disrupts normal flexion–extension. Vertical strain is named for the position of the basisphenoid relative to the occiput, superior or inferior. A superior SBS vertical strain pattern occurs when the sphenoid is moving into relative flexion and the occiput is moving into relative extension about their transverse axes. An inferior SBS vertical strain pattern occurs when the sphenoid is moving into relative extension and the occiput is moving into relative flexion. Therefore, if a physician is palpating a pure superior vertical strain pattern on a supine patient with the vault hold, both index fingers will move inferiorly as the fifth fingers move superiorly while palpation of a pure inferior vertical strain will cause the index fingers to move superiorly as the fifth fingers move superiorly. Vertical strain patterns are considered to be nonphysiologic as a compensatory pattern does not seem to occur. Instead of moving in opposite directions, the sphenoid and occiput are moving in the same direction.

LATERAL STRAINS

Lateral strains or displacement also occur at the SBS and can likewise be superimposed on the above strains. Lateral strain at SBS occurs when both bones rotate in the same direction, clockwise or counterclockwise, around two parallel vertical axes (Fig. 53.4B).

Basisphenoid and basiocciput veer in opposite directions, producing a shearing type of motion. When this strain occurs in utero or during the birth process, it results in a parallelogram-shaped head in the infant. However, this pattern may be found in patients of all ages depending on various mechanical forces or trauma that have occurred. Lateral strain is named for the direction the basisphenoid shifts, right or left. Similar to vertical strain, lateral SBS strains are considered to be nonphysiologic.

In a right lateral strain, the basisphenoid rotates toward the right. Therefore, the right greater wing will move anteriorly and the right lateral angle of the occiput will move anteriorly as the index and fifth fingers of the left hand move posteriorly. When evaluating a supine patient with the vault hold the osteopathic physician may experience the following: physician's right index finger would move anteriorly and slightly to the LEFT, while the right little finger would move anteriorly and to the right. The left

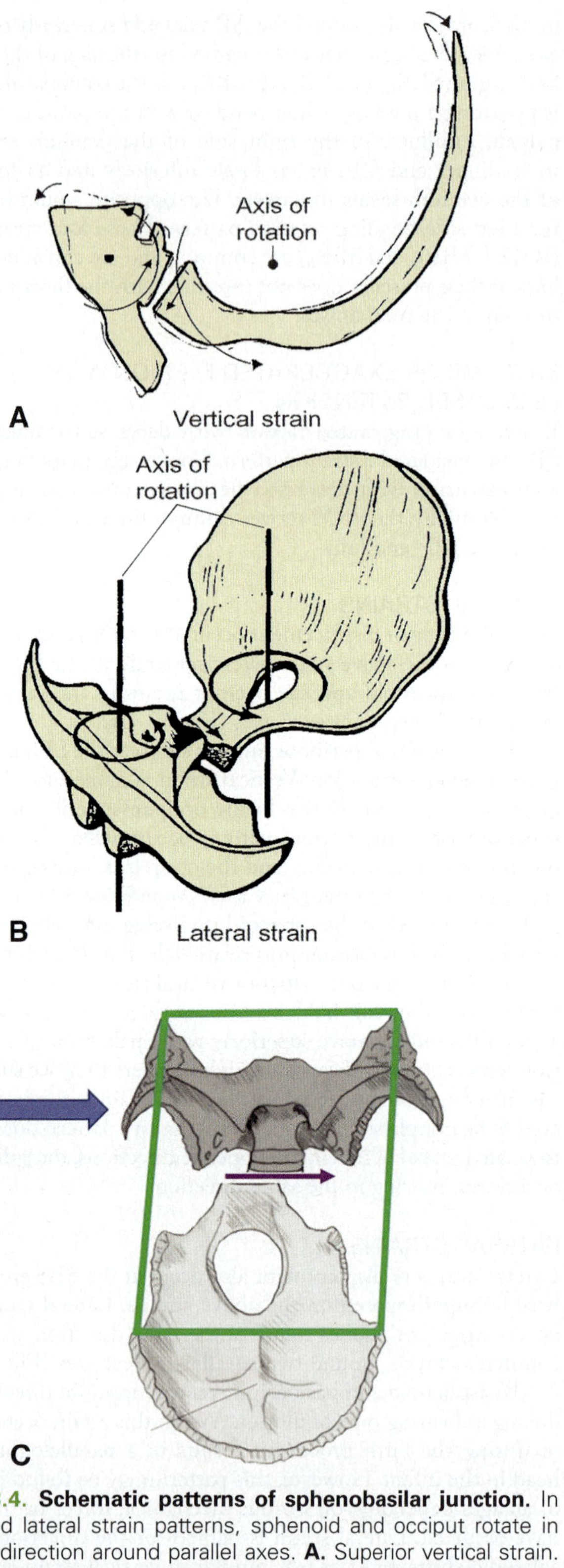

Figure 53.4. Schematic patterns of sphenobasilar junction. In vertical and lateral strain patterns, sphenoid and occiput rotate in the same direction around parallel axes. **A.** Superior vertical strain. As a result of rotation of the bones, the base of the sphenoid is relatively elevated with the base of the occiput relatively depressed. **B.** Right lateral strain. As a result of rotation of the bones, the base of the sphenoid is relatively displaced to the right with the base of the occiput relatively displaced to the left. (Reprinted with permission from Sutherland WG, Wales AL. *Teachings in the Science of Osteopathy*. Sutherland Cranial Teaching Foundation; 1990.) **C.** Lateral shear, displaced from the left. (From ECOP report 2020, with permission.)

index finger would move posteriorly and to the left, while the left little finger would move posteriorly and to the right. The overall result is that, for a RIGHT lateral rotational type strain, the physician's index fingers are moving toward the left, and the little fingers are moving toward the right.

Since publication of FOM4e[165] in 2018, additional features of lateral displacement at the SBS have been discussed by teachers of OCMM to describe a "lateral shear" displacement at the SBS.[164] Lateral strains can be either of a rotational type or a shearing type shown in Figure 53.4C.[166] The AACOM Educational Council on Osteopathic Principles (ECOP) met about this topic and concluded that the rotational type of lateral strain (described above) is most commonly taught as it appears to reflect the original teaching of Sutherland most closely and is well-documented in the most well-known reference on OCMM within the osteopathic profession, OCF, Original Edition, edited by Harold Magoun, DO and approved by Dr. Sutherland.

SBS COMPRESSION

SBS compression is a strain in which the sphenoid and occiput have been forced together to such a degree that physiologic flexion–extension is impaired. Compression varies from mild to moderate to severe and occurs from a force to the back of the head, to the front of the head, or from a circumferential compression (as during birth) that exceeds the resiliency of the tissues.

Strains of the SBS involve the entire cranial and facial structure and influence the position and motion of the sacrum by way of the RTM. The midline bones and paired bones accommodate the strain(s) in the base of the skull. Trauma to the head, face, spine, sacrum, pelvis, or lower extremities is a common strain-producing factor. Pelvic function is affected by a strain in the base of the skull. Likewise, the function of the cranial bones is affected by strain in the pelvis. The body, including the head, truly functions as a unit.

Patient History

Taking the patient's history includes asking leading and pertinent questions to encourage the patient to recall relevant past events and to describe the complaint in some detail. Aside from the usual questions pertaining to heredity, childhood diseases, adult diseases, and surgeries, two other areas for questioning that are pertinent to dysfunction of the craniosacral mechanism are trauma history and information about the delivery and newborn recovery period.

TRAUMA

Obtain the following information about trauma:

1. Age at which the trauma occurred; this includes birth trauma.
2. Type of force, as well as amount, velocity, direction, and the area of impact; vehicular accidents, blows to the face or head, and falls on the tailbone or buttocks are common.
3. Dental history including extractions, orthodontia, malocclusion, bruxism, and TMJ problems.
4. Fractures, concussions, inertial injuries, and coma.
5. Habitual head pressures, such as sleeping positions, thumb sucking, earphones, orthodontic headgear, new dentures, etc.
6. Extremes of temperature: chilling of the face or head may precede Bell palsy; heatstroke or sunstroke may be related to headache.
7. Surgical procedures involving the head such as the mouth gag, the bite block, the bronchoscope or gastroscope, or the anesthetic mask held over the nose–mouth for prolonged periods with a tight headband to keep it in place.
8. Changes in appearance or personality following severe trauma.

Adult patients tend to recall only injuries of the recent past. They may believe that injuries from infancy, childhood, or adolescence are of no importance and thus tend to forget past trauma. The physician may need to ask leading questions to elicit this information. Some patients have amnesia related to trauma to the head and cannot relay accurate information. A family member may be able to give additional history.

HISTORY OF DELIVERY AND NEWBORN PERIOD

If the patient is an infant or child, a more detailed history from the parent(s) is essential. Questions should be asked concerning the:

- Health of the mother during pregnancy
- Number and character of pregnancies
- Details of the delivery
- Appearance and action of the newborn
- Development of the infant

Signs and symptoms compatible with severe forces of labor and delivery are an indication for considering OMT in the care of these patients. The following is a list of signs and symptoms that might indicate that a newborn has experienced severe forces during labor and delivery:

- Distortion of the cranium
- Excessive molding
- Ridging or overriding along any suture
- Difficulty in suckling or swallowing
- Vomiting
- Respiratory distress
- Bradycardia
- Tachycardia
- Abnormal crying
- Strabismus
- Nystagmus
- Spasticity or flaccidity of the limbs
- Opisthotonos
- Drowsiness
- Cyanosis
- Convulsions
- Fever
- Tremors

Abnormal habits indicative of strains of the cranium include:

- Lying with the head turned to one side only
- Head banging
- Constant rubbing of the back of the head against the sheet

Diagnosis by Observation

Look for symmetry or distortion of the osseous structure beneath the soft tissues. Observe the face and head: the shape and contours of the head and face show hereditary influences as well as the combined effect of the forces of labor on the bones. At birth, the sphenoid, temporals, and occiput are composed of several osseous parts with cartilage between them and between the bones to allow for compression and molding of the head during birth. Strains within a bone may occur and are called intraosseous strains.

The flexion type of skull is round in shape, with a wide transverse and a shortened AP diameter, and the temporals in relative external rotation (flared laterally). In this type of skull, the frontals are wide and sloping upward, the cheekbones are wide, and an open mouth view of the maxillary region of the hard palate reveals it to be wide and with a low arch to the vault. All paired structures are in a position of relative external rotation.

The extension type of skull is long and narrow, with temporals in relative internal rotation, frontals narrow with the brow appearing more vertical, orbits and face narrow, and maxillae (hard palate) narrow with a high arched vault. All paired structures are in a position of relative internal rotation.

Note the positioning of the bones. The position of the sphenoid bone influences the position of the peripheral bones of the anterior cranium, which includes the frontals and all bones of the face except the mandible. The position of the occiput influences the position of the bones of the posterior cranium (the parietals and temporals) and in turn, influences the position of the mandible.

With torsion and SBR of the SBS, the facial structures tend to appear asymmetric as they assume a position of relative external rotation on the side of the high wing and a position of relative internal rotation on the side of the low wing. If the sphenoid is rotated on an AP axis, the eyes and orbits will appear unleveled, as will the cheekbones and the maxillae.

Note the relative positioning of landmarks. It is sometimes difficult to determine if the occiput has rotated on the AP axis because it is hidden by hair. As the occiput tilts on this axis, it carries the temporals with it. The temporal on the low side of the occiput is positioned toward relative external rotation, and the temporal on the high side of the occiput is positioned toward relative internal rotation. Therefore, the relative position of the ears gives an indication of the tilt of the occiput. Compare right and left ear lobes to see if they are level, note flaring of the ears. A temporal positioned toward external rotation tends to be more flared; a temporal positioned toward internal rotation tends to be flatter. By combining the findings of the anterior and posterior cranium, the physician is able to arrive at a tentative or working diagnosis of torsion or SBR of the SBS.

Viewing the midline of the face, noting the nose, mouth, and center of the chin, provides additional information. Nasal deviation may indicate the relative position of the maxillae and sphenoid or may indicate past trauma or fracture. The chin (mandible) tends to deviate to the side of the externally rotated temporal bone. Heredity also influences facial characteristics and is a significant consideration for establishing a prognosis.

Strains of the cranial base occur during birth or from trauma. If trauma is induced into a prior strain pattern, the findings of observation are not reliable for diagnosis.

Diagnosis by Palpation

Becoming an expert in the art of palpation for diagnosis and treatment requires repeated experience, patience, and perseverance. These guidelines help improve palpatory skill:

1. Use a light hand contact. Hand contact that is stronger than the force of the inherent motion will interfere with the mechanism to be diagnosed or treated. Do not interject into the patient's PRM.
2. Have a clear visualization of the structure(s) beneath the hands. This requires a detailed study of the anatomy and physiologic motion of each of the bones of the body, including the cranium and face. The design of the articulations between bones, and their mechanical and physiologic relationship is a complex study but is essential in providing accurate diagnosis and successful treatment.
3. Understand that the job of the physician is to assist the patient in obtaining or maintaining optimal health. The physician does not perform the healing; healing comes from within the patient. With knowledge and experience, the physician learns to tune into and be guided by the PRM of the patient to facilitate this

healing process, assisting the patient's own inherent healing capacity to release biomechanical impediments. The automatic processes that promote healing are much more intelligent and efficient in managing the individual's health than any external force or person can be.

PRINCIPLES OF TREATMENT

The aim of treatment with OCMM, as with any osteopathic procedure, is to normalize structure and function. The optimal function of the PRM affects not only the CNS but also every cell and tissue in the body. Regardless of which method or procedure a physician elects to use, this constant cyclic motion is at work behind the scenes, every minute of every hour of every day of every year in an individual's life.

Goals of Treatment

The goals of treatment include:

- Normalizing nerve function, including all cranial and spinal nerves, as well as the ANS
- Counteracting stress-producing factors by normalizing function of the cerebrum, thalamus, hypothalamus, and pituitary body
- Eliminating circulatory stasis by normalizing arterial, venous, and lymphatic channels
- Normalizing CSF fluctuation
- Releasing membranous tension
- Correcting or resolving cranial articular strains
- Modifying gross structural patterns

Some hindrances to treatment are myofascial strains from below the cranium or from the sacrum, local or general infections, nutritional deficiencies, and organic poisons.[5] For optimal management of the patient's health problems, the physician must address nonstructural hindrances to health, in addition to applying OMT.

Balanced Membranous Tension

To use the power or potency of the inherent activity of the PRM within the patient to assist with the release of strains (somatic dysfunctions), it is necessary to understand balanced ligamentous tension and balanced membranous tension.

- Balanced ligamentous tension is used in treating any articulation supported and protected by ligaments.
- Balanced membranous tension refers to the dura mater (RTM) and is used to treat the articulations of the cranium, face, and sacrum.

The point of balanced membranous tension is defined as that point in the ROM of an articulation, where the membranes are poised between the normal tension present throughout the free ROM and the increased tension preceding the strain or fixation that occurs as a joint, which is carried beyond its normal physiologic range.[5] Thus, it is the most neutral position possible under the influence of all the factors responsible for the existing pattern. That is, all attendant tensions have been reduced to the absolute minimum.

This point is unique for each strain that occurs. It is the point at which the inherent force can move through the involved tissues at its maximum efficiency. The physician seeks to position the bones making up the articulation at the point of balanced membranous tension by keen, sensitive, and knowledgeable palpation. Dr. Sutherland expressed this as palpating with seeing, feeling, thinking, and knowing fingers.

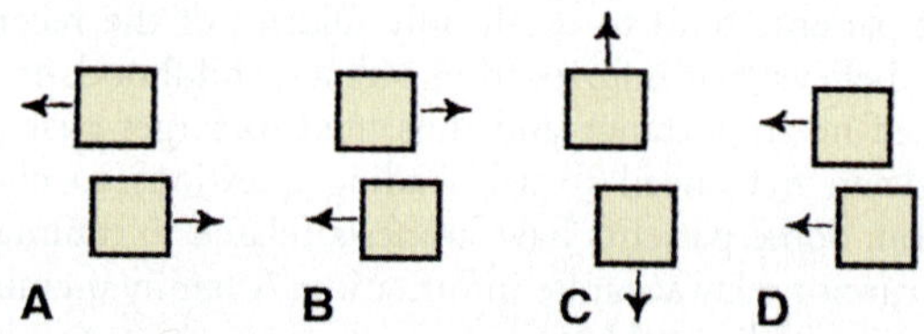

Figure 53.5. Methods for arriving at the point of balanced membranous tension. A. Indirect action (exaggeration). **B.** Direct action. **C.** Disengagement. **D.** Opposite physiologic motion. (From Magoun HI. *Osteopathy in the Cranial Field.* 2nd ed. Journal Publishing Company; 1966, with permission from The Osteopathic Cranial Academy, Indianapolis, IN, https://cranialacademy.org.)

Figure 53.5 illustrates arriving at the point of balanced membranous tension by positioning the components. The squares indicate two bones making up an articulation, and the arrows represent the directions the physician employs for positioning.[5]

Figure 53.5A illustrates indirect action or exaggeration. This procedure is commonly performed on patients from the age of five through adulthood. It is not used in acute trauma to the head, when exaggeration of misalignment may produce or increase intracranial hemorrhage. To employ this method, increase the abnormal relationship at the joint by moving the articulation slightly further in the direction of malalignment.

Figure 53.5B illustrates direct action. This treatment method is employed when exaggeration is not desirable, as in acute trauma and in young children with sutural pattern that has not yet developed. This treatment is also used in the incidence of overriding sutures. The components are gently guided back toward their normal position.

Figure 53.5C illustrates disengagement. This treatment method is used when force or excessive membranous tension impacts the osseous components. Disengagement technique merely separates the opposing surfaces within the anatomic and physiologic limits of permitted motion.

Figure 53.5D illustrates opposite physiologic motion. This method is seldom used but, when needed, is employed to release a strain when a traumatic force has severely violated the physiologic pattern. One component is influenced by direct action; the other is influenced by indirect action. The physician selects the method of choice according to the patient's age and history, in addition to the palpatory diagnosis.

Respiratory cooperation may be used to enhance the effort of inherent motion. The patient is asked to hold their breath in full inhalation or exhalation after the physician has positioned the articulation at balanced ligamentous or membranous tension. Holding the breath at full inhalation is more commonly used, but if the articulation is held toward extension or internal rotation, holding the breath at full exhalation is more effective.

Illustrative Treatment Techniques

EXAMPLE 1

An example would be a case in which the patient reports a history of a fall on their rear end, possibly from a slip on icy pavement.

Diagnosis

Somatic dysfunction of the lumbosacral junction (L5–S1 compression).

Treatment

Treatment is indirect method, using balanced ligamentous tension, exaggeration, and inherent force.

Procedure

1. Position the patient supine.
2. Sit at the side of the table, so that the dominant hand (assume right hand) can be placed under the patient's sacrum.
3. Place the right hand under the sacrum, so that the patient's coccyx rests between the thenar and hypothenar eminences. The fingertips should be placed at the sacral base with the 3rd and 4th digits just below L5 on the patient.
4. Place the left hand perpendicular to the right hand, with the hypothenar eminence barely touching the fingers of the right hand and in firm comfortable palpatory contact with L5.
5. Maintain this position and allow the inherent force to work. Keep the sensing apparatus alert so that it perceives the slow cyclic movement of the PRM. This movement feels like a longitudinal ebb and flow or a subtle pumping effect up and down the spine.
6. Continue to maintain the positioning and observe this cyclic motion; the inherent force is working through the tissues that are maintaining the somatic dysfunction. As they accomplish their task for this articulation at this time, the amplitude of the inherent rhythm lessens and the pumping decreases, and the tissues beneath the palpating fingers seem to soften or melt. Once the tissues have softened, the flexion and extension motion of the sacrum begins to increase. As flexion and extension motion of the sacrum increases toward normal, it may be necessary to gently pull inferiorly on the sacrum before full motion is restored.
7. At this time, cease to hold the articulation in the treatment position. Gently recheck the motion of the articulation to ascertain the therapeutic response. Physiologic motion is restored to varying degrees.

A strain of the sacral base can be treated using the inherent forces and positioning for balanced membranous tension of the RTMs. This technique is applicable for an uncomplicated strain of the sacral base. If a strain of the sacral base is complicated by additional traumatic strains such as a compression in either SI joint, the technique as described will probably not be successful.

If SI joint compression is present, treatment position will vary slightly. If, for example, the patient's left SI joint is compressed, the physician's left hand will be under the sacrum. This hand maintains the same position as for treatment of sacral base compression. However, the physician's other hand (in this case the right hand) would be placed under the ilium, perpendicular to the fingers of the left hand. The fingertips of the right hand would be at the medial border of the left ilium and would barely touch the fifth digit and hypothenar eminence of the left hand. As in step 6, maintain this position while observing the cyclic motion of the PRM. In this case, rather than providing inferior traction, it may be necessary to provide gentle lateral traction until normal balance between the motion of the sacrum and the motion of the ilium is restored.

EXAMPLE 2

Another case is a patient who has been struck on the side of the head, possibly by a baseball bat or fist.

Diagnosis

Somatic dysfunction of the sphenobasilar symphysis is SBR right (SBS is SBR_R).

The sphenoid and occiput have rotated on an AP axis so that the right side of the cranium is relatively inferior and the left side is relatively superior. Concomitant with that position, the greater sphenoid wing and the lateral angle of the occiput on the right side are slightly spread, and the greater sphenoid wing and the lateral angle of the left occiput are slightly approximated.

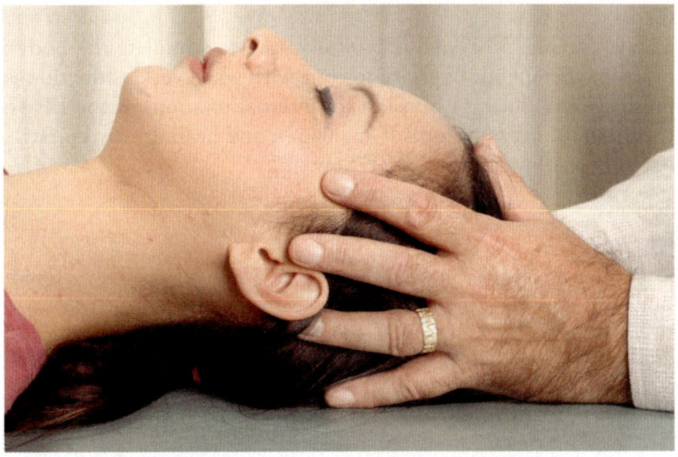

Figure 53.6. Vault hold for contact with the cranium. (Reprinted with permission from Hruby RJ. *Exploring Osteopathy in the Cranial Field.* Author; 2013:36.)

Treatment

Treatment is indirect method, balanced membranous tension, with exaggeration and inherent forces to balance the RTM.

Procedure

1. Position the patient supine.
2. Sit at the head of the table.
3. Place the hands on the lateral sides of the patient's head, with the index fingers contacting the greater wings of the sphenoid, third finger and fourth finger on temporal bone, third finger just anterior to the ear and fourth finger resting on mastoid process and the little fingers contacting the lateral angles of the occiput (vault contact) (Fig. 53.6).
4. Gently palpate the rhythmic activity of the patient's PRM and RTM.
5. Slowly move the right hand slightly inferiorly, with index and fifth fingers spreading slightly, while moving the left hand slightly superior as the fingers approximate slightly. This positioning is slight and must be accurate, being guided by the ease of tension in the membranes within the cranium. With the ease of membranous tension, the inherent forces begin to manifest with increased vigor. The amplitude of the PRM automatically increases.
6. Maintain the positioning and carefully and continuously observe the increased activity of the inherent forces at work within the patient's mechanism. As the inherent forces work through the membranous strain, they gradually cease the increased activity and become quiet. This cessation of the inherent rhythm is called a still point.[13]
7. After the still point occurs, cease to maintain the positioning of the bones and membranes and continue to observe the fluctuant activity by light palpation. The quiet period passes, the rhythmic fluctuation resumes, increasing slowly and steadily in amplitude until it has returned to a more normal flexion–extension of the SBS.
8. Gently remove the hands.

Common OCMM Treatments

There is no substitute for thorough training and practice with regard to OCMM. Well-known and typically utilized treatments based on the principles of OCMM are the compression of the fourth ventricle (CV4) and the V-spread procedures.

CV4

The CV4 (Fig. 53.7A,B) is typically used to stimulate the body's inherent therapeutic capacity to cope with whatever dysfunction is present. By inducing extension (or internal rotation) of the PRM, the inherent capacity for self-regulation and healing may be facilitated by a stimulation of CSF flow.

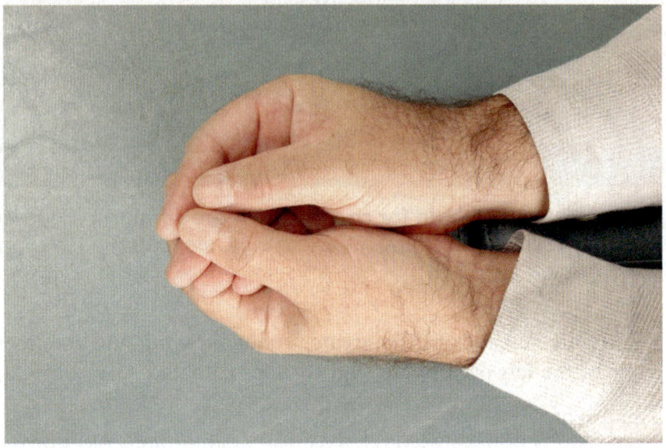

A

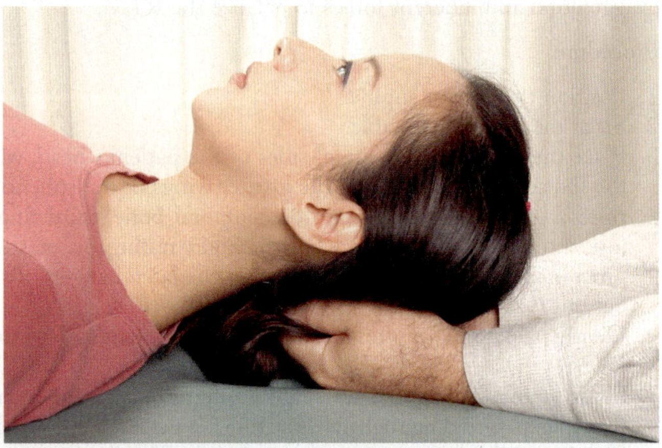

B

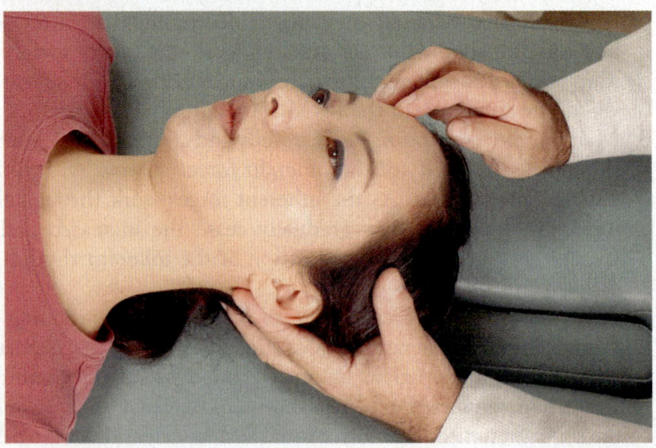

C

Figure 53.7. A. Hand position for compression of the fourth ventricle (CV4) technique. (Reprinted with permission from Hruby RJ. *Exploring Osteopathy in the Cranial Field.* Author; 2013:123.) **B.** Compression of the fourth ventricle (CV4) technique. (Reprinted with permission from Hruby RJ. *Exploring Osteopathy in the Cranial Field.* Author; 2013:123.) **C.** V-spread of the occipitomastoid. (Reprinted with permission from Hruby RJ. *Exploring Osteopathy in the Cranial Field.* Author; 2013:125.)

The technique is as follows:

1. Physician sits at the head of the table.
2. Patient lays supine.
3. With both hands palm up, place one hand in the palm of the other so that the thenar eminences lie parallel to one another. Then slip the hands under the patient's head, permitting the lateral angles of the occiput, medial to the occipitomastoid suture, to rest on the thenar eminences. The thenar eminences provide a cushion for the occiput that should be comfortable for both the patient and physician. The fingers are free and not pressing on the patient's neck. The weight of the head rests on the thenar eminences and thereby gently compresses the lateral angles.
4. Become aware of the cyclic motion of the occiput. Follow it toward extension (i.e., as the hands rock gently toward the physician). Discourage flexion (hands moving away). The amplitude of the motion will become progressively smaller until the still point is reached. The still point may be difficult to detect because it passes so swiftly. However, it is followed by a sense of softening and warmth in the occiput, along with the gentle rocking motion of flexion and extension that should be more easily detectable. At the same time, thoracic respiration should become primarily diaphragmatic and approximate the same cycle as the PRM.
5. Observe the cranial activity to be sure that it remains quiet and then very gently remove the hands and put the patient's head on the table. Figure 53.7 demonstrates the CV4 via the occiput, but it is also possible to accomplish a CV4 via the temporals, parietals, and sacrum.

V-SPREAD

The V-spread (Fig. 53.6C) is a very simple, safe technique for releasing any peripheral sutures such as frontonasal, nasomaxillary, or occipitomastoid. The technique is as follows:

1. Place the index and middle fingers of the ipsilateral hand on either side of the suture. For a linear suture like the occipitomastoid, use the palmar surface of the length of two fingers. For a small suture like the frontonasal, use the fingertips.
2. Place the palm of the other hand on the patient's head at the other end of the longest diameter of the head from the suture (e.g., for the left occipitomastoid), place the hand on the right frontal only. Soon, a gentle impulse will be perceived, coming into the palm of this hand. Now, cluster the fingers at the site of that impulse, thereby localizing the optimum place from which to direct a palpatory sensation of a "fluid wave" to the restricted suture. As long as the suture is restricted, the fluid sensation will "bounce" back, but as soon as it is released, a gentle, easy motion will be felt between the hands.

SBS DECOMPRESSION

SBS decompression is applied to correct a diagnosed SBS compression. The diagnosis is made when the following findings are noted:

- Very small or no amplitude or nonpalpable primary respiratory motion
- Or alternating vertical or lateral strain patterns

Usually, this technique is performed after the peripheral sutures and other somatic dysfunctions are resolved by OMT. The technique is performed as follows:

1. Stand to the side of the supine patient. Grasp the patient's greater wings of the sphenoid at the pterion bilaterally with the

thumb and middle finger pads of one hand, slightly flexing the distal interphalangeal (DIP) joints.
2. The other hand's index, third or fourth finger pads contact the posterior aspect of the patient's upper last molar teeth bilaterally with the DIP joints slightly flexed.
3. With equal force of all four fingers in contact with the patient, lift the sphenoid and maxillae anteriorly (toward the ceiling) until balanced membranous tension is reached with the occiput.
4. Hold until there is a sense of decreased resistance and increased compliance.
5. Recheck the PRM with the vault hold to ensure the compression has resolved and normal SBS motion (flexion/extension) has resumed with an improved or normal motion amplitude and rhythm.
6. Greater effect can be achieved by having a second physician or assistant sitting at the head of the table and, using the occipital–temporal hold, stabilize the occiput and temporal bones while the sphenoid is being lifted away from the occiput by the standing physician. The person stabilizing the occiput can provide feedback to the physician lifting the sphenoid as to whether each of the four fingers is producing equal and balanced forces in the anterior direction; the standing physician can then adjust the forces of each finger to improve a balanced and single vector of force that effectively distracts/decompresses the SBS using balanced membranous tension.

VENOUS SINUS DRAINAGE (VSD) TECHNIQUE

The VSD technique is a relatively safe technique designed to improve overall motion of the cranium and facilitate drainage of the sinuses. Performance of the technique requires appropriate pressure to be transmitted through the bone to the dura which house the sinuses. As glymphatic channels line these venous sinuses, this technique may have the ability to optimize all of these structures. This technique generally consists of seven steps and should be performed after patency of the jugular foramina has been ensured. While the steps may differ in order, the end goal is the same. The order of the steps listed below reflects what Viola Frymann, DO, FAAO, student of W.G. Sutherland, DO, taught.

The technique is performed as follows with the physician sitting at the head of the table with the patient supine.

1. Confluence of sinuses: The physician places the two middle fingers tip to tip with the pads of the fingers supporting the head at the external occipital protuberance, providing the only support for the patient's head. This contact is maintained until the physician senses a "softening" of the bone of this region and the beginning of inherent motion.
2. Occipital sinus: Maintaining a similar relative position, the fingers are moved about a finger's width inferiorly on either side of the midline of the occiput addressing the falx cerebelli and the occipital sinus within. Again, the physician awaits softening of the tissues and the sensation of inherent motion.
3. Condylar decompression: Next, move down the convexity of the occiput toward the foramen magnum. The physician's fingers will now be inclined toward each other at about 45 degrees to the vertical. With a very gentle impulse posteriorly as the pressure is maintained, (think of approximating the wrists), the occiput is decompressed from the atlas, and the condylar parts of the occiput are also released. Wait until softening of the tissues and inherent motion are palpated.
4. Transverse sinus: Approximate the pads of the fifth finger at the external occipital protuberance. The head is then supported by the fingerpads as they line up along the superior nuchal line extending to the inferior lateral angle of the parietals, thus addressing the transverse sinus housed within the tentorium cerebelli.
5. Straight sinus: The patient's head rests on the fingers and the thumbs are placed one on top of another over the sagittal suture close to the vertex. Imagine a line from the thumbs into the center of the head and visualize its intersection with the anterior end of the straight sinus. Maintain these contacts until softening and motion are noted.
6. Superior sagittal sinus: Flex the patient's head and cross the thumbs so that the thumb pads are on either side of the sagittal sinus just superior to the external occipital protuberance. The physician's elbows may be on the table as the patient's head is completely supported by the crossed thumbs. Note that inherent motion is palpable. With the thumbs crossed, apply a gentle distracting force, the right thumb directed toward the left, the left thumb directed toward the right. When softening and motion are palpated, move the thumbs about an inch superiorly and repeat the procedure. Continue step by step along the sagittal suture toward the bregma (the intersection of the sagittal and coronal sutures).
7. Metopic suture: To address the anterior portion of the superior sagittal sinus, place the finger pads on either side of the metopic suture (the midline) of the frontal bone; that is the index finger just anterior to the bregma, the fifth finger above the nasion, and the other fingers between the two. The right fingers are on the right side of the suture, the left fingers are on the left side of the suture. Gentle pressure with slight separation is maintained until softening and physiologic motion is palpated.[167]

FRONTAL LIFT

The frontal lift may be used to aid in the balance of membranous tension. The frontal lift appears to place longitudinal traction on the falx cerebri as it lifts the frontal bone from the sphenoid. While the technique is performed, the physician may feel the sensation that the frontal bone is wobbling from side-to-side while being distracted before it releases and is able to resume its normal relationship. The effective performance of this technique relies on an understanding of the anatomic relationship of the frontal bone to the parietal bone, the greater wing of the sphenoid bone and the temporal bone at the pterion. The frontal bone is the deepest and most medial of all the bones. The principle of the technique is (1) to internally rotate the frontals to disengage them from their related bones (this also narrows the ethmoid notch [OCF, original edition, p. 140]), (2) to lift them anteriorly, and (3) permit them to externally rotate.

The technique may be performed as follows with the physician sitting at the head of the table and the patient is supine.

1. Physician rests elbows on the table. Place the hypothenar eminences on the lateral angles of the patient's frontal bone and interlace the fingers over, but not in contact with, the forehead.
2. Attempt to draw the fingers of one hand from the fingers of the other, yet at the same time gripping the fingers of the one hand with the other utilizing the action of the lumbrical muscles. In this way, the hypothenar eminences exert an influence of internal rotation on the lateral angles of the frontal.
3. Coordinate this action with a lifting of the frontal anteriorly (toward the ceiling) until a balance point is achieved. Wait until the lateral angles move into external rotation.
4. Gently release the hands from the patient's forehead.[167]

PARIETAL LIFT

The parietal lift may be used to aid in the balance of membranous tension. The parietal lift appears to place transverse stress on the tentorium cerebelli. The parietal bone's anterior border is at the coronal suture, which is approximately at the junction of the anterior and middle thirds of the vault. The physician should be aware of the relationship between the parietal and squamous temporal bevels. In internal rotation, the squamous margin of the parietal bone further underrides the squamous portion of the temporal bone, and in external rotation they move laterally.

The technique may be performed as follows with the physician sitting at the head of the table and the patient is supine.

1. The physician rests forearms on the table, and places the fingertips on the inferior border of each of the two parietals just superior to the squamous temporal suture.
2. Cross the thumbs above, but not in contact with the sagittal suture.
3. Firmly press one thumb against another; that is, one thumb presses upward as the other resists this motion by pressing downward. Thus the fingers will approximate and induce internal rotation of the inferior border of the parietal bones.
4. At the same time, lift both hands in a superior direction (toward the physician) until a balance point is achieved. Wait until the parietal bones move into external rotation.
5. Gently release the contact on the parietal bones.[167]

TEMPOROMANDIBULAR JOINT

Disorders of the TMJ may be multifactorial and include but are not limited to acute or repetitive trauma, muscular and/or ligamentous imbalance, and cranial somatic dysfunction. Assessment and treatment may occur with the physician maintaining one position but making shifts in contact in order to address different ligaments and then actual joint itself.

Sphenomandibular Ligament Release

The technique is as follows with the patient: supine and the physician standing at the side of the table opposite to the side being treated. The physician may place their knee on the table to support the patient's head and ensure they are not using excessive pressure during the technique.

1. Position one hand over the forehead so that the greater wings of the sphenoid are being monitored by the thumb on one side and index or middle finger on the other side.
2. Place a gloved thumb on the occlusal surface of the last lower molar on the side of the mouth being treated.
3. Exert slight pressure on the mandible with the gloved thumb so as to move the mandible inferiorly. If there is restriction, or decreased resiliency, the monitoring hand will feel the greater wing of the sphenoid move into a superior direction (i.e., toward extension).
4. If this is the case, use what was the monitoring hand to direct the sphenoid toward flexion while maintaining the inferior pressure on the mandible until the tissue tension is released and physiologic motion is restored.

Stylomandibular Ligament Release

The technique is as follows with the same initial setup as for the sphenomandibular ligament release.

1. Palpate over the temporal bone with one hand by placing the middle finger in the external auditory meatus, the fifth and ring fingers on the mastoid process, and the index finger and thumb grasping the zygomatic arch.
2. Place a gloved thumb on the occlusal surface of the last lower molar on the side of the mouth being treated and wrap the rest of the fingers around the ramus of the mandible.
3. Apply gentle traction on the mandible with the gloved thumb in an inferior, lateral, and anterior direction until the tissues become more compliant and physiologic motion is restored.

TMJ Decompression

The technique is as follows with the same initial setup as for the stylomandibular ligament release.

1. Palpate over the temporal bone with one hand by placing the middle finger in the external auditory meatus, the little and ring fingers on the mastoid process, and the index finger and thumb grasping the zygomatic arch.
2. Place a gloved thumb on the occlusal surface of the last lower molar on the side of the mouth being treated and wrap the rest of the fingers around the ramus of the mandible.
3. Attempt to decompress the TMJ by placing slight anterior–inferior pressure on the mandible.
4. If it will not move easily, apply gentle compression of the head of the mandible into the glenoid fossa until spontaneous decompression occurs.[167]

Treatment procedures of the cranium should be used only by physicians experienced with palpation of the PRM's subtle activity. Guidance by a physician experienced with the function of the PRM and the inherent forces is essential for learning these techniques.

CASE

R.R. is a 26-year-old woman who presented with right-sided facial weakness of 1-week duration, accompanied by a dulled sense of taste and some trouble hearing. She reported that the day before the onset of symptoms, she had been awake all night studying. Her medical history was notable for an incidence of facial weakness that lasted for 1 month when she was 7 years old.

PHYSICAL EXAMINATION

- The physical exam revealed weakness of her right eyelid with delayed blinking, along with right-sided facial droop, and lips that remained flat on the right side when she attempted to smile. The patient's appearance was most notable for facial asymmetry with decreased tone on the right side.
- The structural exam also revealed a side-bending/rotation dysfunction on the right side of the cranium. Cervical vertebrae C2 and C5 were side-bent and rotated right.

DIAGNOSIS

Bell palsy.

TREATMENT

The OMT applied integrated muscle energy, myofascial release, soft tissue, and cranial manipulation.

- The patient's right anterior innominate was treated with muscle energy until symmetry of innominates was achieved.

- Thoracic outlet and respiratory diaphragms were treated with myofascial release, followed by thoracic lymphatic pump.
- Cervical rotation dysfunctions were treated with muscle energy.
- The suboccipital area was treated with soft tissue, occipitoatlantal, and condylar decompression techniques that lead to application of the Galbreath treatment (151) for mandibular drainage, which supports lymphatic drainage and temporal bone-related structure alignment.
- Finally, OCMM was used to balance the cranial intradural tension membranes and to promote symmetry in temporal bone and sacral motion. The cerebellar tentorium served as the focus of this treatment because of its attachments—specifically, its lateral attachments to the temporal bones along the petrous ridge enclosing the superior petrosal sinuses, its posterior attachments to the occipital bone forming the transverse sinuses, and its apical attachment to the cerebral falx forming the straight sinus.

DISCUSSION

The day after the treatment, the patient reported that most of her muscle tone had returned and that her sense of taste had returned to normal. She received a second treatment, and another 1 week after the second treatment, after which she was asymptomatic.

Central to the success of this case is the knowledge of the facial nerve's anatomy as it traverses the temporal bone. The facial nerve exits the cranium through the stylomastoid foramen to give rise to six terminal branches, leading to the muscles of facial expression. This anatomic knowledge allowed for the deduction that the patient's dysfunction was most likely at the chorda tympani. This deduction was also supported by the patient's altered sense of taste and auditory disturbances. For further information on this interesting case, refer to the article upon which it is based.[150]

REFERENCES

1. Educational Council on Osteopathic Principles (ECOP). Glossary of osteopathic terminology. In: Seffinger MA, ed. *Foundations of Osteopathic Medicine*. 4th ed. Wolters Kluwer; 2018:1563–1594.
2. Sutherland AS. *With Thinking Fingers: The Story of William Garner Sutherland*. Cranial Academy. Originally published by Journal Printing Company; 1962:12–13.
3. Northup GW, ed. *Osteopathic Research: Growth and Development*. The Journal of the American Osteopathic Association; 1987:40.
4. DiGiovanna EL. *An Encyclopedia of Osteopathy*. American Academy of Osteopathy; 2001:100.
5. Magoun HI. *Osteopathy in the Cranial Field*. 2nd ed. Journal Printing Company; 1966:23.
6. Lippincott RC. Cranial osteopathy. *Yearb Acad Appl Osteopathy*. 1947:103–108.
7. Lippincott HA. The osteopathic technique of Wm. G. Sutherland, D.O. *Am Acad of Osteopathy*. 1949:1–41.
8. Becker RE, (In: Brooks RE, ed.) *Life in Motion*. Stillness Press; 1997.
9. Becker RE, (In: Brooks R, ed.) *The Stillness of Life*. Stillness Press; 2023.
10. Fulford RC. *Touch of Life*. Gallery Books; 1997.
11. Fulford RC. In: Cisler TA, ed. *Are We On the Path? The Collected Works of Robert C. Fulford, DO, FCA*. The Cranial Academy; 2003.
12. Comeaux Z. *Robert Fulford, DO and the Philosopher Physician*. Eastland Press; 2002.
13. Sutherland WG. In: Wales AE, ed. *Teachings in the Science of Osteopathy*. Rudra Press; 1990.
14. Arbuckle BE. *The Selected Writings of Beryl E. Arbuckle, D.O., FACOP*. American Academy of Osteopathy; 1994.
15. Osteopathic Center for Children. Accessed August 21, 2022. http://www.osteopathiccenter.org/
16. King HH, ed. *The Collected Papers of Viola M Frymann, DO: Legacy of Osteopathy to Children*. American Academy of Osteopathy; 1998.
17. King HH, ed. *Proceedings of International Research Conference: Osteopathy in Pediatrics at the Osteopathic Center for Children in San Diego, CA 2002*. American Academy of Osteopathy; 2005.
18. King HH, ed. *The Collected Papers of Viola M. Frymann, DO: Volume 2: Legacy to Osteopathy*. Osteopathy's Promise to Children; 2021.
19. Lay EM. Osteopathy in the cranial field. In: Ward RC, ed. *Foundations for Osteopathic Medicine*. Lippincott Williams & Wilkins; 1997.
20. DiGiovanna EL, Schiowitz S, Dowling DJ. *An Osteopathic Approach to Diagnosis and Treatment*. 3rd ed. Lippincott Williams & Wilkins; 2005.
21. DeStefano LA. *Greenman's Principles of Manual Medicine*. 4th ed. Wolter Kluwer/Lippincott Williams & Wilkins; 2011.
22. Kuchera ML, Kuchera WA. *Osteopathic Considerations in Systemic Dysfunction*. 2nd Rev ed. Greyden Press; 1994.
23. Heisey SR, Adams T. Role of cranial bone mobility on cranial compliance. In: Thirty-sixth Annual AOA Research Conference Abstracts, 1992, part 2; 1992. Also in: *J Am Osteopath Assoc.* 1992;92(9):1284.
24. Heisey SR, Adams T, Smith MC, Briner B. The role of cranial suture compliance in defining intracranial pressure. In: Thirty-seventh Annual AOA Research Conference Abstracts, 1993, part 2; 1993. Also in: *J Am Osteopath Assoc.* 1993;93(9):951.
25. Norton JM, Sibley G, Broder-Oldack RE. Quantification of the cranial rhythmic impulse in human subjects. In: Thirty-sixth Annual AOA Research Conference Abstracts, 1992, part 2; 1992. Also in: *J Am Osteopath Assoc.* 1992;92(9):1285.
26. Sibley G, Broder-Oldach RE, Norton JM. Inter-examiner agreement in the characterization of the cranial rhythmic impulse. In: Thirty-sixth Annual AOA Research Conference Abstracts, 1992, part 2; 1992. Also in: *J Am Osteopath Assoc.* 1992;92(9):1285.
27. AACOM's Educational Council on Osteopathic Principles. *Glossary of Osteopathic Terminology (Third Edition)*. AACOM. 2023. https://aacom.org/gme/digital-resource-library/digital-resource/glossary-of-osteopathic-terminology-(third-edition)#:~:text=The%20Glossary%20of%20Osteopathic%20Terminology,of%20Osteopathic%20Medicine%20(AACOM)
28. Jealous J. *An osteopathic odyssey*. Tame Prepress; 2015.
29. Blechschmidt E. *Beginnings of Human Life*. Springer-Verlag; 1977.
30. Blechschmidt E, Gasser RF. *Biokinetics and Biodynamics of Human Differentiation*. Charles Thomas Publishing; 1978.
31. Dorland WAN. *Dorland's Illustrated Medical Dictionary*. 26th ed. WB Saunders; 1988.
32. Karki J. *Signal Conditioning Piezoelectric Sensors*. Texas Instruments Application Report SLOA033A; 2000.
33. Becker RE. Craniosacral trauma in the adult. *Osteopath Ann.* 1976;4:43–59.
34. Williams PL, Warwick R, Dyson M, Bannister LH. *Gray's Anatomy*. 37th ed. Churchill-Livingston; 1989.
35. Bates B, Hoekelman RA. *A Guide to Physical Examination*. 3rd ed. JB Lippincott Co.; 1983:149.
36. Heisey SR, Adams T. Role of cranial bone mobility in cranial compliance. *Neurosurgery*. 1993;33(5):869–876.
37. Moskalenko IE, Kravchenko TI, Gaidar BV, et al. [Periodic mobility of cranial bones in man]. *Hum Physiol.* 1999;25(1):51–58.
38. Grietz D, Wirestam R, Franck A, Nordell B, Thomsen C, Ståhlberg F. Pulsatile brain movement and associated hydrodynamics studied by magnetic resonance phase imaging. The Monro-Kellie doctrine revisited. *Neuroradiology*. 1992;34(5):370–380.
39. Poncelet BP, Wedeen VJ, Weiskoff RM, Cohen MS. Brain parenchyma motion: measurement with cine echo-planar MR imaging. *Radiology*. 1992;185(3):645–651.
40. Feinberg DA, Mark AS. Human brain motion and cerebrospinal fluid circulation demonstrated with MR velocity imaging. *Radiology*. 1987;163(3):793–799.
41. DuBolay GH, O'Connell J, Currie J, Bostick T, Verity P. Further investigations on pulsatile movements in the cerebrospinal fluid pathways. *Acta Radiol Diagnost.* 1972;13:496–523.

42. Becher E. Untersuchen über die Dynamic der "Cerebospinalis". *Mitt Grenzgeb Med Chir.* 1922;35:329.
43. O'Connell JAE. Vascular factor in intracranial pressure and maintenance of cerebro-spinal fluid circulation. *Brain.* 1943;66:204–228.
44. Walter BA, Valera VA, Takahashi S, Ushiki T. The olfactory route for cerebrospinal fluid drainage into the peripheral lymphatic system. *Neuropathol Appl Neurobiol.* 2006;32(4):388–396.
45. Hitscherich K, Smith K, Cuoco JA, et al. The glymphatic-lymphatic continuum: opportunities for osteopathic manipulative medicine. *J Am Osteopath Assoc.* 2016;116(3):170–177.
46. Ji S, Zhu Q, Dougherty L, Margulies SS. In vivo measurement of human brain displacement. *Paper presented at: Summer Bioengineering Conference Key Biscayne, FL.* 2003.
47. Kostopoulos DC, Keramidas G. Changes in elongation of falx cerebri during craniosacral therapy techniques applied on the skull of an embalmed cadaver. *J Craniomand Pract.* 1992;10(1):9–12.
48. Zheng N, Chung BS, Li YL, et al. The myodural bridge complex defined as a new functional structure. *Surg Radiol Anat.* 2020:42(2):143–153.
49. Williams PL, ed. *Gray's Anatomy: The Anatomical Basis of Medicine and Surgery*. 38th ed. Churchill Livingston; 1995.
50. Rasmussen TR, Meulengracht KC. Direct measurement of the rhythmic motions of the human head identifies a third rhythm. *J Bodyw Mov Ther.* 2021:24–29.
51. Pritchard JJ, Scott JH, Girgis FG. The structure and development of cranial and facial sutures. *J Anat.* 1956;90(1):73–86.
52. Sabini RC, Elkowitz DE. Significance of differences in patency among cranial sutures. *J Am Osteopath Assoc.* 2006;106(10):600–604.
53. Frymann VM. A study of the rhythmic motions of the living cranium. *J Am Osteopath Assoc.* 1971;70(9):928–945.
54. Moskalenko YE, Cooper R, Crow HJ, Walter G. Variation in blood volume and oxygen availability in the human brain. *Nature.* 1964;202(4926):159–161.
55. Weinstein GB, Demchenko IT, Moskalenko YE. *Biophysical Aspects of Cerebral Circulation*. Pergamon Press; 1980.
56. Moskalenko IE, Frymann V, Weinstein GB, et al. [Slow rhythmic oscillations within the human cranium: phenomenology, origin, and informational significance]. *Hum Physiol.* 2001;27(2):171–178.
57. Moskalenko YE, Frymann VM, Kravchenko T. A modern conceptualization of the functioning of the primary respiratory mechanism. In: King HH, ed. *Proceedings of International Research Conference: Osteopathy in Pediatrics at the Osteopathic Center for Children in San Diego, CA 2002.* American Academy of Osteopathy; 2005:12–31.
58. Hargens AR. Noninvasive intracranial pressure (ICP) measurement. *Space Physiology Laboratory*; 1999. http://spacephysiology.arc.nasa.gov/projects/icp.html
59. Ballard RE, Wilson M, Hargens AR, et al. Noninvasive measurement of intracranial volume and pressure using ultrasound. In: *American Institute of Aeronautics and Astronautics Life Sciences and Space Medicine Conference. Book of Abstracts.* 1996:76–77.
60. Ueno T, Ballard RE, Shuer LM, Cantrell JH, Yost WT, Hargens AR. Noninvasive measurement of pulsatile intracranial pressure using ultrasound. *Acta Neurochir Suppl.* 1998;71:66–69.
61. Ueno T, Ballard RE, Macias BR, Yost WT, Hargens AR. Cranial diameter pulsations measured by non-invasive ultrasound decrease with tilt. *Aviat Space Environ Med.* 2003;74(8):882–885.
62. Nelson KE, Sergueef N, Lipinski CM, Chapman AR, Glonek T. The cranial rhythmic impulse related to the Traube-Hering-Mayer oscillation: comparing laser-Doppler flowmetry and palpation. *J Am Osteopath Assoc.* 2001;101(3):163–173.
63. Sergueef N, Nelson KE, Glonek T. Changes in the Traube-Hering-Meyer wave following cranial manipulation. *Am Acad Osteop J.* 2001;11:17.
64. Nelson KE, Sergueff N, Glonek T. The effect of an alternative medical procedure upon low-frequency oscillation in cutaneous blood flow velocity. *J Manipulative Physiol Ther.* 2006;29:626–636.
65. Nelson KE, Sergueef N, Glonek T. Recording the rate of the cranial rhythmic impulse. *J Am Osteopath Assoc.* 2006;106(6):337–341.
66. Crow WT, King HH, Patterson RM, Giuliano V. Measuring inherent cranial bone motion in humans using MRI. *Poster and Abstract presented at International Conference on Advancements in Osteopathic Research (ICAOR).* 2008.
67. Crow WT, King HH, Patterson RM, Giuliano V. Assessment of calvarial structure motion by MRI. *Osteopath Med Prim Care.* 2009;3:8. http://www.om-pc.com/content/3/1/8
68. ImageJ 1.33u National Institutes of Health, USA. Accessed September 15, 2024. https://imagej.net/
69. Hartman SE, Norton JM. Interexaminer reliability and cranial osteopathy. *Sci Rev Altern Med.* 2002;6:23–34.
70. Cook A. The mechanics of cranial motion—the sphenobasilar synchondrosis (SBS) revisited. *J Bodyw Mov Ther.* 2005;9(3):177–188.
71. Weisl H. The movements of the sacroiliac joint. *Acta Anat.* 1955;23(1):80–91.
72. Kissling RO, Jacob HA. The mobility of the sacroiliac joint in healthy subjects. *Bull Hosp Joint Dis.* 1996;54(3):158–164.
73. Walker JM. The sacroiliac joint: a critical review. *Phys Ther.* 1992;72(12):903–916.
74. Mitchell FL Jr, Pruzzo NA. Investigation of voluntary and primary respiratory mechanisms. *J Am Osteopath Assoc.* 1971;70(10):1109–1113.
75. Mitchell FL Jr. Voluntary and involuntary respiration and the craniosacral mechanism. *Osteopath Ann.* 1977;5:52–59.
76. Pruzzo NA. Lateral lumbar spine double-exposure technique and associated principles. *J Am Osteopath Assoc.* 1970;69(10):1036–1037.
77. Sutherland AS. *With thinking fingers: The Story of Willian Garner Sutherland.* The Cranial Academy; 1962.
78. Woods JM, Woods RH. A physical finding related to psychiatric disorders. *J Am Osteopath Assoc.* 1961;60(8):988–993.
79. Mills MV, Henley CE, Barnes LLB, Carreiro JE, Degenhardt BF. The use of osteopathic manipulative treatment as adjuvant therapy in children with recurrent acute otitis media. *Arch Pediatr Adolesc Med.* 2003;157(9):861–866.
80. Steele KM, Kukulka G, Ilker CL. Effect of osteopathic manipulative treatment on childhood otitis media outcomes. *Poster presented at the American Osteopathic Association 102 Annual Meeting and Scientific Seminar.* 1997: grant # 94-12-400.
81. Degenhardt BF, Kuchera ML. Osteopathic evaluation and manipulative treatment in reducing the morbidity of otitis media: a pilot study. *J Am Osteopath Assoc.* 2006;106(6):327–334.
82. Steele KM, Carreiro JE, Viola JH, Conte JA, Ridpath LC. Effect of osteopathic manipulative treatment on middle ear effusion following acute otitis media in young children: a pilot study. *J Am Osteopath Assoc.* 2014;114(6):436–447.
83. Morin C, Dorion D, Moutquin J-M, Levasseur M. Suture restriction of the temporal bone as a risk factor for acute otitis media in children: cohort study. *BMC Pediatrics.* 2012;12:181.
84. Still AT. *The Philosophy and Mechanical Principles of Osteopathy*. Hudson-Kimberly Publishing Co.; 1902.
85. Whiting LM. Can the length of labor be shortened by osteopathic treatment? *J Am Osteopath Assoc.* 1911;11:917–921.
86. King HH, Tettambel MA, Lockwood MD, Johnson KH, Arsenault DA, Quist R. Osteopathic manipulative treatment in prenatal care: a retrospective case control design study. *J Am Osteopath Assoc.* 2003;103(12):577–582.
87. Gitlin RS, Wolf DL. Uterine contractions following osteopathic cranial manipulation. *J Am Osteopath Assoc.* 1992;92(9):1183.
88. Hensel KL, Buchanan S, Brown SK, Rodriguez M, Cruser DA. Pregnancy research on osteopathic manipulation optimizing treatment effects: the PROMOTE study. *Am J Obstet Gynecol.* 2015;212(1):108.e1–108.e9.
89. Hensel KL, Roane BM. Does compression of the fourth ventricle cause preterm labor? Analysis of data from the PROMOTE study. *J Am Osteopath Assoc.* 2019;119(10):668–672.
90. Frymann V. Relation of disturbances of craniosacral mechanisms to symptomatology of the newborn: study of 1,250 infants. *J Am Osteopath Assoc.* 1966;65(10):1059–1075.
91. Stellwagen L, Hubbard E, Chambers C, Jones KL. Torticollis, facial asymmetry and plagiocephaly in normal newborns. *Arch Dis Child.* 2008;93(10):827–831.
92. Frymann VM. The consequences of being born. In King HH, ed. *Collected papers of Viola Frymann: Volume 2: Legacy to osteopathy.* Osteopathy's Promise to Children; 2021.
93. Frymann VM. Learning difficulties of children viewed in the light of the osteopathic concept. *J Am Osteopath Assoc.* 1976;76(1):46–61.

94. Frymann VM, Carney RE, Springall P. Effect of osteopathic medical management on neurologic development in children. *J Am Osteopath Assoc.* 1992;92(6):729–744.
95. Frymann VM. The osteopathic approach to the child with a seizure disorder. In: King HH, ed. *Proceedings of International Research Conference: Osteopathy in Pediatrics at the Osteopathic Center for Children in San Diego, CA 2002*. American Academy of Osteopathy; 2005:89–96.
96. Lassovetskaia L. Applications of the osteopathic approach to school children with delayed psychic development of cerebro-organic origin. In: King HH, ed. *Proceedings of International Research Conference: Osteopathy in Pediatrics at the Osteopathic Center for Children in San Diego, CA 2002*. American Academy of Osteopathy; 2005:52–59.
97. Hayden C, Mullinger B. A preliminary assessment of the impact of cranial osteopathy for the relief of infantile colic. *Complement Ther Clin Pract.* 2006;12(2):83–90.
98. Pizzolorusso G, Turi P, Barlafante G, et al. Effect of osteopathic manipulative treatment on gastrointestinal function and length of stay of preterm infants: an exploratory study. *Chiropr Man Therap.* 2011;19(1):15.
99. Cerritelli F, Pizzolorusso G, Ciardelli F, et al. Effect of osteopathic manipulative treatment on length of stay in a population of preterm infants: a randomized controlled trial. *BMC Pediatr.* 2013;13:65.
100. Pizzolorusso G, Cerritelli F, Accorsi A, et al. The effect of optimally timed ostreopathic manipulative treatment on length of hospital stay in moderate and late term preterm infants: results from a RCT. *Evid Based Complement Alternat Med.* 2014:22(4):625–631.
101. Cerritelli F, Pizzolorusso G, Renzetti C, et al. A multicenter, randomized, controlled trial of osteopathic manipulative treatment on preterms. *Plos One.* 2015;10(5):e0127370.
102. Lanaro D, Ruffini N, Manzotti A, Lista G. Osteopathic manipulative treatment showed reduction of length of stay and costs in preterm infants: a systematic review and meta-analysis. *Medicine.* 2017;96(12):e6408.
103. Cicchitti L, Di Lelio A, Barlafante G, et al. Osteopathic manipulative treatment in neonatal intensive care units. *Med Sci.* 2020;8(2):24.
104. Manzotti A, Cerritelli F, Lombardi E, et al. Effects of osteopathic treatment versus static touch on heart rate and oxygen saturation in premature babies: a randomized controlled trial. *Compl Therp Clin Pract.* 2020; 39:101116.
105. Pastor-Pons I, Lucha-López MO, Barrau-Lalmolda MB, et al. Efficacy of pediatric integrative manual therapy in positional plagiocephaly: a randomized controlled trial. *Ital J Pediatr.* 2021;47(1):132.
106. Lessard S, Gagnon I, Trottier N. Exploring the impact of osteopathic treatment on cranial asymmetries associated with nonsynostotic plagiocephaly in infants. *Complement Ther Clin Pract.* 2011;17(4): 193–198.
107. King HH, Mai J, Haskell MAM, Wolf K, Sweeney M. Effects of osteopathic manipulative treatment on children with plagiocephaly in the context of current pediatric practice: a retrospective chart review study. *J Osteopath Med.* 2023;124(4):171–177. Submitted and in review.
108. Magoun HI. Osteopathic approach to dental enigmas. *J Am Osteopath Assoc.* 1962;62:34–42.
109. Magoun HI Sr. Dental equilibration and osteopathy. *J Am Osteopath Assoc.* 1975;74(10):981–991.
110. Magoun HI Sr. The dental search for a common denominator in craniocervical pain and dysfunction. *J Am Osteopath Assoc.* 1979;78(11):810–815.
111. Lay EM. The osteopathic management of temporomandibular joint dysfunction. In: Gelb H, ed. *Clinical Management of Head, Neck and TMJ Pain and Dysfunction; A Multidisciplinary Approach to Diagnosis and Treatment.* W.B. Saunders Co.; 1985.
112. Baker EG. Alteration in width of maxillary arch and its relation to sutural movement of cranial bones. *J Am Osteopath Assoc.* 1971;70(6):559–564.
113. Segatto E, Lippold C, Andras V. Craniofacial features of children with spinal deformities. *BMC Musculoskelet Disord.* 2008;9:169.
114. Davis L, Hanson B, Gilliam S. Pilot study of the effects of mixed light touch manual therapies on active duty soldiers with chronic post-traumatic stress disorder and injury to the head. *J Bodyw Move Ther.* 2016; 20(1):42–51.
115. Wetzler G, Roland M, Dietz S-F, Ahern DD. Craniosacral therapy and visceral manipulation: a new treatment intervention for concussion recovery. *Med Acupunt.* 2017;29(4):239–248.
116. Concussion Legacy Foundation. What is Post-Concussion Syndrome (PCS)? Accessed January 28, 2023. https://concussionfoundation.org/PCS-resources/what-is-PCS
117. Patel KG, Sabini RC. Safety of osteopathic cranial manipulative medicine as an adjunct to conventional postconcussion symptom management: a pilot study. *J Am Osteopath Assoc.* 2018;118(6):403–409.
118. Yao SC, Zweibel H, Angelo N, Leder A, Mancini J. Effectiveness of osteopathic manipulative medicine vs concussion education in treating student athletes with acute concussion symptoms. *J Am Osteopath Assoc.* 2020;129(9):607–614.
119. Mazzeo S, Silverberg C, Oommen T, et al. Effects of osteopathic manipulative treatment on sleep quality in student athletes after concussion: a pilot study. *J Am Osteopath Assoc.* 2020;120(9):615–622.
120. Sweeney M, King H, Alexander J, Pung M. The role of osteopathic manipulation in the management of posttraumatic migraine. *Poster presented at American Academy of Osteopathy Convocation March 2020.* Colorado Springs, Co.
121. McCallister A, Brown C, Smith M, Ettlinger H, Baltazar GA. Osteopathic manipulative treatment for somatic dysfunction after acute severe traumatic brain injury. *J Am Osteopath Assoc.* 2016;116(12):810–815.
122. Kashyap S, Brazdzionis J, Savla P, et al. Osteopathic manipulative treatment to optimize the glymphatic environment in severe traumatic brain injury measured with optic nerve sheath diameter, intracranial pressure monitoring, and neurological pupil index. *Cureus.* 2021;13(3):e13823.
123. Huard Y. Influence of the venous sinus technique on cranial hemodynamics. In: King HH, ed. *Proceedings of International Research Conference: Osteopathy in Pediatrics at the Osteopathic Center for Children in San Diego, CA 2002*. American Academy of Osteopathy; 2005:32–36.
124. Roberts B, Makar AE, Canaan R, Pazdernik V, Kondrashova T. Effect of occipitoatlantal decompression on cerebral blood flow dynamics as evaluated by Doppler ultrasonography. *J Osteopath Med.* 2021;121(2):171–179.
125. Vardy TC, Moskalenko Y, Mokhov D, Dombroski RT. Combined bio-impedence and transcranial doppler ultrasonography in Parkinson's patients and neurologically normal ageing subjects. *EC Neurology.* 2020;12(4):01–09.
126. Tamburella F, Piras F, Piras F, Spano B, Tramontano M, Gili T. Cerebral perfusion changes after osteopathic manipulative treatment: a randomized manual placebo-controlled trial. *Front. Physiol.* 2019;10:403.
127. Cerritelli F, Chiacchiarette P, Gambi F, Saggini R, Perrucci MG, Ferretti A. Osteopathy modulates brain-heart interaction in chronic pain patients: an ASL study. *Sci Rep.* 2021;11(1):4556.
128. Cutler MJ, Holland BS, Stupski BA, Gamber RG, Smith ML. Cranial manipulation can alter sleep latency and sympathetic nerve activity in humans: a pilot study. *J Altern Complement Med.* 2005;11(1):103–108.
129. Giles PD, Hensel KL, Pacchia CF, Smith ML. Suboccipital decompression enhances heart rate variability indices of cardiac control in healthy subjects. *J Altern Comple Med.* 2013;19(2):92–96.
130. Henley CE, Ivins D, Mills M, Wen FK, Benjamin BA. Osteopathic manipulative treatment and its relationship to autonomic nervous system activity as demonstrated by heart rate variability: a repeated measures study. *Osteopath Med Prim Care.* 2008;2:7.
131. Purdy WR, Frank JJ, Oliver B. Suboccipital dermatomyotomic stimulation and digital blood flow. *J Am Osteopath Assoc.* 1996;96(5):285–289.
132. Ruffini N, D'Alessandro G, Mariani N, Pollastrelli A, Cardinali L, Cerritelli F. Variations of high frequency parameter of heart rate variability following osteopathic manipulative treatment in healthy subjects compared to control group and sham therapy; randomized controlled trial. *Front Neurosci.* 2015;9:272.
133. Curi ACC, Alves ASM, Silva JG. Cardiac autonomic response after cranial technique of the fourth ventricle (cv4) compression in systemic hypertensive subjects. *J Bodyw Mov Ther.* 2018;22(3):666–672.
134. Fornari M, Camevali L, Sgoifo A. Single osteopathic manipulative therapy session dampens acute autonomic and neuroendocrine responses to mental stress in healthy male participants. *J Am Osteopath Assoc.* 2017;117(9):559–567.
135. Scoppa F, Pirino A, Belloni G, Gallamini M, Messina G, Iovane A, Pirino A. Postural and autonomic modifications following osteopathic manipulative treatment (OMT): comparison between two techniques. A pilot study. *Acta Medica Mediterranea.* 2018;34:431–436.

136. Cerritelli F, Cardone D, Pirino A, Merla A, Scoppa F. Does osteopathic manipulative treatment induce autonomic changes in healthy participants? A thermal imaging study. *Front Neurosci.* 2020;14:887.
137. Roura S, Alvarez G, Sola I, Cerritelli F. Do manual therapies have a specific autonomic effect? An overview of systematic reviews. *Plos One.* 2021;16(12):e0260642.
138. Hanten WP, Olson SL, Hodson JL, Imler VL, Knab VM, Magee JL. The effectiveness of CV-4 and resting position techniques on subjects with tension-type headaches. *J Man Manip Ther.* 1999;7(2):64–70.
139. Miana L, do Vale Bastos VH, Machado S, et al. Changes in alpha band activity associated with application of the compression of fourth ventricular (CV-4) osteopathic procedure: a qEEG pilot study. *J Bodyw Move Ther.* 2013;17(3):291–296.
140. Shi X, Rehrer S, Prajapati P, Stoll ST, Gamber RG, Downey HF. Effect of cranial osteopathic manipulative medicine on cerebral tissue oxygenation. *J Am Osteopath Assoc.* 2011;111(12):660–666.
141. Gerdner LA, Hart LK, Zimmermann MB. Craniosacral still point technique: exploring its effects in individuals with dementia. *J Gerontological Nursing.* 2008;34(3):36–45.
142. Milnes K, Moran RW. Physiological effects of a CV4 cranial osteopathic technique on autonomic nervous system function: a preliminary investigation. *Internat J Osteopath Med.* 2007;10:8–17.
143. Cardoso-de-Mello-E-Mello-Ribeiro AP, Rodríguez-Blanco C, Riquelme-Agulló I, Heredia-Rizo AM, Ricard F, Oliva-Pascual-Vaca Á. Effects of the fourth ventricle compression in the regulation of the autonomic nervous system: a randomized control trial. *Evid Based Complement Alternat Med.* 2015:148285.
144. Lopez D, King HH, Knebl JA, Kosmopolous V, Collins D, Patterson RM. Effect of comprehensive osteopathic manipulation treatment on balance in elderly patients: a pilot study. *J Am Osteopath Assoc.* 2011;111(6):382–388.
145. Fraix M, Gordon A, Graham V, Hurwitz E, Seffinger MA. Use of the SMART balance master to quantify the effects of osteopathic manipulative treatment in patients with dizziness. *J Am Osteopath Assoc.* 2013;113(5):394–403.
146. Alexander J, Kurisu M, Fleming J, King HH. Response of tinnitus to osteopathic manipulation. *Poster and Abstract Presented at Neurology and Integrative Medicine Grand Rounds.* University of California San Diego School of Medicine; 2015.
147. Saggio G, Docimo S, Pilc J, Norton J, Gilliar W. Impact of osteopathic manipulative treatment on secretory immunogloblin A levels in a stressed population. *J Am Osteopath Assoc.* 2011;111(3):143–147.
148. Lee-Wong M, Karagic M, Doshi A, Gomez S, Resnick D. An osteopathic approach to chronic sinusitis. *J Aller Ther.* 2011;2:2.
149. Lintonbon D. A study to investigate the effect of 'Frontal Lift' osteopathic manipulative technique (OMT) in patients with chronic sinusitis. *Am J Biomed Sci Res.* 2019;3:3.
150. Raviv G, Shefi S, Nizani D, Achiron A. Effects of craniosacral therapy on lower urinary tract signs and symptoms in multiple sclerosis. *Complem Ther Clin Pract.* 2009;15(2):72–75.
151. Cordano C, Armezzani A, Veroni J, et al. Osteopathic manipulative therapy and multiple sclerosis: a proof-of-concept study. *J Am Osteopath Assoc.* 2018;118(8):531–536.
152. Terrell ZT, Moudy SC, Hensel KL, Patterson RM. Effects of osteopathic manipulative treatment vs. osteopathic cranial manipulation medicine on Parkinsonian gait. *J Osteopath Med.* 2022;122(5):243–251.
153. King HH, Mills P, Schiehser D, Pung M. Effects of osteopathic manipulative treatment on gait biomechanics in Parkinson's disease. *Mov Disord Clin Pract.* 2024. In preparation.
154. Tobey H, Lucas T, Bledsoe D, et al. Effect of osteopathic cranial manipulative medicine on an aged rat model of Alzheimer disease. *J Am Osteopath Assoc.* 2019;119:713.
155. Tobey H, Lucas T, Paul S, et al. Mechanoceutics alters Alzheimer's disease phenotypes in transgenic rats: a pilot study. *J Alzheimer's Disease.* 2020;74(2):421–427.
156. Anandakrishnan R, Tobey H, Nguyen S, Sandoval O, Klein BG, Costa BM. Cranial manipulation affects cholinergic pathway gene expression in aged rats. *J Osteopath Med.* 2022;122(2):95–103.
157. Greenman PE, McPartland JM. Cranial findings and iatrogenesis from craniosacral manipulation in patients with traumatic brain syndrome. *J Am Osteopath Assoc.* 1995;95(3):182–188; 191–192.
158. Hensel K, ed. *A Teaching Guide for Osteopathic Manipulative Medicine.* American Association of Colleges of Osteopathic Medicine; 2015.
159. Lancaster DG, Crow WT. Osteopathic manipulative treatment of a 26-year-old woman with Bell's palsy. *J Am Osteopath Assoc.* 2006;106(5):285–289.
160. Arnadottir TS, Sigurdardottir AK. Is craniosacral therapy effective for migraine? Tested with HIT-6 questionnaire. *Compl Ther Clin Prac.* 2013; 19(1):11–14.
161. Lund GC, Edwards G, Medlin B, Keller D, Beck B, Carreiro JE. Osteopathic manipulative treatment for the treatment of hospitalized premature infants with nipple feeding dysfunction. *J Am Osteopath Assoc.* 2011;111(1):44–48.
162. Drengler KE, King HH. Inter-examiner reliability of palpatory diagnosis of the cranium. *J Am Osteopath Assoc.* 1998;98(7):387.
163. Upledger JE. The reproducibility of craniosacral examination findings: a statistical analysis. *J Am Osteopath Assoc.* 1977;76(12):890–899.
164. Capobianco JD, Shemon S. Taxonomy of the lateral strain patterns at the sphenobasilar synchondrosis for osteopathic cranial manipulative medicine. *J Am Osteopath Assoc.* 2020;120(1):25–29.
165. Seffinger MA, ed. *Foundations of osteopathic medicine. 4/e.* Lippincott, Williams & Wilkins; 2018.
166. Hruby RJ. Lateral Strains of the Sphenobasilar Synchondrosis: Teaching Their Description and Motion Characteristics to Beginning Learners of Osteopathic Cranial Manipulative Medicine (OCMM). Report of the ad hoc Subcommittee of The Educational Council on Osteopathic Principles (ECOP). 2020.
167. Hruby RJ. *Exploring Osteopathy in the Cranial Field.* 2nd ed. published by the author; 2022.

54 Soft Tissue

WALTER C. EHRENFEUCHTER

KEY CONCEPTS

- Soft tissue techniques are directly applied to the muscular and fascial structures of the body and affect the associated neural and vascular elements.
- Soft tissue preparation facilitates improvement of articular motion. This basic tenet of manipulative intervention has been consistent throughout the history of osteopathic medicine.
- Soft tissue techniques employ a wide range of force applications. It is this characteristic that makes it one of the most versatile technique forms.

DEFINITION

Soft tissue is a direct technique that usually involves the following approaches:

- Lateral stretching
- Linear stretching
- Deep pressure
- Traction and/or separation of muscle origin and insertion

This technique is a form of myofascial treatment[1] and is performed with ongoing monitoring of tissue response and motion changes through palpation.

HISTORY

Soft tissue techniques are among the oldest techniques in the osteopathic medical profession, having been among those employed and taught by Andrew T. Still, DO. Based on descriptions by his students, it is believed that Dr. Still made extensive use of the soft tissue style known as direct inhibitory pressure. Soft tissue techniques or deep directed massage therapies have been known to exist for millennia.

PROPOSED MECHANISM OF ACTION

Soft tissue technique has several proposed mechanisms of action. This approach relaxes hypertonic muscles and reduces spasm. It has been suggested that this is through the technique's mechanical impact on both the alpha and gamma motor neurons that function to set both resting and active muscle tone.

In addition, soft tissue technique stretches and increases the elasticity of shortened fascial structures, improves circulation to local myofascial structures, and improves local tissue nutrition, oxygenation, and removal of metabolic wastes.

Using soft tissue technique, areas of restricted motion, tissue texture changes, and sensitivity are identified. There is improvement of local and systemic immune response. The approach also provides a general state of relaxation and optimizes autonomic tone.

INDICATIONS

As with all osteopathic manipulative treatment, the primary indication is the identification of clinically relevant somatic dysfunction (in this case, of the body's soft tissues), as characterized by tissue tenderness, asymmetry, range of motion abnormality, and/or tissue texture abnormalities, or TART.[2]

Clinical conditions that benefit from soft tissue techniques include:

- Hypertonic muscles
- Excessive tension in fascial structures
- Abnormal somato–somatic and somato–visceral reflexes

Soft tissue techniques are used as an adjunct to additional manipulative treatment to identify other areas of somatic dysfunction. It is important to observe and feel the tissue response to the application of manipulative techniques. Soft tissue techniques can have many effects. Some of these include:

- Providing a general state of relaxation
- Providing a general state of tonic stimulation
- Encouraging blood flow and warmth to an area
- Preparing tissues for other types of manipulation

CONTRAINDICATIONS

- Absolute contraindications[2]
  - Lack of patient consent and/or cooperation is an absolute contraindication for any medical procedure. In addition, if the skin and/or soft tissues are not intact, are traumatized by blunt or sharp force, or there is friable tissue that can be easily disrupted by pressure or strain, it is reasonable to assume that soft tissue manipulative procedures are contraindicated.
  - Cautions and relative contraindications
  - Clinical judgment and consideration for the whole patient is necessary when utilizing any procedural approach. The following categories guide the decision-making regarding caution in the use of soft tissue techniques.
- Skin (disorders that would preclude skin contact)
  - Contagious skin diseases
  - Acute burns
  - Painful rashes
  - Abscesses or cellulitis
  - Skin cancers
- Fascia
  - Acute fasciitis (infectious or autoimmune)
  - Acute fascial tears
- Muscle
  - Acute muscular strains
  - Acute myositis
  - Muscle neoplasms
- Ligament
  - Acute ligamentous sprain
  - Acute ligamentous inflammatory disorders

- Bone
  - Acute fracture
  - Osteomyelitis
  - Primary or secondary bone tumors
  - Osteoporosis
- Joint
  - Septic joint
  - Instability—may be posttraumatic or related to hereditary connective tissue disorders, for example, Ehlers–Danlos syndrome
- Viscera
  - Infection
  - Neoplasm
  - Organomegaly (liver/spleen)
  - Gastric or bowel obstruction or distention
  - Acute or undiagnosed abdominal pain
  - Acute or undiagnosed pelvic pain
- Vascular
  - Hematoma
  - Deep venous thrombosis
  - Coagulopathy

SAFETY AND EFFICACY

Soft tissue techniques are exceptionally safe. The most serious reported reactions to treatment are:

- Ecchymosis
- Acute muscle spasm
- Postprocedure muscle soreness

One of the notable features of this technique is the ability to both diagnose and treat the patient while simultaneously palpating the soft tissue response.[2]

PRINCIPLES OF DIAGNOSIS

Soft tissue dysfunction is identified through layer-by-layer palpation of the soft tissues of the body. The type and duration of soft tissue technique applied is determined by the type of soft tissue dysfunction and the patient's clinical conditions.[2]

PRINCIPLES OF TREATMENT

Soft tissue technique is a passive direct technique with three basic mechanisms in its application.[2] These include traction, kneading (both linear and lateral), and inhibition (deep pressure). Traction, also called stretching, involves longitudinal separation of the origin and insertion of the myofascial structures being treated. Linear kneading can be applied as a pressure parallel to the long axis of the structure. Lateral kneading is a rhythmic lateral stretch of myofascial structures; the origin and insertion are held stationary while a central portion of the structure is stretched, like a bowstring. Inhibition involves sustained deep pressure over a hypertonic myofascial structure.

Other mechanisms used on more superficial fascial structures include variants on techniques developed in the European massage movement, including effleurage, petrissage, tapotement, and skin rolling.

BASIC TREATMENT PRINCIPLES

- The patient should be comfortable and able to relax.
- The physician should also be in a position of comfort to minimize energy expenditure, and to make use of body weight and leverage rather than having to exert muscular force.
- Initially, the applied forces are very gentle and of low amplitude. The force is applied rhythmically, typically 1 or 2 seconds of stretching followed by a similar time frame releasing that stretch.
- As the soft tissues are palpated and are responding to the technique, the physician may increase the applied forces to increase the technique's amplitude. The rate of application typically remains the same.
- The applied forces should be comfortable for the patient. A few patients may experience some discomfort, but it is recognized as positive.
- Care must be taken so that the physician's hands do not create friction by sliding across the patient's skin or by rubbing it. The physician's hand should carry the skin with it as the activating force is applied. Care should be taken to not compress the musculature directly against a bone.
- The technique is continued until the desired effect is achieved. This is typically indicated once the soft tissue's amplitude of excursion has reached a maximum and plateaued at that level.

TYPES OF SOFT TISSUE TECHNIQUES

Parallel Traction

In this type of soft tissue technique, the forces being applied are parallel to the myofascial structures requiring treatment. This may be performed by separating the proximal and distal attachments of the muscle (with both hands moving in opposite directions like a taffy pull) or by anchoring one end of the muscle and pulling on the other (with one hand or structure serving as a stationary anchor, the other one mobile) (Fig. 54.1).

Example of parallel traction: Intermittent cervical traction

POSSIBLE DIAGNOSES

- Hypertonicity of the cervical musculature
- Bulging cervical disk
- Cervical degenerative disk disease
- Somatic dysfunction of cervical spine

TREATMENT POSITION

Patient: Supine on the treatment table.
Physician: Seated at the head of the table.

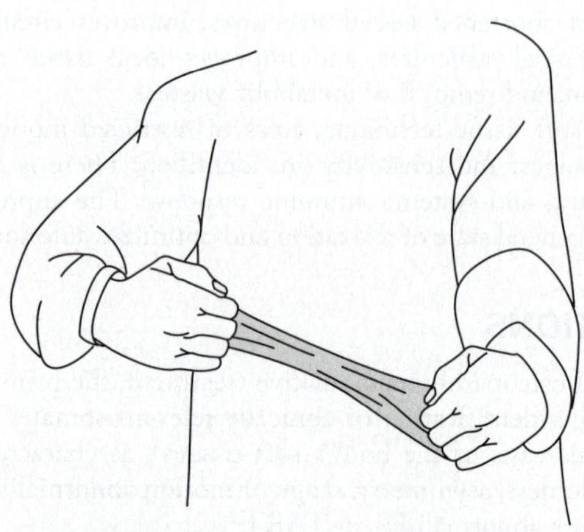

Figure 54.1. The taffy pull.

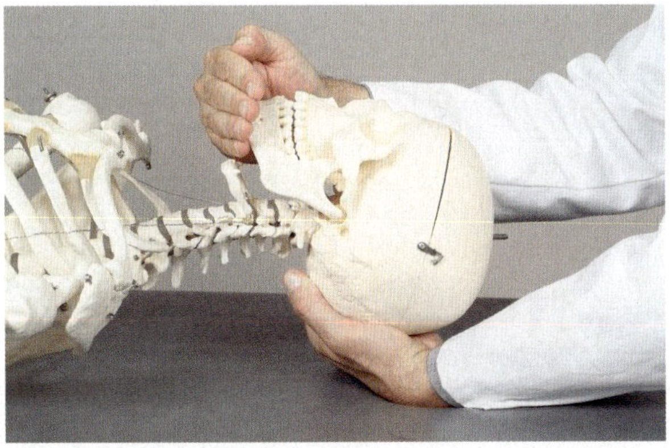

Figure 54.2. Intermittent cervical traction. (Reprinted with permission from Nicholas AS, Nicholas EA. *Atlas of Osteopathic Techniques*. 4th ed. Wolters Kluwer; 2023. Figure 7.1.)

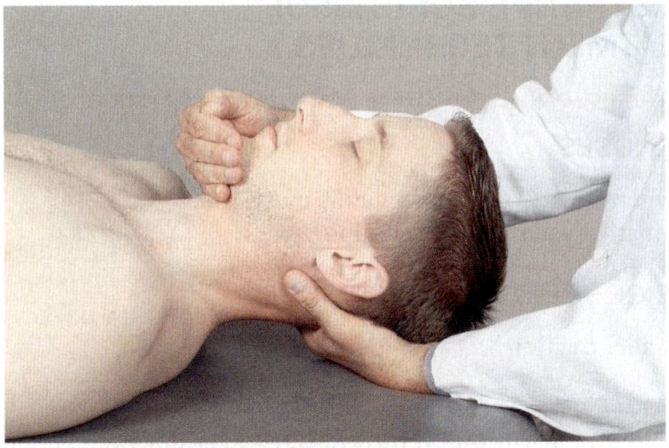

Figure 54.3. Intermittent cervical traction. (Reprinted with permission from Nicholas AS, Nicholas EA. *Atlas of Osteopathic Techniques*. 4th ed. Wolters Kluwer; 2023. Figure 7.2.)

PROCEDURE

1. One of the physician's hands cradles the occiput, with the thumb and index finger spanning the region just inferior to the superior nuchal line.
2. The physician's other hand cradles the chin. (In some patients, this will aggravate a preexisting temporomandibular joint or dental problem—for those cases, an alternative is to place this hand across the patient's forehead.) (Fig. 54.2)
3. Physician applies axial superior traction with both hands simultaneously, maintaining the head and neck in a neutral to slightly flexed position. The occipital hand must not squeeze the occiput, as this will risk compressing the occipitomastoid suture.
4. This technique is applied slowly and rhythmically, with gradually increasing amplitude (Fig. 54.3).
5. The technique is continued until the desired soft tissue or disk response is obtained. This may require anywhere from 2 to 5 minutes.
6. Success of the technique is determined through palpation to reassess the characteristics of the soft tissues that led to the chosen treatment technique. Success may also be determined in part by reassessing the patient's symptomatology.

Perpendicular Traction

In this type of soft tissue technique, the myofascial structure being treated is contacted near its midpoint, between the proximal and distal attachments. A stretching force is applied at right angles to the muscle's longitudinal axis (e.g., like an archer stretching a bowstring) (Fig. 54.4).

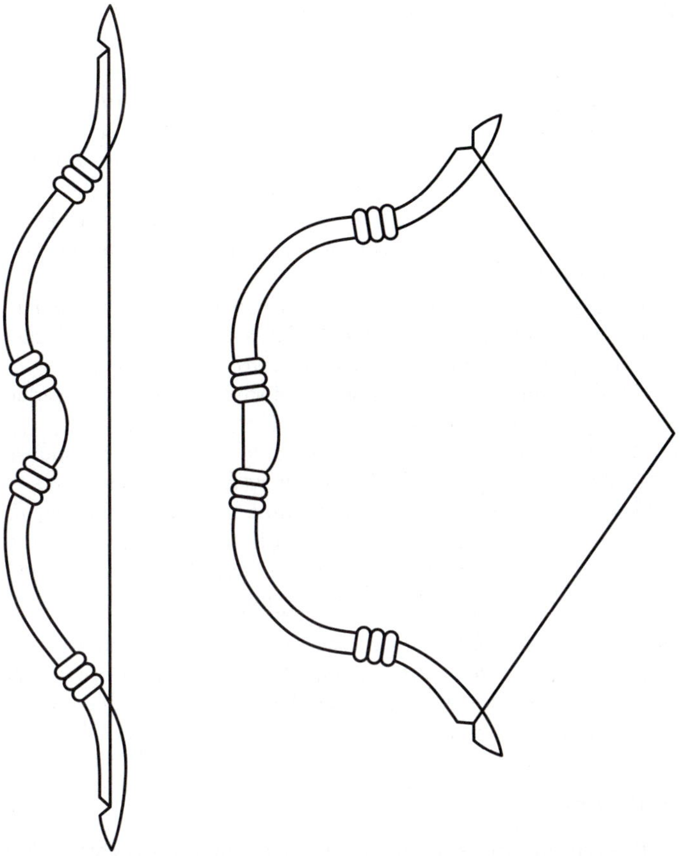

Figure 54.4. The bowstring.

Example of perpendicular traction: Contralateral traction

POSSIBLE DIAGNOSES

- Hypertonicity of the cervical paraspinal musculature
- Somatic dysfunction of cervical spine

TREATMENT POSITION

Patient: Supine on the treatment table
Physician: Standing at the side of the head of the treatment table

PROCEDURE

1. Physician bridges the forehead with one hand to stabilize and control head motion (Fig. 54.5).

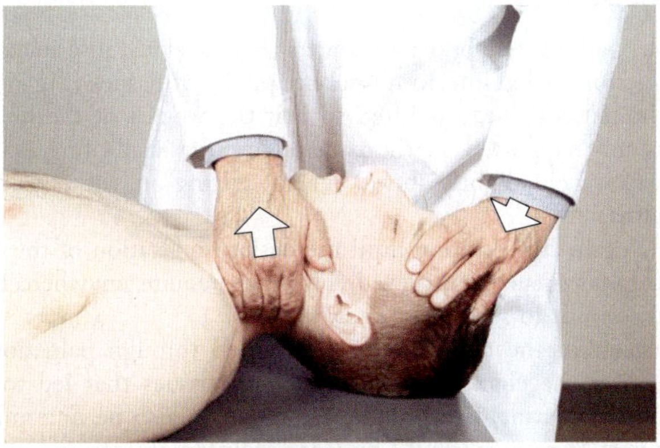

Figure 54.5. Contralateral traction. (Reprinted with permission from Nicholas AS, Nicholas EA. *Atlas of Osteopathic Techniques*. 4th ed. Wolters Kluwer; 2023. Figure 7.13.)

2. The physician's other hand reaches around the side of the neck to contact the cervical paraspinal musculature, just lateral to the spinous processes.
3. While keeping the elbow of the hand in contact with the cervical musculature locked in extension, the physician rotates their upper trunk to draw that arm posteriorly, thus drawing the patient's paraspinal musculature ventrally and laterally. Counterforce must be exerted with the physician's other hand to control the patient's head, and to ensure that minimal cervical extension occurs.
4. Care must be taken not to apply too much pressure to the lateral aspect of the cervical region, as this may provoke bradycardia and hypotension due to a reflex carotid body response.
5. This technique is applied slowly and rhythmically, with gradually increasing amplitude.
6. The technique continues until the desired soft tissue response is obtained. This may require anywhere from 2 to 5 minutes.
7. Success of the technique is determined through palpation to reassess the characteristics of the soft tissues that led to the chosen treatment technique. Success may also be determined in part by reassessing the patient's symptomatology.

Note: By increasing the rotational force, this technique may be converted to an articulatory technique. By adding more of an axial milking motion, it may be used to enhance lymphatic drainage in the cervical lymph node chains.

Inhibition

In this type of soft tissue technique, the myofascial structure being treated is contacted over the musculotendinous portion of the hypertonic muscle with a force directed straight into the muscle. Pressing into a hypertonic muscle belly can be painful and may bruise the muscle; therefore, the pressure should be directed to the musculotendinous junction.

Example: Suboccipital inhibition

POSSIBLE DIAGNOSES

- Hypertonic suboccipital musculature
- Tension headache
- Somatic dysfunction of the cranium and/or cervical spine

TREATMENT POSITION

Patient: Supine
Physician: Seated at the head of the treatment table

PROCEDURE

1. The pads of the physician's fingers are placed just inferior to the superior nuchal line, in the suboccipital soft tissues (Fig. 54.6).
2. The patient's head is lifted so that the weight of the head is entirely supported on the pads of the physician's fingers. The head is held slightly above, but not resting on, the physician's palms.
3. Maintain this position until the desired relaxation of the suboccipital tissues is achieved. This may require anywhere from 30 seconds to several minutes.
4. Success of the technique is determined through palpation to reassess the characteristics of the soft tissues that led to the chosen treatment technique. Success may also be determined in part by reassessing the patient's symptomatology.

Note: This technique is similar in position to the method used by Still to relieve his own headaches using a rope sling.[3]

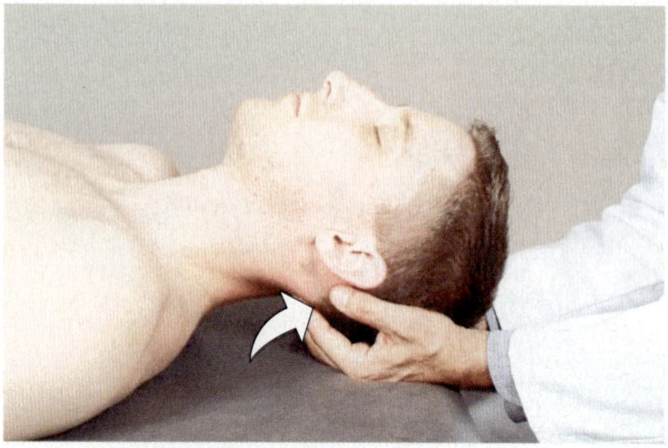

Figure 54.6. Suboccipital inhibition. (Reprinted with permission from Nicholas AS, Nicholas EA. *Atlas of Osteopathic Techniques*. 4th ed. Wolters Kluwer; 2023. Figure 7.19.)

ILLUSTRATIVE SOFT TISSUE TREATMENT TECHNIQUES

Head Region: Temporalis Muscle Soft Tissue

DIAGNOSES

- Hypertonicity of the temporalis muscle
- Somatic dysfunction of cranium

TYPE OF SOFT TISSUE TECHNIQUE

- Parallel traction

TREATMENT POSITION

Patient: Supine, with head turned to place dysfunctional temporalis muscle superiorly
Physician: Seated at the side of the table, facing the patient

PROCEDURE

1. Place one hand beneath the patient's head to prevent excessive head movement (Fig. 54.7).
2. Place the thumb of the other hand approximately 2 cm inferior to the temporal lines in the region of the temporalis muscle that was previously determined to be hypertonic. The remaining fingers extend over the top of the skull.
   a. The one end of the temporalis muscle is anchored by its attachment to the coronoid process.
3. The physician's thumb then exerts a force directly toward the skull until sufficient pressure to engage the musculature is achieved.

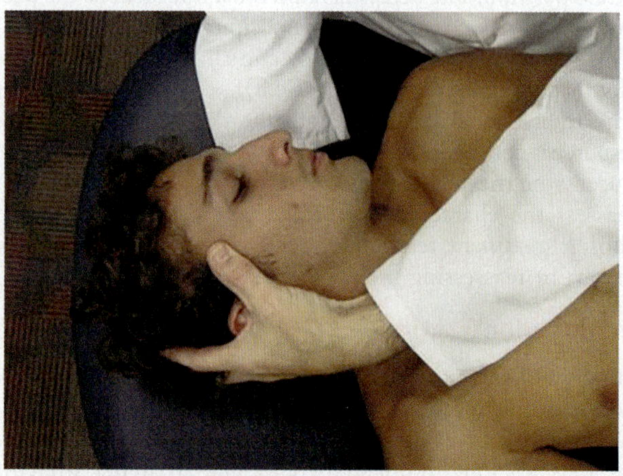

Figure 54.7. Temporalis muscle soft tissue.

4. Exert a tractional force parallel to the muscle fiber direction, toward the top of the skull.
5. Apply this force gently and rhythmically every 1 to 2 seconds. Note the softening of the soft tissue structures as this technique is continued for 1 to 2 minutes. (The time frame is shortened here because of the smaller size of the muscle being treated.)
6. Success of the technique is determined by palpating the previously hypertonic temporalis muscle again.

Cervical Region: Cradling with Traction

DIAGNOSES

- Hypertonicity of the cervical paraspinal musculature
- Somatic dysfunction of the cervical spine

TYPE OF SOFT TISSUE TECHNIQUE

- Parallel traction

TREATMENT POSITION

Patient: Supine
Physician: Seated at the head of the table

PROCEDURE

1. The physician's fingers are placed under the patient's neck bilaterally, with the finger pads contacting the cervical paraspinal musculature overlying the articular pillars, just lateral to the spinous processes (Fig. 54.8).
2. The physician exerts pressure ventrally of sufficient force to engage the soft tissues without extending the cervical spine.
3. The physician pulls the hands superiorly, producing a longitudinal traction.
4. This traction is slowly released.
5. The physician's hands are repositioned along the cervical pillars, and steps 2 to 4 are repeated in a gentle rhythmic manner.
6. This technique is continued for 2 to 5 minutes.
7. Success of the technique is determined by palpating the previously hypertonic cervical musculature.

Thoracic Region: Prone Pressure with Counterpressure

DIAGNOSES

- Thoracic paravertebral muscle hypertonicity
- Somatic dysfunction of the thoracic spine

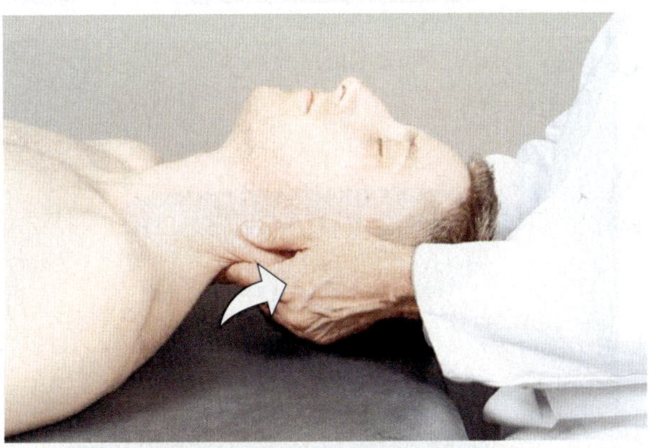

Figure 54.8. Cradling with traction soft tissue technique. (Reprinted with permission from Nicholas AS, Nicholas EA. *Atlas of Osteopathic Techniques*. 4th ed. Wolters Kluwer; 2023. Figure 7.16.)

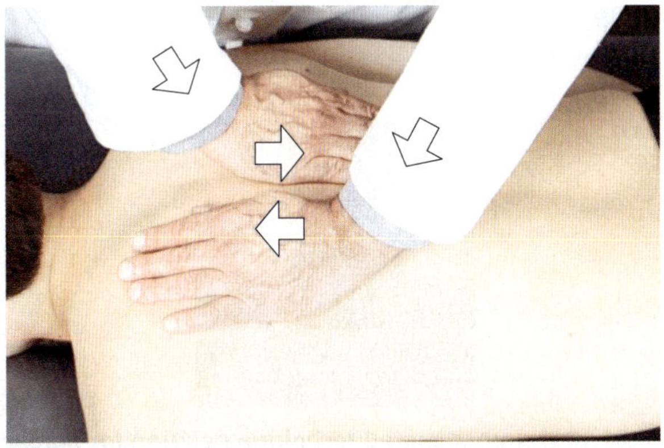

Figure 54.9. Prone pressure with counterpressure soft tissue technique. (Reprinted with permission from Nicholas AS, Nicholas EA. *Atlas of Osteopathic Techniques*. 4th ed. Wolters Kluwer; 2023. Figure 7.50.)

TYPE OF SOFT TISSUE TECHNIQUE

- Parallel traction

TREATMENT POSITION

Patient: Prone with the head turned toward the physician
Physician: Standing at the side of the table, facing the patient's thorax

PROCEDURE

1. Physician places one hand on the patient's spine, with the heel of the hand over the transverse process of the thoracic vertebra at the level of the hypertonic musculature. The fingers of this hand are pointing superiorly (Fig. 54.9).
2. Physician places the other hand on the contralateral side of the patient's spine, with the heel of the hand over the opposite transverse process of that same vertebral segment. The fingers of this hand are pointing inferiorly.
3. Exert sufficient pressure downward toward the table to engage the myofascial structures of the spine.
4. Exert a longitudinal force simultaneously with both hands in opposite directions.
5. This pressure is slowly released.
6. The hands are both repositioned together, either a segment above or below depending upon the needs of the patient.
7. Steps 3 to 6 are repeated in a rhythmic fashion for 2 to 5 minutes.
8. Success of the technique is determined by palpating the previously hypertonic thoracic paravertebral musculature, which should become warmer and less hypertonic.

Lumbar Region: Lumbar Seated Technique for Paraspinal Tissues

DIAGNOSES

- Hypertonicity of the left lumbar paraspinal musculature.
- Somatic dysfunction of the lumbar spine

TYPE OF SOFT TISSUE TECHNIQUE

- Perpendicular traction

TREATMENT POSITION

Patient: Seated, straddling the treatment table with the back to the end of the table.

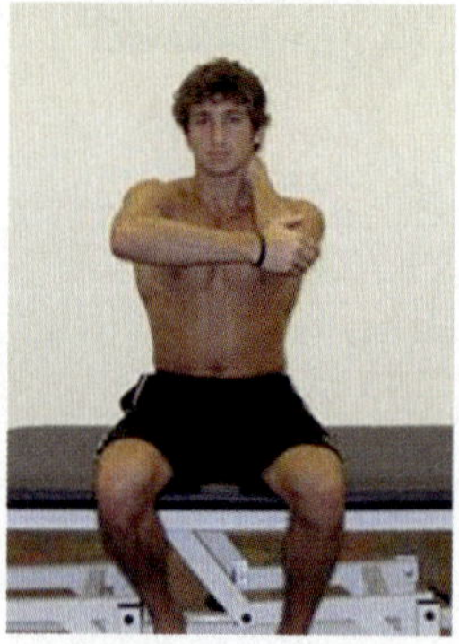

Figure 54.10. Lumbar seated technique position for paraspinal tissues.

Physician: Standing behind the patient opposite the side to be treated. Table height should be adjusted so that the physician stands roughly one head taller than the patient.

PROCEDURE (EXAMPLE, FOR TREATING THE LEFT LUMBAR PARASPINAL MUSCULATURE)

1. The patient's left hand is placed behind the neck. The patient's right hand then grasps the left elbow (Fig. 54.10).
2. The heel of the physician's left hand is placed on the patient's left paraspinal muscle mass, just lateral to the spinous processes.
3. The right arm of the physician is passed in front of the patient (under the right upper arm), with the hand of that arm grasping the patient's left upper arm.
4. Patient leans forward and relaxes so that the weight will be carried by the physician's right arm. The patient will have a natural tendency to rotate the trunk to the right.
5. The physician's left hand carries the hypertonic paraspinal musculature laterally away from the spine. Simultaneously, the physician's body is turned right so that the rotation of the patient's trunk to the right is exaggerated.
6. Traction and rotation are held for a short time, and then released. The natural tension of the soft tissues will return the lumbar column to a position just inside the restrictive barrier (Fig. 54.11).
7. The left hand of the physician is repositioned to engage a different portion of the lumbar paraspinal musculature.
8. Repeat steps 5 to 7 in a rhythmic fashion for 2 to 5 minutes.
9. Success of the technique is determined by palpating the previously hypertonic lumbar musculature, which should be warmer and less hypertonic.

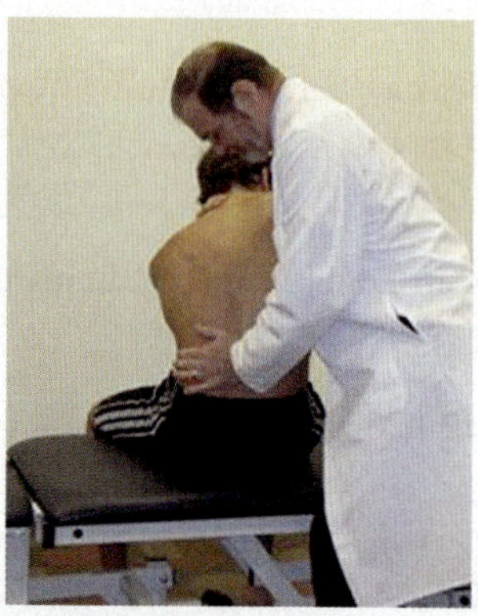

Figure 54.11. Lumbar seated technique position for paraspinal tissues, Step 6 in description.

Sacral Region: Bilateral Thumb Pressure to the Sacral Region

TYPE OF SOFT TISSUE TECHNIQUE

- Parallel traction

DIAGNOSES

- Hypertonicity of the multifidus and erector spinae musculature overlying the sacrum
- Somatic dysfunction of the sacrum

TREATMENT POSITION

Patient: Prone

Physician: Standing at the side of the treatment table at the level of the patient's thighs, facing the head of the patient

PROCEDURE

1. The physician's thumbs are placed on either side of the patient's spinous process of S1 (Fig. 54.12A,B).
2. Gently press down toward the table until sufficient pressure is in place to engage the sacral paravertebral musculature.
   - □ ***Note:*** Care must be taken not to exert excessive pressure, as this will compress the muscle against the bone and cause the patient unnecessary pain that may bruise the soft tissues.
3. The physician slides the thumbs superiorly to the extent permitted by the soft tissues, carrying the skin and musculature with them.
   - □ At the end of longitudinal glide, separate the thumbs slightly, exerting a lateral traction.
   - □ ***Note:*** Do not slide the thumbs over the surface of the skin.

A

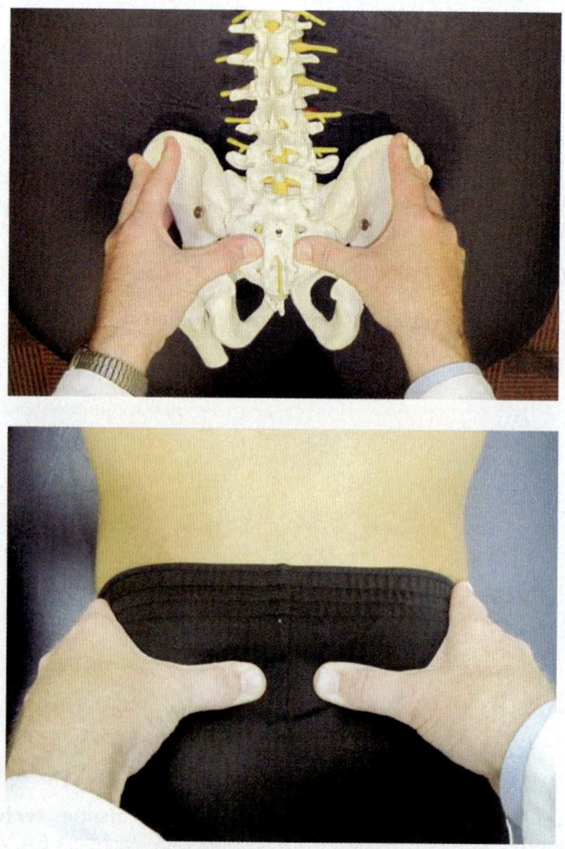

B

Figure 54.12. A and B. Bilateral thumb pressure–sacral region.

4. This position should be held for a short period of time. The tension should then be gradually released.
5. Reposition the thumbs half to one segment lower on the sacrum.
6. Repeat steps 2 to 4 for 2 or 3 minutes.
7. Success of the technique is determined by palpating the tissue tension in the previously hypertonic posterior sacral musculature, which should be less hypertonic.

Pelvic Region: Elbow Pressure to Piriformis Muscle

TYPE OF SOFT TISSUE TECHNIQUE

- Inhibitory pressure

DIAGNOSIS

- Hypertonicity of the piriformis muscle
- Somatic dysfunction of the pelvis

TREATMENT POSITION

Patient: Lateral recumbent with the hypertonic piriformis muscle away from the table

Physician: Standing at the side of the treatment table, facing the patient at the level of the patient's pelvis

PROCEDURE

1. Flex the patient's hips to 45 degrees, and knees to 90 degrees.
2. The hypertonic muscle can be located at the superior posterior corner of the greater trochanter (Fig. 54.13).
3. The olecranon process of the physician's elbow is placed on top of this hypertonic fascicle of muscle (Fig. 54.14).
4. Press gently downward toward the table for 2 to 5 minutes, or until a softening (release) of the muscle is felt.

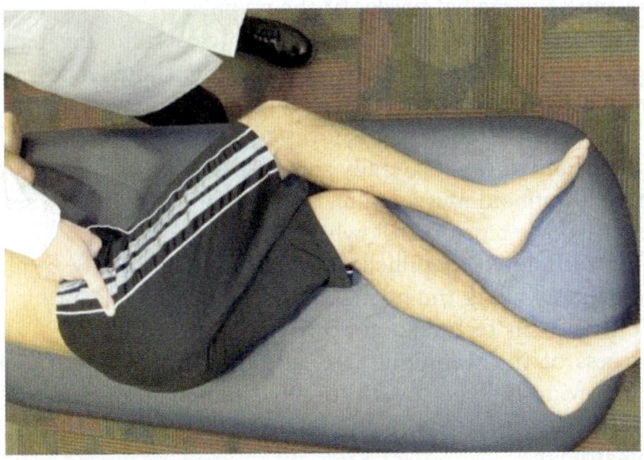

Figure 54.13. **Piriformis muscle technique, step 2 in description.**

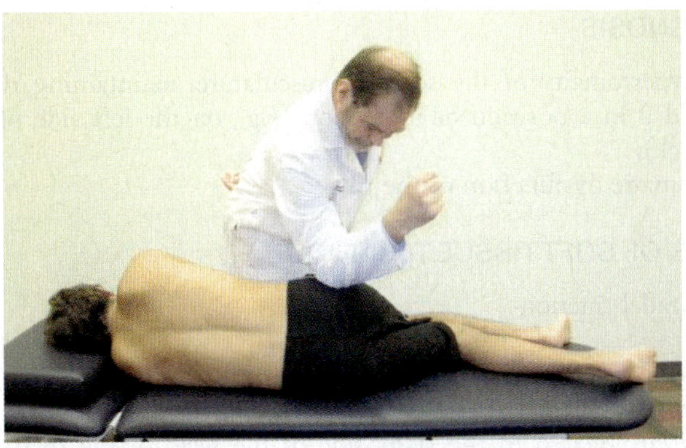

Figure 54.14. **Piriformis muscle technique, step 3 in description.**

   - ☐ ***Note:*** Care should be taken with this technique, as the olecranon is less sensitive to pressure than the hands, and neophytes often exert too much force. Therefore, the thumb of the opposite hand can be used to monitor the softening of the muscle under the pressure applied by the olecranon.
5. Success of the technique is determined by palpating the previously hypertonic piriformis muscle and noting that it is softer, more compliant, and less tender. With the hip held in a neutral position, internal rotation will also be freer following treatment.

Lower Extremity: Plantar Fascia Soft Tissue

DIAGNOSES

- Plantar fasciitis
- Rigid pes planus
- Somatic dysfunction of the lower extremity
- This technique is also helpful for patients in need of general relaxation and sedation

TREATMENT POSITION

Patient: Supine

Physician: Seated at the foot of the treatment table

PROCEDURE

1. Physician places one hand beneath the patient's heel to stabilize the foot (Fig. 54.15).
2. The physician makes a loose fist with the other hand, with the fingers positioned so that a smooth spiraling arc of a surface is created by the proximal phalanges of the fingers (Fig. 54.16).

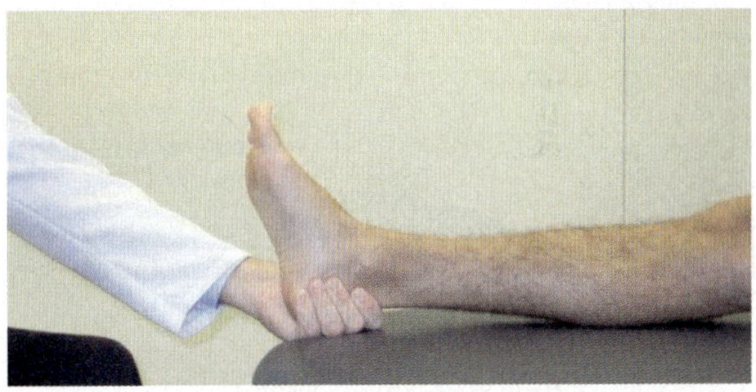

Figure 54.15. **Plantar fascia soft tissue, step 1.**

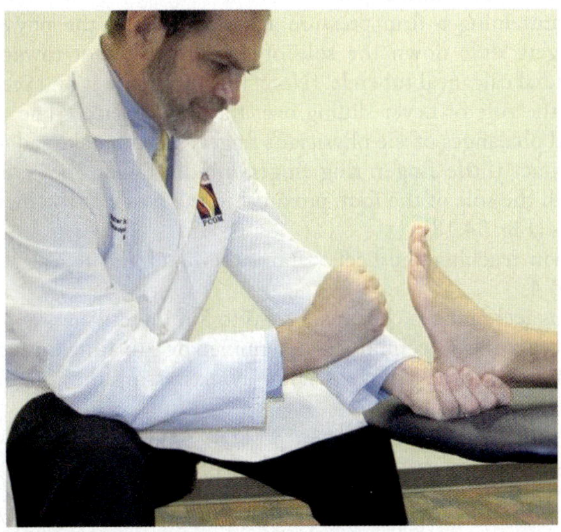

Figure 54.16. **Plantar fascia soft tissue, step 2.**

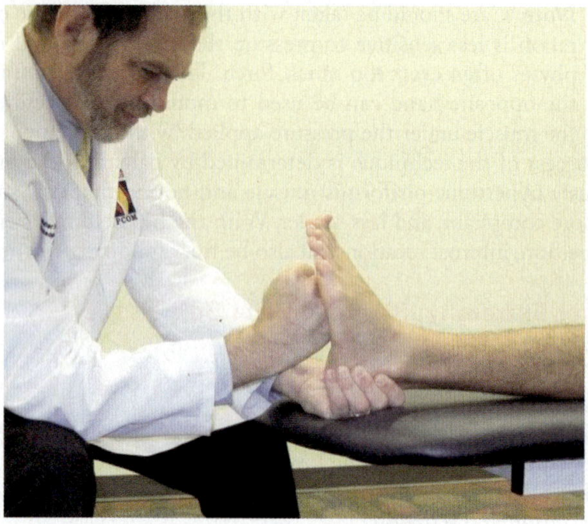

Figure 54.17. Plantar fascia soft tissue, step 3.

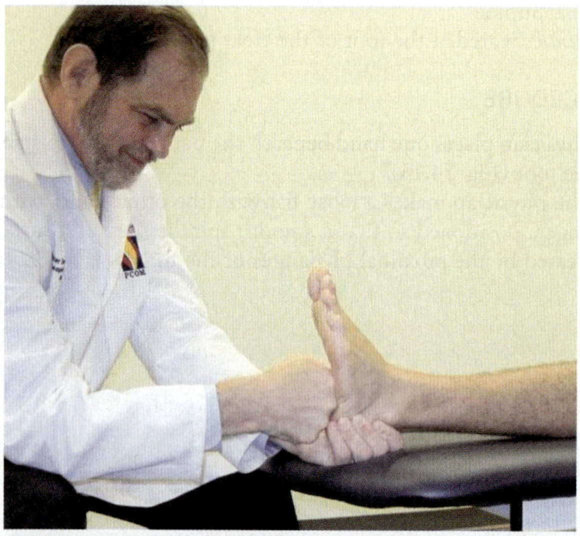

Figure 54.18. Plantar fascia soft tissue, step 4.

3. Physician contacts the sole of the patient's foot just proximal to the heads of the metatarsals, with the proximal phalanx of the little finger (Fig. 54.17).
4. Maintaining a firm pressure against the arch, the physician's fingers slide down the sole of the patient's foot toward the medial calcaneal tubercle. (Note: this technique is an exception to the rule of never sliding over the skin surface.) The proximal phalanges of the physician's fingers should make sequential contact (little finger, ring finger, middle finger, index finger) with the sole of the foot, proximal to the heads of the metatarsals (Fig. 54.18).
5. Upon reaching the heel, remove the hand and repeat steps 3 and 4.
6. This technique is continued for 3 to 5 minutes.
7. Success of this technique is determined by palpating for reduced tension in the plantar fascia, or by reassessing the mobility of the longitudinal arch.

Upper Extremity: Rhomboid Muscle Soft Tissue

TYPE OF SOFT TISSUE TECHNIQUE

- Parallel traction

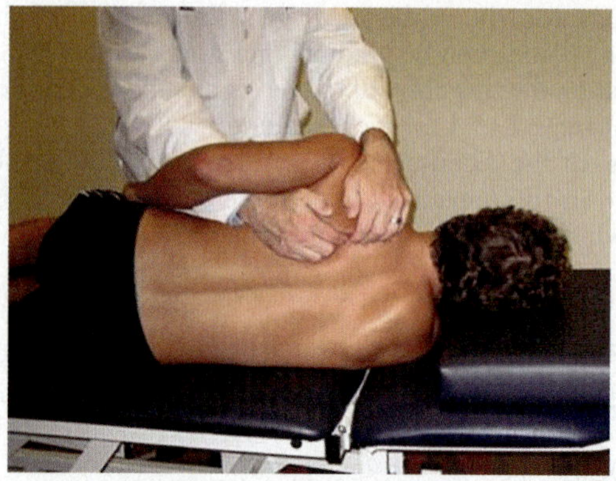

Figure 54.19. Rhomboid muscles soft tissue technique.

DIAGNOSIS

- Hypertonicity of the rhomboid musculature
- Somatic dysfunction of the upper extremity

TREATMENT POSITION

Patient: Lateral recumbent technique, with the rhomboid to be treated away from the table

Physician: Standing facing the patient, at the level of the patient's shoulder

PROCEDURE

1. Extend the patient's shoulder to 45 degrees and have the patient's hand rest on the lateral abdomen (Fig. 54.19).
2. The physician's caudal hand (that closest to the patient's feet) is passed under the patient's arm, with the pads of the fingers grasping the medial border of the scapula.
3. The physician's cephalad hand (that closest to the patient's head) contacts the anterior portion of the shoulder to provide an effective counterforce.
4. This cephalad hand then moves to the medial border of the scapula and draws it laterally and inferiorly, parallel to the fibers of the rhomboid musculature. This position is held for a second, and then the tension is slowly released.
5. This technique is applied slowly and rhythmically, gradually progressing along the medial border of the scapula.
6. Continue this technique for 3 to 5 minutes.
7. Success of the technique is determined through palpation of the previously hypertonic rhomboid musculature. Success may also be determined in part by reassessing the patient's symptomatology.

Rib Region: Scalene Muscle Stretching

DIAGNOSIS

- Hypertonicity of the scalene musculature, maintaining ribs 1 and 2 in a position of inhalation (e.g., on the left side of the neck).
- Somatic dysfunction of the ribs

TYPE OF SOFT TISSUE TECHNIQUE

- Parallel traction

TREATMENT POSITION

Patient: Supine

Physician: Seated to the right side of the head of the treatment table

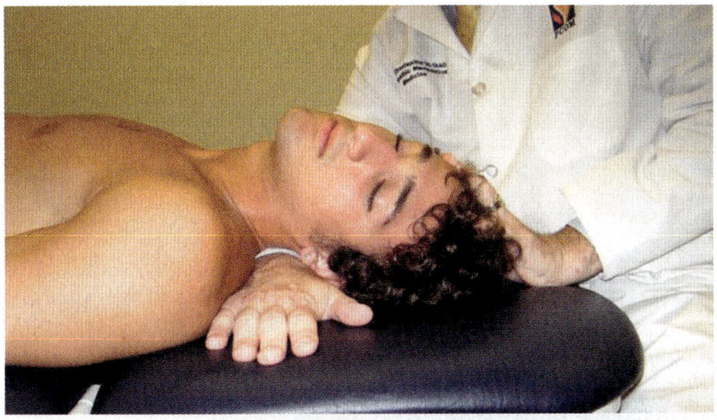

Figure 54.20. Scalene stretching initial position.

PROCEDURE (FOR EXAMPLE OF LEFT INHALED RIBS 1 AND 2 AND HYPERTONIC LEFT SCALENES)

1. Physician's right arm is passed beneath the patient's neck, with the hand adjacent to the patient's left shoulder (Fig. 54.20).
2. Gently, using the physician's left hand, the patient's head is rolled along the physician's right arm, from the physician's right fingers toward the right elbow, until the head is rotated 45 to 60 degrees from the midline.
3. The patient's head is allowed to drop over the physician's forearm, placing the anterolateral cervical musculature on stretch.
   - Physician may have to raise the elbow slightly off the table.
4. Slowly, the physician rolls the head slightly further through the soft tissue restrictive barrier, simultaneously pressing the head gently down toward the table. This position is held for a moment and then released, allowing the head to rise and roll back to just inside the restrictive barrier.
5. This technique is applied slowly and rhythmically, gradually increasing the amount of stretching.
6. Continue this technique for 3 to 5 minutes.
7. Success of the technique is determined by reassessing freedom of motion of the first and second ribs, and by palpating the previously hypertonic scalene musculature. Success is also in part determined by reassessing the patient's symptoms.

Abdominal Region: Lateral Abdominal Wall Soft Tissue

DIAGNOSIS

- Hypertonicity of the lateral abdominal wall musculature
- Somatic dysfunction of the abdomen

TYPE OF SOFT TISSUE TECHNIQUE

- Perpendicular traction or parallel traction, depending upon the muscle layer of interest

TREATMENT POSITION

Patient: Prone

Physician: Standing at the side of the table, on the side opposite of the hypertonic musculature

PROCEDURE

1. The physician wraps one hand around the lateral abdominal wall, making palmar contact as complete as possible (Fig. 54.21).

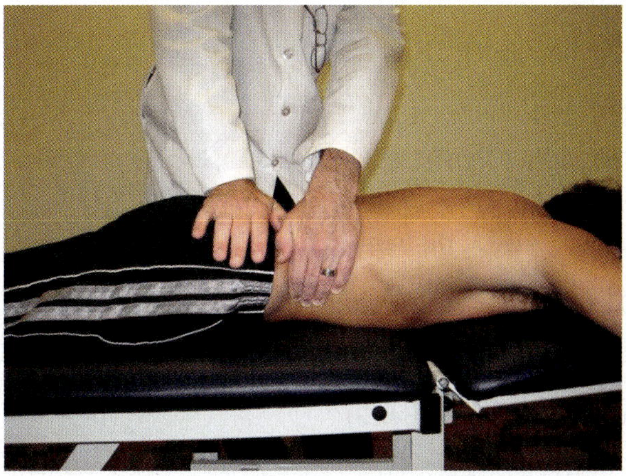

Figure 54.21. Lateral abdominal wall soft tissue technique.

2. The physician's other hand is placed on the patient's iliac crest, with the heel of the hand near the posterior superior iliac spine.
3. The abdominal wall is drawn toward the physician, while simultaneously increasing anterior pressure on the patient's iliac crest to maintain the pelvis in place.
4. This position is held for a second, then released, allowing the abdominal musculature to draw back to its position just inside the restrictive barrier.
5. Reposition the hands slightly on the abdominal wall and repeat.
6. Continue steps 3 to 5 rhythmically for 3 to 5 minutes.
7. Success of the technique is determined by palpating the previously hypertonic abdominal muscles.

CASE VIGNETTE

A 54-year-old man presents to the office with a sore throat and dry cough. He complains of an ulcer on the buccal surface of his left cheek. He admits to having similar ulcers around his mouth in the past. He denies other complaints.

PHYSICAL EXAMINATION

Vital signs are normal. Examination of the buccal mucosa reveals a shallow ulcer with a red border, approximately 2 mm in diameter; tongue is in the midline; there is no tonsillar hypertrophy or erythema; teeth are in good repair. Small left submental node is palpable. CV, pulmonary, abdominal, and neurologic exams are noncontributory. Structural exam reveals rigid, tender, hypertonic paravertebral musculature from the C5–T2 spinal levels bilaterally. Rib 1 on the left is held in inhalation.

DIAGNOSIS

- Acute herpetic stomatitis
- Somatic dysfunction—cervical, thoracic, rib

PLAN

1. Treatment with antiviral medication
2. Soft tissue technique on the hypertonic cervicothoracic musculature
3. Articulatory technique for the inhaled rib dysfunction

SOFT TISSUE TECHNIQUE

Inhibition

TREATMENT POSITION

Patient: Supine
Physician: Seated at the head of the table

PROCEDURE

1. Physician places the pads of the fingers of both hands beneath the cervicothoracic junction, just lateral to the spinous processes (Fig. 54.22).
2. Physician extends the cervicothoracic junction until the musculature is felt to relax under the fingers.
3. Physician then maintains a deep sustained pressure over these muscles until they are further felt to soften (release). This may require anywhere from 30 seconds to several minutes.
4. Success of the technique is determined through palpation to reassess the characteristics of the soft tissues that led to the chosen treatment technique. Success may also be determined in part by reassessing the patient's symptomatology (sore throat and cough).

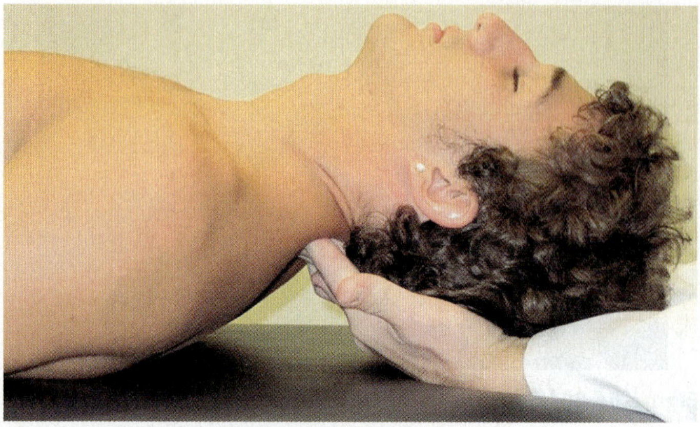

Figure 54.22. Cervicothoracic inhibition technique.

REFERENCES

1. *Glossary of Osteopathic Terminology*. American Association of Colleges of Osteopathic Medicine; 2011:32.
2. Hensel K. *A Teaching Guide for Osteopathic Manipulative Medicine.* 2nd ed. American Association of Colleges of Osteopathic Medicine; 2018: 105–114.
3. Still AT. The autobiography of Andrew Taylor Still. Published by the author; 1908:32.

55

Visceral Manipulation

KENNETH LOSSING ▪ REBECCA E. GIUSTI

KEY CONCEPTS

- Visceral manipulation (also called ventral technique) is a system of diagnosis and treatment directed to the viscera and/or supportive structures to improve physiologic function.
- Impaired or altered mobility/motility of the visceral system is reflected in abnormal motion tests showing change in distensibility of attachments or change in normal viscoelasticity.
- Visceral and pelvic pathologic processes have concomitant spinal effects; for a visceral problem resulting from a somatovisceral reflex, the somatic structure responsible is treated; if a visceral or somatic problem is caused from a viscerosomatic reflex, the viscera responsible is treated.
- In the case of viscerovisceral reflex causing a visceral problem, both involved viscera are treated.
- The following treatments will be discussed; the approach to the viscera from a neurologic standpoint (paraspinal inhibition, also known as colonic stimulation and inhibition of the collateral ganglia); pumps addressing the liver and spleen; the approach to the viscera from a respiratory-circulatory standpoint (cecal, sigmoid, and root of the mesentery lifts); treatment of what may be considered to be reflexogenic zones (the gastroesophageal (GE) junction, pylorus, sphincter of Oddi, and ileocecal valve) and treatment of the main bronchus and lungs.

INTRODUCTION AND DEFINITION

Visceral approach/manipulation (VIS) is defined as an osteopathic method of diagnosis and treatment applied to the viscera and/or the supportive structures to improve physiologic function. Historically, this approach was referred to as ventral techniques.[1]

During osteopathic treatment, the viscera are typically moved toward their fascial attachments to a point of fascial balance.

Direct palpation, evaluation, diagnosis, and treatment of the viscera have existed since the time of Dr. A.T. Still. This valuable approach opens the doors to being able to help a wide range of functional disorders. A visceral dysfunction is defined as "impaired or altered mobility or motility of the visceral system and related fascial, neurological, vascular, skeletal, and lymphatic elements." This is reflected in abnormal motion tests, showing a change in the distensibility of visceral attachments, or a change in their normal viscoelasticity, among other physical findings.

There are different aspects/models of a visceral dysfunction, each equally valid:

- Fascial model—tested with motion testing and fascial pull (listening technique)
- Fluid model—arterial and venous blood, interstitial fluids, and lymphatics can be tested with palpation, Doppler ultrasound, or perfusion studies as necessary
- Respiratory model—excursion of tissue with respiration can be tested with palpation, fluoroscopy, or real-time MRI
- Neurologic model—tested with palpation and motion testing or EMG
- Inherent motion model—tested with palpation/sensing
- Temperature changes/energy/emotions—tested with palpation or thermography

HISTORY

Dr. Still developed osteopathy in the late 19th century. He had been trained as a medical doctor but found that he could treat most diseases by palpating dysfunctional areas and treating them with his hands. He called this new science osteopathy, meaning to "begin with the bones." Finding where the bones are not properly aligned and where they are not moving properly, can guide the physician to the area of the body that needs to be treated, as they reflect where the forces of life are not functioning properly. Notice that Dr. Still "began with the bones" but did not end there. In his writing, he constantly talked about joints, fascia, blood supply, nerves, internal organs, and lymphatic flow. Dr. Still, and his students, treated all of the known medical diseases of the day.

Osteopathic manipulation of the viscera began with Dr. Still. He described treating many different digestive, respiratory, and urogenital complaints.[2] For Dr. Still, almost all medical conditions had an osteopathic treatment, in some cases curative and in some cases supportive. Dr. Still described very few actual techniques in his writings; the most specific information was in his last book, *Research and Practice*, published in 1911. However, thankfully, some of his early students, McConnell[3] and Barber,[4] recorded techniques they learned from Dr. Still.

There are many principles that we can learn from Dr. Still. For instance, when treating appendicitis, he would treat the colon first and then the spine. In treating colic, he treated the spine first and then the colon. Although he never spoke of his rationale, we can presume that there are instances when the primary somatic dysfunction may rest within the viscera and should be treated first or conversely, that the primary somatic dysfunction may reside within the spine.

One of Dr. Still's earliest students, Carl McConnell, MD, DO, graduated from the American School of Osteopathy in 1901 and stayed on as an instructor for some years. Dr. McConnell was very prolific, writing six books and over 250 articles.[3] Among this body of literature, he described direct treatment of all of the viscera, except the lungs and the heart. Dr. McConnell wrote over 10 different articles describing various visceral technique principles. He states:

Those who overlook ventral (visceral) technique are practicing a greatly limited osteopathy. In fact, confining osteopathic adjustment to the posterior plane (no matter how fundamental spinal therapy is) means the neglect of essential factors that even enter into vertebral and pelvic pathology. Structural lesions of the chest, abdomen, and pelvis frequently originate primarily within these cavities. Of course these structural changes present concomitant affects in the spine, and vice versa.

There is no organ of the abdomen and pelvis that cannot be influenced by improving the structural and physiological balance through direct adjustment methods.[3]

One of Dr. Still's most enlightening statements, from an embryologic, physiologic, biologic and technical standpoint, may be this:

It is only the perfection of the organism and the connected oneness that is the keynote to osteopathic practice. Every part has a duty to perform not only for its own maintenance, but also for the health and harmony of the interrelated whole. This is part of the law of supply and demand, which is absolute through all of nature. It is important to know the exact place that each organ and tissue occupies in its normal position. It is only by knowing the normal we are able to detect the abnormal. Each organ seems to be a creator of its own fluid substances. We must know the nerve and blood supply and the drainage.

Dr. Still often told his students that DO stands for "Dig On," encouraging them to expand their view of osteopathy.[5] One of Dr. Still's other early students, William Garner Sutherland, DO, credited Still with the original idea of the cranial concept that Dr. Sutherland later expanded, developed, and taught.[6] While Dr. Sutherland is most known for his work in the cranial area, he never implied that it should be the only area diagnosed or treated. He gave multiple references to treating the viscera (see also Chapter 42 Internal Organ Assessment for Visceral Motion Dysfunction for further details on diagnosing visceral dysfunction).

Jacques Weischenck, DO, wrote one of the first textbooks on visceral technique *Traite d'osteopathie Viscerale* in 1982.[7] His concept of organs having a normal axis of motion during respiration, which becomes perturbed in a dysfunction, was later tested and demonstrated by two of his students, Georges Finet, DO,[8] and Christian Williamae, DO.

The most prolific author, innovator, and teacher of visceral manipulation has been Jean-Pierre Barral. He graduated from the European School of Osteopathy in Maidstone, England, at a time when British osteopathy consisted of spinal diagnosis and treatment. Most of the early American literature was also not easily available. Barral applied the concepts he had learned for the spine in developing visceral approaches. Barral's books,[9] energy, enthusiasm, and love of teaching have resulted in visceral manipulation spreading across the world.

THEORETICAL CONSIDERATIONS

Virtually all forms of organ injury start with molecular or structural alterations in cells, a concept first put forth in the 19th century by Rudolf Virchow, known as the father of modern pathology. We therefore begin our consideration of pathology with the study of the origins, molecular mechanisms, and structural changes of cell injury. Yet different cells in tissues constantly interact with each other, and an elaborate system of extracellular matrix is necessary for the integrity of organs. Cell–cell and cell–matrix interactions contribute significantly in response to injury, leading collectively to tissue and organ injury, which are as important as cell injury in defining the morphologic and clinical patterns of disease.[10]

In order to understand visceral approaches in osteopathy, it will be helpful to review/update some basic science. Advances in biology, embryology, physics, and physiology over the last several years have dramatically changed how scientists view the mechanical forces generated, utilized, and distributed during human life.

In the past, genetics had primacy among proposed explanatory models. During the 1960s, the German embryologist Blechschmidt[11] questioned this idea. Based on the microscopic dissection of very young embryos, he concluded that mechanical forces generated during embryologic cellular growth interact with the environment to change the way the cell functions and what it develops into. Cellular circulation, metabolism, and waste removal start as soon as there are cells. Differential growth patterns between the central nervous system, the vascular system, various organ systems, and the musculoskeletal system, cause tension and compression forces to affect the shape and function of the cells.

Humphrey and Delance state[12]:

It is now known that many cell types express different genes (i.e., perform different functions) in response to even small changes in their mechanical environment.

In the past, the organelles inside of cells were thought to be floating in the intercellular fluid, as a sort of soup. It turns out that this is not the case. The organelles, cellular membrane, and nucleus are all interconnected by microtubules that act like a cellular skeleton and microfilaments that give elastic support to the cell.[13]

With the discovery of integral proteins (integrins) in the cellular membrane, more is known about the mechanical links between the cell, the extracellular matrix, and all tissue systems.[14] Integrins mechanically connect the cell membrane with microfilaments, microtubules, the cell nucleus, and DNA, with the extracellular matrix, transmitting mechanical forces of tension and compression throughout the whole organism.

Visceral ligaments are viscoelastic,[15] that is, they act both like a fluid and like a solid. Visceral ligaments can respond to a "strain" (compression or tension) biomechanically speaking, with both elastic and plastic properties, depending on the amount of force and the amount of time over which the strain is applied. A compression of these viscoelastic ligaments may also affect the vasculature that passes through and supplies the viscera.

A visceral dysfunction of the lungs and airways will have related spinal and rib dysfunctions, cranial dysfunctions, neurologic dysfunctions, lymphatic and other fluid dysfunctions, and temperature imbalances (see Chapter 42 Internal Organ Assessment for Visceral Motion Dysfunction for further discussion). The art of practice is to find the most efficient treatment order and the most effective treatment that the body can accept.

INDICATIONS, CONTRAINDICATIONS, AND COMPLICATIONS

The indications for visceral technique can be categorized into the following:

1. Visceral dysfunctions associated with known medical diagnosis. Almost all medical diagnoses of the viscera have a component that is functional, in other words, can be altered. Since the functional component cannot be recognized with lab or radiologic test, the only way to find out is to treat it. Generally, one to three treatments will reveal if an osteopathic approach is helpful and cost-effective.
2. Visceral dysfunctions are mechanically connected to somatic dysfunction. The viscera are connected to the musculoskeletal

system by connective tissue forming functional chains that connect from head to toe, all of the anatomical structures.

Contraindications to visceral treatment include treating pathologic anatomical disruption and deformities, such as a dissecting abdominal aneurysm, potential internal bleeding, infections uncontrolled by antibiotics, severe pain induced by palpation or manipulation, fractures at the site of treatment and other medical indications for emergent medical workup.

In terms of safety and efficacy, there are no documented adverse effects at this time.[16–18]

Visceral treatment is generally very safe and well tolerated by patients. However, it cannot be stressed enough that the patient should always be approached as a whole. A detailed history and physical should be performed in order to elucidate any contraindications listed above. An emergent situation should be treated accordingly. OMT is not a substitute for warranted emergent medical intervention. Likewise, OMT is often invaluable to a stabilized patient who benefits from improved lymphatic drainage, balance of the autonomic nervous system, reduced symptoms and decreased healing time.

The dosage of OMT will vary depending on the patient and the dysfunction. Hospitalized patients may only be able to tolerate 5 minutes of treatment at a time. Likewise, the frequency may be two to three times daily in acute illness, such as ileus, two to three times weekly for subacute conditions and weekly to monthly for chronic or long-term illnesses. The duration of treatment is determined by re-evaluation of the patient's clinical status and response to treatment.

PALPATION AND DIAGNOSIS

Palpation of the viscera starts with being able to identify the individual organs. This process is addressed in detail in Chapter 42 Internal Organ Assessment for Visceral Motion Dysfunction. The liver, for instance, is easy to identify and palpate for texture, outline, and size. The lungs, however, present some challenges. How is it possible to palpate through the ribcage to feel a lung? Perhaps not as difficult as one might expect, if one remembers Newton's second law: "For every action there is an equal and opposite reaction." In this case, performing a layer palpation on the thorax will reveal skin, superficial fascia, muscles, ribs, endothoracic fascia, pleura, and finally the lungs. As one compresses deeper, each layer will press back into the hand. At each layer, one can palpate for fascial pulling in the direction of tension, dysfunction, and motion test for directions of ease and directions of increased tension, a barrier.

THEORY OF VISCERAL MANIPULATION

Visceral manipulation treats palpable motion dysfunction of viscera to improve physiologic function. This is consistent with the osteopathic theory that states that improved motion leads to improved function. In addition, visceral manipulation applies osteopathic philosophy, principles and practices to visceral dysfunction; this involves addressing related components of the musculoskeletal, neurologic, respiratory, and circulatory systems and application of concepts related to osteopathic cranial manipulative medicine and other OMT approaches as well. In all cases, the theory and principles remain the same; only the area of anatomy changes. The implication, of course, is that by also addressing the viscera, the osteopathic physician is able to address a larger range of medical problems.

PRINCIPLES OF TREATMENT

For a visceral problem resulting from a somatovisceral reflex, the somatic structure responsible is treated. If a visceral or somatic problem is caused by a viscerosomatic reflex, the viscera are treated. In the case of viscerovisceral reflex causing a visceral problem, both involved viscera are treated.

Once the area of the most primary problem is found, it may be addressed by a wide variety of principles and techniques, including short lever arm (direct contact), long lever arm (using a body part as a lever), indirect (in the direction of ease), and direct techniques (in the direction of tension) and various activating forces like respiratory assistance.

As previously mentioned, visceral ligaments are viscoelastic,[15] that is, they have the properties of both a fluid and a solid. Visceral dysfunction can be caused by numerous factors. These may include but are not limited to any of or a combination of trauma, mechanical stress, emotions, chemical imbalances, circulation problems, imbalances in the nervous system, imbalances in circulation of life forces, and hormonal imbalances.

Visceral ligaments can respond to a "strain" (compression or tension) biomechanically speaking, with both elastic and plastic properties, depending on the amount of force and the amount of time over which the strain is applied. In an elastic deformation, the tissue returns to its original shape and configuration once the straining force is removed. In a plastic deformation, the original shape and distensibility are altered, with a resulting storage of force. In a visceral dysfunction, the stress in the ligament has a certain amount of force stored (as potential energy or "potency"), in a certain direction, and that tissue has a certain speed that it will respond to. This results in an altered viscoelasticity curve for that ligament. (The viscosity is more; the elasticity is less.)

Therefore, in visceral dysfunction, applying a force that is exactly matched to the dysfunctional strain in force, direction, and speed, will result in tissue change and its return to a more physiologic normal distensibility. In the process, there is a dissipation of heat, movement of fluid, and a restructuring of the elasticity curve. A dysfunction can be caused by any of or a combination of trauma, mechanical stress, emotions, chemical imbalances, circulation problems, imbalances in the nervous system, imbalances in circulation of life forces, and hormonal imbalances.

The arteries, veins, nerves, and lymphatic channels to the internal organs all go through the visceral attachments (ligaments). If there is increased mechanical tension in the visceral ligaments, the first fluid vessels to become compressed and therefore compromised are those of the least pressure, the lymphatic vessels and veins, leading to a relative edema, with retention of metabolic by-products.

Any occlusion of lymphatic vessels is followed by the abnormal accumulation of interstitial fluid in the affected part, referred to as obstructive lymphedema.[10]

With sustained or increased tension, the arterial vessels can become compressed, leading to decreased nutrition, oxygen, and eventually death.

The goal of treatment is achieving a state of balanced ligamentous tension, balanced mechanical tension, normal motion with respiration, balanced inherent motion, and proper functioning of the viscera through normalization of both the nervous system and fluid, nutrition, and pressure exchange.

EXAMPLES OF TECHNIQUE

The following techniques address the neurologic model of osteopathic care in that the osteopathic physician is not contacting the viscera directly but is affecting the somatic structures related to innervation.

PARASPINAL INHIBITION

This is also known as ileus prevention technique or colonic stimulation (analogous to the rib raising technique in the thoracic spine). In some studies, this technique has been associated with decreased time to flatus and decreased hospital stay after a gastrointestinal surgery.[19,20]

The goal of the technique is to decrease sympathetic hyperactivity of the GI system and restore normal bowel function. Contraindications or cautions may include infection of the region to be treated, presence of incision to that region and thoracolumbar fracture.

Diagnosis

A patient presenting with ileus or at risk for developing an ileus.

Set-up

The patient is supine. The physician is seated at either side of the patient.

Treatment

1. The physician places both hands side by side under the patient's thoracolumbar spine with the fingerpads on the opposite side of the spine contacting the lateral aspect of the erector spinae mass and the thenar and hypothenar eminences contacting the lateral aspect of the erector spinae issue on the side of the patient nearest the physician.
2. The physician then flexes the fingerpads toward the base of the palms, which effectively compresses or approximates the erector spinae masses and draws the thoracolumbar spine into extension.
3. The physician finds a point of tissue tension balance or equalization by adjusting the pressure between the two hands. This may be achieved by moving the forearms closer or farther from the patient's body, and by alternating the pressure between the two hands to match the tension in the paraspinal tissues.
4. Once this balance is achieved the physician maintains this tension on the erector spinae muscles until a sense of release or relaxation is sensed. This usually takes 60 to 90 seconds.
5. These above steps may be repeated until tissue tension at that region is greatly decreased or completely resolved upon reassessment[19,21,22] (Fig. 55.1).

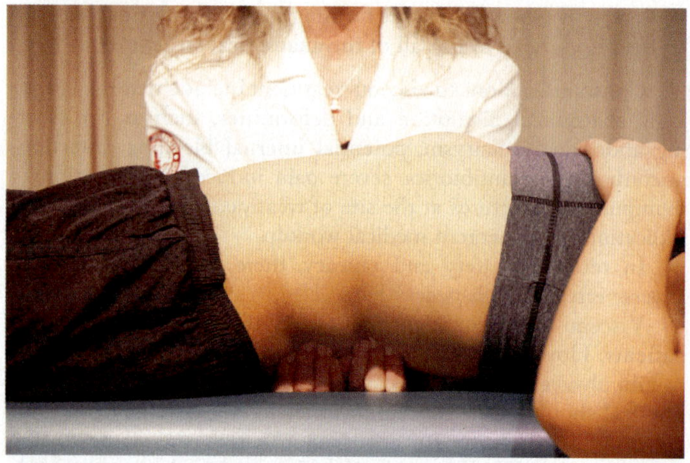

Figure 55.1. Paraspinal inhibition. (Courtesy of Western University of Health Sciences, Pomona, CA, used with permission.)

ASSESSMENT OF COLLATERAL GANGLIA

Diagnosis

1. Patient supine.
2. The physician stands at the patient's side, facing the patient's abdomen.
3. To ensure equal depth of penetration of the tissues when applying pressure to the ganglia, the physician standardizes the length of the fingers of the palpating hand by flexing the longer fingers. The ganglia are located along the patient's midline as follows: the celiac ganglion is located inferior to the xiphoid process; the inferior mesenteric ganglion is located just superior to the umbilicus; the superior mesenteric ganglion is located between those two regions.
4. The physician assesses the tenderness and tension of the soft subcutaneous tissues over each ganglia (celiac, superior mesenteric, and inferior mesenteric) by sensing each region with the palpating hand and applying pressure with the other hand.

If a region or regions over a ganglion is diagnosed as tense or tender, the physician may then apply the collateral ganglia inhibition technique described below[21] (Fig. 55.2).

Collateral Ganglia Inhibition

May be applied to celiac, superior mesenteric, or inferior mesenteric ganglia

Treatment

1. Once an area of increased tension or tenderness is diagnosed as per above, the physician will use the same handhold as described above to contact the midline of the abdomen over the facilitated ganglion.
2. The physician applies posterior pressure to that area until resistance is palpated.
3. The physician instructs the patient to inhale partially (sometimes called "taking a half-breath in") against the physician's applied resistance and instructs the patient to hold that partial inhalation for as long as possible.

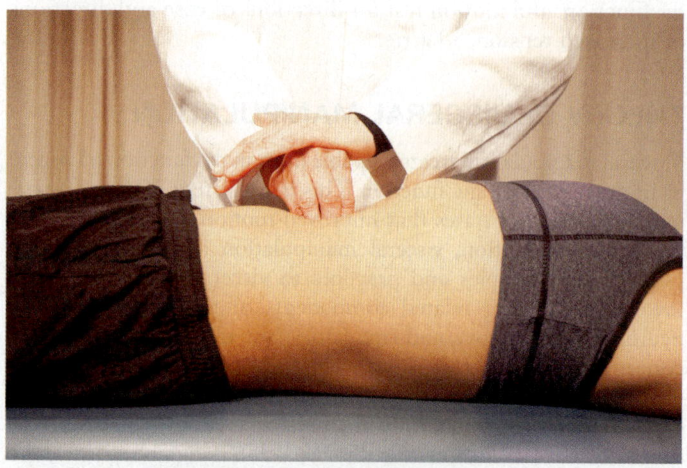

Figure 55.2. Collateral ganglia inhibition. (Courtesy of Western University of Health Sciences, Pomona, CA, used with permission.)

4. As the patient exhales, the physician gently increases their pressure as tolerated by the tissues as they relax, until the next barrier of restriction is met.
5. The physician repeats the above steps until significant decrease or no further tension or tenderness is identified.
6. The physician should reassess by palpating that same region with the initial diagnostic pressure. The patient should no longer report tenderness and the tissues should feel soft and compliant upon palpation.[21]

The following visceral techniques may be categorized as following the respiratory-circulatory model and employ the viscoelastic properties of the targeted viscera and its supporting and/or surrounding tissues.

CECUM AND SIGMOID RELEASES

Diagnosis

Findings of fascial restriction during an abdominal exam or underlying visceral dysfunction determined by history and physical exam.

Set-Up

The patient is supine. The patient's knee on the side to be treated may be slightly flexed to relax the targeted abdominal tissues. The physician stands at the left side of the patient to address the cecum and at the right side of the patient to address the sigmoid.

Treatment

1. The physician contacts the left or right lower quadrant of abdomen with the ulnar edges of their fingers.
2. The physician gently scoops the colon out of the pelvis in line with the attachments in the distal corners of the lower abdomen (sigmoid guided in a diagonal line toward the liver; cecum guided in a diagonal line toward the spleen).
3. The colon and its surrounding tissues are taken gently into this right angle toward their mesenteric attachments until resistance is sensed.
4. The colon may then recede back (recoil) to its corner. The physician follows this recoil and then repeats the above steps three to four times until that aspect of the colon is compliant to motion testing.
5. This technique may also be done as follows: once the physician draws the colon and its surrounding tissues to the point of resistance, the physician instructs the patient to inhale partially and hold their breath until forced to exhale.
6. As the patient exhales, the physician may engage a new restrictive barrier. This cycle of respiration and engaging the new restrictive barrier of the tissues is repeated (generally three to four times) until there is a sense of compliance and relaxation of the involved tissues and structures.
7. To retest, the physician will gently scoop the colon out of the pelvis toward the mesenteric attachments. With this maneuver, no further fascial restriction should be palpated[23] (Figs. 55.3 and 55.4).

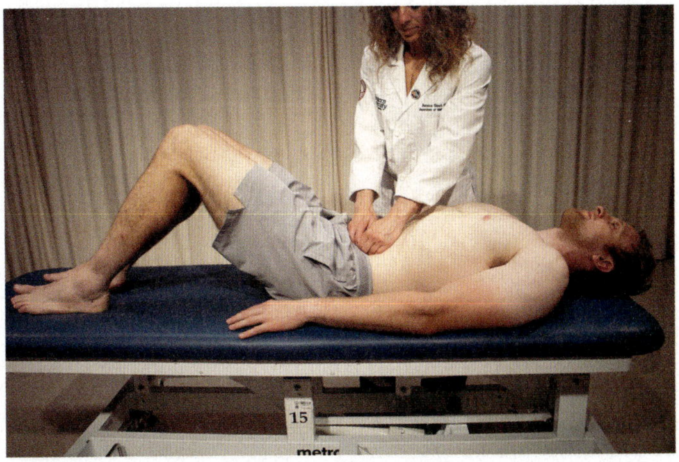

Figure 55.3. Sigmoid release (lateral view). (Courtesy of Western University of Health Sciences, Pomona, CA, used with permission.)

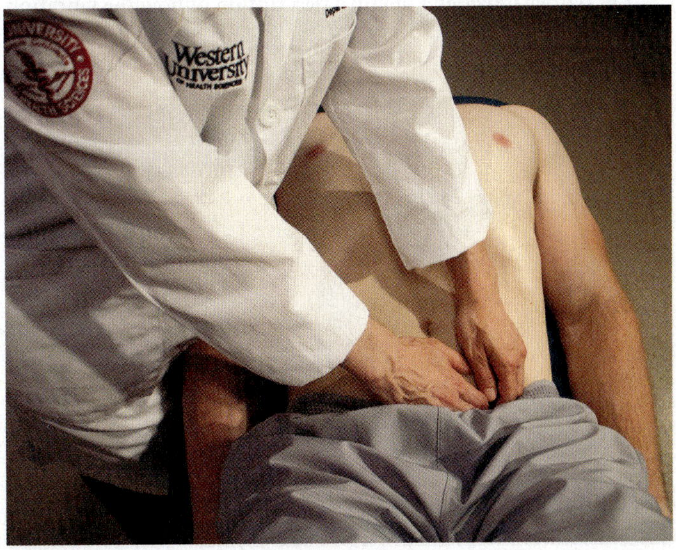

Figure 55.4. Sigmoid release (overhead view). (Courtesy of Western University of Health Sciences, Pomona, CA, used with permission.)

ROOT OF THE MESENTERY RELEASE

Diagnosis

Findings of fascial restriction during an abdominal exam or underlying visceral dysfunction determined by history and physical exam.

Set-Up

Patient supine. The physician stands at the patient's right side.

Treatment

1. The root of the mesentery is roughly at a 45-degree angle, beginning 1 inch cephalad and 1 inch leftward from the umbilicus, ending near the right sacroiliac joint. It is roughly 6 inches long and serves as the attachment of about 30 feet of intestines.
2. The physician contacts the tissues over the root of the mesentery by allowing the ulnar aspects of the hands or the fingerpads to sink into the tissue through anterior parietal peritoneum, greater omentum, and loops of small intestine until the root of the mesentery is palpated as a cord-like structure.
3. The physician then draws the root of the mesentery toward the hepatic flexure until resistance is met.
4. The physician may then use the patient's respiratory cooperation; the patient holds the breath in inhalation as long as possible until forced to exhale at which point the fascia will generally release allowing the physician to engage a new restrictive

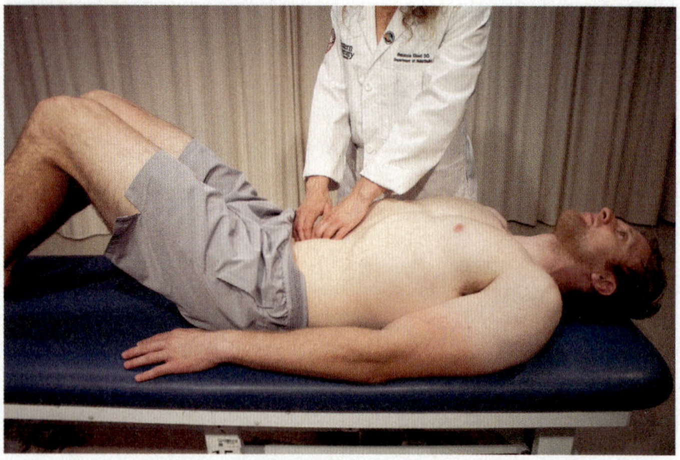

Figure 55.5. Root of the mesentery release (lateral view). (Courtesy of Western University of Health Sciences, Pomona, CA, used with permission.)

barrier. This is repeated five to six times until the root of the mesentery is compliant to motion testing.

5. Instead of employing respiratory cooperation, the physician may choose to hold the tissues to a point of tension until they recoil in which case the physician follows the recoil and repeats this procedure five to six times until the tissues are compliant and relaxed[23] (Figs. 55.5 and 55.6).

PUMPS

The liver and spleen pumps have been described in the 1898 3rd edition of Elmer D. Barber, DO's book, Osteopathy Complete.[4] Dr. Barber was a graduate of the American School of Osteopathy and had been a student of A.T. Still. As part of what appears to be a treatment protocol for "acute and chronic lithemia, biliousness or torpid liver, icterus or jaundice, acute hepatitis, perihepatitis, inflammation, and obstruction of the gall duct and hepatic colic he describes "placing the hand lightly over the liver; vibrate." The vibration may be 2 to 5 minutes depending on the condition and the nature of the tissues.

Dr. Barber provides a detailed description of how the vibration should occur:

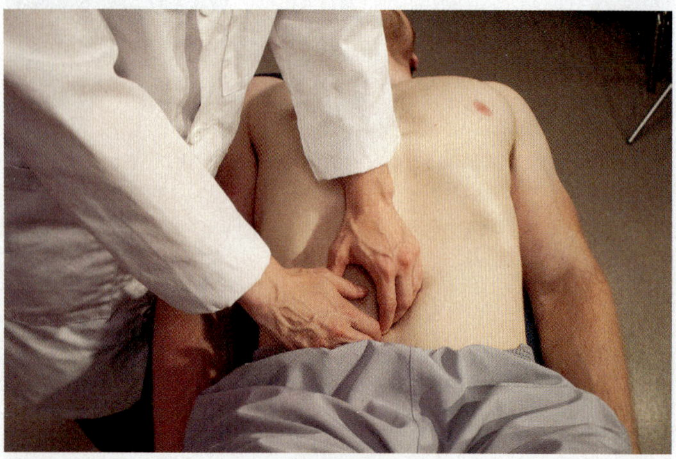

Figure 55.6. Root of the mesentery release (overhead view). (Courtesy of Western University of Health Sciences, Pomona, CA, used with permission.)

"We have recently discovered that vibration administered by the hand quickens, stimulates, strengthens, and assists very materially in reducing congestion and inflammation and is very beneficial in many cases...Vibration should be applied with a loose wrist joint, the whole or part of the palmar surface of the hand or fingers being used. The movement in the wrist-joint are abduction and adduction, while the movements of the elbow are flexion and extension; the hand lies immovable upon the part of the body on which it rests. Through a quick succession of individual movements with a perfectly loose wrist-joint the vibrations are produced. Flexion and extension of the wrist must be carefully guarded against, as this would produce pressure, which would be injurious in many localities. In fact, vibration correctly applied is such a wonderful instrument in relieving pain that we cannot impress this one point too forcibly upon the mind of our readers: *Always vibrate with a loose wrist-joint, using no greater pressure than the weight if the hand,* as the entire benefit to be derived from the treatment is lost if this point is neglected."[4]

"Vibrations might be compared to fine shaking movements in which the whole or part of the palmar surface of the fingers or hand is used....There should be no straining of the muscles in the operator's arm or strong contractions of the muscles of the hand, arm, or shoulder...To further give an idea of how delicately the movements should be made, place a tumbler of water upon a table, and if the vibrations are given absolutely correct upon the same, the water will not move from side to side, but simply quicken in the center. The table should be fairly large to make a fair test."[4]

The physiologic goal of the liver pump has been described as detoxification and mobilization of lymph. Indications have been described as passive hepatomegaly, chronic toxic conditions, epigastric lymphatic congestion. Contraindications or cautions depend on the patient's condition and the skill and knowledge of the physician but may include a friable liver,[21] thoracic cage fractures or dislocations, lymphatic malignancy, traumatic injury to the liver or adjacent organs, and acute hepatitis.

The liver pump is now thought to increase the ability of the Kupffer cells to interact with antigens and toxins in the lymph.[24]

The splenic pump was described by Dr. Barber as part of a treatment protocol for "splenitis, splenic hypertrophy, and tumor of the spleen."

The splenic pump was investigated in 1934 by Yale Castilo, DO, and Louise Ferris-Swift; DO who performed direct splenic stimulation (now known as splenic pump) on patients with acute infectious disease ($N = 100$). Their methodology and investigation were revisited using modern research standards by Noll, Johnson, and Brooks. They confirmed Castilo's and Ferris-Swift's original findings that the performance of the splenic pump was correlated with a posttreatment decrease in circulating erythrocytes, increase in reticulocyte count, phagocytic index, opsonic index, agglutinative power, and serum bacteriolytic power. However, Noll et al. found that 100 compressions, rather than 30 to 40 compressions demonstrated statistically significant changes compared to baseline for leukocyte and reticulocyte counts.[25]

LIVER PUMP: SUPINE

Set-Up

The physician stands at the right side of the supine patient, facing the patient's head.

Treatment

1. The physician passes the left hand underneath the lower ribs and the right hand on the abdominal wall immediately below the costal margin.

2. The patient inhales deeply while the physician identifies the inferior border of the liver with the fingertips of the right hand.
3. As the patient exhales, the physician penetrates the abdominal soft tissue over the liver and underneath the costal margin to access the liver.
4. The patient is instructed to take a deep breath and upon exhalation, the physician applies a vibratory force through the right hand to the liver.
5. This process is repeated, each time with the physician penetrating deeper into the subcostal area gaining more contact with the liver with the goal of reducing liver congestion or any tenderness that may be present.
6. Retest: improved motility and mobility of the liver, increased compliance and softness of the tissues may be noted upon completion.

LIVER PUMP: LATERAL RECUMBENT

Set-Up

The patient is positioned in a left lateral recumbent position with the hips and knees flexed to stabilize the body. The physician is seated on the table behind the thorax facing the patient's feet (Fig. 55.7).

Treatment

1. The patient places the right hand on the back of the physician's right shoulder.
2. The physician places both hands on the lower thoracic cage with the left hand on the anterior aspect and the right hand on the posterior aspect with the thumbs meeting at the axillary line.
3. The physician leans slightly backward to "open" the rib cage by increasing abduction to the patient's arm. The patient is instructed to inhale deeply.
4. As the patient exhales, the physician leans on the thoracic cage with both hands applying a vibratory motion to induce a pumping action to the liver.
5. The process is repeated, each time with the physician penetrating deeper into the subcostal area, gaining more contact with the liver with the goal of reducing liver congestion or any tenderness that may be present.
6. Retest: improved motility and mobility of the liver, increased compliance and softness of the tissues may be noted upon completion.

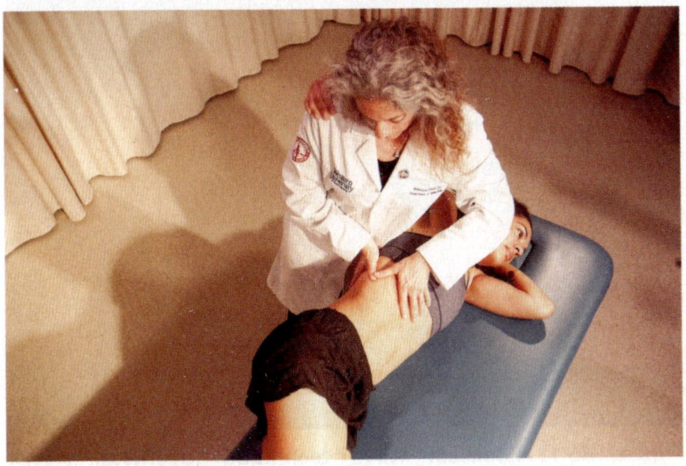

Figure 55.7. Lateral recumbent liver pump. (Courtesy of Western University of Health Sciences, Pomona, CA, used with permission.)

SPLEEN PUMP: SUPINE

Set-Up

The physician stands at the left side of the supine patient, facing the patient's head.

TREATMENT

1. The physician passes their right hand underneath the lower ribs and the left hand on the abdominal wall immediately below the costal margin.
2. The patient inhales deeply while the physician identifies the inferior border of the spleen with the tips of the fingers of the left hand.
3. As the patient exhales, the physician penetrates the abdominal soft tissue over the spleen and underneath the costal margin.
4. The patient is instructed to inhale deeply. As the patient exhales, the physician applies a vibratory force through the left hand to the spleen.
5. This process is repeated, each time with the physician penetrating deeper into the subcostal area gaining more contact with the spleen with the goal of reducing splenic congestion or any tenderness that may be present (Figs. 55.8 and 55.9).
6. Retest: improved motility and mobility of the spleen, increased compliance and softness of the tissues may be noted upon completion.

SPLEEN PUMP: LATERAL RECUMBENT

Set-Up

The patient is positioned in a right lateral recumbent position with the hips and knees flexed to stabilize the body. The physician is seated on the table behind the thorax, facing the patient's feet.

Treatment

1. The patient places the left hand on the back of the physician's left shoulder.
2. The physician places both hands on the lower thoracic cage with the right hand on the anterior aspect and the left hand on the posterior aspect with the thumbs meeting at the axillary line.

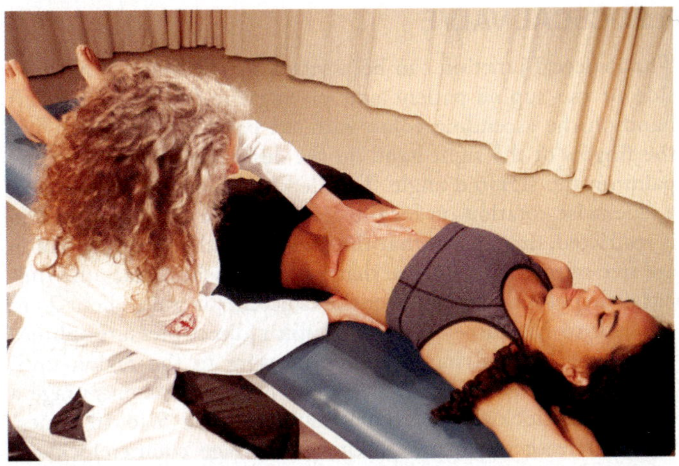

Figure 55.8. Spleen pump view. (Courtesy of Western University of Health Sciences, Pomona, CA, used with permission.)

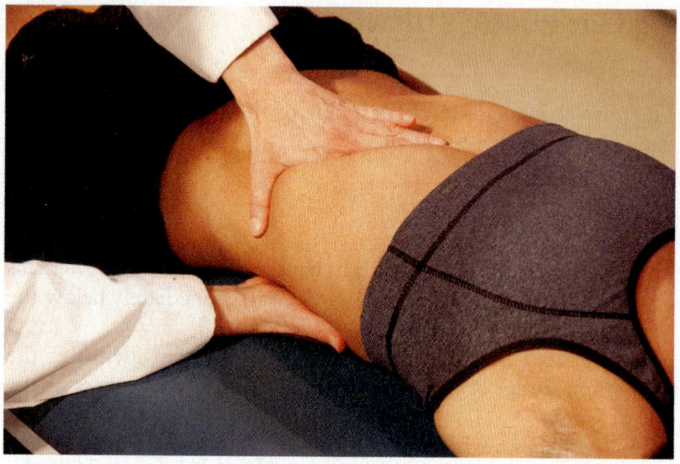

Figure 55.9. Spleen pump view (close up view). (Courtesy of Western University of Health Sciences, Pomona, CA, used with permission.)

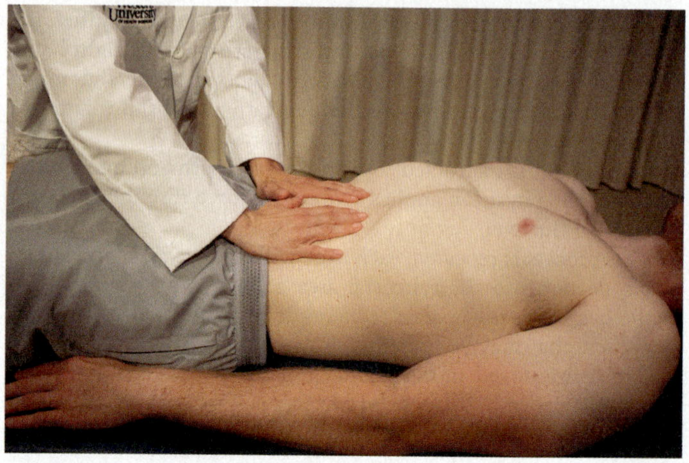

Figure 55.10. Ileocecal valve technique (lateral view). (Courtesy of Western University of Health Sciences, Pomona, CA, used with permission.)

3. The physician leans slightly backward to open the rib cage by increasing abduction to the patient's arm. The patient is instructed to inhale deeply.
4. As the patient exhales, the physician leans on the thoracic cage with both hands, applying a vibratory motion to induce a pumping motion to the spleen.
5. The process is repeated, each time with the physician penetrating deeper into the subcostal area, gaining more contact with the spleen with the goal of reducing splenic congestion or any tenderness that may be present.
6. Retest: improved motility and mobility of the spleen, increased compliance and softness of the tissues may be noted upon completion.

The next techniques listed are performed directly on the structures themselves.

Diagnosis and reassessment of the viscera is often done by what is referred to as "listening." To perform listening, the osteopathic physician places their hands on the patient in a very passive manner in order to gather information. An area of dysfunction will often have less motion than healthy tissue and may "exhibit" a "pulling" sensation toward that region. The physician's hands will be drawn toward that area of dysfunction. Once the region has proper motion and vascular function restored, on reassessment, the physician will no longer feel the "pull."

ILEOCECAL VALVE

The ileocecal junction can be assessed by standing at the right side of the supine patient and placing the fingers of the left hand on the ascending colon with the palm on the cecum and the fingers of the right hand on the descending colon with the palm on the sigmoid angle. The ileocecal junction should have a clockwise rotation on local listening. If the ileocecal junction is restricted, first ensure that the cecum and the ascending colon are free of restriction. Once that is accomplished, place the thenar or hypothenar aspect over the ileocecal junction, about 2 cm superior to McBurney point. Perform a direct pressure sphincter release by applying posterior pressure to the region until resistance is met.[26] Then, release the pressure and encourage a rhythmical clockwise rotational motion (about 5 to 10 cycles) until a release is perceived. Then encourage counterclockwise motion for about 5 to 10 cycles until another release is palpated. This may be followed by an induction technique where the osteopathic physician follows and encourages the inherent motion of the region with greater amplitude until a release is felt[26] (Figs. 55.10 and 55.11).

GASTROESOPHAGEAL (GE) JUNCTION

Barrel states that the purpose of the technique is "to reinforce and relax the gastroesophageal junction by induction focused on this area and to free any fibromuscular restrictions of the junction and surrounding structures."[23] The GE junction may be poorly functioning due to diaphragmatic dysfunction, such as spasm and/or abnormal tension on the hiatus or the stomach being drawn superiorly by intrathoracic pressure.[23]

Indirect Technique

The patient is supine; the physician stands to the right of the patient and places their right hand over the stomach. The thumb is pointed toward the pylorus and the middle finger pointed toward the left clavicle. The physician performs a layer palpation through the abdominal wall to the stomach and assesses for the presence of a fascial pull (listening). The physician takes the stomach in the direction of listening and exaggerates it, until a release is palpated.

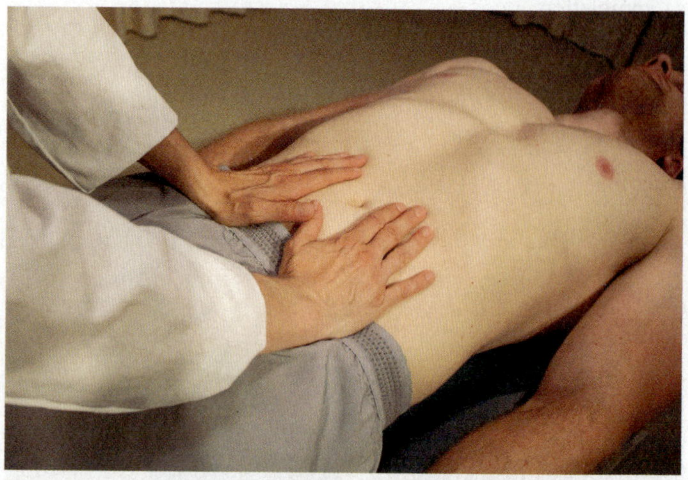

Figure 55.11. Ileocecal valve technique (overhead view). (Courtesy of Western University of Health Sciences, Pomona, CA, used with permission.)

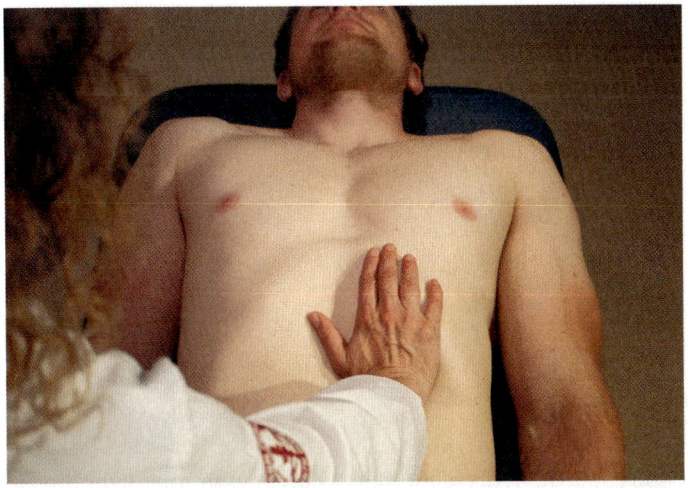

Figure 55.12. Gastroesophageal (GE) junction—indirect technique. (Courtesy of Western University of Health Sciences, Pomona, CA, used with permission.)

This process is repeated as necessary, until the stomach can be motion tested to distend anterior and lateral to the left over 2 cm, without a hard end feel (Fig. 55.12).

Induction Technique

The patient is seated and the physician contacts the left 11th costovertebral articulation posteriorly with one hand and the anterior left 7th costochondral cartilage with the other. The physician compresses the anterior contact toward the posterior one with both hands moving slightly inferiorly. Lateral motions may also be needed. The physician's hands will actively move toward the cardia but induction is utilized by following the tissues. As the tissues releases a feeling of separation between the hands will be palpated indicating the conclusion of the treatment. This technique seems to have an effect on the surrounding structures such as the pericardium, pleura, stomach, and liver[23] (Figs. 55.13 to 55.15).

PYLORUS

Pylorus spasm may arrest gastric mobility and may lead to spasm of the duodenum which can disrupt transit of digestive fluids from the pancreas and gallbladder.[23]

The location of the pylorus can be variable but the osteopathic physician may apply pressure with the thenar or hypothenar eminence of their hand to the region about 6 to 7 cm superior to the umbilicus and slightly to the right of midline.[23] The pylorus usually has a firm palpatory quality and may have a rotational motion. If the pylorus is in spasm it is generally easier to palpate[26] (Figs. 55.16 and 55.17).

Direct Technique

The patient is supine with knees and hips flexed. Using the thenar or hypothenar eminence of the hand on the pylorus, the physician follows the clockwise and counterclockwise rotation about four to six times, drawing the pylorus toward the left at the end of the clockwise rotation (opening) and to the right at the end of counterclockwise rotation (closing). This may be repeated up to 10 to 12 times. Recoil may be used at the beginning of the technique to free up a "frozen" pylorus or at the end of the direct technique. This is accomplished by drawing the pylorus transversely as far to

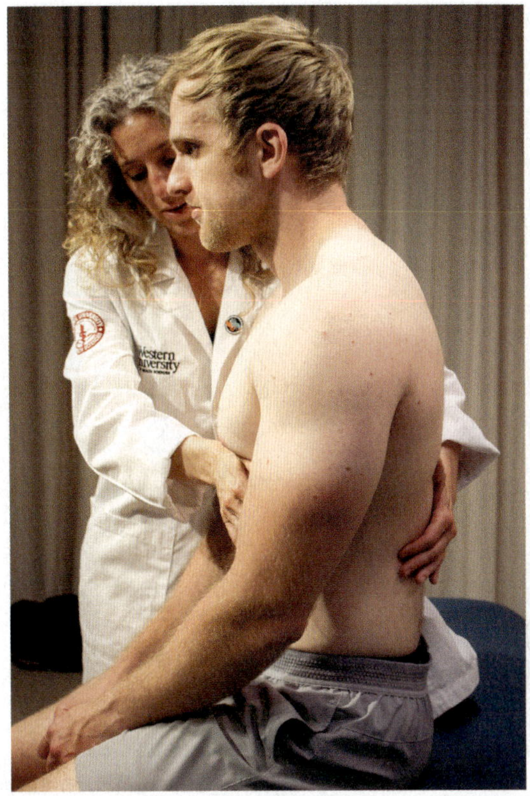

Figure 55.13. Gastroesophageal (GE) junction—induction technique (lateral view). (Courtesy of Western University of Health Sciences, Pomona, CA, used with permission.)

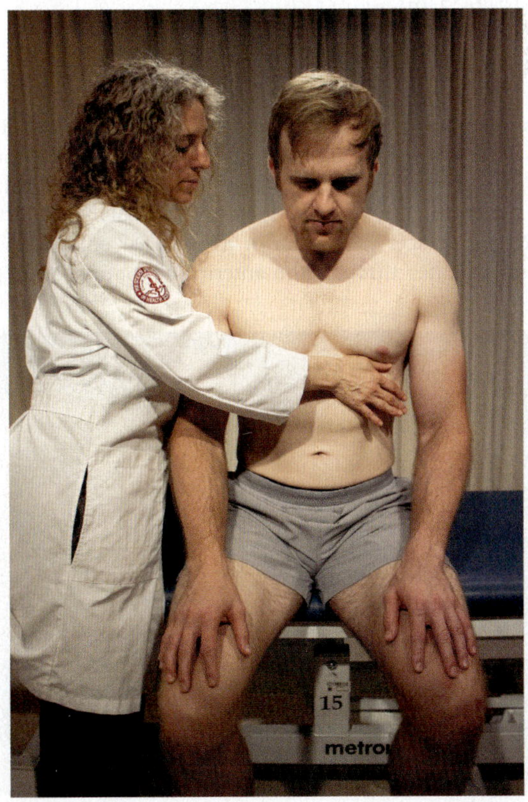

Figure 55.14. Gastroesophageal (GE) junction—induction technique (anterior view). (Courtesy of Western University of Health Sciences, Pomona, CA, used with permission.)

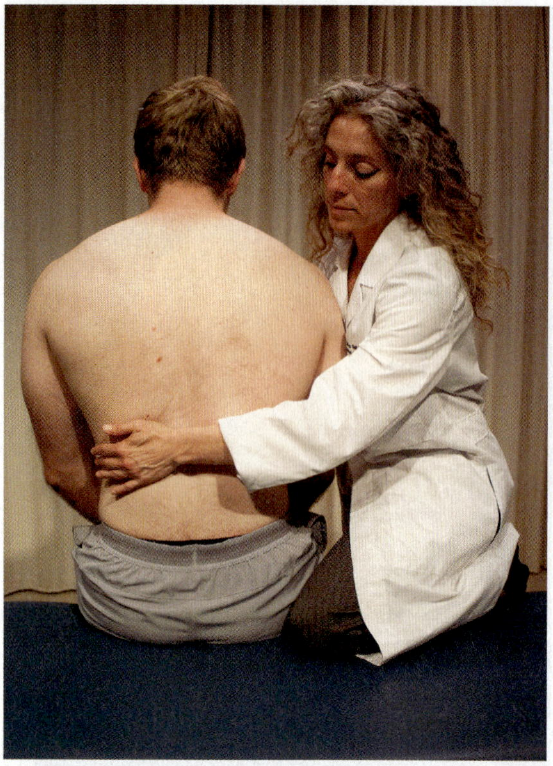

Figure 55.15. Gastroesophageal (GE) junction—induction technique (posterior view). (Courtesy of Western University of Health Sciences, Pomona, CA, used with permission.)

the right and left. Upon completion of the treatment, the pylorus should feel relaxed and may be accompanied by a "whooshing" sound[26] (Fig. 55.18).

SPHINCTER OF ODDI

Treatment of the sphincter of Oddi may decrease transit time of materials of this region and may reduce spasms of its muscular fibers. The sphincter of Oddi is found 2 to 3 fingers' width superior to the umbilicus on the right midclavicular-umbilical line. The physician places the thenar or hypothenar eminence on this point and palpates through the anterior abdominal wall, greater omentum, transverse colon, small intestine, and D2 to induce pressure with a slight clockwise rotation. Sensitivity at the end of palpation may signify dysfunction of the sphincter of Oddi or duodenal papilla. Normal listening of the sphincter should be slow rhythmic clockwise and counterclockwise rotations.[23] Absence of this rotation indicates treatment while counterclockwise motion without clockwise motion indicates that the sphincter is closed. If treatment is indicated, it may be necessary to perform a preparatory transverse technique first. Maintaining pressure on the sphincter, press it medially and laterally along a straight line for three to eight repetitions until a local release occurs. Then follow the clockwise and counterclockwise rotations until a still point is acquired followed by a release (Fig. 55.19).

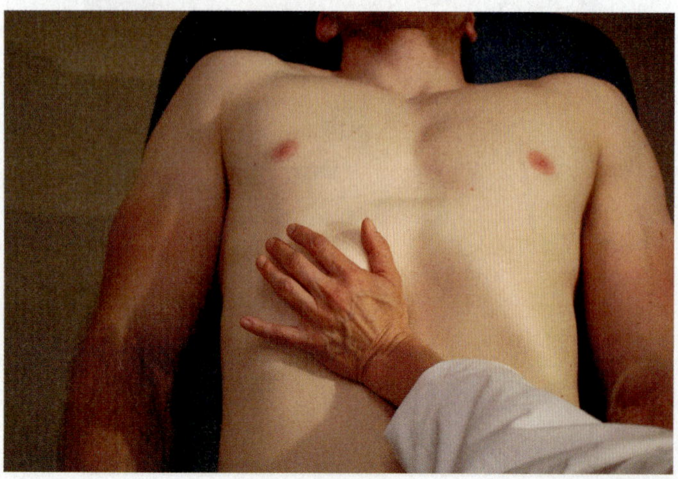

Figure 55.16. Addressing the pylorus with the thenar eminence. (Courtesy of Western University of Health Sciences, Pomona, CA, used with permission.)

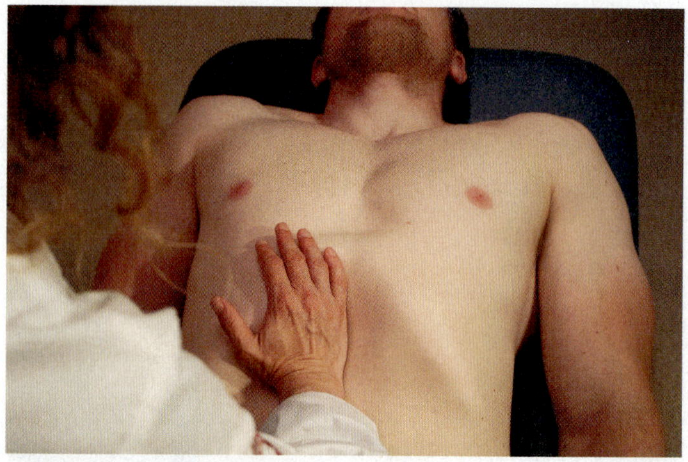

Figure 55.17. Addressing the pylorus with the hypothenar eminence. (Courtesy of Western University of Health Sciences, Pomona, CA, used with permission.)

When considering any organ, one must appreciate all of the functional connections.

The Mainstem Bronchus and Airways

The mainstem bronchus can be appreciated by tractioning the trachea superiorly to tension, and while maintaining the tension, translate it to the left and the right, noting distance, and end feel. If there is no abnormal tension, one should be able to feel the airway distend all the way to the inferior lobes of both lungs. If there is a dysfunction, the distensibility will be less and the "end feel" harder.

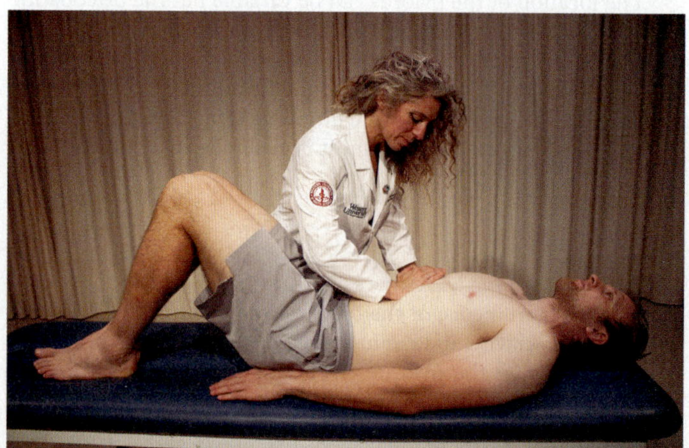

Figure 55.18. Direct treatment of pylorus. (Courtesy of Western University of Health Sciences, Pomona, CA, used with permission.)

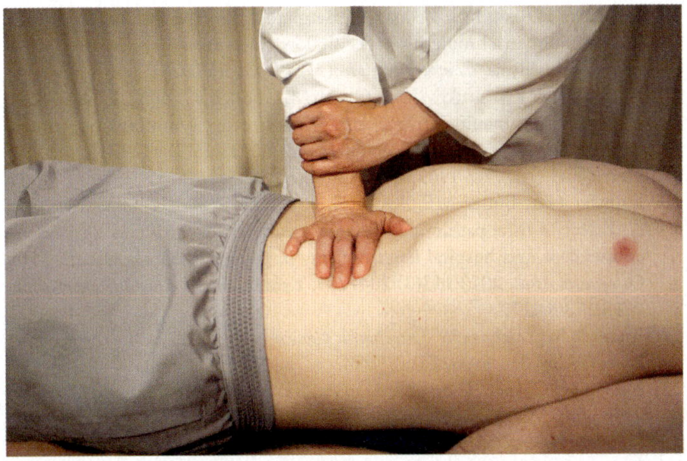

Figure 55.19. Sphincter of Oddi. (Courtesy of Western University of Health Sciences, Pomona, CA, used with permission.)

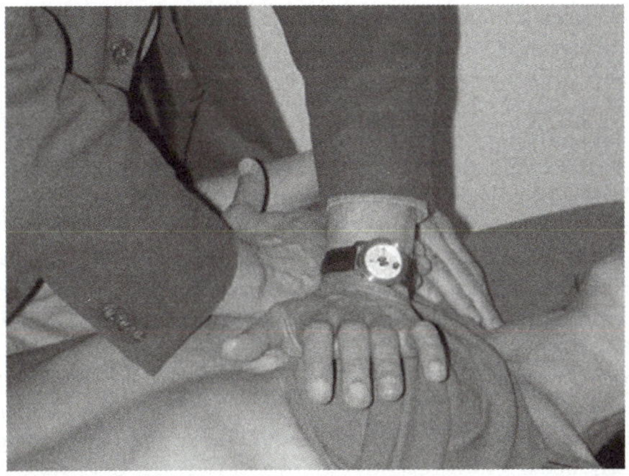

Figure 55.21. Diagnosis and treatment of the bronchi—anterior/posterior approach. (Courtesy of Kenneth Lossing, DO, with permission.)

For instance, if the right airway is in a dysfunction, there will be a shorter tracheal translation to the left, and the end feel will be harder. To mobilize the right airway, traction the trachea superiorly to tension while palpating the second and third rib interspace about 2 to 3 cm from the midline. A slight inward tug will be noted. Using the right thenar eminence at that place, compress posteriorly until a slight feeling of tension is appreciated. Have the patient inhale and exhale, drawing the area inferiorly during each exhale and maintaining tension during the inhale. Typically, within about three breaths, a release will be felt. Recheck the motion testing parameters. Alternative methods of assessing and treating both bronchi are shown in Figures 55.20 and 55.21.

THE LUNGS

To evaluate and treat the right lung, place the patient in the left lateral recumbent position. Place the left hand over the lateral chest wall at the level of ribs 3 to 6. Place the right hand over the left hand. Use the right hand to compress and the left hand to palpate. Pay attention to each layer, skin, adipose, superficial fascia, external muscles, ribs, intercostal muscles, endothoracic fascia, parietal pleura, visceral pleura, and the lung. Feel if the lung is being tractioned superior/inferior, anterior/posterior, or medially/laterally. Motion test in these same directions to reconfirm the findings.

In the plane of the largest restriction, find the direction of ease. Find the midpoint between the restrictive barrier and the physiologic barrier in the direction of ease. Stack the middle point of all three planes, and add a slight compression. A change in the viscoelasticity will be felt as the dysfunction resolves. Recheck fascial pull and motion testing. If these are not fully balanced, take the tissues to the largest remaining barrier, and stack the remaining two planes at their restrictive barriers. Add a slight compression, and wait for the release. When the motion testing is normalized, compress the lung, and release, noting the ease and speed of the return. Assume this speed, compressing and releasing, until a viscoelasticity shift in the tissue is felt.

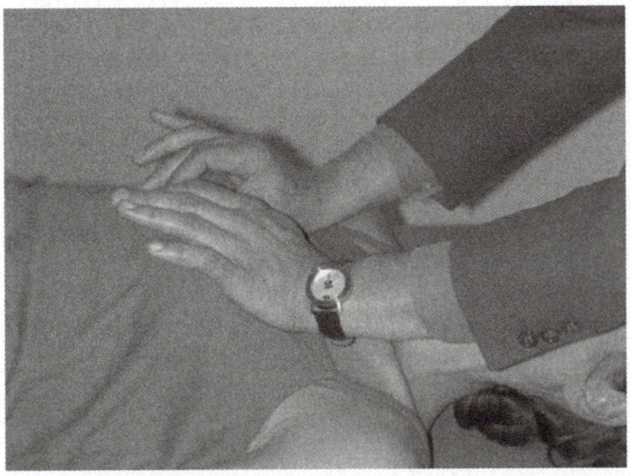

Figure 55.20. Diagnosis and treatment of the bronchi—superior approach. (Courtesy of Kenneth Lossing, DO, with permission.)

CASE STUDIES

CASE STUDY 1

A 45-year-old woman presented to the office with a 2-year history of right flank pain subsequent to a motor vehicle accident. During the accident, her trunk was rotated to the right. Her car was struck from behind. Using general and local listening, it was found that the right kidney was in a second-degree ptosis (dropped inferior more than a centimeter and externally rotated). The kidney was mobilized. On a follow-up visit 1 month later, the patient reported all flank pain to be resolved.

CASE STUDY 2

A 7-year-old female presented to the office with a 6-month history of "tummy aches" and a sensation of acid in her mouth. No other symptoms were present, and her medical history was otherwise normal. Physical exam revealed somatic dysfunction of the left occipitomastoid suture, T6 on the left, and a visceral dysfunction of the GE junction. These areas were treated. On a follow-up visit 1 month later, she reported no "tummy aches" and no instances of acid taste.

REFERENCES

1. Giusti R, ex. ed. *Glossary of Osteopathic Terminology*. 3rd ed. American Association of Colleges of Osteopathic Medicine; 2017.
2. Still AT. *Osteopathy Research and Practice*. Eastland Press; 1992.

3. McConnell CP. *Selected Writings of Carl Philip McConnell, D.O.* Squirrel's Tail Press; 1994.
4. Barber E. *Osteopathy Complete.* Hudson-Kimberly Publishing Co.; 1898.
5. Hildreth A. *The Lengthening Shadow of Dr. Andrew Taylor Still.* Simpson Printing; 1942.
6. Sutherland WG. *Teachings in the Science of Osteopathy.* Rudra Press; 1990.
7. Weischenck J. *Traire D'Osteopathis Viscerale.* Malione; 1982.
8. Finet G, Williame C. *Treating Visceral Dysfunction.* Stillness Press; 2000.
9. Barral JP. *Visceral Manipulation, 1988; Visceral Manipulation II, 1989; The Thorax, 1991; Manual Thermal Evaluation, 1996.* Eastland Press; 1988.
10. Kumar V, Abbas AK, Fausto N, eds. *Robbins and Cotran Pathologic Basis of Disease.* 7th ed. Elsevier; 2005.
11. Blechschmidt E. *The Stages of Human Development before Birth.* W.B. Saunders Company; 1961.
12. Humphrey JD, Delance SL. *An Introduction to Biomechanics.* Springer-Verlag; 2004.
13. Guyton AC, Hall JE. *Textbook of Medical Physiology.* 11th ed. Elsevier Saunders; 2006.
14. Oschman JL. *Energy Medicine: The Scientific Basis.* Churchill Livingston; 2000.
15. Hall S. *Basic Biomechanics.* 4th ed. McGraw Hill; 2004.
16. Tamer S, Öz M, Ülger Ö. The effect of visceral osteopathic manual therapy applications on pain, quality of life and function in patients with chronic nonspecific low back pain. *J Back Musculoskelet Rehabil.* 2017; 30(3):419–425.
17. Dal Farra F, Risio RG, Vismara L, Bergna A. Effectiveness of osteopathic interventions in chronic non-specific low back pain: a systematic review and meta-analysis. *Complement Ther Med.* 2021;56:102616.
18. Lotfi C, Blair J, Jumrukovska A, Grubb M, Glidden E, Toldi J. Effectiveness of osteopathic manipulative treatment in treating symptoms of irritable bowel syndrome: a literature review. *Cureus.* 2023;15(7):e42393.
19. Herman E. *The DO.* 1965;65:163–164.
20. Baltazar GA, Betler MP, Akella K, Khatri R, Asaro R, Chendrasekhar A. Effect of osteopathic manipulative treatment on incidence of postoperative ileus and hospital length of stay in general surgical patients. *J Am Osteopath Assoc.* 2013;113(3):204–209. Erratum in: *J Am Osteopath Assoc.* 2013;113(4):271.
21. Kuchera M, Kuchera W. *Osteopathic Considerations in Systemic Dysfunction.* 2nd ed. Greyden Press, LLC; 1994.
22. Nelson K, Glonek T. *Somatic Dysfunction in Osteopathic Family Medicine.* Lippincott Williams & Wilkins; 2007.
23. Barral J. *Visceral Manipulation II.* Eastland Press; 2001.
24. Remien K, Woo MJ, Vilella RC. Osteopathic manipulative treatment: lymphatic procedures. [Updated 2024 Jan 29]. In: *StatPearls [Internet].* StatPearls Publishing; 2024. https://ncbi.nlm.nih.gov/books/NBK559051/
25. Noll DR, Johnson JC, Brooks JE. Revisiting Castlio and Ferris-Swift's experiments on direct splenic stimulation in patients with acute infectious disease. *J Am Osteopath Assoc.* 2008;108(2):71–79.
26. Barral JP, Mercier P. *Visceral Manipulation, Revised Edition.* Eastland Press; 2005.

56

Still Technique: A Facilitated Indirect Then Direct Method

RICHARD L. VAN BUSKIRK

KEY CONCEPTS

- Still Technique is an osteopathic manipulative method that was recovered by Richard Van Buskirk, DO and redeveloped based on written records from the founder of osteopathic medicine, Dr. Andrew Taylor Still and his students and colleagues.
- Still Technique's history, methodology, a handful of applications and some of the diagnostic methods and findings that emerged from the process of redeveloping this manipulative method are the focus of this chapter.
- Basically, the method starts with placing the restricted tissue in its position of ease, then introducing a vector of light force, and carrying the restricted tissue through neutral and beyond the original restriction.

STILL TECHNIQUE: FACILITATED INDIRECT THEN DIRECT

Still Technique is a redeveloped osteopathic manipulative method that was recovered by the author and redeveloped based on written records from the founder of osteopathic medicine, Andrew Taylor Still, MD and his students and colleagues in the decade before and after the beginning of the twentieth century.[1,2] Still Technique's history, methodology, a handful of applications and some of the diagnostic methods and findings that emerged from the process of redeveloping this manipulative method are the focus this chapter.

One of the primary techniques for musculoskeletal manipulation used by Dr. Andrew Taylor Still had largely disappeared from the toolbox of manipulative methods early in the 20th century. Dr. Still's students referred to this method as "indirect then direct."[3,4] In its most basic form, the method starts with placing a restricted tissue in its position of ease. The position of ease is generally synonymous with the original position of injury and one in which the tissue will be its most relaxed. Introduce a vector of light force, typically either compression or traction, to the restricted tissue. Use the force as a lever along with the intrinsic motion of the tissues to carry the restricted tissue through neutral and beyond the original restriction. Although it was frequently termed "indirect then direct" by Still's students and colleagues, another term frequently applied later was "functional." One could perhaps more accurately term it Dr. Still's "Facilitated Indirect Then Direct" methodology. It is "facilitated" because of the use of a facilitating force introduced or employed by the treating physician. "Indirect then direct" because this is both the nature of the treatment and the historical identifier that came from Dr. Still's students and colleagues.

HISTORY

During the early years of osteopathic medicine, Dr. Andrew Taylor Still apparently used a number of different methods to produce his masterful treatment of musculoskeletal and other medical issues and diseases. Although he is often credited with using what is today termed high-velocity low-amplitude techniques (HVLA),[5] Dr. Still clearly used a different methodology in most cases. In fact, none of the treatments he describes in *Osteopathy Research and Practice*[6] are consistent with HVLA. Carl Phillip McConnell, DO, PhD, a student and subsequently a colleague of Dr. Still at the first osteopathic medical school in Kirksville, Missouri, the American School of Osteopathy, described the "proper method" of manipulative treatment received from Dr. Still as "indirect then direct."[3] Dr. McConnell further described Still's treatment technique in his book, *The Practice of Osteopathy*: "Disengage the articular points that have become locked. Reduce the dislocation by retracing the path along which the parts were dislocated. One can readily see that a dislocated ball and socket joint could be reduced only by the dislocated bone retracing the path through which it left its socket as the capsular ligament would at once prevent its returning to the socket by any path other than that taken when dislocated. This applies to all dislocations to a greater or lesser extent" (3). Nevertheless, Dr. McConnell spent the majority of his text describing the use of HVLA, the first documented descriptions of that manipulative method.

By 1910, Dr. Still's indirect then direct methods were no longer being taught at the founding school, the American School of Osteopathy in Kirksville, Missouri, according to Edith Ashmore, DO.[4] She stated that these "older methods" were no longer being taught because of the difficulty in teaching them. Based on the testimony of a retired DO whose wife was being treated by the author in the late 1990s, there were a few people in Kirksville still using this technology into the 1930s. He graduated from Kirksville in 1920 and was living in Venice, Florida in 1996. He reported that he had tried to convince these osteopathic physicians to teach him these techniques. Unable to do so, he continued to use HVLA throughout his long career.

Versions of Dr. Still's methods were still in use by William Garner Sutherland, DO and George Laughlin DO, Dr. Still's grandson, into the 1940s. Sutherland clearly describes his methods as starting restricted tissues in an indirect or ease position, although he also sometimes describes this as the position of "balanced tension" (e.g., where the tension in the restricted tissue is essentially zero in all directions).[7,8] In his early cranial treatments, Dr. Sutherland was initiating treatment at the ease position, introducing pressure into the tissue and carrying them actively into the position of restriction.[7] He clearly credits his methodology to Dr. Still. Subsequently, he changed his methodology so that after putting the tissue into it ease position, he would introduce slight compression into the tissue to facilitate the "inherent forces" in the tissue to carry it in the direction of restriction and thus back into full mobility. Dr. Sutherland applied the same methodology to both the cranial tissues and the rest of the body. Howard A. Lippincott and Rebecca C. Lippincott were an osteopathic husband and wife team who were close associates of Dr. Sutherland. They wrote down some of Dr. Sutherland's treatments "for the rest of the body" and subsequently published them in the 1949 *Year Book of the Academy of Applied Osteopathy*[9] (the precursor of the American Academy of Osteopathy). These applications are currently documented in Sutherland's posthumous book *Teachings in the Science of Osteopathy*.[10] Taught today as balanced ligamentous tension (BLT) and balanced membranous tension (BMT), the emphasis is on the indirect initial positioning and the initial compression toward the restricted tissue with the patient's intrinsic forces carrying the restricted tissue in the direction of the restriction until the tissue reaches a true balance neutral. Similar principles are utilized in some of the applications presented in *Ligamentous Articular Strain*.[11]

Dr. Laughlin apparently learned a variation of this method from Dr. Sutherland at the first cranial osteopathy course and it became his predominant method of treatment. Although Dr. Laughlin reportedly had difficulty explaining what he was doing, Ed Stiles, DO, FAAO spent several years working with him and derived a methodology that he termed "functional" (Ed Stiles, DO, personal communication). Now identified as part of the Still–Laughlin technology, the method again starts by positioning the patient such that the restricted tissue is in its position of ease. Thereafter, the emphasis is on a form of fascial unwinding driven in part by the permissive force vector generated by the physician and in part by the intrinsic forces of the body from the position of ease through neutral and ultimately including release of the area of restriction.[2]

In the 1980s, Stanley Schiowitz, DO, FAAO developed a novel manipulative treatment method reportedly as a result of his impatience with the length of time it took to perform Counterstrain techniques. As used in his practice, this "new" treatment was fast and efficient. Pressured by his students to teach them the method he developed it into a more systematic approach that came to be called facilitated positional release (FPR). By 1990, Dr. Schiowitz had formulated the treatment to the extent that it was published in the JAOA[12] and taught at national meetings. As published, FPR is primarily an indirect method of treatment utilizing a permissive force directed into the tissue for a few seconds and then carrying the tissue back to true neutral.[13] Actually, as practiced by Dr. Schiowitz and those whom he has directly taught, FPR is a mixed indirect followed by direct treatment, finishing in the position of original restriction.

About the same time that Dr. Schiowitz formally presented FPR, Richard Van Buskirk, DO was redeveloping a manipulative method originally discovered and used by the founder of osteopathic medicine, Dr. Andrew Taylor Still. The methodology was abstracted from a few quotes by one of Dr. Still's students and a colleague at the American School of Osteopathy, Charles Hazzard.[14] The method was given the name Still Technique because of its clear provenance as one of A.T. Still's manipulative techniques. Dr. Van Buskirk published the first modern statement of this recovered method in the *Journal of the American Osteopathic Association* in 1996.[1] Subsequently, more up to date and complete descriptions of the Still Technique and its many applications have been published.[2] Although Dr. Still did in fact write descriptions of manipulative treatments in *Osteopathy Research and Practice*,[6] following his descriptions tended to produce only limited results until the principles abstracted by Dr. Van Buskirk were incorporated. The provenance of the Still Technique has also been validated based on writings by other students of Dr. Still's students and colleagues.[3,4,7,8,14]

Although these four forms of the Facilitated Indirect Then Direct methodology derived from Dr. Still are often thought to be quite distinct, most physicians who practice this form of manipulative medicine find themselves using a blend. Those who use a more physician-active version tend to listen and follow the tissue in a complex dance. Likewise, those who use a more physician-passive form of the original method find themselves amplifying the intrinsic movement, speeding up the resolution.

STILL TECHNIQUE

The abstracted method of the Still Technique has been described and taught by Van Buskirk in various forms since the mid 1990s. Currently the method includes the following steps:

1. Evaluate the affected tissue and place it in its position of ease.
2. Introduce a force vector to the affected the tissue from another part of the body or directly to the affected segment. This compression or traction should be less than 2 lb (1 kg) and optimally much less.
3. Move the affected tissue in a smooth path from its position of ease toward and through the position of its restriction.
4. As the tissue moves through its restriction, a "bump" and/or a click may be felt or heard. Neither is necessary for correction of the somatic dysfunction.
5. Passively move the patient back to neutral and retest.

A relatively new development in Still Technique is that application of the force vector is not necessarily from a distant site as originally described.[1,2] The force vector can be from a distant body part and therefore coupled with the distantly applied movement of the affected tissue (termed a "long lever"). The force vector can also be applied directly to the affected tissue with a distally driven movement of the somatic dysfunctional tissue (termed a "short lever").[15]

As is apparent, Still Technique shares components with a number of other manipulative methods in use in osteopathic medicine today. Its position of ease is comparable to the treatment position of Counterstrain.[16] The restricted position through which the tissue is carried is identical to the positioning for Muscle Energy[17–19] and HVLA.[20]

PHYSIOLOGY OF THE INDIRECT THEN DIRECT TECHNIQUES

The physiologic and anatomical mechanisms thought to underlie the Still Technique have been extensively discussed elsewhere.[2,21] Basically, they are based on the concept that a somatic dysfunction develops and is maintained by a complex interaction of neural elements, particularly the nociceptor and central nervous system repatterning (memory), fascial repair mechanisms and elastic memory, and immunologic, inflammatory, and vascular changes. The Still Technique starts at ease, disarming the neurologic protective mechanisms and relaxing the fascia. The force vector allows repatterning of the neurofascialvascular complex in the same fashion that trauma originally triggered the somatic dysfunction but in a normalizing direction, freeing the tissue from its restriction.

DIAGNOSIS

Diagnostic methods used for the Still Technique are similar to those of Muscle Energy or HVLA,[17–20] although the *Still*

Technique Manual[2] does give a number of practical shortcuts. The definitions of rib and sacral dysfunctions used in Still Technique are different from those commonly in use[2,17–19] although the rib dysfunctions have a lot in common with Greenman's rib diagnoses.[17]

In Still Technique, rib dysfunctions are based on relative positions of the presenting dysfunctional ribs. If a rib angle and anterior costochondral junction are relatively anterior, it is termed an anterior rib. If those landmarks are relatively posterior, it is termed a posterior rib. If the ribs angles are posterior and the costochondral junctions anterior, they are lateral compressed ribs and are sidebent inferior or toward the side of the ribs. If the rib angles are anterior and the costochondral junctions are posterior, they are AP compressed ribs and will be sidebent superior or away from their side of presentation. While anterior and posterior ribs generally present as single rib dysfunctions, the compressed rib dysfunctions present as groups of ribs.

Sacral diagnosis in Still Technique is simpler than in other diagnostic schemes. It is based on the idea that the sacrum has some dysfunctions that are independent from the potential restrictions of the sacroiliac joints. These sacral dysfunctions are assumed to be related to fascial restriction rather than being joint restrictions.[2] Under this rubric, there are four possible restriction types: unilateral, diagonal, bilateral anterior, and bilateral posterior. To test for unilateral and diagonal restrictions, the ILA is evaluated for being tight and presenting inferior and or posterior. The sacral base will ride up in a modified seated flexion test. In the Still Technique version, fingertips are place of the bilateral sacral sulci. The side in which the sulcus rides more superior during the patient's forward flexion is the positive side. When the sacral base and ILA are restricted on the same side it is a *unilateral sacral dysfunction*. When they are restricted over opposite sides, it is a *diagonal sacral dysfunction*.

Bilateral sacral dysfunctions are seen independent of both innominate and the unilateral and diagonal sacral dysfunction. That is, they can be found whether the other types of dysfunctions are present or not. Bilateral sacral dysfunctions are typically the result of an abrupt cessation of downward movement of the pelvis at the ischia, with briefly persistent inferior momentum of the upper body, as in a backward fall or in plopping into a chair. If the upper body was anterior of vertical at the time of injury, the bilateral sacral base will be anterior and restricted from posterior movement. If the upper body was extended posterior at the time of the fall, the bilateral sacral base will be posterior and restricted from anterior movement. They are named for their presenting position or ease.

The concept behind identifying one or more somatic dysfunctions that are primary in a larger pattern of multiple dysfunctions has been around for a long time in osteopathic literature. At different points they have been termed "key lesions," "primary" somatic dysfunctions, and even "area of greatest restriction." This chapter will use the term "key dysfunction" to indicate a localized somatic dysfunction that when treated will result in resolution of that tissue and a number of other somatic dysfunctions that were probably compensatory or secondary. In the spine, key dysfunctions are determined by evaluating for segmental dysfunctions in anterior–posterior, lateral, and rotational planes. If a segmental dysfunction requires movement into ease in all three planes of motion to fully relax, the dysfunctional segment is a Key Dysfunction. If movement into its AP ease is sufficient to relax a segment, that segment is not a key dysfunction. Typically, the rib key dysfunction is attached to the thoracic segmental key dysfunction or is the lowest dysfunctional rib on either side.

CASE STUDY

The patient is a 62-year-old female who presents to the physician's office with a primary complaint of persistent neck pain since falling backward on a ramp about 5 months ago. She denies hitting her head in that fall. Her neck pain is worse when erect and severely limits her ability to bend her neck forward and to turn to the left. Her pain does not affect her sleep. She admits to right shoulder pain and intermittent tingling in her right (dominant) hand and forearm that was not present before her fall.

Since the current increase in neck pain, she has seen her primary care physician, her neurologist, and an orthopedic spine surgeon. She has been treated by physical therapy and her massage therapist with little relief of her pain or restriction. An MRI of her cervical spine revealed a flattened AP curve, multilevel disk degeneration involving the lower cervical vertebrae, facet hypertrophy, and mild to moderate left C4–5 and C5–6 foraminal stenosis.

The patient endorses a history of intermittent, dull, achy, stiff lower back pain located across the base of her spine. Her lower back pain originated in her late 20s with no noted precipitating event. She has been seen by multiple physicians in the past. Prior x-rays of her lumbar spine revealed minimal scoliosis, disk degeneration, and multilevel spondylosis. A lumbar MRI obtained about 18 months ago during an exacerbation of her low back pain with transient right sciatica demonstrated bulging disks at L3–4, L4–5, and L5–S1; hypertrophic facet joints from L2 through L5; and mild central and left L4–5 foraminal stenosis. An orthopedic spine surgeon consulted at the time felt that there was no basis for surgery and sent her to physical therapy after which her symptoms receded.

The patient's history includes premenopausal cyclic headaches. Currently they are rare, once every couple of months, and predominantly left sided. They do not involve any vision changes or prodrome.

Over years she has been prescribed a number of medications for her musculoskeletal pain and headaches including tricyclic and SSRI antidepressants, gabapentin, muscle relaxants, prednisone, nonsteroidal anti-inflammatories, and several different narcotics. Most were ineffective, caused too many side effects or were discontinued after a short time. She has refused any prescription medications for her current episode of neck pain. The only medicine she takes for her current pain is acetaminophen.

She has been married for 36 years, has two adult children, and works full time at a desk job. She describes her private and professional life as satisfying. Normally she goes to yoga three times a week but has limited that since her neck became worse. She tries to walk for at least 30 minutes most days although sometimes her neck pain forces her to stop.

The patient reports medical and surgical history including hypertension, mild osteopenia, an episode of hypothyroidism following her second pregnancy, and an appendectomy. She denies any other constitutional symptoms. She is up to date with her gynecological and physical examinations and is postmenopausal. She has no known allergies. Her current medications include valsartan 160 mg daily and acetaminophen 500 mg as needed. She smoked for 3 years during college but not since. She does not use recreational drugs. She used to drink one to two glasses of wine per week but for the past 5 years has only had a glass of wine during the holidays. Both of her pregnancies resulted in full-term, spontaneous vaginal deliveries.

The patient's family history includes hypertension in both parents and paternal hypercholesterolemia with both parents alive.

On physical examination, the patient is a well-nourished, well-developed woman who appears to be her stated age and is in some distress. Her cardiopulmonary, gastrointestinal, and HEENT examinations are normal. Her neurological examination demonstrates equal and normal tactile, pain, and proprioceptive sensation in all four limbs. Tinel, Phalen, Adson, and Spurling tests are negative for both upper limbs. There is no evidence of weakness in any limb and the straight leg raising test is negative in both lower limbs. Deep tendon reflexes are 2+ and brisk in all four limbs. Cranial nerves 2 through 12 are normal. Gait is normal.

The musculoskeletal exam demonstrates cervical spine limitations with flexion and left sidebending. There is no limitation of range of motion of the right shoulder joint but evidence of muscular tension during passive flexion, abduction, and internal rotation. The rib cage and thoracic spine demonstrate limitation of left sidebending, and the lumbar spine demonstrates minimal scoliosis with a left apex at L3 and limitation of right sidebending. When evaluated supine on the table, there is an apparent leg length discrepancy with the right medial malleolus approximately ¾ inch (2 cm) proximal relative to the left.

Specific musculoskeletal structural findings include Left OA FSlRr, C2 and C4 ESr with C2 being the key cervical dysfunction, elevated left first rib, T2 FSr (key dysfunction), T4 and T8 FSr, and right ribs 2–8 lateral compressed (sidebent right) and left ribs 3, 5, 7 rotated anterior. Lumbar and pelvic evaluation demonstrates L5 NSrRl (key dysfunction), right ASIS and PSIS superior with a positive right seated flexion test (right superior sheared innominate). The sacrum shows a diagonal right somatic dysfunction. There is also clear evidence of bilateral limited sacral motion with flexion but ease with extension of the torso. There is tension and restricted range of motion in the right gluteus maximus and right tensor fascia lata/iliotibial band. A cranial pattern of right sphenobasilar sidebending rotation was noted but not included in treatment planning for the initial treatment session due to a lack of current symptoms.

Diagnosis includes neck pain, cervical and lumbosacral spondylosis without myelopathy, right shoulder pain, lumbosacral strain, acquired short leg, and late effect of a fall from the same level. Additional diagnoses include cervical, rib, thoracic, lumbar, sacral, innominate, and lower limb somatic dysfunctions. The right shoulder pain and restriction of motion are determined to be related to rib restrictions and secondary muscle restrictions and therefore judged to not require direct treatment. The patient is treated with Still Technique. The subsequent course of treatment should involve biweekly treatments for 6 weeks followed by monthly intervals as needed.

TREATMENT

In the following treatments using Still Technique, the treatment versions are those most commonly deployed by the author. Many other approaches can be utilized employing Still Technique and are described in the *Still Technique Manual*.[2]

To treat the C2 cervical somatic dysfunction seen in the case history remember that this key dysfunction was extended, sidebent right, and rotated right:

1. The patient is seated. The physician stands either in front of or behind the patient.

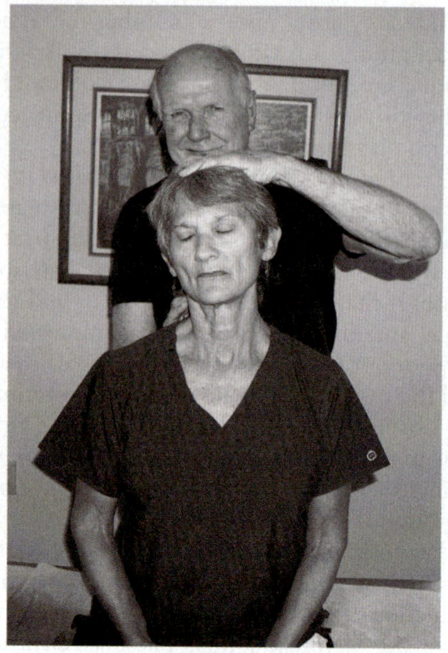

A

Figure 56.1A. C2 extended, sidebent, and rotated right, initial position.

2. The physician's sensing finger is placed on the articular pillar of the affected cervical vertebra (C2). The remainder of the sensing hand supports the head and/or neck.
3. Place the operating hand on the top of the patient's head.
4. The head and neck above the affected spinal segment are then slightly extended with right sidebending and right rotation until the tissues palpably relax.
5. Introduce compression from the operating hand through the top of the head toward the affected segment (long lever) or using the sensing finger directly to the articular pillar of C2 (short lever) (Fig. 56.1A).
6. Rotate the head and neck toward the left and simultaneously reduce the extension in a single smooth vector through neutral and into left rotation and flexion (Fig. 56.1B). Generally, release will be felt sometime between neutral and full left rotation.

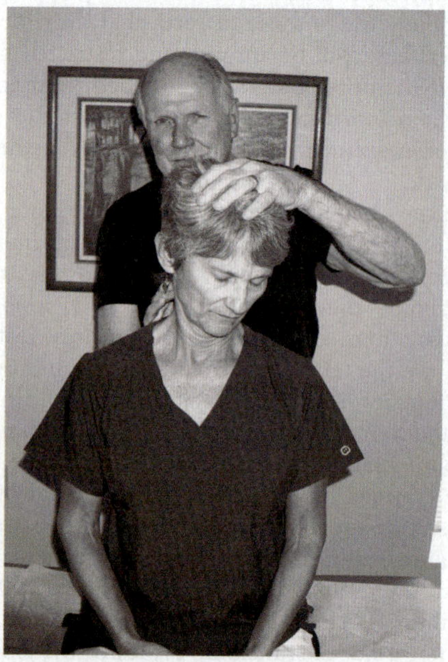

B

Figure 56.1B. C2 extended, sidebent, and rotated right, final position.

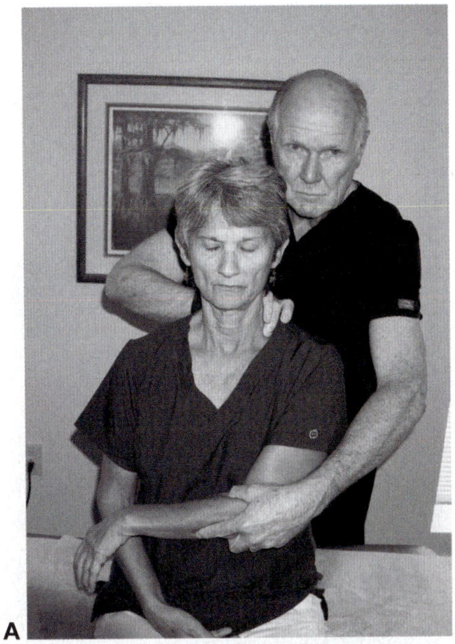

Figure 56.2A. Superior first rib, left, initial position.

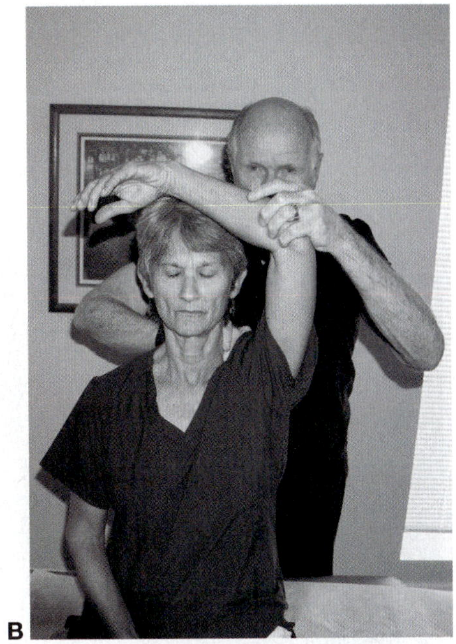

Figure 56.2B. Superior first rib, intermediate position.

7. Once the neck has been rotated past the area where the motion barrier originally was found, release compression and return the neck returned to neutral. Even if no palpable or audible release is noted, the treatment of the somatic dysfunction most likely will have been a success. Reassess motion, position, and tissue texture.

Treating the C2 as a key somatic dysfunction should release both the secondary C4 and OA dysfunctions. Note that this technique easily can be performed with the patient supine.

Treating the superior left first rib starts with an understanding of first rib mechanics. With the head of the first rib at ease in a superior position, the costomanubrial connection will be relatively inferior. There are many Still Technique methods to treat a superior first rib. The one the author uses most of the time is as follows.

1. The patient is seated. Stand in front of or behind the patient.
2. Place the sensing hand so that the index finger is on the affected first rib head.
3. The operating hand encloses the patient's forearm on the side of the superior first rib. The patient's arm is flexed at the shoulder with the forearm in the area of the abdomen (Fig. 56.2A).
4. Introduce compression through the forearm in a vector toward the affected rib head (long lever) or alternately directly on the left rib head by the sensing finger (short lever).
5. Maintaining the compression vector, carry the forearm upward into dorsal extension (Fig. 56.2B).
6. Finally, carry the arm into lateral (Fig. 56.2C) and finish with the arm at the patient's side. Retest.

An alternative treatment with the patient seated starts with positioning the neck flexed and sidebent away from the side of the superior first rib head. This will place that rib at ease. As in the seated cervical treatment above, the operating hand is on the top of the patient's head and the sensing finger on the rib head. Carry the head and neck into the first rib's position of restriction which will be with the neck sidebent to the same side as the affected first rib and extended.

To treat the thoracic segmental dysfunctions we will have the patient remain seated. (This version is usable for all thoracic vertebrae below T1.) The example is the key dysfunction T2FrSr.

1. The patient is seated on a table with the physician standing behind.
2. The sensing hand is that of the same side as the ease of the somatic dysfunction (right transverse process in this case). The pad of the index finger of the sensing hand is placed over the prominent transverse process of the affected segment.
3. Pass the operating arm over the patient's opposite (left) shoulder around the superior chest wall and place the operating hand on the shoulder on the side of the somatic dysfunction (ease). This gives the physician adequate leverage to

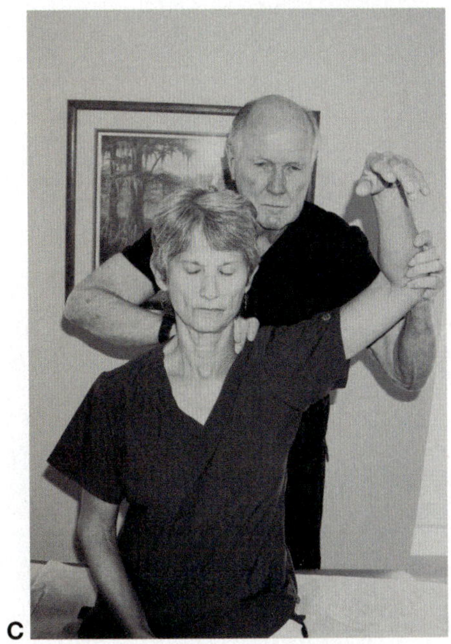

Figure 56.2C. Superior first rib, final position.

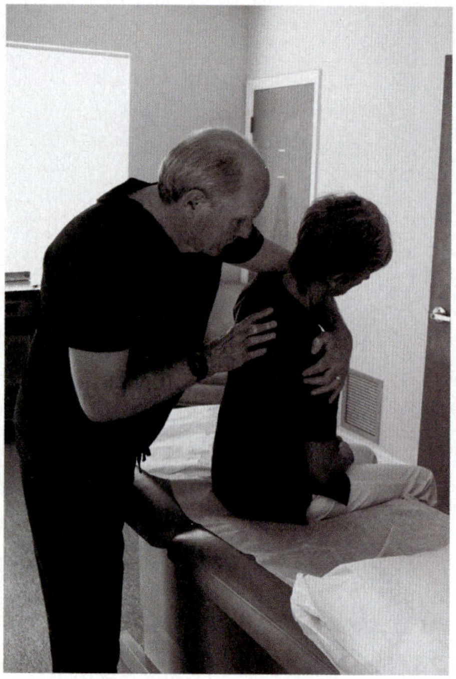

A

Figure 56.3A. T2 FSrRr. Initial position.

introduce the necessary flexion or extension, compression and rotation.

4. The patient's thorax and spine are then flexed (in this case) and rotated toward the side of the somatic dysfunction (right) and compression introduced (Fig. 56.3A).
5. Once the tissues and transverse process have palpably relaxed, the operating arm simultaneously reduces flexion and rotates the spine through neutral into the previously restricted range (left sidebending and rotation with extension) (Fig. 56.3B).
6. Release compression and passively return the patient to neutral. Retest.

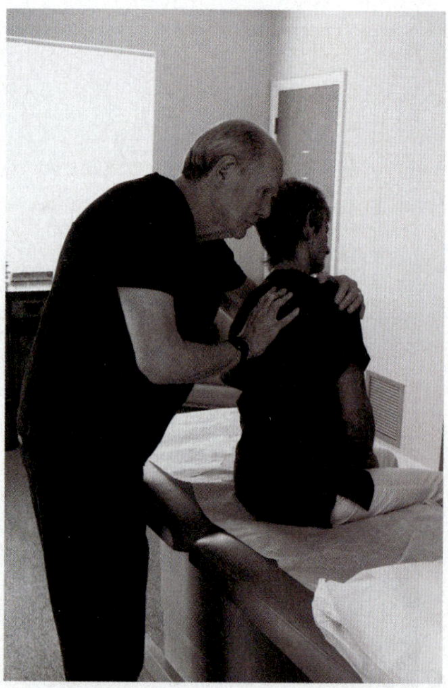

B

Figure 56.3B. T2 FSrRr. Final position.

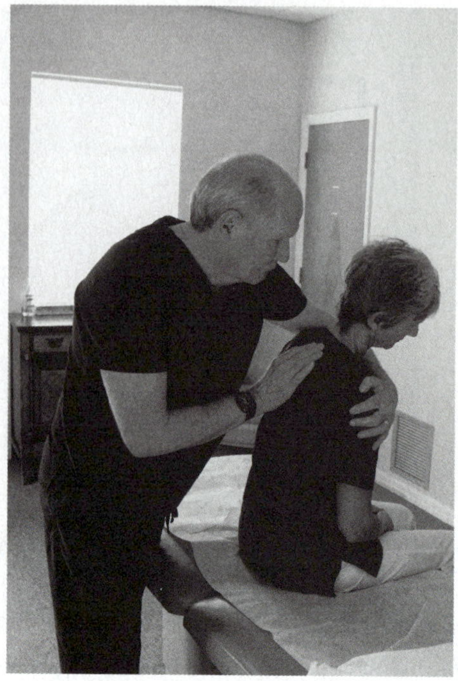

A

Figure 56.4A. Rib 2 lateral compressed right. Initial position.

The right rib 2 was laterally compressed. Assuming this it is most likely the key rib dysfunction, it is treated.

1. The patient is seated. The physician stands behind.
2. The physician's sensing hand is placed with the thumb on the costovertebral junction and additional sensing finger is placed on the right second rib angle. Alternately, the sensing thumb can be placed on the rib angle and an additional finger on the body of the rib in the axillary chest wall.
3. The physician places the operating arm over the patient's opposite shoulder (left) and around the patient's upper chest. The physician's operating hand is placed on the patient's shoulder on the right side.
4. Sidebend the patient toward the right. This will relax the rib and reduce tenderness over the rib. No anterior or posterior rotation is necessary (Fig. 56.4A).
5. Introduce compression from the patient's shoulder toward the rib head (or alternately on the rib itself).
6. Maintaining compression, sidebend the patient toward the left side (Fig. 56.4B).
7. Once release is felt return the patient to neutral. Remove compression. Retest.

As long as the remainder of the rib restrictions resolve after treating rib 2, we advance to treating the lumbar spine and L5 NSrRl.

1. The patient is seated. The physician approaches the patient from behind.
2. The transverse processes and overlying tissues are monitored by the sensing hand.
3. The physician's operating arm is draped around the patient's shoulders and anterior chest. The operating hand is on the patient's shoulder. This allows easy passive movement of the patient's upper body and gives the patient a feeling of safety and support.
4. Since the affected segment is sidebent to the right and rotated to the left (L5N$S_R$$R_L$) the patient's upper body is sidebent to the right down to where the motion isolates into the affected segment and then rotation is induced into the opposite direction (toward the left) (Fig. 56.5A).

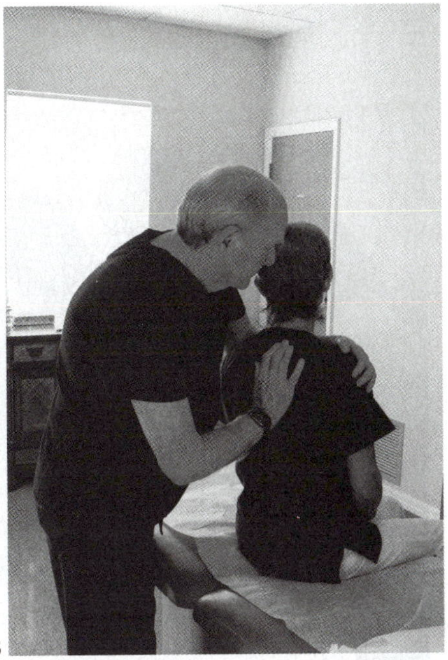

B

Figure 56.4B. Rib 2 lateral compressed right. Final position.

5. Once the tissues have relaxed and the transverse processes are no longer prominent, a vector of force is introduced by the operating hand on the patient's shoulder to and through the affected segment or from the sensing hand directly to L5.
6. Now the physician's operating hand induces sidebending toward the left and rotation toward the right in a smooth arc (Fig. 56.5B).
7. After release remove the force vector and return the patient to neutral. Retest.

The lumbar key dysfunction was L5 NSrRl. As is typically the case when L4 or L5 demonstrate a neutral dysfunction, the sacral dysfunction mimics the L5 finding and is a right diagonal dysfunction. It is treated the same although the focus of the force vector is shifted to the right S1 (sacral sulcus).

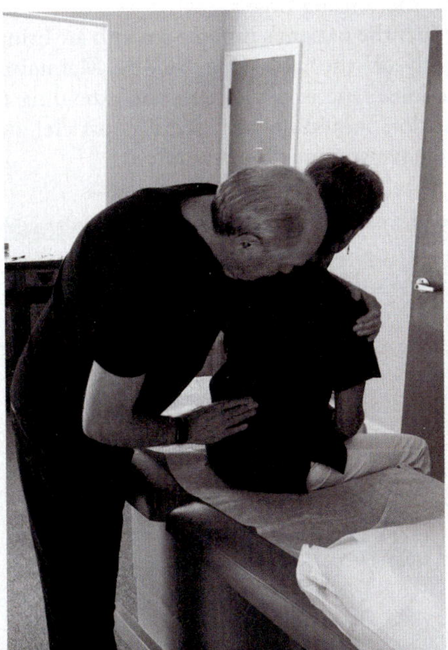

A

Figure 56.5A. L5 NSrRl. Initial position.

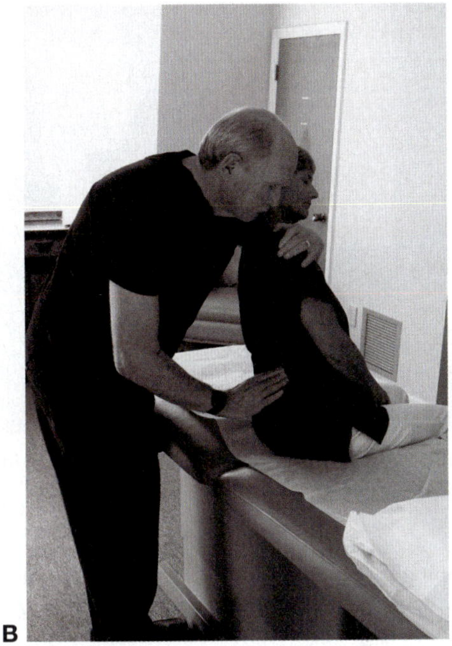

B

Figure 56.5B. L5 NSrRl. Final position.

The right innominate demonstrates what has been classically diagnosed as a superior shear. As Goldman and Van Buskirk discussed,[22] this dysfunction in which the ASIS and PSIS are superior on the same side is better described as a pelvic sidebending with the iliac crest sidebent toward the lumbar spine. This accounts for the amount of apparent leg length discrepancy and does not require severe shearing along the very irregular and peculiarly shaped sacroiliac joint. It also simplifies the mechanics of treatment. For a right superior sheared (or internally sidebent) innominate the treatment is as follows:

1. With patient in the supine position, the right ankle is grasped by the operator and the leg is placed in abduction. This will then bring the innominate into its ease position of superior sidebending (Fig. 56.6A).
2. The sensing digit is on the right sacral sulcus.
3. Light compression or traction is applied from the right leg toward the superior part of the SI joint or alternately to the right SI joint itself.

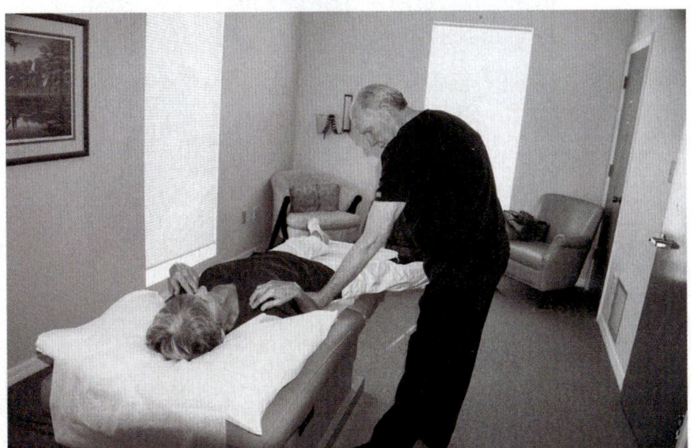

A

Figure 56.6A. Right superior sheared (sidebent) innominate. Initial position.

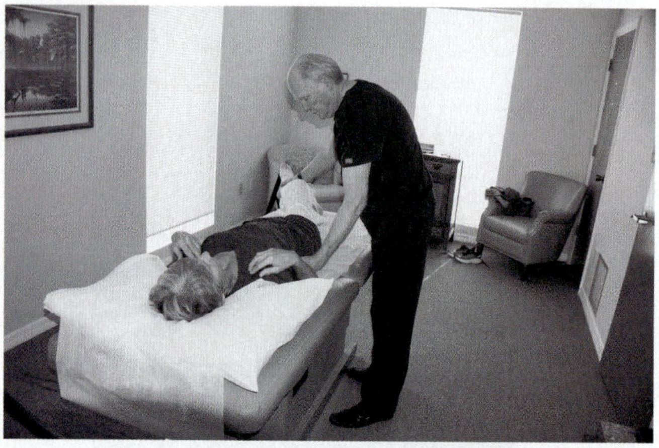
B

Figure 56.6B. Right superior sheared (sidebent) innominate. Final position.

4. Maintaining this compression or traction, the right leg is moved from abduction across midline into adduction (Fig. 56.6B) and then back to neutral. Now retest.

For a bilateral posterior sacral shear, the treatment is as follows:

1. With the patient seated, stand behind the patient.
2. The operating arm is placed across both shoulders similar to the thoracic and lumbar treatments above.
3. Sensing fingers are placed on both sacral sulci.
4. The patient's torso is extended bringing the sacral sulci into ease (Fig. 56.7A)
5. Introduce compression from the shoulders or directly on the sacral sulci.
6. Maintaining the compression force vector, carry the torso into flexion (Fig. 56.7B) which should release the sacrum. Retest.

Finally, we will give an example of treating a muscle using Still Technique. Although any muscle would do, we will use the right gluteus maximus. Again, the method is fairly straightforward. The muscle's ease occurs when it is maximally shortened. Its restriction is in being lengthened.

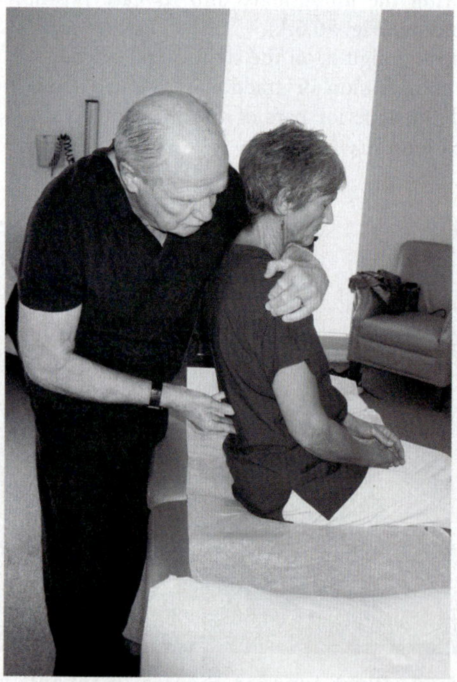
A

Figure 56.7A. Bilateral posterior sacrum. Initial position.

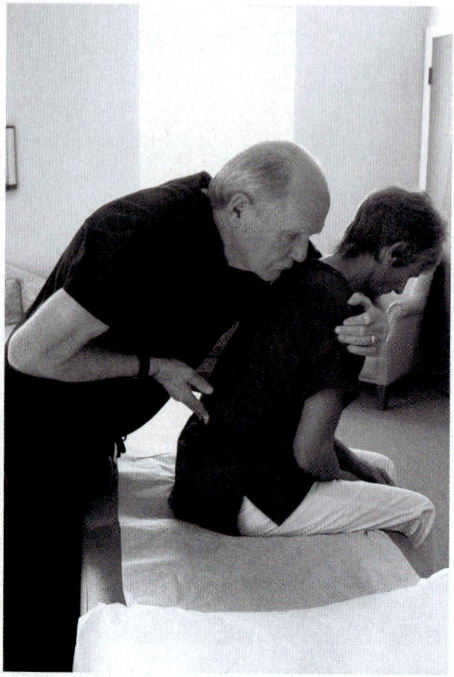
B

Figure 56.7B. Bilateral posterior sacrum. Final position.

1. The patient is supine. The physician stands on the side of the dysfunctional gluteus maximus.
2. The physician's hand closest to the patient's head is placed under the patient's pelvis with a sensing finger on a tenderpoint in the origin of the gluteus maximus.
3. The operating hand flexes the patient's knee and the hip is abducted and flexed until relaxation is felt in the gluteus maximus (Fig. 56.8A).
4. Introduce compression from the knee toward the origin of the gluteus maximus or alternately on the origin of gluteus maximus with the sensing finger.
5. Now adduct the patient's hip in a smooth arc bringing the right hip slightly off the table (Fig. 56.8B). Maintaining compression, the knee's arc is carried inferior, extending the knee. The final position should be with the legs parallel and flat on the table. Remove compression and retest.

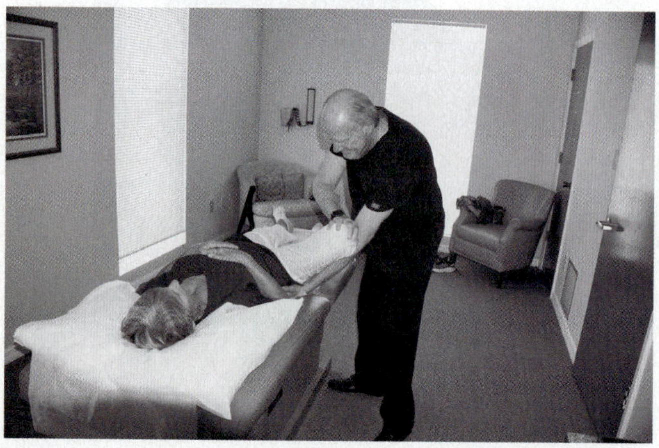
A

Figure 56.8A. Right gluteus maximus dysfunction. Initial position.

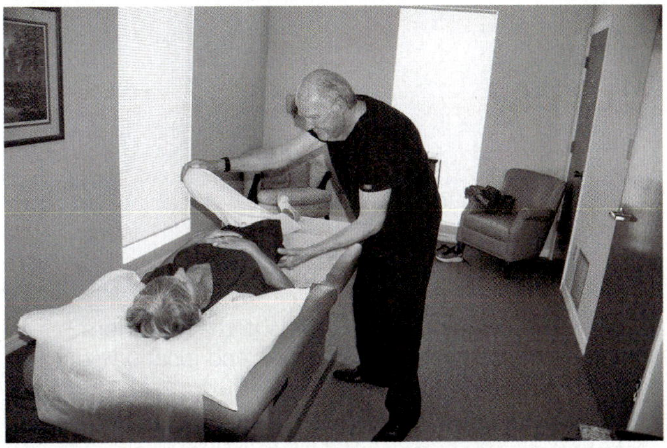

B

Figure 56.8B. Right gluteus maximus dysfunction. Final position.

The tensor fascia lata and iliotibial band somatic dysfunction is treated the same as in sheared innominate except that the focus should be on the hip greater trochanter.

DISCUSSION

The Still Technique is used successfully to treat virtually all tissues of the body, including the cranium, spine, sacrum, pelvis, limbs, muscles, tendons, ligaments and viscera. Its efficacy is only limited by the practitioner's knowledge of functional anatomy. Like most manipulative techniques, it is not advisable to use Still Technique across recent wounds (surgical or otherwise) or bone fractures less than 6 weeks old. Since it utilizes minimal force, it is safe to use in all, from infancy through senescence.

Frequently, we are taught to focus on the patient's area of complaint. Since the patient in our example complained primarily about neck pain, one might approach this case by focusing on the cervical spine and perhaps on the immediately contiguous areas like the thoracic spine and ribs and perhaps on the cranial dysfunctions since she did report a history of headache. However, in doing so there would have been additional somatic dysfunctions in the lower body that were connected to the origin of the patient's worsened cervical pain. In a younger patient, perhaps treating only the upper body might be sufficient. However, given the duration of her symptoms a simple resolution of her problem might not have been possible and certainly would have required treatment of other primary restrictions such as the lumbosacral junction and the bilateral sacral restriction. Further, the patient was older and had significant arthritic changes in both the cervical and lumbosacral spine. Osteoarthritis by itself is not necessarily a source of pain. However, when coupled with somatic dysfunction, arthritis can prolong the symptoms. All of these factors: duration of symptoms, specific trauma, arthritis, and somatic dysfunction distributed throughout the body will likely prolong the time needed for treatment.

My experience has been that treating the whole body is the most successful mechanism to shorten treatment duration. It is also my experience that failing to treat part of the body that has somatic dysfunction may well prevent anything except short term resolution of symptoms, only to have then return at the original site or elsewhere in the untreated body. Therefore, it my habit to treat the whole body each time I treat a patient for somatic dysfunction.

REFERENCES

1. Van Buskirk RL. A manipulative technique of Andrew Taylor Still. *JAOA.* 1996;96:597–602.
2. Van Buskirk RL. *The Still TechniqueManual.* 2nd ed. The American Academy of Osteopathy; 2006.
3. McConnell CP. *The Practice of Osteopathy.* 2nd ed. The Hammond Press; 1900.
4. Ashmore EF. *Osteopathic Mechanics.* Journal Printing Company; 1915.
5. Hildreth AG. *The Lengthening Shadow of Dr. Andrew Taylor Still.* Published by the author; 1938.
6. Still AT. *Osteopathy, Research & Practice.* Kirksville, MO; 1910. (Reprinted by Eastland Press, Seattle, WA, 1992.)
7. Sutherland WG. *The Cranial Bowl.* Free Press, Co.; 1939 (reprinted, 1994).
8. Sutherland WG. Contributions of Thought. Sutherland AS, Wales AL, eds. *The Sutherland Cranial Teaching Foundation.* Ruda Press; 1998.
9. Lippincott HA. *The Osteopathic Technique of Wm. G. Sutherland, DO.* Year Book of the Academy of Applied Osteopathy; 1949. Available as an Appendix in Sutherland, W.G., Teachings in the Science of Osteopathy. Sutherland Cranial Teaching Foundation, Inc., Fort Worth, TX, 1990.
10. Sutherland WG. *Teachings in the Science of Osteopathy.* Sutherland Cranial Teaching Foundation, Inc.; 1990.
11. Speece CR, Crow WT. *Ligamentous Articular Strain.* Eastland Press; 2006.
12. Schiowitz S. Facilitated positional release. *JAOA.* 1990;90:145–146, 151–155.
13. Schiowitz S, DiGiovanna EL, Dowling DJ. Facilitated Positional Release Techniques. In: Ward RC, ed. *Foundations for Osteopathic Medicine.* 2nd ed. Lippincott Williams & Wilkins; 2003:1017–1025.
14. Hazzard C. *The Practice and Applied Therapeutics of Osteopathy.* 3rd rev ed. Journal Printing Co.; 1905.
15. Van Buskirk RL. Introducing short lever Still Technique, a new variant. *AAOJ.* 2020;30(1):31–35.
16. Jones LH. *Strain & Counterstrain.* American Academy of Osteopathy; 1981.
17. Greenman PE. *Principles of Manual Medicine.* 3rd ed. Lippincott Williams & Wilkins; 2003.
18. Mitchell FL Jr., Mitchell PKG. *The Muscle Energy Manual.* Vol. 1,2,3, MET Press; 1995.
19. Mitchell FL Jr., Moran PS, Pruzzo NA. *An Evaluation and Treatment Manual of Osteopathic Muscle Energy Procedures.* Mitchell, Moran, and Pruzzo, Associates, Valley Park, MO; 1979.
20. Walton WJ. *Textbook of Osteopathic Diagnosis and Technique Procedures.* The American Academy of Osteopathy; 1972.
21. Van Buskirk RL. Nociceptive reflexes and the somatic dysfunction: a model. *JAOA.* 1990;90:792–794, 797–809.
22. Goldman SI, Van Buskirk RL. Rethinking superior and inferior sacroiliac shear: a new approach to diagnosis and treatment. *AAOJ.* 2018;28(1): 21–28.

57 Articulatory Procedures

WALTER C. EHRENFEUCHTER

KEY CONCEPTS

- Articulatory techniques involve gentle and repetitive motions through the restrictive barrier.
- Articulatory techniques are one of the most versatile treatment forms available since the physician can use a wide range of force levels and adapt them to a variety of patient body types and locations of dysfunction.
- Many techniques use long lever forces in achieving effects.

CASE VIGNETTE

A 54-year-old man presents to the office with a sore throat and dry cough. He complains of an ulcer on the buccal surface of his left cheek. He admits to having had similar ulcers around his mouth in the past. He denies other complaints.

PHYSICAL EXAMINATION

Vital signs are normal. Exam of the buccal mucosa reveals a shallow ulcer with a red border approximately 2 mm in diameter; the tongue is in the midline; there is no tonsillar hypertrophy or erythema; the teeth are in good repair. Small left submental node is palpable. CV, pulmonary, abdominal, and neurologic exams are noncontributory. Structural exam reveals rigid, tender, and hypertonic paravertebral musculature from the C5 to T2 spinal levels bilaterally. Rib 4 on the left is held in exhalation.

DIAGNOSIS

1. Acute herpetic stomatitis.
2. Somatic dysfunction—cervical, thoracic, and rib.

PLAN

Treatment with antiviral medication
Articulatory technique on the rib dysfunction

ARTICULATORY TECHNIQUE

Dysfunction

Position: Rib 4 on the right is held in exhalation.
Restriction: Rib 4 on the right is restricted in inhalation.

Treatment Position

Patient: Lateral recumbent—patient lying on the right side
Physician: Standing behind the patient at the side of the treatment table

Procedure

1. Physician places left hand posterior to the left iliac crest to stabilize the patient's body (Fig. 57.1).
2. Physician places left knee against the angle of rib 4 on the left and maintains a firm steady pressure (a folded towel or small pillow may be needed between the physician's knee and the patient's rib to minimize patient discomfort) (Fig. 57.2).
3. Physician's right hand grasps the patient's left arm just proximal to the wrist.
4. Physician smoothly carries the left shoulder into a combination of flexion and abduction in order to place the pectoralis minor muscle on passive stretch (Fig. 57.3).
   The tension by the knee, allows the rib to easily articulate (Fig. 57.4).
5. Success of the technique is determined by reassessing the respiratory motion of rib 4. Success may also be determined in part by reassessing the patient's symptomatology (sore throat and cough).

DEFINITION

Articulatory method is a direct, joint-focused group of techniques, which use low-velocity, high-amplitude (LVHA) movements. In performing treatment, the physician gently carries the body region being treated through the restrictive barrier. This may be done as a single movement or repetitively. The repetitive techniques are often referred to as springing. Many articulatory techniques use long lever forces to achieve their effects.

HISTORY

Articulatory techniques are at least as old as the osteopathic profession itself. The only film clip that exists of A.T. Still performing this technique is 9 seconds long and appears to be a shoulder or clavicular articulatory technique.

INDICATIONS

Articulatory technique is indicated when the restrictive barriers to motion appear to be in a joint itself or in the periarticular tissues. It can be used to affect a single joint (e.g., the glenohumeral joint) or an entire region (e.g., the thoracic cage). It is well tolerated by arthritic patients, elderly, or frail individuals, as well as critically

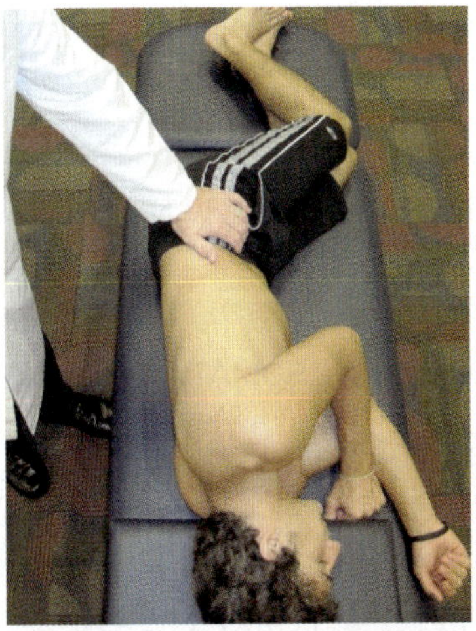

Figure 57.1. **Articulatory technique, upper rib: exhalation dysfunction, step 1.**

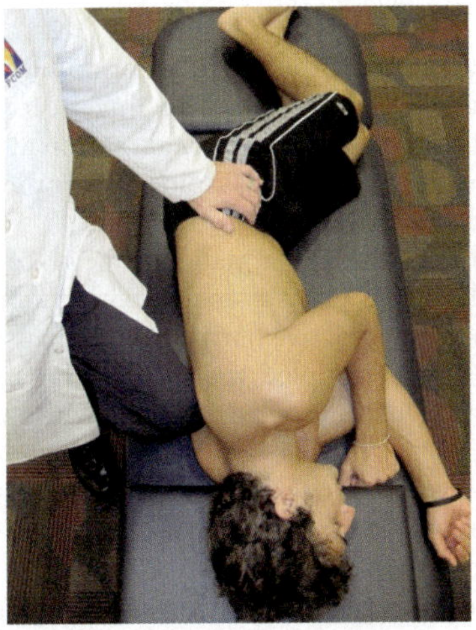

Figure 57.2. **Articulatory technique, upper rib: exhalation dysfunction, step 2.**

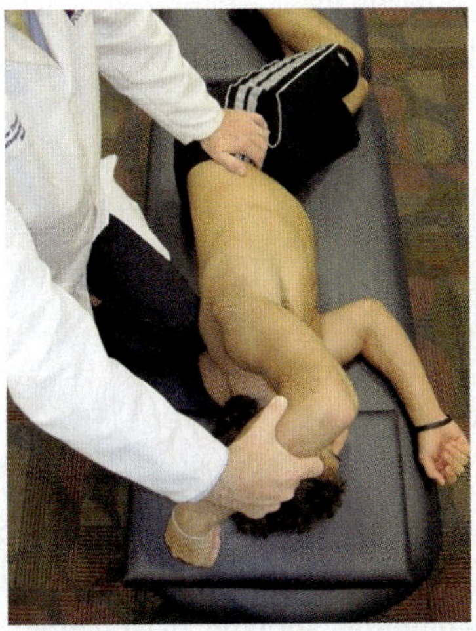

Figure 57.3. **Articulatory technique, upper rib: exhalation dysfunction, step 3.**

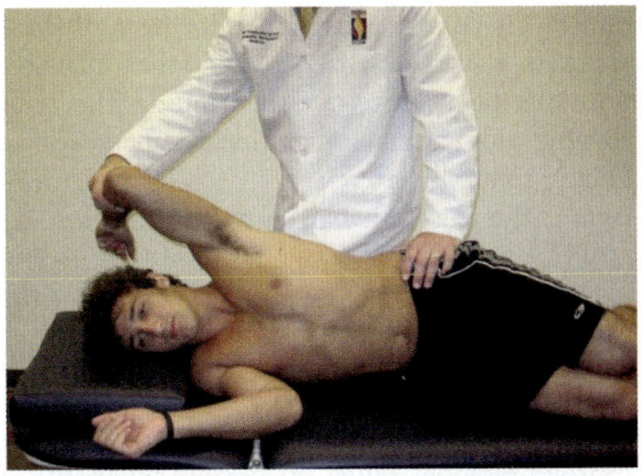

Figure 57.4. **Articulatory technique, upper rib: exhalation dysfunction, step 4.**

ill or postoperative patients. Infants and very young patients, and others unable to cooperate with verbal instructions for other techniques, often derive great benefit from articulatory techniques.

CONTRAINDICATIONS

Absolute Contraindications

Articulatory techniques are contraindicated for use in a region with any of the following conditions:

- Fracture or dislocation
- Neurologic entrapment syndromes
- Serious vascular compromise
- Malignancy
- Infection (e.g., cellulitis, abscess, septic arthritis, osteomyelitis)
- Bleeding disorders

Relative Contraindications

In the upper cervical region, due to the possibility of vertebral artery compromise, it is wise to avoid the combination of repetitive extension and rotation.

BASIC TECHNIQUE PRINCIPLES

1. The patient should be comfortable and able to relax.
2. The physician should also be in a position of comfort to minimize energy expenditure and to make use of body weight and leverage rather than having to exert muscular force.
3. The physician moves the affected joint or body part through its range of motion until the restrictive barrier is engaged.
4. A gentle but firm force is applied, carrying the body region a short distance through the restrictive barrier. The distance is limited by the tissues being treated and the patient's tolerance to pain or fatigue.
5. This force is typically applied rhythmically, consisting of 1 or 2 seconds of stretch followed by a similar time frame releasing the stretch. The joint is permitted to return to a point just short of its restrictive barrier.
6. As the patient responds to the technique, the restrictive barrier will shift position within the physiologic range of motion. For each cycle of the applied technique, the restrictive barrier is re-engaged and the affected body region is carried a short distance farther, through the new barrier to normal motion.
7. The applied forces should be comfortable for the patient. Some patients experience discomfort, but it is recognized by the patient as a good and necessary discomfort.

8. The technique is continued until the location of the restrictive barrier reaches a plateau; that is, no further increase in range of motion can be achieved by continuing the technique or until full physiologic range of motion has been restored to the joint(s) being treated.
9. At no time is the anatomic barrier to joint motion exceeded.

ARTICULATORY TECHNIQUES

Regional

Articulatory techniques may be applied to entire regions of the spine to improve regional range of motion, when the restriction to motion is perceived by the physician to have an articular component to it.

EXAMPLE: CERVICAL SIDEBENDING

Diagnosis

Position: Cervical spine is sidebent to the left.
Restriction: Cervical region is restricted in right sidebending.

Treatment Position

Patient: Lateral recumbent, lying on the side of the positional diagnosis
Physician: Sitting on the side of the table in front of the patient, facing the patient's head

Procedure

1. Physician's left arm places the patient's right shoulder in the physician's left axilla (Fig. 57.5).
2. Physician's left hand grasps the spinous process of T1 to serve as an anchor and a reference for motion.
3. Physician's right hand grasps the patient's head in the left occipitoparietal region and supports it in a position neutral to the rest of the spine.
4. Physician lifts the patient's head up toward the ceiling until motion occurring at the T1 level is palpated. This is the initial restrictive barrier.
5. Physician stretches the cervical spine through this motion barrier, using left hand to anchor T1. The position is held briefly (<1 second). The neck is then returned to a position just away from the restrictive barrier.
6. Rhythmically repeat step 5 as many times as necessary to achieve a full physiologic range of motion for the cervical spine in regional sidebending.
7. If unable to reach full range of motion, continue the technique until there is no further advancement of the restrictive barrier toward the physiologic barrier.
8. Success of the technique is determined by retesting the cervical regional sidebending range of motion.

Segmental

Segmental articulatory techniques are applied to segmental motion restrictions that are perceived to be articular in nature in the vertebral column.

EXAMPLE: SEGMENTAL SOMATIC DYSFUNCTION—C4

Diagnosis

Position: C4 is rotated right and sidebent right.
Restriction: C4 is restricted in left rotation and left sidebending.

Treatment Position

Patient: Supine
Physician: Standing at the head of the treatment table

Procedure

1. Physician's two hands cradle the patient's head (Fig. 57.6).
2. Physician places the pad of the right index or middle finger posterior to the articular process of C4. This is the articulating finger.
3. Physician places pad of the left index or middle finger posterior to the articular process of C5. This finger serves as an anchor and a reference to palpate segmental motion at this level.
4. Physician positions the cervical spine so that the C4/C5 motion segment is in neutral in the sagittal plane.
5. Physician's hands turn the patient's head to the left, until motion reaching the C5 is palpated with the palpating finger. This is the initial restrictive barrier. (Note that sidebending and rotation are always coupled motions to the same side in the C2–C6 region. One cannot be produced without producing the other.)
6. Holding the head and neck stable, physician's right articulating finger exaggerates the rotation/sidebending of C4 to the left. The position is held briefly (<1 second). The C4 segment is then returned to its position just before engaging the restrictive barrier.
7. Rhythmically repeat step 6 as many times as necessary to achieve full physiologic range of motion for C4.
8. If unable to reach full range of motion, continue the technique until there is no further advancement of the restrictive barrier toward the physiologic barrier.
9. Success of the technique is determined by retesting segmental motion at the C4 level.

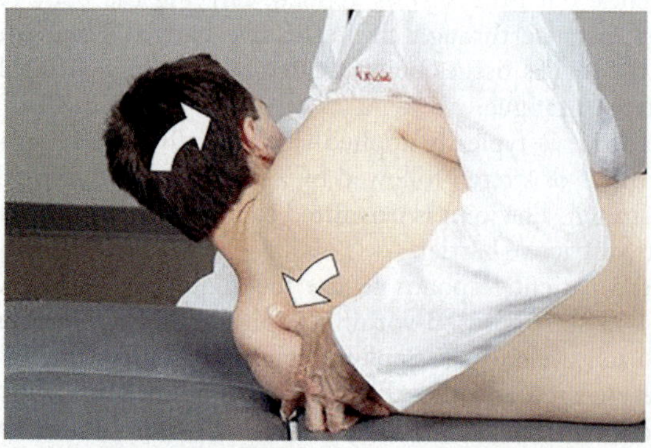

Figure 57.5. Cervical sidebending. (Reprinted with permission from Nicholas AS, Nicholas EA. *Atlas of Osteopathic Techniques*. 3rd ed. Wolters Kluwer; 2016:103.)

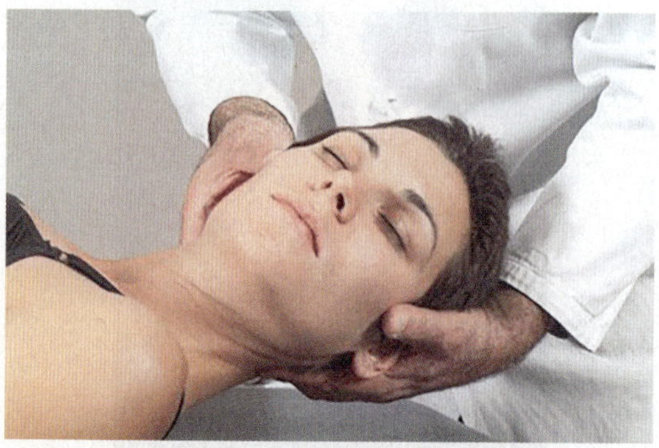

Figure 57.6. Segmental somatic dysfunction: C4. (Reprinted with permission from Nicholas AS, Nicholas EA. *Atlas of Osteopathic Techniques*. 3rd ed. Wolters Kluwer; 2016:365.)

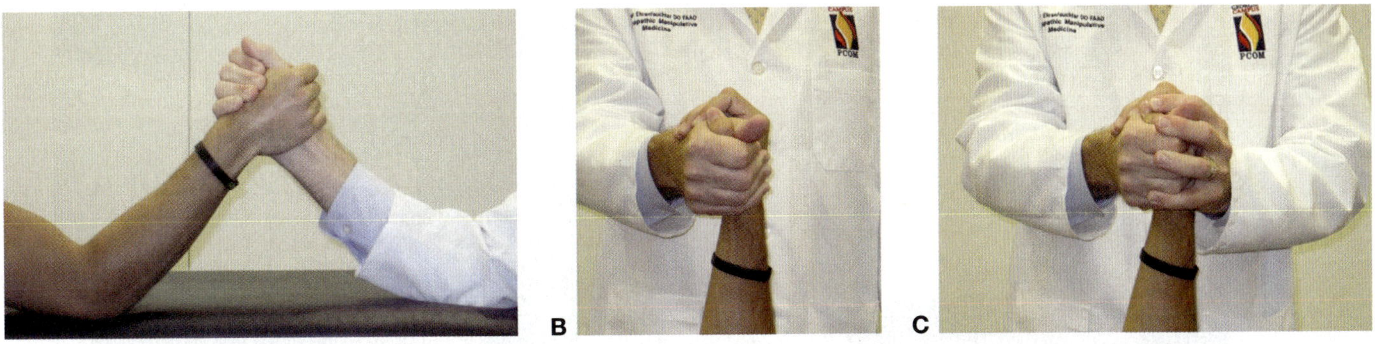

Figure 57.7. **A–C.** Radiocarpal restriction.

Peripheral

Articulatory techniques are especially useful in treating restriction of motion of the peripheral limb joints.

EXAMPLE: RADIOCARPAL JOINT RESTRICTION

Diagnosis

Position: Radiocarpal joint extended

Restriction: Radiocarpal joint restricted in flexion

Treatment Position

Patient: Supine with dysfunctional arm extended toward the ceiling

Physician: Standing at the side of the treatment table on the side of dysfunction

Procedure

1. Physician's hands clasp the patient's hand from both sides. The first hand clasps the patient's hand in a fashion similar to a grip taken in arm wrestling (Fig. 57.7A–C).
2. Physician exerts steady traction upward toward the ceiling. The patient's hand is held pointing vertically toward the ceiling throughout the technique (Fig. 57.8).
3. Physician flexes the patient's wrist to the restrictive barrier by carrying the patient's shoulder toward flexion (Fig. 57.9).
4. Physician carries the radiocarpal joint further into flexion through the restrictive barrier and holds it there for a brief period of time (<1 second). The physician then allows the radiocarpal joint to return to a position just before the restrictive barrier by slightly extending the shoulder (Fig. 57.10).
5. Rhythmically repeat step 4 as many times as necessary to achieve a full physiologic range of motion for the radiocarpal joint.
6. If unable to reach full range of motion, continue the technique until there is no further advancement of the restrictive barrier toward the physiologic barrier.
7. The same techniques can be carried out in radial or ulnar deviation, as well as in circumduction (Fig. 57.11A,B).
8. Success of the technique is determined by retesting the radiocarpal range of motion.

TECHNIQUE EXAMPLES

Head and Suboccipital Somatic Dysfunction

TEMPOROMANDIBULAR JOINT

Diagnosis

Position: Mandible laterally translated to the right

Restriction: Mandible restricted in left lateral translation

Type of Articulatory Technique

Peripheral

Treatment Position

Patient: Supine with the head turned with the side to be treated superior

Physician: Seated at the table, at the side of the head, facing the patient

Procedure

1. Physician places one hand under the patient's head, elevating it slightly (Fig. 57.12).
2. Physician positions the other hand with the third, fourth, and fifth fingers along the posterior border of the ramus of the mandible and the hypothenar eminence along the body of the jaw.
3. Patient opens the mouth slightly.
4. Physician's hand exerts pressure on the patient's jaw, so as to draw the jaw forward at the temporomandibular joint, and deviate the jaw laterally to the left.
5. This traction on the jaw is applied and released in a slow rhythmic pattern and continued for 30 seconds to 2 minutes.

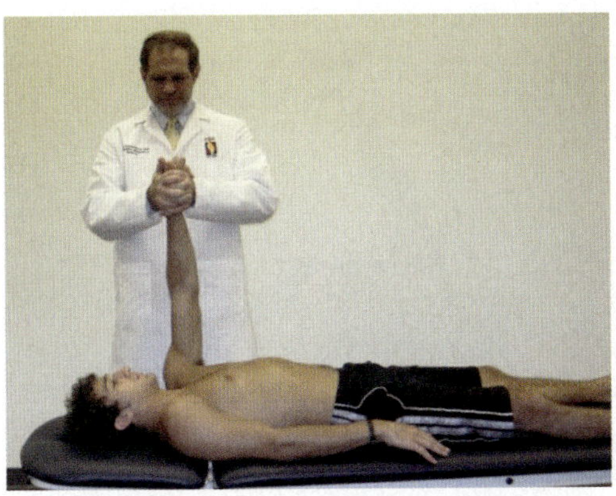

Figure 57.8. **Radiocarpal joint restriction, step 2.**

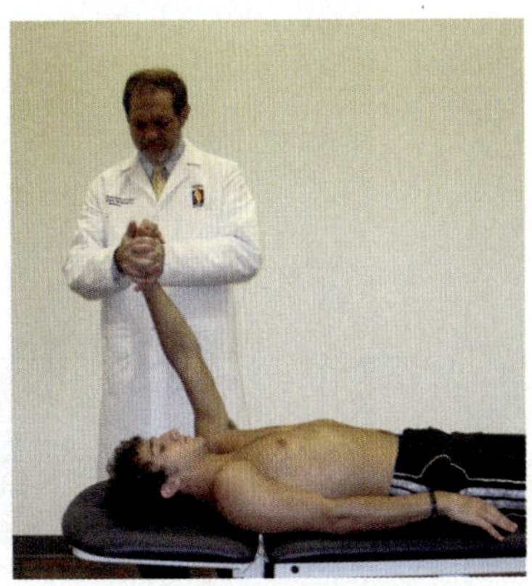

Figure 57.9. **Radiocarpal joint restriction, step 3.**

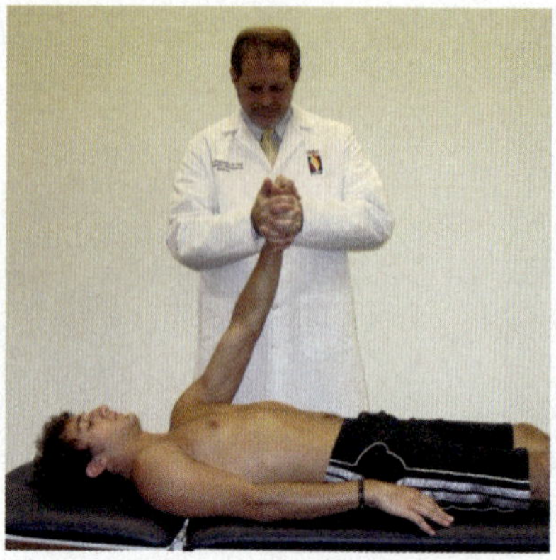

Figure 57.10. Radiocarpal joint restriction, step 4.

6. Success of the technique is determined by reassessing mandibular range of motion in lateral translation.

Cervical Somatic Dysfunction

SEGMENTAL CERVICAL EXTENSION

Diagnosis

Position: C4 flexed (flexed dysfunctions are commonly found following whiplash injuries)
Restriction: C4 restricted in extension

Type of Articulatory Technique

Segmental

Treatment Position

Patient: Supine
Physician: Seated at the head of the treatment table

Procedure

1. Physician places pads of fingers under the patient's neck bilaterally, contacting the C4 articular processes and lateral to the spinous processes (Fig. 57.13).
2. Physician exerts pressure ventrally, of sufficient force to extend C4 on C5 to the initial restrictive barrier.
3. Physician carries C4 through its restrictive barrier into further extension and holds it there for a brief period of time (<1 second). The physician then allows C4 to return to a position just before the restrictive barrier by releasing the extension force.

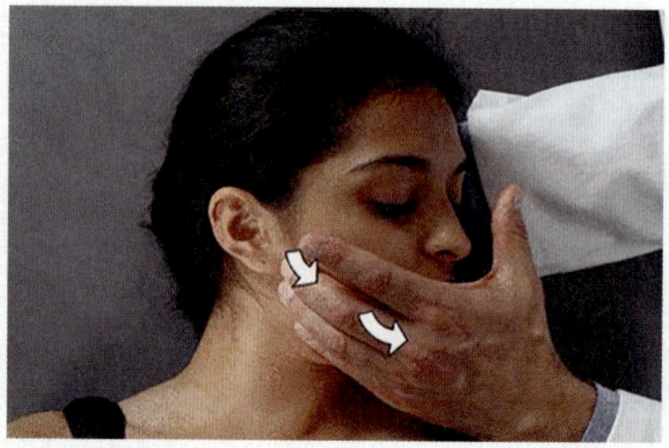

Figure 57.12. Temporomandibular joint articulatory technique. (Reprinted with permission from Nicholas AS, Nicholas EA. *Atlas of Osteopathic Techniques*. 3rd ed. Wolters Kluwer; 2016:511.)

4. Rhythmically repeat step 3 as many times as necessary to achieve a full physiologic range of motion for C4.
5. If unable to reach full range of motion, continue the technique until there is no further advancement of the restrictive barrier toward the physiologic barrier.
6. Success of the technique is determined by retesting the C4 segmental extension.

Thoracic Somatic Dysfunction

THORACIC SIDEBENDING

Diagnosis

Position: T8 sidebent left
Restriction: T8 restricted in the right sidebending

Type of Articulatory Technique

Segmental

Treatment Position

Patient: Prone with the head turned toward the physician
Physician: Standing at the side of the table facing the patient's thorax

Procedure

1. Physician places heel of one hand on the patient's spine, over the transverse process of T8, with fingers pointing superiorly (Fig. 57.14).

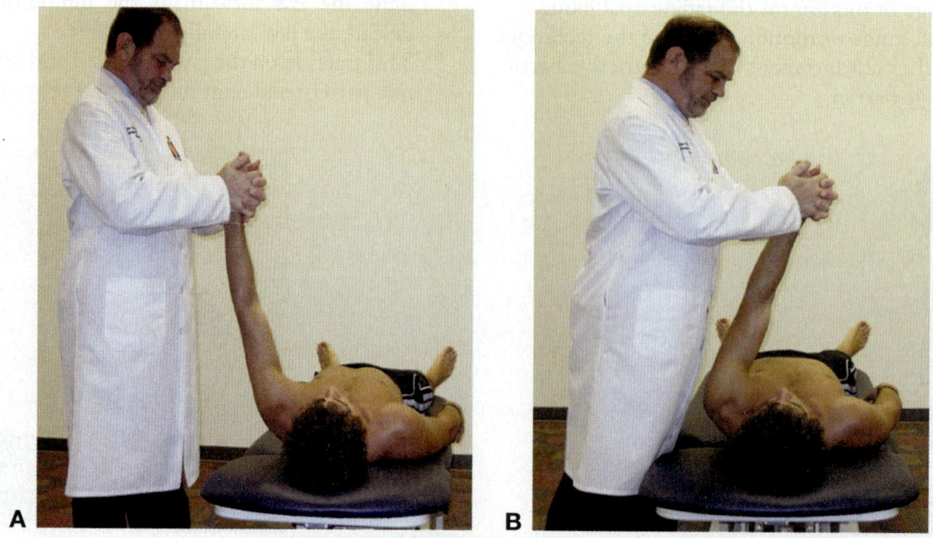

Figure 57.11. A and **B.** Radiocarpal joint restriction, step 7.

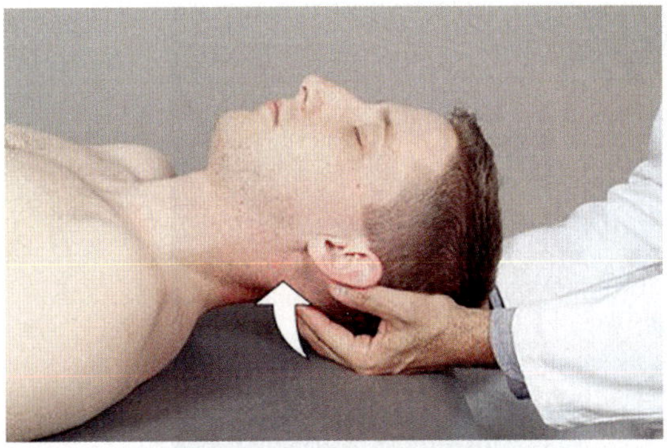

Figure 57.13. Segmental cervical extension articulatory technique. (Reprinted with permission from Nicholas AS, Nicholas EA. *Atlas of Osteopathic Techniques*. 3rd ed. Wolters Kluwer; 2016:92.)

2. Physician places the heel of the other hand on the patient's spine, over the opposite transverse process of T8, with fingers pointing inferiorly.
3. Physician exerts sufficient pressure downward toward the table to produce articular motion of the spine.
4. Once this has been accomplished, physician exerts a longitudinal force simultaneously with both hands to carry T8 through its restrictive barrier and holds it there briefly (<1 second). Physician slowly releases this pressure, allowing T8 to return to a position just before engaging the restrictive barrier.
5. Steps 3 and 4 are rhythmically repeated until full physiologic motion has been restored to T8.
6. If unable to reach full range of motion, continue the technique until there is no further advancement of the restrictive barrier toward the physiologic barrier.
7. Success of the technique is determined by reassessing segmental sidebending at T8.

Lumbar Somatic Dysfunction

LUMBAR REGIONAL ROTATION: SEATED POSITION

Diagnosis

Position: Lumbar region rotated left

Restriction: Lumbar region restricted in right rotation

Treatment Position

Patient: Seated, straddling the treatment table with back to the end of the table.

Physician: Standing behind the patient toward the side opposite the side to be treated. Table height should be adjusted so that the physician stands roughly one head taller than the patient.

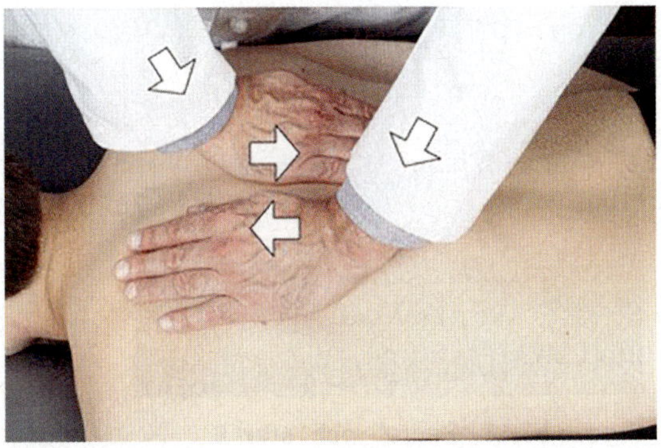

Figure 57.14. Thoracic sidebending articulatory technique. (Reprinted with permission from Nicholas AS, Nicholas EA. *Atlas of Osteopathic Techniques*. 3rd ed. Wolters Kluwer; 2016:102.)

Procedure

1. Patient places the left hand behind the neck and then grasps the left elbow with the right hand.
2. Physician places the heel of the left hand to the left of the patient's spine, overlying the lumbar transverse processes.
3. Physician passes the right arm in front of the patient (under the patient's right upper arm) and grasps the patient's left upper arm.
4. Patient leans forward and relaxes so the physician's right arm carries the patient's weight. The patient will have a natural tendency to rotate the trunk to the right.
5. Physician turns body to the right to exaggerate the rotation of the patient's trunk to the right. Simultaneously, physician's left hand exerts an anterior pressure over the left lumbar transverse processes.
6. Physician holds this rotational force for a short time and then releases it. The natural tension of the soft tissues will return the lumbar column to a position just inside the restrictive barrier.
7. Physician repositions the left hand to engage a different portion of the lumbar spine.
8. Repeat steps 5 to 7 in a rhythmic fashion for 2 to 5 minutes.
9. Success of the technique is determined by retesting lumbar regional range of motion in rotation.

Note: This technique may be converted to a segmental lumbar rotation technique by isolating the forces of the left hand over a single transverse process and by limiting truncal rotation to that amount which specifically articulates that segment.

Sacral Somatic Dysfunction

SACRAL ROCK

Diagnosis

Restriction: Sacral motion with respiration restricted

Treatment Position

Patient: Prone

Physician: Standing at the side of the patient, at the level of the patient's pelvis

Procedure

1. Physician places the heel of one hand on the patient's sacrum at S1, with fingers pointing toward the coccyx (Fig. 57.15A,B).
2. Physician places the heel of the other hand on top of the hand on the sacrum, at the S4/S5 level, with fingers pointing toward the lumbar spine (Fig. 57.16A,B).
3. Patient inhales deeply and the physician's hands follow the sacrum into extension.
4. At the end of inhalation, physician carries the sacrum slightly further into extension and holds it there for a second (Fig. 57.17).
5. Patient exhales and the physician's hands follow the sacrum into flexion.
6. At the end of exhalation, physician carries the sacrum slightly further into flexion and holds it there for a second (Fig. 57.18).
7. Steps 3 to 6 are repeated for 2 or 3 minutes.
8. Success of the technique is determined by reassessing sacral motion.

Pelvic Somatic Dysfunction

POSTERIORLY ROTATED INNOMINATE: MODIFIED SIMS POSITION

Diagnosis

Position: Posteriorly rotated innominate.

Restriction: Innominate is restricted in anterior rotation.

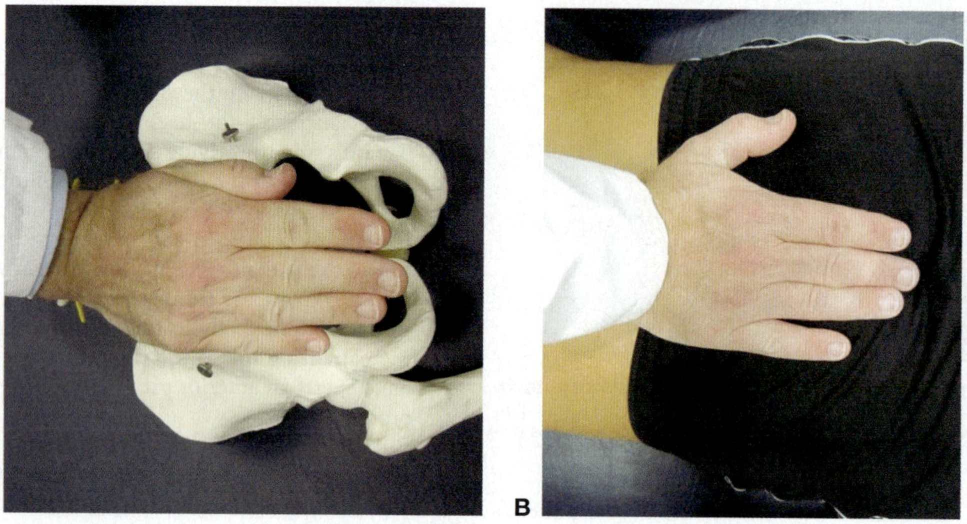

A B

Figure 57.15. **A** and **B.** Sacral rock, step 1.

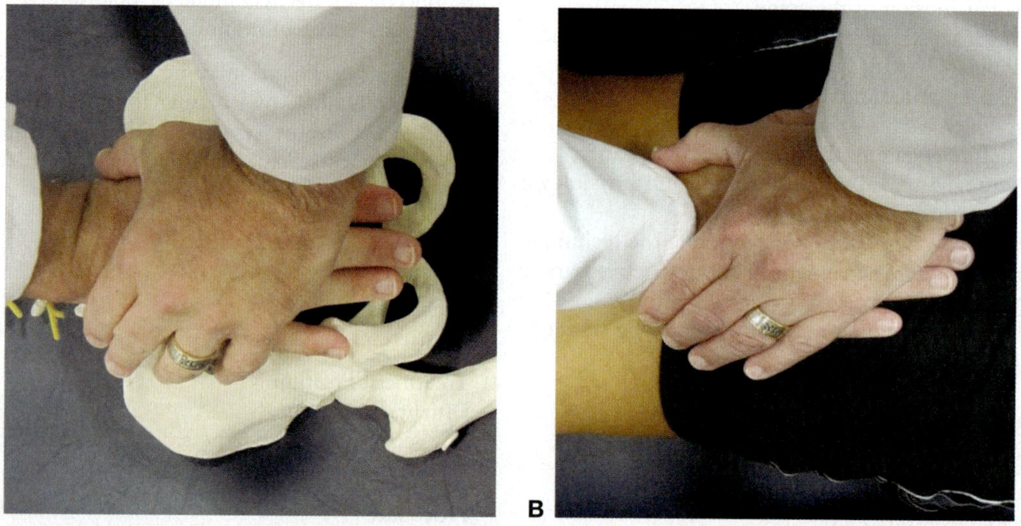

A B

Figure 57.16. **A** and **B.** Sacral rock, step 2.

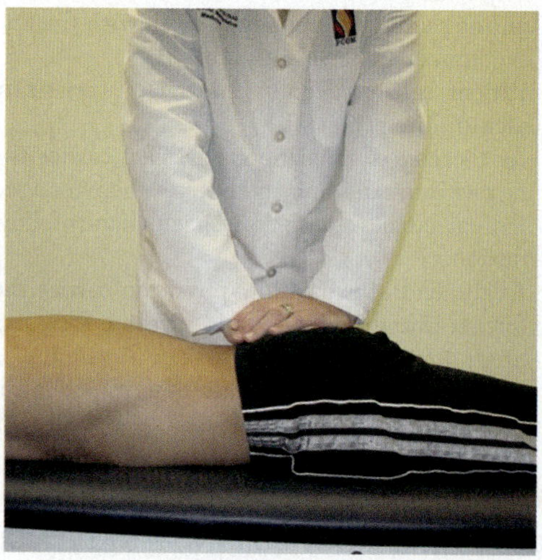

Figure 57.17. Sacral rock, step 4.

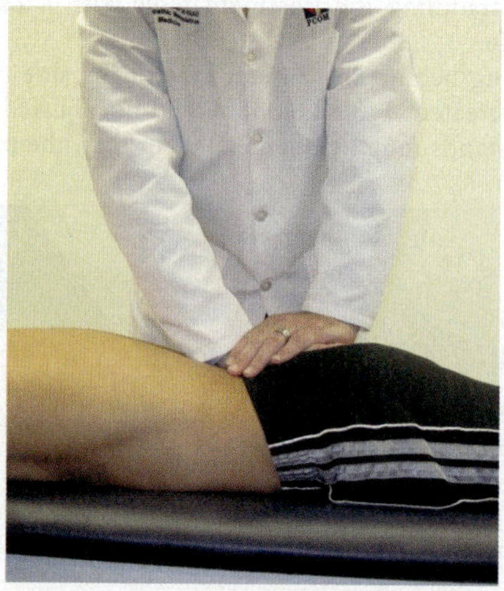

Figure 57.18. Sacral rock, step 6.

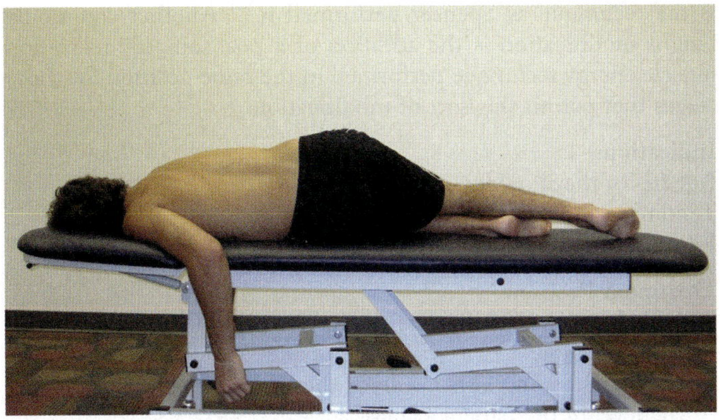

Figure 57.19. Posteriorly rotated innominate—modified Sims position.

Treatment Position

Patient: Modified Sims position with the innominate to be treated away from the table (Fig. 57.19)

Physician: Standing behind the patient at the level of the patient's pelvis

Procedure

1. Physician places the heel of one hand posterior to the patient's posterior superior iliac spine on the side of the dysfunction and exerts a continuous firm force.
2. Physician's other hand grasps the patient's shin just distal to the knee (Fig. 57.20).
3. With a smooth continuous motion, physician performs the following motions:
   A. Flexion of the hip to 100 to 120 (Fig. 57.21, Step 3A)
   B. Abduction of the hip to 25 to 30 degrees (Fig. 57.22, Step 3B)
   C. Extension of the hip to 35 to 40 degrees (Fig. 57.23, Step 3C)
   D. Adduction of the hip to 0 degrees (Fig. 57.24, Step 3D)
   E. Repeat this series of movements three to five times.
   F. Success of the technique is determined by retesting iliosacral motion.

Lower Extremity Somatic Dysfunction

LONGITUDINAL ARCH SPRINGING

Diagnosis

Restriction: Rigidity or reduced motion of the longitudinal arch

Treatment Position

Patient: Supine

Physician: Seated at the foot of the table

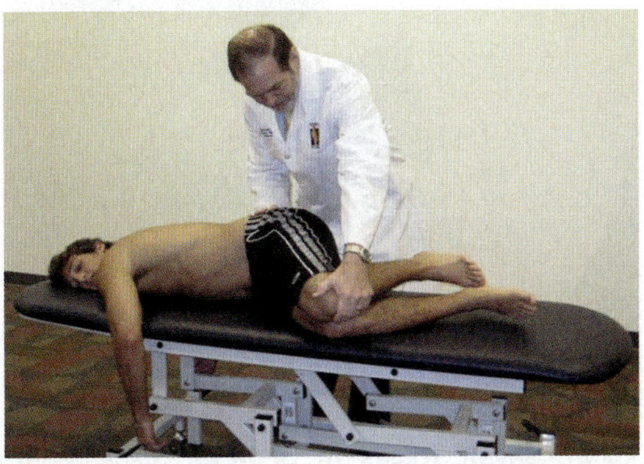

Figure 57.20. Posteriorly rotated innominate—modified Sims position, step 2.

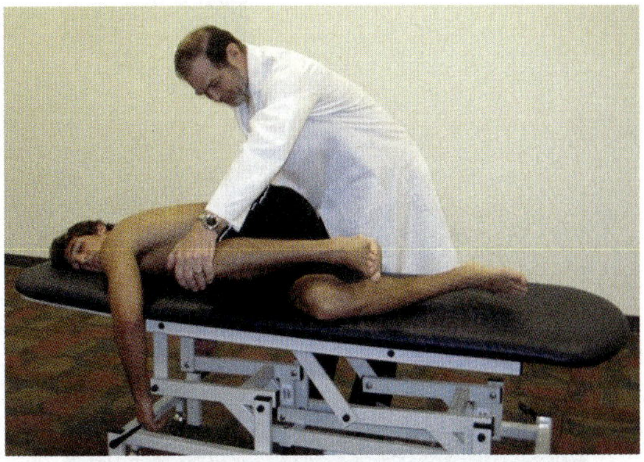

Figure 57.21. Posteriorly rotated innominate—modified Sims position, step 3A: flexion.

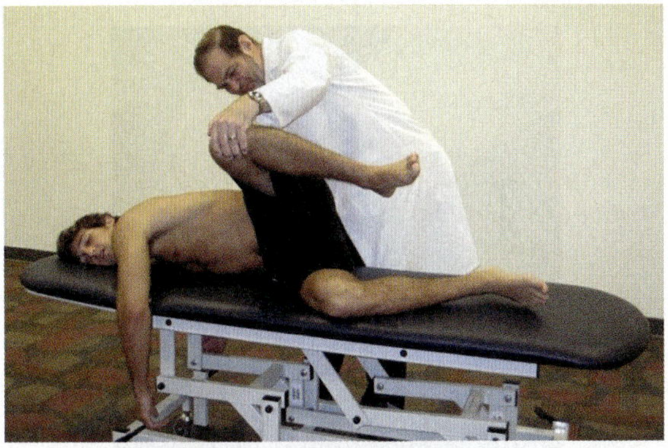

Figure 57.22. Posteriorly rotated innominate—modified Sims position, step 3B: abduction.

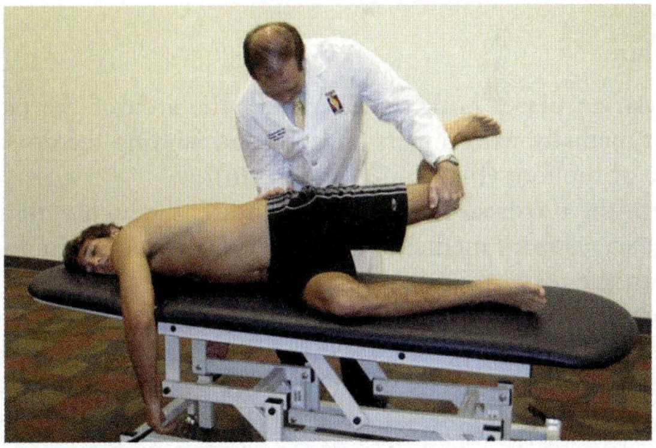

Figure 57.23. Posteriorly rotated innominate—modified Sims position, step 3C: extension.

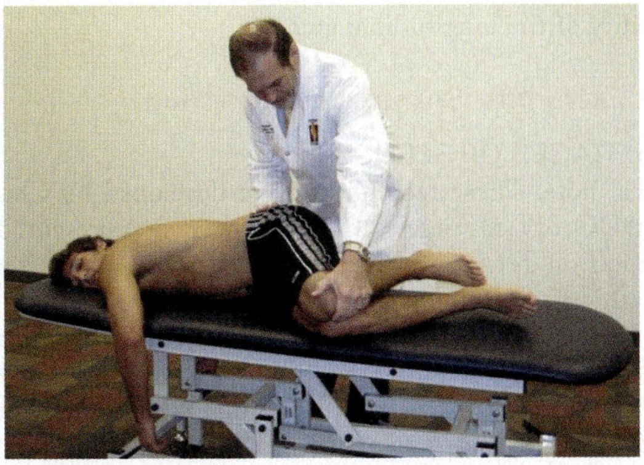

Figure 57.24. Posteriorly rotated innominate—modified Sims position, step 3D: adduction.

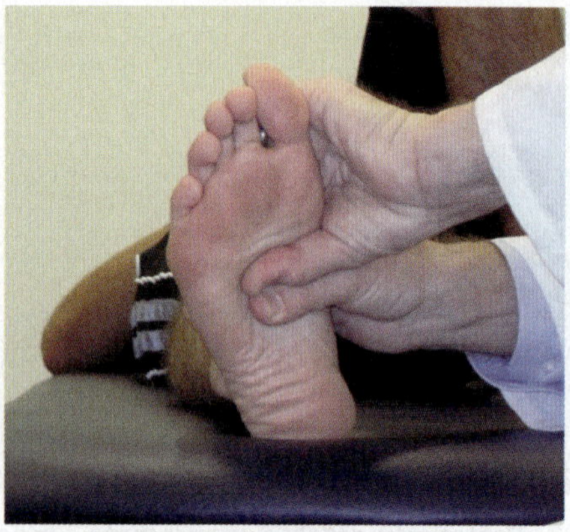

Figure 57.25. Longitudinal arch springing.

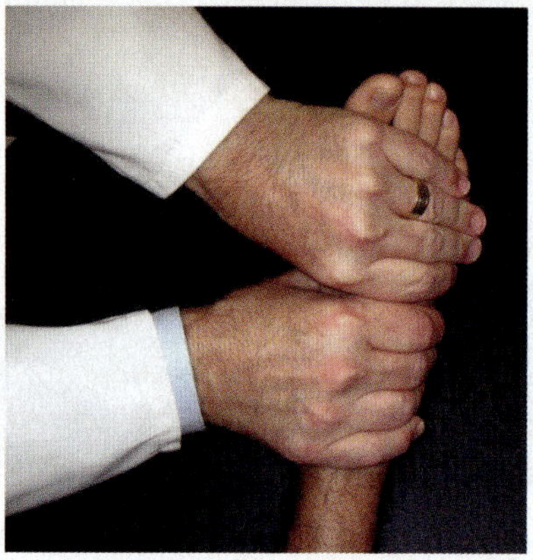

Figure 57.26. Longitudinal arch springing, step 4.

Procedure

1. Physician places both thumbs under the arch of the patient's foot medially, with fingers of each hand fanning the dorsal surface of the foot (Figs. 57.25 and 57.26).
2. With the proximal thumb, physician lifts the arch with a force that wraps from medial to lateral across the top of the foot.
3. With the distal thumb, physician lifts the lateral aspect of the more distal portion of the arch. Physicians hand wraps medially around the patient's foot, creating an arch raising counterforce.
4. Physician's two hands twist in opposite directions with a "wringing" motion, re-establishing the arch. After each wringing motion, physician's thumbs are shifted slightly more proximal or distal on the arch, not twisting the patient's foot in exactly the same way each time.
5. Success of the technique is determined by re-evaluating the mobility of the longitudinal arch.

Upper Extremity Somatic Dysfunction

SEVEN STAGES OF SPENCER

Historical note: These techniques were developed by Charles H. Spencer, DO, of Los Angeles, CA. They were first presented before the Section on Technic at the Portland Session of the American Osteopathic Association Convention, August 1915, and published in the *Journal of the American Osteopathic Association*. The original version of these techniques was largely forgotten, as were the photos and many personal modifications developed by osteopathic physicians over the ensuing years. One of the common modifications of stage 5 was taught by Angus Cathie, DO, in Philadelphia, hence the division of stage 5 into parts 5-A and 5-B. Stage 5-A is the technique as Spencer performed it.[1–4] Another commonly taught modification is the addition of a postisometric relaxation muscle energy technique performed in the same position for those stages that permit this sort of modification.

Indications

Bursitis of the shoulder
Tendinitis and tenosynovitis of the shoulder
Fibrous adhesive capsulitis

Treatment Position

Patient: Lateral recumbent with the shoulder to be treated away from the table

Physician: Standing at the side of the table, facing the patient at the level of the patient's chest

PROCEDURE

Stage 1: Extension

1. Physician uses one hand to stabilize the patient's shoulder girdle, by spanning the scapular spine and clavicle superiorly with the thumb and fingers (Fig. 57.27).
2. Physician's other hand grasps the patient's forearm just distal to the elbow.
3. Physician carries the shoulder into extension until the restrictive barrier is engaged.
4. Physician applies a gentle but firm force carrying the shoulder a short distance through its restrictive barrier, holds it for 1 or 2 seconds, and then releases it. Passive tissue tension will return the shoulder to a position just inside the restrictive barrier. Physician applies this force rhythmically, stretching 1 to 2 seconds, followed by a release of that stretch. Physician continues this rhythmic stretching until no further progress in shoulder extension can be appreciated.
5. Muscle energy modification: Patient flexes the shoulder against the physician's unyielding resistance. This contraction is held for 3 to 5 seconds followed by a second of relaxation before the restrictive barrier is again engaged.
6. Step 5 is repeated three to five times.
7. Success of the technique is determined by retesting shoulder range of motion in extension. Success is determined in part by reassessing the patient's symptoms.

Stage 2: Flexion

1. Physician draws the patient's arm across in front of the body toward flexion. At the same time, physician shifts their feet, turning their body to face the head of the table, with the patient's arm in front of the physician (Fig. 57.28).

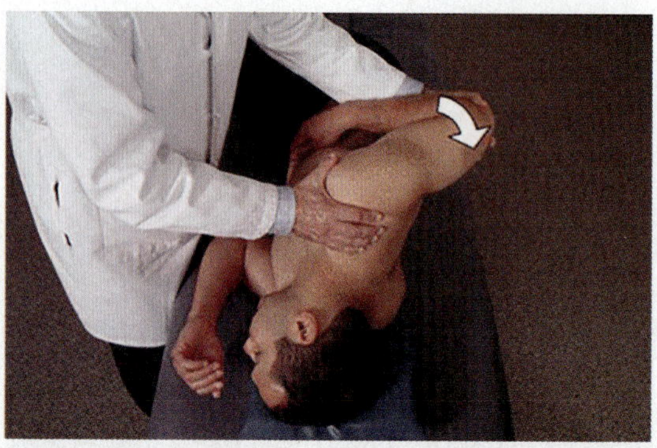

Figure 57.27. Seven stages of Spencer. Stage 1, extension. (Reprinted with permission from Nicholas AS, Nicholas EA. *Atlas of Osteopathic Techniques*. 3rd ed. Wolters Kluwer; 2016:549.)

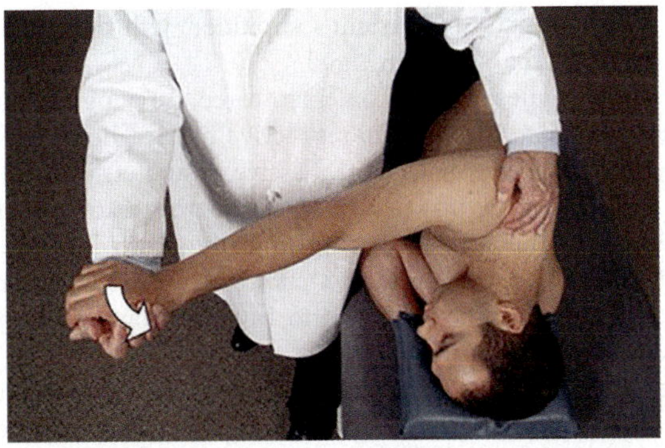

Figure 57.28. Seven stages of Spencer. Stage 2, flexion. (Reprinted with permission from Nicholas AS, Nicholas EA. *Atlas of Osteopathic Techniques*. 3rd ed. Wolters Kluwer; 2016:550.)

2. Physician switches hands and grasps the patient's hand with the hand farthest from the patient.
3. Physician uses the hand closest to the patient to anchor the shoulder girdle, by placing the heel of the hand on the spine of the scapula, with fingers extended over the top of the shoulder to the clavicle.
4. Physician carries the shoulder into flexion until the restrictive barrier is engaged.
5. Physician applies a gentle but firm force carrying the shoulder a short distance through its restrictive barrier, holds it for 1 or 2 seconds, and then releases it. Passive tissue tension will return the shoulder to a position just inside the restrictive barrier. Physician applies this force rhythmically, stretching 1 to 2 seconds, followed by a release of that stretch. Physician continues this rhythmic stretching until no further progress in shoulder flexion can be appreciated.
6. Muscle energy modification: Patient extends their shoulder against the physician's unyielding resistance. This contraction is held for 3 to 5 seconds followed by a second of relaxation before the restrictive barrier is again engaged.
7. Step 5 is repeated three to five times.
8. Success of the technique is determined by retesting shoulder range of motion in flexion. Success is determined in part by reassessing the patient's symptoms.

Stage 3: Compression Circumduction

1. Return to the starting position for stage 1.
2. Physician abducts the patient's shoulder to approximately 90 degrees (Fig. 57.29).
3. Physician very gently compresses the patient's elbow toward the glenoid fossa.
4. Physician starts making small clockwise circles, in a circumduction motion. Physician gradually enlarges these circles, creating larger and larger concentric circles as the patient's condition permits. Physician continues this movement for 15 to 30 seconds.
5. Physician then reverses direction, performing the same maneuver in a counterclockwise direction. There are occasions where a restriction may not be felt in one direction but may become quite evident in the reverse direction.
6. It is not necessary to perform the entire circle every time. If an arc of motion is identified that is particularly restricted, movement can be limited to that restricted arc.
7. Muscle energy modification: None for stage 3.
8. Success of the technique is determined by reassessing circumduction of the shoulder. Success is determined in part by reassessing the patient's symptoms.

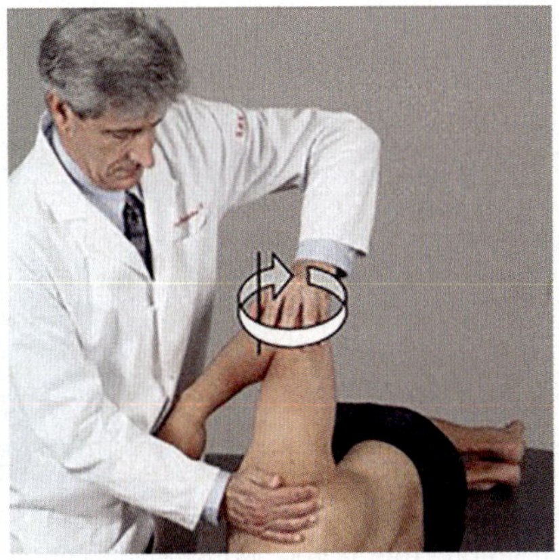

Figure 57.29. Seven stages of Spencer. Stage 3, compression and circumduction. (Reprinted with permission from Nicholas AS, Nicholas EA. *Atlas of Osteopathic Techniques*. 3rd ed. Wolters Kluwer; 2016:551.)

Stage 4: Traction Circumduction

1. Upon completion of stage 3, the physician's hand extends the patient's elbow, grasps the patient's arm at the wrist, and encircles it (physician takes care not to compress any of the neural or vascular structures crossing the wrist joints) (Fig. 57.30).
2. Physician places a gentle traction upward toward the ceiling on the patient's wrist.
3. Physician starts making small clockwise circles, in a circumduction motion. Physician gradually enlarges these circles, creating larger and larger concentric circles as the patient's condition permits. Physician continues this movement for 15 to 30 seconds.
4. Physician then reverses direction, performing the same maneuver in a counterclockwise direction. There are occasions where a restriction may not be felt in one direction but may become quite evident in the reverse direction.
5. It is not necessary to perform the entire circle every time. If an arc of motion is identified that is particularly restricted, movement can be limited to that restricted arc.
6. Muscle energy modification: None for stage 4.
7. Success of the technique is determined by reassessing circumduction of the shoulder. Success is determined in part by reassessing the patient's symptoms.

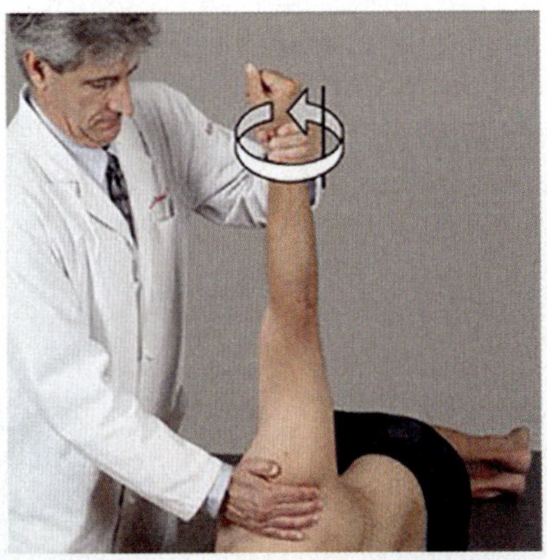

Figure 57.30. Seven stages of Spencer. Stage 4, traction and circumduction. (Reprinted with permission from Nicholas AS, Nicholas EA. *Atlas of Osteopathic Techniques*. 3rd ed. Wolters Kluwer; 2016:552.)

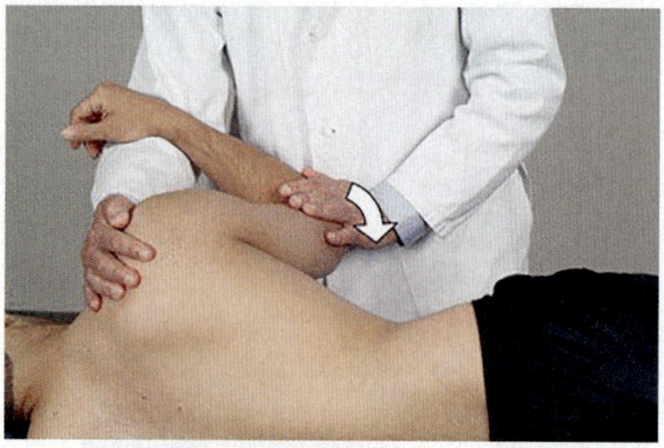

Figure 57.31. Seven stages of Spencer. Stage 5A, adduction and external rotation. (Reprinted with permission from Nicholas AS, Nicholas EA. *Atlas of Osteopathic Techniques*. 3rd ed. Wolters Kluwer; 2016:554.)

Stage 5A: Adduction and External Rotation

1. Return to the starting position for stage 1 (Fig. 57.31).
2. The physician's cephalad forearm (the one stabilizing the shoulder girdle) is positioned at right angles to the long axis of the patient's body, parallel to the surface plane of the table.
3. The patient's arm is slightly flexed with the wrist and hand positioned to rest on the physician's cephalad forearm.
4. Physician's caudad hand exerts gentle pressure at the elbow, adducting the patient's shoulder until the restrictive barrier is engaged.
5. Physician applies a gentle but firm force, carrying the shoulder a short distance through its restrictive barrier, holds it for 1 or 2 seconds, and then releases it. Passive tissue tension will return the shoulder to a position just inside the restrictive barrier. Physician applies this force rhythmically, stretching 1 to 2 seconds, followed by a release of that stretch. Physician continues this rhythmic stretching until no further progress in shoulder adduction can be appreciated.
6. Muscle energy modification: Patient abducts the shoulder against the physician's unyielding resistance. This contraction is held for 3 to 5 seconds followed by a second of relaxation before the restrictive barrier is again engaged.
7. Step 5 is repeated three to five times.
8. Success of the technique is determined by retesting shoulder range of motion in adduction. Success is determined in part by reassessing the patient's symptoms.

Stage 5B: Abduction

1. Return to the starting position for stage 5 (Fig. 57.32).
2. Physician abducts the patient's shoulder with one hand, until the restrictive barrier is engaged.
3. Physician applies a gentle but firm force, carrying the shoulder a short distance through its restrictive barrier, holds it for 1 or 2 seconds, and then releases it. Passive tissue tension will return the shoulder to a position just inside the restrictive barrier. Physician applies this force rhythmically, stretching 1 to 2 seconds, followed by a release of that stretch. Physician continues this rhythmic stretching until no further progress in shoulder abduction can be appreciated.
4. Muscle energy modification: Patient adducts the shoulder against the physician's unyielding resistance. This contraction is held for 3 to 5 seconds followed by a second of relaxation before the restrictive barrier is again engaged.
5. Step 5 is repeated three to five times.
6. Success of the technique is determined by retesting shoulder range of motion in abduction. Success is determined in part by reassessing the patient's symptoms.

Stage 6: Internal Rotation

Note: Patients with severely advanced fibrous adhesive capsulitis may not be able to be placed in position for this technique without significant modification (Fig. 57.33).

1. Physician abducts the patient's shoulder 45 degrees, internally rotates the shoulder 90 degrees (if possible), and then places the dorsum of the patient's hand in the small of the back.
2. Physician reinforces the anterior portion of the patient's shoulder with one hand.
3. Physician gently pulls the patient's elbow forward until the restrictive barrier is engaged.
4. Physician applies a gentle but firm force carrying the shoulder a short distance through its restrictive barrier, holds it for 1 or 2 seconds, and then releases it. Passive tissue tension will return the shoulder to a position just inside the restrictive barrier. Physician applies this force rhythmically, stretching 1 to 2 seconds, followed by a release of that stretch. Physician continues this rhythmic stretching until no further progress in shoulder abduction can be appreciated.
5. Muscle energy modification: Patient pulls the elbow backward against the physician's unyielding resistance. This contraction is held for 3 to 5 seconds followed by a second of relaxation before the restrictive barrier is again engaged.
6. Step 6 is repeated three to five times.
7. Success of the technique is determined by retesting shoulder range of motion in internal rotation. Success is determined in part by reassessing the patient's symptoms.

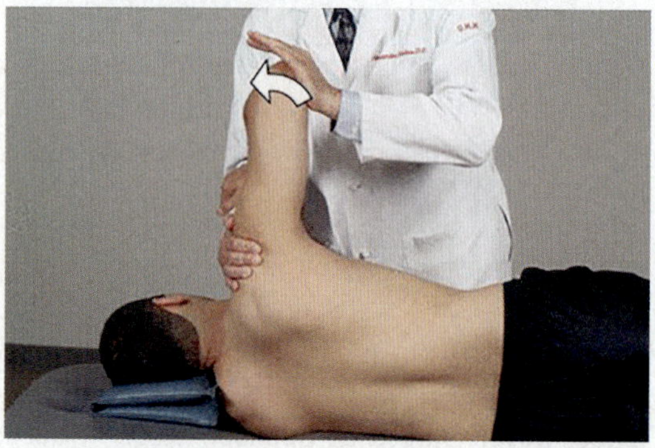

Figure 57.32. Seven stages of Spencer. Stage 5B, abduction. (Reprinted with permission from Nicholas AS, Nicholas EA. *Atlas of Osteopathic Techniques*. 3rd ed. Wolters Kluwer; 2016:553.)

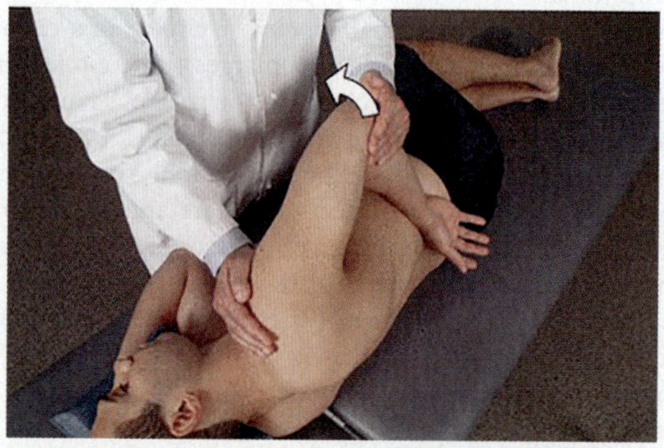

Figure 57.33. Seven stages of Spencer. Stage 6, internal rotation. (Reprinted with permission from Nicholas AS, Nicholas EA. *Atlas of Osteopathic Techniques*. 3rd ed. Wolters Kluwer; 2016:555.)

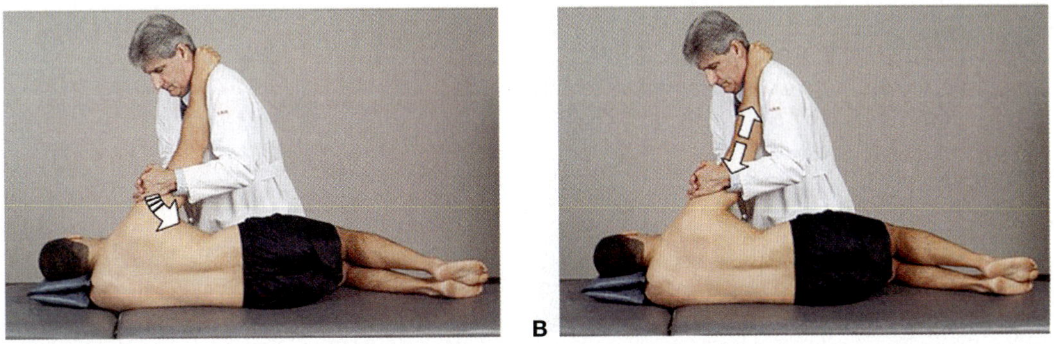

Figure 57.34. **A** and **B.** Seven stages of Spencer. Stage 7, traction. (Reprinted with permission from Nicholas AS, Nicholas EA. *Atlas of Osteopathic Techniques.* 3rd ed. Wolters Kluwer; 2016:556.)

Stage 7: Traction with Inferior Glide

1. Physician turns their torso to face the head of the table (Fig. 57.34A,B).
2. Physician abducts the patient's arm. The patient's hand and wrist are placed on the physician's shoulder which is closest to the patient.
3. With fingers interlaced, the physician's hands are placed just distal to the glenohumeral joint.
4. Physician scoops the patient's humeral head in a caudad direction, parallel to the table, creating a translatory motion toward the inferior edge of the glenoid fossa.
5. Physician applies a gentle but firm force carrying the patient's shoulder a short distance through its restrictive barrier, holds it for 1 or 2 seconds, and then releases it. Passive tissue tension will return the shoulder to a position just inside the restrictive barrier. Physician applies this force rhythmically, stretching 1 to 2 seconds, followed by a release of that stretch. Physician continues this rhythmic stretching until no further progress in shoulder abduction can be appreciated.
6. Muscle energy modification: While the physician maintains caudad traction on the patient's arm, the patient's hand is pressed down against the physician's shoulder. This contraction is held for 3 to 5 seconds followed by a second of relaxation before the restrictive barrier is again engaged.
7. Step 6 is repeated three to five times.
8. Success of the technique is determined by retesting shoulder range of motion. Success is determined in part by reassessing the patient's symptoms.

Rib Somatic Dysfunction

RIB RAISING: SEATED POSITION

Diagnosis

Restriction of motion of ribs 2 to 6. Motion will be created through traction on the pectoralis major muscle. (Motion may be imparted indirectly to rib 1 via its clavicular relations and ribs 7 to 10 through the attachments of the serratus anterior muscle.)

Treatment Position

Patient: Seated on the side or end of the treatment table

Physician: Standing facing the patient with one foot behind the other

Procedure

1. Patient crosses arms, with thumbs hooked into the antecubital fossa (Fig. 57.35).
2. Physician reaches under the patient's arms with both hands and then passes them over the patient's shoulders.
3. The pads of the physician's fingers make contact at the level of the second costotransverse articulation, just lateral to that same joint. Note: At each rib level, the pads of the physician's fingers should be placed between the costotransverse articulation and the angle of the rib.
4. Physician's weight is leaned onto the back foot, drawing the patient toward the physician. Patient's forearms should translate forward, parallel to the floor. At the same time, this should permit the patient's shoulders to drop, increasing the tension on the pectoral musculature and drawing the anterior aspect of the ribs superiorly.
5. Simultaneously, the pads of the physician's fingers press forward to create a gapping pressure at the costotransverse articulations.
6. This position is held for 1 second and then released, allowing the physician's weight to transfer to the more anterior foot and the patient to spring back to a more upright position.
7. The pads of the physician's fingers move down one rib level and repeats. Physician continues this stepwise down the rib cage until the rib levels can no longer be comfortably reached (usually in the range of ribs 6 to 8).
8. Physician reverses the procedure, working back up the rib cage until the second rib is reached again.
9. Success of the technique is determined by retesting the motion of the previously restricted costal levels.

Abdominal: Other Somatic Dysfunctions

LIVER ARTICULATION

Note: In this technique, the liver is considered to articulate with the diaphragm. Inflammatory conditions involving the liver may result in adherence of the liver to the diaphragm with subsequent restriction of diaphragmatic and lower right costal motion.

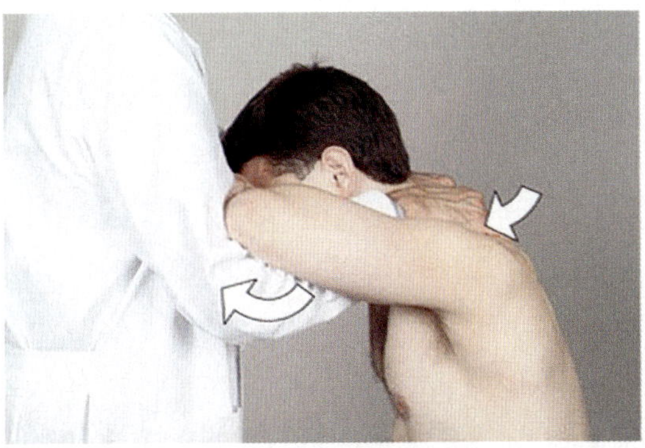

Figure 57.35. **Rib raising, seated position.** (Reprinted with permission from Nicholas AS, Nicholas EA. *Atlas of Osteopathic Techniques.* 3rd ed. Wolters Kluwer; 2016:108.)

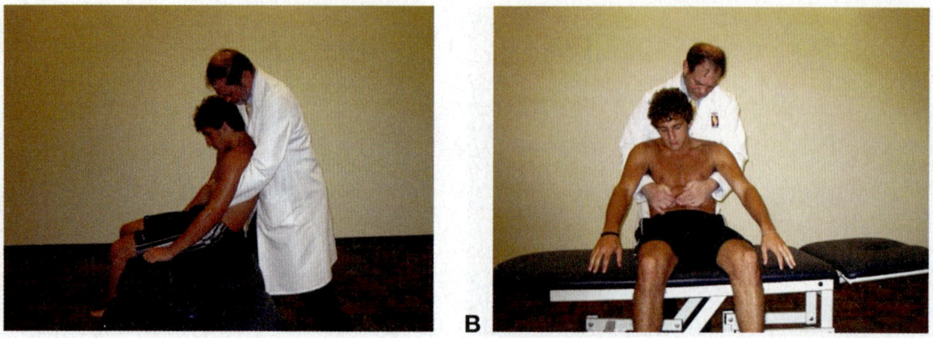

A B

Figure 57.36. A and **B.** Liver articulation.

Diagnosis
Restriction of hepatic motion relative to the diaphragm.

Treatment Position
Patient: Seated on the side of the treatment table
Physician: Standing behind the seated patient

Procedure

1. Physician reaches under the patient's arms, brining finger pads into contact with the patient's abdominal wall 1.5 to 2 inches below the right costal margin (Fig. 57.36A,B).
2. Patient slumps back against the physician, relaxing the abdominal wall.
3. The pads of the physician's fingers exert a posterior pressure and are then curled upward against the inferior surface of the anterior edge of the liver.
4. Patient takes a deep breath.
5. Physician follows the liver edge as it glides slightly down and forward with downward motion of the diaphragm.
6. Patient exhales. Physician again follows the liver edge as it glides superiorly and posteriorly with upward motion of the diaphragm.
7. Physician increases pressure against the liver margin and instructs the patient to breathe deeply again. Try not to allow the liver to move.
8. Patient exhales, and the physician follows the liver as it moves with exhalation.
9. Repeat steps 7 and 8 until no further increase in liver motion is palpable.
10. Success of the technique is determined by reassessing diaphragmatic and right lower costal motion.

SUMMARY

Articulatory techniques span a wide range of force levels and are therefore adaptable to a wide variety of patient body types and locations of dysfunction, making them one of the most versatile techniques available to the osteopathic physician. They can be used alone or in combination with any other manipulative technique.

REFERENCES

1. Spencer H. Shoulder technique. *J Am Osteopath Assoc.* 1916;15:218–220.
2. Spencer H. Treatment of bursitis and tendinitis. *JAOA.* 1926;25:528–529.
3. Patriquin DA. The evolution of osteopathic manipulative technique: the Spencer technique. *J Am Osteopath Assoc.* 1992;92:1134–1136, 1139–1146.
4. Nicholas AS, Nicholas EA. *Atlas of Osteopathic Techniques.* Lippincott Williams & Wilkins; 2008.

58 A Modern Approach to Chapman Reflex Points

CHRISTIAN FOSSUM ▪ MICHAEL L. KUCHERA ▪ WILLIAM H. DEVINE

KEY CONCEPTS

- Identification of gangliform contractions known as "Chapman Reflex Points" is an important consideration in the neurologic–autonomic model of osteopathic health care.
- Gangliform contractions are tender, palpatory tissue texture changes believed to be fascial congestions, resulting from lymph stasis secondary to visceral dysfunction.
- These contractions are generally deep to the skin and subcutaneous tissue, most often lying on the deep fascia or periosteum.
- Sometimes described as neurolymphatic points, their identification may help in differential diagnosis, as well as in a variety of treatment approaches such as vibratory stimulation.

CASE STUDY 1

A 34-year-old female presented to the office with complaints of gastrointestinal (GI) upset, nausea, and vomiting. The nausea and vomiting started suddenly 7 days ago and has continued "on and off." She was seen in the emergency department (ED) 3 days ago, and a diagnosis of early viral gastroenteritis was made. The medicine prescribed had helped the nausea, but the patient continued to experience vomiting, fatigue, and weakness. She complained of abdominal pain that was diffuse and sharp and cramping with eating. She denied fever or chills.

PHYSICAL EXAMINATION

- Lethargic female
- T = 98.0, P = 112, R = 20, and B/P = 110/80 (normal for the patient was 80+/60)

Abdominal Examination

- Suprapubic and subxiphoid tenderness to palpation.
- There was no hepatomegaly.

Structural Exam

- Tender Chapman reflex (CR) on the *anterior sternum* consistent with pylorus
- TART changes in the T5–T9 paraspinal region

Test Results

- The blood sugar was normal at 73 mg/dL.
- The urine dipstick revealed a high specific gravity of greater than 1.030. The pH was 6.0. There were moderate-to-large ketones along with 2+ urobilinogen and a trace of bilirubin.

DIAGNOSIS

Vomiting, unspecified with dehydration
Costal cage somatic dysfunction
Thoracic somatic dysfunction

PLAN

The patient was admitted to the hospital for further workup and rehydration. A complete workup was performed, which included abdominal and pelvic ultrasounds, and an upper GI series. Other than dehydration, all findings were normal except for "mild swelling of the duodenum" on the UGI, which was reported as a "nonspecific finding." Her primary treatment was IV fluid replacement. The patient was discharged on the third hospital day. Her discharge diagnosis was consistent with the clinical perception of vomiting due to a noninfectious gastroenteritis, leading to fluid depletion and dehydration.

Her physician continued weekly treatment for the headaches using cranial osteopathic manipulative medicine. At each of these visits, the patient would report that her GI problem was "getting better." Each time, the CRs on the sternum remained variably tender, which was consistent with a suspected pyloric stenosis.

After 11 weeks of recurrence, the physician performed another comprehensive osteopathic structural examination. Again, there were the TART changes in the T5–T9 and subxiphoid regions and a positive reflex referable to the pylorus. However, the regional CR screen also yielded positive reflexes for "stomach peristalsis" and "stomach acidity." The patient finally admitted that she really had not been able to keep much food down since leaving the hospital.

The patient was referred to an osteopathically focused internist for re-evaluation. Endoscopy revealed pyloric valve swelling and constriction, necessitating the use of a pediatric endoscope to examine the duodenum. A new diagnosis of prepyloric antral ulcer was made.

In this case, CRs identified the problem almost 3 months *before* the definitive diagnosis was made by endoscopic evaluation. Although the original diagnostic workup was negative, only the CRs consistently pointed to the correct diagnosis 2 months prior to re-evaluation. CRs correlated well with the patient's final diagnosis.

DEFINING CHAPMAN REFLEXES

The palpable tissue texture phenomenon known as a *Chapman reflex* has benefited from the historical evolution of its definition and from its integration by different practitioners. Understanding the history allows for greater accuracy in locating, interpreting, and using this somatic finding in the clinical setting. The osteopathic profession currently defines CRs as:

TABLE 58.1

Historical Definitions of Chapman Reflexes

Definition	Author
The original description of *Ganglion-formed* became *Gangliform contracted lymphoid tissue nodules.*	Frank Chapman, DO, 1928
It seemed to me that the lymphatic system had much more profound influence on bodily functions than it had been given credit for... my special plea is on behalf of the lymphatic aspects of disease, which I regard of paramount importance whether they originated in bony lesions, infections, toxins, or other cause.	Frank Chapman, DO, 1937
A Chapman lesion is the result of a lymph stasis in the viscus. This lymph stasis is responsible for the dysfunction of the organ. Both the lymph stasis and the resultant dysfunction are reflexly responsible for the Chapman lesion, due, in part, to nerve impulse and also to a chemical reaction of the lymphoid tissue in which the lesion is found.	Charles Owens, DO, 1944
I believe that it is an autonomic nerve reflex, and that the lesion or nodule is a granulation tissue reaction.	H.L. Samblanet, DO, 1944

> A system of reflex points that present as predictable anterior and posterior fascial tissue texture abnormalities (plaque-like changes or stringiness of the involved tissues) assumed to be reflections of visceral dysfunction or pathology.[1]

This definition encompasses the lymphatic, neuroendocrine, and autonomic response to injury, illness, and disease as palpable and predictable viscerosomatic tissue reflexes found on the anterior and posterior body surface. Historically, definitions of the CR point reflect its structural feel, linking an evolving speculation with the underlying cause for the dysfunction (Table 58.1).

Several mechanisms for the CR points have been proposed by those who value their use empirically. These include:

- Lymphatic abnormalities
- Fibrositis deposits
- Inflamed lymph vessels passing over the ribs and bones
- Inflamed nerve endings
- Inflamed sympathetic nerve filaments around terminal arterioles[2]

Thus, lymphatic, neuroendocrine, and autonomic interactions were considered a part of CRs early on.

HISTORICAL BACKGROUND

Frank Chapman

Early osteopathic practitioners emphasized the role of the nervous system and body fluids in health and disease. Somatic dysfunctions of the musculoskeletal system were considered anatomical abnormalities obstructing these physiologic processes. Through these structure and function considerations, osteopathic manipulation was employed to assist the body's recovery from injuries, illnesses, and disease.[3–7] This was the prevailing philosophy when Frank Chapman (1871–1931) enrolled at the American School of Osteopathy in Kirksville, Missouri. After graduating in 1899, he returned to Galesburg, Illinois, where he practiced until his death.[8]

In 1901, Chapman encountered a patient with severe adenitis, who had a slow response to osteopathic treatment directed to the spine. He noticed that the "groin glands" (inguinal lymphatic nodes) as well as those on the medial side of the thighs were indurated and painful. Chapman decided to gently manipulate to only affect these glands. The patient had improved so much upon his return that subsequent treatment was solely confined to manipulation around these indurated areas. This motivated Chapman to acquire a more detailed understanding of the lymphatic system and its role in health and disease.[9] Building on his osteopathic knowledge, which at that time lacked a detailed discourse on the lymphatic system, Chapman came across *Mechanical Vibratory Stimulation* by Maurice F. Pilgrim, MD. This seminal text described the capacity for mechanical stimulation of reflex centers to influence body fluids and lymphatic drainage, thereby affecting a variety of physiologic functions such as respiration, digestion, secretion, excretion, and muscular metabolism.[9,10] Though Pilgrim's method of treatment differed from that of Chapman's, it likely inspired Chapman's conception of *lymphatically based CRs*.

Encouraged by positive clinical outcomes, Chapman diligently began making observations and case records. He mapped the commonly congested lymphatic areas close to the body surface and referred to them as *neurolymphatic points*, since he believed that they bore a physiologic relation to the lymphatic and nervous system. By the late 1920s, Chapman located over 200 centers on the body surface and established their association with the visceral and endocrine glands.[9] The first chart of these observations was published in his 1929 text *Lymphatic reflexes: a specific method of osteopathic diagnosis and treatment.*[11]

Charles Owens

Charles Owens, DO, was Chapman's brother-in-law and classmate at the American School of Osteopathy. He had little involvement in the development of the CR system until close to Chapman's death. Troubled by an encumbering dizziness, Owens asked for Chapman's clinical opinion. He was intrigued by the way Chapman diagnosed and relieved the ailment. Owens subsequently encouraged Chapman to chart the specific reflex lesion areas for wider use by the osteopathic profession. This task was completed shortly before Chapman's death.[8] Owens then introduced the concept of CRs to the osteopathic community, through an article he penned[12]:

> "In this connection, I am glad to draw attention to the conclusions of an osteopathic physician, Dr. Frank Chapman of Galesburg, IL. As a result of years of research and study, Dr. Chapman advances the idea that in addition to the well-known spinal and sympathetic nervous system, with its controlling nerve centers, there lies within this same system an independent group of gangliform centers which control the activities of the lymphatic system in its relation to the viscera of the body, the knowledge of which enables the practitioner to determine with the utmost precision and accuracy the exact state of the various organs of the body.... That this information will be received with profound interest by that portion of the profession who have given much attention to the spleen and lymph flow in their practices, goes without saying... That the ability to be able to tell his patient, for example,

by the condition of one of these lymphatic centers, that he has a markedly disturbed condition of the hydrochloric secretions of the stomach; or, that the muscular action of the stomach is retarded by the state of another of these same centers, or, that he has a highly acid condition of the blood, due to a stenosis of the pyloric orifice holding the contents of the stomach against normal ejection until, by the continued accumulation of hydrochloric acid, the pylorus is compelled to open and permit some of the stomach content to pass, and do all this by these centers in place of having to resort to test meals, x-rays, etc., is hard to believe."[12]

After Chapman's death, Owens continued to develop the system and organized several postgraduate teaching seminars. He recognized CRs as viscerosomatic tissue reflexes and believed a lymph stasis in the viscus to be the cause for organ dysfunction. He also proposed pelvic girdle somatic dysfunctions as the causative factor, by interfering with blood and nerve supply to the gonads, triggering a cascade of endocrine responses. Owens named this cascade the *pelvic–thyroid* (with adrenals) *syndrome*,[13,14] which was later renamed the *pelvic-thyroid-adrenal*, or *PTA*, *syndrome*.[15] According to Owens, the thyroid was central to this syndrome, since its involvement elicits a widespread metabolic disturbance resulting in:

- Incomplete oxidation in cells
- Body fluids to move slowly
- Lymphatic engorgement leading to retention of toxins

The area of least resistance in the body would develop a local lymph stasis through nerve impulses and chemical reactions of the lymphoid tissue (Owens believed acetylcholine to be involved). This would result in a positive corresponding CR point on the body surface.[16]

In Owens' approach, addressing CRs was proposed to directly affect the disturbed body metabolism through:

- The autonomic nervous system
- The lymphatic system
- The endocrine glands

The treatment would thus help to:

- Normalize endocrine secretions
- Augment flow of body fluids
- Release inhibited trophic (nutritional) centers

Further Dissemination in the Osteopathic Community

Paul E. Kimberly, DO, FAAO, organized the first course on CRs for the osteopathic profession, but it was never offered due to the onset of World War II. In the late 1970s, Kimberly integrated CRs into osteopathic physical examination teachings during his tenure at the Kirksville College of Osteopathic Medicine. Like Chapman and Owens, he described them as *neurolymphatic points*, based on the apparent correlation with tissue texture changes at the anatomic sites, where the cutaneous vascular–lymphatic bundle exited together with the anterior and lateral cutaneous nerves (Figs. 58.1, 58.2, and 58.3A,B).

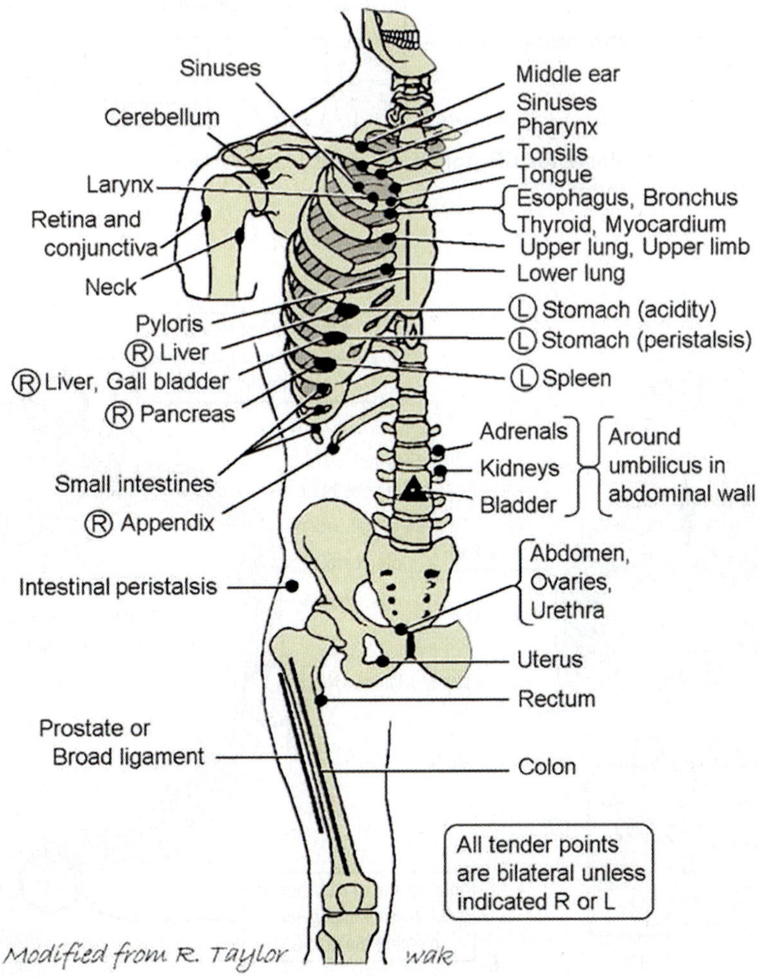

Figure 58.1. Anterior CR points. (Illustration by William A. Kuchera, DO, FAAO, with permission.)

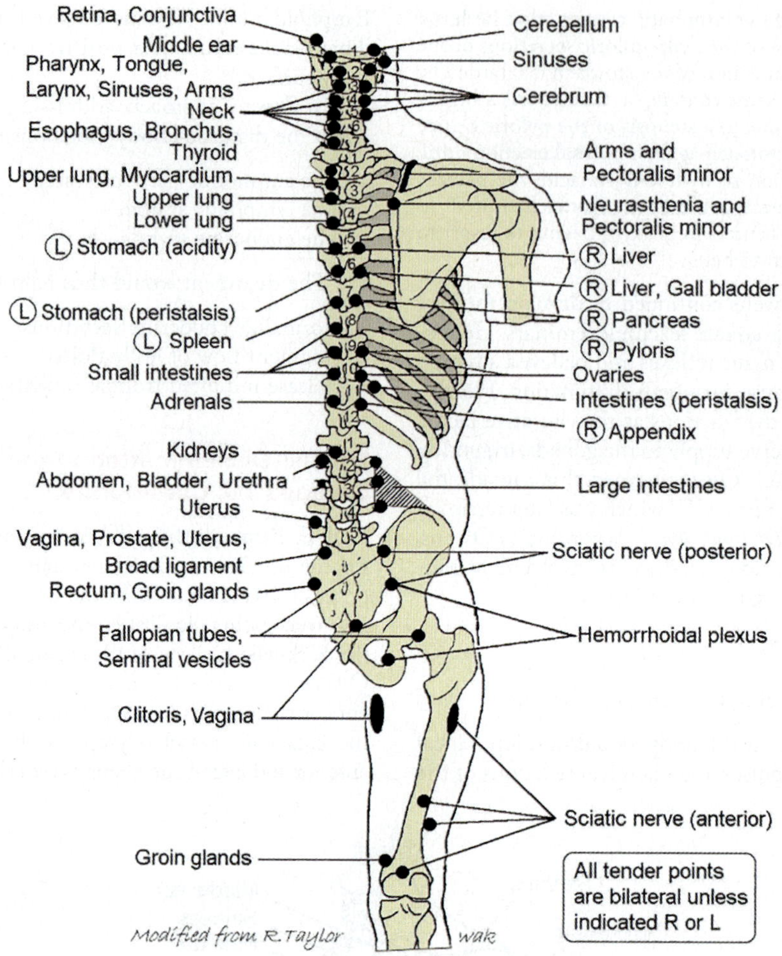

Figure 58.2. Posterior CR points. (Illustration by William A. Kuchera, DO, FAAO, with permission.)

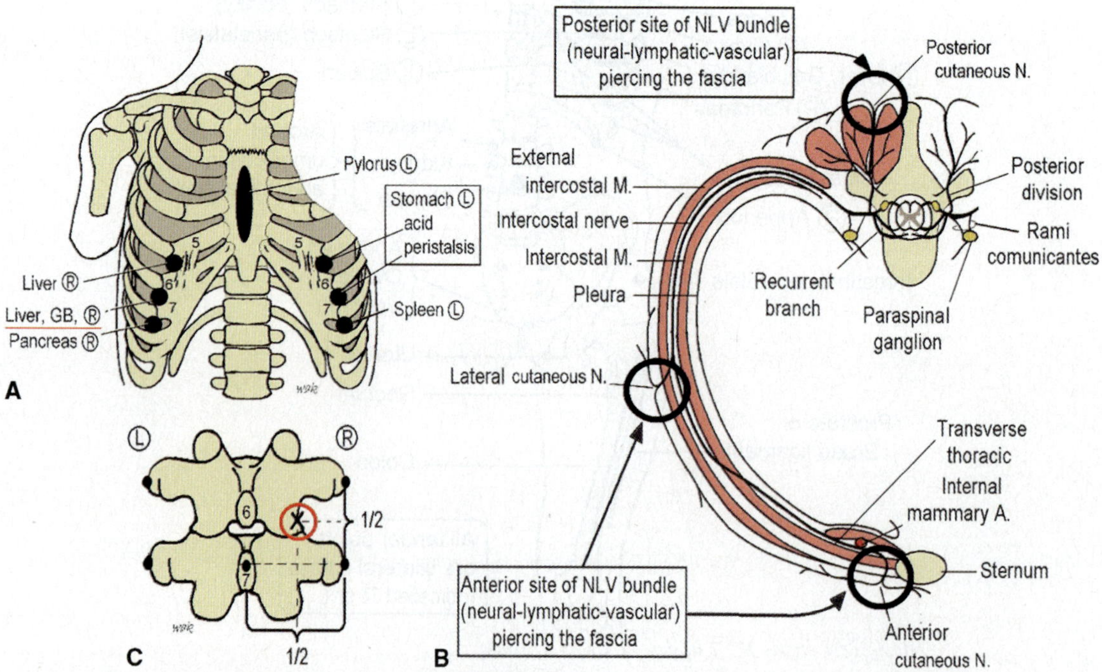

Figure 58.3. A, B, and **C.** Postulated anatomical correlations for CR point locations. (Illustration by William A. Kuchera, DO, FAAO, with permission.)

However, Kimberly presented CRs to his students as viscerosomatic reflexes related to the facilitated segment concept work of his faculty colleagues, Korr and Denslow.

Subsequently, many osteopathic educators described the reflexes as being more highly correlated with the sympathetic nervous system rather than the lymphatic system, indicating its influence on visceral function by acting on some part of a reflex arc.[17] Other authors have classified CRs as part of a viscerosomatic reflex, which points to the consistency in both the location of the CRs and the sympathetic innervation of the dysfunctional organ.[18] One of the authors (MLK) proposes that visceral or viscerosomatic findings may be less reliable when a tissue texture abnormality is defined as a CR, without evidence of a concomitant pattern.[19]

LOCATING AND PALPATING CHAPMAN REFLEXES

CRs are manifested by gangliform contractions, which are believed to be congestions within fascia due to lymph stasis secondary to visceral dysfunction.[20] The types of visceral dysfunction believed to cause positive CRs are[21]:

- Inflammation
- Spasm
- Distention of the viscera

The reflexes are located deep in the skin and subcutaneous areolar tissue, often lying on the deep fascia or periosteum.[22] They are generally found in specific locations, with sizes varying from a "BB" pellet to a pea or from a pinhead to an almond, and have certain recognizable palpatory characteristics,[8,20,22] which Owens described as follows[14]:

- Gangliform
- Edematous
- Ridge-like or ropy
- Fibrospongy
- Shotty

The most useful palpation technique may depend on the location of the CR points (Table 58.2).

TABLE 58.2

Examples of Manual Techniques for Various CR Points

CR Point	Palpatory Technique
Broad ligament (female) and prostate (male)	Deep kneading pressure with lift (should be longitudinal), fingers flexed toward the palm of the hand
Colon	Deep pressure with longitudinal rotary movement; alternative
Ovarian	Treatment approach with percussion hammer[a]
Kidneys	Gentle rotary movement
Adrenals	Deep firm rotary movement
Duodenum	Deep firm rotary movement
Stomach	Gentle but firm rotary movement
Spleen	Firm rotary movement
Small intestine	Firm rotary movement
Eye	Gentle but firm rotary movement
Ear	Gentle but firm rotary movement
Throat, nasal, bronchial	Gentle rotary movement
Pharynx, larynx	Firm rotary movement
Esophagus, tongue	Deep firm rotary movement
Upper and lower lung	Deep firm rotary movement
Arms	Deep firm rotary movement (sometimes steady pressure)
Neuritis of the upper limb	Firm but gentle rotary movement
Cerebellar	Gentle rotary movement
Cerebral	Firm gentle rotary movement
Heart	Firm deep rotary movement
Neurasthenia	Deep firm rotary movement
Atonic constipation	Gentle rotary movement
Appendix	Deep but gentle rotary movement
Urethral	Deep but gentle rotary movement
Cystitis	Firm and deep rotary movement
Sciatic–neuritis	Firm rotary movement
Wry neck	Deep rotary movement
Thyroid	Firm but gentle rotary movement
Gallbladder and liver	Firm but gentle rotary movement

(*continued*)

TABLE 58.2 (*Continued*)

Examples of Manual Techniques for Various CR Points

Examples Using Diagnostically Suited Anterior Points (Palpation should be directed and titrated to reach the tissue depth and location where the tissue texture change resides.)
Intercostal Sites (including sinus, bronchus, stomach): Finger pad directed posterosuperiorly along undersurface of the rib, searching with a deep, firm rotatory movement (examine adjacent sites using a little longitudinal glide along the undersurface of the rib rather than a poking or prodding motion)
Anterior Point Chart: Tip of the floating rib (e.g., appendix)—Deep but gentle rotator stimulation at the tip of the rib using the finger pad
Anterior Point Chart: Abdominal wall (including kidney, bladder)—Compress with finger pad through subcutaneous fat and tissues until reaching the deepest layer of the abdominal wall and there use a deep, firm, rotatory motion
Anterior Point Chart: Pelvis (including the ovary and uterus)—Use deep, firm, rotatory movement approximating the periosteal level of the pelvic bone
Anterior Point Chart: Iliotibial band region (including the colon and prostate)—Deep kneading pressure with lift (should be longitudinal), fingers flexed toward the palm of the hand; finger pads should compress medially approximating the periosteal level of the lateral femur
Posterior Point Chart (Paraspinal): Deep firm rotatory pressure midway between transverse processes of the vertebral segment involved and the segment below; lateral distance from the spinous process is about halfway to the tip of the transverse process ipsilateral to the side of the involved organ. Tissue characteristics will involve more bogginess than the anterior points

Adapted from Owens C. *Chapman's Reflexes Subseries: 7 Folders.* William L. Johnston Collection, Still National Osteopathic Museum; 1943, and Kuchera ML. A pragmatic interpretation of Chapman's reflexes. *J Am Acad Osteopath.* 2008.

[a]Percussion hammer alternative (Kuchera ML, Kuchera WA. *Osteopathic Considerations in Systemic Dysfunction.* 2nd ed. Greyden Press; 1994.).

For instance, in cases where the points are located on the transverse processes of vertebrae, contracted muscles may be overlying the Chapman point, which is often located in the deep fascia or periosteum. Thus, it may be necessary to first relax the overlying muscle to effectively treat the CR point.[14,23] The patient usually feels tenderness ranging from slightly painful to almost unbearably painful. Few patients could even show no tenderness response to firm digital pressure, although the CR point is palpable.[14] It is unknown whether this phenomenon is related to the visceral dysfunction being in early or chronic stages, to the patient's high pain threshold, or to neither. It could simply be a coincidental finding with no clinical relevance.

Historically, pain intensity has been proposed to denote the relative involvement of the related organ and the lack of pain to denote a process of long and very marked involvement.[24] The absence of tenderness in the point has also been suggested to indicate abnormal hypofunction of the associated organ.[25] For a CR point to be positive, both the anterior and posterior CR should be present.[9] The anterior CR is generally recommended for initial diagnosis, since they are more widespread than the posterior CR and have a consistent location. This helps to eliminate the confusion regarding which organ is involved.[24] The presence of a posterior CR confirms the diagnosis of a positive anterior CR.[9] Differentiation of a Chapman point from tissue texture changes described in other systems, however, may require additional historical and palpatory pattern information[19] (see Table 58.2).

When examining for CRs, best results are obtained with:

- The use of a reference chart to identify the location of each CR point
- Well-developed tactile skills to discriminate the findings as either normal or abnormal
- Knowledge of the patient's presenting complaint and medical history

Similarities and Differences between Other Palpably Similar Points

Palpable tissue texture changes appearing in the myofascial tissues have been described and mapped for thousands of years, in the form of acupuncture points. Their clinical use, their interpretation, and even their names are often dependent on the health care provider, who finds and groups them based on the perception of a commonality. Yet between grouping systems (and even within some systems), there are significant differences that distinguish one set of somatic body points from the others.

Chapman Reflexes in Osteopathic Modalities

Osteopathic physicians should attempt to differentiate between various tissue texture abnormalities, including:

- CRs
- Myofascial trigger points (MTrP)
- Tender points as first described by Jones in the counterstrain system
- Points considered by the American College of Rheumatology to be present in fibromyalgia syndrome
- Possibly even some acupuncture points

Based on the similarities among these different somatic or body point systems, they may merely be different views of the same phenomena.[19,26,27] Nonetheless, it is difficult to argue a certain overlap between these discrete clinical findings, since the involved pathophysiologies, patterns of associated signs and symptoms, and clinical implications are often very different (Table 58.3).

Overlap of Chapman Reflex Trigger Points beyond Osteopathic Medicine

One study argued a topographical congruency of 68% (when found within 1.5 cm of each other) between CR points and counterstrain

TABLE 58.3

Chapman Reflex Points, MTrP, and Tender Points

Clinical System	Location	Palpatory Quality	Pain Characteristics	Association	Classic Treatment
Chapman reflexes	Located in soft tissue structures: subcutaneous tissue, fascia, muscle, ligament, and perichondral or periosteal tissue. Mostly in deep fascia or periosteum	Granular feel of tissues overlying the CR. The CR itself is gangliform, contracted, edematous, ridge-like or ropy, shotty, or fibrospongy. Varying in size from a pinhead to that of an almond	Tenderness ranging from slightly painful to almost unbearable. It is well localized under the finger and has an almost sharp quality. No pain radiation.	Viscerosomatic tissue reflex with definite relationship to viscus or gland; pattern of associated somatic dysfunction includes somatic dysfunction in related collateral ganglion, paraspinal tissues (same facilitated segment), and perhaps cranial or sacral referral site of viscus	Rotary stimulation for 20–60 s
MTrP	Central MTrP in fibers in the midportion of muscle. Attachment MTrP in the myotendinous junction. Depth varies with muscles	Distinct nodules (contraction knots) at the MTrP felt in the muscle and a rope-like indulation (taut band)	Localized pain in taut band of the muscle with referred pain to a characteristic distant region based on myofascial referral maps	Local pathophysiology in the muscle exhibiting the MTrP. May cause motion restriction in associated joints; often, stimulation of point causes taut band twitch	Injection, dry needling, ischemic compression, postisometric relaxation (MET), spray and stretch, counterstrain
Tender point	Typically located in tendinous attachments, in the belly of a muscle, or in the ligaments associated with a joint dysfunction	Discrete, small, tense, and edematous, about the size of a fingertip	Exquisitely tender, very localized with no pain radiation. Typically at least four times as tender as the adjacent tissues	Specific muscle or joint somatic dysfunction	Counterstrain

tender points.[28] Another study also alludes to a possible overlap between CR points and acupuncture points.[29] When examining the pathologic associations (e.g., both point systems used for similar conditions) or congruency of a CR point to spatially related acupuncture point, a 20.6% congruency of the anterior points and 44.2% congruency of the posterior points were found.[30] The correlation between MTrP and acupuncture points has also been investigated. A study explored the overlap (positive correlation when points were within 3 cm of each other) between MTrP and acupuncture pain points (Ashi), which showed a 71% correlation based on spatial orientation and pain patterns.[31] The results of these studies should be interpreted with caution, as the definition of correlation or congruency differs between the authors (e.g., 1.5 to 3 cm).

MTrP can also alter neural, autonomic, vascular, and lymphatic activity. A number of MTrP with viscerosomatic and somatovisceral reflex activity have been reported in the literature.[32,33] Several MTrP linked to GI, cardiac, and genitourinary dysfunctions are identical to or in close proximity to the corresponding CR sites. Treatment of MTrP now embraces the use of multiple interventions, from dry needling to osteopathic treatment modalities such as muscle energy and counterstrain. Travell and Simons reported treatment of an MTrP in the lower anterior chest wall, which was diagrammatically consistent with the pattern of palpatory findings an osteopathic physician would report, if celiac ganglion and stomach CR dysfunctions were found. Treatment of this point was reported as such: "(p)ain, which previously had responded to medical therapy for a duodenal ulcer, became unresponsive and persisted until MTrP in the abdominal musculature were found and inactivated."[33]

This system, now termed *applied kinesiology*, was developed in the 1960s by chiropractor George Goodheart. It was initially based on the muscle testing method of physical therapists Kendall and Kendall, which Goodheart applied to the location of Chapman's "neurolymphatic" points. Later, Bennett's points for vascular function were also added to the system, which has since expanded to include acupuncture meridians as well.[34,35]

Further Considerations

A given point in a given system does not need to "read a book" to know where it should or could be; it simply exists. This means that a number of these existing points could end up in multiple systems. Their clinical use and interpretation, along with their names, are often dependent on their discoverer's perceptive. The evolution of CRs is no different. An osteopathic practitioner had grouped the points, with reason from anatomy and physiology, to identify their somatic relationship with underlying visceral or systemic dysfunction. Their clinical diagnostic and therapeutic use is still based on physicians applying them within the major osteopathic models of care, taking into account the risk to benefit ratio.

DIAGNOSTIC UTILITY

Many physicians use CRs as part of a screening or comprehensive osteopathic physical examination. These points are utilized for their contribution to the differential diagnosis and implication of dysfunction of an organ system, rather than for their role as a therapeutic intervention.[19,22] This said, because many modalities can directly treat these points, it is important to perform a complete or focused diagnostic screen prior to any use of physical therapy or preparatory OMT (such as soft tissue massage) that might temporarily reduce their sensitivity or change their tissue texture characteristics. One of the authors (KW) has formulated two principles for using CRs as a diagnostic tool:

1. A nontender CR, *by itself*, indicates nothing. *Never* make a diagnosis based solely on a nontender CR.
2. *Never* ignore or trivialize a tender CR unless there is a good explanation for the findings. This is especially true of a persistently tender reflex.

CRs are more likely to be used selectively from a diagnostic perspective, particularly in the hospital setting. For example, the 30- or 45-second CR screening examinations (Figs. 58.4 and 58.5) are time-effective screens that focus on selected organ systems, in conjunction with other findings in the patient's history and physical examination. The following case study illustrates the use of CRs in diagnosis.

CASE STUDY 2

A 13-year-old female is admitted to the pediatric floor of an osteopathic teaching hospital for complaints of severe lower abdominal/pelvic pain. In her examination, tenderness was found in the RLQ and midline pelvis. Urinalysis was normal. In this age group, the three most likely diagnoses to consider (in no particular order) are as follows:

1. Appendicitis
2. Cystitis
3. Ovarian cysts

DIAGNOSIS

CRs showed bilateral tender reflexes on the anterior/medial pubic bones near the pubic symphysis and unilateral posterior CRs at T9–T10 on the right side only. No other positive CRs were found in that body region (particularly those associated with the right kidney, urinary bladder, or appendix):

- Preoperative diagnosis (without use of CRs): Appendicitis versus right ovarian cyst (50/50 probability).
- Preoperative diagnosis (with use of CRs): Problem with the right ovary involving the entire ovary, both the medial and the lateral halves.
- Postoperative diagnosis: Massive right ovarian cyst obliterating the entire right ovary.

TREATMENT

A right oophorectomy and right salpingectomy were performed. This case illustrates the *high degree of specificity* that can be obtained from diagnosing visceral pathology in certain internal organs. It also shows how CRs are most commonly used as a *differentiator*, after the physician has narrowed the differential diagnosis to two or three possibilities.

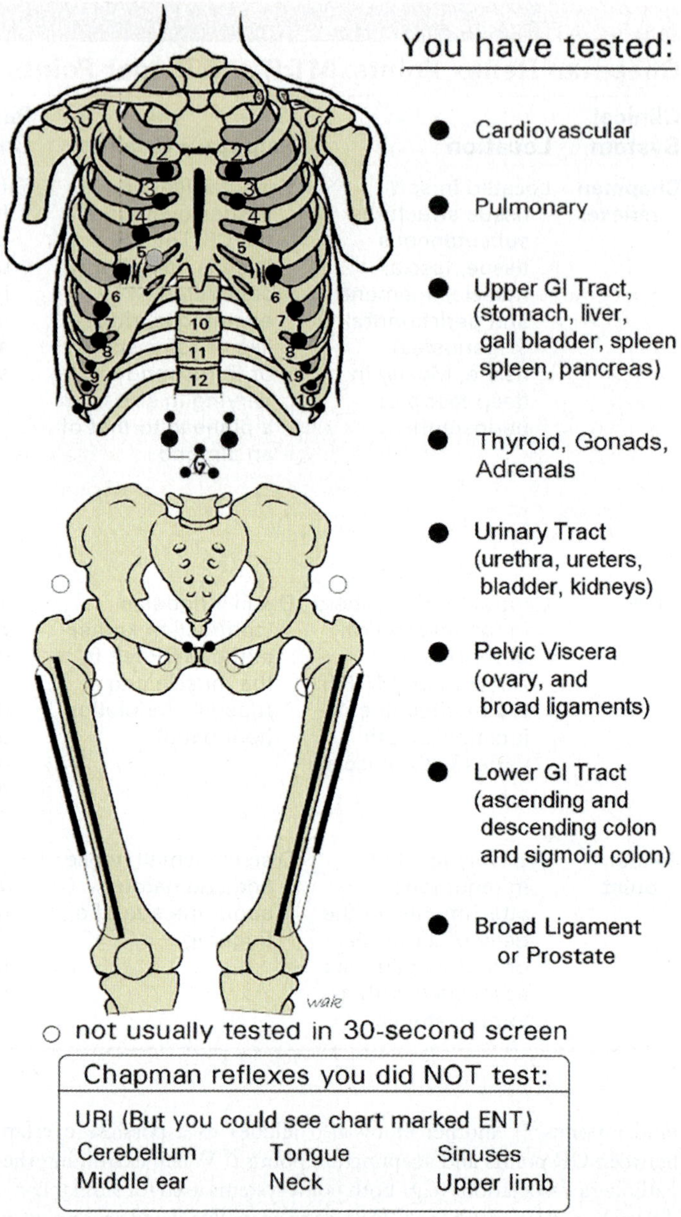

Figure 58.4. A 30-second visceral screen. (Illustration by William A. Kuchera, DO, FAAO, with permission.)

USE OF CHAPMAN REFLEXES

The preoperative prediction of right ovarian involvement was due to all of the patient's discomfort and tenderness to palpation being to the right of midline, in the lower abdominal/pelvic region. As mentioned above, there were bilateral tender Chapman points on the anterior medial pubis, although unilateral posterior CRs were on the right. In the case of paired organs, where only one organ is dysfunctional but the dysfunctional organ is associated with a marked degree of pathology, the physician may occasionally encounter a bilateral Chapman response (especially with the anterior points). Additional palpatory information helpful in the differential diagnosis includes tight, tender superior mesenteric ganglion site (not present when the pubic ramus point is secondary to the AL5 counterstrain point) and somatic dysfunction (especially ERS_R at T10 or T11).

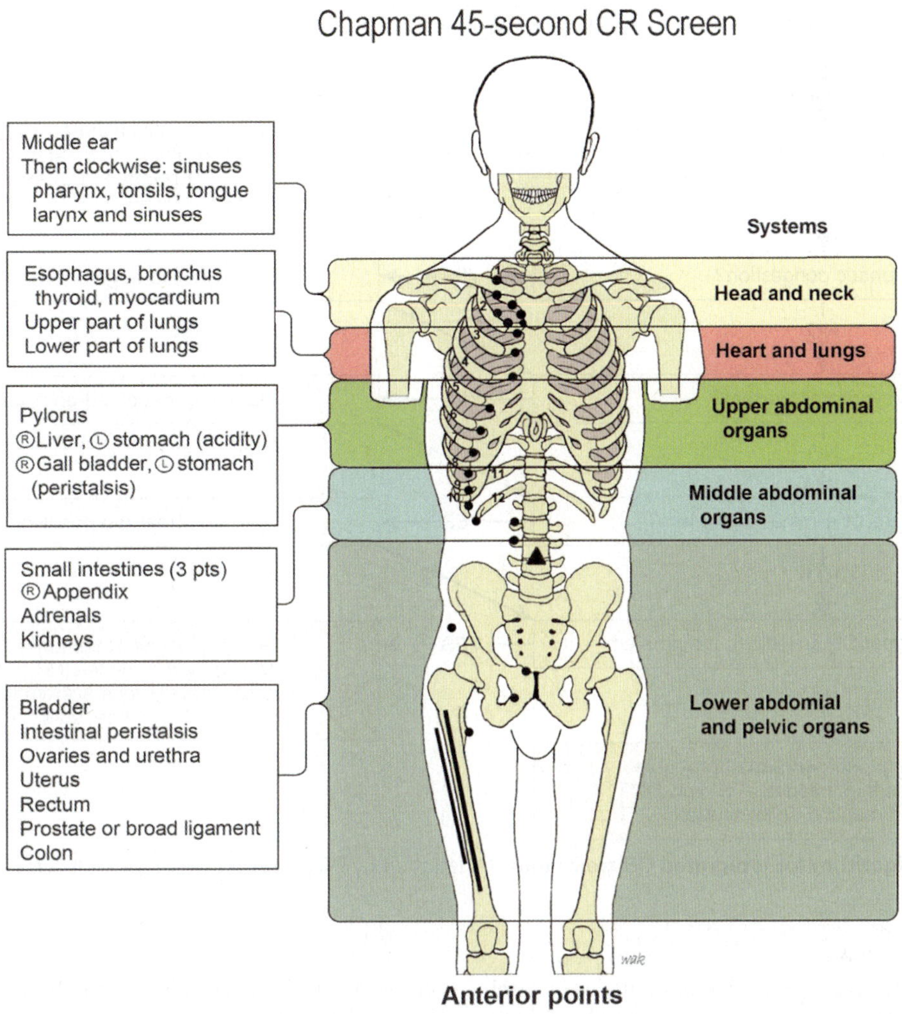

Figure 58.5. A 45-second visceral screen. (Illustration by William A. Kuchera, DO, FAAO, with permission.)

CRs have also been used to augment other forms of osteopathic patient evaluation. Visceral dysfunctions in terms of *mobility* and *motility* are usually detected through careful palpatory evaluation of the body cavities. Because of the depth and partial inaccessibility of some structures, an approximate diagnosis is not uncommon, where the presence (relative severity grading of >1) of CRs can help to determine the dysfunctional structure or to differentiate the relevance between two or more diagnosed dysfunctions.

ANOTHER EXAMPLE

The spinal region of T5–T9 had increased sudomotor activity. There was increased tension in the paravertebral muscles, and motion restrictions indicate a single type II (extended, rotated, and sidebent right) segment within the otherwise type I (sidebent left and rotated right) group curve in this region. These findings, coupled with the predominance of tissue texture change over degree of motion restriction, led to the conclusion of somatic dysfunction being secondary to viscerosomatic reflex activity.

While performing a local listening technique to the abdominal tissue with the patient supine, the palpating hand was drawn toward the upper right abdominal quadrant. Palpation into the quadrant below the border of the ribs revealed tension and tenderness around the liver, gallbladder, sphincter of Oddi, lesser omentum, and hepatic flexure of the colon. There was also tension in the upper third of the linea alba (midline subxiphoid region). Testing the elasticity of the fascial–ligamentous structures, as well as the movement of the structures on their sliding surfaces, indicated visceral dysfunctions involving the lesser omentum, liver, and gallbladder.

The physician found positive CR points for both the liver and the gallbladder. The CR point to the gallbladder was significantly more positive than that of the liver, which led the physician to conclude the gallbladder as the visceral dysfunction responsible for the viscerosomatic reflex activity.

INTEGRATING CHAPMAN REFLEXES IN THE CLINICAL SETTING

Incorporation of CRs does not constitute a stand-alone approach. Its diagnostic and therapeutic usefulness depends on integration with a more comprehensive osteopathic management strategy. The lymphatic system should be addressed by removing obstructions to lymph return and by using techniques to augment lymph flow. Treat somatic dysfunctions of the thorax and pelvis to reduce autonomic interference caused by segmental facilitation. Restore respiratory

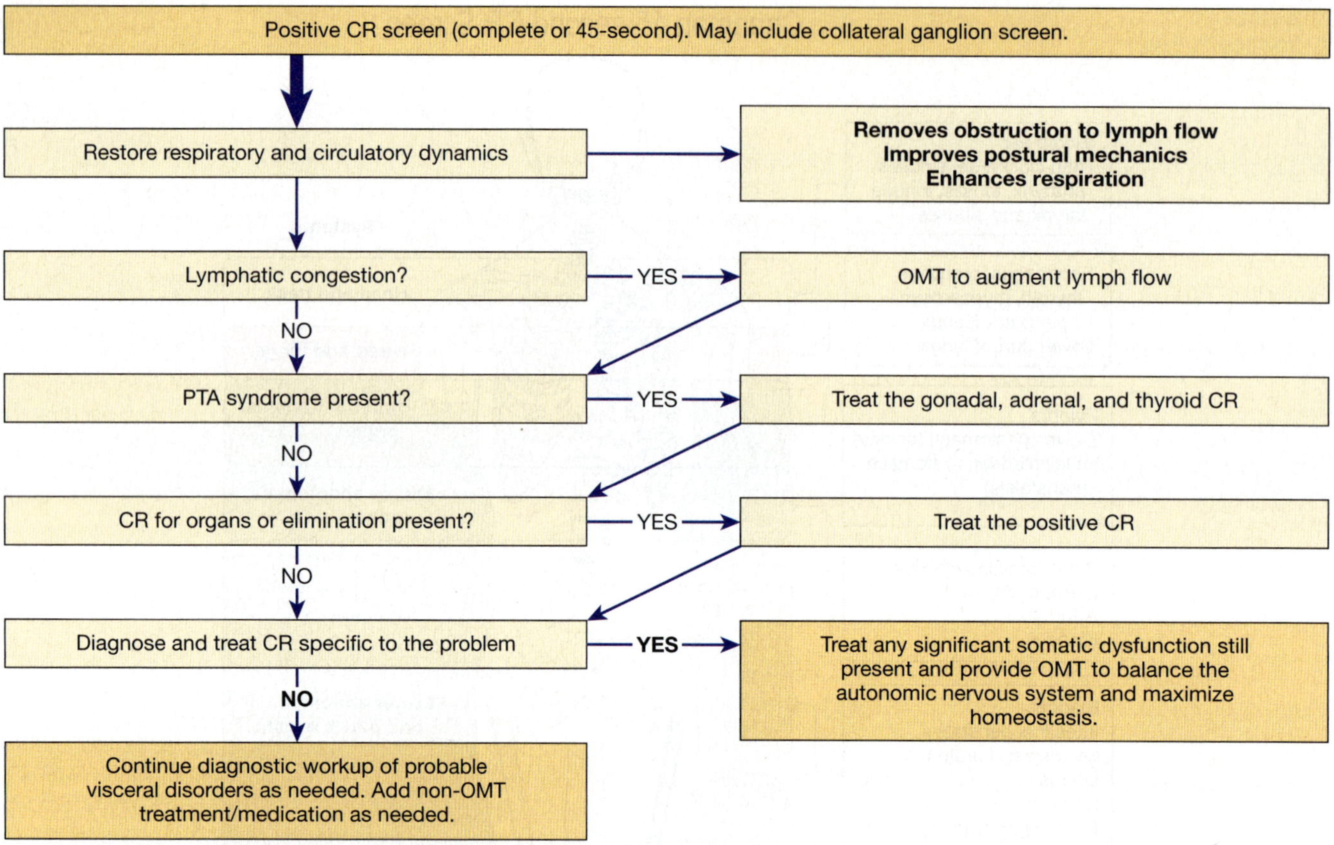

Figure 58.6. Algorithm for integrated CR treatment. (Illustration by William A. Kuchera, DO, FAAO, with permission.)

efficiency by addressing rib cage mechanics and muscles of respiration. Reduce the patient's overall energy expenditure by improving overall biomechanical and postural function. Addressing these factors together with CRs is a useful tool in improving musculoskeletal and systemic function, as well as in reducing the patient's overall allostatic load.

In the original teachings of CRs, the following points were emphasized in diagnosis and treatment[14]:

- Know the exact anatomical location of each CR and its clinical significance.
- Do not overtreat the CR: 15 to 30 or 30 to 60 seconds is sufficient for each center.
- Sequence the treatment:
  1. First, address the biomechanical dysfunctions of the pelvic girdle.
  2. Treat the CR comprising the PTA syndrome.
  3. Treat the CR corresponding with organs of elimination, to reduce load placed on the body from the overall osteopathic treatment.
  4. Treat the CR that is specifically involved.
- Do not forget to assess and treat the lymphatic system, especially the associated regions of impaired lymphatic drainage.
- Articulatory treatment to the axial spine and ribs can be used to reduce and normalize sympathetic activity.
- After reestablishing the "endocrine" balance through CR, other somatic dysfunctions can be treated.

It is important to keep in mind that this recommendation was made in the 1930s and 1940s. Even though the general principles may still be applicable today, the evolution of osteopathic treatment models has allowed for its reinterpretation. Excessive manipulative intervention is now recognized as a potential body stressor. Therefore, procedures employed prior to the use of CR treatment should be administered judiciously, specifically, and with restraint.[25] The algorithm in Figure 58.6 illustrates how CRs could be integrated in a clinical setting.

SPECIFIC TREATMENT USING CHAPMAN REFLEXES

There are several possible approaches commonly employed to treat patients using the CRs (see Table 58.4):

1. Chapman's original recommendation was to start with the anterior points and then proceed to the posterior ones, since treatment of the anterior points greatly aids in the treatment of the posterior points. His protocol also warned against excessive pressure, stating that gentler means will result in quicker relaxation than forceful pressure.[11]
2. If the points are too sensitive to be palpated and treated, myofascial release of the tissue around the gangliform area can help establish drainage more comfortably, which in turn can make it possible to treat the point directly.[9]
3. If the anterior points were too sensitive to treat, performing OMT to the soft tissues posteriorly often decreases or even totally dissipates the related anterior points. The residual change would only need minimal treatment. For this reason, however, it may be important to avoid preparatory soft tissue methods that temporally negate the presence of the anterior points for diagnosis.[18]

TABLE 58.4

Troubleshooting with Chapman Reflexes

Problem	Possible Solution
The CR is too painful to treat.	Treat the myofascial tissues overlying and surrounding the CR with gentle direct or indirect myofascial release. This may help the local drainage of the tissues reducing the sensitivity of the CR. Somatic dysfunctions if present, in segmentally related areas, may also be treated to influence the reflex arc involved in the CR and thereby the sensitivity of the CR (this includes considering treating the related CR on the other side of the body).
There is minimal change in the CR in response to its treatment.	Verify that the tissue texture change is a clinically significant CR and not a different type of somatic change. Both the anterior and the posterior for any given structure along with other clues of visceral and viscerosomatic reflex activity should be present for it to be a positive CR. If they are both present, but still little response in the CR to treatment, evaluate for contributing factors, such as somatic dysfunctions in areas segmentally related to the CR and impaired lymphatic drainage of the area or region where the CR is found.
The effect of the CR treatment is short lived.	When treating CR, the sequencing of the treatment can be important. The overall biomechanical and postural pattern of somatic dysfunction should ideally be treated first, together with OMT strategies to improve respiratory and circulatory dynamics. Then, the PTA syndrome may have to be addressed specifically with CR before attending to the CR correlated with the presenting complaint. Recall that in viscerosomatic reflexes, the pathophysiology lies in the visceral component. Treatment of the somatic end of the reflex may not alone be either adequate or, in some cases, appropriate. Repeated recurrence of a CR warrants further diagnostic or therapeutic action with respect to the underlying visceral cause.
The patient with the CR is extremely ill (also a consideration in certain hospitalized patients).	When treating hospitalized patients, the primary objective is to support the body's physiology through the process of illness and disease. Extensive OTM may not be advisable so as to minimize the energy expenditure of the patient. Treat the CR related to the areas of chief complaint and possibly those that impede the normal homeostatic processes.

PATTERNS OF CHAPMAN REFLEXES IN CLINICAL CONDITIONS

After completing the patient's osteopathic evaluation, the physician will typically sequence the manipulative treatment based on the patient's pattern of dysfunctions. Interaction between dysfunctions through various biomechanical, postural, neurologic (autonomic and somatosensory), and circulatory mechanisms is also crucial. Understanding these interactions typically helps the physician establish the priority and sequence of the treatment. Similarly, when evaluating and treating pain patterns from MTrP, it is important to understand that active trigger points can be maintained by distant satellite MTrP.

A historical analysis of patterns, in positive reflex points palpated and treated in common conditions, illustrates that the early use of CRs was not focused on a single target organ.[14] In many cases, the hormonal–metabolic model was also integrated (Table 58.5).

Similar patterns of CRs as such should be employed in the overall osteopathic management of the patient, rather than as a stand-alone treatment.

RESEARCH RELATED TO CHAPMAN REFLEXES AND THE OSTEOPATHIC CONCEPT

Palpable change in the absence of other objective findings has rendered MTrP and tender points in fibromyalgia patients difficult to instantiate, as is the case with osteopathic points in the CR and counterstrain systems. Nonetheless, there is a growing body of evidence demonstrating a possible basis for such identifiable tissue texture abnormalities, as well as suggestions to coordinate mechanisms that underlie their manifestation.[32,36] Currently, there is limited research investigating the physiologic or chemical characteristics of these specific findings. A number of related studies, however, may be considered in way of interpretation:

- In skin biopsies of patients with fibromyalgia, researchers discovered highly ordered collagen cuffs around terminal nerve fibers that were not found in healthy controls.[37] They termed them *microscars* and concluded that this collagen cross-link, as evident by a decreased collagen metabolism, was needed to maintain the collagen cuffs around nerves in the skin.[38] One proposed explanation for this phenomenon was neurogenic inflammation, which has been demonstrated in the skin of patients with fibromyalgia.[39]
- To investigate the biochemical milieu of MTrP, microdialysis was performed on MTrP. Small volume of fluids were collected from the muscle tissue, at subnanogram levels of solutes.[40,41] Subjects with active MTrP had lower pH levels in the vicinity of their MTrP and significantly higher concentrations of substance P, calcitonin gene–related peptide, bradykinin, serotonin, norepinephrine, tumor necrosis factor-α, and interleukin-1β.[42] Furthermore, continuous nociceptive input from MTrP can increase excitability of dorsal horn neurons, which links peripheral nociceptive events to central sensitization.[43]
- Local tissue findings such as tenderness, edema, and vasodilatation in areas seemingly unrelated to the primary site of dysfunction or injury may be due to neurogenic inflammation, where

TABLE 58.5

Examples of Patterns of CRs in Clinical Conditions

Condition	CRs Involved
Asthma, hay fever, and sinusitis	In hay fever and sinusitis, the sinus CRs are almost always be active. In asthma, the bronchial CR will typically be positive. The duodenal CR is also frequently present in cases of sinusitis, asthma, common colds, influenza, sore throat, and tonsillitis. Consider treating gonadal and thyroid CR for endocrine balance. Treatment may place a load on organs of elimination: Diagnose and treat CR of the spleen, liver, and kidney in preparation for this; CRs for the colon and small intestines are therefore also relevant.
Allergy	Consider treating the whole PTA syndrome; typically the adrenal CR will be involved. For food allergies, check the pancreas CR. In cases where patient regurgitates food, the pyloric CR will be involved.
Diabetes	PTA syndrome and adrenal, pancreas, and duodenum CR are consistently involved. In addition, look for stomach, colon, and kidney CR.
Eyes	In many eye affections, the sinus CR will be involved. In eye strain and conjunctivitis, consider additional examination of liver, small intestine, stomach, and bladder CR.
Digestive disturbances	If present, CR of the gonads, thyroid, and adrenals might best be treated first. Then, special attention is given to the entire digestive tract, CR of the stomach, duodenum, pancreas, small intestines, colon, and liver as well as to organs of elimination: the kidneys, spleen, and colon. Mesenteric releases and other visceral OMT may support treatment.
Inflammatory arthritides	Address the PTA syndrome that is frequently present. CRs of the pancreas and duodenum are also often present, as well as other digestive and eliminative organs. Reestablishing proper lymphatic drainage in conjunction with CR is very important in these cases.
Headaches	If caused by menstrual or menopausal symptoms, treatment to the uterine and ovarian CR may give relief. In blinding, dizzy headache, treatment of the duodenal CR may support the treatment. In gastric headaches (due to central sensitization via vagal afferents), treatment to stomach and pyloric CR may provide relief. Often in cases of vertigo, steady pressure to the cerebellar CR may give relief.

neuropeptides are released from the peripheral terminals of nerves following repeated depolarization. This is referred to as the *axon reflex*. The stimulation of a C-fiber branch from tissue injury and inflammation can result in depolarization. It can also stimulate antidromic activity in other branches unrelated to the site of injury or inflammation through the release of neuropeptides,[44,45] which may explain why tissue texture abnormalities and tenderness can be present in these seemingly unrelated areas.

- Other anatomically localizable, noninflammatory changes in the soft tissues, also thought to be reflexively associated with somatic dysfunctions in the axial spine, have been described. Such tissue texture phenomena are referred to as *irritation zones* and represent small (0.5 to 1.0 cm) soft tissue functional abnormalities that are painful to palpation.[46]

Each of the findings above may not be universally linked to CRs, MTrP, counterstrain, or other such tender point groupings. However, studies like these provide a rationale for better understanding of the relationship between peripheral tissue events, the nervous system, and dysfunction. A few studies showed palpation of the counterstrain, CRs, and MTrP points to have moderate to good reliability.[47–49] They also demonstrated that palpation of tissue texture abnormalities, in combination with pain provocation and the patient's medical history, may be reliable in detecting the presence of such abnormalities.

CLINICAL RELEVANCE OF CHAPMAN REFLEXES

Limited research illustrates the effectiveness of CRs on clinical conditions. One study of hypertensive subjects investigated the effect of treating posterior CRs on the adrenals. Subjects demonstrated a decrease in serum aldosterone levels, lasting 36 hours after treatment.[50] Another study that combined CR treatment with soft tissue techniques reported significant improvement in forced vital capacity, from first pretreatment to last posttreatment. A group of 30 asymptomatic subjects was employed, five of which reported a past history of asthma or bronchitis.[51]

In order to hypothesize how a CR works, it is necessary to consider its potential for modulating autonomic nervous system activity (and its integrated action with the somatomotor and neuroendocrine immune system) and for augmenting lymph flow. Though it is not direct evidence for the clinical benefits of CR, manual techniques that stimulate fluid flow have been proposed to assist repair processes and homeostatic controls in different tissues. This partly explains some of the various effects of manual approaches.[52] When using a fluorescent probe placed in the lower extremity of a rat model, intermittent pressure to the ventral thorax increased the uptake of lymph in the tissues, peripheral to the area in which the technique was applied.[53] In dog models, it was possible to establish the efficacy of thoracic and abdominal lymphatic pump techniques in increasing the net thoracic duct flow.[54] Other studies with dog models also confirmed this effect.[55,56] An additional study reported a significant increase in leukocyte count, in samples taken from the catheterized thoracic duct, which supports the notion that such techniques can enhance immune response.[56]

The stimulation of somatic structures has been shown to influence autonomic function in many experimental studies, using a variety of animal models.[57] Though caution should be exercised when extrapolating such results to humans and clinical conditions, these observations indicate somatosympathetic or somatoautonomic interactions. Related research on the autonomic effects of point-related treatment using electronic acupuncture in humans may also provide insight into the underlying role of the autonomic nervous system.[58]

Additional literature in manual medicine provides evidence for the effect of techniques addressing the spinal zygapophyseal joints, on sympathetic responses. The application of articulatory techniques to the cervical and lumbar spine resulted in the following changes in the sympathetic nervous system[59–68]:

- Sudomotor function
- Cutaneous vasomotor activity
- Cardiac function
- Respiratory function

Sympathoexcitatory effects following manual spinal therapy have also been reported with the mechanical hypoalgesic effect of such intervention in both asymptomatic and symptomatic human subjects. This indicates an activation of the descending pain inhibitory systems from the periaqueductal gray region.[61,69] The same effects have also been reported in animal studies.[70] The effectiveness of OMT in producing favorable autonomic changes was concluded from a combination of suboccipital inhibition, a soft tissue technique applied to the myofascial tissues of the upper cervical spine, and digital strain plethysmography, recording changes in the pulse contour, which demonstrated the occurrence of sympathetic dampening.[71] Studies have further illustrated the influence of OMT on sympathovagal balance (as measured by heart rate variability) in asymptomatic subjects. A shift from the sympathetic to the parasympathetic nervous system was reported in response to myofascial/suboccipital release in the cervical region.[72,73]

Even though these data are not direct evidence for either the mechanisms of action or the clinical effects of CRs, it illustrates the potential for OMT to influence the lymphatic system, as well as the sympathetic and the parasympathetic nervous systems. Much more research is needed to confirm the role of CRs in modulating such activity and the clinical benefits for patients with a variety of conditions.

SUMMARY

CRs have had a long tradition in the osteopathic profession as a diagnostic and therapeutic tool. Their evidence base has grown considerably from the original empirical and anecdotal descriptions and is currently the focus of numerous interexaminer and correlative studies. Nonetheless, despite being linked to specific visceral or systemic conditions, there is a lack of research as to what CRs precisely represent as a tissue texture abnormality. Their somatotopic organization is very predictable and consistent. It is also hypothesized that the lymphatic, autonomic, and neuroendocrine immune systems are involved in the mediation of these reflexes and in the therapeutic action from treating these reflexes. Therefore, successful application of CRs in treatment requires their integration into the overall osteopathic evaluation and management of the patient.

ACKNOWLEDGMENTS

The authors and editors of this chapter would like to acknowledge the scholarly contributions of Dr. Kendall L. Wilson Jr.

REFERENCES

1. Giusti R, Ex ed. *Glossary of Osteopathic Terminology. Educational Council on Osteopathic Principles*. AACOM; 2017.
2. Ketcham AD. *Introduction to Lessons on Chapman Technic*. William L. Johnston Collection, Still National Osteopathic Museum, Typed; 1943:136.
3. Deason WJ. Body fluids—the original osteopathic concept: the influences behind Dr. Still's theories as revealed in his writings and interviews. Part I. *Osteopath Prof.* 1940;7(7):9–11, 43–46; Part 2, 1940;7(8):20–23, 43–45.
4. Hulett GD. *Hulett's Principles*. A.T. Still Research Institute; 1922.
5. Still AT. *Philosophy of Osteopathy*. The Journal Printing Company Ltd; 1899.
6. Still AT. *The Mechanical Principles and Philosophy of Osteopathy*. The Journal Printing Company Ltd; 1902.
7. Still AT. *Osteopathy: Research and Practice*. The Journal Printing Company Ltd; 1910.
8. Samblanet HL. An interpretation of Chapman's reflexes. In: *The Forum of Osteopathy*. American Osteopathic Association; 1944.
9. Lippincott R. Chapman's reflexes. *Osteopath Prof.* 1946:18–22.
10. Pilgrim MF. *Mechanical Vibratory Stimulation: Its Theory and Application in the Treatment of Disease*. Lawrence Press; 1903.
11. Chapman F. *Lymphatic Reflexes: A Specific Method of Osteopathic Diagnosis and Treatment*. Frank Chapman; 1929.
12. Owens C. The endocrine glands, the hormones and the osteopathic lesion. *J Am Osteopath Assoc.* 1930:421–422.
13. Owens C. *An Endocrine Interpretation of Chapman's Reflexes*. Reprint Academy of Applied Osteopathy, Carmel; 1963 (1st edition 1937 by the author).
14. Owens C. *Chapman's Reflexes*, part of William Johnston Collection, Museum of Osteopathic Medicine. 2006;27:1223–1227, ca 1942.
15. Arbuckle BE. Chapman's reflexes charts and notes. In: *The Selected Writings of Beryl E Arbuckle, D.O., F.A.C.O.P.* American Academy of Osteopathy. Plenum Publishing Corp.; 1997:256–264.
16. Owens C. *Mechanical Manipulation and Reflexes in the Treatment of Disease*. Self-published; 1940.
17. Patriquin DA. The evolution of osteopathic manipulative technique: the Spencer technique. *J Am Osteopath Assoc.* 1992;92(9):1134–1136, 1139–1146.
18. Kuchera ML, Kuchera WA. *Osteopathic Considerations in Systemic Dysfunction*. 2nd ed. Greyden Press; 1994.
19. Kuchera ML. An integrated perspective on the differential diagnosis of myofascial points. In: Myers HL, ed. *Compendium Edition, Clinical Application of Counterstrain*. Tucson Osteopathic Medical Association; 2012.
20. Capobianco JD. The neuroendocrine-immune complex illustrated in the work of Dr. Frank Chapman. *J Am Acad Osteopath.* 2004;14(1).
21. Wilson K. *Written Case Studies Presented at Chapman's Think Tank Retreat*. Arizona College of Osteopathic Medicine; 2006.
22. Patriquin D. Chapman's reflexes. In: Ward RC, ed. *Foundations for Osteopathic Medicine*. 2nd ed. Lippincott Williams & Wilkins; 2003.
23. Chapman AH, Owens C. *Lymphatic Reflexes: A Specific Method of Osteopathic Diagnosis and Treatment*. Hinckley-Chapman and Owens; 1932.
24. Brown EA. Clinical aspects of the Chapman's reflexes. In: *Yearbook of the Academy of Applied Osteopathy*. Edwards Brothers Inc.; 1949:112.
25. Mitchell FL Jr. The influence of Chapman's reflexes and the immune reactions. *Osteopath Ann.* 1974;2:12.
26. DiGiovanna EL, Schiowitz S, Dowling D. *An Osteopathic Approach to Diagnosis and Treatment*. 3rd ed. Lippincott Williams & Wilkins; 2005.
27. Northrup T. Role of the reflexes in manipulative therapy. *J Am Osteopath Assoc.* 1941;40(12):521–524.
28. Johns PR. *Comparative Analysis of the Topographical Locations of Chapman's Reflex Points and Jones's Strain-Counterstrain Tender Points*. Thesis, Master Degree. Unitec New Zealand, Carrington, Auckland, New Zealand; 2003.
29. Riley JN, Mitchell FL Jr, Bensky D. Thai manual medicine as reprinted in Wat Pho Epigraphies: preliminary comparisons. *Med Anthropol.* 1981; 5(2):155–194.
30. Kim OB. Comparative analysis of the topographical locations of acupuncture points and Chapman's reflex points. Accessed February 2, 2009. https://www.researchbank.ac.nz/server/api/core/bitstreams/0263d098-eb5e-4566-97f8-2a50d5806b3e/content
31. Melzack R, Stillwell DM, Fox EJ. Trigger points and acupuncture points for pain: correlations and implications. *Pain.* 1977;3:3–23.
32. McPartland JM. Travell trigger points—molecular and osteopathic perspectives. *J Am Osteopath Assoc.* 2004;104(6):244–249.

33. Simons D, Travell G, Simons L. *Travell & Simons' Myofascial Pain and Dysfunction: Upper Half of Body.* Lippincott Williams & Wilkins; 1999.
34. Kendall OH, Kendall FP, Wadsworth GE. *Muscle Testing and Function.* Williams and Wilkins; 1971.
35. Walther DS, Gavin DM, Goodheart G. *Applied Kinesiology: A Synopsis.* Systems DC; 1988.
36. McMakin CR, Oschman JL. Visceral and somatic disorders: tissue softening with frequency-specific microcurrent. *J Altern Complement Med.* 2013;19(2):170–177.
37. Sprott H, Müller A, Heine H. Collagen crosslinks in fibromyalgia. *Arthritis Rheum.* 1997;40(8):1450–1454.
38. Sprott H. Muscles and peripheral abnormalities in fibromyalgia. In: Wallace DJ, Clauw DJ, eds. *Fibromyalgia and Other Central Pain Syndromes.* Lippincott Williams & Wilkins; 2005:101–114.
39. Salemi S, Rethage J, Wollina U, et al. Detection of interleukin 1β (IL-1β), IL-6, and tumor necrosis factor-α in skin of patients with fibromyalgia. *J Rheumatol.* 2003;30:146–150.
40. Shah JP, Danoff JV, Desai MJ, et al. Biochemicals associated with pain and inflammation are elevated in sites near to and remote from active myofascial trigger points. *Arch Phys Med Rehabil.* 2008;89(1):16–23.
41. Shah JP, Gilliams EA. Uncovering the biochemical milieu of myofascial trigger points using in vivo microdialysis: an application of muscle pain concepts to myofascial pain syndrome. *J Bodyw Mov Ther.* 2008;12(4):371–384.
42. Shah JP, Phillips TM, Danoff JV, Gerber LH. An in vivo microanalytical technique for measuring the local biochemical milieu of human skeletal muscle. *J Appl Physiol.* 2005;99(5):1977–1984.
43. Mense S. Peripheral and central mechanisms of musculoskeletal pain. In: Castro-Lopes J, Raja S, Schmelz M, eds. *Pain 2008: An Updated Review.* International Association for the Study of Pain; 2008:55–62.
44. Van Griensven H. *Pain in Practice: Theory and Treatment Strategies for Manual Therapists.* Butterworth and Heinemann/Elsevier; 2005.
45. Willard F. Basic mechanisms of pain. In: Audette JF, Bailey A, eds. *Integrative Pain Medicine: The Science and Practice of Complementary and Alternative Medicine in Pain Management.* Humana Press; 2008:19–62.
46. Dvorak J, Dvorak V, Gilliar W, Scheider W, Spring H, Tritschler T. *Musculoskeletal Manual Medicine.* Thieme; 2008.
47. Hsieh CY, Hong CZ, Adams AH, et al. Interexaminer reliability of the palpation of trigger points in the trunk and lower limb muscles. *Arch Phys Med Rehabil.* 2000;81:258–264.
48. McPartland JM, Goodridge JP. Counterstrain and traditional osteopathic examination of the cervical spine compared. *J Bodyw Mov Ther.* 1997;1(3): 173–178.
49. Washington K, Mosiello R, Venditto M, et al. Presence of Chapman reflex points in hospitalized patients with pneumonia. *J Am Osteopath Assoc.* 2003;103:479–483.
50. Mannino JR. The application of neurological reflexes to the treatment of hypertension. *J Am Osteopath Assoc.* 1978;79:225–231.
51. Lines DH, McMilan AJ, Spehr GJ. Effects of soft tissue technique and Chapman's neurolymphatic reflex stimulation on respiratory function. *J Aust Chiropr Assoc.* 1990;20(1):17–22.
52. Lederman E. *The Science and Practice of Manual Therapy.* 2nd ed. Elsevier Churchill Livingstone; 2005.
53. Dery MA, Yonuschot G, Winterson BJ. The effects of manually applied intermittent pulsation pressure to rat ventral thorax on lymph transport. *Lymphology.* 2000;33(2):58–61.
54. Knott EM, Tune JD, Stoll ST, Downey HF. Increased lymphatic flow in the thoracic duct during manipulative intervention. *J Am Osteopath Assoc.* 2005;105(10):447–456.
55. Downey HF, Durgam P, Williams AG Jr, Rajmane A, King HH, Stoll ST. Lymph flow in the thoracic duct of conscious dogs during lymphatic pump treatment, exercise, and expansion of extracellular fluid volume. *Lymphat Res Biol.* 2008;6(1): 3–13.
56. Hodge LM, King HH, Williams AG Jr, et al. Abdominal lymphatic pump treatment increases leukocyte count and flux in thoracic duct lymph. *Lymphat Res Biol.* 2007;5(2):127–133.
57. Sato A, Sato Y, Schmidt RF. The impact of somatosensory input on autonomic functions. *Rev Physiol Biochem Pharmacol.* 1997;130:1–328.
58. Hsu CC, Weng CS, Te-Sheng Liu TS, Tsai YS, Chang YH. *Am J Chin Med.* 2006;34(1):23–36.
59. Chiu TW, Wright A. To compare the effects of different rates of application of a cervical mobilisation technique on sympathetic outflow to the upper limb in normal subjects. *Man Ther.* 1996;1:198–203.
60. McGuiness JM, Vicenzino B, Wright A. Influence of a cervical mobilisation technique on respiratory and cardiovascular function. *Man Ther.* 1997;2:216–220.
61. Perry J, Green A. An investigation into the effects of a unilaterally applied lumbar mobilisation technique on peripheral sympathetic nervous system activity in the lower limbs. *Man Ther.* 2008;13:492–499.
62. Petersen N, Vicenzino B, Wright A. The effects of a cervical mobilisation technique on sympathetic outflow to the upper limb in normal subjects. *Physiother Theory Pract.* 1993;9:149–156.
63. Slater H, Vicenzino B, Wright A. "Sympathetic Slump": the effects of a novel manual therapy technique on peripheral sympathetic nervous system function. *J Man Manip Ther.* 1994;2:156–162.
64. Sterling M, Jull G, Wright A. Cervical mobilisation: concurrent effects on pain, sympathetic nervous system activity and motor activity. *Man Ther.* 2001;6:72–81.
65. Vicenzino B, Collins D, Wright A. Sudomotor changes induced by neural mobilisation techniques in asymptomatic subjects. *J Man Manip Ther.* 1994;2:66–74.
66. Vicenzino B, Cartwright T, Collins D, et al. Cardiovascular and respiratory changes produced by the lateral glide mobilisation of the cervical spine. *Man Ther.* 1998;3(2):67–71.
67. Vicenzino B, Collins D, Benson H, et al. An investigation of the interrelationship between manipulative therapy-induced hypoalgesia and sympathoexcitation. *J Manipulative Physiol Ther.* 1998;21:448–453.
68. Wright A, Vicenzino B. Cervical mobilisation techniques, sympathetic nervous system effects and their relationship to analgesia. In: Shacklock M, ed. *Moving in on Pain.* Butterworth-Heinemann; 1995:164–173.
69. Hoeger Bement K, Sluka KA. Pain: perception and mechanisms. In: Magee DJ, Zachazewski JE, Quillen WS, eds. *Scientific Foundations and Principles and Practice in Musculoskeletal Rehabilitation.* Saunders Elsevier; 2008:217–237.
70. Skyba DA, Radhakrishnan R, Rohlwing JJ, Wright A, Sluka KA. Joint manipulation reduces hyperalgesia by activation of monoamine receptors but not opioid or GABA receptors in the spinal cord. *Pain.* 2003;106(1–2): 159–168.
71. Purdy WR, Frank JJ, Oliver B. Suboccipital dermatomyotomic stimulation and digital blood flow. *J Am Osteopath Assoc.* 1996;96(5):285–289.
72. Henley CE, Ivins D, Mills M, Wen FK, Benjamin BA. Osteopathic manipulative treatment and its relationship to autonomic nervous system activity as demonstrated by heart rate variability: a repeated measures study. *Osteopath Med Prim Care.* 2008;2:7.
73. Giles PD, Hensel KL, Pacchia CF, Smith ML. Suboccipital decompression enhances heart rate variability indices of cardiac control in healthy subjects. *J Altern Complement Med.* 2013;19(2):92–96.

59 Additional Osteopathic Manipulative Treatment Approaches: Fulford Percussion

RAJIV L. YADAVA

KEY CONCEPTS

- Dr. Fulford included in the definition of somatic dysfunction an area where the "life force is not flowing."
- When mechanical or psychological energy is absorbed into the body, it distorts the bioelectrical matrix of the fascia, bone, and surrounding tissues to create a higher energetic state.
- This distortion can be palpated as a subtle motion restriction, a depression, elevation, or lack of life force along the tissues.
- In order to release the tissue to a more normal state of structure and function, the higher energy state needs to be matched with an equal quantum of energy (Principle of rhythmic balanced interchange[1]).
- With the Fulford percussion vibrator technique, one can amplify what is normally done through the hands alone to save one's energy and deliver it to the tissues.
- Following the release of these high energetic states, healing can begin as the body areas return to a more normal interchange and fluctuation of fluids resulting in a change in structure toward normal.
- During treatment, the percussor applies a specific, mechanical vibratory percussive force coupled with the physician's palpatory feedback, to treat somatic dysfunction.
- The physician's state of mind and thoughts are important components of the treatment; the percussion vibrator amplifies the physician's intent, which allows the energy in the lesion field to be matched and released.

DEFINITION

Fulford percussion is an osteopathic manipulative technique developed by Robert C. Fulford, DO (Fig. 59.1), involving the use of an instrument referred to as a percussor. The percussor applies a specific, mechanical vibratory percussive force to treat somatic dysfunction. It is coupled with the physician's palpatory feedback of the life energies during treatment. This modality is distinct from other massage, vibration, or oscillatory approaches.

Dr. Fulford quietly disapproved of physicians who used the percussor in a modified way. Although he never addressed these individuals directly or publicly, Dr. Fulford felt that they never really understood the philosophy and principles he was teaching. Thus, they changed the way the percussor was used to accommodate their lack of understanding.

HISTORY AND PHILOSOPHY

The history behind the development of Dr. Fulford's percussor helps to facilitate the understanding of its philosophy. Moreover, Dr. Fulford's personal development and level of humanity had much to do with the results he achieved. He achieved excellent clinical results with his hands alone but developed the percussor to save his energy while working 18 hours a day. The lessons he learned from many obstacles he faced in life shaped his future.

Dr. Fulford could not attend medical school in 1929 due to the great depression. This forced him to work at Union Carbide, where he developed an appreciation for subtle motion, after finding that a slight mechanical turn of a dial determined whether pure or impure oxygen was produced. In 1936, he was denied admission to medical school. In 1937, he sustained an injury that awakened an old desire for becoming a physician. He was denied admission into an MD school after repeating organic chemistry at their request and was admitted to Kansas City College of Osteopathic Medicine 2 weeks late. He later recalled that the rejection from the MD school created a desire in him to prove that the MD profession had made a mistake. It was a driving force to make him the best physician he could be. He was fascinated with Dr. A. T. Still's Philosophy of Osteopathy. Dr. Fulford developed an interest in understanding metaphysics, spirituality of all religious philosophies, astrology, yoga, esoteric teachings, and many natural healing arts of the world. This broadmindedness, grounded in medical science and osteopathic anatomy, allowed him to "read between the lines," as he studied the osteopathic writings of Dr. A. T. Still.

In his junior year at Kansas City College, he became interested in Dr. Harold Saxton Burr's research on energy work. Dr. Burr, an anatomist at Yale School of Medicine, published over 90 papers on his experiments measuring energy fields, which raised interest among his colleagues, many of whom then became leaders in science. Dr. Fulford believed that these fields provided a blueprint for all living things and considered them diagnostic for mental as well as physical conditions.

In 1941, a number of physicians left to serve in WWII, which resulted in more work for those that remained in the states, like Dr. Fulford. He also noticed that there was considerably more tension among the patient population after the war began. Patients were more challenging to treat. This reminded him of Union Carbide, where his superintendent would say that where possible, let a motor do the work for you. Accordingly, Dr. Fulford began experimenting with various vibrating motors, but without achieving acceptable results. In the 1940s, however, the Foredom Vibrator flyer arrived in the mail by chance and fulfilled his needs. It allowed manipulative procedures to be performed more easily and effectively after its use.

Dr. Fulford was a student when he met Dr. Sutherland in 1939. His first course was not until 1942, when his interest had once again turned to the energy field. Dr. Sutherland had a profound impact on

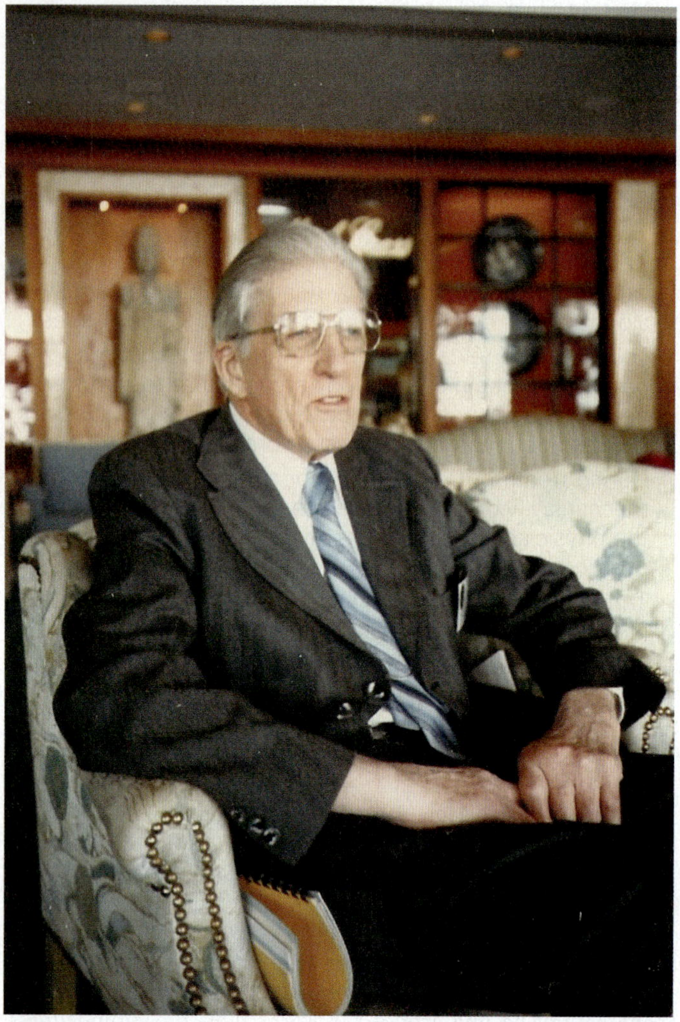

Figure 59.1. Portrait of Robert C. Fulford, DO (1985). Photo courtesy of Sara Saxton, DO, "If you can't project love you're not going to be able to help anyone. You have to have love for other human beings."[9]

his thinking. In Dr. Fulford's own words, "It was a most important day of my life when I had an opportunity to sit in the classroom of Des Moines College back in 1949. Dr. Sutherland was teaching his cranial concept. His ideas were heavily charged with energy and they soon began to work in me like some powerful force."[2]

Dr. Fulford was convinced Dr. Sutherland was aware of the energy fields when Lao Russell, wife of Walter Russell, referred to Dr. Sutherland in her book. In her book, on pages 198 through 199, it mentions a medical condition Walter Russell had for which he consulted Dr. Sutherland. "He consulted the late Dr. William Sutherland, a noted cranial specialist who attached a specially prepared negative to the brain of a dying man. A negative is a photo image that reproduces an image with light portion dark and dark portions as light. At the instant of death, a light flash was recorded on the negative which proved the light was what my husband believed it to be." According to Walter Russell, Dr. Sutherland was a private student of his.

Walter Russell left school at age 10. Through self-education, he became a musician, illustrator, portrait painter, architectural designer, sculptor, business practice advisor for IBM, champion figure skater, natural scientist, philosopher, and author. His writings provided guidance and support for many of Dr. Fulford's ideas regarding osteopathic diagnosis, treatment, and life in general. Though Dr. Fulford met Lao Russell, he never had the opportunity to meet Walter Russell.

Dr. Fulford stated that his understanding of cranial osteopathy as taught to him by Dr. Sutherland was different than what was taught by Sutherland's students after Dr. Sutherland's death. He stated that in the courses he took from Dr. Sutherland, the first week of cranial osteopathy was about anatomy. The second week was taught by Dr. Sutherland himself where Dr. Sutherland would draw a house on the board with all the windows out and floating in the ocean.

According to Dr. Fulford, this house symbolized the human body, and the ocean with its many waves represented the primary respiratory mechanism (PRM) (universal energy). Dr. Fulford further stated this did not correspond with the commentaries made later about the meaning of Dr. Sutherland's recorded lectures. In regard to the PRM, Fulford understood that the terms stood for the following:

- **Primary** is the universal life force expressed as mind, energy, and breath, the breath being the first principle in the cerebral spinal fluid (CSF).
- **Respiratory** is a rhythmic motion of mind energy, fine energies of the CSF, as they motivate and manifest life.
- **Mechanism** is a process, conscious or unconscious, where a result of accomplishment is produced, in this case, where the sensory motor energies relate sensation, experiences, and expression in the world of matter.

In addition to Sutherland's house analogy, Dr. Fulford appreciated two other basic principles:

1. As osteopathic physicians, we should stay close to our maker.
2. The importance of breath in life and healing.

Dr. Fulford was spiritual. He valued the use of meditation and "running the energies through the body" as well as breathing exercises. He credited a breathing exercise for keeping his body alive well into his 90s.

Dr. Fulford observed that many who claim to do cranial work had little or no knowledge of the theory behind the PRM. He states:

> "They know the mechanics of how (PRM) works but little about how consciousness is part of a successful treatment."[2]

When describing the way Dr. Sutherland gave a treatment, Fulford states:

> He sat on a stool, his back straight as a rod and his shoulders level and balanced. The arms extended and appeared as though they were weightless. His eyes were closed; whether he was in a meditative or contemplative state no one will ever know. Then after a few minutes his hands and arms would fly out into space as though they were suddenly given a push outward.[2]

Dr. Fulford's de-emphasis of the cranial rhythmic impulse (CRI) was confusing for some. Though he acknowledged rhythms, he did not focus on any particular rate. Dr. Fulford understood a still point or a fulcrum not as a particular place but as a state of being in which everything is centered. In addition, regarding Dr. Sutherland's writings, Dr. Fulford states:

> In Dr. Sutherland's writings he stresses the mechanics as part of the cranial concept, as an engineer would, and thus he could be understood. But he himself went beyond that in his findings and touch. That was his secret that he could not teach. He tried to leave us his secret when he gave us the phrase, "thinking and knowing fingers . . .[2]

Quoting Dr. Sutherland, Fulford states:

> "...seeing, feeling, thinking fingers...fingers that endeavor to get away from the sensation of physical touch wherein you have knowing touch....by knowing I mean not information gained by the physical sense but a knowledge that comes from getting as far as one can from the physical sense."[2]

In the same way that Dr. Fulford described Dr. Sutherland's inability to directly teach what he knew of osteopathy, Dr. Sutherland described the same of Dr. Still:

> "Dr. Still could not speak of all the things he understood about the living human body. We were not ready to hear him. If you read between the lines in his 'Philosophy of Osteopathy' you will see that this is so."[3]

Around 1949 to 1950, Dr. Fulford along with a number of other DOs left Dr. Sutherland to study with Beryl E. Arbuckle, DO, because of the impressive results she was obtaining.[4] Dr. Fulford said that her treatment of children would cause an autonomic response resulting in perspiration in just a few minutes. She would then move to the next child lying on an adjacent table and do the same, repeating this treatment on patients lying on several tables lined up in a row. She originally met Dr. Sutherland in 1942 and was one of Dr. Sutherland's early trainers for Osteopathy in the Cranial Field courses. Also, she was one of the few physicians who Dr. Sutherland allowed to treat him. Having done more than 250 dissections of fetal cadavers at the Philadelphia College of Osteopathy, she felt that the dural stress bands and bony buttresses should be given more importance before moving on to nonosseous and nonmembranous aspects of cranial osteopathy that Dr. Sutherland was evolving toward at the time. It was not that she did not appreciate the fluid anatomy, but she felt that we must understand what could be verified physically with anatomy before moving on to fluid, potency, and the breath of life aspects of cranial osteopathy Dr. Sutherland was teaching.[4]

Dr. Arbuckle's influence on Dr. Fulford could be seen by the way he firmly put his hands on the cranium. One could also see the use of Dr. Arbuckle's craniometric points in Dr. Fulford's percussion work as well. It is important to point out that Dr. Fulford said that what he was doing was distinct from what Dr. Arbuckle was doing. Dr. Sutherland's communications of the nonphysical aspect of osteopathy, with its mental, emotional, and spiritual implications, could be observed and felt on the patients Dr. Fulford would treat as the fluid forces would move with great vigor under his hands, a phenomenon unique among his peers.

According to Dr. Fulford, the CRI rate and amplitude were not a focus for either Dr. Arbuckle or Dr. Sutherland. They were more focused on the *source* of the phenomena that generated the rate, rhythm, and amplitude.

After 1950, Dr. Fulford met Randolph Stone, DO, with whom he was "good friends." Both men had great interest in matters of spirituality, beyond the boundaries of any particular religion. Influenced by the ancient Ayurvedic medicine of India, Dr. Stone developed polarity therapy. With regard to diagnosis and treatment, Dr. Stone had a greater understanding of polarity than those who practice it today. However, Dr. Fulford did not claim to have acquired this knowledge from Dr. Stone but credited Baron Karl von Reichenbach (1778–1869) instead.

Reichenbach was a chemist, naturalist, geologist, metallurgist, and industrialist known for his discoveries of chemical products extracted from tar. However, he spent his last years researching the energy field, which he called the Odic force.

The number of influences and contacts Dr. Fulford had would be too numerous to name and describe in this short essay. It would be safe to say that he had an almost child-like enthusiasm for knowledge of truth in all matters concerning the understanding of osteopathic medicine and healing. Nothing would be overlooked until it was examined by him and then accepted or discarded.

DIAGNOSIS

Dr. Fulford would say that it takes the mind of a physician (MD/DO/DDS) to understand osteopathy. The knowledge base and experience is not found in other professions. He felt that without the understanding of the interrelationship between structure and function, an accurate diagnosis could not be forthcoming. According to Drs. Still and Fulford, anatomy includes the physiology and chemistry that makes the gross anatomy what it is.

Dr. Fulford's diagnosis valued both the history and physical examination of the patient. In fact, he considered the diagnosis to be more important than the treatment. His holistic approach considered the patient's physical, mental, and emotional states long before it became more common. For any complaint, Dr. Fulford's diagnosis was also unique in that he gave importance to the extremities, abdomen, and anterior chest wall, rather than simply to the spine and cranium. He used both the physical and subtle breath in diagnosis. Not only did he give importance to the breath of the thorax, but he also valued the breath of the whole body, from head to toe. In terms of the patient's history, Dr. Fulford was speaking about trauma to be an important component long before others did in the 1970s. First, birth trauma is reflected in the individual's quality of breathing and is greatly influenced by the first breath the individual took as an infant. Second, physical traumas, and third psychological trauma, are also important particularly if they are early in life. After obtaining the patient's history, Dr. Fulford had already formed most of the diagnosis in his mind. Therefore, the physical exam served to reassure the patient that he acknowledged the area of complaint.

During the physical examination, in addition to looking at structural abnormalities, Dr. Fulford maintained awareness of areas where the "life force was not flowing." Sometimes he began the examination at the foot and ankles and then continued to the knees, hips and pelvis, abdomen, diaphragm, rib cage, upper extremity, shoulder joint, lumbar, thoracic, and cervical vertebrae, and cranium. He could also deviate from any particular order of examination. The goal of the exam was to find restrictions of motion within the joints, by directing attention to the lack of subtle motion in the area being examined. This is different than gross motion testing, where light touch is not an important factor. Here, a light touch is used to appreciate the presence or absence of an underlying lack of motion, reflecting insufficient "life force."

Treatment would many times involve first releasing the "shock" or trauma from the anterior chest and abdomen area after which all other areas of the body could be addressed without much resistance.

MECHANISM OF ACTION

It is likely that multiple mechanisms of action exist to explain Dr. Fulford's use of the percussion vibrator. The device simply amplifies the physician's intent.

Dr. Fulford added and changed many techniques of treatment over the years as he evolved. Many of these techniques would "just come to him," like a gift, out of nowhere. Dr. Fulford's diagnosis and treatment relied on the bioelectric properties of the fascia, bone, and surrounding tissues. When mechanical energy is absorbed into the body, it distorts this bioelectrical matrix and creates a higher energetic state within the tissues. This distortion can be palpated as a subtle motion restriction, a depression, elevation, or lack of life force along the tissues. Since these restrictions can be very subtle, the physician's skill determines how much can be palpated. In the words of Dr. Fulford:

> "When you can feel the placement of a single hair under 18 sheets of paper you are ready to do the cranial work."

In order to release the tissue to a more normal state of structure and function, the higher-energy state needs to be matched with an equal quantum of energy. This may take time, as the cells within the tissue redeposit themselves after partial or full release of potential energy. Tissues are constantly turned over and their chemical components redeposited. For instance, epithelial cells of the gut last around 5 days, but those of the main body of the gut last around 120 days. The epidermis of the skin is recycled every 2 weeks. The liver has a turnover time of 300 to 500 days. The entire human skeleton is replaced every 10 years.[5] The manner in which the tissues are redeposited could also be influenced, at least in part, by the bioelectric field present.[5]

Dr. Fulford believed that mental and emotional trauma can also be absorbed into the memory of the tissue, through these bioelectric phenomena. Thoughts and emotions are known to influence the health and well-being of individuals.[6] "...thought energy is the cause which is in the back of all manifestations, the product is only the effect of thought energy."[7]

Since the percussion vibrator amplifies what is normally done through the hands alone, it increases the amount of energy delivered to the tissues. As mentioned, proper release of the dysfunctional field requires for its high-energy state to be matched through one's intent. Thus, high-impact physical trauma, and intense psychological trauma, can produce and maintain these dysfunctional fields with high-energy states. For instance, if a 100 ft-lb of force is absorbed into the tissues, the physician cannot physically apply the equivalent physical force to release it and must instead rely on their intent. The percussion vibrator amplifies the physician's attention and purity of intent for the release to occur. Dr. Fulford would say empathically that: "Thoughts are things" and "Energy follows thought."

Following the release of these high energetic states, healing can begin as the dysfunctional body areas return to a more normal interchange and fluctuation of fluids restored through the area.

A cursory description to demonstrate its use would be as follows:

- The percussion vibrator is placed on one side of the body part being treated.
- The other side is monitored by the physician's other hand, which is usually on the opposite side of the body part.
- With skillful application of the percussor hand and the monitoring hand, a resonant wave of energy will be created that resonates with the dysfunctional field between the hands.
- To obtain the wave, the speed, direction, pressure, and placement of the percussing hand will vary depending on the area being addressed and the dysfunctional field present.
- The resonating life force will continue until there is a release, relaxation, and flow of the life force through the area.
- Before a release occurs, it is believed that the energy within the resonant wave will match the energy within the dysfunctional field.
- The physician's thought and purity of intent for the patient's well-being are key in releasing the most difficult of dysfunctional areas. The principle of "rhythmic balanced interchange," which was mentioned by Dr. Sutherland and before him Walter Russell, is key to understand this.

Dr. Fulford states:

> "The work of healing will be greatly assisted by tremendous stimulation of the love nature.... We must be sure to pursue genuine healing. Far too often, healing is thought of as relieving stressful symptoms, so we are not bothered by them. As a result, the effort to heal frequently becomes little more than an attack on what is wrong or painful. The healing potential is tapped primarily by learning to identify with the health and using the resources of health to enrich the consciousness and heal the distress as we build up greater health while that which is unhealthy fades away."[2]

A true understanding of this concept requires a background in osteopathic medical training, experience, and guidance from a qualified and properly trained instructor. Dr. Fulford has said many times that "It takes the mind of a physician to understand Osteopathy."

USE AND RESPONSE OF FULFORD PERCUSSION

With discretion, the Fulford percussion vibrator can be used on almost all patients, for any osteopathic dysfunction. Difficult dysfunctions will respond with less treatment time. But rebound symptoms are also more likely to occur with the enhanced tissue response and release. Rebound symptoms can be minimized with experience and skill. Depending on the physician's skill, the frequency of treatment may need to be reduced. Contraindications include areas that require minimal tissue release, such as on cardiac, abdominal, or orthopedic patients within 6 months postoperation, and directly over areas with prosthetic devices such as heart valves and hip replacements. Fulford's percussion vibrator is generally not advised to treat the lumbar, sacral, and lower abdomen areas of pregnant patients. In addition, it should never be used directly over acutely painful areas.

TECHNIQUE

CASE STUDY

A 21-year-old female presents to the office with a complaint of right leg discomfort for the past month. She has an "achiness" of her right leg that radiates into her lateral ankle. She remembers standing on the rung of a ladder for some time to clean her windows. There is no other history of trauma. Past medical/surgical history is negative. She has been using Arnica Montana for relief, but the discomfort returns.

PHYSICAL EXAMINATION

T is 98.8, P 72, R 12, B/P 110/70, Ht 64 in, and Wt 120 lb.

HEENT/CV/Pulmonary/Abdomen/GU—noncontributory.

Neurologic Exam

Neurologic exam is intact.

Structural Exam

Structural exam reveals level landmarks, normal AP curves, and no lateral curves. There is tenderness to palpation along the lateral aspect of the right calf. Lateral malleolar motion is sluggish. There is tension in the interosseous membrane.

Diagnosis

Somatic dysfunction of the lower extremity.

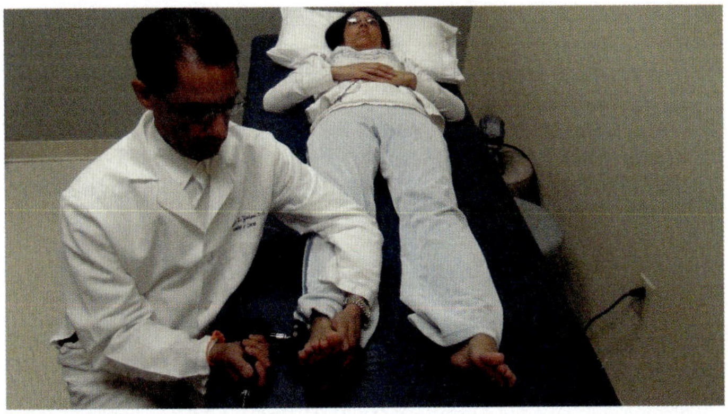

Figure 59.2. **Treatment of the right ankle.**

TREATMENT PLAN

Treatment of the subtle motion restriction with the percussion vibrator.

Example One

Subtle motion restriction is found in the right ankle joint, involving the talus, distal fibula, and tibia (Fig. 59.2).

Percussor speed is lowered because of the area's relative decrease in soft tissue mass. It is placed over the lateral malleolus. Pressure and aim are adjusted for maximum response between the percussing hand and the monitoring hand on the opposite side (over the medial malleolus). The goal is to establish an interchange of life force between the hands. This response will continue until there is a release and the tissue is relaxed. The physician will then once again experience the life force flowing through the area.

Example Two

A restriction in the subtle motion of the left femoral head was found (Fig. 59.3).

The percussor is placed over the right greater trochanter, and the monitoring hand over the left greater trochanter, in accordance with Dr. Fulford's understanding of polarity in diagnosis and treatment. Placing the percussor on the right side of the pelvis allows for more efficient release, even if the restriction is on the opposite side, as is in this case at the left femoral head. This is particularly true when release of the entire pelvis is desired. Percussion speed would be relatively high due to the relative increase in soft tissue in the area. Once the release is achieved at the end of the treatment, the physician should be able to appreciate the flow of energy through the pelvis.

SUMMARY

Regardless of whether or not there exists a theoretical model to support a particular approach, there is much to be gained by the profession by considering it based on clinical experience. Consistent clinical results shape and develop the art over time. Institutional research and explanations have always trailed clinical experience of physicians like Dr. Still. Those who repeatedly witness these events can attest to its clinical significance. Dr. Still states:

> "…we should treat with respect and reverence all truths, great and small….each truth or division as we see it, can only be made known to us by the self-evident fact, which this truth is able to demonstrate by its action."[8]

A

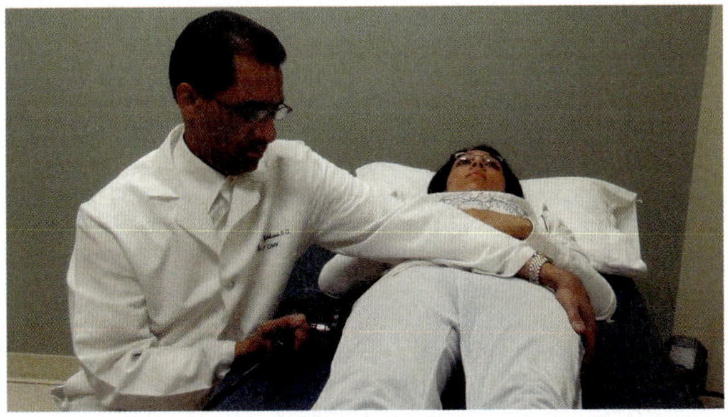

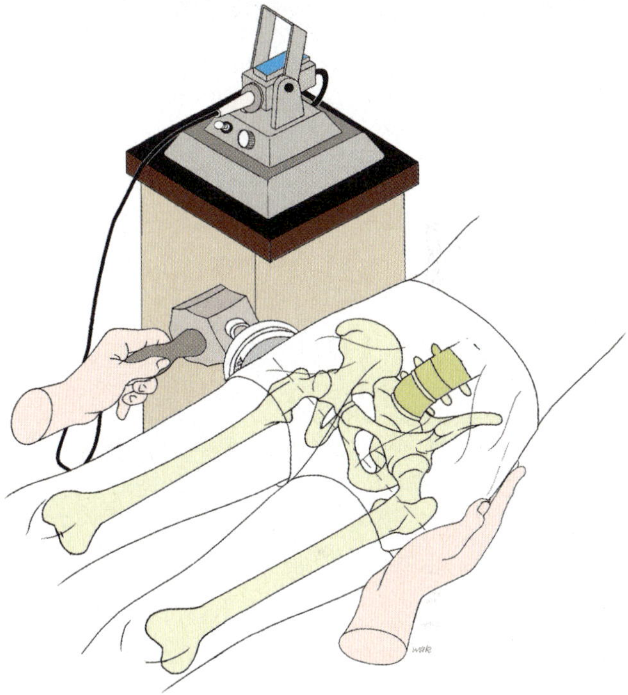

B

Figure 59.3. **A.** Treatment of the left femoral head using polarity concept (i.e., male physician uses percussor vibrator on the right femur of a female patient, even if dysfunction is found on the left). **B.** Drawing of percussion treatment of the femoral head showing underlying skeleton landmarks. (**B**, Courtesy of William A. Kuchera, DO, FAAO.)

No description of Dr. Fulford's work would be complete without mentioning the love that he found necessary to properly carry out diagnosis and treatment. This love for the patient's welfare came across in all his patient encounters. It was reflected in his interactions with friends, as well as with those he preferred to distance himself from. His professional and personal life was a living testimony to that primordial principle of life expressed as love.

Dr. Fulford's treatments created palpatory sensation and results unparalleled among his peers then and now. He spoke of purity of intent that we can all work toward and recreate this sensation and results for ourselves. It is worth repeating what Dr. Fulford said:

> "If you can't project love, you're not going to be able to help anyone. You have to have love for other human beings."[9]

REFERENCES

1. Russell W. *The Secret of Light*. University of Science and Philosophy; 1947.

2. Fulford RC. Are We on the path? *The Collected Works of Robert C. Fulford, D.O.* The Cranial Academy, Inc.; 2003.
3. Sutherland WG. Contributions of thought. *The Collected Writings of William Garner Sutherland, D.O.* 2nd ed. Rudra Press; 1998.
4. Goodman H. *Dr. Arbuckle's Influence on Dr. Fulford.* AAO Presentation; 1999.
5. Wade N. *Your body is younger than you think.* The New York Times; August 2, 2005.
6. Hoffman H. Esoteric osteopathy. *Classic Osteopathic Medical Works.* 1908; 8. https://digitalcommons.pcom.edu/classic_med_works/8
7. Fulford RC. The triune man. Presentation given at AAO convention; March 23, 1988.
8. Still AT. *The Philosophy and Mechanical Principles of Osteopathy.* Hudson-Kimberly Publishing Company; 1902.
9. Fulford RC. *Dr. Fulford's Touch of Life: The Healing Power of the Natural Life Force.* Pocket Books; 1996.

60 Functional Methods

DAVID ELAND ▪ HARRY FRIEDMAN

KEY CONCEPTS

- Functional technique is an indirect osteopathic manipulative treatment (OMT) procedure that uses passive motion to elicit compliance (ease) at a dysfunctional spinal or other joint segment.
- Vital concepts within Functional Methods include the "fundamental unit of somatic dysfunction" and the "mirror-image" motion asymmetries that define it.
- Empiric and scientific deductive processes were used in the development of functional technique, which encompasses an anatomic and physiologic basis (i.e., "the physiology of ease").

FUNCTIONAL METHODS

Functional Methods bring valuable insights into the process of Osteopathic diagnosis and treatment. Though not all of Dr. Johnston's contributions to Osteopathic Medicine will be detailed in this chapter, its careful study will hopefully lead to further exploration of his problem-solving approach, his clinical research, and descriptive papers.

William Johnston, DO's Functional Methods Contributions to Osteopathic Medicine

- Determination of the presence of somatic dysfunction using a standardized (uniform) screening exam that describes the tests and criteria for eliciting positive findings of motion, structure, and tissue.
- Passive motion tests are applied to assess whether resistance to motion occurs sooner in one direction versus the other without regard for end-feel or end-range.
- The use of scanning procedures (repetitive use of one passive motion test over many adjacent segments) to identify a three-segment complex of somatic dysfunction where the central segment behaves exactly opposite to the adjacent segments above and below. These motion responses are palpated and appreciated at the beginning of motion rather than during the mid or end-range of motion.
- Passive motion testing responses reveal unique relationships between the spinal and costal columns in the thoracic cage. Central spinal and unilateral costal responses to passive motion testing that are opposite at the same level are termed "unlinked," while responses that are the same are termed "linked."
- Thoracic cage dysfunctions are treated differently based on if they are linked or unlinked. Upper extremity positioning is used for unlinked dysfunctions, while lower extremity positioning is used for linked ones.
- Development of segmental passive motion testing and assessment of somatic dysfunction to areas where bones are fused across multiple segments (i.e., sternum and sacrum).
- Observation of three-segment units of dysfunction in the sternum (at sterno-chondral articulations) and sacrum (at sacroiliac articulations) exist and are associated with and treated using individual leg positioning.

> *"Tissues about a moving bony part constantly reflect mobile behavior as they comply with demands for movement and positioning of the whole system."*—Charles Bowles, DO

INTRODUCTION

The term "functional" as a descriptor in functional technique diagnosis and treatment is apt. "Functional" incorporates the appreciation and use of organization of movement and muscle function by the central nervous system from the moment movement is contemplated and generated, whether normal or abnormal (somatic dysfunction). Its mechanism includes all the afferent and efferent pathways that control actual motion behavior. This immediacy of response in all tissues of the body and its consistent patterns provide the key to this gentle, effective approach.

HISTORY AND EVOLUTION OF FUNCTIONAL PRINCIPLES

History of Functional Methods

Functional technique dates back to Dr. AT Still. The written record of "functional" is clearest from Hoover to Bowles and Johnston. This chapter's focus will be on the approach as described by Johnston.

Harold V. Hoover, DO, the earliest of the functional proponents, was an osteopathic explorer who practiced a full range of techniques, from "thrust" to cranial. The emphasis in his generation was on the joint lesion. Harrison Fryette, DO, conducted some of the latest and most thought-provoking research, which Dr. Hoover used as a basis for his theory on motion inputs in functional techniques.

Dr. Hoover commented: "let us understand that all technic of correction of joints is applied to and changes only the soft tissue."[1] His definition of soft tissue predated the concept of the "mobile segment."[2] "He explored movement as an independent means of diagnosis and as a guide to treatment." "(a) lesion may be diagnosed in terms of physiological movement and corrected in the same way."[2] Dr. Hoover used the concepts of movement function in diagnosis, palpation of ease and bind in response to motion, soft tissue focus, and then used these ideas in indirect treatment.

The New England Academy of Applied Osteopathy was established after Dr. Hoover taught a course in Massachusetts in 1951. Founding members of the group included Laurence Osborn, DO, Edward B. Sullivan, DO, William Knowles, DO, and Charles Bowles, DO. In the early years, this group had a steady exchange of letters with Dr. Hoover as they researched their topics. Dr. Bowles, formerly an engineer from MIT, was in charge of organizing the educational programs (per personal communication with John Goodridge, DO, October, 2007). Drs. Johnston, Knowles, Osborn, and Sullivan also assisted with these educational programs, as did John Goodridge, DO, from Connecticut, shortly thereafter. They followed Dr. Hoover's lead in working with observable facts, which were carefully distinguished from concepts: "sensation first and idea next (per personal communication with John Goodridge, DO, October, 2007)."[3] This emphasis on "observable fact" has been evident in both Dr. Bowles and Dr. Johnston's writings, as well as in Dr. Johnston's book, *Functional Methods*. As summarized by Dr. Bowles, a key attraction of functional technique in this age of scientific inquiry is that "(w)e have … new ways of looking at old problems, ways that raise new questions that are more amenable to scientific study and understanding."[4]

Inspired by cybernetics, systems theory, and the work of physiologist Irvin Korr, PhD, the group proposed a demand/response–feedback–based explanation for empiric findings and treatment outcomes. Dr. Bowles, in particular, brought the concepts of "demand–response" transactions and "ongoing reciprocal transactions" into the discussions.[5] This built on the work of Korr and John Stedman Denslow, PhD, in the 1940s, which brought attention to the "osteopathic lesion" (somatic dysfunction) as an aberration of neuromuscular function.[6] Consistent with the demand–response paradigm, "a series of continually acting reciprocal transactions,"[5] the evolving concepts guided diagnosis and treatment by focusing on the dysfunctional segment in the context of the entire movement of which it is a part. The first study sessions of the New England Academy developed the concept of "dynamic neutral," referring to a state of consistent ease felt by fingers palpating somatic structures during motion.[3] Unlike the dysfunctional segment, normal function (dynamic neutral behavior) responses are coordinated with the segments above and below.

In 1969, Dr. Johnston, along with Edward G. Stiles, DO, and J. Allan Robertson, DO, collaborated on an article[7] that first introduced segment-to-segment comparison as a way to define the location of a dysfunctional mobile segment. This article is pivotal in introducing the use of the diagnostic "scan" and presaged the use of the term "mirror-image" in 1987.[8]

The immediacy of asymmetric *response to motion* input at a dysfunctional mobile segment supported the idea that dysfunction is comprised of organized, coordinated behavior of vertebral segments opposite in response to the segments above and below (e.g., mirror-image behavior). Diagnostic ease was readily converted into therapeutic motion that promoted ease, facilitating the return to "normal" or dynamic neutral.

Central to Johnston's research was always the differentiation of palpatory fact from conjecture: "(t)here is a need to delineate carefully what is perceived at the hand of the observer and what is conceived in the mind of the observer. Often the relation between the two is tenuous."[10] During a personal communication with chapter authors, he expressed, "Don't let concepts get between your diagnosis and treatment."

Dr. Johnston continued the tradition of scientific inquiry into diagnosis and treatment during his tenure at Michigan State University College of Osteopathic Medicine, from 1973 to his death in 2003. The relationship he formed with the Department of Biomechanics (now the Department of Osteopathic Manipulative Medicine), from 1973 to 1981, particularly influenced his thinking. Dr. Johnston formalized a functional approach to diagnosis, with concepts of screening, scanning, and segmental definition.[6] Several articles in 1987 further defined the nature of a segmental problem using the principles of "segmental definition" in Functional Methods.[9]

In January of 1987, Dr. Johnston first introduced palpable motor changes of visceral reflex origin in the JAOA.[11] These motor changes were distinctly different from Chapman reflexes and any other vertebral correlates with visceral disease. The first edition of *Functional Methods* in 1995 brought the elements of Functional Methods diagnosis and treatment into one place. The 1998 AAO Yearbook then became a complementary resource for all of Dr. Johnston's writings and research.

IMPORTANT FUNCTIONAL CONCEPTS DETAILED

It is important to understand the functional approach's unique concepts to appreciate its implications in diagnosis and treatment. Its application can detect the location of somatic dysfunction, confirm its diagnostic characteristics, guide treatment, and confirm resolution after appropriate treatment. The diagnostic approach outlined by Dr. Johnston pertains to the soma in its primary role as the body's skeletal movement system and a framework of tests for defining the motion characteristics at a dysfunctional mobile segment. According to Dr. Johnston, the diagnosis of a vertebral segment based solely on its position and mobility is not sufficient to understand the movement of that segment. This diagnosis fails to capture important information about how the segment receives stimuli, is controlled by the motor system, and interacts with other parts of the body.[12] To truly understand human movement, one needs to consider the functional dynamics of the entire system, not just individual segments in isolation.[9]

Mobile Segment/Mobile Unit

A single vertebra, along with its adjacent muscular tissue and neural elements, makes up a mobile segment or mobile unit. Dr. Johnston emphasized the role of the mobile segment within a "system" or a group of dynamically related components that operate in concert for the purpose of achieving a specific goal.[9]

Neuroreflexive Nature of Motor Control

The motion of the mobile segment is controlled by spinal reflex neural feedback of information about the quality of the movement from its own adnexal tissues and adjacent segments. As a result of this feedback, the mobile segment's behavior will simultaneously match the demands for movement and positioning of the whole system. Because the adjacent tissues reflect the behavior of this mobile segment, they can be monitored for their palpable expression of compliance with or resistance to the movement being initiated.[6,9] A mobile segment responds to the central demand for active whole-body movement. What emerges is a series of mobile segments or subsystems whose motion is either in or out of coordination with its adjacent segments. When out of coordination, one may appreciate tissue "bind" during motion testing, which reflects disturbed neuromusculoskeletal response at that mobile segment.

Functional technique is based on motion and response to motion at a dysfunctional segment. "If the premise is that there is a disturbance of an organizational nature in the tracking mechanism of a vertebra (mobile segment), then the action that is logical is to manipulate that tracking mechanism until the central switchings fall into their correct sequence again."[14]

William L. Johnston's empiric clinical exploration and research gave birth to two key concepts of functional technique: the "mirror-image motion asymmetry" and the "fundamental unit of somatic dysfunction."[6] Their application can direct the location of somatic dysfunction, confirm the diagnostic characteristics of that dysfunction, guide treatment, and confirm resolution after appropriate treatment.

Mirror-Image Asymmetries

For effective treatment, an accurate diagnosis is necessary to guide the application of the technique. Mirror-image asymmetries can aid in this process by providing an immediate comparison of responses of all adjacent segments. A mirror-image motion asymmetry occurs when signs of asymmetry are opposite at a central segment compared to those of the segments above and below—a three-segment relationship. Somatic dysfunction is characterized by "mirror-image motion asymmetry" between the three elements of the fundamental unit of somatic dysfunction. Mirror-image asymmetries can be found with motions, tissue texture abnormalities, and positions. However, *passive motion* is the diagnostic and therapeutic guide in functional technique (Fig. 60.1).

Vertebral dysfunction is the simplest of this set of findings. This asymmetry is observable by palpation with any motion, whether active (initiated by the patient) or passive (introduced by the physician). As an example, the localized disturbance is noted as "bind" at T3, immediately in response to right trunk rotation and bind at T2 and T4 in response to left trunk rotation (Fig. 60.2).

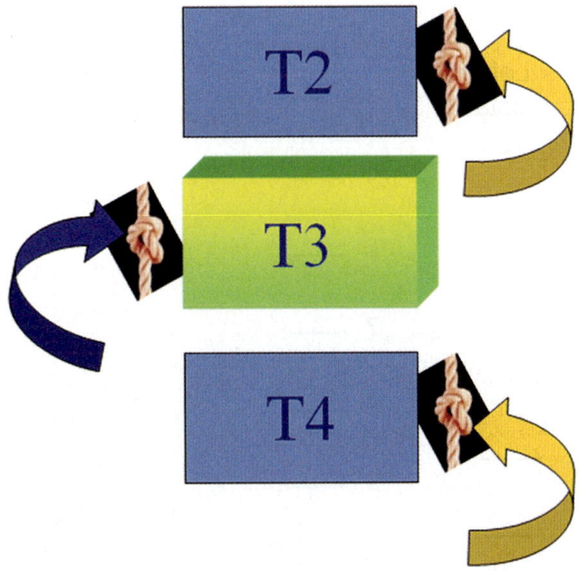

Figure 60.2. Mirror-image asymmetry is illustrated here in a three segment group, the "fundamental unit of dysfunction," exhibiting the characteristics of somatic dysfunction. The *arrows* indicate the direction of motion input initiated from head/neck contact. Knotted rope indicates the palpatory sense of "binding" felt by the palpating hand at the segment.

Fundamental Unit of Segmental Dysfunction

This term utilizes the three-segment relationship described as "mirror-image asymmetries" above. A central primary segment with asymmetric motor function is noted, and adjacent segments exhibit asymmetric motor function that mirrors that of the central segment.[12] Reflex responses among these three segments are mediated through their adnexa and the neural control system. In Functional Methods, palpation of asymmetry throughout a three-segment fundamental unit of segmental dysfunction increases accuracy in locating what Dr. Johnston defines as the "primary dysfunctional segment."

Typically, comparing segment to segment proceeds from above to below and stops when the dysfunctional segment is identified. Implicit in this is the comparison of the segment above the one identified with the identified dysfunctional segment. However, the diagnostic process does not proceed to the segment below for comparison. This leads to the possibility that the segment identified may be one below the actual dysfunctional segment and can be the reason for ineffective treatment—a secondary segment has been treated instead of the primary dysfunctional segment.

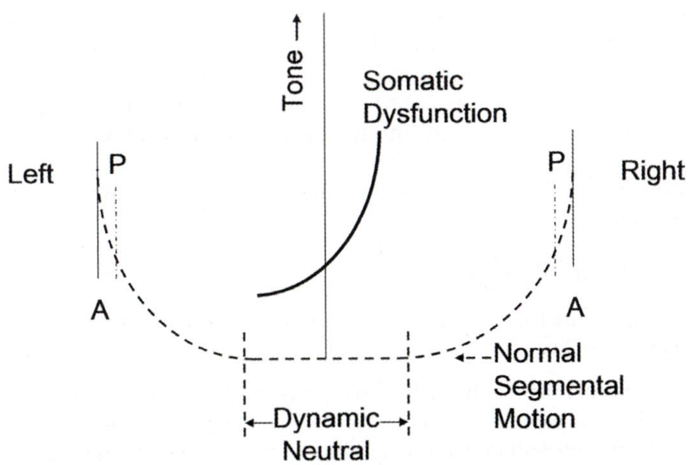

Figure 60.1. It can be seen that resting tone is increased in somatic dysfunction as compared to a normal segment where a "dynamic neutral" is experienced. With somatic dysfunction, any motion input elicits an immediate response of "ease" or "bind" at the monitored segment.

LINKAGE

Linkage is an attempt to make sense of the visceral input and its interplay with the musculoskeletal system in a unique way. "Linkage" is the term Dr. Johnston coined to express the relationship of the rib shaft to the associated vertebra that he found consistently associated with various viscerally-related patient complaints—asthma, cholelithiasis, hypertension, and upper GI disease.

The diagnostic findings for the vertebra and associated rib are unique. Both respond to regional motion input in the same manner, acting as if they were "welded together." This has been interpreted as the nervous system's response to visceral afferent input. The opposite rib does not participate in this dysfunction (Fig. 60.3).

"THE PHYSIOLOGY OF EASE"—Anatomic and Physiologic Principles of Functional Technique

IMMEDIATE RESPONSE

After Irvin Korr, PhD, defined the neural basis for somatic dysfunction, osteopathic physicians gained a better understanding of the tissues' "response" to a (passive or active) motion "demand" at

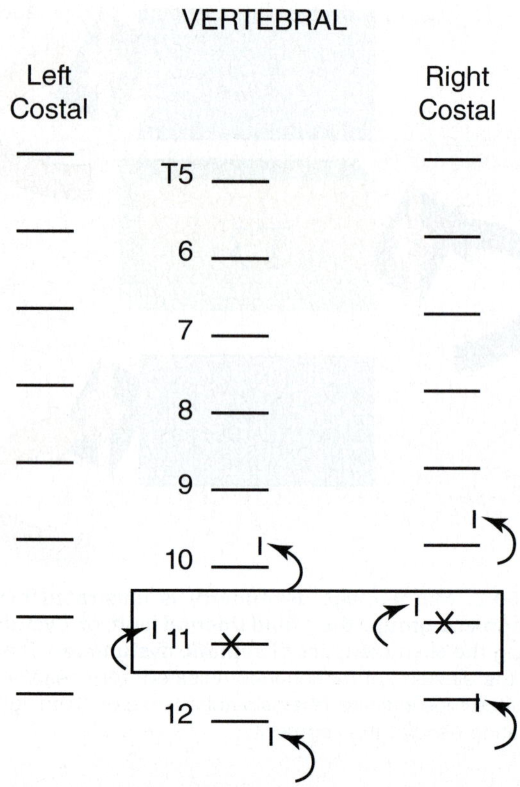

Figure 60.3. This illustration depicts the findings associated with linkage: T11 and right rib 11 have the same response to left rotation—increased resistance/tension. It is valuable to note that the "mirror-image asymmetry" is apparent with linkage as well as the vertebral column, again expressing "fundamental unit of dysfunction" characteristics. (From Johnston WL, Friedman HD, Eland DC. *Functional Methods*. 2nd ed. American Academy of Osteopathy; 2005.)

a dysfunctional vertebral segment or joint.[21] The ideas of *demand–response*[20] and of *organized coordinated behavior of mobile segments in dysfunction* is observed in mirror-image behavior (see Fig. 60.2), as compared to normal function (dynamic neutral). Immediate response can be appreciated in both circumstances. Whether the motion input is active or passive by the physician, the CNS does not wait to organize that motion until it is partially or fully through its reflex arc. The patterned response, modulated through the spinal cord, is not delayed by anything other than nerve conduction velocities (see Fig. 60.1).

The implications for diagnosis and treatment are significant. Functional technique uses the initial *immediate response* to motion input. Therefore, the range of motion is minimal, as is the force applied. Biomechanical leveraging forces and motion sufficient to bring those forces to bear at a barrier for a given segment are unnecessary. Passive regional motion input (PRMI) is a diagnostic technique in which a physician applies a passive force through a region of the body to induce motion, usually using a single elementary motion (such as sidebending, rotation, flexion/extension, translation), in order to assess a monitored segment's response to that regional motion. The motion introduced stays within physiologic motion, and any differences in resistance or ease compared to the segments above and below can indicate dysfunction. This technique is used to evaluate the motion characteristics of a specific segment which then can be taken toward balance and ease, starting from a point where the segment can respond (initial response).[15]

AFFERENT REDUCTION

Johnston used the term "afferent reduction" to describe the neuroreflexive element that plays a role in the effectiveness of functional methods. When there is primary vertebral dysfunction, predictable asymmetries in mirror-image motion indicate the presence of monosynaptic afferent inputs and interneurons as pathways for secondary adaptive behavior to occur in adjacent segments.[6] The reflex basis for these secondary mirror images becomes apparent when all three segments return to motion symmetry following a successful response to a functional manipulative procedure that addresses only the central (primary) dysfunctional segment.[12]

The postulated physiologic basis for the treatment response suggests contributing elements:

1. The spinal cord provides communication pathways that conduct impulses from sensory receptors in both musculoskeletal and visceral tissues. When noxious stimuli are persistent, the afferent bombardment contributes to palpable somatic manifestations of spinal dysfunction. Segmental motion asymmetries develop individuality in their dysfunctional behavior.[12] (See Chapter 13 Somatic Dysfunction, Spinal Facilitation, and Viscerosomatic Integration, for further background and discussion.) Even at rest, when the afferent impulses should be minimal, the dysfunctional segment displays malposition and increased muscular tension as an active source of sensory input.[6]
2. "The physiology of ease" involves local tissue ease, which decreases the afferent bombardment from the segment, at least in part. Initially, this may be due to pressure changes on the nerve endings and the return toward synchronized pattern generation. But local motion, muscle contraction/relaxation responses, and tissue ease all promote lymphatic drainage of local fluid congestion and dispersal of local inflammatory elements.
3. Fluid change that occurs more slowly than the neuroreflexive element may contribute to the prolonged and/or progressive response noted with functional treatment.

As a result of the complex interplay between inputs and the local environment, segmental motion asymmetries develop individuality in their dysfunctional behavior depending on the afferent source, somatic or visceral.[12]

Functional Diagnosis

To apply a functional approach to manipulation, one first has to gather diagnostic information relevant to motion function.[8] To this end, Dr. Johnston often said, "Don't let a concept get between your diagnosis and your treatment."

The goal in Functional Method is to gather information that can be directly translated into treatment. Standardization of procedures is emphasized for that purpose and for purposes of consistency and reproducibility. The following aspects assist in that translation:

Diagnostic Sequence

The examination is broken into steps to facilitate consistency and reproducibility.

1. **Screen/initial approach:** This approach addresses the question, "Is there a problem?" in any of the eight regions of the body.
2. **Scan** determines a more specific location(s) within the region identified by screening through segment to segment tissue texture comparison and ease/bind response to motion inputs.
3. **Segmental definition** determines the nature of the problem at each location identified—segmental ease/bind responses to motion inputs, rotary, and translatory.[7]

"Functional control is executed with a minimum of overall coercion and an absolute absence of coercion or interference at the segment being tested."[16] This principle is expressed in functional methods through the use of "Listening Hand/Motor Hand" contacts and through "Passive Regional Motion Input."

Listening Hand/Motor Hand

The sole purpose of the listening hand is to monitor tissue response at the segment being monitored. For the axial spine, tissue contact is made over the transverse processes/articular pillars with a thumb and finger or two fingers. If not paying close attention, beginners may have these contacts at differing levels.

The motor hand introduces shoulder/trunk rotation with elbow contact (the patient's arms are crossed in front of the body). This hand inputs the motion required as gently and unobtrusively as possible. Only minimal forces are applied for the initial introduction of motion in any one direction. Immediate change in tissue resistance (bind) can be noted at the beginning of motion introduction when the trunk motion is introduced. The motor hand introduces motion as described in the next section.

Passive Regional Motion Input

"[Passive] regional motion input (testing) can be defined diagnostically as a passive force (applied by a physician) through a region(s) of the body to induce motion, usually using a single elementary motion (rotary or translatory), to assess the focus of interest, the mobile segment."[15] Only minimal forces are applied for the initial introduction of motion in any one direction.

MOTION INPUTS

Functional technique is explicit in its recognition of rotary and translatory motions applicable to the axial spine, along with active respiration. (This is a clear example of Michigan State's Biomechanics department's influence on Dr. Johnson's analytic process.) Tests for a functional response using the axial spine as the motion input encompass six degrees of freedom (three rotary motions and three translatory motions) plus active respiration:

- Motion inputs are typically introduced with the motor hand via shoulder/trunk or head/neck contacts.
- Rotary (around an axis):
  1. Flexion/extension
  2. Sidebending
  3. Rotation
- Translatory (within a plane): The incorporation of translation is implicit in advanced applications of other osteopathic treatment approaches.
  1. Lateral/medial to the sagittal plane within the horizontal plane
  2. Superior/inferior to the horizontal plane within the coronal plane
  3. Anterior/posterior to the coronal plane within the sagittal plane
- Active respiration:
  1. Inhalation/exhalation

SUMMARY OF FUNCTIONAL DIAGNOSIS

Monitoring tissues with a gentle touch of the listening hand and observing for changes in tissue texture, followed by an immediate response to a motion input by the motor hand, is an art that requires practice. The motion input is passive and regional in nature, replicating motions that the body can produce. The range of motion is minimal to focus on small changes of interest. Testing involves motions that can replicate the variety of active motions available to the patient (three rotary, three translatory, and respiration for the axial spine). Tissue texture changes and responses to motion input at the segmental level are used to identify mirror-image asymmetries that confirm and characterize segmental somatic dysfunction. Therefore, functional diagnosis always employs more than one test to increase reliability.

PASSIVE REGIONAL MOTION INPUT VERSUS OTHER APPROACHES TO DIAGNOSTIC AND THERAPEUTIC MOTION INPUT

The Functional approach to diagnosis using PRMI is best contrasted with two widely used approaches:

Active regional motion input which, as its name suggests, uses patient-generated motion while the physician monitors the response at the segment being diagnosed.

Passive local motion input where the listening hand and the motor hand are combined. Thumb or finger pressure, usually on a transverse process, induces the motion of interest and monitors response through bilateral contact with a thumb or finger.

Dr. Johnston was familiar with and critiqued both approaches in developing the Functional Method approach. With active regional motion, the concern was reproducibility given that the physician does not control the motion. Alternatively, passive local motion input created an artificial motion that is a motion that the patient could not perform—a person cannot individually rotate T5 to the right in isolation.

FUNCTIONAL METHODS TREATMENT

Functional Method technique is an indirect osteopathic manipulative treatment (OMT) procedure. Thus, motion is applied in the direction that elicits ease in the monitored paraspinal tissues at the level of the dysfunctional segment. Treatment involves continuous refinement of motion through the point of resolution.

If the premise is that there is a disturbance of an organizational nature in the tracking mechanism of a vertebra (mobile segment), then the logical action is to manipulate that tracking mechanism until the central (or neural) switchings fall into their correct sequences again.[14] To achieve this end in Functional Methods, the tools used by the physician are the specific directions of motion (toward ease).[8] The neuroreflexive behavior is the focus rather than the anatomic joint.

FUNCTIONAL METHODS GUIDELINES

Certain procedures help to ensure success in applying this indirect method of manipulation for segmental dysfunction:

1. Prior to motion input, patient positioning may be used to facilitate the ease obtained with motion input and to address aspects of motion ease that are inconvenient or inefficient for a desired treatment.
2. The initial introduction of motion in any one elementary direction is small (not evaluating the range), with minimal forces applied. It is important here to remember this method allows the physician to deal with immediate response guided by CNS organization of responses to inputs.
3. Motion directions are toward a sense of immediately increasing ease. This response manifests a decreasing sense of resistance

to pressure at the fingers monitoring the tense dysfunctional segment.

4. Order of introduction of single elements of rotary and translatory directions of motion inputs are not important, but are introduced sequentially initially. With experience, motion inputs are combined, affecting the control of an eventual "smooth torsion arc" for body movement, leading to the resolution of the dysfunction.
5. The final step of functional procedure involves asking the patient for a specific direction of active respiration, whether inhalation or exhalation, that contributes further to the increasing ease. For example, if requesting inhalation, the subject is asked to slowly take a deep breath and briefly hold it.
   - The ease is then ridden through the opposite phase, exhalation in this example, with further refinement of palpated ease again during the next inhalation.
   - This respiratory attention, added to continuous feedback of decreasing resistance, allows the operator to fine-tune the combination of translatory and rotary directions. The objective is to reach a sense of tissue tension release at the fingertips, which are continually monitoring response at the dysfunctional segment.
6. The release of restraint in the motor mechanism allows a return to midline resting function with dynamic neutral again present, unobstructed by any sense of the resistance previously encountered in the return direction (Fig. 60.4).

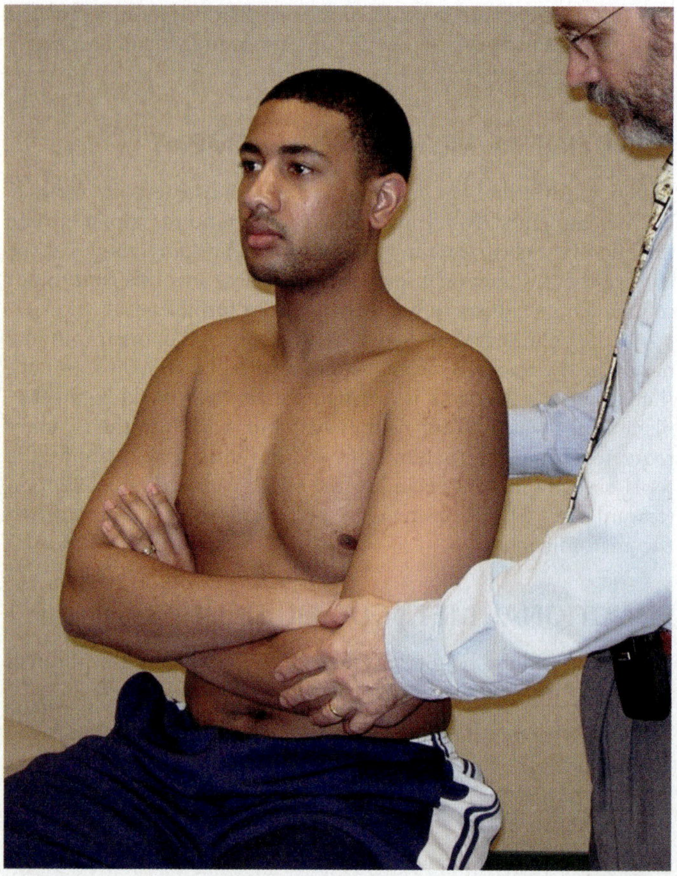

Figure 60.4. Functional Motion input for rotation response: crossed arms, as in the picture, allow full relaxation of the arms and shoulders without the need for muscular effort by the patient. Elbow contact allows for pure rotary motion input by the motor hand (*left*) while the listening hand (*right*) monitors the vertebral segment.

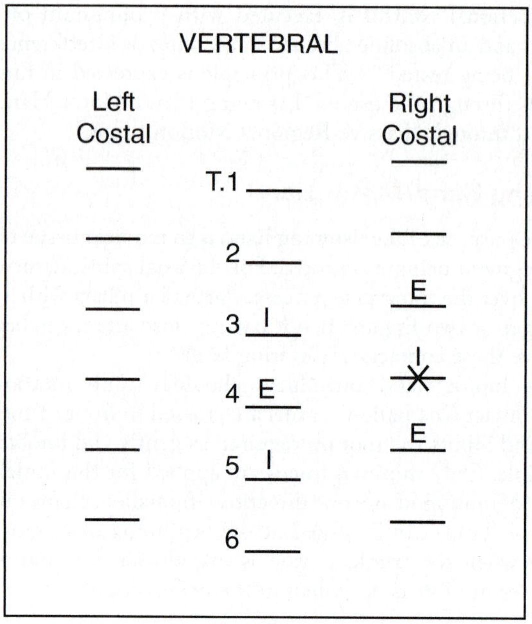

Figure 60.5. Responses to the rotary and translation motion inputs would have the same mirror-image pattern.

FUNCTIONAL METHODS APPROACH TO THE THORACIC CAGE

Unlinked

- Somatosomatic reflex changes exhibit a "mirror-image" phenomenon between the lateral costal and midline spinal columns.
- Thoracic cage motion responses occur in either the left or right lateral costal columns.
- Mirror-image findings are palpated above and below the central segment (rib) as well as in the adjacent central spinal column. A representative unlinked pattern is illustrated in Fig. 60.5.
- Once the central segment has been confirmed, treatment can be carried out in the side-lying position using the ipsilateral upper extremity to introduce motions responding with ease at the central segment being palpated.
- Part 2 of the treatment continues seated with passively induced patient trunk positioning in directions of axial and translatory motion ease (Fig. 60.6A).
- Exhalation and inhalation thoracic cage dysfunctions have predictable motions of ease.

Linked

- Viscerosomatic or somatovisceral reflex changes exhibit a "linkage" phenomenon between the lateral costal and midline spinal columns. Motion responses palpated in either column exhibit identical palpatory responses (Fig. 60.6B).
- Treatment is carried out by introducing ipsilateral lower extremity motions that respond with ease at the central segment of the dysfunction in either a prone or supine position, whichever is associated with a sense of ease at the segment being palpated (prone for ease in posterior translation of shoulders, supine for ease in anterior translation of shoulders).
- Head rotation is toward the side, which produces a sense of ease at the central segment, which is also palpated.
- The operator stands at the same side of the table as the side of the dysfunction and introduces hip flexion/extension, abduction/adduction, internal/external rotation, and cephalad/caudad

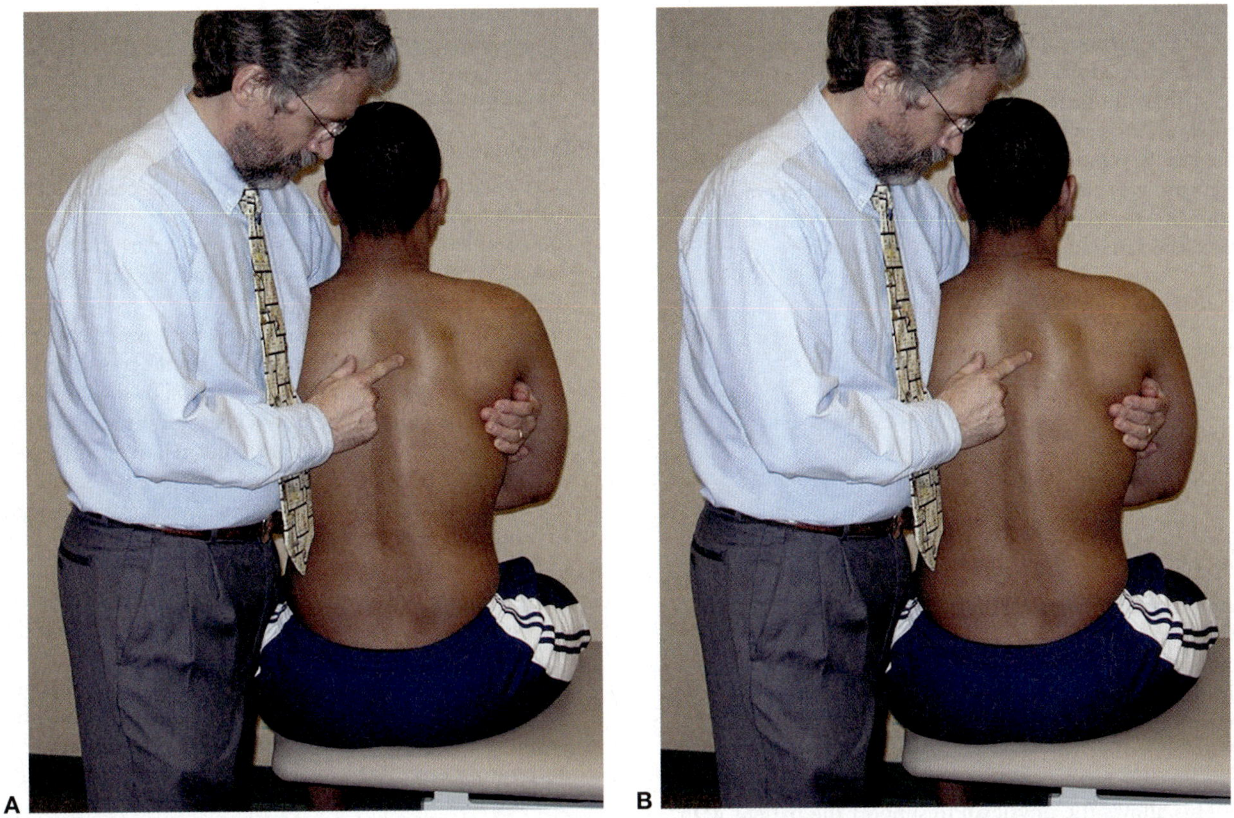

Figure 60.6. **A.** This contact allows patient support and introduction of motion input for rotations and translations. **B.** The physician's left axilla rests upon the patient's left shoulder while the left hand grasps the thorax underneath the patient's right axilla. A gentle hug-like motion allows the physician's trunk to contact the back/left side of the patient for patient support and for control of motion inputs for treatment. Three rotation and three translation motion inputs are input toward ease sequentially during the phase of respiratory ease or as a smooth torsion arc during respiratory ease. (Courtesy of David Eland, DO, FAAO.)

translation, each in the direction responding with ease at the central segment being palpated (Fig. 60.7).

CLINICAL CASE

A 27-year-old male presented to the office with a complaint of sharp interscapular pain. It started 2 days earlier while the patient was lifting weights. He had lifted free weights regularly for 6 months and had just increased the weight for the incline press and the military press. He was nearly finished when he felt a sharp left interscapular pain, at which point he stopped. Over the next 36 hours, the local pain progressed at rest and with activity. The patient mentioned a history of gastroesophageal reflux disease (GERD) in the last year. He had been treating the condition effectively with medication, until a month before the onset of the back symptoms. He had decided to experiment without medication for several months. The reflux symptoms had progressed since. He had no other complaints. The patient was otherwise healthy.

The immediate problem was the weightlifting injury. The 15-minute office visit required a focus on that, but with a follow-up in a week to further evaluate the GERD symptoms.

PHYSICAL EXAM

Vital signs were normal.

HEENT, CV, Pulmonary, Abdominal, and Neurologic Exams

All were normal.

Structural Exam

The fifth thoracic vertebra was extended, rotated, and sidebent to the right. T5 paraspinal tissues felt boggy and slightly warmer. There was associated local muscular hypertonicity focused in the right paraspinal musculature. Traditional positional diagnosis: fifth thoracic extended, rotated, and sidebent left (ER_LS_L).

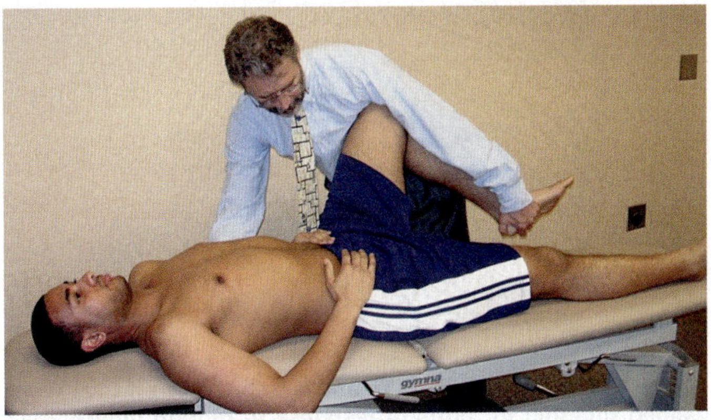

Figure 60.7. **Lower extremity control is easily accomplished with the patient's knee held against the physician's chest by the arm at the axilla.** The motor hand (*left*) grasps the ankle. With this dual contact, all necessary lower extremity motions can be easily accomplished. The right fingerpad contact is easiest on the rib angle of the fifth rib. Both rib and vertebra respond to motion input in the same way, so only one needs to be monitored. (Courtesy of David Eland, DO, FAAO.)

Functional Methods Diagnosis characterizes the somatic dysfunction by the addition of translation and respiratory ease preferences: fifth thoracic response to shoulder/trunk motion input indicates increasing ease with extension, rotation left, sidebending left, translations right, anterior, and inferior. Exhalation ease was also noted. All findings were accompanied by the opposite response at the fourth and the sixth thoracic segments to the same motion inputs.

DIAGNOSIS

1. Thoracic strain
2. Somatic dysfunction—thoracic region

TREATMENT

T5 Example (Fig. 60.8)

Setup

Patient is seated at the end of the table.

1. Patient's arms are crossed, with hands tucked into the opposite elbow crease.
2. Patient's left shoulder is facing the end of the table.
3. Physician faces the patient's left side.
4. Physician's left axilla is draped over the patient's left shoulder. Physician's left forearm is brought across the patient's chest so that the left hand rests just under the patient's right axilla. This allows the physician to support the patient with lateral chest contact to the patient's back. The "gentle hug" also facilitates patient support and relaxation, which in turn permits easy introduction and control of motion inputs.

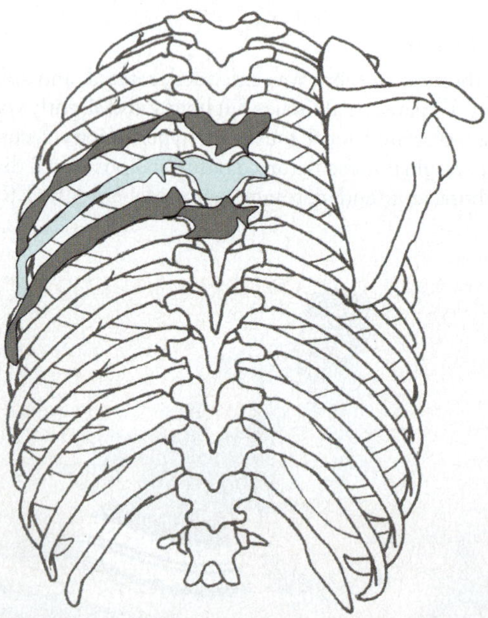

Figure 60.8. With "linkage," T5 and left rib 5 act as if they were welded together in terms of response to motion inputs. They both respond with ease to left sidebending and rotation motion inputs in case 2. The same is true for the other motion inputs and respiration. There is still "mirror-image" response to motion inputs and respiration at the segments above and below, rib and vertebra. (Modified with permission from Johnston WL, Friedman HD, Eland DC. *Functional Methods: A Manual for Palpatory Skills Development in Osteopathic Examination and Manipulation of Motor Function*. 2nd ed. American Academy of Osteopathy; 2005:82–83.)

5. The right (listening) hand contacts the fifth thoracic over the transverse processes, with pads of the thumb and index or middle finger.

Principles of Motion Input

1. Use slight shifting of postural forces to control movement of the patient's body. Three translatory motion inputs can be completed. The patient's hips are relatively fixed by the seated position. Translatory motion inputs are the least familiar to many physicians:
   a. A slight shift in the physician's body weight to the right allows an easy introduction of lateral translation motion input toward ease, as monitored at T5 by the listening hand.
   b. A similar shift of the physician's weight anterior controls the patient's shoulder and trunk relative to the pelvis to initiate anterior translation.
   c. Mild body compression combined with extensive shoulder/trunk contact with the patient introduces inferior translatory motion input.
   d. The initial introduction of each appropriate direction is more important than the extent of range in any one direction alone.
2. The motion inputs Progress, with practice from sequential inputs of the six individual motions during the phase of respiratory ease to an eventual smooth torsional arc riding respiratory ease. Each of the directions will begin to diminish the local tissue resistance monitored during the procedure at T5: sidebending left, right translation, rotation left, translation inferior, extension, and anterior translation.
3. The final element is respiration. Direct a slow inhalation by the patient. During inhalation, refine the rotary and translatory elements of motion input to elicit increasing compliance at the monitored segment. Repeat as needed with sequential or eventually simultaneous motion input. Since exhalation elicited a response of ease at the monitored segment, during exhalation, ride the sense of ease gained during inhalation, that is, increase the eventual motion torsion arc as the patient exhales to maximize the ease or compliance palpated at the dysfunctional segment.
4. The summation of all seven motions and their refinement by the sense of ease palpated at the listening hand's contact over the transverse processes of the fifth thoracic vertebra promotes an eventual release of the holding tensions at the dysfunctional segment. The release allows a return to a central resting position without encountering the previous resistance in these opposing directions.

FOLLOW-UP VISIT

Upon return 1 week later, the acute dysfunction and sharp pain had resolved. GERD symptoms were ongoing.

PHYSICAL EXAM

Musculoskeletal examination revealed that left rib 5 had the same responses to motion input as did T5 (like they were "welded together," "linkage"). Soft tissues overlying T5 and the rib had a warm, boggy feeling, with a deeper fibrotic quality[17] (see Fig. 60.8).

Linkage present at T5 also exhibits resistance to right rotation.[15,18] Linkage is not limited to rotation responses. T5/left rib 5's linked motion asymmetry is typically complete in rotary, translatory, and respiratory tests. Secondary mirror images exist at the adjacent coupled segments.[15] This linkage of vertebral and rib findings is interpreted as the nervous system's response to visceral afferent input: its attempt to make sense of the visceral input and to compensate for this new information as effectively as possible.

Positional Diagnoses

Fifth thoracic extended, rotated, and side-bent left (ER_LS_L). Left rib 5 inhalation dysfunction.

FUNCTIONAL DIAGNOSIS

T5 and left rib 5 "linked": ease with shoulder/trunk extension, rotation, and sidebending left; translation anterior, right, and superior; and inhalation ease. Shoulder/trunk motion inputs for rotary and translational ease during exhalation (the phase of respiratory ease) are accomplished using the same principles used for the "T5 Example." The crucial difference is the involvement of both the left rib and the thoracic vertebra. Since they are "linked," their responses to motion input will be the same and can be monitored from the rib or the vertebra.

LOWER EXTREMITY

The "linkage" finding requires the additional examination of lower extremity responses to motion input while monitoring the rib and/or vertebra. Motion input for the extremities also addresses the six degrees of freedom in regard to the three-dimensional nature of somatic dysfunction. The motions that are readily applied to the lower extremity (inversion/eversion, flexion/extension, adduction/abduction, compression/traction) and, finally, active respiration. This addresses the three-dimensional nature in a manner sufficient to resolve the dysfunction.

DIAGNOSTIC PROCESS (SEE FIG. 60.7)

1. The patient is supine on the table, and the position assists the treatment process.[12] Depending on whether there is a response of ease at the locus of dysfunction in the position chosen, the patient is positioned supine or prone.
2. Physician stands on the left side of the table.
3. Flex the hip and knee of each lower extremity sufficiently to allow the patient's feet to be firmly planted on the table for individual lower extremity testing of motion inputs.[13]
4. The left (ipsilateral) lower extremity is first tested for inversion/eversion to determine whether motion asymmetry is present, as evidenced by the immediate change in ease/bind at T5/left rib 5.
   a. Ease with eversion was found during the follow-up visit.
   b. Other motion tests include flexion/extension, abduction/adduction, and compression/traction, that is, superior/inferior translation.
5. The right (contralateral) lower extremity is tested for inversion/eversion. Increasing resistance is noted in both directions initiated. Since increasing resistance is present in both directions, there are no indicators for introducing motions for the right (contralateral) lower extremity that would assist in easing the linked dysfunction.
   a. Testing of the three remaining motions would yield the same results.
   b. Only the asymmetric responses to left lower extremity motion input provide a basis for treatment input.

Resulting Lower Extremity Functional Diagnosis

The linked fifth thoracic/left rib 5 response to left lower extremity motion input indicates ease with eversion, flexion, adduction, and superior translation (compression) with inhalation. Respiration response is always consistent regardless of motion input—shoulder/trunk or extremity.

Treatment

T5 "LINKAGE" EXAMPLE

1. Spinal motion asymmetries identified by shoulder/trunk motion input are addressed with the patient seated, as in case 1. Improvement is expected, but some resistance will still be apparent when the patient returns to a neutral seated position. Because of the diagnosed linkage, resolution will require treatment using ipsilateral lower extremity motion input. This leads to the second aspect of treatment of linkage—use of lower extremity motion inputs.
2. Lower Extremity—The following sequence details the treatment of this viscerosomatic influence (GERD) using the lower extremity as motion input to elicit responses at T5 and left rib 5 (see Fig. 60.7).
   a. Setup:
      i. Contact the angle of the left fifth rib with the pad of the index finger of the right hand. The left fifth rib, the fifth thoracic, or both can be monitored since they act as though they are "welded together" when linkage is present.
      ii. Physician's left hand holds the patient's left foot next to the physician's left hip. The patient's left knee is positioned in the physician's left axilla for easy motion input.
   b. Principles of Motion Input:
      i. Use slight body shifts to control movement of the left lower extremity.
         1. A slight right sidebending by the physician initiates eversion.
         2. A slight shift toward the patient's head introduces flexion.
         3. A side shift of the physician's body toward the left carries the patient's left foot medially (adduction). Compression from the axillary contact along the axis of the femur initiates superior translation.
         4. An immediate ease response to motion input in each direction of motion is more important than the extent of range in any one direction alone.
      ii. The final element is respiration.
         1. Direct a slow inhalation by the patient.
         2. During exhalation, continue to refine the motions that increase the sense of ease gained during inhalation.
         3. The additional element of increasing ease with exhalation is repeated as needed, with concomitant refinement of the lower extremity motion inputs.
      iii. The summation of all motions and their refinement by the sense of ease palpated at the listening hand's contact with the rib angle of left rib 5 promotes release of the dysfunction. The release allows a return to a central resting position without encountering resistance.
   c. The result is a resolution of the somatic element and its ongoing afferent barrage back to the spinal cord. Facilitation at that level is diminished, reducing potential efferent stimulus to the viscera.

LINKAGE DIAGNOSIS AND TREATMENT SUMMARY

In our evaluation of patient responses to treatment based on diagnoses, we sometimes find an incomplete response to typically performed spinal or rib somatic dysfunction treatment. With the knowledge of "linkage," we can evaluate the dysfunction for the possibility of viscerosomatic influence as the reason for the incomplete resolution, treat appropriately, and further assist our patient's recovery/overall health.

FUNCTIONAL METHODS SUMMARY

A misperception of functional methods became attached to the teaching method as it evolved.

Dr. Johnston broke Functional down into parts that could be taught and consistently applied. He and his predecessors evaluated patients and used the **smooth torsion arc** in treatment.[19] Hoover, Bowles, and Johnston intended to lead others to this smooth, integrated, and efficient clinical experience through practice and synthesis. Therefore, the practitioner should keep the "smooth torsion arc" in mind while reading through the techniques described in this section. Functional technique is not built mechanically out of the parts enumerated here. Practice with the parts/individual motions builds an understanding of the principles inherent in them and create a synthesis that will lead to the "smooth torsion arc" of therapeutic motion in effective treatment.

REFERENCES

1. Little KE, Hoover HV. Respiratory mobilization and molding of the sacrum. In: Northup TL, ed. *Year Book, Academy of Applied Osteopathy*. Edwards Brothers Inc.; 1945:67.
2. Hoover HV. Fundamentals of technic. In: Northup TL, ed. *Year Book, Academy of Applied Osteopathy*. Edwards Brothers Inc.; 1949:40.
3. Johnston WL. Harold Hoover and the CRT. In: Barnes MW, ed. *Year Book, Academy of Applied Osteopathy*. 1969:3–4.
4. Bowles CH. Functional technique: a modern perspective. *J Am Osteopath Assoc*. 1981;80:326–331.
5. Bowles CH. A functional orientation for technic. In: Page LE, ed. *Yearbook, Academy of Applied Osteopathy*. 1955:178.
6. Johnston WL, Friedman HD, Eland DC. *Functional Methods: A Manual for Palpatory Skills Development in Osteopathic Examination and Manipulation of Motor Function*. 2nd ed. American Academy of Osteopathy; 2005:82–83.
7. Johnston WL, Robertson JA, Stiles EG. Finding a common denominator for the variety of manipulative techniques. In: Barnes MW, ed. *Yearbook, Academy of Applied Osteopathy*. 1969:5–15.
8. Johnston WL. Development of a functional orientation for technique. In: Beal MC, ed. *Yearbook, Academy of Applied Osteopathy*. 1987:56.
9. Johnston WL. Segmental definition: parts I. A focal point for diagnosis of somatic dysfunction. *J Am Osteopath Assoc*. 1988;88:99–105.
10. Johnston WL. The role of static and motion palpation in structural diagnosis. In: Beal MC, ed. *Yearbook, Academy of Applied Osteopathy*. 1992:115.
11. Johnston WL, Kelso AF, Hollandsworth DL, Karrat JJ. Somatic manifestations in renal disease: a clinical research study. *J Am Osteopath Assoc*. 1987;87:61.
12. Ward RC, ed. *Foundations for Osteopathic Medicine*. 2nd ed. Lippincott Williams & Wilkins; 2003:1253.
13. Johnston WL, Friedman HD, Eland DC. *Functional Methods: A Manual for Palpatory Skills Development in Osteopathic Examination and Manipulation of Motor Function*. 2nd ed. American Academy of Osteopathy; 2005:55.
14. Bowles CH. A functional orientation for technic—part II. In: Page LE, ed. *Yearbook, Academy of Applied Osteopathy*. 1956:108.
15. Eland DC. Palpatory evidence for viscero-somatic influence upon the musculoskeletal system. *AAOJ*. 2006;16:23.
16. Bowles CH. A functional orientation for technic—part III. In: Barnes MW, ed. *Yearbook, Academy of Applied Osteopathy*. 1957:55.
17. Johnston WL, Friedman HD, Eland DC. *Functional Methods: A Manual for Palpatory Skills Development in Osteopathic Examination and Manipulation of Motor Function*. 2nd ed. American Academy of Osteopathy; 2005:291.
18. Johnston WL, Friedman HD, Eland DC. *Functional Methods: A Manual for Palpatory Skills Development in Osteopathic Examination and Manipulation of Motor Function*. 2nd ed. American Academy of Osteopathy; 2005: Appendix 7.
19. Johnston WL, Friedman HD, Eland DC. *Functional Methods: A Manual for Palpatory Skills Development in Osteopathic Examination and Manipulation of Motor Function*. 2nd ed. American Academy of Osteopathy; 2005:89, 90.
20. Bowles CH. Functional technique: a modern perspective. *J Am Osteopath Assoc*. 1981;80(5):326–331.
21. Korr IM. The neural basis of the osteopathic lesion. *J Am Osteopath Assoc*. 1947;47(4):191–198.

61

Dynamic Strain and the Bioenergetics Model

JAN T. HENDRYX

KEY CONCEPTS

- Dynamic strains or pathologic strain-vectors are abnormal inherent tissue motions associated with somatic, visceral, nervous system, and biofield dysfunctions.
- Effective treatment is accomplished by locating the release point (end point) of the pathologic strain-vector, maintaining contact with or "holding" it through a still point, and waiting until the tissue dysfunction resolves and inherent motion returns to normal.
- The end point may be located on or within the human body or in the biofield surrounding it.
- This osteopathic manipulative technique employs a bioenergetics model rather than a biomechanical or neurophysiologic one.

CASE STUDY

A 28-year-old female presented to the clinic with a complaint of constant refractory lumbar pain after repetitively lifting some heavy objects. Radiologic studies were negative for fracture or diskopathy. The patient underwent 6 weeks of physical therapy employing multiple modalities and exercises. She was subsequently treated by her primary care physician for another month, once or twice a week with integrative forms of osteopathic manipulation. To date, only temporary relief of pain lasting a few hours had been attained.

VITAL SIGNS

Blood pressure 126/70, pulse 88 bpm, and respiration 12 per minute.

PHYSICAL EXAMINATION

Physical examination reveals abnormal tissue texture changes, asymmetry, and restricted gross and segmental range of motion in the L2–L5 region. Marked spasm was present posteriorly in the lumbar paravertebral musculature with exquisite tenderness over the facets and iliolumbar ligaments. Increased palpatory sense of localized vertebral bone density was appreciated indicating possible intraosseous strain. Layer palpation at the level of lumbar dysfunction revealed separate pathologic strain-vectors in both the soft tissues and in the L2, L3, L4, and L5 vertebrae. The straight leg raising test was negative. Lower extremity deep tendon reflexes, sensation, and muscular strength were symmetrical and normal.

DIAGNOSES

1. Lumbar strain
2. Lumbar somatic dysfunction

TREATMENT

The patient was treated solely with dynamic strain-vector release (SVR) to remove key pathologic strains that were not addressed or removed with the other traditional forms of osteopathic manipulative treatment (OMT) or physical therapies. Reassessment revealed a markedly improved lumbar range of motion and complete resolution of tenderness, pain, and dysfunction. One week follow-up evaluation revealed no recurrence of pain symptoms or somatic dysfunction.

THE OSTEOPATHIC MODELS: PATIENT EVALUATION AND TREATMENT

Over the past four decades, six conceptual models of patient functioning, assessment, and care have been developed that are considered central to osteopathic principles and practice. These models provide an osteopathic lens through which the patient can be assessed and treated. They are designated:

1. Biomechanical–Structural
2. Respiratory–Circulatory
3. Neurologic
4. Metabolic–Nutritional (Metabolic–Energy; Metabolic)
5. Behavioral–Biopsychosocial
6. Bioenergetics

These models are supported by anatomical, physiologic, biochemical, immunologic, psychiatric/psychological, and biophysical principles and are discussed in detail elsewhere.[1–4] Figures 61.1 and 61.2 illustrate that the integration and coordination of basic body functions occur through the interface with the neuromusculoskeletal system and are tied to the patient's ability to adapt to numerous environmental stressors and to maintain health.[1–3]

There is some similarity in nomenclature between the metabolic–energy and bioenergetics models. The "metabolic–energy" model (also known as "metabolic–nutritional"[5] or "metabolic"[6]) is described in the previous edition of this book[1,4] in perhaps what might be considered a narrower context than "bioenergetics" model discussed here. Certainly, energy derived from food and metabolism fuels many functions in the human being, from the complete individual to the subcellular level. Energy conversion and conservation are necessary to maintain homeodynamics. Anatomical correlations to the metabolic–energy model are internal organs and endocrine glands. A broader interpretation of energy and its functions in living systems is given below and elsewhere.[2,3,7]

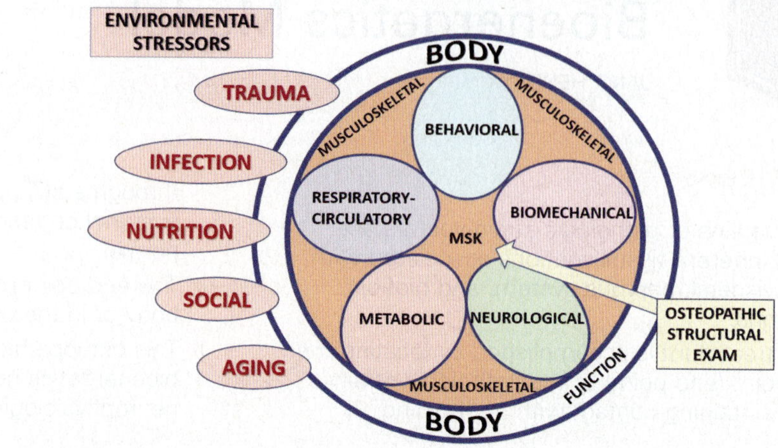

Figure 61.1. Original five (5) models adopted by Educational Council on Osteopathic Principles (ECOP) in 1982. (Courtesy of Jan T. Hendryx, DO, FAAO, and Melodie Chludzinski, DO.)

Bioenergetics Model and the Human Biofield

Healers in different cultures have utilized bioenergetics models of healing for thousands of years. Traditional Chinese Medicine (TCM), for example, which originated in China at least five millennia ago, describes the concept of "qi" (ch'i, energy, or life force).

- The normal flow of qi through the body is thought to maintain homeostasis, homeodynamics, and health, while aberrations in qi flow (deficiencies, excesses, or stagnation) may cause disease.[8]
- Qi can be influenced and normalized by acupuncture, hands-on therapies such as tui na and acupressure, qi gong, martial arts, meditation, appropriate nutrition, and supplemental herbal preparations.

Ayurvedic medicine, which may have existed long before TCM, also emphasizes a similar life force concept, called "prana," that is of vital importance in health on all levels.[9] A therapeutic system called Pranic healing evolved that incorporates these principles.[10] Other examples of systems of healing that use bioenergetics models include:

- Chakra healing[11]
- Energy psychology[12,13]
- Jin Shin Jyutsu[14]
- Marma therapy[15]
- Polarity therapy[16,17]
- Reiki[18]
- Therapeutic touch[19]
- Several models of OMT[2,3]

Rindfleisch has reviewed and summarized these and several other integrative human energy–based (biofield) therapies.[20,21]

Bioenergetics, a component of biophysics,[22] is the study of how endogenous and exogenous energy sources/forms influence and control living systems and their environment. Scientific study of bioenergetics of both plants and animals, including humans, has been prolific and ongoing for at least a century.[23–26]

The *bioenergetics model* seeks to address the bioenergetic nature of the human being in health and disease, striving to maintain and/or support the return to homeodynamics through the application of biophysics principles in the biofield (see definition below).

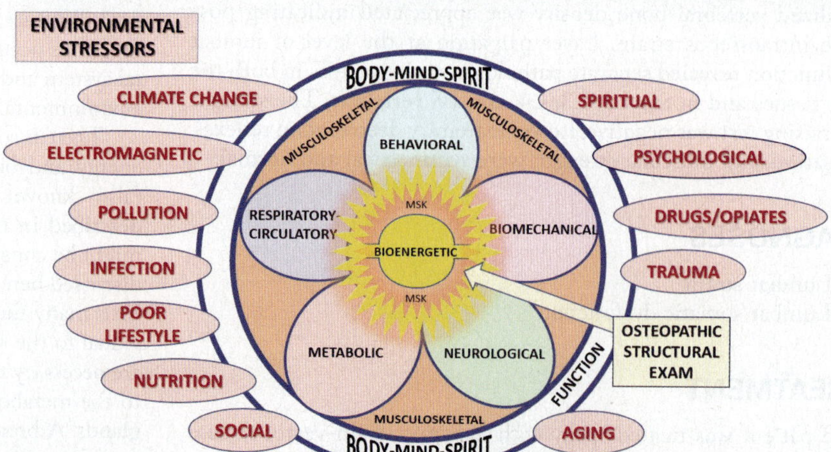

Figure 61.2. Expanded six (6) models to include bioenergetics. (Courtesy of Jan T. Hendryx, DO, FAAO, and Melodie Chludzinski, DO.)

Osteopathic manipulative models and techniques suggested to have a bioenergetic basis include:

- Biodynamics
- Bioelectric Fascial Activation and Release
- Dynamic SVR
- Dynamical Medicine
- Facilitated Oscillatory Release
- Fulford Percussor Treatment (Percussion Hammer)
- Myofascial Release
- Neurofascial Release
- Osteopathic Cranial Manipulative Medicine
- Trauma Vector Release

Bioenergetics may serve as the foundation and integration point for all other osteopathic models of care and can be used to diagnose and treat all levels of dysfunction.[2,3,7]

The original National Center for Complementary and Alternative Medicine (NCCAM) at the National Institutes of Health (NIH) had previously designated and supported research into eight categories of integrative medicine.[2] Disciplines within categories 3 and 4 contained major bioenergetic components.

1. Alternative Systems
2. Botanicals/Herbal Medicines
3. Biofield Therapies (Energy Medicine/Bioelectromagnetics)
4. Manipulative/Manual/Therapeutic Bodywork
5. Movement Therapies
6. Mind–Body Interactions
7. Pharmacologic/Biologic
8. Diet/Nutrition/Lifestyle Changes

These original classifications and descriptors have become more generalized under the categories of Complementary, Alternative, or Integrative Health on the revised National Center for Complementary and Integrative Health (NCCIH) website.[27]

DEFINITIONS OF TERMS

It is important to define several terms related to the bioenergetic model as these terms do not appear in conventional osteopathic resource literature.

Biofield—NCCIH at NIH introduced the term "biofield" in 1992 and defined it as a "massless field, not necessarily electromagnetic, that surrounds and permeates living bodies and affects the body."[28] Since then, numerous publications describing the science behind biofield physics and its role in health and healing have been advanced.[28–34]

In 2002, Rubic described the biofield as "the extremely weak electromagnetic field within and surrounding a living system that may be involved in transmitting electromagnetic bioinformation for regulating homeodynamics."[29] More recently, this definition has been expanded beyond electromagnetism to likely include quantum field phenomena. A deep discussion of quantum physics is beyond the scope of this chapter, but it is thought to underlie other biophysical properties such as coherent states, biophoton emissions, quantum entanglement, and perhaps even consciousness.[28–34]

Biofield therapy—any therapeutic modality that interacts with and alters the biofield and its manifestations.[28–34]

Bioelectromagnetics—study of the interactions between electromagnetic fields and biologic living systems. These fields can be endogenous or exogenous in origin.[22–26]

Bioelectromagnetism—the inherent ability of living cells, tissues, and organisms to produce, emit, and respond to electrical and magnetic fields.[22–26]

Bioelectromagnetic energy fields (bio-EM) can help explain various human-related physiologic functions and interactions such as

TABLE 61.1

Sources of Bioenergy in the Living Human Being

Known	Unknown
Biochemical reactions	Consciousness
Electrochemical polarization and depolarization in the nervous system and conduction through the neuromusculoskeletal system	Inherent motions Primary respiratory mechanism Cranial rhythmic impulse Biodynamic phenomena/Tides/Potency Inspir/expir visceral motions
Ion influx/efflux through membranes (gating mechanisms)	Dynamic and pathologic strain-vectors Trauma vectors
Mechanotransduction	Acupuncture meridian systems
Piezoelectric phenomena	Qi, prana, life force
Blood circulation	Healing biofields
Electromechanical activity of the heart	Subtle energies

nervous system activities, heart rhythms, wound healing, thermal projections, piezoelectric phenomena, and even somatic dysfunction.[2,3,22–34]

Deep consideration of the bio-EM and quantum fields may explain the functioning of living systems from the macroscopic all the way down to microscopic, biochemical, genetic, and pathologic realms. A subtle energy (psychoenergetic) field can also potentially explain interactions between individuals on the consciousness level such as the effects of meditation, intention, attention, and hands-on healing.[30,34] Thus, the states of mind of both the physician and patient are important as they may contribute positively or negatively to the healing encounter. For a more in-depth understanding of biofield phenomena and physics, and their potential roles in homeodynamics and health, please refer to references.[28–34]

Bioenergy—any type of energy produced endogenously by living systems as a result of bioelectromagnetic and other physiologic activities inside all living tissues and cells. Much of this bioenergy manifests in the electromagnetic spectrum ranging from extra low-frequency (ELF) fields (<100 Hz) through 10^{15} Hz (visible light). The heart and brain are the largest producers of electromagnetic fields, respectively.[23,25] The nature and sources of bioenergy are known in some instances and unknown in others (Table 61.1).

HISTORY OF BIOENERGETICS IN THE OSTEOPATHIC PROFESSION

From its early beginnings, the osteopathic profession has had a rich history of exploring and attempting to incorporate the bioenergetics model into patient care. A.T. Still advertised and practiced as a magnetic healer prior to founding osteopathy.[35] In his book, *The Philosophy and Mechanical Principles of Osteopathy*, Dr. Still provided a lengthy discussion of the concept of "biogen" as vital (energetic) force operating through protoplasm to produce living matter.[36] He acknowledged that both electric and magnetic forces in the body are likely important in health.[36,37]

Following the establishment of osteopathy in the late 19th century, generations of DOs would continue to explore bioenergetics in the search for a deeper understanding of healing and for providing better patient care. Table 61.2 provides a summary of individuals who have contributed to the terminology and understanding of osteopathic bioenergetic therapeutics.

TABLE 61.2

Contributors to the Osteopathic Bioenergetics Model

Contributor	Date	Primary Concept(s)	Description/Health
A. T. Still, DO[36,37]	Late 1800s–1917	Osteopathy Biogen	Vital force producing living matter Electric and magnetic forces important in health
J. Martin Littlejohn, MD[38]	1902	Oscillatory rhythms "vibratility" "vital force"	Vibratory properties associated with health and disease
G. D. Hulett, DO[39]	1903	Osteopathic energy model published	Energies Coordination-health Incoordination-disease
C. P. McConnell, DO[40,41]	1938–1939	Biophysics	Emphasized importance of biophysics in understanding pathology and osteopathic therapeutics
W. G. Sutherland, DO[42]	Early 1900s–1954	Osteopathy in the cranial field (OCF) Primary respiratory mechanism (PRM) Potency "Tide"	Inherent motility of brain and spinal cord and fluctuation of cerebrospinal fluid driving forces behind craniosacral motions
Robert Fulford, DO[43]	1940s–1997	Percussion hammer (Percussor treatment)	Human bioenergetics in osteopathic therapeutics
Randolph Stone, DO, DC[16,17]	1950s	Polarity therapy	Electromagnetic wave and polarity imbalances affecting mind-body-spirit
Rollin Becker, DO[44–47]	1964–1965	Bioenergetics in osteopathy	Biodynamic and biokinetic intrinsic energies/forces in health and disease
H. I. Magoun, Sr, DO, FAAO[48]	1966	Osteopathy in the cranial field (book)	Human electrobiology and the cranial concept
Stephen Davidson, DO[49–52]	1987	Neurofascial release (NFR)	Tissue dysfunction model based upon standing waveforms and interference vibratory patterns
Elmer Green, PhD Richard MacDonald, DO[53] John Upledger, DO, FAAO[54]	1980s–2003	Energy cyst	Energetic tissue stagnation patterns secondary to physical, mental, emotional, spiritual trauma
James Jealous, DO[55,56]	1980s–2021	Biodynamics	Expansion of principles from Osteopathy in the cranial field (OCF) model and embryology with experiential journey into the true nature of healing
Carlisle Holland, DO[57–59]	1980s–2023	Dynamical medicine	Biophysics view of tissue dysfunction based upon dynamical systems theory, chaos theory, and fractal principles
Judith O'Connell, DO, FAAO[60,61]	2000	Bioelectric fascial activation and release (BFAR)	Fascial bioresponsive electrical potentials activated for diagnosis and treatment
Zachary Comeaux, DO, FAAO[62]	2000–2003	Vibration and oscillation in osteopathic thought Facilitated oscillatory release (FOR)	Mechanical facilitation of tissue coherent vibrations to normalize function
Jan T. Hendryx, DO Richard L. O'Brien, DO[63]	1999–2003	Dynamic strain-vector release (SVR)	Development of osteopathic system of diagnosis and treatment using the bioenergetics model
R. Paul Lee, DO, FAAO[37,64]	2000–2005	Spiritual dimensions of healing Biophysics Energy	Extracellular matrix (ECM) oscillations and inherent motions; still point transformations and transmutations
Bruno Chikly, MD[65,66]	1990s–2016	Brain manipulation and inherent motion Trauma-vector release	Diagnosis and treatment of brain and biofield abnormalities after trauma
Kenneth E. Nelson, DO, FAAO Thomas Glonek, DO Nicette Sergueef, DO[67–69]	2001+	Oscillatory rhythms in living systems Cranial rhythmic impulse (CRI) correlation to Traube–Hering–Mayer rhythm	In-depth discussions and about many different physiologic rhythms and current research

TABLE 61.2 (Continued)

Contributors to the Osteopathic Bioenergetics Model

Contributor	Date	Primary Concept(s)	Description/Health
Hollis H. King, DO, FAAO, PhD[70]	2011	Osteopathy in the cranial field (OCF), history, applications, research	Primary respiratory mechanism (PRM), cranial motion, synopsis.
Jan T. Hendryx, DO, FAAO[2,3,7]	2014, 2018	Bioenergetics models in osteopathic medicine	Overview of biophysics of living tissues; comparison of SVR and NFR
Jan T. Hendryx, DO, FAAO Ashok Kannan, DO Jessica Prashad, OMS2 Karl Falk, DO[71]	2022	Connecting CV4 cranial manipulation to acupuncture meridian and ANS activities	Bioelectric measurements using the apparatus for meridian identification (AMI)

WHAT IS ENERGY MEDICINE?

Energy medicine can be simply defined as the use of energetic principles and phenomena to diagnose and treat patients. James Oschman, PhD, a researcher and author in the bioenergetics of living systems, argues, "…all medicine is *energy medicine* and that the energetic perspective holds the key to the future of the entire medical enterprise."[25] He has comprehensively reviewed the biophysics, historical background, measurements, and therapeutic uses of energetic phenomena in medicine (including osteopathic) and human performance.[23–25]

Biophysics is an interdisciplinary science using methods of, and theories from, physics to study biologic systems.[22] Biophysics, per se, is not generally a prerequisite course for undergraduate students who prepare to become physicians and/or scientific researchers. Biophysics is also not taught to most medical students in medical school or residency training programs. The importance of biophysics in understanding the driving forces behind life, health, and form and function has, for the most part, been minimized.

Thus, true appreciation of biology, biochemistry, embryology, genetics, pharmacology, medicine, and life itself at deeper levels is extremely limited because biophysics is left out of the curricula. In the bioenergetics model of healing, physics, and energy are reinstated back into the equation, which may be especially important for osteopathic diagnosis and treatment of patients with the hands.

In 1939, Carl Philip McConnell, DO, argued how important it was for the osteopath to recognize the vital role of biophysics in understanding anatomy, physiology, health, and disease.[40] In an article entitled "The Osteopathic Approach," he challenged the osteopathic profession to expand beyond precedence and dogma to learn about and apply biophysics principles so that treatments would truly become individualized, comprehensive, and maximally effective. He wrote, "…keep in mind that osteopathic pathogenesis is preeminently (essentially fundamental) a field of beginning pathology firmly grounded on biophysics. Herein arises the soundness and comprehensiveness of osteopathic science."[41]

THE BIOENERGETICS MODEL AND ENERGY MEDICINE

In medicine, energy concepts provided by the disciplines of physics and biophysics explain the workings of various types of equipment used for diagnosis and treatment of patients (Table 61.3). Besides medical technology applications, physics is used to explain biomechanics of the human body and perhaps even how some forms of biomechanical osteopathic manipulation models work. It would seem, from the examples above, that physics and energy are vital to the diagnosis and treatment of patients.

Energy is defined scientifically as the ability to do work.[72] The first law of thermodynamics states that energy can be neither created nor destroyed. It can only be converted to other forms of energy.[72]

Some familiar forms of energy include:

1. Chemical
2. Electrical

TABLE 61.3

Energy-Based Diagnostics and Treatment Modalities

Diagnostics	"Conventional" Treatment Modalities
Electrocardiography (ECG)	Cardiac defibrillator
Electroencephalography (EEG)	Neurofeedback (EEG biofeedback)
Electromyography (EMG)	Electric/magnetic bone stimulation
Evoked potentials	Electrical stimulation (transcutaneous electrical nerve stimulation; vagal)
Infrared thermographic imaging (thermography)	Light therapy (full spectrum, ultraviolet, laser, infrared)
Holter monitor	Pacemaker
Magnetic resonance imaging (MRI)	Electrocautery
Magnetocardiography (MCG)	Gamma-irradiation
Magnetoencephalography (MEG)	Electromagnetic Stimulation Nervous System (brain, spinal cord)
Positron emission tomography (PET)	Diathermy
Pulse oximetry	Magnatherm therapy
Skin surface electrical potential measuring devices	Music therapy
Superconducting Quantum Interference Device (SQUID) Magnetometry (biomagnetometry)	Radiofrequency rhizotomy
Ultrasound (US)	Ultrasound (US)
X-rays	X-irradiation

3. Gravitational
4. Kinetic (motion)
5. Mechanical
6. Nuclear
7. Potential (stored)
8. Radiant
9. Sound
10. Thermal

Any form of energy can be absorbed by and affect living systems. Living systems also produce, convert, and emit their own energies. Thus interacting with each other and the environment through energy exchange.[21] The entire universe is one big energy conversion system. Humans, being part of the universe, are thus of the same system.

DYNAMIC STRAIN-VECTOR RELEASE: DEFINITIONS, HISTORY, ASSESSMENT, AND TREATMENT

Definitions

Dynamic SVR is a bioenergetics model–based system of osteopathic diagnosis and manipulative treatment developed by this author and Richard O'Brien, DO, in 1999–2000.[63] It is used to effectively treat acute, subacute, or chronic somatic, visceral, neurologic tissue, and bioenergetic dysfunctions that contain dynamic strain or pathologic strain-vectors. SVR is often effective in treating dysfunctions that might not be responsive to other classic models of OMT. It can be applied to any tissue that can be palpated, as well as acupuncture points, meridian systems, and bioenergetic fields.

The efficacy of Dynamic SVR technique relies on the physician's ability to layer palpate to the level of the dysfunctional tissue(s), assess subtle inherent tissue motion for pathologic dynamic strain-vectors located in areas of dysfunction, and then find and treat an SVR point with the nonpalpating hand.

The term "strain" has different meanings depending upon the context. A patient may complain that she strained her back after lifting something heavy. Strain is a medical term that means a stretching or tearing of a muscle or tendon. Muscle strains are graded I, II, or III (mild, moderate, severe) depending upon the severity of tissue damage.[73]

Physics defines strain as a relative change in shape or dimensions of a body or object that is subjected to stress. It is classified as longitudinal, shearing, or volume depending on the direction of the force vectors.[63]

In osteopathic terminology, the concept of strain is expanded beyond orthopedics and muscle to describe other musculoskeletal structures that have tissue distortion with or without deformation or exhibit abnormal inherent motion. Thus, there are defined ligamentous articular, dural membranous and intraosseous strains, various cranial physiologic and pathologic strain patterns of motion, and dynamic strains.[63]

Dynamic strain and *pathologic strain-vector* are related terms. *Dynamic strain* is defined as a palpable distortion of subtle motion in the tissue and/or human biofield that pulls "pathologically" in a certain direction with a certain force (vector) while continuing to move with inherent tissue motion. A single *dynamic strain* ("simple strain") or multiple layers of dynamic strains ("complex strain") can be found in any dysfunctional tissue of the body.[63]

In SVR, a physician initially assesses dysfunctional tissues by palpating for this inherent motion abnormality that is associated with tissue (somatic, visceral, nervous system) dysfunction. Empirically, it has been observed that all dysfunctional tissues can have associated simple or complex strains within them.

Inherent motion is defined as the "spontaneous motion of every cell, organ, system and their component units within the body."[6] These subtle motions occur independently of mechanical respiration and are palpable with a refined sense of touch. The quality, rate, amplitude, and synchronicity of inherent motions are thought to indicate the state of health or disease within an individual. Examples of rhythmic inherent motions in osteopathic terminology include the "tide," cranial rhythmic impulse (CRI), primary respiratory mechanism (PRM), inspiration, expiration, and visceral motions. These topics are covered elsewhere.[70,74,75]

Normally, inherent motion is sensed as back-and-forth motion occurring at a frequency of 8 to 14 cycles/minute, the same as the PRM/CRI. In normal tissues, the subtle oscillatory inherent motion is equidistant from a center point in all planes assessed. One may notice a slight pause in the center of the motion, which is known as the "neutral zone" (Fig. 61.3).

In abnormal dysfunctional tissues exhibiting a dynamic strain, a palpable distortion of motion is appreciated that pulls "pathologically" in a certain direction with a certain force (vector), much

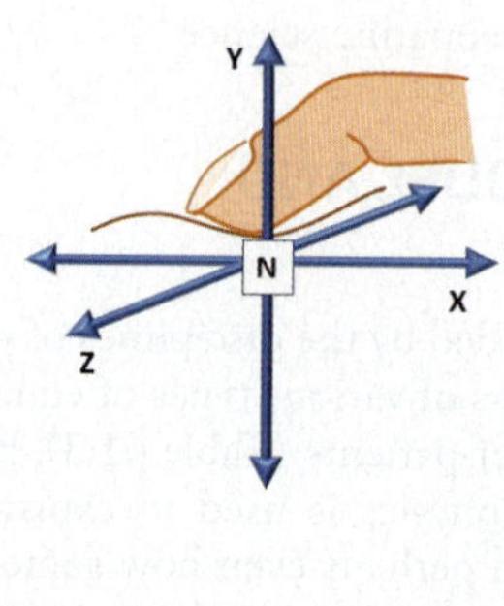

Figure 61.3. Diagram of normal inherent motions in normal tissue. *N*, Neutral zone. (Courtesy of Jan T. Hendryx, DO, FAAO.)

Grouped

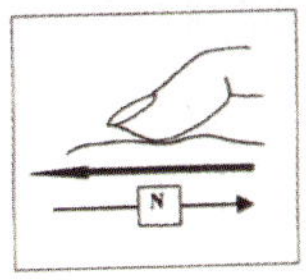

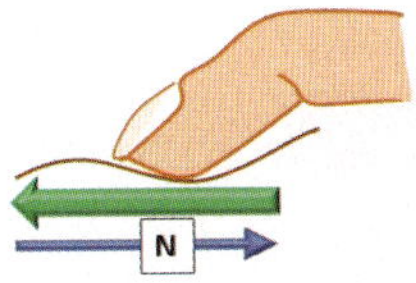

Figure 61.4. Diagram of abnormal inherent motion and pathologic strain-vector. Note there is no neutral zone (N) in the pathologic strain-vector, although one can be appreciated in the reverse motion. The pathologic strain-vector "points" in the direction of the endpoint or release point. (Courtesy of Jan T. Hendryx, DO, FAAO.)

like how a rip current on an ocean beach might be experienced (Fig. 61.4).

Dynamic SVR continues to be expanded and refined. With enhancement of layer palpation skills allowing for the ability to appreciate deeper anatomical structures, it was found that pathologic strain-vectors can be detected in the bone, in the viscera, and even in various regions of the central and peripheral nervous systems, including the autonomics. More recently, it was noted that dysfunctional acupuncture meridian systems and acupuncture points may contain pathologic strain-vectors and can be treated with SVR.

Historical Perspective

SVR was discovered while attempting to treat a middle-aged chronic pain patient who had a cervical fusion and was experiencing severe recurrent neck pain and radiculopathy of the right upper extremity. Five weekly treatment trials of combination therapy, involving integrated forms of OMT and acupuncture, yielded only temporary positive therapeutic responses before symptoms recurred.

The patient was reevaluated to determine whether alternate acupuncture points might be more effective than the ones previously used. According to Chinese medicine theory, different acupuncture points have different hierarchal functions and "qualities."[8] An attempt was made to discern whether there were specific palpatory qualities (texture, tension, temperature, vibration, inherent motion, electromagnetic fields) that might help choose more effective acupuncture points for the treatment of the patient's condition.

The patient's neck was palpated with one hand, while various acupuncture points were gently touched with the other. It was noted that when contact was held at certain acupuncture points on the upper extremity, inherent tissue motion would stop as a still point was induced. The patient's cervical musculature and intraosseous strains would subsequently soften and release. This was often accompanied by a significant decrease in subjective pain.

It was also noted that the pulling sensation ("strain" motions) and tissue tension in both the cervical and upper extremity tissues would change as sequential acupuncture points were palpated along a specific meridian. Analysis of these motion alterations eventually led to the ability to quickly find the release point (end point) of the strain-vector.

Initially, it was thought that the SVR points corresponded primarily to acupuncture points only along the surface of the body. Later, it became apparent that the "tissue pull" of the pathologic strain-vectors actually extended in any direction from the dysfunctional tissue.

In summary, dynamic strain-vectors can be palpated and extend:

- Along the body surface
- Into the body
- Through the body to the opposite surface
- Through the body into the biofield
- Off the body into the biofield without penetrating the body or traveling along the surface

The length of the pathologic strain-vectors from the origin in the dysfunctional tissue to the end point also may vary considerably from a few millimeters to several feet.

Diagnosis and Treatment Using the SVR Model

The steps of diagnosing and treating a patient with SVR are:

1. Locate a somatic, visceral, or energetic dysfunction with the "palpating" hand.
2. Layer-palpate to the correct tissue level of the dysfunction.
3. Appreciate the inherent tissue motion(s) at the dysfunction.
4. Determine in which direction the pathologic strain-vector (dynamic strain) is pulling.
5. Place fingers of the "treating" hand next to the "palpating" hand and move the "treating" fingers/hand in the direction of tissue pull of the pathologic strain-vector.
6. As the "treating" hand is moved toward the *end point* or *SVR point*, note that three phenomena occur:
   a. Tension in the tissue under the "palpating" fingers increases.
   b. A "magnetic" pull occurs between the "palpating" and "treating" fingers (as if there were opposite pole magnets next to each other and the fingers are trying to pull them apart).
   c. The inherent motion under the "palpating" fingers slows and finally stops (still point) once the "treating" fingers reach the exact location of the end point.
7. Wait for the tissue to release after a still point is induced (up to 30 seconds or so).

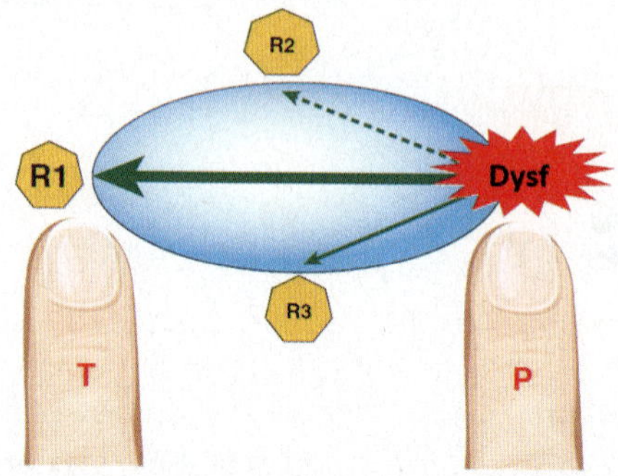

Figure 61.5. An elongated elliptical three-dimensional strain-vector field emanates right-to-left from a tissue dysfunction (Dysf). All *arrows* point in the same general direction of tissue pull or pathologic strain-vector. The *thickest solid arrow* indicates the exact location and direction of the true pathologic strain-vector with R1 being the primary release point (endpoint). When R1 is touched with the treating hand (T), tissue tension at the dysfunction is maximal under the palpating hand (P) as a still point is attained. If the physician moves the treating hand slightly off-center relative to the true pathologic strain-vector, but in the same general direction, tissue under the palpating hand will not tighten as much, although one may be able to attain a still point at alternative endpoints R2 and R3. The thickness of the *arrows* indicates the degree of tissue tension generated under the palpating fingers at the dysfunction as the treating hand moves in the same general direction of the tissue pull toward the release points. (Courtesy of Jan T. Hendryx, DO, FAAO.)

8. Reassess the dysfunctional tissue and the inherent motion to determine if there are any additional layered pathologic strain-vectors remaining.
   a. If tissue inherent motion is normal in all directions and dysfunction is resolved, the treatment is concluded.
   b. If another pathologic strain-vector is present, repeat steps 1 to 8 until all dynamic strains and tissue dysfunction are resolved.

Resolution of all pathologic strain-vectors usually results in reestablishment of normal inherent tissue motion and resolution of the tissue dysfunction and often subjective pain. Although frequently depicted as straight lines to explain concepts and nomenclature, it appears that there may be specific three-dimensional spherical or elongated biofields related to the pathologic strain-vectors (Fig. 61.5).

THE POSSIBLE BIOENERGETIC NATURE OF SOMATIC DYSFUNCTION

To a physician practicing osteopathically, a comprehensive examination of the neuromusculoskeletal system is crucial for accurately diagnosing and appropriately treating a patient. Refined perception of palpatory changes in the motion, position, tension, texture, and temperature of tissues reveals important clues about the status and response of a patient to treatment. Abnormal tissue texture changes, asymmetry, restriction of motion, and tenderness (i.e., T.A.R.T.) are the hallmarks of somatic dysfunction. *Somatic dysfunction* is defined as "impaired or altered function of related components of the somatic (body framework) system; skeletal, arthrodial, and myofascial structures, and related vascular, lymphatic and neural elements."[6]

Common underlying etiologies of somatic dysfunction may include poor body mechanics and posture, muscle imbalances, pelvic shears, abnormal neurologic reflexes, facilitation, emotional stressors, compensation from other areas of the body or visceral dysfunctions, leg length discrepancies, localized sprains and strains, response to trauma and pain, as well as other factors.[76]

Abnormal tissue texture changes palpated in tissues are generally assumed to be maintained by various reflexes in the neuromusculoskeletal system and by biotensegrity imbalances.[77,78] But what about palpatory abnormalities of the viscera? *Visceral dysfunction* is defined as "impaired or altered mobility or motility of the visceral system and related fascial, neurologic, vascular, skeletal and lymphatic elements."[6] What about various components of the nervous system or bone?

Because of the energetic nature of living systems, several key questions arise. Can energetic dysfunctions in the body or biofield cause or contribute to somatic, visceral, or neurologic dysfunction and other health issues? If so, how might these problems manifest? Can bioenergetic osteopathic manipulative techniques be utilized to treat somatic, visceral, or psychological dysfunctions? What are the energetic mechanisms behind these techniques?

Energetic phenomena in the body that can be palpated and utilized in the diagnosis and treatment of somatic or visceral dysfunctions and psychosomatic and other conditions have been previously described and reviewed in depth.[2,3,62]

These include:

- "Listening"[74,75]
- Biodynamic and biokinetic energy fields[44–48]
- Diagnostic pulses[8]
- Energy cysts[53,54]

- Fascial interference patterns[49–52]
- Head and body trauma vectors[65,66]
- Inherent motions and oscillations (nervous system, CRI/PRM, visceral, myofascial, Traube–Hering–Mayer reflex, blood flow)[67–69]
- Pathologic strain-vectors[2,3,7,63]
- Still points[42,48,70]
- Therapeutic pulses[78]
- Thermal projections[74,75]
- Vibratory fields[74]

Holland has made a convincing argument for a biophysics and mathematically based system of an integrative medical system which he terms "dynamical medicine."[57–59,79] Dynamical medicine is based upon a biophysics model and is named for its origin in dynamical systems theory, a branch of science concerned with chaos and fractals. Dynamical systems theory applies to all living systems in all dimensions and describes biologic shapes and processes mathematically.

Sol–gel interconversions have also been theorized to underlie palpatory findings of abnormal tissue texture changes associated with somatic dysfunction.[37,79] Holland has emphasized that all tissues, including the myofascia and extracellular matrix (ECM), are colloidal (a nonprecipitating suspension) in nature and, as such, must follow colloidal physics principles.[57,59] Colloids have special physical properties of being able to exist in either liquid (sol) or solid (gel) forms, depending upon the amount of energy absorbed and stored through their intermolecular bonds. Physical energy transferred to the body secondary to trauma, and even electromagnetic fields, can cause sol–gel interconversions.[57]

Holland has also suggested that somatic dysfunction can be viewed as a "matted fractal" where the energy flow is interrupted.[45] This is similar to the oriental medical concept of a stagnation of wei qi (protective energy) in acupuncture tendinomuscular meridians.[8]

FASCIA AND THE EXTRACELLULAR MATRIX

Andrew Taylor Still placed much emphasis on the fascia and its relationship to health. He wrote, "I know of no other part of the body that equals the fascia as a hunting ground (sic. for health/disease)...By its action we live, and by its failure, we die."[36]

Fascia consists of acellular and cellular components. It is comprised of collagen, elastic, and reticular fibers that are immersed in a sea of colloidal protein aminoglycans. This acellular fiber–colloid component of the fascia is referred to as the *extracellular matrix* or *ECM*. The ECM is a key player in the modulation of cell function and pathophysiology.[37,80]

Cellular fascial components include various leukocytes, macrophages, plasma cells, mast cells, pluripotential cells, fibroblasts, and myofibroblasts. Interestingly, myofibroblasts contain actin and myosin filaments and can provide a contractile force to the fascia.[63] Myofibroblast contraction within the fascia may be important in wound healing and in contributing to the quality of tissue stiffness.[80,81]

Blood vessels penetrate and traverse the fascia to supply tissues with oxygen and nutrients, as well as to drain waste products. Lymphatics are important in immune protection and in the regulation of tissue fluids. Sensorimotor nerves provide afferent and efferent communication locally and at a distance.[80–83]

Fascia provides compartmentalizing and supporting functions as it branches and penetrates deep into tissues. As it envelops and intertwines with the skeletal muscle, it becomes known as *myofascia*. A more in-depth discussion of the fascia can be found in Chapter 7.

Functionally, the ECM has been termed the "living matrix" by Oschman.[23,25,84] He calls it "living" because it is much more than just a passive network of fibers and ground substance holding the body and its organs together. It is dynamically active on many levels of structure and function. The ECM connects into the most intimate reaches of cells through the cell membrane, cytoskeleton, and nuclear matrix. The dynamic nature of the living matrix can be palpated as rhythmic inherent motion that can be influenced by various forms of osteopathic manipulation and bioenergetic fields.

Fascia has three special biophysical properties. These are:

1. Tensegrity
2. Mechanotransduction
3. Piezoelectric

Tensegrity is a term coined by R. Buckminster Fuller as a hybrid of the words "tensional" and "integrity." Tensegrity describes the structure maintained by forces transmitted through a system of interconnected solid struts and flexible cables. A classic example of a tensegrity system is geodesic dome architecture.[83]

In living systems, tensegrity is often referred to as *biotensegrity*. Its principles are key to structure and function on both the macro and micro levels. The human body's macro tensegrity system is composed of bones (struts), muscles, tendons, ligaments, and fascia (cables). The micro tensegrity system is the connection of fascial collagen fibers through the cell membranes to cytoskeletal elements, specifically microtubules (struts), microfilaments, and microfibrils (cables) in the cytoplasm and nucleus. Biotensegrity allows and facilitates the efficient functioning of the human being as an integrated unit.[85]

Collagen fibers in the ECM attach directly to the cellular cytoskeleton through specialized proteins in the cell membrane called integrins. These molecules transmit mechanical forces from the fascia to associated focal adhesions, junctional complexes, and ultimately the cytoskeleton in the interior of the cell by a process known as *mechanotransduction*.[86,87]

Mechanotransduction controls many cellular processes including cell division, differentiation, migration, protein synthesis, DNA and gene expression, immune function, and even pathologic processes.[86–90]

Donald Ingber, MD, PhD, pioneered research into biotensegrity and mechanotransduction over the past several decades and has authored and co-authored numerous peer-reviewed scientific articles on the subjects. From an osteopathic perspective, he has applied these principles in explaining how various forms of manual therapies may influence structure and function down to the cellular level.[83,88,89] Swanson has published an excellent thorough review of biotensegrity and mechanotransduction, including their relevance to osteopathic medicine, education, and research.[85]

Piezoelectric substances accumulate electrical charges in response to the application of mechanical stress. Quartz crystals, bone, collagen, other tissue proteins, cytoskeletal elements, and even DNA are piezoelectric in nature. Piezoelectricity is responsible, for example, for the remodeling of bone due to changes in biomechanical tensions or compressions. A closed grounded loop and fluid salinity in the body allow for electric currents to flow when there is an imbalance in charges. Electrical currents produce corresponding magnetic fields according to the laws of physics. Because of their piezoelectric nature, living tissues thus produce electromagnetic energy fields. These fields extend indefinite distances into and outside of the body. Piezoelectric tissues can also be influenced by external electromagnetic fields which cause them to mechanically respond and change shape. Application of external electricity by certain devices, for example, can alter the palpable tissue texture of stimulated tissues.[23,25,84]

Oschman envisions the human body as a tissue-tensegrity piezoelectric matrix, or liquid crystal under tension.[23] From a biophysics standpoint, these attributes allow the body to react to and create various frequencies and fields of energy over time and instantaneously. The human body also creates other forms of energy including heat, sound, light (photons), chemical, and mechanical.[30–32,34]

EARTHING

An interesting bioelectromagnetic phenomenon that can provide both preventive and therapeutic health benefits to body, mind, and spirit at little to no cost to the patient or health care system is "earthing" or "grounding."[91–93] These terms refer to direct body contact through the skin to the earth or to a grounded conductive device (mat, sheet, pillow) directly connected to the earth. Most of us are familiar with the experience of touching a metal object such as a doorknob and feeling or seeing a spark of static electricity jump from our finger. This is due to an electrical charge difference between the body and the metal.

The normal voltage of a wholly grounded individual is the same as the earth upon which they are in contact. Wearing insulated shoe soles (vs. walking barefoot on the earth) keeps an individual from balancing those charges with negative electrons from the earth. Thus, in a standing nongrounded electron-depleted person, the differences in voltages at ground level can range from a few volts at the feet to 200 volts at the top of the head. Voltages can be much greater in an ungrounded individual elevated in a building two or more stories high.[92]

Fascial/connective tissue ground substance, specifically glycosaminoglycans, are considered to act as "charge reservoirs" capable of storing electrons that keep the body at the same voltage as the earth's surface. This occurs when an individual is directly connected to the earth via bare feet, or by some sort of grounding device such as a specialized mat or sheet.[92]

The clinical significance of this "electron depletion" and, thus, voltage changes in the connective tissue ground substance[37,84] is that it sets the body and organ systems up for numerous potential health-related risks and disease processes. A primary concern of the ungrounded voltage mismatch is an increased inflammatory response through an increase in reactive oxygen species (ROS) throughout the body. Earthing/grounding has been shown to reduce inflammation, free radicals, autoimmune symptoms, chronic pain, stress responses, RBC coagulation, and improve glucose metabolism in Type II diabetics, immune responses to vaccination, sleep, ANS balance toward a more parasympathetic state, and circadian rhythms.[91–93] Earthing has also been shown to increase facial blood flow as measured by thermographic imaging and may even influence inherent muscular rhythmic motions.[94]

People who undergo the earthing process can do it outdoors or indoors. Outdoors, one simply removes the shoes and socks and steps onto the ground barefooted remaining in contact for about 30 minutes. Indoors they can utilize grounded devices discussed above.

OSTEOPATHIC PRINCIPLES AND FINDING HEALTH THROUGH BIOPHYSICS: WHAT'S REALLY GOING ON?

Original research by Denslow, Korr, and others used bioelectromagnetic principles underlying the neurologic model to measure and understand the nature of the "osteopathic lesion" or somatic dysfunction.[95] OMT models have traditionally employed biomechanics (long- and short-levers, fluid mechanics) and neuromuscular reflexes primarily to explain mechanisms of action and efficacy.

However, as mentioned previously, there are multiple osteopathic models that need to be further evaluated perhaps from different nontraditional perspectives (bioenergetic) if we are to understand them mechanistically. This requires an open mind and holistic approach to research, perhaps by looking deeper into and evaluating biofield physics. What are some ways we can explore the biofield and bioenergetic nature of osteopathic manipulative techniques?

Several devices capable of measuring human biofield changes in response to various therapies have been scientifically reviewed.[23,33,34] A recently published osteopathic clinical study on the effects of the OCMM technique, compression of the 4th ventricle (CV4), utilized the apparatus for meridian identification (AMI) to measure bioelectrical activity at acupuncture meridian Ting points. The study found that CV4 significantly reduced ($p < .05$) bioelectrical after-polarization (AP) potential at most meridian Ting points ($p = .00015$) versus Sham ($p = .754$), which indicates a significant shift from ANS sympathetic to parasympathetic activity. It may also demonstrate a connection between OMT and the acupuncture meridian system.[71]

Besides the AMI, another method for measuring the body's overall health and bioenergetic responses to various therapies uses electro-photon imaging through gas discharge visualization (EPI/GDV). Data regarding the body's bioelectromagnetic field can be measured by using technology reminiscent of Kirlian photography.[96] Here, an electrophotonic camera captures corona field images around the fingers/thumbs, and a computer analyzes and correlates the data to the body's energy fields, acupuncture meridian activity, physiologic and psychological parameters, and autonomic responses.[97] Korotkov and colleagues[98] utilized EPI/GDV correlated with blood pressure measurements, pulse rate, and interference electromyograms (EMGs) in a small cohort of 33 patients receiving osteopathic manipulation. Specifics of the osteopathic procedures performed on the "whole body" were not detailed, but subjects were reportedly treated in a similar manner. Twenty participants experienced statistically significant reductions in stress, blood pressure, and pulse within 30 minutes after OMT. In addition, entropy parameter variations were significantly reduced, which indicates harmonization of the bioenergetic fields of the individuals.

Exploration of OMT with these or other biofield devices and methods could offer expanded explanations for efficacy. Perhaps all OMT influences biophysical properties of the body and affects biofields, qi, and the acupuncture meridian system resulting in the physiologic and structural changes observed.[2,3,7] Further investigations are needed.

SUMMARY

Dynamic SVR appears to have efficacy in treating somatic dysfunction through interaction with the human biofield[2,3,7,63] and its oscillations.[99] Other (or all) models of OMT may also have their basis in bioenergetics.

The use of biophysical principles and measurements of human effects from biofield therapies pose unique challenges…and opportunities…to clinicians, researchers, medical students, and traditional Western medical systems (osteopathic, allopathic). These include having an open mind to:

1. Explore nontraditional medical principles and therapies
2. Truly search for and utilize models of healing that are most efficient, safe, and noninvasive

3. Learn how we are connected to and influence our own and our patient's health through consciousness and intention
4. Transcend medical dogma

Knowledge of this integration is crucial to the total holistic approach to patients central to the osteopathic philosophy. Additionally, medicine is now entering an uncertain future in which physicians are mandated to become more proficient, efficient, effective, and prevention oriented. Patients are also awakening to the fact that current conventional medical interventions are often dangerous, costly, and ineffective. The U.S. medical system continues to be the third largest cause of death, after cardiovascular illness and cancer.[100,101] To change this long-term trend, it is vital to employ therapeutics that are effective, efficient, and relatively less expensive and produce the least side effects. The profession needs to identify and treat the root cause of illness, be it of the body, mind, spirit, and/or the energy fields that support them. DOs need to develop, refine, and use their osteopathic skills so that they can adhere to Dr. Still's reminder, "To find health should be the object of the doctor. Anyone can find disease."[102]

REFERENCES

1. Seffinger MA, King HH, Ward RC, et al. Osteopathic philosophy. In: Chila AG, ed. *Foundations of Osteopathic Medicine*. 3rd ed. Wolters Kluwer/Lippincott Williams & Wilkins; 2011:3–22.
2. Hendryx JT. The bioenergetic model in osteopathic diagnosis and treatment: an FAAO thesis. Part 1. *AAO J*. 2014;24(1):12–20.
3. Hendryx JT. The bioenergetic model in osteopathic diagnosis and treatment: an FAAO thesis. Part 2. *AAO J*. 2014;24(2):10–20.
4. Seffinger MA, Ex. ed. *Foundations of Osteopathic Medicine: Philosophy, Science, Clinical Applications, and Research*. 4th ed. Wolters Kluwer; 2018.
5. Hruby RJ, Fraix MP, Giusti RE. Cervicogenic headache. In: Chila AG, ed. *Foundations of Osteopathic Medicine*. 3rd ed. Lippincott Williams & Wilkins; 2011:942.
6. Giusti RE, ed. Educational Council on Osteopathic Principles. *Glossary of Osteopathic Terminology*. American Association of Colleges of Osteopathic Medicine; 2017:30–31, 63,73.
7. Hendryx JT. Dynamic strain. In: Seffinger MA, ed. *Foundations of Osteopathic Medicine: Philosophy, Science, Clinical Applications, and Research*. 4th ed. Wolters Kluwer; 2018:981–990.
8. Helms JM. *Acupuncture Energetics: A Clinical Approach for Physicians*. Medical Acupuncture Publishers; 1995:19–50.
9. Lad V. *Ayurveda: The Science of Self-Healing*. Lotus Press; 1984.
10. Sui CK. *Miracles Through Pranic Healing: Practical Manual on Energy Healing*. Institute for Inner Studies Publishing Foundation, Inc. 2011.
11. Brennan BA. *Hands of Light: A Guide to Healing Through the Human Energy Field*. Bantam Books; 1987.
12. Stoler L. Energy psychology. In: Rakel D, ed. *Integrative Medicine*. 3rd ed. Elsevier; 2011:898–904.
13. Gallo FP. *Energy Psychology: Explorations at the Interface of Energy, Cognition, Behavior, and Health*. 2nd ed. CRC Press; 2005.
14. Burmeister A, Monte T. *The Touch of Healing: Energizing Body, Mind, and Spirit with the Art of Jin Shin Jyutsu*. Bantam Books; 1997.
15. Lad V, Durve A. *Marma Points of Ayurveda*. The Ayurvedic Press; 2015.
16. Stone R. *Polarity Therapy: The Complete Collected Works*, Vol. 1. CRCS Publications; 1986:1–93.
17. Stone R. *Polarity Therapy: The Complete Collected Works*, Vol. 2. CRCS Publications; 1987:1–52.
18. Stein D. *Essential Reiki*. The Crossing Press, Inc.; 1995.
19. Krieger D. *The Therapeutic Touch*. Prentice-Hall, Inc.; 1979.
20. Rindfleisch JA. Biofield therapies: energy medicine in primary care. *Prim Care Clin Office Pract*. 2010;37:165–179.
21. Rindfleisch JA. Biofield therapies. In: Rakel D, Minichiello VJ, eds. *Integrative Medicine*. 5th ed. Elsevier; 2023:921–928.
22. Parke WC. *Biophysics: A Student Guide to the Physics of the Life Sciences and Medicine*. Springer Nature Switzerland AG; 2020.
23. Oschman JL. *Energy Medicine: The Scientific Basis*. 2nd ed. Elsevier; 2015.
24. Oschman JL. *Energy Medicine: The Scientific Basis*. Churchill Livingstone; 2000:1–40.
25. Oschman JL. *Energy Medicine in Therapeutics and Human Performance*. Butterworth/Heinemann; 2003:xxvii, 1–27.
26. Burr HS. *Blueprint for Immortality: The Electric Patterns of Life*. Neville Spearman Publishers; 1972:1–192.
27. NIH. Complementary, Alternative, or Integrative Health: What's In a Name? *National Center for Complementary and Integrative Health (NCCIH)*. Accessed January 10, 2023. https://nccih.nih.gov/health/integrative-health#cvsa
28. Rubik B, Muehsam D, Hammerschlag R, Jain S. Biofield science and healing: history, terminology, and concepts. *Global Adv Health Med*. 2015;4(suppl):8–14.
29. Rubik B. The biofield hypothesis, its biophysical basis and role in medicine. *J Altern Complement Med*. 2002;8(6):703–717.
30. Rein G. Bioinformation within the biofield: beyond bioelectromagnetics. *J Altern Complement Med*. 2004;10(1):59–68.
31. Kafatos MC, Chevalier G, Chopra D, Hubacher J, Kak S, Theise ND. Biofield science: current physics perspective. *Global Adv Health Med*. 2015;4(suppl):25–34.
32. Hammerschlag R, Levin M, McCraty R, et al. Biofield physiology: a framework for an emerging discipline. *Global Adv Health Med*. 2015;4(suppl):35–41.
33. Muesham D, Chevalier G, Barsotti T, Gurfein BT. An overview of biofield devices. *Global Adv Health Med*. 2015;4(suppl):42–51.
34. Rosch PJ, ed. *Bioelectromagnetic and Subtle Energy Medicine*. 2nd ed. CRC Press; 2015.
35. Trowbridge C. *Andrew Taylor Still, 1828-1917*. The Thomas Jefferson University Press. 1991:136.
36. Still AT. *The Philosophy and Mechanical Principles of Osteopathy*. Hudson-Kimberly Publication Co; 1902:248–268, 296–299.
37. Lee RP. *Interface: Mechanisms of Spirit in Osteopathy*. Stillness Press; 2005:35.
38. Littlejohn JM. The physiologic basis of therapeutic law. *J Am Osteopath Assoc*. 1902;2:42–60.
39. Hulettt GD. *A Text Book of the Principles of Osteopathy*. Journal Printing Co; 1903:43–68.
40. McConnell CP. Fundamental fragments. Relatedness. From J Am Osteopathic Assoc 1939. In: Jordan T, Schuster R, eds. *Selected Writings of Carl Phillip McConnell*, DO. Squirrel's Tail Press; 1994:129–130.
41. McConnell CP. The osteopathic approach. J Am Osteopath Assoc. June 1938. In: Jordan T, Schuster R, eds. *Selected Writings of Carl Philip McConnell*, D.O. Squirrel's Tail Press; 1994:28–32.
42. Sutherland WG. Clinical experience in the practice of osteopathy. In: Wales AL, ed. *Teachings in the Science of Osteopathy*. Sutherland Cranial Teaching Foundation; 1990:166–189.
43. Yadava RL. Fulford percussion. In: Seffinger MA, ed. *Foundations of Osteopathic Medicine: Philosophy, Science, Clinical Applications, and Research*. 4th ed. Wolters Kluwer; 2018:997–1002.
44. Becker RE. Diagnostic touch: its principles and applications part I: To feel living function. In: Brooks RE, ed. *Life in Motion*. Rudra Press; 1997:153–165.
45. Becker RE. Diagnostic touch: its principles and applications part II: what a diagnostic touch can do. In: Brooks RE, ed. *Life in Motion*. Rudra Press; 1997:166–179.
46. Becker RE. Diagnostic touch: its principles and applications part III: putting a diagnostic touch to work. In: Brooks RE, ed. *Life in Motion*. Rudra Press; 1997:180–202.
47. Becker RE. Diagnostic touch: its principles and applications part IV: trauma and stress. In: Brooks RE, ed. *Life in Motion*. Rudra Press; 1997:203–216.
48. Magoun HI. *Osteopathy in the Cranial Field*. 2nd ed. Journal Publishing Co; 1966:23–42.
49. Davidson SM. *Neurofascial Release: A Course in Guided Palpation and Treatment*. Practical Publications; 1990:1–20.
50. Malina B. *Neurofascial Release: An Instruction Manual*. Author; 1996:1–28.
51. Davidson SM. *Neurofascial Release Course*. Author; 2001.
52. Davidson SM. *Advanced Neurofascial Release Course: Visceral Manipulation*. Author; 2003.

53. MacDonald RC. "The energy cyst": its ramifications and use in osteopathic manipulative management. *AAO J.* 2003;13(3):16–18.
54. Upledger JE. *Craniosacral Therapy II: Beyond the Dura.* Eastland Press; 1987:212–214.
55. Jealous J. *Biodynamics of Osteopathy.* Accessed January 22, 2023. https://www.jamesjealous.com/courses/postgraduate-biodynamics/Accessed
56. Rubin E, Cohen E. *An Exploration of the Foundations & Principles of the Biodynamic Model of Osteopathy in the Cranial Field.* Authors; 2016.
57. Holland EC. *Holonomics and Relationism: The Principles of Integrative Medicine.* The Holonomic Institute; 2009:2–25.
58. Holland EC. *Viscoelastic and Viscoplastic Axes of Motion in the Cranium: The Biophysics of Cranial Osteopathy (Video).* The Holonomic Institute; 1992.
59. Holland EC. *The Biophysics of Fulford Techniques.* The Holonomic Institute; 2012.
60. O'Connell JA. *Bioelectric Fascial Activation and Release.* American Academy of Osteopathy; 2000:22–25, 59–78.
61. O'Connell JA. Myofascial release. In: Seffinger MA, ed. *Foundations of Osteopathic Medicine: Philosophy, Science, Clinical Applications, and Research.* 4th ed. Wolters Kluwer; 2018:835–863.
62. Comeaux ZJ. Facilitated oscillatory release - a method of dynamic assessment and treatment of somatic dysfunction. *AAO J.* 2003;13(3):30–35.
63. Hendryx JT, O'Brien RL. Dynamic strain-vector release: an energetic approach to OMT. *AAO J.* 2003;10(3):19–29.
64. Lee RP. Spirituality in osteopathic medicine. *AAO J.* 2000;10(4):31–36.
65. Chikly B. *The Inherent Motility of the Brain and Spinal Cord Part 1: Brain Parenchyma, Nuclei and Fluid.* Author; 2010.
66. Chikly B. *Brain Tissue, Nuclei, Fluid and Reticular Alarm System (LDB2).* Author; 2016.
67. Nelson KE, Sergueef N, Lipinski CM, et al. Cranial rhythmic impulse related to the Traube-Hering-Mayer oscillation: comparing laser-Doppler flowmetry and palpation. *J Am Osteopath Assoc.* 2001;101(3):163–173.
68. Nelson KE. The primary respiratory mechanism. *AAO J.* 12(4):25–34.
69. Glonek T, Sergueef N, Nelson KE. Physiological rhythms/oscillations: complementary, alternative and integrative consideration of biorhythms. In: Chila AG, ed. *Foundations of Osteopathic Medicine.* 3rd ed. Wolters Kluwer/Lippincott Williams & Wilkins; 2011:162–190.
70. King HH. Osteopathic Cranial Manipulative Medicine. In: Seffinger MA, ed. *Foundations of Osteopathic Medicine: Philosophy, Science, Clinical Applications, and Research.* 4th ed. Wolters Kluwer; 2018:885–905.
71. Hendryx JT, Kannan A, Prashad J, Falk K. Connecting the dots: alterations in bioelectric activity at acupuncture Ting (Jing-Well) points following CV4 cranial manipulation. *J Osteopath Med.* 2022:1–8.
72. What is energy? U.S. Energy Information Administration. Accessed January 23, 2023. https://www.eia.gov/energyexplained/what-is-energy/
73. Simon RR, Koenigsknecht SJ. *Emergency Orthopedics.* Appleton & Lange; 1987:22.
74. Barral J-P. *Visceral Manipulation.* Eastland Press; 1988:9.
75. Lossing K. Visceral Manipulation. In: Seffinger MA, ed. *Foundations of Osteopathic Medicine: Philosophy, Science, Clinical Applications, and Research.* 4th ed. Wolters Kluwer; 2018:1022–26.
76. DiGiovanna EL. Somatic dysfunction. In: DiGiovanna EL, Amen CJ, Burns DK, eds. *An Osteopathic Approach to Diagnosis and Treatment.* 4th ed. Wolters Kluwer; 2021:12–17.
77. Stiles E. *Biotensegrity and Areas of Greatest Restriction.* Presented at the AOA Convention. Author; 2007.
78. Glover JC, Rennie PR. Strain/Counterstrain. In: Seffinger MA, ed. *Foundations of Osteopathic Medicine: Philosophy, Science, Clinical Applications, and Research.* 4th ed. Wolters Kluwer; 2018:869.
79. Holland EC. *Holonomic Perception: Cognitive Skills, Perceptual Physiology, and Perceptual Transference.* The Holonomic Institute; 2009:12–20.
80. Willard FH, Fossum C, Standley PR. The Fascial System of the Body. In: Seffinger MA, ed. *Foundations of Osteopathic Medicine: Philosophy, Science, Clinical Applications, and Research.* 4th ed. Wolters Kluwer; 2018:80–103.
81. Schleip R, Klingler W, Lehmann-Horn F. Active fascial contractility: fascia may be able to contract in a smooth muscle-like manner and thereby influence musculoskeletal dynamics. *Med Hypotheses.* 2005;65(2):273–277.
82. Schleip R, Naylor IL, Ursu D, et al. Passive muscle stiffness may be influenced by active contractility of intramuscular connective tissue. *Med Hypotheses.* 2006;66(1):66–71.
83. Ingber DE. The architecture of life. *Sci Am.* 1998:48–57.
84. Oschman JL. Charge transfer in the living matrix. *J Bodywork and Movement Therapies.* 2009;13:215–228.
85. Swanson RL. Biotensegrity: a unifying theory of biological architecture with applications to osteopathic practice, education, and research—a review and analysis. *J Am Osteopath Assoc.* 2013;113(1):34–52.
86. Geiger B, Spatz JP, Bershadsky AD. Environmental sensing through focal adhesions. *Nat Rev Mol Cell Biol.* 2009;10(1):21–33.
87. Jaalouk DE, Lammerding J. Mechanotransduction gone awry. *Nat Rev Mol Cell Biol.* 2009;10(1):63–73.
88. Wang N, Tytell JD, Ingber DE. Mechanotransduction at a distance: mechanically coupling the extracellular matrix with the nucleus. *Nat Rev Mol Cell Biol.* 2009;10(1):75–82.
89. Ingber DE. Tensegrity I. Cell structure and hierarchal systems biology. *J Cell Sci.* 2003;116(7):1157–1173.
90. Ingber DE. Tensegrity II. How structural networks influence cellular information processing networks. *J Cell Sci.* 2003;116(8):1397–1408.
91. Chevalier G, Mori K, Oschman JL. The effect of earthing (grounding) on human physiology. *European Biology and Bioelectromagnetics.* 2006:600–621.
92. Oschman JL, Chevalier G, Ober AC. Biophysics of earthing (grounding) the human body. In: Rosch PJ, ed. *Bioelectromagnetic and Subtle Energy Medicine,* 2nd ed. CRC Press. 2015;427–448.
93. Chevalier G, Sinatra ST, Oschman JL, Sokal K, Sokal P. Earthing: health implications of reconnecting the human body to the earth's surface electrons. *J Env and Public Health.* 2012:1–8.
94. Chevalier G. Grounding the human body improves facial blood flow regulation: results of a randomized, placebo-controlled pilot study. *JCDSA.* 2014;4(5):293–308.
95. Peterson B, ed. *The Collected Papers of Irvin M. Korr.* American Academy of Osteopathy. 1979.
96. Kirlian Sd, Kirlian V. Photography and visual observations by means of high-frequency currents. *J Sci Appl Photogr.* 1961;6:397–403.
97. Korotkov K. Science of measuring energy fields. A revolutionary technique to visualize energy fields of humans and nature. In: Rosch PJ, ed. *Bioelectromagnetic and Subtle Energy Medicine,* 2nd ed. CRC Press. 2015; 111–124.
98. Korotkov K, Shelkov O, Shevtsov P, et al. Stress reduction with osteopathy assessed with GDV electrophotonic imaging: effects of osteopathy treatment. *J Altern Complement Med.* 2012;18(3):251–257.
99. Muehsam D, Ventura C. Life rhythm as a symphony of oscillatory patterns: electromagnetic energy and sound vibration modulates gene expression for biological signaling and healing. *Global Adv Health Med.* 2014;3(2):40–55.
100. Starfield B. Is US health really the best in the world? *JAMA.* 2000; 284(4):483–485.
101. Makary MA, Daniel M. Medical error-the third leading cause of death in the US. *Br Med J.* 2016;353:i2139.
102. Still AT. *The Philosophy and Mechanical Principles of Osteopathy.* Hudson-Kimberly Pub Co; 1902:72. Updated Diagrams for Chapter 61, FOM 5, Dynamic Strain and the Bioenergetic Model Hendryx.

62

Progressive Inhibition of Neuromusculoskeletal Structures (PINS)

DENNIS J. DOWLING

KEY CONCEPTS

- PINS is a modality for manually treating persistent or resistant somatic dysfunctions with methodical pressure following discovered patterns.
- PINS is used to decrease tissue tonicity.
- Clinical symptoms are correlated to and directly related to increased dysfunctional tone.
- A steady digital pressure (constant mild/moderate force) is applied to regions of dysfunction.
- The relationship between neuromusculoskeletal structures and underlying visceral organs is considered.
- In order to achieve efficacy and accuracy, a thorough knowledge of the typical and variant courses of nerves, fascial bands, and muscles is required. This knowledge must be augmented by clinical decision-making skills.

CASE STUDY

As a teenager, the author's parents brought him to the family physician for his frequent headaches. Most of the treatments offered had a limited impact or very undesirable side effects. Other apparently related symptoms that accompanied the cephalgia were as follows:

- A boring pain in the right eye
- Increased lacrimation of the ipsilateral greater than the contralateral eye
- Right-sided facial pain
- Nasal congestion that was more pronounced on the ipsilateral side
- Scalp sensitivity that occurred primarily on the ipsilateral side

There was also frequent suboccipital pain that was seemingly related to the onset of the periorbital pain, although no direct connection was initially apparent. Eventually, common precipitating events that lead to the symptoms were discerned:

- Prolonged reading
- Eyestrain due to exposure to bright sunlight
- Dehydration

There were no sensory deficits. Some of the symptoms could occur independently and were usually worsened by stress. The medical diagnosis was migraine headaches with the possibility of cluster elements since they were so frequent and intense.

Since the author had little knowledge of anatomy at the time, he attempted to treat himself by applying manual pressure to various areas of his head. Pressing on the painful sites one at a time brought only temporary relief. The pain could recur almost immediately after releasing the pressure. Adjacent regions of the scalp also developed sensitivity during or after the pressure release. Patterns eventually developed as these secondary and even subsequent points became unmasked. The most successful approach appeared to be the sequential treatment of a series of points. These self-treatments often led to discontinuation of the symptoms, and if done at the first appreciation of the symptoms, prevented the full headache occurrence. Occasionally, this could be applied to other musculoskeletal problems both for himself and others. The pattern included a starting point at the right supraorbital ridge near the trochlear notch and a final one on the ipsilateral side in the suboccipital triangle. This probably involved progressive treatment of the ophthalmic branch of the trigeminal nerve leading from its first superficial appearance upward to the terminal elements of the greater occipital nerve.

Myofascial elements that could simultaneously be involved include the frontalis and occipitalis muscles. Both the nerve and muscle components have a watershed region at the midpoint at the top of the head with shared fibers and the galea aponeurotica, respectively. The point near the orbit was related to the most disturbing symptoms including eye pain. The intervening points represent the connections to the possible origin of the pattern in the suboccipital triangle where muscle spasm of the component muscles impacted the nerves. Both the trigeminal and greater occipital nerves not only innervate the scalp but also the dura mater, a pain-sensitive structure inside the cranium.

Much later, as an osteopathic student and physician, the author began to integrate osteopathic manipulative medicine theory along with his personal clinical observations in treating these apparent linear patterns. This self-treatment was converted into a modality that could be taught to other students of osteopathic manipulative medicine. Gradually, the rationale behind this specialized inhibitory technique, as well as its use beyond the treatment of headaches, became clearer.[1] Also noted were the similarities and differences to other manipulative methods of point or applied pressure techniques. Discussion with other specialists leads to the concept that this could be one method of discovering the "key lesion."

Inhibition

PINS is most closely related to the osteopathic modality of inhibition. The Glossary of Osteopathic Terminology states that inhibition is "…a term that describes steady pressure to soft tissues to effect relaxation and normalize reflex activity".[2] The "steady pressure to soft tissues" is perhaps one of the oldest methods of manual treatment, regardless of the term used to describe it. Classically, inhibition is a constant mild-to-moderate force exerted by the practitioner's fingers, elbow, knee, or even foot on regions of hypertonic muscle. Even though the patient's presenting complaint may be of pain or decreased function, the objective of the treatment is to decrease tissue tonicity. All of the patient's symptoms are assumed to be directly related to this increased dysfunctional tone.[3] Larger, more superficial muscles are the most easily identified, whether they are in the normal–relaxed or hypertonic states. Regional muscles can be selected and treated individually or in pairs.

The patient is typically treated in either the supine or the prone positions. This may facilitate the process by reducing the use of some postural muscles that provide positional support to the trunk and neck. For example, the trapezius can be easily located in the occipital, cervical, shoulder, and upper thoracic regions. Some portion of the muscle can be grasped, pressed, or pinched. A hypertonic muscle is commonly found to be firmer than the same muscle on the opposite side of the body and perhaps even more than its antagonist on the same side. In addition to firmness, greater sensitivity or tenderness may also be noted as pressure is introduced. As long as the applied pressure remains constant, the structures should eventually reflexively relax. With the intention of inhibiting the tension, there should be avoidance of altering the position or amount of pressures, since they are then likely to be stimulatory and not inhibitory.

In regard to inhibition, the relationship between musculoskeletal structures and the underlying visceral organs should also be considered. These organs receive innervations from the same spinal cord segment levels that service the skin, bones, joints, ligaments, and muscles. The sympathetic chain lies just anterior to the rib heads. Dysfunction of the vertebral or rib joints may result in increased stimulation to related visceral and musculoskeletal structures.[4] Acute responses to increased sympathetic activity are the same as for any new injury:

- Redness (rubor)
- Pain (dolor)
- Swelling (tumor)
- Heat (calor)
- Decreased function (functio laesa)[5]

More superficial structures such as the skin and subcutaneous tissue may have a "doughy" consistency, which are typically associated with a sharp and throbbing pain, as noted by the patient.

Chronic sympathetic hyperactivity in the absence of adequate treatment and/or recovery demonstrates altered signs and symptoms that are more associated with chronic dysfunction:

- The muscles may feel fibrotic ("ropy").
- The skin is thinner, paler, and cooler.
- Pain responses can range from relative insensitivity ("anesthetic") to altered sensitivity ("paresthesia") to hypersensitivity.

Applying pressure through a modality such as inhibition may result in a transitory increase in palpatory findings or symptoms, followed by a reflexive reduction of some or all of these components. When the visceral organs are the primary dysfunction, the persistence or recurrence of a musculoskeletal somatic dysfunction may indicate the presence of a viscerosomatic reflex. When a musculoskeletal injury is the etiology, manipulative treatment may more persistently reduce or eliminate all pathologic components.

Inhibitory techniques have a different visceral focus in the suboccipital and sacral region, in that the parasympathetic system dominates over the sympathetic. Somatic dysfunction of the upper cervical, occipital, and sacral regions may result in prolonged inappropriate parasympathetic activity. Inhibition reduces increased regional musculoskeletal tone and congestion and theoretically downregulates the aberrant activity of the more internal mechanisms. The actual effect of treating sympathetic and parasympathetic regions may not be so much increasing or decreasing either, but is more likely a re-setting by normalizing the components.

Accurate application of inhibitory and PINS treatments requires a thorough understanding of the structure and function of all factors related to somatic dysfunction. When correlated with somatic dysfunction findings, treatment patterns may be addressed to several locations in order to reduce all of the relevant dysfunctions.

As a young man, when Andrew Taylor Still suffered from chronic headaches, he treated himself with a rope swing with a blanket slung across it that was lowered to a few inches above the ground. Dr. Still would position his neck with the base of the skull on this support, fall asleep, and then awaken refreshed and pain-free. Whether it was intentional or not, his self-treatment appears to represent an inhibitory treatment as much as a positional intervention.[6] Despite Dr. Still's aversion to defining specific types of treatment, he included descriptions of both inhibition and stimulation methods in his writings.[7]

Likewise, some of Dr. Still's early students described inhibitory techniques and the rationale for their use. In his book, *A Manual of Osteopathy*, Eduard Goetz, DO described this type of technique in the treatment of various somatic and visceral conditions.[8] The accompanying photographs in this small handbook clearly demonstrate inhibition performed on several regions. Importantly, Dr. Goetz recommended that a few minutes of pressure be applied individually to the orbital and suboccipital regions of the head.

A more extensive description of inhibition appears in *The Principles of Osteopathy* by Dain L. Tasker, DO.[9] Dr. Tasker described the rationale for the technique's effectiveness, which was especially crucial since inhibition seemed like a natural phenomenon. Without the adapted or learned ability to perform inhibition, bodily functions such as defecation and urination could not come under conscious and unconscious control. Dr. Tasker explained that the success of physician-applied inhibitory pressure, directed toward decreasing hyperactivity, is not due to the surface pressure but instead to the subsequent initiation or alteration of the reflex arc. The initial response to pressure is essentially a form of stimulation, since it impacts the soft tissue. However, steadily applied pressure diminishes the stimulation, and results in an inhibition in the region, which begins to lessen the dysfunction. This may bring about alterations both deeper and more distant from where the pressure was applied. In citing Hilton's law, "the skin, muscles and synovial membrane of a joint, or the skin, muscles of the abdomen and contents covered by peritoneum, are innervated from the same segment of the cord." According to Tasker, the "overstimulation" caused by inhibition diminishes or eliminates the over-reactivity.

Osteopathic Point and/or Pressure Techniques

There are many types of passive direct and indirect systems in the osteopathic treatment of somatic dysfunction. Some standard points and diagnoses are used as fulcrums and/or monitoring locations in practically all modalities. Constant palpation at these points is one of the best means for an osteopathic physician to experience feedback and monitor success when performing Jones' strain–counterstrain treatment.[10–12] Oftentimes, the patient can also appreciate the alteration.

The muscle spindle sensory organ is embedded into the larger extrafusal muscle. The sensory ends of nerve fibers to these small, intrafusal muscles are stimulated by stretch of any kind, whether static or dynamic. This results in increased alpha motor neuron activity at a single spinal segment, which causes contraction of the whole extrafusal muscle. It is quite successful as a mechanism to prevent tearing and overstretching of the soft tissue, whether dynamic or static, and should decrease as soon as the danger of damage diminishes. However, if the region is underprepared or overwhelmed, the reflex arc can persist longer than is appropriate. The signals from the muscle spindle apparatus continue to fire as if the tissue were being too rapidly stretched or overstretched, even though the overall length of the muscle may be relatively normal or even shortened. The sensitivity of a "tender point" reflects this increased, underlying activity. The external pressure at the tender point often elicits the complaint. However, the positioning during strain–counterstrain shortens the whole muscle, allowing for the spindle reflex mechanism to be reset and for the hypersensitivity to disappear.

Facilitated positional release (FPR)[13] is similar in many respects to counterstrain. Counterstrain is a form of positional release, while FPR utilizes an additional activating force, usually compression or torsion, after the region is initially positioned in neutral. Theoretically, both techniques utilize the same neurophysiologic mechanism: the muscle spindle. According to Richard Van Buskirk, PhD, DO, FAAO, the muscle spindle is also the core activator treated by the Still technique,[13] which also shares many similarities to strain–counterstrain and FPR. Dr. Van Buskirk recovered components of the technique from the writings of Charles Hazzard, DO,[14–16] and of Dr. A.T. Still himself. He subsequently defined the technique as one that uses the initial palpatory diagnosis of dysfunctions to place the region into the somatic dysfunction relative freedoms of motion (i.e., position of ease). The physician then introduces movement past the neutral point, into the restrictive motion barrier directions. This low-velocity, relatively low-amplitude articulatory movement follows the positional treatment of the freedoms. FPR as actually practiced by Stanley Schiowitz, DO, FAAO and many of his students is almost indistinguishable from the Still Technique. They both use a neutral position that is combined with positioning into positions of ease followed by challenges into the restrictive barriers. Both are combination of indirect followed by direct movements. FPR appeared in writings primarily as an indirect technique as the stepwise approach for this element was easier to teach and appreciate.

In the spinal regions, functional technique[17] utilizes diagnostic points to define the somatic dysfunction at that region, relative to its two adjoining vertebrae (the one above and the one below). Somatic dysfunctions are typically detected by percussion and by more specific tests that scan and screen the region.

Elaine Wallace, DO, developed torque unwinding,[1] a concept in which the body is imagined as a collection of adjacent or overlapping cubes. Theoretically, injuries direct vector and/or moment forces into a whole "cube" that is commonly in a state of torsion. When the patient is twisted, the initial force may be initially straight or arced. However, the resultant pathway becomes irregular or more twisted as the patient and region straighten. In this manner, the fascia acts more colloid-like with disruption, adapting to form a memory of the force in the tissues. Torque unwinding treatment involves introducing oscillating rhythmic balancing pressures, directed centrally from two diametrically opposed theoretical cube faces. The therapeutic forces are intended to counteract the residual traumatic ones.

Other variations of myofascial or fascial release techniques[18,19] that utilize point contacts as references, contact points, and/or diagnostic reflections are present in osteopathic literature as follows:

- Triggerband technique: as described by Steven Typaldos, DO,[20] is a method of treating the pathologic cross-linkages of fascial bands by exerting deep pressure along certain connective tissue pathways. This has evolved into treatment with the Fascial Distortion Model.[21]
- Chaitow[22–24] neuromuscular technique: consists mostly of point localization and pressure, followed by deep stroking and/or rolling of the tissue.
- Chapman point treatment[25]: reflects a neurologic/endocrine/lymphatic alteration reflected to specific points on the surface, which are indicative of a possibly latent visceral correlate. Some of these mapped points are similar in both location and correlation to those of acupuncture.

Nonosteopathic Point and/or Pressure Systems

Each of these modalities bears some similarities to typical inhibition and stimulatory techniques of osteopathic manipulation, where the practitioner provides treatment by pressing the patient's soft tissue.

- Cyriax method[26]: The British medical orthopedist James Cyriax, MD, practiced joint mobilization and massage, in which he applied a pinching technique on several locations.
- Trigger point therapy[27]: Developed by Janet Travell, MD, the treatment maps out the relationship between a remote referral region and a damaged myofascial nexus.
  - The methods of treatment can include manual pressure, dry needling, or a combination of saline, sterile water, and anesthetic and steroid agents injected into the trigger point. In addition, a vapo-coolant spray can be directed from the trigger point toward the referral.
- Acupuncture and acupressure[28–31]: Utilizes surface points that represent reflections of energy or chi forces, which are aligned along meridians within the body, at specific point locations.
  - Acupressure generally involves applying pressure as well as circular motions.
  - When treating with acupuncture needles, the practitioner may also burn incense or apply electricity to the outer tip of the acupuncture needles.
- Shiatsu[32]: One of the oldest forms of manual therapy, Shiatsu attempts to reduce the amount of tissue tension present with a typically brief but intense amount of force. Specific treatment patterns are utilized for certain conditions.
- Bonnie Prudden myotherapy[33]: Myotherapy, an apparent variant of the trigger point concept, consists of both primary and satellite points. Both types are treated for short intervals several times per day, over several sessions. Stretching may also be incorporated in both Bonnie Prudden myotherapy and trigger point therapy.
- Rolfing[34]: Ida Rolf, PhD, developed the eponymous system Rolfing. She was sometimes known as "Dr. Elbow," because of her use of the elbow to apply deep forces on regions of the body.
  - This modality utilizes a greater amount of force than is commonly employed in osteopathic inhibition.
  - Approximating ideal symmetry and alignment is heavily emphasized.
  - Followers of Dr. Rolf had made some alterations to the technique and integrated them into other treatments involving movement patterns (Hellerwork, Aston-Patterning).
- Reflexology[35]: The theory involves energetic or visceral components to resonant areas located on the hands, feet, and ear. As with acupuncture, the name of the organ is related more to a theoretical functional contribution to the integrity or energy component of the organ than to the actual physical structure of the viscera.

PINS METHOD

PINS is a modality for treating persistent or resistant dysfunction typically with inhibitory pressure. The points are located using anatomical and clinical knowledge, the involved structures are determined and the sequence of treatment is developed. The physician must thoroughly understand the typical and variant courses of nerves, fascial bands, and muscles among other anatomical components. This knowledge must then be augmented by clinical decision-making skills for greater efficacy and accuracy. The PINS method may also involve:

- Treating contiguous muscles;
- Addressing the overlapping zones where more than one nerve, muscle, or fascial tissue may be contributing to the persistence of somatic dysfunction;
- Developing a sequence of PINS treatment
- When indicated, integrating other osteopathic manipulative techniques

It is not as simple as locating a single sensitive point. Patients may easily note painful areas as well as direct the physician to a point that hurts or is sensitive to pressure. These symptomatic points may indicate a problem but not necessarily the source of the problem.

Shoulder pain can originate in the glenohumeral joint, and specific treatment can be successful in increasing mobility and decreasing discomfort. However, when that is unsuccessful, giving more of the same treatment may not be the answer, and this may prove frustrating to both the patient and the physician. If the shoulder's restricted motion involves a combination of flexion, abduction, and external rotation as well as reduction of scapulothoracic motion with freedoms in the opposite directions, the latissimus dorsi may be in spasm. This muscle attaches in the bicipital groove of the humerus and pulls the arm into extension, internal rotation, and adduction. In other words, the relatively freer motions are directly opposite the restrictions. Treatment may have to exceed this focus, by involving the upper ribs, pectoralis muscles, lower cervical spine, clavicle, thoracic spine, lumbar spine, pelvis, and lower extremity. Fascial planes, and therefore fascial stresses, must also be considered. Often, multiple modalities of manipulation and other forms of treatment may be applied to the location of the shoulder pain without adequately affecting the etiology, in this example, the relatively remote and possibly underappreciated latissimus dorsi.

In PINS, patients can be active participants in their treatment process, especially by offering feedback. They participate in the treatment by describing the amount of pain or other sensitivities in the palpated areas. As the treatment proceeds, the physician takes note of any changes in the tissue and integrates the patient's subjective experience. PINS can be used before or after other methods of treatment, manipulative or otherwise, as part of a more comprehensive treatment regimen.

Procedure

Developing an appropriate diagnostic and treatment protocol using PINS requires the following:

1. The patient usually lies supine or prone. This allows the postural muscles to be in a fairly relaxed state. However, in some regions of the body, treatment can also be given with the patient seated, side lying, or standing.
2. The physician stands or sits near the region to be treated. The fingers of both of the physician's hands should be able to comfortably and accurately contact the patient.
3. The physician examines the patient. Any relationships between the patient's symptoms, somatic dysfunctions, and soft tissue findings should be determined.
4. The different components of the somatic dysfunction using the "STAR"[36] or "TART" mnemonics can be utilized:
   a. [S] Sensitivity changes: Inquire about the patient's subjective responses to palpation, which can include:
      i. *Tenderness* (the second "T" in the "TART" mnemonic)
      ii. Numbness
      iii. Radiation
      iv. Warmth
      v. Irritation
      vi. Throbbing
   b. [T] Tissue texture changes: These can be chronic or acute:
      i. Chronic changes involve:
         1. Prolonged blanching of the skin
         2. Ropy or fibrous texture of the muscles and fascia
         3. Coolness
         4. Dryness
         5. Vascular changes
      ii. Acute changes involve:
         1. Increased redness
         2. Swelling and edema
         3. Moist and/or increased temperature
         Palpation may initially worsen this component.
   c. [A] Asymmetry: Can be noted by visual inspection or palpatory examination.
      i. Theoretically, an imaginary line down the middle of the body should reveal symmetry of one side to the other, in a nondysfunctional condition.
      ii. The nondysfunctional side is used as the standard of expected form.
   d. [R] Restriction of motion: Perhaps the most important determinant of somatic dysfunction and can be measured by quantity or quality:
      i. Quantity—amount of degrees of motion
      ii. Quality—stiffness, tremors, cogwheel rigidity, extraneous movement, etc.
5. The site of subjective pain complaints can be deceptive and may not help in localizing the actual etiology. Pain is a fairly reliable indicator of there being a problem, but it may or may not correlate with the dysfunction. Symptoms may distract the physician from appropriate treatment of other involved components. Tight muscles on one side may be relatively pain-free, while the contralateral stretched muscles may be more "attention-seeking" by eliciting pain or other symptoms.[37]
6. The physician locates a "primary sensitive" point by examining the tissue in the immediate region of the patient's complaint. If a significant point is not found, then the attention should be directed toward widening the search to adjacent areas using knowledge of anatomical relationships.
7. Another point is located by utilizing knowledge of anatomical structures. This may be designated as the "end point" for PINS treatment purposes. It is located either distally or proximally to the primary point, in a structure that links the two points.
   a. Determining this pair of points should require a thorough understanding of muscle origins/insertions, nerve and vascular pathways, and ligamentous attachments. If the primary point is at a muscular origin, then the end point may be at the insertion or oppositely oriented.
   b. Sometimes, one of the points is located in the belly of the muscle. In that case, exploring both ends of the attachments to the bone may reveal the actual location of an end point.

TABLE 62.1

Primary Points, End Points, Connections, and Clinical Conditions

Primary Point	End Point	Connection	Clinical Condition
(a) Supraorbital notch	Suboccipital region	Frontalis–occipitalis muscles Trigeminal–greater occipital nerves (Fig. 62.1)	Tension headache Chronic daily headache Migraine headache
(b) Superior medial scapular border	Base of occiput	Levator scapula (Fig. 62.2)	Cervicalgia
(c) Greater trochanter of the femur	Fibular head	Iliotibial band (Fig. 62.3)	Hip pain Knee pain
(d) Sternum at the second rib	Coracoid process	Pectoralis minor (Fig. 62.4)	Chest pain
(e) Gluteal region	Greater trochanter popliteal region	Piriformis muscle (Fig. 62.5) Sciatic nerve (Fig. 62.6)	Hip pain Sciatica
(f) Xiphoid process	Pubic ramus	Rectus abdominis (Fig. 62.7)	Abdominal pain Nausea
(g) Antecubital region	Wrist	Median nerve (Fig. 62.8)	Carpal tunnel syndrome Double crush syndrome

The midpoint may represent a symptomatic component as part of a series and not the actual end point.

c. Ligaments, which are generally shorter and more fibrous, may also have points that are fairly close together.
d. Fascia encompasses the path between two points, all structures, and may seem to cross other structures. The more specialized the fascia, the more palpable and tendinous it is.
e. Knowledge of superficial and deep nerve pathways is useful when identifying paths that do not appear to correlate with the other structures. Both primary- and end points may be found where a nerve passes out of a foramen, between or through muscles, or around bony protrusions.
   i. Sometimes, if more than one nerve innervates a region, the primary point can be found at the beginning of one nerve and the end point at the beginning of the other nerve. These larger nerves may also share smaller fibers.
   ii When considering the nerve distribution of an extremity, typically one point is found closer to the trunk and the other point closer to the end of the extremity.
f. There are no exhaustive maps of points and sensitive point locations. Likewise, there is no substitution for an excellent working knowledge of functional anatomy.
g. The designated primary point will likely be closer to the patient's symptoms. The end point may also elicit the patient's presenting symptoms or also be sensitive but usually to a lesser extent.
h. Since the entire structure is in dysfunction, all intervening points between the primary and the end points must frequently be addressed. In any case, the two ends of the pattern must first be determined. A patient's complaints of apparently unrelated regions of the body as being related may hint at the location of some components and possible overlapping patterns. Assuming that the patient's knowledge of anatomy is minimal, the physician must be the one to draw the conclusions necessary to begin treatment.

8. Determining these two points, the "primary point" and "end point" is critical to the treatment outcome. This process of selection must be very clear. For the purpose of proceeding in a logical fashion, the point that is more sensitive is designated typically as the "primary point" and can be explained to the patient as the "first point." The other point, found in the region, is then referred to as the "end point." Table 62.1 provides examples of primary and end points. Figures 62.1 to 62.8 are associated with these examples.
9. Determine a muscular, fascial, and/or neurologic pathway between the primary sensitive point and the end point. The line may be curved rather than straight. The direction of treatment may be from distal to proximal, medial to lateral, anterior to posterior, or the reverse of these directions.
10. Knowledge of anatomy is necessary for understanding the connection between the two points, especially for:
    a. Nerve innervations:
       i. Direct connections—The pattern follows the course of a nerve with a connection of a point near the antecubital region of the elbow, to a point along the middle of the forearm near the wrist (median nerve).
       ii. Overlap or "watershed regions" of innervation:
          1. The ophthalmic division of the trigeminal nerve travels from the supraorbital notch, over the frontal region, and to the top of the head.
          2. The greater occipital nerve—Exits the suboccipital region in the occipital sulcus and travels over the

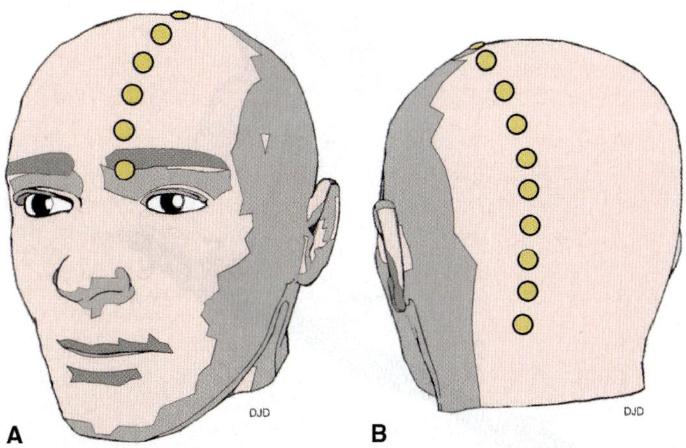

A B

Figure 62.1. **Primary point, supraorbital notch; end point, suboccipital region; connection, frontalis–occipitalis muscles (A), trigeminal–greater occipital nerves (B).** (Courtesy of Dennis J. Dowling, DO, FAAO, with permission.)

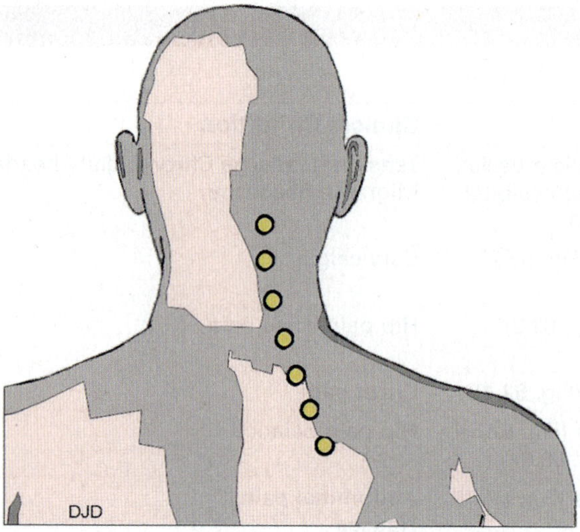

Figure 62.2. Primary point, superior–medial scapular border; end point, base of occiput; connection, levator scapula. (Courtesy of Dennis J. Dowling, DO, FAAO, with permission.)

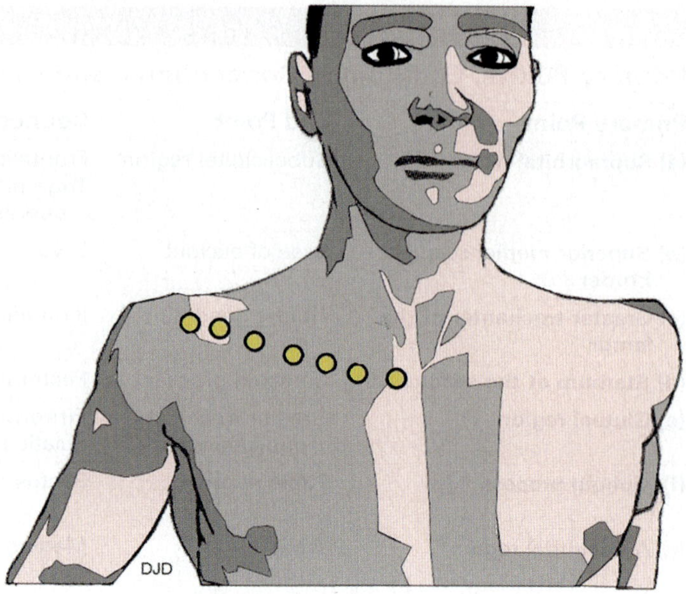

Figure 62.4. Primary point, sternum at second rib; end point, coracoid process; connection, pectoralis minor. (Courtesy of Dennis J. Dowling, DO, FAAO, with permission.)

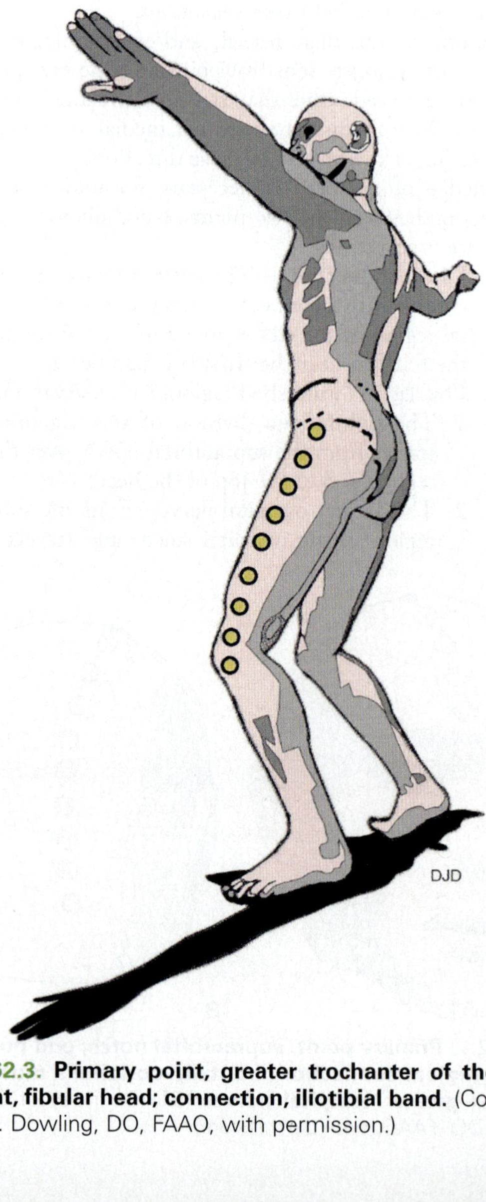

Figure 62.3. Primary point, greater trochanter of the femur; end point, fibular head; connection, iliotibial band. (Courtesy of Dennis J. Dowling, DO, FAAO, with permission.)

occiput to the top of the head. It overlaps in the scalp, near the vertex.

b. Muscle origins and insertions:
   i. Typical—A sensitive point may be found at the medial aspect of the clavicle, and another at the mastoid process, representing involvement of the sternocleidomastoid muscle.

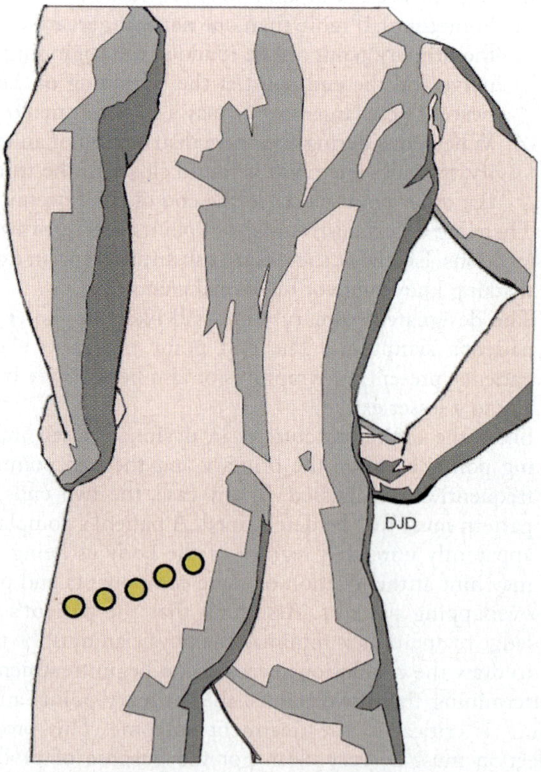

Figure 62.5. Primary point, gluteal region; end point, greater trochanter; connection, piriformis muscle. (Courtesy of Dennis J. Dowling, DO, FAAO, with permission.)

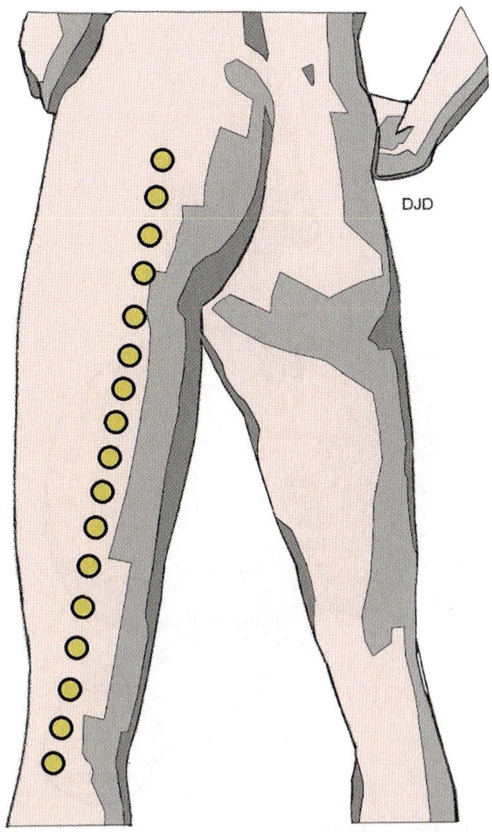

Figure 62.6. **Primary point, gluteal region; end point, popliteal region; connection, sciatic nerve.** (Courtesy of Dennis J. Dowling, DO, FAAO, with permission.)

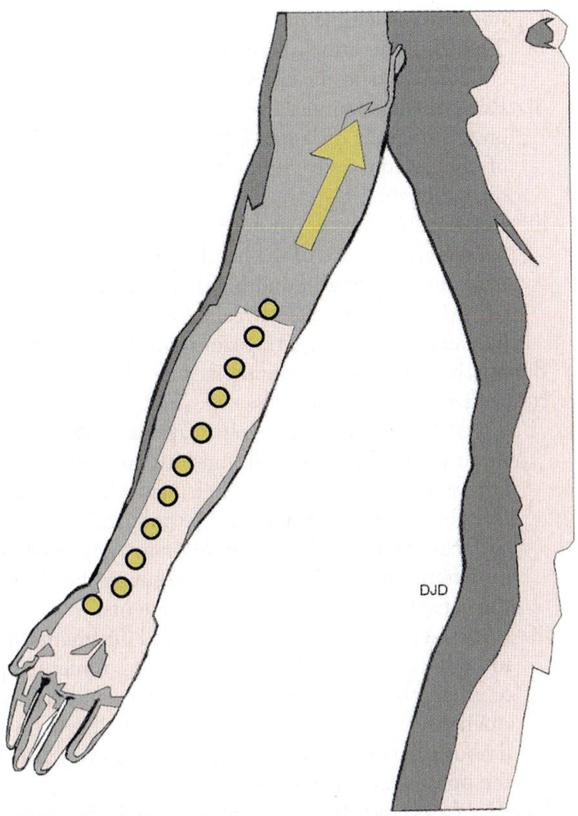

Figure 62.8. **Primary point, antecubital region; end point, wrist; connection, median nerve.** (Courtesy of Dennis J. Dowling, DO, FAAO, with permission.)

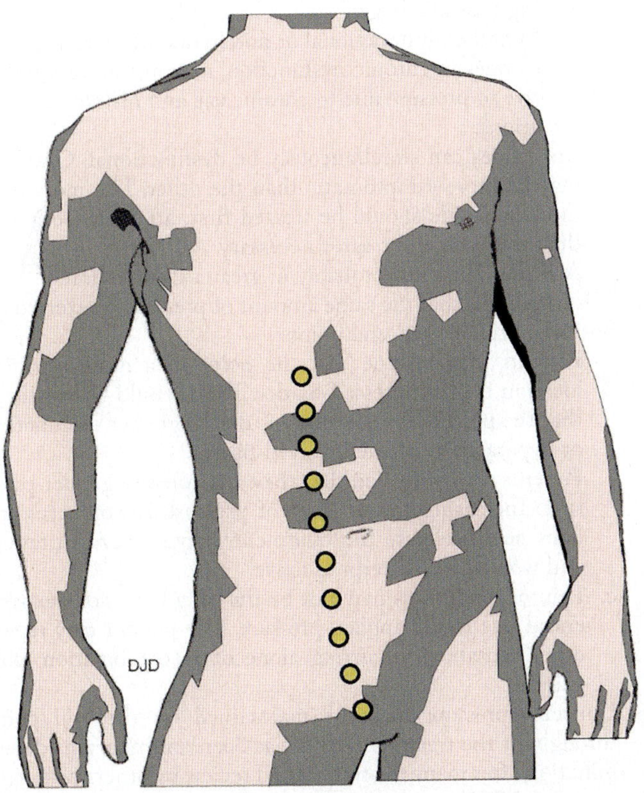

Figure 62.7. **Primary point, xiphoid process; end point, pubic ramus; connection, rectus abdominis.** (Courtesy of Dennis J. Dowling, DO, FAAO, with permission.)

ii. Overlap—The location of a sensitive point on the superoanterior chest may involve intercostal muscles, pectoralis major, and/or pectoralis minor.

iii. Contiguity—The tensor fascia lata and iliotibial band form a continuity for two possible tender points located, respectively, at the greater trochanter and the fibular head. If a terminal point was found near the lateral malleolus instead of the fibular head, then there may be a tensor fascia lata-iliotibial band–peroneal muscle connection.

c. Fascia:

i. Specialized—Interosseous ligaments are actually specialized fascia, connecting the radius and ulna in the arm and the fibula and tibia in the leg. A pattern appearing to overlay their locations may indicate their involvement.

ii. Septums—Even though it is mostly muscular, the diaphragm has fascial components that support and separate, including the central tendon and the crus of the diaphragm. Points found around the lower costal cartilage, the 12th rib, and T10 to T12 may represent a diaphragmatic involvement.

iii. Overlaps—The common thoracolumbar fascia in the back acts as an attachment for muscles, such as the latissimus dorsi. It also overlaps muscles like the quadratus lumborum, iliocostalis, and other erector spinae muscles. Points may be found anywhere within this region and extend to the lateral edge of the 12th rib (quadratus lumborum) or even to the bicipital groove of the humerus (latissimus dorsi).

d. Ligamentous attachments:
   i. Typical—The attachments of either end of the collateral ligaments in the elbow and knee can be considered.
   ii. Relationships to muscles—Specific points can be found on the superior or lateral C7 spinous process. The base of the occiput may represent spinalis muscles or the nuchal ligament.
   iii. Relationships to nerves—The flexor retinaculum and palmar aponeurosis of the hand are related to the median nerve in the forearm and hand. These, in turn, are also related to attachments with at least four bones (pisiform, hamate, scaphoid, and trapezium) of the retinaculum.

e. Bones (they and their components should be considered as connective tissue as well):
   i. Construction of joints—Joint capsules connect two or more bones. They are stronger at the elbow and the knee and are reinforced on their medial and lateral surfaces by collateral ligaments. The anterior and posterior surfaces are relatively weaker and may tighten or loosen in extreme motion. Points may occur in the middle of the capsule and at the bony attachments.
   ii. Lever action—Muscle tendons and ligaments attach to bony prominences. When long-term force is applied to them through activity, they enlarge into tubercles, trochanters, and other processes. Points located at tendinous insertions may also represent contribution from the bony attachments.

f. Vascular (they and their components should be considered as connective tissue as well):
   i. Arteries—Some large arteries travel long distances within the extremities and are responsible for the overall nutrition of the surrounding tissue. Sympathetic nerves also travel with and modify the constriction of the arteries, such as in Raynaud syndrome and in complex regional pain syndromes.
   ii. Veins—The superficial veins often travel with structures such as the nerves. However, be careful when addressing vascular structures with PINS or inhibition, since thrombi and/or phlebitis may be present, exacerbated or created by the sustained pressure.
   iii. Lymphatics—As a secondary drainage system, the lymphatics help move substances, such as immunocompetent cells, in the lymph to all regions of the body and are under intrinsic as well as sympathetic influences. Release of tensions within these structures may result in release of congestion.

11. Press both the primary and end points simultaneously, using the pads of a finger on each hand (Fig. 62.9).

For simplicity and easier comprehension, identify the primary point as the "first point" for the patient. A pound or two of pressure is exerted, which should be enough to elicit the patient's symptoms, and applied equally on both the primary and end points. The patient may initially experience a mild-to-moderate increase in sensitivity. Also, the soft tissue response to the initial pressure should be noted.

   a. Acute dysfunctions may be more sensitive than chronic ones. A hypertonic muscle will usually be more sensitive to pressure than the same muscle on the contralateral side.
   b. Chronic hypertonic muscles will usually be larger than those on the contralateral side.
      i. Larger muscles do not necessarily indicate dysfunction. Asymmetric use, where one side is being used more than the other, will result in the dominant side becoming typically larger.
      ii. Whether dysfunctional or not, frequently used muscles, or ones in chronic dysfunction, may not be very sensitive to pressure due to chronic use and histologic alterations.
   c. Both sides can simultaneously be dysfunctional. One side may be more symptomatic than the other. The more dysfunctional side should be treated first; afterward, evaluate the other side and treat if necessary.
   d. A firmer muscle is probably in greater dysfunction.

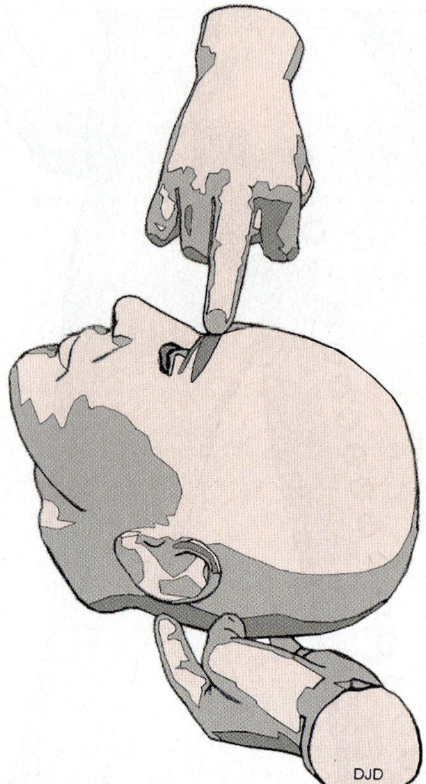

Figure 62.9. Press both the primary point and end point simultaneously using the pad region of a finger on each hand. (Courtesy of Dennis J. Dowling, DO, FAAO, with permission.)

12. It is important that the same amount of pressure be exerted on both the primary and end points:
   a. Patients may assume that the point in a more sensitive location is being pressed harder. They should be reassured that the perceived asymmetry is due to greater dysfunction or hyperactivity of the involved tissue.
   b. Patients may verbalize that they can tolerate greater pressure. Increasing the amount of pressure is not necessary, does not accelerate the treatment, maybe more irritating, and would be counterproductive.
   c. Pain or tenderness may not be the only sensations experienced due to the applied pressure. The patient may report other sensations occurring alone or in combination with pain.

13. Constant pressure must be maintained on the end point throughout the treatment. This has been an important determination after many treatments and review by others who have integrated PINS into their practice. Some have even made discussion that PINS, in general, and the end points are a way of locating "key lesions." The pressure on the point with greater

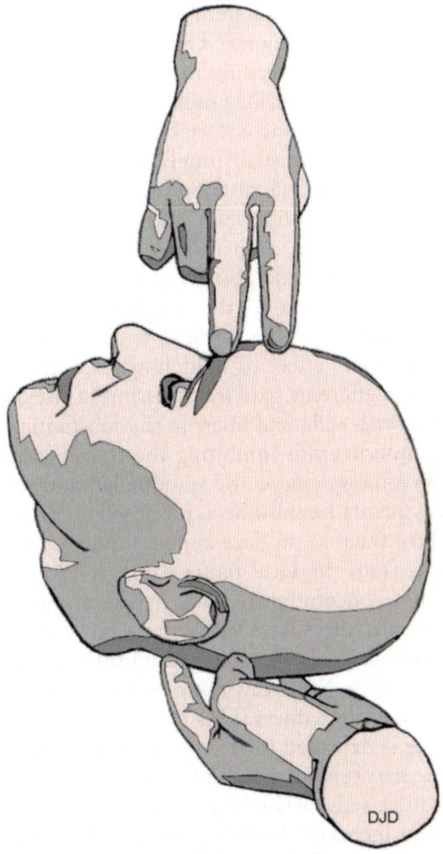

Figure 62.10. One finger remains on the primary point. Use another finger of the same hand to locate a "secondary point." If the middle finger is on the primary point, then use the index finger to palpate the secondary point. (Courtesy of Dennis J. Dowling, DO, FAAO, with permission.)

sensitivity (primary point) represents a type of facilitated component. The patient can give feedback. When inhibition is utilized properly, any increase in sensitivity at a point will likely be transient. It is also common for sensitivity to rapidly decrease, in seconds to minutes, as the tissue accommodates the irritation of the inhibition. Ultimately, it may completely disappear. However, it is very common for contact with the primary point to be held for 20 to 30 seconds before seeking any subsequent intervening points:

a. The primary point's sensitivity does not need to completely abate before searching for subsequent points.
b. One finger remains on the primary point, and often another finger on the same hand is used to locate a "secondary point." If the middle finger is on the primary point, then the index finger is used to palpate the secondary point (Fig. 62.10).
c. The search for a secondary point should be approximately 2 to 3 cm away from the primary point, along an imaginary line connecting the primary- and end points. This typically follows the predicted course of an anatomical structure:
    i. Innervating nerve
    ii. Along the direction of the muscle fibers, bone, and/or blood vessel
    iii. Following fascial planes:
    Because the structures are variable, the secondary point may actually be located along an arc that occurs 2 to 3 cm into the direction of the end point and not in a direct line. Muscles may be more linear in their patterns while nerves and vessels may show "zig-zag" elements
d. The secondary point should be identified as "the second point" for the patient.

14. Exert equal pressure onto both the primary and the secondary points while maintaining the constant pressure on the end point (It is important to attempt to exert the same pressure in order that the patient can make a selection as to which is more sensitive, the primary or the secondary; the end point needs to have pressure throughout the whole treatment with PINS).
15. Request that the patient determine which of the two points (primary vs. secondary or "first vs. second") is more sensitive:
    a. To simplify this for the patient, use a phrase such as "I am pressing on two points that are close together. Please tell me which of the two, the 'first' or the 'second,' is more sensitive." The physician could also say, "I am going to press on another point, close to where my right middle finger is pressing now, and I want you to tell me which one bothers you more."
    b. If the second point is more or equally as sensitive as the first:
        i. Relieve the pressure from the first (primary) point, and then remove it entirely.
        ii. Maintain constant pressure on the new, second (secondary) sensitive point for an additional 20 to 30 seconds. Identify it as the new primary point.
        iii. It is not necessary to wait for the sensitivity at any point to be completely resolved before moving on to the next point. It is more important that each subsequent point is more sensitive than the prior one.
        iv. There can be both increased tension and sensitivity in the new secondary point. With practice, the "secondary" points can be located by palpatory sense of tension alone. A return to a lower level of sensitivity and response baseline usually occurs after a few seconds. The amount of time depends on the soft tissue response.
    c. Before progress can be made, certain points may require further inhibition. When this is complete, a new secondary point may be located where previously there was less sensitivity. If the original or a subsequent "first point" persists as the more sensitive of the two points:
        i. Maintain pressure at the location of the primary point for an additional 20 to 30 seconds.
        ii. Move the finger that was locating the secondary point more laterally or medially from the theoretical connecting line in an arc that is 2 to 3 cm from the primary point. A new located secondary point should have at least the same, if not more sensitivity than the primary point. The anatomical structure (whether muscle, nerve, fascia, etc.) being inhibited may have slight variations in the specific course in this patient.
        iii. Once an equally or more sensitive secondary point is located, relieve pressure from the primary point, and maintain pressure on the new secondary point as described above.
        iv. This secondary point then becomes the new "first" point in the continuing treatment toward the end point.
16. Inhibit the end point with constant pressure, with a finger of the other hand. The patient will often forget that this point is being treated. Continuous treatment is necessary to anchor the dysfunctional tissue, which may lose sensitivity during the process.

17. Repeat the process until an ultimate "second" point is located 2 to 3 cm from the end point.
18. Once the two final points have been treated with inhibition, determine the amount of dysfunction that persists, especially at the end point location. It may have significantly reduced or disappeared completely.
19. All of the intervening points are part of the dysfunction. Therefore, symptoms can persist when the primary point (chief complaint) is treated by another method. It is not so much that it is not a part of the problem but rather one component in a "reverberating circuit."
20. Occasionally, pressure on one of the intervening points between the primary and end points results in a recurrence of the chief complaint, radiation of symptoms from this point to the end point, the primary point, or both. This effectively indicates the continuity of the dysfunction and the need for this thorough treatment. Prior to treatment of the pattern, this possibility can be instructed to the patient. This can be seen as a positive occurrence since it indicates the inclusions and connectivity of the continuum of sensitive points that the patient may not have appreciated previously.
21. Another modality can be used if the dysfunction, including the end point, remains persistent. The end point and overall dysfunction may now be easier to treat than prior. Possibilities include FPR, counterstrain, muscle energy, balanced ligamentous tension techniques, or some other modalities. High velocity low amplitude (HVLA) that was previously difficult to perform may now be easier. Guidelines for determining the appropriate treatment include:
    a. The persistence of the dysfunction or related components after treatment
    b. The ability of the physician to perform other modalities of treatment
    c. The need for or capability of the patient to tolerate additional treatment
    d. The relevant indications and contraindications for such modalities for this patient
22. The conclusion of treatment should be based on palpatory findings, not solely on the patient's subjective complaints. Overtreatment can cause as many problems as under treatment.
23. Patients may limit types of treatment based on prior experience or misconceptions. A patient with no previous difficulties could also have developed a dislike for a particular modality (i.e., "popping" secondary to HVLA). Attempting to coerce a patient into certain forms of treatment would be counterproductive to the therapeutic relationship. It could also be considered illegal (i.e., battery).
24. The somatic dysfunction is always reassessed.
25. Even a relatively comfortable treatment can result in a post-treatment reaction. Inform the patient that reactions can include transient soreness, aches, and fatigue. Ecchymosis may occur in patients prone to bruising or in those with other predisposing factors (i.e., medication). This can also occur with the use of excessive pressure. Generally, all such side effects resolve in 24 to 48 hours.

Possible Mechanism of Action

An important component that distinguishes inhibitory contact from a stimulatory one is the application of a low-level, but constant, pressure to a dysfunctional tissue. The patient may be acutely sensitive at first, with complaints of increased pain, sensitivity, pressure, or some other sensation. However, these reactions decrease and may disappear altogether as the system adapts through accommodation or habituation.[38] This effect may be partly due to the reticular formation's screening mechanisms. The body accommodates other physical stimuli, such as contact with eyeglasses, tight belts, stiff clothing, uncomfortable shoes, as well as constant background auditory and visual stimuli. The spinal cord may act as a mediator or "brake" in this filtering process, when sensory overload[39] occurs. Some stimuli remain relatively subliminal, if not of sufficient quality, duration, or quantity.

Pressure or contact could also act as a possible counterirritant, which inhibits stimulation to the neighboring tissue, and thus reduces the sensitivity of the original tender point. A common example of this is the effect of scratching an itch. Large, rapidly conducting nerve afferents gate transmission in the dorsal horn of the spinal cord, with collateral fibers in the substantia gelatinosa or with adjacent interneurons inhibiting the transmission of pain to the central nervous system via the spinothalamic tract.[40]

Relative ischemia has also been proposed as a theory. Muscles in prolonged contraction produce and accumulate metabolites and waste products from the local tissue damage.[36] Impaired circulation also occurs concomitantly with hyperemia and congestion. Some of these substances have vasoactive effects, which theoretically addresses tissue injury. Trophic and fibrotic changes may occur if the injury persists. Normally, the overlying skin shows a brief blanching followed by redness. This typically fades but can persist when the tissue is damaged for a prolonged time. Applying therapeutic pressure may temporarily aid the ischemia. Though this may not make intuitive sense when considering the amount of nutrient deprivation, the increased ischemia could reduce the nociceptive receptors' capacity to process information. Once this pressure is removed, restored circulation may occur, which flushes the waste products from the region.

A muscle in dysfunction can be hypertonic, even if it appears to be in its neutral position. As the relatively shortened muscle is further stretched, the activity of the muscle spindle mechanisms increases, resulting in a reflexive and prolonged contraction as a means of protection.[39–43] Applying such slow stretching during inhibition introduces a gentle stretch, which allows the stretch receptors to reset.[44] Only a small portion of the tissue may be challenged without upsetting the whole structure. Once this small, localized component is overwhelmed, any adjacent area can subsequently be inhibited with similar results. In general, inhibition, and particularly PINS, are effective methods for addressing a series of irritated pieces. The physician can treat the entire dysfunction by progressively treating all of the involved elements.

The Golgi tendon organ is a sensory mechanism that becomes relatively stretched in muscular contractions where the overall length of the muscle does not change. When a critical amount of tension occurs especially with isometric contraction, the Golgi tendon organ increases its activity, bringing about reflex relaxation of the entire muscle. An inhibitory interneuron, between the afferent nerve ending in the spinal cord and the alpha motor neuron, induces sudden, almost complete muscular relaxation. The pressure from the physician's fingers may create an initial stretch that results in transient contraction, followed by resultant relaxation.[41]

Contraindications and Side Effects

Few contraindications and side effects are associated with the use of PINS. Pressure should not be exerted onto localized inflammations, abscesses, or infections as the integrity of the skin or walled infections may be compromised. It is also necessary to recognize other disease processes that may require nonmanipulative treatment. Metabolic, neoplastic, and autoimmune diseases among others may present symptoms that mimic some neuromusculoskeletal conditions. The presence of somatic dysfunctions does not preclude that the etiology may have visceral origins.

Research

PINS has been studied and found to have significant time effects as compared to baseline ($P < .001$) on several standardly utilized pain, disability, quality of life, and general perception of recovery and compared favorably to another manipulative technique for lumbar radiculopathy.[44,45] The combined use of both techniques in the same protocol was found to be superior to the single use of each technique.[46] PINS was more effective than a positional release treatment in the management of individuals with piriformis syndrome in another study and the effectiveness of both was thought to be enhanced by the inclusion of stretching exercises that were used as adjunct therapies that were included for both groups.[46]

SUMMARY

PINS represent a unique variation on the traditional approach to inhibition and discovering how dysfunction occurs and is maintained. It can be used alone or in combination with other methods of osteopathic manipulation. The effect of other treatment modalities can be enhanced by the use of PINS.

REFERENCES

1. Dowling DJ. Progressive inhibition of neuromuscular structures (PINS) technique. *J Am Osteopath Assoc.* 2000;100(5):285–286, 289–298.
2. *Glossary of Osteopathic Terminology.* AOA Yearbook and Directory of Osteopathic Physicians; 1998.
3. Dowling DJ, Scariati PD. Neurophysiology relevant to osteopathic principles and practice. In: DiGiovanna E, Schiowitz S, eds. *An Osteopathic Approach to Diagnosis and Treatment.* 2nd ed. Lippincott-Raven; 1997:33.
4. Ehrenfeuchter WC. Soft tissue techniques. In: Ward RC, ed. *Foundations for Osteopathic Medicine.* Williams & Wilkins; 1997:781–794.
5. Robbins SL, Kumar V, Cotran RS. *Pathologic Basis of Disease.* 3rd ed. W.B. Saunders Co.; 1984:40.
6. Still AT. *Autobiography of A.T. Still.* Revised ed. Author; 1908:32.
7. Still AT. *The Philosophy and Mechanical Principles of Osteopathy.* Hudson-Kimberly Pub. Co.; 1902:101.
8. Goetz EW. *A Manual of Osteopathy.* 2nd ed. Natures Cure Company; 1909.
9. Tasker DD. *Principles of Osteopathy.* 4th ed. Bireley & Elson Printing Co.; 1916:354–370.
10. Jones LH. *Strain and Counterstrain.* American Academy of Osteopathy; 1981.
11. Jones LH, Kusenose RS, Goering EK. *Jones Strain-Counterstrain.* Jones Strain-Counterstrain Company; 1995.
12. Glover JC, Yates HA. Strain and counterstrain techniques. In: Ward RC, ed. *Foundations for Osteopathic Medicine.* Williams & Wilkins; 1997: 809–818.
13. Dowling, DJ. Facilitated positional release. In: Seffinger MA, ed. *Foundations for Osteopathic Medicine.* 4th ed. Wolters Kluwer; 218: 990–997.
14. Van Buskirk RL. A manipulative technique of Andrew Taylor Still as reported by Charles Hazzard, DO, in 1905. *J Am Osteopath Assoc.* 1996;96(10):597–602.
15. Schiowitz S. Chapter 16. Still technique. In: DiGiovanna E, Schiowitz S, eds. *An Osteopathic Approach to Diagnosis and Treatment.* 2nd ed. Lippincott-Raven; 1997:91.
16. Hazzard C. *The Practice and Applied Therapeutics of Osteopathy.* Journal Printing Co.; 1905.
17. Johnston WL. Functional technique: an indirect method. In: Ward RC, ed. *Foundations for Osteopathic Medicine.* Williams & Wilkins; 1997:795–808.
18. Chila AG. Fascial-ligamentous release: an indirect approach. In: Ward RC, ed. *Foundations for Osteopathic Medicine.* Williams & Wilkins; 1997: 819–830.
19. Ward RC. Integrated neuromusculoskeletal release and myofascial release: an introduction to diagnosis and treatment. In: Ward RC, ed. *Foundations for Osteopathic Medicine.* Williams & Wilkins; 1997:846–849.
20. Typaldos S. Introducing the fascial distortion model. *AAO J.* 1994;4(2).
21. Capistrant T, Harrer G. *The Fascial Distortion Model.* 1st ed. Handspring Publishing Limited. 2021. https://www.perlego.com/book/2789687/the-fascial-distortion-model-philosophy-principles-and-clinical-applications-pdf (Original work published 2021)
22. Chaitlow L. *Osteopathic Self-Treatment.* Thorsons Publishing Group; 1990: 105–119.
23. Chaitow L. *Neuro-Muscular Technique.* Thorsons Publishers Ltd; 1980.
24. Chaitow L. *Modern Neuromuscular Techniques.* Churchill Livingstone; 1996.
25. Owens C. *An Endocrine Interpretation of Chapman's Reflexes.* 2nd ed. Chattanooga Printing and Engraving Co.; 1937.
26. Cyriax J. *Text-Book of Orthopaedic Medicine Volume II: Treatment by Manipulation and Massage.* 6th ed. Harper & Row; 1959.
27. Travell JG, Simmons DG. *Myofascial Pain and Dysfunction: The Trigger Point Manual: The Upper Extremities.* Vol. I. Williams & Wilkins; 1983.
28. Kenyon J. *Acupressure Techniques: A Self Help Guide.* Healing Arts Press; 1988.
29. Cerney JV. *Acupuncture Without Needles.* Parker Publishing Company, Inc.; 1974.
30. Weil A. *Spontaneous Healing.* Ballantine Books; 1995.
31. The Burton Goldberg Group. *Alternative Medicine: The Definitive Guide.* Future Medicine Publishing, Inc.; 1994.
32. Shultz W. *Shiatsu: Japanese Finger Pressure Therapy.* Bell Publishing Company; 1976.
33. Prudden B. *Pain Erasure: The Bonnie Prudden Way.* Ballantine Books; 1980.
34. Dr. Ida Rolf Institute. What is Rolfing? What is Rolfing® Structural Integration? https://www.rolf.org/rolfing.php
35. Facts About Reflexology. https://www.reflexology-usa.net/facts.htm
36. Dowling DJ. S.T.A.R.: a more viable alternative descriptor system of somatic dysfunction. *AAO J.* 1998;8(2):34–37.
37. Bailey HW. Some problems in making osteopathic spinal manipulative therapy appropriate and specific. *J Am Osteopath Assoc.* 1976;75(5): 486–499.
38. Patterson MM. A model mechanism for spinal segmental facilitation. *J Am Osteopath Assoc.* 1976;76(1):62–72.
39. Ganong WF. *Review of Medical Physiology.* Lange; 1995.
40. Stoddard A. *Manual of Osteopathic Practice.* Hutchinson Medical Publications; 1969:238.
41. Buzzell KA. The potential disruptive influence of somatic input. In: Kugelmass IN, ed. *The Physiological Basis of Osteopathic Medicine. The Postgraduate Institute of Osteopathic Medicine and Surgery.* Insight Publishing Company; 1967:39–51.
42. Becker RF. The gamma system and its relation to the development and maintenance of muscle tone. In: Peterson B, ed. *1976 Year Book of the American Academy of Osteopathy.* American Academy of Osteopathy; 1976:26–40.
43. Korr IM. Proprioceptors and somatic dysfunction. *J Am Osteopath Assoc.* 1975;74:638–650. Reprinted in: *1976 Year Book of the American Academy of Osteopathy.* American Academy of Osteopathy; 1976:41–50 and in *The Collected Papers of Irvin M. Korr.* American Academy of Osteopathy; 1979:200–207.
44. Bello B, Danazumi MS, Kaka B. Comparative effectiveness of 2 manual therapy techniques in the management of lumbar radiculopathy: a randomized clinical trial. *J Chiropr Med.* 2019;18(4):253–260.
45. Danazumi MS, Bello B, Yakasai AM, Kaka B. Two manual therapy techniques for management of lumbar radiculopathy: a randomized clinical trial. *J Osteopath Med.* 2021;121(4):391–400.
46. Danazumi MS, Yakasai AM, Ibrahim AA, Shehu UT, Ibrahim SU. Effect of integrated neuromuscular inhibition technique compared with positional release technique in the management of piriformis syndrome. *J Osteopath Med.* 121(8):693–703.

63 Fascial Distortion Model

TODD CAPISTRANT ▪ THOMAS PENTZER ▪ JESSICA PELLETIER

KEY CONCEPTS

- The fascial distortion model is a patient-centered model of diagnosis and treatment in which the patient is considered the expert and directs the clinician.
- Fascial distortions are pathologic alterations of the body's fascia that can manifest as somatic complaints.
- Patients convey these distortions by unconsciously using six constellations of body language and descriptors, which (in conjunction with history and physical exam) guide the treatment.

"The fascial distortion model (FDM) is an anatomical perspective in which the underlying etiology of virtually every musculoskeletal injury (and many neurological and medical conditions as well) is considered to be comprised of one or more of six specific pathological alterations of the body's connecting tissues (fascial bands, ligaments, tendons, retinacula, etc). This model not only allows for strikingly effective manipulative treatments for diverse afflictions such as pulled muscles, fractures, and frozen shoulders, but the results are objective, obvious, measurable, and immediate."

–Stephen Typaldos, DO[1]

INTRODUCTION

The Fascial Distortion Model (FDM) developed from the observations and personal experience of Stephen Typaldos, DO beginning in 1991. Dr. Typaldos encountered a particular patient who refused to leave his office until he treated her. When he admitted that he did not know what to do to help her, the patient guided his treatment of the Star Triggerband.[2] (see Star Triggerband case at the end of the chapter) That treatment stirred the ideas which later formed into the FDM. During his life, Dr. Typaldos produced four editions of a textbook on the FDM. In his initial work, he did not refer to his work as the FDM, but rather by the title "Orthopathic Medicine."[1] He found this title to be confusing to would-be students of the Model and he later felt that the name did not fully reflect what he was developing. By viewing this as a model of thinking, rather than a set of treatment techniques, one is able to visualize how fascia may behave within the human body. Thus, it came to be known as the FDM. Through the perspective of the FDM, the mechanism of many osteopathic techniques can be explained and understood. The development of the FDM occurred over several years, with one distortion at a time being uncovered in Dr. Typaldos' mind. The distortions were identified as he tried to explain what the patient was identifying as their source of pain and what treatment was successful at providing the patient relief. As Dr. Typaldos uncovered new ideas and concepts, these were presented to the osteopathic community via publications in the American Academy of Osteopathy Journal (AAOJ)[3–5] and new editions of his textbook. He presented courses on his new ideas domestically and abroad and many practicing osteopathic physicians attended his presentations.

Dr. Typaldos was very enthusiastic about the success he was having with his new ideas. He felt compelled to share the FDM with his fellow osteopathic physicians. During the development of the FDM he presented his ideas in a very dogmatic way and as a stand-alone concept that superseded much of what was being taught and understood about osteopathic manipulative medicine (OMM). He also embraced a very direct style of treatment that used a significant amount of force with his treatments; the FDM is associated with pain and often bruising. The direct and intense nature of some of the FDM treatments, in part, led to resistance to the FDM being embraced by the osteopathic community. Dr. Typaldos became frustrated with his fellow American osteopathic physicians who were not as enthusiastic and who did not immediately see the importance, benefits, and success that his work was allowing him to achieve with his patients. These frustrations led him to Europe, where the model has been embraced and has a substantial following to this day. Much of the success of the FDM in Europe can be directly tied to the powerful and effective teaching style of Georg Harrer, MD. Dr. Harrer became the leading instructor in Europe for many years and was the main instructor in the United States after the passing of Dr. Typaldos.[6]

Dr. Typaldos passed away early in life at the age of 49 in 2006.[7] He was actively developing the concepts of the FDM at the time of his passing. When he passed away there were no certified instructors of the FDM in the United States. The organization American Fascial Distortion Model Association (AFDMA) took on the mission of spreading his work in the osteopathic community and beyond. Dr. Typaldos felt strongly that the FDM should be a physician-driven model. He envisioned the FDM fundamentally changing how medicine was practiced and felt that it should be included in all aspects of medical training. The AFDMA rigidly adhered to this idea that DOs and MDs should be taught the model above all others. Dr. Harrer was teaching the courses in the United States at the time. Eventually, in 2010, the first group of American FDM instructors took and passed the difficult instructor exam that Dr. Typaldos had left behind. With instructors now located in the United States, the AFDMA was able to arrange more courses in a more cost-effective manner than importing instructors from Europe. With the increased number of courses, awareness of the model began to spread.

An enormous opportunity was presented to the AFDMA by Melicien Tettambel, DO, FAAO, who was the chair of the OMM department at Pacific Northwest University College of Osteopathic

Medicine (PNWU) in Yakima, Washington. She invited the AFDMA to provide brief presentations to the PNWU students and subsequently agreed to host all the FDM modules on the campus. Dr. Tettambel attended these modules, and as a leader in the osteopathic community, she helped shape the path of the FDM to be reintroduced to the American Academy of Osteopathy (AAO) and the remainder of the osteopathic community in America. Dr. Tettambel could see the power of the FDM and felt that FDM helped explain many osteopathic teachings including the field of Osteopathic Cranial Manipulative Medicine.

Over the years since Dr. Typaldos' passing, the concepts originally developed have continued to be supported by the clinical results seen while applying the FDM to patients who are experiencing pain, limited range of motion (ROM), and functional restriction. As the model has continued to spread through the field of osteopathic medicine, more and more research is being performed on the tissue of fascia and the FDM itself. As a natural progression of the FDM, the universality of the concepts contained within the model led the AFDMA to open its courses to more types of medical providers. As a result, FDM courses today include participants from a wide range of medical professions, including physical therapists, athletic trainers, dentists, chiropractors, nurse practitioners, physician assistants, occupational therapists, and more. This expansion into many areas of the medical professions has helped propel the FDM toward Dr. Typaldos' aim to fundamentally change the practice of medicine.

The FDM encourages a practitioner to change perspectives and challenge traditional teachings. In the musculoskeletal world of allopathic medicine, injuries are often seen as being primarily the result of tissues being torn, broken, or inflamed. As medical providers our treatment is designed to correct these underlying causes of pain. Physicians continue to address these issues even when sensitive testing modalities reveal nothing torn, broken, or inflamed. Why is this? It is human nature to match observations within our schemata, even when they are not a perfect match. Physicians are taught early in our medical training that the injuries above are the causes of musculoskeletal pain. When those conditions are not present, the clinician is left with no mental framework or model from which to work. This is where the FDM introduces a new paradigm to illuminate the source of a patient's complaints. The FDM explains many of the pain complaints that do not respond to traditional or standard treatment. By working in the FDM, one can expand their perspective beyond the traditional torn, broken, and inflamed approach, opening avenues for powerful treatment outcomes.

As mentioned above, FDM was originally a very direct and often uncomfortable technique. The intensity required to treat the distortions has evolved over time. The initial approach to treating these distortions was extremely direct and intense, with little attention to the palpation of the distortion and variation of treatment intensity based on tissue texture changes, asymmetry, restriction of ROM, and tenderness (TART) changes. The refinement of the FDM has led to the realization that less force may be required than originally thought, and that the degree of force should be tailored to the individual patient's needs. The intensity of the treatment needed to obtain the desired results is related to the ability of the practitioner to palpate TART changes, the patient's tolerance of the procedure, and the need for a practitioner to function throughout a clinical day. Understanding that the correction of a fascial distortion can be achieved by modulating force while using the proper FDM technique and appreciating TART changes has allowed the treatments to be more acceptable to patients and practitioners who eschew direct treatment styles.

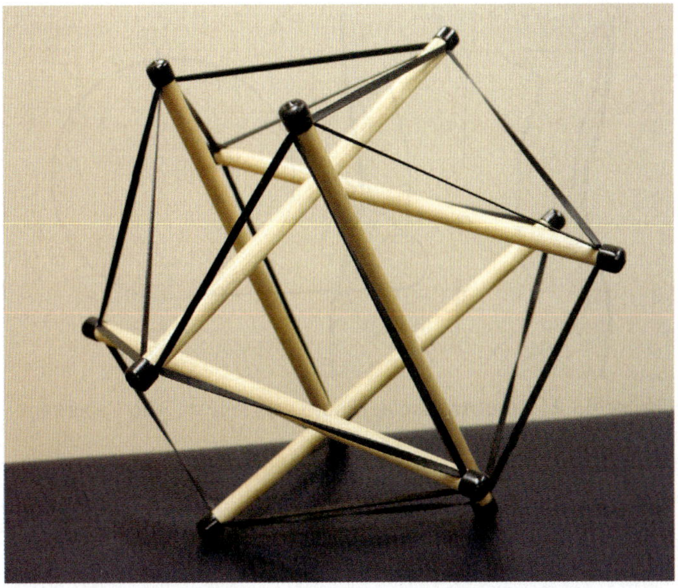

Figure 63.1. Tensegrity model. (Photo by Todd Capistrant.)

TENSEGRITY

The FDM as an osteopathic model is rooted in the importance of fascia as a key component of the concept of tensegrity, the interrelatedness of all anatomic structures of the body that allows it to function as a homogenous physiologic unit. The fascia and associated soft tissues serve as a significant tensional component in the body as a structure.[8] An examination of tensegrity structures (Fig. 63.1) will reveal that the beams within the tensegrity unit do not contact each other directly. Instead, they are connected by cables that exert tension on the beams, maintaining each beam in position relative to each other.[9] Extending this concept of tensegrity to the human body, the soft tissues (loosely defined as fascia) of the body provide the tensional support to keep the beams—in this case, the bones—from directly contacting one another. Any alteration or change to the tension within the fascial structure is associated with an alteration in the tensegrity structure. This concept is known as biotensegrity. As stated in the tenets of osteopathy, structure and function are reciprocally interrelated. Thus, a breakdown in the tensegrity structure can lead to a change in function. This change in function is often associated with a patient's complaint of pain, decreased ROM, or stiffness. Therefore, fascial changes, or distortions, may lead to changes in the structure and function of the body by altering tensegrity.

An excellent example often shared with patients is the tensegrity of a joint, such as the knee. Under the normal tensional structure, the bones of the knee are repelled from one another by the soft tissue tension that surrounds the knee.[10] Just as the beams of the tensegrity model are supported by the flexible portion of the structure, the bones of the body are supported within the fascia. When the tissues are functioning normally, the bones are supported within a tissue matrix and the joint functions without bone impacting other bone. When dysfunctions (or distortions) occur in the soft tissues of the joint, the function of the joint is impacted, potentially damaging soft tissue and causing pain.

FASCIA AS A UNIFYING CONCEPT

In the initial teachings of the FDM, Dr. Typaldos was striving to keep the FDM separate from the classic modalities of osteopathy.

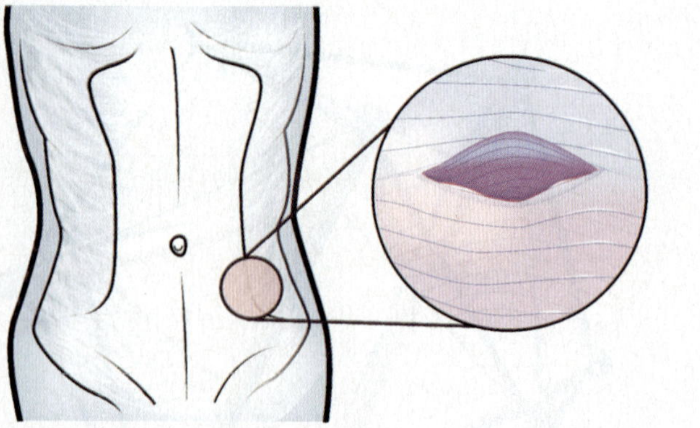

Figure 63.2. **Smooth fascia.** (Photo courtesy of Todd Capistrant.)

However, over the course of the FDM's development and teaching, it has become clear that the FDM's concepts of how the fascia theoretically behaves help elucidate many of the treatment modalities used by osteopathic physicians.

The FDM identifies four types of fascia: banded, smooth, folding, and circular. These fascial types are thought to represent how the fascial matrix responds to forces applied against it; this is a functional concept and not necessarily based on anatomical differences identified in fascia. As the concepts of the FDM continued to evolve, it was understood that since the distortions can occur anywhere in the body, these four fascial types needed to occur anywhere in the body. This means that the fascial matrix has the capacity to behave as any one of these subtypes in response to forces that are applied to the matrix.[1,6]

Smooth Fascia

Smooth fascia (Fig. 63.2) is visualized as sheets of fascia stacked on top of each other in the fascial matrix. These fascial layers slide past one another as the body moves. Any alteration of the matrix's ability to slide and glide is seen as an alteration of the smooth fascia. The Herniated Triggerpoint (HTP) and Tectonic Fixation (TF) are thought to occur in the smooth fascia of the matrix.[6]

Banded Fascia

Banded fascia (Fig. 63.3) is visualized as strong tensional tissue that is resistant to parallel forces, but weak when perpendicular forces are applied to it. One can imagine a cable of fascial tissue, comprised of many filaments. Forces oriented perpendicular to the banded fascia may fray or disrupt the fascial matrix and potentially lead to a distortion of the fascial matrix. Triggerbands (TBs) and Continuum Distortions (CDs) are associated with banded fascia in the FDM.

Folding Fascia

Folding fascia (Fig. 63.4) can be viewed as the embodiment of the fascial matrix's ability to absorb force. The matrix compresses and expands based on force applied to the tissues. A folding distortion (FD) is felt to be an alteration of the matrix's ability to expand and contract. FDs are subdivided into unfolding (uFD) and refolding (rFD) distortions of the folding fascia. The image of an accordion with its pleats able to move back and forth is one way to visualize the folding fascia. Alteration of a pleat can prevent the normal function of the accordion.

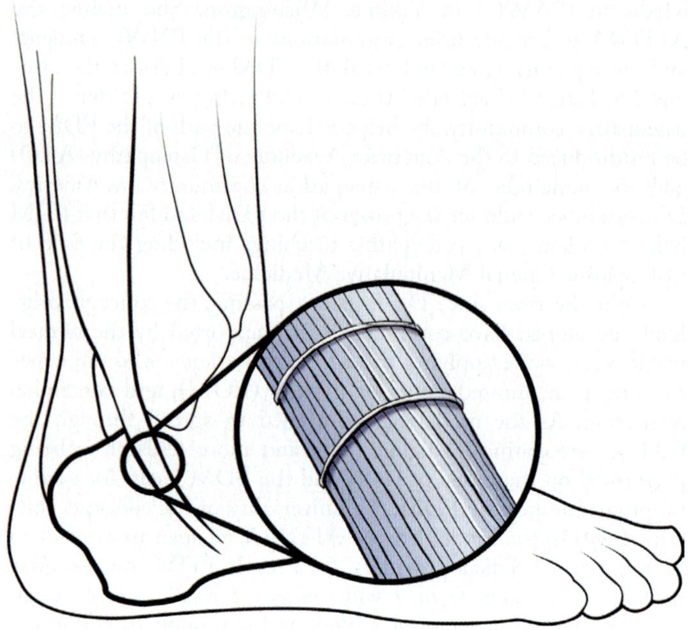

Figure 63.3. **Banded fascia.** (Photo courtesy of Todd Capistrant.)

Coiled Fascia

Coiled fascia (Fig. 63.5) represents the most superficial layer of fascia and is thought to exist just beneath the skin. When behaving as coiled fascia, the fascial matrix is envisioned to contain cylindrical coils of fascia sliding beneath the skin, aligned with the long axis of the body and limbs. When a disruptive force is applied to the matrix, the coils overlap each other, becoming tangled or snarled. External forces generated by restrictive garments, casts, or splints may restrict the coils' ability to slide, causing dysfunction. It is also thought that internal mechanisms such as inflammation may contribute to dysfunction in the circular fascia. Dysfunction of the coiled fascia is identified as a Cylinder Distortion (CyD) in the FDM.

These fascial types can explain and be integrated into traditional osteopathic techniques. For example, indirect techniques such as balanced ligamentous tension (BLT) and facilitated positional release (FPR) can be explained in terms of behaviors of folding fascia. When utilizing high-velocity low-amplitude (HVLA) techniques, the folding fascia mechanism can also be used to assist with treatment.

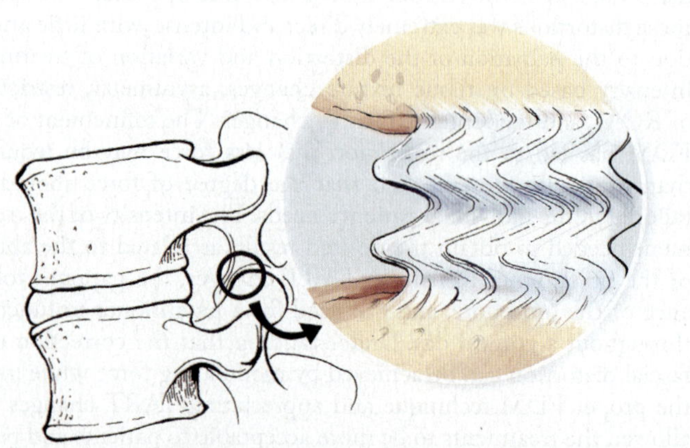

Figure 63.4. **Folding fascia.** (Photo courtesy of Todd Capistrant.)

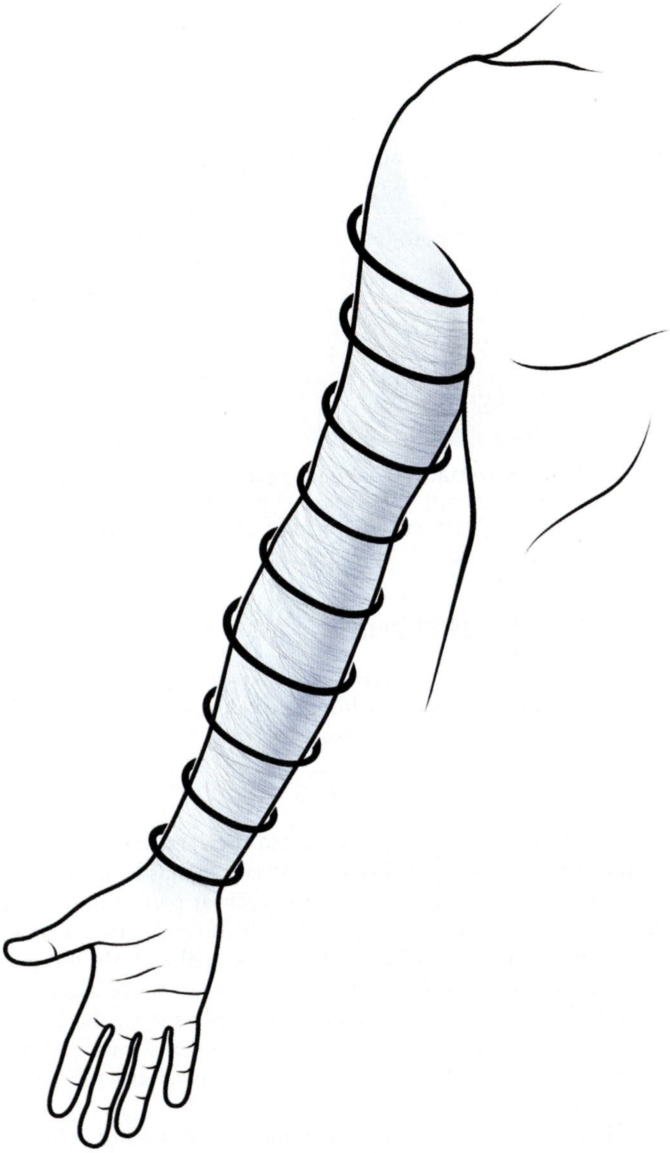

Figure 63.5. **Coiled fascia.** (Photo courtesy of Todd Capistrant.)

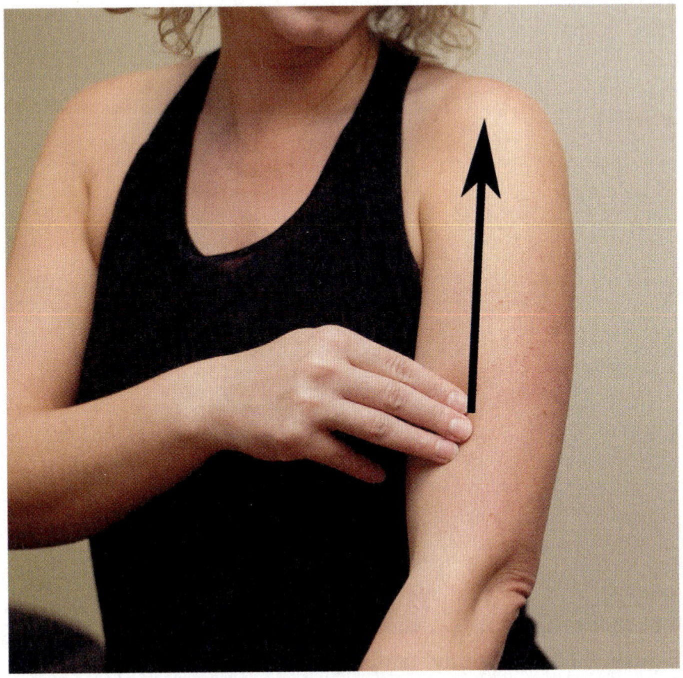

Figure 63.6. **TB body language.** Arrow indicating direction of sweeping fingertips. (Reprinted with permission from Capistrant T, Harrer G, Pentzer T, eds. *The Fascial Distortion Model: Philosophy, Principles and Clinical Applications.* Handspring Publishing; 2021.)

KEY TENETS OF THE FDM

When working within the FDM, there are several key concepts that will guide a practitioner to an accurate FDM diagnosis followed by an effective FDM treatment.

The idea that a patient intuitively knows what needs to happen to their body to improve and restore motion is foundational to the FDM. Patients will often try multiple methods by which to correct their pain. For example, a patient will attempt to reduce an HTP using a tennis ball or a foam roller and will only present for treatment after they have been unsuccessful on their own.

In the FDM it is believed that the patient will use a standard and universal body language (or gestures) to explain their pain.[1,6,11] In addition to the body language, specific words have been identified and associated with each of the distortions. Keen observation and skilled listening are critical to successful implementation of the FDM. FDM practitioners looking to increase their skills and the effective use of FDM in practice will spend considerable time watching and listening to patients as they describe their complaints. This uninterrupted listening allows a physician to connect with the patient. When patients of an FDM practitioner are surveyed, they often report that this is the first time a provider really listened to them (Figs. 63.6 to 63.8).

The goal of the FDM is the removal of the fascial distortions that are inhibiting the normal function of the fascial matrix, which are in turn impeding the body's ability to heal itself. In the FDM, it is believed that correction of fascial distortions eliminates the dysfunction of the fascial matrix, restoring normal function and allowing the patient to resume normal activities.[1,6] This is commonly seen in the FDM treatment of sprains. Upon removing the identified distortions, the patient will demonstrate improved ROM, proprioception, strength, and overall function with noticeable decrease of pain. Since the distortions are no longer present, the patient is allowed to resume normal activities at a much more rapid rate than is often seen with traditional musculoskeletal care.

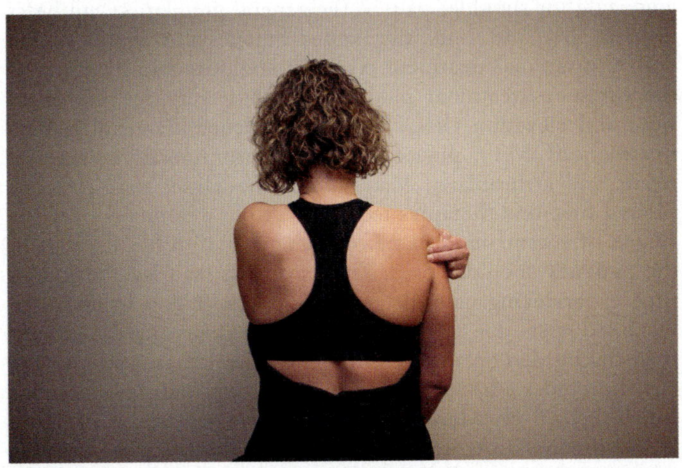

Figure 63.7. **HTP body language.** (Reprinted with permission from Capistrant T, Harrer G, Pentzer T, eds. *The Fascial Distortion Model: Philosophy, Principles and Clinical Applications.* Handspring Publishing; 2021.)

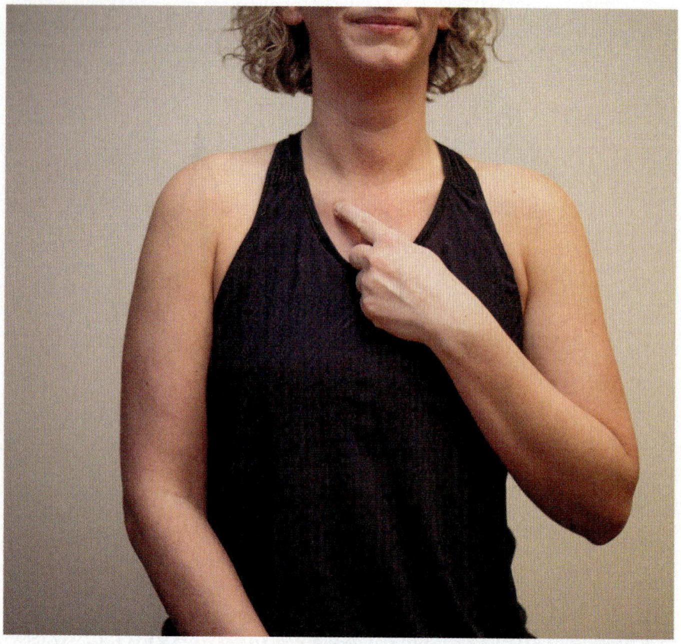

Figure 63.8. CD body language. (Reprinted with permission from Capistrant T, Harrer G, Pentzer T, eds. *The Fascial Distortion Model: Philosophy, Principles and Clinical Applications*. Handspring Publishing; 2021.)

In addition to the body language and verbal description provided by the patient, the mechanism of injury and objective findings on physical exam are combined to guide the practitioner to the clinical FDM diagnosis (which then directs the treatment).

For this chapter, a special emphasis will be placed on demonstrating the use of the FDM in the shoulder region. It is important to understand that the fascial distortions can occur throughout the body and are not limited to the shoulder region. The reader of this chapter should be able to effectively apply the FDM to the shoulder at the completion of this chapter and should also be capable of identifying and treating fascial distortions in other body regions.

Shoulder pain is a very common patient complaint and is frequently seen in the settings of primary care, sports medicine, and orthopedics. One study estimates that the 1-year prevalence rate for shoulder pain in the general population can be as high as 50%.[12] In 2000, the United States spent over 7 billion dollars in annual treatment costs for shoulder pain.[13] Some of the common treatment modalities include rest, ice, compression, and elevation (RICE) therapy, osteopathic manipulative treatment (OMT), physical therapy, joint injections, surgical repair, and arthroplasty. Many of the modalities that are considered first-line therapies require multiple treatments over the course of several months before achieving significant relief of the patient's shoulder pain. This approach may lead to longer time experiencing pain, decreasing quality of life. In addition, increased costs due to more treatment sessions place a greater financial burden on the patient and the healthcare system. The FDM provides a treatment modality that has found tremendous success effectively addressing shoulder pain, reduced ROM, and function complaints in one or two treatment sessions. Patients often experience marked reduction of pain and improved ROM shortly after treatment. This rapid symptomatic improvement decreases pain duration and often leads to fewer treatments and decreased financial burden.

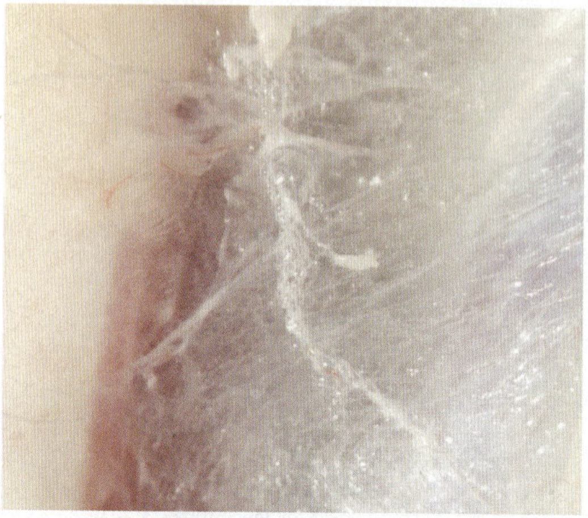

Figure 63.9. Presumed TB in goat fascia. (Reprinted with permission from Capistrant T, Harrer G, Pentzer T, eds. *The Fascial Distortion Model: Philosophy, Principles and Clinical Applications*. Handspring Publishing; 2021.)

FASCIAL DISTORTIONS

The six distortions identified in the FDM are TB, HTP, CD, FD (including unfolding and refolding), CyD, and TF.[1] These are described in the order of their discovery.

Triggerband(s) (TB)

The TB is a twist or wrinkle in the banded fascial matrix (Fig. 63.9). It is thought that the banded type of fascia responds to an external force and no longer functions as a strong linear part of the fascial matrix. A patient experiencing a TB will often describe a pulling, burning, or tightness. The gesture associated with the TB is a sweeping motion of the tip of one or more fingers in the exact linear path of the TB. The exact location is important for the FDM practitioner, as this guides the treatment of the TB. Treatment of a TB should occur exactly where the patient demonstrates their pain (Figs. 63.10 to 63.15).

TBs are noted to start at a point and end at another point. A fascial twist or wrinkle between these two points manifests as a connecting pathway of pain. To treat a TB, the practitioner applies direct pressure focused through the tip of their thumb, visualizing

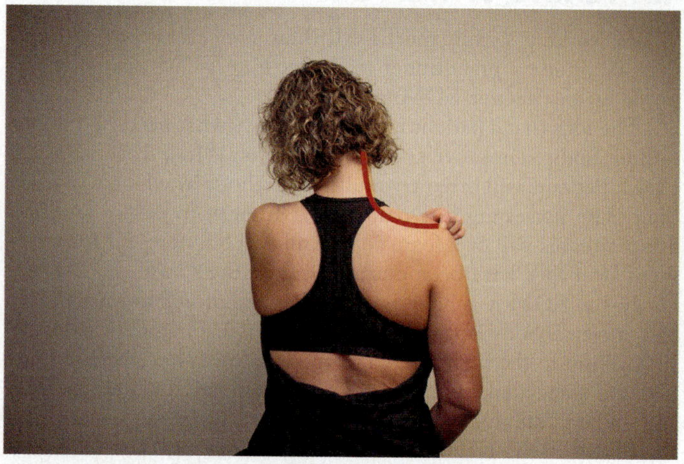

Figure 63.10. Shoulder mastoid TB gesture. (Reprinted with permission from Capistrant T, Harrer G, Pentzer T, eds. *The Fascial Distortion Model: Philosophy, Principles and Clinical Applications*. Handspring Publishing; 2021.)

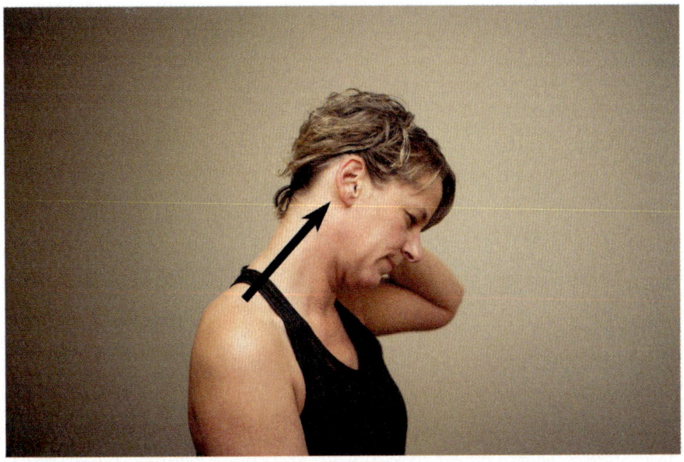

Figure 63.11. Shoulder mastoid TB treatment pathway. (Reprinted with permission from Capistrant T, Harrer G, Pentzer T, eds. *The Fascial Distortion Model: Philosophy, Principles and Clinical Applications*. Handspring Publishing; 2021.)

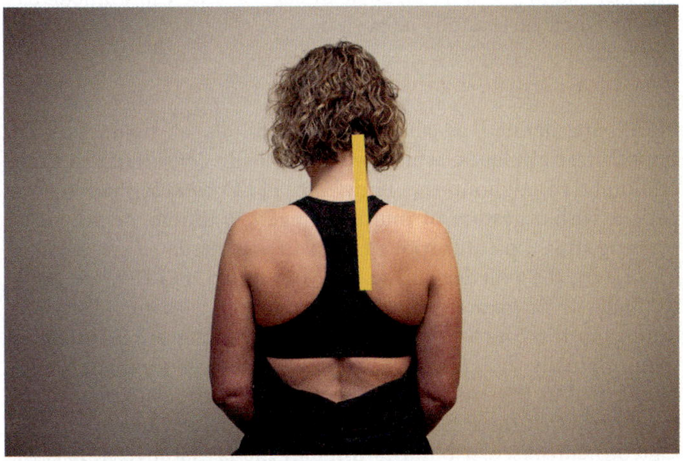

Figure 63.12. Star TB pathway. (Reprinted with permission from Capistrant T, Harrer G, Pentzer T, eds. *The Fascial Distortion Model: Philosophy, Principles and Clinical Applications.* Handspring Publishing; 2021.)

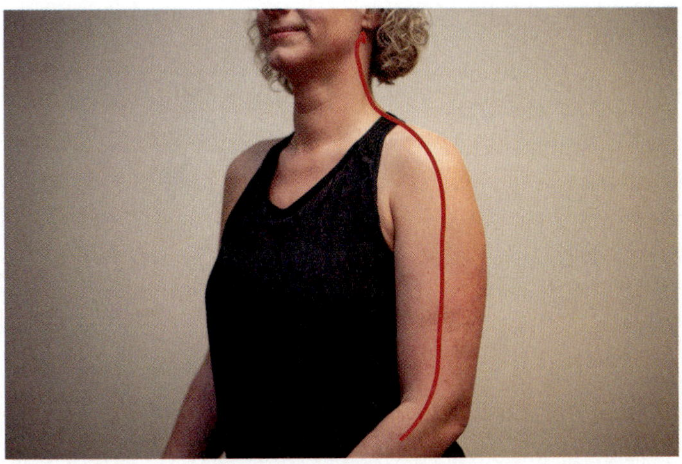

Figure 63.13. Anterior shoulder TB pathway. (Reprinted with permission from Capistrant T, Harrer G, Pentzer T, eds. *The Fascial Distortion Model: Philosophy, Principles and Clinical Applications.* Handspring Publishing; 2021.)

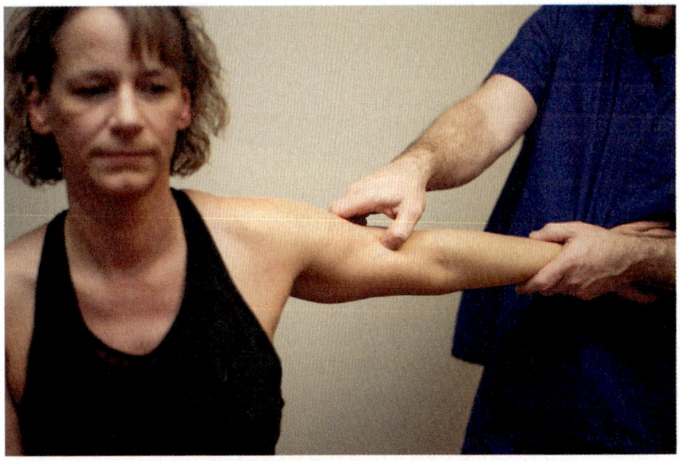

Figure 63.14. Anterior shoulder TB treatment. (Reprinted with permission from Capistrant T, Harrer G, Pentzer T, eds. *The Fascial Distortion Model: Philosophy, Principles and Clinical Applications.* Handspring Publishing; 2021.)

an "ironing out" or "unwinding" of the twisted fascial fibers within the fascial matrix. In the FDM it is believed that the patient will identify the linear path of the TB very specifically, and it is important to apply treatment precisely along that path (Fig. 63.16).

The treatment of the TB can be uncomfortable and may cause bruising. The treatment must occur on exposed, bare skin. Lubrication is not generally indicated when treating a TB. The friction from the tip of the finger through the skin into the fascial matrix is thought to allow the changes in the fascia. The direction of treatment of a TB can be important for its resolution; ideally, the TB should be treated in the direction indicated by the patient. Often a practitioner develops a preferred treatment direction for specific TB. However, if the treatment is not effective, consideration should be given to changing the direction of treatment as well as the amount of pressure applied, targeting the precise depth of the TB.

Another component of TB treatment is the speed with which the thumb is advanced along the presenting TB. The treatment should only occur as fast as the tissues can change under the

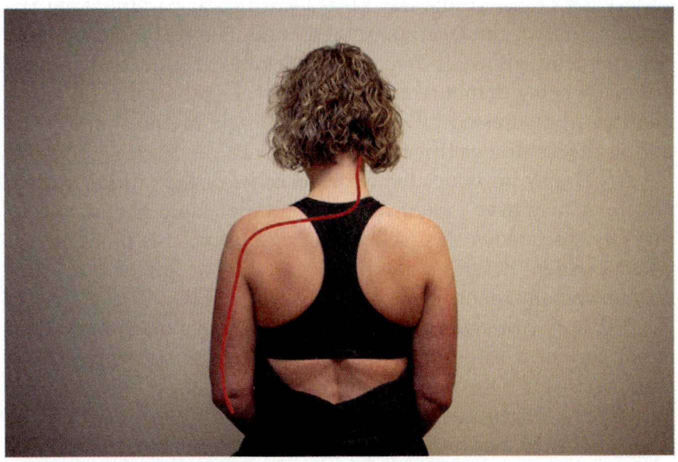

Figure 63.15. Posterior shoulder TB pathway. (Reprinted with permission from Capistrant T, Harrer G, Pentzer T, eds. *The Fascial Distortion Model: Philosophy, Principles and Clinical Applications.* Handspring Publishing; 2021.)

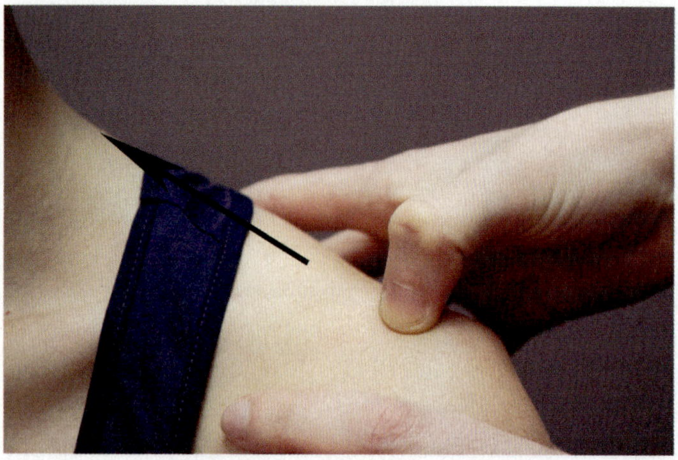

Figure 63.16. Thumb position for TB treatment. (Reprinted with permission from Capistrant T, Harrer G, Pentzer T, eds. *The Fascial Distortion Model: Philosophy, Principles and Clinical Applications.* Handspring Publishing; 2021.)

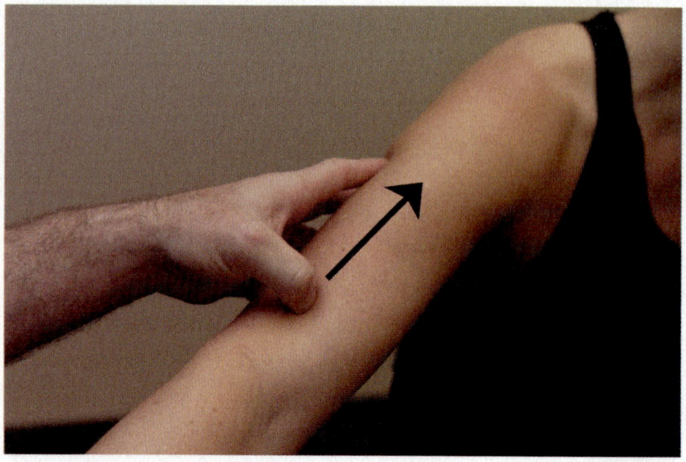

Figure 63.17. Angle of thumb for treating TB—deep. (Reprinted with permission from Capistrant T, Harrer G, Pentzer T, eds. *The Fascial Distortion Model: Philosophy, Principles and Clinical Applications.* Handspring Publishing; 2021.)

pressure of the thumb. It is not uncommon for a TB to be treated too quickly, resulting in inadequate (or failure of) resolution.

TBs are believed to occur wherever a patient identifies the distortion. This means that a practitioner should treat the TB shown by the patient whether or not the patient's TB is one commonly identified. The patient is the expert on their pain and knows where they are feeling the TB.

It is possible to start and stop a TB treatment. This allows for repositioning around clothing such as the bra strap or switching hands if the practitioner's thumb fatigues. When restarting a TB treatment, it is recommended that the thumb be placed a short distance prior to where the treatment was previously stopped before applying a corrective force. This ensures that none of the TB is missed.

The TB is one of the distortions that has undergone significant changes in teaching style since the FDM was initially introduced. Originally, the treatment of a TB was done with significant—often maximal—force, without palpating or appreciating the depth at which a TB was located. Now, practitioners are encouraged to accurately identify the location of a TB and then work to palpate the precise depth of the TB. Treatment utilizes only the necessary depth, force, and speed needed to appreciate TART changes in the underlying fascia. While the TB is identified as painful along the entire course of the treatment, these modulations of force, intensity, and depth allow for much more tolerable treatments than were originally being demonstrated and taught. Depth of the TB treatment can be adjusted by changing the angle of the thumb used during the treatment (Figs. 63.17 and 63.18).

A TB may be associated with weakness of the limb in certain positions, may have loss of motion in one or more planes, and/or may be associated with a lack of proprioception. It is thought that when a patient describes a joint as "unstable" or "giving out," they may be verbally identifying the presence of a TB.

A TB may resolve through a patient's normal movements. If it is not corrected through normal activity such as stretching, a TB may persist for a prolonged period of time. In the FDM, TBs are either acute or chronic. This delineation is not dependent on the passage of time, but instead is based on the presence or absence of inappropriately cross-linked fascial fibers. In the absence of these cross-links, the TB is considered acute, and it may remain acute for any length of time. The development of cross-links renders the TB chronic. These poorly formed cross-links are thought to stabilize the TB, making it more difficult to correct. TBs can immediately resolve when successfully corrected.

Herniated Triggerpoint(s) (HTPs)

HTPs are defined as abnormal protrusions of tissue through smooth fascial planes, which were originally considered to occur randomly throughout the body. An HTP is described by the patient with a gesture of multiple fingers, a thumb, or a knuckle pressing into a painful spot of pain in soft tissue (Figs. 63.19 to 63.22). As the practice of the FDM matured, HTPs were noted to occur with greater frequency at several anatomic locations, leading to the conclusion that these distortions were less random than originally thought. They do occur wherever a patient identifies them, but the predictability of these distortions has led to the hypothesis that these herniations are potentially linked to the passage of neurovascular bundles through the fascial matrix. It is the defect in the matrix caused by the neurovascular bundle that allows the herniation of matrix tissue through another level of the matrix. Patients experiencing an HTP often describe the pain as pinching or catching. The presence of the herniated portion of fascia along

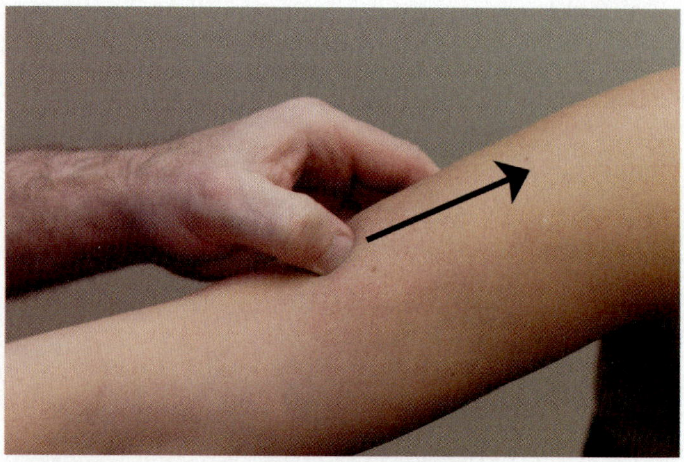

Figure 63.18. Angle of thumb for treating TB—Superficial. (Reprinted with permission from Capistrant T, Harrer G, Pentzer T, eds. *The Fascial Distortion Model: Philosophy, Principles and Clinical Applications.* Handspring Publishing; 2021.)

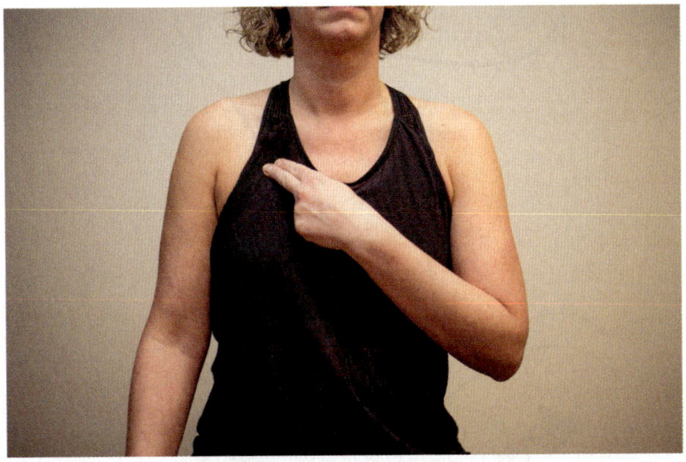

Figure 63.19. Pectoral HTP body language. (Reprinted with permission from Capistrant T, Harrer G, Pentzer T, eds. *The Fascial Distortion Model: Philosophy, Principles and Clinical Applications.* Handspring Publishing; 2021.)

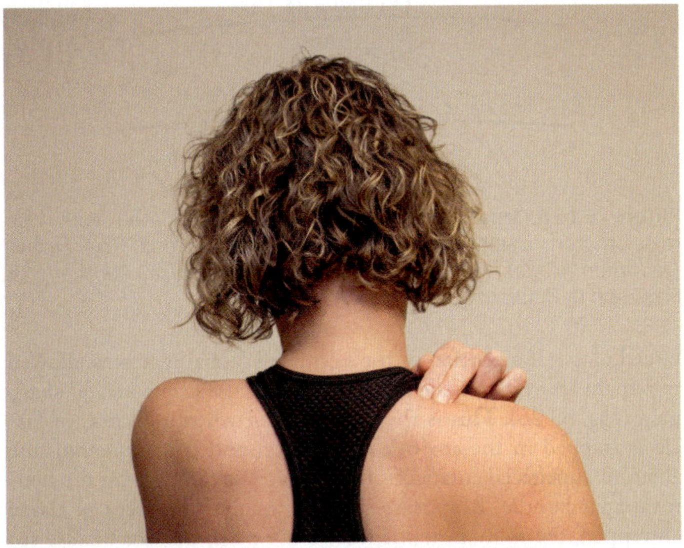

Figure 63.20. Supraclavicular HTP (SCHTP) body language. (Reprinted with permission from Capistrant T, Harrer G, Pentzer T, eds. *The Fascial Distortion Model: Philosophy, Principles and Clinical Applications.* Handspring Publishing; 2021.)

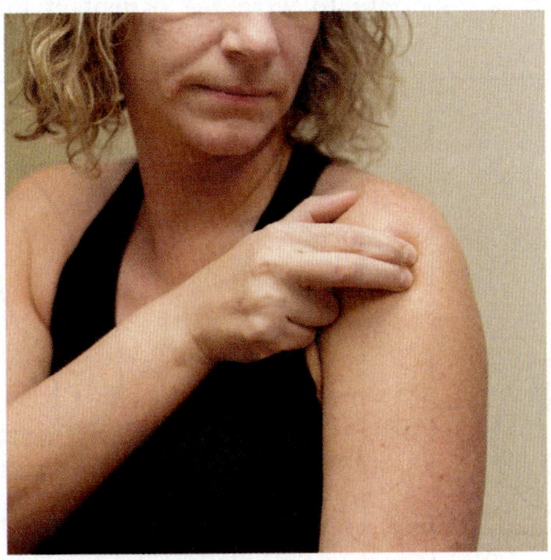

Figure 63.21. Subacromial HTP body language. (Reprinted with permission from Capistrant T, Harrer G, Pentzer T, eds. *The Fascial Distortion Model: Philosophy, Principles and Clinical Applications.* Handspring Publishing; 2021.)

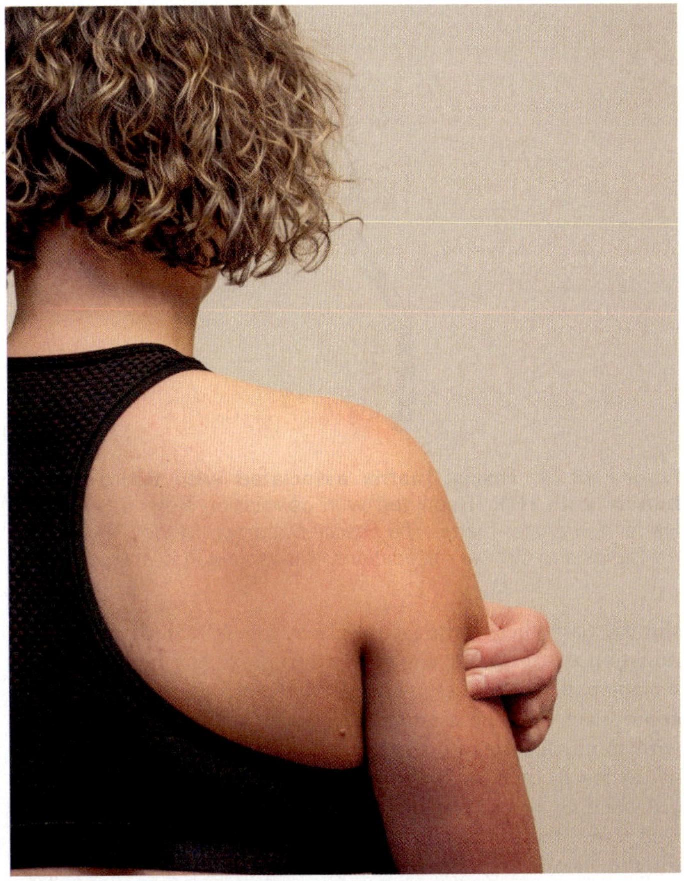

Figure 63.22. Deltoid HTP body language. (Reprinted with permission from Capistrant T, Harrer G, Pentzer T, eds. *The Fascial Distortion Model: Philosophy, Principles and Clinical Applications.* Handspring Publishing; 2021.)

the neurovascular bundle and the altered fascial tension secondary to an HTP may explain many entrapment syndromes seen in patients (Figs. 63.23 and 63.24).

In the treatment of an HTP, the tip of the thumb is used to reduce deeper tissue protruding through a shallower fascial plane. Direct pressure on the tender tissue is increased until a barrier is appreciated and continued pressure or a thrust is then applied to

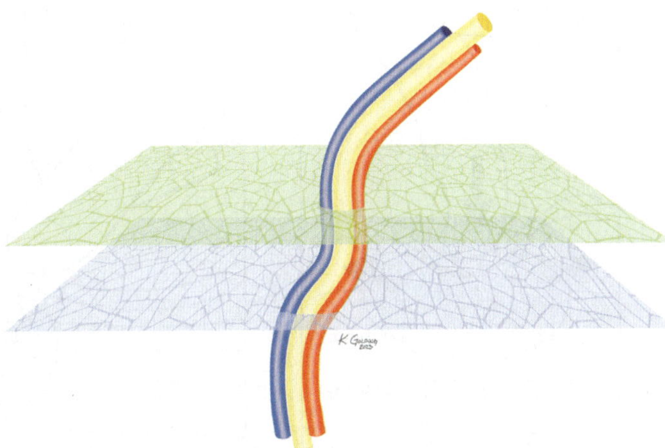

Figure 63.23. Fascial matrix associated with neurovascular bundle without HTP.

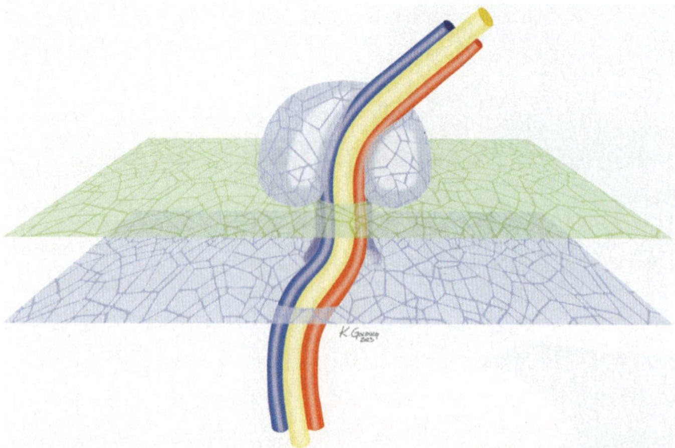

Figure 63.24. Fascial matrix associated with neurovascular bundle with HTP. (Reprinted with permission from Capistrant T, Harrer G, Pentzer T, eds. *The Fascial Distortion Model: Philosophy, Principles and Clinical Applications.* Handspring Publishing; 2021.)

slip the tissue below the fascial plane (Fig. 63.25). Precise determination of treatment angle by palpation of the herniation and seeking patient feedback is critical for the practitioner to apply the appropriate force necessary for reduction of the herniated fascia with minimal discomfort and tissue damage. The normalization of tension in the matrix allows the subsequent closure of the fascial opening through which the tissue protruded. This normalized fascial tension is considered to be the same force responsible for the "floating compression" of tensegrity, not unlike the prestressed cables employed within tensegrity sculptures.[9] The speed with which the layer of tissue closes is thought to be impacted by the health of the fascia and the duration that the herniation has been present.

Occasionally the "stalk" of the HTP may have a twist in it that impacts the ability of the HTP to be reduced. Addressing this rotational component as the practitioner increases the force may assist in decreasing the pain of the treatment.

There are nuances to the speed with which the treatment of an HTP is performed. If the force is applied too quickly, the tissues will rebound or resist the pressure that is being applied, and a successful reduction will not be achieved. After force is applied, it is important to palpate the area of treatment and assure that all elements of the herniated tissue are reduced below the smooth

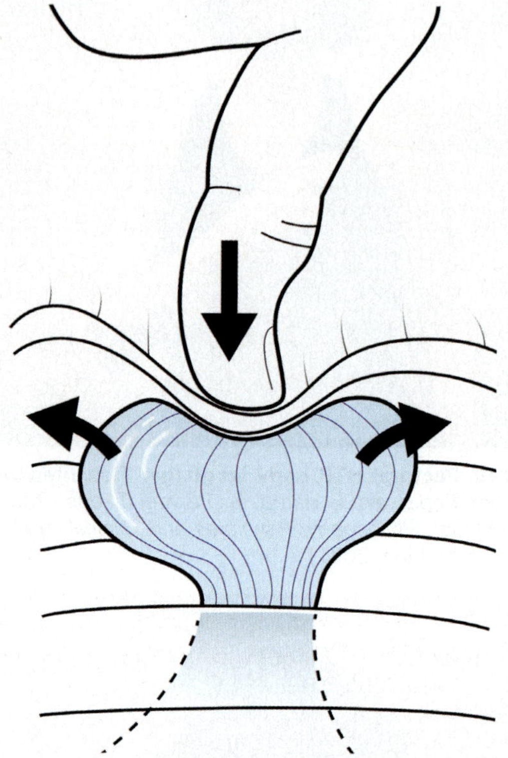

Figure 63.25. Treatment of the SCHTP. (Reprinted with permission from Capistrant T, Harrer G, Pentzer T, eds. *The Fascial Distortion Model: Philosophy, Principles and Clinical Applications.* Handspring Publishing; 2021.)

fascial plane. If a portion of the herniated fascial matrix is allowed to remain above the tissue plane, this can cause exquisite and sharp pain (Fig. 63.26). This is thought to occur when a portion of fascia is trapped in the smooth fascial layer and is compressing the adjacent superficial cutaneous nerve that is traveling with the neurovascular bundle. It appears that the smaller the piece of tissue entrapped, the more potential for severe pain; the exact cause for this is unknown.

Since the HTP involves the neurovascular bundles, including several blood vessels traveling along the course of the nerve, bruising may occur secondary to disruption of these vessels during treatment. It is important to warn the patient of the potential

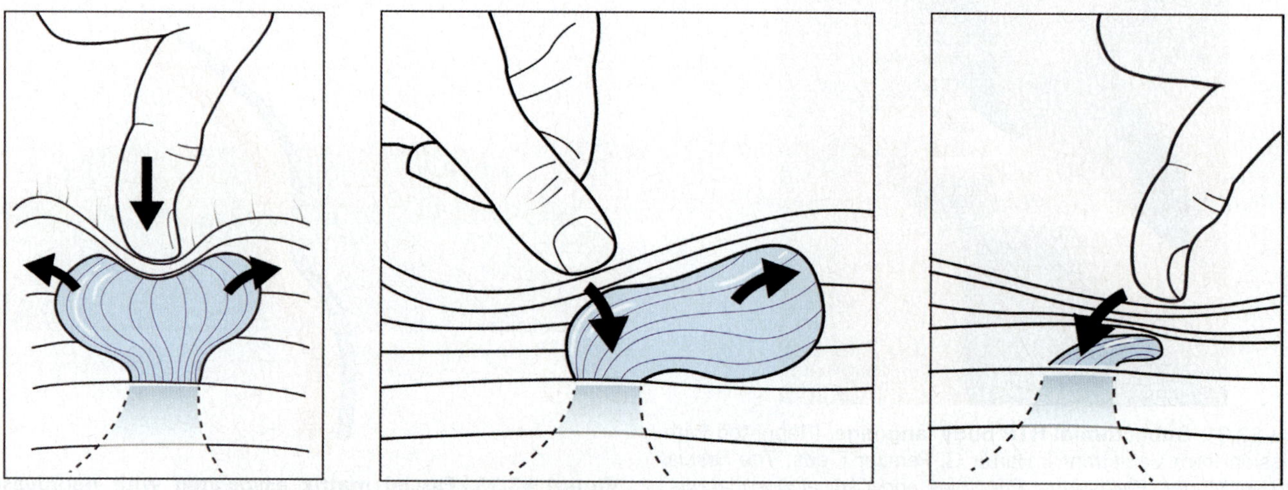

Figure 63.26. Edges of HTP being "tucked under" the fascial layer.

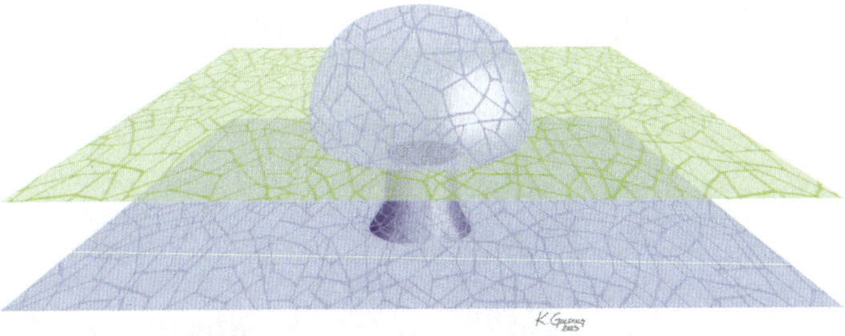

Figure 63.27. **Non-banded HTP.**

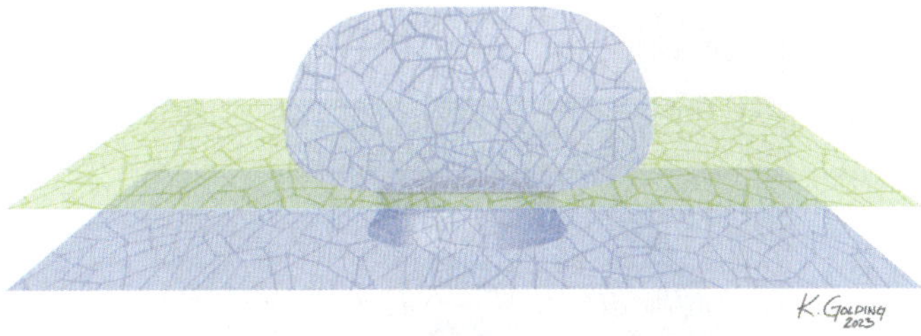

Figure 63.29. **Fascial Rent (side view).**

bruising and soreness that can be associated with the treatment of an HTP. The importance of determining the appropriate angle and depth for a successful and minimally uncomfortable treatment cannot be overstated.

HTPs may occur suddenly secondary to trauma yet may also occur insidiously and without apparent cause or injury. Prolonged sitting, maintenance of one position, or even sleeping can be associated with the development of an HTP.

HTPs are thought to be permanent, meaning they exist until the tissue is forcibly reduced below the fascial plane. An outside force is required to reduce the tissue below the fascial plane in which it has become entrapped. HTPs are often associated with decreased ROM of contiguous joints.

Several subtypes of HTP have been identified. The nonbanded HTP is one that occurs when tissue has pushed up through a layer of the fascial matrix (Fig. 63.27). A banded HTP is one in which there are associated TB in the fascial layer through which the tissue has protruded. It is thought that the existence of these TB could, in part, contribute to the abnormal tension in the matrix that is preventing the herniated tissue from slipping back below the fascial layer. Correction of the associated TB would normalize the tension and thus aid in the reduction of the herniated tissue back below the fascial layer.

Practitioners of the FDM may encounter a large HTP that upon palpation seems to have occurred along an opening of the fascial matrix. This can be visualized as a linear gap in the fascial matrix, allowing underlying tissue to protrude through the opening. This type of HTP is referred to as a fascial rent (Figs. 63.28 and 63.29), and this is treated in a similar fashion to an HTP.

When describing herniations to patients, it is important to avoid words or phrases that induce fear. When describing the fascial rent, it is of value to describe the fascial matrix "opening" or "gapping" rather than "tearing" or "ripping." This can help assuage a patient's fear that the matrix is somehow damaged and unable to be immediately repaired.

Continuum Distortion(s) (CDs)

To understand a CD, one must turn their attention to the sites of the body where there is transition between fascia and bone. Macroscopically, this transition may appear as the junction of two discrete tissue types. Microscopically, this is not a discrete transition, but rather a zone in which the tissues may possess qualities of both bone and fascia. This zone of shared qualities is the continuum. There is a hypothesized calcium flux between the two tissues in which there is a constant shifting between the fascia and bone. The stress placed on this junction determines the direction of flux, rendering the transition site more supple or more robust (depending on where the calcium remains). This transition zone has been identified by researchers at the Technical University of Munich as a protein layer (Fig. 63.30).

A CD occurs when calcium within the transition zone is unable to shift. A sudden force, such as a sprain, alters the continuum so that calcium is unable to move back into bone from the fascia (or out of bone and into the fascia). It is believed that loss of normal calcium flux produces perceived pain precisely at the location of the stuck transition zone. A CD is identified by the patient as a single point of pain, using one finger to specifically locate and identify the location of pain. The gesture is easy to recognize (Fig. 63.31).

When a CD is present, a patient may have the loss of ROM in one plane, often flexion or extension of a joint. CDs appear to occur when the mechanism of injury is sudden, where the continuum is in a state not suited for the sudden application of force and leading to disrupted calcium flux at that site.

Treatment of the CD involves placing the very tip of the thumb directly on the palpable abnormality of the transition zone.

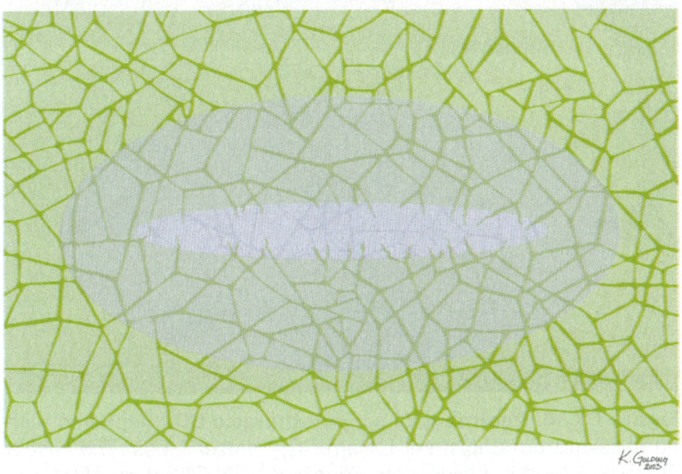

Figure 63.28. **Fascial rent (top view).**

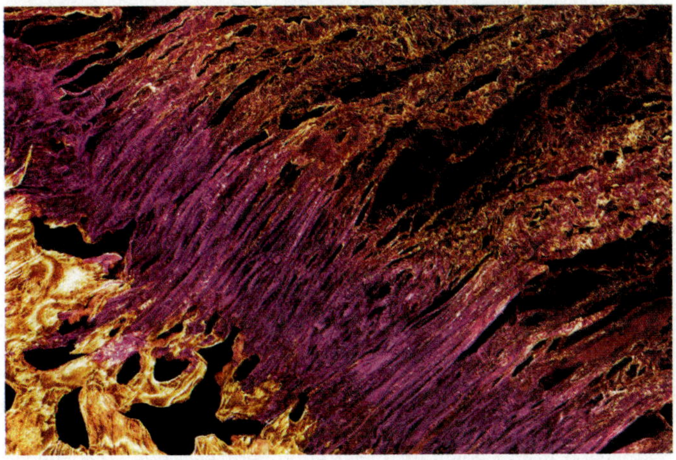

Figure 63.30. **Electron micrograph of CD.** (Courtesy of University of Munich.)

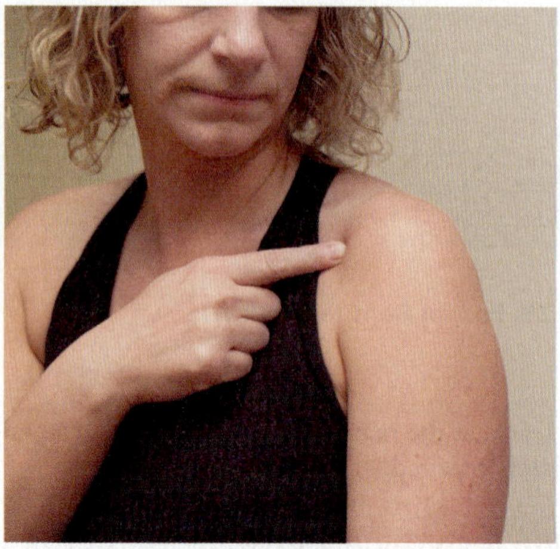

Figure 63.31. AC CD body language. (Reprinted with permission from Capistrant T, Harrer G, Pentzer T, eds. *The Fascial Distortion Model: Philosophy, Principles and Clinical Applications.* Handspring Publishing; 2021.)

This irregularity can vary in size and has been described in several ways. The smallest versions of CD are described as small cortical irregularities; on palpation these CDs feel like a piece of sand or grain of rice on the bony surface. Other CDs are larger and may feel like a lentil or firm nodule on the bony surface. Precise location of this stuck transition zone is possible by asking the patient for guidance. The thumb position of the practitioner can be refined by engaging the patient in directing your efforts to the most painful spot (Fig. 63.32). When treating a CD, the force of the treatment needs to be equal or greater to the force that caused the fibers of the continuum to become stuck. Also, the direction of force needed to correct the CD must be the opposite vector of the injury (Figs. 63.33 and 63.34).

When treating a CD, the practitioner should palpate the small abnormality in the tissue prior to applying a corrective force. As the force is applied, minor adjustments can be made.

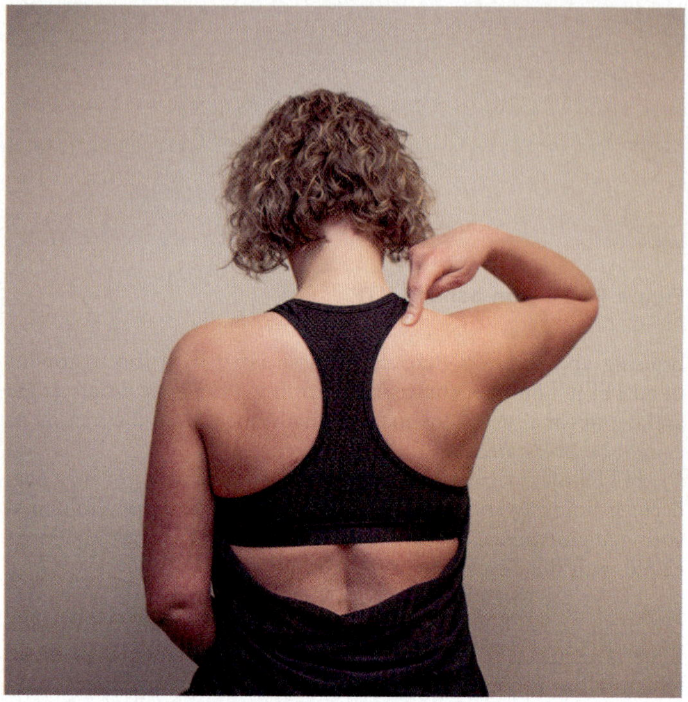

Figure 63.33. Scapulothoracic CD body language. (Reprinted with permission from Capistrant T, Harrer G, Pentzer T, eds. *The Fascial Distortion Model: Philosophy, Principles and Clinical Applications.* Handspring Publishing; 2021.)

The practitioner should palpate for a change in the tissues as the force is increased. This shift or change can be subtle and often missed, resulting in unnecessarily long treatments. Novice practitioners may not have the palpatory skills to appreciate these subtle changes. With force vectors properly aligned, treatment of the CD should require mere seconds. If the practitioner is unable to sense the shift, the treatment time should be limited. Treatment durations no longer than 60 seconds have been suggested; however, if the CD does not shift within the first few seconds of treatment,

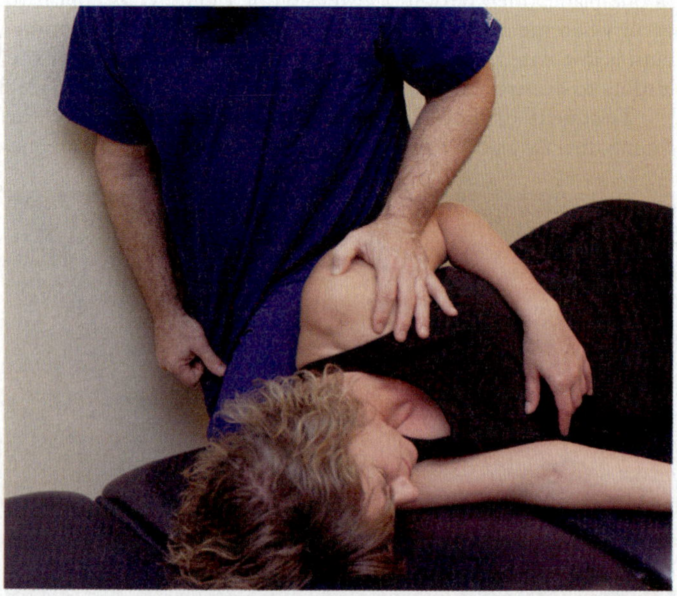

Figure 63.32. Treatment of subacromial CD. (Reprinted with permission from Capistrant T, Harrer G, Pentzer T, eds. *The Fascial Distortion Model: Philosophy, Principles and Clinical Applications.* Handspring Publishing; 2021.)

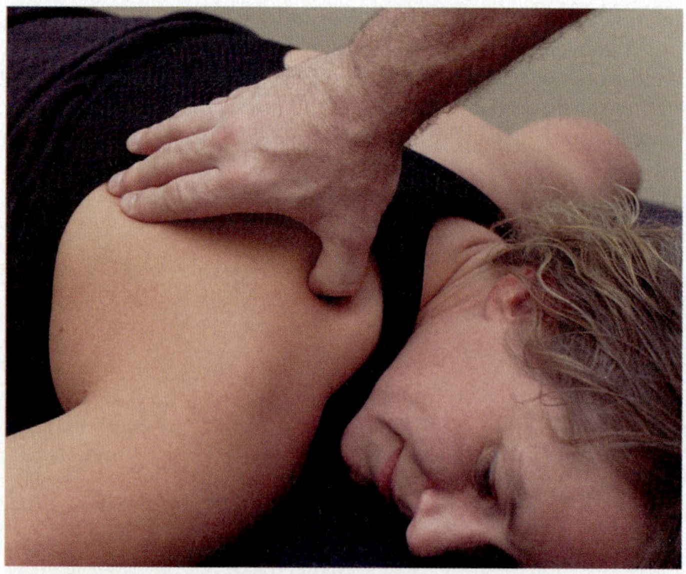

Figure 63.34. Treatment of scapulothoracic CD. (Reprinted with permission from Capistrant T, Harrer G, Pentzer T, eds. *The Fascial Distortion Model: Philosophy, Principles and Clinical Applications.* Handspring Publishing; 2021.)

the practitioner is advised to stop the treatment and reassess the placement of their thumb tip. Pressing for longer than necessary causes undue fatigue of the thumb and unnecessary discomfort for the patient. The practitioner should strive to be able to precisely palpate the CD and to apply only the necessary force to realign the transition zone.

There are two types of CD identified, referred to as everted and inverted CD. Everted CDs are the aforementioned palpable spicules on the cortical bone in which the continuum is thought to be stuck in an osseous state, as calcium is unable to leave the transition zone. Conversely, there are situations where the transition zone is stuck in a state with less calcium present in the continuum; these are referred to as inverted CD. An inverted CD is appreciated as a shallow depression or dip in the bony surface at the site of pain. Inverted CDs are often of similar dimensions to the everted CDs. Treatment of inverted CD can be achieved through the direct pressure technique described above. In addition, a technique that pulls the fibers of the inverted CD out of, or away from, the bone can be used to return the transition zone to normal function.

Given the flux of calcium in the continuum related to physiologic forces, spontaneous resolution of CD through normal physical activity is possible. CDs may appear to come and go based on the patient's activity. Despite the potential for spontaneous resolution, treating CD reduces pain and restores ROM, which speeds the patient's return to normal activity. CDs appear to occur in the banded fascia subtype of the fascial matrix and therefore can be associated with TB.

Folding Distortion(s) (FD)

FDs are thought to occur in folding fascia, which has the ability to compress and expand like the pleats of an accordion or curtain (Fig. 63.35). The compressible and expansile capability of this fascia is thought to absorb force and energy that is applied to the fascial matrix, much like a shock absorber. When the fascial matrix experiences excessive compression, often accompanied by torque, the matrix can remain stuck in the compressed or refolded position. When a force is applied to the fascial matrix that causes an over-expansion of the fascial matrix and torque is applied, the fascia can remain in this over-expanded or unfolded position. Folding fascia is considered to be highly compressible and expansile within physiologic norms; the addition of torque is what causes the matrix to become stuck.

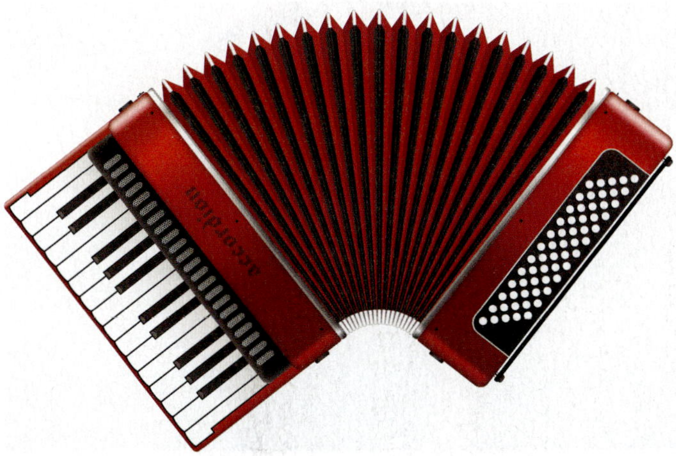

Figure 63.35. FD mechanism. (Reprinted with permission from Capistrant T, Harrer G, Pentzer T, eds. *The Fascial Distortion Model: Philosophy, Principles and Clinical Applications.* Handspring Publishing; 2021.)

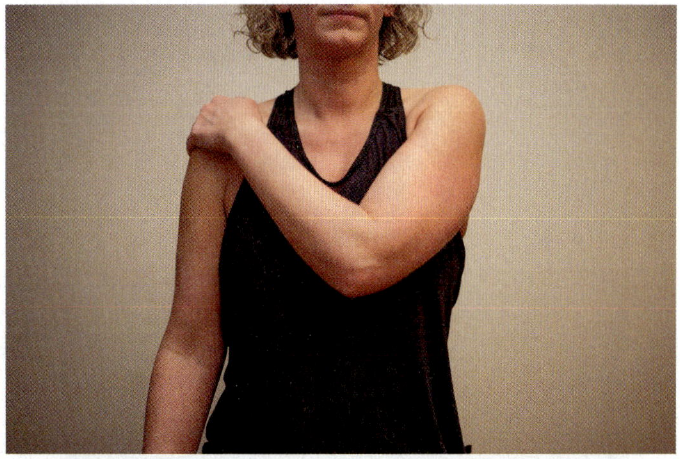

Figure 63.36. Shoulder FD body language. (Reprinted with permission from Capistrant T, Harrer G, Pentzer T, eds. *The Fascial Distortion Model: Philosophy, Principles and Clinical Applications.* Handspring Publishing; 2021.)

The patient experiencing FD will hold or cup the area (Fig. 63.36). They will describe a pain that is located deep within the joint or tissues and they are unable to place a finger on the pain or localize it to a single spot. In addition, patients describing rFD may draw a line across the joint, often using the middle finger to draw this line (Fig. 63.37). Folding injuries cause pain in an area but often do not cause a major loss of ROM.

FDs are thought to occur suddenly, such as in a traumatic event. FDs are thought to remain unchanged until refolded or unfolded and are considered permanent until the mechanism of injury is recreated. FDs are not palpable by the practitioner on examination.

Patients may describe a joint with a FD as feeling "unstable," even though it has never given out (objective joint instability is thought to be related to TB). As they are considered permanent until the mechanism of injury is recreated, these distortions may be present for a long period of time, with the patient describing the pain as something they "have always had."

FD may also be accompanied by effusions, the underlying cause of which is thought to be due to lymphatic drainage impingement by the altered folding fascia. Another theory is that the body utilizes fluid to expand the tissue in an attempt to unfold the fascia.

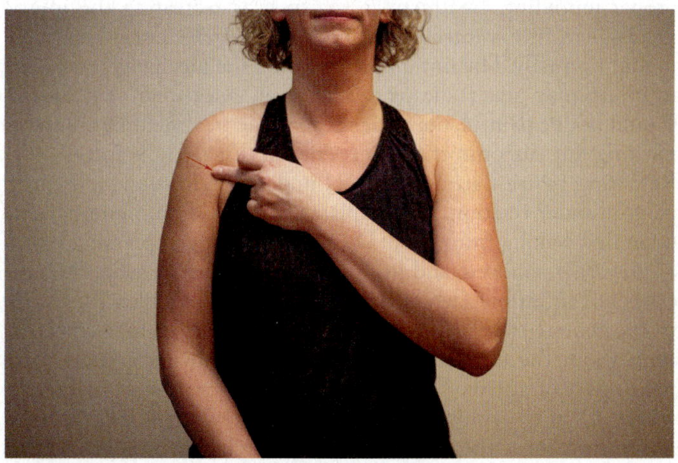

Figure 63.37. rFD body language. (Reprinted with permission from Capistrant T, Harrer G, Pentzer T, eds. *The Fascial Distortion Model: Philosophy, Principles and Clinical Applications.* Handspring Publishing; 2021.)

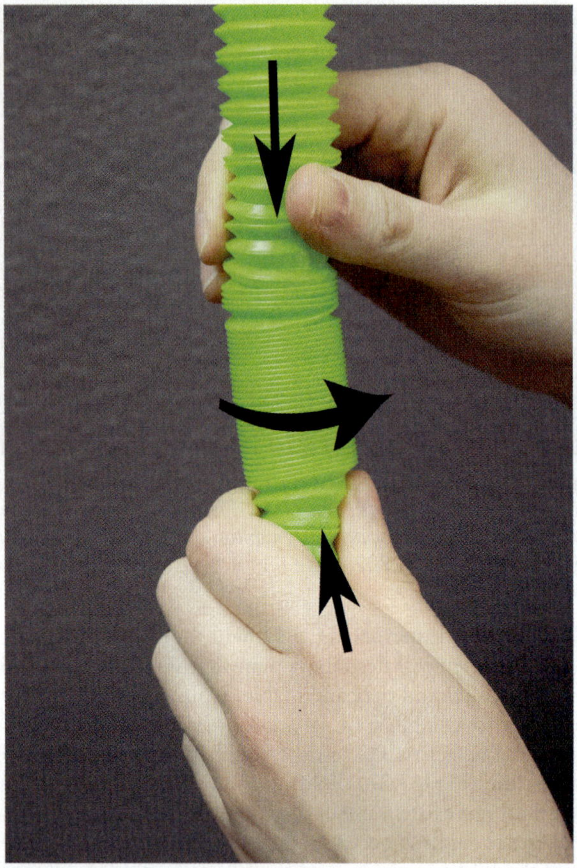

Figure 63.38. rFD mechanism. (Reprinted with permission from Capistrant T, Harrer G, Pentzer T, eds. *The Fascial Distortion Model: Philosophy, Principles and Clinical Applications.* Handspring Publishing; 2021.)

Refolding injuries occur when the fascial matrix is compressed and remains stuck in this compressed state, unable to return to the neutral state (Fig. 63.38). Consider a fall onto an outstretched arm. After a fall like this, a patient may present with pain deep in a joint. When asked where the pain is, they would hold the joint to indicate the area of pain. As an rFD is considered to be misfolding of the fascia in the presence of torque that prevents proper unfolding, treatment is achieved by recreating the injury mechanism in a controlled manner so that the fascia can then unfold normally. The notion of recreating the mechanism that led to injury may give some pause; however, since treatment of FD should not be painful, the patient can guide treatment by communicating any discomfort they experience (Figs. 63.39 and 63.40). Refolding injuries are less painful under compression, and more painful under traction. This explains why rFDs are more painful upon first waking from sleep: During sleep, the compressing effect of gravity is removed, and in the absence of compression, the fascia is left to unfold (tensegrity is attempting to return the fascia to its neutral state). Conversely, this is why rFD may improve throughout the day, as a person is up and moving around with the impact of gravity being exerted on the fascial matrix. People with rFD in the spine find inversion therapy or traction therapy uncomfortable at the level of the refolding injury.

uFDs occur when the fascial matrix is stretched, torque is applied, and the tissue is unable to return to a neutral state (Fig. 63.41). Consider a person walking a dog on a leash. The dog sees something that excites them, causing them to lunge or bolt

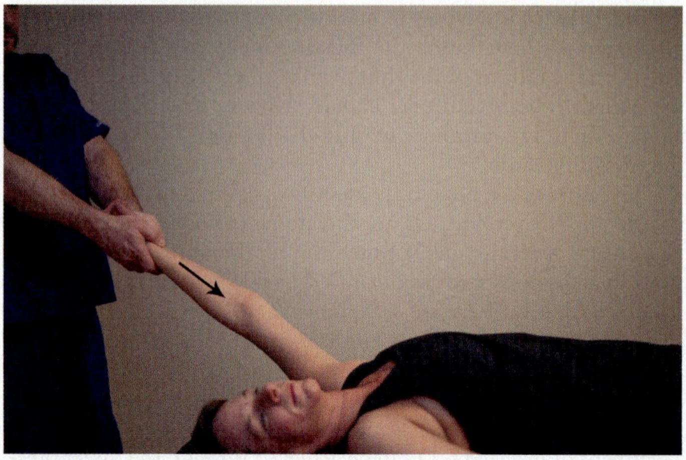

Figure 63.39. rFD treatment shoulder long axis. (Reprinted with permission from Capistrant T, Harrer G, Pentzer T, eds. *The Fascial Distortion Model: Philosophy, Principles and Clinical Applications.* Handspring Publishing; 2021.)

forward until that motion is stopped by the leash. In doing so, the force from the mass of the dog is transmitted to the person's shoulder, which then simultaneously moves in flexion/abduction while receiving rapid traction, producing an uFD. Treatment of FD should never hurt, and again, the patient may help guide treatment by notifying the practitioner of any discomfort during the treatment. uFD will feel better under traction, and treatment will involve applying traction and torque in positions that recreate the injury mechanism (Figs. 63.42 and 63.43).

The complexity of the shoulder joint may make identifying the location and type of the folding injury difficult. One portion of the shoulder fascia can be unfolding while the reciprocal portion of the matrix is refolding. The Frogleg is an easily implemented technique that will assist in identifying and treating FD in the shoulder (Figs. 63.44 and 63.45). While testing the patient in the Frogleg position, it is important to ask the patient if they are experiencing pain, and if so, where their pain is located. If one of the painful distortions—a TB, HTP, or CD—is identified, then these need to be treated and removed before the folding treatment can be performed without pain.

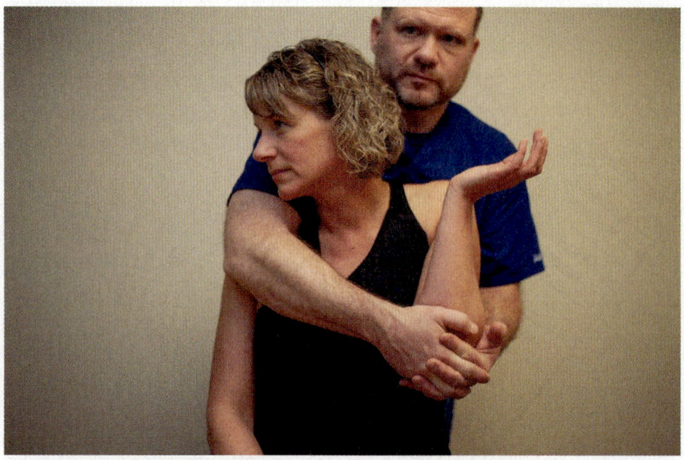

Figure 63.40. rFD shoulder compression. (Reprinted with permission from Capistrant T, Harrer G, Pentzer T, eds. *The Fascial Distortion Model: Philosophy, Principles and Clinical Applications.* Handspring Publishing; 2021.)

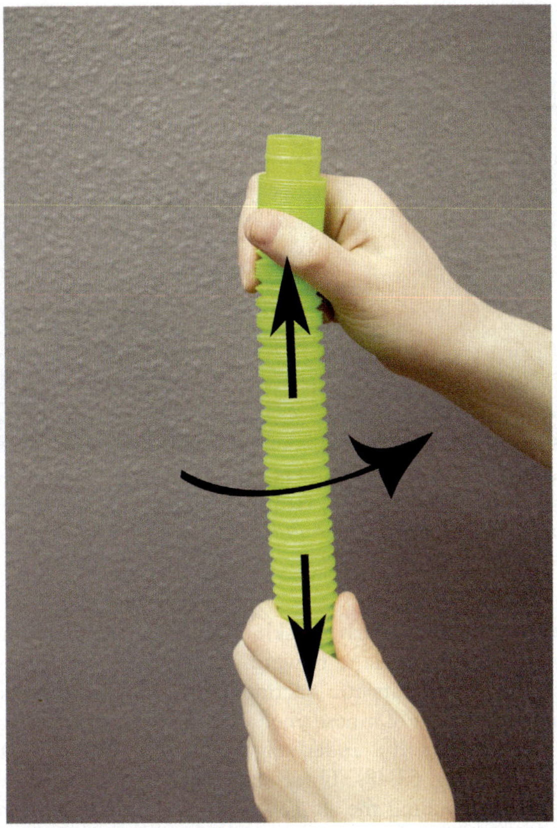

Figure 63.41. **uFD mechanism.** (Reprinted with permission from Capistrant T, Harrer G, Pentzer T, eds. *The Fascial Distortion Model: Philosophy, Principles and Clinical Applications*. Handspring Publishing; 2021.)

Cylinder Distortion(s) (CyD)

CyDs are thought to occur in coiled fascia. The coiled fascia can be visualized as circles or rings of fascia around the body, much like a spring or slinky lying just below the skin. This coiled fascia is considered to be the most superficial fascial type. A CyD might occur when this superficial fascia is restricted and unable to move freely. CyDs are often associated with seemingly bizarre symptoms that include

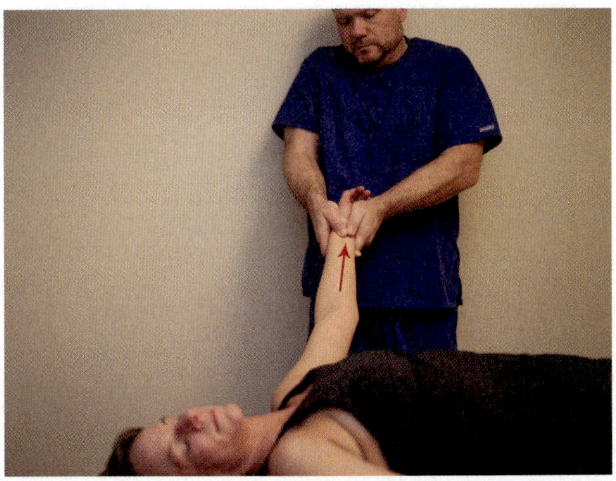

Figure 63.42. **uFD treatment of shoulder long lever.** (Reprinted with permission from Capistrant T, Harrer G, Pentzer T, eds. *The Fascial Distortion Model: Philosophy, Principles and Clinical Applications*. Handspring Publishing; 2021.)

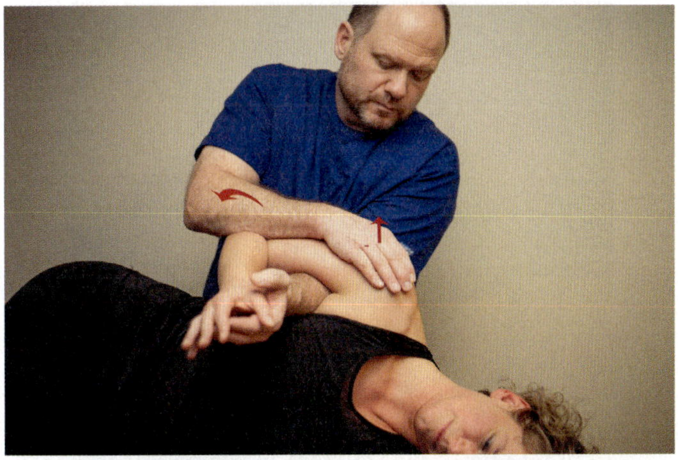

Figure 63.43. **Unfolding treatment "Water Pump" technique.** (Reprinted with permission from Capistrant T, Harrer G, Pentzer T, eds. *The Fascial Distortion Model: Philosophy, Principles and Clinical Applications*. Handspring Publishing; 2021.)

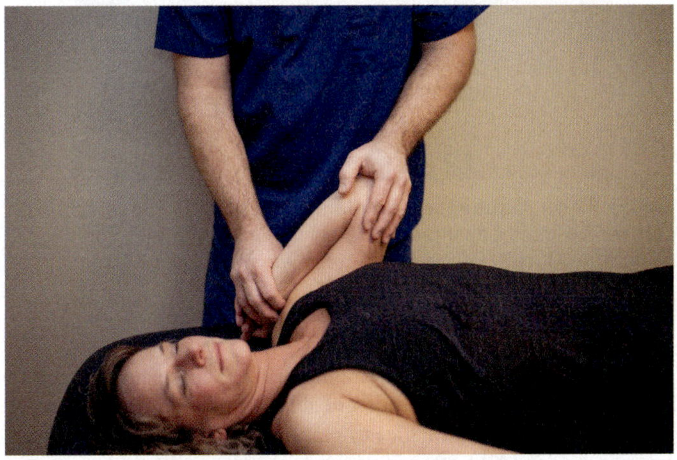

Figure 63.44. **Frogleg treatment of FD.** (Reprinted with permission from Capistrant T, Harrer G, Pentzer T, eds. *The Fascial Distortion Model: Philosophy, Principles and Clinical Applications*. Handspring Publishing; 2021.)

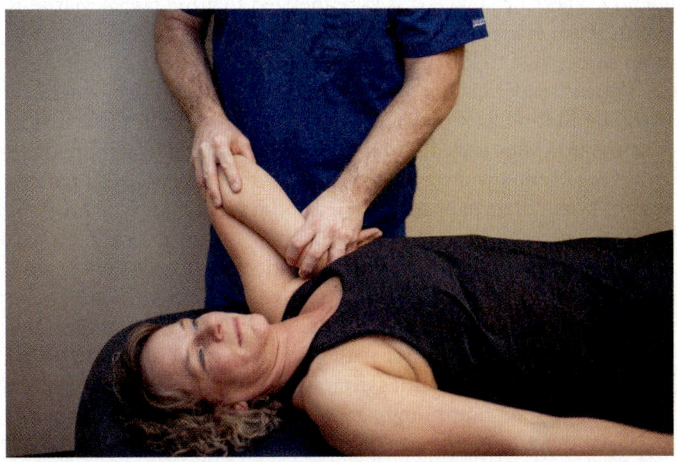

Figure 63.45. **Frogleg treatment of FD.** (Reprinted with permission from Capistrant T, Harrer G, Pentzer T, eds. *The Fascial Distortion Model: Philosophy, Principles and Clinical Applications*. Handspring Publishing; 2021.)

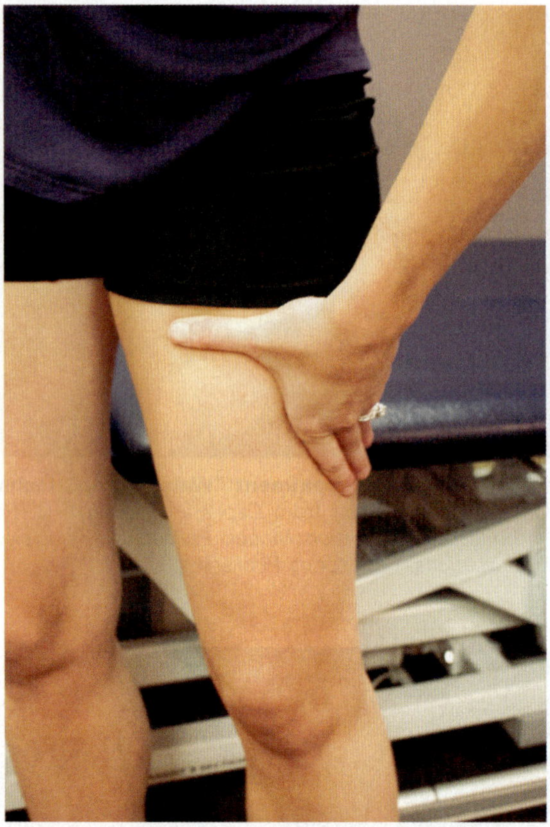

Figure 63.46. Squeegee body language of CyD. (Reprinted with permission from Capistrant T, Harrer G, Pentzer T, eds. *The Fascial Distortion Model: Philosophy, Principles and Clinical Applications*. Handspring Publishing; 2021.)

pain of inexplicable intensity, jumping pain, cramps, pain that comes in the night, pain that is indescribable, numbness, paresthesia, or pain that the patient struggles to pinpoint. The distribution of pain associated with CyD often is not restricted by traditional anatomic distributions such as dermatomes or common referral patterns. One mechanism identified as a possible trigger for the formation of CyD has been linked to the restriction of skin movement on the underlying tissues. This could be due to tight fitting garments, splints, or casts. People who have been diagnosed with fibromyalgia frequently experience CyD. It is hypothesized that the fascial matrix is inflamed or irritated in some manner which makes the fascial matrix more susceptible to kinking of the coiled fascia.

Patients experiencing a CyD often use the hand or fingers in a sweeping motion as if they are trying to wipe water from their skin (Fig. 63.46). They may also demonstrate their pain using repetitive squeezing of the involved area with a hand (Fig. 63.47). If a patient demonstrates their pain with their hand hovering away from their body and not touching the skin, this may represent a CyD. CyD may be painful with active motion and pain-free during passive motion. The presence of CyD should be considered in situations where the pain perceived by the patient is out of proportion to the physical exam findings. These patients may perceive a portion of the body as swollen or edematous even when the area involved appears normal. CyDs are not thought to be palpable by the practitioner.

Treatment of CyD can involve many different techniques, some of which utilize tools applied to the skin and others which use the hands manually applied to the skin. The goal when treating a CyD is to untangle the coiled fascia within the fascial matrix. Many of the techniques that are employed in the treatment of

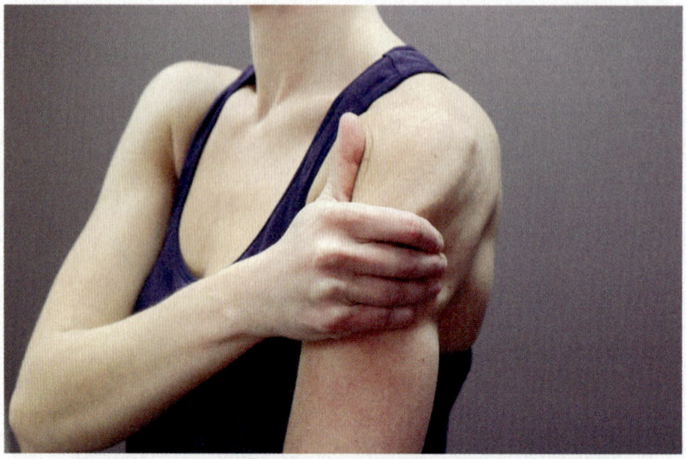

Figure 63.47. Squeezing body language of CyD. (Reprinted with permission from Capistrant T, Harrer G, Pentzer T, eds. *The Fascial Distortion Model: Philosophy, Principles and Clinical Applications*. Handspring Publishing; 2021.)

CyD aim to pull the overlying skin away from the fascial matrix, allowing the coiled fascia to unwind.

The use of therapeutic suction cups sometimes associated with acupressure or Chinese medicine may be utilized to pull the skin away from the underlying fascia while the patient provides motion (Fig. 63.48). These same cups may be used to slide along the skin, pulling the skin away from the underlying tissues (Fig. 63.49). Additional tools that can be employed by the FDM practitioner to treat CyD include clips, clamps, labor assist device vacuum extractors, and even plungers (Fig. 63.50). These tools can be applied to the skin, lifting it away from the underlying fascial matrix, allowing the coils to untangle (Fig. 63.51).

In addition, there are several manual techniques that are used to treat CyD. These include the use of the hand as a squeegee to push the coils, double-thumb technique to separate the coiled fascia, the snakebite to manually untwist the coils, and the tiger claw to lift the skin away from the underlying matrix (Figs. 63.52 to 63.54). Note that these techniques may resemble some of the same gestures the patient was using to describe their pain.

CyDs are the one distortion practitioners may inadvertently cause by overtreating the fascial matrix. They may start suddenly

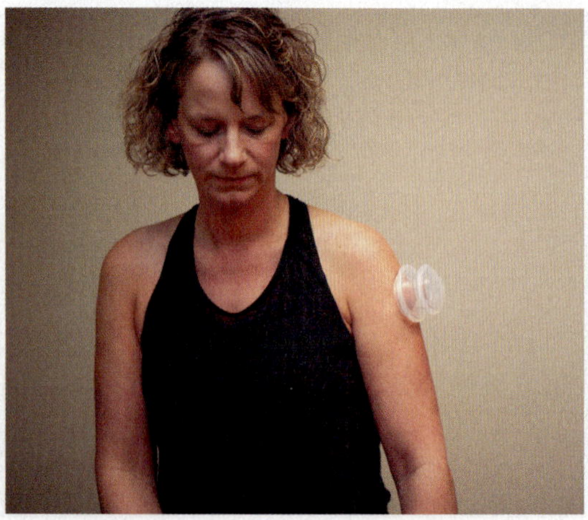

Figure 63.48. Cupping with patient motion. (Reprinted with permission from Capistrant T, Harrer G, Pentzer T, eds. *The Fascial Distortion Model: Philosophy, Principles and Clinical Applications*. Handspring Publishing; 2021.)

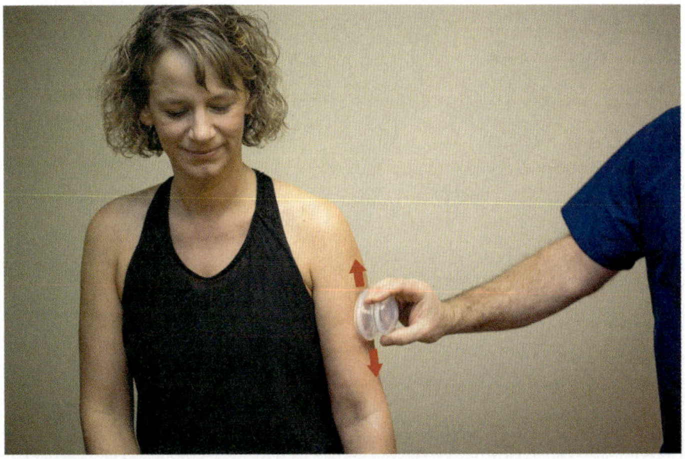

Figure 63.49. Cupping with sliding. (Reprinted with permission from Capistrant T, Harrer G, Pentzer T, eds. *The Fascial Distortion Model: Philosophy, Principles and Clinical Applications*. Handspring Publishing; 2021.)

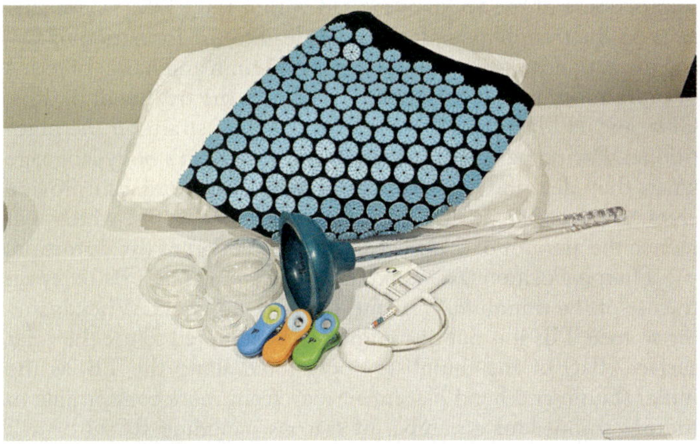

Figure 63.50. CyD treatment tools. (Photo by Thomas Pentzer)

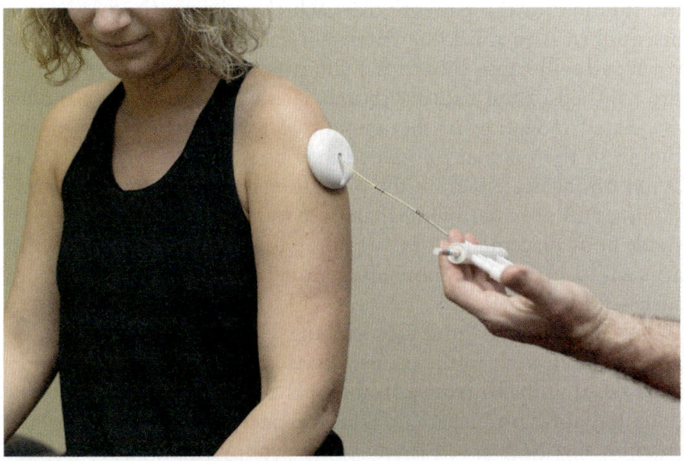

Figure 63.51. CyD treatment with vacuum. (Reprinted with permission from Capistrant T, Harrer G, Pentzer T, eds. *The Fascial Distortion Model: Philosophy, Principles and Clinical Applications*. Handspring Publishing; 2021.)

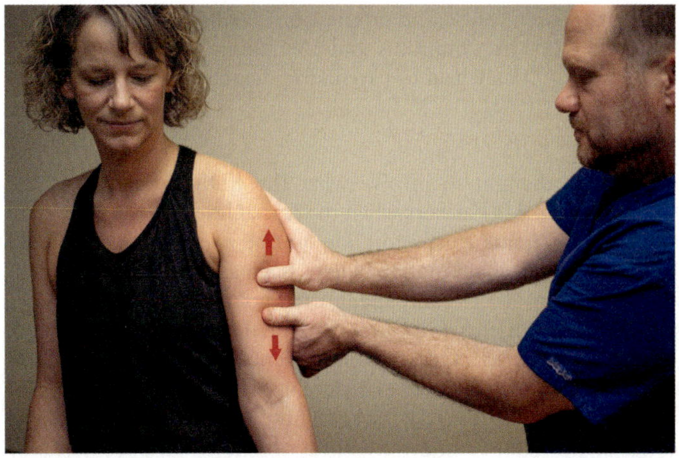

Figure 63.52. Double-thumb treatment. (Reprinted with permission from Capistrant T, Harrer G, Pentzer T, eds. *The Fascial Distortion Model: Philosophy, Principles and Clinical Applications*. Handspring Publishing; 2021.)

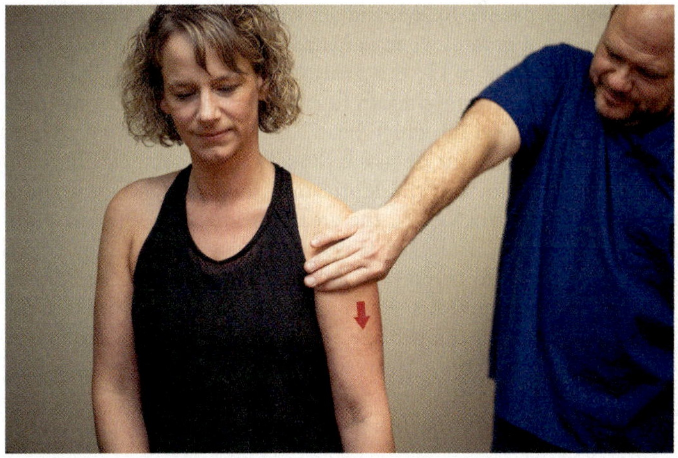

Figure 63.53. Squeegee technique. (Reprinted with permission from Capistrant T, Harrer G, Pentzer T, eds. *The Fascial Distortion Model: Philosophy, Principles and Clinical Applications*. Handspring Publishing; 2021.)

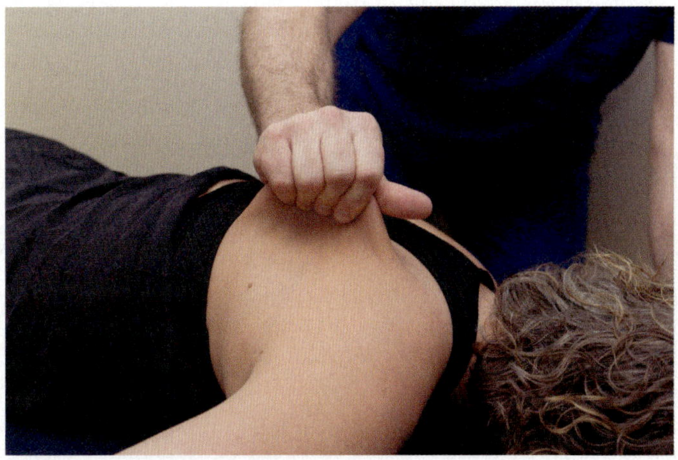

Figure 63.54. Tiger claw. (Reprinted with permission from Capistrant T, Harrer G, Pentzer T, eds. *The Fascial Distortion Model: Philosophy, Principles and Clinical Applications*. Handspring Publishing; 2021.)

without apparent cause, and progression is unknown without treatment. The bizarre symptoms and complaints offered by patients who have CyD may lead to psychiatric diagnoses.

Tectonic Fixation(s) (TF)

The TF is thought to involve what the FDM identifies as the smooth fascia. A TF occurs when the fascial layers in the matrix are stuck together and unable to glide on one another as they would in normal physiologic motion. There is no associated gesture with this distortion other than patient attempts to self-manipulate the affected area. Patients will often describe the area of a TF as stuck or needing to "pop." Occasionally patients will describe the joint as "dry" or "low on oil." TF may develop when something has prevented motion of the fascial matrix. This could be one of the painful distortions that discourages use of the affected body part, or it may be due to physical immobilization imposed by corrective devices such as braces, splints, or slings. A good example of a TF is a frozen shoulder. This condition is often preceded by pain in the shoulder that discourages or prevents movement. In the absence of motion, ground substance does not flow through the matrix and fascial layers become adhered, preventing movement of the joint. There is a global loss of passive ROM, and active ROM reveals a bony end-feel. TF are not painful when palpated.

When treating a TF, the goal of the treatment is to induce movement between the smooth fascial layers. This is the only distortion in the FDM for which heat is thought to aid in treatment. Heat applied to a joint or tissue thought to be tectonically fixed is hypothesized to thin the lubricating fluid (ground substance) of the fascial matrix.[6] Once the area is heated, the affected joint is moved through its ROM (Figs. 63.55 and 63.56). Any other distortions found to be present should be treated. Once the other distortions are removed, a slow tectonic pump of the area is used to apply force at the ends of ROM and to encourage movement of the ground substance between the layers. Applying a gradual increase in pressure at the restrictive barrier helps to increase the movement within the smooth fascial layers.

PRACTITIONER SELF-CARE

As with all osteopathic approaches, proper application of technique is vital for good patient outcomes as well as the health of

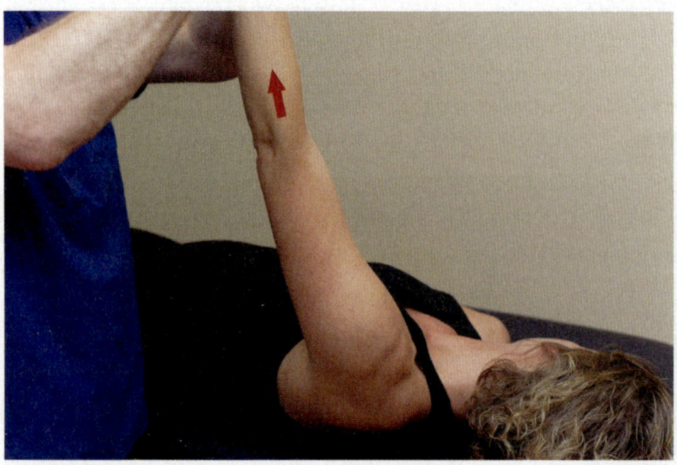

Figure 63.55. Tectonic pump treatment. (Reprinted with permission from Capistrant T, Harrer G, Pentzer T, eds. *The Fascial Distortion Model: Philosophy, Principles and Clinical Applications*. Handspring Publishing; 2021.)

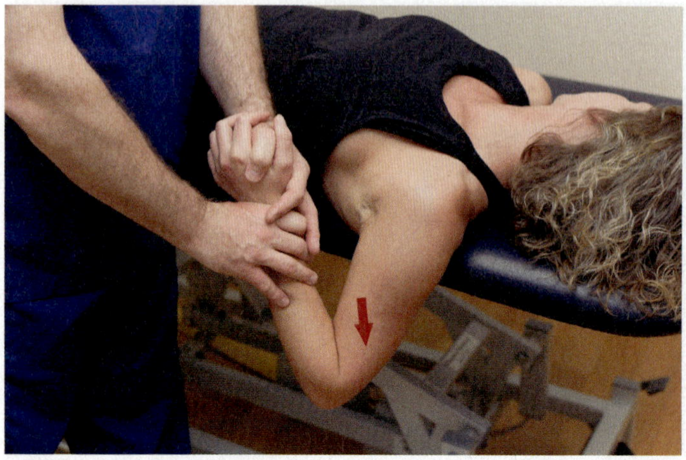

Figure 63.56. Tectonic pump treatment. (Reprinted with permission from Capistrant T, Harrer G, Pentzer T, eds. *The Fascial Distortion Model: Philosophy, Principles and Clinical Applications*. Handspring Publishing; 2021.)

the practitioner and their ability to provide treatments throughout their day and ultimately their career. This is especially so in the case of some of the techniques used within the FDM where reliance on the thumb to apply force can lead to the formation of fascial distortions in the practitioner's own thumb and hand. In terms of prevention, modulating forces applied in the treatment of TBs, CDs, and HTPs play a large role in reducing strain on the practitioner. Paying particular attention to the patient's body language when they describe the location of their distortions can provide clues to proper angle and direction of force to apply, which will reduce the amount of force needed for correction of the distortion.

Thumb Position: As noted above, treatment of TBs relies on the use of the thumb to "iron out" the affected fascia. When learning to treat TBs it is not uncommon to be tempted to use the volar surface (flat) of the thumb to apply force along the TB, as the initial thumb and hand placement may seem more comfortable to the practitioner for a number of reasons including ROM or nail length and/or fear of abrading the patient with one's nail. This is not ideal for a number of reasons. Use of the volar surface results in force being dispersed over a wider area, necessitating more force to achieve the same outcome. Second, the greater surface area of the volar surface leads to a larger amount of friction between the thumb and the patient's skin, which may needlessly increase discomfort. And third, the friction-induced proximal glide of the volar pad will cause substantial strain between the nail plate and the nail bed of the treating thumb, leading to discomfort and an associated reduction in the amount of force applied. Use of the thumb in the manner prescribed may be relatively novel, but it is by no means exempt from the basic fundamentals of patient positioning and provider biomechanics. Ensuring a proper stance and stable body placement along with properly aligned hand, wrist, and arm will contribute to more efficient delivery of force and a more successful treatment.

Nail Care: For those just learning FDM, nail length may be an initial deterrent to the proper positioning and force application with the thumb. To reduce strain on the practitioner nail bed and potential abrasion of patient skin, it is recommended to keep the thumb nails short. If sensitivity in the hyponychium under the free edge of the nail prevents one from trimming the nail back, it may be necessary to gradually reduce the length of the nail over time instead of merely clipping the nail short. Once shortened, many practitioners find the use of a nail file preferable over clipping to keep the thumbnail short, as clipping may leave a sharp edge or accidental removal of too much nail, leading to nail bed irritation.

Patient Clothing: While TB treatment should be done directly on skin, it is possible to apply other treatments through patient clothing, if needed. In such cases, workout clothing or gowns are acceptable options for palpation and treatment. Treating through denim, especially jeans-type garments, should be avoided due to reduction in palpatory localization of the distortion and the dispersion of treatment forces that lead to additional force application and irritation of the practitioner's thumb.

Endurance: Witnessing positive outcomes from patients when first using FDM treatments can be a powerful motivator, and when one starts to recognize distortions with greater frequency, it is compelling to treat every TB, CD, and HTP encountered. Initially, this will result in irritation and soreness of the practitioner's thumb. Instead, it is recommended to start with just a few treatments a day to allow endurance to be built up over time.

TB Thumb: Even with proper position and force modulation, distortions may develop in the hand of the practitioner. Typaldos noted the existence of "triggerband thumb," an rFD in the first metacarpophalangeal joint or the trapeziometacarpal joint, which can be self-treated by refolding the affected joint. TBs and CDs may also develop at times, both easily self-treated with the appropriate techniques.[1,6]

AFTERCARE

Aftercare begins before the treatment, especially for patients who are new to FDM. Discussing the discomfort associated with treatment of some fascial distortions ahead of the treatment can ensure realistic expectations. Establishing rapport with each patient and finding ways to relate posttreatment bruising or soreness in comparison the patient's chronic pain or impeded ROM can provide perspective. Some patients find it helpful to consider it a "good trade," while others consider it "an investment," and yet still others frame the discomfort as compressing a long recovery time into a very short period and "just getting it over with." Inviting the patient to notice a difference between their old pain and the posttreatment discomfort may also be useful. In some cases, "pressure testing" or having the patient recreate the motion that provoked their old pain will provide confirmation that the treatment was successful and allow them to explore this new improvement in a safe space. Contextualizing side effects such as posttreatment discomfort in these or other approaches has been demonstrated to enhance treatment through expectancy effects.[14]

Side Effects: Common side effects associated with the FDM include bruising, swelling, and soreness. In order to reduce the severity of these events, patients are encouraged to use ice (rather than heat, unless they are dealing with a TF);[6] drink plenty of water (as OMT has been shown to be more effective in the euhydrated state)[15]; and use over-the-counter acetaminophen and nonsteroidal anti-inflammatory drugs (NSAIDs) as needed. All patients should be made aware that swelling and soreness should improve over the 24 to 48 hours after treatment with the FDM.[6] Worsening pain would be an unexpected result (and may suggest incomplete reduction of an HTP or development of a new distortion), and the patient should return to see the clinician who performed the FDM.[6] Severe pain that is different from the pain associated with the initial fascial distortion for which they presented for care should warrant re-evaluation by their primary care provider or in the emergency department (ED).[6]

Patients should be cautioned that bruising may take weeks to resolve (longer if they are older or on anticoagulation). If a large hematoma develops, or they develop numbness, weakness, or tingling in a limb treated with the FDM, these would be other indications to seek care from a healthcare professional prudently.[6]

The pseudo-HTP: Following treatment of HTPs that have been present for extended periods of time, it is not uncommon for a bruise or hematoma to form following the disruption of capillaries that have grown through the herniated bit of fascial matrix. This hematoma fills the space once occupied by the HTP and may be misidentified as the HTP having recurred. Palpation of this recurrent HTP may yield a subtle difference—the pseudo-HTP texture is found to be sand-like, or "gritty." Treatment of the pseudo-HTP differs from HTPs in that instead of reducing the tissue below the facial plane, manipulating the pseudo-HTP in a circular motion is done, with a goal of dissipating the hematoma.

Once patients have experienced the FDM, they will often ask what they can do at home to prevent the distortions from returning. If possible, they should be cautioned to avoid any repetitive motion injuries that provoked their initial fascial distortions. If this is not possible (often due to the demands of their work), they should establish regular follow-up with a provider of the FDM. Patients with high healthcare literacy may also be instructed in methods of self-treatment by the FDM provider. They should be shown how to appropriately position their thumb in order to prevent ligament or tendon injury from strain.[6]

Treatment Frequency: In the Model, the goal of all treatments is correction of the distortion. Once the distortion has been corrected, it fundamentally ceases to exist.[1,6] Often simple complaints related to a single distortion may be resolved in one or two visits. In case reports of complex injuries, Typaldos saw patients back in 1 to 2 days for re-evaluation and additional treatment if needed, with a minimum of 2 days being the most common treatment interval, assuming further treatment was needed.[1] TFs are recognized as being the most likely distortion to require repeated visits, often requiring twice-weekly visits over a 6-week period.[6] Practitioners and patients may encounter a phenomenon referred to as "peeling the onion," in which, upon resolution of one distortion, another area of discomfort makes itself known. Several distortions may be treated in one visit, with consideration toward limiting factors including severity of distortions, patient resilience, known response to treatment, and visit length. Current opinion suggests follow up visits for reassessment and additional treatment be no more frequent than once a week (aside from the twice weekly dedicated treatment of a TF), allowing for acute inflammation and hematoma formation to subside.

CURRENT RESEARCH

The FDM is a relatively new domain of OMT; however, research to date has demonstrated the effectiveness of the FDM for back pain, neck pain, extremity pain, and even abdominal wall pain.

Back Pain

One of the most robust studies of the FDM to date[16] was a prospective nonrandomized parallel group trial for low back pain. Seventy seven patients were recruited, and the control group received standard of care. The primary outcome was percent of patients free of symptoms, with secondary outcomes including pain-free ROM, lost work days, use of analgesics, frequency of specialist consultations, and pain scores according to patient diaries. Half of patients were symptom-free at 12 weeks. Though not statistically significant, secondary outcomes included a trend toward missing fewer days of work, using less pain medication, and a faster decline in symptoms in the FDM group.[16]

Neck Pain

A recent pilot study including 90 patients[17] compared the efficacy of a single session of the FDM combined with foam rolling compared to foam rolling alone or no intervention for the management of neck pain. Both the combination of the FDM and foam rolling as well as foam rolling alone were found to produce statistically significant improvements in pain intensity and cervical spine mobility.[17]

Extremity Pain

Numerous studies have investigated the efficacy of the FDM for treating extremity pain. In an unblinded randomized controlled trial (RCT) by Fink et al. in 2012 in which they compared the FDM to passive stretching and ROM, both groups were found to achieve improved ROM, but the FDM group reached this endpoint more rapidly. Pain reduction and functional improvement were also found to be superior in the FDM group.[18] A prospective case control study by Shulze et al. in 2014 investigated the usefulness of the FDM for shin splints and found that half of patients were pain-free at the end of the study.[19] In 2018, Boucher and Figueroa published a case report of a patient whose frozen shoulder resolved completely after two treatment sessions with the FDM.[20] A pilot trial by Boucher and Dewey in 2019 and a subsequent single-arm prospective effectiveness study published by Boucher et al. in 2021 found that the FDM was markedly effective in the treatment of plantar heel pain.[21,22] Their more recent study also identified an anatomical correlate in conjunction with the patients' improvement in symptoms: there was a demonstrated decrease in plantar fascial thickness on ultrasound at 16 weeks compared with baseline after patients were treated with the FDM.[22] Another trial of the FDM published in 2021 by Kim and Kim found no difference in hamstring flexibility when comparing the FDM with static stretching.[23]

Abdominal Wall Pain

In 2023, Pelletier and Boucher published a case report of a patient with chronic abdominal wall pain (CAWP) after abdominoplasty who presented to the ED with a CyD of the abdominal wall induced by wearing an abdominal binder. The CyD completely resolved with the FDM, and her baseline abdominal wall pain—thought to be secondary to chronic HTPs—markedly improved. This study noted a possible anatomical correlate for abdominal wall HTPs known as anterior cutaneous nerve entrapment syndrome (ACNES), in which thoracoabdominal sensory nerves become entrapped and produce CAWP.[24]

RESEARCH LIMITATIONS AND FUTURE DIRECTIONS

The current literature investigating the usefulness of the FDM for the treatment of pain is limited by studies with small numbers, as well as challenges with blinding. Future research must involve high-quality, blinded RCTs with large numbers of patients using well-established OMT sham treatments. Researchers must also investigate the applicability of the FDM in a wider variety of clinical settings, as most of the FDM literature to date has been conducted in the outpatient setting. Critics of the FDM cite the biologic implausibility of the FDM model; thus, strong anatomical correlation data to support the theory of the FDM is needed.[25]

CONCLUSION

The FDM is a relatively novel form of OMT which can be utilized in a rapid fashion to obtain substantial improvements in pain and ROM. This model, developed by Dr. Stephen Typaldos, categorizes somatic dysfunction into six domains—TB, HTP, CD, FD (including unfolding and refolding), CyD, and TF—which are diagnosed based on characteristic patient descriptions and gestures. These verbal descriptions and hand movements are universal and do not differ across cultures. Though research support for the FDM is still in its early stages, evidence to date suggests that this domain of OMT is highly effective for the management of a wide range of acute and chronic pain in any practice setting.

Star Triggerband Story

Why is it called the Star TB? The origin story of the FDM revolves around a fundamental shift in Dr. Typaldos' perspective of the patient's role in their treatment and his role in providing that treatment. As the story goes, Dr. Typaldos was working in his clinic one day when he had a series of patients present with a very similar description and location of pain, consisting of a "pulling" sensation in the thoracic region. These patients described the pain in the thoracic region at about the level of T6 and indicated the pain moved up from there (Fig. 63.57). For the first two of these patients, he gathered a history, performed an examination, and then provided an OMT. In his words, "I cracked their back." The patients expressed little relief with the treatment.

The same day, a third patient demonstrated an identical pattern of pain. Dr. Typaldos was honest with the patient, and he said to her, "I don't know how to fix your pain." He asked her to give him 15 to 20 minutes to see if he could figure this out. Dr. Typaldos was frustrated because he knew he had seen this problem before, and he felt like he had never really helped any patients with similar complaints. He felt that he no longer could blame the

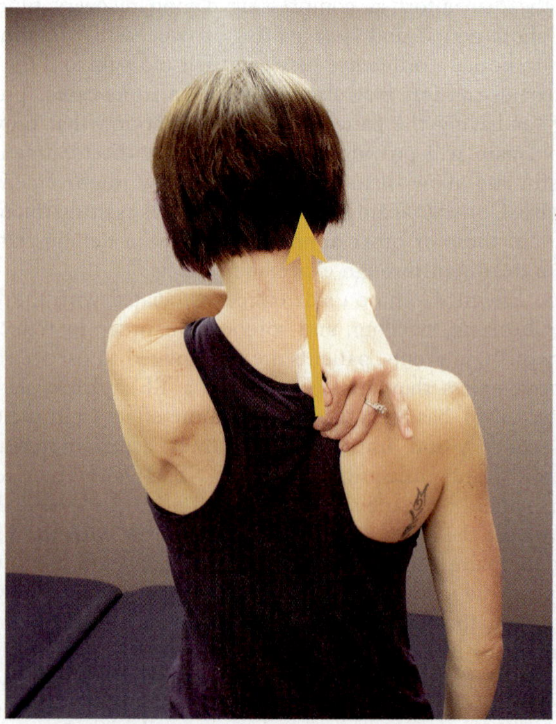

Figure 63.57. Star TB. (Reprinted with permission from Capistrant T, Harrer G, Pentzer T, eds. *The Fascial Distortion Model: Philosophy, Principles and Clinical Applications*. Handspring Publishing; 2021.)

patient, the prescription, the pharmacist, or the physical therapist for the lack of improvement; he could only blame himself. One of his recent realizations was that patients intuitively know what needs to be done to change their pain. He determined that he would allow the patient to show him and tell him how to help her.

Armed with this thought, Dr. Typaldos returned to the room and said he had recuperated, and that he was ready to try and help her. He said, “I have 20 minutes and I want you to talk, and I am going to listen.”

For the next 20 minutes the patient relived the 20-year history of her pain and the unsuccessful attempts that had been made to eliminate it: procedures, office visits, manipulative treatments, and medications. He described this process of listening as painful but necessary. One of the things she said was, “I wish someone would take their thumb and push on my back as hard as they can.”

He replied to her, “I'll do it.”

She was shocked as she said, “Really? Why?”

Dr. Typaldos said, “Because that is what you want me to do.”

She went on to tell him that she had asked so many people to do this and that is what she wanted them to do all along, but they always said “NO.”

So, he took his thumb and pressed on what is now known as the Star TB. The patient stated, “It's moving.”

He said, “What's moving?”

She said, “It's moving.”

Dr. Typaldos said, “What is it?”

She said, “That pain. Stay with it!”

“Stay with what?”

“Stay with that pain. That's it. Stay with it.” He was tracing a pathway up her back and she said, “You're off of it, off to the right, go back.” Thus, she guided him all the way through the treatment. Dr. Typaldos finished the treatment at the mastoid. The patient moved her arm around and said, “This is the best I have felt in 20 years. You're the smartest doctor I have ever been to.”

He replied, “I don't know what I am doing.”

She said, “You're the only one who understands my problem.”

Dr. Typaldos' response was, “I don't understand it. I have no idea what this is.” This was the discovery of the TB treatment in September of 1991.

As Dr. Typaldos moved forward from this experience, he found himself truly listening to patients. He listened and didn't interrupt them as they described their pain. He found himself working within a new framework of listening. He said to himself, “I am going to ignore the things they tell us to pay attention to and pay attention to the things they tell us to ignore.”

Dr. Typaldos began to look at his treatments differently, and the tenets of the FDM were developed. The Star TB is so named because this was the first TB treated, and therefore the “star of the show.”[2,7]

REFERENCES

1. Typaldos S. *FDM: Clinical and Theoretical Application of the Fascial Distortion Model Within the Practice of Medicine and Surgery*. Orthopathic Global Health Publications; 2002.
2. Typaldos S. Recorded lectures from FDM module circa 2004. Lecture presented at: Fairbanks, AK; 2022.
3. Typaldos S. Introducing the Fascial Distortion Model. *AAOJ*. 1994 [cited February 10, 2023];(Spring):14–36. https://afdma.com/articles/introducing-fascial-distortion-model/
4. Typaldos S. Triggerband Technique. *AAOJ*. 1994 [cited February 10, 2023];(Winter):15–33. https://afdma.com//articles/triggerband-technique/
5. Typaldos S. Continuum Technique. *AAOJ*. 1995 [cited February 10, 2023];(Summer):15–19. https://afdma.com//articles/continuum-technique/
6. Capistrant T, Harrer G. Pentzer T, ed. *The Fascial Distortion Model: Philosophy, Principles and Clinical Applications*. Handspring Publishing; 2021.
7. Kasten M. History of the FDM. In: *FDM: An Introduction to the Fascial Distortion Model*. AFDMA; 2010:7–14.
8. Hohenschurz-Schmidt DJ. Tensegrity in the context of the myofascial network: its relevance to osteopathic practice. In: Chila A, Liem T, Tozzi P, eds. *Fascia in the osteopathic field*. Handspring Publishing; 2017:111–117.
9. Snelson K. The Art of Tensegrity. *The International Journal of Space Structures*. 2012. [cited February 1, 2023];27(2,3):71–80. http://kenneths-nelson.net/articles/TheArtOfTensegrityArticle.pdf
10. Levin S, Madden M. In vivo observation of articular surface contact in knee joints. 2005. [cited December 15, 2022]. http://www.biotensegrity.com/resources/in-vivo-obs-knee.pdf
11. Anker S. [thesis]. [Interrater reliability in evaluating the body language based on the Fascial Distortion Model (FDM).] 2011. [cited February 19, 2023]. https://www.osteopathicresearch.com/files/original/1f6774c-75fa60b0b580b6889ab258f07767375ea.pdf
12. Wofford JL, Mansfield RJ, Watkins RS. Patient characteristics and clinical management of patients with shoulder pain in U.S. Primary Care Settings: Secondary data analysis of the National Ambulatory Medical Care Survey. *BMC Musculoskelet Disord*. 2005;6:4.
13. Rodeghero JR, Cleland JA, Mintken PE, Cook CE. Risk stratification of patients with shoulder pain seen in physical therapy practice. *J Eval Clin Pract*. 2016;23(2):257–263.
14. Berna C, Kirsch I, Zion S, et al. Side effects can enhance treatment response through expectancy effects: an experimental analgesic randomized controlled trial. *Pain*. 2017;158(6):1014–1020.
15. Parker J, Heinking KP, Kappler RE. Efficacy of osteopathic manipulative treatment for low back pain in euhydrated and hypohydrated conditions: a randomized crossover trial. *J Am Osteopath Assoc*. 2012;112(5):276–284.
16. Richter D, Karst M, Buhck H, Fink MG. Efficacy of fascial distortion model treatment for acute, nonspecific low-back pain in primary care: a prospective controlled trial. *Altern Ther Health Med*. 2017;23(5):AT5522.
17. Wiaderna K, Selegrat M, Hadamus A. Effect of a single session of facial distortion model manual physiotherapy and a selected foam rolling technique on treatment outcomes in cervical spine overload. Pilot study. *Ortop Traumatol Rehabil*. 2020;22(2):131–141.
18. Fink M, Schiller J, Buhck H. [Efficacy of a manual treatment method according to the fascial distortion model in the management of contracted (“frozen”) shoulder]. *Z Orthop Unfall*. 2012;150(4):420–427.
19. Schulze C, Finze S, Bader R, Lison A. Treatment of medial tibial stress syndrome according to the fascial distortion model: a prospective case control study. *ScientificWorldJournal*. 2014;2014:790626.
20. Boucher JD, Figueroa J. Restoration of full shoulder range of motion after application of the fascial distortion model. *J Am Osteopath Assoc*. 2018;118(5):341–344.
21. Boucher J, Dewey T. Recovery from plantar heel pain through the fascial distortion model: a pilot study. *Postgrad Med*. 2019;131(sup1):1–130.
22. Boucher J, Mooney S, Dewey T, Kirtley RG, Walker T, Rabago D. Manual therapy informed by the fascial distortion model for plantar heel pain: results of a single-arm prospective effectiveness study. *J Altern Complement Med*. 2021;27(8):697–705.
23. Kim JY, Kim SY. A comparison of the effects of static stretching and the fascial distortion model (FDM) on hamstring flexibility. *J Back Musculoskelet Rehabil*. 2021;34(6):1087–1092.
24. Pelletier J, Boucher J. A case of chronic postoperative abdominal wall pain successfully treated with the fascial distortion model. *AAO Journal*. 2023;33(2):60–66.
25. Thalhamer C. A fundamental critique of the fascial distortion model and its application in clinical practice. *J Bodyw Mov*. 2018;22(1):112–117.

64 Integrated General Osteopathic Technique

KENNETH A. RAMEY

KEY CONCEPTS

- JM Littlejohn expanded osteopathic principles by emphasizing the importance of physiology, healing by the body's inherent vital force, and utilizing long-lever oscillatory treatments to encourage nerve function and fluid exchange.
- J Wernham is considered the father of the "Body Adjustment Technique," an essential integrative method of treatment representing Littlejohn's concepts and designed to stimulate the body's inherent ability to self-heal and maintain balance.
- RC Fulford applied concepts using energy medicine models, the impact of birth and first breath, assessment of structural "vitality," and trauma, releasing dysfunction in the body with the Fulford percussion hammer and cranial osteopathy.
- The integrated general osteopathic technique is simple and effective and can be applied to almost any patient including adults and children.

INTRODUCTION

JM Littlejohn, John Wernham, and Robert C. Fulford all described concepts and techniques that allow clinicians to more efficiently and effectively treat their patients. Their contributions have been fused together into an approach called integrated general osteopathic technique (IGOT). This chapter discusses the history, philosophy, and methods for performing integrated general osteopathic technique, and its application into total patient care. General osteopathic techniques use gentle rhythmic oscillation to sequentially treat the body regionally and segmentally, thereby supporting physiologic processes and homeostasis.

HISTORY

John Martin Littlejohn (1865–1947) and John Wernham (1907–2007)

John Martin (JM) Littlejohn was a pivotal Scottish academic who was also a leader in the development of Osteopathy. Born into a family of Reformed Presbyterians in Glasgow, Scotland, he was the son of a preacher.[1] Littlejohn pursued an extensive education at the University of Glasgow, obtaining degrees in the Arts, Divinity, and Laws.[2] In 1888, he suffered a severe concussion and a fractured skull.[1] In 1892, he was awarded the Hunter Gold Medal in Forensic Medicine.[2] That same year, Littlejohn moved to the United States to study at Columbia University in New York. During this time, he had serious bouts of illness and operations on his throat. These medical issues led Littlejohn to seek treatment from Andrew Taylor Still in 1897.[1] This experience profoundly influenced Littlejohn and inspired him to pursue a career as a Doctor of Osteopathy (DO).[1]

Littlejohn later became president of Amity College in Iowa before enrolling at the American School of Osteopathy (ASO) in Kirksville in 1898. By 1899, he had joined the ASO faculty as chair of physiology and was instrumental in teaching students like William G. Sutherland.[1] Littlejohn's academic contributions helped establish Osteopathy as a rigorous discipline rooted in both anatomy and physiology. Littlejohn also applied the principle of the *vital force* as the force that governs the body's physiology within the constraints of environment, diet, exercise, and lifestyle. This concept emphasized the body's inherent ability to self-heal and maintain balance. He viewed the vital force as the animating energy that underlies all physiologic activity. Littlejohn believed that disease arises when this force is disrupted, leading to a loss of harmony within the body's fluids, structures, and functions. His treatments aimed to restore this harmony by addressing both structural and functional imbalances, using techniques that stimulated or inhibited the body's systems as needed. As stated by JF Kemp, DO, Littlejohn considered that health rests on a three-pillared foundation, that is, structure adjustment, function adjustment, and the adjustment of the organism to its environment.[3]

The Littlejohn brothers left Kirksville, MO and began the Chicago College of Osteopathy in 1900. In 1913, JM Littlejohn left Chicago due to personal issues and health concerns and returned to Britain. In 1917, alongside his lifelong friend Dr. FJ Horn, JM Littlejohn founded the British School of Osteopathy.[1] This institution became the first osteopathic school outside the United States and played a crucial role in spreading osteopathic principles across Europe.

Littlejohn's legacy continued through his student John Wernham, who carried forward his teachings at The John Wernham College of Classical Osteopathy in Maidstone, England. John Wernham was also a prominent figure in classical Osteopathy, who dedicated over 70 years to studying, lecturing, and practicing the principles taught by Dr. JM Littlejohn.[2] Wernham's educational contributions were significant, including founding the Maidstone College of Osteopathy in 1984, which was renamed The John Wernham College of Classical Osteopathy in 1996.[2] His influence reached beyond the United Kingdom, as he assisted in establishing osteopathic schools in Canada and Europe. Wernham is considered the father of the "Body Adjustment," an essential integrative method of treatment representing Littlejohn's concept of the General Osteopathic Treatment (GOT).[4] Wernham's techniques were designed to stimulate the body's inherent ability to self-heal and maintain balance, aligning with Littlejohn's concept of the vital force as the animating energy underlying all physiologic activity. This osteopathic treatment encompassed a series of gentle passive rhythmic long lever–based appendicular, pelvic, and spinal mobilization procedures defined by three basic principles: routine, rotation, and rhythm.[4] Wernham stressed that the overriding principle is that the body adjustment (BA) is slow, quiet, gentle, and rhythmic. It focused on the application of physical treatment to address and enhance physiologic processes within the body.[4] While Littlejohn's and Wernham's contributions are celebrated internationally, their techniques remain more widely taught in Britain than in American Osteopathy today.

Robert C. Fulford, DO (1905–1997)

Robert Fulford, DO's philosophy and techniques have been discussed in Chapter 59 Additional Osteopathic Manipulative Treatment Approaches: Fulford Percussion. To reiterate, he organized his diagnostic efforts around energy medicine models, the impact of birth and first breath, assessment of structural "vitality," and the patients' history of physical and emotional trauma.[5–7] One such form of integrating energetic medicine in treating patients was Fulford's application of crystals into his osteopathic treatments. Fulford incorporated refined Vogel-cut quartz crystals into his practice, drawing on the work of Marcel Vogel, PhD, a senior IBM research scientist.[8] The crystals were used as a tool to amplify his intention, thereby enhancing the electromagnetic aspects of his therapeutic approach on the physical body and allowing him to reach deeper into the realms of spirit and mind. This is very consistent with AT Still's description of the triune nature of the individual.[9]

GENERAL PRINCIPLES AND PHILOSOPHY

Background

JM Littlejohn utilized rhythmic body mobilizations and long-lever techniques as part of his GOT, which was used to support physiologic processes and enhance the distribution of forces throughout the body.[10] Littlejohn's approach involved identifying areas of dysfunction while facilitating a fluid continuum in the body.[10] These gentle techniques were applied to the whole body, engaging it globally while working section-by-section to create energy flow throughout.[10] He also emphasized the importance of addressing nerve irritability and the *vital force,* restoring energetic coordination among bodily structures.[10] Littlejohn focused on treating the patient holistically, facilitating healing through supporting the interrelationship of body parts, rather than targeting specific lesions.[10] Littlejohn stated that Osteopathy is a growing discipline, and its path is both innovation and scientific progression; each osteopath can develop their skills by integrating all scientific knowledge with the ultimate goal of observing the body system as a whole.[11–13]

Application

The integrated general osteopathic technique is an amalgamation of three approaches. It is simple and effective and can be applied to almost any patient, including adults and children. The general principle is to treat the body regionally (globally), then address any remaining segmental or specific dysfunction. Treating regionally will result in the clinical resolution of approximately 80% of segmental or specific somatic dysfunctions. The overall goal is to improve the motion and function of the entire patient, encouraging the entire system to integrate as a unit and establish an environment where the body can heal and exist in health. It does not focus on a specific illness or disease. The unity of the human body emphasizes the fact that each body part is in communion; a body area could be affected by a local or distant dysfunction.[13,14]

General osteopathic technique is unique, sequential, and adaptable based upon palpatory feedback. The technique allows for infinite variables specifically adapted to each individual patient's needs and structural and physiologic findings. The overall approach uses fluid circles and rhythmic oscillation to facilitate release. Similar to other osteopathic techniques, GOT improves the motion and function of bones, muscles, and connective tissues, promotes lymphatic drainage, and balances the autonomic nervous system. GOT has been shown to be as efficacious as other osteopathic interventions in patients with anxiety and fibromyalgia.[15,16] The approach integrates the entire body into a harmonious, functional unit. In most instances, the physician is diagnosing and treating simultaneously, which saves considerable time and is advantageous in a busy clinical setting.

Energy Considerations

In 1902, Dr. Littlejohn described an energy field known as "the vital force." It is associated with a palpable vibration, or vibratility, within the individual. He stated that "The vital cycle depends upon vibration. Waves of vibration pass along the tissues, especially from the nerves and the brain to and along the muscle tissues. There is no function of the body that does not have peristaltic or rhythmic vibrations. The power of osteopathic treatment occurs from its effect upon physiological oscillations."[10] When the vital force is depleted, there is a decrease in vibratility, or palpable vibration, both locally and globally within the system. Palpating for a change in this vibratility is another useful way to screen for somatic dysfunction. A successful osteopathic treatment should result in the return of this palpable vibratility, both locally in the area of somatic dysfunction, and globally throughout the entire system.

Likewise, Dr. Fulford taught that "Nothing rests. Everything vibrates. Everything, in some subtle way, moves."[7] He described a life field that is present both within and around the physical body and imparts vitality to the physical body.[7] This includes a component of electromagnetic energy. He referenced Dr. Harold Saxon Burr as describing this as an "organizing field" for the physical body, guiding the atoms and molecules into proper form.[7] In health, this field is strong and freely resonates throughout the individual. Physical, mental, and emotional trauma can result in a local and global depletion of the life field within the individual's system. If persistent, this can manifest as somatic dysfunction and disease. Changes in the life field precede changes in the individual's physiology. Abnormal physiology will not improve until the manifestation of the life field is improved.

Treatment Similarities

Littlejohn and Wernham taught General Osteopathic Technique, or sequential oscillatory articulation, as a means to introduce kinetic energy into the body and facilitate the release of somatic dysfunction. Similarly, Dr. Fulford's Percussion Hammer Techniques incorporate an electric motor to introduce a longitudinal compression wave (standing wave) of kinetic energy into the body to facilitate the release. Listed is the sequence of treatment based upon a Fulford Percussion hammer course taken by the author and editor in 1995[7]: (1) Abdomen and diaphragm, (2) Knee, (3) Ankle, (4) Foot, (5) Hips and trochanters, (6) Pelvis and sacrum, (7) Lumbar and thoracic spine, (8) Ribcage, (9) Shoulders, (10) Elbow, (11) Wrist, (12) Cranial, (13) Cervical spine, (14) Sternum.[7] Interestingly, the treatment sequences between the GOT originally described by Littlejohn, the BA of Wernham and the percussion sequence used by Fulford are quite similar.[12] The end goal of all methods is the same, which is a palpable return of the life force, vibratility, and subsequent physiologic improvement. Through similar treatment sequences, Littlejohn, Wernham, and Fulford all approached the patient from biomechanical and bioenergetic models.

Dr. Littlejohn's biomechanical approach was quite expansive, and he described fascial patterns and interconnections which help account for the local and regional structural and functional effects of his methods. J Gordan Zink, DO also described fascial patterns that can be used in the evaluation and treatment of fascial compensation and decompensation.[17] The fascial patterns described by both individuals favorably respond to the proper application of General Osteopathic Technique.

TECHNIQUE OVERVIEW AND SEQUENCE

Oscillation serves a dual purpose in integrated GOT, functioning as both an assessment tool and a treatment method. When applied to a specific body part, it allows the practitioner to evaluate, treat, and reassess the patient's condition.[4] In line with Littlejohn's teachings, oscillatory technique emphasizes the physiologic aspect of the osteopathic lesion and treatment, rather than just the structural component.[4] By incorporating oscillatory technique into his methods, Wernham developed a comprehensive approach to osteopathic treatment that addresses both structural and functional aspects of the body, emphasizing the importance of treating the patient as a whole. The following structures and regions are addressed in the following order: (1) Abdomen, (2) Lower ribcage, (3) Hips and innominates, (4) Piriformis muscles, (5) Adductor muscles, (6) Lower extremities (knees, ankles/feet), (7) Iliotibial band/lumbar rotation stretch, (8) Hamstrings/psoas major muscles, (9) Sacrum, (10) Lumbars, (11) Thoracics, (12) Ribs, (13) Lumbar and thoracic spine seated, (14) Upper extremity (shoulder, clavicle/thoracic inlet, elbow, wrist, and hand), (15) Neck including OA and suboccipital tissues.

Breathing, Trauma and the Abdomen

Efficient, effortless breathing is vital to health. Unfortunately, many of us either do not know how to, or cannot take a deep breath. When a person undergoes a physical or psychological trauma, one of the first things they do is to inhale and hold it. The abdomen subsequently tightens. This restricts normal diaphragmatic motion. Thereafter, the person cannot breathe properly. When the abdomen tightens and the diaphragm becomes restricted, the entire body frequently becomes tight. The increased tension within the abdominal wall may irritate the three sympathetic ganglia that lie within the abdominal region (celiac ganglion T5–T9, superior mesenteric ganglion T10–T11, and inferior mesenteric ganglion T12–L2), contributing to a somato-somatic reflex in the thoracic and lumbar spine. The sympathetic nerves that innervate the lower extremities arise from spinal cord levels T10–L3.[18] Somatic dysfunction in the low thoracic and upper lumbar areas can facilitate increased sympathetic tone to the lower extremities. This can result in skin, vascular and lymphatic changes, and altered tone of the resting muscles. Dysfunction in this region will frequently cause issues with the psoas major muscles. If a patient has recurring somatic dysfunction in the upper or lower back, despite OMT and the proper performance of stretching exercises, the abdomen and diaphragm may need to be addressed before the somatic dysfunction in these regions favorably responds. In addition, when the abdomen and diaphragm are restricted, the neck muscles may tighten with each breath to assist with rib elevation to allow the patient to breathe more fully. This may result in chronic neck tightness and headaches. This scenario is frequently found in patients with migraine headaches.

Wernham and Fulford both evaluated and treated the abdomen. Dr. Fulford more specifically described how strain patterns are stored in the abdomen and result in restricted diaphragmatic motion.[7] Interestingly, when the abdominal and diaphragmatic restrictions are released, many people will remember the event or feel the emotion associated with the trauma and subsequent restrictions. When this happens, the person needs to deal with emotion in a proper manner, resolve it and this will put them on the road to healing. Many people, however, do not want to deal with these feelings or emotions, attempt to repress or ignore them, and this drives the dysfunction deeper into the body. If you are repeatedly treating a patient's abdomen for the same recurrent dysfunction, they may not be dealing with the emotional contribution to the problem. This needs to be explained to the patient, and they may need to do some psychological homework before the dysfunction will permanently be resolved. After treating the abdomen or diaphragm, inform the patient that they may be tired, sore, achy, and/or moody for several hours or days.

Specific emotions seem to be stored in certain areas of the abdomen. Chinese medicine has described the concept of the visceral brain.[19] Chronic anger is stored in the region of the liver, worry and anxiety in the region of the spleen and stomach, and fear in the region of the kidneys.[19] Dr. Fulford also described a similar concept.[20] This concept may be related to why stress (anxiety) causes ulcers and epigastric pain. If a patient has a restriction over the liver area, ask them if they have been angry about something either recently or for a long time. They may not remember at first, but, in thinking about the question, may return in several days and reveal the source of their negative emotion. If a patient has a chronically tight right psoas or quadriceps muscle, look for a restriction in the liver region. If the left psoas or quadriceps muscle is chronically tight, look for a restriction in the spleen region.

REGIONAL APPLICATION OF TECHNIQUE

Abdomen

Combined Diagnosis and Treatment – Patient Supine

When treating a male patient, stand next to their right side. When treating a female patient, stand next to their left side (mnemonic—"the right man for the job"). According to Dr. Fulford, it has to do with energetic polarities. Clinical experience has supported this concept, and it seems to work better if you follow Dr. Fulford's rule.

The clinician will flex the patient's hips and knees and hold their knees against their chest or body wall with their elbow. Next, the clinician will start in the epigastric area and use one hand to gently palpate for increased tension and tissue texture changes within the abdominal wall. If present, they will apply slight posterior pressure to the abdomen with their free hand. Maintain this pressure while moving the patient's hips and knees in fluid circles (clockwise or counterclockwise, whichever is more comfortable to you) until a release is palpated (tissues soften or tissue texture changes improve). The clinician will work their way down the midline (linea alba) to the pubic symphysis, treating any dysfunction in the above manner (Fig. 64.1).

After treating the midline, the clinician should work their way around the remainder of the abdomen and evaluate and treat the right lower quadrant, right upper quadrant, left upper quadrant, and down the left lower quadrant. Assess each area but only treat areas with significant somatic dysfunction. The goal is to get the entire abdomen integrating and functioning as a unit. Avoid treating around the spleen and lower ribcage if the patient has recently had mononucleosis.

Lower Ribcage

Diagnosis – Patient Supine

Palpate the motion of the lower ribcage. Assess both rotation and translation. Also palpate for restrictions in the abdominal wall

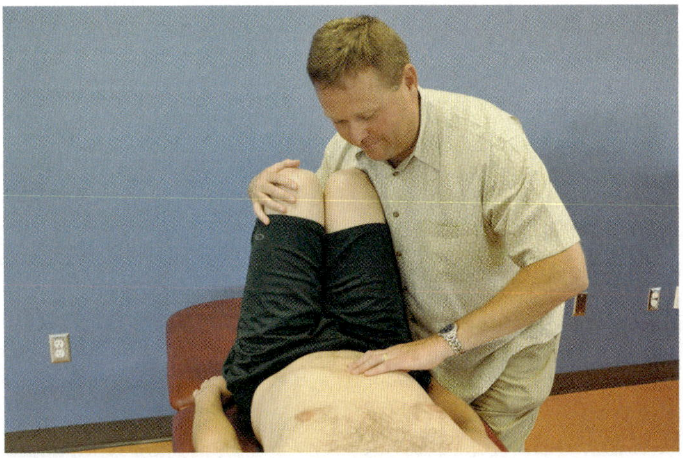

Figure 64.1. Treatment of the abdomen.

underneath the right and left costal margin (area of the liver and spleen).

Treatment – Patient Supine

The clinician will contact the right lower ribcage with their left hand and the left lower ribcage with their right hand. Translate the lower ribcage to the right and left, creating an oscillatory wave that produces motion from the top of the patient's head to the bottom of their feet. Continue until the tissues release and then reassess (Fig. 64.2).

Hips/Innominates

A common dysfunctional pattern is the right anterior/left posterior innominate. It is present in approximately 80% of patients. Treating the anterior/posterior rotation first may result in improvement of any associated innominate shear (superior or inferior) or flare (inflare or outflare). Again, individualize and treat what you find. This technique looks at both innominates as a unit and both sides are treated if dysfunctional. It does not isolate dysfunction to one innominate based on the results of the standing flexion test.

Diagnosis – Patient Supine

The clinician places their left palm over the right ASIS (anterior superior iliac spine) and their right palm over the left ASIS. The clinician will rock the innominates back and forth, one side at a time, toward the table determining any restriction. Next, the clinician will hook their thumbs underneath both ASISs and look at their position. Is the right ASIS more inferior than the left? This is most consistent with a right anterior/left posterior innominate. The clinician can also ask the patient to turn over and assess the position of the posterior superior iliac spines (PSISs).

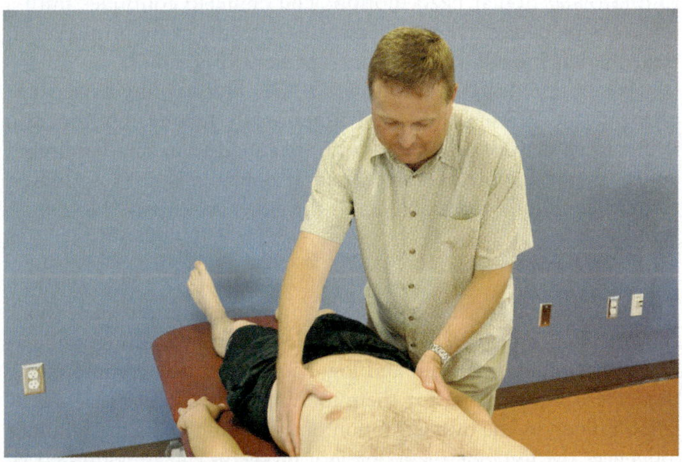

Figure 64.2. Treatment of the lower ribcage.

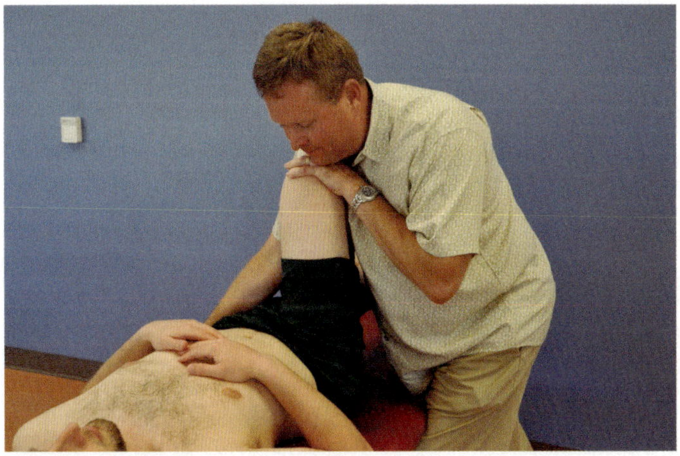

Figure 64.3. Treatment of a right anterior innominate.

Treatment – Right Anterior Innominate – Patient Supine

The clinician will flex the patient's right hip and knee and place their proximal leg against their right shoulder. Next the clinician will stabilize the patient's leg against their right shoulder with their left hand. Next, the clinician will reach their right hand around and under the patient's left innominate and place their fingertips medial to the left PSIS. Now the clinician will use their entire body (not just their arms) to move the right hip through fluid counterclockwise circles (flexion, abduction, and extension). This does not take much force and, according to Littlejohn, movement is approximately a few millimeters past the feather edge of the restrictive barrier. Especially focus on portions of the motion that are the most restricted. Continue until a release is palpated, which usually occurs within ten repetitions (Fig. 64.3).

Treatment – Left Posterior Innominate – Patient Supine

The clinician will flex the patient's left hip and knee and place their proximal leg against their left shoulder. The clinician will stabilize the patient's leg against their left shoulder or chest with their left hand. Now the clinician reaches their right hand under the patient's left innominate and places their fingertips medial to the left PSIS. The clinician uses their entire body to move the patient's left hip through counterclockwise circles (flexion, adduction, and extension). Continue until a release occurs. Reassess both innominates. Has the pelvic rock improved? (Fig. 64.4)

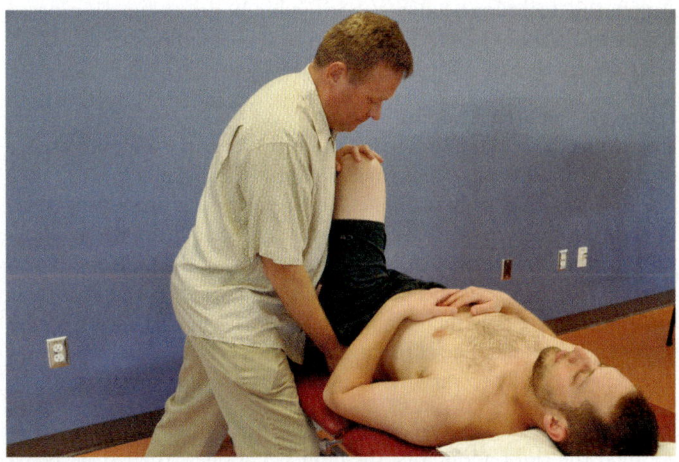

Figure 64.4. Treatment of a left posterior innominate.

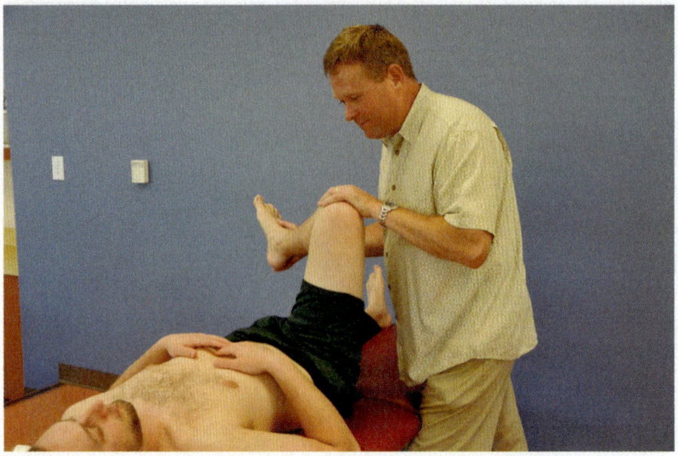

Figure 64.5. **Treatment of the right piriformis muscle.**

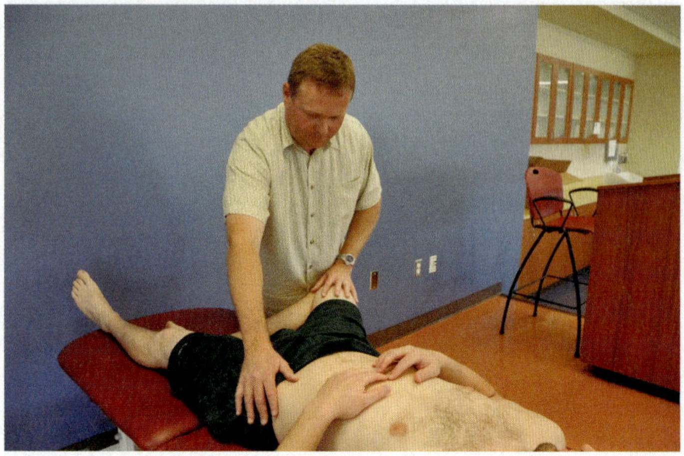

Figure 64.6. **Treatment of the right adductor muscles.**

Piriformis Muscles

The piriformis muscles can be great mischief makers in the pelvis and are frequently associated with pelvic floor and sacral dysfunction (especially the Chicago posterior sacrum). They may also be associated with sciatica. When the hip is extended, the piriformis muscle serves as an external hip rotator and is an abductor when the hip is flexed.

Combined Diagnosis and Treatment – Example – Right Piriformis Muscle Tight – Patient Supine

Stand next to the patient's right side. The clinician diagnoses and treats this area simultaneously. If one side is tight, treat that side and if both sides are tight, treat both sides. Flex their right hip and knee and externally rotate their right hip. The clinician must maintain this external rotation throughout the treatment, or it will not be as effective. Contact the patient's right knee with your left hand and their right ankle (over the lateral malleolus) with your right hand. Keep their right leg close to your body and move their hip in fluid counterclockwise circles (flexion/adduction, abduction, and extension). Continue until a release occurs and reassess (Fig. 64.5).

Adductor Muscles

The adductors are frequently associated with pubic symphysis dysfunction and groin strains. They can also help maintain innominate dysfunction. For example, a tight right adductor can produce a right inferior pubic symphysis shear and contribute to a right anterior innominate. The innominate may not completely respond until the adductor and pubic symphysis dysfunctions are addressed. Again, this technique looks at both pubic bones as functioning as a unit and does not lateralize using the standing flexion test. Both sides are treated in most instances.

Diagnosis – Patient Supine

The clinician places their left middle finger over the superior aspect of the right pubic bone and their right middle finger over the superior aspect of the left pubic bone. Next determine if one side is more inferior. To assess the right adductors, the clinician flexes the patient's right hip and knee and places their right foot on the table medial to their left knee. The clinician uses their right hand to stabilize their left ASIS and places their right hand over the medial aspect of the patient's right knee. The clinician gently abducts their hip by pushing their knee laterally toward the floor and palpates for a restriction.

Treatment – The Treatment Position is the Same

To treat the right adductors, the clinician abducts their right hip a few millimeters past the feather edge of the restrictive barrier. The clinician oscillates the right knee back and forth toward the floor until the adductors release.

Use the same principles to evaluate the left side and treat if a restriction is present. Reassess. Improved motion and symmetry of the pubic bones and innominates should be noted (Fig. 64.6).

Knees

According to Dr. Fulford, during birth, the left knee is frequently tucked underneath the body and is traumatized.[7] A strain pattern may be stored in the knee. The left knee may contain more somatic dysfunction than the right knee, but treatment is based on your evaluation.[7]

Diagnosis – Patient Supine

The tibial tuberosity and the center of the patella should line up. Usually, the tibial tuberosity lies lateral to the center of the patella in the dysfunctional knee. Also assess tension in the iliotibial band, fibular head dysfunction, and external/internal tibial rotation.

Treatment – Patient Supine

The same basic treatment will address any tibial or fibular head dysfunction. To treat the right knee, the clinician stands next to the patient's right side and flexes their right knee and hip. The clinician stabilizes the patient's distal leg against their right lateral ribcage using their right elbow. Next the clinician contacts the proximal leg with both hands and places their fingertips in the popliteal fossa. The clinician uses their body to introduce smooth circles to rotate the knee in a counterclockwise direction (flexion, abduction, or varus force and extension). The varus force is critical to improving fibular head motion. The clinician continues until a release is palpated and then reassesses. Use the same principles to treat the left knee if a restriction is present (Fig. 64.7).

Treatment pearl – according to Dr. Fulford, the knee, diaphragm, and cervical spine are functionally related. Dysfunction in the knee may be associated with dysfunction in the diaphragm and/or cervical spine and vice versa. If one area is not responding to treatment, look for problems in the other two areas.[7]

Ankles/Feet

The talocalcaneal articulation is a very important biomechanical shock absorber. If it is restricted, more force is transmitted during ambulation to the ankle, knee, hip and low back, potentially compromising these areas and predisposing them to injury. The talocalcaneal articulation influences the overall motion of the hindfoot. As the hindfoot influences the forefoot, many forefoot problems can be addressed by improving the motion and function of the talocalaneal articulation.

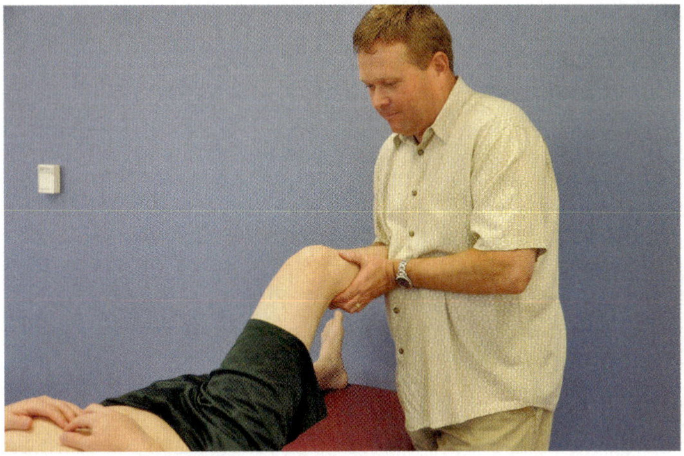

Figure 64.7. Treatment of the right knee.

Diagnosis – Patient Supine
The clinician contacts the foot with one hand and dorsiflexes the ankle. This stabilizes the talus within the ankle mortise. The clinician then cups the calcaneus with their other hand and takes it through inversion/eversion and abduction/adduction. Determine if there is a restriction.

Treatment – Patient Supine
The clinician will use the same hand position as in diagnosis. Maintain ankle dorsiflexion and move the calcaneus through clockwise or counterclockwise circles. This will introduce multiple motions through the talocalcaneal articulation. The clinician continues until a release is palpated and then reassesses (Fig. 64.8).

This technique can be easily modified to treat an anterior/posterior lateral malleolus or any tarsal or metatarsal restriction. It is important to remember the basic principles and adapt them to the specific dysfunction. Many tarsal, metatarsal, or phalangeal dysfunctions will improve when the talocalcaneal articulation is addressed.

Iliotibial Band/Lumbar Rotation Stretch

After the lower extremity is treated, the clinician will reassess for any residual tension within the distal iliotibial band. It may be associated with restriction in the tensor fascia latae or lumbar paraspinal muscles.

Diagnosis – Patient Supine
Palpate for increased tension in the iliotibial band.

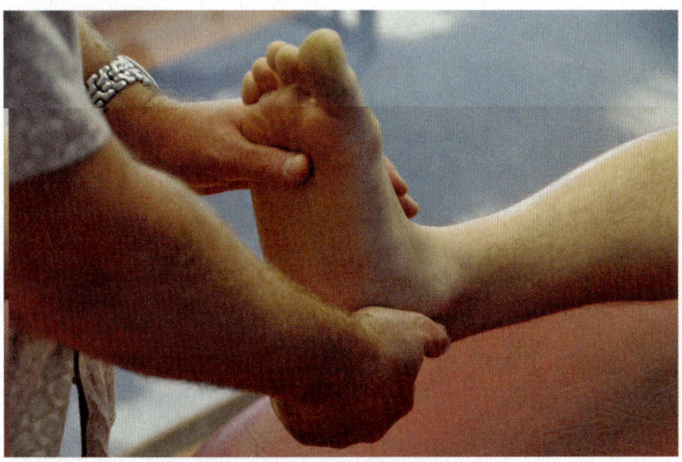

Figure 64.8. Treatment of the right foot.

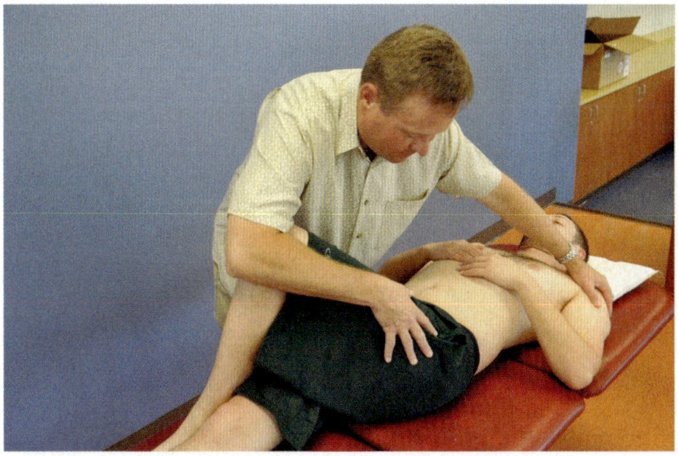

Figure 64.9. Treatment of the left iliotibial band.

Treatment – Patient Supine
If the left iliotibial band is tight, stand next to the patient's right side. The clinician flexes the patient's left knee and hip and places their left foot on the table, lateral to their right knee. The clinician uses one hand to stabilize the patient's left shoulder against the table and contacts the outside of the patient's left thigh with their other hand and forearm. Engage the barrier by gently adducting their left knee. Now the clinician oscillates the knee into the barrier until a release is palpated and then reassesses. The principle is to oscillate into the barrier, not bounce off it (Fig. 64.9).

Hamstrings/Psoas Major Muscles

The hamstring and psoas major muscles are frequently tight, possibly facilitated by somatic dysfunction in the low thoracic and upper lumbar areas.

Diagnosis – Patient Prone
The clinician palpates for increased tension in the hamstring muscles. Many times, the hamstring muscles and psoas major muscles are both tight. The psoas major muscle is tested by lifting the patient's leg and moving the hip into extension. The leg frequently feels heavier on the side of tight psoas major muscles.

Treatment – Patient Prone
To treat the right side, the clinician stands next to the patient's right side. The clinician contacts the patient's right ankle with their left hand and places their right hand over the patient's right low thoracic/upper lumbar paraspinal tissues. The clinician flexes the patient's right knee until the quadriceps muscles are slightly stretched. Now the clinician moves the leg in clockwise circles (flexion, abduction, and extension). The clinician continues until the paraspinal tissues soften and then they reassess both the hamstring and psoas major muscles. Determine if the motion and function have improved (Fig. 64.10).

Mechanism of action – by flexing the knee, the tension is removed from the hamstring muscles, which reduces the nociceptive afferent signals to the thoracolumbar region of the spinal cord. This may reduce facilitation to all structures supplied by this area, including the hamstring and psoas major muscles, resulting in decreased tension in these structures. If there is any residual tension in the psoas major muscle, it can then treat it with muscle energy technique.

Sacrum

Kenneth E. Nelson, DO, FAAO has described the sacrum as the bone of contention, because multiple axes and models of

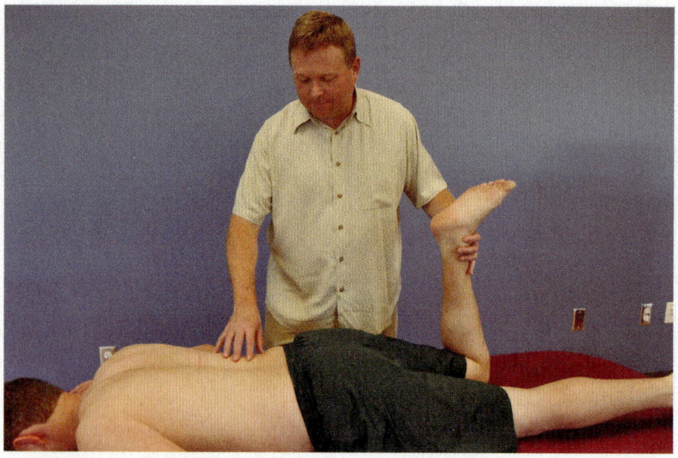

Figure 64.10. **Treatment of the right hamstring and psoas muscle.**

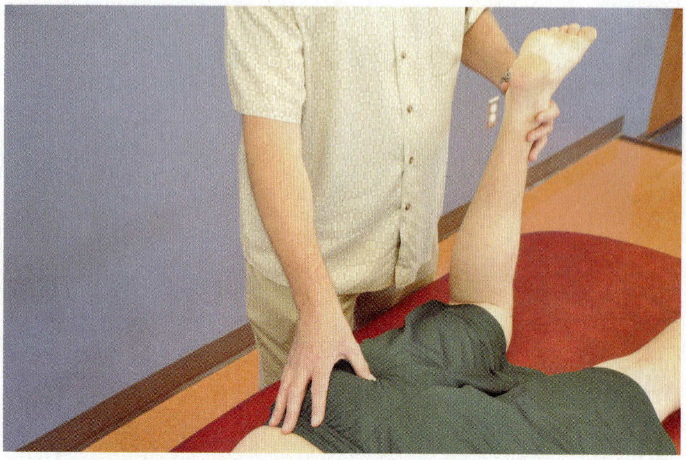

Figure 64.11. **Treatment of the right ILA to ischial tuberosity.**

motion have been described.[21] Regardless of your preferred model, Dr. Robert Kappler encouraged his students and the author to focus on the patient and ask the simple question "why is the sacrum in trouble?"[22]

Sacral motion is influenced by the innominates, lower extremity, and lumbar spine. All of these may need to be addressed before the sacral dysfunction completely resolves. At times, the right upper thoracic spine and ribs may need to be treated before the left side of the sacrum completely releases and vice versa. This model does not localize dysfunction to a single side of the sacrum using the seated flexion test. It is one bone, and both sacroiliac joints are frequently restricted. There are three separate techniques to treat the sacrum.

TECHNIQUE #1 ILA TO ISCHIAL TUBEROSITY – PATIENT PRONE

Diagnosis – Patient Prone

The clinician can use their preferred method, or they can simply cup the sacrum in the palm of their hands. Now the clinician sidebends the sacrum to the left and right determining if a restriction is present. The clinician also assesses the motion and position of the sacral sulci and inferolateral angles (ILAs). Now the clinician palpates for any tension or tissue texture changes from the ILAs down to the ischial tuberosities.

Treatment – Patient Prone

If the right side is tight, stand next to the right side. The clinician places their right thumb over the tight right posterior pelvic tissues. Their left hand contacts the right ankle. The clinician applies a slight anterior and superior pressure with their right thumb. Maintaining this pressure, they move the leg in clockwise circles (flexion of the knee, internal rotation of the hip, and extension of the knee). Treat any tight tissues from the ILA to the medial aspect of the ischial tuberosity (Fig. 64.11).

TECHNIQUE #2 GENERAL SACRAL ARTICULATION ("JIGGLE THE DO-DAD")

Treatment – Patient Prone

The clinician stands next to the patient's right side. The clinician places their palm of their right hand over the sacrum and contacts the right ankle with their left hand. Now, the clinician pulls the ankle toward themselves (internally rotating the hip and gapping the sacroiliac joint) while pushing their right hand away. Now the clinician oscillates their forces and continues applying the technique until the sacral motion improves. The clinician can specifically treat the upper and lower portion of the sacrum by placing their hand over these specific areas and adjusting the amount of flexion at the knee. Then the procedure is repeated on the left side. Reassess for improved sacral motion and function (Fig. 64.12).

TECHNIQUE #3 – CHICAGO POSTERIOR SACRUM ("RAMEY WIGGLE")

Diagnosis – Patient Prone

The Chicago posterior sacrum is a lower pole sacral restriction. The clinician palpates for tissue texture changes over the lower aspects of each sacroiliac joint. The clinician now places their thumbs over the ILAs of the sacrum. Next, the clinician determines by asymmetry and motion testing if one ILA is more posterior/inferior. The side with the tissue texture change and posterior/inferior ILA is known as the posterior sacrum.

Treatment – Example – Right Posterior Sacrum – Patient Prone

The sacrum sidebends and rotates to opposite sides. With a right posterior sacrum, it has rotated right and sidebent left. This technique emphasizes sidebending. Stand next to the patient's right side. The clinician places the heel of their left hand over the right ILA and supports this with their right hand. The clinician now applies an anterior, superior, and medial force to the right ILA to engage the feather edge of the restrictive barrier. The clinician then gently oscillates until the ILA and posterior pelvic tissues soften then reassesses (Fig. 64.13).

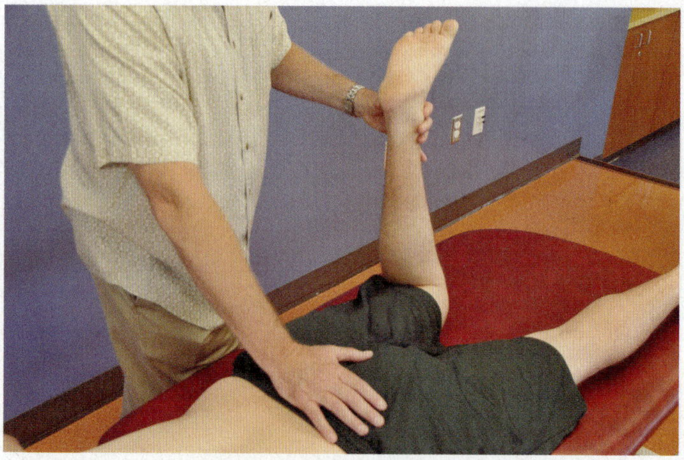

Figure 64.12. **General sacral articulation.**

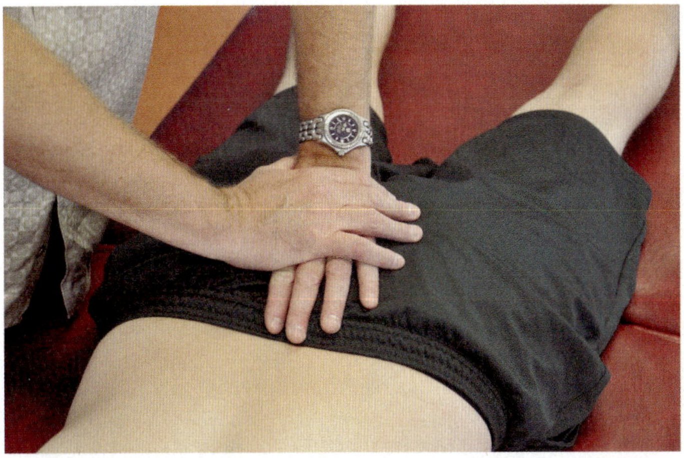

Figure 64.13. Chicago posterior sacrum ("Ramey Wiggle")—patient prone.

Lumbar and Thoracic Spine

This technique begins at L5 and progresses up each vertebra to T1, diagnosing and treating simultaneously. It addresses both side-bending and rotation.

Diagnosis – Patient Prone

To evaluate and treat the right side of the spine, stand next to the patient's right side. The clinician places their left hand over the right ILA of the sacrum. The clinician now places their right thumb on the right side of the spinous process of the vertebrae that they are evaluating. The clinician pushes their left hand to the left (medially) while simultaneously monitoring motion at the spinous process. Motion is introduced through the sacrum. The clinician's right thumb on the spinous process only monitors motion. The clinician then determines if spinal motion is restricted at each subsequent proximal spinal segment. If the motion is restricted, follow the procedure below. If not, move up and evaluate the next vertebrae. Only treat areas with significant motion restrictions.

Treatment – Patient Prone

If a vertebra is restricted, the clinician will oscillate their left hand back and forth by contacting the sacrum until the vertebral motion improves. Remember, motion is introduced through the sacrum and the thumb on the spinous process only monitors motion. Use the same principles to evaluate and treat the opposite side of the spine (Fig. 64.14).

Ribs

The ribs attach to the thoracic vertebrae, and in many cases treating the thoracic spine first will resolve the rib dysfunction. The ribs are treated immediately after the thoracic spine and these techniques work for both mechanical and respiratory rib restrictions and influences pump handle, bucket handle and caliper motions.

Technique – This is a slight variation of the prone technique for the lumbar and thoracic spine

Diagnosis – Patient Prone

To evaluate and treat the left side of the ribcage, stand next to the patient's right side. The clinician places their left hand over the right ILA of the sacrum. They now reach across the midline and place their right thumb over the angle of left first rib. The clinician pushes their left hand on the sacrum medially while monitoring the motion at the rib. Motion is introduced through the sacrum. The clinician's thumb on the rib only monitors motion. Assess the motion of the rib. Significant motion restrictions are treated. If no significant motion restriction is present, move down to the next rib.

Treatment – Patient Prone

The clinician applies a gentle anterior and lateral force to the rib while oscillating back and forth with their left hand on the sacrum until the motion improves. Motion is primarily introduced through the sacrum. The clinicians right thumb located on the involved rib monitors motion and gently disengages it from the thoracic vertebrae. The above principles are then applied to evaluate and treat the right side of the ribcage (Fig. 64.15).

Shoulder

With many shoulder injuries, flexion and abduction are restricted. This technique emphasizes these motions.

Diagnosis – Patient Supine

To evaluate the right shoulder, stand next to the patient's right side. The clinician places their right hand on the anterior portion of the right shoulder to stabilize it. This will help prevent dislocation if the patient has anterior instability. The clinician's other hand will contact the patient's right arm near the elbow. The clinician introduces flexion and abduction of the shoulder evaluating for restriction.

Treatment – Same Position

The clinician introduces counterclockwise circles (emphasizing flexion and abduction) to the right shoulder with their left hand

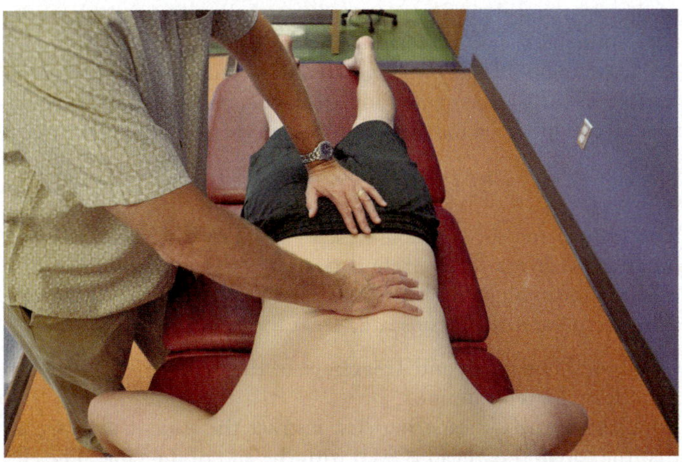

Figure 64.14. Prone treatment of the right side of the spine.

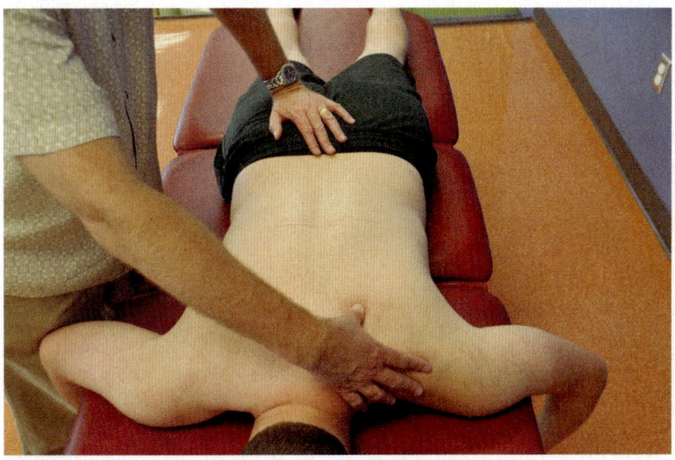

Figure 64.15. Treatment of the left side of the ribcage.

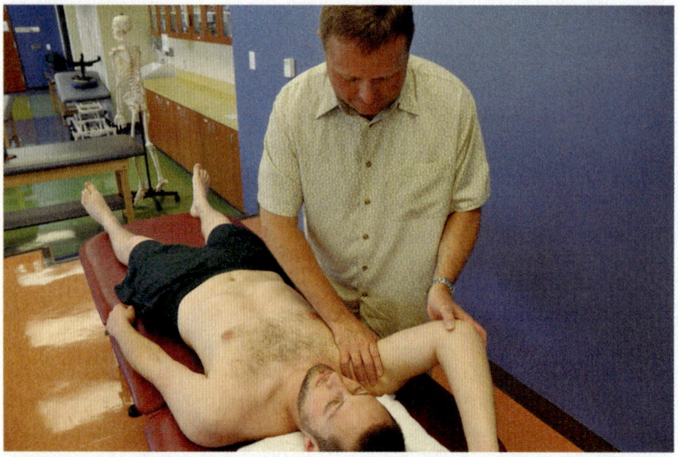

Figure 64.16. Treatment of the right shoulder.

until the motion improves. The clinician's right hand, which is lying over the anterior shoulder, is only there to monitor and help provide stability (Fig. 64.16).

Clavicle/Thoracic Inlet

The thoracic inlet is important to overall lymphatic drainage and clavicular motion influences this area.

Diagnosis – Patient Supine
To assess the right clavicle and right thoracic inlet, the clinician stands next to the patient's right side. The clinician places the patient's right hand against their left upper chest or shoulder and supports it with their left hand. The clinician uses their right hand to palpate the right thoracic inlet, posterior to the sternoclavicular joint (fingers wrap posteriorly and inferiorly over the top of the clavicle). Be careful, as this can be a very tender area. The clinician uses their body to apply and release traction to the right arm and palpates the motion of the clavicle and thoracic inlet. The clinician then moves their right hand laterally and assesses the motion of the thoracic inlet and clavicle from the sternoclavicular joint to the acromioclavicular joint.

Treatment – Patient Supine
The clinician identifies a restriction and applies/releases traction to the right arm until the motion of the clavicle and thoracic inlet improves. The clinician may gently reposition, adjusting their body position to change the force vector and better engage the restrictive barrier. The clinician can utilize the same principles to evaluate and treat the left side (Fig. 64.17).

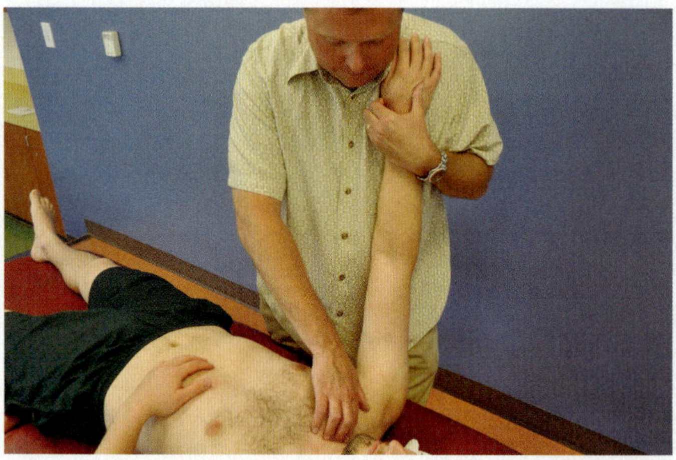

Figure 64.17. Treatment of the right clavicle and thoracic inlet.

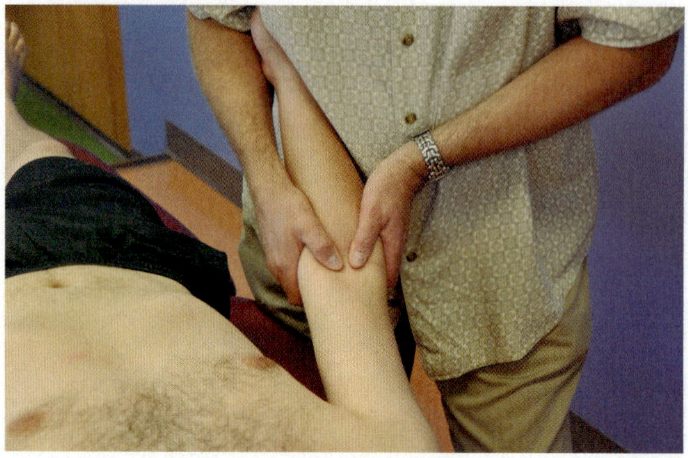

Figure 64.18. Treatment of the right elbow.

Elbow

Diagnosis – Patient Supine
The clinician can utilize standard osteopathic structural examination principles to evaluate for articular dysfunction of the ulna and radius at the elbow. Especially look for an abducted/adducted ulna and/or an anterior/posterior radial head. The same treatment technique will work for all these restrictions.

Treatment – To Treat the Right Elbow, Stand at the Patient's Right Side
The clinician places their hands around the medial and lateral elbow so that their fingertips are over the medial and lateral portion of the olecranon process and their thumbs are over the anterior aspect of the elbow. Next, the clinician uses their body and hands to introduce counterclockwise circles to the elbow (extension, abduction, flexion, and adduction). The varus force is key to releasing the radial head. Continue until the motion improves and reassess (Fig. 64.18).

Wrist/Hand

Diagnosis – Patient Supine
The clinician should assess flexion/extension and abduction/adduction dysfunction of the wrist. In addition, they can also assess increased tension within the transverse carpal ligament.

Treatment – Example – Right Wrist Restricted – Patient Supine
The clinician will contact the medial and lateral aspects of the right wrist with their hands. The clinician's thumbs rest over the dorsum of the wrist and their fingers wrap around the thenar and hypothenar eminences. The clinician uses their thumbs as a fulcrum and applies traction (like a bowstring) to the ventral wrist, stretching the transverse carpal ligament. Move the wrist in fluid counterclockwise circles until the motion improves and reassess (Fig. 64.19).

Neck

The scalene and suboccipital muscles are frequently tight in combination with cervical vertebral restrictions. It is most clinically efficient to simultaneously diagnose and treat. There are three separate techniques to diagnose and treat the neck.

Combined Diagnosis and Treatment of the Scalene Muscles – Patient Supine
To assess the left scalene muscles, instruct the patient to move so that the top of their head is even with the end of the table. The clinician will cup their occiput with their right hand and stabilize the

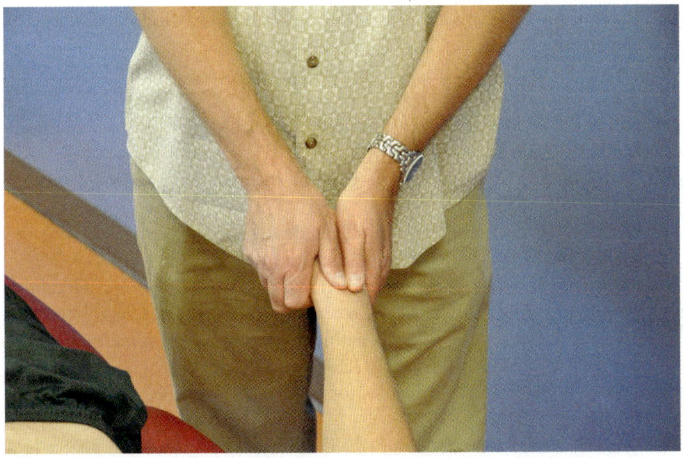

Figure 64.19. **Treatment of the right wrist.**

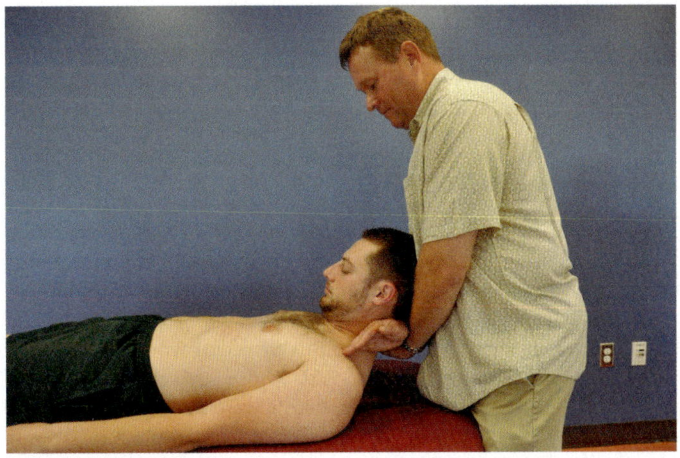

Figure 64.21. **Treatment of the suboccipital tissues.**

patient's left shoulder by applying an inferiorly directed force with their left hand. It is important to maintain this force throughout the evaluation and treatment. Now the clinician will flex the patient's neck and sidebend it to the right (further localization occurs with adding a small amount of rotation). The clinician can rest the back or side of the patient's head against their right hip or abdomen. The clinician can use their body to introduce right sidebending. If the tissues are tight, gently engage the feather edge of the restrictive barrier. The clinician can gently increase right sidebending by oscillating with their body directed toward the patient's feet. Adjust the rate so that the patient's feet move. Continue until a release occurs and then evaluate and treat the right side. This technique also improves the motion and function of the upper thoracic spine and upper ribs (Fig. 64.20).

Combined Diagnosis and Treatment of Posterior Cervical and Suboccipital Tissues – Patient Supine

The clinician will flex the patient's neck and then cross their forearms behind it providing support. Now the clinician rests their hands on the patient's shoulders. The clinician rests the back of the patient's head against their abdomen. The clinician gently uses their body and arms to flex the patient's neck to see if the posterior cervical and suboccipital tissues are tight. If so, the clinician engages the feather edge of the barrier and uses their body and arms to oscillate toward the patient's feet until the tissues release (Fig. 64.21).

Combined Diagnosis and Treatment of the Individual Cervical Vertebrae – Patient Supine

The clinician flexes the patient's neck and allows the back of the patient's head to rest against their abdomen. Beginning at C7, the clinician places their fingertips over the lateral part of the transverse processes (this will assist with translation). The clinician uses their body and arms as a unit to translate C7 to the right and left. If a restriction is found, the clinician will continue translating until the motion improves. If not, they move up to the next vertebrae. Rotation may be incorporated if needed for localization. Once the clinician reaches the OA area, they will place their fingers posterior to the occipital condyles and apply the same principles (Fig. 64.22).

Cranial Mechanism

There is no general osteopathic technique specifically targeting the cranial mechanism. If you treat the rest of the body including the OA and suboccipital area first, many times the cranial mechanism will take care of itself.

Additional Pearls

Any remaining segmental somatic dysfunction can be treated with HVLA technique or another method of choice. The patient can be treated one to two times weekly, depending on their individual

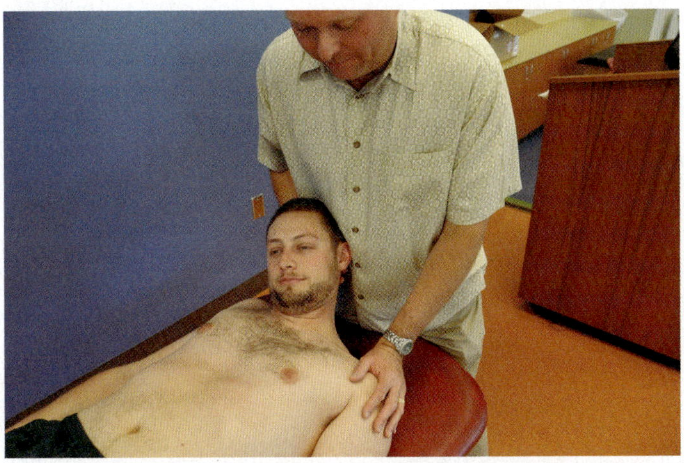

Figure 64.20. **Treatment of the left scalene muscles.**

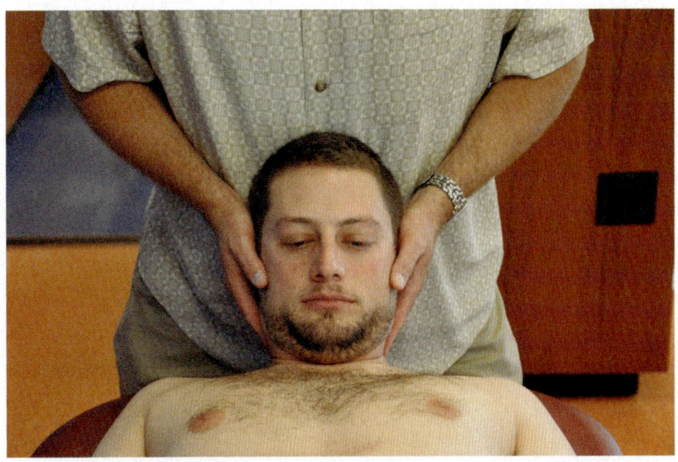

Figure 64.22. **Treatment of the individual cervical vertebrae.**

response, until their motion and function improves and their symptoms resolve. Failure to respond to three to six treatments and/or any progressively worsening neurologic symptoms warrants further evaluation and management.

ACKNOWLEDGMENTS

I would like to dedicate this chapter in memory of my parents, Arnold F. Ramey and Nancy R. Ramey, who always supported and encouraged my Osteopathic education and career. I would like to thank my wife, Lisa R. Ramey, DO, who is supportive of my career and encouraged me in completing this project. I would also like to thank Kurt P. Heinking, DO, FAAO, whose advice and assistance in editing and finalizing this manuscript were invaluable.

REFERENCES

1. Campbell C, Discovering J. *Martin Littlejohn, A Key Figure of Classical Osteopathy*. Lettertec Publishing; 2020.
2. About the John Wernham College of Classical Osteopathy. John Wernham Classical Osteopathy. https://johnwernhamclassicalosteopathy.com/about-the-john-wernham-college-of-classical-osteopathy. Accessed March 19, 2025.
3. Kemp J. The osteopathic general treatment. In: Wernham J, ed. *Classical Osteopathy*. The Osteopathic Institute of Applied Technique; 1996: 67–72.
4. Grolaux PJ, Sparrow TJ, Lalonde F. Traditional osteopathy and the general osteopathic treatment: a historical concept and a modern application. *AAO J*. 2021;31(4):39–46.
5. Comeaux Z. *Robert Fulford, D.O. and the Philosopher Physician*. Eastland Press; 2002.
6. Seffinger MA. *Foundations of Osteopathic Medicine*. 4th ed. Wolters Kluwer; 2018:997–1002.
7. Notes from Dr. *Fulford's Percussion Hammer Course*. Kirksville College of Osteopathic Medicine; April 7–8, 1995.
8. Marcel Vogel Legacy. https://marcelvogellegacy.com. Accessed March 22, 2025.
9. Still AT. *The Philosophy and Mechanical Principles of Osteopathy*. Hudson-Kimberly Publishing Company; 1902:16–17.
10. Littlejohn JM. The physiologic basis of therapeutic law. *J Am Osteopath Assoc*. 1902;2:137–158.
11. Littlejohn JM. Osteopathy an independent system co-extensive with the science and art of healing 1901. *J Am Osteopath Assoc*. 2000;100:14–26.
12. Wernham J. *The Life and Times of John Martin Littlejohn*. The John Wernham College of Classical Osteopathy, 2008 edition, Copyright 1999.
13. Bordoni B, Escher AR Jr. Osteopathic principles: The inspiration of every science is its change. *Cureus*. 2021;13(1):e12478.
14. Korr IM. Osteopathic principles for basic scientists. *J Am Osteopath Assoc*. 1987;87:513–515.
15. Dugailly PM, Fassin S, Maroye L, Evers L, Klein P, Feipel V. Effect of a general osteopathic treatment on body satisfaction, global self-perception and anxiety: a randomized trial in asymptomatic female students. *Int J Osteopath Med*. 2014;17(2):94–101.
16. Albers J, Jäkel A, Wellmann K, von Hehn U, Schmidt T. Effectiveness of 2 osteopathic treatment approaches on pain, pressure-pain threshold, and disease severity in patients with fibromyalgia: a randomized controlled trial. *Complement Med Res*. 2018;25(2):122–128.
17. Seffinger MA. *Foundations of Osteopathic Medicine*. 4th ed. Wolters Kluwer; 2018:706.
18. Dalley AF, Agur AM. *Moore's Clinically Oriented Anatomy*. 9th ed. Wolters Kluwer; 2023.
19. Chia M, Chia M. *Chi Nei Tsang Internal Organ Chi Massage*. Healing Tao Books; 1990:1–2.
20. Cisler TA. *Are We on the Path? The Collected Works of Robert C. Fulford, DO, FCA*. The Cranial Academy; 2003:9.
21. Nelson KE. The sacrum; A bone of contention. *AAO J*. 1997; Winter:17–24.
22. Chila AG. *Foundations of Osteopathic Medicine*. 3rd ed. Wolters Kluwer/Lippincott Williams and Wilkins; 2011:592.

PART FOUR

Osteopathic Considerations in the Specialties

65 Osteopathic Considerations in Primary Care

JAY H. SHUBROOK ▪ KIM PFOTENHAUER

KEY CONCEPTS

The osteopathic primary care physician:

- Provides holistic patient-centered care
- Focuses on primary and secondary prevention
- Offers timely medical interventions when needed
- Provides longitudinal care
- Is always mindful of the integration of structure and function in health and illness
- Is the keystone to an effective health care system

INTRODUCTION

Approximately 938,966 physicians practice in the United States, with approximately 289,309 practicing primary care.[1] In 2021, osteopathic physicians made up 8.3% of all practicing physicians, but they disproportionately represent primary care at 16.4% (https://www.aamc.org/data-reports/workforce/interactive-data/active-physicians-do-degree-specialty-2021). Further, osteopathic medicine is the fastest growing segment of practicing physicians at 16% per year.[2] To a significant degree, the primary care physician's role has defined osteopathic medicine for over 125 years. In the 20th century, more than 70% of osteopathic physicians practiced primary care medicine, whereas at the start of the 21st century, this number hovers between 56% and 58%.[3] Still, while 75% of Americans (including 90% of adults older than 55) reported having a primary care physician in 2019, the country continues to have a shortage of primary care physicians.[4] Osteopathic medicine is poised to help fill this void and better serve medical needs by training primary care physicians of the future.

Osteopathic primary care emphasizes a personal and longitudinal healing relationship between the physician and the patient that is focused on health promotion, disease prevention, and timely interventions (Fig. 65.1). The osteopathic primary care physician helps patients cope with both acute crises and chronic problems, with a goal of restoring and maintaining health by integrating the genetic, anatomic, physiologic, emotional, behavioral, familial, social, cultural, and economic components of each clinical condition. A crucial part of primary care is a focus on primary and secondary prevention of disease as well as the integral interrelationship of structure and function. This approach differs significantly from the limited problem- and system-specific orientation that typifies the medical and surgical specialties.

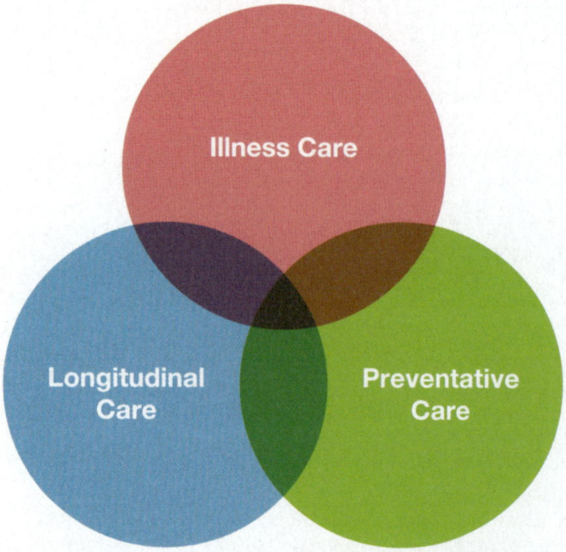

Figure 65.1. The overlapping roles of primary care.

The breadth of knowledge and skill incorporated in osteopathic primary care encompasses most modern medicine. As such, the osteopathic primary care physician tends to be a generalist, recognizing and acknowledging the importance of the details but always attempting to integrate the whole picture. In addition, an effective osteopathic primary care physician is patient centered, utilizing the best aspects of evidence-based medicine to individualize care to fit the specific needs of every patient in the context of their health, family, and cultural beliefs.

For many patients, the primary care physician is the first, and perhaps only, contact with the U.S. health care system. Patients generally present to a primary care physician regarding a routine physical exam or a new complaint. This visit often leads to the early discovery of a medical problem, such as hypertension or diabetes, that has not yet become symptomatic. Thus, in many cases, the primary care physician is the first to diagnose a patient's new health problem.

The primary care physician often provides the primary diagnosis and the majority of the management. Health screening, health maintenance, routine care, chronic disease care, and care for acute, time-limited diseases are generally considered the purview of the primary care physician. Referral to specialists is reserved for cases where the diagnosis is incomplete, the management is beyond an individual physician's knowledge, skills, or experience, or if procedures are required that the primary care physician does not perform.

Even with outside referrals, the primary care physician plays an active and essential role as the bridge between the primary care setting and subspecialty care. Patients expect that the primary care physician will be able to optimize their care by referring them to the best specialist for their particular needs. This requires the primary care physician to know not only the problem but the desires and context in which the patient is experiencing this problem. In short, the primary care physician is the keystone to an efficacious health care team.

In a system with adequate numbers of primary care physicians, the primary care physician will likely make the initial diagnosis, and selectively focused referrals are made to the appropriate specialist(s) when needed, saving time, effort, and money. However, in regions where the number and diversity of specialists are relatively large to the patient population, and there is a paucity of primary care physicians, it is not uncommon for a patient to end up seeing four or five different specialists to obtain a diagnosis and treatment for a specific medical problem. This segmented-care model can expose the best and worst of the U.S. health care system. Patients may receive highly specialized medical attention, but assessment and treatment are typically focused on a subsegment of the health experience. And, if the care is not coordinated or orchestrated effectively, it may overlap in some areas, present gaps in others, or produce treatment plans that may conflict with one another. Treatment of this kind is not cost-effective, nor does it encourage a patient's faith in the effectiveness of the medical care system.

Osteopathic philosophy and principles, as presented in Chapter 1, are utilized in primary care with every patient encounter (Table 65.1). Following these principles, osteopathic primary care has developed with the following defining characteristics:

1. It is an approach that views the patient as a unique, integrated, self-regulating individual, united in mind, body, and spirit. No disease and no attempt to maintain health can be understood in less than the complete context of the individual, including the neuromusculoskeletal system.
2. Disease is viewed as an unnatural state, the natural state being a healthy dynamic balance. Thus, when a fundamentally healthy organism confronts disease, it heals itself. The source of healing is within the patient. It is not the physician who does the healing. The physician helps provide a context in which healing can occur.
3. When disease is present, the osteopathic physician is tasked with discovering, whenever possible, the source or underlying cause of the apparent disease. Treating the patient symptomatically, while possibly useful in self-limiting diseases, is not the desired goal for either the patient or the physician.
4. The osteopathic primary care physician uses all rational and scientific means of diagnosis and treatment methods available to develop and sustain health. This includes palpatory diagnosis and osteopathic manipulative treatment (OMT), medications, surgery, and lifestyle modifications, as appropriate.

TABLE 65.1

Osteopathic Principles and Illustrative Examples

The person is a unit of body, mind, and spirit.	A medical student not sleeping, eating, or exercising well while studying for difficult exams becomes ill with an upper respiratory tract infection.
The body is capable of self-regulating, self-healing, and health maintenance.	A 4-year-old is able to recover from otitis media without the use of antibiotics.
Structure and function are reciprocally interrelated.	A person with a history of rib fractures becomes more susceptible to lower respiratory illnesses.
Rational treatment is based upon an understanding of the basic principles of body unity, self-regulation, and the interrelationship of structure and function.	Effective treatment for musculoskeletal back pain includes osteopathic manipulative treatment, physical therapy, medications, and patient activity such as walking and/or stretching.

OMT can be used throughout the patient's life. For example:

- Newborns with difficulty breastfeeding can benefit from cranial manipulation (see Chapter 53 Osteopathic Cranial Manipulative Medicine, and Chapter 67 Osteopathic Considerations in Pediatrics, for more information).
- Young children with otitis media can recover sooner with manipulative treatment (see Chapter 67 Osteopathic Considerations in Pediatrics for more information).
- In adults, the most common reason to seek manipulative treatment is back pain or injury (see case study in Chapter 66 Osteopathic Considerations in Family Medicine).
- OMT can improve comfort in the pregnant woman and augment labor during childbirth (see Chapter 81 Osteopathic Considerations in Obstetrics).
- In the elderly, OMT has been shown to decrease the length of hospital stay due to pneumonia (see Chapter 68 Osteopathic Considerations in General Internal Medicine and Chapter 69 Osteopathic Considerations in Geriatric Medicine for more information).
- Among primary care physicians, the osteopathic family physician has the unique opportunity to improve health throughout the lives of their patients by using osteopathic manipulation (see Chapter 66 Osteopathic Considerations in Family Medicine for further information).

OSTEOPATHIC PRIMARY CARE AND POPULATION HEALTH

For decades, medicine has been focused on fixing patients with episodic care for defined infectious or traumatic diseases. In contrast, the osteopathic approach, and indeed the future of health care, is committed to helping people, families, and communities prevent and manage chronic disease throughout the life spectrum. Osteopathic primary care physicians strive toward developing and sustaining health in their patient populations rather than more narrowly focusing on eradicating disease. This emphasis on health recognizes that health is not a fixed state. Instead, it is a dynamic, positive interaction affecting all aspects of one's life, circumstances, and needs with ongoing adjustment to maintain the balance. At a family and community level, the osteopathic primary care physician is committed to helping people achieve the healthiest version of themselves.

Criteria for a healthy life include

1. Adequate food, shelter, education, and income
2. Adequate rest and exercise
3. Adequate strength, flexibility, and endurance
4. A mechanically and dynamically balanced neuromusculoskeletal system
5. The ability to maintain functional social and interpersonal relationships
6. Freedom from, or healthy control of, mental impairments and illnesses
7. Emotional and spiritual stability
8. Successful coping strategies that can withstand psychological, interpersonal, and biologic stresses

9. Strong immune responses to biologic and psychosocial challenges
10. Good compensation for long-term genetic, mental, emotional, and disease-related health issues

The uniquely osteopathic contribution to helping patients restore health lies in recognizing that the musculoskeletal system is intimately involved in these criteria. Thus, musculoskeletal diagnosis and treatment is a fundamental and integral part of the methods used by osteopathic primary care physicians to help patients find and maintain health.

REFERENCES

1. AAMC Workforce Report: Physicians by Specialty. Accessed February 21, 2023. https://www.aamc.org/data-reports/workforce/interactive-data/active-physicians-do-degree-specialty-2021
2. Young AJ, Chaudhry H, Pei X, Halbesleben KL, Polk DH, Dugan M. A census of actively licensed physicians in the United States 2014. *J Med Regul.* 2015;101(2):8–23.
3. Membership Directory: American College of Osteopathic Family Physicians and American Osteopathic Board of Family Physicians. 2000–2001:319.
4. Ash Clinical News: Fewer Americans have primary care providers. Accessed February 21, 2023. https://ashpublications.org/ashclinicalnews/news/4901/Fewer-Americans-Have-Primary-Care-Providers

66 Osteopathic Considerations in Family Medicine

JAY H. SHUBROOK ▪ KIM PFOTENHAUER ▪ MICHAEL A. SEFFINGER ▪ JESUS SANCHEZ JR ▪ MARCEL P. FRAIX ▪ PETER ADLER-MICHAELSON

KEY CONCEPTS

The osteopathic family physician:

- Treats the whole person—not just a disease
- Utilizes osteopathic palpatory diagnosis and osteopathic manipulative treatment (OMT)
- Integrates OMT into a comprehensive prevention and treatment plan
- Treats the individual in the context of family and community

INTRODUCTION

Osteopathic medicine emphasizes the dynamic unity of the individual human being and the interlocking aspects of form and function. As such, it would be an error to say that individual organs can have meaningful functions independent from the whole being. Dr. A. T. Still's diagnostic methods involved examining the whole of human anatomy for areas of dysfunction, even at sites well distant from the local manifestation.[1,2] Likewise, the practice of examination of "systems" that span the whole body, such as the circulatory/lymphatic and neural networks, reinforced the osteopathic propensity to treat the whole person.

Today's osteopathic family physicians are trained and certified to practice as primary care physicians in all aspects of health care. In addition, osteopathic family physicians are trained and can be board certified in osteopathic palpatory diagnosis and osteopathic manipulative treatment (OMT). There are two osteopathic physician specialty groups (Osteopathic Family Medicine and Osteopathic Neuromusculoskeletal Medicine) whose certification specifically may include competency in OMT. Osteopathic family physicians assume the responsibility for their patients' comprehensive and continued health care and act as coordinators of individual patient health services. Some osteopathic family physicians may devote particular attention to one or more other fields of specialty practice, such as addiction medicine, geriatrics, adolescent and young adult medicine, sports medicine, sleep medicine, diabetes, obesity, etc.

OSTEOPATHIC FAMILY MEDICINE ROLE IN PRIMARY CARE

Today's osteopathic family physician must be both a generalist and specialist to effectively deal with the broad spectrum and complexity of problems encountered in practice. The family physician specialist is trained in the longitudinal coordination of addressing multiple diverse problems in a holistic patient-oriented system of health care (individual, family, and greater social context). Today's family medicine model implies the presence of personal accessibility, availability for various medical and biopsychosocial problems, and a willingness to coordinate most aspects of continuing personal and family-related health care.[3,4]

Osteopathic family physicians work with patients from womb to tomb. This broad spectrum of care produces several of the unique foci of family medicine:

a. Longitudinal care
b. Care of the individual in the family and social context
c. Care of multiple generations of the same family

These longitudinal, holistic, patient-oriented aspects of care more easily lend themselves to the application of classic osteopathic principles than possibly any other specialty area of medical practice.

THE WHOLE PERSON AND DISEASE

> "To find health should be the object of the doctor. Anyone can find disease."[5]
>
> —A. T. Still, Philosophy of Osteopathy

The tendency to consider disease as the primary concern of health care is pervasive in both popular thinking and the "traditional" medical model. While some attention is given to "preventive medicine," the primary concern continues to be disease diagnosis, treatment, and management. This model seems to imply that disease is the natural state of human beings. In contrast, the general osteopathic model and osteopathic family medicine model, specifically, consider health development and maintenance as the primary focus. According to the osteopathic model, a normal, balanced, and integrated human being can generally avoid infection, even though there is daily exposure to pathogenic organisms. In other words, a person can avoid most diseases when the body is functioning maximally. It is true that even when the body is maintained with structural balance and integrity, there are illnesses that cannot be avoided, such as the common upper respiratory illness. But, with a healthy environment in which stressors are controlled, a person can often readily recuperate.

According to osteopathic principles, when it occurs, a disease is considered a disturbance of the innate dynamic balance of health. Genetic predisposition; inappropriate immune response; dietary insufficiencies or indiscretions; emotional upheavals; familial, social, economic, or environmental stressors; and/or musculoskeletal disturbances can perturb the body's dynamic balance. Many of these factors can, and often do, coexist. Disease occurs when such perturbations, particularly long-term ones, overwhelm the body's natural compensatory mechanisms (see Fig. 66.1).

The body's ability to compensate is such that most individuals maintain what they would characterize as "good health" most of the time, even in the presence of chronic disease. Therefore, it is the objective of the osteopathic family physician to assist and support the patient to restore and maintain the balance of health. In pursuit of that outcome, the primary care objectives extend beyond acute episodes and interventions and into the longitudinal maintenance of health and/or stabilization of disease where it cannot be eliminated.

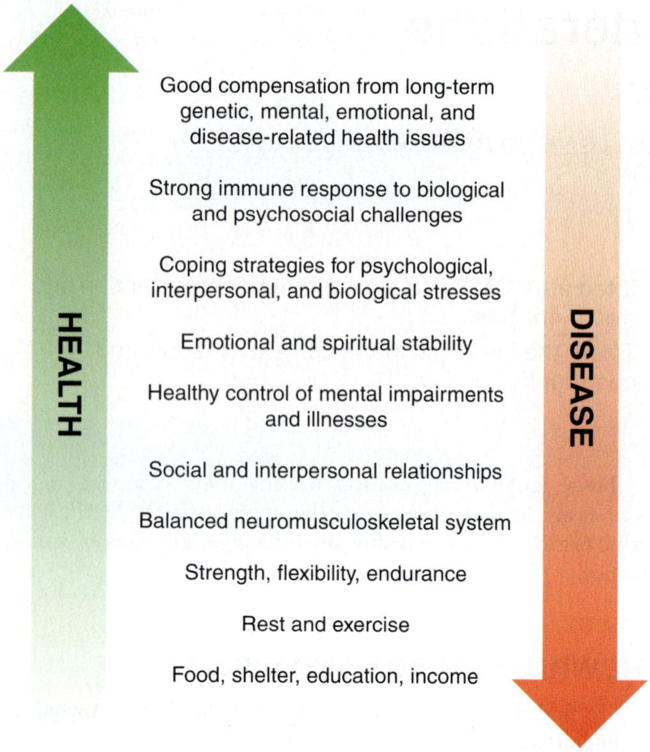

Figure 66.1. Continuum of health to disease.

Most disease has widespread bodily effects. Although it may be convenient to classify a particular disease as limited to a particular organ, it is rare that it does not have repercussions throughout the body. An obvious example is cardiovascular disease, wherein effects are found from the smallest capillaries to the heart itself, thereby affecting the whole body. A similar example is diabetes mellitus, wherein this endocrine disorder has vascular, neural, renal, musculoskeletal, and immunologic effects.

The pathophysiology and management of type 2 diabetes are easily organized by applying the osteopathic principles illustrated in Case 1 and Table 66.1.[5]

CASE 1

Gloria is a 54-year-old Black female with 14 years of type 2 diabetes. She reports that she had gestational diabetes with her third and fourth pregnancies, but in both cases, it resolved after delivery. Then upon her 40-year-old physical, it was determined from a blood test that she had "full-blown" diabetes. She did not feel bad at the time. She checks her glucose three times daily and takes medication and insulin to manage her glucose. She knows she needs to "watch her diet," but her family does not like to eat those "diabetic foods." She intends to walk after work but often is too tired when she gets home. Her glucose readings are often high, and she does not drop low. HbA1c is 9.2%. She admits that her vision is not great and has experienced numbness in both feet. She has also developed carpel tunnel in both wrists. (Discussion in Table 66.1.)

OSTEOPATHIC DIAGNOSIS AND TREATMENT OF DISEASE

Impressive strides have been made in the past 60 years regarding advanced diagnostic testing and imaging. However, the art of history taking and physical examination still provide the best foundation for clinical decision-making. A thorough history and physical often allow physicians to limit the number of additional procedures required to attain a diagnosis. Integrating palpatory

TABLE 66.1

Osteopathic Principles as Applied to Type 2 Diabetes Mellitus

Osteopathic Tenet	Application to T2DM	Supporting Evidence
The body is a unit: the person is a unit of body, mind, and spirit.	Address all three elements for Gloria to help her cope with diabetes management.	40–60% of people with diabetes suffer comorbid pain.[6] Risk of mood disorders increases with duration of diabetes.[7]
The body is capable of self-regulation, self-healing, and health maintenance.	Her poor diet quality, ongoing stress, and lack of physical inactivity are "noxious" stimuli that put her at risk for diabetes. Help Gloria reduce exposure to noxious stimuli by working to improve her diabetes self-management skills.	90–95% of diabetes care is self-care.[8] This care can take up to 3 hr/day.[9] Approximately, 65% adhere to dietary recommendations, and less than 30% adhere to physical activity guidelines.
Structure and function are reciprocally related.	With her chronic hyperglycemia, she has developed tendinopathy and neuropathy, which increases her pain and limits function. When Gloria's MS system is healthy, advise Gloria to be more active. This will ensure that her glucose and lipid transport is maximized.	Skeletal muscle glucose transport is improved during bouts of physical activity.[10–13] Even as little as 1 wk of aerobic training can improve whole-body insulin sensitivity.[14]
Rational treatment is based upon an understanding of the basic principles of body unity, self-regulation, and interrelationship of structure and function.	Osteopathic treatment of Gloria's type 2 diabetes addresses recognition of ongoing exposure to noxious stimuli, need for maximizing musculoskeletal function to improve glucose transport, and recognition of the effects of chronic disease on the mind.	OMT has been shown to treat some of the complications including carpal tunnel syndrome and adhesive capsulitis.[15,16]

Adapted from Shubrook JH Jr, Johnson AW. An osteopathic approach to type 2 diabetes mellitus. *J Am Osteopath Assoc.* 2011;111(9):531–537.

diagnosis into the physical examination and manipulation into the treatment plan gives osteopathic family physicians (and their patients) a unique advantage.

THE ROLE OF PALPATORY DIAGNOSIS AND MANIPULATIVE CARE

A basic osteopathic principle states that the neuromusculoskeletal system is functionally and inextricably linked with all body systems. A corollary of this concept is the explicit statement that disease and musculoskeletal dysfunction are also inextricably linked. This is the fundamental principle behind somatic dysfunction. Somatic dysfunction is a functional impairment with primary manifestation in the neuromusculoskeletal and fascial systems. Although somatic dysfunction may exist in the presence of pathology, it is not in itself pathology.

CASE 2

A 72-year-old male presents with cough, fever, dyspnea, and pleuritic chest pain for the past week. He states that he has had a fever and chills. He states that his cough is productive and that his chest hurts more when he coughs. He denies rhinitis, sore throat, nausea, or vomiting. He has a history of COPD and is currently using an inhaler.

On physical examination, he has a fever, tachycardia, and tachypnea. He has dullness to percussion and decreased breath sounds over the right lower lobe. He also has egophony and increased fremitus. He is diagnosed with pneumonia, and treatment is begun.

What symptoms can be attributed to increased sympathetic response?

Tachycardia and tachypnea can be a result of increased sympathetic response. This is common in acute illnesses. Also, blood vessels can constrict, impeding tissue oxygenation and waste removal.[17] In addition, a viscerosomatic response can be present due to the increased stimulation of the visceral afferent nerve caused by mucosal irritation and lung dysfunction.[18]

What segments are expected to be affected by the sympathetic response?

The most common segments affected are T1–T6. The cough reflex, caused by mucus moving over the bronchial tubes, can also cause exhalation rib somatic dysfunction.[18]

What parasympathetic changes are expected in this patient?

The Hering–Breuer reflex mechanism cannot differentiate between air- and fluid-filled alveoli, limiting the excursion of the diaphragm by the vagus nerve. The carotid body, on the other hand, tries to increase oxygenation, which results in rapid, shallow breathing.[18]

What are the biomechanical concerns in this patient?

In order for the lungs to fill appropriately, each thoracic segment and each costochondral and chondrosternal joint must be able to move without restriction. Particularly, the clavicle and first rib must be flexible to accommodate the mobility of the dome of the lung.[17] Accessory muscles of respiration, such as the scalenes and intercostal muscles, can be restricted due to cough and decreased lung expansion. The diaphragm flattens, causing increasingly shallow breaths and decreased lymphatic movement.[18]

What are the concerns with lymphatic movement?

Flattening of the diaphragm results in decreased lymph movement. This is due to the inability to create a pressure difference between the abdomen and thorax, which acts as a pump. This leads to increased tissue congestion and decreased cardiac output.[18] Poor cellular oxygenation due to lymphatic stasis can decrease the effectiveness of medical therapy.[18]

What osteopathic treatment plan would address the concerns in this patient?

Thoracolumbar treatment can address the mobility of each segment. Rib raising can decrease the sympathetic tone. Doming of the diaphragm can improve air and lymphatic movement. Cervical treatment can improve the function of accessory respiratory muscles. Vagal tone can be addressed by suboccipital decompression. Lymphatic movement can further be improved by treating the thoracic inlet and using the pedal pump.

Discussion: In addition to medication, osteopathic treatment has decreased hospital stays in the elderly with pneumonia.[19] Pneumonia is a multifaceted disease process. Infectious agents create dysfunction in the airways, circulation, and neuroreflexive and lymphatic pathways. Therefore, treatment with antibiotics can be augmented through osteopathic manipulation.

When treating a patient with any health problem, the osteopathic physician determines how to integrate the treatment of somatic dysfunction into the therapeutic protocol by asking the following questions:

1. **How is musculoskeletal dysfunction affecting the ability of the person to function?** Whether one is dealing with activity restrictions due to pain, gait, or other body use disturbances, this is the most obvious manifestation of somatic dysfunction and the most universally treated musculoskeletal issue by osteopathic physicians.
2. **How do musculoskeletal and fascial dysfunctions affect the patient's ability to respond to disease processes?** The mechanical component of somatic dysfunction results in the restriction of motion. For example, consider the compromising effect of thoracic cage somatic dysfunction upon the patient with chronic obstructive pulmonary disease.
3. **How is circulatory stasis affecting the patient?** Efficient movement of the thoracic inlet, thoracic cage, abdominal diaphragm, mesenteries, and the pelvic diaphragm is necessary for optimal low-pressure fluid (lymphatic and venous) dynamics and tissue perfusion. The inefficiency of this mechanism further adds to the tendency for tissue congestion. Somatic dysfunction of the extremities can compromise arterial, venous, and lymphatic flow.
4. **What sympathetic somatovisceral mechanisms are present?** Spinal facilitation associated with thoracic and upper lumbar somatic dysfunction results in increased sympathetic tone in segmentally related structures.
5. **What parasympathetic somatovisceral mechanisms are present?** Spinal facilitation associated with high cervical and sacral somatic dysfunction results in increased parasympathetic tone in segmentally related structures.
6. **What organ-level dysfunctions manifest in musculoskeletal and fascial restrictions and tissue texture changes?** The first three questions address the mechanical effect of somatic dysfunction upon the patient. The fourth and fifth questions deal with the impact of somatovisceral reflexes. Finally, the sixth question relates to what has been termed the viscerosomatic reflexes. See Table 66.2 for further examples.

The first five questions focus on the direct effects of primary somatic dysfunction on general function. Each represents part of

TABLE 66.2

Somatic and Visceral Reflexes with Examples

Question	Reflex	Example
How is the musculoskeletal dysfunction affecting the person's ability to function?	Somatosomatic reflexes	A fall that is causing pain in the patient's hip and shoulder due to a sacral and innominate dysfunction that in turn causes muscle hypertonicity into the upper thoracic spine and ipsilateral shoulder
How are the musculoskeletal and fascial dysfunctions affecting the patient's response to the disease process?	Mechanical somatic dysfunction	A patient with COPD who develops a thoracic somatic dysfunction that decreases his ability to move air
How is circulatory stasis affecting the patient?	Mechanical somatic dysfunction	A patient with a pelvic diaphragm dysfunction after childbirth who complains of lower extremity edema
What sympathetic somatovisceral mechanisms are present?	Somatovisceral	Increased heart rate related to upper rib dysfunction from bronchitis that increases sympathetic activity to the heart
What parasympathetic viscerovisceral mechanisms are present?	Viscerovisceral	Increased vagal tone in a patient with GERD
What organ level dysfunctions are manifesting in musculoskeletal and fascial restrictions and tissue texture changes?	Viscerosomatic	Chronic upper thoracic tissue texture changes in a patient with ischemic heart disease

the most obvious clinical manifestation of the musculoskeletal system's effects on the body's function as a whole. While it may be tempting to restrict musculoskeletal treatment to only those manifestations oriented around the first question, the osteopathic approach will explore and answer all of the questions.

OMT is indicated for specifically treating the neuromusculoskeletal manifestations of somatic dysfunction. OMT is used to increase available motion, modify nervous system activity, improve lymphatic movement, and increase tissue perfusion. OMT is often sufficient for recovery from various conditions, including many that are not specifically musculoskeletal in nature. Part of this effect is undoubtedly due to the interactive effects of the musculoskeletal system on the fascia, circulation, and autonomic nervous system.

Diseases are often the result of structural disorders relating to both the viscera and the somatic system. In current terms, there is close interweaving of visceral, autonomic, neural, immunologic, and musculoskeletal systems. As first propounded by A. T. Still with the profession's founding, the key to restoring health is to enable the body's restorative mechanisms.[1,2] For example, OMT has been shown to have added benefits in the recovery from some viral illnesses, as evidenced by the experience of the osteopathic community in the 1918 influenza epidemic[20] and the general experience of osteopathic physicians over the past 100 years.[7–14] However, it should be noted that formal outcome studies supporting the use of OMT in the treatment of nonmusculoskeletal disease are sparse[9–18] and more studies are needed.

There is a viscerosomatic relationship between dysfunctions in the viscera and the musculoskeletal system (see Chapter 43 for further discussion). Palpatory evaluation of viscerosomatic reflexes has been used as a diagnostic tool by the osteopathic profession for over a century, as demonstrated both clinically and in the laboratory,[21–42] viscerosomatic reflexes are present with a wide variety of disease. These reflexes develop in response to visceral pathology. Although there is considerable overlap in the presentation of these reflexes for various viscera, they can help the osteopathic physician distinguish between various potential diagnoses (see Chapter 6 Autonomic Nervous System for viscerosomatic relationships to spinal levels, Chapter 13 for basic science background, and Chapter 43 for clinical presentations, differentiation, and interpretation of viscerosomatic reflexes). Viscerosomatic reflexes are identifiable as tissue texture abnormality and tenderness in the dermatomes and myotomes that are embryologically and neurologically related to the viscera that stimulate them. They are most easily palpable in the paravertebral soft tissues. A pure viscerosomatic reflex, without concomitant mechanical spinal somatic dysfunction, generally will demonstrate tissue texture abnormality and tenderness proportionate to the degree of visceral pathology in the absence of definitive restriction of motion; that is, the tissue texture abnormality may or may not demonstrate left/right asymmetry, but there will not be vertebral positional asymmetry.

One of the diagnostic challenges of osteopathic musculoskeletal medicine is the differentiation between a viscerosomatic reflex and primary somatic dysfunction. Johnston and Golden have suggested significant differences in the patterns of clinical findings that can help distinguish the two.[42] Viscerosomatic reflexes, like primary somatic dysfunction, cause muscle spasms, tissue tenderness, and pain. For instance, the pudendal nerve (S2–S4), a branch of the pelvic splanchnic nerves, innervates the pelvic diaphragm. Pain in the pelvic floor may be viscerosomatic (pelvic parasympathetic) in origin or simply result from a primary sacropelvic somatic dysfunction. Proper application of OMT should resolve primary somatic dysfunction. Although viscerosomatic reflexes can be affected by OMT, typical viscerosomatic findings will not resolve until the underlying visceral condition is treated. Therefore, failure of somatic dysfunction to respond to properly applied OMT should lead to considering a viscerosomatic etiology. Indeed, evaluation of any somatic dysfunction should include inquiry into segmentally related viscera (see Chapter 43 for further discussion and information).

CASE 3

HPI: A 45-year-old female presents with left shoulder pain. She states the pain began 2 days ago and has been constant. When asked to point to her pain, she has difficulty identifying it with one finger but points to her left shoulder. She cannot recall an injury to her shoulder. She describes it as an achy, burning pain that she rates a 4/10 on a pain scale. She cannot recall anything that makes the pain worse, including movement. She has tried over-the-counter nonsteroidal anti-inflammatory medication, but they have not helped. She denies radiation. She denies shortness of breath, nausea, diaphoresis, and chest pain. Review of systems is otherwise negative.

What are the initial three diagnoses on the differential? A cardiac cause should be considered for anyone with left shoulder pain. Other possible diagnoses include pneumonia, GERD, bursitis, or other musculoskeletal injury. Important items in the HPI that work to elucidate a diagnosis are asking the patient about shortness of breath, nausea, diaphoresis, radiation, and injury.

CASE CONTINUED

Patient History:

Past Medical History: Hyperlipidemia

Past Surgical History: Cholecystectomy at age 40

Medications: Statin

Allergies: None

Family History: Mother, healthy age 67; father, coronary artery disease (CAD) with one stent, alive at age 72

Social history: The patient denies tobacco use, alcohol use, or illicit drug use. She drinks three cups of coffee per day. She is married and has two children. She is an accountant.

The patient has been seen for routine care for years. She is up to date on recommended preventive medicine for her age. Over the past year, she has started walking most days out of the week and has decreased her BMI from 31 to 28.

Does the differential change?

Family history of CAD and the fact that the patient has hyperlipidemia move a cardiac cause up in the differential. It is not known at this point if the hyperlipidemia is controlled.

CASE CONTINUED

Physical Exam:

Vital Signs: BP, 128/82; HR, 72; RR, 12; Ht, 5′3″; Wt, 160 lb; BMI, 28

General: Female with overweight in no acute distress

Cardiac: Regular rate and rhythm on auscultation, normal S1 and S2, no murmurs, rubs, or gallops heard, radial and pedal pulses 2/4 bilaterally

Respiratory: Clear to auscultation bilaterally, no wheezes, rhonchi, or rales

Abdomen: Bowel sounds present, no distention, no tenderness to light or deep palpation, no organomegaly

Musculoskeletal: Full active and passive range of motion of bilateral upper extremity, negative Hawkins', crossover, drop arm, empty can, and Neer tests

Osteopathic structural examination: Left shoulder internal rotation motion restriction, tissue texture abnormalities, and tenderness noted at T5–T7 on the left

EKG: Normal sinus rhythm

What is the top diagnosis?

At this point, a musculoskeletal cause should also be considered. This patient's symptom complex sounds less like a cardiac cause. The pain is constant (not intermittent or associated with activity), there are no associated symptoms (radiation, chest pain, shortness of breath, nausea, or diaphoresis), and an EKG shows a normal sinus rhythm. With her stable vital signs, an infectious cause, such as pneumonia, is less likely.

CASE CONTINUED

Assessment and Plan: On examination of her right shoulder, somatic dysfunction is detected and treated using Spencer techniques (see Chapter 57 Articulatory Procedures). Tissue tenderness at T5–T7 on the left is also detected and treated. She receives stretching exercises for her shoulder and schedules a follow-up in 1 week.

Follow-up: One week later, the patient returns, still complaining of left shoulder pain. She is worried that she is having a heart problem like her father. Again, her examination is normal. When the spine is screened for somatic dysfunction, tissue tenderness T5–T7 on the left is again detected.

Does this change the differential diagnosis?

After treatment only 1 week ago, if somatic dysfunction recurs with a consistent pattern, a viscerosomatic or repetitive motion cause should be considered.

Which system is now the focus of further investigations?

The viscerosomatic reflex that corresponds to T5–T7 is the upper GI system.

CASE CONTINUED

Upon further questioning, the patient admits the pain worsens when she eats certain foods. She has noticed an increase in the pain with spicy foods. GERD is suspected. Lifestyle changes such as decreasing caffeine and sitting upright for 2 to 3 hours after eating are discussed. Her diaphragm is also found to be restricted and responds well to osteopathic treatment. The patient is started on a short course of a proton pump inhibitor. One week later, she reported that her symptoms had resolved at a subsequent visit.

Discussion: What initially presented as a vague complaint was clarified through osteopathic diagnosis and treatment without unnecessary testing. Often, anyone, regardless of age and past medical history, who presents with left shoulder pain, may be sent for a full cardiac workup or even to the emergency room. An osteopathic family physician has the benefit of knowing the patient and her history. Then, through structural diagnosis, the region of the visceral dysfunction can be further pinpointed. Figure 66.2 displays some situations in which OMT would not be appropriate.

Musculoskeletal treatment and palpatory diagnosis are fundamentally safe. There are few specific contraindications for using OMT, although some OMT techniques are relatively contraindicated in some specific circumstances. There are three other reasons why an osteopathic physician might not use OMT on a patient.

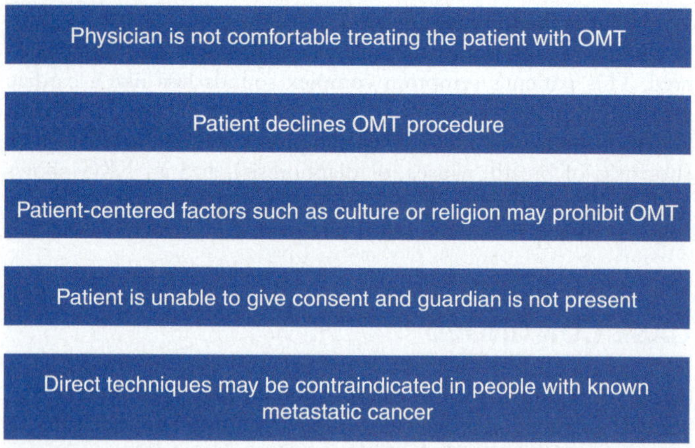

Figure 66.2. Situations in which OMT would not be appropriate.

First, if the physician is uncomfortable performing OMT because of a perceived lack of skill, it is better to refrain from using OMT for complex cases until further training has been obtained. Second, a patient's refusal would be an absolute contraindication for using OMT. Third, the patient's culture may prohibit or limit such treatment in some circumstances. For instance, some religious beliefs prohibit patients from being treated by physicians of the opposite gender. Therefore, it is very important that the osteopathic family physician be sensitive to every individual's psychological, social, and cultural beliefs and orientations.

TREATING THE WHOLE PERSON

It is a fundamental philosophical commitment of the osteopathic profession to treat the whole person: body, mind, and spirit. Patient care consists of many strands: the physical care of the individual, the consideration of emotional health and healing, and recognition of a multitude of influencing factors, including but not limited to family, community, cultural beliefs, work environment, and economic condition. Because of the complexity of the experience of illness, osteopathic family medicine is at its best when integrative thinking and problem-solving are emphasized. This is accomplished by highlighting the importance of interdependent structure and function concepts. For example, recognizing the nervous system's role in integrating the body into a holistic mechanism and the significance that somatic function and dysfunction play in that mechanism greatly facilitates such integrative thinking and problem-solving.[37]

PSYCHOSOCIAL CONSIDERATIONS IN FAMILY PRACTICE

Psychosocial factors must be considered as part of the osteopathic family physician's evaluation protocol. Even the seemingly simple decision to seek health care can often be complicated by marginally understood interactions between a patient's personal, family, cultural, and work-related elements. Economic factors, particularly the availability of insurance, can further complicate a patient's decision-making. An individual's response to psychological, social, and economic factors can lead to significant differences in the decision to seek or not to seek medical care. Some estimates suggest that as many as 60% of a symptomatic population for many diagnosable diseases, such as migraine headaches and back pain, may never see a physician for the complaint.[43] One likely explanation is the overwhelming complexity of our medical care system.

TABLE 66.3

Psychosocial Aspects of Diabetes and Effects on Disease Management

Psychosocial Comorbidity	Disease Management Effects
Depression	Decreased patient adherence to self-care management and medications
Anxiety	Increased patient concern about adverse disease and medication effects
Disease-specific distress	May paralyze patient from engaging in self-care
Disease denial	Prevents patient from getting help and engaging in management
Major life events (i.e., death of a spouse, change in living situation)	May uncover reliance on others and the patient may decompensate during this time

The primary care physician often deals with clearly defined psychological problems such as personality disorders, substance abuse, eating disorders, anxiety, depression, and the disruptive and stressful effects of personal, family, and job-related stressors. There is data to suggest that, except for psychoses, primary care physicians treat more psychological problems than psychiatrists.[3,4,7] Not only do family physicians prescribe appropriate medications for psychologically based problems, but they often provide significant personal and family counseling. Table 66.3 correlates psychosocial comorbidities that may have an effect on chronic disease management using diabetes as an example.

Many patients, some with diseases and many without, complain of problems relating to the body when the core issue may relate more to life stresses, including psychological and interpersonal problems. If the physician overlooks the role of personality and stress-related factors in the patient's complaints, it is unlikely that they will help the patient achieve symptom control or disease cure.

Multisystem somatoform disorders, fatigue, and chronic pain often involve personality and stress-related factors. These disorders frequently include symptoms inconsistent with known diseases or demonstrate objective findings incompatible with the complaints. People who exhibit these problems have very often seen multiple physicians. One of the most telling signs indicating a strong psychological component is the denigration of a previous physician's efforts. It is also worth noting that often these disorders include a significant complaint of musculoskeletal pain that, upon close evaluation by the osteopathic physician, demonstrates little, if any, relevant somatic dysfunction. Their symptoms, however, should not be ignored; instead, the psychological root of the dysfunction should be addressed. This approach embodies treating the whole person, not just a disease.

Finally, it is crucial to remember that most chronic diseases can lead to psychological and social disturbances for both the patient and the family. The role of multiple and chronic stressors in developing psychological disturbances and physical disease has been a recognized component of medicine since Selye's studies in the 1950s.[43] Alternately, failure to recognize the body–mind connection can lead to problems such as poor treatment adherence, acceleration of the disease process, and development of comorbidities, to name a few.

Social Determinants of Health

It is hard to practice osteopathic primary care effectively without having some knowledge and appreciation of the role social determinants of health play in health maintenance and disease management.

"Social determinants of health are conditions in the environments in which people are born, live, learn, work, play, worship, and age that affects a wide range of health, functioning, and quality-of-life outcomes and risks. Conditions (e.g., social, economic, and physical) in these various environments and settings (e.g., school, church, workplace, and neighborhood) have been referred to as 'place.'"[44] Social determinants of health were prioritized in Healthy People 2020 and reaffirmed in Healthy People 2030.[44,45]

Social determinants of health can fall into several categories:

- Economic Stability
  - Employment
  - Food Insecurity
  - Housing Instability
  - Poverty
- Education
  - Early Childhood Education and Development
  - Enrollment in Higher Education
  - High School Graduation
  - Language and Literacy
- Social and Community Context
  - Civic Participation
  - Discrimination
  - Incarceration
  - Social Cohesion
- Health and Health Care
  - Access to Health Care
  - Access to Primary Care
  - Health Literacy
- Neighborhood and Built Environment
  - Access to Foods that Support Healthy Eating Patterns
  - Crime and Violence
  - Environmental Conditions
  - Quality of Housing

When working with your patients, providing a screening tool to assess the Social Determinants of health may be prudent. This lets the patient know you are interested in the nonmedical life challenges that intersect with and affect self-care. Further, by providing the screening, you create the opportunity for you and the patient to discuss ways to handle these determinants while helping with health promotion, disease prevention, and disease management,

TABLE 66.4

Selected and Targeted Use of Medications

Patient Presentation	Osteopathic Treatment Plan
5-year-old patient with otitis media who is otherwise healthy	OMT and pain control with close follow-up. Possibly no antibiotics needed.
35-year-old female with consistent blood pressure readings of 135/85	Discuss with the patient increasing exercise to 150 min/wk to prevent diagnosis of hypertension. DASH diet as effective as a medication.
45-year-old male with a diagnosis of prediabetes	Refer to an evidence-based lifestyle modification program. Lifestyle more effective than medication in preventing type 2 diabetes.
76-year-old male with recent MI with stenting	Refer to cardiopulmonary rehabilitation, encourage follow-up with cardiology, and treat with OMT. Prescribe antithrombic and lipid-lowering medications.

PHARMACOTHERAPEUTICS IN OSTEOPATHIC FAMILY PRACTICE

Early in its history, osteopathic practice employed a holistic approach. Unfortunately, conventional medical practice in the late 19th and early 20th centuries included toxic, ineffective, or addictive chemical compounds such as calomel, morphine, digitalis, whiskey, and laudanum. To his credit, Dr. Still found the use of such drugs repugnant.[1,2,46] His own experience as a physician using the available drugs of the day convinced him that drugs were inevitably harmful. Instead, Dr. Still promoted implementing an appropriate diet, correcting psychological dysfunction, and physical work. While the field of pharmacology for health and disease has significantly advanced, osteopathic practices continue to consider a broad scope of treatment options that include but are not limited to pharmacotherapeutics. While medications are integral and valued elements of osteopathic care, osteopathic physicians are encouraged to be ever mindful of the limitations of all medications, including their side effects and, in the case of antibiotics and antiviral agents, the tendency of drugs to induce resistance in their proposed targets. From both theoretical and practical standpoints, it is crucial that osteopathic family physicians encourage lifestyle modification, remove structural and functional impediments from patients' normal ability to function, and otherwise avoid using medications whenever possible[47] (Table 66.4).

Much of the abuse of pharmacotherapy at the beginning of the 21st century stems from physicians' attempts to ameliorate the symptoms of functional conditions. Even many recognized pathologic conditions, like hypertension, may be thought of as symptoms of an underlying pathophysiology. Osteopathic medicine seeks to affect the underlying physiology through lifestyle modification, OMT, and pharmacotherapeutics when necessary. The osteopathic physician's patient-centered, rather than disease-centered, approach to patient care offers a clear advantage. Many functional symptoms are reduced by the appropriate use of OMT and lifestyle change, thereby decreasing the need to prescribe symptom-suppressing medications. Indeed, the underlying pathophysiology may also be positively affected by reducing drug dosage requirements or enhancing the efficacy of appropriately prescribed drugs.

A prime example is the use of antibiotics to treat self-limiting infections that are generally viral. This practice expends limited resources that might be better used elsewhere and promotes antibiotic resistance in pathogenic bacteria. While this model has been promoted in defense of "evidence-based medicine,"[35] the more general point is that family physicians are strongly positioned to promote a more thoughtful and effective, resource-sparing approach to medicine. This approach balances the needs of the individual against the ultimate needs of the population.

DISEASE MANAGEMENT AND HEALTH RESTORATION

The osteopathic family physician's responsibility is to provide the necessary information and tools with which the patient can recover

BOX 66.1 Goals of Comprehensive Osteopathic Family Medicine

The ultimate purpose of osteopathic medical intervention is to help the patient in the restoration of health. To this end, the physician takes measures to:

- Relieve symptoms
- Remove, or at least diminish, the population of pathogenic organisms when there is infection
- Remove or repair diseased pieces of the body surgically when necessary
- Replace substances no longer produced or absorbed
- Desensitize the body to, or remove from the body, substances that produce imbalance
- Sensitize the body to necessary substances that are being underutilized
- Rebalance the dynamic stability of the body
- Restore emotional and psychosocial stability

health. The physician recommends and, in some cases, performs appropriate interventions. The osteopathic physician also needs to proactively minimize adverse side effects and complications by carefully weighing the risks and benefits of potential therapies. The physician should always recognize that the ultimate decision to participate in any care plan belongs to the patient and that healing is not an act performed by the physician; it is the act of the patient's body, mind, and spirit. Box 66.1 lists the goals of comprehensive osteopathic family medicine.

LONGITUDINAL CARE

It has long been held that a physician's role is to diagnose and treat disease. In contemporary society, disease is considered a relatively acute onset condition responsible for distressing symptoms. The osteopathic family physician, however, deals with specific acute disease episodes and chronic illnesses that may last for decades. Longitudinal care is an important aspect of primary care that distinguishes it from medical and surgical specialties. Primary care physicians typically see patients over many years and for various health care–related incidents. Specialist care, on the other hand, is often episodic and focused on a particular disease. With some long-term diseases, the specialist may see the patient for many visits over many years; however, even in this case, the specialist generally focuses on a single disease or organ system. The family physician, in contrast, may see the same patient from birth to the end of life. Although the family physician can manage many diseases, there are times when a consult from a specialist is warranted. Table 66.5 gives examples of when a referral should be made for the care of a patient with diabetes. Figure 66.3 gives an example of a timeline for the care of a patient who sees a family physician and another specialist, such as a surgeon or subspecialist.

PREVENTIVE HEALTH AND HEALTH MAINTENANCE

As noted previously, osteopathic family physicians emphasize preventive medicine and using homeostatic mechanisms to maintain patient health. This is in accordance with the general osteopathic

TABLE 66.5 Appropriate Referral to Specialist for a Patient with Diabetes

Specialist	When to Refer
Podiatrist	When PAD or neuropathy leads to callusing or need for custom foot care and footwear
Nephrologist	Patients with stage 3B or greater CKD or gross proteinuria
Ophthalmologist	Routine diabetes eye screening
Nutritionist	Recommended at time of diagnosis and at times of major life changes
Diabetes educator	Recommended at time of diagnosis and at times of major life changes
Psychologist/behavioral health	At any time that psychosocial factors disrupt self-care

concept that disease is the effect of a failure to maintain normal compensatory mechanisms in both the body and the environment. This concept explicitly suggests that disease treatment is best achieved by restoring the body's compensatory mechanisms and balance while reducing or eliminating stresses within one's environment. More to the point, it implies that disease is preventable. Thus, the osteopathic physician's fundamental role is to help patients understand and implement a healthy lifestyle. Figures 66.4 and 66.5 provide schematic drawings depicting the interdependence between the various factors related to one's health and illness.

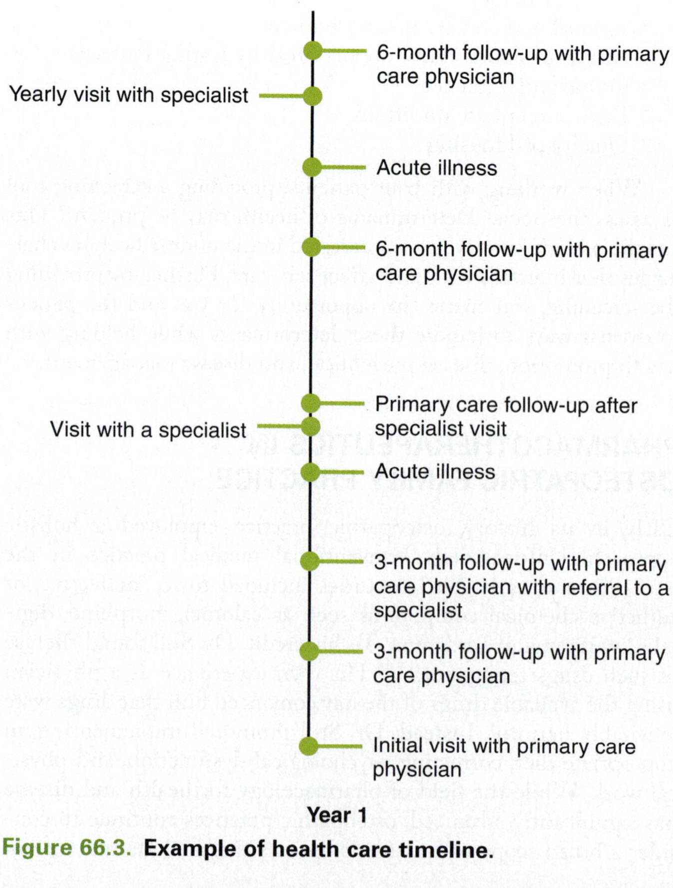

Figure 66.3. Example of health care timeline.

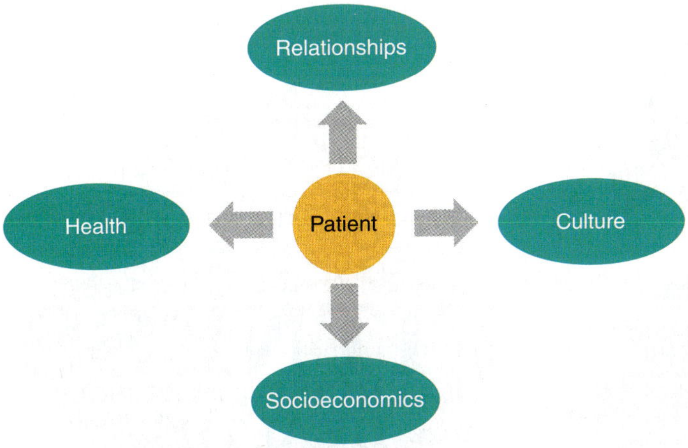

Figure 66.4. Balance between health and illness. During stages of health, the patient is able to maintain relationships, participate in culture, and balance socioeconomic stresses.

FAMILY PHYSICIAN AS OMBUDSMAN

The complexity of the current health care system, coupled with similar complexity in medical diagnosis and treatment, often leaves a patient confused and lost. In this scenario, the osteopathic family physician's role can be an ombudsperson, a health care coordinator, and a facilitator for the complex interactions between the patient, specialists, hospitals and other care facilities, and insurers.

An additional role for the family practice physician in the physician-as-ombudsperson model is that of an interpreter. Patients are often bewildered by the complexities associated with disease, diagnostic tests, and treatment options. The additional information available to patients with internet access and computerized databases only adds to the confusion. The osteopathic family physician can, and should, interpret this information for the patient. Through effective dialogue with the patient, the physician can assist in decision-making to achieve optimal treatment and health.

Finally, the osteopathic family physician must be prepared to deal with questions involving patients' personal and social expectations, economic issues (including affordability of the care proposed by the physician), insurance coverage, and at times religious and health beliefs that may conflict or contradict those of the physician.

Osteopathic family medicine is gaining momentum. Patients and families appreciate a physician who approaches health from a holistic angle, someone who recognizes the complexity of the human condition. Patients and families want a physician who is able to manage and improve health instead of merely identifying disease. As a result, the osteopathic family physician is recognized as a community leader, researcher, and teacher. Whereas once there was a push toward medical and surgical specialties, the pendulum is swinging back as more medical students are pursuing primary care training.

COMMUNITY OUTREACH AND PUBLIC HEALTH

The breadth of knowledge required of the osteopathic family physician and the highly developed communication skills demanded in family medicine make the osteopathic family physician uniquely qualified for private and public health education. As critical members of the community, family physicians advise and act to change policies that will contribute to the improved health of the community. In that light, the osteopathic family physician can be an agent of change.

The osteopathic family physician's commitment to helping patients develop and maintain health often extends beyond office- and hospital-based medical care. For example, teaching patients about the signs and symptoms of potentially important disease manifestations, proper diet and exercise regimens, proper ergonomics on the job and everyday life, appropriate immunizations, and private and public hygiene measures often quickly segues into transmitting the same information to the public.

This concept was demonstrated during the 2020–2023 COVID pandemic. Patients looked to family physicians to navigate the rapidly changing medical information and recommendations. Public health organizations relied on family physicians to discuss immunizations and provide testing to their patients. Osteopathic family physicians were often the first line in triaging and diagnosing those who developed symptoms.

Finally, the osteopathic family physician can provide valuable service to the osteopathic community and the general population by participating in the education of future osteopathic physicians. Whether in the classroom, hospital training programs, or in-office one-on-one training, the unique strengths of osteopathic family practice need to be passed on to future generations of osteopathic physicians.

THE FUTURE OF OSTEOPATHIC FAMILY MEDICINE

While no one can predict the future, many factors at work in the US health care system today will influence family medicine tomorrow. Osteopathic medicine is at the forefront of these changes. The provision of health care will evolve from episodic care of

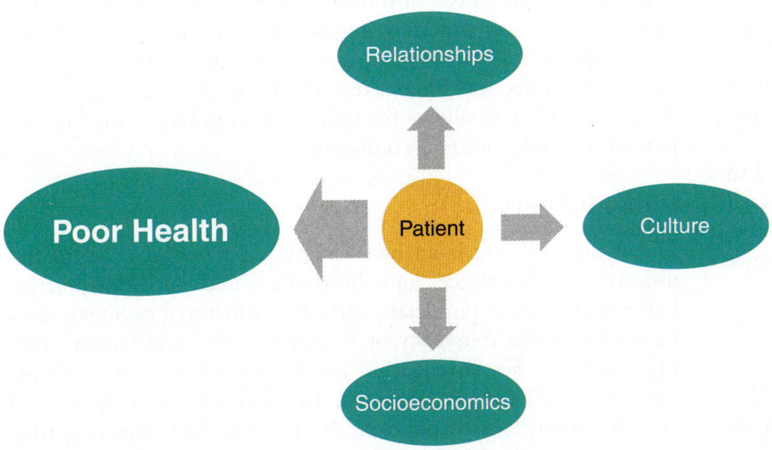

Figure 66.5. When a patient moves away from good health, they expend personal resources and energy that put strains on relationships, cultural participation, and socioeconomic conditions. It is the job of a primary care physician to restore balance while considering all of the factors that impact patient health.

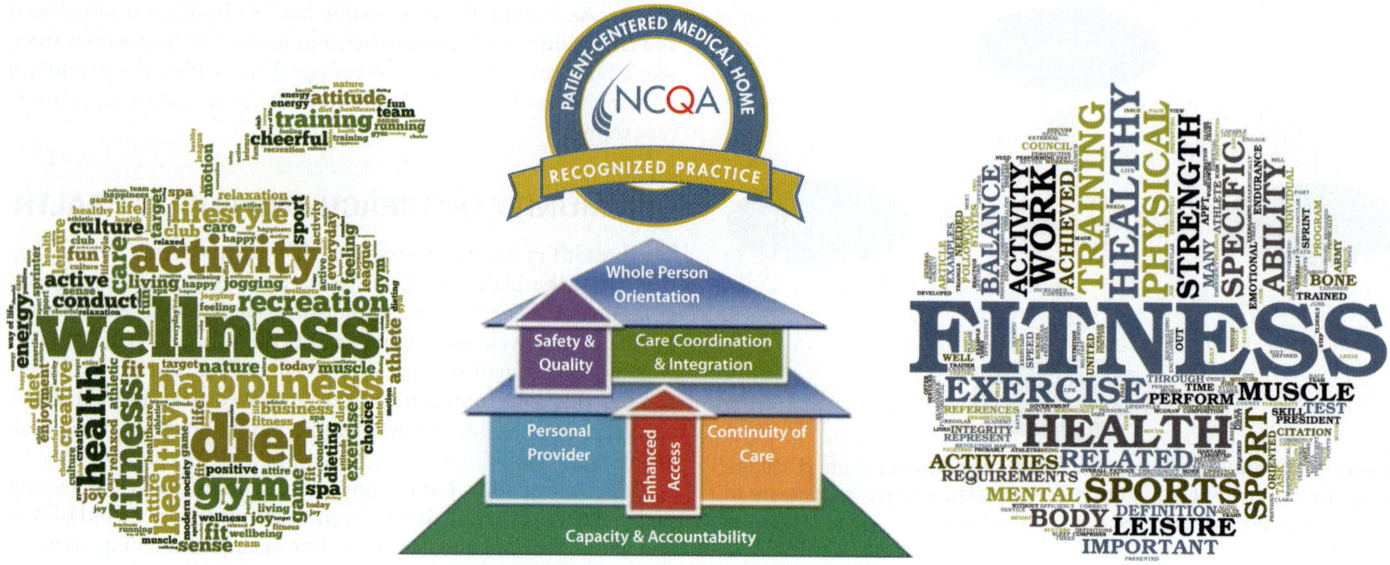

Figure 66.6. The future of family medicine.

isolated problems to long-term chronic disease management with patient-centered longitudinal care. Further, patients will have a greater say in their treatment plans than ever before. This means that individualized treatments are more likely to be adhered to. Health care will no longer be a relationship between one physician and one patient but rather a relationship with a health care team, each contributing to the health of their patients and population. Further, addressing health behavior change will focus on the family, workplace, and community, as few people make health decisions in a vacuum and need the support of those around them to navigate long-term change successfully. Finally, health care payers will finally stop paying for the quantity of care and change the focus to the quality of care. This is crucial as it rewards keeping the patients healthy rather than finding and treating disease. The osteopathic family physician is well-positioned to take the lead in these changes in health care. Figure 66.6 displays symbolic computerized emblems characterizing the future of family medicine.

Telemedicine

One tangible expansion of the health care system resulted from the COVID pandemic. While telemedicine has been used in small programs for 20 years, the use of telemedicine exploded as a result of the restrictions associated with the COVID pandemic. Patients could have acute care, primary care, and other specialty care on a telemedicine platform. Telemedicine can include phone or video visits with programs like Doximity and Doxme. Once felt to be inadequate for care, we have learned that some components of care fit nicely within the telemedicine parameters. This is particularly true when technology allows data to be shared, such as lab values, blood pressure or glucose readings or ambulatory monitors, and continuous glucose monitors.

Telemedicine is most useful for patients who typically need to travel long distances to obtain in-person care or for problem-based rechecks. As the technology improves, it should further enable osteopathic physicians to expand on the physical exam. The future of telemedicine will unfold as regulations evolve.

Growth of Lifestyle Medicine

While osteopathic medicine has consistently recognized the relationship between body homeostasis and prevention of illness, there has been a major increase in focus on lifestyle medicine, especially a significant part of primary care. Lifestyle medicine is a medical specialty that uses therapeutic lifestyle interventions as a primary modality to treat chronic conditions including, but not limited to, cardiovascular diseases, type 2 diabetes, and obesity. The six pillars of lifestyle medicine, as outlined by the American College of Lifestyle Medicine, are as follows: a whole-food, plant-predominant eating pattern, physical activity, restorative sleep, stress management, avoidance of risky substances, and finally, social connection.[48] The modern osteopathic primary care physician has further support to help patients achieve optimal health through healthy habits.

Precision Care

Precision care has become another popular "brand" of medicine. Precision medicine is described as personalized and participatory, allowing it to be preventive and predictive.[49] Much of precision care has been part of routine medical care for a long time. However, the explosion of advances in genetic disease understanding has advanced the modern application of precision medicine. Precision medicine gained greater support after the creation of President Barack Obama's 2015 Precision Medicine Initiative.[50] Precision medicine focuses on the person's health at the molecular, cellular, and organ level. With this focus, we move away from treating the symptoms of established diseases and focus on the causes and disease prevention. The osteopathic physician can use precision medicine techniques to provide a more targeted solution for a given person by leveraging specific genetic findings and biomarkers to obtain improved outcomes. This approach also allows for individualizing treatment for each person for each common condition.

Direct Primary Care

Direct primary care is an increasingly popular alternative to traditional fee-for-service and insurance-based medical practice. Patients and family physicians agree to a structured payment, often regardless of the frequency or length of visits, and without billing insurance. For osteopathic family physicians, direct primary care's benefit is reduced administrative and noncare activities. For patients, access to their physician is improved, and steps to getting to their physician are reduced. In addition, direct primary care creates the opportunity for closer and more continuous communication and care. More physicians who provide direct primary care have a much smaller panel of patients but are essentially "on-call" for those patients 24/7, 365.

CONCLUSIONS

Osteopathic family physicians are uniquely positioned to deal with a broad spectrum of health and disease-related problems, including biologic, social, economic, and cultural influences. The osteopathic family physician will mobilize resources to promote health and healing, including medical and surgical care, osteopathic manipulative care, and psychosocial and general family care. With appreciation for the osteopathic philosophy and its principles, the osteopathic physician is able to provide a uniquely powerful take on family medicine. This includes emphasizing the importance of self-healing and the interdependence of biologic, psychological, and social factors that are so potent in disease development, as well as the recovery and maintenance of health.

REFERENCES

1. Still AT. *Philosophy of Osteopathy*. Published by the author; 1899. Reproduction published by the American Academy of Osteopathy.
2. Still AT. *Osteopathy, Research and Practice*. Author; 1910. Reprinted by Eastland Press; 1992.
3. Rakel RE, Rakel DE. *Textbook of Family Medicine*. 9th ed. Elsevier Health; 2015.
4. Taylor RB, ex. ed. *Family Medicine: Principles and Practice*. 6th ed. Springer-Verlag; 2003.
5. Shubrook JH Jr, Johnson AW. An osteopathic approach to type 2 diabetes. *J Am Osteopath Assoc*. 2011;11(9):531–537.
6. Krein SL, Heisler M, Piette JD, Makki F, Kerr EA. The effect of chronic pain on diabetes patients' self-management. *Diabetes Care*. 2005;28(1):65–70.
7. Egede L. Diabetes, major depression, and functional disability among US adults. *Diabetes Care*. 2004;27(2):421–428.
8. Russel LB, Suh SC, Safford MA. Time requirements for diabetes self-management: too much for many? *J Fam Pract*. 2005;54(1):52–56.
9. Shubrook JH, Klein G, Schwartz FL. *Time Demands for Diabetes Self-Care*. American Diabetes Association Scientific Sessions; 2006.
10. Boon H, Blaak EE, Saris WH, Keizer HA, Wagenmakers AJ, van Loon LJ. Substrate source utilization in long term diagnosed type 2 diabetes patients at rest, and during exercise and subsequent recovery. *Diabetologia*. 2007;50(1):103–112.
11. Wang Y, Simar D, Fiatarone Singh MA. Adaptations to exercise training with skeletal muscle in adults with type 2 diabetes or impaired glucose tolerance: a systematic review. *Diabetes Metab Res Rev*. 2009;25(1):13–40.
12. Suh SH, Palk I-Y, Jacobs K. Regulation of blood glucose homeostasis during prolonged exercise. *Mol Cells*. 2007;23(3):272–279.
13. King DS, Baldus PJ, Sharp RL, Kesl LD, Feltmeyer TL, Riddle MS. Time course for exercise induced alterations in insulin action and glucose tolerance in middle aged people. *J Appl Physiol (1985)*. 1995;78(1):17–22.
14. Winnick JJ, Sherman WM, Habash DL, et al. Short term aerobic exercise training in obese human with type 2 diabetes mellitus improves whole body sensitivity through gains in peripheral, not hepatic insulin sensitivity. *J Clin Endocrinol Metab*. 2008;93(3):771–778.
15. Sucher BM, Hinrichs RN, Welcher RL, Quiroz LD, St Laurent BF, Morrison BJ. Manipulative treatment of carpel tunnel syndrome: biomechanical and osteopathic intervention to increase the length of the transverse carpel ligament: part 2-effect of sec differences and manipulative "priming." *J Am Osteopath Assoc*. 2005;105(3):135–143.
16. Knebl JA, Shores JH, Gamber RG, Gray WT, Herron KM. Improving functional ability in the elderly via the Spencer technique: a randomized, controlled trial. *J Am Osteopath Assoc*. 2002;102(7):387–396.
17. Nelson KE, Glonek T, eds. *Somatic Dysfunction in Osteopathic Family Medicine*. American College of Osteopathic Family Physicians; 2007.
18. Kuchera ML, Kuchera WA. *Osteopathic Considerations in Systemic Dysfunction*. Kirksville College of Osteopathic Medicine Press; 1990.
19. Noll DR, Degenhardt BF, Morley TF, et al. Efficacy of osteopathic manipulation as an adjunctive therapy for hospitalized patients with pneumonia: a randomized controlled trial. *Osteopath Med Prim Care*. 2010;4:2.
20. Smith RK. One hundred thousand cases of influenza with a death rate of one-fortieth of that reported under conventional medical treatment. 1919. *J Am Osteopath Assoc*. 2000;100:320–323.
21. Beal MC. Viscerosomatic reflexes: a review. *J Am Osteopath Assoc*. 1985; 85:786–801.
22. Pearson WM, Hines NH, Polovich CA, et al. Symposium on respiratory diseases—etiology, pathology, diagnosis, and treatment. *J Am Osteopath Assoc*. 1938;36:307–331.
23. Purse FM. Clinical evaluation of osteopathic manipulative therapy in measles. *J Am Osteopath Assoc*. 1961;61:274–276.
24. Rumney IC. Osteopathic manipulative treatment of infectious diseases. *Osteopath Ann*. 1974;2:29–33.
25. Blood HA. Infections of the ear, nose and throat. *Osteopath Ann*. 1978; 6:465–469.
26. Harakal JH. Manipulative treatment for acute upper respiratory disease. *Osteopath Ann*. 1981;9:253–257.
27. Schmidt IC. Osteopathic manipulative therapy as a primary factor in the management of upper, middle, and pararespiratory infections. *J Am Osteopath Assoc*. 1982;81:382–388.
28. Kaluza CL, Sherbin M. The physiologic response of the nose to osteopathic manipulative treatment. *J Am Osteopath Assoc*. 1983;82:654–660.
29. Whiting CA. *Investigation of the Phagocytic Index*. Bull. no.1. AT Still Research Institute. Monford & Co.; 1910:61–63.
30. Measel JW Jr. The effects of the lymphatic pump upon the immune response: I. Preliminary studies on the antibody response to pneumococcal polysaccharide assayed by bacterial agglutination and passive hemagglutination. *J Am Osteopath Assoc*. 1982;82:28–31.
31. Noll DR, Shores JH, Gamber RG, Herron KM, Swift J Jr. Benefits of osteopathic manipulative treatment for hospitalized elderly patients with pneumonia. *J Am Osteopath Assoc*. 2000;100:776–782.
32. Radjieski JM, Lumley MA, Cantieri MS. Effect of osteopathic manipulative treatment on length of stay for pancreatitis: a randomized pilot study. *J Am Osteopath Assoc*. 1998;98:264–272.
33. Beal MC. Viscerosomatic reflexes: a review. *J Am Osteopath Assoc*. 1985; 85:786–801.
34. Beal MC, Morlock JW. Somatic dysfunction associated with pulmonary disease. *J Am Osteopath Assoc*. 1984;84:179–184.
35. Beal MC, Kleiber GE. Somatic dysfunction as a predictor of coronary artery disease. *J Am Osteopath Assoc*. 1985;85:302–307.
36. Korr IM. Sustained sympathicotonia as a factor in disease. In: Korr IM, ed. *The Neurobiological Mechanisms in Manipulative Therapy*. Plenum Publishing Co.; 1978:229–268.
37. Korr IM. The spinal cord as organizer of disease processes: some preliminary perspectives. *J Am Osteopath Assoc*. 1976;76:35–45.
38. Johnston WL, Kelso AF, Babcock HB. Changes in the presence of a segmental dysfunction pattern associated with hypertension: part I. A short-term longitudinal study. *J Am Osteopath Assoc*. 1995;95:243–248, 253–255.
39. Johnston WL, Kelso AF. Changes in the presence of a segmental dysfunction pattern associated with hypertension: part II. A long-term longitudinal study. *J Am Osteopath Assoc*. 1995;95:315–318.
40. Johnston WL, Hill JL, Elkiss ML, Marino RV. Identification of stable somatic findings in hypertensive subjects by trained examiners using palpatory examination. *J Am Osteopath Assoc*. 1982;81:830–836.
41. Johnston WL, Kelso AF, Hollandsworth DL, Karrat JJ. Somatic manifestations in renal disease: a clinical research study. *J Am Osteopath Assoc*. 1987;87:22–35.
42. Johnston WL, Golden WJ. Segmental definition—part IV. Updating the differential for somatic and visceral inputs. *J Am Osteopath Assoc*. 2001;101: 278–283.
43. Selye H. *The Stress of Life*. 2nd ed. McGraw-Hill; 1978.

44. Healthy People 2030. Accessed February 21, 2023. https://www.cdc.gov/nchs/healthy_people/hp2030/hp2030.htm
45. Healthy People 2020. Accessed February 21, 2023. https://www.cdc.gov/nchs/healthy_people/hp2020/hp2020_topic_areas.htm
46. Slawson DC, Shaghnessy AF. Becoming an information master. *J Fam Pract.* 2001;50:51–56.
47. Still AT. *Autobiography of Andrew T. Still.* Author; 1908. Reprinted by the American Academy of Osteopathy; 1989.
48. The pillars of lifestyle medicine. Accessed February 21, 2023. https://lifestylemedicine.org/overview/
49. Jameson JL, Longo DL. Precision medicine—personalized, problematic, and promising. *N Engl J Med.* 2015;372:2229–2234.
50. Precision care initiative. *The White House: President Barack Obama.* Accessed February 21, 2023. https://obamawhitehouse.archives.gov/precision-medicine#:~:text=In%20his%202015%20State%20of,improve%20health%20and%20treat%20disease

67

Osteopathic Considerations in Pediatrics

MARY ANN MAGOUN ▪ ERIC BEVERIDGE ▪ REBECCA E. GIUSTI ▪ ANDREW J. PICCA ▪ JUDITH OH LEONOR ▪ NATALIE HOLLICK PRICE ▪ LUKAS MARTINCIK ▪ KAREN M. STEELE ▪ MIRIAM V. MILLS ▪ MARY ANNE MORELLI HASKELL ▪ JESUS SANCHEZ JR ▪ FRANK SERRECCHIA

KEY CONCEPTS

- Infants, children, and adolescents are dynamically changing entities with differential rates of growth and maturation of component parts.
- As the infant, child, and adolescent mature, their structure changes and, therefore, function between systems and their regulatory mechanisms will vary over time. Therefore, continuous reevaluation of these interrelationships is required.
- The infant, child, and adolescent must be approached and observed for both current and longitudinal changes.
- Fundamental diagnostic and therapeutic principles applied to adults do not always hold true for pediatric patients.

INTRODUCTION

Pediatrics is the art and science of health care that may begin periconceptionally and continue through gestation, infancy, childhood, adolescence, and early adulthood. The concept dates back to Hippocrates, Aristotle, and Galen who acknowledged that this population needs to be viewed and treated differently from a medical perspective.

Through the centuries, the concept of pediatrics evolved. Internationally, Dr. Nils Rosen von Rosenstein (1706–1773) is considered the founder of pediatrics as a medical specialty. Other important dates for the pediatric specialty include:

- The first pediatric hospital—Hopital des Enfants Malades—opened in Paris in 1802.
- Similar hospitals across Europe opened in the 1800s.
- In the United States, the Children's Hospital of Philadelphia opened in 1855, followed by Boston Children's Hospital in 1869.

The principles of pediatrics are clear in that this population ranging from infants to adolescents are not simply miniature adults. They have unique structural concerns with different anatomic proportions, as well as different biochemistry and physiology owing to immature development of body systems, including incomplete myelination of the nervous system, and incomplete bone growth.

All of the above history predates Andrew Taylor Still and his emphasis on the interrelatedness of structure and function, homeostasis, and the body's self-healing capacity. One of his first students, William Garner Sutherland, further described the body's self-healing inherent potency and the cranial concept of the primary respiratory mechanism. Just as the practice of pediatrics as a specialty was taking shape, so was the applicability of osteopathic medicine to pediatric patients.

From a patient's first day of life, the osteopathic pediatrician keeps in mind the interdependence of structure and function and is continually observing and taking note of any evidence of somatic dysfunction that may adversely affect healthy growth and development. The fact that a pediatric patient is a dynamically changing entity with different rates of growth and maturation of component parts demands continuous reevaluation of interrelationships of body systems and their regulatory mechanisms. Fundamental diagnostic and therapeutic principles applied to adults do not always hold true for pediatric patients. Problems that are not addressed early may magnify as they manifest in the growing child with a number of comorbidities.

This chapter will include the application of osteopathic structural examination (OSE) and osteopathic manipulative treatment (OMT) in the evaluation and treatment of a pediatric patient within the framework of the five models of osteopathic care:

1. Biopsychosocial/behavioral
2. Biomechanical/structural/musculoskeletal
3. Respiratory/circulatory
4. Neurologic
5. Metabolic

HISTORICAL LEGACY OF OSTEOPATHIC PEDIATRICS

Since its inception, osteopathic medicine has focused on primary care. Care of the pediatric patient was an integral part of the general osteopathic physician's practice.[1] In his autobiography *Osteopathy: Research and Practice*, A.T. Still presented case studies and principles of osteopathic treatment of infants and children with a wide variety of afflictions, including infectious diseases.[2,3] Osteopathic care, including alleviation of spinal joint restriction and fascial tensions hastened the recovery of ill patients and improved their outcomes.[2]

In 1918, Millard wrote a text on the treatment of poliomyelitis in children with osteopathic methods.[4] In 1939, Watson and Percival, cofounders of the American College of Osteopathic Pediatricians and attending physicians at the Los Angeles County Osteopathic Hospital pediatric unit, reported on the purported benefit of distinctly osteopathic care compared with traditional care of children admitted with pneumonia to a similar in size hospital on the east coast. In a preliminary report, they presented data in support of decreased morbidity and mortality of children under their care.[5]

Special attention, however, has been focused on the newborn since the deleterious effects of uterine forces upon the fetus during labor and delivery were documented by Little in 1862.[6]

- In 1913, Whiting stressed the importance of treating the pregnant mother's somatic dysfunction before delivery, based on data showing decreased labor and delivery time in 223 patients treated with OMT throughout pregnancy.[7]
- In 1954, Arbuckle's publication advocated for correcting the mechanical component of neuromuscular problems in patients diagnosed with cerebral palsy (CP), by treating somatic dysfunction found in newborns as a result of traumatic birth forces upon the cranium.[8]

- Barnes described applications of osteopathic principles and manipulative treatment in the management of common newborn problems.[9] These included:
  - Asphyxia
  - Atelectasis
  - Emesis
  - Brachial plexus injury
  - Colic
  - Bowel problems
  - Clubfoot (pes equinovarus)
- In his 1961 publication, Woods noted that children with psychological disturbances, concentration problems, learning disabilities, and poor performance at school were found to have an increased incidence of cranial somatic dysfunction and a history of an obstetrically complicated delivery.[10,11] Such children showed demonstrable improvements upon resolution of somatic dysfunction with OMT.[12,13]
- Sutherland lectured on how birth trauma to the occiput could potentially affect the vagus nerve (CN X) and cause vomiting and irritability in the newborn.[14] Potential causes may include:
  - Compression or distortion of the jugular foramen (Fig. 67.1) whose contents include:
    - CNs IX, X, and XI
    - Pars nervosa from CN IX, pars vascularis from CN X, and Arnold nerve from CN XI
    - Jugular bulb
    - Posterior meningeal branch of the ascending pharyngeal arteries
  - Compression or distortion of the hypoglossal canal (Fig. 67.1)—CN XII
  - Compression or distortion of the occipital condyles (Fig. 67.2)
- Frymann's examination of 1,250 newborns investigated this proposed relationship between cranial structure and neurologic dysfunction.[15] Her survey supported Sutherland's postulate of vagal nerve irritability found in strain patterns of developing newborn occiput. Frymann continued to participate in several clinical research studies and lectures worldwide and founded the Osteopathic Center for Children and Osteopathy's Promise to Children Foundation in San Diego, CA.[16]
- In 2000, in a meta-analysis of outcomes data regarding osteopathic care of obstetric patients, King found that prenatal OMT improved postnatal outcomes (less meconium staining of amniotic fluid, need for forceps, and caesarian sections).[17]

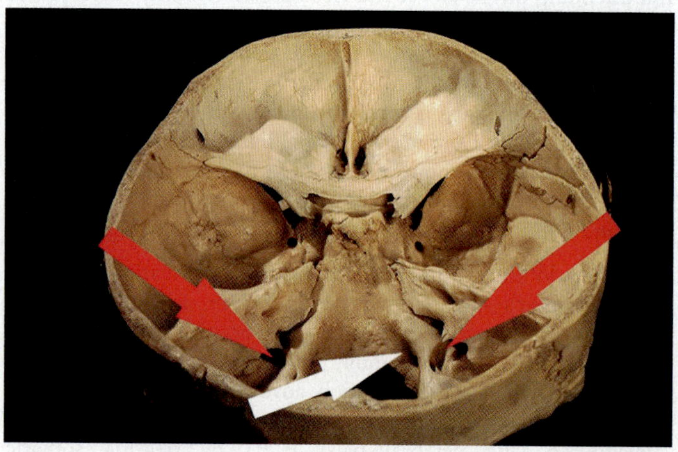

Figure 67.1. Posterior superior view of internal cranial base (calvaria removed) on cadaver skull demonstrating location of jugular foramina (*red arrows*) and hypoglossal canal (*white arrow*). (Courtesy of Western University of Health Sciences.)

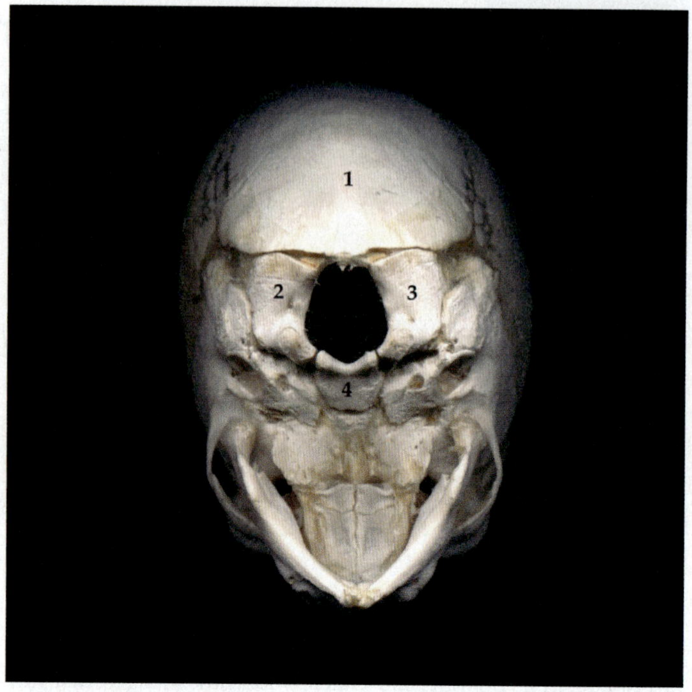

Figure 67.2. Inferior view of external base of cadaver fetal skull labeling the four parts of the occiput at birth. *1*, Squamous occiput; *2* and *3*, Lateral masses with condylar parts; *4*, Basiocciput. (Courtesy of Mary Ann Magoun, DO.)

OMT IN PRIMARY CARE

Preventive Care

The pediatrician focuses on primary, secondary, and tertiary prevention.[18]

1. Primary prevention refers to prevention of a disease process, such as dietary guidance and immunizations.
2. Secondary prevention is aimed at identification of subclinical disease before the development of overt symptoms (e.g., at the time of the interim history, physical, and structural examination). In this way, intervention can arrest clinical progression or eliminate the disease.
3. Tertiary preventive practices consist of identification and alleviation of disease or disorder through therapeutics and/or rehabilitation.

OMT is efficacious as primary and secondary intervention for asymptomatic somatic dysfunction, as well as tertiary intervention in the symptomatic pediatric patient. Regularly scheduled visits with the pediatrician for routine care provide sufficient time for primary and secondary prevention of pertinent lifestyle-related disease processes.

POINTS TO INCLUDE AT VISIT

- Infant and child development
- Accident prevention
- Nutrition
- Discipline
- Parenting

SPECIFIC OSTEOPATHIC CONSIDERATIONS

Addressing structural problems can facilitate healthy development and prevent the progression of developmental issues. Therefore, a "wait and see" approach is not an effective solution for a pediatric patient with developmental abnormalities. Infants should be evaluated shortly after delivery for the effects of birth trauma. Structural problems in the pediatric population should be treated early to prevent problems at a later date.[19]

Furthermore, children should receive osteopathic treatment at regular intervals. During times of rapid growth and development, and as they learn to climb, walk, and run, periodic treatments may be beneficial. They should be treated at the first sign of illness to facilitate healing. When behavioral or academic issues surface, it is important to perform a complete OSE.

Orthodontia

As children mature, some require orthodontic care. OMT can help free any structural restrictions in the face, palate, and jaw as well as contributing factors from the axial spine. During orthodontic care, OMT can help alleviate headaches and general discomfort. It may also be beneficial for the orthodontist and osteopathic physician to work in collaboration during this process to ensure optimization of the interrelatedness of the patient's structure and function.

Sports Injuries

Exercise is a key component of the healthy lifestyle practices recommended to pediatric patients and their families. Whether or not it is within the context of organized sports, physical activity inevitably poses some degree of risk for injury in the developing child. OMT can prevent injuries and alleviate somatic dysfunction arising from sports injuries and overuse phenomena.[20,21]

OSTEOPATHIC EVALUATION OF THE PEDIATRIC PATIENT

Osteopathic Pediatric Structural Examination

The osteopathic pediatrician incorporates a thorough OSE as part of the overall care of pediatric patients.

- The content and goals of such an examination differ little from that used when evaluating adult patients. See Chapter 27 for an example of the osteopathic history and physical examination.
- Tissue texture and tone have greater significance than range of motion (ROM) in infants and young children due to ligamentous laxity, which tends to exaggerate ROM.
- Children are best evaluated by examining ROM regionally, rather than by segmental testing of individual vertebral units.
- Manner of examination must be minimally threatening to the infant or child.
  - It is often helpful to engage young children (i.e., infant to 5 years of age), or children with developmental delay, in play to elicit cooperation.
  - Utilize the fine art of distraction (Fig. 67.3).
- Useful information about the infant's or child's structural and functional status can be gained by observing them sitting, lying, nursing, crawling, walking, and interacting with the environment.

Osteopathic Newborn Examination

A systematic approach to evaluation is used by most osteopathic pediatricians. In addition to a comprehensive physical examination, the osteopathic structural evaluation pays particular attention to the cranium and sacral regions. This examination pertains to premature infants as well as full-term infants.[22]

CRANIUM

1. Assess visually, checking for signs of gross structural asymmetry.
   - Head asymmetry may indicate a possible strain pattern, condylar compression, and/or suture/fontanelle abnormalities.
   - The infant's head is examined from above, noting any occipital flattening with asymmetrical anterior placement of the pinnae and frontal bones on the ipsilateral side. Found asymmetry is referred to as plagiocephaly, originating from Greek "crooked head" (Fig. 67.4).

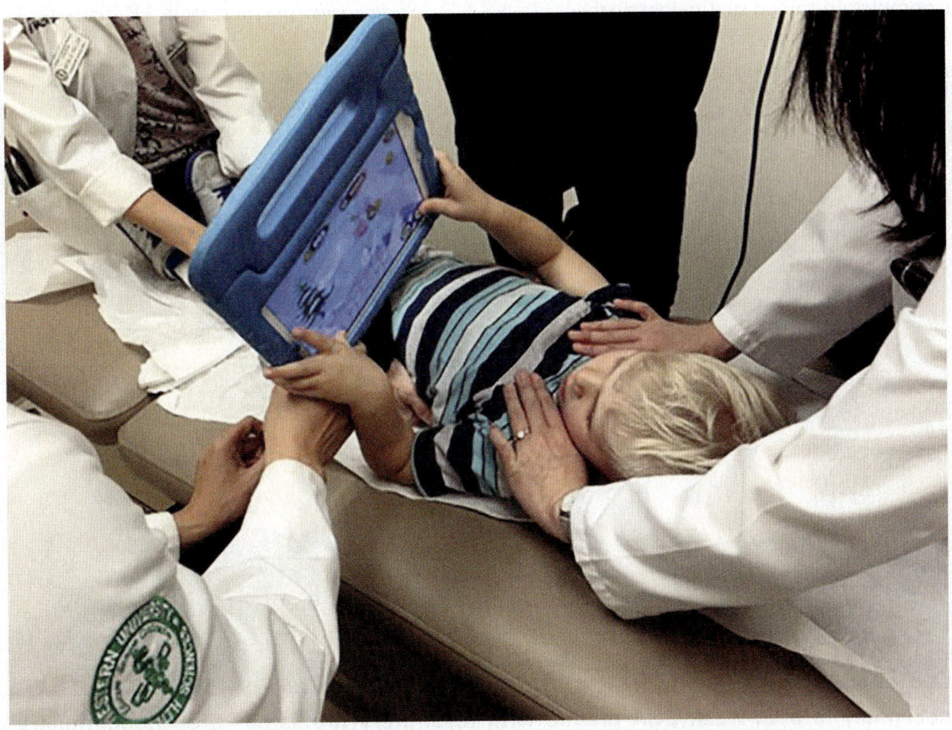

Figure 67.3. The fine art of distraction. (Courtesy of Mary Ann Magoun, DO.)

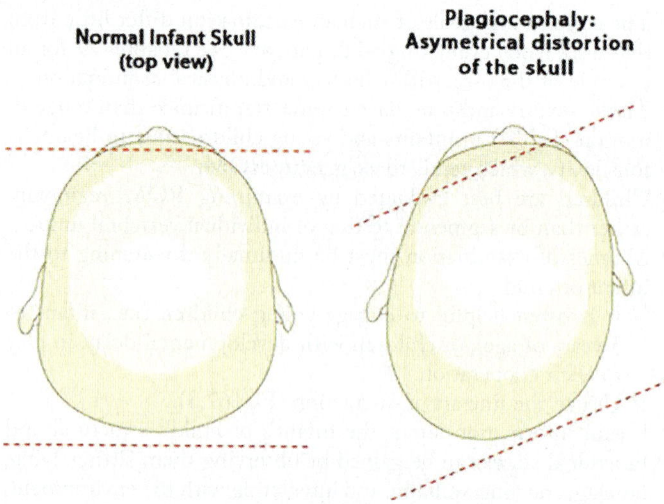

Figure 67.4. Normal/plagiocephaly. (Courtesy of T.S. Magoun.)

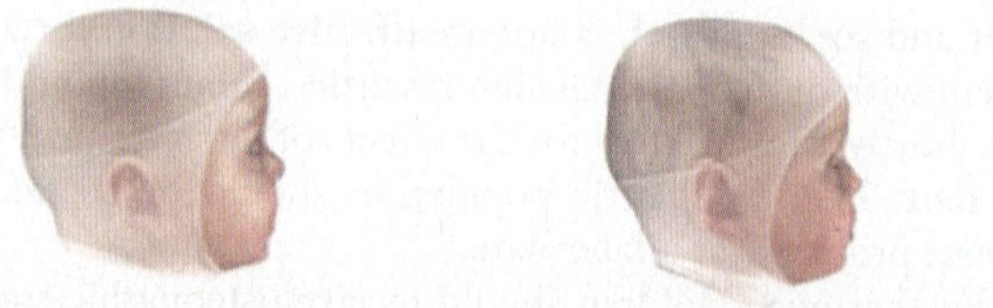

Figure 67.5. Plagiocephaly in an infant. Notice flattening of the occiput from prolonged supine position on a ventilator in the hospital as a newborn. (Computerized image courtesy of Mary Ann Magoun, DO.)

- □ Facial asymmetry should also be noted, including positioning of the eyes, nose, ears, and loss of nasal labial folds.
- □ Asymmetry of the neck may also be seen and is usually associated with head asymmetry (Torticollis is a condition in which the neck muscles cause the head to sidebend and/or rotate to either side usually involving the sternocleidomastoid muscle [SCM] which sidebends the head one way and rotates the opposite.).

2. Palpate for asymmetry.
   - □ All sutures and fontanelles are evaluated.
   - □ Assess for overriding, approximated, or spread sutures.
3. Assess cranial motion.
   - □ The infant's cranial motion may be difficult to feel.
     - Placing a gloved finger into the mouth to encourage sucking often aids in evaluating cranial motion with the other hand.
     - If the cranial motion can be palpated equally, this is generally a sign of symmetry in the cranial mechanism.
   - □ An occipital hold can also be used to further assess cranial motion.
     - Cradle the occiput in the hands, and gently place the tips of the index fingers on the mastoid process of the temporal bones. As there is no bony mastoid process at birth, the attachment of the SCM can be used as the palpatory landmark.
4. Intraoral exam
   - □ Should include the relationship of the maxilla with the mandible, assessment of the labia and lingula frenula, and lingual protrusion and motion.
   - □ Note if asymmetry is present. This may be indicative of a cranial strain pattern, which is described in Chapter 53 Osteopathic Cranial Manipulative Medicine.
     - A lateral strain of the sphenobasilar synchondrosis (SBS) is often found and may be related to transient tachypnea of the newborn and other respiratory irregularities.[17,23] This strain pattern with an accompanying parallelogram head is common in very premature infants on ventilators for a prolonged period as seen in (Figs. 67.5 to 67.7).

Key Concept: Differential Diagnosis

1. *Deformational (positional) plagiocephaly* (Fig. 67.8) versus *craniosynostosis*—premature closure of one or more sutures (Fig. 67.9).
2. *Scaphocephaly*—increased AP diameter (Figs. 67.10 and 67.11).

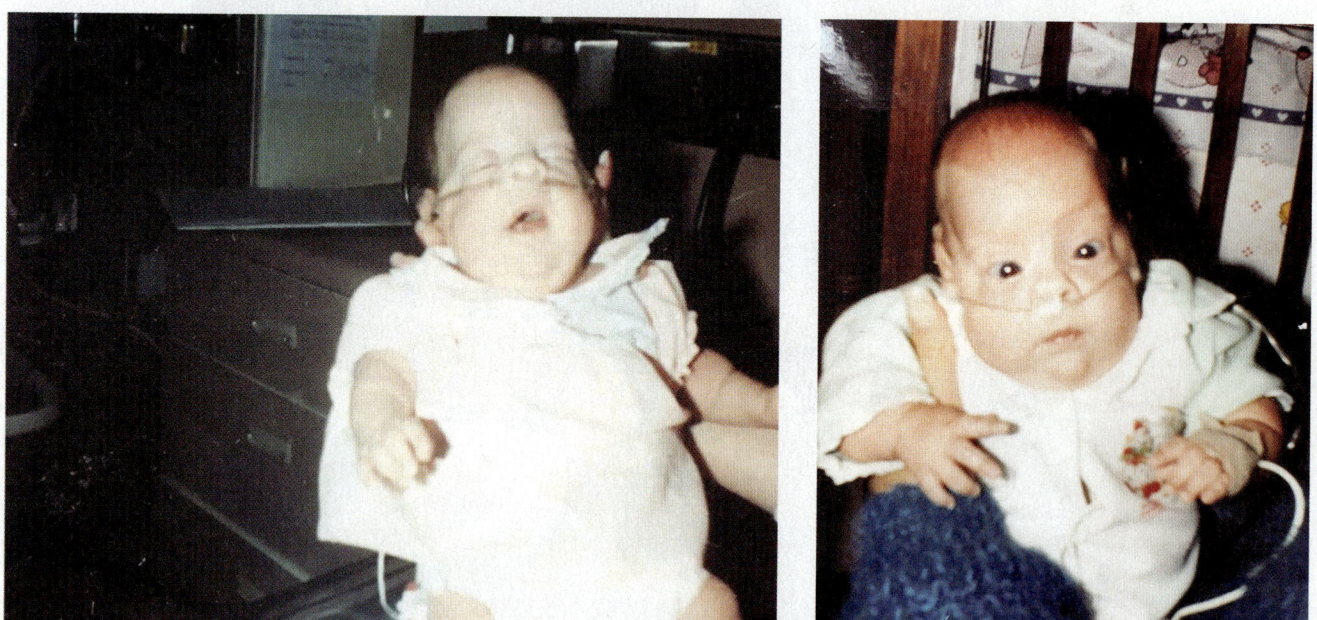

Figure 67.6. Plagiocephaly in a 24-week EGA premie with respiratory problems—bronchopulmonary dysplasia (BPD). (Courtesy of Mary Ann Magoun, DO.)

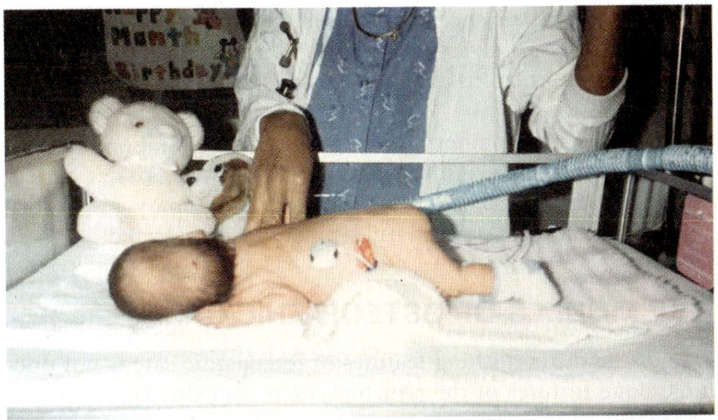

Figure 67.7. Plagiocephaly in a 24-week EGA premature infant with very–low-birth weight of 600 g and Apgar scores of 4/8/9. (Courtesy of Mary Ann Magoun, DO.)

3. *Brachycephaly*—increased bifrontal diameter, flattened occiput. This may also be attributed to genetic and/or metabolic causes (Fig. 67.12). Trisomy 21 is a prime example. The majority of cases of brachycephaly are mild with this condition, but regardless of severity, early intervention is always best.

THE SACRUM

The sacrum of the infant should be examined for lumbosacral compression and torsion patterns. Intra- and interosseous strains in the sacrum are oftentimes clinically related to strain patterns in the cranium through the reciprocal tension membrane (RTM).[24] The spinal dural attachments at C2–C3 and S2 may transmit reciprocal mechanical strain forces between the sacrum, cervical spine, and cranium, through the intracranial dural membranes (see Chapter 38 for further discussion).

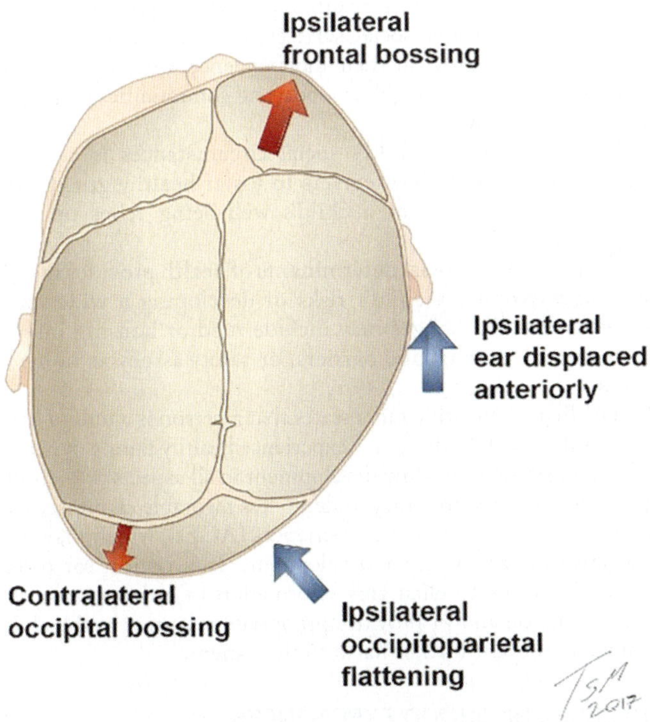

Figure 67.8. Diagram of deformational plagiocephaly. (Courtesy of T.S. Magoun.)

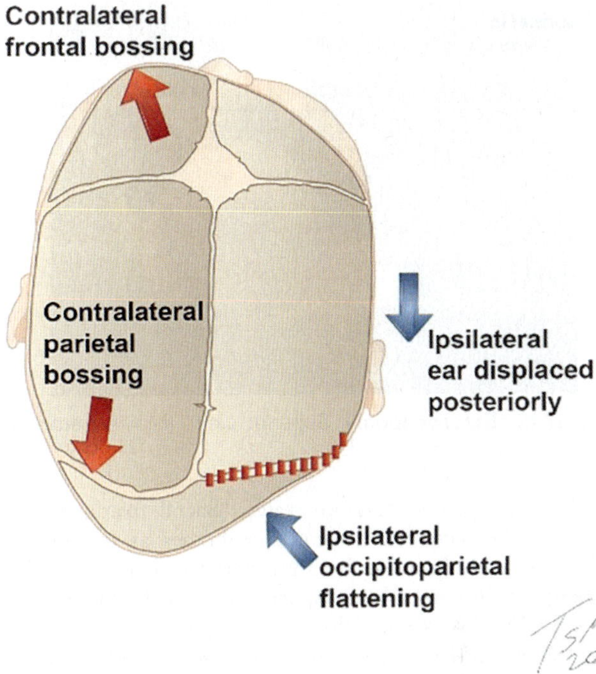

Figure 67.9. Unilambdoid synostosis. (Courtesy of T.S. Magoun.)

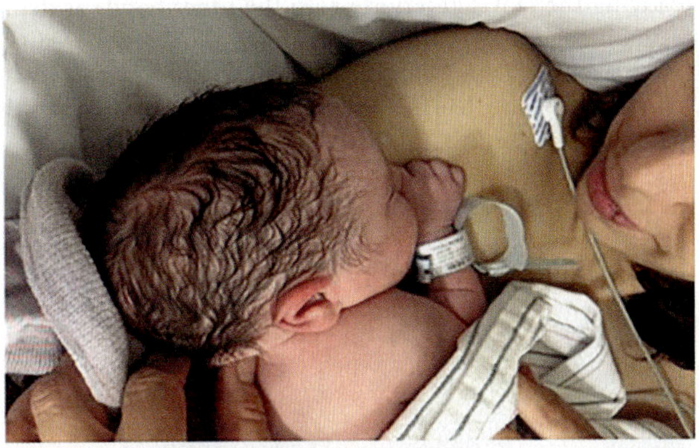

Figure 67.10. Scaphocephaly at birth. (Courtesy Mary Ann Magoun, DO.)

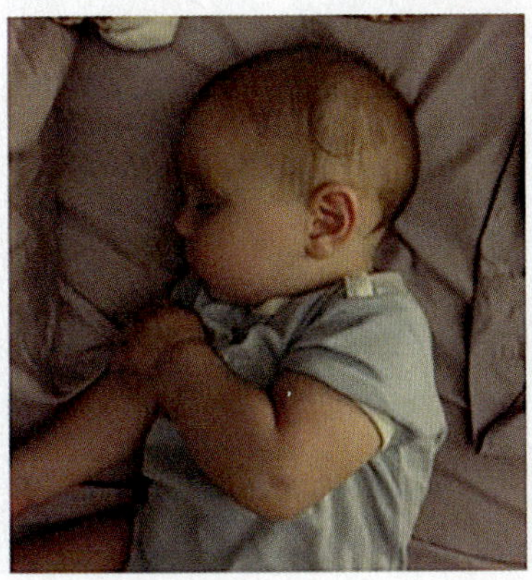

Figure 67.11. Scaphocephaly 4 months post-OMT. (Courtesy of Mary Ann Magoun, DO.)

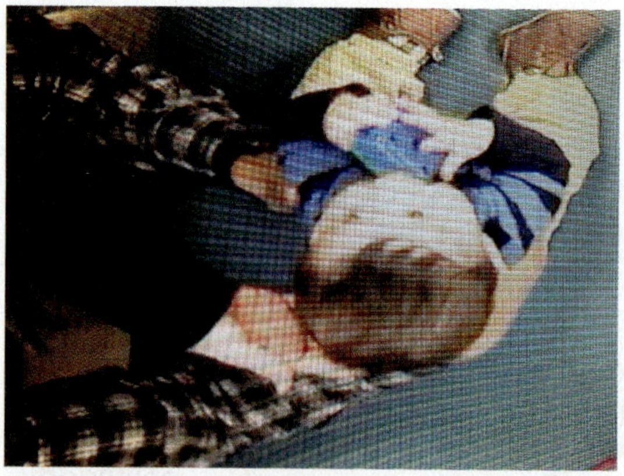

Figure 67.12. Brachycephaly. Superior view. (Movie frame courtesy of Mary Ann Magoun, DO.)

- As the child grows, Magoun states, "Sacral fixations can so influence the reciprocal tension membranes as to cause disturbances in the head such as interference with venous sinus drainage of the cerebral hemispheres or with the fluctuation of the CSF. With locking of the sacroiliac joint on one side there may well be locking of the sphenobasilar or occipitomastoid on that side also."[24]

Palpatory Examination

1. To assess the motion of the sacrum, sit next to the infant or child and place two fingers or a hand under the sacrum while steadying the pelvis anteriorly with the other hands as demonstrated in Figure 67.13.
2. Check for symmetry between the two sides of the sacrum.
   - □ One side may feel lower, indicating rotation around an anteroposterior axis.

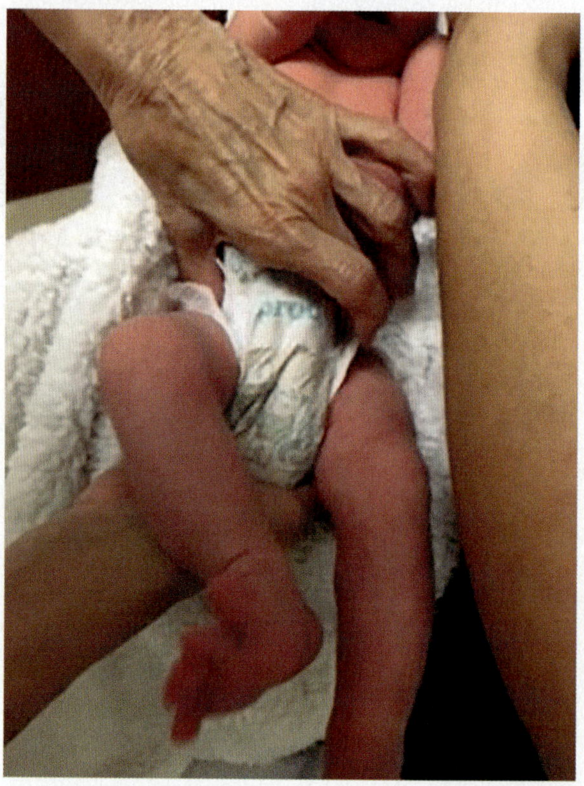

Figure 67.13. Palpating the sacrum in a supine newborn child. (Courtesy of Mary Ann Magoun, DO.)

   - □ If the base of the sacrum feels anterior on one side, it is rotated about a vertical axis.
3. Note any restrictions in regional motion evidenced by abnormal static position.
4. The primary respiratory mechanism (intrinsic motion not postural) should be symmetric around a transverse axis at S2. As the patient grows, the amplitude of the primary respiratory mechanism increases and can be more easily palpated.

FIVE MODELS OF OSTEOPATHIC CARE

One of the distinguishing features of osteopathic care is not only the unique features of the structural exam, but the lens by which osteopathic physicians elicit a history, diagnose, formulate an assessment, and generate an individualized plan for each patient. This lens includes the four osteopathic tenets and the five models of osteopathic care: biopsychosocial, biomechanical/structural, respiratory/circulatory, neurologic, and metabolic. Each will be discussed as they pertain to the pediatric patient.

1. Biopsychosocial Model

This model actually starts in utero, as throughout gestation, the fetus is affected by the mother's health. The birth process itself is also critical. Did this patient have a relatively easy birth or was trauma involved, possibly sensitizing the sympathetic nervous system from the first day of life? Once born, children are inherently situated within social connections, which set the stage for their growth and development. Because of a child's intrinsic vulnerability, these relationships can profoundly impact the course of their life, with effects, both positive and negative, across all domains of their health.

During early years of development, the parent–child dyad functions as a single unit, although the child and the parent remain individuals. Early parent–infant bonding is vital to healthy child development. When bonding is incomplete or dysfunctional or poses a threat to the child's health and survival, appropriate intervention by health and social service professionals is warranted. Even as children grow in their independence, their relationships with caregivers, peers, neighborhoods, and communities play a pivotal role in their lives.

Learning about a child's social circumstances is a crucial step in partnering with caregivers to foster healthy growth and development as much of a child's well-being relies on their caregivers.

Recognition of social determinants of health provides insight into understanding a child's risks of developing a wide range of conditions. Challenges may include food or housing insecurity, financial or language barriers, or safety issues at home or school.

The first osteopathic tenet states that a person is a unit of body, mind, and spirit. Children may experience healthy family dynamics which contribute to healthy development in all aspects of their life. However, some children may undergo less favorable circumstances, known as adverse childhood experiences (ACEs), which may have a negative impact on their development. It is critical for osteopathic physicians to elicit this information in order to stop this course of action and/or provide appropriate resources to the child/family and prevent further harm to the patient.

ADVERSE CHILDHOOD EXPERIENCES

It is well understood that the circumstances of a child's growth and development can affect the trajectory of their lifelong health.

Indeed, this motivates much of the preventative care that characterizes pediatrics. Growing evidence continues to illuminate the negative downstream effects of traumatic events early in life. Exposure to childhood emotional, physical, or sexual abuse, as well as household dysfunction, has been linked to numerous impairments across the lifespan. These ACEs have been linked to a greater prevalence of a wide variety of disease, including coronary artery disease, cancer, depression, and drug abuse.[25] In addition, mental health problems, teen pregnancies, physical inactivity, and smoking have been linked to these early childhood events.[26] The potential impacts of ACEs across all domains of a child's current and future health are extensive. Thus, early identification and intervention are paramount.

Identification of these traumatic events relies on thorough history gathering and examination, which may include regular screening for children facing toxic stress. The pediatrician's role in intervention may include connecting families with community resources—particularly with culturally competent mental health professionals—and advocating beyond the office setting for increased access to these services.[27] In addition to these interventions, efforts are being made to identify entities that support the resilience of children as they process the variety of stressors that may impact their lives. One important protective factor is a child's access to safe, stable, and nurturing relationships (SSNRs). These relationships between a child and their parents or other supportive adults have been shown to mitigate the negative health and social impacts of ACEs.[28] Thus, promoting the development of a child's SSNRs can foster their inherent protective and healing mechanisms in the face of ACEs. Recent investigation into additional environmental factors affecting the long-term impacts of ACEs has identified the important role of safe and supportive neighborhoods in weakening the association between ACEs and overall health status.[29] This growing collection of research supports the critical role of the pediatrician in leading community-based prevention and intervention efforts to combat the significant risks associated with childhood toxic stress.

ELICITING A HISTORY UTILIZING THE BIOPSYCHOSOCIAL MODEL OF OSTEOPATHIC CARE

Osteopathic physicians are trained to search for the underlying cause of an illness or, at a minimum, the anatomic, structural, and functional contributors, including the presence of somatic dysfunction, to a disease process. Thus, the importance of an accurate, detailed history, with special attention to trauma history, including birth trauma and associated physical, environmental, and emotional events that lead to such trauma, cannot be overstated. As stated above, childhood traumas and/or ACEs tend to have far-reaching and long-term effects as children are in their formative stages of growth and development.

Additionally, understanding both the personality and the nature of a child's mental health may illuminate important dynamics at play regarding behavioral choices that may impact their health and development, such as diet, activity level, hobbies, screen time, sleep, etc.

In the evaluation and treatment of children, the pediatrician is trained to elicit a thorough detailed history from the parent or guardian, especially in the case of infants and/or children who cannot speak for themselves. History gathering is tailored to each encounter with the understanding that eliciting information about a child's social environment may provide critical insight into the child's overall health.

From the perspective of the biopsychosocial model, the chief complaint may be viewed with reference to any preceding history of trauma, exposures, travel, or changes in the social environment. When applicable, social issues are addressed, with particular attention to:

- The stability and safety of the child's home and family life
- History of substance, physical, or emotional abuse among family members

Intake, especially at the initial visit, should include pregnancy history and birth history.

- Pregnancy history:
  - ☐ Trauma to mother
  - ☐ Psychological state of mother during and after the pregnancy
  - ☐ Planned or unplanned pregnancy
  - ☐ Twins or multiple births
  - ☐ Medications, alcohol, or illicit drugs used by mother
- Birth history:
  - ☐ Gestational age
  - ☐ Duration of labor, rupture of membranes
  - ☐ Mode of delivery (vaginal, Caesarean)
  - ☐ Use of anesthesia
  - ☐ Delivery complications
  - ☐ Apgar score if available
  - ☐ Presence of caput succedaneum or any cranial molding, as well as any abnormalities from delivery. Normal delivery mechanics are illustrated in Figure 67.14.
- Delivery
  - ☐ Was there need for a cesarean section? If so, why?
  - ☐ Was there a period of uterine inertia?
  - ☐ Was there meconium aspiration?
  - ☐ Was the first breath vigorous?
  - ☐ Did the baby require stimulation or resuscitation?
  - ☐ Did the baby have a lusty cry?
- Post delivery
  - ☐ Was the baby able to establish nursing in the first 24 hours?
- History of any of the following behaviors can indicate cranial base somatic dysfunction:
  - ☐ Difficulty in latching or learning to suck
  - ☐ Excessive crying or inconsolability
  - ☐ Arching of the back or repeatedly throwing the head back in early infancy
  - ☐ Excessive vomiting or spitting up

Intake should also include the following:

- History of previous illness, allergies, and surgeries
- Family history (seeking to identify presence of possible genetic disorders)
- History of accidents and trauma—force, direction, and location of trauma
- Treatment received
- Occurrence of changes in behavior or personality
- Social history, diet, feeding position, feeding type (breast or bottle), home environment, and safety of patient (e.g., appropriate car seats). Please see the section on HEEADDSSS for possible questions related to these.
- Developmental history with emphasis on the age of pertinent milestones and any regression (Table 67.1)
  - ☐ Examples of screening tools include Ages and Stages Questionnaire (ASQ), Modified Checklist for Autism in Toddlers (M-CHAT R/F), Denver Developmental Screening Test II (DDST-II); Early Screening Inventory-Revised (ESI-R), Infant Toddler Developmental Assessment (IDA), and PEDS: Developmental Milestones Measurements (PEDS:DM) for children 0 to 8 years.

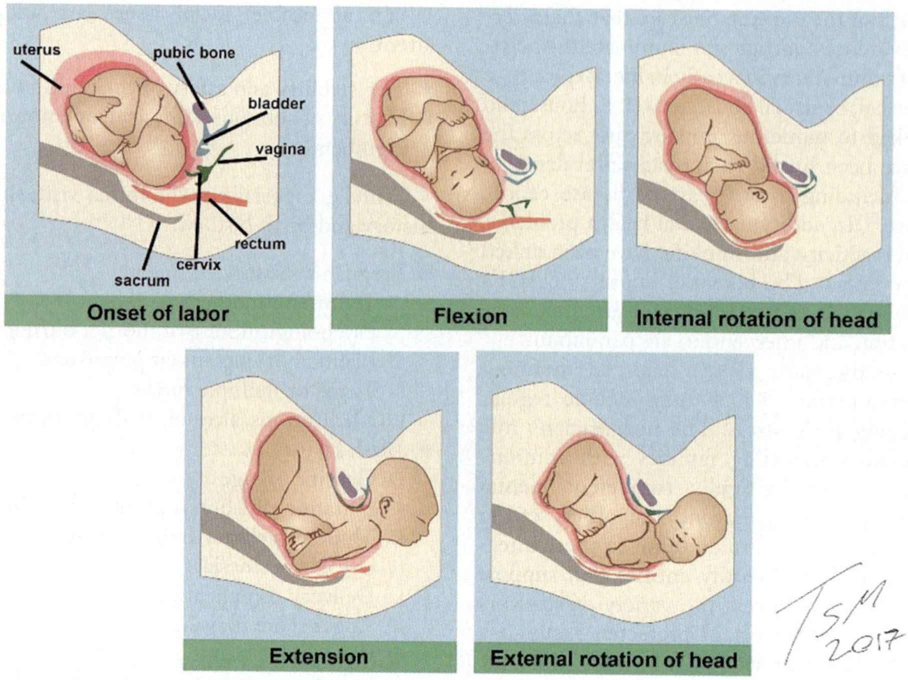

Figure 67.14. Normal delivery. (Courtesy of T. S. Magoun.)

TABLE 67.1

General Developmental Milestones Ages 1 Month to 5 years

Age	Gross Motor	Fine Motor	Language	Social
1 mo	Elevates head momentarily from prone position	Tight fist grasp	Responds to sounds	Prefers the human face
3 mo	Steadily holds head up in midline	Hands held open at rest, reaches for objects	Coos	Anticipates feeding
4–5 mo	Rolls over	Hand-to-hand transfer	Laughs	Visually explores environment
6 mo	Sits up	Raking grasp	Babbles	Stranger recognition
9 mo	Crawls, pulls self to standing position	Immature pincer grasp, holds bottle	Waves bye-bye, understands "no"	Plays games "pat a cake"
12 mo	Walks	Mature pincer grasp	Uses single words	Begins to imitate actions
18 mo	Runs	Scribbles, three-block tower	Combines two words	Copies parent tasks
24 mo	Walks up/down steps	Draws a line, removes shoes and pants, seven-block tower	Follows two-step commands, uses two-word sentences	Parallel play
3 y	Rides tricycle	Draws circle, undresses self completely	Vocabulary at least 250 words, uses three-word sentences	Gender identity, full name, and age
4 y	Jumps, hops on one foot, alternates feet going up and down stairs	Draws square or plus sign, dresses self completely	Knows songs, poems, and colors	Plays cooperatively with others
5 y	Skips, jumps over object	Draws triangle	Writes name, some letters, and numbers	Plays games and understands rules

- Dental history (extractions and any other procedures)
- Personality development and any psychiatric assessment (Tables 67.2 to 67.4)

HEADDSSS-PSYCHOLOGICAL SCREENING TOOL FOR ADOLESCENTS

The HEEADDSSS (sometimes referred to as HEADSSS or HEEADDSS) assessment is a psychosocial screening tool designed for the adolescent population. The American Academy of Pediatrics (AAP) and other organizations recommend using this assessment in order to address risk behaviors.[33] This acronym is designed to help the provider remember to ask questions pertaining to the following items; **H**ome environment, **E**ducation and **E**mployment, **E**ating and **E**xercise, **A**ctivities, **D**rugs/Alcohol/Smoking, **D**iet, (**D**epression), **S**uicidal Ideation/Depression, **S**exual activity, and **S**afety.

TABLE 67.2

Major Influences on Personality Development in Children

- Inherited physiologic patterns known as temperament
- Parental practices and personality
- Quality of schools attended
- Relationships with peers
- Ordinal position within the family
- Historical era in which late childhood and early adolescence are spent

Adapted from Kagen J. The role of parents in children's psychological development. *Pediatrics.* 1999;104(1 suppl):164–167.

This should be provided to an adolescent with and without a parent or caregiver in the room so that the patient has an opportunity to speak freely. It is important to explain confidentiality to both the patient and the family and what that entails before beginning the assessment, specifically that the physician will only disclose what is shared by the patient to their caregivers/parents with the patient's expressed permission unless there is a concern about the patient causing harm to themselves or others.[34]

Listed below are sample questions that may be used during the assessment that can be tailored to each patient depending on the responses received. The bolded items have been identified as those to potentially use if there is less time for the assessment or as possible opening questions in each category.[34]

- H: Home environment
- Possible questions to ask:
  - □ **Tell me about your parents and/or caregivers.**
  - □ Who lives at home with you? Where do you live? How long? Do you have your own room?
  - □ How many brothers and sisters do you have and what are their ages? Are your brothers and sisters healthy?
  - □ Are there any new people living in your home?
  - □ Are your parents healthy? What do your parents do for a living?
  - □ What are the rules like at home?
  - □ How do you get along with your parents, your siblings? What kinds of things do you and your family argue about the most? What happens in the house when there is a disagreement?
  - □ Is there anything you would like to change about your family?[34]
  - □ Do you feel safe at home?
  - □ Are there pets in the home?
  - □ Does anyone smoke inside the house around you?
  - □ Are there guns and weapons inside the home? If so, where are they stored?

TABLE 67.3

Common Psychiatric Disorders in School-Age Children

- Separation anxiety disorder
- Attention deficit hyperactivity disorder[32]
- Learning disorders
- Oppositional defiant disorder

TABLE 67.4

Standardized Questionnaires for Use in Identifying Psychiatric Disorders in Children and Adolescents[30]

- Pediatric symptom checklist-17
- Generalized Anxiety Disorder (GAD-7)
- Screen for Child Anxiety Related Disorders (SCARED)
- Beck depression inventory (age 13 and older)
- Child Depression Inventory (CDI)[31]
- Child Behavior Checklist (CBCL)
- Strengths and Difficulties Questionnaire (SDQ) (age 2–17)[33]
- Patient Health Questionnaire Modified for Adolescents (PHQ9M)
- Columbia Depression Scale

- E: Education
- Possible questions to ask:
  - □ **How are you doing in school?**
  - □ **Are you in school?** If yes, what school? What grade are you in?
  - □ Any recent changes in school?
  - □ How are you doing in school? What grades are you getting?
  - □ What subjects do you like/dislike?
  - □ **What do you like best and least about school?**
  - □ What were your most recent grades? Are these the same or different from the past? Have you ever failed or repeated any years? Have you ever had to remediate a class?
  - □ Are you in mainstream classes or a special education program?
  - □ Do you have an individualized learning plan (ILP)?
  - □ How many hours of homework do you do daily?
  - □ What do you want to do when you finish school? Any future plans/goals?
  - □ Tell me about your study habits.
  - □ Do you work now? How much? Have you worked in the past?
  - □ How do you get along with teachers, employers?
  - □ How do you get along with your peers?
  - □ Have you ever been teased, attacked, or bullied?[34]
  - □ Who or what is your support system?
- E: Eating and Exercise:
- Possible questions to ask:
  - □ **Do you have any struggles with eating or body image?**
  - □ What do you like and not like about your body?
  - □ How would you describe your eating habits? Does your weight or body image cause you any stress?
  - □ Have there been any recent changes in your weight or body?
  - □ Tell me about any exercise that you do or get in your daily routine.
  - □ What do you think would be a healthy diet? How does that compare with your current eating patterns?
  - □ What would it be like if you gained/lost 10 pounds?
  - □ Have you ever taken pills or supplements that you hoped would bring about changes in your body?[34]
  - □ Do you feel that you diet frequently or feel the need to control your eating?
  - □ Do you feel that you snack throughout the day? If so, what is your favorite snack food?
  - □ Does your weight or body shape cause any stress? If so, can you tell me about it?[35]

- A: Activities
- Possible questions to ask:
  - ☐ Do you participate in any school-related activities, clubs, sports, music, art, or dance?
  - ☐ Do you participate in any of those outside of school?
  - ☐ **Do you have any other activities, hobbies, or interests outside of school?**
  - ☐ Are most of your friends from school or somewhere else? Are they the same age as you?
  - ☐ Who do you go to with problems?
  - ☐ Do you hang out with mainly people of your same sex or a mixed crowd?
  - ☐ Do you have one best friend or a few friends? Do you have a lot of friends?[36]
  - ☐ Do you spend time with your family? What do you do with your family?
  - ☐ How do you spend your evenings? Weekends? Do you go to parties?
  - ☐ Do you have a religious affiliation, belong to a church, or practice some kind of spiritual belief?
  - ☐ How much TV do you watch a day? Do you have a favorite show(s)?
  - ☐ How much time do you spend online? What types of things do you use the internet for?
  - ☐ Do you play video games? If, yes, how often?
  - ☐ Do you read for fun? What do you read?
  - ☐ What is your favorite music?
  - ☐ Do you spend a lot of time on social media? Do you have an account that your parents/caregivers are unaware of? If so, what do you use it for?
- D: Diet
- Possible questions to ask:
  - ☐ Are you vegan, vegetarian, or pescatarian?
  - ☐ Do you have any food allergies or sensitivities?
  - ☐ How many fruits and vegetables do you consume in a day?
  - ☐ How much protein do you eat in a day? What kinds of protein do you eat?
  - ☐ Do you eat sweets? If so, how many?
  - ☐ How much water do you drink a day?
  - ☐ Do you drink caffeinated beverages? If so, how many a day?
  - ☐ Do you drink soda? Do you drink juice? If yes, how much per day? What kind?
  - ☐ How often do you eat fast food and/or junk food (chips, etc.)?
- D: Drugs
- Possible questions to ask:
  - ☐ **Do you do drugs?**
  - ☐ Do you take drugs; over-the-counter (OTC), prescription, designer, street/recreational?
  - ☐ Some young people experiment with drugs, alcohol, or cigarettes. Have you or your friends ever tried them? What have you tried?
  - ☐ When you go out with your friends or to party, do most of the people that you hang out with drink or smoke? Do you? How much and how often?
  - ☐ Does any of your family members drink, smoke, or use other drugs? If so, how do you feel about this—is it a problem for you?
  - ☐ Have you or your friends ever tried any other drugs? Specifically, what? Have you ever used a needle?
  - ☐ Do you regularly use other drugs? How much and how often?
  - ☐ Do you or your friends drive when you have been drinking?
  - ☐ Have you ever been in a car accident or in trouble with the law, and were any of these related to drinking or drugs?
  - ☐ How do you pay for your cigarettes, alcohol, or drugs?[34]
- S: Suicidal ideation/depression (note that these could be split into separate categories)
- Possible questions to ask:
  - ☐ **Are you currently feeling suicidal or that you want to harm yourself?**
  - ☐ Do you ever have thoughts about hurting yourself, or wishing that you didn't exist? How have you handled such feelings in the past?
  - ☐ Have you felt stressed or anxious more than usual lately?
  - ☐ Are you having trouble sleeping?
  - ☐ Tell me about a time when someone picked on you or made you feel uncomfortable.
  - ☐ Does it seem that you have lost interest in things that you used to really enjoy? Can you tell me more about that?
  - ☐ Do you find yourself spending less time with friends and people you care about?
  - ☐ Would you rather just be by yourself most of the time?
  - ☐ Have you ever tried to kill yourself, or planned to kill yourself but didn't follow through?
  - ☐ Have you ever had to hurt yourself (by cutting yourself, for example) to calm yourself down or make yourself feel better?
- S: Sexual activity
- Possible questions to ask:
  - ☐ **Have you ever had sex?**
  - ☐ What does sex mean to you?
  - ☐ If you have had sex, was it a good experience? Are you comfortable with sexual activity?
  - ☐ **Tell me about your boyfriend/girlfriend.**
  - ☐ Are you involved in a relationship? Have you been involved in a relationship? How was that experience for you?
  - ☐ How would you describe your feeling towards guys or girls? How do you see yourself in terms of sexual preference, that is, gay, straight, or bisexual?
  - ☐ How many sexual partners have you had?
  - ☐ Do you use contraception? Type and how often (10%, 50%, or 70% of the time)?
  - ☐ Have you ever been pregnant or had an abortion?
  - ☐ Have you ever had a discharge or sore that you are concerned about? Have you ever been checked for a sexually transmitted disease (STD)? What can you tell me about STDs and their prevention?
  - ☐ Have you ever had a pap smear?
  - ☐ Do you have any concerns about hepatitis or AIDS?
  - ☐ Have you had an experience in the past where someone did something to you that you did not feel comfortable with or that made you feel disrespected?
  - ☐ If someone abused you, who would you talk to about this? How do you think you would react to this?
  - ☐ For females: ask about menarche, last menstrual period (LMP), and menstrual cycles. Also inquire about breast self-examination (BSE) practices.
  - ☐ For males: ask about testicular self-examination (TSE) practices.[34]
- S: Safety
- Possible questions to ask:
  - ☐ **Do you feel that you make wise decisions with regard to keeping yourself safe?**
  - ☐ Have you ever made decisions that could have put you at risk of being harmed? How do you decide if a person/situation is safe for you?
  - ☐ Who do you go to with problems?
  - ☐ Have you ever been seriously injured? (How?) How about anyone that you know?

- □ Do you always wear a seatbelt in the car?
- □ Have you ever met in person (or plan to meet) with anyone that you first encountered online?
- □ When was the last time you sent a text message while driving?
- □ Have you ever ridden with a driver who was drunk or high?
- □ Is there a lot of violence at your home? School? Neighborhood? Among friends?
- □ Have you ever been picked on or bullied? Is that a current problem?
- □ Have you gotten into physical fights at school or in your neighborhood? Does that still happen?
- □ Have you ever felt you had to carry a knife, gun, or other weapon to protect yourself? Do you still feel that way?
- □ Have you ever been locked up/incarcerated?[34]

There are great references on how to conduct this assessment as well as wrap it up within the reference section of this chapter for those wishing further information.

When conducting the assessment and when performing the wrap-up, great care must be taken to remain sensitive to the patient's needs and psyche as pediatric patients may perceive or internalize sensitive issues differently. It is also best to avoid reiterating previous diagnoses, as they reinforce the feeling of the patient being negatively labeled by the health care system. Therefore, to build a patient's trust and elicit the most appropriate information, a "strength-based approach" may be used.[35]

This approach:

1. Identifies positives or strengths during the assessment that can be encouraged or used to motivate the patient to create a change.
2. Promotes resilience by identifying examples of past difficulties that the patient has successfully overcome.
3. Utilizes praise when warranted as many adolescents have not heard praise from an adult.
4. Uses reflective listening and pause, allowing the patient time to confirm or further elucidate their thoughts.
5. Creates a culture of trust, comfort, respect, and nonjudgment. Consider phrases such as "I want you to be comfortable coming to me for your health information."
6. Allows the physician to share concerns and allows the patient to reflect on their choices. For example, "I am concerned that your alcohol use could be a barrier to your goal of having a career as a teacher."[35]

Any issues about the patient's safety and concerns about suicidal ideations must be addressed immediately.

The biopsychosocial model is also incorporated into the physical and osteopathic structural exam which will provide insight into underlying issues or conditions including nutrition status, evidence of nonaccidental trauma (NAT), presence of viscerosomatic reflexes and Chapman reflexes, and somatic dysfunction that may be contributing to pain and cognitive and sensory (visual, auditory, etc.) impairments.

2. Biomechanical–Structural Model

MUSCULOSKELETAL DEVELOPMENT

- The bony development of children is guided by the various activities in which the child engages. Mechanical stresses mold bone to grow to accommodate these stresses. Bony development is largely complete by the time of vertebral ossification, around 25 years of age. Initially, the infant cranium constitutes 20.8% of the infant's body surface area (using Boyd's formula to calculate) and 25% of the length.
  - □ The head circumference doubles in size during the first year of life.
  - □ By 6 years of age, the skull reaches 90% of adult size and, at the same time, constitutes only one-eighth of the body size (vs. 25% at birth).
- The ribs begin primarily as cartilage and are oriented horizontally in infants.
  - □ Increased compliancy facilitates the birth process.
  - □ As the infant starts to use abdominal muscles and pulls to a stand, the angulation of the ribs shifts downward (e.g., rectus abdominis originating at the xiphoid process attaching at the pubic symphysis).
  - □ As the child grows and ambulates, the ribs slowly progress toward their final "bucket handle" and "pump handle" motions.
- The sacrum is composed of five modified vertebrae with cartilaginous articulations at birth. These articulations have maximum mobility in the infant and ossify throughout adolescence.
- At birth, the ilium is composed of three bones: the iliac bone, ischium, and pubis. These are partially cartilaginous at birth with fibrous articulations.
- Growth plates are present at joints and in the long bones.
- Long bones constitute a minimum of the body surface area in the infant but become more significant as the child grows.
- A normal ROM in the joints should be present in the neonate. Variable factors possibly affecting ROM include ligamentous laxity, abnormal neuromuscular conditions, and prematurity.

CRANIUM

The infant cranium is a complex structure at birth. The bones of the infant skull are composed of small areas of ossification formed within cartilage at the base and within membrane at the vault (Fig. 67.15). They are connected by dense fibroelastic tissues (referred to as sutures) that allow for maximal motion and compressibility during the birth process. Sutures will override (overlap) to accommodate passage through the birth canal with the least

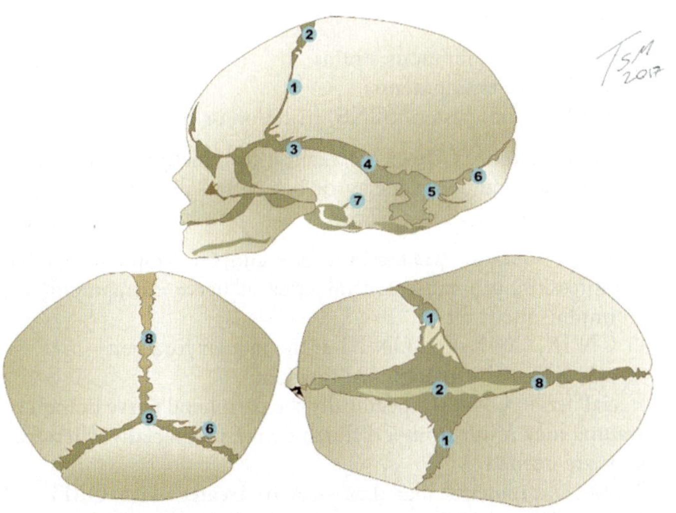

Figure 67.15. Illustration of the fetal skull. 1, coronal suture; 2, anterior fontanelle; 3, anterolateral (sphenoid) fontanelle; 4, parietomastoid suture; 5, posterolateral fontanelle (occipitomastoid); 6, lambdoid suture; 7, external auditory meatus; 8, superior sagittal suture; 9, lambda. (Courtesy of T.S. Magoun.)

resistance. They are designed to withstand the intense rotational and corkscrew-like forces of uterine contractions (up to 100 mm Hg psi).

Optimally, the first deep breath of life should reexpand the sutures, once again allowing free movement of the cranial bones. Being put to the breast to suckle (driving the motion of the sphenoid via the pterygoid plates) will also aid in restoring normal mechanics to the cranium. However, sometimes cranial somatic dysfunction persists or is unable to self-correct. This is evidenced by palpation of tension within the dural membranes and/or restricted motion of the cranial bones.

- The cranial bone most likely to be affected is the occipital bone due to the compressive forces of labor.
- The occipital bone is in four parts at birth (see Fig. 67.2). Fusion of the individual parts occurs sequentially.
- This gives the osteopathic pediatrician a window of opportunity in which to effect a change to assist in normal development.

According to the osteopathic cranial concept, these membranous attachments determine how the cranial bones move in relation to each other and the sacrum (see Chapter 53). As the infant matures, the cranial bones ossify and the flexible articulations of the occiput and parietal bones interdigitate, limiting motion. The cranial bones are enveloped in fascial membrane; the dura and pia mater and arachnoid.

- The dura mater has reflections that form:
  - ☐ Falx cerebri
  - ☐ Falx cerebelli
  - ☐ Tentorium cerebelli
- The duplication over the petrous temporal bone forms the petrosphenoid ligament.
- CN III courses above the petrosphenoid ligament, CN IV pierces it, and CN VI courses under it. Dysfunction of the temporal bone may cause impingement to these cranial nerves yielding ocular manifestations such as:
  - ☐ Dysconjugate gaze
  - ☐ Uneven tracking
  - ☐ Esophoria and exophoria
  - ☐ A fixed esotropia or strabismus

As previously mentioned, a baby or child with plagiocephaly (a misshapen skull) from a traumatic birth may suffer from a variety of disorders related to[6,11,15]:

- Intracranial membranous strains
- Cranial nerve entrapments
- Central nervous system (CNS) irritation or compression

Manifestations of these mechanical dysfunctions can be general, as in developmental delay or behavioral disorders, or more specific, as shown in Table 67.5.

- A single somatic dysfunction, for example, occipital condylar compression, can cause several signs of nerve entrapment due to impingement of:
  - ☐ CN IX, CN X, and CN XI at the jugular foramen
  - ☐ CN XII at the hypoglossal foramen
- Facial nerve (CN VII, specifically the peripheral nerve branches) trauma may result from a difficult delivery, especially when forceps are needed.
- Nerve entrapments like these can be treated with OMT.[37–40] Osteopathic cranial manipulative medicine has been noted empirically to facilitate restoration of normal eye position and movement.[23,37]
- Residual dysfunctions may have a relation to neurobehavioral development.

TABLE 67.5

Manifestations of Cranial Nerve Entrapment Dysfunctions

Area of Damage	Symptoms
Pyramidal Tracts	Opisthotonic posturing
CN VI	Lateral rectus weakness and nystagmus
CN VII	Peripheral: flaccid paralysis to face with loss of nasolabial fold Central: eye cannot completely close, smooth forehead
CN X	Excessive vomiting
CN XI	Colic, torticollis
CN XII	Difficulty with tongue movement in suckling

Sphenobasilar and intracranial strain patterns may produce:

- Plagiocephaly
- Tension on the tentorium cerebelli (CN III, CN IV, and CN VI as discussed above)

Cranial strain patterns in children do not necessarily manifest as neurologic deficits. Patients may be asymptomatic or have generalized complaints, ranging from allergies to severe head pain. Treatment of cranial traumatic birth injuries may include:

- O-A and condylar decompression with gentle posterolateral traction (Fig. 67.16).
- Gentle sacral traction for lumbosacral compression
- Release of the cranial membranous strain patterns with sutural restrictions

OCMM for infants and young children typically involves gentle but firm direct OMT that consists of distracting and guiding the cranial bones into their respective restrictive motion barriers and maintaining them in that position until a release is felt.

- This requires very little force.
- Release restrictions as soon as the infant is physiologically stable, such as those who may be in the pediatric intensive care unit (PICU).

COSTAL CAGE

Costal cage somatic dysfunction may be the result of:

- A direct traumatic force to the area
- Muscle imbalance

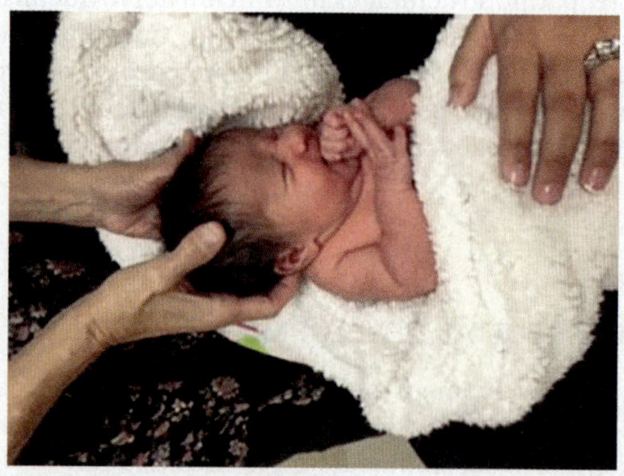

Figure 67.16. O-A and condylar decompression with gentle posterolateral traction. (Courtesy Mary Ann Magoun, DO.)

TABLE 67.6

Thoracic and Rib Cage Somatic Dysfunction Treatment with OMT

Medical Conditions Predisposing to Rib Somatic Dysfunction	Proposed Protocol for Treating Rib Somatic Dysfunction
Cystic fibrosis	Relieve muscle spasm with inhibition, counterstrain, or muscle energy
Asthma	Treat rib/segment with indirect OMT Still technique
Alpha-1 antitrypsin deficiency	HVLA if appropriate (older child/ teenager)
Scoliosis	Relieve diaphragm motion restrictions

- A spasm secondary to a nonrhythmic breathing mechanism (e.g., cough)

In normal breathing, air movement is accomplished by unrestricted movement and mobility of the diaphragm. The coordinated contraction of the diaphragm is mediated via the phrenic nerve and nerve fibers that exit from the midcervical area (C3–C5). Thus, cervical or thoracic somatic dysfunction can predispose a patient to rib dysfunction. There are also numerous medical conditions predisposing children to somatic dysfunction of the rib and thoracic regions. A selection of these conditions, along with a proposed protocol for treating them with OMT, is provided in Table 67.6. Rib fractures in children are rare. See Box 67.1 for further information.

VERTEBRAL SPINE

Torticollis

Torticollis may be congenital, present shortly after birth or it may present at any time during childhood. The differential diagnosis includes a cervical dislocation of the vertebra or spinal cord tumor, which would have associated structural and neurologic findings including sensory deficits. If there is a high clinical index of suspicion of the above, the patient would require an emergent MRI and neurosurgery consultation. However, the majority of torticollis is due to muscular strain and is amenable to OMT. Torticollis may arise as a functional compensation for strabismus or be associated with plagiocephaly.[41]

Congenital torticollis may result from a strain induced by in-utero lie or delivery. It often involves the scalene muscles with associated dysfunction of rib mechanics and palpable hypertonicity of the scalenes. The craniocervical junction, especially the occiput and condyles, is typically involved and there may be irritation of the spinal accessory nerve. Trauma during the birthing process such as large size, difficult delivery, or shoulder dystocia can cause a hematoma of the SCM resulting in palpable swelling of the muscle and then subsequently, its fibrosis and shortening.[41]

Older pediatric patients with torticollis usually have a shortening or contracture of the SCM on one side, with the head tilted toward and rotated away from that side (Fig. 67.17). These cases generally respond well to OMT.

In chronic torticollis, there may be a pattern of long-standing O-A dysfunction with lateral and, possibly, vertical strain patterns of the cranium.

- These may be the result of abnormal intrauterine positioning or an abnormal birth event/position.
- There may be a history of shoulder dystocia at birth.
- Due to the very shallow condyles at birth, there may be side slippage of the occiput on the atlas.
- Differential diagnosis includes a cervical malformation or Klippel–Feil anomaly, C3–C4 or C5–C6 fusion with Sprengel deformity—a hypoplastic scapula.

Treatment of torticollis should address the primary strain within the overall complex. Balanced ligamentous tension to address the articular dysfunction of the cervical area, balanced membranous techniques for cranial somatic dysfunction, myofascial release, and facilitated positional release may all be beneficial.[41]

BOX 67.1 Rib Fractures in Children

- It is rare for children to sustain rib fractures since their ribs are flexible and well calcified with good cartilaginous articulations.
- Infants with posterior rib fractures should always be suspected of having suffered abuse (NAT).
- Fractured ribs have nodular calcified areas at the costotransverse articulation adjacent to the spinal column. Radiographically, the fractures are often at various stages of calcification.
- Posterior rib fractures are the result of the infant being held and shaken. The cartilage absorbs the force anteriorly, but posteriorly, the ribs have bony articulations with the transverse processes and are relatively inflexible.
- Such infants present with severe to moderate pain with breathing. They have tenderness and fullness over the affected rib that becomes worse with either inhalation or exhalation.

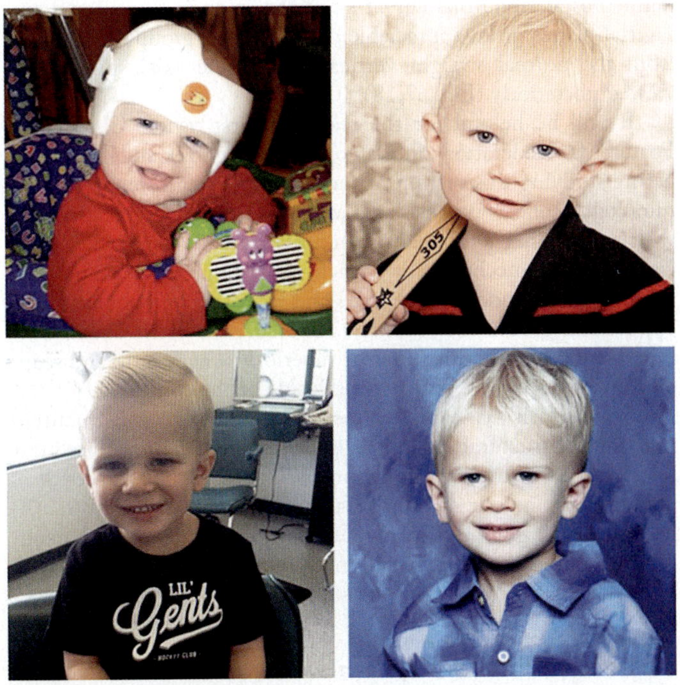

Figure 67.17. Torticollis resolving over time, initially as an infant with helmet, followed by OMT. (Photos courtesy of Mary Ann Magoun, DO.)

Other modalities to address somatic dysfunction related to torticollis include:

- Inhibition of tender points, counterstrain if the patient is able to cooperate or relax, and indirect techniques. Techniques can be modified so that the area is positioned until the physician appreciates a fascial softening.
- Muscle energy techniques
  - Match the existing tension for 3 to 5 seconds, creating an isometric contraction, followed by 3 seconds of rest for repolarization/recovery. Then gently take to a new barrier.
  - For infants, as the mother is cuddling, the point of contact may be her hand or even cheek to encourage rotation into the restrictive barrier.
- The use of anti-inflammatory medication and muscle relaxants may be necessary, with the child returning in 24 to 48 hours for further OMT and evaluation.
- Teach parents techniques to stretch the SCM. During periods of accelerated growth, patterns of torticollis may recur. Therefore, inform the parents of this possibility and encourage a return visit to the clinic or reinitiation of stretches if they see signs of recurrence.
- Parental and/or patient education on feeding position, sleep position, and rest positions may be beneficial.
- During future well-child visits, asymmetry should be rechecked and balanced.

Figure 67.17 displays a 3-year-old boy who received helmet therapy for plagiocephaly twice, initially at 5 months of age and then again at 14 months of age. The mother sought out treatment that would address the entire body that was recreating the torticollis. The patient responded well to OMT and continues to receive treatment.

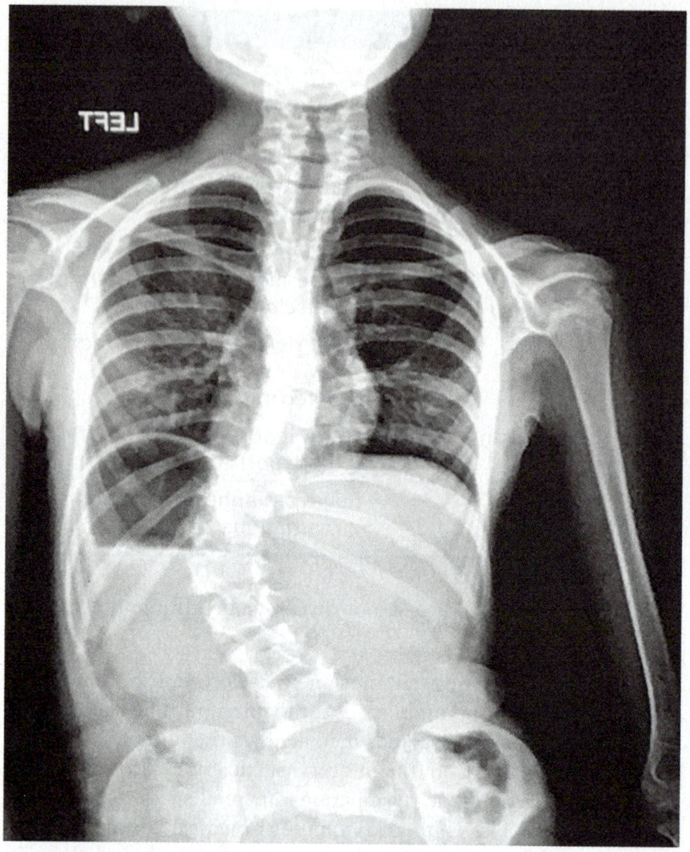

Figure 67.18. Example of scoliosis shown on a radiograph of a child, posterior view. (Courtesy of Mary Ann Magoun, DO.)

Scoliosis

Scoliosis is one of the most common orthopedic deforming problems in children.[42] It is a major concern for pediatrics, as it may adversely affect optimal growth. Scoliosis seen in childhood is defined as an abnormal curvature of the spine in the coronal and sagittal planes or an appreciable deviation of a group of vertebrae from the normal straight vertical line of the axial spine when viewed posteriorly (Fig. 67.18).

It will be helpful for the reader to first review Chapter 92 Postural Considerations in Osteopathic Diagnosis and Treatment before studying this section of the chapter. Using osteopathic terminology, scoliosis is considered as consisting of a lateral curvature with a rotational component in accordance with the Fryette principles (type I mechanics, in which neutral spinal mechanics are prominent and sidebending [SB] and rotation components are to opposite directions, i.e., NSxRy). The curve is often bound by a type II segment inferiorly and/or superiorly. There is rib and scapular involvement; ribs spread on the side of the convexity.

Scoliosis is categorized as structural or nonstructural/functional. Structural scoliosis is either congenital or acquired due to trauma. Nonstructural/functional scoliosis may be the result of poor posture, muscle spasms, or a short leg. It is common in athletes, dancers, gymnasts, and skaters whose routines or choreography is one sided, creating an imbalance, and also in those with heavy backpacks slung over one shoulder.

Structural Scoliosis

Structural scoliosis usually presents in childhood, notably in infancy (congenital). Early detection and intervention are extremely important. Congenital anomalies of the spine, which are secondary to neuromuscular disorders, are diagnosed with postural radiographs. Without early intervention and detection, structural scoliosis may continue to worsen after growth plates have fused.

Key features of structural scoliosis:

- Diagnosed with postural radiographs
- Fixed, unable to correct with lateral bending in the forward flexed position
- May contain compensatory curves superior or inferior to fixed area

Congenital Scoliosis

Congenital scoliosis is caused by anomalies of the spine involving fusion or abnormal development of the spine (incomplete formation or hemivertebrae, failure of separation of vertebra). These vertebral anomalies and malalignments may include:

- Cystic masses
- Hemangiomata (Klippel–Trenaunay–Weber)
- Sinus tracts
- Hyperpigmentation–neurofibromatosis
- Congenital hip dysplasia
- Lumbosacral dysgenesis

Congenital scoliosis found on initial newborn exam may be indicative of a syndrome or neuromuscular disorder and often is associated with organ involvement. Therefore, further genetic/metabolic and neurologic workup is warranted. Congenital associations include:

- Occipitocervical problems
- Arnold–Chiari malformations
- Syringomyelia
- Klippel–Feil syndrome/Sprengel deformity (hypoplastic scapula)

Functional (Nonfixed, Acquired) Scoliosis

The etiology of most abnormal spinal curves is idiopathic and multifactorial. There are many reasons functional scoliosis can occur. Etiologies stemming from a cellular level could include the inability of the spine to resist ordinary functional stresses (inherent weakness), skeletal or musculoskeletal metabolic deficiencies, and secondary to central and peripheral neurologic mechanisms. Other underlying etiologies include:

- Pelvic obliquity/sacral unleveling from a short leg (which in itself can be either functional or structural, such as after a healed leg fracture; see Box 67.2 and Chapter 92 for further discussion)
- Somatic dysfunction involving cranial membranous strain patterns—a "cranial scoliosis" with cranial base unleveling
- Osteomalacia
- Spine inflammation or irradiation
- Compensatory and noncompensatory fascial patterns
- Changes in muscle tone/hypertrophy/atrophy
- Poor posture or repetitive movements
  - □ Backpacks (one shoulder)
  - □ Athletes, gymnasts, dancers: asymmetrical overuse patterns
  - □ Study positioning habits
- Unilateral paraspinal muscle spasm
- Psoas syndrome
- Herniated lumbar disks
- Sciatic nerve irritation
- Unilateral flatfoot/hyperpronation
- Tibial torsion/knee deformity

BOX 67.2 Leg Length Discrepancy in Children

Leg Length Discrepancy, whether anatomical or acquired, may drive the evolution of the scoliosis (see Chapter 92 for further discussion). There are multiple causes related to leg length discrepancy, including the following:

- Somatic dysfunction
  - □ Innominates, sacrum
- Fractures
  - □ Involving growth plate
  - □ Femoral or tibial fractures with overgrowth
- Growth plate injury
  - □ Aseptic necrosis
  - □ Osteomyelitis
  - □ Septic arthritis
- Neurotropic
  - □ Hemiparetic cerebral palsy
  - □ Peripheral nerve
  - □ Polio
- Inflammatory/vascular
  - □ Juvenile rheumatoid arthritis
  - □ Large hemangioma
- Syndromes
  - □ Neurofibromatosis
  - □ McCune–Albright
  - □ Beckwith–Wiedemann
  - □ Klippel–Trenaunay–Weber
  - □ Hereditary—autosomal dominant with incomplete penetrance is multifactorial

Idiopathic Scoliosis

Idiopathic scoliosis is by far the most common type of scoliosis, with three subgroups. It accounts for 80% to 85% of all cases—including both structural and functional types. The incidence is 4% of all curves. Only 0.3% need treatment as it is usually self-correcting, nonprogressive, or subclinical. There are no primary structural anomalies. The three subgroups are:

1. Infantile:
   - □ Before age 3, not congenital, 80% resolve spontaneously
   - □ Curves greater than 30 degrees have propensity to progress.
   - □ Single curve; if greater than 30 degrees or progressing, consider a brace (orthopedics consult).
   - □ No fusion recommended for idiopathic infantile scoliosis.
   - □ Assess for and treat plagiocephaly and occipitocervical obliquity with OMT.
2. Juvenile—onset 3 to 9 years of age; occurrence is 12% to 21%.
3. Adolescent—10 years old and above, painless and asymptomatic, undetected by parents (rarely see their kids this age without clothes on). School screening: seventh grade for girls and eighth grade for boys.

Degrees of Severity

Cobb angle measurements:

- Mild: 5 to 20 degrees
- Moderate: 20 to 45 degrees
- Severe: 50 degrees or greater. Will start to have systemic effects on viscera, respiratory function; greater than 75 degrees will affect cardiac function.
- Clinical guidelines for management using full scoliosis films with grid—Cobb angles
  - □ If curve is less than 10 degrees, repeat in 6 months.
  - □ If curve is 10 to 20 degrees, repeat in 4 months.
  - □ If curve is greater than 20 degrees, refer directly to orthopedics.
  - □ If curve increase is greater than 5 degrees, refer directly to orthopedics.
  - □ If curve is less than 20 degrees, OMT, physical therapy, taping and bracing (Milwaukee or Boston) are all appropriate modalities of treatment. They may be continued if curvature increases, the referral process to Orthopedics is lengthy and/or surgery is decided against.
  - □ If curve is greater than 40 degrees, surgery will be needed which may consist of placement of Harrington rods, Luque fixation, and Cotrel–Dubouset technique Surgical correction of scoliosis continues to evolve[43] and is categorized as dynamic and static.[44]

Major Types

- Double major curve (S). This is the most common and tends to have a dextro thoracic curve and levo lumbar curve. The vertebrae at the crossover points are subject to degeneration.
- Single thoracic (C) curve (dextro) is the second most common.
  - □ Single lumbar curve is the third most common. It is usually painless and its cause is multifactorial: genetic, subtle CNS dysfunction (proprioception/vibratory)

Identifying Scoliosis during Physical Osteopathic Structural Examination

- Five signs during screening and regional exam are strong indicators of scoliosis.[45]
  - □ Asymmetrical shoulder levels
  - □ Winged scapula

- ☐ Unequal waistline
- ☐ Unequal space between arms and torso
- ☐ Palpable lateral curvature of the spine

As Assessed by the Spinous and Transverse Processes

- Adams test—forward bending, asymmetric rib angle prominence
- Cranial assessment for plagiocephaly
- Growth potential (growth charts), Tanner staging/Risser grading, curve magnitude at time of diagnosis, and location of curve (thoracic tends to progress faster) are important components to chart in the medical record.
- See Chapter 92 for postural assessment for scoliosis.

Findings of Respiratory/Circulatory Model

Scoliosis may lead to unbalanced/asymmetric thoracic and pelvic diaphragms, impaired homeostasis of the lower extremities resulting in venous/lymphatic congestion or swelling. Achilles tendonitis or rupture may occur.

Red Flags or Findings Suggestive of Pathology

- Pain
- Extreme stiffness–hypertonicity
- Paresthesias—neurologic signs and symptoms
- Thoracic curves extending into the C-spine
- Left-sided thoracic curves
- Right-sided lumbar curves

Other Possible Findings

- Plagiocephaly
- Postural changes
- Compensatory increased lumbar lordosis
- Increased posterior load on vertebrae
- Unilateral quadratus lumborum spasm
- L-spine sidebent (SB) ipsilateral
- T/L junction SB ipsilateral and rotation contralateral
- L/S junction SB contralateral and rotation ipsilateral
- 20% to 30% will have anomalies of the urinary tract, especially renal.[46]

For example, unilateral agenesis of the kidneys

- Increased incidence of congenital heart disease associated with caudal regression
- Agenesis of the lumbosacral spine
- Congenital anomalies: unilateral or bilateral, for example, sacralization of L5 or lumbarization of S1
- Foot deformities (equinovarus)
- Lower extremity joint contractures

Diagnosis

- Determine underlying cause (as mentioned previously, early intervention is key, which can only begin upon accurate diagnosis of the underlying problem).

Progression

- Females have a higher risk of progression (10 times more) than males. They tend to have greater curvatures than males which are more likely to progress than smaller curvatures.[45]
- Studies indicate that low levels of vitamin D and/or melatonin may be associated with progression of scoliosis.[45] Vitamin D levels were lower in adolescent idiopathic scoliosis (AIS) patients and levels were negatively correlated with Cobb angle.
- Osteopenia in both their axial and peripheral skeleton has been shown to occur in around 30% of AIS patients.
- Several studies show a relationship between elevated platelet calmodulin levels and scoliosis progression. Lowe et al. suggest the platelet changes are related to paraspinous muscle activity and that calmodulin acts as a systemic mediator of contractile tissues.[47–49]
- A curve >40 degrees at Sanders Stage 7 (SS7) is at high risk for progressing to a curve measuring >50 degrees or requiring surgery. However, patients with curves below this threshold still have potential to make clinically significant progression after skeletal maturity. Follow-up of patients beyond SS7 is essential for curves measuring >40 degrees.[50]
- Asynchronous neuro-osseous growth of the spinal column and cord has also been suggested to play a role in AIS.[51] The thoracic spine is longer anteriorly than posteriorly in AIS patients, a phenomenon known as relative anterior spinal overgrowth (RASO) or an uncoupled neuro-osseous growth.[51–56] This is likely due to the secondary increased anterior intervertebral disk height.[55] The longitudinal growth of the vertebral bodies in AIS patients is disproportionate and faster than in age-matched controls and mainly occurs by endochondral ossification. On the other hand, the circumferential growth by membranous ossification is slower in both the vertebral bodies and pedicles.[57]
- The Hueter–Volkmann theory suggests that increased pressure on a vertebral epiphyseal growth plate impedes its rate of growth, whereas decreased pressure across the plate accelerates its growth.[58] The theory suggests that on the concave side of the curve, the epiphyseal plates have abnormally high pressures which lead to decreased rates of growth, whereas on the convex side, the pressure is less, thus leading to accelerated growth.[59]
- Stokes et al. later proposed their "vicious cycle" hypothesis whereby asymmetric loading causes vertebral wedging during growth in progressive scoliosis curves. Their hypothesis implies that regardless of the initial cause of scoliosis, mechanical factors increase significantly during periods of rapid adolescent growth, when risk of curve progression is greatest.[54,60]
- S curves tend to worsen with time more than C curves. Thoracic curves tend to worsen more than cervical or lumbar; but, they tend to be fixed/structural.

Poor Prognosis

- Worst prognosis associated with unilateral unsegmented bar, which needs spinal fusion as further growth will increase the deformity[61]
- Diminished potential for longitudinal growth of the spine
- Multiple hemivertebrae on same side of spine: usually require spinal fusion
- Isolated hemivertebrae: close monitoring
- Overall 50% of congenital etiologies will require surgery

Treatment

Scoliosis may be managed by surgical or conservative management. Lesser curvatures that do not compromise the cardiopulmonary system are managed with conservative treatment.

Conservative treatment is comprised of OMT, exercise and stretching programs, proper footwear, and bracing. The initial focus should be addressing postural decompensation.

Exercise:

- Appropriate exercise such as pilates can improve flexibility and strength of the trunk and promote expansion of the costal cage. Sports such as soccer and basketball can improve neuromotor control and thus provide support and stabilization to the spine.[62,63] Unilateral sports or activities should be approached with caution. Other forms of exercise have evolved in order to address scoliosis such as the Schroth and Lyon method.[64]

Osteopathic Manipulative Treatment

The goal is to increase intrinsic sustaining forces of the musculoskeletal system, enhance circulatory/respiratory, and balance muscles (neural input) with direct and indirect techniques.

- ME and MFR may be used to relieve spasm and contracture by addressing the rotational component of the transition areas, the SB component of type I curves and type II segments within the curve or acting as a transition zone.
- BLT—costotransverse articulations and crossover points of S-curve.
- HVLA is useful for type II segments found superiorly, inferiorly, and within the curves as well as for the type I functional curves.
- Balanced ligamentous and membranous tension and osteopathic cranial manipulative medicine techniques help to relieve primary and secondary strain patterns that course throughout the body, including the cranium.[65]

Bracing

The use of a brace will not cure but may halt progression of the scoliosis. The brace places repetitive loads to trigger remodeling where curvature has occurred. The efficacy increases with compliance; it must be worn day and night. In teens, the biopsychosocial model is critical if the patient is concerned about appearance or being "different" in front of their peers. If necessary, the brace may be removed to participate in sports; however, unequal loading may generate compensatory issues. Bracing continues to evolve and improve.

Some examples of braces available:

- Thoracolumbar orthotic (TLO).
  - ☐ Underarm, low profile, around rib cage, lower back, and hips
  - ☐ Not helpful if there is a C-spine component
  - ☐ Liked better by teenagers
- Milwaukee brace—full torso
  - ☐ Neck ring, rests for chin and back of the head
  - ☐ Flat bar in the front and two flat bars in the back
- Both are cumbersome and increase incidence of somatic dysfunction above and below the level of the brace.
- Others include the Boston, Triac, Cheneau and Cheneau Light, Charleston and Dynamic derotational brace[64]

Surgery

Surgery for scoliosis likewise continues to improve with the goal being a flexible and supported functional spine.

- Spinal fusion
  - ☐ Posterior screws appear to be more effective than hybrid.
  - ☐ Vertebral segments are fused together.
- Metal rods—now expandable with magnets
- Hooks and screws to single segment or several
- Bone grafting[44]

SOMATIC DYSFUNCTION FOUND IN PEDIATRIC POPULATIONS

The pediatric population is susceptible to somatic dysfunction just as adults are. The below provides a brief overview of somatic dysfunction from the structural/biomechanical model of osteopathic care.

Lumbosacral somatic dysfunction

Lumbosacral somatic dysfunction is often symptomatic if induced from a fall or hyperextension injury.

- Athletes who experience fall injuries include gymnasts, dancers, ice-skaters, skateboarders, and those who participate in a wide range of sports such as basketball, soccer, and hockey players.
- It can also be the result of "overuse" with a pre-existing structural problem, such as the presence of a short leg, scoliosis, and spondylolysis sometimes accompanied by spondylolisthesis.
- Patients with lumbosacral somatic dysfunction may present with pain in the low back or hip or even lower extremity.
- If neurologic findings are present, radiographs may be taken, including oblique lumbar views. If imaging is within normal limits treatment may begin and is directed toward relieving the acute problem.
- Initial relaxation of muscle spasm using the following may alleviate symptoms: counterstrain, soft tissue relaxation, trigger point inhibition and/or muscle energy.

SACRAL SOMATIC DYSFUNCTION

Physiologic sacral nutation (anterior movement of the sacral base) occurs about a transverse axis at S2.

- Toddlers have an accentuated lumbar lordosis due to inadequate abdominal musculature. This induces bilateral sacral nutation.
- As growth and development continue into adolescence, the sacrum undergoes unusual stresses secondary to rapid phases of growth and physical activities.
- Sacral and lumbar somatic dysfunctions may respond well to both direct and indirect OMT procedures.
- When the child has recurrent dysfunction, exercises and stretching may be prescribed to maintain the treatment.

UPPER EXTREMITIES

Shoulder dystocia and fractured clavicles may occur from a traumatic birth and may be accompanied by an associated nerve root palsy (Table 67.7). Clavicle fractures are diagnosed with a defect to the lateral aspect of the clavicle, with palpable crepitus upon elevation of the shoulder. These fractures are treated initially with immobilization in a clavicle restraint for 3 to 4 weeks. In infants, MFR and BLT may be used. In older children, Spencer technique and counterstrain may be used to increase ROM and decrease pain.

The elbow is an area of vulnerability for the child because of the confluence of growth plates.

Supracondylar fractures are the most common fracture of the elbow in the pediatric population, usually resulting from a

TABLE 67.7

Brachial Palsies

Associated Nerve Root	Symptoms	Prognosis	Proposed Treatment
C5–C6	Arm extended, internally rotated		
C7–C8 and T1	Additional paralysis of the hand, ipsilateral ptosis, and miosis	90% resolve spontaneously within first year, unless nerves are severed. Better prognosis if upper arm is involved	Gentle handling, avoidance infant lying on affected side, splint hand in physiologic position, indirect OMT. Avoid HVLA

fall on an outstretched hand with the elbow in full extension.[66] Supracondylar fractures are the result of significant forces and involve the growth plates. Therefore, they must be identified and treated properly to avoid residual growth and functional problems.

- Gartland classification plays a fundamental role in decision making regarding management and prognosis. Recent literature recommends conservative management for non- or minimally displaced fractures (long arm cast with the elbow in 60 to 90 degrees of flexion for approximately 3 weeks.)
- The preferred treatment for displaced Gartland II and Gartland III fractures is closed reduction and percutaneous fixation with lateral pins.[66]
- OMT may be used during the immobilization process to improve lymphatic drainage and promote healing. Once the immobilization phase is complete, OMT that promotes ROM such as articulatory and muscle energy may be used as well.
- The radial head is vulnerable to dislocation secondary to a sudden jerk to the arm resulting in a "nursemaid's" elbow.
    - These injuries are treated with initial positioning in pronation/extension to a sudden supination/flexion position, with pressure over the radial head at the antecubital area. BLT and ME may also be useful in addressing somatic dysfunction of the radial head.

Children may sustain overuse injuries resulting in lateral or medial epicondylitis. These entities are more common in adolescents whose growth plates have closed.

- These are best treated with rest, ice, and anti-inflammatory medication. Counterstrain and treatment of trigger points may decrease associated symptoms.

Depending on the skeletal maturity of the child, what may seem similar to a tendinopathy of the wrist extensor or flexor tendons is an apophysitis, commonly called "little league elbow."

- Treatment of this physeal injury is similar to other apophysites, primarily focusing on rest and strengthening exercises with gradual return to play. OMT for compensatory patterns of somatic dysfunction may be beneficial in facilitating the child's healing process as well as the development of healthy ergonomics and proper for in their respective sport.

Wrist injuries present with pain over the wrist with flexion and are often the result of repeated forces on the dorsiflexed hand.

- They are seen in gymnasts, volleyball players, cheerleaders, and string instrument/piano players.

Distal radius fractures are the most common fracture in the pediatric population and while scaphoid fractures are uncommon, they are the most common carpal bone to be fractured in this population.[67] Fractures have continuous pain with tenderness to percussion or vibration directly over the fractured carpal bone. If a fracture is suspected by history or testing, imaging should be obtained prior to attempting manipulation. Treatment may require surgical intervention, thumb spica casting, ice, rest, modification of precipitating behavior, and OMT.

However, somatic dysfunction can result from displaced carpal bones or stress fractures of the carpals. Patients may present with a "catch" or pain of the wrist with dorsiflexion and/or experience a continuous ache.

The dislocated or displaced scaphoid may respond to:

- HVLA, rotation in a figure of eight, and then sudden flexion with pressure over the scaphoid with the thenar eminence
- BLT
- If median nerve entrapment/inflammation occurs, counterstrain, myofascial release, stretching exercises and nocturnal splinting may be appropriate.

Fingers and toes are prone to compression or "jamming" injuries, the result of a sudden force to the end of the digits resulting in pain and swelling over the proximal or distal joints.

- The physician should always perform motion testing to ensure that the tendons are intact and not avulsed from the bone at their points of insertion.
- Once it has been established that there is no fracture via examination or imaging, the injury can be treated with simple techniques such as traction, articulatory, balanced ligamentous tension, still technique, myofascial release, and lymphatic drainage.

LOWER EXTREMITIES

Leg length discrepancy (LLD) is a common and underrecognized condition in the pediatric population.[68] Incidence in the asymptomatic pediatric population is between 85% and 90%.[69] LLD can be categorized as functional or acquired.

- Acquired LLD may be caused by trauma (fractures along the physis [Salter–Harris fractures can disrupt growth rate], infection (osteomyelitis extending to the physis), inflammation (juvenile idiopathic arthritis), neoplasms, radiation, or other idiopathic causes, such as Blount disease or Legg–Perthes disease.[68]
- Functional LLD refers to apparent asymmetry of the lower extremity, without physical shortening or lengthening of the osseous components of the lower limb.[70] Functional LLD can occur anywhere from the superior aspect of the ilium to the inferior aspect of the foot and/or result from pelvic obliquity related to adaptive soft tissue shortening, joint or muscle contractures, ligamentous laxity, or axial malalignment.[70]
- In contrast, structural LLD is a primary disorder with true shortening or lengthening of one extremity.

LLDs <20 mm are generally asymptomatic and likely represent a normal variant. However, LLDs affect the normal biomechanics of the overall body and result in functional alterations, including posture and gait abnormalities.[68] Treatment may include internal shoe or heel lifts, external lifts, physical therapy, and OMT. OMT may help reduce an unlevel sacral or cranial base, correct functional scoliosis, resolve associated or contributing somatic dysfunction, and continue to optimize a patient's structure and function in the case of anatomical scoliosis or a structural or acquired LLD.

Spiral fractures of the long bones are indicative of child abuse unless the history of injury is sufficient to explain the fracture.

HIP DYSPLASIA

Infants may be born with hip dysplasia, which occurs more commonly among infants in the breech position during the third trimester.[71]

- The hips will dislocate with Ortolani and Barlow testing (Fig. 67.19A and B).
    - Ortolani test: The femoral head is gently lifted over the labrum and into the socket.
    - Barlow test: In the case of a reduced hip that is unstable, the Barlow test dislocates the hip as the femur is gently adducted with the hip flexed. The physician gently applies pressure over the medial proximal femur and, while doing so, can feel the femoral head slip out of the socket. As the hip is dislocated, gentle pressure on the thigh or knees gives the feeling

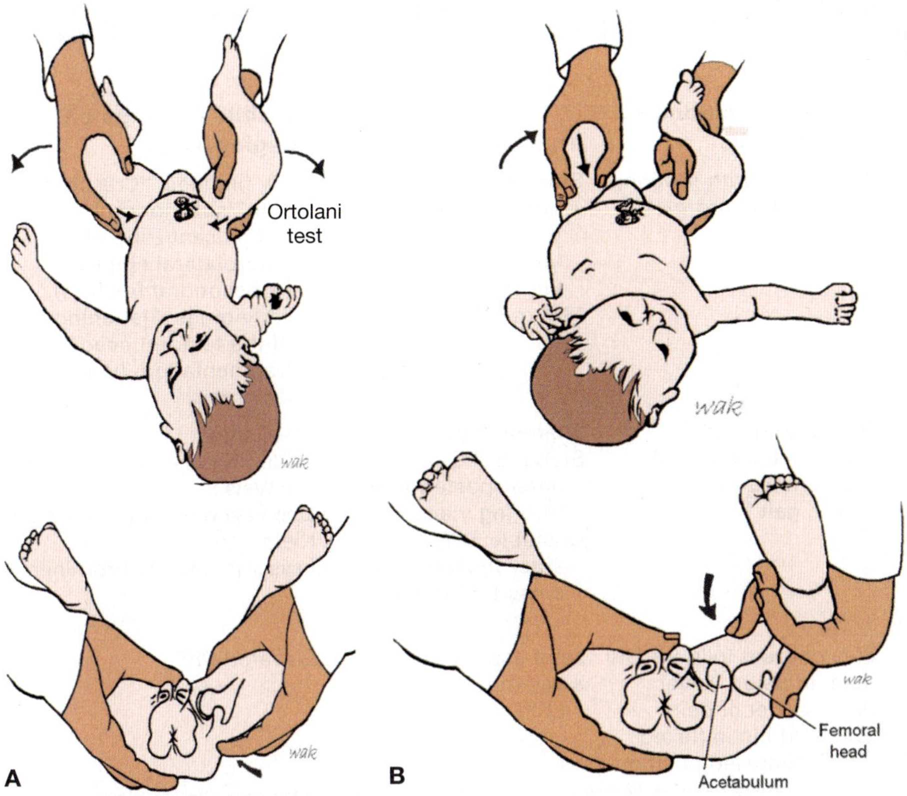

Figure 67.19. Assessing for congenital hip dysplasia in the newborn infant. A. Ortolani test. **B.** Barlow test. (Illustration by William A. Kuchera, DO, FAAO, with permission.)

that the head is not articulating with the socket but that there is a soft endpoint as the pressure is applied. Moreover, the thigh appears shorter.

- Asymmetrical leg creases are also usually noted on physical exam.
- These infants should have hip ultrasounds performed by experienced radiologists at 2 weeks of age.
  - If the hips can be dislocated, they should be placed in a Pavlik harness and referred to an orthopedic surgeon.[72]
  - If they remain undetected until 4 months of age or later, plain films should be ordered with bilateral frog-leg positioning.

PAIN IN THE LOWER EXTREMITY

In children presenting with pain in the lower extremity, the source can be from any area below the waist. They often cannot localize the pain specifically. Osteopathic physicians should address somatic dysfunction with appropriate OMT and prescribed exercises if indicated.

HIP AND KNEE PAIN

Significant red flags for which the physician must be vigilant are listed in Table 67.8.

LEGG–CALVE–PERTHE DISEASE (LCPD)

LCPD is an idiopathic osteonecrosis or idiopathic avascular necrosis of the capital femoral epiphysis of the femoral head usually occurring between the ages of 3 to 12 years old, with the highest rate of occurrence at 5 to 7 years.[76] It occurs more commonly in males and has four stages; necrosis, fragmentation (where the body reabsorbs the bone), reossifcation (osteoblastic activity reestablishes the femoral epiphysis), and remodeling where the new femoral head may be enlarged or flattened.[77] Synovitis and arthritic changes may occur and lead to permanent damage.[78]

Patients present with a limp that is often painless. If pain is present, it may be localized to the hip or referred to the knee, thigh, or abdomen. As the condition progresses, pain typically worsens with activity. Physical exam often reveals the following:

- Gait evaluation: In the acute phase, an antalgic gait is noted with a short-stance phase secondary to pain in the weight-bearing leg. The chronic phase is often marked with a Trendelenburg gait or an inferior pelvic tilt away from the affected hip during the swing phase.
- Decreased internal rotation and abduction of the hip
- Restricted motion to passive extension, abduction, and internal rotation of the hip
- Pain on rotation referred to the anteromedial thigh and/or knee
- Atrophy of thighs and buttocks from pain leading to disuse (abductor and hamstring muscles may have atrophied from disuse and inhibition)
- Afebrile
- LLD[78,79]

The goals of treatment include pain and symptom management, restoration of hip ROM and mechanics, and containment of the femoral head in the acetabulum without further deformation. Referral to an experienced pediatric orthopedist is recommended. This condition may be addressed operatively or nonoperatively. Nonoperative measures include activity restriction, protective weight bearing until ossification is complete, and NSAIDs for comfort.[80] The synovitis may be additionally addressed with non–weight-bearing lymphatic and fluid techniques to improve vascular function.[78] Current literature does not seem to support the use of orthotics, braces, or casts.[81] It is important to inform parents and patients that the treatment process may last several months to years depending on the age of the patient at the time of the diagnosis and the extent of damage to the femoral head.[78]

TABLE 67.8

Possible Etiologies for Hip Pain

Condition	Age and Predominant Sex	Significant Findings May Include:	Imaging	Possible Findings on Imaging/Labs
Legg–Calve–Perthe disease (LCPD)[73]	3–12 Male	Often pain with motion; Trendelenburg gait; Afebrile	Standard anteroposterior pelvis and frog-leg lateral (Lauenstein) views MRI may be warranted	Early findings: "Crescent sign" subchondral radiolucent zone of the anterolateral epiphysis (subchondral fracture) Late findings: Flattening of the femoral head, fragmentation, healing (sclerosis)
Slipped capital femoral epiphysis (SCFE)[74]	8–15 Male	Pain with motion; Affected hip usually externally rotated with gait	Bilateral hip: Stable SCFE: anteroposterior and frog-leg views Unstable SCFE: anteroposterior and cross-table lateral views	Steel sign Widening of growth plate or physis Decreased epiphyseal height Klein line Lesser trochanter prominence
*Septic arthritis	50% of cases <2 years old	80% of cases follow a URI Joint effusion; Fever Acute onset of pain Will hold hip in flexed and abducted position	Joint aspiration X-ray may rule out LCPD and SCFE	Elevated CRP

*Emergent surgical condition.[75]

SLIPPED CAPITAL FEMORAL EPIPHYSIS (SCFE)

Slipped capital femoral epiphysis (SCFE) is the most common hip disorder in adolescents, usually occurring between 8 and 15 years of age. SCFE is defined as the posterior and inferior slippage of the proximal femoral epiphysis on the metaphysis (femoral neck), which occurs through the epiphyseal plate (growth plate).[82,83] Its etiology is unknown and is likely multifactorial but has been associated with obesity, growth spurts, and less commonly endocrine disorders such as hypothyroidism, growth hormone supplementation, hypogonadism, and panhypopituitarism.

SCFE is classified as stable (patient able to ambulate with or without crutches) or unstable (unable to ambulate even with crutches).[84,85]

Physical exam findings may reveal an antalgic gait with an obligate external rotation of the affected lower extremity. Passive motion may be tolerated but with hip flexion there is limited internal rotation.[86] Patients may also complain of knee pain. Acute changes require immediate referral and evaluation by an orthopedic surgeon due to the risk of avascular necrosis, chondrolysis, femoroacetabular impingement, and malunion.[85] However, patients with preslippage benefit from conservative treatment including osteopathic evaluation and treatment. OMT with the goal of minimizing somatic strains, and improving lymphatic and vascular function is also beneficial to patients with chronic SCFE.[86] For those patients requiring surgery, osteopathic evaluation and treatment is an important component of the postoperative rehabilitation.

OTHER CONDITIONS CAUSING HIP AND KNEE PAIN

Hip and knee pains commonly present in children involved with sports and repetitive activities involving the lower extremity.

Examples include gymnastics, dance, ice skating, and soccer.

- A common cause of somatic dysfunction at the knee and hip is related to abnormal body mechanics. For example:
  - Ballet requires continual external rotation of the hip. If done incorrectly (as it commonly is), ballet dancers will apply a torquing force to the knee, resulting in abnormal lower extremity mechanics. This results in knee pain (Fig. 67.20).
  - Children sitting in a "crisscross" or "W position" for prolonged periods may also exert an excessive force exerted on the fibular head.

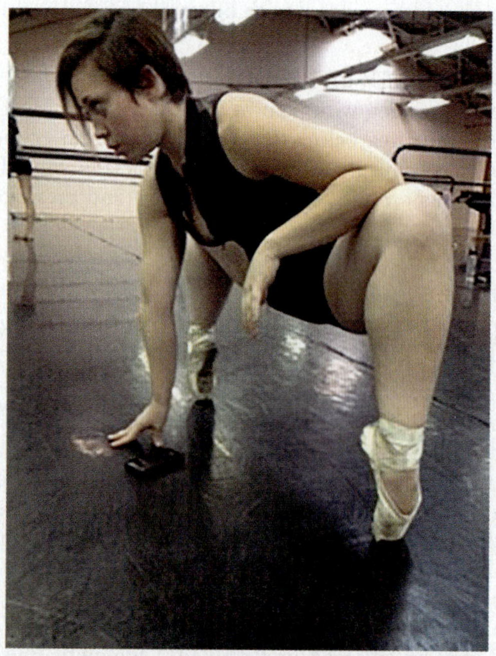

Figure 67.20. Ballet, external rotation of the hip (torquing force to the knee). (Courtesy of Mary Ann Magoun, DO.)

The child's knee is a dynamic area of growth and development that is especially prone to stress injuries.

- Osgood–Schlatter disease presents in adolescence during a pubertal growth spurt, where the rate of long bone growth is faster than that of the muscular attachments (most notably, the quadriceps).
  - Patients may exhibit pain and swelling over the patellar tendon insertion site.
  - Ice, rest, and NSAIDs are commonly used in treatment.
  - It is important to consider treatment of pelvic and lower extremity somatic dysfunction to further address tensile forces exacerbating the symptoms.
- Young children with fever, knee pain, and effusion can have septic arthritis.
  - If this is suspected, aspiration and culture of the fluid, blood counts and cultures, and radiographs should all be obtained.
  - Antibiotics are warranted if the condition is determined to be septic.

ANKLE AND FOOT PAIN

Similar to adults, inversion ankle sprains are common in children participating in sports.

- If a fracture is suspected, imaging should be obtained prior to manipulation, including a stress view, to rule out involvement of the growth plate. If the radiographs are negative for fracture, treatment may include appropriate OMT (e.g., BLT, MFR, lymphatic drainage, treatment for any compensatory changes that may have occurred throughout the body), NSAIDs, ice, and elevation.

Commonly, toddlers and children have ligamentous laxity of the calcaneonavicular (spring) ligament, which, instead of supporting the longitudinal arch, allows it to drop, creating a flexible flatfoot and hyperpronation.[87] Shoes with proper arch support may counter this effect and assist in the maintenance of osteopathic treatment of associated somatic dysfunction.

Ballet requires an additional mention. Ballet dancers' training utilizes extreme plantar flexion, especially with the use of "pointe shoes." This displaces the talus anteriorly over the calcaneus, restricting the talocrural joint in dorsiflexion (Fig. 67.21).

In skeletally immature children, repetitive stress through the plantar fascia and heel cords may injure the calcaneal growth plates. This inflammation of the growth plate is known as calcaneal apophysitis, or Sever disease, and commonly presents as heel

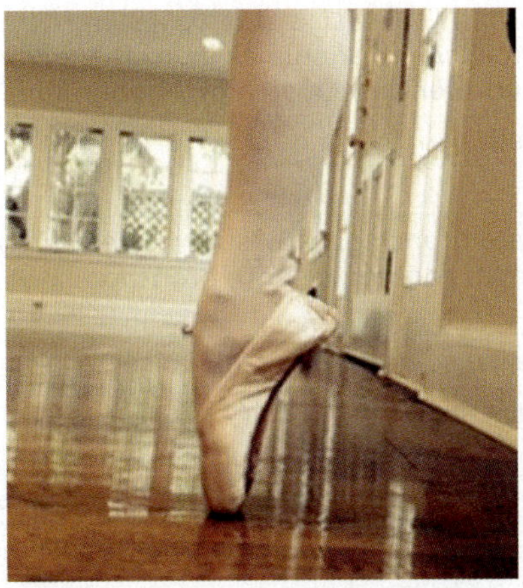

Figure 67.21. Ballet, extreme plantar flexion (displaces the talus anteriorly over calcaneus). (Courtesy of Mary Ann Magoun, DO.)

TABLE 67.9

Benefits of OMT to Joints

Techniques	Benefits
Lymphatics/pumping	Maximize circulation of nutrients, removal of waste
CV4, rib raising	Balance autonomics, ensures adequate circulation
Diaphragm mobility, O-A mobilization	Optimize fluid movement

pain. In addition to activity modification, stretching exercises, and OMT, it is important to select footwear that provides adequate hindfoot support.

In summary, it is important to consider the following with respect to lower extremity conditions and somatic dysfunction:

- Injuries may be prevented with stretching exercises and orthotics when structural problems are identified.
- In children, sports injuries are complicated by the presence of growth plates and hyperflexible joints.
- Physical therapy rehabilitation should be offered to the competitive child athlete for complete healing and protection from further injury.
- OMT is beneficial to restore and improve joint function and overall health (Table 67.9).

GROWING PAINS (BENIGN NOCTURNAL LIMB PAINS [BNLP])

Growing pain is the most common cause of musculoskeletal pain in early childhood.[88] It occurs in children 4 to 12 years of age[89] and is defined as aching in the lower legs, usually at night, without associated joint swelling. Pain may be exacerbated by vigorous activity.

- The etiology remains poorly understood but it may be worsened with exertion. There may be a concomitant fascial strain due to rapid growth.
- It is a diagnosis of exclusion and history and physical exam are necessary to exclude the possibility of a serious issue such as osteomyelitis or osteosarcoma.[89]
- Physical examination includes assessment of gait, posture, pelvic and sacral somatic dysfunction, and LLD.

Treatment may include:

- Fascial mobilization (with use of counterstrain and MFR)
- Addressing any specific areas of somatic dysfunction
- Instructions on stretching and any activity modification
- Reassurance that this is a self-limiting condition
- Massage of limb by parent or caregiver
- Stretching of hamstrings, quadriceps, and calves
- OTC medication such as acetaminophen and/or ibuprofen[89]

3. Respiratory/Circulatory Model

MECHANICS OF PEDIATRIC RESPIRATORY SYSTEM

Due to differences in anatomy, children are more prone to developing certain respiratory problems as compared to adults.

- The upper airway and nose account for the majority of airway resistance in adults, but in children, it is the lower airway.
- In children younger than 5 years, the lower airway resistance is greater than in adults, which plays a major role in pediatric

TABLE 67.10

Child Airway Resistance Factors

- Softer, looser, more compressible tissues
- Small airway muscles incompletely developed
- Recruiting accessory muscles leads to airway collapse
- Small thoracic volume secondary to short, narrow airways

pulmonary diseases such as asthma, pneumonia, and bronchiolitis (Table 67.10).

- Poiseuille law: Airway resistance is inversely proportional to the fourth power of the radius—the smaller the radius, the higher the resistance, the less air can flow unless the force of breathing is increased. Thus, if a child who has a 4-mm bronchiolar tube radius is reduced by half to 2 mm by edema, or bronchospasm, the resistance will increase 16-fold. If the same amount of reduction (one-half) of airway radius occurs in the adult airway that has an 8-mm radius initially, there is still 4-mm radius remaining, thus 16 times less resistance compared to the child's.

The patency of the upper airway is maintained by the genioglossus muscle.

- It pulls the base of the tongue and hyoid bone anterior when it contracts, dilating the upper airway and opposing the negative pressure exerted by the diaphragm.
- Suppression of the genioglossus muscle and other upper airway muscle activity may occur with sleep or severe esophageal reflux leading to further resistance of a child's airway.

The cartilaginous ribs of the infant facilitate the birth process and are twice as compliant as adult ribs.

- Infant ribs articulate linearly with the spinal column and sternum, creating a horizontal orientation of the ribs when compared to adults.
- Due to this horizontal orientation, the intercostal muscles of the infant primarily stabilize the chest wall because they lack the leverage to lift and expand the ribs.
- The diaphragm is especially important in the child for its role in generating changes in tidal volume. The diaphragm muscle fibers insert horizontally (vs. oblique orientation in adults) on the inner surfaces of the ribs to accomplish this.
- Breathing is the only subconscious vital function that can be raised to a conscious level. Proper breathing helps the nervous system relax while shallow, spasmodic breathing signals alarm.[90]

OSTEOPATHIC APPROACH TO THE PEDIATRIC PATIENT WITH RESPIRATORY TRACT INFECTIONS

Injury, lack of sleep, poor nutrition, and social stress can predispose a child to be more susceptible to viral infections.

See Table 67.11 for symptoms of upper respiratory tract infection and approaches to treatment, including use of OMT.

Acute otitis media is the most common infectious disease of children less than 2 years of age.[91]

Epidemiology

- Most common reason for doctor visits in the first 5 years of life (30 million visits per year)
- Most prevalent disease after respiratory illness in children
- Affects 20% of infants in the United States

Risk Factors

Risk factors associated with increased incidence of otitis media

Nonmodifiable:

- Less than 5 years old
- Male sex
- Family history of ear infections
- Low birth weight (less than 2.5 kg [5 lb 8 oz])
- Premature birth (before 37 weeks gestation)
- Prior ear infections
- White ethnicity
- Recent viral upper respiratory tract infection

TABLE 67.11

Examples of Symptomatic Care for Upper Respiratory Tract Infections (URI) Which Are Usually Self-Limiting and Resolve Naturally in Short Course

Common Symptoms with Upper Respiratory Tract Infection	Common Treatments for URI
Fever	Increase fluids, CV4 OMT, provide pharmacologic agents as indicated, e.g., antibiotics if bacterial cause, acetaminophen or ibuprofen to reduce high temperature or cephalgia
Cough	OMT, antitussives medication if indicated
Erythema	Increase fluids
Wheezing	OMT to decrease airway resistance, dilate bronchioles through increased sympathetic activation; home remedies (oxygen mist, cool air, steam); bronchodilator medication as indicated
Rales	OMT to mobilize lung congestion, increase costal cage compliance
Retractions of accessory muscles of respiration	OMT to rest tired muscles, improve efficiency of respiratory effort
Nasal flaring	OMT to reduce airway resistance, increase sympathetic tone to dilate bronchioles
Increased respiratory rate	OMT to reduce costal cage compliance, dome thoracic diaphragm to increase its efficiency

Treatment of symptoms can decrease the morbidity and increase patient comfort and may shorten the course of illness. Children with underlying chronic diseases benefit most from lessening the burden of illness to their already compromised health status.

Potentially modifiable:

- Exposure to tobacco smoke or environmental air pollution
- Factors that cause crowded living conditions (e.g., cold seasons, low socioeconomic level, daycare/school)
- Gastroesophageal reflux disease (GERD)
- Lack of breastfeeding
- Pacifier use after 6 months of age
- Supine bottle feeding[92]

Etiology

Etiology of middle ear infections

1. Viral
2. Bacterial—the three most common are:
   - ☐ *Streptococcus pneumoniae*
   - ☐ *Haemophilus influenzae*
   - ☐ *Moraxella catarrhalis*[92]

Eustachian Tube (Figs. 67.22–67.23)

The incidence of otitis media in young children is a reminder of the osteopathic tenet "structure and function are interrelated." The early anatomy of the eustachian tube plays a key role in the development of otitis media.

- It is a short canal on the lateral wall of the pharynx, connecting the middle ear to the nasopharynx.

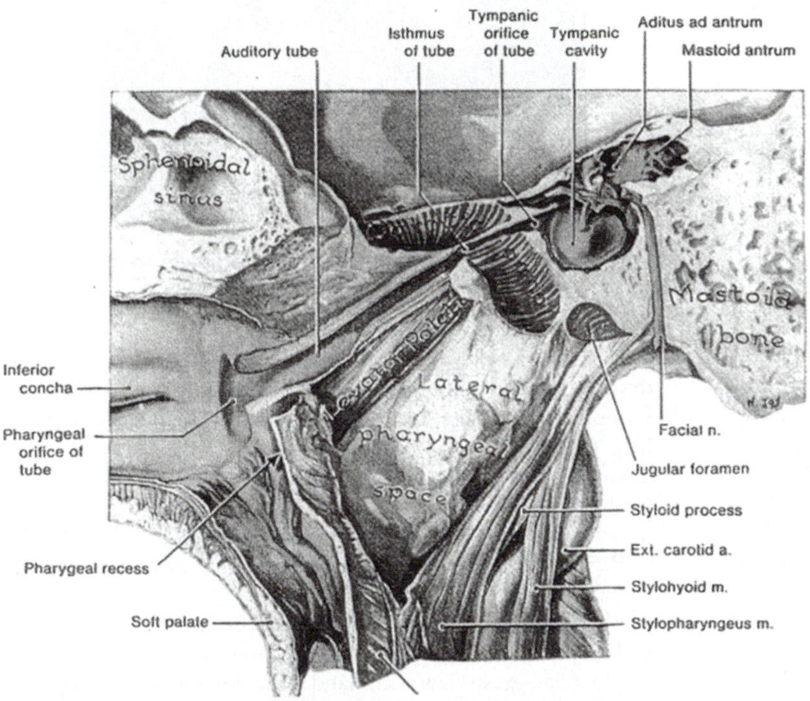

Figure 67.22. Interior view of relationship of ET to adjacent structures in the adult. (From Centers S, Morelli MA, Vallad-Hix C, Seffinger MA. General Pediatrics. In: Ward RC, ed. *Foundations for Osteopathic Medicine*. 2nd ed. Lippincott Williams & Wilkins; 2003:315–316.)

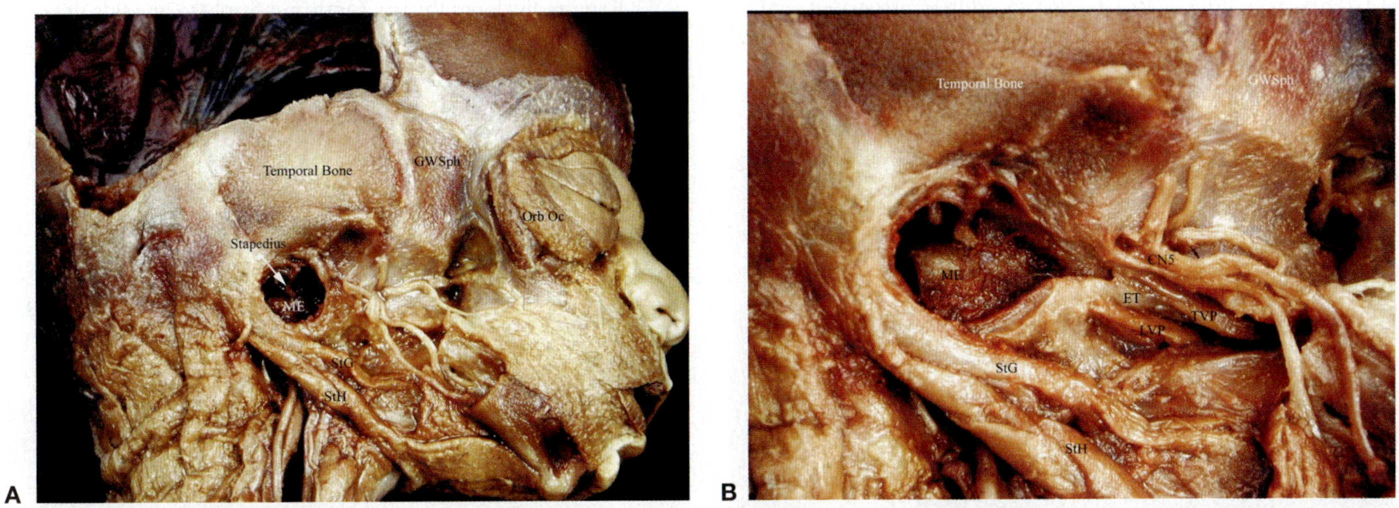

Figure 67.23. A. Lateral view of neonatal dissection. The mandible and zygoma bones have been cut and the muscles of mastication removed. The TM has collapsed, revealing the middle ear (ME) and malleus. The styloglossus (StG) and stylohyoid (StH), orbicularis oculi (ORbOc), mandibular branch of the trigeminal (V3), and greater wing of the sphenoid (GWSph) are labeled. **B.** Close-up of area indicated by the arrow in (**A**). The lateral aspect of the temporal bone has been drilled away to reveal the ET surrounded by the tensor veli palatine (TVP) and levator veli palatini (LVP) muscles. Note the relative size of the muscles as compared to the ET. The middle ear (ME), styloglossus (StG), stylohyoid (StH), greater wing of the sphenoid (GWSph), and ophthalmic branch of the trigeminal nerve (V3) are labeled. (Used with permission from the Willard/Carreiro Collection, University of New England.)

- Lined with ciliated epithelial cells, it helps move secretions from the middle ear to the nasopharynx.
- Equilibration between the middle ear and atmospheric pressures occur via the eustachian tube with assistance from yawning, sucking, and swallowing.
- In children 0 to 4 years of age, the decreased length and horizontal orientation make them more prone to eustachian tube collapse.
- As the facial bones lengthen in the growing child, the eustachian tube orients more obliquely, allowing for better drainage of the middle ear, thus decreasing the risk for acute otitis media.

Eustachian Tube Dysfunction

- This may result from contributory muscle imbalance of the tensor tympani, posterior pharyngeal, medial pterygoid, and digastric muscles.

Temporal Bone Dysfunction

- Temporal bone dysfunction may result from birth trauma, a direct blow, and muscle imbalance such as a hypertonic SCM.
- Dysfunction leads to impaired drainage of the middle ear causing fluid stasis, accumulation, and inflammation. This blocks the eustachian tube predisposing the child to otitis media.
  - Impaired mobility of the petrous portion of the temporal bone is a common structural finding in children with otitis media.

Inefficient, Uncoordinated Suckling

- This may result from possible irritation/compression of the hypoglossal (CN XII) nerve at the hypoglossal canal and/or irritation/compression of the glossopharyngeal (CN IX) nerve at the jugular foramen.
- Tongue thrusting or unfavorable nipple position on the hard palate may drive internal rotation of the palatine bones. This may contribute to either reflux of milk into the eustachian tube or obstruction of the eustachian tube.

Treatment of Otitis Media

In combination with appropriate supportive care and antibiotics (if necessary), the following techniques may be utilized:

- Cranial techniques (Fig. 67.24) to address associated cranial somatic dysfunctions such as condylar decompression, temporal bone rocking, and V-spread.

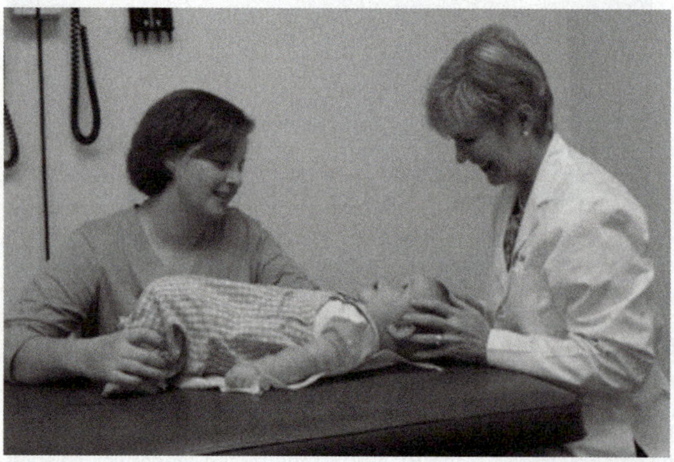

Figure 67.24. Child receiving osteopathic manipulative treatment for AOM with parent nearby, utilizing OCMM technique. (Photo courtesy of Dr. Steele.)

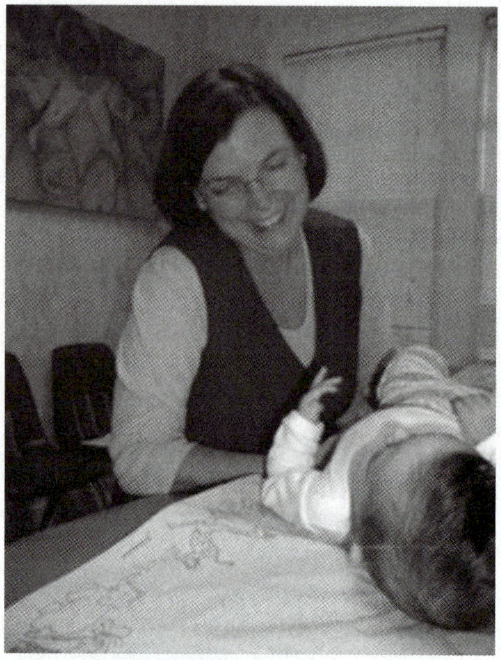

Figure 67.25. Child receiving OMT of the pelvis to assist with function of middle ear drainage. (Photo courtesy of Dr. Mills.)

- Pelvic and sacral techniques may be useful to address cranial dysfunction due to the reciprocal tension membrane (Fig. 67.25)
- Lymphatic drainage techniques to increase fluid movement (Fig. 67.26)
- Thoracic inlet release
- Galbreath technique, also known as mandibular drainage was first described by William Galbreath, DO in 1929[93] (Fig. 67.27):
  - Patient lying supine with unaffected side against pillow for stability.
  - Physician's contralateral hand stabilizes head.
  - The patient is asked to relax the mandible.
  - Physician grasps jaw with hand with one or two fingers pressing on condyle.
  - Repeatedly draws the jaw gently but firmly to one side drawing the condyle inferiorly and medially for about 3 to 4 seconds before releasing it.[93]

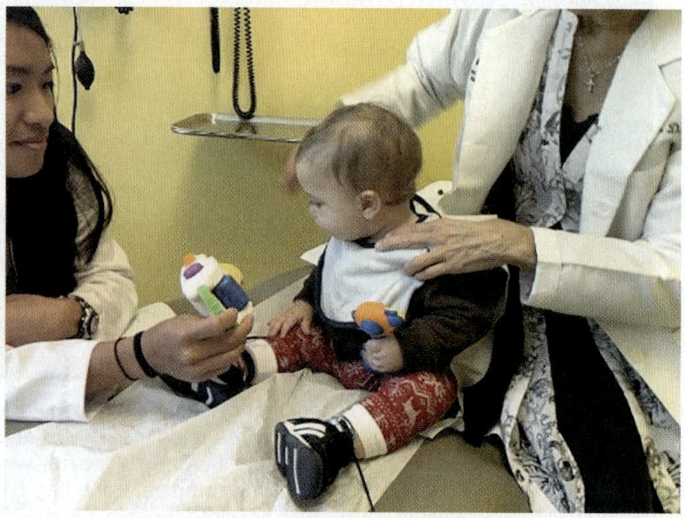

Figure 67.26. Lymphatic drainage techniques. (Courtesy of Mary Ann Magoun, DO.)

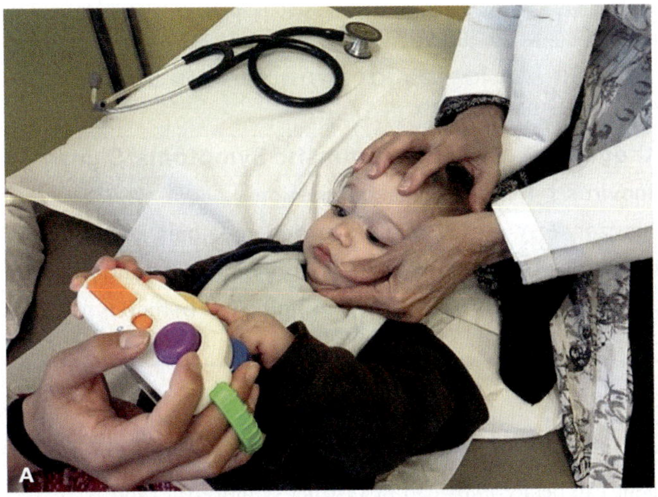

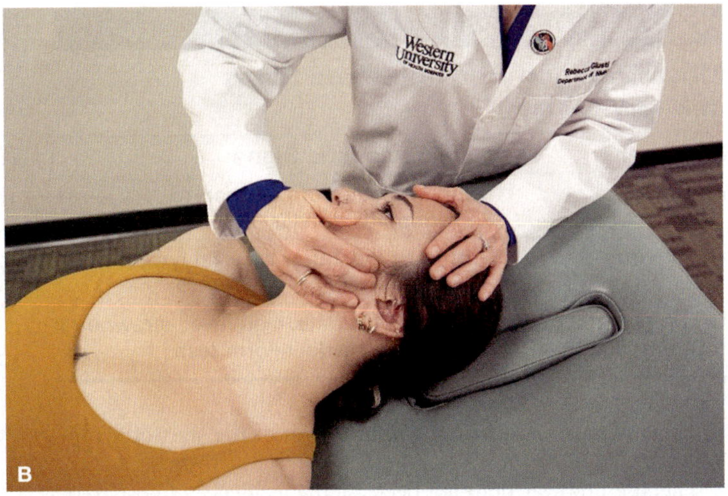

Figure 67.27. A. Galbreath technique—mandibular drainage. (Courtesy of Mary Ann Magoun, DO.) **B.** Galbreath technique on older child or adult. (Photo courtesy of Western University of Health Sciences, Pomona, CA, with permission.)

- □ "In this way, the condyle of the mandible is used to relax and normalize all of the soft structures which lie in close relation to the eustachian tube" thus likely facilitating the drainage of the eustachian tube. Galbreath went on to state that the time required to relax the mandibular articulation to the extent that its condyle may be used to affect the eustachian tube varied by patient but the "desired results can be obtained in 10 or 20 minutes."[93]
- Auricular drainage (Fig. 67.28):
  - □ Physician's treatment hand is placed such that the base of "V" formed between the 3rd and 4th digits is just inferior to the patient's external auditory canal (EAC) as depicted in Figure 67.29.
  - □ Other hand stabilizes the patient's head.
  - □ Perform a gentle but firm clockwise movement several times, followed by a counterclockwise movement.

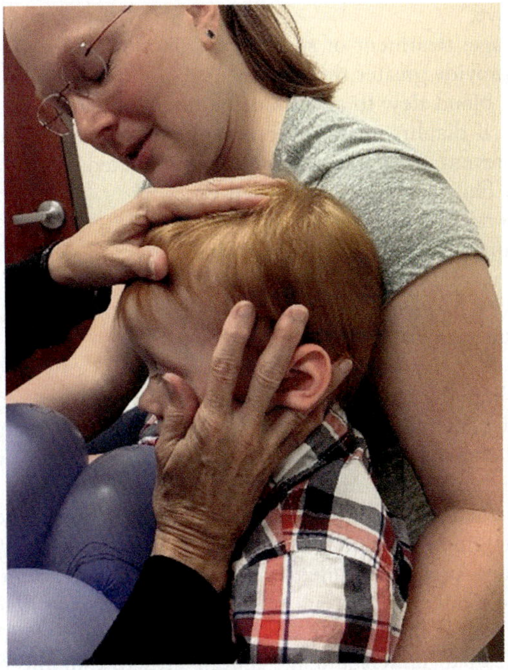

Figure 67.28. Auricular drainage. (Courtesy of Mary Ann Magoun, DO.)

PHARYNGITIS

Pharyngitis is one of the most common complaints in children, representing about 5% of all pediatric visits (Table 67.12).

If a bacterial pathogen is suspected, a culture and rapid antigen test should be obtained.[94]

- Culture-positive disease requires antibiotic treatment to prevent rheumatic fever.

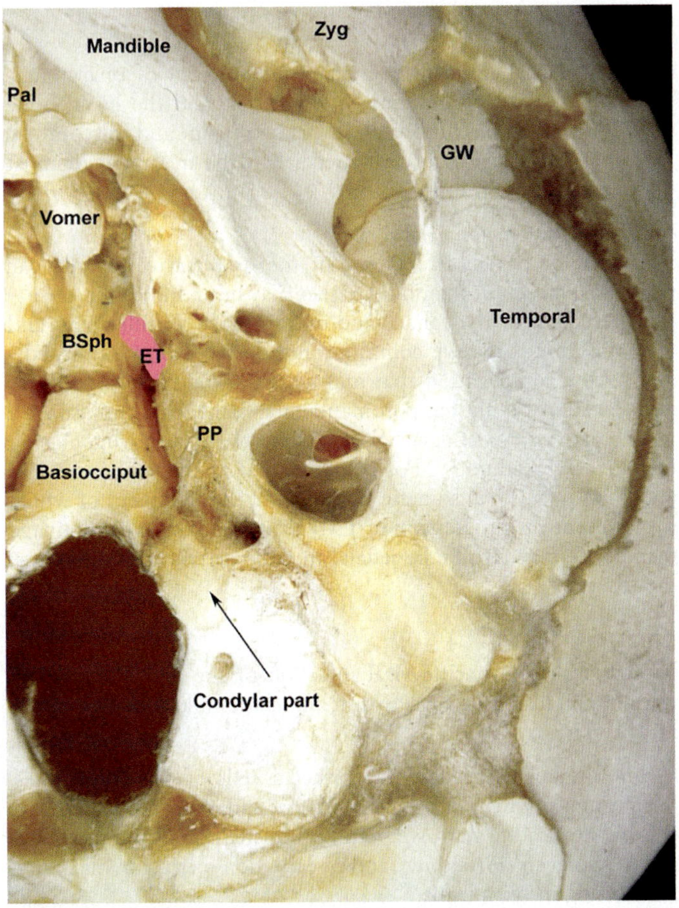

Figure 67.29. Photograph showing location of ET between petrous portion of the temporal bone and the basisphenoid. (Used with permission from the Willard/Carreiro Collection, University of New England.)

TABLE 67.12

Most Common Etiologies and Signs of Pharyngitis

Pathogen	Characteristic Signs
Rhinovirus	Inflammation of the pharynx, adenoids, tonsils
Adenovirus	Rhinitis, posterior cervical lymph node inflammation
Group A β-hemolytic Streptococcus	Tonsillar exudate, high fever, strawberry tongue, scarlatiniform rash

- Therapy must be initiated within 9 days of the start of symptoms.
- Therapy, however, does not decrease the incidence of poststreptococcal glomerulonephritis.

Structural findings may include:

- Inflammation of the posterior pharyngeal muscles
- Cervical lymphadenopathy
- Cervical somatic dysfunction
- Restriction in the physiologic motion of the clavicles, thoracic outlet, and diaphragm
- Hypertonicity of the SCM and elevation of the first rib
- Restricted hyoid motion
- Hypertonic medial pterygoid

Treatment

OMT may be helpful in the symptomatic relief of pharyngitis. Techniques targeting anterior cervical fascia and the hyoid bone may help with resolution of associated pain and discomfort. Lymphatic drainage may be beneficial in the treatment of most upper respiratory infections.

Surgical Intervention

Recurrent or chronic infections of the oropharynx, middle ear, paranasal sinuses, or lymphoid tissues may be an indication of surgical resection of the tonsils and/or adenoids. Tonsillectomy and adenoidectomy are very common procedures performed in pediatrics. One complication that may occur during these procedures is dislocation of the temporomandibular joint with the use of a mouth gag, a surgical device used to keep the mouth from closing during the procedure.[95,96] Postoperative OSE of the temporal bones and TMJ may reveal somatic dysfunction, the treatment of which may prevent the progression of TMJ sequelae. Lymphatic drainage techniques may also be beneficial in patients who undergo these procedures.

BRONCHIOLITIS

Bronchiolitis is an acute viral infection of the lower respiratory tract in children up to age two. It can cause mild to severe respiratory distress.

- The organism invades the epithelial cells of the bronchioles, causing sloughing of the cells, edema, and increased mucus.[97]
- This can lead to narrowing and overdistention of the small airways, uneven air trapping, and a ventilation–perfusion mismatch resulting in hypoxemia.[97]
- The diagnosis is based on:
  - □ Clinical presentation
  - □ Age of the child
  - □ The time of year[98]

TABLE 67.13

Common Etiologies for Bronchiolitis and Related Symptoms

Pathogen	Characteristic Symptoms/Signs
Rhinovirus	Nasal congestion
Influenza	Cough, diarrhea, myalgias
Adenovirus	Pharyngeal erythema and congestion
Mycoplasma	Bullous myringitis (air behind tympanic membrane)

- The incidence of bronchiolitis increases in winter and spring and is most commonly caused by a number of viruses. These pathogens can be accompanied by distinct symptoms (Table 67.13).
- As noted above, in children under 5 years, lower airway resistance is much greater than in adults.
  - □ These changes in airway resistance make bronchiolitis a challenge in the young infant.
  - □ In addition, the muscles in the small airways may not be completely developed, making bronchodilator therapy potentially less efficacious.

Treatment

Treatment of bronchiolitis includes adequate hydration, respiratory care, and use of antibiotics (if indicated) for secondary bacterial infection. OMT may be used to aid in relief of respiratory symptoms; however, robust clinical trials have yet to be reported.[99] Regions to screen and assess include the following:

1. Cervical region: somatic dysfunction of the O-A and A-A junctions may affect parasympathetic tone via the vagus nerve while somatic dysfunction of C3–C5 may affect motor innervation to the thoracoabdominal diaphragm by way of the phrenic nerve. OMT may include O-A decompression and myofascial release to areas of cervical somatic dysfunction. Depending on the age of the child, Still technique, ME, and BLT may also be effective.
2. Rib cage: treatment of somatic dysfunction of the costal cage may provide greater thoracic excursion and motion thus facilitating blood flow to and from the lungs, enhanced thoracoabdominal diaphragmatic motion, enhanced lymphatic drainage and prevention of and clearing of accumulated bronchial secretions. This may be accomplished via:
   - □ Rib raising
   - □ Scapula release
   - □ Intercostal fascial release
   - □ Thoracoabdominal diaphragm release
   - □ Clavicular release

   Note: Rib raising in an infant or small child can be done by encircling the rib cage with both hands; the finger pads are placed bilaterally on the posteroinferior rib angles and apply lateral and superior traction. Recall that the ribs are oriented in a more horizontal plane in children versus adults.
3. Thoracoabdominal diaphragm: restoring thoracoabdominal diaphragmatic motion assists in generating changes in tidal volume and pressure gradients. The posterior crural attachments can be treated with lateral traction of the heads of ribs 11 and 12, as well as the upper lumbar segments. It is important for the physician to understand the unique structure of the pediatric thoracoabdominal diaphragm when addressing it with OMT (Figs. 67.30 and 67.31).

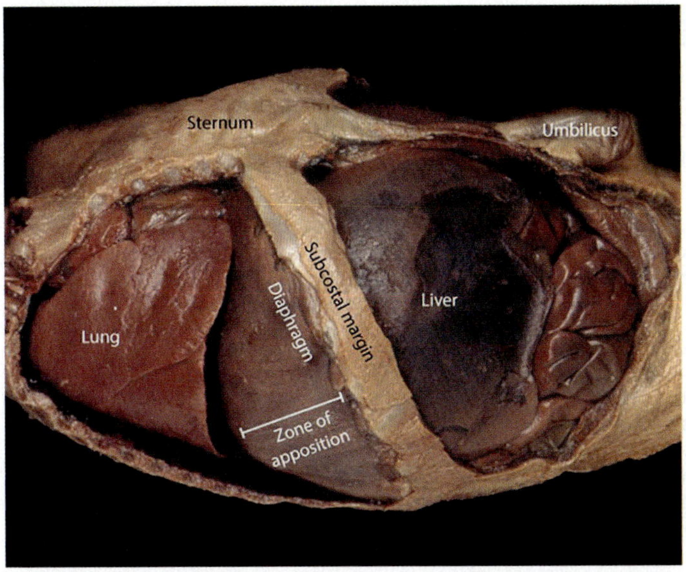

Figure 67.30. Dissection of term infant, right lateral view. The ribs 1 through 9 have been removed as has the right lateral abdominal wall to reveal the dome of the diaphragm draping the superior surface of the liver. The zone of apposition lies between the dome of the diaphragm and its inferior attachment and represents the length of inferior excursion possible during inhalation. (Used with permission from the Willard/Carreiro Collection, University of New England.)

4. Sacrum: The second sacral segment serves as a dural attachment as part of the RTM with superior attachments to foramen magnum and C2. Tethering or restriction of the sacrum may alter its motion as well as the structures superior to it, affecting the quality of respiration. Treatment may include gentle decompression; the physician places two fingers under the sacrum and applies inferior traction matching the forces encountered.

Bronchiolitis may lead to recurrent airway obstruction symptoms[100] and many pharmacologic agents have limited effectiveness;[101] the search continues for the most effective treatment. The comprehensive osteopathic approach to addressing the pathophysiology and related somatic dysfunctions is usually of great assistance to patients with this condition.

OSTEOPATHIC APPROACH TO THE PEDIATRIC PATIENT WITH ASTHMA

Asthma is a common chronic disease in children and is a frequent admitting diagnosis in children's hospitals, disproportionately

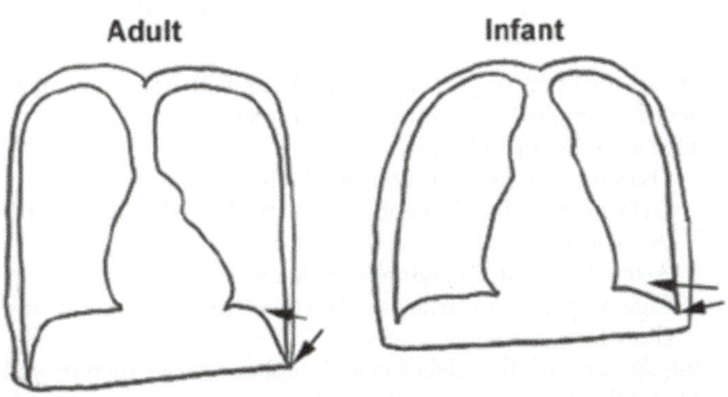

Figure 67.31. Schematic diagram comparing zone of apposition in the infant with that of the adult. The flattened diaphragm and widened thoracic cage contribute to the decreased zone.

TABLE 67.14

Factors That May Precipitate an Asthma Attack

Factor	Example
Exercise	Running, physical education classes, sports
Respiratory infections	Flu, bronchiolitis, croup, etc.
Weather changes	Including wind and changes in temperature/humidity
Allergens	Pollens, mold, spores, house dust, mites, animal dander, food
Irritants	Tobacco, smoke, air pollution, aerosol sprays, strong odors
Gastroesophageal reflux	Stomach acid or contents irritating the esophagus, eliciting viscerovisceral reflex bronchospasm
Medications	Aspirin, nonsteroidal anti-inflammatory drugs, β-blockers
Emotional	Anxiety, fear, stress

affecting non-Hispanic Black children.[102] Unlike pharyngitis or otitis media infection, which resolves in days, an asthma exacerbation may take weeks to resolve. Due to this prolonged period of illness, asthma is a leading cause of school (and parental work) absenteeism. Parents are required to stay home with their children, providing nebulized treatments and administering medications.

Asthma is a lung disease characterized by:

1. Airway obstruction or narrowing that is usually reversible
2. Airway inflammation
3. Bronchial hyper responsiveness[103]

The clinical manifestations of asthma—wheezing, dyspnea, and cough—are the result of airway obstruction that may develop gradually or abruptly. The diameter of the airway lumen determines the amount of obstruction and is influenced by a number of factors including airway smooth muscle contraction and hypertrophy. Bronchial smooth muscle is innervated by the vagus nerve (CN X), and vasovagal reflexes can cause bronchoconstriction. Therefore, in asthma, bronchial spasm and increased bronchial secretions can be caused by overactivity of the bronchial branches of the vagus nerve. In considering the differential diagnosis in patients with signs and symptoms of asthma, it is important to identify the underlying cause or trigger. A number of factors may precipitate an asthma attack (Table 67.14).

Management of Children with Asthma (Table 67.15)

The most effective approach toward treating a child with asthma is multifaceted.

- Treat the underlying pathophysiology:
  - ☐ Bronchoconstriction
  - ☐ Inflammation
  - ☐ Increased secretions
  - ☐ Medications include beta-agonists, corticosteroids (inhaled, oral, IV), leukotriene antagonists, muscarinic antagonists, antibiotics (for superimposed bacterial infection), and mucolytic agents.
- Environmental control and allergen reduction to reduce known triggers:
  - ☐ Reduce dust and potential for dust mites—drapes, stuffed animals, and carpets.

TABLE 67.15

Asthma Management Recommendations National Asthma Education and Prevention Program

	<5 Years Age	>5 Years Age
Mild intermittent asthma: 2 or less days per week and 2 or less nights per month	Treat as needed only, not daily	Treat as needed only
Mild persistent asthma: for >2 d/wk but less than once daily and >2 nights per month	Daily low-dose inhaled corticosteroid, OR cromolyn or leukotriene receptor antagonist	Preferred: Daily low-dose inhaled corticosteroid Alternative: Cromolyn, LTRA, nedocromil, or sustained release theophylline
Moderate persistent asthma: daily and 1 night per week	<5 years age; medium-dose inhaled corticosteroid; medium-dose inhaled corticosteroid + either long-acting inhaled beta-2 agonist or leukotriene receptor antagonist; OR medium-dose inhaled corticosteroid only; medium-dose inhaled corticosteroid + long-acting inhaled beta-2 agonist in recurring severe exacerbations	>5 years: low- to medium-dose inhaled corticosteroid + long-acting inhaled beta-2 agonist; increase corticosteroid and add long-acting inhaled beta-2 agonist in recurring severe exacerbations
Severe persistent asthma: continuous or repeatedly during the day and frequent at night	High-dose inhaled corticosteroid + either long-acting inhaled beta-2 agonist or leukotriene receptor antagonist; oral corticosteroid PRN	High-dose inhaled corticosteroid + long-acting inhaled beta-2 agonist; oral corticosteroid PRN

Adapted from Centers for Disease Control and Prevention. Key clinical activities for quality asthma care: recommendations of the National Asthma Education and Prevention Program. *MMWR Recomm Rep.* 2003;52(RR-6):1–8.

- ☐ Use of hypoallergenic pillows, sheets, and mattress covers.
- ☐ Use of air purifier.
- Avoid exposure to tobacco smoke, toxic chemicals, cleaners, and pesticides.
- Maintain a well-balanced diet and hydration:
  - ☐ Increase fluid intake to account for known increased insensible water losses
  - ☐ Avoid known food allergens
  - ☐ Encourage exclusive breastfeeding in the first 3 months of life to decrease the incidence of children developing reactive airway disease.[104]
- Breathing exercises:
  - ☐ Breathing exercises help strengthen peripheral and accessory muscles that aid breathing.
  - ☐ Expiratory exercises are beneficial due to pathologic air-trapping caused in asthmatics.
  - ☐ A game can be created out of blowing a pinwheel.

A rationale for OMT in children with asthma:

- The physician should focus on balancing the autonomic nervous system, which may entail stimulation of the sympathetic nervous system, particularly T1–T6, to aid in bronchodilation. Key segments of restriction are usually found at T2, T3, and T4.[105,106] Address the vagus nerve activity by treating somatic dysfunction at the cranial base.
- Address somatic dysfunction of the ribs and costal cage to further improve respiratory mechanics. Rib raising is an effective technique and can also be taught to parents and caregivers.
- Address structural restrictions, which may influence circulatory system function.
- Viscerosomatic reflexes should be addressed, as well as somatosomatic and somatovisceral reflexes to decrease the overall allostatic load on the body.
- Once the asthma exacerbation has resolved, remaining somatic dysfunction with segmental facilitation may predispose the patient to another exacerbation.
- After an acute attack, it is important to treat somatic dysfunction related to all aspects of the primary and secondary respiratory system to aid the body's inherent healing capacity (Table 67.16 and Box 67.3).
- A randomized clinical trial of 140 asthmatic pediatric patients with asthma demonstrated an improvement in peak expiratory flow in the short term from OMT[107]; however, in another trial, a standardized OMT protocol did not demonstrate benefit[108]; long-term outcome studies have not been reported.

As a historical note, A.T. Still had great success in relieving asthma and hay fever. He attributed his success to correcting spinal somatic dysfunctions, especially of the third and fourth thoracic vertebrae.[2,3] The presence of somatic dysfunction at this spinal segment is most likely due to a viscerosomatic reflex. It is also one of the spinal segments from which the sympathetic nervous system innervates the lungs.

4. Neurologic Model

The nervous system of the pediatric patient is a dynamic, expanding, and integrated system that ultimately affects all other vital systems of the body.

- Proper function of this system is dependent upon an unimpeded, physiologic, and integrated structure.
- This structure includes the:
  - ☐ Osseous case that surrounds the brain and spinal cord
  - ☐ Delicate fascial and membranous coverings that lie beneath the osseous covering
  - ☐ Arterial, venous, and lymphatic channels
  - ☐ Ligamentous and articular structures that both limit and allow for motion
- Impairment of this delicate and multifaceted structure will impair function.

There are three main principles that govern sensory neural development.

TABLE 67.16

Areas to Check for Somatic Dysfunction in Asthmatic Patient

Area of Potential Dysfunction	Rationale for Assessing the Area
T1–T5	Sympathetic innervation to the lungs
Upper thoracic vertebrae, ribs, sternum	Structural component of respiration
Occiput, temporal bones; O-A junction, vagus nerve	Fourth ventricle, origin of sympathetic drive/respiratory center in brain; parasympathetic innervation to the lungs
Accessory muscles of respiration; fascia	Often hypertonic and congested with metabolites; soft tissue enveloping the lungs
Thoracic diaphragm	Used in all phases of breathing
Cranial–sacral mechanism	Central nervous system aspect to respiration
T10–L2	Sympathetic innervation to the kidneys, adrenal glands

BOX 67.3 Factors that Affect Breathing Difficulties

From an osteopathic perspective, the following areas may contribute to or exacerbate the patient's breathing difficulties.

1. Upper thoracic vertebrae, ribs, sternum
2. T1–T6 because of sympathetic innervation to the lungs
3. Occipitoatlantal junction and the course of the vagus nerve that supplies parasympathetic input to the pulmonary tree
4. Accessory muscles of respiration
5. Anterior cervical fascia
6. Thoracic diaphragm (The diaphragm is enervated by the phrenic nerve from the cervical plexus [C3–C5], and its mobility is influenced by the lower six ribs, L1–L2, and the sternum.)
7. Chapman reflexes for the lungs, sinuses, and adrenal glands
8. The cranial–sacral mechanism
9. T10–L2 and the lower ribs

1. The sequence of development is the same in all children[109–111] (Table 67.1).
   - At birth, primitive reflexes (including Moro, startle, palmar/plantar grasp, and Babinski) should be elicited, representing normal neurologic development.
   - As neuronal development proceeds, the well-organized newborn will initially have an atonic neck reflex (fencing pose) at 1 to 4 months, which will lead to the ability of the infant to roll back to front at 5 months.
   - From 6 to 8 months, the infant will begin to first crawl and then creep. The myelination and developmental stimulation in the areas of the pons and midbrain mediate this phenomenon.
   - Standing and walking begin at 9 to 12 months as the cortex begins to develop.
2. Primitive reflexes must be extinguished before corresponding voluntary movements can be obtained.
   - Primitive reflexes generally fade by 4 to 5 months of age. If these reflexes persist, the child should be evaluated for neurologic abnormalities.
3. The rate of milestone achievement may not be parallel in all areas of development.

Gross motor, fine motor, social, and language skills may exhibit varying degrees of advancement. Children who are inefficient in their ability to receive, process, store, and utilize information through their five senses may not have been able to appropriately integrate or pattern sensory information from their body or the environment (Table 67.17).

- These developmental inefficiencies are thought to be the result of a nervous system that has not been able to properly integrate or regulate input from the senses or proprioceptors. A number of studies show that brain growth and development occur at predetermined chronologic ages (e.g., rapid growth occurs between 3 months of fetal life to about 2 to 3 years postnatally).
- Lack of appropriate sensory integration arises from nonsequential, or lack of, attainment of developmental milestones. This may occur if there is prolonged interruption of normal infant development due to lack of stimulation.
   - Forced deprivation of external stimuli may lead to developmental delays.

TABLE 67.17

Presentation of Children with Sensory Neural Developmental Disorders

	Hyperesthesia	Hypoesthesia
Definition	An abnormal increased response to sensory stimulation	Abnormal decreased response to sensory stimulation
Typical behaviors	• Refusal to wear certain types of clothing • Exhibition of extreme irritability from tags on clothing • Potential refusal certain textured food or in some cases all solid food	• Extremely increased pain threshold • Potential exhibition of self-mutilating behavior in order to receive tactile pain stimulation • Potential to constantly run the hands across the carpet or to seek various forms of vibration to receive deep joint stimulation
Common aversions	Vibratory stimulation	

- Critically ill children with prolonged hospitalization are also at risk.
- An example of nonsequential development would be seen in a child who progresses from a sitting position to a standing position/walking without ever crawling or creeping.

- Discrepancies in motor–sensory organization may lead to problems in the areas of learning, socializing, and behaving.
  - An example would be lack of vestibular stimulation (turning head from side to side), which further decreases the integration of motor, vision, and hearing afferent fibers within the superior colliculus and thalamus.
  - This may lead to lack of crawling in the child, and possibly predispose them to gait abnormalities and depth perception difficulties.

Evaluation of children from a neurodevelopmental approach can give valuable clues in developing a management plan, including the utilization of OMT.

- In neurologically compromised children, manipulation directed toward the autonomic nervous system may positively affect the sensory responses and sensory integration of the CNS.
- Both neurologically compromised and uncompromised children show marked improvement in standard neurodevelopmental profiles upon receiving OMT compared with a control group.[112]

Common Conditions Related to the Neurologic Model of Osteopathic Care

COLIC

Colic is defined as a benign condition hallmarked by inconsolable crying, irritability, and screaming that lasts for 3 hours or more without an apparent cause in an otherwise healthy and well-fed infant. Infants with colic often experience these symptoms in the evening, display grimacing or facial expressions of discomfort, leg-drawing, and abdominal tension.[113]

Colic may be the result of immaturity of both the CNS and gastrointestinal system in which it is difficult for the systems to differentiate between a constant barrage of non-noxious and noxious stimuli.[114]

Structural exam may reveal:

- Somatic dysfunction of the upper cervical, cranial-cervical, and/or cranial base[115]
- SBS strain patterns such as lateral or vertical strain SBS patterns
- Significant membranous restrictions with poor cranial motion
- Sacral base restriction
- Abnormally shaped heads with one eye appearing “more shallow” than the other and placed inferiorly
- Torticollis

These infants may respond to release of the sacral restrictions and with treatment of possible vertical and lateral SBS strain patterns.

- The strains are treated with direct, gentle remolding of any parietal and frontal abnormalities and carrying the greater wings of the sphenoid into normal position.
- Somatic dysfunction of the O-A joint should be addressed; O-A decompression may be effective.

APNEA OF PREMATURITY

Apnea of prematurity (AOP) is frequently defined as a pause in breathing lasting more than 20 seconds, or more than 10 seconds with accompanying bradycardia and/or oxygen desaturations in an infant born before 37 weeks gestation.[116] AOP is one of the most common diagnoses in the Neonatal Intensive Care Unit (NICU),[116] affecting almost half of infants before 32 weeks gestation and nearly all whose birthweight is below 1,000 g.[117]

Along with acute morbidities such as cyanosis and chronic intermittent hypoxia, this condition may have a negative impact on later health, particularly on the CNS, which is highly sensitive to hypoxia.[118] Children born prematurely are much more likely to suffer from poor neurodevelopmental outcomes than those born at term[119–123] and some studies have suggested that this could in part be related to the frequency of apneic events and desaturations they experience in early life.[124,125]

AOP may be associated with spitting up. The gastroesophageal reflux stimulates vagal activity resulting in bradycardia and constriction of the airways.

Structural exam findings:

Infants and children with a history of AOP may present with the following findings on structural exam:

- Marked reduction in the primary respiratory motion.
- Cranium held in extension, with temporal bones fixed in internal rotation.
  - Infants that have been intubated tend to have highly arched palates, secondary to the lack of maturity of diaphragm activation and lung function, as well as the mechanical effects of the endotracheal tube. The high-arched palate further drives cranial extension, which may lead to narrowed airways. This decreased diameter makes clearance of secretions more difficult, possibly predisposing to mucous plugs and apnea.
- The foramen magnum may be narrowed, which can lead to distention of the fourth ventricular due to impaired CSF drainage. The brain stem may experience minimal disruption leading to abnormal modulation of homeostasis, causing apnea and bradycardia.
- Restrictions at the craniocervical junction and condylar region and interosseous strains in the cranial base.[126]

Treatment includes release of any cranial base dysfunction and associated sacral restriction with restoration of balance to the autonomic nervous system. Another major focus of treatment is to restore physiologic brain stem activity. If appropriate, the physician should address any functional tissue strain patterns that may interfere with the functional relationship between the diaphragm and esophageal sphincter and the reflux and vagal response.[127]

CLOSED HEAD INJURIES

Closed head injuries may be related to accidental trauma (e.g., during sports, during a whiplash-type injury, fall, etc.) or NAT. Inertial injuries can result in concussion and postconcussion syndrome. Patients may present with a history of a blow to the head or a sudden change in directional forces, resulting in a brief loss of consciousness or disorientation, with or without neck pain. Pediatric considerations in closed head injuries include:

- Children have flexible necks and relatively large heads.
- Their neurologic system is still developing and the membranes are highly vascular.[128]
  - Structural findings may include cervical spasm, diminished primary respiratory mechanism, and somatic dysfunction of the cranium, cervical, thoracic, lumbar, pelvis, and sacral regions.

Prior to treatment, children should be evaluated for traumatic brain injuries and any emergent conditions should be appropriately addressed.[129]

- Closed head injuries may be treated with a wide range of osteopathic techniques including counterstrain or muscle energy OMT to the cervical somatic dysfunctions.
- Cranial osteopathic manipulative medicine such as balanced membranous tension, venous sinus drainage, and CV4 may all enhance the primary respiratory mechanism and restore normal physiologic structure and function.

LEARNING DISORDERS AND DIFFICULTIES

Learning disorders are increasingly common among children of all ages. Children with learning difficulties may present with the following osteopathic findings, and those with associated hyperactivity may have more severe findings.

- Visual tracking disturbance and lateral strains of the SBS
- Compression of the SBS
- Cranial dysfunction may arise in these children from sacral compression or other distant areas of the body.
- The occipital condyles and the foramen magnum are often compressed, resulting in pyramidal and autonomic disturbances.

Suggested treatment modalities may include:

- Condylar decompression and release of basilar compression may improve symptomatology.
- Directing a fluid wave from the occipital sinus to glabella (frontal cortex—area of executive function) can be very calming.
- Treatment of the underlying cause of the child's symptoms is essential.
- Nutrition and diet should be explored for allergies and sensitivities.
- If there are associated visual disturbances, neurodevelopmental therapy or developmental optometric training may be necessary once the underlying somatic dysfunctions are corrected (vision therapy).

Nonspecific learning difficulties were addressed in the following study, in which 209 children between the ages of 4 and 14, diagnosed with learning difficulty, were evaluated by OSE.[11]

- Seventy-two percent of the children with a learning difficulty diagnosis had a significant past history of birth trauma compared to only 28% in the control group.
- Labor lasting more than 24 hours was highly associated with learning difficulty.
- Eye–motor coordination and visual perception imbalances were highly associated with children experiencing difficulty.
- Lateral strains of the SBS may be especially implicated in oculomotor disturbances.
  - These dysfunctions may be a result of intrauterine pressure or early postnatal or perinatal trauma displacing the axis of the orbit.
  - This can cause changes of tension in extraocular eye muscle resulting in eye muscle imbalance.
  - These distortions would also change membranous, fascial, neural, and venous relationships.

CEREBRAL PALSY

CP is a group of neurologic disorders of postural control and movement due to a nonprogressive defect or lesion of the developing brain. It appears in infancy or early childhood and usually permanently affects body movement and muscle coordination. CP is caused by damage to or abnormalities inside the developing brain that disrupt the brain's ability to control movement and maintain posture and balance.[130] Common causes of CP include prematurity, intraventricular hemorrhage, especially in premature infants, congenital abnormalities, and perinatal hypoxic–ischemic injury resulting in cortical damage. The location and extent of insult in a child with CP will determine how they are able to learn and develop new compensatory movement strategies (Table 67.18). While CP is the leading cause of childhood disabilities in the United States, it doesn't always cause profound disabilities.[130,131] There are several forms of CP including spastic, extrapyramidal, atonic, cerebellar, dyskinetic, ataxic, and mixed.

TABLE 67.18

Possible Classifications of Cerebral Palsy

Etiology	Genetic, Infectious, Malformation, Infarction, a Hypoxic-Ischemic Injury
Site of brain injury	Cortical, subcortical, periventricular white matter, cerebellar
Body distribution	Monoplegia, diplegia, quadriplegia
Physiologic type	Spastic, atonic, dystonic, dyskinetic, ataxic, or mixed
Severity	Mild, moderate, or severe

CP clinical presentation:

- At birth, infants may have an abnormality of suckling, swallowing, alertness, and/or breathing patterns.
- If seizure activity is present, untreated seizure disorders may contribute to increased muscular tone.
- Hypoxic–ischemic encephalopathy may cause generalized hypotonia and abnormal primitive reflexes in the postnatal period.
- Earliest signs of spasticity include resistance to passive movement. When spasticity is severe, the child may develop contractures, which affect limb functionality.

Osteopathic Treatment of Cerebral Palsy

Goals of osteopathic treatment include:

- To decrease pain and limit progression of contractures, hip dislocations, and scoliosis.[132] Overall, this may assist in improving functionality.
- Effect changes in the proprioceptive input from joints, connective tissues, and muscle to help the patient maintain balance.
- Alleviate abnormal or stressful inputs resulting from compensatory changes (somatic dysfunction and/or muscle spasm that has arisen secondarily) to allow the patient to create new motor strategies that improve the patient's ability to perform motor planning and execute movement.[132]

Some approaches and considerations in this population include:

- Strain–counterstrain and balanced ligamentous and other indirect techniques are appropriate for all ages.[132]
- OMT aimed at passive or isometric muscle stretch, such as muscle energy techniques, can be effective.[132]
- Alleviating biomechanical stresses with osteopathic manipulation may help the child by normalizing input to joint afferents and balancing agonist–antagonist muscle tone.
- Using OCMM and/or MFR to relieve compensatory somatic dysfunction that affects the overall level of muscle tone and motor control in the child with CP, assists in improving the child's ability to perform motor planning and execute movement, as demonstrated in a clinical trial comparing OMT to acupuncture therapy and waitlist control groups[133]; however, in another trial, use of "cranial osteopathy" alone did not

demonstrate improvement in motor function, pain, or sleep in children aged 5 to 12 years with CP.[134]

- Patients with CP require consistent osteopathic treatment in order to maintain a lowered afferent drive. Osteopathic treatment is especially important at every growth spurt.
  - Of historical note, Beryl Arbuckle, DO, treated patients from around the world at her Osteopathic Cerebral Palsy Institute from 1953 to 1967.[8]
  - One example of the magnitude of addressing somatic dysfunction with OMT in this critical period of development was found in a twin who suffered severe prenatal birth trauma from uterine crowding and being lodged in his mother's pelvis for several months before delivery.
    - At 10 months, he was diagnosed with CP and was so stiff that he was unable to sit.
    - With weekly OMT, his flexibility increased markedly. He was soon able to sit without aid, crawl, and creep, and began to walk by 18 months.

5. Metabolic

THE PEDIATRIC GASTROINTESTINAL SYSTEM

The gastrointestinal system is one of the most important systems in physiologic maintenance of health in pediatric patients. It is fundamental for proper growth and development.

- Gastrointestinal complaints are commonly seen by osteopathic pediatricians.
- The enteric nervous system parallels the CNS in density and quantity of neurons. The system can be surgically separated from the CNS and maintain its physiologic function.
- A.T. Still attributed many childhood diseases to dysfunction of the enteric nervous system.[3]

GASTROESOPHAGEAL REFLUX DISEASE (GERD)

GERD in newborns often presents as frequent emesis or spitting up shortly after feeding and may be associated with failure to thrive, apnea, and bradycardia. In toddlers and older children, it may present as pain, chronic cough, recurrent pneumonia, wheezing, or anorexia.[135]

- These children may have a significant increase in their gag reflex.
- They often have a history of abnormal delivery events including:
  - Face presentation
  - Vacuum extraction
  - Augmentation with oxytocin
  - Prolonged labor
- These events may place abnormal stress on the cranial base leading to symptoms

Structural exam findings may include the presence of viscerosomatic reflexes usually found from T5 to T7, diaphragmatic restrictions, strains at the thoracolumbar junction, altered respiratory mechanics of the thorax, strains or compression of the occipitoatlantal region and cranial findings suggesting vagal irritation.[136] Sacral somatic dysfunction and compression of the fourth ventricle due to foramen magnum asymmetry may also be found. Cranial somatic dysfunction may lead to abnormal stimulation of CN IX, CN X, and CN XI. The increased vagal tone is responsible for:

- Bronchospasm
- Bradycardia
- Alteration of the emesis reflex pathway

This is best treated by releasing the O-A restriction but may require treating the sacral base restriction simultaneously. The physician should place the pads of the middle fingers over the condyles at the base of the skull and then apply gentle traction in an outward and upward direction until the tissue softens. Gentle sacral traction may help facilitate release of the O-A somatic dysfunction. Addressing viscerosomatic reflexes could potentially mediate continued symptoms through neurologic mechanisms. Fluid techniques may be used for cranial somatic dysfunction and premature and newborns may benefit from BLT and balanced membranous techniques.[137]

CONSTIPATION

Constipation in young children is a common complaint. A detailed history should be taken to determine the cause. Using the following questions may assist in determining if the constipation is from an organic cause, such as a congenital or a genetic anomaly (e.g., Hirschsprung's or cystic fibrosis):

- Has the constipation been present since birth?
- Did the infant stool within 24 hours of delivery?
- Was there a meconium ileus?
- Is the child potty trained? (withholding syndrome)
- Is there pain with defecation?
  - Pain may lead to the cycle of constipation.
  - A child who is afraid of pain associated with a bowel movement will willfully not stool.
- What is the child's dietary intake? This includes:
  - Milk and cheese consumption
  - Carbohydrates
  - Fiber
  - Fruits and vegetables
  - Free water intake
- Has the constipation been controlled with juice or fruits?
- What is the child's bowel hygiene and medication history?
  - Has a bowel regimen been attempted?
- Has there been trauma?
  - Blood in stool, anal fissures, fall/physical activity history?
  - NAT/sexual abuse?
- In older children, examine for psychosocial components such as "Is there a fear of public restrooms or asking permission in a classroom setting?"

Constipation and many of its causative factors may be treated effectively with OMT.

- The physician should be careful to examine for autonomic imbalance and pay close attention to the A-A and O-A joints. Recall that vagus nerve involvement can contribute to autonomic imbalance. Assess for pelvic and sacral somatic dysfunction as well as altered mechanics of the lower thoracic and upper lumbar segments, likely related to viscerosomatic reflexes and/or autonomic modulation of lower gut motility.[138]
- Both the pelvic and abdominal diaphragms should be addressed. The external anal sphincter has deep and superficial portions, both of which are extensions of the perineal body of the pelvic diaphragm.[139] In children with chronic constipation, the anal canal is positioned more obliquely which may affect optimal functioning of the external sphincter.[140]
- Lumbosacral decompression and rhythmic sacral pumping and rocking may be effective.
  - Older children can lie supine with their sacrum over a small 5-inch pilates ball.
  - Instruct them to arch their lower back and suck their belly button in. This rocks the sacrum about a transverse axis.
  - They can lift each hip anteriorly to rock the sacrum about a vertical axis.

- If visceral restriction is present:
  - The patient assumes the prone knee-to-chest position, and the physician gently lifts the intestines from the pelvis, engaging restriction. This may assist in restoring free unimpeded motion and blood flow to the intestine.
  - Treating the child with fascial release of the colon may be helpful.

DIARRHEA

Diarrhea in the infant and child is common and may respond to OMT. The underlying cause must first be addressed. Acute diarrhea, most often caused by viruses, must be differentiated from chronic diarrhea, which could have multiple causes.[141] Infectious diarrhea should be differentiated from the noninfectious type.

Regardless of cause, somatic dysfunction is often found.

Supportive care is essential for all types and causes of diarrhea.

- This should include adequate hydration and dietary modifications.
- OMT may be used to address the autonomic imbalance of the vagus nerve (at the cranium, O-A joint, and upper cervical complex) and the parasympathetic plexus (sacrum), which may be beneficial in reducing symptoms. If present, structural somatic dysfunction of the diaphragms and pelvic bowl should be treated with various techniques as tolerated by the child.
- Overall, treatment may assist in restoring proper structure and function to the area.

CYSTIC FIBROSIS

As a prime example of the metabolic model, cystic fibrosis is a genetic disorder of exocrine gland function, predominantly affecting the pulmonary and gastrointestinal systems.

- The cystic fibrosis transmembrane conductance regulator (CFTR) gene codes for an ABC transporter-class ion channel protein that conducts chloride and bicarbonate ions across epithelial cell membranes. A structural mutation in the CFTR alters the function of salt regulation throughout the body and leads to dysregulation of epithelial lining fluid transport in the lung, pancreas, and other organs.
- Numerous types of mutation in the CFTR gene are responsible for the syndrome and its variations. This leads to:
  - Decreased water into the lumen, creating viscous mucus that obstructs airways, promoting infection.
  - Impaired transport of bicarbonate (HCO3-) in the ductal lumen of the pancreas which is required to maintain alkalinity and keeps the pancreatic enzymes (large proteins) soluble. Without sufficient bicarbonate (creating an acidic environment), the macromolecules precipitate out in the ductal lumina resulting in obstruction and damage.

Common findings in cystic fibrosis are as follows:

- Absence of vas deferens in male
- Biliary cirrhosis
- Chronic airway obstruction
- Chronic sinusitis
- Failure to thrive
- Gastrointestinal manifestations
- Nasal polyps
- Pancreatic insufficiency
- Recurrent lung infection

Osteopathic treatment is used to support the body's attempt to compensate and respond to the syndrome. Tissue strains and restriction of the facial and respiratory mechanics are often present in children with cystic fibrosis. OMT aims to restore the mechanics decrease any obstructions of sinus drainage in the head and neck and optimize the neuroendocrine immune system, pulmonary lymphatic function, and respiratory mechanics. Techniques that exacerbate hyperinflation of the lungs should be avoided.[142]

CHILDHOOD OBESITY

Obesity in early life continues to grow as a public health challenge. This disease is linked with numerous long-term health problems and is associated with the emergence of comorbidities formerly seen in older populations, such as hypertension, type 2 diabetes mellitus, and nonalcoholic fatty liver disease, among others. Childhood obesity is increasing in prevalence, such that approximately 40% of today's young adults experienced obesity or overweight before leaving primary school.[143,144]

This poses a significant threat to the lifelong health of children and their communities.

The etiology of this disease is multifactorial, including genetic and psychosocial causes, but the most common cause is a positive energy balance due to caloric intake in excess of caloric expenditure. Therefore, lifestyle interventions, including dietary modifications and increased physical activity, remain the cornerstone of treatment.[145] The osteopathic pediatrician is uniquely situated to address this multifactorial disease through the five models of osteopathic care. With movement being a central component of optimizing the health of children experiencing obesity or overweight, OSE and utilization of OMT may help facilitate the necessary increase in physical activity.

CONCLUSION

New challenges are presenting themselves in pediatrics.

- The number of multiple births has risen as a product of infertility interventions, thus producing challenges that result from two or more fetuses sharing the uterus.
- The following are also being identified:
  - Autistic spectrum disorders
  - Behavioral issues
  - Developmental delay
  - Infectious disease
  - Learning difficulties
  - Lifestyle-related diseases
  - Psychiatric Illnesses
- As many major adult disease processes likely have roots in childhood, optimizing the earliest years of health is critical.

The future of pediatrics will focus heavily on primary care and preventive medicine.

Lifestyle diseases that affect the majority of the population can be prevented or minimized by providing anticipatory guidance in epidemiologically important areas such as:

- Dietary counseling for control of obesity, hypercholesterolemia, and metabolic syndromes
- Drug, alcohol, and tobacco avoidance
- Accident prevention

Osteopathic structural diagnostics and OMT can be significant modalities for primary, secondary, and tertiary disease prevention in the pediatric population. Although one systematic review of OMT for various pediatric conditions demonstrated the need for more high-quality, robust randomized clinical trials to assess the effectiveness of OMT,[146] another systematic review and meta-analysis demonstrated that OMT reduces duration of hospitalization and costs in preterm infants.[147] As primary care physicians viewing the patient from the osteopathic lens of the four tenets and five models of osteopathic care, osteopathic pediatricians are ideally positioned to have a positive impact on the health and well-being of their patients.

Osteopathic pediatricians are responsible for systematically investigating and documenting applications of osteopathic concepts and principles during the early stages of child development. Osteopathic treatment of the child will continue to be comprehensive as physicians strive to optimize childhood health, wellness, and growth in their communities.

REFERENCES

1. Bomboy RP. *The Golden Anniversary History of the American College of Osteopathic Pediatricians, 1940–1990.* American College of Osteopathic Pediatricians; 1990.
2. Still AT. *Autobiography of A.T. Still.* American Academy of Osteopathy; 1908.
3. Still AT. *Osteopathy: Research and Practice.* Eastland Press; 1992. Originally published in Journal Printing Co.; 1910.
4. Millard FP, ed. *Poliomyelitis.* Journal Printing Co.; 1918.
5. Watson JO, Percival EN. Pneumonia research in children at Los Angeles County Osteopathic Hospital. *J Am Osteopath Assoc.* 1939;39(3):153–159.
6. Arbuckle BE. Effects of uterine forces upon the fetus. *J Am Osteopath Assoc.* 1954;53:499–508.
7. Whiting LM. Can the length of labor be shortened by osteopathic treatment. *J Am Osteopath Assoc.* 1911;11:917–921.
8. Arbuckle BE. *The Selected Writings of Beryl E. Arbuckle, D.O., F.A.C.O.P.* The National Osteopathic Institute and the Cerebral Palsy Foundation; 1977. Currently available through American Academy of Osteopathy.
9. Barnes M. Osteopathic treatment of infants. *J Am Osteopath Assoc.* 1941; 40:242–243.
10. Upledger JE. The relationship of craniosacral examination findings in grade school children with developmental problems. *J Am Osteopath Assoc.* 1978;77:738–754.
11. Frymann VM. Learning difficulties of children viewed in the light of the osteopathic concept. *J Am Osteopath Assoc.* 1976;76:46–61.
12. Woods RH, Woods JM. A physical finding related to psychiatric disorders. *J Am Osteopath Assoc.* 1961;60:988–993.
13. Woods RH. Structural normalization in infants and children with particular reference to disturbances of the central nervous system. *J Am Osteopath Assoc.* 1973;72(9):903–908.
14. Wales AL. Teachings in the science of osteopathy. In: Sutherland WG, ed. *Transcribed Lectures of William Garner Sutherland, D.O.* Rudra Press; 1990.
15. Frymann VM. Relation of disturbances of craniosacral mechanisms to symptomatology of the newborn: study of 1250 infants. *J Am Osteopath Assoc.* 1966;65:1059–1075.
16. King HH, Frymann VM. *The Collected Papers of Viola M. Frymann: Legacy of Osteopathy to Children.* American Academy of Osteopathy; 1998.
17. King HH. Osteopathic manipulative treatment in prenatal care: evidence supporting improved outcomes and health policy implications. *J Am Osteopath Assoc.* 2000;10:25–33.
18. Behrman RE, Kliegman RM, Jenson HB, Nelson WE. *Nelson Textbook of Pediatrics.* 16th ed. WB Saunders; 2001.
19. Greenman PE. Structural abnormalities of children. *J Am Osteopath Assoc.* 1971;71:157.
20. Zago J, Amatuzzi F, Rondinel T, Matheus JP. Osteopathic manipulative treatment versus exercise program in runners with patellofemoral pain syndrome: a randomized controlled trial. *J Sport Rehabil.* 2020;30(4):609–618.
21. Brumm LF, Janiski C, Balawender JL, Feinstein A. Preventive osteopathic manipulative treatment and stress fracture incidence among collegiate cross-country athletes [published correction appears in J Am Osteopath Assoc. 2014 Apr;114(4):236]. *J Am Osteopath Assoc.* 2013;113(12):882–890.
22. Cerritelli F, Martelli M, Renzetti C, Pizzolorusso G, Cozzolino V, Barlafante G. Introducing an osteopathic approach into neonatology ward: the NE-O model. *Chiropr Man Therap.* 2014;22:18.
23. Frymann VF. The expanding osteopathic concept. In: *Academy of Applied Osteopathy Yearbook.* 1967; 67:50–62. Reprinted in King HH, ed. The Collected Papers of Viola M. Frymann, DO: Legacy of Osteopathy to Children. American Academy of Osteopathy; 1998.
24. Magoun HI Sr. *Osteopathy in the Cranial Field.* Journal Printing Co.; 1951.
25. Felitti VJ, Anda RF, Nordenberg D, et al. Relationship of childhood abuse and household dysfunction to many of the leading causes of death in adults: the adverse childhood experiences (ACE) study. *Am J Prev Med.* 1998;14(4):245–258.
26. Shonkoff JP, Boyce WT, McEwen BS. Neuroscience, molecular biology, and the childhood roots of health disparities: building a new framework for health promotion and disease prevention. *JAMA.* 2009;301(21): 2252–2259.
27. Garner AS, Shonkoff JP; Committee on Psychosocial Aspects of Child and Family Health; Committee on Early Childhood, Adoption, and Dependent Care; Section on Developmental and Behavioral Pediatrics. Early childhood adversity, toxic stress, and the role of the pediatrician: translating developmental science into lifelong health. *Pediatrics.* 2012;129(1):e224–e231.
28. Srivastav A, Strompolis M, Kipp C, Richard CL, Thrasher JF. Moderating the effects of adverse childhood experiences to address inequities in tobacco-related risk behaviors. *Health Promot Pract.* 2020;21(Suppl 1): 139S–147S.
29. Srivastav A, Richard C, McRell AS, Kaufman M. Safe neighborhoods and supportive communities protect children from the health effects of adverse childhood experiences (ACEs). *J Child Adolesc Trauma.* 2022;15(4): 977–986.
30. American Academy of Pediatrics. *Screening Tools: Pediatric Mental Health Minute Series.* Accessed April 2, 2024. https://www.aap.org/en/patient-care/mental-health-minute/screening-tools/
31. Kovacs M. *Children's Depression Inventory.* 2nd ed. (CDI-2). Multi-Health Systems; 2010.
32. Riglin L, Agha SS, Eyre O, et al. Investigating the validity of the strengths and difficulties questionnaire to assess ADHD in young adulthood. *Psychiatry Res.* 2021;301:113984.
33. Schmitt C, Koh J, Borzutzky C, Wu S. HEADSS UP: predictors for completion of adolescent psychosocial screening by inpatient pediatric residents. *Pediatrics.* 2021;147(3):566.
34. BC Children's Hospital. *HEADSS Assessment Guide.* Accessed April 2, 2024. http://www.bcchildrens.ca/youth-health-clinic-site/documents/headss20assessment20guide1.pdf
35. Contemporary Pediatrics. *HEEADSSS 3.0: The Psychosocial Interview for Adolescents Updated for a New Century Fueled by Media.* 2014. Accessed April 2, 2024. https://www.contemporarypediatrics.com/view/heeadsss-30-psychosocial-interview-adolescents-updated-new-century-fueled-media
36. Kip EC, Udedi M, Kulisewa K, Go VF, Gaynes BN. Barriers and facilitators to implementing the HEADSS psychosocial screening tool for adolescents living with HIV/AIDS in teen club program in Malawi: health care providers perspectives. *Int J Ment Health Syst.* 2022;16(1):8.
37. Magoun HI, ed. *Osteopathy in the Cranial Field.* 3rd ed. Journal Printing Co.; 1976.
38. Magoun HI Sr. Entrapment neuropathy in the cranium. *J Am Osteopath Assoc.* 1968;67:643–652.
39. Magoun HI Sr. Entrapment neuropathy of the central nervous system, part II. Cranial nerves I-IV, VI-VIII, XII. *J Am Osteopath Assoc.* 1968;67:779–787.
40. Magoun HI Sr. Entrapment neuropathy of the central nervous system, part III. Cranial nerves V, IX, X, XI. *J Am Osteopath Assoc.* 1968;67: 889–899.
41. Carreiro EJ. *An Osteopathic Approach to Children.* 2nd ed. Churchill Livingstone Elsevier; 2009:247.
42. Herring JA. *Tachdjian's Pediatric Orthopaedics: From the Texas Scottish Rite Hospital for Children.* Elsevier Health Sciences; 2013.
43. Galbusera F, Cina A, Panico M, Bassani T. The importance of curve severity, type and instrumentation strategy in the surgical correction of adolescent idiopathic scoliosis: an in silico clinical trial on 64 cases. *Sci Rep.* 2021;11(1):1799.

44. Block AM, Tamburini LM, Zeng F, et al. Surgical treatment of pediatric scoliosis: historical origins and review of current techniques. *Bioengineering (Basel)*. 2022;9(10):600.
45. Addai D, Zarkos J, Bowey AJ. Current concepts in the diagnosis and management of adolescent idiopathic scoliosis. *Childs Nerv Syst*. 2020; 36(6):1111–1119.
46. Lorente R, Mariscal G, Lorente A. Incidence of genitourinary anomalies in congenital scoliosis: systematic review and meta-analysis. *Eur Spine J*. 2023;32(11):3961–3969.
47. Lowe TG, Burwell RG, Dangerfield PH. Platelet calmodulin levels in adolescent idiopathic scoliosis (AIS): can they predict curve progression and severity? *Eur Spine J*. 2004;13(3):257–265.
48. Kindsfater K, Lowe T, Lawellin D, Weinstein D, Akmakjian J. Levels of platelet calmodulin for the prediction of progression and severity of adolescent idiopathic scoliosis. *J Bone Joint Surg*. 1994;76(8):1186–1192.
49. Lowe T, Lawellin D, Smith D, et al. Platelet calmodulin levels in adolescent idiopathic scoliosis. *Spine*. 2002;27(7):768–775.
50. Grothaus O, Molina D, Jacobs C, Talwalkar V, Iwinski H, Muchow R. Is it growth or natural history? Increasing spinal deformity after sanders stage 7 in females with AIS. *J Pediatr Orthop*. 2020;40(3):e176–e181.
51. Cheung CSK, Lee WTK, Tse YKT, et al. Abnormal peri-pubertal anthropometric measurements and growth pattern in adolescent idiopathic scoliosis: a study of 598 patients. *Spine (Phila Pa 1976)*. 2003;28(18): 2152–2157.
52. Somerville EW. Rotational lordosis; the development of single curve. *J Bone Joint Surg Br*. 1952;34-B(3):421–427.
53. Roaf R. The basic anatomy of scoliosis. *J Bone Joint Surg Br*. 1966;48(4): 786–792.
54. Fadzan M, Bettany-Saltikov J. Etiological theories of adolescent idiopathic scoliosis: past and present. *Open Orthop J*. 2017;11(1):1466–1489.
55. Brink RC, Schlösser TPC, van Stralen M, et al. Anterior-posterior length discrepancy of the spinal column in adolescent idiopathic scoliosis-a 3D CT study. *Spine J*. 2018;18(12):2259–2265.
56. Lao L-F, Shen J-X, Chen Z-G, Wang Y-P, Wen X-S, Qiu G-X. Uncoupled neuro-osseous growth in adolescent idiopathic scoliosis? A preliminary study of 90 adolescents with whole-spine three-dimensional magnetic resonance imaging. *Eur Spine J*. 2011;20(7):1081–1086.
57. Guo X, Chau WW, Chan YL, Cheng JCY. Relative anterior spinal overgrowth in adolescent idiopathic scoliosis. Results of disproportionate endochondral-membranous bone growth. *J Bone Joint Surg Br*. 2003;85(7):1026–1031.
58. Stokes IA, Mente PL, Iatridis JC, Farnum CE, Aronsson DD. Enlargement of growth plate chondrocytes modulated by sustained mechanical loading. *J Bone Joint Surg Am*. 2002;84(10):1842–1848.
59. Stokes IAF. Analysis and simulation of progressive adolescent scoliosis by biomechanical growth modulation. *Eur Spine J*. 2007;16(10):1621–1628.
60. Stokes IA, Burwell RG, Dangerfield PH; IBSE. Biomechanical spinal growth modulation and progressive adolescent scoliosis–a test of the 'vicious cycle' pathogenetic hypothesis: summary of an electronic focus group debate of the IBSE. *Scoliosis*. 2006;1:16.
61. Li C, Fu Q, Zhou Y, Yu H, Zhao G. Surgical treatment of severe congenital scoliosis with unilateral unsegmented bar by concave costovertebral joint release and both-ends wedge osteotomy via posterior approach. *Eur Spine J*. 2012;21(3):498–505.
62. Rrecaj-Malaj S, Beqaj S, Krasniqi V, Qorolli M, Tufekcievski A. Outcome of 24 weeks of combined schroth and pilates exercises on Cobb angle, angle of trunk rotation, chest expansion, flexibility and quality of life in adolescents with idiopathic scoliosis. *Med Sci Monit Basic Res*. 2020;26: e920449.
63. McMaster ME, Lee AJ, Burwell RG. Physical activities of patients with adolescent idiopathic scoliosis (AIS): preliminary longitudinal case-control study historical evaluation of possible risk factors. *Scoliosis*. 2015;10:6.
64. Karimi MT, Rabczuk T. Scoliosis conservative treatment: a review of literature. *J Craniovertebr Junction Spine*. 2018;9(1):3–8.
65. Feely RA, Kapraun HE. Progressive infantile scoliosis managed with osteopathic manipulative treatment. *J Am Osteopath Assoc*. 2017;117(9):595–599.
66. Micheloni GM, Novi M, Leigheb M, Giorgini A, Porcellini G, Tarallo L. Supracondylar fractures in children: management and treatment. *Acta Biomed*. 2021;92(S3):e2021015.
67. Williams AA, Lochner HV. Pediatric hand and wrist injuries. *Curr Rev Musculoskelet Med*. 2013;6(1):18–25.
68. Applebaum A, Nessim A, Cho W. Overview and spinal implications of leg length discrepancy: narrative review. *Clin Orthop Surg*. 2021;13(2): 127–134.
69. Beal MC. A review of the short-leg problem. In: Peterson B, ed. *Posture Balance and Imbalance*. American Academy of Osteopathy; 1983:26–42.
70. Brady RJ, Dean JB, Skinner TM, Gross MT. Limb length inequality: clinical implications for assessment and intervention. *J Orthop Sports Phys Ther*. 2003;33(5):221–234.
71. Mulpuri K, Song KM, Goldberg MJ, Sevarino K. Detection and nonoperative management of pediatric developmental dysplasia of the hip in infants up to six months of age. *J Am Acad Orthop Surg*. 2015;23(3): 202–205.
72. Vaquero-Picado A, González-Morán G, Garay EG, Moraleda L. Developmental dysplasia of the hip: update of management. *EFORT Open Rev*. 2019;4(9):548–556.
73. Laine JC, Martin BD, Novotny SA, Kelly DM. Role of advanced imaging in the diagnosis and management of active Legg-Calvé-Perthes disease. *J Am Acad Orthop Surg*. 2018;26(15):526–536.
74. Peck D. Slipped capital femoral epiphysis: diagnosis and management. *Am Fam Physician*. 2010;82(3):258–262.
75. Xu G, Spoerri M, Rutz E. Surgical treatment options for septic arthritis of the hip in children. *Afr J Paediatr Surg*. 2016;13(1):1–5.
76. Leroux J, Abu Amara S, Lechevallier J. Legg-Calvé-Perthes disease. *Orthop Traumatol Surg Res*. 2018;104(1S):S107–S112.
77. Dustmann HO. Atiologie und pathogenese der epiphysennekrose im kindesalter am beispiel der hüfte (etiology and pathogenesis of epiphyseal necrosis in childhood as exemplified with the hip). *Z Orthop Ihre Grenzgeb*. 1996;134(5):407–412.
78. Carreiro EJ. *An Osteopathic Approach to Children*. 2nd ed. Churchill Livingstone Elsevier. 2009:260–261.
79. Dobbe AM, Gibbons PJ. Common paediatric conditions of the lower limb. *J Paediatr Child Health*. 2017;53(11):1077–1085.
80. Nguyen N-A, Klein G, Dogbey G, McCourt JB, Mehlman CT. Operative versus nonoperative treatments for Legg-Calvé-Perthes disease: a meta-analysis. *J Pediatr Orthop*. 2012;32(7):697–705.
81. Hardesty CK, Liu RW, Thompson GH. The role of bracing in Legg-Calve-Perthes disease. *J Pediatr Orthop*. 2011;31(2 Suppl):S178–S181.
82. Loder RT. Slipped capital femoral epiphysis. *Am Fam Physician*. 1998; 57(9):2135–2142, 2148–2150.
83. Gholve PA, Cameron DB, Millis MB. Slipped capital femoral epiphysis update. *Curr Opin Pediatr*. 2009;21(1):39–45.
84. Loder RT, Richards BS, Shapiro PS, Reznick LR, Aronson DD. Acute slipped capital femoral epiphysis: the importance of physeal stability. *J Bone Joint Surg Am*. 1993;75(8):1134–1140.
85. Loder RT. Slipped capital femoral epiphysis in children. *Curr Opin Pediatr*. 1995;7(1):95–97.
86. Carreiro EJ. *An Osteopathic Approach to Children*. 2nd ed. Churchill Livingstone Elsevier; 2009:260.
87. Boerum DHV, Sangeorzan BJ. Biomechanics and pathophysiology of flat foot. *Foot Ankle Clin*. 2003;8(3):419–430.
88. Pavone V, Vescio A, Valenti F, Sapienza M, Sessa G, Testa G. Growing pains: what do we know about etiology? A systematic review. *World J Orthop*. 2019;10(4):192–205.
89. Lehman PJ, Carl RL. Growing pains. *Sports Health*. 2017;9(2):132–138.
90. Firshein RN. *Reversing Asthma*. Warner Books; 1996.
91. Jamal A, Alsabea A, Tarakmeh M, Safar A. Etiology, diagnosis, complications, and management of acute otitis media in children. *Cureus*. 2022; 14(8):e28019.
92. Gaddey HL, Wright MT, Nelson TN. Otitis media: rapid evidence review. *Am Fam Physician*. 2019;100(6):350–356.
93. Galbreath WO. Acute otitis media: including its postural and manipulative treatment. *JAOA*. 1929;28:377–379.
94. Robinson JL. Paediatrics: how to manage pharyngitis in an era of increasing antimicrobial resistance. *Drugs Context*. 2021;10:2020-11-6.
95. Kundi NA, Mehmood T, Abid O. Application of mouth gag and temporomandibular joint pain and trismus in tonsillectomy. *J Coll Physicians Surg Pak*. 2015;25(4):268–270.

96. Maini S, Osborne JE, Fadl HMS, Spyridakou C, Ogunyemi L, Hill P. Temporomandibular joint dysfunction following tonsillectomy. *Clin Otolaryngol Allied Sci*. 2002;27(1):57–60.
97. Meissner HC. Bronchiolitis. *Principles and Practice of Pediatric Infectious Diseases*. 2018:234–237.e1.
98. Panitch HB. Bronchiolitis in infants. *Curr Opin Pediatr*. 2001;13(3): 256–260.
99. Belcastro MR, Backes CR, Chila AG. Bronchiolitis: a pilot study of osteopathic manipulative treatment, bronchodilators, and other therapy. *J Am Osteopath Assoc*. 1984;83(9):672–676.
100. Kattan M. Epidemiologic evidence of increased airway reactivity in children with a history of bronchiolitis. *J Pediatr*. 1999;135(2 Pt 2):8–13.
101. Bertrand P, Aranibar H, Castro E, Sanchez I. Efficacy of nebulized epinephrine versus salbutamol in hospitalized infants with bronchiolitis. *Pediatr Pulmonol*. 2001;31(4):284–288.
102. Johnson CC, Chandran A, Havstad S, et al. US childhood asthma incidence rate patterns from the echo consortium to identify high-risk groups for primary prevention. *JAMA Pediatr*. 2021;175(9):919–927.
103. Brusasco V, Crimini E, Pellegrino R. Airway hyperresponsiveness in asthma: not just a matter of airway inflammation. *Thorax*. 1998;53: 992–998.
104. Gdalevich M, Mimouni D, Mimouni M. Breast-feeding and the risk of bronchial asthma in childhood: a systematic review with meta-analysis of prospective studies. *J Pediatr*. 2001;139(2):261–265.
105. Nelson KE, Glonek T, eds. *Somatic Dysfunction in Osteopathic Family Medicine*. Lippincott Williams & Wilkins; 2007.
106. Pottenger FM. *Symptoms of Visceral Disease*. 5th ed. Mosby; 1938.
107. Guiney PA, Chou R, Vianna A, Lovenheim J. Effects of osteopathic manipulative treatment on pediatric patients with asthma: a randomized controlled trial. *J Am Osteopath Assoc*. 2005;105(1):7–12.
108. Brady NS. Efficacy of a standardized osteopathic manipulative therapy protocol on pulmonary function and symptomatology in moderate persistent asthmatic children. *Ann Allergy Asthma Immunol*. 2010;105(5): A36–A37.
109. Waller JD. CDC and AAP just changed developmental milestone guidelines for the first time in decades. Motherly. February 11, 2022. Updated January 17, 2023. Accessed April 2, 2024. https://www.mother.ly/health-wellness/cdc-aap-developmental-milestones/#:~:text=Adding%20checklists%20for%20ages%2015,your%20attention%2C%20age%204%20months
110. Centers for Disease Control and Prevention. CDC's Developmental Milestones. 2023. Accessed April 1, 2024. https://www.cdc.gov/ncbddd/actearly/milestones/index.html
111. Zubler JM, Wiggins LD, Macias MM, et al. Evidence-informed milestones for developmental surveillance tools. *Pediatrics*. 2022;149(3):e2021052138.
112. Frymann VM, Carney RE, Springall P. Effect of osteopathic medical management on neurological development in children. *J Am Osteopath Assoc*. 1992;92:729–744.
113. Walker WA, Durie PR, Hamilton JR, Barr RG. Colic and gas. In: Walker WA, Durie PR, Hamilton JR, eds. *Pediatric Gastrointestinal Disease: Pathophysiology, Diagnosis and Management*. Decker; 1991:55–61.
114. Carreiro EJ. *An Osteopathic Approach to Children*. 2nd ed. Churchill Livingstone Elsevier; 2009:234.
115. Carreiro EJ. *An Osteopathic Approach to Children*. 2nd ed. Churchill Livingstone Elsevier; 2009:235.
116. Eichenwald EC; Committee on Fetus and Newborn, American Academy of Pediatrics. Apnea of prematurity. *Pediatrics*. 2016;137(1).
117. Henderson-Smart DJ. The effect of gestational age on the incidence and duration of recurrent apnoea in newborn babies. *Aust Paediatr J*. 1981;17(4):273–276.
118. Williamson M, Poorun R, Hartley C. Apnoea of prematurity and neurodevelopmental outcomes: current understanding and future prospects for research. *Front Pediatr*. 2021;9:755677.
119. Pierrat V, Marchand-Martin L, Arnaud C, et al. Neurodevelopmental outcome at 2 years for preterm children born at 22 to 34 weeks' gestation in France in 2011: EPIPAGE-2 cohort study. *BMJ*. 2017;358:j3448.
120. Stoll BJ, Hansen NI, Bell EF, et al. Trends in care practices, morbidity, and mortality of extremely preterm neonates, 1993–2012. *JAMA*. 2015;314(10):1039–1051.
121. Jarjour IT. Neurodevelopmental outcome after extreme prematurity: a review of the literature. *Pediatr Neurol*. 2015;52(2):143–152.
122. Balain M, Oddie S. Management of apnoea and bradycardia in the newborn. *Paediatr Child Heal*. 2014;24:17–22.
123. Stephens BE, Vohr BR. Neurodevelopmental outcome of the premature infant. *Pediatr Clin North Am*. 2009;56(3):631–646, Table of Contents.
124. Janvier A, Khairy M, Kokkotis A, Cormier C, Messmer D, Barrington KJ. Apnea is associated with neurodevelopmental impairment in very low birth weight infants. *J Perinatol*. 2004;24(12):763–768.
125. Poets CF. Apnea of prematurity: what can observational studies tell us about pathophysiology? *Sleep Med*. 2010;11(7):701–707.
126. Carreiro EJ. *An Osteopathic Approach to Children*. 2nd ed. Churchill Livingstone Elsevier; 2009:94.
127. Carreiro EJ. *An Osteopathic Approach to Children*. 2nd ed. Churchill Livingstone Elsevier; 2009:218.
128. Araki T, Yokota H, Morita A. Pediatric traumatic brain injury: characteristic features, diagnosis, and management. *Neurol Med Chir (Tokyo)*. 2017;57(2):82–93.
129. Nadel F, Corwin D, Jacobstien C, Lavelle J, Scribano P. Emergency Department Clinical Pathway for the Evaluation/Treatment of Children with Acute Head Trauma. Children's Hospital of Philadelphia. 2010. Updated March, 2023. Accessed April 3, 2024. https://www.chop.edu/clinical-pathway/head-trauma-acute-clinical-pathway
130. Cerebral Palsy. National Institute of Neurological Disorders and Stroke. Accessed April 3, 2024. https://www.ninds.nih.gov/health-information/disorders/cerebral-palsy
131. Carreiro EJ. *An Osteopathic Approach to Children*. 2nd ed. Churchill Livingstone Elsevier; 2009:290–293.
132. Carreiro EJ. *An Osteopathic Approach to Children*. 2nd ed. Churchill Livingstone Elsevier; 2009:296–297.
133. Duncan B, McDonough-Means S, Worden K, Schnyer R, Andrews J, Meaney FJ. Effectiveness of osteopathy in the cranial field and myofascial release versus acupuncture as complementary treatment for children with spastic cerebral palsy: a pilot study. *J Am Osteopath Assoc*. 2008;108(10):559–570.
134. Wyatt K, Edwards V, Franck L, et al. Cranial osteopathy for children with cerebral palsy: a randomised controlled trial. *Arch Dis Child*. 2011;96(6):505–512.
135. Carreiro EJ. *An Osteopathic Approach to Children*. 2nd ed. Churchill Livingstone Elsevier; 2009:230.
136. Carreiro EJ. *An Osteopathic Approach to Children*. 2nd ed. Churchill Livingstone Elsevier; 2009:232.
137. Carreiro EJ. *An Osteopathic Approach to Children*. 2nd ed. Churchill Livingstone Elsevier; 2009:233.
138. Carreiro EJ. *An Osteopathic Approach to Children*. 2nd ed. Churchill Livingstone Elsevier; 2009:237.
139. Carreiro EJ. *An Osteopathic Approach to Children*. 2nd ed. Churchill Livingstone Elsevier; 2009:236.
140. Carreiro EJ. *An Osteopathic Approach to Children*. 2nd ed. Churchill Livingstone Elsevier; 2009:236–237.
141. Viegelmann GC, Dorji J, Guo X, Lim HY. Approach to diarrhoeal disorders in children. *Singapore Med J*. 2021;62(12):623–629.
142. Carreiro EJ. *An Osteopathic Approach to Children*. 2nd ed. Churchill Livingstone Elsevier; 2009:221.
143. Ogden CL, Fryar CD, Martin CB, et al. Trends in obesity prevalence by race and Hispanic origin-1999–2000 to 2017–2018. *JAMA*. 2020;324(12):1208–1210.
144. Cunningham SA, Hardy ST, Jones R, Ng C, Kramer MR, Narayan KMV. Changes in the incidence of childhood obesity. *Pediatrics*. 2022; 150(2):e2021053708.
145. Kumar S, Kelly AS. Review of childhood obesity: from epidemiology, etiology, and comorbidities to clinical assessment and treatment. *Mayo Clin Proc*. 2017;92(2):251–265.
146. Posadzki P, Lee MS, Ernst E. Osteopathic manipulative treatment for pediatric conditions: a systematic review. *Pediatrics*. 2013;132(1):140–152.
147. Lanaro D, Ruffini N, Manzotti A, Lista G. Osteopathic manipulative treatment showed reduction of length of stay and costs in preterm infants: a systematic review and meta-analysis. *Medicine (Baltimore)*. 2017;96(12):e6408.

68 Osteopathic Considerations in General Internal Medicine

MAXWELL ROUSE ▪ MINDY A. CHILMAN MCCOMB ▪ BRIAN E. KAUFMAN

KEY CONCEPTS

- Physicians who practice internal medicine are known as internists, and most general internists practice as primary care providers or hospitalists.
- A distinction of internal medicine is the emphasis on the diagnosis and management of complex medical problems.
- Although osteopathic internists have much in common with their MD colleagues, there are cultural differences between the two professions.
- When complex systems fail, they present as complex health problems. One set of signs and symptoms may represent more than one disease process.
- Second to musculoskeletal problems, osteopathic manipulative treatment's (OMT) greatest potential application may be for the treatment of infectious disease.

INTRODUCTION

General internal medicine is the clinical specialty that deals with complex diseases and "internal" organ system disorders. Physicians who practice internal medicine are known as internists, and most general internists practice as primary care physicians or hospitalists. While family medicine offers cradle-to-grave care (see Chapter 66 Osteopathic Considerations in Family Medicine), most internists focus on adult medicine. A small number of internists have completed a combined internal medicine and pediatrics residency program, and of these, 82% report seeing both adults and children in clinical practice.[1] Internists are dedicated to disease prevention and diagnosis as well as the management of both acute and chronic disorders. A distinction of internal medicine is an emphasis on the diagnosis and management of complex medical problems. This requires an in-depth knowledge of diagnostics, pathophysiologic processes, and disease interactions. The emphasis within general internal medicine is on depth of knowledge on a broad scale.

The residency training period for general internal medicine is 3 years. The American College of Osteopathic Internists (ACOI) is the organization representing internal medicine within the osteopathic profession, whereas the American College of Physicians (ACP) is the organization representing allopathic internal medicine. The ACOI was formed in 1923 for those osteopathic physicians primarily interested in the diagnosis and treatment of diseases of the internal organs. Internal medicine is a rapidly growing specialty within the osteopathic profession. In 1984, only 4.7% of practicing DOs self-identified as general internal medicine specialists, but by 2022, the percentage had grown to 19%.[2] Internists practice in a wide range of clinical settings, including hospitals, offices, home care, hospice care, subacute rehabilitation, and long-term care.

Within internal medicine, there are a number of subspecialty areas. Most internists who subspecialize have specialty-based practices, although some do function as primary care physicians. One exception is geriatric medicine, which is typically practiced as a primary care subspecialty similar to pediatrics. The ACOI subspecialty sections include:

- Allergy/immunology
- Cardiology
- Critical care medicine
- Endocrinology
- Gastroenterology
- Geriatric medicine/palliative care medicine
- Hematology/oncology
- Infectious diseases
- Nephrology
- Pulmonary diseases/sleep medicine
- Rheumatology

An internist who manages patients primarily in the hospital is called a hospitalist, although not all hospitalists are internists. The term hospitalist was coined in 1996. The number of practicing adult hospitalists has grown by more than 50% from 2012 to 2019.[3] See Section XI: Chapters 70 to 82 for osteopathic considerations within selected subspecialties.

DISTINCTIVENESS OF OSTEOPATHIC INTERNAL MEDICINE

Osteopathic internists have much in common with their MD colleagues. They see the same types of patients, read the same textbooks, journals, and medical literature; they use the same laboratory and radiologic diagnostic procedures and prescribe the same medications. DO and MD internists practice alongside each other and have collaborative practice arrangements. They both follow the same clinical practice guidelines and community standards of practice. The standard medical management of heart failure, hypertension, diabetes, pneumonia, chronic obstructive pulmonary disease, and other disorders is essentially the same for MD and DO internists. This commonality has recently been affirmed by the move to a single graduate medical education accreditation system.[4]

However, there are distinct differences between MD and DO internists and cultural differences between the two professions. Graduates of osteopathic medical schools are more likely to choose a primary care specialty. Osteopathic tradition asserts that to be a good subspecialist, one must first be a good generalist who can readily deal with "whole person" concepts. Osteopathic internists understand that problems within one body system impact the whole body. There is also evidence that osteopathic principles

TABLE 68.1

Axioms from the Osteopathic Toolbox

Axiom	Comments
Find it, fix it, and leave it alone.	This is an axiom attributed to Dr. Still. It stresses the importance of identifying the cause of the problem (find it) and then developing a rational treatment plan (fix it). The last part (leave it alone) recognizes the body's inherent capacity for healing and the need to give the body time to heal. Each treatment plan needs an adequate therapeutic trial period to see if it will work. It is also a warning against overtreatment or changing the care plan too frequently. Taken together, the axiom lays out a simple orderly process for patient care.
You treat what you find.	Dr. Still taught his students that the body itself shows you what to do and what needs to be done. Still illustrated this by telling his class he was going to draw a pig, but actually drew a turkey. Then he asked, "How many of you diagnosed a pig?" The axiom is a warning against being misled by previously assigned diagnostic labels and encourages healthy skepticism of accepted conventions.
If you talk with your patients long enough, they will tell you what is wrong with them.	This axiom is attributed to Dr. Max Gutenshon, who was known for his diagnostic abilities. He believed patients have an inherent sense of what is wrong with them. Dr. Gutenshon said he would find out about the patient's family, encourage a conversation, and then something they would say would ring a bell in his knowledge and he would know what was wrong with them.
First, try to blame it on the medications.	Medications frequently cause side effects and adverse reactions. Whenever a patient presents with a new medical problem, always look at the medication list for the cause. Because the body is constantly changing, the proximity of starting a medication does not always correlate with the development of adverse side effects. Medication intolerance can develop many months or even years after it was initially started.

Noll DR, Sthole HJ, Cavalieri TA. Axioms, osteopathic culture, and a perspective from geriatric medicine. *J Am Osteopath Assoc.* 2013;113(12):908–915.

influence patient–physician communication styles.[5,6] Osteopathic principles and practices essentially constitute a toolbox of concepts useful for enhancing the application of medical knowledge to improve patient care, principles that make the application of clinical knowledge more effective. Many of these principles in the osteopathic toolbox are crystallized into easily remembered axioms that are a rich aspect of the osteopathic profession's culture and heritage.[7] Examples of osteopathic axioms useful in patient care are listed in Table 68.1. Because osteopathic medicine is founded on a philosophy instead of specific manipulation techniques, how distinctive an individual DO internist is from their MD counterpart depends upon how well the internist implements osteopathic principles in day-to-day practice. Osteopathic principles are not exclusive secrets known only to DOs, but tend to be universal truths available to everyone. Thus, it is possible for an MD internist to also practice osteopathically. Osteopathic philosophy is discussed further in Chapter 1 Philosophy of Osteopathic Medicine.

Another distinctive aspect of osteopathic internists is training in palpation of the neuromusculoskeletal system. When knowledgeably applied, utilization of palpation in diagnosis and treatment reflects the physician's sensitivity to both the osteopathic philosophy and its concepts (see Chapter 1). Much can be discerned from touching the patient during a physical exam. Muscle tone in Parkinson disease is distinctly different than normal. Individuals with pyelonephritis have muscle tenderness over the costovertebral angles. Chapman reflex points have a sensitivity and specificity of 69% for acute pneumonia.[8] Inflammation in an organ frequently causes a viscerosomatic reflex manifesting as tissue texture changes and tenderness in the neuromusculoskeletal system. These changes provide valuable diagnostic clues.[9] (For a more detailed discussion, see Chapter 43 on Chapman reflex points and viscerosomatic reflexes.) The value of an internist knowing the musculoskeletal tissue texture changes for diagnostic purposes is summed up by Dr. Max Gutensohn, one of the profession's early internists whose diagnostic skills were legendary.[10]

"I always felt that with my training, I could diagnose some diseases just by touching the patient—by the referral from the organ to the spine…I could feel it by the somatic process in the back. I used manipulation for diagnosis on about 20% of my patients."[10]

MANAGING PATIENTS WITH COMPLEX PROBLEMS

In the clinical setting, patients often present with signs and symptoms that are neither obvious nor classic (i.e., they are not found in the textbooks). From an osteopathic principle perspective, the human body is analogous to a complex machine capable of self-regulation and healing. Dr. Still's writings are filled with imagery of the osteopathic physician as a master mechanic who reasons how the machine works in all its many complex systems. When complex systems fail, they present as complex health problems. One set of signs and symptoms may represent more than one disease process. For the internist, this is the rule rather than the exception. An individual with hypertensive cardiovascular disease often presents with multiple comorbidities such as diabetes, emphysema due to smoking, and a variety of neck and shoulder-related complaints associated with somatic dysfunction. Each condition interdependently affects the others. The osteopathic internist's role is to understand and knowledgeably deal with these relationships.

How do internists best manage complexity? A key principle for managing complexity is crystallized by Dr. Still's axiom, "We know that if we ever know the whole, we must first know the parts." This is superficially similar to methodologic reductionism, which is the scientific effort to understand complex systems by systematically reducing them to ever simpler component parts. Reductionism has been criticized for its tendency toward fragmentation and loss of context; the offered solutions in the literature are to remember organizing principles or holism.[11,12] Thus, reductionism fails when the goal of knowing the whole is forgotten, which is the central point of the axiom, "We know that if we ever know the whole, we must first know the parts."

	Comments
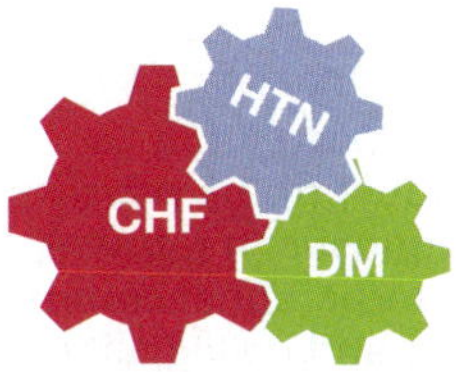	The patient presents with a wide range of symptoms and problems, often representing more than one medical problem.
	The internist separates out the problems for clarity and considers each. This is often represented by an active problem list.
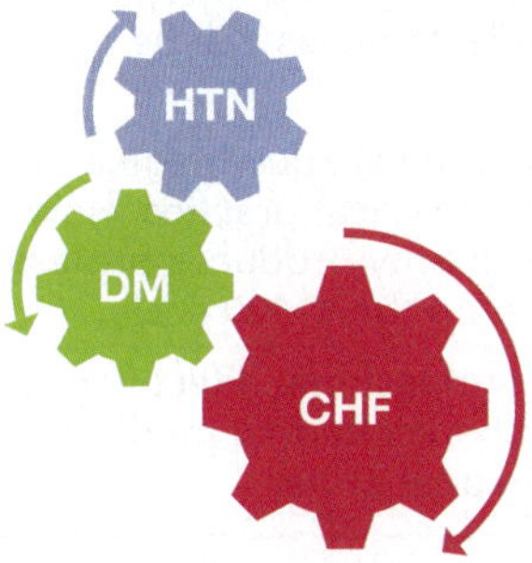	Then, like a master engineer, the internist puts the pieces together and develops a treatment plan that complements the whole. The treatment plan should minimize side effects and potential complications.

Figure 68.1. Managing complex multisystem disorders. HTN, hypertension; DM, diabetes mellitus type II; CHF, congestive heart failure.

A useful tool for breaking complex problems down into "the parts" is the problem-oriented medical record, which was developed by Dr. LL Weed.[13] The centerpiece of the problem-oriented medical record is the problem list.[14] To know the parts, the internist assesses the patient's presenting complaints, symptoms, history, physical findings, and diagnostic tests to create an active problem list. From the problem list, it is a relatively easy step to develop a treatment for each problem that considers how each problem and its treatment affect the others. In other words, the internist systematically breaks the presenting problem(s) down into its component parts, generating a hierarchical problem list. A determination is then made as to how each element relates to the total picture. Some problems will carry more weight than others. By taking this systematic approach, a rational treatment plan can be developed that works for the patient as a whole (Fig. 68.1). Active medical problem lists should be maintained by regularly removing inactive and resolved problems so as not to clutter up the picture with irrelevant information.

When developing a care plan, a series of circumstantial questions should always be kept in mind. These questions are summarized in Figure 68.2.

1. How is each problem affecting the others? In a laboratory experiment, scientists strive to create simple or "perfect" problems in which all the variables are eliminated except for the one under study. However, in clinical practice, physicians must deal with "imperfect" problems which have many confounding variables. For example, an acute worsening of chronic kidney disease will promote fluid retention and trigger congestive heart failure (CHF) in an individual with pre-existing left ventricular dysfunction due to prior myocardial infarction. Worsening CHF often leads to hypoperfusion, further impacting kidney function and setting up a fatal feedback loop. When developing a treatment plan, the internist must consider how renal disease affects the patient's heart disease and vice versa.
2. How does the treatment affect each problem? It is rare for a medication to have only one local effect. A useful drug for one problem may have harmful consequences for another. For example, antimuscarinic medications for bladder spasms work well for urge incontinence, but worsen cognitive function and can trigger acute confusion in patients with dementia.
3. How does the treatment affect the patient? Treatments of all types do more than alter biologic systems and modify faulty physiology. They also have side effects that may impact the patient. For example, many selective serotonin reuptake inhibitors help depression, but in some individuals cause a vague dizzy sensation, which the patient may find intolerable. Few patients will comply with a treatment plan if it causes them discomfort.
4. How does the patient affect the treatment? Treatment must be acceptable on both a personal and cultural level. Patients may reject blood products based on their religious beliefs or reasons of conscience. Too commonly, treatments are inaccessible to the patient because of costs. Dosing schedules affect compliance; once daily medications are likely to be taken more consistently than those requiring multiple doses a day.

The 1954 consensus statement on the osteopathic concept affirmed that the practice of medicine is both an art and a science. The science of medicine represents the sum of the physician's knowledge about basic sciences, diagnostics, treatments, and technical skills with procedures. The art of medicine involves the application of knowledge through interpersonal skills such as communication, bedside manner, and collegiality with other health care professionals. A physician's professional effectiveness can be described as the product of knowledge and interpersonal skills. Those who are strong in one but weak in the other are greatly

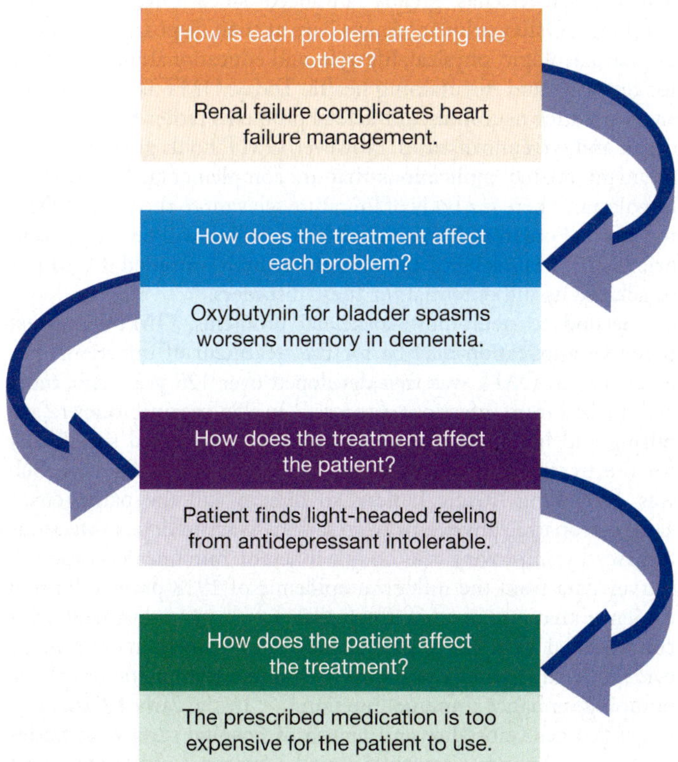

Figure 68.2. Considerations in complexity.

TABLE 68.2

A Model of Physician Effectiveness

Medical Knowledge 1–10 scale		Interpersonal Skills 1–10 scale		Professional Effectiveness 1–100 scale	Comments
	×		=		The professional effectiveness is the product of the physician's medical knowledge (basic science, diagnostic, treatment, and procedure skills) and the physician's interpersonal communication skills (communication, bedside manner, and collegiality).
10	×	1	=	10	If a physician has perfect medical knowledge but extremely poor interpersonal skills, then the physician's professional effectiveness will be low.
1	×	10	=	10	If a physician has low medical knowledge but perfect interpersonal skills, then the physician's professional effectiveness will also be low.
5	×	5	=	25	If a physician has modest medical knowledge and interpersonal skills, the physician's professional effectiveness will be moderately low.
7 6 8 7	× × × ×	7 8 5 8	= = = 	49 48 40 56	Most physicians develop both strong medical knowledge and interpersonal skills for the successful medical practice. However, having above-average scores for both only produces professional effectiveness scores in the midrange on the 1–100 scale.
9	×	9	=	81	To score in the upper quartile on the professional effectiveness scale, a physician needs to have both exceptional medical knowledge and exceptional interpersonal skills.

diminished in their professional effectiveness. Only those who excel in both make exceptional physicians. This concept is explored in Table 68.2.

OSTEOPATHIC MANIPULATIVE TREATMENT IN THE PRACTICE OF INTERNAL MEDICINE

Medical science has greatly advanced since OMT was first developed. Osteopathic internists have at their disposal a full range of pharmacologic, physical, lifestyle, and educational interventions for restoring and maintaining health. Today, OMT is most extensively used for neuromusculoskeletal problems rather than internal organ and systemic diseases. However, OMT holds great potential for many related applications that are complementary to conventional care. There is a body of literature relevant to the use of OMT for internal organ and systemic diseases, which will be reviewed in brief. More basic science and clinical research is needed if OMT is to achieve its full potential for these disorders.

Second to neuromusculoskeletal problems, OMT's greatest potential application may be for the treatment of infectious diseases. When OMT was first developed over 125 years ago, most people died from infectious diseases.[15] In that preantibiotic era, rib raising and lymphatic pump techniques were created specifically for the treatment of pneumonia.[16,17] In 1907 while Paul Ehrlich was developing "magic bullets" to directly kill the pathogens,[18] early osteopathic physicians were seeking ways to defeat infectious diseases by improving the body's inherent immune response.[19,20] Survey data from the influenza epidemic of 1918 provide limited evidence that osteopathic treatment was an improvement over conventional care. Early mechanistic studies in humans provide evidence that rhythmic pumping techniques (lymphatic or splenic pumping) enhance immune function.[21–24] In the early 1930s, clinical outcomes (mortality and length of hospital stay) were better in the Los Angeles County Hospital segregated osteopathic unit relative to the larger allopathic unit.[25]

Immobility in the elderly is associated with a ninefold increased risk of death from pneumonia,[26] and the simple act of getting a patient with pneumonia out of bed for 20 minutes from the first day of hospitalization shortens their length of hospital stay.[27] OMT in the acute care setting has the potential to reverse the effects of immobility. Bed-bound patients who cannot get out of bed can have body parts and fluids mobilized using lymphatic pump and other osteopathic manipulative techniques.

Pneumonia is the classic example of an infectious disease responsive to OMT and has the best evidence. At the beginning of the antibiotic era, Kline compared the outcomes of children hospitalized for respiratory tract infections who received OMT in the form of rib raising, antibiotics only, or both rib raising and antibiotics.[28] Those who received only rib raising had the longest mean length of hospital stay, those who received only antibiotics had a shorter mean length of stay, and those who received both rib raising and antibiotics had the shortest mean length of stay.[28] The differences were most striking in the subgroup hospitalized for pneumonia.[28] Interestingly, a similar pattern was shown in a recent rat model study. In the "no antibiotic and no lymphatic pump" group, no animals cleared *Streptococcus pneumoniae* from the lungs after 96 hours. However, in the "lymphatic pump only" group, 13% cleared the bacteria, in the "antibiotic only" group, 25% cleared the bacteria, and in the "lymphatic pump plus antibiotic" group, 63% cleared the bacteria.[29] These studies suggest that OMT has a potential role in boosting the effectiveness of antibiotics and enhancing antibiotic stewardship.[30]

Three separate clinical trials of OMT in the elderly hospitalized for pneumonia have consistently shown that OMT added to standard care using antibiotic therapy reduces the mean length of hospital stay relative to antibiotic use only.[31–33] These clinical trials suggest the magnitude of reduction in length of hospital stay is related to the duration of OMT treatment. In other words, when the length of stay is long, the patient receives more "doses" of OMT during the hospital stay and the magnitude of reduction is greater. If this proves to be correct, then OMT's best opportunity for improving outcomes is when hospital stay is likely to be long or when OMT can be extended to the subacute care setting where many seniors today complete their recovery.

OMT is well tolerated even in severely ill, frail elderly patients. In the Multicenter Osteopathic Pneumonia Study in the Elderly (MOPSE) trial, adverse side effects were limited to post-treatment musculoskeletal soreness for 22% of the conventional care plus OMT group, 7% of the conventional care plus light-touch group, and 7% of the conventional care only group.[31] Only one subject withdrew from the study because of musculoskeletal discomfort.

There is also evidence that OMT reduces mortality in pneumonia. In the pilot study, which enrolled 21 elderly patients hospitalized for pneumonia, there were no deaths in the OMT group and two deaths in the control group.[32] In the follow-up study enrolling 58 individuals, one person in the OMT group and three persons in the control group died.[33] In the MOPSE trial, of 318 patients who received the protocol as intended, no one died in the OMT group, three died in the light-touch group, and 8 died in the conventional care only control group, with statistical significance between the OMT and conventional care only groups.[31] Subgroup analysis shows that seniors hospitalized for pneumonia aged 75 and older have the greatest reduction in mortality from OMT.[34] Subgroup analysis also shows that those with the higher severity of pneumonia (Pneumonia Severity Index of IV or V) have higher mortality reductions from OMT.[34] Those younger than 75 years who received OMT had the greatest reductions in length of hospital stay.[34] In other words, seniors with pneumonia who are very old or very ill are more likely to survive if they receive OMT, while younger seniors with pneumonia who receive OMT are likely to recover faster and leave the hospital sooner if they receive OMT.

ACKNOWLEDGMENTS

The authors and editors of this chapter would like to acknowledge the scholarly contributions of Dr. Donald R. Noll for prior editions of this chapter.

REFERENCES

1. Frohna JG, Melgar T, Mueller C, Borden S. Internal medicine-pediatrics residency training: current program trends and outcomes. *Acad Med.* 2004; 79(6):591–596.
2. *2022 Osteopathic Medical Profession Report.* American Osteopathic Association; 2022.
3. Lapps J, Flansbaum B, Leykum LK, Bischoff H, Howell E. Growth trends of the adult hospitalist workforce between 2012 and 2019. *J Hosp Med.* 2022;17(11):888–892.
4. Buser BR, Swartwout J, Gross C, Biszewski M. The single graduate medical education accreditation system. *J Am Osteopath Assoc.* 2015;115(4): 251–255.
5. Noll DR, Ginsberg T, Elahi A, Cavalieri TA. Effective patient-physician communication based on osteopathic philosophy in caring for elderly patients. *J Am Osteopath Assoc.* 2016;116(1):42–47.
6. Carey TS, Motyka TM, Garrett JM, Keller RB. Do osteopathic physicians differ in patient interaction from allopathic physicians? An empirically derived approach. *J Am Osteopath Assoc.* 2003;103(7):313–318.
7. Noll DR, Sthole HJ, Cavalieri TA. Axioms, osteopathic culture, and a perspective from geriatric medicine. *J Am Osteopath Assoc.* 2013;113(12): 908–915.
8. Washington K, Mosiello R, Venditto M, Simelaro J. Presence of Chapman reflex points in hospitalized patients with pneumonia. *J Am Osteopath Assoc.* 2003;103(10):479–483.
9. Dinnar U, Beal MC, Goodridge JP, et al. Classification of diagnostic tests used with osteopathic manipulation. *J Am Osteopath Assoc.* 1980;79(7):451–455.
10. Gutensohn MT, Blondefield P. *Dr. Max.* A. T. Sill University of Health Sciences; 2010.
11. Chummun H. Reductionism and holism in coronary heart disease and cardiac nursing. *Br J Nurs.* 2006;15(18):1017–1020.
12. Wolkenhauer O, Green S. The search for organizing principles as a cure against reductionism in systems medicine. *FEBS J.* 2013;280(23): 5938–5948.
13. Weed LL. Medical records that guide and teach. *N Engl J Med.* 1968; 278(12):652–657.
14. Wright A, Sittig DF, McGowan J, Ash JS, Weed LL. Bringing science to medicine: an interview with Larry Weed, inventor of the problem-oriented medical record. *J Am Med Inform Assoc.* 2014;21(6):964–968.
15. Yoshikawa TT. Antimicrobial resistance and aging: beginning of the end of the antibiotic era? *J Am Geriatr Soc.* 2002;50(7 suppl):S226–S229.
16. Noll DR, Degenhardt BF, Fossum C, Hensel K. Clinical and research protocol for osteopathic manipulative treatment of elderly patients with pneumonia. *J Am Osteopath Assoc.* 2008;108(9):508–516.
17. Miller CE. The specific cure of pneumonia. *J Am Osteopath Assoc.* 1927; 27(9):35–38.
18. Zaffiri L, Gardner J, Toledo-Pereyra LH. History of antibiotics. From salvarsan to cephalosporins. *J Invest Surg.* 2012;25(2):67–77.
19. Lane MA. *Dr. A. T. Still, Founder of Osteopathy.* The Osteopathic Publishing Co.; 1918.
20. Miller CE. Osteopathic treatment of acute infections by means of the lymphatics. *J Am Osteopath Assoc.* 1920;19:494–499.
21. Whiting CA. Investigations of the opsonic index. *J Am Osteopath Assoc.* 1912;12(9):20–21.
22. Castlio Y, Ferris-Swift L. The effect of direct splenic stimulation on the cells and antibody content of the blood stream in acute infectious diseases. *Coll J Kansas City Coll Osteopath.* 1934;18(7):196–211.
23. Measel JW Jr. The effect of the lymphatic pump on the immune response: I. Preliminary studies on the antibody response to pneumococcal polysaccharide assayed by bacterial agglutination and passive hemagglutination. *J Am Osteopath Assoc.* 1982;82(1):28–31.
24. Noll DR. Revisiting Castlio and Ferris-Swift's experiments testing the effects of splenic pump in normal individuals. *Int J Osteopath Med.* 2005; 8:124–130.
25. Reinsch S, Seffinger MA, Tobis J. *The Merger: M.D.s and D.O.s in California.* Xlibris Corporation; 2009.
26. Wawruch M, Krcmery S, Bozekova L, et al. Factors influencing prognosis of pneumonia in elderly patients. *Aging Clin Exp Res.* 2004;16(6): 467–471.
27. Mundy LM, Leet TL, Darst K, Schnitzler MA, Dunagan WC. Early mobilization of patients hospitalized with community-acquired pneumonia. *Chest.* 2003;124(3):883–889.
28. Kline CA. Osteopathic manipulative therapy, antibiotics, and supportive therapy in respiratory infections in children: comparative study. *J Am Osteopath Assoc.* 1965;65(3):278–281.
29. Hodge LM, Creasy C, Carter K, Orlowski A, Schander A, King HH. Lymphatic pump treatment as an adjunct to antibiotics for pneumonia in a rat model. *J Am Osteopath Assoc.* 2015;115(5):306–316.
30. Noll DR. The potential of osteopathic manipulative treatment in antimicrobial stewardship: a narrative review. *J Am Osteopath Assoc.* 2016; 116(9):600–608.
31. Noll DR, Degenhardt BF, Morley TF, et al. Efficacy of osteopathic manipulation as an adjunctive treatment for hospitalized patients with pneumonia: a randomized controlled trial. *Osteopath Med Prim Care.* 2010; 4:2.
32. Noll DR, Shores J, Bryman PN, Masterson EV. Adjunctive osteopathic manipulative treatment in the elderly hospitalized with pneumonia: a pilot study. *J Am Osteopath Assoc.* 1999;99(3):143–146, 151–152.
33. Noll DR, Shores JH, Gamber RG, Herron KM, Swift J Jr. Benefits of osteopathic manipulative treatment for hospitalized elderly patients with pneumonia. *J Am Osteopath Assoc.* 2000;100(12):776–782.
34. Noll DR, Degenhardt BF, Johnson JC. Multicenter osteopathic pneumonia study in the elderly: Subgroup analysis on hospital length of stay, ventilator-dependent respiratory failure rate, and in-hospital mortality rate. *J Am Osteopath Assoc.* 2016;116(9):574–587.

69 Osteopathic Considerations in Geriatric Medicine

SARAH E. ROSS ▪ JANICE A. KNEBL

KEY CONCEPTS

- Geriatric medicine has been an undersubscribed primary care specialty.
- Osteopathic principles improve patient care in the elderly. Understanding clinical concepts of self-healing capacity, risk versus benefit, and individualization of care is a useful tool for managing multiple comorbidities that commonly occur in the elderly.
- Biologic changes of normal aging make seniors vulnerable to multiple comorbidities and geriatric syndromes.
- Comprehensive care for older adults using an age-friendly health systems approach includes medical, functional, psychological, and social components (Fig. 69.1).
- The Medicare Annual Wellness Visit provides an opportunity to assess and act upon the 4Ms of age-friendly care: What Matters, Medication, Mentation, and Mobility.

INTRODUCTION

Older adults, defined as those over the age of 65, require a special approach to medical care and treatment. Elderly individuals have needs stemming from normal aging physiology, the psychosocial impact of aging, and age-related diseases and syndromes. The approach to the care of the elderly must be interprofessional and holistic; it must be driven by the goals of preventive care, health maintenance, and optimizing function. Osteopathic medicine is ideally suited to provide an approach to clinical care of older adults aimed at achieving these goals.

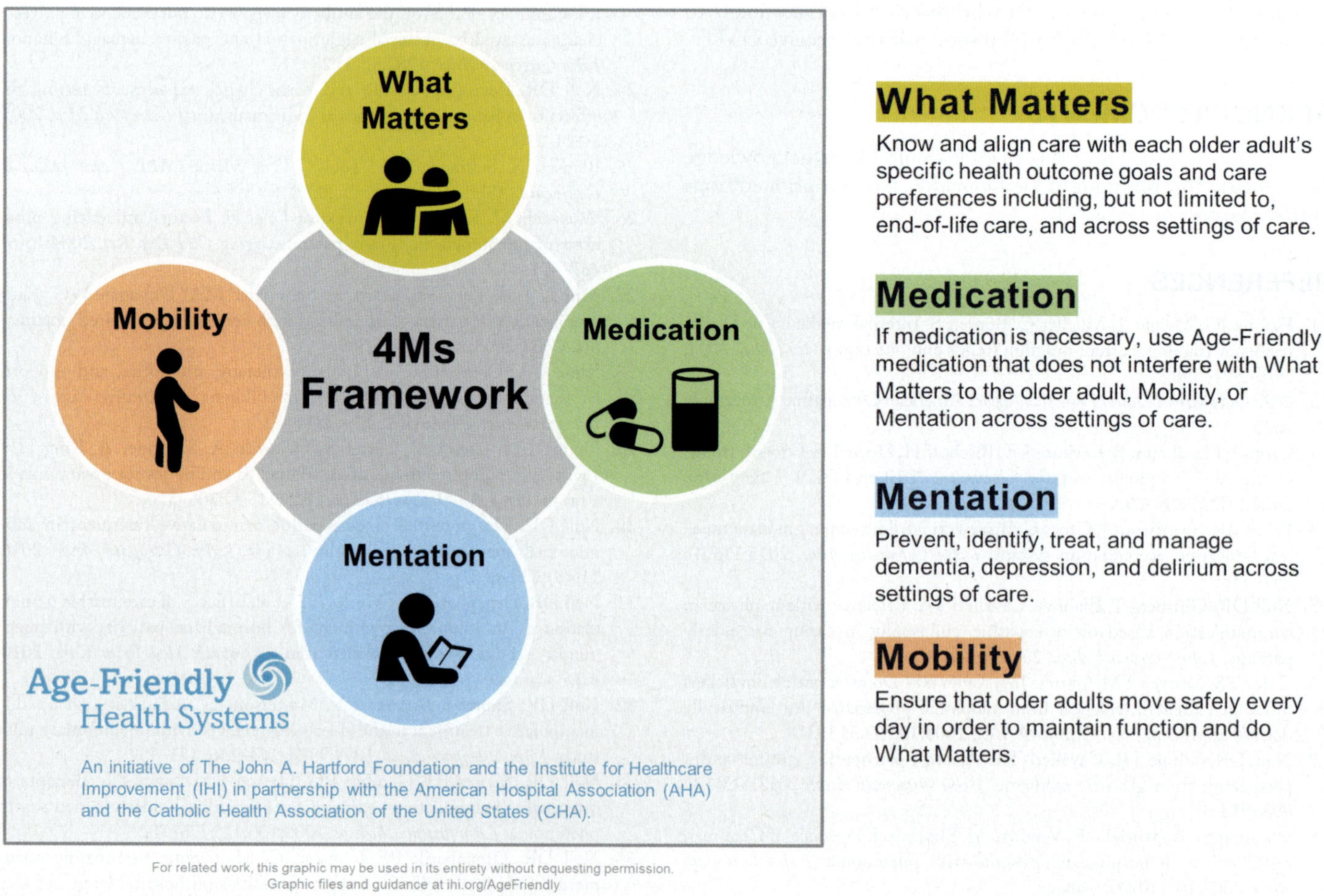

Figure 69.1. Age-friendly health systems 4Ms framework. (From ihi.org/AgeFriendly. Reprinted with permission from Institute for Healthcare Improvement.)

HISTORICAL PERSPECTIVE

In 1909, the term "geriatrics" was coined by Ignatz Nascher from *geras* (old age) and iakrikos (relating to the physician).[1,2] The new name was patterned off the term pediatric. Geriatrics is one of a few health care specialties defined by a stage of human development, similar to pediatrics, neonatology, and adolescent medicine. Geriatrics is the field of medicine pertaining to care for the elderly and their unique and complex health issues. The term gerontology is the field of science pertaining to the study of the aging process and should not be confused with geriatrics. Geriatric medicine is a relatively young specialty. The American Geriatrics Society was founded in 1942, the first fellowship training programs began in the 1980s, and the American Board of Internal Medicine first offered a certificate of added qualification in geriatrics in 1988.[1] The National Institute of Aging promulgated the geriatric imperative in the 1970s and 1980s. It called for health care professions to respond to unmet clinical needs of the elderly.[3]

Today, a graduate of medical school can complete a residency in either family medicine or internal medicine and then complete a fellowship in geriatrics for either one or two years in order to become eligible to take a Certificate of Added Qualifications in Geriatrics from their original certifying board either osteopathic, the American Board of Osteopathic Family Practice or the American Board of Osteopathic Internal Medicine or allopathic, the American Board of Family Medicine or the American Board of Internal Medicine.

Within the United States, most geriatricians practice as primary care specialists rather than being geriatrics consultants, they practice in:

- Ambulatory medical care clinics
- Home-based primary care
- Hospital
- Postacute and long-term care settings (including assisted living settings)
- Hospice/palliative care

In 2021, life expectancy at birth in the United States for the total population was 76.1 years—73.2 years for males and 79.1 years for females.[4] In the United States, the population aged 65 and older numbered 54.1 million in 2019. They represented 16% of the population, more than one in every seven Americans, and is expected to grow to 21.6% of the population by 2040.[5] Worldwide 8.5% of the globe's population was 65 years or older in 2015, and by 2030, one in six people in the world will be aged 60 years or over.[6,7] The "advanced aged," those over age 85, are the most rapidly growing segment of the US population and in most countries.[6,8] By the year 2050, it is projected that there will be 1 million centenarians in the United States. With the elderly as the highest users of health care resources, these demographic changes will have an impact on the cost of health care.[8] However, the numbers of geriatricians in clinical practice are relatively few and dramatically inadequate to cover this growing population. Currently, there are only 7,454 certified geriatricians and 8,220 full-time practicing geriatricians with a projection of need for 12,320 geriatricians by 2030.[9] Given the aging demographic reality and dearth of geriatricians, all primary care practitioners will need to become knowledgeable and skilled in care for older adults.

THREE OSTEOPATHIC PRINCIPLES IN GERIATRICS

Healing Capacity

A core principle of osteopathic medicine is that each individual has an inherent capacity for self-healing and homeostasis is maintained by self-healing and self-regulating processes. These inherent systems are constantly bringing the body back toward homeostasis. Whenever homeostasis is disrupted, the body is in a state of instability or decompensation. If a state of decompensation continues for too long, then body systems progressively fail and the patient will eventually die. Much of clinical practice is simply learning treatments or strategies designed to move the patient back to a state of homeostasis. For example, if the blood pressure is too high, there are lifestyle changes and/or medications to lower it, and if the blood pressure is too low, there are treatments or other interventions to raise it back toward an optimal homeostasis. Osteopathic physicians work with the body's self-healing capacity to bring an individual toward health.

Aging has been defined as the progressive decline and deterioration of functional properties at the cellular, tissue, and organ level that lead to a loss of homeostasis, decreased ability to adapt to internal or external stimuli, and increased ability vulnerability to disease and mortality.[10] So with advancing age, an individual's self-healing capacity tends to diminish. A primary reason for this is that normal aging reduces the physiologic reserve of many organ systems. For example, glomerular filtration rates, pulmonary function, and cellular immunity all decline with aging. The second reason is that chronic disease or comorbid medical problems tend to greatly increase with advancing age. Table 69.1 illustrates the principle that with increasing age an individual's inherent healing capacity tends to be diminished.

The clinical significance of diminished intrinsic self-healing capacity is that physicians have less room for error. An individual with a robust physiologic reserve or self-healing capacity can withstand an iatrogenic event much more easily than an individual with diminished physiologic reserves or self-healing capacity. For example, any patient with volume overload heart failure can be overdiuresed causing volume depletion, resulting in renal failure. Any dehydrated patient can be given too much fluid too quickly, which could result in heart failure. What is distinctive about frail elderly, is that the margin for error is more narrow because the self-healing capacity is often reduced. An individual's response to any particular medication and potential adverse drug reactions are unpredictable, but the consequences in the elderly are often greater. There is wisdom in the axiom that prescriptions treatments for older adults should "start low and go slow" or start a lower doses be advanced slowly. Particular caution should be taken when treating physiologically stable advanced age older adults, especially centenarians because the inherent forces keeping them from decompensation are reduced.

Risk Versus Benefit

Universally, physicians consider the risks versus the benefits of any therapeutic intention. Because of reduced self-healing capacity, this becomes especially important in caring for older adults. Many times, the potential burdens of a treatment are simply not worth the potential benefits. When considering risk or burden versus the benefit, the whole person needs to be considered, in addition to the acceptability of the patient. Many treatments may be good for a particular symptom, but not advantageous for the whole person'

TABLE 69.1

Physiology of Aging and Clinical Impact

Age-Related Change	Clinical Predisposition
Body Composition and Conformation	
Decreased height	
Decreased lean body mass	Changes in pharmacokinetics
Decreased body water	
Increased body fat	
Aging Skin	
Thinning and sparseness of hair	Baldness
Hair follicles produce less melanin	Graying hair
Thin, fragile, wrinkled skin	Propensity to injury
Capillary fragility	Senile purpura
Decreased subcutaneous fat	Pressure sore
Atrophy of sweat glands	Difficulty in body temperature regulation
Decreased response to pain sensation and temperature	Accidents
Aging Eyes	
Loss of elasticity of lens	Presbyopia
Increased density of lens	Cataracts
Change in aqueous kinetics	Glaucoma
Decreased pupillary size	Falls and accidents
Sluggish light reflex	
Decreased color vision	
Increased glare sensitivity	
Aging Mouth and Teeth	
Loss of lingual papillae	Loss of interest in food
Poor taste sensation	Malnutrition and weight loss
Atrophy of olfactory bulbs and decline in sensation of smell	Decreased appetite Increased risk of gas poisoning
Resorption of gum and bony tissue surrounding teeth and bone of mandible	Loss of teeth and periodontal disease
Aging Ears	
Decrease in cerumen glands	Drier cerumen
Atrophy of cochlear hair cells	Presbycusis
Loss of auditory neurons	Presbycusis
Aging Cardiovascular System	
Increase in blood pressure	Hypertension
Aorta and large arteries lose elasticity and systemic vascular resistance increases	Left ventricular hypertrophy
Decreased baroreceptor reflex activity	Orthostatic hypotension
Calcification and sclerosis of heart valves	Valvular stenosis, endocarditis
Calcification and sclerosis of conduction system	Conduction abnormalities
Altered cardiac output	Decreased hemodynamic response to stress
Decreased heart rate	Decreased response to stress
Aging Respiratory System	
Calcification of costal cartilages	Decreased secretion clearance
Decline in alveolar surface area	Effects of hypoxemia
Alteration in pulmonary function tests	
Decreased vital capacity	Increased risk of pulmonary complications
Decreased maximum breathing capacity	
Increased residual volume	
Decreased PaO_2	
Aging Renal System	
Progressive loss of renal mass	Alteration in drug pharmacokinetics
Decrease in renal blood flow	
Decreased tubular function	Greater tendency toward dehydration
Decrease in creatinine clearance	Increased risk of adverse drug reactions

TABLE 69.1 (Continued)

Physiology of Aging and Clinical Impact

Age-Related Change	Clinical Predisposition
Aging Nervous System	
Decrease in brain weight	Drug toxicities, delirium
Alteration in CNS neurotransmitters	
Decrease in memory	"Benign senile forgetfulness"
Decreased reaction time	Decreased IQ scores
Altered sleep with decreased deep sleep and increased wakefulness	Increased sleep disturbances
Decreased vibratory sense	Altered gait
Decreased righting reflex	Falls, accidents
Increased postural instability	Falls, accidents
Altered gait	Falls, accidents
Aging Musculoskeletal System	
Loss of muscle mass	Decreased strength
Loss of bone mineral density	Osteoporosis
	Fractures
Osteoarthritis	Symptomatic arthritis
Aging Hematologic System	
Decreased lymphocyte production	
Decreased bone marrow cellularity	
Decreased hematopoietic functional reserve	Predisposition for anemia
Aging Endocrine System	
Impaired glucose tolerance	Diabetes mellitus
Increased insulin resistance	
Decreased estrogen	Menopause, predisposition to osteoporosis, and coronary artery disease
Aging immune System	
Decreased T-cell function	Predisposition to infections and malignancies
Decreased antibody production to new or old antigen	Predisposition to infection
Increased autoantibodies	Predisposition to autoimmune disorders
Aging Gastrointestinal System	
Decreased gastric HCl production	Altered drug absorption
Colonic motility diminished	Constipation
Decreased calcium absorption	Osteoporosis
Decreased hepatic biotransformation	Altered pharmacokinetics
Decreased hepatic albumin synthesis	Altered pharmacokinetics
Aging Genitourinary System	
Decreased bladder capacity	Urinary incontinence
Alterations in pelvic support	
Enlarged prostate gland	Prostate obstruction
Diminished vaginal and cervical secretion	Pruritus, dyspareunia
Decrease in sexual response	Fear of impotence

health. For example, an older adult who develops a severe pruritic allergic rash may be prescribed diphenhydramine, which is a reasonabe treatment for this problem; however, if the strong anticholinergic properties of this pharmacologic treatment cause acute confusion, the treatment is not good for the whole person. Likewise, many medications for bladder outlet obstruction may cause orthostatic hypotension. While the medication may greatly reduce nocturia, the benefit can be negated by the orthostatic-related fall and subsequent hip fracture.

The individual's estimated life expectancy must be considered when weighing risks and benefits of therapies. How long does the treatment need to be given to provide a benefit and will the patient live long enough to see the benefit. This is particularly important when considering if the intervention is for primary or secondary prevention since it generally takes longer to see a benefit in primary prevention than for secondary prevention. Statin therapy is a good example of this. The guidelines for statin therapy are more aggressive for those who have had an atherosclerotic event (secondary prevention) than for those who are low risk or have no history of an atherosclerotic event (primary prevention). Many clinical practice guideline recommendations for preventative health screening have an upper age limit because shortening life expectancy limits the benefit of testing. Goals of care can also change with advancing age and chronic disease. The goals of care for an individual with a terminal chronic illness, such as advanced dementia, may shift from a health-restorative approach to a palliative care and comfort approach.

Individualization

Another osteopathic principle important in geriatrics is individualization. Dr. Still could never bring himself to write a manual of treatment techniques because he believed every case was different. Two important but competing approaches to patient care are standardization versus individualization. Clinical practice guidelines represent the impulse to improve patient care through standardization of best practices. There is no question that working toward consensus and standardizing treatment based on the best clinical evidence improves patient care. On the other hand, individual variation in response to treatment is a significant reality. Much of the art of clinical practice is balancing these two seemingly contradictory principles. In the geriatric population, there are, more often than not, atypical presentations of disease, patients have multiple comorbid medical problems, and patients more frequently have combinations of disorders for which no clinical trial has ever studied. Clinical trials frequently try to exclude various comorbidities to avoid confounding variables, but this may limit the studies generalizability for an individual patient. Some seniors are physiologically young relative to their chronologic age, and others are physiologically much older than their chronologic age. Thus, an individualized approach to patient care is particularly important in geriatrics.

THE AGING PROCESS AND CLINICAL PRACTICE

Aging is a diverse, complex phenomenon that requires the physician to become aware of both normal and pathologic age-associated changes. While we might view older adults as a homogeneous group, there are actually tremendous variations in the cognitive, physical, functional, behavioral, and emotional aspects of aging. To this end, physicians must be aware of both normal and pathologic changes linked to late-life development. A holistic perspective is especially advantageous when dealing with complex medical, psychosocial, and end-of-life issues. A holistic perspective always asks if the intervention will benefit the whole person. Because seniors often have complex medical, psychosocial, and end-of-life issues, geriatricians often utilize a multidisciplinary approach.

The definition of "older adult" depends upon the context in which it is given. The establishment of Medicare in 1965 provided the cutoff at age 65, an age at which individuals could receive full Medicare and Social Security benefits. Gerontologists have used a broader definition, considering age 60 as the beginning of late life. In contrast, some cultures equate the term "old" with what the Western world would consider middle age, that is, age 45. In other words, there is no set universally accepted age at which an individual becomes elderly. However, geriatricians have divided late life into young–old (ages 65 to 75), older–old (ages 75 to 85), and oldest–old (age 85+).[11] The young–old are similar to middle-aged adults; possibly still working, married, relatively healthy, and active. The older–old have some health problems and challenges with daily living activities; the oldest–old are often frail and in need of long-term care and supportive services.

Cellular Changes Associated with Aging

There are a number of possible explanations for why cells decline resulting in aging of the organism. Although no single theory is generally accepted, researchers currently view the impact of environment upon genetic substrate as a possible reason for such variability in the aging process. Below are descriptions of some of the cellular aging theories:

- The Hayflick limit theory purports that the aging process is driven by loss of molecular fidelity rather than genes. Aging is considered a molecular disorder with an escalating loss of molecular fidelity that ultimately exceeds repair and turnover capacity and increases vulnerability to pathology or age-associated disease.[12]
- Telomere shortening is another theory of cellular aging. Telomeres serve to camouflage chromosome ends from the DNA damage response machinery. Telomerase activity is required to maintain telomeres. One consequence of telomere dysfunction is cellular senescence, a permanent growth arrest state. The introduction of telomerase is proposed as a method to combat aging via cell therapy and a possible method to regenerate tissue.[13]
- The free radical theory of aging proposes that reactive oxygen species cause aging. Chronic states of oxidative stress exist in cells even under normal conditions. However, an imbalance leads to a steady-state accumulation of oxidative damage in a variety of macromolecules that increases during aging, resulting in a progressive loss in the functional efficiency of various cellular processes.[14]
- Genes may also impact the aging process. Developmental genetics theorists propose that aging is genetically programmed and controlled by influences in the second half of life. Both oxidative stress and DNA methylation are possible regulators of gene expression. Examples of genetic influences in aging are
  - apolipoprotein (ApoE-4) in the development of Alzheimer disease
  - coronary heart disease
  - longevity[15]
- Inflammation may be linked to cellular aging. A large number of studies have documented changes in zinc metabolism in experimental animal models of acute and chronic inflammation and in human chronic inflammatory diseases. In particular, modification of zinc plasma concentration and intracellular disturbance of antioxidant intracellular pathways have been found to be associated with age-related inflammatory diseases, like atherosclerosis. Zinc deficiency in individuals genetically predisposed to a dysregulation of inflammation response may play a crucial role in causing adverse events and in reducing the probability of successful aging.[16]
- Other aging theories focus on inflammation and evolution. Chronic inflammatory conditions (as demonstrated by increased homocysteine and plasma cholesterol levels) may shorten the life span by causing cellular damage and diverting resources.[17]
- Evolutionary theories include the notion that genes that are adaptive in early life may be harmful later in life when natural selection is not operative.

As noted in the possible explanations of cellular aging above, it appears that cellular aging can be grouped into three broad themes: First, the random damage that accumulates over time, such as misfolded proteins, telomere attrition, DNA mutations, and oxidative damage to membrane lipids. Second, are the ramifications of accumulated damage, such as mitochondrial dysfunction, loss of stem cells, immnosenescence, and accumulation of senescent cells. Third, are the endogenous pathways that attempt to repair damage and maintain function, for example by recycling damaged proteins (autophagy) or repairing DNA damage.[10]

BODY COMPOSITION CHANGES

With normal aging, there is an increase in body fat, a decrease in lean body mass, and body water content. This may be protective from an evolutionary standpoint, providing body with calorie reserves to withstand periods of illness.[18] Because of the increase in total body fat, drugs that are lipid soluble have prolonged half-lives. This alternation in pharmacokinetics must be accounted for when prescribing or evaluating treatment regimes. For example, while diazepam (Valium) has a half-life of 20 hours in a 20-year-old, the half-life in an 80-year-old may be 80 to 100 hours.[19] In addition, the volume of distribution of many medications changes as a result of these shifts in body composition, and creatine-based determinations can overestimate renal clearance in older adults. Water soluble medications have higher concentrations in older adults because of lower water content and reduced volume of distribution.[10]

SKIN CHANGES

Skin changes are well-known markers of aging. In youth, the epidermis interdigitates with dermis whereas with aging the interdigitations flatten, resulting in reduced contact between epidermis and dermis, decreased nutrient transfer, and increased skin fragility. There is also slower turnover of epidermal cells which may account for slower rate of wound healing and there is also lower number of immune antigen-presenting cells (such as Langerhans) which may cause reduced cutaneous immune surveillance which may affect the quality of wound healing and influence the potential for infection. The aging dermis has a decrease in ground substance which leads to wrinkling and atrophy and the decrease in collagen and elastin causing haphazard, fragmented fiber orientation which leads to decreased elasticity and gives the appearance of laxity and atrophy. Aging is also associated with decreased lipids in top skin layer, which leads to dryness and roughness and decreased barrier function. Dermatologic care of older adults requires an awareness of these cutaneous changes of aging and the effects of cumulative UV radiation exposure, as well as knowledge of the common tumors, inflammatory conditions, and infections seen in this population.[10] Skin changes associated with aging cause contribute to easy bruising, skin tears, changes in body temperature regulation, and pressure sores.[20] Adequate nutrition and mineral supplementation, management of shear forces, body positioning, and physical health are a few of the many critical components of good skin care management in late life.

SENSORY CHANGES

Hearing and vision decline with normal aging. Vision changes include loss of elasticity of the lens resulting in presbyopia. Many older adults experience a variety of visual perceptual problems resulting from aging-related changes in the optics of the eye and degeneration of the visual neural pathways. These problems consist of impairments in visual acuity, contrast sensitivity, color discrimination, temporal sensitivity, motion perception, peripheral visual field sensitivity, and visual processing speed,[21] with the most common vision problems being the diminished contrast sensitivity, slowed adaptation to darkness (resulting in reduced light sensitivity at night), and slowed visual processing.[10] Visual changes can make it more difficult to read, encouraging older adults to use back lighting as well as large-print materials to accommodate these changes. Vision loss also makes it harder for older adults to prepare a meal or to get outside their home environment.[10]

Hearing diminishes with well-documented loss of auditory neurons and cochlear hairs and thickening and less elasticity of the tympanic membrane.[10,22] The resulting presbycusis, which literally means "old age hearing," is bilateral sensorineural hearing loss which causes a more pronounced hearing loss in the high frequencies and can also lead to misunderstanding of information and conversations. It becomes increasingly difficult to hear conversation with background ambient noise, making conversation in a crowd quite difficult. An older adult may withdraw from social situations as a way to deal with hearing loss and may suffer from negative psychological effects such as loss of self-esteem, family discord, and depression. Epidemiologic studies suggest associations between hearing loss and cognitive impairment and between hearing loss and falls. Overall, hearing loss can have profound effects on quality of life.

Taste and smell change with aging. In general, both young and elderly confuse salty and sour much more than they confuse sweet and sour.[23] Changes in taste can impact diet and nutrition, causing decreased food intake and enjoyment in eating. The sense of smell is more impaired by aging than is the sense of taste.[24] As with taste, if smell is impaired, the older adult may be less likely to enjoy the smell of food and the impact of smell on digestion and appetite.

BRAIN CHANGES

Age-related neuron changes such as the number and functioning of sensory neurons, the number of motor neurons, and the ability of neurons to grow branches of both axons and dendrites decrease underlie some of the observed declines in cognitive and physical function. These also include subtle changes within the cortex such as alterations in receptors, loss of dendrites, and spine and myelin dystrophy, as well as alterations in synaptic transmission.[25] Loss of brain weight with cerebral atrophy, volume loss, and microvascular changes in the white matter, has been demonstrated on MRI. Both whole-brain metabolism and frontal lobe metabolism decrease significantly with age (38% and 42%, respectively), whereas cerebellar metabolism does not show a significant decline with age.[26] In normal aging, many elderly individuals demonstrate increased time to recall memories. In dementia, the cognitive losses are progressive, are of greater magnitude, and are considered to be pathologic, not part of normal aging.

MUSCULOSKELETAL CHANGES

Age-related changes to the musculoskeletal system have tremendous impact on the older adult. Muscles achieve peak force in women in their 40s, and then force trends downward for those in their 50s and 60s, with significant reductions by the 70s. Tactile acuity, vibration sensitivity, and joint position sense for a non–weight-bearing toe-matching task were significantly reduced by the 40s or 50s, with further reductions by either the 60s or 70s.[27] Lean body mass decreases with age, caused in part by loss of muscle tissue. Average rates of muscle mass decline are 15% per decade between the ages of 50 and 60 and increase up to 30% after 60 years of age. Muscle tissue is replaced more slowly with aging and may be replaced with a tough fibrous tissue. Sarcopenia, the geriatric syndrome of reduced skeletal muscle mass and strength, is one of the most important causes of immobility decline, functional decline, and loss of independence in older adults.[10]

Bone mass (or density) decreases with aging with bones becoming more brittle, height decreases by shortening of the trunk and spine as intervertebral disks gradually lose fluid and become thinner, and vertebrae lose some of their mineral content. Overall, this decreased muscle mass and demineralization contribute to falls and fractures as well as spontaneous compression and stress fractures. Decreased mobility and pain associated with osteoarthritis can lead to social isolation and the inability to complete activities of daily living (ADLs). The osteopathic physician's holistic philosophy and manipulative therapy are well suited for musculoskeletal issues, relieving pain, and improving mobility.

CARDIOPULMONARY CHANGES

The aging heart increases in size and weight, mostly because of increasing thickness of the left ventricular wall.[10] Calcification and sclerosis of arteries and heart valves can affect blood pressure and hemodynamic response to exertion. The main changes in the cardiovascular system include loss of large artery compliance, dysfunction of some of the systems modulating resistance vessel tone, increased activity of the sympathetic nervous system, and reduced hemodynamic responses to inotropic agents.[28] Pacemaker cells are lost at a rate of 10% per decade, potentially leading to bradycardia, sinus arrest, or tachy–brady syndrome.[10] These changes may contribute to fatigue, decreased endurance, and depression.

The structural changes associated with the pulmonary system and aging result in a loss of chest wall compliance (increased stiffness), leading to increase work of breathing. The lung parenchyma loses its supporting structure, causing dilation of air spaces: "senile emphysema." Respiratory muscle strength decreases with age and can impair effective cough, which is important for airway clearance. The lung matures by age 20 to 25 years, and thereafter, aging is associated with progressive decline in lung function. The alveolar dead space increases with age, affecting arterial oxygen without impairing carbon dioxide elimination.[29] There is a decline in alveolar surface area, a decrease in vital capacity, and a decrease in the partial pressure of arterial oxygen. These changes may contribute to the experience of shortness of breath, decreased exercise tolerance, and lower pulmonary reserve.

LIVER CHANGES

Several age-related changes in the liver have been documented, including a decline in liver mass and liver blood flow, an increase in the hepatic dense body compartment (lipofuscin), moderate declines in the phase I metabolism of certain drugs, shifts in the expression of a variety of proteins, and diminished hepatobiliary functions. Other subtle changes (e.g., muted responses to oxidative stress, reduced expression of growth regulatory genes, diminished rates of DNA repair, telomere shortening) may contribute to reduced hepatic regenerative capacity, shorter postliver transplant survival, and increased susceptibility to certain liver diseases in the elderly.[30] Metabolic clearance of drugs by the liver may be reduced in older adults placing them at a greater risk for increased drug–drug interactions, adverse drug events, and delirium.

RENAL CHANGES

The function of the kidney as well as its morphology changes markedly with age. The glomerular filtration rate falls progressively, independent of overt pathology. Glomerular, vascular, and accompanying parenchymal changes occur.[31] The number of nephrons is reduced, and creatinine clearance declines. This impacts the kidney's ability to clear drugs. Care must be taken when prescribing drugs that are cleared through the kidney as drug toxicity may result quite rapidly. In addition, as chronic kidney disease is quite prevalent in late life, special care should be taken with drug prescribing and dosing to avoid kidney-related drug toxicity.

IMMUNOLOGIC CHANGES

With increasing age, the competence of the immune system to fight infections and tumors declines. The older immune system requires more stimulus and more time to become activated, produces less primary and secondary responses, and loses memory cells faster.[10] Age-dependent changes have been mostly described for human CD8 T cells.[32] Antibody production and B-cell function decrease and autoantibodies increase with age. These changes may account for the higher rate of infection, decreased vaccine efficiency, reactivation of latent infections, autoimmune disease, poorly regulated inflammatory responses, and perhaps malignancy with age.

Psychological Changes Associated with Aging

Most older adults experience significant transitions as they age, which necessitates psychological adjustment. Late life has been described as a season of change and loss. Older adults are faced with a variety of predictable transitions including retirement, reduction in income, loss of spouse, death of friends and peers, loss of health, and change of living environment. The elder may experience a shift from an internal locus of control to an external one, as many life changes occur outside of one's control.

A number of developmental theorists have addressed the psychological issues associated with aging. Erickson identified the last stage of aging as "integrity versus despair." In this stage, the older adult is faced with looking back on their life and determining meaning and value in their history. Regrets for mistakes, losses, and life events left undone can create bitterness and frustration. Erickson believes that successful resolution of this stage results in wisdom. High levels of extraversion and low levels of neuroticism are associated with reduced risk of mortality in old age, and these associations are mediated in part by personality-related patterns of cognitive, social, and physical activity.[33] Older adults who are more outgoing may be able to weather the changes associated with late life more flexibly than those who are more introverted. Anxiety also appears to play a role in survival in that elders with low levels of anxiety appear to survive longer than those with high levels of anxiety.

Overall, there is importance in socialization as we age and this provides cognitive engagement and stimulation, can reduce loneliness, and add to our social support network. In fact, socialization is vital for older adults providing a sense of meaning and connectedness.[10]

COMPREHENSIVE AND AGE-FRIENDLY GERIATRIC CARE

The major focus of geriatric care is optimizing function, avoiding institutionalization, and maintaining the older adult in the community. The geriatric multidisciplinary assessment is defined as a multidimensional interdisciplinary process focused on determining a frail elderly person's medical, psychological, and functional capacity in order to develop a coordinated and integrated plan for treatment and long-term follow-up.[34] Team members may include a geriatrician, nurse practitioner, social worker, dietician, pharmacist, psychiatrist, physical therapist, and other medical specialties. The domains addressed in a comprehensive geriatric assessment include competency and communication, functional status, physical status, nutrition, mobility, symptoms and distress, psychological/social status, spiritual issues, care services, and quality of life.[35]

While the model of a comprehensive geriatric assessment has been the approach to care used by geriatricians and geriatric care teams, the age-friendly health systems 4Ms framework provides a simplified approach to care of the older adult for the primary care provider. Moreover, the Medicare Annual Wellness Visit, created in 2011, provides a structured opportunity for assessing and addressing the 4Ms of age-friendly care, including screening for dementia, depression, and fall risk, reviewing healthcare maintenance tasks, and discussing healthcare priorities and preferences.[36] The interdisciplinary team can support completion of the Medicare Annual Wellness Visit and models utilizing registered nurses to lead this type of visit have been studied.[37] Primary care physicians in the office setting must be proficient in geriatric assessment as they will be the medical professionals caring for the majority of older adults as the population ages.[38] Addressing what matters, medication, mentation, and mobility at each encounter with an older adult allows the opportunity to identify and address age-related challenges and disease states.

Components of the Medical Assessment

In caring for older adults, a thorough understanding of the different medical and social issues is needed before a comprehensive plan can be developed. Physicians should be mindful of atypical presentations in the elderly. Examples include abdominal pain from a ruptured diverticulum that often presents with less pain and less inflammation in an older adult relative to a younger person. Depression may present as memory loss or somatic complaints in the elderly rather than overt sadness. Drug interactions are more serious for older adults, because of effects related to polypharmacy and drug interactions that may occur.

In caring for older adults, physicians may need to allow additional time for older adult patients due to physical or cognitive impairments or complex medical history. Obtaining collateral history from informants such as children or caregivers becomes very important when memory loss is an issue. Insight into deficits, safety, functional limitations, and symptoms is often absent with the development of memory loss, and so caregivers are relied upon to provide an accurate history and assist with implementing the care plan. Patients or their caregivers should be encouraged to bring all medications or an accurate list to each office visit as medication adherence and confusion surrounding medication management may need to be addressed. Table 69.2 outlines areas that should be part of geriatric assessment and age-friendly care. Functional status should be assessed in older adults, including basic ADLs such as dressing, toileting, bathing, continence, feeding, and transferring. Independent ADLs should also be assessed including housekeeping, laundry, finances, cooking, medication management, transportation, and telephone use. The individual's ability to complete affects the level of care needed, including decisions related to a move to residential care or increased support in the current residence.

TABLE 69.2

Components of the History of Age-Friendly Care

What matters
- Advanced directives

Medication
- Medications and polypharmacy issues
- Assessing for use of high-risk medications
- Assessing for medication side effects

Mentation
- Mood/affect
- Cognitive functioning and memory
- Hearing status
- Vision status

Mobility
- Fall risk
- Osteoarthritis
- Osteoporosis
- Status of feet/gait

Other important areas
- Nutrition
- Swallow difficulties
- Dentition/dentures
- Pressure Injuries
- Mistreatment
- Infections
- Bowel and bladder control

ASSESSING AND ACTING ON WHAT MATTERS

All patients deserve care that meets their needs, and needs and priorities for health care evolve as patients get older. Incorporating the individual's goals and priorities into their care plan is an important part of age-friendly care. Conversations about "What Matters" to the older adult include identifying the older adult's preferred language, preferences for how they would like to be addressed, cultural considerations, health beliefs, and social/family support. Identifying patient preferences allows the physician to provide care that is in alignment with patient priorities. "What Matters" conversations also encompass advanced care planning. Primary care physicians should provide opportunities for the older adult to express their wishes for end-of-life care and complete medical directives. Advance care planning is part of the Medicare Annual Wellness Visit.

ASSESSING AND ACTING ON MEDICATION

A review of all medications the older adult takes should be part of every visit. Assessing the patient's medications for high-risk medication allows for discussion of discontinuing medications that may be causing harmful side effects. When presented with a new symptom in an older adult, always try to blame the medications, as you can often improve how a patient feels by discontinuing an offending medication.[39] Because adverse side effects can develop months to even years after the initial start of a medication, length of use should never exclude a medication for review.

ASSESSING AND ACTING ON MOBILITY

The osteopathic physician should help their patients keep active and moving. Falls are a significant source of morbidity in older adults, and staying mobile helps reduce the risk of falls. For falls and gait issues, the "Timed Up and Go" test[40] can be a helpful assessment of balance and ambulation (Table 69.3).

ASSESSING AND ACTING ON MENTATION

Given that age is the greatest risk factor for developing dementia, performing a mental status examination regularly is helpful in identification of new-onset cognitive impairment. Appearance

TABLE 69.3

The Timed Up and Go Test

Directions: Patients wear their regular footwear and can use a walking aid, if needed. Begin by having the patient sit back in a standard armchair and identify a line 3 m, or 10 ft away, on the floor.

- First instruct the patient as follows—When I say "Go," I want you to: 1. Stand up from the chair. 2. Walk to the line on the floor at your normal pace. 3. Turn. 4. Walk back to the chair at your normal pace. 5. Sit down again.
- On the word "Go," begin timing.
- Stop timing after patient sits back down.
- Record time.

Note: An older adult who takes ≥12 seconds to complete the Timed Up and Go Test is at risk for falling and requires further assessment.

TABLE 69.4

The Geriatric Depression Scale

Scoring system: Answers indicating depression are highlighted. Each bold-faced answer counts as one (1) point.	
1. Are you basically satisfied with your life?	Yes/**no**
2. Have you dropped any of your activities and interests?	**Yes**/no
3. Do you feel that your life is empty?	**Yes**/no
4. Do you often get bored?	**Yes**/no
5. Are you in good spirits most of the time?	Yes/**no**
6. Are you afraid that something bad is going to happen to you?	**Yes**/no
7. Do you feel happy most of the time?	Yes/**no**
8. Do you often feel helpless?	**Yes**/no
9. Do you prefer to stay in your room rather than going out?	**Yes**/no
10. Do you feel you have more problems with memory than most?	**Yes**/no
11. Do you think it is wonderful to be alive?	Yes/**no**
12. Do you feel worthless the way you are now?	**Yes**/no
13. Do you feel full of energy?	Yes/**no**
14. Do you feel that your situation is hopeless?	**Yes**/no
15. Do you think that most people are better off than you?	**Yes**/no

Score >5 = Probable Depression Score______.

can inform the clinician about self-neglect and dementia issues. Orientation and short-term memory assessment are invaluable tools to understand whether a patient will be able to live independently and comply with complex medical treatments. Mood assessment is critical to evaluate for any level of depression that may impair functioning or quality of life. The Geriatric Depression Scale[41] (Table 69.4) can be used for older adults without cognitive impairment. For patients with cognitive decline in which one suspects dementia, the Cornell Scale for Depression in Dementia[42] may be used to assess the cognitively impaired patient for depression (Table 69.5).

Assessment of cognitive function should include a standardized tool (Table 69.6). The mini-mental state examination (MMSE)[43] is one such cognitive examination frequently used as both a baseline and an outcomes measure of cognitive decline. Although the current recommendations by the United States Preventive Services Task Force state that the evidence is insufficient to recommend for or against screening for cognitive impairment in older adults, implementation of Medicare Annual Wellness Visits has been shown to increase rates of dementia diagnosis.[44]

PHYSICAL EXAMINATION OF THE OLDER ADULT PATIENT

The geriatric patient should have a physical examination as part of their geriatric assessment. The components of the physical examination are not unlike those of a younger adult with special attention being focused on issues associated with aging. The osteopathic physician should be mindful of modesty issues with older adults and sensitively examine them in a warm comfortable environment. Table 69.7 outlines issues to focus on with respect to each area of the physical examination.

APPLYING THE 4Ms FRAMEWORK TO PATHOLOGIC CHANGES IN OLDER ADULTS

Older adults can be at a higher risk for pathologic changes associated with aging. Advancing age can allow more time to develop new health challenges and age is a significant risk factor for several conditions, including dementia. Changes to social networks and shifts in priorities for health care also occur with advancing age. Important to the care of older adults is knowing about their social supports and assessing what matters to them. It is also important to recognize problems related to depression, anxiety, dementia, delirium, psychosis, polypharmacy, and falls.

What Matters: Social Supports and Care Priorities

Humans are social creatures, and socialization is beneficial across the lifespan. Late-life transitions, such as loss of a spouse or retirement, can lead to major shifts in the individual's social support network. Social networks work as buffers for stresses and moderate losses. Older adults who lose their social networks due to death, changes in location, or illness tend to not do as well physically or psychologically as those adults whose lives are more stable. Those with a strong ability to adapt and evolve by maintaining or obtaining supportive connections despite major life transitions also do well. Assessing the older adult's social support network is critical to understanding the nature and scope of support available to them as this may impact their ability to live independently in the community. The osteopathic physician will want to understand components of support and social determinants of health including financial, educational, environmental, community context, and health care access. This is critical to help the patient access appropriate services as well as to guide treatment and therapy decisions. The interprofessional team can be more effective at assessing and addressing social determinants of health and social support than any single health professional may be. Assessing social determinants of health and care preferences allows the physician to advocate for appropriate care for their patient.

As older adult's psychosocial and medical challenges evolve, their priorities for health care may change. If the osteopathic physician is to provide individualized care, assessing patient priorities becomes vital to guide medical decision making. Older adults with multiple chronic conditions receive a lot of care, which may be burdensome and may not be in alignment with what matters most to them. It is beneficial to develop a comfort level by discussing risks and benefits of care options and potential tradeoffs. For example, an older adult may prefer not to use insulin to treat diabetes due to the care burden of multiple glucose checks and insulin shots and may be comfortable with the tradeoff of potential risk of higher sugars in order to avoid that care burden. For those of an advanced age, evidence-based guidelines may not exist for their age group or their compilation of chronic conditions. Especially in these situations where practice guidelines may not be easily applicable to the patient, adjusting care based on goals and preferences is paramount.

Mentation: Depression, Anxiety, Dementia, Delirium, and Psychosis

DEPRESSION

Depressive symptoms are prevalent in late life with many older adults presenting with subsyndromal depressive symptoms that may not meet DSM-V criteria for major depression. Minor depression continues to impact functioning significantly and has been associated with increased use of health services, excess disability, and poor health outcomes. Major depressive disorder is found in

TABLE 69.5

The Cornell Scale for Depression in Dementia

a	0	1	2	**A. Mood-related signs**
				1. Anxiety: anxious expression, rumination, worrying
				2. Sadness: sad expression, sad voice, tearfulness
				3. Lack of reaction to present events
				4. Irritability: annoyed, short tempered
a	0	1	2	**B. Behavioral disturbance**
				5. Agitation: restlessness, hand wringing, hair pulling
				6. Retardation: slow movements, slow speech, slow reactions
				7. Multiple physical complaints (score 0 if gastrointestinal symptoms only)
				8. Loss of interest: less involved in usual activities (score only if change occurred acutely, i.e., in <1 mo)
a	0	1	2	**C. Physical signs**
				9. Appetite loss: eating less than usual
				10. Weight loss (score 2 if >5 lb in 1 mo)
				11. Lack of energy: fatigues easily, unable to sustain activities
a	0	1	2	**D. Cyclic functions**
				12. Diurnal variation of mood: symptoms worse in the morning
				13. Difficulty falling asleep: later than usual for this individual
				14. Multiple awakenings during sleep
				15. Early morning awakening: earlier than usual for this individual
a	0	1	2	**E. Ideational disturbance**
				16. Suicidal: feels life is not worth living
				17. Poor self-esteem: self-blame, self-deprecation, feelings of failure
				18. Pessimism: anticipation of the worst
				19. Mood congruent delusions: delusions of poverty, illness, or loss

Score______. Score >12 = probable depression. Score ratings should be based on symptoms and signs occurring during the week before interview. No score should be given if symptoms result from physical disability or illness. Scoring system: a, unable to evaluate; 0, absent; 1, mild to intermittent; and 2, severe.

6% to 10% of older adults in the community, with up to 40% having minor depression or depressive symptoms. Rates are higher in nursing facilities with 12% to 20% of nursing home residents having major depressive disorder.[10] Table 69.8 describes the symptoms associated with major and minor depression[45] in the elderly. When assessing mentation and depression, the osteopathic physician must be mindful of suicide risk in the older adult. Assessing for suicide risk factors will help identify those who need additional attention. These risk factors for suicide in older adults include previous attempts, suicidal thoughts or a wish to be dead, recent losses, hopelessness, treatment nonadherence, impulsive behaviors, substance abuse, and perceived burden on family or others.

Depression is treatable in late life and should not be considered merely a normal reaction to loss. Antidepressants may be helpful for symptom management of sleep disturbance, weight changes, and depressed mood. Care must be taken in dosing due to decreased renal and liver clearance, generally using lower dosages to reduce the risk of toxicity. A variety of selective serotonin reuptake inhibitors or noradrenergic–serotonergic reuptake inhibitors may be used safely in older adults. It is important to remember that benefits may not be seen for 4 weeks and treatment for up to 12 weeks may be needed before remission is achieved. Frequent visits with the physician to both monitor for side effects and provide encouragement in waiting for antidepressant response are encouraged.

Psychotherapy is helpful in managing depression and coping with major life transitions or losses. Cognitive behavioral, interpersonal, and supportive therapies are helpful for the older adult.[46] Used in combination with antidepressant medication, psychotherapy can provide additional help in dealing with the adjustment to life changes as well as problem solving. Exercise reduces depressive symptoms and the osteopathic physician should help older adults with depressive symptoms find ways to increase their physical activity.

ANXIETY

There is significant overlap between depression and anxiety in late life. Anxiety may manifest itself as panic, generalized anxiety, or simple phobias. Feeling nervous or restless may be signs of anxiety, but in the older patient, anxiety may be closely tied to medical illness. Pulmonary disorders such as chronic obstructive pulmonary disease can create hypoxia and mimic the signs and symptoms of anxiety. Cardiac disease has also been associated with anxiety in older adults.[47]

Although often used, benzodiazepines can be highly problematic for older individuals. This class of drug is associated with falls, delirium, and even depression. A better choice to manage anxiety is the use of a selective serotonin reuptake inhibitor. Benzodiazepine use should be short term and of low potency in order to reduce risks associated with these medications.

TABLE 69.6

Mini-Mental State Examination

Orientation	Maximum Score
1. What is the (year) (season) (date) (day) (month)?	5
2. Where are we? (state) (country) (town) (hospital) (floor)	5
Registration Ask the patient if you may test his or her memory. Then say the names of three unrelated objects, clearly and slowly. After you have said all three, ask the patient to repeat. This first repetition determines the score (0–3), but keep saying them until the patient can repeat all three, up to six trials.	3
Attention and Calculation Ask the patient to begin with 100 and count backward by 7, stop after 5 subtractions 93, 86, 79, 72, 65. If the patient cannot do serial 7s, ask them to spell the word WORLD backward.	5
Recall Ask the patient to recall the three items repeated above.	3
Language	
Naming: Show the patient a wristwatch and pencil and ask the name.	2
Repetition: Repeat the phrase "No ifs, ands, or buts" after you.	1
Three-Stage Command: Give the patient a blank paper and ask them to take the paper in the right hand, fold it in half, and put it on the floor. One point for each part correctly executed.	3
Reading: On a blank page of paper, print "CLOSE YOUR EYES." Ask the patient to do what it says.	1
Writing: Give the patient a blank piece of paper and ask them to write a sentence that must contain a subject and a verb.	1
Copying: Ask the patient to copy the figure of intersecting pentagons. All 10 angles must be present and 2 must intersect to form a four-sided figure.	1

SCORING:

MAXIMUM 30

Mild impairment MMSE 21–29; moderate MMSE 10–20; severe MMSE < 9.

Cognitive behavioral therapy has been demonstrated to be highly effective for the management of anxiety.[48] Learning to deal with irrational thoughts, developing strategies for replacing negative thoughts with positive ones, and helping a patient find solutions for overwhelming worries are all practical functions of psychotherapy.

DEMENTIA—MAJOR NEUROCOGNITIVE DISORDER

Dementia is a degenerative disease characterized by short-term memory loss, disorientation, word-finding difficulties, apraxia, and agnosia with significant functional decline. In 2013, the American Psychiatric Association renamed this diagnosis as either minor or

TABLE 69.7

Key Components of the Geriatric Physical Examination

Vital Signs
- Assess for orthostatic hypotension (blood pressure sitting and standing)
- Assess temperature
- Monitor weight with each visit

Skin
- Evaluate for common skin lesions in aging including lentigo, senile keratosis, senile purpura, pressure sores, or evidence of falls

Head
- Assess vision and eye movements, evidence for cataracts
- Assess hearing
- Evaluate skull for trauma with a history of falls
- Examine patient for cerumen impacting ear canal
- Auscultate for carotid bruits

Cardiopulmonary System
- Evaluate for systolic ejection murmurs (common secondary to aortic valve changes associated with aging)
- Presence of peripheral pulses
- Assessment for leg edema
- Auscultate for bibasilar rales and possible atelectasis secondary to immobility

Abdomen
- Assess hernias
- Deep palpation for aortic size
- Palpate for enlarged bladder
- Rectal examination and assessment for stool in blood
- Prostate examination in men

Musculoskeletal
- Evaluate gait
- Assess posture
- Range of motion of upper and lower extremities
- Feet evaluation for ulcers and nail care
- Osteopathic structural evaluation of muscle and joint for somatic dysfunction

Neurological Examination
- Evaluate vibration (may be normal in older adults)
- Reflexes (ankle reflex may be absent in normal older adult)
- Observe for asymmetrical test results (could be suggestive of stroke)
- Minimental state examination to evaluate cognition (Table 69.6)

TABLE 69.8

Symptoms Associated with Major and Minor Depression

Major Depressive Disorder

- Depressed or irritable mood for >2 wks
- Five or more of the following symptoms >2 wks that impair social, occupational, or other important areas of functioning:
  - Diminished interest or pleasure
  - Significant weight change
  - Insomnia or hypersomnia
  - Psychomotor agitation or retardation
  - Fatigue
  - Feelings of worthlessness or guilt
  - Diminished ability to concentrate
  - Recurrent thoughts of death

Minor Depression

Presence of 2–5 symptoms of major depressive disorder. In addition, these symptoms may also be associated with minor depression:

- Increased somatic preoccupation
- Anergic, anhedonia
- Isolation
- Pessimistic attitude
- Fatigue
- Increased emotional sensitivity
- Increased mood reactivity

major neurocognitive disorder. Alzheimer disease is the most common type of dementia and an estimated 6.7 million Americans age 65 and older have Alzheimer.[49] Patients with dementia require increased supervision and care due to safety concerns related to memory loss and cognitive impairments.

A number of behavioral issues can arise with dementia. These include psychosis, depression, agitation, and physical aggression. Personality changes may also occur leading the individuals responding with irritability or aggression that is out of character. These behavioral issues can be particularly troublesome to caregivers and are the place where the osteopathic physician, considering the impact of mind–body–environment, can help provide psychoeducation, behavioral strategies to minimize excessive stimulation, and support for the family caregivers.[50] Pharmacologic treatment for the management of dementia currently includes acetylcholinesterase and glutamate inhibitors.[49] Newer treatments of amyloid beta-directed monoclonal antibody therapy through intravenous infusion have yet to prove that clinically meaningful benefits outweigh the risk of significant side effects.[52] Antidepressants can be helpful in the management of depression in dementia. Atypical antipsychotics have been used in the management of agitation and psychosis in dementia; however, they have come under scrutiny for increased risk of cerebrovascular risk and sudden death.[53]

DELIRIUM

Delirium is characterized by an acute confusional state, in which the patient has fluctuating sensorium, attentional deficits, waxing and waning levels of alertness, and intermittent psychosis. The phrase "acute mental status change" or "altered mental status" are essentially other terms for delirium. Older adults are at a higher risk for delirium, and its manifestation may be frightening for family members witnessing an abrupt change in the patient. Underlying dementia, functional impairment, and medical comorbidity also predispose an individual to develop delirium. Delirium may result from many sources including medications or medication withdrawal, infection, electrolyte imbalance, hypoxia, and reduced sensory input (i.e. hearing or vision loss).

Tools such as the Confusion Assessment Method diagnostic algorithm can aid in accurate detection of delirium.[54] Important interventions for consideration include addressing modifiable risk factors such as sensory impairment by providing eyeglasses or hearing aids, and removing potentially offending medications such as anticholinergics, benzodiazepines, or opioids. Osteopathic physicians should work to identify the medical and environmental causes of delirium. Providing psychoeducation to caregivers and family is also an important component in trying to aggressively anticipate the problem of delirium in the older adult.

PSYCHOSIS

Older schizophrenics have more multiple medical problems as a result of chronic illnesses due to poor lifestyle choices as well as lack of health care. Interestingly, the overt symptoms of hallucinations, delusions, and paranoia tend to lessen with age. Elderly patients may be at greater risk for tardive dyskinesia and parkinsonian side effects of antipsychotic medications.[55] Psychosis may result from schizophrenia, mood disorders, dementia, or organic etiologies. Since new-onset psychosis in older individuals is much more likely to be related to an organic etiology, it requires a thorough medical workup. In persons living with dementia, behavioral and mood disturbances can occur, which may include psychosis.

Medication: Reducing Risks of Polypharmacy

Older adults can experience significant morbidity associated with inappropriate prescribing and overprescribing. Polypharmacy has been linked to negative clinical outcomes such as frailty, hospitalizations, adverse drug events, and mortality. Polypharmacy is typically defined as the routine use of five or more medications and is very common in older adults.[56] The classes of medications most frequently associated with preventable adverse drug events include antidiabetics, anticoagulants and antiplatelet agents, cardiovascular drugs, diuretics, antipsychotics, and nonsteroidal anti-inflammatory medications (NSAIDs). Each patient encounter should include a thorough review of the patient's active medications, looking for opportunities to discontinue medications that may be harmful or unnecessary. In the outpatient setting this can prove challenging for individuals who follow with multiple prescribers, use multiple pharmacies, or have transitioned from one care setting to another.

The goal of addressing polypharmacy is avoidance of adverse drug events, drug–drug interactions, and drug–disease interactions. The larger picture of prescription optimization is to ensure that every prescription has an appropriate indication and chronic diseases are being appropriately managed per evidence-based guidelines. To this end, tools such as the Beers Criteria, Medication Appropriateness Index, and STOPP/START Criteria are available. The Beers Criteria are a list of potentially inappropriate medications that should be avoided or used with caution in older adults. The Medication Appropriateness Index evaluates individual medications using 10 criteria to determine appropriateness. STOPP (Screening Tool of Older Persons' Prescriptions) and START (Screening Tool to Alert to Right Treatment) are criteria to guide medication review for optimization, including discontinuing medications with high risk or indications not supported and starting medications that may have been inappropriately omitted.[57] Medication optimization is an ongoing process that ties back into what matters most to the individual with respect to their goals of therapy and priorities related to chronic conditions, symptom management, and overall health.

Mobility: Reducing Fall Risks

Accidental falls are the most common cause of fatal and nonfatal accidental injury for those aged 65 years and older.[58] About 30% of community-dwelling seniors age 65 years or older fall at least once per year.[59,60] While most falls do not cause major injury, 10% to 20% of falls result in fracture or more serious injury or head trauma.[10] Given the prevalence and significant morbidity, finding interventions that prevent falls is a high priority at the Center for Disease Control and Prevention (CDC),[61] the National Institute of Health (NIH), National Institute on Aging (NIA), and the Patient-Centered Outcomes Research Institute (PCORI).[62,63]

Causes of falls are generally multifactorial, with risks related to the individual such as age, chronic disease, or medications, and risks external to the individual such as environmental hazards or risk-taking behaviors. Falls in older adults are a major geriatric syndrome because falls are common and represent a complex clinical problem with a significant public health impact.[20] The CDC maintains a Web site promoting fall prevention through their Stopping Elderly Accidents, Deaths, and Injuries (STEADI)—Older Adult Fall Prevention program.[64] The STEADI program recommends a simple but comprehensive algorithm for determining risk and steps for management by primary care physicians.[65] A key component of this algorithm is a referral to an exercise program because physical interventions designed to improve gait and balance have shown the most promise for preventing falls.[66,67] Reducing an older adult's risk of falls includes reducing that individual's risk factors. This can include addressing impaired balance,[68,69] correcting vitamin D deficiency, or implementing exercise or physical therapy interventions.[59] Additional modalities that have been evaluated for their benefits to fall risk reduction include Tae chi programs and other types of exercise programs which generally provide benefits in fall risk reduction in community-dwelling or nonfrail seniors.[65,70–74] Overall, interventions aimed at reducing falls can be difficult to study and there is a need to research improved and more practical protocols.

It has been posited that OMT has great potential to enhance the effectiveness of exercise for falls prevention and there is a growing body of supportive research. Studies have shown that older adults with somatic dysfunction and restricted motion can benefit from OMT.[75] OMT can be used to address dizziness and was shown to improve balance scores, both directly after treatment and a week later.[76] Other studies have shown positive outcomes for OMT to help prevent falls in older adults,[77] reduce postural sway,[78] and improve gait in Parkinson disease.[79,80]

Several studies have demonstrated that manual therapies can improve gait, balance, and dizziness.[81–84] Clinical trials of OMT in Parkinson disease have clearly demonstrated immediate improvement in gait measures following just one OMT session.[85] Thus, manipulation interventions that improve musculoskeletal function have potential to improve gait and balance and prevent fall-related injuries in older adults.

CONCLUSION

Many principles that have guided osteopathic medicine for decades are the same principles that are at the heart of geriatric medicine. The whole-person approach of osteopathic medicine is essential to geriatric care and involves an interprofessional team to help address complex medical and psychosocial challenges. Utilizing the age-friendly 4Ms framework can help ensure that the important areas of what matters, mentation, medication, and mobility are considered. The primary care setting is the best forum in which to implement age-friendly care and a personalized approach to caring for the older adult, adapting care to what matters to them. A primary care focusing on preventive care has been a true strength of osteopathic medicine and is vital to holistic geriatric care. The integral relationship of structure to function is a core principle of osteopathic medicine and is epitomized in the philosophy of geriatric care, with a primary aim of optimizing function. Osteopathic physicians are uniquely qualified to meet the health care needs of older adults.

ACKNOWLEDGMENTS

The authors and editors of this chapter would like to acknowledge the scholarly contributions of Drs. Donald R. Noll, Thomas A. Cavalieri, Bruce Bates, Marilyn R. Gugliucci, and Jeffrey Tsai for prior editions of this chapter.

REFERENCES

1. Forciea MA. Geriatric medicine: history of a young specialty. *Virtual Mentor*. 2014;16(5):385–389.
2. Nascher I. Geriatrics. *NY Med J*. 1909;90:358–359.
3. Butler RN. Geriatrics and internal medicine. *Ann Intern Med*. 1979; 91(6):903–908.
4. CDC/National Center for Health Statistics. August 31, 2022. Accessed January 30, 2025. https://www.cdc.gov/nchs/pressroom/nchs_press_releases/2022/20220831.htm
5. Administration for Community Living. 2020 profile of older Americans. U.S. Department of Health and Human Services; 2020. Accessed January 30, 2025 https://acl.gov/sites/default/files/Aging%20and%20Disability%20in%20America/2020ProfileOlderAmericans.Final_.pdf
6. World Health Organization. Ageing and Health Fact Sheet; 2024. https://www.who.int/news-room/fact-sheets/detail/ageing-and-health.
7. He W, Goodkind D, Kowal P. *An Aging World: 2015, International Population Reports;* March 2016. US Census, US Department of Commerce, Economics and Statistics, Administration; US DHHS.
8. Kramarow EA, Lentzner HR, Rooks RN, Weeks JD, Saydah SH. *Health, United States, 1999 With Health and Aging Chartbook*. Centers for Disease Control and Prevention; 1999.
9. AGS Website: Geriatrics Workforce by the numbers. https://www.americangeriatrics.org/geriatrics-profession/about-geriatrics/geriatrics-workforce-numbers. July 2022.
10. Harper MG, Lyons WL, Potter JF. *Geriatrics Review Syllabus*. American Geriatrics Society; 2022.
11. Craik FIM, Salthouse TA, eds. *The Handbook of Aging and Cognition*. 3rd ed. Psychology Press and Taylor and Francis Group; 2008.
12. Hayflick L. Biological aging is no longer an unsolved problem. *Ann N Y Acad Sci*. 2007;1100:1–13.
13. Shawi M, Autexier C. Telomerase, senescence and ageing. *Mech Ageing Dev*. 2008;129(1–2):3–10.
14. Muller FL, Lustgarten MS, Jang Y, et al. Trends in oxidative aging theories. *Free Radic Biol Med*. 2007;43:477–503.
15. Hamet P, Tremblay J. Genes of aging. *Metabolism*. 2003;52(10):5–9.
16. Vasto S, Mocchegiani E, Candore G, et al. Inflammation, genes and zinc in aging and age related diseases. *Biogerontology*. 2006;7(5–6):315–327.
17. Mattson MP. Gene-diet interactions in brain aging and neurodegenerative disorders. *Ann Intern Med*. 2003;139(5 pt 2):441–444.
18. Zafon C. Oscillations in total body fat content through life: an evolutionary perspective. *Obes Rev*. 2007;8(6):525–530.
19. Murry JB. Effects of valium and Librium on human psychomotor and cognitive functions. *Genet Psychol Monogr*. 1984;109(2D Half):167–197.
20. Inouye SK, Studenski S, Tinetti ME, Kuchel GA. Geriatric syndromes: clinical, research, and policy implications of a core geriatric concept. *J Am Geriatr Soc*. 2007;55(5):780–791.

21. Jackson GR, Owsley C. Visual dysfunction, neurodegenerative diseases, and aging. *Neurol Clin.* 2003;21(3):709–728.
22. Frisina RD, Walton JP. Age-related structural and functional changes in the cochlear nucleus. *Hear Res.* 2006;216:216–223.
23. Stevens JC, Cain WS. Changes in taste and flavor in aging. *Crit Rev Food Sci Nutr.* 1993;33(1):27–37.
24. Winkler S, Garg AK, Mekayarajjananonth T, Bakaeen LG, Khan E. Depressed taste and smell in geriatric patients. *J Am Dent Assoc.* 1999; 130(12):1759–1765.
25. Dickstein DL, Kaboso D, Rocher AB, Luebke JI, Wearne SL, Hof PR. Changes in the structural complexity of the aged brain. *Aging Cell.* 2007;6(3):275–284.
26. Tumeh PC, Alavi A, Housenia M, et al. Structural and functional imaging correlates for age-related changes in the brain. *Semin Nucl Med.* 2007; 37(2):69–87.
27. Low Choy NL, Brauer SG, Nitz JC. Age-related changes in strength and somatosensation during midlife: rationale for targeted preventative intervention programs. *Ann N Y Acad Sci.* 2007;1114:180–193.
28. Moore A, Mangoni AA, Lyons D, Jackson SH. The cardiovascular system. *Br J Clin Pharmacol.* 2003;56(3):254–260.
29. Sharma G, Goodwin J. Effect of aging on respiratory system physiology and immunology. *Clin Interv Aging.* 2006;1(3):254–260.
30. Floreani A. Liver diseases in the elderly: an update. *Dig Dis.* 2007; 25(2):138–143.
31. Martgin JE, Sheaff MT. Renal ageing. *J Pathol.* 2007;211(2):198–205.
32. Czesnikiewicz-Guzik M, Lee WW, Cui D, et al. T cell subset-specific susceptibility to aging. *Clin Immunol.* 2008;127(1):107–118.
33. Steunenberg B, Beekman AT, Deeg DJ, Kerkhof AJ. Personality and the onset of depression in late life. *J Affect Disord.* 2006;92(2–3):243–251.
34. Langhorne P. Comprehensive geriatric assessment for older hospital patients. *Br Med Bull.* 2005;71:45–50.
35. Arseven A, Chih-Hung C, Arseven OK, Emanuel LL. Assessment instruments. *Clin Geriatr Med.* 2005;21:121–146.
36. Colburn JL, Nothelle S. The medicare annual wellness visit. *Clin Geriatr Med.* 2018;34(1):1–10.
37. Farford BA, Baggett CL, Paredes Molina CS, Ball CT, Dover CM. Impact of an RN-led medicare annual wellness visit on preventive services in a family medicine practice. *J Appl Gerontol.* 2021;40(8):865–871.
38. Tatum Iii PE, Talebreza S, Ross JS. Geriatric assessment: an office-based approach. *Am Fam Physician.* 2018;97(12):776–784.
39. Noll DR, Sthole HJ, Cavalieri TA. Axioms, osteopathic culture, and a perspective from geriatric medicine. *J Am Osteopath Assoc.* 2013;113(12): 908–915.
40. Moncada LVV, Mire LG. Preventing falls in older persons. *Am Fam Physician.* 2017;96(4):240–247.
41. Yesavage JA. Geriatric depression scale. *Psychopharmacol Bull.* 1988;24(4): 709–711.
42. Alexopoulos GS, Abrams RC, Young RC, Shamoian CA. Cornell scale for depression in dementia. *Biol Psychiatry.* 1988;23(3):271–284.
43. Scott J, Mayo AM. Instruments for detection and screening of cognitive impairment for older adults in primary care settings: a review. *Geriatr Nurs.* 2018;39(3):323–329.
44. Lind KE, Hildreth K, Lindrooth R, Morrato E, Crane LA, Perraillon MC. The effect of direct cognitive assessment in the Medicare annual wellness visit on dementia diagnosis rates. *Health Serv Res.* 2021;56(2):193–203.
45. Rapaport MH, Judd LL, Schettler PJ, et al. A descriptive analysis of minor depression. *Am J Psychiatry.* 2002;159:637–643.
46. Miller MD. Using interpersonal therapy (IPT) with older adults today and tomorrow: a review of the literature and new developments. *Curr Psychiatry Rep.* 2008;10(1):16–22.
47. Kloner RA. Natural and unnatural triggers of myocardial infarction. *Prog Cardiovasc Dis.* 2006;48(4):285–300.
48. Gorenstein EE, Papp LA. Cognitive-behavioral therapy for anxiety in the elderly. *Curr Psychiatry Rep.* 2007;9(1):20–25.
49. Alzheimer's disease facts and figures. *Alzheimers Dement.* 2022;18(4): 700–789.
50. Ouldred E, Bryant C. Dementia care: part 2: understanding and managing behavioural challenges. *Br J Nurs.* 2008;17(4):242–247.
51. Van Marum RJ. Current and future therapy in Alzheimer's disease. *Fundam Clin Pharmacol.* 2008;22(3):265–274.
52. Alexander GC, Karlawish J. The problem of aducanumab for the treatment of Alzheimer disease. *Ann Intern Med.* 2021;174(9):1303–1304.
53. Schneider LS, Dagerman K, Insel PS. Efficacy and adverse effects of atypical antipsychotics for dementia: meta-analysis of randomized, placebo-controlled trials. *Am J Geriatr Psychiatry.* 2006;14(3):191–210.
54. Oh ES, Fong TG, Hshieh TT, Inouye SK. Delirium in older persons: advances in diagnosis and treatment. *JAMA.* 2017;318(12):1161–1174.
55. Correll CU, Schenk EM. Tardive dyskinesia and new antipsychotics. *Curr Opin Psychiatry.* 2008;21(2):151–156.
56. Pazan F, Wehling M. Polypharmacy in older adults: a narrative review of definitions, epidemiology and consequences. *Eur Geriatr Med.* 2021; 12(3):443–452.
57. Halli-Tierney AD, Scarbrough C, Carroll D. Polypharmacy: evaluating risks and deprescribing. *Am Fam Physician.* 2019;100(1):32–38.
58. Santos-Lozada AR. Trends in deaths from falls among adults aged 65 years or older in the US, 1999–2020. *JAMA.* 2023;329(18):1605–1607.
59. Michael YL, Whitlock EP, Lin JS, Fu R, O'Connor EA, Gold R. Primary care-relevant interventions to prevent falling in older adults: a systematic evidence review for the U.S. Preventive Services Task Force. *Ann Intern Med.* 2010;153(12):815–825.
60. Stevens JA, Mack KA, Paulozzi LJ, Ballesteros MF. Self-reported falls and fall-related injuries among persons aged > or = 65 years—United States, 2006. *MMWR Morb Mortal Wkly Rep.* 2008;57(9):225–229.
61. National Center for Injury Prevention and Control, Centers for Disease Control and Prevention, U.S. Department of Health and Human Services. *CDC Injury Research Agenda, 2009–2018.* U.S. Department of Health and Human Services; 2009:47.
62. Cire B. NIH, PCORI announce major award to prevent falls injuries in older people. 2014. Accessed January 30, 2025. https://www.nia.nih.gov/news/nih-pcori-announce-major-award-prevent-falls-injuries-older-people
63. National Institute on Aging. Division of Geriatrics and Clinical Gerontology Research Goals. 2016. Accessed December 11, 2016. https://www.nia.nih.gov/research/dgcg/dgcg-research-goals
64. CDC. Stopping Elderly Accidents, Deaths and Injuries (STEADI)—Older adult falls preventions. 2016. Accessed December 11, 2016. https://www.cdc.gov/steadi
65. Phelan EA, Mahoney JE, Voit JC, Stevens JA. Assessment and management of fall risk in primary care settings. *Med Clin North Am.* 2015; 99(2):281–293.
66. El-Khoury F, Cassou B, Charles MA, Dargent-Molina P. The effect of fall prevention exercise programmes on fall induced injuries in community dwelling older adults: systematic review and meta-analysis of randomised controlled trials. *BMJ.* 2013;347:f6234.
67. Gillespie LD, Robertson MC, Gillespie WJ, et al. Interventions for preventing falls in older people living in the community. *Cochrane Database Syst Rev.* 2012(9):CD007146.
68. Rubenstein LZ, Josephson KR. The epidemiology of falls and syncope. *Clin Geriatr Med.* 2002;18(2):141–158.
69. Rubenstein LZ, Josephson KR. Falls and their prevention in elderly people: what does the evidence show? *Med Clin North Am.* 2006;90(5):807–824.
70. Church J, Goodall S, Norman R, Haas M. An economic evaluation of community and residential aged care falls prevention strategies in NSW. *N S W Public Health Bull.* 2011;22(3–4):60–68.
71. Leung DP, Chan CK, Tsang HW, Tsang WW, Jones AY. Tai chi as an intervention to improve balance and reduce falls in older adults: a systematic and meta-analytical review. *Altern Ther Health Med.* 2011;17(1):40–48.
72. Hill KD, Hunter SW, Batchelor FA, Cavalheri V, Burton E. Individualized home-based exercise programs for older people to reduce falls and improve physical performance: a systematic review and meta-analysis. *Maturitas.* 2015;82(1):72–84.
73. Uusi-Rasi K, Patil R, Karinkanta S, et al. Exercise and vitamin D in fall prevention among older women: a randomized clinical trial. *JAMA Intern Med.* 2015;175(5):703–711.
74. Sherrington C, Whitney JC, Lord SR, Herbert RD, Cumming RG, Close JC. Effective exercise for the prevention of falls: a systematic review and meta-analysis. *J Am Geriatr Soc.* 2008;56(12):2234–2243.
75. Fraix M. Role of the musculoskeletal system and the prevention of falls. *J Am Osteopath Assoc.* 2012;112(1):17–21.
76. Fraix M, Gordon A, Graham V, Hurwitz E, Seffinger MA. Use of the SMART Balance Master to quantify the effects of osteopathic manipulative

treatment in patients with dizziness. *J Am Osteopath Assoc.* 2013; 113(5):394–403.

77. Cavalieri TA, Miceli DL, Goldis M, Masterson EV, Forman L, Pomerantz SC. Osteopathic manipulative therapy: impact of fall prevention in the elderly. *J Am Osteopath Assoc.* 1998;98(7):391.
78. Lopez D, King HH, Knebl JA, Kosmopoulos V, Collins D, Patterson RM. Effects of comprehensive osteopathic manipulative treatment on balance in elderly patients: a pilot study. *J Am Osteopath Assoc.* 2011;111(6):382–388.
79. Yao S. Effect of osteopathic manipulative medicine on Parkinson disease. 2015. Accessed November 17, 2016. https://clinicaltrials.gov/ct2/show/NCT02107638?term=sheldon=yao&rank=1
80. Bellumori M, Uygur M, Knight CA. High-speed cycling intervention improves rate-dependent mobility in older adults. *Med Sci Sports Exerc.* 2017;49(1):106–114.
81. Noll DR. Management of falls and balance disorders in the elderly. *J Am Osteopath Assoc.* 2013;113(1):17–22.
82. Hawk C, Cambron JA, Pfefer MT. Pilot study of the effect of a limited and extended course of chiropractic care on balance, chronic pain, and dizziness in older adults. *J Manipulative Physiol Ther.* 2009;32(6):438–447.
83. Hawk C, Pfefer MT, Strunk R, Ramcharan M, Uhl N. Feasibility study of short-term effects of chiropractic manipulation on older adults with impaired balance. *J Chiropr Med.* 2007;6(4):121–131.
84. Strunk RG, Hawk C. Effects of chiropractic care on dizziness, neck pain, and balance: a single-group, preexperimental, feasibility study. *J Chiropr Med.* 2009;8(4):156–164.
85. Wells MR, Giantinoto S, D'Agate D, et al. Standard osteopathic manipulative treatment acutely improves gait performance in patients with Parkinson's disease. *J Am Osteopath Assoc.* 1999;99(2):92–98.

70 Osteopathic Considerations in Rheumatology

KEN BAXA ▪ ADAM GRUNBAUM ▪ CAMERON BRAZ

KEY CONCEPTS

- Musculoskeletal conditions are common, costly, and have a tremendous impact on society.
- Rheumatologists diagnose and treat a variety of musculoskeletal medical conditions that affect not only joints, but organs and connective tissues as well.
- Inflammatory arthritis, osteoarthritis, soft tissue injury, crystalline arthropathies, connective tissue diseases, and fibromyalgia are some of these conditions that will be covered in this chapter.
- Patients with these conditions can benefit from a management plan guided by osteopathic principles and practices.

INTRODUCTION

Rheumatology is the subspecialty of internal medicine and pediatrics that focuses on the medical evaluation and treatment of the musculoskeletal system. Rheumatologists are specialists who devote themselves to the diagnosis and management of autoimmune, inflammatory, and noninflammatory medical problems related to soft tissues and joints. Patients with a potential inflammatory joint or connective tissue disease are often referred to rheumatologists for diagnosis and, if indicated, treatment. Patients with advanced joint destruction, whether from osteoarthritis (OA), inflammatory disease, or trauma, are typically referred to orthopedic surgeons for surgical treatment, including joint replacement. Patients with inflammatory arthropathies complicated by extra-articular disease manifestations may benefit from additional specialist consultation. This review of rheumatology is introductory, and in no way exhaustive. Drawing from Bernard Rubin's material in the first edition of this text,[1] this chapter highlights the integration of osteopathic principles with management of rheumatic and other musculoskeletal problems.

EPIDEMIOLOGY

Musculoskeletal disorders are the leading source of pain and disability globally but are especially prevalent in the industrialized nations including the United States.[2] Musculoskeletal complaints affect approximately 33% of the North American population and are frequently cited as among the most common reasons for patient visits to physicians; on average one out of every five primary care physician visits is related to these complaints. The social and economic impact of these conditions is enormous. The Arthritis Foundation reports that there are more than 100 different forms of arthritic diseases.[3] Clinically, they account for more impairment and functional limitation among middle-age and older adults than any other disease category.[4]

Prevalence is highest among older adults, but all age groups are affected. A North American study of patients over age 65 showed that musculoskeletal symptoms, including knee trouble, back trouble, and unspecified joint pain, were more common in this population than in any other group.[5] Prevalence rates increase with age and are rare under age 18.[6] Among those over age 65, arthritic diseases are among the leading causes of physician visits. Patient surveys document that many individuals aged 75 and over report having arthritis.[7] Racial and ethnic differences in the prevalence, treatment, and outcome of different forms of arthritis have been reported.[8] In patients with systemic lupus erythematous, studies have found African Americans to have a higher prevalence, more severe disease, and poorer outcomes due to than Whites.[8]

A 2019 analysis of Global Burden of Disease (GBD) data showed that approximately 1.71 billion people live with musculoskeletal conditions, including low back pain, neck pain, fractures, other injuries, OA, amputation, and rheumatoid arthritis (RA).[9] Musculoskeletal conditions are also the biggest contributors to years lived with disability (YLDs) worldwide with approximately 149 million years, accounting for 17% of all YLDs worldwide.[2] In 2016, the top causes of YLDs in the United States included low back pain (no. 1), other musculoskeletal disorders (no. 4), neck pain (no. 6), OA (no. 12), and RA (no. 20).[10] Projections based on data from 2010 to 2012 estimate that by 2040 one in four adults (78 million) will have doctor-diagnosed arthritis.[2]

In addition to causing substantial physical suffering for individuals with these conditions, the rising monetary costs are significant. Work loss and rehabilitation contribute to indirect costs, accounting for anywhere from 50% to 76.5% of all medical costs. Regarding patients with the most common rheumatic diseases, like RA, OA, and fibromyalgia (FM), studies have documented much higher-than-expected direct medical costs when compared with patients of similar ages without arthritis. Patients with OA, for example, lost $71.3 billion in annual earnings; those with RA lost $7.9 billion.[2] Not surprisingly, those with the most severe and disabling diseases incur the highest costs.[11] In the United States alone, the annual costs have been estimated to be $874 billion, 5.7% of the annual US GDP.[12]

Due to the prevalence of nearly one-third of the population and significant disability associated with musculoskeletal conditions, there is global need for rehabilitation.[13] The World Health Organization (WHO) launched the Rehabilitation 2030 initiative in 2017 to draw attention to the profound unmet need for rehabilitation worldwide.[13] Osteopathic physicians with their knowledge and skills in musculoskeletal conditions hold an important role in the future management of these patients.

PATIENT EVALUATION AND PROBLEM-SOLVING (ALSO SEE CHAPTERS 27, 28, 30, AND 31)

Because of their additional training in the use of palpatory skills, osteopathic physicians are exceptionally qualified to evaluate patients presenting with musculoskeletal complaints. Along with empathetically sensitive interviewing and other examination methods, these skills are useful for establishing trusting relationships. More precisely, defined and described patient problems can be identified with these special skills.

Younger patients often assume that rheumatic diseases are afflictions of older patients. They are also apt to assume that their problems are self-limited or curable when they are not. On the other hand, many physicians either miss or delay a diagnosis of rheumatologic disease, which can create some devastating long-term consequences. It is crucial to educate oneself in these disease processes. Similarly, educating patients while coordinating treatment will help prevent long-term disease complications and disability.

Establishing a precise history is vital for a correct diagnosis. In general, patients seek help for pain, pain equivalents, depression, and anxiety. Painful sensations have many elements. Some are physiologic, but many are perceptually driven; that is, they are learned behaviors. Feelings of helplessness and hopelessness are common in this population, particularly among those who make frequent physician visits (see Chapter 74 Chronic Pain Management and Chapter 79 Osteopathic Considerations in Psychiatry for further information). Pain equivalents include unpleasant (not necessarily painful) sensations such as itching, aching, stiffness, burning, and nausea. The history should include detailed inquiry about the patient's motivation for coming to the doctor, especially in the absence of pain or pain equivalent.[14] Consequently, successful treatment depends on an understanding of a diagnosis and an interpretation of expected pain relief. In short, clear, understandable explanations are the keys for long-term success.

History Taking[14] (Also See Chapter 27)

Key questions during the medical history of a patient with rheumatologic complaints that help to differentiate between various possible diagnoses may include the following:

- In general, do the symptoms raise the possibility of systemic disease(s) or local conditions? Keep in mind that a localized condition may affect multiple sites.

Common questions for systemic questioning may include:

- What joints or other structures are involved?
- What is the pattern of involvement?
- In what order does joint involvement occur?
- How fast does it occur?
- At what time of the day does it start?
- If joint involvement is painful, severity is graded by whether it interferes with function of the affected extremity or with sleep and work.
- Is involvement self-limited, migratory, additive or progressive?
- If limited, how long do episodes last? Are they migratory or progressive?

Migratory means that the process subsides completely before moving to another apparently normal joint.

Progressive means that the first joint stays afflicted as the pathologic process moves on to additional joints.

- Has the problem been treated previously?
- What was done and for how long?
- What was the prior response to treatment?
- What was its effect on the disease?
- Were there any medication adverse effects?
- Lastly, a thorough review of systems should be asked, indicating if there is presence or absence of: associated headaches, dry eyes or dry mouth, parotid swelling, inflammatory eye disease, sore throat, difficulty swallowing, skin rashes, joint swelling, morning stiffness, digit swelling, inflammation and pain at insertion sites of tendons and ligaments, longstanding cough or difficulty breathing, chest pain at rest or worsens with respiration, palpitations, numbness or tingling, recurring fever, abnormal weight loss, history of blood clots, seizure, stroke, miscarriage, unexplained hair loss, mucosal lesions, or swollen lymph nodes. (All of which could be indications of rheumatologic disease process.)

The duration of morning stiffness serves as a convenient, nonspecific index of inflammatory activity. Typically, it is directly proportional to the severity of the inflammatory process. Variations in duration are used to evaluate inflammation and responses to treatment. For example, the duration of morning stiffness can serve as a more precise assessment than the erythrocyte sedimentation rate (ESR) for rheumatoid inflammation. Sixty minutes or more of morning stiffness can be characteristic of inflammatory arthritis. The morning stiffness is brought about by a rise in proinflammatory cytokines such as IL-6, which is released by CD4 T-cell lymphocytes that cycle with the patient's circadian rhythm.[15]

If a structure is severely inflamed, motion usually causes pain unless there are neurologic problems that interfere with nociception. In general, pain arises from stimulation of free, unmyelinated nerve endings in synovial, capsular, periosteal, ligamentous, or tendinous regions. Mechanical irritation and inflammation are common causes. For example, both pain and numbness occur in association with nerve entrapments in the carpal tunnel. Other common sites are the suprascapular nerve in the shoulder and radicular syndromes arising from arthritic and degenerative changes in the neck and back. Intermittent muscle spasm and chronically increased muscle tone can occur in this group of patients as well.

As joint involvement advances, disuse muscle atrophy occurs rapidly in affected muscles, often within a few days. Diffuse, systemic rheumatic diseases may also demonstrate characteristic muscle pathology. For example, upper limb involvement commonly causes clumsiness of varying types, with loss of hand strength as a common complaint. Morning stiffness, swelling, pain, neuropathy may also occur. Difficulty rising from a chair or climbing and descending stairs signals both hip girdle and lower limb involvement.[16]

Depression is common in individuals with chronic arthritis and chronic pain. Two types are common: primary and reactive. Primary depression can occur with FM patients, over 95% of whom are women. Living alone, having maladaptive thoughts, and expressing more functional limitations are particularly common in about half of these patients.[17] The high occurrence of depression in FM patients, as well as response to treatment with some antidepressants, has led to consideration of common pathophysiologic mechanisms and to the possible classification of FM as one of the family of affective spectrum disorders along with major depressive disorder.[18]

Reactive depression, on the other hand, is common with rheumatic diseases, which tend to create long-term problems due to mounting frustration with loss of personal autonomy (see Chapters 16, 17, 18, and 79 for further discussion on reactive depression). The problem frequently arises or is aggravated with the onset of pathologic fatigue. Emotional lability, manifesting as crying, having morbid thoughts, temperamental outbursts, or withdrawal, is common under these circumstances. These symptoms often disappear as the disease remits.[14] There has been a direct link between long-standing OA and trends toward depressed mood through ongoing concerns and complications from chronic pain and disability.[19]

Several questionnaires are available for long-term evaluation: the Stanford Health Assessment Questionnaire, Functional Disability Index, and Arthritis Impact Measurement Scales. These instruments document the patient's functional status with results comparable to traditional measures of disease-related joint activity, such as tender-point count, radiographic joint erosion score, and ESR.[20]

Other historic cues, such as chorea or "growing pains" in childhood, may aid in differentiating rheumatic fever or juvenile idiopathic arthritis (JIA) in an adult patient. A history of recent exposure to ticks or viral illness may clarify an otherwise obscure arthritis. Clues about prior skin rashes, family history, and kidney stones can also help guide work up.

Other important areas for evaluation would be obtaining a sexual history, history of recent streptococcal infection, colitis, or gastrointestinal infection, in a patient suspected of having gonorrheal arthritis or reactive arthritis, previously known as Reiter syndrome. Diabetes is often associated with adhesive capsulitis of the shoulders, Dupuytren contracture, nerve entrapment, peripheral neuropathy, and OA.

A family history can be helpful in differentiating systemic lupus, RA, psoriasis, and ankylosing spondylarthritis since all have been found to have some familial inheritance.[19,21] The stability of family life and job security are also important points to establish.

Hobbies should be recorded because these are often dealt with in designing a treatment program. Current drug use, including alcohol and tobacco, and medication changes (recent or new) should be noted.

Mental status examinations are important to establish the patient's level of emotional health, cognitive acuity, and reality testing. Organic brain disease, including dementia, Alzheimer disease, and late effects related to brain injury, is a particularly important consideration when assessing treatment compliance issues.[14]

PHYSICAL EXAMINATION (SEE ALSO CHAPTER 27, 28, 29, AND 30)

Palpation

A standard, disciplined routine examination of the musculoskeletal system is essential. Several excellent monographs are available to provide more detailed descriptions.[22,23]

Osteopathic physicians utilize their hands and fingers as important physical examination tools. Having additional knowledge and skills in using palpatory diagnosis, osteopathic physicians are particularly suited for this work. A working knowledge of both topographic and functional anatomy is essential to know when sensing structures under a palpating hand. This integration of knowledge and skill allows the clinician to have an enhanced, precise diagnostic ability. Various mechanical devices exist and are useful for quantifying tenderness, joint swelling, and skin temperature. Yet, none are as useful as trained fingers. A typical peripheral joint and spinal screening examination should take 5 to 6 minutes, on average.

Joint and muscle tenderness are nonspecific, but very sensitive signs of trouble. Some experts use a great deal of force, other clinicians take a gentler approach. In general, inexperienced practitioners tend to use too little force when evaluating superficial structures. On the other hand, some experts, such as McCarty,[24,25] recommend force sufficient to blanch the thumbnail to rule out active disease (when examining areas that are not obviously inflamed). If tenderness is present, then either a low pain threshold or pathologic change may be responsible. Fortunately, tenderness due to an inflammatory cause usually coexists with more specific findings, such as swelling, crepitus, and increased local heat. In patients with symptoms of widespread pain, typically reported in the muscles and joints, and findings of multiple tender points in characteristic soft tissue locations, a clinical diagnosis of FM is likely.[26]

Areas of tenderness can be "compared" by applying similar pressure over nearby areas. Patients with heightened pain sensitivity may be tender everywhere on the body. Another technique to assess if joint pain is intra-articular or extra-articular is called "stressing" a joint. In this technique, pain associated with passive range of motion would be more revealing of intra-articular pathology, whereas pain with active range of motion and added resistance could clue the clinician in to extra articular pathology as well as bursa involvement.

For example, the anterior tibia may be tender in older subjects for unknown reasons. Bone tenderness may also be present in severe osteoporosis and other forms of systemic bone disease. In all presentations, a careful exam to discern the quality and potential source of the patient's discomfort or pain should occur.

Range of Motion

Passive joint motion testing embraces a set of common and familiar osteopathic palpatory procedures. It is used to evaluate all peripheral, spinal, and pelvic mechanics for altered tissue tension, asymmetry, restricted motion capability, and tenderness (TART). It is also a method for eliciting pain and assessment for crepitation and joint contractures.

Swelling

Swelling of joints, bursae, and tendons is always abnormal. Unlike tenderness, swelling specifically indicates organic disease. Swelling is most often due to underlying inflammation and can be due to synovial thickening, increased volume of joint fluid, or local edema. If thickened tissue is felt, particularly in multiple areas, synovium is probably thickened, owing either to inflammatory proliferation or to storage of abnormal material, such as in RA, systemic lupus, crystalline arthritis, or amyloidosis. Synovial thickening in a tendon sheath, common in reactive arthritis (Reiter syndrome) or psoriatic arthritis (PsA), produces a sausage-like swelling of the digits, known as dactylitis. Dactylitis is included in the CASPAR criteria as one of the hallmarks of PsA.[27] In general, synovial swelling is most pronounced on extensor surfaces of joints, where the capsule is more distensible.

Effusions are particularly common in large weight-bearing joints. Thus, fluid is often found in the knee and is less common in the hip, where it is also more challenging to assess. It is even less common in ankles, upper limbs, hands, and wrists because of their tighter capsules. Nodular swelling that has a firm/boney-like presentation over peripheral joints is commonly a signal of osteophytes and OA. Less frequently, they mark the presence of rheumatoid nodules, which tend to be less firm, mobile, and generally lie more on extensor surfaces of affected joints and commonly felt on the dorsum of hands and elbows when present.

Clinically, a pathologic nodule cannot be accurately identified without a biopsy. Most turn out to be synovium herniated through defects in the joint capsule and are most associated with RA or systemic lupus erythematosus (SLE). Nodule biopsy is not generally recommended unless the underlying disease etiology is difficult to identify, a separate infectious or noninfectious process is expected, or more concerning acute findings with pain are present.

Other Clinical Findings

Increased skin temperature is a common, and usually nonspecific, finding (see TART above). Sometimes, crepitus (joint noises) occurs during passive range-of-motion testing. Generally, the finer the crepitus, the more clinically significant it is. Sometimes, tendons will snap over joint surfaces and bony prominences. Typically, the noise is due to tendons snapping over bony prominences. This snapping is not always consistent with an acute disease process but is a common concern for patients.

DIFFERENTIAL DIAGNOSIS AND USE OF DIAGNOSTIC TOOLS

The general category in which a problem falls is usually obvious from the history and physical examination. To pinpoint the diagnosis, however, laboratory examination, including gross and microscopic joint fluid analysis, radiologic study, specialized tests, and occasionally biopsy for microscopy are often indicated.[28]

Routine laboratory tests include complete blood count, chemistry panel, sedimentation rate, C-reactive protein (CRP), and urinalysis. Synovial fluid examination in selected individuals commonly provides useful diagnostic information, looking for presence of inflammation, infectious etiology, and crystal analysis. Autoantibody and immune complex assays are indicated when specific inflammatory rheumatic diseases are suspected.

One must be alert to diagnostic pitfalls. Patients with RA can have a positive antinuclear antibody titer, positive rheumatoid factor (RF) antibodies, positive cyclic citrullinated protein (CCP) antibodies, and, in some instances, have none of the associated antibody titers present. Persons can have RF present in the absence of RA as the likelihood of false-positive RF increases with age. An elevated sedimentation rate is sensitive for the presence of any type of inflammation or infection, and not just specific to autoimmune or rheumatic diseases. An abnormal creatine phosphokinase (CPK) value may indicate, but is not specific to, the diagnosis of various types of myopathies.[1]

Radiographic examination is important for differentiating inflammatory from noninflammatory disorders. X-ray imaging is used to diagnose and stage disease progression and can be used to follow progress once therapy has been instituted. In general, joint inflammation, whether from long-term infection, crystalline arthritis, or an autoimmune process, can lead to osteopenia and joint erosions with irreversible joint damage. On the other hand, noninflammatory degenerative diseases frequently cause an increase in bone density because of subchondral sclerosis, osteophyte formation, and bridging of joint spaces.

Ultrasound (US), magnetic resonance imaging (MRI), and computerized tomography (CT) are also helpful to differentiate musculoskeletal conditions and are often used following initial radiographs.

INFLAMMATORY ARTHROPATHIES

Inflammatory arthropathies are conditions characterized by inflammation of the joints and often other tissues. These include RA, PsA, ankylosing spondylitis (AS), JIA, and SLE, among others. RA and PsA are among the most common inflammatory arthropathies and are important causes of disability in adults.[29,30]

Rheumatoid Arthritis

RA is a systemic inflammatory disease with its primary manifestation in the synovium that results in substantial disability, morbidity, and premature death.[31–33] Early diagnosis and treatment to prevent joint destruction and deformity is therefore of critical importance for patients with RA. The diagnosis of RA is considered in any patient with polyarticular inflammatory arthritis of greater than 6 weeks of duration, with or without the presence of RF or CCP antibody titer, with evidence of inflammation, especially if the hands and feet are involved in a symmetric fashion.[34]

Taking an accurate history and performing a thorough physical exam are crucial in the diagnosis of RA. This is because there are no pathognomonic serologic tests or imaging. However, biologic markers can provide diagnostic and prognostic information supporting the diagnosis. The most used biomarkers include a specific, detectable IgM protein called RF, anti–cyclic citrullinated protein antibody (anti-CCP), and acute phase reactants like ESR and CRP. Despite the naming convention, RF is slightly less specific and sensitive than anti-CCP. In addition, emerging evidence has shown that anti-CCP, and RF to some extent, can aid in predicting the course of disease and response to specific therapies. While these markers are helpful in several RA patients, their nonspecific nature makes them less than ideal. Ongoing research is looking into new biologic markers for future use.[35]

The hallmark of the disease is a chronic, symmetric polyarthritis that typically affects the hands, wrists, and feet initially and later may involve any joint lined by a synovial membrane, most frequently the knees, ankles, hips, elbows, and shoulders (Fig. 70.1).[34] Although RA primarily involves the synovium, features of systemic disease are also present in almost all patients, ranging in severity from fatigue, low-grade fevers, keratoconjunctivitis, mild-to-moderate anemia, serositis (pleural or pericardial effusions), and severe multisystemic vasculitis. Fortunately, recent pharmacologic advances with disease-modifying antirheumatic drugs (DMARDs), biologic agents (bDMARDs) such as tumor necrosis factor (TNF)-α inhibitor therapy, and targeted synthetic disease modifying drugs such as Janus kinase (JAK) inhibitors are significantly improving treatment outcomes.[36]

Below is the listed 2010 American College of Rheumatology (ACR)/European League against Rheumatism classification criteria for RA.

Target populations to be tested are patients who:

1. Have at least one joint with definitive clinical synovitis or swelling
2. With synovitis not better explained by another disease

Classification criteria for RA, a score of ≥6/10 points is needed for classification of a patient as having definite RA.

		Score
A.	**Joint Involvement**	
a.	1 large joint	0
b.	2–10 large joints	1
c.	1–3 small joints (with or without involvement of large joints)	2
d.	4–10 small joints (with or without involvement of large joints)	3
e.	>10 joints (at least one joint must be a small joint)	4
B.	**Serology/Lab Testing**	
a.	Negative RF and negative ACPA	0
b.	Low positive RF or low positive ACPA	1
c.	High positive RF or high positive ACPA	2
C.	**Acute Phase Reactants (at least one test result is needed for classification)**	
a.	Normal CRP and normal ESR	0
b.	Abnormal CRP or abnormal ESR	1
D.	**Duration of symptoms**	
a.	<6 weeks	0
b.	≥6 weeks	1

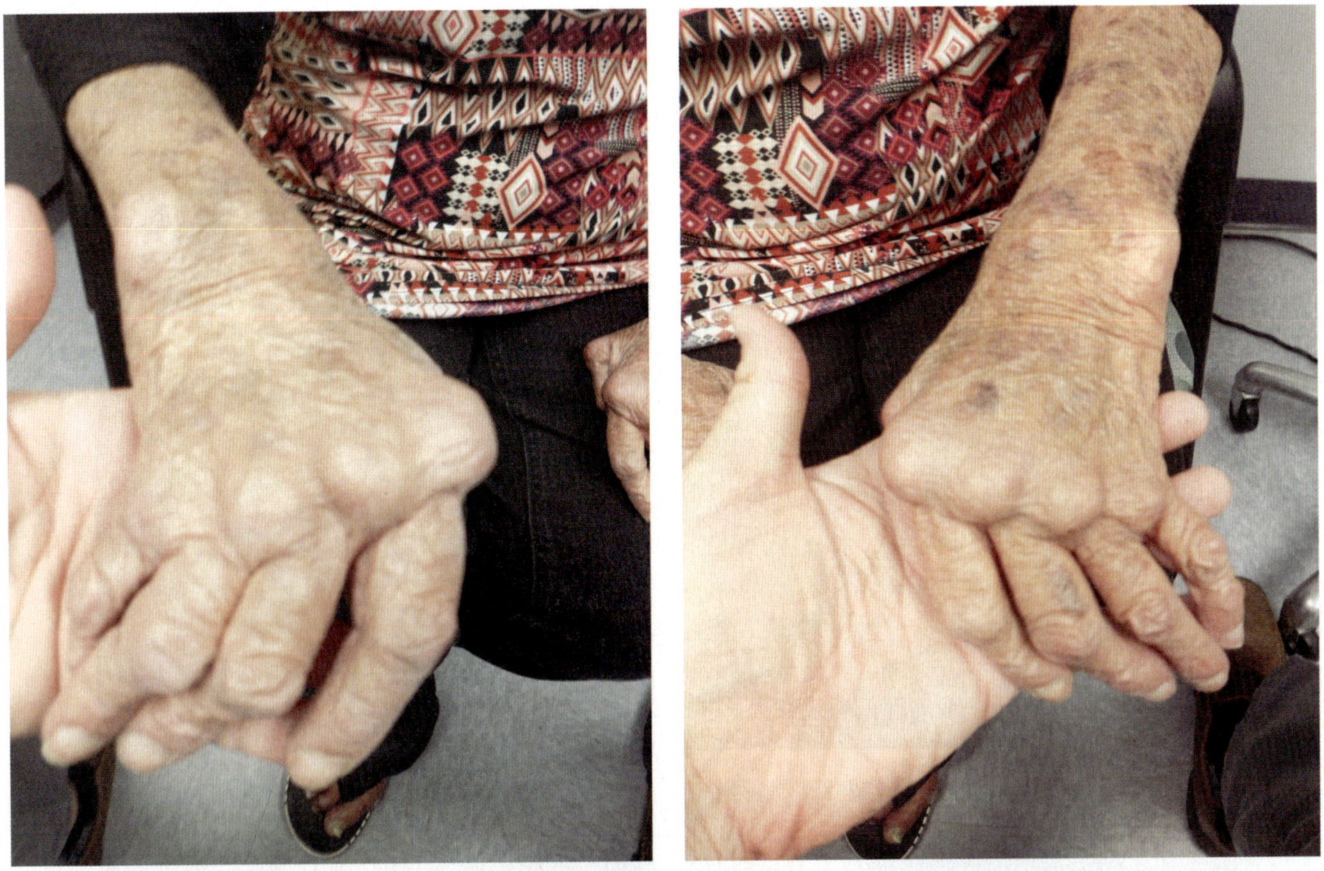

Figure 70.1. Severe rheumatoid arthritis of a 72-year-old female. Note the metacarpal phalangeal joint synovial thickening, the subluxation of the metacarpal phalangeal joints with ulnar deviation of the second through fifth metacarpal phalangeal joints. This is typical of advanced joint changes seen in rheumatoid arthritis.

The 6-week recommendation for diagnosis is very helpful, but as you can see from the criteria not necessary for the diagnosis of RA. Due to the fact that there are many other causes of symmetric polyarthritis (viral and others) that often mimic RA, this requirement strengthens the diagnosis.[34,37] All physicians caring for patients with musculoskeletal conditions should be familiar with the latest criteria for diagnosing the various diseases and clinical entities that manifest as symptoms of joint pain and evidence of swelling.

The principal measures used to assess response to treatment and remission for RA are composite, multidimensional outcome measures that incorporate clinical and laboratory data, functional assessment, patient-reported symptoms, and patient-reported global assessments.[38] The goals of RA treatment include reducing joint pain and swelling, preventing deformity, maintaining quality of life, and limiting extra-articular disease manifestations.[39] Nonpharmacologic treatments include physical and occupational therapy, exercise, patient education, and psychosocial interventions.[40] Medications used for short-term symptom relief include nonsteroidal anti-inflammatory drugs (NSAIDs) and low-dose glucocorticoids; the latter may be administered orally, intramuscularly, or intra-articularly. Both classes of medication can provide symptom relief within days. DMARDs are typically prescribed under the supervision of a rheumatologist and include methotrexate, leflunomide, hydroxychloroquine, and sulfasalazine. Biologic DMARDs include anti-TNF agents (adalimumab, certolizumab pegol, etanercept, golimumab, infliximab), and non-TNF biologics (abatacept, rituximab, tocilizumab). A final class of DMARDs includes JAK-inhibitors, of which tofacitinib is the primary agent used for RA. With DMARDs, clinical improvement is typically expected within 3 to 6 months of starting therapy.[41] Surgery is indicated for intractable pain, severe loss of motion, or functional impairment that exists despite medical management.[40]

While pharmacologic treatments for RA can substantially improve symptoms, they also have associated toxicities that are important to consider.[42] During both acute and chronic phases of the RA process, osteopathic physicians can also offer patients treatment of associated somatic dysfunction with gentle, indirect osteopathic manipulative procedures. Osteopathic treatment must be used with caution to not worsen a flare or cause increased pain.

Seronegative Spondyloarthropathies

In patients presenting with symmetrically or asymmetrically distributed inflammatory peripheral/extremity arthritis, with or without spinal joint involvement (axial involvement), a diagnosis of seronegative spondyloarthropathy should be considered.

The seronegative spondyloarthropathies are characterized by sacroiliitis, peripheral inflammatory arthritis, enthesitis, dactylitis, bursitis, tendonitis, a duration of longer than 12 weeks, and often the absence of serum RF.[7] There is an association with the HLA-B27 allele in many cases, although the presence of this genetic marker is neither diagnostic nor predictive of spondyloarthropathies. Examples of seronegative spondyloarthropathies include juvenile and adult AS, reactive arthritis (Reiter syndrome), spondylitis associated with chronic inflammatory bowel disease (also known as enteropathic arthritis), undifferentiated spondylarthritis, and PsA (Fig. 70.2A–C).

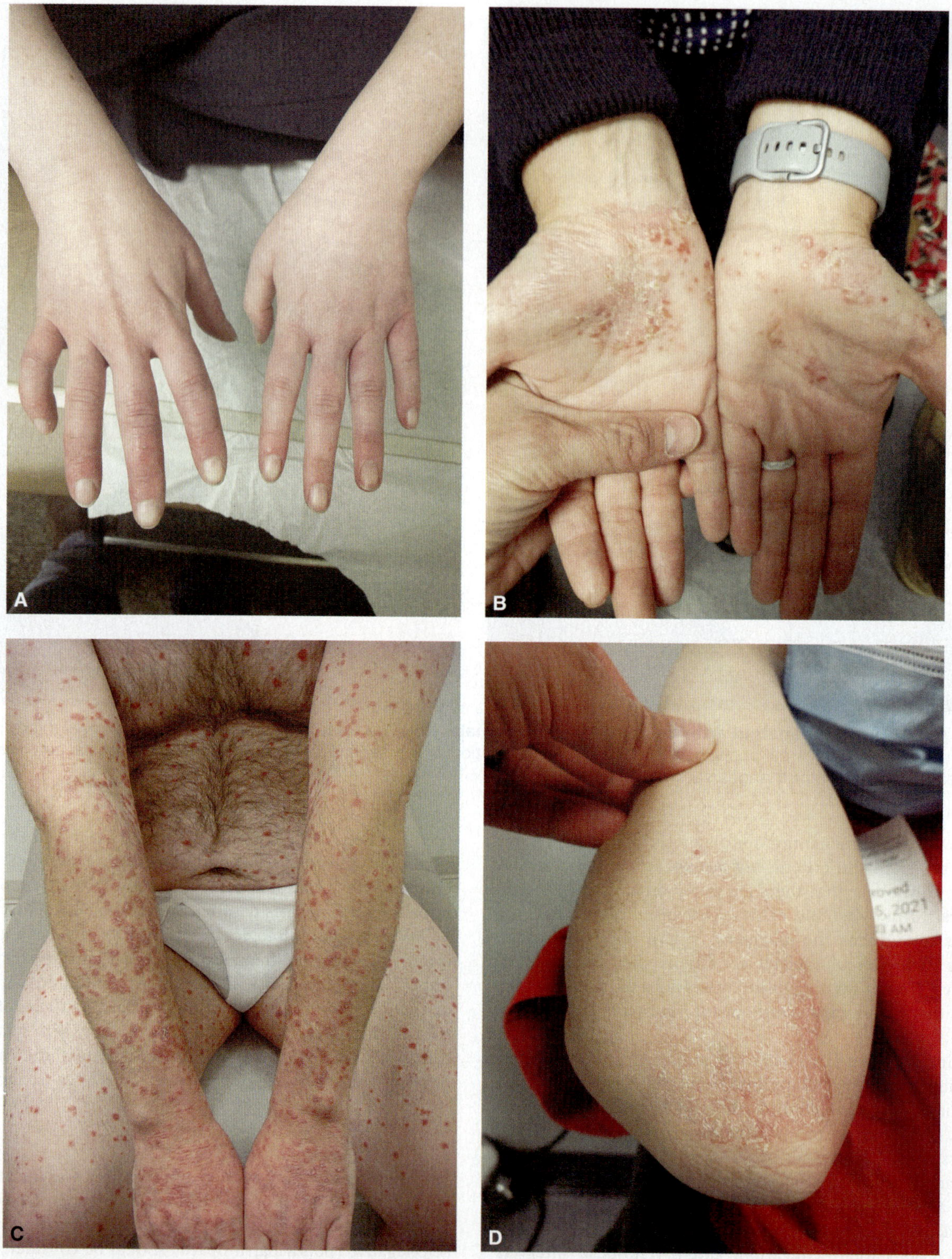

Figure 70.2. Figure A reveals swelling of the digits of the second, third, fourth metacarpal phalangeal joints, causing characteristic changes, can be seen in different forms of spondylarthritis, i.e., psoriatic arthritis (PsA). Figure B reveals palmar pustular psoriasis, which can be seen in PsA. Figure C reveals an example of disseminated guttate psoriasis. Figure D reveals findings characteristic of common plaque psoriasis seen on the extensor surface of the left elbow, seen in a patient with PsA.

The 2010 update of criteria for axial spondylarthritis by the Assessment of Spondylarthritis International Society (ASAS) in patients with back pain of >3 months' duration and age of onset <45 years of age is:

- Sacroiliitis on imaging by x-ray or MRI with the addition of one spondylarthritis feature

OR

- HLA B27 positive testing with the addition of two or more spondylarthritis features.

Spondylarthritis features: inflammatory back pain (morning stiffness >60 minutes), arthritis, enthesitis (heel), uveitis, dactylitis (Fig. 70.2D), psoriasis, Crohn disease/ulcerative colitis, good response to NSAIDs, family history of spondylarthritis, + HLA B27, elevated CRP.

Sacroiliitis on imaging: active (acute) inflammation on MRI of the pelvis showing sacroiliitis; or definite radiographic sacroiliitis.

Some forms of reactive arthritis follow enteric infection with such organisms as *Yersinia, Shigella, Salmonella, and Campylobacter*. All share similar clinical manifestations. The prevalence of sacroiliitis is high, along with extra-articular manifestations, including uveitis and, occasionally, oral ulcers.[7]

Chronic low back pain and stiffness are typically the first symptoms of AS.[43–45] Since onset is usually insidious rather than abrupt, patients often cannot date when symptoms first began or precisely localize the areas affected.[46] Complaints of alternating pain, first in one buttock and then the other, occasionally with radiation down the posterior thigh, can be elicited from some patients and probably represent sacroiliac involvement. Often these symptoms are incorrectly ascribed to hip disease or sciatica.

Because low back discomfort is such a common malady in the population at large, much attention has been directed at attempting to differentiate inflammatory from noninflammatory back pain.[43] Characteristically, inflammatory back symptoms are suggested by prominent stiffness and pain in the morning with stiffness lasting greater than 60 minutes, or after other periods of rest (gelling phenomenon) that improve with exercise. Such symptoms are most likely to reflect AS in a person younger than 45 years. Additional historic data suggesting AS include back pain that forces the individual out of bed at night or is not relieved by lying down, as well and may have concomitant chest wall pain.[44] Enthesitis, especially involving Achilles or plantar tendon insertions and causing heel pain, may appear alone or with arthritis.[47,48]

Treatment generally includes a combination of medications, physical therapy (PT), exercise, and lifestyle modifications. NSAIDs are often the first-line treatment for managing symptoms. DMARDs like sulfasalazine may be prescribed to help slow the progression of AS and reduce joint inflammation. In more severe cases, or when NSAIDs and DMARDs are ineffective, biologic medications may be considered. Examples include TNF-α inhibitors (such as adalimumab, etanercept, and infliximab), IL-17 inhibitors (such as secukinumab and ixekizumab), and IL-23 inhibitors (such as ustekinumab). Biologics target specific immune system molecules to reduce inflammation and improve symptoms. PT and osteopathic management are helpful for maintaining strength, flexibility and mobility of the spine and other affected joints.[49]

Juvenile Idiopathic Arthritis

JIA is the most common pediatric rheumatologic disorder and is classified by subtype according to International League of Associations for Rheumatology criteria.[50] It is characterized by progressive joint destruction and serious systemic manifestations. JIA, known outside of North America as juvenile chronic arthritis, occurs in patients younger than 18 years of age and persists for at least 6 weeks. Approximately 250,000 children in the United States have JIA.[51] JIA takes many forms, including oligoarthritis, polyarthritis, systemic, enthesitis-related arthritis (ERA), PsA, and undifferentiated arthritis.

Oligoarticular JIA is characterized by inflammation of up to four joints that begins as asymmetrical arthritis predominantly affecting the joints of the lower extremities, such as knee and ankle. There is a high frequency of positivity to antinuclear antibody (ANA) and a high risk of chronic uveitis.[50]

Polyarticular JIA (pJIA) affects five or more large/small joints and is hallmarked by injury to the metacarpophalangeal joints and wrists.[50]

Systemic JIA (sJIA) manifests not only with widespread joint arthritis, but also with a significant range of systemic inflammation symptoms. Approximately 10% of sJIA patients present systemic symptoms with associated macrophage activation syndrome (MAS), a potentially life-threatening condition.[50]

PsA often proceeds as oligoarthritis or RF-negative polyarthritis and more commonly involves the small joints accompanied by dactylitis, psoriatic rash and/or nail pitting. Psoriatic JIA itself is described as a heterogeneous disease where children <6 years are more likely to be female, ANA-positive, and predisposed to chronic uveitis, with arthritis of wrists and small joints of the hands and feet.[50]

ERA resembles oligoarthritis, affecting the joints of the lower limb in association with enthesitis. Due to the association with lower limb and sacroiliac joints, enthesitis, uveitis, and the association with HLA-B27, it may also belong to the group of spondyloarthropathies.[50]

Although the exact cause of JIA is unknown, there are complex interactions between immune cell populations. A triggering of a pathophysiologic cascade occurs involving proinflammatory cytokines and abnormal activation of T-cells, B-cells, natural killer (NK) cells, dendritic cells (DC), macrophages, and neutrophils. This process causes joint destruction and systemic complications.[52]

Environmental factors, infectious agents, vaccinations, antibiotics, vitamin D deficiency, stress, and trauma have been proposed as risk factors. Infectious viruses (Epstein-Barr virus, Parvovirus B, Rubivirus, Hepatitis B virus) and bacteria (*Salmonella* spp., *Shigella* spp., *Campylobacter* spp., *S. pyogenes, B. henselae, M. pneumoniae, Chlamydophila pneumonia*) have been reported as causal factors provoking JIA.[53] Gastrointestinal infection leading to loss of gut microbiome diversity and disrupted tryptophan metabolism increases the risk of ERA.[54] Several studies have documented genetic associations to JIA.[50]

Clinical symptoms, family history, laboratory markers, and instrumental examinations (US and MRI) are used to determine JIA subtype. Physical examination findings are paramount and include signs of arthritis (pain, tenderness, stiffness, and swelling of synovial joints) and extra-articular findings (such as rash, lymphadenopathy, dactylitis, nail changes). Laboratory tests for HLA-B27, RF, or anti-CCP antibody identifies the subtype of JIA and the risk of bone erosions and joint damage.

Therapeutic intervention begins at diagnosis with NSAIDs followed by disease-modifying antirheumatic drugs (DMARDs, most often methotrexate) and/or intra-articular corticosteroid injections. Local corticosteroid joint injections are effective in synovitis and may be a first-line treatment for oligoarthritis alone or in addition to DMARDs.

Systemic administration of high dose corticosteroids provides good short-term effect, especially in sJIA patients, but has no influence on the long-term disease outcome.

The ACR recommends early use of DMARDs, specifically methotrexate, leflunomide and/or sulfasalazine.[55] A broad range of DMARDs such as T-cell inhibitors, anti–TNF-α agents, IL-1, and IL-6 blockers, and JAK inhibitors have significantly improved the clinical management of JIA. Administration of biologic agents has decreased the mortality rate of JIA from 1% to 4% in the 1970s to 0.3% to 1% in 2016.[56] TNF-α inhibitors are recognized as the most effective drugs for the treatment of JIA with influence on pain, stiffness, growth, and quality of life.[50] Early, aggressive treatment of JIA was shown to be beneficial with 40% of patients achieving clinically inactive disease within 6 months.[57] With only 20% to 25% of patients achieving complete remission, there is still room for improvement in these therapies.[58]

Patients with positive antinuclear antibodies or HLA-B27 are at risk for iridocyclitis. Iridocyclitis is a specific type of anterior uveitis, where inflammation is concentrated in the iris (iritis) and also extends into the ciliary body (cyclo). Therefore, iridocyclitis is essentially a subtype of anterior uveitis. JIA-associated uveitis is one of the main causes of vision loss in childhood. Regular ophthalmologic visits with thorough slit lamp examinations are necessary. Half of these patients suffer from active uveitis in adulthood.[59] Older patients with pauciarticular JIA who are HLA-B27 positive might also have a form of juvenile AS manifested by sacroiliitis and asymmetric lower extremity arthritis, of whom are also at risk for iridocyclitis.[1]

Crystal-Induced Arthritis

Crystal-induced arthritis primarily includes gout and pseudogout. The latter is classified as calcium pyrophosphate deposition disease (CPPD). Gout is the most common form of inflammatory arthritis, more so than RA, and should be included in the differential of any inflammatory arthritis workup. Crystalline arthritis manifestations are typically monoarticular; however, they can be polyarticular and mimic other types of inflammatory arthritis as they progress.

Gout mainly affects middle-aged and older men. Gout is caused by the buildup of uric acid crystals in the joints. Uric acid is a natural waste product that is normally excreted through the kidneys. In individuals with gout, there is either an overproduction of uric acid or impaired excretion, leading to high levels of uric acid in the blood (hyperuricemia). When uric acid levels become excessively high, urate crystals can form and accumulate in the joints, particularly in the big toe, but also in other joints like the ankle, knee, wrist, and fingers. Gout attacks are characterized by sudden and severe joint pain, swelling, redness, and warmth. These attacks can be triggered by dietary factors, alcohol consumption, or other factors that increase uric acid levels. Gout can be perpetuated by genetic predisposition to hyperuricemia, diet, renal disease, hospitalization, malignancy, and medications like thiazide diuretics.[7] Following joint aspiration, polarized microscopy of synovial fluid identifies the monosodium urate crystals in gouty arthritis.[1,60,61]

Pseudogout (CPPD) is caused by the deposition of calcium pyrophosphate crystals in the joint spaces. These crystals are different from the uric acid crystals seen in gout. Similar to gout, pseudogout can lead to acute joint inflammation with symptoms such as pain, swelling, and redness. It can affect various joints, including the knees, wrists, and ankles. Pseudogout is more common in older individuals and may be associated with other medical conditions.

Treatment for crystalline-induced arthritis typically involves NSAIDs and/or corticosteroids that are often prescribed to reduce pain and inflammation during acute attacks. Indomethacin and colchicine are medications used to prevent and manage gout attacks. For recurrent or severe gout, medications that lower uric acid levels, such as allopurinol and febuxostat, may be prescribed. Dietary modifications, such as reducing intake of foods high in purines (which can contribute to uric acid buildup) and alcohol, are often recommended for gout management.

DEGENERATIVE ARTHRITIS

Osteoarthritis

OA comprises a family of degenerative joint disorders characterized by clinical and radiographic findings. OA is a slowly evolving articular disease characterized by the gradual development of joint pain, stiffness, and limitation of motion.[62] At present, the terms OA, osteoarthrosis, and degenerative joint disease are used interchangeably.

OA is the most common form of arthritis, affecting more than 30 million Americans.[63] OA is the most common cause of disability for people older than 65 years. OA has a huge economic impact, in terms of productivity (single greatest cause of days lost from work) and cost of treatment (chronic use of analgesics and anti-inflammatory drugs).[64] Age is one of the strongest risk factors for OA of all joints. It is most common in older people; before age 45 more men than women have OA, while after age 45 it is more common in women.[65] Women are more likely than men to have OA, and their OA tends to be more severe.[66] The etiology of the disorder is still not clearly understood, OA has been shown to be a family of disorders with the cartilage as a target organ. Newer concepts of pathogenesis suggest that OA is not an inevitable sequence of aging itself and raise the possibility of rational preventive and therapeutic approaches in the future.[62] Degeneration of the cartilage is the most prominent pathologic change. Both experimental[67] and clinical[68] studies have shown mild-to-moderate synovitis, although inflammatory changes may be absent early.[69] Although OA is often benign, severe degenerative changes often cause serious disability.

Biomechanical factors play a central role, while risk factors, such as age, weight, trauma, and occupation act as major variables. With more severe disease, pain may be persistent and interfere with normal activities of daily living. Chronic loss of restorative sleep with attendant increases in pain reports is common in this group.

Pain is the predominant symptom and initially often involves only one joint. Others tend to occur as time passes. The pain is most often described as a deep ache that is frequently accompanied by joint stiffness after periods of inactivity, such as on rising in the morning and after sitting. Morning stiffness and pain does not regularly last more than 30 to 45 minutes. Pain is aggravated by using the involved joints and may radiate or be referred to surrounding structures. In the early stages, it is commonly relieved by rest. Joint tenderness and crepitus on movement may also be present; there are no systemic symptoms.[70]

In the early stages of the disease, pain may be absent, but advanced disease may have grinding or locking with joint motion or buckling that signals instability of joints. Pain is present in patients with advanced disease, and overuse of muscle groups (locally and distant) can lead to the development of pain syndromes.[70]

OA can be defined pathologically, radiographically, or clinically. Radiographic OA has long been considered the reference standard.[66] Patients may have radiographic OA without evidence of clinical OA. Below is the Kellgren and Lawrence classification system.[71]

- Grade 0 (none): definite absence of x-ray changes of OA
- Grade 1 (doubtful): doubtful joint space narrowing and possible osteophytic lipping

- Grade 2 (minimal): definite osteophytes and possible joint space narrowing
- Grade 3 (moderate): moderate multiple osteophytes, definite narrowing of joint space, and some sclerosis and possible deformity of bone ends
- Grade 4 (severe): large osteophytes, marked narrowing of joint space, severe sclerosis, and definite deformity of bone ends

OA is deemed present at grade 2 although of minimal severity.[71]

Because no treatment can currently prevent or ameliorate the basic disease process or its progression, medical treatment is aimed at relieving pain and improving function. Guidelines recommend nondrug therapies as first-line treatments for chronic low back pain and OA pain.[72,73] Nonpharmacologic therapy includes patient education, weight loss if clinically indicated, PT, an organized low-impact exercise program, and assistive devices as needed. Osteopathic manipulative treatment (OMT) provided for associated somatic dysfunction is a component of conservative care. A recent study demonstrated that OMT and exercise treatment together improved function and provided more pain relief than exercise treatment alone.[74] In past studies it has been suggested that a combination of manual PT and supervised exercise provided functional benefits in knee OA patients. These benefits included improving pain and stiffness[75] and delaying or reducing the need for total knee replacement and steroid injections.[76–78]

Progressive OA may result in reduced mobility and the resultant systemic complications of immobility and deconditioning. The osteopathic physician needs to encourage their patients to stay physically fit and emotionally supported. There is moderate to strong evidence suggesting that exercise therapy and psychosocial interventions are effective for relieving pain and improving function for many patients with OA pain.[79–81]

Medications, especially NSAIDs, are typically recommended as second-line or adjunct therapy. Pharmacologic therapy often begins with analgesic medications or topical analgesics and NSAIDs as needed. Intra-articular injections of corticosteroids can relieve pain, but the effect is of limited duration. A systematic review of intra-articular corticosteroid injections found evidence of pain reduction for up to 6 weeks following injection.[82] Orthopedic intervention is largely reserved for situations that cannot be controlled with more conservative therapy.[64] Osteopathic manipulative techniques may also benefit rheumatologic patients who undergo joint replacements. Manual lymphatic drainage (MLD) techniques performed in the early postoperative stages following total knee arthroplasty may improve active knee flexion for up to 6 weeks postoperatively.[83] However, some study results are mixed, as MLD did not demonstrate a significant difference in pain intensity post total knee arthroplasty versus those in a control group.[84]

The most effective treatment for patients with rheumatologic conditions is a multidisciplinary approach combining the skills of many providers and clinicians. A holistic osteopathic approach includes supporting the patient's body, mind, and spirit through integrating multiple participants such as the primary care physician, rheumatologist, physiatrist, orthopedist, physical therapist, occupational therapist, psychologist, psychiatrist, clergy, nurse/nurse coordinator, dietitian, and social worker.

NONARTICULAR RHEUMATISM

Fibromyalgia

Primary FM has been defined as chronic, widespread musculoskeletal pain and tenderness at 11 of 18 specified sites established by the ACR initially proposed in 1990.[85] Qualitatively, the FM tender point count has been referred to as a "sedimentation rate" for distress.[86] In 2010, the ACR did not require tender point examination but based on the following three conditions being met: (1) Widespread pain index (WPI) score >7 with symptom severity scale >5 or WPI score of 3 to 6 and symptom severity scale >9, (2) symptoms present for at least 3 months, and (3) there is no disorder that would otherwise explain the patient's symptoms. The symptom severity scale was based on 19 different criteria including estimate of degree of fatigue, waking unrefreshed, and cognitive symptoms in general can help with clinical diagnosis. To note, in 2016, revised criteria for FM included the important statement that "A diagnosis of fibromyalgia is valid irrespective of other diagnoses. A diagnosis of fibromyalgia does not exclude the presence of other clinically important illnesses." This stresses the importance to know that FM can coexist with other disease processes, that is, autoimmune diseases, inflammatory arthritis, metabolic derangements, and mechanical disease processes.[87]

FM affects about 5% of the world population and approximately 2% of US and Canadian citizens have FM.[88] The incidence is higher in women than in men, and the age range in which FM generally appears is between 30 and 35 years.[88] On a typical day, a primary care physician may see several patients with this diagnosis.

The absence of signs of connective tissue or other musculoskeletal diseases is implicit in this definition, and to note, can coexist with such disease processes. Because of its subjective nature and its frequent association with disturbed sleep, chronic fatigue, headaches, and irritable bowel syndrome, the validity of classifying FM as a (rheumatic) disease rather than a "syndrome of being out of sorts" has been challenged.[89–96]

The exact cause of FM is not fully understood, but it is believed to involve a combination of genetic, environmental, and psychological factors. To date, no definitive pathology has been found in the muscles of FM patients. The pathophysiologic factors of FM are being studied and determined. According to current theories, it appears to be a central sensitization and pain-processing problem in the brain and spinal cord.[88] Therefore, FM is considered a central sensitivity syndrome. The main biochemical alterations observed in FM are dysfunctions in mono-aminergic neurotransmission, leading to elevated levels of excitatory neurotransmitters, such as glutamate and substance P, and decreased levels of serotonin and norepinephrine in the spinal cord at the level of descending anti-nociceptive pathways.[88] Although central sensitization plays an important role in FM, it is even more important to understand the initial cause; that is, the persistent nociceptive input associated with tissue damage, including peripheral sensitization. Increasing evidence indicates that the neurogenic-derived inflammatory processes occurring in the peripheral tissues, spinal cord, and brain are also responsible for the pathophysiology of FM.[97–99]

Psychosocial factors seem to play a large role in the development of the disease. According to several studies, the prevalence of psychiatric comorbidities, such as anxiety disorders and depression, among patients with this pathology reaches 60% in certain subpopulations.[100] Patients with FM may appear anxious and depressed. Studies have shown that they may feel dissatisfied with several aspects of their lives. Strong evidence has been given for an association between FM and major depressive disorder. Nevertheless, the specific characteristics of anxiety and depression have not been identified consistently in psychological testing. On the other hand, it has been suggested that chronic pain and fatigue of any cause regularly engender anxiety and depression.[101,102] The efficacy of SNRIs and other double-acting antidepressants, such as mirtazapine, suggests that neurotransmission dysfunction of both serotonin and norepinephrine exists in FM.[103]

Despite their subjectivity, symptoms of FM tend to be constant over many years. Decreased threshold to pain on pressure over certain sites and increased skin fold tenderness have led to numerous attempts to demonstrate localized peripheral abnormalities and to speculation that FM is a disorder of pain modulation within both the central and peripheral nervous systems.[86,104]

There are no irrefutable biochemical, immunologic, or anatomic abnormalities detected in FM. However, studies of biopsied muscle samples have found decreased levels of adenosine triphosphate and phosphocreatine both at rest and after exercise.[105] These findings have been confirmed by magnetic resonance spectroscopy in a small number of patients.[106] Other findings, such as decreased regional cerebral blood flow with low cerebrospinal fluid metabolite levels, have been cited as evidence for functional dysregulation of central pain pathways.[107–109]

An osteopathic approach to patients with FM uses a patient-centered, health-oriented methodology that includes manual diagnosis and OMT in conjunction with medication, counseling, and nutritional recommendations. This offers a multidimensional holistic approach to the multifaceted challenges FM patients face[110] (see Chapter 104). Current research on OMT demonstrates mixed or inconclusive findings.[111,112] However, recent studies on spinal manipulation[113] and myofascial release[114,115] have shown promise for effective treatment for the patients' pain, sleep, quality of life, and functionality. In addition to these nonpharmacologic methods, current research supports physical exercise and psychological treatments (including cognitive behavioral therapy and mindfulness) to improve pain, sleep, and depression as well as mind–body exercises to improve fatigue.[116]

RHEUMATIC DISEASE MANAGEMENT

Management of rheumatic diseases relies on an accurate diagnosis. Once a diagnosis is established, the evolving evidence that most rheumatic diseases are neither benign nor inevitably disabling should inform interventions and recommendations for treatment. As with many other chronic conditions, such as diabetes mellitus and hypertension, rheumatologic diseases are treated to a target or treatment goal. For rheumatologic diseases, this focuses on aiming for low disease activity or remission as well as quality-of-life issues with strategies designed to prevent adverse outcomes to the extent possible. Fortunately, both medical personnel and the public have a much better understanding of these situations than they did only a few years ago. The good news is that, with proper care, most patients with rheumatic diseases can function at quite high levels with only a minor impact on their daily lives.

Nonpharmacologic Treatments[1]

Nonpharmacologic therapies for rheumatic diseases are often rewarding, generally providing an assistive role. Along with improving general physical fitness, both PT and occupational therapy are fundamental components of treatment for both rheumatic and nonrheumatoid disorders.

No single modality has proven to be the most successful. However, treatment of the somatic component of any arthritic process by administration of appropriately chosen manipulative treatment is often helpful in relieving both pain and emotional distresses.[117] Manipulative techniques also supplement other adjunctive measures. Indirect approaches are particularly useful, including counterstrain, myofascial release, and functional techniques (see Chapters 46 to 64). Exercise, muscle strengthening, weight management, and nutritional guidance, along with general home and workplace considerations, are also factored in, including appropriate ergonomic advice.

Both OA and FM have proven to be particularly responsive to osteopathic manipulative methods. Medical management generally focuses on symptom management because, until recently, no single intervention has been proven to cure the primary disease processes, including DMARDs and biologic treatments. NSAIDs are particularly useful, and their generic forms are inexpensive.

A carefully graded, incremental exercise program is essential. If the regimen advances too quickly, symptoms may worsen, threatening compliance. Importantly, advise each patient that worsening pain is a warning sign that exercise tolerance has been reached.[118] Symptomatic relief commonly also occurs using both heat and cold.

Many supplements, dietary nutrients, and varying forms of exercises have been studied with varying outcomes for different disease processes. These topics can be difficult to navigate, and a reliable source for information is often welcomed. A good resource of well documented results from complementary and integrative health topics can be reviewed at https://www.nccih.nih.gov/. This is routinely and regularly updated based on new findings/research.

Pharmacologic therapies for rheumatic conditions vary, both in direct targeted treatment to specific disease processes as well as symptomatic treatment. Some work nonspecifically, others focus on underlying physiology targeting specific parts of the immune system. Below we will cover medications with an understanding of how they work, potential side effects, and what disease processes they are commonly used for.

Anti-inflammatory Drugs[119]

NSAIDs are supplemental to the treatment of most rheumatic diseases. They work via inhibition of cyclooxygenase activity of prostaglandin synthase 1 and 2. This can directly decrease production of inflammatory markers, erythema, hyperalgesia, and reduce fever. They are useful as both analgesic and anti-inflammatory agents, are generally inexpensive, and most have generic counterparts. As with any NSAID, their safety monitoring for cardiovascular disease, cerebrovascular disease, renal failure, gastrointestinal side effects, contraindications, correct dosing, and unique implications to each NSAID are of significant concern, raising the importance in making the correct decision for the most appropriate therapeutic choice.

Salicylates are also inexpensive and generally well tolerated in the short term. In general, larger doses are required than those used for primary analgesia. A constant blood level of 20 to 30 mg/dL is needed, which for most patients requires between 3 and 6 g of aspirin daily. All patients should be monitored for toxic blood levels and side effects, including tinnitus, deafness, and gastrointestinal intolerance. Recent evidence suggests that the latter occurs more often when *Helicobacter pylori* infection is present. Eradication of the *H. pylori* then allows for the safer use of these products.[120]

Overt gastrointestinal tract hemorrhage or ulceration is infrequent, but when it occurs, it dictates discontinuation of the drug and exploration for H. pylori infection.[120] This is caused by inhibition of prostaglandin endoperoxide synthase, which is a major source of gastric prostaglandin production, affecting intestinal ulcerations and delays in gastric ulcer healing.[121] In most cases, concomitant administration of proton pump inhibitors significantly reduces NSAID-induced gastrointestinal toxicity.[119] NSAIDs have the potential to cause acute kidney injury, abnormalities in maintaining appropriate systemic pH levels, nephrotic syndrome, papillary necrosis, electrolyte abnormalities, and fluid retention. Thus, patients with long-term NSAID use must be monitored appropriately.[122]

Corticosteroids

Glucocorticoids are potent medications, discovered in 1949 by Drs. Hench and Kendall, of whom both won the Nobel prize in 1950. Glucocorticoids are used parenterally, orally, intra-articular, inhaled, intradermal, intralesional for the purposes of this section. The mainstay of their use in rheumatology is for their suppressive effects on the inflammatory cascade and modification of the immune response. Like NSAIDs, they also suppress production of prostaglandins and interleukins through inhibition of phospholipase A2. This reduces proinflammatory cytokines like IL-10, IL-6, IL-1, COX-2, etc. Corticosteroids also upregulate enzymes that downregulate bradykinin, causing vasoconstriction and reducing swelling and pain. Clinically, they can be very effective in reducing pain, swelling, and inflammation, but their use should also be limited to as little as reasonably possible due to concurrent side effects of both acute and chronic use.[123]

Local injection of corticosteroids into affected joints and myofascial trigger points often produces dramatic symptomatic and functional improvements. Unfortunately, long-term side effects make them less desirable choices, except for the unresponsive patient with aggressive autoimmune/inflammatory conditions and joint disease that threatens loss of functional abilities. Oral prednisone is commonly helpful in this group of patients. Higher doses are necessary for patients with neuropathy, nephropathy, acute vasculitis, pleuritis, pericarditis, scleritis, central nervous system involvement, organ failure, and related conditions.[119]

Complications from acute and chronic use of glucocorticoids include but are not limited to:

- Glucose intolerance and development of insulin resistance
- Suppression of growth and can act as antagonists to growth hormone in pediatric use
- Osteonecrosis of the hip, or any bone for that matter
- Risk of cataract formation, glaucoma, choroidopathy
- Skin changes including easy bruising, impaired wound healing, hirsutism, and striae
- Gastric and peptic ulcer disease, bowel perforation
- Weight gain though water retention and potential cushingoid effects
- Increased risk of fungal infection, bacterial infection, opportunistic infections
- Increased risk of developing hypertension
- Abnormal hormone regulation through decrease in follicular stimulating hormone and luteinizing hormone, and depressed thyroid stimulating hormone and testosterone levels
- Mental disturbances, psychosis, irritation, insomnia, aggravation, restlessness
- Progression of osteoporosis
- Inhibited response to vaccinations, allergy skin testing with higher doses of glucocorticoids
- Sodium and electrolyte imbalances

Although helpful, noting its potential side effects, corticosteroid use should be monitored appropriately.

DISEASE-MODIFYING THERAPIES

DMARDs,[119] also known as disease-modifying antirheumatic drugs, work by changing the course of a disease for at least 1 year through sustained improvement of physical function, improving inflammation in joints with synovitis, and have been shown to slow or prevent progression of irreversible joint damage.[124] Conventional DMARDs include antimalarials, methotrexate, penicillamine, leflunomide, minocycline, and sulfasalazine. They are commonly used in such conditions as RA, PsA, AS, systemic sclerosis, systemic lupus, Sjogren syndrome, vasculitis, inflammatory bowel disease, myositis, uveitis, and certain forms of cancer as well.

Hydroxychloroquine (Plaquenil), an antimalarial-based DMARD, is administered 200 mg once or twice daily at a dose no more than 5 mg/kg/d. It tends to be the least toxic of all DMARDs and can work as monotherapy or in combination with other immunosuppressive medications. This drug may cause retinal lesions, maculopathy, or retinopathy, with loss of vision, making regular annual ophthalmologic evaluations a necessity. The proposed mechanism of hydroxychloroquine is that it inhibits intracellular toll-like receptor 9, which leads to decreased production of NFkB activation, cytokine reduction, and decreased inflammatory response. It has no increased risk of severe infections, hepatotoxicity, or renal dysfunction, but must be monitored for anemia, leukopenia, myopathy, and cardiomyopathy.

Methotrexate is one the most widely used, best evidenced, and effective form of long-term therapy for RA and other rheumatologic diseases. Methotrexate works through a complicated intracellular polyglutamation, inhibiting 5 AICAR transformylase, thymidylate synthetase, and dihydrofolate reductase, which causes anti-inflammatory and antiproliferative effects as a result. An oral or subcutaneous dosage of 2.5 to 25 mg once weekly is usually effective. A therapeutic response usually occurs within several weeks as the medication takes time to build up intracellularly and make immunomodulatory changes. It can be used for a wide variety of autoimmune and inflammatory conditions, including RA, PsA, AS, systemic sclerosis, systemic lupus, Sjogren syndrome, vasculitis, inflammatory bowel disease, myositis, and uveitis; it is touted as a steroid-sparing medication. Side effects include hepatotoxicity with a possibility of cirrhosis, bone marrow suppression, increased susceptibility to infections, poor wound healing, oral ulcers, hair loss, and potentially life-threatening pneumonitis. It is teratogenic. Methotrexate may cause more rheumatoid nodules to form as well. Simultaneous treatment with folic acid 1 mg/day reduces methotrexate toxicity without impairing efficacy and improves tolerance while reducing side effects.

Leflunomide (Arava), a pyrimidine antagonist that selectively inhibits dihydroorotate dehydrogenase, decreases synthesis of pyrimidines. This can decrease activated B- and T-lymphocytes and is used commonly in long-term treatment of RA or when methotrexate may not be well tolerated. Thus, it is commonly used with the same diseases that methotrexate is indicated for as an alternative option when appropriate. Side effects can include gastrointestinal irritation, skin rash, cytopenias, hepatotoxicity, hypertension, dyslipidemia, weight loss, pneumonitis, neuropathy, and is teratogenic/category X.

Sulfasalazine is a DMARD that has a two-part function, one as an antimicrobial, and as an active form of 5 aminosalicylic acid, providing anti-inflammatory properties. It is proposed that its anti-inflammatory effects come from upregulation of adenosine-like methotrexate. It is more commonly used in mild to moderate disease processes, with RA, sJIA, reactive arthritis, PsA, AS, and enteropathic arthritis. Side effect includes gastrointestinal changes, rash, headache, azoospermia, agranulocytosis, hemolysis (more with G6PD deficiency), pulmonary changes, and hypersensitivity reactions in those with an allergy to sulfa-based medications. It is safe to use in pregnancy.[125]

Minocycline has also been found to be effective in RA.[126] As a tetracycline antibiotic, it has some anti-inflammatory benefits. It can be a good choice for patients of comorbidities like COPD, for example, with a lower side effect profile of hyperpigmentation, dizziness, and photosensitivity. It is more commonly used in patients with low disease activity.

Gold salts, rarely used, are given in weekly intramuscular injections. It is not commonly used due to its severe side effect manifestations including bone marrow suppression (usually leukopenia or thrombocytopenia), renal damage with proteinuria, and nephrotic syndrome. Although it had a propensity to induce remissions if patients could tolerate the medication, it has fallen out of favor as more effective and better tolerated treatments have become available but is listed for its historical significance.

Penicillamine is no longer used due to concerns about inefficacy. Like gold salts, however, its effects begin slowly. Bone marrow and kidney toxicity are more common side effects. It also has the potential for inducing other autoimmune diseases, such as myasthenia gravis, Goodpasture syndrome, and lupus erythematosus. As a result, both gold salts and penicillamine are rarely used today.

Immunosuppressive agents, such as azathioprine, cyclophosphamide, chlorambucil, and cyclosporine, have been used to treat especially severe, unremitting RA, SLE, scleroderma, lupus nephritis, vasculitis, myositis, and uveitis. These medications also can be used in interstitial lung diseases related to autoimmune diseases. Monitoring safety is very important with use of these medications.

Biologic therapies including etanercept (Enbrel), a soluble recombinant TNF-α receptor inhibitor, have been approved for severe RA management. This class of drugs have proven to be highly effective in slowing progression of RA with a favorable risk to benefit ratio with more than 20 years now that they have been part of the treatment landscape. Infliximab (Remicade), a chimeric TNF-α receptor antagonist, is also available via intravenous infusion every 4 to 8 weeks. Additional anti-TNF agents available include adalimumab (Humira), certolizumab (Cimzia), and golimumab (Simponi). Additional therapies which target the IL-6 receptor (tocilizumab and sarilumab) and JAK inhibition (tofacitinib, baricitinib, and upadacitinib) are available for treatment.[127,128] Rituximab,[125] a CD20 B-cell depletion medication, and Abatacept,[129] a CD 80/86 costimulatory T-cell inhibitor, are two other classes of biologic agents that have demonstrated efficacy in RA. These agents are used typically after treatment failures with methotrexate and anti-TNF receptor antagonists.

Biologic therapies are approved for including belimumab[130] and anifrolumab,[131] as well as IL1 inhibitors which have therapy indications for RA, JRA.[132]

Surgery

Surgical joint replacement has been a major benefit for thousands of disabled arthritis sufferers. Prosthetic devices for hip and knee joints generally give excellent results, and devices for ankle, elbow, and shoulder replacement are improving. Joint replacement is indicated when pain has failed to respond to nonoperative management and is limiting functions and activities of daily living. The greatest benefit generally seen from surgery and joint replacement is pain relief.

OSTEOPATHIC MANIPULATIVE TREATMENT: EFFECTIVENESS AND RESEARCH

Arthritis patients appear to experience improved quality of life when offered OMT, as opposed to more traditional pharmacologic therapy. Research studies involving large numbers of patients followed for months or years have not yet been done. The long-term benefits of OMT are unknown, however older clinical trials have demonstrated the short- and intermediate-term benefit of manual therapies in patients with rheumatologic conditions.[133–138] Recent evidence for OMT in FM, OA, and AS are promising.[74,115]

CONCLUSION

Osteopathic principles and concepts described throughout this text are particularly useful when working with arthritic patients of all types. Palpatory diagnosis and manipulative treatment are particularly applicable for this population.

Except for infectious arthritis, no rheumatic disease can truly be cured. By combining appropriate neuromusculoskeletal and laboratory diagnoses with carefully selected pharmacologic therapy and manipulative treatment, the patient can experience both symptomatic and functional improvements, including an improved sense of well-being. Administering care and comanagement with a rheumatologist can benefit this patient group both with diagnostics and with treatment.

Continued clinical research is important for patient management and regarding the benefits of OMT in this population.

ACKNOWLEDGMENTS

The authors and editors of this chapter would like to acknowledge the scholarly contributions of Drs. J. Michael Finley, J. Michael Wieting, William Foley, Kurt P. Heinking, James A. Lipton, and Beth A. Valashinas for prior editions of this chapter.

REFERENCES

1. Rubin B. Osteopathic considerations in the clinical specialties—rheumatology. In: Ward RC, ed. *Foundations of Osteopathic Medicine*. 1st ed. Lippincott Williams & Wilkins; 1995.
2. National Academies of Sciences, Engineering, and Medicine; Health and Medicine Division; Board on Health Care Services; Committee on Identifying Disabling Medical Conditions Likely to Improve with Treatment. Chapter 5, Musculoskeletal disorders. In: *Selected Health Conditions and Likelihood of Improvement with Treatment*. National Academies Press (US); 2020. https://www.ncbi.nlm.nih.gov/books/NBK559512/
3. Decker JL. American Rheumatism Association nomenclature and classification of arthritis and rheumatism (1983). *Arthritis Rheum*. 1983;26:1029–1032.
4. Haber LD. Disabling effects of chronic disease and impairment. II. Functional capacity limitations. *J Chronic Dis*. 1973;26(3):127–151.
5. Verbrugge LM. From sneezes to adieux: stages of health for American men and women. *Soc Sci Med*. 1986;22(11):1195–1212.
6. Lawrence RC, Helmick CG, Arnett FC, et al. Estimates of the prevalence of arthritis and selected musculoskeletal disorders in the United States. *Arthritis Rheum*. 1998;41(5):778–799.
7. Felson D. Epidemiology of the rheumatic diseases. In: Koopman WJ, ed. *Arthritis and Allied Conditions: A Textbook of Rheumatology*. 14th ed. Lippincott Williams & Wilkins; 2001.
8. Obana KK, Davis J. Racial disparities in the prevalence of arthritis among Native Hawaiians and Pacific Islanders, Whites, and Asians. *Hawaii J Med Public Health*. 2016;75(6):155–161.
9. Cieza A, Causey K, Kamenov K, Hanson SW, Chatterji S, Vos T. Global estimates of the need for rehabilitation based on the Global Burden of Disease study 2019: a systematic analysis for the Global Burden of Disease Study 2019. *Lancet*. 2021;396(10267):2006–2017.
10. Mokdad AH, Ballestros K, Echko M, et al. The state of US Health 1990–2016: burden of diseases, injuries, and risk factors among US states. *JAMA*. 2018;319(14):1444–1472.
11. Yelin E, Callahan LF. The economic cost and social and psychological impact of musculoskeletal conditions. National Arthritis Data Work Groups. *Arthritis Rheum*. 1995;39(11):1351–1362.

12. Malik KM, Beckerly R, Imani F. Musculoskeletal disorders a universal source of pain and disability misunderstood and mismanaged: a critical analysis based on the U.S. model of care. *Anesth Pain Med.* 2018;8(6):e85532.
13. Rehabilitation 2030 initiative. World Health Organization. https://www.who.int/initiatives/rehabilitation-2030
14. McCarty DJ. Differential diagnosis of rheumatic disease: analysis of signs and symptoms. In: Koopman WJ, ed. *Arthritis and Allied Conditions: A Textbook of Rheumatology.* 14th ed. Lippincott Williams & Wilkins; 2001.
15. Gibbs JE, Ray DW. The role of the circadian clock in rheumatoid arthritis. *Arthritis Res Ther.* 2013;15:205.
16. Csuka ME, McCarty DJ. Simple method for measurement of lower extremity muscle strength. *Am J Med.* 1985;78:77–81.
17. Okifuji A, Turk DC, Sherman JJ. Evaluation of the relationship between depression and fibromyalgia syndrome: why aren't all patients depressed? *J Rheumatol.* 2000;1:212–219.
18. Gracely RH, Ceko M, Bushnell MC. Fibromyalgia and depression. *Pain Res and Treat.* 2012;2012:486590. Accessed August 28, 2017.
19. Hawker GA, Gignac MA, Badley E, et al. A longitudinal study to explain the pain-depression link in older adults with osteoarthritis. *Arthritis Care Res (Hoboken).* 2011;63(10):1382–1390.
20. Gordon DA. Approach to the patient with musculoskeletal disease. In: Goldman L, Bennett JC, eds. *Cecil Textbook of Internal Medicine.* 21st ed. WB Saunders; 2000.
21. Criswell LA, Pfeiffer KA, Lum RF, et al. Analysis of families in the Multiple Autoimmune Disease Genetics Consortium (MADGC) Collection: the PTPN22 620W allele associates with multiple autoimmune phenotypes. *Am J Hum Genet.* 2005;76(4):561–571.
22. Polley HF, Hunder GG. *Rheumatologic Interviewing and Physical Examination of the Joints.* 2nd ed. WB Saunders; 1978.
23. Doherty M, Doherty J. *Clinical Examination in Rheumatology.* Wolfe; 1992.
24. McCarty DJ Jr, Gatter RA, Phelps P. A dolorimeter for quantification of articular tenderness. *Arthritis Rheum.* 1965;8:551–559.
25. McCarty DJ Jr, Gatter RA, Steele AD. A twenty-pound dolorimeter for quantification of articular tenderness. *Arthritis Rheum.* 1968;11:696–698.
26. Goldenberg DL. Diagnostic and therapeutic challenges of fibromyalgia. *Hosp Pract (Off Ed).* 1989;24(9A):39–52.
27. Yamamoto T. Optimal management of dactylitis in patients with psoriatic arthritis. *Open Access Rheumatol.* 2015;7:55–62.
28. Shmerling RH, Liang MH. Laboratory evaluation of rheumatic diseases. In: *Primer on the Rheumatic Diseases.* 10th ed. Arthritis Foundation; 1993:64–66.
29. Merola JF, Espinoza LR, Fleischmann R. Distinguishing rheumatoid arthritis from psoriatic arthritis. *RMD Open.* 2018;4(2):e000656.
30. Sangha O. Epidemiology of rheumatic diseases. *Rheumatology (Oxford).* 2000;39(Suppl 2):3–12.
31. Scott DL, Symmons DP, Coulton BL, Popert AJ. Long-term outcome of treating rheumatoid arthritis: results after 20 years. *Lancet.* 1987;1:1108–1111.
32. Pincus T, Brooks RH, Callahan LF. Prediction of long-term mortality in patients with rheumatoid arthritis according to simple questionnaire and joint count measures. *Ann Intern Med.* 1994;120(1):26–34.
33. Wolfe F, Mitchell DM, Sibley JT, et al. The mortality of rheumatoid arthritis. *Arthritis Rheum.* 1994;37(4):481–494.
34. O'Dell JR. Rheumatoid arthritis: the clinical picture. In: Koopman WJ, ed. *Arthritis and Allied Conditions: A Textbook of Rheumatology.* 14th ed. Lippincott Williams & Wilkins; 2001.
35. Puentes-Osorio Y, Amariles P, Calleja MÁ, Merino V, Díaz-Coronado JC, Taborda D. Potential clinical biomarkers in rheumatoid arthritis with an omic approach. *Auto Immun Highlights.* 2021;12(1):9.
36. Guidelines for the management of rheumatoid arthritis. American College of Rheumatology Ad Hoc Committee on Clinical Guidelines. *Arthritis Rheum.* 1996;39(5):713–722.
37. Aletaha D, Neogi T, Silman AJ, et al. 2010 rheumatoid arthritis classification criteria: an American College of Rheumatology/European League against rheumatism collaborative initiative. *Arthritis Rheum.* 2010;62(9):2569–2581.
38. Felson DT, LaValley MP. The ACR20 and defining a threshold for response in rheumatic diseases: too much of a good thing. *Arthritis Res Ther.* 2014;16(1):101.
39. Wasserman AM. Diagnosis and management of rheumatoid arthritis. *Am Fam Physician.* 2011;84(11):1245–1252.
40. Rindfleisch JA, Muller D. Diagnosis and management of rheumatoid arthritis. *Am Fam Physician.* 2005;72(6):1037–1047.
41. Kavanaugh A, Klareskog L, van der Heijde D, Li J, Freundlich B, Hooper M. Improvements in clinical response between 12 and 24 weeks in patients with rheumatoid arthritis on etanercept therapy with or without methotrexate. *Ann Rheum Dis.* 2008;67(10):1444–1447.
42. Aletaha D, Smolen JS. Diagnosis and management of rheumatoid arthritis: a review. *JAMA.* 2018;320(13):1360–1372.
43. Calin A, Porta J, Fries JF, Schurman DJ. Clinical history as a screening test for ankylosing spondylitis. *JAMA.* 1977;237(24):2613–2614.
44. Blackburn WD Jr, Alarcon GS, Ball GV. Evaluation of patients with back pain of suspected inflammatory nature. *Am J Med.* 1988;85(6):766–770.
45. Gran JT. An epidemiologic survey of the signs and symptoms of ankylosing spondylitis. *Clin Rheum Dis.* 1985;4:161–169.
46. Arnett FC. Ankylosing spondylitis. In: Koopman WJ, ed. *Arthritis and Allied Conditions: A Textbook of Rheumatology.* 14th ed. Lippincott Williams & Wilkins; 2001.
47. Ball J. The enthesopathy of ankylosing spondylitis. *Br J Rheumatol.* 1983;22(4 suppl 2):25–28.
48. Olivieri I, Barozzi L, Padula A. Enthesopathy: clinical manifestations, imaging and treatment. *Baillieres Clin Rheumatol.* 1998;12:665–681.
49. Seiler M, Vermeylen B, Poortmans B, Feipel V, Dugailly PM. Effects of non-manipulative osteopathic management in addition to physical therapy and rehabilitation on clinical outcomes of ankylosing spondylitis patients: a preliminary randomized clinical trial. *J Bodyw Mov Ther.* 2020;24(4):51–56.
50. Zaripova LN, Midgley A, Christmas SE Beresford MW, Baildam EM, Oldershaw RA. Juvenile idiopathic arthritis: from aetiopathogenesis to therapeutic approaches. *Pediatr Rheumatol Online J.* 2021;19:135.
51. Singsen BH. Rheumatic diseases of childhood. *Rheum Dis Clin North Am.* 1990;16:581–599.
52. Mellins ED, Macaubas C, Grom AA. Pathogenesis of systemic juvenile idiopathic arthritis: some answers, more questions. *Nat Rev Rheumatol.* 2011;7(7):416–426.
53. Rigante D, Bosco A, Esposito S. The etiology of juvenile idiopathic arthritis. *Clin Rev Allergy Immunol.* 2015;49:253–261.
54. Mistry RR, Patro P, Agarwal V, Misra DP. Enthesitis-related arthritis: current perspectives. *Open Access Rheumatol.* 2019;11:19–31.
55. Ringold S, Weiss PF, Beukelman T, et al. 2013 update of the 2011 American College of Rheumatology recommendations for the treatment of juvenile idiopathic arthritis: recommendations for the medical therapy of children with systemic juvenile idiopathic arthritis and tuberculosis screening among children receiving biologic medications. *Arthritis Care Res (Hoboken).* 2013;65(10):1551–1563.
56. Momah T, Ray L. Juvenile idiopathic arthritis: old disease, new tactics. *J Fam Pract.* 2019;68(2):E8–E13.
57. Blazina Š, Markelj G, Avramovič MZ, Toplak N, Avčin T. Management of juvenile idiopathic arthritis: a clinical guide. *Paediatr Drugs.* 2016;18(6):397–412.
58. Selvaag AM, Aulie HA, Lilleby V, Flatø B. Disease progression into adulthood and predictors of long-term active disease in juvenile idiopathic arthritis. *Ann Rheum Dis.* 2016;75(1):190–195. https://doi.org/10.1136/annrheumdis-2014-206034.
59. Barišić Kutija M, Perić S, Knežević J, Juratovac Z, Vukojević N. Complication and prognosis of juvenile idiopathic arthritis associated uveitis in the era of modern immunomodulatory treatment. *Psychiatr Danub.* 2019;31(Suppl 1):44–49.
60. McCarty DJ. Coexistent gout and rheumatoid arthritis. *J Rheumatol.* 1981;8:253–254.
61. Lawrence RC, Hochberg MC, Kelsey JL, et al. Estimates of the prevalence of selected arthritic and musculoskeletal diseases in the United States. *J Rheumatol.* 1989;16:427–441.
62. Moskowitz RW, Holderbaum D. Clinical and laboratory findings in osteoarthritis. In: Koopman WJ, ed. *Arthritis and Allied Conditions: A Textbook of Rheumatology.* 14th ed. Lippincott Williams & Wilkins; 2001.
63. Arthritis Foundation. Arthritis by the numbers: book of trusted facts & figures. 2018. Accessed January 10, 2020. https://www.arthritis.org/

getmedia/e1256607-fa87-4593-aa8a-8db4f291072a/2019-ABTN-final-March-2019.pdf

64. Schnitzer TJ. Osteoarthritis (degenerative joint disease). In: Goldman L, Bennett JC, eds. *Cecil Textbook of Internal Medicine.* 21st ed. WB Saunders; 2000.
65. National Institute of Arthritis and Musculoskeletal and Skin Diseases. Osteoarthritis. 2016. Accessed November 15, 2019. https://www.niams.nih.gov/health-topics/osteoarthritis
66. Zhang Y, Jordan JM. Epidemiology of osteoarthritis. *Clin Geriatr Med.* 2010;26(3):355–369.
67. Moskowitz RW, Goldberg VM, Berman L. Synovitis as a manifestation of degenerative joint disease: an experimental study. *Arthritis Rheum.* 1976;19:813.
68. Goldenberg DL, Egan MS, Cohen AS. Inflammatory synovitis in degenerative joint disease. *J Rheumatol.* 1982;9:204–209.
69. Myers SL, Brandt KD, Ehrlich JW, et al. Synovial inflammation in patients with early osteoarthritis of the knee. *J Rheumatol.* 1990;17:1662–1669.
70. Frontera WR, Silver JK, Rizzo TD. *Essentials of Physical Medicine and Rehabilitation.* 4th ed. Elsevier; 2019.
71. Kellgren J, Lawrence J. Radiological assessment of osteo-arthrosis. *Ann Rheum Dis.* 1957;16(4):494–502.
72. Bannuru RR, Osani MC, Vaysbrot EE, et al. OARSI guidelines for the nonsurgical management of knee, hip, and polyarticular osteoarthritis. *Osteoarthritis Cartilage.* 2019;27(11):1578–1589.
73. Qaseem A, Wilt TJ, McLean RM, Forciea MA. Noninvasive treatments for acute, subacute, and chronic low back pain: a clinical practice guideline from the American College of Physicians. *Ann Intern Med.* 2017;166(7):514–530.
74. Altınbilek T, Murat S, Yumuşakhuylu Y, İçağasıoğlu A. Osteopathic manipulative treatment improves function and relieves pain in knee osteoarthritis: a single-blind, randomized-controlled trial. *Turk J Phys Med Rehabil.* 2018;64(2):114–120.
75. Moss P, Sluka K, Wright A. The initial effects of knee joint mobilization on osteoarthritic hyperalgesia. *Man Ther.* 2007;12:109–118.
76. Deyle GD, Henderson NE, Matekel RL, Ryder MG, Garber MB, Allison SC. Effectiveness of manual physical therapy and exercise in osteoarthritis of the knee. A randomized, controlled trial. *Ann Intern Med.* 2000;132:173–181.
77. Iudica AC. Can a program of manual physical therapy and supervised exercise improve the symptoms of osteoarthritis of the knee? *J Fam Pract.* 2000;49:466–467.
78. Abbott JH, Robertson MC, Chapple C, et al. Manual therapy, exercise therapy, or both, in addition to usual care, for osteoarthritis of the hip or knee: a randomized controlled trial. 1: clinical effectiveness. *Osteoarthritis Cartilage.* 2013;21:525–534.
79. Fransen M, McConnell S, Hernandez-Molina G, Reichenbach S. Exercise for osteoarthritis of the hip. *Cochrane Database Syst Rev.* 2014;2014:CD007912.
80. Fransen M, McConnell S, Harmer AR, Van der Esch M, Simic M, Bennell KL. Exercise for osteoarthritis of the knee. *Cochrane Database Syst Rev.* 2015;1:CD004376.
81. Pedersen BK, Saltin B. Exercise as medicine—evidence for prescribing exercise as therapy in 26 different chronic diseases. *Scand J Med Sci Sports.* 2015;25(suppl 3):1–72.
82. da Costa BR, Hari R, Juni P. Intra-articular corticosteroids for osteoarthritis of the knee. *JAMA.* 2016;316(24):2671–2672.
83. Ebert JR, Joss B, Jardine B, Wood DJ. Randomized trial investigating the efficacy of manual lymphatic drainage to improve early outcome after total knee arthroplasty. *Arch Phys Med Rehabil.* 2013;94:2103–2111.
84. Fujiura T, Nagasawa H, Wakabayashi H. Effect of manual lymph drainage for up to 10 days after total knee arthroplasty: a randomized controlled trial. *Phys Ther Res.* 2020;23(1):39–46.
85. Wolfe F, Smythe HA, Yunus MB, et al. The American College of Rheumatology 1990 criteria for the classification of fibromyalgia. Report of the multicenter criteria committee. *Arthritis Rheum.* 1990;33:160–172.
86. Ball EV. Non-articular rheumatism. In: Goldman L, Bennett JC, eds. *Cecil Textbook of Internal Medicine.* 21st ed. WB Saunders; 2000.
87. Wolfe F, Clauw DJ, Fitzcharles MA, et al. 2016 revisions to the 2010/2011 fibromyalgia diagnostic criteria. *Semin Arthritis Rheum.* 2016;46(3):319–329.
88. Siracusa R, Paola RD, Cuzzocrea S, Impellizzeri D. Fibromyalgia: pathogenesis, mechanisms, diagnosis and treatment options update. *Int J Mol Sci.* 2021;22(8):3891.
89. Bennett RM. Fibromyalgia and the facts. Sense or nonsense. *Rheum Dis Clin North Am.* 1993;19:45–59.
90. Granges G, Littlejohn GO. A comparative study of clinical signs in fibromyalgia/fibrositis syndrome, healthy and exercising subjects. *J Rheumatol.* 1993;20:344–351.
91. Powers R. Fibromyalgia: an age-old malady begging for respect. *J Gen Intern Med.* 1993;8:93–105.
92. Waylonis GW, Heck W. Fibromyalgia syndrome. New associations. *Am J Phys Med Rehabil.* 1992;71:343–348.
93. Veale D, Kavanagh G, Fielding JF, Fitzgerald O. Primary fibromyalgia and the irritable bowel syndrome: different expressions of a common pathogenetic process. *BMJ.* 1991;30:220–222.
94. Littlejohn GO. A database for fibromyalgia. *Rheum Dis Clin North Am.* 1995;21:527–557.
95. Jacobsen S, Petersen IS, Danneskiold-Samsøe B. Clinical features in patients with chronic muscle pain with special reference to fibromyalgia. *Scand J Rheumatol.* 1993;22:69–76.
96. Yunus MB, Masi AT, Aldag JC. A controlled study of primary fibromyalgia syndrome: clinical features and association with other functional syndromes. *J Rheumatol.* 1989;16:62–71.
97. Slade GD, Conrad MS, Diatchenko L, et al. Cytokine biomarkers and chronic pain: association of genes, transcription, and circulating proteins with temporomandibular disorders and widespread palpation tenderness. *Pain.* 2011;152:2802–2812.
98. Sturgill J, McGee E, Menzies V. Unique cytokine signature in the plasma of patients with fibromyalgia. *J Immunol Res.* 2014;2014:938576.
99. Mendieta D, De la Cruz-Aguilera DL, Barrera-Villalpando MI, et al. IL-8 and IL-6 primarily mediate the inflammatory response in fibromyalgia patients. *J. Neuroimmunol.* 2016;290:22–25.
100. Epstein SA, Kay G, Clauw D, et al. Psychiatric disorders in patients with fibromyalgia. A multicenter investigation. *Psychosomatics.* 1999;40:57–63.
101. Hudson JI, Pope HG Jr. The relationship between fibromyalgia and major depressive disorder. *Rheum Dis Clin North Am.* 1996;22(2):285–303.
102. Goldenberg D, Mayskiy M, Mossey C, Ruthazer R, Schmid C. A randomized, double-blind crossover trial of fluoxetine and amitriptyline in the treatment of fibromyalgia. *Arthritis Rheum.* 1996;39(11):1852–1859.
103. Moret C, Briley M. Antidepressants in the treatment of fibromyalgia. *Neuropsychiatr. Dis. Treat.* 2006;2:537–548.
104. Vecchio E, Lombardi R, Paolini M, et al. Peripheral and central nervous system correlates in fibromyalgia. *Eur J Pain.* 2020;24(8):1537–1547.
105. Jacobsen S, Bartels EM, Danneskiold-Samsøe B. Single cell morphology of muscle in patients with chronic muscle pain. *Scand J Rheumatol.* 1995;20(5):336–343.
106. Van-Denderen JC, Boersma JW, Zeinstra P, Hollander AP, van Neerbos BR. Physiological effects of exhaustive physical exercise in primary fibromyalgia syndrome (PFS): is PFS a disorder of neuroendocrine activity? *Scand J Rheumatol.* 1995;21(1):35–37.
107. Jacobsen S, Jensen KE, Thomsen C, Danneskiold-Samsoe B, Henriksen O. 31P magnetic resonance spectroscopy of skeletal muscle in patients with fibromyalgia. *J Rheumatol.* 1994;19(10):1600–1603.
108. Russell IJ, Vaeroy H, Javors M, Nyberg F. Cerebrospinal fluid biogenic amine metabolites in fibromyalgia/fibrositis syndrome and rheumatoid arthritis. *Arthritis Rheum.* 1995;35(5):550–556.
109. Russell IJ, Michalek JE, Vipraio GA, Fletcher EM, Javors MA, Bowden CA. Platelet 3H-imipramine uptake receptor density and serum serotonin levels in patients with fibromyalgia-fibrositis syndrome. *J Rheumatol.* 1994;19(1):104–109.
110. Seffinger MA. An osteopathic approach to fibromyalgia. *Pract Pain Manag.* 2010;10(5). Accessed June 29, 2017. https://www.practicalpainmanagement.com/pain/myofascial/fibromyalgia/osteopathic-approach-fibromyalgia

111. Coste J, Medkour T, Maigne JY, Pérez M, Laroche F, Perrot S. Osteopathic medicine for fibromyalgia: a sham-controlled randomized clinical trial. *Ther Adv Musculoskelet Dis*. 2021;13:1759720X211009017.
112. Schulze NB, de Melo Salemi M, de Alencar GG, Moreira MC, de Siqueira GR. Efficacy of manual therapy on pain, impact of disease, and quality of life in the treatment of fibromyalgia: a systematic review. *Pain Physician*. 2020;23(5):461.
113. Ince B, Kara M, Erdem I, Yurdakul OV, Erden T, Aydın T. Effectiveness of spinal manipulation in addition to pharmacological treatment in fibromyalgia: a blinded randomized trial. *PM R*. 2023;15(3):342–351.
114. Ughreja RA, Venkatesan P, Gopalakrishna DB, Singh YP. Effectiveness of myofascial release on pain, sleep, and quality of life in patients with fibromyalgia syndrome: a systematic review. *Complement Ther Clin Pract*. 2021;45:101477.
115. Dal Farra F, Chiesa A, Risio RG, Vismara L, Bergna A. Fast improvements in functional status after osteopathic manipulative treatment based on myofascial release in patients with moderate or severe fibromyalgia: a retrospective study. *J Complement Integr Med*. 2021;20:779–787.
116. Kundakci B, Kaur J, Goh SL, et al. Efficacy of nonpharmacological interventions for individual features of fibromyalgia: a systematic review and meta-analysis of randomised controlled trials. *Pain*. 2022;163(8):1432–1445.
117. Tettambel MA. Osteopathic treatment considerations for rheumatic diseases. *J Am Osteopath Assoc*. 2001;101(4 Suppl Pt 2):S18–S20.
118. Lozada CJ, Altman RD. Management of osteoarthritis. In: Koopman WJ, ed. *Arthritis and Allied Conditions: A Textbook of Rheumatology*. 14th ed. Lippincott Williams & Wilkins; 2001.
119. Arnett FC. Rheumatoid arthritis. In: Goldman L, Bennett JC, eds. *Cecil Textbook of Internal Medicine*. 21st ed. WB Saunders; 2000.
120. Huang JQ, Sridhar S, Hunt RH. Role of *Helicobacter pylori* and nonsteroidal anti-inflammatory drugs in peptic ulcer disease: a meta-analysis. *Lancet*. 2002;359:14–22.
121. Schmassmann A, Peskar BM, Stettler C, et al. Effects of inhibition of prostaglandin endoperoxide synthase-2 in chronic gastro-intestinal ulcer models in rats. *Br J Pharmacol*. 1998;123(5):795–804.
122. Whelton A, Hamilton CW. Nonsteroidal anti-inflammatory drugs: effects on kidney function. *J Clin Pharmacol*. 1991;31(7):588–598.
123. Ericson-Neilsen W, Kaye AD. Steroids: pharmacology, complications, and practice delivery issues. *Ochsner J*. 2014;14(2):203–207.
124. Benjamin O, Goyal A, Lappin SL. Disease modifying anti-rheumatic drugs (DMARD). In: *StatPearls [Internet]*. StatPearls Publishing; 2022. Updated July 4, 2022. https://www.ncbi.nlm.nih.gov/books/NBK507863/
125. Choi J, Fenando A. Sulfasalazine. In: *StatPearls [Internet]*. StatPearls Publishing; 2022. Updated November 11, 2022. https://www.ncbi.nlm.nih.gov/books/NBK557809/
126. Tilley BC, Alarcón GS, Heyse SP, et al. Minocycline in rheumatoid arthritis. A 48 weeks, double blind, placebo controlled trial. MIRA Trial Group. *Ann Intern Med*. 1995;122(2):81–89.
127. Bijlsma JW, Welsing PMJ, Woodworth TG, et al. Early rheumatoid arthritis treated with tocilizumab, methotrexate, or their combination (U-Act-Early): a multicentre, randomised, double-blind, double-dummy, strategy trial. *Lancet*. 2016;388(10042):343–355.
128. Lee EB, Fleischmann R, Hall S, et al; ORAL Start Investigators. Tofacitinib versus methotrexate in rheumatoid arthritis. *N Engl J Med*. 2014;370(25):2377–2386.
129. Blair HA, Deeks ED. Abatacept: a review in rheumatoid arthritis. *Drugs*. 2017;77(11):1221–1233.
130. Davidson A. The rationale for BAFF inhibition in systemic lupus erythematosus. *Curr Rheumatol Rep*. 2012;14(4):295–302.
131. Furie RA, Morand EF, Bruce IN, et al. Type I interferon inhibitor anifrolumab in active systemic lupus erythematosus (TULIP-1): a randomised, controlled, phase 3 trial. *Lancet Rheumatol*. 2019;1(4) e208–e219.
132. Gabay C. IL-1 inhibitors: novel agents in the treatment of rheumatoid arthritis. *Expert Opin Investig Drugs*. 2000;9(1):113–127.
133. Fiechtner JJ, Brodeur RR. Manual and manipulation techniques for rheumatic disease. *Med Clin North Am*. 2002;86(1):91–103.
134. Vernon H. Manipulation/manual therapy in the treatment of osteoarthritis. *J Arthritis*. 2013;2:e107.
135. Tucker WE. Treatment of osteoarthritis by manual therapy. *Br J Clin Pract*. 1969;23(1):38.
136. Rubin B. Management of osteoarthritic knee pain. *J Am Osteopath Assoc*. 2005;105(4):S23–S28.
137. Gamber RG, Shores JH, Russo DP, Jimenez C, Rubin BR. Osteopathic manipulative treatment in conjunction with medication relieves pain associated with fibromyalgia syndrome: results of a randomized clinical pilot project. *J Am Osteopath Assoc*. 2002;102(6):321–325.
138. Castro-Sánchez AM, Aguilar-Ferrándiz ME, Matarán-Peñarrocha GA, Sánchez-Joya Mdel M, Arroyo-Morales M, Fernández-de-las-Peñas C. Short-term effects of a manual therapy protocol on pain, physical function, quality of sleep, depressive symptoms, and pressure sensitivity in women and men with fibromyalgia syndrome: a randomized controlled trial. *Clin J Pain*. 2014;30(7):589–597.

71 Osteopathic Considerations in Cardiovascular Medicine

KURT P. HEINKING ▪ KELLY RYCHTER

KEY CONCEPTS

- Patients with cardiovascular (CV) conditions represent the largest component of internal medicine, and cardiovascular disease (CVD) is the leading cause of mortality in the United States and worldwide.[1,2]
- The osteopathic physician traditionally focuses on health while controlling the disease process to obtain the maximal health capacity of each patient.
- A comprehensive approach to patients with CVD requires the incorporation of evidence-based guidelines and an emphasis on primary and secondary disease prevention through lifestyle modification.[1]
- The components of a CV screening evaluation are the history, physical examination, and risk assessment. Further additional components can then include blood tests, echocardiography, stress tests, chest x-ray, electrocardiogram (EKG), and a cardiac CT or MRI.
- The history and physical exam are crucial for determining if the patient is having a life-threatening event and for risk-stratifying patients. Proper risk factor stratification allows targeted interventions.[3]
- Heart failure (HF) is a leading cause of CV morbidity and mortality worldwide despite the advances in therapies and prevention, and the most common causes of HF are ischemic heart disease (IHD) and systemic arterial hypertension, both are preventable.[1]
- Atrial fibrillation (AF) is the most common sustained cardiac arrhythmia worldwide and one of the most common cause of admission to the hospital.[4]
- Physical activity in patients with peripheral artery disease (PAD) is associated with a decrease in all-cause and CV mortality, however, chronic limb-threatening ischemia (CLTI) despite treatment has an amputation rate of up to 20% at 12 months and over 50% of all CLTI patients die within 5 years after presentation.[5]
- In patients with stable coronary artery disease (CAD), coronary artery bypass graft (CABG) surgery and percutaneous transluminal coronary angioplasty (PTCA) do not prevent myocardial infarction (MI).[6]
- Having a quality diet that emphasizes the intake of vegetables, fruits, nuts, whole grains, lean vegetables or animal protein, and fish was associated with an 18% to 26% lower all-cause and CVD mortality risk.[7]
- Adults should engage in at least 150 minutes of accumulated moderate-intensity physical activity per week or 75 minutes of vigorous-intensity physical activity per week.[8]
- Hypertension is the leading preventable risk factor for CVD and all-cause mortality worldwide.[9]
- The Osteopathic management approach for CV patients should not only specifically address the disease process but engage the patient with shared decision making and consider the patients' physical, mental, and spiritual health in their journey toward improving wellness.
- A holistic approach to patients with CVD recognizes that a multifactorial disease process requires a comprehensive therapeutic plan including progressive aerobic exercise, weight loss, control of hypertension and diabetes, cessation of cigarette smoking, treatment of somatic dysfunction, reduction of serum cholesterol, dietary modifications, and control of stress.
- Osteopathic treatment assists in the resolution of accompanying somatic dysfunction improving the patient's musculoskeletal functioning and pain. Osteopathic manipulative treatment (OMT) helps adults increase their physical activity, restoring homeostasis and reducing their overall CV risk.
- Mental health and CV health are interconnected. It is important to address mental health in comprehensive CV care.

OVERVIEW

Patients with CV conditions represent the largest component of internal medicine, and CVD is the leading cause of mortality in the United States and worldwide.[1,2] Cardiology is captivating and encompasses a broad spectrum with robust opportunities for care spanning the spectrum from prevention to intervention. The Strategic Plan from the American Heart Association (AHA) for 2020, articulated the goal "by 2020 to improve the CV health of all Americans by 20%, while reducing deaths from CVD and stroke by 20%."[2] To achieve these goals, the AHA recommended (a) prevention (b) decreasing risk factors for CVD early in life, and (c) to balance individualized risk with population-level approaches. It is estimated that one-third of CV deaths may be preventable through healthy lifestyle choices including diet and physical activity.[2,10] The osteopathic physician should educate and encourage all patients to reduce their CV risk through diet, exercise, smoking cessation, weight control, and stress management.

The management approach for patients should address the disease process and consider their physical, mental, and spiritual health in their journey toward improving wellness.[11]

The goal of this chapter is to present a brief review of common CV conditions and how the application of the osteopathic approach can benefit the CV patient. Although biological, physiologic, pathophysiologic, and clinical data to support an osteopathic approach will be presented, it should be noted that osteopathic medicine is both an art and a science. Therefore, we must rely on the medical evidence, yet utilize the osteopathic clinical experience and skills passed down from past generations for the good of the patient. This integrates science and art, so we can follow evidence-based guidelines and choose to implement osteopathic approaches that are proven or have biologic and pathophysiologic plausibility. Osteopathic considerations also include a holistic patient-centered philosophy, focusing on finding the health of a patient. This includes a biopsychosocial approach, addressing pertinent somatic dysfunction and enhancing the patient's emotional and spiritual life. Somatic dysfunction can accompany CVD, and if present, is thought to have functional implications. OMT is not used to treat CVD, rather it is integrated into the comprehensive treatment of patients with CVD who also have somatic dysfunction. Osteopathic principles embrace a unique aspect in the realm of CV care which fosters a more comprehensive and patient-centered approach to CV well-being.

Application of Osteopathic Tenets/ Philosophic Principles

Since the time of AT Still, the osteopathic profession has taught and stressed the importance of the following basic tenets and philosophic principles applied in all branches of medicine. Despite suggested modifications, these tenets are still upheld and taught today.[12] These include:

1. The body is triune, comprised of body, mind, and spirit
2. The body has its own inherent capacity to heal
3. The body's structure and function are interrelated
4. Rational treatment is based on these principles

These tenets can be viewed in the context of the patient with CVD. As CVD is a spectrum of long-term intrinsic and extrinsic factors, the principles can be applied at various times and in various ways throughout the patient's life.

Body: Dietary Considerations[10]

A suboptimal diet is responsible for an estimated one in five premature deaths globally from 1990 to 2016.[13] Having a quality diet was associated with an 18% to 26% lower all-cause and CVD mortality risk in the Women's Health Initiative Observational Study (from 1993 to 2010).[7] The literature supports calorie restriction for cardiometabolic benefit, specifically for improvements in insulin sensitivity, blood glucose, and inflammation.[13,14] The Mediterranean diet is associated with reduced CV mortality in individuals with CVD, whereas the dietary approaches to stop hypertension (DASH) eating plan is associated with a reduced risk of CAD.[15] Low-carbohydrate and Mediterranean diets are superior to low-fat diets in maintaining weight loss.[14] Some trials that examine macronutrient composition for weight loss reported greater long-term benefit for individuals consuming higher amounts of protein and fat compared to those who consumed higher amounts of carbohydrates.[16,17] Eating marine fish rich in long-chain omega-3 fatty acids, is thought to reduce arrhythmias, thrombosis, inflammation, blood pressure, as well as favorably modify the lipid profile.[18] Eating a low (1 serving/wk) or moderate fish consumption (2 to 4 servings/wk) has a significantly beneficial effect on the prevention of CHD mortality.[18] Nuts and legumes are beneficial because they contain unsaturated fat, fiber, micronutrients, and phytochemical content.[19] Low-to-moderate daily alcohol consumption (i.e., <15 to 20 g/day, 1 to 2 standard drinks) is associated with a reduced risk of CV disease and mortality, whereas greater amounts of alcohol consumption and a binge pattern of drinking have been linked to an increased risk.[20] Moderate alcohol intake has been shown to increase HDL-C, apolipoprotein A1, adiponectin, and decrease fibrinogen levels.[21] Higher consumption of sugar-sweetened beverages has been associated with risk of CVD in a dose-dependent relationship.[22] Regular consumption of coffee has been consistently associated with lower risk of CVD, with the greatest risk reduction occurring at around 3 to 5 cups per day conferring an 11% lower risk.[23] Tea has likewise been reported to be inversely associated with CVD incidence.[24]

Body: Physical Activity

Physically inactive adults should be counseled that any increase in physical activity is associated with a reduction in CV risk (grade A evidence).[25,26] To guide patients and clinicians, The Physical Activity Guidelines for Americans[25] describes the major research findings on the health benefits of physical activity. A summary of their recommendations and findings include:

- Regular physical activity reduces the risk of many adverse health outcomes.
- Some physical activity is better than none.
- For most health outcomes, additional benefits occur as the amount of physical activity increases through higher intensity, greater frequency, and/or longer duration.
- Most health benefits occur with at least 150 minutes (2 hours and 30 minutes) a week of moderate-intensity physical activity, such as brisk walking. Additional benefits occur with more physical activity.
- Adults should also do muscle-strengthening activities that are moderate or high intensity and involve all major muscle groups on 2 or more days a week, as these activities provide additional health benefits.
- Both aerobic (endurance) and muscle-strengthening (resistance) physical activity are beneficial.
- Health benefits occur for children and adolescents, young and middle-aged adults, older adults, and those in every studied racial and ethnic group.
- The health benefits of physical activity occur for people with disabilities.
- The benefits of physical activity far outweigh the possibility of adverse outcomes.
- Children and adolescents should do 60 minutes (1 hour) or more of physical activity daily.
- Of note emerging evidence suggests extreme exercise, characterized by long-term, high-volume, high-intensity training may induce deleterious CV adaptations in some individuals. While this does not apply to most individuals it is still worth considering.[27]

Osteopathic physicians have a unique role in helping patients achieve these physical activity goals due to their training in musculoskeletal medicine. Keeping the patients physically functioning at a higher level by the reduction of somatic dysfunction can improve their compliance with the above recommendations.

Body: Air Pollution

Air pollution containing harmful particles and toxins significantly increases the risk of CVD. Ambient particulate matter smaller than 25 μm and household air pollution from cooking represent the leading environmental risk factors for premature CVD and mortality.[28]

Mind

Mental stress is an emerging risk and prognostic factor for CAD and stroke, independent of conventional risk factors.[29] The relationship between chronic stress with increased risk of CAD is mainly due to acceleration of atherosclerosis. Transient myocardial ischemia, defined as mental stress-induced myocardial ischemia (MSIMI)[29] can occur in patients with and without significant coronary obstruction. The clinical consequences may be angina, MI, arrhythmias, and left ventricular (LV) dysfunction. Conversely, illnesses, especially heart disease, result in negative emotions which can also affect the disease progression and outcome. In addition, MI and heart failure (HF) activate inflammatory pathways that not only accelerate atherosclerosis but also contribute to neurologic changes and cognitive dysfunction.[30] Positive emotions are thought to decrease the CV reactivity to stress, heart rate (HR), blood pressure, development of arrhythmias, thrombogenesis, and the risk of developing CAD.[31,32]

Spirit

The link between the heart and spirit goes back thousands of years. Religion and spirituality are among the most important cultural factors that give structure and meaning to human values, behaviors, and experiences.[1] Spirituality is a concept broader than religion and is primarily a dynamic, personal, and experiential process. There are many definitions of spirituality (see the spirituality Chapters 19 and 20). One definition is that spirituality is the aspect of humanity that refers to the way individuals seek and express meaning and purpose and the way they experience their connectedness to the moment, to self, to others, to nature, and to the significant or sacred.[33] Just as physical and mental health impact spiritual health, spiritual health impacts physical and mental health. Emotional and spiritual suffering can have profound physical consequences. One example of this is Takotsubo cardiomyopathy (see Chapter 20). Research on the links between spirituality and CV health is mixed. One survey found that 94% of patients regard their spiritual health and their physical health as equally important.[34] The implications of this for clinical practice have recently been reviewed.[35] Studies have found that religious involvement is associated with less CVD. Of 16 studies examined in a 2001 review,[36] 12 found that religious involvement was associated with less CVD or CV mortality. Religious involvement is associated with health-promoting behaviors, such as more exercise,[37] proper nutrition,[38] regular seat belt use,[39] smoking cessation,[37] and greater use of preventive services.[40] The role of intercessory prayer on cardiac patients is less clear: A randomized, controlled trial conducted on coronary care unit patients showed no significant effect.[41] Religious practices were found to have no impact on postdischarge survival in patients with acute coronary syndrome (ACS).[42] Multiple studies exploring the impact of prayer on various health outcomes have been done with mixed results; a Cochrane review in 2009 concluded there is no correlation, though it is unlikely to be harmful.[43]

A recent study in 2022 demonstrated that higher levels of religiosity/spirituality were independently associated with beneficial effects on CV health in African American patients.[44] The researchers found improvement in multiple American Heart Association Life's Simple 7 (LS7) indicators. They recommended reinforcement of religiosity/spirituality in lifestyle interventions to decrease overall CVD risk. They commented that spirituality in the lives of African American adults may serve to address CV health disparities through sociocultural understanding and the strategic development of culturally relevant lifestyle interventions.[44]

The Body Has Its Own Inherent Capacity to Heal

The clinical course of many patients with heart disease is characterized by exacerbation and remission. Many patients return to virtually normal functional status, even after catastrophic experiences with MI or decompensation due to HF. CAD provides a clear example of inherent self-regulating and self-healing properties.[45] A century ago, the rule of the artery was supreme. The dramatic role of revascularization therapy for acute MI makes this rule no less true today.[1] Knowledge of self-regulation and self-healing forces at the arterial and arteriolar level forms the rational basis for the treatment of MI, angina pectoris, and congestive HF. Research over many years has demonstrated that lifestyle modifications, which is a form of inherent self-healing, can lower cholesterol, and slow or reverse the progression of atherosclerosis.[46–48] Another example of the body's inherent capacity to heal is demonstrated by angiogenesis and remodeling in response to the development of atherosclerosis. An older report demonstrated that LV myocytes can regenerate following acute MI.[49] Currently, there is research occurring on the different cellular phenotypes and complex pathways implicated in injury, remodeling, and regeneration of the myocardium after MI.[50]

The early practitioners of osteopathic medicine believed that the body produced its own medicine for healing, especially if there was normalization of structural abnormalities that affected circulation, the lymphatics, and nerve function. The challenge for osteopathic physicians is to determine when and which of the body's inherent production of endogenous substances is beneficial and needs to be supported.

The Body's Structure and Function are Interrelated

The osteopathic physician should help patients attain a high-quality, longer life free of preventable disease, disability, injury, and premature death. This can be done by creating social and physical environments that promote good health, and healthy behaviors across all life stages. Regarding CV disease, the Healthy People 2020 initiative[51] demonstrated that Americans had improved upon, met, or exceeded 50% or more of their trackable objectives regarding heart disease, stroke, nutrition, and weight status. These findings were strongly correlated with improved physical activity. Results from a recent study show that chronic diseases, particularly CV and musculoskeletal disorders, correlate with faster degradation of physical capability in the elderly.[52] The association between CV and musculoskeletal health may be a significant contributor to early retirement due to CV and musculoskeletal deterioration.[53] Although physical fitness and exercise capacity represent important prognostic markers for the general population,[54] as many of one-fourth of patients with HF,[55] and coronary heart disease (CHD)[56] have functional limitations caused by the musculoskeletal system.[57]

A recent comprehensive review of the literature found that there is high-quality evidence that people with chronic musculoskeletal pain are 1.91 times more likely to also report having a CVD. Regarding specific types of CVDs, a review found moderate-quality evidence that chronic musculoskeletal pain is probably associated with ischemic heart disease.[58] Palpatory findings and myofascial trigger points have been related to cardiac ischemia and arrythmias.[59]

Specific Conditions

A recent study demonstrated that CVD risk factors strongly predict the risk of developing carpal tunnel syndrome, medial and lateral epicondylitis, and rotator cuff tendinopathy.[60] For example, CVD risks, such as tobacco use and obesity, are associated with rotator cuff tears presumably due to a mechanism of impaired blood supply to the relatively avascular central zone of the rotator cuff tendons.[60]

Prevalent osteoarthritis (OA) was associated with self-reported heart disease, particularly angina, and congestive HF in both men and women, after controlling for established risk factors for these conditions.[61] Chronic longstanding reflex mechanisms affecting the heart may be seen in cervical and thoracic OA.[62,63] When there is a change in structure, functional changes follow. Over a prolonged period, somatovisceral structural changes can be related to changes in physiology and can lead to pathology. A classic yet extreme example of this is severe thoracic scoliosis leading to pulmonary and CV changes.[64]

Improving the patients musculoskeletal functioning and pain so they can lead an active lifestyle and reduce their CV risk is critical.[1]

PHYSIOLOGIC CONSIDERATIONS IN THE CARDIOVASCULAR SYSTEM

The following section will review some of the fundamental physiologic considerations of the CV system and how they are applied to the conditions that are discussed later in this chapter.

Cardiac Cycle[65] (Fig. 71.1)

The cardiac cycle describes the path of the blood through the heart. It runs in the following order:

- Atrial contraction and closure of the mitral valve
- Isovolumetric phase
- Opening of the aortic valve
- Ejection phase (rapid and reduced ejection), emptying of the left ventricle
- Closure of the aortic valve
- Isovolumetric relaxation
- The opening of the mitral valve
- Filling phase (rapid and reduced filling) of the left ventricle

Cardiac Function

To understand patients with IHD and/or HF, it is important to review the basic physiologic relationships of cardiac output (CO) stroke volume (SV), preload, afterload, and their relationships to ejection fraction (EF). The CO is the amount of blood ejected from the left ventricle, and normally it is equal to the venous return. The formula is CO = stroke volume (SV) × heart rate (HR). CO also equals the rate of oxygen consumption divided by the difference in arterial and venous oxygen content.[65] The SV is the amount of blood pumped out of the heart with each contraction. The SV increases with increased contractility, increased preload, and decreased afterload.[65]

As blood returns to the heart, it applies a pressure (preload) to the ventricle due to the amount of end-diastolic volume (EDV). The Frank–Starling law describes how the heart attempts to equalize CO with venous return. As venous return increases, there is a larger EDV in the left ventricle, which stretches the ventricle causing a proportionally larger contraction force. This contraction force produces a larger SV leading to a larger CO, thus equalizing CO with venous return.[65] The Frank–Starling curve explains the relationship between SV/CO and left ventricle end-diastolic pressure (LVEDP).

Afterload is the pressure that the LV pressure must exceed to push blood forward or by the minimum amount of pressure needed to open the aortic valve, which is equivalent to the diastolic blood pressure (DBP). Thus, DBP is one of the better ways to index afterload. In chronic hypertension, there is an increase in afterload which leads to concentric hypertrophy of the heart and eventual left-sided diastolic HF. Finally, the EF is equal to SV/EDV. EF of the left ventricle is an index for contractility. A normal EF is greater than 55%.[65]

Electrical Activity

The heart is unique in that it has cardiac muscle cells and conducting cells that can initiate their own electrical potential and spread from cell to cell (auto rhythmicity). The electrical conduction system is composed of the sinoatrial (SA) node, atrioventricular (AV)

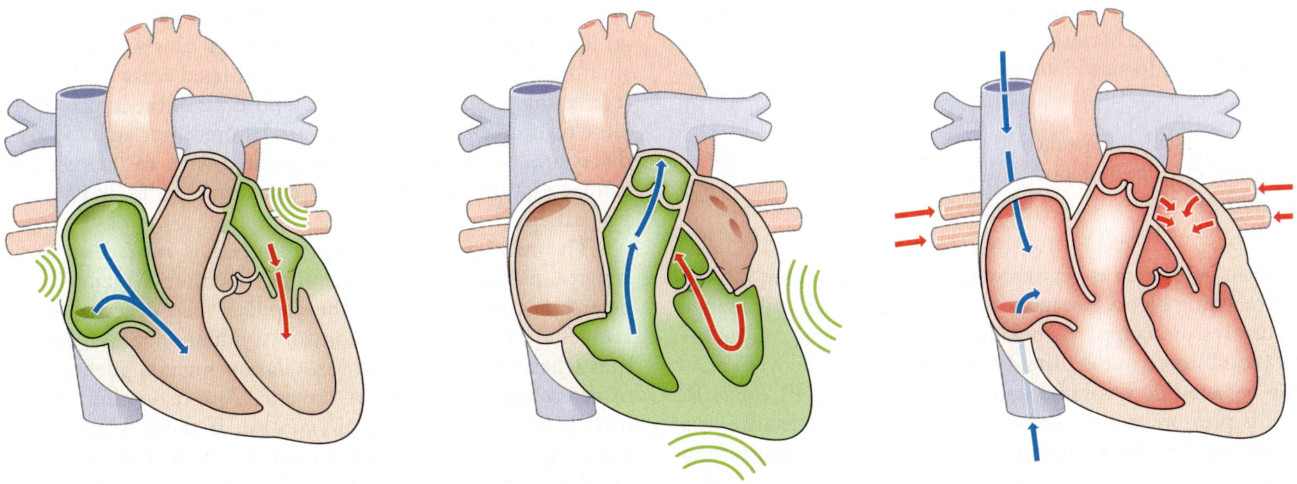

Atrial systole
Contraction of atria pumps additional blood into the ventricles.

Ventricular systole
Contraction of ventricles pumps blood into aorta and pulmonary arteries.

Complete diastole
Atria fill with blood, which flows directly into the relaxed ventricles.

Figure 71.1. The cardiac cycle describes the path of the blood through the heart.

node, AV bundle left and right bundle branches in the Purkinje fibers. The SA node is known as the pacemaker and initiates the sinus rhythm. The impulse spreads through the atria and internodal pathways down to the AV node. Once an impulse reaches the AV node there is a delay of approximately 100 ms that allows the atria to complete pumping their blood. The normal path of transmission for the conductive cells is the SA node, internodal pathways, AV node, AV bundle of His, bundle branches, and Purkinje fibers. The action potential for the conductive cells consists of a prepotential phase with a slow influx of Na^+ followed by a rapid influx of Ca^{2+} and outflux of K^+.[66] The contractile cells of the heart have an action potential with an extended plateau phase that results in an extended refractory period (250 to 300 ms). This refractory period allows the heart to follow the electrical cycle and pump blood effectively.

Occasionally, an area of the heart other than the SA node will initiate an impulse known as an ectopic focus or ectopic pacemaker. An ectopic focus may be stimulated by localized ischemia; exposure to certain drugs, including caffeine, digitalis, or acetylcholine; elevated stimulation by both sympathetic or parasympathetic divisions of the autonomic nervous system (ANS); and several pathologic conditions.[66] For example, in AF, an initiating trigger excites an ectopic focus in the atria, most commonly around the area of the pulmonary veins, and allows for an unsynchronized firing of the electrical impulses.[67] The ectopic focus in AF has been found to be related to electrical remodeling occurring in the atrial cardio myocytes.[67] In this situation, the patient would have an irregularly irregular pulse on clinical examination and an abnormal electrical pattern prior to the QRS complex, on the EKG.

Blood Pressure

DBP is the lowest pressure in an artery at the beginning of the cardiac cycle while the ventricles are relaxing and filling. DBP is directly proportional to total peripheral resistance (TPR) and the elasticity of the aorta during systole. Systolic blood pressure (SBP) is the peak pressure in an artery at the end of the cardiac cycle while the ventricles are contracting. Pulse pressure is the difference between SBP and DBP. Pulse pressure is proportional to SV and inversely proportional to arterial compliance. Thus, the stiffer the artery, the larger the pulse pressure. Mean arterial pressure (MAP) is the average pressure in the arteries throughout the cardiac cycle.[65]

Five factors influence blood pressure:

1. CO
2. Peripheral vascular resistance
3. Volume of circulating blood
4. Viscosity of blood
5. Elasticity of vessels walls

The venous system is very compliant and contains up to 70% of the circulating blood. Because of its compliance, a small change in venous pressure (support stockings, OMT, walking) can mobilize the blood stored in the distal lower extremities. There is a relationship between flow, volume, and pressure. Flow = (P1 – P2)/R, where P is pressure, and R is resistance. Increasing resistance in a vessel, such as the constriction of an arteriole, causes a decrease in blood flow.[65]

This same formula can be used to study pulmonary vasculature. However, in this situation, F represents CO, P1 represents pulmonary artery pressure (PAP), P2 represents left atrial pressure (LAP), and R is pulmonary vascular resistance (PR); CO = (PAP – LAP)/PR.[65] A Swan–Ganz catheter helps to measure both PAP and LAP, allowing for the measurement of PR and, thus, the etiology of pulmonary hypertension.[65] The Swan–Ganz catheter tip lies in the main pulmonary artery, where the balloon can be inflated for measurement of the pulmonary capillary wedge pressure (PCWP).[68] In most cases, the PCWP is also an estimate of left ventricular end-diastolic pressure (LVEDP). The normal PCWP is between 4 and 12 mm Hg. Elevated levels of PCWP might indicate severe LV failure or mitral stenosis.[68] In cardiogenic shock, there is an increase in PCWP because there is a backup of blood; the heart is not able to pump blood forward because it is not able to overcome the afterload. In hemorrhagic shock, there is a loss of blood, thus a loss in total volume. Because there is a loss of volume, there is a decrease in pressure and, therefore, a decrease in PCWP.

Regulation

The regulation of the CV system is complicated. Animal studies have identified both neural and endocrine pathways, by which the central nervous system adjusts CO and peripheral vascular resistance to changing physiologic demands. The outflow of these pathways is coordinated by various central nervous regions based on afferent information from baroreceptors, chemoreceptors, nociceptors, and circulating hormones, and is modulated by physiologic and behavioral states.[69]

The nervous system regulates the CV system with the help of baroreceptors and chemoreceptors. The baroreflex control of circulatory homeostasis occurs on a negative feedback basis. Baroreceptors are in the carotid sinus and the aortic arch and respond to changes in blood pressure. These receptors respond quickly through the vagus nerve and glossopharyngeal nerves respectively. When blood pressure decreases there is less stretch on these baroreceptors and a subsequent decrease in signaling. This causes an increase in sympathetic activity causing vasoconstriction, an increase in HR, and a subsequent increase in blood pressure.[65]

There are also both central and peripheral chemoreceptors. The central chemoreceptors in the brainstem measure pH and carbon dioxide changes in the cerebral spinal fluid. The peripheral chemoreceptors in the carotid body and aortic arch respond to changes in oxygen levels, carbon dioxide levels, and the pH of the blood. If the carbon dioxide level increases, the oxygen level decreases, and the pH drops. This will stimulate the chemoreceptors causing an increased RR.[65] Hypoxia of the lungs causes vasoconstriction, shunting blood away from poorly ventilated areas of the lung and redirecting perfusion to ventilated portions of the lung.[65] There is a close relationship between reduced baroreceptor activity and heart disease that was found to be associated with an increased risk of cardiac mortality and sudden cardiac death (SCD) in post-MI and HF patients.[70]

The regulation of the vascular bed is related to metabolic activity, perfusion, and autonomic function. Metabolic activity determines blood flow in the capillary bed because some substances are vasoactive and control vasodilation. Some compounds that when in excess cause vasodilation include adenosine, nitric oxide, oxygen, and carbon dioxide. Autoregulation of vascular beds is also under myogenic control. If there is an increase in perfusion to the arterioles, the vascular smooth muscle is stretched which then reflexively causes it to constrict.[65] In addition to these considerations, the sympathetic nervous system (SNS) innervates the skin, hair follicles, and blood vessels. In this state of increased sympathetic tone (fight-or-flight response) to a peripheral vascular bed, vasoconstriction would occur. Increasing sympathetic tone to the skin and hair follicles aids in the regulation of body temperature.[65]

Neural Regulation

Advances in neuroanatomical, neurophysiologic, and functional imaging studies have provided insight into the central and peripheral mechanisms of neural control of cardiac function in humans.[70] The neural control of the heart is accomplished throughout a multilevel neural network within the central nervous system and peripheral extracardiac and cardiac ganglia that exert their influence via the sympathetic and parasympathetic nervous systems (PNS). There is also an intrinsic cardiac nervous system that processes sensory information and provides efferent input to the myocardium under the tonic modulation of the extrinsic sympathetic and parasympathetic input.[70]

The Sympathetic and Parasympathetic Nervous System (ANS)

The ANS helps the body to adapt to changes in the internal and external environment. The ANS works with the hypothalamic–pituitary–adrenal axis, and both are affected by the circadian rhythm, and levels of circulating hormones.

SYMPATHETIC NERVOUS SYSTEM

The SNS is often referred to as the "fight-or-flight" system because it becomes active in response to stress, excitement, or situations requiring increased CO. When the SNS is activated, it releases the neurotransmitter norepinephrine, which binds to beta-adrenergic receptors in the cardiac muscle cells. This binding leads to an increased HR (chronotropy), increased contractility (inotropy), and dilation of the coronary arteries, which allows for greater blood flow to the heart muscle. These actions collectively prepare the body for increased physical activity. The SNS also controls the heart by promoting adrenal medullary release of adrenaline (epinephrine).

The superficial cardiac plexus is responsible for this. It lies just beneath the arch of the aorta and is made up of sympathetic nerve fibers. These fibers originate from the sympathetic trunks. Since the SNS has thoracolumbar outflow, the spinal segments that affect the heart are between T1 and T5. Sustained sympathetic tone may predispose the patient to tachyarrhythmias, cause coronary vasoconstriction, and impair revascularization following MI.[71] Therefore, it is thought that treatment of somatic dysfunction between the T1 and T5 is important to try to ameliorate local sensitization of the sympathetic nerves and spinal cord.

Stimulation of the SNS may be proarrhythmic, particularly in conditions of acute myocardial ischemia, while vagal nerve stimulation may reduce the potential for lethal arrhythmias.[70] Optimal function of these mechanisms is important. Research has shown that sympathetic–parasympathetic imbalance and impairment of baroreflex control of HR are factors in the development of HF.[72] Chronic stress produces withdrawal of coping mechanisms, and an "hyperarousal state," characterized by chronic sympathetic and hypothalamic–pituitary–adrenocortical system activation. The consequences of this overactivity have been referred to as "excessive allostatic load," which is thought to be consequential in CVDs.[73]

PARASYMPATHETIC NERVOUS SYSTEM

The PNS is often referred to as the "rest and digest" system because it promotes relaxation and helps conserve energy. It primarily uses the neurotransmitter acetylcholine to slow down the HR (negative chronotropy) and decrease contractility (negative inotropy). Activation of the PNS is especially important during periods of rest and recovery. The PNS has cranial and sacral outflow.

The parasympathetic preganglionic neurons involved in the control of cardiac function are in the nucleus ambiguus (within the medulla oblongata), reticular formation, and the dorsal motor nucleus of the vagus nerve.[74] The primary parasympathetic innervation of the heart comes from the deep cardiac plexus. This plexus is located near the AV septum, close to the AV node. It consists of parasympathetic (vagal) nerve fibers that originate from the vagus nerve. Parasympathetic postganglionic fibers innervate the cardiac conduction system and the atrial and ventricular myocardium. Parasympathetic activity also lengthens AV conduction time and decreases atrial and ventricular contractility. There is a predominance of vagal over sympathetic cardiac modulation at rest.

Cardiac function can be profoundly altered by the reflex activation of cardiac autonomic nerves. The physiologic advantage of reciprocal baroreflex control of the heart by sympathetic and parasympathetic nerves is that it allows for rapid and large compensatory responses.[75] Interestingly, chemoreceptor stimulation evokes parasympathetic and sympathetic co-activation, as in the diving reflex, where sympathetic-mediated vasoconstriction occurs with profound vagally mediated bradycardia. This causes maximal oxygen conservation while at the same time maintaining an adequate perfusion pressure for the brain and the heart.[75]

Central Sensitization and the "Facilitated Segment"[76]

Excessive or aberrant sensory information from cardiac disease enters the thoracic spinal cord segments T1–T5. Over time, this neural input will cause excitation of the entire segmental spinal cord level. The segmental spinal cord will have a lower threshold of excitation, therefore any information coming into that level will be magnified as it is sent to the brain to be processed. In addition, the local somatic structures also innervated by that same segmental level will be influenced by this neural sensitization, which can create palpable tissue texture abnormalities in the related dermatome, sclerotome, or myotome.

Biologic Rhythms

Biologic rhythms, including circadian rhythms and ultradian rhythms, can significantly affect the heart's function and CV health. These rhythms influence various aspects of heart physiology and function. Circadian rhythms are daily, approximately 24-hour cycles that regulate various physiologic processes in the body. Ultradian rhythms are shorter biologic cycles that occur multiple times within a 24-hour period.

Circadian rhythms are primarily influenced by the body's internal biologic clock and external cues such as light and darkness. Blood pressure and HR tend to follow a circadian pattern, with higher levels during the daytime and lower levels during the nighttime.[1] Circadian rhythms can affect the release of hormones like cortisol, which can have indirect effects on the heart by influencing blood pressure and inflammation. Research suggests that the risk of CV events like heart attacks and strokes is higher in the morning hours due to the combination of increased blood pressure, HR, and clotting factors during this time.[1] The increase in morning incidence of acute ischemic coronary events has been attributed to an increase in catecholamines and sensitivity of vascular receptors, increasing coronary vasomotor tone, and increasing myocardial oxygen demand, all of which lower the threshold for ischemia.[77]

Ultradian rhythms contribute to heart rate variability (HRV), which is the variation in the time intervals between successive heartbeats. Higher HRV is generally associated with better CV health, and disruptions in ultradian rhythms can lead to reduced HRV. Somatic dysfunction of the suboccipital region is thought to affect the vagus nerve and when treated can improve HRV.[78] There are also ultradian variations in blood pressure, such as the dipping of blood pressure during sleep, which can affect the heart's workload and influence its function. The various stages of sleep have different effects on HR, blood pressure, and cardiac workload. Disruptions in sleep patterns can impact CV health.

Overall, disruptions in biologic rhythms, such as those caused by shift work, irregular sleep patterns, or lifestyle factors, can contribute to an increased risk of CV problems, including hypertension, arrhythmias, and heart disease.

PATIENT ASSESSMENT

Screening for heart disease is an essential component of every comprehensive evaluation performed by a family practitioner, surgeon, anesthesiologist, or internist (see Fig. 71.2). The components of a CV screening evaluation are the history, physical examination, and risk assessment. Further additional components can then include blood tests, echocardiogram, stress tests, chest x-rays, EKG, and a cardiac CT or MRI.

History

When a patient presents with symptoms referable to the CV system, the physician must first determine if the patient is having a life-threatening event. The physician must rapidly assess the situation and determine if emergent intervention is necessary. Taking an accurate history has a dual purpose: to obtain important medical information and to establish a relationship between the patient and the physician. Since the management of most CV conditions involves lifestyle changes recommended by the physician, the initial history may also be considered as the first step in establishing the foundation for later risk factor modification programs.

The history of the CV patient should include the following elements:

CARDIAC RISK FACTORS

- Age
- Gender (risk in males > females)
- Obesity
- Smoking (quantify in pack-years)
- Hypertension
- Hypercholesterolemia
- Diabetes
- Family history (parent or sibling with a history of heart disease before age 55 for males or 65 for females)

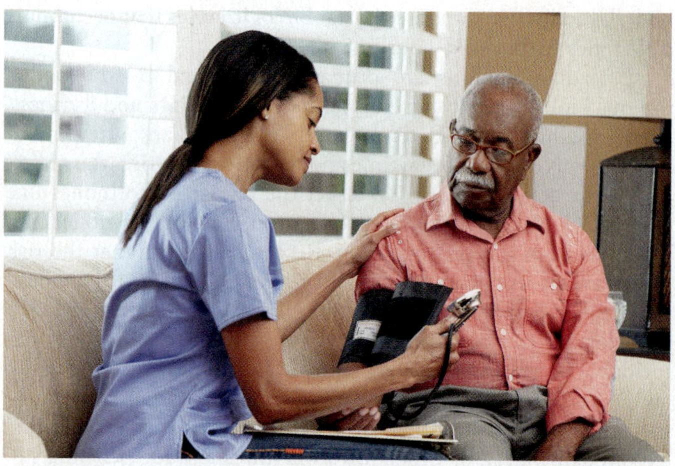

Figure 71.2. (Reprinted with permission from Eliopoulos C. *Gerontological Nursing.* 10th ed. Wolters Kluwer; 2022:28. Figure 3-1.)

CARDIAC HISTORY

- Angina
- MI
- Ischemic heart disease
- Valvular heart disease
- Cardiac surgery bypass
- AF or other rhythm disturbance
- Rheumatic fever
- Endocarditis
- Pericarditis, myocarditis, COVID
- CVA or TIA

SOCIAL HISTORY

- Alcohol consumption
- Illicit drug use
- Patient's employment
- Stress

CHEST PAIN

Definition

Chest pain is a common complaint and encompasses a broad differential diagnosis that includes several life-threatening causes. A workup must focus on ruling out serious pathology before a physician considers more benign causes. An initial assessment is recommended to triage patients effectively on the basis that the pain may be due to cardiac ischemia. Chest pain should not be described as atypical, because it is not helpful in determining the cause and can be misinterpreted as being benign. Instead, it should be characterized as cardiac, possibly cardiac, or noncardiac as the terms are more specific.[79]

It is vitally important to remember that symptoms are cues for patients that a problem exists. Symptoms also trigger clinicians to obtain EKGs, and subsequent clinical decision-making. There are many cardiac and noncardiac causes of chest pain. Visceral pain tends to be dull in nature and poorly defined as to location. Somatic pain, on the other hand, can be sharp or dull, and is more localized. Pleural and peritoneal pain is typically sharp and localized. This is because the parietal pleura and peritoneum are somatically innervated.

Classic symptoms of angina from an ACS are left-sided substernal chest pressure radiating to the neck and left shoulder/arm, that occur with exertion, and are improved with rest or nitroglycerin. Even though chest pain is a sensitive symptom of ACS, it is not very specific.

Epidemiology

After injuries, chest pain is the second most common reason for adults to present to the emergency department (ED) in the United States and accounts for >6.5 million visits, which is 4.7% of all ED visits.[79] Although the cause of chest pain is often noncardiac, CAD affects >18.2 million adults in the United States and remains the leading cause of death for men and women, accounting for >365,000 deaths annually.[79] The lifetime prevalence of chest pain in the United States is 20% to 40%, and women experience this symptom more often than men.[79] Of all ED patients with chest pain, only 5.1% will have an ACS and more than half will ultimately be found to have a noncardiac cause.[79]

Classification

ATYPICAL CHEST PAIN

Atypical chest pain signifying angina pectoris may be present in a minority of patients with IHD/ACS. Atypical pain is frequently described as epigastric or back pain which is a burning, stabbing, or sensation of indigestion.[80,81] Atypical symptom presentations are more common in women than men, contributing to a lower likelihood of a diagnosis and treatment.[82] Other authors have demonstrated that evidence suggests that although sex differences in symptoms exist, they are modest and do not contribute significantly to risk stratification.[81]

SILENT ISCHEMIA

It is not uncommon for patients with CAD to have undiagnosed episodes of silent ischemia. It was published in the Framingham study that approximately 25% of infarctions may be silent or unrecognized due to an atypical presentation. This includes unusual somatic chest wall pain, or previously experienced somatic pain due to the possibility of facilitation of local spinal cord segments.[1]

NONCARDIAC CHEST PAIN

In approximately one-third of patients who present with chest discomfort, no cardiac cause is found, and these patients are labeled as having noncardiac chest pain. Many of the cases are attributed to the upper GI tract, based on clinical history and examination findings.[1] The typical investigations do not identify the cause of the pain. An accurate abdominal exam and palpatory examination can help determine if the GI tract is involved in the patient's condition.

SYMPTOMS RELATED TO LOCUS OF ISCHEMIA

The relationship between the myocardial region of ischemia or infarction and the pattern of distribution of angina has been studied. Studies on the distribution of cardiac pain by intracoronary injection of adenosine are discussed by Rogers in Foundations for Osteopathic Medicine second edition.[1] For all patients with Q-wave MI, pain location, radiation, duration, and severity were similar.

- Gastrointestinal symptoms aka "fatal gastritis" was more common with inferior wall MI.[1]
- In a study of palpatory findings of musculoskeletal changes with MI, abnormalities of paraspinal soft tissue texture were more often associated with anterior than with inferior MI.[1]

ASYMPTOMATIC CORONARY PATIENTS

At least 25% of coronary patients have an MI without any prior symptoms.[84] Therefore, the search for a coronary patient with subclinical disease who could potentially benefit from intensive primary prevention efforts is critically important (see Fig. 71.3).

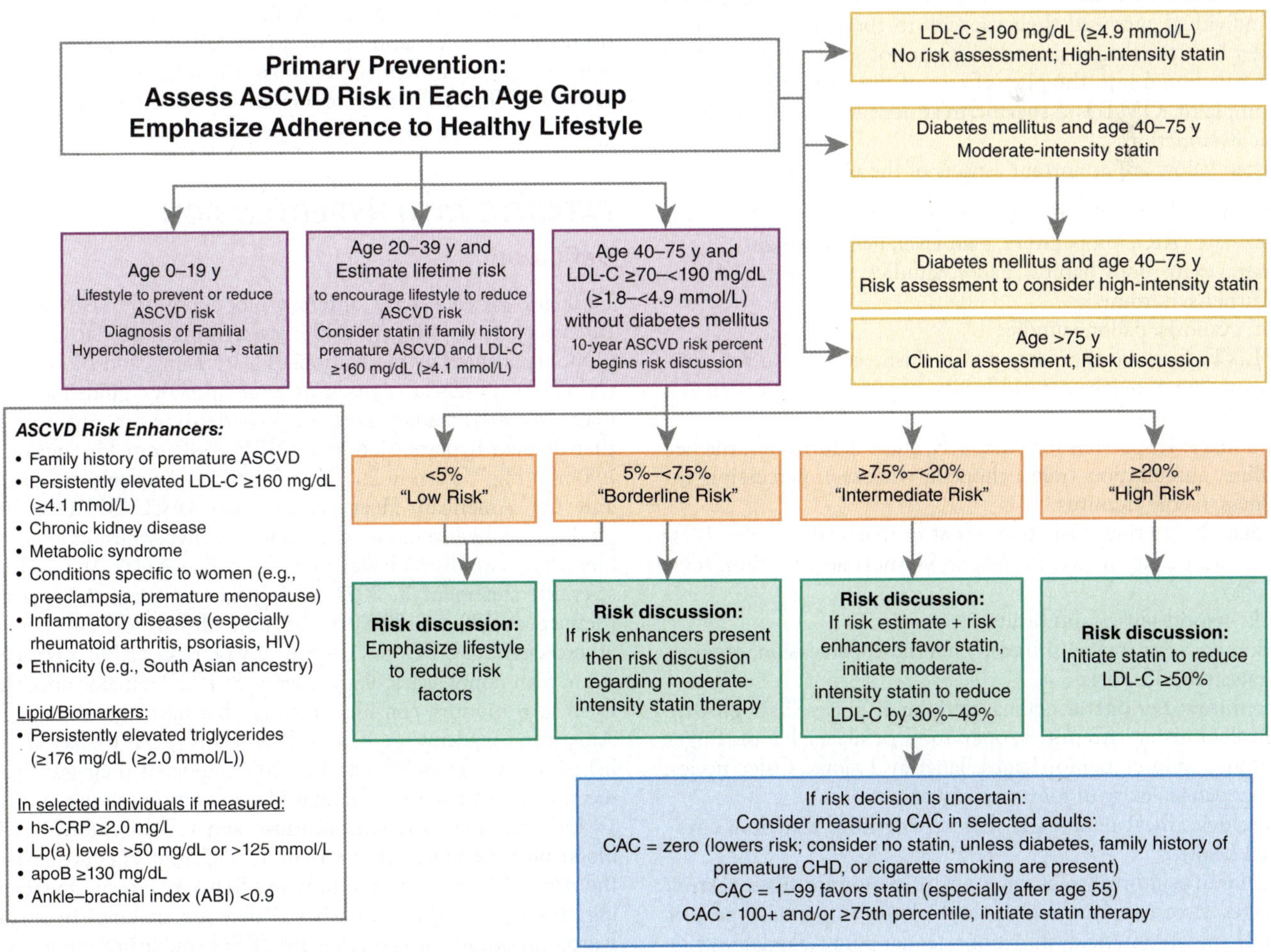

Figure 71.3. (Reprinted with permission from Tucker RG. *Karch's Focus on Nursing Pharmacology*. 9th ed. Wolters Kluwer; 2023. Figure 47.2.)

Defining a patient's risk of having a coronary event is important for the clinician. There are many office-based approaches for screening patients, to better define their coronary event risk.[1,85] Asymptomatic adults are stratified as low risk (about 35% of patients). They are reassured of this status by their physician and then retested in about 5 years.

- Intermediate-risk patients may benefit from noninvasive testing for further risk assessment. Tests would include the ankle-brachial blood pressure index, CT scanning, and exercise stress testing.
- High-risk patients (about 25% of patients) are candidates for intensive risk factor intervention.

Physical Examination

Based on observation of the patient, the patient may be placed into one of two categories: stable or unstable. If the patient is unstable (unconscious or semiconscious, abnormally low, or high blood pressure, brady or tachyarrhythmia, respiratory distress), the first action is ABC's—airway, breathing, circulation, obtain the automated external defibrillator (AED) and to activate the emergency medical services (EMS). If the patient is stable, there is time to incorporate the aspects of the physical exam necessary for that patient. Osteopathic physicians also diagnose the musculoskeletal component of the patient's chief complaint or clinical presentation. For this, a structural and palpatory examination for somatic dysfunction is performed. If somatic dysfunction is found, the type, location, and severity need to be correlated to the patient's condition. Somatic dysfunction becomes clinically more significant as an individual ages and their capacity to compensate decreases. Consider how the diagnosis and treatment of somatic dysfunction may be integrated into the plan of care of the patient with a cardiac complaint. OMT is a specific treatment for the diagnosis of somatic dysfunction.

Listed below are important aspects of the physical exam:

- Vitals: Blood pressure (BP), pulse: rate, rhythm, character, respiratory rate (RR), temperature, pain level, height, weight
- General exam: body habitus, pallor, jaundice, evidence of Marfan or Turner syndrome
- Skin: cyanosis, pallor, jaundice
- HEENT: face xanthomata, mylar flush, corneal arcus, fundoscopy, thyromegaly, carotid bruits, jugular venous distension (JVD)
- Pulmonary: Inspection for scars, RR, chest deformities, trachea midline, auscultation (rales, rhonchi, wheezes), percussion for dullness, tactile fremitus
- Cardiac: Inspection, palpation, point of maximal impulse, lifts/heaves, auscultation (S1, S2, S3, or S4, murmurs, rhythm, rubs, gallops)
- Neck: carotid pulses and bruits
- Abdomen: scars, bowel sounds, tenderness, percussion, organomegaly, pulsatile aorta
- Extremities: peripheral edema, peripheral pulses, hair growth, scars, cool distal extremities, open sores or ulcers, hands: finger clubbing, splinter hemorrhages, Janeway lesions, Osler nodes, sweaty palms, laxity of joints, vein observation
- Neurologic: focal neurologic deficits, cognitive function, emotional health
- Structural: standing structural exam, palpation for tissue texture changes, viscerosomatic reflexes and Chapman points, type 1 or type II spinal somatic dysfunctions, tender points, fascial restrictions, rib dysfunction.

Diagnostics

- Fasting glucose, glycosylated hemoglobin
- Renal function, LFTs, TFT
- Lipid profile
- Cardiac enzymes
- ESR or CRP
- 12-lead EKG
- Chest x-ray
- Spirometry
- Echocardiogram
- Ankle-brachial index
- Cardiac stress test
- Cardiac catheterization
- Cardiac MRI
- Coronary CTA
- CT calcium scoring

Somatic Dysfunction and OMT

The role of OMT for patients suffering from chest pain is not clear as there are only a few studies on the topic. Some studies examined the paraspinal musculature and soft tissue for a segmental somatic expression of a cardiac visceral disturbance.[86,87] Somatic dysfunction in those who had confirmed acute MI found tissue texture changes in the upper thoracic region.[88] Palpatory findings are supported by multiple studies and are accepted in the osteopathic community as a viscerosomatic reflex indicating underlying cardiac dysfunction.[89–92] A case study also demonstrated resolved chest pain and shortness of breath in an individual who had a negative work-up for MI.[93] OMT can be used preventatively to decrease the total amount of stress (allostatic load) created by somatic dysfunction in body areas thought to influence cardiac function.[94] The treatment of somatic dysfunction with OMT has been shown to affect the blood vessels as well.[95]

PATIENTS WITH HYPERTENSION

Definition

Different societies have different blood pressure (BP) guidelines. In history, from 1977 to 2003 seven Joint National Committees (JNC) sponsored by the National Heart, Lung, and Blood Institute (NHLBI), produced consensus multispecialty guidelines on the diagnosis and management of hypertension. It was the JNC7 that defined hypertension as an SBP ≥140 mm Hg and/or DBP ≥90 mm Hg.[96] Then in 2017 the American Academy of Cardiology and the American Heart Association (ACC/AHA) published guidelines which most notably redefined hypertension as sustained blood pressure over 130/80 mm Hg.[97] The AHA/ACC released a scientific statement in 2021 stating that for stage 1 hypertension (defined as 130 to 139/80 to 89 mm Hg) in low-risk adults (no atherosclerotic CVD or 10-year CVD risk <10%) management starts with nonpharmacologic therapy.[97] If BP remains uncontrolled for 3 to 6 months, consider starting pharmacologic therapy.[97] The American Academy of Family Physicians (AAFP) has also published its own guidelines and in 2022, updated their guidelines to recommend treating to a standard blood pressure target of less than 140/90 mm Hg to reduce all-cause and CV mortality.[98] A lower blood pressure target of less than 135/85 mm Hg further reduces the risk of MI but not mortality, and the AAFP recommends treating this lower target with shared decision making. In 2023, the European Society of Hypertension (ESH) published guidelines that aligned with the guidelines from the American Heart Association from 2017, however, they also included essential recommendations on hypertension in children, adolescents, and the transition to young hypertensive adult individuals.[99] The ESH guidelines also provided guidance on hypertension in the demographic and clinical conditions listed below:

- Children/adolescents and transition to adulthood
- Young patients
- Sex-related differences
- Pregnancy and puerperium
- PAD
- Aortic aneurism
- Valvular heart disease
- Treatment of hypertension in acute cerebrovascular diseases
- Hypertensive emergencies/urgencies
- Perioperative hypertension
- Obesity
- COVID-19
- Chronic inflammatory diseases
- Hypertension in oncology
- Baroreflex failure and dysautonomia
- Glaucoma

Epidemiology

Hypertension is known as the "silent killer" because patients with high blood pressure generally don't feel sick or know that they have it. Hypertension is the most prevalent CV disorder in the world and according to the World Health Organization (WHO) and is a leading cause of death worldwide. According to the WHO[100]:

- An estimated 1.28 billion adults aged 30 to 79 years worldwide have hypertension, most (two-thirds) living in low- and middle-income countries.
- An estimated 46% of adults with hypertension are unaware that they have the condition.
- Less than half of adults (42%) with hypertension are diagnosed and treated.
- Approximately one in five adults (21%) with hypertension have it under control.
- Hypertension is a major cause of premature death worldwide.
- One of the global targets for noncommunicable diseases is to reduce the prevalence of hypertension by 33% between 2010 and 2030.
- Hypertension especially affects patients living in low-income and middle-income countries.

In 2019, the global age-standardized average prevalence of hypertension in adults aged 30 to 79 years was reported to be 34% in men and 32% in women.[101] There is a strong relationship between hypertension and an increased risk of CAD, HF, stroke, and progression of chronic kidney disease. This applies to all age groups and all ethnicities.[98]

Classification[102]

- Essential hypertension (>90% of cases)
  - Hypertension (aka essential hypertension) does not have one specific cause but does have a complex multifaceted pathophysiology.
- Secondary hypertension.
  - Has a specific cause; Treatment is directed at lowering blood pressure and treating the cause.
  - Common causes are listed below
    - Kidney diseases
    - Endocrine diseases
    - Coarctation of the aorta
    - Preeclampsia or eclampsia
    - Acute stress
    - Obstructive sleep apnea
    - Increased intravascular fluid volume
    - Diseases of the nervous system
    - Drugs
    - Toxic substances
  - Clinical reasons to suspect secondary hypertension
    - Younger patients (<40 years) with grade 2 or 3 hypertension or hypertension of any grade in childhood
    - Sudden onset of hypertension in individuals with previously documented normotension
    - Acute worsening of BP control in patients who were previously well controlled by treatment
    - True resistant hypertension
    - Hypertensive emergency
    - Clinical features of the above causes

Pathophysiology[102]

The pathophysiology of primary (essential) hypertension is complex and still developing. The hallmark mechanism is an increase in systemic vascular resistance commonly found in most hypertensive patients. However, what exactly causes the increase in systemic vascular resistance is multifactorial based on genetic and environmental factors. Left untreated, this pathophysiologic process can become the "silent killer" and lead to heart disease, stroke, and kidney failure.[103] Listed below are some of the current pathophysiologic considerations that are at play in patients with hypertension.

Genetic Factors

It is known that there is a strong heritable component to hypertension with heritability estimates ranging from 25% to 60% in the general population.[104] Substantial data also indicates that elevated blood pressure and its accompanying substantial CV risks are largely secondary to the interplay between genetics and environment.[104] Genome-wide association studies (GWASs) and whole-exome sequencing techniques have revealed many potential blood pressure–related pathways, but consistent associations with hypertension are infrequent to rare.[104]

Environmental Factors[105]

- Noise
- Cold ambient temperatures
- High altitude
- Increase in average BP as distance from the equator increases
- Fine particulate matter (pm) air pollution
- Persistent organic pollutants, metals (i.e., lead, cadmium, mercury), and facial cold-water exposure

Pathophysiologic Mechanisms[106]

- Alterations in the renin–angiotensin–aldosterone system (RAAS)
- Central and peripheral autonomic vascular regulation
- Excess sodium intake
- Endothelin system
- Nitric oxide
- Natriuretic peptides
- Genetic factors
- Gut intestinal dysbiosis and sodium sensitivity

- Inflammation mediated by the immune system
- Oxidative stress and reactive oxygen species (ROS)
- Gender differences; racial, ethnic, and environmental factors

The interaction of all these mechanisms makes the study of hypertension complex and gives rise to why diet, lifestyle, and multiple medications can work synergistically with the greatest effect on the patient.

Natural History/Risk Factors

The relation between BP and the risk of CVD is direct, graded, and continuous over a wide range, apparently beginning at 115 mm Hg systolic and 75 mm Hg diastolic.[107] Experimental and clinical data support the fact that there are differences between primary and secondary forms of hypertension and that they have different prognostic implications and may require different therapeutic approaches.

Some risk factors of hypertension include:

- A family history of hypertension, CVD, kidney disease, or stroke
- A personal history of smoking
- A personal history of alcohol consumption
- A personal history of sedentary lifestyle, weight gain
- A personal history of erectile dysfunction
- A personal history of snoring, sleep apnea
- A personal history of excessive stress at work or at home
- Being a long-term cancer survivor
- A personal history of having hypertension in pregnancy or preeclampsia
- A personal history of recreational drug use or substance abuse

Diagnosis

The evaluation of patients with hypertension has four main components: (1) Identify the cause, (2) Assess for target organ damage, (3) Evaluate the response to therapy, (4) Identify CV risk factors and comorbid disorders.[108] Because of the variability of BP, an elevation of office BP (SBP ≥130 mm Hg or DBP ≥80 mm Hg) should be confirmed by at least two to three visits. Office-based blood pressure evaluation is the most well-studied and recommended method to accurately record blood pressure. However, it can be confirmed by at-home measurements, and ambulatory blood pressure measurements. Home blood pressure cuffs can be brought to the office and can be checked against the office-based sphygmomanometer. Hypertension can be diagnosed during the hypertensive urgency or emergency when there is significantly elevated blood pressure and or the CV risk is high. There are risk stratification systems based on the Framingham study, which can estimate the 10-year risk of both fatal and nonfatal CAD by the presence of hypertension. It is important to determine secondary causes of hypertension such as renovascular, coarctation, pheochromocytoma, mineral corticoid excess, primary aldosteronism, sleep apnea, and thyroid disease.[108] European guidelines on CVD prevention published the SCORE guidelines and in 2021 the SCORE 2 guidelines which estimate an individual's 10-year risk of fatal and nonfatal CV events.[109]

History

Obtaining an accurate history is important in the evaluation of patients with hypertension. It is important to know if the patient already has an existing diagnosis of hypertension and when this diagnosis was made. The duration of hypertension can be correlated with end-organ damage. There are several questions to consider including: What workups have been done as well as what treatments? Was the patient compliant with treatment and was it effective? Has the patient's blood pressure been stable, increasing, or decreasing and have there been any hypotensive episodes? Does the patient have any associated symptoms referable to the CV system such as chest pain, shortness of breath with exertion, palpitations, peripheral edema? Have there been current antihypertensive medications or lifestyle changes? Are they a smoker? Do they drink alcohol? Have they ever had an emergency room visit, TIA, stroke, or other CV issue due to their hypertension? What is their diet like?

Physical Exam

The physical examination should begin with an evaluation of vital signs, including height, weight, level of pain (if present), and body habitus. The physical examination should evaluate for end-organ damage (see Fig. 71.4). A detailed CV examination should include auscultation of the heart, carotid arteries, renal arteries, and lungs. Examination of pulses should include palpating the carotid, aortic, femoral, radial, popliteal, posterior tibial, and dorsalis pedis pulses. Capillary refill, clubbing of the fingertips, and nail beds should also be evaluated. The neurologic exam should be performed to look for any focal deficits, and/or cognitive decline. The eye/funduscopic exam should be performed to look for visual loss, retinal hemorrhages, A–V nicking, and disk edema. It is important to evaluate the endocrine system for signs of Cushing disease, acromegaly, diabetes, and thyroid disease. The abdominal exam should also involve palpation of the kidneys especially if there is a family history of polycystic kidney disease. The musculoskeletal exam should be evaluated for tissue texture changes or other signs of somatic dysfunction, especially at the OM suture, cervical spine, T1–T4, sternum, ribs 6 to 12, xiphoid, L1–L3, and restriction of the diaphragm.[89]

Laboratory Studies/Diagnostics

The following lab studies and diagnostic tests should be considered in the evaluation of the patient with primary hypertension. Patients with secondary hypertension have more specific diagnostics needed in their evaluation.

- Fasting glucose, hemoglobin A1c
- Comprehensive metabolic panel
- Fasting lipid panel
- Complete blood count (CBC)
- Thyroid-stimulating hormone
- Urinalysis
- 12-lead EKG
- Ankle-brachial index
- Magnesium

Treatment

The goals in the treatment of hypertension are to reduce CV risks and to prevent complications such as HF, CAD, chronic kidney disease, and stroke. Lowering blood pressure reduces CV risks; maintaining SBP of less than 130 mm Hg demonstrably prevents complications in patients with HF, diabetes, CAD, stroke, and other CVDs.[110]

Additionally, untreated hypertensive patients had increased risk of all-cause, CVD-specific, heart disease-specific, and cerebrovascular disease-specific death.[111] No significant differences were identified between normotensives, and treated and controlled hypertensives, thereby supporting primary and secondary prevention efforts.[111]

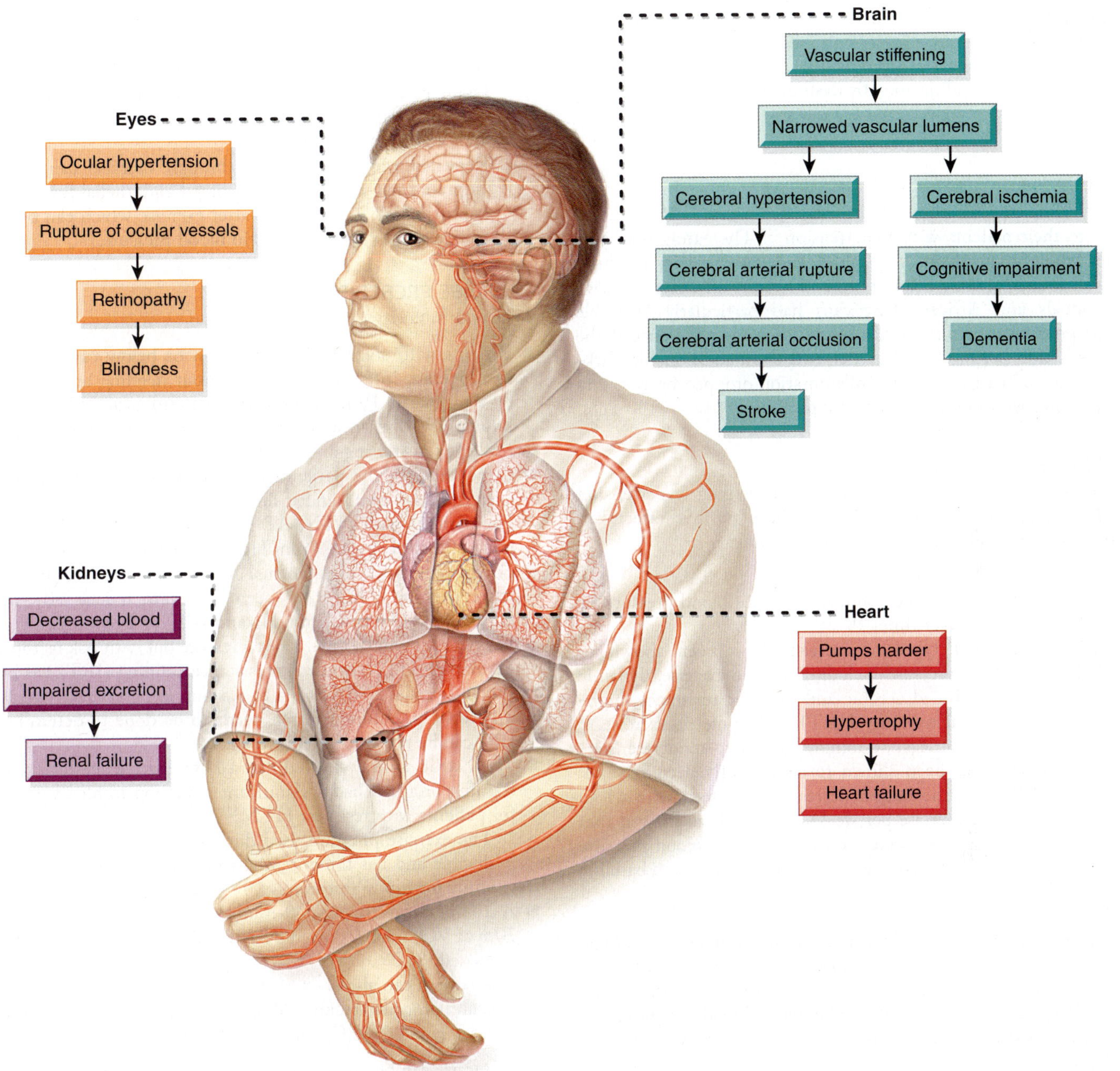

Figure 71.4. Effects of hypertension on target organs. (Modified from Anatomical Chart Company. *Hypertension.* Wolters Kluwer; 2016.)

Even with significant research and published guidelines on management of hypertension, worldwide BP guidelines are not being well implemented. The US National Ambulatory Medical Care Survey indicates that in 41.7 million primary care visits (2005 to 2012) in patients with SBP ≥140 mm Hg or DBP ≥90 mm Hg, new antihypertensive medication was only initiated in 7 million (16.8%).[112] Reasons for failing to initiate or intensify antihypertensive therapy include lack of time, workflow constraints, concern about side effects, lack of knowledge to make pharmacologic agent and/or dosing decisions, and uncertainty about the patient's out-of-office BP. Another major cause of uncontrolled BP is suboptimal adherence to the antihypertensive regimen, including failure to (1) initiate pharmacotherapy, (2) take medications as frequently as prescribed, and (3) persevere on therapy long-term.[113] Barriers to the achievement of a high level of adherence include limited access to care, cost, social determinants of health, complex medication regimens, inconvenient medication dosing and frequency, behavioral factors, and adverse effects of medications in asymptomatic patients.[114]

Lifestyle Changes and Nonpharmacologic Methods of Lowering Blood Pressure[115]

- Eating a heart-healthy diet with less salt
- Getting regular physical activity
- Maintaining a healthy weight or losing weight
- For adults with type 2 diabetes mellitus (DM), lifestyle changes are crucial.

- Limiting alcohol
- Not smoking
- Getting 7 to 9 hours of sleep daily
- Having corresponding somatic dysfunction treated

Diet and Exercise

DIET

Many clinicians recommend the evidence-based DASH eating plan to their patients with hypertension.[116] The eating plan features whole grains, fruits, vegetables, and low-fat dairy products as well as fish, poultry, beans, nuts, and healthy oils. Hypertensive individuals and African Americans had particularly favorable blood pressure reductions to the DASH diet, and adherence to the diet was high (>90%) for all participants.[116] In addition, biomarkers linked to heart injury and inflammation dropped by 18% and 13%, respectively, compared with a typical diet.[116]

EXERCISE

Exercise can play a significant role in managing hypertension (HTN). Regular physical activity can have positive effects on blood pressure and overall CV health including:

- Lowering blood pressure:
  - Exercise alone has been shown to reduce blood pressure by 5 to 7 mm Hg over time.[89,117]
  - Many different types of exercises have been shown to decrease blood pressure including aerobic exercise, dynamic resistance, combined aerobic and dynamic resistance, high-intensity interval training (HIIT), and isometric exercise.[118] A minimum of at least 30 minutes of low-to-moderate exercise weekly has been shown to significantly decrease SBP and DBP with the largest decrease being seen with 61 to 90 minutes of exercise per week. Meta-analysis showed that aerobic exercise has been shown to decrease blood pressure irrespective of age, frequency of exercise sessions, and baseline BMI.[119]
- Weight management:
  - For patients with hypertension, chronic responses to aerobic training (AT) include a decrease in body mass index (BMI), body weight, waist circumference, and percentage of body fat. There tends to be a greater reduction of blood pressure associated with larger amounts of weight loss after AT.[119]
- Improved CV function:
  - Having high cardiorespiratory VO_2 max has been shown to be protective over the progression of prehypertension to hypertension. Resistance training is safe for people who are at high risk for major cardiac disease by increasing hemodynamic functions and functional capacity of the heart. This can include increasing SV via increasing LV contraction as well as increasing coronary collateralization and decreasing systemic vascular resistance.[119] These cardiac changes help reduce incidences of cardiac ischemia.
- Stress reduction:
  - Exercise helps alleviate stress and tension.
  - Regular exercise can also decrease oxidative stress within the body which can reduce inflammation as well.[119]
- Improved insulin sensitivity:
  - Regular aerobic physical activity will decrease blood glucose in the long run by increasing insulin sensitivity. The benefits of losing weight with regular aerobic activity along with improved insulin sensitivity will help patients decrease their blood pressure even further.[119]
- Reduced sodium sensitivity:
  - Regular exercise will reduce renal sympathetic activity and can help with sodium sensitivity. The benefit of decreasing blood pressure with regular exercise will also decrease the renal baroreflex which can also reduce sodium sensitivity.[119]
- Enhanced endothelial function:
  - Repeated physiologic stress through exercise can lead to "supranormal" nitric oxide–mediated endothelial function for approximately 1 to 2 hours after exercise which can be protective against any increases in blood pressure.[119]

EXERCISE PRESCRIPTION

Type and Intensity:

- Patients with stage I[119] hypertension or below can start low-to-moderate–intensity exercise without needing an evaluation by a physician. Patients who have symptomatic HTN or have known CV disease should be evaluated with an exercise stress test prior to starting an exercise program.[119]
- Depending on the patient's blood pressure, different types of exercises are recommended for reducing blood pressure.[120]
- For patients with HTN, AT has been shown to reduce SBP most effectively by 4.49 mm Hg and DBP by 2.53 mm Hg.[118]
- For patients with high normal blood pressure, dynamic resistance training (DRT) has been shown to reduce SBP most effectively by 3.0 to 4.7 mm Hg and DBP by 2 to 3.8 mm Hg.[121]
- For patients with normal blood pressure but with risk factors for developing HTN, isometric resistance training (IRT) has been shown to reduce SBP by 5.4 to 8.3 mm Hg and DBP by 1.9 to 3.1 mm Hg. Future research needs to be done to determine if IRT can be recommended over AT.
- The EnRicH study showed that a 1- to 2-week aerobic exercise training program had a significant reduction in blood pressure for patients with resistant HTN.[121]
  - The exercise program used during the study is easily reproducible and has the potential to be applied to a larger-scale study for future research.
- A 10-minute warm-up, 40-minute aerobic exercise at 50% to 70% of VO_2 max, followed by a 10-minute cool down has been proposed.[119]
- The patient can also start at 20 minutes of exercise at 50% VO_2 max and progress weekly with alternating increases of 5 minutes to session and 5% VO_2 max to intensity of exercise.[119]

Exercise can be a valuable part of a comprehensive strategy to manage and control hypertension. The osteopathic-created exercise plan will be individualized depending on the patient and their structural and functional factors. The goal is to tailor the exercise program to the patient's needs, goals, and capabilities. Progression should promote a safe and effective benefit in lowering blood pressure and improving overall health and well-being.

Risk Scores

An important consideration for starting blood pressure-lowering treatment is one's CV risk. The best-known risk profile is the Framingham Risk Score for CHD, published in 1998. This widely used risk score uses age, sex, total and HDL-cholesterol, smoking, and SBP to estimate the 10-year risk of CHD, cerebrovascular disease, PAD, and HF.[122] Patients with a higher Framingham score have a higher CV risk and a more profound absolute risk reduction with treatment, leading to a lower number needed to treat.[122] Based on the success of the Framingham Heart Study, other scores were created from various cohorts.

In 2012, the US Department of Health and Human Services (HHS), The Centers for Disease Control and Prevention, and the Centers for Medicare and Medicaid Services (CMS), initiated *Million Hearts*, a national public–private initiative with a goal of preventing 1 million heart attacks and strokes by 2017.[123] The implementation of these strategies included the "ABCS"—aspirin therapy in appropriate patients, blood pressure control, cholesterol management, and smoking cessation.[123] Following this initiative, the Million Hearts Tool has been developed to assist clinicians and patients to understand risk, monitor patients' risks over time, and quantify potential benefits of preventive therapies based on high-quality evidence. Using the tool, individuals at low absolute predicted risk for atherosclerotic cardiovascular disease (ASCVD) in the near term (<10 years) are recommended for all appropriate lifestyle modifications, and those at higher predicted risk receive lifestyle counseling as well as consideration for immediate drug therapy.[124] In 2013, the ACC/AHA risk assessment guidelines developed new multivariable equations (the "Pooled Cohort Equations") to provide sex- and race-specific estimates of ASCVD risk.[124]

Based upon this work and screening tools, clinicians currently use risk reduction scores to help them determine treatment initiation based upon the medical evidence. Many of these are accessible as apps on the physician's mobile device. This is important because patients with a higher ASCVD risk score have a higher CV risk and a more significant risk reduction with treatment.[125] Because the Framingham score was initially done in one community in the 1970s, the AHA/ACC developed the Pooled Cohort Equations by assembling more contemporary, diverse cohorts to assist with atherosclerotic CVD evaluation among Black Americans.[126] Many risk tools have been created worldwide, and many of these now are aligned with specific populations. These tools include the SCORE (Europe), QRISK (UK), and PREDICT (New Zealand) scores. Many of these scores discriminate comparably well but all tools seem to overestimate the risk of developing CVD, among men, women, and all four race/ethnic groups.[126]

Pharmacotherapy

There are multiple classes of antihypertensive medications used for the treatment of HTN; the most recommended classes used as first-line for treatment are:

- Thiazide-type diuretics
- Calcium channel blockers (CCBs)
- Angiotensin-converting enzyme (ACE) inhibitors and angiotensin II receptor blockers (ARBs)

Other Classes of antihypertensive medications include:

- Diuretics
- Beta-blockers
- Alpha-blockers
- Alpha-2 receptor agonists
- Combined alpha and beta-blockers
- Vasodilators

Contraindications to Antihypertensives[110]

- Thiazide type diuretics are contraindicated if the patient is anuric, and in patients with sulfonamide allergies.
- Nondihydropyridine CCBs are contraindicated in patients with HF with reduced EF, patients with sick sinus syndrome, and patients with second- or third-degree AV blockade.
- ACE inhibitors are contraindicated in patients with a history of previous hypersensitivity to ACE inhibitors, history of ACE inhibitor-related angioedema, other types of angioedema, pregnancy, or the use of Aliskiren (renin inhibitor).
- Beta-blockers, especially nonselective beta-blockers, are contraindicated in asthmatic patients.
- Loop diuretics are contraindicated in patients with hypersensitivity to sulfonamides, anuric patients, and patients with hepatic coma.
- Potassium-sparing diuretics are contraindicated in patients with advanced chronic kidney disease and hyperkalemia.
- Clonidine is contraindicated in patients with hypersensitivity to alpha-2 agonists and should be avoided in patients with depression and recent MIs.
- Hydralazine is contraindicated if the patient has a history of hydralazine allergy. In patients with CAD, hydralazine can stimulate the SNS. In patients with rheumatic mitral valve disease, PAP can increase due to hydralazine treatment.
- Minoxidil is contraindicated in pregnant and breastfeeding females and patients with hypersensitivity to minoxidil.
- Contraindications to alpha-blockers include patients with a history of orthostatic hypotension and patients on phosphodiesterase inhibitors.

Osteopathic Implication

The musculoskeletal system plays an important role in health and disease of the CV patient. OMT has been used in the treatment of hypertension for over 100 years, utilizing a variety of approaches and treatment modalities. Early osteopathic researchers such as Louisa Burns studied the cardiac viscerosomatic reflexes in dogs. She found that stimulation of the visceral pericardium causes a reflex muscle contraction in the second through sixth intercostal muscles.[127] Burns also studied the converse somatovisceral reflexes and found that treatment of the upper thoracic segments caused a decrease in SBP.[127] These early studies suggested that somatic dysfunction in the upper thoracic spine and ribs (T1–T5) is felt to affect the function of the cardiac sympathetic nerves to the heart.

Mechanisms

Korr and Patterson[76] discussed/demonstrated the connection between increased sympathetic tone, spinal facilitation, and cardiac viscerosomatic reflexes. Increased sympathetic tone is associated with increased HR, contractility, and blood pressure. A study performed by Yates et al.[128] demonstrated that treatment targeting the T1–T5 segments showed a decrease in BP in patients with elevated BP. Cardiac sympathetic nerves cause dilation of the coronary arteries and accelerate the HR.[129] OMT is thought to decrease sympathetic outflow from sympathetic preganglionic neurons and sympathetic chain ganglia by treating somatic dysfunction in the thoracic spine and ribs, respectively.[130]

The cardiac innervation by the PNS is primarily through the vagus nerve. The vagus nerve travels from the medulla, through the jugular foramen between the occipital and temporal bones, where it descends through the neck and eventually integrates into the cardiac plexus. Magoun[131] explains that occipitomastoid (OM) suture compression is often implicated in vagal dysfunction, thereby affecting cardiac function. The function of the vagus nerve is important when there is an elevation of blood pressure. With elevated blood pressure, the afferent neurons are stimulated in the carotid sinus and aorta, and this stimulation causes reflex activity of the vagus nerve to slow HR.[128] Potential mechanisms of how OMT works involve modulating the ANS through decreasing sympathetic outflow and/or increasing parasympathetic outflow in the patient.[129] Suboccipital release has been found to alter autonomic CV function and improve HR variability.[78]

In addition to autonomics, the heart's close relationship with the diaphragm makes the biomechanical model of osteopathy very applicable to the role of OMT in addressing hypertension. The parietal pericardium has an external fibrous layer that is continuous superiorly with the great vessels and visceral fascia of the neck and inferior with the central tendon of the diaphragm. The pericardium's attachment to the diaphragm at the central tendon via the pericardiophrenic ligaments is a firm, and direct connection.[89,132] During inspiration, the heart descends along with the diaphragm's descent and flattening as the ribcage widens in anterior–posterior and lateral views. The diaphragm descends 1.5 cm with normal inspiration, and as much as 7 cm with deep inspiration, something that is taken advantage of for obtaining quality chest x-rays.[89,132]

Additionally, major vessels such as the aorta, inferior vena cava, and lymphatic vessels pass through the diaphragm. Sutherland[133] described the important role that diaphragmatic motion plays with lymphatic and venous return through the negative pressure is creates in the thoracic cavity. Frymann[134] described how diaphragmatic dysfunction can "increase the burden of the left ventricle and decrease venous return" by creating a sphincter-like effect on these major vessels. These anatomic connections and influences discussed by Sutherland and Frymann place an increased interest in diaphragmatic dysfunction when it comes to managing hypertension in patients.

Clinical Studies

An older study by Northrup evaluated and treated 100 hypertensive patients with OMT. He found an average drop of 33 mm Hg systolic and 9 mm Hg diastolic.[135] In 1979, Mannino demonstrated a blood pressure decrease of 15 mm Hg systolic and 8 mm Hg diastolic and a decrease in aldosterone levels by treating posterior adrenal gland Chapman reflex points at the T11 and T12 segments.[129,135,136] A clinical study diagnosing and treating cardiac Chapman points has not been formally done, despite observational evidence.[89] Beal published a paper describing a specific pattern of palpatory findings in CV patients in 1983.[87,129,137] Following these findings, in a series of publications, Johnston et al. noted a reproducible pattern of somatic dysfunction at the C6, T2, and T6 levels in most patients with hypertension.[129,137] Johston also described a "linkage pattern" of motion characteristics of the involved ribs for patients who had viscerosomatic reflexes.[129,137] This palpatory pattern persisted in hypertensive patients but resolved in nonhypertensive patients at multiple year follow-ups.

Prieto et al.[89] published a 2020 review article looking at the role OMT may play in managing hypertension and how it relates to the different models of osteopathy.[89] Prieto recognized key areas of focus when utilizing OMT, including "OM suture, cervical spine, T1–T4, sternum, ribs 6–12, xiphoid, L1–L3, and restriction of the diaphragm."

Another study performed by Cerritelli et al.[95] showed how OMT can be used to manage hypertension when applied to patients in a holistic fashion, rather than targeting individual key somatic dysfunctions. This study used various techniques, including fascial, cranial, and balanced ligamentous tension techniques to address a variety of somatic dysfunctions found in patients at the time of their appointment. This study demonstrated that over the course of 1 year, patients receiving bimonthly OMT were found to have improvements in both SBP and blood vessel intima-media wall thickness, which may serve as a contributor to atherosclerosis and plaque development.[95] They proposed that these findings may be a result of decreased production of inflammatory factors produced by tissues associated with somatic dysfunction and/or the improved functionality of the SNS.[95]

Other treatment modalities such as cranial osteopathic manipulative medicine (addressing central mechanisms) and Chapman point treatment (for reflexes from the heart and adrenal glands) have been proposed to play a role in the treatment of hypertension.[138]

Overall, there is a need for robust research on this topic, the use of OMT and providing an osteopathic approach to patient care may provide a significant and underutilized method for addressing hypertension in patients. OMT can be applied to both specific somatic dysfunctions and as a general approach to patient care.

PATIENTS WITH ISCHEMIC HEART DISEASE

Definition

Ischemic heart disease is also known as coronary artery disease (CAD) and coronary heart disease. It is the most common cause of heart disease.[139] It is commonly due to atherosclerosis of a coronary artery that develops plaque and narrows its lumen, potentially restricting flow. CAD can be classified as stable or unstable, depending on the clinical manifestations of the disease. The ACSs represent a spectrum of conditions that hold in common the presence of plaque fissuring, which has been described as the cause of acute MI and unstable angina, as well as sudden ischemic death.[1,140]

Epidemiology

The World Health Organization reported that in 2019, IHD led to 8.9 million deaths, accounting for 16% of total deaths worldwide.[141] IHD continues to be a leading cause of morbidity and mortality in the United States. A study published in JAMA Cardiology in 2022 analyzed data from the Behavioral Risk Factor Surveillance System (BRFSS) from 2011 to 2018 and found that the prevalence of self-reported CHD remained relatively stable, with an overall decline in age-standardized IHD mortality rates.[142]

Classification of CAD

The classification of CAD is largely based on if it stable or unstable. If unstable, the EKG findings, clinical presentation, and progression are used.[143]

Stable CAD: Chronic coronary syndromes

- Stable angina pectoris.
- Vasospastic angina (Prinzmetal variant angina).
- Microvascular angina (syndrome X).
- Angina is associated with myocardial bridging of coronary arteries.

Unstable CAD: Acute coronary syndromes (ACSs).
Based on initial electrocardiographic (EKG) findings:

- Non–ST-segment elevation ACS.
- ST-segment elevation ACS.

Based on clinical manifestations, biochemical markers of myocardial necrosis, and EKG:

- Unstable angina (UA).
- Non–ST-segment elevation myocardial infarction (NSTEMI).
- ST-segment elevation myocardial infarction (STEMI).
- Unspecified myocardial infarction (MI)
- SCD.

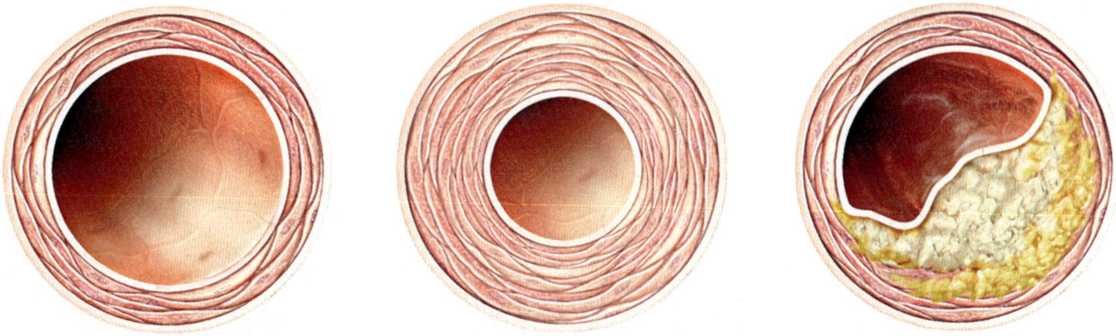

Figure 71.5. Hypertension. Potential complications of hypertension. Arteriosclerosis and atherosclerosis. Sustained hypertension damages blood vessels. If blood vessels are subjected to high blood pressure for an extended period of time, they can thicken and harden, making them less flexible. This condition is called arteriosclerosis. Also, if excessive amounts of fat are found in the blood, the arteries can accumulate fatty deposits called plaques. This buildup, called atherosclerosis, causes the vessels to narrow or become obstructed. (Asset provided by Anatomical Chart Co.)

Based on the evolution of EKG features:

- Q-wave MI.
- Non–Q-wave MI.

Pathophysiology

The pathophysiologic processes that underlie the development of the atherosclerotic lesion begin as a fatty streak and develop into a complex obstructive lesion that characterizes ischemic heart disease (see Fig. 71.5).[1,144–146]

The histopathologic events associated with the transformation of stable atheroma into one of the ACSs are now well-defined from autopsy, cardiac catheterization, and intravascular ultrasound studies. They include plaque fissure and/or rupture, and the subsequent development of thrombus on pre-existing plaques.

Braunwald proposed an etiologic approach to management of unstable angina.[140] He described five different, but not mutually exclusive, causes of angina:

- Nonocclusive thrombus on pre-existing plaque
- Dynamic obstruction (coronary vasoconstriction)
- Progressive mechanical obstruction
- Inflammation and/or infection
- Secondary angina pectoris (unstable angina precipitated by conditions extrinsic to the coronary vascular bed, such as thyrotoxicosis, anemia, hypotension, etc.)

This type of unstable angina represents approximately 75% of those patients described in the Braunwald classification.[140] There are two main components to the vulnerable atherosclerotic plaque: the lipid-rich core, and the meshwork of extracellular-matrix proteins that form the fibrous cap. The vulnerable atherosclerotic lesion, although not necessarily stenotic at angiography,[147] may be prone to disruption because of its softness caused by a high lipid content and macrophage-dependent chemical properties.

Chronic minimal injury to the arterial endothelium is physiologic and is often the result of a disturbance in the pattern of the blood flow at bending points and near bifurcations in the arterial tree. In addition to these local shear forces, endothelial dysfunction occurs. Endothelial dysfunction is a systemic pathologic condition that can be broadly defined as an imbalance between vasodilating and vasoconstricting substances produced by the endothelium adversely affecting its function.[148] Endothelial dysfunction can result from and/or contribute to several disease processes, such as DM, hypercholesterolemia, and hypertension, and environmental factors, such as smoking tobacco products and exposure to air pollution.[149] Active disruption of atherosclerotic plaques releases shed particles and may be a major contributor to the initiation of the coagulation cascade. In addition, endothelial cells (ECs) have been found to be present in circulation with a higher frequency in patients with ACS compared with control patients, or those with stable effort angina.

There is also a connection between systemic inflammation and CHD. DeJongste and Horst,[150] describe the toxic effects of shear stress, oxidized low-density lipoprotein (LDL), sensitized lymphocytes, and infections, viruses and bacteria on the CV system, and the body's response in terms of increased C-reactive protein (CRP), acute-phase proteins, IL-1, IL-6, and other immunologic markers of inflammation.[89,150] Systemic inflammation has been gaining momentum as a contributor to chronic disease.[89,126]

Imbalance between the myocardial oxygen demand and supply is most frequently due to occlusion of a coronary artery by a thrombus formed on a ruptured atherosclerotic plaque.[143] Unstable angina most frequently results from rupture of an eccentric plaque. The resulting thrombus reduces coronary blood flow, but occlusion is not complete, so myocardial necrosis does not occur. A NSTEMI is the result of the same process but is associated with myocardial necrosis causing an elevation of troponin levels, due to subendocardial ischemia (see Fig. 71.6). In STEMI, the thrombus usually causes a complete and sudden occlusion of a coronary artery. Necrosis starts to develop within 15 to 30 minutes of the cessation of blood flow and spreads from the subendocardium to the epicardium[143] (see Fig. 71.7).

Myocardial Injury Versus MI

Myocardial injury is defined as elevation of cardiac troponin values >99th percentile. Patients with MI have troponin elevations, ischemic signs or symptoms, and evidence of typical findings on EKG. They may also have new regional wall motion abnormalities. In some situations, myocardial injury is associated with MI, as per the definitions specified below (Clinical markers of ischemia must be present).

Types of MI include[143]:

- Type 1: MI caused by atherothrombotic event precipitated by plaque erosion or plaque rupture with thrombus formation.
- Type 2: Ischemic myocardial injury, usually in the setting of coronary atherosclerosis, from oxygen supply–demand mismatch without plaque erosion or rupture
- Type 3: SCD with new ischemic EKG changes or ventricular fibrillation

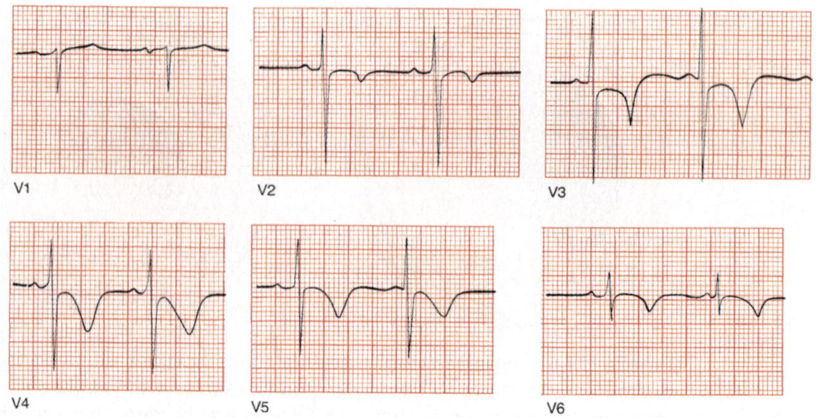

Figure 71.6. (Reprinted with permission from Thaler MS. *The Only EKG Book You'll Ever Need.* 10th ed. Wolters Kluwer; 2022:280.)

- Type 4:
  - 4a: Percutaneous coronary intervention (PCI)–related MI
  - 4b: In-stent thrombosis
  - 4c: In-stent or balloon angioplasty restenosis
- Type 5: Coronary artery bypass graft (CABG)–related MI

Similarly, cross-sectional, and longitudinal epidemiologic surveys have clearly identified the role of risk factors in the development of coronary atherosclerosis, which have been summarized in various reports.[1,151–153]

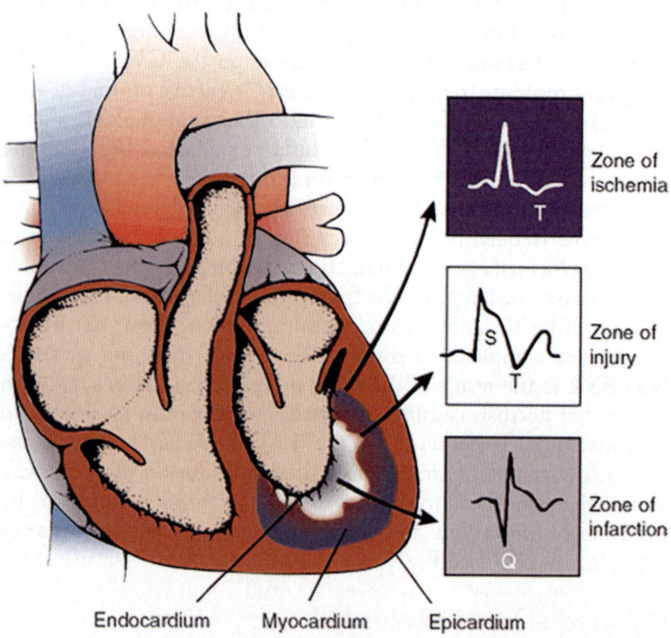

Figure 71.7. Electrocardiogram (EKG) changes associated with myocardial ischemia. The initial effects of ischemia create an inverted T wave in the EKG. The distinctive ST segment elevation in ischemic myocardium is associated with myocardial injury. The apparent zero baseline of the EKG before depolarization is below zero because of partial depolarization of the injured area. After depolarization (during the action potential plateau), all areas are depolarized and true zero is recorded. Because zero baseline is set arbitrarily (on the EKG recorder), a depressed diastolic baseline (TP segment) and an elevated ST segment cannot be distinguished. Regardless of the mechanism, this is referred to as an elevated ST segment. The EKG of a patient with acute myocardial infarction produces a Q wave in association with ST segment elevation. (Reprinted with permission from Bell DR. Electrical activity of the heart. In: Rhoades RA, Bell DR, eds. *Medical Physiology: Principles for Clinical Medicine.* 4th ed. Wolters Kluwer Health/Lippincott Williams & Wilkins; 2013:227–247. Figure 12.18.)

Natural History

Chronic, stable CAD, chronic angina, and chronic silent ischemia commonly result from increases in myocardial oxygen demand that outstrips the ability of stenosed coronary arteries to supply the needed blood flow. Atherosclerotic lesions can progress slowly for decades before they become symptomatic.

In a matter of moments, atherosclerotic lesions become symptomatic, with three manifestations: angina pectoris, MI, and SCD.[1] Angina is the only symptomatic presentation of IHD in which there is neither permanent morbidity nor mortality, giving the physician the greatest opportunity to do the best for the patient.[1]

In unstable angina, there is an abrupt reduction in coronary flow. A small erosion or fissuring of an atherosclerotic plaque may lead to an acute change in plaque structure and a reduction in coronary blood flow, resulting in exacerbation of angina.[154] Transient episodes of thrombotic vessel occlusion at the site of plaque injury may occur, leading to angina at rest. This thrombus is usually labile and results in temporary vascular occlusion, lasting only 10 to 20 minutes.[1,146,154] In non–Q-wave MI, more severe plaque damage results in more persistent thrombotic occlusion, lasting up to 1 hour. The sudden total or near total occlusion of a coronary artery usually occurs at the site of stenosis that was previously not hemodynamically significant, or at least not critical.[1,146,154] The arterial lesion of unstable angina and MI is a complex eccentric plaque angiographically, which histologically represents a ruptured plaque with a superimposed thrombus. Depending on whether it is a Q-wave (STEMI) or non–Q-wave (non-STEMI) infarction, the treatment is slightly different. This pathophysiologic feature defines the therapeutic role of thrombolytic agents for patients with ST-segment elevation MI, and the use of antiplatelet agents (aspirin, heparin, platelet glycoprotein IIb/IIIa receptor-blocking agents) in non–Q-wave MI.[154]

Diagnosis

Patients will often present with retrosternal chest pain and shortness of breath. Chest pain will often be described as "pressure-like," "a heaviness," or "a tightness." It can be burning, or sharp as well. Often patients will report discomfort as opposed to actual pain. The pain will often radiate to the jaw or arms, and both the left and right sides can be affected.[155] Constitutional symptoms such as nausea, epigastric symptoms, vomiting, diaphoresis, dizziness, and palpitations may also be present. Exertion may worsen pain, and rest can ease the pain. Nitroglycerin and aspirin administration may also improve the pain. Unstable angina may not completely resolve with these reported relieving factors. Patients may also present with an increase in episodes of chest pain that take longer to resolve or have increased in severity.[155]

On physical examination, HR may be increased secondary to a high sympathoadrenal discharge. An irregular pulse may be present due to ventricular ectopy, an accelerated idioventricular rhythm, ventricular tachycardia, AF or flutter, or other supraventricular arrhythmias. Bradyarrhythmia's may also be present. Blood pressure may be initially elevated due to peripheral arterial vasoconstriction from an adrenergic response to pain and ventricular dysfunction.[1] Hypotension may be seen in right ventricular MI or severe LV dysfunction.[1] RR may be increased due to pulmonary congestion or anxiety and coughing, wheezing, and frothy productive sputum may occur.

Other findings suggestive of a high-risk situation include[155]:

- Dyskinetic apex
- Elevated jugular venous pressure (JVP)
- Presence of S3 or S4
- New apical systolic murmur
- Presence of rales and crackles
- Hypotension

Treatment

The major treatment goals for patients with unstable angina are to control chest discomfort, relieve ischemia, and prevent the development of acute MI. Lifestyle modifications, with or without medications to lower cholesterol, can slow or reverse the progression of atherosclerosis.[46–48] The presence of collateral circulation and limiting the duration of myocardial ischemia, thrombolysis, and vasoconstriction resolution are all important factors in preventing the development of infarction. The strategy to treat MI includes reducing the extent of infarction, preventing reinfarction, and protecting against deleterious effects of ventricular remodeling. Guidelines for the diagnosis and treatment of angina have been developed and clinical practice guidelines (CPGs) have been published based on scientific and clinical evidence.[156] In 2023, CPGs for the management of patients with chronic CAD were also published.[156] The guidelines review in depth the following topics[156]:

- General team-based approach
- Patient education
- Shared decision making
- Social determinants of health
- Guideline-directed management and therapy
- Nutrition, including supplements
- Mental health considerations
- Tobacco products
- Alcohol and substance use
- Sexual health and activity
- Lipid management
- Blood pressure management
- SGLT-2 inhibitors and GLP-1 receptor agonists
- Weight management
- Cardiac rehabilitation
- Physical activity
- Environmental exposures
- Medical therapy to prevent events and manage symptoms
- Antiplatelet therapy and oral anticoagulation
- Beta-blockers
- Renin–angiotensin–aldosterone inhibitors
- Colchicine
- Immunizations
- Medical therapy for relief of angina
- Management of refractory angina
- Chelation
- Revascularization
- Special populations

The following are key takeaways from the guidelines to help guide clinicians regarding chronic coronary disease (CCD)[157]:

- The CCD guideline emphasizes team-based, patient-centered care that considers social determinants of health along with associated costs while incorporating shared decision making.
- Lifestyle modification and nonpharmacologic therapies, including healthy dietary habits and exercise, are recommended for all patients with CCD.
- Patients with CCD who are free from contraindications are encouraged to participate in habitual physical activity, including activities to reduce sitting time and increase aerobic and resistance exercise.
- Cardiac rehabilitation for eligible patients provides significant CV benefits, including decreased morbidity and mortality outcomes.
- Use of sodium–glucose cotransporter 2 inhibitors and glucagon-like peptide-1 receptor agonists is recommended for select groups of patients with CCD, including groups without diabetes.
- Long-term beta-blocker therapy is not recommended to improve outcomes in patients with CCD in the absence of MI in the past year, LV EF ≤50%, or another primary indication for beta-blocker therapy.
- Either a calcium channel blocker or beta-blocker is recommended as first-line antianginal therapy.
- Statins remain the first line for lipid lowering in patients with CCD.
- Several adjunctive therapies (e.g., ezetimibe, proprotein convertase subtilisin/kexin type 9 [PCSK9] inhibitors, inclisiran, bempedoic acid) may be used in select populations. Although clinical outcomes data are not yet available for novel agents such as inclisiran and bempedoic acid.
- Shorter durations of dual antiplatelet therapy (DAPT) are safe and effective in many circumstances, particularly when the risk of bleeding is high, and the ischemic risk is not high.
- The use of nonprescription or dietary supplements, including fish oil and omega-3 fatty acids or vitamins, is not recommended in patients with CCD given the lack of benefit in reducing CV events.
- Routine periodic anatomic or ischemic testing without a change in clinical or functional status is not recommended for risk stratification or to guide therapeutic decision making in patients with CCD.
- Because of the lack of long-term safety data and risks of sustained use, e-cigarettes are not recommended.
- In patients with CCD and lifestyle-limiting angina despite guideline-directed management and therapy and with significant coronary artery stenoses, revascularization is recommended to improve symptoms.
- In patients with CCD who require revascularization for multivessel CAD with complex and diffuse CAD (e.g., SYNTAX score >33), it is reasonable to choose CABG over PCI to improve survival.
- Finally, studies are needed to assess which interventions lead to effective guideline implementation in clinical practice.
- Research is needed to assess the effect of a new guideline release at the patient, clinic, hospital, health care system, and community levels.

Exercise

Exercise can be an essential component of managing chronic coronary artery disease (CAD), also known as coronary heart disease (CHD) or ischemic heart disease. Exercise has several benefits for individuals with chronic CAD:

- Improved CV health: Regular exercise can improve CV health in several ways. It strengthens the heart muscle, making it more efficient at pumping blood. It can also help reduce blood pressure, improve cholesterol levels, and improve blood vessel function. These improvements can lead to a reduced risk of further heart complications.[158]
- Increased exercise tolerance: Exercise helps individuals with CAD build endurance and improve their exercise tolerance. This means they can engage in physical activities with less discomfort and fatigue.
- Reduced angina symptoms: For many people with CAD, angina (chest pain or discomfort) is a common symptom. Regular exercise can help reduce the frequency and severity of angina episodes by improving blood flow to the heart muscle and enhancing the heart's efficiency via angiogenesis. Angiogenesis is increased because of the shear stress placed within the endothelium of blood vessels leading to an increase in various growth factors. The development of these collateral circulations will reduce the frequency of anginal symptoms from occurring.[158]
- Weight management: Maintaining a healthy weight is crucial for individuals with CAD, as excess weight can worsen the condition. Exercise, combined with a balanced diet, can help with weight management.[158] Weight management will also help control the patient's other comorbidities which can slow the progression of CAD.
- Stress reduction: Exercise can reduce stress and anxiety, which are risk factors for CAD. Managing stress through exercise and other relaxation techniques can have a positive impact on heart health. In a study comparing stress relief with endurance training, relaxation, and no activity, the endurance training group showed decreased levels of cortisol, HR, and HR variability. The relaxation showed decreased cortisol levels. This showed that both kinds of exercise can help with reducing stress in an individual's life.[159]
- Blood sugar control: Regular physical activity can help control blood sugar levels, which is important for individuals with diabetes, a common comorbidity in CAD patients. Exercise will increase insulin sensitivity which can help patients manage their diabetes more easily.
- Reduction in risk factors: Exercise can help control risk factors associated with CAD, such as obesity, hypertension, and diabetes.[160] Regular exercise can also improve risk factors by the modulation of the ANS leading to better cardiac function and vascular resistance. It can also help improve lipid profiles, reducing the risk of further plaque buildup in coronary arteries. Regular exercise has shown some signs of being able to regress coronary stenosis from plaque formation, while inactive people will have a higher rate of stenosis progression.[158]

Here are some key considerations for individuals with chronic CAD when incorporating exercise into their routine:

- Medical evaluation: Before starting or intensifying an exercise program, individuals with CAD should undergo a medical evaluation by a healthcare provider.[120] This assessment will help determine the type and level of exercise that is safe and appropriate, considering individual health conditions and any specific limitations. There are various combinations of exercise prescriptions, so each one must be tailored for the individual patient taking into consideration the patient's history, risk factors, and goals.[120]
- Medication management: If prescribed, medications to manage CAD (such as antiplatelet drugs, beta-blockers, or statins) should be taken as directed and managed in conjunction with exercise. There have been insufficient studies to show that prophylactic use of beta-blockers or aspirin will decrease exercise-related acute cardiac events.[159]
- Exercise type and intensity: When starting any training regimen, patients should always start at a lower intensity and gradually increase the intensity over time or as tolerated.[158] Low-to-moderate-intensity aerobic exercises are typically recommended for individuals with CAD. Activities like brisk walking, cycling, swimming, and stationary biking are good choices. Strength training exercises may also be included to improve muscle strength.
- Monitoring: Monitoring HR and blood pressure during exercise is important to ensure that the intensity is within safe limits. A gradual warm-up and cool-down period before and after exercise can help prevent sudden changes in HR and blood pressure.
- Lifestyle modifications: In addition to exercise, individuals with CAD should adopt a heart-healthy diet, quit smoking (if applicable), and manage stress as part of their overall CAD management strategy.

Exercise can play a crucial role in managing chronic CAD by improving CV health, reducing angina symptoms, and addressing risk factors associated with the condition. Starting an exercise regimen can be dangerous for individuals with CAD who have been inactive due to the increased risk of causing an adverse cardiac event.[161] The absolute contraindications for entry into inpatient and outpatient exercise training are unstable angina, resting SBP >200 mm Hg, resting DBP >100 mm Hg, moderate to severe aortic stenosis, acute systemic illness or fever, uncontrolled tachycardia (>100 bpm), symptomatic congestive HF, third-degree heart block without a pacemaker, active pericarditis or myocarditis, recent embolism, thrombophlebitis, resting ST segment displacement (>3 mm), uncontrolled diabetes and orthopedic problems that would prohibit exercise.[162] To help transition individuals into incorporating regular physical activity into their lives, it's essential for the osteopathic physician to understand these guidelines and tailor a program that meets individual needs and limitations.

Somatic Dysfunction and OMT

It is important for the clinician to recognize and diagnose an MI and treat it with an evidence-based standard of care. However, in patients with associated significant somatic dysfunction, the use of OMT as an adjunct treatment for an MI patient may be beneficial and needs to be clinically researched. Historically, studies have related palpatory findings of the axial skeleton and the angiographic status of the coronary arteries,[63,87] with palpatory findings in patients with MI.[88] Because cardiac pain is transmitted to the spinal cord by sympathetic afferent nerves, palpable viscerosomatic reflexes have been found in the areas of T1–T5.[83,85]

Treatment of somatic dysfunction can potentially decrease sympathetic tone to the heart and great vessels, and this may reduce the risk of myocardial ischemia and tachyarrhythmias. The lymphatics are under sympathetic control and have a unique role following MI. It is known that after MI, lymphatic vessel density increases during the healing process, most likely to drain excessive fluid and allow immune cells into the area.[163] Treatment of the autonomics and lymphatics to the heart following MI could have the potential to enhance lymphangiogenesis and improve myocardial fluid balance, attenuate cardiac inflammation, and help to preserve a healthy cardiac microenvironment and cardiac homeostasis after MI.[163]

In addition to local effects, the role of OMT for patients suffering from CCD is aimed at helping decrease the amount and severity of somatic dysfunction that adversely impairs their day-to-day activities. Because lifestyle changes are paramount for patients to make, osteopathic physicians can contribute to patients' success by keeping their musculoskeletal system functioning optimally. The use of OMT can be used preventatively to decrease the allostatic load of somatic dysfunction in body areas thought to influence cardiac function.[73]

PATIENTS WITH HEART FAILURE

Definition

In response to the necessity for a consensus definition of HF, in 2020 a writing committee across 14 countries and 6 continents assembled the following consensus definition. HF is a clinical syndrome with symptoms and/or signs caused by a structural and/or functional cardiac abnormality and corroborated by elevated natriuretic peptide levels and/or objective evidence of pulmonary or systemic congestion.[164]

HF is a clinical syndrome caused by abnormal cardiac structure and function which most of the time results in a reduced CO, and increased intracardiac pressures at rest or during exertion. High-output cardiac failure is a much less common form of HF. The clinical syndrome of HF may result from a disorder of the pericardium, myocardium, endocardium, heart valves, or great vessels.[1] In HF the heart cannot produce enough CO for the demands of the body's systems. Because of these unmet systemic demands, the patient will present with symptoms such as orthopnea, peripheral edema, abdominal swelling, fatigue, and shortness of breath. Clinical signs include elevated JVP, pulmonary crackles, and pitting edema[165] (see Fig. 71.8).

In addition to the presenting symptoms and clinical signs, the diagnosis of HF needs to be confirmed by an elevated natriuretic peptide level, abnormal chest x-ray, or abnormal echocardiogram. Hospitalized patients may have abnormalities seen on right heart catheterization.[166] The term "HF" has replaced the term "congestive HF" because many patients with HF do not manifest pulmonary or systemic congestion.[1]

Epidemiology

HF is a significant public health problem worldwide with a prevalence of over 5 to 6 million patients in the United States and approximately 26 million patients worldwide.[167–170] It is a leading cause of CV morbidity and mortality worldwide despite the advances in therapies and prevention. There was a decline in the rate of decrease of heart disease (HD) mortality between 2011 and 2014 and a decrease in age-adjusted mortality associated with HD and CHD.[171] However, because there is a concomitant rapid increase of adults aged 65 years and older, there has been a steady, substantial increase in the total number of HD deaths. Due to the projected 44% increase in the number of adults aged 65 years and older from 2017 to 2030 alone, the prevalence of patients with HF is increasing and can be expected to create significant challenges for health care professionals and the health care industry.[171] Another confounding variable is that the incidence rates of obesity and diabetes are also expected to increase, and the increased prevalence rates of these may further elevate the prevalence of HF.[172] As a result, HF remains a substantial and growing public health burden. According to available data in Europe and the United States, the prevalence of HF ranges from 1% to 14%. When all adults are included, HF is considered a chronic debilitating disease regardless of age.[172] The prevalence of HF increases with age.[173] In addition, HF is the main cause of hospitalization in individuals over 64 years of age.[174] The treatment of HF is important for improving the prognosis of patients and reducing health system expenditures.[172,175]

HF costs the US healthcare system nearly 31 billion dollars every year, and since the population is aging, it is projected to increase to 50 billion by 2030.[176] Patients with HF experience fourfold higher overall 2-year healthcare expenditure compared with individuals without HF.[176]

The Framingham heart study estimated the prevalence of HF to be 8 per 1,000 in men aged 50 to 59 years of age however as high as 66 per 1,000 men in ages 80 to 89 years of age.[170,177,178] Having a higher blood pressure and basal metabolic index (BMI) leads to a higher lifetime risk.[178] HF patients are older, more frequently have hypertension, and are overweight. Epidemiologic data from Medicare beneficiaries hospitalized for HF suggested a 30-day readmission risk of 25% and a 1-year mortality risk of 37%.[170]

Classification

Many CPGs have suggested classification systems for HF. The reader must also understand that clinically, HF may also be classified as LV, right ventricular, or biventricular failure, systolic HF with reduced ejection fraction (HFrEF), or diastolic HF with preserved ejection fraction (HFpEF), depending on the predominant symptoms. High-output HF refers to clinical HF

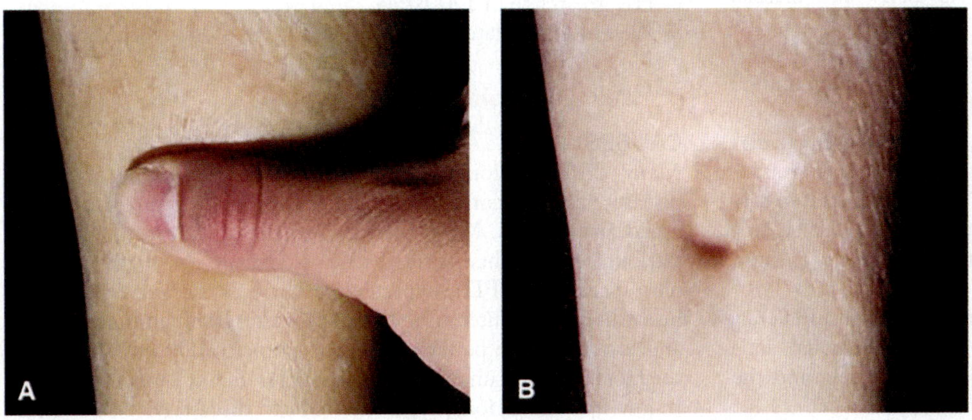

Figure 71.8. Pitting edema of the leg. **A.** In a patient with congestive heart failure, severe edema of the leg is demonstrated by applying pressure with a finger. **B.** The resulting "pitting" reflects the inelasticity of the fluid-filled tissue. (Reprinted with permission from McManus BM, Allard MF, Yanagawa R. Hemodynamic disorders. In: Rubin R, Strayer DS, Rubin E, eds. *Rubin's Pathology: Clinicopathologic Foundations of Medicine*. 6th ed. Wolters Kluwer Health/Lippincott Williams & Wilkins; 2012:281. Figure 7-25.)

occurring due to increased CO and hyperdynamic states, which may not always be associated with an underlying structural heart disease.

Currently, there are four classification systems utilized.

The first classification system is from the American Heart Association (AHA) and the American College of Cardiology (ACC). They recommend classification as listed below.[170]

ACC/AHA Stages of Heart Failure[170]

- At risk:
  - Stage A—at high risk for HF without structural HF
- Asymptomatic:
  - Stage B—structural HF without signs and symptoms of HF
- Symptomatic:
  - Stage C—structural HF with current or prior signs and symptoms of HF
  - Stage D—refractory HF

New York Heart Association

The second classification system is from the New York Heart Association (NYHA). It classifies HF into four classes based on HF symptoms and functional limitations[179]:

- Class I: asymptomatic LV dysfunction with no limitations on physical activity or symptoms.
- Class II: mild symptoms with slight limitation of physical activity. Ordinary activities lead to symptoms.
- Class III: moderate symptoms with marked limitation of physical activity. Less than ordinary activities lead to symptoms.
- Class IV: severe symptoms at rest.

Classification Based Upon Left Ventricular Ejection Fraction

The third classification system is based upon LVEF, which is defined as SV (end-diastolic volume minus end-systolic volume) divided by the EDV. Differentiation between these types is important in diagnosis and management.

Heart Failure With Reduced Ejection Fraction (HFrEF)[170]

- HFrEF: EF less than or equal to 40%
  - Almost all patients with HFrEF have concomitant diastolic dysfunction; in contrast, diastolic dysfunction may occur in the absence of systolic dysfunction.
  - It represents approximately half of all HF cases. The most common etiology of HFrEF is CAD and arterial hypertension.
  - Maladaptive changes after myocardial injury lead to pathologic remodeling of the ventricle with dilatation and impaired contractility.
  - Other causes include viral infection, alcohol abuse, valvular heart disease, chemotherapy (e.g., doxorubicin or trastuzumab), peripartum cardiomyopathy, "idiopathic" dilated cardiomyopathy, and genetic cardiomyopathies. In HFrEF, this is mediated by a maladaptive left ventricle, abnormal calcium homeostasis, and myocardial fibrosis.
  - These changes lead to the progression of mitral insufficiency and pulmonary hypertension causing neurohormonal activation of the renin–angiotensin–aldosterone system and the SNS.

Heart Failure With Preserved Ejection Fraction (HFpEF)[170]

- HF with preserved EF (HFpEF): EF is greater than or equal to 50%
  - HFpEF is less understood and is increasing in prevalence.
  - Patients are more likely to be older, female, and obese, and have a better prognosis than those with HFrEF.
  - They are less likely to have CHD and more likely to have hypertension, AF, and sleep apnea.
  - Pathophysiology involves heterogeneous factors

Heart Failure With Mid-Range EF (HFmrEF)[170]

- EF is 41% to 49% per European guidelines and 40% to 49% per the US guidelines.
  - A new class of HF was introduced by the 2016 European Society of Cardiology (ESC) guidelines.
  - Also called HFpEF-borderline

Heart Failure With Improved EF (HFimpEF)[170]

- Symptomatic HF with a baseline LVEF ≤40%, a ≥10-point increase from baseline LVEF, and a second measurement of LVEF >40%

Framingham Classification[170]

The fourth classification system is based upon the Framingham study. It developed criteria for the diagnosis of congestive HF which was based upon major and minor criteria. They also included diagnostics. For a person to have HF they would need to meet two major criteria *or* meet one major and two minor criteria concurrently. They are listed below:

Major Criteria

- Paroxysmal nocturnal dyspnea (PND)
- Orthopnea
- Elevated JVP
- Rales
- S3
- Cardiomegaly on chest x-ray
- Pulmonary edema on chest x-ray

Minor Criteria

- Peripheral edema
- Night cough
- Dyspnea on exertion
- Hepatomegaly
- Pleural effusions
- HR greater than 120 BPM
- Weight loss greater or equal to 4.5 kg in 5 days with diuretic

Causes/Pathophysiology

CAUSES

Many different conditions can cause HF, including systemic diseases, cardiac conditions, medical treatments, pregnancy, and hereditary defects. More than two-thirds of all cases of HF are attributable to ischemic heart disease, chronic obstructive pulmonary disease (COPD), hypertensive heart disease, and rheumatic heart disease.[170] The cause of HF also varies between high-income and lower-income patients.[180] For example, IHD and COPD are the most common underlying causes of HF in high-income regions. In low-income regions, hypertensive heart disease, rheumatic heart disease, cardiomyopathy, and myocarditis are the primary causes of HF, according to a systemic analysis for the Global Burden of Disease Study.[181]

Often the causes of HF are multifactorial, including features of hypertension, ischemic heart disease, and volume overload. Together, these factors cause systolic dysfunction with depression of contractility and a depressed EF/CO. Other possible causes of HF include congenital heart disease, myocarditis, infiltrative disease, peripartum cardiomyopathy, human immunodeficiency virus (HIV), connective tissue disease, amyloidosis, substance abuse, long-standing alcohol use, obesity, DM, hyperthyroidism, pulmonary hypertension, constrictive pericarditis, pulmonary embolism, and chemotherapies.[170] There are instances where the patient has a "high-output" HF with hyperdynamic circulation. These include severe anemia, thyrotoxicosis, large systemic arteriovenous fistulas, advanced cirrhosis, polycythemia or secondary erythrocytosis, Paget disease, beriberi, carcinoid syndrome, or pregnancy.

Cardiomyopathies are a heterogeneous group of heart muscle diseases and an important cause of heart failure (HF). They include dilated (DCM), hypertrophic (HCM), restrictive (RCM), arrhythmogenic right ventricular (ARVC), and nonclassified cardiomyopathies. Current knowledge of incidence, pathophysiology, and natural history of HF in cardiomyopathies is limited.[182] Cardiomyopathies are defined as pathologic myocardial processes and dysfunction that are a direct consequence of CV abnormalities other than valvular heart disease, systemic hypertension, congenital heart disease, and atherosclerotic CAD.[170]

PATHOPHYSIOLOGY

The pathophysiology of HF is complex and includes structural, neurohumoral, cellular, and molecular mechanisms' activation to maintain physiologic functioning. The performance of LV function and SV is under the control of preload (venous return and ventricular EDV), myocardial contractility, and afterload (the impedance during ejection from the aorta and wall stress).[170]

HF causes activation of neurohormones and substances to maintain perfusion of vital organs: SNS, renin–angiotensin–aldosterone system (RAAS), antidiuretic hormone, and other vasoactive substances (brain natriuretic peptide [BNP], nitric oxide, and endothelin).[170]

The degree of activation of neurohormonal mechanisms appears to depend on the severity and acuteness of cardiac impairment as well as the status of extracellular fluid volume.[183] Local autocrine and paracrine systems in blood vessels and myocardium may also contribute to the long-term regulation of vascular tone and play a role in the pathogenesis of ventricular remodeling, dilation, and progressive HF.[184] Besides these neurohormonal effects, HF also affects the kidneys, gastrointestinal system, and skeletal muscle.

HF causes decreased carotid baroreceptor response, which in turn increases sympathetic nervous activity (SNS) and leads to increased cardiac contractility and heart rate, vasoconstriction, and increased afterload. Activation of the RAAS in response to low renal perfusion from HF causes salt/water retention and increases preload. RASS activation increases angiotensin II, which leads to vasoconstriction and more salt and water retention, which further stresses the ventricular wall and causes dilatation, worsening ventricular function, and further HF. Together, these compensatory mechanisms cause negative remodeling of the heart (inflammation, apoptosis, hypertrophy, and fibrosis) and worsening LV function.[170]

Another hypothesis proposed by Rogers[185] states that abnormal skeletal muscle function in HF patients results in activation of muscle ergoreceptors which causes an increase in sympathetic activation. Patients will develop increased ventilation, exertional fatigue, and breathlessness.[185] Patients with obesity and an elevated BMI due to muscle mass (not waist circumference) were found to do better than lean patients.[186] Studies indicated that muscle mass may confer a favorable prognosis and that skeletal muscle mass and muscle strength may be protective against CVD and HF.[186] It is thought that the cardioprotective effect may be due to skeletal muscles secreting anti-inflammatory and cardioprotective cytokines.[185]

Natural History/Prognosis

The natural history and prognosis of HF are determined by the underlying disease process, the treatment undertaken, and the patients' comorbidities. Some causes of HF may be spontaneously reversible, such as peripartum cardiomyopathy, alcoholic cardiomyopathy, or viral myocarditis. Life expectancy for a person with HF has substantially improved over time, due to evidence-based care, yet patients with HF have a poor prognosis. A 2019 meta-analysis estimated that the 1-, 2-, 5-, and 10-year survival rates of all-type HF are 87%, 73%, 57%, and 35%, respectively.[187] Age is also a factor as the 5-year survival rate for people under 65 years of age was around 79%, while the rate was about 50% for those 75 and over.[170]

The natural history of HF is characterized by a progressive course of the condition, leading to worsening symptoms and potential complications over time. Progression can be influenced by several factors, including the underlying cause of HF, the individual's overall health, and the effectiveness of treatment. HF often develops because of underlying heart conditions, such as CAD, hypertension, valvular heart disease, or cardiomyopathy. In the early stages, individuals with HF may have underlying heart disease but no noticeable symptoms of HF. At this point, the focus is on identifying and managing risk factors, such as controlling blood pressure and addressing CAD. As HF progresses, symptoms typically develop. Common symptoms include fatigue, exertional shortness of breath, swelling in the legs and ankles, and reduced exercise tolerance. As it progresses, patients can easily decompensate, often triggered by factors such as infections, uncontrolled hypertension, alcohol or drugs, obstructive sleep apnea, kidney failure, and dietary/or medication noncompliance. During these episodes, symptoms can worsen suddenly, leading to hospitalization for management. In cases where HF continues to progress despite treatment, it may reach an advanced stage. Advanced HF is characterized by severe and debilitating symptoms, frequent hospitalizations, and a reduced quality of life. The need for hospitalization and rehospitalization are important markers for a poor prognosis. A 2017 study reported that the 5-year life expectancy is poor among all patients admitted to the hospital with HF regardless of their EF, with the estimated 5-year mortality at 75.4%.[188] Poor prognostic factors in chronic HF include S3 gallop, DM, hyponatremia, decreased LVEF, high NYHA functional class, reduced cardiac index, and increased pulmonary artery capillary wedge pressure.[189] End-stage HF is the most severe form of the condition. It is marked by a substantial decline in heart function and a poor prognosis. Individuals in this stage may require advanced therapies, such as mechanical circulatory support devices (e.g., ventricular assist devices) or heart transplantation.[57] The mortality rate is higher in HFrEF than HFmrEF and HFpEF, according to the OPTIMIZE-HF trial.[170] SCD accounts for up to 50% of all deaths among patients with HF.

Diagnosis

The diagnosis of HF is typically based on a combination of clinical evaluation, medical history, physical examination, and various diagnostic tests. There are no single definitive criteria. There is a broad differential diagnosis of HF, which includes but is not limited to bacterial pneumonia, COPD, liver cirrhosis, acute kidney injury (AKI), idiopathic pulmonary fibrosis, nephrotic syndrome, pulmonary embolism, respiratory failure, primary pulmonary hypertension, anemia, and venous insufficiency.

Listed below are established symptoms, signs, and diagnostics.

1. Symptoms: The presence of typical symptoms associated with HF is a crucial component of the diagnosis. Common symptoms include:
   - Shortness of breath (dyspnea), especially with exertion or when lying flat.
   - PND usually awakens the patient from sleep and usually takes at least 30 minutes to resolve.
   - Fatigue and weakness.
   - Impaired exercise tolerance.
   - Swelling in the legs, ankles, feet, or abdomen (edema).
   - Rapid or irregular heartbeat.
   - Persistent cough, wheezing, or nocturnal cough.
   - Sudden weight gain due to fluid retention.
   - Right ventricular failure produces more systemic congestion including peripheral dependent edema, abdominal pain, anorexia, nausea, constipation, oliguria, malabsorption, and cachexia.
2. Clinical signs: It is important to check vital signs and assess volume status during each clinic visit.[170]
   - LV failure
     - Crackles in the lungs.
     - S3 gallop rhythm
     - Displaced apical impulse
   - Right ventricular failure
     - Right ventricular heave
     - Enlarged and tender liver
     - Elevated JVP
     - Kussmaul sign (increased JVP during inspiration)
     - Peripheral edema (swelling in the extremities)
     - Ascites
     - Sacral edema
   - Biventricular failure
     - Pale and cool skin of the extremities
     - Diaphoresis
     - Tachycardia
     - Third heart or fourth heart sound (diastolic HF)
3. Diagnostic tests:
   - Echocardiogram: An echocardiogram is a key diagnostic test. It uses ultrasound to provide images of the heart's structure and function. It can help assess the heart's EF and detect structural abnormalities.
   - Blood tests:
     - CBC
       - Anemia, infection
     - Complete metabolic panel (CMP)
       - Hyponatremia, hypo/hyperkalemia, renal function, hepatic function
     - B-type natriuretic peptide (BNP)[190,191]
       - Natriuretic peptides are recommended to exclude HF but not to establish HF diagnosis.
       - NPs have a very high negative predictive value of 0.94 to 0.98 and can exclude the diagnosis of HF but cannot confirm the diagnosis.
       - BNP has 70% sensitivity and 99% specificity for HF diagnosis.
     - N-terminal pro B-type natriuretic peptide (NT-proBNP)
       - NT-proBNP, not BNP, is used for these purposes in patients on ARNIs.
       - NT-proBNP has 99% sensitivity and 85% specificity.
     - Lipids
     - TSH, free T4
       - Hypo/hyperthyroidism
       - Should be checked in all patients older than 65 years of age
   - Electrocardiogram (EKG):
     - Is necessary for all patients with suspected HF, however, it is usually nonspecific. It helps rule out HF if completely normal, with a sensitivity of 89% but low specificity.[192] Abnormal EKG increases the likelihood of HF diagnosis.[193]
     - EKG can reveal clues about the underlying etiology: ischemic heart disease, arrhythmia, conduction disturbances, or ventricular hypertrophy.
   - Chest x-ray:
     - Usually reveals an enlarged cardiac silhouette, and pulmonary congestion.
     - May have pleural effusions, and Kerley B-lines (interstitial edema)
   - Echocardiography[170,194]
     - Is a key diagnostic study in HF and is usually performed in patients with suspected HF as it allows assessment of (1) LV systolic function (2) LV diastolic function (3) Structural heart disease (4) valvular heart disease, (5) pericardial effusion.
     - Echocardiogram also helps to assess LVEF in HFrEF to guide evidence-based medical and device therapies.
   - Computed tomography (CT) scanning
     - Is not routinely indicated in the diagnosis and management of HF, and the role of imaging modalities other than a transthoracic echocardiogram (TTE) was restricted in the 2016 ESC guidelines. Cardiac CT can help to evaluate the coronary arteries in patients with HF with low to intermediate pretest probability of CAD.
   - Cardiac magnetic resonance imaging (cMRI)
     - cMRI is particularly useful when differentiating between various forms of cardiomyopathy, cardiac tumors, pericardial disease, and congenital heart disease and evaluating the right ventricle.
   - Coronary angiography[170,195]
     - Coronary angiography is indicated in patients with suspected ischemic heart disease, history of unexplained cardiac arrest, severe ventricular arrhythmias if myocardial ischemia is suspected as a cause, HF that is treatment resistant or of unknown etiology, or prior to elective cardiac surgery.
     - It is also indicated in patients with HF and angina symptoms or ischemic changes on EKG or noninvasive testing. Indications also include worsening HF symptoms without a clear cause.
   - Stress nuclear imaging
     - May be an acceptable option for assessing ischemia in patients presenting with HF who have known CAD and no angina unless they are ineligible for revascularization.[170]

4. Functional classification
   - Healthcare providers may use functional classification systems, such as the NYHA classification or the ACC/AHA stages of HF, to further characterize the severity and impact of HF symptoms on daily life.
   - There are also multiple electronic scoring tools to assist the clinician in evaluating the HF patient.[196,197]
   - Many heart risk calculators classify a patient's risk of CVD as:
     - Low: Less than a 5% risk.
     - Borderline: A 5% to 7.4% risk.
     - Intermediate: A 7.5% to 19.9% risk.
     - High: More than a 20% risk.
   - Clinicians may also utilize the Framingham clinical criteria[198] to help diagnose HF.
   - The Framingham Heart Study criteria are 100% sensitive and 78% specific for identifying patients with congestive HF.[198]
   - However, the Framingham clinical criteria have low specificity but excellent sensitivity to exclude the diagnosis of HF in the absence of specific signs and symptoms.[170]
   - Some authors criticize the Framingham equations used in current risk scoring methods because they overpredict the risk of mortality from CHD by 47%.[199]

Treatment

Since CAD is preventable, and hypertension is imminently treatable, most cases of HF are potentially preventable.[1] Treatment of HF starts with the prevention of overt HF by controlling the risk factors. Hypertension is a significant risk factor. The SPRINT trial found that intensive blood pressure control (SBP under 120 mm Hg) was more beneficial for the prevention of CVDs than standard treatment (SBP goal of less than 140 mm Hg).[200] Controlling blood glucose and weight management are critical factors in risk factor modification. Recent studies have shown that sodium–glucose cotransporter-2 (SGLT-2) inhibitors reduced mortality and HF hospitalization in patients with type 2 diabetes.[201] For prevention to be beneficial, the physician must identify those conditions and behaviors that are associated with an increased risk of HF before patients show any evidence of structural heart disease (stage A). This is where osteopathic physicians can utilize their unique skill set to help patients become more physically active, manage stress, and make healthier choices in their diets. Encouraging them to care for their body, mind, and spirit will help them improve their risk factors at an early stage. This will reduce their chance of HF decompensation, and in turn the impact of HF on public and individual health.

Treatment of HF is indicated in all patients with LV dysfunction (diastolic or systolic) regardless of symptoms. The goal of treatment is to improve survival and symptoms, reduce the hospital length of stay and HF readmissions, decrease morbidity, prevent organ damage from HF, and prevent symptoms of asymptomatic LV dysfunction. Treatment of HF includes[170]:

- Definitive treatment of the underlying condition (e.g., coronary revascularization, valvular surgery)
- Long-term treatment of HF
- Treatment of HF exacerbations
- Continued management of underlying conditions and risk factors

Treatment of HF can fall into several categories: nonpharmacologic therapy, pharmacologic therapy, devices and nonsurgical interventions, and invasive strategies.[170]

NONPHARMACOLOGIC MANAGEMENT

Nonpharmacologic therapy is indicated for all types of HF regardless of EF. Nonpharmacologic management of HF plays a crucial role in improving the quality of life and reducing symptoms for individuals with this condition.

Here are some general nonpharmacologic approaches for managing HF[170]:

- Low-sodium diet:
  - Limiting sodium intake to 2 to 3 g/day is critical because excess salt can lead to fluid retention and worsen HF symptoms. Limiting processed foods, canned soups, and restaurant meals can help achieve this. Fluid restriction:
    - In some cases, fluid intake may need to be restricted to about 2 liters per day to prevent fluid overload.
- Daily weight monitoring:
  - Patients are often advised to weigh themselves daily and report any sudden weight gain to their healthcare provider. An increase of >2 kg in body weight over 3 days may indicate fluid retention caused by HF. Daily weight and diuretic dosing adjustments are needed for sudden weight changes.
- Cardiac rehabilitation:
  - Supervised exercise programs can help patients gradually build CV fitness and strengthen their hearts.
- Aerobic exercise:
  - Engaging in regular, moderate-intensity aerobic exercise, such as walking or swimming, can improve overall CV health.
  - Aerobic exercise training in clinically stable patients with HF includes regular moderate physical activity: 30 minutes of aerobic exercise at least three times a week. This can reverse LV remodeling in stable patients.
  - Participation in interval or continuous training programs is recommended in HF regardless of LVEF values if the patient is clinically stable and physical activity does not lead to exhaustion or trigger new HF symptoms.
  - Isometric exercise is not recommended.
- Treatment of somatic dysfunction
  - Decreasing the amount of spinal facilitation to the heart, kidneys, and adrenal glands
  - Resolving viscerosomatic reflexes
  - Improving function of the diaphragm, breathing mechanics, and ribs
  - Normalizing vagal tone
- Lifestyle modifications:
  - Smoking cessation: Quitting smoking is essential because smoking damages the CV system and worsens HF.
  - Alcohol moderation: Limiting alcohol intake or abstaining completely may be necessary,
- Weight management:
  - Achieving and maintaining a healthy body weight can reduce the workload on the heart and improve heart function.
  - Reduce body weight in obese patients, especially those with a BMI >35 kg/m^2.
  - Improve nutrition in patients with features of malnutrition (BMI <22 kg/m^2, <90% of ideal body weight).
- Symptom management:
  - Elevating the head during sleep: Using extra pillows or an adjustable bed to keep the head elevated can help reduce nighttime symptoms like shortness of breath.
  - Pacing activities: Patients should learn to balance rest and activity, taking breaks as needed to prevent overexertion.

- Emotional and mental health support:
  - Psychosocial support: Dealing with a chronic condition like HF can be emotionally challenging. Support groups, counseling, and therapy can help patients cope with stress and anxiety.
  - Stress reduction: Learning stress-reduction techniques, such as meditation or deep breathing exercises, can improve overall well-being.
- Compliance with medication and medical appointments:
  - It's crucial for patients to take their prescribed medications as directed and attend regular medical check-ups to monitor their condition.
  - For patients with HF who have recently been hospitalized, nurse home visits, nurse case management, and outpatient disease management/HF clinics should be considered, as they reduce all-cause mortality and readmissions.
- Devices and surgical interventions:
  - In some cases, devices like pacemakers or implantable cardioverter defibrillators (ICDs) may be recommended to help manage HF.
  - Surgical interventions such as heart valve repair or replacement may be necessary for some patients.
- Education and self-management:
  - Patients and their caregivers should receive education about HF, its management, and how to recognize and respond to worsening symptoms.
  - Nonpharmacologic management should always be individualized based on the patient's specific condition and needs.
  - Caution is advised when traveling to altitudes >1,500 m above sea level or to hot and humid climates. In the case of long-distance journeys, air travel is preferred overland travel.
- Prevention
  - Annual influenza and pneumococcal vaccination; severe acute respiratory syndrome coronavirus 2 (SARS-CoV-2) vaccination according to local regulations.
  - Diagnosis and treatment of clinically significant depression.
- Drugs that can adversely affect HF[170]:
  - NSAIDs, including cyclooxygenase-2 (COX-2) inhibitors
  - Glucocorticoids (increase fluid retention and risk of hypokalemia)
  - Class I antiarrhythmic drugs (particularly class Ia and Ic agents)
  - Tricyclic antidepressants (TCAs)
  - Dronedarone is contraindicated in patients with symptomatic or recent decompensation requiring hospitalization or NYHA class IV HF
  - Nondihydropyridine calcium channel blockers (avoid in patients with HFrEF)
  - Alpha-1-blockers
  - Moxonidine (increases the risk of death)
  - Metformin should be avoided in patients with contraindications.
  - Thiazolidinediones (rosiglitazone, pioglitazone)
  - Anthracyclines

EXERCISE

Exercise plays a crucial role in the management and rehabilitation of individuals with HF. Appropriate exercise can have several benefits for people with HF:

- Improved CV fitness:
  - There have been some meta-analyses that show regular exercise can induce reverse cardiac remodeling in patients with HF.[159] Improved LV function can decrease bouts of HF exacerbations.
- Strengthening of skeletal muscles:
  - Regular exercise can improve exercise tolerance by making skeletal muscles more efficient at oxygen extraction without affecting the LV function.[202]
- Enhanced quality of life: From the HF:
  - A Controlled Trial Investigating Outcomes of Exercise Training (HF-ACTION) trial, the patients enrolled in the exercise groups had improved quality of life when compared to patients in the control group.[204]
- Weight management:
  - Body mass index can be affected with regular exercise as it affects an individual's metabolic rate.
  - Cardiorespiratory fitness has an inverse relationship with rates of HF hospitalizations.[202]
- Exercise prescription:
  - From a 2016 meta-analysis evaluating the effectiveness of different training exercises, there was no significant difference in cardiopulmonary exercise test parameters between any of the training modalities tested.[202] The general standard training modality for patients with chronic HF remains to be moderate continuous training. Still, each exercise prescription needs to be tailored to everyone's needs and capability.
  - Individualized exercise plans:
    - Each patient with HF needs to be appropriately assessed before starting a training regimen. Some of these assessments include risk stratification, functional capacity, or any other comorbidities.[203]
  - Monitoring:
    - In an outpatient setting, many forms of aerobic exercise can be measured using a cycle ergometer or treadmill, which is typically seen within cardiac rehab facilities.[203]
  - Type of exercise:
    - Different types of exercises include aerobic/endurance training, strength or resistance training, and mobility or flexibility exercises. Any combination of exercises has been shown to help with improving symptoms of HF. Aerobic training and HIIT have been shown to potentially be more efficient for training since they place a greater challenge upon the patient's cardiopulmonary, metabolic, and peripheral systems. Resistance training is an effective method for increasing muscle mass and strength which can be a good complement to aerobic exercise training.[203]
  - Intensity:
    - The most studied type of exercise involves continuous AT starting at around 40% to 50% of VO_2 max. The intensity can slowly be increased as the patient's fitness improves.[203]
  - Progression:
    - Patients with HF who do not perform regular exercise should be cautious about starting an exercise regimen too intensely too quickly. Since it takes time for the body to adjust to a training regimen, the progression of a training program should happen only as the patient's fitness starts to improve as well.[203]
  - Safety:
    - According to the American Heart Association, "exercise training is recommended as safe and effective for patients with HF who are able to participate to improve functional status."[204] For patients just starting a training regimen, their exercise prescriptions should be tailored for them and supervised by an exercise therapist to ensure that they are doing the program correctly. They should also be starting at a lower intensity and frequency, and gradually increase in both intensity and frequency as they become more physically conditioned.

TABLE 71.1

Summary of Six Randomized Controlled Trials of the Benefits of Endurance Training in Patients with Heart Failure and Preserved Ejection Fraction

Trial	Number of Subjects (*n*)	Intensity	Length of Training Program (wk)	Major Conclusions
Smart et al. (2012) (19)	ET = 12 Cnt = 13	60–70% peak VO_2	16	↑ Peak exercise capacity ↔ QOL
Alves et al. (2012) (20)	ET = 20 Cnt = 22	70–75% HRmax for 3–5 min (five to seven intervals)	24	↑ Peak METS ↑ Rest LVEF ↓ L atrial pressure ↓ LV stiffness
Haykowsky et al. (2012) (21)	ET = 22 Cnt = 18	40–70% HHR	16	↑ Peak exercise capacity ↑ Peak HR
Edelmann et al. (2011) (13) (EX-DHF)	ET = 44 Cnt = 20	50–70% HRmax, 60–65% PeakVO_2, 1repetition max	12	↑ Peak exercise capacity ↑ 6MWD ↑ Self-reported physical function
Kitzman (2010) (14)	ET = 24 Cnt = 22	40–70% HRR	16	↑ Peak exercise capacity ↑ 6MWD ↑ Physical QOL
Gary (2006) (15)	ET = 15 Cnt = 13	40–60% HRmax	12	↑ 6MWD ↑ Physical QOL

The mean age of participants ranged from 63 to 70 years, with a mean ejection fraction greater than 55.5%. Frequency of training in all trials ranged from two to three sessions/week, for a duration between 15 and 60 minutes/session. Training modalities included walking, treadmill, and stationary cycling, with inclusion of resistance training only in the EX-DHF trial.

6MWD, 6-minute walk distance; Cnt, control group; ET, endurance training; HR, heart rate; HRR, heart rate reserve; HRmax, maximum heart rate maximum; LV, left ventricle; LVEF, left ventricle ejection fraction; MET, metabolic equivalents; QOL, quality of life.

Used with permission of American Osteopathic Association from Rogers FJ, Gundala T, Ramos JE, Serajian A. Heart failure with preserved ejection fraction. *J Am Osteopath Assoc.* 2015;115(7):432–442; permission conveyed through Copyright Clearance Center, Inc.

Exercise is a valuable component of the management and rehabilitation of HF (see Table 71.1). However, it should be cautiously approached and tailored to the individual's specific needs and abilities. Structural and functional factors are incorporated to tailor the exercise program to the patient's needs and capabilities. There should be a slow progression to maximal intensity to promote a safe and effective setting for the patient's overall health and well-being.

PHARMACOLOGIC TREATMENT

Pharmacologic treatment of HF is based on the type of HF present, medical evidence, the status and comorbidities of the patient, the patient's current medications, and adverse effects of the treatment itself.

General Principles of Pharmacotherapy[165,170,205–208]

Here are some common classes of medications used in the pharmacologic management of HF:

- Angiotensin-converting enzyme inhibitors (ACEIs): Examples: enalapril, lisinopril, ramipril
  - Mechanism: These drugs block the effects of angiotensin II, a hormone that constricts blood vessels and causes the heart to work harder. By dilating blood vessels and reducing the heart's workload, ACE inhibitors improve heart function.
  - ACEIs: Initiate these in patients with acute MI with HF, an LVEF ≤40% post-MI (regardless of HF), those with HFrEF who are intolerant to ARNIs.[165,170]
- ARBs: Examples: losartan, valsartan, candesartan[165,170]
  - Mechanism: ARBs work similarly to ACE inhibitors by blocking the effects of angiotensin II, but they act at a different point in the pathway. They are used when ACE inhibitors are not tolerated.
  - ARBs are typically initiated in patients who do not tolerate ACEIs because of persistent cough or angioedema. Approximately 10% of patients develop a cough with ACEIs.
- Beta-blockers: Examples: metoprolol, carvedilol, bisoprolol[165,170,205]
  - Mechanism: Beta-blockers reduce the HR and decrease the heart's workload. They can improve symptoms and reduce the risk of HF progression.
  - Beta-blockers: Evidence supports the use of bisoprolol, carvedilol, and extended-release metoprolol. They should be used in patients with NYHA classes II to IV and LVEF ≤40% or in patients with asymptomatic systolic LV dysfunction.[205]
- Diuretics: Examples: furosemide (loop diuretic), hydrochlorothiazide (thiazide diuretic)[161,166]
  - Mechanism: Diuretics help eliminate excess fluid from the body, reducing fluid buildup in the lungs and extremities, which is common in HF.
  - Diuretics are used in patients with symptoms of volume overload and then continued at the lowest dose that prevents water retention. Loop diuretics are generally the first-line agents in managing volume overload, particularly in symptomatic HF.
- Mineralocorticoid antagonists (MRAs): Examples: spironolactone, eplerenone[165,170]
  - Mechanism: These drugs block the effects of aldosterone, a hormone that can lead to sodium and water retention.
  - MRAs (eplerenone, spironolactone) should be used in patients with (1) LVEF ≤40% and NYHA classes II to IV

(2) LVEF ≤40%, recent MI, and HF symptoms or diabetes. Do not use MRAs in pregnant patients.[170]

- Angiotensin receptor neprilysin inhibitors (ARNIs): Examples: sacubitril/valsartan (Entresto)[170]:
  - Mechanism: This medication combines an angiotensin receptor blocker (ARB) with a neprilysin inhibitor. It helps relax blood vessels and reduce strain on the heart while increasing the levels of beneficial peptides.
  - ARNIs: Initiate these as first-line therapy in both ambulatory and hospitalized patients with HFrEF without prior exposure to an ACEI or ARB, provided there are no contraindications.[165] Use ARNIs preferentially over ACEIs or ARBs in patients with HFrEF (LVEF <40%) who are symptomatic.[165]
- Digoxin:
  - Mechanism: Digoxin increases the strength of the heart's contractions and can help control HR in certain cases. It is less commonly used today than in the past but may still be considered for some patients.
  - Digoxin reduces the frequency of hospitalization with no survival benefit.
  - Digoxin has been associated with a higher absolute risk of all-cause death in women than in men. Research is warranted to further ascertain the safety of digoxin use in female patients with HF.
- Hydralazine/isosorbide dinitrate[165,170]:
  - Mechanism: This combination of medications can help dilate blood vessels, reduce afterload on the heart, and improve symptoms, especially in individuals who cannot tolerate ACE inhibitors or ARBs.
  - A fixed-dose combination of hydralazine (or dihydralazine) and isosorbide dinitrate: In patients with LVEF ≤35% (or LVEF ≤45% and LV dilation), this may be considered an alternative to the ACEI/ARNI/ARB if none of these agents are tolerated due to renal dysfunction or hyperkalemia.
- Selective I_{funny} (IF), or funny current, channel inhibitor[206]: Example: ivabradine
  - Mechanism: Ivabradine reduces HR by specifically inhibiting the pacemaker current in the heart. It can be considered in patients with a reduced EF who have a high HR despite optimal therapy with other medications.
  - This drug reduces the HR by having selective effects on the sinus node, in patients with LVEF ≤35%, preserved sinus rhythm ≥70 beats/min, and NYHA classes II to IV.
- Anticoagulants and antiplatelet agents[165,170]:
  - Medications like warfarin or newer oral anticoagulants (e.g., apixaban, rivaroxaban) may be prescribed to prevent blood clots and reduce the risk of stroke in certain HF patients with AF. Antiplatelet agents like aspirin may be considered for specific indications.
  - Antithrombotic treatment should be used in patients with additional indications such as paroxysmal or persistent AF or atrial flutter, intracardiac thrombus, or a history of peripheral embolism.
- Sodium–glucose cotransporter 2 (SGLT-2) inhibitors[165,170]:
  - SLGT-2 inhibitors are agents classically used in the treatment of type 2 DM. Recently these drugs, mainly dapagliflozin and empagliflozin, have been shown to significantly reduce the risk of CV death and hospitalization due to HF in patients with HFrEF, with or without type 2 DM. They have been shown to decrease the risk of hospitalization in HF with mildly reduced EF and HFpEF (NYHA class II to IV symptoms, LVEF >40%) in comparison with placebo. Notably, these benefits were demonstrated regardless of diabetes history.[165]
- Guanylate cyclase (sGC) stimulator: Example: vericiguat[165,170]
  - Augments nitric oxide production[208]
  - sGC stimulator may be considered as a second-line agent in addition to guideline-directed medical therapy (GDMT) in selected patients with HFrEF (LVEF ≤45%), HF hospitalization within the previous 6 months, and worsening symptoms.

TREATMENT OF HFrEF: FIRST-LINE AGENTS

GDMT is the cornerstone of pharmacologic therapy for patients with HFrEF and consists of the four main drug classes: renin–angiotensin system inhibitors, evidence-based β-blockers, MRAs, and SGLT-2 inhibitors.[170] The recommendation for use of GDMT is based on the results of multiple major randomized controlled trials demonstrating improved clinical outcomes. The effect is most beneficial when medications from the four main drug classes are used in conjunction.[207] Initiation of GDMT is multifactorial and should be driven by the unique qualities and comorbidities of each patient. Symptomatic patients should be started on all four major classes of HF therapy as soon as possible, with further titration to target dosages used in clinical trials during the early outpatient period, to improve patient outcomes and reduce healthcare burden.[207] These pharmacologic advancements have reduced the rates of mortality and hospitalization in patients with HFrEF.[208] These drugs are also important in LVAD recipients in relation to lowering the risk of complications as well as improving myocardial recovery.[208] A combination of diuretics is used for volume overload to improve symptoms, but they do not improve survival and routine use of loop diuretics without volume overload may even increase mortality.[170]

Hospitalizations for acute HF serve as an opportune time to initiate or optimize HF therapies. In the multinational Safety, tolerability, and efficacy of up-titration of guideline-directed medical therapies for acute HF (STRONG-HF) trial, reduced HF readmissions and all-cause mortality with early initiation and rapid up-titration of HF were seen using GDMT.[209] There is limited evidence to support the order in which medications should be added in the outpatient setting.

Pharmacologic Treatment of HFpEF and HFmrEF[165,170]

There are no disease-modifying therapies for HFpEF or HFmrEF that improve outcomes compared to HFrEF agents. Unfortunately, the current therapies for HFrEF have failed to demonstrate the same benefit for HFpEF. Spironolactone has been shown to reduce HF hospitalization rates in HFpEF, but no treatment has demonstrated improved survival.[210] Treatment focuses on controlling BP using beta-blockers, ACEIs or ARBs. There are no studies to determine the impact of revascularization on symptoms or outcomes, specifically in patients with HFpEF.[170]

There is no convincing data to date for treatments that reduce morbidity or mortality in patients with HF with EF. Nonetheless, the current standard of practice includes:

- Optimal treatment of the underlying condition: This may involve rate control in the setting of AF, treatment of sleep apnea with continuous positive airway pressure, and strict control of hypertension.
- Restriction of sodium and fluid intake
- Beta-blockers have not been adequately tested in HFpEF, but they are used to improve LV filling.
- RAAS inhibitors: ACEIs, ARBs, MRAs, and ARNIs may be used to reduce the risk of HF hospitalization.[170]
- SGLT-2 inhibitors
- Diuretics are used in patients with symptoms of fluid retention.

CLINICAL PRACTICE GUIDELINES

The following are key points to remember taken from the 2021 Update to the 2017 ACC Expert Consensus Decision Pathway for Optimization of HF Treatment[164]:

- For patients with newly diagnosed Stage C HFrEF, a beta-blocker, ACEI/ARB/ARNIs should be started in any order.
- Only guideline-recommended beta-blockers (i.e., carvedilol, metoprolol succinate, or bisoprolol) should be used in patients with HFrEF.
- Diuretics should be added as needed and the dose should be titrated to achieve decongestion.
- After initiation of beta-blocker and angiotensin antagonist, addition of an aldosterone antagonist should be considered with close monitoring of electrolytes.
- SGLT-2 inhibitors should also be considered for HFrEF with NYHA class II o IV patients.
- For persistently symptomatic Black patients despite above therapies, hydralazine, and isosorbide dinitrate should be considered.
- An ideal time to consider therapy optimization is during hospitalization for HFrEF.
- Outpatient adjustment of therapies should be considered every 2 weeks to achieve GDMT within 3 to 6 months of initial diagnosis.
- Surgical treatment is recommended for patients with severe primary chronic mitral regurgitation.
- Hyperkalemia and/or abnormal renal function are common barriers to achieving target medication doses.
- Socioeconomic barriers pose a major barrier to use of ARNI, SGLT-2 inhibitors, and ivabradine.
- For patients with recovery of LVEF to >40%, GDMT should be resumed in the absence of a defined, reversible cause.
- Repeat echocardiograms should be considered in the context of change in clinical status or other high-risk features only. Measuring BNP or NT-proBNP is useful for risk assessment and decision making.
- Right heart catheterizations should be considered when symptoms persist despite adequate diuretic dose, worsening renal function, or those with repeated hospitalizations.
- Referral to an HF specialist should be considered in symptomatic patients needing inotropes, persistently elevated natriuretic peptides, end-organ dysfunction, EF ≤35%, ICD shocks, and recurrent hospitalizations.
- Delivering care for HF requires a team-based approach. Medication adherence should be assessed regularly.
- Goals of care should be addressed during the illness and expectations should be calibrated to guide timely decisions.

DEVICE THERAPY[170]

Specific medical devices are often used in addition to medications and other treatments when HF symptoms persist or worsen. Device therapy can help regulate the heart's rhythm, improve its pumping ability, and enhance overall heart function. Before proceeding with device therapy, patients should be treated with ACEI/ARB plus Beta-blockers for at least 3 months and then the LVEF should be reassessed. If the EF remains less than or equal to 35%, the recommendation is a referral for device therapy. Here are some common types of device therapy for HF:

- Implantable cardioverter-defibrillator (ICD):
  - An ICD is a small, implantable device that continuously monitors the heart's rhythm. It can detect and treat life-threatening ventricular arrhythmias, such as ventricular tachycardia and ventricular fibrillation, by delivering electrical shocks or pacing impulses as needed. ICDs can prevent SCD in individuals with HF who are at risk of dangerous arrhythmias.
  - They are indicated as primary prevention (preventing SCD in individuals without a history of sustained ventricular arrhythmias) for those with reduced EF, usually ≤35% and for those following an infarction who meet specific criteria.[211]
  - They are also used in secondary prevention (preventing recurrent life-threatening arrhythmias in individuals with a history of sustained ventricular arrhythmias (VT), cardiac arrest, or near-fatal arrhythmias).
  - These devices have been shown to reduce SCD and are typically considered in patients receiving optimal pharmacotherapy for ≥3 months, after revascularization (where indicated), and with >1-year life expectancy of good functional status.[211]
  - The ESC 2016 guidelines recommend ICD for primary prevention in symptomatic HF (NYHA II-III) with LVEF ≤35% despite ≥3 months of GDMT in ICM (IA) or NIDCM (IB).[211]
- Cardiac resynchronization therapy (CRT):
  - CRT devices, often called biventricular pacemakers, are implanted to improve the coordination of the heart's contractions. They have three leads: one in the right atrium, one in the right ventricle, and one in the left ventricle. By pacing both ventricles simultaneously, CRT can help the heart pump blood more efficiently and improve symptoms.[170]
  - CRT is primarily indicated for individuals with moderate–severe HF who have a reduced LV ejection fraction (typically ≤35%) and those with left bundle branch block or significant intraventricular conduction delays.[211]
  - The ESC 2016 guidelines recommend CRT for symptomatic HF with sinus rhythm and LVEF ≤35% despite GDMT with left bundle branch block and a QRS duration ≥150 ms (I-A) or 130 to 149 ms (I-B).[211]
- Left ventricular assist device (LVAD):
  - LVADs are mechanical pumps implanted in the chest and attached to the left ventricle and aorta. They are used in advanced HF when the heart is unable to pump blood effectively. LVADs assist the heart by pumping blood directly from the left ventricle into the aorta, taking over much of the heart's pumping function.[170]
  - LVADs are indicated when individuals have significant symptoms and (ACC/AHA) Stage D HF with an EF <25%.[170]
  - LVADs can be used as a bridge to a heart transplant or as destination therapy for individuals who are not eligible for heart transplantation.
- Intra-aortic balloon pump (IABP):
  - IABPs are temporary devices inserted into the aorta to assist the heart in pumping blood. They inflate and deflate in synchrony with the heart's rhythm, improving coronary artery perfusion and reducing the workload of the heart.
  - IABPs are typically indicated in cases of cardiogenic shock, resulting from various causes, such as acute MI, severe HF, or complications during cardiac surgery.
  - IABPs may be considered to provide circulatory support following MI, during procedures such as PCI, and as part of bridge therapy in severely ill patients.
- Pacemakers:
  - While pacemakers are primarily used to treat bradyarrhythmias, they can also be helpful in some HF cases. They may be used with CRT devices to manage HF with conduction system abnormalities.

- Device therapy for HF is typically recommended based on an individual's specific condition and response to other treatments. These devices can significantly improve the quality of life and prognosis for many people with HF, especially those with advanced or complex forms of the condition.

- PCI
  - PCI is a minimally invasive procedure commonly used to relieve symptoms of angina and improve blood flow in cases where coronary artery blockages are causing reduced blood supply to the heart.
  - PCI can also be performed in certain cases of ACS to quickly restore blood flow to the affected artery and prevent further damage to the heart.
  - In patients with STEMI, rapid PCI and administration of ACEI, beta-blockers, mineralocorticoid receptor antagonists (MRAs), and statins can reduce HF hospitalization and mortality.[212]
- Coronary revascularization (CABG)
  - Coronary revascularization is usually done in patients with HF caused by ischemic heart disease, who have suitable anatomy and have symptoms of angina.
  - CABG is indicated when there are severe blockages or narrowing in multiple coronary arteries that cannot be adequately treated with PCI or angioplasty. These blockages often involve critical or high-risk coronary vessels such as the left anterior descending artery (LAD).
  - CABG is also considered when there are blockages in all three main coronary arteries, or two vessels with concerning features, or if there is concomitant valvular disease.[170]
  - In diabetic individuals with CAD, CABG may be preferred over PCI in certain cases, as it has been shown to have better long-term outcomes in this population.
- Heart transplant
  - Heart transplantation is indicated for individuals with end-stage HF who have advanced to stage D, as defined by the ACC/AHA HF classification system.[170]
  - It is typically considered when there is severe LV dysfunction, often characterized by a LVEF of 20% or less, and when HF symptoms do not improve or worsen despite optimal medical therapy.[170]
  - Heart transplant is also considered in patients with ventricular arrhythmia, or congenital heart disease that remains uncontrolled despite drug, device, or alternative surgical therapy.[213]
  - In cases where a patient's HF is so severe that their life expectancy is estimated to be less than 2 years without transplantation.
  - The evaluation process for heart transplantation is comprehensive and individualized, involving assessments by a multidisciplinary team.
  - Data from the registry of the International Society of Heart and Lung Transplantation indicates a current 1-year survival of 84.5% and 5-year survival of 72.5%; subsequently, survival decreases linearly by approximately 3.4% per year.[170,214]

Complications

Common complications of HF include:

- Fluid retention (Edema):
  - HF often causes fluid to build up in the lungs and extremities, leading to symptoms like shortness of breath, swelling of the legs and ankles, and weight gain.
- Acute decompensated HF (ADHF):
  - Sudden worsening of HF symptoms can occur, leading to severe shortness of breath, extreme fatigue, and fluid overload.
- Arrhythmias:
  - HF can disrupt the heart's electrical system, leading to irregular heart rhythms (arrhythmias).
  - Atrial fibrillation (AF) can be a cause or a consequence of HF and may be present in 10% to 50% of chronic HF patients, and those patients with HF and AF have a poor prognosis.[170]
  - Ventricular arrhythmias like ventricular tachycardia and ventricular fibrillation can be life threatening.[215]
- Cardiogenic shock:
  - In severe cases, HF can lead to cardiogenic shock, where the heart cannot pump enough blood to meet the body's needs. This is a critical condition requiring intensive medical intervention.
- Kidney problems:
  - Reduced blood flow and fluid retention can strain the kidneys, leading to impaired kidney function or AKI.
  - Renal function may get worse in both acute and chronic HF, and that predicts poor prognosis, and even a small transient rise in creatinine will be clinically relevant.[216]
- Liver congestion:
  - Congestion in the right side of the heart can affect liver function, potentially leading to liver congestion or cirrhosis.
- Pulmonary hypertension:
  - Elevated pressure in the pulmonary arteries (pulmonary hypertension) can occur because of chronic HF, further complicating the condition.
- Cognitive impairment:
  - In some cases, reduced blood flow to the brain can lead to cognitive impairment, memory problems, and difficulty concentrating.
- Depression and anxiety:
  - Living with a chronic illness like HF can lead to emotional distress, including depression and anxiety.
- Increased risk of blood clots:
  - HF, especially when associated with AF, can increase the risk of blood clots, which can lead to stroke or other thromboembolic events.
  - There is a high relative risk for DVT and PE in patients with HF, especially those who are under 60 years of age.[217]
- End-stage HF:
  - Over time, HF can progress to a point where the heart's function becomes severely compromised, and advanced therapies or heart transplantation may be necessary.
- Gastrointestinal symptoms:
  - Some people with HF may experience digestive problems, including a feeling of fullness, loss of appetite, nausea, and abdominal discomfort.
- Frailty:
  - Chronic illness and reduced physical activity can lead to frailty, making it harder for individuals with HF to perform daily activities.
  - In end-stage cases, hospice care and hospice nurses can work with the patient and their family to provide comfort care. These interprofessional collaborations will optimize patient outcomes in HF cases.

Somatic Dysfunction and OMT

There are currently very few studies looking into the efficacy of OMT on HF. Historically, lymphatic techniques have shown improvement in lymphatic flow and respiratory function in patients with respiratory infections[218,219] and are well tolerated by patients.[220] These results with respiratory complaints have shown promise in potentially helping individuals with HF to decrease fluid overload and increase respiratory function.[221] A recent case study demonstrated that lymphatic techniques decreased patient's pain and increased exercise tolerance postcardiac transplantation[222] further providing evidence for lymphatic treatment. Another study looking specifically at HF showed techniques aimed at normalizing autonomic function increased brachial blood flow and stimulated the vagal system to help decrease excessive sympathetic stimulation that is present in individuals with HF.[223] Research looking into other techniques, such as myofascial release, has shown less success with no significant changes in blood flow or cardiopulmonary performance when compared with control trials.[224,225] With this mixed evidence, future research elucidating which techniques are most helpful for patients with HF would be beneficial to provide direction for the osteopathic physician's treatment plans.

PATIENTS WITH ATRIAL FIBRILLATION (AF)

Definition

AF is a supraventricular tachyarrhythmia with uncoordinated atrial electrical activation and consequently, ineffective atrial contraction, resulting in a loss of atrial contractility and irregular ventricular response.[4] The subsequent ventricular rate depends on AV nodal conduction properties, and typically ranges from 120 to 160 beats/min. The rate can exceed 200 beats/min in some cases, or may be excessively slow, resulting in an irregular ventricular rate.

The diagnosis of AF requires rhythm documentation with an EKG tracing showing AF. The minimum duration of an EKG tracing of AF required to establish the diagnosis of clinical AF is at least 30 seconds of a rhythm strip or on an entire 12-lead EKG.

Electrocardiographic characteristics of AF include:

- Irregularly irregular R–R intervals (when AV conduction is not impaired)
- Absence of distinct repeating P waves
- Irregular atrial activations.

AF is the most common type of cardiac arrhythmia. It is due to abnormal electrical activity within the atria of the heart, causing them to fibrillate. This arrhythmia may be paroxysmal (less than 7 days) or persistent (more than 7 days). Due to its rhythm irregularity, blood flow through the heart becomes turbulent and has a high chance of forming a thrombus, which can ultimately dislodge and cause a stroke. AF is the leading cardiac cause of stroke.[226]

Epidemiology

Worldwide, AF is the most sustained cardiac arrhythmia in adults.[4] The prevalence of AF has been increasing and generally increases with age. The current estimation is that in the United States, 6 to 12 million people will suffer from this condition by 2050, and in Europe, 17.9 million people will have AF by 2060.[227] Although the worldwide prevalence of AF is approximately 1%, it is found in approximately 9% of individuals over the age of 75. At the age of 80, the lifetime risk of developing AF jumps to 22%.[226] AF is more commonly seen in White individuals compared to Black individuals and men compared to women. Women with AF are more often symptomatic than men with AF, with greater symptom severity.[4] Women with AF have a greater stroke severity and higher permanent disability rates than men with AF.[4] Female sex is an age-dependent stroke risk modifier rather than a risk factor. AF is associated with substantial morbidity and mortality, thus portending significant burden to patients, societal health, and health economy.[4] The incidence of AF in ACS ranges from 2% to 23% and the risk of new-onset AF is increased by 60% to 77% in MI patients. AF may be associated with an increased risk of STEMI or non–STEMI ACS.

Classification[4,226]

- First diagnosed AF
  - A condition when AF was not diagnosed before irrespective of its duration or presence/severity of symptoms.
- Paroxysmal AF
  - A condition when the episodes terminate spontaneously or within 7 days of treatment. But they may recur with an unpredictable frequency.
- Persistent AF
  - A condition when the AF is continuous and lasts for more than 7 days and fails to terminate spontaneously.
- Long-standing AF
  - A condition when the continuous AF lasts more than 12 months.
- Permanent AF
  - A condition when no further treatments are attempted to restore or maintain normal sinus rhythm.
- Nonvalvular AF
  - A condition in the absence of rheumatic mitral valve disease, mitral valve repair, or a prosthetic heart valve.

AF can also be classified as valvular or nonvalvular. Valvular typically involves moderate to severe mitral stenosis or artificial mechanical valves. It's important to note that the congestive HF, hypertension, age, DM, prior stroke or TIA or thromboembolism, vascular disease, age, sex category (CHA2DS2-VASc) score is used for both valvular and nonvalvular AF. However, for patients with valvular AF, there are additional considerations, such as the presence of mechanical heart valves, which could impact the choice of anticoagulation therapy. Anticoagulation for patients with mechanical heart valves can be more complex and challenging compared to anticoagulation for patients with AF alone.[4,226]

Warfarin, a vitamin K antagonist, has traditionally been used for anticoagulation in patients with mechanical heart valves. These patients typically require higher levels of anticoagulation to prevent clot formation. The target international normalized ratio (INR) range for patients with mechanical heart valves is generally higher than that for patients with AF. The optimal INR range varies depending on the type and location of the valve.[4,226]

AF can also be classified as clinical or subclinical. Subclinical AF, also known as subclinical atrial tachyarrhythmia, refers to a type of AF that doesn't cause noticeable symptoms and therefore often goes undetected by the person experiencing it. In typical cases of AF, individuals experience symptoms like palpitations, shortness of breath, fatigue, dizziness, and chest discomfort. However, in subclinical AF, these symptoms may be absent or very mild, making it challenging to diagnose without specific monitoring methods. Subclinical AF can still be significant because even though it lacks overt symptoms, it is associated with an increased risk of complications, particularly stroke.[4,226]

Diagnosing subclinical AF (atrial high-rate episodes/subclinical AF) often involves the use of continuous monitoring devices, such as:

- Holter monitor: This portable device records your heart's electrical activity continuously over a period of 24 hours to 7 days.
- Event monitor: This is worn for a longer period (weeks to months) and can be triggered by the individual when they experience symptoms or suspect an irregular heartbeat.

- Implantable loop recorder: A small device is implanted under the skin and can continuously monitor heart rhythms for months to years. It's often used for detecting infrequent or subclinical arrhythmias.
- Smartphone applications: Some smartphone apps are designed to detect irregular heart rhythms using the phone's built-in sensors. These can be useful for long-term monitoring.
- Wearable devices: Some fitness trackers and smartwatches have built-in HR monitors that can detect abnormal heart rhythms and alert the user.

It is important for clinicians to understand that the classification of AF does not change the decision to anticoagulate.[4,226] During AF, blood may pool in the atria, increasing the risk of blood clot formation. If a clot forms and travels to the brain, it can cause a stroke.

Causes/Risk Factors

Risk factors for AF include advanced age, high blood pressure, underlying heart and lung disease, congenital heart disease, and increased alcohol consumption. Symptoms vary from asymptomatic to symptoms such as chest pain, palpitations, tachycardia, shortness of breath, nausea, dizziness, diaphoresis, and generalized fatigue.[226]

- Advanced age
- Congenital heart disease
- Underlying heart disease—valvular disease, CAD, structural heart disease, atrial ischemia
- Increased alcohol consumption
- Hypertension—systemic or pulmonary
- Endocrine disorders—diabetes, pheochromocytoma, and hyperthyroidism
- Genetic factors
- Neurologic disorders—subarachnoid hemorrhage or stroke
- Hemodynamic stress—mitral or tricuspid valve disease, LV dysfunction, pulmonary embolism
- Obstructive sleep apnea
- Inflammation—myocarditis and pericarditis
- Pulmonary disorders—pneumonia, pulmonary embolism

For many risk factors (e.g., age), stroke risk is a continuum. Risk factors are dynamic and, given the elderly AF population with multiple (often changing) comorbidities, stroke risk needs to be reevaluated at each clinical review.[4]

Pathophysiology

Typically, an initiating trigger excites an ectopic focus in the atria, most commonly around the area of the pulmonary veins, and allows for an unsynchronized firing of electrical impulses leading to fibrillation of the atria.[226] Cardiac remodeling, particularly of atria, results in structural and electrical changes that eventually become the cause of deranged rhythm in AF. Structural remodeling is caused by the changes in myocytes and the extracellular matrix, and fibrous tissue deposition also plays a major role in some etiologies. Tachycardia and shortening of the refractory period can lead to electrical remodeling.[226] Some research has shown evidence of genetic causes of AF involving a gene mutation affecting membrane stability.[228] Obesity causes left atrial enlargement and this fatty infiltration in the left atrium is where the pulmonary veins enter (see Fig. 71.9). This anatomical location is the target for many ablation procedures.[57] In critically ill patients and those with severely impaired LV systolic function, AF is often precipitated/exacerbated

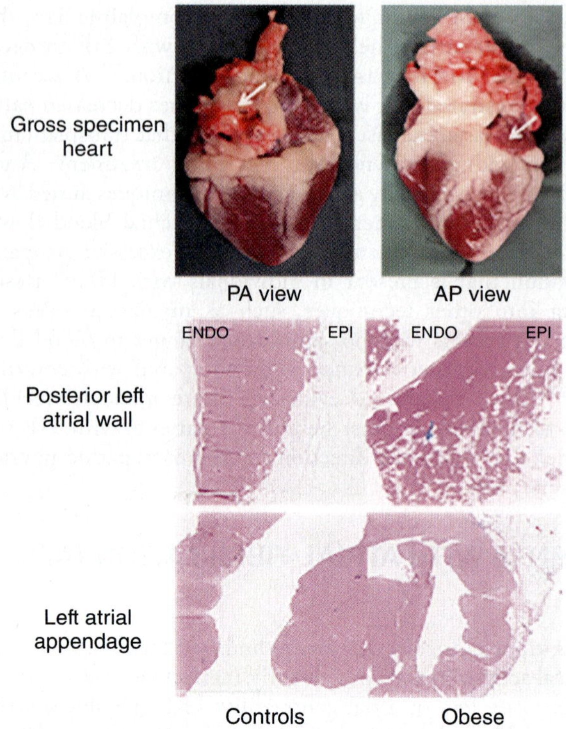

Figure 71.9. Epicardial fat: novel substrate for AF in chronic obesity. Top. Gross specimen of sheep heart after removal of parietal pericardium with pericardial fat. PA view: *arrow* points to epicardial fat adjacent to the LAPW. AP view: *arrow* points to the LAA, which has very little epicardial fat. **Middle and Bottom.** Representative H&E stained sections (1.25×) of the LAPW and LAA, respectively, from control and obese groups. *Arrow* shows infiltration of atrial musculature with fat cells. AF, atrial fibrillation; AP, anterior–posterior; ENDO, endocardial; EPI, epicardial; H&E, hematoxylin and eosin; PA, posterior–anterior. (Reprinted from Mahajan R, Lau DH, Brooks AG, et al. Electrophysiological, electroanatomical, and structural remodeling of the atria as consequences of sustained obesity. *J Am Coll Cardiol.* 2015;66(1):1–11. Copyright © 2015 American College of Cardiology Foundation. With permission.)

by increased sympathetic tone. Methods to decrease sympathetic tone, including OMT, may be beneficial. It is also important to identify and correct precipitating factors and secondary causes to enhance treatment.[4] The most common site for an embolus to form is the atrial appendage. The thrombus can dislodge and embolize the brain and other parts of the body.

Natural History

The natural history of AF can vary widely among individuals and is influenced by factors such as age, underlying health conditions, lifestyle, genetics, and more. AF can start suddenly or develop gradually. The initial triggers might include conditions like high blood pressure, heart valve disease, thyroid disorders, alcohol consumption, and certain heart surgeries. AF can become paroxysmal, occurring intermittently, and stopping on its own, or become permanent. At this point, cardioversion (using electrical shock or medications) might be needed to reset the heart's rhythm and control the rate. If AF continues for more than a year without reverting to normal sinus rhythm, despite medical intervention, it is considered long-standing, leading to various complications, and an increased risk of stroke. Complications can include HF, decreased exercise tolerance, and a reduced quality of life. Progression to persistent/permanent AF is associated with adverse CV events, hospitalizations, and death.[4]

Some individuals may experience infrequent episodes of AF and remain relatively stable, while others might progress to more frequent and sustained episodes. Treatment options include medication to control HR and rhythm, anticoagulation therapy to prevent blood clots and stroke, and catheter ablation to restore a normal heart rhythm. Cerebral vascular accidents (CVA) can lead to severe morbidity and mortality. CVA risk can be reduced significantly by anticoagulation and control of the rate/rhythm. Other complications include heart disease and HF.[4] Evidence shows that rhythm control does not offer a survival advantage over rate control. Patients with AF have multiple admissions and anticoagulation-related complications over their lifetime. In addition, the management of AF is prohibitively expensive, with most of the financial burden borne by the patient.[226]

Diagnosis

The diagnosis of AF includes an EKG rhythm strip of AF for at least 30 seconds, or the entire 12-lead EKG demonstrating these characteristics findings:

- Irregularly irregular R–R intervals (when AV conduction is not impaired),
- Absence of distinct repeating P waves, and
- Irregular atrial activations.

The history and physical exam are crucial for diagnosing and risk-stratifying patients with AF. Proper risk factor stratification and medical/surgical therapy can decrease the risk of stroke and HF significantly.[3] AF risk stratification involves assessing an individual's likelihood of developing complications associated with AF, particularly stroke. The most used risk stratification tool for AF-related stroke is the CHA_2DS_2-VASC score.[229] This scoring system considers various clinical factors to estimate the risk of stroke in AF patients.[4,226]

- Congestive HF (1 point): Individuals with HF have an increased risk of stroke.
- Hypertension (1 point): High blood pressure is a significant risk factor for stroke.
- Age 75 years or older (2 points): Advanced age increases stroke risk.
- DM (1 point): Diabetes is associated with an elevated risk of stroke.
- Stroke or transient ischemic attack (TIA) (2 points): A history of stroke or TIA indicates a higher risk of future stroke.
- Vascular disease (1 point): Presence of other vascular diseases like PAD, CAD, or aortic plaque increases stroke risk.
- Age 65 to 74 years (1 point): This age range is associated with a slightly increased risk of stroke.
- Sex category (female) (1 point): Women have a slightly elevated risk compared to men.

The total score ranges from 0 to 9. The higher the score, the greater the estimated risk of stroke. Based on the CHA2DS2-VASc score, the following guidelines[4,226] are often used for stroke prevention strategies:

- Score 0: Low risk (male) or very low risk (female). Anticoagulation therapy is generally not recommended, but individualized assessment is important.
- Score 1: Generally low risk. Consideration of anticoagulation therapy should be individualized based on clinical judgment.
- Score 2 or higher: Moderate to high risk. Anticoagulation therapy, such as with oral anticoagulants like warfarin or direct oral anticoagulants (DOACs), is typically recommended to reduce the risk of stroke.

It is important to note that risk stratification is a dynamic process, and individual factors, preferences, and bleeding risks should be considered when making treatment decisions. The CHA2DS2-VASc score provides a guideline for clinicians to assess stroke risk in AF patients, but the final decision on treatment should be made through shared decision making between the patient and their healthcare provider.

History

A complete history should focus on cardiopulmonary symptoms such as palpitations, chest pain, shortness of breath, increased lower extremity swelling, dyspnea on exertion, and dizziness. In addition, history taking should identify risk factors such as hypertension, history of valvular, structural, or ischemic heart disease, obstructive sleep apnea, obesity hypoventilation syndrome, smoking, alcohol intake, illicit drug use, history of rheumatic fever/heart disease, history of pericarditis, and hyperlipidemia.[226] It is important to determine if this is the first episode of AF, a recurrent episode, and the duration of the problem. Questions to ask may include:

- If recurrent, what triggers are present?
- Have they needed to go to the ER or be admitted in the past?
- Do they need ablation?
- Have their medications been changed recently?

The osteopathic physician will also inquire about stress, anxiety, social support, job satisfaction, and the patient's home life. Evaluating the patient's lifestyle, diet, exercise habits, and hobbies is also helpful.

Physical Exam

A physical exam should always begin with the assessment of airway breathing and circulation as it is going to affect the decision making regarding management. On general physical examination, patients may be tachycardic with an irregularly irregular pulse. The HR usually ranges from 110/min to 140/min (see Fig. 71.10). Extremities should be evaluated for edema, peripheral pulses in both upper and lower extremities, and integumentary signs of peripheral vascular disease (PVD), such as hair loss and skin breakdown.[226]

The physical exam should focus on identifying the cause of AF.

- HEENT: Examining the neck of the patient may determine if there is a goiter or a carotid bruit.
- Pulmonary: The pulmonary examination may reveal signs of HF in the form of crackles, and the presence of wheezing may indicate antecedent pulmonary diseases such as asthma and/or COPD.
- CV: A CV exam should consist of careful auscultation of all four cardiac posts and palpation of apical impulse, with murmurs indicating underlying valvular pathology. AF has an irregularly irregular rhythm.
- Abdominal: An abdominal exam should consist of palpating the aorta and listening for abdominal bruits. Moreover, hepatomegaly and abdominal distension may indicate HF.
- Neurologic: A careful examination of the central and peripheral nervous system may reveal signs of prior TIA or cerebrovascular accident.[226]
- Extremities: Look for peripheral edema, decreased hair growth and shiny skin, decreased pulses, varicosities, and open sores or ulcers.
- Structural: A screening structural exam should screen for forward head position, increased upper thoracic kyphosis, and

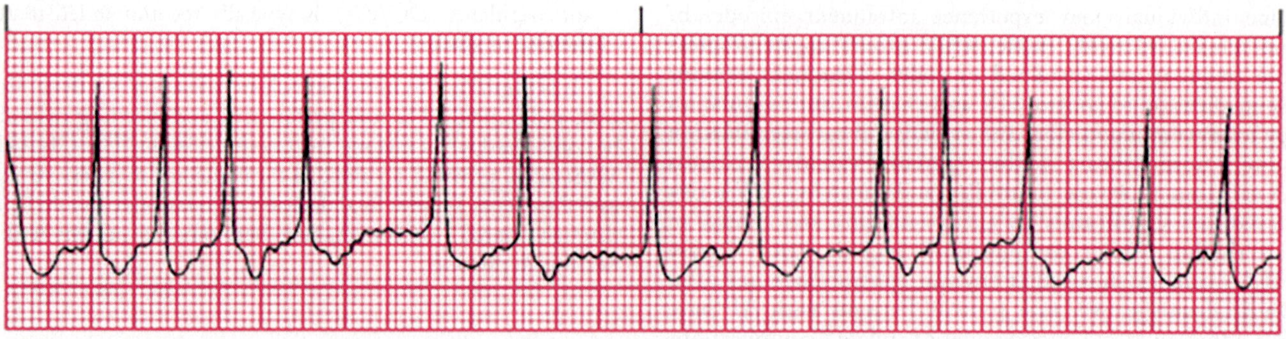

Figure 71.10. Recognizing atrial fibrillation. The following rhythm strip shows atrial fibrillation: Rhythm: irregular; rate: atrial—indiscernible; ventricular—130 beats/min; P-wave: absent; replaced by fine fibrillatory waves PR interval: indiscernible QRS complex: 0.08-second T wave: indiscernible QT interval: unmeasurable; other: none. (Reprinted with permission from *Lippincott's Nursing Advisor 2009.* Wolters Kluwer Health/Lippincott Williams & Wilkins; 2009. Figure 49.1.)

scoliosis that would potentially affect somatic structures related to the heart. Since the heart embryologically descends from the neck and pulls its fascia with it into the chest, postural fascial strains of the neck, clavicles, and thoracic inlet may influence fascial tensions on the pericardium (Biomechanical model).

- Somatic dysfunction: Evaluate for TART changes over the left upper thoracic region; FRS and ERS dysfunctions of the upper thoracic spine can cause facilitated spinal segments in the T1–T4 region. Dysfunction of ribs 1 to 5, trigger points in the pectoral muscles, and cardiac-related Chapman reflexes points are also findings in patients with AF.

Differential Diagnosis[226]

Differential diagnoses include:

- Atrial flutter
- Atrial tachycardia
- Multifocal atrial tachycardia
- Wolf–Parkinson–White syndrome
- AV nodal reentry tachycardia.

Diagnostics

The diagnostic evaluation of AF patients should include a complete medical history and physical examination, EKG, labs, chest x-ray, and echocardiogram. Clinicians should evaluate concomitant conditions such as AF pattern, stroke risk, AF-related symptoms, thromboembolism, and LV dysfunction.

A 12-lead EKG is necessary in all AF patients, to establish the diagnosis of AF, assess ventricular rate during AF, and check for the presence of conduction defects, ischemia, or signs of structural heart disease[4] (see Fig. 71.11). Laboratory tests should include thyroid and kidney function, serum electrolytes, full blood count, cardiac biomarkers, and BNP. It is important to evaluate the patient for pulmonary embolism (with the d-dimers test or spiral CT scan) because the right heart strain can lead to AF. A chest x-ray is important for ruling out pulmonary causes, cardiomegaly, occult disease, infections, and pneumothorax. A transthoracic echocardiography (TEE) is typically performed to evaluate LV size and function, LA size, valvular disease, and right heart size and systolic function.[4]

Screening Tools/Smartwatches

Mobile health technologies are rapidly developing for AF detection and other purposes. When AF is detected by a screening tool, including mobile or wearable devices, a single-lead EKG tracing of ≥30 seconds or 12-lead EKG showing AF analyzed by a physician with expertise in EKG rhythm interpretation is necessary to establish a definitive diagnosis of AF.[4]

Treatment

Primary prevention of AF refers to the implementation of preventive measures for patients at risk but without previous documentation of AF. This strategy relies on the identification and management of risk factors and comorbidities predisposing to AF, before the development of atrial remodeling and fibrosis.[4] For example, proper management of hypertension and HF may prevent AF by reducing atrial stretch.[4]

The management of AF in the acute setting depends on hemodynamic stability and risk stratification. In cases where the patient is hemodynamically unstable, it is recommended to carry out immediate cardioversion with anticoagulant therapy. TEE is generally recommended before any cardioversion.[226]

AF With Rapid Ventricular Response

If there is evidence of rapid ventricular response, a beta-blocker or calcium channel blocker should be used for rate control. Typically, an IV bolus is administered to the patient and then they are

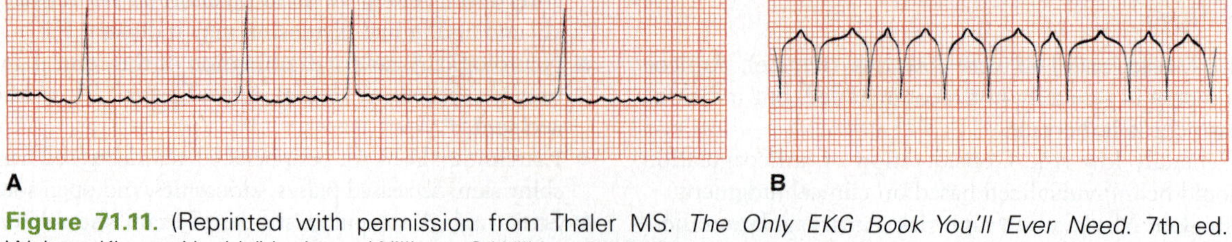

Figure 71.11. (Reprinted with permission from Thaler MS. *The Only EKG Book You'll Ever Need.* 7th ed. Wolters Kluwer Health/Lippincott Williams & Wilkins; 2012:130.)

started on a drip if symptoms do not resolve. First-line medications include diltiazem and/or beta-blockers. Digoxin can be considered for rate control but is not advised as a first-line agent pertaining of its adverse effects and tolerance. Amiodarone can also be given as a rhythm control agent but is also not a first-line option in the acute setting. In any case, if the decision to start amiodarone is made, cardiology should be consulted before its administration.[226]

Pre-Existing AF

In the case of pre-existing AF, the patient should be risk stratified using the CHADs-2-Vasc score, which is helpful in estimating the risk of stroke per year. If the patient receives a 0 score, it is considered "low risk," and anticoagulation is not recommended in such cases. If the patient receives a score of 1, falling in the "low–moderate" risk category; the providers should consider anticoagulation. If the patient receives a score of greater than 2, they are in the "moderate–high" risk category, and anticoagulation therapy is indicated.[226] Patients are usually evaluated for their risk of bleeding if anticoagulation is started. Bleeding risk scores have been used but have limitations and population-based studies suggest that the benefits of stroke prevention generally outweigh the risks of bleeding.[226]

Summary of Current Guidelines for AF Management[4,226]

- In all patients with AF, the CHA2DS2-VASc score is recommended to assess stroke risk.
- In patients with AF and elevated CHA2DS2-VASc score of 2 or more, oral anticoagulation is recommended.
- Females with the absence of AF risk factors and males with CHA2DS2-VASc of 1 or 0 have a low stroke risk.
- Non-vitamin K oral anticoagulants (NOACs) (apixaban, dabigatran, edoxaban, and rivaroxaban) are recommended over warfarin, except for patients with moderate to severe MS or with a mechanical heart valve in place.
- Obtain renal and liver function before initiating non-vitamin K oral anticoagulants.
- Aspirin is not recommended in patients with low CHA2DS2-VASc scores.
- Idarucizumab is recommended for dabigatran reversal if there is an urgent procedure or bleeding. Andexanet alfa is recommended for the reversal of rivaroxaban and apixaban-associated bleeding.
- Percutaneous left atrial appendage occlusion is recommended in AF patients with a risk of stroke who have contraindications to long-term anticoagulation.
- If the duration of AF is more than 48 hours or if the time is unknown, start anticoagulation and maintain INR between 2 and 3 or commence a factor Xa inhibitor for at least 3 weeks before and at least 4 weeks after cardioversion.
- Rate control is an integral part of AF management and is often sufficient to improve AF-related symptoms. The primary indication for rhythm control is reduction in AF-related symptoms and improvement of quality of life.
- Catheter ablation is a well-established treatment for prevention of AF recurrence in patients with a low EF. When performed by appropriately trained operators, catheter ablation is a safe and superior alternative to antiarrhythmic drugs (AADs) for maintenance of sinus rhythm and symptom improvement.
- Recommend controlling risk factors of obesity, hypertension, and EtOH use in patients with AF.
- Left atrial appendage occlusion devices now have additional safety and efficacy data in patients with long-term contraindications to anticoagulation.

When to Use NOAC/DOAC Anticoagulation?

Non-vitamin K antagonist oral anticoagulants (NOACs), also known as direct oral anticoagulants (DOACs), are a newer class of anticoagulant medications developed as alternatives to warfarin. They are indicated for various medical conditions where anticoagulation therapy is needed. NOACs are commonly indicated for stroke prevention in patients with nonvalvular AF who have risk factors for stroke.[230] They are often used as an alternative to warfarin in these patients. Different NOACs, such as dabigatran, rivaroxaban, apixaban, and edoxaban, have been studied and approved for various indications. The annual rate of major hemorrhage for warfarin is 1.2% per year and NOACs have a significantly lower risk of intracerebral hemorrhage and thus carry a class 1A recommendation.[230] See below:

Annual Rate of Major Hemorrhage
Warfarin: 1.2%/year
NOACs

- Dabigatran:
  - ☐ 110 μg (0.23%)
  - ☐ 150 μg (0.30%)
- Rivaroxaban 20/15 μg (0.50%)
- Apixaban 5/2.5 μg (0.33%)
- Edoxaban
  - ☐ 30 μg (0.26%)
  - ☐ 60 μg (0.39%)

Cardioversion

The decision to choose cardioversion for AF depends on several factors, including the patient's symptoms, the duration of the AF episode, underlying heart conditions, and the potential risks and benefits of the procedure. There are two main types of cardioversions: electrical cardioversion and pharmacologic (chemical) cardioversion.

- Acute symptomatic AF: Cardioversion may be considered in patients with acute, symptomatic AF who are experiencing severe symptoms such as palpitations, shortness of breath, chest pain, dizziness, or fainting.
- Recent-onset AF: In cases of recent-onset AF (AF that started within the last 48 hours), cardioversion can be used to restore a normal heart rhythm and prevent the condition from becoming chronic. In some cases, patients might undergo cardioversion even beyond 48 hours if certain conditions are met.
- Hemodynamic instability: Patients with AF who are hemodynamically unstable, meaning their blood pressure is severely affected and they are experiencing significant symptoms, may require immediate cardioversion to restore a normal rhythm.
- Failed rate control: If attempts at controlling the HR in AF using medications are unsuccessful or not well tolerated, cardioversion might be considered as an option.
- Elective cardioversion: In cases of persistent or long-standing persistent AF (AF lasting longer than 7 days or of unknown duration), elective cardioversion may be chosen if the patient and healthcare provider believe that restoring a normal rhythm could improve the patient's quality of life and reduce symptoms.
- Anticoagulation: Before cardioversion, especially if it's performed more than 48 hours after the onset of AF, patients may

need to be adequately anticoagulated to reduce the risk of blood clot formation and subsequent stroke. The decision to anticoagulate and the duration of anticoagulation depend on the patient's CHA2DS2-VASc score and other risk factors for stroke.
- Underlying conditions: Cardioversion may be avoided or carefully considered in patients with certain underlying heart conditions, such as valvular heart disease or significant structural heart abnormalities.

Interprofessional Care

AF is best managed by an interprofessional team to improve outcomes. Complex patients would benefit from a multidisciplinary team that includes relevant specialists, their primary care physician, nurses, pharmacists, and therapists. Involvement of the patient and their family members is integral to the success of AF management.[4] Part of the osteopathic approach and philosophy is to engage the patient with shared decision making, exploring their thoughts on management of their condition, and accepting their values, goals, and preferences. Empathetic listening and respecting their viewpoint can tailor their treatment to their needs while simultaneously preventing the risk of death, stroke, and major bleeding.

Patient Education

Patient knowledge about AF, its risks, and treatment options are often limited, particularly when first diagnosed.[4] Clinicians should not assume the patient understands their condition. Instead, clinicians should ask them what their understanding is, and then provide education.

It is important for multiple clinicians to contribute to educating the patient on how to adhere to treatment and the potential consequences of nonadherence, in addition to managing the patient's expectations of treatment goals. This fosters compliance and improves safety.[4] Treatment burden can be overwhelming for patients with multiple chronic illnesses, especially when they must take multiple medications daily, and frequently visit multiple healthcare providers.

The simple Atrial fibrillation Better Care (ABC) holistic pathway ("A" Anticoagulation/avoid stroke; "B" Better symptom management; "C" Cardiovascular and Comorbidity optimization) streamlines integrated care of AF patients across different specialties. Compared with usual care, implementation of the ABC pathway has been associated with lower risk of all-cause death, stroke/major bleeding, CV death, first hospitalization, and lower health-related costs.[4]

Exercise

Exercise can be beneficial for individuals with AF. However, patients with AF must approach exercise with some caution and under the guidance of a healthcare provider, as there are specific considerations to keep in mind. Benefits of exercise for AF include the following:

- Improved CV health:
  - Exercise may reduce the risk of AF-related complications and improve the heart's ability to tolerate and recover from episodes of irregular heart rhythm. It has been shown that patients who have symptomatic AF, are overweight, and obese have a 9% reduction in AF recurrence over a 4-year follow-up for each one metabolic equivalent incremental gain in fitness.[231]
- Weight management:
  - Engaging in regular physical activities can help decrease the percentage of visceral fat within the body, which will in turn reduce the risk of AF.[232] Additionally, having a lower sympathetic drive along with structural remodeling from regular physical activity can potentially reduce the risk of AF.[232]
- Stress reduction:
  - Exercise can help reduce stress and anxiety, which are known triggers for AF episodes in some individuals.
- Better sleep:
  - Regular physical activity can promote better sleep, and adequate sleep is essential for managing AF symptoms and overall heart health. Regular exercise can help with weight management as stated above, which can also help patients with sleep apnea.[232]

Considerations for Exercising with Atrial Fibrillation

- Medical evaluation:
  - Before starting or intensifying an exercise program, individuals with AFib should undergo a thorough medical evaluation to determine the type and level of exercise that is safe and appropriate. AF is unique in that it shows a J-shaped distribution where patients who are sedentary and patients who are extreme athletes are at a high risk of having AF.[231]
- Medication management:
  - The goal of medications for the treatment of AF is to control the HR or control the rhythm. Beta-blockers or calcium channel blocks are medications that can help control the rate in patients with AF, while some physicians will use antiarrhythmic drugs initially.[233] Depending on the risk factors, ablation can be recommended as an initial treatment. Anticoagulation should be considered if the patient is at high risk of developing an embolic stroke.[234]
- Exercise type and intensity:
  - Low-to-moderate–intensity aerobic exercises are generally recommended for individuals with AF. Activities like walking, cycling, swimming, and gentle dancing can be good choices. High-intensity exercise outside of a prescribed training regimen can trigger AF episodes in some individuals. It is helpful to recommend exercises that the patient will enjoy ensuring compliance with regularly performing the activity.[231]
- Monitoring:
  - Some individuals may be advised to wear an HR monitor during exercise to ensure that their HR stays within a safe range. Smart watches contain an HR monitor which patients can use to track their HR as well.
- Hydration and electrolyte balance:
  - Maintaining proper hydration and electrolyte balance is essential for heart health and may help reduce the risk of AF episodes.
- Avoiding triggers:
  - Identify and avoid any specific triggers that exacerbate AF symptoms. There has been no evidence to date that "suggests exercise training within current guidelines exacerbates AF."[231]
- Gradual progression:
  - Have patients start slowly and gradually increase the duration and intensity of exercise.

In summary, exercise can have several benefits for individuals with AF, including improved CV health, stress reduction, and better weight management. However, it is essential to exercise safely and consider individual factors, including the severity of AF and any specific triggers.

Somatic Dysfunction and OMT

The role of somatic dysfunction and OMT in those with AF has not been widely studied, although there has been some research to support its use alongside the current treatment regimens to help resolve symptoms.

Osteopathic medicine can be used to help lower a patient's blood pressure, which can indirectly lower the risk of developing AF since hypertension is a risk factor. Postganglionic nerves from T1 to T4 are the origin of the SNS that targets CV function.[89] It has been found that patients with hypertension tend to have somatic dysfunction of their upper thoracic vertebrae.[137] OMT of these segments can lower blood pressure in patients with elevated blood pressure.[128] The 2009 Cerritelli study demonstrated that 1 year of OMT reduced blood pressure through its effects on the intima-media thickness (IMT) on arterial walls. Measurements demonstrated that compared to the control group, the OMT group had a smaller IMT that resulted in "vasodilation" of the blood vessel due to the larger arterial diameter; these effects resulted in a lower blood pressure reading in those with hypertension.[95]

Like the effects seen in hypertension, the treatment of somatic dysfunction and the application of OMT can be used to benefit patients with AF. Osteopathic medicine has thoroughly explored the idea of the relationship between visceral systems and somatic presentations known as "viscerosomatic reflexes." Stress on the viscera can have a physical manifestation at a site distant from the affected viscera. The location of these sites is related segmentally to the body through origins in embryonic development. Commonly tissue texture change, asymmetry, restriction of motion, tenderness, and somatic dysfunction are found near the left upper four thoracic vertebrae posteriorly in patients' cardiac conditions.[88,89,161] Ultimately, the identification of these somatic manifestations can help with further diagnosis and treatment of underlying visceral disease. The 2018 Tabina study demonstrated that treatment of these thoracic somatic dysfunctions was found to reduce the paroxysms of AF, number of atrial extrasystoles, and decreased symptoms which improved the quality of life in individuals with AF.[235]

Further research regarding the utilization of OMT in those with cardiac dysfunction focuses on its impact on HRV. HRV is influenced by the sympathetic excitation and vagal inhibition of the SA node which results in beat-to-beat fluctuations in heart rate. Those with dominant sympathetic influence are found to have low-frequency (LF) HRV, while those with dominant parasympathetic influence are found to have high-frequency (HF) HRV.[236] A patient with LF-HRV holds an unfavorable prognostic marker for cardiac disease and treatment is aimed at increasing HRV. Multiple studies have demonstrated that treatment with OMT after introducing a stressor was significantly associated with higher HF-HRV values, indicative of countering the sympathetic response of the body and promotion of vagal tone, and lowered the LF/HF ratios.[237–240] This concept can be applied to patients with AF while considering that HRV in those with AF is primarily influenced by vagal tone.[241] The right vagus portion of the cardiac plexus innervates the SA node and, during times of excess stimulation, is thought to contribute to sinus bradycardia, while the left vagus portion innervates the AV node, and in extreme stimulation is felt to contribute to AV block.[242,243] OMT targeting the upper cervical and thoracic regions can help normalize parasympathetic and sympathetic tone, which together will help increase HF–HRV ratios to promote better cardiac prognoses.[239]

Traditional treatment and management of AF should include the diagnosis and treatment of related somatic dysfunction. It is plausible that supplementation of OMT to the standard of care could help prevent the development of this arrhythmia and promote a better prognosis in those who have already been diagnosed. Further research on this topic needs to be undertaken.

PERIPHERAL ARTERY DISEASE

Definition

PAD is a chronic, atherosclerotic disease of the peripheral vasculature resulting in limb-associated complications such as intermittent claudication (IC), ischemic rest pain, ischemic ulcer, gangrene, and functional impairment.[244] PAD typically affects the abdominal aorta, iliac arteries, lower limbs, and occasionally the upper extremities.[245] Early identification and risk factor modification are essential to improve the outcomes in patients with PVD.[246] PAD causes IC. IC represents peripheral ischemia distal to stenosis in the setting of exertion. This supply–demand mismatch is often a result of stenosis, thus insufficient vasodilatory response may result in symptoms that are relieved by rest.[244]

Epidemiology

PAD affects nearly 200 million people worldwide including approximately 40 to 45 million Americans. The disease is uncommon in younger populations; however, the incidence increases sharply, with over 20% of people over 80 years old having PAD. Gender differences are somewhat conflicting, with women being more likely to have atypical and late presentations with intrinsically lower ABI values.[246] African Americans have approximately two to three times the rate of PAD as compared to non-Hispanic Whites. PAD is also two times more common in populations with a lower educational level and lower income.[246] In addition to these statistics, PAD treatment in Blacks remains suboptimal despite a high incidence of PAD and complications in this population.[244] Blacks who have a high burden of disease are less likely to receive evidence-based treatment, and have higher rates of complications, including they are two to four times more likely to undergo amputation when compared with non-Hispanic Whites.[244]

Causes/Risk Factors

PAD is a type of PVD that is primarily driven by progressive atherosclerotic disease caused by multiple risk factors, including smoking, diabetes, prior CAD, and a sedentary lifestyle. When present, PAD results in the reduction of major organ blood flow and end-organ ischemia.[246]

Risk factors include[246]:

- Tobacco use
- DM
- Hypertension
- HIV
- High cholesterol
- Age more than 50 years
- Elevated homocysteine levels
- BMI greater than 30
- Family history of CVD
- Black race

Of the above risk factors, smoking is associated with the highest risk of PAD development with an odds ratio of 2.7 (95% CI 2.4–3.1). The history of CVD and diabetes are also significant risk factors with odds ratios of 2.6 (95% CI 2.2–3) and 1.9 (1.7–2.1), respectively.[247]

Classification

The 2020 Global Vascular Guidelines (GVGs) have recommended a transition in terminology from "critical limb ischemia (CLI)" to the more descriptive term of "chronic limb-threatening ischemia," (CLTI) which objectively includes patients with ischemic rest pain or tissue loss due to atherosclerotic arterial disease.[248] This is important because although CLTI represents less than 10% of all PAD patients, it comes with a considerable burden in terms of morbidity, mortality, and socio-economic costs. Despite treatment, the amputation rate is up to 20% at 12 months,[5] while over 50% of all CLTI patients die within 5 years after presentation. The guidelines provide a framework for evidence-based revascularization (EBR).[248]

Structured decision making is determined via three dimensions in a framework known as PLAN (patient risk, limb status, and anatomical pattern).

- Patient risk
  - The vascular quality initiative prediction model (VQI) for determining overall patient risk
- Limb status
  - Wound, ischemia, and foot infection (WIfI)
  - This (WIfI) classification system has four grades of severity for each of the following: wound, ischemia, and presence of infection.[249]
  - The wound grade is based on the presence of gangrene or ulcers (or both).
  - The ischemia grade is based on ABI, arterial systemic pressure, and toe pressures.
  - The infection grade is based on signs and symptoms of infection.
- Anatomical pattern[250]
  - Uses the global limb anatomic staging system (GLASS)
    - The glass staging is a structured framework for assessing the severity and extent of PAD in the lower extremities. GLASS staging evaluates the separately scoring the femoropopliteal (FP) and infrapopliteal (IP) segments based on criteria such as stenosis severity, lesion length, and the overall burden of atherosclerotic disease.
  - Determining the anatomical pattern is considered a valuable tool for guiding clinical decisions regarding revascularization strategies and for improving research quality.
  - The physician must identify the target artery pathway (TAP), which is the preferred IP artery for revascularization.

This classification framework helps surgeons determine the chance of successful revascularization. The anatomic and limb risk stagings combine to provide an idea of the success of revascularization and to provide a recommendation for treatment including: "no revascularization," "endovascular," "indeterminate," or "open bypass."[249]

- Stage I: Average complexity disease: technical failure <10% AND >70% 12-month limb-based patency (LBP).
- Stage II: Intermediate complexity disease: technical failure <20% AND 12-month LBP 50% to 70%.
- Stage III: High complexity disease: technical failure >20%; OR <50% 12-month LBP.

Pathophysiology

PAD typically affects the lower extremity vascular beds, but larger arteries such as the abdominal aorta and iliac arteries are frequently involved. More severe disease can involve multilevel and/or diffuse disease. The pathophysiology of atherosclerosis is a complex inflammatory response with the involvement of various vascular cells, thrombotic factors, and cholesterol and inflammatory molecules. Atherosclerosis has two significant factors in its pathogenesis: cholesterol deposition and chronic inflammation. When these two factors are present there are three general stages which include (1) formation of the fatty streak, (2) induction of atheroma, and (3) development of the atherosclerotic plaques.[251] Tobacco smoke increases EC permeability by formation of ROS, which enables atherosclerosis to settle within vessel walls.[244] ROS and reactive nitrogen species (RNS) damage the cellular function of lipids, proteins, and carbohydrates, causing lipoprotein (LDL) oxidation.[246,251] Oxidized LDL (ox-LDL) initiates the development of atherosclerosis by inducing EC dysfunction, increasing leukocyte adhesiveness, and inducing the expression of leukocyte and monocyte adhesion molecules.[251] Monocytes, T-lymphocytes, and mast cells are taken up into vascular wall intima by these adhesion molecules. Through other mediators, macrophages uptake ox-LDL molecules to form lipid-laden foam cells. Yellow foam cells aggregate on the arterial walls and cause the development of fatty streaks.[251] A fibrous atherosclerotic plaque cap is formed from the fatty streak due to proliferation and migration of smooth muscle cells (SMCs).

At advanced stages of atherosclerosis, macrophages, and T-lymphocytes in the atherosclerotic plaque cap secrete proteolytic enzymes such as metalloproteinase to reduce the stability of the fibrous cap and lyse the fibrous cap extracellular matrix. A rupture of the fibrous cap leads to coagulation process, blood clot formation, and thrombus formation.[251] As the plaque continues to accumulate, it further compromises the lumen which can lead to critical narrowing of the artery. As narrowing progresses and obstructs the artery, collateral circulatory beds frequently develop to preserve distal perfusion and tissue viability. These collateral circulatory pathways are unable to match the blood supply and result in oxygen delivery that is unable to match oxygen demand.[246] The most severe form of PAD is CLI, which is defined as limb pain at rest or impending limb loss. Arterial thrombosis is secondary to progressive atherosclerotic disease and thrombosis represents 40% of acute limb ischemia (ALI) cases.[252] ALI is a vascular emergency with an immediate physician consultation required for the preservation of limb viability.

Diagnosis

The diagnosis of PAD can be sufficiently made based on a thorough history, evaluation of patient risk factors, clinical presentation, and physical exam findings including the ABI[246] (see Fig. 71.12). If arteries at the ankle cannot be compressed or if the ABI is >1.40, use alternative methods (e.g., toe-brachial index [TBI] or Doppler). Diagnosis of PVD can be difficult due to the increasing prevalence of similar conditions and the large number of patients having an asymptomatic or atypical presentation.[253] CLI is diagnosed in a patient with chronic ischemia with pain at rest, necrosis, or ulceration (Fontaine classification stages III and IV or Rutherford stages 4–6).[254]

Differential diagnosis of pain:

Neurological

- Nerve root compression
- Spinal stenosis
- Peripheral neuropathy
- Nerve entrapment

Musculoskeletal

- Medial tibial stress syndrome
- OA
- Muscle strain
- Baker cyst

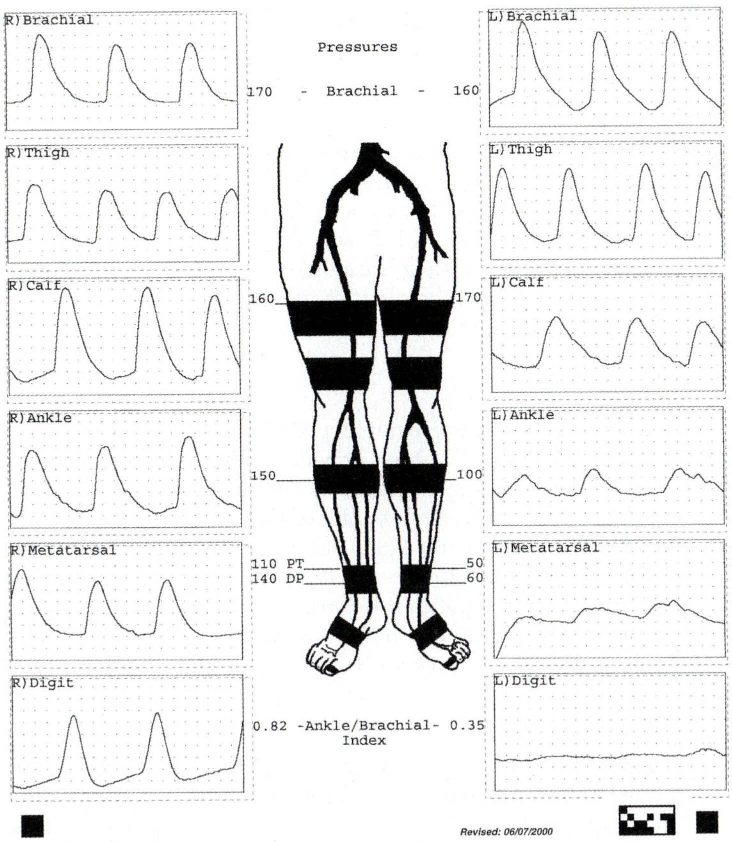

Figure 71.12. Noninvasive assessment (ankle-brachial index [ABI], segmental limb pressures, and pulse volume recordings [PVR]) of lower extremity arterial circulation, in 73-year-old male with known peripheral vascular disease. ABI—Right ABI is mildly reduced at 0.82 (140/170), left ABI is severely reduced at 0.35 (60/170). Segmental limb pressures and PVRs—Right-sided segmental-limb pressures show a 10-mm Hg drop in gradient between the upper thigh, upper calf, and ankle. There is no segmental drop >20 mm Hg, so one is unable to determine the level of disease causing the mild decrease in ABI. Note that the upper thigh pressure is less than the brachial pressure, raising a suspicion for aortoiliac disease. However, the PVR at this site appears normal suggesting that there is no significant aortoiliac disease. The remaining PVRs on the right side also appear normal. Left-sided segmental limb pressures show significant (i.e., >20 mm Hg) drops in pressure between the upper thigh and the upper calf, and between the calf and the ankle, suggesting the presence of significant, left-sided, superficial femoral and popliteal artery disease, and below-knee disease. The metatarsal PVR tracings show marked diminution in amplitude, and the digit PVR tracing is flat, suggesting severe small-vessel disease in the left foot. (Reprinted with permission from Casserly IP, Sachar R, Yadav JS. *Manual of Peripheral Vascular Intervention.* Lippincott Williams & Wilkins; 2005. Figure 2.1.)

Vascular

- Chronic venous insufficiency
- Thrombophlebitis
- Deep venous thrombosis
- Raynaud phenomenon
- Thromboangiitis obliterans (Buerger disease)

Differential Diagnosis of Arterial Narrowing

There are multiple other nonatherosclerotic causes of lower extremity arterial narrowing or occlusion that can present as chronic lower limb ischemia.[254] Some of these include:

- Peripheral emboli from the heart (arrhythmias, valvular heart disease)
- Peripheral emboli from proximal arteries (plaque or aneurysms)
- Large-vessel vasculitis
- Thromboangiitis obliterans (Buerger disease)
- Radiation injury (especially in iliac arteries following pelvic irradiation).
- Trauma
- External iliac artery endofibrosis (cyclist hip pain)
- Popliteal artery entrapment
- Coarctation of the aorta
- Fibrous dysplasia, and anomalous development of the lower extremity vasculature

History

Early PAD is asymptomatic. With time, patients develop easy fatigability of the limbs, increased sensitivity to cold, and paresthesia. They usually seek medical attention because of IC. IC is the most classic symptom of PAD and is characterized by an exercise-induced cramping sensation with associated fatigue, weakness, and or pressure. Patients may not have rest pain, so asking about discomfort while ambulating is a more useful screening question. Symptoms are exacerbated by leg elevation and relieved by placing the limb in a dependent position. Paresthesia's, lower extremity weakness, stiffness, and cool extremities may also be present.[246] Claudication pain usually involves large muscle groups of the lower extremity, such as the buttocks, thighs, and most frequently the calf. Severe narrowing or occlusion of the aorta, iliac arteries, or both may present as Leriche syndrome, which is defined as IC, absent femoral pulses, and erectile dysfunction.[246] In advanced stages patients complain of foot pain, leg pain, or both occurring at night (often relieved by hanging the limb over the side of a bed) or pain at rest.[254]

Atypical

Atypical pain is characterized by pain unrelated to physical activity, pain that occurs both at rest and with exertion, and pain lasting longer than 10 minutes after exercise cessation.[246,255] Pseudoclaudication refers to neuropathic pain observed in patients with spinal stenosis and can be differentiated from PAD with a thorough history and physical examination. Patients with pseudoclaudication tend to have pain characterized by weakness and paresthesias irrespective of the degree of their physical activity. It is usually relieved by sitting down or changing body positioning rather than resting.[246,255]

Physical Exam

The physical examination begins when the patient walks into the room, as there may be gait and station clues regarding their clinical condition. Patients with spinal stenosis and neurogenic claudication of their legs are flexed forward and prefer to slump. Examination of the limbs should involve assessment for pulselessness, pallor, muscular atrophy, cool or cyanotic skin, pain with palpation, abnormal capillary refill time, pallor with leg elevation, rubor, dependent edema, and auscultation of bruits in major vessels including the femoral and popliteal arteries. Lower extremity ulcers may be arterial, venous, neuropathic, or a combination of two or more. The skin of a patient with PVD will have decreased hair growth and the skin will appear shiny and smooth. Looking at the nails is important as they may be dystrophic, have tar sustaining, or have clubbing. There may also be scars from previous surgeries, either orthopedic or vascular, which will be important to determine. Advanced disease may manifest as nonhealing ulcers or gangrene. Ulcers secondary to arterial insufficiency are tender and typically have ragged borders with a dry base and pale or necrotic centers.[246]

The CV exam needs to include an examination of the peripheral pulses to determine rate, rhythm, and strength. All palpable pulses should be assessed and compared bilaterally. Palpate the carotid arteries and auscultate for bruits. On the lower extremities, pulse is assessed on the following arteries: the dorsalis pedis artery (on the dorsum of the foot between the first and second metatarsal bone; not palpable in 8% of healthy persons), posterior tibial artery (behind the medial malleolus), popliteal artery (in the popliteal fossa), and femoral artery (in the groin, just below the inguinal ligament).[254]

Chest auscultation should be performed to evaluate for pulmonary diseases such as COPD, wheezing, decreased breath sounds, and crackles indicative of HF/fluid overload. Cardiac auscultation should evaluate heart sounds and murmurs. Abdominal examination can evaluate for an enlarged aorta, bruits of the aorta or the renal arteries as well as bruits from the area of iliac bifurcation, just below the umbilicus.

Structural and palpatory findings may be found anywhere in the body, Especially, including myofascial restrictions of the lower extremities and popliteal spaces, pelvic somatic dysfunction, and segmental somatic dysfunctions of the lower thoracic and upper lumbar spine.

DIAGNOSTIC STUDIES

ABI

Measurement of the ABI is a cost-effective noninvasive objective measure for PAD diagnosis (see Fig. 71.12). The ABI is obtained by measuring the systolic ankle pressure ratio to the systolic brachial pressure.[246] The ankle pressure of each leg is then divided by the highest systolic pressure of either brachial artery. A normal ABI ratio ranges from 0.9 to 1.2, and values less than 0.9 are diagnostic of PAD. Patients who are older with stiff noncompressible blood vessels may have an elevated ankle-brachial index (ABI >1.3). Individuals with abnormally high ABI ratios have higher all-cause mortality compared to normal ABI ratios.[246] Further diagnostic evaluation for these patients often warrants a TBI, which is the comparison of the toe systolic pressure to the higher systolic brachial pressure. A normal TBI is >0.7; lower values indicate the possibility of lower limb ischemia.[246,254]

Duplex US

If the patient has an abnormal ankle or toe brachial index ordering an arterial duplex ultrasound with B-mode and spectral waveform analysis is a safe and cost-effective method of determining PAD location, stenosis severity, and length of stenosis or occlusion. It provides an accurate assessment of lesion stenosis, hemodynamic severity, and plaque characteristics. Doppler ultrasonography can be used in routine follow-up postprocedure for surveillance of patency. This diagnostic modality can assist in decision making when further intervention is contemplated.[246,254]

Stress Testing

For patients who have borderline ABI values and if there are doubts based on the history and physical a treadmill stress test can be helpful to objectively assess the claudication distance. An ABI may be performed before and afterward. If pain forcing the patient to interrupt testing is caused by ischemia, the ankle pressure after exercise will be significantly lower than before exercise (often <50 mm Hg).[254]

MRA/CTA

Magnetic resonance angiography (MRA) or computed tomography angiography (CTA) both provide excellent high-quality vascular imaging (see Fig. 71.13). The advantages of MRA include the ability to identify small runoff vessels that sometimes may not be seen. Compared with digital subtraction angiography (DSA), MRA has 90% sensitivity and 97% specificity in identifying hemodynamically significant lesions.[246] CTA has similar diagnostic accuracy to MRA with both imaging techniques being useful for determining candidacy for bypass surgery versus angioplasty.[246]

Arteriography

Arteriography is still considered the gold standard and is performed in the case of diagnostic doubts or more commonly during therapeutic endovascular procedures such as angioplasty (with or without stenting).[254]

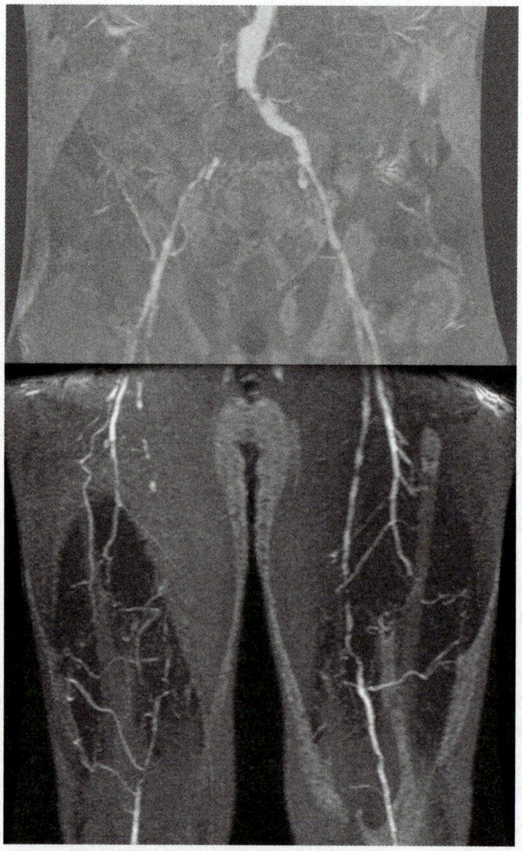

Figure 71.13. (Reprinted with permission from Pedrajas FG, Schneider PA. Percutaneous femoral–popliteal reconstruction techniques: antegrade approaches. In: Dalman RL, Mulholland MW, eds. *Operative Techniques in Vascular Surgery*. Wolters Kluwer; 2015:267.)

Natural History

Patients with PAD have a variable disease presentation and course with some patients remaining asymptomatic and others progressing to arterial ulceration, claudication, resting limb ischemia, and limb loss.[256] The presence or absence of PAD symptoms is a major defining feature of this condition with drastically different clinical outcomes.[244]

The overall prognosis of patients with PVD must consider patient risk factors, CV health, and disease severity. In terms of limb health at 5 years, nearly 80% of patients will have stable claudication symptoms. Only 1% to 2% of patients will progress to CLI in 5 years. Sequelae requiring amputation carries a mortality of ≤50% at 1 year.[244]

Patients with PAD have an increased rate of ischemic stroke, MI, and CV death. Patients with CAD and PAD have a much higher risk of CV mortality than CAD alone.[244] Approximately, 20% to 30% of patients with PAD will die within 5 years, with 75% of those deaths attributed to CV causes. PAD is a progressive systemic disease with poor long-term outcomes. Although symptoms of claudication remain stable for many years, these patients are at high risk of fatal and nonfatal CV events.[246]

Treatment

Treatment strategies can be subdivided into lifestyle modification, medical management, endovascular therapies, and surgical interventions.[244] Interprofessional coordination is necessary for identifying patients at risk of disease, preventing secondary progression, and assisting patients with various treatment options for their disease. This includes involvement of family physicians, internists, nurses, cardiologists, pharmacists, CV surgeons, podiatrists, and PT/OTs.

A holistic treatment strategy is established on an individual basis depending on the severity of disease as well as the patient's general condition, age, activity level (including type of occupation), and comorbidities. Management includes[254]:

- secondary prevention of CVDs
- treatment aimed at improving walking distance, and rest pain
- treatment of associated somatic dysfunction to assist with daily functioning

To achieve these goals, initial treatment of PAD includes risk factor modification, antiplatelet therapy, and exercise. However, since patients with PAD are at increased risk of CAD mortality (relative risk = 6.6), CV mortality (relative risk = 5.9), and all-cause mortality (relative risk = 3.1), the addition of medical, interventional, and surgical options are many times required to achieve symptomatic control and reduce risks of having a CV event.[246]

Medical Management

Medical management can be broken down into lifestyle modifications including diet, exercise, stress management and smoking cessation, and pharmacologic treatment. Pharmacologic treatment includes cholesterol reduction, antiplatelet therapy, anticoagulation, peripheral vasodilators, and blood pressure control.[244] Relative to CAD, PAD is an undertreated condition.[244]

Patient management for the desired outcomes is based on a holistic approach that includes nonpharmacologic lifestyle modification and pharmacologic management, such as:

- Smoking cessation
- Ambulatory blood pressure monitoring
- Medication and exercise therapy compliance
- Cholesterol management through diet and statin therapy
- Weight reduction
- HbA1c goal of less than 7% (or more for significant comorbid conditions or hypoglycemia)
- Regular follow-up with an interprofessional team

Lifestyle Modifications[254]

SMOKING

Smoking cessation reduces the risk of PAD progression, CV events including MI and stroke, and CLI. Smoking is a major risk factor for PAD as it constricts blood vessels and reduces blood flow. Quitting smoking can significantly improve blood circulation and overall vascular health. Multidisciplinary efforts to intervene with smoking can be effective. In one randomized trial of 124 patients, an intensive intervention group, which included cognitive behavioral counseling, motivational interviewing, and pharmacologic therapy, resulted in a significantly higher rate of cessation than verbal advice alone.[244] According to guidelines, bupropion is equivalent in efficacy to varenicline for smoking cessation purposes. Nicotine replacement therapy is also recommended as a therapy to aid smoking cessation. A recent Cochrane Review on the safety and efficacy of 136 nicotine replacement therapy trials found that all varieties of nicotine replacement therapy (gum, patch, lozenge, spray) effectively increase the rate of cessation. Combined nicotine replacement therapy, for example, using a nicotine patch and gum, is also felt to be more effective than use of a single agent alone. The impact that these interventions can have on smoking cessation efforts was sufficient to make these interventions class IA recommendations for the PAD patient.[244]

HEALTHY DIET

A balanced diet rich in fruits, vegetables, whole grains, lean proteins, and healthy fats can help maintain a healthy weight and improve CV health. Reducing sodium intake helps manage blood pressure.

REGULAR EXERCISE

Engaging in regular physical activity, as advised by a healthcare provider, can help improve circulation, lower blood pressure, and maintain a healthy weight. Physical activity in patients with PAD decreases all-cause mortality and walking, swimming, and low-impact exercises are often recommended[57] (Table 71.2). The ACC/AHA provides a class 1A recommendation for supervised exercise therapy (SET) for patients with claudication.[257] SET for symptomatic PAD is also reimbursable by most insurances. Improvements in walking performance can be dramatic. However, referral and participation in SET remain very low, and thus SET is vastly underutilized.[257]

Meta-analysis from nine studies with 391 participants showed overall improvement in pain-free walking distance in the exercise group compared with the no-exercise group (MD 82.11 m, 95% CI 71.73–92.48, $P < .00001$, high-quality evidence). Data also showed benefit from exercise in improved maximum walking distance (MD 120.36 m, 95% CI 50.79–189.92, $P < .0007$, high-quality evidence), as revealed by pooling data from 10 studies with 500 participants. Improvements were seen for up to 2 years.[244] (Lane)

- Meta-analysis also showed that SET programs appear to be even more effective than home-based therapy with similar adherence rates.[244,258]
- The duration of benefit from exercise therapy is prolonged well beyond the completion of the program, ≤7 years following a 28-week supervised program.[244,258]

TABLE 71.2

A Practical Home Exercise Program for Patients with PAD

Frequency
3–5 days per week
Modality
Treadmill (this program can be adapted for walking outside)
Method
1. Begin at 2 mph and a grade of 0 (flat).
2. Try not to hold onto the treadmill. Use the side panels for balance only.
3. Stop the treadmill completely when pain is 3–4 on claudication discomfort scale.[a]
4. When the discomfort has ceased, resume exercise at the same intensity.
5. Repeat rest–exercise cycles.
6. Progress to a higher workload when able to walk for 8 min without having to stop for leg symptoms. (a) Increase speed by 0.2 mph each time when able to walk for 8 min. (b) Once able to walk at 3.4 mph, or reach a speed at which can no longer be kept up, begin increasing the grade by 1%.
Duration
The total exercise period, including rest periods, should equal 45 min/day.
Tips for Success
1. Do not continue walking past 3–4 on claudication pain/discomfort scale. This way, the pain/discomfort should go away in 2–5 min. If walking is continued until severe pain is reached, lactic acid will be built up in the muscles, and it will take much longer for the pain to go away.
2. When at 3–4 on pain/discomfort scale, stop walking completely. Do not slow down, but stop and stand on the treadmill until the discomfort is gone.
This works if it is done! Not only will this improve walking performance, decrease discomfort, and improve quality of life, this type of program is also beneficial for the heart, blood pressure, and lipid (cholesterol and triglyceride) levels.

[a]Claudication pain scale: 1 = no pain or discomfort; 2 = onset of claudication; 3 = mild pain or discomfort; 4 = moderate pain or discomfort; 5 = severe pain or discomfort.

PAD, peripheral artery disease.

From Olin JW, White CJ, Armstrong EJ, Kadian-Dodov D, Hiatt WR. Peripheral artery disease: evolving role of exercise, medical therapy, and endovascular options. *J Am Coll Cardiol.* 2016;67(11):1338–1357. Adapted by permission from Nature: Weinberg MD, Lau JF, Rosenfield K, Olin JW. Peripheral artery disease. Part 2: medical and endovascular treatment. *Nat Rev Cardiol.* 2011;8(8):429–441. Copyright © 2011 Springer Nature.

- Several studies have shown improvements in flow-mediated dilation following exercise therapy, but not all trials demonstrated success.[244,258]
- Exercise therapy does not have a clear effect on mortality or amputation rates.[244,258]
- A Cochrane Review found supervised exercise programs resulted in ≈150 m increases in walking distance or ≈30% to 35% increase, which was sustained at 6 months.[244,259]

WEIGHT MANAGEMENT

Maintaining a healthy weight is essential for managing PAD. Excess weight can put additional stress on the CV system and contribute to reduced blood flow.

CONTROLLING BLOOD SUGAR LEVELS

It's crucial to manage blood sugar levels through proper medication, diet, and exercise. High blood sugar can damage blood vessels and exacerbate PAD. Diabetic patients have a higher risk for complications with invasive CV procedures. Diabetes is a risk factor for symptomatic and asymptomatic PAD by 1.5 to 4-fold, respectively, and a hemoglobin A1c target of less than 7% should be achieved with less stringent goals for individuals with extensive comorbidities.[246,260]

BLOOD PRESSURE

The 2016 ACC/AHA guidelines for lower extremity PAD give antihypertensive therapy a class IA recommendation for patients with PAD and suggest that blood pressure management should be in accordance with current hypertension guidelines.[244] According to current 2017 ACC/AHA guidelines on hypertension, antihypertensive medication is recommended for patients with CVD and SBP >130 mm Hg or DBP >80 mm Hg.[97]

Mortality benefits were seen with a treated SBP of 135 to 145 mm Hg and treated DBP of 60 to 90 mm Hg with higher mortality observed in low systolic and high SBP ranges, supporting the paradigm that blood pressure management in PAD is a balance between limb perfusion and risk factor modification.

FOOT CARE

Proper foot care is important for individuals with PAD, and Diabetes, as reduced blood flow can lead to slower wound healing. Frequent foot examinations for ulcers, sores, cuts, or blisters are important. Elevating the legs when sitting or lying down can help improve blood circulation in the lower extremities. Cold temperatures can lead to vasoconstriction and reduced blood flow. Extremities should be kept warm and protected from extreme cold.

STRESS MANAGEMENT

Chronic stress can contribute to poor CV health. Patients who undergo open-heart surgery or have amputations have a higher incidence of depression. Depression screening can help identify high-risk individuals which allows for timely support, treatment, and improved overall well-being.

MEDICATION COMPLIANCE

A common cause of recurrence of IC, failure of lifestyle modifications, and worsening of metabolic parameters is due to poor medication compliance and lack of appropriate follow-up. Therefore, it is important for patients with CVD to have regular medical care visits to monitor the progression of PAD and adjust the treatment plan as necessary.

Pharmacotherapy

Pharmacologic therapy for IC management can be offered to patients who have not benefited from exercise therapy and risk factor modification.

STATINS

Statin therapy appears to suppress progression of this disease. Statin therapy has been effectively shown to reduce CV events, all-cause mortality, and reduce the need for revascularization and should be routinely used in patients with PAD. The Heart Protection Study Collaborative Group provided the first randomized controlled trial data on statin therapy in PAD.[244] Moderate-intensity statin therapy with simvastatin reduced peripheral vascular events (defined as noncoronary revascularization, amputation, aneurysm repair, and death from PAD) by 17% in a prespecified PAD group.[244] Since the Heart Protection Study, multiple retrospective studies corroborated the finding that statin therapy reduces the rate of amputation with relative risk reductions between 18% and 35%. Patients taking nonstatin lipid therapy did not share a reduction in lower extremity amputation rates. There was also a dose response with respect to statin intensity with high-intensity statin therapy resulting in a greater reduction of limb loss. The idea that statin therapy reduces the risk of vascular events outside the periphery is supported by meta-analyses.[261,262] Despite robust evidence showing a reduction in vascular events, meta-analysis did not demonstrate an overall reduction in mortality.[261,262] While current guidelines suggest the use of high-intensity statin therapy,[244] the ACC/AHA considers PAD to be equivalent to a history of MI or stroke with respect to cholesterol-lowering therapies.[244] The ACC/AHA recommends all patients with symptomatic PAD to be on high-intensity statin. In addition, individuals with PAD and another major atherosclerotic CVD event (or two minor risk factors) should be treated to an LDL-C of <70 with a class I recommendation.[244]

Cholesterol-lowering therapies are less frequently prescribed in Blacks even when indicated by the guidelines.[112,113] Black women appear to have even lower rates of guideline-based statin use.

EZETIMIBE

The ACC/AHA cholesterol guidelines recommend the use of ezetimibe in the management of very-high–risk patients with LDL-C >70 despite maximally tolerated statin therapy and select non–very-high-risk patients with similarly resistant cholesterol levels.[244] This indicates that ezetimibe without statin therapy is not sufficient in the management of PAD.

PCSK9 INHIBITORS

Although quite expensive, patients in a prespecified symptomatic PAD group had a reduction of 42% in major adverse limb events such as ALI, major amputation, or urgent peripheral revascularization for ischemia.[263] This reduction was seen regardless of the intensity of statin therapy without excess adverse events. The addition of alirocumab therapy to statins did not alter superficial femoral artery plaque volume, calf perfusion, or 6MWD despite significant LDL lowering.[263]

ANTIPLATELET THERAPY

To prevent CV incidents, every patient should receive long-term treatment with an antiplatelet agent. Platelet activity is instrumental to the development of complications from CVD, and PAD is no exception. Not only is platelet adherence an initial step toward atherosclerotic disease but platelet activity is abnormal in PAD. PAD is associated with platelet hyperaggregability and increased adhesion with higher expression of surface protein, P-selectin.

ACETYLSALICYLIC ACID

Use acetylsalicylic acid (ASA) 75 to 150 mg/day; if this is contraindicated, use clopidogrel 75 mg/d or ticlopidine 250 mg bid. However, multiple trials failed to show a reduction in CV events for aspirin in patients with asymptomatic PAD, including the Aspirin for Asymptomatic Atherosclerosis Trial, which compared 100-mg aspirin to placebo in 3,350 patients with a follow-up time of >8 years.[259,260] These results are in line with emerging data suggesting that aspirin is not effective in the primary prevention of CV mortality.[244,264–267] Aspirin has historically been shown to be effective for symptomatic PAD.[268] Evidence supported this in 2007 with the CLIPS (Critical Leg Ischemia Prevention Study), which evaluated the use of low-dose aspirin (81 mg) in 366 patients with symptomatic and asymptomatic PAD and found a 64% relative risk reduction in major vascular events: ischemic stroke, MI, and vascular death ($P = .022$).[269] More recent studies show that patients with lower extremity PAD with high-risk limb presentations (or high-risk comorbidities) are at increased risk of major adverse vascular events. For these patients, treatment with rivaroxaban and aspirin in combination compared with aspirin alone led to a large absolute reduction in vascular risk.[270] Clinicians should consider this combination in patients who are not at high bleeding risk and have high-risk limb presentations.[270]

CLOPIDOGREL

The P2Y12 receptor inhibitor clopidogrel has been compared with aspirin in the CAPRIE trial (Clopidogrel Versus Aspirin in Patients at Risk for Ischemic Events), which remains the only trial data with a subgroup analysis comparing these two antiplatelet agents.[271] The results were impressive: they found almost a 25% reduction in the primary endpoint of vascular death, nonfatal MI, or cerebrovascular accident in patients with clopidogrel over aspirin. Compared with the other subsets in the trial, the prespecified symptomatic PAD group benefited the most. Single-agent antiplatelet therapy is a 2016 ACC/AHA class Ia recommendation; however, the guidelines do not recommend clopidogrel over aspirin despite the results of this subgroup analysis.[244]

In 2017, the Examining Use of Ticagrelor in Peripheral Artery Disease (EUCLID) trial compared clopidogrel to ticagrelor in almost 14,000 symptomatic PAD patients. The primary endpoint of CV death, MI, or ischemic stroke was not significantly different (10.6% vs. 10.8%) between the two agents.[272]

DUAL ANTIPLATELET THERAPY

The CHARISMA trial (Clopidogrel for High Atherothrombotic Risk and Ischemic Stabilization, Management, and Avoidance) compared DAPT to single antiplatelet therapy and included patients with PAD. The primary outcomes of the trial were stroke, death, bleeding, and MI, but the authors found no significant difference in outcome between DAPT and single antiplatelet therapy in the general trial population.[273] However, a posthoc subgroup analysis on PAD patients alone showed DAPT therapy resulted in a statistically significant 15% relative risk reduction in the primary endpoint.[244]

WARFARIN

The OASIS (Organization to Assess Strategies for Ischemic Syndromes) and WARIS-II (Warfarin, Aspirin, or Both After Myocardial Infarction) trials found the combination of warfarin and aspirin was better than aspirin alone at preventing major adverse CV events in this patient population The WAVE trial (Warfarin Antiplatelet Vascular Evaluation) investigated the use of warfarin anticoagulation in combination with aspirin for patients with symptomatic PAD (81.8% of the total trial population), subclavian disease, and carotid disease.[274] The trial found no significant difference in the occurrence of major adverse CV events between patients receiving combination of aspirin and warfarin therapy alone.[274] Furthermore, they found a significant increase in the amount of major bleeding events, including intracranial hemorrhage.[274]

CILOSTAZOL

The ACC/AHA guidelines include cilostazol, a class IA recommendation, in the treatment of symptomatic claudication. A systematic Cochrane Review of 15 trials concluded that cilostazol increases exercise tolerance compared with placebo. Of note, cilostazol is contraindicated in patients with HF as medications in this class may be associated with excess mortality. Cilostazol is infrequently used and should only be considered in otherwise medically optimized patients with refractory claudication who can tolerate the medication.

The COMPASS trial (Cardiovascular Outcomes for People Using Anticoagulation Strategies) published in late 2017 demonstrated improved mortality with low-dose rivaroxaban in combination with aspirin for patients with PAD.[275]

Patients ≥75 years old with PAD are at heightened ischemic and bleeding risk after revascularization. No excess harm with respect to major, intracranial, or fatal bleeding was seen in older patients, and benefits were observed. This suggests that low-dose rivaroxaban combined with aspirin should be considered in PAD after revascularization.[276] The Heart Protection Study found a 22% relative risk reduction in the first major vascular event with moderate-intensity statin therapy while the COMPASS trial showed a 28% relative risk reduction in the primary outcome with the use of low-dose rivaroxaban and aspirin.[277]

ACE/ARB

Several prospective and retrospective studies have shown a reduction in mortality with ACE inhibitor and ARB over other antihypertensive agents.[278,279] As a result, both the European Society of Cardiology and ACC/AHA guidelines give a class II recommendation for ACE inhibitor or ARB for PAD. Nevertheless, a posthoc subanalysis of the ALLHAT (Antihypertensive and Lipid-Lowering Treatment to Prevent Heart Attack Trial) and a prespecified subgroup analysis of VALUE (Valsartan Antihypertensive Long-Term Use Evaluation) did not show a significant reduction in primary endpoints of fatal or nonfatal MI and major adverse CV events, respectively, with ACE inhibitor or ARB over other antihypertensive classes in subgroup analysis of patients with symptomatic PAD.[280–282] Certainly, control of hypertension is an important facet of medical therapy in PAD, but it remains to be seen whether ACE inhibitor or ARB offer benefits beyond blood pressure control in PAD.

Invasive Procedures

Patients who have debilitating symptoms unresponsive to risk factor modification and exercise and pharmacologic therapy may be candidates for endovascular, surgical, or combined endovascular and surgical intervention. Indications for intervention include individuals with incapacitating claudication interfering with daily activity and limb salvage in patients with CLI manifested by ischemic pain at rest, ulceration, and gangrene.[246] The decision on surgical versus percutaneous intervention is dependent on many factors, including the patient's functional status and surgical risk, skills of the operator, anatomic location and extent of disease, presence of multifocal vascular lesions, and patient preference.[246] An interprofessional team approach involving an internist, interventionalist, and vascular surgeon should be undertaken for personalized patient care to improve outcomes and patient satisfaction.[246] Clinicians can use Figure 71.14 to appreciate the differences between percutaneous and surgical (bypass) patency rates.

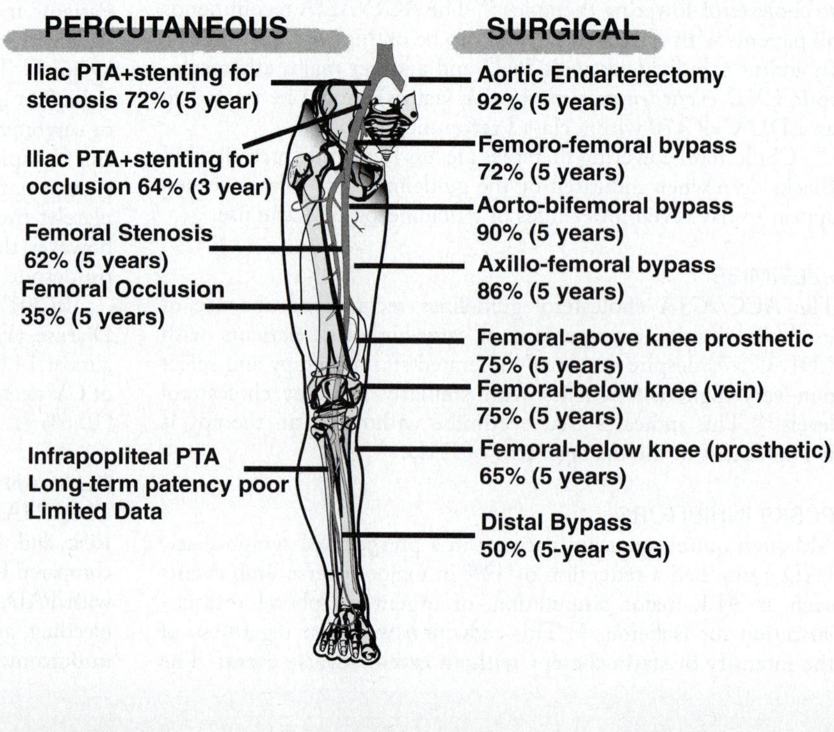

Figure 71.14. Patency rates for percutaneous and bypass procedures in intermittent claudication. (Source: Data adapted from Intermittent Claudication in Transatlantic Inter-Society Consensus [TASC]. Management of peripheral arterial disease. *J Vasc Surg.* 2000;31:S54–S122.)

Endovascular Procedures

Advances in endovascular therapies have broadened the options for treating PVD percutaneously. Endovascular procedures are recommended in patients who have not responded to lifestyle changes, exercise, and pharmacologic therapy and who have debilitating symptoms.[249]

Endovascular treatment offers a lower-risk alternative to open surgery in many patients with multiple comorbidities. Noninvasive physiologic tests and arterial imaging precede an endovascular intervention and help to localize the disease and plan the procedure. The timing and need for revascularization are related to the three main clinical presentations[283]:

- Claudication
- CLI
- ALI

In general, endovascular treatments have greater long-term durability for aortoiliac disease than femoral popliteal disease. Balloon angioplasty and stenting are the mainstays of endovascular therapy. There are also newer innovations such as drug-eluting stents and drug-coated balloons (DCBs). Patients receiving endovascular procedures need a structured surveillance plan for follow-up care. This includes intensive treatment of CV risk factors to prevent MI and stroke, which are the main causes of death. Limb surveillance aims to identify restenosis and new disease beyond the intervened segments, both of which may jeopardize patency and lead to recurrent symptoms, functional impairment, or a threatened limb.[283]

Indications for invasive treatment (percutaneous endovascular treatment or surgical treatment)

- Critical lower limb ischemia (Fontaine stages III and IV, Rutherford stages 4–6)
- Patients without CLI but with moderate to severe claudication (Fontaine stage IIb, Rutherford stages 2–3) not improved by medical management, are a good procedural risk and are determined to have anatomy favorable for successful intervention.
- In patients with extensive tissue loss (Rutherford stage 6), consideration may be given to proceed to primary amputation without revascularization.

Percutaneous Transluminal Angioplasty

Following diagnostic angiography, one of the mainstays of endovascular therapy is percutaneous transluminal angioplasty (PTA). This involves placing a wire intraluminally beyond the target lesion and then expanding the inserted balloon at the lesion to the appropriate pressure which leads to fracture of the lesion and stretching of the arterial wall. Several angioplasty balloons beyond the standard balloon are available. These include cutting balloons (CBs), cryoplasty balloons, focal pressure balloons, and DCBs.

Endovascular Stents

Currently, stents are predominantly composed of nitinol, nickel, and titanium, stainless steel, or cobalt chromium. Balloon-expandable stents are mounted onto a delivery system over an angioplasty balloon. These devices are rigid to prevent movement and allow for precise placement. However, balloon-expandable stents may become deformed because of external compression. Often, these can be used in iliac, subclavian, mesenteric, and renal arteries.[284]

Atherectomy

Although balloon angioplasty and stenting have provided a strong base for endovascular therapy, atherectomy developed as an additional option for anatomic locations not normally amenable to stents, including the common femoral artery and popliteal artery. Atherectomy has become widely adopted across specialties with four main methods of function: directional, rotational, orbital, and laser atherectomy.[249] Directional atherectomy functions using a carbide cutting blade with varying sizes to customize to the type of lesion. Rotational atherectomy uses a metallic drill that, with high-speed rotation, can be used on a variety of different plaques, including calcified and soft thrombus. Orbital atherectomy is similar to rotational atherectomy and uses an abrasive diamond-coated crown that rotates to grind debris down to particles small enough not to cause problematic distal embolization. Finally, laser atherectomy uses highly focused light to ablate lesions by direct contact and with minimal surrounding thermal damage. Although atherectomy has been widely adopted, large numbers of randomized controlled trials studying atherectomy techniques against PTA are still lacking.[249]

Lithoplasty

Among other new technologies currently under investigation is the Shockwave Lithoplasty System (Shockwave Medical, Fremont, CA, USA), which adapts technology used in the treatment of renal calculi. This technology uses a catheter-guided balloon that produces powerful acoustic shockwaves to disrupt plaque while reducing vessel wall injury.[249,285]

Revascularization Surgery

Revascularization surgery for CLI is a critical intervention aimed at limb salvage and reducing mortality. The choice between endovascular and surgical revascularization strategies is complex and depends on the patient's specific clinical situation. Meta-analyses have compared the outcomes of endovascular-first and surgery-first revascularization strategies for CLI, with findings suggesting no significant difference in overall survival or amputation-free survival between the two approaches.[286] These findings underscore the importance of individualized treatment plans and the need for ongoing research to optimize revascularization strategies for patients with CLI.

Decreasing CV Risk: Postprocedure Antiplatelet Therapy

The efficacy of DAPT for patients with PAD after lower-limb intervention remains controversial. Currently, the prescription of DAPT after an intervention is not fully recommended in guidelines due to limited evidence. However, a study in 2023 demonstrated that DAPT in PAD patients after intervention was associated with lower rates of all-cause mortality, and major amputation when follow-up was for more than 1 year.[287] DAPT was not associated with major bleeding events when compared with monotherapy but was associated with a higher rate of minor bleeding as a complication.[287]

Somatic Dysfunction and OMT

OMT has consistently shown its effectiveness in improving clinical outcomes for PAD, both through anecdotal evidence and scientific research.[288,289] PAD is characterized by the accumulation of atherosclerosis in peripheral blood vessels, leading to flow restrictions and impairments in the adaptability of these vessels to tissue requirements.[289]

In PAD, the limitations of blood flow to resulting organs and tissues cause downstream complications. A primary goal of medical management involves promoting blood flow in affected vessels, whether that be through medication or surgery.[289] Studies have demonstrated the utility of OMT for this objective. In the lower extremity, osteopathic evaluation and treatment of fascial restrictions have been shown to increase blood flow and decrease vascular resistance in arterial vessels.[288] Similar findings have been demonstrated through use of more complete and thorough OMTs, showing improvements in brachial flow-mediated vasodilation and inflammatory markers over a period of 6 months.[289] These measured improvements in vascular function and flow due to OMT highlight the implications and utility of OMT in treatment of PAD.

Osteopathic philosophy has long embraced lymphatic treatments to aid various healing processes. Lymphatic flow plays a vital role in eliminating waste products, inflammatory mediators, and excess fluid. Therefore, lymphatic treatments have become a focal point in addressing PVD.[290,291] Lymphatic techniques such as the abdominal pump and thoracic pump have demonstrated their ability to increase lymphatic flow in the thoracic duct, as observed directly in canines.[290] Furthermore, lymphatic OMT has been found to stimulate an immune response, as demonstrated by both canine and human studies showing increased recruitment of various leukocytes following trials of OMT.[291] The lymphatic system is integral to the normal function of the body, but it is also an important part of the body's healing capabilities and adaptation to injury. PAD impairs the process of wound healing, and further complications of the disease include development of chronic, nonhealing wounds. Treatment with osteopathic manipulation promotes wound healing through many proposed mechanisms, but especially by augmenting the function of the lymphatics.[291] This underscores the profound significance of lymphatic OMT for treatment of PAD.

To improve lymphatic and vascular flow, graded exercise therapy is a core facet of PAD management to help alleviate symptoms. However, adherence to graded exercise therapy can be difficult for patients especially due to the exacerbation of symptoms that many experience. Regular OMT in patients with PAD has demonstrated improvements in patients' quality of life over time, as well as increased walking times and participation in graded exercise therapy.[289] Not only is OMT an effective adjuvant therapy for PAD, but it can also enhance patients' abilities to engage in further therapeutic modalities.

PATIENTS WITH CORONARY ARTERY BYPASS GRAFTS

Introduction

CABG surgery is used to treat atheromatous obstructions in the coronary arteries that are limiting the supply of oxygen-rich blood to the heart (see Fig. 71.15). During the procedure healthy blood vessels from other parts of the body are connected to the coronary blood vessels above and below the blocked artery, creating a new route for blood to flow bypassing the diseased section of the artery. Bypass surgery can markedly reduce or relieve chest pain for most people and improve CV function. Appropriately selected patients receiving CABG have increased survival benefits compared to those receiving medical therapy or PCI alone.[292–294]

In traditional "open heart" CABG, your heart is stopped, and a heart-lung bypass machine takes over the job of pumping blood throughout the body. This is still the most common approach, but several new surgical approaches are now being developed that may reduce the discomforts and risks associated with traditional bypass surgery. Known as "minimally invasive bypass surgery" and "off-pump surgery," these approaches, called "off-pump" procedures, may be an option for some people.[293,294]

The conduits used as bypass grafts are routinely the left internal mammary artery (LIMA) and the saphenous vein grafts (SVG) out of the lower extremities. Other conduits that may be grafted include the right internal mammary artery (RIMA), the radial artery, and the gastroepiploic artery. The type and location of the grafts depend on the patient's anatomy and the location of the

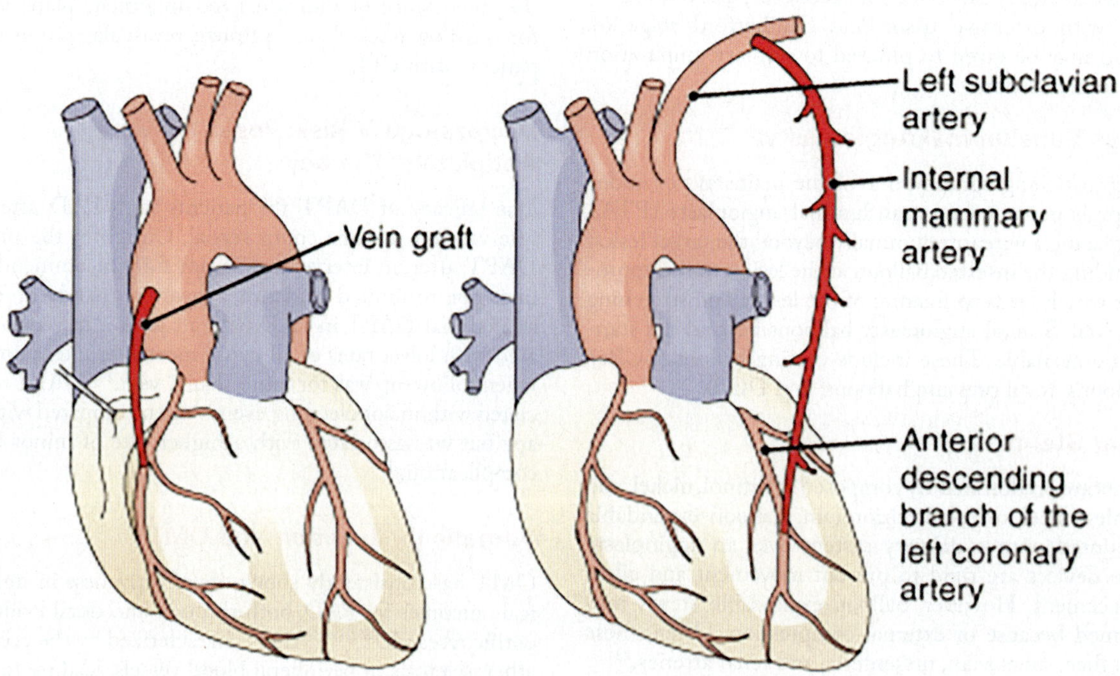

Figure 71.15. Coronary artery bypass graft. A portion of the saphenous vein or internal mammary artery is typically used to bypass a portion of an occluded coronary artery. A portion of the radial artery can also be used in some cases. (Reprinted with permission from *Lippincott's Nursing Advisor 2013*. Wolters Kluwer Health/Lippincott Williams & Wilkins; 2013. Figure 37.1.)

arteries that are occluded. Typically, the LIMA is grafted to the LAD artery, and the other conduits are used for the other occluded arteries.[294,295]

Epidemiology

Almost 400,000 CABG surgeries are performed each year making it the most performed major surgical procedure, but surgical trends have decreased as the use of alternative options such as medical treatment and PCI have increased.[294] CAD and consequently CABG are more common in older adults. Men have traditionally had higher rates of CAD, but the gap has been narrowing. Women tend to develop CAD about 10 years later than men, often due to hormonal protection until menopause.[296]

Anatomy[237]

The coronary arteries are a crucial part of the CV system, supplying oxygenated blood to the myocardium. These arteries branch off the aorta and ensure that the heart receives the nutrients and oxygen it needs to function properly. The anatomy of the coronary arteries involves several main branches and segments:

- Left main coronary artery (LMCA): The LMCA originates from the aorta and quickly divides into two main branches:
  - LAD artery: The LAD branches further into diagonal branches. This artery supplies blood to the anterior wall of the left ventricle and a significant portion of the interventricular septum (the wall separating the ventricles).
  - Circumflex artery: The circumflex artery branches into obtuse marginal branches. This artery runs around the left side of the heart in the AV groove. It supplies blood to the left atrium and the lateral and posterior walls of the left ventricle.
- Right coronary artery (RCA): The RCA also originates from the aorta and supplies blood to the right atrium, right ventricle, and parts of the AV septum. It has several branches, including:
  - Right marginal artery: This artery supplies the lateral wall of the right ventricle.
  - Posterior descending artery (PDA) or posterior interventricular artery: This artery runs along the posterior interventricular sulcus and supplies the posterior walls of both ventricles.

The coronary arteries are divided into segments based on their locations and the areas they supply:

- Proximal segment: This segment is closest to the aorta and typically experiences the highest shear forces. It's also where atherosclerotic plaques tend to develop.
- Mid segment: This segment is in the middle portion of the artery and is less prone to atherosclerotic changes compared to the proximal segment.
- Distal segment: This segment is farther away from the aorta and is responsible for supplying blood to smaller branches and capillaries within the myocardium.

It's important to note that variations in coronary artery anatomy are common among individuals. Some people might have additional branches or variations in the way the arteries are distributed. The coronary circulation can be divided into left-dominant, right-dominant, and co-dominant systems depending on which artery supplies the interventricular septum and PDA. In a left-dominant system, the PDA is supplied by the circumflex artery, whereas, in a right-dominant system, the PDA is supplied by the RCA. Co-dominant arterial supply has the PDA supplied by both the RCA and circumflex arteries simultaneously. Knowledge of these variations is essential for cardiac surgeons and interventional cardiologists, as they perform procedures like CABG and angioplasty.

Proper functioning of the coronary arteries is vital. Blockages in any of the coronary arteries cause a corresponding defect in myocardial perfusion, ischemia and, if unrepaired, can lead to permanent infarct or damage to the myocardium.

Indications/Clinical Practice Guidelines

CABG is usually performed when other interventions, such as lifestyle changes, medications, and less invasive procedures like angioplasty and stenting, have not been effective in managing severe CAD. CABG may also be indicated for individuals with multiple or complex blockages. CABG is generally recommended when there are high-grade blockages in any of the major coronary arteries and/or PCI has failed to clear the blockages. Class 1 recommendations from the 2011 ACCF/AHA guidelines are as follows[293,294]:

- Left main disease greater than 50%
- Three-vessel CAD of greater than 70% with or without proximal LAD involvement
- Two-vessel disease: LAD plus one other major artery
- One or more significant stenosis greater than 70% in a patient with significant anginal symptoms despite maximal medical therapy
- One vessel disease greater than 70% in a survivor of SCD with ischemia-related ventricular tachycardia

The 2021 ACC/AHA/SCAI Clinical Practice Guideline for Coronary Artery Revascularization provided an update and consolidated the 2011 and 2015 guidelines. They added consideration of using a patient-centric disease approach.[297] Listed below is a summary of those guidelines.[297]

- Treatment decisions regarding coronary revascularization in patients with CAD should be based on clinical indications, regardless of sex, race, or ethnicity.
- If possible, coronary revascularization should be performed by a multidisciplinary heart team. For patients with significant left main disease, surgical revascularization is indicated to improve survival relative to that likely to be achieved with medical therapy.
- There is also evidence for a mortality benefit of revascularization in patients with stable ischemic heart disease, and triple-vessel CAD.
- The use of a radial artery as a surgical revascularization conduit is preferred versus the use of a saphenous vein.
- Revascularization decisions in patients with diabetes and multivessel CAD should undergo surgical revascularization with a heart team approach.
- Treatment decisions for patients undergoing surgical revascularization of CAD should include the calculation of a patient's surgical risk with the Society of Thoracic Surgeons score.

Surgical treatment may be recommended for different situations[294]:

- Stable angina: People with chronic stable angina may require CABG if they develop persistent and intolerable symptoms despite optimal medical treatment.
- Extensive disease: People with extensive CHD, including narrowing of the LMCA, multiple narrowed coronary arteries, and poor EF, generally live longer when they undergo CABG as compared with people who have medical therapy or PCI.
- Left main disease greater than 50%
- Three-vessel CAD of greater than 70% with or without proximal LAD involvement

- Two-vessel disease: LAD plus one other major artery
- Future risk of cardiac event: Patients with a high risk for a future cardiac event based on a stress test showing poor exercise capacity, failure to raise blood pressure during exercise, or severely limited blood flow to multiple areas of the heart.
- Unstable angina: People who develop unstable angina may be candidates for CABG or stenting. Angina is considered unstable if it becomes more frequent, occurs with less exertion or at rest, is more severe, lasts longer, or fails to respond to appropriate medication.
- After MI: People who have acute MI complications such as a leaky heart valve, cardiogenic shock requiring mechanical support, or a coronary anatomy that is unfavorable or not feasible with PCI may undergo CABG.

Contraindications to CABG include:

- Patient refusal
- Coronary arteries incompatible with grafting
- Absence of viable myocardium to graft

Surgery is not always the best option for everyone. The final decision regarding the best choice of treatment depends upon several factors, including the benefit versus risk of surgery, the severity of the symptoms and cardiac disease, and patient comorbidities.

Procedure

Conventional CABG is performed while the person is under general anesthesia. The surgery generally takes 3 to 6 hours. The patient is sterilely prepped and draped. An anesthesiologist may place an arterial line for invasive monitoring of the patient's blood pressure before induction of general anesthesia. After general anesthesia is induced and the patient is intubated, a central line for venous access and a pulmonary artery catheter may be placed followed by insertion of a transesophageal echocardiography transducer. The surgeon performs a median sternotomy, to open the chest and gain access to the heart. If the internal mammary artery is being used, it is separated from the chest wall; if a vein or radial artery is being used, it is removed from the leg or arm. The patient is placed on a cardiopulmonary bypass (CPB) machine so that the surgeon can attach the bypass vessel to the diseased coronary artery. After starting CPB, the heart is arrested using high potassium-containing cardioplegia so the surgeon can anastomose the harvested conduits to the coronary arteries distal to the blockages.[294] The surgeon sews one end of the graft onto the aorta and the other end to a part of the coronary artery beyond the narrowing, hence bypassing the diseased area. After the surgeon anastomoses the distal portions, the conduits are attached to new ostia created in the proximal aorta. The surgeon can check the grafts for both blood flow and competence as well as checking for bleeding from the anastomosis sites. After that, the chest is closed using sternal wires, and the patient is transferred to the intensive care unit for monitoring of hemodynamic stability and extubation.

Choice of Graft

Generally, blood vessels can be obtained from four areas of the body: the chest, leg, arm, and abdomen. In general, arterial grafts rarely develop stenosis (narrowing) and have an improved long-term patency compared with vein grafts. In addition, people with arterial grafts tend to have better survival, fewer reoperations, a lower rate of MI, and less recurrent angina, as compared with vein grafts.

Internal Thoracic Artery Grafts

Left internal thoracic (or mammary) artery (ITA) grafts have emerged as the preferred bypass graft due to their excellent graft patency and close proximity to the LAD artery. They are often referred to as LIMA grafts (LIMA grafts). Internal thoracic arteries (internal mammary arteries) grafts are not fully removed from their original position. These grafts remain connected to their natural site of origin, and only the distal end is separated from the chest wall. This end is then attached to one of the coronary arteries. The LIMA is generally the first choice for a graft, as it has been shown to improve outcomes since it remains patent longer having a patency rate exceeding 90% at 10 years.[294,298]

Saphenous Vein Grafts

SVG are still the most widely used in coronary bypass surgeries. Saphenous grafts are the most convenient, however most prone to occlusion. The occlusion develops in approximately 50% of people. Some occlusions occur as early as months after surgery, while others develop within 5 to 7 years. Saphenous vein conduits are harvested from legs and grafted from the ascending aorta to the coronary artery beyond the obstructive lesion. Right coronary grafts are usually anastomosed to the RCA or PDA. Left coronary grafts are usually anastomosed to LAD artery, left circumflex, obtuse marginal, or diagonal branches. Most grafts are directly sutured to the aorta, however, recently aortovenous connector devices are being increasingly used.[293,298]

Radial Artery

Radial arteries are taken from the inner forearm. The long-term outcome with these arteries is also excellent and almost equivalent to that of the ITA. There are usually only minimal changes in hand function after removal of the radial artery for CABG, which manifest as a small amount of forearm numbness and tingling, but generally no change in motor function, and the symptoms are self-limited.[298]

Recovery/Postoperative Care

Immediately after surgery, the patient spends one to two days in an intensive care unit. Family members can visit periodically during this time. For the first 1 to 2 days continuous monitoring occurs to evaluate heart rate and rhythm, blood pressure, temperature, and breathing rate; monitoring is gradually discontinued as the person recovers. The patient is extubated when they're awake and able to breathe on their own; this usually occurs a few hours after the surgery. Patients will have an IV as well as a Foley catheter initially until they are able to ambulate and go to the bathroom. Patients will have drainage tubes in their chest that will typically be removed within 1 to 3 days following the surgery. Patients will have midline sternal pain and be typically placed on a patient-controlled anesthesia pump. When continuous monitoring is no longer required patients will be moved to a stepdown unit. Most patients can sit in a chair the day after the surgery and start walking within 1 to 2 days following surgery. It is common for patients to have a decreased appetite and be constipated following the surgery. Patients who had a saphenous vein harvested may have pain and swelling of the involved leg. Patients can wear compressive stockings to assist with this as well as early ambulation. Patients who underwent CABG had a higher risk of new onset of depression compared to sex- and age-matched controls in the general population.[299] The risk of depression was especially pronounced in younger patients during the first 5 years after surgery.[299] This may be related to poor sleep in the hospital, the stress of surgery, and many other predisposing factors. Most people recover in the hospital for 4 to 5 days after surgery.

Before leaving the hospital, it is important for the patient and family to participate in and understand the discharge plan. People who do not have complications or a prolonged hospital stay are usually able to return to desk work within 4 to 6 weeks. Complete recovery from surgery often takes 2 to 3 months. Care after bypass surgery aims to reduce the risk factors for heart disease and includes strategies to help patients and family members stop smoking, control high blood pressure, improve cholesterol levels, begin exercising regularly, reduce weight if necessary, and reduce stress. Some of these changes can be made by adjusting lifestyle habits through diet and exercise. However, lifestyle changes alone may not be adequate, and medications are often needed.[293] Most people who have had bypass surgery are sent home with prescriptions for aspirin therapy, beta-blockers, nitrates, ace inhibitors, and statins. Patients should avoid heavy lifting and extremes of shoulder movement for 6 to 8 weeks after surgery. Most surgeons recommend avoiding driving for at least 4 weeks.

CABG Risks/Complications

Although uncommon, there are several complications that can occur after CABG surgery. Frail patients with significant comorbidities, who are undergoing urgent or repeat CABG, require mechanical support prior to surgery, or need combined cardiac procedures, are at higher risk. The complications of CABG include stroke, wound infection, graft failure, renal failure, postoperative AF, and death. The stroke rate of CABG has been reported at 1% to 2% depending on the characteristics of the patient and their risk factors for stroke including advanced age, prior stroke, aortic atherosclerosis, PAD, perioperative AF, and diabetes.[292] Chronic pain following CABG procedures continues to be a major problem in recovery, contributing to the development of additional complications. Surgery involving the upper thoracic vertebrae (specifically T1–T5) and pain activates the SNS which increases the demand for cardiac function leading to further cardiac complications which include tachycardia, arrhythmia, and myocardial ischemia.

Exercise

Exercise is a crucial component of the recovery process following CABG surgery. Aerobic exercise begun early after cardiac surgery significantly improves functional and aerobic capacity. A systematic review identified all studies reporting safety and efficacy outcomes of aerobic exercise commenced within 2 weeks of cardiac surgery.[300] This meta-analysis was performed comparing functional, aerobic, and safety outcomes in patients receiving early postoperative aerobic exercise compared with usual postoperative care.[300] There was no significant difference in adverse events rates between the two groups (odds ratio 0.41, 95% CI 0.12–1.42, $P = .16$). Although more studies are needed, this study supports safety outcomes of aerobic exercise commenced early after cardiac surgery. Engaging in a structured exercise program post-CABG can have several benefits, including:

- Improved cardiovascular health:
  - ☐ Osailan, 2020 showed that patients had improved resting SBP and DBP after going through a structured cardiac rehabilitation exercise program.[301] Early rehabilitation has also shown an increase in left ventricular ejection fraction (LVEF) as well as decreased left ventricular end-diastolic diameter (LVEDDD) and left ventricular end-systolic diameter (LVESD).[302] This is important because reduced blood pressure in post-CABG patients acts as secondary prevention for any future complications that can occur from hypertension. Improving LVEF will also ensure adequate perfusion throughout the body and through the grafted vessel as well. The combination of improved CV health paired with other secondary preventions can lower the incidence of cardiac ischemia.
- Enhanced lung function:
  - ☐ Shan et al. showed that their exercise groups demonstrated increased distance traveled during the 6-minute walk test (6MWT), increased VO_2 max, and anaerobic threshold (AT).[302] Their pulmonary exercise program started after the patient was extubated, which shows that early intervention can help patients recover quicker and return to normal activity. Because of the early intervention, it resulted in a shorter hospital stay after leaving the ICU, which further reduced costs for the patients and the healthcare system.
- Reduced risk of complications:
  - ☐ A study in China showed that patients who underwent cardiac rehab after a CABG had a decreased incidence of pulmonary infection and hypoxemia compared to the control group.[302] Having fewer incidences of complications is also good for the patient because it reduces costs and hospitalization time.
- Weight management:
  - ☐ Reduction of weight will help decrease blood pressure, which is important for the secondary prevention of heart disease. Weight management should be done in conjunction with cardiac rehab because it can help control other comorbidities the patients may already have.
- Improved mood and mental health:
  - ☐ Shan et al. also demonstrated that the patients reported improvements in their physical function, general health, and emotional state.[302] The authors speculated that the early exercise program allowed patients to regain their function quicker which helped them return to their normal lives and improve their mental state. This is important since having a CABG done can be mentally taxing to the patient.
- Enhanced functional capacity:
  - ☐ A structured exercise program for CABG patients has been shown to improve heart rate recovery (HRR) and peak heart rate during the incremental shuttle walking test (ISWT).[301] These patients were also able to increase their maximum speed and maximum total distance during the ISWT. This means that these patients can tolerate higher levels of exercise post-CABG. Improved functional capacity of the heart especially after surgery will help patients return to normal activity quicker than patients who do not undergo cardiac rehabilitation.
- Exercise prescription:
  - ☐ Medical supervision: Depending on a patient's risk factors, they could be at increased risk of having heart-related complications with exercise; therefore, a trained clinician should work with the patient to assess and develop an exercise training regimen that is safe and beneficial for the patient.[293]
  - ☐ Timing: Pulmonary rehab can be started with some breathing exercises the moment the patient is extubated after the CABG.[302] From there, patients can be assessed to have an exercise training program developed. Once the patients get discharged from the hospital, the patient can follow up with their program several times a week in an outpatient facility to allow the patients to sleep at home.[293] Giving them that

flexibility can make sure that patients are compliant with the rehab program.

- Gradual progression: A structured cardiac rehabilitation program can provide a safe and effective framework for post-CABG exercise.
- Monitoring: For patients who are at higher risk for complications, they can exercise at a facility where an EKG can be monitored during exercise and advanced life support equipment is available nearby.[293] Patients who are not at high risk could be allowed to exercise without supervision.
- Types of Exercise: Aerobic exercises like walking, cycling, and swimming are typically recommended for post-CABG patients. Strength training exercises can also be included to improve muscle strength. Patients try exercises that they like since it will increase the likelihood that they will continue to exercise even after their official exercise program ends.
- Frequency: Initially, this may involve several short sessions per day. The patient can increase exercise frequency as tolerated. If they are going to an outside facility, it can limit how often their sessions are due to transportation, time, or availability.
- Lifestyle modifications: The patient should still be counseled on reducing other cardiac risk factors including eating a healthy diet, cessation of smoking, managing diabetes, reducing stress, and treating high blood pressure.[293] Having these other risk factors well-controlled can help slow the progression of heart disease.
- Medication management: Heart rate and blood pressure post-CABG can partially be controlled with beta-blockers.[301] Using both exercise and medications can be beneficial because they help control the other comorbidities that patients can still have after having a CABG done.

The osteopathic-created exercise plan will vary from person to person, depending on the individual and their structural and functional factors. The goal is to tailor the exercise program to the patient's needs, capabilities, and progress to promote a safe and effective benefit to their overall health and well-being.

Somatic Dysfunction and OMT

Osteopathic manipulative medicine including OMT techniques addressing somatic dysfunction in the postoperative patient can have clinical benefits. Following a median sternotomy, patients who had received postoperative OMT for associated somatic dysfunction demonstrated an accelerated clinical recovery, improvement of respiratory function, an improved pain threshold, and an earlier discharge, compared to control groups not subjected to the OMT.[91,222] There are several mechanisms that can explain why the use of OMT resulted in improvement in patients following CABG. There has been a strong correlation of somatic dysfunction found in the upper thoracic vertebrae (T1–T4 on the left), the upper ribs, and C2 dysfunctions in those with known CVD.[91]

In a 2013 study,[91] patients were voluntarily enrolled and randomized into one of three groups: (1) standardized daily OMT and conventional postoperative care (the OMT group), (2) daily time-matched placebo OMT and conventional postoperative care (the placebo group), or (3) conventional postoperative care only (the control group). Specific OMT techniques used were thoracic inlet myofascial release, standard rib raising (with paraspinal muscle stretch to the L2 vertebral level), and soft tissue cervical paraspinal muscle stretch (with suboccipital muscle release). Primary outcome measures included time to discharge, time to postoperative bowel movement, and functional assessment scores. Although not statistically significant, researchers found that a daily postoperative OMT protocol improved functional recovery of patients who underwent a CABG operation.[303] OMT facilitated shorter postoperative recovery times, improved gastrointestinal motility, and optimized basic mobility and activities of daily living. Some of these effects are thought to be due to balancing the sympathetic and PNSs function and improving lymphatic drainage. Utilizing gentle techniques such as balanced ligamentous tension of thoracic vertebrae, indirect myofascial release of the sternum, rib raising, and myofascial release of the suboccipital joint allows for correction of those dysfunctions while also normalizing autonomic tone.[304] Fascial techniques can restore the mobility of the tissue and decrease the stimulation of somatic afferents in the spinal cord which can then attenuate the nociceptive response leading to an increased pain threshold.[91,303] Techniques targeting the thoracic outlet, pelvic floor, and thoracic diaphragm allow for improved lymphatic flow, decreased risk of fluid mismanagement, and restoration of normal respiratory function to help relieve fluid accumulation.[304] Researchers suggest that OMT has immediate, beneficial hemodynamic effects after CABG surgery when administered while the patient is sedated and pharmacologically paralyzed.[304] The use of OMT has also been shown to decrease thoracic pain at 12 weeks postoperative and up to 1 year thereafter.[305] In another randomized study on OMT in poststernotomy patients, OMT treatment decreased the level of perceived pain, and substantially improved the functional capacity in terms of inspiratory volumes.[303] Also observed was a reduced hospital stay of 2 days, in the OMT-treated group.[303]

The use of OMT in CABG patients includes risks such as arrhythmia, cerebrovascular accident, displacement of intravenous lines and pacer wires, and reopening of surgical incisions. However, studies reviewed have reported no adverse effects from OMT.[222,303–305] The OMT benefits include increased quality of care for patients, decreased cost, a noninvasive approach, safe treatments, and statistically significant reduction in CABG postoperative complications. The use of OMT should be added to the standard of care as an addition to the traditional cardiorespiratory rehabilitation therapies following surgery with the first session of OMT beginning 1-week post-CABG.[303]

Outcomes and Challenges

CABG surgery can improve a patient's chances of survival, especially in cases where the CAD is severe or extensive. Yet, there is some controversy in the published literature regarding major adverse cardiovascular and cerebrovascular events (MACCE) associated with PCI versus CABG.[306] Large, randomized studies in patients with stable IHD have shown that an initial strategy of revascularization by PCI or CABG plus GDMT was not different than GDMT alone in reducing ischemic CV events.[307–309] In addition, there are some challenges for women undergoing CABG surgery, according to a large study led by investigators at NewYork-Presbyterian/Weill Cornell Medical Center. The analysis showed that, without adjusting for differences in age and other health factors that influence risk, the female bypass patients have a roughly 30% to 40% higher risk of dying following coronary artery bypass surgery than men.[310] A recent 7-year-long study performed at the Tehran Heart Center in Iran showed a higher risk of all-cause mortality and MACCE in diabetic patients undergoing isolated CABG. Therefore, short- and long-term measures should be taken to improve the CABG outcomes in this patient population.[311]

The outcomes after CABG surgery can vary based on several factors, including the patient's overall health, the extent of CAD, how patent the graft remains over time, the surgical technique used, and the quality of postoperative care. Outcomes can vary widely from person to person. Outcomes are also dependent on patients making significant lifestyle changes. CABG surgery is often successful in relieving angina and dyspnea. About 95% of people who have narrowing of several arteries have improvement or complete relief of their angina immediately after surgery. About 85% to 90% of people remain angina-free 1 to 3 years after surgery, and about 75% of people remain angina-free or free of major coronary events at 5 years after surgery.[293] Overall, CABG surgery has been shown to be effective in improving outcomes and quality of life for many individuals with significant CAD.

SUMMARY

The osteopathic approach to the CV patient is based upon primary prevention, risk factor reduction, and implementation of homeostatic support to the patient's body, mind, and spirit. A holistic approach to the patient with CVD requires a comprehensive management plan that involves all aspects of the patient's life. Addressing lifestyle factors is of paramount importance to prevent, improve, and resolve many CV conditions. These include multifactorial risk factor modifications including components of progressive regular exercise, weight loss, control of hypertension and diabetes, smoking cessation, dietary modification with lowering of cholesterol and fats, and the management of stress. It is important for osteopathic physicians to evaluate, address, and treat the patient's emotional concerns and mental health. Providing psychological support and resources are key features in successful treatment of the patient with CVD. Clinicians should also consider the social determinants of health that may affect the patient's treatment decisions.

The most important way to prevent atherosclerotic vascular disease, HF, and AF is to promote a healthy lifestyle throughout life. All adults should consume a healthy diet that emphasizes the intake of vegetables, fruits, nuts, whole grains, lean vegetable or animal protein, and fish and limit the intake of trans fats, red meat and processed red meats, refined carbohydrates, and sweetened beverages. For adults who are overweight and obese, counseling and caloric restriction are recommended for achieving and maintaining weight loss. Adults should engage in at least 150 minutes per week of accumulated moderate-intensity physical activity or 75 minutes per week of vigorous-intensity physical activity.[8] For adults with type 2 DM, glucose control through lifestyle changes, such as improving dietary habits and achieving exercise recommendations, are crucial.

All adults should be assessed at every healthcare visit for tobacco use, and those who use tobacco should be assisted and strongly advised to quit. Adults who are 40 to 75 years of age and are being evaluated for CVD prevention should undergo 10-year ASCVD risk estimation and have a clinician–patient risk discussion before starting on pharmacologic therapy.

Aspirin should be used infrequently in the routine primary prevention of ASCVD because of lack of net benefit.[244,266,267]

Statin therapy is the first-line treatment for primary prevention of ASCVD in patients with elevated LDL cholesterol levels (≥190 mg/dL), those with DM, those who are 40 to 75 years of age, those with PAD, and those determined to be at sufficient ASCVD risk.[157,244]

Nonpharmacologic interventions are recommended for all adults with elevated blood pressure or hypertension. For those requiring pharmacologic therapy, the target blood pressure should generally be <130/80 mm Hg. To guide clinicians there are many CPGs with detailed information for patient management including extensive published literature on pharmaceutical management.

Osteopathic manipulative medicine recognizes the unity of body, mind, and spirit, in the health and wellness of the patient. Osteopathic treatment of somatic dysfunction has been shown to be beneficial for patients with CV conditions. The use of OMT has also been correlated with physician empathy.[312] The osteopathic hands-on patient approach is a vital component that helps physicians maintain a more open-hearted connection with their patients. Osteopathic medicine recognizes the structure and function interrelationship, which is where offering OMT and lifestyle modifications can help guide patients toward optimal health along with standard of care using appropriate medications and procedures. Frequent encouragement of patients toward a healthier diet, and avoiding/minimizing toxins such as tobacco, alcohol, and other drugs strengthen the self-healing properties of the body. Osteopathic philosophy is patient centered but also involves environmental influences and therefore should consider environmental pollution, environmental conditions, and world events, as they also affect long-term health. Finally, to ensure that treatments remain rational, the profession should continue to pursue high-quality research on OMT, beginning with case studies of what practicing DOs encounter, as well as robust clinical trials examining larger effects, and systematic reviews to examine overall risks and benefits of the unique the osteopathic approach.[89]

ACKNOWLEDGMENTS

The authors of this chapter would like to acknowledge the scholarly contributions of Dr's. Felix J. Rogers and Brian Kaufman for prior editions of this chapter.

The authors of this chapter would like to acknowledge the scholarly contributions of Dr. Andy Kotis.

The authors of this chapter would like to acknowledge the editorial contributions of Dr. Michael Terzella.

The authors of this chapter would like to acknowledge following student(s) Emily Daly, Ryan Schultz, Jason Vo, Jordan Barry, and Reem Darwish for contributions to this chapter.

REFERENCES

1. Rogers FJ. An osteopathic perspective on cardiology. In: Ward RC, ed. *Foundations for Osteopathic Medicine*. 2nd ed. Lippincott, Williams and Wilkins; 2003:345–369.
2. Rippe JM. Lifestyle strategies for risk factor reduction, prevention, and treatment of cardiovascular disease. *Am J Lifestyle Med*. 2018;13(2): 204–212.
3. McManus DD, Rienstra M, Benjamin EJ. An update on the prognosis of patients with atrial fibrillation. *Circulation*. 2012;126(10):e143–e146.
4. Hindricks G, Potpara T, Dagres N, et al. 2020 ESC Guidelines for the diagnosis and management of atrial fibrillation developed in collaboration with the European Association for Cardio-thoracic Surgery (EACTS): the task force for the diagnosis and management of atrial fibrillation of the European Society of Cardiology (ESC) developed with the special contribution of the European Heart Rhythm Association (EHRA) of the ESC. *Eur Heart J*. 2020;42:373–498.
5. Abu Dabrh AM, Steffen MW, Undavalli C, et al. The natural history of untreated severe or critical limb ischemia. *J Vasc Surg*. 2015;62:1642–1651.
6. Forrester J. Angioplasty versus thrombolytic therapy in acute myocardial infarction. Whose time (for testing) has come. *Circulation*. 1997;96: 1360–1362.
7. George SM, Ballard-Barbash R, Manson JE, et al. Comparing indices of diet quality with chronic disease mortality risk in postmenopausal women in the Women's Health Initiative Observational Study: evidence to inform national dietary guidance. *Am J Epidemiol*. 2014;180(6):616–625.

8. *Physical Activity Guidelines for Americans.* 2nd ed. U.S. Department of Health and Human Services; 2018. https://health.gov/sites/default/files/2019-09/Physical_Activity_Guidelines_2nd_edition.pdf
9. GBD 2017 Risk Factor Collaborators. Global, regional, and national comparative risk assessment of 84 behavioural, environmental, and occupational, and metabolic risks or clusters of risks for 195 countries and territories, 1990–2017: a systematic analysis for the Global Burden of Disease Study 2017. *Lancet.* 2018;392:1923–1994.
10. Yu E, Malik VS, Hu FB. Cardiovascular disease prevention by diet modification: JACC health promotion series. *J Am Coll Cardiol.* 2018;72(8): 914–926.
11. Sin NL. The protective role of positive well-being in cardiovascular disease: review of current evidence, mechanisms, and clinical implications. *Curr Cardiol Rep.* 2016;18(11):106.
12. Rogers FJ, D'Alonzo GE Jr, Glover JC, et al. Proposed tenets of osteopathic medicine and principles for patient care. *J Am Osteopath Assoc.* 2002;102(2):63–65.
13. Abajobir AA, Abate KH, Abbafati C, et al. Global, regional, and national comparative risk assessment of 84 behavioural, environmental and occupational, and metabolic risks or clusters of risks, 1990–2016: a systematic analysis for the Global Burden of Disease Study 2016. *Lancet.* 2017;390:1345–1422.
14. Shai I, Schwarzfuchs D, Henkin Y, et al. Weight loss with a low-carbohydrate, Mediterranean, or low-fat diet. *N Engl J Med.* 2008;359:229–241.
15. Lopez-Garcia E, Rodriguez-Artalejo F, Li TY, et al. The Mediterranean-style dietary pattern and mortality among men and women with cardiovascular disease. *Am J Clin Nutr.* 2014;99(1):172–180.
16. Skov AR, Toubro S, Rønn B, Holm L, Astrup A. Randomized trial on protein vs carbohydrate in ad libitum fat reduced diet for the treatment of obesity. *Int J Obes.* 1999;23:528.
17. Layman DK, Evans EM, Erickson D, et al. A moderate-protein diet produces sustained weight loss and long-term changes in body composition and blood lipids in obese adults. *J Nutrition.* 2009;139:514–521.
18. Zheng J, Huang T, Yu Y, Hu X, Yang B, Li D. Fish consumption and CHD mortality: an updated meta-analysis of seventeen cohort studies. *Public Health Nutr.* 2012;15:725–737.
19. Afshin A, Micha R, Khatibzadeh S, Mozaffarian D. Consumption of nuts and legumes and risk of incident ischemic heart disease, stroke, and diabetes: a systematic review and meta-analysis. *Am J Clinical Nutr.* 2014;100:278–288.
20. Piano MR. Alcohol's effects on the cardiovascular system. *Alcohol Res.* 2017;38(2):219–241.
21. Brien SE, Ronksley PE, Turner BJ, Mukamal KJ, Ghali WA. Effect of alcohol consumption on biological markers associated with risk of coronary heart disease: systematic review and meta-analysis of interventional studies. *BMJ.* 2011;342:d636.
22. Xi B, Huang Y, Reilly KH, et al. Sugar-sweetened beverages and risk of hypertension and CVD: a dose-response meta-analysis. *Br J Nutr.* 2015; 113:709–717.
23. Ding M, Bhupathiraju SN, Satija A, van Dam RM, Hu FB. Long-term coffee consumption and risk of cardiovascular disease: a systematic review and a dose-response meta-analysis of prospective cohort studies. *Circulation.* 2014;129(6):643–659.
24. Mittleman MA, Mostofsky E. Physical, psychological and chemical triggers of acute cardiovascular events: preventive strategies. *Circulation.* 2011;124:346–354.
25. U.S. Department of Health and Human Services. 2008 Physical Activity Guidelines for Americans. Office of Disease Prevention and Health Promotion Publication No. U0036. October 2008. Accessed January 12, 2024. http://health.gov/paguidelines/pdf/paguide.pdf
26. Sattelmair J, Pertman J, Ding EL, Kohl HW, Haskell W, Lee IM. Dose response between physical activity and risk of coronary heart disease: a meta-analysis. *Circulation.* 2011;124(7):789–795.
27. Eijsvogels TMH, Aengevaeren VL. Exercise at the extremes: unraveling the mechanisms of deleterious cardiovascular adaptations. *JACC Basic Tranl Sci.* 2022;7(7):694–696.
28. Vaduganathan M, Mensah GA, Turco JV, Fuster V, Roth GA. The global burden of cardiovascular diseases and risk: a compass for future health. *J Am Coll Cardiol.* 2022;80(25):2362–2371.
29. Vancheri F, Longo G, Vancheri E, Henein MY. Mental stress and cardiovascular health-part I. *J Clin Med.* 2022;11(12):3353.
30. Thackeray JT, Hupe HC, Wang Y, et al. Myocardial inflammation predicts remodeling and neuroinflammation after myocardial infarction. *J Am Coll Cardiol.* 2018;71:263–275.
31. Boehm JK, Kubzansky LD. The heart's content: the association between positive psychological well-being and cardiovascular health. *Psychol Bull.* 2012;138:655–691.
32. Pressman SD, Cohen S. Does positive affect influence health? *Psychol Bull.* 2005;131:925–971.
33. Puchalski C, Ferrell B, Virani R, et al. Improving the quality of spiritual care as a dimension of palliative care: the report of the consensus conference. *J Palliat Med.* 2009;12(10):885–904.
34. King DE, Bushwick B. Beliefs and attitudes of hospital in patients about faith healing and prayer. *J Fam Pract.* 1994:39:349–352.
35. Mueller PS, Pleveak DJ, Rummans TA. Religious involvement, spirituality, and medicine: implications for clinical practice. *Mayo Clin Prox.* 2001:76:1225–1235.
36. Koenig HG, McCullough ME, Larson DB. *Handbook of Religion and Health.* Oxford University Press; 2001.
37. Strawbridge WJ, Shema SJ, Cohen RD, Kaplan GA. Religious attendance increases survival by improving and maintaining good health behaviors, mental health, and social relationships. *Ann Behav Med.* 2001:23:68–74.
38. Wallace JM Jr, Forman TA. Religion's role in promoting health and reducing risk among American youth. *Health Educ Behan.* 1998;25:721–741.
39. Oleckno WA, Blacconicre MJ. Relationship of religiosity to wellness and other health-related behaviors and outcomes. *Psychol Rep.* 1991:68: 819–826.
40. Comstock GW, Partridge KB. Church attendance and health. *J Chronic Dis.* 1972:25:665–672.
41. Aviles JM, Whelan E, Hernke DA, et al. Intercessory prayer and cardiovascular disease progression in a coronary care unit population: a randomized controlled trial. *Mayo Clin Proc.* 2001:76:1192–1198.
42. Abu HO, Lapane KL, Waring ME, et al. Religious practices and long-term survival after hospital discharge for an acute coronary syndrome. *PLoS One.* 2019;14(10):e0223442.
43. Roberts L, Ahmed I, Davison A. Intercessory prayer for the alleviation of ill health. *Cochrane Database Syst Rev.* 2009;2009(2):CD000368.
44. Brewer LC, Bowie J, Slusser JP, et al. Religiosity/spirituality and cardiovascular health: the American Heart Association life's simple 7 in African Americans of the Jackson Heart study. *J Am Heart Assoc.* 2022;11:e024974.
45. Davies MJ, Thomas A. Thrombosis and acute coronary lesions in sudden cardiac ischemic death. *N Engl J Med.* 1984;310:1137–1140.
46. Ornish DM, Brown SE, Scherwitz LW, et al. Can lifestyle changes reverse coronary atherosclerosis? The lifestyle heart trial. *Lancet.* 1990; 336(8708):129–133.
47. Haskell WL, Alderman EL, Fair JM, et al. Effects of intense multiple risk factor reduction on coronary atherosclerosis and clinical cardiac events in men and women with coronary artery disease: the Stanford Coronary Risk Intervention Project (SCRIP). *Circulation.* 1994;89(3):975–990.
48. Pitt B, Mancini GBJ, Ellis SG, Rosman HS, Park JS, McGovern ME. Pravastatin limitation of atherosclerosis in the coronary arteries (PLAC I): reduction in atherosclerosis progression and clinical events. *J Am Coll Cardiol.* 1995;26(5):1133–1139.
49. Beltrami AP, Urbanek K, Kajstura J, et al. Evidence that human cardiac myocytes divide after myocardial infarction. *N Engl J Med.* 2001; 344:1750–1757.
50. Lodrini AM, Goumans MJ. Cardiomyocytes cellular phenotypes after myocardial infarction. *Front Cardiovasc Med.* 2021;8:750510.
51. Healthy People 2020. Accessed January 12, 2024. https://health.gov/sites/default/files/2021-03/21%20HP2020EndofDecadeSnapshot2.pdf
52. Juopperi S, Sund R, Rikkonen T, Kröger H, Sirola J. Cardiovascular and musculoskeletal health disorders associate with greater decreases in physical capability in older women. *BMC Musculoskelet Disord.* 2021;22:192.
53. Ras J, Soteriades ES, Smith DL, Kengne AP, Leach L. Association between cardiovascular and musculoskeletal health in firefighters. *J Occup Environ Med.* 2023;65(7):e496–e505.
54. Blair SN, Kohl HW III, Barlow CE, Paffenbarger RS Jr, Gibbons LW, Macera CA. Changes in physical fitness and all-cause mortality. A

prospective study of healthy and unhealthy men. *JAMA*. 1995;273:1093–1098.
55. Bitter V, Weiner DH, Yusuf S, et al; SOLVD Investigators. Prediction of mortality and morbidity with a 6-minute walk test in patients with left ventricular dysfunction. *JAMA*. 1993;270:1702–1707.
56. Mark DE, Shaw L, Harrell FE Jr, et al. Prognostic value of a treadmill score in outpatients with suspected coronary artery disease. *N Engl J Med*. 1991;325:849–853.
57. Rogers FJ. Osteopathic considerations in cardiovascular medicine. In: Seffinger MA, ed. *Foundations for Osteopathic Medicine*. 4th ed. Wolters Kluwer; 2018:1229–1244.
58. Oliveira CB, Maher CG, Francium MR, et al. Co-occurrence of chronic musculoskeletal pain and cardiovascular diseases: a systematic review with meta-analysis. *Pain Medicine*. 2020;21(6):1106–1121.
59. Simons DG. Cardiology and myofascial trigger points: Janet G. Travell's contribution. *Tex Heart Inst J*. 2003;30(1):3–7.
60. Hegmann KT, Thiese MS, Wood EM, et al. Cardiovascular disease risk factors predict the development and numbers of common musculoskeletal disorders in a prospective cohort. *J Occup Environ Med*. 2023;65(8):e527–e533.
61. Rahman MM, Kopec JA, Cibere J, Goldsmith CH, Anis AH. The relationship between osteoarthritis and cardiovascular disease in a population health survey: a cross-sectional study. *BMJ Open*. 2013;3:e002624.
62. Salalnikas RG, Gradauskas L. Cervical osteochondrosis and angina pectoris. In: Blužas J, ed. *Ischemic Heart Disease: Diagnosis, Clinical Manifestations, and Prevention*. Kaunas: Institute of Cardiology; 1993:139–142.
63. Cox JM, Gideon D, Rogers FJ. Incidence of osteophytic lipping of the thoracic spine in coronary heart disease: results of a pilot study. *J Am Osteopath Assoc*. 1983;82(11):837–838.
64. Tsiligiannis T, Grivas T. Pulmonary function in children with idiopathic scoliosis. *Scoliosis*. 2012;7:7.
65. Chaudhry R, Miao JH, Rehman A. Physiology, cardiovascular. In: *StatPearls*. StatPearls Publishing; 2023. https://www.ncbi.nlm.nih.gov/books/NBK493197
66. Cardiac muscle and electrical activity. 2022. Accessed May 13, 2022. https://med.libretexts.org/@go/page/755
67. Nesheiwat Z, Goyal A, Jagtap M. Atrial fibrillation. In: *StatPearls*. StatPearls Publishing; 2023. https://www.ncbi.nlm.nih.gov/books/NBK526072
68. Nair R, Lamaa N. Pulmonary capillary wedge pressure. In: *StatPearls*. StatPearls Publishing; 2023.
69. Manuel J, Färber N, Gerlach DA, et al. Deciphering the neural signature of human cardiovascular regulation. *eLife*. 2020;9:e55316.
70. La Rovere MT, Porta A, Schwartz PJ. Autonomic control of the heart and its clinical impact. *Front Physiol*. 2020;11:582.
71. Kuchera M, Kuchera W. Osteopathic considerations in cardiovascular disorders. In: Kuchera M, Kuchera W, eds. *Osteopathic Considerations in Systemic Dysfunction*. 2nd rev ed. Greyden Press; 1994:53–78.
72. Floras JS, Ponikowski P. The sympathetic/parasympathetic imbalance in heart failure with reduced ejection fraction. *Eur Heart J*. 2015;36(30):1974–1982.
73. Guidi J, Lucente M, Sonino N, Fava GA. Allostatic load and its impact on health: a systematic review. *Psychother Psychosom*. 2020;90(1):11–27.
74. Hopkins DA, Bieger DJ, Steinbusch WM. Vagal efferent projections: viscerotopy, neurochemistry and effects of vagotomy. *Prog Brain Res*. 1996;107:79–96.
75. Silvani A, Calandra-Buonaura G, Dampney RA, Cortelli P. Brain–heart interactions: physiology and clinical implications. *Phil Trans R Soc A*. 2016;374:20150181.
76. Korr I. Spinal cord as organizer of disease processes. *J Am Osteopath Assoc*. 1976;76(1):35–45.
77. Chi JS, Kloner RA. Stress and myocardial infarction. *Heart*. 2003;89(5):475–476.
78. Giles PD, Hensel KL, Pacchia CF, Smith ML. Suboccipital decompression enhances heart rate variability indices of cardiac control in healthy subjects. *J Altern Complement Med*. 2013;19(2):92–96.
79. Writing Committee Members; Gulati M, Levy PD, Mukherjee D, et al. 2021 AHA/ACC/ASE/CHEST/SAEM/SCCT/SCMR Guideline for the Evaluation and Diagnosis of Chest Pain: Executive Summary: a report of the American College of Cardiology/American Heart Association Joint Committee on Clinical Practice Guidelines. *J Am Coll Cardiol*. 2021;78(22):2218–2261.
80. Greenslade JH, Cullen L, Parsonage W, et al. Examining the signs and symptoms experienced by individuals with suspected acute coronary syndrome in the Asia-Pacific region: a prospective observational study. *Ann Emerg Med*. 2012;60:777–785.
81. DeVon HA, Rosenfeld A, Steffen AD, Daya M. Sensitivity, specificity, and sex differences in symptoms reported on the 13-item Acute Coronary Syndrome Checklist. *J Am Heart Assoc*. 2014;3:e000586.
82. Ferry AV, Anand A, Strachan FE, et al. Presenting symptoms in men and women diagnosed with myocardial infarction using sex-specific criteria. *J Am Heart Assoc*. 2019;8:e012307.
83. DeVon HA, Mirzaei S, Zègre-Hemsey J. Typical and atypical symptoms of acute coronary syndrome: time to retire the terms? *J Am Heart Assoc*. 2020;9(7):e015539.
84. Myerburg RJ, Kessler KM, Castellanos A. Sudden cardiac death: epidemiology, transient risk, and intervention assessment. *Ann Intern Med*. 1993;119:1187–1197.
85. Greenland P, Smith SC, Grundy SM. Improving coronary heart disease risk assessment in asymptomatic people. Role of traditional risk factors in non-invasive cardiovascular tests. *Circulation*. 2001;104:1863–1867.
86. Cox M, Gorbis S, Dick L, Rogers JC, Rogers FJ. Palpable musculoskeletal findings in coronary artery disease. Results of a double blind study. *J Am Osteopath Assoc*. 1983;82:831–836.
87. Beal MC. Palpatory testing for somatic dysfunction in patients with cardiovascular disease. *J Am Osteopath Assoc*. 1983;82:822–831.
88. Nicholas AS, DeBias DA, Ehrenfeuchter W, et al. A somatic component to myocardial infarction. *Br Med J*. 1985;291:13–17.
89. Prieto H, Pena N, Shubrook JH, Talsma J. Hypertension: an osteopathic perspective. *AAO J*. 2020;30(2):27–34.
90. Beal MC. Viscerosomatic reflexes: a review. *J Am Osteopath Assoc*. 1985;85(12):53–68.
91. Wieting JM, Beal C, Roth GL, et al. The Effect of osteopathic manipulative treatment on postoperative medical and functional recovery of coronary artery bypass graft patients. *J Osteopath Med*. 2013;113(5):384–393.
92. King HH, Jänig W, Patterson MM. *The Science and Clinical Application of Manual Therapy*. Elsevier Health Sciences; 2010.
93. Berkowitz MR. Application of osteopathic manipulative treatment to a patient with unremitting chest pain and shortness of breath undergoing "Rule-Out Myocardial Infarction" protocol for one week. *Int J Osteopath Med*. 2012;15(2):73–77.
94. McEwen BS. Protective and damaging effects of stress mediators. *N Engl J Med*. 1998;338(3):171–179.
95. Cerritelli F, Carinci F, Pizzolorusso G, et al. Osteopathic manipulation as a complementary treatment for the prevention of cardiac complications: 12-Months follow-up of intima media and blood pressure on a cohort affected by hypertension. *J Bodyw Mov Ther*. 2011;15(1):68–74.
96. Seventh Report of Joint National Committee on Prevention, Detection, Evaluation, and Treatment of High Blood Pressure. National Heart, Lung, and Blood Institute. Accessed January 12, 2024. https://www.nhlbi.nih.gov/health-topics/seventh-report-of-joint-national-committee-on-prevention-detection-evaluation-and-treatment-high-blood-pressure
97. Whelton PK, Carey RM, Aronow WS, et al. 2017 ACC/AHA/AAPA/ABC/ACPM/AGS/APhA/ASH/ASPC/NMA/PCNA guideline for the prevention, detection, evaluation, and management of high blood pressure in adults: executive summary: a report of the American College of Cardiology/American Heart Association Task Force on Clinical Practice Guidelines. *Circulation*. 2018;138(17):e426–e483.
98. News Staff, AAFP News. AAFP issues new clinical practice guideline on hypertension. *Ann Fam Med*. 2023;21(2):190–191. https://www.aafp.org/dam/AAFP/documents/journals/afp/AAFPHypertensionGuideline.pdf
99. Mancia Chairperson G, Kreutz Co-Chair R, Brunström M, et al. 2023 ESH Guidelines for the management of arterial hypertension The Task Force for the management of arterial hypertension of the European Society of Hypertension Endorsed by the European Renal Association (ERA) and the International Society of Hypertension (ISH). *J Hypertens*. 2023;41(12):1874–2071.

100. Campbell NRC, Paccot Burnens M, Whelton PK, et al. 2021 World Health Organization guideline on pharmacological treatment of hypertension: Policy implications for the region of the Americas. *Lancet Reg Health Am.* 2022;9:100219.
101. NCD Risk Factor Collaboration (NCD-RisC). Worldwide trends in hypertension prevalence and progress in treatment and control from 1990 to 2019: a pooled analysis of 1201 population-representative studies with 104 million participants. *Lancet.* 2021;398(10304):957–980.
102. Gupta S, Brimble KS, Guyatt G, Mathew A, Januszewicz A, Prejbisz A. *Essential Hypertension. McMaster Textbook of Internal Medicine.* Medycyna Praktyczna. Accessed January 2, 2025. https://empendium.com/mcmtextbook/chapter/B31.II.2.20.1
103. Centers for Disease Control and Prevention. Cardiovascular diseases. Accessed January 12, 2024. https://www.cdc.gov/globalhealth/healthprotection/ncd/cardiovascular-diseases.html
104. Manosroi W, Williams GH. Genetics of human primary hypertension: focus on hormonal mechanisms. *Endocr Rev.* 2019;40(3):825–856.
105. Brook RD, Weder AB, Rajagopalan S. Environmental hypertensionology: the effects of environmental factors on blood pressure in clinical practice and research. *J Clin Hypertens.* 2011;13(11):836–842.
106. Saxena T, Ali AO, Saxena M. Pathophysiology of essential hypertension: an update. *Expert Rev Cardiovasc Ther.* 2018;16(12):879–887.
107. Lewington S, Clarke R, Qizilbash N, Peto R, Collins R; Prospective Studies Collaboration. Age-specific relevance of usual blood pressure to vascular mortality: a meta-analysis of individual data for one million adults in 61 prospective studies. *Lancet.* 2002;360(9349):1903–1913.
108. Nelson KE, Glonek T. *Somatic Dysfunction in Osteopathic Family Medicine.* 1st ed. LWW; 2006:263.
109. SCORE2 Working Group and ESC Cardiovascular Risk Collaboration. SCORE2 risk prediction algorithms: new models to estimate 10-year risk of cardiovascular disease in Europe. *Eur Heart J.* 2021;42(25):2439–2454.
110. Khalil H, Zeltser R. Antihypertensive medications. In: *StatPearls.* StatPearls Publishing; 2023.
111. Zhou D, Xi B, Zhao M, Wang L, Veeranki SP. Uncontrolled hypertension increases risk of all-cause and cardiovascular disease mortality in US adults: the NHANES III Linked Mortality Study. *Sci Rep.* 2018;8(1):9418.
112. Milman T, Joundi RA, Alotaibi NM, Saposnik G. Clinical inertia in pharmacological management of hypertension: a systematic review and meta-analysis. *Medicine (Baltimore).* 2018;97:e11121.
113. Burnier M, Egan BM. Adherence in hypertension: a review of prevalence, risk factors, impact and management. *Circ Res.* 2019;124:1124–1140.
114. Carey RM, Wright JT Jr, Taler SJ, Whelton PK. Guideline-driven management of hypertension: an evidence-based update. *Circ Res.* 2021; 128(7):827–846.
115. Arnet DK, Blumenthal RS, Albert MA, et al. 2019 ACC/AHA guideline on the primary prevention of cardiovascular disease: a report of the American College of Cardiology/American Heart Association Task Force on clinical practice guidelines. *Circulation.* 2019;140:e596–e646.
116. Conlin PR. The dietary approaches to stop hypertension (DASH) clinical trial: implications for lifestyle modifications in the treatment of hypertensive patients. *Cardiol Rev.* 1999;7(5):284–288.
117. Pescatello LS, MacDonald HV, Lamberti L, Johnson BT. Exercise for hypertension: a prescription update integrating existing recommendations with emerging research. *Curr Hypertens Rep.* 2015;17(11):87.
118. Edwards JJ, Deenmamode AHP, Griffiths M, et al. Exercise training and resting blood pressure: a large-scale pairwise and network meta-analysis of randomised controlled trials. *Br J Sports Med.* 2023;57(20):1317–1326.
119. Sharman JE, La Gerche A, Coombes JS. Exercise and cardiovascular risk in patients with hypertension. *Am J Hypertens.* 2015;28(2):147–158.
120. Hanssen H, Boardman H, Deiseroth A, et al. Personalized exercise prescription in the prevention and treatment of arterial hypertension: a Consensus Document from the European Association of Preventive Cardiology (EAPC) and the ESC Council on Hypertension. *Eur J Prev Cardiol.* 2022;29(1):205–215.
121. Lopes S, Mesquita-Bastos J, Garcia C, et al. Effect of exercise training on ambulatory blood pressure among patients with resistant hypertension: A randomized clinical trial. *JAMA Cardiol.* 2021;6(11):1317–1323.
122. D'Agostino RB, Vasan RS, Pencina MJ, et al. General cardiovascular risk profile for use in primary care. *Circulation.* 2008;117:743–753.
123. Frieden TR, Berwick DM. The "Million Hearts" initiative–preventing heart attacks and strokes. *N Engl J Med.* 2011;365:e27.
124. Lloyd-Jones DM, Huffman MD, Karmali KN, et al. Estimating longitudinal risks and benefits from cardiovascular preventive therapies among medicare patients: the million hearts longitudinal ASCVD risk assessment tool: a special report from the American Heart Association and American College of Cardiology. *Circulation.* 2017;135(13):e793–e813.
125. Brouwer TF, Collard D, van den Born BH. Blood pressure lowering treatment and the Framingham score: do not fear risk. *J Clin Hypertens (Greenwich).* 2019;21(12):1821–1822.
126. Ridker PM. The pooled cohort equations 3 years on. *Circulation.* 2016; 134:1789–1791.
127. Burns L. Viscero-somatic and somato-visceral spinal reflexes. *J Am Osteopath Assoc.* 1907;7:52–60.
128. Yates RG, Lamping DL, Abram NL, Wright C. Effects of chiropractic treatment on blood pressure and anxiety: a randomized, controlled trial. *J Manipulative Physiol Ther.* 1988;11(6):484–488.
129. Nelson KE, Glonek T. *Somatic Dysfunction in Osteopathic Family Medicine.* 2nd ed. LWW; 2015:290–292.
130. Spiegel AJ, Capobianco JD, Kruger A, Spinner WD. Osteopathic manipulative medicine in the treatment of hypertension: an alternative, conventional approach. *Heart Dis.* 2003;5(4):272–278.
131. Magoun H. *Osteopathy in the Cranial Field.* The Sutherland Cranial Teaching Foundation; 2006.
132. Ganong W. *Review of Medical Physiology.* 20th ed. Lange Medical Books/McGraw-Hill; 2001.
133. Sutherland W. *Contributions of Thought.* 2nd ed. Sutherland Cranial Teaching Foundation; 1998.
134. Frymann V. The osteopathic approach to cardiac and pulmonary problems. *J Am Osteopath Assoc.* 1978;77(9):668–673.
135. Northup TL. Manipulative management of hypertension. *J Am Osteopath Assoc.* 1961;60:973–978.
136. Mannino JR. The application of neurologic reflexes to the treatment of hypertension. *J Am Osteopath Assoc.* 1979;79:225–231.
137. Johnston WL, Kelso AF. Changes in the presence of a segmental dysfunction pattern associated with hypertension: 2. A long-term longitudinal study. *J Am Osteopath Assoc.* 1995;95:315–318.
138. Ioudina M, Toder E, Muyot A, Salloum L, Boo S, Concepcion J. Cardiovascular responses to selected cranial osteopathic manipulations in hypertensive patients. *FASEB J.* 2018;32(S1):lb321.
139. Centers for Disease Control and Prevention. Coronary Artery Disease (CAD). Accessed January 12, 2024. https://www.cdc.gov/heartdisease/coronary_ad.htm
140. Braunwald E. Unstable angina. An etiologic approach to management. *Circulation.* 1998:98:2219–2222.
141. Zhang L, Tong Z, Han R, et al. Global, regional, and national burdens of ischemic heart disease attributable to smoking from 1990 to 2019. *J Am Heart Assoc.* 2023;12:e028193.
142. Khan MA, Hashim MJ, Mustafa H, et al. Global epidemiology of ischemic heart disease: results from the global burden of disease study. *Cureus.* 2020;12(7):e9349.
143. Hijazi W, Jolly SS, Budaj A, Beręsewicz A, Undas A; Ischemic Heart Disease (IHD). *McMaster Textbook of Internal Medicine.* Medycyna Praktyczna; 2023. Accessed July 30, 2023. https://empendium.com/mcmtextbook/chapter/B31.II.2.5
144. Schwartz SM, Campbell GR, Campbell JH. Replication of smooth muscle cells in vascular disease. *Circulation Res.* 1986:58:427–444.
145. Geer JC. Fine structure of human aortic intimal chickening fatty streaks. *Lab Invest.* 1965;14:1764–1783.
146. Fuster V, Badimon I, Badimon JJ, Chesebro JH. The pathogenesis of coronary artery disease and the acute coronary syndromes. *N Engl J Med.* 1992:326:242–250, 310–318.
147. Ambrose JA, Winters SL, Stern A, et al. Angiographic morphology, and the pathogenesis of unstable angina pectoris. *J Am Coll Cardiol.* 1985:5:609–616.
148. Kolluru GK, Bir SC, Kevil CG. Endothelial dysfunction and diabetes: effects on angiogenesis, vascular remodeling, and wound healing. *Int J Vasc Med.* 2012;2012:918267.
149. Cai H, Harrison DG. Endothelial dysfunction in cardiovascular diseases: the role of oxidant stress. *Circ Res.* 2000;87(10):840–844.

150. DeJongste MT, Ter Horst GJ. Mediators of inflammation in patients with coronary artery disease. In: Ter Horst GJ, ed. *The Nervous System and the Heart.* Humana; 2000:467–487.
151. Expert Panel on Detection, Evaluation and Treatment of High Blood Cholesterol in Adults. Executive summary of the third report of the national cholesterol education program (NCEP) expert panel on detection, evaluation, and treatment of high blood cholesterol in adults (Adult Treatment Panel III). *JAMA.* 2001;285:2486–2497.
152. Grundy SM. National cholesterol education program: second report of the expert panel on detection, evaluation, and treatment of high blood cholesterol in adults. *Circulation.* 1994:89:1329–1445.
153. Ross R. Atherosclerosis- an inflammatory disease. *N Engl J Med.* 1999; 340(2):115–126.
154. Davies MJ, Thomas AC. Plaque fissuring: the cause of acute myocardial infarction, sudden ischemic death, and crescendo angina. *Br Heart J.* 1985;53(4):363–373.
155. Goyal A, Zeltser R. Unstable angina. In: *StatPearls [Internet].* StatPearls Publishing; 2023. https://www.ncbi.nlm.nih.gov/books/NBK442000/
156. Writing Committee Members; Virani SS, Newby LK, Arnold SV, et al. 2023 AHA/ACC/ACCP/ASPC/NLA/PCNA guideline for the management of patients with chronic coronary disease. *J Am Coll Cardiol.* 2023;82(9):833–955.
157. Mukherjee D. 2023 Multisociety guideline for managing chronic coronary disease: key perspectives. Latest in cardiology. 2023. https://www.acc.org/Latest-in-Cardiology/ten-points-to-remember/2023/07/17/19/06/2023-guideline-for-chronic-coronary-disease-gl-ccd
158. Winzer EB, Woitek F, Linke A. Physical activity in the prevention and treatment of coronary artery disease. *J Am Heart Assoc.* 2018;7(4):e007725.
159. Franklin BA, Rusia A, Haskin-Popp C, Tawney A. Chronic stress, exercise and cardiovascular disease: placing the benefits and risks of physical activity into perspective. *Int J Environ Res Public Health.* 2021;18(18):9922.
160. Akyuz A. Exercise and coronary heart disease. *Adv Exp Med Biol.* 2020; 1228:169–179.
161. Thompson PD, Franklin BA, Balady GJ, et al; American Heart Association Council on Nutrition, Physical Activity, and Metabolism; American Heart Association Council on Clinical Cardiology; American College of Sports Medicine. Exercise and acute cardiovascular events placing the risks into perspective: a scientific statement from the American Heart Association Council on Nutrition, Physical Activity, and Metabolism and the Council on Clinical Cardiology. *Circulation.* 2007;115(17):2358–2368.
162. Bracker MD. Cardiac rehabilitation. In: Sallies RE, Massimino F, eds. *Essentials of Sports Medicine.* 1st ed. Mosby-Year Book Inc; 1997:2–7.
163. Liu X, Oliver G. New insights about the lymphatic vasculature in cardiovascular diseases. *F1000Res.* 2019;8:F1000 Faculty Rev-1811.
164. Bozkurt B, Coats AJ, Tsutsui H, et al. Universal definition and classification of heart failure: a report of the Heart Failure Society of America, Heart Failure Association of the European Society of Cardiology, Japanese Heart Failure Society and Writing Committee of the Universal Definition of Heart Failure. *J Card Fail.* 2021;27:387–413.
165. Malik A, Brito D, Vaqar S, et al. Congestive heart failure. In: *StatPearls [Internet].* StatPearls Publishing; 2023. https://www.ncbi.nlm.nih.gov/books/NBK430873/
166. Kim IC, Yoo BS. Multidimensional approach of heart failure diagnosis and prognostication utilizing cardiac imaging with biomarkers. *Diagnostics (Basel).* 2022;12(6):1366.
167. Writing Group Members; Mozaffarian D, Benjamin EJ, Go AS, et al. Executive summary: heart disease and stroke statistics–2016 update: a report from the American Heart Association. *Circulation.* 2016;133(4):447–454.
168. Benjamin EJ, Blaha MJ, Chiuve SE, et al. Heart Disease and Stroke Statistics-2017 Update: a report from the American Heart Association. *Circulation.* 2017;135(10):e146–e603.
169. Ponikowski P, Anker SD, AlHabib KF, et al. Heart failure: preventing disease and death worldwide. *ESC Heart Fail.* 2014;1(1):4–25.
170. Hajouli S, Ludhwani D. Heart failure and ejection fraction. In: *StatPearls [Internet].* StatPearls Publishing; 2023. https://www.ncbi.nlm.nih.gov/books/NBK553115/
171. Sidney S, Go AS, Jaffe MG, Solomon MD, Ambrosy AP, Rana JS. Association between aging of the US population and heart disease mortality from 2011 to 2017. *JAMA Cardiol.* 2019;4(12):1280–1286.
172. Lan T, Liao YH, Zhang J, et al. Mortality and readmission rates after heart failure: a systematic review and meta-analysis. *Ther Clin Risk Manag.* 2021;17:1307–1320.
173. Abhayaratna WP, Smith WT, Becker NG, Marwick TH, Jeffery IM, Mcgill DA. Prevalence of heart failure and systolic ventricular dysfunction in older Australians: the Canberra Heart Study. *Med J Aust.* 2006;184:151–154.
174. Jencks SF, Williams MV, Coleman EA. Rehospitalizations among patients in the Medicare fee-for-service program. *J Vasc Surg.* 2009;50(1):234.
175. Giamouzis G, Kalogeropoulos A, Georgiopoulou V, et al. Hospitalization epidemic in patients with heart failure: risk factors, risk prediction, knowledge gaps, and future directions. *J Card Fail.* 2011;17(1):54–75.
176. Wang SY, Valero-Elizondo J, Ali HJ, et al. Out-of-pocket annual health expenditures and financial toxicity from healthcare costs in patients with heart failure in the United States. *J Am Heart Assoc.* 2021;10(14): e022164.
177. Ho KK, Pinsky JL, Kannel WB, Levy D. The epidemiology of heart failure: the Framingham Study. *J Am Coll Cardiol.* 1993;22(4 Suppl A): 6A–13A.
178. Huffman MD, Berry JD, Ning H, et al. Lifetime risk for heart failure among White and Black Americans: cardiovascular lifetime risk pooling project. *J Am Coll Cardiol.* 2013;61(14):1510–1517.
179. Bennett JA, Riegel B, Bittner V, Nichols J. Validity, and reliability of the NYHA classes for measuring research outcomes in patients with cardiac disease. *Heart Lung.* 2002;31(4):262–270.
180. Yusuf S, Rangarajan S, Teo K, et al. Cardiovascular risk and events in 17 low-, middle-, and high-income countries. *N Engl J Med.* 2014;371(9): 818–827.
181. Savarese G, Becher PM, Lund LH, Seferovic P, Rosano GMC, Coats AJS. Global burden of heart failure: a comprehensive and updated review of epidemiology. *Cardiovasc Res.* 2023;118(17):3272–3287.
182. Seferović PM, Polovina M, Bauersachs J, et al. Heart failure in cardiomyopathies: a position paper from the Heart Failure Association of the European Society of Cardiology. *Eur J Heart Fail.* 2019;21(5):553–576.
183. Benedict CR, Johnstone DE, Weiner DH, et al. Relation of neurohumoral activation to clinical variables and degree of ventricular dysfunction: a report from the Registry of Studies of Left Ventricular Dysfunction. SOLVD Investigators. *J Am Coll Cardiol.* 1994;23(6):1410–1420.
184. Drau VJ. Contributions of neuroendocrine and local autocrine-paracrine mechanisms to the pathophysiology and pharmacology of congestive heart failure. *Am J Cardiol.* 1982;62:76E–81E.
185. Rogers FJ. The muscle hypothesis: a model of chronic heart failure appropriate for osteopathic medicine. *J Am Osteopath Assoc.* 2001;101(10): 576–583.
186. Kamiya K, Masuda T, Matsue Y, et al. Complementary role of arm circumference to body mass index in risk stratification of heart failure. *JACC Heart Fail.* 2016;4(4):265–273.
187. Jones NR, Roalfe AK, Adoki I, Hobbs FDR, Taylor CJ. Survival of patients with chronic heart failure in the community: a systematic review and meta-analysis. *Eur J Heart Fail.* 2019;21(11):1306–1325.
188. Solomon SD, Dobson J, Pocock S, et al. Influence of nonfatal hospitalization for heart failure on subsequent mortality in patients with chronic heart failure. *Circulation.* 2007;116(13):1482.
189. Ouwerkerk W, Voors AA, Zwinderman AH. Factors influencing the predictive power of models for predicting mortality and/or heart failure hospitalization in patients with heart failure. *JACC Heart Fail.* 2014; 2(5):429–436.
190. Dassanayaka S, Jones SP. Recent developments in heart failure. *Circ Res.* 2015;117(7):e58–e63.
191. Roberts E, Ludman AJ, Dworzynski K, et al. The diagnostic accuracy of the natriuretic peptides in heart failure: systematic review and diagnostic meta-analysis in the acute care setting. *BMJ.* 2015;350:h910.
192. Mant J, Doust J, Roalfe A, et al. Systematic review and individual patient data meta-analysis of diagnosis of heart failure, with modelling of implications of different diagnostic strategies in primary care. *Health Technol Assess.* 2009;13(32):1–207, iii.
193. Kelder JC, Cramer MJ, van Wijngaarden J, et al. The diagnostic value of physical examination and additional testing in primary care patients with suspected heart failure. *Circulation.* 2011;124(25):2865–2873.

194. Agha SA, Kalogeropoulos AP, Shih J, et al. Echocardiography, and risk prediction in advanced heart failure: incremental value over clinical markers. *J Card Fail.* 2009;15(7):586–592.
195. Yancy CW, Jessup M, Bozkurt B, et al. 2013 ACCF/AHA guideline for the management of heart failure: a report of the American College of Cardiology Foundation/American Heart Association Task Force on Practice Guidelines. *Circulation.* 2013;128(16):e240–e327.
196. https://medicalcriteria.com/web/category/criteria/cardiology/ Accessed January 2, 2025.
197. https://www.mdcalc.com/ Accessed January 2, 2025.
198. McKee PA, Castelli WP, McNamara PM, Kannel WB. The natural history of congestive heart failure: the Framingham study. *N Engl J Med.* 1971;285:1441.
199. Brindle P, Emberson J, Lampe F, et al. Predictive accuracy of the Framingham coronary risk score in British men: prospective cohort study. *BMJ.* 2003;327:1267–1270.
200. SPRINT Research Group; Wright JT, Williamson JD, Whelton PK, et al. A randomized trial of intensive versus standard blood-pressure control. *N Engl J Med.* 2015;373(22):2103–2116.
201. Pradhan A, Vohra S, Vishwakarma P, Sethi R. Review on sodium-glucose cotransporter 2 inhibitor (SGLT2i) in diabetes mellitus and heart failure. *J Family Med Prim Care.* 2019;8(6):1855–1862.
202. Cattadori G, Segurini C, Picozzi A, Padeletti L, Anzà C. Exercise and heart failure: an update. *ESC Heart Fail.* 2017;5(2):222–232.
203. Dibben GO, Hannay JR, Taylor RS. Exercise training in heart failure. *Heart.* 2024;110(5):373–381.
204. Morris JH. Exercise training and heart failure: a review of the literature. 2019;5(1):57–61.
205. Masarone D, Martucci ML, Errigo V, Pacileo G. The Use of β-blockers in heart failure with reduced ejection fraction. *J Cardiovasc Dev Dis.* 2021;8(9):101.
206. Kim Y, Boucher M, Argáez C. Ifunny channel inhibitors: an emerging option for heart failure. In: *CADTH Issues in Emerging Health Technologies.* Canadian Agency for Drugs and Technologies in Health; 2016–2021: 151.
207. Vishram-Nielsen JKK, Tomasoni D, Gustafsson F, Metra M. Contemporary drug treatment of advanced heart failure with reduced ejection fraction. *Drugs.* 2022;82(4):375–405.
208. Patel J, Rassekh N, Fonarow GC, et al. Guideline-directed medical therapy for the treatment of heart failure with reduced ejection fraction. *Drugs.* 2023;83(9):747–759.
209. Mebazaa A, Davison B, Chioncel O, et al. Safety, tolerability and efficacy of up-titration of guideline-directed medical therapies for acute heart failure (STRONG-HF): a multinational, open-label, randomised, trial. *Lancet.* 2022;400(10367):1938–1952.
210. Pitt B, Pfeffer MA, Assmann SF, et al. Spironolactone for heart failure with preserved ejection fraction. *N Engl J Med.* 2014;370(15): 1383–1392.
211. Ponikowski P, Voors AA, Anker SD, et al. 2016 ESC Guidelines for the diagnosis and treatment of acute and chronic heart failure: the Task Force for the Diagnosis and Treatment of Acute and Chronic Heart Failure of the European Society of Cardiology (ESC)Developed with the special contribution of the Heart Failure Association (HFA) of the ESC. *Eur Heart J.* 2016;37(27):2129–2200.
212. Wong EC, Fordyce CB, Wong G, et al. Predictors of the use of mineralocorticoid receptor antagonists in patients with left ventricular dysfunction post-ST-segment-elevation myocardial infarction. *J Am Heart Assoc.* 2021;10(14):e019167.
213. Heart Failure Society of America; Lindenfeld J, Albert NM, Boehmer JP, et al. HFSA 2010 comprehensive heart failure practice guideline. *J Card Fail.* 2010;16(6):e1–e194.
214. Lund LH, Edwards LB, Kucheryavaya AY, et al. The registry of the International Society for Heart and Lung Transplantation: thirty-first official adult heart transplant report–2014; focus theme: retransplantation. *J Heart Lung Transplant.* 2014;33(10):996–1008.
215. Xiao YF. Cardiac arrhythmia and heart failure: from bench to bedside. *J Geriatr Cardiol.* 2011;8(3):131–132.
216. Udani SM, Koyner JL. The effects of heart failure on renal function. *Cardiol Clin.* 2010;28(3):453–465.
217. Beemath A, Stein PD, Skaf E, Al Sibae MR, Alesh I. Risk of venous thromboembolism in patients hospitalized with heart failure. *Am J Cardiol.* 2006;98(6):793–795.
218. Yao S, Hassani J, Gagne M, George G, Gilliar W. Osteopathic manipulative treatment as a useful adjunctive tool for pneumonia. *J Vis Exp.* 2014;(87):50687.
219. Earley BE, Luce H. An introduction to clinical research in osteopathic medicine. *Prim Care.* 2010;37(1):49–64.
220. Chin AJ, Fischione AD, Shilian R, et al. Tolerance of rib raising among hospitalized patients: a pilot study. *J Osteopath Med.* 2019;119(1):19–23.
221. Remien K, Vilella RC. Osteopathic manipulative treatment: lymphatic procedures. In: *StatPearls.* StatPearls Publishing; 2023.
222. Bordoni B, Morabito B, Simonelli M, et al. Osteopathic approach with a patient undergoing cardiac transplantation: the five diaphragms. *Int Med Case Rep J.* 2019;12:303–308.
223. Amatuzzi F, Gervazoni Balbuena de Lima AC, Da Silva ML, et al. Acute and time-course effects of osteopathic manipulative treatment on vascular and autonomic function in patients with heart failure: a randomized trial. *J Manipulative Physiol Ther.* 2021;44(6):455–466.
224. Thomaz S, Cipriano G, Cahalin L, et al. Osteopathic manipulative treatment/myofascial release upon the resistive index/blood pressure in heart failure. *Arch Phys Med Rehabil.* 2017;98(10):89.
225. Thomaz S, Cipriano G, Cahalin L, et al. Osteopathic manipulative treatment (OMT) and circuit resistance training (CRT) in heart failure. *Arch Phys Med Rehabil.* 2017;98(10):88–89.
226. Nesheiwat Z, Goyal A, Jagtap M, et al. Atrial fibrillation (nursing). In: *StatPearls.* StatPearls Publishing; 2023.
227. Lippi G, Sanchis-Gomar F, Cervellin G. Global epidemiology of atrial fibrillation: an increasing epidemic and public health challenge. *Int J Stroke.* 2021;16(2):217–221.
228. Markides V, Schilling RJ. Atrial fibrillation: classification, pathophysiology, mechanisms and drug treatment. *Heart.* 2003;89(8):939–943.
229. Camm AJ, Kirchhof P, Lip GY, et al. Guidelines for the management of atrial fibrillation: the Task Force for the Management of Atrial Fibrillation of the European Society of Cardiology (ESC). *Eur Heart J.* 2010;31(19):2369–2429.
230. January CT, Wann LS, Calkins H, et al. 2019 AHA/ACC/HRS Focused Update of the 2014 AHA/ACC/HRS Guideline for the Management of Patients with atrial fibrillation: a report of the American College of Cardiology/American Heart Association Task Force on Clinical Practice Guidelines and the Heart Rhythm Society. *J Am Coll Cardiol.* 2019;74(1):104–132.
231. Elliott AD, Mahajan R, Pathak RK, Lau DH, Sanders P. Exercise training and atrial fibrillation. *Circulation.* 2016;133(5):457–459.
232. Sepehri Shamloo A, Arya A, Dagres N, Hindricks G. Exercise and atrial fibrillation: some good news and some bad news. *Galen Med J.* 2018;7: e1401.
233. Wołowiec Ł, Grześk G, Osiak J, et al. Beta-blockers in cardiac arrhythmias-Clinical pharmacologist's point of view. *Front Pharmacol.* 2023;13:1043714.
234. Weiss BD, Walling A. Fitness-related cardiac arrhythmias. *Am Fam Physician.* 2019;99(2):78–79.
235. Tabina A, Leleka E, Mazalskiy K. Results of osteopathic treatment of patients with paroxysmal atrial fibrillation. *J Bodyw Mov Ther.* 2018; 22(4):858.
236. Stauss HM. Heart rate variability. *Am J Physiol Regul Integr Comp Physiol.* 2003;285(5):R927–R931.
237. Carnevali L, Lombardi L, Fornari M, Sgoifo A. Exploring the effects of osteopathic manipulative treatment on autonomic function through the lens of heart rate variability. *Front Neurosci.* 2020;14:579365.
238. Carnevali L, Cerritelli F, Guolo F, Sgoifo A. Osteopathic manipulative treatment and cardiovascular autonomic parameters in rugby players: a randomized, sham-controlled trial. *J Manipulative Physiol Ther.* 2021; 44(4):319–329.
239. Henley CE, Ivins D, Mills M, Wen FK, Benjamin BA. Osteopathic manipulative treatment and its relationship to autonomic nervous system activity as demonstrated by heart rate variability: a repeated measures study. *Osteopath Med Prim Care.* 2008;2:7.
240. Ruffini N, D'Alessandro G, Mariani N, Pollastrelli A, Cardinali L, Cerritelli F. Variations of high frequency parameter of heart rate variability

following osteopathic manipulative treatment in healthy subjects compared to control group and sham therapy: randomized controlled trial. *Front Neurosci.* 2015;9:272.

241. Khan AA, Lip GYH, Shantsila A. Heart rate variability in atrial fibrillation: the balance between sympathetic and parasympathetic nervous system. *Eur J Clin Invest.* 2019;49(11):e13174.
242. Moore K, Dalley AF, Agur AMR. *Clinically Oriented Anatomy.* 9th ed. Wolters Kluwer; 2022.
243. Kuchera ML, Kuchera WA. *Osteopathic Considerations in Systemic Dysfunction.* Rev 2nd ed. Greyden Press; 1994.
244. Bevan GH, White Solaru KT. Evidence-based medical management of peripheral artery disease. *Arterioscler Thromb Vasc Biol.* 2020;40(3): 541–553.
245. Tendera M, Aboyans V, Bartelink ML, et al; ESC Committee for Practice Guidelines. ESC Guidelines on the diagnosis and treatment of peripheral artery diseases: document covering atherosclerotic disease of extracranial carotid and vertebral, mesenteric, renal, upper and lower extremity arteries: the Task Force on the Diagnosis and Treatment of Peripheral Artery Diseases of the European Society of Cardiology (ESC). *Eur Heart J.* 2011; 32(22):2851–2906.
246. Gul F, Janzer SF. Peripheral vascular disease. In: *StatPearls.* StatPearls Publishing; 2023.
247. Sampson UKA, Fowkes FGR, Naidoo NG, Criqui MH. Peripheral artery disease. In: Prabhakaran D, Anand S, Gaziano TA, Mbanya JC, Wu Y, Nugent R, eds. *Cardiovascular, Respiratory, and Related Disorders.* 3rd ed. The International Bank for Reconstruction and Development/The World Bank; 2017.
248. Conte MS, Bradbury AW, Kolh P, et al. Global vascular guidelines on the management of chronic limb-threatening ischemia. *Eur J Vasc Endovasc Surg.* 2019;58:S1–S109.e33.
249. Lazar A, Morrissey N. Recent advances in endovascular treatment of peripheral arterial disease. *F1000Res.* 2020;9:F1000 Faculty Rev-122.
250. Wijnand JGJ, Zarkowsky D, Wu B, et al. The Global Limb Anatomic Staging System (GLASS) for CLTI: improving inter-observer agreement. *J Clin Med.* 2021;10(16):3454.
251. Malekmohammad K, Bezsonov EE, Rafieian-Kopaei M. Role of lipid accumulation and inflammation in atherosclerosis: focus on molecular and cellular mechanisms. *Front Cardiovasc Med.* 2021;8:707529.
252. Olinic DM, Stanek A, Tătaru DA, Homorodean C, Olinic M. Acute limb ischemia: an update on diagnosis and management. *J Clin Med.* 2019;8(8):1215.
253. Dhaliwal G, Mukherjee D. Peripheral arterial disease: epidemiology, natural history, diagnosis and treatment. *Int J Angiol.* 2007;16(2):36–44.
254. Szalay D, Frołow M, Leśniak W, Bodzoń W. Lower extremity peripheral artery disease (PAD). In: *McMaster Textbook of Internal Medicine.* Medycyna Praktyczna; 2023. Accessed January 2, 2025. https://empendium.com/mcmtextbook/chapter/B31.II.2.27.1
255. McDermott MM, Greenland P, Liu K, et al. Leg symptoms in peripheral arterial disease: associated clinical characteristics and functional impairment. *JAMA.* 2001;286(13):1599–1606.
256. Krishna SM, Moxon JV, Golledge J. A review of the pathophysiology and potential biomarkers for peripheral artery disease. *Int J Mol Sci.* 2015;16(5):11294–11322.
257. Ehrman JK, Gardner AW, Salisbury D, Lui K, Treat-Jacobson D. Supervised exercise therapy for symptomatic peripheral artery disease: a review of current experience and practice-based recommendations. *J Cardiopulm Rehabil Prev.* 2023;43(1):15–21.
258. Lane R, Harwood A, Watson L, Leng GC. Exercise for intermittent claudication. *Cochrane Database Syst Rev.* 2017;12(12):CD000990.
259. Bendermacher BLW, Willigendael EM, Teijink JAW, Prins MH. Supervised exercise therapy versus non-supervised exercise therapy for intermittent claudication. *Cochrane Database Syst Rev.* 2006:CD005263.
260. American Diabetes Association. 2. Classification and diagnosis of diabetes. *Diabetes Care.* 2016;39(Suppl 1):S13–S22.
261. Mihaylova B, Emberson J, Blackwell L, et al; Cholesterol Treatment Trialists' (CTT) Collaborators. The effects of lowering LDL cholesterol with statin therapy in people at low risk of vascular disease: meta-analysis of individual data from 27 randomised trials. *Lancet.* 2012;380: 581–590.
262. Aung PP, Maxwell HG, Jepson RG, Price JF, Leng GC. Lipid-lowering for peripheral arterial disease of the lower limb. *Cochrane Database Syst Rev.* 2007:CD000123.
263. Rrapo-Kaso E, Loffler AI, Petroni GR, et al. Alirocumab and plaque volume, calf muscle blood flow, and walking performance in peripheral artery disease: a randomized clinical trial. *Vasc Med.* 2023;28(4):282–289.
264. Belch J, MacCuish A, Campbell I, et al; Prevention of Progression of Arterial Disease and Diabetes Study Group; Diabetes Registry Group; Royal College of Physicians Edinburgh. The prevention of progression of arterial disease and diabetes (POPADAD) trial: factorial randomised placebo-controlled trial of aspirin and antioxidants in patients with diabetes and asymptomatic peripheral arterial disease. *BMJ.* 2008;337:a1840.
265. Fowkes FG, Price JF, Stewart MC, et al. Aspirin for prevention of cardiovascular events in a general population screened for a low ankle brachial index: a randomized controlled trial. *JAMA.* 2010;303:841–848.
266. McNeil JJ, Nelson MR, Woods RL, et al; ASPREE Investigator Group. Effect of aspirin on all-cause mortality in the healthy elderly. *N Engl J Med.* 2018;379:1519–1528.
267. ASCEND Study Collaborative Group; Bowman L, Mafham M, Wallendszus K, et al. Effects of aspirin for primary prevention in persons with diabetes mellitus. *N Engl J Med.* 2018;379:1529–1539.
268. Antithrombotic Trialists' Collaboration. Collaborative meta-analysis of randomised trials of antiplatelet therapy for prevention of death, myocardial infarction, and stroke in high-risk patients. *BMJ.* 2002;324:71–86.
269. Catalano M, Born G, Peto R; Critical Leg Ischaemia Prevention Study (CLIPS) Group. Prevention of serious vascular events by aspirin amongst patients with peripheral arterial disease: randomized, double-blind trial. *J Intern Med.* 2007;261:276–284.
270. Kaplovitch E, Eikelboom JW, Dyal L, et al. Rivaroxaban and aspirin in patients with symptomatic lower extremity peripheral artery disease: a subanalysis of the COMPASS randomized clinical trial. *JAMA Cardiol.* 2021;6(1):21–29.
271. CAPRIE Steering Committee. A randomised, blinded, trial of Clopidogrel Versus Aspirin in Patients at Risk of Ischaemic Events (CAPRIE). *Lancet.* 1996;348:1329–1339.
272. Hiatt WR, Fowkes FG, Heizer G, et al; EUCLID Trial Steering Committee and Investigators. Ticagrelor versus clopidogrel in symptomatic peripheral artery disease. *N Engl J Med.* 2017;376:32–40.
273. Bhatt DL, Steg PG, Miller M, et al; REDUCE-IT Investigators. Cardiovascular risk reduction with icosapent ethyl for hypertriglyceridemia. *N Engl J Med.* 2019;380:11–22.
274. Anand S, Yusuf S, Xie C, et al; Warfarin Antiplatelet Vascular Evaluation Trial Investigators. Oral anticoagulant and antiplatelet therapy and peripheral arterial disease. *N Engl J Med.* 2007;357:217–227.
275. Mega JL, Braunwald E, Wiviott SD, et al; ATLAS ACS 2–timi 51 Investigators. Rivaroxaban in patients with a recent acute coronary syndrome. *N Engl J Med.* 2012;366:9–19.
276. Krantz MJ, Debus SE, Hsia J, et al. Low-dose rivaroxaban plus aspirin in older patients with peripheral artery disease undergoing acute limb revascularization: insights from the VOYAGER PAD trial. *Eur Heart J.* 2021;42(39):4040–4048.
277. Heart Protection Study Collaborative Group. Randomized trial of the effects of cholesterol-lowering with simvastatin on peripheral vascular and other major vascular outcomes in 20,536 people with peripheral arterial disease and other high-risk conditions. *J Vasc Surg.* 2007;45:645–654; discussion 653–654.
278. Armstrong EJ, Chen DC, Singh GD, Amsterdam EA, Laird JR. Angiotensin-converting enzyme inhibitor or angiotensin receptor blocker use is associated with reduced major adverse cardiovascular events among patients with critical limb ischemia. *Vasc Med.* 2015;20:237–244.
279. Feringa HH, van Waning VH, Bax JJ, et al. Cardioprotective medication is associated with improved survival in patients with peripheral arterial disease. *J Am Coll Cardiol.* 2006;47:1182–1187.
280. Zanchetti A, Julius S, Kjeldsen S, et al. Outcomes in subgroups of hypertensive patients treated with regimens based on valsartan and amlodipine: an analysis of findings from the VALUE trial. *J Hypertens.* 2006;24: 2163–2168.
281. Piller LB, Simpson LM, Baraniuk S, et al; ALLHAT Collaborative Research Group. Characteristics and long-term follow-up of participants

with peripheral arterial disease during ALLHAT. *J Gen Intern Med.* 2014;29:1475–1483.

282. ALLHAT Officers and Coordinators for the ALLHAT Collaborative Research Group. The antihypertensive and lipid-lowering treatment to prevent Heart Attack Trial. Major outcomes in high-risk hypertensive patients randomized to angiotensin-converting enzyme inhibitor or calcium channel blocker vs diuretic: the Antihypertensive and Lipid-Lowering Treatment to Prevent Heart Attack Trial (ALLHAT). *JAMA.* 2002;288:2981–2997.
283. Thukkani AK, Kinlay S. Endovascular intervention for peripheral artery disease. *Circ Res.* 2015;116(9):1599–1613.
284. Baerlocher MO, Kennedy SA, Rajebi MR, et al. Meta-analysis of drug-eluting balloon angioplasty and drug-eluting stent placement for infrainguinal peripheral arterial disease. *J Vasc Interv Radiol.* 2015; 26(4):459–473.e4.
285. Holden A. The use of intravascular lithotripsy for the treatment of severely calcified lower limb arterial CTOs. *J Cardiovasc Surg (Torino).* 2019;60(1):3–7.
286. Mufarrih SH, Khan MS, Qureshi NQ, et al. An endovascular- versus a surgery-first revascularization strategy for chronic limb-threatening ischemia: a meta-analysis of randomized controlled trials. *Am J Cardiol.* 2024;214:149–156.
287. Tsai SY, Li YS, Lee CH, et al. Mono or dual antiplatelet therapy for treating patients with peripheral artery disease after lower extremity revascularization: a systematic review and meta-analysis. *Pharmaceuticals (Basel).* 2022;15(5):596.
288. Jardine WM, Gillis C, Rutherford D. The effect of osteopathic manual therapy on the vascular supply to the lower extremity in individuals with knee osteoarthritis: a randomized trial. *Int J Osteopath Med.* 2012; 15(4):125–133.
289. Lombardini R, Marchesi S, Collebrusco L, et al. The use of osteopathic manipulative treatment as adjuvant therapy in patients with peripheral arterial disease. *Man Ther.* 2009;14(4):439–443.
290. Knott EM, Tune JD, Stoll ST, Downey HF. Increased lymphatic flow in the thoracic duct during manipulative intervention. *J Am Osteopath Assoc.* 2005;105(10):447–456.
291. Anglund DC, Channell MK. Contribution of osteopathic medicine to care of patients with chronic wounds. *J Am Osteopath Assoc.* 2011;111(9): 538–542.
292. Serruys PW, Morice MC, Kappetein AP, et al. Percutaneous coronary intervention versus coronary-artery bypass grafting for severe coronary artery disease. *N Engl J Med.* 2009;360(10):961–972.
293. Arosty JM. Patient education: recovery after coronary artery bypass graft surgery (CABG) (Beyond the Basics). UpToDate. Accessed January 15, 2024. https://www.uptodate.com/contents/recovery-after-coronary-artery-bypass-graft-surgery-cabg-beyond-the-basics
294. Bachar BJ, Manna B. Coronary artery bypass graft. In: *StatPearls [Internet].* StatPearls Publishing; 2023. https://www.ncbi.nlm.nih.gov/books/NBK507836
295. iData Research. How many cardiac surgeries are performed each year? Accessed August 9, 2022. https://idataresearch.com/over-900000-cardiac-surgeries-performed-every-year-in-the-united-states
296. Alexander JH, Smith PK. Coronary-artery bypass grafting. *N Engl J Med.* 2016;375:e22.
297. Writing Committee Members; Lawton J, Tamis-Holland J, Bangalore S, et al. 2021 ACC/AHA/SCAI guideline for coronary artery revascularization: a report of the American College of Cardiology/American Heart Association Joint Committee on Clinical Practice Guidelines. *J Am Coll Cardiol.* 2022;79(2):e21–e129.
298. Jha P, Ranchod A, Weerakkody Y, et al. Coronary artery bypass graft. Accessed January 2, 2025. Radiopedia.org. https://radiopaedia.org/articles/coronary-artery-bypass-graft?lang=us
299. Stenman M, Jeppsson A, Pivodic A, Sartipy U, Nielsen SJ. Risk of depression after coronary artery bypass grafting: a SWEDEHEART population-based cohort study. *Eur Heart J Open.* 2022;2(2):oeac015.
300. Doyle MP, Indraratna P, Tardo DT, Peeceeyen SC, Peoples GE. Safety and efficacy of aerobic exercise commenced early after cardiac surgery: a systematic review and meta-analysis. *Eur J Prev Cardiol.* 2019;26(1):36.
301. Osailan A, Abdelbasset WK. Exercise-based cardiac rehabilitation for postcoronary artery bypass grafting and its effect on hemodynamic responses and functional capacity evaluated using the Incremental Shuttle Walking Test: a retrospective pilot analysis. *J Saudi Heart Assoc.* 2020;32(1):25–33.
302. Shan R, Zhang L, Zhu Y, et al. Effect of early exercise rehabilitation on cardiopulmonary function and quality of life in patients after coronary artery bypass grafting. *Contrast Media Mol Imaging.* 2022;2022:4590037.
303. Racca V, Bordoni B, Castiglioni P, Modica M, Ferratini M. Osteopathic manipulative treatment improves heart surgery outcomes: a randomized controlled trial. *Ann Thorac Surg.* 2017;104:145–152.
304. O-Yurvati AH. Hemodynamic effects of osteopathic manipulative treatment immediately after coronary artery bypass graft surgery. *J Am Osteopath Assoc.* 2005;105(10):475–481.
305. Roncada G. Osteopathic treatment leads to significantly greater reductions in chronic thoracic pain after CABG surgery: a randomised controlled trial. *J Bodyw Mov Ther.* 2020;24(3):202–211.
306. Mehaffey JH, Hayanga JWA, Kawsara M, et al. Contemporary coronary artery bypass grafting vs multivessel percutaneous coronary intervention. *Ann Thorac Surg.* 2023;116(6):1213–1220.
307. Spertus JA, Jones PG, Maron DJ, et al. Health-status outcomes with invasive or conservative care in coronary disease. *N Engl J Med.* 2020; 382:1408–1419.
308. Weintraub WS, Spertus JA, Kolm P, et al. Effect of PCI on quality of life in patients with stable coronary disease. *N Engl J Med.* 2008;359: 677–687.
309. Writing Committee Members; Dehmer G, Grines C, Bakaeen FG, et al. 2023 AHA/ACC clinical performance and quality measures for coronary artery revascularization: a report of the American College of Cardiology/American Heart Association Joint Committee on performance measures. *J Am Coll Cardiol.* 2023;82(11):1131–1174.
310. Gaudino M, Chadow D, Rahouma M, et al. Operative outcomes of women undergoing coronary artery bypass surgery in the US, 2011 to 2020. *JAMA Surg.* 2023;158(5):494–-502.
311. Pezeshki PS, Masoudkabir F, Pashang M, et al. 7-year outcomes in diabetic patients after coronary artery bypass graft in a developing country. *BMC Cardiovasc Disord.* 2023;23:248.
312. Rizkalla MN, Henderson KK. Empathy and osteopathic manipulative medicine: is it all in the hands? *J Osteopath Med.* 2018;118(9):573–585.

72 Osteopathic Considerations in Pulmonology

JORDAN L. BARRY ▪ KURT P. HEINKING

KEY CONCEPTS

- Osteopathic pulmonology is patient-centered and considers the interaction between body, mind, and spirit.
- Osteopathic approaches have significantly contributed to the understanding of prevention and treatment of lung diseases, including pneumonia, chronic obstructive pulmonary diseases, lung cancer, respiratory distress syndrome, and postoperative pulmonary complications.
- Osteopathic pulmonology considers costal cage mechanics, neurocirculatory integration, and lung structure and function in its approach to the patient.
- The presence of somatic dysfunction can impair these structure and function relationships, potentially impairing gas exchange, local metabolism, and the effective pumping mechanism for lymphatic drainage.
- Osteopathic physicians and researchers have documented the benefit of the application of osteopathic manipulative treatment (OMT) for somatic dysfunction, pulmonary function, and lymphatic drainage.

INTRODUCTION

Pulmonology, a subspecialty of Internal Medicine, refers to the study of lung diseases and has continued to expand. From the earliest studies on diseases including tuberculosis (TB) to the more recent COVID-19 pandemic, knowledge and treatment of diseases of the pulmonary system have evolved greatly over time. The field of pulmonology itself continues to expand, especially with further growth in the practice of interventional pulmonology. Technologic advances including spirometry, flexible bronchoscopy, and the use of the mechanical ventilator outside of the operating room have widened the scope of practice.

While its focus primarily spans a single organ, the field of pulmonology is intertwined with numerous body systems. Through its function in conjunction to these other body systems, the respiratory system serves as a pinnacle example of osteopathic medicine, principles, and practice. Due to this interconnected nature, osteopathic physicians have contributed to the evolution of the field since the beginning of pulmonary medicine. Osteopathic training further prepares its physicians with knowledge of the body as a whole and its intricate interconnected mechanisms. This training is especially advantageous with the evolution of pulmonology to encompass further specialization into areas including critical care and sleep medicine. The number of osteopathic physicians practicing in these specialties has grown, and the practices of critical care and sleep medicine also require understanding of the body as a whole.

An osteopathic approach to the pulmonary patient places primary consideration on the patient and is not solely focused on the disease process. Equally important as treating the disease adequately is supporting the host through the life changing factors that occur with chronic pulmonary disease. Almost every aspect of the patient's life can be affected by pulmonary disease; this is especially true when facing barriers to normal daily activity or decreased physical activity. Many patients with pulmonary conditions may feel a loss of autonomy due to their disease processes, leaving them feeling powerless and without control. In addition to medical management, osteopathic physicians can encourage patient involvement by teaching a maintenance program of exercises (stretching, range of motion, or strengthening) directly related to the musculoskeletal manifestations of their illness. This may afford them a way to improve their own condition, decrease their pain, improve their outlook, and relieve some of their fears and anxieties.

There is a significant interrelationship of structure and function between the pulmonary system and the musculoskeletal system. For optimal lung functioning, movement of the thoracic cage, ribs, and spinal joints should be unrestricted and coordinated. This is also true between the coordinated movement of the abdominal diaphragm and accessory muscles of respiration. Proper neural, hormonal, vascular, and lymphatic functioning is critical not only for gas exchange but for disease prevention. Somatic dysfunction can alter these neural, vascular, lymphatic, and structural elements, worsening any underlying pathophysiologic process. Knowing this information, the informed osteopathic physician can create a management plan that includes medical or surgical management, emotional support, and treatment of associated somatic dysfunction. Treatment of associated somatic dysfunction has been shown not only to reduce pain and immobility, but also improve mortality in patients with inflammatory and infectious diseases involving the lungs.[1]

Please review Chapter 15 Anatomy, Mechanics, and Physiology of Pulmonary Respiration, as many concepts will be discussed throughout the chapter.

PATIENT ASSESSMENT

Observation

The physical examination of the pulmonary patient begins with observation of the patient's general appearance. It is important to determine if the patient appears acutely ill, is uncomfortable or anxious, or has difficulty talking or moving. Signs of acute hypoxemia include restlessness, tachypnea, cyanosis, and use of accessory muscles. In young children or infants, clinicians should be aware of nasal flaring as an additional sign of respiratory distress. One characteristic position that some patients may assume to help decrease their work of breathing in signs of distress is the "tripoding" position. This position involves a patient sitting or standing upright, leaning forward, often resting their upper extremities on a surface in front of them or on their lower extremities, and extending their neck. Other physical exam findings such as peripheral edema and jugular venous distention may suggest cardiopulmonary conditions affecting the lungs, indicating need for further intervention.

In some chronic pulmonary conditions, the chest and rib cage may take on characteristic appearances. In chronic obstructive pulmonary disease (COPD), patients can develop adaptations and scarring due to the chronic nature of their condition. In patients with emphysema, destruction of lung tissue and trapping of air within the lungs causes many patients to develop an outwardly expanded chest (in the anterior–posterior direction) in which relaxation on exhalation is limited. This is often called a "barrel chest" appearance.[2] In addition, respiratory distress and increased work of respiration can lead to accessory muscle use. Patients requiring constant use of these muscles to compensate for decreased effectiveness of the primary muscles of breathing, including the diaphragm, may develop hypertrophy of the accessory muscles.

Eliciting Patient History

In any patient, a detailed history of health and illness is of utmost importance to obtain. Patients with pulmonary conditions are no exception. However, a patient in acute pulmonary distress may present with symptomatic barriers (i.e., shortness of breath, wheezing, cough) or require prompt treatment (i.e., ventilation or other assistive respiration devices) which prevent acquisition of a full history. In any case, detailed review of medical records and discussions with other members of the team or companions of the patient can be helpful to obtain baseline history. In assessing the chief complaint, a detailed determination of the character and frequency of symptoms is obtained. These may include cough, dyspnea, chest pain, wheezing, hemoptysis, and sputum production. It is important to differentiate whether this is an acute condition, an acute exacerbation of a chronic condition, or a recurrent chronic condition.

Eliciting a history of present illness in pulmonary conditions requires specific questioning. Respiratory symptoms to elicit include cough, dyspnea, difficulty with inhalation or exhalation, hemoptysis, fever, disordered sleep, congestion, sinus pressure, postnasal drip, and changes in vision, hearing, or swallowing.

Potential for infection must be determined, whether this be environmental or social. For example, a practitioner must consider any exposure of the patient to infection, such as recent social contact of the patient or environmental exposures. The patient should be asked about any recent illnesses of other people who live in their home or with whom they spend their time, and age groups of these individuals. Exposure risk includes consideration of any societal pulmonary conditions particular to their geographic location (i.e., fungal infections endemic to areas of the United States). Likewise, recent and remote travel history must be obtained to stratify other potential risk of endemic infection or environmental exposures. Occupational history is also important due to exposure to particulate matter, toxins, fumes, smoke, or infectious agents. Any of these environmental exposures may contribute to their pulmonary condition. Smoking status and other drug use should be reviewed with the patients, including information about length of smoking history, amount smoked, form of smoking, and attempts to quit.

Practitioners should inquire about family history of lung disease or lung cancer, exposure to secondhand smoke, or rheumatologic diseases. Other medical conditions and body systems should be reviewed, especially within the cardiac system due to its close relationship and dependence on the pulmonary system. In addition, the history of any allergies and reactions to allergens, allergy testing results, or episodes of atopic dermatitis is important to obtain, as these may be related to pulmonary conditions such as asthma. It is important to review the patient's medications including over-the-counter drugs and supplements, as some may have respiratory side effects. Patients should be asked about their sleep history, including sleep latency, duration, quality, and symptoms they may experience including shortness of breath, cough, sleep apnea, snoring, or daytime sleepiness. While this information is important for assessment of many pulmonary conditions, pulmonologists also manage patients with snoring, narcolepsy, and sleep apnea. Complete history also includes information on previous respiratory illnesses, surgeries, emergency room visits, intubations, hospitalizations, and any ongoing treatment, both gathered from the patient and from prior consultations or studies.

Physical Examination

In osteopathic medicine, a physical exam should be thorough and encompass all body systems to gain knowledge of the whole patient. This includes inspection, auscultation, palpation, percussion, musculoskeletal assessment, and special tests. All of this information will be useful in diagnosis and treatment of a patient.

The physician should observe and evaluate the vital signs for evidence of respiratory distress including hypertension, tachycardia or bradycardia, tachypnea, hypoxia, and restlessness of the patient. The cardiopulmonary exam should focus on the quality, location, and character of breath sounds, including volume on auscultation, unilateral/bilateral/upper/lower, presence or absence of sounds (pneumothorax or pleural effusion) and any adventitious sounds (pleural friction rubs, crackles). Upon cardiac auscultation, signs of pulmonary hypertension, such as a loud pulmonic second heart sound (P2) may be heard.[3] Percussion over the lung fields can reveal areas of dullness (consolidation) or hyper-resonance (hyperinflation). Percussion can help detect the presence and level of pleural effusion. Palpation is used to determine the presence of any tactile fremitus (changes in the vibrations transmitted through the lungs indicating underlying lung pathology). Palpation should be performed posteriorly over the thoracic transverse processes and rib angles for tissue texture changes. Tissue texture changes that feel edematous may be related to viscerosomatic reflexes from the pulmonary system.

In addition to palpating for viscerosomatic reflexes, rib motion, and tactile fremitus, trained osteopathic physicians can palpate subtle motion of the lower respiratory tract. Bordoni et al. describes how to place the hands for an effective osteopathic assessment of the tracheal, bronchial, and pulmonary structures. Understanding how to perform palpation of the lung areas and related somatic structures is a fundamental tool for applying osteopathic manual medicine techniques in the clinic.[4]

Structural Examination

The structural exam can provide useful information in the pulmonary patient. If the patient can stand upright, evaluation should include anatomic landmarks for significant postural asymmetry (please see Chapter 30 on the screening and regional structural exam). If the patient cannot stand but can sit, palpation and observation used together should evaluate the thoracic spine, ribs, clavicles, head position, and sternum. This portion of examination can identify abnormalities such as deformity of the sternum including pectus excavatum or carinatum, indicating possible underlying connective tissue disorder. Scoliosis in the thoracic region is important to evaluate and monitor, as severe cases of kyphoscoliosis can cause restrictive lung disease.

Hospitalized or bedridden patients should be assessed differently. In the supine position, the physician can obtain useful information by palpating the pectoral girdle, lower ribcage, abdomen, and pelvis for asymmetry, fascial preference, and tenderness.

Extremities should be evaluated for edema, clubbing, cyanosis, nail changes, skin turgor, and motion restrictions.

The Integrated Examination

An integrated systems-based evaluation can save time and integrate components from the review of systems, physical examination, and osteopathic structural examination. Following evaluation of the chief complaint and history of present illness, it is important to consider all the patient's vitals, weight changes, pain level, pulse oximetry, and intake and output. The efficient clinician will integrate palpation for T.A.R.t. changes during their physical examination, including in supine-laying hospitalized patients. It can be time-effective to question the patient regarding symptoms referable to the review of systems while examining or palpating that region. An example of an integrated approach is listed below.

HEENT

Perform a thorough exam of the eyes, ears, nose, throat, and sinuses. Physical exam findings to observe may include allergic "shiners," blue or erythematous nasal turbinates, cyanosis, pursed lip breathing, and oropharyngeal narrowing (evaluated by Mallampati score) (see Fig. 72.1). The Mallampati score, also known as the Mallampati classification, is a medical tool used in the assessment of obstructive sleep apnea and airway obstruction.[5]

When examining the lymph nodes in this region, the physician can concurrently evaluate for anterior and poster cervical counterstrain points and cervical tissue texture changes over the facet joints. Palpate for hypertrophy or atrophy of the scalene muscles, which act as accessory muscles of respiration and frequently become overused in patients with pulmonary disease. To evaluate the thyroid, stand behind the seated patient and ask them to take a sip of water as you palpate the thyroid gland for asymmetry, nodules, and enlargement. As this can be a sensitive examination for some patients, take extra care to practice consent before contact. Examine the thoracic inlet, uppermost thoracic vertebrae, clavicles, and bilateral first ribs for symmetry and T.A.R.t changes.

CARDIAC

The cardiac exam begins with observation of the patient's posture, ease of respiration, skin color, and peripheral edema. Ask about chest pain/pressure, shortness of breath, palpitations, and fatigue. Following auscultation of the listening posts, assess the anterior chest wall for counterstrain points, Chapman points, and rib asymmetry. Palpation and auscultation of the carotid pulses can be followed by palpation of anterior structures of the neck for fascial mobility and tenderness. Evaluation of pulses and peripheral edema of the legs may be coupled with palpation of myofascial restriction behind the knees and tibiofibular and ankle motion.

PULMONARY

A thorough pulmonary exam begins with observation for sequelae of pulmonary disease such as barrel chest, scars, cyanosis, cough, wheezing, conversational dyspnea, prolonged expiration, jugular venous distension (JVD), and retractions or paradoxical movement (more common in children). Ask the patient about fatigue, shortness of breath, cough, phlegm, pain, hemoptysis, fatigue, and sleep disturbance. Auscultate for breath sounds (noting asymmetry, diminished, or absence of sounds), rales, rhonchi, wheezing, or abnormal locations of normal breath sounds. When present, these signs may lead the clinician to further palpatory and/or diagnostic assessment. Palpation for tactile fremitus over a potential area of consolidation can provide clinical confirmation or guide the clinician to order imaging. However, palpation can also discern the presence of myofascial and rib dysfunctions, which may be the primary cause of the clinical issue or associated with the patient's condition. Palpation over the rib angles for puffy tissue texture changes can reveal the presence of viscerosometic reflexes, whose location and severity can be correlated to the patient's condition.

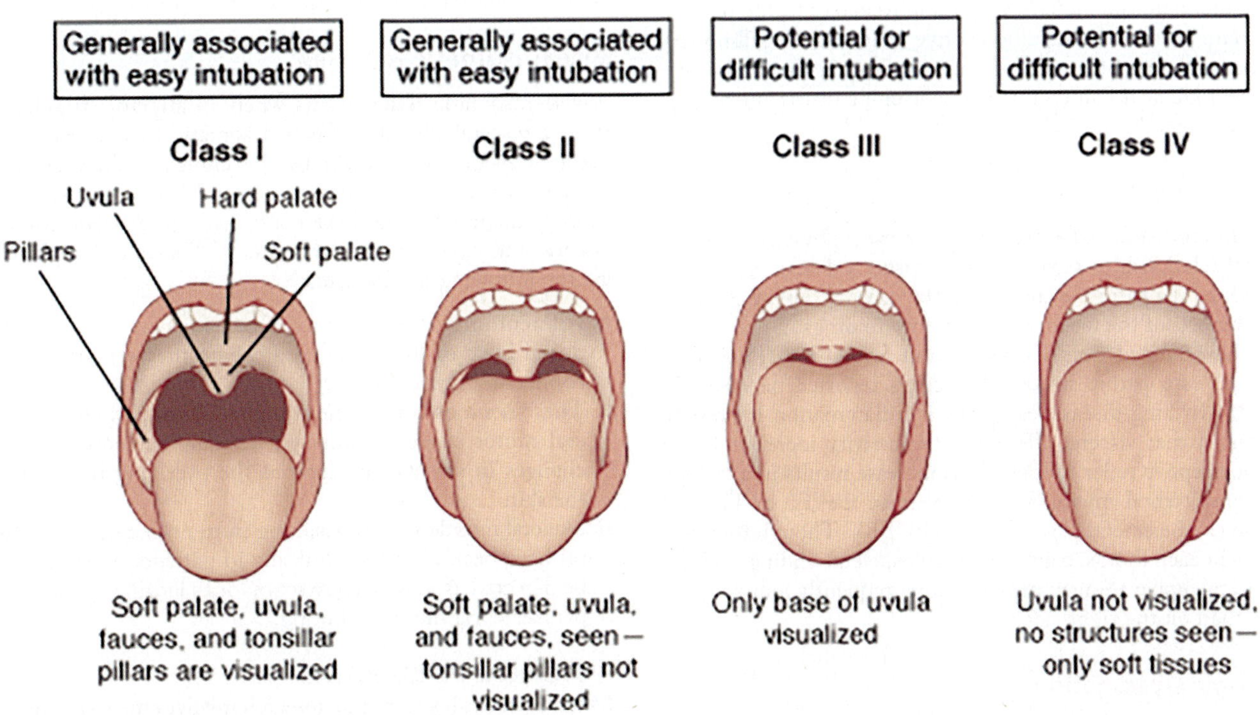

Figure 72.1. Mallampati score. Understanding the Mallampati score. To evaluate a patient for ease of endotracheal intubation, you must determine a Mallampati score, which is based on the amount of visualization of the pharyngeal airway.

Palpation of the abdominal diaphragm and its attachments can provide useful insight on pulmonary function.

GI

The gastrointestinal evaluation, like other examinations, depends on observation, inspection, auscultation, palpation, and percussion. Symptoms to elicit include changes in the patient's appetite, bowel habits, weight, diet, or elimination. Pay particular attention for signs of chronic disease such as ascites, jaundice, hepatomegaly, splenomegaly, abdominal scars, and weight gain or weight loss. Following auscultation of the abdomen, and during palpation, evaluate the abdominal wall for viscerosomatic reflexes along the midline. These areas of localized tension and tissue texture change are thought to be viscerosomatic reflexes from the celiac, superior mesenteric, and inferior mesenteric ganglia. According to Dr. Fulford, tension along the linea alba was a key area that he described as an "energy sink," in which shock from trauma was stored in the somatic structures (see Chapter 59 Additional Osteopathic Manipulative Treatment Approaches: Fulford Percussion). Jones counterstrain points and Chapman points for the small bowel are also located in this area. Palpation under each hemidiaphragm can be performed for tissue tension and texture changes, potentially indicating diaphragm restriction. Advanced palpation of the abdominal viscera can be performed according to procedures in Chapters 42 and 43. If restricted to a supine examination of the patient, the clinician can reach both hands around either side of the patient's torso to contact the thoracic paraspinals. By applying an anterior springing force to the spinal segments, the clinician can determine spinal motion restrictions, muscle tension, and tissue texture change in the thoracic area. The gastrointestinal examination plays a significant role in evaluation of many pulmonary conditions (i.e., cystic fibrosis) or acute conditions affecting all body systems (i.e., after antibiotic use for pulmonary infection).

SOMATIC DYSFUNCTION

The presence of significant somatic dysfunction can potentially alter or potentiate the underlying pathophysiology of the pulmonary system. Sustained sympathetic drive related to the pulmonary condition and areas of somatic dysfunction can be factors in producing neurogenic inflammation and worsening disease pathogenesis (see Chapters 6 and 12).[6]

Spinal Segmental Relationships

Due to interest and expertise of osteopathic physicians, spinal segmental relationships associated with visceral disease have been identified by palpatory examination by several investigators.[7,8] Clinical reports of the location of palpatory findings in pulmonary patients have ranged from C3 to C4 and from T2 to T9, with a majority of osteopathic structural findings reported between T4 and T6.[7–11] In lung disease, especially if inflammation is present, it is thought that visceral afferent nerve activity increases based on the nociceptive reflex model.[9] This increase results in a change in the paravertebral muscular anatomy from the T1 to T7 cord levels and can be extended as low as T9 or T10.[7] Though there are two lungs in each thorax, palpable musculoskeletal findings of lung disease in the upper thoracic area are more frequently found on the left side than on the right side.[9]

Neurologic Dysfunction

The cervical paravertebral area is another common area of somatic dysfunction in respiratory disease. Areas of somatic dysfunction and spinal facilitation could interfere with phrenic nerve function (C3–C5) and diaphragmatic function. During states that increase sympathetic tone in the lung, hypersympathetic effects are speculated to occur. Increased sympathetic tone results in lung vasoconstriction with regional hypoperfusion and airway epithelial hyperplasia. This hyperplasia leads to an increase in goblet cells and luminal secretions, contributing to pulmonary symptoms.[12]

Diaphragm and Thoracic Inlet Dysfunction

Diaphragmatic function may be stressed by the relative immobility of the ribs and spine, as influenced by viscerosomatic reflexes in the thoracic area. The increased workload on the diaphragm could result in enhanced fatigability. In patients who compensate by recruitment of the secondary muscles of respiration (often apparent in patients with advanced respiratory disease), fatigue of the scalene muscles and sternocleidomastoid muscle may result in dysfunction of the upper thoracic rib cage, including the first rib. This mechanical disruption likely further impairs breathing efficiency. See Chapter 15 Anatomy, Mechanics, and Physiology of Pulmonary Respiration, for further discussion of the mechanics of respiration.

Chapman Points

Chapman points related to the pulmonary system are located in specific areas and have distinct palpatory characteristics. For the upper lung, the anterior Chapman point is found in the third intercostal space at the sternocostal junction, while the posterior point is located at the intertransverse space between the T3 and T4 vertebrae, midway between the spinous and transverse processes. For the lower lung, the anterior point is in the fourth intercostal space at the sternocostal junction, and the posterior point is at the intertransverse space between T4 and T5, midway between the spinous and transverse processes. These points are palpable as small, discrete, smooth nodules, approximately 2 to 3 mm in diameter. When compressed, they can cause sharp, nonradiating pain indicative of potential internal dysfunction or pathology of the lungs.

Viscerosomatic Reflexes

A viscerosomatic reflex occurs when an afferent stimulus arising from a visceral disorder affects a somatic tissue, producing palpatory changes determined by the clinician. They are typically located in the subcutaneous tissues and have a puffy, doughy, or rubbery quality. Studies have confirmed the existence of somatovisceral and viscerosomatic reflexes.[13,14] They are thought to occur via the following mechanisms:

- Afferent impulses from visceral receptors are transmitted to the dorsal horn of the spinal cord, where they synapse with interconnecting neurons.
- These neurons convey the stimulus to sympathetic and peripheral motor efferent pathways, resulting in sensory and motor changes in skeletal muscle and the overlying tissue, including the skin.
- Skeletal muscle spasms resulting from nociceptive visceral stimuli have been observed clinically in patients. These spasms can be detected as muscle contraction or as localized tenderness and paravertebral muscle splinting.

HISTORICAL PERSPECTIVE

Much historical osteopathic research involves the evaluation of visceral reflexes. In a 5-year, double-blind study of 5,000 hospitalized patients who were examined for evidence of somatic dysfunction and its relationship to diagnosis, most visceral diseases appeared to have more than one region with an increased frequency of segmental findings.[15] Unpaired viscera were also found to have an increased frequency of findings on the side of the dysfunctional viscera, and the number of spinal segments involved appeared to be related to the duration and severity of the disease.[15]

Subsequently, research has gone on to explore osteopathic involvement in pulmonary disease. Kelso and colleagues observed an increased incidence of palpatory findings in the cervical spine in patients with upper airway diseases, while upper thoracic involvement was seen in patients with lower respiratory disease.[16] In a study by Beal and Morlock, 40 patients with a diagnosis of pulmonary disease, mainly COPD were examined for evidence of somatic dysfunction. A prevalence of spinal changes was found in the T2–T7 paraspinal area. The somatic dysfunction generally involved two or more adjacent spinal segments, deep muscle splinting, and resistance to a compression motion test.[9] Other investigators have reported similar findings in patients with respiratory disease.[17–20] Nicholas evaluated 10 patients with respiratory disease and found an increased incidence of paravertebral muscle tension at C4–C7 and T2–T9 bilaterally.[19] The majority of findings were seen in the spinal segments T1–T9.[20]

PATHOPHYSIOLOGY

Generally, related palpatory findings of somatic dysfunction are located at the level of the segmental sympathetic autonomic nerve supply of the dysfunctional viscera (see Chapter 6 Autonomic Nervous System, for discussion about the autonomic nerve supply to the lungs). With lung irritation or a disease process, such as an infection, visceral afferents carry information to the seven upper thoracic cord segments. With prolonged stimulation of the thoracic cord segments, the spinal cord can undergo facilitation (sensitization). Facilitated segments of the spinal cord have been found to have low reflex thresholds causing them to discharge easily (see Chapter 13 Somatic Dysfunction, Spinal Facilitation and Viscerosomatic Integration). Such facilitation is thought to excite the internuncial neurons and resultant somatic motor efferent nerves producing palpatory changes and a viscerosomatic reflex. These reflexes allow the physician to palpate the paravertebral musculature and discern tissue texture changes indicating lung dysfunction.

It is possible that presymptomatic signs of visceral disease may be evident in the somatic system. The intensity and the extent of the tissue response differ among individuals and disease states.[8,14] For example, somatic dysfunction has been shown to be greater in patients with cardiac disease who present with symptoms of severe pain than in patients with pulmonary disease, who are more apt to present with symptoms of dyspnea.[9,14]

Just as viscerosomatic reflexes can create somatic dysfunction that affects pulmonary function, osteopathic physicians have postulated how a somatovisceral reflex may disturb the costal cage, therefore disturbing lung mechanics and pulmonary gas exchange. This would contribute mechanistically to perceived symptoms of dyspnea, as well as contribute to regional discomfort or pain for the patient. Treatment of somatic dysfunction by appropriate osteopathic manipulative intervention helps relieve dyspnea or other symptoms.

DIAGNOSTIC STUDIES

Technologic advances in pulmonary and medical testing have improved osteopathic pulmonology practices. These tests improve the ability to diagnose and treat pulmonary conditions, as well as correlate disease history and osteopathic findings to gather a more complete picture of the patient. Different diagnostic studies contribute to the pulmonary care of patients in various ways. These include sleep studies, tuberculin skin tests, cultures, labs, chest x-rays (CXRs), computed tomography (CT) scans and pulmonary function testing (PFT), PET scans, and bronchoscopy reports.

Sleep Studies

The sleep study, also known as a polysomnogram, is a comprehensive test that monitors various bodily functions during sleep to diagnose sleep disorders. Sleep studies are recommended for individuals experiencing symptoms of excessive daytime sleepiness, snoring, difficulty breathing during sleep, narcolepsy, or abnormal nighttime behaviors. The primary purpose of a sleep study is to diagnose a range of sleep-related conditions, including sleep apnea, restless legs syndrome, narcolepsy, insomnia, and behaviors such as sleepwalking and REM sleep behavior disorder. Following screening for these conditions by a physician in office, diagnosis necessitates thorough investigation through a sleep study.[21–23]

This noninvasive diagnostic procedure provides a detailed picture of sleep quality and identifies disruptions. Sleep studies are typically conducted overnight in specialized sleep centers or labs that are designed to resemble a comfortable hotel room. Participants are connected to sensors used to monitor brain waves (EEG), eye movements (EOG), muscle activity (EMG), heart rate (electrocardiogram [ECG]), breathing patterns, and oxygen levels in the blood. Sleep architecture (the amount of time spent in each sleep stage) is assessed by looking at different sleep stages throughout the night, including REM and non-REM sleep. Any disruptions in these patterns or to sleep architecture, the number of apneas (breathing stops) and hypopneas (shallow breathing), and O_2 desaturation per hour of sleep are recorded. A high apnea to hypopnea index suggests obstructive sleep apnea, while frequent awakenings and reduced deep sleep may indicate insomnia or another sleep disorder.[21–23]

Infectious Disease Screening

TUBERCULOSIS SCREENING: MANTOUX TEST VERSUS QuantiFERON GOLD

The Mantoux skin test, also known as the tuberculin skin test (TST), and the QuantiFERON Gold blood test (QFT-Gold) are both used to detect TB infection. They differ significantly in their methodology, accuracy, and convenience.[24]

The Mantoux skin test involves injecting a small amount of tuberculin into the skin and requires the patient to return to the health care provider 48 to 72 hours later to have the results read. Interpretation of the skin test is somewhat subjective by palpation and observation. It can vary based on the reader, potentially leading to false-positive results, especially in individuals who have been vaccinated with the Bacillus Calmette–Guérin (BCG) vaccine or who have had previous TB skin tests. The skin test has a sensitivity of 79% and specificity of 97%, but specificity can be as low as 59% in BCG-vaccinated patients.[24]

In contrast, the QuantiFERON Gold blood test is an interferon-gamma release assay (IGRA) that requires only one patient visit for a blood draw, with results typically available within 24 hours. It provides objective results that are not affected by the BCG vaccine or previous TB tests, thus reducing the likelihood of false positives. The QuantiFERON Gold Plus, an updated version of the test, has been optimized to detect TB-specific antigens that elicit CD8 and CD4 T-cell responses, allowing for a more accurate and comprehensive assessment of cell-mediated immune responses to TB infection. This test is over 97% accurate at detecting TB infection. The QuantiFERON Gold Plus test is considered the new gold standard for TB testing by most clinicians due to its higher accuracy rates, efficiency, and the elimination of follow-up visits, which can save time and resources for both patients and clinics.[24] The CDC recommends the use of TB blood tests, like QuantiFERON, for people who have received the BCG vaccine and for those who may have difficulty returning for a second appointment to read the Mantoux skin test.[25]

While both tests aim to detect TB infection, the QuantiFERON Gold blood test offers greater specificity, convenience, and accuracy, making it a preferred choice for TB testing in adults, especially in those with prior BCG vaccination or a history of TB exposure.[24,25]

Pulmonary CT Scans

CT scans are highly valuable in the imaging and assessment of various pulmonary conditions due to their ability to provide detailed cross-sectional images of the chest, including the lungs, airways, and surrounding structures.

CT SCANS FOR INTERSTITIAL LUNG DISEASE

CT scans, particularly high-resolution CT (HRCT), are considered the most important radiologic modality for detecting, analyzing, and diagnosing diffuse interstitial lung diseases. HRCT can provide high morphologic detail of both normal and abnormal lung parenchyma, which is essential for accurate diagnosis and management of interstitial lung diseases. The ability to visualize the lungs in detail allows for the identification of characteristic patterns associated with specific lung diseases, which can be crucial for early intervention and treatment.[26]

CT SCANS FOR COPD

CT imaging can be used quantitatively to provide precise measurements of lung, airway, and vessel volumes, which correlate with traditional PFTs. This quantitative analysis is particularly useful in COPD, where CT can assess airway wall thickness, detect air trapping on expiratory scans, and evaluate the extent of emphysema. In addition to its diagnostic capabilities, CT scanning is routinely used to evaluate a wide range of acquired and congenital lung abnormalities, including pneumonia, tumors, and chronic lung diseases.[27]

CT SCANS FOR LUNG CANCER

Lung Cancer Screening

High-quality, low-risk screening tools are essential in prevention and early diagnosis of treatable cancers. Early detection is paramount in combating lung cancer, a disease often diagnosed at advanced stages when treatment options are limited. Low-dose CT (LDCT) has emerged as a powerful tool in lung cancer screening, offering a lower-exposure, noninvasive screening method for detection in high-risk individuals. By using LDCT scans for screening, physicians can identify lung cancers at their earliest stages when interventions are most effective.[28,29]

LDCT scans are particularly important in lung cancer screening for high-risk populations such as smokers and exsmokers.[28] In 2019, there were about 2.26 million new cases globally of tracheal, bronchus, and lung cancer. Of those who died from tracheal, bronchus, or lung cancer in 2019, smoking contributed to an estimated 64.2% of deaths.[29] Current and past smokers are at a higher risk of mortality due to lung cancer. The U.S. Preventive Service Task Force (USPSTF) currently recommends yearly LDCT scans for lung cancer screening in all patients ages 50 to 80 with a 20-pack-year smoking history who are current smokers or who have quit within the past 15 years.[30] Pack-year-history is determined by multiplying the number of packs of cigarettes smoked per day by the number of years smoking (i.e., 1/2 pack per day for 30 years = 15 pack-year history). These guidelines attempt to help detect cancer at earlier stages when treatment is more likely to be successful. Along with a discussion with their physician about minimizing risk factors (i.e., smoking cessation) and encouraging healthy lifestyle habits, LDCT as a screening tool serves a significant role in prevention of mortality from lung cancer.[28,30]

Management and Monitoring Using CT

CT imaging plays a pivotal role in the modern management of cancer, particularly in guiding biopsies, monitoring tumor response to treatment, and planning radiation therapy. The precision of CT imaging allows for accurate targeting during biopsies, ensuring that tissue samples are obtained from the most relevant areas of a tumor.[31] This accuracy is crucial for diagnosing and staging cancer, which in turn informs treatment planning. In the realm of treatment monitoring, CT scans are instrumental in evaluating the effectiveness of therapies such as radiation therapy and chemotherapy by providing detailed images of tumor size and structure over time.[32] Furthermore, CT imaging is indispensable in radiation therapy planning, where it aids in delineating the tumor boundaries and surrounding critical structures to optimize the delivery of radiation doses.[33] CT angiography (CTA) is used to assess the blood vessels in the chest, enhancing the detection of vascular abnormalities with the aid of contrast material. The integration of CT with positron emission tomography (PET) has enhanced the ability to differentiate between treatment effects and residual or recurrent disease, particularly in the context of head and neck cancers. This synergy between CT and PET in PET/CT imaging modalities has improved the precision of radiation therapy planning, biopsy guidance, and the monitoring of tumor response.

PET Scan

PET scans can identify metabolic activity of lung tissues, offering a unique perspective beyond the structural insights provided by CT or MRI scans. This functional imaging capability is crucial for distinguishing between malignant and benign lung nodules, thereby aiding in the accurate diagnosis of lung cancer. PET scans utilize 18F-fluorodeoxyglucose (FDG), a glucose-based tracer that detects metabolically active cancer cells.[34,35] When combined with CT, PET/CT provides a three-dimensional image that highlights areas of rapid metabolic activity, aiding in identification of malignant masses. In the management of lung cancer, PET scans play a pivotal role in evaluating the effectiveness of treatments, such as chemotherapy, radiation therapy, or surgery.[34,35] By comparing pre- and posttreatment PET images, clinicians can assess the metabolic activity of cancer cells, providing insights into the treatment's success in reducing or eliminating the tumor. This approach is particularly valuable for adjusting treatment plans based on the tumor's response, optimizing patient outcomes. PET/CT imaging has been shown to have greater accuracy than conventional imaging modalities in some scenarios, making it a valuable noninvasive method for investigating lung cancer (see Fig. 72.2).[36] Additional information about cancer treatment can be found in Chapter 76 Osteopathic Considerations in Oncology.

Beyond lung cancer, PET scans have been explored in various nononcologic lung diseases, such as TB and pulmonary fibrosis. In TB, PET scans can monitor disease activity and response to antimycobacterial therapy, potentially guiding the duration of treatment. Similarly, in pulmonary fibrosis, PET imaging can assess the extent of disease and inflammatory activity, offering a noninvasive means to monitor disease progression and response to therapy.[36,37]

In addition, PET/CT is used in characterizing various inflammatory conditions of the lungs, including pneumonia, lung abscess,

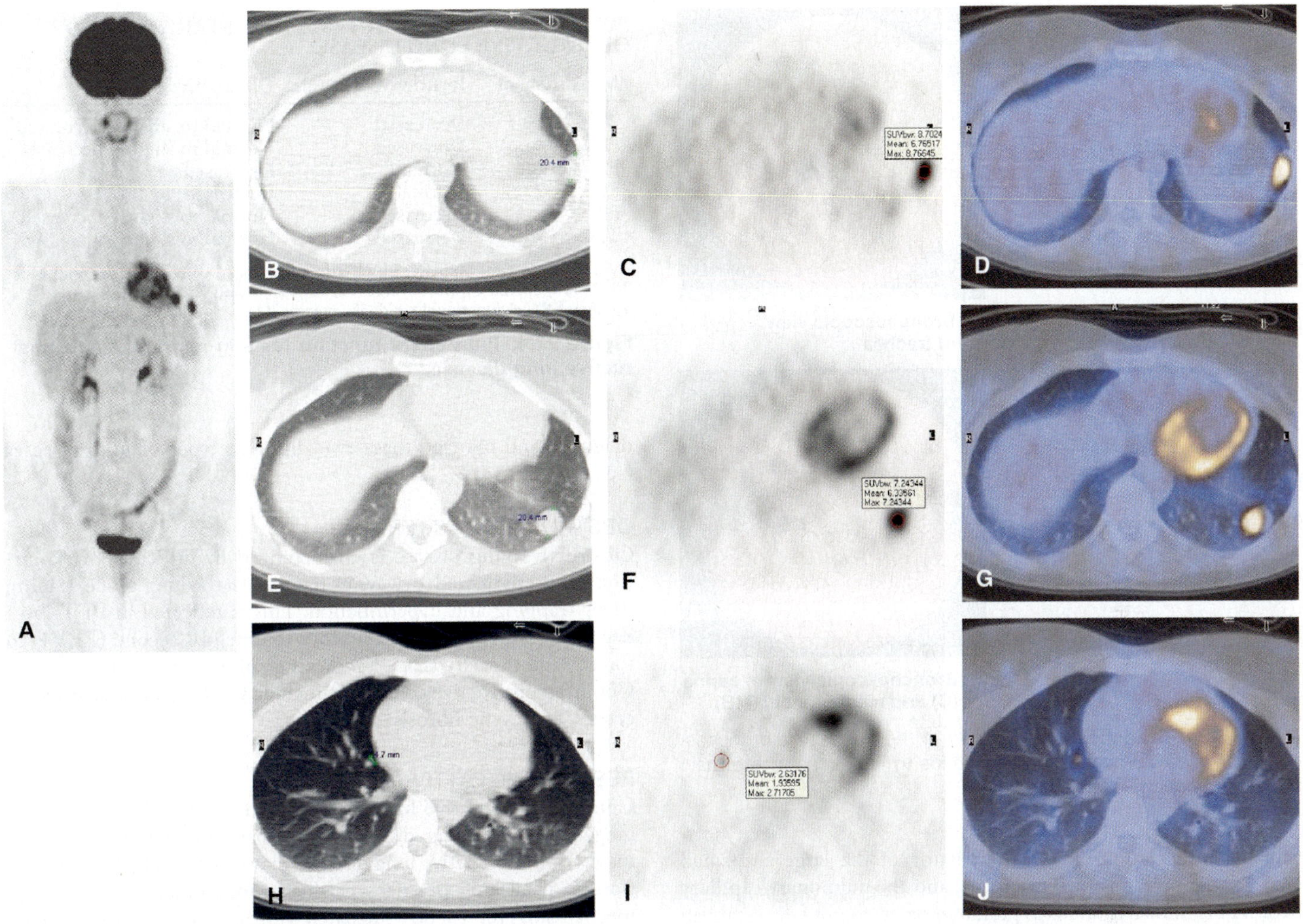

Figure 72.2. PET CT pulmonary metastasis. A 30-year-old woman 8 years after resection of a malignant melanoma with a subcutaneous metastasis of the right lower arm. A right-sided axillary lymph node metastasis was known. PET/CT was performed for whole-body staging. Three months after the resection of the axillary metastasis, a follow-up PET/CT examination was performed. No residual tumor or recurrence was found in the right axilla. MIP image (**A**), corresponding PET section (**C, F, I**), and corresponding PET/CT images (**D, G, J**), respectively, show a strongly increased FDG accumulation in the lung lesions. Transaxial CT sections demonstrate an increase in volume of the lung metastases in the left lung and a new metastasis in the right lung (**B, E, H**).

and sarcoidosis, providing valuable information on disease activity and assisting in predicting disease progression.[38] The combination of PET and CT imaging (PET/CT) provides comprehensive information by merging metabolic and anatomical data, improving the accuracy of lung cancer staging and the assessment of other pulmonary conditions.[35,36]

Bronchoscopy

Bronchoscopy is a critical diagnostic and therapeutic tool in the management of various pulmonary conditions, offering direct visualization of the airways with the ability to perform tissue biopsy, aspiration, and therapeutic interventions. Its role in diagnosing, staging, and managing lung diseases, particularly lung cancer, has been significantly enhanced by technologic advancements and the integration of complementary imaging modalities (see Fig. 72.3).

For diagnostic use, bronchoscopy allows for collection of tissue samples through biopsy forceps, brushes, or needles, facilitating histopathologic examination of lung lesions. This capability is crucial for the accurate diagnosis of lung cancer, infectious diseases like TB, and inflammatory conditions such as sarcoidosis.[39] The advent of endobronchial ultrasound (EBUS) has further expanded the diagnostic utility of bronchoscopy, enabling the visualization and biopsy of mediastinal and hilar lymph nodes for cancer staging without the need for more invasive surgical procedures.[40]

In the staging of lung cancer, EBUS-guided transbronchial needle aspiration (TBNA) has become a standard practice, offering a minimally invasive method to obtain samples from lymph nodes and assess the extent of disease spread. This technique has improved the accuracy of lung cancer staging, which is essential for determining the most appropriate treatment strategy.[40]

Therapeutically, bronchoscopy is employed in the management of airway obstructions, whether due to tumors, foreign bodies, or stenosis. Techniques such as laser therapy, stent placement, and balloon bronchoplasty can be performed during bronchoscopy to relieve obstructions and improve symptoms. In addition, bronchoscopy facilitates the delivery of localized treatments, including brachytherapy for lung cancer and thermoplasty for severe asthma.[39]

Pulmonary Function Testing

PFT measures various aspects of lung function, including the capacity, volume, and flow rates of air exhaled and inhaled, which are essential for diagnosing conditions such as asthma, COPD, and interstitial lung disease.[41] PFTs are noninvasive and provide

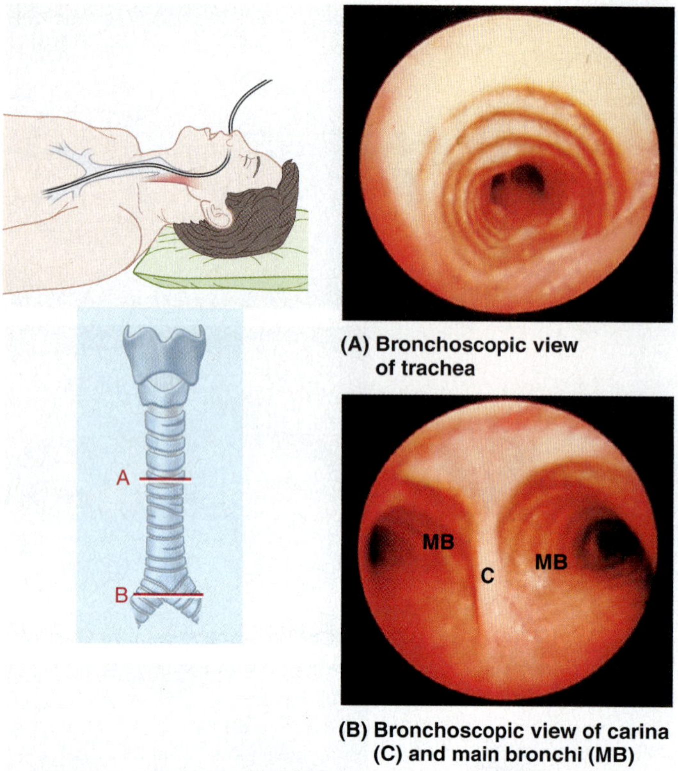

Figure 72.3. Bronchoscopy. A. View of the trachea via bronchoscopy. **B.** View as bronchoscope descends to the carina where main bronchi branch off.

valuable information on the functioning of the large and small airways, the pulmonary parenchyma, and the pulmonary capillary bed.[41] This information helps pulmonologists to not only establish a diagnosis by identifying patterns of abnormalities specific to different respiratory diseases, but also to monitor the progression of diseases and the effectiveness of treatments over time. In addition, PFTs are used in the preoperative evaluation of patients to assess the risk of lung diseases and to guide decisions regarding further treatment and intervention. Obstructive and restrictive lung diseases are two distinct categories of pulmonary disorders that can be differentiated through PFT results. Restrictive syndromes account for about 20% of pulmonary syndromes, while obstructive syndromes are the majority (80%).[42] Pulmonologists use these PFT results, alongside other diagnostic tools, to accurately diagnose and manage these two different types of lung diseases (see Fig. 72.4).

PULMONARY FUNCTION TESTS IN RESTRICTIVE AND OBSTRUCTIVE LUNG DISEASE

Measurement	Restrictive disease	Obstructive disease
FVC	Decreased	Normal to slightly decreased
FEV1	Decreased	Normal to slightly decreased
FEV1/FVC	Normal	Decreased
FEF 25–75%	Normal	Decreased
FRC	Decreased	Normal to slightly increased
TLC	Decreased	Normal to slightly increased

FVC = forced vital capacity; FEV1 = forced exhaled volume in 1 second; FEF 25–75% = forced expiratory flow between 25% and 75% of total exhaled volume; FRC = functional residual capacity; TLC = total lung capacity.

Figure 72.4. Pulmonary function tests in restrictive and obstructive lung disease.

OBSTRUCTIVE PATTERN

Obstructive lung disease is characterized by difficulty of expiration due to narrowed airways or damage to the lung tissue, leading to air trapping and hyperinflation. This is reflected in PFTs by a decreased ratio of forced expiratory volume in 1 second (FEV1) to forced vital capacity (FVC), indicating an obstruction in airflow.[43] Common obstructive conditions include COPD, asthma, bronchiectasis, and cystic fibrosis.

RESTRICTIVE PATTERN

Conversely, restrictive lung disease is characterized by a reduced lung volume, causing difficulty of expansion of the lungs with inspiration. Restrictive lung diseases may be caused by the destruction of distal lung parenchyma due to inflammation, toxins, and mechanisms yet to be elucidated (intrinsic conditions) as well as extraparenchymal conditions (extrinsic causes).[42] Some external mechanisms include neuromuscular diseases, pleural disorders, obesity, scoliosis, sternocostal or costovertebral fusion, and fusion or deviation of the thoracic vertebra.[42] These conditions cause stiffness in the lungs or chest wall, or weakened respiratory muscles. PFTs in restrictive lung disease typically show a normal or increased FEV1/FVC ratio because both FEV1 and FVC are reduced proportionally, but the total lung capacity (TLC) is decreased, indicating a restriction in lung expansion (see Fig. 72.5). Conditions such as interstitial lung disease, sarcoidosis, and neuromuscular diseases are associated with restrictive lung patterns.

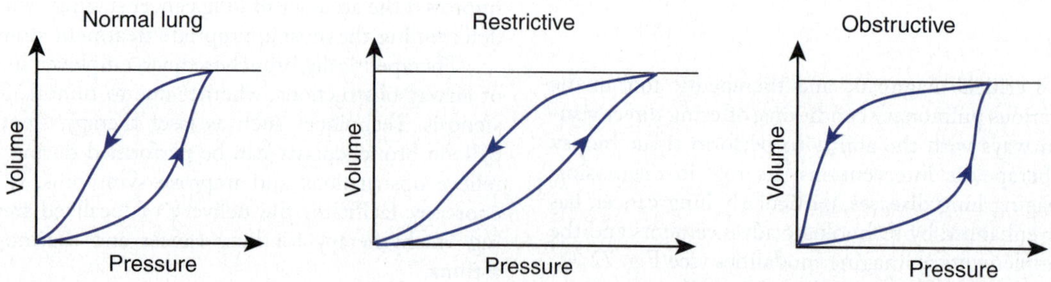

Figure 72.5. Work of breathing during breathing cycle in a normal lung, a restrictive, and an obstructive lung. Pressure is plotted on the x-axis, and volume is plotted on the y-axis. Work equals force times distance and is represented by the *blue* area of the pressure–volume curve. The area above the curve represents of work of breathing during inspiration. Note that with a restrictive disorder, the inspiratory work of breathing is increased. In an obstructive disorder, less work is required to bring air in because of the loss of elastic recoil. However, airway resistance is increased during expiration, which requires more energy to force air out in an obstructive lung disorder.

EFFECT OF OMT ON PFTs

In a 2014 study, Kocchar et al. evaluated the effects of osteopathic manipulative treatment (OMT) on pulmonary function in healthy adult males, comparing baseline PFTs to measurements taken 10 minutes and 24 hours after treatment of specific somatic dysfunctions with OMT. This was compared to a control group (quiet reading) protocol. Of those treated with OMT, 75% of the subjects in the OMT group were found to have somatic dysfunction in the C2–C7, T5–T9, ribs, and L1–L5 regions. After OMT, upper thoracic excursion increased from 5.7 ± 0.5 to 6.3 ± 0.5 cm ($P = .03$) and FVC increased from 5.13 ± 0.20 to 5.24 ± 0.19 L ($P = .02$) at 24 hours. OMT treatment of subjects with rib dysfunction significantly improved FVC at 24 hours ($P = .02$). Their data demonstrated that OMT can increase upper thoracic excursion and lung volumes. These data support the possibility that OMT can improve pulmonary function in patients with extrinsic restrictive lung disease.[44]

Other studies have aimed to build upon knowledge of the impact of OMT on respiration. In healthy patients, Stepnik et al. applied an OMT intervention including supine thoracic thrust manipulation, sternal pump and sternal recoil, and diaphragm stretch in a sitting position compared to placebo interventions. These techniques demonstrated change in peak expiratory flow (PEF) as measured by spirometer, but not in FEV1 or FVC. These results appear to indicate improved respiratory function after OMT intervention as measured by PEF, but not overall lung health as measured by FEV1 or FVC20.[45]

DIFFERENTIAL DIAGNOSIS OF LUNG DISEASE

Acute Pulmonary Conditions

A differential diagnosis for a patient with acute lung disease encompasses a broad range of conditions, reflecting the complexity and diversity of diseases that can affect the lungs. Many conditions can present with similar symptoms, such as dyspnea, cough, and hypoxemia, making a thorough clinical evaluation, including history, physical examination, and diagnostic testing essential for accurate diagnosis and appropriate management. A differential of acute pulmonary diseases can include the following considerations[3,46,47]:

- Acute respiratory distress syndrome (ARDS)
- Aspiration pneumonitis and pneumonia
- Asthma
- Atelectasis
- Bronchitis
- Cardiac conditions
- Pulmonary embolism
- Pneumonia
- Exacerbation of COPD
- Pulmonary hemorrhage
- Drug reactions
- Acute noncardiogenic pulmonary edema
- Other infections

Chronic Pulmonary Conditions

A differential diagnosis for a patient with chronic lung disease involves considering a variety of conditions that can present with similar symptoms, such as dyspnea, cough, and sputum production. It is important to conduct a thorough clinical evaluation supplemented by appropriate investigations, such as spirometry, chest imaging, and possibly blood tests, to accurately diagnose the underlying cause of chronic lung disease and differentiate it from other conditions with similar presentations. A differential of chronic pulmonary diseases can include the following considerations[3,48–50]:

- Asthma
- Congestive heart failure (CHF)
- Bronchiectasis
- Alpha1-antitrypsin (AAT) deficiency
- Asthma-COPD overlap syndrome (ACOS)
- Chronic bronchitis
- Bronchiolitis obliterans
- Chronic asthma
- Coronary artery disease
- Lung cancer
- Cor pulmonale
- Interstitial lung diseases
- Anxiety and depression
- Granulomatous lung disease

CLINICAL CONDITIONS

Asthma

Asthma is a reactive airway disease that continues to increase in prevalence The complications of this condition, its chronicity, and complexity in management leads to many emergency department visits and hospital stays for patients when not well-controlled, especially in the pediatric population.[51] The symptoms of asthma can be incredibly cumbersome for patients, and osteopathic physicians have long been involved in the treatment of this condition. Asthma is characterized by acute and reversible airway inflammation. Asthma is a condition closely linked to environmental factors and certain triggers, particularly exposure to tobacco smoke and inhaled particulates. Despite the lack of a cure or definitive preventive measures, effective treatments are available. Asthma encompasses a diverse group of diseases with various phenotypes, influenced by both genetic predispositions—such as a personal or family history of atopy (a tendency toward allergies, often manifesting as eczema, hay fever, or asthma)—and environmental factors, including exposure to tobacco smoke and other irritants.[52] The 2018 Asthma Guideline Update introduced new recommendations aimed at enhancing the care of those with asthma, which was further refined in a 2020 update by an expert panel.[53,54] This update focused on six key areas: intermittent use of inhaled corticosteroids (ICSs), the addition of long-acting muscarinic antagonists (LAMAs), the use of fractional exhaled nitric oxide (FeNO) for diagnosis and monitoring, strategies for mitigating indoor allergens, the safety and efficacy of immunotherapy, and bronchial thermoplasty.[53,54] These guidelines are built upon the foundational work of the 2007 National Asthma Education and Prevention Program Expert Panel Report 3 (EPR-3).[55]

CAUSES/EPIDEMIOLOGY

The prevalence of asthma varies globally, affecting approximately 15% to 20% of the population in developed countries and 2% to 4% in less developed regions. It is notably more prevalent among children, with up to 40% experiencing wheezing at some point. The etiology of asthma is complex and not fully understood, particularly in predicting which children with pediatric asthma will continue to experience symptoms into adulthood. While up to 40% of children may experience wheezing, only about 1% of adults are diagnosed with asthma. When wheezing is reversible with beta-2 agonists, it is classified as asthma, regardless of lung function test results.[52]

Asthma is far from a benign condition; it is responsible for approximately one death per 100,000 individuals in certain countries. Mortality rates are influenced by several factors, including age over 40, a history of smoking more than 20 pack-years, blood eosinophilia, an FEV1 between 40% and 70% of the predicted value, and significant reversibility of symptoms. The disease not only leads to loss of productivity due to missed work and school days, but also results in numerous hospital admissions, thereby increasing health care costs. Poorly managed asthma can severely impair quality of life, rendering it a disabling condition. In children, asthma is more commonly observed in boys, with a male to female ratio of 2:1, until puberty, at which point the ratio evens out to 1:1. Post puberty, females exhibit a higher prevalence of asthma, especially in adult-onset cases occurring after the age of 40. The prevalence of asthma also tends to be higher at the extremes of age, which may be attributed to increased airway responsiveness and lower levels of lung function. Notably, about 66% of asthma cases are diagnosed before the age of 18 years, and nearly half of these children experience a reduction in severity or complete remission of symptoms during early adulthood. While up to 40% of children may experience wheezing, only about 1% of adults are diagnosed with asthma.[52]

PATHOPHYSIOLOGY

The pathologic process is initiated when an individual inhales an irritant (such as cold air) or an allergen (like pollen), leading to airway inflammation and increased mucus production due to bronchial hypersensitivity. This results in a marked increase in airway resistance, most noticeably during expiration. Without prompt intervention, asthma can become increasingly difficult to manage as excessive mucus production hinders the effectiveness of inhaled medications in reaching the airway mucosa, and the inflammation becomes more severe (see Fig. 72.6).

CLINICAL PRESENTATION

As discussed previously, patients with asthma often report symptoms such as wheezing or coughing, which can worsen due to allergies, physical activity, or cold temperatures. Symptoms for patients with asthma frequently vary throughout the day, with many individuals with asthma experiencing coughing spells during the night while remaining symptom-free during the day. Acute asthma exacerbations may be accompanied by mild chest pain (see Fig. 72.7). It is common for asthmatic patients to also have a history of other atopic conditions, including eczema and hay fever.[52] The atopic triad refers to the tendency for asthma, allergies, and eczema to occur together.

A patient with asthma can present with a benign physical exam when stable. However, the findings during an exam can vary largely especially if a patient is undergoing an acute exacerbation at the time of assessment. On observation, patients in an exacerbation often present with paroxysmal or persistent cough, accessory muscle use, nasal flaring, cyanosis, or hyperinflation of the chest due to air trapping. During such exacerbations, patients may exhibit a fine hand tremor as a side effect of salbutamol (a medication commonly used in asthma treatment).[52] Vital signs may include tachypnea, tachycardia, and decreased O_2 saturation. Auscultation typically reveals a bilateral expiratory wheeze. In cases of life-threatening asthma, the chest may sound silent due to the inability of air to enter or exit the lungs, accompanied by signs of systemic hypoxia. As discussed previously in this chapter, patients in respiratory distress may adopt a forward-leaning posture to help open their airways, often called the "tripod" position. Children nearing respiratory arrest might present as drowsy, unresponsive, cyanotic, and confused, with possible wheezing absence and bradycardia, indicating severe respiratory muscle fatigue.[52] Life-threatening asthma, characterized by its lack of response to systemic steroids and beta-2 agonist nebulization along with clinical examination findings, requires prompt identification due to its high mortality risk.[52]

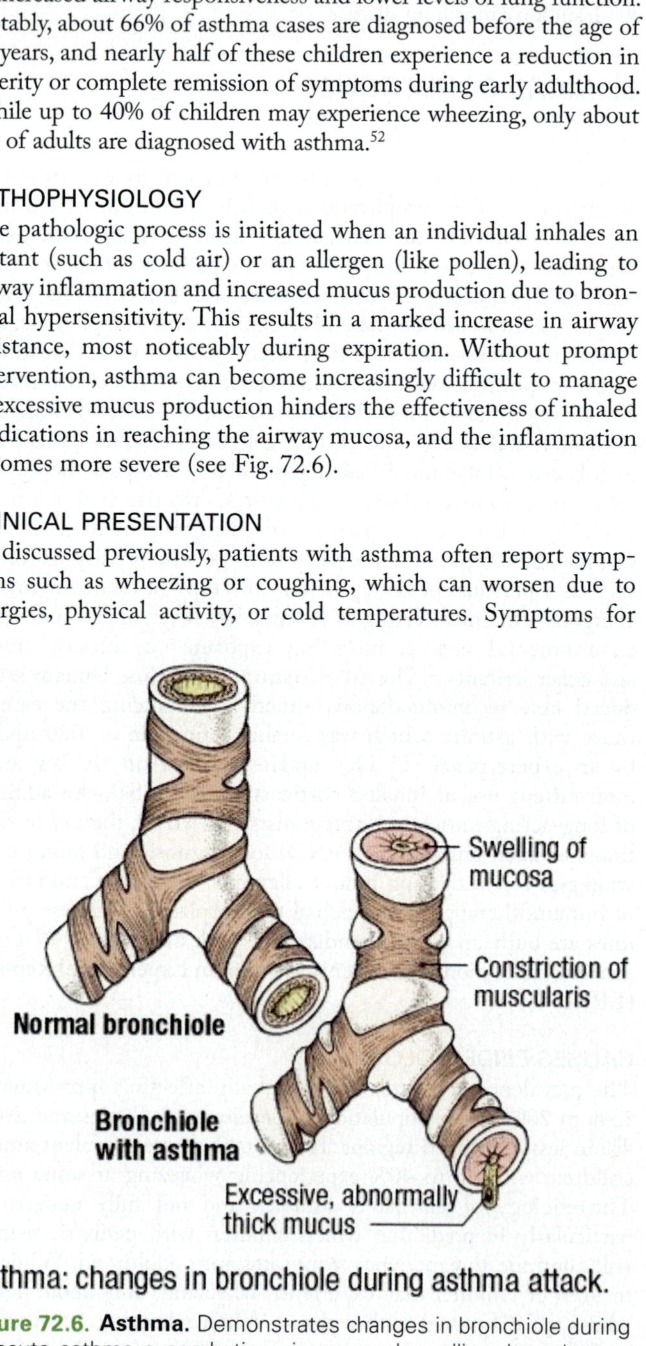

Figure 72.6. Asthma. Demonstrates changes in bronchiole during an acute asthma exacerbation via mucosal swelling, bronchoconstriction, and changes in mucus production.

DIAGNOSIS

There is no single definitive test for diagnosing asthma; a diagnosis of asthma requires integrating information on symptoms and clinical course, as well as testing. Initial testing for asthma should include spirometry with bronchodilator administration, with the expected result for a patient with asthma revealing an obstructive pattern, marked by a reduced FEV1/FVC ratio. This pattern is expected to have partial or complete improvement of spirometry results on reversibility testing through administration of a short-acting beta-2 agonist (SABA) inhaler to the patient. An improvement in FEV1 of 12% or 200 mL from the baseline is indicative of reversibility and is diagnostic for bronchial asthma.[52,53]

When the diagnosis is still uncertain based on history, physical examination, and spirometry, or if an individual cannot perform spirometry, FeNO can be a useful adjunct measurement. FeNO is used as a biomarker of type 2 inflammation. Type 2 inflammation, also known as eosinophilic inflammation in the airway, is characterized by airway immune responses mediated primarily by eosinophils, mast cells, basophils, type 2 helper T lymphocytes, group 2 innate lymphoid cells, and immunoglobulin E (IgE)–producing B cells.[56]

As a marker of airway inflammation, FeNO results alone are not diagnostic; results need to be interpreted in conjunction with other available clinical and diagnostic information.[53] Clinicians should be aware that some individuals with asthma have low levels of FeNO and some individuals without asthma have high levels of FeNO. FeNO testing involves minimal patient effort (exhaling into a monitoring device) and few adverse effects and can be performed by most individuals aged 12 years or older. However, because specialized equipment and trained personnel are required, FeNO testing is typically available only in a subspecialty setting,

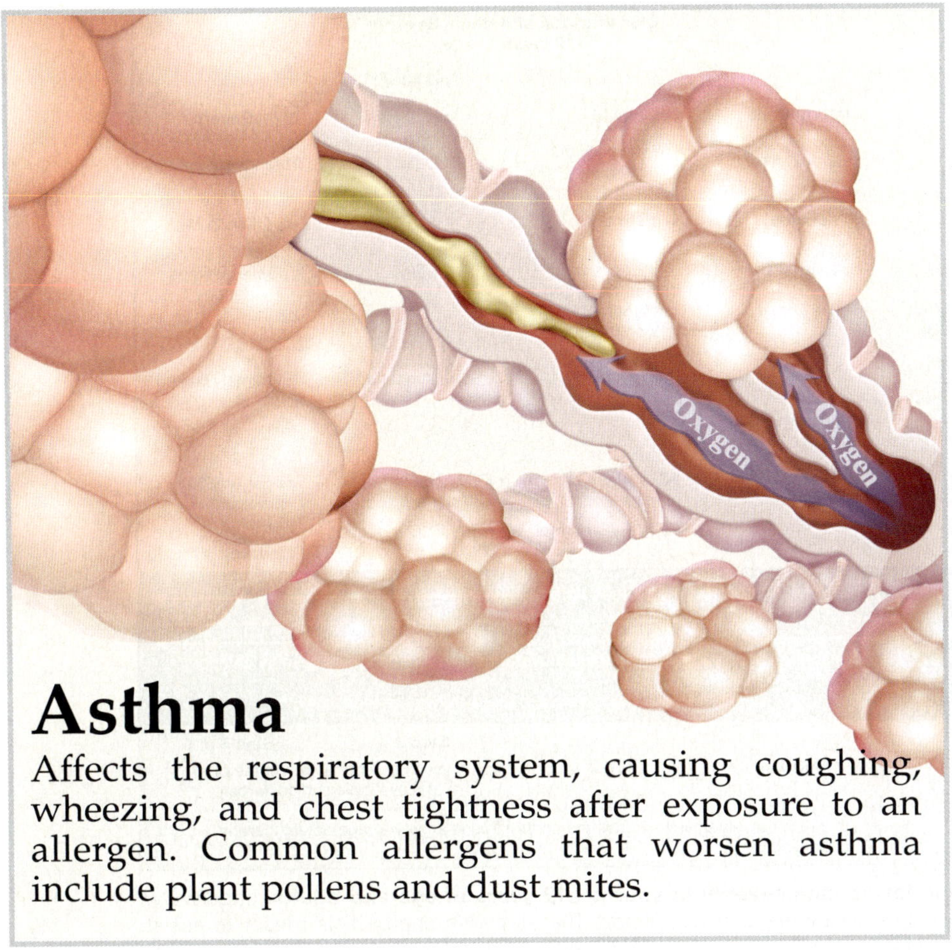

Figure 72.7. Depiction of how inflammation and mucus production in an asthmatic can impact oxygen delivery to alveoli.

which may limit access. Expert panels have determined clinical utility of FeNO in selecting medications, monitoring treatment, and monitoring disease activity in individuals aged 5 years or older.[53,57]

PEF measurement is widely used to document the response to therapy, though it is effort-dependent and may not be reliable in all patients.[52] In cases where airway hyper-reactivity needs to be confirmed, a methacholine or histamine challenge test may be necessary, but this should only be conducted by trained professionals. Exercise spirometry can be helpful in identifying exercise-induced bronchoconstriction.[52]

DISEASE MONITORING

FeNO testing is recommended as part of an ongoing asthma monitoring and management strategy to choose and/or adjust anti-inflammatory therapy. A monitoring frequency of every 2 to 3 months is recommended. The FeNO thresholds to use to adjust anti-inflammatory therapy and reduce the risk of exacerbations are not clearly established. FeNO is not recommended for use alone to predict future exacerbations or assess exacerbation severity. Other clinical information should include history, clinical findings, and spirometry.[53]

In assessing the severity of an asthma attack and for monitoring potential deterioration, pulse oximetry is a valuable tool. However, due to a lag in measurement and the physiologic reserve in many patients, it is important to recognize that a decline in oxygen saturation (pO_2) as measured by pulse oximetry is a late sign, often indicating that the patient is severely ill or close to respiratory arrest.[52] Peak flow measurements are also used to assess asthma severity. Results should be compared against a nomogram as well as the patient's personal baseline. Acute asthma attacks are categorized by their severity, which correlates with specific percentages of the patient's expected peak flow (Fig. 72.8).

Laboratory tests are also a crucial part of diagnosis and management of asthmatic patients. Recent research suggests that sputum eosinophil levels may be useful in guiding treatment. In addition, some patients may exhibit elevated serum IgE levels.[52,58] While eosinophilia is a common finding, it is not exclusive to asthma. Standard asthma therapy includes the use of the bronchodilator salbutamol, also known as albuterol in the United States. At high doses or with repeated administrations of this medication, it is crucial to monitor kidney function with urea and electrolytes. Salbutamol can cause a temporary shift of potassium into cells, potentially leading to transient hypokalemia. In severe cases, arterial blood gas analysis may show hypoxemia and respiratory acidosis.[52]

For additional monitoring, an ECG may display sinus tachycardia, which could be a result of the asthma itself, the use of salbutamol, or theophylline treatment. A CXR is crucial, particularly if there is a concern about a foreign body, potential infection, or other risks. For patients with recurrent symptoms that are unresponsive to treatment, a chest CT scan may be warranted.[52]

TREATMENT

Asthma management has evolved significantly, with current guidelines recommending a comprehensive approach that encompasses both pharmacologic and nonpharmacologic strategies. According to the National Asthma Education and Prevention Program's expert panel, high-quality asthma care involves not only the initial

Components of Severity		Classification of Asthma Severity ≥12 years of age			
			Persistent		
		Intermittent	Mild	Moderate	Severe
Impairment Normal FEV_1/FVC: 8–19 y 85% 20–39 y 80% 40–59 y 75% 60–80 y 70%	Symptoms	≤2 days/wk	>2 days/wk but not daily	Daily	Throughout the day
	Nighttime awakenings	≤2x/mo	3–4x/mo	>1x/wk but not nightly	Often 7x/wk
	Short-acting beta$_2$-agonist use for symptom control (not prevention of EIB)	≤2 days/wk	>2 days/wk but not daily, and not more than 1x on any day	Daily	Several times per day
	Interference with normal activity	None	Minor limitation	Some limitation	Extremely limited
	Lung function	• Normal FEV_1 between exacerbations • FEV_1 >80% predicted • FEV_1/FCC normal	• FEV_1 >80% predicted • FEV_1/FVC normal	• FEV_1, >60% but <80% predicted • FEV_1/FVC reduced 5%	• FEV_1 <60% predicted • FEV_1/FVC reduced >5%
Risk	Exacerbations requiring oral systemic corticosteroids	0–1/y (see note)	≥2/y (see note) →		
		← Consider severity and interval since last exacerbation. → Frequency and severity may fluctuate over time for patients in any severity category. Relative annual risk of exacerbations may be related to FEV_1.			
Recommended Step for Initiating Treatment		Step 1	Step 2	Step 3 and consider short course of oral systemic corticosteroids	Step 4 or 5
		In 2–6 wk, evaluate level of asthma control that is achieved and adjust therapy accordingly.			

Figure 72.8. NHLBI classification for asthma severity in youths ≥12 years of age and adults. http://www.nhlbi.nih.gov/health-pro/guidelines/current/asthma-guidelines Notes: The stepwise approach is meant to assist, not replace, the clinical decision making required to meet individual patient needs. Level of severity is determined by assessment of both impairment and risk. Assess impairment domain by patient's/caregiver's recall of previous 2 to 4 weeks and spirometry. Assign severity to the most severe category in which any feature occurs. At present, there are inadequate data to correspond frequencies of exacerbations with different levels of asthma severity. In general, more frequent and intense exacerbations (e.g., requiring urgent, unscheduled care, hospitalization, or ICU admission) indicate greater underlying disease severity. For treatment purposes, patients who had ≥2 exacerbations requiring oral systemic corticosteroids in the past year may be considered the same as patients who have persistent asthma, even in the absence of impairment levels consistent with persistent asthma.

diagnosis and treatment to achieve asthma control, but also long-term, regular follow-up care to maintain control. Proper asthma treatment focuses on symptom reduction and minimizing future risk. This includes reducing frequency and intensity of symptoms and future exacerbations, as well as reducing medication side effects. Achieving and maintaining asthma control requires the provision of appropriate medication, addressing environmental triggers, patient education on self-management, regular monitoring, and adjustment of therapeutic regimen as needed.[59] These recommendations are corroborated by the Global Initiative for Asthma (GINA), emphasizing personalization of asthma management, including escalation or de-escalation of therapy; assessment of inflammatory biomarkers to guide treatment; a written asthma plan; management of comorbid conditions; and nonpharmacologic strategies for symptom relief.[60]

Management of asthma requires an interprofessional and collaborative approach. During each visit, medication compliance should be reinforced.[52,61] Environmental exposures can play a significant role in the pathogenesis of asthma. Prioritizing environmental control is crucial for prevention of recurrent attacks, with allergen avoidance notably enhancing quality of life. This includes avoidance of triggers such as tobacco, dust mites, animals, and pollen. Therefore, this lifestyle modification can help significantly with symptoms and disease progression. In addition, weight reduction among obese asthmatics leads to improved control of asthma.[52] Evidence shows that educating patients about their condition, including monitoring techniques, medication compliance and inhaler use, and environmental adjustments, improves outcomes.[52,61]

PHARMACOLOGIC THERAPY FOR MANAGING ASTHMA IN INDIVIDUALS AGED 12 YEARS OR OLDER

Medical management of asthma has changed since initial therapy guidelines were released, with recommended therapies evolving from trials including the BADGER trial (Best Add-on Therapy Giving Effective Responses) and Salmeterol Multicenter Asthma Research Trial (SMART), among other randomized controlled trials. Current treatment includes bronchodilators such as beta-2 agonists, muscarinic antagonists, and anti-inflammatories such as ICSs.[52] Beta-2 agonists (such as salbutamol, salmeterol, or albuterol) are designed to alleviate inflammation and relax the bronchial muscles, thereby reducing mucus production. Muscarinic receptor antagonists (like ipratropium bromide) can also be beneficial in reducing inflammation and relaxing bronchial musculature. Although complete resolution is the theoretical goal in asthma management, in practice, the effectiveness of these treatments is not always verified through testing.[52,53]

The 2020 Asthma Management Guidelines by the National Heart Lung and Blood Institute (NHLBI), highlight the importance of using ICSs for recurrent wheezing or persistent asthma, the addition of LAMAs with ICSs for long-term management, and avoidance of indoor asthma triggers. They also advocate for immunotherapy in some cases of allergic asthma, the use of FeNO tests for asthma diagnosis and management, and bronchial thermoplasty for selected adults with persistent asthma.[59]

The GINA 2021 Executive Summary stresses personalized, continuous care to minimize symptoms and prevent exacerbations. It advises against managing asthma solely with SABA and recommends that all patients 6 years or older with asthma should be treated with ICS-containing therapy, with frequency depending on asthma severity. This report recommends the use of Maintenance-and-Reliever Therapy (MART) for patients with moderate to severe asthma. MART combines ICS and formoterol in the same inhaler, allowing for both anti-inflammatory treatment and bronchodilation simultaneously (see Fig. 72.9).[60]

Single Maintenance and Reliever Therapy (SMART)

The 2020 Asthma Guideline Update recommends SMART as the preferred daily controller therapy and as the preferred as-needed rescue therapy.[53] As discussed above, this therapy allows for concomitant use of ICSs to treat inflammation in addition to formoterol, a long-acting beta agonist with the goal of inducing bronchodilation. This recommendation has since been supported by numerous organizations.[54,62] The trial from which the SMART recommendation was derived used formoterol as the long-acting beta-2 agonist (LABA). Compared with other currently available LABAs, formoterol has a rapid onset of action and a dose range that allows for patient use more than twice daily. SMART is used with a single inhaler containing both formoterol and an ICS (see Fig. 72.9).[53]

Use of Long-Acting Muscarinic Antagonists

Add-on LAMA therapy is recommended for many individuals aged 12 years or older with uncontrolled asthma as a secondary alternative to SMART. LAMA therapy is recommended for long-term asthma control in the ambulatory setting and not to treat acute asthma in the emergency department or inpatient setting. Addition of a LAMA to ICS–LABA therapy is also recommended for more severe asthma management. However, LAMA therapy is not recommended for use in individuals with or at risk of urinary retention or glaucoma.[53]

NEWER THERAPIES

Immunotherapy (both subcutaneous and sublingual) refers to treatments used to attenuate the IgE-mediated allergic clinical response associated with asthma. Immunotherapy consists of therapeutic administration of exogenous aeroallergens with the goal of attenuating that individual's asthmatic response. Before initiating immunotherapy, individuals with asthma need to demonstrate allergic sensitization to the allergen by either (1) immediate hypersensitivity skin testing, followed by assessment 15 to 20 minutes later for a wheal-and-flare reaction to the allergens tested or (2) laboratory testing to measure the blood level of (aeroallergen) antigen-specific IgE antibody. Allergen immunotherapy is administered by subcutaneous injection (subcutaneous immunotherapy [SCIT]) of the allergen or sublingually (sublingual immunotherapy [SLIT]) in the

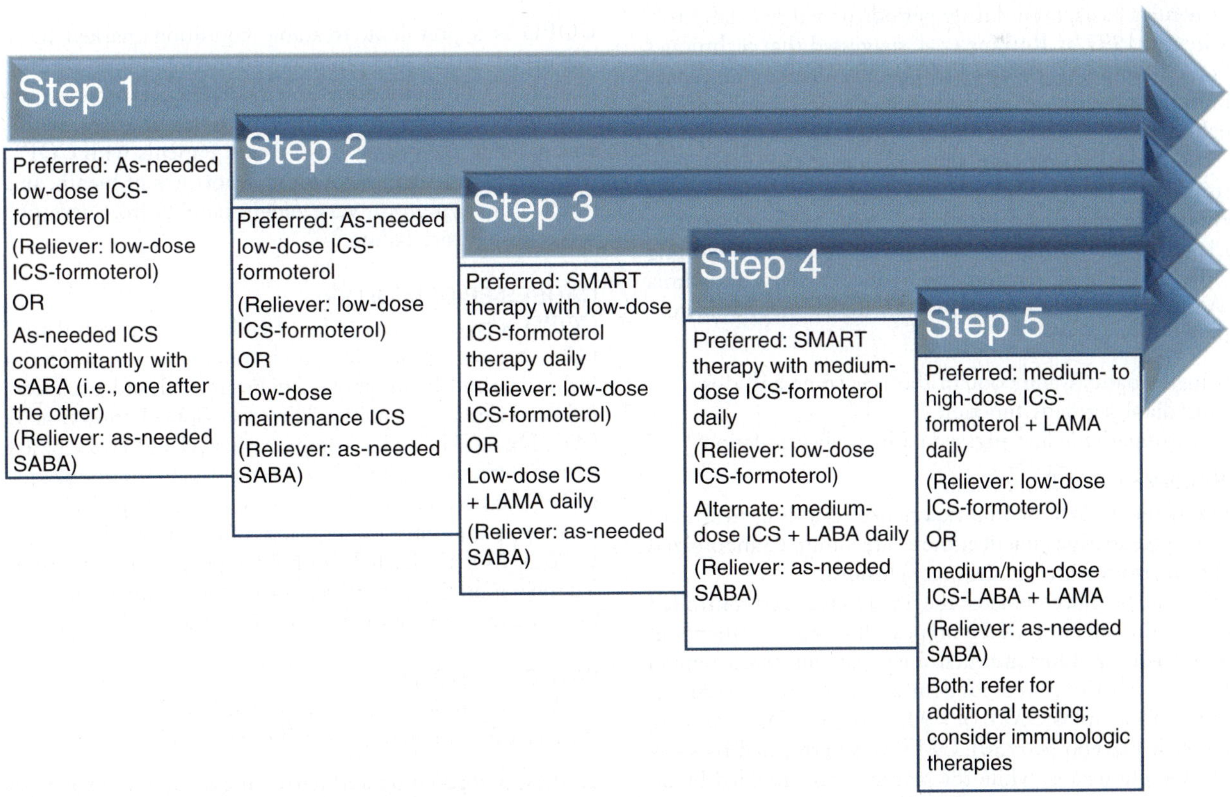

Figure 72.9. Treatment guidelines for persistent asthma with controller and preferred reliever. The preferred reliever for all the above therapies is as-needed low-dose ICS formoterol. Alternative therapies can be found in the GINA updates 2022. Using ICS-formoterol as reliever reduces the risk of exacerbations compared with using a SABA as a reliever.[60] ICS, inhaled corticosteroid; LABA, long-acting beta-2 agonist; LAMA, long-acting muscarinic antagonist. Adapted from the 2022 Global Initiative for Asthma (GINA). (Created by author Jordan Barry based on reference 60.)

form of aqueous drops or tablets. SCIT is recommended in individuals aged 5 years or older with mild to moderate persistent asthma whose asthma worsens following acute exposure on a seasonal basis. Monoclonal antibody therapy is indicated for patients with moderate to severe asthma who have a positive skin test. Monoclonal antibody therapy acts by binding to specific target molecules that mimic antibodies found in the body. Through this mechanism, they can lower IgE levels, which in turn decreases histamine production. However, the cost of the injections is high.[52,53]

Bronchial thermoplasty is a relatively new technique that delivers thermal energy to the airway wall, reducing the narrowing of the airways. Several studies show that this therapy can reduce emergency visits and days missed from school; however, this therapy is not recommended at this time.[52,53]

OSTEOPATHIC MANIPULATIVE TREATMENT IN ASTHMA

Historical Perspective

Early osteopathic research involving asthma has documented much anecdotal evidence supporting various aspects of treatment, including OMT. Many papers emphasized environmental control measures for treatment of asthma, including those as early as 1902.[63,64] These included recommendations for avoidance of irritant gases and dusts, structural findings associated with reactive airway disease, and how OMT is effective in attenuating the chronic symptoms of this disease.[65] The first known clinical study of manipulation and pulmonary disease was performed by Wilson.[66]

Studies by Wilson and Kline in the mid-20th century continued to build on knowledge of OMT and pulmonary disease. These studies emphasized the benefits of OMT in improving thoracic mobility, diaphragmatic function, and overall respiratory mechanics. Kline strongly urged physicians to continue manipulative treatment on a regular basis, even during periods of asthma stability.[67] Later research in 1999 by Rowane et al. suggested that techniques such as thoracic lymphatic pump (TLP) could enhance vital capacity and immune function, complementing medical interventions like bronchodilators. These techniques were also suggested to promote mobility of the rib cage and function of the diaphragm. Incorporating soft tissue techniques and diaphragm release, along with methods like pursed-lip breathing, aligns with osteopathic psychosocial and biomechanical models to optimize breathing function, alleviate muscle tension, and reduce anxiety in asthma patients. According to Schend et al., OMT for asthma has historically targeted three areas[68]:

- Addressing somatic dysfunction of thoracic spine and ribs
- Improving diaphragmatic function
- Balancing sympathetic and parasympathetic dysregulation[68]

Modern Studies on OMT in Asthma

While there is much documented experience regarding treatment of asthma in osteopathic practice, there are limited randomized controlled trials from which to draw conclusions.

In 2005, Guiney et al. conducted the first randomized controlled trial evaluating the effect of OMT on peak flow measurements in children with asthma. One hundred forty patients (ages ranged from 5 to 17) with asthma were randomly assigned to two groups: standard medical care plus OMT ($n = 90$) or standard medical care with light touch placebo ($n = 50$). OMT was performed by various osteopathic physicians, while the placebo was provided by an allopathic physician. Osteopathic techniques included rib raising, muscle energy for ribs, and myofascial release (MFR). The OMT group showed a statistically significant improvement of 7 L/min to 9 L/min for PEF rates (95% confidence interval). Full PFTs, long-term follow-up, and larger sample size were recommended.[69]

Following this study, multiple systematic searches and reviews have documented that this study was considered to have inconclusive yet favorable evidence for OMT in treating pediatric asthma.[70,71] More robust clinical research is necessary to help guide clinicians in their management decisions of pediatric patients with asthma.

Intervention with OMT has historically been shown to decrease respiratory rate and increase tidal volume (VT) after treatment.[72–74] A study by Jones et al. in 2020 investigated the effect of OMT on pulmonary function testing in pediatric asthma patients. The study included children ages 7 to 18 with a diagnosis of asthma who were receiving routine care at a primary care asthma clinic and had undergone baseline spirometry. Participants were randomized to either an OMT or a control group. The OMT group was treated with rib raising and suboccipital release in addition to standard asthma care, while the control group received standard care alone. OMT was performed by trained osteopathic pediatric residents. Following the intervention, a second PFT was administered to both groups. Patients who received OMT had greater improvement in all spirometry results (FVC, FEV1, FVC/FEV1, and forced expiratory flow 25% to 75%) compared to the control group; however, these changes were not statistically significant. The benefits of OMT on short term spirometry results in pediatric asthma patients remain unclear.[75]

The cost and time burden of asthma exacerbation is costly, with repeated trips to the emergency room or urgent clinics brought on by triggers.[76] When treated with OMT, length of hospital stay is reported to be reduced by nearly one day when OMT is used as a treatment modality for acute asthma exacerbation. It has been suggested that substantial cost savings would occur as well.[77]

COPD

COPD is a prevalent, treatable condition marked by a gradual decline in airflow and pulmonary function due to chronic inflammation.[78,79] This inflammation-mediated deterioration stems from long-term exposure to harmful particles or gases, with cigarette smoke being the primary risk factor. Patients with COPD experience symptoms such as coughing, shortness of breath, and sputum production. Symptoms vary widely, ranging from asymptomatic to severe respiratory failure.[78,79]

CAUSES/EPIDEMIOLOGY

COPD is typically caused by extended contact with damaging particles or gases. In addition to cigarette smoke, contributing factors include second-hand smoke, environmental and occupational hazards, and a genetic condition known as alpha-1 antitrypsin deficiency (AATD). AATD is a less common cause, characterized by a deficiency in antiproteases, making lung tissue more susceptible to damage. COPD predominantly affects smokers and individuals over the age of 40. It is the third-leading cause of death and disease globally.[78–80] In 2015, COPD affected 174 million people and was responsible for 3.2 million deaths worldwide, though these numbers likely underestimate the true prevalence due to frequent underdiagnosis.[78,79]

PATHOPHYSIOLOGY

COPD is comprised of multiple pulmonary pathologic processes that are often interconnected. These include[80]:

1. Airway thickening and narrowing leading to expiratory airflow obstruction
2. Chronic mucus hypersecretion leading to chronic cough and phlegm production
3. Dilation of distal airspaces and destruction of alveolar walls, also known as emphysema[80]

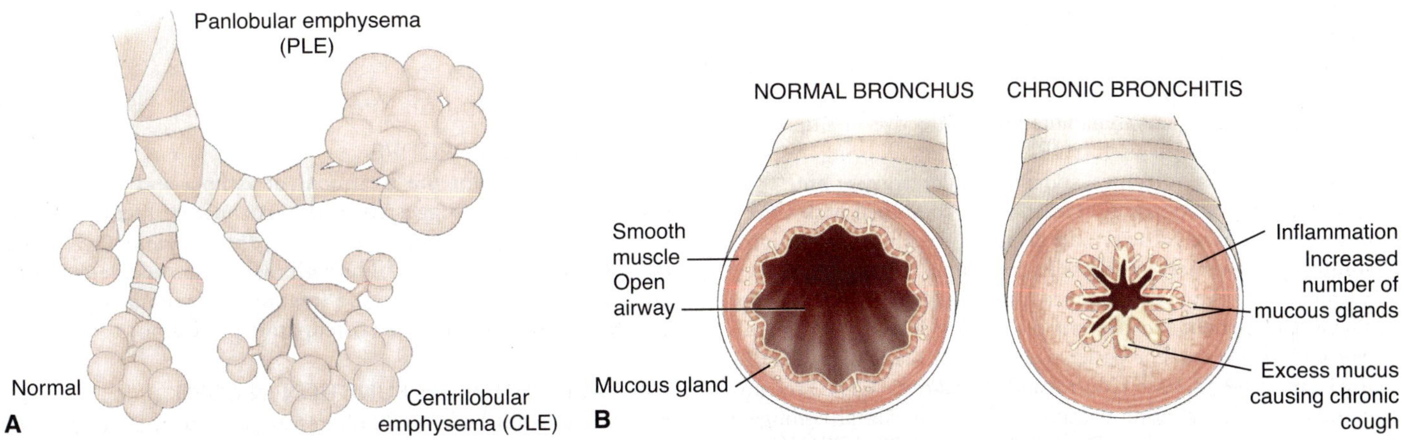

Figure 72.10. Changes in the airways with chronic obstructive pulmonary disease (COPD). A. Example of alveolar changes in COPD. **B.** Airway changes in bronchitis.

Chronic inflammation from COPD leads to airway narrowing and reduced lung elasticity, causing symptoms and potential complications. For instance, lung hyperinflation, visible in imaging studies, results from air becoming trapped due to airway collapse during exhalation. This trapping of air not only causes difficulty with exhalation, but also leads to CO_2 retention. As COPD advances, the amount of gas exchange occurring in the lung declines, resulting in hypoxia. This hypoxic state induces widespread pulmonary vasoconstriction, which may lead to the development of pulmonary hypertension[78,79] (see Fig. 72.10).

CLINICAL PRESENTATION

Patients with COPD often experience chronic and progressive shortness of breath, coughing, and sputum production. Additional symptoms can include wheezing and a sensation of chest tightness, with symptoms often becoming more pronounced in the winter. While a history of smoking is common among COPD patients, some patients may have had exposure to second-hand smoke, occupational and environmental hazards, or a family history of respiratory conditions. COPD typically manifests in adulthood.[78,79]

Emphysema and chronic bronchitis are both forms of COPD, often presenting with different patient characteristics and symptoms. Emphysema has classically been associated with the adage of "pink puffer," describing a patient with pursed-lip breathing, a barrel-chest-appearance due to hyperinflation of the lungs, and a minimal cough. This is because emphysema primarily affects the alveoli, impairing oxygenation, resulting in breathlessness and a chronic cough.[80,81] Chronic bronchitis has been historically linked to the adage of the "blue bloater" phenotype. Patients with this condition may appear cyanotic, with a bluish discoloration of the skin due to insufficient oxygenation, hence the term "blue." This disease process causes a productive cough with excessive mucus production, and patients may exhibit signs of right-sided heart failure such as peripheral edema. The "bloater" term refers to the tendency of these patients to retain fluid, a possible consequence of chronic hypoxia and hypercapnia causing pulmonary hypertension and right heart strain.[81]

DIAGNOSIS

Patients exhibiting symptoms consistent with COPD, especially those with known risk factors, should undergo a thorough evaluation. Spirometry is the cornerstone of COPD diagnosis, confirming the condition when the ratio of the FEV1 to the FVC (FEV1/FVC) is less than 0.7.[79] Additional assessments may include a 6-minute walk test to evaluate exercise capacity, laboratory tests to check for infections or blood disorders, and radiographic imaging to visualize lung structure.[57,79]

Spirometry is typically conducted before and after the administration of an inhaled bronchodilator, which may be a SABA, a short-acting anticholinergic, or a combination of both.[78,79] Pulmonary function tests (PFTs), such as spirometry, is crucial not only for diagnosing COPD but also for staging and monitoring disease progression.

The Global Initiative for Chronic Obstructive Lung Disease (GOLD) is a comprehensive program initiated by the World Health Organization (WHO) and the National Heart, Lung, and Blood Institute (NHLBI). The 2019 GOLD report introduced a simplified method for evaluating patients and selecting initial COPD treatments, including the refined ABCD assessment tool, which helps health care providers determine the severity of the disease.[79] The diagnosis of COPD can be supported by the steps listed below[79,82]:

- Once COPD is confirmed with spirometry (FEV1/FVC <0.7), the FEV1 measurement is used to determine the severity of the disease, categorized into GOLD classifications 1 to 4.
- The COPD Assessment Test (CAT) scores eight functional parameters to gauge the disease's impact on a patient's daily life.
- The 6-minute walk test, conducted indoors along a flat, straight path, typically 100 feet in length, measures the distance a patient can walk in 6 minutes to assess submaximal functional capacity.
- Laboratory tests often include a complete blood count to screen for infection, anemia, or polycythemia and a CXR may reveal signs of hyperinflation, diaphragm flattening, and an increased anterior–posterior diameter of the chest.
- A CT scan of the chest can show centrilobular emphysema and, in some cases, bullae in the subpleural regions.[79,82]

TREATMENT

The primary objectives of COPD treatment are to manage symptoms, enhance quality of life, minimize the frequency of exacerbations, and reduce mortality risk. Treatment strategies encompass both nonpharmacologic and pharmacologic approaches.[79]

Nonpharmacologic Approaches

- Smoking Cessation: All patients should be counseled on the benefits of smoking cessation. In current smokers with COPD, smoking cessation has been shown to improve and slow the rate of decline of pulmonary function testing.[83]

- Pulmonary Rehabilitation: Guidelines have recommended patients be enrolled in pulmonary rehabilitation after hospitalization for COPD. Studies have demonstrated decreased mortality in patients enrolled in pulmonary rehabilitation after hospital discharge.[84] Pulmonary rehabilitation is effective at improving symptoms for patients with COPD, including relieving dyspnea, increasing exercise tolerance, and improving quality of life.[84,85] In addition, pulmonary rehabilitation, when combined with OMT, improved exercise capacity and decreased residual lung volume compared to pulmonary rehabilitation alone.[86]
- Vaccinations: Annual influenza vaccinations are advised for all COPD patients to prevent respiratory infections that can worsen the disease. For patients aged 65 or older with COPD, the Centers for Disease Control and Prevention (CDC) recommends the routine administration of pneumococcal conjugate vaccines (PCVs), specifically PCV15 or PCV20. If PCV15 is used, it should be followed by a dose of the pneumococcal polysaccharide vaccine (PPSV23) at least 1 year later. However, if PCV20 is used, an additional dose of PPSV23 is not needed.[87] There are certain circumstances in ages 19 to 64 in which a pneumococcal conjugate vaccine is recommended, such as having a congenital or acquired immunodeficiency and iatrogenic immunosuppression.

Pharmacologic Treatments

The medication regimen for COPD may include:

- Bronchodilators such as beta-2 agonists, antimuscarinics, and methylxanthines to dilate the airways.
- ICSs to reduce pulmonary inflammation.
- Systemic glucocorticoids for managing acute exacerbations.
- Phosphodiesterase-4 (PDE4) Inhibitors to decrease inflammation.
- Antibiotics for treating or preventing bacterial infections that can trigger exacerbations.[79]

Management of Acute Exacerbations

The severity of an exacerbation, as previously discussed, determines whether treatment occurs in an outpatient or inpatient setting. Mild exacerbations may be managed outpatient with bronchodilators, corticosteroids, and antibiotics. Moderate to severe exacerbations require inpatient care, often involving oxygen therapy and bronchodilator treatment using a SABA with or without a short-acting muscarinic antagonist (SAMA). Antibiotics are considered if a bacterial infection is suspected. Oxygen therapy may range from nasal cannula to mechanical ventilation based on the exacerbation's severity.[79]

Long-Term Assessment and Surgical Interventions

For long-term management, treatment should be personalized and comprehensive, incorporating proper medical management with optimization of quality of life for patients. One useful tool for assessment of patient status is the BODE index. The BODE index is a multidimensional grading system developed to predict survival in patients with COPD. It encompasses four components:

- Body mass index (BMI)
- Obstruction measured by FEV1
- Dyspnea assessed using the modified Medical Research Council (MMRC) dyspnea scale
- Exercise capacity evaluated through the 6-minute walk test.[88]

This comprehensive approach allows for a more accurate assessment of a COPD patient's health status and prognosis compared to traditional methods that primarily focus on lung function. The BODE index has been shown to correlate with the quality of life in stable COPD patients, highlighting its utility not only in predicting survival but also in assessing the impact of COPD on patients' daily lives.[89]

Osteopathic Manipulative Treatment in COPD

HISTORICAL PERSPECTIVE

The use of OMT for the treatment of asthma and other forms of COPD has been suggested in the osteopathic literature from as early as 1902, when the *Journal of the American Osteopathic Association* first appeared.[63,64] Through many years and generations of osteopaths, the knowledge and treatment of pulmonary disease has been intertwined with the osteopathic profession.

OMT ON PULMONARY FUNCTION IN COPD

In a study published in 2008, researchers at the A. T. Still University of Health Sciences—Kirksville College of Osteopathic Medicine reported that a protocol used to treat elderly patients with COPD resulted in worsening of air trapping during the 30 minutes immediately after the OMT session. The OMT group also had a statistically significant increase in the residual volume and TLC compared with the sham group. However, most subjects (82% OMT group; 65% sham group) reported breathing better after treatment. Results suggested a worsening of air trapping during the 30 minutes immediately following one multitechnique OMT session relative to the sham group.[90]

In a follow-up study, Noll et al. attempted to determine the immediate effects of four osteopathic techniques on pulmonary function measures in patients over age 50 with COPD relative to a minimal-touch control protocol. Subjects received five, single-technique treatment sessions: minimal-touch control, TLP with activation, TLP without activation, rib raising, and MFR. Results indicated that in patients with COPD, TLP with activation, TLP without activation, rib raising, and MFR mildly worsened pulmonary function measures immediately posttreatment relative to baseline measurements. The activation component of the TLP technique also appeared to increase posttreatment residual volume. Despite adverse changes in pulmonary function measures, patients with COPD continued to subjectively report benefit from osteopathic manipulation.[91]

Raguckas et al. published a systematic review of the evidence on osteopathic considerations in COPD. They determined that incorporating OMM into the treatment of COPD demonstrated an inconsistent impact on objective pulmonary measures, but improvement was noted when patient assessment of symptoms was included. They recommended larger studies that minimize bias, incorporate patient-oriented measures, and evaluate the effect on acute exacerbations as the next steps to build the body of evidence regarding the utilization of OMM in COPD.[92]

In a subsequent randomized control trial, Buscemi et al. evaluated the efficacy of OMT in patients with moderate-to-severe COPD. Patients were assessed using spirometry, the CAT and a 6-minute walking test (6MWT). The main goals were to improve the quality of life of patients with stable moderate-to-severe COPD, and to revise the parameters of the assessment tests, such as spirometry and 6MWT. The osteopathic approach to treatment focused on treatment of the maxillary sinuses, vertebral–pleural ligaments, phrenic nerves, ribs, pleura, lungs, bronchi, subclavian muscles, and trapezoid and conoid ligaments. Patients of the OMT group improved in all tests compared to the control group. The results showed that the patients with COPD who received the conventional pharmacologic treatment in association with the OMT therapy demonstrated a good response to the osteopathic treatment, thus leading to significant improvements in their health and daily lives.[93]

OMT IN CONJUNCTION WITH OTHER THERAPIES

In a 2013 study, the effects of soft tissue, direct technique spinal manipulation (high-velocity low-amplitude) of the thoracic region, and exercise were evaluated on adults diagnosed with moderate COPD. The outcomes included FVC, chronic respiratory questionnaire scores, plus distance and speed walked in a 6-minute walk test. Patients were randomly assigned to one of three groups: soft tissue + spinal manipulation + exercise ($n = 5$), soft tissue + spinal manipulation ($n = 4$), or soft tissue alone ($n = 5$). Treatments lasted no longer than 30 minutes, with eight sessions performed over a 4-week period. The group who received a combination of all modalities (soft tissue + spinal manipulation + exercise) demonstrated significantly improved lung capacity and walking distance at the end of the trial; furthermore, walking distance, walking speed, and dyspnea scores significantly improved with soft tissue + spinal manipulation compared with soft tissue treatment alone. Limitations of the study included a narrow age range of participants and the lack of a no-treatment control group.[94]

Another possible adjunct therapy includes pulmonary rehabilitation. A study by Zanotti et al. examined the effects of OMT paired with pulmonary rehabilitation on patients more than 65 years old with stage III COPD via PFT over 4 weeks. The primary outcomes of the study were residual volume on pulmonary function testing and exercise capacity as measured by the 6-minute walk test. Patients were randomly assigned to either pulmonary rehabilitation + OMT or pulmonary rehabilitation + sham treatment. OMT included a structural examination followed by treatments tailored to examination findings, while sham treatment included light touch. After 4 weeks of treatment, patients' 6-minute walk test distance increased significantly more in the pulmonary rehabilitation + OMT group compared to the pulmonary rehabilitation + sham treatment group. Pulmonary rehabilitation + OMT also significantly decreased residual volume more than pulmonary rehabilitation + sham treatment.[86]

In 2019, Krus-Johnston et al. published a review of past studies (2008–2013) and came to the conclusion that osteopathic manipulative therapy (OMTh) has an unclear impact on residual volume in patients with COPD; however, OMT combined with pulmonary rehabilitation or exercise is associated with improved pulmonary function, symptoms, walking distance, and walking speed versus sham treatments.[95]

Pneumonia

GENERAL CONSIDERATIONS

Pneumonia is defined as an acute infection of the lung parenchyma caused by one or more coinfecting pathogens affecting the air sacs, or alveoli, of the lungs, causing them to accumulate fluid or pus, leading to symptoms such as cough, shortness of breath, fever, and difficulty breathing.[96] Pneumonia remains a significant health concern globally, with an estimated 5.6 million cases of community-acquired pneumonia (CAP) occurring annually in the United States alone.[97] *Streptococcus pneumoniae* is known for causing pneumococcal pneumonia that infects over 900,000 Americans annually.[97] Pneumonia is a leading cause of infectious disease mortality, particularly among the geriatric population, accounting for nearly half of infectious disease-related deaths.[98] CAP has an overall incidence of approximately 10 to 12 cases per 1,000 persons per year in the United States, and is the seventh leading cause of death.[98] The prevalence and impact of pneumonia are influenced by factors such as advanced age, pre-existing health conditions, recent surgery, and lifestyle factors such as smoking and excessive alcohol consumption. Immunocompromised patients, such as those with HIV/AIDS or those undergoing transplantation, are at increased risk for opportunistic infections, including pneumonia caused by atypical pathogens.[99,100] These factors can impair host defenses, causing an exudative inflammation of the lung. The complexity of lung infections is further underscored by the fact that exacerbations of conditions like COPD and cystic fibrosis are often polymicrobial, involving multiple bacteria and even viruses, rather than being caused by a single pathogen.[99,100]

CATEGORIZATION OF PNEUMONIA[101]

Pneumonia is categorized based on various criteria including the setting in which it was acquired, the area of the lung affected, the immune status of the patient, and the causative pathogens.

ANATOMIC CLASSIFICATION

Anatomically, pneumonia can be classified as lobar pneumonia, which affects a single lobe of the lung, or bronchopneumonia, which involves multiple areas.

Lobar pneumonia involves the acute bacterial infection of a large portion of a lobe or an entire lobe of the lung. Lobar pneumonia is most commonly caused by *Streptococcus pneumonia*.[102] The consolidation in lobar pneumonia is more uniform, and it often involves one or two entire lobes of the lung. While bronchopneumonia tends to present with patchy findings on imaging, lobar pneumonia typically shows more extensive and homogenous consolidation on chest radiographs[102] (see Fig. 72.11).

Bronchopneumonia, also known as *lobular* pneumonia, is characterized by a patchy consolidation of inflammation that originates around the bronchi and bronchioles and then spreads to adjacent areas of the lung, often affecting multiple lobes. It is typically associated with a variety of bacteria, including *Streptococcus pneumoniae*, *Haemophilus influenzae*, and *Staphylococcus aureus*, and is more common in the extremes of life.[102]

MICROBIOLOGIC CLASSIFICATION

Pneumonia can be caused by bacterial, viral, fungal, mycobacterial, or parasitic agents, although identifying the specific pathogen can be challenging and often requires advanced diagnostic techniques.

IMMUNE STATUS OF THE PATIENT

Pneumonia can also be categorized by the immune status of the patient, distinguishing between infections in immunocompetent versus immunocompromised individuals.

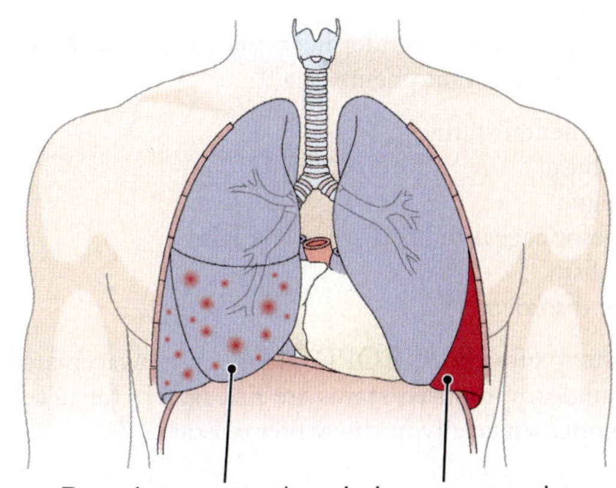

Figure 72.11. Bronchopneumonia versus lobar pneumonia. In bronchopneumonia (right lung), patchy areas of consolidation occur. In lobar pneumonia (left lung), an entire lobe is consolidated.

Diagnosis

Prior to evaluating the patient for pneumonia, it is important for clinicians to follow universal precautions and wear appropriate personal protective equipment (PPE). When gathering a complete history, evaluate progression of illness, obtain vaccination history, perform a complete physical exam and assess for any progression of illness. Patients with pneumonia typically present with new or worsening respiratory symptoms such as fever, cough, purulent sputum, tachypnea, and impaired oxygenation. Symptoms often include cough, fever, chills, dyspnea, and chest pain. The clinical presentation can vary, making it essential to differentiate the type of pneumonia and any other respiratory condition.

Diagnosis of CAP typically involves a combination of clinical assessment, laboratory tests, and imaging. Sputum samples and blood cultures are recommended for patients with severe CAP to identify the causative pathogen, although the yield from blood cultures is generally low.

The diagnosis of pneumonia often involves chest radiography to confirm the presence of an infection in the lung tissue, supported by the patient's clinical presentation and laboratory findings.[97] Once diagnosed, clinicians may use the Pneumonia Severity Index (PSI) and CURB-65 which are among the tools used to assess the severity of pneumonia and guide decisions regarding the need for hospitalization or intensive care.[107,108]

HISTORY AND CLINICAL FEATURES

The clinical presentation of pneumonia can vary widely, but typically includes symptoms such as cough, fever, chills, fatigue, dyspnea, and pleuritic chest pain. The severity of these symptoms can range from mild to life-threatening, necessitating careful assessment and management.

When taking a history, the osteopathic clinician should explore the patient's potential exposures, risks of aspiration, host factors, and presenting symptoms. Certain pathogens are associated with various exposures (See Box 72.1).[104]

Common Exposures

- Contaminated air-conditioning: Legionella pneumonia.
- Crowded spaces, such as jails, and shelters: *Streptococcus pneumonia,* Mycobacteria, Mycoplasma, and Chlamydia.
- Exposures to animals, such as cats, sheep, and cattle: *Coxiella burnetii.*
- Exposure to birds such as chickens, turkeys, and ducks: *Chlamydia psittaci.*

Host Factors

It is also important to consider host-related issues that predispose the patient to aspiration pneumonia[104]:

- Altered mental status
- Drug abuse
- Dysphagia
- Gastroesophageal reflux disease (GERD)
- Alcoholism
- Seizure disorder

A history of asthma, COPD, smoking, nonvaccinated status, and immunocompromised status are risk factors for development of pneumonia, especially in the winter season.

PHYSICAL EXAM

Physical examination may reveal signs of lung consolidation such as decreased breath sounds, crackles, and in some cases, pleural rub. Other signs include tachypnea, productive cough, and an increased work of breathing (See box 72.2). Similarly, inpatients may present with increased temperature, increased respiratory rate, and physical signs like crackles, rigors, decreased pulse oximetry, and abnormal breath sounds upon auscultation.[104,109] In addition, findings such as dullness to percussion, egophony, and increased fremitus are relatively uncommon but highly specific for pneumonia, aiding in its diagnosis.[110] In children, the physical exam findings that are most reliable are wheezing, retractions, and respiratory rate.[111]

Structural findings may include chronic postural changes such as a barrel chest as seen in COPD, or increased kyphosis/kyphoscoliosis as seen in the elderly. It is common for patients with pneumonia to utilize accessory muscles of breathing such as the scalene, abdominal, and intercostal muscles. These muscles may be tight and tender from overuse. Specific motion restrictions of the ribs include a lack of symmetric pump/bucket handle motion, and a lack of compliance to compression. The ribs may be held in a position of exhalation due to repeated, forceful coughing. It is common to palpate tension and tenderness along the Linea alba, as these patients use their abdominal muscles to assist with the work of breathing. The abdominal diaphragm and its associated ribs and spinal segmental attachments may be tight, restricted, and tender. Chapman reflex points may be located anteriorly along the sternum and ribs or posteriorly along the upper to mid thoracic spinal segments between the spinous and transverse processes (see Chapter 58 A Modern Approach to Chapman's Reflex Points). Puffy tissue texture changes can be palpated along the rib angle at the spinal level, on the side of the associated pneumonia.[112]

BOX 72.1 Infectious Agents in Pneumonia[101,103–106]

Some common causes are listed below:

Common causes of viral pneumonia[101]

- Respiratory syncytial virus (RSV)
- Influenza virus types A and B
- Parainfluenza virus
- Adenovirus (less common)
- Coronaviruses (e.g., SARS-CoV-2, which causes COVID-19 pneumonia)

Most common causes of post-viral pneumonia[103,104]

- *Streptococcus pneumoniae*
- *Staphylococcus aureus*
- *Haemophilus influenzae*
- *Moraxella catarrhalis*
- Methicillin-resistant *Staphylococcus aureus*
- *Pseudomonas aeruginosa*

Most common causes of atypical pneumonia[105]

- *Mycoplasma pneumoniae*
- *Chlamydia pneumoniae*
- *Legionella pneumophila*
- *Chlamydia psittaci*

Most common causes of atypical pneumonia, fungal[106]

- Coccidioidomycosis
- Histoplasmosis
- Blastomycosis
- *Pneumocystis jirovecii*
- Cryptococcus
- Aspergillus
- Mucormycosis

BOX 72.2 Pneumonia Physical Exam Findings[104]

Specific sputum characteristics suggesting certain bacterial causes[104]:

- Rust-colored sputum: *Streptococcus pneumoniae*
- Green sputum: Pseudomonas or Haemophilus
- Red currant–jelly sputum: Klebsiella
- Foul-smelling and bad-tasting sputum: Anaerobic bacteria

Key physical findings on examination include the following[104]:

- Increased temperature (usually more than 38 °C or 100.4 °F)
- Decreased temperature (less than 35 °C or 95 °F)
- Increased respiratory rate (more than 18 breaths/min)
- Increased heart rate (more than 100/min)
- Cyanosis
- Percussion sounds vary from flat to dull
- Tactile fremitus
- Crackles, rales, and bronchial breath sounds are heard during auscultation
- Tracheal deviation
- Lymphadenopathy
- Pleural rub
- Egophony

Associated findings[104]:

- Bradycardia (less than 60/min) (Legionella)
- Dental disease (Anaerobes)
- Impaired gag reflex (Aspiration)
- Bullous myringitis (Mycoplasma)

LABORATORY EVALUATION[104]

Patients with pneumonia commonly also have laboratory indicators of infection, including elevated white blood cell (WBC) counts and C-reactive protein levels.

- Pulse oximetry of less than 92% indicates severe hypoxia.
- Blood cultures should be obtained before administering antibiotics but are only positive in 40% of cases.
- Sputum evaluation may reveal more than 25 WBC per low-power field and less than 10 squamous epithelial cells.
- An elevated CRP predicts a serious infection.

IMAGING

Radiographic features, while not always specific, play a crucial role in diagnosis. CXR is a fundamental imaging tool in the diagnosis and management of pneumonia, offering critical insights into the various forms of this condition. Pneumonia can manifest in several radiographic patterns on CXR, including lobar pneumonia, bronchopneumonia, interstitial pneumonia, and atypical pneumonia.[113] Each of these patterns provides clues about the causative agent and the severity of the infection, aiding clinicians in tailoring the most appropriate treatment strategies (see Fig. 72.12).

- Lobar pneumonia is characterized by homogeneous consolidation affecting one or more lung lobes, often accompanied by air bronchograms—air-filled bronchi visible against the background of pus-filled alveoli. This pattern is typically associated with bacterial infections, particularly *Streptococcus pneumoniae*.[113,114]
- Bronchopneumonia, on the other hand, presents as patchy consolidation across multiple lung lobes, reflecting the diffuse bronchial distribution of the infection, commonly seen in cases caused by *Staphylococcus aureus* or *Haemophilus influenzae*.[113]
- Interstitial pneumonia shows a more reticular or nodular pattern on CXR, indicative of viral or mycoplasma infections.
- Atypical pneumonia, which is caused by less common pathogens and may present with less defined radiographic features,

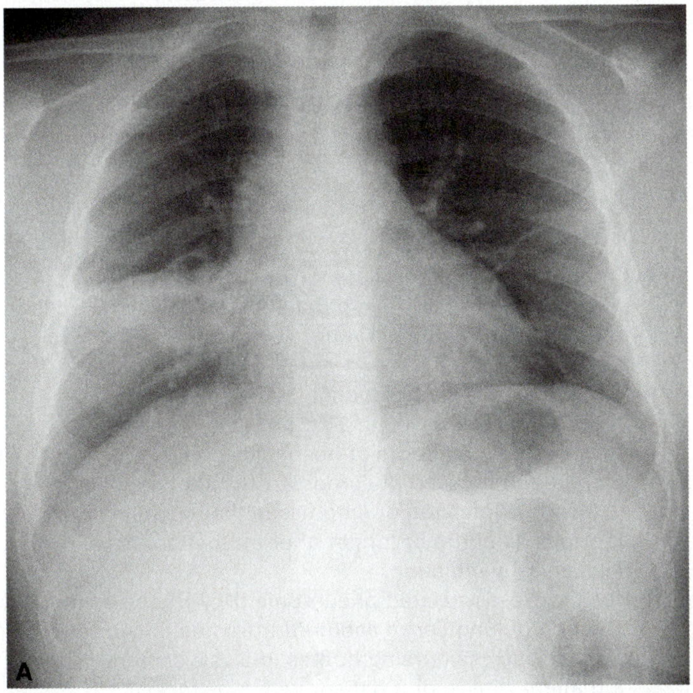

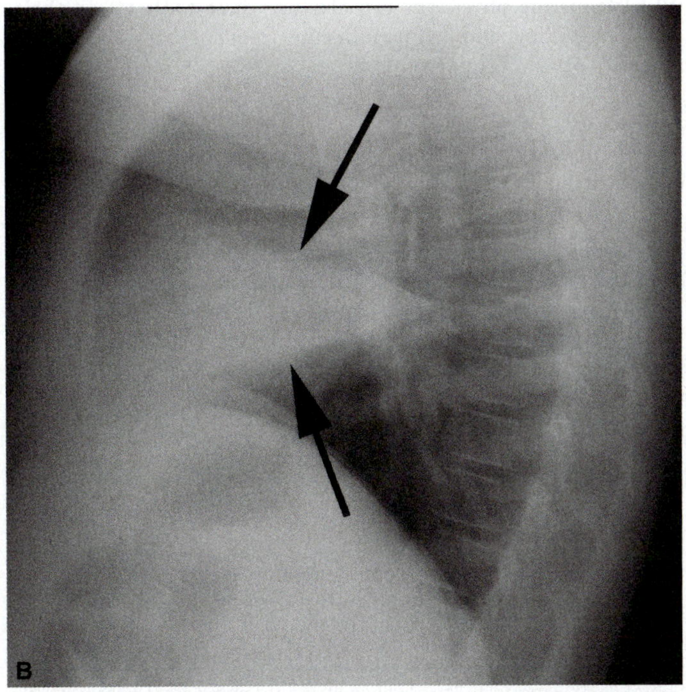

Figure 72.12. Right middle lobe pneumonia. Lobar pneumonia presenting with complete opacification of the right middle lobe on the frontal (**A**) and lateral (**B**) radiographs (*arrows*).

including ground-glass opacities or a more diffuse infiltrative pattern.[113,115]

- The radiologic diagnosis of HAP requires demonstrating new or progressive lung infiltrates, which can be challenging due to the variability in x-ray appearances and the presence of underlying lung condition.
- Patients presenting very early in the course of the disease may have negative findings on chest radiography.[3,116] After treatment, CXR findings generally lag behind clinical features and may take 6 to 12 weeks to resolve.[104]

Management of Pneumonia: General Guidelines

Pneumonia is a common condition affecting patients worldwide, requiring treatment both inside and outside the hospital. Making the decision whether to admit an ill patient to the hospital, or to provide treatment from an outpatient setting can be challenging. There are important, nonnegligible risks associated with each. Longer time in the hospital increases the risk of complications with further drug-resistant pathogens, immobility, and inactivity, among other things.[108] However, the decision to send a patient home to recover without supervision or the additional resources of the hospital should be carefully considered.

Currently, many providers use criteria for cases of CAP such as CURB-65/CRB-65 and PSI to assist in this decision-making. These assessment tools are used to determine risk of mortality from pneumonia and aid in choosing a site of care (Table 72.1).

While CURB-65 criteria are useful for risk stratification for mortality of pneumonia patients, the acquisition of blood urea nitrogen (BUN) levels poses a barrier for outpatient physicians without access to lab results. Further studies have suggested that CRB-65 can serve as a similar tool in situations without the ability to measure BUN.[117] The PSI takes into account more factors including demographic factors, coexisting illnesses, physical examination findings, and laboratory/radiographic findings, each assigned various point values.[118] This method also splits patients into different classes based on various risks of mortality. Osteopathic physicians can also use these tools to aid their decision-making and help guide the frequency and choice of modality of OMT intervention.

STANDARD OF CARE

Osteopathic treatment of pneumonia has many therapeutic options, including antibiotics, bronchodilators, steroids, respiratory and physical therapy, OMT, oxygen, hydration, body positioning, mechanical ventilation, immunotherapy, and psychological support. Treatment of pneumonia was forever altered by the discovery of antibiotics. As the mainstay of curative treatment for pneumonia, the selection of antibiotics used by physicians in hospitals or outpatient is specific to the patient, suspected causes, and characteristics of the infection before determination of susceptibilities by culture.[108] However, drug resistance of bacterial strains to antibiotics is an emerging problem. Therefore, methods to augment conventional medical treatment are needed. The osteopathic pulmonologist who diagnoses and treats corresponding somatic dysfunction has another tool to augment conventional medical treatment. By incorporating the concept of structure and function and using OMT, respiratory therapy, and physical therapy, they can help the patient clear secretions and improve their clinical condition.

Treatment should target the suspected pathogens causing the pneumonia. However, potential for community antibiotic resistance should be considered, and steps should be taken for the clinician to use universal precautions so as not to spread the infection to others and further contribute to spread of disease and/or resistance.

TABLE 72.1

CURB-65 Criteria for Pneumonia Risk Stratification[101]

Criteria	+1 for Each
Confusion	Mental Test Score of ≤8; new disorientation in person, place, or time
Urea	>7 mmol/L
Respiratory rate	≥30/min
Blood pressure	Low systolic (<90 mm Hg) or diastolic (≤60 mm Hg)
65	Age ≥65 years

Score: (0–1) = mortality low, likely suitable for home treatment; (2) = mortality intermediate, consider hospital supervised treatment; (3 or more) = mortality high, manage in hospital as severe pneumonia.[101]

A CLOSER LOOK: CAP VERSUS HAP

This section will discuss in more detail CAP and hospital-acquired pneumonia (HAP), two common conditions osteopathic physicians treat on a frequent basis (See Box 72.3).

Community Acquired Pneumonia

CAP is defined as pneumonia that is not acquired in a hospital or a long-term care facility. CAP is the most common type of pneumonia and is the most common cause of hospital admissions among adults in the United States and is associated with substantial health care costs.[97,98] It was responsible for an estimated 50,000 deaths in 2010 in the United States alone, a figure that likely underestimates the true impact due to indirect causes of death related to pneumonia. The disease is a leading cause of death worldwide, surpassing deaths from TB, HIV, and malaria combined.[98] Vaccination,

BOX 72.3 Pneumonia Classification by Setting[104]

Pneumonia can be categorized based on the setting in which it was acquired.[104]

- Community-acquired pneumonia (CAP): The acute infection of lung tissue in a patient who has acquired it from the community or within 48 hours of the hospital admission.
- Hospital-acquired pneumonia (HAP): The acute infection of lung tissue in a nonintubated patient develops after 48 hours of hospitalization.
- Ventilator-associated pneumonia (VAP): A type of nosocomial infection of lung tissue that usually develops 48 hours or longer after intubation for mechanical ventilation.
- Health care–associated pneumonia (HCAP): The acute infection of lung tissue acquired from health care facilities such as nursing homes, dialysis centers, outpatient clinics, or a patient with a history of hospitalization within the past 3 months.

especially in children, has led to a decrease in pneumonia-related deaths globally.

The clinical presentation of CAP can vary significantly. The disease's presentation can be particularly challenging to diagnose in previously healthy patients, those with comorbid conditions, and those with atypical pathogens[104,109] (see Fig. 72.13). Early and accurate diagnosis is essential for effective management and improving patient outcomes.

The most common cause of CAP is *S. pneumoniae*, viral pathogens like influenza, followed by *Klebsiella pneumoniae, Haemophilus influenzae,* and *Pseudomonas aeruginosa*.[104,109,119] For outpatient treatment, the recommended antibiotics include macrolides (such

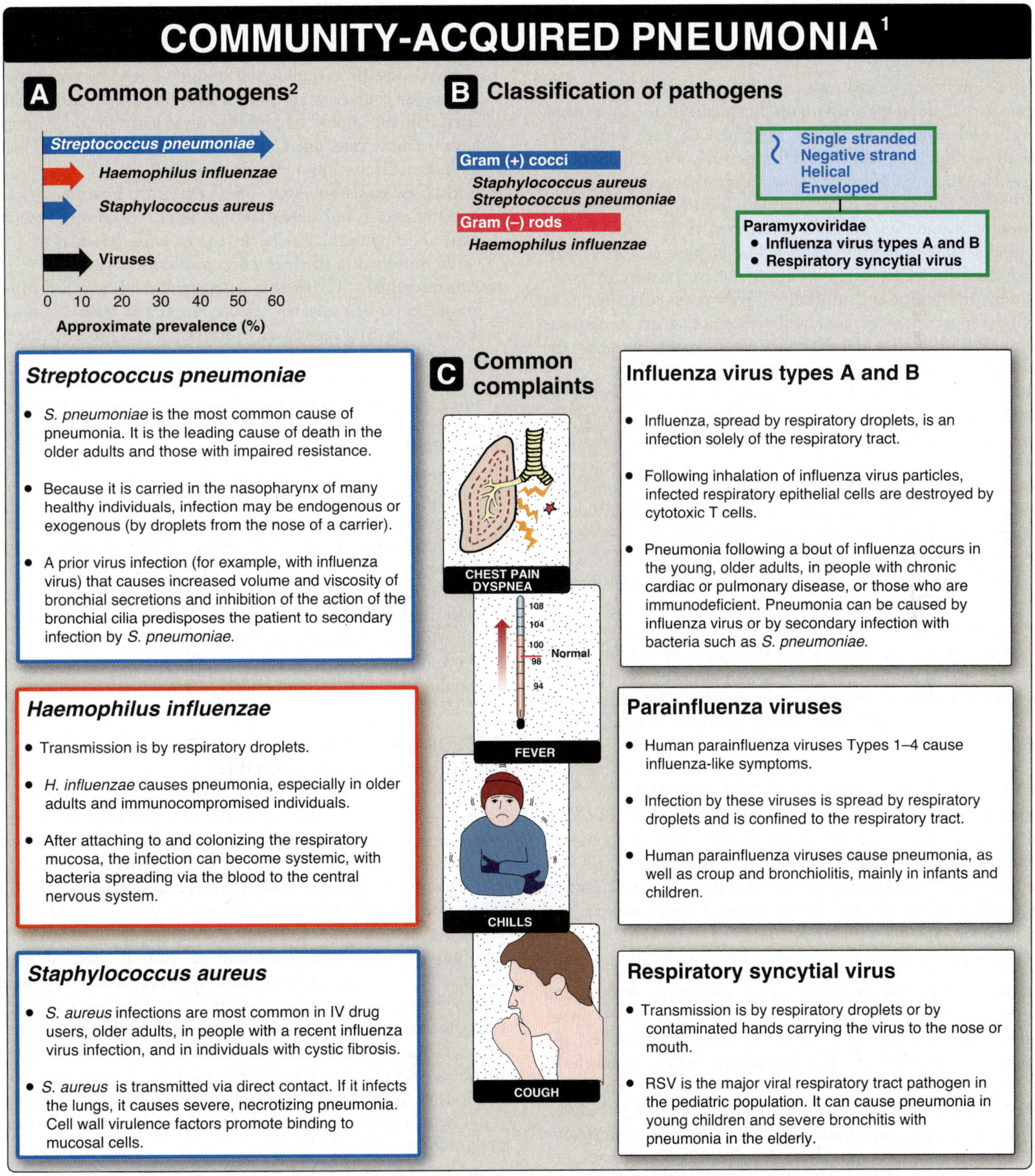

[1]Disease may be "typical" or "atypical." "Typical" pneumonia is characterized by shaking chills, purulent sputum, and x-ray abnormalities that are proportional to the physical signs. "Atypical" pneumonia is characterized by insidious onset, scant sputum and x-ray abnormalities greater than predicted by physical signs.
[2]Additional causes of community-acquired pneumonia are described in Box 72.1.

Figure 72.13. Community-acquired pneumonia (CAP). Characteristics of CAP including (**A**) common pathogens, (**B**) classifications of pathogens, and (**C**) common complaints.

as azithromycin) or doxycycline for previously healthy adults without recent antibiotic use.[109,120] For patients with comorbidities such as chronic heart, lung, liver, or renal disease, diabetes, alcoholism, malignancies, or immunosuppressing conditions, a combination therapy that includes a beta-lactam (like high-dose amoxicillin or amoxicillin–clavulanate) and a macrolide, or a respiratory fluoroquinolone alone, is advised.[109,120] Inpatient treatment for CAP requires more aggressive therapy including a respiratory fluoroquinolone or a beta-lactam antibiotic plus a macrolide.[109,120]

HAP

HAP is a significant health care concern and is characterized by pneumonia that develops in patients hospitalized for more than 48 hours, excluding those already intubated or with ventilator-associated pneumonia (VAP). HAP particularly affects patients in intensive care units (ICUs) and those requiring mechanical ventilation.[121] The condition is more prevalent among elderly patients and those with underlying health conditions, making them more susceptible to developing pneumonia. The incidence of HAP significantly contributes to increased hospital stays, health care costs, and patient morbidity and mortality. HAP poses a challenge in terms of diagnosis, management, and prevention, given its association with high morbidity and mortality rates, especially among the elderly and those with compromised health statuses.[121]

The diagnosis of HAP is primarily clinical, supported by radiologic evidence of new or progressive lung infiltrates. Diagnosis also involves identifying potential risk factors such as older age, depressed consciousness, aspiration, previous antibiotic treatment, and coexisting conditions that may predispose patients to pneumonia. Microbiologic testing, including sputum and blood cultures, is recommended to identify the causative pathogens. The most common causes are methicillin-resistant *Staphylococcus aureus* (MRSA) and *Pseudomonas aeruginosa*, with a notable concern for antibiotic-resistant strains.[104,122]

Treatment of HAP includes aggressive broad-spectrum antibiotics with coverage against all likely pathogens, as recommended by international guidelines.[121] This treatment should especially target MRSA and *Pseudomonas aeruginosa*, which are common in hospital settings, and treatment should consider local antibiotic resistance and patient-specific risk factors.[121,123]

CLINICAL PRACTICE GUIDELINES: CAP, HAP, VAP

The latest guidelines for the management of CAP, HAP, and VAP emphasize a strategic approach that balances effective treatment with the prevention of antibiotic resistance. They all emphasize a tailored approach to diagnosis, treatment, follow-up, consideration of the severity of the disease, the presence of comorbidities, and local patterns of antimicrobial resistance.[124]

Key recommendations from these guidelines include:

- Empirical Antibiotic Therapy: The guidelines recommend empirical antibiotic therapy tailored to the severity of pneumonia, potential exposure to drug-resistant pathogens, and the presence of comorbidities. For outpatients without comorbidities, monotherapy with a macrolide (azithromycin, clarithromycin) or doxycycline is suggested. For patients with comorbidities, broader-spectrum coverage is recommended, such as monotherapy with a respiratory fluoroquinolone (levofloxacin, moxifloxacin) or combination therapy with a beta-lactam (amoxicillin–clavulanate or a cephalosporin) plus a macrolide or doxycycline.[106,124] The patient's response to therapy should be assessed within 48 to 72 hours; if there is no clinical improvement, consider modification of antibiotic regimen.
- Severity Assessment: Severity of CAP should dictate the appropriate setting for patient care (outpatient, inpatient, or ICU). Tools such as the PSI or CURB-65 help guide these decisions.[124]
- Diagnostic Testing: Routine is not recommended for all patients. Instead, these tests are advised for patients with severe CAP, those who are hospitalized, or those with risk factors for specific pathogens like MRSA or *P. aeruginosa*. Testing for influenza and other respiratory viruses is recommended during periods of community viral spread.[124,125]
- Treatment Duration: Recommended duration of antimicrobial treatment for CAP is a minimum of 5 days; however, a 7-day course of antimicrobial therapy is widely recommended. Prolonged courses of antibiotics have not shown additional benefits. Patients should be afebrile for at least 48 to 72 hours and have no more than one CAP-associated sign of clinical instability before discontinuing antibiotics.[106,124]
- Early De-escalation: Appropriate empirical treatment should be initiated early, and de-escalation based on culture results and clinical response is crucial to increase the chance of survival while minimizing the impact on antibiotic resistance.[126]
- Antimicrobial Stewardship: Antimicrobial stewardship programs minimize adverse effects associated with antimicrobial use, such as drug resistance and toxicity, and promote the use of cost-effective treatments.
- Training health care workers in recommended preventive measures, such as adequate hand hygiene and proper management of respiratory devices, is vital to reduce the incidence of HAP and VAP. The development of protocols and policies for these preventive strategies is encouraged.
- Assessment of Risk Factors for Multi-Drug–Resistant (MDR) Organisms: Identifying patients at risk for infections caused by MDR organisms is a key component of the management strategy.
- Follow-up Imaging: Routine follow-up chest imaging is not universally recommended but may be considered for patients with persistent symptoms or signs of illness to evaluate for complications or alternative diagnoses.[124]
- Prevention: Vaccination against pneumococcal disease and seasonal influenza is recommended as a key preventive measure for CAP.[127]

OSTEOPATHIC MANIPULATIVE TREATMENT IN PNEUMONIA MANAGEMENT

OMT has been shown through preliminary evidence and historical experience to have utility in treating respiratory conditions and improving patient infection–related outcomes. Smith's report on the osteopathic treatment of influenza patients in 1918, although not rigorous by today's scientific standards, described a 10% mortality rate for patients with pneumonia who received OMT as compared to 33% for those with standard medical care.[128] The addition of osteopathic treatment to current medical management can help optimize treatment of pneumonia in patients.[101] Osteopathic manipulative medicine, when used in treating infection, has been associated with decreased bacterial counts in lung tissue, changes in immunologic profiles as shown by inflammatory markers, shorter durations of IV antibiotics, decreased rates of respiratory failure and death, and enhanced patient satisfaction.[129]

There are four main goals of initial manipulative treatment for pneumonia:

1. Reduce parenchymal lung congestion
2. Reduce sympathetic hyper-reactivity to the parenchyma of the lung
3. Increase mechanical thoracic cage and diaphragmatic motion
4. Enhance the body's lymphatic clearance of the infection

The mainstay of osteopathic treatment for respiratory infection has been focused on enhancing patient homeostasis by impacting lymphatic flow. In adjunct to medical antibiotic therapy, use of lymphatic pump technique has demonstrated improvements in outcomes for patients including reducing the use of intravenous antibiotics, duration of hospitalization, rate of ventilator-dependent respiratory failure, and overall mortality rate.[1,130,131] The suspected mechanisms include decreasing pathogenic presence in the pulmonary space by mobilizing fluids and immune cells and increasing the humoral response.[132,133]

One of the more recent advances in osteopathic research includes studies conducted by Noll et al.[134] Initially, Noll et al. discovered that, in a small group of patients older than 60 years of age with acute pneumonia, OMT was effective in reducing the duration of antibiotic use and the duration of significant leukocytosis.[134] Based on the results of this initial small trial, a large, comprehensive multisite study, the Multicenter Osteopathic Pneumonia Study in the Elderly (MOPSE) trial was performed. On execution, the MOPSE trial was performed on 387 patients, age 50 years and older, meeting criteria for pneumonia on hospital admission. Each participant received conventional care and was split into one of three groups receiving (1) adjunct OMT protocol, (2) light touch protocol, or (3) conventional care only. Patients in the OMT group received OMT from an accomplished specialist. They received these interventions twice daily, using the following protocol for the OMT group, with each treatment session lasting about 20 minutes:

- Thoracolumbar soft tissue
- Rib raising
- Doming of the diaphragm with MFR
- Cervical spine soft tissue
- Suboccipital decompression
- Thoracic inlet MFR
- TLP
- Pedal pump

The light touch protocol involved light touch to the same body regions for about the same length of time. In participants 50 to 74 years old, results demonstrated that adjunctive OMT for pneumonia reduced length of stay from 4 days to 2.9. In addition, in patients 75 and older, adjunctive OMT significantly lowered in-hospital mortality rates significantly.[1]

These studies have demonstrated that OMT adjuvant to conventional medical care in patients hospitalized with pneumonia can reduce the use of intravenous antibiotics[135] duration of hospitalization, rate of ventilator-dependent respiratory failure, and overall mortality rate.[1,90,91,134]

Pulmonary function can also be enhanced for patients in the hospital postoperatively. OMT has been shown to accelerate the recovery of preoperative values of FVC and FEV1 of postoperative patients with atelectasis.[135]

OMT in Children and Infants

A review study by Roland et al. examined the role of OMT in the neonatal intensive care unit (NICU). The study explored how the use of OMT can be used to not only prevent hospital and community acquired pneumonia but has been shown to aid in the recovery process by enhancing innate immunity and maximizing the effects of antibiotics. Techniques such as lymphatic pump, diaphragm manual release, balanced ligamentous tension (BLT), MFR, and cranial manipulation have been shown to be safe in neonates and can prove useful when treating infants with pneumonia, asthma, and other respiratory diseases.[136] Belcastro and colleagues investigated OMT in the treatment of bronchiolitis in infants. They studied 12 infants between the ages of 2 and 11 months with a clinical diagnosis of bronchiolitis. They randomly assigned each infant to a treatment scheme, comparing OMT with postural drainage and bronchodilator therapy with placebo. Data was limited due to the small number of patients; however, this study established a research protocol and discussed the treatment of bronchiolitis from an osteopathic standpoint.[137] More studies are needed to verify the anecdotal and limited scientific support for OMT in treatment of respiratory infection in infants.[136]

COMPLICATIONS

Most patients respond with improvement within 48 to 72 hours; however, if they fail to improve within 72 hours, another cause should be suspected.[104] In patients with advanced age, lung disease, immunosuppression, infection with aggressive gram-negative organisms (*Klebsiella*), and other comorbidities, the outcomes are usually poor. Complications are respiratory failure, sepsis, multiorgan failure, coagulopathy, and exacerbation of pre-existing comorbidities. When pneumonia is left untreated, it carries mortality more than 25%.[104]

PREVENTION OF PNEUMONIA

The osteopathic clinician should have a firm understanding of the current vaccine' roles in preventing pneumococcal pneumonia and highlight the importance of integrating vaccination into holistic health care programs for older adults and those at increased risk. There is a significant amount of evidence supporting the efficacy and critical role of pneumococcal vaccines in preventing pneumonia, with ongoing research into expanding serotype coverage.[87] At the time of this writing, there are multiple vaccines that help prevent pneumonia especially for those patients with comorbid conditions. The choice between these vaccines depends on the individual's age, health status, and previous vaccination history, with PCV15 and PCV20 offering broader serotype coverage. The reader is guided to the CDC for the most updated recommendations on vaccination. In summary, Table 72.2 shows vaccine options and uses in the prevention of pneumococcal disease.[138]

Pneumonitis

Pneumonitis refers to inflammation of lung tissue, which can be caused by infection, noninfectious factors such as airborne irritants, certain cancer treatments, or various drugs. The inflammation triggered by these conditions can lead to symptoms such as dyspnea, cough, and fatigue. In severe cases, the inflammation may result in irreversible lung damage. This damage often leaves the patient with persistent symptoms long after the infection or inciting event has occurred. It also reduces the immune defense of the lungs by impairing airway and mucus clearance, increasing the risk for secondary bacterial infections.[103] This can result in ongoing interstitial damage, visible as a ground glass appearance on CXR, and eventually fibrotic changes seen on CT scans of the chest (see Fig. 72.14).

CAUSES OF PNEUMONITIS

Pneumonitis can develop as a result of inflammatory lung disease, which encompasses a variety of conditions. These inflammatory conditions produce a complex immune response, involving both the innate and adaptive immune systems. COPD, ARDS, and severe asthma are characterized by innate neutrophilic inflammation.[38] Other inflammatory lung diseases include bronchiectasis, where chronic infection leads to inflammation and damage to the airways, and sarcoidosis, which is characterized by granulomatous

TABLE 72.2

Available Pneumococcal Vaccines[138]

PCV 13 (Prevnar 13)	PPSV23	PCV15 (Vaxneuvance)	PCV20 (Prevnar 20)
Previously a staple in pneumococcal vaccination, PCV13 is now less emphasized in the latest guidelines. It is still available and can be used if it is the only pneumococcal conjugate vaccine available and the recipient would otherwise go unvaccinated.	This vaccine continues to be recommended for adults aged 65 y and older and for those aged 19–64 y with certain underlying health conditions. It is recommended following vaccination with PCV13 or PCV15 (1 y later) but is not recommended for those who have previously received PCV20.	Approved for use in adults and children as young as 6 weeks, PCV15 includes the 13 serotypes found in PCV13 plus an additional two serotypes (22F and 33F). For adults, PCV15 is recommended to be followed by PPSV23 1 y later. This sequence is advised to enhance the breadth of protection against pneumococcal disease.	This vaccine, covering 20 serotypes, is recommended for adults aged 19 y and older, including those previously vaccinated with PCV13 or PPSV23. PCV20 offers a broader range of protection and simplifies the vaccination schedule as no additional doses of PPSV23 are needed after PCV20 administration.

inflammation with infiltration of activated lymphocytes and macrophages.[38] Pulmonary fibrosis, another inflammatory lung condition, results from scarring or thickening of the lungs, affecting oxygen exchange.

A wide range of infections, both bacterial and viral, can cause inflammation of the lung parenchyma and associated interstitial edema. Alveolar macrophages, crucial in host defense against viral and bacterial pathogens, encounter pathogens in the resting lung. They engage in phagocytosis and killing, antigen presentation, and recruitment of other cell types. Viral respiratory infections can impair macrophage phagocytic function and monocyte chemotaxis to the lung early after infection.[103] Post–viral pneumonitis, a postinflammatory reaction to infection, can persist longer than the infection itself. This differs from hypersensitivity pneumonitis, where the body forms antigen-specific IgG antibodies.[139] With subsequent exposures to the antigen, the body develops episodic lung inflammation and immune complex formation with an influx of neutrophils. These mechanisms contribute to increased inflammation in the lungs, and therefore increase risk of pneumonitis development.

COVID-19

COVID-19, also known as coronavirus disease 2019, is an infectious disease caused by the severe acute respiratory syndrome coronavirus 2 (SARS-CoV-2). The virus was first identified at the end of 2019 as the cause of a cluster of pneumonia cases in Wuhan, China and quickly spread, leading to a global pandemic. COVID-19 has posed a more recent challenge for all osteopathic physicians, but most significantly pulmonologists.[140]

The spread of COVID-19 has been characterized by rapid transmission during close contact through respiratory droplets produced by coughing, sneezing, or talking, with the potential for aerosol and contact spread, although the latter is considered less common. Increased transmission occurs in poorly ventilated and crowded indoor settings, contributing to community transmission. The risk of severe illness and death from COVID-19 is higher in older adults, people with underlying health conditions, and those who are unvaccinated. Genetic factors and comorbidities such as hypertension, diabetes, and obesity have been identified as risk factors for severe disease, highlighting the role of host factors in disease progression. The epidemiologic understanding of COVID-19 continues to evolve as new variants of the virus emerge and as public health measures adapt in response to changing infection dynamics.[141]

Diagnosis is critical for not only patient management but also for implementing public health measures to control the spread of the virus. Guidelines for diagnosing COVID-19 continue to evolve and are updated routinely by the CDC. Currently, diagnosing relies on molecular diagnostic tests, with the Infectious Diseases Society of America (IDSA) strongly recommending nucleic acid amplification tests (NAATs) for symptomatic individuals suspected of having COVID-19, due to their high sensitivity and specificity. The CDC also emphasizes the importance of PCR tests, a type of NAAT, for their ability to provide a more reliable negative test result compared to

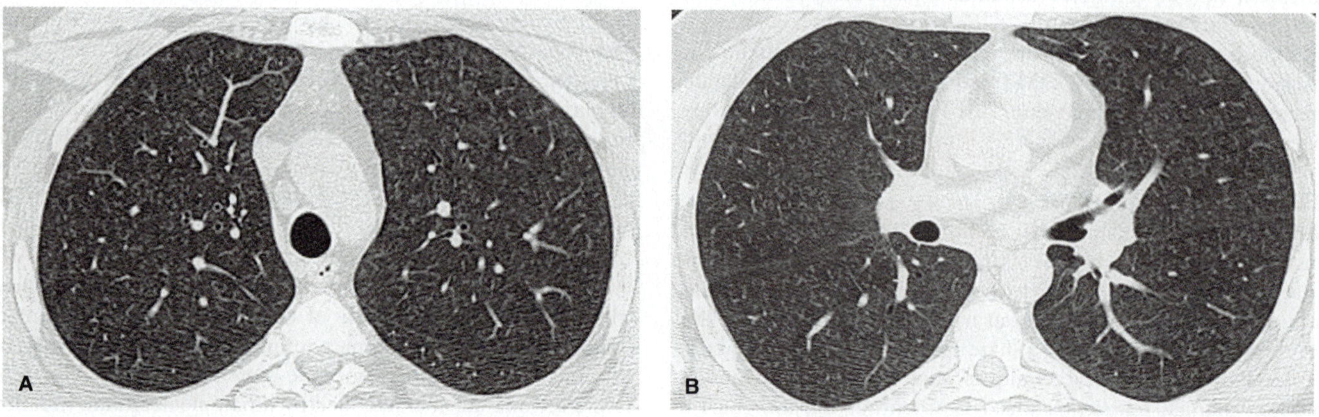

Figure 72.14. Hypersensitivity pneumonitis. A. 35-year-old man presents with progressive dyspnea after installing a hot tub. **B.** Sequential CT images show diffuse centrilobular nodules and scattered ground glass opacities. Lung biopsy confirmed hypersensitivity pneumonitis, presumed secondary to hot tub exposure ("Hot Tub Lung").

antigen tests, which are rapid but less sensitive. In addition to molecular and antigen tests, antibody tests can be used for public health surveillance or to test for conditions associated with COVID-19, but they should not be used to diagnose a current infection.

Often, COVID-19 leads to flu-like symptoms requiring no severe medical intervention, and physicians suggest ample rest and hydration to support the immune defense against the virus. Outpatient evaluation will often include a PFT, ongoing imaging such as CXR or CT, and oxygen evaluation. Oral antivirals have been authorized for use in nonhospitalized patients at high risk for severe disease. If symptoms progress to severe dyspnea (dyspnea at rest and interfering with the ability to speak in complete sentences), oxygen saturation on room air of less than 90% regardless of the severity of dyspnea, or concerning alterations in mentation, the patient must be evaluated in the Emergency department.[142] These severe cases requiring hospitalization can include treatment options such as antiviral medications, immune modulators, and supportive care. In critical cases, patients may require oxygen support, mechanical ventilation or Bi-PAP, bronchodilation, or even extracorporeal membrane oxygenation (ECMO) to assist with heart and lung function. Convalescent plasma therapy, which uses the antibody-rich plasma from recovered COVID-19 patients, may also be considered for individuals with weakened immune systems.

OSTEOPATHIC MANIPULATIVE TREATMENT IN COVID-19

In addition to pharmacologic or procedural interventions, studies have shown nonpharmacologic alternatives, including OMT, have improved pulmonary function and alleviated symptom burden in those with inflammatory lung conditions. In cases of persistent hypoxia, simply having patients lay in a prone position has shown improvements in V/Q matching and therefore improvements in oxygenation. A meta-analysis of COVID-19 patients demonstrated that prone position improved PaO_2/FiO_2 ratio with better SpO_2 than supine position.[143] If positioning alone has shown favorable outcomes, a combination with OMT and other treatment regimens may improve patient recovery by enhancing the innate systems of healing and improve responsiveness to further interventions.

Regarding those with chronic inflammatory diseases (CID), several trials were conducted aiming to measure the effects of manipulative therapies on patients affected by CID. A literature review of 10 studies involving a total of 386 subjects was analyzed. A similar osteopathic approach was found across several studies which included a cranio-sacral focus executed through BLT, muscle energy, MFR, and still techniques. Results suggest a beneficial effect of OMT due to improvement in PFT values and interestingly, positive outcomes in the pediatric population. Although some results showed inconsistent data on the effect of OMT in the treatment of medical conditions potentially associated with CID, OMT appears to be a safe approach for adjunctive treatment.[144]

ARDS is most associated with sepsis, leading to severe morbidity and mortality for hospitalized patients, especially in vulnerable populations such as newborns and geriatrics. One historic 1967 study exists, in which OMT was used in the treatment of respiratory distress syndrome in newborns. A rib-raising technique was used, and a variety of treatment end-point variables were assessed. Results showed the death rate in the study group was lower than that found using historical controls, suggesting favorable use of OMT for newborns with ARDS.[145] Geyer-Roberts et al. describes a proposal for the utility of OMT in treatment of sepsis-associated ARDS in the geriatric population. This includes promotion of circulation, optimization of physiologic movement, reduction of pain, and improved patient comfort.[61] Overall, more research is needed to understand the effect of OMT on patients with respiratory distress syndrome.

The emergence of novel pathogens, such as SARS-CoV-2, without available initial drug treatments or vaccines further underscores the need for nonpharmacologic adjunctive measures for infection management.[129] With further understanding of the disease process of COVID-19, there is more evidence for therapeutic mechanisms of OMT through modulation of inflammation and various body systems including neurologic, respiratory, and gastrointestinal.[146] Researchers at Penn State College of Medicine conducted a study, designed as a feasibility-oriented retrospective observational cohort study, which assessed the adjunctive use of OMT in hospitalized patients experiencing respiratory distress due to SARS-CoV-2 infection. Patients received daily OMT treatments, including rib raising, abdominal diaphragm doming, thoracic pump, and pedal pump. The study found that 90% of patients accepted OMT and reported greater ease of breathing, and high satisfaction, with few negative effects and no adverse events. Although no significant differences were observed in secondary outcomes, patients who received OMT tended to have fewer hospital days compared to controls.[147]

Another osteopathic study was conducted to evaluate the immune response following COVID-19 vaccination. Participants were randomized into either a control group or an OMT intervention group, with both groups receiving the Pfizer mRNA COVID-19 vaccine. OMT techniques applied included MFR of the thoracic inlet, pectoral traction, diaphragm release with MFR, splenic pump, and thoracic pump, performed the day of and the day following each vaccination session. Anti-spike IgG immunoglobulin titers were measured at multiple time points postvaccination to assess immune response. The study found that subjects in the OMT group exhibited a trend toward higher-average anti-spike IgG levels, particularly significant at 1 week after the second vaccine dose in COVID-19 subjects. In addition, while both groups reported similar rates of symptomatic breakthrough infections, the OMT group experienced a significantly shorter duration of symptoms and medication usage. The study concluded that OMT is a safe adjunct to COVID-19 vaccination, potentially enhancing immune response and reducing the impact of breakthrough infections, though it noted the need for larger studies to confirm these findings.[148]

Overall, the use of OMT in those with pulmonary disease is safe, can shorten recovery time, and reduce symptoms in patients with inflammatory lung conditions. Techniques in these patients often includes thoracic and lymphatic pump techniques to enhance airway clearance and improve circulation, rib-raising techniques to help with lung movement and reduce restriction, and combined rehabilitation with chest physical therapy to enhance pulmonary function.

PREVENTION OF POSTOPERATIVE PULMONARY COMPLICATIONS

Pulmonary complications are a frequent cause of postoperative morbidity. Osteopathic physicians have classically treated patients with manipulative treatment, both preoperatively and postoperatively, to prevent respiratory complications from occurring.[149] Atelectasis, a collapsed or airless segmental lung condition, is a common pulmonary complication. Surgeries commonly associated with the development of lung atelectasis include high abdominal surgery and thoracic surgery. Aggressive pulmonary toilet measures, including patient-generated incentive spirometry, have been important in reducing the incidence of this complication postoperatively. It has been shown that OMT can enhance the effects of incentive spirometry following abdominal surgery.[150] Sleszynski and Kelso studied the effects of thoracic pump administered on the first postoperative day in patients who had undergone cholecystectomy. They compared this manipulative modality with the use of incentive spirometry in the prevention of atelectasis. The patients treated with thoracic pump had similar occurrences of atelectasis to those patients treated with incentive spirometry. However, the patients treated with thoracic pump had an earlier recovery and a quicker return toward preoperative values for FVC and forced expiratory volume in the first second than did patients treated with incentive spirometry.[151]

In addition, other pulmonary complications may result from interference with the structures involving the respiratory system. For example, patients who undergo a median sternotomy can often have postoperative rib fractures, atelectasis, and ileus. Dickey described numerous postoperative complications associated with median sternotomy and the value of osteopathic interventions performed both pre- and postoperatively.[152] OMT may be useful to help manage these issues. In Italy, OMTh showed some benefit in patients in a rehabilitation program after sternotomy for cardiac surgery. Eighty poststernotomy adult inpatients were randomly assigned to receive either a standardized cardiorespiratory rehabilitation program alone (control group) or combined with OMTh. Pain intensity and respiratory functional capacity were quantified by the visual analogue scale score and by a standardized breathing test, at the start and end of rehabilitation. At the start of rehabilitation, the control group and the OMTh group had similar visual analogue scale median scores and mean inspiratory volumes. At the end of rehabilitation, the OMTh group had a lower visual analogue scale median score ($P < .01$) and higher mean inspiratory volume ($P < .01$). The analgesic drug intake, depression, and anxiety were similar in the two groups. The hospitalization period was shorter in the OMTh group than in the control group ($P < .05$). The authors concluded that the combination of standard care with OMTh is effective in inducing pain relief and functional recovery and significantly improves the management of patients after heart surgery with sternotomy.[153]

Hospitalized, bedridden patients are prone to develop venous stasis and deep venous thrombosis. In addition to intermittent compression stockings and early ambulation, prophylactic rib elevation, thoracic pump, and pedal pump techniques are clinically useful in the prevention of venous stasis. They should play a role in prophylaxis of deep venous thrombotic disease and pulmonary embolism for patients at bed rest. Research supports this concept as the osteopathic pedal pump technique, when utilized on those without leg lymphedema, has been shown to reduce lower limb volume as measured by the volumetric water gauge. Further studies are warranted, especially in persons with excess lower-extremity edema, lymphedema, or venous stasis.[154]

Osteopathically, it is important to recognize that these surgeries often involve a musculoskeletal component, even without postoperative pulmonary complications. Moreover, a prolonged hospital stay due to the occurrence of a pulmonary complication enhances the probability of patients developing musculoskeletal dysfunction and needing OMT and therapies to recover fully.

THE PULMONARY PATIENT AND THE FIVE MODELS OF OSTEOPATHY

A tenet of osteopathic medicine states that structure and function are reciprocally interrelated, and this serves as a core principle of the understanding of osteopathy. As such, rational treatment of patients with pulmonary conditions must follow the same principle. Alterations, compensations, or dysfunction of the structures related to the pulmonary system impact its function. An osteopathic approach to pulmonary patients including OMT has been taught and published since the days of Still.[149] From early writings on approaches to pulmonary patients and their own clinical experience, Kuchera and Kuchera[12] published a staged application of OMT to be used in pulmonary patients to complement the standard of care. Osteopathic approaches are based upon foundational anatomy and physiology. Though medical management has evolved significantly since this time, the treatment of somatic dysfunction has a significant anatomic and physiologic role in achieving homeostasis.[112] Both generalized and specific localized somatic dysfunction can have effects on the pulmonary patient and may be effectively treated through applying the five models of osteopathic care.[155]

Biomechanical Model

For the thorax to function, the complex of costovertebral articulations, intervertebral facet joints, and the resulting mobility of the spinal column needs to function unrestricted to accommodate lung expansion.[112] In addition, the costochondral and chondrosternal joints must be mobile, including the clavicle and first rib, to allow for expansion of the lung.[112] Thoracolumbar somatic dysfunction, scoliosis, iliopsoas dysfunction, and abdominal diaphragm dysfunction all may adversely affect generation of an adequate contraction to produce proper intrathoracic pressure changes.[112] Normally, contraction of the diaphragm and movement of the thoracic cage during respiration produce pressure gradients between the thoracic and abdominal cavities that allow for effective lymphatic drainage and venous return to the heart.

The effects of these biomechanical factors can be understood by considering a patient with scoliosis. A patient with kyphoscoliosis has lateral displacement and rotation of the vertebral bodies, seen as a paravertebral prominence that is visualized during the Adams forward bending test. When the curvature is significant, kyphoscoliosis affects the mechanics of respiratory muscles, chest compliance, and increases the work of breathing at rest, during exercise, and sleep. In addition, thoracic cage distortion leads to extrinsic restrictive lung disease from the diminution of lung volume on the concave side, where the ribs impinge on the lung.[156] In severe cases, scoliosis can even lead to pulmonary hypertension and respiratory failure.[157] Scoliosis can lead to a restrictive lung disease pattern, characterized by decreased lung volumes, including TLC. Lung function abnormalities become detectable when the Cobb angle exceeds 50 to 60 degrees.[157] The severity of these abnormalities correlates with the Cobb angle, and larger curves (70 to 80 degrees) are associated with more significant clinical impairment.[157]

A systematic review and meta-analysis published in the Spine Journal in 2022 revealed a statistically significant inverse relationship between thoracic Cobb angle and pulmonary function parameters such as FVC and TLC. The study found that for each increase in the Cobb angle, there was a corresponding decrease in predicted pulmonary function.[158] In addition to lateral spinal curvature, anterior–posterior curves may also play a role in the pulmonary patient as shown by Doran and colleagues.[159] In their experience, many patients have an increased lumbar lordosis in the initial physical examination that manipulation can decrease. Experiments were performed to establish the reproducibility and variability of a table that they constructed to quantify the degree of lumbar lordosis. Once the reliability of their measurement table was determined, they recruited young adult volunteers. They assessed how OMT would affect respiratory function. Following manipulative treatment, which often successfully decreased the lumbar lordotic curvature, there was a corresponding decrease in respiratory rate and an increase in VT. The Doran group concluded that one of the significant factors that correlates with impairment of respiration is the lumbar lordotic curve, and OMT can alter this curve to favorably affect the mechanics of respiration.[159]

Structural factors not only include spinal joints but also the fascia and connective tissues. Distensibility of the horizontal diaphragms (tentorium cerebelli, thoracic inlet, thoracoabdominal, and pelvic floor) and the fascial elements of the accessory muscles of respiration is required for optimal respiration.[112] Treating dysfunction of the abdominal diaphragm through procedures such as re-doming of the diaphragm and MFR, can help restore optimal respiratory motion. To completely address the abdominal diaphragm, the diaphragm crura insert on the lumbar spine at the level of L1–L3. If the crura are hypertonic, treating the spinal segments of L1–L3 can also be beneficial, encouraging normal thoracic diaphragm motion.[112,160] In addition to the horizontal diaphragms, recruitment of the accessory muscles of respiration can occur from coughing or labored breathing.[161] Patients with respiratory infections, asthma, COPD, and cystic fibrosis can develop cervical, thoracic spinal, or rib dysfunction, resulting in chronic cervical or thoracic pain.[19] According to Yao[160] and Nelson,[112] treating the first ribs, clavicles, C7–T4 spinal segments, and scalene muscles helps to release the thoracic inlet fascia, enhancing respiratory motion and lymphatic drainage. This is due to the anatomy of the superior thoracic aperture, where the suprapleural membrane (Sibson fascia) attaches to the internal border of the first rib and the transverse process of C7 vertebra.[162] Treating the T1–T4 region and their ribs also can affect sympathetic tone to the head, neck, and bronchi which may improve drainage and clearance of microorganisms.[112,160]

Respiratory-Circulatory Model

Considering the respiratory-circulatory model, proper blood flow and lymphatic drainage through the lungs are considered important for the maintenance of normal homeostatic function. Somatic dysfunctions of the ribs, thoracic inlet, thoracic spine, and thoracoabdominal region can prevent full excursion during respiration and negatively impact the intrathoracic pressure which in turn, can decrease lymph drainage.[112] Osteopathic physicians have long been concerned with optimizing lymphatic drainage from tissues. Maintenance of proper lymphatic drainage is thought to encourage tissue activity and metabolism and plays an important role in promoting a stable immunologic environment (see Chapter 14 Anatomy and Physiology of the Lymphatic System). Moreover, increasing lymphatic flow helps improve removal and filtering of inflammatory mediators, fluid, and waste products from interstitial spaces. This is imperative when treating patients with edema or infections.

The right side of the head, neck, and portions of the lung drain into the right lymphatic duct, while the left side of the head, neck, portions of the lung, and the rest of the body drain into the left lymphatic duct, or thoracic duct.[12,160] Restricted fascia in the neck and upper thorax should also be treated.[160] Opening restricted fascia in the neck and thoracic inlet with myofascial techniques facilitates lymph drainage so lymph can freely return to the venous circulation to aid drainage to and from areas of infection.

The thoracic duct conducts most of the lymphatic flow, delivering about 1.38 mL/kg/h of lymph to the venous system.[163] The thoracic inlet, abdominal diaphragm, and pelvic diaphragm are all considered interdependent diaphragms which work in unison, creating intrathoracic and intra-abdominal pressure gradients; somatic dysfunction in any of these regions can adversely influence this respiratory circulatory pump and lymphatic flow.[4] Impairments in this system are commonly seen in bedridden and hospitalized patients suffering from respiratory infection. Small improvements in the ability of the pump function of the diaphragm may have profound effects on lymphatic fluid drainage and circulation.[135,164] This idea has been supported by Knott et al. who studied the impact of the thoracic and abdominal pump techniques on thoracic duct lymphatic flow in canines compared to movement generated from physical activity. They found a significant increase in thoracic duct flow during both abdominal and thoracic pump techniques, as well as through physical activity.[164]

Metabolic Model

Considering the metabolic model, proper respiratory movement is essential for fighting infection and for reducing healing time. Tissue congestion has been found to cause impairment of leukocyte migration, toxin and waste removal, and delivery of medication, thereby decreasing the effectiveness of medical therapy.[164,165] OMT can address myofascial restrictions with the goal of improving tissue congestion, resolving inflammation, and removing metabolic waste products.[160]

As discussed previously, patients with COPD can benefit from pulmonary rehabilitation in combination with sessions of OMT to improve exercise capacity and reduce residual volume.[86] This is in distinction to other studies by Noll and was attributed to a decrease in airway resistance. The authors hypothesized that a decrease in airway resistance could be due to improving chest wall and diaphragm mobility.[86] Osteopathic physicians use manipulative treatments such as rib raising, diaphragm relaxation, thoracic inlet release, and thoracic pump to resolve somatic dysfunction and significantly enhance fluid movement and lymphatic drainage. Lymphatic pump has been proposed to prevent venous stasis throughout the body and to enhance fluid movement from the parenchyma of the lung. In the metabolic model, this clearance of toxic waste products and improvement of fluid movement in the body is of utmost importance in management of many conditions, especially in the pulmonary system. This is thought to have both a preventive and therapeutic influence on disease (see Chapter 78 Osteopathic Considerations and Approaches in the Acutely Ill or Hospitalized Patient for further details). As discussed in the MOPSE protocol, which relies heavily on lymphatic OMT, treatment of patients with OMT may help augment use of antibiotics and shorten length of stay in the hospital due to respiratory infection.[1]

Neurologic Model

In a patient with pulmonary disease, the osteopathic physician should consider neurologic influences in the pathophysiology of the disease state and attempt to return the patient to homeostasis. Neurologic influences on the pulmonary patient include the sympathetic and parasympathetic nervous system, the phrenic and vagus nerves, and viscerosomatic reflexes.

SYMPATHETIC AND PARASYMPATHETIC NERVOUS SYSTEM

The sympathetic fibers of the pulmonary plexuses are postsynaptic fibers. Their cell bodies (sympathetic ganglion cells) are in the paravertebral sympathetic ganglia of the sympathetic trunks.[162] Vertebral and rib somatic dysfunction in these regions are thought to influence the sympathetic nervous system due to fascial connections of the rib heads to the sympathetic chain ganglia.[12,112] The sympathetic fibers act in an inhibitory fashion on bronchial muscle (*bronchodilator*) and on the alveolar glands of the bronchial tree, provide motor innervation to the pulmonary vessels (*vasoconstrictor*).[162] Somatic dysfunction in the upper thoracic spine causing facilitation of those spinal segments can increase sympathetic activity, further augmenting effects on the target tissues. Increased sympathetic tone leads to an increase in heart rate, airway epithelial hyperplasia, increased luminal secretions, thick mucus, poor ciliary function, and bronchodilation which results in pulmonary congestion.[12] Rib raising is a paravertebral technique that targets the rib angles to inhibit and normalize sympathetic ganglia, and can be used even in patients who are severely ill.[12,112] According to the Clinically Oriented Learning Scenarios (COILS) published by AACOM, by performing OMT to the facilitated cord segments T2–T7 using paraspinal inhibition and active rib raising, the patient will expectorate a significant quantity of sputum and clinically improve.[166]

The parasympathetic fibers conveyed to the pulmonary plexus are presynaptic fibers from the vagus nerve (CN X). The vagus nerve exits the skull via the jugular foramen and has pulmonary branches, which are categorized into anterior and posterior groups. The anterior bronchial branches are distributed on the anterior surface of the root of the lung. The anterior bronchial group combined with filaments from the sympathetic nervous system forms the anterior pulmonary plexus. The posterior group, with filaments from the third and fourth (and occasionally first and second) thoracic ganglia of the sympathetic trunk, forms the posterior pulmonary plexus.[162] Somatic dysfunction of the upper cervical region (C0–C3) can influence the vagus nerve, causing changes in parasympathetic effects.[112] The parasympathetic fibers provide motor to the smooth muscle of the bronchial tree (*bronchoconstriction*), inhibition to the pulmonary vessels (*vasodilation*), and secretory effects to the glands of the bronchial tree (*secretomotor*).[162] Increased parasympathetic tone leads to thin watery secretions, runny nose, postnasal drip, and relative bronchiole constriction.[12,112] OMT to the suboccipital region, such as occipitoatlantal release, is thought to normalize tensions and decrease tissue congestion near the jugular foramen.[112] Treatment in this region has been shown in preliminary studies to effect vagally mediated heart rate variability (HRV).[167] The vagal effects on the pulmonary system are still to be determined; however, according to the COILS published by AACOM, authors discuss performing OMT to the upper cervical somatic dysfunction and occipitomastoid sutures to help normalize parasympathetic function from the vagus nerve in patients with COPD.[166]

VISCERAL AFFERENT FIBERS

There are also both nociceptive and reflexive visceral afferent fibers. The *visceral afferent fibers* of the pulmonary plexuses conduct subconscious sensations associated with reflexes that control function. The reflexive visceral afferent fibers have cell bodies in the sensory ganglion of the vagus nerve (CN X) and accompany the parasympathetic fibers. Afferents from the trachea also accompany the parasympathetic fibers to the sensory ganglion of the vagus nerve. Somatic dysfunction (and subsequent OMT) of structures around the vagus nerve may influence this control and reporting system of the pulmonary tract as well.[162]

The nociceptive afferents conduct pain impulses in response to painful or injurious stimuli, such as chemical irritants, ischemia, or excessive stretch. The nociceptive afferent fibers from the visceral pleura and bronchi accompany the sympathetic fibers through the sympathetic trunk to the sensory ganglia of upper thoracic spinal nerves.[162] Therefore, somatic dysfunction (and subsequent OMT) of structures around the sympathetic chain ganglia may influence nociceptive reporting of the pulmonary tract.

THE PHRENIC NERVES

The phrenic nerves, originating from the C3–C5 spinal nerves, play a crucial role in the respiratory system by providing the primary motor innervation to the diaphragm. The phrenic nerves also carry sensory fibers that innervate the central part of the diaphragm, the pericardium, and the mediastinal part of the parietal pleura.[162] Each side of the diaphragm is innervated by its respective (left and right) phrenic nerve, which is essential for the rhythmic contraction and relaxation of the diaphragm during respiration. The nerve descends from the neck, passing anterior to the root of the lung and between the fibrous pericardium and mediastinal parietal pleura, before reaching the diaphragm. Dysfunction of the phrenic nerve can manifest as shortness of breath, especially during physical activities or when lying flat. Dysfunction of the phrenic nerve can lead to persistent or intractable hiccups.[162] Lung cancer or trauma involving a phrenic nerve may result in paralysis of one half of the diaphragm (hemidiaphragm)[162] Somatic dysfunction of the C3–C5, region may impair the function of the phrenic nerve and its target tissues (pleura, diaphragm) and also produce sensory symptoms in the C3–C5 dermatomes of the ipsilateral supraclavicular region (top of the shoulder of the same side).

INTERCOSTAL NERVES

The costal pleura and the peripheral part of the diaphragmatic pleura are supplied by the *intercostal nerves*, which mediate the sensations of touch and pain. The intercostal nerves, arteries, and veins course parallel to the ribs just inferior to the costal grooves (thus sheltered by the inferior margins of the overlying ribs). The anterior ramus of most thoracic spinal nerves is simply the intercostal nerve for that level, except for the first and second intercostal nerves which have unique anatomical characteristics. The intercostal nerve, artery, and vein course in the intercostal spaces, parallel to the ribs, and supply the intercostal muscles, integument, and parietal pleura.[162] Somatic dysfunction that alters the position and motion of the ribs (especially inhaled or exhaled dysfunctions) can affect the intercostal neurovascular bundle and its supplied structures. Likewise, patients with pleuritic conditions may develop painful somatic dysfunction of the ribs. Inhaled rib dysfunctions can occur with hyperinflation and are related to extended thoracic spinal segments. Inhaled rib dysfunctions may cause anterior chest pain with inhalation. Exhaled rib dysfunctions can occur with sneezing or coughing and are related to flexed thoracic spinal segments. Patients with exhaled rib dysfunctions may feel unable to take in a full breath.

REFERRED PAIN AND VISCEROSOMATIC REFLEXES

Referred pain from the pulmonary system can be seen in various regions and is important to consider when palpating for somatic dysfunction and viscerosomatic reflexes (see Box 72.4). Viscerosomatic reflexes are localized, visceral stimuli that produce patterns of reflex responses in segmentally related somatic structures. In addition, viscerosomatic reflexes are a palpatory manifestation of disturbed physiology. When the abhorrent stimulation to the segmental spinal cord from an injured, diseased, or inflamed tissue/organ is significant or prolonged, it creates palpable tissue texture changes in various anatomic locations (dermatome, myotome, sclerotome) (see Chapter 13 Somatic Dysfunction, Spinal Facilitation, and Viscerosomatic Integration). Viscerosomatic reflexes often associated with respiratory illness are generally found in the upper thoracic region for sympathetic reflexes and in the upper cervical region for parasympathetic reflexes. These palpable tissue changes tend to have a puffy quality and a rubbery end-feel (see Chapter 13 Somatic Dysfunction, Spinal Facilitation, and Viscerosomatic Integration). When the effects of viscerosomatic reflexes are prolonged, multiple segments can be involved, and a group curve can develop.[6,112]

BOX 72.4 Referred Pain

Viscerosomatic Referral Patterns:

- Visceral pleura is relatively insensitive to pain because it receives no somatic nerve fibers for general sensation.[162]
- Parietal pleura is somatically innervated, which typically causes pleural pain to be sharp and localized.[162]
  - The costal part of the parietal pleura may refer pain to dermatomes supplied by the same spinal (posterior root) ganglia and spinal cord segments.[162]
  - The costal and peripheral parts of the diaphragmatic pleura refer pain to the dermatomes of the thoracic and abdominal walls.[162]
  - The mediastinal and central diaphragmatic areas of the parietal pleura refer pain to the root of the neck and over the shoulder (C3–C5 dermatomes).[162]

Chapman reflexes represent another method of recognizing viscerosomatic effects. Chapman reflexes tend to manifest as small (2 to 3 mm), nodular masses that are palpable as gangliform contractions of fascia with distinct tissue texture abnormalities and pinpoint, and nonradiating tenderness (see Chapter 58 A Modern Approach to Chapman Reflex Points). As viscerosomatic reflexes, they are typically found anteriorly and posteriorly in locations that are segmentally related to visceral innervation. Manipulative treatment of Chapman reflexes can provide a beneficial somatovisceral effect. They are treated with rotatory pressure through the clinician's finger for approximately 30 seconds. Table 72.3 lists their general locations.

BEHAVIORAL MODEL

Psychophysiological factors can affect both biomechanical and biochemical respiratory processes and can have a pronounced influence on the development of dysregulated breathing. Breathing is one of the few regulatory systems in our body that allows for both conscious and unconscious control and it is profoundly affected by stress in both our external and internal environments.[168] Acute and chronic stress can directly affect respiration, often leading to hyperventilation characterized by shallow and rapid breathing. Hyperventilation can result in hypocapnia and associated symptoms such as dizziness, tingling sensations, numbness, and heightened anxiety.[168,169] Patients under stress and fear of their own pulmonary condition have a heightened perception and appraisal of their breathlessness and dyspnea.[168] Stress can also impact respiration by triggering the activation of the sympathetic nervous system and the release of stress hormones like cortisol, which can contribute to additional respiratory changes. Patients with chronic pulmonary diseases such as asthma and COPD often experience significant emotional challenges from their illness and changes in their activities of daily living. Physical limitations imposed by the disease, such as difficulty breathing and reduced ability to engage in daily activities, can lead to feelings of isolation and helplessness. Moreover, patients may develop physical changes including postural adaptations, muscle hypertrophy, or muscle atrophy. Osteopathic physicians can impact these patients' physical and emotional health by incorporating OMT and through considering the psychological impact of the patient's condition and environment in their treatment. This includes evaluation of the patient's support system, the patient's trust in the health care team, fear of hospitalization, and other factors that may psychologically impact the patient's outcomes.[160]

TABLE 72.3

Location of Chapman's Reflexes

Locations of Pulmonary Chapman Reflexes		
Bronchi	Anterior	Intercostal space between ribs 2 and 3 adjacent to sternum
	Posterior	Across the face of the transverse process of the T2, midway between spinous process and transverse process
Upper lung	Anterior	Between ribs 3 and 4 near sternum
	Posterior	Between the transverse processes of T3 and T4 midway between the spinous process and transverse process
Lower lung	Anterior	Between ribs 4 and 5 near sternum
	Posterior	Between the transverse processes of T4 and T5 midway between the spinous process and the transverse process

When chronic pulmonary patients have chronic pain as a comorbidity, they can adopt shallow breathing, muscle stiffness, and heightened levels of alertness. Chronic pain has been associated with alterations in respiratory muscle strength and functioning, leading to dysregulated biochemical and biomechanical respiratory outcomes. Patients with kinesiophobia, (the fear of movement), tend to have an increased respiratory rate, shallow breathing patterns, and reduced oxygen saturation levels.[168,170] These changes can heighten the likelihood of individuals avoiding deep breaths, refraining from exertion or movement, and assuming an inefficient posture for breathing.[168]

In addition to chronic pain, chronic upper respiratory infections in patients with asthma and COPD have also been correlated, corresponding with an increase in anxiety and depression.[160,171] Clinicians should screen for depression and anxiety and have a low threshold to involve consultation from behavioral medicine specialists. The severity and chronicity of respiratory infections correlates with impairments in well-being, quality of life, and sleep.[160,172] This is a perfect opportunity for osteopathic physicians to encourage the patient on postural awareness, support their emotional health and treat dysfunctional structure–function relationships.

SUMMARY

The respiratory system is a beautifully designed pump whose chief purpose is to exchange CO_2 for oxygen in the respiratory process. Diseases or conditions affecting any component of pulmonary physiology generally disrupts the entire pulmonary system. Since all tissues of the body require metabolic gas exchange, this can cause systemic problems and thoroughly impact quality of life.

In any osteopathic examination of patients, a thorough patient evaluation is necessary. Within this evaluation, it is necessary to determine whether the patient is presenting for an acute condition, an acute exacerbation of a chronic condition, or a recurrent chronic condition. A thorough pulmonary exam begins with a detailed history of present illness with relevant questioning. During the subsequent physical exam, the efficient osteopathic physician will incorporate observation for sequela of pulmonary disease and palpation for T.A.R.t. changes concurrently with a standard exam. Laboratory, technical, and imaging modalities of assessment have improved the diagnosis and management of pulmonary conditions and allow for improvement in overall patient care. These tests are important in the care of patients with pulmonary conditions and should be correlated with the other components of the osteopathic exam.

Pulmonary conditions are often classified into two categories: obstructive lung disease and restrictive lung disease. In obstructive lung disease, patients have trouble exhaling air from the lungs due to narrowed airways or damage to the lung tissue, leading to air trapping and hyperinflation. Conversely, restrictive lung disease is characterized by reduced lung volume, leading to difficulty with inspiration.

Among obstructive diseases, asthma has a predominant role in chronic lung disease worldwide. Guidelines continue to evolve as superior medical therapy is discovered, and standard of care should be followed to prevent worsening of patients' conditions. Most notable in asthma care is the addition of ICSs in rescue and maintenance therapy, which has been shown to produce superior outcomes in disease management for patients. COPD, another obstructive lung disease, is also increasing in prevalence in the world as more is being discovered about this condition. Continuing guidelines support the use of a multifaceted approach to care, emphasizing regular follow-up and monitoring of symptoms, as well as improved communication and discussions with patients on adherence to treatment regimen. Moreover, studies have demonstrated the benefits of OMT in symptom management of COPD and especially improvement in outcomes when combined with other therapies such as pulmonary rehabilitation. The practice of osteopathic medicine works in parallel with treatment of obstructive lung disease, as has been shown since the first publications in the field of osteopathic medicine. From anecdotal evidence, to preliminary observations, to small-scale studies, to continuing larger trials, the role of OMT in management of obstructive lung disease is substantial and continues to evolve.

Diagnosis, treatment, and prevention of pulmonary infection are complex areas of pulmonology and infectious disease, as evidenced by continual adaptation of guidelines and the need for continued studies on proper therapy. This could not have been more evident than during the recent COVID-19 pandemic, which required novel medications for treatment and prevention along with refined protocols for evidence-based treatments. In hospitalized pneumonia patients, OMT has been shown to improve numerous outcomes. One study, the MOPSE trial, showed that OMT can reduce the use of intravenous antibiotics, duration of hospitalization, rate of ventilator-dependent respiratory failure, and overall mortality rate.[1] Similar outcomes have been found in COVID-19 patients. In one study, 90% of patients with COVID accepted OMT and reported greater ease of breathing, higher satisfaction, and stayed fewer days in the hospital with few negative effects and no adverse events.[147]

Somatic dysfunction can affect the pulmonary patient and may be effectively treated through applying the five models of osteopathic care. The osteopathic standard of care for pulmonary patients is patient-centered and involves the incorporation of evidence-based methodologies implemented through a holistic philosophy and applied via medical management, emotional/spiritual support, and manual treatments to support the patient's innate ability to heal.

ACKNOWLEDGMENTS

The authors and editors of this chapter would like to acknowledge the scholarly contributions of Drs. Gilbert D' Alonzo Jr, Samuel L. Krachman, William Foley, Hugh Ettlinger, and Jane E. Carreiro for prior editions of this chapter.

The authors and editors of this chapter would like to acknowledge the scholarly contributions of Richard Lovy, DO.

The authors and editors of this chapter would like to acknowledge the editorial contributions of Drs. Kimberly McKinnon, Alyssa Hart, and Haley Koth.

The authors and editors of this chapter would like to acknowledge the scholarly contributions of the following students: Reem Darwish, Ryan Schultz, and Alyssa Kampen.

REFERENCES

1. Noll DR, Degenhardt BF, Johnson JC. Multicenter osteopathic pneumonia study in the elderly: subgroup analysis on hospital length of stay, ventilator-dependent respiratory failure rate, and in-hospital mortality rate. *J Am Osteopath Assoc.* 2016;116(9):574–587.
2. Cassart M, Gevenois PA, Estenne M. Rib cage dimensions in hyperinflated patients with severe chronic obstructive pulmonary disease. *Am J Respir Crit Care Med.* 1996;154(3):800–805.
3. Differential diagnosis: pulmonary. University of Washington School of Medicine. Accessed April 5, 2024. https://depts.washington.edu/physdx/pulmonary/diffdx.html
4. Bordoni B, Escher AR. Palpation of the respiratory system in osteopathic manual medicine: from the trachea to the lungs. *Cureus.* 2021;13(9):e18059.
5. Stutz EW, Rondeau B. Mallampati score. In: *StatPearls.* StatPearls Publishing; 2023. Accessed April 7, 2024. http://www.ncbi.nlm.nih.gov/books/NBK585119/
6. Korr I. Sustained sympathicotonia as a factor in disease. In: Peterson B, ed. *The Collected Papers of IM Korr.* American Academy of Osteopathy; 1979:77–89.
7. Beal M. Viscerosomatic reflexes: a review. *J Am Osteopath Assoc.* 1985;(85):786–801.
8. Hansen K, Schliack H. *Segmental Innervation.* Theime; 1962.
9. Beal MC, Morlock JW. Somatic dysfunction associated with pulmonary disease. *J Am Osteopath Assoc.* 1984;84(2):179–183.
10. Pottenger FM. *Symptoms of Visceral Disease.* CV Mosby Co; 1938.
11. Bhagat BD, Young PA, Biggerstaff DE. *Fundamentals of Visceral Innervation.* Charles C Thomas; 1977.
12. Kuchera WA, Kuchera ML. *Osteopathic Considerations in Systemic Dysfunction.* 2nd ed. Greyden Press; 1992.
13. Koizumi K, Brooks CM. The integration of autonomic system reactions: a discussion of autonomic reflexes, their control and their association with somatic reactions. *Ergeb Physiol.* 1972;67:1–68.
14. Beal MC. Palpatory testing for somatic dysfunction in patients with cardiovascular disease. *J Am Osteopath Assoc.* 1983;82(11):822–831.
15. Kelso AF. A double-blind clinical study of osteopathic findings in hospital patients: progress report. *J Am Osteopath Assoc.* 1971;70(6):570–592.
16. Kelso AF, Larson NJ, Kappler RE. A clinical investigation of the osteopathic examination. *J Am Osteopath Assoc.* 1980;79(7):460–467.
17. Long F. Study of the segmental incidence of certain spinal changes in various disorders. *Osteopath Dig.* 1940;(6):11–13.
18. Deming G, Kruener V. Study of the segmental incidence of certain spinal palpatory findings in disorders of the respiratory tract. *J Am Osteopath Assoc.* 1943;(43):264–267.
19. Nicholas NS. Correlation of somatic dysfunction with visceral disease. *J Am Osteopath Assoc.* 1975;75(4):425–428.
20. Miller W. Treatment of visceral disorders by manipulative therapy. In: *The Research Status of Spinal Manipulative Therapy.* US Department of Health, Education, and Welfare; 1975:295–301.
21. Sleep Study (polysomnography). Cleveland Clinic. Accessed April 5, 2024. https://my.clevelandclinic.org/health/diagnostics/12131-sleep-study-polysomnography

22. Fry A, Rehman A. Sleep studies. Sleep Foundation. 2020. Accessed April 5, 2024. https://www.sleepfoundation.org/sleep-studies
23. What happens in a sleep study? Johns Hopkins Medicine. 2021. Accessed April 5, 2024. https://www.hopkinsmedicine.org/health/wellness-and-prevention/what-happens-in-a-sleep-study
24. Smart A. TB testing—the differences between QuantiFERON Gold, QuantiFERON Gold Plus and PPD skin testing. NMS Health. 2018. Accessed April 5, 2024. https://nmshealth.com/quantiferon-gold-plus-compared/
25. CDCTB. Tuberculosis (TB)—testing for TB infection. Centers for Disease Control and Prevention. 2023. Accessed January 2, 2025. https://www.cdc.gov/tb/testing/?CDC_AAref_Val=https://www.cdc.gov/tb/topic/testing/tbtesttypes.htm
26. Nishino M, Itoh H, Hatabu H. A practical approach to high-resolution CT of diffuse lung disease. *Eur J Radiol.* 2014;83(1):6–19.
27. Iwasawa T, Matsushita S, Hirayama M, Baba T, Ogura T. Quantitative analysis for lung disease on thin-section CT. *Diagnostics.* 2023;13(18):2988.
28. Low-dose CT lung cancer screening FAQ. American College of Radiology. Accessed April 5, 2024. https://www.acr.org/Clinical-Resources/Lung-Cancer-Screening-Resources/FAQ
29. GBD 2019 Respiratory Tract Cancers Collaborators. Global, regional, and national burden of respiratory tract cancers and associated risk factors from 1990 to 2019: a systematic analysis for the Global Burden of Disease Study 2019. *Lancet Respir Med.* 2021;9(9):1030–1049.
30. USPSTF Recommends Lung Cancer Screening with Low-dose CT. American Academy of Family Physicians. Accessed April 7, 2024. https://www.aafp.org/news/health-of-the-public/20210325uspstflung-cancer.html
31. Lung cancer screening (PDQ®)—Health Professional Version. 2024. Accessed May 9, 2024. https://www.cancer.gov/types/lung/hp/lung-screening-pdq
32. Alcantara P, Martínez BC, García-Esquinas MG, Belaústegui LG, Bustos A. Evaluation of tumor response after stereotactic body radiation therapy for lung cancer: role of 18F-fluorodeoxyglucose positron emission tomography/computed tomography. *J Clin Transl Res.* 2020;6(4):155–167.
33. Alhilali L, Reynolds AR, Fakhran S. Osteoradionecrosis after radiation therapy for head and neck cancer: differentiation from recurrent disease with CT and PET/CT imaging. *AJNR Am J Neuroradiol.* 2014;35(7):1405–1411.
34. PET scans for lung cancer: how accurate are they? MyLungCancerTeam. Accessed April 5, 2024. https://www.mylungcancerteam.com/resources/lung-pet-scan
35. Lung PET scan. MedlinePlus Medical Encyclopedia. Accessed April 5, 2024. https://medlineplus.gov/ency/article/007342.htm
36. Capitanio S, Nordin AJ, Noraini AR, Rossetti C. PET/CT in nononcological lung diseases: current applications and future perspectives. *Eur Respir Rev.* 2016;25(141):247–258.
37. Chen DL, Ballout S, Chen L, et al. Consensus recommendations on the use of 18F-FDG PET/CT in lung disease. *J Nucl Med.* 2020;61(12):1701–1707.
38. Vass L, Fisk M, Lee S, Wilson FJ, Cheriyan J, Wilkinson I. Advances in PET to assess pulmonary inflammation: a systematic review. *Eur J Radiol.* 2020;130:109182.
39. Mahmoud N, Vashisht R, Sanghavi DK, Kalanjeri S. Bronchoscopy. In: *StatPearls.* StatPearls Publishing; 2024. Accessed April 5, 2024. http://www.ncbi.nlm.nih.gov/books/NBK448152/
40. Practical approach to interventional bronchoscopy© presentations. Bronchoscopy International. Accessed April 5, 2024. https://bronchoscopy.org/practical-approach-presentations/
41. Ranu H, Wilde M, Madden B. Pulmonary function tests. *Ulster Med J.* 2011;80(2):84–90.
42. Martinez-Pitre PJ, Sabbula BR, Cascella M. Restrictive lung disease. In: *StatPearls.* StatPearls Publishing; 2024. Accessed April 7, 2024. http://www.ncbi.nlm.nih.gov/books/NBK560880/
43. David S, Edwards CW. Forced expiratory volume. In: *StatPearls.* StatPearls Publishing; 2024. Accessed May 10, 2024. http://www.ncbi.nlm.nih.gov/books/NBK540970/
44. Kochhar K, Hines P, Heinking K, Henderson K. Somatic dysfunction and effect of OMT on pulmonary function in healthy adult male subjects (871.7). *FASEB J.* 2014;28.
45. Stępnik J, Kędra A, Czaprowski D. Short-term effect of osteopathic manual techniques (OMT) on respiratory function in healthy individuals. *PLoS ONE.* 2020;15(6):e0235308.
46. Berliner D, Schneider N, Welte T, Bauersachs J. The differential diagnosis of dyspnea. *Dtsch Ärztebl Int.* 2016;113(49):834–845.
47. Buschulte K, Cottin V, Wijsenbeek M, Kreuter M, Diesler R. The world of rare interstitial lung diseases. *Eur Respir Rev.* 2023;32(167).
48. Understanding the Differential Diagnosis of COPD Why the exclusion of other causes is needed. Verywell Health. Accessed April 5, 2024. https://www.verywellhealth.com/differential-diagnosis-of-copd-914739
49. Price DB, Yawn BP, Jones RCM. Improving the differential diagnosis of chronic obstructive pulmonary disease in primary care. *Mayo Clin Proc.* 2010;85(12):1122–1129.
50. Celli BR, Fabbri LM, Aaron SD, et al. Differential diagnosis of suspected chronic obstructive pulmonary disease exacerbations in the acute care setting: best practice. *Am J Respir Crit Care Med.* 2023;207(9):1134–1144.
51. Asthma's effect on the nation. Centers for Disease Control and Prevention. 2023. Accessed January 2, 2025. https://www.cdc.gov/asthma/national-surveillance-data/healthcare-use.htm
52. Hashmi MF, Tariq M, Cataletto ME. Asthma. In: *StatPearls.* StatPearls Publishing; 2024. Accessed April 7, 2024. http://www.ncbi.nlm.nih.gov/books/NBK430901/
53. Cloutier MM, Dixon AE, Krishnan JA, Lemanske RF, Pace W, Schatz M. Managing asthma in adolescents and adults: 2020 Asthma Guideline Update from the National Asthma Education and Prevention Program. *JAMA.* 2020;324(22):2301–2317.
54. Expert Panel Working Group of the National Heart, Lung, and Blood Institute (NHLBI) administered and coordinated National Asthma Education and Prevention Program Coordinating Committee (NAEPPCC); Cloutier MM, Baptist AP, Blake KV, et al. 2020 Focused Updates to the Asthma Management Guidelines: a report from the National Asthma Education and Prevention Program Coordinating Committee Expert Panel Working Group. *J Allergy Clin Immunol.* 2020;146(6):1217–1270.
55. National Heart, Lung, and Blood Advisory Council Asthma Expert Working Group. *Expert Panel Report 3: Guidelines for the Diagnosis and Management of Asthma.* National Institutes of Health/National Heart, Lung, and Blood Institute. 2007. https://www.nhlbi.nih.gov/sites/default/files/media/docs/EPR-3_Asthma_Full_Report_2007.pdf
56. Fahy JV. Type 2 inflammation in asthma—present in most, absent in many. *Nat Rev Immunol.* 2015;15(1):57–65.
57. Dweik RA, Boggs PB, Erzurum SC, et al; American Thoracic Society Committee on Interpretation of Exhaled Nitric Oxide Levels (FENO) for Clinical Applications. An official ATS clinical practice guideline: interpretation of exhaled nitric oxide levels (FENO) for clinical applications. *Am J Respir Crit Care Med.* 2011;184(5):602–615.
58. Mangattu Parambil PB, Mohapatra AK, Behera D, Subhankar S, Jagaty SK, Singh P. Determination of sputum eosinophil count and serum absolute eosinophil count in patients with bronchial asthma and its correlation with disease severity and response to treatment. *J Fam Med Prim Care.* 2023;12(9):2053–2057.
59. Asthma management guidelines: focused updates 2020. NHLBI, NIH. Accessed May 12, 2024. https://www.nhlbi.nih.gov/health-topics/asthma-management-guidelines-2020-updates
60. Rurey K. New: Global Initiative for Asthma 2021 Executive Summary on asthma management and prevention. Global Initiative for Asthma. 2021. Accessed April 7, 2024. https://ginasthma.org/new-global-initiative-for-asthma-2021-executive-summary-on-asthma-management-and-prevention-2/
61. Geyer-Roberts E, Lacatusu DA, Kester J, Foster-Moumoutjis G, Sidiqi M. Preventative management of sepsis-induced acute respiratory distress syndrome in the geriatric population. *Cureus.* 2023;15(2).
62. 2022 GINA Main Report. Global Initiative for Asthma. Accessed May 12, 2024. https://ginasthma.org/gina-reports/
63. Forbes H. Bronchial asthma. *J Am Osteopath Assoc.* 1902;(1):106–109.
64. Coffman K. Asthma. *J Am Osteopath Assoc.* 1902;(1):188–190.
65. Burns L. Clinic reports from the Pacific College of Osteopathy. *J Am Osteopath Assoc.* 1912;(11):1054–1056.
66. Wilson P. Experimental work in asthma at the Peter Bent Brigham Hospital. *J Am Osteopath Assoc.* 1925;(25):212–214.

67. Kline JA. An examination of the osteopathic management of bronchial asthma. *AAO Yearbook*. 1959:127–131.
68. Schend J, Rowane M, Sanan N, Hostoffer SR. An osteopathic modular approach to asthma: a narrative review. *J Osteopath Med*. 2020;120(11): 774–782.
69. Guiney PA, Chou R, Vianna A, Lovenheim J. Effects of osteopathic manipulative treatment on pediatric patients with asthma: a randomized controlled trial. *J Am Osteopath Assoc*. 2005;105(1):7–12.
70. Parnell Prevost C, Gleberzon B, Carleo B, Anderson K, Cark M, Pohlman KA. Manual therapy for the pediatric population: a systematic review. *BMC Complement Altern Med*. 2019;19(1):60.
71. Posadzki P, Kyaw BM, Dziedzic A, Ernst E. Osteopathic manipulative treatment for pediatric conditions: an update of systematic review and meta-analysis. *J Clin Med*. 2022;11(15):4455.
72. Murphy AJ. Preliminary studies of the influence of pulmonary and thoracic mobilization procedures on pulmonary function. *J Am Osteopath Assoc*. 1965;64:951–952.
73. Murphy AJ. Continuation of the study of the effect of thoracic mobilization on the distribution of 131 I MAA in the lungs. *J Am Osteopath Assoc*. 1971;70(10):1057–1058.
74. Murphy A. Comparison of nitrogen washout curves from human experiments and from a mathematical model of the lung. *J Am Osteopath Assoc*. 1971;(70):1057–1058.
75. Jones LM, Regan C, Wolf K, et al. Effect of osteopathic manipulative treatment on pulmonary function testing in children with asthma. *J Osteopath Med*. 2021;121(6):589–596.
76. Castillo JR, Peters SP, Busse WW. Asthma exacerbations: pathogenesis, prevention, and treatment. *J Allergy Clin Immunol Pract*. 2017;5(4): 918–927.
77. Fitzgerald M, Stiles E. Osteopathic hospitals' solution to DRGs may be OMT. *The DO*. 1984;(25):97–101.
78. Singh D, Agusti A, Anzueto A, et al. Global strategy for the diagnosis, management, and prevention of chronic obstructive lung disease: the GOLD Science Committee report 2019. *Eur Respir J*. 2019;53(5):1900164.
79. Agarwal AK, Raja A, Brown BD. Chronic obstructive pulmonary disease. In: *StatPearls*. StatPearls Publishing; 2023. Accessed April 7, 2024. http://www.ncbi.nlm.nih.gov/books/NBK559281/
80. Forey BA, Thornton AJ, Lee PN. Systematic review with meta-analysis of the epidemiological evidence relating smoking to COPD, chronic bronchitis and emphysema. *BMC Pulm Med*. 2011;11(1):36.
81. Emphysema vs. chronic bronchitis: understanding the differences. National Emphysema Foundation. Accessed April 7, 2024. https://www.emphysemafoundation.org/index.php/about-uss/privacy/83-copd-emphysema-articles/428-emphysema-vs-chronic-bronchitis-understanding-the-differences
82. Shaker SB, Dirksen A, Bach KS, Mortensen J. Imaging in chronic obstructive pulmonary disease. *COPD*. 2007;4(2):143–161.
83. Scanlon PD, Connett JE, Waller LA, et al. Smoking cessation and lung function in mild-to-moderate chronic obstructive pulmonary disease: the Lung Health Study. *Am J Respir Crit Care Med*. 2000;161(2):381–390.
84. Lindenauer PK, Stefan MS, Pekow PS, et al. Association between initiation of pulmonary rehabilitation after hospitalization for COPD and 1-year survival among Medicare beneficiaries. *JAMA*. 2020;323(18):1813–1823.
85. Puhan MA, Gimeno-Santos E, Cates CJ, Troosters T. Pulmonary rehabilitation following exacerbations of chronic obstructive pulmonary disease. *Cochrane Database Syst Rev*. 2016;12(12):CD005305.
86. Zanotti E, Berardinelli P, Bizzarri C, et al. Osteopathic manipulative treatment effectiveness in severe chronic obstructive pulmonary disease: a pilot study. *Complement Ther Med*. 2012;20(1–2):16–22.
87. Pneumococcal vaccine recommendations. CDC. 2023. Accessed May 12, 2024. https://www.cdc.gov/vaccines/vpd/pneumo/hcp/recommendations.html
88. Celli BR, Cote CG, Marin JM, et al. The body-mass index, airflow obstruction, dyspnea, and exercise capacity index in chronic obstructive pulmonary disease. *N Engl J Med*. 2004;350(10):1005–1012.
89. Kamath S, Kumar A, Panda SK, Samanta RP. Correlation of BODE index with quality of life in stable chronic obstructive pulmonary disease (COPD) patients—a prospective study. *J Fam Med Prim Care*. 2020;9(11):5606–5613.
90. Noll DR, Degenhardt BF, Johnson JC, Burt SA. Immediate effects of osteopathic manipulative treatment in elderly patients with chronic obstructive pulmonary disease. *J Am Osteopath Assoc*. 2008;108(5):251–259.
91. Noll DR, Johnson JC, Baer RW, Snider EJ. The immediate effect of individual manipulation techniques on pulmonary function measures in persons with chronic obstructive pulmonary disease. *Osteopath Med Prim Care*. 2009;3:9.
92. Christina Raguckas DO, Jonathan Ference P, Gretta A, Gross DO. Osteopathic considerations in obstructive pulmonary disease: a systematic review of the evidence. *Osteopath Fam Physician*. 2016;8(3):28–40. Accessed April 7, 2024. https://www.acofp.org/news-and-publications/journal/search-results?searchQuery=Osteopathic%20considerations%20in%20obstructive%20pulmonary%20disease
93. Buscemi A, Pennisi V, Rapisarda A, Pennisi A, Coco M. Efficacy of osteopathic treatment in patients with stable moderate-to-severe chronic obstructive pulmonary disease: a randomized controlled pilot study. *J Complement Integr Med*. 2019;17(1):/j/jcim.2019.17.issue-1/jcim-2018-0128/jcim-2018-0128.xml.
94. Engel RM, Vemulpad SR, Beath K. Short-term effects of a course of manual therapy and exercise in people with moderate chronic obstructive pulmonary disease: a preliminary clinical trial. *J Manipulative Physiol Ther*. 2013;36(8):490–496.
95. Krus-Johnston A, Mirocha N. Does OMT reduce symptoms of obstructive pulmonary disorders? *Evidence-Based Pract*. 2019;22(9):21.
96. Mackenzie G. The definition and classification of pneumonia. *Pneumonia (Nathan)*. 2016;8:14.
97. Lutfiyya MN, Henley E, Chang LF, Reyburn SW. Diagnosis and treatment of community-acquired pneumonia. *Am Fam Physician*. 2006; 73(3):442–450.
98. Wunderink RG. Community-acquired pneumonia. *Infect Dis*. 2017: 251–257.e1.
99. Mosenifar Z. Viral pneumonia clinical presentation. Medscape. 2023. https://emedicine.medscape.com/article/300455-clinical
100. File TM Jr. Patient education: pneumonia in adults (beyond the basics). *UpToDate*. 2024. Accessed January 2, 2025. https://www.uptodate.com/contents/pneumonia-in-adults-beyond-the-basics#H13
101. Lim WS, van der Eerden MM, Laing R, et al. Defining community acquired pneumonia severity on presentation to hospital: an international derivation and validation study. *Thorax*. 2003;58(5):377–382.
102. Pahal P, Rajasurya V, Sharma S. Typical bacterial pneumonia. In: *StatPearls*. StatPearls Publishing; 2023. Accessed May 13, 2024. http://www.ncbi.nlm.nih.gov/books/NBK534295/
103. Prasso JE, Deng JC. Postviral complications: bacterial pneumonia. *Clin Chest Med*. 2017;38(1):127–138.
104. Sattar SBA, Nguyen D, Sharma S. Bacterial pneumonia. In: *StatPearls*. StatPearls Publishing; 2024. Accessed May 13, 2024. http://www.ncbi.nlm.nih.gov/books/NBK513321/
105. Atypical Pneumonia | CDC. Published September 30, 2022. Accessed May 13, 2024. https://www.cdc.gov/pneumonia/about/index.html
106. Fungal community-acquired pneumonia. CDC. 2023. Accessed May 13, 2024. https://www.cdc.gov/fungal/diseases/community-acquired-pneumonia/index.html
107. Gamache J. Bacterial pneumonia clinical presentation: history, physical examination, risk stratification. *Medscape*. Accessed April 7, 2024. https://emedicine.medscape.com/article/300157-clinical
108. Kaysin A, Viera AJ. Community-acquired pneumonia in adults: diagnosis and management. *Am Fam Physician*. 2016;94(9):698–706.
109. Ramirez J. Overview of community-acquired pneumonia in adults. *UpToDate*. Published April 5, 2024. https://www.uptodate.com/contents/overview-of-community-acquired-pneumonia-in-adults
110. Watkins RR, Lemonovich TL. Diagnosis and management of community-acquired pneumonia in adults. *Am Fam Physician*. 2011;83(11):1299–1306.
111. Florin TA, Ambroggio L, Brokamp C, et al. Reliability of examination findings in suspected community-acquired pneumonia. *Pediatrics*. 2017;140(3):e20170310.
112. Nelson KE, Glonek T. *Somatic Dysfunction in Osteopathic Family Medicine*. 2nd ed. Lippincott Williams & Wilkins; 2015.
113. Das D, Howlett DC. Chest X-ray manifestations of pneumonia. *Surgery*. 2009;27(10):453–455.

114. Jones J, Bell D, Hacking C, et al. Pneumonia (summary). Radiopaedia. 2015.
115. Amanullah S. Typical bacterial pneumonia imaging: practice essentials, radiography, computed tomography. *Medscape*. 2023. Accessed April 7, 2024. https://emedicine.medscape.com/article/360090-overview
116. Ramirez JA. Overview of community-acquired pneumonia in adults. *UpToDate*. 2024. Accessed January 2, 2025. https://www.uptodate.com/contents/overview-of-community-acquired-pneumonia-in-adults/print
117. Bauer TT, Ewig S, Marre R, Suttorp N, Welte T; CAPNETZ Study Group. CRB-65 predicts death from community-acquired pneumonia. *J Intern Med*. 2006;260(1):93–101.
118. Fine MJ, Auble TE, Yealy DM, et al. A prediction rule to identify low-risk patients with community-acquired pneumonia. *N Engl J Med*. 1997;336(4):243–250.
119. Baer S. Community-acquired pneumonia (CAP): practice essentials, overview, etiology of community-acquired pneumonia. *Medscape*. 2022. Accessed April 7, 2024. https://emedicine.medscape.com/article/234240-overview?form=fpf
120. Davis D, Thadhani J, Choudhary V, et al. Advancements in the management of severe community-acquired pneumonia: a comprehensive narrative review. *Cureus*. 2023;15(10):e46893.
121. Plata-Menchaca EP, Ferrer R. Current treatment of nosocomial pneumonia and ventilator-associated pneumonia. *Rev Espanola Quimioter*. 2022;35(Suppl 3):25–29.
122. Russell CD, Koch O, Laurenson IF, O'Shea DT, Sutherland R, Mackintosh CL. Diagnosis and features of hospital-acquired pneumonia: a retrospective cohort study. *J Hosp Infect*. 2016;92(3):273–279.
123. Niederman MS, Craven DE, Chastre J, et al. Treatment of hospital-acquired pneumonia. *Lancet Infect Dis*. 2011;11(10):728.
124. Metlay JP, Waterer GW, Long AC, et al. Diagnosis and treatment of adults with community-acquired pneumonia. An official clinical practice guideline of the American Thoracic Society and Infectious Diseases Society of America. *Am J Respir Crit Care Med*. 2019;200(7):e45–e67.
125. Metlay JP, Waterer GW. Update in adult community-acquired pneumonia: key points from the new American Thoracic Society/Infectious Diseases Society of America 2019 guideline. *Curr Opin Pulm Med*. 2020;26(3):203–207.
126. Kalil AC, Metersky ML, Klompas M, et al. Management of adults with hospital-acquired and ventilator-associated pneumonia: 2016 Clinical Practice Guidelines by the Infectious Diseases Society of America and the American Thoracic Society. *Clin Infect Dis*. 2016;63(5):e61–e111.
127. Losier A, Dela Cruz CS. New testing guidelines for community-acquired pneumonia. *Curr Opin Infect Dis*. 2022;35(2):128–132.
128. Smith RK. One hundred thousand cases of influenza with a death rate of one-fortieth of that officially reported under conventional medical treatment. 1919. *J Am Osteopath Assoc*. 2000;100(5):320–323.
129. Lesho E, McKeown A, Laguio-Vila M. The rationale for including osteopathic manipulative treatment in the management of infections: a hermeneutic review. *Expert Rev Anti Infect Ther*. 2022;20(1):23–31.
130. Miller C. The lymphatic pump, its application to acute infections. *J Am Osteopath Assoc*. 1926;25:443–445.
131. Gjikolaj B, Morabito B, Castellan A. Efficacy of osteopathic manipulative treatment (OMT) with lymphatic pump treatment (LPT), adjuvant to conventional antibiotic therapy in hospitalized patients with pneumonia: a systematic review of randomized controlled trials (RCTs). 2022; 6(01).
132. Measel JW Jr. The effect of the lymphatic pump on the immune response: I. Preliminary studies on the antibody response to pneumococcal polysaccharide assayed by bacterial agglutination and passive hemagglutination. *J Am Osteopath Assoc*. 1982;82(1):28–31.
133. Creasy C, Schander A, Orlowski A, Hodge LM. Thoracic and abdominal lymphatic pump techniques inhibit the growth of *S. pneumoniae* bacteria in the lungs of rats. *Lymphat Res Biol*. 2013;11(3):183–186.
134. Noll DR, Shores J, Bryman PN, Masterson EV. Adjunctive osteopathic manipulative treatment in the elderly hospitalized with pneumonia: a pilot study. *J Osteopath Med*. 1999;99(3):143–152.
135. Hodge LM. Osteopathic lymphatic pump techniques to enhance immunity and treat pneumonia. *Int J Osteopath Med IJOM*. 2012;15(1): 13–21.
136. Roland H, Brown A, Rousselot A, et al. Osteopathic manipulative treatment decreases hospital stay and healthcare cost in the neonatal intensive care unit. *Medicines*. 2022;9(10):49.
137. Belcastro MR, Backes CR, Chila AG. Bronchiolitis: a pilot study of osteopathic manipulative treatment, bronchodilators, and other therapy. *J Am Osteopath Assoc*. 1984;83(9):672–676.
138. Kobayashi M, Farrar JL, Gierke R, et al. Use of 15-valent pneumococcal conjugate vaccine and 20-valent pneumococcal conjugate vaccine among U.S. adults: updated recommendations of the Advisory Committee on Immunization Practices—United States, 2022. *MMWR Morb Mortal Wkly Rep*. 2022;71.
139. Chandra D, Cherian SV. Hypersensitivity pneumonitis. In: *StatPearls*. StatPearls Publishing; 2024. Accessed February 15, 2024. http://www.ncbi.nlm.nih.gov/books/NBK499918/
140. Pietersen PI, Konge L, Jørgensen R, Stolz D, Farr A, Laursen CB. Pulmonologists' work and clinical life during the COVID-19 pandemic: a society-led survey. *Breathe (Sheff)*. 2022;18(1):220001.
141. Gandhi R, Meyerowitz E, McIntosh K. COVID-19: epidemiology, virology, and prevention. *UpToDate*. Accessed April 7, 2024. https://www.uptodate.com/contents/covid-19-epidemiology-virology-and-prevention
142. Cascella M, Rajnik M, Aleem A, Dulebohn SC, Di Napoli R. Features, evaluation, and treatment of Coronavirus (COVID-19). In: *StatPearls*. StatPearls Publishing; 2024. Accessed April 7, 2024. http://www.ncbi.nlm.nih.gov/books/NBK554776/
143. Chua EX, Zahir SMISM, Ng KT, et al. Effect of prone versus supine position in COVID-19 patients: a systematic review and meta-analysis. *J Clin Anesth*. 2021;74:110406.
144. Cicchitti L, Martelli M, Cerritelli F. Chronic inflammatory disease and osteopathy: a systematic review. *PloS One*. 2015;10(3):e0121327.
145. Bailey W. Evaluation of rib raising technique in respiratory distress syndrome. *J Am Osteopath Assoc*. 1963;(62):924–928.
146. Jacob B, Sawhney M, Sridhar A, et al. Potential therapeutic effects of adjunct osteopathic manipulative treatments in SARS-CoV-2 patients. *J Osteopath Med*. 2023;123(7):343–349.
147. Study signals osteopathic manipulative treatment may be beneficial in treating COVID-19. Penn State Health News. 2022. Accessed April 7, 2024. https://pennstatehealthnews.org/2022/07/osteopathic-manipulative-treatment-covid19/
148. Martinez E, Loveless B, Crone P, Szurmant H, Fuchs S, Sanchez J. Serological assessment of the effectiveness of osteopathic manipulative to augment the Covid-19 vaccine immune response. *J Investig Med*. 2023:41–41.
149. Still G. Advantages and necessity of osteopathic post-operative treatment. *J Am Osteopath Assoc*. 1919;18:481–486.
150. Pratt-Harrington D, Neptune-Ceran R. The effect of osteopathic manipulative treatment in the post abdominal surgical patient. *AAOJ*. 1995;Fall:9–13.
151. Sleszynski S, Kelso A. Comparison of thoracic manipulation with incentive spirometry in the prevention of post-operative atelectasis. *J Am Osteopath Assoc*. 1993;93:834–845.
152. Dickey JL. Postoperative osteopathic manipulative management of median sternotomy patients. *J Am Osteopath Assoc*. 1989;89(10):1309–1314, 1319–1322.
153. Racca V, Bordoni B, Castiglioni P, Modica M, Ferratini M. Osteopathic manipulative treatment improves heart surgery outcomes: a randomized controlled trial. *Ann Thorac Surg*. 2017;104(1):145–152.
154. Adams JS, Parikh SH, Goodwin BJ, Noll DR. Does the osteopathic pedal pump reduce lower limb volume in healthy subjects? *J Osteopath Med*. 2023;123(4):201–206.
155. Seffinger MA, ed. *Foundations of Osteopathic Medicine*. 4th ed. Wolters Kluwer; 2018.
156. Vitale MG, Matsumoto H, Bye MR, et al. A retrospective cohort study of pulmonary function, radiographic measures, and quality of life in children with congenital scoliosis: an evaluation of patient outcomes after early spinal fusion. *Spine (Phila Pa 1976)*. 2008;33(11):1242.
157. Tsiligiannis T, Grivas T. Pulmonary function in children with idiopathic scoliosis. *Scoliosis*. 2012;7(1):7.
158. Kempen DHR, Heemskerk JL, Kaçmaz G, et al. Pulmonary function in children and adolescents with untreated idiopathic scoliosis: a systematic review with meta-regression analysis. *Spine J*. 2022;22(7):1178–1190.

159. Doran J, Freiburger L, Zink G, Kilmore M. Relationship of osteopathic manipulative treatment, lordosis, and respiration. 1982;82:139–140.
160. Yao S, Mikhail N, Koutsouras G, Coombs A, Terzella MJ. Osteopathic considerations in the infections of the respiratory tract. *Osteopath Fam Physician*. 2017;9(1). Accessed January 2, 2025. https://www.acofp.org/docs/default-source/ofp/vol-13-no-5-(2021)-september-october-2021/osteopathic-considerations-in-pneumonia.pdf?sfvrsn=eddcc73f_0
161. Hadjikoutis S, Wiles CM, Eccles R. Cough in motor neuron disease: a review of mechanisms. *QJM*. 1999;92(9):487–494.
162. Dalley AF, Agur AMR. *Moore's Clinically Oriented Anatomy*. 9th ed. Wolters Kluwer; 2023.
163. Ilahi M, St Lucia K, Ilahi TB. Anatomy, thorax, thoracic duct. In: *StatPearls*. StatPearls Publishing; 2023. Accessed February 11, 2024. http://www.ncbi.nlm.nih.gov/books/NBK513227/
164. Knott EM, Tune JD, Stoll ST, Downey HF. Increased lymphatic flow in the thoracic duct during manipulative intervention. *J Am Osteopath Assoc*. 2005;105(10):447–456.
165. Anglund DC, Channell MK. Contribution of osteopathic medicine to care of patients with chronic wounds. *J Am Osteopath Assoc*. 2011;111(9):538–542.
166. Clinical osteopathically integrated learning scenarios (COILS). AACOM. Accessed May 15, 2024. https://www.aacom.org/medical-education/teaching-and-learning/competency-curriculum-resources/clinical-osteopathically-integrated-learning-scenarios
167. Carnevali L, Lombardi L, Fornari M, Sgoifo A. Exploring the effects of osteopathic manipulative treatment on autonomic function through the lens of heart rate variability. *Front Neurosci*. 2020;14:579365.
168. Niwa S, Fila-Pawłowska K, Van den Bergh O, Rymaszewska J. Respiratory dysfunction in persistent somatic symptoms: a systematic review of observational studies. *J Psychosom Res*. 2024;181:111607.
169. Macnaughton J. Making breath visible: reflections on relations between bodies, breath and world in the critical medical humanities. *Body Soc*. 2020;26(2):30–54.
170. Bränström H, Fahlström M. Kinesiophobia in patients with chronic musculoskeletal pain: differences between men and women. *J Rehabil Med*. 2008;40(5):375–380.
171. Katotomichelakis M, Simopoulos E, Zhang N, et al. Olfactory dysfunction and asthma as risk factors for poor quality of life in upper airway diseases. *Am J Rhinol Allergy*. 2013;27(4):293–298.
172. Juniper EF, Guyatt GH, Dolovich J. Assessment of quality of life in adolescents with allergic rhinoconjunctivitis: development and testing of a questionnaire for clinical trials. *J Allergy Clin Immunol*. 1994;93(2):413–423.

73 Osteopathic Considerations in Neurology

MITCHELL L. ELKISS ▪ KURT P. HEINKING ▪ RAYMOND J. HRUBY ▪ MARCEL P. FRAIX ▪ REBECCA E. GIUSTI

KEY CONCEPTS

- Headaches, including migraine, cluster, cervicogenic, and tension type, are common disorders seen by neurologists as well as primary care practitioners. Osteopathic structural evaluation and manipulative treatment (OMT) are useful in both differentiating and treating these disorders.
- Spinal disorders affecting the spinal cord and peripheral nerves are considered in the differential diagnosis of neck and back pain and need to be distinguished from somatic dysfunction.
- Peripheral entrapment neuropathies are often amenable to OMT.
- Neurologic tests help to determine likely causes of clinical neuropathology and are essential components of both complete and focal neurologic examinations.

INTRODUCTION

The specialty of neurology deals with the structure, function, disease, and dysfunction of the neuromusculoskeletal system. The neuromusculoskeletal system includes the brain, spinal cord, peripheral and autonomic nervous systems, as well as the muscular system. The early development of osteopathic medical concepts emphasized the role of the nervous system as an integrator of function between the various systems of the body.[1] This chapter provides an overview of neurology as practiced by osteopathic physicians, focusing on some common neurologic disorders in which the application of osteopathic concepts is straightforward. The syndromes of headaches and peripheral nerve entrapments are addressed specifically. Other conditions seen by neurologists are addressed in various chapters in this textbook, for example:

- Nociception and chronic pain in Chapters 11, 74, and 93
- Application of the five models of osteopathic care to patients with acute neck or low back pain in Chapter 66 Osteopathic Considerations in Family Medicine
- Dementia in Chapter 69 Osteopathic Considerations in Geriatric Medicine
- Spinal cord injuries and quadriplegia in Chapter 75 Osteopathic Considerations in Physical Medicine and Rehabilitation
- Low back pain in Chapter 84 Osteopathic Considerations in Orthopedics and Chapter 93 Osteopathic Considerations in the Patient with Low Back Pain
- Closed head injuries and concussion in athletes in Chapter 87 Osteopathic Considerations in Sports Medicine

OVERVIEW

The central nervous system (CNS) is unique in the human organism. It allows us the potential to pursue rational thought, experience the deepest emotional states, perform complex motor functions with little or no conscious attention, and have mechanisms for integrating a multitude of highly regulated bodily functions. The system includes segmental mechanisms for regulating sensory, motor, and reflex functions. It includes primitive brain centers responsible for posture, locomotion, and visceral sensing and regulation, more evolved systems of personality and feeling, and the most evolved system with the capacity for human mindfulness. All functions of the human organism are under some form of neural control; therefore, the maintenance of normal nervous system activity is essential for health. Relevant to the osteopathic physician is the intimate relation between the nervous system and manifestations of somatic dysfunction.[2] Although the nervous system is discussed in its component parts, it is important to remember that the subtotal of nervous system activity is a complex of electrophysiologic and neurochemical phenomena, demonstrating features of phasic or dynamic activity superimposed on tonic or static activity at multiple levels of the nervous system and resulting in the complex neurobiology of humans.

The structure of the nervous system can be clinically divided into reasonably circumscribed areas that correspond to specific neurologic functions. For purposes of discussion, these divisions are the:

- Brain, including the cerebral cortex, basal ganglia, cerebellum, and brainstem
- Spinal cord
- Peripheral nerves and muscles

These areas are discussed more comprehensively in other texts.[3]

The cerebral cortex contains the primary motor system for the initiation of conscious motor activity, the primary sensory system for the appreciation of conscious sensory input, and the centers for memory, speech, and visuospatial integration. Lesions in these areas produce contralateral defects in motor and sensory functions. Compromise of the dominant hemisphere disturbs speech and language functions, while nondominant hemispheric disruption influences visuospatial processing and the potential for visual imagery.

The basal ganglia are intermediate nuclear structures that act as relay stations between the other sensorimotor control systems. The primary clinical functions of the basal ganglia include the inhibition of spinal segmental reflexes, such that resting muscles can remain at rest. They control automatic and associated movements that occur without conscious processing (e.g., swinging the arms while walking or smiling while talking). Disorders of the basal ganglia typically produce:

- Tremors at rest 3 to 4 Hz
- Rigidity
- Loss of associated movements
- Posture disturbances

The cerebellum functions to match proprioceptive input (state of the muscles and joints) with cortical output (motor intent) to control muscles during movement to ensure smooth motor transitions and to maintain posture and balance. The cerebellum has an increasingly recognizable role in disorders of executive function, language, and affect.

Clinical disorders of the cerebellum classically manifest as:

- Tremor increasing during intentional movement
- Postural abnormalities
- Imbalance
- Ataxia

The brainstem acts as a connection between the:

- Cerebral cortex
- Basal ganglia
- Cerebellum
- Spinal cord

All impulses traveling into or out of the CNS are transmitted through the brainstem, which contains the nuclei of the cranial nerves and the autonomic centers. From here, impulses are transmitted out to the periphery through each segmental spinal cord level.

Each spinal cord level contains a set of nerve roots and is a processor, organizer, and distributor of sensory, motor, and autonomic impulses. Each spinal segment contains the anterior horn cells from which the peripheral motor nerves arise and the dorsal horns where sensory neurons enter. In essence, the motor roots supply all the muscles related to that segment (myotome) and similarly receive the sensory input from that segment (dermatome). The peripheral nerves transmit impulses to the muscles for movement and contain the sensory fibers for:

- Pain
- Temperature
- Touch
- Proprioception

The autonomic nervous system, sympathetic and parasympathetic, controls the visceral functions of the body. With rapidity and intensity, the autonomic nervous system can influence visceral functions. Each autonomic pathway comprises a preganglionic and postganglionic neuron. Preganglionic sympathetic neurons originate in the intermediolateral column of the thoracolumbar spinal cord and exit through the ventral roots and spinal nerve to pass into one of the chain ganglia. They either synapse or pass through to one of the outlying sympathetic ganglia. From the sympathetic chain ganglia or the outlying ganglia, postganglionic neurons originate and course to their organ of destination. The parasympathetic division originates in the brainstem and the sacral spinal cord. Their preganglionic neurons pass uninterrupted to the organ that is to be controlled. The postganglionic neurons are located in the wall of the target organs.

These summary descriptions of the anatomy of the nervous system illustrate that each of these systems is interdependent and exerts its ultimate effect in either the facilitation or inhibition of the spinal cord segments.[4] The nervous system continually receives information about the organism's internal and external environment through the afferent sensory system arising from the musculoskeletal system and the viscera. This information is processed centrally, transmitted throughout the CNS, and stored as learned or retained information. The nervous system output is transmitted through the efferent limb to the somatic and visceral compartments of the body. It is through the motor unit that the dominant effects of the motor system are manifested and through the peripheral autonomic system that efferent nervous functions are played out on the viscera. Through this process, the neuromuscular system helps to preserve and maintain total body functional integrity. The neuromuscular system generates action within the physical universe in support of the whole organism. Consider the physical manifestations of running, fighting, gathering food, eating, breathing, playing, and caring for one another as examples of maintaining total body functional integrity through the work of the neuromusculoskeletal system.

Practically speaking, the assumption of the upright stance involves an intricate interaction of the basic neurologic centers, with reference to the:

- Descending supraspinal pathways
- Cooperation of the basal ganglia and cerebellum
- Limbic system
- Lobes of the neocortex

This evolutionary accomplishment frees the human hands for manipulation of its environment and for further development. Biomechanical dysfunction can be a consequence of an imperfect adaptation to the continually changing center of gravity associated with an upright stance. The neuromusculoskeletal system provides the human with its behavioral repertoire; from complex athletic feats, simple postural maintenance, and locomotion to the segmental dysfunction of the neuromusculoskeletal system resulting in somatic dysfunction. Further discussion of these concepts as they relate to somatic dysfunction can be found in Chapter 13 Somatic Dysfunction, Spinal Facilitation, and Viscerosomatic Integration.

Perceptions and feelings can influence the state of the body's muscular activity, the autonomic activity, and the capacity of its homeostatic mechanisms to respond to exogenous allostatic influences—including the ability to respond to osteopathic manipulative treatment (OMT). Neuroendocrine mechanisms allow the affective tone of individuals, their feeling state, and their personality to have an impact on their neuromusculoskeletal system. These mechanisms can be localized to the:

- Limbic system
- Hypothalamus
- Pituitary gland
- Neuroendocrine circuits

In the early stages of somatic dysfunction, continued afferent barrage (nociceptive, proprioceptive, autonomic) and a widening zone of involvement maintain the state of chronic facilitation, also known as central sensitization. With chronic somatic dysfunction, a more lasting mechanism must be at work. Sustained patterns of excitability and synaptic transmission become learned behavior in the spinal cord and brain.[5] The facilitated segment is the focus of efferent neuronal hyperexcitability. Metaphorically speaking, the zone of somatic dysfunction continues to represent the squeaky wheel. Additional local or general afferent stimulation results in an increased somatic and sympathetic efferent outpouring to those tissues innervated through the facilitated segment, manifesting as increased signs and symptoms of somatic dysfunction (see also Chapter 13).

The osteopathic point of view considers wellness, or health, a positive state. It appreciates the organizational unity, inherent healing capacity, and self-regulating ability of the human body. Concern for the interrelationship between structure and function is crucial.

PERSONAL APPROACH TO NEUROLOGIC DIAGNOSIS

When patients present with variable complaints of pain, sensory disturbance, or weakness, it is the neurologist's job to answer three questions.

1. Is there a neurologic abnormality?
2. Can the neurologic abnormality be localized?
3. Can a differential diagnosis be generated for the abnormality in question?

For example, if a patient presents with neck or back pain, the physician attempts to localize the symptom by history. An effort is made to differentiate spinal cord disorders, nerve root syndromes, or vertebral disorders.

When taking the history, it is necessary to know the patient's past personal history of illness, trauma, and surgery. Knowing the family history is valuable as a potential source of hereditary or constitutional susceptibility. The general history explores the psychosocial background of the patient and their family and includes a search into the history of abuse (substance, physical, sexual, and emotional). Inquire into the patient's:

- Nutrition
- Work
- Exercise habits
- Sleep patterns
- Potential risk exposures

A mental status examination to evaluate the higher cortical functions and arousal system should be followed by a complete neurologic examination. This examination includes evaluation of the cranial nerves and the motor and sensory system. Test coordination and gait. Motor examination includes an assessment of:

- Muscle tone
- Muscle strength
- Muscle bulk
- The activity of the associated myotendinous reflexes

Sensory examination includes tests of:

- Light touch
- Pain
- Temperature
- Vibration
- Proprioception

In addition to a routine neurologic examination, perform a systematic musculoskeletal and structural examination on patients with spinal complaints, including:

- Inspection of the patient walking and standing, from an anterior, posterior, and lateral view, looking for static and kinetic structural asymmetries
- Performance of the standing flexion test
- Performance of the standing side bending test
- Performance of the seated flexion test
- Assessment of seated trunk rotation
- Assessment of seated side bending
- Seated cervical assessment for flexion, extension, side bending, and rotation
- Supine rib assessment for structural asymmetries and inhalation and exhalation motion restrictions
- Supine upper extremity assessment for structural asymmetries, tissue texture changes, and quality and quantity of motion
- Supine and prone lower extremity assessment for structural asymmetries, tissue texture changes, and quality and quantity of motion

The musculoskeletal structural examination provides structural signs of asymmetry (e.g., scoliosis, an increase in kyphosis or lordosis, or significant deviation from balanced gravitational centering). In addition, the limbs and vertebral complex can be assessed for characteristics of motion by adding a palpatory examination of the soft tissue (muscles, ligaments, tendons, deep and superficial fascia, and the subcutaneous structures). The site of the primary musculoskeletal problem can often be determined. It is possible to know what biomechanical problems are helping to create, maintain, and aggravate the primary problem. In the areas of clinical interest, make the soft tissue examination, the motion testing, and the static structural examination sufficiently precise to identify the local elements of dysfunction.

The musculoskeletal findings are often secondary to another disorder of the musculoskeletal system, a reaction to internal disease, or a compensatory response to the presence of pain. Assessing the patient more thoroughly allows an inclusive diagnosis with the possibility of a more extensive treatment program, increasing the potential for success. The ability to exclude the more unusual and potentially morbid conditions can only result from such an osteopathic neurologic evaluation. In addition, this approach offers the ability to choose among multiple and costly diagnostic possibilities.

HEADACHES

Headaches are one of the most frequent presenting complaints to both the general practitioner and the neurologist. Table 73.1 represents the current International Headache Society classification of headaches.[6] This classification is useful for establishing a clinical diagnosis of headache type; good scientific models exist for only some of the headache types, and there could be overlap between categories of headache in each patient. Most headaches are mixed tension type and migraine. This presentation is complicated by the multifactorial nature of headache, including these features:

- Physical
- Psychological

TABLE 73.1

International Headache Society Classification of Headaches

1. Migraine
2. Tension-type headache
3. Trigeminal autonomic cephalalgias (TACs)
4. Other primary headache disorders
5. Headache attributed to trauma or injury to the head and/or neck
6. Headache attributed to cranial or cervical vascular disorder
7. Headache attributed to nonvascular intracranial disorder
8. Headache attributed to substance or its withdrawal
9. Headache attributed to infection
10. Headache attributed to disorder of homeostasis
11. Headache or facial pain associated with disorder of the cranium, neck, eyes, ears, nose, sinuses, teeth, mouth, or other facial or cervical structures
12. Headache attributed to psychiatric disorder
13. Painful cranial neuropathies and other facial pains
14. Other headache disorders

From Headache Classification Committee of the International Headache Society (IHS). The International Classification of Headache Disorders, 3rd edition (beta version). *Cephalalgia.* 2013;33(9):629–808. Copyright © 2013 International Headache Society. Reprinted by permission of SAGE Publications, Inc.

- Familial
- Ethnic
- Cultural

The osteopathic physician is uniquely trained to evaluate the headache patient and to manage diagnostic and therapeutic resources.

Pain can result from noxious stimulation of the eyes, ears, mouth, and nasal cavities. Pain-sensitive intracranial structures include the venous sinuses and their tributaries, the dura (particularly at the base of the brain), and the arteries of the pia-arachnoid and dura mater. Some extracranial structures are also pain sensitive, including the:

- Skin
- Subcutaneous tissues
- Fascia
- Muscles
- Arteries
- Nerves
- Cranial periosteum
- Regional articulations

Acute head pain is often the result of dysfunction, displacement, or encroachment on one of the above structures. Cranial nerves V, VII, IX, and X and upper cervical nerve roots II and III convey impulses from the head and face. The afferent signal is carried along A-delta and C fibers of the peripheral nervous system, predominantly within the trigeminal spinal tracts terminating in laminae I, II, V, and X of the spinal cord. The nociceptor fibers transmit synaptically using glutamate, substance P, calcitonin gene-related peptide (CGRP), and other neuropeptides.[7]

A description of the quality and location of the headache is useful in establishing a cause. Investigate these questions:

- Does it pound like a vascular headache or squeeze like a tension headache?
- Does it localize to the region of the extracranial arteries, sinuses, teeth, tendinomuscular attachments, temporomandibular joint, or cervical vertebrae?
- What are the severity and the time course of the pain?
- Is there an acute, severe onset, as is typically seen in subarachnoid hemorrhage?
- Is it chronic and nagging, more typical of tension-type headache?
- Does it tend to recur stereotypically like migraine?

For example, migraines often occur in the morning and rarely last more than a day or two. Cluster headaches typically occur at night and rarely last for more than 30 to 120 minutes. Tension headaches can last for weeks or months.

The associated features of a headache include its relation to:

- Menstruation
- Activities
- Head position
- Time of day
- Exercise
- Sleep habits
- Environmental toxicity
- Food and drink intake

It is important to know the age of onset, relevant family history, and exacerbating and relieving factors. A psychosocial assessment and thorough history and physical examination can reveal the symptoms and signs of anxiety, depression, or anger that can increase and heighten pain awareness.

The physical examination of these patients includes a thorough general examination and a comprehensive neurologic examination, including:

- Mental state
- Cranial nerves
- Strength
- Reflexes
- Coordination
- Sensation
- Appropriately detailed musculoskeletal assessment

The musculoskeletal assessment is most rewarding for patients with chronic or acute recurring headaches.

The neuromusculoskeletal assessment includes active and static body analysis. Observe and palpate the:

- Facial and mandibular attachments
- Temporomandibular joints
- Temporalis
- Masseter
- Occipitofrontalis
- Buccinators
- Pterygoid muscles

Evaluate the levels of muscle contraction and local tenderness with direct superficial and deep cervical palpation from the skin to the synovial joints. Assess rotational characteristics of the head, cervical, and upper thoracic regions, as well as the basioccipital attachments at the atlas for anterior, lateral, and posterior asymmetry. In addition, carry out a screening of the total musculoskeletal system. The screening can include evaluation of:

- Leg length and lower extremity symmetry
- Sacropelvic base analysis
- Cranial rhythmic activity and suture mobility analysis
- Presence and severity of tender points and trigger points (TrPs)

In clinical practice, the relationship between symptoms and signs and the ability to reproduce the painful symptoms during the examination are helpful in clinical localization. This is particularly true for the biomechanical syndromes, such as[8–10]:

- Temporomandibular joint syndrome
- Malocclusive dental syndromes
- Cervical spine syndromes (spondylosis, disk degeneration, facet dysfunction)
- Cranial neuralgias
- Cranial suture syndrome
- Short-leg syndrome
- Nerve encroachment syndrome
- Myofascial pain syndromes

This type of evaluation supplies information that can be essential to formulating comprehensive therapeutic objectives.

In addition to primary headache syndromes, a wide variety of neurologic and systemic disorders may present with headaches. These disorders must be considered when evaluating the patient while establishing a working differential diagnosis, before proceeding with any therapeutic intervention. Table 73.2 is a collection of some of those conditions, highlighting clinical, diagnostic, and therapeutic features.

Consider further diagnostic studies, magnetic resonance imaging (MRI), computerized tomography, electroencephalography, cerebral angiography, blood and cerebrospinal fluid analysis, and neurologic consultation when the patient has new or evolving neurologic complaints or when they do not respond promptly and appropriately to osteopathic medical management.

TABLE 73.2

Headaches Resulting from Systemic Disease or Primary Neurologic Disorder

Disorder	Pathophysiology	Clinical Features	Paraclinical Features (lab, x-ray, etc.)	Treatment
Glaucoma[11]	Increased intraocular pressure	Dilated pupil, disturbed vision, general headache	Abnormal tonometry	Medication, surgery
Cerebral aneurysm, ruptured or unruptured[12]	Berry aneurysm, hypertension	Explosive headache, nuchal rigidity, abnormal neurologic signs	Blood in the CSF, abnormal angiogram	Neurosurgery
Temporal arteritis[13]	Inflammation	Throbbing headache, >55 year old, tender temporal artery, blurred vision, jaw claudication	Elevated ESR, positive biopsy for arteritis	Glucocorticoids
Optic neuritis[14]	Inflammation, demyelination	Orbital pain, loss of vision, worse with eye motion, papillitis	Abnormal visual evoked response, abnormal MRI	Glucocorticoids
Dissection of carotid or vertebral arteries[15–17]	Drugs, trauma	Severe, local pain, tender artery, Horner syndrome	Angiogram, ultrasound, MRI, MRA	Surgery, anticoagulants
Temporomandibular joint syndrome, internal derangement, myofascial[18]	Joint degeneration, muscular imbalance	Pain in jaw, click in joint, locking of joint, pain with lateral or vertical movement, tight muscles	Abnormal MRI	Dental, physical therapy, exercise
Trigeminal neuralgia[19]	Irritation of CN-5, vascular loop, mechanical	Sharp, stabbing pain in trigeminal zone, triggers: wind, eating, chewing	Rarely abnormal MRI	Medication (anticonvulsants), neurosurgery
Herpes zoster trigeminalis cervicalis	Infection	Burning pain hypersensitive rash/vesicles	Virus identification	Antiviral therapy
Meningitis encephalitis	Usually infection, bacterial, viral, etc.	Nuchal rigidity acute headache, fever, signs of infection	(+) CSF pleocytosis, low glucose, high protein	Antibiotics, corticosteroids, supportive therapy
Sinusitis, facial osteomyelitis[20]	Infection	Nasal obstruction, tender bone, fever	Leukocytosis, abnormal CT/MRI	Antibiotics
Intracranial hypertension from a mass	Traction, displacement of painful structures, block of CSF, hydrocephalus	Recent onset, headache, worse at rest papilledema	Abnormal CT/MRI	Glucocorticoids, furosemide, mannitol, neurosurgery
Benign intracranial hypertension[21]	Altered CSF dynamics	Young, female, obesity, hormone fluctuating, sight papilledema	Increased CSF pressure, small ventricles, enlarged blind spot	Glucocorticoids, acetazolamide, CSF removal, neurosurgery
Exertional headache, strain, lift, cough, exercise, coitus[22]	Posterior fossa mass, Chiari malformation, migraine variant	Abrupt, severe, lasts 15–20 min, men > women	CT/MRI	If no mass, precede activity with NSAIDs
Normal pressure hydrocephalus	Communicating, block in CSF absorption	Ataxia, incontinence, dementia	Hydrocephalus, cisternography	Ventricular shunt, CSF removal
Myofascial pain syndrome[10]	Trauma	Bands, nodules, trigger points, poor sleep	—	OMT, spray/stretch, needling

CN, cranial nerves; CSF, cerebrospinal fluid; CT, computed tomography; ESR, erythrocyte sedimentation rate; MRA, magnetic resonance angiography; MRI, magnetic resonance imaging; NSAIDs, nonsteroidal anti-inflammatory drugs; OMT, osteopathic manipulative treatment.

Therapeutic success can be optimized by multimodality evaluation and treatment. The behavioral model can suggest whether cognitive, behavioral, or psychotherapeutic assessments and intervention are needed. The neurologic and metabolic models attempt to describe the problem neurochemically and offer a logical interventional protocol based on differential pharmacotherapeutic profiles (such as serotonergic, dopaminergic, noradrenergic, glutamatergic, GABAergic [refers to something related to or involving the neurotransmitter gamma-aminobutyric acid], cholinergic). The biomechanical model provides a rational basis for choosing among OMT methods (i.e., direct action, indirect action, or myofascial techniques).

Furthermore, therapies directed at enhancing the self-healing capacities of an individual are important in the overall therapeutic formulation as discussed in Chapter 17 Mind-Body Medicine and Chapter 21 Lifestyle Medicine—Osteopathic Perspectives.

- Nutritional evaluation and counseling
- Evaluation and education in sleep hygiene
- Instruction and prescription of appropriate relaxation and stress reduction therapies
- The use of therapeutic exercise

- The promotion of a positive attitude through education about the nature of headaches, the realistic objectives of management, and the use of positive visual imagery

Migraine Headaches

Migraine headaches are a common cause of functional disability in the United States. The annual cost of lost productivity in the United States has been estimated to range from $1.2 billion to $17.2 billion.

PRESENTATION

Migraine headaches are frequently described as a unilateral, throbbing, pounding pain following a vascular distribution of the superficial or deep cerebral vessels and lasting for several hours. They can radiate to the opposite side. They may be associated with:

- Nausea
- Vomiting
- Diarrhea
- Vertigo
- Dizziness
- Tremors
- Photophobia (light sensitivity)
- Phonophobia (sound sensitivity)
- Sweating
- Chills

Migraines may be preceded by:

- Scotomas (blind spots in the eyes)
- Photopsia (flashing lights)
- Vertigo
- Paresthesia (abnormal sensations)
- Visual, olfactory, and auditory hallucinations
- Syncope (passing out)

Migraine headaches are recurrent and vary widely in intensity, frequency, and duration. The initial episode most often occurs during puberty but can occur at any age between 5 and 40 years. Migraine can begin in childhood, adolescence, or adulthood. In women, it can be associated with hormonal fluctuation. For some patients, tenderness, tightness, pain, and limitation of motion in the suboccipital and cervical musculature accompany their migraine. Characteristically, migraine is relieved by sleep.

Migraine headaches may be triggered by[23]:

- Head injury or other traumas
- Stress
- Hormone fluctuations
- Fasting
- Oversleeping and under sleeping
- Vasoactive substances in foods (wine, cheese, cold foods)
- Changes in weather and temperature (bright light, poor ventilation)
- Physical stimuli smoking, caffeine, perfume scents

MECHANISMS

Migraine headaches are thought to occur by the following general mechanism[23]:

- The production of migraine symptoms involves two major events: vasoconstriction and vasodilation.
- The cerebral blood vessels can be divided into two major systems: the innervated (adrenergic) system and the noninnervated arterial system.
  - □ The large innervated vascular system consists of the arteries at the base of the brain and the pial arteries. These have a rich adrenergic nerve supply and respond to catecholamines.
  - □ The noninnervated vascular system consists of the parenchymal arteries and the terminal high-resistance arteries. They respond to local metabolic factors.
- Trigger factors (listed above) produce unilateral cerebral *vasoconstriction* via the adrenergic nervous system. Platelets systemically aggregate and release serotonin, which augment vasoconstriction of these adrenergically innervated blood vessels. The overall result is vasoconstriction with a reduction in cerebral blood flow. When blood flow is sufficiently reduced, an aura develops with symptoms occurring in the brain region affected by the vasoconstriction. The vasoconstriction phase causes local anoxia and acidosis and a systemic drop in serotonin. Serotonin sensitizes the pain receptors in the blood vessels.
- In response to local metabolic factors (anoxia and acidosis), the vessels of the noninnervated arterial system dilate, increasing cerebral blood flow and promoting local vasomotor changes resulting in a combined dilation of the innervated extracranial and intracranial arteries on the same side. This *vasodilation*, along with the *sensitization* of pain fibers, produces the pain of migraine. Vasodilation is not autonomic—it is humoral.

A trigeminal vascular reflex may also explain some of the events seen in the production of migraines.[23]

- Afferent pain fibers from the cortex, thalamus, hypothalamus, and cervical roots C1–C3 communicate with the spinal nucleus of the trigeminal nerve.
- These impulses can then travel via the facial nerve (CN VII) to produce parasympathetic dilation of the internal and external carotid arteries.
- Stimulation of the trigeminal ganglion, through vasodilation of the internal carotid, can also produce edema in the dura.[23]
- Pain perception is increased when the effects of this dilation feed back into the spinal nucleus of the trigeminal nerve.

When the biologically sensitive nervous system is confronted with trigger factors (listed above) that can provoke a migraine, the neurochemical balance of the nervous system changes, and symptoms, recognized as *prodromal*, may occur. This change progresses until the migraine threshold is crossed and an area in the brainstem called the "migraine generator" is activated. This may initiate a wave of spreading neuronal depression across the cortex activating trigeminal afferents and the vascular structures they innervate.

- As branches of the first division of the trigeminal nerve are activated, neuropeptides are released at the neurovascular junction. The neuropeptides produce a sterile inflammation of the meningeal arteries associated with platelet aggregation and release of serotonin, which may potentiate the migraine process.
- Bidirectional conduction transmits nerve impulses back into the CN V nucleus located in the brainstem. These impulses are then routed to various neurons in the thalamus and cerebral cortex. The upper cervical spinal cord gets involved through this nucleus too, and that explains the neck pain that is often involved with migraine and their relief using occipital nerve blocks.
- Brainstem reflexes are activated that produce migraine-associated symptoms, including nausea, vomiting, photophobia, and phonophobia.
- Autonomic, parasympathetic activation occurs via the facial nerve and results in nasal congestion, rhinorrhea, and lacrimation.
- Pain in the face over the sinus cavities is also common and may be due to CN V2 activation.

- Researchers have found evidence of breakdown products of serotonin in the urine of those who have just experienced a migraine headache. They have also found that injecting anyone with a *serotonin-depleting chemical* can produce a migraine headache, even if the person has never had a migraine in the past. Medications (e.g., sumatriptan and other 5HT-1d receptor agonists) are effective in treating a migraine headache even during the attack.[23]

A more detailed description of the series of events, and potential complications, during migraine headaches follows:

- Disordered neurogenic control of the craniocerebral circulation accompanies the attack.[24]
- The trigeminal vascular system (the trigeminal neuron whose unmyelinated axon surrounds a cephalic blood vessel) functions in pain transmission and in promoting inflammation in the affected blood vessels via the neurochemical activity of substance P.[25]
- Cerebral, meningeal, basilar, and vertebral arteries can be affected through the trigeminal, vagal, and upper cervical axons, which all converge in the trigeminal nucleus caudalis of the brainstem and upper cervical spinal cord.[26,27]
- The inflammatory response is associated with norepinephrine and serotonin release from brainstem origin, and histamine, adenosine, and bradykinin of local origin. CGRP and adenylate cyclase-activating polypeptide (PACAP) are also involved.[28]
- As depicted in Figure 73.1, several factors play a role in migraine cephalgia, including gene polymorphisms, menstrual cycle, pregnancy, medications, and other chemicals.
- When the migraine is triggered, the intrinsic brainstem noradrenergic system (from the locus coeruleus) is activated, triggering enhanced neuronal firing in the susceptible cerebral cortex. This firing in the cerebral cortex generates a spreading wave of cortical depolarization that ultimately reaches pain-sensitive blood vessels, resulting in depolarization of the associated trigeminovascular axon.
- This depolarization triggers a sterile inflammatory reaction through the release of substance P, CGRP, the activation of mast cells, and prostaglandin synthesis.[24,25,28]
- Migraine can be accompanied by an aura consisting of neurologic changes, typically in a vascular distribution, lasting from 10 to 90 minutes, that mimics and sometimes results in transient cerebral ischemia.
- In rare cases, the neurologic aura resolves, and the migraine becomes complicated as the patient suffers cerebral infarction.
- The most common auras are ocular and can involve scintillating scotomata or flashing lights, often occurring in jagged lines—the so-called fortification spectrum.[29] The visual phenomena can be multicolored and typically changes size, shape, and distribution during the evolving aura. The aura usually precedes the actual headache but can occur during and even after. On occasion, the aura is separate from the headache component, or the headache can be absent.[30]
- Multifocal neurologic symptoms can occur in the basilar artery distribution (the Bickerstaff syndrome) and include[31]:
  - □ Cranial nerve changes
  - □ Dysarthria
  - □ Facial paresthesia
  - □ Ataxia
  - □ Vertigo
- In the middle cerebral artery distribution, migraine can have manifestations of hemiparesis, hemisensory loss, or aphasia. In general, the migraine aura presents with visual phenomena of occipital lobe origin, atypical for cerebrovascular insufficiency.

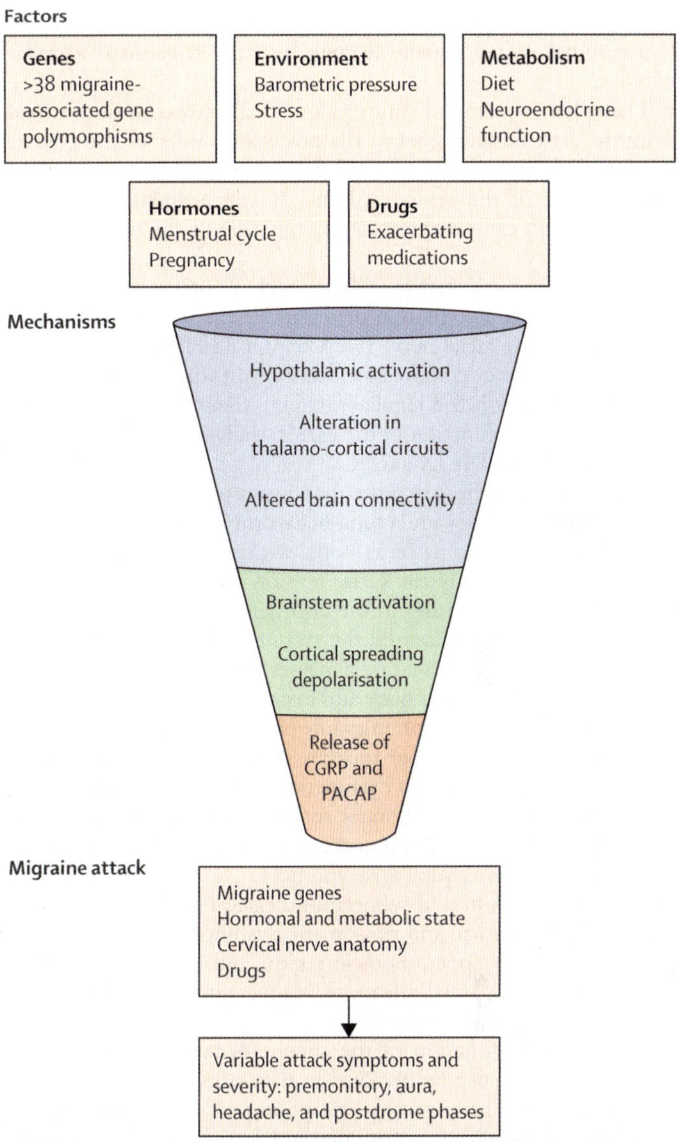

Figure 73.1. Factors and mechanisms involved in migraine cephalgia. CGRP, calcitonin gene-related peptide; PACAP, pituitary adenylate cyclase–activating polypeptide. (Reprinted from Charles A. The pathophysiology of migraine: implications for clinical management. *Lancet Neurol.* 2018;17(2):174–182. Copyright © 2017 Elsevier. With permission.)

- A clue to migraine symptoms is its gradual progression of symptoms over multiple minutes, unlike the rapid march of a focal seizure or the sudden onset of cerebral vessel thrombosis or embolism.

Somatic dysfunction in the upper thoracic spine is thought to increase the level of sympathetic tone to the innervated blood vessels of the head. Increased sympathetic tone produces vasoconstriction and a resultant decrease in cerebral blood flow. This results in a relative anoxia and may lower the threshold for vasodilation, thereby contributing to the production of migraine symptoms. Intracranial dysfunction affecting the cortex, thalamus, and hypothalamus and upper cervical spine dysfunction affecting cervical nerve roots C1–C3 may result in the transmission of afferent pain stimuli to the spinal nucleus of the trigeminal nerve.

- The trigeminal nerve courses through various portions of the sphenoid bone. An elevated greater wing of the sphenoid (torsion) may apply dural pressure resulting in irritation of the trigeminal nerve, thereby feeding into the trigeminal vascular reflex.

- The sphenosquamosal suture is a vertical cranial suture formed by the articulation between the posterior border of the greater wing of the sphenoid bone and the anterior border of the squamous part of the temporal bone. A sphenosquamosal suture compression can compromise the function of the middle meningeal artery.
- Dysfunction of the temporal bone, such as internal rotation, can result in reflex vasodilation of the internal and external carotid arteries via the facial nerve (see Chapter 32 Head Region)
- Occipitomastoid compression can result in reduced venous drainage through the jugular foramen, thereby producing congestion and dysfunction in the cortex, thalamus, and hypothalamus as well as CNs IX and X.
- Migraine headaches are more than just a problem with the cranial structures. They are a total body problem:
  - Myofascial strain patterns stored within the abdomen or elsewhere in the body can cause tension changes on the base of the skull contributing to the disorder.
  - Excessive tension around the sacrum and coccyx can pull on the dura and posterior fascial planes, contributing to increased tension in the upper back and neck.
  - Patients with common migraine or mixed tension-type headaches often have upper thoracic somatic dysfunction associated with (autonomic) dysfunction to the head and neck.
  - An extended upper thoracic somatic dysfunction (type II) is typically acutely painful and can maintain muscle tension in the head, suboccipital area, and neck.
  - It is common to find suboccipital cervical dysfunction related to upper thoracic and rib somatic dysfunction.[32]
  - Treating the upper thoracic region and ribs with counterstrain or myofascial release techniques improves suboccipital tissue texture abnormality.
  - Somatic dysfunction of the sphenoid, temporal bones, and occiput may also be involved in trigeminal dysfunctions and headaches. The trigeminal ganglion provides sensory nerves from the forehead and upper and lower jaw. According to Magoun,[8] normal movement of the temporal bones is critical, especially in migraine patients.

DIAGNOSTICS

On initial presentation of migraine, it is not always possible to be certain of the diagnosis, and a well-designed differential diagnostic process is appropriate (Table 73.2). Although the risk of aneurysm, brain tumor, arteriovenous malformation, or vasculitis is slight, enhanced brain computed tomography, MRI, or cerebral angiography is useful to exclude these possibilities and should be used if the diagnosis is uncertain.[33]

TREATMENT

Migraine can acutely respond to vasoactive drugs, such as sumatriptan, other triptans, CGRP antagonists, CGRP receptor blockers, dihydroergotamine, ergotamine, isometheptene, and even caffeine. The serotonin 1D receptor agonists (e.g., sumatriptan or dihydroergotamine) and the anti-CGRP agent (e.g., erenumab) are particularly effective in aborting a migraine. Simple agents like aspirin or acetaminophen are often combined with barbiturates and/or narcotics. Other nonsteroidal anti-inflammatory drugs (NSAIDs) are also used with variable success. The parenteral use of phenothiazines is helpful, but, unfortunately, they are frequently associated with unacceptable side effects.[34]

When migraine headaches are frequent or severe, the prophylactic use of medications is indicated. Medications used regularly to help prevent migraines include beta-blockers (e.g., propranolol), calcium channel blockers (e.g., verapamil), tricyclic antidepressants (e.g., amitriptyline), selective serotonin reuptake inhibitors, (fluoxetine), antihistamine/antiserotonin drugs (cyproheptadine), CGRP antagonists (e.g., erenumab), CGRP receptor blockade (e.g., rimegepant), ergot derivatives (e.g., methysergide), anticonvulsants (e.g., topiramate, valproic acid), and botulinum toxin. Potential targets for new treatments are outlined in Figure 73.2.[28]

Nonpharmacologic approaches, including OMT, are often valuable. Osteopathic management of migraine can include OMT. In the active phase of migraine though, vigorous treatment can increase blood flow to an already inflamed vascular bed, thereby explaining the clinical exacerbation that can follow treatment. Gentle therapy with indirect techniques, distal techniques, venous and lymphatic drainage techniques are likely to be more helpful during the attack. Because of the prominent autonomic involvement, evaluate and treat at the sympathetic sites of lower cervical and upper thoracic vertebrae, associated ribs, and myofascial attachments. Treatment can be directed at:

- Joints and dural strain patterns of the head, neck, and sacrum
- Hypertonic or hypotonic muscles of the head, neck, and shoulders
- Myofascial restrictions of the head, neck, and shoulders
- Tender points in the head, neck, and shoulder regions

OMT will enable many patients to either reduce the dosage or frequency of their medication. Remember, it is difficult to treat a patient during an acute migraine with OMT alone. Treatment of a patient with a migraine disorder with OMT between migraines can reduce the severity and frequency of their acute migraine attacks, but the immediate treatment of an acute migraine in progress is usually pharmacologic.

Some patients, when treated with OMT, may only occasionally require NSAIDs or acetaminophen for rare minor headaches. Does OMT work when the patient is actively having a migraine headache? Usually, it is possible to provide some relief while the patient is having a migraine headache. It does take some time, however, for the inflammatory mediators and other chemicals involved in migraine headaches to be removed from the head by the venous and lymphatic circulation. It is best to treat the patient with OMT in between migraine headaches when the focus can be on prevention.

Most patients will be placed on a home exercise program that focuses on stretching exercises to reduce the amount of tension in the body (especially in the upper back and neck) and to help return balance to the body. OMT is used to improve motion in the body. The patient's responsibility is to maintain the improvements by performing the prescribed home exercises. Stretches seem especially important. Less often, weak muscles need strengthening.

Behavioral techniques like biofeedback, relaxation therapy, and programs that teach stress reduction and coping skills have also been successfully used to reduce the frequency and severity of migraine attacks.[35] These must be learned before they can be successfully deployed. They cannot be learned in the throes of a migraine. For some patients, musculoskeletal triggers or prodromes exist for their migraines.[36,37]

The possible role of musculoskeletal triggers is further suggested in posttraumatic migraine. In such cases, trauma to the skull, cervical spine, or myofascial elements is followed by a unilateral, throbbing migraine.[8,38] These headaches can recur for days, weeks, and months. OMT can be used to modify triggers arising from bony, ligamentous, and myofascial structures. In practice, OMT

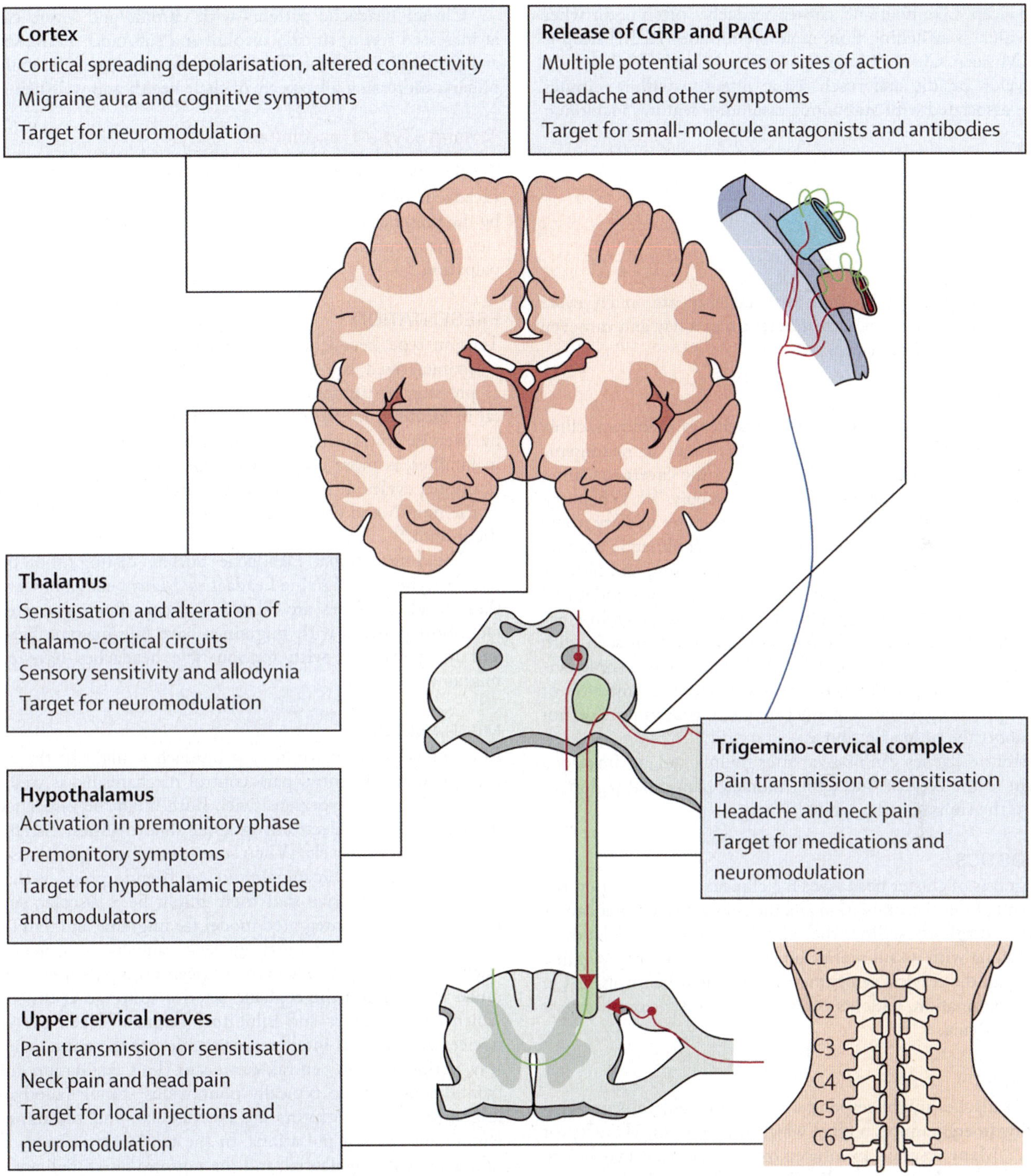

Figure 73.2. Mechanisms in migraine cephalgia and potential targets for treatment. CGRP, calcitonin gene-related peptide; PACAP, pituitary adenylate cyclase–activating polypeptide. (Reprinted from Charles A. The pathophysiology of migraine: implications for clinical management. *Lancet Neurol.* 2018;17(2):174–182. Copyright © 2017 Elsevier. With permission.)

is especially useful between migraine events, when the patient is more tolerant of manipulation.

Applications of local heat, cold, massage, acupressure, trigger point therapy, acupuncture, traction, or local anesthetic blockade can be used in these regions that typically harbor tender points referring pain to the headache zone. These applications might help to decrease the afferent activity from the painful site and reduce the primary and secondary muscle spasms. It helps reduce the afferent load on the neurons of the trigeminal nucleus caudalis.

Cluster Headaches

PRESENTATION

Cluster headache is a rare, severe, and distinctive vascular syndrome characterized by attacks that tend to occur daily for weeks at a time only to vanish again for months or years. Approximately 20% of patients develop a chronic form, called chronic paroxysmal hemicrania or hemicrania continua.[39] Headaches tend to occur at certain times of the day; most notably, they develop 2 to 3 hours after going to sleep. Like migraine, cluster headaches often occur when the individual is switching from rapid eye motion (REM) sleep to non-REM sleep. Cluster headaches tend to be periorbital in location, develop rapidly and reach severe intensity within minutes. They are associated with autonomic vasomotor features including:

- Ptosis
- Miosis
- Conjunctival injection
- Unilateral lacrimation
- Rhinorrhea
- Nasal congestion

Distinct from migraine, cluster headaches are much more common in men. They can occur several times a day and can even awaken the sufferer from sleep.

MECHANISMS

Although the exact cause of cluster headaches is unknown, clinicians believe that cluster headaches are the result of neurogenic inflammation affecting the vascular plexus of the cavernous sinus, its tributaries, and its autonomic nervous supply.[40,41] When the headaches occur during changes between the stages of sleep, there is a physiologic shift from parasympathetic, cholinergic activity to sympathetic, aminergic (catecholamine, serotonin, and norepinephrine) activity.[42] Positron emission topography has identified the posterior hypothalamic gray matter to be a key area in cluster headache. Hypothalamic dysfunction has also been seen with magnetic resonance spectroscopy.[43,44] Although there is some evidence of histamine playing a role, as a subcutaneous injection of histamine provokes attacks in many patients, antihistamines do not alter or abort the headache course.

Cluster headaches can be seen after trauma and, at times, can refer pain to the cervical and upper thoracic paraspinal region, as well as to the suprascapular region.[45,46]

DIAGNOSTICS

The diagnosis of cluster headaches is a clinical one based upon the history and physical examination and the ruling out of other causes with neuro-diagnostics. Since the carotid–cavernous vasculature is involved along with its autonomic innervation, the pterygopalatine ganglion and the cervical sympathetic ganglia may be involved. On physical examination, patients often have a tender carotid artery, called carotidynia.

TREATMENT

Cluster headaches might respond acutely to parenteral sumatriptan or dihydroergotamine, both of which are serotonin 1D receptor agonists.[47] Many respond to inhaled oxygen via facial mask (5 to 7 L/min for 5 to 10 minutes). Prophylactically, beta-blockers, calcium channel blockers, and tricyclic antidepressants are used along with short courses of high-dose steroids or NSAIDs. For the more chronic cluster, lithium is a potent therapy. OMT may help these patients by balancing the autonomic nervous system, by reducing venous congestion of the head, and by encouraging relaxation. OMT is best directed to the:

- Upper thoracic spine and ribs (sympathetic innervation to the head and neck)
- Cervicothoracic spine (cervical ganglia)
- Associated soft tissues of the suboccipital region (venous congestion)
- Relevant craniofacial structures (branches of the trigeminal nerve and parasympathetic innervation)

Cluster headache patients with chronic and severe cases are at increased risk of suicide, alcohol and substance abuse, smoking, and peptic ulcer disease. Therefore, treatment must be multidisciplinary, addressing all aspects of their health and well-being.

Tension-Type Headaches

Tension-type headaches are classified by the International Headache Society as episodic or chronic. They are further divided by the presence or absence of involvement of the pericranial muscles. Involvement can be demonstrated by electromyography or palpation.[48,49]

PRESENTATION

Tension-type headache is the most frequent headache type. It is characterized by mild-to-moderate intensity pain, described as pressing or tightening, typically bilateral, and usually occipital in location. In distinction from migraine, it is not aggravated by exercise or routine physical activity. Like migraine, it runs in families, is more common in women, and can be affected by hormonal cycles. It is episodic if it occurs less than half the days of the month and chronic if it occurs more than half the days of the month.[50]

The International Headache Society distinguishes between tension-type and migraine headaches. Many believe, however, that these headache types are related disorders along a spectrum. In fact, most patients with migraines have tension-type headaches, and many patients with tension-type headaches have episodic migraines.

MECHANISMS

Both migraine and tension-type headaches might be the result of abnormalities in central pain control mechanisms, as well as trigeminal neuronal hypersensitivity. Both might be associated with muscle tenderness, electromyographic abnormalities, and abnormal platelet serotonin levels. When severe, they both can be associated with depressed cerebrospinal fluid and β-endorphin levels.[50]

Clinicians theorize that there might be a vascular, supraspinal, and myogenic integrated model for migraine and tension-type headache.[51] The trigeminal nucleus caudalis is a major relay nucleus for head and neck pain. Nociceptive inputs from the pericranial muscles and the cephalic arteries converge at this nucleus, which has excitatory and inhibitory outputs. When the afferent nociceptive signal is intense, sensitization of the entire pain pathway, peripheral and central, can occur. This facilitation creates a painful sensitivity to typically nonnoxious stimuli (allodynia). In migraines, the nociceptors are perivascular, and the nonnoxious stimuli are vascular pulsations. In the tension-type headache, the nociceptors are myofascial, and the nonnoxious stimuli are muscle contractions. In either case, supraspinal facilitation is likely to be present and neuronal sensitization can occur.

DIAGNOSTICS

Neurologists have modified the classification of the International Headache Society to include chronic daily headache, which is further differentiated as a daily or near-daily type of headache with superimposed migraine. Patients with chronic headaches are prone to overusing multiple drugs and have a high rate of treatment failure. Headaches can be the primary cause, as in transformed migraine, chronic tension-type headache, new daily headache, or hemicrania continua. Or secondary causes of chronic daily headache can exist, including posttraumatic headache, cervical spine dysfunction, medication overuse, vascular disorders,

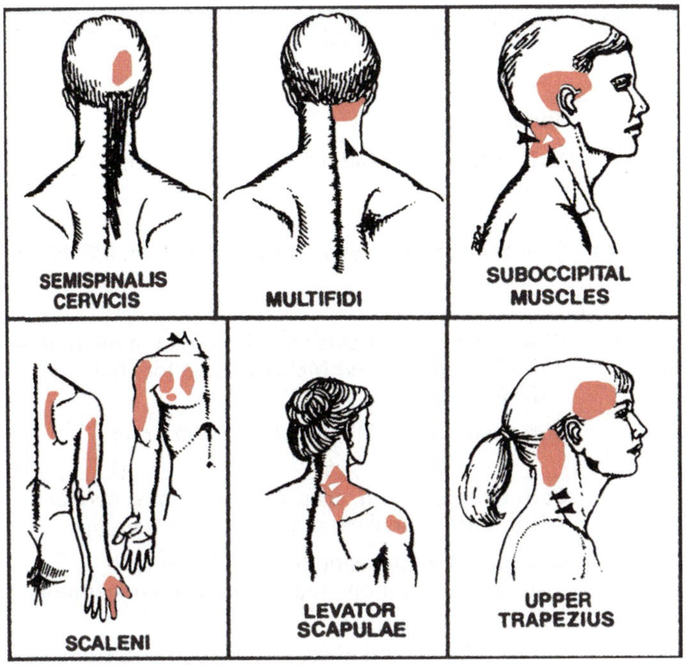

Figure 73.3. Myofascial trigger points in the head, neck, and upper extremity regions. (Illustration courtesy of William A. Kuchera, DO, FAAO, with permission.)

and nonvascular intracranial disorders.[36,52–54] Frequently, an episodic problem becomes chronic because of analgesic medication overuse.

TREATMENT

Treatment begins with a close look to identify any medication overuse, drug dependency, or depression, which require specific intervention. Inquire for a history of emotional, physical, or sexual abuse, and incorporate that information into the treatment rationale. Every effort is made to identify and eliminate potential sources for triggers, such as the:

- Teeth
- Jaw
- Sinuses
- Cranial and cervical bones
- Joints
- Ligaments
- Associated myofascial structures (myofascial TrPs are depicted in Fig. 73.3).

Patients with headaches require specific personalized interventions. Physical, psychological, and pharmacologic therapies can operate synergistically.[55] Reviewing the neuroanatomy of the upper cervical region clarifies how somatic dysfunction in that region can cause headaches (Box 73.1).

Effectiveness of OMT in the management of frequent episodic tension-type headaches was assessed in a 2014 single-blind randomized placebo-controlled pilot study.[56] In this study, 40 patients were randomly allocated to either an experimental group (OMT) or a control group (sham therapy measuring cranial rhythmic impulse). The study consisted of three separate periods:

- One month of baseline
- One month of treatment
- Three months of follow-up

BOX 73.1 Dorsal Rami of the Upper Cervical Nerves

Understanding the anatomy of the dorsal rami of the cervical nerves is important in understanding how somatic dysfunction at C2 and C3 may be related to tension headaches and "occipital neuritis." The greater and lesser occipital nerves have been implicated in the production of tension headaches, so this region is a common area of OMT. These branches of the dorsal rami of the upper cervical segments pierce through the fascia just below the superior nuchal line. Tension in this fascia has been implicated to cause compression and irritation of the greater occipital nerve.

- The *greater occipital nerve* is the medial branch of the dorsal ramus of the second cervical nerve. It ascends between the muscles of the suboccipital triangle and the semispinalis capitis. The greater occipital nerve pierces the semispinalis capitis and the trapezius near their attachments to the occipital bone and ascends on the back of the scalp with the occipital artery.
- The greater occipital nerve supplies the skin of the occipital part of the scalp lateral to the median line and as far superiorly as the vertex of the skull.
- Its lateral branches communicate with those of the lesser occipital nerve.
- The greater occipital nerve gives off muscular branches to semispinalis capitis and joins with *occipitalis tertius*, the cutaneous branch of the third cervical nerve. The *occipitalis tertius* supplies the skin of the upper part of the back of the neck, near the median line, and the skin of the scalp over the external occipital protuberance.

The cutaneous branches of the cervical plexus are *the lesser occipital, the great auricular, the transverse cervical, and the supraclavicular nerves.*

- The lesser occipital nerve (C2, sometimes also C3) ascends in the neck along the posterior border of the sternocleidomastoid muscle. It pierces the superficial layer of cervical fascia near the insertion of the muscle and divides into branches, which supply the skin and subcutaneous tissue of the scalp behind and above the ear and of the upper portion of the cranial surface of the ear.
- The *great auricular nerve* (C2, C3) arises in the posterior triangle at the lateral border of the sternocleidomastoid muscle. It travels below the lesser occipital nerve and crosses obliquely in a course toward the ear and the angle of the mandible.

Upon the study's completion, the OMT group had[56]:

- Significant reduction in headache frequency by 40% at 1 month after the end of treatment and by 50% at 3 months after treatment ($P < .001$)
- A 45% reduction in the use of over-the-counter medication at 3 months after treatment ($P < .001$)
- A 20% reduction in pain intensity at 3 months after treatment ($P < .001$)

TABLE 73.3

Treatment Algorithm for Tension-Type Headache

Treatment Plan	Objective	Technique
Treat upper thoracic and rib dysfunctions	Eliminate upper thoracic dysfunction involved in perpetuating the pain; balance autonomic tone	Soft tissue, MFR, ME, FPR, counterstrain, HVLA, rib raising
Treat cervical dysfunction, particularly involving the occiput, C1, and C2	Eliminate dysfunctional cervical mechanics and soft tissue tension involved in exacerbating the pain	Soft tissue, suboccipital release MFR, FPR, ME, HVLA
Treat cranial dysfunction including TMJ dysfunction	Eliminate cranial strain patterns affecting the trigeminal neurovascular system	Direct and indirect osteopathic cranial manipulative medicine; MFR and ME technique for TMJ dysfunction
Treat the lumbar, sacrum, and pelvis	Eliminate compensatory or contributing strain patterns from below	Soft tissue, MFR, ME, HVLA, counterstrain
Address postural mechanics	Reduce exacerbating factors	Core strengthening, scapular retractions, cervical isometric exercises, proprioceptive training
Stress reduction counseling	Reduce exacerbating factors while enhancing overall well-being	One-on-one counseling to identify specific stressors and individualize stress management strategies
Health promotion and disease prevention	Reduce risk of future illness; enhance overall well-being	Smoking cessation, weight management, exercise, and nutrition counseling; health screening

FPR, facilitated positional release; HVLA, high-velocity low-amplitude; ME, muscle energy; MFR, myofascial release; TMJ, temporomandibular joint.

OMT may be an adjunctive modality to medical management or an alternative for patients who are at increased risk of or intolerant to adverse drug effects or simply are not compliant with drug regimens.[56] Further clinical trials are warranted. An osteopathic treatment algorithm for tension-type headache using OMT is outlined in Table 73.3.

In headache management, the presence of somatic dysfunction is systematically identified and handled with OMT. Cervical vertebral segmental disorders, local and regional myofascial disorders, and craniosacral disorders are common.[57,58]

Note: Exercise particular care regarding high-velocity, low-amplitude (HVLA) manipulation of the cervical spine. Infrequently, cervical HVLA manipulation has been reported to aggravate a herniated intervertebral disk or a spinal cord injury[59]; most critically, cervical spinal (HVLA) manipulation therapy has been associated with the following in the vertebrobasilar distribution of the posterior circulation[60–62]:

- Vertebral artery laceration
- Intimal dissection
- Thrombosis
- Thromboembolic brain/brainstem infarction

Most of the complications of cervical spinal manipulation therapy (HVLA) have been seen with hyperextension and hyperrotation of the upper cervical segments, often in the course of a thrusting (HVLA) technique,[63] although many reported cases of cervical artery dissection and stroke are of spontaneous origin and causation by HVLA is controversial.[11,64-73] In one study, associations between chiropractic and primary care physician/provider visits and stroke were similar and likely due to patients with early cervical artery dissection–related symptoms seeking care prior to developing their strokes[12] (see Chapters 49 High-Velocity Low-Amplitude (HVLA) Thrust and 95 Effectiveness and Safety of Osteopathic Manipulative Treatment for further discussion).

Pharmacologic therapy is best served with a clearly limited (symptomatic) regimen to prevent drug-induced headaches. Preventive therapy usually begun with a tricyclic antidepressant, is especially useful when there is an associated sleep disturbance. More recently, sodium valproate and topiramate have been found to have prophylactic value in chronic daily headaches.

Nonpharmacologic therapies are also prescribed. Patients can be evaluated and educated regarding proper sleep hygiene. A therapeutic exercise program should be customized to the patient. Nutritional evaluation and recommendations need to be discussed. Relaxation strategies and personalized visual imagery techniques can be taught to each patient. It is important to involve the patient as an active participant in their own therapy.

Being able to assess the patient more completely permits a more comprehensive diagnosis. Multifactorial problem assessment allows the formulation of a more thorough and multifaceted treatment program, increasing the potential for success. The osteopathic approach offers a successful model for an integrated multidimensional treatment with the patient as the focus and the physician as the facilitator.[13,58]

SPINAL DISORDERS

The practice of neurology frequently involves problems affecting the spine. This can involve the spinal column and its structural elements (spondylopathy), the nerve roots (radiculopathy), and even the spinal cord (myelopathy).

The spinal column includes the:

- Vertebral body
- Intervertebral disk
- Facet joints
- Ligaments
- Myotendinous structures

Presentation

The symptom of **vertebral bone** or ligamentous disease is usually pain. Typically, patients complain of deep, aching pain in the affected region of the spine. Often, the pain is worse in certain positions or with certain activities. For example, patients with intervertebral disk disease commonly complain that their back pain is worse with prolonged sitting or standing, whereas acute problems are made worse with activity and improved with rest. The pain can refer locally to paraspinal segments. This referral pattern most likely has to do with nociceptors converging on a common dorsal horn projection neuron.[15] In the cervical region, the pain can involve the upper arm, shoulder, and scapulothoracic region. In the lumbar region, it involves the low back, hip, and upper leg. Numbness, weakness, and other neurologic symptoms are notably absent when only the bone and ligamentous vertebral elements are affected.

Patients with **radiculopathy** might complain of pain, numbness, tingling, or other sensations that typically are described as radiating from proximal to distal.

- In the cervical region (C2–T2), the radiation is in a dermatomal pattern in the posterior cranial region, neck, upper torso, and upper extremity.
- In the thoracic region, the radiation is in a dermatomal pattern in the chest or abdomen.
- In the lumbosacral region (L1–S5), it is in a dermatomal pattern in the low back, buttock, and low extremity.

Because the pain is generated in the nerve root, patients describe a variety of pain sensations, including electric, burning, stabbing, dull, sharp, or tearing pain. Patients also describe impulses of pain with coughing, sneezing, lifting, or moving the bowels. The pain is often worse with positions that either compress the nerve root (side bending of the spine) or stretch the nerve root (forward bending of the spine). The pain can be relieved by maneuvers that take the pressure or stretch off the nerve root. Spinal stenosis can produce radicular symptoms because of intermittent ischemia to the nerve roots, typically related to walking (neurogenic claudication).

When the motor fibers are affected, patients with radiculopathy can complain of weakness localized to the muscles innervated by the segmental myotome.

- In the lumbosacral region, the nerves supplying bladder, bowel, and sexual function can be affected; with bilateral involvement patients might complain of urinary hesitancy or retention, constipation, or sexual dysfunction.

The pain of **spinal tract** origin is diffuse and referred to dermatomes of several segments below the level of the lesion. The location of motor and sensory complaints depends on the area of the spinal cord involved.

- Unilateral lesions of the spinothalamic tract cause contralateral numbness to pain and temperature, whereas lesions of the posterior columns cause ipsilateral loss of position sense, light touch, and vibration.
- Bilateral lesions of the sensory fibers result in bilateral sensory disturbances below the level.
- Limb weakness results when there is an abnormality in the anterior horn cells or corticospinal tracts.
  - The weakness can be accompanied by atrophy if it is in the lower motor neurons or spasticity if in the upper motor neurons.
  - Bladder, bowel, and sexual functions are often compromised.

Mechanisms

The pathophysiology of **spinal column disorders** often involves a degenerative process, such as spondylosis of the vertebral body, which is typically seen in association with degeneration of the intervertebral disk. The degeneration ultimately affects the adjacent related facet joints and results in strain on the facet joints, ligaments, and myotendinous structures. Trauma and time commonly underlie this process.

The spinal column can also be affected by malignancy arising in the bone or, more commonly, from secondary metastasis of systemic cancer. Infection of the spinal column can result from systemic infection, such as mycobacterial, fungal, or bacterial sepsis. Spinal pathologic conditions can also occur with osteoporosis and other metabolic abnormalities of the bone, or from less common arthritic diseases, such as ankylosing spondylitis or rheumatoid arthritis. Disease processes adjacent to the spine can also result in spinal column destruction, including paraspinal tumors and abscesses.

The spinal **nerve roots** are vulnerable due to their location within the spinal canal. They are exposed to trauma from:

- Extruding disks
- Fractured bone fragments
- Spinal and paraspinal tumors
- Degenerative changes in the vertebral elements
- Intraspinal ligaments
- Frank avulsions

In addition, the nerve roots lack the tight endothelial junction of the blood–brain barrier which makes them vulnerable to:

- Infection (e.g., herpes zoster, syphilis)
- Neoplastic invasion
- Inflammatory demyelination (e.g., Guillain–Barré syndrome)
- Toxic exposure to chemotherapy agents
- Myelography contrast agents
- Anesthetic agents

The nerve roots are also susceptible to vascular insufficiency in the form of:

- Vasculitis
- Diabetes mellitus
- Radiation exposure

Spinal cord syndromes can result from an intrinsic pathologic condition or from injury to the spinal cord from extrinsic compression.

- Intrinsic spinal cord pathologic conditions include:
  - Myelitis, typically of viral origin
  - Vasculitis
  - Multiple sclerosis
  - Neoplasms of the glial elements of the cord
  - Nutritional deficiencies can also result in degeneration of the spinal cord (e.g., subacute combined degeneration from cobalamin deficiency)
  - CNS degenerative diseases affecting the spinal cord include upper motor neuron disease and multisystem degeneration
  - The spinal cord is vulnerable to ischemia if there is disruption in the anterior spinal artery circulation
  - Severe spinal trauma can result in hemorrhage or laceration of the spinal cord
- Extrinsic compression of the spinal cord can result from the same conditions that cause nerve root compression:
  - Tumors that are primary or metastatic in the spinal canal
  - Epidural infection:
    - When the spinal cord is compressed from epidural tumor or infection, the spinal cord symptoms are typically preceded by vertebral pain.

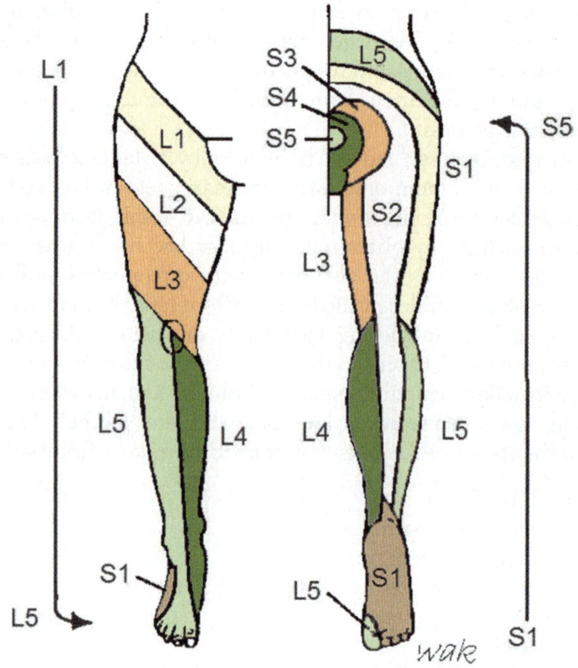

Figure 73.4. Dermatomal or radicular (nerve root) sensory distribution in the anterior and posterior right lower extremity. (Illustration courtesy of William A. Kuchera, DO, FAAO, with permission.)

- Hematoma
- Compression fractures of the vertebral bodies can result in subluxation and spinal cord compression

Diagnostics

On physical examination, assess the patient's gait and posture, and motion for signs of asymmetry, abnormalities, or lack of coordination. Observe for muscle atrophy, sarcopenia, or hypertrophy. Observe the skin for discolorations, surface abnormalities, abnormal hair growth or loss, and signs of excessive dryness or sweating. Test sensation with pain, temperature, vibration, and touch. With radiculopathy, the sensory loss is dermatomal, and the margins of sensory loss are not well demarcated, as in peripheral nerve lesions (Fig. 73.4). The motor deficits are in muscle groups with a common myotome innervation. The weakness of individual muscles is usually partial rather than complete. Because the ventral roots contain the lower motor neurons, radicular weakness is often associated with fasciculations, decreased muscle tone and bulk, and decreased reflexes.

- Muscle strength is assessed by isolating the muscle(s) to be tested and providing a counterforce to the patient's active contraction of that muscle. Strength is graded on a scale of 0 to 5 as listed in Table 73.4. Test muscle strength for all of the major muscle groups of the upper and lower extremities.
- Deep tendon reflexes (DTRs) are graded in terms of amplitude and the presence or absence of clonus on a scale of 0 to 4 as listed in Table 73.5.
  - In the upper extremities, the root innervation is evaluated with the DTRs of the biceps (predominantly C5), brachioradialis (predominately C6), and triceps (predominately C7) (see Table 73.6).
  - In the lower extremities, the root innervation is evaluated with the DTRs of the quadriceps at the patella tendon (predominantly L4), biceps femoris (predominantly L5), and gastrocnemius at the Achilles tendon (predominantly S1) (Table 73.7).

TABLE 73.4

Standard Method for Recording Motor Strength

5/5	Normal	Complete range of motion against gravity with full resistance
4/5	Good	Complete range of motion against gravity with some resistance
3/5	Fair	Complete range of motion against gravity
2/5	Poor	Complete range of motion with gravity eliminated
1/5	Trace	Evidence of slight contractility; no joint motion
0	Zero	No evidence of contractility

- Unilateral sacral root lesions can cause numbness but usually do not affect muscle control. However, when bilateral sacral roots are involved, the rectal sphincter can become weak.

Provocative maneuvers can be of great diagnostic value in patients with radiculopathy.

- In cervical or lumbar nerve root compression syndromes, side bending of the involved spine can narrow the intervertebral foramina and increase radicular complaints (Spurling sign). Conversely, applying manual traction to the cervical or lumbar region usually offers relief.
  - Cervical radiculopathy can often be ruled out using the Spurling maneuver. This is a test of nerve root compression or irritation. This maneuver is designed to provoke the patient's symptoms. The test is done in three stages, each of which is more provocative. If symptoms are produced, one does not proceed to the next stage. The first stage involves compression with the head in neutral. The second stage places the head in extension and then adds compression. The final stage places the head into side bending away from the affected side and then toward the affected side which adds compression. A positive test is indicated by dermatomal pain down the arm in the distribution of the nerve root indicating nerve root compression.
  - The Spurling test has a sensitivity of 55% and a specificity of 98%; thus, it is not as useful as a screening test, but it is clinically useful in helping to confirm cervical radiculopathy.[16] The high sensitivity of the neck tornado test (Choi test) (85%) indicates that there are few false-negative results, and thus fewer cases of disease are missed, making it a potentially good screening test. In addition, its positive predictive value is excellent when compared to cervical MRI diagnosis of nerve root compression.[16]
- Babinski sign is elicited by firmly stroking the lateral aspect of the plantar foot from proximal to distal with the pointed end of

TABLE 73.5

Standard Method for Recording Amplitude of a Reflex

0	Absent
1/4	Decreased but present
2/4	Normal
3/4	Brisk with unsustained clonus
4/4	Brisk with sustained clonus

TABLE 73.6

Deep Tendon Reflexes of the Upper Extremity

Reflex	Biceps	Brachioradialis	Triceps
STIMULUS Site	Biceps tendon	Brachioradialis tendon or just distal to the musculotendinous junction	Distal triceps tendon above the olecranon process
Typical response	Biceps contraction	Flexion of the elbow and/or pronation of the forearm	Elbow extension/muscle contraction
Central nervous system correlate	C5–C6	C5–C6	C7–C8

the handle of the reflex hammer. A normal reaction is for the toes to plantar flex. A positive sign is extension of the great toe with spreading of the remaining toes. This indicates an upper motor neuron lesion.

- The Hoffmann sign can be elicited by placing the patient's middle phalanx of the third digit across the DIP joint of the examiner's third digit on the dominant hand, with the palm facing down. Next, by placing the patient's third digit in slight extension, the DIP joint is "flicked" downward by the examiner's thumb. An involuntary flexion of the DIP joints of the patient's thumb and little finger is a positive test.
- Superficial reflexes, for example, cremasteric reflex (L1–L2) in males, are assessed when history and physical examination indicate possible involvement.
- Stretching the nerve roots of the sciatic nerve with the straight leg raising test can provoke radicular symptoms (Lasègue sign).
- Manual compression of the external jugular veins causing an increase in intraspinal pressure and aggravating radicular symptoms in either the upper or lower extremity can be a sign of nerve root compression (Naffziger sign).

Many diagnostic tools are available for evaluating the functional and structural aspects of nerve roots.

- MRI offers the best noninvasive view of the nerve roots and surrounding structures.
- Computerized tomography has some value when bone details are needed.
- Invasive myelography, with the instillation of intrathecal contrast, continues to have a role diagnostically, especially when combined with postmyelogram computerized tomography.
- Sometimes, it is important to evaluate the cerebrospinal fluid for signs of infection, inflammation, neoplasia, or hemorrhage by determining the cell count along with protein, glucose, and microbiologic studies.

The functional status of nerve roots can be tested with nerve conduction studies that include antegrade and retrograde response to stimulus (F responses and H reflexes).

TABLE 73.7

Deep Tendon Reflexes of the Lower Extremities

Reflex	Patellar	Achilles
Stimulus site	Patellar tendon	Achilles tendon
Typical response	Knee extension	Ankle plantar flexion
Central nervous system correlate	L3, L4	S1

- Nerve conduction studies and electromyography can reveal the presence of radiculopathy, but the abnormalities detected are a function of the severity and chronicity of the lesion.
- Electrophysiologic testing of the nerve roots can also be done with somatosensory evoked potentials.

Treatment

Treatment is directed to the underlying cause of the symptoms; palliative care with analgesics is indicated for patient comfort and pain control. OMT for somatic dysfunction can augment the analgesic effect, mobilize congestion and edema, and balance autonomic function.

Myelopathy

PRESENTATION

Patient complaints depend on the site of the lesion. There can be deficits in sensation, motion, strength, balance, gait, and/or problems with defecation or micturition.

MECHANISMS

Trauma to the spinal cord from herniated disks, penetrating objects, shearing or compression high-impact forces, and metastatic cancer are common causes of extrinsic myelopathy. Viral infections or autoimmune diseases such as multiple sclerosis can lead to transverse myelitis, an intrinsic myelopathy.

DIAGNOSTICS

The physical findings in myelopathy classically reveal a sensory level. Spinothalamic-mediated pain and temperature and dorsal column–mediated touch, vibration, and position sense are disturbed below the level of spinal cord disturbance. Typically, this affects pain and temperature beginning several segments below the actual level of the lesion. Usually, both sides are affected. Because primarily upper motor neurons are involved, the motor examination reveals a spastic increase in motor tone and an increase in the muscle stretch reflexes below the level of the lesion. Muscle weakness is diffuse and can be mild, moderate or severe. The distribution of weakness reflects the pathologic condition in the anterior horn cells or corticospinal tracts. Depending on the level of the lesion, the patient can have positive Babinski signs and ankle clonus in the lower extremities and/or positive Hoffman signs in the upper extremities. Sphincter tone can be increased or decreased. Gait can be disturbed by spasticity, weakness, or sensory ataxia. Patients with dorsal column sensory loss lose their balance and fall when asked to stand unaided with their eyes closed (Romberg sign). If the patient's neck is flexed, they can experience an electric sensation traveling the spinal cord and the extremities (Lhermitte sign), which is the result of stretching the long dorsal column fibers. Confirmatory diagnosis is with MRI.

TREATMENT

Treatment for traumatic spinal cord injuries is supportive, including surgery to stabilize the spine to prevent further damage to the spinal cord. Viral or immune-mediated myelitis can respond to corticosteroids if diagnosed and treated early. Tumors can be debulked or removed with radiation and surgery.

Radiculopathy

PRESENTATION

Patients commonly complain of unilateral leg pain with or without back pain, typically in a dermatomal distribution, with or without the following:

- Muscle weakness
- Paresthesia (e.g., tingling, numbness, burning, gnawing, or sharp-shooting pain)
- Muscle atrophy
- Antalgic gait
- Imbalance
- Knee or ankle instability
- Frequent trips and falls

MECHANISMS

Lumbar radiculopathy is one of the most common radiculopathies. Lumbar radiculopathy may be caused by a herniated nucleus pulposus, osteoarthritic spur, advanced spondylolisthesis, or a mass lesion.

DIAGNOSTICS

Regardless of the cause, there are relatively predictable structural and functional effects that need to be evaluated in the lower extremities. History and physical exam findings will uncover patterns of lower extremity motor and sensory changes, pain, and reflex changes as well as muscle weakness, lack of muscle tone, atrophy, predisposition to myofascial TrPs, and imbalance. The diagnosis of lumbar or upper sacral radiculopathies by electromyography focuses on the discovery of denervation, fasciculation, and fibrillation potentials in patterns of lower extremity muscles sharing a common involved nerve root (myotome).

L4 radiculopathy is suspected when there is a reduction of the patellar deep tendon reflex, dysesthesia in the L4 distribution, and patterns of weakness, cramping, or TrPs in those muscles innervated by the L4 nerve root, such as the quadriceps and tibialis anterior. Often, a patient exhibiting these symptoms will complain that a knee gives way or that climbing stairs is difficult.

L5 radiculopathy is associated with a decrease in the biceps femoris deep tendon reflex; it is suspected when there is dysesthesia in the L5 distribution and patterns of weakness, cramping, or TrPs in the gluteus medius and ankle dorsiflexors, such as tibialis anterior, extensor hallucis, and extensor digitorum brevis. This patient may often complain of tripping over carpets or "small cracks in the sidewalk" because of a foot drop. The patient may have difficulty walking on the heels due to a loss of dorsiflexion on the symptomatic side.

An S1 radiculopathy is suspected when there is a decreased Achilles reflex, numbness over the lateral aspect of the calf muscle, and weakness of the foot evertors. It is not uncommon to find myofascial TrPs in the intrinsic foot muscles, gastrocnemius/soleus complex, and gluteal muscles. This is the most common radiculopathy, often resulting from a herniated disk between L5 and S1. The patient may have difficulty walking on the toes due to weakness of plantar flexion on the symptomatic side.

Acute lumbosacral radiculopathies are capable of disturbing efficient gait and have a significant impact on the bioenergetic and biomechanical structure–function models of osteopathic care. Even after their resolution, chronic changes such as atrophy and residual lower extremity muscle weakness can continue to disturb efficient gait. Muscles in the radicular myotome are at high risk of developing TrPs.

TREATMENT

Although radiculopathy from herniated lumbar disks can resolve spontaneously over a period of 3 to 12 months, several modalities can help to alleviate or palliate symptoms and improve lower limb function and quality of life:

- Physical therapy
- Electrotherapeutics
- OMT for related somatic dysfunctions
- Analgesics
- Neuroleptics
- Antidepressants
- Anesthetic blocks
- Ankle foot orthotic

Surgery may be necessary if neurologic deficits progressively worsen or do not improve (see Chapter 93 for discussion).

When specific disease of the spinal column is identified, institute appropriate treatment. When there is structural weakness, supportive bracing can be used. Physical therapies are often valuable. Therapeutic exercise regimens are a critical component of all comprehensive recovery plans. Employ nutritional assessment and supplementation as needed. Use medications with analgesic, anti-inflammatory, and bone-supportive properties. Anesthetic blocks of locally irritable structures (nerve roots or facets) can be effective for pain control.

As discussed in Part Three: The Somatic Component of this text, a common pathophysiologic process affecting the spinal column is somatic dysfunction, which is treated with OMT. Somatic dysfunction can affect single segments or multiple spinal segments and accompany any of the spinal column pathologies. It is critical to distinguish somatic dysfunction that is amenable to OMT from spinal pathology that requires medication, surgery, or other primary therapies to restore health. Although treating the somatic component of spinal or visceral diseases can ameliorate symptoms, and potentially reduce the allostatic burden of the disease or help the patient restore homeostasis, identifying the underlying cause of the somatic dysfunction is essential to care for the patient competently and thoroughly. If somatic dysfunction is the primary problem, OMT alleviates it and resolves the signs and symptoms completely. Chapters 46 to 64 introduce a variety of OMT procedures used to alleviate somatic dysfunction throughout the body (also see Chapter 95 for more information regarding safety and efficacy of OMT for somatic dysfunction).

OMT can be used to treat the somatic component of spinal pathologies as part of a comprehensive management plan. A prospective study conducted in 2011 found OMT for chronic pain management in spinal cord injury patients to be an effective and feasible treatment, especially for patients in whom available drugs are not an option.[17] Patients treated with both medications and OMT experienced significantly higher pain relief than patients being treated either with medications or OMT alone.[17]

Osteopathic treatment plans are best derived after the more comprehensive nature of an osteopathic neurologic evaluation. The examination can yield information local to the area of chief complaint, as well as more general information on the effects of interrelated problems. For example, a person with mechanical low back pain could have an associated visceral disease (such as endometriosis) that can contribute viscerosomatically to the physical findings that the patient presents. Likewise, a similar low back pain could be related to a problem with the foot or leg. By identifying contributing elements, a more complete diagnostic understanding can be reached, and a more comprehensive treatment undertaken.

Standard treatment of radiculopathy is appropriately directed to the specific pathologic condition involved. For example, antiviral agents are used for herpes zoster infection or antineoplastic agents for carcinomatous radiculopathy. For degenerative spine conditions causing radiculopathy, physical measures to reduce compression and deformation with traction, physical therapy, and therapeutic exercise are beneficial. Attempting to decrease inflammation with oral corticosteroids or nonsteroidal anti-inflammatory medication is reasonable, though not always effective. Corticosteroids, along with anesthetic agents, for example, lidocaine, introduced into the epidural space, usually lumbar but occasionally thoracic or cervical, are effective at reducing radicular pain from herniated disks impinging upon spinal nerves causing radiculitis, but not alleviating any underlying structural spinal stenosis.[18,19] Patients are given extensive education about provocative aspects of their lifestyle, work, and habits with a goal of minimizing aggravating factors. If persistent radiculopathy causes progressive sensory or motor findings, or pain that cannot be controlled, surgical decompression is advisable. When the cauda equina is affected, a particular urgency exists to diagnose and decompress. In these cases, a delay in treatment can be associated with a marked increase in morbidity with lingering bladder, bowel, sexual, and lower extremity dysfunction.

Specific intervention with OMT must be undertaken gently and cautiously for patients with radiculopathy. Any treatment position or manipulative procedure that increases nerve root compression or deformation can be potentially injurious. Nonetheless, in educated, trained, and careful hands, the use of knowledgeably applied gentle manipulative forces might improve conditions for the nerve root and could potentially affect arterial, venous, and lymphatic circulation, as well as improve local biomechanical factors. At the least, OMT can be useful in alleviating some of the secondary musculoskeletal reactions that develop in the face of nerve root pathologic conditions.

ENTRAPMENT NEUROPATHIES

Entrapment neuropathies represent a localized injury or irritation to one of the peripheral nerves. They are caused by the mechanical effects of the impinging adjacent tissues. The typical anatomic causes include entrapment within the fibro-osseous tunnels where the nerve changes course against fibrous and muscular bands. Entrapment can be precipitated by repetitive or acute trauma; once the trauma occurs, the local anatomic configuration often causes a repetition of the mechanical injury. This local anatomic configuration can result in local compressive injury to the neural elements. The neural elements at risk include both the axon and the associated myelin. It can compromise local circulation, including arterial, venous, and lymphatic influences. Table 73.8 represents specific sites of nerve entrapment.[20,21]

Bell Palsy

PRESENTATION

Symptoms of Bell palsy may be mild or quite severe. Inability to smile, pucker the lips or kiss, keep liquids in the mouth, drooling, close one eyelid, and raise an eyebrow are common complaints. Severe symptoms of unilateral facial paralysis and ineffective tear production sometimes progress to corneal ulcerations.

MECHANISMS

Idiopathic peripheral facial paralysis, known commonly as "Bell palsy," is caused by an inflammation and compression of the facial nerve and results in unilateral paralysis or paresis of the muscles of

TABLE 73.8

Sites of Nerve Entrapment and Treatments

Nerve	Site of Entrapment	Treatment
Median	Carpal tunnel, pronator teres, anterior interosseous syndrome	OMT, splint, exercise, surgery
Ulnar	Elbow, cubital tunnel, canal of Guyon, thoracic outlet	OMT, exercise, surgery
Radial	Supinator muscle	OMT, exercise, surgery
Brachial	Thoracic outlet scalenes, pectoralis minor, cervical rib	OMT, exercise, surgery
Sciatic	Pelvic outlet piriformis muscle	OMT, exercise, surgery
Posterior tibial	Tarsal tunnel	OMT, exercise, surgery
Common peroneal	Fibular head	OMT, exercise, surgery
Obturator	Obturator foramen	OMT, exercise, surgery
Femoral	Pelvic brim inguinal ligament	OMT, exercise, surgery
Ilioinguinal	Abdominal wall	OMT, exercise, surgery
Intercostal	Rib cage	OMT, exercise, surgery
Trigeminal	Foramen ovale, foramen rotundum petrosphenoid ligament, Meckel cave	OMT, surgery
Cranial nerves II–VI	Orbital apex, exit foramina, reciprocal tension membrane, cavernous sinus	OMT, surgery
Cranial nerves VIII–XII	Basisphenoid, basiocciput, jugular foramina, hypoglossal canal	OMT, surgery
Cranial nerves VII and VIII	Temporal bone, internal auditory meatus	OMT, surgery
Cranial nerve I	Ethmoid, cribriform plate, sphenoid, lesser wing	OMT, surgery

OMT, osteopathic manipulative treatment.

facial expression. It is the most common facial mononeuropathy. The condition affects up to 40 in 100,000 persons, with onset typically occurring between the ages of 15 and 50 and over 70 years of age.[22,74,75] Bell palsy affects men and women at a roughly equal rate of occurrence; however, there is an increased prevalence during pregnancy, in patients with diabetes, hypothyroidism, and concurrent upper respiratory tract infections.[22,74,75] Etiology is unknown; however, some patients may have an underlying infection, for example, herpes simplex virus I or Lyme disease.[22,75]

DIAGNOSTICS

Physical signs of Bell palsy include drooping of the corners of the mouth, indistinct skin folds and facial creases, and an unfurrowed forehead. They are unable to fully close their affected eye. The clinical presentation is worrisome as Bell palsy has signs resembling a stroke. When patients eat, food may collect between their teeth and lips, and they may drool from the corner of their mouth. Smiling may reveal a marked contrast between the two sides of the face, with the affected side drawn without wrinkles. Depending on where the lesion occurs in the osseous facial canal, a patient's taste reception in the anterior two-thirds of the tongue may be altered. A patient may also experience pain in or behind the ear and hyperacusis. Bell phenomenon—the upward movement of the eye on attempted closure of the lid due to weakness of the orbicularis oculi—is a pathognomonic sign.[22]

TREATMENT

Many patients recover spontaneously within 1 to 3 weeks, with standard of care being administration of oral corticosteroids with an antiviral medication, for example, acyclovir within 3 days of onset.[22,74,75] Protection of the affected eye with an eyepatch, from dryness, wind, and foreign objects must be part of the management plan. Understanding the anatomy of the facial nerve and facial canal is important prior to treating patients with OMT. When using OMT to treat a patient who has Bell palsy, knowledge of the anatomy of the facial nerve as it traverses the temporal bone is important in understanding the nature of symptoms. The facial nerve travels through the internal acoustic meatus, located in the petrous portion of the temporal bone. It travels through the temporal bone via the facial canal. When the nerve becomes inflamed and swollen, it can become further entrapped in the facial canal and on rare occasions, require surgical decompression. Here lies the geniculate ganglion, which supplies taste to the anterior tongue and cutaneous sensation of the external acoustic meatus. Branches of the facial nerve include:

- The greater petrosal nerve
- The stapedius nerves
- The nerve of the chorda tympani

The petrosal nerve provides parasympathetic innervation of the lacrimal gland. The stapedius nerve innervates the stapedius muscle, allowing dampening of loud sounds, and the chorda tympani supplies taste to the anterior two-thirds of the tongue and parasympathetic innervation of the submandibular and sublingual glands. The facial nerve exits the cranium through the stylomastoid foramen to give rise to six terminal motor branches leading to the muscles of facial expression.

The treatment plan should include treatment of the whole person, not just the face and head. OMT can decrease the severity of symptoms and help speed recovery. Dysfunction of the sacrum, upper thoracic, cervical spine, and cranial mechanism can contribute to impaired lymphatic drainage from the facial canal, leading to inflammation of the facial nerve. Start by treating the patient's lymphatic system by freeing up restrictions found in four key diaphragms: the thoracic outlet, respiratory diaphragm, suboccipital diaphragm, and cerebellar tentorium.

- Begin lymphatic drainage by starting at the endpoint of the drainage, that is, around the thoracic duct, at the thoracic inlet, by using myofascial release of the supraclavicular fascia and the thoracic pump technique.
- The respiratory diaphragm is treated to allow for deeper breathing, thus creating greater pressure gradients to aid in lymphatic flow.
- Primary respiratory mechanism and osteopathic cranial manipulative medicine are used to release restrictions in the cranial base, occiput, and cerebellar tentorium, which attaches to the temporal bone and allows for physiologic temporal motion.
- Osteopathic physicians commonly find restricted ipsilateral motion of the temporal bone and upper cervical restrictions in patients with Bell palsy.[76]
- Another area commonly restricting temporal motion is at the occipitomastoid suture. Look for a compression of the occipitomastoid maintaining an internally rotated temporal bone on the side of facial paralysis.

A particularly osteopathic approach to the cranial neuropathies can be based on the writings of Sutherland as outlined by Magoun.[76] In this text, the anatomy of the nerves and their relationship to dural investments, nearby vasculature, bony foramina, and osseoligamentous structures are elaborately described. The naturally mobile aspect of these cranial and intracranial structures was appreciated. Sutherland and Magoun recognized the potential for vulnerability to mechanical distortion and compression with the resultant production of symptoms, often directly localized to individual cranial nerves. Such symptoms can be related to trauma, developmental phenomena, inflammation, or ischemia.

Carpal Tunnel Syndrome

PRESENTATION

The patient complains of pain and paresthesia in the thumb, index, and long finger.

- Aching can spread proximally to the arm and forearm.
- Early, the pain is transient; later, it becomes permanent.
- Commonly, it is worse at night or during provocative activities.
- In the earliest stages, a shake of the hand can restore circulation and relieve symptoms.
- Later, immobilization with a splint can relieve symptoms.
- Vague weakness, often described as dropping things or trouble with buttons, is common.

MECHANISMS

Carpal tunnel syndrome is the result of entrapment of the distal branches of the median nerve as it passes through the carpal tunnel. The tunnel is formed by the carpal bones and the carpal ligaments. The contents of the tunnel are flexor tendons and the median nerve. Either strong flexion or extension of the wrist can impact the median nerve. There can be acute compression with mechanical deformation and ischemic change. Chronic progressive compression can result in vascular compromise.

- The first effect of increased compression is an obstruction of venous return from the nerve, which leads to increased capillary distension and further increases in intratunnel pressure. This continues to self-amplify in a cyclic fashion, impairing nutrition to the nerve. The large, myelinated fibers are the most vulnerable.

At this stage, symptoms appear with pain and paresthesia, usually transient and reversed by restoring proper circulation.
- Progressively, the capillary circulation is sufficiently slowed to create endoneurial edema, epineurial edema, and intratunnel edema. This edema can still be reversed if adequate decompression is obtained.
- In the final stages, there is arterial insufficiency and increasing mechanical deformation, resulting in nerve fiber destruction, muscle atrophy, and ultimate fibrous replacement.

Carpal tunnel can be caused by trauma to the wrist, hypertrophic arthritis, or thickening of the flexor retinaculum. Hypertrophic neuropathy, local edema, ganglion cysts, and tenosynovitis can all compromise the carpal tunnel. Predisposing systemic diseases include:

- Hypothyroidism
- Diabetes mellitus
- Pregnancy
- Leukemia
- Paraproteinemia
- Gout

DIAGNOSTICS

The diagnosis depends on a careful history to differentiate local disease from systemic disease. With systemic disease, the symptoms are often bilateral. History is important in understanding predisposing biomechanical factors. These factors are often related to work, hobbies, or chronically repeated behaviors.

Physical examination reveals a sharply demarcated median nerve sensory deficit, confined to the palm, often splitting along the long finger or ring finger. Motor examination reveals a weakness of the thumb abductor, thumb opposer, and distal thumb flexor. In the more advanced stages, atrophy of the thenar eminence is evident. Phalen test, forced wrist flexion, can reproduce the pain and paresthesia. Tinel sign is often positive, with percussion of the nerve at the wrist producing a tingling into the hand/finger.

Phalen Test

The Phalen test is used in the diagnosis of carpal tunnel syndrome. Attempt to elicit or reproduce symptoms by flexing the patient's wrist to its maximum degree and holding it in that position for at least 1 minute (Fig. 73.5).

Tinel Sign

The Tinel sign is used in the diagnosis of carpal tunnel syndrome. Attempt to elicit or reproduce pain or tingling in the distribution of the median nerve by tapping over the transverse carpal ligament.

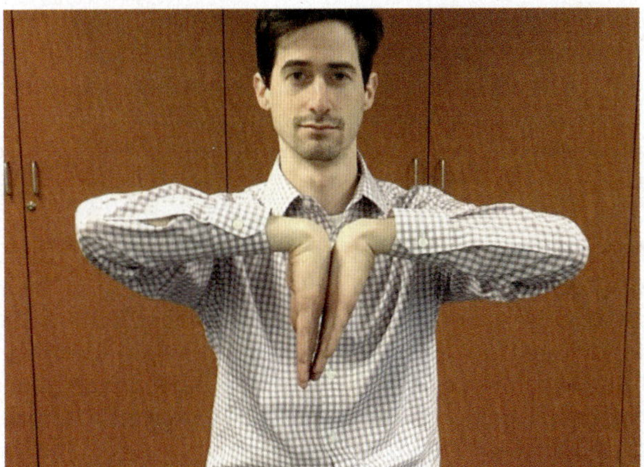

Figure 73.5. Phalen test for carpal tunnel syndrome. (Photo courtesy of Dr. Heinking, with permission.)

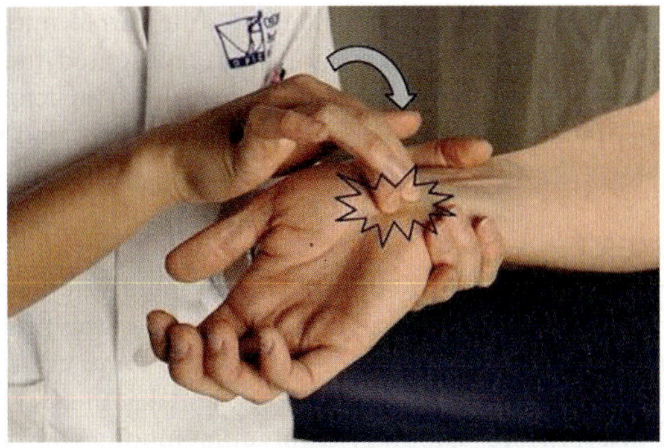

Figure 73.6. Tinel sign at the wrist for carpal tunnel syndrome. A positive Tinel sign (abnormal) is when the patient experiences pain and paresthesias (tingling, numbness) along the distribution of the median nerve. (Photo and illustration courtesy of Western University of Health Sciences, Pomona, CA, with permission.)

The sensory distribution of the median nerve in the hand consists of the palmar surfaces of part of the thumb, the index finger, the middle finger, and the lateral half of the ring finger (Fig. 73.6).

Modified Allen Test

The modified Allen test can be used to determine if there is a vascular etiology to the hand pain, for example, from ischemic compression of the radial or ulnar arteries (Fig. 73.7A,B).

1. After elevating the patient's affected hand, have the patient make a fist, then compress both radial and ulnar arteries, and have the patient open the fist. The palm should become pale due to ischemia, indicating the compression test is able to produce ischemia.
2. Upon release of one artery at a time, the palm should turn red within 15 seconds, typically less than 5 seconds, demonstrating perfusion from the patent artery. If compression of one of the arteries alone causes pallor, then the other is obviously not patent and likely compressed or diseased. This is a positive test and requires further evaluation for underlying etiology.

Electrodiagnostic tests are helpful in corroborating the diagnosis and quantifying the degree of abnormality. The finding of prolonged distal median nerve motor and/or sensory latencies is an early sign of demyelination. Axonal involvement and degeneration are demonstrated by the appearance of neurogenic atrophy on electromyography. The electromyogram can be useful to rule out more

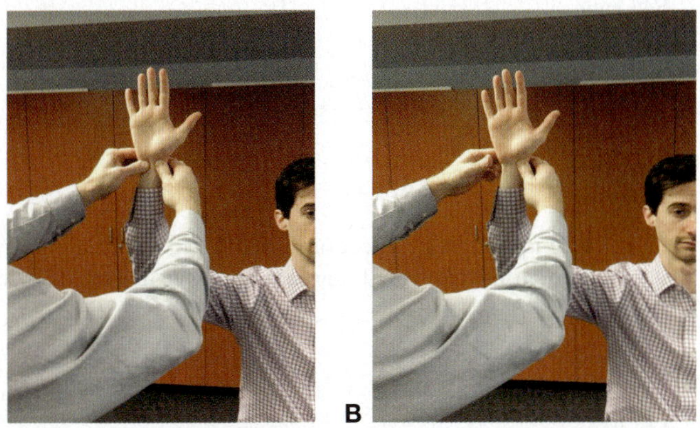

A B

Figure 73.7. Modified Allen test for vascular assessment of the hand. After the patient makes a fist, compress both radial and ulnar arteries. **A.** Upon opening the palm while compression is maintained on both arteries, the palm should be pale. **B.** Release one artery at a time to assess for patency of the contralateral artery. Compression of one artery alone should not produce pallor.

proximal lesions, such as a radiculopathy. The carpal tunnel itself may be demonstrated on plain radiogram, computed tomogram, and even better with MRI, which can reveal the structural consequences of anatomic compression. Recently, ultrasound is being used to assess the carpal tunnel as well.

TREATMENT

The standard treatment has consisted of immobilization with wrist splints, especially during sleep, and avoidance of the provocative activities related to carpal tunnel syndrome. Home exercise program to stretch tight muscles, tendons, and ligaments. Physical therapy, acupuncture, cupping, ergonomic modifications are all worth considering. Perineural infiltration with local anesthetics and corticosteroids can also be used. When conservative measures fail, surgical decompression is the appropriate treatment.[77]

The osteopathic neurologist begins with a more thorough evaluation. Not only is the biomechanical function of the wrist examined, but the biomechanics of the fingers, hand, forearm, elbow, arm, shoulder, cervical and thoracic spine, and rib cage are also assessed. This assessment is performed in the context of a complete osteopathic structural examination.

- Restrictive lesions along the upper extremity and shoulder girdle can influence circulation (venous, lymphatic, and arterial) and mechanical deformation of the median nerve that begins at the nerve root, runs through the brachial plexus, and terminates in the median nerve that runs through the arm and forearm before passing through the carpal tunnel.
- Whole-body mechanical issues, like slumped posture, can influence the local conditions of the carpal tunnel. The veins and lymphatics drain proximally into the superior vena cava and thoracic duct. Mechanical dysfunction in the rib cage and cervicothoracic region are as relevant as the mechanics of the arm itself.
- Arterial insufficiency can be affected similarly at multiple levels.
- The sympathetic component, often understated, can be influenced from the root of the neck, where the sympathetic ganglia is found, through the upper extremity itself.

The treatment, then, is to treat general structural problems with OMT and exercise. Manipulation releases biomechanical barriers to nerve and vascular functions at the:

- Neck
- Upper back
- Shoulder
- Rib cage
- Thoracic inlet and outlet
- Upper arm
- Forearm
- Wrist
- Hand
- Fingers

The techniques can be direct or indirect, and numerous examples of osteopathic treatment approaches have been proposed, including[78–80]:

- Myofascial release
- Muscle energy
- HVLA
- Articulatory
- Functional techniques

Sucher[78] has demonstrated a model for clinically, electrophysiologically, and graphically evaluating carpal tunnel syndrome. He has shown the pathologic changes on neurologic examination, through distal nerve latency studies, and by obtaining MRI images of the carpal tunnel to measure its volume. He then proceeds to treat these patients with OMT. He retests his patients and demonstrates objective changes in neurologic findings, distal nerve latencies, and carpal tunnel volume, as measured by MRI. Sucher[79] presents strong evidence for the therapeutic value of osteopathic management techniques and specific stretches. A recent clinical pilot study did demonstrate some benefit in reducing pain and improving function in nine patients (six females) with CTS after 6 weekly treatments of OMT; however, aside from an increase in carpal tunnel length as measured by ultrasound, no widening of the carpal tunnel or improved function of the median nerve conduction velocity was found.[81] Further clinical trials are warranted.

Thoracic Outlet Syndrome

Another syndrome of nerve entrapment is thoracic outlet syndrome (TOS).

PRESENTATION

Patients present with pain, tingling, coolness, dysesthesia, and numbness of the affected upper extremity. The typical presentation is numbness extending along the ulnar aspect of the hand. The pain is usually worse with the arm elevated or abducted (white hand syndrome). TOS can be associated with pain, weakness, and a lack of endurance of the arm musculature.

MECHANISMS

TOS refers to a group of signs and symptoms produced by compression of the neurovascular bundle in the region of the thoracic outlet. It has been called cervical rib syndrome, scalenus anticus syndrome, costoclavicular space syndrome, and hyperabduction syndrome. Although compression can affect the subclavian artery or vein, most cases also involve the lower trunk of the brachial plexus. TOS may be associated with abnormal cervical ribs and most often with disturbed myofascial relations.

Compression can occur typically in three areas:

1. Over the slope of the first rib
2. In the triangle made by the anterior and middle scalene muscles
3. Under the pectoralis minor muscle

If fibrous bands are present with fibro-osseous cervical rib rudiments, compression can occur there as well. The etiology of the compression may be multifactorial. The most common area of compression is between the anterior and middle scalene muscle. Many patients with this condition have significant muscular tension in their scalenes due to overuse (asthma, COPD), stress, poor posture, orthopedic shoulder issues, poor abdominal breathing, or underlying cervical instability. Some **serious** causes include Pancoast tumor, lymphadenopathy or malignancy, fracture, cervical spinal stenosis, subclavian thrombosis, and peripheral vascular disease.

DIAGNOSTICS

Physical findings include sensory loss, particularly in the ulnar distribution. Weakness of intrinsic, ulnar innervated muscles is a late finding in TOS. Provocative tests are helpful to diagnose and localize the syndrome. At the site of entrapment, there might be localized tenderness. For example, with symptoms elicited on isometric scalene contraction, the entrapment can be localized to the scalene triangle and is associated with localized tenderness of the brachial plexus at this site. When hyperabduction with extension is the culprit, the site of entrapment is often the tendon of the pectoralis minor and local pectoral hypertonicity and tenderness is typically present. Sometimes, a bruit of the subclavian artery can be auscultated at the site of its compression.[82] The Adson test is usually positive.

Adson Test

The Adson test is used to determine the state of the subclavian artery, which may be compressed by an extra cervical rib or by tightened anterior and middle scalene muscles. To perform the Adson test, take the patient's radial pulse at the wrist. Continue to feel the pulse while abducting, extending, and externally rotating the arm. Then, instruct the patient to take a deep breath, and turn the head toward the side being tested. Marked diminution or absence of the radial pulse indicates compression of the subclavian artery.

Electrodiagnostic confirmation is frequently difficult. Prolonged nerve conduction velocity across the thoracic outlet can be demonstrated; in more advanced cases, axonal involvement might be encountered on electromyography. Somatosensory evoked potentials of the upper extremity can be localizing.[83] Imaging of the region in question is best attempted with MRI; however, MRI findings are frequently inconclusive. Simple cervical spine radiographs will reveal the presence of cervical ribs.

TREATMENT

Standard management includes exercises to improve posture, reduce mechanical stress, lengthen shortened muscles, strengthen weakened antagonist muscles, and avoid symptom-producing circumstances. Analgesics, anti-inflammatory agents, muscle relaxants, and physical therapies are used. Progressive stretching and strengthening exercise programs are included when indicated. When conservative measures fail, surgical intervention remains but is reserved for only the most severe cases who have signs and symptoms of progressive nerve damage.

Osteopathic management of TOS includes appropriate structural evaluation with particular attention to the cervical, thoracic, costal, scapular, and brachial mechanical relationships.[84] In comparison with carpal tunnel, the TOS involves a more widely affected area. It is therefore more difficult to define the inciting event and to establish targeted therapy. Evaluation of posture reveals a high incidence of posture with head forward and with rounded, upward, and anterior displaced shoulders.[84] Evaluation of the workstation and of the patient's hobbies and habits can reveal a subset of behaviors that are underlying the dysfunctional process. OMT consisting of myofascial-releasing maneuvers to the restrictive musculoskeletal structures can be useful.[85–87] When they are only temporarily useful and symptoms return when the patient resumes their unaltered lifestyle, efforts to modify the patient's life circumstances are employed. These efforts include modification and elimination of occupational and avocational mechanical stressors and the promotion of postural awareness with training in postural modification. The most important long-term aspects are the identification of the specific biomechanical restrictors and the prescription and training of the patient in the performance of self-administered stretching exercises.[85–87] As a general concept, the temporary beneficial response to manipulative therapies can be understood using this model. When the pathologic process involves chronically acquired, well-learned maladaptive somatic behaviors, it is not surprising that a single manipulation does not eradicate such a process. Multiple strategies are necessary. Patient education, instruction, and performance in a protracted therapeutic exercise program are often most useful. In this way, the neuromusculoskeletal system can be reeducated.

Meralgia Paresthetica

PRESENTATION

Meralgia paresthetica is a condition characterized by a burning, tingling, or numbness sensation over the anterior lateral aspect of the thigh.

MECHANISMS

It is an entrapment mononeuropathy of the lateral femoral cutaneous nerve and may be caused by injury, compression, or disease. The nerve becomes entrapped about 1 cm medial to the anterior superior iliac spine (ASIS). Meralgia paresthetica is a consequence of jeans, belts, or garments that are too tight, excess abdominal adiposity, or pelvic somatic dysfunctions affecting the lateral femoral cutaneous nerve as it passes under the inguinal ligament, near its attachment at the ASIS.

DIAGNOSTICS

There is decreased sensation to light touch and/or pin prick in the lateral femoral cutaneous dermatome distribution. Somatic dysfunction may involve the L2 or L3 vertebral units, the psoas muscle, the innominate, or the fasciae of the thigh or innominate.

TREATMENT

Decompression of the nerve with loose clothing alleviates the condition if caused by tight pants. OMT resolves not only the somatic dysfunctions but often also relieves the symptoms associated with this condition if the inciting behavior (tight clothing) is eliminated as well.

Sciatica Neuralgia

PRESENTATION

In most commonly affecting patients between ages 30 to 50, sciatica neuralgia is characterized by sudden onset of unilateral sharp and aching pain that radiates from the buttock to the posterolateral thigh and leg to the plantar and lateral foot. It often occurs after physical activity that strains the lower back but can occur slowly over time in cases of degenerative joint or disk disease. Some patients have pain in the anterolateral thigh if the compression is from an L4 disk herniation. Rarely, the pain can be bilateral. It can last as short as 2 weeks, or 4 to 6 months, rarely up to a year, but usually resolves spontaneously. The patient typically limps and may have a foot drop.

MECHANISMS

The sciatic nerve is derived from the spinal nerve roots of the fourth and fifth lumbar and first two sacral spinal nerves. It is comprised of the peroneal and tibial nerves as they exit the lumbosacral plexus. Inflammation or compression anywhere along its course gives rise to sciatica neuralgia. Compression of the sciatic nerve most commonly occurs close to the spinal column from fragments of herniated nucleus pulposus or osteoarthritic bony growths at the L4–L5 or L5–S1 levels (see "Radiculopathy" section above). Though uncommon, a posterolateral compression can occur at the L3–L4 level. Local inflammation occurs at the site of compression. Both nerve roots can be simultaneously compressed in cases of central disk herniation, spinal stenosis, or spondylolisthesis. In a small percentage of patients, the sciatic nerve passes through the piriformis muscle. If the muscle contracts for a prolonged period (spasm), it can compress the sciatic nerve enough to cause reversible symptoms once the muscle relaxes. In most individuals, it passes under the piriformis muscle; however, in approximately 10% of the U.S. population, the peroneal portion of the sciatic nerve passes through the piriformis muscle (Fig. 73.8). When the piriformis is the etiology of the sciatic pain, patients complain of

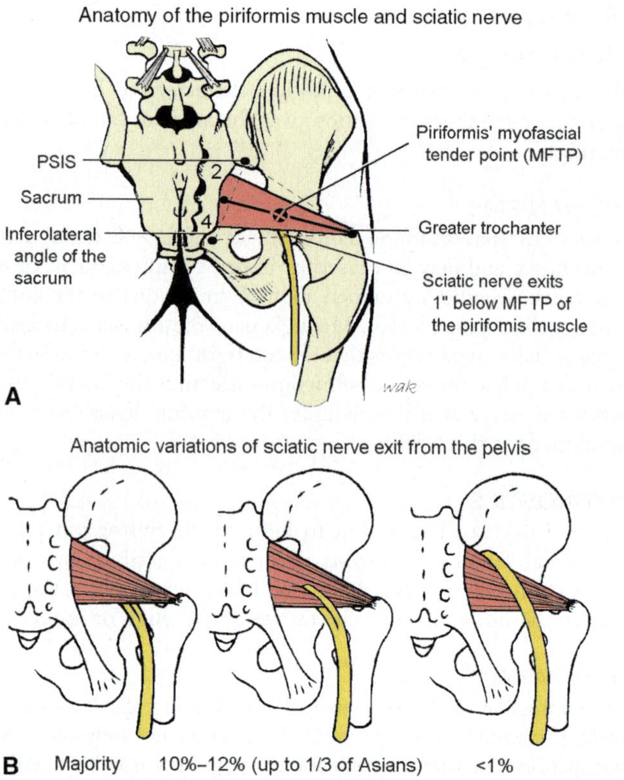

Figure 73.8. A, B. Piriformis structure–function relationships. (Illustration courtesy of William A. Kuchera, DO, FAAO, with permission.)

posterior thigh pain stopping at the knee (see Chapter 93 for more information on the piriformis syndrome).

DIAGNOSTICS

DTRs are diminished or absent depending on the nerve root involved. The straight leg raising test is the most sensitive test although not specific (see Chapters 84 and 93 for description of this and other orthopedic tests used to diagnose lumbar disk herniation). MRI of the lumbar spine identifies the site of compression. There are nonspinal causes and conditions that simulate sciatica, but they are not common.[88]

TREATMENT

Pain management with medication and physical therapy is standard. Long-term use of opioid medication is no longer a standard therapy due to abuse potential. Corticosteroids provided locally may help diminish inflammation. Pregabalin and other neuroleptics have been used to decrease radicular pain symptoms. Surgery is indicated to decompress the nerve from a herniated disk (see Chapter 84 Osteopathic Considerations in Orthopedics for further discussion). OMT may be helpful if used judiciously to treat associated somatic dysfunctions, especially if the piriformis is involved.

LOWER LEG AND FOOT ENTRAPMENT NEUROPATHIES

Peroneal Nerve Entrapment

PRESENTATION

Paresthesia or pain in the feet in the distribution of the peroneal nerve.

MECHANISMS

The remainder of the nerve supply in the thigh, leg, and foot is derived from the posterior tibial and common peroneal (common fibular) nerves. A vulnerable site for entrapment or trauma exists as the common peroneal nerve (common fibularis nerve) passes behind the fibular head (Fig. 73.9). The tibial nerve supplies the posterior compartment of the leg and the muscles of the foot. The deep peroneal nerve supplies the anterior compartment of the leg with sensation to the webbing between the first and second toes. The superficial peroneal nerve supplies the lateral compartment of the leg as well as the skin on the anterolateral side of the leg and the dorsum of the foot.

DIAGNOSTICS

Physical examination reveals decreased sensation of the dorsum of the affected foot and/or at the web between the great and second toes.

TREATMENT

OMT to the fibular head is often effective in treating this entrapment.[89]

Figure 73.9. Superficial and deep peroneal nerve distribution. (Illustration courtesy of William A. Kuchers, DO, FAAO, with permission.)

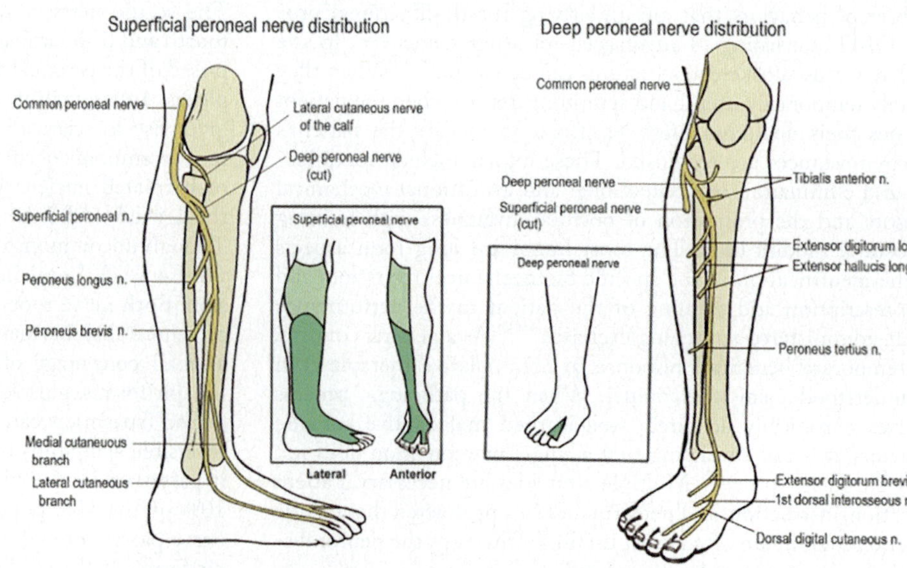

Tarsal Tunnel Syndrome

PRESENTATION

Pain is felt anywhere along the bottom of the foot.

MECHANISMS

The posterior tibial nerve runs through the tarsal tunnel—a narrow space that lies on the inside of the ankle next to the ankle bones. The tunnel is covered with a thick ligament, the *flexor retinaculum*, that protects and maintains the structures, which includes the posterior tibial nerve, contained within the tunnel; therefore, compression of the posterior tibial nerve at this site is referred to as *tarsal tunnel syndrome*. This syndrome is often associated with diabetes, back pain, or arthritis. It can also be caused by an injury to the ankle, such as a sprain, or by a growth, abnormal blood vessels, or scar tissue that press against the nerve. A flat foot increases the risk of developing tarsal tunnel syndrome because the outward tilting of the heel (hindfoot valgus) can produce strain on the medial ankle structures (flexor retinaculum) and cause compression of the nerve.

DIAGNOSTICS

Physical exam findings can be supported by ultrasound or MRI of the tarsal tunnel.

TREATMENT

Treatment for tarsal tunnel syndrome includes in-shoe orthotics designed to help redistribute weight and take pressure off the nerve or corticosteroid injections. Tarsal tunnel syndrome caused by known conditions, such as tumors or cysts, might respond better to surgery than when the cause is not known.

Morton Neuroma

PRESENTATION

Patients complain of distal foot or toe pain, usually in the third and fourth toes, aggravated by walking and wearing tight shoes.

MECHANISMS

Morton neuroma is an enlarged nerve that usually occurs in the interspace between the third and fourth metatarsals where the local pain is worsened by wearing tight shoes and by walking.

DIAGNOSTICS

Morton neuroma can be diagnosed by palpating this interspace and squeezing the forefoot from side to side to recreate the patient's pain or to palpate an audible click (*Mulder sign*).

TREATMENT

Changing shoes, decreasing walking, and injecting local corticosteroids is usually curative. In refractory cases, surgery may be indicated. OMT can be used to decrease edema and related muscle spasms.

CONCLUSION

Assessing the patient's neuromusculoskeletal system more completely generates a more comprehensive diagnosis. This fosters a prescription for a multifaceted treatment program that increases the potential for success. An additional advantage includes the ability to exclude more unusual yet potentially serious causes of chronic pain. Furthermore, it offers the osteopathic neurologist the tools to rationally choose among the multiple (and costly) diagnostic and therapeutic possibilities. The osteopathic approach offers a successful model for integrated multidimensional treatment with the patient as the focus and the physician as the facilitator.

REFERENCES

1. Still AT. *Autobiography of A. T. Still*. Author; 1897.
2. Denslow JS. Neural basis of the somatic component in health and disease and its clinical management. *J Am Osteopath Assoc*. 1972;72:149–156.
3. Brodal A. *Neurological Anatomy in Relation to Clinical Medicine*. Oxford University Press; 1981.
4. Kandel E, Schwartz J, Jessell T. *Principles of Neural Science*. Elsevier Science; 1991:326–380.
5. Denslow JS. Pathophysiologic evidence for the osteopathic lesion: the known, unknown, and controversial. *J Am Osteopath Assoc*. 1975;74:415–421.
6. Headache Classification Committee of the International Headache Society (HIS). *The International Classification of Headache Disorders*. 3rd ed (beta version). Cephalalgia; 2013;33(9):629–808.
7. Jessell T, Kelly D. Pain and analgesia. In: Kandel E, Schwartz J, Jessell T, eds. *Principles of Neural Science*. Elsevier Science; 1991:389–392.
8. Magoun HI Sr. Trauma: a neglected cause of cephalgia. *J Am Osteopath Assoc*. 1975;74:400–410.
9. Lay EM. Osteopathic management of trigeminal neuralgia. *J Am Osteopath Assoc*. 1975;74:373–389.
10. Travell JG, Simons DG. *Myofascial Pain and Dysfunction: The Trigger Point Manual*. Williams & Wilkins; 1983.
11. Nielsen SM, Tarp S, Christensen R, Bliddal H, Klokker L, Henriksen M. The risk associated with spinal manipulation: an overview of reviews. *Syst Rev*. 2017;6(1):64.
12. Cassidy JD, Boyle E, Cote P, et al. Risk of carotid stroke after chiropractic care: a population-based case-crossover study. *J Stroke Cerebrovasc Dis*. 2017;26(4):842–850.
13. Elkiss M. *Chronic Headache Pain, An Osteopathic Perspective*. Testimony before the Agency for Health Care Policy and Research; October 31, 1995. Transcript of Open Forum, Duke University, Durham, NC.
14. Simon RP, Aminoff MJ, Greenberg DA, eds. *Clinical Neurology*. 10th ed. McGraw-Hill; 2018.
15. Jessell T, Kelly D. Pain and analgesia. In: Kandel E, Schwartz J, Jessell T, eds. *Principles of Neural Science*. Elsevier Science; 1991:388–389.
16. Park J, Park WY, Hong S, et al. Diagnostic accuracy of the neck tornado test as a new screening test in cervical radiculopathy. *Int J Med Sci*. 2017;14(7):662–667. http://www.medsci.org/v14p0662.htm
17. Arienti C, Daccò S, Piccolo I, Redaelli T. Osteopathic manipulative treatment is effective on pain control associated to spinal cord injury. *Spinal Cord*. 2011;49(4):515–519.
18. Manchikanti L, Knezevic NN, Boswell MV, Kaye AD, Hirsch JA. Epidural injections for lumbar radiculopathy and spinal stenosis: a comparative systematic review and meta-analysis. *Pain Physician*. 2016;19(3):E365–E410.
19. Chou R, Hashimoto R, Friedly J, et al. Epidural corticosteroid injections for radiculopathy and spinal stenosis: a systematic review and meta-analysis. *Ann Intern Med*. 2015;163(5):373–381.
20. Sunderland S. *Nerves and Nerve Injuries*. Churchill Livingstone; 1978:653–1021.
21. Magoun HI. *Osteopathy in the Cranial Field*. The Journal Printing Co; 1966:95, 184, 207, 251, 259, 294.
22. Zandian A, Osiro S, Hudson R, et al. The neurologist's dilemma: a comprehensive clinical review of Bell's palsy, with emphasis on current management trends. *Med Sci Monit*. 2014;20:83–90.
23. Diamond S. *Clinical Symposia: Head Pain, Diagnosis and Management*. Ciba-Geigy Corp., 1994.
24. Welch KM. Migraine. A biobehavioral disorder. *Arch Neurol*. 1987;44:323–327.
25. Moskowitz MA. The neurobiology of vascular head pain. *Ann Neurol*. 1984;16:157–168.
26. O'Connor T, van der Kooy D. Pattern of intracranial and extracranial projections of trigeminal ganglion cells. *J Neurosci*. 1986;6:2200–2207.
27. Brodal A. The cranial nerves. In: *Neurological Anatomy in Relation to Clinical Medicine*. Oxford University Press; 1981:508–513.
28. Charles A. The pathophysiology of migraine: implications for clinical management. *Lancet Neurol*. 2017;17(2):174–182.

29. Boles DB. Visual field effects of classical migraine. *Brain Cogn.* 1993;21:181–183.
30. Pederson DM, Wilson WM, White GL Jr, Murdock RT, Digre KB. Migraine aura without headache. *J Fam Pract.* 1991;32:57.
31. Bickerstaff ER. Basilar artery migraine. *Lancet.* 1961;1:1520.
32. Brindise JP, Nelson KE, Kappler RE. Association between cervical and thoracic somatic dysfunction among second year osteopathic medical students. *J Am Osteopath Assoc.* 2014;114(7):540–548.
33. Blend R, Bull J. The radiological investigation of migraine. In: Smith R, ed. *Background to Migraine: First Migraine Symposium.* Heinemann Medical Books Ltd; 1967:110.
34. Ong JJY, De Felice M. Migraine treatment: current acute medications and their potential mechanisms of action. *Neurotherapeutics.* 2017;15(2):274–290.
35. Davidoff RA. Trigger factors and non-pharmacologic approaches. In: *Migraine: Manifestations, Pathogenesis, and Management.* FA Davis Co; 1995:183–193.
36. Kidd RF, Nelson R. Musculoskeletal dysfunction of the neck in migraine and tension headache. *Headache.* 1993;33(10):566–569.
37. Blau J, MacGregor EA. Migraine and the neck. *Headache.* 1993;33(10):88–91.
38. Weiss H, Stern B, Goldberg J. Post-traumatic migraine: chronic migraine precipitated by minor head or neck trauma. *Headache.* 1991;31:451–456.
39. Kudrow L. Cluster headaches new concepts. *Neurol Clin.* 1983;2:369–384.
40. Hardebo J. How cluster headache is explained as an intracavernous inflammatory process lesioning sympathetic fibers. *Headache.* 1994;34:125–126.
41. Gawel M, Krajewski A, Luo Y, Ichise M. The cluster diathesis. *Headache.* 1990;30:652–655.
42. Graham J. Cluster headache: the relation to arousal, relaxation, and autonomic tone. *Headache.* 1990;30:145–148.
43. Goadsby PJ. Pathophysiology of cluster headache: a trigeminal autonomic cephalgia, *Lancet Neurol.* 2002;4:251–257.
44. Lodi R, Pierangeli G, Tonon C, et al. Study of hypothalamic metabolism in cluster headaches by proton MR spectroscopy. *Neurology.* 2006;66(8):1624–1626.
45. Sanin L, Mathew N, Ali S. Extratrigeminal cluster headache. *Headache.* 1993;33:369–370.
46. Mathew N, Rueveni V. Cluster-like headache following head trauma. *Headache.* 1988;28:297–299.
47. Hardebo J. Subcutaneous sumatriptan in cluster headache. *Headache.* 1993;33:18–21.
48. Langemark M, Olesen J. Pericranial tenderness in tension headache: a blind, controlled study. *Cephalalgia.* 1987;7:249–255.
49. Schoenen J, Jamart B, Gerard P, Lenarduzzi P, Delwaide PJ. Exteroceptive suppression of temporalis muscle activity in chronic headache. *Neurology.* 1987;37:1834–1836.
50. Silberstein S. Tension-type headaches. *Headache.* 1994;34:S2–S7.
51. Olesen J. Clinical and pathophysiological observations in migraine and tension-type headache explained by integration of neural, vascular, and myofascial inputs. *Pain.* 1991;46:125–132.
52. Meloche J, Bergeron Y, Bellavance A, Morand M, Huot J, Belzile G. Painful intervertebral dysfunction: Robert Maigne's original contribution to headache of cervical origin. The Quebec Headache Study Group. *Headache.* 1993;33:328–334.
53. Michler R, Bovim G, Sjaastad O. Disorders in the lower cervical spine. A cause of unilateral headache? A case report. *Headache.* 1991;31:550–551.
54. Hack G, Koritzer R, Robinson W, Hallgren RC, Greenman PE. Anatomic relation between the rectus capitis posterior minor muscle and the dura mater. *Spine (Phila Pa 1976).* 1995;20:2484–2486.
55. Olesen J, Rasmussen B. Management of acute nonvascular headache: the Danish experience. *Headache.* 1990;30:541–543.
56. Rolle G, Tremolizzo L, Somalvico F, Ferrarese C, Bressan LC. Pilot trial of osteopathic manipulative therapy for patients with frequent episodic tension-type headache. *J Am Osteopath Assoc.* 2014;114(9):678–685.
57. Miller HC. Head pain. *J Am Osteopath Assoc.* 1972;72:135–143.
58. Kuchera ML. Osteopathic principles and practice/osteopathic manipulative treatment considerations for cephalgia. *J Am Osteopath Assoc.* 1998;98(suppl):S14–S19.
59. Vick DA, McKay C, Zengerle CR. The safety of manipulative treatment: review of the literature from 1925 to 1993. *J Am Osteopath Assoc.* 1996;96:113–115.
60. Raskind R, North CM. Vertebral artery injuries following chiropractic cervical spine manipulation: case reports. *Angiology.* 1990;41:445–452.
61. Powell FC, Hanigan WC, Olivero WC. A risk/benefit analysis of spinal manipulation therapy for relief of lumbar and cervical pain. *Neurosurgery.* 1993;33:73–79.
62. Hart RG, Easton JD. Dissections of cervical and cerebral arteries. *Neurol Clin.* 1983;1:155–182.
63. Okawara S, Nibbelink D. Vertebral artery occlusion following hyperextension and rotation of the head. *Stroke.* 1975;5:23.
64. Di Fabio RP. Manipulation of the cervical spine: risks and benefits. *Phys Ther.* 1999;79:50–65.
65. Haldeman S, Kohlbeck FJ, McGregor M. Risk factors and precipitating neck movements causing vertebrobasilar artery dissection after cervical trauma and spinal manipulation. *Spine (Phila Pa 1976).* 1999;24:785–794.
66. Smith WS, Johnston SC, Skalabrin EJ, et al. Spinal manipulative therapy is an independent risk factor for vertebral artery dissection. *Neurology.* 2003;60:1424–1428.
67. Rubinstein SM, Peerdeman SM, van Tulder MW, Riphagen I, Haldeman S. A systematic review of the risk factors for cervical artery dissection. *Stroke.* 2005;36:1575–1580.
68. Carlesso LC, Gross AR, Santaguida PL, Burnie S, Voth S, Sadi J. Adverse events associated with the use of cervical manipulation and mobilization for the treatment of neck pain in adults: a systematic review. *Man Ther.* 2010;15:434–444.
69. Carnes D, Mars TS, Mullinger B, Froud R, Underwood M. Adverse events and manual therapy: a systematic review. *Man Ther.* 2010;15:355–363.
70. Haynes MJ, Vincent K, Fischhoff C, Bremner AP, Lanlo O, Hankey GJ. Assessing the risk of stroke from neck manipulation: a systematic review. *Int J Clin Pract.* 2012;66:940–947.
71. Puentedura EJ, March J, Anders J, et al. Safety of cervical spine manipulation: are adverse events preventable and are manipulations being performed appropriately? A review of 134 case reports. *J Man Manip Ther.* 2012;20:66–74.
72. Biller J, Sacco RL, Albuquerque FC, et al; American Heart Association Stroke Council. Cervical arterial dissections and association with cervical manipulative therapy: a statement for healthcare professionals from the American Heart Association/American Stroke Association. *Stroke.* 2014;45:3155–3174.
73. Church EW, Sieg EP, Zalatimo O, Hussain NS, Glantz M, Harbaugh RE. Systematic review and meta-analysis of chiropractic care and cervical artery dissection: no evidence for causation. *Cureus.* 2016;8(2):e498.
74. Madhok VB, Gagyor I, Daly F, et al. Corticosteroids for Bell's palsy (idiopathic facial paralysis). *Cochrane Database Syst Rev.* 2016;7(7):CD001942.
75. Gagyor I, Madhok VB, Daly F, et al. Antiviral treatment for Bell's palsy (idiopathic facial paralysis). *Cochrane Database Syst Rev.* 2015;(11):CD001869.
76. Magoun HI. *Osteopathy in the Cranial Field.* 3rd ed. Northwest Printing; 1976:27–28, 269.
77. Sunderland S. The carpal tunnel syndrome. In: *Nerves and Nerve Injuries.* Churchill Livingstone; 1978:711–723.
78. Sucher BM. Palpatory diagnosis and manipulative management of carpal tunnel syndrome. *J Am Osteopath Assoc.* 1994;94:647–663.
79. Sucher BM. Myofascial manipulative release of carpal tunnel syndrome: documentation with MRI. *J Am Osteopath Assoc.* 1993;93:1273–1278.
80. Siu G, Jaffe JD, Rafique M, Weinik MM. Osteopathic manipulative medicine for carpal tunnel syndrome. *J Am Osteopath Assoc.* 2012;112:127–139.
81. Burnham T, Higgins DC, Burnham RS, Heath DM. Effectiveness of osteopathic manipulative treatment for carpal tunnel syndrome: a pilot project. *J Am Osteopath Assoc.* 2015;115:138–148.
82. Sunderland S. Disturbances of brachial plexus origin associated with unusual anatomical arrangements in the cervico-brachial region: the

thoracic outlet syndrome. In: *Nerves and Nerve Injures*. Churchill Livingstone; 1978:901–917.
83. Synek VM. Diagnostic importance of somatosensory evoked potentials in the diagnosis of thoracic outlet syndrome. *Clin Electroencephalogr*. 1986; 17:112–116.
84. Sucher BM. Thoracic outlet syndrome—a myofascial variant: part I. Pathology and diagnosis. *J Am Osteopath Assoc*. 1990;90:686–704.
85. Sucher BM. Thoracic outlet syndrome: a myofascial variant. II. Treatment. *J Am Osteopath Assoc*. 1990;90:810–812, 817–823.
86. Sucher BM, Heath DM. Thoracic outlet syndrome: a myofascial variant. III. Structural and postural considerations. *J Am Osteopath Assoc*. 1993; 93:334, 340–345.
87. Dobrusin R. An osteopathic approach to conservative management of thoracic outlet syndromes. *J Am Osteopath Assoc*. 1989;89:1046–1050, 1053–1057.
88. Ropper AH, Zafonte RD. Sciatica. *N Engl J Med*. 2015;372:1240–1248.
89. Lavelle JM, McKeigue ME. Musculoskeletal dysfunction and drop foot: diagnosis and management using osteopathic manipulative medicine. *J Am Osteopath Assoc*. 2009;109:648–650.

74 Chronic Pain Management

MITCHELL L. ELKISS ▪ JOHN A. JEROME

KEY CONCEPTS

- Pain is an unpleasant sensory, emotional, and musculoskeletal experience.
- Acute pain is a symptom; chronic pain is a disease.
- The pain neuromatrix is nested in the central nervous system, where modulation, transmission, and transduction of noxious stimulation occur.
- The musculoskeletal, immune, neurologic, and endocrine (MINE) systems interact as one "supersystem" in response to nociception.
- Body unity and structure/function interrelationships guide osteopathic thinking regarding chronic pain management.
- Stress dysregulates the MINE supersystem, predisposing one to chronic pain.
- Chronic pain results from a sustained loss of a system's ability to function normally regarding its own self-regulation and/or its normal regulatory role in interacting with other systems.
- Osteopathic assessment of chronic pain is dynamic, patient focused, and comprehensive.
- The standard of care of osteopathic pain management is based on an integration of the five models.

INTRODUCTION

In the evaluation and management of patients with chronic pain, osteopathic medicine offers a particularly illustrative example of its unique diagnostic and therapeutic potential. The principles that have defined osteopathic philosophy and practices can be readily recognized as central to the diagnosis and treatment of patients with chronic pain.

In osteopathic medicine, emphasis is placed on evaluating, not just the painful region of the patient, but the "person who is in pain," taking into consideration the general health of their body, their relations with family and close associates, as well as their cultural background. In this manner, the pain syndrome "sufferer" is seen as nested in ever-expanding circles of influence. Each element in this nested array represents a diagnostic vector capable of affecting other elements, at every other level (Fig. 74.1).

Chronic pain management has been formally studied only since the late 20th century. In that time, the profession has come to understand the profound influence that noxious peripheral stimuli can have on the musculoskeletal, immune, and endocrine systems as well as on the central nervous system (CNS).

- In the spinal cord, brainstem, and forebrain regions, synaptic organization and function can change rapidly, in response to acute nociceptive input.[1]
- Such changes can range from the molecular to the gross structural levels, involving alterations in gene expression and protein synthesis.
- These immediate responses can be transient or long term, and, unfortunately, given the right circumstances, can become permanent.
- Certainly, one of the most profound findings in the research on pain is the dynamic or plastic nature of pain and its pervasive influence on body physiology and behavior.[2]

Therefore, it is important to keep in mind, when evaluating a patient in pain that:

- The process is dynamic and may rapidly evolve in catastrophic directions.
- Detailed and repeated examinations are required to monitor the situation.
- Treatment protocols must have both a strong evidence-based grounding and the patient's confidence to succeed.

PAIN IS AN UNPLEASANT SENSORY, EMOTIONAL, AND MUSCULOSKELETAL EXPERIENCE

Pain is always subjective. Everyone learns the application of the word through experiences related to injuries in their early life. Pain is the experience that we associate with actual or potential tissue damage. It is always unpleasant and therefore an emotional experience. Many people report pain in the absence of apparent tissue damage or any pathophysiologic cause; usually, this happens for psychological reasons. This definition avoids tying pain to the stimulus. Activity induced in the nociceptor and nociceptive pathways by noxious stimulus is not actually pain until it is interpreted/processed by the patient's psychological and physiologic state.

American Osteopathic Association's House of Delegates resolved in 1997 and reaffirmed every 5 years thereafter, a position paper on chronic pain management. Chronic pain is defined as:

> "A pain state in which the cause of the pain cannot be removed or otherwise definitively treated and which in the generally accepted course of medical practice, no relief or cure of the cause of the pain is possible or none has been found after reasonable efforts."[3,4]

Osteopathic physicians recognize a duty and a responsibility to treat patients suffering from chronic pain. Certainly, the differences between acute pain and chronic pain represent qualitatively different experiences for both patient and physician.

It is understood that nociception is related to the process of detecting real or potential tissue damage.

- Specialized A-delta and C fibers (nociceptors) respond to a variety of noxious stimuli. They convert the chemical, mechanical, or thermal stimuli into altered neuronal activity. This is largely

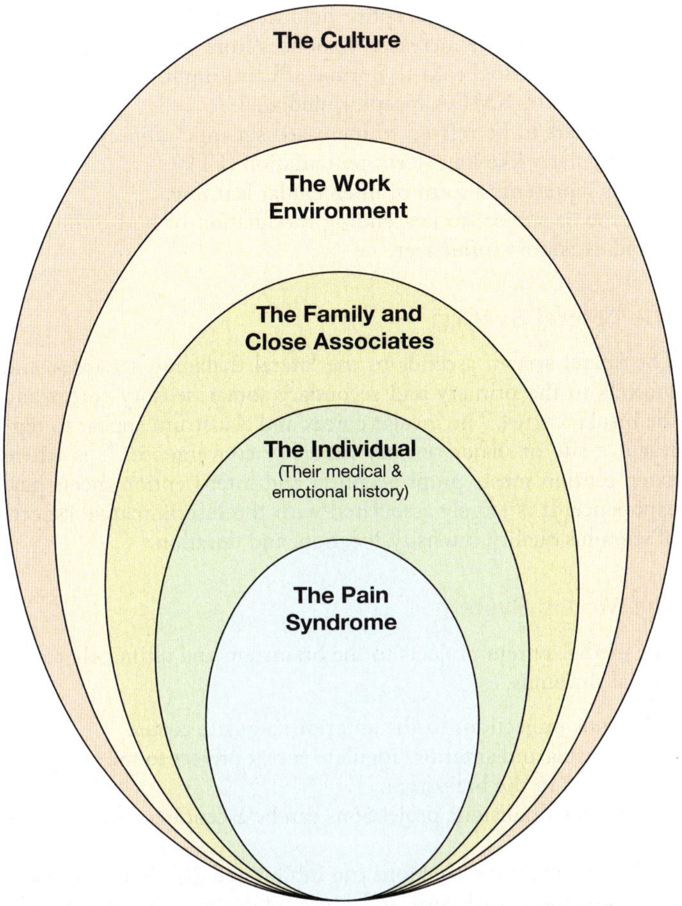

Figure 74.1. The nested spheres of influence on the pain syndrome.

transmitted to the dorsal horn in segment-derived, organized, receptive patterns.

- The nociceptor responses themselves are affected by local chemical and neural activity. In their normal state, they respond to energies capable of damaging cells. In abnormal states, they can demonstrate altered response characteristics associated with hyperalgesia and painful responses to noninjurious stimuli, known as allodynia.
- Nociception can be disrupted or enhanced by descending modulation from the brain and brainstem.
- In chronic pain, there is a bias toward greater nociceptive facilitation and less inhibition.

Pain is the response to nociception. When the system is healthy, it represents offensive nociceptive-driven activity in the spinal cord and brain. When the system is not healthy, it may represent impaired function of the peripheral nervous system (PNS) or CNS. Pain may be experienced even when there is no noxious stimulus (i.e., phantom limb pain).[5,6] Therefore, pain is a perception. This perception is part of a greater pain experience.

Suffering is a negative affective experience and response to pain. It is seen in association with pain and other psychic states (i.e., "a broken bone can cause pain… while the suffering of a broken heart may often be inconsolable"). Suffering is associated with activity in specific brain regions. It, too, is under the influence of ascending and descending influences. It is a feeling. This feeling is part of a greater pain experience. It frequently leads to pain-related behaviors. Often it is this suffering that is the primary concern driving a patient to seek health care.

ACUTE PAIN

Acute pain is a symptom. It is usually associated with a well-defined biologic cause and a rapid onset that alerts the possibility of tissue damage. It usually vanishes as healing occurs. Acute pain follows an injury to the body and implies a natural healing process of short duration. It is only expected to persist as long as the tissue pathology itself.

Acute pain is often, but not always, associated with objective physical signs of:

- Increased cardiac rate
- Increased systolic and diastolic blood pressure
- Increased pupil diameter
- Striated muscle tension
- Decreased gut motility
- Decreased salivary flow
- Decreased superficial capillary flow
- Fear and/or anxiety
- Releases of glycogen, adrenaline, and noradrenaline

These are collectively understood as the triggered alarm response and the initiation of secondary stages of resistance/healing that can lead to recovery.

- These changes in nociceptive activity have been assumed to be roughly proportional to the intensity of a noxious stimulus.
- The enormous biologic value of acute pain is to promote a rapid orientation to the noxious stimulus and to promote reactions to minimize or escape the damage being done by the noxious stimulus.
- Some pain fosters rest, protection, and care of the injured area during healing, thereby promoting recuperation.
- In other situations, acute pain can be suppressed temporarily in the service of a greater circumstance.
- These examples can be seen on the battlefield, the athletic field, and in emergency, crisis situations as anyone might experience.[5]

The overall behavioral signs of acute pain are agitation and the emerging flight-or-fight reaction. Patients with acute pain are anxious about the pain's intensity, meaning, and impact on themselves and their lifestyles.[6] This is rapidly followed by the resistance phase during which the organism resists a compromise of its homeostasis. Through allostatic actions of the integrated musculoskeletal (M), immune (I), neural (N), and endocrine (E) systems, the person is led toward recovery.

Unfortunately, and rather often, pain persists after initial healing. It may persist after all conventional medical treatments and drugs have been tried to little or no avail. A constant barrage of erratic nociceptive impulses into the brain provides no new or useful information, but the adverse signal continues to reach consciousness.

- As an example, a patient with a failed back surgery 2 years postoperatively does not need to experience pain every time they move their spine to remind them that they have scar tissue, adhesions, and functional changes in the structure of their back.
- Since they are no longer in the acute healing phase, the information provided by this type of repetitive noxious stimulation may lead to central sensitization, with musculoskeletal, immunologic, neurologic, endocrinologic disturbances, and abnormalities of regional cerebral blood flow[7] and metabolism.

CHRONIC PAIN

Chronic pain is a disease that can affect both the structure and the function of the CNS.[8] Pain patients imaged with functional magnetic resonance imaging (f-MRI), positron emission tomography (PET), single-photon emission computed tomography (SPECT), and magnetoencephalography (MEG) have revealed changes in neural processing that differentiates chronic pain from acute pain.[9–11]

- In patients with irritable bowel syndrome[12] with chronic pain, there is cortical thinning, and cell loss in the anterior cingulate cortex and anterior insula. Similar changes are also seen in chronic tension headache[13] and chronic back pain.[3] In addition, effects are seen on thalamic and prefrontal gray matter density, as well as on ascending and descending pain-modulating pathways.[14]
- In the fibromyalgia syndrome, there is an altered sensitivity to stimulation, with sensitization in pain-related neural activity.[15] There is a relative excess of glutamate and a deficiency of GABA.[16,17]
- In migraine sufferers, there has been a reported thickening of the somatosensory cortex.[18]

It is also reasonable to consider that a person's inherent structural/functional neural capacity may predispose them to the development of chronic pain. Genetically determined or acquired disturbances in the neural circuitry affecting the following all help create a pain neuromatrix:

- Neurotransmitter production and metabolism
- Receptor morphology and function
- Ion channel structure and function
- Disturbances of the neurons, their cell bodies and metabolism, their axons, their transmission properties, their structure and function, the tracts in which they run, the nuclei that they form, and their neuronal/glial interactions.

The pain neuromatrix is nested in the CNS, where modulation, transmission, and transduction of noxious stimulation occur.

At the basic biochemical level, when noxious stimulation of muscle afferent C fibers is prolonged and persistent, excitatory amino acid and neurotransmitters are released in greater amounts and for longer periods.[19] The resulting activation of *N*-methyl-D-aspartate (NMDA) receptors and the release of substance P, both centrally and peripherally, lead to hyperexcitability of PNS and CNS neurons with expansion of the size of the painful area beyond the original site of damage. This peripheral and central sensitization, the enlargement of peripheral pain receptor fields,[20] allows noxious sensations to be experienced as more painful (hyperalgesia),[21] and even non-noxious sensations as painful (allodynia).

Hyperalgesia

Hyperalgesia occurs at the site of tissue damage as an increased sensitivity to heat or mechanical stimulation. This primary hyperalgesia is due to peripheral sensitization.[22]

- Such is one way in which a healthy peripheral nerve can be chronically activated at its periphery.
- For heat, it has been linked to sensitization of the peripheral terminals of the primary pain afferents.[23]
- The primary afferent can also be sensitized by descending noradrenergic and serotonergic systems that work directly, in the spinal cord, on the primary afferent's central terminals (presynaptic), and on the segmental interneurons to increase their sensitivity in chronic pain states.

Secondary hyperalgesia occurs around the site of tissue damage, manifesting as an increased sensitivity to mechanical stimulation only. This secondary hyperalgesia is due to central sensitization.

- It is in this enlarged receptive field that mechanical stimulation elicits abnormally increased responses from second-order afferents in the spinal cord to normal afferent input.
- It is, in part, NMDA receptor mediated.
- It appears to be related to increased synaptic efficacy, which is molecularly like long-term potentiation (LTP).
- This represents a form of intercellular learning.
- It, too, is subject to descending modulation of both inhibitory and excitatory influences.

The Lateral System

The lateral system ascends to the lateral thalamus, synapses, and projects to the primary and secondary somatosensory cortex and the insular cortex. The insular cortex and claustrum appear to represent a site of major sensory modality convergence. It is where exteroception meets proprioception and interoception meets past experience. It is largely associated with the discriminative aspects of stimulus quality, intensity, location, and duration.

The Medial System

The medial system projects to the brainstem and ultimately to the medial thalamus.

- It sends projections to the anterior cingulate cortex.
- The insula and anterior cingulate cortex project to the amygdala and then to the brainstem.
- From the brainstem, projections can be ascending and descending.
- The descending projections can inhibit and disinhibit the activities in the spinal cord and lower brainstem and in this way contribute to primary and secondary hyperalgesia.

The medial nociceptive system has been associated with general arousal, emotional, autonomic, and motor responses, leading the drive state to end the painful problem. Here, afferent sensory information is linked to efferent autonomic and gross motor actions of defense and avoidance. This activity may be studied with objective measures of chemical levels, neural activity, and gross behaviors.

The patient's experience of pain is influenced by experience, memory, and expectation and is cortically and subcortically mediated. The way a person feels and thinks about their pain condition can affect the way they process and cope with pain. Cognitive elements promote modulation of the medial and lateral ascending nociceptive systems and provide a connection to the conscious experience.[24]

The Endogenous Opioid System

The endogenous opioid system is richly represented at all levels of the neural axis involved in pain processing. It is part of the parallel distributed and integrated endogenous system for relieving pain. It is part of the medicine chest to which A. T. Still referred. It, however, can be inadequate in states of chronic pain. Ironically, the long-term use of exogenous opioids can inhibit the body's capacity to respond to pain. The chronicity of pain is associated with structural and functional changes at multiple levels of the neural axis.[14] It can involve changes in:

- Excitability
- Lowered thresholds and higher gain in the system
- Changes in receptors
- Channel-mediated changes

- Second messenger effects
- Transduction and translational effects at the cellular level
- Changes in synaptic efficacy[9]

This form of LTP is part of the neural basis for learning, known as *plasticity*.

Plasticity

Plasticity means that the nervous system has the capacity to change its structure/function in response to environmental demands.[25,26] Maladaptive plasticity[14,27] at several levels of the nervous system is the biology behind the continuation of pain long after the original offending event has passed, depriving pain of its functional role of protection, withdrawal, adaptation, and functional recovery.[14,28–30] Plasticity can also be influenced by and can certainly influence the development of depression and anxiety.[31–33]

When pain results in the activation of peripheral nociceptive afferents, there is tremendous activity in the brain. Pain perception requires a brain. "No brain, no pain." Proceeding from the peripheral receptive fields associated with the pain, there is an activation of limbic, autonomic, brainstem, and spinal cord networks of modulation.[34,35]

PARALLEL NEURAL NETWORKS

Parallel neural networks of processing pain information are responsible for the pain behaviors resulting from the peripheral activation of nociceptors.[6,7] These parallel networks are always represented in some ratio to each other. The ratios vary as the *symptoms* of acute pain become the *disease* of chronic pain.[35]

It is important for the osteopathic physician to recognize that a systems network understanding of chronic pain would not be complete without consideration of the structural/functional *interactions* of the musculoskeletal, immune, neurologic, and endocrine (MINE) systems in response to nociception (Table 74.1).

TABLE 74.1

Pathologic Contributors to Pain

Pathologic Process	Clinical Examples
Malignant	Primary, metastatic, paraneoplastic
Degenerative	Trauma, wear and tear, apoptotic
Inflammatory	Immune mediated, organ effects
Immunologic	Antibodies, interleukins, tumor necrosis factor, etc.
Respiratory, circulatory	Local, regional, global
Energy, metabolic	Local, regional, global
Endocrine	Hormones, releasing factors
Infection	Local, regional, global
Somatic dysfunction	Local, regional, global
Trauma	Severity, complexity
Neurogenic	Neoplasm, infarction, demyelination, trauma, infection, degenerative, migraine
Psychogenic	Somatoform, depression, anxiety, hypervigilance, personality disorder, malingering, catastrophizing

The MINE systems interact as one "supersystem" in response to nociception.

Chapman talks about a system of "reciprocal, neural, endocrine, and immune interactions"[34,35] in the human response to pain and stress.

- In this, he posits a coherent model of interacting systems with global and local features.
- From there, complex pain behaviors emerge as immune (I), neurologic (N), and endocrine (E) interactions (i.e., INE system).
- Chapman's comprehensive, systematic review of the immune-neural-endocrine systems as they respond to pain and stress is a clear elaboration of principles, which are characteristic of osteopathic medical thinking.
- This, then, joins the works of Denslow and Korr, as further demonstration of the underlying biologic, anatomic, and physiologic mechanisms of human functioning (see Chapter 13 Somatic Dysfunction, Spinal Facilitation, and Viscerosomatic Integration)
- When Chapman describes his INE system, he calls it a "nested system." It provides a nest for the INE systems and is itself nested in a larger, more complex system. That is, it is nested, nurtured and nurturing, and defended and defending a greater system.
- This greater system is the neuromusculoskeletal system whose activity is crucial to our survival. The musculoskeletal system is the primary body machinery, the "machinery of life" (see "Korr's Explication of Osteopathic Principles" in Chapter 1 Philosophy of Osteopathic Medicine).[36]

There is an interdependent interaction of these four systems:

1. Musculoskeletal (M)
2. Immune (I)
3. Neurologic (N)
4. Endocrine (E)

As they interact in response to nociception, they form a *MINE system* that is continually adjusting to incoming information from both internal and external environments.

Many of the behavioral responses of the MINE system can be observed and measured.

- The behaviors occur at levels of scale, from the molecular to the cellular, to the whole human level.
- The responses represent both incoming information about the outer world and outward-directed responses designed to meet and satisfy the needs and drives of that person to decrease their pain.
- The four individual systems that comprise the MINE system demonstrate feedback effects that can be both facilitating and inhibiting.
- They show connectivity, through their common shared receptors and their associated ligands.
- Neurotransmitters, peptides, hormones, cytokines, and endocannabinoids are the biochemical messengers, responsible for some of the interactive crosstalk between these four systems.

The final pain effects of the MINE system interactions vary depending on where, when, and how they are expressed and reinforced by the environment. Pain inhibitory or excitatory systems and MINE feedback and feed-forward mechanisms are all at work. Though elements within each individual MINE system can be reduced to relatively simple observable physical/chemical activity, their coordinated interactive efforts create a more complex system of observable pain behaviors (Fig. 74.2).

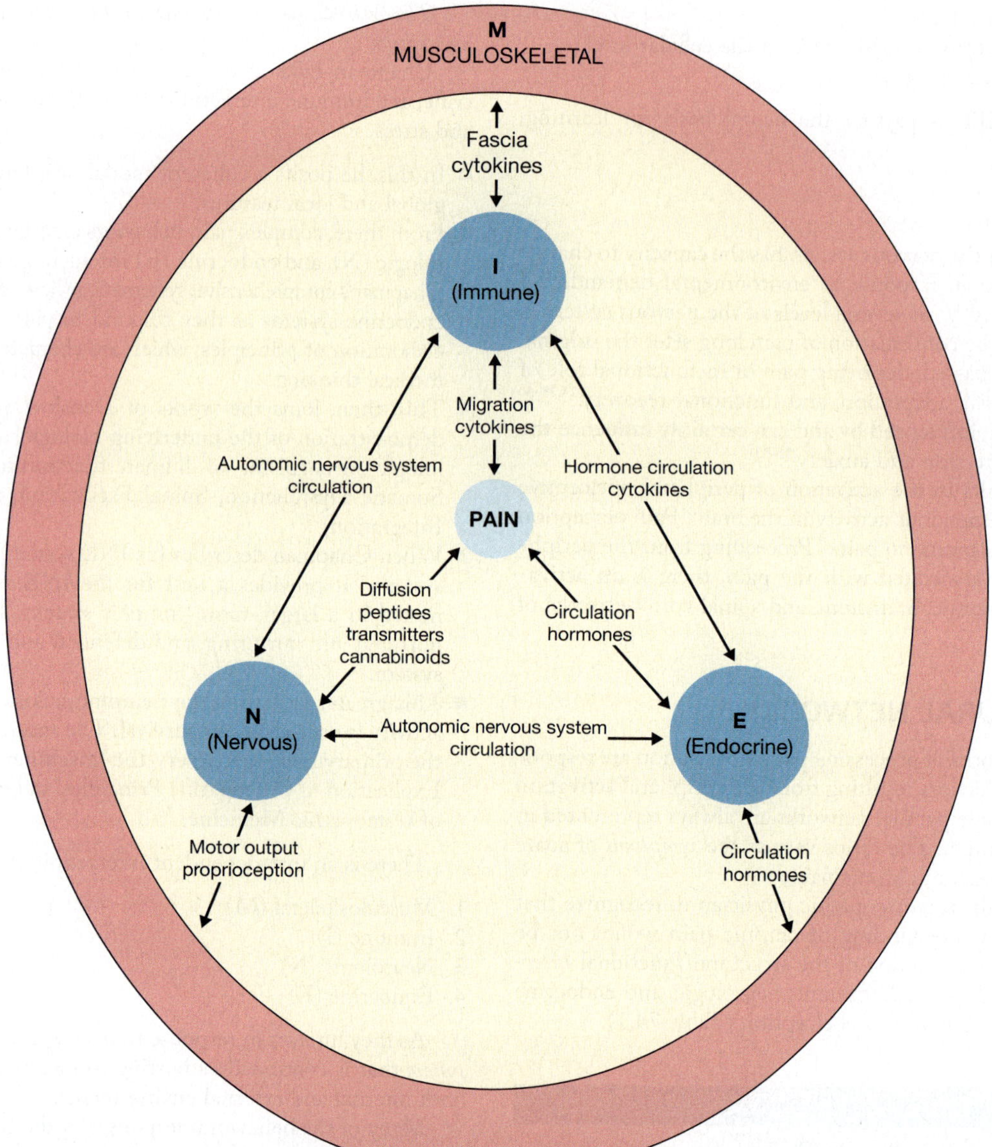

Figure 74.2. MINE supersystem in response to nociceptive input.

- For example, measurements can be made of afferent nociceptive activity in the:
  - ☐ Primary afferent neurons
  - ☐ Ascending secondary afferents
  - ☐ Brainstem
  - ☐ Subcortical and cortical neurons
  - ☐ Hormone levels and endocrine activity
  - ☐ Immune systems expression of cytokines
- The freeze, fight, or flight response, the endocrine aspect of stress response, and the inflammatory reaction are examples of more complex pain behaviors.
- Even more complex is the individual's ability to recognize danger and avoid it and run or fight as needed.
- The ability to fight off infection, the ability to recover from abuse or trauma, and the capacity to suffer are representative behaviors of even greater complexity.

These coordinated complex whole-body behaviors are based upon simple principles occurring at every level of the system.

Dysregulation within the MINE system also has individual components that can be measured, modeled, and understood. The multitude of possible states and phases, for each of the four systems, from the level of the molecules to patient perception and behavior, represents all the possibilities for healing or obstruction.

> "Remove all obstruction; and when it's intelligently done, nature will kindly do the rest." (A. T. Still, see Chapter 1 Philosophy of Osteopathic Medicine)

The human pain management system is thus characterized as dynamic. The dynamics of these systems are very sensitive to initial nociceptive conditions. Even though many parameters can be measured and monitored, in the face of apparent deterministic anatomic, physiologic, and pathophysiologic principles, there is still an inherent unpredictability. Therefore, with nociception there is unpredictability in patient pain experience and behavior. Pain behaviors in the patient often appear random, nonlinear, or chaotic; yet these behaviors are characteristic of dynamic systems.

For example, consider someone bending over to tie their shoelaces daily for years without event; until one day when they cannot straighten back up due to acute low back pain (LBP)! What was different that day? Complexity and sometimes random emergence of chronic pain behaviors, in this complex pain system, is natural.

Body unity and structure/function interrelationships guide osteopathic thinking regarding chronic pain management.

Each of the MINE subsidiary systems has an inherent capacity for self-regulation, self-learning, and health maintenance. Any of these subsidiary systems can also break down. Chronic pain, therefore, is likely an effect or consequence of system breakdowns or dysregulation.

Sometimes, it is easy to understand why a patient might be hurting. While other times, it is less easy to explain how a particular set of circumstances might result in a patient's unique pain expression and experience. Understanding this dynamic pain system's extreme sensitivity to initial and/or prolonged nociceptive conditions makes it understandable that some people will experience chronic pain.[29,34]

The idea of holistic, interactive, nested systems, such as the MINE supersystem, is an idea consistent with osteopathic philosophy.

- The MINE system has properties greater than the sum of its individual subsidiary systems.
- It explains how individuals can live and adapt, respond to, and survive stressful painful situations.
- The MINE system also explains how they can mount a defensive response to a stressor/pain crisis, recover from that response, survive, and maintain health.
- The four systems themselves:
  - □ are interdependent
  - □ show reciprocity of structure and function
  - □ demonstrate self-regulation
  - □ produce and maintain the necessary biologic products to sustain their own continued existence

Homeostasis serves to regulate the internal resources ready to be called upon when stressed by pain.

From a system's analysis, homeostasis exists as an attractor, or home base from which the body maintains its internal balance.

Allostasis is the set of adaptive reactions that help the individual maintain homeostasis in the face of any number of stressors.

Pain, trauma, illness, aging, excess, or deficiency can all call forth a stress response. This is a mobilization of internal resources to meet stressor challenges.

- First, there is an alarm response, which is accompanied by both immediate stressor resistance and a slower-forming recovery response.
- In fact, a critical part of the recovery response is its ability to down-regulate the initial pain defensive response when the threat is over. This avoids overactivity of the defensive catabolic responses of active resistance and permits self-mediated recovery and return to health.
- The defensive response turns itself on and then turns itself off, when it is appropriate.
- If the stressor prevails, exhaustion results. If the individual prevails, recovery occurs.
- The range of an individual's biopsychosocial responses, as well as their ability to tolerate pain intrusion and still maintain homeostasis, helps to define their level of health.

Failure to self-manage pain symptoms might occur if the defensive response is inadequate or excessive. Such a recovery response is associated with clinical symptoms as seen in chronic pain, especially in the musculoskeletal system.

Stress dysregulates the MINE, predisposing one to chronic pain.

Dysregulation in the MINE system's ability to respond to stress, at any of its component sites or its numerous interfaces, compromises one's overall ability to heal or recover from pain/stress. Nociception can create dysregulation and become chronic pain due to any of the following:

- Extraordinary stress
- Compounding comorbidities
- Confounding social stressors
- Intrinsic system vulnerability (Consider patients who have suffered abuse: physical, sexual, emotional, or verbal)

The musculoskeletal system is ultimately involved in all pain processes and management.

One factor essential to understanding the MINE system is an appreciation of the musculoskeletal (M) system.

- This system is uniquely available for observation and palpation.
- The INE systems are nested within the musculoskeletal system.
- The musculoskeletal system executes the freeze, flight, or the fight, and maneuvers in the external world to secure the necessary objects of sustenance, food, drink, and breath.
- Through movement, it allows seeking behaviors, interpersonal behaviors, and collective communal behaviors.
- It is built upon basic behaviors reiterated at cellular, tissue, and organism levels.
- This system also shows feedback, and feed-forward mechanisms.
- It is interactive with the other systems, not only through a common chemical language but also through a network of mechanical linkages that can affect pain-coping behaviors.[32]

Mechanical transducers include muscle, tendon, ligament, bone, fascia, extracellular matrix, and fibroblasts.

- The transmission occurs along planes of physical connection.
- The patterns of connection can be described as mechanical, anatomical, neurologic, circulatory, and/or biomolecular.
- The effects will include skeletal muscle behavior, segmental, regional, and global.
- They may be seen in coordinated and patterned motor system responses (i.e., fight or flight).
- They may be seen in the transformation of fibroblasts to myofibroblasts when they are under mechanical stress (i.e., wound healing).[32]
- Similarly, the behavior of bone in response to stress loading is a dynamic process.

The musculoskeletal system is body wide in its presence and in its purpose.

- There is fractal-like, reiteration at every scale:
  - □ From the cytoskeleton to the integrins to the intercellular connective tissues
  - □ From the osteon to the bones
  - □ From the myofibril to the muscle groups
  - □ From the local fascia to the entire body of fascia
- There is complexity and there is predictability in the musculoskeletal system.
- It is a part of the body's essential response to pain and stress.
- The musculoskeletal system interacts with the following systems:
  - □ Immune
  - □ Nervous
  - □ Endocrine
  - □ Respiratory

- Circulatory
- Digestive
- Eliminative

The musculoskeletal system responds to pain/stress.

The musculoskeletal system is the active agent of how muscles tense, contract with a purpose, and relax, when the stress has passed.

- This system affects the nervous system through a proprioceptive stream of information, complementing the flow of nociceptive, afferent information.
- It affects the endocrine system through its complex relationship with the sympathetic–adrenal–medullary (SAM) axis and the hypothalamic–pituitary–adrenal (HPA) systems.
- The musculoskeletal system affects the immune system, particularly by enabling the movement of cells and their products along the fascial networks, which are responsible for mounting immune responses.

The immune system responds to pain/stress with an inflammatory response.

Tissue trauma elicits an elaboration of immune active molecules at the site of trauma and systemically, triggering both the acute, inflammatory response at the site of injury, along with a more global acute phase reaction, which has been dubbed, the "sickness response." Proinflammatory cytokines and immune cells (lymphocytes, granulocytes, neutrophils, and macrophages) are "circulated" through blood vessels and lymphatics and along fascial networks. (See Chapter 12 The Role of Inflammation in Healing and Homeostasis, for further discussion.) The combined effects of cytokines, lymphoid tissue, and immune cells affect the body's internal homeostasis.

- The immune system interacts with the nervous system.
  - Nociceptor activation causes release of substance P and neurokinase A at the site of the disturbance. These are immune-stimulating, proinflammatory neuropeptides.
  - Neurogenic inflammation is a part of the initiating mechanism and propagation of the immune defensive response.
  - This inflammatory response is sensitive to sympathetic enhancement from primary nociceptor activation.
- The immune system interfaces with the endocrine system.
  - This is accomplished largely by cytokines, such as interleukins 1 and 6, and their receptors that are found throughout the HPA and the SAM.
- The immune system affects the musculoskeletal system via the structure and function of tissues that are responding to potential invasion.
  - These are local, mechanical, anatomic, and neurologic in their pattern of organized, coordinated involvement.

Features of tissue texture abnormalities, both acute and chronic, can be associated with the primary pain response of reactive nervous, immune, and endocrine systems.

The nervous system responds to pain/stress.

Tissue trauma, anticipated or perceived, elicits transduction, transmission, coordination, and activation of a system-wide adaptive response.

- When wounds occur and primary afferent nociceptors (PANs) are aroused, their signal activity increases, and they contribute to their own peripheral responsivity by producing peripheral neurogenic inflammation in concert with the immune system.
- These nociceptors and immune system elements show connectivity in the periphery, where they participate in the acute inflammatory reaction, a part of the acute phase reaction.
- Peripheral sensitization is the result, with additional neural contribution from the sympathetic-mediated peripheral effects.

Dorsal horn (central) sensitization refers to the lowered threshold and increased responsiveness, which occurs in secondary afferents from severe or protracted nociceptive stimulation by glutamate and NMDA receptor mechanisms.

- Inhibitory and excitatory influences from segmental, multisegmental, and descending mechanisms help determine the afferent sensitivity of ascending transmission.
- The sites of relay and response of the ascending neural message are central connections in the:
  - Thalamus
  - Hypothalamus
  - Locus coeruleus (LC)
  - Solitary nucleus (visceral)
  - Hippocampus
  - Amygdala
  - Periaqueductal gray (PAG)
  - Cerebellum
- Further projection to the insula and anterior cingulate cortex appears to represent convergent sites for affective (amygdala), motivational (LC), and primary sensory processing.
- Multiple sensory modalities are integrated and coordinated.
- Of course, the somatosensory cortex is activated. Descending influences may be inhibitory or excitatory.
- The presence of inadequate inhibition or excessive excitation can explain a circumstance in which chronic pain may develop.

In the alarm response, a stage of defensive arousal, the hypothalamus, amygdala (affective intensity), and PAG (negative affect, pain modulation) are engaged. They coordinate their sensory inputs with emotional content and cognitive meaning, with the goal of driving behaviors that favor survival. They connect with higher-order cortical structures and lower-order brainstem and subcortical elements to foster learning and ultimate mastery.

Emotional regulation (ER) is the ability to monitor and regulate one's own emotions. Beginning with gut feelings (interoception), then emotional labeling (limbic), leading to regulation of those emotions (prefrontal cortex), and finally leading to words and behavior.

- The nervous system's alarm response affects the endocrine system via the HPA axis and the SAM axis.
- The nervous system also affects the immune system.
  - The vagal nerves have an afferent role and an efferent role in mediating inflammatory responses by modulating cytokine levels. Vagal nerve afferent activity is necessary for interoceptive awareness.
- The nervous system affects the musculoskeletal system.
  - Acutely, in stress it shunts blood to the skeletal muscles and away from the viscera (sympathetic).
  - In recovery, it shifts to a resting state, decreasing skeletal muscle shunting, and becomes more supportive of visceral, vegetative processes (parasympathetic).

The endocrine system is seen to respond to stress in fast defensive arousal and in the slower process of recovery.

Hormones variably affect the nervous system.

- At the level of the LC, noradrenergic engagement occurs.
- Through the HPA, the hypothalamic periventricular nucleus, and the pituitary, adrenal effects are reinforced or restrained.
- Corticotrophin-releasing hormone (CRH), pro-opiomelanocortin, as a precursor for adrenocorticotrophic hormone (ACTH),

and glucocorticoids, are involved in a feedback-dependent response system. This affects adrenocortical behavior through glucocorticoid (cortisol) release.

- The LC, noradrenergic axis, affects adrenal medullary behavior through release of epinephrine, norepinephrine, and neuropeptide Y.
- Through the effects of CRH and its receptors CRH-1 and CRH-2, the endocrine system initiates defensive arousal and recovery, respectively.

The endocrine system affects the immune system through its effects on cytokines.

- HPA axis activation affects the cytokines differentially, at times encouraging inflammation, and other times encouraging recovery and resolution of inflammation.

The endocrine system also affects the musculoskeletal system.

- Through an activated sympathetic state of arousal, there is shunting of blood to the necessary fight or flight participants. This is the musculoskeletal system.

Other nested systems responding to stress include the visceral, arterial, venous, lymphatic, and respiratory/circulatory systems.

These nested systems are also intra-active and interactive.

- Their communication is via the holistic musculoskeletal, circulatory, and nervous systems.
- They share many of the same properties and demonstrate similar feedback and feed-forward modulation.
  - The feed-forward aspect allows the ability to mount a rapidly accelerating and amplified response when needed.
  - The feedback aspect is part of a process of deceleration that helps control the acute, defensive reactions and prevent their excesses.
- Excesses or deficiencies, in positive and negative feedback, create the potential for dysregulation. These dysregulatory mechanisms can also be related to the problem of chronic pain.
  - This can occur when the fast immediate arousal state does not yield to the slow response recovery phase, or when the response to the stressor fails to readjust to the normal level after the stress has passed.
  - Hypervigilance and hyperreactivity continue as the systems fail to hear the all-clear signal[25] and back off.
  - It can occur when the classic changes in cortisol and HPA axis regulation fail to occur.
  - Disturbances in the coordination of the elements involved in the MINE system can result in circumstances predisposing to chronic pain.

Chronic pain results from a sustained loss of a system's ability to function normally regarding its own self-regulation and/or its normal regulatory role interacting with other systems.

Impaired connectivity of the following can lead to pain system dysregulation:

- Neuromusculoskeletal system
- Autonomic nervous system
- The LC, the endocrine, HPA, and SMA axes
- Immune cytokines

Coordination of the MINE system is disrupted when the mechanisms of interaction are impaired. This can lead to an inadequate recovery. In this same vein, the system and its set points can be altered by experience such as seen in both post-traumatic stress disorder (PTSD)[30,33] and chronic pain.

Autonomic Dysregulation

Autonomic dysregulation is first manifested by loss of inter r-wave intervals on ECG.

- This electrophysiologic variable typically fluctuates in association with inhalation and exhalation (respiratory sinus arrhythmia).
- This heart rate variability (HRV) is modulated by the vagal nerve and reflects the balance of sympathetic and parasympathetic activity.
- Its presence is a sign of health and stress-managing capacity.
- Its absence is a sign of autonomic dysregulation and portends a lesser capacity to respond and recover from stress/pain.

Sensory Dysregulation

Sensory dysregulation can lead to chronic pain.

- Excessive facilitation, as in the phenomenon of wind-up, can lead to a sensitized state and chronic pain.
- Deficient inhibition at any level of the neural axis can lead to a chronic pain predisposition.

The Default Mode Network (DMN) dysregulation of Raichle shows changes in function and structural distribution of brain activity in patients with chronic pain compared to healthy controls.[33] The insula and somatosensory cortex (SSII) are more tightly connected to the DMN when there is pain. The anterior insula becomes more connected as the individual thinks of their pain, rates their pain, or when their pain increases.[37]

The neuroendocrine and biochemical systems, and their set point changes, contribute to the suffering and misery associated with chronic pain. It is as though these patients continue to experience the memory of pain and are unable to stop.

Endocrine Dysregulations

Endocrine dysregulations, as they affect the HPA axis and cortisol release, can be measured and correlated with diurnal fluctuations and in the response to dexamethasone suppression and/or corticotrophin stimulation.

- This informs the clinician as regards the inherent endocrine capacity to respond to stress.
- When disturbed, as in depression, it can lead to an increased incidence of dysregulation and chronic pain.

Immune System Dysregulation

Immune system dysregulation is exemplified in the complex relation of Th1, proinflammatory, and Th2, anti-inflammatory cytokines.

- Th1/Th2 ratios can be measured and can be quantified as a sign of dysregulation.
- Glucocorticoids and catecholamines can locally stimulate Th1 changes but globally have a Th2 effect.
- This suggests that they can promote local inflammation while maintaining generalized, opposing, anti-inflammatory effects.
- An inadequacy of Th1 response, as seen in the chronically stressed, may reflect a compromised ability to respond to stress.

A pattern of objective clinical signs[9] also emerges with dysregulation as the patient in chronic pain now reports:

- Sleep disturbance
- Decreased libido
- Irritability

- Depression
- Decreased activity level
- Deterioration in interpersonal relationships
- Change in work status
- Increased preoccupation with health and physical function

Over time, patients in chronic pain become hypervigilant to all incoming stimuli, their behavior regresses, and they demand pain control (including opiates) from the medical community at any cost. The environment around the patient in chronic pain also often reinforces these ongoing pain behaviors. The pain behaviors are expressed through the musculoskeletal system and are integrated into the patient's lifestyle.

> *Every aspect of human life is acted out by the body's muscles and joints*...These are the body parts that act together to transmit and modify force and motion...Everything man does to express his aspirations and convictions can be perceived by others only through his bearing and demeanor and utterances, and these are composites of myriads of finely controlled motions.
>
> —I. M. Korr (See "Korr's Explication of Osteopathic Principles" in Chapter 1 Philosophy of Osteopathic Medicine)[36]

The result is that chronic pain becomes the focal point of an individual's life. This leads to demoralization and suffering. The outcome of dysregulation is the refractory, enduring pain experience commonly referred to as the "chronic pain syndrome."

The person in pain expresses structural changes and functional disturbances, associated with their unique thoughts, feelings, and pain behaviors, through the musculoskeletal and visceral systems. Immunologic, neurologic, and endocrine systems are also continually responding to the moment-by-moment changes of the musculoskeletal system, in response to prolonged pain. It is inevitable that continuous, redundant pain has profound consequences on the patient's mind, body, and spirit.

An osteopathic model of pain goes beyond the biologic level of sensory modalities and neurologic transmissions to include dynamic interactions among and within the mind, body, spirit, and social environment to describe each patient's unique pain presentation.[38]

For the osteopathically trained physician, pain is more than sensation and perception (Fig. 74.3). It is fundamentally recognized that nociception sets in motion a conscious and unconscious awareness of discomfort, thoughts, emotions, and dysregulation of the MINE systems, which are displayed throughout the musculoskeletal system.

- Over time, the social environment (i.e., family, culture, work, etc.) responds to the pain, suffering, and system dysregulation to further shape and reinforce each unique and highly individualized aspect of the individual's pain presentation.[39,40]
- This model, which builds on the biopsychosocial model[41] and Loeser's conceptual model of pain,[42] emphasizes the critical role of system dysregulation.[31]
- More importantly, it recognizes the central role of the neuromusculoskeletal system that is ultimately involved in all pathophysiologic processes, regardless of where or how they originate.

OSTEOPATHIC ASSESSMENT OF CHRONIC PAIN IS DYNAMIC, PATIENT FOCUSED, AND COMPREHENSIVE

For both assessment and reassessment of the pain management plan and review of the patients' pain scores and functional capacities,[43–45] osteopathic evaluation includes a complete:

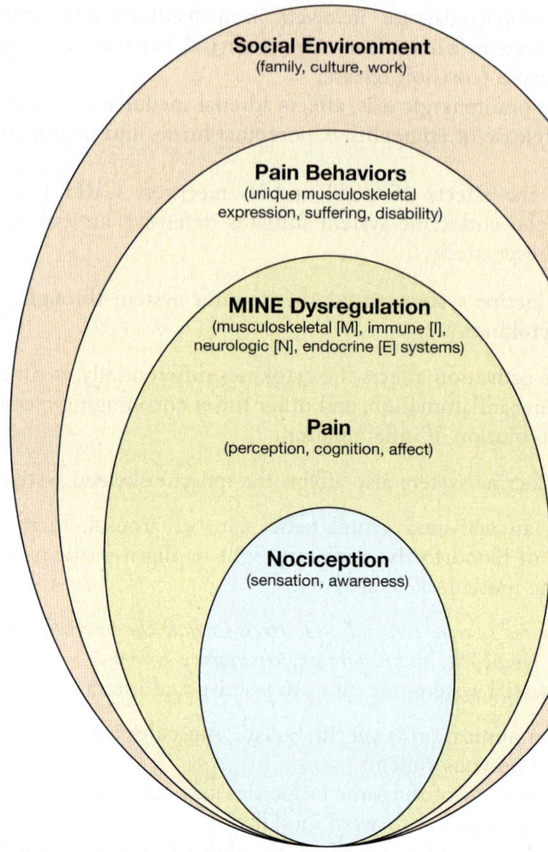

Figure 74.3. Osteopathic model of pain.

- Biopsychosocial history
- Physical examination
- Osteopathic structural examination
- Neurologic examination
- Follow-up visits
- Imaging/testing (Table 74.2)

The osteopathic physician recognizes that the palpatory examination provides clues to the underlying pain generators.

- Pain generators may be confirmed by an effective therapeutic response, even temporarily, to manual correction through osteopathic manipulative treatment (OMT): "somatic dysfunction may be causative, reflective, reactive or perpetuating, or a combination."[43]
- Osteopathic thinking requires more than assessing somatic dysfunction and relying on pain intensity scores.
- Comprehensive osteopathic assessment and care for patients with chronic pain considers:
  - □ Patient's moods
  - □ Patient's beliefs about pain
  - □ Patient's coping efforts
  - □ Patient's biopsychosocial resources[40]
  - □ Response of the family members
  - □ The impact of pain on the patient's functional quality of life (QOL)

> *The patient reporting the pain must be evaluated, not just the pain.*[40]

The general medical history holds many keys to understanding chronic pain. The past medical history includes a childhood and early life history, a history of previous or current medical

TABLE 74.2

Investigations to Support History and Physical Examination

Categories of Tests	Examples of Tests
Psychometric testing	Formal neuropsychologic evaluation, MPQ
Diagnostic imaging	X-ray, computerized tomography (CT), MRI
Functional diagnostic imaging	Isotope scan, PET, blood oxygen level–dependent MRI (BOLD-MRI), fluoro-deoxyglucose-PET (FDG-PET), O2-PET, ultrasound (US)
Neurophysiologic testing	Electroencephalography (EEG), MEG, electromyography (EMG), nerve conduction velocity (NCV), evoked potentials (EP), quantitative sensory testing, vibration threshold
Fluid testing (serology)	Blood, urine, feces, cerebrospinal fluid (CSF)
Tissue testing (histology)	Nerve biopsy, tissue biopsy
Cellular testing (cytology)	Morphology, function, energy, transformation
Molecular testing	Immunologic, hormonal, neurotransmitters
Genetic testing	HLA testing, inherited disorders
Diagnostic anesthetic blockade	Nerve blocks, facet blocks, epidural blocks

conditions, trauma, and abuse.[33,46] Of particular importance is a history of dysregulations of the MINE system, the:

- Musculoskeletal system
- Immunologic system
- Nervous system
- Endocrine system

Active listening is essential for both understanding pain and developing trust.

Chronic pain management begins with careful listening and observations, is followed by a physician-guided examination, and is completed with a review of the historical record. The patient is seen as a whole person affected within many spheres of influence. The patient has sought help from the physician because their sense of health and well-being is challenged. There is hurt. What has been tried for pain relief has failed. Fear of the worst outcome, or fear that the physician will not find anything physically wrong to account for the pain and state "the pain is in your head," becomes overwhelming.

As a physician, remember to deliver this simple message:

> "I know you have pain. I believe that your pain is real. I want to know all about you and the pain you are experiencing. I will treat your pain in parallel with the necessary investigations to exclude serious underlying pathology. The goal is to identify the reasons for the pain, to restore function, and to reduce your pain to the lowest possible level."

A common mnemonic of OPQRST (onset, pain, quality, radiation, severity, temporal) is a good starting point for the focused pain history.

Pain

The most frequently used pain assessments are single-item verbal rating scales with 0 being "no pain" and 10 being "unbearable pain." These assessments rely on patients' self-reported experience of pain intensity or unpleasantness. A great deal of information is available about the psychometric qualities and properties of single-item, numeric, rating scales. A systematic review of clinical and randomized controlled clinical trials shows them to be reliable and valid.[47]

In addition to pain scores' intensity, multidimensional measurements of affective response, coping, function, QOL, and analgesic use allow a more comprehensive approach to measuring pain and function.[45,48] These measures are designed to assess:

- Ability to engage in functional activities such as walking, sitting, lifting, and performing ADL
- An overall sense of satisfaction
- QOL

Quality

What does the pain feel like? Is it throbbing with your heartbeat, is it a steady pressure, is it a dull ache, or it is sharp like an ice pick stabbing?

One of the most frequently used pain assessment instruments is the McGill Pain Questionnaire (MPQ).[49–51] This instrument has three parts:

1. A descriptive scale (pain intensity)
2. A front and back of a drawing, of a human figure, on which patients indicate the location of their pain.
3. A pain-rating index based on patient selection of adjectives from 20 categories of words reflecting sensory, affective, and cognitive components of pain.

The MPQ provides a great deal of information in less than 5 minutes (Fig. 74.4) with good test/retest reliability.[52,53]

Radiation

Where is the pain, and to where does it travel or refer? (See pain drawing on MPQ.) Look for dermatomal patterns, peripheral nerve distribution patterns, or CNS patterns.

Severity (Intensity)

How bad it is; sometimes the pain intensity score and behavioral observations can be corroborating or contradictory (i.e., 10/10 but the patient looks comfortable, or 2/10 and looks dreadful).

Pain Intensity and Duration

Another useful clinical parameter of pain assessment is a pain intensity–time curve. These can be graphed. Basically, over a 24-hour period, how does the pain wax and wane? This line of questioning can be valuable. For example:

- A subarachnoid hemorrhage is likely to produce severe pain rapidly.
- Meningitis may take hours or days to reach maximum intensity.
- A muscle tension headache patient may describe maximal pain continuously over days, weeks, and months.

It is useful to understand and classify pain by its intensity and persistence over time. This can lead to differential diagnoses based on differential anatomy, physiology, and pathology (Table 74.3).

McGILL PAIN QUESTIONNAIRE

PATIENT'S NAME ____ DATE ____ TIME ____ AM/PM

PRI: S ____ A ____ E ____ M ____ PRI(T) ____ PPI ____
(1-10) (11-15) (16) (17-20) (1-20)

1 FLICKERING ___
QUIVERING ___
PULSING ___
THROBBING ___
BEATING ___
POUNDING ___

2 JUMPING ___
FLASHING ___
SHOOTING ___

3 PRICKING ___
BORING ___
DRILLING ___
STABBING ___
LANCINATING ___

4 SHARP ___
CUTTING ___
LACERATING ___

5 PINCHING ___
PRESSING ___
GNAWING ___
CRAMPING ___
CRUSHING ___

6 TUGGING ___
PULLING ___
WRENCHING ___

7 HOT ___
BURNING ___
SCALDING ___
SEARING ___

8 TINGLING ___
ITCHY ___
SMARTING ___
STINGING ___

9 DULL ___
SORE ___
HURTING ___
ACHING ___
HEAVY ___

10 TENDER ___
TAUT ___
RASPING ___
SPLITTING ___

11 TIRING ___
EXHAUSTING ___

12 SICKENING ___
SUFFOCATING ___

13 FEARFUL ___
FRIGHTFUL ___
TERRIFYING ___

14 PUNISHING ___
GRUELLING ___
CRUEL ___
VISCIOUS ___
KILLING ___

15 WRETCHED ___
BLINDING ___

16 ANNOYING ___
TROUBLESOME ___
MISERABLE ___
INTENSE ___
UNBEARABLE ___

17 SPREADING ___
RADIATING ___
PENETRATING ___
PIERCING ___

18 TIGHT ___
NUMB ___
DRAWING ___
SQUEEZING ___
TEARING ___

19 COOL ___
COLD ___
FREEZING ___

20 NAGGING ___
NAUSEATING ___
AGONIZING ___
DREADFUL ___
TORTURING ___

PPI
0 NO PAIN
1 MILD
2 DISCOMFORTING
3 DISTRESSING
4 HORRIBLE
5 EXCRUCIATING

BRIEF ___	RHYTHMIC ___	CONTINUOUS ___
MOMENTARY ___	PERIODIC ___	STEADY ___
TRANSIENT ___	INTERMITTENT ___	CONSTANT ___

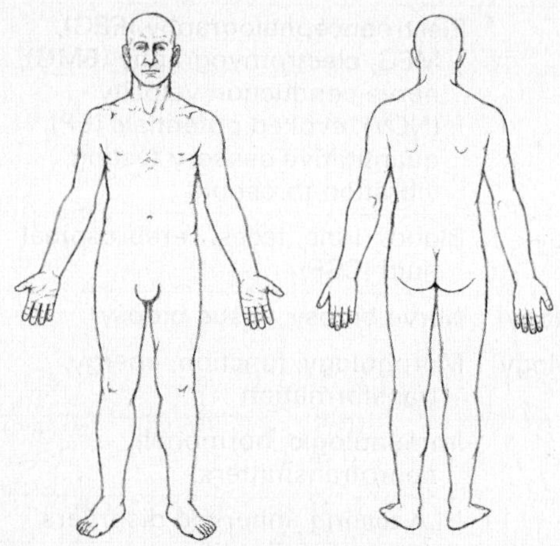

E = EXTERNAL
I = INTERNAL

COMMENTS:

The descriptors fall into four major groups: sensory, 1 to 10; affective, 11 to 15; evaluative, 16; and miscellaneous, 17 to 20. The rank value for each descriptor is based on its position in the word set. The sum ofthe rank values is the pain rating index (PRI). The present pain intensity (PPI) is based on a scale of 0 to 5.

Figure 74.4. McGill Pain Questionnaire.

TABLE 74.3

Assessment/Diagnosis: Temporally Defined

Temporal Character	Clinical Examples
Acute	Trauma, illness
Acute, recurring	Migraine
Subacute	Longer-lasting insult or time to resolution
Chronic	LBP, neck pain, daily headache, fibromyalgia, irritable bowel syndrome
Chronic, progressive	Malignancy, degenerative, inflammatory
Chronic with acute recurrences	Spondylosis

THE BEHAVIORAL MODEL

The patient is queried regarding the impact of pain on affective state and functional capacities.

What is the mood?

- Is it depressed, anxious, angry, or fearful?
- What is the history of these feelings?
- To what degree and in what ways is the patient suffering?

What is the impact on their cognitive state? (Use pain-coping skills)

- What is their self-image, and how has it been affected by pain?

What is the impact on the patient's ADL?

- Is there an ability to eat, dress, wash, and toilet?
- Is there an ability to do the shopping, cooking, and cleaning?
- Is there an ability to work?
- Is the patient completely unable to work, or have a limited ability to work?
- Is the patient using disability insurance income or seeking to be classified as disabled?
- Is disability insurance income activated?
- Has there been an effect on mobility?
- Is there an ability to walk, bend, stand, sit, or lie without pain?
- Is there an ability to exercise?
- What is the prepain activity or exercise level, and has it changed because of the pain?
- Has the pain affected self-esteem or personal feelings?
- How has the pain affected diet and nutrition?
- Has there been a loss of appetite?
- Has the pain affected the availability of healthy food choices, or are there physical impediments to eating?
- Lifestyle changes and high-risk choices such as increased alcohol use, substance use, lack of exercise, and comfort eating are other important factors.

How is sleep?

- Is there insomnia? (i.e., trouble falling asleep, staying asleep, staying awake, or getting enough rest?)
- Is sleep restorative? (i.e., does it provide a feeling of being refreshed upon awakening?)

What is the impact on family life?

- How have family dynamics and interpersonal relationships been affected?
- Is there a family history that is relevant?
- Are there family members with autoimmune, migraine, degenerative disk disease, connective tissue disease, substance abuse, or other abuses?
- Who are the caregivers?

What is the impact on the community?

- Has there been a change in the patient's role in the community?
- Does the patient derive caregiving from the community?
- What is the cultural stigma or stereotype associated with admitting, showing, or seeking treatment for pain?

What are the economic implications of the pain?

- Is the patient missing work, losing wages, receiving, or seeking disability payments?
- What is the degree of health care utilization?
- Is the patient seeking medicolegal redress?

What are the environmental stressors?
Is there:

- Poverty?
- Malnutrition?
- Dysfunctional living circumstances?
- Toxic exposure?
- Substance abuse?
- High-risk behavior?

Ultimately, the behavioral model assesses the pain and its impact on the patient's *QOL*.

Osteopathic Physical Examination

The osteopathic physician is uniquely trained to evaluate the musculoskeletal system. Through observation, palpation, and motion testing, key information is gathered. The neurologic/musculoskeletal system is known as reflector and effector of the entire organism and all its systems. The combination of this information with the general physical exam and appropriate evidence-based test results provides the osteopathic physician with a comprehensive data set. This allows for a complete biopsychosocial evaluation of:

- Pain
- Physical functioning
- System dysregulations
- Adaptive response patterns

The osteopathic physical examination is patient-focused and solution-oriented. It can allow a connection to the patient, otherwise unavailable. The musculoskeletal system is not just for securing a diagnosis. It provides an avenue for treatment that can target the nociceptors, the pain experience, the suffering, and the pain behaviors. Armed with the knowledge of anatomy, physiology, and pathologic physiology, a dynamic, interactive, systems analysis can be made. Specific diagnostic considerations include the following:

- Ongoing tissue injury
- Effects of neurologic processing
- Presence and degree of suffering
- Cognitive and affective disruptions
- Musculoskeletal manifestations
- Premorbid, and subsequent, adaptive responses

The diagnostic systems analysis will typically describe multiple axes of dysfunction. This leads directly to an integrated diagnostic assessment and a proactive treatment plan.

TABLE 74.4

Assessment/Diagnosis: Location Defined

Anatomic Location	Clinical Examples
Visceral	Liver, lung
Vascular	Large vessel, small vessel
Muscular	Muscle, myofascial pain syndrome
Skeletal	Bone, joint, capsule, ligament, tendon
Nervous system	Cortical, thalamic, brainstem, spinal cord, peripheral nerve, autonomic nervous system
Other	Skin, eyes, ears, nose, mouth

Biomechanical/Musculoskeletal Examination

The formal biomechanical/musculoskeletal examination is integral and distinctive to osteopathic medicine.

- Besides the obvious orthopedic aspects of the examination, the characteristic evaluation for static structural asymmetry, tissue texture abnormalities, and restriction of motion has become an integral part of the osteopathic examination.
  - Static asymmetry looks at posture, spinal curvature, and limb asymmetry.
  - Tissue texture abnormalities and motion restrictions can be examined in local, regional, and even global fashion.
- In this part of the examination, it is important to be mindful of what the patient's major pain complaints might be.
  - Be sure to examine where it hurts.
  - How does it look, how does it feel, how does it move?
  - Knowing exactly where it hurts also suggests any number of associated mechanical, anatomical, and neurologic associations, visceral and somatic, that can augment the biomechanical examination and its contribution to a comprehensive diagnosis (Table 74.4).
- Patients in pain are sometimes not touched by their doctors.
  - Sometimes, their painful areas are not directly examined and, as a result, their complaints are not fully understood, and the physician's formulations are not believed.

THE NEUROLOGIC MODEL

The neurologic examination is particularly relevant in evaluating patients in pain. This is designed to ferret out those patients with irritation of a previously healthy nervous system from those with disorders of the nervous system that might be predisposing to painful states.

Always when evaluating the holistic nervous system, both peripheral, central, and autonomic the questions to be answered are:

1. Is there something wrong?
2. Where is it localized?
3. What is causing it?

It begins with an evaluation of the patient's level of arousal and content of consciousness.

- Is the patient bright and alert, or are they dull and sluggish?
- Is the patient making sense?
- Is the patient demanding, delirious, demented, or encephalopathic?
- Is the mood appropriate to the complaints?

Particular attention to the cranial nerves is obviously appropriate in pain complaints of the head, face, and the special sensory organs. The eyes, ears, nose, and mouth are known to be richly innervated and very sensitive. The following are all evaluable:

- Smell
- Sight
- Eye movements
- Facial strength
- Facial sensation
- Hearing
- Taste
- Speech
- Swallowing

Sensory Examination

Sensory testing is designed to evaluate the peripheral nerves, spinothalamic, and dorsal column pathways, from their peripheral elements to their central pathways and connections. Further testing is aimed at evaluating cortical and subcortical components of sensory processing. Obviously, in pain conditions, sensory processing is hugely relevant. An attempt to recognize a pattern of sensory dysfunction is sought.

- Is there altered sensation in the territory of a peripheral nerve, or is it the territory of a nerve root with dermatomal features?
- Do the small fibers that respond to pinprick and temperature react differently than the larger fibers that respond to touch, vibration, and proprioception? Sometimes, this can point to a disorder of the peripheral nerves such as a small fiber neuropathy. These conditions are known to have an association with peripheral neuropathic pain.
- Is there a sensory level suggestive of a spinal cord etiology?
- Is there a hemi somatic distribution of sensory changes suggesting a central source?
- Are there dissociations of sensory deficits?
  - For example, is there loss of pain and temperature with preservation of touch as in syringomyelia?
  - Is there loss of pain and temperature on one side of the body with loss of touch on the other as in hemi section lesions of the spinal cord?
  - Are there deficits in touch and proprioception with sparing of pinprick sensation, as in dorsal column disorders such as vitamin B_{12} deficiency or multiple sclerosis?
  - Does the sensory loss include the face on one side and the arm and leg on the other side, suggestive of brainstem pathology?
  - Does the sensory loss involve the face, arm, and leg on the same side, suggesting a disorder at the level of the thalamus or sensory cortex?
  - These central lesions have long been known to be the cause of central pain syndromes, such as thalamic pain syndrome or parietal pain syndrome. Whether from cerebral infarction, neoplasm, trauma, or demyelinating disease, they can represent vexing conditions to manage.

Armed with a pin, tuning fork, and a wisp of cotton, the sensory evaluation is pursued. Not just patterned disturbances are relevant. Sometimes, the patients' responses themselves are illuminating.

- Is there evidence of allodynia, hyperpathia, or hyperalgesia indicating unusual sensitivity to stimuli?
- Is there evidence of sensory loss in areas that are reported as painful, so-called, anesthesia dolorosa?

- Is there pain in parts that are no longer there, as in phantom pain syndrome?
- Are there dissociations between the ability to feel and localize painful stimuli and the ability to manifest appropriate affect or cognitive correlates? This can be seen in some cerebral hemispheric disorders.

It is particularly important to assess the sensory status in the area or areas of complaint.

- Is it normal or abnormal?
- If abnormal, is there greater or lesser sensitivity?
- Is there indifference?
- If the sensory exam is abnormal, do the sensory findings correlate with the pain in some way?
- Is there a pattern of sensory loss, suggesting a neurologic localization?

Motor Examination

The motor examination begins with a casual examination as the patient walks into the physician's office, moves about the examination room, describes their pain problem, and participates in the examination process, passively and actively.

- Because pain is at least part of the problem, pay particular attention toward the patient's signs of protective behaviors, such as limping or hobbling.
- Look for and document signs of suffering, such as grimacing, moaning, or crying.
- Sad, anxious, and angry affective behaviors are part of the casual motor examination, as are observations of the cognitive behavioral manifestations, like resigned, slumped shouldered, head drooped, slow-moving postural adjustments.
- This is an important opportunity to broaden the osteopathic impressions regarding the entirety of the burden that has befallen the patient.

The formal testing of the motor system includes passive tests of motor tone looking for flaccidity, spasticity, or rigidity, as well as atrophy, or fasciculations. In patients with pain, there may be guarding, which must be considered. Likewise, in active testing of strength, pain may limit effort or willingness to exert a particular action or many different actions. This is best recorded as pain-limited strength testing. Testing for strength can be done both regionally and locally. So, while testing general arm and leg raising, grip, and toe wiggle may be enough for a screening exam; sometimes a meticulous muscle-by-muscle, limb-by-limb, and trunk exam must be conducted, particularly, if there are pain complaints, associated with symptoms of weakness, cramping, spasms that can be localized. In those cases, the more thorough version of motor examination is mandated.

Furthering the motor examination requires tests of the reflexive properties of the body, which include the segmental, monosynaptic myotatic reflexes.

- These tendon reflexes can be obtained from most myotendinous junctions but are usually tested at elbow, wrist, hand, knee, and ankle.
- Their hypo- or hyperreactivity must be ascertained.
- Is there a pattern to the reflex and motor findings?
- Is there a problem in the muscles generally with proximal weakness and normal reflexes?
- Is there distal weakness and reflex loss due to neuropathy?
- Is there weakness in one side of the body involving the leg, arm, and face with hyperactive reflexes on that same side suggesting a CNS disorder?

Some reflexes are usually not present in adults and are considered pathologic when present.

- Plantar responses that are extensor (Babinski sign) and thumbs that flex with middle finger flicking (Hoffman sign) are signs of upper motor neuron deficiency.
- Palms that grasp when stroked, chins that twitch when the palm is stroked, loss of extinction to glabellar tapping, rooting, and sucking signs are generally hemispheric deficiency signs.

Somewhere, the physician should also be collating this information with what was already obtained in the mental, cranial nerve, and sensory exams.

Cerebellar/Motor Examination

The cerebellar testing includes an assessment of:

1. Gait and posture
2. Coordination
3. Balance

The cerebellum has a great capacity for learning and remembering. Mostly what it learns is how to balance and move. In general, signs of imbalance are in the body proper but may include affect and cognition.

Balance is what is sought when we are seeking health.

- The patient stands, walks, eyes open, eyes closed, along an imaginary tightrope.
- The patient is instructed to stand on one leg, or touch one finger at a time first to the tip of the nose and then to the tip of the physician's finger at a distance of the length of the patient's outstretched arm as the physician moves the finger into four distinct quadrants, and/or to sit and move one heel downward along the other leg from the knee to the ankle without removing it from the surface of the leg.
- Rapidly alternating motions can be tested, including finger and foot tapping.
- The qualities of speech and eye movements are also assessed.

Eighty percent of the neurons of the CNS are in the cerebellum, which occupies only 10% of its volume. It has a prominent role in the nervous system's contribution to health or disease. Its activities are, for the most part, not consciously appreciated. It is becoming clear that the cerebellum is involved in all manners of dysfunctions, including pain, somatic dysfunction, affective, and executive dysfunction.[54]

AUTONOMIC MODEL

Autonomic testing has largely been performed earlier in the examination. The following are likely noted by now:

- Heart rate
- Respiratory rate
- Blood pressure
- State of the pupils
- Tears and saliva
- Color and temperature of the limbs
- Associated sudomotor activity
- Sweaty and clammy features

The presence of "goose flesh" due to piloerection or skin mottling has already been observed during the general physical, but here is reformulated in the context of overall autonomic behavior.

- Is the pattern sympathetic driven, sympathetic exhausted, or parasympathetic in nature?
- Is it generalized or regional?

The evaluation of the skin provides the most external opportunity for evaluation and can lead to important observations about regional, dermatomal, or local problems. For the skin to be adequately examined, the patient needs to be gowned and draped, and consent obtained prior to examination.

- The tuft of hair over the midline lower back may overlie a neural tube closure defect like a spina bifida.
- The blistered rash over a single dermatome can be the presentation of herpes zoster or shingles.

The fascial system, another of the body's holistic systems, is an organizing tissue like no other.

- It is continuous from top to bottom, front to back, inside to outside.
- It invests every tissue type, from its outermost coverings to its deepest cellular structures.
- In its investments, it is found to be continuous.
- Current research has now revealed intracellular and intercellular linkage through this same fascial system.
    - Connective tissue, collagen, integrins, cytoskeletons are the levels of scale in which the reiterated properties of mesodermal derivatives serve as a principal organizer for the multitude of the body's structures and functions.
- As a mechanical force transducer, a mechanical force transmitter, and an effector tissue, the fascial system impacts immunologic, neurologic, endocrinologic, and, of course, musculoskeletal functions and structures.
- Many of its functions will be discussed elsewhere, but its evaluation of patients suffering pain can be uniquely rewarding.
    - It can reveal biomechanical linkages between internal and external structures as well as information regarding the patient's unique constellation of painful parts.

THE RESPIRATORY/CIRCULATORY MODEL

The respiratory/circulatory testing demands a thorough examination of both the cellular and the whole-body adequacy of oxygen, blood, lymph, interstitial fluid, and cerebrospinal fluid dynamics.

- Good health requires the maintenance of adequate arterial, venous, lymphatic, cerebrospinal, and interstitial fluid dynamics.
- The cardiovascular exam evaluates the very essence of circulatory function, from the pump to the pipes.
- Every region must be considered for the adequacy of its blood supply and the health of its components.
    - Is there leg pain from claudication?
    - Is it due to peripheral vascular disease?
    - Is it due to neurogenic claudication, because of spinal stenosis?

The "rule of the artery" must always be considered. This is one of the holistic systems of the body that reaches every single cell and influences every single function.

- Is their head pain associated with an indurated, tender superficial temporal artery?
- Is their acute LBP associated with an abdominal bruit and loss of pedal pulses?

In some texts, the respiratory system is considered as part of a cardiorespiratory system. But it merits its own consideration as another of the holistic systems of the body.

- The adequacy of breath, and the dependence on adequate oxygenation, again, can be seen to affect every organ, every system, every cell, and cellular function.
- The examination considers the patients' color, their respiratory effort and capacity, as well as its adequacy.
- Signs of chronic insufficiency like clubbing of the fingers raise concerns about more widespread problems.
- Ultimately, the adequacy of the cardiorespiratory system is vital to the essential well-being of the individual.

In managing pain, optimization of respiratory and circulatory structure and function is critical.

- Of course, this involves auscultation, palpation, and observation of the thoracic space.
- Examination of the heart, lungs, lymphatic structures, great and small vessels, diaphragm, and thoracic inlet comprise the test.

There are palpable reactions of the musculoskeletal system to stress/pain.

Touching the patient's pain is more than a euphemism. It is an experience for doctors and patients alike (see Chapter 9 The Physiology of Touch).

- It is an opportunity to validate a patient-centered subjective experience with more objective physical data.
- A physician will always feel more confident in diagnosis when the patient's symptoms are reproducible. This is not always possible even with a meticulous and comprehensive examination. Sometimes, the examination process is straightforward; other times, it remains elusive.
- Patients feel better understood when examined and touched in ways that inform the physician regarding the nature of the pain.

Understanding the generators and mechanisms of a painful process enhances the therapeutic options. Therefore, understanding what actions exacerbate or initiate the pain is essential.

- Ask the patient to demonstrate the behaviors, positions, movements, and activities that influence the pain.
- Pay attention to what worsens and what improves the symptoms.

At some point in the examination, if it has not already occurred, provocative testing is pursued. This means attempting to reproduce or aggravate the pain.

- If the clinical scenario suggests nerve root compression, then intervertebral foraminal compression with vertebral side bending and extension may exacerbate the nerve root symptoms.
- A straight leg raising test that causes pain to radiate down the leg suggests nerve/nerve root entrapment that is affected by the neurofascial stretch.
- Compression or traction on peripheral nerves that reproduces symptoms can be diagnostic of conditions like:
    - Thoracic outlet syndrome
    - Carpal tunnel syndrome
    - Cubital tunnel syndrome
    - Tarsal tunnel syndrome
    - Piriformis syndrome
- Skeletal percussion can help identify a bony source of pain, such as fracture or metastasis.
- Visceral palpation can identify a visceral source of pain.

Palpation of the myofascial system, systematically seeking tender points, can reveal:

- The trigger points of myofascial pain syndrome
- Chapman's points of neurolymphatic dysfunction

- The muscles, tendons, ligaments, skeletal, and connective tissue generators of pain

At times, the relationship between the tender points and the pain complaint is obvious. The patient sprained an ankle, and the talofibular ligament is tender. Other times it is less obvious; the appendix is inflamed, and the abdominal wall is tender. The relationship between the tender places and the pain complaints is usually related to their segmental, autonomic, and central relations.

The pattern of tenderness may reveal patterns of musculoskeletal involvement that involve multiple structures. This pattern can be analyzed to reveal whole-body patterns of myofascial strain and trauma.

- It provides an opportunity to correlate the patterns of dysfunction with the biomechanical/musculoskeletal behaviors of origin.
- Such analysis can reveal the somatic and visceral traumatic vectors underlying the strain.

Even more important than the attempts to increase pain are the efforts to reduce pain.

- Besides asking the patient to demonstrate what helps relieve their pain, maneuvers such as distraction or compression are performed.
- Attention to the functional anatomy and neurology of the maneuvers can reveal keys to diagnosis as well as treatment.
- OMT, as will be described in greater detail in this text, is the osteopathic approach to this process.
  - For example, the confirmation of a cervical origin to a headache by relieving it using manual cervical distraction provides useful diagnostic information.
  - In addition, it provides critical understanding that can be translated into therapeutic strategy.

BEHAVIORAL MODEL

The psychological examination has been ongoing and largely completed by now.

- Has the patient been anxious, tense, fearful, angry, worried, or depressed?
- Is there catastrophizing[55] about the pain? (i.e., Does the patient dramatically express the pain in terms of a catastrophic event?)
- Is the belief in the pain so firmly maintained as to disagree with logic or rational argument?[56]
- Does the patient express fear of pain or movement (i.e., kinesiophobia)[57] and avoid activity?

Patients who catastrophically (mis)interpret the pain are prone to become fearful and consequently engage in protection (e.g., escape/avoidance) behaviors, such as guarding and resting.

- Paradoxically, these behaviors will increase pain and pain disability rather than reducing them.[58]
- There are many patients with musculoskeletal pain who avoid physical activities unnecessarily because of the fear that movement can be harmful.
- As a result of inactivity and withdrawing, the patient may feel helpless, have little initiative to comply, and become clinically depressed.[59]

Pain sets in a still joint. Depression sets in a still person.

Motion is a basic function of life. In fact, prolonged bed rest is no longer recommended for the management of LBP; it is ineffective and may even delay recovery. Recent guidelines encourage the patient to continue to stay active, continue ordinary activities, and work as normal, as this leads to faster recovery and lower risk of chronic pain and disability.[45,48]

The osteopathic physician remembers that pain is a complex, subjective perceptual phenomenon with intensity, quality, time course, personal impact, and meaning—"That you assess the person, not just see the pain."[60,61]

- Persons experiencing nociception display a large range of reactions that are indicative of pain, distress, fear, anger, depression, and/or suffering.
- Their autonomic arousal, muscle tension, endocrine, immune, and neurologic reactions add to the pain behaviors.
- Pain behaviors further develop and change through learning and are molded by past painful experiences.[62,63]

It is important not to mistake these pain behaviors as being synonymous with malingering. Malingering is a conscious purposeful effort to defraud and fake symptoms of pain for financial and/or emotional gain. In many cases, chronic pain behaviors do not automatically correlate with conscious deception, but rather they are behaviors that are unintended and result either from unrelieved pain or environmental reinforcement. Most patients who display pain behaviors are not aware of them nor are they consciously motivated to obtain reinforcements from others. There is little support for the contention of outright faking of pain or that the process of malingering is widespread.[60]

FORMULATION AND EXECUTION OF OSTEOPATHIC PAIN MANAGEMENT

Proper therapy depends upon a proper diagnosis.

- The diagnostic process is multivariate, and it is reasonable to conclude that therapeutic plans are best conceived as offering benefit at multiple levels.
- The diagnosis must include relevant medical diagnoses, including medical, affective, cognitive, and behavioral comorbidities.
- It must include an understanding of the involved nociceptive mechanisms, peripheral and central.
- Finally, the diagnosis must include an understanding of the biopsychosocial impact on the patients' function and QOL.
- Our targets, therefore, are the peripheral, spinal, and forebrain structures and their functions. They include the MINE systems.
- Additional targets include:
  - Comorbidities
  - Psychiatric
  - Social
  - Behavioral
  - Medical
- In all patients, with or without chronic pain, general advice is offered regarding:
  - Proper nutrition
  - Levels of activity and exercise
  - Sleep and rest
  - The importance of creating and maintaining thoughts of wellness[64]

The Osteopathic Pain Management Plan Is Evidence Based and Comprehensive

Osteopathic treatment decisions are based on systematic reviews and evidence-based considerations (Table 74.5).[65]

TABLE 74.5

Pain-Related Behavior Management

Type of Intervention	Clinical Examples
OMT	Direct, indirect
Meditation	Mindfulness meditation, self-hypnosis, Tai Chi
Visual imagery	Guided, self-guided. Distraction and visualization training
Behavioral therapies	Functional recovery programs (Fordyce), operant conditioning, interdisciplinary pain programs
Exercise	Healthy activity, prescribed stretch, strengthening, endurance, balance training

- Their therapeutic prescription, after reviewing all the evidence on nonpharmacologic therapies for chronic pain (>4 weeks duration) when compared to placebo, sham, or no treatment, found *good evidence* for:
  - Spinal manipulation
  - Exercise
  - Cognitive behavioral therapy
  - Interdisciplinary rehabilitation
- The only nonpharmacologic therapies with *fair-to-good evidence* of efficacy for acute pain (<4 weeks duration) are superficial heat and spinal manipulation.[66]
- Cold therapy has been used regularly as an immediate treatment to induce analgesia and decrease swelling following acute soft tissue injuries, however, there is still controversy in the literature of its beneficial effects. Randomized controlled trials (RCTs) with good methodologic quality are still needed in the future to evaluate the effects of different cryotherapy modalities.[67]
- The choice and sequencing of these therapies and the methods of tailoring therapy to the unique individual patient is the true art of osteopathic care.

The therapeutic plan is aimed at removing noxious influences, at any level or location. Concurrently, efforts at optimizing structure and function are the objective goals for moving toward health. The inherent vitality and capacity for wellness of the patient is the focus of therapy. From the molecular, cellular, systemic, and regional perspectives, therapeutic strategies are conceived.

- They are often stratified.
- First, the physician will try treatment A and, if not successful, will change to treatment B.
- They are typically multifaceted.
- Sometimes, they are additive and even synergistic, that is, treatments A and B are given together.
- In this way, they represent a microcosmic, multidisciplinary, therapeutic plan.
- Of course, in some situations, multiple different healthcare providers are involved in delivering and coordinating the plan.
- This represents the true interdisciplinary therapeutic team.

In some cases, there is clear synergy of therapies. The total amount of therapeutic efficacy is greater than the sum of the individual therapeutic efforts. Likewise, the idea that interdisciplinary management can offer synergistic therapeutic opportunities has led to the creation of interdisciplinary pain management centers treating both pain and disability. This is often not understood by third-party payers.

The osteopathic mission through both OMT and the doctor–patient relationship is to restore postural and mechanical alignments and manage myofascial strain, to encourage the patient's innate ability to heal.[65,68] Osteopathic thinking has long considered pain as a symptom closely linked to biopsychosocial factors and somatic dysfunction.

In addition to neuromuscular factors triggering nociception and the initial report of pain, biopsychosocial factors often worsen and perpetuate the pain experience.

- Osteopathic physicians need to approach patients in chronic pain with support and empathy while drawing heavily from the expertise and communication skills of their pain specialist colleagues.
- Caring for chronic pain often warrants an interdisciplinary approach, blending osteopathic thinking, and the best evidence-based knowledge about biopsychosocial treatments.[69,70]
- The goal is to assist the patient's internal healing and their ability to mount an allostatic response. Each therapeutic prescription needs to be individualized.

Biopsychosocial Interventions Decrease Suffering

Much of the disabling nature of chronic pain thus stems from cognitive and affective factors and cannot be fully explained by objective physical measures alone (Table 74.6).[71,72] Osteopathic interventions are biopsychosocial, and they target nociception in an attempt to decrease distress and increase functioning (Table 74.7).[61]

Four systematic reviews[73–76] and a meta-analysis[77] of RCTs of specific measurement domains such as pain expression, functional activity level, health related QOL, and depression substantiate the critical need for treating the psychological factors of chronic pain.

- Specifically, these RCTs showed cognitive–behavioral treatments (Table 74.8) were moderately superior to no treatment, placebo, and wait-list controls.
- Positive effects of psychological interventions when compared to these various control groups were noted for pain intensity, pain-related interference, health-related QOL, and depression.

TABLE 74.6

Psychological Factors that Interfere with Pain Relief

Number of failed surgeries
Length of pain duration
History of smoking/alcohol overuse/medication failures/substance abuse
Job dissatisfaction/disability payments
Unhealthy food choices/obesity
Stress, anxiety, depression, fear, or panic associated with pain
Personality disorders, hypervigilance, somatization
Catastrophic misinterpretations of bodily sensations
Fear of movement, lack of exercise
History of physical, emotional, sexual abuse
Insomnia, nonrestorative sleep

TABLE 74.7

Management of Suffering

Type of Intervention	Clinical Examples
OMT	Direct, indirect
Cognitive and behavioral therapy	Psychotherapy, cognitive restructuring, hypnosis, motivational interviewing, relaxation therapy, acceptance and commitment (ACT) therapy
Relaxation	Biofeedback, progressive relaxation
Breathing exercise	Yoga, Tai Chi, diaphragmatic breathing
Medication	Opiates, antidepressants, anticonvulsants, NSAIDs, acetaminophen, anxiolytics
Surgery	Ablation, deep brain stimulation

- Cognitive, behavioral, and self-regulatory treatments were specifically found to be efficacious in decreasing suffering.[77]

The robust nature of these studies should encourage confidence in osteopathic physicians as they offer advice and counsel to their patients experiencing chronic pain in the areas of:

TABLE 74.8

Common Components of Cognitive–Behavioral Treatment of Chronic Pain

Strategy	Focus of Treatment
Cognitive restructuring	Self-statement reanalysis to change pain behaviors and distressing thoughts and to decrease anxiety linked to pain and movement
Challenging irrational beliefs	Catastrophizing, all or none thinking, negative predicting, selectively focusing on pain, overgeneralizations, jumping to conclusions, fatalistic viewpoints
Motivating patients	Reduce social isolation, improve communication and problem-solving skills, and reinforce attainable outcome expectancy
Desensitize patients	Pacing activities, goal setting, muscular relaxation training
Reinforce activity	Operant and respondent conditioning
Teach self-management	Breathing techniques, biofeedback, imagery training, distraction techniques. Acceptance and commitment (ACT) counseling
Educate on mind/body/spirit	To understand body unity and our inherent capacity for self-regulation, self-learning, and the importance of healthy lifestyle choices
Relapse prevention	Pain-coping skills, support groups, family interventions, caregiver support/education, breakthrough pain rescue planning

- Pain catastrophizing[55]
- Fear avoidance[62]
- Managing biopsychosocial comorbidities[78]
- Reinforcing pain pertinent and applicable conversations[79]
- Promotion of pain self-management and self-healing.[80]

The strength of osteopathic medicine in managing chronic pain comes through talk and touch. Nothing can be more powerful.

Exercise Is Treatment for Chronic Pain

The body is designed to move. At every stage of life and health, there is a range of activities that can be realized. There is a minimum, and there is a maximum. Within this window of physicality is the domain of exercise and conditioning. Outside of this window is the realm of atrophy and injury.

In 2003, the Centers for Disease Control (CDC) presented information on over 200,000 individuals in the United States and found less than half engage in activities that fulfill the CDC's minimal recommendations for exercise.[81]

Exercise significantly enhances physical and psychological health,[82,83] contributes to antidepressant and anxiolytic effects,[84–88] and benefits sleep.[89]

- Prescriptive exercises can begin to teach the patient to think about health-oriented behaviors.
- Exercise affects:
  - Posture
  - Balance
  - Flexibility
  - Strength
  - Coordination to promote optimal structure and function
- Over time, exercise promotes lessening of tension and stress as the patient learns to support their own health.
- Exercise also has an important impact on the respiratory/circulatory and metabolic/energy systems.

Metaregression analysis found the best outcomes for exercise, incorporating the following elements[90]:

- Individualized regimens
- Supervision
- Stretching
- Strengthening

When exercise included these features, compared to no treatment, pain scores went down nearly 20% and function scores improved by 60%! The standard exercise course includes:

- Educating the patient
- Clearly defined goals
- A program of 30 minutes performed once or twice daily, beginning with low-stress activities (walking, aquatic exercise, stationary bike with rest breaks)
- Encouraging self-management[91]

Mindfulness meditation, muscle relaxation, cognitive behavioral therapy, and diaphragmatic breathing exercises can also be taught along with an exercise prescription.[92–94] OMT can provide a window into pain relief giving solace and comfort while the patient is in the physician's hands.[95,96] It is likely that maladaptive pain states can be partially characterized by excessive suffering.[97] To this end, helping the patient feel calm allows their intrinsic systems to function more optimally.

Suffering can be relieved, at least temporarily. The reduction of suffering is part of the process of altering pathologic activity in the limbic and autonomic domain. Once the lack of value of suffering has been realized, like getting the attention of those around, including caregivers and health professionals, its value quickly diminishes.

Osteopathic medicine is at its most essential level a mechanism for changing pain-related behaviors.[65,68]

- From the OMT effects on segmental, regional, and global neuromusculoskeletal activity, to its calming limbic and autonomic effects, it is attempting to change behaviors.
- At the whole-person level, OMT affords the patient an opportunity to function and feel better.
- Even if only transient, OMT permits the patient a glimpse of their capacity for having less pain.

Educating the patient to gain understanding and self-manage pain is therapeutic.

Enabling the patient to understand their pain generators and pain management strategies allows them to self-manage their symptoms. The patient is empowered by accurately understanding the causes, treatments, and prognoses relative to their pain. Listening to the patient and educating is the art of the true Osteopathic Physician.

Active listening skills and sound advice can help the patient maintain reality-based expectations for course and outcome.

- Patient education can be conducted one-on-one but can also be carried out in small group sessions (8 to 10 patients).
  - Clinical trials show this group model helps to increase activity levels and effectively apply pain self-management skills.[98]
- In addition, pain support groups are an extremely powerful and low-cost strategy for educating larger numbers of patients with chronic pain.[99]
  - The goal is to help patients cope with and adjust to their pain and condition.
  - In support groups, patients reconceptualize the meaning of their pain, their cognitive and emotional appraisals, and problem-solving strategies.[100]
  - They review how their pain impacts themselves and their lifestyle and identify the events in the environment that reinforce their pain behaviors and musculoskeletal reactions.
- If not taught in a group therapy model, the following concepts form at least an outline for teaching coping strategies within the doctor–patient relationship.

These concepts are also the foundational ideas for the advice given to the patients on how to think about and manage their pain.[48] Patients who must "live with the pain" are taught to hold the following ideas as true:

1. My pain is real. It occurs in my body, and I have a reaction to it in my head.
2. I accept that I may need outside help to control my pain, and I refuse to quit or give in to the pain and the deterioration it causes.
3. At times, my pain has had an overwhelming influence on my life, but I believe that I can choose how I react to it.
4. My best efforts and those of the medical community have not stopped my pain. This is not necessarily a fault of mine or a shortcoming of medicine. I will no longer fight with myself about this or blame medicine. No fight, no blame.
5. I will recognize some aspects of my coping with the pain that I am doing well and will also admit to myself mistakes that I have made.
6. I will forgive myself unconditionally for my past mistakes and forgive others whom I perceive are responsible for my pain and troubles.
7. I will fix any mistakes I've made struggling to live with the pain.
8. I will go forward with the hope that the pain will someday pass or be relieved and, at the same time, recognize that I have to cope with the pain that I have.
9. I will strive for higher goals, making pain a side issue, to be managed as necessary.
10. I now recognize there is more to my life than struggling with pain.
11. With this knowledge, I will separate myself from my pain management program or doctor, with the complete understanding that I may return at any time.
12. I understand that I have more important goals in my life than coping with the pain and I will strive toward them as my mission.

Remembering that "Pain runs in front of the skillful surgeon's scalpel or anesthesiologist's needle," a laudable goal, if possible, is to find and block nociception.

To control acute pain, anesthetic blockade of neural transmission to virtually any part of the body can temporarily be achieved by direct application of local anesthetics (nerve blocks), such as procaine, lidocaine, tetracaine, or bupivacaine. In some severe cases, substances that destroy neural tissue, such as phenol, can be injected (neurolytic block) in an effort to permanently obliterate the neural transmission mechanisms.

Diagnostically, nerve blocks can help determine specific pathways of involvement that aid in the differential diagnosis, of the site or transmission mechanisms, of a given pain. Prognostically, they partially predict the probable effectiveness of neurolytic or neurosurgical procedures. Interestingly, the pain-relieving effects of local anesthetics can often exceed the duration of the chemical blockade of neural transmission.

- The reason for this is not completely understood.
- It might be a result of decreasing sympathetic reflexes and skeletal muscle tension.
- Perhaps it results from the creation of pain-free time during which the patient can restructure their cognitive and emotional processing routines or learn new behavior patterns that help in coping with pain, or possibly the activation of a placebo response.

The treatment of acute pain adequately may help prevent some cases of chronic pain. For example, the following represent ways of preventing the unnecessary experience of pain using:

- Topical anesthesia before starting an IV
- Adequate local anesthesia before an invasive procedure
- Nitrous oxide with dental procedures

Chronic pain requires chronic care.

Medications for chronic pain involve three main categories:

1. Nonopioid analgesics: aspirin, salicylate salts, acetaminophen, and nonsteroidal anti-inflammatory drugs (NSAIDs)
2. Opioid analgesics
3. Analgesic adjuvants

These drugs are prescribed according to the World Health Organization's analgesic ladder.[101] It involves choosing among these three groups based primarily on pain intensity.

- Many mild-to-moderate acute pains readily respond to nonopioid analgesics alone; they are the obvious first choice.

- Some moderate-to-severe pains may require combining the nonopioid analgesics with a low-dose opioid preparation, the second step in the analgesic ladder.
- The third step is the addition of a time-released opioid preparation to the nonopioid analgesics.

At any of these three steps, analgesic adjuvants might also be useful.

The American Pain Society (APS) and the International Association for the Study of Pain outline several important concepts to remember when choosing drugs to manage chronic pain:

1. Analgesia should be integrated into a comprehensive patient evaluation and management plan.
2. The emotional and cognitive aspects of pain must be recognized and treated.
3. Individualize route, dosage, and schedule.
4. Administer analgesics on a regularly predetermined time schedule.
5. Recognize and treat side effects.
6. Do not use placebos to assess the nature of pain.
7. Watch for the development of tolerance.
8. Use analgesic adjuvants.
9. Block pain transmission whenever possible.
10. Consider a multimodal approach that applies both pharmacologic and nonpharmacologic therapies.

It is important to remember that, for chronic pain, management with medication taken "as needed" is often insufficient. Adequate management of chronic pain is better accomplished using time-contingent, long-acting medications with adequate medication for breakthrough pain.[102] This also frees the patient from constantly thinking about how much pain there is and wondering when medication should be used.

When narcotics are a part of the medication regimen,[103,104] special communication and contracting between physician and patient also becomes necessary. Monitoring benefits, side effects, and possible inappropriate drug use becomes a part of standard osteopathic pain management.[105]

- Finally, one must remember that opioids can also activate proprioceptive mechanisms, creating *opioid-induced hyperalgesia*[106] through distinct cellular mechanisms such as spinal dynorphin, glutamatergic activity, and descending facilitation[107,108]
- Diminished opioid analgesic efficacy may be opioid tolerance.[109]
- These complex pain management patients may require opioid rotation, adding adjunctive medications, combining an NMDA receptor antagonist, or a trial of opioid tapering.[108–111]

Interdisciplinary rehabilitation is the osteopathic standard of care for complex chronic pain management.

The APS and the American College of Physicians (ACP) released the clinical practice guidelines for treating back pain and recommended *interdisciplinary rehabilitation* and exercise therapy for chronic LBP patients.[111]

- The advantages and benefits of an interdisciplinary approach to managing pain, especially when it is chronic, are well documented.[73]
- Treatment in interdisciplinary pain rehabilitation programs is considered the premier treatment for chronic pain.[6,98,112]
- As reported by Flor et al.,[69] behavioral outcomes, including return to work, were significantly better, for interdisciplinary, compared with unimodal treatments. Their analyses extend these findings by demonstrating that interdisciplinary treatments were superior to other treatments at improving work-related outcomes at both short-term and long-term follow-up.
- Using local treatments to reduce noxious stimulation can be multidimensional.
- Physical measures such as heat and cold, topical agents, local injections of anesthetics, acupuncture, and transcutaneous electrical nerve stimulation (TENS) all can be seen as affecting nociception locally.
- Systemic medications that have local effects include NSAIDs, narcotics, channel/receptor blockade (sodium, calcium, glutamate), and the expanding list of anti-inflammatory agents targeting recently discovered elements of the inflammatory cascade (tumor necrosis factor, leukotrienes, interleukins, etc.)
- As the nociceptive signal is processed rostrally, additional sites of intervention become available.

For the most updated guidelines for the management of chronic lower back pain, please see Chapter 93 Osteopathic Considerations in the Patient with Low Back Pain.

OMT throughout the stages of treatment, as a strategy, can address primary causes and secondary manifestations of pain and, in so doing, can enhance healing capacity. It fosters an individualization of treatment designed to influence health restoration, recovery, and disease prevention (Table 74.9).

Special considerations arise when there is damage to the peripheral, autonomic, or CNS (neuropathic pain). The traditional treatments may be less effective as the nature of pathophysiology between them is different. The following can be part of a well-timed, coordinated option in an evolving interdisciplinary treatment plan:

- Peripheral blockade with local anesthetics, affecting sodium channels.
- Anticonvulsants with effects on glutamate and NMDA transmission
- SNRI antidepressants, affecting NE and 5-HT
- Opiates

TABLE 74.9

Management of Nociceptive Activity

Type of Intervention	Clinical Examples
OMT	Direct, indirect
Anesthesia	Local, regional, sympathetic
Medication, systemic	NSAID, opiates, pregabalin, gabapentin, lamotrigine, acetaminophen
Medication, local	Lidocaine, NSAID, OTC topical
Surgery	Removal, repair, restoration, ablation, stimulation
Biofeedback	EMG, temperature, galvanic skin response (GSR), EEG
Physical therapy	Heat, cold, laser, ultrasound, electrical stimulation, traction, exercise, balance
Acupuncture	With or without electrical stimulation, local, systemic

In this interdisciplinary model, the patient, as leader, in partnership with the physician creates a healthcare team. Using appropriate consultants and caregivers, coordinated pain management can be delivered. Part of the process of team building involves consulting healthcare providers in:

- Pain management
- Anesthesiology
- Pain psychology/psychiatry
- Osteopathic manipulative medicine
- Rehabilitation medicine
- Physical and occupational therapy
- Orthopedics
- Neurosurgery
- General surgery
- Gynecology
- Oncology
- Otolaryngology
- Neurology
- Internal medicine
- Endocrinology
- Immunology
- Pharmacology
- Addictionology
- Behavioral medicine/social workers
- Sleep medicine
- Dentists
- Any other subspecialty required

Coordinated nursing services are also appropriate when medical acuity or complexity requires a protracted need for health services.

The fact that anything ever heals is a reminder of the miracle of life. From a simple paper cut that heals without much thought, to a pelvic fracture that requires surgery and thoughtful rehabilitation, there is represented a spectrum of the ongoing manifestation of one of osteopathy's guiding principles.

- A broken bone is likely to heal relatively quickly in a healthy person. A "broken heart may be inconsolable."
- A sprained ankle might take longer to heal if the patient is misbehaving or suffers from comorbidities that interfere with healing.
- A more serious injury, with greater tissue injury, or with more systems or sites of involvement, is likely to take longer to rehabilitate, even in a healthy person.

Most healing is less than perfect, leaving its mark, a scar, a memory on the mind, on the body, and on the spirit.

By integrating the five models, the osteopathic perspective seeks to restore optimal structural and functional relations.

A comprehensive palpatory examination and a review of psychosocial factors are required for optimal chronic pain management.[43] The neuromusculoskeletal system is the primary source of pain in many patients with neck, low back, spine, and extremity conditions. Therefore, here, again, is a setting where OMT can be of therapeutic value.

The CDC, APS, and the ACP clinical practice guidelines recommend heat, spinal manipulation, and time to allow the natural healing processes to occur,[76,74] as mainstays for treatment of LBP. Neck and low back syndromes are often related to disturbances of muscle, tendon, ligament, joint capsule, joint, or disk. Appropriate use of OMT can encourage healing and health maintenance. By optimizing structure and function, the patient course can be positively affected.

In chronic pain states, whether primary or secondary, there are always manifestations of somatic dysfunction, compensatory structural adaptations, and altered sense of self-confidence for healing.

- OMT, at this level, is useful by promoting afferent reduction through:
  - ☐ Direct and indirect techniques
  - ☐ Muscle relaxation
  - ☐ Improved mobility
- This includes attempts at balancing muscle tension and identifying and treating pain-generating compensatory musculoskeletal processes.
- For example, a patient with a limp, from a musculoskeletal or neurologic pathology, may secondarily develop LBP. Treating back pain helps treat the compensatory process and may suggest preventive strategies. These treat aspects of the pain arising remotely.

There are times when surgical intervention, removing the inflamed gallbladder, decompressing the nerve root, etc., is the clear and best option.

- Anesthesiologic interventions like trigger point injections, nerve blocks, sympathetic nerve blocks, and even spinal cord stimulators can be of selective utility.
- Currently, deep brain stimulation also exists as an extreme option for extreme circumstances.
- Surgical procedures can influence the suffering aspect of pain and leave the pain experience otherwise intact. Through ablation and deep brain stimulation of structures like the thalamus, hypothalamus, and amygdala, this can be accomplished.
- Due to its invasive nature, it is usually reserved for patients with complex and prolonged clinical courses.

Still, it is the patient who must be up to the healing process to fully benefit.[105]

The goal of chronic pain management is, "Wellness," fostered by self-regulation, self-healing, and health maintenance.

This notion of wellness refers to the balance and recuperative capacity of an individual (Fig. 74.5).

- It takes into effect inherited constitution, acquired conditions through illness, injury, and abuse, as well as the restorative and healthful aspects of an individual.
- Their nutrition, exercise regimen, sleep habits, state of mind, support system, and willingness to enter health-oriented partnerships with doctors and others help determine their reservoir for health.[64]
- This includes their ability to recover from or successfully live with a variety of chronic conditions. It reflects the vulnerability of any given individual to develop pathology in response to a variety of stressors.
- These pathologies can manifest as organ pathology, musculoskeletal dysfunction, and/or system dysregulation.

Osteopathic chronic pain management is a true art and true science.

Chronic pain, like so many other conditions, often cannot be cured. Patients can learn to live successfully despite chronic pain, however:

- This requires the patient and practitioner forming a therapeutic alliance, a partnership for health.
- In this context, medical investigations can be conducted, and psychological and sociologic information can be gathered, all to educate the patient and the practitioner.

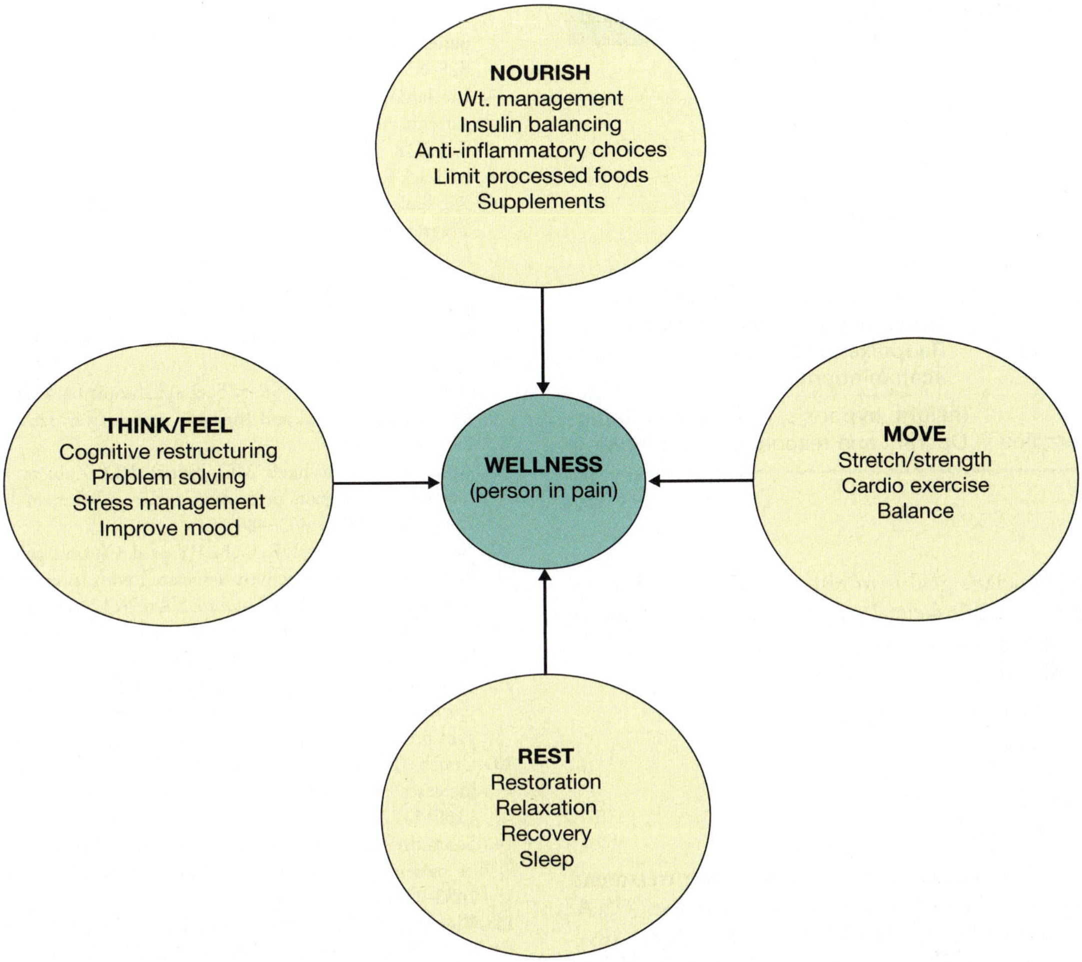

Figure 74.5. Wellness is appreciated through multiple interacting systems.

- Treatment begins by educating the patient about their unique:
  - Constitutional predisposition
  - Heredity
  - Effects of trauma and illness
  - Lingering learned behavioral/neurophysiologic traits on how they contribute to their burden of pain.
- Then, in healing fashion, this information is slowly reformulated into a workbook of health-restoring activities. This workbook includes counsel on:
  - Nutrition
  - Exercise
  - Rest and sleep
  - Mental attitude
- This advice includes recommendations regarding traditional medical care, traditional osteopathic manipulative medical care, and whatever care of the future whose evidence-based value is yet to be proved.

With the growing knowledge of the MINE correlates of chronic pain experience and behavior, a more comprehensive, individualized program for traveling toward wellness can be offered. Whether it is a nanobot delivery/repair system or new biochemically targeted molecules, physicians are prepared to critically evaluate biomedical research of the future, as well as the past and present.

Utilizing the osteopathic precepts of *self-healing* and a *self-contained medicine chest*, physicians and patients are drawn toward interventions that encourage the expansion and enhancement of these inherent capacities.

- Recognizing the primacy of structure/function reciprocity and having the neuromusculoskeletal system readily accessible for evaluation enable osteopathic physicians to enjoy unique access to biologically relevant physical diagnostic information, thereby creating a more complete patient-centered evaluation.
- As a logical corollary, it also allows an avenue of OMT intervention that is uniquely well tailored and therapeutically useful to the chronic pain patient.

Pain management tests the skills of all physicians. Whether it is the symptom of acute pain or the disease of chronic pain, proper management is dependent on proper assessment.

- The more multifactorial and biopsychosocial the evaluation can be and the more comprehensive and patient-focused the treatment plan, the greater the decrease in reported pain scores and the better the QOL at 2-year follow-up.[75,76,79]
- Being comprehensive and incorporating the five models ensures the patient feels heard and thoroughly understood.
- At many levels, the patient feels "touched" by the osteopathic physician.

As an important aside, this collaborative doctor–patient relationship allows the osteopathic *physician* to participate in the patients' healing process, and in so doing, will help them heal themselves. Physicians are certainly not immune to the problems of chronic pain. In this way, the focus of caring for oneself is encouraged, which unfortunately is generally not well supported at the professional or institutional level.

TABLE 74.10

Management of Pain Perception

Type of Intervention	Clinical Examples
OMT	Direct, indirect
Education	Information about pain and self-management
Exercise	Stretch, balance, strengthen
Medication	Opiates, Tricyclic antidepressants, Norepinephrine and Serotonin Reuptake Inhibitor, cannabinoids, acetaminophen
Cognitive and behavioral therapies	Insight, hypnosis, relaxation training Operant and respondent conditioning

SUMMARY

In summary, the physician's goal is to restore both physical functioning and adaptive musculoskeletal responses through the simultaneous use of physiologic and psychological interventions.[64,112,113] When managing chronic pain, it is routine to use:

- Osteopathic manipulative techniques
- Exercise prescription
- Sleep monitoring
- Nutritional support
- Psychological counseling

Combining the five models into a comprehensive treatment approach increases the chances of a successful outcome.[69,114] A treatment plan that simultaneously addresses the biologic, psychological, and social factors of chronic pain is more likely to succeed and decreases chronic pain perception and behavior (Table 74.10).[107–110,115–117]

Pain is the most common element in the symptoms presented to physicians. But as so eloquently stated by John Loeser[97]:

> *"It is suffering, not pain, that brings patients into doctor's offices in hopes of finding relief."*

Astounding developments in our understanding of the mechanisms of nociception should not cause us to lose sight of our patients' goals. Chronic pain is far more than a sensory process. We must maintain the biopsychosocial model of chronic pain if we are to provide effective health care to our patients. Understanding the components of pain facilitates this goal. Suffering is an emergent property of the human brain and is dependent upon consciousness…

Successful management of chronic pain depends on much more than knowledge. Knowledge must be teamed with keen observation, patience, and compassion. Many physicians have come to believe that treating chronic pain and suffering, with all their biopsychosocial elements, reflects both the true art and the true science of osteopathic medicine. This is truly a labor of body, mind, and spirit.

REFERENCES

1. May A. Chronic pain may change the structure of the brain. *Pain.* 2008; 137(1):7–15.
2. Gatchel RJ, Robinson RC, Peng YB, Benitez OJ, Noe C. The brain and pain: what have we learned using fMRI? *Pract Pain Manage.* 2008; 8(5):28–40.
3. D'Alonzo GE Jr, Bgorkman-Stipp K. AOA adopts policies on treatment of patients in pain: an overview. *J Am Osteopath Assoc.* 2005;105(11 Suppl 5): S29–S31.
4. Licciardone VC. The unique role of osteopathic physicians in treating patients with low back pain. *J Am Osteopath Assoc.* 2004;104(11 Suppl 8): S13–S18.
5. Melzack R. The gate control theory 25 years later. New perspectives on phantom limb pain. In: Bond MR, Charlton JE, Woolf CJ, eds. *Pain Research and Therapy: Proceedings of the 6th World Congress on Pain.* Elsevier; 1991.
6. Jerome JA. Transmission of transformation? Information processing theory of chronic human pain. *Am Pain Soc J.* 1993;2(3):160–171.
7. Raichle ME, MacLeod AM, Snyder AZ, Powers WJ, Gusnard DA, Shulman GL. A default mode of brain function. *Proc Natl Acad Sci U S A.* 2001;98:676–682.
8. Apkarian AV, Sosa Y, Sonty S, et al. Chronic back pain is associated with decreased prefrontal and thalamic gray matter density. *J Neurosci.* 2004; 24:10410–10415.
9. Apkarian AV, Bushnell MC, Treede RD, Zubieta J-K. Human brain mechanisms of pain perception and regulation in health and disease. *Eur J Pain.* 2005;9:463–484.
10. Baliki MN, Chialva DR, Geha PY, et al. Chronic pain and the emotional brain: specific brain activity associated with spontaneous fluctuations of intensity of back pain. *J Neurosci.* 2006;26:12165–12173.
11. Craig AD. Interoception: the sense of physiological condition of the body. *Curr Opin Neurobiol.* 2003;13:500–505.
12. Davis KD, Pope G, Chen J, Kwan CL, Crawley AP, Diamant NE. Cortical thinning in IBS: implications for homeostatic, attention, and pain processing. *Neurology.* 2008;70:153–154.
13. Couch JR, Lipton RB, Stewart WF, Scher AI. Head or neck injury increases the risk of chronic daily headache. *Neurology.* 2007;69: 1169–1177.
14. Schmidt-Wilcke T, Leinisch E, Straube A, et al. Gray matter decreases in patients with chronic tension type headache. *Neurology.* 2005;65: 1483–1486.
15. Vierck CJ Jr. Mechanisms underlying development of spatially distributed chronic pain(fibromyalgia). *Pain.* 2006;124:242–263.
16. Harris R, Sundgren PC, Craig AD, et al. Elevated insular glutamate in fibromyalgia is associated with experimental pain. *Arthritis Rheum.* 2009;60(10):3146–3152.
17. Mawla I, Ichesco E, Zöllner HJ, et al. Greater somatosensory afference with acupuncture increases primary somatosensory connectivity and alleviates fibromyalgia pain via insular g-aminobutyric acid: a randomized neuroimaging trial. *Arthritis Rheum.* 2020;73(7):1318–1328.
18. Alexandre FM, Granzlera C, Snyder J, Hadjikhani N. Thickening in the somatosensory cortex of patients with migraine. *Neurology.* 2007;69: 1990–1995.
19. Urban MO, Gebbart GF. Central mechanisms in pain. *Med Clin North Am.* 1999;83(3):585–596.
20. Allemer SR, Bradley LA, Crofford LJ, Moldofsky H, Chrousos GP. The neuroscience and endocrinology of fibromyalgia. *Arthritis Rheum.* 1997;40(11):1928–1939.
21. Bennett RM. Emerging concepts in the neurobiology of chronic pain: evidence abnormal sensory processing in fibromyalgia. *Mayo Clin Proc.* 1999;74(4):385–398.
22. Treede RD. Pain and hyperalgesia: definitions and theories. In: Cervero F, Jensen TS, eds. *Handbook of Clinical Neurology.* Vol. 81. Elsevier B.V.; *Pain.* 2006:3–10.
23. Johnstone T, van Reekum CM, Urry HL, Kalin NH, Davidson RJ. Failure to regulate: counterproductive recruitment of top-down prefrontal-subcortical circuitry in major depression. *J Neurosci.* 2007;27(33):8877–8884.
24. Argyropoulos GPD, van Dun K, Adamaszek M, et al. The cerebellar cognitive affective /Schmahmann syndrome: a Task Force paper. *Cerebellum.* 2020;19(1):102–125.
25. May A, Hajak G, Ganbbauer S, et al. Structural brain alterations following 5 days of interventions: dynamic aspects of neuroplasticity. *Cereb Cortex.* 2007;17:205–210.
26. Draganski B, Gaser C, Volker B, Schuierer G, Bogdahn U, May A. Neuroplasticity: changes in grey matter induced by training. *Nature.* 2004;427:311–312.

27. Flor H, Nikolajsen L, Staehelin Jensen T. Phantom limb pain: a case of maladaptive CNS plasticity? *Nat Rev Neurosci.* 2006;7:873–881.
28. Woolf CJ, Salter MW. Neuronal plasticity: increasing the gain in pain. *Science.* 2000;288:1765–1769.
29. Flor H. Cortical reorganization and chronic pain: implications for rehabilitation. *J Rehabil Med.* 2003;35(suppl 41):66–72.
30. Bedi US, Arora R. Cardiovascular manifestation of post-traumatic stress disorder. *J Natl Med Assoc.* 2007;99:642–649.
31. Jerome JA. Information processing theory of chronic pain [bulletin]. *Am Pain Soc J.* 1992;1:7–10.
32. Langevin HM. Connective tissue: a body-wide signaling network? *Med Hypotheses.* 2006;66(6):1074–1077.
33. Roth RS, Geisser ME, Bates R. The relationship of post-traumatic stress symptoms to depression and pain in patients with accident related chronic pain. *J Pain.* 2008;9(7):588–596.
34. Chapman CR, Tuckett RP, Song CW. Pain and stress in a systems perspective: reciprocal neural, endocrine, and immune interactions. *J Pain.* 2008;9(2):122–145.
35. Loeser JD. Pain as a disease. In: Cervero F, Jensen TS, eds. *Handbook of Clinical Neurology.* Vol. 81 Elsevier B.V.; *Pain.* 2006;(3rd ser):11–20.
36. Korr IM. An explication of osteopathic principles. In Ward RC ed. *Foundations for Osteopathic Medicine.* 1st ed. Williams and Wilkins; 1997: 7–12.
37. Napadow V, Harris R. What has functional connectivity and chemical neuroimaging in fibromyalgia taught us about the mechanisms and management of 'centralized' pain? *Arthritis Res Ther.* 2014;16(5):425.
38. Gatchel RJ, Maddrey AM. The biopsychosocial perspective of pain. In: Raczynski J, Leviton L, eds. *Healthcare Psychology Handbook.* Vol. II. American Psychological Association Press; 2004.
39. Gatchel RJ. *Clinical Essentials of Pain Management.* American Psychological Association; 2005.
40. Turk DC, Monarch ES. Biopsychosocial perspective on pain. In: Turk DC, Gatchel RJ, eds. *Psychological Approaches to Pain Management: A Practitioners Handbook.* 2nd ed. Guilford; 2002.
41. Engel GL. The need for a new medical model: a challenge for biomedicine. *Science.* 1977;196(4286):129–136.
42. Loeser JD. Concepts of pain. In: Stanton-Hicks J, Boaz R, eds. *Chronic Low Back Pain.* Raven Press; 1982.
43. Kuchera ML. Osteopathic manipulation medicine consideration in patient with chronic pain. *J Am Osteopath Assoc.* 2005;105(4):S29–S36.
44. Turk DC, Melzack R. *Handbook of Pain Assessments.* 2nd ed. The Gilford Press; 2001.
45. Litcher-Kelly L, Martino SA, Broderick JE, Stone AA. A systematic review of treatment outcomes in chronic pain clinical trials: IMMPACT recommendations. *Pain.* 2008;9:105–121.
46. Baliki MN, Geha PY, Apkarian AV, Chialvo D. Beyond feeling: chronic pain hurts the brain, disrupting the default-mode network dynamics. *J Neurosci.* 2008;28:1398–1403.
47. Turk DC, Dworkin RH, Revicki D, et al. Identifying important outcome domains for chronic pain clinical trials: an IMMPACT survey of people with pain. *Pain.* 2008;137:276–285.
48. Kerns RD, Rosenberg R. Predicting responses to self-management treatments for chronic pain: application of the pain stages of change model. *Pain.* 2000;84:49–55.
49. Holroyd KA, Holm JE, Keefe FJ, et al. A multi-center evaluation of the McGill Pain Questionnaire: results from more than 1700 chronic pain patients. *Pain.* 1992;48:310–311.
50. Pearce J, Morley S. An experimental investigation of the construct validity of the McGill Pain Questionnaire. *Pain.* 1989;39:115–121.
51. Melzack R. The McGill Questionnaire: major properties and scoring methods. *Pain.* 1975;1:277–299.
52. Melzack R. The short-form McGill Pain Questionnaire. *Pain.* 1987;30: 191–197.
53. Reading AE, Everitt BS, Sledmere CM. The McGill Pain Questionnaire: a replication of its construction. *Br J Clin Psychol.* 1982;21:339–349.
54. Marek S, Siegel JS, Gordon EM, et al. Spatial and temporal organization of the individual human cerebellum. *Neuron.* 2018;100(4):977–993.
55. Petrini L, Arendt-Nielsen L. Understanding pain catastrophizing: putting pieces together. *Front Psychol.* 2020;11:603420.
56. Eccleston C, Crmbez G. Worry and chronic pain: a misdirected problem solving model. *Pain.* 2007;132:233–236.
57. Neblett R. Pain Catastrophizing: an historical perspective. *J Appl Biobehav Res.* 2017;22:e 12086.
58. Schutze R, Rees C, Smith A, Slater H, Campbell JM, O'Sullivan P. How can we best reduce pain catastrophizing in adults with chronic noncancer pain? A systematic review and meta-analysis. *J Pain.* 2018;19: 233–256.
59. Kuchera ML, Jerome JA. Adults with chronic pain and depression. In: Chila AG, ed. *Foundations of Osteopathic Medicine.* 3rd ed. Lippincott Williams & Wilkins; 2011:903–909.
60. Jensen M, Turk D. Contributions of psychology to the understanding and treatment of people with chronic pain: why it matters to all psychologists. *Am Psychol.* 2014;69:105–118.
61. Nielson WR, Weir R. Biopsychosocial approaches to the treatment of chronic pain. *Clin J Pain.* 2001;17(4 Suppl): S114–S127.
62. Serrano-Ibanez E, Lopez-Martinez A. The behavioral inhibition and activation systems and function in patients with chronic pain. *Personal Individ Differ.* 2019;138:56–62.
63. Fordyce WE. Environmental factors in the genesis of low back pain. In: Bonica JJ, Liebeskind JE, Albe-Fessard DG, eds. *Advances in Pain Research and Therapy.* Vol. 3. Raven Press; 1979:659–666.
64. Oken BS. Complementary and alternative medicine: overview and definitions. In: Oken BS, ed. *Complimentary Therapies in Neurology: An Evidence Based Approach.* The Parthenon Publishing Group; 2004:1–7.
65. Task Force on the Low Back Pain Clinical Practice Guidelines. American osteopathic association guidelines for osteopathic manipulative treatment (OMT) for patients with low back pain. *J Am Osteopath Assoc.* 2016;116(8):536–549.
66. Chou R, Huffman LH; American Pain Society; American College of Physicians. Nonpharmacologic therapies for acute and chronic low back pain: a review of the evidence for an American Pain Society/American College of Physicians clinical practice guideline. *Ann Intern Med.* 2007;147(7):492–504.
67. Wang ZR, Ni GX. Is it time to put traditional cold therapy in rehabilitation of soft-tissue injuries out to pasture? *World J Clin Cases.* 2021;9(17):4116–4122.
68. Franke H, Franke JD. Osteopathic manipulative treatment for nonspecific low back pain: a systematic review and meta-analysis. *BMC. Muscloskeletal Disord.* 2014;15:286.
69. Flor H, Fydrich T, Turk D. Efficacy of multidisciplinary pain treatment center: a meta-analytic review. *Pain.* 1992;49(2):221–230.
70. Gatchel R, Okifuji A. Evidence based scientific data documenting the treatment and cost effectiveness of comprehensive pain programs for chronic nonmalignant pain. *J Pain.* 2006;7(11):779–793.
71. Koechlin H, Coakley R, Schechter N, Werner C, Kossowsky J. The role of emotional regulation in chronic pain; a systematic literature review. *J Psychom Res.* 2018;107:38–45.
72. Sullivan M, Rogers W, Kirsch I. Catastrophizing, depression and emotional regulation for pain and emotional distress. *Pain.* 2001;91:147–154.
73. Guzman J, Esmail R, Karjalainen K, Malmivaara A, Irvin E, Bombardier C. Multidisciplinary rehabilitation for chronic low back pain: systematic review. *BMJ.* 2001;322:1511–1516.
74. Morley S, Eccleston C, Williams A. Systematic review and meta-analysis of randomized controlled trials of cognitive behavior therapy for chronic pain in adults, excluding headache. *Pain.* 1999;80:1–13.
75. van Tulder MW, Ostelo R, Vlaeyen JWS, Linton SJ, Morley SJ, Assendelft WJ. Behavioral treatment for chronic low back pain: a systematic review within the framework of the Cochrane Back Review Group. *Spine.* 2001; 26:270–281.
76. van Tulder MW, Koes BW, Bouter LM. Conservative treatment of acute and chronic nonspecific low back pain: a systematic review of randomized controlled trials of the most common interventions. *Spine (Phila Pa 1976).* 1997;22:2128–2156.
77. Hoffman BM, Papsa RK, Chatkoff DK, Kerns RD. Meta-analysis of psychological interventions for chronic low back pain. *Health Psychol.* 2007;26(1):1–9.
78. Gatchel RJ. Comorbidity of chronic pain and mental disorders: the biopsychosocial perspective. *Am Psycho.* 2004;59:795–805.

79. Burns JW, Day MA, Thorn BE. Is reduction in pain catastrophizing a therapeutic mechanism specific to cognitive behavioral therapy for chronic pain? *Transl Behav Med.* 2012;2:22–29.
80. Kerns RD, Habib S. A critical review of the pain readiness to change mode. *J Pain.* 2004;5:357–367.
81. Centers for Disease Control and Prevention (CDC). Strength training among adults aged >/=65 years–United States, 2001. *Morb Mortal Wkly Rep.* 2004;53(2):25–28.
82. Jordan J, Holden M, Mason E, Foster N. Interventions to improve adherence to exercise for chronic musculoskeletal pain in adults. *Cochrane Database Syst Rev.* 2010;210(1):CD005956.
83. Booth J, Mosley GL, Schitenwolf M, Cashin A, Davies M, Hubscher M. Exercise for chronic musculoskeletal pain: a biopsychosocial approach. *Muscloskeletal Care.* 2017;15(4):413–421.
84. Dimeo F, Bauer M, Varahram I, Proest G, Halter U. Benefits from aerobic exercise in patients with major depression: a pilot study. *Br J Sports Med.* 2001;35(2):114–117.
85. Dunn A, Trivedi M, Kampert J, Clark CG, Chambliss HO. Exercise treatment for depression: efficacy and dose response. *Am J Prev Med.* 2005;28(1):1–8.
86. Fox K. The influence of physical activity on mental well-being. *Public Health Nutr.* 1999;2(3A):411–418.
87. Paluska SA, Schwenk TL. Physical activity and mental health: current concepts. *Sports Med.* 2000;29(3):167–180.
88. Strohle A, Feller C, Onken M, Godemann F, Heinz A, Dimeo F. The acute antipanic activity of aerobic exercise. *Am J Psychiatry.* 2005;162: 2376–2378.
89. Salmon P. Effects of physical exercise on anxiety, depression, and sensitivity to stress: a unifying theory. *Clin Psychol Rev.* 2001;21(1):33–61.
90. Hayden JA, van Tulder MW, Tomlinson G. Systematic review: strategies for using exercise therapy to improve outcomes in chronic low back pain. *Ann Intern Med.* 2005;142:776–785.
91. O'Conner SR, Tully MA, Ryan B, et al. Walking exercise for chronic musculoskeletal pain: systematic review and meta-analysis. *Arch Phys Med Rehabil.* 2015;96(4):724–734.
92. Greeson JM. Mindfulness Research Update: 2008. *Complement Health Pract Rev.* 2009;14(1):10-18.
93. Turk DC, Gatchel RJ, eds. *Psychological Approaches to Pain Management: A practitioner's Handbook.* 3rd ed. Guilford Publications; 2018.
94. Ruben R, Vega R, Jensen M, Miro J. Neurofeedback for pain management: a systematic review. *Front Neurosci.* 2020;14:671.
95. Licciardone JC, Schmitt ME, Aryal S. Empathy in medicine osteopathic and allopathic physician interpersonal manner, empathy, and communication style and clinical status of their patients: a pain registry based study. *J Am Osteopath Assoc.* 2019;119(8):499–510.
96. Anderson GB, Lucente T, Davis AM, Kappler RE, Lipton JA, Leurgans S. A comparison of osteopathic spinal manipulation with standard care for patients with low back pain. *N Engl J Med.* 1999;341(19):1426–1431.
97. Loeser JD. Pain and suffering. *Clin J Pain.* 2000;16(suppl 2):S2–S6.
98. Turk DC, McCarberg B. Non-pharmacological treatments for chronic pain: a disease management contest. *Dis Manage Health Outcomes.* 2005; 13(1):19–30.
99. Leo RJ. *Concise Guide to Pain Management for Psychiatrists.* American Psychiatric Publishing, Inc; 2003.
100. Turk DC. A cognitive-behavioral perspective on treatment of chronic pain patients. In: Turk DC, Gatchel RJ, eds. *Psychological Approaches to Pain Management: A Practitioner's Handbook.* Guilford Press; 2002:138–158.
101. Vargas-Schaffer G. Is the WHO analgesic ladder still valid? Twenty-four years of experience. *Can Fam Physician.* 2010;56(6):514–517.
102. Rasor J III, Harris G. Opioid use for moderate to severe pain. *J Am Osteopath Assoc.* 2005;5(6):2–7.
103. Dowell D, Haegerich TM, Chou R. CDC Guideline for Prescribing Opioids for Chronic Pain—United States. http://www.cdc.gov/drugoverdose/prescribing/guideline.html
104. American Society of Anesthesiologists Task Force on Chronic Pain Management; American Society of Regional Anesthesia and Pain Medicine. Practice guidelines for chronic pain management: an updated report by the American Society of Anesthesiologists Task Force on Chronic Pain Management and the American Society of Regional Anesthesia and Pain Medicine. *Anesthesiology.* 2010;112(4):810–833.
105. Galluzzi KE. Management of neuropathic pain. *J Am Osteopath Assoc.* 2005;105(suppl 4):S12–S19.
106. Mao J. Opioid-induced hyperalgesia. Pain clinical updates. In: *International Association for the Study of Pain.* Vol. XVI, Issue 2, Elsevier Science B.V.; 2008.
107. Vanderah TW, Ossipov MH, Lai J, Malan TP Jr, Porreca F. Mechanisms of opioid-induced pain and antinociceptive tolerance: descending facilitation and spinal dynorphin. *Pain.* 2002;92:5–9.
108. Mao J. Opioid-induced abnormal pain sensitivity: implications in clinical opioid therapy. *Pain.* 2002;100:213–217.
109. Angst MS, Clark JD. Opioid-induced hyperalgesia: a qualitative systematic review. *Anesthesiology.* 2006;104:570–587.
110. Baron MJ, McDonald PW. Significant pain reduction in chronic pain patients after detoxification from high-dose opioids. *J Opioid Manag.* 2006;2:277–282.
111. Chou R, Qaseem A, Snow V, et al; Clinical Efficacy Assessment Subcommittee of the American College of Physicians; American College of Physicians; American Pain Society Low Back Pain Guidelines Panel. Diagnosis and treatment of low back pain: a clinical practice from the American College of Physicians and the American Pain Society. *Ann Intern Med.* 2007;147:478–491.
112. Morris DB. The challenges of pain and suffering. In: Jensen TS, Wilson PR, Rice AS, eds. *Clinical Pain Management: Chronic Pain.* Arnold; 2003.
113. Loeser J, Turk DC. Multidisciplinary pain management. In: Loeser JD, Butler SD, Chapman CR, Turk DC, eds. *Bonica's Management of Pain.* 3rd ed. Williams & Wilkins; 1990:2069–2079.
114. Fusco G, Hruby R, Lunghi C, Tozzi P. *The Five Osteopathic Models: Rationale, Application, Integration - From an Evidence-Based to a Person-Centered Osteopathy.* 1st ed. Handspring Publishing; 2017.
115. Friedrich M, Gittler G, Arendasy M, Friedrich KM. Long term effect of a combined exercise and motivational program on the level of disability of patients with chronic low back pain. *Spine.* 2005;30:995–1000.
116. Sullivan MJ, Stanish WD. Psychologically based occupational rehabilitation: the Pain-Disability Prevention Program. *Clin J Pain.* 2003;19:97–104.
117. Berry PH, Chapman CR, Covington EC, et al. *Pain: Current Understanding of Assessment Management and Treatments.* National Pharmaceutical Council and the Joint Commission on Accreditation of Healthcare Organizations; 2001.

75 Osteopathic Considerations in Physical Medicine and Rehabilitation

MARCEL P. FRAIX ▪ J. MICHAEL WIETING ▪ NICHOLAS C. ELWERT

KEY CONCEPTS

- The philosophy of Physical Medicine and Rehabilitation (PM&R) is in alignment with the tenets of osteopathy.
- The history of PM&R has fostered a holistic, patient-centered, and multidisciplinary approach to patient care.
- Identifying disability and maximizing each patient's functional status is a key consideration for PM&R physicians.
- The osteopathic PM&R physician seeks to comprehensively assess a patient and provide treatment to maximize their physical, mental, and emotional recovery from illness or injury.
- The five models of osteopathic care are well suited for PM&R physicians who must often care for patients with complicated conditions unique to the specialty, such as a spinal cord injury.

INTRODUCTION

The specialty of PM&R is, at its core, in alignment with the tenets of osteopathic medicine; PM&R physicians, or "physiatrists," have a goal to restore and enhance the physical function and quality of life of their patients. This restoration of function often addresses the physical structure of the musculoskeletal and nervous systems. Treatment is employed to maximize the inherent healing capacity of the body and enhance the overall quality of a patient's life. Physiatrists practice in both inpatient and outpatient settings and address a diversity of conditions, including musculoskeletal conditions with sports medicine care and bracing, spinal cord and brain injuries, stroke, amputations along with possible prosthetic needs, neuromuscular diseases, cancer, and cardiac and pulmonary disease. They may see pediatric and adult patients, including those affected by cerebral palsy and spina bifida. Broadly speaking, the specialty can be divided into two categories:

- Physical medicine: Diagnosis and treatment of musculoskeletal injuries and pain syndromes, including acute and chronic musculoskeletal diseases, sports and occupational injuries, and degenerative diseases.
- Rehabilitation medicine: Comprehensive rehabilitation of neurologic and musculoskeletal conditions, such as stroke, brain injury, and spinal cord injury. The physiatrist often practices rehabilitation medicine while directing a collaborative team of medical rehabilitation professionals including, but not limited to, physical and occupational therapists, rehabilitation nurses, rehabilitation and neuropsychologists, speech–language pathologists, social workers/discharge planners, case managers, and others.

The types of PM&R subspecialization and the scope of practice within these areas are illustrated in Tables 75.1 and 75.2. Regardless of their area of focus, however, PM&R physicians stress a patient-centered, humanistic approach to patient care that considers the biopsychosocial model. They strive not only to provide accurate diagnoses and efficacious treatment but also to see patients in the context of their social roles and relationships and how this impacts their disease process.[1] The patient or person is not just the body, but rather a unit of body, mind, and spirit.

HISTORY OF PHYSICAL MEDICINE AND REHABILITATION

Physical methods of healing date to ancient times. Hippocrates used traction and leverage to treat spinal deformities, and heliotherapy and hydrotherapy were recognized and used in Roman times. However, the specialty of PM&R did not become a recognized American medical specialty until 1947. An influential figure in this process was Frank H. Krusen, MD, who is recognized as the "Father of physical medicine" and helped establish the foundation for residency training in the specialty in the United States after moving to the Mayo Clinic in 1936.[2,3] Key events in the development of the specialty included circumstances in which large numbers of individuals were impacted by disability.[4–7] These included the following:

- World War I: Army Medical Corps referred to the importance of the use of physical and occupational therapies in the rehabilitation of wounded and other disabled persons in World War I. After the war, empirical trials provided evidence that physical methods were useful to augment traditional medical care.
- World War II: American society became more aware of the need for advanced treatment and rehabilitation care for disabled persons due to large numbers of soldiers returning from war with injuries and disabilities that had previously proved fatal. After World War II, Dr. Howard Rusk, a traditionally trained internist, and military physician, noted that inactive, nonphysically involved rehabilitation in convalescence resulted in functional deterioration in soldiers recovering from trauma or disease. As a result, the military had unprecedented numbers of soldiers who were not allowed to return to active duty. Dr. Rusk carried out a controlled experiment that demonstrated a dramatically improved return of strength, endurance, and overall function with an aggressive, patient-centered approach to rehabilitation.
- Polio epidemic: Prior to the Salk vaccine, 40,000 new cases of polio were reported each year from 1951 to 1955, one-third of which resulted in disabling paralysis.

In the osteopathic profession, the specialty of rehabilitation medicine began in the late 1940s in response to osteopathic physicians who were interested in structural diagnosis, manipulation,

TABLE 75.1

Subspecialty Training/Fellowship with ABMS or AOA Board Certification

Subspecialty Training	Scope of Patient Care
Brain injury medicine	Traumatic and nontraumatic brain injury and their associated complications (i.e., spasticity, cognitive impairment)
Interventional spine and musculoskeletal medicine	In-depth multidisciplinary training for advanced evaluation and management of acute and chronic spinal and musculoskeletal disorders
Neuromuscular medicine	Disorders affecting the motor neuron, peripheral nerve, neuromuscular junction, and muscle fiber (i.e., amyotrophic lateral sclerosis, myasthenia gravis, muscular dystrophy)
Pain medicine	Pharmacologic and interventional management of somatic and/or neuropathic pain associated with a variety of disorders (i.e., musculoskeletal and spinal conditions, cancer)
Pediatric rehabilitation medicine	Evaluation and treatment of conditions that result in impairment and disability in the pediatric population (i.e., cerebral palsy, spina bifida, brain injury, neuromuscular disease)
Spinal cord injury medicine	Traumatic and nontraumatic spinal cord injury and their associated complications (i.e., spasticity, neurogenic bowel and bladder)
Sports medicine	Assessment and treatment of sports-related disorders (i.e., ligament and tendon injuries, concussion), exercise prescription, and on-field management

TABLE 75.2

Newer Subspecialty Training/Fellowship without ABMS or AOA Board Certification

Subspecialty Training	Scope of Patient Care
Cancer rehabilitation	Diagnosis and management of neuromuscular and musculoskeletal impairments related to cancer
Electrodiagnostic medicine	Development of skills related to the electrodiagnostic evaluation of patients affected by neuromuscular disease
Multiple sclerosis research	Advanced training in diagnosis and management of multiple sclerosis and closely related disorders along with related research
Neurorehabilitation	Exposure to patients primarily affected by spinal cord and traumatic brain injury and stroke
Occupational and environmental medicine	Evaluation and management of job-related disorders, including preventive medicine, clinical care, and education
Parkinson disease and movement disorder	Advanced clinical and research training in patient care and interventions for Parkinson disease and other movement disorders.
Spasticity management	Expert clinical training in the diagnosis and treatment of spasticity and its complications
Stroke	Assessment and management of patients affected by stroke, including stroke syndromes, spasticity, and cognitive disability

and the rehabilitation process. It became evident that an additional level of care was needed, and the osteopathic profession developed the practice affiliate, the American Osteopathic College of Rehabilitation Medicine, in 1954. The American Osteopathic Association added physiatry as a specialty in 1954. The prevailing attitude within the osteopathic profession at that time was that specifying "Physical Medicine" was a redundancy, as osteopathic training at that point emphasized treatment oriented to physical medicine, as opposed to allopathic medical schools, which neglected it. Thus, the osteopathic profession elected to designate the specialty as Rehabilitation Medicine which was later the osteopathic specialty and its affiliate College renamed as Physical Medicine and Rehabilitation and the American Osteopathic College of Physical Medicine and Rehabilitation, respectively, in 2001. The American Osteopathic Board of Rehabilitation Medicine (renamed the American Osteopathic Board of Physical Medicine and Rehabilitation) was organized in 1954 to provide a credentialing mechanism for osteopathic physicians in the specialty of physiatry.

DISABILITY AND FUNCTION

A central tenet of PM&R is addressing disability that results from injury or disease, which is accomplished by restoring or maximizing a patient's function. To accomplish this, physiatrists look to measure a patient's improvement in terms of performing a task with the treatment provided. This tracking of function has historically been incorporated since World War II, and PM&R physicians have continued to improve functional assessments to enable them to be more valid, reliable, and reproducible. Instruments or tools are frequently used in the rehabilitation setting to set goals, develop therapeutic interventions, and monitor patient progress. These are often useful when evaluating the efficacy of treatment in complex conditions such as spinal cord injury, stroke, and traumatic brain injury. They are also helpful when attempting to determine if a patient can successfully return home or reintegrate into the community or workplace after suffering illness or injury.[8] Examples of commonly used assessments are included in Table 75.3.

TABLE 75.3

Assessment Tools Used in PM&R

Assessment Tool	Domain of Assessment
Functional Independence Measure (i.e., FIM), Barthel Index, Patient-Specific Functional Scale	Evaluate the ability of patients to perform activities of daily living (i.e., dressing, bathing, eating) and their level of independence
Standardized Form 36, Community Integration Questionnaire, Reintegration to Normal Living Index	Assess quality of life and community reintegration of patients
Glasgow Coma Scale, Mini Mental Evaluation, Mini-Addenbrookes Cognitive Examination, Neuropsychological Assessment	Evaluate cognition and orientation, including memory, attention, learning capacity, language perception, and executive functioning
Peak Aerobic Capacity, Shuttle Walk Test, Step Test, Six Minute Walk Test, VO_2max, or Maximal Oxygen Uptake	Assess functional capacity in terms of aerobic metabolism
Visual Analog Scale, McGill Pain Questionnaire, Pain Disability Questionnaire	Pain severity and how it relates to function
Bordeaux Verbal Communication Scale, NIH Stroke Scale, Fugl-Meyer Assessment of Motor Recovery, Stroke Impact Scale	Evaluate severity and function in stroke patients
Coma Recovery Scale, Rancho Los Amigos Scale, Galveston Orientation Amnesia Tests, Agitated Behavior Scale	Assess severity and function in patients with brain injury
Ashworth Scale, Modified Ashworth Scale, Tardieu Scale, Modified Tardieu Scale	Used to assess the degree of spasticity in patients
Functional Capacity Evaluation, Targeted Functional Assessment	Assess global functional tolerance of workers safe performance
Multi-Directional Reach Test, Get up and Go Test, Timed Get up & Go test, Berg Balance test, Performance Oriented Mobility Assessment	Evaluate balance, predict fall risk, and determine treatment of balance dysfunction
Palliative Performance Scale, Fatigue Scale, Karnofsky Performance Scale, de Morton Functional Assessment Tool	Assess fatigue, functional performance, and quality of life in severely ill, cancer, and terminally ill patients

ASSESSMENT AND MANAGEMENT BY THE OSTEOPATHIC PHYSIATRIST

As is the case with any physician, the osteopathic physiatrist must understand the basic pathophysiology inherent in a patient's disease process. At the same time, the physiatrist stresses a comprehensive approach to evaluation that considers the whole patient, especially when appreciating the secondary effects of injury and illness and how they can negatively impact a patient's function.[9] While the assessment performed by a physiatrist contains the components inherent in any history and physical examination, it emphasizes factors that impact a patient's illness and disability along with their physical and psychological recovery.[10] These factors include the following:

- Biologic
- Psychological
- Behavioral
- Sociocultural
- Occupational
- Environmental

The physiatric history will encompass traditional components such as the chief complaint and history of present illness along with medical, surgical, social, and family histories. However, it will also emphasize the functional status of a patient, both at home and in the community setting, and how it may be impacted by the patient's disease process or illness. Therefore, a functional history is included and typically contains the following points:

- Mobility (ambulation, manual, or power wheelchair)
- Activities of daily living (dressing, bathing, and hygiene activities)
- Household and community activities
- Assessment of cognition, communication, vocational and avocational status
- Need for assistive devices

Traditionally speaking, the physiatrist determines physical deficits and their functional impact, since identification of functional problems allows the determination of functional goals that become the basis for developing a therapeutic management strategy.[11] This process identifies the following key aspects:

- Impairment (loss or abnormality of psychological, physiologic, or anatomical structure or function)
- Disability (a restriction resulting from an impairment of the ability to perform an activity in the manner that is considered "normal")
- Handicap (disadvantage resulting from the fulfillment of a societal role that is considered "normal" for an individual)

Though patients may have multiple impairments, these might not cause disabilities or handicaps unless they affect the patient's ability to function in the home or community. Physiatrists have recently adopted the World Health Organization's International Classification of Function (ICF), which allows for a better understanding of how a patient's diagnosis impacts their function and quality of life. An appreciation of the activity limitations and participation restrictions associated with one or more disorders, as well as how this may impact the roles of a patient in the home, workplace, and community, is gained. The ICF views functioning and disability as a complex interaction between the health condition of the individual and contextual factors (i.e., environmental,

TABLE 75.4

Glasgow Coma Scale

Grade	Eye Response (E)	Verbal Response (V)	Motor Response (M)
1	Does not open eyes	Makes no sounds	Makes no movement
2	Opens eyes in response to painful stimulus	Incomprehensible sounds	Extension to painful stimulus (i.e., decerebrate posture)
3	Opens eyes to verbal stimulus	Utters incoherent words	Abnormal flexion to painful stimulus (i.e., decorticate posture)
4	Opens eyes spontaneously	Confused but disoriented	Flexion or withdrawal to painful stimulus
5	N/A	Oriented, converses normally	Localizes to painful stimulus
6	N/A	N/A	Obeys commands

and personal factors).[12,13] This provides a picture of "the person in their world" and is relevant regardless of age, gender, or culture. It uses the following domains to measure health and disability at the individual or population level:

- Body function and structure
- Activities related to tasks and actions performed by an individual and participation in life situations
- Information regarding the impact of environmental factors

As with the history performed by the osteopathic physiatrist, the physical examination contains many of the cardinal elements inherent in any physical exam, including assessment of the cardiovascular, respiratory, gastrointestinal, and genitourinary systems. With most PM&R patients, however, there is often additional emphasis placed on evaluation of the neurologic and musculoskeletal systems. Neurologic conditions are frequently encountered in the inpatient and outpatient settings. Key elements of the neurologic examination may include assessing for level of consciousness using the Glasgow Coma Scale (Table 75.4) in patients with brain injuries, or various reflexes and upper and lower motor neuron signs (Table 75.5) in patients with stroke, multiple sclerosis, and spinal cord injury. Detailed sensory and motor strength testing is an essential part of the physical examination, and special attention is often given to the integrity of nerve root levels and their respective dermatomes and myotomes. Additionally, physiatrists typically pay close attention to the evaluation of gait in terms of a patient's stride length, balance, and walking speed. Abnormal gait patterns are commonly seen by the physiatrist and yield useful information in terms of potential neuromuscular dysfunction (Table 75.6).

TABLE 75.5

Upper and Lower Motor Neuron Signs

	Upper Motor Neuron	Lower Motor Neuron
Physical Examination Findings	Hyperreflexia, pathologic reflexes (i.e., Babinski response), increased tone and reflexes, spastic weakness, clonus	Hyporeflexia, absent reflexes, decreased tone and reflexes, flaccid weakness, atrophy of muscles
Anatomical Site of Involvement	Prefrontal cortex through the internal capsule to the brainstem and spinal cord	Anterior horn cell through the peripheral nerve

Key components of the musculoskeletal system evaluation include inspection and palpation, active and passive range of motion of joints, and specific provocative maneuvers to test the integrity of joint-related structures, including muscles, tendons, and ligaments. Some of the commonly employed maneuvers are listed in Table 75.7 and can be used when evaluating conditions affecting the spine and upper and lower extremities joints. Several of these tests are shown in Figures 75.1 to 75.7.

Once the PM&R-focused history and physical examination is completed, the physiatrist establishes functional goals and measures progress with instruments such as those noted in Table 75.3. Additional testing may be employed to further clarify a diagnosis or delineate the extent of a disease process, including the use of electrodiagnostic testing and imaging studies. Electrodiagnostic evaluation (i.e., nerve conduction studies and electromyography) is frequently integrated into the history and physical examination by physiatrists to assess the integrity of muscles and nerves. This allows for the delineation of conditions causing weakness and sensory loss, affecting either the peripheral nervous system or muscle fibers. It also facilitates more accurate prognostication and can be useful with conditions such as peripheral neuropathy, myopathy, neuromuscular junction disease (i.e., myasthenia gravis), or amyotrophic lateral sclerosis. Additionally, imaging studies, including conventional radiographs, diagnostic ultrasound, magnetic resonance imaging, or computerized tomography, are utilized, especially when evaluating conditions affecting the nervous and musculoskeletal systems.

Given the comprehensive, team-centered approach of physiatrists, treatment can be broad and entail a variety of approaches including management with medication as well as treatment modalities that are more commonly used in the specialty of PM&R. Medications frequently used are those that treat pain and inflammation, spasticity, and cognitive issues. Interventional procedures may be utilized to reduce acute and chronic joint- or nerve-related pain, including peripheral and spinal joint injections and epidural injections (Table 75.8). In the acute inpatient rehabilitation setting, emphasis is placed on an interdisciplinary approach to patient care, and the services of physical and occupational therapists along with speech–language pathologists are an integral part of treatment, especially in those patients with a spinal cord injury, traumatic brain injury, or stroke. Along these lines, physical modalities, including heat, cryotherapy, electrotherapy, and ultrasound, are often employed as part of the treatment plan. Therapeutic exercise can be prescribed for a variety of conditions, to improve physical and mental well-being and cardiovascular function and to reduce pain. Orthoses are used to support

TABLE 75.6

Common Gait Abnormalities

Gait Abnormality	Description	Condition/Anatomic Involvement
Trendelenburg	Waddling-type gait with swaying of the trunk toward the weight-bearing lower extremity	Weakness of the gluteus medius and minimus muscles due to injury of the superior gluteal nerve or a myopathy
Hemiplegic	Accentuated lower extremity extension which results in circumduction and hiking of the hip to increase clearance of the foot and toes	Lesions of upper motor neurons resulting in hemiplegia and spasticity (i.e., stroke)
Myopathic	Broad-based waddling-type gait with accentuation of lumbar extension	Weakness of the proximal lower extremity and pelvic girdle muscles (i.e., myopathy)
Steppage	Lifting of the affected lower extremity higher than normal to assist in clearance of the foot, which tends to slap on the floor during heel strike	Injury or disease of the peripheral nervous system affecting the fibular nerves (i.e., radiculopathy, mononeuropathy at the fibular head, lumbar plexopathy)
Scissoring	Flexion of the hips and legs that results in a crouched-type stance with knees and thighs crossing past midline due to hypertonicity of the hip adductor muscles	Conditions affecting the corticospinal tracts (i.e., spinal cord injury, cerebral palsy)
Ataxic	Broad-based gait with irregularity of stride length and increased sway of the body	Dysfunction of the cerebellum or loss of sensory function

TABLE 75.7

Common Musculoskeletal Examination Maneuvers

Test	Description
Spurling test	Passive sidebending and extension of the cervical spine to compress the nerve root affected by cervical spine radiculopathy
Hoffmann sign	Passive flexion of the distal phalanx of the middle finger results in flexion and adduction of the thumb and index finger, which may be indicative of compression/injury of the central nervous system
Adson test	Decrease or disappearance of the radial pulse with inspiration and extension and rotation of the head to the ipsilateral side; may be indicative of thoracic outlet syndrome
Empty can or supraspinatus test (see Fig. 75.2)	Resisted downward pressure of the shoulder placed in internal rotation and abduction causes weakness and pain in patients with injury of the supraspinatus muscle or tendon
Neer sign	Forward flexion of the arm placed in internal rotation causes pain due to impingement of the rotator cuff
Yergason test	Resisted supination of the forearm with the elbow placed in 90 degrees of flexion causes pain with the long head of the biceps along the bicipital groove
Apprehension test (see Fig. 84.29)	Pain with passive abduction of the externally rotated shoulder that may be indicative of injury to the glenoid labrum
Resisted wrist extension (Cozen test) (see Fig. 75.3)	Pain at the lateral elbow with resisted wrist extension in patients with lateral epicondylitis
Finkelstein test (see Fig. 75.4)	Ulnar deviation at the wrist with the thumb in the palm of the hand causes pain over the distal radius in patients with de Quervain tenosynovitis
Carpal compression test (Phalen test) (see Fig. 73.5)	Pressure over the median nerve within the carpal canal reproduces pain and/or numbness when the median nerve is affected by carpal tunnel syndrome
Straight leg raise test (see Fig. 84.15)	The supine patient's leg is passively flexed with the knee in extension reproducing symptoms associated with lumbar disk herniation
Patrick (FABER) test (see Fig. 84.21)	The hip of the supine patient is placed in flexion, abduction, and external rotation, and the knee is depressed as the contralateral anterior superior iliac spine (ASIS) is stabilized; anterior hip (groin) pain indicates hip joint pathology (i.e., osteoarthritis), and low back pain may be indicative of sacroiliac joint dysfunction
Thomas test (see Fig. 84.20; for variation, see Fig. 75.5)	The supine patient's hip is flexed to the chest, and if the contralateral hip elevates off the table, contracture of this hip may be present
Lachman test (see Fig. 75.6); anterior drawer test (see Fig. 75.7)	Pressure is applied to the proximal tibia while the femur of the supine patient is stabilized, and the knee joint is maintained in 15 degrees of flexion; excessive anterior translation of the tibia can be present in patients with injury of the anterior cruciate ligament; the anterior drawer test does not stabilize the femur
Thompson test	With the patient in a prone position and their foot hanging off the examination table, the calf muscles are squeezed; no plantar flexion is indicative of injury or rupture of the Achilles tendon

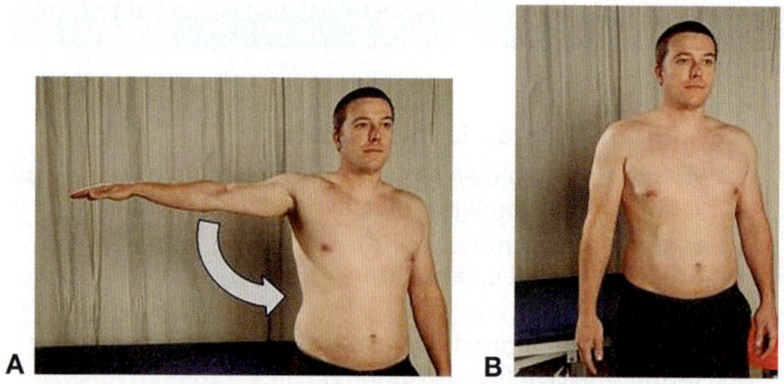

Figure 75.1. Drop arm test for supraspinatus muscle injury. This is an active test that the physician observes from the anterior view. **A.** After abducting the arm to 90 degrees, (**B**) the patient is instructed to slowly drop the arm to their side. A positive test is the inability to control the movement and the arm drops rapidly to the side, indicating weakness of the supraspinatus muscle. (Photo and illustration courtesy of Western University of Health Sciences, Pomona, CA, with permission.)

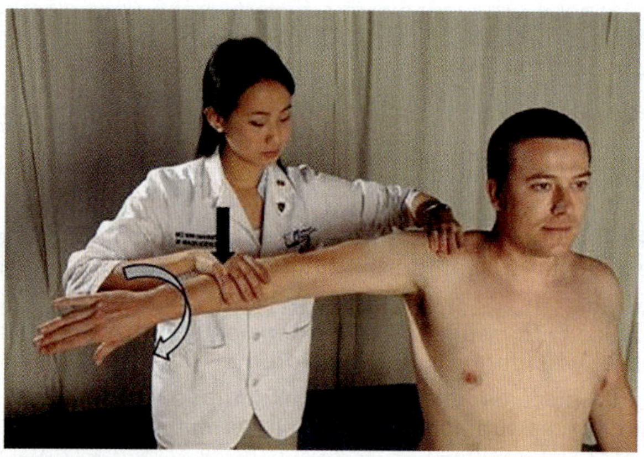

Figure 75.2. Empty can test for supraspinatus muscle injury. The patient tries to resist the physician's attempt to challenge the muscle, which is isolated by abducting the shoulder to 90 degrees and internally rotating it as if emptying the contents of a canned beverage. (Photo and illustration courtesy of Western University of Health Sciences, Pomona, CA, with permission.)

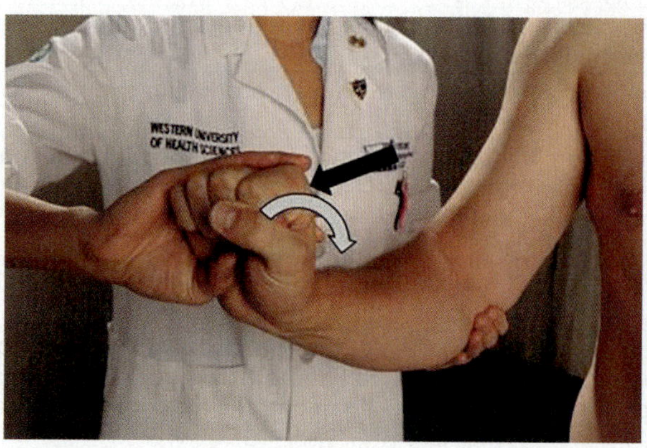

Figure 75.3. Cozen test for lateral epicondylitis. (Photo and illustration courtesy of Western University of Health Sciences, Pomona, CA, with permission.)

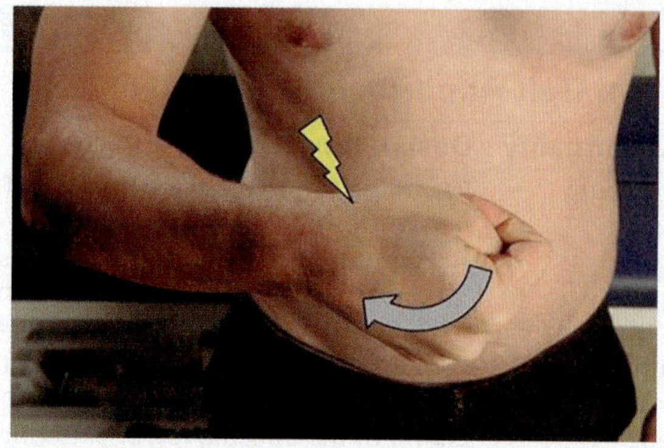

Figure 75.4. Finkelstein test for de Quervain tenosynovitis. The patient holds their distal thumb across the palm by a closed fist and the wrist is adducted (ulnar deviated) rapidly, in effect stretching the abductor and extensor pollicis tendons. Pain elicited along the distal radial head area is indicative of tenosynovitis. (Photo and illustration courtesy of Western University of Health Sciences, Pomona, CA, with permission.)

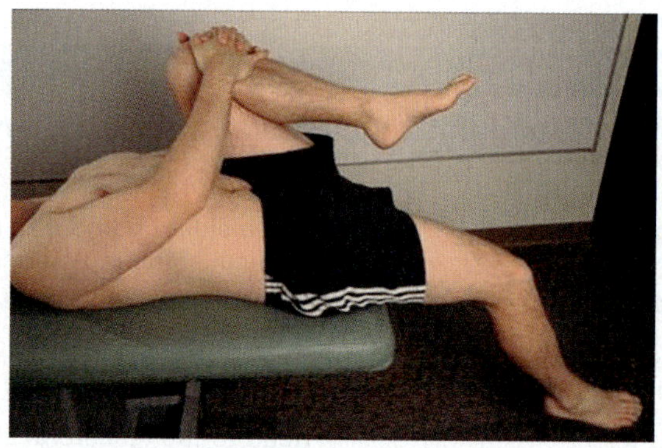

Figure 75.5. A variation of the Thomas test for psoas muscle hypertonicity with one leg off the table to allow hip extension. If the posterior thigh is unable to touch the table, a hypertonic ipsilateral psoas muscle is likely the reason. (Photo courtesy of Western University of Health Sciences, Pomona, CA, with permission.)

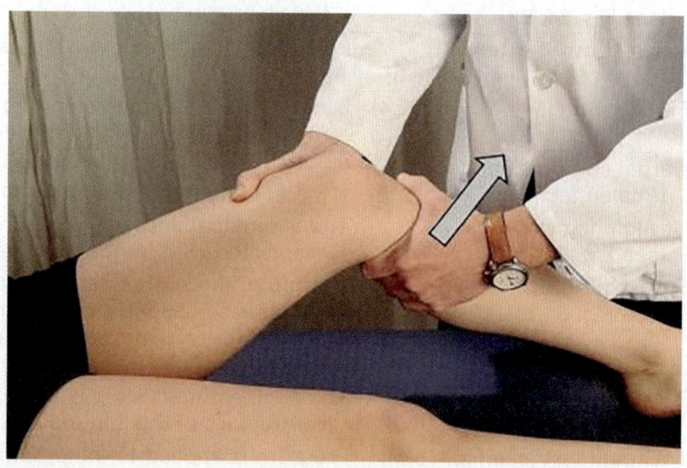

Figure 75.6. Lachman test for cruciate ligament tear/knee joint instability. The physician stabilizes the femur while pulling the tibia anteriorly to test for a tear or rupture of the anterior cruciate ligament. Pushing the tibia posteriorly tests the posterior cruciate ligament. (Photo and illustration courtesy of Western University of Health Sciences, Pomona, CA, with permission.)

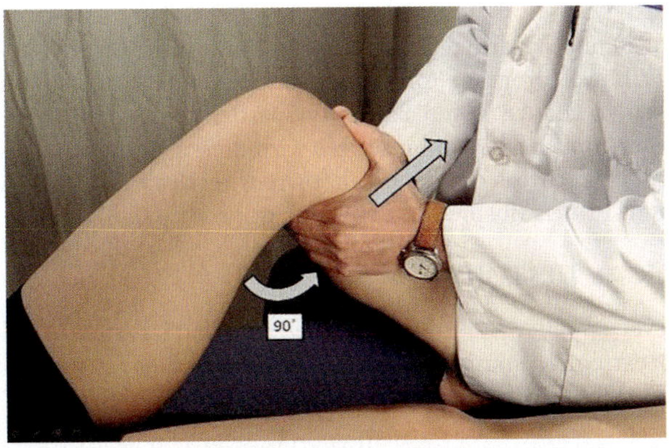

Figure 75.7. Anterior knee drawer test for anterior cruciate ligament tear. In this variation, the physician sits on the patient's foot to stabilize the ankle while pulling the tibia anteriorly. (Photo and illustration courtesy of Western University of Health Sciences, Pomona, CA, with permission.)

the limbs and spine and allow for more normal, pain-free motion, and prostheses are used to replace a missing body part and allow for enhanced ambulation and/or the ability to perform activities of daily living (Table 75.9).

OSTEOPATHIC APPROACH TO PHYSICAL MEDICINE AND REHABILITATION

The inter-relationship between structure and function is one of the fundamental principles of osteopathic medicine. Given a physiatrist's emphasis on reducing functional impairment, it is not difficult

TABLE 75.8

Types of Injections and Spinal Procedures Used in PM&R

Medication	Description
Peripheral joint injection	Anesthetic agent and/or corticosteroid are injected into joints (i.e., glenohumeral, knee) as both a diagnostic and therapeutic means by which to reduce pain and inflammation and improve mobility
Epidural steroid injection	Anesthetic and corticosteroid are injected into the epidural space using an interlaminar or transforaminal approach in order to treat radicular pain
Zygapophyseal (i.e., facet) joint injection	Injection of the facet joint or the nerve fibers innervating them with anesthetic and corticosteroid; allows for the identification and treatment of pain emanating from the spinal facet joints
Radiofrequency neurotomy or ablation	Uses radiofrequency current to denervate the nerve fibers innervating the facet joints when they are a generator for spinal spine
Diskography	Injection of contrast dye into the intervertebral disk to localize the disk as a potential source of pain
Dorsal column spinal cord stimulator	Implantable neuromodulation device that interferes with transmission of signals within the nerves of the dorsal columns, thereby reducing a patient's pain

TABLE 75.9

Examples of Orthotic and Prosthetic Devices

Device	Description
Wrist hand orthosis (WHO)	Used to protect the joints of the wrist and hand while providing neutral alignment; some devices provide support for weak wrist extensors and allow for flexion of the fingers (i.e., tenodesis); can be used in patients with peripheral nerve and spinal cord injuries
Knee orthosis (KO)	Provides support of the knee joint in any plane of motion, especially in patients with hyperextension (i.e., genu recurvatum) or ligamentous injury (i.e., ACL tear)
Ankle foot orthosis (AFO)	Stabilizes the foot and ankle during ambulation in patients with weakness or paralysis, especially in ankle dorsiflexion; helpful in patients with lower extremity weakness and spasticity due to stroke or neuromuscular disease
Cervical orthosis (CO)	Allows for stabilization of the cervical spine and some degree of restriction with flexion, extension, rotation, and sidebending of the spine; used postoperatively or with ligamentous injury but not spinal instability
Halo vest cervical thoracic orthosis (CTO)	Consists of a rigid device with pins that allow for external fixation to the skull; used in the management of unstable cervical spine fractures
Cervical–thoracic–lumbar–sacral orthosis (CTLSO)	Provides full support of the spine and used as a measure to prevent or slow the progression of scoliosis
Transfemoral or above-knee amputation (AKA) prosthesis	Oftentimes used following an amputation due to trauma, tumor, or vascular disease to maintain ambulation; includes a socket, suspension system, knee and ankle unit, and prosthetic foot
Transtibial or below knee amputation (BKA) prosthesis	Oftentimes used following amputation due to peripheral vascular disease; as with a transfemoral prosthesis, includes a socket, suspension system, ankle unit and prosthetic foot, but no knee unit
Transhumeral or above elbow amputation prosthesis	Used commonly after traumatic amputation; includes a socket, suspension and cable control system, elbow and forearm unit, and terminal device that simulates hand function; may use an externally powered or myoelectric system in lieu of a cable control system
Transradial or below elbow amputation prosthesis	As with the transhumeral prosthesis, it is commonly used after amputation due to trauma; includes a socket, suspension and cable control system, and terminal device; may also use an externally powered or myoelectric system in lieu of a cable control system

to see why osteopathic physicians gravitate toward the specialty of PM&R and how osteopathic structural evaluation and treatment can be integrated into the practice of a physiatrist. In fact, according to the Association of American Medical Colleges (AAMC), PM&R has the second highest percentage (31.9%) of Accreditation Council for Graduate Medical Education (ACGME) residents and fellows with a Doctor of Osteopathic Medicine degree by specialty, eclipsing postgraduate training programs in Emergency Medicine, Pediatrics, and Obstetrics & Gynecology.[14] In terms of practicing PM&R physicians, 14.4% are osteopathic physicians, only second to Family Medicine (16.3%).[14] The evaluation performed by a physiatrist focuses on the musculoskeletal and neurologic systems of the human body. Therefore, assessing for somatic dysfunction can be seamlessly integrated, and an appreciation for how it contributes to functional impairment is gained. Using osteopathic manipulative medicine (OMM), somatic dysfunctions are assessed and treated, resulting in improved motion, health, and function of the patient. Osteopathic medicine stresses the interrelated nature of the human body and looks at the patient as a whole unit of body, mind, and spirit. This approach toward patient care aligns well with the patient-centered, interdisciplinary approach of PM&R. It is also helpful when treating patients who are affected by complex diseases and injuries that impact multiple organ systems, such as a spinal cord injury or a traumatic brain injury.

THE FIVE MODELS OF OSTEOPATHIC CARE IN PHYSICAL MEDICINE AND REHABILITATION

The osteopathic physiatrist can utilize the five models of osteopathic care in the evaluation and treatment of patients with conditions commonly encountered in PM&R. These models include the biomechanical/structural, respiratory/circulatory, neurologic, metabolic, and behavioral/biopsychosocial models which are central to osteopathic principles and practice. As noted previously, physiatrists utilize the biopsychosocial model for patient care and emphasize evaluation of the neurologic and musculoskeletal systems. The five models of osteopathic care integrate with the physiatrist's humanistic and multifaceted approach to the evaluation and management of patients. While the five models' approach can be utilized in a multitude of PM&R-related conditions, it will be instructive to use it in the context of a patient with a spinal cord injury affecting multiple organ systems leading to significant psychological and social implications. Additionally, it is a condition that requires a multidisciplinary approach to patient care and is primarily the purview of PM&R physician specialists.

CASE VIGNETTE

A 33-year-old right hand–dominant male, with a past medical history of a C7 spinal cord injury, returns to the clinic for a follow-up with a new complaint of right shoulder and arm pain. He originally sustained his spinal cord injury as the result of a motor vehicle accident at 24 years of age. He reports that his right shoulder pain is worse with activity, particularly when performing transfers to and from a manual wheelchair. There is no significant loss of strength in the right upper extremity, but the pain does intermittently radiate into the forearm and hand with a tingling sensation. The pain is improved with rest and does not interfere with sleep. The patient performs intermittent self-catheterization for his neurogenic bladder and a daily bowel program for a neurogenic bowel. He uses oral baclofen to reduce lower extremity spasticity which, at times, can be uncomfortable and interfere with dressing and transfers. He reports no areas of skin breakdown or respiratory difficulty, although he was hospitalized the year prior for pneumonia.

MEDICAL HISTORY

C7 level spinal cord injury; neurogenic bladder and bowel; lower extremity spasticity; history of pneumonia; history of urinary tract infection.

SURGICAL HISTORY

Cervical spine fusion

FAMILY HISTORY

His mother and father are in good health, and there is no significant, contributory, family history.

SOCIAL HISTORY

The patient lives in a ground-level apartment with wheelchair access. He is single, works as a computer programmer, and reports no tobacco use and occasional use of alcohol in social settings.

FUNCTIONAL HISTORY

He is independent with most of his activities of daily living, including bathing, toileting, upper body dressing, and grooming, but does use adaptive equipment and needs occasional assistance with lower body dressing. He can perform transfers independently and uses a manual wheelchair for mobility in both home and community settings. He can operate a motor vehicle with adapted hand controls.

MEDICATIONS

Baclofen 20 mg orally three times daily; docusate 100 mg three times daily; senna two tablets daily; bisacodyl suppository once daily after breakfast.

ALLERGIES

No history of drug or food allergies.

REVIEW OF SYSTEMS

General

He reports no fever, chills, or night sweats; denies loss or gain of weight, changes in appetite, and fatigue.

HEENT

No sore throat or dysphagia; no sinusitis; no auditory changes, tinnitus, or vertigo; no seasonal allergies

Respiratory

No dyspnea: occasional difficulty clearing secretions due to impaired ability to generate a strong cough with paralyzed intercostal muscles

Cardiovascular

No chest pain or palpitations

Gastrointestinal

Neurogenic bowel, no hematochezia, melena, or hemorrhoids

Genitourinary

Neurogenic bladder; no urinary tract infection within the past 6 months; no hematuria

Nervous

Intermittent tingling in the right upper extremity, but no persistent changes in baseline sensory function; no change in upper extremity motor strength

Musculoskeletal

Right upper extremity pain; no swelling of joints; no fractures

Dermatologic

No areas of skin breakdown or pressure sores

Psychological

Denies depression or anxiety

PHYSICAL EXAM

Vital Signs

Temperature: 37 °C; pulse 76/min; respirations 16/min; blood pressure 105/70; pain 2/10

General

Well-nourished male in no acute distress; alert and oriented to person, place, and time; sitting in a manual wheelchair

HEENT

Sclera clear; visual acuity is 20/20; auditory canals are clear and tympanic membranes intact; oropharynx shows no exudate or erythema; no cervical lymphadenopathy

Respiratory

Diminished inspiratory and expiratory effort with decreased lung sounds; no rales, rhonchi, or wheezing

Cardiovascular

Regular without murmurs; no lower extremity edema

Genitourinary

No erythema, sores, or ulceration of the penis

Neurologic

Cranial nerves II to XII are grossly intact; motor strength is 5/5 with shoulder abduction, elbow flexion and extension, and wrist extension, but hand intrinsic strength is absent as well as lower extremity strength; sensation is intact to pinprick and light touch at the C7 dermatome, but absent below this level; muscle stretch reflexes are brisk in the lower extremities bilaterally with sustained ankle clonus; spasticity in the lower extremities is present with increased tone throughout the entire range of motion of the hip, knee, and ankle.

Musculoskeletal

Decreased right glenohumeral joint flexion and abduction; Neer sign and supraspinatus testing are positive; Spurling and carpal compression testing are negative; atrophy of the hand intrinsic musculature is present.

Osteopathic

Cranial examination shows restricted motion of the right occipitomastoid suture; cervical spine demonstrates decreased active and passive range of motion in all planes, especially with left sidebending and rotation; there is hypertonicity of the cervical paraspinal and trapezius muscles; OA RrSl; AA Rr; T1-3 RrSl; Rib 1 inhalation lesion on the right side.

Dermatologic

No areas of skin breakdown or pressure sores over the sacrum, ischial tuberosities, or greater trochanters; some friable skin over the left upper extremity

DIFFERENTIAL DIAGNOSIS

The major considerations for the patient's right upper extremity pain include the following:

- Rotator cuff tendinopathy/impingement
- Acromioclavicular joint osteoarthritis
- Bicipital tendonitis
- Cervical radiculopathy
- Brachial plexopathy
- Ulnar mononeuropathy at the elbow or wrist
- Median mononeuropathy at the wrist
- Syringomyelia

Patients with a spinal cord injury, both paraplegic and tetraplegic, are at high risk for developing upper extremity musculoskeletal pathology due to overuse. They must rely on their upper limbs for mobility, including transfers and operating a wheelchair, which is not necessary for those who can ambulate. Increased use of the upper extremities also predisposes this patient population to focal mononeuropathies (i.e., compression of nerves) at the wrist and elbow. Finally, syringomyelia, a fluid-filled syrinx within the spinal cord, must be considered since patients who have experienced trauma to the spinal cord are at increased risk for developing it. Syringomyelia presents with pain in the upper extremities in those with cervical spinal cord injury. The patient depicted in Figure 75.8 had a traumatic lower cervical spinal cord injury. His left upper extremity can be seen fixed with the forearm supinated and the wrist extended due to spastic paralysis from restraints used while being treated in the early stages of his management. Notice the profound muscle atrophy and friable skin in the left upper extremity. A patient with a spinal cord injury is highly susceptible to pressure sores and skin infections, especially in areas of bony prominence. Increased pressure over a bony prominence predisposes the skin to potential pressure sore formation. Upper extremity pain could also be due to referred pain from pneumonia, which often requires aggressive treatment and hospitalization. It is important to be vigilant to inspect for and rule out infection in this patient population.

OSTEOPATHIC MANAGEMENT USING THE FIVE MODELS OF OSTEOPATHIC CARE

Biomechanical/Structural Model

This spinal cord–injured patient's motion, posture, and gait are all significantly compromised. Immediately following the patient's injury, the focus would entail maintaining range of motion and

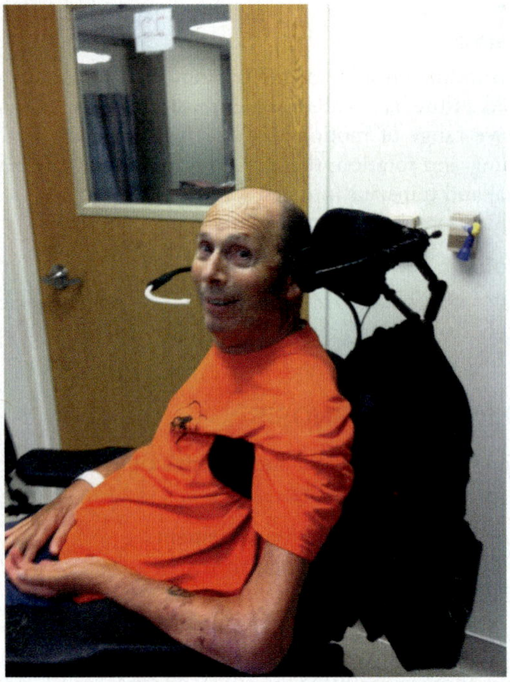

Figure 75.8. A tetraplegic patient with immobile left upper extremity from restraints used to hold arm steady during first few weeks of treatment after traumatic complete lower cervical spinal cord injury, notice skin friability and muscle atrophy of the left arm. (Photo courtesy of Randi Levin-Dubey taken of her late husband Larry Dubey while at a doctor's appointment during his rehabilitation, with permission.)

preventing contracture. In the inpatient rehabilitation setting, restoration of motion and function are maximized depending on the degree of neurologic recovery. This pertains to complete or incomplete spinal cord injuries, which are differentiated by the amount of motor or sensory function remaining below the level of injury. The rehabilitation team, including the physiatrist and physical and occupational therapists, evaluates the patient's neurologic level of injury and sets goals for mobility and to what degree the patient can ultimately perform activities of daily living independently or with assistance. Once discharged from the acute inpatient rehabilitation setting, the patient will continue to make gradual progress regaining strength and maximizing function. However, the patient is at risk for developing secondary musculoskeletal complications from altered body mechanics and the increased demands placed on upper extremities. Aspects or functions of the musculoskeletal system that are actually or potentially impacted, and treatment considerations, include the following.

- Strength and range of motion
  - Loss of strength or range of motion results from injury to the spinal cord itself and lack of continuity with lower motor neurons or subsequent conditions, including spasticity (i.e., hypertonicity of muscle fibers due to loss of descending inhibition of muscle stretch reflexes) or contracture of joints.
  - In the acute care setting, treatment includes passive motion of affected joints in the upper and lower extremities using physical and occupational therapy to maximize range of motion and prevent contracture. This allows for the optimization of function as the patient recovers strength and function (i.e., mobility and the ability to perform activities of daily living). Indirect OMM techniques, including counterstrain and myofascial release, may be useful in this setting.
- Mobility
  - The level of spinal cord injury, and whether it is complete or incomplete, determines the patient's level of mobility. Mobility is the ability to move and not synonymous with ambulation. The patient may lose his ability to walk but maintains the capacity for mobility, especially with the use of an assistive device such as a wheelchair. For patients with complete spinal cord injuries, the ability to ambulate is typically lost. However, incomplete, and lower spinal level injuries can have variable outcomes. In fact, many individuals who are motor incomplete (i.e., maintain some degree of motor activity below the level of injury) recover the ability to ambulate.[15]
  - This patient, with a higher spinal level of injury can maintain mobility and independence with the use of a manual wheelchair. Patients with lower spinal levels and incomplete injuries can recover the ability to ambulate, both with and without the use of assistive devices (i.e., canes, crutches, or orthotics for the lower extremities). Energy demands should be taken into consideration since a patient's gait pattern may be less efficient and place additional stress on the cardiovascular and respiratory systems.[16,17]
- Posture
  - Spinal cord injury, particularly affecting the cervical and thoracic spine, impairs the sitting balance of patients and the ability to maintain alignment of the spine. This is due to loss of paraspinal muscle strength and can result in scoliosis, especially in pediatric patients since they have the potential for continued bone growth.
  - Treatment considerations include bracing and consideration of an appropriately timed spinal fusion (in the pediatric population) with supportive seating systems and wheelchairs for the adult spinal cord injury population. This patient would benefit from a seating system for his manual wheelchair that maximizes his spinal alignment as well as reduces the risk of developing pressure injuries.
- Upper extremity function
  - Patients with a spinal cord injury who are nonambulatory require the use of their upper extremities, not only for performing activities of daily living such as feeding, dressing, and grooming, but also to perform transfers (i.e., movement from a bed to a wheelchair, wheelchair to a chair or toilet) and allow for mobility (i.e., propulsion of a manual wheelchair). This places additional stress on joints of the upper extremities and leads to an increased risk of developing overuse-related shoulder, elbow, and wrist conditions, including rotator cuff tendinopathy and carpal tunnel syndrome.[18–20]
  - Special attention must be given to minimizing stress on the joints of the upper extremities, maximizing ergonomic efficiency, and treating conditions early. This allows for decreased pain and the ability to perform upper extremity activities while maintaining the capacity for continued mobility. As with any patient suffering from an upper extremity musculoskeletal condition, somatic dysfunction should be evaluated and treated with OMM to reduce pain and improve function.[21]

Respiratory/Circulatory Model

This spinal cord–injured patient's respiratory function can be significantly impacted due to a disruption of muscles that allow for respiration, including the diaphragm and intercostal muscles. The alteration of respiratory mechanics leads to insufficient oxygenation of tissues, reduced venous and lymphatic return, and impaired immune system function, all of which predisposes a patient to developing complications such as pneumonia. After spinal cord injury, the cardiovascular system is also affected. Patients with autonomic imbalance to the vascular endothelium and stasis of blood flow can develop hypercoagulability predisposing them to the development of venous thromboembolism (Virchow triad). Aspects or functions of the respiratory and cardiovascular systems that are impacted and treatment considerations include the following:

- Respiratory capacity
  - The patient has a cervical spinal cord injury and is tetraplegic, which causes the development of a pattern of restrictive lung disease in which lung volumes, including forced vital capacity (FVC), decrease which predisposes him to develop respiratory illness, including atelectasis and pneumonia. Pneumonia is, in fact, the leading long-term cause of mortality in patients with spinal cord injury.[22]
    - The tetraplegic patient in Figure 75.8 passed away from pneumonia in his sleep at home while being treated with oral antibiotics.
    - His family shared his story and photo hoping it would help educate future physicians and caregivers.
    - It is vital for physicians and caregivers to be attentive to and aggressively manage seemingly mild infections in this highly vulnerable patient population.
  - Mechanical ventilation is required in patients suffering spinal cord injury at the C1–C3 levels. Patients with injury above the C3 level may also be candidates for phrenic nerve pacing. Many injuries at the level of the lower cervical spine or thoracic spine do not require long-term mechanical ventilation. Techniques enhancing the patient's ability to cough may be useful in improving secretion clearance. Assessing and treating thoracic spine somatic dysfunction as well as using OMM techniques to facilitate remaining costal cage motion may be helpful in improving respiratory efficiency.[23,24]
- Venous thromboembolism (VTE)/deep venous thrombosis (DVT)
  - Immobility after spinal cord injury predisposes patients to the development of VTE/DVT. This may also be precipitated by the presence of trauma (i.e., endothelial injury or fracture) or pre-existing vascular disease. VTE/DVT is more common in patients whose injuries are complete and result in tetraplegia. Complications of VTE/DVT include pulmonary embolus which is the third leading cause of death in acute spinal cord injury.[25,26]
  - Given the high risk for the development of VTE/DVT following spinal cord injury, chemoprophylaxis with low–molecular-weight heparin is typically started 72 hours after injury. This may be combined with mechanical prophylaxis, including external pneumatic compression devices. Duration of treatment varies depending on the level and completeness of the spinal cord injury. Current recommendations suggest a minimum of 3 months or after completion of inpatient rehabilitation. OMM, including lymphatic techniques, can be utilized in patients affected by edema or poor venous return but would be contraindicated in the presence of DVT.[26]

Neurologic Model

Spinal cord injury can be traumatic (i.e., fracture of the spinal column) or nontraumatic (transverse myelitis, spinal stenosis with myelopathy, spinal cord tumor, etc.) in nature. Regardless of type, there is usually significant involvement of the central nervous system and spinal cord tracts, including the corticospinal and spinothalamic tracts. Along with alteration of motor and sensory function, spinal cord injuries also impact the sympathetic nervous system and result in a dysregulation of sympathetic activity. The above alterations in the nervous system result in a multitude of potential complications unique to the spinal cord–injured patient, including development of pressure ulcers from impaired sensation, neurogenic bowel and bladder, spasticity, and autonomic dysreflexia. This patient does not have a history of autonomic dysreflexia but must manage his neurogenic bladder with intermittent catheterization and his neurogenic bowel with a bowel program, which includes a stool softener (e.g., docusate) and stimulant suppository (e.g., bisacodyl). He does not have significant neuropathic pain but does have spasticity affecting the lower extremities, for which he takes oral baclofen. The osteopathic physiatrist must be aware of these potential complications and treat them in a comprehensive fashion.[27,28]

- Spasticity and hyperreflexia
  - Spasticity is often defined as a velocity-dependent increase in muscle tone and resistance to stretch, which results from a loss of descending inhibition within the spinal cord. It causes disinhibition of muscle stretch reflexes and the reemergence of primitive reflexes. While this may be readily apparent in the skeletal muscle of the patient with a spinal cord injury, spasticity also affects the muscle tissue of organs such as the bladder resulting in hyperactivity of the detrusor muscle and development of neurogenic bladder.[29,30]
  - Treatment is aimed at reducing spasticity that interferes with function, including performing transfers and activities of daily living, or that causes contracture or pain. This may include the use of oral medications such as baclofen, to act as a GABA agonist, injection with botulinum toxin to block the presynaptic release of acetylcholine, or implantation and use of an intrathecal baclofen pump.[31–33]
- Autonomic dysreflexia
  - This condition, unique to patients with spinal cord injuries, is due to increased sympathetic activity that is no longer inhibited by descending control due to interruption by the injury. It usually presents in patients injured at or above the T6 level. Symptoms and signs include elevated blood pressure, bradycardia, sweating and flushing above the level of spinal cord injury, piloerection, and pupillary constriction.[34–36]
  - Initial management of autonomic dysreflexia, considered a medical emergency, includes sitting the patient in an upright position and finding the noxious stimulus potentially responsible for the increased afferent activity and facilitated sympathetic response. The most common stimulus for autonomic dysreflexia is from the bladder, either an infection or distension. Other etiologies include the bowel (fecal impaction) or even tight clothing. If a satisfactory reduction in blood pressure is not achieved, after addressing these issues, medications used to treat the elevated blood pressure including nitroglycerin paste, clonidine, nifedipine, hydralazine, and others can be used.[22,37]
- Pain
  - Patients with a spinal cord injury are frequently affected by pain (i.e., 60% to 80%) which can interfere with function and is somatic or neuropathic in nature. Somatic pain is frequently reported in the upper extremities and can be the result of overuse injuries of the musculoskeletal system, including rotator cuff tears, tendonitis, and myofascial pain. Neuropathic pain is usually the result of direct injury to the peripheral or central nervous system and may include carpal tunnel syndrome, cervical radiculopathy, or post-traumatic syringomyelia.[38,39]

- Successfully treating pain in patients with a spinal cord injury requires accurate localization of pain generator(s) and a comprehensive approach that may include physical therapy, medications (oral and/or intrathecal), interventional procedures, psychological counseling, and manual medicine.[40,41] OMM has been shown to be a feasible treatment option in patients with a spinal cord injury who suffer from pain and can be used in patients for whom medication may be contraindicated or in combination with medication when indicated.[41,42]

Metabolic/Nutritional Model

Metabolic and nutritional concerns are important in post-injury management and long-term quality of life. Surveillance should be done after the injury, and adequate nutrition should be maintained long term to promote health and maximize healing, in both healthy and affected tissues, especially in the setting of possible pressure injury development. Hypercalcemia and superior mesenteric artery (SMA) syndrome are conditions that the osteopathic physiatrist should assess for in this patient during an acute inpatient rehabilitation setting and beyond. Fortunately, this patient has not developed a pressure sore and has been vigilant with limiting pressure to areas prone to the development of pressure injuries, including the ischial tuberosities and sacrum.

- Hypercalcemia
  - Hypercalcemia affects as many as 10% to 20% of spinal cord–injured patients, especially adolescent males. Patients present with symptoms classically associated with hypercalcemia (i.e., "bones, stones, and psychic overtones") as well as dehydration, confusion, and renal impairment, and can often be vague and insidious in nature. It is thought to be due to reduced mechanical stimulation of bone formation. Patients who are immobilized following injury, or other conditions associated with limited movement (stroke, amputee, etc.) can undergo bone resorption.[43]
  - Treatment typically consists of intravenous fluid hydration, early mobilization as possible, and medication aimed at inhibiting osteoclast activity, if necessary.
- SMA syndrome
  - SMA syndrome is a condition in which the third portion of the duodenum is compressed by the SMA and the aorta, causing obstruction of the gastrointestinal tract with associated epigastric abdominal pain, distention, and postprandial nausea, and vomiting that is worse in the supine position. Rapid weight loss is a contributing factor that can precipitate compression of the duodenum.[44]
  - Symptoms can be alleviated by eating smaller meals more frequently, positional eating, and occasionally, use of fluid resuscitation, nasoenteric tubes and feedings, or total parenteral nutrition.
- Pressure injuries
  - Up to 80% of patients affected by a spinal cord injury develop a pressure injury during their lifetime. Pressure injuries commonly develop over bony prominences, including, but not limited to, the sacrum, ischium, heels, and trochanters. They develop due to a combination of factors that include ischemia, direct pressure over bony prominences, and friction.[45,46]
  - Prevention and treatment of pressure injuries include adequate and frequent pressure relief and optimal nutrition to promote the integrity and healing of muscle, skin, and connective tissues.[47]

Behavioral/Biopsychosocial Model

A spinal cord injury is a life-altering event that impacts not only the ability of a patient to perform activities of daily living and work, but also their sense of self and relationships within their home and community. A core principle of rehabilitation is viewing the patient as more than just their physical being and facilitating the successful reintegration of the patient into their life. Psychological issues, including depression, posttraumatic stress disorder, and anxiety must be recognized following a spinal cord injury along with assessing how they may interfere with the process of reintegration. Fortunately, this patient is not suffering from current psychological issues, and he has adapted to his injury, returning to living independently. He is working full-time and driving a motor vehicle with adapted hand controls.

- Depression
  - Depression occurs in approximately 20% to 40% of spinal cord–injured patients with the highest incidence occurring during the acute phase of their rehabilitation. Suicide is the leading cause of mortality in younger age groups and is highest in those who are paraplegic and suffer incomplete versus complete injuries.[48–50]
  - Early recognition of depression is important to minimize interference with the rehabilitation process. This can include medication and psychological counseling. Encouraging an optimistic outlook is helpful for optimizing longer-term outcomes and successfully reintegrating into the home and community. Fostering relationships and a support network, as well as maximizing independence, including the ability to drive, are useful since they promote a return to work and school and other activities.[51]

SUMMARY

The philosophy of PM&R as a specialty closely aligns with fundamental osteopathic tenets. PM&R physicians, or physiatrists, aim to maximize patients' physical function and quality of life. The osteopathic approach emphasizes the interrelated nature of structure and function. The osteopathic physiatrist performs a comprehensive patient-focused evaluation that considers all factors impacting a person's physical, functional, and psychological recovery. This approach aligns closely with osteopathic medicine, which views the person as a unit of body, mind, and spirit. The relationship between osteopathic medicine and PM&R potentially explains why so many osteopathic physicians choose this specialty as a career. A central tenet of PM&R is addressing the disability that results from injury or disease, which is accomplished by restoring or maximizing a patient's function. To accomplish this, physiatrists must measure a patient's improvement in terms of performing o tasks with the treatment provided. Physiatrists address a variety of conditions, especially those affecting the musculoskeletal and nervous systems. Their comprehensive patient-centered approach lends itself to addressing the disability resulting from conditions such as stroke, spinal cord, and traumatic brain injury. Complicated illnesses and injuries such as spinal cord injury affect multiple organ systems and require a multidisciplinary approach, that is supported by the five models of osteopathic care.

ACKNOWLEDGMENTS

The authors and editors of this chapter would like to acknowledge the scholarly contributions of James A. Lipton, DO, FAOCPMR,

FAAO, to prior editions of this chapter and to the specialty of PM&R and Osteopathic Medicine in the U.S. Navy Medical Corps and civilian settings.

REFERENCES

1. Sandel E. *The Philosophical Foundations of Physical Medicine and Rehabilitation*. American Academy of Physical Medicine & Rehabilitation. Accessed November 1, 2017. http://www.aapmr.org
2. Opitz JL, Folz TJ, Gelfman R, Peters DJ. The history of physical medicine and rehabilitation as recorded in the diary of Dr. Frank Krusen: part 1. Gathering momentum (the years before 1942). *Arch Phys Med Rehabil.* 1997;78(4):442–445.
3. Folz TJ, Opitz JL, Peters DJ, Gelfman R. The history of physical medicine and rehabilitation as recorded in the diary of Dr. Frank Krusen: part 2. Forging ahead (1943–1947). *Arch Phys Med Rehabil.* 1997;78(4):446–450.
4. Gelfman R, Peters DJ, Opitz JL, Folz TJ. The history of physical medicine and rehabilitation as recorded in the diary of Dr. Frank Krusen: part 3. Consolidating the position (1948–1953). *Arch Phys Med Rehabil.* 1997;78(5):556–561.
5. Peters DJ, Gelfman R, Folz TJ, Opitz JL. The history of physical medicine and rehabilitation as recorded in the diary of Dr. Frank Krusen: part 4. Triumph over adversity (1954–1969). *Arch Phys Med Rehabil.* 1997;78(5):562–565.
6. AAPMR History Preservation Committee. *The History of the Specialty of Physical Medicine and Rehabilitation*. American Academy of Physical Medicine & Rehabilitation. Accessed November 1, 2017. http://www.aapmr.org
7. Halstead LS. A brief history of postpolio syndrome in the United States. *Arch Phys Med Rehabil.* 2011;92(8):1344–1349.
8. Reppel A, Dawodu S. *Conceptual Models of Disability*. American Academy of Physical Medicine & Rehabilitation. Accessed November 1, 2017. http://www.aapmr.org
9. Frontera WR, Joel AD. *Physical Medicine & Rehabilitation: Principles and Practice.* 5th ed. Wolters Kluwer/Lippincott Williams & Wilkins Health; 2010. Chapter 1: Clinical Evaluation; Chapter 2: Physical Examination.
10. Stanton DF, Wieting JM. Osteopathic medicine, and the role of manipulation in the treatment of chronic pain. In: Anchor KN, Felicetti TC, eds. *Disability Analysis in Practice.* Kendall Hunt; 1999:112–113.
11. World Health Organization. *International Classification of Impairments, Disabilities, and Handicaps: A Manual of Classification Relating to the Consequences of Disease.* World Health Organization; 1980.
12. Stucki G, Melvin J. The International Classification of Functioning, Disability and Health: a unifying model for the conceptual description of physical and rehabilitation medicine. *J Rehabil Med.* 2007;39(4):286–292.
13. *Towards a Common Language for Functioning, Disability, and Health: The International Classification of Functioning, Disability and Health.* World Health Organization; 2002.
14. Association of American Medical Colleges. Physician specialty data report. 2020.
15. van Middendorp JJ, Hosman AJ, Donders AR, et al; EM-SCI Study Group. A clinical prediction rule for ambulation outcomes after traumatic spinal cord injury: a longitudinal cohort study. *Lancet.* 2011;377(9770):1004–1010.
16. AlHuthaifi F, Krzak J, Hanke T, Vogel LC. Predictors of functional outcomes in adults with traumatic spinal cord injury following inpatient rehabilitation: a systematic review. *J Spinal Cord Med.* 2017;40(3):282–294.
17. Consortium for Spinal Cord Medicine. Outcomes following traumatic spinal cord injury: clinical practice guidelines for health-care professionals. *J Spinal Cord Med.* 2000;23(4):289–316.
18. Bayley JC, Cochran TP, Sledge CB. The weight-bearing shoulder. The impingement syndrome in paraplegics. *J Bone Joint Surg Am.* 1987;69(5):676–678.
19. Liang HW, Wang YH, Pan SL, Wang TG, Huang TS. Asymptomatic median mononeuropathy among men with chronic paraplegia. *Arch Phys Med Rehabil.* 2007;88(9):1193–1197.
20. Davidoff G, Werner R, Waring W. Compressive mononeuropathies of the upper extremity in chronic paraplegia. *Paraplegia.* 1991;29(1):17–24.
21. Paralyzed Veterans of America Consortium for Spinal Cord Medicine. Preservation of upper limb function following spinal cord injury: a clinical practice guideline for health-care professionals. *J Spinal Cord Med.* 2005;28(5):434–470.
22. Reeves RK, Brubaker M, Kirshblum SC. Rehabilitation of spinal cord injury. In Frontera WR, DeLisa JA, Basford JR, Bockenek WL, Chae J, Robinson LR, eds. *DeLisa's Physical Medicine and Rehabilitation: Principles and Practice.* 6th ed. Lippincott Williams & Wilkins; 2020:449–500.
23. Consortium for Spinal Cord Medicine. Respiratory management following spinal cord injury: a clinical practice guideline for health-care professionals. *J Spinal Cord Med.* 2005;28(3):259–293.
24. DiMarco AF, Takaoka Y, Kowalski KE. Combined intercostal and diaphragm pacing to provide artificial ventilation in patients with tetraplegia. *Arch Phys Med Rehabil.* 2005;86(6):1200–1207.
25. Aito S, Abbate R, Marcucci R, Cominelli E. Endogenous risk factors for deep-vein thrombosis in patients with acute spinal cord injuries. *Spinal Cord.* 2007;45(9):627–631.
26. Piran S, Schulman S. Thromboprophylaxis in patients with acute spinal cord injury: a narrative review. *Semin Thromb Hemost.* 2019;45(2):150–156.
27. Consortium for Spinal Cord Medicine. Bladder management for adults with spinal cord injury: a clinical practice guideline for health-care providers. *J Spinal Cord Med.* 2006;29(5):527–573.
28. Clinical practice guidelines: neurogenic bowel management in adults with spinal cord injury. Spinal cord medicine consortium. *J Spinal Cord Med.* 1998;21(3):248–293.
29. Finnerup NB. Neuropathic pain and spasticity: intricate consequences of spinal cord injury. *Spinal Cord.* 2017;55:1046–1050.
30. Sahai A, Cortes E, Seth J, et al. Neurogenic detrusor overactivity in patients with spinal cord injury: evaluation and management. *Curr Urol Rep.* 2011;12(6):404–412.
31. Walker HW, Lee MY, Bahroo LB, Hedera P, Charles D. Botulinum toxin injection techniques for the management of adult spasticity. *PM R.* 2015;7(4):417–427.
32. de Sousa N, Santos D, Monteiro S, Silva N, Barreiro-Iglesias A, Salgado AJ. Role of baclofen in modulating spasticity and neuroprotection in spinal cord injury. *J Neurotrauma.* 2022:39(3–4):249–258.
33. Khan F, Amatya B, Bensmail D, Yelnik A. Non-pharmacological interventions for spasticity in adults: an overview of systematic reviews. *Ann Phys Rehabil Med.* 2019;62(4):265–273.
34. Hagen EM. Acute complications of spinal cord injuries. *World J Orthop.* 2015;6(1):17–23.
35. Eldahan KC, Rabchevsky AG. Autonomic dysreflexia after spinal cord injury: systemic pathophysiology and methods of management. *Auton Neurosci.* 2018;209:59–70.
36. Hou S, Rabchevsky AG. Autonomic consequences of spinal cord injury. *Compr Physiol.* 2014;4(4):1419–1453.
37. Consortium for Spinal Cord Medicine. Acute management of autonomic dysreflexia: individuals with spinal cord injury presenting to health-care facilities. *J Spinal Cord Med.* 2002;25(1):S67–S88.
38. Saulino M. Spinal cord injury pain. *Phys Med Rehabil Clin N Am.* 2014;25(2):397–410.
39. Felix ER. Chronic neuropathic pain in SCI: evaluation and treatment. *Phys Med Rehabil Clin N Am.* 2014;25(3):545–571, viii.
40. Mehta S, McIntyre A, Janzen S, Loh E, Teasell R; Spinal Cord Injury Rehabilitation Evidence Team. Systematic review of pharmacologic treatments of pain after spinal cord injury: an update. *Arch Phys Med Rehabil.* 2016;97(8):1381–1391.e1.
41. Boldt I, Eriks-Hoogland I, Brinkhof MW, de Bie R, Joggi D, von Elm E. Non-pharmacological interventions for chronic pain in people with spinal cord injury. *Cochrane Database Syst Rev.* 2014;(11):CD009177.
42. Arienti C, Daccò S, Piccolo I, Redaelli T. Osteopathic manipulative treatment is effective on pain control associated to spinal cord injury. *Spinal Cord.* 2011;49(4):515–519.
43. Maynard FM. Immobilization hypercalcemia following spinal cord injury. *Arch Phys Med Rehabil.* 1986;67(1):41–44.
44. Desai MH, Gall A, Khoo M. Superior mesenteric artery syndrome—a rare presentation and challenge in spinal cord injury rehabilitation: a case report and literature review. *J Spinal Cord Med.* 2015;38(4):544–547.

45. Gélis A, Dupeyron A, Legros P, Benaïm C, Pelissier J, Fattal C. Pressure ulcer risk factors in persons with SCI: Part I: acute and rehabilitation stages. *Spinal Cord.* 2009;47(2):99–107.
46. Gélis A, Dupeyron A, Legros P, Benaïm C, Pelissier J, Fattal C. Pressure ulcer risk factors in persons with spinal cord injury part 2: the chronic stage. *Spinal Cord.* 2009;47(9):651–661.
47. Consortium for Spinal Cord Medicine Clinical Practice Guidelines. Pressure ulcer prevention and treatment following spinal cord injury: a clinical practice guideline for health-care professionals. *J Spinal Cord Med.* 2001;24 (1):S40–S101.
48. Khazaeipour Z, Taheri-Otaghsara SM, Naghdi M. Depression following spinal cord injury: its relationship to demographic and socioeconomic indicators. *Top Spinal Cord Inj Rehabil.* 2015;21(2):149–155.
49. Kraft R, Dorstyn D. Psychosocial correlates of depression following spinal injury: a systematic review. *J Spinal Cord Med.* 2015;38(5):571–583.
50. Tran J, Dorstyn DS, Burke AL. Psychosocial aspects of spinal cord injury pain: a meta-analysis. *Spinal Cord.* 2016;54(9):640–648.
51. Perkes SJ, Bowman J, Penkala S. Psychological therapies for the management of co-morbid depression following a spinal cord injury: a systematic review. *J Health Psychol.* 2014;19(12):1597–1612.

76 Osteopathic Considerations in Oncology

JENNIFER A. BELSKY ▪ KATIE KERRIGAN

KEY CONCEPTS

- This chapter focuses on the care of the patient with cancer using osteopathic philosophy and principles.
- Several malignancies involving bone and soft tissue structures, the central nervous system (CNS), or the peripheral nervous system which should be included in the differential diagnosis of musculoskeletal disorders.
- These malignancies have clinical manifestations in the musculoskeletal system including: back, extremity, joint, and muscle pain with occasional skin involvement.
- CNS malignancies can have unique presentations and include both cerebral and indirect paraneoplastic malignancies, which often display elements of viscerosomatic-type oncologic responses.
- Osteopathic tenets are applicable to all components of cancer care and are involved in the diagnosis, treatment options, and education to patients and families.
- Providing supportive care for patients with cancer includes symptom and pain relief, blood and blood products, and general supportive care.
- Many cancers are caused by lifestyle choices or environmental toxicities that can be prevented.
- Pediatric and adolescent young adult cancer presentations can vary from adult, with unique presentations and intense treatment options.
- The osteopathic approach, including indications and contraindications for osteopathic manipulative treatment, and stress management issues are addressed.

Osteopathic physicians do not treat disease, they treat patients.[1]

—Philip E. Greenman, DO

Care more particularly for the individual patient than for the special features of the disease.[2]

—Sir William Osler

INTRODUCTION

Medical and pediatric oncology are a subspecialty of internal medicine or pediatrics and represents unique branches of medicine dealing with the incidence, prevention, diagnosis, and medical management of malignancy. Cancer is the second leading cause of mortality in the United States in adults, and a top five leading cause of mortality in children.[3] The field of study surrounding oncology is constantly changing due to rapid progress of cancer research in diagnosis and treatment over the past 50 years. Oncology has grown as a specialty over the years with the advent of subspecialty fellowships since the mid-1960s. This 3-year training program is taken after completion of 3 years of training in general internal medicine or pediatrics.

Patients traditionally present to primary care physicians (PCPs) or surgeons, and if concern for malignancy arises, patients are referred to oncologists for further workup and management. In most cases, the oncologist will serve as the guide for a patient's care through the maze of cancer diagnosis, surgical and radiation treatment, and/or delivery of chemotherapy, immunotherapy, and, when necessary, end-of-life and palliative care.

Significant advances leading to cure and long, functional disease-free intervals are now commonplace.

ONCOLOGY

The patient with a cancer diagnosis presents a complex series of events for the PCP. The clinical manifestations of this heterogeneous family of diseases are diverse with a wide range of initial symptoms depending on cancer type and location. Presenting symptoms may be secondary to altered structure or function at the primary site of tumor involvement or due to involvement of a secondary site with metastatic disease. Rarely, paraneoplastic syndromes may create bizarre presenting signs and symptoms of an undiagnosed malignancy, usually through generation of hormones or auto-antibodies which attack the normal structure and function of tissues.

Patients with cancer, as in all persons with chronic disease, are first and foremost human. As cancer affects all ages from birth to elderly, patients have unique challenges to consider as treatment options are developed. They are human beings with families, with thoughts, feelings, hopes, and dreams. They often have parents, children, friends, and colleagues. These are not cancer patients but people living with cancer. Children diagnosed with cancer are pulled from school and routine social environments with their lives upended. Discussion surrounding treatment options must be carefully individualized. Patients must be offered choices and personal autonomy to make the appropriate individualized care plan. Regardless of treatment choice, patients must always be offered oncologic care, even if the disease is incurable. This supportive care will include prevention and treatment of pain, emotional and mental support, and in the case of end-of-life, can encompass other symptoms as they arise through the process of dying. This will include supporting the person's fullest level of functioning at home with family and loved ones,

In many cases, there arrives a time in the course of a disease when no further curable treatment is available. Focus can shift to palliative care. This is a significant opportunity for the caregiving physician and multidisciplinary support team. Although treatment of the whole person is the foundation of the physician's interactions with the patient, it is especially important to emphasize this aspect of the relationship when you can no longer treat the disease.

THE WHOLE PATIENT: DEFINITION

Throughout this chapter, the reader will see several times the phrase "*whole patient*." The context in which this is used refers to a person or human being together with a disease and not only an illness to be diagnosed and managed. The individual may have personal, social, financial, and spiritual concerns in addition to a constellation of potential issues that may or may not be disease related, and the treating oncologist must be aware of this and incorporate it into treatment decision making. This defines the "whole patient" and, although a humanistic quality to be strived for by all physicians, is especially linked to the osteopathic, "holistic" philosophy associated with treating a fully integrated/interrelated system.

Review Chapter 17 Mind–Body Medicine, Chapter 21 Lifestyle Medicine—Osteopathic Perspectives, and Chapter 80 Osteopathic Considerations in End-of-Life Care as the concepts discussed in this chapter dovetail with those addressed therein.

OSTEOPATHIC PHILOSOPHIC PRINCIPLES OF CARE OF THE PATIENT WITH CANCER

Traditional cancer therapy may include surgery, radiation therapy, drug, and/or immune therapy. Osteopathic physicians must continue to use these modalities when applicable, while being ever mindful that it is a person being cared for rather than a tumor. Patient decisions and actions are often based on their thoughts, feelings, and perceptions. It is vital for osteopathic physicians to use joint decision making with patients and families as they navigate the initial diagnosis, treatment, and outcome of their disease.

To Treat or Not to Treat

Many physicians assume that all cancer must be treated, whether or not there are effective therapeutic options. Remember that the clinician should treat every patient, but it is not necessary to treat every cancer. In many cases, equal benefit can be provided to the patient with careful understanding and supportive therapy. Transparent and honest communication with the patient is key to having tough conversations surrounding shared decision making. A life-threatening disease, such as metastatic renal cell cancer, can be discussed in a positive and optimistic fashion. The patient can be informed regarding the unpredictable natural history of the disease, which can have long-term stable control in some patients. Immunotherapeutic treatments can be discussed and offered if the patient is an appropriate candidate. The patient, however, must be reassured that the physician will be available throughout the treatment course. Patients must be reassured that as symptoms of their cancer or side effects of treatment arise, they need not be uncomfortable. They should be reassured that the physician will discuss all decisions regarding therapy with them and assist them in decision making. The physician must inform and support the family if the patient wishes. Throughout the discussion, which may become more repetitious and personal as the relationship develops, therapeutic and empathic touch of the patient is important. The patient must leave the physician after each visit confident that a partnership has developed.

Touching as Communication

Physical touch is a nonverbal important communication tool that is often underutilized with patients. Patients have voiced that the only time a physician has touched them in the past was in the process of physical examination. Patients with cancer feel comforted by an appropriate touch of a hand or even, on occasion, a tear shed with theirs. Touching is a nonverbal communication with the patient that says, "I recognize you as a whole person, not only a diseased body or an interesting case." Recognition of the *whole person* encompassing the cancer is to recognize the integration of all body systems. This offers the consideration that no system can alone become diseased or healthy without impact or benefit to the whole person or other systems. They must all get well and survive together. The basic osteopathic philosophy emphasizes the need to treat the person as a whole. This approach must consider the patient with the disease as well as the patient's environment. During the COVID-19 global pandemic, many cancer patients were forced to receive care via telehealth, significantly impairing the benefits of nonverbal communication like touch.

Osteopathic physicians are well known for their excellent physician exam skills and their ability to connect through physical touch while treating dysfunction. Palpatory diagnosis and treatment of neuromusculoskeletal dysfunctions have been hallmarks of this profession from its inception and play a key role in cancer diagnosis and care.

METASTASIS TO NEUROMUSCULOSKELETAL STRUCTURES

Within this chapter, cancer will be discussed with an emphasis on its manifestations/effects on the neuromusculoskeletal system. The relationship of the neurostructural presentation of a patient with malignancy versus a nonneoplastic structural lesion can be interesting and deceiving. Back pain is the most common musculoskeletal complaint seen in primary care practice.[4] Often the cause is a somatic dysfunction and is amenable to osteopathic manipulative treatment (OMT) (see Chapters 65, 84, 93, and 95). When other concerning symptoms are present, including those that are refractory to medications, systemic correlating symptoms, or progression of pain despite optimal treatment, further investigation is required to rule in or out more consequential diagnoses. For examples:

- A 72-year-old female had chronic midback pain that progressively worsened over the past 3 weeks, was refractory to NSAIDs, and associated with dyspnea and sleep disruption. She went to the emergency department and was given a muscle relaxant and a narcotic analgesic. She was instructed to see her PCP if her pain did not improve in a couple of days. Two days later, her unrelenting pain led to a visit to her PCP. During that visit and on physical examination, she was found to have a hard and noncompliant right T11 and T12 vertebrae and ribs to springing palpation. In addition, the area had tender hypertonic muscles that did not relax with soft tissue treatment. An x-ray of the area revealed the absence of T11 and T12 vertebral bodies and the heads of the associated ribs, which were replaced by tumor. She was ultimately diagnosed with multiple myeloma (see below).
- A 57-year-old male with prostate cancer was taken by his wife by wheelchair to the emergency department complaining of back pain and sudden onset of right leg weakness and difficulty with ambulation. His physical exam showed back muscle spasms and tenderness with motor deficits in the right lower extremity extensors. CT of his spine showed two areas of metastatic cancer compressing his spinal cord.

Bone metastases are common in patients with advanced solid tumors.[5] Cancers particularly associated with bone metastases include (Table 76.1)[5]:

- Prostate and breast (65% to 75% of patients)
- Lung (30% to 40%)
- Kidney (20% to 32%)[5,6]

TABLE 76.1

Primary Malignancies, Which Commonly Metastasize to the Vertebral Column and Spinal Cord, Listed in Descending Order of Frequency

Vertebrae	Spinal Cord
Breast	Lung
Prostate	Breast
Lung	Colon
Kidney	Sarcoma
Thyroid	

- They are often associated with skeletal-related events (SREs)[7]:
  - □ Pathologic fracture
  - □ Spinal cord compression
  - □ Hypercalcemia

Untreated, SREs may occur every 3 to 6 months[7] and can lead to considerable burden on patients, their families and caregivers, and the health care system.[8] Thus, early detection and treatment are warranted.[9] Early detection usually starts with a high degree of suspicion on the part of the PCP and oncologist. A signal of possible bone metastasis may be a complaint of increased pain and need for stronger opioid analgesic required to alleviate it.[10] Bone metastasis is associated with decreased survival in breast[11] and prostate[12] cancers but not necessarily in renal cancer, for example, which may be partly due to advanced treatments with immunotherapy that prolong survival.[6] Treatment of bone metastasis with bisphosphonates or receptor activator of nuclear factor kappa-B ligand (RANKL) inhibitor, denosumab in addition to radiation and chemotherapy, may reduce SREs which could affect both morbidity and mortality.[9,13]

Neuromusculoskeletal metastasis may occur in the spine, producing back pain to soft tissue areas as:

- A mass
- A compression of the spinal cord
- Nerve root producing peripheral neuropathic symptoms

Central nervous system (CNS) signs and symptoms can also be produced due to direct metastasis or paraneoplastic effects (hypercalcemia).

Diagnostic methods of bone metastasis include[14]:

- Radiographs (x-ray)
- Scintigraphy
- Positive emission tomography
- Magnetic resonance imaging
- Biopsy:
  - □ Liquid
  - □ Fine needle
  - □ Open
  - □ Core needle
  - □ CT or MRI guided
- Biomarkers are still experimental but hold a promise[15]

Some tumors do not present with symptoms in the organ system as would be expected. For example, in renal cancer, the systemic manifestations may include:

- Anemia or erythrocytosis
- Fever of unknown origin
- Weight loss
- Hypercalcemia

All of the above may occur in the absence of metastatic disease. The hypercalcemia is often a paraneoplastic syndrome related to production of ectopic parathyroid hormone–like substance from the tumor (parathyroid hormone–related protein or PTHrP) (see below re: hypercalcemia).

CASE IN POINT: PLASMA CELL NEOPLASM (MULTIPLE MYELOMA)

This disease is the most common primary tumor to involve medullary bone and may often be overlooked in a patient presenting with back pain. The incidence of myeloma is between two to four per 100,000 population with a higher rate in Blacks than Whites.[16] This is a neoplasm of plasma cells, a type of B-lymphocyte, resulting in overproduction of monoclonal immunoglobulins. They can be detected in blood and urine as M-protein on a protein electrophoresis. The diagnostic characteristics of this neoplasm include:

- Bone marrow plasmacytosis
- Monoclonal immunoglobulin detection
- Anemia
- Bone pain
- Hypercalcemia

Often, the symptoms are vague and nonspecific. Typical lytic "punched out" bone lesions may be absent, and a diffuse osteoporosis pattern may be seen on radiograph. Plasma cell tumors may originate in extramedullary sites as well.

- They have been known to arise in almost any organ with the upper air passages (nasal sinuses, nose, nasopharynx, tonsil) being the most frequent extramedullary sites.
- These tumors may also arise in the skin and subcutaneous tissue, thereby presenting as soft tissue masses.

At least two-thirds of patients present with the skeletal symptom of bone pain, especially in axial skeleton.

- Pathologic fractures are common.
- Spinal cord compression and nerve root compression are common complications of this disease and may produce radicular pain.
- Peripheral neuropathies may occur as a result of amyloid deposition in nerves or perineural vasculature.

Other clinical problems common in the patient with myeloma include hypercalcemia.

- The progressive confusion and drowsiness in these patients may resemble CNS disease.
- GI symptoms of nausea, vomiting, and constipation together with polyuria may signal the onset of hypercalcemia (see below re: paraneoplastic syndromes for further discussion).

A hyperviscosity syndrome is also a complication of myeloma, especially immunoglobulin M (IgM) myeloma, and is due to a change in concentration, size, and shape of the monoclonal globulin.

- If the serum viscosity relative to water rises above four, symptoms occur. These may include:
  - □ Cephalalgia
  - □ Visual disturbance
  - □ Fatigue

- Vertigo
- Nystagmus
- Paresis
- Eventually confusion and coma

This combination of symptoms may closely resemble CNS metastasis.

Attempts should be made to diagnose myeloma earlier than presentation with pathologic fracture. Early clues may be:

- Anemia
- Proteinuria
- Rouleaux formation on a peripheral smear report
- A report of bone demineralization

Myeloma usually enters a chronic phase that is easily responsive to steroids and alkylating drugs.

- Fluid hydration is beneficial for the renal complications and in preventing hyperviscosity.
  - Hyperviscosity is treated by plasmapheresis and specific chemotherapy including steroids and alkylating agents.
- Pathologic fractures may be surgically treated with orthopedic fixation.
- Impending fractures and spinal cord/nerve root compression should be irradiated.
- Maintaining activity and ambulation is essential in treatment of this disease.
- Eventually, the patients enter an acute phase characterized by bone marrow infiltration by plasma cells resulting in pancytopenia and potential infectious complications.
- Infection and renal failure are often terminal events.
- Although no cure has been discovered for this devastating disease, immunotherapeutics have shown some promising results[17]

The manifestations of metastasis to neuromusculoskeletal structures discussed within this section will be divided into three categories:

- Musculoskeletal
- CNS
- Peripheral nervous system

Metastasis can often influence the presentation within these systems. The major conduits of metastasis from internal organs to the neuromusculoskeletal structures involve[18]:

- Direct tumor extension
- Lymphatic dissemination
- Hematogenous dissemination

In the 1940s, Batson described the anatomy of the vertebral venous plexus, a system of valveless vessels extending along the spine and forming anastomoses with veins extending from the brain to the pelvis. He demonstrated extensive retrograde–antegrade vascular flow potential in this venous system as related to posture and abdominal pressure.[19,20] This system that now carries his name has been thought to be a primary conduit involved in the spread of prostate and breast cancer to the vertebral spine. Prostate cancer metastasis to the bone may also involve recruitment and reprogramming of bystander and dormant cells by a population of metastasis-initiating cells.[21] The bone microenvironment is a unique and fertile soil, called the "metastatic niche," for cancer metastasis, and tumor cells modify the bone microenvironment during cancer invasion and expansion through the recruitment and modulation of osteoclasts, osteoblasts, immune cells, vascular elements, bone matrix, and neuronal processes.[22,23]

Musculoskeletal System

BACK PAIN

The bony skeleton is the most common metastatic site of malignancy.[5] Over 80% of the metastatic tumors to the skeleton originate from breast, prostate, lung, kidney, and thyroid cancers which present as metastases in the spine.[5,23] Metastatic bone disease in the spine may be lytic (clastic or destructive) or blastic (sclerotic) or a mixture of both. Metastatic bone disease is much more common than primary bone tumors. Back pain is often the first indication of metastatic disease.

- Back pain may be present for varying periods of time before the onset of neurologic signs or symptoms, which usually occur secondary to compression of a nerve root or the spinal cord.
- The origin of back pain may be difficult to localize in the skeletal system due to the vagaries of diagnostic tests available (see Ref. 12 for review). For example:
  - Radiographs do not visualize osseous changes as early as radionuclide scans.
  - Scans depend on osteoblastic activity for demonstration of abnormalities.
  - Actual loss of bone density of at least 50% is required to demonstrate metastasis by radiograph.
  - Nuclear medicine bone scans do not detect osteoclastic lesions.
  - In the older adult patient, a reactive or inflammatory process such as arthritis or degenerative vertebral disease can mimic the metastatic process and create a false-positive bone scan. Therefore, bone scan abnormalities require radiographic, CT, or MRI confirmation of metastases.
  - Two procedures are often indicated for comparison prior to a definitive diagnosis and initiation of treatment. CT and MRI, which have a greater degree of resolution, are often helpful in detection of otherwise silent lesions.
  - Often, with a high index of clinical suspicion and without imaging documentation, localization by specific sensory or dermatomal level can focus an area to permit treatment by radiation therapy.
- In evaluation of the patient with back pain, one must always consider malignancy, especially prostate cancer in a man over 55 years of age.
  - Additional systemic manifestations may include weight loss, pain unrelated to motion or position, and pain unresponsive to analgesic medications.
  - Oftentimes, there is an urgency in considering spinal metastasis so that appropriate therapy and maintenance of neurologic function can be maintained in patients with spinal cord compression.

JOINTS

The joints may be involved with malignancy by either a primary tumor or metastatic process to the bone or synovium. This presents as a picture of asymmetric arthritis or diffuse articular changes caused by an indirect, humoral-related process as in hypertrophic osteoarthropathy. Examples include:

- Leukemia in children
- Lung cancer
- Renal cancer
- Hypertrophic pulmonary osteoarthropathy (HPOA) from lung carcinoma

MUSCLE AND SKIN

A wide spectrum of skin, muscle, and connective tissue manifestations are associated with previous, current, or undiagnosed malignancy. These may be secondary to direct or metastatic involvement or secondary to paraneoplastic effect. Metastatic soft tissue or muscle masses can occur and have been reported in any anatomic area. These may produce pain and alter function due to muscle or nerve compression or invasion. These masses may occasionally be small, deep-seated, and not readily detected. Two rheumatologic diseases have a high degree of association with malignancy:

- Dermatomyositis
- Polymyositis

These conditions may precede the malignancy by days or years. The skin manifestations, when present, include a purplish erythema. The predominant clinical complaint is a progressive proximal muscular weakness developing over weeks to months. Muscle biopsy, elevated erythrocyte sedimentation rate, and muscle enzymes, and abnormal electromyogram (EMG) all play a role in the diagnosis. This syndrome is often labeled carcinomatous myopathy or neuromyopathy due to the diminished to absent deep tendon reflexes. The predominant associated malignancies are lung, gastric, and ovarian cancer.

Acanthosis nigricans, a hyperpigmented, hyperkeratotic skin lesion in intertriginous or flexor areas of axillary, neck, or anogenital areas, is often associated with gastric carcinoma or other abdominal malignancies.

Asymmetric shoulder girdle and arm pain may occasionally present as a structural problem simulating cervical nerve root irritation or brachial plexopathy, as in thoracic outlet syndrome. This may be seen in lung cancer with apical involvement and brachial plexus compression by a superior sulcus (Pancoast) tumor.

OCCULT MALIGNANCY PRESENTING WITH MUSCULOSKELETAL SYMPTOMS

Children

Cancer in children is more insidious than in adults and may mimic musculoskeletal disease, developmental processes, or childhood psychological problems.[24] Occult cancer in children presenting with musculoskeletal symptoms is an especially poignant example of why a high index of suspicion should be triggered when a child presents with disproportionate pain levels or an "atypical" pattern of arthritis that is not characteristic of a specific rheumatic disease. Although underlying neoplasm is found in less than 1% of such patients complaining of musculoskeletal symptoms,[25] cancer kills more children than any other disease.[24] Although primary bone cancer is more common in children than in adults, metastasis occurs with a variety of cancers, including neuroblastoma, rhabdomyosarcoma, teratoma–teratocarcinoma, Wilms tumor, retinoblastoma, lymphoma, and a few others.[26]

In an oncologic study on 1,254 children with cancer presenting with rheumatologic complaints, there were six cases of acute lymphoblastic leukemia, two cases of lymphoma, one case of Ewing sarcoma, and one case of neuroblastoma.[25] In a retrospective survey of 29 children ultimately diagnosed with malignancy and referred to a pediatric rheumatology clinic, provisional diagnoses included[27]:

- Juvenile rheumatoid arthritis (12 children)
- Nonspecific connective tissue disease (4 children)
- Diskitis (3 children)
- Spondyloarthropathy (3 children)
- Systemic lupus erythematosus (2 children)
- Kawasaki disease (2 children)
- Lyme disease, mixed connective tissue disease, and dermatomyositis (1 child each)

The final diagnoses were 13 cases of leukemia, six neuroblastoma, three lymphoma, three Ewing sarcoma, and one each of ependymoma, thalamic glioma, epithelioma, and sarcoma. The children, between the ages of 1 and 15 years (19 boys and 10 girls), had symptoms or signs of:

- Musculoskeletal pain (82%)
- Fever (54%)
- Fatigue (50%)
- Weight loss (42%)
- Hepatomegaly (29%)
- Arthritis (25%)

Features that suggested malignancy included:

- Nonarticular "bone" pain (68%)
- Back pain (32%)
- Bone tenderness (29%)
- Severe constitutional symptoms (32%)
- Features "atypical" of most rheumatic diseases (48%).

The "atypical" features:

- Night sweats (14%)
- Ecchymoses and bruising (14%)
- Abnormal neurologic signs (10%)
- Abnormal masses (7%)
- Ptosis (3%)

Adults

Malignant neoplasms in the adult are associated with a wide variety of paraneoplastic hematologic syndromes. The most frequently recognized are[28]:

- Hypertrophic osteoarthropathy
- Carcinomatous polyarthritis
- Dermatomyositis/polymyositis
- Paraneoplastic vasculitis

Lesser-known associations are[28]:

- Fasciitis
- Panniculitis
- Erythema nodosum
- Raynaud phenomenon
- Digital gangrene
- Erythromelalgia
- Lupus-like syndromes

Paraneoplastic musculoskeletal manifestations of malignancy may coincide, follow, or antedate the diagnosis of cancer or herald its recurrence. The clinical course parallels that of the primary tumor, and treatment of the underlying malignancy often results in the regression of the rheumatic disorder. Rheumatic manifestations suggesting a hidden cancer include[28]:

- Rapid onset of an unusual inflammatory arthritis
- Clubbing or diffuse bone pain in a patient 50 years or older
- Chronic unexplained vasculitis
- Refractory fasciitis
- Raynaud syndrome unresponsive to vasodilator therapy
- Rapidly progressing digital gangrene
- Lambert–Eaton myasthenic syndrome

Management of paraneoplastic rheumatic syndromes consists in control of the underlying cancer; symptomatic treatment of the rheumatic syndrome with nonsteroidal anti-inflammatory drugs, disease modifiers, cyclo-oxygenase-2 inhibitor, or glucocorticoid; and appropriate osteopathic manipulative techniques.

Central Nervous System

LEPTOMENINGEAL CARCINOMATOSIS

Leptomeningeal carcinomatosis is seen most often in breast cancer (12% to 35%), lung cancer (10% to 26%), melanoma (5% to 25%), gastrointestinal cancer (4% to 14%), and cancers of unknown primary (1% to 7%).[24] In these patients, a variety of diagnoses may precede the diagnosis of leptomeningeal disease, including[29]:

- Cerebral tumor
- Meningitis
- Psychoses
- Polyneuritis

This manifestation of systemic malignancy may occur as a presenting symptom. The presenting symptoms often include.[29]

- Low back pain
- Nonspecific leg pain (radicular)
- Headache
- Mental status change
- Extremity weakness
- Neck pain
- Nuchal rigidity
- Nausea and vomiting

MRI with gadolinium enhancement is the radiologic technique of choice.[29] The diagnosis is confirmed by finding malignant cells in the cerebral spinal fluid (CSF) as well as elevated CSF protein and low CSF glucose levels.[29] Leptomeningeal carcinomoatosis may be misdiagnosed as "musculoskeletal somatic dysfunction" based on vague presenting signs and symptoms.

INTRACRANIAL MALIGNANCY

Malignant disease may occur in the brain either as a primary tumor or as metastasis from an extracranial primary site. The symptoms noted are referable to the region of the brain involved, but 90% of patients at the time of diagnosis have significant impairment in one or more neurocognitive domains (memory, fine motor coordination, executive functions, and speech).[30]

Cancers of the lung, breast, and melanoma most often spread to the brain. Baseline brain MRI as a staging and screening modality is recommended in non–small cell lung cancers and small-cell lung cancers (SCLCs), as well as in melanoma.[31] Treatment depends on the clinical situation. Examples include[30]:

- Extensive intracranial dissemination often results in the use of whole brain radiotherapy (WBRT), whereas smaller, more isolated lesions may be amenable to stereotactic techniques (SRS).
- Surgical therapy is limited to selected situations (true solitary lesions) in metastatic brain disease.
- Treatment of the underlying systemic disease is also essential, for example, trastuzumab (monoclonal antibody against HER2-positive breast cancer).
- Multimodal approaches, which include WBRT, radiosurgery, surgery, and systemic and local medical therapies, have become more common in patients with brain metastases.

INDIRECT PARANEOPLASTIC SYNDROMES

Various syndromes have been described that may indirectly affect the CNS; the most common are encephalomyelitis, limbic encephalitis, and subacute cerebellar degeneration.[32] CSF analysis and serum onconeural antibody detection are used in diagnosis of these syndromes.[32] They can present with neurologic signs of dementia or cerebellar dysfunction.

A number of endocrinologic manifestations of malignancy occur in which there are indirect CNS signs. These are not a result of metastasis but due to polypeptide hormone–like substances or cytokines produced by the primary tumor. These hormones are autonomous in their production and not regulated by normal hormonal feedback control. The three most frequent of these syndromes are Cushing syndrome, syndrome of inappropriate antidiuretic hormone (SIADH), and nonmetastatic hypercalcemia (see below under neoplastic syndromes).

Peripheral Nervous System

This section will discuss the direct and remote effects of the malignant process from the standpoint of symptoms related to peripheral motor or sensory nerve involvement in the extremities. Although it is acknowledged that many of these problems have their origin within the CNS, oftentimes the end effects manifest themselves peripherally in the extremities. Therefore, these considerations will occur from the point of signs and symptoms rather than origin.

REMOTE PERIPHERAL MANIFESTATIONS

Peripheral neurologic problems are common in many patients with cancer. The most frequent etiology of these problems is direct invasion by primary or metastatic tumor. However, neuropathic symptoms (carcinomatous neuropathy) due to remote effects of the malignancy on the peripheral nervous system can occur uncommonly. Therefore, in addition to the discussion of the myasthenic syndrome and sensory motor polyneuropathy, this section will describe spinal cord disease with nerve root and plexus involvement.

Myasthenic syndrome, also known as Lambert–Eaton syndrome, is particularly associated with SCLC. This disorder is characterized by proximal pelvic girdle muscle weakness as the initial symptom, followed by proximal muscle weakness of the upper extremities, as well as gradual onset of fatigue, weight loss, slurred speech, difficulty swallowing, droopy eyelids, double vision, difficulty chewing, neck weakness, and autonomic symptoms such as dry mouth, male impotence, and constipation.[33]

- Other muscle symptoms may occur, and other tumors may be associated.
- Circulating immunoglobulin G antibodies against presynaptic P-/Q-type voltage-gated calcium channels (VGCCs) modulate expression of functional VGCC and thereby inhibit neurotransmission.[34]
- This syndrome is unlike myasthenia gravis in that the EMG muscle potential and clinical strength improve with repeated stimulation or with exercise.[35,36]
- The Tensilon test (diagnostic for myasthenia gravis by instant relief of muscle weakness after edrophonium administration) is not responsive as it is with myasthenia gravis.
- Treatment of this disorder rests essentially with treatment of the primary malignancy (SCLC) and amifampridine.[33]

Mixed sensory motor polyneuropathy may also be associated with cancer, particularly those of small-cell lung, breast, and ovarian origin.[37] The involvement produces distal extremity muscle weakness and wasting of muscles associated with distal sensory loss and areflexia. Many patients also present with distal limb pain. Most patients have onconeural antibodies (e.g., anti-Hu, anti-Yo, anti-Ri).[37,38] EMG studies have shown motor denervation more often than sensory, and nerve conduction studies have shown axonal/neuronal pattern to be most frequent, followed by axonal/demyelinating and demyelinating patterns.[38] Treatment of the underlying cancer, and addressing symptoms with plasmapheresis, immunomodulation with IVIG, immunosuppression with corticosteroids, or chemotherapy, may be useful.[37,38]

SPINAL CORD COMPRESSION

Epidural metastasis and spinal cord compression occur in 5% to 10% of patients with cancer.[39,40] The vertebral bodies are the most common sites of bone metastasis, which may lead to fractures, vertebral collapse, and/or compressive involvement of the spinal cord and nerves. This subject is of importance because of the frequency with which it occurs and the devastating effects that result if the signs and symptoms are not recognized in a timely fashion. It is common for patients with vertebral metastasis to present to emergency rooms or PCPs with low back pain and have this approached as a structural or somatic problem. It is of ultimate importance that spinal cord compression, which is a true oncologic emergency, be considered clinically and evaluated carefully. Certain clinical presentations and warning clues should direct the physician's attention to this consideration, including[39]:

- Age over 50 years
- Recent weight loss
- Presence of lymphadenopathy
- Pain nonresponsive to previous treatment measures
- Neurologic deficits in a patient with a history of malignancy (especially prostate, lung, breast, and multiple myeloma)

Constans and colleagues report on a review of 600 cases of spinal metastases with neurologic manifestations and note that 53% had thoracic spine localization, 32% lumbosacral spine localization, and 15% cervical spine localization.[39] Therefore, it appears appropriate to recommend radiographic evaluation for patients with thoracic back pain without a known etiology. This recommendation, however, does not apply to patients with lower back discomfort, the most common back pain complaint seen by PCPs. In Constans' review, the most common primary tumor in men was in the lung (19.17%) and in women was in the breast (53.31%).[39]

The primary presenting symptom of spinal cord compression is back pain, which in most cases is localized to the involved area of vertebral damage. In reported series in which radiographic and surgical findings are noted, osteolytic lesions are usually present (71%), with osteoblastic lesions in 21% and mixed lytic–blastic lesions in 8%.[39] The back pain may have been present for days to weeks. The progression of symptoms to motor weakness, numbness (sensory loss), and finally bladder or rectal dysfunction (autonomic loss) will create concern for the patient. The entire process may have a variable rate of progression. The significant pathophysiologic process is related to spinal cord and nerve infarction due to arterial or venous occlusion by the compression process. As the progression of neural compression occurs, the symptom focus shifts from that of back pain to localization of neurologic symptoms in the extremities with pain, weakness, or numbness. Radiculopathy, identified by pain referred from the primary spinal site, dermatomal sensory changes, and altered deep tendon reflexes, is common, especially in the lower extremities. This process may be bilateral or unilateral. If bilateral, it is not unusual for one side to progress more rapidly than the other side. Occasionally, an entire nerve plexus (cervical or lumbar plexopathy) may be involved, producing pain, or aching in a single extremity only, without a dermatomal pattern.

The anatomic site of the radiculopathy or plexopathy may be determined by the primary tumor. Most cervical spinal cord compression is noted with lung cancer (40%), followed by breast cancer. Brachial plexus involvement occurs most often in association with lung cancer. Apical or superior sulcus tumors of the lung commonly predispose to brachial plexopathy resulting in arm and hand symptoms of pain, swelling, and loss of function. Lumbar plexopathy is most often associated with pelvic tumors, especially colorectal cancer and sarcomas.[41] The symptom complex presented is generally the same as with spinal cord compression, with pain the first and predominant symptom. The pain is radicular in approximately 85% of cases.[41] Plexopathy in the lumbar area can also present as unilateral or bilateral lower extremity symptoms. Specific areas of paresis, paresthesia, or pain can help localize tumor involvement to a specific portion of the plexus.

Diagnostic tests beyond plain x-ray are needed to localize the tumor and plan therapy. MRI is the modality of choice in spinal cord compression. When suspicion exists for spinal cord or plexus compression, diagnostic imaging studies should be performed quickly so that neurosurgery and/or radiation oncology consultation can ensue.

Treatment for suspected spinal cord compression is high-dose dexamethasone. It is administered as soon as the diagnosis is suspected and before diagnostic studies are completed. The beneficial effect of steroids may be only short term and may result in pain relief by relieving inflammatory edema. Steroid administration is usually continued through the immediate therapy period and then tapered. Definitive therapy requires surgical laminectomy and/or radiotherapy. Surgery is preferred in radioresistant tumors (renal carcinoma) or in cases of tumor recurrence after previous radiation. Combinations of radiation therapy and surgery have shown improved outcomes compared to radiation therapy alone.[40] The responses are variable and must be judged by the degree of symptoms and neurologic deficit with which the patient presents at diagnosis. Most patients with significant paresis or paraplegia at diagnosis will not regain neurologic function. Patients who maintain neurologic function at diagnosis will generally retain function after therapy.[42]

OTHER CAUSES OF PERIPHERAL NEUROPATHY

Other phenomena may produce peripheral neuropathy with direct tumor or paraneoplastic involvement. Neurotoxic chemotherapy, primarily vinca alkaloids, cisplatin, and taxanes can cause direct damage to axons and result in paresthesia, muscle weakness, and hyporeflexia.[43] Although the majority of peripheral neuropathy manifestations affect the upper and lower extremities, the autonomic consequences can include constipation, vocal cord paralysis, and neurogenic bladder. Peripheral neuropathic symptoms are common and can often be a cause of treatment cessation. Thus, it is imperative to closely monitor and treat symptoms as they arise with both pharmacologic, and nonpharmacologic interventions including OMT, cryotherapy, and additional complementary techniques.[1,2] Other neuropathic effects have been reported such as neuronal deposition of amyloid in multiple myeloma or hemorrhage into nerves in leukemia.

In conclusion, it is not uncommon for malignant tumors to present at onset or through the course of disease progression with neurologic, muscular, or skeletal symptomatology. Often, the symptoms may mimic somatic dysfunction with or without accompanying neurologic components.

PARANEOPLASTIC SYNDROMES

Paraneoplastic syndromes are rare but may be the presenting symptom in advanced malignancies. Lung cancers are the most common tumor type to produce paraneoplastic syndromes, and they can be present in early or widespread disease. Paraneoplastic syndromes include[37]:

- Cushing syndrome
- SIADH
- Nonmetastatic hypercalcemia (PTHrP)
- HPOA
- Subacute cerebellar degeneration
- Dementia syndromes
- Peripheral neuropathies
- Polymyositis
- Dermatomyositis
- Hematologic abnormalities

Any of these syndromes may present as altered CNS function and may create difficulty in discussing appropriate treatment options and decisions. The first four on the list will be discussed in more depth. The others were mentioned briefly above (see literature review for further information).[37]

Cushing Syndrome

The ectopic adrenocorticotropic hormone (ACTH) syndrome (Cushing syndrome) is most commonly associated with neuroendocrine lung tumors, especially SCLC and bronchial carcinoid tumors. In SCLC, 25% of patients have either the clinical syndrome or significant elevations of ectopic-produced ACTH.[37] Corticoid excess produces the clinical manifestations including:

- Muscle weakness
- Hypokalemia
- Edema
- Hyperglycemia
- Hypertension
- Altered mental status/confusion

The same syndrome may occur in other tumors as well. The most effective therapy is treatment of the primary tumor, typically with aggressive multi-agent chemotherapy.[37] The following medications can be used to inhibit steroid production[37]:

- Ketoconazole
- Mitotane
- Metyrapone
- Aminoglutethimide

In addition:

- Antihypertensive agents and diuretics for hypertension.
- Octreotide, which blocks the release of ACTH.
- Etomidate, which inhibits aspects of steroid synthesis, decreases serum cortisol levels in patients who are unable to take oral medications.
- When medical therapy is not successful, adrenalectomy may be considered.

Syndrome of Inappropriate Antidiuretic Hormone

The SIADH also occurs most commonly in lung cancer, especially in SCLC. The hormone arginine vasopressin (AVP) is produced in high quantities by the tumor. The major laboratory features are:

- Hyponatremia
- Reduced serum osmolality
- Increased urine osmolality relative to serum

The clinical symptoms include:

- Altered mental status
- Confusion
- Lethargy
- Psychosis
- Seizures
- Coma

This may mimic a primary CNS tumor. Vasopressin receptor antagonists are generally considered only after failure of fluid restriction.[37]

Hypercalcemia

Hypercalcemia is the most frequent metabolic complication associated with malignancy. It occurs commonly with:

- Breast
- Lung
- Renal carcinomas
- Prostate
- Head/neck cancers
- Multiple myeloma

This entity occurs in approximately 10% of all patients with cancer. There are four principal mechanisms of hypercalcemia in cancer patients[37]:

1. Secretion of PTH-related protein (PTHrP) by tumor cells (80%), most common with squamous cell carcinomas of the lung or head/neck.
2. Upon binding to PTH receptors in the bone and kidney, PTHrP regulates bone resorption and renal handling of calcium and phosphate.
3. Directly from osteolytic activity at sites of skeletal metastases (29%), breast cancer, multiple myeloma, and lymphomas.
4. Tumor secretion of vitamin D, lymphomas, or in association with ectopic tumor secretion of PTH.

Hypercalcemia may present as GI, renal, neurologic, or cardiovascular symptoms.

The GI system effects include:

- Nausea
- Emesis
- Anorexia
- Constipation

The renal manifestations include:

- Polyuria
- Polydipsia
- Late effect of nephrocalcinosis

Cardiovascular effects include:

- Significant echocardiographic alterations
- Arrhythmias, typically through effect on the QT interval
- Hypertension
- A marked increase in digitalis sensitivity

Neurologic effects include:

- Depression
- Lethargy
- Hyporeflexia
- Progressive stupor and eventual coma
- Possibly death

Treatment should begin promptly and include intravenous hydration, cessation of calcium-containing products, discontinuation of medications that contribute to hypercalcemia (e.g., vitamin D, thiazide diuretics, calcium-containing antacids, and lithium), and anticancer therapy.[37] Selected use of drugs includes[37]:

- Osteoclast inhibitors such as mithramycin
- Calcitonin
- Bisphosphonates
- Corticosteroids
- Hemodialysis for patients with renal or cardiac disease for which the above treatments may not be tolerated

Hypertrophic Pulmonary Osteoarthropathy

HPOA is an infrequently encountered musculoskeletal paraneoplastic manifestation and consists of digital clubbing, increased periosteal activity in the tubular bones, arthralgias, and join effusions. The hallmark of the disease is abnormal proliferation of the skin, soft tissues, and osseous tissues in the most distal aspects of the extremities.

- The joints most frequently involved are the knees, ankles, and wrists; metacarpal–phalangeal and proximal interphalangeal joints may also be involved.
- Vascular endothelial growth factor, platelet-derived growth factor, and prostaglandin E2 are likely involved in producing a symmetric clubbing of fingers and toes, periostitis of long bones, and polyarthritis resembling rheumatoid arthritis.[37]
- The clinical presentations are pain, tenderness, and swelling of the affected joints.
- A classic finding is periosteal tenderness and radiographic evidence of periosteal elevation.
- About 10% of patients with lung cancer have HPOA.[37]
- Serologic tests are normal; that is, inflammatory markers and rheumatoid factor are negative.
- Primary treatment is treatment of the underlying disease, with secondary options include bisphosphonates, opiate analgesics, nonsteroidal anti-inflammatory drugs, and localized palliative radiation.[37]

While the previously noted endocrine syndromes, except for PTHrP production, are particularly common with SCLC, osteoarthropathy is most commonly seen with non–small cell lung cancer. Lung cancer should be included as a part of the differential diagnosis in all patients with paraneoplastic syndromes.

A VISCEROSOMATIC-TYPE ONCOLOGIC RESPONSE

Cachexia

Cancer cachexia, also known as "wasting syndrome," occurs in about half of cancer patients and is characterized by a chronic skeletal muscle and adipose tissue loss that is resistant to nutritional support. There is alteration in carbohydrate, protein, and fat metabolism. Cachexia is responsible for the reduction in muscle strength and quality and length of life of many cancer patients.[44] The following proinflammatory and procachectic factors produced by the tumor cells are involved in this debilitating and lethal process[44]:

- Interleukin-1 (IL-1)
- IL-6
- IL-8
- Interferon (IFN)-γ
- PTHrP
- Macrophage migratory factor (MIF)
- Tumor necrosis factor-alpha (TNF-α):
  - □ TNF-α has a direct catabolic effect on skeletal muscle and causes wasting of the muscle by the induction of the ubiquitin–proteasome system (UPS).
  - □ TNF-α is involved in insulin resistance and is responsible for the increase in gluconeogenesis, loss of adipose tissue, and proteolysis while causing decrease in protein, lipid, and glycogen synthesis.
  - □ TNF-α is involved in the formation of IL-1 and increases the uncoupling of protein-2 (UCP-2) and the UCP-3 expression in skeletal muscle in the cachectic state.

TNF-α can serve as an example of a potential viscerosomatic antineoplastic response. TNF-α represents an excellent model in oncology of a somatic response to stimulation of a viscera or organ system by invasion of tumor or infection. The response provides evidence for the self-regulatory and self-protective healing capacity of the somatic structure.

PRESENTATION, DIAGNOSIS, AND TREATMENT OF CANCER IN THE PEDIATRIC AND YOUNG ADULT (AYA) PATIENT

Cancer is among the top leading cause of overall mortality in the United States in children in adolescents. Children are not little adults, and present with a unique challenge to diagnose and manage. Although cancer in children and adolescents is rare and much less common than adults, it is the leading cause of death by disease past infancy among children in the United States. The most common cancer diagnosis in children and adolescents (ages 0 to 19 years) in the United States are leukemias, lymphomas, brain, and CNS tumors. Amongst adolescent young adult (AYA) aged 15 to 19 years, the most common cancer diagnoses include brain and other CNS tumors, lymphoma, leukemia, thyroid cancer, gonadal germ cell tumors, and malignant bone tumors (NCI). Differences between adult and pediatric cancers include childhood cancers[42]:

- Tend to be more aggressive and progress more rapidly; however, chance of recovery is higher in childhood cancer treatments
- Are detected at a later stage at time of diagnosis (80% vs. only 20% of adults have metastatic disease at presentation)
- Genomes have few genetic mutations compared to adult cancer genomes, and are not strongly linked to lifestyle or environmental risk factors
- Current methods for treatment are exceedingly more toxic than adult therapies due to a number of factors
- Are biologically different than their adult counterparts, even within the same disease entity

Cancer in Children and AYAs Presents Differently than in Adult Patients

The PCP has a daunting task of interpreting often vague complaints from a child with challenges during physician exam of attention and cooperation on behalf of the patient. Due to obvious communication barriers in younger children, cancer is often diagnosed in more advanced stages than compared to adult cancers. Unique clues can help determine a possible diagnosis of malignancy, particularly in diagnosing leukemia in young children. The following should trigger the PCP to think more about starting a workup for possible malignancy:

- Limping or refusal to bear weight in the lower extremity
- Petechiae or bruising in atypical areas (abdomen, face, back)
- Fever >100.4 °F for more than 5 days
- Unexplained lump, firmness, or swelling of a lymph node with matted, fixed on appearance (particularly pathognomonic in the finding of supraclavicular lymphadenopathy)
- Headaches with warning signs including wakens the patient from sleep, associated vomiting or weight loss, or changes in patient ability to walk
- Weight loss

Any of the above findings should prompt the physician to consider adding additional laboratory orders including complete blood count with differential to assess white blood cells, hemoglobin, and platelets to look for signs of leukemia, brain imaging if a warning sign with headache is present to assess for the possibility of a brain mass, and/or an ultrasound if a concerning lymph node is palpated on exam.

Oncologic Emergencies in Pediatric and AYA Cancer

The PCP should be aware of common oncologic emergencies and their presentation in children and AYAs. As mentioned previously, cancers in children tend to present more aggressively and progress more rapidly than adult cancers, which leave them particularly vulnerable to emergent conditions secondary to cancer progression. Emergencies that necessitate immediate intervention include superior vena cava syndrome, spinal cord compression, brain herniation, and hyperleukocytosis. Emergencies with the potential for adverse consequences to the child include leukopenia, coagulopathy, anemia, tumor lysis syndrome, and hypercalcemia. As many of these emergencies are resultant of large anterior mediastinal masses and other space occupying lesions, a chest x-ray should always be included in the workup of a patient with suspected leukemia or lymphoma. Patients with concern for an oncologic emergency should be sent to the closest emergency department for further management including aggressive IV fluid hydration to prevent hyper viscosity sequelae from hyperleukocytosis and close monitoring of electrolyte and renal function for tumor lysis syndrome (Table 76.2).

ETHICS OF PRESENTATION OF DIAGNOSTIC AND TREATMENT OPTIONS TO THE PATIENT

Several challenges arise after a cancer diagnosis. When discussing the finding of malignancy or the effectiveness of treatment, it important to present the patient and their family with facts and transparency about the prognosis. It may not be unusual that protective family members request that the patient not be informed of the diagnosis, but it is often themselves that these families are protecting. This is particularly true and challenging when the diagnosis involves a child; however, most children are astute, and can perceive the stress and anxiety surrounding their parents and physician conversations. The patient perspective is important about how and when to receive bad news. Patients universally have responded that information given over time with space to ask questions is more useful than longer more in-depth medical conversations. However, additional information need not be offered all at one time unless requested. Patients and families need honesty, and the transparency of their physician is a key component. Optimism may not always relate to effectiveness of treatment or longevity but must offer assurance of comfort, symptom control, and lack of physician abandonment if no further curative treatment is available. Therefore, the physician must:

- Tell the truth, never lie.
- Remember that all of the truths are not necessary during each conversation unless asked specifically.
- Offer optimism and reassurance.

Relating the diagnosis of cancer to the patient and discussing the disease, prognosis, and diagnostic and treatment options must be done with knowledge and understanding of the perceptions of the patient. This aspect of patient care is extremely significant. As an osteopathic physician, one has a distinct advantage in these discussions because of the osteopathic philosophy of treating the *whole patient* rather than only the disease. Most patients continue to perceive a future with cancer as a short, lonely, painful, and helpless prospect. The initial discussion with the patient may be by the oncologist or the PCP. The philosophy used when presenting a cancer diagnosis to the patient and family is based on hope, realistic goal setting, honesty, integrity, and the knowledge that the individual is more than their disease.

TABLE 76.2

Pediatric Oncologic Emergencies Caused by Mass Lesions

Emergency	Signs and Symptoms	Laboratory/Radiology	Oncologic Conditions
Superior vena cava syndrome	Shortness of breath, facial swelling, syncope	Anterior mediastinal mass	Non-Hodgkin lymphoma, T-cell leukemia, teratoma, thyroid cancer, thymoma, Hodgkin disease, sarcoma, neuroblastoma
Spinal cord compression	Back pain, radicular pain, leg weakness or paralysis, extremity weakness, neck pain	MR imaging: epidural mass Radiograph: lytic lesion	Neuroblastoma, sarcoma, lymphoma, leukemia, astrocytoma, ependymoma, metastases
Increased intracranial pressure	Headache	CT scanning/MR imaging: mass	Brain tumor
Brain herniation	Morning vomiting, diplopia, ataxia, Cushing triad, increase in head size, cerebrovascular accident	Hydrocephalus, hemorrhage, thrombus	Brain metastasis, CNS leukemia, abscess
Massive hepatomegaly	Huge liver, cardiorespiratory failure	Coagulation studies	Neonatal stage 4S neuroblastoma

Reprinted from Kelly KM, Lange B. Oncologic emergencies. *Pediatr Clin North Am.* 1997;44(4):809–830.

It is important to inform the patient and family that the diagnosis is malignancy or cancer. The patient should be asked whether or not to include their spouse or family in the initial discussion. In most instances, a strong suspicion already exists, and the patient may prefer familial support. It is important to sit with the patient and discuss the diagnosis in a supportive, unhurried fashion. Furthermore, having the presence and assistance from a multidisciplinary team of social works, psychologists, and therapists can be incredibly helpful. The understanding and support offered at this time will set the tone and pattern for the remainder of the treatment relationship with the patient. A fully informed, trusting, and cooperative patient will, in most cases, remain cooperative and trusting.

Cure versus Control

The physician should ask the patient and their family what they have been told before beginning a discussion. After informing the patient about the diagnosis, a distinction should be made for the patient about cure of disease and control of disease based on realistic expectations of available options. Patients and families need an opportunity to think, ask questions, discuss, and express feelings. They may feel abandoned if they are hurried through a brief one-sided discussion, informed they will be referred to an oncologist, and sent on their way before they can ask questions. Speak in lay language no matter what the educational level of the patient. Stress that something positive can be done for the patient. The greatest fear of the patient is that they will be told there is nothing that can be done. Even in the case of a medically untreatable cancer, the patient can be given hope of support, comfort, and caring. If surgery, radiation, or chemotherapy is available and to be offered, the patient is informed but always with the knowledge that general supportive care and symptom management will be available concurrently if needed. In the event of metastatic disease or a terminal diagnosis, the physician should stress the potential long-term control options utilizing palliative chemotherapy or radiation. Indicate that the purpose of the systemic therapy is to at least stabilize the disease at present levels and prevent further growth or spread. Throughout the entire interaction, an atmosphere of concern for the *whole patient* rather than only interest in the disease should be created. Throughout the course of the conversation, do not hesitate to provide physical touch through hand holding. Patients and families have indicated that this seems to convey even more sincerity in caring about the *whole patient* than any level of discussion.

Often when discussing therapy, especially chemotherapy, a patient may be very resistant to discuss treatment options due to previous unfounded "horror stories." It is appropriate to be aggressive in encouraging chemotherapy when there is high likelihood is of beneficial effect. Otherwise, therapy, including investigational or cooperative group protocols, can be offered in an objective manner while informing the patient of all benefits and risks. If the patient is strongly opposed to the uncertain benefit of a treatment program, reassure the patient and allay any guilt. This can be done by informing the patient and family that, in many malignancies, there is no definite right or wrong therapy. The right choice is the choice that leaves the patient and family comfortable with their decision and does not create conflict between patient and family, especially in the later phases of the disease process. The physician must support the patient's choices, unless proven benefit is being deprived by the choice made by the patient. This may not apply at the time of initial discussion and therapy presentation but later when searching for a subsequent therapy or when choosing to discontinue an ineffective or toxic therapy. The support by the physician of the patient's choices reaffirms the care and importance of the patient in the total treatment of the disease.

Discussion of prognosis is important but may be avoided at the initial consultation with the patient. Address this question by a statement indicating the need to wait to observe the response of the planned treatment. The presence or absence of a response and type of response will influence and may change prognosis.

Often during the initial presentation, it is helpful to sit beside or across from the patient. Closeness to the patient, body language, and verbal communication consistent with an empathic discussion of support and concern, and the agreement to work as a partner in treating the patient, all help to create an integral relationship between patient and physician. A focus on the *whole patient,* rather than just the disease, is incredibly important for creating the foundation of this complex relationship.

Patients who have been treated with the holistic philosophy discussed may have improved longevity and function over comparable patients who have been treated with only an objective, rigid, scientific philosophy of an investigational study without personalization.

SUPPORTIVE CARE OF THE PATIENT WITH CANCER

The supportive care that the patient may require at certain times during their illness carries an equal weight to the specific antineoplastic therapy used. At the time of progressive disease, patient decline, or elective cessation of therapy, supportive care is of paramount importance.

Supportive care consists predominantly of three categories:

1. Symptom control and pain relief
2. Blood and blood products
3. Medical and psychosocial care

The latter category includes infection prevention and treatment, nutrition support, and rehabilitative support and may also include mental health, legal, and pastoral care support, all of which are components of hospice care.

The discussion on medical management of pain control, use of blood and its products, nutrition, and infection therapy will be limited here. These subjects are well reviewed and documented in the medical literature. Rather, these subjects will be reviewed from the philosophic viewpoint of a medical oncologist with an osteopathic background and experience.

Symptom and Pain Relief

Symptoms other than pain and discomfort are important to address for the cancer patient. Anxiety and apprehension may be addressed by spending time in discussion with the physician, social worker, nurse, psychiatrist, or psychologist. Pain should always be treated, and physicians should acknowledge additional fears to help mitigate. Many traditional modalities are available to treat pain including analgesics and various delivery methods to improve effectiveness (intrathecal or intraventricular injections, continuous infusion pumps, self-delivery pumps, etc.). In addition, neurosurgical procedures such as cordotomy and rhizotomy are available as well as anesthetic blocks. Scientific data are limited but available to support integrative modalities in selected patients to alleviate anxiety and pain symptoms. Simple, gentle, soft tissue manipulation without any pressure or thrust can be safe and effective, especially in late-stage, inactive, and bed-bound patients. The procedure permits the physician to touch the patient and commit time to care for the patient in addition to the disease.

Blood and Blood Products

Red blood cell transfusions to correct anemia, granulocyte colony stimulating factor injections during prolonged neutropenia, and platelet transfusions to prevent bleeding during bone marrow suppression are all supportive measures that are occasionally needed. These may be needed during periods of disease complications or during toxicity from systemic therapy. This support is often lifesaving. However, continued support with expensive or scarce blood products must be balanced with the benefit to be attained in end-stage patients in the terminal phase of the disease process.

General Supportive Care

Nutritional support for patient with malignancy is essential whether the patient is actively pursuing life-saving treatment or not. Malnutrition is part of a general failure-to-thrive syndrome commonly associated with cancer. The patient may need other supportive cares such as antibiotics, blood products, and psychosocial support in order to assist with nutrition. In addition, nutritional counseling with a dietician and nutritional supplements may be helpful. Total parenteral nutrition administered through percutaneous or surgically placed venous access may also be used for hospitalized patients for whom the enteral approach is not possible due to intestinal or other specific circumstances.

Anti-infective therapy can be lifesaving during periods of increased risk, such as granulocytopenia after chemotherapy. It may also be provided as combination antibiotic therapy to treat documented infection, sepsis, or fever during granulocytopenia. Specific antimicrobial therapy is guided by culture and sensitivity results.

Mobility and bowel or bladder functions are areas of general supportive care not only for the patient with cancer but also for any geriatric patient or patient who is critically ill. All patients can be encouraged to be mobilized out of bed as much as possible. A positive attitude on the part of the patient can be maintained to a greater degree with increased mobility. This may lessen stress and anxiety and even support the immune system in its attack on the disease. In addition, mobilization enhances venous blood return and reduces the risk of:

- Venous thrombosis
- Decubitus ulceration
- Edema
- Constipation

Many patients with cancer have prolonged periods of bed rest due to bone pain, pathologic fracture, or paraplegia due to spinal cord compressive disease. In these patients, mobilization is essential to maintain even minimal functional ability. If assisted ambulation is possible, it should be encouraged. If ambulation is impossible due to pain, fracture, weakness, or neurologic deficit, sitting in a chair may be possible. For the totally bed-bound patient, side-to-side moving with mild soft tissue manipulation can be offered.

Bowel function can be maintained with appropriate hydration, nutrition, and activity. Stool softeners and other medications or maneuvers such as manual (suppository or digital) stimulation can be used if patients without neutropenia or thrombocytopenia. Constipation can provide significant discomfort to an immobile patient. Several studies in the pediatric and adolescent populations have demonstrated the safety, feasibility, and potential efficacy of OMT for the treatment of constipation.[45] Specifically mesenteric lift and sacral rocking for opioid-induced constipation.

Bladder function and control are also essential for patients confined to bed. If incontinence is present, an indwelling catheter can be useful, yet should be limited in times of neutropenia due to infection risk.

Rehabilitative care is often an essential element in symptomatic and supportive management of the patient with cancer. Rehabilitation may include physical, occupational, and speech therapy. This may be indicated after management of spinal cord compression syndrome, cerebral metastasis, and head and neck malignancies.

Hospice care is widely recognized and used as an effective modality in the care of terminally ill persons for both children and adults. Hospice focuses on meeting the needs of the patient and the family after effective therapy for the disease is no longer available. The hospice philosophy is focused on effective pain and symptom management while also meeting other physical, social, emotional, and spiritual needs with the aid of a multidisciplinary team of specialists in each area. The patient is maintained in an environment of warmth and caring with family, in the home, except when this is not possible. Dealing with pain and preparation for death is very difficult or impossible for some physicians and represents a deficiency in medical training. Hospice meets this need, so death can be accepted as a natural phase of life (see Chapter 80 Osteopathic Considerations in End-of-Life Care for further discussion).

STRESS OF DISEASE AND TREATMENT OF THE PATIENT AS MODULATORS OF BIOLOGIC RESPONSE

Psychoneurobiology refers to the interrelationship between emotions, the CNS, and somatic cellular biologic responses. There is little argument that the immune system plays a significant role in the initiation and course of malignant disease. The role of T- and B-cell lymphocytes and helper, suppressor, and natural killer (NK) cells together with interferons have all been extensively reviewed in the literature. It appears that the connection between the CNS and the systemic response to illness is often mediated by the endocrine system with the assistance of cortisol, the endogenous opiates (endorphins and enkephalins), and other steroids and hormones that can regulate some aspects of cellular biologic response. Nerve endings have been demonstrated within lymphoid organs (nodes and spleen). In addition, receptors have been demonstrated on the surface of lymphocytes for hormones such as ACTH. Cancer is a type of stressor that can alter the biologic response in terms of enhanced or suppressed output or function of substances including interferon, NK cells, etc. and produce further suppression of an already suppressed immune system (see Chapter 12 The Role of Inflammation in Healing and Homeostasis for further details).

Alterations in the emotional state and spirit of the patient with cancer, assisted by the physician through optimism, support, and empathy, can result in an enhanced biologic response (see Chapter 20 Spirituality and Health Care for further details). Recognition and treatment of the *whole person* can produce this alteration in the patient's emotional status. The oncologist often encounters a patient with advanced metastatic disease who, without specific antitumor therapy can continue to live and function while waiting for important life event to occur (i.e., a child to graduate, a marriage, or the birth of a grandchild). The emotional state and the will to live seem to have the ability to affect the biologic behavior of the disease and the well-being of the patient.

OSTEOPATHIC MANIPULATIVE TREATMENT FOR THE PATIENT WITH CANCER

Many osteopathic physicians have mistakenly believed that manipulative treatment is contraindicated for the patient with cancer.

TABLE 76.3

Manipulative Techniques Bearing Consideration and Potential Caution

Thrust near bone/joint cancer
Lymphatic pumps
Effleurage
Any technique in immediate vicinity of cancer

While this may be true for some techniques, other techniques can be helpful for:

- Relieving pain
- Improving visceral function
- Reducing tension and stress
- Improving the doctor–patient relationship through touch

This section will review the contraindications, indications, and specific techniques for OMT in the patient with cancer.

Osteopathic Manipulative Treatment for Oncologic Conditions

While OMT in general is not contraindicated (see Table 76.3), treatment of the area immediately surrounding a cancer has historically been contraindicated because of the theoretical risk of hematogenous spread. This is particularly true for the vertebral column where the Batson venous plexus, a system of valveless vessels anastomosing with brain and pelvic veins, provides a two-way route of metastasis. Therefore, OMT for the entire vertebral column is contraindicated when there is known or suspected vertebral tumor. A primary or metastatic vertebral cancer should be suspected when there is acute back pain associated with systemic symptoms such as:

- Fever
- Chills
- Night sweats
- Fatigue
- Weight loss

Persistent back pain despite adequate treatment also raises a possibility of vertebral tumor. And, of course, back pain in a patient with another known cancer or a suspected cancer at a site that commonly metastasizes to the spinal column should raise the index of suspicion (see Table 76.1).

Two types of manipulative techniques do pose risk when used for the patient with cancer. High-velocity, low-amplitude (HVLA) techniques have been reported to cause pathologic rib fractures in patients with osteoporosis. Presumably, these thrust techniques could result in fracture of a rib or other bones weakened by primary or metastatic tumor. Therefore, HVLA technique is contraindicated for joints associated with bones that have known or possible cancer.[46] As many conditions require steroids for treatment, indirect techniques are preferred over any direct techniques in patients with cancer.

Lymphatic pump and effleurage have a role in helping with edema and swelling during cancer treatment. The theoretical risk of metastasis via lymphogenous spread exists, however, it has not been fully investigated yet. In contrast, some hypothesize that these techniques could be advantageous in the era of immunotherapy to help spread therapy throughout the body and into cancer regions. These techniques should be used at physician discretion after taking many factors into account[47–49]:

- Passive limb exercise
- Prior cortisone therapy
- Extent of local disease
- Lymphatic invasion and obstruction

This potential for lymphatic metastasis appears to be due to normal lymphatic transport of cells and lymph node efficiency at filtering and disseminating such cells.[50–52] Interestingly, abdominal lymphatic pump technique in the murine model demonstrated enhanced immunity and decreased tumor formation in the lung.[53] Tissue massage has been demonstrated to stimulate lymph transport and to reduce lymphedema.[54,55] Physical-based therapies have been shown to reduce connective tissue inflammation and fibrosis and theoretically may have direct beneficial effects on cancer spreading and metastasis.[56] This effect was not demonstrated in patients with osteosarcoma or in the murine model osteosarcoma, where massage therapy of the tumor area prior to diagnosis led to poor prognosis.[57] Manual lymphatic drainage is safe and effective at aiding in reduction of mild-to-moderate upper extremity edema in breast cancer patients who are post surgery and radiation therapy.[58] Massage therapy has also been shown to be similar to light touch and attention at improving pain and mood in patients with advanced cancer.[58] Further randomized clinical trials are needed to better elucidate mechanisms and effectiveness of manual forms of manipulation in cancer patients.

The balance of evidence cited here suggests that lymphatic pumps and effleurage should be applied with caution in patients with cancer. Passive lymphatic treatment can be substituted for active lymphatic pumps and effleurage when lymphatic metastasis is a concern. Myofascial techniques for the thoracic inlet and abdominal diaphragm as well as pectoral traction can be safely applied in patients with cancer with pneumonia, lymphedema, or other problems for which a lymphatic pump or effleurage might have otherwise been considered.[59,60]

Indications for Osteopathic Manipulative Treatment in the Oncology Patient

OMT, if judiciously applied, can be a very valuable tool for the care of oncology patients, who have the same potential for noncancer somatic dysfunction and pain as others, but with more psychological stress (Table 76.4). In addition, the patient with cancer may be saddled with postsurgical pain as well as cancer pain. Furthermore, the terminally ill patient may have immobility-related visceral dysfunction amenable to OMT.

For patients with known cancer, the primary indication for OMT is musculoskeletal pain associated with somatic dysfunction but not directly related to the tumor. The somatic dysfunction can be unrelated to or secondary to the cancer or its treatment. For

TABLE 76.4

Indications for Osteopathic Manipulative Treatment in Patients with Cancer

Indications
Pain and somatic dysfunction
Constipation
Atelectasis
Pneumonia
Postsurgical lymphedema

instance, a patient who underwent median sternotomy and resection of a lung cancer may develop thoracic and intercostal pain from a pre-existing somatic dysfunction made worse by the surgery, a viscerosomatic reflex from the lung to the thoracic spine, or surgical trauma to the costovertebral or costochondral joints. The choice of techniques for treating somatic dysfunction in the patient with cancer and musculoskeletal pain is highly individualized and depends on age, severity of illness, previous injuries, other diseases, and time since surgery. In general, indirect methods, such as myofascial release and counterstrain techniques, are more applicable when there is acute or severe illness and with advancing age. Direct methods such as HVLA and muscle energy should be reserved for the stable patient and when metastasis to the area being treated has been definitively ruled out.

OMT is also indicated for prevention or treatment of immobility-related complications in the bedridden patient who is terminally ill with cancer. Prolonged immobility can cause constipation or atelectasis predisposing to pneumonia. To prevent and treat atelectasis or constipation, thoracolumbar soft tissue and rib-raising treatment can be applied daily, in many cases by family members instructed to do these techniques at home. The initiation of rib raising should be preceded by treatment of significant vertebral and rib somatic dysfunction to prevent exacerbation of visceral facilitation.

Pain, immobility and its consequences, and postsurgical lymphedema are common problems in patients with cancer that can be readily treated with OMT. An additional benefit of treatment is an improved sense of well-being, which many patients report. It is entirely possible that this period of well-being is due to enhancement of the immune system with elevated output of cellular immune substances, NK cells, or endogenous opiates. OMT has been found to induce a rapid increase in the levels of cytokines such as IL-8, MCP-1, MIP-1a, and notably G-CSF, in healthy individuals.[61] Further clinical trials are warranted to measure serum and CSF levels of various cytokines in response to OMT in cancer patients.

COMPLEMENTARY AND ALTERNATIVE MEDICINE IN ONCOLOGY

While scientifically rigorous and objective research is lacking in the use of alternatives in cancer treatment, several modalities have been used anecdotally for discomfort or symptom control and general immune enhancement. These include acupuncture and static magnets for control of discomfort, better rest, and reduced need for analgesics. Massage and other relaxation techniques may assist in stress reduction. Herbal products are often considered by patients, and brought to their oncologist for discussion, however these must be used with caution, considering potential drug interactions with prescribed pharmaceuticals and potential false hope for patients.

LIFESTYLE AND CANCER PREVENTION

Most adult cancers have been linked to behaviors or environmental toxins, with the remaining genetically related. As discussed in Chapter 21 Lifestyle Medicine—Osteopathic Perspectives, the following are the cornerstones of the foundation of cancer prevention as well as improved quality of life and decreased mortality in patients with cancer[62–72]:

- Smoking cessation
- Exercise
- Healthy diet and nutrition
- Weight control
- Elimination of environmental toxin exposure
- Stress management

In contrast, most childhood and AYA cancers do not have a preventable cause and are often a sporadic or germline mutation associated with a genetic predisposition syndrome.

CONCLUSION

The osteopathic physician has a special opportunity and obligation to treat the patient with cancer as a *whole person*, not just a disease. Osteopathic physicians are uniquely poised, with our emphasis on touch and healing, to provide patients with cancer and their families the management and support they need.

ACKNOWLEDGMENTS

The authors and editors of this chapter would like to acknowledge the past contributions of Drs. Michael I. Opipari, Augustine L. Perrotta, and David R. Beatty for prior editions of this chapter.

REFERENCES

1. Greenman PE. The osteopathic concept in its second century: is it still germane to specialty practice? *J Am Osteopath Assoc.* 1976;75:589–595.
2. Bean RB, Bean WB. *Sir William Osler Aphorism from His Bedside Teachings and Writings.* Henry Schuman, Inc; 1950.
3. https://bmcprimcare.biomedcentral.com/articles/10.1186/s12875-023-01976-z. Accessed January 11, 2023.
4. Haas, R., Gorelik, A., Busija, L, et al. Prevalence and characteristics of musculoskeletal complaints in primary care: an analysis from the population level and analysis reporting (POLAR) database. *BMC Prim Care* 2023;24:40.
5. Coleman RE. Metastatic bone disease: clinical features, pathophysiology and treatment strategies. *Cancer Treat Rev.* 2001;27:165–176.
6. Woodward E, Jagdev S, McParland L, et al. Skeletal complications and survival in renal cancer patients with bone metastases. *Bone.* 2011;48:160–166.
7. Coleman RE. Clinical features of metastatic bone disease and risk of skeletal morbidity. *Clin Cancer Res.* 2006;12:6243s–6249s.
8. Carter JA, Ji X, Botteman MF. Clinical, economic and humanistic burdens of skeletal-related events associated with bone metastases. *Expert Rev Pharmacoecon Outcomes Res.* 2013;13:483–489.
9. Brodowicz T, Hadji P, Niepel D, Diel I. Early identification and intervention matters: a comprehensive review of current evidence and recommendations for the monitoring of bone health in patients with cancer. *Cancer Treat Rev.* 2017;61:23–34.
10. von Moos R, Body JJ, Egerdie B, et al. Pain and analgesic use associated with skeletal-related events in patients with advanced cancer and bone metastases. *Support Care Cancer.* 2016;24:1327–1337.
11. Cetin K, Christiansen CF, Særke C, Jacobsen JB, Sørensen HT. Survival in patients with breast cancer with bone metastasis: a Danish population-based cohort study on the prognostic impact of initial stage of disease at breast cancer diagnosis and length of the bone metastasis-free interval. *BMJ Open.* 2015;5:e007702.
12. Howard LE, De Hoedt AM, Aronson WJ, et al. Do skeletal-related events predict overall survival in men with metastatic castration-resistant prostate cancer? *Prostate Cancer Prostatic Dis.* 2016;19:380–384.
13. Jehn CF, Diel IJ, Overkamp F, et al. Management of metastatic bone disease algorithms for diagnostics and treatment. *Anticancer Res.* 2016;36:2631–2637.
14. Łukaszewski B, Nazar J, Goch M, Łukaszewska M, Stępiński A, Jurczyk MU. Diagnostic methods for detection of bone metastases. *Contemp Oncol (Pozn).* 2017;21(2):98–103.

15. D'Oronzo S, Brown J, Coleman R. The role of biomarkers in the management of bone-homing malignancies. *J Bone Oncol.* 2017;9:1–9.
16. https://www.ajmc.com/view/spotlighting-health-disparities-for-black-americans-with-multiple-myeloma-and-potential-solutions. Accessed January 14, 2023.
17. D'Agostino M, Boccadoro M, Smith EL. Novel immunotherapies for multiple myeloma. *Curr Hematol Malig Rep.* 2017;12:344–357.
18. Alizadeh AM, Shiri S, Farsinejad S. Metastasis review: from bench to bedside. *Tumour Biol.* 2014;35(9):8483–8523.
19. Batson OV. The function of the vertebral veins and their role in the spread of metastases. *Ann Surg.* 1940;112(1):138–148.
20. Batson OV. The role of the vertebral veins in metastatic processes. *Ann Intern Med.* 1942;16:3845.
21. Ziaee S, Chu GC-Y, Huang JM, Sieh S, Chung LWK. Prostate cancer metastasis: roles of recruitment and reprogramming, cell signal network and three-dimensional growth characteristics. *Transl Androl Urol.* 2015;4(4):438–454.
22. Weilbaecher KN, Guise TA, McCauley LK. Cancer to bone: a fatal attraction. *Nat Rev Cancer.* 2011;11(6):411–425.
23. Ren G, Esposito M, Kang Y. Bone metastasis and the metastatic niche. *J Mol Med (Berl).* 2015;93(11):1203–1212.
24. Starling KSA, Shepherd DA. Symptoms and signs of cancer in the school age child. *J Sch Health.* 1977;47(3):144–146.
25. Cabral DA, Tucker LB. Malignancies in children who initially present with rheumatic complaints. *J Pediatr.* 1999;134(1):53–57.
26. Leeson MC, Makley JT, Carter JR. Metastatic skeletal disease in the pediatric population. *J Pediatr Orthop.* 1985;5(3):261–267.
27. Trapani S, Grisolia F, Simonini G, Calabri GB, Falcini F. Incidence of occult cancer in children presenting with musculoskeletal symptoms: a 10-year survey in a pediatric rheumatology unit. *Semin Arthritis Rheum.* 2000;29(6):348–359.
28. Fam AG. Paraneoplastic rheumatic syndrome. *Baillieres Best Pract Res Clin Rheumatol.* 2000;14(3):515–533.
29. Le Rhun E, Taillibert S, Chamberlain MC. Carcinomatous meningitis: leptomeningeal metastases in solid tumors. *Surg Neurol Int.* 2013;4(4): S265–S288.
30. Soffietti R, Rudà R, Trevisan E. Brain metastases: current management and new developments. *Curr Opin Oncol.* 2008;20(6):676–684.
31. Gavrilovic IT, Posner JB. Brain metastases: epidemiology and pathophysiology. *J Neurooncol.* 2005;75(1):5–14.
32. Zoccarato M, Gastaldi M, Zuliani L, et al. Diagnostics of paraneoplastic neurological syndromes. *Neurol Sci.* 2017;38(2):237–242.
33. Schoser B, Eymard B, Datt J, Mantegazza R. Lambert-Eaton myasthenic syndrome (LEMS): a rare autoimmune presynaptic disorder often associated with cancer. *J Neurol.* 2017;264(9):1854–1863.
34. Titulaer MJ, Lang B, Verschuuren JJ. Lambert–Eaton myasthenic syndrome: from clinical characteristics to therapeutic strategies. *Lancet Neurol.* 2011;10:1098–1107.
35. Lambert EH, Eaton LM, Rooke ED. Defect of neuromuscular condition associated with malignant neoplasms. *Am J Physiol.* 1956;187:612.
36. Lambert EH, Rooke ED. Myasthenic state and lung cancer. In: Brain WR, Norris FH, eds. *The Remote Effects of Cancer on the Nervous System.* Grune & Stratton; 1965:67–80.
37. Pelosof LC, Gerber DE. Paraneoplastic syndromes: an approach to diagnosis and treatment. *Mayo Clin Proc.* 2010;85(9):838–854.
38. Fanous I, Dillon P. Paraneoplastic neurological complications of breast cancer. *Exp Hematol Oncol.* 2016;5:29.
39. Constans JP, de Divitiis E, Donzelli R, Spaziante R, Meder JF, Haye C. Spinal metastases with neurological manifestations. Review of 600 cases. *J Neurosurg.* 1983;59(1):111–118.
40. Sciubba RJ, Petteys MB, Dekutoski CG, et al. Diagnosis and management of metastatic spine disease. A review. *J Neurosurg Spine.* 2010;13:94–108.
41. Jaeckle KA, Young DF, Foley KM. The natural history of lumbosacral plexopathy in cancer. *Neurology.* 1985;35:8–15.
42. https://treehousegenomics.ucsc.edu/2017/11/28/did-you-know-that-childhood-cancer-is-very-different-than-adult-cancer/. Accessed January 14, 2023.
43. Kerckhove N, Collin A, Condé S, Chaleteix C, Pezet D, Balayssac D. Long-term effects, pathophysiological mechanisms, and risk factors of chemotherapy-induced peripheral neuropathies: a comprehensive literature review. *Front Pharmacol.* 2017;8:86.
44. Patel HJ, Patel BM. TNF-α and cancer cachexia: molecular insights and clinical implications. *Life Sci.* 2017;170:56–63.
45. Belsky JA, Stanek JR, Rose MJ. Investigating the safety and feasibility of osteopathic medicine in the pediatric oncology outpatient setting. *J Osteopath Med.* 2022;122(8):423–429.
46. Kuchera WA, Kuchera ML. *Osteopathic Principles in Practice.* 2nd ed. KCOM Press; 1992:295.
47. Schmidt JD, McLaughlin AP, Saltzstein SL, Garcia-Reyes R. Risk factors for the development of distant metastases in patients undergoing pelvic lymphadenectomy for prostatic cancer. *Am J Surg.* 1982;144(1): 131–135.
48. Stoker TA. The effect of cortisone therapy and limb exercise on the dissemination of cancer via the lymphatic system. *Br J Cancer.* 1969;23(1): 132–135.
49. Yamagata K, Kumagai K. Experimental study of lymphogenous peritoneal cancer dissemination: migration of fluorescent-labelled tumor cells in a rat model of mesenteric lymph vessel obstruction. *J Exp Clin Cancer Res.* 2000;19(2):211–217.
50. Gendreau KM, Whalen GF. What can we learn from the phenomenon of preferential lymph node metastasis in carcinoma? *J Surg Oncol.* 1999;70(3):199–204.
51. Sleeman JP. The lymph node as bridgehead in the metastatic dissemination of tumors. *Recent Results Cancer Res.* 2000;157:55–81.
52. Verhoeven D, Buyssens N. Macrophages and carcinoma cells migrate at the same pace to the lymph nodes. *Lymphology.* 1989;22:141–143.
53. McCauley L, Pedrueza M, Zhang X, Jones H, Hodge L. Lymphatic pump treatment enhances pulmonary immunity and protects against solid tumor formation in the rat lung. *J Immunol.* 2011;186(1):161.14.
54. Potapov IA, Abisheva TM. [The action of massage on lymph formation and transport]. *Vopr Kurortol Fizioter Lech Fiz Kult.* 1989;5:44–47.
55. Wozniewski M. Value of intermittent pneumatic massage in the treatment of upper extremity lymphedema. *Pol Tyg Lek.* 1991;46(30–31):550–552.
56. Langevin HM, Keely P, Mao J. Connecting (T)issues: how research in fascia biology can impact integrative oncology. *Cancer Res.* 2016;76(21):6159–6162.
57. Wang J-Y, Wu P-K, Chen PC-H, et al. Manipulation therapy prior to diagnosis induced primary osteosarcoma metastasis—from clinical to basic research. *PLoS One.* 2014;9(5):e96571.
58. Ezzo J, Manheimer E, McNeely ML, et al. Manual lymphatic drainage for lymphedema following breast cancer treatment. *Cochrane Database Syst Rev.* 2015;(5):CD003475.
59. Kutner JS, Smith MC, Corbin L, et al. Massage therapy versus simple touch to improve pain and mood in patients with advanced cancer: a randomized trial. *Ann Intern Med.* 2008;149(6):369–379.
60. Kuchera ML, Kuchera WA. *Osteopathic Considerations in Systemic Dysfunction.* 2nd ed. KCOM Press; 1992:28.
61. Walkowski S, Singh M, Puertas J, Pate M, Goodrum K, Benencia F. Osteopathic manipulative therapy induces early plasma cytokine release and mobilization of a population of blood dendritic cells. *PLoS One.* 2014; 9(3):e90132.
62. Stamatakis E, Lee IM, Bennie J, et al. Does strength-promoting exercise confer unique health benefits? A pooled analysis of data on 11 population cohorts with all-cause, cancer, and cardiovascular mortality endpoints. *Am J Epidemiol.* 2018;187:1102–1112.
63. Vainshelboim B, Chen Z, Lee YN, et al. Cardiorespiratory fitness, adiposity, and cancer mortality in men. *Obesity (Silver Spring).* 2017;25(2): S66–S71.
64. Vainshelboim B, Müller J, Lima RM, et al. Cardiorespiratory fitness, physical activity and cancer mortality in men. *Prev Med.* 2017;100:89–94.
65. Schmid D, Leitzmann MF. Cardiorespiratory fitness as predictor of cancer mortality: a systematic review and meta-analysis. *Ann Oncol.* 2015; 26(2):272–278.
66. Lee MK, Kim JY, Kim DI, et al. Effect of home-based exercise intervention on fasting insulin and adipocytokines in colorectal cancer survivors: a randomized controlled trial. *Metabolism.* 2017;76:23–31.
67. Zimmer P, Trebing S, Timmers-Trebing U, et al. Eight-week multimodal exercise counteracts a progress of chemotherapy-induced peripheral neuropathy and improves balance and strength in metastasized colorectal

cancer patients: a randomized controlled trial. *Support Care Cancer.* 2018;26:615–624.

68. Stout NL, Baima J, Swisher AK, et al. A systematic review of exercise systematic reviews in the cancer literature (2005–2017). *PM R.* 2017;9(9S2):S347–S384.
69. Jayasekara H, English DR, Haydon A, et al. Associations of alcohol intake, smoking, physical activity and obesity with survival following colorectal cancer diagnosis by stage, anatomic site and tumor molecular subtype. *Int J Cancer.* 2018;142:238–250.
70. Kushi LH, Doyle C, McCullough M, et al; American Cancer Society 2010 Nutrition and Physical Activity Guidelines Advisory Committee. American Cancer Society Guidelines on nutrition and physical activity for cancer prevention: reducing the risk of cancer with healthy food choices and physical activity. *CA Cancer J Clin.* 2012;62:30–67.
71. Katzke VA, Kaaks R, Kühn T. Lifestyle and cancer risk. *Cancer J.* 2015;21(2):104–110.
72. Key TJ, Appleby PN, Spencer EA, et al. Cancer incidence in British vegetarians. *Br J Cancer.* 2009;101:192–197.

77 Osteopathic Considerations in Endocrinology

DENISE K. BURNS ▪ MICHAEL A. SEFFINGER ▪ MARY BANIHASHEM

KEY CONCEPTS

- Endocrine disorders adversely affect basic life functions, including:
  - ☐ Musculoskeletal structure and function
  - ☐ Reproduction
  - ☐ Growth and development
  - ☐ Energy management
  - ☐ Preservation and stabilization of the internal environment (homeostasis)
  - ☐ Behavioral health
  - ☐ OMT is a safe and effective treatment option in patients with endocrine disorders.
- Osteopathic philosophy and tenets provide a framework for addressing health problems involving the endocrine system. The musculoskeletal system is an integral part of the endocrine system as both a secretory and an end organ, with autocrine, endocrine, and paracrine functions.
- Musculoskeletal exercise is critical to health restoration and maintenance. There are important musculoskeletal manifestations of endocrine disorders detectable by palpatory examination and radiologic studies.
- Osteopathic manipulative treatment (OMT) is indicated to treat somatic dysfunction in patients with endocrine disorders to improve physiologic function and quality of life. There are important contraindications to selective OMT procedures in patients with certain endocrine disorders, for example, osteoporosis.

INTRODUCTION

- The endocrine system comprises glands and tissues that produce hormones for regulating and coordinating vital bodily functions. The hypothalamus produces several releasing and inhibiting hormones that act on the pituitary gland, stimulating the release of pituitary hormones.
- Several of the pituitary hormones act on various glands located throughout the body.
- Other hormone-producing glands throughout the body include the adrenal glands, which primarily produce cortisol; the gonads (i.e., ovaries and testes), which produce sex hormones; the thyroid, which produces thyroid hormone; the parathyroid, which produces parathyroid hormone; and the pancreas, which produces insulin and glucagon.
- Many of these hormones are part of regulatory hormonal cascades involving a hypothalamic hormone, one or more pituitary hormones, and one or more target gland hormones.
- Endocrine information is transmitted in the form of structurally specific chemical messengers, hormones, and received by equally specific chemical structures, the cell receptors.
- The endocrine system participates in the control and integration of bodily processes that are fundamental to human life:
  - ☐ Musculoskeletal structure and function
  - ☐ Reproduction, growth, and development
  - ☐ Energy management
  - ☐ Preservation and stabilization of the internal environment (homeostasis)
  - ☐ Behavioral health
- The traditional view of hormones and endocrine glands considers a hormone as an information-carrying molecule, secreted in small amounts by a specific gland and transported in the blood to a distant site, where it exerts its biologic effect. Certain nontraditional hormones and hormone-like substances are secreted by the organs themselves. Examples of this include atrial natriuretic peptide (ANP), prostaglandin, renin, erythropoietin, myokines, and active metabolites of vitamin D.
- Responses to internal and external events are modulated through negative and positive feedback mechanisms with homeostasis of the internal environment, the internal milieu, as a major goal. Homeostasis of the internal environment is a primary goal of endocrine physiology.
- The rate of hormone secretion is modulated according to changes in the internal environment. The relationship between hormones and the internal environment is completely interactive: changes in the internal environment affect hormone secretion, and changes in hormone concentration influence the composition of the internal environment milieu.
- The body structure or external environment also influences the internal environment milieu.
- The secretion of a hormone is typically controlled by a self-regulating servomechanism designed to match circulating concentrations of the hormone to the momentary needs of the individual. Two essential features of the control scheme are readily apparent.
- First, the systemic concentration of the hormone, or of some variable related to the hormone, such as a metabolite, must be monitored.
- Second, this information must be returned to the endocrine organ. The secretion of the hormone is adjusted up or down according to the nature of the information received: inhibitory, negative feedback or stimulatory, positive feedback. Negative feedback mechanisms are inherently self-limiting.
- In all cases, the rate of hormone secretion is tightly coupled to demands for the hormone. The temporal pattern of changes in the secretory rate and circulating concentration of the hormone also influence hormone activity.
- This chapter will focus on the musculoskeletal component of common endocrine problems seen in primary care medical practice using osteopathic principles and practice. The

basic science mechanisms, current diagnostic methodology, and treatment options of endocrine disorders can be found in the latest edition of standard internal medical textbooks such as *Harrison's Principles of Internal Medicine* or clinical endocrinology texts and therefore will not be reiterated herein. Complex endocrine disorders or presentations are deftly handled by practicing internists and endocrinologists in each local community and should be consulted when specialty care is indicated.

OSTEOPATHIC PHILOSOPHY AND PRINCIPLES APPLIED TO PATIENTS WITH ENDOCRINE DISORDERS

- Osteopathic philosophy includes its tenants; the body is a unit that is self-healing and self-regulating and structure and function are interrelated. Osteopathic medicine is a health-oriented, patient-centered approach to patient care. The body is inherently self-regulating and self-healing.
- For the endocrine system to function optimally, the body must function as a unit. The endocrine system relies on other organ systems to distribute its hormones released. A.T. Still developed a predominantly mechanistic theory on how disorders of the vital body fluids (i.e., blood, lymph, cerebrospinal fluid [CSF], hormones) and their flow occur.
- He postulated that bones, muscles, membranes, organs, nerves, blood, and lymph are interlinked harmoniously. If these mechanical disturbances were eliminated, the unhindered flow could be restored. He believed that health is based on structural integrity and develops when the flow of body fluids is unhindered. Obstructions of these fluids or their neural control centers can lead to disturbances in the flow.[1] These concepts provided by Still led to the saying "the rule of the artery is supreme."
- Endocrine function is highly dependent on cardiovascular function. This is most obvious in that hormones rely on the cardiovascular system (CVS) as a means of transport to distant sites. While the endocrine system clearly depends on cardiovascular function, hormones have a major influence on the CVS:
  - □ Catecholamines have well-known actions on the heart and vasculature.
  - □ Adrenergic cardiac fibers influence myocardial contractility and rhythm.
  - □ Adrenergic vasoconstrictor fibers are a dominant influence on systemic vascular resistance.
  - □ Catecholamines of adrenal medullary origin and several other hormones also influence the CVS, for example:
    - Vasopressin and angiotensin are vasoconstrictors.
    - Thyroid hormones affect heart rate.
    - Thyroid hormones and aldosterone increase the force of ventricular contraction.
- In addition to these direct actions, endocrine mechanisms (the renin–angiotensin–aldosterone system, antidiuretic hormone, ANP) are an important component in the regulation of whole-body fluid and electrolyte metabolism, the extracellular fluid (ECF) and blood volume and, indirectly, the cardiovascular function.
- The endocrine mechanisms serve to maintain fluid homeostasis and cardiovascular function under normal conditions and to protect cardiovascular function against the consequences of challenges such as water deprivation or hemorrhage. A wide variety of external stimuli, or changes in the external environment, alter the activity of the endocrine system by means of multisynaptic neural pathways.
- Auditory stimuli activate the hypothalamic–pituitary axis (HPA) and increase cortisol secretion. Light cycles influence endocrine rhythms, and groups of females living together may develop synchronous periods of gonadotropin secretion and ovarian function.
- Just as the nervous system influences endocrine activity, hormones have significant effects on neural activity. The endocrine effects can range from actions on single neurons to alterations of complex mental activity and behavior. BNP and vasopeptide are examples of these interactions.
- Insulin secretion is a typical example: although glucose and other metabolites stimulate release of the polypeptide, β-cell innervation (sympathetic and parasympathetic) modulates the secretory response.
- Gonadal and adrenocortical steroids affect the activity of the hypothalamic neurons that control the anterior pituitary. They thus play a major role in regulating pituitary–gonadal and pituitary–adrenocortical activity. Moreover, both types of steroids influence complex patterns of neural activity.
- The actions of the thyroid amines on the development and function of the CNS are especially profound. For example, infantile hypothyroidism (cretinism) is associated with retarded mental development. The earlier the condition appears and the longer it goes untreated, the more severe the effects, culminating in irreversible damage to the brain.

FINAL COMMON PATH

This exquisite interrelationship of neural, vascular, and endocrine function is sometimes referred to as the final common path.

- Neural influences predominate in the regulation of anterior pituitary hormone secretion. It is well known that adrenocorticotropic hormone (ACTH) secretion is related to photoperiod.
- Growth hormone secretion is associated with sleep stages. Light, odor, auditory, and tactile stimuli as well as emotional disturbances influence gonadotropin secretion and reproductive function.
- Historically, the (older) endocrine literature referred to the anterior pituitary as a gland under neural control but lacked a nerve supply. For a time, the relationship between anterior pituitary and CNS function presented a conceptual difficulty, since the adenohypophyseal secretory cells are not innervated.
- Although the anterior pituitary is innervated by vasomotor fibers, the physical link between the CNS and the anterior pituitary is *not neural but vascular*, consisting of a specialized arrangement of vessels, alternatively known as the pituitary portal vessels or the hypothalamic–hypophyseal portal vessels. In brief, the anterior pituitary is regulated by neurohormones that are produced in the hypothalamus and transported to the pituitary in the portal venous blood.
- The portal vessels originate in a capillary network (primary plexus) located in the hypothalamus. The capillaries coalesce to form the pituitary portal veins, which enter the anterior pituitary and give rise to a secondary capillary plexus.
- The hypothalamic neurohormones, hypophysiotropic hormones, are produced by neurons that terminate in the hypothalamus in close contact with the primary capillary plexus.
- The neurohormones enter the portal venous blood and are delivered to the anterior pituitary.
- Somatic dysfunction of the cranium may alter sphenobasilar motion and membranous motion characteristics affecting the dynamic diaphragmatic sellae and the delicate pituitary portal circulation. Generalized dysfunction of the HPA may occur.

Processes Regulated by Hormones

- Hormones are involved in regulating the most fundamental aspects of human life. Indeed, hormones play a vital role regarding the survival of the species. That role includes:
  - ☐ Reproduction
  - ☐ Growth and development
  - ☐ Internal environment maintenance
  - ☐ Energy metabolism

Reproduction

- Hormones produced by the hypothalamus (gonadotropin-releasing hormone or GnRH), the pituitary (FSH, LH, prolactin [PRL], growth hormone), and the gonads (androgens, estrogens, progestogens) interact to regulate reproductive function. Reproductive competence requires the ability to produce gametes (ova, sperm) and the ability to unite the gametes by attracting and mating with members of the opposite sex. There are several aspects of this process:
  - ☐ Gamete formation (e.g., spermatogenesis, oogenesis)
  - ☐ Mating ability (e.g., growth, development, maintenance of the reproductive tract)
  - ☐ Mutual attractiveness (e.g., male, and female phenotype, pattern of sexual behavior)
- All are influenced by or totally depend on reproductive hormones. After conception, maternal support for the developing fetus (pregnancy) is hormone dependent, and in mammals, even after birth, hormones continue to play a role in nurturing the infant during lactation.

Growth and Development

- The regulation of intrauterine growth is poorly understood. Surprisingly, hormones that have dramatic effects on the neonate (growth hormone, thyroid hormone) appear to have little influence on fetal growth. Somatomedins and other growth factors, including muscle-derived myokines, undoubtedly play a role in prenatal growth, but further research must be done to clarify that role.
- The regulation of postnatal growth is better understood. In addition to a number of nonhormonal factors, such as nutrition, hygiene, and general health, normal growth and development depend on the interplay of several hormones, including:
  - ☐ Growth hormone and the somatomedins
  - ☐ Thyroid hormone
  - ☐ Insulin
  - ☐ Cortisol
  - ☐ Gonadal steroids
- Imbalances in the secretion of these hormones, excesses, as well as deficiencies, dramatically affect growth, especially if the imbalance occurs during the normal growing period.
  - ☐ Hyposecretion of growth hormone produces dwarfism.
  - ☐ Hypersecretion of growth hormone leads to gigantism.
  - ☐ Thyroid hormone deficiency impairs growth of the body and has devastating effects on the development of the CNS and mental capacity.
  - ☐ Cortisol or the gonadal steroids in excess slow or even arrest growth and lead to short adult stature.

Internal Environment

- Many, and in a broad sense all, hormones participate in the defense of the internal environment. Although no aspect of the internal environment is unimportant to health and well-being, certain features are regulated and guarded especially closely by functional groups of hormones. These include:
  - ☐ Ionic composition (Na^+, K^+, and H^+) of the body fluids, most notably the blood and CSF (the renin–angiotensin–aldosterone system, ANP, insulin, and other hormones)
  - ☐ Volume of the body fluids, especially the ECF volume and the blood volume (ADH, the renin–angiotensin–aldosterone system, ANP, cortisol, and others)
  - ☐ Plasma level of calcium and phosphate ions (PTH, 1,25-[OH]2-D3, calcitonin, and others)
  - ☐ Structural integrity and function of body tissues, including bone, muscle, and adipose tissue (growth hormone and the somatomedins, PTH, 1,25-[OH]2-D3, gonadal steroids, insulin, glucagon, cortisol, and others)
  - ☐ Direction and rate of flow of metabolic energy

Energy Metabolism

- The hormonal regulation of energy metabolism allows the body to meet its need for a constant supply of energy despite the intermittent intake of food. Even at rest, vital bodily processes must be maintained. There is a significant metabolic "cost of living," the basal metabolic rate. On the other hand, the intake of energy (calories contained in food) is sporadic; the consumption of excess food (caloric intake exceeds momentary needs) is interspersed with periods of fasting. To resolve this problem, excess energy is stored in a form that is readily mobilized and available for use when necessary. The metabolic flow in both directions, storage, and retrieval, is directed and controlled by hormones.
- During the period when exogenous fuels are available, insulin is of primary importance. The polypeptide stimulates the uptake and metabolism of glucose (glycolysis) and promotes the storage of small metabolites in their respective macromolecular forms (i.e., glucose as glycogen, amino acids as protein, and free fatty acids as triglyceride). When exogenous fuels are not available, several hormones, most notably glucagon and cortisol, collaborate to mobilize energy from endogenous storage sites. Glucagon stimulates the hydrolysis of glycogen (glycogenolysis) and triglyceride (lipolysis). It increases the formation of new glucose from noncarbohydrate sources (gluconeogenesis). Cortisol stimulates gluconeogenesis and mobilizes amino acids (gluconeogenic precursors) from protein depots. Ghrelin and leptin influence energy balance, fuel utilization, and body weight by affecting appetite.
- The importance of the hormonal controls is dramatically illustrated in clinical conditions such as diabetes mellitus and Addison disease (cortisol deficiency).
  - ☐ The absence of insulin leads to a metabolic profile that in many respects resembles that seen in long-term food deprivation (starvation) and, if left untreated, death.
  - ☐ In the absence of cortisol, gluconeogenesis is so seriously impaired that short periods of food deprivation, even an overnight fast, pose a serious threat to life.
- Skeletal muscle myokines and bone endocrine factors have autocrine, paracrine, and endocrine functions that affect energy metabolism (see below "Metabolic Model" section for further discussion), for example:
  - ☐ Myokines increase glucose uptake, improve lipolysis, stimulate angiogenesis, reduce adiposity, and are involved with bone growth and degradation.
  - ☐ Lack of exercise reduces muscle mass and induces sarcopenia and obesity.
  - ☐ Bone-derived fibroblast growth factor (FGF)23, osteocalcin, and sclerostin have wide-ranging effects on mineral and energy metabolism.

Osteopathic Diagnosis and Treatment

- Osteopathic philosophy and principles applied to the patient with an endocrine disorder directs the physician to search for the underlying cause of the disease, treat it, and assist the patient in restoring their health.
- Disease is considered an effect, and identifying the underlying cause is key to effective healthcare. Still states that "local shocks affect the whole system, the nerve and blood supply to every part of the body. They disable or confuse the secretory and excretory systems and the fluids retained become deadly poisons."[1]
- If the underlying cause cannot be found, further medical workup must be done including evaluation and management of other organ systems which may be causing secondary effects in the endocrine system.
- If there are mechanical, vascular, lymphatic, neurologic, metabolic, and/or behavioral etiologies, these should be addressed, and alleviated if possible.
- Osteopathic palpatory diagnosis and treatment are used to aid in the diagnosis and management of all patients, including those with endocrine disorders. The procedure of OMT is indicated by the presence (cause or etiology) of somatic dysfunctions palpated on the physical examination (TART findings) as it relates to restoring normal physiologic processes and homeostasis.
- The OMT techniques chosen to treat the patient, should be based on several factors including acute or chronic somatic dysfunction present, the severity of the patient's health, limitations of treatment position, indications, and contraindications for OMT based on the patient's health status, physical location of the patient and patient consent. The osteopathic techniques should be directed as dictated by the five osteopathic treatment models of care.

APPLICATION OF THE FIVE MODELS OF OSTEOPATHIC CARE TO PATIENTS WITH ENDOCRINE DISORDERS

- There are five models of osteopathic patient care that are used to help focus the doctor and patient on determining the cause of the illness and the pathways needed to restore and maintain health. These are the biomechanical, neurologic, behavioral, respiratory/circulatory, and metabolic models. They are based on osteopathic philosophy and its four tenets. They focus the discussion on healthy physiologic function as the primary outcome of treatment (Fig. 77.1).
- Using these models of osteopathic care, various endocrine dysfunctions can be viewed from the perspective of the role of the musculoskeletal system in health and disease, providing the osteopathic physician with unique avenues for diagnosis and treatment, including the appropriate use of OMT. Osteopathic palpatory diagnosis and treatment are used to aid in the diagnosis and management of all patients, including those with endocrine disorders. OMT is used as indicated by the diagnosis (cause or etiology) and addresses somatic dysfunction found on physical examination as it relates to restoring normal physiologic processes and homeostasis.

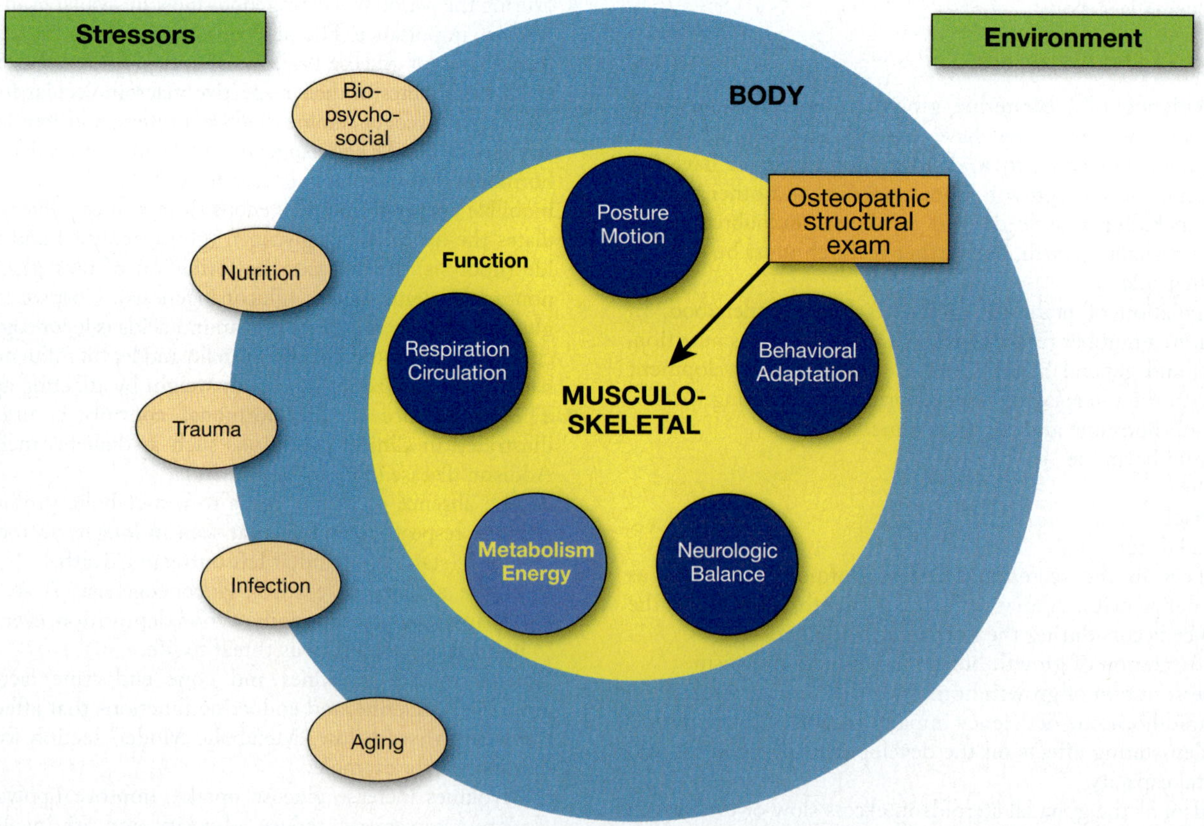

Figure 77.1. The five models of osteopathic care. The musculoskeletal system makes up over 80% of the body's mass (*yellow center*) and is involved with all body functions (*dark blue circles* inside the body, which is depicted as the larger circle, encompassing all other circles). Environmental stressors (*outer yellow circles*) challenge the body to maintain homeostasis. The endocrine system is critical for maintaining homeostasis, metabolic functions, and energy balance. Its functions are also involved with all other body functions. The osteopathic structural examination assesses the musculoskeletal system in terms of its role in each of the main body functions, to identify somatic dysfunction that impairs normal physiologic functions. (From Seffinger MA. Osteopathic considerations in endocrinology. In: Seffinger MA, ed. *Foundations of Osteopathic Medicine: Philosophy, Science, Clinical Applications, and Research*. 4th ed. Wolters Kluwer; 2018:1308. Figure 43F.1.)

- A thorough history and physical exam including review of systems should be completed. The patient with an endocrine disorder often presents with a vague complaint of being fatigued, stating "I feel tired all the time." The physician then begins the process of investigation to determine the underlying cause.
- Often, the exact cause of an endocrine disorder cannot be found. Occasionally, it is a mechanical (musculoskeletal system or connective tissue) obstruction to blood flow or lymphatic drainage to or from an endocrine organ or altered neuronal control of an endocrine organ. Most commonly, it is an autoimmune malfunction that destroys the anatomy and physiology (structure and function) of an endocrine organ. What triggered this autoimmune reaction or dysfunction? Was it a trauma or a virus or a stressed immune system that has malfunctioned? Perhaps, a neurologic dysfunction from an anatomical derangement of the musculoskeletal system should be a consideration. Was it influenced by a genetic predisposition, deleterious behavior, use of toxic substances, environmental toxins, or a spiritual practice or cultural belief system?
- Limiting and hence controlling the pathologic process with medication, radiation, and/or surgery, is a contemporary management plan. Enhancing or aiding the body's production of the hormone by diet, medication, exercise, OMT, and stress management may be helpful when the endocrine organ or system is not functioning maximally or efficiently and is not diseased beyond the abilities of compensatory or self-healing mechanisms to restore health.
- Behavioral therapy may be indicated in the treatment of a chronically ill patient with depression and anxiety. A pilot study by Abrahams et al. demonstrated a decrease in serum biomarkers such as cortisol levels associated with stress as well as serum cytokines with the use of OMT.[2]
- Examples of stress-related treatments include a specific focus on the suboccipital and thoracic regions which are associated with increased heart rate variability, improved autonomic homeostasis, decreased muscular tension, and reduced perception of stress.[3,4] Rib-raising treatment has been shown to reduce sympathetic output which results in parasympathetic predominant state—otherwise understood as a relaxed state.[5] Compression of the fourth ventricle (CV4) influences ANS function and has been shown to alter the physiologic parameters of blood flow velocity, heart rate, blood pressure, and cerebral tissue oxygenation.[6]
- For patients who need palliative care, the use of OMT may be indicated. Some endocrine disorders, or their treatments, cause structural and functional alteration in muscles and bones, and thus specific osteopathic manipulative techniques may be relatively or absolutely contraindicated in patients with some endocrine disorders.

Somatic Dysfunction, Research, and Endocrine Dysfunction

- Somatic dysfunctions are defined by the ECOP/AACOM Glossary of Osteopathic Terminology as "impaired or altered function of related components of the body framework system: skeletal, arthrodial and myofascial structures, and related vascular, lymphatic and neural elements." Early osteopathic research with animal models discovered that cervical and thoracic vertebral joint dislocation and fixation led to pathophysiological changes in the HPA[7]:
  - Vasoconstriction (dilation)
  - Diapedesis (tissue congestion)
  - Edema:
    - Increased CSF
    - Increased intracranial pressure
  - Petechial hemorrhages
  - Fibrosis then ischemia
  - Behavioral changes
- This encouraged osteopathic physicians to treat spinal somatic dysfunction with hopes to prevent endocrine organ dysfunction. However, OMT is directed at all tissues that are dysfunctional or involved in dysfunction, not just the spine. The goal of OMT for somatic dysfunction related to endocrinopathies is to remove somatic or visceral dysfunction that is impeding normal physiologic functions, to improve blood supply, venous and lymphatic drainage, and autonomic nervous system (ANS) balance to and from endocrine organs to help patients restore homeostasis.[8] Korr states that "One of the most reliable of the hypotheses (relating the nervous system to somatic dysfunction) is that the entire nervous system-from the highest centers of the brain to the peripheral neurons-is involved in all somatic dysfunction and in every manipulative treatment."[9] He further states that "the personality of the patient influences the nature, site, and clinical impact of somatic dysfunction." He further states, "the participation of the endorphins, other neuropeptides, and other neuroendocrine mechanisms is almost certainly involved."[9]
- An international study in Brain Science by M. Tramontano et al. in 2020 presented evidence that OMT showed a distinct functional and reversible connectivity rearrangement of the supraspinal locomotor network, consisting of the premotor cortex, basal ganglia, and midline cerebellum, as well as the emotional/autonomic network, with specific activation of the amygdala and posterior cingulate cortex (PCC) associated with autonomic activity.[6]
- Along the lines of the research reported by Burns in the early half of the 20th century,[7] more recently, Berkowitz et al.[10] reported about a patient who had cervical spine joint dysfunction from a breakdown of a previous spinal fusion at the C5–C7 vertebrae, which seemingly correlated to her development of hypothyroidism with resolution of the hypothyroidism only after surgical refusion of the unstable cervical spine. This case example demonstrated the principle of somatovisceral reflexes in which musculoskeletal dysfunction adversely affects neurologically related organ function.
- A subgroup analysis of a large, randomized placebo-controlled clinical trial investigating the efficacy of OMT for patients with low back pain showed that patients with diabetes initially had higher pain levels and higher severity levels of somatic dysfunction on osteopathic structural examination. Upon treatment with OMT, this subgroup also had significantly decreased pain levels, and their blood TNF-α levels were also decreased.[11,12] Further studies are ongoing to delineate the relationship between low back pain, somatic dysfunction, and TNF-α levels in diabetic patients.

Musculoskeletal Manifestations of Endocrine Disorders

- Musculoskeletal manifestations of endocrine disorders can be discerned by palpatory examination[13–15] and radiologic studies (see below). Endocrine disorders often manifest in changes in the soft tissues in the region of the diseased organ but also have systemic manifestations affecting the entire musculoskeletal system, for example:
  - Atraumatic soft tissue swelling, muscle wasting, or myopathies of proximal limb muscles (thyroid disease)

- □ Atraumatic joint immobility (Charcot joint) and peripheral neuropathy (diabetes mellitus)
- □ Soft tissue calcifications and atraumatic bone pain without palpable somatic dysfunction (primary hyperparathyroidism)

- When performing the osteopathic structural examination, these findings should alert the astute physician that an underlying endocrine disorder may be the etiology, and not a primary mechanical somatic dysfunction.
- Some osteopathic considerations when viewing the patient with endocrinopathies from the perspective of the metabolic model include the topics of:
  - □ Radiographical effects of hormone deficiency or excess on the musculoskeletal system
  - □ Muscles and bones as endocrine organs
  - □ Nutrition and dietary supplements used to enhance endocrine functions

Radiographical Evidence of Hormone Excess or Deficiency on the Musculoskeletal System

Radiologic findings in the musculoskeletal system are listed below, organized by glandular endocrine disorder[16]:

Pituitary Disorders

- Gigantism causes the following:
  - □ Increased longitudinal bone growth leading to excessive height
- Acromegaly causes the following:
  - □ Coarsened facial features with frontal bossing and mandibular prognathism (Fig. 77.2)
  - □ Spade-like terminal tufts and widened phalanges
  - □ Joint space widening early but premature osteoarthritis
  - □ Soft tissue hypertrophy, including heel pad thickening
  - □ Median neuropathy, trigger finger

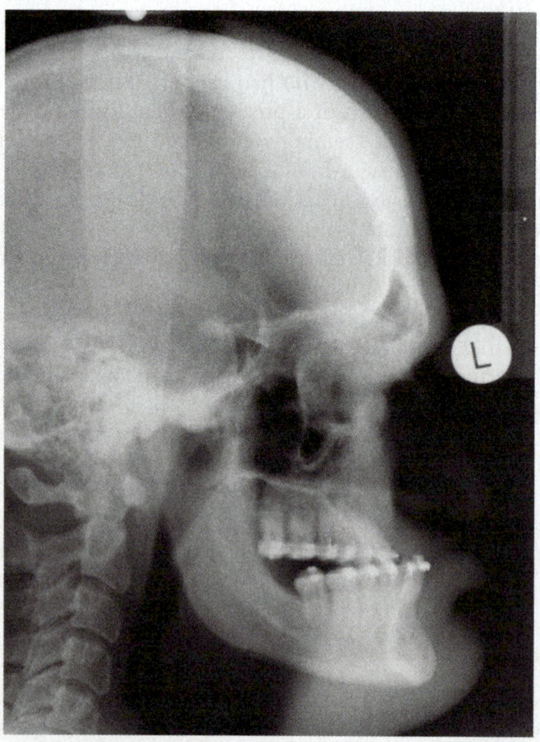

Figure 77.2. Lateral cephalometric radiograph. Mandibular prognathism caused by acromegaly—a surgical orthodontic case. (Reprinted from Gosau M, Vogel C, Moralis A, Proff P, Kleinheinz J, Driemel O. Mandibular prognathism caused by acromegaly—a surgical orthodontic case. *Head Face Med.* 2009;5:16. http://creativecommons.org/licenses/by/2.0)

Thyroid Disorders

- In hyperthyroidism, muscle atrophy can be seen and palpated. Also, look for signs of:
  - □ Myopathy with atrophy and fatty infiltration.
  - □ Acropachy—soft tissue swelling and clubbing of the fingers; radiograph shows periostitis of metacarpal bones: lacy, periosteal new bone formation along the shafts of the phalanges.
  - □ Pretibial myxedema and ophthalmopathy.
  - □ Shoulder adhesive capsulitis (frozen shoulder syndrome).
- In hypothyroidism, look for:
  - □ Irregular or stippled epiphyses
  - □ Delayed bone maturation
  - □ Proximal muscle myopathy
  - □ Carpal tunnel syndrome

Parathyroid Disorders

- Primary hyperparathyroidism causes the following:
  - □ Bone resorption (osteoporosis)
  - □ Soft tissue calcifications (Fig. 77.3)
  - □ Brown tumors
- In pseudo- and pseudohypoparathyroidism from Albright hereditary osteodystrophy, look for the following:
  - □ Metacarpal and/or metatarsal shortening (usually fourth/fifth)

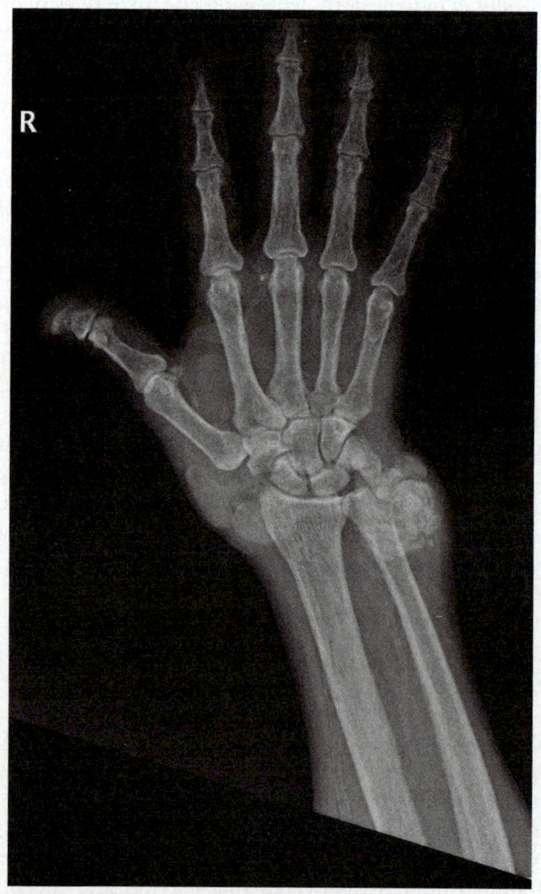

Figure 77.3. Frontal x-ray of the left wrist: Large soft tissue calcifications are seen on the ulnar side in the left distal forearm with overlying soft tissue bulging. (Case courtesy of Naim Qaqish, Radiopaedia.org, rID: 82116.)

- □ Short middle and distal phalanges with coned epiphyses
- □ Short stature, rounded facies, central obesity
- □ Subcutaneous calcifications

Adrenal and Renal Disorders

- Hypercortisolism (Cushing disease or side effect of long-term corticosteroid medication) causes:
  - □ Osteopenia and osteoporosis with insufficiency fractures
  - □ Osteonecrosis
  - □ Muscle wasting
- Renal osteodystrophy causes the same findings as found in hyperparathyroidism plus:
  - □ Osteosclerosis, including "rugger-jersey" spine (Fig. 77.4)
  - □ Osteomalacia with Looser zones (pseudo-fracture sites commonly affecting the scapula, pubic rami, and proximal femurs)
  - □ "Tumoral" calcinosis
- Diabetes mellitus causes the following:
  - □ Neuropathic arthropathy
  - □ Osteomyelitis and septic arthritis
  - □ Insufficiency fractures
  - □ Myonecrosis
  - □ Adhesive capsulitis
  - □ Dupuytren contracture
  - □ Charcot joint

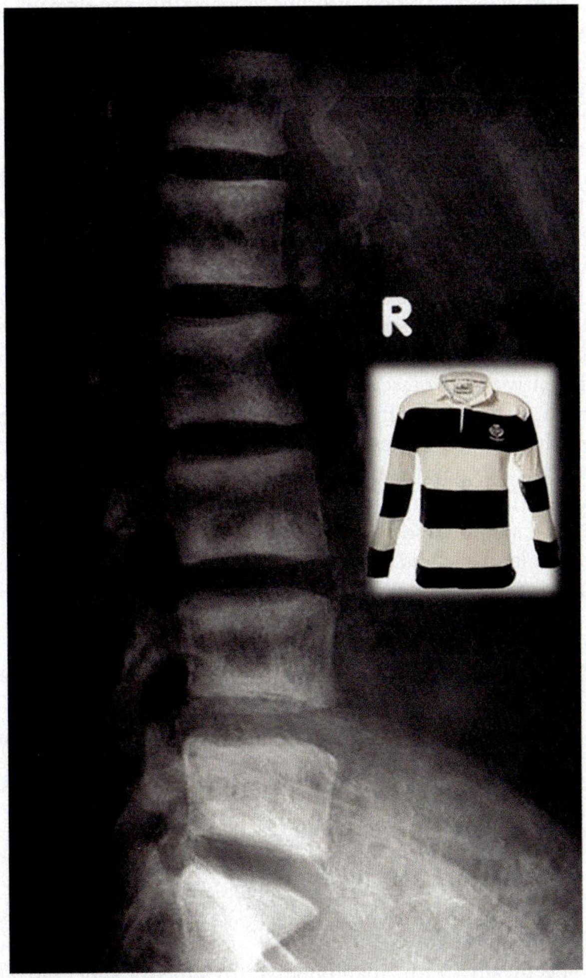

Figure 77.4. Adrenal/Renal disorders—Osteosclerosis and "rugger-jersey" spine. (Case courtesy of Ian Bickle, Radiopaedia.org, rID: 39481.)

Muscles and Bones as an Endocrine Organ

- **Myokines and Metabolism**
  Muscle function is not limited to the generation of power, locomotion, posture, and breathing. Skeletal muscle is an endocrine organ that secretes myokines that have paracrine, autocrine, and endocrine activities that affect total body metabolism.[17–27]
  - □ Paracrine activities affect local neurons, Schwann cells, blood vessels, bone, tendon, and muscles (e.g., IL-6, Ang1, BDNF, FGF-2, CTRP3, CTRP15, FGF-2, LIF, CT-1, VEGFA, PDEF, LRP4, CNTFRa).
  - □ Autocrine activities affect the muscles (e.g., myostatin, BDNF, IGF-1, FGF-2, FGF21, adiponectin, TRP1, CTRP5, CTRP15, ghrelin, musclin, irisin, visfatin, apelin, LCN13, IL-6, CNTF, CT-1, oncostatin M).
  - □ Endocrine activities affect distant organs (e.g., myostatin, BDNF, FGF21, adiponectin, CTRP1, CTRP12, CTRP15, ghrelin, irisin, visfatin, apelin, LCN13, IL-6, CT-1, oncostatin M).
- **Myokines and Homeostasis**
  - □ Myokines have various roles in homeostasis including[17–27]:
    - Shivering (temperature regulation)
    - Skeletal muscle is the most important organ for the maintenance of body temperature besides nonshivering thermogenesis by brown adipose tissue.
    - Energy storage, glycolysis, and gluconeogenesis
    - Skeletal muscle stores triglycerides and glycogen, especially in athletes.
    - Anaerobic glycolysis and breakdown of skeletal muscle tissue during starvation release lactate and amino acids, respectively, some of which subsequently are utilized to fuel hepatic (mainly alanine and lactate) and renal (mainly glutamine) gluconeogenesis.
    - Mediation of communications between the muscle and liver, adipose tissue, brain, and other organs involved in lipid and glucose metabolism.
    - Glucose and Lipid Metabolism & Inflammation
    - Myokines affect muscle mass and myofiber switching and have profound effects on glucose and lipid metabolism and inflammation, thus contributing to energy homeostasis and the pathogenesis of obesity, diabetes, and other diseases. IL-6, IL-8, IL-15, and brain-derived neurotrophic factor are some examples:
    - IL-6 increases glucose uptake and fatty acid oxidation locally in skeletal muscle, enhancing insulin secretion, which further increases glucose uptake into muscle cells and stimulates hepatic glucose output and fatty acid release from adipose tissue providing energy substrates for the exercising muscle.
    - Angiogenesis and Neovascularization
    - IL-8 attracts primary neutrophils, associates with the CXC receptor 2 (CXCR2), and thereby promotes angiogenesis.
    - IL-8 mRNA levels in skeletal muscle are elevated after exercise, and IL-8 plasma levels are increased after eccentric muscle contractions, perhaps promoting exercise-induced neovascularization of muscle tissue.
    - IL-15 has anabolic effects on skeletal muscle and shrinks adipose tissue.
    - Brain-derived neurotrophic factor (BDNF) is found in skeletal muscle and is thought to be involved in myogenesis, satellite cell activation, and skeletal muscle regeneration.
- **Myokines and inflammation**
  - □ IL-6 releases from skeletal muscle in response to exercise[19]:

- Increases circulating levels of several potent anti-inflammatory cytokines such as IL-1RA and IL-10, suggesting that IL-6 may also have anti-inflammatory properties (opposite the effect of macrophage-secreted IL-6).
- Very high-intensity exercise triggers systemic inflammation.
- Proinflammatory cytokines secreted by adipose tissue (adipokines) are overly secreted in obesity (e.g., TNF-α, IL-1β and macrophage IL-6, chemokine C–C motif ligand 2, and plasminogen activator inhibitor-1) and promote diabetes and cardiovascular disease.
- Exercise-induced myokines (e.g., interleukin-15, brain-derived neurotrophic factor, leukemia inhibitory factor, irisin, FGF21) counteract inactivity and obesity-induced proinflammation and promote anti-inflammation.[27]

- ☐ Growth and development
  - Stimulate bone growth[28,29]
  - Stimulate appropriate fetal growth and development[30]
  - Stimulate glucose utilization, insulin sensitivity, and muscle growth[17–27]

INDICATIONS FOR OMT IN PATIENTS WITH ENDOCRINE DISORDERS

- Somatic dysfunction related to the following:
  - ☐ Viscerosomatic or somatovisceral reflexes including "Chapman reflexes," for example, adrenal points have been associated with complaints of fatigue and malaise upon rising in the morning.
  - ☐ Endocrine organ blood flow or lymphatic drainage
  - ☐ Compensatory changes to organ disease or dysfunction
  - ☐ Dysfunction in one or more of the five models of osteopathic care
- Physiologic dysfunction related to somatic dysfunction; restore homeostasis.

OMT for the Endocrine Patient

Osteopathic manipulation would likely restore glandular perfusion, function, and increased health. By alleviating musculoskeletal restrictions, enhancement of self-regulatory and self-healing mechanisms can be fostered. A complement of techniques can be used to best address the somatic dysfunctions present in the patient.

Thyroid Gland

- Hypothyroidism /Hashimoto Thyroiditis
  Hypothyroidism is a condition characterized by low levels of thyroid hormone, which can manifest in a variety of ways due to the hormone's role in many metabolic processes.[31,32] The clinical presentation of hypothyroidism can be subtle and nonspecific, with different symptoms present in different patients. Typical features such as cold intolerance, puffiness, decreased sweating, and skin changes may not always be present. Other symptoms can include fatigue, weight gain, decreased appetite, dry skin, hair loss, sleepiness, muscle pain, joint pain, depression, emotional lability, mental impairment, forgetfulness, impaired memory, inability to concentrate, constipation, menstrual disturbances, impaired fertility, decreased perspiration, and paresthesias and nerve entrapment syndromes.[31,32] The diagnosis of hypothyroidism is primarily based on laboratory tests that measure the levels of thyroid hormones (T3 and T4) and thyroid-stimulating hormone (TSH) in the blood.[31,32] If TSH levels are above the reference range, the next step would be to measure free thyroxine (T4). Subclinical hypothyroidism, also referred to as mild hypothyroidism, is defined as normal serum levels of free T4 and triiodothyronine (T3) with a slightly high serum TSH concentration. The management of hypothyroidism mainly involves thyroid hormone replacement, typically with levothyroxine monotherapy.[31,32] It's important to note that thyroid replacement treatment can exacerbate co-existing adrenal insufficiency, and a comprehensive workup for other differentials is recommended for unresolved symptoms in the presence of biochemical euthyroidism. The treatment goals for hypothyroidism are to reverse clinical progression, restore hormone levels, and resolve contributing somatic dysfunction.[32]
- The goal of medical management is to:
  - ☐ Balance hormonal levels
  - ☐ Increase innate glandular function
  - ☐ Decrease organ system strain
  - ☐ Restore homeostatic mechanisms
- Common therapeutic interventions include hormone replacement therapy, trigger point therapy, diet modification, stress reduction, surgery, and radioactive iodine therapy. The goal of OMT is to resolve somatic dysfunction and its implications on body health.
- Dr. Still relates the etiology and treatment of the thyroid gland to the malposition of the clavicles, scapula, sternum, and that of the cervical spine, first and second ribs as a possible cause for the backup of blood or other fluids within the thyroid gland resulting in inflammation and thyroiditis. He states that the loss of the normal anatomic relationship between these structures interferes with the proper function of nerves, lymphatic drainage, and blood vessels ultimately leading to disease. In addition, malfunction of the structures that drain the organs from noxious elements hinder the natural healing processes of the body. It follows that the removal of these structural obstructions would allow the return of optimal performance of the thyroid gland.[1]
- Consideration of structural and functional features of the thyroid may suggest potential routes through which OMT could have a positive influence on glandular function.
- The hypothalamic–pituitary–thyroid axis can function more efficiently if myofascial, neurologic, lymphatic, and articular structures anatomically related to the thyroid gland act harmoniously. In those cases where the disease has been prolonged and thyroid gland has been inflamed and edematous due to chronic infectious or autoimmune insult (thyroiditis), osteopathic manipulation may be able to prevent irreversible damage to the gland such as fibrosis and atrophy.[33]
- Early intervention with OMT in a patient is ideal and may help to preserve the glands' function.
- Regions to target with OMT:
  - ☐ Cranium–cranial base, OM suture, temporal bones, dural membranes
  - ☐ Cervical-OA, AA, C2, hyoid, suprahyoid, infrahyoid muscles, pretracheal fascia, trigger points in sternocleidomastoid, trapezius muscles, thyroid gland proper
  - ☐ Ribcage-upper ribs
  - ☐ Sternum, thoracic outlet, T1–T4 spinal levels, Chapman points T2, thoracoabdominal diaphragm
  - ☐ Upper extremity
- Cranial region:
  - ☐ Specifically, with manipulative treatment, sphenoid bone mobilization is used to increase vascular nutrition to and from the pituitary gland and cranial base manipulation via base spread can be used to augment sphenobasilar motion.[33]

- ☐ Occipital bone mobilization, parasympathetic output and myofascial attachment strains at the foramen magnum and cervical regions below can be addressed.
- ☐ Temporal bone balancing can affect the thyroid cartilage attachments via the stylohyoid ligaments and stylopharyngeus muscle groups. Vagotonic and allergic reactions with resultant histamine release are due in many cases to insufficient vascular supply to and from the pituitary gland can be augmented via sphenoid manipulation and its relations to dural and the deep cervical fascial. Sphenobasilar motion restriction exists from excessive cranial membranous tension and cranial fluid congestion.[33]

- Cervical region:
  - ☐ This is in direct correlation with the upper cervical spine restriction (OA and AA joints), dural tug, and anterior cervical fascial tug. Milking of the thyroid gland can be done by a gentle lift away from the gland anteriorly and squeezing motion towards the inlet as described by Still. This can be repeated until a positive change is felt.
  - ☐ Occipitoatlantal and atlantoaxial joint somatic dysfunctions from autonomic tone abnormalities and vagal tone can be enhanced by osteopathic cranial manipulation which can help with the constipation commonly seen in hypothyroid patients.[33,34]
  - ☐ Pretracheal myofascial release can also be augmented by techniques such as tracheal mobilization, thyroid mobilization, cricoid mobilization, hyoid bone mobilization, and anterior cervical soft tissue mobilization. The arteries, lymph vessels, and veins of the thyroid gland run within this fascial layer.
  - ☐ Treatment of the anterior cervical tissues helps alleviate the goiter and hoarseness and recurrent laryngeal nerve alterations.[1]
  - ☐ Fluid mobilization techniques can be utilized locally and distally, using drainage enhancement techniques such as cervical effleurage and cervical paravertebral muscular inhibition. These will allow soft tissue relaxation and optimal vascular flow.
- Thoracic and rib cage:
  - ☐ Vertebral somatic dysfunction correction, sternal lymphatic pump, thoracic outlet release, sternal release, and T1/first rib release can all help restore vascular flow. Because of the proximity of the sternoclavicular joints to the thyroid, clavicular somatic dysfunction should be treated to ensure venous and lymphatic drainage of the thyroid gland. Elevation of the first rib unilaterally and or bilaterally will cause unilateral and or bilateral supraclavicular bogginess.
- Chapman points:
  - ☐ Chapman points, which are abnormal gangliform contractions induced from hypersympathetic tone, result in edema and myofascial thickening (tender points).[34] These points lie deep in the skin in deep fascia or periosteum. They are typically paired reflex points having an anterior and a posterior component. Anterior points can be palpated and tenderness at the 2nd intercostal space anteriorly is a common finding and is associated with a thyroid Chapman point.[34]
  - ☐ In thyroid disease, posterior Chapman points are palpated at and around the T2 spinous process. Treatment to these points can improve lymphatic drainage and help to normalize sympathetic tone to the thyroid gland, which in turn can affect thyroid function. Cardiovascular flow can also be enhanced. Sympathetic supply can be normalized to promote maximum vascular patency using osteopathic techniques that will treat the superior, middle, and inferior cervical sympathetic ganglia and upper thoracic spine.[34]
  - ☐ It is important to treat cervical and upper thoracic muscle hypertonicity, segmental dysfunction at the T2 level, and associated first and second rib somatic dysfunction. This is thought to decrease sympathetic tone to structures of the head and neck, including the thyroid.
- Sacral mobilization, which enhances cranial motion via the core link, can be enhanced with sacral rocking techniques.[33,34]

Adrenal Gland

- Addison disease
- Cushing syndrome
- Adrenal hyperplasia
- Polycystic ovary syndrome (PCOS)

Adrenal gland disorders encompass a range of conditions that occur when the adrenal glands produce either too much or too little of certain hormones. These disorders can significantly impact the body's ability to maintain essential life functions, such as responding to stress, controlling blood pressure, and managing blood sugar levels.[35,36] One common adrenal gland disorder is adrenal insufficiency, also known as Addison disease. This condition arises when the adrenal glands do not produce enough hormones, particularly cortisol and sometimes aldosterone. Symptoms can range from mild nonspecific symptoms to life-threatening shock conditions. The decrease in adrenal function may be masked until stress or illness triggers an adrenal crisis.[36,37]

Another common disorder is Cushing syndrome, which is caused by an excess of cortisol in the body. This can result from long-term use of steroid medicines. Symptoms can include hypertension, headache, tachycardia, fatigue, proximal muscle weakness, and polyuria.[35,38]

Congenital adrenal hyperplasia (CAH) is an autosomal recessive disorder, which is caused by a deficiency of one of the enzymes necessary for adrenal steroid production, especially cortisol. This deficiency leads to excessive secretion of ACTH with resultant bilateral adrenal hyperplasia.[35,38] The most common enzyme deficiency in CAH is 21-hydroxylase. Depending on the residual enzymatic activity governed by the genetic mutation, 21-hydroxylase deficiency CAH is classified as either classical (salt wasting or simple virilizing) or nonclassical.[39] In classical 21-hydroxylase deficiency CAH, there is an accumulation of 17-hydroxyprogesterone which is shunted into the intact androgen pathway and may lead to prenatally virilized external genitalia in females as early as 9 weeks of gestation.[39] Impaired cortisol synthesis leads to chronic elevations of ACTH via the negative feedback system, causing overstimulation of the adrenal cortex and resulting in hyperplasia and over-secretion of the precursors to the enzymatic defect. The imbalance of hormones the body needs to function may mean too little cortisol, too little aldosterone, excess androgens, or a combination of these imbalances.[40] Although CAH is not curable, patients can go on to lead normal lives if they receive adequate care and treatment. Physicians are urged to recognize the physical characteristics of CAH in newborns (e.g., atypical genitalia) and to refer such cases to appropriate clinics for full endocrine evaluation.

- The goal of medical management is to:
  - ☐ Balancing of the ANS
  - ☐ Restore glandular function
  - ☐ Normalize hormonal levels
- Regions to target with OMT:
  - ☐ Cranium—SBS, OM suture, dural membranes, posterior parietal lift
  - ☐ Cervical—OA, AA, C3–C5

- Thoracic spine-thoracic outlet, T9–T11 Thoraco-abdominal diaphragm, Chapman points at T11
  - Abdomen—Chapman point 1′ out and 2″ up from umbilicus
  - Ribcage—Ribs 1–5, 9, 10, 11, and 12 bilaterally
  - Lumbar spine—L1–L3
- Goal:
  - Downregulation of sympathetic tone and upregulation of parasympathetic tone is the key goal.
- Cranium
  - The PCC, an area posterior to the midline of the brain, is a critical node of the central autonomic network which controls preganglionic sympathetic and parasympathetic motoneurons. This area has important involvement in the control of parasympathetic functioning.[6] To achieve this goal, the CV4 technique, parietal lift, sutural decompression, balanced membranous tension and SBS decompression techniques can be utilized.[6] The hypothalamic–pituitary–thyroid axis can function more efficiently if myofascial, neurologic, lymphatic, and articular structures anatomically related to the adrenal gland act harmoniously.
- Thoracic Spine
  - In addition, the action of OMT to balance the autonomics from T9 to T11 has favorable effects on the adrenal glands.[33] An example of this would be inhibitory rib raising techniques, applied to the costotransverse articulations with the objective of inhibiting the viscerosomatic reflex, freeing local joint restrictions and influencing the sympathetic ganglia's nerve supply to the adrenal gland. The focus of manipulative treatment is directed to the theoretical association between OMT and the ANS, which is being supported by emerging empirical evidence obtained through physiologic measures of ANS activity.[3]
- Abdomen/Chapman points
  - Chapman reflex for the adrenal glands is palpated on the anterior aspect of the patient, lateral and superior to the umbilicus and 11 o'clock and 1 o'clock relative positions and posteriorly T11 and T12 intertransverse space.[33,34]
  - These reflexes are found to be gangliform contractions and are mediated by a sympathetic arm of the ANS causing an excessive tissue congestion and lymphatic stasis. They are points used both diagnostically and to treat by breaking this cycle through a somatovisceral pathway to restore the autonomic balance. Treatment is achieved by gentle rotatory movement over the point for approximately 15 to 30 seconds until the edema or hypercongested points of the gangliform contractions has resolved.
- Diaphragm and ribs
  - The diaphragm is key to circulate fluids to and from the adrenal glands.[34] "The cause of nerve irritation must be found and removed before the channels can relax and open sufficiently to admit the passage of the obstructed fluids." – A.T. Still.[1]
  - The hemidiaphragms can be treated with direct or indirect myofascial release techniques and BLT can be used to free up the 11th and 12th rib motion, which dictates posterior diaphragm motion. The diaphragms anchoring tensions in the thoracolumbar junction can affect adrenal sympathetic spinal levels causing spinal facilitation and nerve irritability.

OVARIES

Polycystic ovarian syndrome

PCOS is a complex hormonal condition that affects approximately 1 in 10 women of reproductive age.[41] It is characterized by menstrual dysfunction, anovulation, and signs of hyperandrogenism.[42] PCOS is a condition in which the ovaries produce an abnormal excess amount of androgens, that are usually present in women in small amounts. Somatic dysfunction may play a role in the pathogenesis by increasing sympathetic tone to the ovarian vasculature, thereby reducing blood supply to the ovaries. This contributes to long-term health risks for cardiovascular disease and promotes PCOS pathogenesis. The term PCOS describes the numerous small cysts (fluid-filled sacs) that form in the ovaries. When ovulation doesn't happen, the ovaries can develop many small cysts. The exact cause of PCOS is not fully understood, but it is believed to result from abnormal function of the hypothalamic–pituitary–ovarian (HPO) axis.[42] It is also associated with insulin resistance and hyperinsulinemia, which can be amplified by obesity.[42] The major features of PCOS include inappropriate gonadotropin secretion, raised plasma testosterone levels, and the presence of polycystic ovaries.[42] The ovaries in PCOS are enlarged bilaterally and have a smooth, thickened capsule that is avascular. On microscopic examination, hyperplasia of the theca stromal cells surrounding arrested follicles is a striking feature.[42] PCOS is a genetically heterogeneous syndrome, with the genetic contributions remaining incompletely described.[42] However, it is estimated that up to a third of women with PCOS have a female relative with the condition, suggesting a genetic link. PCOS is associated with a range of symptoms, which can vary in severity and change at different life stages. Common symptoms include irregular or absent periods, excessive hair growth on the face or body, skin conditions such as acne and skin tags, hair loss, reduced fertility, stress, anxiety, depression, weight problems, and sleep problems. PCOS is also linked to several long-term health risks, including type 2 diabetes, cardiovascular disease, endometrial cancer, and sleep apnea.[41,43] Women with PCOS have higher rates of these conditions compared to women without PCOS.[43] Diagnosis of PCOS requires at least two of the following three features: oligo-ovulation or anovulation manifested as oligomenorrhea or amenorrhea, hyperandrogenism or hyperandrogenemia, and polycystic ovaries as defined on ultrasonography.[42] Nonpharmacologic therapies can include advocating for a healthy lifestyle, OMT and weight loss. Targeted therapy includes hormone replacement and other supportive medications. Nonpharmacologic approaches such as lifestyle modifications like weight loss and exercise can sometimes reverse the reproductive and metabolic features of PCOS.[43] Osteopathic medicine can offer effective treatment of the sympathetic tone and ovarian blood flow in these women.[44–46] Improvements in sympathetic tone after OMT suggest that weekly manipulation of Chapman point and viscerosomatic reflexes can be a useful adjunctive therapeutic option for women with PCOS.[47] Pharmacotherapeutic interventions are designed to reduce insulin levels and ovarian androgen production, ultimately correcting sex hormone–binding globulin (SHBG) levels.[43]

- The Goal of Medical Management:
  - Balance hormonal levels
  - Increase innate glandular function
  - Decrease organ system strain
  - Restore homeostatic mechanisms
- Body Regions to target with OMT:
  - Cranium—SBS, OM suture
  - Cervical—OA, AA joints, C3-C5
  - Thoracic spine—Chapman points (Ovary: T9–T11 transverse processes)
  - Thoracoabdominal diaphragm
  - Pelvis—Pubic bone
  - Pelvic floor

- Cranium
  - SBS treatment has effects on the sphenoid motion and dural tensions hence the HPA axis. Gonadotropin-releasing hormone (GNRH) is released from the hypothalamus and subsequently gonadotropic hormones, FSH and LH, and prolactin, from the pituitary gland. The ovaries then secrete estrogen and progesterone. Androstenedione and testosterone are also secreted by the ovaries and adrenal glands in abnormal amounts in PCOS. Since the vagus nerve innervates the ovaries, treatment aimed at the cranial base (OM suture decompression), and upper cervical spine can help upregulate parasympathetic tone.[47]
- Thoracic cage and ribs
  - Weekly manipulation of Chapman points and rib-raising for viscerosomatic reflexes associated with the ovaries, adrenal glands, and heart have been most effective to control and treat symptoms associated with PCOS.[47] Sympathetic supply can be normalized to promote maximum vascular patency using osteopathic techniques such as rib raising.
- Chapman points
  - The Chapman points for the ovary are located anteriorly at the upper to lower border of the pubic bone and the posterior point for the ovary is located at T9 and T11 transverse processes and the outer ovary is the T10 and T11 intertransverse points.[34] Treatment to these points can relieve vasoconstriction and improve venous and lymphatic drainage and help to normalize sympathetic tone to the ovary, which in turn can affect ovarian function. Cardiovascular flow can also be enhanced.
- Thoracoabdominal and pelvic diaphragms
  - Thoracoabdominal and pelvic diaphragms should be treated to ensure adequate pelvic circulation. Barral discusses the importance of good mobility and lack of restrictions in the tubo-ovarian motion. Visceral manipulation may also be helpful for patients with PCOS.[48]

PANCREAS

Diabetes Mellitus

Diabetes is a metabolic disorder characterized by the presence of chronic hyperglycemia either immune-mediated (type 1 diabetes mellitus [T1DM]) insulin resistance (type 2 diabetes mellitus [T2DM]) gestational or others. Diabetes is associated with a high prevalence of comorbidities. Morbidity from diabetes is a consequence of both macrovascular disease (atherosclerosis) and microvascular disease (retinopathy, nephropathy, and neuropathy). The pancreas has both digestive and hormonal functions. It is both an exocrine gland producing pancreatic enzymes that are secreted into the duodenum and an endocrine gland producing insulin and glucagon that are released as hormones in the blood. The enzymes secreted by the exocrine gland in the pancreas help break down carbohydrates, fats, proteins, and acids in the duodenum. The head of the pancreas is intimately connected to the duodenum and penetrated by the termination of the bile duct. The insulin-producing function of the pancreas is more commonly stressed and ultimately compromised. As a result, the pancreas produces inadequate amounts of insulin to meet the body demands or insulin resistance is present where the body cells fail to respond to insulin despite higher levels.

Type 1 Diabetes Mellitus

- In T1DM, the disease onset may be abrupt, and early diagnosis and clinical intervention are essential for preventing and/or reducing complications. The clinical presentation can vary, but common symptoms include increased thirst, frequent urination, increased hunger, unexplained weight loss, fatigue, blurred vision, and nausea. In some cases, T1DM may present with diabetic ketoacidosis (DKA), an acute metabolic complication characterized by hyperglycemia, hyperketonemia, and metabolic acidosis. DKA may manifest with nausea, vomiting, and abdominal pain, and can lead to cerebral edema, coma, and death.
- Current guidelines for the management of T1DM includes a multifaceted approach that requires a combination of insulin therapy, glucose monitoring, lifestyle modifications, and psychosocial support.[49] However, insulin therapy is the cornerstone of management. Most people with T1DM should be treated with a multiple daily injection regimen of prandial insulin and basal insulin or continuous subcutaneous insulin infusion.[50] The American Association of Clinical Endocrinology (AACE) recommends using the percentage of time in range (%TIR) and below range (%TBR) as a starting point for the evaluation of the quality of glycemic control.[50] Insulin injected subcutaneously is the first-line treatment of T1DM. The different types of insulin vary with respect to onset and duration of action. Short-, intermediate-, and long-acting insulins are available. Short- and rapid-acting insulins are the only types that can be administered intravenously (IV). Human insulin currently is the only species of insulin available in the United States; it is less antigenic than the previously used animal-derived varieties. The ADA also recommends that psychosocial care should be integrated with a collaborative, patient-centered approach and provided to all people with diabetes, with the goal of optimizing health outcomes and health-related quality of life.[49,50]

Type 2 Diabetes Mellitus

- In T2DM, disease onset is insidious, and diagnosis is often delayed. Some people with T2DM have no symptoms. The most common symptoms include increased thirst, frequent urination, increased hunger, unexplained weight loss, fatigue, blurred vision, slow-healing sores, and frequent infections. It's also worth noting that some people with T2DM may experience areas of darkened skin, usually in the armpits and neck.
- Current guidelines for the management of T2DM recommend a comprehensive approach that includes lifestyle modifications, pharmacologic interventions, glucose monitoring, and patient education.[51]
- Healthy eating, regular physical activity, and weight management are essential components of T2DM management. A balanced diet, portion control, and carbohydrate counting can help maintain blood glucose levels. Engaging in at least 150 minutes of moderate-intensity physical activity per week is recommended by the current CDC guidelines. Medications such as metformin, sulfonylureas, meglitinides, thiazolidinediones, DPP-4 inhibitors, GLP-1 receptor agonists, and SGLT2 inhibitors may be prescribed to help control blood glucose levels. The choice of medication depends on the individual patient's needs and the specific characteristics of each drug.[51] Regular monitoring of blood glucose levels are crucial for managing T2DM. Diabetes self-management education and support (DSMES) is a key intervention for patients with T2DM. DSMES programs help patients understand how diet, physical activity, and medication affect their glucose levels and how these levels relate

to acute and chronic complications.[52] These efforts may temporarily improve glucose control, but they are less effective in stopping the progression of this serious disease.

Clinical Practice Guidelines

- For a more comprehensive review of diabetes, the reader is referred to the following clinical practice guidelines.
- "Recent Updates to Clinical Practice Guidelines for Diabetes Mellitus" – This article discusses the American Diabetes Association (ADA) updates to the Standards of Medical Care in Diabetes.[53]
- "Standards of Medical Care in Diabetes—2022 Abridged for Primary Care Providers" – This abridged version of the ADA's Standards of Medical Care in Diabetes includes the most current evidence-based recommendations for diagnosing and treating adults and children with all forms of diabetes.[54]
- "American Association of Clinical Endocrinology Clinical Practice Guideline: Developing a Diabetes Mellitus Comprehensive Care Plan—2022 Update" – This guideline includes 170 updated and new evidence-based clinical practice recommendations for the comprehensive care of persons with diabetes.[55]

Comorbidities

- T1DM and T2DM are associated with various comorbidities, which can impact the management and progression of the disease.
  - Comorbidities of T1DM include[56]:
    - Autoimmune thyroid disorders
    - Celiac disease
    - Vitamin B12 deficiency
    - Obesity (although not strictly a comorbidity, it has significant implications for treatment and development of complications)
  - Comorbidities of T2DM include[57]:
    - Hypertension
    - Ischemic heart disease
    - Chronic kidney disease (CKD)
    - Chronic obstructive pulmonary disease (COPD)
    - Depression
- It is important to note that the presence of these comorbidities can influence osteopathic management diabetes and its progression. Identifying and treating these comorbidities should also be an integral part of the care provided by the osteopathic physician and diabetes healthcare team.
  - Goals of Osteopathic Medical Management:
    - Normalize pancreatic function
    - Enhance homeostasis of the endocrine system
    - Normalize neurologic tone
    - Balance hormone secretion
- Body Regions to target with OMT:
  - Cranium–OM suture, SBS, cranial venous drainage techniques
  - Cervical–OA, AA Joints, C3-C5
  - Thoracic–Thoraco-abdominal diaphragm, thoracic outlet (left), Chapman points–right medial T7 interspace, right T7 TP, T10-T12 (renal and adrenal), and T1-T5 (heart)
  - Ribcage–Ribs 1–5,7–12 bilaterally
  - Abdomen–Celiac, superior mesenteric periaortic ganglia
  - Lower extremities– Foot and ankle
  - Upper extremities–Shoulder elbow, wrists
  - Pelvis–Pelvic floor, innominates
- Structure and function are reciprocally interrelated.[1] Viscerosomatic manifestations of diabetes mellitus influence the local and distal regions of the body.[33]
- Insults to the cranium, central and peripheral nervous system, spine, ribcage, upper and lower extremities soft tissues (fascia, muscle, tendons) and end-organ dysfunction can result. OMT can serve as an effective adjunct to the current methods of T2DM management.[33] The musculoskeletal system, which substantially influences the individual's ability to maintain homeostasis and health can be positively influenced by OMT.
- The sympathetic nervous system plays a significant role in decreasing insulin secretion.[33] The vagus nerve controls the parasympathetic nerve supply to the pancreas. Sympathetic innervation of the pancreas originates from the sympathetic preganglionic neurons in the thoracic and upper lumbar segments of the spinal cord.
- Musculoskeletal manifestations in diabetes are numerous. The musculoskeletal system is vulnerable to insults due to compromised circulation; poor wound healing, fibrosing conditions of multiple joints (hands, ankle, and shoulders), and comorbid states.[33] Musculoskeletal examination should be performed regularly on this patient population. The more advanced the disease, the more frequent the evaluation and treatment. Microscopically, the musculoskeletal manifestations are due to abnormal collagen deposition in the periarticular connective tissues. In addition, glycosylation increased hydration and abnormal collagen matrices may be involved.
- Patients with higher random blood sugar levels demonstrated increased tissue fullness and bogginess as demonstrated by two of three measurements that reached statistical significance.[15]
- The findings suggested that increased fluid level shifts into the extracellular compartment were due to increased glucose levels. Renal and cardiac pathology may also play a role in this process.
- Patients with diabetes have increased joint biomechanical forces, soft tissue thickening, muscle wasting, and polyneuropathy. Changes in the soft tissue, joints, and fascial structures over time may initiate somatic dysfunction in the form of TART changes.[33]
- The musculoskeletal exam should include the determination of viscerosomatic reflexes from the pancreas and upper GI system, cranium, heart, kidneys, and eyes. Spinal somatosomatic reflexes should be diagnosed and treated.[33] Dysfunction of the sympathetic nervous system leads to neuropathy and neuroarthropathy. The cranial base may present with strain patterns emanating from the midbrain, medulla, and hypothalamus. Other organs of the endocrine system should be screened and treated if necessary.
- Vagal reflexes may cause suboccipital soft tissue tension and OA and AA joint somatic dysfunction. Phrenic nerve irritation would likely result in midcervical somatic dysfunction.
- Gait alterations especially in diabetic neuropathy patients reduce the joint movement at the ankle during walking. Fascial distortion is a complication with associated fibrosis in commonly affected areas. This reduces ankle joint motion (net joint force plus combined with muscle force) including higher metabolic expenditure during walking. The diabetic foot undergoes abnormal plantar pressure, resulting in a thickened Achilles and plantar fascia. A rigid foot develops with abnormal loading under the forefoot. One of the more critical foot problems that can result from diabetic neuropathy is Charcot arthropathy. This condition is the result of undetected injuries to the bones of the foot, which can lead to significant deformity and disability.

- OMT using a combination of articulatory, BLT, HVLA, OCMM, and Spencer Muscle Energy Techniques can be used safely and effectively in diabetic patients. Lymphatic techniques circulate body fluids and enhance immunity.

CONTRAINDICATIONS FOR OMT IN PATIENTS WITH ENDOCRINE DISORDERS

- Patients with diabetes are more prone to gout and osteoporosis.[15,33] HVLA OMT is contraindicated in patients with severe osteoporosis or of an acutely inflamed or infected joint. Many endocrinopathies can cause osteoporosis (see above for examples). Long-time use of corticosteroid medications causes osteoporosis. Caution should be exercised in using OMT at the site where there is evidence of tissue friability or damage when the endocrine disorder causes skin, connective tissue, muscle, or bone disease or dysfunction, that is, when the muscles, joints, and bones are not anatomically or physiologically normal due to disease such as in the case of a Charcot joint in diabetics.
- OMT can be used distal to that site to improve arterial blood flow and venous and lymphatic drainage and improve neurologic function. OMT is a procedure that requires a diagnosis of somatic dysfunction or a condition that is amenable to OMT, such as congestion or swelling, so lack of a diagnosis, a rational management plan, and/or goals of treatment would also be a contraindication because there is no clear indication for using it.

CONCLUSION

Osteopathic philosophy, its tenets, and the five models of osteopathic care help organize the scientific knowledge regarding the endocrine system's role in metabolic aspects of homeostasis. The musculoskeletal system is an integral part of the endocrine system as both a secretory and an end organ, with autocrine, paracrine, and endocrine functions. Skeletal muscle exercise is critical to total body metabolic homeostasis and health. There are important musculoskeletal manifestations of endocrine disorders detectable by palpatory examination and radiologic studies. OMT is indicated to treat somatic dysfunction in patients with endocrine disorders in order to improve physiologic function. There are important contraindications to selective OMT procedures in patients with certain endocrine disorders, for example, osteoporosis. A nutritious diet, regular exercise, restorative sleep, effective stress management, and elimination of toxic exposures are the keystones to efficient endocrine-related metabolic functions at all levels.

REFERENCES

1. Still AT. *Still Osteopathy Research and Practice*. Eastland Pr; 1992.
2. Abraham C, Sloan SNB, Coker C, et al. Osteopathic manipulative treatment as an intervention to reduce stress, anxiety, and depression in first responders: a pilot study. *Mo Med.* 2021;118(5):435–441.
3. Rechberger V, Biberschick M, Porthun J. Effectiveness of an osteopathic treatment on the autonomic nervous system: a systematic review of the literature. *Eur J Med Res.* 2019;24(1):36.
4. Singh A, Petrides JS, Gold PW, Chrousos GP, Deuster PA. Differential hypothalamic-pituitary-adrenal axis reactivity to psychological and physical stress. *J Clin Endocrinol Metab.* 1999;84(6):1944–1948.
5. Henderson AT, Fisher JF, Blair J, Shea C, Li TS, Bridges KG. Effects of rib raising on the autonomic nervous system: a pilot study using noninvasive biomarker. *J Am Osteopath Assoc.* 2010;110(6):324–330.
6. Tramontano M, Cerritelli F, Piras F, et al. Brain connectivity changes after osteopathic manipulation treatment: a randomized manual placebo-controlled trial. *Brain Sci.* 2020;10(12):969.
7. Burns L. *Pathogenesis of Visceral Disease Following Vertebral Lesions.* American Osteopathic Association; 1948.
8. Downing CH. *Osteopathic Principles in Disease.* Richard J. Orozco; 1935.
9. Korr IM. Somatic dysfunction, osteopathic manipulation treatment, and the nervous system: a few facts, some theories, many questions. *J Am Osteopath Assoc.* 1986;86(2):109–114.
10. Berkowitz MR. Resolution of hypothyroidism after correction of somatovisceral reflex dysfunction by refusion of the cervical spine. *J Am Osteopath Assoc.* 2015;115(1):46–49.
11. Licciardone JC, Kearns CM, Hodge LM, Minotti DE. Osteopathic manual treatment in patients with diabetes mellitus and comorbid chronic low back pain: subgroup results from the osteopathic trial. *J Am Osteopath Assoc.* 2013;113(6):468–478.
12. Licciardone JC, Kearns CM, Hodge LM, Bergamini MVW. Associations of cytokine concentrations with key osteopathic lesions and clinical outcomes in patients with nonspecific chronic low back pain: results from the osteopathic trial. *J Am Osteopath Assoc.* 2012;112(9):596–605.
13. Nelson KE, Mnabhi AKS, Glonek T. The accuracy of diagnostic palpation: the comparison of soft tissue findings with random blood sugar in diabetic patients. *Osteopath Fam Physician.* 2010;2(6):165–169.
14. Tarr R, Nelson K, Vatt R, Richardson D. Palpatory findings associated with the diabetic state. *J Am Osteopath Assoc.* 1985;85(9):604–605.
15. Licciardone JC, Fulda KG, Stoll ST, Gamber RG, Cage AC. A case-control study of osteopathic palpatory findings in type 2 diabetes mellitus. *Osteopath Med Prim Care.* 2007;1:6.
16. Boswell SB, Patel DB, White EA, et al. Musculoskeletal manifestations of endocrine disorders. *Clin Imaging.* 2014;38(4):384–396.
17. Pratesi A, Tarantini F, Di Bari M. Skeletal muscle: an endocrine organ. *Clin Cases Miner Bone Metab.* 2013;10(1):11–14.
18. Iizuka K, Machida T, Hirafuji M. Skeletal muscle is an endocrine organ. *J Pharmacol Sci.* 2014;125(2):125–131.
19. Schnyder S, Handschin C. Skeletal muscle as an endocrine organ: PGC-1α, myokines and exercise. *Bone.* 2015;80:115–125.
20. Ahima RS, Park HQ. Connecting myokines and metabolism. *Endocrinol Metab.* 2015;30:235–245.
21. Kostrominova TY. Role of myokines in the maintenance of whole-body metabolic homeostasis. *Minerva Endocrinol.* 2016;41(4):403–420.
22. Karstoft K, Pedersen BK. Skeletal muscle as a gene regulatory endocrine organ. *Curr Opin Clin Nutr Metab Care.* 2016;19(4):270–275.
23. Giudice J, Taylor JM. Muscle as a paracrine and endocrine organ. *Curr Opin Pharmacol.* 2017;34:49–55.
24. Dalamaga M. Interplay of adipokines and myokines in cancer pathophysiology: emerging therapeutic implications. *World J Exp Med.* 2013;3(3):26–33.
25. Li F, Li Y, Duan Y, Hu CA, Tang Y, Yin Y. Myokines and adipokines: involvement in the crosstalk between skeletal muscle and adipose tissue. *Cytokine Growth Factor Rev.* 2017;33:73–82.
26. Kalinkovich A, Livshits G. Sarcopenic obesity or obese sarcopenia: a cross talk between age-associated adipose tissue and skeletal muscle inflammation as a main mechanism of the pathogenesis. *Ageing Res Rev.* 2017;35:200–221.
27. So B, Kim HJ, Kim J, Song W. Exercise-induced myokines in health and metabolic diseases. *Integr Med Res.* 2014;3(4):172–179.
28. Brotto M, Bonewald L. Bone and muscle: interactions beyond mechanical. *Bone.* 2015;80:109–114.
29. Guo B, Zhang ZK, Liang C, et al. Molecular communication from skeletal muscle to bone: a review for muscle-derived myokines regulating bone metabolism. *Calcif Tissue Int.* 2017;100(2):184–192.
30. Dubé C, Aguer C, Adamo K, Bainbridge S. A role for maternally derived myokines to optimize placental function and fetal growth across gestation. *Appl Physiol Nutr Metab.* 2017;42(5):459–469.
31. Patil N, Rehman A, Jialal I. Hypothyroidism. [Updated 2023 Aug 8.] In: *StatPearls [Internet].* StatPearls Publishing; 2023. https://www.ncbi.nlm.nih.gov/books/NBK519536/
32. Orlander P. Hypothyroidism. *Medscape.* Updated October 4, 2024. Accessed November 19, 2024. https://emedicine.medscape.com/article/122393-overview
33. DiGiovanna E, Burns DK, Amen C. *An Osteopathic Approach To Diagnosis and Treatment.* 4th ed. Wolters Kluwer; 2020.

34. Nguyen B, Bordoni B, *Physiology, Chapman's Points.* StatPearls Publishing; 2022.
35. National Library of Medicine. Adrenal gland disorders. *MedlinePlus.* Updated January 19, 2024. Accessed November 19, 2024. https://medlineplus.gov/adrenalglanddisorders.html
36. National Institute of Diabetes and Digestive and Kidney Diseases. Adrenal insufficiency & Addison's disease. Updated September 2018. Accessed November 19, 2024. https://www.niddk.nih.gov/health-information/endocrine-diseases/adrenal-insufficiency-addisons-disease
37. Huecker MR, Bhutta BS, Dominique E. Adrenal insufficiency. [Updated 2023 Apr 9.] In: *StatPearls [Internet].* StatPearls Publishing; 2023. https://www.ncbi.nlm.nih.gov/books/NBK441832/
38. Kay S. Pediatric adrenal gland disorders. *Medscape.* Updated April 16, 2024. Accessed November 19, 2024. https://emedicine.medscape.com/article/940347-overview
39. Yau M, Khattab A, Yuen T, New M. Congenital adrenal hyperplasia. In: Feingold KR, Anawalt B, Blackman MR, et al., eds. *Endotext.* MDText.com, Inc.; 2022.
40. Mayo Clinic Staff. Congenital adrenal hyperplasia. Mayo Clinic. Updated March 22, 2024. Accessed November 19, 2024. https://www.mayoclinic.org/diseases-conditions/congenital-adrenal-hyperplasia/symptoms-causes/syc-20355205
41. Office on Women's Health. Polycystic ovary syndrome. U.S. Department of Health & Human Services. Updated February 22, 2021. Accessed November 19, 2024. https://www.womenshealth.gov/a-z-topics/polycystic-ovary-syndrome
42. Lucidi R. Polycystic ovarian syndrome. *Medscape.* Updated November 27, 2023. Accessed November 19, 2024. https://emedicine.medscape.com/article/256806-overview
43. Ndefo UA, Eaton A, Green MR. Polycystic ovary syndrome: a review of treatment options with a focus on pharmacological approaches. *P T.* 2013;38(6):336–355.
44. Henley CE, Ivins D, Mills M, Wen FK, Benjamin BA. Osteopathic manipulative treatment and its relationship to autonomic nervous system activity as demonstrated by heart variability: a repeated measured study. *Osteopath Med Prim Care.* 2008;2:7.
45. Merklin R. *Suprarenal Gland Drainage.* American Journal of Anatomy; 1966
46. Uchida S, KagitaniF. Autonomic nervous regulation of ovarian function by noxious somatic afferent stimulation. *J Physiol Sci.* 2015; 65(1):1–9.
47. Davis SE, Hendryx J, Menezes C, et al. Weekly osteopathic manipulative treatment to improve measure of sympathetic tone in women with poly cystic ovaries syndrome: a randomized, controlled pilot *study. J Am Osteopath Assoc.* 2020;120(5):310–321.
48. Barral J. *Visceral Manipulation.* Eastland Press; 2006.
49. Holt RIG, DeVries JH, Hess-Fischl A, et al. The management of type 1 diabetes in adults. A consensus report by the American Diabetes Association (ADA) and the European Association for the Study of Diabetes (EASD). *Diabetes Care.* 2021;44(11):2609–2652.
50. Khardori R. Type 1 diabetes mellitus guidelines. *Medscape.* Updated December 13, 2023. Accessed November 19, 2024. https://emedicine.medscape.com/article/117739-guidelines
51. Mahler RJ, Adler ML. Clinical review 102: Type 2 diabetes mellitus: Update on diagnosis, pathophysiology, and treatment. *J Clin Endocrinol Metab.* 1999;84(4):1165–1171.
52. Davies MJ, Aroda VR, Collins BS, et al. Management of hyperglycemia in type 2 diabetes, 2022. A consensus report by the American Diabetes Association (ADA) and the European Association for the Study of Diabetes (EASD). *Diabetes Care.* 2022;45(11):2753–2786.
53. Yu J, Lee SH, Kim MK. Recent updates to clinical practice guidelines for diabetes mellitus. *Endocrinol Metab (Seoul).* 2022;37(1):26–37.
54. American Diabetes Association. Standards of medical care in diabetes—2022 abridged for primary care providers. *Clin Diabetes.* 2022;40(1):10–38.
55. Blonde L, Umpierrez GE, Reddy SS, et al. American Association of Clinical Endocrinology clinical practice guideline: Developing a diabetes mellitus comprehensive care plan—2022 update. *Endocr Pract.* 2022; 28(10):923–1049.
56. Zaharia OP, Lanzinger S, Rosenbauer J, et al. Comorbidities in recent-onset adult type 1 diabetes: a comparison of German cohorts. *Front Endocrinol (Lausanne).* 2022;13:760778.
57. Nowakowska M, Zghebi SS, Ashcroft DM, et al. The comorbidity burden of type 2 diabetes mellitus: patterns, clusters and predictions from a large English primary care cohort. *BMC Med.* 2019;17(1):145.

78

Osteopathic Considerations and Approaches in the Acutely Ill or Hospitalized Patient

HUGH M. ETTLINGER

KEY CONCEPTS

- An osteopathic structural examination provides clues to the medical/surgical diagnosis of an acutely ill or hospitalized patient.
- An individualized osteopathic manipulative treatment plan is designed at each visit for each acutely ill or hospitalized patient, specifically directed toward dysfunction discovered during a musculoskeletal structural examination, and appropriate for the patient's condition.
- Osteopathic manipulative treatment is directed toward improving physiologic function for support and assistance to the patient recovering from an illness or other acute stress and is directed toward the underlying pathophysiology of the disease process.

INTRODUCTION

The science of osteopathy is applicable to the full spectrum of medical and surgical problems. Osteopathic evaluation and treatment, integrated into the care of the acutely ill or hospitalized patient, are based on an understanding of the mechanical and functional aspects of the body's viscera and systems, including the respiratory, circulatory, immune, and autonomic nervous systems. This chapter specifically presents a template for an osteopathic structural evaluation that investigates body physiology related to a patient's disease processes, not just the mechanics of the neuromusculoskeletal system, and, as such, becomes an invaluable part of the physical examination. It presents the general principles upon which the treatment plan is based and suggests manipulative treatment techniques that apply these principles. The resulting treatment plan is a natural extension of the structural examination. The osteopathic treatment that is administered supports the patient and assists in their recovery from illness or other acute stress. A unique and individualized treatment plan must be designed for each acutely ill hospitalized patient at each visit.

THE STRUCTURAL EXAMINATION

Accurate diagnosis is the key to appropriate treatment of any patient with any disease process. For this reason, a basic structural examination should be performed on all hospital patients. The structural examination offers the osteopathic physician additional clues that assist in the overall assessment of a patient's condition and the development of an appropriate treatment plan. The hospital structural examination is a variation of the general structural examination described in Chapter 30. The American Osteopathic Association (AOA) has designed a standardized hospital structural examination form for use in all osteopathic services (Fig. 78.1).

This examination consists of required and optional parts. The required section, which includes static symmetry, both anteroposterior (AP) and lateral, and regional screen for tissue tension, fulfills the requirements of a basic musculoskeletal examination. This part of the examination is described in Chapter 30 and adaptations must be made for the condition of the patient; some patients are unable to sit, stand, or walk.

This author strongly recommends that the focused examination described herein be carried out in the acutely ill patient, as it will provide clues to the diagnosis and overall condition of the patient. It assesses the function of the patient's major organ systems. Also, if an osteopathic manipulative treatment (OMT) is to be performed on a hospitalized patient, a focused musculoskeletal examination is required. Notes regarding the focused examination can be recorded in the "optional" region of the standardized form, for later dictation with the physical examination or the progress notes. The aspects of this focused structural examination will be described in detail in this chapter.

The Five Models of Osteopathic Care

Using the five models, which are organized to focus the osteopathic physician on the physiologic functions that require special attention when developing and administering a management plan for a patient, facilitates construction of an organized approach to the acutely ill or hospitalized patient. A review of Chapter 26 would serve as a valuable foundation for understanding the rationale behind the treatments discussed in this chapter. Improving neurological, respiratory–circulatory, biomechanical, and metabolic functions using OMT procedures that have been found to be safe and effective are presented in this chapter.

Assessing for Segmental Facilitation

Reflex somatic dysfunction provides important clues to the presence of acute and/or chronic disease.[1–8] The information gathered is combined with the rest of the physical examination to reach a working differential diagnosis. See Chapter 43 Clinical Assessment: Viscerosomatic, Somatosomatic, Somatovisceral Reflexes; Counterstrain Points, Myofascial Trigger Points, and Chapman Reflexes for further details.

Assessing Breathing

Breathing is one of the most fundamental processes in human physiology. Respiration is responsible not only for the movement of air but is also directly involved with venous and lymphatic circulation. A focused evaluation and treatment of the thorax are indicated in all respiratory diseases, such as asthma and pneumonia. Thoracic function also has an impact in less obvious situations,

Osteopathic Musculoskeletal Examination of the Hospitalized Patient

Examiner: *(print)* ______________________

Chief Complaint: ______________________

Required

For Coding Purposes only

Ant. / Post. Spinal Curves:	I	N	D
Cervical Lordosis	▯	▯	▯
Thoracic Kyphosis	▯	▯	▯
Lumbar Lordosis	▯	▯	▯

I = increased; N = normal; D = decreased

Scoliosis (Lateral Spinal Curves)

▯ None
▯ Functional
▯ Mild
▯ Moderate
▯ Severe

sitting ▯
standing ▯
prone / supine ▯
lat. recumb. ▯
unable to examine ▯

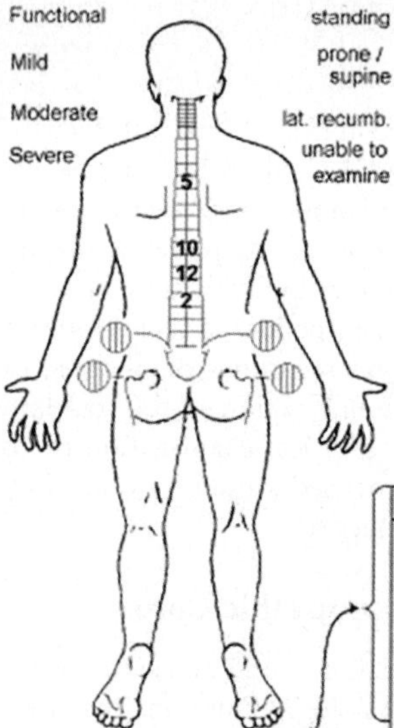

Assessment Tools:

▯ T = Tenderness
▯ A = Asymmetry
▯ R = Restricted Motion
▯ Active
▯ Passive
▯ T = Tissue Texture Change

Severity Key:

0 = No SD or background (BG) levels
1 = Minor TART more than BG levels
2 = TART obvious (R & T esp.) + / - symptoms
3 = Symptomatic, R and T very easily found, "key lesion"

Optional Worksheet

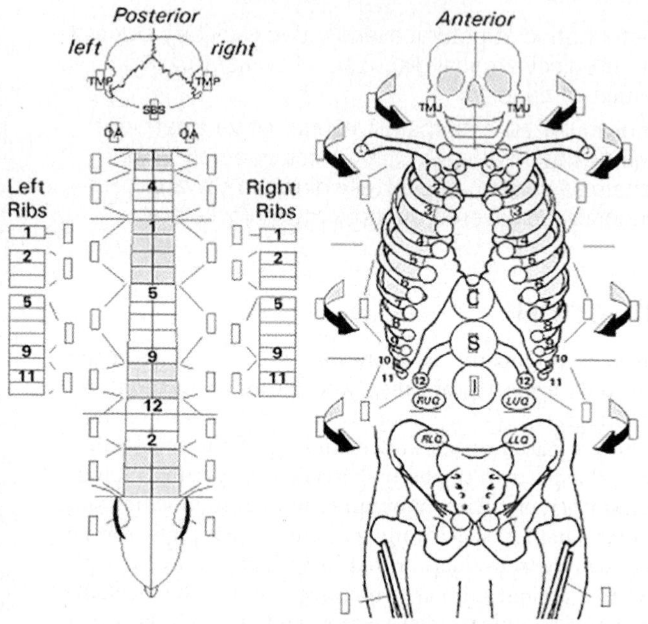

Abbreviation Key:

OA Occipitoatlantal joint
Sympathetic ganglia:
C Celiac
S Superior mesenteric
I Inferior mesenteric
TMJ Temporomandibular joint
TMP Temporal bone
SBS Sphenobasilar symphysis

Region Evaluated	Severity 0	1	2	3	Specific of Major Somatic Dysfunctions
Head	▯	▯	▯	▯	
Neck	▯	▯	▯	▯	
Thoracic T1-4	▯	▯	▯	▯	
T5-9	▯	▯	▯	▯	
T10-12	▯	▯	▯	▯	
Lumbar	▯	▯	▯	▯	
Pelvis / Sacrum	▯	▯	▯	▯	
Pelvis / Innominate	▯	▯	▯	▯	
Extremity (lower) R	▯	▯	▯	▯	
Extremity (lower) L	▯	▯	▯	▯	
Extremity (upper) R	▯	▯	▯	▯	
Extremity (upper) L	▯	▯	▯	▯	
Ribs	▯	▯	▯	▯	
Other / Abdomen	▯	▯	▯	▯	

Major Correlations with:

▯ Traumatic	▯ Rheumatological
▯ Orthopedic	▯ EENT
▯ Neurological	▯ Cardiovascular
▯ Viscero-somatic	▯ Pulmonary
▯ Primary Ms-Skeletal	▯ Gastrointestinal
▯ Activities of daily living	▯ Genitourinary
▯ Other ____	▯ Congenital

Other: ______________________

Signature of the examiner: ______________________ *Date of Examination:* ______________

Signature of the examiner (s) ______________________ *Date of Examination:* ______________

05A2X.PCX MLK/WAK Version 8: 032803

Official form of the American Osteopathic Association and the Educational Council on Osteopathic Principles—1993

Figure 78.1. **The American Osteopathic Association standardized hospital structural examination form.** (Used with permission from the AOA and Natalie Nevins. Available for download via the academyofosteopathy.org website.)

such as the postoperative abdominal surgery patient, whose most likely complication will be pulmonary, or the lower extremity cellulitis patient, whose body depends on diaphragmatic respiration for proper drainage of the infection. There are few, if any, acutely ill patients who do not warrant a focused examination of their respiratory mechanism.

The structural examination of the thorax can reveal a great deal about the underlying condition of the respiratory system.

- Breathing may be divided into an inhalation and exhalation phase. Restricted motion in one phase may suggest one pathology over another.
- Pneumonia will reduce the excursion of the thorax toward inhalation locally, over the area of consolidation, whereas asthma and other obstructive diseases will reduce the excursion of the thorax toward exhalation.
  - This finding may help differentiate the patient with a primary asthmatic attack from one whose asthmatic attack was triggered by pneumonia.
- Osteopathic principles can help the clinician differentiate patients with chronic obstructive pulmonary disease (COPD) from congestive heart failure (CHF). These conditions often coexist in the same patient and may present similarly with shortness of breath and crackles in the lung bases.
  - If the present exacerbation is due primarily to CHF, there will be restriction of the lower thorax to inhalation, and the exhalation phase will be relatively effortless.
  - If the present exacerbation is due primarily to COPD, the patient will have dramatic limitation in exhalation, and the exhalation phase will be active and prolonged (the patient will work to get the air out).
- This effort by the patient is easily observed by placing the finger pads or palm in contact with the patient's skin, just below the costal margin.

Structural examination of the thorax should be performed along with auscultation and percussion in the physical examination of the cardiac and respiratory systems. The structural examination includes evaluation of the entire spine, the pelvis, and the sacrum, which move, in addition to the ribs, during respiration and contribute to the overall shape change of the thoracic cavity.[9,10] The excursion of the thorax produces the volume and subsequent pressure changes that produce the movement of air and fluids. See Chapter 15 Anatomy, Mechanics, and Physiology of Pulmonary Respiration for further information.

- Compliance of the thorax is a separate, important functional parameter of respiration related to the structural evaluation of respiration, as it more accurately reflects the work of breathing, especially in obstructive and restrictive pulmonary disease.
- The clinical difference between excursion and compliance may be understood by comparing the difference between an otherwise healthy patient with COPD, who will have a limited but adequate excursion of a very stiff, noncompliant thorax, and a patient with no pre-existing pulmonary disease going into acute respiratory failure due to exhaustion of the respiratory musculature.
  - The latter patient will have a very limited excursion of their thorax but may have a compliant spine and rib cage.
  - Comparing excursion (by monitoring movement during respiration) to compliance (by motion testing the spine and rib cage) will yield a much more complete picture of the respiratory system than reviewing either of these factors alone.

The length and tone of the respiratory musculature, including the diaphragm, will complete the structural examination of the respiratory system.

- Evaluate the muscles, both during contraction (inhalation) and at rest (end exhalation).
- Evidence of respiratory muscle fatigue and failure should be obtained during this part of the examination.
  - Intercostal retractions may be observed during the evaluation of rib excursion.
  - Paradoxical motion of the lower ribs (inward movement during inhalation), an indicator of a flattened, tense diaphragm, may be observed during evaluation of the excursion of the lower rib cage.
  - Paradoxical movement of the abdomen (inward movement of the abdomen during inhalation), a sign of impending respiratory failure, may be observed with a hand below the costal margin.
  - A less obvious sign of diaphragm fatigue may be noted with the same contact, as the effort or force of contraction during inhalation will be reduced as the diaphragm fatigues.

See Table 78.1 for summary of these clinical pearls.

Focused Structural Examination of the Thorax

UPPER THORAX

Patient is supine. Doctor is sitting at the head or side of the bed.

1. *Sternum.* Evaluate general movement of the sternum, both inhalation and exhalation. Also, test for hinge motion of the sternomanubrial joint during inhalation and exhalation.
2. *Clavicle.* Evaluate a sense of posterior/superior movement of the clavicle with inhalation and an anterior/inferior movement during exhalation. Also, evaluate inferior movement at the sternoclavicular (SC) joint during upward shrug of the shoulders and its relative superior movement during return to resting state. Evaluate rotation on its long axis during forward flexion of the shoulder. Palpate for a normal slight movement of the acromioclavicular (AC) joint during adduction of the arm across the chest.
3. *First rib.* Evaluate when examining the clavicle.
4. *Ribs 2 through 6.* Evaluate pump handle motion of the upper ribs with hands lateral to the sternum; evaluate middle ribs with thumbs approaching the xiphoid and finger pads over the midaxillary line; evaluate bucket handle motion with hands below the breasts.
5. *Musculature.* Evaluate the tension of the scalene, sternocleidomastoid, and trapezius muscles when evaluating the clavicle and first rib. Evaluate the intercostal muscles when evaluating rib motion. Evaluate the paravertebral musculature, particularly those with rib attachments.

LOWER THORAX AND DIAPHRAGM

1. *Ribs 6 through 10.* Evaluate bucket handle motion at the midaxillary line, thumbs along the costal margin to evaluate any degree of AP motion.
2. *Costal margin.* Rest thumbs along the costochondral margins. Evaluate angle and motion.
3. *Twelfth rib.* Most easily found just lateral to the lateral edge of the erector spinae musculature. Compare the right and left 12th rib angles and motion and note that it should move down with inhalation as opposed to other ribs that move up with inhalation.

TABLE 78.1

Clinical Pearls

	Patient	Findings
Compare	1. Paradoxical movement of lower ribs 2. Paradoxical movement of the abdomen	1. Inward movement of these ribs during inhalation; indicates *flattened tense diaphragm.* 2. Inward movement of the abdomen during inhalation; indicates *impending respiratory failure.*
Compare	1. Sign of impending respiratory failure 2. Sign of a *flattened, tense abdominal diaphragm*	1. Paradoxical movement of the abdomen during breathing 2. Paradoxical movement lower ribs
Compliance of the rib cage		The ease with which the rib cage will move
Compare	1. Poor excursion 2. Poor compliance	1. Evaluated by movement of the rib cage during breathing (i.e., poor observed motion) 2. Evaluated by motion testing of the rib cage and sternum (i.e., poor motion tests)
Sign: abdominal *diaphragmatic fatigue*		Force of diaphragmatic contraction is reduced during inhalation
Compare	1. Obstructive lung disease 2. Pneumonia	1. Dramatic limitation of exhalation; patients use active effort to exhale. 2. Restricted local (area of pneumonia) rib cage excursion during inhalation; relatively relaxed exhalation.
Compare	1. Congestive heart failure patient 2. Chronic obstructive pulmonary disease acute exacerbation	1. Limited excursion to inhalation; exhalation with no active effort 2. Forced or active exhalation
Compare	1. Chronic COPD (no acute exacerbation) 2. Health person going into ARF	1. Poor compliance, good excursion 2. Good compliance, poor excursion
A manipulative technique is appropriate when		1. It addresses the underlying physiology and mechanics 2. It is appropriate for the present condition of the patient 3. It brings about changes expected when applying efficient treatment to accomplish a specific physiologic goal
The work of breathing		A quantitative measure of the energy required by the body to overcome the resistance of the lung parenchyma and chest wall and accomplish inhalation and exhalation
35–60% of thoracic duct lymphatic flow is due to		The response and effects of respiratory movements

COPD, chronic obstructive pulmonary disease.

4. *Diaphragm.* Direct palpation of the diaphragm can be difficult due to its position under the rib cage. Its motion can be evaluated in several ways.
   a. With a hand just below the costal margin, the superior/inferior motion of the anterior and lateral parts of the diaphragm may be evaluated. This will allow evaluation of the anterior and lateral aspects of the diaphragm but will not yield information about the posterior aspect. These regions do not necessarily operate together, as in the vomiting reflex, where the anterior and lateral contractions produce the forces for regurgitation; simultaneously, the crura must relax to maintain patency of the gastroesophageal junction. The motion of the diaphragm should be differentiated from the motion of the abdominal wall.
   b. The motion of the 12th rib closely parallels the excursion of the posterior part of the diaphragm.
   c. The lumbar spine will reflect the tension in the posterior aspect of the diaphragm through the attachment of the crus to the first three lumbar vertebrae. When tense, the crura will flatten the upper lumbar vertebra. This will be noted as flattening or reversed lordosis statically, and resistance to upward spring or compression, at levels L1–L3. This is easily accomplished with the patient in the supine position.
   d. With a hand above and below the lower thorax, the superior/inferior motion of the diaphragm may be distinguished from the lateral excursion of the ribs.

The Abdomen

Evaluation of the container should accompany the classic palpatory evaluation of the abdomen. The shape of a container will affect the function of its contents. The abdomen has a roof, a floor, and anterior and posterior walls.

- The *diaphragm* is the roof of the abdomen; the liver, spleen, and supporting mesenteries are suspended from it.
- The *pelvic diaphragm* is the floor. It, along with the shelf created as the posterior abdominal wall crosses the pelvic brim at the level of the pectinate line, supports the abdominal and pelvic viscera from below.
- The *iliopsoas and quadratus lumborum* make up the posterior abdominal wall. The insertion of iliopsoas on the lesser trochanter of the femur involves the hip in abdominal and pelvic function.
- The *abdominal wall* is its anterior boundary.

SKELETAL CONSIDERATIONS

The sacrum, pelvis, hip joint, lumbar spine, lower six ribs, and thoracic vertebrae form the structural and functional framework to which the soft tissue container of the abdomen is attached and supported. All should be evaluated for motion restriction and/or altered position.

The diaphragm should be evaluated with emphasis on its lower attachments to the 12th rib and lumbar spine. When the diaphragm becomes tense, it flattens and carries the 12th ribs inferiorly at their tips. The lumbar spine will become flattened and resist anterior pressure in the supine patient. The same relative positions will be adopted when the diaphragm has a fascial "drag" placed on it, although the resistance encountered will be of a lesser degree and different quality. Rarely will the diaphragm be displaced superiorly from a dysfunction.

The movement of the pelvic diaphragm may be inferred by the magnitude and intensity of the consequent nutation/counternutation movement of the sacrum occurring during respiration. Although this movement may be more obvious with the patient prone, supine evaluation is often necessary in the acutely ill or hospitalized patient. A two-handed contact from the side of the patient, one hand contacting the sacral base and the other on the sacral apex, may be used for this evaluation. More direct evaluation of the tension and movement of the pelvic diaphragm may be performed with a contact in the ischiorectal fossae. These regions are found just medial and slightly posterior to the tip of the ischial tuberosities (Fig. 78.2). The pelvic diaphragm will move inferiorly with inhalation and superiorly with exhalation.

The quadratus lumborum may be palpated anterior and lateral to the erector spinae mass in the lumbar spine. Its edge is usually discernible beginning just below the tip of the 12th rib. The psoas major is a deeper, more medial flank muscle that is more difficult to palpate directly. The increased amount of muscle tone observed and the combination of upper lumbar somatic dysfunction and external hip rotation on the same side may infer tension. The tendon of the iliopsoas is directly palpable just below the inguinal ligament on the floor of the femoral triangle. The iliopsoas tendon is usually tense, full, and tender when the muscle is in spasm. One can often sense the tension in the entire iliopsoas with one hand contacting the tendon in the femoral triangle and the other under the upper lumbar attachments. Only the iliopsoas travels anteroinferolaterally here. Jones has also described anterior abdominal tender points related to spasm of the iliopsoas muscle (see Chapter 47 Strain–Counterstrain).

PALPATION

Palpation is an essential part of any abdominal examination. However, extra care must be taken to avoid exacerbation of the patient's pain, as the resultant guarding by the patient will interfere with the examiner's ability to gather reliable information.

Light Palpation

It is useful to begin the abdominal examination with light palpation and in a region of the abdomen distant from the patient's chief complaint of pain or discomfort. This will help secure the patient's comfort and cooperation and can yield information not obtainable with deep palpation.

- *Involuntary guarding by the patient.* Involuntary guarding, present without any actual or perceived stimulation of the discomfort, should be distinguished from voluntary guarding due to actual or perceived exacerbation of pain induced by the examination. This determination is an essential part of the abdominal examination and is most accurately evaluated with light palpation, as many healthy individuals will guard with deep palpation.
- *Ptosis.* Dr. Still often taught that there is a sag of the abdominal contents into the pelvis resulting in physiologic consequences. He writes:

"The caecum and the transverse and sigmoid flexure are often forced from their normal positions and piled into the pelvis, dragging the uterus and small intestine down with the caecum and obstructing all possible chance for the fluids of the small intestine to pass through the ileocecal valve and reach the colon."[11]

Sag of the abdominal contents and the mesenteries that support them may be evaluated by comparing the resistance to normal limits with the right and left sides, produced by a gentle lift just

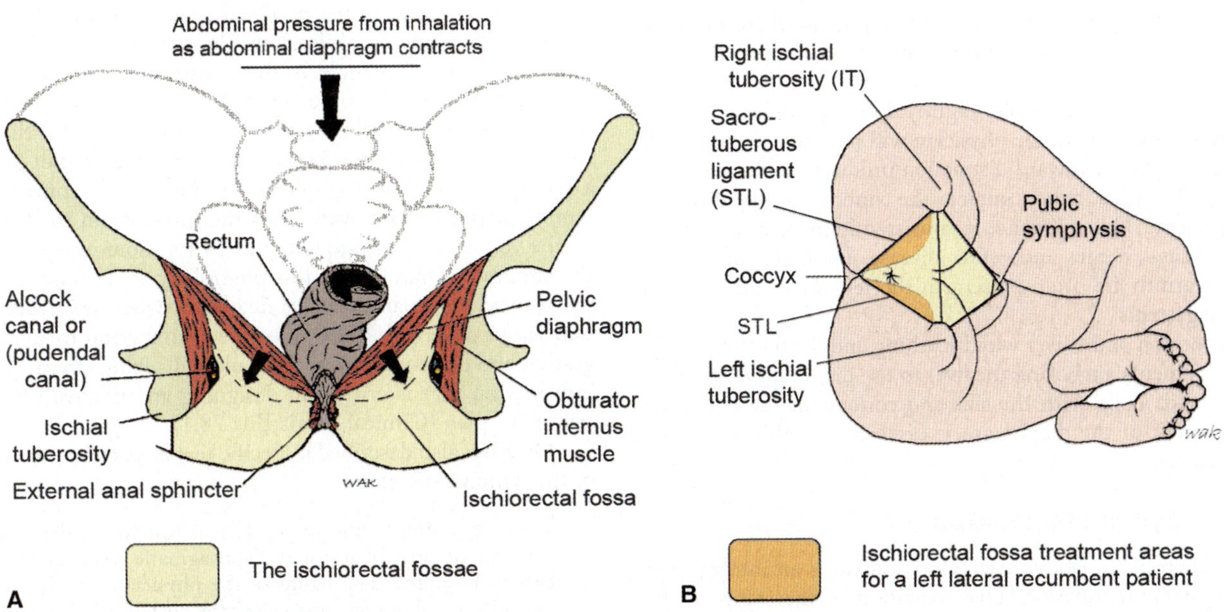

Figure 78.2. The ischiorectal fossa and pelvic diaphragm. A. The *broken line* depicts the pelvic diaphragm during inhalation. **B.** The ischiorectal fossa as it would appear in a lateral recumbent patient. (Illustration by William A. Kuchera, DO, FAAO, used with permission.)

superior to each inguinal ligament. This quick test should be part of the light palpatory examination.

- *Congestion.* A sense of fullness and/or congestion will often be evident over areas of acute inflammation, such as cholecystitis or diverticulitis. It may be accompanied by a palpable sense of warmth. This somewhat subtle finding will be much more difficult to identify during deep palpation. There may also be a subcutaneous puffiness palpable deep to the epigastric region of the abdomen, a terminal drainage site related to the abdomen.
- *Tenderness.* Tenderness is a subjective symptom but can usually be identified accurately during light palpation. Identifying the tender area early in the examination and leaving that area for evaluation near the end of the examination will help maximize patient cooperation for the bulk of the early abdominal examination. The area of the patient's tenderness can be evaluated in depth at the end of the abdominal examination.

Deep Palpation

Deep palpation must be carefully performed. Slow, deliberate movements will minimize discomfort and voluntary guarding. Never palpate with your fingertips. Always use your finger pads.

- Palpation with one hand over the other may be more comfortable for the patient and enhance palpatory sensing.
- The finger pads of a relaxed hand rest on the patient and receive information while the other hand, resting on top, exerts gentle, steady pressure to reach the desired depth.
- The abdomen is classically divided into four quadrants for palpation. The epigastrium and suprapubic areas may be considered separately.
- The examiner should always keep a clear mental picture of all significant anatomic structures in the area being palpated. Although many viscera are not palpable in normal conditions, in pathologic situations they may become discernible and offer clues to an accurate working diagnosis.
- Several examples, which this author has found to be useful in practice, are presented, but the possibilities of abdominal palpation are far greater than just these examples.
  - The tip of the gallbladder capsule is often palpable in cases of acute cholecystitis, with associated fullness, congestion, and often warmth overlying it. When present, these signs are more accurate than the Murphy sign of right upper quadrant tenderness.
  - The stomach is palpable slightly left and inferior to the xiphoid. Sometimes, the physician will note that the stomach resists gentle downward distraction produced with one hand, while the other hand contacts the xiphoid to stabilize the diaphragm. This resistance is consistently present in patients with hiatal hernia and reflux disease. Fullness, congestion, and warmth are often present in the left upper quadrant in acute gastritis.
  - The motion of the liver with breathing and the tension within the ligaments anchoring the liver to the diaphragm should be evaluated, along with the size and contour of the liver. The movement of the diaphragm is essential for efficient portal circulation.[12]

The Fluid (Lymph) Mechanism

The evaluation of the body's circulatory system is an integral part of any physical examination. The evaluation of the status of the lymphatic circulation is indicated in any inflammatory process, as the lymphatic system is responsible for the drainage of inflammatory exudates and is integral in the progression and resolution of an inflammatory process (see Chapters 12, 14 for further information). Millard was the first osteopathic physician to discuss the evaluation of the lymphatic system in the physical examination. He said:

> "For every congested tissue, there is a corresponding lymph disturbance. Wherever pus is present there is enlargement in the nearest nodes. The lymph stream ebbs and flows according to the amount of blockage and nodular involvement at certain points."[13]

Dr. Millard considered it possible to differentiate disease processes by the location, degree, and quality of lymph node enlargement. He also described a principle that is important in the treatment of lymph congestion:

> The lymph stream is readily checked in many ways. The lymph vessels are pliable and readily compressed.[13]

In the evaluation of lymphatic function, one must investigate tissue tension along the course of lymphatic drainage, with an emphasis on the regions where lymph vessels are most vulnerable to altered tissue tension. This is most often the place where lymph node aggregations are found.

J. Gordon Zink, a student of Dr. Millard, continued to develop methods for the evaluation of lymph function and dysfunction. He called attention to the congestion produced in the regions of lymph nodes when there was dysfunction of the lymph system, with or without frank edema, and the supraclavicular congestion found with dysfunction of the thoracic duct and "terminal lymph drainage from the head and neck."

In the management of hospitalized patients, who often have areas of significant inflammation, supraclavicular congestion can often be seen on exam, and has at times, in our experience, reduced noticeably following treatment. There are also times, particularly in situations of severe inflammation, where the finding of supraclavicular congestion would be an expected finding, and its absence is an indicator of significant downstream obstruction. This has led this author to the concept of tracking congestion along the course of drainage to identify the areas of greatest obstruction. For example, in acute cellulitis of the lower leg, lymph will travel through several vulnerable areas: the popliteal space, the femoral triangle, under the crus of the diaphragm, and finally the thoracic inlet. If congestion is found in the popliteal area and inguinal region, but not at the diaphragm or inlet, it would indicate significant obstruction at the femoral triangle. In these situations, it is common to see the upstream areas become congested, including the supraclavicular area, following effective treatment. In the view of this author, the finding of congestion in these areas is therefore not necessarily a pathologic finding. Lymph nodes function to concentrate the lymph, giving off free water into the interstitium to be absorbed by the venous system (see Chapter 14 for more information), and the congestion may reflect this physiology. It becomes pathologic when it occurs to an excessive degree, or when upstream congestion is not observed. Regardless, the examination for lymph congestion and obstruction is simple, and will yield extremely valuable information that is critical to designing an effective Osteopathic treatment plan (Clinical Pearls Box 78.1).

Dr. Zink also described a specific test he used in the evaluation of the lymphatic system:

> There is a simple but very practical test to confirm better circulation, because of restored diaphragmatic respiration, when the patient is supine. The hands of the physician are placed high on the patient's abdomen, just below the costal arch. Firm pressure is used downward toward the table and cephalad, as if to "raise" or "redome" the diaphragm. The patient should experience a sensation of "warmth" or "heat" in the lumbar and sacral area.[10]

BOX 78.1 Clinical Pearls: Examining for Lymph Congestion/Obstruction

- Lower Extremity—Popliteal space, inguinal area (femoral triangle), subdiaphragmatic area, supraclavicular space
- Upper Extremity—Axilla, supraclavicular space
- Abdomen/Pelvis—Mesenteries, subdiaphragmatic space, supraclavicular space
- Thorax—Mediastinal fascia, supraclavicular space
- Head Neck—Jugulo-digastric area, supraclavicular space

W.G. Sutherland introduced the concept of fluid fluctuation in his description of the primary respiratory mechanism.[14] The movement of interstitial fluids is important in the process of cellular respiration (the cellular exchange of gases), as well as the exchange of nutrients and waste products.

- Motion of the interstitial fluids occurs in response to intrinsic, rhythmic motions of the body, including pulse, respiration, and the primary respiratory mechanism.
- Interstitial fluid fluctuation may be evaluated passively, by the presence or absence of these inherent forces in the region of the body being evaluated.
- They can also be actively evaluated by assessing the response of the tissue and its fluid matrix to local or general lymph pump techniques aimed at fluctuating the interstitial fluid.

The evaluation of the static and dynamic findings of the lymphatic circulation is important in the overall physical evaluation of the circulatory system (see Table 78.1).

APPROACHING THE ACUTELY ILL HOSPITALIZED PATIENT

Osteopathic treatment in the hospital setting is most effective when it addresses underlying physiologic mechanisms of the disease and supports the physiologic response of the host who has the disease.

- Although the manipulative treatment is ultimately based on the findings of the structural examination, these findings should be interpreted with consideration of the body's response to the disease process and directed toward supporting the body's physiologic processes.

This section will present a variety of conceptual models from which treatment plans should evolve. Techniques will be described to provide examples of how some of the underlying principles may be achieved but should not be construed as the best or only way to treat an area or problem. One cannot overemphasize the importance of designing treatments for the individual. There is, therefore, no such thing as a technique for asthma, CHF, or any disease, nor is there a manipulative technique for reducing segmental facilitation, improving respiratory/circulatory function, or any other physiologic process. A variety of techniques can be employed for any of these treatment goals. Any technique is appropriate if it addresses the underlying physiology and mechanics, is appropriate for the present condition of the patient, and brings about the changes a physician expects to see from application of an efficient treatment to accomplish a specific physiologic goal.

Inflammation

Inflammation is the generalized response to injury and disease. It is the hallmark of most acute illnesses.

- Inflammation involves the vascular system, the immune system, the nervous system, and the connective tissues.
- It is essential to the initial response of the body to the disease process, as well as the healing process.
- During any inflammatory process, increased capillary permeability allows a tremendous efflux of protein into the interstitial spaces, producing an exudative swelling.
- This exudate can only be drained through the lymphatics.
- The lymphatic system is an integral part of the progression and ultimate resolution of inflammation.
  - Besides draining areas of infection and injury, lymphatic drainage carries antigen to the nodes, where immune stimulation takes place to produce T-cells and B-cells.
  - Nodal efferents provide migration routes for these cells to enter the primary circulatory system.
  - The lymphatics are the only vascular system permeable to large particles, fats, and proteins.
  - In a normal function, the lymphatics remove the proteins, which leak into the interstitium from the capillaries, maintaining a delicate osmotic balance and keeping the interstitial environment pristine.
  - In addition, there is evidence that lymphatic drainage is necessary for the removal and deactivation of the chemical and immune mediators, which control inflammatory processes, making the lymphatics central in the progression and resolution of the process itself.[15–18]
  - Diseases including pancreatitis, asthma, rheumatoid arthritis, and even myocardial infarction will depend on lymphatic drainage for resolution.

The large efflux of protein and water from the capillary bed leaves a very high concentration of erythrocytes, which pack into the small venules producing local venous stasis.[17] This makes the lymphatic system the only source of fluid drainage from an inflamed tissue. The tissue becomes saturated when the small hydrostatic gradient that produces capillary filtration is met by the increased interstitial pressure that the swelling tissue produces. At this point, the rate of blood supply will equal the rate of lymphatic drainage.

Inflammation and healing are aspects of one continuous process, guided by the same group of cells. Cellular activity will shift from proinflammatory to healing as the proportion of relative controlling mediators shifts their activity. Although this progression is related to the production of mediators, one must consider the role of the efficient breakdown and removal of these mediators in the progression and resolution of any inflammatory process.

- Prolonged inflammation leads to poor healing, smoldering infections, chronic inflammatory processes, and eventually tissue destruction.
- There is evidence that lymphatic drainage is involved in the removal and breakdown of histamine, bradykinin, prostaglandins, and leukotrienes (including cytokines).
- See Chapter 14 Anatomy and Physiology of the Lymphatic System and Chapter 12 The Role of Inflammation in Healing and Homeostasis for further information.

As proinflammatory mediators are removed, those that stimulate fibroblasts and macrophages will predominate, and the healing process will ensue. Residual (interstitial plasma) protein from the inflammatory exudate will also stimulate fibroblasts to produce collagen. As with the inflammatory phase, rapid and efficient removal of these elements is essential to a physiologic healing process.

- A prolonged healing phase will lead to excess collagen production, fibrous adhesions, and eventually tissue fibrosis.
- The lymphatic system is responsible for the removal of most, if not all, of the inflammatory exudate.
- It has been shown that lymphatic drainage is involved in controlling the rate of collagen production, both during the healing process and in the pathogenesis of diseases that result in tissue fibrosis.
- Diseases such as cirrhosis of the liver, interstitial lung diseases, and atherosclerosis have been linked to impaired lymphatic function.[19]

The lymphatic system is vulnerable to somatic dysfunction, and its dysfunction is responsive to OMT. The function of the lymphatic system should be evaluated and treated as part of the osteopathic treatment of any patient with an inflammatory process.

Segmental Facilitation

Often, the consequences of facilitation create physiologic imbalance that interferes with the body's response to a challenge. Segmental facilitation is a consequence of many acute diseases, especially those producing pain and/or inflammation.[20–27] One osteopathic treatment goal is to remove somatic dysfunctions of related segments to reduce their somatic contribution to the facilitated spinal cord segments. Another goal might be to improve the general function of the nervous system. See Chapter 43 Clinical Assessment: Viscerosomatic, Somatosomatic, Somatovisceral Reflexes; Counterstrain Points, Myofascial Trigger Points, and Chapman Reflexes for discussion on the importance of assessing for the presence of segmental facilitation. Osteopathic manipulative techniques useful in the acutely ill or hospitalized patients that are designed to reduce the effects of segmental facilitation are presented below.

Neuroendocrine Immune Considerations

The hypothalamus, and the neuroendocrine immune system that it controls, is at the center of the body's response to the almost unlimited variety of challenges from the body's external and internal environments. It is central to the maintenance of homeostasis in the face of these challenges and deeply involved in the body's response to virtually all acute illnesses. The hypothalamus exerts immense influence on the central functioning of the autonomic nervous system, the pituitary gland, and, through it, by way of the autonomic nervous system and adrenal glands, the entire endocrine system, and the immune system. The physiology of the hypothalamic–pituitary axis is also vulnerable to the neurophysiologic effects brought about by the mechanical dysfunctions resulting from somatic dysfunction.

Information about the local functioning within the body is monitored by the hypothalamus in several ways. The ability of the hypothalamus to respond to internal and external changes will depend on the accuracy of its inputs.

- The hypothalamus receives a large input from the nociceptive system, via the spinohypothalamic tract.[28] Spinal cord facilitation will exaggerate this source of input, affecting the degree and quality of the response.
- The hypothalamus also receives input about levels of inflammation and immune activity in the body from circulating leukotrienes, delivered to the systemic circulation by the lymphatics.[18]
    - □ Levels of circulating leukotrienes are monitored by circumventricular organs in the third and fourth ventricles.[29]
    - □ This system will operate at maximum effectiveness when circulation and fluctuation of cerebrospinal fluid are undisturbed. Reduced rate and amplitude of the primary respiratory mechanism will reduce the fluctuation of the cerebrospinal fluid.
- The pituitary gland sits within the sella turcica of the sphenoid. The hypothalamus is just above, in close relation to the body of the sphenoid and sphenobasilar junction.
- The pituitary gland has a portal circulation, similar to the portal circulation of the liver. The liver is situated against the undersurface of the diaphragm and is anchored to it, and the respiratory movement of the diaphragm provides the motive power for its circulation. The pituitary gland has a similar anatomic relation to the diaphragma sella. The diaphragma sella continues into the sella turcica. It completely surrounds the pituitary gland and blends with its capsule.[30]
    - □ The diaphragma sella is a continuation of the anterior reaches of the tentorium cerebelli.
    - □ The movement of the sphenoid and the tentorium cerebelli would, therefore, alternately change the shape of the gland with the phases of the primary respiratory mechanism, pumping the fluid within it.
    - □ It has been suggested that the portal circulation of the pituitary is bidirectional; the backward movement from the pituitary gland to the hypothalamus is theorized to be important to the feedback regulation of the hypothalamic–pituitary axis.[30]
        - This is also a possible mechanism for the central distribution of corticotropin-releasing factor (CRF), which has far-reaching effects on the central nervous system.
        - The alternating movement of the primary respiratory mechanism would explain the ability of this circulation to move in alternating directions.
    - □ W.G. Sutherland described the importance of the motion of the sphenoid to the functioning of the pituitary gland.[31]
    - □ It is important to consider treatment of somatic dysfunctions of the cranium, including the sphenobasilar area, in the management of the acutely ill hospitalized patient.

Approach to the Thorax

Sutherland writes:

> "The diaphragm is the 'piston' to the big 'combustion cylinder' of the body. Its crura are the 'legs' that lead down from the piston to the 'crankshaft' in the lumbar vertebrae. Its ligamenta arcuata are the 'piston rings.' The lungs might represent the 'combustion chamber' to the cylinder while the nasal region the 'carburetor,' while the 'ignition' and 'self-starter' might be found somewhere in the 'cranial bowl'."[31]

The thorax contains the heart, lungs, and mediastinum and its contents. These structures are related anatomically by their fascial attachments. The fibrous pericardium blends inferiorly into the central tendon of the diaphragm; this relation is important to diaphragmatic function. The fibrous pericardium attaches to the sternum via the sternopericardial ligaments, and is continuous superiorly with the mediastinal fascia, which blends with the anterior cervical fascia at the inner aspect of the clavicles and manubrium. The anterior cervical fascia, including the pretracheal fascia, has attachment to the hyoid bone and mandible before finally hanging from the cranial base. This continuity must be considered in any approach to manipulative treatment of the thorax, neck, or cranium.

Breathing is largely a mechanical process by which intrathoracic pressure changes are created via the action of skeletal musculature on the spine and bony thorax. It also produces pressure gradients between the thoracic and abdominal cavities. This process is critical to the movement of both air and fluids throughout the body. A detailed look at the mechanics involved will offer insight as to how osteopathic treatment may improve the efficiency and effectiveness of breathing in the acutely ill patient, an important consideration whether or not the patient is suffering directly from a respiratory problem.

The physical action of producing negative intrathoracic pressure requires a definable amount of energy, referred to as the work of breathing. Although difficult to quantify, increased work of breathing is clinically relevant since many pulmonary problems dramatically alter the work of breathing.

- Restrictive lung diseases, by their very nature, increase the work of breathing.
- West considers increases in work of breathing an important factor in the pathophysiology of COPD.[32]
- In the pathophysiology of asthma, patients progress to respiratory stage three and ultimately to respiratory failure due to an inability to maintain a state of hyperventilation caused by fatigue and the eventual exhaustion of the respiratory musculature. This failure is directly related to increased work of breathing in patients with acute asthma.
- The work of breathing is a quantitative measure of the energy required by the body to overcome the resistance of the lung parenchyma and chest wall and accomplish inhalation and exhalation.
- Compliance is the ease with which tissues are stretched (moved). Overall pulmonary compliance is the combination of compliance of the parenchyma, airway compliance and resistance (secretions), and compliance of the musculoskeletal structures of the thorax.
- Compliance with one or more of these is reduced in all of the above diseases, contributing to the overall increased work of breathing.
  - □ Restrictive diseases directly reduce lung elasticity, reducing parenchymal compliance. Obstructive diseases reduce compliance through reduced airway compliance (bronchospasm) increased airway resistance and a variety of other factors.

Somatic dysfunction, by its definition, will reduce the compliance of the bony thorax in patients with pulmonary diseases and increase the work of breathing. Somatic dysfunction of the thoracic spine and ribs has been noted by several sources.[5] The general shape changes of the thorax in COPD (barrel chest) can produce dramatic changes in chest wall compliance. These are obvious on osteopathic structural examination and, in addition to the specific dysfunctions noted in association with pulmonary disease, actually stand out. General techniques will be described to address general compliance issues, as well as more specific techniques for individual somatic dysfunctions. Osteopathic treatment to improve the compliance of the thorax will not necessarily directly alter the parenchymal pathology, especially for those with chronic lung disease. However, it will improve issues such as exercise tolerance, giving the patient the ability to function with their disease. West notes the effect of the work of breathing on exercise tolerance of the chronic lung patient.[33]

In addition to general changes in compliance of the bony thorax, specific somatic dysfunctions may influence the function of the respiratory mechanism that goes beyond the small changes in compliance they invariably produce.

- The movement of a typical rib during breathing operates in conjunction with the orientation of its costotransverse and costovertebral joints (Fig. 78.3).
- Rotation of the thoracic vertebrae with somatic dysfunction will not only create resistance to movement but will change the orientation of the costotransverse and costovertebral articulations, produce thoracic fascial torsions, and further impair the ability of the muscles to move the rib during inhalation.

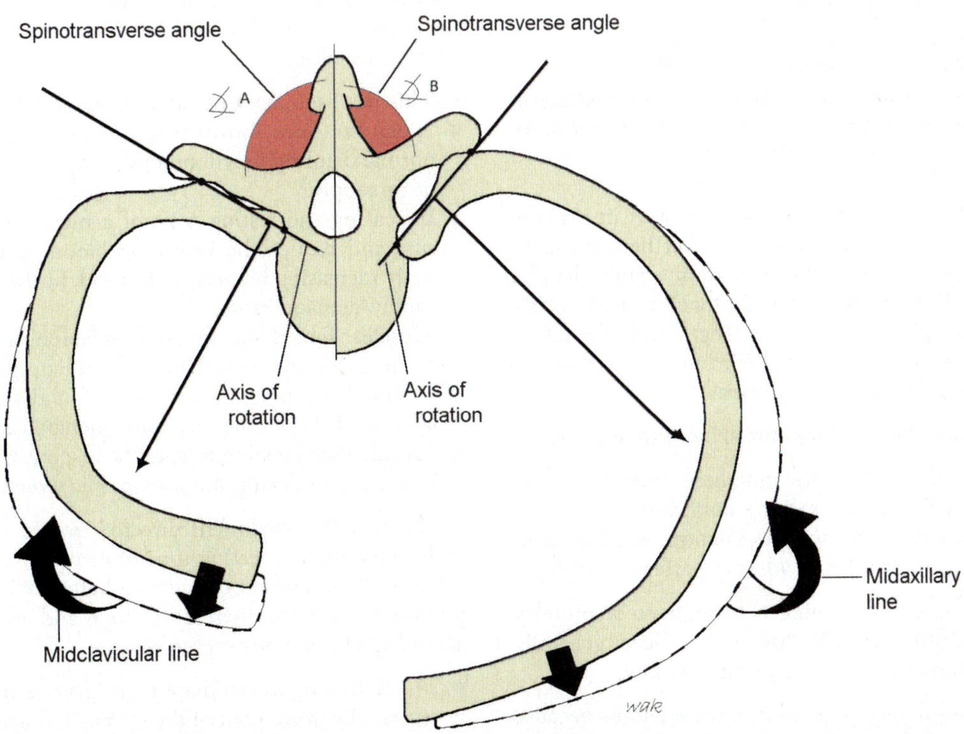

Figure 78.3. The orientation of the costotransverse and costovertebral articulations helps determine the direction of movement of a rib with respiration. (Illustration by William A. Kuchera, DO, FAAO, used with permission.)

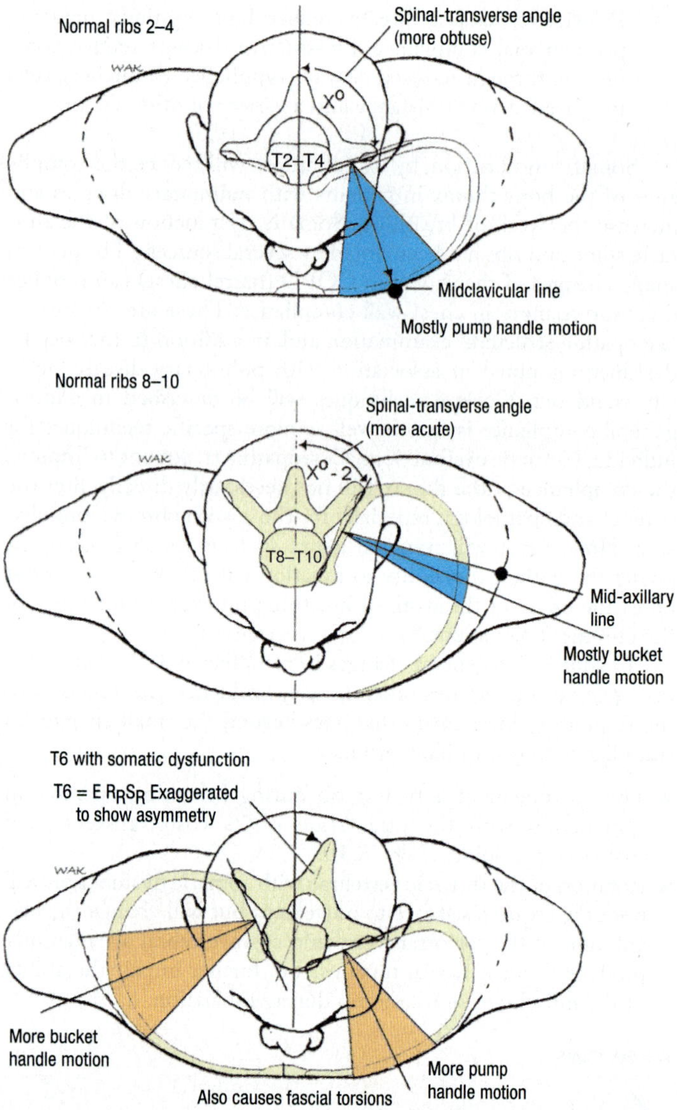

Figure 78.4. Vertebral rotation will change the orientation of the rib and the movement of that rib produced with respiration. (Illustration by William A. Kuchera, DO, FAAO, used with permission.)

- With rotation of thoracic vertebral units involved in somatic dysfunction, a rib with a predominantly bucket handle movement might become oriented to move more in a pump handle movement (Fig. 78.4). Lumbar somatic dysfunction, particularly in the upper lumbar spine, will alter the length and orientation of the crura and may, thereby, impair their function in connection with the contraction of the diaphragm.

Cathie describes movement of the entire spine with respiration.[9]

- During inhalation, all spinal curves straighten, including rotation of the sacrum with the base moving posteriorly.
- The reverse movement occurs with exhalation. Somatic dysfunction anywhere in the body may adversely affect breathing.

Increases in the work of breathing contribute to respiratory muscle fatigue. Respiratory muscle fatigue has been generally implicated in the pathophysiology of respiratory failure.

- Obstructive diseases produce respiratory muscle fatigue because of the effects of hyperinflation.[34]
- Muscular fatigue has been long understood as the immediate factor leading to the demise of the patient with acute asthma. Their muscles of inspiration exhaust, and the patient can no longer hyperventilate to maintain adequate air exchange.
- Respiratory muscle fatigue is also important in COPD and has led to the identification of chronic respiratory muscle fatigue in the pathophysiology of lung disease.[35]
- Respiratory muscle fatigue has also been implicated in diverse problems such as pulmonary edema, lung shock, and difficulties weaning patients off ventilators.[35,36]

Increasing the compliance of the thorax will reduce the load on the respiratory muscles and may reduce the likelihood of fatigue in both acute and chronic conditions. Osteopathic treatment may also be used to improve the function and efficiency of the respiratory musculature.

Respiratory muscles, like all skeletal musculature, operate on the principle of their length–tension relationship. In this relationship, muscles will develop a far stronger contraction at a longer resting tone.

- Consider the typical physical changes associated with exacerbations of obstructive lung disease, such as a flattened diaphragm visualized on radiograph or the hypertonicity of accessory muscles, such as the sternocleidomastoid.
- These are indications of shortened musculature that will have a reduced contractile force in the face of an increased workload. In the case of chronic obstructive lung disease, the barrel-type changes in the thorax will actually prevent inspiratory muscles from returning to full resting length during exhalation.
- Likewise, increased tone in the inspiratory musculature may prevent the thorax from fully assuming the position of exhalation, contributing to the overall shape change of the thorax.
- In addition to altering the length–tension curve, increasing the resting tone of the respiratory musculature will alter its blood supply and oxygen supply/demand ratio.

Muscles get most of their blood supply during their resting or diastolic phase. The increased tone during contraction increases the pressure within the muscle and shunts blood away via nonnutritive arterioles.

- This has been demonstrated in the diaphragm.[35]
- It has also been shown that increased demand in an otherwise normal diaphragm will produce oxygen demand that is in excess of its supply.[35]
- Increasing the resting tone of a muscle will increase its pressure and reduce the incoming blood supply while simultaneously increasing its oxygen demand, further stressing the oxygen supply/demand ratio.
- Muscles forced to function anaerobically are as much as 15 times less efficient than those utilizing aerobic metabolism.[37]
- Fatigued diaphragms have been found to have high levels of lactic acid, indicating anaerobic metabolism.[35]
- The increased resting tone of the inspiratory musculature should be identified during the osteopathic structural examination.

Osteopathic treatment directed toward increasing the length and decreasing the resting tone of inspiratory musculature is indicated in the treatment of acute and chronic lung disease. The diaphragm is prone to increase in tone and associated flattening in acute and chronic obstructive disease.

- The flattening of the diaphragm may become severe enough to reverse the movement of the lower ribs during inspiration, called paradoxical rib motion.
- This will reduce the transverse diameter of the chest and greatly reduce the efficiency of the entire respiratory mechanism.

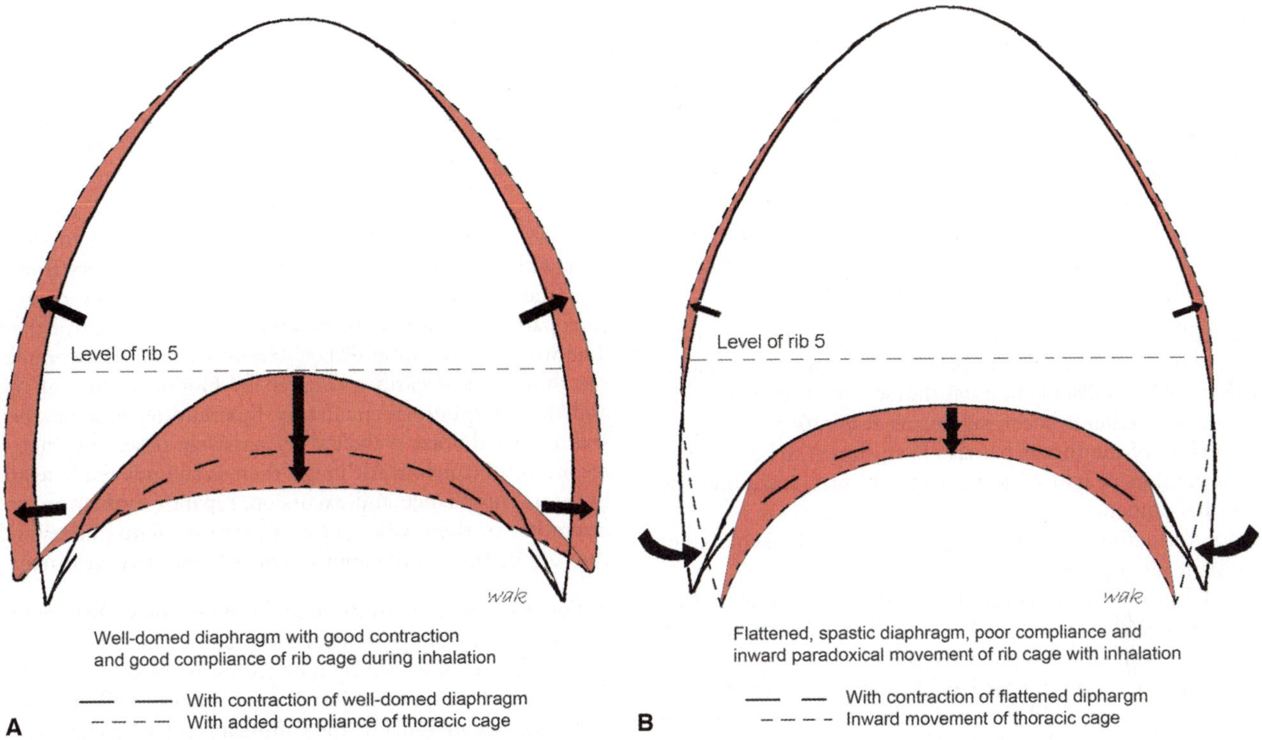

Figure 78.5. The mechanical effects of contraction of the diaphragm. A. Normal excursion of a compliant thoracic rib cage with contraction of a well-domed diaphragm. **B.** Reduced excursion of thoracic cage and even the possibility of paradoxical motion of the lower rib cage with contraction of a flattened abdominal diaphragm. (Illustration by William A. Kuchera, DO, FAAO, used with permission.)

- In osteopathic literature, restoration of the length and vertical orientation of the diaphragm is called doming of the diaphragm.
- Doming of a flattened diaphragmatic muscle will increase the pressure gradients that it is able to produce between the thoracic and abdominal regions and can help reverse paradoxical rib motion and improve the function of the diaphragm as well as the respiratory mechanism as a whole (Fig. 78.5).

Addressing the mechanics of breathing, including the work of breathing, the compliance of the thorax and spine, both specifically and generally, and the function and efficiency of the respiratory musculature will have far-reaching applications in the treatment of acute and chronic respiratory diseases.

The physiologic impact of respiration is not limited to the exchange of air. The negative pressures produced by thoracic excursion are important to the function of the circulatory system as well. The role of respiratory movements on inferior vena caval and portal circulations has been extensively studied. Breathing has a tremendous influence on both the inferior vena cava and portal return[12] (Fig. 78.6).

- During inspiration, the negative intrathoracic pressure produced dramatically increases the flow in the inferior vena cava, while, simultaneously, the compression of the liver by the descent of the diaphragm virtually eliminates hepatic flow.
  - During this time, blood flows into the liver, so its pressure increases.
- During exhalation, the vena cava loses its pressure gradient and flow decreases substantially.
  - This is balanced by the large portal flow from the pressurized portal veins of the liver, as the diaphragm lifts off.
  - Return to the heart remains somewhat balanced. However, the composition of the blood differs greatly between these two phases of the respiratory cycle.
- The effect of respiration on central venous flow is greatest in supine, nonactive patients, who lose the effects of the peripheral pumps created by muscle contraction.
  - Zink noted this when he presented his model of respiratory/circulatory function.[10]
  - This encompasses many acutely ill hospital patients, who are bedridden most, if not all, of the time during their convalescence.
  - Patients with CHF demonstrate a clinical application of this concept. These patients develop fluid congestion in their liver and lower extremities. They consistently have substantial restrictions on their diaphragmatic excursion, as can be determined by structural examination. Treatment of the diaphragm

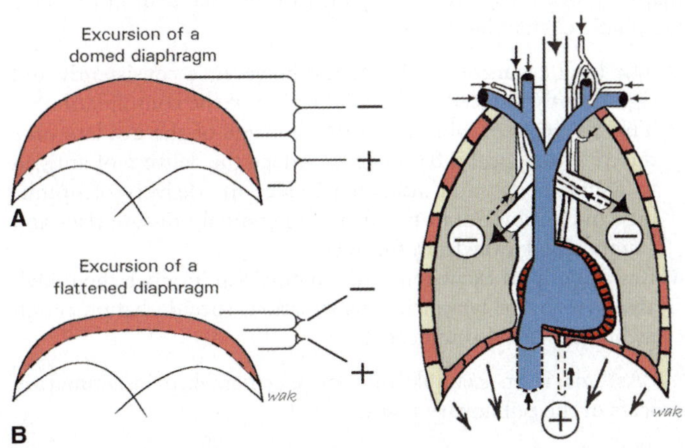

Figure 78.6. A. The excursion of the diaphragm has a powerful influence on venous and lymphatic return. **B.** This effect is reduced when the resting diaphragm is flattened. (Illustration by William A. Kuchera, DO, FAAO, used with permission.)

improves the overall circulatory function, and venous back pressure is reduced, decreasing afterload on the heart.

The action of the diaphragm and thorax also has a major influence on the function of the lymphatic system. This is the second aspect of the "respiratory/circulatory" model. Zink's original model described the role of respiration, with its action on central venous flow and pressure, as they influence the emptying of the thoracic duct into the junction of the internal jugular and brachiocephalic veins. This idea has since been confirmed with studies measuring thoracic duct flow in relation to respiratory excursion.

- A variety of studies have measured the role of respiration in the movement of thoracic duct lymph; estimates from these studies show that 35% to 60% of the total thoracic duct drainage is in response to movements occurring during respiration.[38–42]
- The excursion of the thorax has also been shown to be involved in the formation of lymph in a variety of areas, including the lungs and abdomen.
  - Lymph formation is a critical step in the overall mechanics of lymphatic circulation.
  - A small but significant uphill hydrostatic gradient exists that must be overcome for fluid to move from the interstitium into the initial, blind lymphatic vessel.[38]
  - The excursion of the thorax has been shown to be the primary force moving fluid from the pulmonary interstitium to the initial pulmonary lymphatics.
  - The expansion of the pulmonary interstitial tissue, to which the initial lymphatics are tethered by anchoring filaments, increases the volume of the initial lymphatic vessel and produces a temporary pressure gradient for filling the initial lymph vessels.
  - Exhalation then closes the vessel and moves the lymph forward, past the first valve, and into the contractile part of the vessel.
  - The respiratory cycle then produces a pump that initiates the process of lymph formation.
  - All initial lymphatics have anchoring filaments and will therefore respond to respiratory movements to the degree that they occur in the area.
  - The initial lymphatics in the abdomen and pelvis respond significantly to respiratory excursions.

The clinical significance of this mechanism is considerable. Lobar pneumonia is an example of an intrapulmonary inflammatory process that will greatly increase the demand on the local lymphatic circulation.

- The local excursion of the thorax, however, is consistently and significantly reduced in the local region of the consolidation.
- This discrepancy will reduce the drainage of the exudate produced by the local inflammation, reduce the delivery of antigen to lymph nodes, and ultimately reduce the delivery of immunity and antibiotics to the area as interstitial pressure rises and shunts blood away from the area.
- Restoring local excursion of the thorax will improve the body's ability to move lymph in this situation; specific lymph pump techniques are also indicated.[41,42]

Asthma is an example of a more generalized inflammatory process of the pulmonary tissues.

- This disease produces a significant, overall restriction of the thorax to the exhalation phase of respiration, reducing both local drainage of lymph from the small airways and central lymph drainage through the thoracic duct.
- This physiologic model should also be considered in patients who have had a thoracotomy and/or sternotomy.
- These procedures produce intrathoracic inflammation, while simultaneously will dramatically reduce the patient's ability to produce excursion of the thorax in the postoperative period, reducing regional drainage.

The work of breathing, with its mechanical considerations associated with respiration, and its respiratory/circulatory function, with its role in the body's response and recovery from disease (especially inflammatory processes), must be considered in the osteopathic evaluation and treatment of any disease of the thorax. The work of breathing directs one to consider the compliance of the thorax, most easily evaluated by motion testing of the spine and ribs. Respiratory/circulatory function depends on the excursion of the thorax, evaluated by passively observing the patient's respiratory excursion. Although there is an undeniable relationship between compliance and excursion, separate evaluation, and consideration of these will lead to a more accurate understanding of the patient and a more appropriate and effective treatment plan.

- For example, a relatively strong and healthy COPD patient may have a relatively good excursion, but a much-reduced thoracic compliance, best seen by motion testing of the ribs and thorax.
- Alternately, a patient just out of surgery will have a greatly reduced excursion, but the compliance may be relatively good.
- These two situations will lead to very different treatment programs.
- The ability to address both compliance and excursion of the thorax is essential to appropriately applying OMT in the management program of patients with a wide variety of diseases.

An important clinical scenario that ties together all the above concepts is the weaning of patients off a ventilator. Mechanical ventilation, even for relatively short periods, impacts the respiratory musculature, compliance of the lungs and chest wall, fluid dynamics of the thorax, and the work of breathing. This, in turn, impairs the functioning of the respiratory system, and ultimately can make weaning from the ventilator extremely difficult, and can potentially lead to chronic ventilator dependence.

The respiratory muscles, unlike most other skeletal muscles, never have rest periods during life. They will therefore weaken, and atrophy relatively quickly compared to other skeletal muscles. This has been shown to occur when a patient is on a ventilator, and the respiratory musculature is given prolonged rest. Biopsy and ultrasound studies have shown the diaphragm to atrophy by more than 20%, and as much as 57% during mechanical ventilation, and these changes have been seen to occur in as little as 18 hours after intubation.[43–45] This atrophy has been shown to weaken diaphragmatic contraction by more than 50%.[45]

Mechanical ventilation also alters fluid dynamics, as it removes the negative intrathoracic pressure necessary for venous and lymphatic drainage, replacing it with a positive pressure. This has been shown to reduce venous return, consequently reducing cardiac output and pulmonary blood volume.[46]

Lymphatic drainage is also impaired during mechanical ventilation, especially when PEEP is utilized. One study showed an improvement in thoracic lymph drainage by 70% with spontaneous breathing, compared to mechanical ventilation with PEEP.[47]

Another showed a reduction in pleural lymph drainage with mechanical ventilation.[48]

Although not quantified in studies, there is a reduced compliance and excursion of the entire spine, ribcage, sternum, and pelvis observable in mechanically ventilated which is consistently

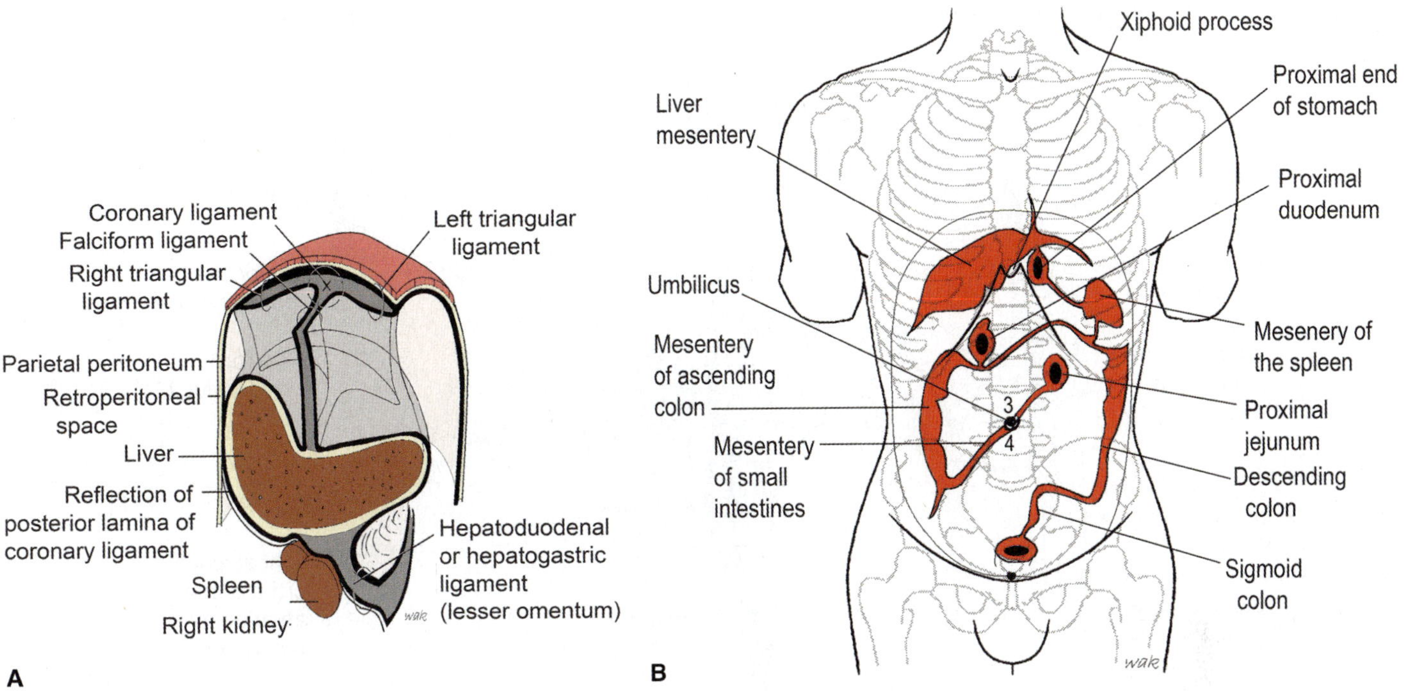

Figure 78.7. **A.** The attachments of the liver to the diaphragm. These are firm and allow the diaphragm to strongly influence portal circulation. **B.** The attachments of the abdominal mesenteries. These provide support for the abdominal viscera as well as providing the pathways for their neurovascular supply. (Illustration by William A. Kuchera, DO, FAAO, used with permission.)

present, and often quite severe, significantly increasing the work of breathing.

When taken together, these consequences of mechanical ventilation serve to create a powerful barrier to extubation and the return to spontaneous breathing, one that increases the longer someone is on a ventilator. The increased fluid load will increase surface tension, predisposing to atelectasis, and increasing both airway and pulmonary parenchymal resistance, while simultaneously increasing the volume of fluid in the alveolar interspaces, impairing gas exchange between the alveolus and capillaries. The changes in the compliance of the thorax will place a significantly increased workload on what quickly becomes weakened, atrophied respiratory muscles, leading to the frequent "failed" weaning trials, when mechanical must be resumed as the respiratory muscles fatigue. OMT can be an important part of the weaning process, reducing the work of breathing as the patient undertakes the process of progressively increasing their strength, until they are able to transition to spontaneous breathing, and be extubated. Also of note is that although edema often occurs throughout the body, the most effective "lymph pump" in a patient who is ventilated is supporting their wean, and working to restore spontaneous breathing, thereby restoring the patient's intrinsic lymph pump, and a physiologic situation much more favorable to fluid return.

Approach to the Abdomen/Pelvis

The abdomen and pelvis form a single space, even though anatomists separate this space into two divisions. The abdomen, viewed as a single space, functionally contains, supports, and influences the function of the GI and the genitourinary viscera.

- The lower ribs and their thoracic vertebral attachments, lumbar spine, sacrum, and pelvic bones form the osseous components of this container.
- The diaphragm, anterior and posterior abdominal walls, and pelvic diaphragm are the myofascial components.
- The abdominal diaphragm is as integrated into the function of the abdomen as it is in the thorax.
- The diaphragm forms the roof of the abdomen and suspends the liver, stomach and spleen, and colon via direct ligamentous attachments (Fig. 78.7).
- Flattening of the diaphragm, which may result from increases in its resting tone, airway obstruction, or sag from fascial strain and drag, will allow sag of these viscera as well as those suspended beneath them.

The posterior attachments of the diaphragm, which lie within the abdomen, are mechanically important. They provide the stable fulcrum necessary for effective contraction.

- The crura blend with the anterior longitudinal ligament of the upper lumbar spine, usually L1–L3.[49] Posterolaterally, the lumbocostal arches extend across the posterior abdominal wall to the tips of the 12th ribs on either side. The medial lumbocostal arch is a thickening of the psoas major fascia (Fig. 78.8). Its medial aspect blends with the crus of the diaphragm. It then crosses over the psoas muscle and is laterally attached to the front of the transverse process of the first lumbar vertebra near its tip. Here, it blends with the lateral lumbocostal arch. The lateral lumbocostal arch is a thickening of the quadratus lumborum fascia. Medially, it is attached to anterior surface of the tip of the transverse process of the first lumbar vertebra. It then crosses over the quadratus lumborum muscle and is attached laterally to the lower border of the 12th rib.
- Together, the lumbocostal arches and the right and left crus of the diaphragm, attaching to the lumbar spine, form a continuous series of five arches, which integrates the function of the diaphragm and posterior abdominal wall.
- Mechanical support for the contraction of the diaphragm comes from the crural anchors to the lumbar spine and from the depression and stabilization of the 12th rib through the contraction of the quadratus and tension in the lumbocostal arches.

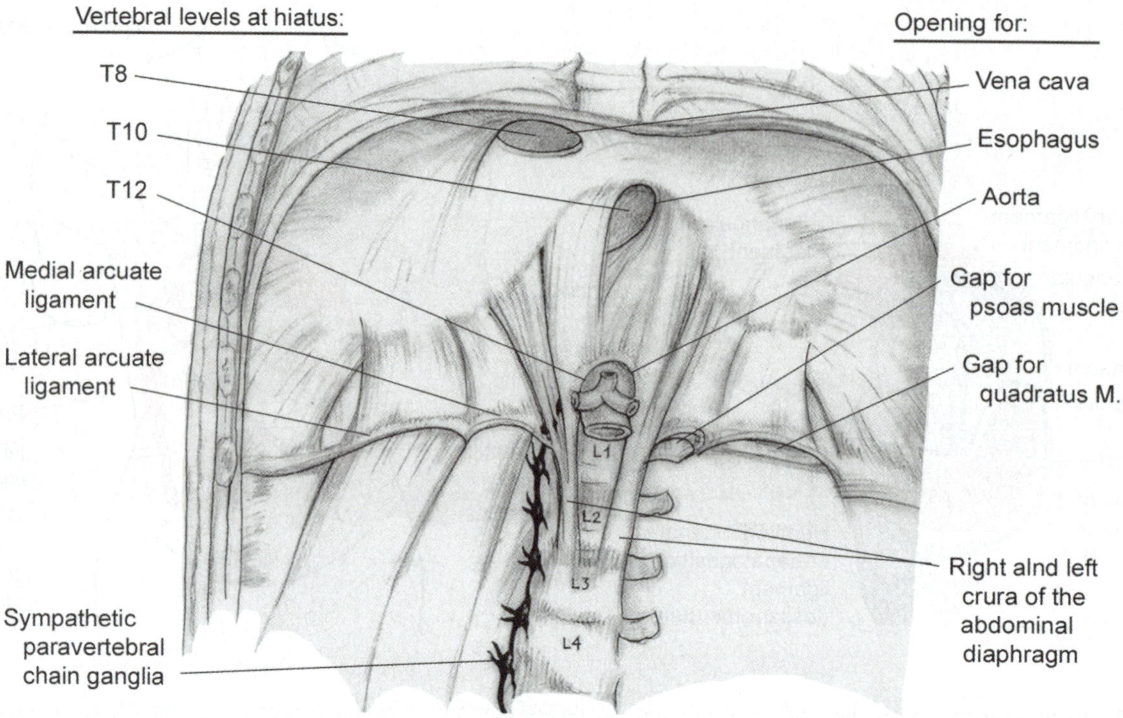

Figure 78.8. The abdominal surface of the diaphragm. The crura and lumbocostal arches blend, forming a continuous series of arches, which anchors the diaphragm posteriorly to the 12th ribs and lumbar spine. (Illustration by William A. Kuchera, DO, FAAO, used with permission.)

- The continuity of the posterior abdominal wall to the pelvic brim and to the lesser trochanter of the hip allows these more remote, but important, mechanical anchors to also be included as supports for diaphragmatic contraction.

Evaluation and treatment of somatic dysfunctions of the crura and lumbocostal arches via the 12th ribs and lumbar spine will have a major impact on the excursion and physiologic function of the diaphragm.

The diaphragm has openings for the passage of numerous structures between the thorax and abdomen (see Fig. 78.8).

- The esophagus passes through a loop in the right crus that acts as the most substantial functional portion of the gastroesophageal sphincter.[49]
  - Dysfunction of the crus is often present in patients with gastroesophageal reflux and hiatal hernia.
  - The right crus is stronger, broader and longer than the left, and originates from the anterolateral surface of the first three lumbar vertebral bodies and their disks. The left crus arise from similar surfaces of the upper two lumbar vertebrae and their disks.[49]
  - The medial margins of the two crura meet in the midline and form the median arcuate ligament and the boundaries of the aortic hiatus.[49]
  - Somatic dysfunction in these regions can alter tension of the crus and OMT may be helpful in the management of patients with these problems.
- The aorta and the cisterna chyli, or beginning of the thoracic duct, pass between the right and left crus.
- During pulmonary respiration, the potential effect of the phasic contraction of the crura may influence normal central lymph flow, through the thoracic duct. If there is increased tension in the crura, the potential for obstruction of central lymph flow must be considered.
- The sympathetic chain with its paraspinal ganglia passes through the medial lumbocostal arch. Several authors have implicated that altered tension of the fascia surrounding the chain ganglia influences the function of the sympathetic chain ganglia.[4,25,31]

The passage beneath the lumbocostal arch is a small, tight space vulnerable to altered tension of the psoas and/or diaphragm.

- The inferior vena cava passes through the tendinous portion of the diaphragm near its apex. Unequal tension in the diaphragm, either side to side or front to back, can draw the central tendon off-center and alter the size, shape, and position of this opening, interfering with passage of blood through the diaphragm. As stated by Dr. Still:

> "He cannot expect blood to quietly pass through the diaphragm if impeded by muscular constriction around the aorta, vena cava, or thoracic duct. The diaphragm can and is often pulled down on both the vena cava and thoracic duct, obstructing blood and chyle (lymph) from returning to [the] heart."[50]

In this regard, one must consider the potential deleterious effects of altered tension in the diaphragm on venous and lymphatic circulation as an additional consideration, using treatment according to the respiratory circulatory model. The diaphragm, on a variety of levels, is intimately involved in the function of the GI system, the circulatory system, and the nervous system.

The iliacus, psoas, and quadratus lumborum constitute the posterior abdominal wall. The role of the posterior abdominal wall in the mechanical function of the diaphragm has been discussed, particularly the lumbocostal arches. The posterior abdominal wall is also involved in support of the abdominal viscera.

- The psoas fascia blends with the fascia of the kidney and is the primary support for this organ.
- The iliopsoas forms a shelf as it crosses the pelvic brim, and this helps to support the cecum and sigmoid colon. Increased tension

in this region will reduce the overall support of the colon and may predispose to sag of the viscera and the mesenteries.

- The posterior abdominal wall is also the site for most of the posterior mesenteric root attachments (see abdominal mesenteries shown in Fig. 78.7), and this further increases its importance as support of the abdominal viscera.
- The ureter travels along the medial aspect of the psoas in the abdomen. It is not surprising that psoas spasm is a common finding in nephrolithiasis and pyelonephritis.
- The deep abdominal lymph nodes also travel in relation to the iliopsoas as they ascend from the inguinal area to the diaphragm.
- The tendon of iliopsoas also forms the floor of the femoral triangle where the inguinal lymph vessels and the femoral veins cross into the pelvis and abdomen.
- The psoas major has an anatomic/functional relationship with the medial arcuate ligament and continues with the thoracic diaphragm and the endothoracic fascia: the psoas major muscle exerts influence on the dynamics of respiratory function and holds a functional relationship between the diaphragm and the pelvic floor.[51]

The pelvic diaphragm forms the floor of the abdominopelvic cavity. Its muscular attachments include the pubic symphysis, the ischial tuberosities, and the coccyx and sacral apex.

- In addition to supporting the pelvic viscera, including the prostate in the male, the pelvic diaphragm forms the external anal sphincter and has an opening for the passage of the urethra and, in the female, the vagina.
- Sensory nerves in the pelvic diaphragm are part of the reflex control mechanism for urination.
- In addition to its roles in the function of the bladder and rectum, the pelvic diaphragm has a role in respiration.[52]
    - The pelvic diaphragm descends with the abdominal diaphragm during inhalation, creating space for the descending abdominal viscera (Fig. 78.9).
    - Clinically, there is tension palpable with its descent.
    - The pelvic diaphragm may act in conjunction with the anterior abdominal wall, lengthening under tension to control the descent of the diaphragm and stabilize abdominal pressure.
    - The abdominal diaphragm will lose the important fulcrum created by the resistance of the viscera if abdominal pressure is reduced by poor tone of the abdominal wall or dysfunction of the pelvic diaphragm.
    - If abdominal pressure is allowed to rise, the increased resistance reduces the effectiveness of the diaphragm and reduces inferior vena cava flow.
        - One of the problems occurring after abdominal surgery is the reduced ability of the abdominal wall to participate in this process.
        - The role of the pelvic diaphragm becomes heightened in the postsurgical patient, and freedom of the sacrum and pelvic diaphragm is essential in this situation.

The integrated function of the diaphragm, pelvic diaphragm, and abdomen, occurring as the patient breathes, plays a significant role in the prognosis of the postsurgical patient. Two of the most common complications from abdominal surgery are atelectasis and pneumonia.[53]

- The patient is predisposed to these complications by the shallow, costal breathing that is so common in postoperative cases.
- Although usually considered to be one of the effects of pain, it has been shown that intraoperative epidural injection, completely blocking postoperative pain, does nothing to alter the limited and dysfunctional diaphragmatic breathing pattern.[54]
- Other explanations for the pattern of altered postsurgery diaphragmatic breathing include the effects of the somatovisceral reflex produced by the incision and the altered abdominal wall function.

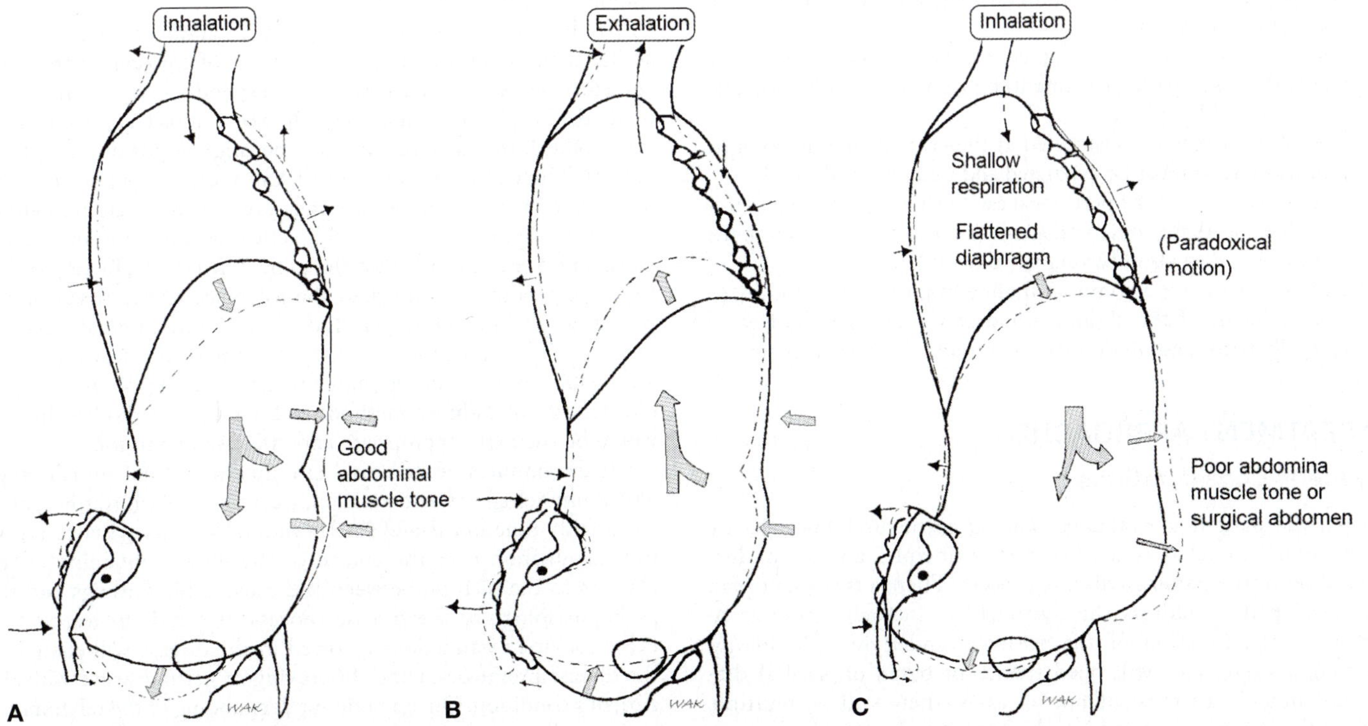

Figure 78.9. **A and B.** Relative movements and function of the abdominal diaphragm, pelvic diaphragm, abdominal wall, spine, and sacrum occurring during respiration. **C.** The effect of a significant abdominal surgical incision or presence of poor abdominal tone on the physiologic movements occurring during breathing. (Illustration by William A. Kuchera, DO, FAAO, used with permission.)

- A midline abdominal incision extending from the xiphoid to the pubic bone will produce bilateral reflex facilitation from the T5–T7 region (including ribs) all the way to the L2–L3 area.
  - This includes the entire attachment of the diaphragm, including the crura, and disproportionately increases the lower thorax workload and limits its excursion.
  - The coordinated action of the abdominal wall and diaphragm is impaired.
  - The abdominal incision alters the tone and reactivity of the abdominal wall, impairing its ability to help control inhalation.
- Osteopathic treatment of the lower thorax and lumbar spine will improve compliance of these tissues, thereby reducing the resistance against which the diaphragm must push.
  - It will simultaneously reduce sympathetic outflow to the entire GI tract and thereby reduce the chance of postoperative ileus, another common postoperative complication.
  - Treatment of the sacrum and pelvis with a focus on maximizing the excursion of the pelvic diaphragm will help compensate for the reduced ability of the abdominal wall to participate in the coordinated control of inhalation.

Respiration also plays a role in abdominal lymph circulation. The role of breathing in the central movement of lymph has already been discussed. Respiration also exerts a powerful influence on the formation of lymph in the abdomen[55]; only peristalsis is more influential.[56] The postsurgical abdomen, particularly when peritonitis is present, responds with a tremendous inflammatory process. At the same time, the two most powerful factors in the abdomen related to the accumulation of lymph and the reduction of lymphatic flow are (1) impaired breathing and (2) the absence of peristalsis.[55,56] Osteopathic treatment to promote lymph formation and flow is important to the immediate healing process.

- The inability to clear inflammatory exudate increases the potential to produce the most common long-term complication of abdominal surgery, adhesions.
- Most diseases of the abdomen are inflammatory and will respond to osteopathic treatment to promote the formation and propulsion of lymph.
- Lymph flow may be obstructed at the crura of the diaphragm, and this region must be evaluated and treated if indicated.
- Lymph vessels exit the peritoneal cavity via the mesenteric roots and drag on these mesenteries will increase the tension at the root, which may also obstruct the flow of lymph.
- Mesenteric drag is a common finding in postsurgical and medical problems of the abdomen and pelvis and may be treated carefully with mesenteric lifts, to promote the flow of lymph.

TREATMENT APPROACHES

General Considerations

First, the patient is evaluated, and the structural findings are interpreted in relation to the above principles and an understanding of the patient's disease process. Then, a treatment plan is developed to address the dysfunctions in such a way as to improve the function of the patient's underlying physiology. Often, a single area will need treatment based on several different models. In most, if not all cases, there will be multiple physiologic issues that can be addressed simultaneously through a treatment process. For example, an area of the thoracic spine and ribs may be facilitated in a patient who has a dysfunctional breathing pattern and central lymph congestion. In such a case, the ribs need only be treated once to accomplish all three treatment goals, as the choice of technique is one that is consistent with accomplishing all three goals. Furthermore, the techniques described in each of the treatment areas that follow may or may not be the proper choice for any patient, even if they have the same diagnosis. The choice of technique is based on the effect desired and the condition of the patient. Sometimes, it is the combination of techniques in a particular sequence that best achieves the desired physiologic effects.

It is important to keep the treatment within the capabilities of the patient. It is often difficult, if not impossible, to know what those capabilities are before initiating the treatment. It is also difficult to know in advance which techniques will be effective and well tolerated. Therefore, in the acutely ill patient, it is often best to apply a focused manipulative treatment, in a minimal effective time frame, and then recheck later to see how the patient responds. At that time, the type and dosage of treatment for that patient can be better formulated. The most effective way to consistently provide a safe and effective treatment is to monitor the effect of a chosen technique on the patient while it is being performed, sensing how the tissues are reacting to the technique and modifying the technique, as indicated, as it is being applied. A common mistake of the inexperienced practitioner is to place all their attention on the procedural aspects they are performing and not sense the dynamic nature of the patient's tissue changes occurring during the treatment process. By paying attention to the patient and the palpated tissues as the treatment is performed, several things become possible. The technique and the forces involved may be continuously adjusted to the response of the tissue, making the treatment more effective. This is particularly useful in deciding between a direct and indirect method of treatment in a particular area. The initial impression may be to perform a direct method treatment, but as the tissue barriers are engaged, the response of the tissue may suggest that an indirect approach should be performed instead.

If the initial impression suggests an indirect approach, but as the tissue is positioned into its point of freedom there is no palpatory sense that the tissues are responding to the treatment method, the physician may need to use a direct approach or at least recheck the diagnosis and/or the original positioning of the patient. The choice between direct and indirect approaches is an important one; indirect approaches are, by their nature, gentler than direct approaches. Since the activating force for an indirect treatment comes from within the patient, it is virtually impossible to give a treatment more than the tolerance of the tissue or the patient as a whole. However, since they require internal forces to generate the therapeutic response, sometimes the sickest patients are unable to generate enough force to accomplish the desired effect from an indirect method, and a direct method technique would be the more appropriate and effective one to use.

If the findings of structural examination do not initially suggest a physiologic treatment plan, treatment to arbitrarily reduce somatic dysfunction *should not be initiated.* It is far wiser to repeat the examination over the course of the illness, obtaining added clues as to the relation between the osteopathic findings and the pathophysiology of the disease process. It stands to reason that those somatic dysfunctions involved in the disease will change as the disease progresses, either improving or getting worse with the patient's condition. Once a better understanding of the relationship between the somatic dysfunction and disease process is achieved, a physiologic treatment plan to assist that patient's recovery from their disease will be apparent and should be initiated.

Segmental Facilitation

A viscerosomatic reflex is produced when nociceptor input from inflamed viscera reaches a level great enough to produce facilitation of the interneurons of the spinal cord on which they converge. Spread of the impulses within the facilitated cord segment to involve the somatic neurons and the resulting muscle spasm produces a palpable, segmental somatic dysfunction, which, in turn, stimulates somatic nociceptors. This somatic nociceptive input converges on the same spinal cord segment and involves the interneurons of the original visceral input, creating a positive feedback loop, which further increases the reflex output to segmentally related viscera and soma. The goal of osteopathic treatment is to remove the added somatic input, reduce the overall firing of the segmental interneurons, and remove the potentially devastating, self-perpetuating effects of a positive feedback loop. There is no definitive technique for reducing segmental facilitation; any procedure that normalizes the somatic tissues and reduces the nociceptive input will work. Treatment is based on the condition and responsiveness of the patient. However, several guidelines should be followed when designing a treatment program to reduce segmental facilitation. The remainder of this chapter presents these guidelines and manipulative treatment techniques that have been found useful in treating patients with acute segmental facilitation.

NOCICEPTION

Viscerosomatic and somatovisceral reflexes are initiated through pain-carrying fibers. Rapid movements at the vertebral unit, and of course painful maneuvers, have been shown to create a sympathetic motor outburst from the related and also distant facilitated spinal cord segments. Pain experienced at the segment will create further facilitation. Vigorous or painful procedures should be avoided when treating to reduce segmental facilitation, especially in acute situations.

ORDER OF TREATMENT

Neurons in facilitated segments have a low threshold and often fire off, even to signals passing through the spinal cord from other regions. Treatment of the facilitated areas first will help prevent these segments from excessively firing impulses to their related viscera in response to treatment given in another region. Extremely reactive segments may require several treatments before other body areas can be effectively treated, although this is unusual. Gentle, deliberate procedures used throughout the entire treatment will minimize this effect.

FREQUENCY OF TREATMENT

Facilitated segments are often the result of acute visceral processes. The underlying disease will reproduce facilitation at the segments, often quite rapidly. Frequent treatment, even more than once daily, is indicated. As the process improves, treatment frequency may decrease.

ARTICULAR TISSUES

Although the most obvious signs of acute segmental facilitation are found in the soft tissues, remember that treatment is directed to those tissues sending somatic nociceptive information back into the spinal cord. The muscle has a low concentration of nociceptors, whereas a joint capsule has the second highest, next to the skin. Treatment directed toward articular tissues may have a greater effect on the segmental facilitation than soft tissue techniques, such as myofascial releases or counterstrain. The techniques presented will all be directed toward the tension in articular segments.

SKELETAL/FASCIAL RELATIONS

Traditional focus has been on the areas immediately surrounding the sympathetic chain ganglia as these have an increased clinical importance in the treatment of segmental facilitation. Patriquin suggests an effect of respiratory motion on the functioning of the chain ganglia.[4] Kuchera and Kuchera discuss the fascial relation of the ganglia with the rib head.[25] Johnston also focuses on the costovertebral junction in his discussion of the diagnosis of viscerosomatic reflexes.[7] Sutherland discusses the relationship between anterior vertebral ligamentous and fascial tension and autonomic function.[31] Although the known physiology of reflex phenomena focuses on the nociceptor input as the cause of segmental facilitation, and both somatic and visceral motor (via the chain ganglia) as the effects, one cannot deny the improved clinical response when the application of manipulative treatment is directed more specifically to the somatic dysfunctions and paraspinal fascial and ligamentous tissues in the anatomic location of the chain ganglia related to the patient's visceral dysfunction. The sacral plexus lies anterior to the sacrum. The lumbar chain ganglia lie anterior to the bodies of the lumbar vertebrae, medial to the edge of psoas. The thoracic chain ganglia lie anterior to the heads of the ribs. The cervical ganglia lie anterior to the cervical transverse processes.

SPECIFIC MANIPULATIVE TREATMENT TECHNIQUES

All the techniques described here are direct methods; they engage a restrictive barrier and involve the application of an activating force. They are especially applicable to the hospital patient and may be used to produce a wide variety of physiologic effects. Force should always be introduced gradually, with attention to the patient and the patient's response, and maintained at the level that matches or balances the resistance or tension felt in the tissues.

Indirect method techniques may also be used in the treatment of acute segmental facilitation and should be considered especially in patients whose tissues are sensitive or reactive to the application of outside forces. Indirect technique, on the other hand, will not always work, because the acutely ill patient may not be able to generate the inherent forces necessary to affect a good response to the treatment process.

Paravertebral Ganglia Techniques

DIRECT RIB RELEASE

Position

1. The patient is supine. The physician is seated at the side of the patient.
2. One hand of the physician identifies a single rib to be treated. The other hand extends under the patient to the spinous process and identifies the two segments with which a typical rib articulates. This is most easily done by gently springing the rib medially while monitoring the spinous process.
3. Contact the two vertebrae at the spinous processes and simultaneously carry the rib and two vertebrae laterally. This will disengage the costovertebral articulation.

FIRST RIB/STELLATE GANGLION TECHNIQUE

The stellate ganglia sit just anterior to the heads of the first ribs.

Position

1. The patient is supine. The physician is seated or standing at the head of the bed.

2. The physician contacts the posterior aspects of the first ribs at the angle with the thumbs of each hand.
3. The physician simultaneously applies gentle lateral traction to both ribs, gradually increasing until the traction force is equal to the resistance found in the tissues.
4. Traction is held at this level until release is felt.

SUBOCCIPITAL DECOMPRESSION

The superior cervical ganglion and vagus nerve are related to the occipital–atlantal and suboccipital tissues.

Position

1. The patient is supine. The physician is seated at the head of the bed.
2. The physician places the finger pads in the patient's suboccipital sulcus (groove) on both sides.
3. The physician carries their elbows medially, placing superior and lateral traction on the suboccipital tissues.
4. The physician simultaneously places gentle traction on the occiput. The force of the physician's traction matches the resistance of the tissues.
5. This position is held until release of both sides is felt.

LUMBAR GANGLIA TECHNIQUE

Position

1. The patient is supine with their arms crossed over their chest. The physician is seated at the side of the patient.
2. The physician makes a fist with the fingers of the cephalad hand, leaving the thumb extended.
3. The physician slides that hand under the patient's upper lumbar spine, fitting the lumbar spinous processes in the depression between the distal phalanges and the base of the hand.
4. The physician applies a gentle superior lift with the cephalad hand, the knuckles, and base of the hand maintaining even pressure on the respective transverse processes.
5. With the caudad hand on the patient's elbows, the physician uses downward pressure into the bed (or treatment table) to closely control the lift of the fingers, balancing the lift to the resistance felt in the tissues.
6. This positioning is held until release is felt.

Sacral Plexus Techniques

SACROILIAC DECOMPRESSION

Position

1. The patient is supine. The physician is seated at the side of the patient.
2. The physician contacts the medial aspect of the posterior superior iliac spine and associated medial ilium with the finger pads of one or both hands.
3. The physician leans back, with the arms as straight as possible to create the traction with their shoulders and trunk, rather than with the forearms.
4. The physician's traction equally matches the resistance that is palpated.
5. The physician holds until yielding or release is felt.
6. This process is repeated on the other side.

SACRAL TECHNIQUE

Position

1. The patient is supine with the arms crossed over the chest. The physician is seated at the side of the patient.
2. The physician contacts the sacrum in the midline, with the caudad hand on the inferior lateral angle near the sacral apex and the cephalad hand on the sacral base above the level of S2. Alternately, the physician may use only one hand and spread the fingers so that some rest above and the others rest below the S2 sacral vertebra.
3. The physician's fingers, contacting the patient's sacrum, are gently lifted anteriorly. The physician's arms are resting on the bed or tabletop, and the degree of lift is controlled by applying downward pressure on the elbows and upward pressure with the fingers.
4. This position of lift is held until a yielding or release is felt.

Collateral (Prevertebral) Ganglia Inhibition Techniques

ABDOMINAL GANGLIA INHIBITION

The celiac and the superior mesenteric and inferior mesenteric ganglia may be treated by the same method, altering the hand position on the abdomen for the different ganglia. The celiac area is below the xiphoid, the inferior mesenteric just above the umbilicus, and the superior mesenteric halfway between.[a]

Position

1. The patient is supine. The physician stands at the side of the patient.
2. The physician's finger pads of one or both hands are lined up along the patient's midabdominal line, contacting the skin over the collateral ganglion that is to be inhibited[a] (Fig. 78.10).
3. The physician applies a gentle, downward pressure until the resistance of the underlying tissues is felt and its resistance is matched.
4. This pressure is held until a softening or release is felt.

CERVICAL GANGLIA INHIBITION

Although the cervical ganglia are situated more like the collateral (paravertebral) ganglia, the cervical ganglia functions more like prevertebral ganglia, having their spinal origin in the thoracic spinal cord.

Position

1. The patient is supine. The physician is seated at the head of the bed or table.
2. The physician's finger pads contact the articular pillars of the patient's cervical spine on both sides.
3. The physician gently lifts the finger contacts in an anterior and superior direction until articular (not soft tissue) resistance is perceived and matches the degree of lift.
4. This amount of lift is held until release is sensed.

Thoracic and Costal Cage Region Techniques

The treatments described here are designed to increase thoracic compliance and excursion. Choice of method in clinical situations will depend primarily on the condition and tolerance of the patient. One will encounter patients limited to the supine position, such as the postoperative thoracotomy patient, and those limited to sitting, such as the patient with COPD. Adaptability in applying treatment techniques is key to giving an effective treatment.

---

[a]This technique should not be attempted in the postoperative patient with a midline abdominal incision.

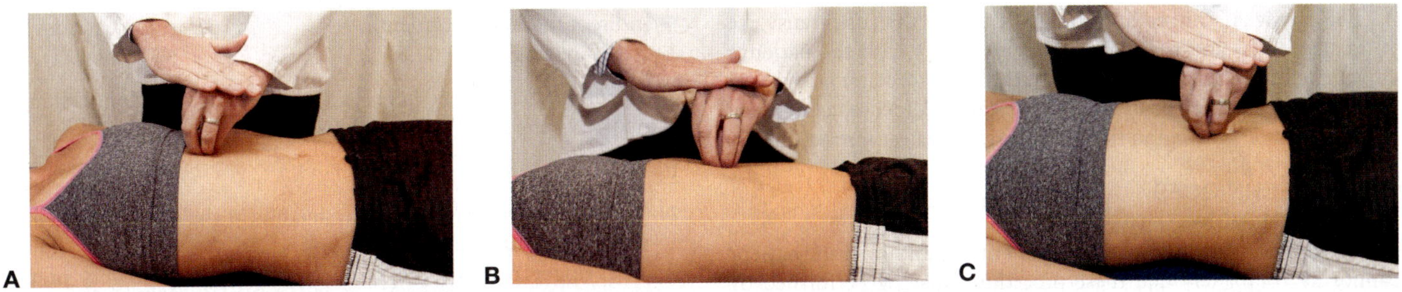

Figure 78.10. **Abdominal ganglia inhibition technique.** Use one hand to apply controlled pressure and the other to contact and assess tissue tension and response to the pressure. **A.** Celiac ganglia. **B.** Superior mesenteric ganglia. **C.** Inferior mesenteric ganglia. (Courtesy of Western University of Health Sciences, Pomona, CA, used with permission.)

Appropriate caution must always be exercised when working with acutely ill patients. Autonomic and lymphatic considerations should also be applied to the thorax. They are described elsewhere in the chapter.

SEATED TECHNIQUES

In acute respiratory illness, or CHF, the patient is sometimes unable to lie down for treatment. Seated techniques are particularly useful in these situations. All procedures described may be done very gently or more forcefully depending on the particulars of the case. Care must always be exercised when using force in an acutely ill hospitalized patient.

TRANSLATION OF THE SPINE

Since the heads of ribs two through ten articulate with a vertebral unit, rather than a single vertebral segment, the motion of the thoracic spine is intimately involved with rib motion and thoracic compliance.

Position

1. The patient is seated. The physician stands at the left side of the patient.
2. The patient's left hand is placed on the right shoulder.
3. The physician places their left hand over the patient's hand and right shoulder while allowing the left axilla to rest lightly on the patient's left shoulder for patient control.
4. The physician's right palm is placed over the patient's left paravertebral tissues near the T10–T12 region.
5. The physician simultaneously leans on the patient's left shoulder and places a right lateral translatory force on the spine via the left axillary and right-hand contacts.
6. The physician moves the hand contact and the apex of the translation superiorly, and the right lateral translatory force to the spine is repeated until the entire hemithorax is mobilized. A focused effort may be placed on the region with the greatest restriction.
7. The physician then moves to the patient's right side, positions of the patient's arms and the physician's arms and hands are reversed, and the other side of the thorax is treated with translation to the left.

Note: This mobilization by spinal translation can also be carried into the lumbar region of the body.

ROTATION AND RIB RAISING

Position

1. The patient is seated. The physician stands on the left side of the patient.
2. The patient's left hand is placed on the right shoulder.
3. The physician places their left hand over the patient's hand and right shoulder while allowing their left axilla to rest lightly on the patient's left shoulder for control of the patient.
4. The physician's right palm is placed over the patient's lower right rib cage with the thenar eminence in the area of the tenth rib angle.
5. The physician simultaneously produces a right anterolateral translatory force as the patient's body is rotated to the left.
6. The right-hand contact with the patient's right rib angles is moved superiorly, and the right anterolateral translatory force and left rotation of the spine are repeated until the entire hemithorax is mobilized. A focused effort may be placed on the region with the greatest restriction.
7. The physician then moves to the patient's right side, positions of the patient's arms and the physician's arms and hands are reversed, and the left side of the thorax is treated in a similar manner.

RIB RAISING

Position

The patient is seated with arms crossed in front of the chest. The physician stands facing the patient. Shorter physicians treating taller patients may modify this to patients' arms crossed and placed over the physician's shoulder.

1. The patient's arms are supported on the physician's chest, and the physician's hands reach around the patient to contact the patient's rib angles on both sides (Fig. 78.11).
2. The physician leans so that gentle extension of the patient's thoracic spine occurs and simultaneously carries the contact with the patient's ribs, anteriorly and superiorly.

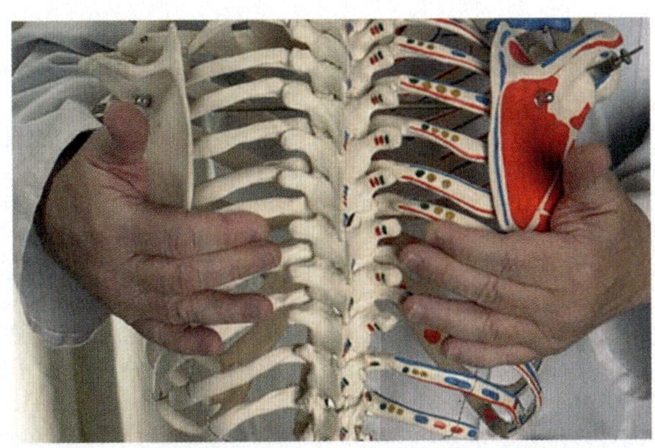

Figure 78.11. **For seated rib raising OMT, the physician's hands contact the rib angles, as shown on a skeleton model.** (Courtesy of Western University of Health Sciences, Pomona, CA, used with permission.)

3. The physician's finger tips are just lateral to the costotransverse joints (CTJs) and their fingers are in contact with the patient's rib angles superiorly and/or inferiorly. The procedure is repeated until all the patient's ribs have been treated. A focused effort may be placed on any region that exhibits the greatest restriction.

SUPINE TECHNIQUES

Mobilizing the Ribs

This is rib raising coordinated with patient respiration. If the patient cannot lie completely flat, these procedures may be performed by elevating the head of the bed or emergency room stretcher to a more comfortable angle. These techniques are useful in the stable acute asthmatic patient, who reacts with further increased difficulty in breathing, even when very light pressure is applied to the rib cage. These techniques may be adapted to both pump and bucket handle motion. It is best to begin in the area of greatest rib restriction and continue up and/or down the entire thorax until all ribs are treated. By coordinating the procedure to the patient's respiratory rhythm, you can avoid any challenge to the patient's breathing. Used in this way, any of these treatment techniques will immediately lessen the patient's work of breathing and can be used even in patients with the most acute respiratory problems.

- Direct method
  - ☐ Bucket handle ribs

This technique is most useful for lower rib restrictions.

Position

1. The patient is supine. The physician is at the side of the table, facing the patient.
2. The physician's finger pads of the cephalad hand contact rib angles posteriorly, and the finger pads of the caudad hand contact costochondral junction on the same side. The thumbs make a broad contact with rib shafts across the midaxillary line.
3. The physician monitors the patient's breathing with light finger contact until the patient's breathing rhythm is familiar.
4. Then, as the patient begins to inhale, the physician's hands turn in the same direction, moving both thumbs cephalad, exaggerating the inhalation motion of the bucket handle–type ribs.
5. As the patient begins to exhale, the physician's hands also turn in the opposite direction to exaggerate the exhalation motion of these ribs.

Note: The entire hand and palm should be in contact with the rib cage to broaden the surface area of contact.

- Pump handle ribs

Position

1. The patient is supine. The physician is seated at the side of the table, facing the patient.
2. The physician's finger pads of the cephalad hand contact a pump handle rib posteriorly at its rib angle.
3. The physician's caudad hand contacts the same rib anteriorly with its finger pads across the rib's costochondral junction. The palm of this hand is lifted to avoid the breast of a female patient.
4. The physician monitors the patient's breathing with light finger contact until the rhythm of the patient's breathing is familiar.
5. As the patient begins inhalation, the physician's caudal finger pad contacts move superiorly, while the finger pad contacts of the cephalad hand simultaneously move inferiorly to exaggerate the inhalation motion of the pump handle rib.
6. As the patient begins exhalation, there is reversal of the physician's hand movements to exaggerate the exhalation motion of the pump handle rib.

- Indirect method treatment
  - ☐ Rib raising

This method is described here for a single rib dysfunction, although it may be applied to a group of ribs.

Position

1. The patient is supine. The physician is at the side of the bed or table, facing the patient.
2. The finger pads of the index and/or middle fingers of the physician's cephalad hand contact the restricted rib posteriorly across its angle.
3. The physician's index and/or middle fingers of the caudad hand contact the same rib anteriorly across the patient's costochondral junction.
4. The physician's thumb pads should contact the shaft of that rib at its midaxillary line for added control.
5. The patient's inhalation and exhalation are monitored as the physician gently encourages the rib to move in the direction of its freedom. This is carried to the point of ligamentous balance (point of greatest ease) and held there.
6. Adjustments in cephalad/caudad, anterior/posterior, and traction/compression may need to be carried out by passive motion testing and added to bring about the best-balanced positioning of the rib.
7. Respiratory cooperation may be added by asking the patient to hold their breath in the direction associated with the greatest freedom.
8. The positioning is held in ligamentous balance until release is felt.
9. The rib motion is re-evaluated during active inhalation and exhalation.

STERNAL MOBILIZATION

The mediastinal fascia is continuous with the fibrous pericardium of the heart and central tendon of the diaphragm. The fibrous pericardium of the heart is attached to the sternum via the superior and inferior sternopericardial ligaments. A sternal release may be used to mobilize this important fascial mechanism.

Position

1. The patient is supine. The physician is seated at the head of the table.
2. The physician's anterior hand contacts the sternum and manubrium, and the palm of their posterior hand is placed posteriorly across the patient's spinous processes, approximately in the T1–T6 region.
3. The physician's sternal contact moves the patient's sternum through its six motions—superior, inferior, lateral to the right, lateral to the left, clockwise rotation, and counterclockwise rotation—determining its directions of restriction in motion.
4. The hand of the physician's spinal contact will always be moved in the direction that is opposite to the sternal restrictions.
5. As the patient continues to breathe normally, each sternal preference is held at its motion barrier until release occurs. Rather than doing each motion separately, the sternal restrictions can be taken to their restrictive barrier and each "stacked upon the other" and the composite held until release occurs.

Note: This can also be performed as an indirect method technique. To do this, the sternal motions are stacked, or each is separately carried to the point of ligamentous balance and held at that balance while intrinsic forces release the dysfunction. Respiratory force can be added to hasten release by having the patient hold their breath in the phase that produces the most ligamentous relaxation.

Abdominal Treatment Techniques

The abdomen follows the principle that the shape of a container will affect the function of its contents. The abdomen has a roof, a floor, and anterior and posterior walls. The diaphragm is the roof of the abdomen; the liver, spleen, and supporting mesenteries are suspended from it. The pelvic diaphragm is the floor. It supports the abdominal and pelvic viscera, along with the shelf created as the posterior abdominal wall crosses the pelvic brim. The iliopsoas and quadratus lumborum make up the posterior abdominal wall. The insertion of iliopsoas on the lesser trochanter of the femur involves the hip in abdominal and pelvic function. The aforementioned structures are usually treated before directly treating the viscera. The autonomic relationships and lymphatic drainage of the abdomen and pelvis should also be considered. See Chapter 55 Visceral Manipulation for more techniques.

DIRECT HIP RELEASE

Position

1. The patient is supine. The physician is at the side of the table on the side of the leg to be treated.
2. The physician's cephalad hand contacts the patient's hip behind the greater trochanter for monitoring.
3. The physician's caudad hand holds the leg so it can be maneuvered.
4. The physician's caudad hand induces abduction/adduction and internal/external rotation to find the point of balanced tension of the hip joint.
5. While monitoring with the cephalad hand, the physician's caudad hand places the patient's ankle into the axilla to control the patient's leg position. The caudad hand then moves up to or above the knee to create a fulcrum.
6. The distal part of the patient's extremity is taken medially to create lateral traction at the femoral head and held in that position.
7. When lateral release is felt, the physician applies inferior traction on the patient's leg and holds that until another release is felt.

PELVIC DIAPHRAGM RELEASE

Position

1. The patient is in the lateral recumbent position with the legs and knees flexed. The physician stands behind the patient. This may also be done with the patient in the supine position with the physician standing by the patient on the side that is to be treated. *The physician should explain the procedure to the patient and that contact will be made near an intimate area before proceeding.*
2. The extended fingers of the physician's caudad hand contact the ischial tuberosity of the patient on the dysfunctional side. The fingers are then moved at a point that is just medial and slightly caudad to the tuberosity; the finger pads may stay in contact with the medial aspect of the tuberosity.
3. The physician's fingertips and rigid fingers are then gently but firmly advanced, medial to the sacrotuberous ligaments, into the ischiorectal fossa until the resistance of the pelvic diaphragm (on that side) is initially palpated (see Fig. 50.20 in Chapter 50 Lymphatic Drainage Procedures).
4. At that point, the excursion of the pelvic diaphragm is monitored during the patient's respiratory efforts.
5. Then, the fingers are held at the point of tissue tension (*not lifted to produce more tension*). They simply resist the downward movement of the pelvic diaphragm that occurs as the patient inhales slowly and deeply.
6. The physician's fingers follow the pelvic diaphragmatic tension cephalad as the patient exhales slowly and completely.
7. Steps 5 and 6 are repeated until the maximal amount of diaphragmatic lift (muscular tension release) has occurred.
8. The patient is turned to the opposite lateral recumbent position. With the physician behind the patient, the other half of the pelvic diaphragm is released in a similar manner.

POSTERIOR ABDOMINAL DIAPHRAGMATIC RELEASES

Releasing the Lumbar Spine/Crura

Position

1. The patient is supine, and the physician is at the side of the table facing the patient.
2. The physician evaluates T12–L3 for somatic dysfunction or increased paraspinal tissue tension.
3. The physician then contacts the spinous processes on either side of the vertebral unit that has somatic dysfunction.
4. The vertebral unit is moved in directions that exaggerate its freedom of motion—flexion/extension, rotation, and right or left side bending.
5. These directions of freedom may be individually held at their point of ligamentous balance, or each direction of motion preference might be stacked, one upon the other, and released.
6. Release occurs as the tissues are held at their point of ligamentous balance.
7. Respiratory effort of the patient may be added to hasten the release. This is performed by asking the patient to hold their breath in the respiratory cycle that is sensed to be accompanied by the greatest relaxation of the tissues.

Releasing the 12th Ribs/Arcuate Ligaments

Position

1. The patient is supine. The physician is at the side of the patient to be treated.
2. The physician contacts the patient's 12th rib near midshaft. *Note:* Doubling finger contact may provide better control. Remember, the 12th rib does not have a rib angle.
3. The physician applies traction to the 12th rib in a direction between the horizontal and the long axis of the 12th rib; settle on the composite direction that maximizes the perception of "tension in the lumbocostal arches," matching the traction force with resistance found in the tissues.
4. The rib is held in this position of traction until release is felt. This may occur as a change in the long axis of the rib rather than just a simple decompression.
5. The physician walks to the other side of the patient, and the technique is repeated for the other 12th rib.

Anterolateral Abdominal Diaphragm Releases

Position

1. The patient is seated. The physician stands behind the patient.
2. The physician reaches around the patient and contacts the soft tissues just below the costal margin (chondral masses) with the finger pads of both hands.
3. The patient is asked to slouch as the physician supports the patient's back with their chest. This allows the physician's fingers to advance medially and superiorly around the costal margin.
4. The excursion of the abdominal diaphragm during respiration is monitored.
5. The physician's finger placements gently resist the downward motion of the diaphragm as the patient inhales and follow the diaphragm superiorly as the patient exhales. Note: *Do not push upward against the diaphragm.*

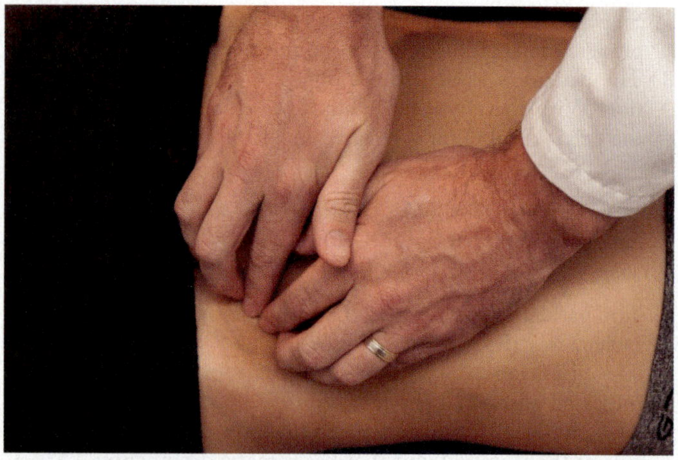

Figure 78.12. Abdominal lift for the left lower quadrant internal organs and fascial attachments. (Courtesy of Western University of Health Sciences, Pomona, CA, used with permission.)

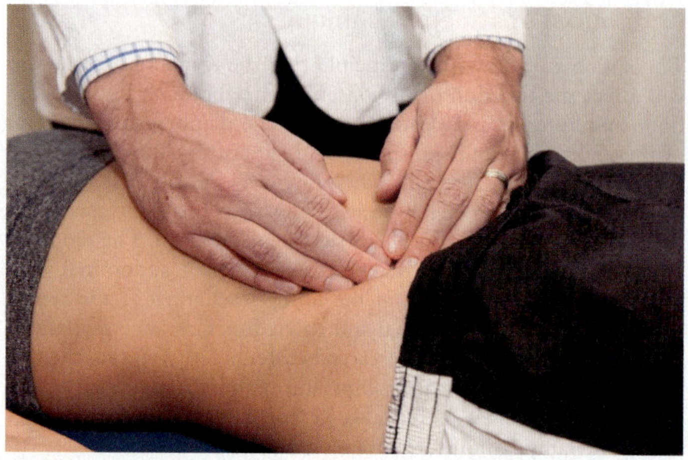

Figure 78.13. Abdominal lift for the right lower quadrant internal organs and fascial attachments. (Courtesy of Western University of Health Sciences, Pomona, CA, used with permission.)

6. Step 5 is repeated, as the patient continues to take slow, deep breaths, until a release is felt.
7. The fingers of the physician's hands are then moved medially or laterally until the entire anterolateral surface of the diaphragm has been treated.

ABDOMINAL LIFTS

Abdominal lifts provide a safe, simple means of addressing ptosis and congestion of the abdominal viscera and its mesenteries. More specific treatment techniques for the viscera should not be attempted until palpatory skill and anatomic familiarity with the abdomen have been studied and achieved.

Position

1. The patient is supine with the knees bent to 90 degrees and the feet are flat on the table. The physician stands at the side of the patient that is to be treated.
2. The physician contacts the lower left quadrant of the abdomen just superior to the inguinal ligament and gently inserts the finger pads into the patient's abdomen (Fig. 78.12).
3. The physician then gently lifts the patient's abdominal contents obliquely toward the right upper quadrant until slight tension is palpable.
4. The tissues are then held in this position until a release is felt and the contents can be moved slightly further toward the patient's right upper quadrant. *Note:* The physician should be attentive so that the lift occurs to the internal organs and not just the anterior abdominal wall.
5. Steps 3 and 4 are repeated until the patient's maximal release has been accomplished.
6. For the right lower quadrant, repeat steps 1 to 5, lifting vertically toward the *right* upper quadrant (Fig. 78.13). *Note:* A minor vibration may be transmitted to the abdomen by the physician's finger contacts and be substituted for the lift. Also, respiratory force may accentuate and hasten the release of a lift. Respiratory force is instituted by asking the patient to take a partial breath in and hold it until they must breathe. Just as the patient must take a breath, the physician will notice a release of the tissues.

Lymph Mobilization

STIMULATING THE MOVEMENT OF LYMPH

Osteopathic treatment to enhance lymph flow is described elsewhere in this text. In this chapter, the concept of interstitial fluid fluctuation was introduced in relation to lymph formation and flow. Techniques to stimulate the formation of lymph using this principle were taught by Anne Wales, DO, and will be presented here as an addition to those presented in Chapter 50 Lymphatic Drainage Procedures. The respiratory mechanism, as well as any areas of restriction along the course of drainage, should be treated before stimulating the formation and movement of lymph.

Osteopathic treatment designed to stimulate formation and movement of lymph is based on an understanding of the physiology and mechanics of lymph formation and propulsion. A limiting factor in lymphatic drainage is the movement of fluid from the interstitium into the initial lymphatic vessels. This is the formation of lymph. There are no inherent hydrostatic or osmotic gradients to drive this process. Fluid fluctuation and rhythmic movement in the immediate environment of the initial lymphatic vessels form lymph. These actions form the physiologic basis for most of the following lymphatic techniques. Successful treatment depends upon creating a rhythmic fluctuation of extracellular fluid. This movement of fluid can be palpated and monitored from the hand contact on the patient and must be differentiated from the tissue movements monitored during treatment on the musculoskeletal tissues. The movement of the body's fluids in response to the treatment is the key.

Propulsion of lymph is dependent on several factors. Stretch receptors located in the distal end of lymphatic vessels, responsive to the formation of lymph, begin the peristaltic contraction of smooth muscle in the wall of the lymph vessels. The thin and pliable lymphatic vessels are also responsive to external pressures, such as skeletal muscle contraction in muscle adjacent to the vessel. The relative importance of these factors differs in different areas.

LATERAL FLUCTUATION AT THE KNEE

Position

1. The patient is supine. The physician stands at the side of the patient to be treated.
2. The physician flexes the patient's knee to 90 degrees and the hip to 45 degrees; the patient's foot is resting flat on the table.
3. The physician's caudad hand gently holds the dorsum of the patient's foot and ankle.
4. The physician's cephalad hand rests on top of the patient's knee.
5. The physician gently moves the patient's leg medially and laterally at the knee to find the position of greatest ease.
6. At that point of ligamentous balance, a small medial, lateral excursion is initiated and maintained.

LATERAL FLUCTUATION AT THE FOREARM

Position

1. The patient is seated. The physician sits facing the patient.
2. The physician grasps the hand of the patient on the affected side as if to make a handshake.
3. The physician's other hand supports the patient's elbow, keeping it at 90 degrees.
4. The patient's forearm is supinated and pronated to find the point of greatest ease.
5. From this point of ligamentous balance, a gentle, rhythmic pronation/supination excursion is initiated to fluctuate fluid.

ABDOMINAL LYMPH STIMULATION

Abdominal lymphatics reside in the mesenteries of the abdomen. Dr. W.G. Sutherland described the use of a transmitted vibration to stimulate the movement of abdominal and thoracic lymph. The effect of the vibration is to produce a wave like that produced by a pebble landing in the center of a pond. The transmitted vibration to the abdomen will also act to lift the mesenteries in a very gentle manner. This can be useful in acute situations, such as the immediate postoperative period. These specific techniques were demonstrated by Dr. Wales and are based on this concept.

Position

1. The patient is supine with knees bent to relax the abdominal wall. The physician stands at the right side of the patient.
2. A physician contacts the patient's left lower abdomen just superior to the inguinal ligament, placing one hand over the other.
3. The tissues are gently lifted superomedially until the first sense of resistance is palpable.
4. A transmitted vibration is directed toward the cisterna chyli—a point that would be approximately posterior to halfway between the xiphoid process and the umbilicus, slightly to the right of center. This point will be approximately perpendicular to the suspension of the mesentery of the descending colon.
5. A palpatory sense of decongestion or lift of the mesenteries indicates successful treatment.
6. The physician walks to the left side of the patient and contacts the right lower abdomen in the same manner, and steps 3 through 5 are repeated for the right side of the patient.

THORACIC DUCT TECHNIQUE

Dr. Sutherland likened the thoracic duct to a siphon, indicating a functional significance to the turn located at its superior end, that allows it to drain downward into the superior aspect of the subclavian vein. The thoracic duct may be stimulated with a transmitted vibration at its proximal and distal ends.

Position

1. The patient is supine, and the physician stands on the right side of the patient.
2. The physician contacts the patient's abdomen just below the costal margin and to the right of center, in the area overlying the cisterna chyli. Use the contact of one hand over the other hand.
3. The physician induces a transmitted vibration directed toward the cisterna chyli.
4. Then, the physician contacts the left anterior chest wall at the second or third intercostal space, near the midclavicular line, using the one-hand-over-the-other-hand contact.
5. The physician transmits a vibration of tissues directed posteriorly and slightly laterally.
6. A perceived change in the quality of the deep tissues or a sense of decongestion may become apparent as the treatment proceeds.

CONCLUSION

Osteopathic treatment of the acutely ill or hospitalized patient is designed to support and enhance the underlying physiology of a patient as they recover from an illness or other severe stress. Care must be taken to ensure that the treatment is appropriate and within the physical capabilities of the patient to respond appropriately. Specialist level of intervention may be indicated in unusual and challenging cases, but many cases can be treated effectively by osteopathic physicians, residents, and students if the principles described in this chapter are followed. The structural examination findings, along with knowledge of the pathophysiology of the disease process and individual patient's condition, are combined to form a unique treatment plan for each patient, at each visit.

ACKNOWLEDGMENTS

Special thanks to the guidance, hard work, valuable suggestions, and drawings of William Kuchera, DO, FAAO. This chapter is better because of his efforts.

REFERENCES

1. Korr IM, Wright HM, Thomas PE. Effects of experimental myofascial insults on cutaneous patterns of sympathetic activity in man. *Acta Neuroveg (Wien)*. 1962;23(22):329–355.
2. Nicholas AS, DeBias DA, Ehrenfeuchter W, et al. A somatic component to myocardial infarction. *Br Med J (Clin Res Ed)*. 1985;291(6487):13–17.
3. Denslow JS, Korr I, Krems AD. Quantitative studies of chronic facilitation in human motoneuron pools. *Am J Physiol*. 1947;150:229–238.
4. Patriquin DA. Viscerosomatic reflexes. In: Patterson MM, Howell JN, eds. *The Central Connection: Somatovisceral and Viscerosomatic Interaction*. University Classics, Ltd.; 1992.
5. Beal MC, Morlock JS. Somatic dysfunction associated with pulmonary disease. *J Am Osteopath Assoc*. 1984;82:179–183.
6. Beal MC. Palpatory testing for somatic dysfunction in patients with cardiovascular disease. *J Am Osteopath Assoc*. 1983;82:822–831.
7. Johnston WL. Segmental definition: III. Definitive basis for distinguishing somatic findings of visceral reflex origin. *J Am Osteopath Assoc*. 1988;88:347–353.
8. Beal MC. Viscerosomatic reflexes: a review. *J Am Osteopath Assoc*. 1985; 85(12):53–68.
9. Cathie A. Physiological motions of the spine as related to respiratory activity. In: Barnes MW, ed. *AAO Yearbook*. American Academy of Osteopathy; 1974:59–60.
10. Zink JG. Applications of the osteopathic holistic approach to homeostasis. In: Barnes MW, ed. *AOA Yearbook*. American Academy of Osteopathy; 1973:37–47.
11. Still AT. *The Philosophy and Mechanical Principles of Osteopathy*. Hudson-Kimberly Publishing Co; 1902:155.
12. Rabinovici N, Navot N. The relationship between respiration, pressure and flow distribution in the vena cava and portal and hepatic veins. *Surg Gynecol Obstet*. 1980;151(6):753–763.
13. Millard FP. *Applied Anatomy of the Lymphatics*. The Journal Printing Co; 1922:26.
14. Sutherland WG. *Teaching in the Science of Osteopathy*. Rudra Press; 1990.
15. Hurley JV. Inflammation. In: Staub NC, Taylor AE, eds. *Edema*. Raven Press; 1984:463–488.
16. Atkinson TP. Histamine and serotonin. In: Gallin JI, Goldstein I, Snyderman R, eds. *Inflammation: Basic Principles and Clinical Correlates*. Raven Press; 1992:196.
17. Movat HZ. *The Inflammatory Reaction*. Elsevier; 1985.
18. Olszewski WL, Pazdur J, Kubasiewicz E, Zaleska M, Cooke CJ, Miller NE. Lymph drainage from foot joints in rheumatoid arthritis provides insight into local cytokine and chemokine production and transport to lymph nodes. *Arthritis Rheum*. 2001;44(3):541–549.

19. Witte CL, Witte MH. Lymphatics in the pathophysiology of edema. In: Johnston MG, ed. *Experimental Biology of the Lymphatic Circulation.* Elsevier; 1985:167–188.
20. Van Buskirk R. Nociceptive reflexes and somatic dysfunction: a model. *J Am Osteopath Assoc.* 1990;90(9):792–794, 797–809.
21. Schmidt RF. Neurophysiologic mechanisms of arthritic pain. In: Patterson MM, Howell JN, eds. *The Central Connection: Somatovisceral and Viscerosomatic Interaction.* University Classics, Ltd.; 1992.
22. Talman WT. The central nervous system and cardiovascular control in health and disease. In: Low PA, ed. *Clinical Autonomic Disorders.* Little, Brown and Company; 1993.
23. Korr IM. Sustained sympathicotonia as a factor in disease. In: Korr IM, ed. *The Neurobiologic Mechanisms in Manipulative Therapy.* Plenum Publishing Co; 1978:229–268.
24. Qing-Gong F, Chandler MJ, McNeill DL, Foreman RD. Vagal afferent fibers excite upper cervical neurons and inhibit activity of lumbar spinal cord neurons in the rat. *Pain.* 1992;51(1):91–100.
25. Kuchera M, Kuchera W. *Osteopathic Considerations in Systemic Dysfunction.* 2nd ed. Greyden Press; 1994.
26. Rosero HO, Greene CH, Debias DA. Correlation of palpatory observations with the anatomical locus of acute myocardial infarction. *J Am Osteopath Assoc.* 1987;87:118–122.
27. Wilson P. The osteopathic treatment of asthma. *J Am Osteopath Assoc.* 1946;45(11):491.
28. Geisler GJ. Studies of spinal cord neurons that project directly to the hypothalamus. In: Willard FH, Patterson MM, eds. *Nociception and the Neuroendocrine Immune Connection.* University Classics, Ltd.; 1994.
29. Dinarello CA. Role of interleukin-1 and tumor necrosis factor in systemic responses to infection and inflammation. In: Gallin JI, Goldstein I, Snyderman R, eds. *Inflammation: Basic Principles and Clinical Correlates.* 2nd ed. Raven Press; 1992.
30. Williams PL, ed. *Gray's Anatomy.* 38th ed. Churchill-Livingstone; 1995:1883.
31. Sutherland WG. *Contributions of Thought.* 2nd ed. Rudra Press; 1998:339.
32. West JB. *Pulmonary Pathophysiology: The Essentials.* 4th ed. Williams & Wilkins; 1992:74.
33. West JB. *Respiratory Physiology: The Essentials.* 5th ed. Williams & Wilkins; 1995.
34. Roussos C, Macklem PT. Inspiratory muscle fatigue. In: Ayvazizn LF, ed. *Handbook of Physiology, Section III. The Respiratory System, Vol. III. The Mechanics of Breathing, Part II.* American Physiological Society; 1986:521.
35. Grassino A, Macklem PT. Respiratory muscle fatigue and ventilatory failure. *Annu Rev Med.* 1984;35:625–647.
36. Cohen C, Zagelbaum G, Gross D, Roussos C, Macklem PT. Clinical manifestations of inspiratory muscle fatigue. *Am J Med.* 1982;73:308–316.
37. West JB, ed. *Best and Taylor's Physiologic Basis of Medical Practice.* 12th ed. Williams & Wilkins; 1991:95–96.
38. Aukland K, Reed RK. Interstitial mechanisms in the control of extracellular fluid volume. *Physiol Rev.* 1993;73:1–78.
39. Browse NL, Lord RS, Taylor A. Pressure waves and gradients in the canine thoracic duct. *J Physiol.* 1971;237:401–413.
40. Dumont AE. The flow capacity of the thoracic duct-venous junction. *Am J Med Sci.* 1975;269(3):292–301.
41. Hodge LM. Osteopathic lymphatic pump techniques to enhance immunity and treat pneumonia. *Int J Osteopath Med.* 2012;15(1):13–21.
42. Hruby RJ, Martinez ES. The lymphatic system: an osteopathic review. *Cureus.* 2021;13(7):e16448.
43. Tobin MJ, Laghi F, Jubran A. Narrative review: ventilator-induced respiratory muscle weakness. *Ann Intern Med.* 2010;153(4):240–245.
44. Levine S, Nguyen T, Taylor N, et al. Rapid disuse atrophy of diaphragm fibers in mechanically ventilated humans. *N Engl J Med.* 2008; 358(13):1327–1335.
45. Hooijman PE, Beishuizen A, Witt CC, et al. Diaphragm muscle fiber weakness and ubiquitin–proteasome activation in critically ill patients. *Am J Respir Crit Care Med.* 2015;191(10):1126–1138.
46. Cherniack RM, Cherniack L. *Respiration in Health and Disease.* 3rd ed. Saunders; 1983.
47. Frostell C, Blomqvist H, Hedenstierna G, Halbig I, Pieper R. Thoracic and abdominal lymph drainage in relation to mechanical ventilation and PEEP. *Acta Anaesthesiol Scand.* 1987;31(5):405–412.
48. Moriondo A, Mukenge S, Negrini D. Transmural pressure in rat initial subpleural lymphatics during spontaneous or mechanical ventilation. *Am J Physiol Heart Circ Physiol.* 2005;289(1):263–269.
49. Sirasanagandla SR, Nayak SB, Bhat KM, et al. Duplicated right crus of the diaphragm: a cadaveric case report. *J Can Chiropr Assoc.* 2014;58(1):39–44.
50. Still AT. *Philosophy of Osteopathy.* Author; 1899:36.
51. Siccardi MA, Tariq MA, Valle C. Anatomy, bony pelvis and lower limb: psoas major. In: *StatPearls [Internet].* StatPearls Publishing; 2024. https://www.ncbi.nlm.nih.gov/books/NBK535418/
52. Bordoni B, Zanier E. Anatomic connections of the diaphragm: influence of respiration on the body system. *J Multidiscip Healthc.* 2013;6: 281–291.
53. Kelkar KV. Post-operative pulmonary complications after non-cardiothoracic surgery. *Indian J Anaesth.* 2015;59(9):599–605.
54. Simonneau G, Vivien A, Sartene R, et al. Diaphragm dysfunction induced by upper abdominal surgery. *Am Rev Respir Dis.* 1983;128(5):899–903.
55. Drake RE, Gabel JC. Diaphragmatic lymph vessel drainage of the peritoneal cavity. *Blood Purif.* 1992;10:132–135.
56. Schmid-Schonbein GW. Microlymphatics and lymph flow. *Physiol Rev.* 1990;70(4):987–1028.

79 Osteopathic Considerations in Psychiatry

TIMOTHY E. BLUMER

KEY CONCEPTS

- The biopsychosocial context in which psychiatric medicine functions is coherent with osteopathic tenets and the osteopathic approach to patient care.
- Osteopathic philosophy is part of the comprehensive psychiatric formulation of a patient.
- Categorical and dimensional are two main systems of classification of psychiatric conditions.
- Therapeutic alliance plays a significant role in the overall treatment impact.
- Use the RULE for motivational listening to trigger the individual's own motivation for change and hence improve health.
- The osteopathic-oriented psychiatrist can utilize osteopathic manipulative medicine as part of patient management keeping in mind issues of transference and professional boundaries.
- Psychological approaches to mind–body syndromes include mindfulness meditation, cognitive-behavioral therapy, and therapeutic writing techniques.

CASE VIGNETTE

A 35-year-old female presented to the emergency department complaining of suicidal ideation with a plan and was admitted to the inpatient psychiatric unit for further assessment and treatment. She had a history of the following, all of which started after a traumatic brain injury (TBI) secondary to a motor vehicle accident (MVA) 4 years earlier:

- Depression
- Posttraumatic stress disorder (PTSD)
- Alcohol abuse
- Multiple suicide attempts
- Daily migraine headaches

The patient:

- Lost consciousness during the MVA >30 minutes
- Had open wounds on her jaw requiring repair with plastic surgery
- Required hospitalization at that time due to cerebral edema and concussion

She was able to function well prior to the TBI, describing herself as "happy and upbeat." Immediately after the MVA she:

- Became depressed
- Was unable to maintain focus
- Started having daily migraine headaches and tremors
- Became hyper somnolent, sleeping episodically up to 22 hours per day for 1 to 2 weeks per episode
- Was unable to work
- Reported waking up with bilateral periorbital headaches daily, with associated:
  - Nausea
  - Photophobia
  - Phonophobia
  - Osmophobia
  - Electric-shock-like sensations in the temporal area
- There was minimal relief of the headaches with position changes and medication.
- Had impaired concentration and cognition since the MVA, previously reading voraciously, and upon presentation, struggling to read three pages before needing to rest, symptoms consistent with a severe TBI.

The patient had previously taken:

- Sumatriptan and Ibuprofen as abortive treatment
- Topiramate for preventive treatment for her migraine headaches with minimal relief
- Venlafaxine, citalopram, and amitriptyline for depression

Upon admission, the patient was on:

- Duloxetine, bupropion, and lithium for depression
- Diazepam and gabapentin for anxiety related to PTSD
- Prazosin for nightmares related to PTSD
- Trazodone for sleep
- Topiramate for migraine prevention
- Cyclobenzaprine for muscle spasms

Yet, none of her symptoms were controlled, leading her to desperation secondary to pain, and a sixth suicide attempt via medication overdose.

During the hospitalization, her diagnosis of depression was clarified as depressive disorder due to another medical condition, with major depressive like episode, as her depression was determined to be secondary to the previous TBI.

Upon admission:

- Aripiprazole (5 mg daily) was started to augment the activity of the antidepressant medication.
- Bupropion and hydroxyzine (25 mg four times daily as needed) were started later in the hospitalization to treat PTSD-related anxiety. Bupropion was changed from the immediate release to the XL formulation and reduced from a total daily dose of 450 to 300 mg to be given in the morning.
- Duloxetine was decreased from 60 mg twice daily to 60 mg once daily, which seemed to improve the patient's sleep pattern.

Initially, Sumatriptan and Topiramate, the patient's home migraine medications, were available to her and she had been using more than the recommended doses of these medications without relief. The patient took the Sumatriptan daily until after her second osteopathic manipulative treatment (OMT) treatment, at which time she found no need for either medication for headache relief.

Cognitively, the patient initially scored a 19/30 on the Montreal Cognitive Assessment (MoCA), indicating moderate cognitive impairment. On the day prior to discharge:

- On a subsequent MoCA, scored a 29/30 (normal, no cognitive impairment)
- Was able to follow a conversation much better than previously
- Was able to read seven pages at a time (formerly 1 to 3)
- Scored a 51 on the Texas Functional Living Scale,[1] suggesting she can live independently without issue

The Osteopathic Neuromusculoskeletal Medicine service was consulted on day four of her hospital stay, and she was treated for 7 of her 12 days of hospitalization.

- Upon her initial Osteopathic evaluation, she was experiencing:
  - Daily migraines
  - Poor concentration
  - An active sense of hypervigilance
  - Tremors
  - Insomnia
  - A profound sense of hopelessness with positive suicidal ideation
- She related that all of these symptoms she developed progressively after her TBI and reported that she "didn't recognize herself" after her MVA.
- On her initial osteopathic exam, she was noted to have:
  - Severe sphenobasilar synchondrosis (SBS) compression
  - Decreased central nervous system (CNS) motility
  - Very high sympathetic tone
  - A generally tremulous system
- She was able to tolerate:
  - Very gentle osteopathy in the cranial field (OCF)
  - Balanced membranous tension (BMT)
  - Balanced ligamentous tension (BLT)
  - Myofascial release (MFR)
- During her first osteopathic treatment, her migraine resolved completely despite only tolerating a small treatment length. That night, she was able to sleep a full 9 hours (previously 1–3 hours/night) and awoke the next morning without a headache for the first time in years, followed by her typical headache prodrome 2 hours later, so she took one preventative Sumatriptan, then underwent her second OMT treatment.
- At her second exam, with more relative motion in her cranium and improving sympathetic tone, she was noted to have a dural strain of C2, cerebellar fullness with an inferior membranous strain of the tentorium cerebelli. She again responded well to treatment (same modalities as above).
- She never developed a full migraine, slept 7 to 9 hours nightly, and remained headache free for the remainder of her hospitalization.
- Attention to the following were all important aspects of her treatment as her examinations evolved, and her serial treatments unfolded to treat the interconnected compensatory patterns sustained after her initial unphysiologic trauma.
  - Her sacral motion
  - Dural strain to her coccyx
  - Diaphragmatic motion
  - Abdominal congestion
  - Anterior thoracic myofascial strain
  - Mandibular periosteal fibrosis
- She noted:
  - Progressively decreasing "brain fog" each day
  - A "brighter" affect
  - More hope
  - Increasing recognition of her "former self"
- This profound change was reflected in her:
  - Daily interactions with other staff and peers
  - Art and collages
  - Balanced autonomic nervous system (ANS)
  - Improved cranial motion, circulation, and lymphatic drainage on osteopathic exam

The patient's depression improved significantly during her hospitalization.

- Per clinical observation and patient's report:
  - Her affect brightened
  - She isolated less
  - Her anxiety improved
  - Her suicidal thinking resolved
- Per the patient, her suicidal thoughts were mostly caused by her migraines and inability to function with impaired cognition and hypersomnia.
  - Once the migraines were adequately treated, and she was able to think clearly and sleep usually about 8 hours per night, her depression improved, and she was no longer suicidal.
  - Except for starting aripiprazole and hydroxyzine, the patient's treatment revolved around decreasing dosages of and discontinuing medications along with receiving OMT.
  - The patient's resolution of migraines seemed mostly related to treatment with OMT as she had tried Sumatriptan in the past with minimal relief.
  - Her improvement in mood seemed to be due to a combination of medication changes and OMT along with the usual care received in the inpatient psychiatry unit (participation in the therapeutic milieu, group and individual psychotherapy, psychoeducation, etc.).

She was discharged with:

- Medications as discussed above.
- Follow-up with mental health (individual and group), primary physician, osteopathic neuromusculoskeletal medicine.
- The suggestion to initiate physical therapy with balance training and vestibulo-ocular reflex rehabilitation.[2]

BRIEF HISTORY OF PSYCHIATRY

Psychiatric medicine from its inception has focused on understanding the individual from a biologic, cognitive, emotional, psychological, and social standpoint all within the context of that individual's daily life and interpersonal interactions.

- Treatment strategies were focused on assisting the individual find mental and emotional health to improve their functioning and interactions within their lives.
- Although not stated in the osteopathic terms, the philosophy certainly follows the four basic tenets of osteopathic medicine.
- Psychiatric medicine as practiced today is typically a "hands-off" field of medicine.

It is helpful to understand the origin and history of psychiatric medicine to better understand the challenges of developing an integrative psychiatric model that includes the provision of osteopathic manipulative medicine (OMM).

- Although mental disorders were recognized and specialized hospitals were set up as early as the eighth century, modern psychiatry as a field of medicine started in the early 1800s.
- The term "psychiatry" was first coined by the German physician Johanne Christian Reil in his paper "On the term of medicine and its branches, especially with regard to the rectification of the topic in psychiatry."
  - During this time, psychiatrists treated those individuals with mental illness that were confined to asylums.
  - The treatment of individuals with mental health disorders outside of asylums was provided the neurologists, treating "conditions of the nerves."
- One neurologist from the early 1900s, Sigmund Freud, changed the direction and care of mental health disorders at the time through his theories on the unconscious etiology of "nervous disorders."
  - Out of his understanding of this unconscious cause of mental health disorders, he developed the process of psychoanalysis.
  - This may be considered the first "true" treatment for individuals living in the community with mental disorders.
- The foundation of psychoanalysis requires the physician/therapist to be a "blank slate" on which the patient can make conscious that which had previously been hidden or unconscious through the process of free association, fantasies, and dreams.
  - This style of treatment and theory dominated psychiatric thinking and practice into the first half of the 20th century.
  - The idea of the blank slate remains an aspect of current psychiatric training and practice although the theories of Freud have been modified over the years by his contemporaries with new therapies being developed and researched, such as cognitive behavioral therapy and many others.

Biologic psychiatry developed on its own path.

- By the mid-1900s, insulin coma therapy and electroconvulsive therapy (ECT) were being utilized for schizophrenia and mood disorders.
- The medication revolution started in 1954 with the introduction of Chlorpromazine for schizophrenia.
- The first paper on the antidepressant Imipramine was published in 1958.
- With the advent of medications, the role and practice of psychiatry began its transformation into a primary care specialty.

The contemporary psychiatrist is a blend of the old and new, both the psychoanalytic and neurobiologic, however, it is still very much "hands off."

- Psychiatrists are taught how to look at an individual using a wholistic framework.
- One common framework is the biopsychosocial formulation although there are several formulation models that are available.

BIOPSYCHOSOCIAL FORMULATION

The biopsychosocial formulation is a synthesis or understanding of an individual from the following perspectives:

1. Biologic
   - Neuropsychiatric
   - Genetic
   - Physiologic
2. Psychological
   - Strengths
   - Vulnerabilities
   - Defense strategies
   - Drives both conscious and unconscious
   - Transference
   - Countertransference
   - Others
3. Social
   - How the individual sees and is seen in their community/social group
   - Relationships within family/social group
   - Work
   - Religion
   - Ethnicity
   - Socioeconomic class
   - Others

The purpose of the formulation is to avoid an overly narrow approach to a patient and their specific needs.

- The psychiatrist needs to weigh and balance the various components of the biopsychosocial formulation to develop the initial treatment plan.
- This plan is adjusted as the formulation changes over time and with greater understanding of the individual.

Osteopathic philosophy is part of the comprehensive psychiatric formulation of a patient.

- The goal of osteopathic medical treatment is to provide patients with the tools they need to restore and maintain their natural, self-healing state.
- The four basic tenets of osteopathic medical philosophy that are a mainstay of thinking of the osteopathically trained psychiatrist include[3,4]:
  1. The body is completely united; the person is a fully integrated being of body, mind, and spirit.
  2. The body is capable of self-regulation, self-healing, and health maintenance.
  3. Structure and function are reciprocally interrelated.
  4. Rational treatment is based on an understanding of these three principles.
- These tenets complement and fit within the framework of the biopsychosocial formulation.
- This certainly includes the consideration for OMT by the primary care psychiatric physician.

NOSOLOGY

Psychiatry, like other fields of medication, relies on diagnostic criteria for the diagnosis and hence treatment of mental health disorders.

- There are different models of classification for phenomena that can be evaluated in terms of their utility for purposes, rather than requiring forced choices between one model as right versus other models as wrong.
- Some models are designed to represent relations among phenomena without representing causes of the phenomena.
- Other models are designed to represent the causes of phenomena.
- In psychiatry, there are two main systems of classification:
  1. Categorical
  2. Dimensional

The categorical approach is the approach to classifying mental disorders involving assessment of whether an individual has a disorder, based on symptoms and characteristics typical of the disorder.

- Categorical approaches are based on underlying principles and assumptions including:
  1. A mental disorder can be diagnosed from specific symptoms that are shown during a mental health assessment.
  2. Thoughts, feelings, and behavior can be organized into categories representing disorders.
  3. All or nothing principle (so the individual either has a diagnosable mental disorder or does not have a diagnosable disorder).
- Strengths for using the categorical approach include:
  - Helping communication
  - Allowing for a diagnosis
- Weaknesses of using the categorical approach include:
  - Low inter-rater reliability
  - Lots of overlap between symptoms which can make diagnosis tricky
  - Stigma
  - Labeling

The dimensional approach is the approach to classifying mental disorders that quantifies a person's symptoms or other characteristics of interest and represents them with numerical values on one or more scales or continuums, rather than assigning them to a mental disorder category.

- Diagnosis then becomes not a process of deciding the presence of a symptom or disorder but the degree to which a particular characteristic is present.
- Instead of making judgments, the dimensional approach asks the question "how much?"
  - Lower scores equate to lower impairment
  - Higher scores equate to higher impairment
- A dimensional approach focuses on the EXTENT in which a person has a disorder.
- Strengths of using the dimensional approach include:
  - More detailed information on each symptom
  - Takes into account a wider range of factors (more than categorical approaches)
  - Creating a profile instead of labeling
- Weakness of using the dimensional approach include:
  - Time consuming
  - No standard inventory to compare scores, making diagnosis difficult

Both the diagnostic and statistical manual of mental disorders (DSM) and the international classification of disease (ICD) systems rely extensively on a categorical approach, but also note the dimensional nature of syndromes and symptoms. Neither is well tested outside of a handful of societies.

PRINCIPLES OF PSYCHIATRIC THERAPEUTIC TECHNIQUES

Therapeutic Alliance and Working Alliance

Therapeutic alliance is a term typically used within the mental health field and is considered to have a significant impact on the overall treatment.

- The concept was first described by Freud as "friendly affectionate feelings," referring to positive transference within the context of psychoanalytic therapy.
- The concept has been expanded by many others since that time.

In other fields of medicine, terms such as working alliance are used.

- There is no specific definition of working alliance, although there are generally accepted concepts.
- This includes a collaborative relationship in which there is overall agreement between the patient and physician on:
  - The goals of treatment
  - The type(s) of intervention
  - The commitment of everyone, their confidence in each other, and their "liking" of one another.
- The working alliance develops and changes over time.

Research has identified the importance of the patient–physician relationship on adherence to medical treatment and hence treatment outcomes[5,6]

- De Vries et al.[7] found patient satisfaction and working alliance to be a function of the physician's self-regulation and the physician's stress within the oncology care setting.
- Medical service payors now understand that patient satisfaction, often influenced by the quality of the patient–provider relationship, significantly impacts patient outcomes.

The osteopathic physician is patient centered and places high value on the working alliance for the betterment of their patients. Some basic skills for a working alliance include:

- Listening thoughtfully to the patient's words and meaning, nonjudgmental attitude toward patient and the patient's difficulties
- Recognizing that the patient is an expert on their difficulties and the "best fit" for their treatment
- Setting clear boundaries
- Being genuine
- Having a positive regard for the patient

Motivational Interviewing (MI)

MI was first described in 1983 as a brief intervention for problematic alcohol use.

- In the 1990s, MI began to be used for other health concerns.
- Since that time, there have been clinical trials utilizing MI for a range of medical conditions including diabetes, hypertension, and others.
- Motivational interviewing had a significant and clinically relevant effect in approximately three out of four studies, with an equal effect on physiological (72%) and psychological (75%) diseases.[8]
- The underlying principle of MI is to trigger the individual's own motivation for change, and hence improve health.

There are four principles of MI:

1. Resist
2. Understand
3. Listen
4. Empower [RULE][9]
   - **R**—Patients often know what the best solution would be but are ambivalent about the necessary change. It is important the physician resists (**Resist**) the urge to convince patients what is best for them.
     - The physician's attempt to convince the patient only leads to increased defensiveness toward change.
     - Often, the most successful intervention is helping the patient voice the arguments for change.
     - The physician helps the patient move through their ambivalence to make positive change in their lives.

    - In a very time-limited setting, it may be more productive to ask a patient why they would want to make a change rather than telling them they should.
    - Likewise, it is often more productive to ask how they might make the change rather than giving them a list of changes.
  - U—A very active process, often called reflective listening, requires the physician to be interested in, have empathy toward, and understand (**Understand**) the patients concerns, values, and motivations.
    - The physician then must be able to accurately reflect this understanding back to the patient.
    - This allows for a joint understanding surrounding the presenting complaint, through which the next step can be taken.
  - L—Listening (**Listen**) is the basis for understanding, resisting, and empowering.
  - E—Empower (**Empower**) patients; support their hope for change, so they believe that change is possible and that it can make a difference in their health.
    - The physician can bring the patient's expertise into the consultation allowing for a strong working alliance and improved outcomes.

This author encourages physicians and other health care professionals to learn more about MI. Books and courses are available to the medical professional. One such book is Motivational Interviewing in Health Care, by Stephen Rollnick, 2008 the Guilford Press.

Transference, Professional Boundaries, and Osteopathic Manipulative Medicine

One concern raised for the use of OMM by the psychiatrist is the issue of transference, and how this will impact the overall recovery of the patient.

- Transference is the redirecting of thoughts, feelings, and desires toward a new object (individual).
- These desires, feelings, and thoughts are often out of conscious awareness of the patient.
- The blank slate prominent in psychoanalytic work allows a space for the transference to occur, and to be worked through, resulting in the resolution of symptoms in the patient.
- Transference is typically only with therapists and psychiatrists, but this phenomenon can and does occur in many day-to-day interactions and relationships.
- Physicians in other specialties such as family practice and internal medicine learn to use transference for the benefit of the patient. They may not provide interpretations of the transference as a psychoanalyst, but rather use it to aid engagement in the treatment process.[10]

The role of the psychiatrist has changed to a much more biologic model. Hence, the day-to-day practice of the contemporary primary care psychiatric physician looks more like that of a family practice physician than that of the psychoanalyst.

- This suggests the psychiatrist can be aware of and use the transference in a manner used by other primary care specialties.
- This allows the psychiatrist to broaden their therapeutic interventions, including the use of OMM.
- The psychiatrist's training allows for a better understanding of the patient and their defense structure (coping styles), and thus how to maintain appropriate boundaries in the care of the patient.

Boundaries are another issue raised for the use of OMM by the psychiatrist.

- A boundary violation occurs when a health care professional's behavior goes beyond appropriate professional limits.
- They generally arise when a personal interest displaces the professional's primary commitment to the patient's welfare, in ways that harm the patient or the patient–clinician relationship.[11]
- Boundaries are a concern for all physicians and are taught from the start of their medical training.

Health care professionals should beware of interacting with any patient in ways that could reasonably be expected to:

- Create awkward situations for either party
- Compromise the professional's primary commitment to patient welfare
- Call the professional's objectivity into question

Professionals should critically examine their own actions by considering the following[11]:

- "Is this activity a normal, expected part of practice for my profession?"
- "Might engaging in this activity compromise my relationship with this patient? With other patients? With my colleagues? With my institution? With the public?"
- "Could this activity cause others to question my professional objectivity?"
- "Would I want my other patients, other professionals, or the public to know that I engage in such activities?"

An osteopathic physician is trained in OMM/OMT during medical school and starts their specialty training after graduation.

- It is appropriate for a physician trained in OMM to use those skills with patients, keeping in mind the professional boundaries of the profession.
- As psychiatric medicine continues to transform into a primary care specialty with a much broader and interactive focus, OMM can become an integrated component of psychiatric care as it is in other primary care fields.

OMM and Primary Care Psychiatry

Why the primary care psychiatric physician should recommend OMM as one of the recommendations developed out of a comprehensive biopsychosocial formulation:

- There is theoretical and research evidence to support OMM as an adjunctive treatment in a comprehensive treatment plan, based on a biopsychosocial formulation for an individual with mental health issues.
- Several targets for OMM for such patients include:
  - Chronic pain
  - Hypothalamic–pituitary–adrenal axis (HPA) dysregulation
  - Chronic stress
- Chronic pain is associated with the development of depression/mental health issues, sleep issues, and cognitive disturbance.[12]
  - Research using positron emission tomography of patients with chronic neuropathic pain shows a shift of acute pain activity in the sensory cortex to regions such as the anterior cingulate gyrus associated with affective-motivational processing.[13]
  - The anterior cingulate gyrus is an important area of consideration in mental health due to its association with depression, anxiety, and executive functions.[14]
  - For more information on psychoneuroimmunology, see Chapter 16.

Management of Mind–Body Syndromes (Functional Neurologic Disorder)

- Functional neurologic disorder (FND) is a prevalent condition that leads to persistent and disabling neurologic symptoms, affecting a wide range of functions including movement control, awareness (like epileptic seizures), sensation, and is often accompanied by chronic pain, fatigue, and cognitive issues.[15]
- FND, also known as conversion disorder or functional neurologic symptom disorder, primarily manifests through neurologic symptoms without a recognized neurologic cause.[16] Historically, it was believed that psychological distress manifested as physical symptoms in FND. Modern diagnostic approaches allow for an inclusive diagnosis by identifying specific neurologic signs unique to FND, without the need to prove the presence or absence of psychological stressors.[17]
- According to the American Psychiatric Association Diagnostic and Statistical Manual of Mental Disorders (DSM-5-TR), for a diagnosis, there must be evidence that physiologic functions remain intact despite neurologic symptoms.[18] It's possible for patients to have symptoms without a medically explained condition, provided they exhibit certain psychobehavioral characteristics such as excessive behaviors or health-related anxieties.[16]
- FND predominantly affects young and middle-aged adults and can lead to significant disability. Early diagnosis and access to evidence-based rehabilitation and psychological treatments are crucial for recovery, although not all patients may respond to existing treatments.[19]
- Effective management of FND usually requires a multidisciplinary team approach, involving neurologists, psychiatrists, physical therapists, occupational therapists, speech therapists, and other specialists tailored to the patient's symptoms.[15,17,19] This collaborative care is essential because FND symptoms lie at the crossroads of neurology and psychiatry, necessitating integrated treatment strategies.

Current treatment approaches to patients with unexplained symptom complexes consist of[15,17,19]: (These modalities are all successful in many patients; however, certain patients do not respond and appear to require alternative approaches.)

Pain medications

- Modulators of pain perception, such as pregabalin and gabapentin
- Exercise
- Osteopathic manipulation
- Physical therapy/rehabilitation strategies

Psychological approaches (typically consist of cognitive behavioral therapy and stress reduction)

- Studies using mindfulness meditation have shown a reduction in pain for patients with chronic musculoskeletal pain[20] and fibromyalgia.[21,22]
- Cognitive-behavioral therapy, which works in part by reducing psychosocial stress, has also been shown to be effective in chronic musculoskeletal pain.[23–26]
- Finally, studies using therapeutic writing techniques in fibromyalgia have shown reductions in pain comparable to standard pharmacologic therapy.[27,28]

One model for treatment of these "mind–body syndromes" consists of the following steps.

1. First, each patient is asked to read The Mindbody Prescription by Dr. Sarno.[29] This gives the patient a basic understanding of how physical symptoms, which are real, located in the body and often severe, can be caused by conscious and unconscious emotional turmoil.
2. Second, each patient has a 60-to-90-minute office visit to rule out any physical disorders that require conventional medical attention, and to search for patterns of psychosomatic symptoms across their lifespan, beginning in childhood.
   - □ It is important to listen carefully to the patient's life story and to help them uncover stressors and emotional reactions that have triggered such psychosomatic symptoms.
   - □ It is useful to help the patient understand the role of conditioned responses that trigger the neurologic pathways that have developed over time (e.g., certain positions, activities, weather changes, foods, and locations).
   - □ It is necessary to explain the physiologic pathways between the emotional centers of the brain (amygdala) and the ANS, which creates the physiologic substrates of pain and other symptoms (e.g., sensitized nerve pathways), to help them understand the role of the unconscious mind in producing emotions that can produce significant physical symptoms despite being suppressed.
   - □ It is critical to normalize and destigmatize psychosomatic disorders and accept them as a part of being "human," and to explain how simple psychological techniques can alter the vicious cycle of pain and offer hope that their symptoms are curable.
3. An important step in the treatment process is patient participation in a 4-week seminar. Participants receive a workbook and instructions for performing:
   - □ Specific therapeutic writing exercises to help express emotions and better cope with prior and current stressors.
   - □ Specific meditative exercises based on mindfulness meditation developed for this purpose.
   - □ Specific declarative and affirmative sentences that are spoken to oneself as a method for disrupting patterns of neurologic connections that promote symptoms.
   - □ Exercises to develop and carry out activities that previously caused symptoms or are pleasurable and desirable.
4. Finally, follow-up is conducted to develop a plan on the response obtained to this program.
   - □ Patients may require individual psychotherapy as an adjunct to the program.
   - □ The program is also available on the internet[30] and in a self-help book.[31]

In 1976, Ivan Illich warned of the potential iatrogenic consequences of a classification of disease that labels patients.[32]

- When patients with psychosomatic disorders are labeled as having degenerative disk disease based on an MRI or as having fibromyalgia based on an arbitrary classification system, the stage is set for a vicious cycle, exacerbating symptoms and psychological status.
- Eugene Carragee also warned of this process occurring in patients with back pain, "ill-considered attempts to make a diagnosis on the basis of imaging studies may reinforce the suspicion of serious disease, magnify the importance of nonspecific findings, and label patients with spurious diagnoses."[33]

The tremendous advances in biomedical technology over the past several decades have led to an overemphasis on the biologic while ignoring the psychological and the social causes of common symptoms.

- In addition, there has been a surge in expenditure for complementary and alternative treatments.
- An alternative nosology of disease has been created by this movement and includes labels such as:
  - Chronic yeast infection
  - Chronic food allergies
  - Deficiencies of natural hormones, gastric acid, or various nutritional supplements
- Such "diagnoses" can have similar effects to medical labeling, that is, turning a person with functional symptoms due to stressors into a patient with a "disease."

Application to Patient Care

Therefore, during routine patient care, it is critical for physicians to be aware of the probability that psychosomatic disorders will occur in most people during their lifetime. A careful history and physical examination should include investigation into the potential for both organic and functional disorders; that is, examining not only for signs of nerve root compression, tumor, or infection, but also determining the psychological and social factors that may have led to this set of symptoms at this point in a person's life.

The most important question to ask is "What was happening in your life at the time these symptoms began?"

- For patients who present with the new onset of headaches, bowel or bladder symptoms, or painful conditions that are not determined to have a clear pathologic basis, some amount of probing regarding stressors and underlying emotions may be required to uncover feelings of:
  - Guilt
  - Fear
  - Resentment
  - Anger
- Careful listening is important to validate the suffering of the patient and to reassure the patient that their condition is taken seriously.
- Listening for and probing to obtain the psychosocial context of this point in a patient's life will:
  - Allow the physician to understand the potential contribution of psychosocial factors in the illness.
  - Serve as starting point for understanding and potentially curing those ailments that are purely functional.

It is critical to inform the patient with a psychosomatic illness that they are "not crazy," but that these conditions commonly occur in many people.

- If the patient feels they are being told, "It's all in your head," they will be less likely to improve.
- It is better to tell patients that all symptoms have a cause, and it is vital to get to the root cause of the symptoms to cure them.

A careful psychosocial history with emphasis on their childhood stressors as well as their adult stressors is necessary to uncover potential root causes. Looking carefully for temporal relationships between stressors (even mild stressors can precipitate significant symptoms if they trigger an emotional response connected to childhood stressors) is important to confirm a psychosomatic etiology.

Once a psychosomatic condition is diagnosed, the management should consist of the following:

- Avoid excessive rest and disability.
- Encourage routine activities and exercise as tolerated.
- Reassure about the lack of serious disease and inform the patient that they do have a condition. One useful term is "mind–body syndrome." Emphasize how physiologic mechanisms in the brain and body create this vicious cycle, and that their symptoms are very real, but they are curable.
- Avoid excessive testing and excessive referral to specialists who may be likely to reinforce the suspicion of serious disease.
- Explain the results of nonspecific test findings (such as degenerative disk changes) as findings that are within the range of normal.
- Consider a referral to a physician, psychologist, or counselor who can help the patient understand and cope with their childhood and adult stressors.
- Consider resources, such as books by Dr. John Sarno referenced above.

A tremendous amount of money is spent on the diagnosis and treatment of psychosomatic disorders. Many people will have physical and psychological symptoms at some time in their life due to psychological states.

- If psychosomatic disorders were widely recognized by the lay public and medical professionals (both traditional and alternative), there would be:
  - Increased potential for alleviation of common symptoms
  - Decreased medical costs
  - Prevention of chronic symptom complexes
- The treatment of these disorders requires:
  - A careful history
  - Judicious use of diagnostic tests to rule out serious pathologic processes
  - Attention to past and current psychosocial stressors and reactions to these stressors
  - Validation of the real nature of the symptoms ("It's not all in your head")
  - Explanation of the psychophysiological basis of functional symptoms
  - Brief educational and psychological interventions
- In this way, patients are empowered to:
  - Gain control over their symptoms
  - Understand themselves better
  - Obtain tools to improve their psychological states

DIAGNOSIS AND TREATMENT OF DEPRESSION, BIPOLAR DISORDER, GENERALIZED ANXIETY DISORDER, AND ATTENTION-DEFICIT HYPERACTIVITY DISORDER

Major Depressive Disorder[18,34]:

- Lifetime prevalence (average): 5% to 17%
- Male-to -female ratio: 1: 1.5 to 1:3, with women being more likely to experience MDD than men
- Differential diagnosis (limited)
  - Bipolar disorder, depressed episode
  - Mood disorder due to a medical condition
  - Substance/medication-induced mood disorder
  - Adjustment disorders
  - Sadness/grief
- Comorbidity:
  - Substance use disorders
  - Panic disorder
  - Obsessive compulsive disorder
  - Anorexia nervosa/bulimia nervosa
  - Borderline personality disorder

DIAGNOSTIC CRITERIA (DSM5-TR)[18]

- The word "depression" refers to a syndrome in which a variety of signs and symptoms occur.
- Typically, there is a change from previous adequate emotional functioning to a depressed mood and a loss of pleasure in life's usual activities referred to as a state of anhedonia.
- The depressed person feels sad or empty most of the time and often experiences impairment in interpersonal, social, or occupational functioning.
- Conceptually, these symptoms may be grouped as disturbances in:
  - Emotions, depressed mood most of the day, nearly every day as indicated by either subjective report, for instance:
    - Feels sad, empty, hopeless
    - Insomnia or hypersomnia nearly every day
    - Loss of interests/pleasure
    - Worthlessness or guilt
    - **Note:** In children and adolescents, can be irritable mood
  - Ideation:
    - Worthlessness/guilt
    - Death/suicide
  - Neurovegetative or somatic symptoms:
    - Sleep
    - Appetite/weight
    - Psychomotor
    - Energy
    - Concentration
- If five or more of these symptoms are present for more than 2 weeks, a diagnosis of *major depressive disorder (MDD)* is considered and *persistent depressive disorder*, if more than over 2 years.
- These symptoms (all but depressed mood) may be more readily recalled using the acronym "SIG: E CAPS"
  - Sleep
  - Interest
  - Guilt
  - Energy
  - Concentration
  - Appetite
  - Psychomotor

MEASUREMENT OF DEPRESSION

The diagnosis and management of depression in a patient can be facilitated through numerous self-administered inventories, such as:

- The Zung Depression Scale[35,36] for ages ≥18 years
- The Beck Depression Inventories[37,38] for ages ≥15 years
- The MMPI Depression Scale[39,40] for ages ≥18 years
- Children's Depression Inventory 2[41] for ages ≥7 years
- These inventories provide reliable and valid measures of the severity of depression. The patient can initially be tested for a baseline measure and then repeatedly tested with the same instrument to measure progress.

More recently developed structured interviews such as the PHQ-9,[42,43] a 9-item self-report instrument assessing the nine symptoms of DSM-5 major depression, is feasible to use, reliable, and valid in primary care settings for adults and youth.

TREATMENT

It is based on the biopsychosocial formulation utilizing the Osteopathic Five Model approach.

A. Metabolic:
  a. Nutrition
    i. Omega-3 fatty acid
      1. Omega-3 fatty acids have been found to be useful in treating depression.
      2. A meta-analysis published in Translational Psychiatry in 2019 demonstrated an overall beneficial effect of omega-3 polyunsaturated fatty acids (PUFAs) on depression symptoms, with specific formulations containing high levels of eicosapentaenoic acid (EPA) showing clinical benefits at dosages of ≤1 g/day.[44]
      3. Additionally, observational studies have indicated that omega-3 supplementation can significantly improve depressive symptoms when used alongside conventional antidepressant treatments.[45]
    ii. L-Methylfolate
      1. L-Methylfolate is useful in treating depression, particularly in certain groups of patients.
      2. L-Methylfolate has been shown to be beneficial as both a monotherapy[46] and as an adjunctive therapy[47] in the treatment of MDD.
      3. The effectiveness of L-methylfolate in treating depression may be particularly pronounced in individuals with variations in the MTHFR gene, which affects the metabolism of folate.[47]
    iii. N-Acetylcysteine (NAC)
      1. N-AC has been used in the treatment of paracetamol overdose for more than 30 years.[48]
      2. N-AC has shown potential in treating depression, although the results from studies have been mixed. NAC is of interest in psychiatric treatment due to its antioxidant, anti-inflammatory, and glutamate modulation activities.[48]
  b. Pharmacologic
    i. When looking at pharmacologic treatment of depression we typically start with one medication titrating to a reasonable or standard dose then wait a period of 3 to 4 weeks then re-evaluate. If there is a limited response the dose of the single medication is serially increased to the maximum dose at 3-to-4-week intervals. If the first medication at a full dose for a full 4-to-6-week trial is not effective, we then discontinue the first medication and start a trial of the second medication. If there is a moderate response to a single medication at the full dose and time, we may choose to add a second antidepressant agent that targets different neurochemicals to augment the response. Beyond this, a referral to a psychiatrist or medical specialist who specializes in mental health would be advised.
    ii. A treatment protocol such as the Psychopharmacology Algorithm Project at Harvard South Shore Program can be used effectively for management of major depressive disorders. The Harvard algorithm is a nuanced and comprehensive tool with up-to-date research-based recommendations.[49]
    iii. Antidepressants were once thought to not exert their effects for 2 to 4 weeks. Current data suggest all antidepressants show a pattern of response with rapid improvement in the first 1 to 2 weeks.
    iv. The most common mistake in prescribing antidepressants is use of a dose that is too low and for a duration that is too short. Although the medication is started at

a low dose, the medication should be raised every 3 to 4 weeks to the maximum dose or adverse effects prior to considering the trial unsuccessful.
v. Once remission is obtained the medication should be continued for a minimum of 6 to 9 months after a single episode.
vi. Maintenance therapy appears to be safe and effective for chronic depression.

c. Switching strategies:
i. Sertraline, escitalopram, or bupropion
ii. Venlafaxine or mirtazapine
iii. S-Adenosylmethionine or St. John's wort

d. Augmentation strategies:
i. Nutritional support or light therapy
ii. Atypical antipsychotic (aripiprazole, quetiapine, risperidone)
iii. Bupropion or mirtazapine
iv. Lithium
v. Thyroid supplementation (T3)

B. Neurologic and behavioral:
a. Psychological therapies: cognitive therapy, interpersonal therapy, behavioral therapy
i. The combination of psychotherapy and pharmacotherapy is suggested by research for MDDs[34]
b. Vagal nerve stimulation
c. Transcranial magnetic stimulation (TMS)
d. Sleep deprivation
e. Sleep hygiene program
f. Phototherapy
g. ECT
h. Pain control

C. Biomechanical:
a. OMT addressing the biomechanical aspects of somatic dysfunction in psychiatric patients may be beneficial to improve their pain, motion, and movement.
b. The historical and modern evidence points to the potential benefits of OMT for patients with mental health disorders, although the current literature indicates a need for more robust research to firmly establish its efficacy in psychiatry. Positive effects of OMM on psychiatric symptoms have been published for anxiety and depression, tension headache, chronic pain, fibromyalgia, and irritable bowel syndrome, suggesting that OMM could serve as an adjunct treatment in these cases.[50] Despite the growing presence of osteopathically trained psychiatrists, the direct application of OMT in treating psychiatric conditions remains underexplored, with existing studies facing limitations such as small sample sizes and a lack of comprehensive research on a wide range of mental illnesses.

D. Respiratory/Circulatory/Lymphatic:
a. Recent studies have highlighted the significant role of exercise in treating depression, emphasizing its therapeutic effects across various age groups, predominantly among individuals aged 18 to 65 years. Exercise, whether as a standalone therapy, an adjunct, or in combination with other treatments, has shown comparable benefits to traditional depression treatments.[51]
b. Recommendations suggest aerobic or mind–body exercises, conducted three to five times per week at moderate intensity for durations of 4 to 16 weeks, with individualized, supervised group exercise protocols.[51]
c. High-intensity low-volume (HILV) or moderate continuous aerobic training (MCT) regimes have been shown to reduce depressive symptoms.[52]

Bipolar Disorder

- Lifetime prevalence: (0% to 2.4%)
- Male-to-female ratio: 1.1:1
  - The mean age at onset of the first manic, hypomanic, or major depressive episode is approximately 18 years for bipolar I disorder.
- Differential diagnosis
  - MDD
  - Generalized anxiety disorder (GAD)
  - PTSD
  - Substance/medication-induced disorder
  - Mood disorder due to a medical condition
  - Personality disorder such as borderline personality disorder
- Comorbidity:
  - Anxiety disorders; panic attacks, social phobia
  - Attention-deficit hyperactivity disorder (ADHD)
  - Substance use disorders
  - Metabolic syndrome and migraine

DIAGNOSTIC CRITERIA (DSM5-TR)[18]

BIPOLAR I DISORDER

A. Criteria have been met for at least one manic episode (Criteria A–D under "Manic Episode" above).
B. The occurrence of the manic and major depressive episode(s) is not better explained by schizoaffective disorder, schizophrenia, schizophreniform disorder, delusional disorder, or other specified or unspecified schizophrenia spectrum and other psychotic disorder.

For a diagnosis of bipolar I disorder, it is necessary to meet the following criteria for a manic episode. The manic episode may have been preceded by and may be followed by hypomanic or major depressive episodes.

MANIC EPISODE

A distinct period of abnormally and persistently elevated, expansive, or irritable mood and abnormally and persistently increased activity or energy, lasting at least 1 week and present most of the day, nearly every day (or any duration if hospitalization is necessary).

A. During the period of mood disturbance and increased energy or activity, three (or more) of the following symptoms (four if the mood is only irritable) are present to a significant degree and represent a noticeable change from usual behavior:
a. Inflated self-esteem or grandiosity.
b. Decreased need for sleep (e.g., feeling rested after only 3 hours of sleep).
c. More talkative than usual or pressure to keep talking.
d. Flight of ideas or subjective experience that thoughts are racing.
e. Distractibility (i.e., attention too easily drawn to unimportant or irrelevant external stimuli), as reported or observed.
f. Increase in goal-directed activity (either socially, at work or school, or sexually) or psychomotor agitation (i.e., purposeless non–goal-directed activity).
g. Excessive involvement in activities that have a high potential for painful consequences (e.g., engaging in unrestrained buying sprees, sexual indiscretions, or foolish business investments).

B. The mood disturbance is sufficiently severe to cause marked impairment in social or occupational functioning or to necessitate hospitalization to prevent harm to self or others, or there are psychotic features.

C. The episode is not attributable to the physiologic effects of a substance (e.g., a drug of abuse, a medication, or other treatment) or another medical condition.
D. Note: A full manic episode that emerges during antidepressant treatment (e.g., medication, ECT) but persists at a fully syndromic level beyond the physiologic effect of that treatment is sufficient evidence for a manic episode and, therefore, a bipolar I diagnosis.

Note: Criteria A–D constitutes a manic episode. At least one lifetime manic episode is required for the diagnosis of bipolar I disorder."

MEASUREMENT OF MANIA

The diagnosis and management of bipolar disorder in a patient can be facilitated through self-administered inventories, such as the:

- Mania Rating Scale (MRS)[53] for ages ≥18 years
- The Young Mania Rating Scale YMRS[53] for ages 4 to 18 years
- K-SADS Mania Rating Scale (KMRS)[54] for ages 4 to 18 years

These inventories provide reliable and valid measures of the severity of mania.

HYPOMANIC EPISODE

A. A distinct period of abnormally and persistently elevated, expansive, or irritable mood and abnormally and persistently increased activity or energy, lasting at least 4 consecutive days and present most of the day, nearly every day.
B. During the period of mood disturbance and increased energy and activity, three (or more) of the following symptoms (four if the mood is only irritable) have persisted, represent a noticeable change from usual behavior, and have been present to a significant degree:
   a. Inflated self-esteem or grandiosity.
   b. Decreased need for sleep (e.g., feeling rested after only 3 hours of sleep).
   c. More talkative than usual or pressure to keep talking.
   d. Flight of ideas or subjective experience that thoughts are racing.
   e. Distractibility (i.e., attention too easily drawn to unimportant or irrelevant external stimuli), as reported or observed.
   f. Increase in goal-directed activity (either socially, at work or school, or sexually) or psychomotor agitation.
   g. Excessive involvement in activities that have a high potential for painful consequences (e.g., engaging in unrestrained buying sprees, sexual indiscretions, or foolish business investments).
C. The episode is associated with an unequivocal change in functioning that is uncharacteristic of the individual when not symptomatic.
D. The disturbance in mood and the change in functioning are observable by others.
E. The episode is not severe enough to cause marked impairment in social or occupational functioning or to necessitate hospitalization. If there are psychotic features, the episode is, by definition, manic.
F. The episode is not attributable to the physiologic effects of a substance (e.g., a drug of abuse, a medication, or other treatment) or another medical condition.

Note: A full hypomanic episode that emerges during antidepressant treatment (e.g., medication, ECT) but persists at a fully syndromic level beyond the physiologic effect of that treatment is sufficient evidence for a hypomanic episode diagnosis. However, caution is indicated so that one or two symptoms (particularly increased irritability, edginess, or agitation following antidepressant use) are not taken as sufficient for diagnosis of a hypomanic episode, nor necessarily indicative of a bipolar diathesis.

Note: Criteria A to F constitute a hypomanic episode. Hypomanic episodes are common in bipolar I disorder but are not required for the diagnosis of bipolar I disorder.

MAJOR DEPRESSIVE EPISODE (AS LISTED ABOVE)

TREATMENT

It is based on the biopsychosocial formulation utilizing the Osteopathic Five Model approach.

A. Metabolic
   a. Nutrition
      i. Nutraceuticals (PUFAs 1,000 mg EPA/day, St. John's wort, lysine, magnesium) are tolerable and accessible and may be useful as potential adjunctive treatments for bipolar disorder.[55]
      ii. Nutraceuticals targeting neuroinflammation or mitochondrial activity may have the most potential for the depressive phase.[56]
   b. Pharmacologic
      i. When looking at pharmacologic treatment of depression we typically start with one medication titrating to a reasonable or standard dose then wait a period of 2 to 4 weeks then re-evaluate. Based on response a change to a different mood stabilizing agent is recommended. Beyond this, a referral to a psychiatrist or medical specialist who specializes in mental health would be advised.
      ii. A treatment protocol such as the Psychopharmacology Algorithm Project at Harvard South Shore Program can be used effectively for management of bipolar disorder. The Harvard algorithm is a nuanced and comprehensive tool with up-to-date research-based recommendations.[57] Clarifying the bipolar presentation, (manic, mixed presentation, etc.), will allow a more targeted approach to pharmacologic treatment.
      iii. Consider lithium in regimen for its antisuicidal and neuroprotective effects as the first line treatment of bipolar disorder, manic.
      iv. Avoid use of two second-generation antipsychotics at the same time.
      v. Use of antidepressant medications in bipolar depression is typically the LAST option and only if on an adequate dose of a mood stabilizer first.
   c. Typical first-line interventions for bipolar disorder, manic presentation:
      i. Lithium
      ii. Quetiapine or another second-generation antipsychotic
      iii. Divalproex sodium
   d. Typical first-line interventions for bipolar disorder, mixed presentation:
      i. Quetiapine or another second-generation antipsychotic
      ii. Add divalproex sodium (Depakote)
      iii. Add lithium
      iv. Other second-generation antipsychotic agents, carbamazepine, haloperidol (first-generation antipsychotic)
   e. Typical first-line interventions for bipolar disorder, depressed presentation

i. Lithium
ii. Second-generation antipsychotic agents; quetiapine, lurasidone, cariprazine
iii. Anticonvulsants; di-valproate

f. Commonly used combinations of medication for bipolar disorder:
i. Atypical antipsychotic agent (quetiapine, lurasidone, cariprazine) with a mood stabilizer (lithium, di-valproate, carbamazepine)

B. Neurologic and behavioral:
a. Psychological therapies: cognitive therapy, interpersonal therapy, behavioral therapy
b. The combination of psychotherapy and pharmacotherapy is suggested by research for MDDs.[34]
c. ECT in bipolar depression is used in patients unresponsive to lithium or other mood stabilizers.

C. Biomechanical:
a. OMT may be helpful. No research data to support

D. Respiratory/Circulatory:
a. Exercise—no data to support effectiveness for core symptoms of bipolar disorder

Generalized Anxiety Disorder

- Lifetime prevalence: (5%)
- Male-to-female ratio: 1:2
- Differential diagnosis
  - ☐ Other anxiety disorders
  - ☐ Anxiety disorder due to a medical condition
  - ☐ PTSD
  - ☐ Substance/medication-induced disorder
  - ☐ Personality disorder such as borderline personality disorder
- Comorbidity:
  - ☐ Insomnia
  - ☐ Other anxiety disorders
  - ☐ PTSD
  - ☐ MDD
  - ☐ Bipolar disorder (depressed or manic)
  - ☐ Substance use disorders

DIAGNOSTIC CRITERIA (DSM5-TR)[18]

A. Excessive anxiety and worry (apprehensive expectation), occurring more days than not for at least 6 months, with several events or activities (such as work or school performance).

B. The individual finds it difficult to control the worry.

C. The anxiety and worry are associated with three (or more) of the following six symptoms (with at least some symptoms having been present for more days than not for the past 6 months):
a. Note: only one item is required in children
b. Restlessness or feeling keyed up or on edge
c. Being easily fatigued
d. Difficulty concentrating or mind going blank
e. Irritability
f. Muscle tension
g. Sleep disturbance (difficulty falling or staying asleep, or restless, unsatisfying sleep)

D. The anxiety, worry, or physical symptoms cause clinically significant distress or impairment in social, occupational, or other important areas of functioning.

E. The disturbance is not attributable to the physiologic effects of a substance (e.g., a drug of abuse, a medication) or another medical condition (e.g., hyperthyroidism).

F. The disturbance is not better explained by another mental disorder (e.g., anxiety or worry about having panic attacks in panic disorder, negative evaluation in social anxiety disorder [social phobia], contamination or other obsessions in obsessive-compulsive disorder, separation from attachment figures in separation anxiety disorder, reminders of traumatic events in PTSD, gaining weight in anorexia nervosa, physical complaints in somatic symptom disorder, perceived appearance flaws in body dysmorphic disorder, having a serious illness in illness anxiety disorder, or the content of delusional beliefs in schizophrenia or delusional disorder).

MEASUREMENT OF ANXIETY

The diagnosis and management of anxiety disorders in a patient can be facilitated through numerous self-administered inventories, such as:

- Hamilton Anxiety Rating Scale (HAM-A)[58] for ages ≥18 years
- Beck Anxiety Inventory[59] for ages ≥18 years
- Screen for Child Anxiety Related Disorders (SCARED)[60] for ages 8 to 18 years
- State-Trait Anxiety Inventory for Children (STAIC)[61] for ages 9 to 12 years

These inventories provide reliable and valid measures of the severity of anxiety in adults and children.

TREATMENT

It is based on the biopsychosocial formulation utilizing the Osteopathic Five Model approach.

A. Metabolic
a. Nutrition
i. PUFAs meta-analyses of randomized controlled trials (RCTs) yield mixed findings.[62,63]
ii. Past preliminary research on anxiety; reported a statistically significant reduction in the severity of anxiety with 2.1 g/day EPA (dose ratio of 85.6% EPA to total EPA + DHA), compared to placebo.[64]

b. Pharmacologic
i. GAD can be thought of as a long-term disorder so stop and plan prior to starting any treatment.
ii. A treatment that combines psychotherapy, supportive measures, and pharmacologic interventions is likely to be the most successful.
iii. Cognitive behavioral therapy has significant research to support its use in anxiety disorders.
iv. Individuals with GAD require a significant amount of the clinician's time as part of their treatment.
v. Medications most often used for GAD.
vi. Benzodiazepines (for short-term use—less than 2 weeks only)
vii. As with depression we start with monotherapy and maximize the dose of medication. The specific dose and time to see clinical response varies based on the medication. As with depression we often try several monotherapies prior to using combined medications.
viii. A treatment protocol such as the Psychopharmacology Algorithm Project at Harvard South Shore Program can be used effectively for management of GAD. The Harvard algorithm is a nuanced and comprehensive tool with up-to-date research-based recommendations.[34]
ix. First-line treatment includes use of the selective serotonin reuptake inhibitor (SSRI) medications. If the first does not demonstrate clinical response try another

SSRI agent, then consider use of duloxetine or a serotonin-norepinephrine reuptake inhibitor (SNRI) agent.
x. Second-generation antipsychotic agents (quetiapine and risperidone) are typically reserved as third-line agents. Other second-generation agents have not been adequately studied as monotherapy for GAD.
xi. Commonly used combinations of medication for GAD:
1. Augment with hydroxyzine
2. Augment with short-term benzodiazepine (1 to 2 weeks)
3. Augment with pregabalin

B. Neurologic and behavioral:
a. Psychological therapies: Cognitive behavioral therapy
b. The combination of psychotherapy and pharmacotherapy is suggested by research for MDDs.[34]

C. Biomechanical:
a. OMT

D. Respiratory/Circulatory:
a. Exercise—no data to support effectiveness for core symptoms of GAD
b. Breathwork for relaxation[65]

Attention-Deficit Hyperactivity Disorder (ADHD)

- Lifetime prevalence: 5% children
  2.5% adults
- Male to Female ratio: 2:1 in children
  1.6:1 in adults
- Adult presentation:
  - ☐ Poor time management
  - ☐ Trouble initiating and completing tasks
  - ☐ Trouble with multitasking
  - ☐ Procrastination
  - ☐ Avoiding activities that demand attention in adults
  - ☐ Adults cope with their symptoms and tend to adapt to them by self-selecting active lifestyles and using support staff
  - ☐ All cases of "full" adult ADHD are preceded by childhood-onset ADHD
  - ☐ Many adults with ADHD had their childhood ADHD overlooked
- Differential diagnosis
  - ☐ Age-appropriate behaviors
  - ☐ Oppositional defiant disorder
  - ☐ Specific learning disabilities
  - ☐ Intellectual disabilities
  - ☐ Autism spectrum disorder
  - ☐ Reactive attachment disorder
  - ☐ Anxiety disorders
  - ☐ Depressive disorders
  - ☐ Bipolar disorder
  - ☐ Disruptive mood dysregulation disorder
  - ☐ Substance use disorders
  - ☐ Personality disorders
  - ☐ Psychotic disorders
- Comorbidity:
  - ☐ Conduct disorder
  - ☐ Disruptive mood dysregulation disorder
  - ☐ Specific learning disorders
  - ☐ Obsessive compulsive disorder
  - ☐ Tics/tic disorders/Tourette disorder
  - ☐ Anxiety disorders
  - ☐ Depressive disorders
  - ☐ Autism spectrum disorders

DIAGNOSTIC CRITERIA (DSM5-TR)[18]

A. A persistent pattern of inattention and/or hyperactivity-impulsivity that interferes with functioning or development, as characterized by inattention and/or hyperactivity/impulsivity.

B. Inattention: Six (or more) of the following symptoms have persisted for at least 6 months to a degree that is inconsistent with developmental level and that negatively impacts directly on social and academic/occupational activities:
Note: The symptoms are not solely a manifestation of oppositional behavior, defiance, hostility, or failure to understand tasks or instructions. For older adolescents and adults (age 17 and older), at least five symptoms are required.
a. Often fails to give close attention to details or makes careless mistakes in schoolwork, at work, or during other activities (e.g., overlooks or misses details, work is inaccurate).
b. Often has difficulty sustaining attention in tasks or play activities (e.g., has difficulty remaining focused during lectures, conversations, or lengthy reading).
c. Often does not seem to listen when spoken to directly (e.g., mind seems elsewhere, even in the absence of any obvious distraction).
d. Often does not follow through on instructions and fails to finish schoolwork, chores, or duties in the workplace (e.g., starts tasks but quickly loses focus and is easily sidetracked).
e. Often has difficulty organizing tasks and activities (e.g., difficulty managing sequential tasks; difficulty keeping materials and belongings in order; messy, disorganized work; has poor time management; fails to meet deadlines).
f. Often avoids, dislikes, or is reluctant to engage in tasks that require sustained mental effort (e.g., schoolwork or homework; for older adolescents and adults, preparing reports, completing forms, reviewing lengthy papers).
g. Often loses things necessary for tasks or activities (e.g., school materials, pencils, books, tools, wallets, keys, paperwork, eyeglasses, mobile telephones).
h. Is often easily distracted by extraneous stimuli (for older adolescents and adults, may include unrelated thoughts).
i. Is often forgetful in daily activities (e.g., doing chores, running errands; for older adolescents and adults, returning calls, paying bills, keeping appointments).

C. Hyperactivity and impulsivity: Six (or more) of the following symptoms have persisted for at least 6 months to a degree that is inconsistent with developmental level and that negatively impacts directly on social and academic/occupational activities:
Note: The symptoms are not solely a manifestation of oppositional behavior, defiance, hostility, or a failure to understand tasks or instructions. For older adolescents and adults (age 17 and older), at least five symptoms are required.
a. Often fidgets with or taps hands or feet or squirms in seat.
b. Often leaves seat in situations when remaining seated is expected (e.g., leaves his or her place in the classroom, in the office or other workplace, or in other situations that require remaining in place).
c. Often runs about or climbs in situations where it is inappropriate. (Note: in adolescents or adults, may be limited to feeling restless.)
d. Often unable to play or engage in leisure activities quietly.
e. Is often "on the go," acting as if "driven by a motor" (e.g., is unable to be or uncomfortable being still for extended time, as in restaurants, meetings; may be experienced by others as being restless or difficult to keep up with).
f. Often talks excessively.

g. Often blurts out an answer before a question has been completed (e.g., completes people's sentences; cannot wait for turn in conversation).
h. Often has difficulty waiting his or her turn (e.g., while waiting in line).
i. Often interrupts or intrudes on others (e.g., butts into conversations, games, or activities; may start using other people's things without asking or receiving permission; for adolescents and adults, may intrude into or take over what others are doing).

D. Several inattentive or hyperactive-impulsive symptoms were present prior to age 12 years.
E. Several inattentive or hyperactive-impulsive symptoms are present in two or more settings (e.g., at home, school, or work; with friends or relatives; in other activities).
F. There is clear evidence that the symptoms interfere with, or reduce the quality of, social, academic, or occupational functioning.
G. The symptoms do not occur exclusively during the course of schizophrenia or another psychotic disorder and are not better explained by another mental disorder (e.g., mood disorder, anxiety disorder, dissociative disorder, personality disorder, substance intoxication, or withdrawal).

MEASUREMENT OF ADHD

The diagnosis and management of ADHD in a patient can be facilitated through numerous self-administered inventories, such as the:

- ADHD Rating Scale-IV (ADHD-RS-IV)[49] for ages 5 to 18 years
- National Institute for Children's Health Quality (NICHQ) Vanderbilt Assessment Scale[66] for ages 6 to 12 years
- Conners Comprehensive Behavior Rating Scale (CBRS)[67,68] for ages 6 to 18 years
- Adult ADHD Self-Report Scale (ASRS v1.1)[69,70] for ages ≥18 years
- ADHD Rating Scale—5[71] for Children and Adolescents: Checklists, Norms, and Clinical Interpretation.

TREATMENT

It is based on the biopsychosocial formulation utilizing the Osteopathic Five Model approach.

A. Metabolic Model
  a. Evaluation for hyperthyroidism
  b. Nutrition
    i. PUFAs
    ii. An intake of 550 mg EPA fatty acid and 225 mg DHA fatty acid per day for 8 weeks is associated with less marked impulsive behavior in children with ADHD.[72]
    iii. High protein diet
  c. Pharmacologic
    i. Treatment typically starts with one of the stimulant medications. Start at low dose of medication then increase every week to clinical response, adverse effects, or maximum dose. Based on response the medication is maintained at the effective dose or a new medication is started in the case of lack of response or adverse effects. This medication is then titrated as the first medication. If needed a third stimulant medication is utilized. After the stimulant medications other medications such as the alpha agonists or combination medications, stimulant with an alpha agonist, are utilized.
    ii. A treatment protocol such as the one listed by the American Academy of Family Physicians may be utilized.[73]
    iii. Follow medication response with standardized rating scales such as the Vanderbilt or the ADHD VI rating scales (both are available to use at no cost), see above for additional resources.
    iv. Commonly used combinations of medication for ADHD (see Fig. 79.1)
      1. Augmentation with alpha-adrenergic agent
      2. Augmentation with bupropion
      3. Augmentation with venlafaxine

B. Neurologic model
  a. Decrease central stimulation
  b. Improve sleep patterns
  c. Involve special senses like art or music
C. Behavioral model
  a. Psychological therapies: cognitive therapy, social skills therapy, parent management training
  b. School Interventions: individual educational plan (IEP), 504 plan
D. Biomechanical:
  a. OMT may be helpful.[74,75]
E. Respiratory/Circulatory:
  a. Encouraging 30 to 60 minutes of exercise or play daily can improve attention, executive function, and motor skills.[76]

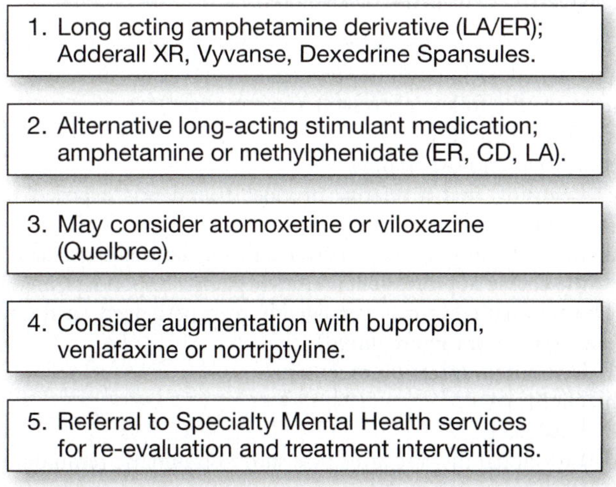

Figure 79.1. ADHD Algorithm. (Adapted from American Academy of Family Physicians; Overview of Treatment Recommendations for Adult ADHD, September 5, 2019. Loskutova N, et al.)

Posttraumatic Stress Disorder

- Lifetime prevalence: (8.7%)
- Sex ratio: PTSD is more prevalent among females than among males across the lifespan.
- Differential diagnosis
  - □ Adjustment disorders
  - □ Other anxiety disorders including obsessive compulsive disorder
  - □ MDD
  - □ Personality disorders
  - □ Dissociative disorders
  - □ Conversion disorders
  - □ Psychotic disorders
- Comorbidity:
  - □ MDD
  - □ Bipolar disorder
  - □ Other anxiety disorders
  - □ Substance use disorders
  - □ Traumatic brain injury

DIAGNOSTIC CRITERIA (DSM5-TR)[18]

A. The person was exposed to death, threatened death, actual or threatened serious injury, or actual or threatened sexual violence, in the following way(s): (one required)
   a. Direct exposure
   b. Witnessing the trauma
   c. Learning that a relative or close friend was exposed to a trauma
   d. Indirect exposure to aversive details of the trauma, usually in the course of professional duties (e.g., first responders, medics)

B. The traumatic event is persistently re-experienced, in the following way(s): (one required)
   a. Unwanted upsetting memories
   b. Nightmares
   c. Flashbacks
   d. Emotional distress after exposure to traumatic reminders
   e. Physical reactivity after exposure to traumatic reminders

C. Avoidance of trauma-related stimuli after the trauma, in the following way(s): (one required)
   a. Trauma-related thoughts or feelings
   b. Trauma-related reminders

D. Negative thoughts or feelings that began or worsened after the trauma, in the following way(s): (two required)
   a. Inability to recall key features of the trauma
   b. Overly negative thoughts and assumptions about oneself or the world
   c. Exaggerated blame of self or others for causing the trauma
   d. Negative affect
   e. Decreased interest in activities
   f. Feeling isolated
   g. Difficulty experiencing positive affect

E. Trauma-related arousal and reactivity that began or worsened after the trauma, in the following way(s): (two required)
   a. Irritability or aggression
   b. Risky or destructive behavior
   c. Hypervigilance
   d. Heightened startle reaction
   e. Difficulty concentrating
   f. Difficulty sleeping

F. Symptoms last for more than 1 month. (Required)

G. Symptoms create distress or functional impairment (e.g., social, occupational). (Required)

H. Symptoms are not due to medication, substance use, or other illnesses. (Required)

I. Two specifications of PTSD
   a. Dissociative specification.
      i. In addition to meeting criteria for diagnosis, an individual experiences high levels of either of the following in reaction to trauma-related stimuli:
      ii. Depersonalization. Experience of being an outside observer of or detached from oneself (e.g., feeling as if "this is not happening to me" or one were in a dream).
      iii. Derealization. Experience of unreality, distance, or distortion (e.g., "things are not real").
   b. Delayed specification.
      i. Full diagnostic criteria are not met until at least 6 months after the trauma(s), although onset of symptoms may occur immediately.

MEASUREMENT OF PTSD

The diagnosis and management of PTSD in a patient can be facilitated through numerous self-administered inventories, such as:

- PTSD Checklist—Civilian Version (PCL-C) (greater than 18 years of age)
- This inventory provides reliable and valid measures of the severity of PTSD in adults.

TREATMENT

It is based on the biopsychosocial formulation utilizing the Osteopathic Five Model approach.

A. Metabolic
   a. Nutrition
      i. PUFAs 1,000 mg EPA/day
   b. Pharmacologic
      i. A treatment protocol such as the Psychopharmacology Algorithm Project at Harvard South Shore Program can be used effectively for management of ADHD. The Harvard algorithm is a nuanced and comprehensive tool with up-to-date research-based recommendations.[77]
      ii. First-line treatments are the SSRI medications followed by an alternative SSRI, SNRI, or mirtazapine.
      iii. If nightmares or nighttime arousals consider prazosin.
      iv. If psychosis is present consider use of an antipsychotic agent.
   c. Table of commonly used augmentation for PTSD:
      i. Augmentation for hyperarousal symptoms
         1. Clonidine, quetiapine, risperidone
      ii. Augmentation for re-experiencing symptoms
         1. aripiprazole, lamotrigine, quetiapine, risperidone, topiramate
         2. augmentation for avoidance symptoms:
         3. aripiprazole, lamotrigine

B. Neurologic and behavioral:
   a. Psychological therapies: trauma-focused cognitive behavioral therapy, cognitive processing therapy, trauma informed therapy
   b. Mind–body practices[78,79]:
   c. A 2017 Meta-analysis of 19 studies found that meditation and yoga are promising complementary approaches in the treatment of PTSD among adults and warrant further study.[80]

C. Biomechanical:
   a. Consider OMT for associated somatic dysfunction—No specific studies were found utilizing OMT for PTSD.[75]

D. Respiratory/Circulatory:
   a. Exercise—a systematic review and meta-analysis found a small but significant effect of exercise on depressive symptoms, a larger effect on sleep, and quality of life.[81]
   b. Breathwork for relaxation—part of mind–body practices noted above.

Obsessive Compulsive Disorder

- Twelve-month Prevalence: (1.2%)
- Sex ratio: In adulthood females are slightly greater than males/ in childhood males more common than females
- Differential diagnosis
  - ☐ Anxiety disorders
  - ☐ MDD
  - ☐ Eating disorders
  - ☐ Tic and stereotyped movements
  - ☐ Psychotic disorders
  - ☐ Obsessive compulsive personality disorder
- Comorbidity:
  - ☐ Other anxiety disorders
  - ☐ Depressive disorders

- ☐ Bipolar disorder
- ☐ PTSD
- ☐ Schizoaffective disorder
- ☐ Tourette disorder

DIAGNOSTIC CRITERIA (DSM5-TR)[18]

A. Presence of obsessions, compulsions, or both:
   a. Obsessions are the recurrent and persistent thoughts, urges, or images that are intrusive and cause distress or anxiety.
   b. Compulsions are the repetitive behaviors or mental acts that a person feels compelled to do to relieve the anxiety caused by the obsessions. The individual attempts to ignore or suppress obsessions or compulsions or to neutralize them with some other thought or action (i.e., by performing a compulsion).

B. Obsessions or compulsions are time-consuming (taking up more than 1 hour per day) or cause clinically significant distress or impairment in social, occupational, or other important areas of functioning.

C. The disturbance is not attributable to the physiologic effects of a substance (e.g., a drug of abuse, a medication) or another medical condition (e.g., head trauma).

D. The disturbance is not better explained by the presence of another mental disorder (e.g., panic disorder with agoraphobia, separation anxiety disorder, body dysmorphic disorder, trichotillomania [hair-pulling], skin picking disorder, hoarding disorder, autism spectrum disorder, ADHD).

E. Determine if the patient has
   a. Good or fair insight
   b. Poor insight
   c. Absent insight/delusional beliefs

MEASUREMENT OF OCD

1. Yale-Brown Obsessive Compulsive Disorder Checklist (Y-BOC)—The short form Y-BOC can be utilized to track symptom response.[82]
2. This checklist is typically utilized by a clinician specializing in the treatment of OCD.

TREATMENT

It is based on the biopsychosocial formulation utilizing the Osteopathic Five Model approach.

A. Metabolic
   a. Nutrition
      i. PUFAs 1,000 mg EPA/day
   b. Pharmacologic
      i. A treatment protocol such as the Psychopharmacology Algorithm Project at Harvard South Shore Program can be used effectively for management of ADHD. The Harvard algorithm is a nuanced and comprehensive tool with up-to-date research-based recommendations.[83]
      ii. First-line treatments are the SSRI medications; fluoxetine, sertraline, or fluvoxamine.
      iii. Each trial of medication must be at an adequate dose and for 8 to 12 weeks.
      iv. Pharmacogenetic testing for "rapid metabolizer" may be helpful for choice of SSRI medication and/or dosing strategies.
      v. Augmentation strategies include memantine, lamotrigine, NAC, riluzole, topiramate, and others.
      vi. TMS is an option for augmentation, is FDA-approved, and has been widely used as an alternative treatment. However, the most effective parameters, targets, and stimulation frequencies remain controversial, and high-quality RCTs are needed.[84]
      vii. Many novel agents have been looked at for OCD. Referral to a clinician specializing in treatment of OCD for use of these agents is recommended.

B. Neurologic and behavioral:
   a. Psychological therapies: exposure response prevention (ERP) therapy is the therapy of choice for addressing OCD.[85]
   b. ERP involves exposing individuals to the thoughts, images, objects, and situations that trigger their anxiety and obsessions, while simultaneously teaching them to refrain from engaging in the compulsive behaviors typically performed to alleviate their distress.[85]
   c. The combination of psychotherapy and pharmacotherapy is suggested by research.[86]

C. Biomechanical:
   a. Consider OMT for associated somatic dysfunction—No specific studies were found utilizing OMT for PTSD.[75]

D. Respiratory/Circulatory:
   a. Regular exercise as small RCTs have shown that exercise and health-related behaviors may be beneficial to patients with OCD. However, a large systematic review and meta-analysis is needed to estimate potential efficacy.[87,88]

SUMMARY

The psychiatric profession has roots in both the medical "hands on" world and psychoanalytic thinking. The contemporary psychiatrist is a blend of the old and new. The biopsychosocial formulation is the foundation for understanding a patient and development of a comprehensive treatment plan to address the patient's specific needs. The Osteopathic five-model concept is a biopsychosocial formulation that can be effectively used by the psychiatrist trained in osteopathic approaches. The therapeutic or working alliance between the patient and physician is the underlying foundation for effective implementation of the treatment plan derived from the five-model formulation. Contemporary osteopathic psychiatrists have many tools to assist patients including biologic, psychological, and manual medicine. This requires the primary care osteopathic psychiatric physician to have a clear understanding of transference, professional boundaries, and communication skills. With this understanding, skill, and medical knowledge, the contemporary primary care osteopathic psychiatrist will be able to provide comprehensive and effective care to those who seek care.

ACKNOWLEDGMENTS

Case by: Allison Abresch-Meyer, DO. The author and editors of this chapter would like to acknowledge the editing and scholarly contributions of Yunting Tang and Kurt P. Heinking.

REFERENCES

1. Cullum CM, Saine K, Chan LD, Martin-Cook K, Gray KF, Weiner MF. Performance-based instrument to assess functional capacity in dementia: the Texas Functional Living Scale. *Neuropsychiatry Neuropsychol Behav Neurol.* 2001;14(2):103–108.
2. Hall CD, Herdman SJ, Whitney SL, et al. Vestibular rehabilitation for peripheral vestibular hypofunction: an updated clinical practice guideline from the academy of neurologic physical therapy of the American Physical Therapy Association. *J Neurol Phys Ther.* 2022;46(2):118–177.

3. American Osteopathic Association; Chila AG, Carreiro JE, eds. *Foundations of Osteopathic Medicine*. 3rd ed. Lippincott Williams & Wilkins; 2010.
4. DiGiovanna EL, Schiowitz S, Dowling DJ. *An Osteopathic Approach to Diagnosis and Treatment*. Lippincott Williams & Wilkins; 2005.
5. Fuertes JN, Boylan LS, Fontanella JA. Behavioral indices in medical care outcome: the working alliance, adherence, and related factors. *J Gen Intern Med.* 2009;24(1):80–85.
6. Jones A, Vallis M, Cooke D, Pouwer F. Working together to promote diabetes control: a practical guide for diabetes health care providers in establishing a working alliance to achieve self-management support. *J Diabetes Res.* 2016;2016:2830910.
7. De Vries AMM, Gholamrezaee MM, Leeuw IMV, et al. Patient satisfaction and alliance as a function of the physician's self-regulation, the physician's stress, and the content of consultation in cancer care. *Psychooncology.* 2017;26(7):927–934.
8. Rubak S, Sandbæk A, Lauritzen T, Christensen B. Motivational interviewing: a systematic review and meta-analysis. *Br J Gen Pract.* 2005; 55(513):305–312.
9. Rollnick S, Miller WR, Aloia MS. *Motivational Interviewing in Health Care: Helping Patients Change Behavior*. The Guilford Press; 2008.
10. Zinn WM. Transference phenomena in medical practice: being whom the patient needs. *Ann Intern Med.* 1990;113(4):293–298.
11. Walther R, Douglas SP, Mozdzierz GJ, Poon P, Fox E. *Ethical Boundaries in the Patient-Clinician Relationship. Report by the National Ethics Committee of the Veterans Administration*. National Center for Ethics in Health Care. National Ethics Committee; 2003.
12. Fine PG. Long-term consequences of chronic pain: mounting evidence for pain as a neurological disease and parallels with other chronic disease states. *Pain Med.* 2011;12(7):996–1004.
13. Hsieh J-C, Belfrage M, Stone-Elander S, Hansson P, Ingvar M. Central representation of chronic ongoing neuropathic pain studied by positron emission tomography. *Pain.* 1995;63(2):225–236.
14. Stevens FL, Hurley RA, Taber KH. Anterior cingulate cortex: unique role in cognition and emotion. *J Neuropsychiatry Clin Neurosci.* 2011;23(2): 121–125.
15. Gilmour GS, Nielsen G, Teodoro T, et al. Management of functional neurological disorder. *J Neurol.* 2020;267(7):2164–2172.
16. O'Neal MA, Baslet G. Treatment for patients with a functional neurological disorder (conversion disorder): an integrated approach. *Am J Psychiatry.* 2018;175(4):307–314.
17. Espay AJ, Aybek S, Carson A, et al. Current concepts in diagnosis and treatment of functional neurological disorders. *JAMA Neurol.* 2018;75(9): 1132–1141.
18. American Psychiatric Association. *Diagnostic and Statistical Manual of Mental disorders*. 5th ed. American Psychiatric Association; 2013.
19. Aybek S, Perez DL. Diagnosis and management of functional neurological disorder. *BMJ.* 2022;376:o64.
20. Plews-Ogan M, Owens JE, Goodman M, Wolfe P, Schorling J. A pilot study evaluating mindfulness-based stress reduction and massage for the management of chronic pain. *J Gen Intern Med.* 2005;20(12): 1136–1138.
21. Kaplan KH, Goldenberg DL, Galvin-Nadeau M. The impact of a meditation-based stress reduction program on fibromyalgia. *Gen Hosp Psychiatry.* 1993;15:284–289.
22. Astin JA, Berman BM, Bausell B, Lee W-L, Hochberg M, Forys KL. The efficacy of mindfulness meditation plus Qigong movement therapy in the treatment of fibromyalgia: a randomized controlled trial. *J Rheumatol.* 2003;30(10):2257–2262.
23. Kole-Snijders AM, Vlaeyen JW, Goossens ME, et al. Chronic low-back pain: what does cognitive coping skills training add to operant behavioral treatment? Results of a randomized clinical trial. *J Consult Clin Psychol.* 1999;67(6):931–944.
24. McCarberg B, Wolf J. Chronic pain management in a health maintenance organization. *Clin J Pain.* 1999;15:50–57.
25. Johansson C, Dahl J, Jannert M, Melin L, Andersson G. Effects of a cognitive-behavioral pain-management program. *Behav Res Ther.* 1998; 36(10):915–930.
26. Haugli L, Steen E, Laerum E, Nygard R, Finset A. Learning to have less pain—is it possible? A one-year follow-up study of the effects of a personal construct group learning programme on patients with chronic musculoskeletal pain. *Patient Educ Couns.* 2001;45(2):111–118.
27. Broderick JE, Junghaenel DU, Schwartz JE. Written emotional expression produces health benefits in fibromyalgia patients. *Psychosom Med.* 2005;67(2):326–334.
28. Gillis ME, Lumley MA, Mosley-Williams A, Leisen JCC, Roehrs T. The health effects of at-home written emotional disclosure in fibromyalgia: a randomized trial. *Ann Behav Med.* 2006;32(2):135–146.
29. Sarno JE. *The Mindbody Prescription: Healing the Body, Healing the Pain*. Warmer Books; 1999.
30. Schubiner H. Mind body syndrome. https://unlearnyourpain.com/mind-body-syndrome/. Accessed November 21, 2024.
31. Schubiner H. *Unlearn Your Pain*. Sheridan Books, Inc.; 2009.
32. Illich I. *Medical Nemesis: The Expropriation of Health*. Pantheon; 1976.
33. Carragee EJ. Clinical practice. Persistent low back pain. *N Engl J Med.* 2005;352(18):1891–1898.
34. Sadock BJ, Sadock VA, Ruiz P. *Kaplan & Sadock's Synopsis of Psychiatry*. 11th ed. Wolters Kluwer; 2015, Chapters 8, 9.
35. Zung WWK. A self-rating depression scale. *Arch Gen Psychiatry.* 1965; 12:63–70.
36. Zung WWK. A rating instrument for anxiety disorders. *Psychosomatics.* 1971;12(6):371–379.
37. Beck AT. *Depression: Clinical, Experimental and Theoretical Aspects*. Harper & Row; 1967.
38. Beck AT. *Cognitive Theory and Emotional Disorders*. International Universities Press; 1976.
39. Hathaway SR, McKinley JC. *MMPI Manual*. Psychological Corp.; 1943.
40. Dahlstrom WG, Welsh GS. *An MMPI Handbook*. University of Minnesota Press; 1972.
41. Bae Y. Test review: children's depression inventory 2 (CDI 2). *J Psychoeduc Assess.* 2012;30(3)304–308.
42. Spitzer RL, Williams JBW, Kroenke K, et al. *PRIME-MD Clinical Evaluation Guide*. New York State Psychiatric Institute, Biometrics Research Dept.; 1994.
43. Spitzer RL, Williams JB, Linzer M, et al. Utility of a new procedure for diagnosing mental disorders in primary care. The PRIME-MD 1000 study. *JAMA.* 1994;272(22):1749–1756.
44. Liao Y, Xie B, Zhang H, et al. Efficacy of omega-3 PUFAs in depression: a meta-analysis. *Transl Psychiatry.* 2019;9(1):190.
45. Mehdi S, Manohar K, Shariff A, et al. Omega-3 fatty acids supplementation in the treatment of depression: an observational study. *J Pers Med.* 2023;13(2):224.
46. Hardin A, Baldwin-Sayre C. L-methylfolate as monotherapy for treatment-resistant depression: a case study. *Integr Med (Encinitas).* 2020;19(4): 14–18.
47. Maletic V, Shelton R, Holmes V. A review of L-methylfolate as adjunctive therapy in the treatment of major depressive disorder. *Prim Care Companion CNS Disord.* 2023;25(3):22nr03361.
48. Dean O, Giorlando F, Berk M. N-acetylcysteine in psychiatry: current therapeutic evidence and potential mechanisms of action. *J Psychiatry Neurosci.* 2011;36(2):78–86.
49. Giakoumatos CI, Osser D. The psychopharmacology algorithm project at the Harvard South Shore Program: an update on unipolar nonpsychotic depression. *Harv Rev Psychiatry.* 2019;27(1):33–52.
50. Bowes MR, Speicher MR, Tran L-AT, Santiago PN. Osteopathic manipulative medicine and its role in psychiatry. *Cureus.* 2023;15(10): e47045.
51. Xie Y, Wu Z, Sun L, et al. The effects and mechanisms of exercise on the treatment of depression. *Front Psychiatry.* 2021;12:705559.
52. Hanssen H, Minghetti A, Faude O, et al. Effects of endurance exercise modalities on arterial stiffness in patients suffering from unipolar depression: a randomized controlled trial. *Front Psychiatry.* 2018;8:311.
53. Young RC, Biggs JT, Ziegler VE, Meyer DA. A rating scale for mania: reliability, validity and sensitivity. *Br J Psychiatry.* 1978;133(5): 429–435.
54. Axelson D, Birmaher BJ, Brent D, et. al. A preliminary study of the kiddie schedule for affective disorders and schizophrenia for school-age children mania rating scale for children and adolescents. *J Child Adolesc Psychopharmacol.* 2003;13(4):463–470.

55. Appleton KM, Voyias PD, Sallis HM, et al. Omega-3 fatty acids for depression in adults. *Cochrane Database Syst Rev*. 2021;11(11):CD004692.
56. Ashton MM, Berk M, Ng CH, et al. A systematic review of nutraceuticals for the treatment of bipolar disorder. *Can J Psychiatry*. 2021;66(3):262–273.
57. Wang D, Osser DN. The psychopharmacology algorithm project at the Harvard South Shore Program: an update on bipolar depression. *Bipolar Disord*. 2020;22(5):472–489.
58. Hamilton M. The assessment of anxiety states by rating. *Br J Med Psychol*. 1959;32:50–55.
59. Beck AT, Epstein N, Brown G, Steer RA. An inventory for measuring clinical anxiety: psychometric properties. *J Consult Clin Psychol*. 1988;56(6):893–897.
60. Monga S, Birmaher B, Chiappetta L, et al. Screen for child anxiety-related emotional disorders (SCARED): convergent and divergent validity. *Depress Anxiety*. 2000;12:85–91.
61. Reynolds CR. Concurrent validity of What I think and feel: the revised Children's Manifest Anxiety Scale. *J Consult Clin Psychol*. 1980;48(6):774–775.
62. Su K-P, Tseng P-T, Lin P-Y, et al. Association of use of omega-3 polyunsaturated fatty acids with changes in severity of anxiety symptoms: a systematic review and meta-analysis. *JAMA Netw Open*. 2018;1(5):e182327.
63. Kelaiditis CF, Gibson EL, Dyall SC. Effects of long-chain omega-3 polyunsaturated fatty acids on reducing anxiety and/or depression in adults; a systematic review and meta-analysis of randomised controlled trials. *Prostaglandins Leukot Essent Fatty Acids*. 2023;192:102572.
64. Kiecolt-Glaser JK, Belury MA, Andridge R, Malarkey WB, Glaser R. Omega-3 supplementation lowers inflammation and anxiety in medical students: a randomized controlled trial. *Brain Behav Immun*. 2011;25(8):1725–1734.
65. Jerath R, Crawford MW, Barnes VA, Harden K. Self-regulation of breathing as a primary treatment for anxiety. *Appl Psychophysiol Biofeedback*. 2015;40(2):107–115.
66. Becker SP, Langberg JM, Vaughn AJ, Epstein JN. Clinical utility of the Vanderbilt ADHD diagnostic parent rating scale comorbidity screening scales. *J Dev Behav Pediatr*. 2012;33(3):221–228.
67. Conners K, Pitkanen J, Rzepa SR. *Conners Comprehensive Behavior Rating Scale*. Encyclopedia of Clinical Neuropsychology; 2011.
68. Conners CK, Sitarenios G, Parker JD, Epstein JN. The revised Conners' Parent Rating Scale (CPRS-R): factor structure, reliability, and criterion validity. *J Abnorm Child Psychol*. 1998;26(4):257–268.
69. van de Glind G, van den Brink W, Koeter MWJ, et al. Validity of the adult ADHD Self-Report Scale (ASRS) as a screener for adult ADHD in treatment seeking substance use disorder patients. *Drug Alcohol Depend*. 2013;132(3):587–596.
70. Gray S, Woltering S, Mawjee K, Tannock R. The adult ADHD Self-Report Scale (ASRS): utility in college students with attention-deficit/hyperactivity disorder. *PeerJ*. 2014;2:e324.
71. DuPaul GJ, Power TJ, Anastopoulos AD, Reid R. ADHD rating scale—5 for children and adolescents: Checklists, norms, and clinical interpretation. 2nd ed. New York, NY: Guilford Press; 2016.
72. Martin ISM, Vilar EG, Rojo SS, et al. Impulsiveness in children with attention-deficit/hyperactivity disorder after an 8-week intervention with the Mediterranean diet and/or omega-3 fatty acids: a randomised clinical trial. *Neurologia (Engl Ed)*. 2022;37(7):513–523.
73. Loskutova N. *Overview of Treatment Recommendations for Adult ADHD*. American Academy of Family Physicians; 2019.
74. Accorsi A, Lucci C, Granchelli C, et al. Effect of osteopathic manipulative therapy in the attentive performance of children with attention-deficit/hyperactivity disorder. *J Am Osteopath Assoc*. 2014;114(5):374–381.
75. Bohlen L, Shaw R, Cerritelli F, Esteves JE. Osteopathy and mental health: an embodied, predictive, and interoceptive framework. *Front Psychol*. 2021;12:767005.
76. Sun W, Yu M, Zhou X. Effects of physical exercise on attention deficit and other major symptoms in children with ADHD: a meta-analysis. *Psychiatry Res*. 2022;311:114509.
77. Bajor LA, Ticlea AN, Osser DN. The psychopharmacology algorithm project at the Harvard South Shore Program: an update on posttraumatic stress disorder. *Harv Rev Psychiatry*. 2011;19(5):240–258.
78. Kim SH, Schneider SM, Kravitz L, Mermier C, Burge MR. Mind-body practices for posttraumatic stress disorder. *J Investig Med*. 2013;61(5):827–834.
79. Hilton L, Maher AR, Colaiaco B, et al. Meditation for posttraumatic stress: systematic review and meta-analysis. *Psychol Trauma*. 2017;9(4):453–460.
80. Gallegos AM, Crean HF, Pigeon WR, Heffner KL. Meditation and yoga for posttraumatic stress disorder: a meta-analytic review of randomized controlled trials. *Clin Psychol Rev*. 2017;58:115–124.
81. Björkman F, Ekblom Ö. Physical exercise as treatment for PTSD: a systematic review and meta-analysis. *Mil Med*. 2022;187(9–10):e1103–e1113.
82. du Mortier JAM, Visser HAD, van Balkom AJLM, et al. Examining the factor structure of the self-report Yale-Brown Obsessive Compulsive Scale Symptom Checklist. *Psychiatry Res*. 2019;271:299–305.
83. Beaulieu AM, Tabasky E, Osser DN. The psychopharmacology algorithm project at the Harvard South Shore Program: an algorithm for adults with obsessive-compulsive disorder. *Psychiatry Res*. 2019;281:112583.
84. Liang K, Li H, Bu X, et al. Efficacy and tolerability of repetitive transcranial magnetic stimulation for the treatment of obsessive-compulsive disorder in adults: a systematic review and network meta-analysis. *Transl Psychiatry*. 2021;11:332.
85. Nezgovorova V, Reid J, Fineberg NA, Hollander E. Optimizing first line treatments for adults with OCD. *Compr Psychiatry*. 2022;115:152305.
86. Fineberg NA, Baldwin DS, Drummond LM, et al. Optimal treatment for obsessive compulsive disorder: a randomized controlled feasibility study of the clinical-effectiveness and cost-effectiveness of cognitive-behavioural therapy, selective serotonin reuptake inhibitors and their combination in the management of obsessive-compulsive disorder. *Int Clin Psychopharmacol*. 2018;33(6):334–348.
87. Abrantes AM, Brown RA, Strong DR, et al. A pilot randomized controlled trial of aerobic exercise as an adjunct to OCD treatment. *Gen Hosp Psychiatry*. 2017;49:51–55.
88. Bottoms L, Pons MM, Fineberg NA, et al. Effects of exercise on obsessive-compulsive disorder symptoms: a systematic review and meta-analysis. *Int J Psychiatry Clin Pract*. 2023;27(3):232–242.

80 Osteopathic Considerations in End-of-Life Care

KAREN J. NICHOLS

KEY CONCEPTS

- End-of-life decisions should be the result of the collaboration and mutual informing of the patient, the patient's family, and the physicians; each sharing their own expertise to help the patient make the best possible decisions, often in the worst possible circumstances.
- A significant opportunity is presented for offering each patient the most complete expression of osteopathic medicine's philosophy and practice.
- Physicians must respect and accommodate patient needs in communicating prognosis.
- Physicians must also respect family members' needs in order to understand the dying process and grief.
- Student–physician interaction with the dying may be the ideal training ground for young doctors.

INTRODUCTION

Death reminds us of our fragility and sameness: we all die. Caring for the dying is a gift. Death is not so much denied but invisible.

Death should be understood to be a relational and spiritual process rather than simply a physiologic event.[1]

The opportunity and ability to employ all the facets of being an osteopathic physician is never more needed than at the end of a patient's life. When there is no more surgical intervention possible or advisable, when there are no more tests and studies to conduct, when there is no more medication that can turn the tide of the inevitable decline, then the physician moves fully into utilizing their most important tool, the physician–patient relationship for psychological support.

End-of-life care is filled with demands and challenges that all physicians must deal with at some point. No discipline in medicine escapes the issues of end-of-life care. Ironically and unfortunately for their patients, physicians in those disciplines that are perceived as relatively immune to routinely dealing with end-of-life issues find themselves least prepared when these issues inevitably arise. Further, a very interesting phenomenon that occurs not infrequently is that the student physician who has taken the time to establish a rapport through caring may be the first physician the patient will turn to with questions and concerns at end of life. The wise medical student will learn the principles of end-of-life care to be able to assist patients.

PRINCIPLES OF END-OF-LIFE CARE

To clarify the requirements for proper care, The Milbank Memorial Fund published a set of "Principles for Care of Patients at the End of Life: An Emerging Consensus among the Specialties of Medicine."[2] The American Osteopathic Association (AOA) End-Of-Life Care Advisory Council prepared an osteopathic version of these principles, which was approved by the AOA House of Delegates in 2000 with subsequent reviews and updates since.[3,4]

RESEARCH INTO END-OF-LIFE CARE

The landmark study—"A controlled trial to improve care for seriously ill hospitalized patients: The study to understand prognoses and preferences for outcomes and risks of treatments (SUPPORT)"—gave the first clear understanding of how patients and families viewed their end-of-life care experiences.[5]

- The phase I observation stage revealed and documented shortcomings in communication, frequency of aggressive treatment, and the characteristics of hospital death. It documented the following:
  - A strong indictment of the medical care system discovering that only 47% of physicians knew when their patients preferred to avoid cardiopulmonary resuscitation.
  - 46% of do-not-resuscitate (DNR) orders were written within 2 days of death.
  - 38% of patients who died spent at least 10 days in an intensive care unit.
  - For 50% of conscious patients who died in the hospital, family members reported moderate-to-severe pain at least half of the time.
- Unfortunately, the phase II intervention stage of the study did not demonstrate any improvement in care or patient outcomes. The study's conclusions recommended greater individual and society commitment and more proactive and forceful measures to fill the gaps identified.[5]

Many subsequent studies have sought to study the quality of end-of-life care and to understand the perception of both physicians and patients/families about expectations and knowledge of end-of-life care issues.

- The persistent lack of patients' knowledge of options at the end of life was studied by Silveira et al.[6]
- Of the 1,000 patients surveyed, there were 728 respondents.
- Only 23% to 46% of those responding demonstrated an appropriate awareness of four areas relevant to end-of-life care.

All research points to the importance of more education of physicians and patients about end-of-life care issues.

GOALS OF CARE

The most important issue that needs to be addressed in dealing with patients at end of life is to determine their goals of care. For example:

1. What does the patient perceive as appropriate care at the end of life?

2. How does the patient wish to see themself living out the final days of life?
3. What does the patient see as the acceptable limits of their existence given the constraints of the current medical condition?

These open-ended questions take the emphasis from "which procedure to perform" and move it to "how do you want to spend your final days?" The patient who states that they want every measure employed to keep themselves alive every possible minute regardless of being aware of their surroundings leads the physician to create a very different care plan than one for the patient who states that they want to spend the final days at home out of pain surrounded by loved ones. End-of-life decisions should be the result of the collaboration and mutual informing of the patient, the patient's family, and the physicians, each sharing their own expertise to help the patient make the best possible decision, often in the worst possible circumstances.

Patients and families also need to understand that the goals of care can and should change as the disease progresses.

> "Initially, patients might hope that the cancer responds to chemotherapy or surgery. When disease control is no longer possible, patients might hope to live pain free, achieve closure on personal issues or die surrounded by friends and family."[7]

Adults with decision-making capacity should be informed of their choices, and they have the legal and ethical right to make their own decisions about their life, including the right to refuse recommended life-sustaining medical treatment. This position honors the patient's autonomy and liberty as guaranteed in the U.S. Constitution. This right exists even when the physician disagrees with the patient's decision.[4]

Patients without decision-making capacity can have their choices adhered to by physicians who follow a previously executed advance directive described below. The principle of "best interests" (what would the reasonable and informed patient select) is invoked if the individual's wishes are not known. Quality of life should be viewed from the patient's perspective in all these decisions because quality of life can only be self-determined. Extreme caution must be exercised when trying to determine what constitutes quality of life for another person as research has shown that patients consistently assess their quality of life to be better than their caregivers think their patients do.[4]

The overriding issue is not what the family or friends want for the patient at end of life, but rather what would the patient want for themselves. If the noncognitive patient were to awaken for only 15 minutes and be able to fully understand the circumstances, what decisions would the patient make? If the answer is unclear, society should err on the side of life. If the answer is clear, then refusal to follow the patient's wishes is unethical and illegal.[4]

ADVANCE CARE PLANNING

Ideally, every person who comes to the hospital or care setting would have completed some type of document that falls under the category of "advance care planning." This approach was the impetus for the "Patient Self-determination Act of 1991," which requires that every person entering a facility that receives Medicare/Medicaid funding must be asked whether they have executed such a document or wishes to do so.

- Provision of care is not predicated upon the existence or absence of such a document; the only requirement is that the patient or family is aware that such information is available and that such a document could be created.
- Advance care planning documents generally include living wills or durable medical powers of attorney for health care affairs (proxy designation for health care affairs) and can be self-executed with or without the aid of an attorney.
- This medical power of attorney is separate and distinct from the legal power of attorney, and neither implies the presence or intent of the other. Such documents are available from many organizations and are also online.
- These documents carry the weight of law but can be superseded by the patient at any time.
- Living wills document the desired treatments but leave much room for interpretation when the situation doesn't match the directives, so a combination of a living will and a durable medical power of attorney may be best.

When the physician, patient, and family have had these conversations earlier and are in agreement, there is less need for such documentation. However, when that is not the case, these documents can assist in settling disagreements. Ultimately, if agreement cannot be reached, the hospital ethics committee can be called upon to assist with these deliberations (Table 80.1).

Sample living wills and durable medical powers of attorney can be downloaded from several Internet sites, using the search term: **living will form**.

WHOLE PATIENT ASSESSMENT

Nowhere is the principle of assessing the whole patient more important than at end of life. Whole patient assessment does not imply that the physician will be employing futile treatment. It implies that the patient approaching the end of their life is to be accorded the same well–thought-out evaluation and care as any other patient.

- A patient dying from heart failure develops a fever. The fever is not caused by heart failure and may be an indication of an easily treatable problem.
- Pedal edema in a patient with respiratory failure without cor pulmonale cannot be assumed to be due to respiratory failure.
- A patient at the end of life may have incorrect assumptions about symptoms and be denied simple and appropriate care just because they are "dying anyway."

A proper patient assessment does not have to be painful, costly, onerous, or futile. It just has to be thoughtful and appropriate.

TABLE 80.1

Differences between Living Will and Power of Attorney

	Living Will	Durable Medical Power of Attorney for Health Affairs	Power of Attorney
Purpose	Guidance about my end-of-life preferences	Who gets to make the actual decision about my end of life when I can't	Who can act on my behalf for legal and financial decisions
Limitations	None	Medical decisions only	Legal/financial decisions only

SYMPTOM MANAGEMENT

Closely tied to the approach of whole patient assessment is the requirement to provide proper symptom management. When whole patient assessment does not reveal a treatable cause for a specific symptom, there are appropriate interventions for those symptoms. The types of symptoms most frequently encountered as part of the end-of-life process that may not be indicative of another medical cause include the following:

- Anorexia
- Cachexia
- Constipation
- Decubitus ulcers
- Diarrhea
- Dyspnea
- Edema
- Fatigue
- Fluid balance problems
- Insomnia
- Nausea
- Odors
- Skin integrity
- Vomiting
- Weakness

The physician caring for the patient with such symptoms at end of life should reference the American College of Physicians (ACP) Clinical Practice Guidelines[8] and Education for Physicians on End-of-Life Care (EPEC).[9]

PAIN MANAGEMENT

Another aspect of patient care at the end of life, which bears special mention, is proper pain management. The key concept about how much medication to provide to control pain is: "it takes as much as it takes." Many of the restrictions and guidelines about dosing pain medication do not apply at end of life for anyone other than a narcotic-naive patient.

- The principle of "start low and go slow" applies to every patient until the appropriate level of pain relief has been achieved.
- The concept of pain management is that pain medication should never be administered on a "prn" basis but as a continuous infusion to maintain a baseline of pain control. This level of control may have to be supplemented at times of unavoidable painful processes, or if the level of pain steadily escalates, but the patient should never be allowed to experience unrelieved pain.
- There is no need to prevent addiction at the end of life. Medication tolerance may be seen, expected, and properly managed with increased dosing though.
- The proper usage of narcotics at the end of life in a person who is or was addicted to narcotics prior to acquiring the terminal illness requires thoughtful planning, but no such person should ever be denied narcotics for the purposes of providing adequate pain relief.

DOUBLE EFFECT OR SECONDARY EFFECT AND TERMINATION SEDATION

Subtopics under pain management are the related principles of terminal sedation, and double effect or secondary effect.

Terminal Sedation

- It is possible that a patient can be in so much pain at end of life, particularly with such diagnoses such as bone metastasis after the patient has passed the limits of radiation, that the patient's pain may be uncontrolled by any current intervention.
- At that point, it is appropriate to present the option of controlling that pain by medicating the patient into a coma. The patient makes the decision about whether this is what they want to do, and if this is their choice, then when to induce the coma.
- The patient is kept comfortable though not cognizant of the surroundings.
- The appropriate level of pain medication dosing is determined by monitoring the patient's blood pressure, respiratory rate, and heart rate to see the response of the body to the effects of the pain medication.
  - Another natural response to uncontrolled pain that can be helpful in this assessment is grimacing.
  - Monitoring how the body naturally responds to the relief of pain allows for appropriate adjustments in dosage, increasing to control the pain, and decreasing the dosage if the current medication level appears to be too strong for the body's present pain level.
- Such a required level of pain medication may result in the patient dying sooner than without that level of pain medication.
- The sheer anxiety of unrelieved pain can trigger counterregulatory hormones that can act to prolong life.
- Relief of that level of pain may decrease those same counterregulatory hormones to the level that the life processes are no longer stimulated, and the patient may die sooner.

Double or Secondary Effect

- The concept of double effect or secondary effect indicates that the primary and intended effect was to ease pain, and not to kill the patient.
- A well-designed study in a hospice population found no association between percentage of change in dose of opioids and time until death.[10]
- The primacy of the intent of maintaining pain control is evident by the proper monitoring as described above under *Terminal Sedation*.

VOLUNTARILY STOPPING, EATING, AND DRINKING

Another option some patients elect to employ at an earlier stage in the dying process, is to voluntarily stop eating and drinking (VSED). This occurs when a mentally capable patient initiates this decision to refuse foods and fluids of any kind to advance the time of their death.

HOSPICE AND PALLIATIVE CARE

The hospice concept of providing comfort when cure is no longer possible was initiated in England and quickly spread to the United States beginning in the 1970s. Although the number of patients who die while being cared for by hospice has been rising slowly, patients generally do not spend enough time in these programs to experience all the potential benefits. Such benefits include the following:

- Provision of medications and durable medical equipment
- A major focus on aggressive pain management

BOX 80.1 Palliative Care[11]

- Palliative care may be considered at any time during serious illness.
- Effective communication is critical in assisting the patient and their family.
- Insurance companies reimburse for palliative care like consultative services.
- Palliative care may be provided by the patient's primary care provider.
- Palliative care may be provided in many hospital and outpatient settings.

- Counseling services both before and up to a year following death for the family
- Outpatient medical support and inpatient care for extremely demanding situations

More recently, palliative care programs have been developing across the United States to provide the expertise and standards of practice developed by hospice to patients who have needs for symptom control and supportive care earlier in their illness. All hospice programs fall under the umbrella of palliative care; however, *palliative care* is (see Box 80.1):

- Indicated beyond the specific time limits of and criteria for hospice
- Generally anticipated to apply to the specific diagnoses
- Limited to the last 6 months of life

The focus of *hospice* is to work toward death with dignity employing an entire team of professionals bringing the needed expertise to the entire galaxy of end of life (Box 80.2).

According to anecdotal experience, while designed to improve the quality of patients' lives as they fight their disease, good palliative care may help to increase life expectancy in certain diagnoses.[9,11]

TRANSITIONS OF LIFE

In the November 3, 1999 issue of *JAMA*, Thomas Finucane, MD, eloquently points out another challenging aspect of assisting patients as they move toward the end of their lives.[12] It is the process of "moving through the transition from gravely ill and fighting death to terminally ill and seeking peace, shifting the goals of treatment from cure or longer survival to preservation of comfort and dignity."

Two conflicting issues clash here. The dying patient desperately wants to live as long as possible, as healthy as possible, able to enjoy life and people, and without pain. When this is no longer possible, the patient also wants death to come swiftly, peacefully, and painlessly at the last possible minute. The physician also wants this scenario for every patient. The problem is that we do not have the ability to predict the future and give patients a precise, reliable date and time when death will come. Ironically, many chronically ill patients never experience a time during which they are clearly dying of their disease; "the sickest patients are not necessarily the ones who die first."[12]

The result is that the patient chooses to accept a less and less "ideal" quality of life, adjusting to more and more incapacitation and pain in exchange for one more day, and yearning for this day not to be the last. Some patients seem to accept death's coming easily, accepting the future, even choosing not to eat and drink. For many others, however, hope (no matter how faint) persists so strongly that surrender to the inevitable end of life is more excruciating than the pain and the struggle. Openly discussing this struggle to shift goals may be the only way to avoid a time where "do everything you can, doctor," in life becomes "why did this have to drag on so long?" after death as the family reflects on the course of the final illness.[12]

- This point is confirmed by a significant study of prognosis from George Washington University and the Department of Veterans Affairs published in *JAMA*.[13]
- The study looked at seriously ill hospitalized patients with advanced chronic obstructive pulmonary disease, congestive heart failure, or end-stage liver disease.
- It found that the recommended clinical prediction criteria are not effective in identifying a population with a prognosis for survival of 6 months or less.[13]

While we may not be able to predict the exact day of demise, we can predict that all indications point to the fact that the time is so short that hospice and palliative care is the best way to proceed, even though the patient and family may not be eager to hear that recommendation. The following words from the attending physician may be useful in the discussion[7]:

> "Do you think it is time to consider a different type of treatment that focuses on your symptoms? I'll be here with you no matter what you decide."

Another approach might be:

> "I want to provide intense, coordinated care with a team of professionals who will treat your symptoms and help you stay comfortable."

BOX 80.2 End-of-Life Care and Hospice[11]

- End-of-life care can incorporate either curative or supportive aspects of treatment.
- In serious medical conditions it may be difficult to know if the care provided is end of life, or life sustaining.
- Patients may enroll in Hospice through their insurance company when there is less than 6 months of life expectancy.
- Hospice provides comprehensive comfort care, emotional support, and education throughout the dying process.
- Hospice services can occur in the hospital, rehabilitation facility, or patients' home.

LEGAL MYTHS AND REALITIES

A significant barrier to proper care is lack of understanding on the part of the physician about legal issues at the end of life. Many physicians are not aware of the underlying principles regarding actual legal concerns. The body of law known as right-to-die cases extends ordinary treatment refusal doctrine to end-of-life decisions. The courts have affirmed a right to refuse life-sustaining treatment. Making a distinction between what treatment is life sustaining and what is not is the difficulty though. Meisel, Snyder, and Quill published a well-written set of "Seven legal barriers to end-of-life care: myths, realities and grains of truth," for the ACP–American Society of Internal Medicine End-of-Life Care Consensus Panel.[14]

COMMUNICATING BAD NEWS

One of the major challenges at end of life is that of telling a patient that they are at the end of life. Every physician must communicate uncomfortable information or give the family/patient bad news at some time in the process of providing medical care. It is important to develop the skill of delivering this type of information. Most people want to know such information, and delivering it well strengthens the patient–physician relationship. The patient/family not only learns the information, but also learns that the physician who doesn't shy away from the hard issues can be trusted to tell the truth. Delivering such information thoughtfully fosters collaboration between the physician and the patient/family as they then have time to plan and cope.

One admonition, or words of wisdom, passed down from A. T. Still, is that the physician should not deny hope to the patient. Some cultures are accustomed to not knowing the precise diagnosis of the patient's condition for fear that the patient may believe that death is near and give up hope. In these families, a significant other may request that the doctor not tell the patient what the diagnosis is (see Family Requests to Withhold Information section below). Maintaining hope is one of the purposes of religious or spiritual beliefs (see Chapter 20 for further discussion on spiritual aspects of health care).

A series of excellent questions on this topic come from Atul Gawande in his book "Being Mortal."

What is your understanding of where you are and of your illness?
What are your fears or worries for the future?
What are your goals and priorities?
What outcomes are acceptable to you?
What are you willing to sacrifice and me not?
And later, what would a good day look like?[15]

COMMUNICATION PROTOCOL

There is a seven-step protocol that has been developed as part of the program "Education for Physicians on End-of-Life Care (EPEC)" that is recommended as an effective approach to communicating bad news.[9] These steps may need to be modified by the urgency of the situation. The emergency department setting with an elderly demented patient quickly approaching their final minutes dictates a different pace than in the office setting talking to an alert patient who needs to be advised of a condition with a long prognosis. The specific wording of the questions from Atul Gawande (above) fit into this protocol structure.

1. Know yourself. Whether they know it or not, physicians communicate their own emotional responses in the most subtle ways, so it is important to be aware of your own responses.
2. Create a plan. Allot adequate time without interruption. Plan what to say after confirming the medical facts. Don't delegate this job. Create an environment that is conducive to conversation.
3. Establish what the patient already knows. The patient may already have suspected the worst.
4. How much does the patient want to know? There can be various patient preferences, either declining to know the details or choosing to designate someone else to communicate on their behalf. This varies with race, ethnicity, culture, religion, socioeconomic status, age, and developmental level.
5. Say the information and stop to allow the patient/family time to process. Avoid a monologue, jargon, and euphemisms, and pause frequently.
6. Be prepared for emotions. Some may respond with tears, anger, or anxiety, and others may experience denial, blame, guilt, fear, detachment, or shame.
7. Plan for the next steps in the process of the disease and approach.

There is an additional service that has developed recently, the death doula/midwife. It has developed based on the concept of the birth doula/midwife. The death doula is a community worker who assists/supports in the death process. The death doula movement has a specific aim to "bring dying home" in our communities as we (the doula movement) believe it is all of our business and not the sole preserve of experts and professionals.[16]

FAMILY REQUESTS TO WITHHOLD INFORMATION

If the family anticipates the worst and requests that information not be told to the patient, the physician still has a legal obligation to tell the patient. The family needs to discuss the reason for their fears of the information being shared. It is always the physician's responsibility to tell the truth to the patient, but it may be necessary to assist the family in working through their issues so that they see the importance of telling the truth and understand why it is not fair to the patient not to have this information. It may be appropriate to talk to the family and the patient at the same time.

LANGUAGE BARRIERS

When language is a barrier, the best approach is to obtain a translator as the family members who may be able to translate may have difficulty with the medical terms and concepts or may feel compelled to modify the news to protect the patient. A family translator may also not want to be the one to be the first to have to utter the words that will bring such dismay.

COMMUNICATING PROGNOSIS

When the physician is asked about prognosis and timing of death, it is helpful to find out why the patient wants to know. There may be a specific event coming up that the patient wishes to plan for, or the reasons for asking may be very ill-defined. The "planner" patient will want more details. Avoiding precise answers is appropriate, indicating that the prognosis is either in hours instead of days, days instead of weeks, weeks instead of months, or months instead of years. Precise answers can be perceived as a guarantee that no physician is able to provide.

THE TIME TO WITHDRAW INTERVENTIONS

Another aspect of communication that can be unexpectedly challenging is when the time comes for the invoking of the patient's wishes to withdraw interventions. It is unkind and unwise to ask the family, "Do you want us to take your family member off the ventilator now?" This approach puts the family member in the position of having to "make the decision to let Mom die," and actually having to say those words, when in reality that decision was already made by the patient some time ago.

A better approach is to tell the family,

> "As we have discussed repeatedly, your mother indicated in her living will that when we got to this point, she did not want life support continued, so we think it is time to take her off the ventilator, which we can do at 6 PM tomorrow."

Allowing plenty of time for that information to sink in and for the family to respond guides the rest of the treatment plan and timing.

WITHHOLDING AND WITHDRAWING TREATMENT

As was indicated in the "legal myths and realities" section, there is much misinformation about the difference between withholding and withdrawing treatment. In my experience in seminar after seminar that I have personally presented on end-of-life care topics, when I have polled physicians about which choice seems to be "harder" for the physician to perform, the results always indicate that physicians feel that choosing to withdraw treatment is more difficult to handle psychologically than withholding treatment. Nevertheless, all sources agree that there is no difference legally, morally, or ethically as the end result is the same, death of the patient.[9] If the treatment is initially withheld, there is no possibility of determining whether or not it may have been successful.

On the other hand, if the specific treatment is instituted and is determined not to be successful, there is often significant reluctance to remove that treatment. This reluctance is based upon the fact that when the treatment is removed, the patient will likely die sooner than if the treatment had been continued, so the appearance is created that removing the treatment was the event that killed the patient. On the contrary, there is no question that the disease process kills the patient. The treatment was shown to be ineffective in reversing the disease process and therefore was futile. The best approach to this difficult situation is to explain prospectively that a specific treatment will be instituted as a time-limited trial, with the time specified, usually 48 to 72 hours. At the appointed time, depending upon the natural course of the disease process and the chosen treatment, the issue is then revisited. Either the treatment is successful and is no longer needed, or the treatment is achieving desired results, and a new time-limited plan is created, or the treatment is unsuccessful with no reason to continue and a plan to remove the treatment is created. The time-limited trial combines the advantages and avoids as much as possible the disadvantages of these two approaches to patient treatment.

Withholding and withdrawal are beneficent omissions—neither negligent omissions nor, unlike delivering a lethal substance, are they acts done with the intention of ending a life. And we have "withdrawal aversion."[17] Because they are unable to make a distinction between an "intention to cause death" and an "intention to allow natural death," some clinicians equate withdrawal of life-sustaining treatments with euthanasia and are reluctant to withdraw treatments, even when the law permits it.[18] A fuller understanding of withholding or withdrawing treatment (see Table 80.2) will assist more clinicians in guiding their patients in the most effective direction.

ARTIFICIAL NUTRITION AND HYDRATION

Providing such support at end of life may at times be beneficial; however, sometimes this intervention may be excessively burdensome and may actually prolong the dying process. The use of artificial nutrition and hydration involves a medical procedure with potential side effects and complications. That fact is also the reason that the proper terminology is to use the technical medical phrase "artificial nutrition and hydration," not "providing food and water." A decision not to provide or to discontinue this intervention may pose some significant challenges particularly for families. Physicians need to assist patients and families to understand the role of artificial nutrition and hydration at the end of life, which is to provide temporary support to allow time for other interventions to have a chance to work. Families also need to understand that as body processes shut down, loss of the sensations of hunger and thirst are part of the dying process. Research has shown that discontinuing such support does not contribute to suffering, but those concerns may persist.[4]

DO NOT (ATTEMPT) RESUSCITATION STATUS (DNR/DNAR)

This status is indicated for most patients when it is anticipated that there is only a short length of life remaining. It means that the physician continues to provide all comfort care and when the patient slips into the final minutes of life, nothing is done to stop that process. Sometimes physicians who have been reluctant to write an actual DNR order will indicate that any code procedure should be "slow" (when full resuscitative efforts are not expended with the pretense that they are). This is not appropriate as it represents an attempt to deceive, which is an ethical violation.[4] Even in optimal circumstances, code procedures are not successful in most patients, so any "restricted" code order (chemical code, do not intubate, no compressions) is even less likely to be successful, therefore seldom indicated.

Obtaining patient/family permission for a DNR status order can be very challenging. Following the principles in the paragraph "communicating bad news" will be helpful. A suggested sequence of discussion can be as follows:

TABLE 80.2

Withholding versus Withdrawing Treatment

	Withholding	Withdrawing
Positive	The patient will never experience the potential downsides of the treatment	The patient will be given a chance to see if the treatment might work
Negative	The patient will never experience the possible benefits of the treatment	It may feel more difficult to remove the treatment even if ineffective
No difference	If you don't start treatment, THE PATIENT DIES	If you start treatment and it is ineffective, THE PATIENT DIES

1. Gently introduce the topic of end of life, such as "It looks like your disease isn't really responding to treatment."
2. Let the patient/family respond about their thoughts, feelings, and impressions.
3. Introduce the next statement such as "We have all been working to meet your needs and want to be sure we follow your wishes in the event your time is near."
4. Again, let the patient/family respond.
5. Ask the question, "Have you thought about what is most important to you in how you want to spend your final hours?"
6. If there is no clear direction from the patient/family, another question could be "In the event your heart stops, do you want to be kept alive on machines?"
7. It is always best to focus on the patient's goals of care. Having the patient explain their last-hour wishes can also lead to the question, "So it sounds like you want your last hours to be quiet and peaceful and free of pain, with no machines to prolong the inevitable?"
8. The best approach is to be osteopathic and focus on the whole person, letting the dialogue flow from your human-to-human relationship. It is important never to take away hope and to acknowledge that if the clinical situation improves, a change in DNR status can be made.

Families have specific needs at this time, as well as the patient, that is, the need to understand the dying process, the need to have cultural and religious differences understood and honored, the need to process grief. The osteopathic physician understands the important contribution of the family to the patient's overall well-being.

SUDDEN ILLNESS

A particularly difficult aspect of end-of-life care arises when the terminal illness/trauma occurs suddenly without warning and especially in an otherwise healthy and/or young person. All the principles of good communication apply. The physician must be aware that the level of understanding about the terminal illness including the options and pathway ahead will likely be minimal. Determining the approach to care will be a delayed "process" and may be much more contentious as the terminal nature of the illness is complicated by the unexpected nature of the situation. The grief and anger that result from the sudden and unplanned nature of the illness are almost inevitable. Frequently, the physician has never met that new patient and/or family until this event; so, this fact further complicates patient care as there is no basis for trust in the physician–patient relationship. The best approach is always to be as open as possible, provide as much information as possible, and never withhold partial information waiting for more definitive testing. It is also appropriate to err on the side of life to allow families time to process the grief. The assistance of social workers and other support staff as well as any of the patient's or family's personal trusted advisors, especially including spiritual advisors, is incredibly valuable in this situation.

MEDICAL FUTILITY

A further aspect of sudden illness but also of other terminal illnesses is the issue of medical futility. Present-day medical care has not been well served by the media where every illness is solved at the conclusion of the movie or the TV show. There is a very high expectation by the American public that with sufficient consultations, testing, and interventions, every patient can be saved, for the present day. Also, the lack of medical knowledge in the general population complicates this issue, as there is often little understanding of basic anatomic and physiologic principles. The physician is often faced with a demand/expectation that a particular intervention should be instituted, when there is no possibility that the intervention is appropriate or indicated for the diagnosis. An excellent example is that of the individual who has suffered a severe crush injury to the chest in a motor vehicle accident, which has created a diminished cardiac output that has prevented adequate perfusion of the kidneys, resulting in kidney failure. The demand for a kidney transplant in this situation is a request for a medically futile procedure. While technically feasible, a kidney transplanted into this setting of inadequate perfusion is also doomed to fail. The best approach is a thorough explanation, assistance from social workers, and a willingness to understand, acknowledge, and tolerate the frustration of the person requesting the futile intervention.

PHYSICIAN-ASSISTED SUICIDE AND PHYSICIAN-ASSISTED DEATH

Currently in flux is the issue of physician-assisted suicide (PAS). PAS refers to the situation in which the physician prescribes a drug that the patient self-administers in a lethal dose; this is in contrast to euthanasia, in which the physician administers the lethal dose. While Oregon, Washington, Vermont, California, Colorado, Hawaii, Montana, Maine, New Jersey, New Mexico, and Washington, DC, currently (2022) allow the full legal provision of PAS, other state legislatures are also addressing this issue in various forms. It is recommended to contact your state osteopathic medical licensing board for the most up to date status of this law. The general provisions of the Oregon law, which was the first to be passed, require verification of terminal status without clinical depression, a waiting period between a repeated request for PAS, and the ability to swallow the specified prescribed barbiturate in liquid form.

The Oregon Death with Dignity Act (DWDA) is the oldest such legislation in the United States, thus has generated the most data. Since the law passed in 1997, a total of 3,712 people have received prescriptions under the DWDA and 2,454 people (66%) have died ingesting the medications. The 2022 annual report (the most recent report) reports the following: Demographic characteristics of DWDA patients in 2022 were like those of previous years: most patients were age 65 years or older (85%) and White (96%). The most common diagnosis was cancer (64%), followed by heart disease (12%) and neurologic disease (10%). During 2022, DWDA deaths accounted for an estimated 0.6% of total deaths in Oregon. As in previous years, the three most frequently reported end-of-life concerns were decreasing ability to participate in activities that made life enjoyable (89%), loss of autonomy (86%), and loss of dignity (62%). The section of the survey of patients who have received DWDA prescriptions that asks about their reasons for participating in the DWDA process allows the selection of more than one factor. It is important to note that "inadequate pain control, or concern about it" has been included by those patients who completed the survey as one of the items in the list of "end-of-life concerns" for only 28% of those who chose to obtain prescriptions under DWDA.[19]

The osteopathic oath specifically states, "I will give no drugs for deadly purposes, though it be asked of me." The AOA opposes the practice of PAS. Such a practice puts the physician in the position of deciding as to whether to be on the side of working to save a patient or on the side of working to kill a patient. No physician should have to make that decision, and no patient should wonder if the physician is weighing that option. In a survey of 988 terminally ill patients by Emanuel and associates in 2000, identified factors associated with a patient being less likely to consider euthanasia or PAS were "feeling appreciated, being aged 65 years or older, and being African American." Factors associated with being more likely to consider euthanasia or PAS were "depressive symptoms, substantial care-giving needs, and pain."[20] Foley[21] makes the strong point that competent care for the dying can relieve the concern of those patients' considering PAS, and this approach should be advocated in preference to PAS. Additional perspectives on this topic come from outside of the United States.[22]

There is also a move to change the descriptive title of this practice from PAS to physician-assisted death (PAD).[23,24] Another proposed term is medical aid in dying (MAID). These proposed changes would appear to be an attempt to camouflage the fact that when the patient takes the prescribed medication for its intended purpose, the patient is dying by suicide and the physician assisted that suicide by providing the means. PAS (where the physician provides the means and the patient acts) is also clearly differentiated from euthanasia (where the physician provides the means and completes the act for the patient).

There is no question this is a highly emotionally charged issue with strong opinions on both sides. The most important takeaway is that the patient deserves excellent care, regardless of their choices, up to and including at end of life.

CHANGING PERSPECTIVES ON DEATH AND LIFE

When A. T. Still was a practicing physician, most care was provided in the patient's home. The physician had immediate access to information on the resources available to provide care to the patient. As physicians became busier and long horse (and buggy) rides into the countryside were too time-consuming, the provision of care gradually shifted to having the patient come to the doctor's office. With the development of hospitals, beginning in the doctor's office/home for the sicker patients, patients were again seen outside their home setting. Efficiency was gained. However, the appreciation of the fuller picture of the patient's life was certainly lost.

Then came the COVID pandemic. The initial thought in the early days of the pandemic was that COVID would have a universal effect on all people. That was certainly not what happened. As we come to better understand the social determinants of health, there is a corollary of social determinants of death with similar components. Social determinants of health and social determinants of death determine not only how people live but also how they die. Poor deaths often follow poor lives.[1]

And further, COVID has changed the death and dying experience. The COVID pandemic experience has made death prominent in daily media reports and health systems. People died the ultimate medicalized deaths, often alone but for masked staff in hospitals and ICUs, unable to communicate with family except electronically. This situation has further fueled the fear of death, reinforcing the idea of health care services as the custodian of death. The pandemic has reminded us that we are part of nature and not in control of nature.[1]

Climate change...environmental destruction, and attitudes about death in high-income countries have similar roots—our delusion that we are in control of, and not part of, nature. Large sums are being invested to dramatically extend life, even achieve immortality, for a small minority in a world that struggles to support its current population. Health care and individuals appear to struggle to accept the inevitability of death. Were it a country, health care would be the world's fifth largest emitter of greenhouse gases.[1]

In high-income countries, between 8% and 11.2% of annual health expenditures for the entire population is spent on the less than 1% who die in that year. Some of this high expenditure is justified, but there is evidence that patients and health professionals hope for better outcomes than are likely, meaning treatment that is intended to be curative often continues for too long.[1]

STUDENTS AND END-OF-LIFE CARE

To what degree should students be involved in this process? Should students restrict participation to information gathering? If so, are there key elements to determine? How do they record their findings (this information does not exactly fit in the SOAP note)? Should students ever introduce discussion in this area? If so, are there limits to how they advance the information that they gain? Who is the recipient of the information they gather: attending case worker, hospital chaplain, or potential hospice person? This is a provocative series of questions to which the answer is yes, no, maybe, sometimes, and even "I don't know." After learning how to diagnose and treat disease, the student on clinical rotation starts to experience the biggest challenge to being a physician, how to translate all that knowledge into real patient care. The patient who cannot understand, refuses to listen, chooses not to follow the instructions, or hides the true problem out of fear is still the patient who needs care. The physician must learn that they are frequently part of the trigger or reason the patient acts and responds in the way that they do. The physician–patient relationship is ultimately the strongest tool the physician has to help the patient. The student physician cannot wait to learn to work in this relationship until after completion of residency.

On the other hand, the student physician is still a student working under the attending physician's license. The best guidance this author can provide is to include the following question in every history and physical,

> "Have you made anyone aware of your wishes for the end of your life through some tool like a living will?"

The answer is to be precisely documented as stated by the patient, in the notes section of the chart in the appropriate manner with the rest of the history and physical information such as "last tetanus shot, last mammogram, last colonoscopy, etc." This simple question opens the door for the patient to walk through if desired. If the patient is not ready to discuss this topic, the answer will indicate it is time to move to the next topic. The student is not expected to probe any further, to answer questions, or to counsel the patient. The student is expected to bring to the attention of the attending physician (or designee such as a resident) if the patient requests further discussion or information. The student should function like a conduit to carry information and concerns from the patient to the attending physician who can assess the situation and decide what orders are appropriate, including a possible DNR status. The patient will set the tone, indicate the depth and length of the conversation, indicate whether further questions are appropriate, or whether the patient just wants a willing listener. Many times, the patient has been waiting for a physician to broach this topic. Two leaders in end-of-life care, Dr. Susan Block and Dr. J. Andrew Billings, have studied the student–physician interaction with the dying and suggest that end-of-life care may be the ideal training ground for young doctors.[25]

SUMMARY

By giving time, attention, and compassion as people die, we connect with them and with our shared fragility, pushing us to acknowledge our interdependence and understand what is at the core of human relationships.[1] Although the challenges of patient care at end of life are daunting, it is a truly rewarding time to care for patients. Every one of our patients and each of us will pass through this experience. It can be handled well or be given short shrift. It may be the only opportunity to bring to bear all the best that osteopathic medicine has to offer, honoring the patient as a whole person and calling upon each osteopathic physician to create the milieu for the use of everything we have learned. To share this time with a patient and make their last days comfortable and meaningful is a true gift, a reciprocal gift that the patient and physician give each other. The physician who welcomes and embraces the interaction at end of life is touched in ways that won't be forgotten by the patient, the family, or the physician.

REFERENCES

1. Sallnow L, Smith R, Ahmedzai SH, et al; Lancet Commission on the Value of Death. Report of the Lancet Commission on the value of death: bringing death back into life. *Lancet.* 2022;399:837–884.
2. Cassel CK, Foley KM. *Principles for Care of Patients at the End of Life: An Emerging Consensus among the Specialties of Medicine.* Milbank Memorial Fund; 1999.
3. Nichols KJ. Approach to optimal care at end of life. *J Am Osteopath Assoc.* 2001;101:586–593.
4. The American Osteopathic Association End of Life Care Advisory Committee. End of Life Care Policy, approved by the American Osteopathic Association House of Delegates, reaffirmed as amended 2016. Accessed May 21, 2017. https://osteopathic.org/index.php?aam-media=/wp-content/uploads/past-resolutions/H419-A2023-SR-Policy-Statement-on-End-of-Life-Care-Resolution-and-white-paper-wACTION.pdf
5. Connors AF Jr, Dawson NV, Desbiens NA. A controlled trial to improve care for seriously ill hospitalized patients. The study to understand prognoses and preferences for outcomes and risks of treatments (SUPPORT). *JAMA.* 1995;274:1591–1598.
6. Silveira MJ, DePiero A, Gerrity MS, Feudtner C. Patients' knowledge of options at the end of life: ignorance in the face of death. *JAMA.* 2000;284:2483–2488.
7. Ngo-Metzger Q, August K, Srinivasan M, Liao S, Meyskens FL Jr. End-of-life care: guidelines for patient-centered communication. *Am Fam Physician.* 2008;77(2):167–174.
8. Qaseem A, Snow V, Shekelle P, et al; Clinical Efficacy Assessment Subcommittee of the American College of Physicians. Evidence-based interventions to improve the palliative care of pain, dyspnea, and depression at the end of life: a clinical practice guideline from the American College of Physicians. *Ann Intern Med.* 2008;148:141–146.
9. Education for physicians on end-of-life care (EPEC) trainers' PowerPoint slides. Accessed May 21, 2017. bioethics.northwestern.edu.>programs>epec
10. Portenoy RK, Sibirceva U, Smout R, et al. Opioid use and survival at the end of life: a survey of a hospice population. *J Pain Symptom Manage.* 2006;32:532–540.
11. American Association of Critical-Care Nurses. Palliative care in acute & critical care settings. Accessed February 18, 2024. Aacn.org/clinical-resources/palliative-end-of-life
12. Finucane TE. How gravely ill becomes dying: a key to end-of-life care (editorial). *JAMA.* 1999;282:1670–1672.
13. Fox E, Landrum-McNiff K, Zong Z, Dawson NV, Wu WA, Lynn J. Evaluation of prognostic criteria for determining hospice eligibility in patients with advanced lung, heart, or liver disease. SUPPORT Investigators. Study to understand prognoses and preferences for outcomes and risks of treatment. *JAMA.* 1999;282:1638–1645.
14. Meisel A, Snyder L, Quill T; American College of Physicians–American Society of Internal Medicine End-of-Life Care Consensus Panel. Seven legal barriers to end-of-life care: myths, realities, and grains of truth. *JAMA.* 2000;284:2495–2501.
15. Gawande A. *Being Mortal. Illness, Medicine and What Matters in the End.* Profile Books; 2015.
16. End of Life Doula UK. What is an end of life doula? Accessed January 22, 2022. https://eol-doula.uk/what-is-an-end-of-life-doula/
17. Wilkinson D, Butcherine E, Savulescu J. Withdrawal aversion and the equivalence test. *Am J Bioeth.* 2019;19:21–28.
18. Kitzinger J, Kitzinger C. Why futile and unwanted treatment continues for some PVS patients (and what to do about it). Case study, context, and policy recommendations. *Int J Mental Health Capacity Law.* 2017;129:84–149.
19. 2022 Data Summary. https://www.oregon.gov>documents>year25
20. Emanuel EJ, Fairclough DL, Emanuel LL. Attitudes and desires related to euthanasia and physician-assisted suicide among terminally ill patients and their caregivers. *JAMA.* 2000:284:2460–2468.
21. Foley KM. Competent care for the dying instead of physician-assisted suicide. *N Engl J Med.* 1997;336:54–58.
22. Emanuel, EJ, Onwuteaka-Philipsen BD, Urwin JW, Cohen J. Attitudes and practices of euthanasia and physician-assisted suicide in the United States, Canada, and Europe. *JAMA.* 2016;316(1):79–90.
23. Statement on physician-assisted dying. Accessed November 20, 2024. https://aahpm.org/advocacy/where-we-stand/pad/
24. National Academies of Sciences, Engineering, and Medicine. *Physician-Assisted Death: Scanning the Landscape: Proceedings of a Workshop.* The National Academies Press; 2018.
25. Block S, Billings JA. Nurturing humanism through teaching palliative care. *Acad Med.* 1998;73(7):763–765.

81 Osteopathic Considerations in Obstetrics

ANITA SHOWALTER

KEY CONCEPTS

- Somatic dysfunction is more common in pregnancy, including low back pain and other musculoskeletal problems.
- Physiologic adaptations, such as center of gravity shifts, increased fluids, and hormonal changes, increase the incidence of somatic dysfunction in pregnancy.
- Physicians should be familiar with indications and contraindications for osteopathic manipulative treatment (OMT) during pregnancy.
- Evaluation and treatment of the lumbosacral spine and pelvis should be done in preparation for labor and birth.
- Osteopathic care includes evaluation and treatment for somatic dysfunction including performing a structural examination, identifying viscerosomatic reflexes, skeletal changes, and biomechanical changes in each trimester of pregnancy and postpartum.

> An up-to-date osteopath must have a masterful knowledge of anatomy and physiology. He [sic] must have brains in osteopathic surgery, osteopathic obstetrics, and osteopathic practice.
>
> —A.T. Still, MD, DO[1]

AN OSTEOPATHIC APPROACH TO CARE OF THE PRENATAL PATIENT

It is important to consider the role of the osteopathic physician in obstetrics following the four tenets of osteopathic practice.

- Obstetrics is a branch of medicine dedicated to the normal physiologic process of birth.
- With each pregnancy, the physician cares for two patients:
  1. The obstetric patient
  2. The fetus
- Before the advent of modern obstetric care, both mother and fetus were at higher risk of morbidity and mortality.
- While modern medical advances continue to increase the safety of pregnancy and childbirth worldwide, osteopathic manipulation can further contribute to normalizing the normal physiologic processes of pregnancy, thereby increasing benefits for the patient, the fetus, and the mother–baby dyad (see Box 81.1).
  1. For optimal outcomes to be appreciated, the osteopathic physician must also consider the psychological impact of the transition from patient to mother.
  2. This chapter will review each trimester and phase of parturition with special considerations the osteopathic physician should address.

BOX 81.1

"To find health should be the object of the doctor. Anyone can find disease."

—A.T. Still, MD, DO[1]

FIRST TRIMESTER

Preconception and Prenatal Care

Ideally, each woman anticipating pregnancy would have a preconception visit to address the following:

- A health inventory, to identify modifiable risk factors
- Care to optimize chronic health conditions
- Review medications in order to change or discontinue those with potential adverse effects

If a preconception visit is missed, the same information is gathered at the initial prenatal visit (ideally after the first or second missed menstrual period).

Pre-existing Somatic Dysfunction

The initial prenatal evaluation includes a physical exam.[2]

- In addition to performing a traditional pelvic examination, the osteopathically trained obstetrician may perform a palpatory structural examination to identify somatic dysfunction that could affect the outcome of pregnancy.
  - Asymmetry of bony landmarks, joint motion tests, tissue texture changes, and local tenderness (TART findings) are used to confirm areas of somatic dysfunction.
  - Palpatory examination of the paraspinal tissues is performed to identify areas of tissue texture changes that represent viscerosomatic reflex sites.[3]
  - Spinal segmental sites for somatic dysfunction associated with visceral disease are related to the autonomic nervous system supply and can be used to diagnose and help treat underlying disease.[4]
  - Identification of Chapman points may assist in diagnosis of underlying and pre-existing conditions that may be confounded by early pregnancy symptoms (see Table 81.1 and Box 81.2).

The hormonal changes of pregnancy may cause decompensation of long-standing somatic dysfunction, causing pain or other

TABLE 81.1

Chapman SNS "Lymphatic" Reflex Centers Pertinent to Pregnancy

Groin gland	Irritated clitoris and vaginismus
Broad ligament of the uterus	Uterus
Salpingitis	Leukorrhea
Ovaries	Abdominal tension
Urethra	Kidneys
Adrenal points (as the adrenals lie on the kidney)	

symptoms that complicate pregnancy. The goal is early identification and treatment.

Changes in Circulation and Fluids

An understanding of the many physiologic changes in pregnancy explains variations in lab values and physiologic adaption to the demands of a growing fetus:

- Total body water content increases about 6 to 8 L.
  - Two-thirds of the extra fluid is located in the extravascular space.
  - Plasma volumes begin to rise by 6 weeks' gestation, continuing to increase through 32 to 34 weeks.
- Hemodilution of red blood cells results in physiologic anemia.
- Cardiac output begins to increase by 10 weeks' gestation, reaching maximum levels by 20 to 24 weeks[5]
  - Oxygen consumption is increased during exercise.
  - Peak cardiac output is reached earlier in pregnancy than in a nonpregnant state.

To address lymphatic function, osteopathic techniques can be used to remove restrictions.

- Thoracic and pelvic diaphragms should operate in harmony to achieve optimal function of the thoracic diaphragm as a lymphatic pump.
- These relationships will be markedly stressed as the pregnancy progresses.

Hormonal Changes

Early pregnancy symptoms are primarily caused by the hormones of the corpus luteum.[6] These hormones include the following:

- Progesterone
- 17-Hydroxyprogesterone
- Relaxin
- Estradiol

RELAXIN

The effect of relaxin on tissues makes this hormone of special interest to the osteopathic physician. Relaxin:

- Has a role in implantation and cervical and uterine relaxation.
  - Reaches peak concentrations by about 10 weeks' gestation then declines.
  - Can contribute to cervical shortening and increased risk of preterm labor when present in excess.
- Plays a role in endothelial relaxation and the increased glomerular filtration rate of pregnancy.[7]
- Is known to have a softening effect on ligamentous tissue; however, its role in human parturition remains controversial. Some researchers have found a relationship between serum relaxin levels and pelvic girdle pain, but the findings are not consistent.[8]
- Causes lengthening of the fibers of the symphysis pubis in pregnancy but does not cause significant pain independently of other factors.
- Is involved in pubic symphysis distension during pregnancy and delivery.
  - There is an association between pelvic pain and increased pubic symphysis distension.
  - The degree of distension does not relate to the severity of pain for the individual patient. Other factors are thought to be primarily contributing to the pain.[9]

Nausea and Vomiting in Early Pregnancy

In the first trimester of pregnancy, hyperemesis ("morning sickness") is a common complaint affecting 50% to 80% of pregnant women.

- The precise cause of the nausea and vomiting remains unclear.
  - It has been postulated that morning sickness provides a protective effect by encouraging maternal avoidance of noxious substances during the most critical time of fetal organogenesis.
  - Research shows that patients experiencing nausea and vomiting in pregnancy have improved outcomes unless the symptoms are severe.[10]
- Conservative treatment of mild nausea and vomiting may include the following:
  - Treatment of viscerosomatic reflexes by addressing Chapman points[11,12] (see Box 81.3)

BOX 81.2

The genitourinary system will be changing significantly as pregnancy progresses. It is possible that pre-existing Chapman points could cause problems, as forces, both endocrine and mechanical, increase with advancing pregnancy. See Table 81.1 for Chapman SNS "lymphatic" reflex centers for this system. Note that changes in the *clitoris and vaginismus* points can be associated with formation of the *neurasthenia* and *insomnia* points. Also, the Chapman ovary points differentiate at two levels of the thoracic spine.

BOX 81.3 Clinical Pearl

Treatment of Chapman points may be done in the following way: Hold the posterior point with one finger and the anterior point(s) with fingers of the other hand, sensing that there is no allowed motion between these two points, and then allow the primary respiratory mechanism to resolve this limitation of motion. This has been found to be more effective in resolving viscerosomatic issues than treating either point separately.

  - Evaluation and treatment of C2 and T5–T9[13]
  - Cranial manipulation
  - Vitamin B[14]
  - Delayed release doxylamine and pyridoxine[15]
- When medications are indicated because of the severity of nausea and vomiting, those with optimal side effect profiles are preferred. Medications may have varying safety profiles and should be used cautiously when conservative methods have failed, or electrolyte imbalance demands a more aggressive approach.

Exercise

Many women request information about exercise at their first prenatal visits and should be counseled about the health benefits of exercise throughout pregnancy. Benefits of exercise include the following:

- Reduction in cesarean rates
- Appropriate maternal and fetal weight gain
- Improved management of gestational diabetes
- Improved psychological well-being[16,17]

Regular exercise routines may need to be modified to accommodate the physical changes of pregnancy and to reduce the risk of injury to the patient and fetus.

- The American College of Obstetricians and Gynecologists recommends moderate exercise of 20 to 30 minutes daily during pregnancy and through the postpartum period.
- Moderate exercise rarely raises heart rate or core temperature enough to be concerning.
- Strenuous exercise should be avoided because of the increased oxygen demands of pregnancy and risk of injury.
- Physicians should evaluate the patient for risk factors that may make exercise contraindicated, but these are rare, so continued activity should be encouraged for most patients.[18]

Spotting

Spotting is common in the first trimester of pregnancy and can be very anxiety provoking; thus, prompt evaluation for viability and ruling out ectopic pregnancy is important.

- Undiagnosed vaginal bleeding is a contraindication of OMT.
- Bed rest has not been shown to improve outcomes when spotting is encountered in early pregnancy.[19]
- Normal activity may be encouraged, but the patient should be advised to avoid strenuous activity when bleeding is present.

Breastfeeding Education

Exclusive feeding of human milk is the preferred method of nutrition for infants through 6 months of age.

- The combination of nutrients is easily digested and gives the infant the appropriate balance of proteins, vitamins, and minerals.
- Human milk is known to have very low levels of iron, yet most is absorbed.
- In addition, there are many trace substances that continue to be isolated that improve growth and development of the infant.
- Cow's milk binds to iron; therefore, formulas made from a cow's milk must have additional iron added for absorption of its protein base.
- Supplemental iron may lead to constipation and colic.

The benefits of breastfeeding are well-known for both the immediate and future health of the infant and the patient.

- According to the American Academy of Pediatrics, benefits of breastfeeding include the following:
  - Protective effect against:
    - Respiratory illnesses
    - Ear infections
    - Gastrointestinal diseases
    - Allergies including asthma, eczema, and atopic dermatitis
  - Reduced rate of sudden infant death syndrome (SIDS) by over a third
  - Reduction in adolescent and adult obesity by 15% to 30%[20]
- Educating and encouraging breastfeeding early and throughout the pregnancy during prenatal visits will help prepare the patient.

SECOND TRIMESTER

Changes in Maternal Structure and Biomechanics

As the fetus develops, the uterus begins to rise out of the pelvis by about 12 weeks' gestation, and by 16 weeks, it is midway between the pubic bone and the umbilicus.

- The patient usually becomes aware of fetal motion between 16 and 20 weeks' gestation, as well as stretching pains above the pubic symphysis.
- If the patient has had abdominal or pelvic surgery or has had a medical condition prone to adhesion formation such as endometriosis or pelvic inflammatory disease, pain may occur because of stretching of previously formed adhesions. Fascial release (direct or indirect) and visceral manipulation may provide some relief.
- Round ligament pain may respond to anterior counterstrain point treatment at L3–L5.

Physiologic shortness of breath is thought to be related to hormones and mechanical changes in pregnancy.[21]

- Oxygenation remains normal even though the patient feels short of breath unless another pathologic process is in place.
- Osteopathic techniques such as rib raising, rib/thorax myofascial release, and doming of the diaphragm may give symptomatic relief.

Low Back Pain

More than two-thirds of pregnant patients experience low back pain and one-fifth experience pelvic pain, which increases with advancing pregnancy.

- Pain interferes with activities of daily living, work, and sleep.
- Exercise programs have been shown to improve pain and dysfunction.
- The addition of osteopathic manipulation has been shown to improve pain and disability more than prenatal care alone.[22]

As the center of gravity changes with the growing uterus, increased stresses are realized in the tissues of the lumbar spine and pelvic ligaments.

- In a study of patients with lumbosacral pain during late pregnancy and after pregnancy, palpatory examination showed that the most frequently irritated ligaments were[23]
  - Interspinous (60%)
  - Iliolumbar (40%)
  - Sacroiliac (36%)

BOX 81.4 OMT Protocol

Part I: Patient lateral recumbent
1. Bilateral hip circumduction
2. Lumbosacral joint decompression
3. Pelvic diaphragm (assessment and treatment)
4. Lumbar soft tissue treatment
5. Rib raising (assessment and treatment)
6. Thoracic diaphragm (assessment and treatment)
7. Thoracic soft tissue treatment
8. Cervical somatic dysfunction diagnosis
9. Cranial somatic dysfunction diagnosis

Part II: Patient seated
1. Thoracic inlet (assessment and treatment)
2. Cardinal ligament dysfunction diagnosis (assessment and treatment)

The Sacroiliac Joint

The sacroiliac (SI) joint is the largest synovial joint in the body and contributes to the stability and mobility of the pelvis. Dysfunction of the SI joint is implicated in low back pain and pelvic girdle pain, especially in pregnancy when hormonal changes may cause increased laxity of the ligaments.[24]

- SI joint dysfunction has the potential to have broad consequences in the musculoskeletal system, including cranial function through the dural attachments to the sacrum.
- Successfully addressing SI dysfunction requires a global evaluation and treatment of the musculoskeletal system. Researchers have described a 15-minute evaluation and osteopathic treatment protocol that is appropriate for the pregnant patient[25] (see Box 81.4).

During the second trimester, the growing uterus rising out of the pelvis begins to shift the patient's center of gravity and contributes to increased somatic dysfunction.

- Osteopathic techniques can be effectively used to identify and treat specific areas of somatic dysfunction with better outcomes than exercise alone in reducing pain and disability.
- The patient may be treated in whichever position is best tolerated. The usual positions used may be modified to accommodate the enlarging abdomen.
- Almost any type of treatment modality (direct or indirect treatments) can be used, depending on the physician's skill and patient acceptance; for further information, (see Sections VIII and IX for OMT technique procedures).

Carpal Tunnel Syndrome

Although complaints related to skeletal changes continue in the second trimester, another frequent area of musculoskeletal symptoms during pregnancy is pain in the hands and wrists. Carpal tunnel syndrome:

- Symptoms[26] often include the following:
  - Numbness
  - Tingling
  - Pain at night
  - Sparing of the fifth digit
- Occurs most frequently[27]:
  - In the second trimester
  - In patients with excessive edema
  - In women with fluid retention
- In pregnancy, virtually always resolves completely soon after delivery, although it may not resolve while a patient is breastfeeding.[28]

Palliative management is indicated for patients who are sufficiently symptomatic to warrant any treatment.

- The following has been reported to be helpful[29]:
  - Nighttime splinting of the wrist to support it in neutral
  - Slight dorsiflexion
  - OMT treatment for 6 weeks
- Sucher has demonstrated improvement in nerve conduction studies and magnetic resonance imaging changes resulting from osteopathic myofascial release treatment.[30,31]

THIRD TRIMESTER

Changes in Maternal Structure and Biomechanics

In the last 3 months of pregnancy, gravitational effects on the uterus and its contents accentuate abdominal fascial drag on inguinal tissues, causing pressure on the venous and lymphatic return flow from the lower extremities and on the inferior vena cava. The pregnant woman may find it difficult to lie in a supine position without experiencing nausea or dizziness due to hypotension from inferior vena cava compression.

During the third trimester, the mechanical and structural changes in the woman become maximal. As a result, the following biomechanical changes may be noted:

- Loss of balance
- Gait changes
- Low back pain
- Pelvic pressure
- Constipation
- Leg edema
- Hemorrhoids
- Reflux esophagitis

Specific palpatory structural examination to identify gastrointestinal viscerosomatic reflexes for treatment may be helpful.

- Somatic dysfunction found on osteopathic structural examination can be resolved using various OMT procedures:
  - Myofascial or soft tissue osteopathic treatment may mobilize fluids from extremities to the systemic circulation.
  - Treatment of the pelvic diaphragm to lift pelvic contents may relieve constipation.
  - Treatment of the midthoracic spine may relieve gastrointestinal complaints.
  - Ischial tuberosity spread may aid treatment of hemorrhoids and pelvic pressure.
- Osteopathic evaluation and treatment to relieve somatic dysfunction in the third trimester should include spinal segmental levels of T10–L2, the sympathetic nerve supply that influences adrenal and ovarian function, as well as uterine contractility.
  - Gitlin and Wolf describe cases of uterine contractions in a small group of women with term pregnancies following use of osteopathic cranial manipulation.[32]
  - Additional case histories pertaining to osteopathic management of pregnancy, with discussion of treatment techniques, may be found in *Osteopathy in the Cranial Field.*[33]

Low Back Pain

With maximum structural changes and pressure on the pelvic tissues from the growing uterus, patients in the third trimester complain most frequently of low back and pelvic girdle pain.

- This complaint is so common that women may be told it is "normal" to have low back pain in pregnancy.
- Symptoms can become severe and significantly interfere with ability to perform daily activities, sleep, and work.

Two studies of interest published in English literature assessed the effect of OMT on alleviating low back pain in the third trimester.

One study looked at outcomes of 144 patients recruited in the third trimester, at about 30 weeks' gestation, and randomly assigned to one of three groups[34]:

1. Routine prenatal care ($n = 49$)
2. Prenatal care plus placebo (ultrasound without an energy source) ($n = 48$)
3. Routine prenatal care plus OMT ($n = 49$)

OMT or placebo treatment was provided at the routine prenatal visit.

- OMT
  - □ Treated areas include the following:
    - Cervical, thoracic, and lumbar spine
    - Thoracic outlet and clavicles
    - Ribcage and diaphragm
    - Pelvis and sacrum
  - □ OMT was provided to each region until a tissue response was noted for a total of 20 minutes.
  - □ The following techniques were used:
    - Soft tissue
    - Myofascial release
    - Muscle energy
    - Range-of-motion mobilization
- Placebo
  - □ Utilized an ultrasound wand that was moved in a circular motion over clothes in the same regions as OMT was applied in the intervention group.
- Results showed significantly decreased pain and disability in patients treated with OMT or placebo over routine prenatal care alone.
  - □ A secondary analysis of this study using the Cochrane Back Review Group Criteria for assessing significant and clinically relevant treatment effects demonstrated that the OMT group had a medium to large treatment effect in preventing progressive back-specific dysfunction.[35]

The second study was a prospective randomized clinical trial (PROMOTE study) that measured back pain and function in 400 third-trimester obstetrical patients at three ambulatory clinics, of which 136 were treated with OMT.[36]

- The patients were randomly assigned to one of three groups:
  1. Routine prenatal care
  2. Routine prenatal care plus placebo ultrasound wand without ultrasonic waves
  3. Routine prenatal care plus OMT
- OMT
  1. Treated areas include the following:
     - □ Cranium
     - □ Cervical, thoracic, lumbar spine
     - □ Pelvis and sacrum
     - □ Abdominal and pelvic diaphragm
  2. OMT was provided to each region until adequate tissue response was noted for a total of 20 minutes.
  3. The following techniques were used:
     - □ CV4
     - □ Articulation
     - □ Soft tissue
     - □ Myofascial release
     - □ Muscle energy
     - □ Placebo
       - The study utilized a deactivated ultrasound wand that was moved in a circular motion over clothes in the same regions as OMT was applied in the intervention group.
- Results showed the OMT group had less severe pain scores and higher level of back-related functioning as compared to the usual care-only group.[36]
- A secondary analysis of the PROMOTE study data was published in 2016. It analyzed the safety of OMT during the third trimester by looking at labor and delivery outcomes.[37] The results suggested that the OMT protocol given during the third trimester of pregnancy as applied in the PROMOTE study is safe regarding labor and delivery outcomes.[37]
- Another secondary analysis of the PROMOTE study data was published in 2019 and demonstrated that the application of CV4 as part of an OMT protocol during the third trimester was safe and caused neither a higher incidence of preterm labor nor the development of high-risk status.[38] In addition, there were no adverse health outcomes for the mothers, their fetuses, or newborns.[38]

Uterine Irritability

Braxton Hicks contractions are the disorganized contractions that increase in frequency in normal pregnancies from about 30 weeks to delivery, often called false labor.

- Preterm labor occurs when the contractions become organized and begin to make cervical change. It can be difficult to distinguish Braxton Hicks contractions from preterm labor when labor is early.
- Risk factors for preterm labor include the following:
  - □ Infections within the pelvis that increase uterine contractility
  - □ Increased uterine distension such as multiple gestation and polyhydramnios
- The osteopathic physician should consider that the following could contribute to uterine irritability:
  - □ Inflammation of the pelvic floor tissues
  - □ Pelvic asymmetry
  - □ Pelvic floor dysfunction
- Anecdotal evidence suggests that gentle treatment of the pelvic floor with a pelvic floor (diaphragm) release in addition to addressing structural asymmetry may decrease frequency of false labor contractions.

Perinatal and Hemodynamic Outcomes

Osteopathic philosophy teaches that improved structural symmetry, joint motion, and decreased sympathetic activity enhance arterial, venous, and lymphatic circulation. One study suggests fewer adverse outcomes in pregnancy when OMT is applied during prenatal care.[39]

- This was a retrospective chart review of 321 randomly selected pregnant patients at four medical centers in which MD and DO obstetricians cared for patients.[39] In total, 160 patients received OMT at routine prenatal visits.

- The "usual care" and "usual care plus OMT" groups were compared for the following outcomes of pregnancy:
  - □ Preterm labor
  - □ Meconium-stained amniotic fluid
  - □ Cord prolapse
  - □ Cesarean delivery
  - □ Forceps-assisted vaginal delivery
- There were significantly fewer incidences of preterm labor and meconium-stained fluid in the usual care plus OMT group. These are important outcomes that can greatly affect morbidity and mortality.[39]
- Preterm labor carries a great toll of morbidity and mortality as well as a significant financial burden for patients, hospitals, and third-party payers.
- While the mechanisms for improved outcomes with OMT are not known, it is possible that OMT improves arterial blood supply, venous drainage, and lymphatic flow, thereby reducing the likelihood of subclinical infections and inflammation that could result in preterm labor.
  1. Meconium-stained fluid is thought to be related to stress of the fetus, usually from hypoxia or a matter of maturity in a postdate fetus.[39]
  2. Two mechanisms of action could reduce meconium. First, improved circulation by reducing tensions surrounding uterine blood supply could improve oxygenation to the fetus, thus reducing stress.
  3. Second, a symmetric pelvis ready to receive the fetus, aligned in the longitudinal plane, could help labor occur at the proper time, reducing postdate deliveries.

In another OMT study looking at hemodynamic outcomes, 100 subjects (PROMOTE study participants) were recruited at 30 weeks' gestation.[40] They were assessed for the effect of OMT on hemodynamic changes in the third trimester. Subjects were randomized into one of three treatment groups: OMT, placebo ultrasound, or time control.

- After the prenatal visit, patients were placed on a tilt table.
  - □ Heart rate, blood pressure, and heart rate variability were measured supine and after a 60-degree tilt.
  - □ Heel-raise exercises were used to actively return blood to the circulation.
  - □ Each OMT group participant received a 20- to 30-minute standardized set of hands-on treatments to her head, neck, abdominal diaphragm, back, pelvis, sacrum, and pelvic diaphragm. Techniques used included soft tissue, articulatory, myofascial release, and muscle energy.
  - □ Placebo ultrasound group participants received a 20-minute subtherapeutic ultrasound systematically administered over the same major body regions as addressed by the OMT.
  - □ The routine prenatal care with OMT group showed an increase in blood pressure with heel-raise exercises, but no effect on heart rate variability or on the response to head-up tilt alone.[40]
  - □ Since the heart rate variability remained constant, the change in blood pressure was theorized to be more of a structural alteration than one of a change in autonomic control.
  - □ OMT can have some acute benefits for hemodynamic regulation in pregnant women that could impact the incidence or severity of common complaints such as lower extremity edema, varicose veins, and hemorrhoids.[40]

More studies are needed to explore how OMT in routine prenatal care could provide a cost-effective method of significantly improving perinatal outcomes.

Edema

The gravid uterus is situated in the pelvis, so in the upright position, it compresses the venous and lymphatic return from the lower extremities to the central circulation.

- When patients stand for extended periods of time, lower extremity edema may develop.
- Osteopathic treatment to relieve restrictions of the soft tissues permits improved venous and lymphatic return.
- Following the principles of lymphatic treatment, addressing restrictions of the thorax, ribs, and diaphragm will improve lymphatic flow to the general circulation through optimization of the thoracic cage as a central lymphatic pump.[41]

Hemorrhoids

Hemorrhoids are a frequent complaint in pregnancy.

- Contributory factors include the following:
  - □ Increased venous stasis because of the weight of the gravid uterus
  - □ Increased straining because of the frequency of constipation in pregnancy
  - □ Iron supplementation
- Treatment to improve lymphatic and venous drainage and balance pelvic floor tensions, such as the ischial tuberosity spread, may improve symptoms.[41]

PREPARATION OF THE PATIENT FOR LABOR

Pelvic Examination

After the 36th or 37th week of gestation, prior to active labor, pelvic examination is performed to evaluate fetal size, presentation, and pelvic outlet accommodation for the fetus.

- At this time, the patient may describe "lightening" or the descent of the fetal presenting part in the pelvis.
  - □ This is accompanied by increased pelvic pressure and a sensation of decreased midepigastric fullness.
  - □ The patient feels more "room" to breathe.
- An assessment of the patient's chances for delivering vaginally can be made by interpreting the examination of the "true pelvis" (inlet, midpelvis, and outlet).
  - □ The pelvic inlet:
    - Is bounded anteriorly by mentally constructing a line from the iliopectineal lines, along the pectineal eminence and pubic crest, to the symphysis.
    - Is bounded posteriorly by the sacrum at the level of termination of the iliopectineal lines. The sacral base is not included, as it is superior to this territory.
    - Has a plane with a flat surface bounded similarly but usually inclined horizontally (with the patient in a standing position), at a 40- to 60-degree angle.
  - □ The pelvic outlet is bound by the pubic symphysis, ischial tuberosities, and coccyx.
  - □ The midpelvis contains all structures between the pelvic inlet and outlet.
- While the physical examination may provide clues about the adequacy of the pelvis, it is important to note that the fetal cranial bones are separated by membrane or cartilage and are not approximated.
  - □ Yet, their edges are smooth, providing ability to mold throughout labor in response to the forces of the contracting uterus to decrease the head diameter, as the fetus traverses the pelvis.

- Additionally, the effect of relaxin on the symphysis pubis provides some mobility to expand and increase the pelvic area.
- It is not possible to adequately predict ability to successfully deliver vaginally without a trial of labor, even with the use of pelvic CT.[42]
  - Furthermore, while ultrasound measurements are frequently done to determine fetal size and probability of vaginal delivery, there is a 15% to 20% error in estimated fetal weight during the second and third trimester.[43]

Forces of Labor on the Pelvic Floor

Despite a great variation in individual features of the bony pelvis, the birth canal is curved anteriorly in nearly all women (Fig. 81.1).

- To be born, the fetal presenting part must negotiate both the pelvic curve and any narrow areas that may be present in the pelvis.
- Other maternal and fetal variables to contend with during labor are the quality of uterine contractions, head molding ability, and head flexion capability.
- Most normal labor requires minimal intervention.

Osteopathic structural evaluation of the patient in labor should focus on the lumbosacral spine and pelvis, especially on mobility of the sacrum and symmetry.

- Asymmetry of the pelvis and sacral base unleveling can contribute to an asynclitic (asymmetric) presentation.
- Poor abdominal muscle tone may prevent direction of the fetus through the pelvis in the longitudinal plane.

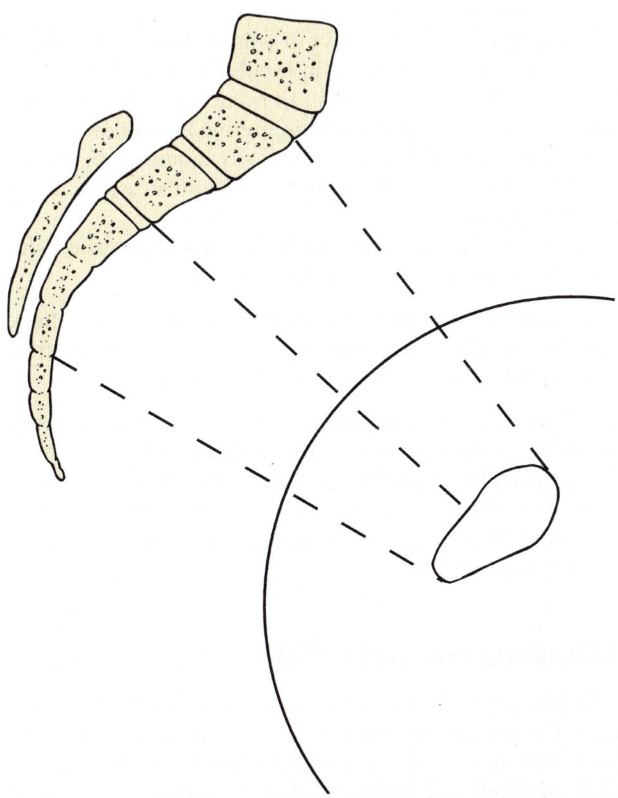

Figure 81.1. Axis of the pelvis, seen on the sagittal section. Note that the curve is relatively straight throughout the inlet but curves anteriorly in the midpelvis. The *dashed lines* indicate planes of the pelvic inlet, midpelvis, and outlet, top to bottom. (Reprinted with permission from Scott JR, Disaia PJ, Hammond CB, Spellacy WN. *Danforth's Obstetrics and Gynecology*. 7th ed. J.B. Lippincott; 1994:105–128.)

Manipulative management considerations might include gentle techniques (such as soft tissue or myofascial stretching) that cooperate with natural forces of labor.

- Patients in latent or active labor may not tolerate active or aggressive manual procedures.
- Treating of the:
  - Pelvis to correct asymmetry of the anterior superior iliac spines will increase the pelvic inlet diameter.
  - Thoracolumbar spine with soft tissue techniques may regulate uterine contractions via sympathetic influence.[44]
  - Sacral base dysfunction may influence cervical dilation.
  - Cranial motion has been shown to influence uterine contractions.[45]
- Positioning of the patient can assist longitudinal vectors for fetal descent, such as use of the lateral recumbent position with pillows to support the abdomen when the fetus has assumed an oblique lie.

A posterior sacral base provides ample space throughout the course of fetal descent; however, the fetal occiput may maintain the posterior position at delivery.

- If the sacral base is restricted anteriorly in its lower portion, the occiput tends to rotate into the anterior pelvis, usually maintaining the occiput anterior position for delivery.
- If the entire sacrum persists in an anterior position throughout its long axis (i.e., a flat pelvis), the head descends through the midpelvis in the transverse position.
- Sometimes a cesarean section becomes necessary for delivery because the head cannot descend any further or cannot rotate for a vaginal delivery.
- OMT of the maternal pelvis with the objective of addressing sacral motion restrictions may assist the labor and birth process.

Despite the variety of pelvic types and distortions, the fetal head may traverse the pelvis uneventfully, if the pelvis is large enough to accommodate the size of the infant[46] (see Fig. 81.2).

- The most deleterious conditions are those encountered when an average-sized head attempts to squeeze through an average-sized android, or "funnel" pelvis in which the spines are prominent, sidewalls convergent, lower sacrum anterior, and subpubic arch narrow.
  - When the subpubic arch is wide, the occiput may position itself with ease.
  - If the arch is narrowed, the occiput remains posterior, in the area of the sacrum.
- With prolonged maternal pushing, in addition to possibly unsatisfactory placement of the maternal legs in stirrups, the following may occur[47,48]:
  - Iliac dysfunction
  - Sacral base restriction
  - Back and leg pain with resultant neuropathy
  - Pubic symphysis separation
  - True rupture of the ligaments supporting the symphysis pubis (rare but does occur)

Pain Relief in Labor

Modern obstetrical practice provides relief of painful contractions in labor with the use of narcotic analgesia and/or epidural anesthesia. Understanding the effects of these agents is important in determining risk/benefit ratios for the patient.

- Fast-metabolizing narcotic analgesia agents are frequently used in labor and delivery units. In addition to some pain relief,

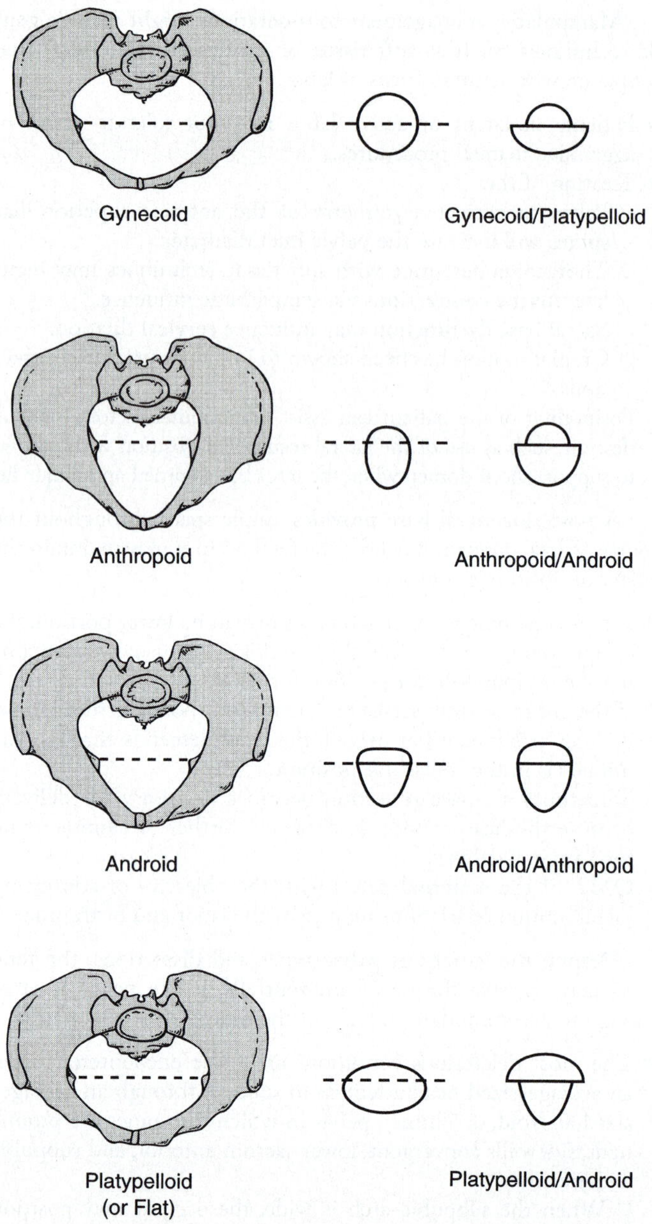

Figure 81.2. Pelvis types. The four "classic types," as defined by Caldwell–Moloy classification of pelvic types are shown in the left column. The shapes of the pelvic space for each type are shown in the center column. "Mixed" pelvic types are shown in the third column; these are named by the posterior shape first, followed by the anterior shape.

they cause relaxation in the patient, which also reduces pain sensation.
  - While the most commonly used medications will clear the patient's system rapidly, the time taken to completely metabolize in the fetus is not known. Of most immediate concern is the known risk of these medications to reduce neonatal respiratory effort after delivery and may require reversal with naloxone.
  - The effect of narcotics on imprinting normal newborn reflexes such as rooting, latching on, and crawling of the neonate to the breast to initiate suckling is not well understood.
- Many studies report poorer rates of successful breastfeeding and delayed onset of lactation when narcotics are given during labor.[49]
- Other studies also question the effect of narcotics on the developing brain and future risk for substance abuse.
  - Two studies found a dose-dependent relationship between opiate and nitrous oxide exposure during labor and future risk of substance abuse.
  - The more often the mother was dosed during her labor, the more likely the offspring was to have substance abuse issues as an adult.[50,51]

Epidural anesthesia has become a preferred method of pain relief for labor.

- Because narcotics are given in the epidural space, much less medication reaches the fetus.
- Several studies have shown similar rates of successful breastfeeding with patients receiving epidurals compared to patients without pain medications during labor.[52,53]
- While epidural anesthesia provides pain relief with minimal fetal exposure to narcotics, common side effects include the following:
  - Hypotension
  - Decrease in the intensity and frequency of contractions
  - Increased risk of operative vaginal delivery
  - Need for bladder catheter
- More serious complications include the following:
  - Spinal headache after inadvertent entry into the dural space
  - Subdural hematoma
  - A high epidural, requiring intubation
- Additional fluids given to correct hypotension can lead to:
  - Fluid overload
  - Edema
  - Pulmonary edema
- The epidural decreases:
  - The patient's ability to move to assist fetal descent in the pelvis
  - The urge to push to assist in expulsion of the fetus
- Fetal heart rate abnormalities can occur secondary to hypotension and the resulting decrease in uterine blood flow.
- Contractions often decrease in intensity, requiring oxytocin augmentation to improve them, and may begin a cascade of subsequent interventions.
  - Oxytocin decreases the available oxygen perfusion during contractions and can cause fetal distress.

Conversely, if a patient is exhausted or overly tense, the relief an epidural provides may permit the patient to rest, regain strength, and successfully participate in a vaginal delivery.

- OMT in labor has been used successfully to assist patients in obtaining delivery without analgesia or anesthesia.[53]
- The osteopathic physician is uniquely poised to:
  - Promote the benefits of physiologic birth in normal cases
  - Educate the patient regarding risks and benefits of any medical procedure

MANAGING THE DELIVERY

It is important to encourage patients regarding their upcoming delivery that the female body is uniquely designed to handle the task. The astute physician can help the patient navigate her transition to motherhood without damaging herself or her infant in many cases.

- Alignment of the fetus in the pelvis in the occiput anterior position can make the delivery easier.
  - A.T. Still taught a technique to physically align the fetus in the longitudinal plane.[54]

- The hands and knees positioning of the patient allows gravity to help move the fetal back anteriorly, encouraging the head to rotate to the occiput anterior position.
- The cervical spine has more range of motion in extension than flexion, making the occiput anterior position preferred for navigating the pelvic curve.
- The psoas muscle can push the fetus forward, especially in cases where the patient has an exaggerated lumbar curve.
- Flattening the lumbar spine relaxes the psoas and allows the fetus to drop into the pelvis. Possible positions to accomplish this include:
  - Squatting
  - Sitting on a birthing (exercise) ball
  - Reclining in bed in the McRoberts position with hips and knees flexed.
- Squatting opens the pelvis 1.1 cm more in the transverse diameter and 0.6 cm in the A/P diameter than other positions.[55]
- The upright position for labor speeds the labor process and reduces complications.[56]

- Osteopathic physicians had a reputation for performing deliveries without lacerations.
  - The physician must understand the properties of fascia, and that the perineal tissue is designed to stretch under gentle pressure but will tear if the force is too aggressive.
  - Slow the delivery over the perineum if fetal heart tones are stable.
  - Support the perineum during delivery to help prevent laceration.
  - Patient's relaxation of buttocks and thighs permits more stretching of the tissue.
  - Rather than having the patient push the baby out, have her "breathe" the baby out.
  - Perineal tissue will blanche before it tears. Watch the integrity of the tissue and direct the patient to allow time for stretching.
- Make sure the focus is on the patient, the baby, and her support persons.
  - Dim delivery room lights and keep the room quiet, unless a procedure is needed, to aid in relaxation of the mother.
  - Delay routine procedures that can wait until after bonding and breastfeeding have occurred.

Breast Crawl

The World Health Organization promotes using the "breast crawl" after birth to improve proper latch-on and breastfeeding initiation, and to decrease infant mortality. UNICEF and WHO strongly recommend initiating breastfeeding within a half-hour of birth as part of the Ten Steps to Successful Breastfeeding program.[57]

In industrialized countries, infant survival is less of an issue, yet successful breastfeeding has been shown beneficial for many health issues including the following[58]:

- Protection from infections and illnesses including diarrhea, otitis media, and pneumonia
- Reduced risk of developing asthma
- Decreased risk of obesity (for infants breastfed for 6 months)
- Reduced risk of SIDS
- Decreased risk of breast and ovarian cancers (for mothers who breastfeed)

The principle of the breast crawl includes understanding that the infant's inborn reflexes will guide the neonate to crawl to the nipple and latch on spontaneously within 30 minutes of delivery when left undisturbed on the maternal abdomen, in most cases.[59]

- After delivery and before clamping the cord, the infant is dried and placed on the maternal abdomen and covered for warmth.
- The infant will begin to crawl to the nipple by propelling forward, pushing with feet and arms.
- Given sufficient time, the infant will spontaneously latch onto the nipple and begin to suckle without assistance.
- The effort exerted reinforces the infant's suckling reflexes, corrects latch on, and establishes better feeding patterns.

Immediate and prolonged skin-to-skin contact has been shown to benefit breastfeeding outcomes, increase cardiorespiratory stability, and decrease infant crying and has no apparent short- or long-term negative effects.[60]

Delayed Cord Clamping

When managing a normal labor and delivery, the osteopathic physician should be mindful of normal physiologic function and carefully determine when intervention is appropriate.

- In the case of clamping of the umbilical cord after delivery, the physician should be aware of why the cord pulses and why it stops spontaneously and question whether it is appropriate to intervene and clamp the cord before postnatal circulation has been established.
- In utero, the fetal lungs are fluid filled, and amniotic fluid is breathed in and out as the fetus practices diaphragmatic activity prior to birth.
- After birth, it is necessary for the fetal lungs to clear the fluid. This happens quickly, but not instantaneously.
- The pulsing cord provides oxygenation through a central line to the fetal circulation while fluid is absorbed, allowing for transition time.

The first breath brings about rapid physiologic changes in the neonate.

- Pulmonary arterial pO_2 increases and pCO_2 decreases. This results in:
  - Pulmonary vascular dilation
  - Decreased pulmonary vascular resistance
  - Constriction of the ductus arteriosus
- When the umbilical blood flow ceases, the ductus venosus closes.
- Increased right-sided pressures result in closure of the foramen ovale, and transition to postnatal circulation is completed.[61]
- At this time, the neonate has received the portion of the placental blood that is necessary for homeostasis and a transfusion of the stem cells within the umbilical cord.

A growing body of research confirms significant benefit to the neonate by receiving the placental transfusion rather than immediately clamping the umbilical cord.

- A delay of 30 to 120 seconds in the preterm infant had the following positive effects[62]:
  - Less need for blood transfusion
  - Better circulatory stability
  - Less intraventricular hemorrhage (all grades)
  - Lower risk for necrotizing enterocolitis
- When the effects of delayed cord clamping were studied in the term infant, the primary outcome noted for the delayed clamping was significantly improved iron stores in the early months of infant life, but there was also a higher risk of need for phototherapy in the early neonatal period.[63]

POSTPARTUM MANAGEMENT

Decreased Morbidity and Mortality

The osteopathic physician can maximize a successful labor and delivery experience for the mother.

- The patient may need treatment of residual somatic dysfunction in the postpartum period.
- The most obvious challenge is to assist the postpartum patient in returning the pelvis, axial skeleton, and the supporting soft tissues to their pregravid state; this can be expedited by using OMT.
- OMT may reduce morbidity and mortality due to complications of labor and delivery.[64,65]

Pubic Dysfunction

Forces of labor on the pubic symphysis can increase the risk of postpartum somatic dysfunction.

- These include the following:
  - Lateral traction during delivery of a large fetus
  - Unequal pressure against the legs when in McRoberts position
  - Risk of trauma when a patient with an epidural cannot feel when the legs are past the normal physiologic barrier
- The patient may experience:
  - Pinching midpubic pain
  - Low pelvic pain with ambulation
  - Inability to bear weight
- Structural examination may reveal:
  - A vertical pubic shear
  - Anterior/posterior pubic shear
  - Pubic symphysis diaphysis
- Appropriate treatment early in the postpartum period will greatly reduce the patient's disability and speed recovery.

VERTICAL SHEAR

Vertical shear is the most common pubic symphysis dysfunction and responds well to osteopathic manipulation.

- The shear is identified by noting vertical displacement from one side to the other on the superior border of the symphysis.
- The patient will not need much treatment force in the immediate postpartum period, as the pelvis is still very mobile.
- A gentle leg tug on the more superior side will often be sufficient for treatment, or muscle energy can be used on the contralateral side to elevate that pubic bone.

ANTERIOR/POSTERIOR SHEAR

Anterior/posterior pubic shear is much less common and causes much more disability and pain.

- Diagnosis is performed by palpation of the pubic rami at equidistance from the symphysis on the anterior portion of the bone.
- Compare the anterior/posterior symmetry. The side of dysfunction will be exquisitely tender in acute injury.
- Treatment may include muscle energy to move the posterior hemipelvis anterior.
- Treatment should also include myofascial release of the suprapubic tissues, as they also are under strain.

PUBIC SYMPHYSIS DIAPHYSIS

Pubic symphysis diaphysis involves rupture of part or all of the symphysis ligaments. This causes extreme instability, difficulty weight bearing, and pain.

- X-rays are useful in diagnosis by showing a widening of the symphysis.
- Patients are given a walker to assist in ambulation, and use of a trochanter belt gives additional support to aid healing. When a trochanter belt is not available, a long strip of linens can be used by tying firmly horizontally around the pelvis at the level of the trochanters, gluteus maximus, and pubic symphysis.
- Regular osteopathic treatment can shorten the convalescent period. Treatment should focus on correcting any asymmetry and relieving fascial strains in the surrounding tissues.

Hand and Wrist Complaints

CARPAL TUNNEL SYNDROME

Although carpal tunnel syndrome usually occurs in the second or third trimesters, Wand reports its development in 18 patients, not during pregnancy but while they were nursing.[66] These symptoms resolved when breastfeeding ceased. Snell and coworkers report similar findings in five patients in the puerperium and attribute the problem to fluid retention caused by the hormone prolactin.[67]

DE QUERVAIN TENOSYNOVITIS

Another frequently encountered cause of pain in the hand and wrist is de Quervain tenosynovitis, which results from compression and irritation of the extensor pollicis brevis and abductor pollicis longus tendons as they pass through the first dorsal compartment of the wrist, near the styloid process of the radius.[68]

- Fluid retention has been suspected as an initiator of this problem, which is intensified using the hand and fingers and by movement of the wrist.[69,70]
- The following can aggravate the condition and lead to persistent symptoms:
  - Infant care activities[69]
  - Breastfeeding[70,71]

Low Back Pain

Although back pain is the most common complaint of expectant mothers, persistent back pain can also become a problem during the postpartum period.

- Russell and associates have investigated factors associated with long-term backache after childbirth in 299 patients, especially those factors that may have been associated with epidural anesthesia during labor.[72]
  - They concluded that, although new long-term backache was reported by the women given epidural analgesia in labor, the pain tended to be postural and not severe.
  - No differences existed in the nature of the backache between those who did or did not receive epidurals during labor.
- Although back pain during or after pregnancy may be common, it should not be dismissed on the basis that it is a normal accompaniment of pregnancy.
- The lumbosacral spine should be evaluated for extended segmental dysfunction.
- Back pain can also be addressed by normalizing structures passing through the obturator canal.

Breast Engorgement/Mastitis

Proper initiation of breastfeeding and nursing on demand with frequent suckling makes problems of breast engorgement and mastitis less probable. They remain, however, very common postpartum problems.

- Lymphatic techniques addressing the thorax and breasts can help relieve engorgement and speed healing in cases of mastitis.
- Patients should be educated on breastfeeding frequently, every 2 to 3 hours, and alternating which side the infant suckles first.
- If mastitis does occur, breastfeeding is not contraindicated, and frequent suckling will help to drain plugged ducts.
- A warm compress to the breast while feeding is helpful.
- If antibiotics are deemed necessary, many antibiotics to cover the skin flora most often associated with mastitis are safe to use while nursing.

Pseudosciatica and Chapman Reflexes

Hip and leg pain, whether from sciatic nerve compression pain or from other causes, is common in pregnancy and can occur during childbirth. Janet Travell described a condition called "pseudosciatica"[73] in which radiating leg pain is caused by gluteus minimus trigger points without signs of sciatic nerve compression.

The genitourinary system might exhibit the presence of Chapman points, either as a pre-existing condition and becoming more symptomatic through the forces of pregnancy or developed as an acute response to those forces or to an infection.

- The genitourinary system is thought of as beginning with the groin gland points as "these reflexes are very important in establishing drainage in all cases of infections involving the pelvic organs or that occur in the feet and legs."[12]
- The genitourinary points include the irritated:
  - ☐ Clitoris and vaginismus
  - ☐ Uterine fibroma
  - ☐ Broad ligament
  - ☐ Uterus
  - ☐ Urethra
  - ☐ Ovaries
  - ☐ Abdominal tension
  - ☐ Leukorrhea
  - ☐ Salpingitis
  - ☐ Kidney
  - ☐ Adrenal points
  - ☐ Urinary bladder
- Chapman relates presence of the irritated clitoris and vaginismus point to the development of the neurasthenia point,[12] which involves the state of not only "extreme nervousness" but also insomnia.
- Some of Frank Chapman's descriptions of these points bring a deeper osteopathic insight into physiologic understanding of the medical condition.
  - ☐ For instance, the physiologic description of the broad ligament points or reflex center is of "a contraction or apparently callous state of the tissues in the female indicates a lymphatic congestion of the broad ligament, even to the extent of an inflammation of the ligament. Because of this irritation, there may be an abnormal position of the uterus."[12]
  - ☐ Activation of these broad ligament Chapman points has the potential to create hip/leg pain or "pseudo sciatica." For more detailed discussion (see Chapters 43 and 58 regarding, Viscerosomatic Reflexes and Somatosomatic Reflexes, Jones Tenderpoints, Trigger Points, and Chapman Reflexes).

INDICATIONS AND CONTRAINDICATIONS FOR USE OF OMT DURING PREGNANCY

The indications and contraindications for use of OMT during pregnancy are listed in Table 81.2.

TABLE 81.2

Indications and Contraindications for Osteopathic Manipulative Treatment During Pregnancy

Indications
- Somatic dysfunction during pregnancy
- Scoliosis or other structural condition associated with pregnancy
- Edema, congestion, or other pregnancy-associated condition amenable to osteopathic manipulative treatment

Contraindications
- Undiagnosed vaginal bleeding
- Threatened or incomplete abortion
- Ectopic pregnancy
- Placenta previa
- Placental abruption
- Preterm premature rupture of membranes
- Preterm labor (relative contraindication)
- Prolapsed umbilical cord
- Eclampsia and severe preeclampsia
- Surgical or medical emergencies (other than those listed above)

CASE VIGNETTE

OBSTETRICAL PATIENT WITH PELVIC AND LEG PAIN

A 33-year-old G4P3 at 36 weeks' gestation presented to labor and delivery triage with complaint of constant low pelvic pain and sciatica (posterior leg pain to the plantar foot) on her right side.

- She was anxious and experienced increased pain with any motion of her lower extremities. The pain:
  - ☐ Had been present for about a month
  - ☐ Was rated 7 out of 10
  - ☐ Was greatest on her right SI area and in the right groin
  - ☐ Was worse with walking and lying supine
- The patient had been sleeping in a recliner for the past month because of difficulty finding a comfortable position in bed.
- She had been referred to physical therapy but could not tolerate the sessions. Her physician's plan was to refer her to physical therapy again after delivery.
- The pregnancy had been uncomplicated except for her pain, and all three previous deliveries were vaginal.
- The patient complained of occasional nausea for which she took an antacid. The review of systems was otherwise normal.

A nonstress test was performed.

- Fetal heart tones were in the 150 seconds with moderate variability, and no decelerations were noted, a category 1 reading.
- No contractions were seen.
- The abdomen was soft, and no uterine tenderness was appreciated.

An osteopathic structural examination was performed.

- Anterior superior iliac spine (ASIS) was inferior on the right, and pelvic compression test showed more restriction on the right than the left. Posterior superior iliac spine (PSIS) was superior on the right. Thus, she had an anterior right innominate rotation.

- A vertical pubic shear was noted, inferior on the right.
- There was soft tissue tenderness in the right groin with induration that had a "bubble wrap" texture.
- An articulatory technique was used to address the iliac rotation bilaterally. Leg pull was used to correct the pubic shear. After these two techniques were done, the patient began to appear more relaxed.
- Direct myofascial release was done in the region of the sacrum.
- The SI joints were taken through a range of motion in a direct articulatory technique, and the patient's partner was instructed on how to perform the maneuver at home.
- Next, the tender groin area was treated with direct myofascial release. There was a sensation of "popping" the bubble wrap.
- Tissue texture normalization was appreciated as the pain decreased.
- After the treatment, the patient rated her pain 4 out of 10 and she was able to move more freely in the bed and ambulate with less pain.

Recommendations on discharge were:

- To seek osteopathic treatment weekly until time of delivery, then request referral for osteopathic treatment.
- Physical therapy
- Core strengthening exercises postpartum

TEACHING POINTS

- Somatic dysfunction can contribute to disability during pregnancy.
  - Symptoms of sciatica often improve with correction of somatic dysfunction.
- Pubic shear is very common in pregnancy, especially around the 30th to 32nd week, and causes pain with weight bearing and walking.
  - The pannus progressively overhangs the groin as pregnancy advances, compromising proper drainage of fluids in the dermal layer, and causing significant discomfort.
  - Myofascial release and lymphatic techniques improve drainage and can resolve induration, normalize tissue texture, and relieve pain.
  - Pregnancy support belts may also be beneficial.
  - SI range of motion exercises can be taught to patients and their partners to correct SI dysfunction, as well as relieve pain and tissue congestion.
- Patients are greatly comforted when they recognize the pain is treatable and is from a structural cause.
  - Patients become motivated to exercise and improve core strength when osteopathic manipulation demonstrates a structural etiology of pain.

CONCLUSION

A systematic approach by the osteopathic obstetrician who has been trained to identify and treat somatic dysfunction may reveal underlying sources of discomfort. In this situation, OMT may be used to affect a more comfortable, healthy, and enjoyable child-bearing experience.

REFERENCES

1. Still AT. *The Philosophy and Mechanical Principles of Osteopathy*. Hudson-Kimberly Publishing Co; 1902.
2. AAP Committee on Fetus and Newborn and ACOG Committee on Obstetric Practice. *Guidelines for Perinatal Care (7)*. American Academy of Pediatrics; 2012. ProQuest ebrary. 2016: 95–161.
3. Kuchera ML, Ettlinger H, Seffinger MA. Chapter 31: assessing for viscero-somatic reflexes and somato-somatic reflexes, Jones tenderpoints, trigger points and Chapman reflexes. In: ExSeffinger ed. *Foundations of Osteopathic Medicine*. 4th ed. Wolters Kluwer; 2018.
4. DiGiovanna EL, Schiowitz S. *An Osteopathic Approach to Diagnosis and Treatment*. JB Lippincott Co.; 1992:459.
5. Hacker NF, Gambone JC, Hobel CJ. *Essentials of Obstetrics and Gynecology*. 6th ed. Elsevier; 2016.
6. Taylor RN, Badell ML. Chapter 16: the endocrinology of pregnancy. In: Gardner DG, Shoback D, eds. *Greenspan's Basic & Clinical Endocrinology*. 9th ed. McGraw-Hill; 2011.
7. Cunningham F, Leveno KJ, Bloom SL, et al. Maternal physiology. In: Cunningham F, Leveno KJ, Bloom SL, et al., eds. *Williams Obstetrics*. 25th ed. McGraw-Hill; 2013. Accessed August 03, 2018. http://accessmedicine.mhmedical.com.proxy.pnwu.org/content.aspx?bookid=1918&sectionid=138822592
8. Aldabe D, Ribeiro DC, Milosavljevic S, Bussey MD. Pregnancy-related pelvic girdle pain and its relationship with relaxin levels during pregnancy: a systematic review. *Eur Spine J*. 2012;21:1769–1776.
9. Bjorklund K, Bergstorm S, Nordstrom ML, et al. Symphyseal distention in relation to serum relaxin levels and pelvic pain in pregnancy. *Acta Obstet Gynecol Scand*. 2000;79:269–275.
10. Flaxman SM, Sherman PW. Morning sickness: a mechanism for protecting mother and embryo. *Q Rev Biol*. 2000;75(2):113–148.
11. Beal MC. Viscerosomatic reflexes: a review. *J Am Osteopath Assoc*. 1985; 85(12):786–801.
12. Owens C. *An Endocrine Interpretation of Chapman's Reflexes*. 2nd ed. Chattanooga Printing & Engraving Co; 1937.
13. Taylor GW. The osteopathic management of nausea and vomiting of pregnancy. *J Am Osteopath Assoc*. 1949;48:581–582.
14. Smith CA, Armour M, Ee C. Complementary therapies and medicines and reproductive medicine. *Semin Reprod Med*. 2016;34:67–73.
15. Madjunkova S, Maltepe C, Koren G. The delayed-release combination of doxylamine and pyridoxine (Diclegis/Diclectin) for the treatment of nausea and vomiting of pregnancy. *Paediatr Drugs*. 2014;16(3): 199–211.
16. Poyatos-León R, García-Hermoso A, Sanabria-Martínez G, Alvarez-Bueno C, Sanchez-Lopez M, Martinez-Vizcaino V. Effects of exercise during pregnancy on mode of delivery: a meta-analysis. *Acta Obstet Gynecol Scand*. 2015;94(10):1039–1047.
17. Hinman SK, Smith KB, Quillen DM, Smith MS. Exercise in pregnancy: a clinical review. *Sports Health*. 2015;7(6):527–531.
18. Committee Opinion. *Physical Activity and Exercise During Pregnancy and the Postpartum Period. Number 650*. American College of Obstetricians and Gynecologists Compendium of Selected Publications; 2015.
19. Aleman A, Althabe F, Belizán JM, Bergel E. Bed rest during pregnancy for preventing miscarriage. *Cochrane Database Syst Rev*. 2005;(2):CD003576.
20. Section on Breastfeeding. Breastfeeding and the use of human milk. *Pediatrics*. 2012;129(3):e827–e841.
21. Burdon J. Breathlessness and pregnancy. *Aust Fam Physician*. 2000;29(5): 451–452.
22. Liddle SD, Pennick V. Interventions for preventing and treating low-back and pelvic pain during pregnancy. *Cochrane Database Syst Rev*. 2015;(9): CD001139.
23. Barczyk K, Eliasz G, Sipko T, Grygier D. The occurrence of strain symptoms in the lumbosacral region and pelvis during pregnancy and after childbirth. *J Manipulative Physiol Ther*. 2010;33(5):370–377.
24. Vleeming A, Schuenke MD, Masi AT, Carreiro JE, Danneels L, Willard FH. The sacroiliac joint: an overview of its anatomy, function and potential clinical implications. *J Anat*. 2012;221(6):537–567.

25. Morimoto K, Harrington A, Nelson C, Loveless B. Osteopathic approach to sacroiliac joint pain in pregnant patients. *J Osteopath Med.* 2022;122(5): 235–242.
26. Johnston JC, Deune E. Chapter 6: approach to the patient with hand, wrist, or elbow pain. In: Imboden JB, Hellmann DB, Stone JH, eds. *Current Diagnosis & Treatment: Rheumatology.* 3rd ed. McGraw-Hill; 2013.
27. Meems M, Truijens S, Spek V, Visser LH, Pop VJM. Prevalence, course and determinants of carpal tunnel syndrome symptoms during pregnancy: a prospective study. *BJOG.* 2015;122(8):1112–1118.
28. Zyluk A. Carpal tunnel syndrome in pregnancy: a review. *Pol Orthop Traumatol.* 2013;78:223–227.
29. Burnham T, Higgins DC, Burnham RS, Heath DM. Effectiveness of osteopathic manipulative treatment for carpal tunnel syndrome: a pilot project. *J Am Osteopath Assoc.* 2015;115(3):138–148.
30. Sucher BM. Myofascial manipulative release of carpal tunnel syndrome: documentation with magnetic resonance imaging. *J Am Osteopath Assoc.* 1993;93:1273–1278.
31. Sucher BM. Palpatory diagnosis and manipulative management of carpal tunnel syndrome. *J Am Osteopath Assoc.* 1994;94:647–663.
32. Gitlin RS, Wolf DL. Uterine contractions following osteopathic cranial manipulation—a pilot study. *J Am Osteopath Assoc.* 1992;92:1183.
33. Magoun H. *Osteopathy in the Cranial Field.* Journal Printing Company; 1966.
34. Licciardone JC, Buchanan S, Hensel KL, King HH, Fulda KG, Stoll ST. Osteopathic manipulative treatment of back pain and related symptoms during pregnancy: a randomized controlled trial. *Am J Obstet Gynecol.* 2010;202(1):43.
35. Licciardone JC, Minotti DE, Gatchel RJ, Kearns CM, Singh KP. Osteopathic manual treatment and ultrasound therapy for chronic low back pain: a randomized controlled trial. *Ann Fam Med.* 2013;11(2):122–129.
36. Hensel KL, Buchanan S, Brown SK, et al. Pregnancy research on osteopathic manipulation optimizing treatment effects: the PROMOTE study a randomized controlled trial. *Am J Obstet Gynecol.* 2015;212(1):108.
37. Hensel KL, Roane BM, Chaphekar AV, Smith-Barbaro P. PROMOTE Study: safety of osteopathic manipulative treatment during the third trimester by labor and delivery outcomes. *J Am Osteopath Assoc.* 2016;116(11):698–703.
38. Hensel KL, Roane BM. Does compression of the fourth ventricle cause preterm labor? Analysis of data from the PROMOTE study. *J Am Osteopath Assoc.* 2019;119(10):668–672.
39. King HH, Tettambel MA, Lockwood MD, Johnson KH, Arsenault DA, Quist R. Osteopathic manipulative treatment in prenatal care: a retrospective case control design study. *J Am Osteopath Assoc.* 2003;103(12):577–582.
40. Hensel KL, Pacchia CF, Smith ML. Acute improvement in hemodynamic control after osteopathic manipulative treatment in the third trimester of pregnancy. *Complement Ther Med.* 2013;21:618–626.
41. Nelson KE, Glonek T. Somatic Dysfunction in Osteopathic Family Medicine. *American College of Osteopathic Family Physicians.* 2nd ed. Wolters Kluwer, Chapter 13 The Female Patient, Obstetrics; 2015: 127–141.
42. Maharaj D. Assessing cephalopelvic disproportion: back to the basics. *Obstet Gynecol Surv.* 2010;65(6):387–395.
43. Gupta S, Roman AS. Chapter 11: imaging in obstetrics. In: DeCherney AH, Nathan L, Laufer N, Roman AS, eds. *Current Diagnosis & Treatment: Obstetrics & Gynecology.* 11th ed. McGraw-Hill; 2013.
44. Guthrie RA, Martin RH. Effect of pressure applied to the upper thoracic versus lumbar areas for inhibition of lumbar myalgia during labor. *J Am Osteopath Assoc.* 1982;82:247–251.
45. Frymann V. Relation of disturbances of cranio-sacral mechanisms to symptomatology of the newborn: study of 1250 infants. *J Am Osteopath Assoc.* 1966;65:1059–1075.
46. Whiting L. Osteopathic prevention of certain complications of labor and the puerperium. *J Am Osteopath Assoc.* 1945;44:495–498.
47. McCormick J. Some variations can be made in the "obstetrical workshop." *J Am Osteopath Assoc.* 1944;44:195–197.
48. Jacobson B, Nyberg K, Grönbladh L, Eklund G, Bygdeman M, Rydberg U. Opiate addiction in adult offspring through possible imprinting after obstetric treatment. *BMJ.* 1990;301(6760):1067–1070.
49. Lind JN, Perrine CG, Li R. Relationship between use of labor pain medications and delayed onset of lactation. *J Hum Lact.* 2014;30(2): 167–173.
50. Nyberg K, Allebeck P, Eklund G, Jacobson B. Socio-economic versus obstetric risk factors for drug addiction in offspring. *Br J Addict.* 1992; 87(12):1669–1676.
51. Loubert C, Hinova A, Fernando R. Update on modern neuraxial analgesia in labour: a review of the literature of the last 5 years. *Anaesthesia.* 2011;66:191–212.
52. Wilson MJA, MacArthur C, Cooper GM, et al.; on behalf of the COMET Study Group UK. Epidural analgesia and breastfeeding: a randomized controlled trial of epidural techniques with and without fentanyl and a non-epidural comparison group. *Anaesthesia.* 2010;65:145–153.
53. Smallwood CR, Borgerding CJ, Cox MS, et al. Osteopathic manipulative treatment (OMT) facilitates a natural drug-free childbirth for a primigravida patient: a case report. *Int J Osteopathic Med.* 2013;16:170–177.
54. Still AT. *The Philosophy and Mechanical Principles of Osteopathy.* Osteopathic Enterprise; 1902.
55. Hemmerich A, Bandrowska T, Dumas GA. The effects of squatting while pregnant on pelvic dimensions: a computational simulation to understand childbirth. *J Biomech.* 2019;87:64–74.
56. Lawrence A, Lewis L, Hofmeyr GJ, Styles C. Maternal positions and mobility during first stage labour. *Cochrane Database Syst Rev.* 2013;(10): CD003934.
57. *Ten Steps to Successful Breastfeeding.* Updated May 28, 2013. Accessed March 7, 2017. http://www.tensteps.org/ten-steps-successful-breastfeeding.shtml
58. *The Surgeon General's Call to Action to Support Breastfeeding.* Health Benefits of Breastfeeding. Updated January 20, 2011. Accessed March 7, 2017. http://www.surgeongeneral.gov/library/calls/breastfeeding/factsheet.html
59. *The Breast Crawl.* Updated October 26, 2016. Accessed March 7, 2017. http://www.breastcrawl.org
60. Moore ER, Anderson GC, Bergman N, Dowswell T. Early skin-to-skin contact for mothers and their healthy newborn infants. *Cochrane Database Syst Rev.* 2012;5(5):CD003519.
61. Davis RP, Mychaliska GB. Neonatal pulmonary physiology. *Semin Pediatr Surg.* 2013;22(4):179–184.
62. Rabe H, Diaz-Rossello JL, Duley L, et al. Effect of timing of umbilical cord clamping and other strategies to influence placental transfusion at preterm birth on maternal and infant outcomes. *Cochrane Database Syst Rev.* 2012;(8):CD003248.
63. McDonald SJ, Middleton P, Dowswell T, Morris PS. Effect of timing of umbilical cord clamping of term infants on maternal and neonatal outcomes. *Cochrane Database Syst Rev.* 2013;2013(7):CD004074.
64. King HH. Osteopathic manipulative treatment in prenatal care: evidence supporting improved outcomes and health policy implications. *Am Acad Osteopathy J.* 2000;10:25–33.
65. Hitchcock ME. Osteopathic care in pregnancy. *Osteopath Ann.* 1976;4: 405–411.
66. Wand JS. Carpal tunnel syndrome in pregnancy and lactation. *J Hand Surg Br.* 1990;15B:93–95.
67. Snell NJ, Coysh HL, Snell BJ. Carpal tunnel syndrome presenting in the puerperium. *Practitioner.* 1980;224:191–193.
68. Heckman JD, Sassard R. Musculoskeletal considerations in pregnancy. *J Bone Joint Surg Am.* 1994;76:1720–1730.
69. Schned ES. De Quervain tenosynovitis in pregnant and postpartum women. *Obstet Gynecol.* 1986;68:411–444.
70. Schumacher HR Jr, Dorwart BB, Korzeniowski OM. Occurrence of De Quervain's tendonitis during pregnancy. *Arch Intern Med.* 1985;145: 2083–2084.
71. Johnson CA. Occurrence of De Quervain's disease in postpartum women. *J Fam Pract.* 1991;32:325–327.
72. Russell R, Groves P, Taub N, et al. Assessing long term backache after childbirth. *BMJ.* 1993;306:1299–1303.
73. Travell JG, Simons DG. *Chapter 9: Myofascial Pain and Dysfunction, The Trigger Point Manual.* 1st ed. Vol. 2. Lippincott Williams & Wilkins; 1992.

82 Osteopathic Considerations in Gynecology

ANITA SHOWALTER

KEY CONCEPTS

- Knowledge of pelvic anatomy and physiology are essential to properly diagnosing pelvic conditions and pelvic dysfunctions.
- Multiple organ systems may contribute to pelvic pain syndromes.
- Osteopathic evaluation of pelvic pain and dysfunctions include somatic and visceral etiologies as well as behavioral considerations.
- Osteopathic treatment includes osteopathic manipulative treatment (OMT), and medical and surgical management as appropriate.

INTRODUCTION

> What diseases does woman have that man does not have? Such diseases as belong to the womb and its appendages…It matters not whether the cause is far remote or in close proximity to the uterus; we must find it, or we will be found in the antediluvian tribe of speculum cranks of all the blind female doctors' ages.
>
> —A.T. Still, MD, DO[1]

The osteopathic obstetrician–gynecologist has the opportunity to integrate the influences of the musculoskeletal system into the management of a variety of health care concerns experienced by female patients.

- The following are keys to osteopathic diagnosis and management of somatic dysfunction:
  - Knowledge of anatomy and physiology of the reproductive system and pelvis
  - Expertise in palpation
- Because of the broad scope of gynecology, this chapter does not address all diagnostic and treatment topics involving the female reproductive system. Instead, it:
  - Focuses on the most common disorders presenting to the gynecologist
  - Proposes an osteopathic perspective on the evaluation and management plan for the patient

PELVIC ANATOMY

Evaluation of pelvic pain requires extensive knowledge of the anatomy and physiology of the female pelvis.

- The concept of visceral convergence is important in evaluation of pelvic pain.[2] There is significant overlap of sensory fibers with visceral afferents in the pelvis, so pain is broadly referred and is often sensed on the abdominal wall.
- The patient may not be able to localize pain, so a thorough understanding of pelvic anatomy will help the physician identify possible visceral or somatic sources of pain and determine if pain is likely to be from a gynecologic or other origin.
- If associated symptoms of the gastrointestinal tract, urinary tract, or other organ system are present, consultation with another specialist to complete the patient workup may be indicated.
- Although standard references[3] completely discuss the anatomy of the female pelvis, salient points helpful to osteopathic physicians are summarized here to assist in understanding causes of somatic dysfunction (Fig. 82.1).

Skeletal System

The bony structure of the pelvis includes the sacrum and paired ilia that are continuous with the paired pubic bones.

- Three joints connect these bones, the paired sacroiliacs and the pubis symphysis.
- Strong ligamentous attachments lend stability to the pelvis while permitting enough motion for ambulation.
- The sacroiliac joints have ligamentous fibers arranged in a herringbone fashion while the pubic symphysis has transverse fibers (Fig. 82.2).

Fibers are oriented to contribute to joint stability in normal range of motion.

- Knowledge of fiber orientation will also help the physician understand vectors of positioning and force used during osteopathic manipulation.
- In effect, this anatomic arrangement creates a bony circle with three points of mobility, the two sacroiliac joints and pubic symphysis.
- Asymmetry at any point in this unit causes associated dysfunction and tenderness at the others (Fig. 82.3).

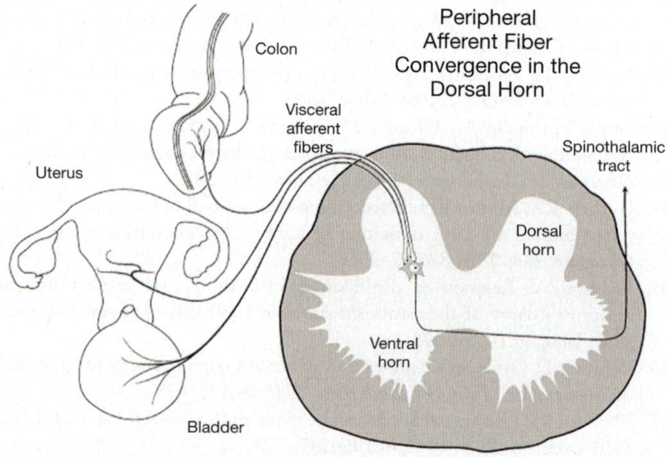

Figure 82.1. Afferent convergence. Afferent fibers from multiple viscera are in close proximity to each other as well as in proximity to the somatic afferents. This provides an understanding for how viscerovisceral and viscerosomatic reflexes occur. (Used with permission from the Willard/Carreiro Collection, University of New England.)

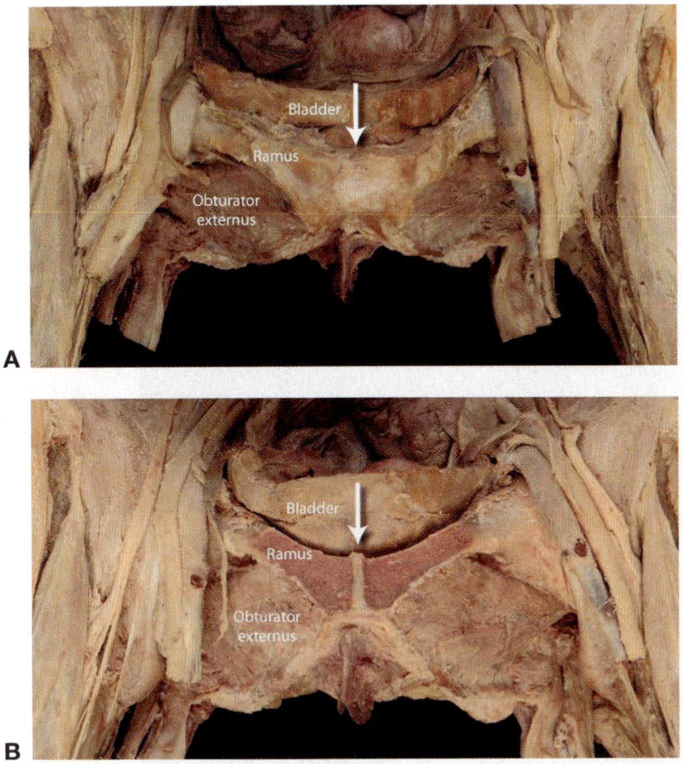

Figure 82.2. **A.** The pubic symphysis dissected from anterior tissues showing the orientation of the bladder and obturator externus. **B.** Frontal section of the pubic ramus to show the ligamentous articulation of the pubis symphysis. (Used with permission from the Willard/Carreiro Collection, University of New England.)

The skeleton provides the:

- Bony framework for the pelvis
- Suspension of the fascia, muscles, and viscera from the pelvic sidewalls

Any asymmetry of the bony pelvic structure may contribute to:

- Planes of pelvic diaphragm tension
- Corresponding compromise of vasculature, lymphatics, and neural function
- Subsequent alteration of the homeostatic mechanisms of the pelvic viscera

Pelvic Muscles

The pelvic floor consists of the levator ani muscles and pelvic diaphragm complex.[4] It contains the:

- Visceral pelvic fascia
- Pelvic diaphragm
- Urogenital anal triangles with superficial and deep genital muscles
- Sphincters of the urethra

The pelvic floor performs three important functions:

1. Supportive
2. Sphincteric
3. Sexual

The pelvic floor, in conjunction with the pelvis bones, muscles, and connective tissues, provides support of the pelvic organs against gravity and any increases in abdominal pressure.

- The muscles maintain proper orientation of the viscera for normal function.
- Support and tone for vaginal walls are also provided.
- Sphincteric function aids in control of perineal openings for micturition and defecation and maintains urinary and fecal continence.

Pelvic floor muscles help prevent urinary incontinence by increasing intraurethral pressure and stabilizing endopelvic fascia during sphincter contraction.[5]

- A functional pelvic floor:
  - ☐ Stabilizes the proximal urethra
  - ☐ Improves severe lower tract symptomatology
  - ☐ Assists in the ability to delay urination via bladder reflex inhibition[6]
- The pelvic floor muscles must relax to permit defecation and contract to control stool and flatus.
- After defecation, they contract to expel stool and help prevent fecal incontinence by maintaining the appropriate anorectal angle.[6]

The sexual function of the pelvic floor consists of contraction of perivaginal muscles during coitus to enhance sexual activity.

- The muscles respond reflexively during orgasm.
- Decreased pubococcygeal strength and awareness impede sexual response.[7]

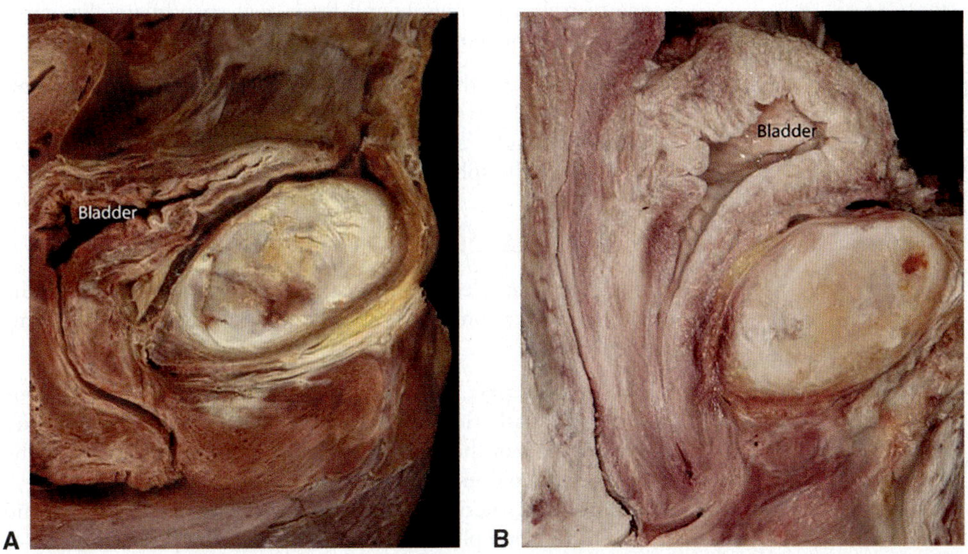

Figure 82.3. **A, B.** Sagittal views of the pubic symphysis, bladder, and uterus. Note the position of the bladder superior to the symphysis, with room for expansion into the abdominal cavity with distension. Also note orientation of the uterus posterior to the bladder, with the vesicouterine pouch between. (Used with permission from the Willard/Carreiro Collection, University of New England.)

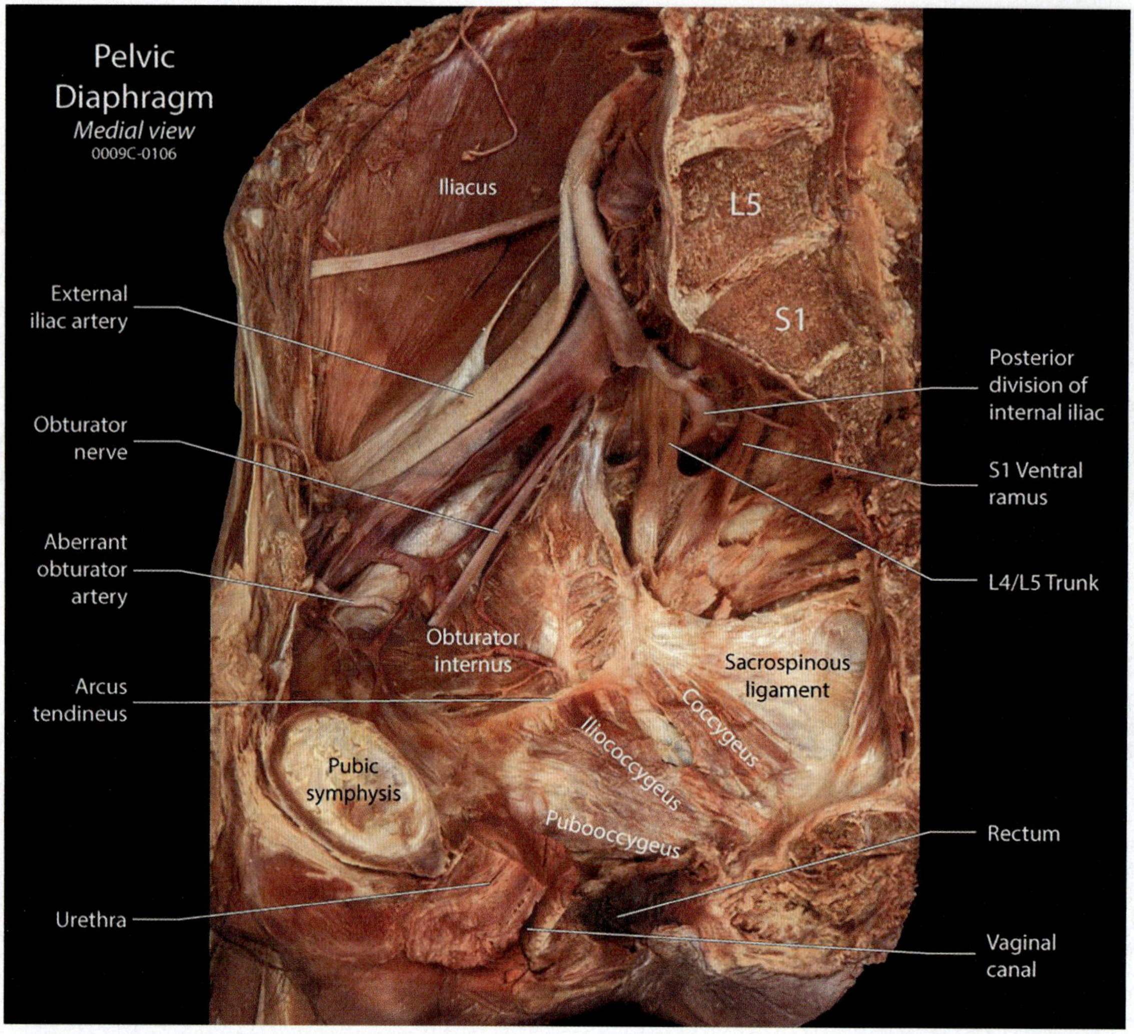

Figure 82.4. Pelvic diaphragm, medial view. Note the levator ani muscles, the pubococcygeus, and iliococcygeus. These muscles form a funnel that gives lateral and interior support to the urethra, vagina, and rectum and forms the floor of the pelvis. (Used with permission from the Willard/Carreiro Collection, University of New England.)

- The bulbocavernosus muscle and levator ani group have sphincter function for vaginal closure (Fig. 82.4).

The levator ani group forms the deepest layer of striated muscles.

- This group is laterally bordered by the:
  - □ Arcus tendineus
  - □ Piriformis muscle
  - □ Obturator internus muscle
- The fascia of this group is continuous with these pelvic diaphragm muscles.
- The anterior pubic portion of the levator ani muscles includes the pubococcygeus, with puborectalis and pubovaginalis portions.
- The iliococcygeus forms the posterior iliac portion. The coccygeus muscle lies adjacent but more superior to the levator ani group and assists the levator ani in its supportive function.
- Weakness in the levator muscles and damage to fascial integrity can lead to vaginal and visceral prolapse and fecal incontinence (Fig. 82.5).

The perineum can be divided into the urogenital triangle regions and the anal triangle regions[3] (Tables 82.1 and 82.2).

- Superficial external genital muscles form a figure eight around the vagina and urethra and around the anus.
- The urogenital triangle is covered superiorly by the levator ani muscles.
- The perineal membrane is a strong fascial platform without a similar structure in the anorectal triangle. It is also incorporated transversely with muscle and fascia that span bilaterally across the ischiopubic rami.

The female urethral sphincters are the striated sphincter urethrae and distal intrinsic and external sphincters included in the urogenital triangle. The levator ani and the compressor urethrae muscles assist the sphincters in urethral closing.[8]

Pelvic Innervation

The striated muscles of the vaginal introitus and skin of the perineum receive somatic motor and sensory fibers from the lumbosacral plexus.

- The pelvic viscera are supplied by the autonomic plexuses, conveying sympathetic and parasympathetic nerves to these organs.
- Ventral roots of the lumbar and sacral nerves originate from the lumbosacral plexuses.
- The obturator nerve, the lumbosacral trunk (of the plexus), and the entire sacral plexus lie in proximity to the pelvic organs.

A

B

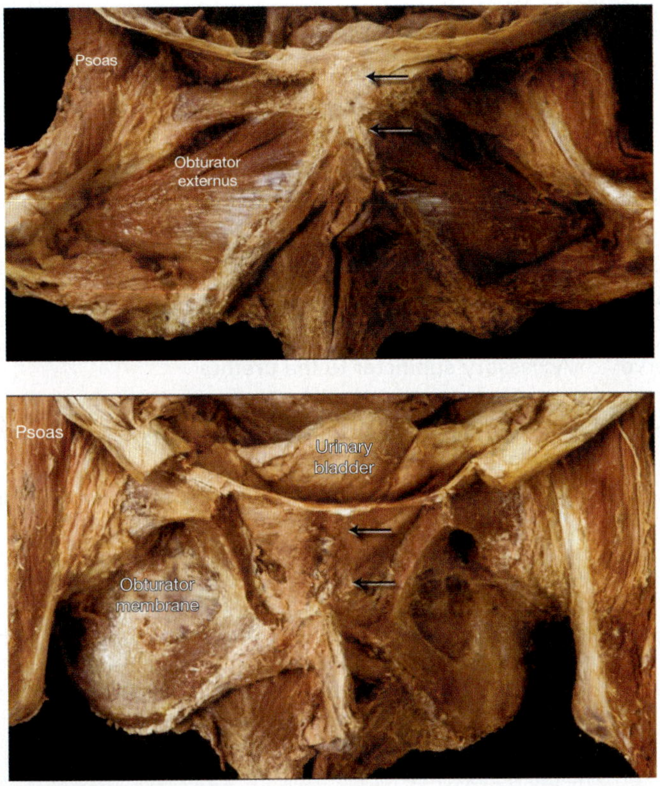

Figure 82.5. A. Pubic symphysis and obturator externus. **B.** The obturator externus was removed to reveal the obturator membrane, and the pubic rami were sectioned in the coronal plane to reveal fibers of the posterior pubic ligament and fascia. *Arrows* identify the pubic symphysis. (Used with permission from the Willard/Carreiro Collection, University of New England.)

- Only particular branches of the plexuses are directly involved in pelvic innervation (Table 82.3).

Muscular contraction and vasoconstriction are mediated by sympathetic innervation, whereas muscle relaxation and vasodilation are caused by parasympathetic innervation.

TABLE 82.1

Pelvic Diaphragm (The Pelvic Floor and Walls)

Muscle	Action
Levator ani	
Anterior pubic portion	
Pubococcygeus (pubovisceral)	Supports the pelvic viscera
Pubovaginalis	Sphincter of vagina and urethrae
Puborectalis	Loops around rectum, elevates, and helps constrict anal canal
Posterior iliac portion	
Fibococcygeus	Assists in support of pelvic viscera
Coccygeus ischiococcygeus	Flexes coccyx, assists in support of pelvic viscera, and stabilizes the sacroiliac joint
Obturator internus	Lateral or external rotator of hip
Piriformis	External rotator of hip, stabilizes hip joint

TABLE 82.2

Urogenital and Anal Triangles

Muscle	Action
Urogenital triangle region (superficial layer)	
Ischiocavernosus ischial tuberosity	Erection of clitoris
Bulbocavernosus (bulbospongiosus)	Vaginal sphincter and assists in erection of clitoris
Superficial transverse perineals	Anchors perineal body
Urogenital triangle region (deep layer)	
Upper portion	
Sphincter urethrae (rhabdosphincter)	Constrict urethral lumen
Lower portion (deep transverse perineal)	
Urethrovaginal sphincter	
Compressor urethrae	Compresses ventral wall, assists incontinence mechanism
Anal triangle region	
External and sphincter	
Subcutaneous part Superficial part Deep part	Voluntary sphincter of the anal canal and assists the puborectalis

- Most autonomic fibers enter the pelvis via the superior hypogastric plexus, which runs from the fourth lumbar vertebra to the hollow of the sacrum.
- It descends into the base of the broad ligament to join the parasympathetic fibers from the pelvic plexuses.
- The motor fibers and accompanying sensory nerves arrive at the pelvic plexus from S2 to S4 by way of the pelvic splanchnic nerves.
- The sensory nerves from the uterus, which escort the sympathetic nerves to enter the cord at T11 and T12, cause referred pain to the abdomen.
- Afferent nerves from the cervix, S2–S4, refer pain to the lower back and lumbosacral regions.

Autonomic innervation to the pelvic organs includes these sensory fibers:

- Sympathetic
- Parasympathetic
- Motor
- Visceral

The following are supplied by the inferior hypogastric plexus:

- Uterus
- Vagina
- Ureter
- Bladder
- Rectum

Visceral afferent pain pathways of the ovary, fallopian tube, uterus, and cervix connect with the spinal cord at the level of T11–T12.

- Pain is referred to corresponding skin dermatomes, usually from the lower abdomen.

TABLE 82.3

Urethral, Anorectal, and Pelvic Floor Innervation in the Female

Muscles	Innervation	Function
Deep Perineal Pouch		
Striated (external) urogenital sphincter	Perineal branch of the pudendal nerve S2–S4	Voluntarily compresses the membranous urethra for continence, relaxes during micturition
Internal urethral sphincter	Sympathetic hypogastric nerves T11–L2	Smooth muscle contraction under autonomic control
Deep transverse perineal	Perineal branch of the pudendal nerve S2–S4	Stabilizes the perineal body
Compressor urethrae	Perineal branch of the pudendal nerve S2–S4	Accessory sphincter to the urethra
Sphincter urethrovaginalis	Perineal branch of the pudendal nerve S2–S4	Accessory sphincter to the urethra, may also assist in closing the vagina
External anal sphincter	Branch of the pudendal nerve	Voluntary muscle aids in continence when constricted and relaxes for defecation
Internal anal sphincter	Autonomic nervous system	Involuntary contraction with peristalsis
Pelvic Diaphragm		Contributes to formation of the pelvic floor
Levator ani group	Direct branch of S3, S4, inferior rectal nerve, perineal nerve, S2–S4 (variations noted in cadavers)	Supports pelvic viscera, maintains the angle between the rectum and anal canal, reinforces the external anal sphincter, functions as a vaginal sphincter
Puborectalis	Direct branches of S3–S5	
Pubococcygeus	Branch of the pudendal	
Iliococcygeus	Direct Branch S3–S5	
Coccygeus	Direct branch of S3, S4	Pulls the coccyx forward after defecation
Pelvic Sidewalls		
Obturator	Obturator nerve L5–S1	Lateral rotation of extended hip, abduction of flexed hip
Piriformis	Branches L5, S1, S2	Lateral rotation of extended hip, abduction of flexed hip

- Sacral plexus injury can cause disabling changes of a motor or sensory nature, as Beal[9] discusses in his review of viscerosomatic reflexes (Fig. 82.6).

The genitofemoral nerve (L1–L2) traverses across the belly of the psoas major muscle to the anterior thigh to supply the labia majora.

Injury results in sensory changes.

- The obturator nerve (L2–L4) supplies motor branches to the adductor muscles of the:
  - □ Leg
  - □ Hip
  - □ Knee joint
  - □ Medial thigh
- Injury results in loss of:
  - □ Thigh adduction
  - □ Internal and external rotation
  - □ Senses to these areas (Fig. 82.7)

Lymphatics and Circulation

Circulation and lymphatic drainage of the female reproductive system are closely integrated.

- The blood supply to the ovary is derived from the ovarian artery off the abdominal aorta, and the ovarian branch of the uterine artery.
- Veins accompany the arteries as plexiform vessels. Those on the left converge to form the left ovarian vein that drains into the inferior vena cava.
- Lymphatic drainage of the ovary proceeds from the hilum of the ovary to the lumbar nodes.

The fallopian tubes derive their blood supply from the ovarian artery, as well as from the uterine artery.

- Venous drainage is into the ovarian or uterine veins.
- Lymphatic drainage is into the lumbar lymph nodes, accompanying the ovarian lymphatics.

The blood supply to the uterus originates from the internal iliac arteries through the uterine arteries.

- Each uterine artery gives off a cervical branch.
- The vessel terminates by communicating with the ovarian artery.
- Venous return is from the uterine plexus, which communicates with the vaginal plexus and the ovarian plexus, forming the uterine vein that empties into the internal iliac vein.

Lymphatic drainage is divided.

- The body of the uterus is drained by the:
  - □ Lumbar nodes
  - □ Superficial inguinal nodes
  - □ External iliac nodes

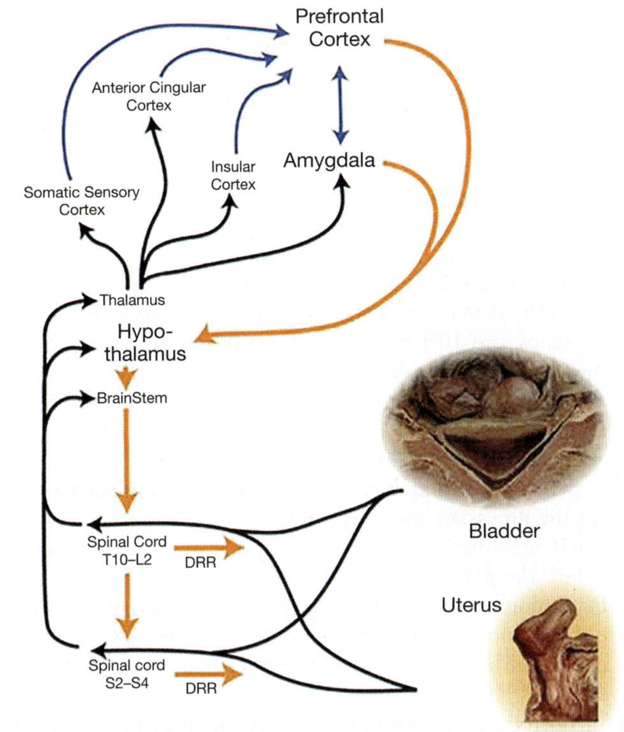

Figure 82.6. Diagram showing innervation of the uterus and bladder. Note that these structures can receive dorsal root reflexes (DRRs) through the afferent fibers. This gives rise to cross-sensitization where dysfunction of one organ can influence the surrounding organs. This principle makes localization of visceral pain challenging. (Used with permission from the Willard/Carreiro Collection, University of New England.)

- The cervix is drained by the:
  - External and internal iliac nodes
  - Sacral nodes

The vagina is supplied by the vaginal branch of the uterine artery.

- Inferior vesical and middle rectal arteries send branches to the vaginal wall.
- The internal pudendal artery supplies the lower vaginal wall.
- Venous return is through a vaginal plexus, which joins the uterine plexus to form the uterine veins and empty into the internal iliac vein.
- Sacral nodes and superficial inguinal nodes drain the lower portion of the vagina; the upper vault drains into the external iliac, internal iliac, or common iliac nodes (Fig. 82.8).

GYNECOLOGIC PATIENT EVALUATION: HISTORY AND PHYSICAL EXAMINATION

Patient visits to the gynecologist are most often for:

- Health maintenance examinations
- Menstrual irregularities
- Endocrine issues
- Sexual dysfunction or for pain

This chapter focuses on the osteopathic evaluation and treatment of pelvic pain.

- Women having pain often present to a gynecologist as a first step in beginning investigation of their symptoms.

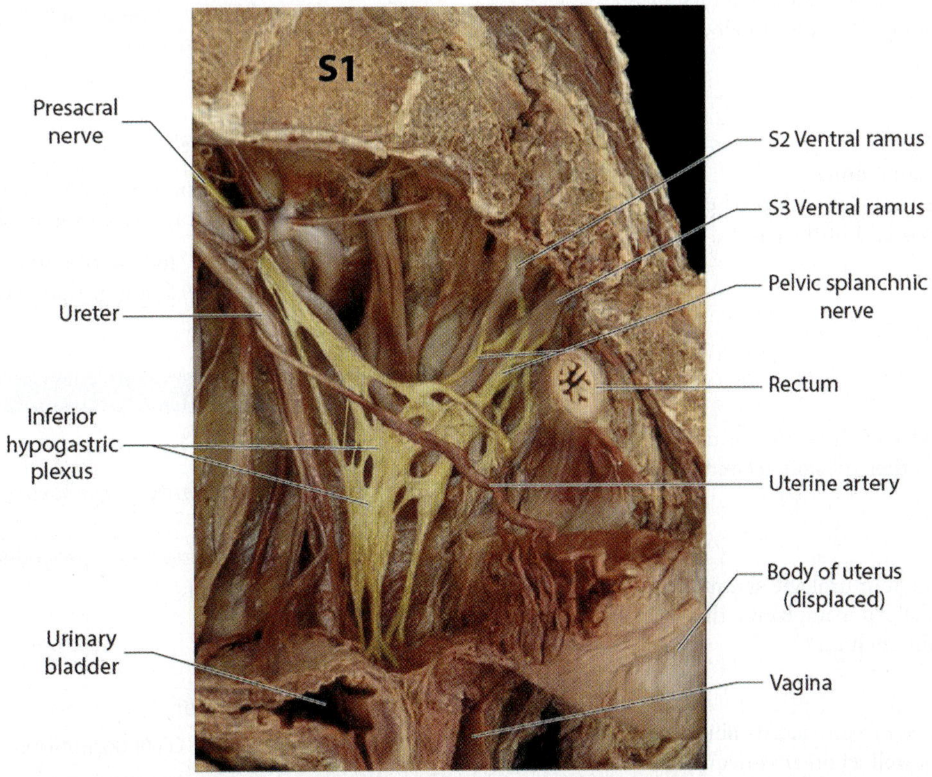

Figure 82.7. The inferior hypogastric plexus, pelvic nerves, ureter, and branches of the uterine artery. Understanding the relationship of the ureter to the uterine artery is critical to avoid ureteral damage in pelvic surgery. (Used with permission from the Willard/Carreiro Collection, University of New England.)

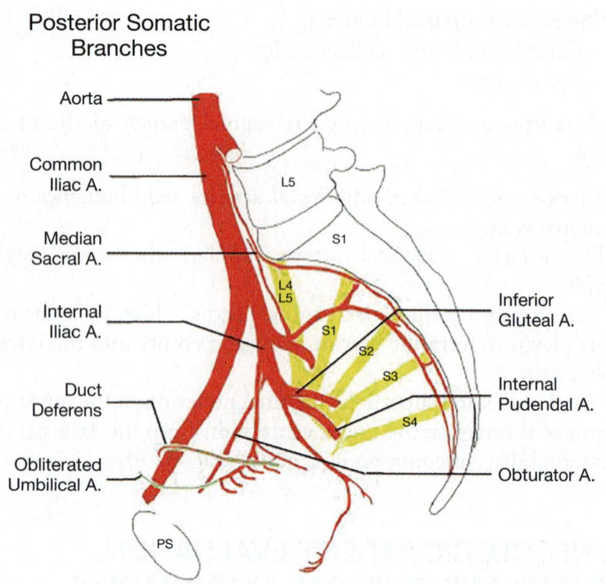

Figure 82.8. Blood supply to the pelvic muscles. (Used with permission from the Willard/Carreiro Collection, University of New England.)

- When the chief complaint is for pain, the history should include description of pain with reference to:
  - Onset
  - Localization
  - Quality
  - Intensity
  - Radiation
  - Duration
  - Aggravating factors and alleviating factors
- In addition to gynecologic sources of pain, pelvic pain may be:
  - Gastrointestinal
  - Urologic
  - Neurologic
  - Somatic
  - From a psychosomatic source
- Questions regarding the relationship of pain to the following may give clues to the origin of the pain:
  - Menstrual cycle
  - Bowel movements
  - Urination
  - Sexual activity
  - Physical activity
  - Trauma
- Similar painful episodes in the recent or distant past should be explored, along with other possible related somatic complaints, such as:
  - Anorexia
  - Weight gain
  - Other gastrointestinal or urologic symptoms[10]
- Also note musculoskeletal complaints that may or may not accompany pelvic pain, such as:
  - Low back pain
  - Headache
- Ascertain the influence of pain and its ability to disrupt activities of daily living, as well as other concurrent events that may have occurred with the acute onset of pain. Examples include the following:
  - Cramps with IUD placement
  - Sexual trauma
  - Falls
  - Strain from lifting heavy objects[11]

Whereas acute pelvic pain may be of sudden onset and localize within 24 hours, chronic pelvic pain differs in both duration and location.

- Chronic pain:
  - Has been present for 6 months
  - Is diffuse and intermittent in nature
  - Involves no organic pathologic findings
- Up to 40% of women presenting with this complaint undergo laparoscopy and 10% to 12% undergo hysterectomy.[12,13]
- Some women may have associated stressors, such as:
  - Depression over pregnancy loss
  - Employment issues
  - Problems in personal relationships[14]
- The perceptions that both the patient and her partner have about the illness are also important.
  - Elicit information about medications or other attempts to relieve the pain.
  - Psychological evaluation may become necessary but should not preclude other diagnostic studies, especially when the pain itself becomes the disease rather than a symptom of the disease.[10,15]
- A full obstetric and gynecologic history should be taken including inquiries about other factors in the patient's history (Table 82.4).

The surgical history should include not only pelvic procedures but also any other operations, such as:

- Orthopedic
- Urologic
- Neurologic

The medical history should include conditions that could manifest as pelvic pain, such as:

- Colitis
- Interstitial cystitis
- Bladder pain syndrome[16]

To avoid guarding, the physical examination should focus on careful and gentle palpatory evaluation of the abdomen.

- Attempt to reproduce and localize the pain during the pelvic examination to discover findings that may correspond to specific pathology.[17]

TABLE 82.4

Important History in Pelvic Pain Patients

Age at menarche, regularity of menses, presence of dysmenorrhea
Obstetric history, deliveries, and procedures
History of trauma or falls
Infertility
Infection and STIs
Methods of contraception
Endometriosis, or other GYN conditions
Gynecologic surgery and procedures
Last pelvic examination
Abnormal pap test history or HPV

- Consider endometriosis if the uterus is fixed and if there is uterosacral nodularity that is also tender to palpation.[18]
- Note if the cervix is laterally displaced on bimanual examination.[19] A displaced cervix could indicate either asymmetry of pelvic floor tensions or adnexal masses.
- Tender adnexal enlargement may suggest:
  - An ovarian cyst
  - Torsion
  - Ectopic pregnancy
  - Infection
- A backache may be the result of uterine prolapse or uterine fibroids.[20]

Palpatory structural examination may guide the physician to address neuromuscular hyperactivity or inappropriate somatovisceral reflex activity.[21]

- This is achieved by evaluating:
  - Spinal curves
  - Unlevel sacral base or lower extremities
  - Paravertebral muscle contractions
  - Somatic dysfunction from the cranial base to the feet
- Particular emphasis should be placed on the identification of somatic dysfunction of the:
  - Sacrum
  - Lumbar spine
  - Pelvic and respiratory diaphragms
- Localization of counterstrain tender points may be used to treat pain caused by asymmetric muscle tensions.
- Identification of Chapman reflex points may render clues about pelvic organ dysfunction.
- A postural x-ray study may confirm palpatory findings of scoliosis or other structural imbalances such as leg length discrepancy.
- When somatic dysfunction is identified and there are no contraindications to osteopathic manipulation, osteopathic manipulation may improve symptoms and reduce the number of diagnostic tests needed.

Consider psychological evaluation if an obviously traumatic event is directly associated with the onset of pain or if there is concomitant neurosis, psychosis, or aberrant behavior.[22]

- Patients with chronic pelvic pain may have secondary depression as a consequence to their pain.
- A multidisciplinary approach to treatment of chronic pelvic pain has been shown to provide improvement in psychological distress and pain-related disability.[23]

DIFFERENTIAL DIAGNOSIS OF PELVIC PAIN

Dysmenorrhea

Painful menstruation, or dysmenorrhea, can be classified as primary or secondary based on when it occurs in relation to menarche and if organic pelvic disease is present.

Primary dysmenorrhea usually appears within 6 to 12 months of menarche and may be a feature of ovulatory cycles.

- Dysmenorrhea may be caused by:
  - Uterine contractions or ischemia
  - Psychological factors (which may alter pain perception)
  - Cervical factors (cervical stenosis has been cited as a painful stimulus)[24–26]
- Primary dysmenorrhea affects up to 93% of young women and can lead to absenteeism from school or work. One-third to one-half of adolescents with primary dysmenorrhea miss school or work each month.[27]

TABLE 82.5

Treatment Options for Primary Dysmenorrhea

Treatment Options for Primary Dysmenorrhea
Nonsteroidal anti-inflammatory drugs (NSAIDs)[28]
Combination estrogen–progestin contraception, oral, transdermal patch, or vaginal ring
Calcium channel blockers
Progestogens, oral, intramuscular, implantable, or levonorgestrel intrauterine device
Osteopathic manipulative treatment[29–31]
Gonadotropin-releasing hormone (GnRH) agonists[32]

Women with dysmenorrhea may have increased frequency or duration of uterine contractility.

- Cramping usually begins a few hours before menses and can persist for hours or longer.
- The pain is localized to the lower abdomen and back.
- It may also be associated with:
  - Nausea
  - Fatigue
  - Dizziness
  - Headache
  - Altered bowel habits (Table 82.5)

Osteopathic treatment may reduce the severity of pelvic pain.

- Relief can be accomplished by:
  - Treating Chapman points in the iliotibial band
  - Addressing somatic dysfunction at the level of T10–L2 (sympathetics) and dysfunction at S2–S4 (parasympathetics)
- To relieve edema, lymphatic drainage should be enhanced at the:
  - Abdominal diaphragm
  - Thoracic inlet
  - Lower extremities[33]
- Self-treatment may include the knee–chest position to temporarily lift the uterus out of the pelvis.
- If a patient fails to respond to medical and/or OMT, consideration should be given to a secondary cause of dysmenorrhea. Laparoscopy and/or hysteroscopy with endometrial curettage may be performed to exclude pelvic disease.

Secondary dysmenorrhea is caused by a disorder in the reproductive organs. It is not limited to menstrual pain, is less related to the first day of bleeding, develops in women 30 to 40 years of age, and may be associated with other symptoms.

- These symptoms may include the following:
  - Dyspareunia
  - Infertility
  - Abnormal bleeding[34]
- Table 82.6 summarizes possible causes of primary and secondary dysmenorrhea.
- Management focuses on the treatment of specific underlying disease or somatic dysfunction. Some of these diseases are discussed in the following sections (Table 82.6).

Premenstrual Syndrome

Premenstrual problems have been formally described since 1931 by Frank.[35] See Table 82.7 for common symptoms of premenstrual syndrome (PMS) (Table 82.7).

TABLE 82.6

Clinical Features of Primary and Secondary Dysmenorrhea

Primary Dysmenorrhea
Initial onset—within 2 years of menarche.
Pain—cramplike, lasting 48–72 hours after onset of menses; strongest in intensity over lower abdomen. May radiate to back or inner thigh.
Associated symptoms—nausea and vomiting, fatigue, diarrhea, lower backache, headache.
Pelvic examination findings—normal.
Secondary Dysmenorrhea
Endometriosis—pain occurs in premenstrual or postmenstrual phase or may be continuous. Patient may experience dyspareunia or premenstrual spotting or have cul-de-sac nodularity on examination. Age of onset in the 20s or 30s.
Pelvic inflammation—initially pain may be menstrual but may extend into premenstrual phase with subsequent cycles. Patient may have intermenstrual bleeding, dyspareunia, and pelvic tenderness.
Fibroids, adenomyosis—pain is a dull, heavy ache in pelvis. Uterus enlarged on examination and may be tender.
Ovarian cysts—unilateral tenderness, radiating into thigh. Adnexal enlargement on examination.
Pelvic congestion—dull, ill-defined ache that worsens premenstrually but improves with menses. Patient may have history of sexual dysfunction.

The term "premenstrual syndrome" was first used by Greene and Dalton in 1953[36] because many symptoms also occur around the time of ovulation, or midcycle.

- Approximately 5% to 10% of women experience severe PMS symptoms that interfere with normal daily life.
- Other women may have more severe depression or mood swings that are mentally and physically debilitating.
- Premenstrual dysphoric disorder is a psychiatric diagnosis used to distinguish those patients who have augmented PMS signs or symptoms.[37]

The cause of PMS has not been entirely determined.[38] Table 82.8 lists proposed hypotheses that attempt to explain the syndrome.

- Most healthy women report occasional symptoms before menses.

TABLE 82.7

Common Symptoms of Premenstrual Syndrome

Symptom
Bloating of abdomen or pelvis
Weight gain
Irritability
Mood swings
Depression
Fatigue
Difficulty concentrating

TABLE 82.8

Proposed Hypotheses for Causes of Premenstrual Syndrome

Abnormal estrogen secretion
Excess or deficiency of progesterone
Excess or deficiency of cortisone, androgens, or prolactin
Excess or deficiency of prostaglandin
Excess of antidiuretic hormone
Abnormality of endogenous opiates or melatonin secretion
Deficiencies of vitamins A, B1, B6, or minerals such as magnesium
Hypoglycemia
Hormone allergy
Menstrual toxin
Psychological, social, evolutionary, and genetic factors

- The syndrome is associated with ovulation and, therefore, does not occur before puberty, during pregnancy, or after menopause. Nor does it occur in anovulatory women.
- Menstruation is incidental, as cyclic symptoms continue to be bothersome if the ovaries are still present in a woman who has had a hysterectomy.
- Extensive metabolic and psychological studies have yet to identify a specific abnormality, but serotonergic neurotransmission dysfunction has been implicated.[39]
- Treatment options for PMS are summarized in Tables 82.8 and 82.9.

Endometriosis

Endometriosis is a benign condition in which endometrial glands and stroma are present outside the endometrial cavity.

- Other locations include the following:
  - ☐ Ovary
  - ☐ Bowel
  - ☐ Bladder
  - ☐ Peritoneum
  - ☐ Sites outside the pelvic boundaries
- Endometriosis is a challenge to gynecologists because it is a diagnostic and surgical enigma.[43]

TABLE 82.9

Treatment Options for Premenstrual Syndrome

Treatment
Medication to suppress cyclic ovarian activity
Psychotherapy to develop coping skills
Diuretics to reduce bloating
Diets with reduced fat, caffeine, or salt to reduce irritability or water retention
Pyridoxine may lessen cramps but causes neuropathy in high doses[40]
Supplements such as vitex (chasteberry) and calcium have been shown to reduce symptoms[41]
Osteopathic manipulative treatment[42]

- It is estimated to be present in 6% to 11% of asymptomatic women, in between 20% and 50% of infertile women, and from 40% to 50% in women with pelvic pain.
- In one study, endometriosis was noted in approximately 60% of adolescents undergoing laparoscopy for dysmenorrhea or chronic pelvic pain.[44]

The characteristic triad of symptoms associated with endometriosis is dysmenorrhea, dyspareunia, and dyschezia.

- Secondary dysmenorrhea first appears or escalates in the late 20s or early 30s.
- If endometriosis is associated with obstructive genital anomalies, severe dysmenorrhea may occur at menarche.[45,46]

Dyspareunia is generally associated with deep coitus.

- This can irritate the following structures:
  - Endometrial implants located in the cul-de-sac.
  - Uterosacral ligaments
  - Portions of the posterior vaginal fornix
- On pelvic examination, the cul-de-sac may feel gritty and be exquisitely tender to the touch.[82]

Dyschezia is experienced with uterosacral, cul-de-sac, and rectosigmoid colon involvement.

- As stool passes between the uterosacral ligaments, the patient experiences pain.
- This symptom is highly characteristic and is more common with endometriosis than with chronic salpingo-oophoritis, a condition sometimes otherwise mistaken for endometriosis.[48]

If the ovarian capsule is involved with endometriosis, ovulatory pain and midcycle vaginal bleeding may be reported by the patient.

- However, the nature of pelvic pain caused by endometriosis is variable.
- Some investigators have found that the degree of pain is inversely proportional to the extent of the disease.[49] Minimal endometriosis in the cul-de-sac may be more painful than a large ovarian endometrioma that can expand freely into the abdominal cavity.
- Frequently, pelvic examination yields no signs of endometriosis.

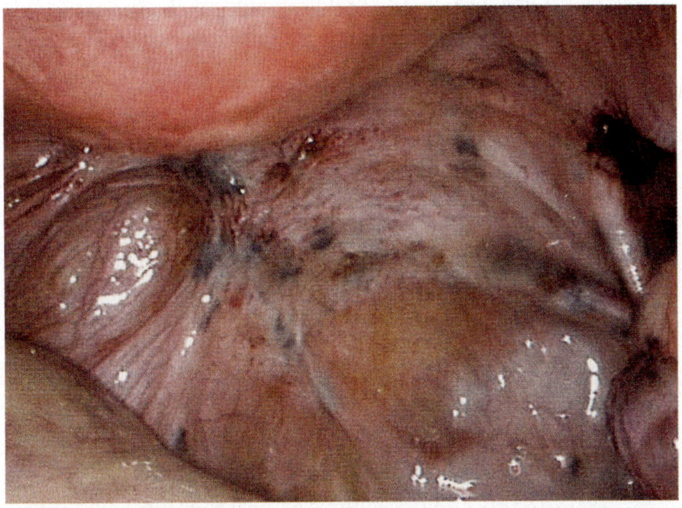

Figure 82.9. Classic powder-burn lesions of endometriosis on the pelvic peritoneum as seen on laparoscopy. (From Beckmann CRB, Ling FW, Herbert WNP, et al. *Obstetrics and Gynecology.* 7th ed. Lippincott Williams & Wilkins; 2014.)

TABLE 82.10

Management Considerations in Endometriosis

Certainty of the diagnosis
Severity of symptoms
Extent of the disease
Preservation of fertility
Compromised function of the gastrointestinal and/or urinary tracts

The diagnosis of endometriosis should be suspected in an afebrile patient with the previously mentioned characteristic endometriosis symptom triad.

- This involves the following:
  - A firm, fixed, tender adnexal mass
  - Tender nodularity in the cul-de-sac and uterosacral ligaments
- Pelvic ultrasound may indicate an adnexal mass of complex echogenicity.
- The definitive diagnosis is made by:
  - The characteristic gross findings of "blueberry" spots, chocolate cysts, or "powder burns" (Figure 82.9).
  - Histologic findings of endometrial tissue at laparoscopy or laparotomy[50,51]

The presence of interstitial cystitis with endometriosis has been termed the "evil twins' syndrome," and the two diseases may be found together in up to 80% of cases.[52]

- One study found both diseases in 65% of patients undergoing diagnostic laparoscopy for chronic pelvic pain and bladder hydrodistension to diagnose interstitial cystitis (Table 82.10).
- This emphasizes the importance of being aware of endometriosis, interstitial cystitis and ovarian cysts as possible etiologies of chronic pelvic pain, especially if hysterectomy is being considered for treatment (Figs. 82.9 and 82.10).

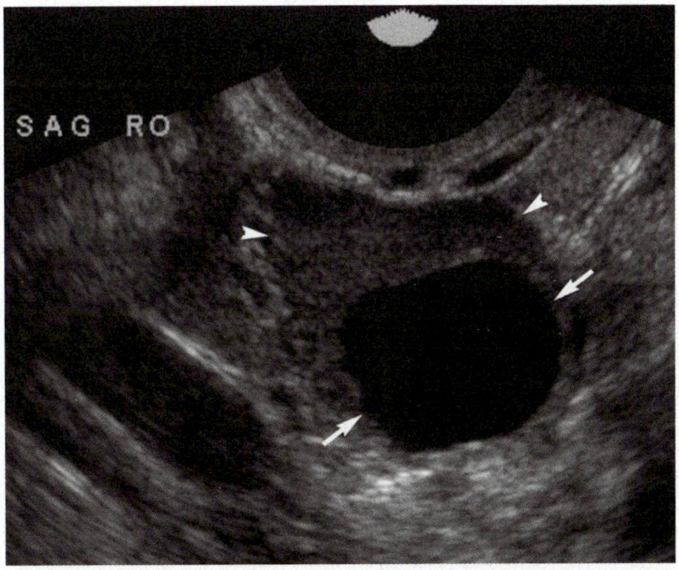

Figure 82.10. Ultrasound image of a simple ovarian cyst. *Arrows* identify ovarian tissue. (From Beckmann CRB, Ling FW, Herbert WNP, et al. *Obstetrics and Gynecology.* 7th ed. Lippincott Williams & Wilkins; 2014.)

It is appropriate to treat endometriosis presumptively once other etiologies have been ruled out, since it may be missed visually on diagnostic laparoscopy.

- Nonsteroidal anti-inflammatories have not been effective.
- Effective treatments in reducing pain include the following:
  - Short-term gonadotropin-releasing hormone (GnRH) agonist suppression of the cycle
  - GnRH antagonist suppression of the cycle
  - Ovulation suppression with oral contraceptives
  - Implantable prostaglandins and levonorgestrel intrauterine devices[53]
  - Fertility is preserved by involution of implants.
  - However, when a palpable endometrioma is present, the likelihood of a complete response to medical therapy is small.[54]
  - If the patient becomes pregnant, ovulation suppression secondary to the hormones of pregnancy, and continued suppression if lactating, permit involution of the implants.
  - When regular menstrual cycles resume, the disease again progresses.

If future fertility is a consideration, pursue conservative surgery.

- Such surgery includes the following:
  - Resection of the disease
  - Lysis of adhesions
  - Ovarian resection
  - Ablation of small lesions[50]
- If reproductive capacity is not a concern, total abdominal hysterectomy with bilateral salpingo-oophorectomy may be considered.
- Surgical menopause may be managed with hormone replacement therapy.

Osteopathic treatment considerations for menstrual disorder pain include "rocking" of the sacral base for parasympathetic inhibition[33] and treatment of somatic dysfunction of the thoracolumbar spine, particularly T10–L2.[29]

- Mobilization of the respiratory diaphragm should improve respiration and circulation of body fluids.
- Treatment of the pelvic diaphragm relieves pelvic congestion and edema of the lower extremities.
- Because the menstrual cycle is controlled by neuroendocrine system feedback, cranial base or vertebral strain may interfere with endocrine function.

Ovarian Pain

Ovarian cysts that are slow growing are usually asymptomatic, but pain may occur as a result of rapid distension of the ovarian capsule.

- Mittelschmerz is pain midcycle thought to be from ovulation.
- Ovaries are just anterior to the area in which the psoas courses through the pelvis.
- Some women may develop recurrent hemorrhagic ovarian cysts that cause pain and dyspareunia.
- Impaired blood supply to the ovaries has been implicated, especially after previous pelvic surgery, such as partial oophorectomy or hysterectomy.[55]
- Bimanual examination reveals an adnexal enlargement with tenderness.
- Ultrasound may determine whether the cystic structure is complex or contains clear fluid.
- An ovary or ovarian remnant may become retroperitoneal secondary to inflammation or previous surgery[56] (Fig. 82.10).

Osteopathic treatment considerations exist for ovarian pain.

- These include the following:
  - Treatment of somatic dysfunction of the thoracolumbar junction
  - Assessment of sacral imbalance and leg length discrepancy
  - Identification of Chapman reflex areas
- Mobilization of the spine addresses aberrant somatovisceral reflex pathways.
- Additional treatment of the sacral base and leg length discrepancies may mechanically affect and improve blood supply to the ovaries and the pelvis.
- Chapman reflex areas identify possible related somatic dysfunction of the reproductive system and gastrointestinal tract.

Uterine Pain

Uterine position and orientation in the pelvis is rarely the cause of pelvic pain. Deep dyspareunia may occasionally be associated with retroversion, whereby:

- The pelvic nerves are irritated by stretching of the uterosacral ligaments.
- Pelvic veins become congested from uterine heaviness and position[57]

A tender uterus that is noted on pelvic examination to be fixed in retrogression should arouse suspicions of other intraperitoneal pathology.

- Laparoscopy is indicated to evaluate all pelvic structures for such pathology as:
  - Endometriosis
  - Pelvic inflammatory disease (PID)
  - Adhesions
- Pelvic heaviness and low back pain may be present with advanced degrees of uterine prolapse.
- Before deciding on hysterectomy as a course of treatment, some of these symptoms may be remedied by use of a pessary.
  - Low back pain may respond to osteopathic treatment of the pelvic diaphragm or myofascial trigger points in the vaginal floor or rectum.
  - Application of deep inhibitory pressure may relieve back or pelvic pain in addition to identifying and treating pelvic and lower extremity somatic dysfunction[58] (Fig. 82.11).

Under normal conditions, the chief characteristic of uterine support is its mobility, and any loss of this mobility or changes associated with altered positional relationships are important diagnostic signs.

- The structures involved in uterine support are the:
  - Levator muscle and fascia of the pelvic floor
  - Paracervical and paravaginal tissues, which extend outward from the vagina to the pelvic walls, and which include the cardinal and uterosacral ligaments, and the round ligaments that assist in holding the uterus in its anterior position.
- Of these, the cardinal ligament is the most important.
  - This structure consists of a loose meshwork of connective tissue, which cannot be palpated when it is relaxed, but forms a very firm ligament when the area is under tension.
  - Under tension, the cardinal ligament can contribute to lateral deviation of the cervix.
- When these findings are encountered, the osteopathic physician should consider performing a structural examination of the pelvis.
  - Any TART findings should be treated and corrected.
  - Then myofascial techniques, counterstrain, or balancing ligamentous tension may be used to normalize the cardinal ligament tensions and restore the cervix to its normal midline position.

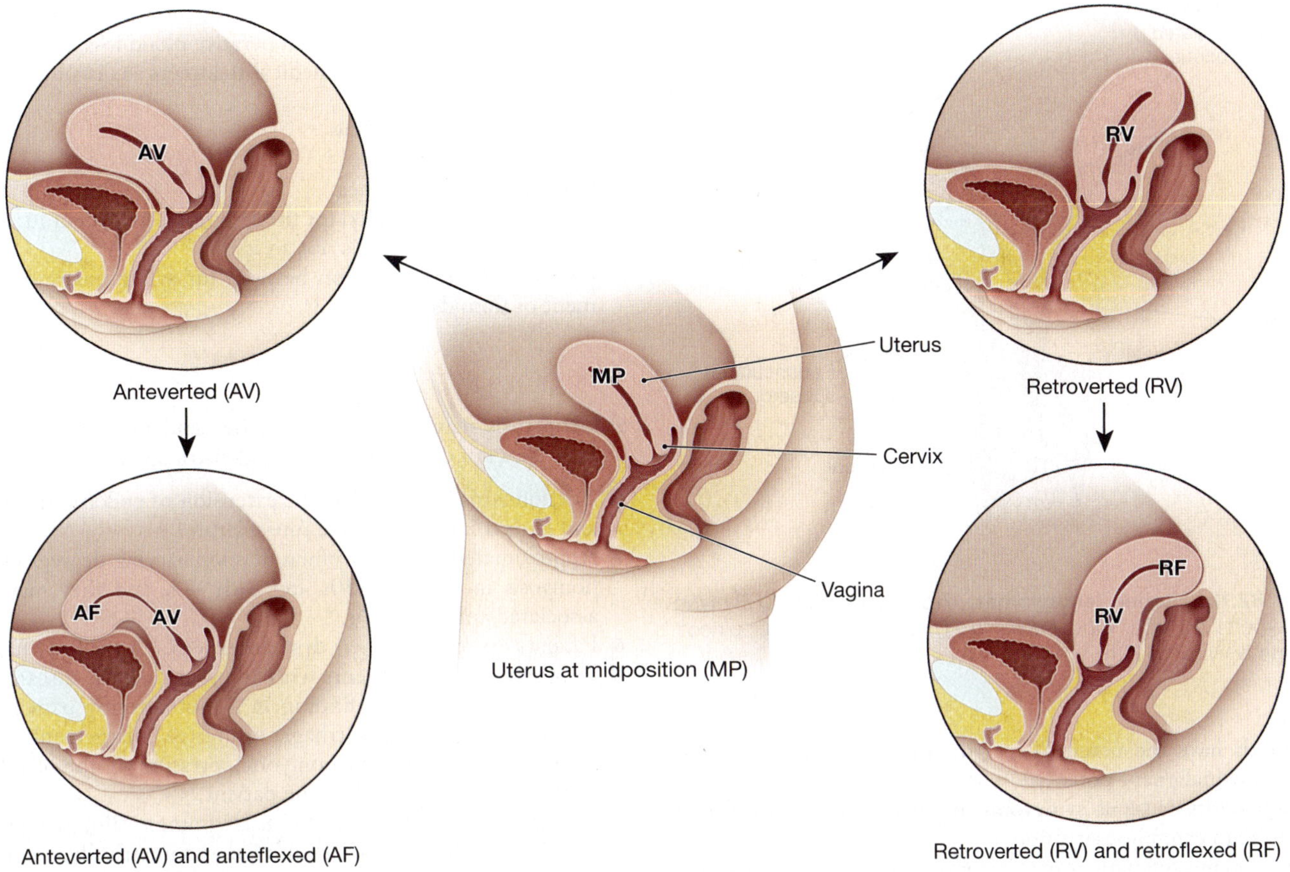

Figure 82.11. Uterine positions. (From Beckmann CRB, Ling FW, Herbert WNP, et al. *Obstetrics and Gynecology*. 7th ed. Lippincott Williams & Wilkins; 2014.)

Pelvic Congestion Syndrome

The concept of pelvic congestion syndrome has a variety of proponents.

- This syndrome has been described in multiparous women who have pelvic vein varicosities and congested pelvic organs.[57]
- Pain is worse premenstrually and is aggravated by:
  - Fatigue
  - Standing
  - Sexual intercourse
- In the clinical examination, the uterus is mobile, usually retroverted, soft and boggy, and slightly enlarged.
  - There may be associated menorrhagia and urinary frequency.[58]
  - Dilated veins may be seen on venographic studies.[59]
- Additional and independent factors other than venous congestion may be involved, as some women with pelvic varicosities have no pain.
- Surgery may be beneficial when congestion is secondary to blockage. Stent placement may provide significant improvement in selected patients.[60]
- Structural and postural evaluation with palpatory examination of somatic dysfunction of the lumbar spine and pelvis may elucidate areas for osteopathic treatment to relieve muscle distress and improve circulation to the pelvis.

Sometimes a tender uterus is encountered without an obvious etiology.

- Pelvic cultures may be negative, there is no history to suspect sexually transmitted infections, and there are no recent procedures as a risk factor for endometritis.
- These patients should be examined for possible somatic dysfunction that may contribute to uterine congestion and pain.
- Structural examination with treatment of identified TART findings may resolve the uterine tenderness.

The pelvic diaphragm can be treated by several different osteopathic techniques.

- Myofascial release can be done with an external approach to address the pelvic floor.
- The pelvic floor may also be evaluated and treated with an internal approach vaginally.
- When preparing to do internal treatment with counterstrain on the pelvic floor, the patient is usually examined in the dorsal lithotomy position.
- A tender point may be identified with gloved finger on the perineum or in the vagina contacting the muscle layer. The point is monitored while the patient's ipsilateral foot is placed on the physician's shoulder.
- The physician can induce flexion and extension by moving toward or away from the patient.
- Internal and external rotation can be controlled by using the other (nonexamining) hand.
- Position of ease is held for 90 seconds while the monitoring finger notes the usual tissue pulsation while treating.
- Recheck pain level after treatment.

Uterine Leiomyomas (Fig. 82.12)

Uterine leiomyomas (fibroids) are smooth muscle tumors of the uterus that are a common indication for major surgery in women.

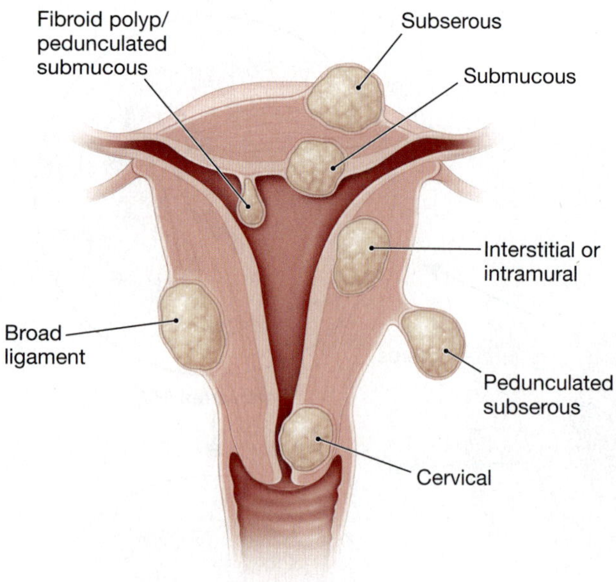

Figure 82.12. Uterine leiomyomas. (From Beckmann CRB, Ling FW, Herbert WNP, et al. *Obstetrics and Gynecology*. 7th ed. Lippincott Williams & Wilkins; 2014.)

- Fibroids have the potential to grow to an enormous size but have low malignant potential.
- The majority cause no symptoms and may require no treatment other than careful observation.
- Occasionally, the patient may become aware of a lower abdominal fullness or mass above the pubic symphysis.
- Symptoms develop insidiously as the fibroid competes with neighboring organs for space in the pelvis (Table 82.11).

Other causes of pain are the result of:

- Fibroid infarction with degeneration
- Torsion on the fibroid's pedicle
- Compression of pelvic nerves
- Occasional protrusion of a submucous leiomyoma through the cervix, causing stretching pain akin to that of vaginal childbirth

Management of this condition includes addressing the patient's desire for preserving future fertility, along with careful observation.

- Myomectomy may be performed to maintain the uterus for future pregnancy.
- Menorrhagia may be controlled by:
  - Uterine curettage
  - Endometrial ablation

TABLE 82.11

Symptoms Associated with Uterine Leiomyomas

Pressure
Congestion
Bloating
Urinary frequency or retention
Dysmenorrhea
Backache

- GnRH agonists have been used to shrink myomas to enhance fertility, as well as reduce intraoperative blood loss; however, the fibroids will return when medical treatment is discontinued.
- Oral contraceptives also:
  - Reduce menstrual flow
  - Preserve fertility
  - Control dysmenorrhea
- Hysterectomy is reserved for the symptomatic patient for whom reproductive capability is not an issue.
- Osteopathic treatment can be used for symptomatic management of fibroids (Fig. 82.13).

Adenomyosis

Adenomyosis may cause dysmenorrhea and menorrhagia, but it usually does not cause chronic intermenstrual pain.

- Adenomyosis is defined as the extension of endometrial glands and stroma into the uterine musculature.
- Approximately 15% of women develop varying degrees of adenomyosis in their late 30s and early 40s, and they may have associated endometriosis.[34]
- Patients express that their dysmenorrhea is of a colicky nature.
- In 30% to 40% of patients with adenomyosis, the disease is an unexpected pathologic finding in a hysterectomy patient who did not experience menorrhagia or uterine enlargement.[49]
- In the case of a large adenomyoma, pressure on the bladder or rectum may be reported by the patient.
- On pelvic examination, the uterus is symmetrically enlarged, but occasionally the uterus may enlarge asymmetrically, suggesting the presence of a fibroid. However, the adenomyomatous uterus is softer than a uterine myoma.

Treatment depends on the specific symptoms and on the exclusion of other uterine pathologic conditions.

- Menorrhagia and dysmenorrhea, if not too severe, may be treated palliatively with:
  - NSAIDs
  - COX-2 inhibitors
  - Oral contraceptives
  - GnRH agonists[28]
- Osteopathic management consists of treating somatic dysfunction of the following that may be influenced by posture:
  - Lumbar spine
  - Pelvis
  - Pelvic diaphragm
  - Muscles of the anterior abdominal wall
- Recent research on adenomyectomy has shown promise in uterine sparing procedures that remove foci of adenomyosis and leave the rest of the uterus.
  - This may be considered in patients wishing to maintain fertility.[61]
  - Otherwise, hysterectomy may be indicated.
  - The ovaries may be preserved if they are normal and if the patient is not menopausal (Fig. 82.14).

Pelvic Inflammatory Disease

PID comprises a constellation of inflammatory disorders of the upper genital tract (Table 82.12). The two most common conditions of PID in the nonpregnant patient are:

1. Salpingo-oophoritis
2. Tubo-ovarian abscess

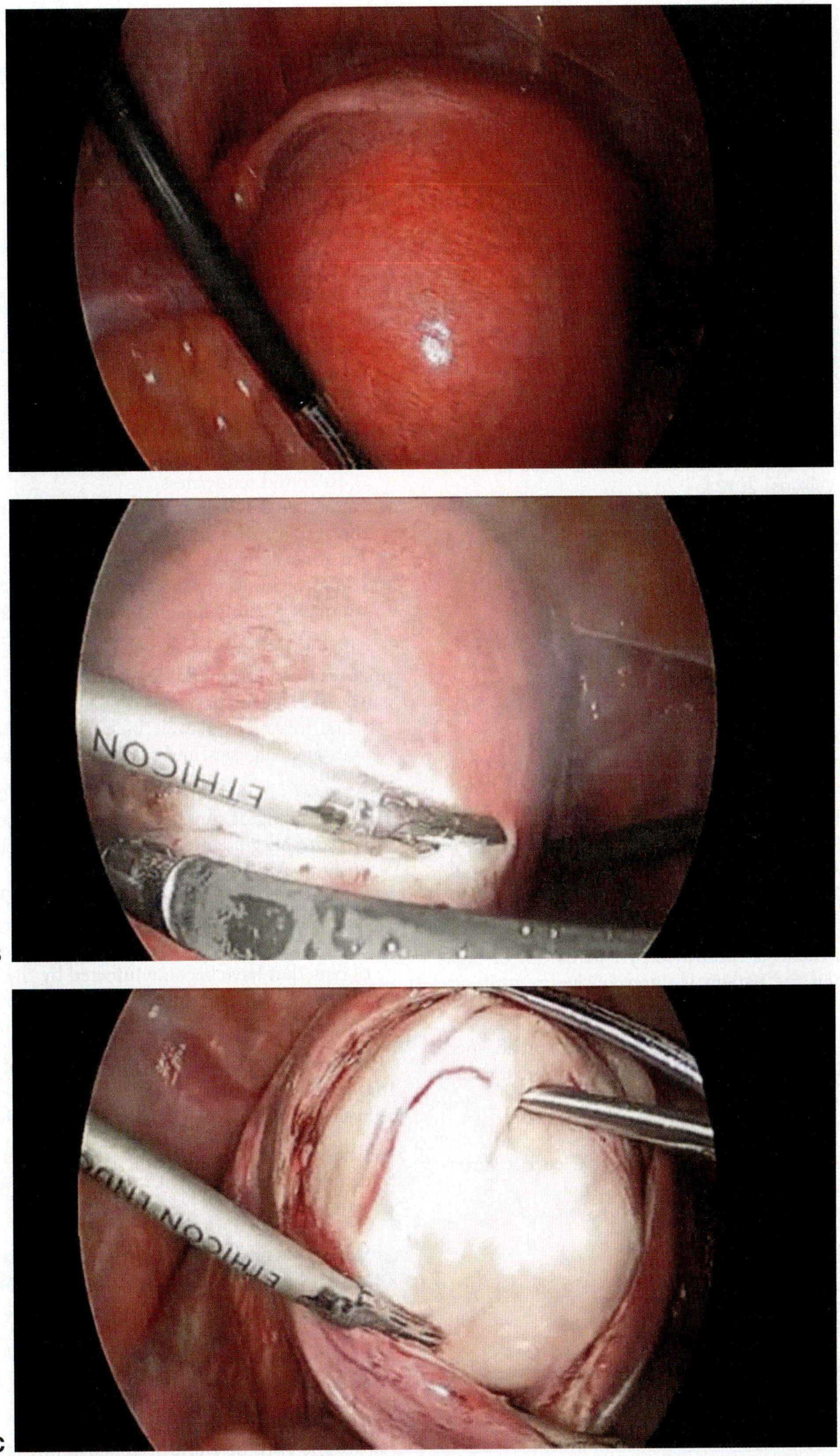

A B C

Figure 82.13. Laparoscopic myomectomy. A. Laparoscopic view of the uterine fundus. **B.** The fundal myometrium is dissected with laparoscopic instruments. **C.** The fibroid tissue dissected and the fundal defect reapproximated. (From Berek JS. *Berek & Novak's Gynecology*. 15th ed. Lippincott Williams & Wilkins; 2012.)

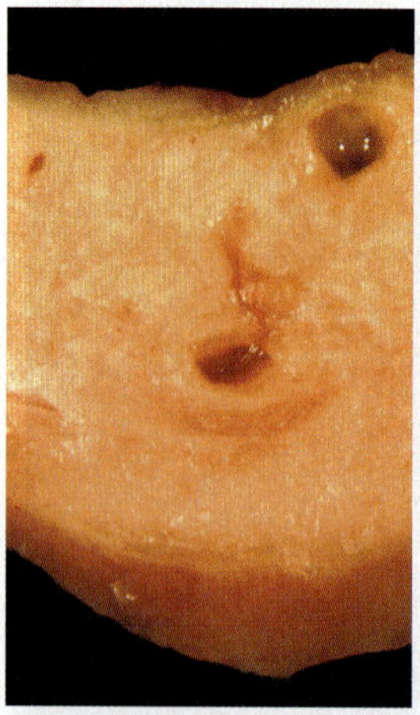

Figure 82.14. Adenomyosis. This gross pathology specimen shows foci of adenomyosis within the myometrium. (From Reichert RA. *Diagnostic Gynecologic and Obstetric Pathology: An Atlas and Text.* Lippincott Williams & Wilkins; 2012.)

The diagnosis of acute salpingo-oophoritis is often made inappropriately.[62,63]

- The patient usually presents with:
  - ☐ Lower quadrant abdominal pain that is frequently bilateral
  - ☐ The start of menstrual period
  - ☐ Nausea
  - ☐ Dysuria
  - ☐ Purulent vaginal discharge
- Abdominal examination reveals generalized tenderness without palpable masses.
- Bimanual examination reveals cervical motion tenderness and bilateral adnexal tenderness.
- Usually, there are no adnexal masses.
- Differential diagnoses include those conditions that can cause unilateral or bilateral pain [63] (Table 82.13).

The definitive diagnosis is confirmed by laparoscopy or laparotomy, especially when the patient is unresponsive to antibiotic therapy.

- If surgery is not indicated, empirical treatment with broad-spectrum antibiotics may be initiated on an outpatient or inpatient basis until the infectious agent is identified.[64]
- Medication alterations are then based on laboratory results.

Patients with acute tubo-ovarian abscess experience a variety of symptoms.

- These include the following:
  - ☐ Severe pain in the low abdomen/pelvis
  - ☐ High fever
  - ☐ Nausea and vomiting
  - ☐ Impending septic shock

TABLE 82.12

Conditions Associated with PID

Endometritis
Salpingitis
Tubo-ovarian abscess
Pelvic peritonitis
Adhesions

TABLE 82.13

Differential Diagnoses Associated in PID without a Pelvic Mass

Acute appendicitis
Urinary tract infection
Adnexal torsion
Endometriosis
Hemorrhagic corpus luteum cyst
Ectopic pregnancy
Somatic dysfunction

- Abdominal examination reveals:
  - ☐ Marked tenderness with muscular rigidity
  - ☐ A pelvic mass
  - ☐ Rebound tenderness
- Bimanual pelvic examination is extremely difficult because of the abdominal pain.
- An adnexal mass may be discovered.
- It may be easier during a rectal examination to recognize a pelvic mass possibly directed into the cul-de-sac (Table 82.14).

Laboratory results of any vaginal cultures confirm the infectious cause. Ultrasound may demonstrate adnexal pathology or cul-de-sac flocculation.

The treatment plan includes hospitalization with intravenous hydration, analgesics, and systemic antibiotics.

- Abscesses may resolve without need for acute surgical intervention. Timing of surgical intervention requires clinical judgment.
- Ultrasound guidance can be used to drain abscesses percutaneously to avoid surgery.
- Should the patient not respond to 72 hours of multiagent broad-spectrum antibiotics and have persistent spiking fevers, urgent surgery may be necessary to remove affected pelvic organs that have become infected by the ruptured abscess.
- Drainage and lavage of the peritoneal cavity may conserve pelvic organs (Fig. 82.15).

Chronic PID may cause pain because of recurrent exacerbation that requires antibiotic therapy or because of hydro salpinges and adhesion formation around the tubes, ovaries, and intestines.

- Endometriosis is the most frequently encountered differential diagnosis, particularly if there is no well-documented history of acute infection.

TABLE 82.14

Differential Diagnosis in PID with a Pelvic Mass

Septic incomplete abortion
Uterine rupture
Acute appendicitis with possible rupture
Peritonitis with or without abscess formation
Diverticular abscess (in left-sided pain)
Adnexal torsion
Perforated peptic ulcer
Pancreatitis
Mesenteric artery thrombosis

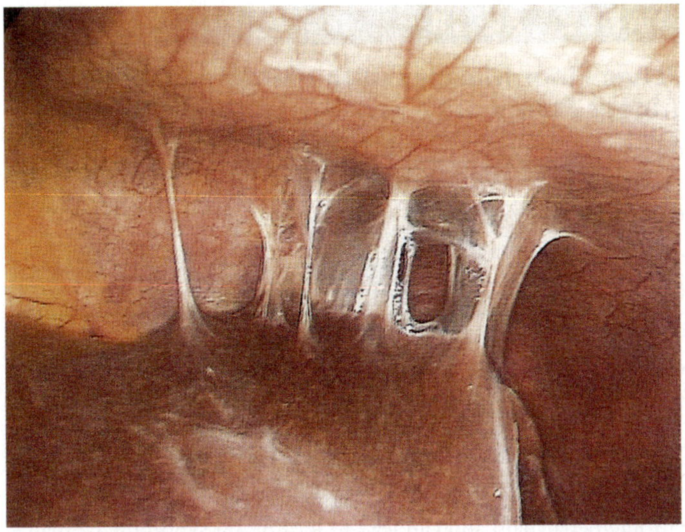

Figure 82.15. Perihepatitis (Fitz–Hugh–Curtis syndrome). Adhesions between the liver and the diaphragm are evidence of perihepatitis caused by chlamydial infection. (Casanova R, Connolly AM, Goepfert AR, Hueppchen NA, Weiss PM. *Beckmann and Ling's Obstetrics and Gynecology*. 9th ed. Lippincott Williams and Wilkins; 2024.)

- Before ascribing pain symptoms to adhesions, the physician should note adhesions specifically in the area of pain localization.
- Some patients with extensive pelvic adhesions may be asymptomatic.
- Laparoscopy or laparotomy may be required to identify the adhesions.

Osteopathic considerations for treatment of PID:

- These include evaluation and treatment of somatic dysfunction:
    - □ At T11–L2 to improve circulation
    - □ At the sacrum and related pelvic bones to balance the nervous system and to improve body fluid circulation/lymphatic drainage
- In cases of chronic PID, osteopathic treatment to stretch pelvic adhesions may be useful.

PELVIC FLOOR DYSFUNCTION

Pelvic floor dysfunction can contribute to many conditions (Table 82.15).

- These problems are underreported, embarrassing, and undertreated.[65]
- Symptoms of these problems may limit a woman's activities of daily living.
- Pelvic floor dysfunctions are often preventable; emphasis should be placed on prevention through education and exercise before problems arise.[66]

TABLE 82.15

Conditions Associated with Pelvic Floor Dysfunction

Conditions
Urinary stress incontinence
Fecal incontinence
Sexual dysfunction
Pelvic relaxation
Levator ani syndromes

Women are twice as likely as men to be incontinent.

- Denial is common because many patients believe that it is an inevitable result of childbirth and aging.
- Involuntary loss of urine during physical activity is called stress incontinence.
- Nygaard et al.[67,68] studied the relationship between exercise and incontinence and found that 82% of regularly exercising women experience some degree of incontinence. Of 326 women, 22% were nulliparous.
- High-impact exercises (running and jumping) resulted in even more episodes of incontinence than did low-impact activities.
- Women who frequently exercised addressed their incontinence by wearing protective pads, staying close to a toilet, and limiting fluid intake.[69]

Urogynecologic dysfunctions have multifactorial causes that require medical evaluation and urodynamic testing.

- When an evaluation indicates muscle dysfunction, an osteopathic physician may gain additional insight from understanding interrelationship between structure and function of the pelvic structures.
- Successful manipulative treatment and exercise depend on the condition of the sensory and motor system of the patient.
- A routine pelvic examination may identify poor performance of pelvic floor musculature.
- Further examination should include visual inspection of the perineum during a pelvic floor contraction to note:
    - □ Whether the proper muscles are contracting and relaxing
    - □ Muscle strength or pain using digital palpation
    - □ A cystocele, rectocele, or poorly repaired episiotomies
    - □ Uterine or vaginal prolapse

Pelvic relaxation with decrease in normal pelvic floor support can occur with congenital or developmental weakness of the supportive structures, or when pelvic structures (especially the pudendal nerve) are damaged during childbirth.[70]

- Even if the pelvic floor muscles are not damaged in vaginal delivery, the muscles must accommodate the passage of the fetus through the pelvis.
- Scar tissue may limit muscle contractility.[71]
- Postpartum patients are often afraid to recondition the perineum because of pain, and they may fail to perform the Kegel exercises taught in childbirth classes.[72]
- Manipulative treatment can be very beneficial in improving muscle tone and general nervous and circulatory function, particularly in correcting associated postural imbalance. Nervous system dysfunction may be affected by uterine displacement and sacral base dysfunction.[57]

The fascia and support structures are also influenced by menopause and aging.[73]

- Changes in the pelvic floor from chronic constipation and straining during defecation can lead to anorectal incontinence with outstretched perineum and sphincter denervation.[74]
- Chronic cough strains the muscles of the pelvic floor.[75]
- Kegel exercises, developed in the 1950s, were meant to address early stages of pelvic relaxation, not to prevent the need for surgery.[72]
- More recent research has developed comprehensive pelvic floor training programs that can aid in correcting early pelvic floor dysfunction, although they remain underutilized. The mechanism by which these exercises alleviate dysfunction is not fully understood, but many patients report benefits from regular

TABLE 82.16

Symptoms Associated with Pelvic Floor Hypertonus Dysfunction

Dysmenorrhea
Dyspareunia
Sexual dysfunction
Voiding difficulty
Urinary frequency/urgency

contraction and relaxation of isolated muscle groups to increase motor recruitment abilities.[60]

Hypertonus dysfunctions of musculoskeletal and urogynecologic systems are known as the levator ani syndrome.[76]

- The primary symptom is poorly localized pain.
- The pain may be located:
  - In perivaginal or perirectal area
  - In lower abdominal quadrants
  - In the pelvis
  - In suprapubic or coccyx regions
  - Down the posterior thigh
- Vulvar or clitoral burning may sometimes be present.
- More specific symptoms reported by women with hypertonus dysfunction include those in Table 82.16.[76]

Tissues of the pelvic floor can be evaluated by turning the finger pads posteriorly during bimanual evaluation of the pelvis, then serially sweeping the levator ani muscles and their fascia to evaluate tensions. Tension myalgia of the pelvic floor is a spectrum of diagnoses of various syndromes of pelvic musculature.

- These include the following:
  - Piriformis syndrome
  - Levator ani syndrome
  - Coccygodynia
  - Vaginismus[78]
- Other diagnoses with a component of hypertonus dysfunction include those listed in Table 82.17.[79,80]

Chronic Pelvic Pain

Chronic pelvic pain is the second most common complaint in gynecologic practice and is defined as continual pain of more than 6 months' duration.

- Thorough evaluation should be performed to determine if the chronic pain is from visceral origin.

TABLE 82.17

Conditions Causing Pelvic Floor Hypertonus Dysfunction

Chronic low back pain
Endometriosis
Chronic pelvic pain with negative surgical findings
Painful bladder syndrome
Urethral syndrome
Sphincter dyssynergia

TABLE 82.18

Pelvic Floor Muscles with Identified Travell Trigger Points

Coccygeus
Levator ani
Obturator internus
Adductor magnus
Piriformis or oblique abdominals

- Research has uncovered a cross-organ viscerovisceral convergence induced by inflammation and modulated through the hypogastric nerve. This finding could explain the frequency in which multiple organ systems are involved in chronic pelvic pain syndromes.[81]

Musculoskeletal postural dysfunction has been implicated in chronic pelvic pain and can lead to levator ani syndrome by maintaining inefficient holding patterns of muscles that contribute to the persistence of pain.[80,82,83]

- Somatic dysfunction of the pelvis, if untreated, may cause hypertonus as a result of restriction of motion of pelvic joints and their related structures.
- Myofascial pain syndromes create pain, tenderness, and autonomic phenomena from myofascial trigger points. Travell and Simons[84] have identified trigger points in muscles of the pelvic floor (Table 82.18).

A pubic shear is a frequently identified somatic dysfunction in the vertical plane and is easily corrected with osteopathic treatment.

- Anterior/posterior shears are much less common but can cause significant pain when present.
- Imbalance of tensions on the pelvic floor is a likely finding.
- After correction of the structural asymmetry, soft tissue techniques, such as myofascial release of the suprapubic tissues and pelvic diaphragm release, can significantly improve symptoms.

These pelvic muscle somatic dysfunctions may be treated with bimanual relaxation of muscle contractions.

- The vaginal palpating digits may apply inhibitory pressure or use principles of counterstrain or myofascial technique to achieve release of tension or spasm.
- Identification of Chapman reflex points may also direct the osteopathic physician to treat related somatic dysfunction within the pelvis.[85]

OTHER ORGANIC CAUSES OF PELVIC PAIN

Because the uterus and fallopian tubes share the innervation of the lower intestinal tract, pelvic pain can be nongynecologic in origin.

- During history and physical examination, the physician should ask questions to ascertain whether associated symptoms may indicate a nongynecologic origin to the pain.
- Table 82.19 describes symptoms that may aid the gynecologist in directing referral to another specialist for evaluation.

Osteopathic consideration exists for treatment of this condition.

- Treatment involves addressing somatic dysfunction of the following to improve circulation and enhance lymphatic drainage:
  - Thoracolumbar spine
  - Pelvis
  - Lower extremities

TABLE 82.19

Symptoms Suggesting Need for Specialist Referral

Gastrointestinal conditions	
	Bloating
	Flatus
	Burping
	Diarrhea
	Constipation
Urinary tract	
	Dysuria
	Frequency
	Hesitancy
Neurologic	
	Pain that follows known nerve pathways
	Paresthesias
	Weakness
Psychological	
	History of trauma
	History of sexual/physical abuse

- Findings of tender Chapman reflex points aid with differential diagnosis.[85]

Low back pain of neuromuscular origin usually increases with activity and stress.

- Chronic low back pain without lower abdominal pain is seldom of gynecologic origin.[86]
- Occasionally, a pelvic mass accompanied by neuromuscular symptoms may be revealed during surgical exploration to be a neuroma or bony tumor.[87]

Dosing Intervals

Patients with somatic dysfunction in acute conditions generally respond well to osteopathic treatment.

- After a successful treatment, if pain returns within 24 hours, there is concern that the somatic dysfunction may be viscerosomatic.
- Patients should be instructed to notify the physician if the pain returns immediately as a more thorough workup is in order.
- For patients with chronic pain, long-standing somatic dysfunction is more challenging to treat.
- After a successful treatment, the goal is to have the patient return about the time symptoms recur.
- With each subsequent successful treatment, the benefit should remain longer.

CONTRAINDICATIONS

Contraindications to osteopathic treatment of the gynecology patient follow usual contraindications for adult women. Table 82.20 outlines contraindications to OMT.

GYNECOLOGIC SURGERY

Gynecology is a surgical specialty, but osteopathically trained gynecologists develop an in-depth appreciation of the architecture and engineering of the pelvis that impacts their practice.

TABLE 82.20

Contraindications to OMT for the Gynecology Patient

Absolute Contraindications	
	Surgical emergency
	Undiagnosed bleeding
Medicolegal issues	
	Lack of informed consent (language barrier)
Relative Contraindications	
	Patients with diseases causing bone fragility should not be treated with high velocity low amplitude (HVLA) or forceful techniques
	Cancer diagnosis (concern for tumor seeding)
Caution	
	Very ill patients should only be treated for brief periods

- Through use of skilled palpatory evaluation of a patient's internal and external body structure, there is an opportunity to diagnose, treat, and prevent dysfunction that has been influenced by the musculoskeletal system.
- When a patient has a condition that does not respond to conservative measures, surgery may be indicated.
- When surgery is necessary, osteopathic principles can be utilized to improve patient outcomes.
- Using a minimally invasive approach preserves body integrity and reduces surgical complications[88]
- Robotic surgery is now accepted for benign gynecologic disease. While outcomes for robotic and laparoscopic cases are similar, robotics permits a minimally invasive approach for complicated patients who may not have been candidates for routine laparoscopy[89]
- Enhanced Recovery After Surgery (ERAS) protocols seek to reduce the anabolic stress of surgery and have been shown to decrease complications and length of hospital stay.[89,90]

GYNECOLOGY PATIENT CASE PRESENTATION

A 38-year-old G2P2 female presented to a gynecologist as a referral from the emergency department. The patient:

- Presented lying in a fetal position sobbing on the examination table.
- Rated her pain 10/10 and described the pain as cramping with intermittent stabbing pains, low and diffuse in the pelvis.
- Had been seen emergently multiple times in the past 6 weeks for severe pelvic pain.
- Recently relocated and had not yet established care with a physician.

The patient had a hysterectomy 8 years earlier for endometriosis and pelvic pain.

- Her pain did not resolve, so a unilateral oophorectomy was later performed.
- When the pain continued, the other ovary was subsequently removed.
- She was not placed on hormone replacement because of concern for stimulating the endometriosis with exogenous hormones.
- Later, a fourth surgery, laparoscopy with adhesiolysis was done.
- Her pain continued.

The patient was separated from her husband. She believed that her pelvic pain and dyspareunia contributed to failure of the marriage.

The patient's medications included oxycodone received in the emergency department.

- She denied any other health issues.
- Her two children were both delivered at term via cesarean delivery.

Physical examination of the patient was very difficult because of her significant pain.

- Inspection of the external genitalia revealed erythematous tissue, but no discrete lesions.
- Attempt to insert a speculum was unsuccessful because of discomfort.
- The patient had voluntary guarding and did not appear to have involuntary guarding.
- An ultrasound performed at one of her emergency department visits was available, which showed no uterus or ovaries and no pelvic or adnexal masses or cysts.
- A decision was made to begin investigation with a diagnostic laparoscopy since a significant acute event could not be ruled out and to perform a thorough examination under anesthesia.

Diagnostic laparoscopy was performed.

- Pelvic examination under anesthesia revealed no abnormalities.
- Laparoscopy revealed adhesions of the small bowel on the vaginal cuff, which were gently sharply and bluntly dissected.
- The rest of the small bowel was adhesed in a block. Those adhesions were not addressed.

On return, the patient stated that her pain had decreased to 7/10. An osteopathic approach with structural evaluation and gentle treatment was described and the patient consented.

- Structural exam revealed:
  - A sacral torsion
  - ASIS asymmetry
  - A vertical and anterior/posterior pubic shear
- The following areas were treated:
  - Pelvis
  - Sacrum
  - Pubic symphysis
- After structural treatment was completed, the perineal erythema decreased.
- The patient then permitted full examination.
  - Counterstrain technique was used for tender points found in the tissues of the pelvic diaphragm intravaginally.
  - Myofascial release was performed on the suprapubic tissues.
- The patient's pain was 4/10 after the treatment.

The patient was instructed to call when the pain returned.

- The treatment effect lasted about 3 days.
- The patient was seen urgently so treatment could be given before there was opportunity for the underlying somatic dysfunction patterns to reestablish.
- She was treated serially over a period of several months with gradually increasing intervals between treatment and she was given exercises to strengthen the pelvic floor.
- In addition, prolotherapy was used to stabilize the pubic symphysis and sacroiliac joints.
- After 6 months, the patient was pain free and sought assistance to discontinue her narcotic use and counseling for her family stresses.

Case Study Teaching Points

- Anterior/posterior pubic shear causes significant pelvic floor dysfunction and pain.
- Visible inflammation can be secondary to somatic dysfunction.
- The patient had proven endometriosis, but her pain was also likely musculoskeletal prior to her first surgery.
- Prior to surgery, when there is not a life-threatening condition, a trial of OMT may save health care dollars and morbidity when somatic dysfunction is present.
- Chronic pelvic pain is not only disabling for the patient but also causes significant psychosocial stress.
- A multidisciplinary approach is often needed to address the many issues common to chronic pelvic pain patients.

CONCLUSION

Osteopathic gynecologists are well equipped to manage the complex symptoms and syndromes their patients may present with. Using osteopathic principles and carefully listening to the patient will help the physician address the patient's concerns. Excellent palpatory skills developed by osteopathic physicians assist in identifying sources of pain and somatic dysfunction and assess treatments. Being instrumental in aiding a patient with a difficult diagnosis to an improved state of health is a great reward for the osteopathic gynecologist.

REFERENCES

1. Still AT. *The Philosophy and Mechanical Principles of Osteopathy*. Hudson-Kimberly Publishing Co; 1902. Churchill-Livingstone Elsevier; 2012: 208–262.
2. Spitznagle TM, Robinson CM. Myofascial pelvic pain. *Obstet Gynecol Clin North Am*. 2014;41(3):409–432.
3. Drake RL. Chapter 5 pelvis and perineum. In: Drake R, Drake RL, Vogl W, Mitchell AWM, eds. *Gray's Basic Anatomy*. Churchill Livingstone; 2012.
4. DeLancey J, Richardson AC. Anatomy of genital support. In: Benson JT, ed. *Female Pelvic Floor Disorders*. WW Norton; 1992.
5. Hoffman BL, Schorge JO, Bradshaw KD, Halvorson LM, Schaffer JI, Corton MM. Anal Incontinence, Anorectal Disorders, and Rectovaginal Fistula. In: Hoffman BL, Schorge JO, Halvorson LM, Hamid CA, Corton MM, Schaffer JI. eds. *Williams Gynecology*. 4e. McGraw-Hill Education; 2020. Accessed September 18, 2024. https://accessmedicine.mhmedical.com/content.aspx?bookid=2658&sectionid=225559812
6. Spence-Jones C, Kamm MA, Henry MM, Hudson CN. Bowel dysfunction: a pathogenic factor in uterovaginal prolapse and urinary stress incontinence. *Br J Obstet Gynaecol*. 1994;101:147–152.
7. Graber B, Kline-Graber G. Female orgasm: role of pubococcygeus muscle. *J Clin Psychiatry*. 1979;40:348–351.
8. Barrett KE, Barman SM, Boitano S, Brooks HL. Renal function & micturition. In: Barrett KE, Barman SM, Boitano S, Brooks HL, eds. *Ganong's Review of Medical Physiology*. 25th ed. McGraw-Hill; 2016.
9. Beal MC. Viscerosomatic reflexes: a review. *J Am Osteopath Assoc*. 1985; 185:786–801.
10. Walker E, Katon W, Harrop-Griffiths J, Holm L, Russo J, Hickok LR. Relationship of chronic pelvic pain to psychiatric diagnoses and childhood sexual abuse. *Am J Psychiatry*. 1988;145:75–80.
11. Smith RP. Identifying the causes of pelvic pain. *Female Patient*. 1993;18:41–51.
12. Chung MK, Chung RP, Gordon D. Interstitial cystitis and endometriosis in patients with chronic pelvic pain: the "Evil Twins" syndrome. *JSLS*. 2005;9(1):25–29.
13. Chung MK, Jarnagin B. Early identification of interstitial cystitis may avoid unnecessary hysterectomy. *JSLS*. 2009;13(3):350–357.
14. Perez-Stable EJ, Miranda J, Muñoz RF, Ying YW. Depression in medical outpatients: under-recognition and misdiagnosis. *Arch Intern Med*. 1990; 150:1083–1089.
15. Harrop-Griffith J, Katon W, Walker E. The association between chronic pelvic pain, psychiatric diagnosis, and childhood sex abuse. *Obstet Gynecol*. 1988;71:589–594.
16. Clemons J, Arya LA, Myers DL. Diagnosing interstitial cystitis in women with chronic pelvic pain. *Obstet Gynecol*. 2001;97:S7–S8.

17. Barbieri RL. Evaluating pelvic pain using Barbieri's triad. *OBG Management.* 2000;12:26–39.
18. Barbieri RL, Propst AM. Physical examination findings in women with endometriosis: uterosacral ligament abnormalities, lateral cervical displacement, and cervical stenosis. *J Gynecol Tech.* 1999;4:1–3.
19. Propst AM, Storti K, Barbieri RL. Lateral cervical displacement is associated with endometriosis. *Fertil Steril.* 1998;70:568–570.
20. Rapkin AJ, Reading AE. Chronic pelvic pain. *Curr Probl Obstet Gynecol.* 1991;49:99–106.
21. Burrows EA. Disorders of the female reproductive system. In: Hoag JM, Cole WV, Bradford S, eds. *Osteopathic Medicine.* McGraw-Hill; 1969: 676–684.
22. Wood DP, Wiesner MG, Reiter RC. Psychogenic chronic pelvic pain, diagnosis, and management. *Clin Obstet Gynecol.* 1990;33:179–195.
23. Twiddy H, Lane N, Chawla R, et al. The development and delivery of a female chronic pelvic pain management programme: a specialised interdisciplinary approach. *Br J Pain.* 2015;9(4):233–240.
24. Pickles VR. A plain-muscle stimulant in the menstruum. *Nature.* 1957; 180:1198–1199.
25. Rosenwaks Z, Seegar-Jones G. Menstrual pain: its origin and pathogenesis. *J Reprod Med.* 1980;25:207–212.
26. Barbieri RL. Stenosis of the external cervical os: an association with endometriosis in women with chronic pelvic pain. *Fertil Steril.* 1998;70:571–573.
27. De Sanctis V, Soliman A, Bernasconi S, et al. Primary dysmenorrhea in adolescents: prevalence, impact and recent knowledge. *Pediatr Endocrinol Rev.* 2015;13(2):512–520.
28. Minjarez DA, Schlaff WD. Update on the medical treatment of endometriosis. *Obstet Gynecol Clin North Am.* 2000;27:641–651.
29. Boesler D, Warner M, Alpers A, Finnerty EP, Kilmore MA. Efficacy of high velocity, low amplitude manipulative techniques in subjects with low back pain during menstrual cramping. *J Am Osteopath Assoc.* 1993;93:203–214.
30. Chapman JD. Progress in scientifically proving the benefits of OMT in treating symptoms of dysmenorrhea. *J Am Osteopath Assoc.* 1993;93:196.
31. Hitchcock ME. The manipulative approach to the management of primary dysmenorrhea. *J Am Osteopath Assoc.* 1976;75:109–118.
32. Lapp T. ACOG issues recommendations for the management of endometriosis. American College of Obstetricians and Gynecologists. *Am Fam Physician.* 2000;62:1431–1434.
33. Kuchera M, Kuchera W. *Osteopathic Considerations in Systemic Dysfunction.* Greyden Press; 1994:139–142.
34. Hacker NF, Gambone JC, Hobel CJ. *Chapter 21. Hacker and Moore's Essentials of Obstetrics and Gynecology.* 6th ed. WB Saunders; 2016.
35. Frank RT. The hormonal causes of pre-menstrual tension. *Arch Neurol Psychiatry.* 1931;26:1053–1064.
36. Greene R, Dalton K. The premenstrual syndrome. *BMJ.* 1953;1:1007–1014.
37. Steiner M, Born L. Diagnosis and treatment of premenstrual dysphoric disorder: an update. *Int Clin Psychopharmacol.* 2000;3:S5–S17.
38. Frackiewicz EJ, Shiovitz TM. Evaluation and management of premenstrual syndrome and premenstrual dysphoric disorder. *J Am Pharm Assoc (Wash).* 2001;41:437–447.
39. Steiner M, Romano SJ, Babcock S, et al. The efficacy of fluoxitine in improving physical symptoms associated with premenstrual dysphoric disorder. *BJOG.* 2001;108:462–468.
40. Herbal treatment for PMS? *Harv Womens Health Watch.* 2001;8:7.
41. Labruzzo B, Chasuk R, Kendall S. Which complementary therapies can help patients with PMS? *J Fam Pract [serial online].* 2009;58(10):552–559.
42. Starzinski M. Pre-menstrual syndrome: update and osteopathic approach to treatment. *Osteopath Ann.* 1987;14:39–42.
43. Perry CP. Criteria that indicate endometriosis is the cause of chronic pelvic pain. *Obstet Gynecol.* 1999;93:473.
44. Janssen EB, Rijkers AC, Hoppenbrouwers K, Meuleman C, D'Hooghe TM. Prevalence of endometriosis diagnosed by laparoscopy in adolescents with dysmenorrhea or chronic pelvic pain: a systematic review. *Hum Reprod Update.* 2013;19(5):570.
45. Wolfman WL, Kreutner K. Laparoscopy in children and adolescents. *J Adolesc Health.* 1984;5:261–265.
46. Hall JE. Menstrual disorders and pelvic pain. In: Kasper D, Fauci A, Hauser S, eds. *Harrison's Principles of Internal Medicine.* 19th ed. McGraw-Hill; 2015.
47. Wellbery C. Diagnosis and treatment of endometriosis [published correction appears in Am Fam Physician 2000 May 1;61(9):2614]. *Am Fam Physician.* 1999;60(6):1753–1768.
48. Moore JG, Binstock MA, Growdon WA. The clinical implications of retroperitoneal endometriosis. *Am J Obstet Gynecol.* 1988;158:1291–1298.
49. Adamson G. Diagnosis and clinical presentation of endometriosis. *Am J Obstet Gynecol.* 1990;162:568–569.
50. Ranney B. Endometriosis I. Conservative operations. *Am J Obstet Gynecol.* 1970;107:743–753.
51. Revised American Fertility Society classification of endometriosis. *Fertil Steril.* 1985;43:351–352.
52. Al-Shaiji TF, Alshammaa DH, Al-Mansouri MM, Al-Terki AE. Association of endometriosis with interstitial cystitis in chronic pelvic pain syndrome: Short narrative on prevalence, diagnostic limitations, and clinical implications. *Qatar Med J.* 2021;2021(3):50.
53. Brown J, Farquhar C. Endometriosis: an overview of Cochrane Reviews. *Cochrane Database Syst Rev.* 2014;(3):CD009590.
54. Prentice A, Deary AJ, Goldbeck-Wood S, Farquhar C, Smith SK. Gonadotrophin-releasing hormone analogues for pain associated with endometriosis. *Cochrane Database Syst Rev.* 2000;(2):CD000346.
55. Dicker RC, Greenspan JR, Strauss LT, et al. Complications of vaginal and abdominal hysterectomy in the United States. The collaborative review of sterilization. *Am J Obstet Gynecol.* 1982;144:841–848.
56. Pettit PD, Lee RA. Ovarian remnant syndrome: diagnostic dilemma and surgical challenges. *Obstet Gynecol.* 1988;71:580–583.
57. Taylor HC Jr. Vascular congestion and hyperemia: their effect on structure and function of the female reproductive system: parts I and II. *Am J Obstet Gynecol.* 1949; 57:211–221.
58. Taylor HC. Pelvic pain based on a vascular and autonomic nervous system disorder. *Am J Obstet Gynecol.* 1954;57:1177–1196.
59. Harris RD, Holtzman SR, Poppe AM. Clinical outcome in female patients with pelvic pain and normal pelvic US findings. *Radiology.* 2000;216: 440–443.
60. Daugherty SF, Gillespie DL. Venous angioplasty and stenting improve pelvic congestion syndrome caused by venous outflow obstruction. *J Vasc Surg Venous Lymphat Disord.* 2015;3(3):283–289.
61. Chong GO, Lee YH, Hong DG, Cho YL, Lee YS. Long-term efficacy of laparoscopic or robotic adenomyomectomy with or without medical treatment for severely symptomatic adenomyosis. *Gynecol Obstet Invest.* 2016;81:346–352.
62. Stones RW, Mountfield J. Intervention for treating chronic pelvic pain in women. *Cochrane Database Syst Rev.* 2000;(4):CD000387.
63. Toth A. Alternative causes of pelvic inflammatory disease. *J Reprod Med.* 1983;28:699–702.
64. American College of Obstetricians and Gynecologists (ACOG). *Technical Bulletin 153: Antimicrobial therapy for gynecological infections.* The American College of Obstetricians and Gynecologists; 1991.
65. Cotton P. Physicians hear about incontinence. *JAMA.* 1990;264(18): 2361–2362.
66. Pope CS, Rabin J. Urinary incontinence: evaluation and non-surgical management. *Female Patient.* 2001;26:41–47.
67. Nygaard I, DeLancey JO, Arnsdorf L, Murphy E. Exercise and incontinence. *Obstet Gynecol.* 1990;75:848–851.
68. Nygaard I, Thompson FL, Svengalis SL, Albright JP. Urinary incontinence in elite nulliparous athletes. *Obstet Gynecol.* 1994;84:183–187.
69. Wallace K. Female pelvic floor functions, dysfunctions, and behavioral approaches to treatment. *Clin Sports Med.* 1994;13:459–481.
70. Sampselle CM, Miller JM, Mims BL, Delancey JO, Ashton-Miller JA, Antonakos CL. Effect of pelvic muscle exercise on transient incontinence during pregnancy and after birth. *Obstet Gynecol.* 1998;91:406–412.
71. Fitzpatrick M, O'Herlilhy C. The effects of labour and delivery on the pelvic floor. *Best Pract Res Clin Obstet Gynaecol.* 2001;15:63–79.
72. Kegel A. Early genital relaxation: new technique of diagnosis and nonsurgical treatment. *Obstet Gynecol.* 1956;8:545–550.
73. Fantl JA, Bump RC, Robinson D, McClish DK, Wyman JF. Efficacy of estrogen supplementation in the treatment of urinary incontinence. *Obstet Gynecol.* 1996;88:745–749.
74. Halligan S, Bartram CR. Evaculation, proctography, combined with positive contrast peritoneography to demonstrate pelvic floor hernias. *Abdom Imaging.* 1995;20:442–445.

75. Swami SS, Abrahams P. Urge incontinence. *Urol Clin North Am.* 1996;23:417–425.
76. Salvati E. The levator syndrome and its variant. *Gastroenterol Clin North Am.* 1987;16:71–78.
77. Klock SC. Female sexuality and sexual counseling. *Curr Probl Obstet Gynecol Fertil.* 1993;16(3):101–135.
78. Sinaki IM, Merritt J, Stillwell GK. Tension myalgia of the pelvic floor. *Mayo Clin Proc.* 1977;52:717–722.
79. Benson JT. *Female Pelvic Floor Disorders: Investigation and Management.* WW Norton; 1992.
80. King PM. Musculoskeletal factors in chronic pelvic pain. *J Psychosom Obstet Gynaecol.* 1991;12:87–98.
81. Winnard KP, Dmitrieva N, Berkley KJ. Cross-organ interactions between reproductive, gastrointestinal, and urinary tracts: modulation by estrous stage and involvement of the hypogastric nerve. *Am J Physiol Regul Integr Comp Physiol.* 2006;291:R1592–R1601.
82. McCandless S, Mason G. Physical therapy as an effective change agent in the treatment of patients with urinary incontinence. *J Miss State Med Assoc.* 1995;36:271–274.
83. Cammu H, Nylan MV. Pelvic floor exercises in genuine urinary stress incontinence. *Int Urogynecol J.* 1997;8:297–300.
84. Travell J, Simons D. *Myofascial Pain and Dysfunction: The Trigger Point Manual. The Lower Extremities.* Vol 2. Lippincott Williams & Wilkins; 1992.
85. Owens C. *An Endocrine Interpretation of Chapman's Reflexes.* 2nd ed. Chattanooga Printing & Engraving Co; 1937.
86. Holley R, Richter H, Wang L. Neurologic disease presenting as chronic pelvic pain. *South Med J.* 1999;92:1105–1107.
87. Malinak LR. Operative management of pelvic pain. *Clin Obstet Gynecol.* 1980;23:191–200.
88. Sehnal B, Klat J, Herboltova P, et al. Comparison of complications in very obese women undergoing hysterectomy—abdominal vs laparoscopic approach with short- and long-term follow-up. *Eur J Obstet Gynecol Reprod Biol.* 2022;276:148–153.
89. Wijk L, Udumyan R, Pache B, et al. International validation of Enhanced Recovery After Surgery Society guidelines on enhanced recovery for gynecologic surgery. *Am J Obstet Gynecol.* 2019;221(3):237.e1–237.e11.
90. Ljungqvist O, Scott M, Fearon KC. Enhanced recovery after surgery: a review. *JAMA Surg.* 2017;152(3):292–298.

83 Osteopathic Considerations in Patients with Head, Eyes, Ears, Nose, and Throat Disorders

SHAN SHAN WU ▪ ROBERT W. HOSTOFFER

KEY CONCEPTS

- Osteopathic principles and practices in disorders of the head, eyes, ears, nose, and throat (HEENT) region relies on a detailed understanding of the underlying anatomy and physiology.
- This chapter focuses on osteopathic perspectives in understanding the pathophysiology, making the diagnosis, and providing treatment options for common HEENT problems seen in primary care settings, including rhinosinusitis, allergic conjunctivitis and rhinitis, otitis media, vertigo, acute tonsillitis and pharyngitis, and temporomandibular joint (TMJ) disorders.
- The five models of osteopathic care are useful for developing osteopathic management plans for patients with HEENT disorders, for example, rhinosinusitis and dizziness.

INTRODUCTION

The head, eyes, ears, nose, and throat (HEENT) are not a system unto themselves; they are parts of at least three different systems. Primary cranial disorders are discussed in Chapter 53 Osteopathic Cranial Manipulative Medicine. This chapter mainly focuses on the disorders of the ears, nose, and throat as they relate to the head and neck regions. It also describes the structure and function of the eyes as ocular disturbances often coexist with the various disorders of the nose and throat. In addition, the TMJ disorders will be addressed.

Their grouping together as a specialty (HEENT) is likely due to their sharing of several factors, including:

- Having a respiratory mucosal lining (ears, nose, and throat)
- Containing organs of special senses
- Having internal connections to each other
- Being in the head and neck

The nose, paranasal sinuses, mouth, and throat function in the respiratory system as passageways for air. The nose and paranasal sinuses filter the inspired air. Olfaction is the special sense of the nose. The special senses of hearing and balance are housed in the ears. The mouth and throat function as part of the digestive system in chewing, swallowing, and the special sense of taste. The throat and mouth also aid in speech.

Due to the diverse nature of this area, various symptoms arise, and different modalities are used to treat disorders of the HEENT. Symptoms range from infectious processes to vertigo to difficulty swallowing or talking. Preventing and treating these problems depend on an appreciation of the existing physiologic functions and anatomical relationships.

HEENT problems are commonly encountered in the primary care setting. These include but are not limited to allergic conjunctivitis, allergic rhinitis, otitis media, sinusitis, and tonsillitis. Treating this area from an osteopathic perspective uses the basic concepts of structure–function relationship and the body's inherent healing capacity. These common problems serve as examples of how to approach the HEENT patient osteopathically.

The respiratory system demonstrates the remarkable health maintenance systems within the body. With an understanding and appreciation of normal anatomy and function, the physician can effectively treat HEENT patients to enhance the ability for recovery and the natural resistance to disease.

It is the responsibility of the osteopathic physician to consider the specific needs of the patient and design an individualized treatment plan in favor of promoting the body's ability to regulate itself toward health.

- **Patient education** increases patient awareness of medication abuse, pollutants, humidification, and allergies (see Chapter 24 Environmental Issues for further discussion).
- **Osteopathic manipulative treatment** (OMT) has been used historically and empirically for many years to treat HEENT problems commonly encountered in primary care.[1–3]
  - This treatment is based on the musculoskeletal system's impact on circulatory flow to and from all the tissues of the body and its effects on physiologic function by way of the autonomic nervous system.
  - Promoting lymphatic circulation plays an important role in reducing swelling and inflammation, as well as in stimulating the immune system.
  - Studies have shown physiologic function of various organs to be affected by noxious somatic afferent stimulation.[4,5]
  - Clinical experience has shown that incorporation of musculoskeletal treatment in the management of HEENT patients improves recovery time and reduces incidence of recurrence and complications.[6,7]
- **Medical intervention** can be accomplished in the most beneficial way when consideration is made of the natural forces at work to maintain homeostasis. Medications, surgery, and allergy desensitization can be most effective when based on specific diagnoses and combined with patient education and appropriate musculoskeletal treatment.

General knowledge of myofascial anatomy, lymphatic circulation, and autonomic nervous supply to the head and neck can enhance osteopathic treatment of patients with HEENT problems. Specific attention to each organ's unique aspects of anatomy, built-in mechanisms for health, and predisposing factors for disease will enhance treatment of specific conditions. Prior to reading this chapter, it would be helpful to review head and neck anatomy:

Chapters 32 and 33 for general regional anatomy, Chapter 7 regarding fascia, Chapter 14 for lymphatic drainage, Chapter 6 for autonomic nervous system innervations, and Chapter 23 for the ecology of the microbiome.

NOSE AND PARANASAL SINUSES

Nervous System Regulation

There are some key points regarding the nervous system's involvement in sinus pathophysiology worthy of remembering when considering diagnosis and management plans for patients with sinus congestion and disease.

SYMPATHETIC NERVOUS SYSTEM

- Sympathetic fibers to the head arise from the upper thoracic segments of the cord (T1–T4).
- Preganglionic fibers ascend from there to the superior cervical ganglion, located in the upper cervical area, where they synapse.
- Postganglionic fibers from the superior cervical ganglion join the internal carotid plexus, becoming part of the deep petrosal nerve and the nerve of the pterygoid canal (see Fig. 32.8).
- Sympathetic supply to the nose and paranasal sinuses passes without synapsing through the sphenopalatine ganglion in the pterygopalatine fossa.
- They continue with the parasympathetic fibers to the nose and sinuses.
- The sympathetic nervous system produces vasoconstriction in the nose and increased nasal airway patency.
- Norepinephrine is the primary neurotransmitter of the sympathetic system in the nose.
- Blood supply to the nasal mucosa is regulated primarily through the sympathetic nervous system.
- Unopposed sympathetic stimulation leads to vasoconstriction accompanied by drying of the mucosa.

PARASYMPATHETIC NERVOUS SYSTEM

- Parasympathetic supply to the nose originates from the superior salivary nucleus.
- Its preganglionic fibers form part of the superficial greater petrosal nerve (CN VII), which joins the deep petrosal nerve, forming the nerve of the pterygoid canal (vidian nerve).
- After passing through the pterygoid canal, the fibers synapse in the sphenopalatine ganglion (see Figs. 32.6 and 32.7).
- The sphenopalatine ganglion is suspended in the pterygopalatine fossa, bordered by the pterygoid process, maxilla, palatine bone, and floor of the sphenoid.
- The parasympathetic postganglionic nerves modulate their effect by integrating inhibitory and stimulatory channels.
- Postganglionic fibers are distributed to the nasal mucosa from the sphenopalatine ganglion along with the sensory and sympathetic fibers.
- Nasal mucus production is predominantly regulated by parasympathetic nerve fibers, but sympathetic fibers also reach the glands.
- Stimulation of parasympathetic fibers generally increases goblet cell secretions. The action of the parasympathetic nervous system on the upper respiratory mucosa is stimulation of the glandular epithelium with production of mucus, rich in:
    - Glycoproteins
    - Lactoferrin
    - Lysozymes
    - Secretory leukoprotease inhibitor
    - Neural endopeptidase
    - Secretory IgA
- Tobacco smoke and other pollutants adversely affect mucociliary clearance by inactivating cilia.[8,9]
- The quantity and composition of the mucus are influenced by various factors, such as:
    - Temperature
    - Humidity
    - Oxygen concentration
    - Pollution
    - Irritants

NEUROMODULATORS

Neuromodulators such as substance P (SP) also appear to influence the function of the submucosal glands[10] via a cystic fibrosis transmembrane conductance regulator (CFTR)–dependent mechanism.[11]

Common Pathophysiology

Inflammation is a common cause of disease in the nose and paranasal sinuses (see Chapters 12, 15 and 16 for background information) (Table 83.1).

The inflammatory process can be initiated by:

- Infections (viral, bacterial, fungal)
- Allergies (food or inhalants)
- Irritants (chemical or mechanical)

Inflammation is accompanied by swelling of the mucosa, excessive mucus production, and decrease in ciliary motility.

Symptoms include:

- Obstructed breathing
- Pain
- Rhinorrhea
- Epistaxis
- Anosmia

TABLE 83.1

Common Disorders of the Nose and Paranasal Sinuses

Disorder
Epistaxis
Nasal fractures
Acute rhinitis
Allergic rhinitis
Nonallergic vasomotor rhinitis
Atrophic rhinitis
Polyposis
Deviated nasal septum
Unilateral nasal discharge Foreign body Choanal atresia Malignancy Head trauma
Sinusitis

Prolonged inflammation predisposes to recurrent infection and changes, such as thickening of the mucous membranes and inhibition of cilia. These conditions impede the normal airflow and functioning of the mucosa. Poor venous and lymphatic circulation from the area can cause inflammatory mediators to remain in the tissues longer and prolong the inflammatory reaction.

Nasal obstruction and abnormal airflow may be due to:

1. Venous and lymphatic congestion causing engorgement of the mucosa, commonly seen in allergic rhinitis or upper respiratory infections
2. Structural defects, such as polyps or deviated septum

Changes in the mucosa and in airflow patterns have an adverse effect on the cleaning, humidifying, and temperature control of the air, as well as on the oxygen concentration in the sinuses. Sinusitis may result from prolonged derangement of airflow.

Obstructions due to mucosal changes are responsive to activities that alter sympathetic nerve discharge:

- Vigorous physical exercise has been shown to improve nasal function for up to 60 minutes by reducing nasal airflow resistance and nasal blood flow.[12]
- In a group of 12 subjects serving as their own controls, osteopathic manipulation resulted in significant improvement of nasal function, as measured by nasal pressure curves.[13]
- Addressing somatic dysfunction with osteopathic manipulation adds to patient comfort and aids the normal healing process.[6,7]

Tissue changes in the upper thoracic and upper cervical areas would be expected to accompany sympathetic motor dysfunction of the nose and paranasal sinuses. Chronic conditions and progression of disease can be prevented by decreasing congestion and promoting good airflow.

Rhinosinusitis

DIAGNOSIS

"Rhinosinusitis" is the preferred term instead of "rhinitis" when there is simultaneous inflammation of the nasal cavity with that of the sinus cavity.[14]

- Rhinosinusitis is the inflammation of at least one paranasal sinus and nasal cavity.
- It can be acute, with symptoms lasting less than 12 weeks, or chronic, with symptoms greater than 12 weeks.
- In some literature, acute rhinosinusitis is defined as having symptoms that resolve within 4 weeks with the additional term of subacute rhinosinusitis having symptoms between 4 and 12 weeks.[15]
- Recurrent acute rhinosinusitis is when there are at least three acute episodes in a year.

ACUTE RHINOSINUSITIS

Clinical Manifestations

- Anosmia
- Cough
- Fever
- Headache
- Nasal congestion
- Pain in the face or head
- Postnasal drainage
- Clear or purulent rhinorrhea and discharge

Physical Examination

Examination of the nose may reveal:

- Blood-tinged, erythema or crusting of the nasal mucosa
- Engorged turbinates
- Deviated septum
- Discolored nasal and oropharyngeal secretions
- Nasal polyps
- Sinus tenderness on palpation
- Decreased light transmission upon transillumination of the sinuses (this is not a definitive test)

The posterior oropharynx may demonstrate signs of postnasal drainage such as:

- Cobblestone appearance of lymphoid hyperplasia
- Pharyngeal edema
- Purulent secretions
- Osteopathic findings on physical examination
  - Numerous studies describe accompanying cervical soft tissue hypertonia with varying degrees of motion dysfunction.[1,16,17]
  - Localized, small areas of tenderness and tissue tension corresponding to Chapman reflex points have been noted in the suboccipital area and inferior to the clavicle, over the first rib.[18] Various other somatic dysfunctions occur unique to the individual patient.

Labs and/or Imaging

- Patient may have an elevated white blood cell count on the complete blood count (CBC), or leukocytosis, if the inflammation is caused or superimposed by a bacterial infection.
- X-ray of the head or computed tomography (CT) of the sinuses are usually not recommended for acute rhinosinusitis, as most are resolved within 12 weeks and/or after pharmacotherapy.

CHRONIC RHINOSINUSITIS

Chronic rhinosinusitis can develop if the cause of inflammation persists and steps are not taken to restore the conditions favoring normal physiologic function. Symptoms are milder than the ones in the acute phases with nasal congestion and olfactory disturbances more pronounced. In addition to the findings on physical examination of the patient with acute rhinosinusitis, effusion of the middle ear may be found on otoscopy (Fig. 83.1A,B).

It is important to determine whether infectious agents, allergens, or irritants are the primary etiology. Local structural deformities causing poor aeration of the sinuses may be predisposing to persistent infection. Decreased venous and lymphatic return can contribute to continued congestion and poor healing. CT of the sinuses is the imaging modality of choice for chronic rhinosinusitis. It can delineate an anatomic blockage at the ostiomeatal complex, which suggests the need for functional endoscopic surgery.

Treatment/Management

Treatment falls under several categories:

- Patient education/compliance
- Medication
- Musculoskeletal
- Surgical

Once the underlying pathophysiologic process has been determined, management in the four areas can be tailored to the patient's needs, keeping in mind the general goals of reducing edema and inflammation, promoting sinus drainage, and controlling infection.[19,20]

History is helpful in identifying patients with hypersensitivity to allergens, such as pollen or pet dander, or overexposure to common chemicals, such as formaldehyde and petroleum products. Chemical irritants, with tobacco smoke as the most prevalent, can cause inflammation of the respiratory mucosa. Smokers suffer from frequent inflammatory conditions of the nose and paranasal sinuses. Children living in a home where tobacco smoke is present

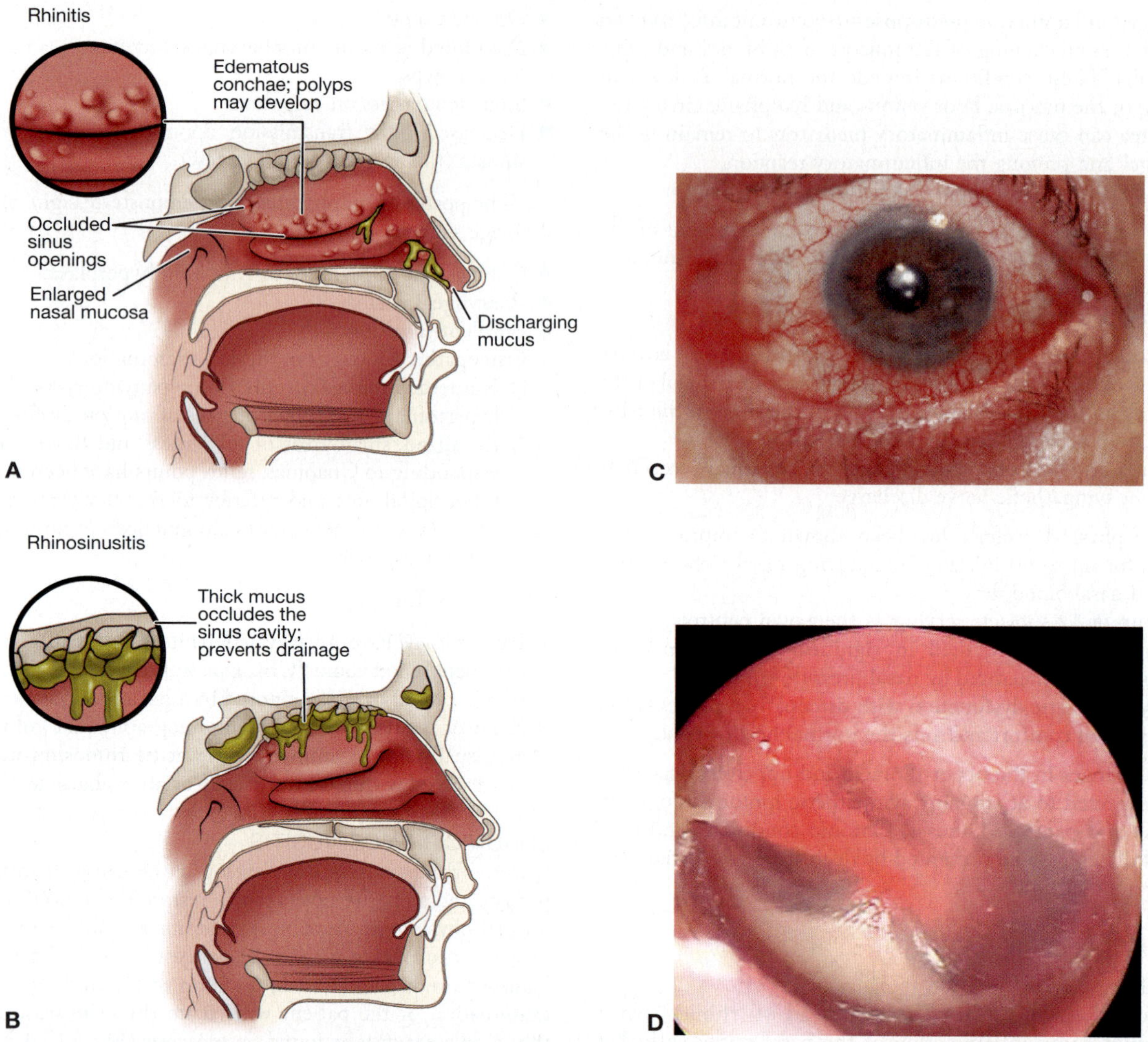

Figure 83.1. **A, B.** Pathophysiologic processes in rhinitis and rhinosinusitis. Although pathophysiologic processes are similar in rhinitis and rhinosinusitis, they affect different structures. **A.** In rhinitis, the mucous membranes lining the nasal passages become inflamed, congested, and edematous. The swollen nasal conchae block the sinus openings, and the mucus is discharged from the nostrils. **B.** Rhinosinusitis is also marked by inflammation and congestion, with thickened mucous secretions filling the sinus cavities and occluding the openings. (Reprinted with permission from Hinkle JL, Cheever KH. *Brunner & Suddarth's Textbook of Medical-Surgical Nursing*. 14th ed. Wolters Kluwer; 2018:554. Figure 22-1.) **C.** Allergic conjunctivitis. (Photo courtesy of Leonid Skorin Jr.) **D.** Videoendoscopy of one of the various middle ear states: acute otitis media with fluid level. (Courtesy of Alejandro Hoberman, MD, Children's Hospital of Pittsburgh of UPMC.)

are at high risk for developing respiratory disorders.[18] Patient education is essential and often needs to be ongoing. Judicious use of nicotine supplements and smoking cessation programs are helpful for some patients. Increasing awareness of potential exposure to allergens and irritants is often sufficient treatment; however, some cases require substantial lifestyle and occupation changes.

Promoting mucociliary clearance is essential to the overall treatment and prevention of complications. Patients should be instructed to drink warm, clear fluids to hydrate the mucous membranes and increase mucociliary clearance.[12] Dairy products are believed to thicken secretions in some patients and may not be recommended, especially in those with refractory symptoms.

When medications are used, they should be selected for specific reasons. Inflammation due to bacterial infection should be treated with appropriate antibiotics.

The most common bacteria involved in acute bacterial rhinosinusitis are:

- *Streptococcus pneumoniae*
- *Haemophilus influenzae*
- *Moraxella catarrhalis*

In chronic rhinosinusitis, anaerobes and *Staphylococcus aureus*, especially methicillin-resistant *Staphylococcus aureus*, may also be encountered.[21]

Pharmacotherapy

- Antibiotics such as amoxicillin–clavulanate and, for penicillin-allergic individuals, doxycycline, levofloxacin, and moxifloxacin are recommended for the treatment of acute bacterial rhinosinusitis.[22]

- Intranasal corticosteroids can be added to antibiotics especially if there is a history of atopy or nasal polyps and are often used as monotherapy for chronic rhinosinusitis. They help reduce edema and inflammation, thus promoting sinus drainage and increase nasal patency.
- A short course of oral corticosteroids may be recommended for an acute exacerbation of chronic rhinosinusitis.
- Oral and topical decongestants may be helpful in treating congestion and swelling, but both can lead to rebound swelling of the mucosa, which is known as "rhinitis medicamentosa"; therefore, they should be used short term in acute sinusitis.[23]
- Mucoactive agents, such as guaifenesin, hypertonic saline, and saturated solution of potassium iodide (SSKI), that alter the character, production, or movement of mucus may be helpful.[12]

If patient has a history of atopy, such as asthma or allergic rhinitis, antihistamines and cysteinyl leukotriene blockers may be of added benefit. No controlled clinical trials of antihistamines in rhinosinusitis exist, nor is histamine known to play a role in this disease.[12,20,24] Antihistamine side effects of overdrying the mucosa and slowing ciliary motion should be considered before use of these medications. For patients with concomitant allergic disease, the availability of antihistamines with less significant anticholinergic effects, such as loratadine, desloratadine, cetirizine, and fexofenadine, has made it possible to avoid some of these complications. See case study for further discussion.

Osteopathic Manipulative Treatment

The rationale for the use of osteopathic manipulation in sinus disease is to regulate myofascial constraint on venous and lymphatic flow and to alter somatovisceral reflexes to the sinuses.[19] Muscle activity is a recognized mechanism of increasing lymphatic flow.

- OMT to the neck, specifically those techniques involving muscle action (such as muscle energy and myofascial techniques), should contribute to increased lymphatic flow from the head.
- Because lymphatic channels are embedded in the cervical fascia, soft tissue technique treatment (see Chapters 50 and 54) to the cervical area may also serve to promote lymphatic circulation. The expected result would be reduced swelling of the sinus and nasal mucosa.
- Direct and indirect pressure techniques over the sinuses and sphenopalatine ganglion are described for assisting drainage of the sinuses.[18] With some of the lymphatic drainage leaving the nose and entering the lymphatics of the skin, direct pressure in this area would be expected to encourage lymphatic circulation.
- Rhythmic motion of the cranial bones as part of the cranial rhythmic impulse may be a significant factor in promoting sinus drainage. Following this line of thinking, treatment of dysfunctional motion patterns, particularly involving the maxillae, sphenoid, ethmoid, and frontal bones, should be part of sinusitis treatment (see Chapter 53).
- Ultimately, lymphatic fluid from the head and neck must enter the central circulation in the area of the subclavian and internal jugular veins. Somatic dysfunction of the structures in this area, including the upper ribs, upper thoracic spine, and clavicles, should be considered as a potential impediment to lymphatic flow (see Fig. 32.14).

The observation of somatovisceral reflexes by Sata and Schmidt[4,5] suggests the modulation of visceral function with various somatic stimuli. Somatic stimuli associated with somatic dysfunction of cervical and upper thoracic areas could impact the sympathetic vasomotor tone to the sinus area. One of the goals of OMT to this area would be to improve blood flow by altering the somatic component of this somatovisceral reflex.

Surgery

Obstruction due to local structural abnormalities may exist and needs to be evaluated on physical examination and, at times, with further diagnostic tests (CT and nasal endoscopy). In the presence of structural abnormalities, such as deviated septum, nasal polyps, enlarged turbinates, or obstruction of the sinus ostia, if conservative therapy fails to control recurrent infections, a surgical approach may be indicated.

Allergic Rhinitis

DIAGNOSIS

Allergic rhinitis is the inflammation of the nasal mucosa. It is an IgE-mediated reaction and consists of two steps:

1. The initial sensitization of allergen to nasal mucosa, results in specific IgE production, or antigen-specific IgE, with high-affinity receptor to mast cells and basophils.
2. The subsequent exposure to same allergens causes release of both preformed and newly synthesized mediators. This step consists of an early- and late-phase response[25]:
   - The early phase occurs within minutes due to preformed mediators and is characterized by itching, rhinorrhea, and sneezing.
   - The late phase occurs within hours after cellular influx of basophils, eosinophils, neutrophils, and mononuclear cells in addition to more mast cells, characterized by nasal congestion.[26]

Allergic rhinitis shows seasonal variation or seasonal allergic rhinitis, or annual recurrent or perennial allergic rhinitis.

Common allergens of seasonal allergic rhinitis include pollen from:

- Trees
- Grasses
- Weeds
- Ragweeds

Year-round symptoms suggest indoor allergens. Common allergens of perennial allergic rhinitis include:

- Cockroaches
- Dust mites
- Feathers
- Molds
- Pet dander

Clinical Manifestations

- Itching
- Rhinorrhea (anterior and posterior)
- Nasal congestion
- Sneezing
- Ocular symptoms often coexist such as ocular pruritus, increased lacrimation, and redness of the conjunctiva.

Physical Examination

- Engorgement of the turbinates, which appear pale or violaceous rather than erythematous, as in infectious rhinitis
- Nasal polyps as semitranslucent, gray to yellow-brown, boggy masses of mucosa
- Signs of chronic rhinorrhea and postnasal drainage with increased secretions from the nasal, lacrimal, and submandibular glands due to parasympathetic hyperactivity[27]

- Osteopathic findings on physical examination
  - Dysfunction of the facial, glossopharyngeal, and vagus nerve
  - Cranial, thoracic, and cervical somatic dysfunction

While the history and symptoms guide the clinician to making the diagnosis of allergic rhinitis, allergy testing is necessary for definitive diagnosis and treatment. Allergy tests such as skin prick/intradermal testing or fluorescence enzyme immunoassay, for example, ImmunoCAP, can determine the specific allergen and thus provide a target for treatment.

TREATMENT/MANAGEMENT

Addressing the specific allergic cause is essential to effective and lasting treatment. Obtaining a thorough history is important as it cues the clinician in on the suspected allergen as well as revealing other atopic disorders such as asthma. Studies have shown strong association between allergic rhinitis, chronic rhinosinusitis, and asthma, demonstrating the concept of "united airway disease" where the upper and lower airway are viewed as a single organ and its disorders share a connection.[28] Management of allergic rhinitis can potentially reduce the exacerbation and severity of asthma.

The primary treatment is avoidance of known allergens. Environmental control is an important part of treating HEENT disease with an allergic etiology. For dust mite allergy, this includes using high-efficiency particulate arrestance (HEPA) filters on noncarpeted floor, dehumidifiers, and air conditioners, pillows and mattress cover with plastic or fine woven fabric and washing linens in hot water every 1 to 2 weeks.[29] For pollen allergy, avoiding prolonged exposure outdoors during days of high pollen count minimizes symptoms. Removal of the offending allergen when it comes to pet dander allergy can be nonpractical and emotionally difficult for patients but limiting exposure to pet dander such as removing pet from bedroom or bathing pet/using pet wipes regularly can be beneficial.

Chemical, inflammatory mediators also travel to the nasal mucosa and induce a non–IgE-mediated inflammatory response causing the symptoms of allergic rhinitis. Reducing swelling by promoting venous and lymphatic circulation and decreasing the concentration of chemical, inflammatory mediators in the interstitial tissues is particularly important in managing the disease. Avoidance of inciting allergens and particulate matters requires educating and encouraging the patient who may become discouraged by the demanding lifestyle changes.

Allergic rhinitis can also be managed by pharmacotherapy and osteopathic manipulative medicine and treated by allergen-specific immunotherapy (AIT).

Pharmacotherapy

- Nasal saline
  - Intranasal nasal saline is offered through different delivery systems, such as spray or irrigation.
  - It moisturizes dry nasal passages and enhances the clearing of the mucus.
- Antihistamines
  - Antihistamines block the effects of histamine, preventing pruritus, vasodilation, and bronchoconstriction.
  - Selective H1 antihistamines minimize the mucosal drying effect of anticholinergics and offer a safer option for treating the allergic component of HEENT problems.[12]
  - First-generation H1 antihistamines have sedative effects.
  - Second-generation H1 antihistamines have minimal sedative effects.
  - Intranasal H1 antihistamines, such as azelastine and olopatadine, the latter also exhibiting mast cell inhibiting properties, have a direct interaction with the nasal mucosa with faster onset of action than oral antihistamines.[30]
- Decongestants
  - Oral decongestants mainly alleviate nasal congestion and often are combined with an oral antihistamine for maximal relief of symptoms.
  - Intranasal decongestants, such as phenylephrine and oxymetazoline, have a faster onset of action than oral decongestants, however with a higher risk of rebound congestion, or rhinitis medicamentosa.[31,32]
  - They can be considered for up to 3 to 5 days of use in those with severe mucosa edema which inhibits the delivery of other intranasal agents.[32]
- Corticosteroids
  - Intranasal corticosteroids are indicated in moderate to severe cases or if symptoms persist despite use of other agents.
  - They are highly effective in reducing the local inflammation and associated symptoms.
  - They may require from 3 days to 2 weeks of regular use for symptomatic improvement.
  - A short course of oral steroids of about 5 to 7 days should be used cautiously and reserved for severe and/or recalcitrant cases.
- Mast cell stabilizer
  - Sodium cromoglycate (cromolyn sodium) has a suppressive effect on other inflammatory cells.
  - It is best used prophylactically for allergic rhinitis and may also require regular use over 1 to 2 weeks for benefits to become apparent.[33]
- Leukotriene inhibitor
  - Montelukast is an oral leukotriene receptor antagonist that is reserved for severe symptoms or in patients with intolerance to alternative therapies as serious neuropsychiatric events have been reported.

Osteopathic Manipulative Treatment

Osteopathic manipulative techniques with soft tissue and myofascial release of the corresponding area of somatic dysfunction can be used, such as supraorbital and infraorbital massage and nasion gapping. Techniques targeting lymphatic drainage such as periauricular drainage and Chapman reflex for ear and/or sinuses can also be implemented. Cranial OMT including CV4 technique and occipitoatlantal release are used for decreased cranial rhythm impulses and vagus nerve, respectively.[27]

ALLERGEN-SPECIFIC IMMUNOTHERAPY

AIT such as subcutaneous immunotherapy (SCIT) is a definitive treatment. AIT is the only curative therapy for allergic rhinitis and has shown to be effective in altering immunologic response. It improves the quality of life and decreases the use and cost of medications.

There are two ways AIT can be performed:

1. SCIT requires regular subcutaneous injections of the allergen, from the initial weekly injections (build-up phase) to the maintenance monthly injections (maintenance phase). A duration of at least 3 to 5 years of continuous SCIT is required for the treatment to be effective.[34]
2. Sublingual immunotherapy (SLIT) is given in a liquid form, and it is more effective at treating patients with a single environmental allergen. This procedure also requires a long-term commitment with efficacy shown when therapy is continued for at least 3 years.[34]

EYES

Common Pathophysiology

Besides visual impairments such as loss of acuity, accommodation, or color vision caused by primary disorders of the eyes, ocular disease and symptoms can also arise due to somatic dysfunction and associated head and neck disorders.

Orbital bone restriction, through fascial connections, contributes to venous and lymphatics stasis, which leads to dysfunction of the ocular tissues of the eyelids, conjunctiva, cornea, lacrimal glands, optic nerves, and extraocular muscles[35] and causes or worsens disorders of the head and neck.[36] Obstruction to the jugular foramen due to occipital bone dysfunction, for example, occipitomastoid compression, can lead to poor or obstructed flow of venous drainage and subsequent buildup of pressure to the orbit.[37]

Due to the proximity to the sinuses and its thin bony structure, the medial portion of the orbit is prone to pathologic thinning. It is susceptible to the spread of infection, inflammation, and neoplasms from the sinuses.

The nasolacrimal canal holds the nasolacrimal duct, which connects the lacrimal sac to the inferior nasal meatus. This anatomical link may explain the association of allergic rhinitis with allergic conjunctivitis.

Allergic Conjunctivitis

DIAGNOSIS

Allergic conjunctivitis is an IgE-mediated hypersensitivity reaction. It is caused by the exposure of the allergen, or antigen, to the conjunctival epithelium. It is followed by the release and infiltration of inflammatory mediators such as histamine, tryptase, and arachidonic acid metabolites, to the site of exposure.[38]

Based on the occurrences of symptoms, allergic conjunctivitis, like allergic rhinitis, is classified as either seasonal, with symptoms predominately during the spring or fall, or perennial, with year-round symptoms.

A personal and family history of atopy should also be obtained due to its association with allergic rhinitis, atopic dermatitis, and asthma.[39]

Clinical Manifestations

- Watery eyes
- Ocular pruritus
- Periorbital swelling
- The visual acuity is preserved in both seasonal and perennial allergic conjunctivitis

Physical Examination (Fig. 83.1C)

- Conjunctival injection
- Edema of the lid and conjunctiva
- Ocular discharge, usually white and stringy
- Mast cells and eosinophils predominate within the conjunctival epithelium in histology
- Osteopathic findings on physical examination include:
    - Orbital bone dysfunction (any of the seven bones that constitute the orbit)
    - Occipital bone dysfunction
    - Cranial strain patterns
    - Head and neck muscle dysfunction (cervical, occipital, and sternocleidomastoid muscle) affecting lymphatic drainage

TREATMENT/MANAGEMENT

Avoidance of known allergen is paramount in the management of allergic conjunctivitis. Patient education on the identified allergen and the use of topical lubricating agents such as artificial tears limit exposure to allergens and reduce the amount of already exposed allergens.[40]

Topical antihistamines, mast cell stabilizers, and antiallergic agents targeting various pathways, or multimodal agents are used to mediate the hypersensitive, inflammatory response. For refractory or severe ocular symptoms, topical vasoconstrictors, nonsteroidal anti-inflammatory drugs (NSAIDs), and corticosteroids may be used and referral to an ophthalmologist is generally recommended. Moreover, AIT may be beneficial in severe cases of allergic conjunctivitis.

Osteopathic Manipulative Treatment

Evidence-based literature concerning manual manipulation in general (OMT, massage therapy, and chiropractic work) and conjunctivitis remains limited. Sherman et al. cited the dearth of literature for osteopathic manipulation in ophthalmologic conditions including keratoconjunctivitis sicca and cephalgia from asthenopia, or eye strain, and provided descriptions and rationale for each disorder.[41] In keratoconjunctivitis sicca, or dry eye syndrome, the sphenopalatine ganglia release has been found to induce lacrimation by applying pressure to the parasympathetic sphenopalatine ganglia, thus stimulating the trigeminal nerve.[41] In allergic conjunctivitis, the opposite symptom of watery eyes occurs.

There remain no published studies to date on the direct effect of OMT on allergic conjunctivitis.

- Hom and Bielroy postulated the possibility of using techniques to normalize the parasympathetic tone under the ocular neurogenic inflammation phenomenon.[42]
    - They noted that ocular neurogenic inflammation may be direct, through the progression of electromagnetic potential, or indirect, through the stimulation of neurotransmitter release.
    - Mast cells degranulate, thereby releasing histamine that activates sensory receptors. The brain receives sensory information from the conjunctiva and then releases more histamine from the conjunctival substantia propria. This process is termed neurogenic inflammation.
    - Understanding the role of neurogenic inflammation and histamine release provides a rationale for osteopathic application of using OMT to normalize parasympathetic activity.
- As the allergic inflammatory response plays a key role in the pathogenesis and the resulting clinical manifestations of allergic conjunctivitis, OMT may be used to reduce lymphatic congestion.
    - The osteopathic technique of effleurage can promote lymphatic drainage and reduce the swelling that is accompanied by the inflammatory process.
    - Effleurage over the eyelid and periorbital area is often beneficial in cases where edema is present in the eyelid and/or sclera.[43]
    - This technique is contraindicated in patients who wear contacts or have foreign body in eyes.[43]
- In addition, the "naso-ocular reflex" suggests OMT benefiting nasal conditions, that is, allergic rhinitis, will also provide ocular relief.
    - The nasolacrimal duct links the structures of the nose and the eyes, and thus a relationship between the nose and the eyes exists.[44]
    - The naso-ocular reflex implies that tear production and conjunctival erythema result from nasal stimulation.[45,46]
    - Both the physiologic response and manual manipulation affecting these pathways remain valuable areas of future research.

TABLE 83.2

Common Disorders of the Ear

Hearing loss Sensorineural Conductive
External canal obstruction Impacted cerumen Exostoses/chondromas Foreign bodies
External otitis Bacterial Fungal
Otitis media Acute With effusion
Mastoiditis
Tinnitus
Vertigo/dizziness

EARS

Common Pathophysiology

The ear is subject to numerous types of disorders involving the external, middle, or inner ear (Table 83.2). It can be affected by infection and inflammation and by neurologic and vascular problems. Pain, hearing loss, vertigo, and tinnitus are some symptoms associated with these processes. The sensory innervation to the ear is derived from the:

- Trigeminal
- Facial
- Glossopharyngeal
- Vagal
- Upper cervical nerves

Therefore, otalgia is frequently a result of referred pain from other areas of the head and neck. Temporomandibular joint (TMJ) dysfunction and cervical dysfunction are common causes of ear pain.

The external ear is subject to infections, especially if persistently exposed to a moist environment. The vestibular function of the inner ear can be disturbed because of infection or neurologic or vascular impairment. Hearing loss can be due to various disturbances in the middle ear or due to neurologic deficits. Chronic exposure to loud noise contributes to hearing loss (sensorineural) by traumatic damage to the receptors in the cochlea. Infectious and inflammatory processes in the eustachian tube and middle ear are common causes of temporary hearing loss and ear pain.

Auditory (Eustachian) Tube Dysfunction

ETIOLOGY AND PATHOPHYSIOLOGY

- Upper respiratory infections and allergy, with mucosal inflammation and lymphoid hyperplasia, may lead to eustachian tube dysfunction.
- Persistent obstruction of the auditory tube pressure-equalizing system results in increasing negative pressure and decreased ventilation in the middle ear.
- Under these conditions, nasopharyngeal secretions and microorganisms could be aspirated into the middle ear, impairing drainage, and causing infection.
- Reflux of nasopharyngeal contents into the middle ear is more likely when swallowing occurs in the supine position.
    - ☐ Conventional non- or undervented feeding bottles have been associated with increased incidence of otitis media[47] (see Chapter 67 Osteopathic Considerations in Pediatrics for further discussion, including case presentation and literature review).
- The lowered PaO_2 impedes granulocyte formation, and bacterial colonization frequently results.
- Factors such as enlarged adenoids can aggravate the pooling of secretions in the middle ear.

Middle ear effusion can accompany acute infections and persist over several weeks or months. It is usually associated with temporary hearing loss and, when present over extended periods, may lead to delays in receptive and expressive language development that can persist into late childhood and early teens.[48,49] Attendance at day-care programs, exposure to environmental allergens, and second-hand tobacco smoke increase the risk of middle ear infections.[50]

Otitis Media

DIAGNOSIS

Infection of the middle ear, or otitis media, is among the most common childhood diseases encountered in primary care. The incidence may be increasing with larger numbers of children attending day-care centers. Acute otitis media often follows an upper respiratory infection.

ACUTE OTITIS MEDIA

Clinical Manifestations

- Otalgia
- Hearing loss
- Fever
- Purulent drainage
- Irritability, insomnia, and tugging at the ear in children

Physical Examination

- Bulging and erythematous tympanic membrane, not only including the pars tensa, but also the pars flaccida (Fig. 83.1D)
- Decreased mobility of tympanic membrane with pneumatic otoscopy

CHRONIC OTITIS MEDIA

After resolution of the acute infection, effusion may persist in the middle ear.

Clinical Manifestations

- Painless hearing loss
- Postnasal drainage
- Tenderness below pinna near angle of the jaw (if accompanied by eustachian tube dysfunction)

Physical Exam

- Persistent effusion (may have presence of bubbles or air–fluid level)
- Dull, often retracted tympanic membrane
- Inflammation of nasopharyngeal mucosa
- Lymphadenopathy
- Osteopathic findings on physical exam:
    - ☐ Cervical soft tissue tenderness
    - ☐ Upper thoracic tenderness
    - ☐ Cranial dysfunction, particularly involving the temporal bones, is frequently seen[2,36]

The presence of fluid that is of a noninfectious etiology may also be present in the middle ear, or otitis media with effusion (OME). OME often occurs after an episode of acute otitis media or after an upper respiratory tract infection due to inflammatory changes or eustachian tube dysfunction. Vestibular disturbances, for example, dizziness, arise in chronic OME (see below).

TREATMENT/MANAGEMENT

Recognizing the causes of eustachian tube dysfunction is critical to the treatment and prevention of otitis media. Allergic manifestations, such as red, itchy eyes and persistent, clear nasal discharge, suggest further allergic workup. Dietary questions regarding food intolerances or infant colic may suggest the influence of food sensitivities. Control of the allergic aspect of inflammation needs to be considered and discussed with the patient or the patient's family.

Current clinical practice guidelines for OME (indicated for patients 2 months through 12 years of age) from HEENT specialists include the following[51]:

- Strong recommendations
  - □ Perform pneumatic otoscopy to document the presence of middle ear effusion with pneumatic otoscopy when diagnosing OME in a child and to assess for OME in a child with otalgia, hearing loss, or both.
  - □ Obtain tympanometry in children with suspected OME whom the diagnosis is uncertain after performing pneumatic otoscopy.
  - □ Children with OME who are not at risk may be managed with watchful waiting for 3 months from the date of diagnosis.
  - □ Recommend against using intranasal or systemic steroids for treating OME.
  - □ Recommend against using systemic antibiotics for treating OME.
  - □ Recommend against using antihistamines, decongestants, or both for treating OME.

Enlarged tonsils or adenoids are a cause of poor auditory tube drainage. Swallowing and chewing open the auditory tube and can be suggested as exercises for patients to help clear middle ear effusion.[52] Allergy, as well as infection, may play a role in the enlargement of these lymphoid organs. If acute bacterial infection is the cause, it should be appropriately treated with antibiotics, considering the common pathogens—*S. pneumoniae, H. influenzae,* and *Streptococcus pyogenes.*

Informing patients and families about practices that predispose them to ear problems is part of total patient care. In the well-baby examination, the opportunity often exists to discuss infant feeding and avoidance of bottle feeding in the supine position. It is appropriate to encourage parents to protect their children from passive tobacco smoke.

There are conflicting views regarding treatment of acute otitis media.[53] It is generally held that prolonged hearing loss, especially in certain developmental stages, is detrimental to development of language and, possibly, reading skills. Therefore, attention needs to be paid to recurrent or chronic otitis media.

Osteopathic Manipulative Treatment

Several manipulative techniques have been described to specifically address improved lymphatic and venous drainage from the head and neck.[16,54,55] Osteopathic manipulation for the treatment of general respiratory infections should include techniques to[56]:

1. Increase lymphatic flow
2. Address viscerosomatic and somatovisceral reflexes
3. Improve thoracic cage motion
   - □ Galbreath mandibular drainage is easily performed and may provide considerable benefit in reducing the congestion that leads to a chronic condition.[54,55]
   - □ Normalizing cervical muscle tone by treating specific cervical somatic dysfunction or using soft tissue techniques may allow for improved lymphatic drainage from around the auditory tube. Infectious processes benefit from improved blood flow, which is necessary for healing and delivery of medications.
   - □ Arterial blood flow to the ears should be optimized by addressing the effect of somatic dysfunction in the upper thoracic and cervical areas on vasomotor tone. Techniques such as rib raising, and lymphatic pump can provide a more general approach to increasing lymphatic circulation and reducing congestion and inflammation in the ears.
   - □ Treatment of specific rib dysfunctions may offer a longer-lasting improvement in lymphatic flow.
   - □ Treatment of temporal bone and TMJ dysfunction (especially the medial pterygoid muscle dysfunction) may restore normal exit of fluids from the middle ear through the eustachian tube.

Recent studies provide evidence of clinical improvement in children with acute otitis media regarding decreased use of antibiotics, decreased number of infections, decreased need for surgical tube placement, and improved tympanograms.[57]

Vertigo

RELEVANT FUNCTIONAL ANATOMY AND PHYSIOLOGY

Balance is a whole-body experience that depends on the interaction of and processing of information from multiple sources. There are three primary sensory inputs to the balance system:

1. Vestibular (inner ear)
2. Visual
3. Proprioceptive

Central processing of balance-related information takes place in the vestibular nuclear complex and cerebellum. Motor output, primarily to the eyes and postural muscle, helps the body react to balance issues (Fig. 83.2).

VESTIBULAR SYSTEM

The vestibular system consists of the bony and membranous labyrinth, including its blood and nerve supply.

- The bony portion contains peri lymphatic fluid (somewhat like cerebral spinal fluid), in which the membranous structures are suspended. The bony complex is housed in the temporal bones bilaterally and consists of the following as depicted in Figure 83.3.
- Cochlea (responsible for hearing)
- Semicircular canals
  1. The semicircular canals are three in number, each having a widened end called the "ampulla" where the sensory hair cells that are sensitive to rotational movement of the head are located.
  2. The semicircular canals are oriented perpendicular to each other, like the floor and two adjacent walls of a rectangular room.
  3. Pairing of the bilateral structures, in mirror image fashion, allows detection of motion in any direction.
  4. Their arrangement corresponds closely to the pulling directions of the extraocular muscles.
  5. Information from the semicircular canals helps the eyes remain still in space as the head moves, making clear vision possible.

Figure 83.2. Sensorimotor integration for balance—sensory input, central processing, and motor output.

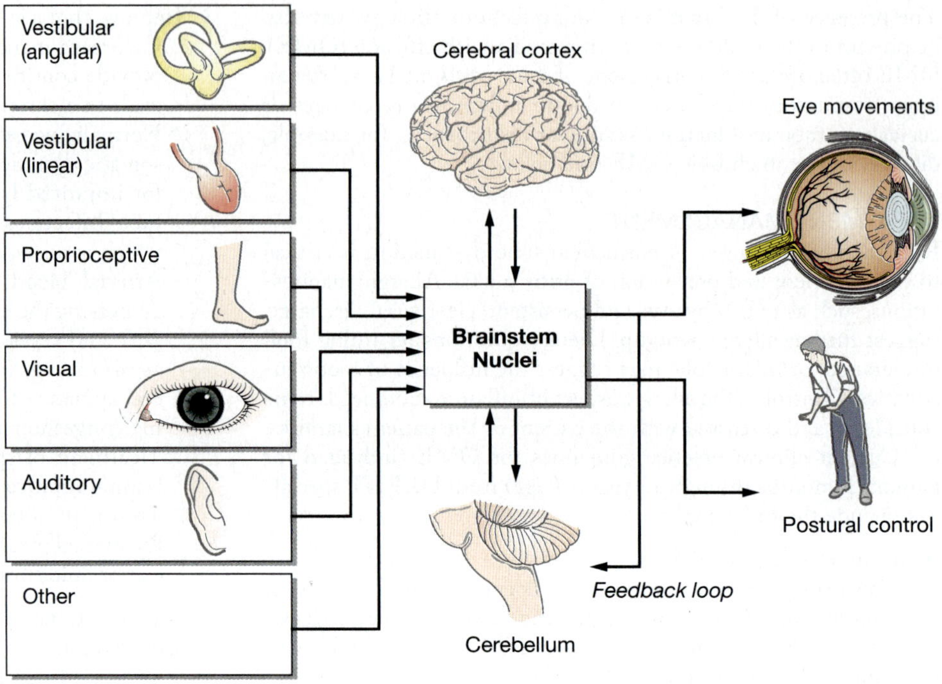

- Central chamber or vestibule
- The membranous labyrinth contains endolymphatic fluid (similar to intracellular fluid) and specialized sensory hair cells, responsible for the neural firing of the labyrinth (Fig. 83.4).
  1. The utricle and saccule are sensory organs of the membranous labyrinth.
  2. They are located in the vestibule and contain calcium carbonate crystals called otoconia, in addition to sensory hair cells.
  3. Their arrangement (the saccule is vertical, while the utricle is horizontal) along with the mass of the otoconia makes these otolithic organs sensitive to gravity and linear acceleration (Fig. 83.5).

Afferent signals from the labyrinth are carried by the vestibular nerve, which courses along with the cochlear nerve, facial nerve, and labyrinthine artery, through the internal auditory canal of the petrous portion of the temporal bone. The vestibular nerve enters the brain stem at the pontomedullary junction, and its information goes to the cerebellum and vestibular nuclear complex.

Arterial blood supply to the labyrinth is from the vertebral basilar system. The labyrinthine artery usually is a branch of the anterior inferior cerebellar artery but may be a direct branch from the basilar. Its branches supply the cochlea, semicircular canals, utricle, saccule, ampulla, and vestibular nerve. There is no collateral circulation, making the labyrinth very susceptible to ischemia and disruption of blood flow.

Figure 83.3. Vestibular complex housed in temporal bones.

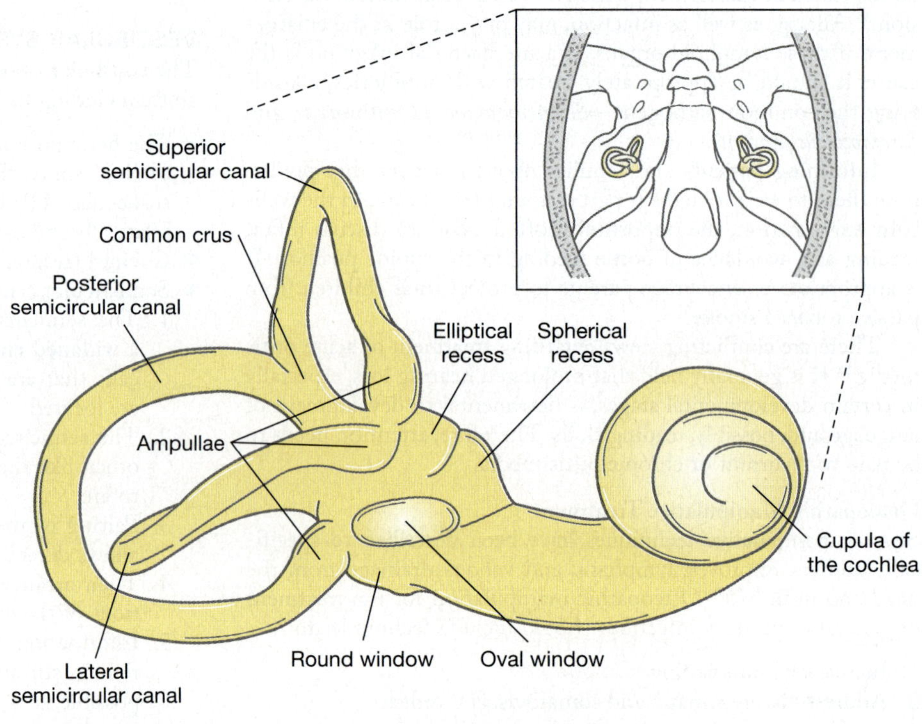

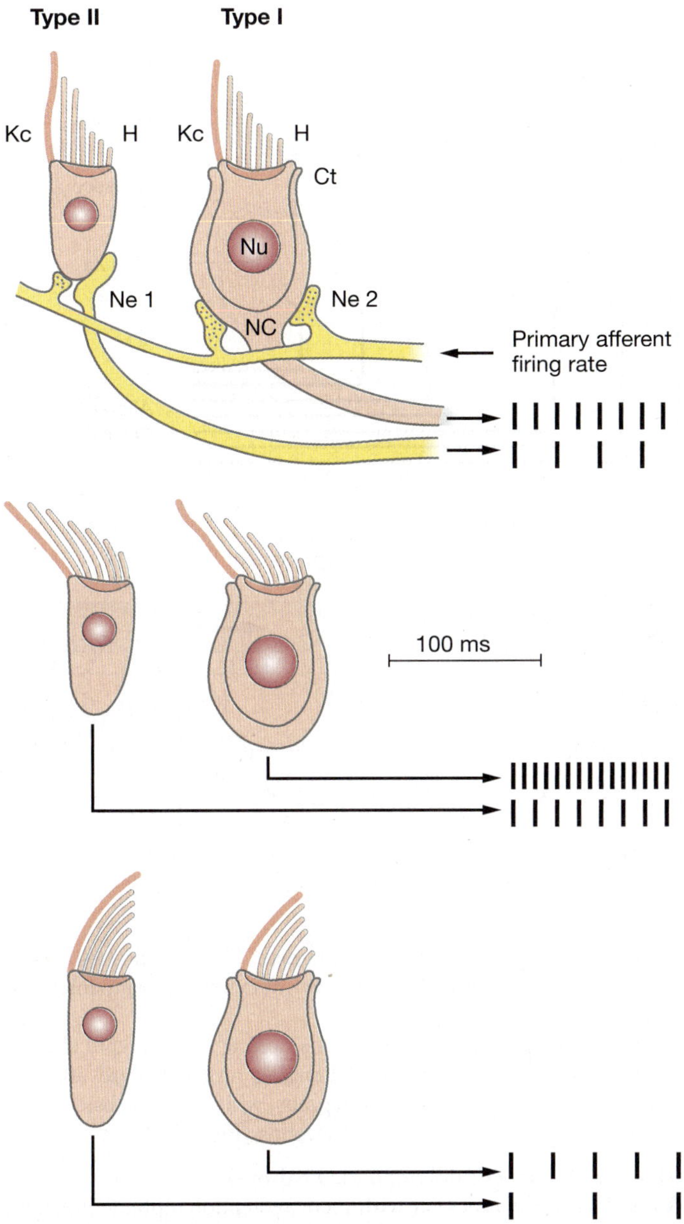

Figure 83.4. Specialized, sensory hair cells of the membranous labyrinth are deflected during head movement.

VISUAL AND PROPRIOCEPTIVE SYSTEMS

- Visual information is processed along with that from the vestibular system and all the proprioceptors of the body to determine position in space.
- Proprioceptive input from postural muscles, related fascia, joints, and ligaments is all interpreted, but information from the ankles and neck is especially important in balance control.

CENTRAL PROCESSING

- The vestibular nuclear complex (four major and seven minor nuclei) in the pons and medulla is the primary processor of the information from the above sources. It provides fast and direct connection between incoming information and motor output response.
- The cerebellum serves as an adaptive processor:
  - Acts as a modulator and monitor
  - Fine tunes and make adjustments to the system
  - Regulates various reflexes responsible for balance. This is due to interactions between the vestibular nuclear complex and the cerebellum.

The balance function of the brain stem and cerebellum depends on symmetrical, accurate, and consistent information from its sensory sources. It can, however, compensate for some missing information by using information from other sources. Generally, compensation is possible if two of the three sources are functioning properly, even though this may require some adaptation over time.

REFLEXES

Vestibulo-Ocular Reflex

Using information from the semicircular canals and otoliths (saccule and utricle), the vestibulo-ocular reflex (VOR) provides clear vision during head motion. Motor impulses to the extraocular eye muscles generate eye movement compensatory to head movement.

Vestibulospinal Reflex

The vestibulospinal reflex (VSR) is more complex than the VOR as it functions to stabilize the body and prevent falling. Motor impulses are sent to skeletal muscles, in response to information reaching the vestibular nuclear complex and cerebellum. This information is then used to carry out strategies to maintain upright posture. These may include several complex interactions such as:

- Stepping forward
- Flexing the ankles
- Grabbing a stable object

Vestibulocollic Reflex

Vestibulocollic reflex (VCR) acts to stabilize the neck in response to vestibular output. This reflex could explain the neck pain sometimes experienced with diseases of the inner ear. This would be considered a viscerosomatic reflex.

Cervico-Ocular Reflex

Stimuli from neck ligaments, muscles, and joints cause a responsive movement of the eyes. This cervico-ocular reflex (COR) interacts with the VOR. Normally, the gain of the COR is very low.

DIAGNOSIS

The complaint of dizziness is common, especially in the primary care and emergency department setting. Dizziness is used by patients to describe a variety of symptoms including:

- Light-headedness
- Feeling faint, weak, or unsteady
- Sensation that the room is spinning
- Giddiness or the feeling that one's head is spinning
- Vertigo or the sensation of movement, usually spinning, rotating, or whirling.

Vertigo is associated with dysfunction in the vestibular system. Disequilibrium, imbalance, or unsteadiness only occurs when walking or standing and may or may not be accompanied by vertigo.

Certain conditions or dysfunctions have warranted specific names and are associated with distinct presentations that will be discussed below:

- Cervicogenic vertigo
- Acute labyrinthitis
- Benign paroxysmal positional vertigo (BPPV)
- Meniere disease
- Acoustic neuroma
- OME

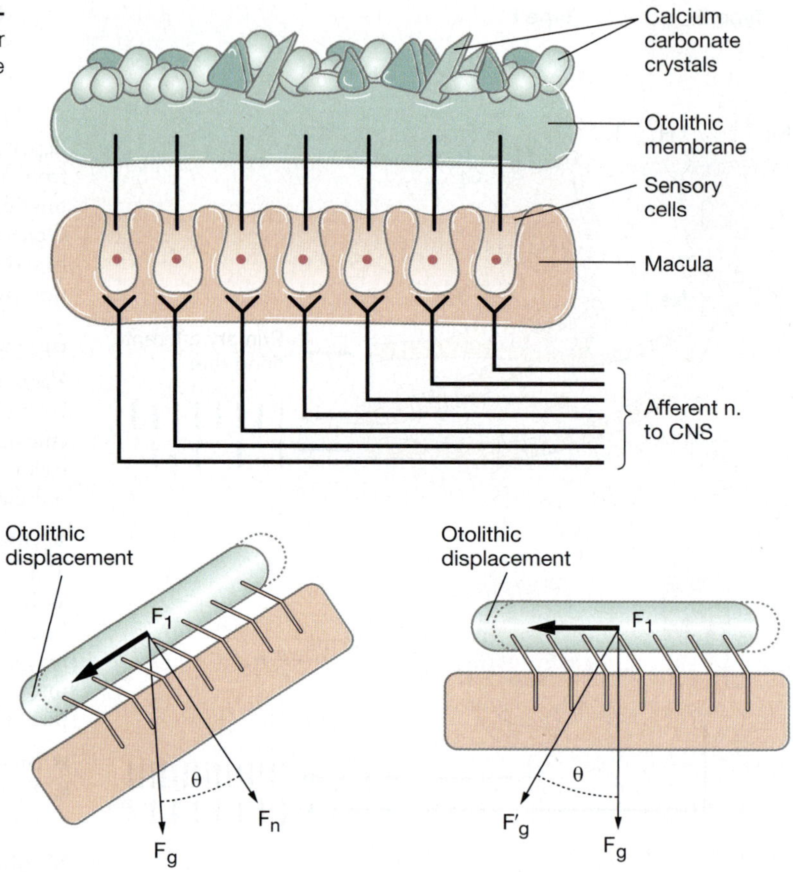

Figure 83.5. **Otolithic membrane in the utricle and saccule is embedded with calcium carbonate crystals.** Linear acceleration or change with respect to gravity causes the membrane to shift and trigger underlying hair cells.

Cervicogenic Vertigo

Many people have reported symptoms of dizziness, unsteadiness, and imbalance following neck injury, especially with whiplash-associated disorder (WAD). The symptoms are concurrent with neck pain and stiffness and are made worse by neck movement. There is no accompanying hearing loss or tinnitus, but nausea may occur. Somatic dysfunctions are typically found in the head, cervical and thoracic regions, and the lumbar, sacral, pelvic, costal cage, and extremities regions in cases of postwhiplash injury, as depicted in the case study below.

Acute Labyrinthitis

Inflammation or infection of the inner ear may occur alone or in combination with a viral or, less commonly, a bacterial infection. In acute labyrinthitis, the patient complains of sudden onset of severe vertigo. It is accompanied by:

- Hearing loss
- Tinnitus
- Nausea
- Vomiting
- Nystagmus

The acute episode lasts 24 to 48 hours. The condition slowly resolves with several days of disequilibrium and motion-induced vertigo, followed by slow improvement over several weeks.

Benign Paroxysmal Positional Vertigo

BPPV is thought to be caused by debris in the endolymph of the posterior semicircular canal. It presents with episodic vertigo brought on by changes in head position. Patients often report rolling over in bed or rapid neck extension precipitating symptoms. The episodes last 30 seconds to 2 minutes and will subside even if the offending position is maintained. There is no associated hearing loss or tinnitus, but rotatory nystagmus accompanies the vertigo.

Performing the Dix–Hallpike positioning test—a rapid change from sitting to lying, with head hanging turned toward affected side—brings on vertigo and nystagmus, which then subside after holding the position for 10 to 40 seconds (Fig. 83.6).

Ménière Disease (Endolymphatic Hydrops)

A disorder of the inner ear with increased endolymphatic pressure, Ménière disease, can cause devastating vestibular symptoms and hearing loss.

- Initial symptoms:
    - ☐ Pressure in the ear
    - ☐ Reduced hearing
    - ☐ Tinnitus
- Secondary symptoms:
    - ☐ Severe vertigo
    - ☐ Nausea
    - ☐ Vomiting

Severe symptoms can last 30 minutes to 24 hours. Intensity of symptoms diminishes over several days. Unsteadiness may persist for weeks. Hearing loss and tinnitus may gradually improve, or sensorineural loss may be permanent. As the disease progresses, attacks continue with continuation of hearing loss, but the severity of vertigo may decrease.

Acoustic Neuroma (Vestibular Schwannoma)

Schwannoma of the eighth cranial nerve causes unilateral sensorineural hearing loss and tinnitus. Vertigo, when it occurs, is not an early symptom and is usually short lived, replaced by a sense of

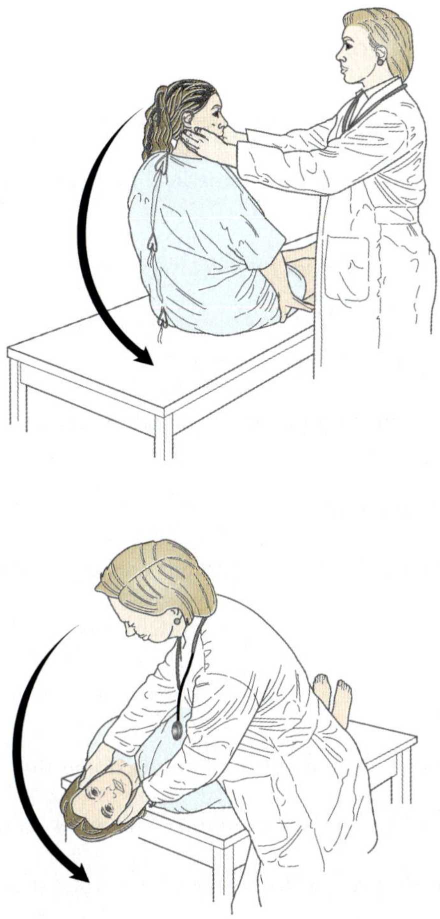

Figure 83.6. Dix–Hallpike maneuver for detecting BPPV.

imbalance or disequilibrium. Suspicion of acoustic neuroma should be followed up with an MRI of the internal auditory canal with gadolinium contrast.

Otitis Media with Effusion

OME is the presence of fluid in the middle ear without acute ear infection. Acute otitis media is a rapid onset of inflammation of the middle ear usually caused by viral or bacterial infection. OME may occur after an episode of acute otitis media or an upper respiratory infection due to an inflammatory response or impaired eustachian tube function. Its presenting symptom may only be dizziness.

TREATMENT/MANAGEMENT

- *Cervicogenic vertigo*—Manual therapy and exercises have been shown to be effective (see case study).
- *Acute Labyrinthitis*—Self-limiting; symptomatic treatment; OMT may reduce duration.
- *BPPV*—Self-limiting and responds to vestibular exercises and particle repositioning maneuvers (see Fig. 83.7 and Box 83.1).
- *Meniere disease*—Medical or surgical management may include:
  - □ Medication: Betahistine, diuretics, or transtympanic injection of corticosteroids or gentamicin (see case study for further discussion).
  - □ Surgery: Endolymphatic sac surgery, vestibular neurotomy, and labyrinthectomy
- *Acoustic neuroma*—Surgical removal
- *OME*—Self-limiting; symptomatic treatment; OMT may reduce duration (see case study Chapter 100 for further information).

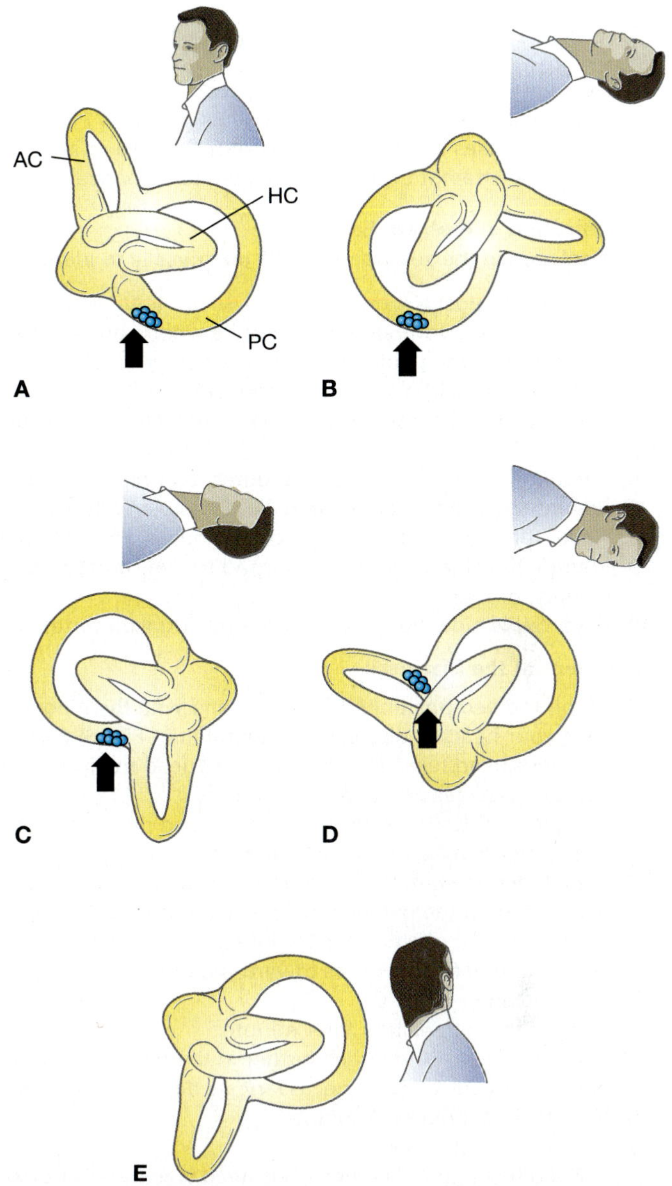

Figure 83.7. Particle repositioning treatment for BPPV may be performed by physician and taught to patients. A to **E** depict the steps used to move the particle as explained in Box 83.1. AC, anterior (superior) canal; HC, horizontal canal; PC, posterior canal.

THROAT/PHARYNX

Common Pathophysiology

A variety of pathologic processes can occur in the pharynx (Table 83.3), but infection is the most common. Group A beta-hemolytic streptococci and viruses are the common infectious agents. *Neisseria gonorrhoeae, Mycoplasma,* and *Chlamydia trachomatis* are also considerations. Viral infections may cause ulcerative lesions of the tongue, lips, or buccal mucosa. Herpes simplex virus is responsible for herpes labialis or cold sores.

Oral candidiasis (thrush) is commonly encountered in:

- Denture wearers
- Patients on corticosteroids or broad-spectrum antibiotics
- Diabetics
- Immunocompromised patients (as by acquired immunodeficiency syndrome [AIDS], chemotherapy, or local radiation)

BOX 83.1 Patient Education: Self-Treatment of Dizziness from BPPV

- These instructions accompany the illustrations in Figure 83.7. Refer to these diagrams while reading these instructions.
- These exercises can be best done with the help of an assistant.
- If on initial attempt of these exercises the response is too severe to continue, the prescribed medication may be used.

Identification of Problem Ear

The first step in the self-treatment of dizziness is to identify the side of the poorly functioning ear. This is done as follows:

1. Identify the position on a firm bed where you can lie back without hitting anything.
2. Identify where your shoulders will lie when you lie back in the bed.
3. Place a midsized pillow on the bed where your shoulders will land when you lie back in the bed.
4. Position yourself in the bed as above.
5. Lower yourself with your shoulders contacting the pillow and your head contacting the bed and your head turned to the left.
6. Remain in that position for 2 minutes, and record your feelings.
7. Repeat the above maneuver in No. 5; however, this time turn your head to the right.
8. Again remain in that position for 2 minutes, and record your feelings.
9. Identify the side your head is turned to, which produced the most uncomfortable feelings whether they be dizziness, anxiety, or fear.
10. Record this side that produced the most uncomfortable feelings.

Treatment of the Dizziness

1. Sit on the bed positioned as above and with the pillow positioned as above.
2. Turn your head 45 degrees as illustrated in Figure 83.7 (Letter A).
   - If your head turned to the right produced the most uncomfortable feelings, turn to the right before doing the maneuver described in No. 5 above.
   - If your head turned to the left produced the most uncomfortable feelings, turn to the left before doing the maneuver described in No. 5 above (Letter B).
3. Rapidly lie down in the bed turning your head to the above position, as described in No. 5 above, with your shoulders positioned on the pillow and your head touching the bed.
4. Remain in that position for 1 minute.
5. Turn your head 90 degrees toward the opposite side (45-degree angle but to the other side) without raising your head, as depicted in Letter C.
6. Remain in that position for 1 minute.
7. Turn your head 90 degrees further in the direction you are presently turned (so you will be looking down at an angle), and move your body as necessary, as depicted in Letter D.
8. Hold this position for 1 minute.
9. Sit up in this manner:
   - Keep facing the direction your head was turned as depicted in Letter E.
   - Hang your feet off the bed in preparation to stand up.
   - Place your chin on your chest, and slowly sit up, keeping your chin on your chest throughout the sitting up motion.
10. Remain in that sitting position for 1 minute.
11. Do not lie flat for 24 hours. A semirecumbent position is best (recliner position).
12. Assume normal activity after 24 hours.

TABLE 83.3

Common Disorders of the Throat

Disorder
Pharyngitis
Tonsillitis
Epiglottiditis
Infectious mononucleosis
Thrush
Peritonsillar abscess
Laryngitis

Acute Tonsillitis/Pharyngitis

DIAGNOSIS

Clinical Manifestations

- Edema
- Inflammation
- Pain
- Sore throat, particularly in children
- Accompanied by fever, odynophagia, and tender adenopathy
- Hoarseness, cough, rhinorrhea, and coryza more often associated with viral infection

PHYSICAL EXAM

- Typically, exudative secretions with bacterial infection
- Typically, serous secretions with viral infection

The appropriateness of using certain tests to identify group A beta-hemolytic streptococci infections is being questioned.[31] Latex agglutination antigen tests and solid-phase enzyme-linked immunosorbent assay (ELISA) provide quick, but only moderately sensitive, screens for streptococcal infection. Although more sensitive, throat cultures take longer for results to become available.

Because all group A beta-hemolytic streptococcal pharyngitis cases should be treated to prevent more serious sequelae, individual decisions for diagnosis and treatment should be considered:

- Local prevalence of resistant streptococcal infections
- Patient history
- Potential for compliance
- Availability and reliability of the laboratory

Differential diagnosis includes infectious mononucleosis, diphtheria, fungal infections, and pharyngeal manifestations of systemic disease.

Treatment/Management

Symptomatic treatment (viral and bacterial infection) includes:

- Analgesics
- Anti-inflammatory agents
- Saltwater gargling
- Osteopathic manipulation

Antibiotics (bacterial infection) include:

- Group A beta-hemolytic streptococcal pharyngitis requires a 10-day course of oral antibiotics or a single intramuscular dose of benzathine penicillin G.
- Penicillin V potassium and cephalosporins are also effective.
- Erythromycin and azithromycin are reasonable alternatives for individuals who are allergic to penicillin.

Tonsillar hypertrophy, anterior cervical lymphadenopathy, and pharyngeal exudates may be present in a patient with pharyngitis.[58] An uncommon but serious complication of pharyngitis is Lemierre syndrome. This syndrome is characterized by septic thrombophlebitis of the jugular vein with showering of distant septic emboli. It is caused by the spread of bacteria from the pharynx and peritonsillar tissue via lymphatic vessels.[59] Thus, recognition, prompt treatment, and management aimed at reducing swelling and improving lymphatic flow are imperative to the health of the patient.

Osteopathic Manipulative Treatment

Osteopathic manipulation to improve lymphatic flow by likely stimulating the immune response can be particularly helpful in providing symptomatic relief.[7,56]

- The Galbreath technique of mandibular drainage reduces tonsillar congestion and may offer pain relief and reduce the chance of lymphatic congestion around the eustachian tube (Fig. 67.24).
- Improving lymphatic circulation by addressing any somatic dysfunction of the upper ribs, thoracic inlet, clavicle, cervical, and upper thoracic spinal areas not only reduces swelling but also stimulates the immune response.
    - □ OMT can be targeted at addressing the prevertebral fascia and the hyoid bone in acute uncomplicated pharyngitis.[57]
    - □ Chronic pharyngitis may be a symptom of GERD, mouth breathing, and allergic sequelae. OMT using lymphatic drainage techniques (Chapter 50) and osteopathic cranial manipulative medicine (Chapter 53) will encourage drainage and circulation.
    - □ Schander et al. designed a canine study to quantitatively measure the effect of repeated lymphatic techniques. The study showed an increase in thoracic duct lymph (TDL) flow, leukocyte count, total leukocyte and interleukin-8 (IL-8) flux, keratinocyte-derived chemoattractant, nitrite, as well as superoxide dismutase (SOD). Schander suggests the use of lymphatic pump treatment to repeatedly stimulate the immune system.[60]
    - □ Healing may also be enhanced by addressing sympathetic, vasomotor control affected by somatic dysfunction of the upper thoracic and upper cervical (superior cervical ganglion) areas.
    - □ Rib raising may decrease sympathetic tone, improving secretions and vasoconstriction (see Chapters 57 and 78).
    - □ Cranial techniques addressing the sinuses may improve postnasal drip (see Chapter 53).
- Presumably, improved arterial flow would also increase the tissue levels of prescribed antibiotics or other medications.

OSTEOPATHIC APPROACH TO HEAD AND NECK SOMATIC DYSFUNCTIONS USING OMT

The major goals in treating patients with somatic dysfunction in the head and neck regions using OMT are akin to other regions:

- Restore proper biomechanics (structure–function relationships)
- Assist venous and lymphatic circulation
- Promote arterial flow
- Normalize spinal reflexes affecting function
- Relieve pain

It is reasonable to expect that the use of musculoskeletal diagnosis and treatment in these patients will help the patient feel better, assist in healing, and improve overall resistance to disease.

As a guide, evaluate and treat somatic dysfunction from central body areas to the periphery, allowing for free flow of venous and lymphatic fluids. The rationale for treating somatic dysfunction in the upper thoracic and cervical spine is to decrease somatic stimulation in the area of the sympathetic outflow and ganglia supplying the head and neck.

Improving venous and lymphatic flow through the cervical and thoracic inlet areas (Fig. 43.11) is essential for draining the congestion in the head region. An attempt is made to decrease myofascial tension in the areas through which lymphatic and venous vessels pass from the head to where they enter the central circulation at about the level of the first rib.

- Superficial drainage techniques (effleurage) applied to the face from medial to lateral decrease tissue congestion in the anterior sinus regions.
- The mandibular drainage technique described by Galbreath[55] is an effective lymphatic drainage procedure for the ear, auditory canals, and throat (Fig. 67.24). It is used along with cervical soft tissue (Chapter 54) and mobilization procedures for the clavicle, first rib and upper thoracic spine, lymphatic and venous drainage from the head through the superior thoracic aperture region back to central circulation.
- Lymphatic pump techniques are intended to stimulate general lymphatic flow by affecting intrathoracic pressures (see Chapter 50). Their use is described in the osteopathic literature regarding treatment of infectious disease.[19,54,56]
- Cranial treatment, using OCMM (Chapter 53) and soft tissue techniques (Chapter 54) including suboccipital inhibitory pressure, is especially indicated in sinus disease and middle and inner ear conditions (Fig. 54.6).

For relieving pain and normalizing reflexes, along with other techniques as described in Section VIII, Chapters 47, 49 to 54, Chapman reflexes and Jones tender points (Chapter 43) should also be addressed[60] (see Chapter 58 A Modern Approach to Chapman Reflex Points). Counterstrain techniques (Chapter 47) are used to treat Jones tender points.

Addressing TMJ disorders with OMT is covered in the following section.

Temporomandibular Joint Disorder

TMJ disorder is the most common nondental orofacial pain condition seen in primary care clinical practice.[61]

- Affects both women and men (3.3:1 ratio).
- Age range (mean) 20 to 60 years old (30 to 40); younger patients have more myofascial pain with or without disk displacement; older patients greater than 50 have more arthritis-related joint dysfunction.
- Half of the patients present with myofascial pain in or around the TMJ.
- Prevalence is estimated to be between 6% and 12% in the general population.[62]

Diagnostic criteria on physical examination include at least one of the following, with combinations common[62–65]:

- Myofascial pain upon digital palpation
- Decreased motion
- Clicking sound upon movement (disk displacement)
- Deviation of the jaw upon movement
- Crepitus or radiologic findings of arthritis

Differential diagnosis includes[65]:

MYOFASCIAL PAIN

- Malocclusion
- Bruxism
- Fibromyalgia
- Myopathy
- Emotional stress (leads to bruxism and myofascial strain)

INFLAMMATORY ARTHRITIS

- Rheumatoid arthritis
- Ankylosing spondylitis
- Psoriatic arthritis
- Gout
- Infectious arthritis

NONINFLAMMATORY/DEGENERATIVE ARTHRITIS

- Osteoarthritis
- Trauma
- Surgery
- Cartilage/bone disorder

MECHANICAL DYSFUNCTION

- Disk displacement
- Somatic dysfunction

Osteopathic perspectives on TMJ disorder include:

- Basic anatomical structures and mechanics of TMJ motion are depicted in Figures 83.8 to 83.13.
- The TMJ is a ginglymoarthrodial (hinge-like) joint with a unique biconcave intra-articular disk; it is one of the most complex joints in the body.

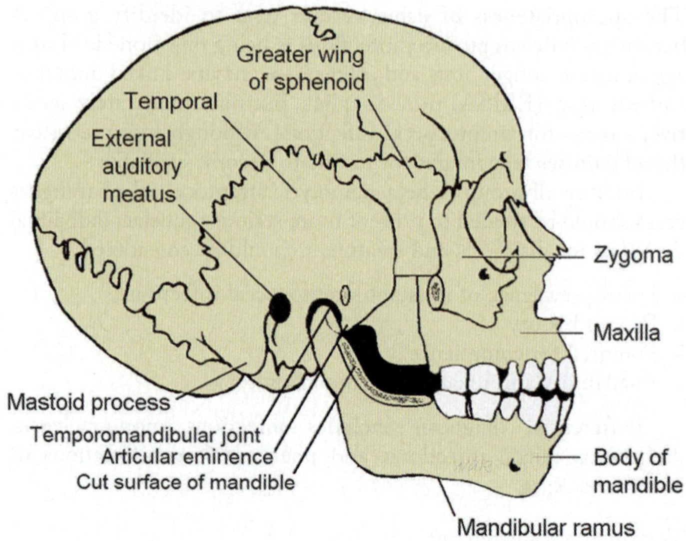

Figure 83.8. Illustration of the lateral view of the right cranium with focus on the temporomandibular joint. (Courtesy of William A. Kuchera, DO, FAAO, with permission.)

- Embryologic origin of the mandible (Meckel cartilage from the mandibular part of the first branchial arch) and its ligaments (from the middle ear ossicles and cervical fascia) links the TMJ mechanics to the temporal bone, as well as the sphenoid bone medially and the cervical region inferiorly.[36]
- The Meckel cartilage forms the template for the malleus (middle ear ossicle) and the jaw, linking the mandible to the middle ear via the remnant anterior malleolar ligament (AML).[66]

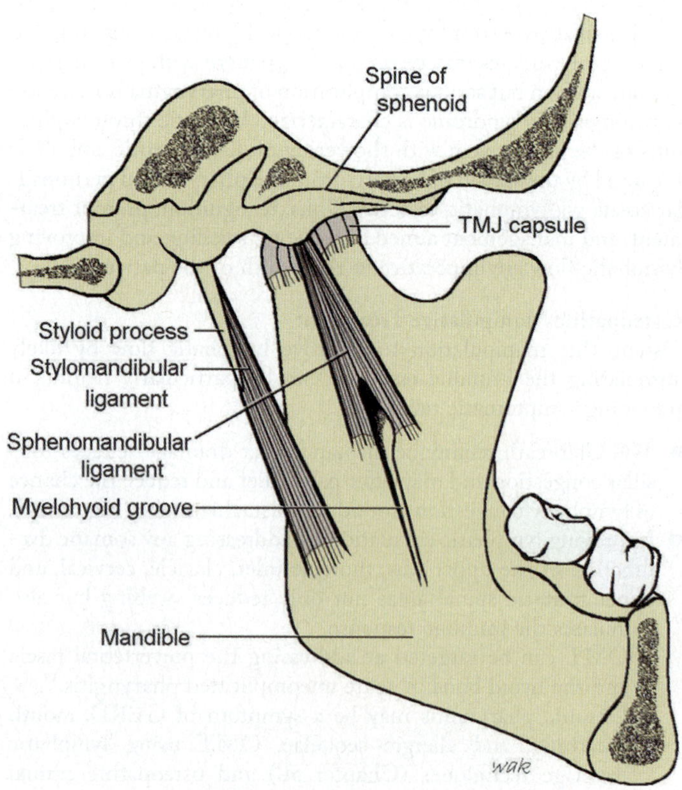

Figure 83.9. Illustration of the medial view of the left mandible focusing on the sphenomandibular and temporomandibular ligaments. (Courtesy of William A. Kuchera, DO, FAAO, with permission.)

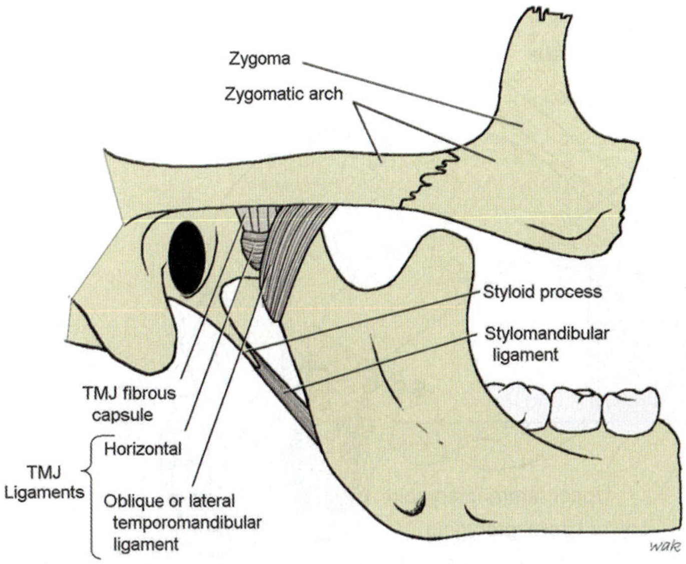

Figure 83.10. Illustration of the lateral view of the right temporomandibular joint with focus on the capsular ligaments. (Courtesy of William A. Kuchera, DO, FAAO, with permission.)

- Another remnant of the Meckel cartilage forms the sphenomandibular ligament, which has fibrous connections to the AML.[67]
- The diskomalleolar ligament (DML) limits the intra-articular disk movement through its attachment to the malleus.[68]
  - The connective tissue surrounding the DML has nociceptors, for example, calcitonin-gene–related peptide (CGRP), protein gene product (PGP) 9.5, and SP receptor nerve fibers, surrounding the numerous local blood vessels.
  - The intra-articular disk slides along with the condyles, tethered posteriorly by the DML, which also assists in tracking the mandible as it retracts into the infratemporal fossa upon closing the mouth.
- The mandible is formed partly within membrane (rami and bodies) and partly in cartilage (condyles and chin) in two parts, united at birth by a fibrous midline symphysis that ossifies during the first year of life. It is primarily subject to the mechanics of the temporal bones.
  - Its mechanics can be considered in terms of the relationship between each articular condyle in the infratemporal fossa and the ipsilateral temporal bone.
  - Therefore, the mandibular condyles can be considered to internally and externally rotate, along with the temporal bones. For example, as the left temporal bone internally rotates, the ipsilateral mandibular condyle also internally rotates within the infratemporal fossa.
  - The condyles are inferior to the axes of the temporal bone, which run diagonally through the petrous portions, dividing the squamous portions superiorly from the mastoid processes and infratemporal fossae inferiorly.
  - As each mandibular condyle is essentially level with its respective ipsilateral mastoid process, its movements are in the same direction as its ipsilateral mastoid process, as both are inferior to the axis of rotation for the ipsilateral temporal bone.
    - As the temporal bone externally rotates, the ipsilateral mandibular fossa moves posteriorly and medially.
    - Internal rotation allows the ipsilateral mandibular fossa to move anteriorly and laterally.
    - The mandible will deviate toward the side of the externally rotated temporal bone or away from the side of the internally rotated temporal bone.
- The stylomandibular ligament connects the angle of the mandible to the styloid process of the temporal bone, and the sphenomandibular ligament connects the lingula (medial aspect) of the mandible to the spine of the sphenoid.
  - Sphenoid dysfunction can affect the TMJ through its direct articulation with the temporal bone or by its articulation with the mandible through the sphenomandibular ligament.

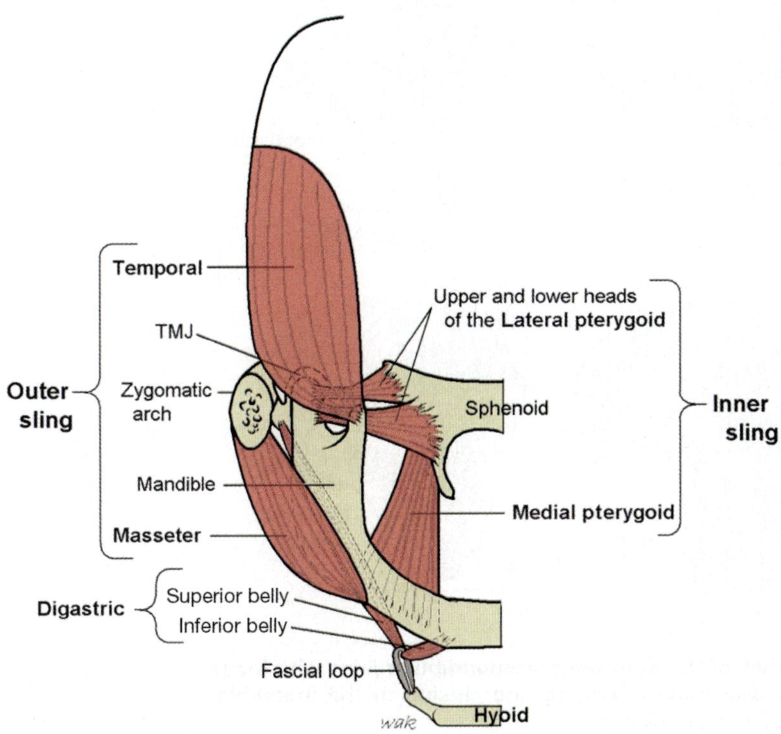

Figure 83.11. Illustration of the muscles of the right temporomandibular joint. (Courtesy of William A. Kuchera, DO, FAAO, with permission.)

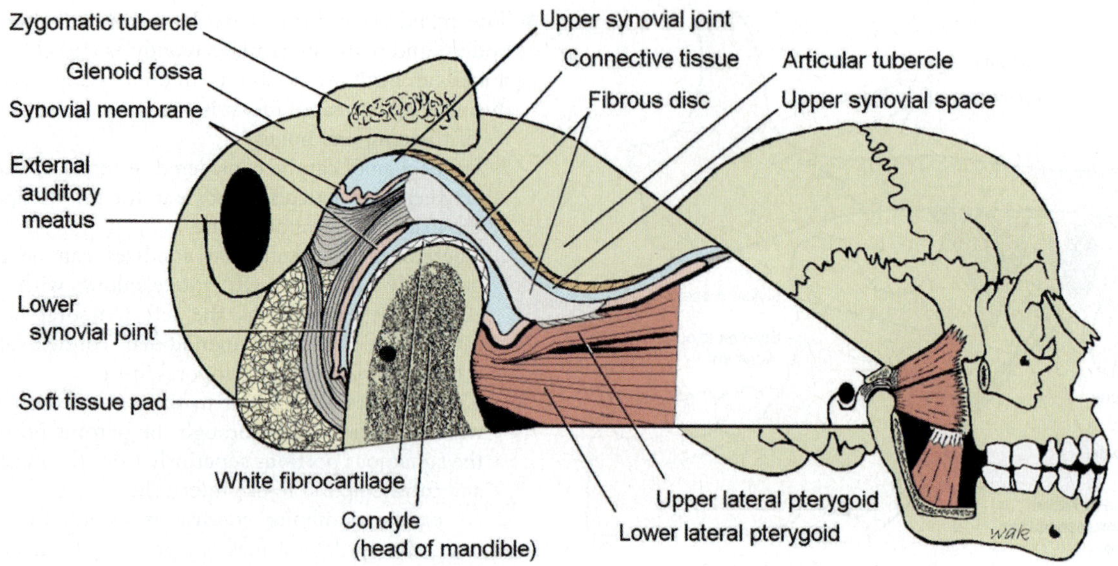

Figure 83.12. Illustration of the lateral view of the right temporomandibular joint with focus on the intra-articular structures. (Courtesy of William A. Kuchera, DO, FAAO, with permission.)

- Lateral, or external, and medial, or internal, pterygoid and hyoid muscle imbalances lead to tissue degeneration and disk displacements, motion dysfunction, and myofascial pain.[69]
  - The suprahyoid muscles (mylohyoid, geniohyoid, and digastric muscles) provide a hinge-like movement to open the mouth.
  - Anterior condylar glide (and protrusion) is provided by the inferior division of the lateral pterygoid muscles assisted by the medial pterygoid muscles.
  - Closing the mouth is accomplished by the temporalis, masseter, and medial pterygoid muscles.
  - Lateral displacement (grinding movement) activates the ipsilateral temporalis and the contralateral medial and lateral pterygoids and masseter muscles.
  - Much of the pathophysiology of temporomandibular joint disorder (TMD) is likely due to imbalance and dysfunction of the superior and inferior heads of the lateral pterygoid muscles.
  - Stress, anxiety, and depression are often associated with TMD by increasing masticatory muscle hypertonicity.
  - Asymmetric tension of the jaw muscles, bruxism, and malocclusion will affect the position and motion of the cranium.

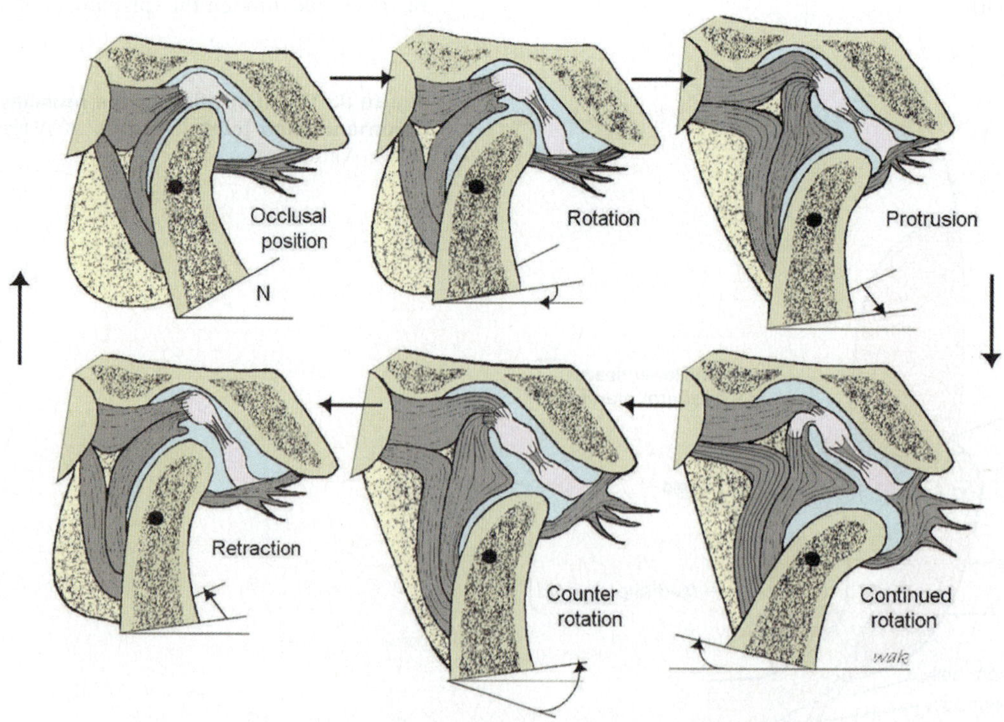

Figure 83.13. Illustration of the lateral view of the right temporomandibular joint with focus on the mechanics of the intra-articular disk during opening and closing of the mandible. (Courtesy of William A. Kuchera, DO, FAAO, with permission.)

- Total body evaluation for distal somatic dysfunction, including the rest of the cranium, spine, pelvis, and extremities is essential to address contributing factors that affect TMJ dysfunction.[70]
- Swallowing opens the eustachian tube while clenching the teeth.

OSTEOPATHIC STRUCTURAL EXAMINATION OF THE TMJ

- While facing the seated patient, palpate the patient's TMJs bilaterally, and observe for lateral tracking of the mandible away from midline as the mouth is slowly actively opened and closed.
  - A deflection of the jaw to one side may occur in a C- or S-shaped pattern.
  - While testing jaw ROM, palpate for clicking or popping of the joint as well as crepitus.
  - Sometimes, the jaw will become locked when opening or closing.
- Assess the temporal bones for internal or external rotation.
- Assess the sphenoid and temporal bones for displacement when passively depressing the patient's jaw with a gloved thumb internally placed upon the posterior mandibular molar teeth.
- The temporal bones motion and position are affected by the occiput.
- The position and motion of the occiput, temporals, and mandible are affected not only by conditions of the HEENT region, but also by postural balance.
- Assess the spine, pelvis, and extremities for somatic dysfunction, especially for scoliosis, short leg, and pelvic or occipital obliquity.[70–73]
- Assess for myofascial trigger points in the muscles of mastication (see Chapter 43).

IMAGING

When considering the workup of patients with TMJ, laboratory and imaging studies generally are not indicated. MRI of the TMJ, although costly, is the study of choice if[71]:

- Articular or meniscal pathology is suspected.
- An endoscopic or surgical procedure is contemplated.
- There is a history of traumatic injury to the TMJ.

If the patient has associated tinnitus, hearing loss, or other neurologic complaints, an MRI of the brain should be ordered.

TREATMENT, INCLUDING OMT

Treatment needs to address the pathology present, the exacerbating factors, and the presenting symptoms. Improving somatic dysfunction of the cranium, upper cervical, and upper thoracic region is of great benefit in TMJ patients. These are common regions of dysfunction in these patients; however, somatic dysfunction of any region may contribute to the TMJ patient through the continuity of the fascia. Addressing postural factors such as short leg, scoliosis, and pelvic obliquities aid in the recovery of TMD.

Dysfunction of the occiput and atlas are commonly associated with the temporal bone. Tender points located in the soft tissues between the ramus of the mandible and the mastoid process are commonly found. Sometimes referred to as atlas counterstrain points, treatment of this area with counterstrain, effleurage, or the William Galbreath technique is useful. Articular dysfunction of the occiput on atlas usually has an upper thoracic component maintaining it. The occiput dysfunction will return if adequate treatment of the upper thoracic is neglected.[74]

Somatic dysfunction and myofascial trigger points (see Chapter 43 for more information) are closely related and potentiate one another. Emotional stress may be associated with clenching of the teeth and may produce myofascial trigger points in the masseter and pterygoid muscles. Pain control is most important to prevent chronic pain syndrome and help to restore normal neurologic function.

- Pain is usually controlled with medications; however, using OMT to reduce tension in the jaw muscles, decrease swelling and inflammation, and improve drainage of tissue congestion can reduce pain and decrease the need for medication.
- NSAIDs can reduce inflammation and control pain,[75] especially after dental procedures.
- The muscle relaxant cyclobenzaprine, corticosteroids, and hyaluronate injections have been shown to be effective for short-term pain relief associated with TMD.[75]
- Intramuscular botulinum toxin type A[74,76] and platelet-rich plasma injections have shown effectiveness in TMD.[76,77]
- Gabapentin and its analog pregabalin may provide pain relief for central or peripheral sensitization, that is, chronic pain syndrome.
- Any chronic painful condition, such as chronic TMJ syndrome, will worsen any pre-existing anxiety or depression. Therefore, treatment should include stress management, relaxation techniques for the face and neck, as well as medications when necessary (see Chapter 18 Stress Management for further discussion).

Exercise sheets and other resources can be obtained online from the TMJ Association. The key to relaxing jaw muscles is keeping the teeth slightly apart, which can be accomplished during sleep using an intraoral night splint or occlusal orthotics.[78] OMT should be given before and after fitting for occlusal splints and before and after restorative dentistry.[71] With long-standing dysfunction, the joint capsule may stretch, making the joint unstable.

- In this instance, injection of a proliferating agent into the joint (prolotherapy) may tighten the capsule and help normalize motion (see Chapter 89 for further information).

SUMMARY

This chapter focused on osteopathic perspectives in understanding the pathophysiology, making the diagnosis, and providing treatment options for common HEENT problems seen in primary care settings, including rhinosinusitis, allergic conjunctivitis and rhinitis, otitis media, vertigo, acute tonsillitis, pharyngitis, and TMJ disorders. Osteopathic principles and practices provide a framework to guide the osteopathic physician in managing patients with various disorders of the HEENT.

ACKNOWLEDGMENTS

The authors and editors of this chapter would like to acknowledge the past contributions of Drs. Harriet H. Shaw, Michael B. Shaw, and Kathleen Gibbons for prior editions of this chapter.

REFERENCES

1. Blood HA. Infections of the ear, nose and throat. *Ost Ann.* 1978;6(11):14–18.
2. Woods DE. Management of ENT problems. *Ost Ann.* 1980;8(5):31–41.
3. Moser RJ. Sinusitis, the effective osteopathic manipulative procedures in the management thereof. *Yearbook of Selected Papers. Academy of Applied Osteopathy.* 1953:15–16.
4. Sato A. Reflex modulation of visceral functions by somatic afferent activity. In: Patterson MM, Howell JN, eds. The Central Connection: Somatovisceral/Viscerosomatic Interaction. *Proceedings of 1989 American Academy of Osteopathy International Symposium.* University Classics; 1992:53–72.
5. Sato A, Schmidt RF. The modulation of visceral functions by somatic afferent activity. *Jpn J Physiol.* 1987;37(1):1–17.

6. Pintal WJ, Kurtz ME. An integrated osteopathic treatment approach in acute otitis media. *J Am Osteopath Assoc.* 1989;89(9):1139–1141.
7. Schmidt IC. Osteopathic manipulative therapy as a primary factor in the management of upper, middle, and pararespiratory infections. *J Am Osteopath Assoc.* 1982;81(6):382–388.
8. Wasserman SJ. Ciliary function and disease. *J Allergy Clin Immunol.* 1984;73:17–19.
9. Cikojević D, Krnić M, Marčina S. [Influence of smoking on the nasal mucosa mucociliary transport.] *Acta Med Croatica.* 2014:68(3):247–251.
10. Wagenmann M, Naclerio RM. Anatomic and physiologic considerations in sinusitis. *J Allergy Clin Immunol.* 1992;90(3):419–423.
11. Choi JY, Khansaheb M, Joo NS, et al. Substance P stimulates human airway submucosal gland secretion mainly via a CFTR-dependent process. *J Clin Invest.* 2009;119(5):1189–1200.
12. Zeiger RS. Prospects for ancillary treatment of sinusitis in the 1990s. *J Allergy Clin Immunol.* 1992;90(3 Pt 2):478–495.
13. Kaluza CL, Sherbin M. The physiologic response of the nose to osteopathic manipulative treatment: preliminary report. *J Am Osteopath Assoc.* 1983;82(9):654–660.
14. Peters AT, Spector S, Hsu J, et al; Joint Task Force on Practice Parameters, representing the American Academy of Allergy, Asthma and Immunology, the American College of Allergy, Asthma and Immunology, and the Joint Council of Allergy, Asthma and Immunology. Diagnosis and management of rhinosinusitis: a practice parameter update. *Ann Allergy Asthma Immunol.* 2014;113(4):347–385.
15. Rosenfeld RM. Clinical practice. Acute sinusitis in adults. *N Engl J Med.* 2016;375(10):962–970.
16. Harakal JH. Manipulative treatment for acute upper-respiratory diseases. *Ost Ann.* 1981;9(7):30–37.
17. Hoyt WH III. Current concepts in management of sinus disease. *J Am Osteopath Assoc.* 1990;90(10):913–919.
18. Cathie AG. The sino-bronchial syndrome. *Yearbook of Selected Papers.* Academy of Applied Osteopathy; 1968:9–11.
19. Shrum KM, Grogg SE, Barton P, Shaw HH, Dyer RR. Sinusitis in children: the importance of diagnosis. *J Am Osteopath Assoc.* 2001;101(5): S8–S13.
20. Rudmik L, Soler ZM. Medical therapies for adult chronic sinusitis a systematic review. *JAMA.* 2015;314(9):926–939.
21. Brook I, Foote PA, Hausfeld JN. Increase in the frequency of recovery of methicillin-resistant Staphylococcus aureus in acute and chronic maxillary sinusitis. *J Med Microbiol.* 2008;57(Pt 8):1015–1017.
22. Chow AW, Benninger MS, Brook I, et al; Infectious Diseases Society of America. IDSA clinical practice guideline for acute bacterial rhinosinusitis in children and adults. *Clin Infect Dis.* 2012;54(8):e72–e112.
23. Knipping S, Holzhausen HJ, Goetze G, Riederer A, Bloching MB. Rhinitis medicamentosa: electron microscopic changes of human nasal mucosa. *Otolaryngol Head Neck Surg.* 2007;136(1):57–61.
24. Runkle K. Decongestants, antihistamines and nasal irrigation for acute sinusitis in children. *Paediatr Child Health.* 2016;21(3):143–144.
25. Prussin C, Metcalfe DD. 5. IgE, mast cells, basophils, and eosinophils. *J Allergy Clin Immunol.* 2006;117(2 suppl Mini-Primer):S450–S456.
26. Dvoracek JE, Yunginger JW, Kern EB, Hyatt RE, Gleich GJ. Induction of nasal late-phase reactions by insufflation of ragweed-pollen extract. *J Allergy Clin Immunol.* 1984;73(3):363–368.
27. Channell M, Mason D. Chapter 53: rhinitis, allergic. *The 5-minute Osteopathic Manipulative Medicine Consult.* Lippincott Williams & Wilkins; 2008.
28. Yii ACA, Tay TR, Choo XN, Koh MSY, Tee AKH, Wang D-Y. Precision medicine in united airways disease: a "treatable traits" approach. *Allergy.* 2018;73(10):1964–1978.
29. Wilson JM, Platts-Mills TAE. Home environmental interventions for house dust mite. *J Allergy Clin Immunol Pract.* 2018;6(1):1–7.
30. Kaliner MA. Azelastine and olopatadine in the treatment of allergic rhinitis. *Ann Allergy Asthma Immunol.* 2009;103(5):373–380.
31. Graf P. Long-term use of oxy- and xylometazoline nasal sprays induces rebound swelling, tolerance, and nasal hyperreactivity. *Rhinology.* 1996; 34(1):9–13.
32. Dykewicz MS, Wallace DV, Amrol DJ, et al. Rhinitis 2020: a practice parameter update. *J Allergy Clin Immunol.* 2020;146(4):721–767.
33. Naclerio RM. Allergic rhinitis. *N Engl J Med.* 1991;325(12):860.
34. Cox L, Nelson H, Lockey R, et al. Allergen immunotherapy: a practice parameter third update. *J Allergy Clin Immunol.* 2011;127(1):S1–S55.
35. Chen L. Ocular lymphatics: state-of-the-art review. *Lymphology.* 2009; 42(2):66–76.
36. Magoun HI. *Osteopathy in the Cranial Field.* 3rd ed. The Journal Printing Co.; 1976.
37. Heinking KP, Kappler RE, Ramey KA. Head and suboccipital region. In: Chila AG, Ex., ed. *Foundations of Osteopathic Medicine.* 3rd ed. Lippincott Williams & Wilkins; 2011:495.
38. Burks AW, Holgate S, O'Hehir R, et al. Middleton's allergy: principles and practice. In: Barney NP, ed. *Allergic and Immunologic Disease of the Eye.* 9th ed. Elsevier Saunders; 2020:605–623.
39. Rich R, ed. *Clinical Immunology: Principles and Practice.* 4th ed. Elsevier Saunders; 2013:558–563.
40. Bielory BP, O'Brien TP, Bielory L. Management of seasonal allergic conjunctivitis: guide to therapy. *Acta Ophthalmol.* 2012;90(5):399–407.
41. Sherman T, Qureshi Y, Bach A. Osteopathic manipulative treatment to manage ophthalmic conditions. *J Am Osteopath Assoc.* 2017;117(9): 568–575.
42. Hom MM, Bielory B. The anatomical and functional relationship between allergic conjunctivitis and allergic rhinitis. *Allergy Rhinol.* 2013;4(3): e110–e119.
43. Kuchera ML, Kuchera WA. *Osteopathic Considerations in HEENT Disorders.* Greyden Press, LLC; 2012:50.
44. Baroody FM, Foster KA, Markaryan A, deTineo M, Naclerio RM. Nasal ocular reflexes and eye symptoms in patients with allergic rhinitis. *Ann Allergy Asthma Immunol.* 2008;100(3):194–199.
45. Philip G, Baroody FM, Proud D, Naclerio RM, Togias AG. The human nasal response to capsaicin. *J Allergy Clin Immunol.* 1994;94(6):1035–1045.
46. Lanier BQ, Abelson MB, Berger WE, et al. Comparison of the efficacy of combined fluticasone propionate and olopatadine versus combined fluticasone propionate and fexofenadine for the treatment of allergic rhinoconjunctivitis induced by conjunctival allergen challenge. *Clin Ther.* 2002;24:7:1161–1174.
47. Brown CE, Magnuson B. On the physics of the infant feeding bottle and middle ear sequela: ear disease in infants can be associated with bottle feeding. *Int J Pediatr Otorhinolaryngol.* 2000;54(1):13–20.
48. Updike C, Thornburg JD. Reading skills and auditory processing ability in children with chronic otitis media in early childhood. *Ann Otol Rhinol Laryngol.* 1992;101(6):530–537.
49. Bennett KE, Haggard MP, Silva PA, Stewart IA. Behaviour and developmental effects of otitis media with effusion into the teens. *Arch Dis Child.* 2001;85(2):91–95.
50. Froom J, Culpepper L. Otitis media in day-care children. A report from the International Primary Care Network. *J Fam Pract.* 1991;32(3): 289–294.
51. Rosenfeld RM, Shin JJ, Schwartz SR, et al. Clinical practice guideline: otitis media with effusion (update). *Otolaryngol Head Neck Surg.* 2016; 154(1):S1–S41.
52. Honjo I, Okazaki N, Kumazawa T. Opening mechanism of the eustachian tube. *Ann Otol Rhinol Laryngol.* 1980;89(3):25–27.
53. Thomas NM, Brook I. Otitis media: an update on current pharmacotherapy and future perspectives. *Expert Opin Pharmacother.* 2014;15(8): 1069–1083.
54. Greenman PE. Fascial considerations in treatment of the head and neck. *Ost Ann.* 1975;3(2):34–42.
55. Galbreath W. Manipulative structural adjustive treatment in middle ear deafness. *J Am Osteopath Assoc.* 1925;24:741.
56. Rumney IC. Osteopathic manipulative treatment of infectious diseases. *Ost Ann.* 1974;2:29–33.
57. Mills MV, Henley CE, Barnes LL, Carreiro JE, Degenhardt BF. The use of osteopathic manipulative treatment (OMT) as adjunctive therapy in children with recurrent acute otitis media. *Arch Pediatr Adolesc Med.* 2003;157(9):861–866.
58. Kelley PM, Tempero RM. Lymphatic vessel hypertrophy in inflamed human tonsils. *Lympat Res Biol.* 2010;8(2):121–126.
59. Righini CA, Karkas A, Tourniaire R, et al. Lemierre syndrome: a study of 11 cases and literature review. *Head Neck.* 2014;36(7):1044–1051.

60. Schander A, Padro D, King HH, Downey HF, Hodge LM. Lymphatic pump treatment repeatedly enhances the lymphatic and immune systems. *Lymphat Res Biol.* 2013;11(4):219–226.
61. Owens C. *An Endocrine Interpretation of Chapman's Reflexes.* Academy of Applied Osteopathy; 1963.
62. Lipton JA, Ship JA, Larach-Robinson D. Estimated prevalence and distribution of reported orofacial pain in the United States. *J Am Dent Assoc.* 1993;124:115–121.
63. Manifredin D, Guarda-Nardini L, Winocur E, Piccotti F, Ahlberg J, Lobbezoo F. Research diagnostic criteria for temporomandibular disorders: a systematic review of axis I epidemiological findings. *Oral Surg Oral Med Oral Pathol Oral Radiol Endod.* 2011;112:453–462.
64. Schiffman E, Ohrbach R, Truelove E, et al; International RDC/TMD Consortium Network, International Association for Dental Research; Orofacial Pain Special Interest Group, International Association for the Study of Pain. Diagnostic criteria for temporomandibular disorders (DC/TMD) for clinical and research applications: recommendations of the International RDC/TMD Consortium Network* and Orofacial Pain Special Interest Group†. *J Oral Facial Pain Headache.* 2014;28(1):6–27.
65. Liu F, Steinkeler A. Epidemiology, diagnosis, and treatment of temporomandibular disorders. *Dent Clin N Am.* 2013;57:465–479.
66. Sencimen M, Yalçin B, Doğan N, et al. Anatomical and functional aspects of ligaments between the malleus and the temporomandibular joint. *Int J Oral Maxillofac Surg.* 2008;37(10):943–947.
67. Alkofide EA, Clark E, el-Bermani W, Kronman JH, Mehta N. The incidence and nature of fibrous continuity between the sphenomandibular ligament and the anterior malleolar ligament of the middle ear. *J Orofac Pain.* 1997;11(1):7–14.
68. Arai H, Sato I. Anatomical study of the human discomalleolar ligament using cone beam computed tomography imaging and morphological observations. *Okajimas Folia Anat Jpn.* 2011;88(3):89–101.
69. Butts R, Dunning J, Perreault T, Mettille J, Escaloni J. Pathoanatomical characteristics of temporomandibular dysfunction: where do we stand? (Narrative review part 1). *J Bodyw Mov Ther.* 2017;21:534–540.
70. Hruby RJ. The total body approach to the osteopathic management of temporomandibular joint dysfunction. *J Am Osteopath Assoc.* 1985;85: 502–510.
71. McPartland J. The patient with temporomandibular joint pain and dysfunction. In: Nelson K, Glonek T, eds. *Somatic Dysfunction in Osteopathic Family Medicine.* 2nd ed. Lippincott Williams & Wilkins; 2015.
72. Saccucci M, Tettamanti L, Mummolo S, Polimeni A, Festa F, Tecco S. Scoliosis and dental occlusion: a review of the literature. *Scoliosis.* 2011; 6:15.
73. Végh A, Fábian G, Jianu R, Segatto E. Orofacial characteristics of adolescents with diagnosed spinal disorders. *Biomed Tech (Berl).* 2012;57(1): 65–69.
74. Brindise J, Nelson K, Kappler R. Association between cervical and thoracic somatic dysfunction among second-year osteopathic medical students. *J Am Osteopath Assoc.* 2014;114(7):540–548.
75. Häggman-Henrikson B, Alstergren P, Davidson T, et al. Pharmacological treatment of orofacial pain—health technology assessment including a systematic review with network meta-analysis. *J Oral Rehabil.* 2017;44: 800–826.
76. Ataran R, Bahramian A, Jamali Z, et al. The role of botulinum toxin a in treatment of temporomandibular joint disorders: a review. *J Dent (Shiraz).* 2017;18(3):157–164.
77. Bousnaki M, Koidis P. Platelet-rich plasma for the therapeutic management of temporomandibular joint disorders: a systematic review. *Int J Oral Maxillofac Surg.* 2018;47:188–198.
78. Fernández-González FJ, Cabero-López J, Brizuela A, et al. Efficacy of selective grinding guided by an occlusal splint in management of myofascial pain: a prospective clinical trial. *Open Dent J.* 2017;11:301–311.

84 Osteopathic Considerations in Orthopedics

JOSEPH P. BRINDISE ▪ KURT P. HEINKING ▪ MICHAEL L. KUCHERA

KEY CONCEPTS

- The study of orthopedics is integral to understanding osteopathic medicine.
- Applications of osteopathic philosophy and principles to patients commonly seen by the osteopathic orthopedic surgeon are exemplified by the following examples:
  - Developmental dysplasia of the hip
  - Hip fracture in the geriatric population
  - Osteoarthritis of the knee
  - Shoulder instability
  - Low back pain
- Osteopathic manipulative treatment is efficacious for resolving or reducing somatic dysfunction–related acute or chronic low back pain; therefore, diagnosing and treating lumbar, sacral, and pelvic somatic dysfunction in patients with low back pain is presented in detail.
- Exercises for patients with low back pain are important to prescribe as part of a comprehensive treatment plan.
- Orthopedic tests are used in conjunction with the osteopathic structural examination to assess for muscle, ligamentous, joint, and bone pathology that may be amenable to surgery, physical therapy, and rehabilitation.

INTRODUCTION

The study of orthopedics is an integral part of osteopathic education. After residency, osteopathic orthopedic surgeons make up one of the specialty colleges in the osteopathic profession. Orthopedics is the specialty of medicine concerned with the preservation of the health and restoration of function of the skeletal system and its associated structures (i.e., spinal and other bones, joints, and muscles).[1] Orthopedic training is essential to the osteopathic physician; orthopedic knowledge extends the ramifications of somatic dysfunction into the structural and anatomic–pathologic arena. Orthopedic knowledge is vital in the differential diagnosis of patients presenting with musculoskeletal complaints; it offers unique insights into the diagnosis and treatment of traumatic and nontraumatic diseases of the musculoskeletal system. Many osteopathic orthopedic physicians specialize in sports medicine or devote a portion of their practice to this field. They have skills and a special perspective in treating structural and functional problems arising from sports injuries. Through prevention and rehabilitation, they want to encourage maximum function within the athlete's structure.

The emblem of the orthopedic society is based on an 18th-century drawing by Nicholas Andry (Fig. 84.1) that depicts a tree curved and twisted by the winds and weather, held upright by a series of ropes and splints.[2] This image continues to influence the orthopedic community. By molding the growing skeleton, orthopedic physicians help a child grow into a straighter and more functional adult. The etymology of the term orthopedics reflects this perspective as well: *Ortho* means to straighten, and *pedic* refers to the pediatric population. The osteopathic orthopedic physicians, with their emphasis on structure–function interrelationships, understand and respect this perspective.

The field of orthopedics has subsequently been divided into orthopedic medicine and orthopedic surgery. Beginning in the 1930s, James Cyriax, MD, a British orthopedist, applied the concept of interrelated structure and function and developed a diagnostic and treatment system that is now known as orthopedic medicine, in contradistinction to orthopedic surgery. He authored a series of original papers and the definitive text, *Textbook of Orthopaedic Medicine*, which describes the importance of making a precise anatomic diagnosis based on:

- Joint range of motion patterns and their end feel
- Referred pain patterns
- Differentiation of contractile and inert structures
- Understanding of selective tension

He also created his own system of manual techniques to be incorporated into treatment.

Until his death in 1989, Cyriax believed that the intervertebral disk and dura was the source of almost all spinal pain. While alive, his influence and his dogmatic teaching did not allow alternative ideas to compete.[3] Since his death, however, orthopedic medicine in North America has expanded its paradigm to embrace an understanding of myofascial and ligamentous pain. The American Association of Orthopedic Medicine (AAOM) and the Canadian Association of Orthopaedic Medicine (CAOM) consist of MDs and DOs who find value in Cyriax's commitment to making a specific anatomic diagnosis using standardized physical examination of the somatic system and who wish to emphasize conservative management of orthopedic cases. These organizations embrace the diagnosis of somatic dysfunction and use manipulative techniques in their treatment regimens; since 1992 one or the other has acted as a North American representative of the international organization of fully licensed physicians interested in manual medicine. AAOM officially adopted the Glossary of Osteopathic Terminology to maintain consistency in their discussions of diagnoses amenable to manipulation. Treatment tools in orthopedic medicine include the following:

- Manual manipulation (including osteopathic manipulative treatment [OMT])
- Prolotherapy
- Trigger point therapy
- Orthotics
- Exercise prescription
- Commitment to an orthopedic perspective

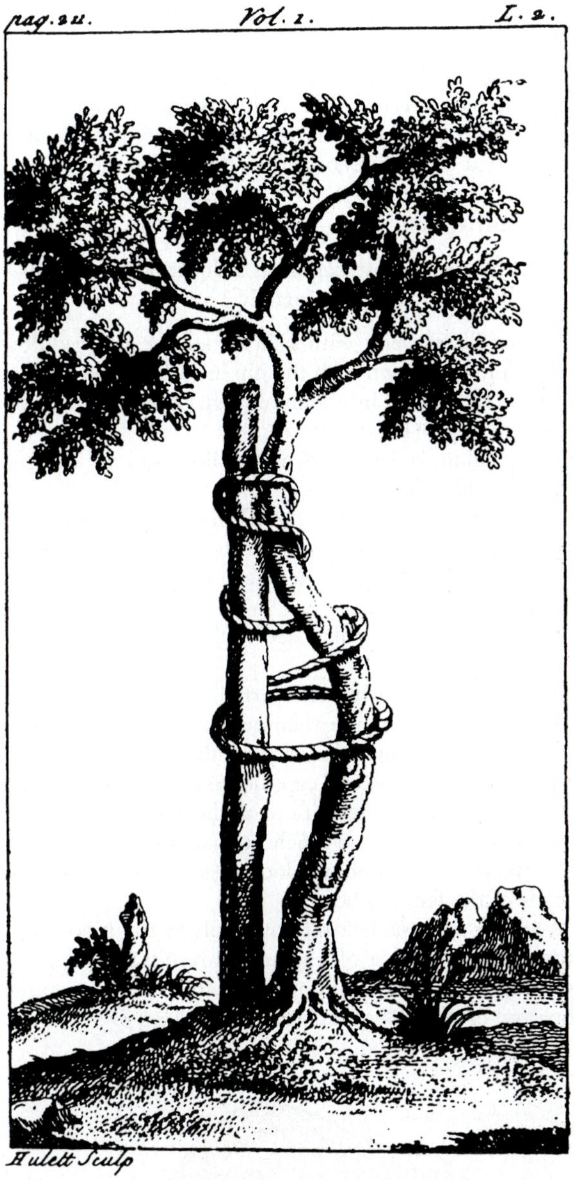

Figure 84.1. An important basic orthopedic principle is embodied in the figure of the tree. The bone is not an inert, calcified, fibrous material. It is a growing, plastic, dynamic structure with an active metabolism that responds to a wide variety of stimuli and is as truly alive as any other structure in our bodies. "Just as the twig is bent, the tree's inclined," wrote Alexander Pope. (From Peltier LF. *Orthopedics: A History and Iconography*. Norman Publishing; 1993. Art from Andry N. L'Orthopedie. Paris: La veuve Alix, 1741.)

Orthopedic surgery in the osteopathic profession is almost as old as the profession itself. At the American School of Osteopathy (ASO) in Kirksville, Missouri, at the beginning of the 20th century, George Laughlin, DO, was gaining acclaim as an orthopedic surgeon by applying European techniques to perform bloodless surgery on congenital hip dislocations and in other orthopedic cases. The surgical team at the ASO at this time also included Andrew Taylor Still, MD, DO, who is credited with revolutionizing the practice of surgery by osteopathy by employing OMT in preoperative and postoperative care.[4] Research on the efficacy of the osteopathic approach for reducing postoperative surgical complications with OMT was carried out many years later by another Kirksville orthopedic surgeon, Edward Herrmann, DO.[5]

The osteopathic orthopedic specialist has been influenced by adherence to the principles of osteopathic medicine. Even if most of the time in orthopedics is spent in busy mechanical pursuits, equally important moments are spent practicing as an osteopathic physician. In this sense, the orthopedist approaches patient care with a keen awareness that the orthopedic problem is but one part of an entire medical and social paradigm. It is in these moments of interaction with internists, family practitioners, and patients' family members that the osteopathic orthopedist brings into play much of their osteopathic orientation. One of the goals in osteopathic orthopedics is to inculcate this attitude of wholeness in treatment; lest the specialists in training take the easy route and forget that their area of expertise is only part of the whole.

An osteopathic physician treating an orthopedic problem adjusts or modifies the approach in a manner that may or may not be different from that of a nonosteopathic physician. Osteopathic orthopedic surgeons are in the subsection of orthopedic surgeons who have been trained osteopathically, but they are essentially surgeons. The thought processes of surgeons, different from those of nonsurgeons and internists, involve an approach to problem solving that has an immediacy based on the need for urgent decision making.

Orthopedics, both surgical and nonsurgical, deals with the diagnosis and treatment of traumatic and nontraumatic diseases of the musculoskeletal system. One of the aspects that may make orthopedics alluring today is the tremendous advance in the ability of physicians to diagnose and surgically treat and thus modify diseases and problems that, in the past, could only be watched as they progressed. What differentiates the orthopedist from other physicians and surgeons includes often lengthy technical procedures using saws, drills, and metallic implants, as well as the activities associated with fracture reduction and casting, juxtaposed to delicate repairs of tendons and nerves under magnification. Before a surgical procedure, the orthopedic surgeon performs appropriate diagnostic examinations and tests and formulates a treatment protocol. If the patient is a surgical candidate, they are optimized for surgery from both a mental and physical standpoint. The patient care team tries to identify and reduce all comorbid modifiable risk factors to help improve patient safety and outcomes. After surgery, prevention of complications, education about postoperative nutrition, and rehabilitation necessitate a wide range of physician knowledge and skills.

In the hospital, the surgeon faces a bewildering, ever-changing number of possible procedures and implants with differing materials and engineering designs. The surgeon must also work closely with the medical managers and hospital administrators who control the expenditures for this technology. Ultimately, these procedures and tests are done for and on people who are not growing properly, have suffered traumatic injury, have developed arthritis, or have intractable pain.

INTEGRATED OSTEOPATHIC ORTHOPEDIC EXAMINATION

The integrated osteopathic examination is detailed in Chapters 27, 29 to 31, 42, 43, and 92, but certain principles bear summary here. Recognition of referred pain patterns from nerve roots, peripheral nerves, myofascial trigger points, and ligamentous structures is a prerequisite for the integrated osteopathic orthopedic examination. A neurologic screening examination is also important for differential diagnosis and prognosis in patients referred for orthopedic evaluation.

Use of selective tension in the examination relies on the observation that normal structures are painless and/or strong when stressed; inflamed or strained structures are painful or weak. Orthopedic examination employs selective tension to evaluate muscle, meniscal, tendinous, and ligamentous structures, and functions, looking for evidence of inflammation or strain. The physician isolates somatic structures and gently but specifically stresses them, looking for pain, weakness, and crepitus. The McMurray meniscal test and Yergason test are examples of this form of examination (see "Specific Orthopedic Tests" section).

The orthopedic physical examination of the somatic system evaluates specific joint characteristics, including range of motion and the end feel associated with major and minor joint motions. Often the same test of joint motion allows for structural and dysfunctional interpretations: Excessive motion and/or a sloppy endpoint to the motion may suggest a ligamentous laxity or ligamentous tear, while a restrictive barrier at the end of motion testing may suggest adhesion or somatic dysfunction. It is important to recall that, in somatic dysfunction, the restrictive barrier appears in one combination of directions and is absent in the opposite combination of directions; the barrier is also reversible with manipulation. Restriction in all directions is characteristic of a capsular pattern seen in pathologic conditions such as adhesive capsulitis of the shoulder, commonly known as "frozen shoulder," arthritis, or the fibrotic reaction to trauma, scar tissue from prior surgery, or overwhelming stress. In such structural diagnoses, somatic dysfunction is also often secondarily present and can be appropriately treated to the patient's benefit. After the secondary somatic dysfunction is treated, the primary structural barrier characteristics remain.

This chapter is intended for generalists and primary care physicians and reviews a few types of orthopedic diseases while discussing how the orthopedist sees these problems biologically, mechanically, and socially. The chapter discusses what may be distinctive aspects of an osteopathic practitioner's approach to five commonly seen orthopedic problems:

- Developmental dysplasia of the hip (DDH)
- Geriatric hip fractures
- Osteoarthritis of the knee
- Instability of the shoulder
- Low back pain (LBP)

DEVELOPMENTAL DYSPLASIA OF THE HIP

The term dysplastic hip is used for the abnormality in appearance and congruity of the child's hip. The proper terminology is DDH, which implies that dysplasia may occur not only at birth but also after birth. Congenital dysplasia implies that all dysplastic hips are present at birth. If that were the case, then all should be recognizable at birth. Some hips, however, are normal at birth but become dysplastic in the extrauterine environment. It is important that the physician routinely examine the well baby's hips at regular office visits as this is one of the most common orthopedic disorders in newborns.

- The physician should check the child's hips for symmetry, leg length, and equality of abduction at the first postpartum office visit, at 6 weeks of age, and at 6 months of age.
- The final examination is at 1 to 2 years of age, when standing and walking ability and balance are included.

Early Presentation

The osteopathic physician, in examining the child at the time of birth and afterward, first evaluates the whole child. In so doing, the physician looks for dysmorphic features that may be associated with multiple anomalies: the child who has cardiac or gastrointestinal abnormalities, failure to thrive, supernumerary digits, or the inability to bend limbs after delivery.[6] DDH can be associated with "packing" deformities such as congenital muscular torticollis, metatarsus adductus, and congenital knee dislocation.[7–9] In addition, one should consider that a child with multiple congenital anomalies may have abnormalities of the musculoskeletal system that occurred at the same moment in embryogenesis.

Late Presentation

A typical case of a late, unrecognized dislocation presents in a child of early walking age, at approximately 1 year.

- Such a toddler presents with a shortened leg or a waddling gait.
- As the child has grown with the hip in a dislocated position, the femur has progressed into a more valgus position at the femoral neck–shaft angle (Fig. 84.2).
- The acetabulum is deformed and shallow, and the cartilaginous lip, or labrum, is defective.
    - Moreover, the acetabulum, which has not been stimulated by the femoral head acting within its cartilaginous tissues, has grown dysplastic with a deficient outer anterior or anterolateral rim.
    - In spastic cerebral palsy, acetabular deficiency is typically posterosuperior.[10]
- The axis of the femur has anteverted, or rotated anteriorly, and developed into a straighter than normal, or valgus, axis.
- Due to these anatomic relationships, the femur is now too long relative to the muscular and capsular tissues surrounding the hip. Thus, forced, manual reduction of the femoral head into the acetabulum, can place too much pressure on the growing bones and occlude the surrounding blood vessels, resulting in avascular necrosis of the femoral head.
    - Avascular necrosis is a serious insult to the blood supply of the articular surface of a joint and results in collapse of the underlying subchondral bone with fractures that cannot heal because of the lack of nutrition.

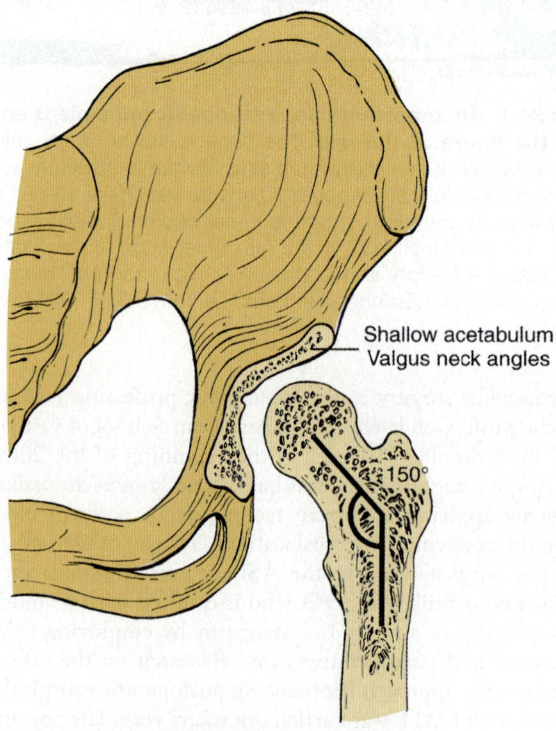

Figure 84.2. **Long-standing hip dislocation.**

Physical Examination and Diagnosis

Instability of the hip is one of the more common problems in newborn children.[11] To evaluate hip stability, the physician observes any abnormalities in skin creases or gluteal folds, leg lengths, and inequalities, and watches for spontaneous motion and activities. The physician evaluates the hip while passing it through a range of motion, checks to see if there is easy and full abduction, and feels the placement and fluidity of motion of the femoral head in the acetabulum (the ball in the socket). An abnormality discovered in any of these observations or tests points to a problem.

Most physicians know the Ortolani sign, which is a palpable sensation of a rapid motion of the femoral head or a "clunk" felt as the dislocated head is reduced into the hip socket from its dislocated position. Here, as Figure 84.3 shows, the femoral head is gently lifted over the labrum and into the socket. In the case of a reduced hip that is unstable, the Barlow test, as shown in Chapter 67, dislocates the hip as the femur is gently adducted with the hip flexed. The physician gently applies pressure over the medial proximal femur and, while doing so, can feel the femoral head slip out of the socket. As the hip is dislocated, gentle pressure on the thigh or knees gives the feeling that the head is not articulating with the socket but that there is a soft endpoint as the pressure is applied. Moreover, the thigh appears shorter. A positive result in any of these tests, performed routinely in the neonatal examination, suggests further studies or treatment. It should be noted that Barlow and Ortolani are rarely positive after 3 months of age due to soft tissue contractures that occur about the hip. After 3 months of age, leg length discrepancy predominates and limited hip abduction is a more sensitive test once contractures have begun to occur. When the child is over 1 year of age and walking, pelvic obliquity, Trendelenburg gait, and toe walking become more obvious. These tests are performed easily and simply by the osteopathic physician and are examples of the pre-eminence of a physical examination and the significance of palpatory findings in the evaluation. In the early period of neonatal development, these physical examination tests are more significant than are most imaging modalities, although the use of diagnostic ultrasonography increases the accuracy and sensitivity of the diagnosis of the dysplastic hip. Ultrasonography is especially useful with abnormalities in the development of the soft tissues of the acetabular region, which are not visualized on x-ray films.[12] It is recommended to perform an ultrasound in patients with suspicious physical exam findings at 3 to 4 weeks of age or to detect silent DDH in high-risk infants from 6 weeks to 4 to 6 months of age.[13] During treatment, various images such as ultrasound, x-ray studies, and computed tomography (CT) scans can be used to assess the accuracy and adequacy of the treatment as the child grows or to confirm the physical diagnosis.

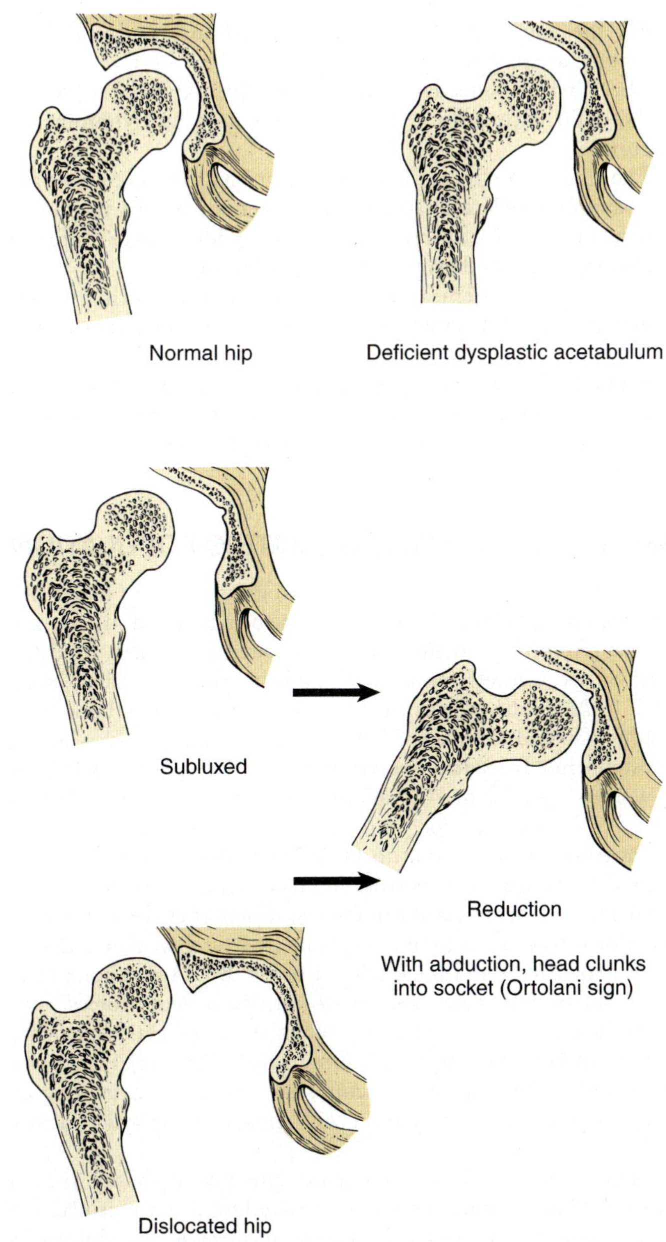

Figure 84.3. Ortolani sign.

Treatment

Treatment of developmentally dysplastic and dislocated hips involves the application of a fundamental osteopathic precept: that growth and maturation of the skeleton follow function. A properly positioned joint with good, easy motion and adequate blood supply and muscle balance grows and develops normally. The orthopedist's goal in the treatment of the dysplastic hip is to place that hip in a position whereby normal stimulation for growth of the acetabulum and proximal femur occurs. One can use external position devices such as casts or braces, or one can make structural internal changes operationally to reconstruct the alignment of the bones so that they are allowed to grow and mature in an improved position.

In most cases, a dislocated or dislocatable hip can be either reduced shortly after birth or, if not reducible, held in a position in which the proximal femur is heading or pointing toward and centered over the triradiate cartilage, the middle portion of the acetabulum.

- Many orthopedists use a Pavlik harness or spica casting to hold such a hip in a position of flexion and abduction (Fig. 84.4).
  - The principle is of essential importance: placing the hip within the socket in a stable position allows the body to continue to nourish the hip socket and allows its normal growth over a period of time.
  - Pavlik himself stated, "With the help of stirrups, we want to achieve suitable flexion of the hips, and nonviolent unforced abduction of the hips with simultaneous facilitation of movement in the hip joints. Centralization of the femoral heads in the acetabulum results spontaneously."
  - While this has proven successful in most cases, there is still controversy regarding when to apply and how to define if the treatment is successful.

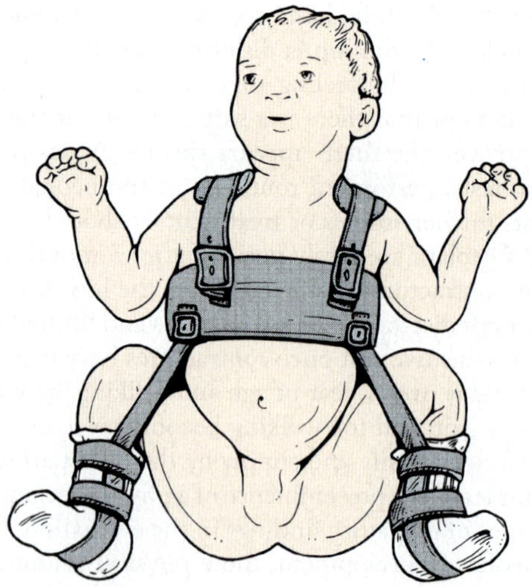

Figure 84.4. Pavlik harness.

- One may use ultrasonography or magnetic resonance imaging (MRI) as well as CT scans to help determine adequacy of reduction and position.
- The risk of complications such as femoral palsy from tight straps over the femoral nerve above the knee or of avascular necrosis from constriction of the epiphyseal blood supply is rare.[14–16]

The second form of treatment for the growing child involves the realignment of the proximal femur and acetabulum to center the growing femoral head within the acetabulum. The operative treatment for this condition is shown in Figure 84.5.

This operation requires the following:

1. The inferior and superior sides of the hip joint, which include the femur and the acetabulum, be addressed simultaneously.
2. In the femur, a shortening, varus osteotomy allows the femoral head to be reduced without undue pressure and changes the neck–shaft angle to a more normal degree from its valgus position.
3. In the acetabulum, a more horizontal socket is formed by either placing a bone graft at the rim or performing an osteotomy above the rim and bending the growing cartilage.
4. If the femoral head is kept reduced into the acetabulum and held there while the tissues heal, it stimulates joint growth and encourages continued normal development over time.

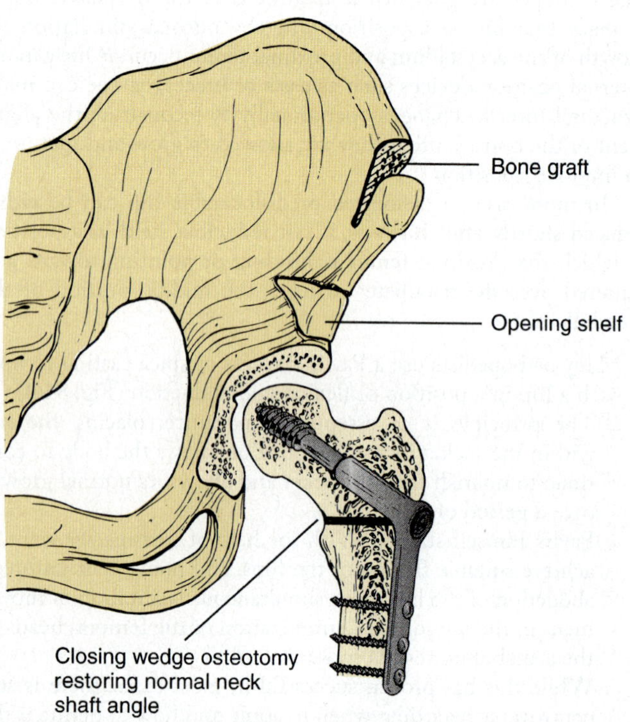

Figure 84.5. Open correction of late deformity.

Bones and joints are plastic and develop because of the forces that are applied to them. One of the joys of treating young people is to watch the growing child mature over time. The physician can guide this development in many ways. The old saying, "As the twig is bent, so grows the tree," implies a molding of the whole person. This image continues to influence the orthopedic community: by molding the growing skeleton, orthopedists help children grow into straighter, more functional adults.

The physician who treats the child with a dysplastic hip is not only treating a mechanical problem in a child but also a child in a family, a small member of a complicated social structure.

- For the young child, nutritional, educational, and emotional support are paramount.
- The physician needs to encourage the parents to provide the child with sufficient protein, minerals, and vitamins for growth.
- The physician also needs to encourage the parents to continue to supply intellectual stimuli or the school system to provide homebound instruction when these children have difficulty attending classes during treatment and recovery.
- Ensure that parents, siblings, and other nurturing family members provide emotional support to the child in a cast or in bed.
- A family with a child with hip dysplasia worries that the child will not walk and be active in life. They need encouragement that the child will probably be able to enjoy a lifestyle not unlike that of their friends.

HIP FRACTURE IN THE GERIATRIC POPULATION

One of the drawbacks of aging is the progressive loss of bone mineral density (BMD) and bone mass universally noted in men and women. According to the National Center for Health Statistics (part of the Centers for Disease Control and Prevention), from 2017 to 2018, the prevalence of osteoporosis and low bone mass in adults 50 and older was 55.7%.[17] Low bone mass is also known as osteopenia. In general, postmenopausal osteoporosis is highest in women aged 50 to 70 years of age, senile osteoporosis begins after 70 years of age for both men and women, and secondary osteoporosis, which is due to underlying disease or medication, begins at any age. Osteoporosis and osteopenia are bone quantity problems, not bone quality problems. Bones that develop osteopenia or osteoporosis have a resultant structural weakness due to the loss of BMD and bone mass. Loss of BMD and bone mass in weight-bearing bones that must withstand heavy forces, such as the hip, are prone to fracture. When the structural inadequacy of the hip bone is joined with diminished visual acuity, balance, and coordination, falls and fractures are common. In treating an aging population, the physician will encounter geriatric fracture problems.

The patient with a hip fracture presents with not only a postural–biomechanical problem to solve but also a personal and social problem. The personal upheaval in lifestyle and abilities as well as the severe economic hardships to the injured person and their family profoundly influences all caregivers, illustrating a major problem for public health providers. The number of aging persons with hip fractures is huge, and the costs of treatment for the fracture and its associated morbidity are staggering.

- It is estimated that 260,000 to 300,000 Americans suffer hip fractures annually.
- By 2040, it is projected that more than 500,000 geriatric hip fracture will occur annually in the United States.[18]
- The annual economic burden is estimated at $5.69 billion to the U.S. health care system.[19]
- If a disease becomes a public health problem when it affects a significant portion of the population, it is incumbent on the public and on physicians to attempt to prevent or control the disease rather than simply treat the disease as it occurs.

Presentation

Often the patient is elderly who presents after a fall with hip pain and difficulty bearing weight on the affected leg.

Physical Examination and Diagnosis

Upon observation, the patient's leg may be externally rotated and appear shorter than the unaffected side. Pain on palpation is often elicited in hip fractures. Imaging is invaluable for diagnosing hip fractures including x-rays of the pelvis, hip, and femur.

Treatment

In the aging population, fractures of the hip are of multiple types and are somewhat dependent on the forces that act through the hip. These fractures are described according to their bony anatomic location involving the femoral head, femoral neck, intertrochanteric, or subtrochanteric regions. They can further be classified as intracapsular or extracapsular fractures which have some treatment implications.

Figure 84.6 represents the types of fracture and the treatment options. Each particular type of fracture has its own treatment approach. Fractures of the proximal femur are generally classified as intracapsular (occurring within the joint) or extracapsular (which are usually intertrochanteric), in which the fracture line goes between or through the greater and lesser trochanters. Those fractures that are extracapsular and within the intertrochanteric or subtrochanteric regions generally heal with stable internal fixation such as sliding compression screw or cephalomedullary nail. Fractures involving the femoral head and neck, which are intracapsular, generally are treated with internal fixation or more commonly partial or total hip replacement. The younger the patient, the more the physician should attempt to bring the bones to a physiologic healing using internal fixation, as opposed to hip replacement, and attend to total body postural considerations (see Chapter 92).

The blood supply to the femoral head is precarious. Simply aligning the bones and holding them together does not necessarily ensure healing. Just as in the growth of the immature skeleton, healing of fractures requires adequate oxygenation, nutrition, and blood supply. For any patient with a displaced femoral neck fracture, the risk of avascular necrosis is high; nevertheless, with adequate protection and/or internal fixation and limited weight bearing, union can occur. The surgeon may try to reestablish circulation to the femoral head through a revascularization procedure, such as a muscle pedicle bone graft, in which a pedicle of bone attached to a blood supply is rotated into the proximal femur.

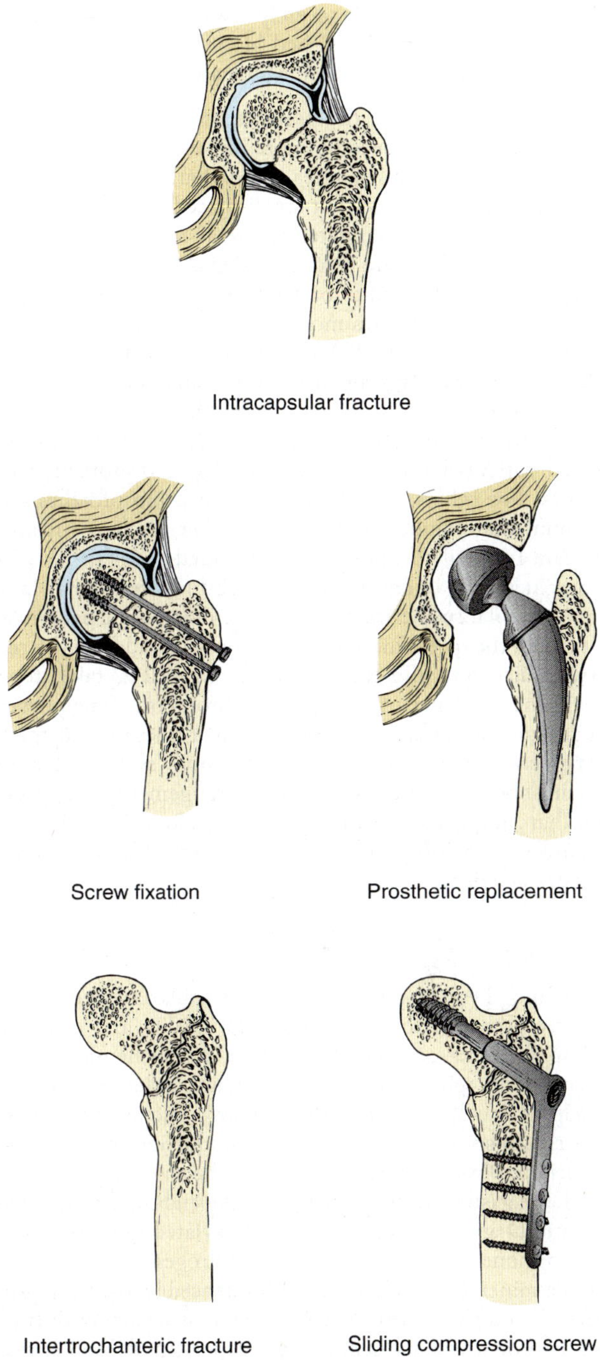

Figure 84.6. Fractures of proximal femur.

One method one of the authors (Richard A. Scott) has used with success is the transfer of a pedicle of bone from the trochanteric region attached to the quadratus femoris muscle along with its large artery.

- This pedicle is implanted into the femoral head and neck.
- For younger patients, the surgeon tries to avoid prosthetic hip joint replacement, which is the alternative to internal fixation of the fracture.
- The younger the patient, the more likely it is that a prosthesis will fail before the patient has completed their active weight-bearing life. If the prosthesis fails then additional surgery to revise or replace the implant is generally required.
- To recapitulate, nondisplaced femoral neck fractures should be treated with internal fixation in the hope that healing will occur.

- However, if the fracture is severely displaced or if there appears to be a high risk of diminished blood supply to the femoral head, a prosthetic replacement is indicated.

As a person ages and the bone becomes more osteoporotic, femoral neck fractures become more impacted or displaced, and the treatment protocol separates those that are stable or minimally displaced from those that are displaced. For the first group, internal fixation with cannulated screws is recommended; in the latter group, prostheses are recommended. As a person ages more and the ability to ambulate or even get out of bed disappears, the protocol again becomes more complex because the physician needs to weigh the costs of hospital and surgical treatment and the high mortality rates against the possible alleviation of the acute fracture pain. A period of immobilization with traction may be sufficient for fibrous healing in very old or cognitively impaired patients because it allows turning and protection from bed sores. For others, a replacement with a hip prosthesis may allow immediate ambulation and an earlier discharge from the acute care hospital to home or an extended care facility with a lessened incidence of contractures, decubitus ulcers, heart failure, and pneumonia. In the treatment of the older adult patient with hip fracture, the osteopathic physician needs to address the respiratory, cardiac, and alimentary systems, as well as take steps to decrease the incidence of deep venous thrombosis. The physician must realize that after a trauma, such as a fracture and fracture surgery, derangements occur in all of the body systems. The physician must be vigilant and treat these derangements as they occur rather than simply pay attention to the hip alone. Mobilization of the thoracic spine often increases cardiorespiratory function and stimulates activity.

Prevention

Osteopathic physicians need to use their skills and knowledge to help society in an effort to increase the quality and quantity of life. Hip fractures occur partly because of biochemical changes associated with aging. The physician should understand how they can help older adults maintain their bony structure and integrity. The basic substrates needed for bone production include protein and calcium. Physicians understand that the absorption of calcium through the gastrointestinal tract partly depends on the interaction of vitamin D and its various active hydroxylated forms with circulating hormones such as calcitonin and estrogen.

Bone mineral production also is influenced by the basic principle that if an organ or structure is not used, it wastes away. If bone is not used or stressed, calcium is not deposited. A limb at rest or not stressed by gravity, as in a space station astronaut or in a person on bed rest, quickly becomes osteopenic.

- A physician can help patients maintain bone production by ensuring dietary and supplemental control of essential vitamins, minerals, and hormones.
- Patients should be encouraged to exercise, particularly weight-bearing exercise.
- Regular loading of the appendicular and axial skeleton is the best way to enhance sustained mineral production.
- All bone will not be maintained strong enough not to fracture, despite these measures.
- The home and workplace must be made safer. Obstacles that may cause one to trip and fall should be removed.
- Finally, the balance and agility of the older adult should be evaluated regularly, and appropriate steps taken to prevent sarcopenia, orthostatic hypotensive episodes, and/or vision loss.

The incidence of hip fractures is increasing as the population ages. This is a population that is nutritionally and hormonally depleted. Moreover, it is a population that has forgotten to walk. Regulation of these factors as well as decreasing the extrinsic risk factors in the environment helps decrease the number of hip fractures.

- One of the ways in which the physician can decrease the risk of fractures is to decrease the amount of sedatives and drugs that can impair balance.
- A novel method for increasing stamina and balance has been proposed by Wolf. Based on a study performed by the National Institute of Aging, Wolf recommends that older adults practice the ancient Chinese exercise, Tai Chi.[20]

Dual-energy x-ray absorptiometry (DXA) can be used to screen and monitor BMD and predict risk of future fracture due to osteoporosis. Adults who have a fracture after the age of 50 years should have a DXA to assess their BMD per the National Osteoporosis Foundation.[21] The osteopathic physician has a major role in helping the individual patient as well as the population at risk for these fractures. In the treatment of a patient with a hip fracture, the goal is to control pain and return the patient to a nonhospital environment. How the physician treats or recommends treatment depends on the anatomic type of fracture as well as on the physiologic status of the patient.

OSTEOARTHRITIS OF THE KNEE

To examine and treat the arthritic knee requires that one understand how arthritis affects the whole body. Arthritis is joint inflammation. An arthritic problem can be the result of a degenerative "wear and tear" process, systemic disorder that may be immunologically based, the effect of infection, or a metabolic disorder such as rickets. It can be a late effect of trauma such as a fall, a vehicular accident, or a sports-related ligamentous injury. Before evaluating the joint in question, the physician must first ascertain if there is a systemic cause for arthritis. Often the different types and presentations of the various forms of arthritis are recognizable with a thorough history and physical examination.

Patient History and Presentation

A careful history allows the physician to recognize that a young woman who presents with morning stiffness and symmetric polyarticular disease might have rheumatoid arthritis.

- It allows for the assumption that a middle-aged man with a history of recurrent great toe pain associated with dietary indiscretions, who presents with a hot, inflamed knee joint, probably has gout.
- Examination of the gowned patient forces even the most casual examiner to recognize advanced psoriatic skin changes in an arthritic patient.

To paraphrase one of the tenets of osteopathic medicine, a patient's disease affects their entire body system. It is appropriate and necessary that the osteopathic physician understand the relationship of an arthritic joint to the whole patient.

The most common kind of knee arthritis that presents to the orthopedist is degenerative osteoarthritis of the knee which is a wearing out or progressive loss of the articular cartilage. This is most commonly seen in the medial compartment of the knee. This is usually the result of repeated minor articular trauma or wear.

Physical Examination of the Knee

Observe the patient's standing posture. Knee wear and tear is oftentimes coupled with a normal varus or mild bowlegged body habitus.

- As shown in Figure 84.7A, in this presentation, a line of weight bearing from the center of the axis of the femur passing to the center of the ankle joint passes inside of or medial to the center of the knee. In this case, the vast amount of forces and stresses that pass through the knee pass entirely through the medial compartment or through the medial femoral condyle and tibial plateau.

Disabling unilateral medial knee arthritis displays a dysmorphic enlarged knee upon observation and palpation. It has other effects as well. The patient with a painful joint has an antalgic gait: they limp. Limping causes a twisting motion to the joints above and below the painful joint.

- A common problem with limping is an imbalance in the sacroiliac articulation with a resultant somatic dysfunction in this joint. Therefore, evaluating the pelvic and sacral mechanics is indicated.
- Often, as the knee bows medially, an effective leg length difference occurs that may need to be addressed with a lift, indicating the need to assess for leg length inequality. (Discussion of assessment and treatment for leg length inequality are found in Chapters 92 and 93.)

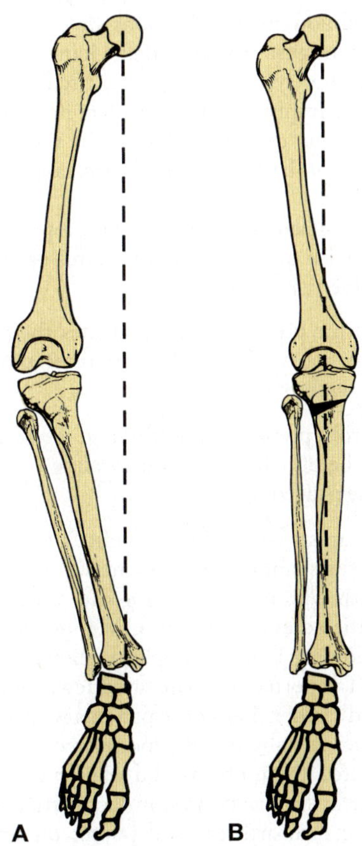

Figure 84.7. Genu varum. A. A lower extremity with extreme genu varum in which the weight-bearing line from the hip to the foot passes medial to the knee joint. **B.** A limb after a high tibial osteotomy in which the weight-bearing line passes through a point lateral to the center of the knee joint.

- In addition, patients with pronated feet increase the stresses over the medial knee joint, so be sure to assess for foot pronation in the standing position.
- With pain, the patient fails to exercise and becomes deconditioned; the entire cardiopulmonary status may deteriorate if left unattended. Thus, the heart and lungs should be examined and assessed for signs of deconditioning.
- Many patients with pain cannot work as hard at their jobs and their hobbies as they would like and become depressed. Therefore, assess for signs of depression.

The following tests are examples of those used commonly to assess the integrity of the knee ligaments and meniscus. Test descriptions and photos demonstrating these procedures can be found in the section on orthopedic tests.

- McMurray test
- Drawer and Lachman tests
- Patella apprehension test
- Varus and valgus tests
- Anterior ankle drawer test (often with knee dysfunction, there is also ankle dysfunction and vice versa)

Management

If there has been an injury to the ligaments or cartilage of the knee, with time and the increase of stresses, there is increasing wear and debris in the joint. Optimizing treatment requires some understanding of how articular cartilage is nourished, what steps can be taken to decrease the wear debris or particulate gravel in the knee, and how to diminish stresses in the medial joint.

- The articular surface, or the cartilaginous weight-bearing element of a joint, is made up of a matrix of water-heavy proteins with few living chondrocytes present.
- This anatomic area has no direct blood flow.
- The metabolites necessary for the nutrition and repair of the cartilage pass into the structure through the sponge-like cartilage.
- With pressure from weight bearing or muscle contracture, the cartilage surfaces collapse, pushing the fluid into the joint.
- As the pressure is relieved, the joint fluid seeps back into the cartilaginous matrix, bringing the necessary metabolites and oxygen required for cell life.
- Therefore, it is important to maintain the motion and normal stresses to the knee.

As part of the treatment of the patient with knee osteoarthritis, the osteopathic physician needs to encourage motion and activities, such as:

- Low-impact aerobics
- Water exercise
- Repetitive low-stress activities such as walking, bicycling, swimming, and use of elliptical trainers

Routine exercise is important for sustaining the metabolic demand of the cartilaginous matrix; however, overuse may cause serious problems.

- Activities including eccentrically loaded high-stress activities, twisting, and torquing are not recommended due to increased stress and shearing forces across the joint and on the ligaments.
- In addition, damage to the articular cartilage due to previous trauma and aging can cause irregularities of the cartilage which may be easily torn with compression and shearing forces.

Assisting the patient to obtain and maintain a body weight within normal limits also helps to diminish the stresses in the joint. The tibiofemoral joint reaction forces are three to four times body weight with walking and climbing. The patellofemoral joint reaction forces are two to three times body weight with descending stairs and up to seven times body weight with squatting. Weight loss can have a pronounced effect in easing a patient's joint discomfort by decreasing their joint reactive forces. Adjunctive treatments may also be helpful, such as:

- The use of a custom orthosis in the shoe often changes the dynamics, relieves pain, and allows the patella to track more normally in the patella–femoral trochlear groove.
- Counseling and the use of antidepressant medications may be helpful for addressing the emotional and socioeconomic stress of debilitating injury.

At the present time in the development of orthopedic implants, laboratory-designed and manufactured biomaterials do not have the same degree of biologic function as normal tissues. They are not self-reparative. They have different moduli of elasticity than the human tissues; they do not bend the same amount with force as do human bones. The result of this is increased stress at the interface between the implant and the biologic tissue.

- Particles of wear debris that occur normally with time, particularly those of the high-density polyethylene that serves as the bearing surface in most prostheses, are read by the host cells as foreign.
- This causes an intense foreign body reaction of releasing biologically active mediators in turn causing the body to resorb the bone surrounding the implant. This results in weakening the junction between the prosthesis and the bone and allowing loosening, pain, and fracture to occur.

The options for the surgeon treating osteoarthritis are limited because no surgical implant can guarantee a relief of pain. In young patients, replacement arthroplasty should be avoided for as long as possible. Treatment is recommended case by case based on the understanding of that patient's physiology, age, life requirements, and goals, as well as on knowledge and experience with the types of treatment available.

One of the simplest treatments is the application of a knee brace ("unloader brace") that applies pressure to the tibia below and the femur above, thereby increasing the forces applied over the lateral joint line.

- For many, the brace is successful for pain relief, although it may be cumbersome to apply and bulky under clothes.

For those who have an angular deformity that is severe and painful, osteotomy may realign the mechanical problems associated with genu varum. As depicted in Figure 84.7B, a simple form of osteotomy removes a wedge of bone from the lateral proximal tibia.

- If this wedge is properly calculated, when the osteotomy heals, the center of gravity or the forces acting through the knee pass through the lateral joint, thus diminishing the forces through the arthritic medial joint.

For many, as an adjunct to or substitute for osteotomy or bracing, arthroscopy may afford relief. If there is a degree of effusion and torn tissues with multiple loose particles floating inside the knee joint, debridement or vacuuming of the knee can wash out the offending particles. While this is not curative, for many it affords a long period of pain relief.

For those whose knee joint is not a candidate for osteotomy and whose lifestyle and physiologic age are appropriate, joint replacement arthroplasty is indicated.

- Joint replacement arthroplasty requires adherence to a host of mechanical constraints.
- The joint must be in a normal and mechanically sound position, and the components need to be securely fixated to the bones of the knee joint.
- There are many options, ranging from the unicompartmental hemiarthroplasties that simply replace the damaged medial compartment to constrained systems in which the design attempts to substitute for damaged ligaments.

The osteopathic physician needs to understand some of the features of the implants and the physiologic changes that occur with implant arthroplasty.

- The risks of deep venous thrombosis are high.
  - ☐ Precautions are necessary, ranging from early activity and external compression devices to pharmacologic agents for the prevention of venous thromboembolism such as vitamin K antagonists (e.g., warfarin), indirect thrombin inhibitors (e.g., low–molecular-weight heparins and unfractionated heparin), direct thrombin inhibitors (e.g., dabigatran), direct factor Xa inhibitors (e.g., rivaroxaban), and antiplatelet agents (e.g., aspirin).
- The risk of infection, both early and late, although not abundant, is disastrous when it occurs.
  - ☐ The risks are diminished through good surgical and sterile techniques, as well as with the use of appropriate antibiotics.
  - ☐ Scheduled follow-up examinations are essential.
  - ☐ The physician must recognize that a joint implant is a foreign body. With any systemic infection, circulating bacteria may adhere to the implant and cause a late infection.
    - The judicious use of antibiotics in the face of systemic infections or bacteremia may decrease the incidence of infection.
    - Many physicians recommend the prophylactic use of antibiotics with oral surgical procedures or at other times of predictable risk for bacteremia.

The osteopathic physician who evaluates the patient for total joint arthroplasty must address the variety of problems that are involved in knee arthritis.

- Weight control, physical conditioning, exercise, and proper nutrition are helpful to encourage healing and maximize the gains from the procedure.

Physical therapists have shown benefit of manual therapy and exercises in reducing pain and delaying need for surgery in patients with osteoarthritis who met criteria for knee arthroplasty.[22,23]

A study of the adjunctive use of OMT in the early postoperative period following joint arthroplasty showed that those who underwent OMT reported less pain, used fewer analgesic medications, and walked farther than those patients who were not manipulated.[24] However, a subsequent randomized placebo-controlled clinical trial refuted these claims, did not find OMT efficacious post hip or knee arthroplasty, and, in fact, patients in the OMT cohort with knee osteoarthritis had poorer outcomes post knee arthroplasty such as increased length of stay and decreased rehabilitation efficiency.[25] More recently, in 2020, a prospective comparative study was published showing that standardized preoperative OMT was found to be effective in reducing pain in the first month after total knee arthroplasty for osteoarthritis and significantly reduced opioid consumption during the first postoperative week.[26] Additional studies are needed to further develop objective measures and assess the outcome of patients who have undergone total knee arthroplasty and treated with OMT perioperatively.

INSTABILITY OF THE SHOULDER

Injuries to the ligamentous structures of the major joints are common. The average layperson and general practitioner understand that a sprained ligament is painful and causes swelling and edema. All respect the need for rest, ice, compression, and elevation (RICE) and protection of the injured joint until healing has occurred. This section of the chapter discusses injuries of the shoulder joint as a model for sprains, or ligamentous injuries, the biomechanical changes that occur with sprains, and recognition of laxity of ligaments with instability or tightness of joint structures causing adhesions. The spectrum flows from those joints unable to be maintained within normal physiologic ranges and those unable to have normal physiologic motion. The goal of this section is to introduce the student to the osteopathic approach to the joint, to understand the biomechanical aspects of joint stability, and to review possible mechanisms of treatment.

The osteopathic physician needs to be able to recognize the unstable and the dislocated shoulder. Many physicians see patients with shoulder problems soon after a traumatic episode, such as an auto accident or sports-related injury. Other times, weeks may pass after an injurious event before the patient presents to the physician with pain and instability. Physicians also need to be able to recognize the unusual dislocation that occurs after seizure or electric shock.

Sprains are either acute or chronic. The acute injury is associated with tearing of structures, the chronic with stretched or inadequate structures. Instability is also characterized by degree: complete dislocation versus subluxation or subtle instability, such as is found in the "dead shoulder" of baseball pitchers who have pain associated with the overhead pitching motion.[27] Instabilities are also diagnosed by direction: anterior, posterior, inferior, and multidirectional. A most interesting case of fracture dislocation was reported in which the humeral head was not seen on radiograph and was found in the retroperitoneum.[28] In addition, there have been humeral fracture dislocation cases described with intrathoracic humeral head migration.[29,30] While this incomplete list of classification may seem daunting, it should not, as the physician should cover these aspects in the history and physical examination of the patient.

Presentation and History

As in other areas of the orthopedic structural examination, the physician should *listen, look,* and *feel.* One can often learn more about the structure by finding out how and when the initial injury occurred, how often it has happened, and what the shoulder or joint looks or looked like when it was injured than from sophisticated images.

As a case example, a common presentation to the emergency room is of a middle-aged, cachectic alcoholic man with seizure history and multiple comorbidities. He presents postictally complaining of pain over the front of his shoulder and holds his arm protectively. Radiographic examination is negative.

Physical Examination

The physical examination is diagnostic. If the shoulder is posteriorly dislocated, there is a palpable hollowness anteriorly, and as the elbow is brought posterior to the midaxillary line with gentle pressure on the humeral head, the examiner can feel the shoulder return to its normal position. Often the reverse examination of the shoulder that has spontaneously reduced will allow the physician to feel the head slide out of the joint. The patient examined long after the original injury will often have symptoms when the arm is circumducted.

Specific orthopedic tests to identify ligamentous laxity, inflammation, sprain, or damage include the following:

- Apprehension test of the shoulder
- Biceps load test
- Drop arm test
- Apley scratch test

These tests are described and photos demonstrating them can be found in the Orthopedic Tests section.

Diagnosis

Imaging, such as MRI and ultrasonography, is helpful to confirm a clinical diagnosis. In our society, a corroborative image may be necessary prior to invasive treatment. Imaging, however, often lacks specificity and sensitivity. Sometimes the readily obtained radiographs are not helpful.

Posterior dislocations account for 5% of all acute dislocations. Nearly half are missed at the initial presentation. They are mentioned because the examination is diagnostic just as in the other directions of instability. The interested reader can read more about these problems in a textbook that details shoulder problems[31] (Fig. 84.8).

Many factors are associated with joint stability. Problems with the osseous structures are common static factors. These include abnormal version of either glenoid or humerus; crushed glenoid, in which the defect in the structure allows the humeral head to slide out of the joint; and the Hill–Sachs lesion, wherein

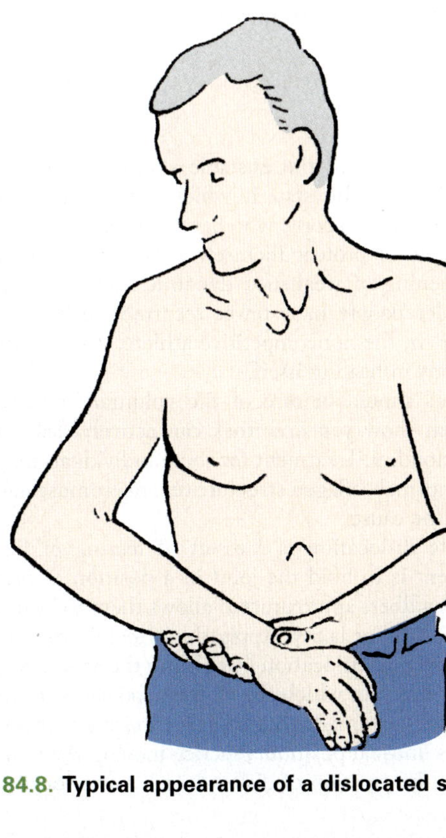

Figure 84.8. Typical appearance of a dislocated shoulder.

a defect or grooved fracture in the humeral articular surface induces recurrent instability. The ligaments are thickenings of the capsular structure, which provide stability in the multiple positions in which the shoulder can be moved. The ligaments are mostly type I collagen. The strength, aging characteristics, and repair mechanisms of torn ligaments are important factors in the healing process.

Thickening of the capsule on the periphery of the joint results in the formation of the labrum, or lip. The labrum has an essential stabilizing force for the shoulder in increasing its depth, as the joint is inherently unstable. Arthroscopic visualizations, anatomic dissections, and MRI imaging have helped us understand the anatomy and function of the ligamentous structures. The small amount of fluid within the joint acts as a fluid membrane allowing sliding or slipping but inhibiting separation. This force is analogous to that of two wet glass plates that will slide on each other easily but are difficult to separate.[32]

The study of what makes the shoulder stable continues, but the answers are elusive. The interested reader is referred to the studies of Soslowsky and colleagues on contact areas of the glenohumeral joint and to the recent analysis of the role of the labrum in centralization of the humeral head by Halder and others.[33,34]

The many muscles around the shoulder are essential to stability, provide dynamic restraints, and are important in dysfunction. The rotator cuff muscles, long head of the biceps, and the periscapular muscles all play a role in shoulder stability. The primary biomechanical role of the rotator cuff is stabilizing the glenohumeral joint by compressing the humerus against the glenoid and acts as a humeral head depressor. If torn, the shoulder may displace. If healed and tightened too much, they can cause adhesions. The osteopathic examiner should palpate and test the function of the various muscles of the shoulder girdle. Treatment then can be directed toward stretching the fibrosed muscle and exercising the weak or lax muscle. Electromyographic studies may help to ascertain if there is a neuromuscular etiology to dysfunctional shoulder girdle. In a high-performance, throwing athlete, these can be augmented with video of the throwing motion that can help in planning treatment.

Treatment

The goal of treatment of the unstable shoulder is to bring the patient to a painless, stable state in which they can carry out normal life functions. Most people who have dislocated their shoulder have learned how to protect themselves from recurrent dislocations. Strengthening of weakened dynamic stabilizers will often assist this. Older people have fewer recurrent dislocations than younger people. In the noncompetitive athlete, it is often prudent to assist the body in healing itself.

Practitioners should beware of the voluntary recurrent dislocator who can show you how they can actively dislocate their shoulder like Houdini. Treatment for these individuals may not be rewarding. Abnormal collagen structure or a neuromuscular abnormality may be the cause.

If the acute dislocation is a result of tearing of fibers, the goal of treatment is to hold the joint in a position of protection. Keeping the torn fibers approximated allows them to heal with the least amount of scar or laxity. Apply the principle to our case of seizure with posterior dislocation by holding the arm in a thoracobrachial cast or brace in which the elbow is posterior to the chest wall and the arm is externally rotated. It is intuitive to maintain the shoulder in this unusual position. Practice moving the arm around and reduplicate the position of dislocation; a posterior dislocation occurs often when the arm is extended forward, and a large force directs the humeral head out the back of the joint. It is then obvious that reversing these positions would tend to keep the shoulder in a "reduced" position. Recent information has demonstrated that the position that approximates the torn fibers of the joint capsule in an "anterior" dislocation (the most common type of dislocation seen) is not what we most commonly use. Normally, a "reduced" anterior dislocation is kept in an arm sling with the arm internally rotated. Itoi and coresearchers found, with the use of MRI, that the torn anterior capsule was most closely approximated with the arm held at 90 degrees of external rotation.[35] This can be a difficult position in which to hold the patient. Protection while healing is the precaution to take to allow the body to heal its injured tissues in the best way. Athletes can be protected from reinjury with braces. Hockey players may benefit from straps that inhibit the checking opponent from lifting their arm overhead, which may be an unstable position.

A tear of the labrum may not heal. A tear of the labrum at the anterior portion of the glenoid is called a Bankart lesion. If this is found in a recurrent dislocator or in a young athlete with an acute dislocation, then surgical repair may be necessary. Surgery of the shoulder to repair instability is either open, through larger incisions, or more commonly arthroscopically. During shoulder arthroscopy, the surgeon inserts a small camera, called an arthroscope, into the shoulder joint. The camera is used to visualize the shoulder joint and associated anatomic structures and specially designed surgical instruments are used to facilitate repair through small incisions. The results of acute repair of Bankart lesions are promising. In recurrent instability, the goal of treatment is to strengthen weak structures and stretch tight structures. Nonoperative means are preferred. If surgery is necessary, there are multiple means for reconstruction of joints.

One can divide the means of surgical reconstruction into simplistic categories. Surgery is either open or arthroscopic. Bones can be osteotomized where the angle or version is incorrect or grafted where there is a defect. Tissues torn from their origin are sewn, nailed, or screwed back into position. Tucks or plication is used to tighten up lax structures. Energy sources such as heat, thermal, electrical, or light and chemical are used to scar or shrink loose collagen structures. Prolotherapy has shown some benefit in stabilizing joints that have ligamentous laxity (see Chapter 89 for further information on prolotherapy).

Orthopedic surgeons enjoy the challenges and excitement of these varied innovative procedures. These techniques, however, are beyond the scope of this chapter. Of more importance is recognition of what the practitioner can do to help the injured joint. In summary, the practitioner must, with careful attention to palpatory skills, define the position of stability and begin a program to strengthen the rotator cuff muscles that will help hold the joint in a reduced position. More commonly, we are faced with a tight joint. The syndrome known as adhesive capsulitis ("frozen shoulder") is poorly understood and should be differentiated from other conditions such as subscapularis myofascial trigger points.

- Some link it to an inflammatory condition of the synovial lining of the joint.
- In diabetics, it may be part of the diabetic arthropathy which affects joint mobility, where changes in the collagen structure occur because of metabolic changes in glucose metabolism.
- Spencer technique (see Chapter 57 Articulatory Procedures) has been used by osteopathic physicians for over a century, and muscle energy techniques (see Chapter 51) have been used for

over 50 years, both with acclaimed clinical success at improving shoulder pain and motion dysfunction from adhesive capsulitis, impingement syndrome, and shoulder muscle restrictions. Recent randomized clinical trials have demonstrated that these procedures improve shoulder range of motion and functional ability.[36–38]

LOW BACK PAIN

The most frequently seen problem for general orthopedists today is LBP and it is ubiquitous in the population. LBP is secondary only to upper respiratory tract infection, "the common cold," as cause to visit the doctor's office. LBP affects more than 80% of the population in their lifetime.[39,40] The costs of treatment, the expenses of failed work, and the problems frequently associated with blame and the legal system make the treatment of LBP one of urgency. LBP is associated with $100 billion in annual health care expenditures.[41] The patient and family need to have a return-to-work schedule and sense of normalcy restored; society needs some surcease from the huge costs necessitated by the disability structure. Every physician sees the patient with acute disabling back pain who is unable to walk and unrelieved of discomfort. From the orthopedist's point of view, the urgency to relieve pain and disability quickly makes a dispassionate evaluation and treatment plan impossible. The new technologic advances in imaging and surgical techniques have led many patients to believe that a rapid, easy, risk-free surgical treatment is available. It is the surgeon's duty to convey to the patient, in no uncertain terms, that no surgery is risk-free or without the risk of complication. There is nothing that cannot be made worse with surgery if the surgery is not performed for the right reasons and in the right way. In addition, surgery may not be in the patient's best interest, despite being indicated based on pathology, if the patient will be unable to tolerate the procedure due to their medical and/or mental status. Everyone has known someone who, following back surgery, did not get better but may have gotten worse. The litigants would have us believe it is because of faulty technique, lack of informed consent, delay in diagnosis, or delay in treatment.[42] Spine surgeons are still evolving techniques, materials, and methods to find out which patients with LBP can benefit from which procedure. Other surgeons often do not want to examine, evaluate, or treat the patient with acute or chronic back pain because such patients are often difficult and demanding.

The osteopathic orthopedic surgeon approaches the patient with LBP with a systematic protocol. The primary objective for all physicians and surgeons is to define a distinct diagnosis founded on accurate anatomic and pathologic basis. The great problem for surgeons in general and for orthopedists in particular is to identify appropriate surgical pathologic conditions. Most back pain does not need to be treated surgically. In a great percentage of patients with LBP, the final diagnosis is idiopathic. This means essentially that nobody knows what the cause of the disease is. Some estimates indicate that more than 50% of all patients with LBP do not have a firm, accurate, anatomically defined reason for their pain. To operate is problematic if the diagnosis is uncertain.

Spine surgeons realize that for people with the same pathologic diagnosis, the long-term result of surgical and nonsurgical treatment may be the same. The outcome in equivalent groups of patients with diskogenic LBP may be similar, and not clinically significantly different, for those who have undergone lumbar fusion surgery and those treated nonsurgically with structured physical therapy.[43] This does not mean that the patient with a frank neurologic deficit, weakness, numbness, and intractable pain over the ipsilateral dermatome should not be operated on. The immediate results of pain relief and neurologic recovery usually outweigh the fact that later, after the settling down of the disk space and the degenerative changes that occur in the surrounding structures, the postsurgical patient may subsequently have episodes of back and buttock pain. The spine surgeon must approach each patient who has been referred with back pain, with or without radiating leg pain, on an individual basis and construct a treatment plan based on the patient's needs and wants. Just because there may be surgical pathology does not necessarily mean surgery will be best for the patient.

The orthopedic spinal surgeon who evaluates the patient referred by the family practitioner, emergency room physician, internist, or family members first must understand the reasons for referral. People may want to believe that back pain that is severe enough to make the bearer nauseous, that has defied the palliative or curative modalities that often prove successful, and that is unrelieved by narcotic medications, rest, and anti-inflammatory shots, pills, and emollients must be a surgical disease. If pain is the anathema of life, then those who suffer and complain have an urgent imperative to seek the services of the surgeon. Patients and physicians are eager believers in the curative possibilities of the newer technologies. If MRI shows a bulging disk and a person has back pain, many assume excision of the disk will relieve the pain; however, this does not always prove true. The fact that the patient may not improve following surgery does not necessarily mean that the surgeon was inept. Many times, the acute episode is but one point in time of an ongoing process.

Asymptomatic herniations in the lumbar spine are common.[44] A systematic review identified that many imaging findings of degenerative spine disease have a high prevalence among asymptomatic individuals. All imaging findings examined had an increased prevalence with increasing age. Disk bulge prevalence increased from 30% of those 20 years of age to 84% of those 80 years of age. Over 50% of asymptomatic individuals 30 to 39 years of age have disk degeneration, height loss, or bulging. Some findings (disk degeneration and signal loss) were present in nearly 90% of individuals 60 years of age or older. These findings suggest that many imaging-based degenerative features may be part of normal aging and unassociated with LBP, especially when incidentally seen. These imaging findings must be interpreted in the context of the patient's clinical condition.[45] It is impossible for the person suffering severe intractable back pain to think rationally about the nature of their pain. As compassionate as the physician–surgeon may be, it is their job to review the possible causes of back pain (Table 84.1) to be able to outline the appropriate steps to best understand and treat the acute episode.

LBP is so ubiquitous that its definition is elusive. In the context of this chapter, LBP is that symptom complex in which the person experiencing pain describes it as encompassing the area of the lumbar spine and the associated musculature of the lumbar spine, as well as the sacrum and buttocks. Pain in the lumbar spine may be of local origin or may be referred. Disorders causing LBP may compress spinal nerve roots. If this occurs, the patient may experience radiating leg pain, numbness or weakness indicating a lumbar radiculopathy. Lumbar radiculopathy produces these symptoms in the sensory (dermatome) and muscle (myotome) areas specific to the involved nerve root. The specific pattern of symptom involvement act like a map to help the physician diagnose the spinal pathology causing the condition. There are large lists of entities that can be associated with back pain. Often, they serve as diagnostic guides in which the observer–physician

TABLE 84.1

Posterior, Middle, and Anterior Spinal Elements Related to Back Pain

Elements	Possible Etiologies
Posterior Elements—Most Common	
Spinous process, transverse processes, lamina, pedicles, ligaments, and joining capsule, intervertebral joints	Somatic dysfunction—TART[a] Especially the "dirty half-dozen." Age-related and activity-related strains—arthritis, overuse. Severe or chronic twists. Strains and sprains. Spondylosis, overuse, or chronic trauma. Spondylolisthesis. Severe trauma and twists. Fractures of pedicle, transverse process, or spinous process[b]
Middle Elements	
Central spinal canal, meninges, spinal cord, and nerves	Compression of the spinal canal or nerve root Cauda equina syndrome[b] Intrinsic Intradural tumors Meningeal infections Extrinsic pressure through foramen and/or the thecal sac Metastatic tumors Ruptured disk with contents free in the spinal canal Neurofibromas Spurs or other symptoms of aging or degenerative conditions (osteoarthritis) Benign tumors or fibromas Reflex etiologies—visceral dysfunctions and diseases
Anterior Elements	
Posterior longitudinal ligament, vertebral body, anterior longitudinal ligament, and intervertebral disk	Compression fractures of the vertebral body. Vascular causes—abdominal aneurysm Traumatic disk disruption with pressure on nerve root or thecal sac. Infection

[a]Glossary of osteopathic terminology. *AOA Yearbook and Directory.* American Osteopathic Association; 2000:869.

[b]Emergency.

finds an easy way to choose tests for diagnostic possibilities. For instance, most people with back pain do not have myeloma. To run a gamut of blood and urine tests on an otherwise healthy 30-year-old to rule out myeloma is not reasonable until the more common and statistically significant clinical entities have been differentiated.

Tests should be chosen with regard to their pretest probability using the test to help firm up a diagnosis only after a careful history has been elicited and a physical examination has explored abdominal, pelvic, and spinal structures. In *Acute Low Back Problems in Adults*,[46] a clinical practice guideline published by the U.S. Department of Health and Human Services, the authors have included a series of red flags that help alert the examiner to responses or findings that merit detailed evaluation.

The authors provide 5 algorithms for the diagnosis and management of patients with low back pain. These include:

A1: Initial assessment of acute low back symptoms
A2: Treatment of acute low back problems on initial and follow-up visits
A3: Evaluation of the slow to recover patient (limitations > 4 weeks)
A4: Surgical considerations for the patient with persistent sciatica
A5: Further care of acute low back problems

Their first algorithm (Fig. 84.9) outlines an approach to assessing LBP symptoms. Throughout the patient evaluation and while considering the diagnostic tests and therapeutic regimens, the physician should be continually asking if there is some reason for this pain outside of or beyond the spinal area. The red flags that suggest a serious underlying conditions include:

- Age of 50 years or older
- Previous history of cancer
- Unexplained weight loss
- Failure to improve with 1 month of therapy
- No relief with bed rest

For a patient suffering from a known trauma or with a history of corticosteroid use, fracture is suspected. Intravenous drug abuse, urinary tract infection (UTI), or skin infection in a patient with back pain suggests osteomyelitis or diskitis. Sciatica suggests disk herniation. Neurogenic claudication, the symptom of increasing leg pain or weakness that is eased with forward flexion or rest, suggests spinal stenosis.[46] Guidelines regarding methods to use in identifying red flags in patients with LBP are continually being updated.[47–50]

History and Physical Examination

As in most areas of medical care, the history is of primary importance. A quiet listening attitude on the part of the physician may encourage the patient to be frank and more open. The algorithm for the evaluation of back pain is so large that one item or another from the history given by the patient leads the physician interviewer to follow one pathway in their continued questioning and

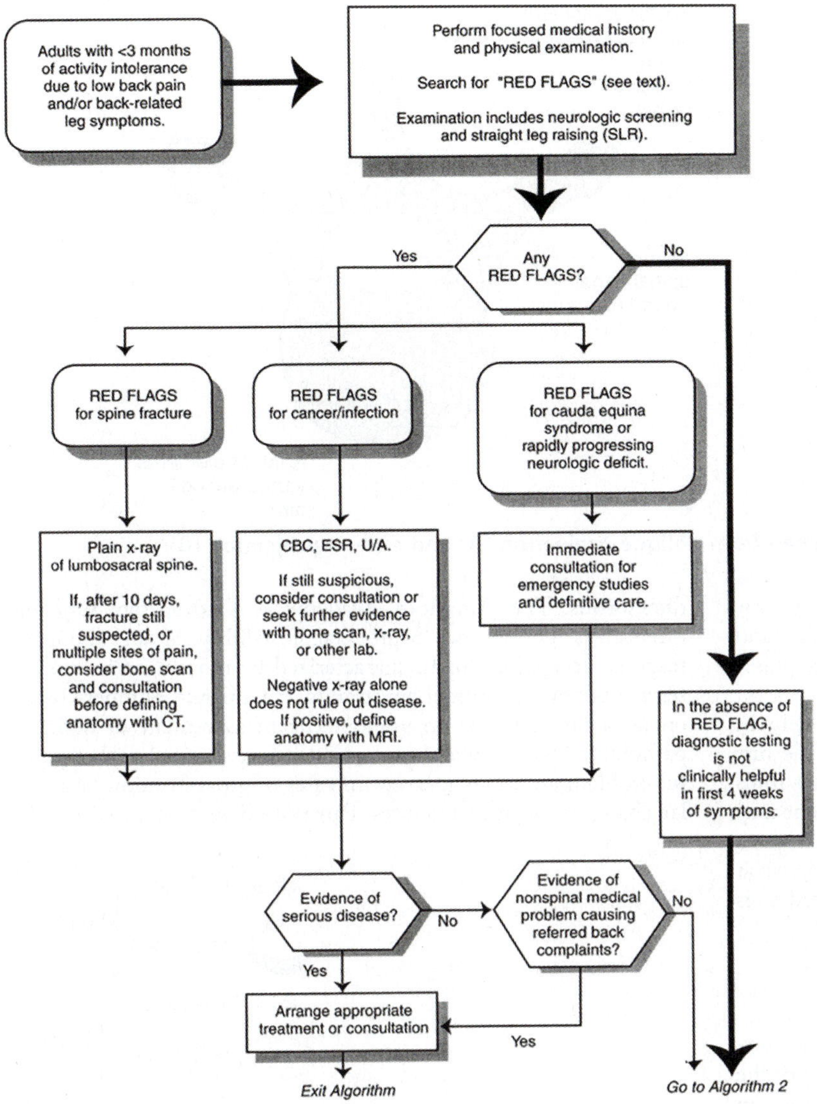

Figure 84.9. Algorithm (A1) for assessing the patient with low back pain. Initial assessment of acute low back pain symptoms. CT, computed tomography; CBC, complete blood count; ESR, erythrocyte sedimentation rate; U/A, urine analysis. (From Bigos S, Bowyer O, Braen G, et al. *Acute low back problems in adults. Clinical Practice Guideline, Quick Reference Guide Number. 14.* U.S. Department of Health and Human Services, Public Health Service, Agency for Health Care Policy and Research. AHCPR Pub. No. 95-0643. 1994.)

in test ordering. Examples of questions that can help guide the examiner include:

- When did the pain begin?
- When is it worse?
- What aggravates the pain?
- What relieves the pain?
- Have other family members had similar problems?
- Was the onset associated with a traumatic episode?
- Is litigation pending?

Although many of the tests are essential to confirm a diagnosis, the physical examination is crucial. Physical examination includes

1. Observation
2. Palpation and manual motion testing
3. Neuromuscular examination
4. Vascular assessment

Much of the physical examination can be performed quickly and concurrently while distracting the patient. All require that the patient be gowned so that their back and legs can be observed and palpated. Examination of a fully clothed patient is inadequate.

Observe the patient while they move from chair to examining table and note ability to get off and on the examining table with or without assistance. Note the gait to ascertain if limp, foot drag or drop, or lurch exists. Note the use of an assistive device, cane, or walker, as well as any alteration of muscle mass, tone, or atrophy, and the presence of any scars.

Palpation of the back and limbs can be performed in multiple positions. Note the tone of the muscles and the turgor of the skin in the extremities. Examine the spine in standing and supine positions, noting areas of discomfort, pain provocation, asymmetries, or muscle spasm. As the spine is placed through ranges of motion, note individual segments with abnormal findings, and make measurements of the ranges of rotation, side bending, and flexion. Perform percussion of the spinous process and palpation of contiguous areas such as ischial tuberosity, greater trochanter, iliolumbar ligament, and groin.

The neuromuscular examination tests motor power, particularly the strength of the ankle and toe flexors and extensors, knee extensors and flexors, hip flexors, gluteal muscles, and rectal tone. The ability to stand on toes or heels unassisted is a sensitive evaluator of leg strength and the presence of intact S1, L5, and L4 nerve roots. Test for absent, present, or hyperesthetic sensation in legs, thighs, back, and perineum. Check deep tendon reflexes as well as the presence of clonus or a Babinski reflex. Assess the presence or absence of pressure on the nerve roots in the lumbar spine using the straight leg–raising maneuver, which can be performed with the patient sitting and supine. This maneuver is performed as the patient flexes

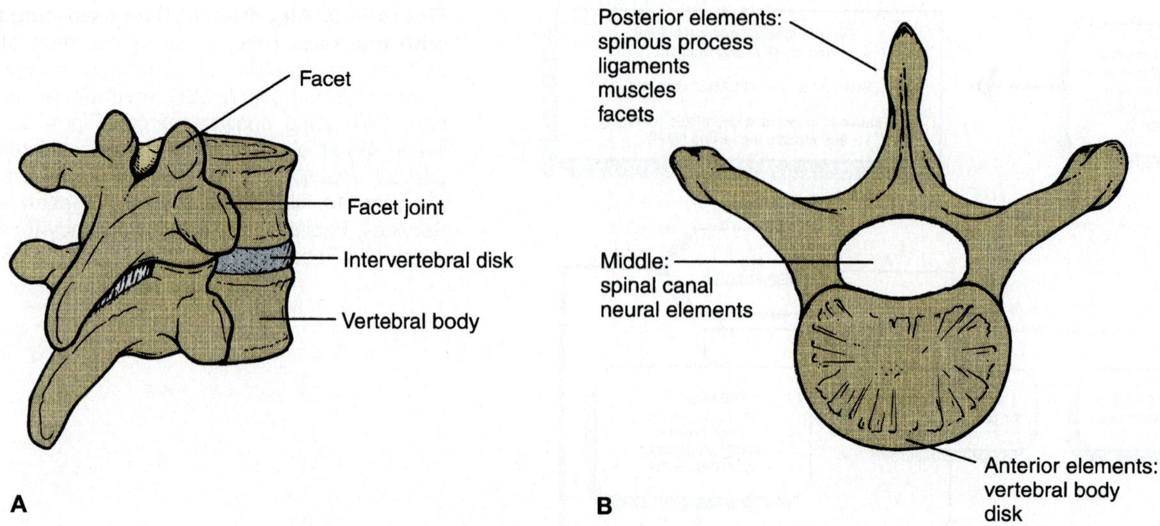

Figure 84.10. Functional spinal unit (FSU) seen from oblique projection (A) and end-on projection (B).

the hip while keeping the knee extended. Record symptom provocation in the form of back or ipsilateral or contralateral thigh and leg pain. Vascular assessment includes palpation of peripheral pulses and auscultation of abdominal, iliac, and femoral vessels.

Multiple tests and signs can elicit symptoms and help in the diagnosis. Examination of contiguous joints, such as the hip, may elicit a cause of referred pain. Frequently, the examiner finds patients with exaggerated complaints. Sometimes the patient may appear hysterical, to magnify the symptoms or to be a malingerer. Careful recording of these findings will help the examiner arrive at a meaningful conclusion. Waddell and colleagues have listed tests and suggested evaluation for those with atypical findings.[51]

Pathophysiology

The study of LBP begins with an anatomic and pathologic consideration of the basis for pain. The basic structural element of the spine is the functional spinal unit (FSU). The FSU is the motion segment and is the smallest segment of the spine that exhibits biomechanical characteristics like those of the entire spine. It consists of two adjacent vertebrae, the intervertebral disk, facet joints, and the connecting ligamentous tissues.[52] How an FSU behaves depends on the structure of each of the elements and its characteristics, strength, flexibility, and responses to stress. Each FSU is part of the entire axial skeleton from the inion to the coccyx, and each has a mechanical role to support the mass of the body as it moves in space and time.

The anatomic basis for disease encourages our understanding of the FSU. Disease can emanate from the bony structure, the synovial joints, and the ligaments constraining the adjacent vertebra. Moreover, disease can be caused by problems with the intervertebral disk.

Figure 84.10 shows the anatomic basis of the FSU. The FSU contains the elements of contiguous spinal vertebrae, their connecting disks, and the associated ligaments and muscles. The posterior elements consist of the spinous processes, ligaments, muscles, and facet joints. The middle segment contains the bony spinal canal and its contents, the neural elements, fat, and vasculature. The anterior elements include the vertebral bodies and the disk. In thinking about the spine as a source of pain, remember this anatomic image.

Figure 84.11 describes the type of motions the FSU undergoes in response to applied forces. This is a three-dimensional image. There are various definitions of segmental instability in three dimensions. The American Academy of Orthopedic Surgeons offers this definition: "Segmental instability is an abnormal response to applied loads, characterized by movement in motion segments beyond normal constraints".[53] Concrete numbers based on an x-ray study or on goniometric measurement to define a pathologic instability and prove that it is associated with a painful problem are lacking, except in cases of gross luxation or angular change as seen in fractures. Palpatory diagnosis, in which the

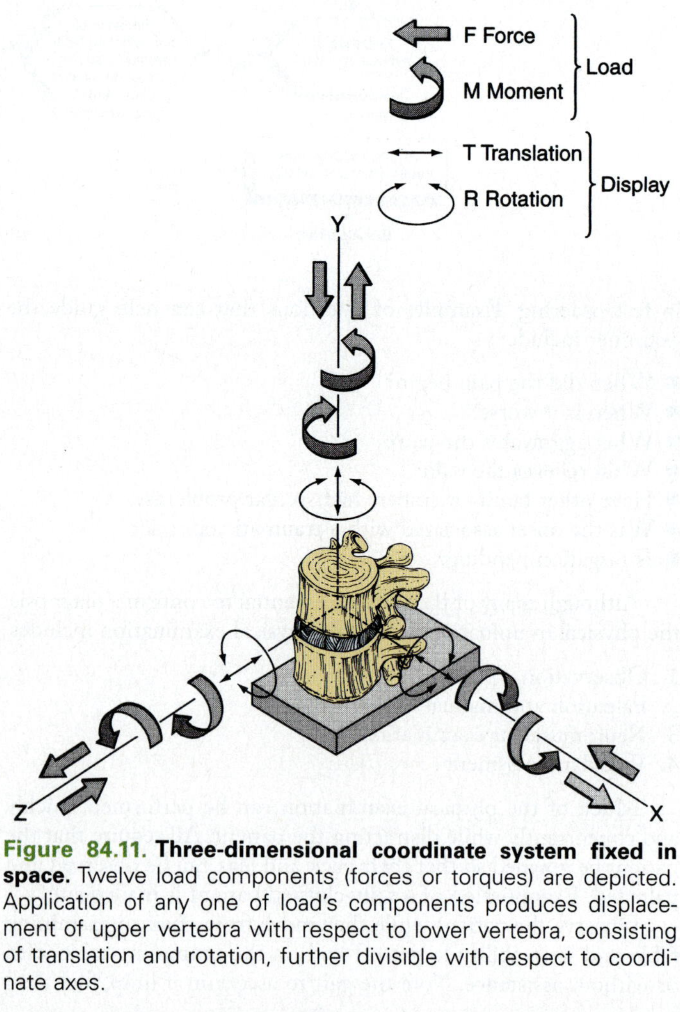

Figure 84.11. Three-dimensional coordinate system fixed in space. Twelve load components (forces or torques) are depicted. Application of any one of load's components produces displacement of upper vertebra with respect to lower vertebra, consisting of translation and rotation, further divisible with respect to coordinate axes.

endpoint of vertebral motion is ill defined and either restricted from normalcy or lacking uniformity, offers meaningful data to the examining physician.

The stability of the osseous spine depends on three zones, consisting of the anterior, middle, and posterior elements. This model, devised after a retrospective analysis of spinal fractures in the thoracic and thoracolumbar spine, has been widely adapted for use by spinal surgeons to arrange the thought processes in a more logical manner.[54] This discussion centers on the problems of the bony and soft tissue structures. The three columns as described by Denis include the posterior, middle, and anterior as follows[54]:

- The posterior column is formed by all structures posterior to the posterior longitudinal ligament which includes the posterior bony arch along with the posterior ligamentous complex:
  - □ Pedicles
  - □ Lamina
  - □ Facet joints
  - □ Spinous process
  - □ Posterior ligamentous complex (supraspinous and interspinous ligaments, facet capsules, and ligamentum flavum)
- The middle column is formed by the:
  - □ Posterior one-third of the vertebral body and annulus
  - □ Posterior vertebral wall
  - □ Posterior longitudinal ligament
- The anterior column is formed by the:
  - □ Anterior longitudinal ligament
  - □ Anterior two-thirds or the vertebral body and annulus

Denis designed his classification in an attempt to better understand the biomechanical changes found in the common and often devastating thoracic and thoracolumbar fractures. In his retrospective study, he described fractures at risk for neurologic compromise based on injury of the middle column. Although fractures of the low back or lumbar and lumbosacral spine are uncommon, the risk of damage to neural elements from middle column disruption in the lumbar spine is less because the cord usually stops above this area. The bony spinal canal is larger, and the cauda equina can be remarkably resistant to compressive damage from fracture fragments. For the anatomic basis of LBP, the arbitrary separation of the spine into three segments is helpful. It allows the physician to focus on the anatomic element that is the pain generator, as shown in Table 84.1.

Gunnar Andersson has divided the spine into anterior and posterior segments for ease in isolating causes of disease.[55] This author has labeled the central spinal canal as the middle column to isolate those entities that can cause back pain and may be present in the spinal canal alone (Fig. 84.10B). Entities that may cause acute back pain in the anterior spine include:

1. Fractures
2. Invasive diseases of the vertebral body and disk, which include
   - □ Tumor
   - □ Infection
   - □ Traumatic disk disruption
     - The Schmorl node or herniation of the disk through the vertebral end plate often characterizes traumatic disk disruption.
     - The disk has often been implicated as the major source of spinal pain.
     - Certainly, as the disk ages, undue stresses may be placed on the facet joints and arthritic spurs may compress into the spinal canal. However, in the normal spine, the disk under load bulges as a viscoelastic shock absorber (Fig. 84.12).

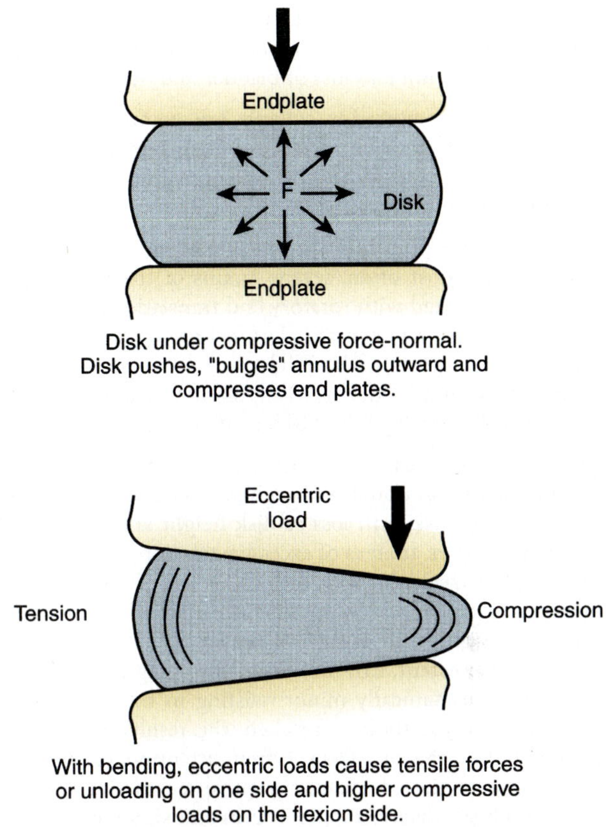

Figure 84.12. Disk stresses. F, force.

- The normal disk behaves in a viscoelastic manner under pressure. During bending (flexion, extension, lateral bending), one side of the annulus is subjected to compression, while the other side is put under tensile load.
- Although it is normal for the disk to bulge in a degenerated state or with a deficient annulus, the disk can herniate or protrude through the ligament and irritate, compress, or damage the neural structures.

Diseases of the middle column include those that compress the contents of the spinal canal; these can be either extrinsic or intrinsic to the canal.

- Extrinsic examples are
  - □ Fragments of bone or disk that are herniated into or compress the thecal sac
  - □ Neurofibromas or metastatic tumor masses that have entered the canal through the neural foramina and caused compression of the canal
- Intrinsic compression examples are
  - □ Intradural tumors
  - □ Extradural benign tumors or fibromas
  - □ Meningeal infections
  - □ Sequestered disk when free within the spinal canal

Any narrowing of the spinal canal causes stenosis, a constricting and narrowing of the space available for the spinal nerves and the cauda equina.[56]

- Most often, spinal stenosis is a problem caused by bony changes, which are usually developmental and associated with aging and degenerative changes.
- These changes of stenosis rarely occur because of genetic problems, as in the case of the achondroplastic dwarf whose ossification has prevented the development of a large enough spinal canal.

- The cauda equina syndrome is a syndrome of LBP, characterized by involvement of the sacral nerves causing numbness around the perineum and loss of bladder and bowel function.[55]

Changes in the posterior column are common and often related to age or activity. The posterior elements contain the major motion segments of the spinal column including the apophyseal joints and the spinous processes.

- Fractures of the posterior elements may be associated with severe trauma; most often, severe sprains of the posterior elements are associated with rotatory and translational forces.
- Fractures, sprains, and somatic dysfunction are part of a spectrum of derangements of the FSU.
  - Mechanical means such as manipulation or traction provide proper realignment of the FSU in these conditions.

The patient with acute LBP often has a combination of preexisting problems associated with aging.[57] Such changes involve desiccation of the disk with loss of disk height and elasticity, the development of spurs at areas of excessive traction, and inflammation of the apophyseal joint with the production of synovial hypertrophy. For many patients, combinations of factors work together to summate the pain load at each of the areas that generate LBP. Low-grade, yet constant, LBP caused by the aging process may be increased by a mechanically minor twisting in the posterior elements. When the threshold is reached, the resulting pain drives the patient to see the physician. Often, attention to the posterior elements with the use of manipulative techniques spares the expense of multiple diagnostic procedures and surgeries.

Spondylolysis is the most common structural problem in pediatrics; it often is not diagnosed until radiologic examination is performed on the adult patient. Spondylolysis is a defect in the pars interarticularis, the bony bridge between the two facet joints; it is most often developmental or caused by a structural weakness (see sagittal plane postural gravitational strain discussion in Chapter 92). It may also be caused by an acute fracture, as in the case of the gymnast who repetitively stresses the area in hyperextension activities or in the contact athlete who acutely loads the spine in lordosis (see Chapter 87 for sports medicine considerations in spondylolysis). Although the radiologic findings in the oblique, lumbar spinal x-ray view might suggest a more serious problem, most patients with acute LBP and spondylolysis do get better.

With progressive motion, a vertebra can move or slip on the inferior vertebra; this is called spondylolisthesis. This can be due to structural defects such as a spondylolysis as described above or more commonly can be a result of degenerative changes. The intervertebral disk degeneration leads to facet degeneration and ligamentous laxity. The degenerative changes and ligamentous laxity leads to microinstability which causes further degeneration and eventual macroinstability and a resultant spondylolisthesis. The L4–5 level is most commonly affected.

Differential Diagnosis

The thought processes involved in diagnosis require separating into definable groups the different known entities with which acute and chronic back pain are associated. One of the ways to separate the different types of back pain is to ask a few elementary questions:

1. Is the pain intrinsic or extrinsic to the spine?
2. Does the pain emanate from some deranged structure in the spine, or is it directed to the spine from a distant or contiguous area?
3. Is the nature of the pain related to an injury, an inflammatory condition, an infection, a congenital anomaly, or compression of a neurologic structure?

The extrinsic causes of back pain are associated with viscerogenic and vasculogenic causes. Any visceral disease can manifest as back pain. The pain associated with pancreatitis is classic for irresolvable, unrelenting paroxysms of back discomfort. Prostatitis, renal colic from infection or an obstructed ureter, colitis, or perforated viscus, and metastasis of cancer from the colon, ovary, or other contiguous organs may all present as back pain. Most often, a quick but deliberate palpatory examination of the abdomen and rectum differentiates these entities.

Vasculogenic causes of back pain can be associated with vascular claudication. Usually, vascular claudication presents with leg pain, particularly in the calves, during exertion and relieved with rest. Vascular claudication is most commonly caused by peripheral arterial diseases, however, it can be caused by other vascular etiologies. The vasculogenic cause of LBP that is the most urgent is that of the abdominal aortic aneurysm. This is not an uncommon entity in the elderly population prone to atherosclerosis; therefore, the physician should palpate and auscultate the abdomen. It is also important to assess all anatomic structures when looking at advanced images of the spine such as with MRI or CT, as many times the aorta can be seen, and an abdominal aortic aneurysm can be diagnosed and treated if necessary.

Of the myriad other causes of back pain, those that are systemic in origin tend to act directly on the spine rather than from a distant focus. There are systemic diseases of inflammation, infection, and metastasis that cause back pain. Of the inflammatory diseases, arthritides are the most important; that which presents most insidiously is ankylosing spondylitis, one of the spondyloarthropathies. The diagnosis is difficult in the patient who has not developed the classic, late radiologic changes but who presents with severe episodic nontraumatic LBP and stiffness in bending. For this patient, the appropriate blood studies may help confirm the diagnosis. The other seronegative spondyloarthropathies and the inflammatory bowel diseases present with back pain for which the treatment is nonsurgical.

Infections of the spine have been rare, but they may become more prevalent in the near future as viral diseases increase in a population with primary and secondary immunosuppression. In the proper host, any organism, if unchecked, can invade the paravertebral tissues, disk, or vertebral body. The paravertebral plexus of veins of Batson, for example, drains the organs of the pelvis and has been implicated as the conduit down which clusters of tumor cells or aggregates of bacterial organisms pass. These cells may then grow as a metastatic site in a vertebral body or in the epidural space. An awareness of the problem leads to appropriate differential diagnosis followed by controlled biopsy, aspiration, and culture.

Multiple myeloma is an example of a tumor that spreads to bone, particularly the marrow-rich vertebral body. Myeloma and all myeloproliferative diseases are systemic diseases that tend to grow in the vertebral body, rendering it structurally weak and ready to fracture even with minimally applied force. The more common tumors to spread to bone are:

- Breast
- Prostate
- Kidney
- Thyroid
- Lung

If faced with a middle-aged patient with LBP and radiographic suggestions of a metastatic bone tumor, first ascertain whether the more common tumors have become metastatic. There are multiple tumors, benign and malignant, primary, and metastatic, that can cause back pain. Figure 84.13 is an algorithm for diagnosis of spine tumors as proposed by James Weinstein, DO, a tertiary spine

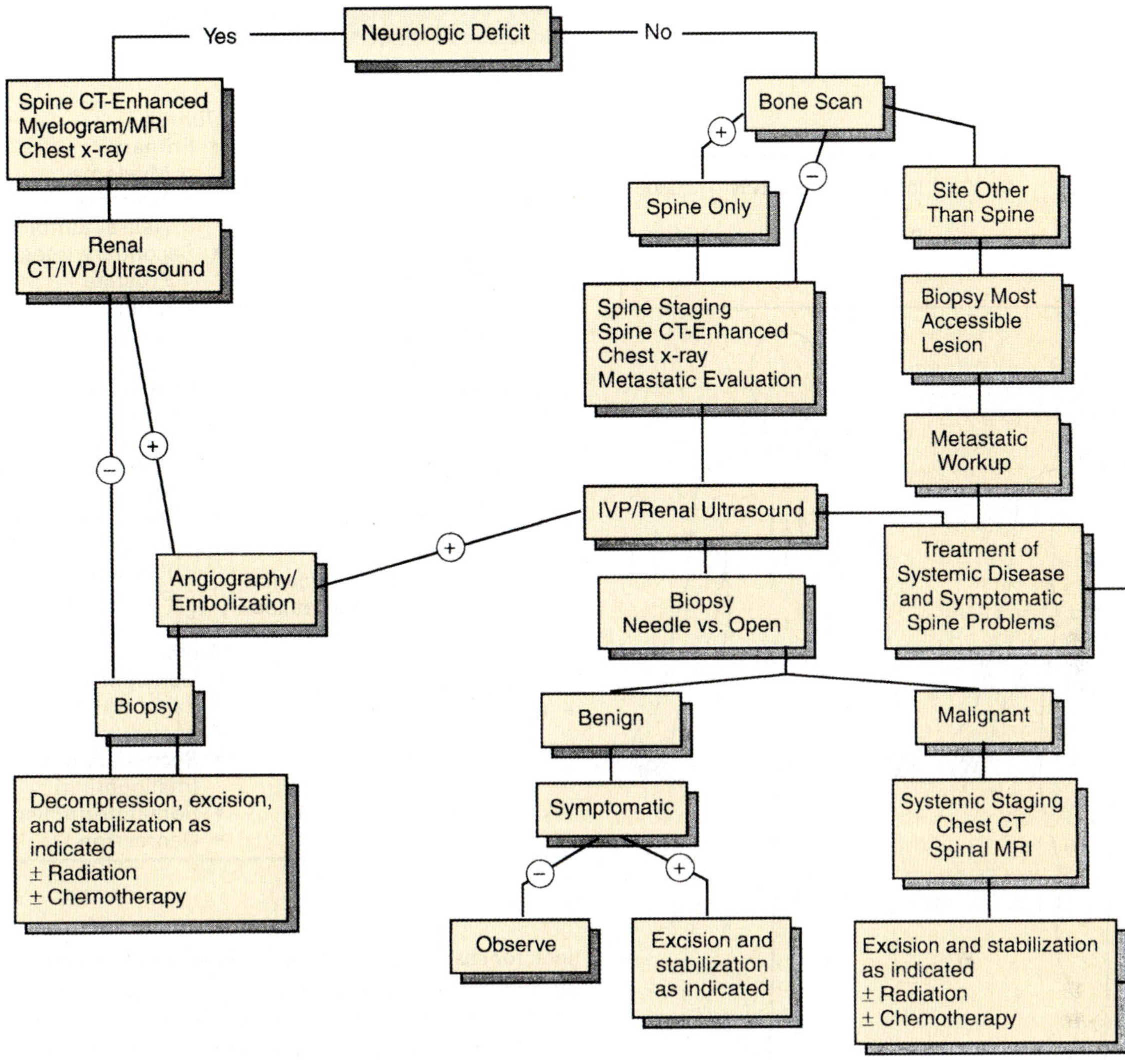

Figure 84.13. Algorithm of approach to spine tumors. (Reprinted with permission from Weinstein J. Differential diagnosis and surgical treatment of primary benign and malignant neoplasms. In: Frymoyer JW, Ducker TB, eds. *The Adult Spine: Principles and Practice*. Raven Press; 1991:851.)

specialist.[58] (See Chapter 76 for further information regarding primary spinal cancer or metastasis to the spine.)

The physician and orthopedist evaluating the patient with LBP must include tumor as a possible cause of the pain, realizing that it is an uncommon cause. All of the following should alert the physician that there may be a remote source of the LBP:

- Malaise
- Fevers
- Weight loss
- Increased incidence of infections
- Change in stool character
- Blood in urine, sputum, or feces

A history of night or rest pain greater than pain with activity also is suggestive of tumor spread to bone. Of the various tests performed in physical examination, the most important is that of percussion. In tumor and infection of the spine, percussion of the spinous process of the affected vertebra causes severe pain out of proportion to that which might be expected. The physician who meets a patient whose LBP is a sign of metastatic disease may not find the diagnosis unexpected, although such a diagnosis usually startles the patient and the family. Patients with a somatoform disorder or psychogenic pain are not rare. Sometimes, there are clues indicating a psychosomatic or hypochondriac pain pattern, such as frequent trips to the hospital or multiple operations, which may suggest some nonorganic cause of back pain. Hysterical paralysis, reputed to be common in Freud's time, is rarely encountered today. Nevertheless, all physicians see patients with "executive back pain" or back pain caused or amplified by the stresses of life. The terminology used by people to describe their symptoms is often suggestive of nonorganic pain. "My fellow worker gives me a headache," "My job is a pain in the buttocks," or "I feel like I'm carrying the weight of the world on my shoulders" are all examples of the kind of metaphors used by patients in describing their somatic complaints. These may suggest there are additional factors in back pain not associated with structural lesions. It is helpful to include in the patient history form a pain drawing in which the patient pencils in the anatomic site of their pain (Fig. 84.14). For those who have psychosomatic pain, characteristic patterns of nonanatomic pain radiation are present.[59] Just as it is important for the examining orthopedist to remember that metastatic disease is an omnipresent possibility and that a careful history and physical examination directs them to that possibility, it is equally important to remember that the mentally ill patient can have disease. Patients with psychoses and neuroses also have infections, tumors, fractures, and diskogenic disease.[60]

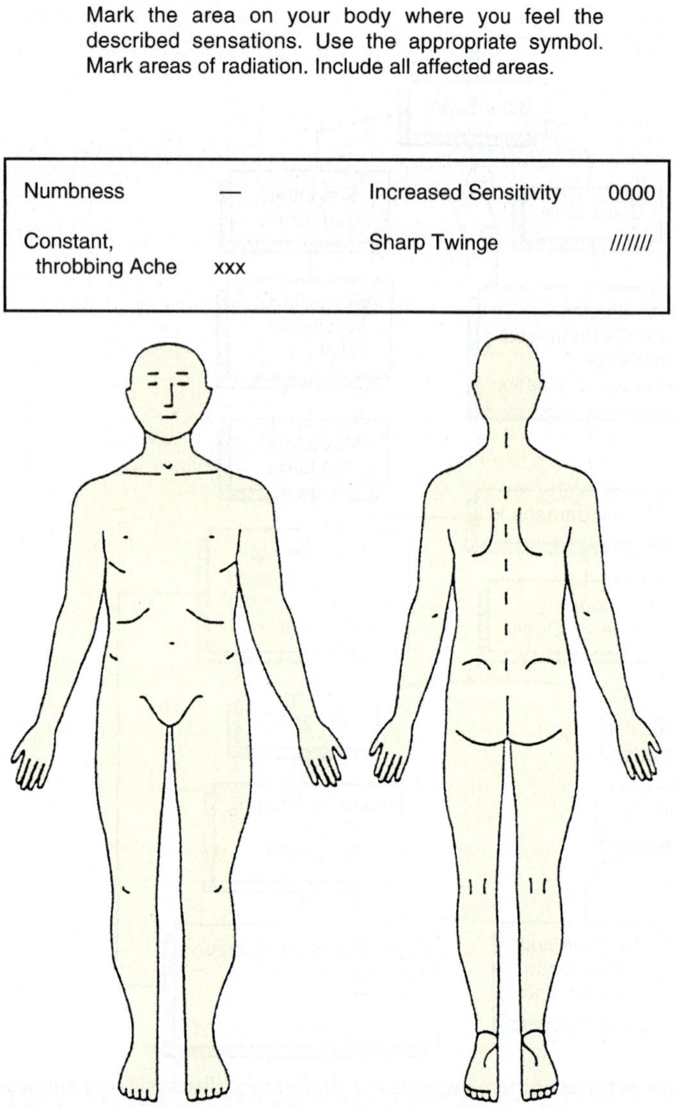

Figure 84.14. Pain drawing used by patients to depict severity, type, and location of pain. (Adapted from Bigos S, Bowyer O, Braen G, et al. Acute low back problems in adults. *Clinical Practice Guideline, No. 14.* US Department of Health and Human Services; December 1994. Public Health Service, Agency for Health Care Policy and Research. AHCPR publication 95-0642.)

Table 84.2 organizes the differential diagnosis of LBP into two basic categories of mechanical or nonmechanical pathology.

Physical Examination

The physical examination of the patient with lower back pain begins when the patient walks into the room. The patient's posture, demeanor, and gait are important in deciding the etiology of their pain. Patients who have a unilateral psoas spasm and back pain related to this may have a flexed forward posture to one side. In addition, patients with significant stress and depression may be bent forward with slumped shoulders and a flat affect. Patients who walk with a limp may have a radiculopathy, osteoarthritis of the hip/knee, or leg length inequality. The physical examination should confirm the physician's suspicions based on the history. In addition to examination of other body systems, the osteopathic orthopedist should perform a standing structural examination,

TABLE 84.2

Causes of Back Pain

Mechanical
- Spinal arthritis
- Degenerative disk disease
- Facet arthritis
- Fracture
- Spondylolysis
- Spondylolisthesis
- Congenital
  - Genetic malformations
  - Achondroplasia

Nonmechanical

Viscerogenic
- Renal colic
- Inflammatory bowel disease
- Endometriosis

Vasculogenic
- Aortic aneurysm
- Ischemic spinal claudication
- Epidural venous anomalies

Infection
- Diskitis
- Herpes zoster
- Osteomyelitis

Tumor
- Primary
  - Myeloma
  - Sarcoma
  - Neural tumor
- Secondary (metastatic)
  - Prostate
  - Lung
  - Breast
  - Kidney

Rheumatologic
- Seronegative spondyloarthropathy
  - Ankylosing spondylitis
  - Psoriatic arthritis
  - Reiter syndrome
  - Behçet syndrome
  - Fibromyalgia
  - Polymyalgia rheumatica
- Rheumatoid arthritis

Metabolic
- Osteoporosis
- Paget disease

Biopsychosocial
- Secondary gain (malingering)
- Somatoform disorder
- Depression

look for changes in anatomic landmarks and scoliosis. Active range of motion testing, followed by passive range of motion testing of the lumbar spine, pelvis, and hips, is important. Palpation of the soft tissues and joints for tenderness, tissue texture change, and restricted motion guide the physician in developing a differential diagnosis.

- Bony point tenderness may indicate a fracture.
- A prominent spinous process may be seen with a vertebral compression fracture or spondylolisthesis.
- A tuft of hair over the L5 region may indicate spina bifida occulta.
- A vesicular rash that is unilateral may be due to shingles.
- Pain with a posteroanterior glide of L4 or L5 might indicate a spondylolisthesis.
- Restricted hip extension and internal rotation may indicate hip arthritis or iliopsoas spasm.
- A positive straight leg raising sign may indicate a lumbar radiculopathy.

Specific orthopedic tests used to assess the patient with LBP with or without radiculopathy include the following:

- Straight leg raising (SLR) test
- Bragard test
- Contralateral SLR test
- Nachlas test
- Slump test
- Schober test
- Thomas test

These and other tests are described and photos demonstrating some of them can be found in the section on Orthopedic Tests.

Management

Most often, the orthopedist is encouraged to believe that the referring generalist has evaluated the possibility of nonlocalized origin of back pain. Although the orthopedist runs through a checklist of nonlocalized possibilities during the interview and examination of the patient, the thoughts center on the kinds of problems that are mechanical or structural and might require some form of operative intervention. Most acute LBP improves over a period of rest or over time. Many patients can be assisted by manipulative treatment. Both acute and chronic LBP related to somatic dysfunction are amenable to OMT (see Chapters 93 and 94, for further information on safety and effectiveness of OMT for patients with LBP and Chapter 99 for a case presentation on acute LBP).

Over the last 25 years, there have been major efforts to understand the nature of back pain. What are the sites or pain generators that transmit nociceptive impulses?[61] Operating orthopedists are attempting to develop surgical designs to stabilize the unstable spine, as well as to define what stability is.[62] They have also been refining approaches and tools to decompress the stenotic spine or entrapped nerve root.

New technologies and materials are expanding the physician's ability to manage back pain and spinal conditions both surgically and nonsurgically. For patients with chronic LBP without spinal nerve impingement, the pain generators are thought to come from pain receptors innervating the zygapophyseal facet joints, spinal ligamentous and myofascial structures, or the disrupted annular fibers of the intervertebral disk. This "diskogenic" back pain, at times confirmed by a provocative diagnostic injection into the disk itself, has eluded surgical therapy short of removing the functioning but painful disk or fusing the FSU to obliterate irritant motion. Percutaneous corticosteroid injections and chemical, electrothermal, or laser disk procedures have been used with some benefit. There are ongoing studies evaluating effectiveness of various surgical procedures, as well as biologic and biomechanical studies to design and build appropriate implants, which might enable the maintenance of stability and normal spinal unit motion[63–77]:

- Disk herniations resulting in sciatica that do not respond to conservative measures often drive a patient who is suffering to seek a surgical alternative. Removal of the offending disk material that is compressing nerves concordant with the patient's symptoms is generally accepted to bring pain relief to 90% of properly selected patients. Surgical treatment was associated with greater improvement than nonsurgical treatment at 5 years.[78]
- A variety of surgical techniques for open diskectomy, microdiskectomy, percutaneous, and endoscopic techniques exist.
- Open diskectomy or microdikectomy is considered the standard; microdiskectomy can be performed as outpatient surgery or, if in the hospital setting, enables a shorter hospital stay and return to work.

OSTEOPOROTIC VERTEBRAL COMPRESSION FRACTURES

The vertebral bodies are among the most common sites of osteoporotic fractures and, hence, back pain in older adults, particularly in postmenopausal women of European descent. Rates of vertebral fracture approaching 25% of women over 70 years of age and 50% over 80 years of age have been reported.[79] There are 700,000 vertebral compression fractures annually in the United States causing 70,000 hospitalizations and $15 billion in annual costs.[80] Increased back pain and the resulting functional limitations are a significant cause of medical visits, costs, morbidity, and mortality.[81] Several medical therapies have emerged in the prevention and treatment of these causes of back pain, for example[81]:

- Bisphosphonates (e.g., alendronate) increase bone mass by inhibiting the normal bone resorptive process.
- Selective estrogen receptor modulators (e.g., raloxifene) and parathyroid hormone derivatives (e.g., teriparatide) increase bone density.
- Vitamin D and calcium supplements increase the substrate available for bone formation.
- Calcitonin can be used for 4 weeks to help alleviate pain associated with compression fracture if initiated within 5 days of fracture.[82]
- Bracing may help provide symptomatic relief, however, studies have not shown that brace use accelerates fracture healing, affects the devolvement of postfracture kyphotic deformity, or changes long-term clinical outcomes.[83]

Surgical treatment of intractable back pain from vertebral compression fractures has previously necessitated major open procedures.

- Initially, anterior surgical approaches to the spine were necessary to attempt to restore height to the vertebral body, thus restoring the normal contour of the spinal column.
- The morbidity associated with this type of invasive procedure, especially in the patient age group associated with osteoporotic fractures, has limited it as a feasible option for treating pain alone.

Vertebroplasty and kyphoplasty have developed as reasonable and effective treatments for intractable pain secondary to osteoporotic vertebral compression fractures.[84,85]

- Considered to be minimally invasive surgeries, the operations are performed percutaneously under fluoroscopic guidance and involve injection of cement (e.g., polymethylmethacrylate [PMMA]).
- Both procedures reduce pain and disability and can help maintain and/or improve alignment.
- Cement augmentation can facilitate early mobilization and reduce the length of hospital stay.
- Cement augmentation is most beneficial for patients with acute pain (<3 months) secondary to acute/subacute compression fractures confirmed by imaging (such as bone edema seen on MRI or bone activity on bone scan) and associated functional limitations after failing a trial of nonoperative management.
- Vertebroplasty:
  - Injection of bone cement into a fractured vertebral body.
  - Imparts stability by eliminating micromotion after the cement cures.
  - Has higher rates of cement extravasation and associated complications than kyphoplasty.
- Kyphoplasty:
  - Uses an inflatable balloon or mechanical device to create a cavity and allow for the cement to be injected with less pressure and less risk for cement extravasation.
  - The expansion of the balloon or mechanical device can aid in restoring height to the fractured vertebra.

The vertebra is then injected with cement and the cement imparts stability and eliminates micromotion.

Patients with spinal deformities, for example, scoliosis, and neurologic deficits along with vertebral compression fractures present challenges that require innovative approaches.[86] Numerous substances have been used, and are continually being developed and studied, to enhance bone growth and increase stability and longevity of vertebral compression fracture repair.[87]

SPINAL FUSION

A variety of degenerative spinal conditions causing pain and neural compromise (e.g., degenerative disk disease, spinal arthritis, degenerative scoliosis, spinal stenosis, degenerative spondylolisthesis) are often refractive to other therapies and are amenable to surgery to relieve pain and improve function. Most procedures involve fusion of the involved FSUs as the common final step. Similar to other procedures to cease motion across a joint, spine surgeons have tried a variety of methods to achieve bony fusion and remove pain by obliterating motion. The most common method of lumbar fusion is posterior lumbar fusion. The addition of an interbody fusion, fusion across the intervertebral disk space, can be achieved posteriorly through a posterolateral interbody fusion (PLIF) or a transforaminal interbody fusion (TLIF). In addition, an interbody fusion can be achieved via an anterior-based approach with an anterior lumbar interbody fusion (ALIF), oblique lumbar interbody fusion (OLIF), or lateral lumbar interbody fusion (LLIF). Each approach takes advantage of a different anatomical corridor to reach the spine.[88]

Basics of posterior spinal fusion necessitate removing cartilage from the opposing facet joint surfaces along with decortication of the posterior elements, placing bone graft material and then holding the segments in a relatively motionless position by external bracing or internal hardware, and waiting months for transplanted bone to complete the osseous bridge across the motion segments, achieving fusion. The difficulty of obtaining a solid fusion in the best of circumstances is best appreciated considering confounding factors. These include:

- Patient compliance with an uncomfortable brace
- Pre-existing medical conditions that hamper bone graft incorporation
- Corticosteroid use
- Smoking (a proven detriment to the local environment necessary for fusion to occur)

The intervertebral surfaces and disk space have become another common site for fusion, especially when preforming minimally invasive spinal surgery. This is known as interbody fusion. Traditionally the posterolateral bony surfaces of the vertebra (transverse process, pars, lamina) have been exposed and bone graft applied over successive levels to create the fusion mass. By removing a portion or all of the already degenerated disk and applying bone graft into that potential space, a greater surface area for fusion is available, increasing the likelihood of achieving arthrodesis.

Interbody fusion is usually supplemented by interbody devices such as bone spacers or prosthetic devices, known collectively as "cages." These interbody devices are inserted into the disk space in place of the degenerated disk, maintaining or even restoring the disk space height, while awaiting bony growth to bridge the space. Material commonly used for the interbody devises are bone, metal such as titanium, carbon fiber, and polyetheretherketone (PEEK). Proposed benefits of interbody device usage are placement of graft material along the weight-bearing axis of the spine, improved spinal alignment, indirect decompression of the neural foramen by increasing disk height, increased fusion rates, improved reduction of spondylolisthesis and improved restoration of lordosis.[89]

Spinal surgeons who deal with major complex curves in adolescents and adults with scoliosis must approach the skeleton in total as they plan their surgery to balance the weight of the body over the sacrum with an instrumented spinal fusion. The geometric designs require four-dimensional (4D) analyses using the *x*, *y*, and *z* axes as well as spatiotemporal deformity prediction to calculate the appropriate postoperative apex of thoracic kyphosis or lumbar lordosis in order to achieve an anatomically correct spinal curvature.[90] Approaches to each patient are individualized. For example, the approach to a 14-year-old with a 75-degree right main thoracic idiopathic scoliotic curve is different from that of a 40-year-old with a 75-degree thoracic kyphotic deformity resulting from Scheuermann disease and is different from that of a 60-year-old with a 50-degree degenerative lumbar scoliosis, positive sagittal imbalance, and associated spinal stenosis and radiculopathy. Both short- and long-fusion approaches are used in adults with degenerative scoliosis; incidence of pulmonary complications is less with short fusion.[91]

NONSURGICAL APPROACHES TO PATIENTS WITH LOW BACK PAIN

There are various nonsurgical management approaches for patients with nonspecific LBP. Systematic reviews, meta-analyses, and evidence and expert panel-based clinical practice guidelines are continually being updated that address these approaches.[92–94]

In general, the following are recommended:

- Provide information about prognosis, warning signs, and advise to remain active
- Patient education, different types of supervised exercise, and physical therapy
- Aerobic exercise
- Cognitive behavioral therapy in conjunction with physical therapy

Not recommended interventions include:

- Bed rest
- Traction
- Oral or IV steroids

The following interventions or therapies are recommended by some but not all national guidelines:

- Acetaminophen
- Acupuncture
- Antidepressants
- Non-steroidal anti-inflammatory drugs
- Topical capsicum on short-term basis (<3 months)
- Massage
- Muscle relaxants
- Opioid analgesics
- Spinal manipulation (low evidence)
- Yoga

The North American Spine Society (NASS) recently, in 2020, released Evidence-Based Clinical Guidelines for Multidisciplinary Spine Care: Diagnosis and Treatment of Low Back Pain. In their guidelines, they made recommendations for patients with acute LBP, spinal manipulative therapy (SMT) results in similar outcomes to no treatment, medication, or modalities. Periodically, short-term improvement is statistically better, but clinical significance is uncertain. For patients with chronic LBP, there is conflicting evidence that outcomes for SMT are clinically different than no treatment, medication, or modalities.[94] For patients with lumbar disk herniation with radiculopathy, the NASS guidelines recommend spinal manipulation and a course of physical therapy–directed exercises as optional for symptomatic relief.[63] Epidural steroid injections (transforaminal or interlaminar) are also recommended for short-term relief. Care should be taken not to delay surgery, if indicated, too long with nonsurgical symptomatic care since surgery within 6 months to 1 year of onset of disk herniation provides faster recovery and improved long-term functional outcomes, although chronic low back and/or leg pain symptoms may persist.[63]

The American Osteopathic Association 1A level evidence-based national guideline (based on a systematic review of high-quality randomized clinical trials) recommends OMT for somatic dysfunction related to acute, subacute, or chronic LBP.[95] See Chapter 93 for details regarding the osteopathic manual approach to diagnosing and addressing somatic dysfunction in patients with LBP.

SUMMARY

Despite the exciting approaches and materials now available, surgery is only useful to try to stabilize or decompress the spine. Most of the time, surgery is unnecessary. Just as treatment for disorders of the growing skeleton is directed toward helping the patient's body mature under guidance, in most cases of acute LBP, restoration of nutrition, strength, and normal intersegmental motion alleviates pain. The use of algorithms or flow charts, although not foolproof, offers the clinician and the patient the greatest opportunity not to miss causes of back pain that are dangerous and life threatening, such as fractures or tumors, or are unusual, such as aneurysms or vertebral osteomyelitis/diskitis. Most often, based on history and presentation, these life-threatening diseases that can be associated with back pain are ruled out. Nonoperative treatment consists of patient education and encouragement that the body will heal, exercise and physical therapy to restore strength, and at times medication for symptomatic relief and manipulation to restore segmental normalcy.

SPECIFIC ORTHOPEDIC TESTS (ORGANIZED BY CHIEF COMPLAINT)

Low Back Pain With or Without Lower Extremity Radiculopathy

1. STRAIGHT LEG RAISING (SLR) TEST (LASÈGUE TEST)

The classic test of sciatic nerve (L1–L5, S1) irritation is the SLR test (Fig. 84.15). Its purpose is to stretch the sciatic nerve and the dura around the sciatic nerve as it exits the intervertebral foramen in cases where there is swelling due to disk herniation causing impingement.

- The SLR test is done by raising the leg with the knee extended.
- When the sciatic nerve is stretched and its nerve roots and corresponding dural attachments are inflamed, the patient experiences pain along its anatomic course to the posterior lower leg, ankle, and foot.
- The test is performed with the patient in the supine position and the hip medially rotated and adducted; with the knee extended, the examiner flexes the hip until the patient complains of pain in the back of the symptomatic leg.
- Symptoms should not be produced in the lower leg until the leg is raised to 30 to 35 degrees. Initiation of the radicular pain at a lower angle of leg elevation (i.e., 30 degrees) is associated with a larger disk protrusion documented at the time of surgery.[96]
  - □ Until 30-degree elevation, there is no dural movement.
  - □ Between 30 and 60 to 70 degrees, tension is applied to the dura and nerve roots.
  - □ Symptoms produced at elevations above 70 degrees may represent nerve root irritation but may also be related to mechanical LBP secondary to muscle strain or joint disease.[96]

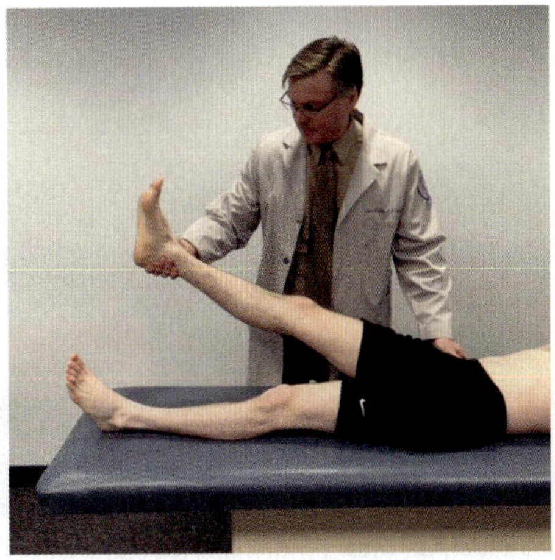

Figure 84.15. Straight leg raising (SLR) test. (Photo courtesy of Dr. Heinking, with permission.)

- The test is considered positive when the patient's radicular symptoms are reproduced.
- The diagnostic accuracy of the SLR test is limited by its low specificity.
  - □ The diagnosis of a radiculopathy should not be based on an SLR test alone but on the totality of evidence from all the physical findings.

2. BRAGARD TEST

A modification of the SLR test, called Bragard test, involves dorsiflexion of the patient's ankle (Fig. 84.16).

- As the leg is lowered back toward the table, until the patient experiences no pain, the examiner then dorsiflexes the ankle.
- If the dorsiflexion movement of the ankle reproduces the patient's symptoms, then the test is positive indicating a radiculopathy.[97]

3. CONTRALATERAL STRAIGHT LEG RAISING TEST

A positive contralateral SLR test is when the clinician lifts the uninvolved leg and the patient experiences radicular symptoms down the involved leg.

- A positive contralateral SLR test is less sensitive but more specific than the SLR test for disk herniation.[96]

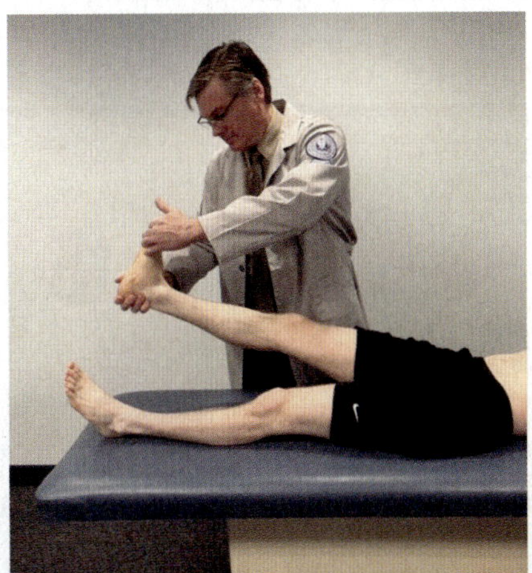

Figure 84.16. Bragard test. (Photo courtesy of Dr. Heinking, with permission.)

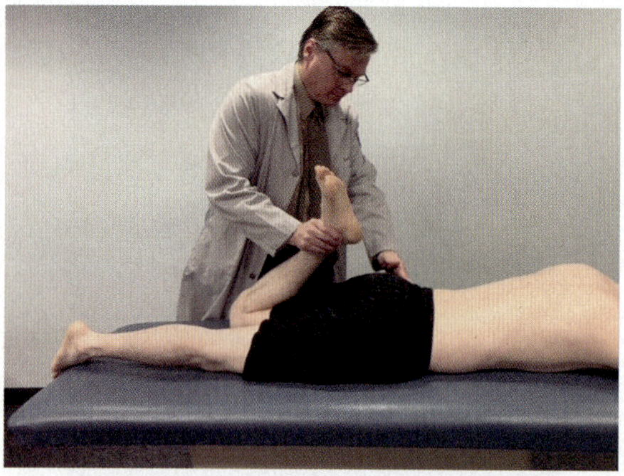

Figure 84.17. Nachlas test. (Photo courtesy of Dr. Heinking, with permission.)

4. NACHLAS TEST (PRONE KNEE BENDING TEST)

For "high" disks (L2–L3 and L3–L4), dural irritability is checked by the *Nachlas test*, which assesses irritation of the roots of the femoral nerve—L2 and L3 (Fig. 84.17).[96,97]

- With the patient prone, the L2 to L3 nerve roots are stretched by bending the knee until the heel reaches the ipsilateral buttocks.
- In patients who cannot achieve this, the examiner should flex the patient's knee as far as possible and then passively elevate the thigh up from the examining table.
- The flexed knee position should be maintained for 45 to 60 seconds.
- The test is positive if unilateral pain is reproduced in the lumbar area, buttocks, and/or posterior thigh.[97]
- If unilateral pain is produced in the front of the thigh (femoral stretch test), this indicates tight quadriceps muscles or stretching of the femoral nerve.[97]

5. SLUMP TEST

The slump test adds more specificity to the SLR test by placing more dural tension on the affected nerve roots.

- The seated patient is asked to slump all the way forward and extend the neck (Fig. 84.18A,B).
- If no symptoms are produced by this position, the examiner then holds the patient's head down (keeping the patient's shoulders slumped) to see if patient's pain is produced.

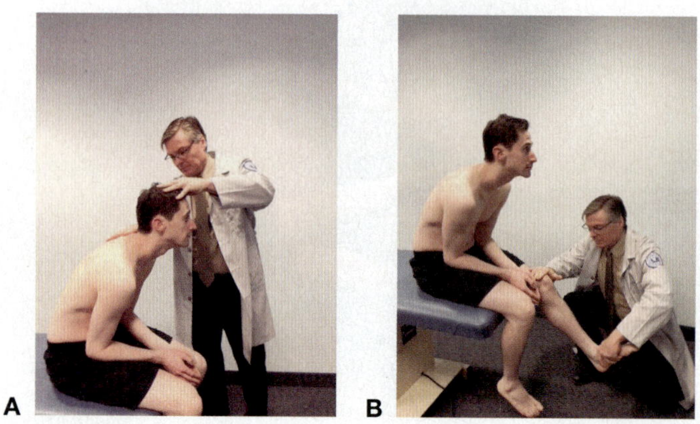

Figure 84.18. A and **B**. Slump test. (Photo courtesy of Dr. Heinking, with permission.)

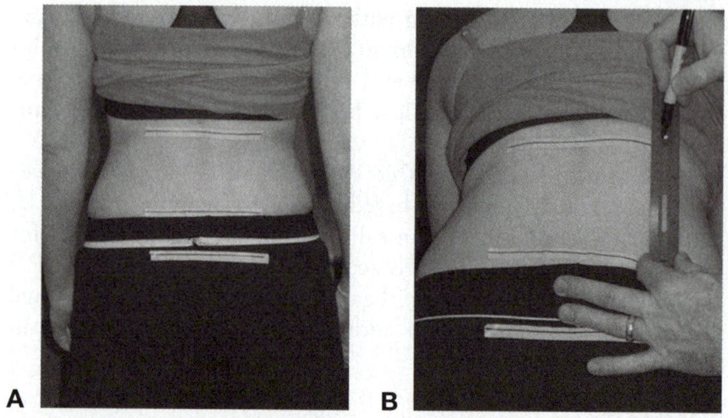

Figure 84.19. Schober test. A. Upright distance marked. **B.** Measurement of new distance after forward bending. (Photo courtesy of Dr. Heinking, with permission.)

- If no pain is present, the clinician extends one of the patient's knees.
- If still no symptoms are produced, then the clinician should passively dorsiflex the patient's foot.[97]
- Each of these provocative maneuvers applies more tension causing impingement of the dura and spinal cord or nerve roots.

6. SCHOBER TEST

Schober test is typically used to measure the amount of lumbar flexion (Fig. 84.19A,B).

1. A point between the sacral dimples (level of S2) is marked with a horizontal line.
2. The second point is marked 5 cm below this line.
3. A third point 10 cm superior to the sacral dimples is also marked.
4. The patient is asked to bend forward, and the distance is measured.
5. Patients with less than 4 cm of movement have decreased lumbar flexion.
6. Lumbar extension can also be measured in this fashion.
7. Patients with spondyloarthropathies have abnormal measurements and an abnormal Schober test.[97]

7. CAUDA EQUINA SYNDROME

Cauda equina syndrome is a condition of spinal nerve root compression, usually by a massive disk protrusion, fracture, or tumor that results in bowel and/or bladder dysfunction.

- *Cauda equina syndrome requires emergent management and surgical decompression within 48 hours or permanent neurologic damage can ensue.*

Although there is not one single test to determine cauda equina syndrome, the clinician needs to be aware of this medical emergency.

- In suspected cases, sensory loss of the perineum (saddle anesthesia) and decreased anal sphincter tone are found. If these findings are present, additional tests and emergency management must be undertaken.

8. TESTS FOR MALINGERING

To evaluate patients with these functional disorders, a list of physical signs was developed by Waddell and colleagues.[96] Any of the individual signs count as one if positive. A finding of three or more of the five types is clinically significant. Isolated positive signs are ignored. The physical signs include:

1. Tenderness tests: Nonanatomic/nonorganic tenderness
2. Stimulation tests: Simulated movements that don't produce pain but are based on those that do, thus the patient may think it is supposed to be painful, for example, thoracic, or LBP elicited with vertical pressure on the skull of a patient who is standing.
3. Distraction tests: Positive tests which are negative when rechecked with the patient distracted, for example, the SLR test.
4. Regional tests: Motor or sensory changes that are not associated with neuroanatomy, for example, numbness in the forearm in the supinated and pronated positions.
5. Overreaction assessment: The patient overreacts to a normal stimulus.

9. TESTING THE ABDOMINAL DIAPHRAGM

This test is for the diagnosis of abdominal diaphragmatic dysfunction or testing for evidence of flattening of the dome of the diaphragm. Diaphragm somatic dysfunction can occur in relationship to upper lumbar dysfunction.

- The physician grasps the lateral sides of the patient's lower rib cage and tests for right and left rotational preference of the deep fasciae.
- Freedom of rotation in both directions is a negative test.
- The patient is instructed to "Take a deep breath in and out."
- At this point, if the patient has a flattened diaphragm, movement can be detected on only one side of the thoracoabdominal region.

10. HIP DROP TEST

This test is a screening procedure to determine how well the lumbar spine compensates for sacral base declination. It is performed by having the patient bear weight on one leg by flexing the contralateral knee, which in effect lowers the ilium ("drops the hip") on the flexed knee side. The physician is positioned to observe the degree of drop of the hip and lumbar spine response from the posterior view.

- *Negative test:* The iliac crest on the unsupported side drops 20 to 25 degrees, and there is a smooth lumbar curvature toward the weight-bearing side of the body.
- *Positive test:* The iliac crest *does not* drop 20 to 25 degrees on the non–weight-bearing side, and there is an angled, uneven, or poor lumbar spinal curve toward the weight-bearing side. A positive test indicates that the lumbar and/or thoracolumbar spine has difficulty side bending toward the weight-bearing side of the body (i.e., the side *opposite* the positive test).

11. THOMAS TEST

The Thomas test for psoas tension (hip flexion contracture) is the standard evaluation tool in physical therapy and orthopedics (Fig. 84.20). Patients are tested in the supine position.

- The patient lies supine on the examination table and holds the uninvolved knee to the chest while allowing the involved extremity to lie flat on the table. Holding the knee to the chest flattens out the lumbar lordosis and stabilizes the pelvis.
- If the iliopsoas muscle is shortened, or a contracture is present, the lower extremity on the involved side will be unable to fully extend at the hip (i.e., the thigh and popliteal region will not lay flat on the table).
- Degrees of hip flexion can be measured with a goniometer.
- The Thomas test is a "positional test" and, unlike the prone evaluation of hip extension, provides limited "end feel."

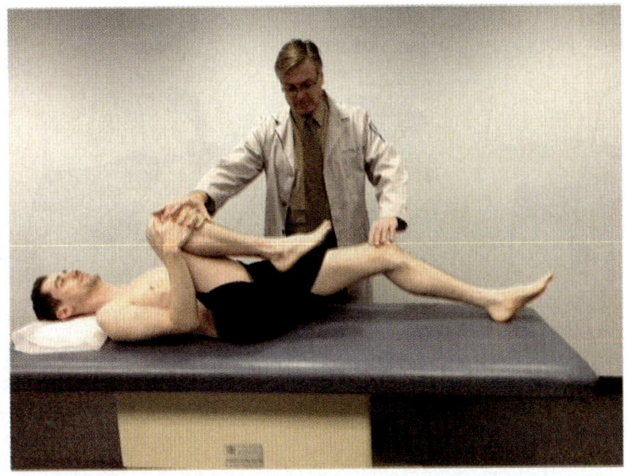

Figure 84.20. Thomas test for psoas hypertonicity. Also commonly performed with patient at end of table. (Photo courtesy of Dr. Heinking, with permission.)

Hip Pain or Dysfunction

1. PATRICK "FABERE" TEST

The Patrick test assesses both hip joint for pathology, for example, osteoarthritis, and ipsilateral sacroiliac joint pathology, for example, sacroiliitis or joint dysfunction. FABERE stands for the movements involved in testing the hip joint as follows:

- With the patient supine, stand aside the patient on the side of the hip being tested.
- While stabilizing the contralateral hip at the ASIS with one hand, passively Flex the hip being tested, then ABduct, Externally Rotate, and, finally, extend it by depressing the knee toward the floor (Fig. 84.21).
- The test may reproduce back or buttock pain from sacroiliitis or severe SI joint dysfunction; groin pain is often indicative of hip joint pathology (e.g., osteoarthritis).

2. OBER TEST

The Ober test assesses for iliotibial band tightness due to tensor fascia lata (TFL) muscle hypertonicity.

- With the patient in the lateral recumbent position on the unaffected side, the physician stands behind the patient, flexes the leg being tested to 90 degrees at the hip and knee, and then abducts and extends the leg by supporting it underneath the knee and at the ankle (Fig. 84.22). Some place one hand on the patient's ipsilateral hip to stabilize it while using the other hand to move the leg being tested.
- Gently allow the knee to adduct (drop toward the table).
- If the TFL is hypertonic, the leg will be suspended above the table, indicating a positive test.
- If the knee drops easily toward the table, then it is a negative test.

Knee Pain or Dysfunction

1. McMURRAY TEST

The McMurray test assesses for medial, lateral, or posterior meniscus injuries. In these tests, start with the patient's knee fully flexed while the patient is supine. One hand palpates the knee at the medial and lateral joint line while the other hand holds the foot to control external and internal rotation of the foot and tibia (Fig. 84.23B).

- For the **McMurray medial meniscal test**:
  - □ The leg is flexed to 90 degrees.
  - □ The foot and tibia are externally rotated.

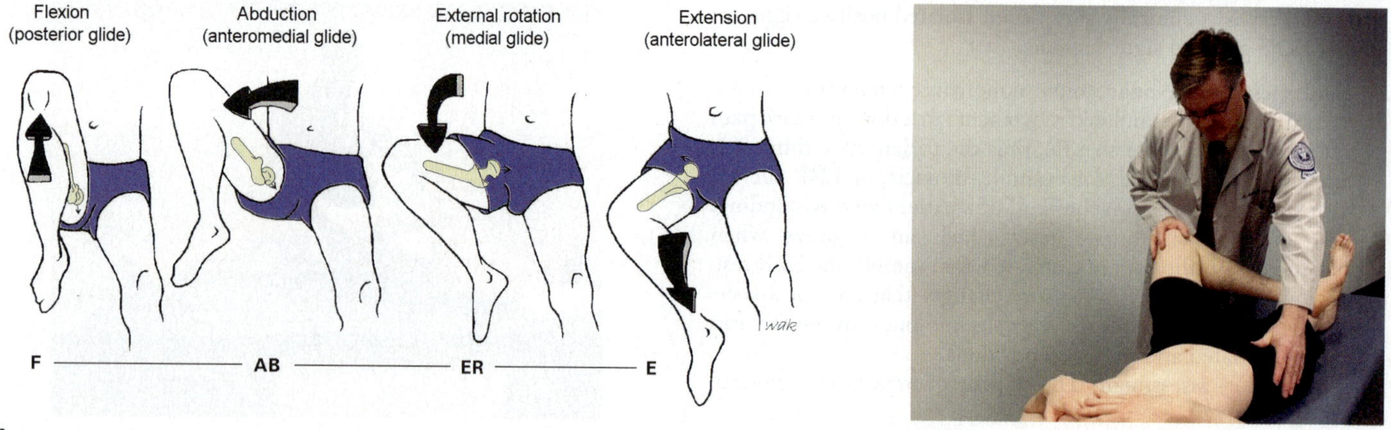

A B

Figure 84.21. A. Patrick FABERE test of the right hip. (Illustration by W. A. Kuchera, DO, FAAO, with permission; photo courtesy of Dr. Heinking, with permission.) **B.** FABERE test of the left hip. (Photo courtesy of Dr. Heinking, with permission.)

- □ Place the tibia into abduction (genu valgus) while externally rotating the foot.
- □ While holding this positioning, the leg is slowly extended.
- □ Pain with a palpable "click" constitutes a positive test.

- For the **Fouche variation for lateral and posterior meniscus injuries:**
  - □ The leg is flexed to 90 degrees.
  - □ The foot and tibia are internally rotated.
  - □ Place the tibia into adduction (genu varus).
  - □ While holding this positioning, the leg is slowly extended.
  - □ Pain with a palpable "click" constitutes a positive test.
- Note that starting with the leg extended and reversing the steps essentially constitute Steinmann I meniscal signs.

2. THESSALY TEST

This test assesses for meniscal tears with the patient in the standing position (weight-bearing on the affected knee).[98]

- The patient stands on the affected leg with the foot flat on the floor.
- The physician holds the patient's hand for support while the patient initially flexes the weight-bearing knee to 5 degrees of flexion.

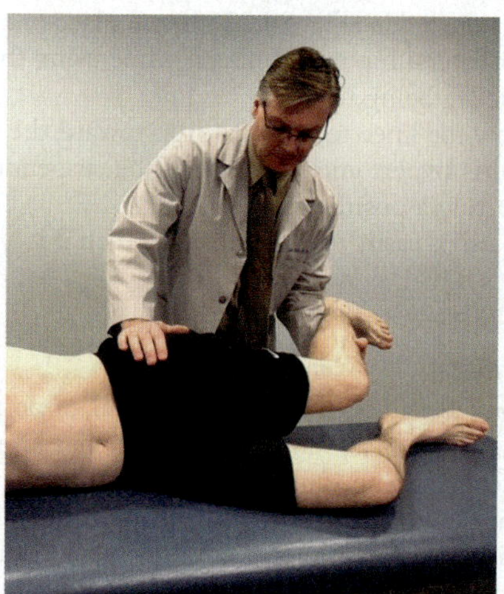

Figure 84.22. Ober test for iliotibial band hypertonicity. (Photo courtesy of Dr. Heinking with permission.)

- The patient actively twists at the knee, making sure to rotate specifically internally and externally at the knee joint rather than at the pelvis or back.
- Although reproduction of pain symptoms indicates a positive test, stressing the affected knee further increases the validity of the test. Reassess with the patient flexing the weight-bearing knee to 20 degrees while actively twisting at the knee joint.
- Reproduction of pain symptoms localized to the knee joint line, with more pain with the knee flexed at 20 degrees rather than 5 degrees, indicates a positive test and a high likelihood of a meniscal tear.

3. DRAWER AND LACHMAN TESTS

Drawer and Lachman tests at the knee joint assess for integrity of the cruciate ligaments. Stability of the anterior cruciate ligament is assessed with an anterior drawer test (knee flexed 90 degrees) or, with greater specificity, a Lachman test (knee flexed up to 30 degrees). Stability of the posterior cruciate ligament is checked with a posterior drawer or Lachman test (Fig. 84.24).

- The patient is supine, and the physician stands distal to the patient's knee being tested.
- The physician stabilizes the ankle for the drawer tests or the femur for the Lachman tests.
- The knee being tested is passively flexed to 90 degrees for the drawer tests and 20 to 30 degrees for the Lachman tests.
- To test the integrity of the anterior cruciate ligament, gently but firmly pull the tibia anteriorly; to test the integrity of the posterior cruciate ligament, push the tibia posteriorly.
- Decreased or lack of resistance to the maneuver (the tibia glides easily without restriction in the direction of the force) indicates a positive test and a torn cruciate ligament.

4. PATELLA APPREHENSION TEST

Patella apprehension test assesses for patella or patellar tendon injury or dislocation (Fig. 84.25).

- With the patient resting supine, the physician passively flexes the knee being tested (using a pillow or wedge or resting the patient's leg on one thigh while sitting on the table—not depicted in image; Fig. 84.25).
- Gently grasping the patient's patella between the thumbs and index fingers of both hands, the physician glides the patella laterally while observing the patient's facial expression for signs of

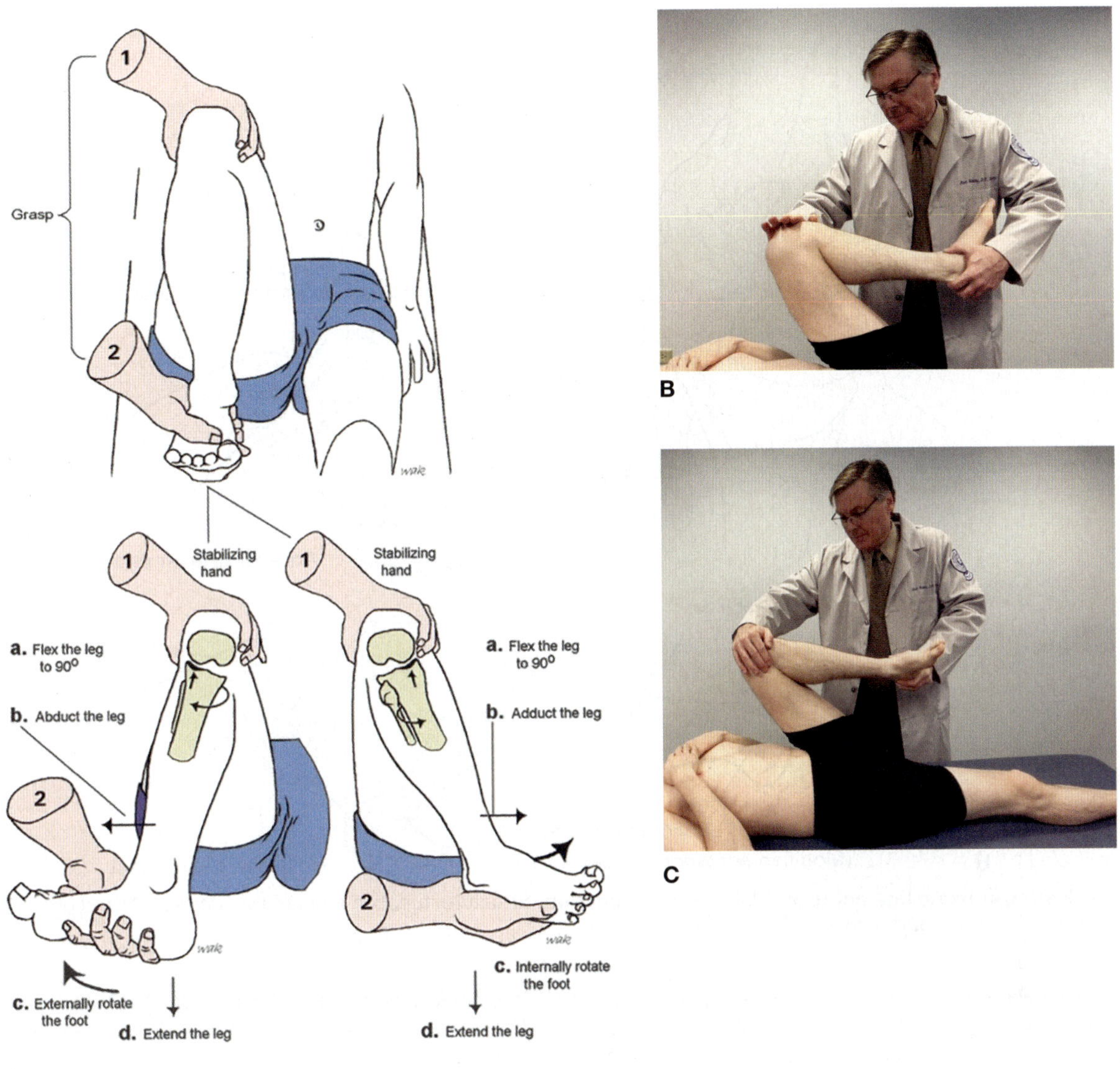

Figure 84.23. Meniscal diagnostic tests. A. For the **McMurray medial meniscal test** (depicted on the left), the leg is flexed to 90 degrees (*a*); the foot and tibia are externally rotated (*b*); place the tibia into abduction (genu valgus) while externally rotating the foot (*c*); while holding this positioning, the leg is slowly extended (*d*). For the **Fouche variation for lateral and posterior meniscus injuries** (depicted on the right), the foot and tibia are internally rotated, the two hands (*c*) place the tibia into adduction (genu varus), and while holding this positioning, the leg is slowly extended. Pain with a palpable "click" constitutes a positive test. (Illustration by W. A. Kuchera, DO, FAAO, with permission.) Photos show diagnostic positions for assessing for integrity of the medial meniscus (**B**) and lateral meniscus (**C**). (Photos courtesy of Dr. Heinking, with permission.)

apprehension (positive test) and/or the patient's ipsilateral thigh muscle reflexively contracting in attempt to protect the patella from dislocation.

5. VARUS AND VALGUS TESTS

Varus and valgus stress tests at the knee joint assess for integrity of the lateral and medial collateral ligaments, respectively (Fig. 84.26).

- With the patient supine, stand aside the patient at the level of the affected knee.
- Stabilize the patient's knee joint by placing one hand on the distal femur and the other on the tibia of the affected knee.
- Passively flex the affected knee joint to 30 degrees, and adduct the tibia while inducing a lateral glide, which puts a localized stress on the lateral collateral ligament.
- Pain symptoms at the site of the tested ligament indicate a positive test for a torn or sprained lateral collateral ligament.
- Passively flex the affected knee joint to 30 degrees, and abduct the tibia while inducing a medial glide, which puts a localized stress on the medial collateral ligament.
- Pain symptoms at the site of the tested ligament indicate a positive test for a torn or sprained medial collateral ligament.

Ankle Pain or Dysfunction

1. ANTERIOR ANKLE DRAWER TEST

The anterior ankle drawer test assesses for anterior tibiotalar ligamentous tear and ankle instability (Fig. 84.27).

- With the patient seated on the treatment table, the physician sits facing the patient's leg and uses one hand to grasp and stabilize

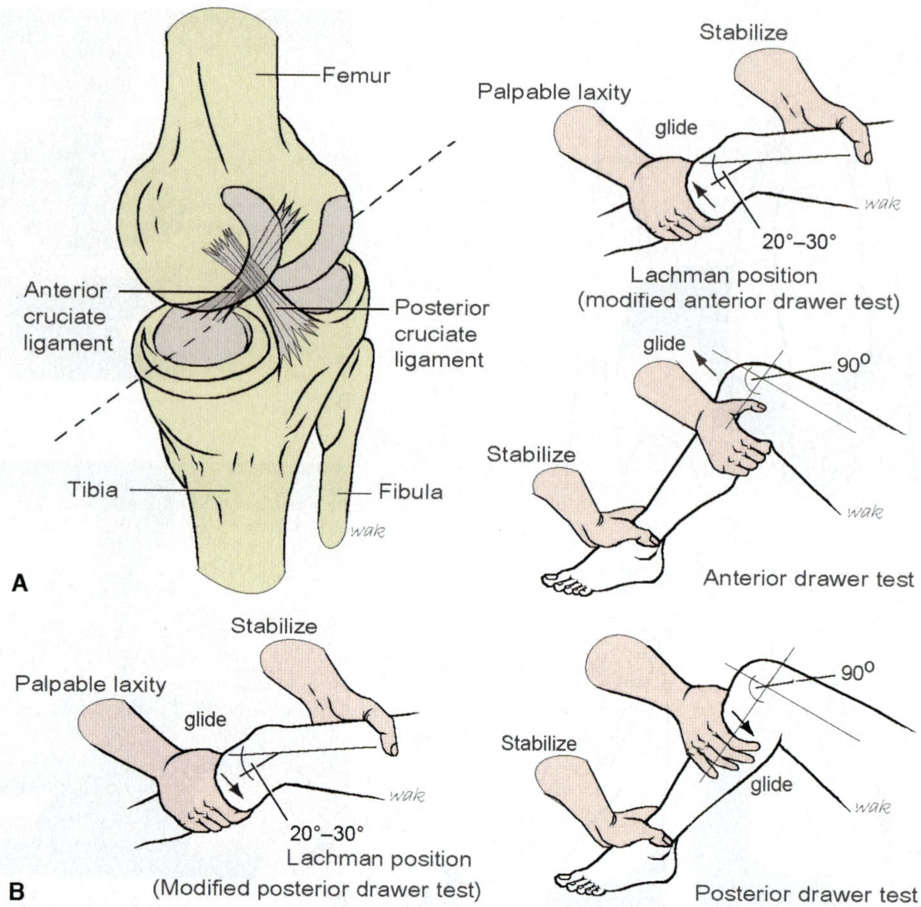

Figure 84.24. Testing cruciate ligaments and A-P glide dysfunction. Structure–function tests of the anterior (**A**) and posterior (**B**) cruciate ligaments using the Lachman and drawer tests.

the patient's tibia while the other hand cups the patient's ipsilateral calcaneus (along with the talus) and pulls anteriorly, as if trying to open a drawer, parallel to the ground.

- Increased joint laxity indicates ligamentous tear and dislocation of the tibia upon the talus.

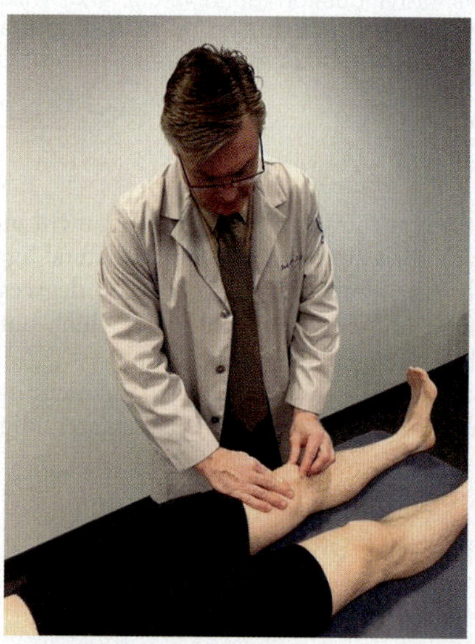

Figure 84.25. Patella apprehension test for patella or patellar tendon injury. (Photo courtesy of Dr. Heinking, with permission.)

2. DORSALIS PEDIS PULSE ASSESSMENT

Dorsalis pedis pulse assessment is essential when assessing the lower extremities for fractures, dislocations, compartment syndromes, and traumatic soft tissue injuries to ensure vascular integrity (Fig. 84.28).

Shoulder Pain or Dysfunction

1. APPREHENSION TEST OF THE SHOULDER

The shoulder apprehension test assesses for shoulder instability (Fig. 84.29). The patient sits on the treatment table, while the physician stands behind the patient but positioned to be able to observe the patient's facial expression in response to the challenge test of the integrity of the glenohumeral joint.

- The physician stabilizes the scapula at the acromioclavicular joint with the palm of one hand over the spine of the scapula and fingers over the acromion and coracoid processes.
- The other hand grasps the patient's forearm at the wrist, abducts the patient's arm to 90 degrees, flexes the elbow, and externally rotates the humerus.
- If the patient grimaces and appears apprehensive (of the shoulder being dislocated), the test is positive and indicates laxity of the shoulder joint anteriorly, which is the most common type of dislocation.

2. BICEPS LOAD TEST

The biceps load test assesses for biceps long head or glenoid labrum injury, commonly found in recurrent shoulder dislocations (Fig. 84.30).

- The patient rests in the supine position.

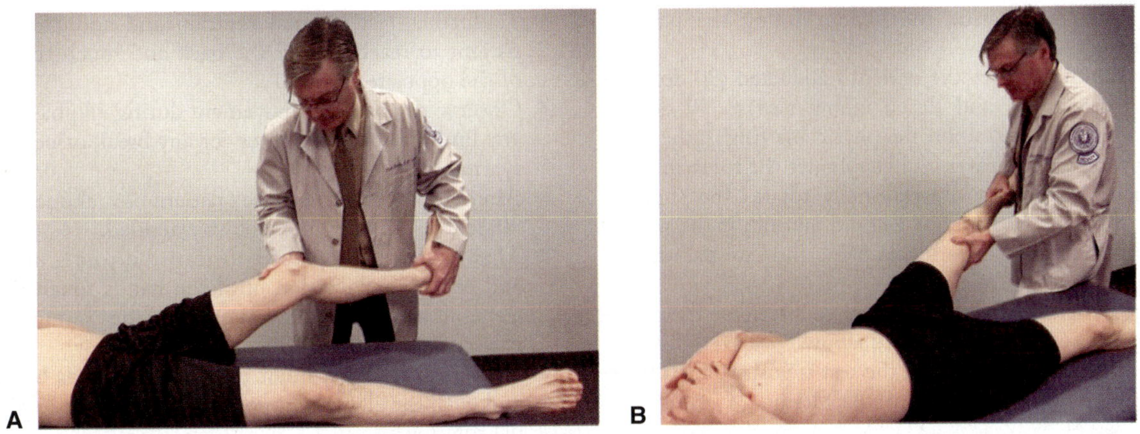

Figure 84.26. **A.** Valgus stress assessing for medical collateral ligament sprain or tear. **B.** Varus stress assessing for lateral collateral ligament sprain or tear. (Photos courtesy of Dr. Heinking, with permission.)

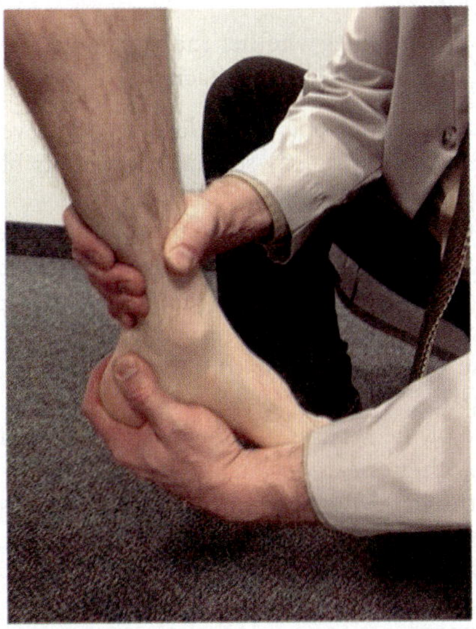

Figure 84.27. **Anterior ankle drawer test for ligamentous tear.** (Photo courtesy of Dr. Heinking, with permission.)

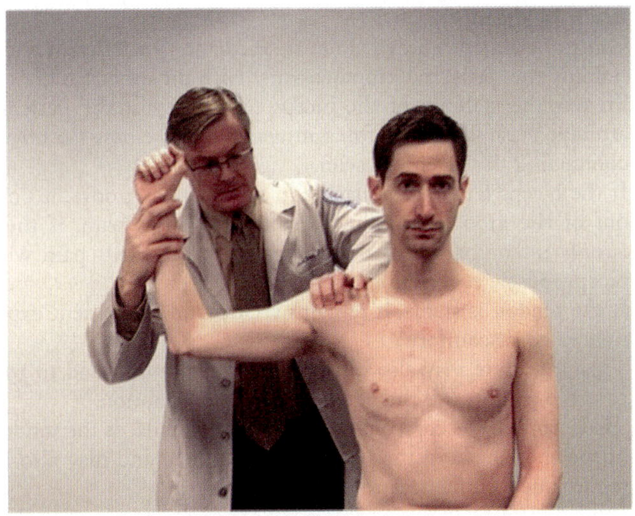

Figure 84.29. **Apprehension test for shoulder instability.** (Photo courtesy of Dr. Heinking, with permission.)

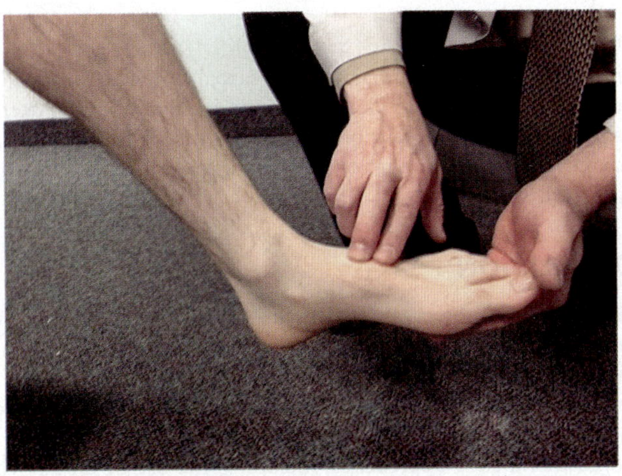

Figure 84.28. **Dorsalis pedis pulse assessment.** (Photo courtesy of Dr. Heinking, with permission.)

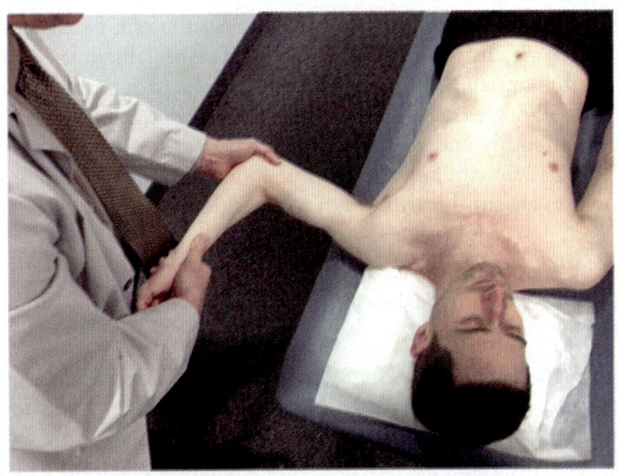

Figure 84.30. **Biceps load test for biceps long head or glenoid labrum injury.** (Photo courtesy of Dr. Heinking, with permission.)

- The physician stands aside the patient facing the patient's shoulder being tested.
- While one hand stabilizes the patient's abducted (90 degrees), externally rotated arm and flexed elbow, also to 90 degrees (which can be supported upon the physician's thigh), the other hand grasps the patient's wrist and supinates the forearm.
- The physician then passively externally rotates the shoulder to localize force at the superior glenoid labrum; if the patient appears apprehensive or experiences pain, stop external rotation at that point.
- Instruct the patient to resist with equal counterforce the physician's attempt to extend the patient's elbow.
- If apprehension or pain increases, the test is positive for a superior labral anterior and posterior (SLAP) lesion.

3. YERGASON TEST

The Yergason test determines whether the biceps tendon is stable (held in place by the transverse humeral ligament) in the bicipital groove. It will also identify bicipital tendonitis.

- With the patient standing or seated, instruct the patient to flex the elbow to 90 degrees, adducting the arm flush against the torso.
- Grasp the patient's flexed elbow in one hand to stabilize it while holding the ipsilateral pronated wrist with the other hand.
- To test the stability of the biceps tendon, resist the patient's attempt to supinate the forearm and flex the elbow (in effect, contracting the biceps muscle).
- If the biceps tendon is unstable in the bicipital groove, it pops out of the groove, and the patient experiences pain; if there is only inflammation of the tendon, this test elicits pain with biceps muscle contraction.
- If the tendon is stable, it remains secure, and the patient experiences no discomfort.
- This procedure may also be performed using one hand to palpate the tendon and the other hand to resist motion.[96]
- Also examine the coracoid process of the scapula, as the tendon of the short head of the biceps attaches there and may also be tender due to inflammation.

4. DROP ARM TEST

The drop arm test detects whether there are any tears in the rotator cuff, particularly full-thickness tears in the supraspinatus.

- First, with the patient standing, instruct the patient to fully abduct the arm.
- Then instruct the patient to slowly lower the arm to the side.
- If there are any tears in the rotator cuff (especially in the supraspinatus muscle), the arm drops to the side from a position of about 90 degrees abduction. The patient is not able to lower the arm smoothly and slowly no matter how many attempts. Also, if the patient can hold the arm in abduction, a gentle tap of the forearm causes the arm to fall to the side.[96]

5. APLEY SCRATCH TEST

The Apley scratch test is used to evaluate the range of shoulder motion.

- With the patient standing, first, to test abduction and external rotation, ask the patient to reach behind their head and touch the superior medial angle of the opposite scapula.
- To test the range of internal rotation and adduction, instruct the patient to reach in front of the head and touch the opposite acromion.
- To further test internal rotation and adduction, instruct the patient to reach behind the back and touch the inferior angle of the opposite scapula.
- Observe the patient's movement during all phases of testing for any limitation of motion or for any break of normal rhythm or symmetry.
- Alternatively, instruct the patient to abduct the arms to 90 degrees, keeping the elbows extended.
- Then instruct the patient to turn the palms up in supination and continue abduction until the hands touch overhead. This tests full bilateral abduction and provides instant bilateral comparison.
- Next, instruct the patient to place the hands behind the neck, and push the elbows out posteriorly to test abduction and external rotation.
- Finally, test adduction and internal rotation by instructing the patient to place the hands behind the back as high as they will go to scratch the inferior angle of the scapula.[96]

Hand Pain or Dysfunction

1. ALLEN TEST

The Allen test determines whether the radial and ulnar arteries are supplying the hand to their full capacity.

- Instruct the patient to open and close the fist several times and then squeeze the fist tightly so that the venous blood is forced out of the palm.
- The physician occludes the patient's radial artery with the thumb of one hand and using the same hand's index and middle fingers occludes the patient's ulnar artery by pressing both arteries against the underlying respective bones.
- Instruct the patient to open the hand; the palm of the hand should be pale.
- Release one of the arteries at the wrist while maintaining pressure on the other one.
- Normally, the hand flushes immediately. If it does not react or flushes very slowly, the released artery is partially or completely occluded. Test both arteries.[96]

2. PHALEN TEST

The Phalen test is used in the diagnosis of carpal tunnel syndrome (see Chapter 73 Osteopathic Considerations in Neurology). Attempt to elicit or reproduce symptoms by flexing the patient's wrists, back-to-back, to maximum degree and holding it in that position for at least 1 minute (Fig. 73.7).

3. TINEL SIGN

Tinel sign is used in the diagnosis of carpal tunnel syndrome (see Chapter 73 Osteopathic Considerations in Neurology). Attempt to elicit or reproduce pain or tingling in the distribution of the median nerve by tapping over the transverse carpal ligament (Fig. 73.8).

CONCLUSION

This chapter is not meant to discuss in any detail the surgical aspects of orthopedic treatment, even though these are the more exciting avenues for the surgeon. Acknowledgment and respect for the whole person and the inherent healing capacity, the interdependent relationship of structure and function, and the need for rational therapeutic approaches, including the use of OMT when indicated, form the foundation of the osteopathic approach to orthopedic medical and surgical problems. And so, the reader is led back to the first illustration in this chapter, in which Andry likened the orthopedic surgeon to the gardener who nurtured his fruit trees so that, by gentle, steady guidance, they grew strong and straight. Andry espoused principles of orthopedic medicine that will always stay in favor.

ACKNOWLEDGMENTS

The authors and editors of this chapter would like to acknowledge the past contributions of Dr. Richard A. Scott for prior editions of this chapter.

REFERENCES

1. *The New Encyclopaedia Britannica: Micropedia*. Vol VIII. Encyclopedia Britannica, Inc; 1987:1017.
2. Andry N. *L'Orthopedie. Paris: La veuve Alix; 1741, as referenced in Peltier L. Orthopedics: A History and Iconography*. Norman Publishing; 1993:22.
3. Cyriax JH. Lumbago: the mechanism of dural pain. *Lancet*. 1945;ii:427.
4. Walter GW. *The First School of Osteopathic Medicine*. Thomas Jefferson University Press; 1992:63.
5. Herrmann E. *Precepts and Practice*. The DO; 1965:163–164.
6. Goldberg MJ. *The Dysmorphic Child: An Orthopedic Perspective*. Raven Press; 1987.
7. von Heideken J, Green DW, Burke SW, et al. The relationship between developmental dysplasia of the hip and congenital muscular torticollis. *J Pediatr Orthop*. 2006;26(6):805–808.
8. Håberg Ø, Foss OA, Lian ØB, Holen KJ. Is foot deformity associated with developmental dysplasia of the hip? *Bone Joint J*. 2020;102-B(11):1582–1586.
9. Johnson E, Audell R, Oppenheim WL. Congenital dislocation of the knee. *J Pediatr Orthop*. 1987;7(2):194–200.
10. Hosseinzadeh P, Baldwin K, Minaie A, Miller F. Management of hip disorders in patients with cerebral palsy. *JBJS Rev*. 2020;8(3):e0148.
11. Staheli LT. *Fundamentals of Pediatric Orthopedics*. Raven Press; 1992.
12. Hensinger RN. The changing role of ultrasound in the management of developmental dysplasia of the hip (DDH). *J Pediatr Orthop*. 1995;15(6):723–724.
13. Shaw BA, Segal LS; SECTION ON ORTHOPAEDICS. Evaluation and referral for developmental dysplasia of the hip in infants. *Pediatrics*. 2016;138(6):e20163107.
14. Pavlik A. Stirrups as an aid in the treatment of congenital dysplasia of the hip in children. *J Pediatr Orthop*. 1989;9:157–159.
15. Mostert A, Pulp N, Castelein R. Results of Pavlik harness treatment for neonatal hip dislocation as related to Graf's sonographic classification. *J Pediatr Orthop*. 2000;20:306–310.
16. Laor T, Roy DR, Mehlman CT. Limited magnetic resonance imaging examination after surgical reduction of developmental dysplasia of the hip. *J Pediatr Orthop*. 2000;20(5):572–574.
17. Sarafrazi N, Wambogo EA, Shepherd JA. Osteoporosis or low bone mass in older adults: United States, 2017–2018. *NCHS Data Brief*. 2021;(405):1–8.
18. Swenning T, Leighton J, Nentwig M, Dart B. Hip fracture care and national systems: the United States and Canada. *OTA Int*. 2020;3(1):e073.
19. Adeyemi A, Delhougne G. Incidence and economic burden of intertrochanteric fracture: a Medicare claims database analysis. *JB JS Open Access*. 2019;4(1):e0045.
20. Wolf SL, Coogler CE, Green RC, Xu T. Novel interventions to prevent falls in the elderly. In: Perry HM III, Morley JE, Coe RM, eds. *Aging and Musculoskeletal Disorders: Concepts, Diagnoses, and Treatment*. IW Springer Publishing Co Inc; 1993:178–195.
21. LeBoff MS, Greenspan SL, Insogna KL, et al. The clinician's guide to prevention and treatment of osteoporosis. *Osteoporos Int*. 2022;33:2049.
22. Deyle GD, Henderson NE, Matekel RL, Ryder MG, Garber MB, Allison SC. Effectiveness of manual physical therapy and exercise in osteoarthritis of the knee. A randomized, controlled trial. *Ann Intern Med*. 2000;132(3):173–181.
23. Bove AM, Smith KJ, Bise CG, et al. Exercise, manual therapy, and booster sessions in knee osteoarthritis: cost-effectiveness analysis from a multicenter randomized controlled trial. *Phys Ther*. 2018;98(1):16–27.
24. Jarski RW, Loniewski EG, Williams J, et al. The effectiveness of osteopathic manipulative treatment as complementary therapy following surgery: a prospective, match-controlled outcome study. *Altern Ther Health Med*. 2000;6:77–81.
25. Licciardone JC, Stoll ST, Cardarelli KM, Gamber RG, Swift JN Jr, Winn WB. A randomized controlled trial of osteopathic manipulative treatment following knee or hip arthroplasty. *J Am Osteopath Assoc*. 2004;104(5):193–202.
26. Barral P, Klouche S, Barral N, Lemoulec YP, Thés A, Bauer T. Preoperative osteopathic manipulative therapy improves postoperative pain and reduces opioid consumption after total knee arthroplasty: a prospective comparative study. *J Am Osteopath Assoc*. 2020;120(7):436–445.
27. Andrews JR, Zarins B, Wilk KE, eds. *Injuries in Baseball*. Lippincott-Raven; 1998.
28. Wirth MA, Jensen KL, Agarwal A, Curtis RJ, Rockwood CA Jr. Fracture-dislocation of the proximal part of the humerus with retroperitoneal displacement of the humeral head. A case report. *J Bone Joint Surg Am*. 1997;79(5):763–766.
29. Harman BD, Miller NG, Probe RA. Intrathoracic humeral head fracture-dislocation. *J Orthop Trauma*. 2004;18(2):112–115.
30. Frodl A, Eberbach H, Senbaklavaci Ö, Schmal H, Jaeger M. Fracture dislocation of the humerus with intrathoracic humeral head fragment—A case report and review of the literature. *Trauma Case Rep*. 2021;37:100592.
31. Nicholson GP, ed. *Orthopedic Knowledge Update: Shoulder and Elbow 5*. American Academy of Orthopedic Surgeons; 2020.
32. Cole BJ, Warner JJP. Anatomy, biomechanics, and pathophysiology of glenohumeral instability. In: Ianotti JP, Williams GR, eds. *Disorders of the Shoulder: Diagnosis and Management*. Lippincott Williams & Wilkins; 1999:207–232.
33. Soslowsky LJ, Flatow EL, Bigliani LU, Pawluk RJ, Ateshian GA, Mow VC. Quantitation of in situ contact areas at the glenohumeral joint: a biomechanical study. *J Orthop Res*. 1992;10(4):524–534.
34. Halder AM, Kuhl SG, Zobitz ME, Larson D, An KN. Effects of the glenoid labrum and glenohumeral abduction on stability of the shoulder joint through concavity compression. *J Bone Joint Surg Am*. 2001;83-A(7):1062–1068.
35. Itoi E, Sashi R, Minagawa H, Shimizu T, Wakabayashi I, Sato K. Positions of immobilization after dislocation of the glenohumeral joint. A study with use of magnetic resonance imaging. *J Bone Joint Surg Am*. 2001;83-A(5):661.
36. Knebl JA, Shores JH, Gamber RG, Gray WT, Herron KM. Improving functional ability in the elderly via the Spencer technique, an osteopathic manipulative treatment: a randomized, controlled trial. *J Am Osteopath Assoc*. 2002;102(7):387–396.
37. Moore SD, Laudner KG, McLoda TA, Shaffer MA. The immediate effects of muscle energy technique on posterior shoulder tightness: a randomized controlled trial. *J Orthop Sports Phys Ther*. 2011;41(6):400–407.
38. Curcio JE, Grana MJ, England S, et al. Use of the Spencer technique on collegiate baseball players: effect on physical performance and self-report measures. *J Am Osteopath Assoc*. 2017;117(3):166–175.
39. Baliga S, Treon K, Craig NJ. Low back pain: current surgical approaches. *Asian Spine J*. 2015;9(4):645–657.
40. Ibrahim T, Tleyjeh IM, Gabbar O. Surgical versus non-surgical treatment of chronic low back pain: a meta-analysis of randomised trials. *Int Orthop*. 2008;32(1):107–113.
41. Katz JN. Lumbar disc disorders and low-back pain: socioeconomic factors and consequences. *J Bone Joint Surg Am*. 2006;88(Suppl 2):21–24.
42. Jackson KL, Rumley J, Griffith M, Linkous TR, Agochukwu U, DeVine J. Medical malpractice claims and mitigation strategies following spine surgery. *Global Spine J*. 2021;11(5):782–791.
43. Bydon M, De la Garza-Ramos R, Macki M, Baker A, Gokaslan AK, Bydon A. Lumbar fusion versus nonoperative management for treatment of discogenic low back pain: a systematic review and meta-analysis of randomized controlled trials. *J Spinal Disord Tech*. 2014;27(5):297–304.
44. Herzog RJ. Magnetic resonance imaging of the spine. In: Frymoyer J, ed. *The Adult Spine: Principles and Practice*. Raven Press; 1991:475.

45. Brinjikji W, Luetmer PH, Comstock B, et al. Systematic literature review of imaging features of spinal degeneration in asymptomatic populations. *AJNR Am J Neuroradiol.* 2015;36(4):811–816.
46. Bigos S, Bowyer O, Braen G, et al. Acute low back problems in adults. *Clinical Practice Guideline, No. 14.* AHCPR publication 95–0642. Agency for Health Care Policy and Research, Public Health Service, US Department of Health and Human Services; 1994.
47. Chou R, Qaseem A, Snow V, et al; Clinical Efficacy Assessment Subcommittee of the American College of Physicians; American College of Physicians; American Pain Society Low Back Pain Guidelines Panel. Diagnosis and treatment of low back pain: a joint clinical practice guideline from the American College of Physicians and the American Pain Society. *Ann Intern Med.* 2007;147(7):478–491.
48. Clinical Guideline Subcommittee on Low Back Pain; American Osteopathic Association. American Osteopathic Association guidelines for osteopathic manipulative treatment (OMT) for patients with low back pain. *J Am Osteopath Assoc.* 2010;110(11):653–666.
49. Downie A, Williams CM, Henschke N, et al. Red flags to screen for malignancy and fracture in patients with low back pain. *Br J Sports Med.* 2014;48(20):1518.
50. Verhagen AP, Downie A, Popal N, Maher C, Koes BW. Red flags presented in current low back pain guidelines: a review. *Eur Spine J.* 2016;25(9):2788–2802.
51. Waddell G, McCulloch JA, Kummel E, Venner RM. Non-organic physical signs of low back pain. *Spine (Phila Pa 1976).* 1980;5:117–125.
52. White AA, Panjabi MM. *Clinical Biomechanics of the Spine.* 2nd ed. J.B. Lippincott Co; 1990:45.
53. American Academy of Orthopedic Surgeons. A glossary on spinal terminology. Quoted in: Frymoyer J, Pope MH. *Segmental instability. Semin Spine Surg.* 1991;3(2):109.
54. Denis F. The three-column spine and its significance in the classification of acute thoracolumbar spine injuries. *Spine (Phila Pa 1976).* 1983;8:817–831.
55. Andersson GB, McNeil T. *Lumbar Spine Syndromes, Evaluation and Treatment.* Springer-Verlag; 1989.
56. Mirkovic S, Garfin SR. Spinal stenosis: history and physical examination. In: Schafer M, ed. *Instructional Course Lectures.* Vol 43. American Academy of Orthopedic Surgeons; 1994:435–439.
57. Frymoyer JW, Gordon SL, ed. *New Perspectives on Low Back Pain.* American Academy of Orthopedic Surgeons; 1989:217–241.
58. Weinstein J. Differential diagnosis and surgical treatment of primary benign and malignant neoplasms. In: Frymoyer JW, ed. *The Adult Spine: Principles and Practice.* Raven Press; 1991;41:851.
59. Ransford AO, Cairns D, Mooney V. The pain drawing as an aid to the psychological evaluation of patients with low-back pain. *Spine.* 1976;1(2):127–134.
60. Stein D, Floman Y. Psychologic approaches to the management and treatment of chronic low back pain. In: Weinstein JN, Wiesel SW, eds. *The Lumbar Spine.* WB Saunders; 1990:811–827.
61. King AI, Cavanaugh J, Fairbank J, et al. Diagnosis and neuromechanisms. In: Weinstein JN, Wiesel SW, eds. *The Lumbar Spine.* WB Saunders; 1990:74–162.
62. Weinstein J, LaMotte R, Rudevile B. Nerve. In: Frymoyer JW, Gordon SL, eds. *New Perspectives on Low Back Pain.* American Academy of Orthopedic Surgeons; 1989;4:35–110.
63. Kreiner DS, Hwang SW, Easa JE, et al; North American Spine Society. An evidence-based clinical guideline for the diagnosis and treatment of lumbar disc herniation with radiculopathy. *Spine J.* 2014;14:180–191.
64. Manchikanti L, Abdi S, Atluri S, et al. An update of comprehensive evidence-based guidelines for interventional techniques in chronic spinal pain. Part II: guidance and recommendations. *Pain Physician.* 2013;16(2 suppl):S49–S283.
65. Onyia CU, Menon SK. The debate on most ideal technique for managing recurrent lumbar disc herniation: a short review. *Br J Neurosurg.* 2017;22:701–708.
66. Brouwer PA, Brand R, van den Akker-van Marle ME, et al. Percutaneous laser disc decompression versus conventional microdiscectomy for patients with sciatica: two-year results of a randomised controlled trial. *Interv Neuroradiol.* 2017;23(3):313–324.
67. Di Martino A, Russo F, Denaro L, Denaro V. How to treat lumbar disc herniation in pregnancy? A systematic review on current standards. *Eur Spine J.* 2017;26(suppl 4):496–504.
68. Lackey A, Phan K, Mobbs R. A systematic review and meta-analysis of outcomes in hybrid constructs for multi-level lumbar degenerative disc disease. *J Clin Neurosci.* 2016;34:23–29.
69. Kamson S, Trescot AM, Sampson PD, Zhang Y. Full-endoscopic assisted lumbar decompressive surgery performed in an outpatient, ambulatory facility: report of 5 years of complications and risk factors. *Pain Physician.* 2017;20(2):E221–E231.
70. Jha RT, Syed HR, Catalino M, Sandhu FA. Contralateral approach for minimally invasive treatment of upper lumbar intervertebral disc herniation: technical note and case series. *World Neurosurg.* 2017;100:583–589.
71. Phan K, Xu J, Schultz K, et al. Full-endoscopic versus micro-endoscopic and open discectomy: a systematic review and meta-analysis of outcomes and complications. *Clin Neurol Neurosurg.* 2017;154:1–12.
72. Huliyappa HA, Singh RK, Singh SK, et al. Transdural herniated lumbar disc disease with muscle patch for closure of durotomy—a brief review of literature. *Neurol Neurochir Pol.* 2017;51(2):149–155.
73. Choi K-C, Lee DC, Shim H-K, Shin S-H, Park C-K. A strategy of percutaneous endoscopic lumbar discectomy for migrated disc herniation. *World Neurosurg.* 2017;99:259–266.
74. Awe OO, Maltenfort MG, Prasad S, Harrop JS, Ratliff JK. Impact of total disc arthroplasty on the surgical management of lumbar degenerative disc disease: analysis of the Nationwide Inpatient Sample from 2000 to 2008. *Surg Neurol Int.* 2011;2:139.
75. Delamarter R, Zigler JE, Balderston RA, Cammisa FP, Goldstein JA, Spivak JM. Prospective, randomized, multicenter Food and Drug Administration investigational device exemption study of the ProDisc-L total disc replacement compared with circumferential arthrodesis for the treatment of two-level lumbar degenerative disc disease: results at twenty-four months. *J Bone Joint Surg Am.* 2011;93(8):705–715.
76. van den Eerenbeemt KD, Ostelo RW, van Royen BJ, Peul WC, van Tulder MW. Total disc replacement surgery for symptomatic degenerative lumbar disc disease: a systematic review of the literature. *Eur Spine J.* 2010;19(8):1262–1280.
77. Chou R, Loeser JD, Owens DK, et al; American Pain Society Low Back Pain Guideline Panel. Interventional therapies, surgery, and interdisciplinary rehabilitation for low back pain: an evidence-based clinical practice guideline from the American Pain Society. *Spine.* 2009;34(10):1066–1077.
78. Atlas SJ, Keller RB, Chang Y, Deyo RA, Singer DE. Surgical and nonsurgical management of sciatica secondary to a lumbar disc herniation: five-year outcomes from the Maine Lumbar Spine Study. *Spine (Phila Pa 1976).* 2001;26(10):1179–1187.
79. Melton LJ III, Kan SH, Frye MA, Wahner HW, O'Fallon WM, Riggs BL. Epidemiology of vertebral fractures in women. *Am J Epidemiol.* 1989;129:1000–1011.
80. Gass M, Dawson-Hughes B. Preventing osteoporosis-related fractures: an overview. *Am J Med.* 2006;119(4 Suppl 1):S3–S11.
81. Stevenson M, Jones ML, De Nigris E, Brewer N, Davis S, Oakley J. A systematic review and economic evaluation of alendronate, etidronate, risedronate, raloxifene and teriparatide for the prevention and treatment of postmenopausal osteoporosis. *Health Technol Assess.* 2005;9(22):1–160.
82. Savage JW, Schroeder GD, Anderson PA. Vertebroplasty and kyphoplasty for the treatment of osteoporotic vertebral compression fractures. *J Am Acad Orthop Surg.* 2014;22(10):653–664.
83. Kim HJ, Yi JM, Cho HG, et al. Comparative study of the treatment outcomes of osteoporotic compression fractures without neurologic injury using a rigid brace, a soft brace, and no brace: a prospective randomized controlled non-inferiority trial. *J Bone Joint Surg Am.* 2014;96(23):1959–1966.
84. Chandra RV, Maingard J, Asadi H, et al. Vertebroplasty and kyphoplasty for osteoporotic vertebral fractures: what are the latest data? *AJNR Am J Neuroradiol.* 2018;39:798–806.
85. Gu CN, Brinjikji W, Evans AJ, Murad MH, Kallmes DF. Outcomes of vertebroplasty compared with kyphoplasty: a systematic review and meta-analysis. *J Neurointerv Surg.* 2016;8:636–642.
86. Alpantaki K, Dohm M, Korovessis P, Hadjipavlou AG. Surgical options for osteoporotic vertebral compression fractures complicated with spinal deformity and neurologic deficit. *Injury.* 2018;49:261–271.

87. Kadam A, Millhouse PW, Kepler CK, et al. Bone substitutes and expanders in spine surgery: a review of their fusion efficacies. *Int J Spine Surg*. 2016; 10:33.
88. Mobbs RJ, Phan K, Malham G, Seex K, Rao PJ. Lumbar interbody fusion: techniques, indications and comparison of interbody fusion options including PLIF, TLIF, MI-TLIF, OLIF/ATP, LLIF and ALIF. *J Spine Surg*. 2015;1(1):2–18.
89. Cole CD, McCall TD, Schmidt MH, Dailey AT. Comparison of low back fusion techniques: transforaminal lumbar interbody fusion (TLIF) or posterior lumbar interbody fusion (PLIF) approaches. *Curr Rev Musculoskelet Med*. 2009;2(2):118–126.
90. Sudo H. Four-dimensional anatomical spinal reconstruction in thoracic adolescent idiopathic scoliosis. *JBJS Essent Surg Tech*. 2022;12(1):e21.00038.
91. Phan K, Xu J, Maharai MM, et al. Outcomes of short fusion versus long fusion for adult degenerative scoliosis: a systematic review and meta-analysis. *Orthop Surg*. 2017;9(4):342–349.
92. Stochkendahl MJ, Kjaer P, Hartvigsen J, et al. National Clinical Guidelines for non-surgical treatment of patients with recent onset low back pain or lumbar radiculopathy. *Eur Spine J*. 2018;27:60–75.
93. Qaseem A, Wilt TJ, McLean RM, et al. Noninvasive treatments for acute, subacute, and chronic low back pain: a clinical practice guideline from the American College of Physicians. *Ann Intern Med*. 2017;166(7): 514–530.
94. Kreiner DS, Matz P, Bono CM, et al. Guideline summary review: an evidence-based clinical guideline for the diagnosis and treatment of low back pain. *Spine J*. 2020;20(7):998–1024.
95. Task Force on the Low Back Pain Clinical Practice Guidelines. American Osteopathic Association Guidelines for Osteopathic Manipulative Treatment (OMT) for patients with low back pain. *J Am Osteopath Assoc*. 2016;116(8):536–549.
96. Waddell G, McCulloch JA, Kummel ED, Venner RM. Nonorganic physical signs in low back pain. *Spine (Phila Pa 1976)*. 1980;5(2):117–125.
97. McGee DJ. *Orthopedic Physical Assessment*. 4th ed. Saunders-Elsevier; 2006.
98. Harrison BK, Abell BE, Gibson TW. The Thessaly test for detection of meniscal tears: validation of a new physical examination technique for primary care medicine. *Clin J Sport Med*. 2009;19(1):9–12.

85 Osteopathic Considerations in Emergency Medicine

BILL D. HAMPTON

KEY CONCEPTS

- Emergency medicine as a specialty is responsible rapidly diagnosing and stabilizing life- or limb-threatening conditions.
- A favorable or unfavorable response to OMM does not rule out a life-threatening condition.
- "Red Flags" are historical and/or physical exam features that suggest the presence of serious illness or injury.
- Patients will self-select a clinical venue based on perceived severity of symptoms, prior health care experiences, and convenience.

GENERAL CONSIDERATIONS

The first consideration in any patient being considered for osteopathic manipulative medicine (OMM) should be to determine if the patient has a musculoskeletal component (TART changes) related to their complaint. In the emergency department (ED), determining the presence of an emergency medical condition must precede this question. Until the workup of a life-threatening problem is definitively answered, the OMM skillset must emphasize diagnosis over treatment. If this priority is kept well in mind, OMM is an extremely useful tool in the diagnostic and therapeutic approach of the astute clinician.

One of the most important things OMM can contribute to the Emergency Physician is to encourage the physician to routinely palpate various tissues across all ages and physical complaints. This habit will develop and refine a mental repository of how certain conditions "feel" beneath the physician's hands. A skillful chef uses senses beyond simply smell and taste throughout the cooking process. What is the sound the skillet makes when ingredients are added? How quickly does the bread color change while it is baking? How does the steak feel as it moves from rare to well done? The analogy is that when the physician who has regularly palpated their patients is confronted with something that they have never felt before, one can quickly identify something uncommon and potentially of a serious nature.

A favorable response to OMM does not rule out an emergency medical condition, any more than a favorable response to antipyretics or analgesics rules out a serious illness or injury. Oftentimes there is the belief that a patient's response to a particular therapy is helpful in diagnosing the underlying condition. This mistake has been well documented in EM literature. A response to milk of magnesia does not rule-out a myocardial infarction.[1] The improvement of pediatric fever in response to antipyretics does not rule-out a serious bacterial infection.[2] The improvement of a patient's headache with acetaminophen or ibuprofen does not eliminate the possibility that the patient has serious underlying pathology.[3] Osteopathic manipulative medicine when done skillfully and in a goal-directed fashion is likely to improve a patient's complaints. Because regardless of the proximate cause, there is often a musculoskeletal component to most disease processes. This response to treatment, however, cannot be safely used to exclude life-threatening conditions. Neither does a treatment failure indicate the presence of a serious medical condition. The OMM modality may not have been appropriate for that patient and their complaint.

This chapter is organized in a head-to-toe fashion discussing common ED complaints, some important diagnostic considerations, a comparison of common ED complaints that overlap with musculoskeletal diagnoses, and how good osteopathic palpatory skills can be applied to help refine the differential diagnosis.

HEADACHE

A chief complaint of headache accounts for a significant number of all ED visits. Of these, the vast majority will have a benign etiology, which means seeing enough cases of serious causes of headaches to become proficient in diagnosing those instances is very challenging and, indeed, a career-long endeavor.[4] The following discussion will focus on what are described as "red flags" in a patient with a complaint of headache. These are historical factors in a chief complaint of headache, that when present should elicit a thoughtful pause. The physician should carefully evaluate this patient and consider that they may have serious pathology and warrants an expanded diagnostic evaluation, specifically advanced imaging, and laboratory testing. Where the patient presents (e.g., family medicine clinic, urgent care, ED) should not dictate the workup. The patient's history and physical examination are what drives the evaluation, not the locale.

Any alteration in the patient's level of consciousness or normal mentation should immediately prompt an expansive workup as this may be associated with serious pathology such as malignancy, infection, space-occupying process, or vascular etiology. Also of concern is a "first-worst headache," meaning that the patient has never had a similar headache before, or this headache is of a much greater severity than the previous. A useful question to assess for chronicity, pattern, and frequency of headaches is "When was the last time you had a headache like this?" Another good question is "When is the last time you sought medical attention for a headache?" An answer of "never" to either question warrants an expanded evaluation (Table 85.1).[5]

There are several diagnoses that can have distinctive palpatory findings to help the physician when confronted with a headache complaint.[4] Giant cell/temporal arteritis may have reproducible tenderness with palpation over the scalp or one or both temporal arteries, but the presence or absence of this finding is quite variable.[6] Trigeminal neuralgia (tic douloureux) is distinct from other headaches as symptoms can reliably be provoked (in 97% of patients in one study) with physical maneuvers such as gently touching the face (79%), talking (54%), chewing (44%), or brushing one's teeth (31%).[7] While there is a great deal of variation (due to when a patient presents in their illness), neck stiffness associated with meningeal irritation from intracranial hemorrhage or meningitis has palpatory findings quite distinct from somatic dysfunction.

TABLE 85.1

Red Flags in Headache

Red Flags in Headache
Systemic symptoms including fever
Neoplasm history
Neurologic deficit (including decreased consciousness)
Sudden or abrupt onset
Older age (onset after 65 yrs)
Pattern change or recent onset of new headache
Positional headache
Worse with Valsalva maneuvers (sneezing, coughing, or exercise)
Presence of papilledema
Progressive headache and atypical presentations
Pregnancy or puerperium
Painful eye with autonomic features
Posttraumatic onset of headache
Pathology of the immune system such as HIV

Given a lack of objective criteria to measure, the exact degree of somatic dysfunction cannot be quantified. Sinusitis will often present with TART findings in the distribution of the infection. However, given this condition's overlap with other upper respiratory infections, the best diagnostic approach appears to be the physician's overall impression instead of the presence or absence of discrete physical findings.[8] Mastoiditis, an uncommon but known complication from otitis media, will reliably present with pain and tenderness over the postauricular region. Palpation of this area is, therefore, a key component to making that diagnosis.[9]

TRAUMATIC NECK PAIN

If a physician assumes that anyone presenting with neck pain following trauma has either a cervical spine fracture or blunt carotid vascular injury, then the thoroughness of the evaluation and the care taken to thoroughly examine the patient and obtain relevant imaging will follow.

Blunt cerebrovascular injury (BCVI) can mislead even a seasoned emergency physician. It most frequently follows a significant acceleration/deceleration mechanism of injury, where the workup will logically follow based on the clinical presentation. However, it is the young person with no significant medical history who may present with vague neurologic symptoms (paresthesias, weakness, sensory disturbances) following a history of minor trauma where the diagnosis can be overlooked. Sometimes the trauma will not be recalled or connected to the presenting complaint as symptoms may have developed hours to days later. While BCVI most commonly results from high-velocity trauma, a variety of low-velocity precipitating events have been cited in the literature including yoga, a forceful sneeze, chiropractic cervical manipulation, gymnastics, etc.[10] An adage in emergency medicine is "the eyes cannot see what the mind does not know." In this specific diagnosis, simply having an awareness of it and a tendency to believe the patient (instead of applying a psychiatric diagnosis to a chief complaint that seems implausible) will often lead the physician down the correct path of diagnosis.

The cervical spine tends to fracture in age-based patterns. For example, a high cervical fracture (C1 or C2) is more common finding among elderly patients due to the overall stiffness of the cervical spine.[11] A relatively low-energy trauma can be enough to

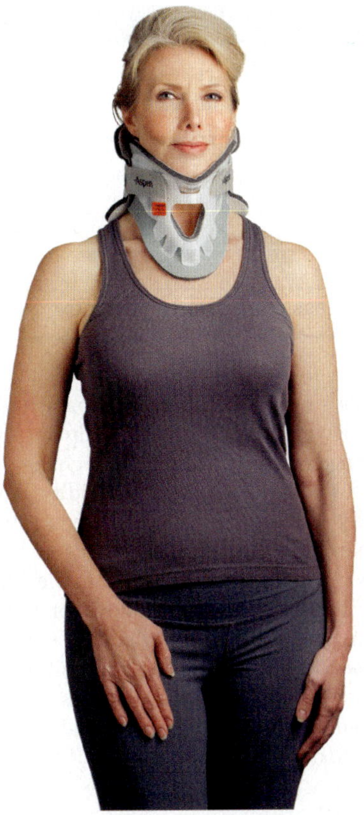

Figure 85.1. Cervical immobilization with a hard collar. (Courtesy of Aspen Medical Products, Irvine, CA.)

cause this injury, specifically a simple ground-level fall with closed head injury. Contrast this with the adult spine who is more likely to sustain a midcervical (C3–C5) fracture.

Pediatric patients tend to have an age-based distribution of injuries. In general, SCIWORA (spinal cord injury without obvious radiographic abnormality) tends to present almost exclusively in young children. This is due to relatively smaller cervical vertebrae, weaker neck muscles, and in the very young, the disproportionately larger and heavier head. In children less than 8 years of age, upper cervical spine injuries and ligamentous injuries are more common. After 8 years of age, cervical spine injuries usually involve the lower cervical spine (C5-C7) and tend to be vertebral fractures instead of ligamentous injuries.[12]

Suspicion of cervical spine injury doesn't mean to neglect palpation of the cervical spine. However, it would be wise to postpone range of motion testing until confirmative imaging can be obtained. Removing the cervical collar (if present) and carefully palpating the cervical spine in a patient who can provide the physician with subjective feedback can be valuable in assisting in the diagnosis (see Fig. 85.1). Palpation can provide a clue of where to look more closely at imaging studies and may help identify other clinically important injuries that would otherwise be obscured. These include burns, abrasions, contusions, and even lacerations (that will obviously not show up on radiographic imaging).

NONTRAUMATIC NECK PAIN

There is often an overlap of neck complaints in patients with serious intracranial pathology. Severe nontraumatic neck pain must at least suggest to the physician the possibility of intracranial pathology. Subarachnoid hemorrhage, meningitis, and intracranial abscess all may present with a complaint of neck pain.[4]

TABLE 85.2

Red Flags in Neck Pain

Gait disturbance
Unexpected weight loss
Night sweats
Fever
Intractable pain
Exquisite tenderness over a vertebral body

In the author's clinical experience, subarachnoid hemorrhage and meningitis have dramatic cervical palpatory findings. There is a stark difference between tissue texture changes due to somatic dysfunction versus patients with nuchal rigidity. True neck stiffness feels dramatically distinct from TART. The extent of the affected tissues is extensive and diffuse. There tends to be less segmental findings and more global restricted motion. Flexion and extension are particularly impacted (major motions of the cervical spine) much more than would be found in simple somatic dysfunction. Additionally, most patients with somatic dysfunction of the cervical spine do not appear acutely ill. Patients with simple somatic dysfunction should have largely normal vital signs and an overall lack of systemic toxicity (Table 85.2).[13]

CHEST PAIN

Due to the potential of a life-threatening etiology, a complaint of chest pain is often referred to the ED for urgent evaluation. Indeed, a chief complaint of chest pain encompasses 5% of all ED visits.[14] Given the frequency of the chief complaint, the emergency physician needs to be adept in not only evaluating emergency causes of chest pain, but other non–life-threatening problems. The emergency medicine axiom for chest pain is "think worst first." Only when the physician is convinced that there is no life-threatening condition present, should musculoskeletal diagnoses be entertained. The following discussion will focus on the taxonomy of musculoskeletal conditions that can cause chest pain (Table 85.3).[15]

There are numerous conditions that can cause chest pain. The following is not meant to be comprehensive, and diagnoses that would be characterized as rheumatologic conditions (e.g., fibromyalgia, spondylarthritis), traumatic injuries (e.g., rib fractures, pulmonary contusion, pneumothorax), and infectious etiologies (*Herpes zoster*) are entirely excluded. This discussion should give the osteopathic physician an expanded taxonomy to explain the patient's symptoms once other more serious conditions have been confidently excluded. Telling a patient what they don't have is unlikely to satisfy them. Patients want to give a name to their symptoms, to understand what is causing the discomfort, and to know how long it will last and what can be done to make it better.

TABLE 85.3

Historical Features in Chest Pain

Concerning	Reassuring
Described as "pressure"	Described as "sharp" or "stabbing"
Exertional pain	Unrelated to exertion
Associated nausea and/or vomiting	Reproducible with palpation
Similar to previous coronary artery disease	Pain is positional
Presence of diaphoresis	Pleuritic pain
Radiation of chest pain (especially bilaterally or to the right side)	Distinctly localized chest pain limited to a discrete area

Upper Chest Wall Pain

Costochondritis is cited most frequently as the cause of chest wall pain.[16] This may be due to familiarity and comfort with the term "costochondritis" as opposed to actual disease prevalence. Other descriptors include costosternal syndrome and anterior chest wall syndrome. Essentially this is reproducible, regional pain at the costochondral or costosternal junction. These tender points (not to be confused with the osteopathic use of that term) lack other traditional findings of inflammation (erythema, warmth, or swelling). Despite the frequency with which this diagnosis is assigned, the literature is less revealing as to why some patients develop this and others do not. Similarly suggested treatments for costochondritis (NSAIDs, injections, ice, stretching, etc.) are mostly anecdotal and not supported by strong evidence.[17] A careful history of how the pain began and an osteopathic musculoskeletal exam focused on the thoracic spine are likely to be of greatest benefit to the patient.

Tietze syndrome is distinguished from costochondritis by having palpable swelling of sternoclavicular, costosternal, or costochondral junctions. This may follow a respiratory infection with significant cough. It most commonly presents at the level of the second or third ribs.[17]

Lower Chest/Rib Pain

There are multiple names to describe lower chest pain thought to be of a musculoskeletal nature: Rib-tip syndrome, slipping rib, twelfth rib, and clicking rib. Like upper chest wall pain, these are tender areas reproducible with palpation or other maneuvers. The area of complaint similarly lacks erythema, objective swelling, or redness. A purported reason for this syndrome is hypermobility of the lower ribs, exacerbated by trauma such as twisting or lifting. Patients with this diagnosis tend to be females (average age of mid-40s). Like upper chest wall pain, no strong evidence supports one treatment modality over another. Symptomatic care is advised, and symptoms persist in as many as 70% of patients at 4 years.[17]

Precordial Catch Syndrome

This is a common, albeit not well understood, cause of episodic chest pain particularly in children or young adults. Like the other chest wall etiologies, it too has multiple names including precordial catch and Texidor twinge. First described in 1955 by Miller and Texidor, it is characterized by sharp, stabbing, or needle-like pain of a discrete area (one or two fingertips), of abrupt onset, lasting between 30 seconds and 3 minutes.[18] With regard to duration, there are case reports of symptoms lasting as long as 90 minutes.[19] The symptoms tend to occur at rest, are made worse with deep breathing, and lack any other associated symptoms (e.g., palpitations, syncope, vomiting, cough, fever). Similarly, there should be no abnormal physical exam findings on exam. As previously discussed, simply giving the condition a name, and explaining its benign nature is one of the most therapeutic actions an osteopathic physician can offer to a patient and his/her family.

Other Less Commonly Described Chest Wall Syndromes

Sternalis syndrome is basically giving a name to tenderness over the sternum that has no other explanation such as arthritis, trauma, etc. Xiphodynia (xiphoidalgia) is similar tenderness that is isolated to the xiphoid process. Expectantly, symptoms can be exacerbated by coughing, activity, eating a large meal, bending, twisting, etc.[17]

Spontaneous sternoclavicular subluxation is exactly what it describes: a spontaneous, atraumatic subluxation of the SC joint. Found almost exclusively in women aged 40 to 60 years, it tends to occur on the dominant hand side and is found following moderate to heavy repetitive work.[17]

Posterior Causes of Chest Wall Pain

Thoracic disk herniations occur with significantly less frequency than lumbar disk herniations. This uncommon condition is reported most frequently in adults in their 40s, who often describe "band-like" chest pain. This is a tricky diagnosis but should be considered when patients report one-sided pain in a dermatomal distribution.[17]

Snapping scapula syndrome is upper back pain due to dysfunction of the scapulothoracic joint. It is most commonly found in individuals who participate in overhead throwing activities but may present following a single, forceful incident. The osteopathic physician will feel and/or hear crepitus with an examination of the affected side. In addition to the audible and/or palpable crepitus (giving the condition its name), patients may report pain along the medial scapular border, either at the superior-medial angle or at the inferior pole. Treatment ranges from conservative to surgical.[20]

BACK PAIN

Back pain is another extremely common ED complaint, averaging approximately 3% of all ED visits.[21] In most instances, imaging is unnecessary and largely unhelpful. This recommendation should be ignored at the extremes of age, however, as back pain among pediatric patients raises concern for congenital abnormality or other organic pathology. Back pain is not an uncommon symptom among pediatric patients, but a pediatric patient presenting to the ED for the evaluation of nontraumatic back pain should be regarded as potentially significant as this is relatively uncommon, in one study occurring a rate of 4/1,000 consecutive visits.[22] Elderly back pain (depending on which source is cited beginning either at age 55 or 65 years) is also statistically more likely to be of a more serious nature due to an increasing prevalence of malignancy, the higher incidence of serious intra-abdominal pathology, and the overall fragility of vertebral bodies from osteoporosis.[23]

Correlation does not imply causation. Remember, something always happens prior to symptom onset. The osteopathic physician must be especially careful of this when dealing with musculoskeletal complaints. While an inciting incident may have caused somatic dysfunction, it is also possible that the patient has sought their own explanation and is relating a clinical narrative that seems to make the most sense to them. Furthermore, TART can accompany back pain due to metastatic cancer. There may be tissue texture changes found in a patient with a rupturing abdominal aortic aneurysm. This is not to suggest that everyone with a musculoskeletal complaint needs CT or MRI, but careful consideration and great care should be undertaken before simply assigning a musculoskeletal diagnosis due to the presence of TART. To learn more about intra-abdominal pathology as it pertains to lower back pain (e.g., Abdominal aortic aneurysm) please see Chapter 93 Osteopathic Considerations in the Patient with Low Back Pain.

TABLE 85.4

Red Flags in Back Pain

Age less than 18 or greater than 50
Symptom duration greater than 6 wks
History of trauma
Systemic symptoms such as fever, chills, or weight loss
Unremitting pain
Neurologic deficits such as hyper or hyporeflexia, weakness of either lower extremity, saddle anesthesia, or decreased anal sphincter tone
Medical history of immunocompromise such as chemotherapy, immunomodulators, history of solid organ transplant, etc.
Intravenous drug use

A number of "red flag" features must be considered when evaluating a patient in the emergency department for back pain. These are listed in the accompanying table. A brief explanation as to what makes them red flags follows (Table 85.4).[24]

Back pain at less than 18 years of age raises concerns for a congenital abnormality that may predispose the pediatric patient to instability and/or vertebral injury. Older than 50 years of age is a threshold for concern for malignancy causing pain. Most back pain resolves between 4 and 6 weeks' duration.[25] Pain that does not resolve within this time frame suggests a more sinister etiology such as malignancy or infection. Accompanying constitutional symptoms (fever, chills, weight loss, nocturnal pain, etc.) implies serious pathology until it has been thoroughly evaluated and excluded. Conditions that increase a patient's risk for malignancy or infection (e.g., solid organ transplant, immunocompromised state, IVDU) must be pursued similarly. Lastly, somatic dysfunction does not cause substantial neurologic findings! There should not be weakness, sensory deficits, or bowel or bladder dysfunction in any patient with simple musculoskeletal back pain. In the clinic setting or the ED, a systematic and careful physical examination looking specifically for these deficits should be undertaken even if the patient does not disclose these symptoms in their history of the chief complaint.

While a patient may complain of back pain, the problem may actually be due to pathology in the abdomen. Clinical examples of abdominal pathology presenting as a chief complaint of back pain include abdominal aortic aneurysm, retroperitoneal hemorrhage, pancreatic cancer, acute cholecystitis, and psoas abscess. Think of the abdomen as the anterior back, and the back as the posterior abdomen. Keeping a three-dimensional model in mind when evaluating a patient (in the same way that always examining the joint above and the joint below in any orthopedic complaint) can often provide valuable clinical findings that may otherwise be overlooked.

ABDOMINAL PAIN

Abdominal pain is the most common ED chief complaint, accounting for as many as 10% of all patient visits.[26] In the ED evaluation of the patient presenting with abdominal pain, this author advises trainees that there are only two causes of abdominal pain: surgical and everything else. This classification is useful as the treatment pathways are largely distinct from one another, as well as conceptualizing the evaluation and management of the patient. Despite

TABLE 85.5

Abdominal Pain Red Flags

Abrupt onset of pain (especially when accompanied by nausea and vomiting)
Elderly patients (age greater than 60 yrs)
Pregnancy
Previous abdominal surgeries (especially bariatric surgery)
Recent GI procedure (upper endoscopy, colonoscopy)
Immunocompromised state
History of vascular disease
History of cancer (especially abdominal/pelvic malignancy)

the expansive use of advanced imaging, a formal diagnosis is never found for this chief complaint.[26] However, deciding whether or not a surgical problem is present is extremely relevant in a patient's disposition (as most surgical patients require admission). Like other ED complaints, a few important characteristics should alert the osteopathic physician that a more serious etiology may be the cause of the presenting complaint, and an expansive workup should be considered (Table 85.5).[27]

Pain is not the same as tenderness. Pain is a patient's subjective experience or description of a complaint. Tenderness is a physical finding elicited by the physician that assists in clarifying location, dimensions, radiation, and quality of the affected tissues. There is not a significant number of life-threatening abdominal complaints attributable to musculoskeletal etiology. However, a careful discussion of the palpatory findings and provocative tests in evaluating a patient with an abdominal complaint is highly relevant. While entire surgical textbooks are devoted to examination of the abdomen, the reader is referred to Chapter 86 Osteopathic Considerations in General Surgery to clarify the physician's approach when presented with an abdominal complaint.

JOINT PAIN

A discussion of joint injuries, complaints, and bedside diagnostic maneuvers is covered in Chapter 84 Osteopathic Considerations in Orthopedics.

MUSCLE PAIN

Diffuse or widespread muscle pain (myalgias) often accompanies viral syndromes. Isolated muscle pain usually is due to an injury such as a contusion or a strain. Two emergency medical muscular complaints deserve further discussion here, however.

Compartment Syndrome

Compartment syndrome in an extremity depends upon two factors: the presence of a closed anatomic space (the compartment) and an injury or exertional activity that would generate the cascade of swelling and consequent neurovascular compromise. Classically, this is taught as the Six Ps: pain out of proportion, pain with passive stretch, pallor, paresthesia, paresis/paralysis, poikilothermia, and pulselessness. Of these signs and symptoms, pain out of proportion to exam presents earliest, and pulselessness will present last, if at all. Untreated, this condition can progress to Volkmann's ischemic contracture (Fig. 85.2). The most common site for this to occur is in the anterior compartment of the lower leg and secondarily, the forearm. Fractures of the tibia and a crush injury to the limb are of specific concern for developing compartment syndrome. It is important to note that open fractures can still develop compartment syndrome as the skin laceration is inadequate to relieve the deeper muscle compartment pressure. Young men are the most affected population, likely due to overall musculature and preponderance for inciting activities or injuries.[28]

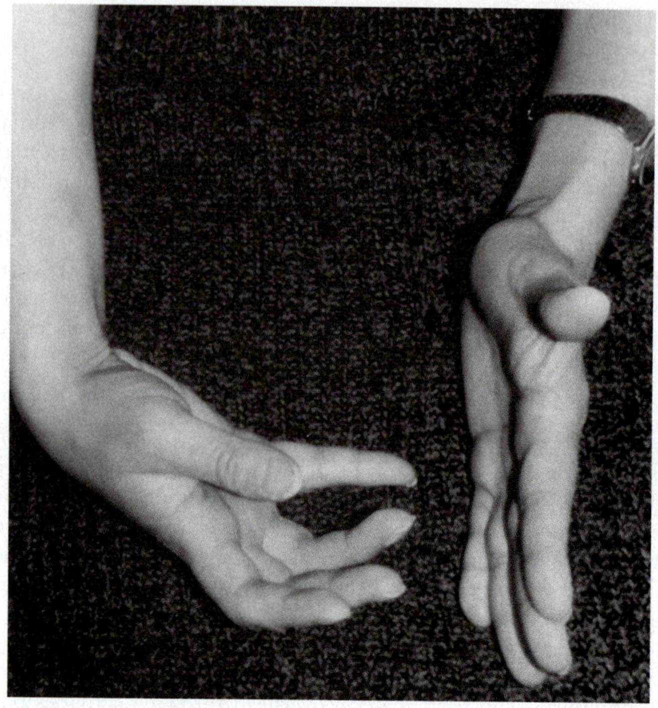

Figure 85.2. Untreated compartment syndrome of the right upper extremity. (Reprinted with permission from Bucholz RW, Heckman JD. *Rockwood and Green's Fractures in Adults.* 5th ed. Lippincott Williams & Wilkins; 2002.)

Radiographic imaging is of limited use in diagnosing compartment syndrome. CPK levels >4,000 in patients with a lower leg fracture are indicative of compartment syndrome in most cases. Palpation of the suspected limb is also, unfortunately, unreliable. Measuring the pressure of the suspected compartment is the only accepted diagnostic modality. This can be done with a commercial product such as the Stryker system or using an arterial line set-up. Either a compartment pressure of >30 mm Hg or a delta pressure (i.e., diastolic blood pressure minus the compartment pressure) of <30 mm Hg can be diagnostic and indicative of the need for emergent fasciotomy, the only accepted treatment for this condition.[29]

Psoas Abscess

Psoas muscle abscess is a very tricky diagnosis to make given the variety of clinical presentations, the lack of specific signs or symptoms, its ability to affect all ages and genders, and the lack of history or physical findings to either rule-in or rule-out the diagnosis. Although a classic triad of fever, pain, and limited hip movement is described in the literature, in clinical practice these three symptoms are only present in about one-third of cases. Of these symptoms, pain is reportedly present 91% of the time, and fever 75% of the time. Because the psoas muscle transverses the lumbar vertebrae and inserts on the lesser trochanter of the femur, the patient may present with abdominal pain (usually lower instead of upper). Unilateral flank pain may be a psoas abscess and although less common, may present in a bilateral fashion. Given the adjacent anatomy, pain may radiate to the groin, hip, posterior or anterior thigh. Given the psoas muscle's role in hip flexion, there may be decreased range of motion of the affected side (particularly in hip extension) and/or an antalgic gait. As this is an infectious process, a variety of symptoms such as fever, chills, weight loss, anorexia, or nausea may also be present. Intravenous drug use is the most associated risk factor for psoas abscess (47%). The history of recent abdominal or retroperitoneal surgery is the second most common (37%). Any underlying immunosuppression such as malignancy, HIV, solid organ transplant, diabetes, etc. can increase a patient's risk for psoas abscess. Spinal instrumentation as well as adjacent trauma or infections can also predispose to psoas abscess.[30]

The following are key things to keep in mind when presented with a patient in whom a diagnosis of psoas abscess is suspected. Examine both sides of the patient thoroughly, keeping in mind a bilateral presentation is possible but uncommon. Laboratory testing neither confirms nor excludes the diagnosis. As the aphorism correctly states, "The white blood cell count is the last refuge of the intellectually destitute." Pyuria may be seen with this given the proximity of the ureter to the psoas muscle. Markers of inflammation such as C-reactive protein, erythrocyte sedimentation rate, and/or procalcitonin are likely to be elevated. The gold standard diagnostic test for psoas abscess is a CT scan of the abdomen and pelvis. MRI could theoretically be used as well, however, this modality usually has much less real-time availability than computed tomography. Any patient with either suspected or confirmed diagnosis is recommended to be started on intravenous antibiotics to cover gram-positive organisms as well as bacteria found within the gut. At the time of this writing, all patients diagnosed with a psoas abscess should be admitted to the hospital.[30]

CONCLUSION

There is significant overlap in the types of patients with musculoskeletal complaints that present to the ED as well as an OMM clinic. Keep in mind that patients select venues based on their perceived severity of illness, prior experience, as well as simple convenience. It is equally likely that an emergency medical condition can present to an OMM practice as to an ED. A careful history and physical exam and a low threshold for referral or advanced imaging and labs is indicated in the patient with historical risk factors (immunosuppression and IVDU in particular) or with symptoms atypical for musculoskeletal complaints (especially fever and tachycardia).[31] Osteopathic manipulative medicine treatment failure or success cannot rule in or rule out an underlying disease process. The more patients the physician assesses and treats, the greater the chance of success in recognizing and acting upon abnormal palpatory findings.

ACKNOWLEDGMENTS

The editor of this chapter would like to acknowledge the contributions of student Amanda Bernett.

REFERENCES

1. Simpson FG, Kay J, Aber CP. Chest pain—indigestion or impending heart attack? *Postgrad Med J.* 1984;60:338–340.
2. Wing R, Dor MR, McQuilkin PA. Fever in the pediatric patient. *Emerg Med Clin North Am.* 2013;31(4):1073–1096.
3. Edlow JA, Panagos PD, Godwin SA, Thomas TL, Decker WW; American College of Emergency Physicians. Clinical policy: critical issues in the evaluation and management of adult patients presenting to the emergency department with acute headache. *Ann Emerg Med.* 2008;52(4):407–436.
4. Walker LE. Headache. *Rosen's Emergency Medicine: Concepts and Clinical Practice.* 16:151–157.e1.
5. Do TP, Remmers A, Schytz HW, et al. Red and orange flags for secondary headaches in clinical practice: SNNOOP10 list. *Neurology.* 2019;92(3):134–144.
6. Narváez J, Nolla-Solé JM, Narváez JA, Clavaguera MT, Valverde-García J, Roig-Escofet D. Musculoskeletal manifestations in polymyalgia rheumatica and temporal arteritis. *Ann Rheum Dis.* 2001;60(11):1060–1063.
7. Di Stefano G, Maarbjerg S, Nurmikko T, Truini A, Cruccu G. Triggering trigeminal neuralgia. *Cephalalgia.* 2018;38(6):1049–1056.
8. Wyler B, Mallon WK. Sinusitis update. *Emerg Med Clin North Am.* 2019;37(1):41–54.
9. Fort GG. Mastoiditis. *Ferri's Clinical Advisor.* 2025:691.e7–691.e8.
10. Biffl WL, Moore EE, Elliott JP, Brega KE, Burch JM. Blunt cerebrovascular injuries. *Curr Probl Surg.* 1999;36(7):505–599.
11. Southerland LT, Fath JJ. Geriatric trauma. *Rosen's Emergency Medicine: Concepts and Clinical Practice.* 179:2325–2330.e2.
12. Baumann F, Ernstberger T, Neumann C, et al. Pediatric cervical spine injuries: a rare but challenging entity. *J Spinal Disord Tech.* 2015;28(7):E377–E384.
13. Karnath Bernard M. Identifying the musculoskeletal causes of neck pain. March 28, 2012. http://www.rheumatologynetwork.com/articles/identifying-musculoskeletal-causes-neck-pain. Last accessed November 25, 2024.
14. Brown JE. Chest Pain. *Rosen's Emergency Medicine: Concepts and Clinical Practice.* 22:202–210.e2.
15. Swap CJ, Nagurney JT. Value and limitations of chest pain history in the evaluation of patients with suspected acute coronary syndromes [published correction appears in JAMA. 2006 May 17;295(19):2250]. *JAMA.* 2005;294(20):2623–2629.
16. Klinkman MS, Stevens D, Gorenflo DW. Episodes of care for chest pain: a preliminary report from MIRNET. Michigan Research Network. *J Fam Pract.* 1994;38:345–352.
17. Wise CM, Fenton J. Major causes of musculoskeletal chest pain in adults. UpToDate. October 28, 2024. Last accessed November 25, 2024.
18. Gumbiner C. Precordial catch syndrome. *South Med J.* 2003;96(1):38–41.
19. Kumar N, Pasi R, Chacham S, Verma PK. Texidor's twinge a rare cause of benign paroxysmal chest pain. 2020.
20. Merolla G, Cerciello S, Paladini P, Porcellini G. Snapping scapula syndrome: current concepts review in conservative and surgical treatment. *Muscles Ligaments Tendons J.* 2013;3(2):80–90.
21. Edwards J, Hayden J, Asbridge M, Magee K. The prevalence of low back pain in the emergency department: a descriptive study set in the Charles V. Keating Emergency and Trauma Centre, Halifax, Nova Scotia, Canada. *BMC Musculoskelet Disord.* 2018;19(1):306.
22. de Inocencio J. Musculoskeletal pain in primary pediatric care: analysis of 1000 consecutive general pediatric clinic visits. *Pediatrics.* 1998;102(6):E63.
23. Della-Giustina D. Evaluation and treatment of acute back pain in the emergency department. *Emerg Med Clin North Am.* 2015;33(2):311–326.
24. DePalma, MG. Red flags of low back pain. *JAAPA.* 2020;33(8):8–11.
25. Maher C, Underwood M, Buchbinder R. Non-specific low back pain. *Lancet.* 2017;389(10070):736–747.
26. National Center for Health Statistics. *National Hospital Ambulatory Medical Care Survey: 2020 Emergency Department Summary Tables.* Centers for Disease Control; 2020.
27. Martinez JP. Abdominal pain. *Rosen's Emergency Medicine: Concepts and Clinical Practice.* 23:211–220.
28. Torlincasi AM, Lopez RA, Waseem M. Acute compartment syndrome. [Updated 2023 Jan 16]. In: StatPearls [Internet]. Treasure Island (FL): StatPearls Publishing; 2024 Jan-. Available from: https://www.ncbi.nlm.nih.gov/books/NBK448124. Last accessed November 25, 2024.
29. Lily H. Extremity compartment syndrome. In: Mattu A, Swadron S, ed. *CorePendium.* CorePendium, LLC. Accessed January 31, 2023. https://www.emrap.org/corependium/chapter/recqDLYW7YLB8TxBj/Extremity-Compartment-Syndrome#h.vkf94kx406h8
30. Coronel M-K E, Burk C. Psoas abscess. In: Mattu A, Swadron S, ed. *CorePendium.* CorePendium, LLC. Accessed January 31, 2023. https://www.emrap.org/corependium/chapter/recm1YNZ1OljUOUDM/Psoas-Abscess#h.v0msimuvscas
31. Wolf E, Stern S. Costosternal syndrome: its frequency and importance in differential diagnosis of coronary heart disease. *Arch Intern Med.* 1976;136(2):189–191.

86 Osteopathic Considerations in General Surgery

JANET KRETTEK

KEY CONCEPTS

- Surgical treatment is most effective by following osteopathic tenets.
- The art of surgery is integrating the scientific knowledge of the disease process with the whole-person approach.
- Treatment is not rote for a disease process, but formulated for each individual's overall state of health and well-being.
- Work with the body's mechanisms to return it to its homeostatic state.

Dr. Still "*Osteopathy is a scientific knowledge of anatomy and physiology in the hands of a person of intelligence and skill, who can apply that knowledge to the use of man when sick or wounded...*"[1]

INTRODUCTION

Surgery, like OMT, is a modality that combines the knowledge of anatomy and physiology together in treating the patient. It is a very intimate form of treatment, considering one is entering their body. Therefore, one must be at their most respectful. Surgical treatment can be significantly impactful, whether positive or negative. Body, mind, and spirit are very important in the care of surgical patients and must be considered and addressed prepared prior to, during surgical treatment, and postoperatively.

The difference between allopathic and osteopathic surgical treatment may not be obvious to the casual observer. The difference starts philosophically and in one's manner of composing a diagnostic and treatment plan. This chapter will review osteopathic considerations used preoperatively, operatively, and postoperatively. Treatment plans for surgical patients will be considered using a holistic approach, including the use of OMT.

Surgeons consider the use of injury/force to lead to a cure of disease: removing an obstruction (lysis of adhesions for a small bowel obstruction, removing the gallbladder and stones in cholecystitis), repair of anatomy (hernia repair), or removal of an overgrowth (colon cancer, skin cancer). These treatments are based on the tenets of osteopathic medicine using the interrelationship of structure and function, treating the structure allows the body to self-heal and return to its homeostatic balance.

PREOPERATIVE CONSIDERATIONS

A complete history and physical exam are the basis for one's diagnosis and assist in designing the treatment plan. A diagnosis is not an endpoint in itself. One must understand the whole person and how this diagnosis fits into the rest of this individual. How are their comorbidities affecting this diagnosis? The treatment plan is influenced by comorbidities, diet, functional capacity, habits (smoking, alcohol use), psychological, religious, and social issues.

DIAGNOSIS OF SOMATIC DYSFUNCTION

An osteopathic physician is trained to detect changes in the soma. The heightened palpatory skills of the astute examiner offer insight into abdominal processes. The training to detect and distinguish various tissue texture changes their chronicity and depth in somatic dysfunctions allows the physician to detect the layers of the abdomen to discern the source of the discomfort and the amount of pain at each level. For example, detecting an abdominal rectus hematoma from an intra-abdominal process.

Viscerosomatic Reflexes

One portion of the exam to include is the nonvisceral portion, the soma. Viscerosomatic reflexes are segmentally predictable dermatomal and myotomal responses to inflammatory visceral pathology. The location of the reaction identifies the involved organ, and the intensity of the tissue texture abnormality indicates the degree of visceral inflammation. Neoplastic lesions that are not specifically innervated may not produce a viscerosomatic response commensurate with the severity of the disease process. However, if significant pressure, stretch, and or inflammatory reaction of the involved organ (or surrounding tissues) is present, a viscerosomatic reflex is likely to be produced. Visceral disease can also be reflected in the soma either in a referred fashion (shoulder pain with pneumoperitoneum) or in a viscerosomatic reflex. Disease can affect the soma and mimic a visceral disorder. Each area must be examined well, and each finding must be incorporated with the history to reach a working diagnosis and differential diagnoses.

The tissue texture change of the viscerosomatic reflex (sympathetic or parasympathetic), is most readily palpated in the paravertebral soft tissues of the spinal level, that innervates the structure responsible for the reflex. General visceral afferent, nociceptive neurons return to the spinal cord in the same nerves that carry the efferent autonomic fibers. The reflexes lateralize to the paravertebral soft tissues on the same side of the body where the viscus is located. Midline organs produce bilateral reflex reactions. The location of these palpatory findings is often at the same spinal level that the patient may report referred pain. Consequently, cholecystitis results in a right-sided response in the area of T5–T10, appendicitis produces tissue texture abnormality at T12 on the right, the dermatomal level of McBurney point, and pancreatitis produces a bilateral reaction in the mid thoracic, T5–T9, region.

Viscerosomatics give an extra indicator towards diagnoses, not a diagnosis in itself. Using the viscerosomatic patterns, an osteopathic physician is able to come closer to a diagnosis than without. For example, in the case of right-sided abdominal pain the differential diagnoses being considered may be cholecystitis, appendicitis, right colon diverticulitis, ovarian torsion, ovarian cyst rupture, renal lithiasis. Particularly in pregnancy, the intra-abdominal anatomy may be shifted, making diagnosis more complicated. Noting if there are any somatic dysfunctions, whether they are acute or chronic, and their position can indicate which viscera are affected. A roaming somatic dysfunction from T10 to T11 to S1 may be following along the path of a moving kidney stone. Whereas a T8 dysfunction on the right with shoulder blade discomfort may indicate cholecystitis. Chronic tissue texture changes may alert physicians to other pathology, such as aT2 lesion in the patient who forgot to mention their chronic asthma.

SOMATOSOMATIC REFLEXES

When examining the whole person, one is screening for clues of disease. Some findings will lead to delving deeper into specific, directed tests to confirm or refute the working diagnosis. At times the findings may lead to more distal exams that appear unrelated. For example, a patient with inguinal pain without findings of a hernia, may lead you to consider a hip disorder, possibly caused by a poor gait from a foot disorder. Keep an open mind and avoid cognitive bias in your diagnosis.

SOMATOVISCERAL REFLEXES

Though not as common, somatic dysfunction can cause visceral symptoms. An example is a patient post cholecystectomy who continues to have nausea, dyspepsia, and right upper quadrant pain that does not resolve until the chronic somatic dysfunction at T8–T9 is addressed.

Circulatory Considerations

The term "circulatory" connotes that there is a circle, an ebb and flow. The flow must be examined in each direction for health. Arterial flow is often the focus; however, all forms of circulation are important. Arterial circulation delivers nutrients and oxygen to the tissues. From the pump, the heart, through the large and small arteries and arterioles, and into the capillaries, the flow must be assessed. Delivery of nutrients and oxygen feeds the growing, repairing tissue. However, the flow of waste out of an area is just as significant. If the venous and lymphatic systems do not clear the waste, healing/homeostasis cannot be obtained. Consider food delivery to your home, but sewer and trash retrieval systems are not working. The buildup of waste over a rather short time could be quite disturbing and unhealthy. An inadequate cranial rhythmic impulse (CRI) gives the same concern for the neurologic system, including the brain. Without proper flow of CSF debris may accumulate which diminishes function.

Stasis is our nemesis. Without free-flowing fluids, infection develops as the removal of bacteria/viruses is not performed. Static blood is prone to clotting in an arterial or venous system. Cancer can grow if the lymphatics are unable to carry deformed/malignant cells away from the tissues to be destroyed. Brain function slows or malfunctions without enough flow of cerebral spinal fluid.

These systems not only need to be evaluated but optimized prior to surgical treatment. This approach may include further studies to check vascular flow or as simple as having the patient increase their stretching and walking daily to improve flow.

Pulmonary Considerations

As with the circulatory system, an exchange of oxygen and carbon dioxide along with other waste products must be considered prior to going to the OR. Particularly patients undergoing sedation or general anesthesia, are susceptible to compounding respiratory difficulties as they decrease one's respiratory drive. This may last for merely a few hours or for days depending on intraoperative time, pain, and postoperative needs for ventilation. A full pulmonary consultation may be required for those with chronic lung disease. For lesser concerns, OMT alone may be in order, thoracic myofascial release, treatment of the thoracoabdominal diaphragm, and/or rib-raising to prepare the patient for surgery.[2–4]

Prehabilitation

Major surgery has been compared to a 5K race. Before taking on a race, one prepares their body and mind through rigorous training. Patients undergoing surgery experience a reduction in functional status postoperatively.[5] Prehabilitation decreases the surgical stress response and increases the preparedness of the patient to undergo planned surgical insult.[6] Prehabilitation is performed preoperatively resulting in less need for rehabilitation and often provides better overall results.[5]

Habits are hard to make and break. On average, it takes 8 weeks to change a habit, so addressing these concerns well in advance of surgery is important. Smoking cessation prior to surgery is worthwhile. The best timing is 2 months prior to surgery, since the lungs take that long to rebuild cilia and cleanse the area enough to prevent major coughing after anesthesia. Even decreasing the amount smoked is helpful. In significant doses, alcohol is a poison, though it can be pleasurable, when taken in small amounts. There is no level of alcohol that is necessarily healthy, however, when taken in smaller amounts, less than 7 ounces per week, negative effects are minimized. If able, abstinence for 2 weeks prior to surgery is optimal.[5,6]

Marijuana has not been well studied in the United States due to its federal restrictions. However, it is known to have more damaging effects on the lungs when smoked. Cessation for 2 weeks is preferred and will improve one's anesthetic response, thus decreasing complications from increased dosage of anesthetic.

Diet is probably the greatest factor in health and disease. Obtaining appropriate proportions of macronutrients and micronutrients is the goal. Food is medicine. Unfortunately, our world is oversupplied with over-processed foods which are abundant in calories, but low in micronutrients. Whole foods, and low-processed diets with the least amount of pesticide/herbicide residue is best, including an abundance of fruits and vegetables in a rainbow of colors. Adequate amounts of fiber and water in the diet will improve bowel movement and help to prevent postoperative constipation.[7]

Sleep issues can often be accounted for by poor sleep hygiene and inadequate stress management. We heal at a faster rate during sleep. Though the stresses our ancestors dealt with are different than ours, our society seems to have more difficulty dealing with what we have today. Managing to align sleep habits with the recommended practices before surgery will improve healing after.

Stress is significant in most people's lives, though it affects some more than others, depending on their ability to cope with their stressors. Evaluation of the patient's stress level and social stressors gives the surgeon an idea of what can and cannot be addressed. Examples include changes in marital status, living situation, caregiving of children or elders, job changes with insurance changes, or incarceration. Knowing which resources are available can improve the situation. Positive stress management techniques can help one manage their response to these stressors to decrease their sympathetic state. Healing is more effective in a parasympathetic state. Cognitive behavioral therapy and mindfulness-based therapies can assist patients in preparation for their surgery.

Physical activity is important on a daily basis. Overall aerobic activity is appropriate to prepare for most major surgeries. Walking, running, biking, swimming, and dancing are all able to increase metabolism and stimulate circulation in a manner that will prepare the body for the trauma of surgery and anesthesia. Patients are encouraged to start at the level they are at the first preop visit and increase in small increments to keep the challenge at a rate of being able to talk while exercising but breathing noticeably harder. Specific exercises may be helpful for orthopedic surgery to tone or strengthen the surrounding muscles, tendons, and fascia involved.

SURGICAL TREATMENT

Indications for surgical treatment may be clear for some diagnoses. A hernia cannot be repaired at this time without surgery. However, there are alternative options for other disease processes that can be considered when looking at the individual. For example, an elderly, bed-bound woman living in a nursing home may not be a good candidate for cholecystectomy and may respond better to ursodiol orally. Patients with acalculous cholecystitis may opt to follow a healthier diet and botanicals to change their bile composition and/or undergo visceral manipulation. Gallbladder manipulation can change the fascial tensions around the cystic duct and allow for improved drainage.

Appendicitis, once thought to be a purely operative diagnosis, is now treated more frequently nonoperatively, at least as an initial option. In this case, visceral manipulation with antibiotics may optimize treatment. Still in its infancy in the United States, studies are still needed to evaluate this combination, however, theoretically, and philosophically it is appropriate.[8]

OMT is appropriate preoperatively to prepare the patient for elective surgery. Treatment should be targeted to optimize the patient's status, decrease pain, and improve function for postoperative healing. Rib-raising, thoracic fascial release, and visceral manipulation allow for improved pulmonary function. Treating viscerosomatics for other nonsurgical disease processes, such as cardiac, pulmonary, endocrine function will allow the body to balance itself. Increased sympathetic tone lowers the pain threshold. By treating the autonomics, one can help the patient return to a more balanced state, which then decreases the patient's sensation of pain. Treating a VS reflex at this point may or may not have much effect if the underlying pathology cannot be treated but via surgery. There may be a temporary relief of pain with OMT without surgery, however, usually the VS reflex returns since the underlying cause has not been addressed. OMT to areas that will allow the patient to improve their mobility will be an asset towards healing postoperatively.

Midcervical (C3, C4, C5) somatic dysfunction is associated with increased postoperative pulmonary complications. This has been described as a somatovisceral mechanism. It most likely represents a somatosomatic reflex in which the cervical somatic dysfunction effects the thoracoabdominal diaphragm through the phrenic nerve, and the resultant dysfunction predisposes the patient to develop pulmonary complications. The use of OMT preoperatively to reduce midcervical somatic dysfunction has been shown to significantly decrease postoperative pulmonary complications.[5]

OMT to a diseased site scheduled for surgery may or may not help. The cause is NOT somatic dysfunction, but a reaction to the visceral disease. Until the cause is treated, OMT is not doing more than symptomatic treatment for a short period of time. If that is the intention and both the physician and the patient understand this, then it is worthwhile.

PREPARATION CONSIDERATIONS

Using a holistic approach, all comorbidities have been addressed and optimized, the patient's nutrition and exercise level are in a healthy balance, their habits have been ameliorated and life circumstances prior to surgery are ideal. Education of the patient and their family/supporters is important to understand what to expect and anticipate. Knowledge is power. Knowing what to expect allows one to feel they have some control over the situation. A review of the preoperative testing and visits leading up to the day, what to do and avoid the day prior to and into the day of the surgery, and what takes place the day of and after the surgery gives a patient some understanding of what is taking place and why. Explain what to expect postoperatively, such as the level of pain to expect and how to treat it, and who to call if there are any concerns. It is important to ensure that the patient understands that they will have someone supporting them at all times so they do not feel scared, abandoned, or alone. Teach them how to care for themselves and the incision, including any restrictions and how long these are in effect.

This is the time to touch on spiritual aspects. Facing a serious illness is often when people ask bigger questions. Give them a space to ask and reflect. Help them identify where they can turn to find their answers and have resources you can share. Empathize with a patient while establishing the surgeon's role and boundaries of the professional relationship with the patient.

Intraoperative Considerations

The patient needs to feel comfortable and confident with the surgeon and the surgical team. Ensure the atmosphere is patient-centered with conversation including the patient, music to the patient's liking, and temperature to the patient's comfort. Having a positive mindset before general anesthesia and upon awakening colors patients' experience and belief in their recovery.

The patient must be placed in a position of comfort for them as well as a position wherein the surgeon can easily reach the area of operation. For example, when positioning a patient in stirrups for a pelvic or rectal procedure, ensure symmetry of position. Asymmetric placement of the lower extremities may result in sacropelvic somatic dysfunction postoperatively.[9]

To step back, remember that the surgeon's ergonomics is part of the equation. Working in an uncomfortable position for a length of time may taint the surgeon's ability to withstand a long case or day full of cases. The surgeon is responsible for ensuring the table height is correct for all those at the operating table, using steps as needed. Ensure arms are relaxed without elevating the shoulders, particularly for laparoscopic cases. Robotics allow the surgeon the best ergonomic position.[10]

Pain starts with a noxious stimulus. If one can prevent pain, then a pain reflex loop can be prevented before it begins. The use of local anesthesia with or without the use of general/regional anesthesia will block the C-fibers to prevent the pain reflex from the start of the procedure. Inject the tissue prior to making an incision. Local anesthetics can be used postoperatively, too, as needed, with fewer side effects than narcotics.[11,12]

Considering that structure and function are related, it follows that one respects the tissue of the patient while operating. Correct use of the instruments and exertion of force on the tissues requires an understanding of each layer and type of tissue encountered, so as to work with the body while removing an obstructing or malignant segment. The surgeon must take care to respect the tissue, retracting gently and smoothly and only as needed. Students must be taught how to touch the different tissues to avoid injury. Surgery

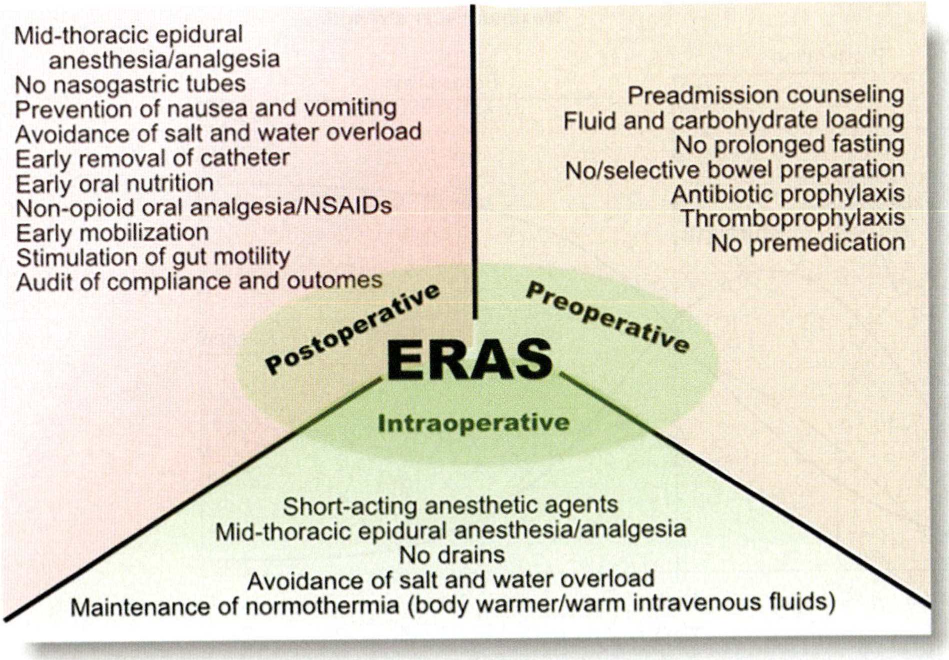

Figure 86.1. Enhanced recovery after surgery (ERAS). (From Steenhagen E. Enhanced recovery after surgery: it's time to change practice! *Nutr Clin Pract.* 2016;31(1):18–29. Reprinted from Varadhan KK, Lobo DN, Ljungqvist O. Enhanced recovery after surgery: the future of improving surgical care. *Crit Care Clin.* 2010;26(3):527–547. Copyright: © 2010 Elsevier. With permission.)

by its nature is a destructive and forceful means to a healing end and must be used in a very conscious, controlled manner.[13,14]

The surgical approach to the patient is important. The less tissue disturbed, the better. Minimally invasive surgery has been revolutionary in decreasing postoperative pain and discomfort. Robotic surgery has improved some types of surgery beyond laparoscopy.[15] The healing process is the same for the visceral tissues as well as the disturbed layers and cannot be rushed. When less-invasive surgical approaches are used, then the risk for many complications are decreased, such as the amount of pain, pulmonary complications such as pneumonia and atelectasis, and ileus. However, the body still endures the stress of surgery and hernias can still occur if healing time is not allowed for the patient's recovery.

The body can balance its fluids better than a physician can. Administration of fluids is a balancing act, knowing what fluids to give, in what circumstances, and what route. Oral administration is the best route. Surgical protocols are catching up to this understanding in the Enhanced Recovery After Surgery (ERAS) protocols, giving patients carbohydrate-rich oral fluids up to 2 hours prior to major surgery (see Figure 86.1).[16] This allows the patient to be orally hydrated, needing less IVF intraoperatively, plus stimulates the bowels to decrease postoperative ileus. The patient is therefore able to take fluids orally immediately after surgery, preventing the need for salt-rich IVF. With this approach, patients are able to return to their homeostatic selves at a much faster rate with fewer complications (Fig. 86.1).[16]

POSTOPERATIVE CONSIDERATIONS

Having set the patient to succeed, the path must now be reinforced and followed up. Pain control is very important at this time. Monitor the patient for signs of pain and discomfort. The most obvious reason is to decrease human suffering, but there are other reasons that are not as obvious. By treating the patient's pain early, the pain cycle can be broken, and viscerosomatic and somatosomatic reflexes interrupted. If it is left unchecked, pain can be much harder to manage on the second or third postoperative day since the patient's pain tolerance is lowered due to hyperactivity of the sympathetic nervous system. When the pain is lessened or obliterated, the patient can take deeper breaths and increase their activity, thus improving the pulmonary, lymphatic, gastrointestinal, and cranial systems. This has a virtuous spiraling effect to a better recovery. An ice pack is a simple form of pain control that has few side effects. It should be avoided with grafts. Higher doses of acetaminophen and NSAIDs used in a staggered fashion can cover postoperative pain in most instances. This allows multiple mechanisms of pain relief to be utilized. Narcotics and their derivatives are most useful in the first few days. Diminished gastrointestinal motility is of secondary importance to pain control, but one of the reasons that narcotics are used in a stepwise fashion for pain control, used only early on if the other forms of pain medications are not adequate. Do not be concerned at this time with the possibility of starting an addiction. Addiction will not be initiated by adequate treatment of postoperative pain in a controlled fashion. Teach the patient how to use ice packs, distractions, and medications. Ensure they understand that their pain level should NOT be at a "0" on the pain scale, but at a "3–4." The pain should not be noticeable when sitting still and distracted by reading material, TV, or conversation.[16]

Recall that the first phase of healing, the inflammatory stage, takes place over the first 3 postoperative days. One can change the intensity of this phase with ice, rest, elevation, anti-inflammatory medications, and OMT, but it still takes place (Fig. 86.2).[17]

On postoperative day 4, the diuresis phase begins, in which the patient will now lose the retained fluids from the intra and extracellular spaces, including the surgical site. This is a time to ensure the renal and circulatory functions are at their peak. Eight to twelve liters of fluid are picked up by the lymphatic system daily. Two to four liters are returned to the venous circulation via the thoracic duct. The remainder is returned via capillary exchange in the lymph nodes.

During the diuretic phase, the fluid load increases. At this time, thoracic cage mobility is imperative, not only for efficient respiration, but also for returning lymph to the general circulation. The thoracic duct terminates into the left subclavian vein; therefore, mobility of the thoracic outlet is critical to prevent obstruction to the flow of lymph.[18]

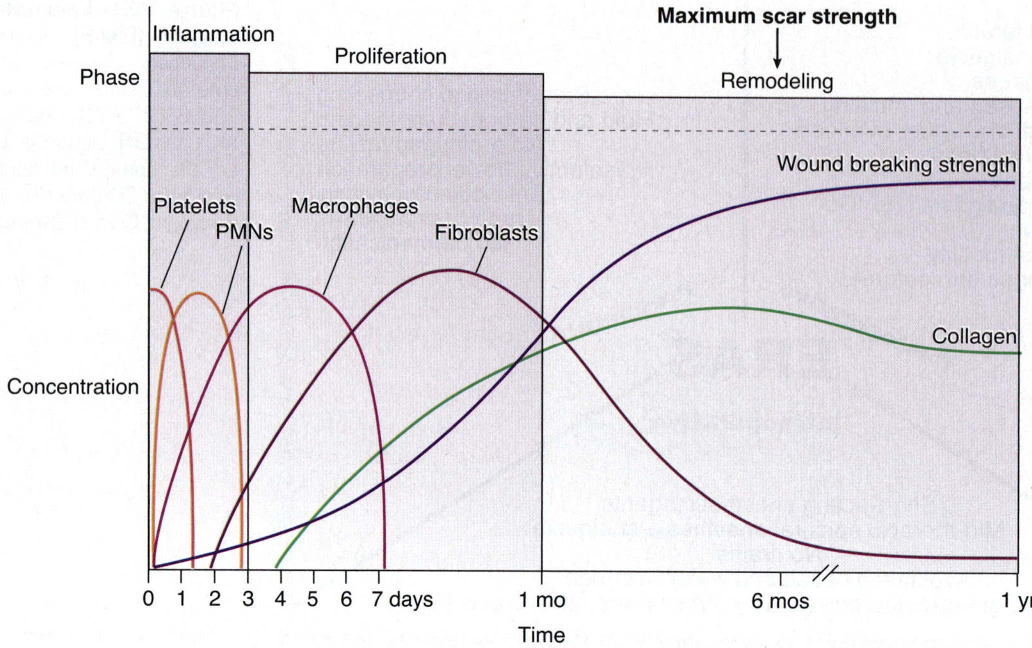

Figure 86.2. Wound healing. (Reprinted with permission from Copeland AW, Fraser S, Holder-Haynes JG, Lewis B. Wounds and wound healing. In: Lawrence PF, Smeds MR, O'Connell JB, eds. *Essentials of General Surgery and Surgical Specialties*. 6th ed. Wolters Kluwer; 2019:69. Figure 7-1.)

To assist the hospitalized patient to homeostasis, an osteopathic physician can use their hands to treat or stimulate the patients' intrinsic mechanisms for returning to a point of balance. The first few days are concentrated on the overall health of the patient. General anesthesia causes the alveoli to collapse, and this process is not well reversed when on a ventilator or when bed bound. Chest and abdominal procedures will cause splinting due to incisional pain and contribute to diminished inspiration.

Pulmonary Considerations

Respiratory motion results, through the motion of the diaphragm, in alternating negative and positive intrathoracic pressure simultaneously coupled with alternating positive and negative intra-abdominal pressure. This two-chambered pump mechanism and the unidirectional flow that results from the presence of valves in the lymphatic vasculature pulls the lymph centrally into the venous circulation. Enhancing thoracic cage mobility preoperatively is directed at reducing lymphatic congestion postoperatively as well as reducing the incidence of pulmonary stasis.

Lymphatic flow occurs as the result of lymphatic vasomotion augmented by movement of structures surrounding the lymphatic vasculature.[18] It can also be improved using OMT.

Cephalic traction on the anterior axillary folds of the supine patient pulls the thoracic cage into the position of inhalation from above. This takes out the accessory muscle use and the patient focuses on diaphragmatic breathing.

The diaphragm may be treated directly or indirectly depending on the area of incision and the areas of restriction. Consider the multiple origin and insertion points of the diaphragm when evaluating its function as it is a broad muscle and any of these areas that are restricted can trigger the rest of the muscle to spasm or function inadequately. Use of accessory muscles of respiration may indicate somatic dysfunction of the diaphragm. The function of the mesenteric plexus is affected by dysfunction of the diaphragm.[19]

The CRI has been demonstrated to be synchronous with the Traube–Hering (baroreflex) oscillation in blood flow velocity and pressure. This fluctuation in sympathetic tone may also be a driving force behind lymphatic vasomotion and is a possible explanation for how cranial manipulative procedures, such as CV-4, affect the patient. Treating the primary respiratory mechanism may stimulate the glymphatic system to eliminate accumulated waste developed by the nervous system from the stress of surgery as well as balance the autonomic nervous system.[19]

Pre-existent spinal (and to a lesser extent, appendicular) somatic dysfunction should be identified and treated. Spinal somatic dysfunction results in spinal cord–level segmental facilitation with somatovisceral effects. High cervical and sacropelvic dysfunction results in parasympathetic somatovisceral reflexes. Consider techniques such as occipitoatlantal release. Use of this technique at the beginning of a treatment session may relax the patient enough to allow other areas to balance themselves. Sacropelvic techniques are useful to stimulate urinary function, particularly in cases of postanesthetic urinary retention. Thoracolumbar dysfunction results in sympathetic somatovisceral reflexes and so should be addressed. Treatments such as modified rib-raising, paraspinal inhibition, or lumbosacral decompression will help with the return of or improve GI function.[20,21]

Know that touch is powerful. Though science does not know the full scope of how this process, this exchange works, this form of communication is able to be felt by all and described by few. Osteopathic physicians should ensure that they are holding good intentions towards the patient and are not hurried or distracted in a projected manner as OMT is performed.

As a patient, moving oneself is hard to motivate, but is well rewarded. This is particularly true after surgery when one is fatigued, in pain, and uncomfortable. However, simple exercises and walking are quite therapeutic. The act of walking moves fluids via the venous, lymphatic, and CSF systems through muscular motion, stimulates deeper breathing and increases heart rate which moves the lymphatics and increases the exchange of gases, and increases arterial supply, respectively. Walking stimulates the GI tract which stimulates the immune system and the psychoneurologic system, thus decreasing the risk of ileus, improving digestion, decreasing risk of infection, and improving mood and outlook towards recovery. Deeper breathing will also stimulate the parasympathetic nervous system which will improve wound healing and overall recovery. The sooner the patient returns to their home, their place of comfort, even if not in complete harmony, the sooner they will be able to be healthier.[22]

Most surgical procedures are now performed on an outpatient basis. There are few postoperative surgical patients in the hospital these days. This does not relieve us of our duty to act as physicians and educators for their postoperative period. Teach the patient at discharge how to care for themselves and when to check-in. Or check-in with the patient a day or two postoperatively to ensure they understand the plan and their questions are answered. This preventative ounce is worth a pound of cure and a good night's sleep.

EARLY VERSUS LATE OMT

Osteopathic surgeons work with the body and listen to the tissues, to determine how the body is returning to its state of balance. Experience teaches one to listen to the body's cues, when looking at the overall disease process and concomitant disorders. If the body had a severe attack in that area and it is still inflamed, then treating the viscerosomatic reflex may not give the intended relief. As the body recovers and the inflammation decreases, the viscerosomatic reflex may now respond to treatment. It may be difficult to discern if the healing process has progressed to the point that the viscerosomatic reflexes will respond to OMT, trial of OMT and the area's response can be the best test. For example, a woman who has four children with gallbladder attacks worsening over the years with each one and now could not ignore the problem any longer, may not respond to treatment of her viscerosomatic reflex immediately after surgery, but will respond to OMT first 4 to 6 weeks postop.

Not all of the surgeon's patients go to the OR. Some are monitored and treated nonoperatively. For example, small bowel obstruction or ileus are often treated similarly, monitoring the course, and allowing the body to return to self-heal. This still requires treatment and OMT is a great adjunct. Localized edema around the obstruction or more extensive edema found with ileus can be treated via techniques of modified rib-raising, OA release for the parasympathetic system, and lymphatic techniques to improve the flow of fluids. Recall that the fluids in this area are lymph heavy. Deep breathing and techniques that encourage this will help move these fluids. Walking, of course, is a clear choice for self-healing. Relief of pain will also decrease the sympathetic outflow; thus, treatment of any somatic dysfunction will be helpful.

WOUND MANAGEMENT

In the first few days postoperatively, the inflammatory stage, the wound seals and becomes fluid resistant, but not "waterproof" thus showering is allowed after 24 hours, but swimming and soaking of the area are not allowed for 2 to 3 weeks, after the proliferative stage has completed. During this time the wound is undergoing granulation, angiogenesis, contracting, and epithelialization. Warmth can help stimulate the vasculature to improve the healing process at this stage. Gentle manipulation towards the wound is appropriate, but tension, pulling against the wound at this point may cause dehiscence or widening of the scar. For instance, post-lumpectomy surgery of the breast, a supportive postoperative brassiere is worn for 2 to 3 weeks to decrease tension on the wound as well as to decrease seroma formation. So-called dead space allows room for fluid accumulation. The natural reaction to an injury, such as surgery, is to place fluid in that space to neutralize the acidic milieu caused by the inflammatory substances. Gentle pressure/compression, similar to that of a gentle hug, encourages the body to absorb this fluid. Drains can be used to assist in this process, particularly in areas that cannot be externally compressed, such as intra-abdominally. However, there are associated risks with this, such as infection, and newer protocol, such as the earlier mentioned ERAS protocol discourage this as a routine practice, saving it for particular needs, such as draining an abscess, and leaving them in for the shortest possible time. In the maturation phase of wound healing, the tissue is modeling and remodeling according to the patient's movements, the tensions placed on the tissue. This phase lasts 12 to 24 months. During this time, OMT can be utilized to assist in the relaxing of the tissue, particularly, myofascial techniques, to allow the patient to remodel this area. OMT improves fluid movement and motion of the tissues to allow the body to return to homeostasis.[23]

COMPLICATIONS

Prevention is the best medicine. This is a maxim to use in surgical care. Complications are much harder to deal with than their prevention. Protocols, checklists, screening, gentle, appropriate care, and communication are all helpful, however, complications may still occur. A short list includes infection, bleeding, injury to other structures, atelectasis, pneumonia, thromboembolism, pulmonary embolism, and death. Despite all the miracles of modern medicine, the rate of complications ranges from 4% to 43%. This is a fact that the surgeon must accept while striving to improve. Lifelong learning is required. Acceptance, yet maintaining one's empathy, allows the surgeon to assist the patient in dealing with the problem while also treating the complication.[24]

Looking at patients from an osteopathic perspective, one is able to treat in a holistic fashion with the anticipation of a healthier, happier, more functional patient outcome (Table 86.1).

Patient Case A

MJ is a 35-year-old woman, G1P0 in 39 weeks gestation who presents with RUQ abdominal pain and indigestion that has been intermittent and at a pain level of 3 to 4 until last night when the pain awoke her from sleep and is now at a 9/10 on the pain scale. Her pain wraps around her back and she is nauseated, though she

TABLE 86.1

Postoperative Complications of Major Surgical Procedures

- Wound infections
- Intra-abdominal sepsis (peritonitis)
- Subphrenic and subhepatic abscess
- Empyema
- Mediastinitis
- Pneumonia
- Acute respiratory insufficiency (including adult respiratory distress syndrome [ARDS])
- Renal failure
- Postoperative jaundice
- Postoperative ileus
- Bowel obstruction
- Acute gastric hemorrhage
- Multiple organ failure
- Myocardial infarction

hasn't vomited. She ate ice cream before going to bed. This has not caused her problems in the past however, she noticed that fried chicken and French fries caused her indigestion recently, and she stopped eating them.

Past medical history includes UTI during pregnancy, no past surgical history, family history (FH)- her mother and sister had their gallbladders removed after their pregnancies, lives with her fiancé, 15 pack-year tobacco history which is stopped upon learning she was pregnant. Denies use of any medications or substances since pregnancy. She's an administrative assistant at your institution and has health insurance coverage.

Exam reveals. Are well-developed, morbidly, obese, well-hydrated gravid woman in significant pain. Patient is a good historian.

Temp is 99.1, pulse 110, BP 140/85.

Pertinent positives on exam include mild rales in the right base, mild tachycardia, tenderness in the right upper quadrant, difficult to discern a Murphy due to the patient's gravid state. Tenderness on the right over T8. With acute on chronic tissue checks or changes.

Laboratory review shows a normal white blood count, mildly elevated liver function tests. Ultrasound reveals 3 mm, nonthickened, gallbladder wall with gallstones and a normal common bile duct.

The assessment is biliary colic, in a gravid patient.

Considerations: There are two patients, and both must be considered. The primary patient is the mother as she is sustaining both. There is no evidence of infection and delivery is imminent in the next 2 weeks. The patient may be monitored for the development of cholecystitis or gallstone pancreatitis and treated for her pain, with the anticipation of surgery postpartum. Microscopic cholecystectomy is less invasive and tolerated better. It would not be able to be performed at this stage of pregnancy. Were the patient to develop acute cholecystitis the options would be cholecystostomy with delayed cholecystectomy versus open cholecystectomy.

Patient's pain can be treated with an OA release to increase parasympathetic output, OMT to T8 to decrease the visceral somatic input, and use of acetaminophen as needed. Counseling concerning avoidance of fatty foods and fasting should be provided. The patient may delay surgery until the patient is ready postpartum.

Patient was able to return home and followed up 4 weeks later, with a beautiful boy in her arms. She had no further significant episodes, however, she had a few minor episodes of right upper quadrant abdominal pain with indigestion after sampling ice cream again. Laparoscopic cholecystectomy was performed 8 weeks postpartum without incident.

Six weeks postop the patient complains of mild pain along her 8th rib. That hasn't been resolved since her first episode. OMT is applied to this area with good resolution and no recurrence.

SUMMARY

Surgery, like OMT, is a modality that combines the knowledge of anatomy and physiology together in treating the patient. Body, mind, and spirit are very important in the care of surgical patients and must be considered and addressed in preparation for, during, and after surgery. The treatment plan is influenced by a complete history and physical exam to assess a patient's individual comorbidities, diet, functional capacity, habits (smoking, alcohol use), mental health, spirituality, and social needs. Evaluation of the patient's stress level and stressors gives the surgeon an idea of what can and cannot be addressed. OMT is appropriate preoperatively to prepare the patient for elective surgery. Treatment should be targeted to optimize the patient's status, decrease pain, and improve function for postoperative healing. Patients undergoing surgery experience a reduction in functional status postoperatively. Considering that structure and function are related, it follows that one respects the tissue of the patient while operating.

The surgeon must take care to respect the tissue, retracting gently and smoothly and only as needed. In the first few days following surgery, patients are in the first phase of healing, the inflammatory stage. One can change the intensity of this phase with ice, rest, elevation, anti-inflammatory medications, and OMT. Treatments such as modified rib-raising, paraspinal inhibition, or lumbosacral decompression will help with the return of or improve GI function. Be mindful that complications are much harder to deal with than their prevention. Looking at patients from an osteopathic perspective, one is able to treat in a holistic fashion with the anticipation of a healthier, happier, more functional patient outcome.

ACKNOWLEDGMENTS

The author and editors of this chapter would like to acknowledge the past contributions of Drs. Constance Cashen, Sydney P. Ross, and Christina Bohr for prior editions of this chapter.

REFERENCES

1. Still, AT, Webster, G. *Sage Sayings of Still: Selected from the Writings of Dr. A.T. Still.* Wetzel Publishing Co.; 1935.
2. Henderson AT, Fisher JF, Blair J, Shea C, Li TS, Bridges KG. Effects of rib raising on the autonomic nervous system: a pilot study using noninvasive biomarkers. *J Am Osteopath Assoc.* 2010;110(6):324–330.
3. Chin AJ, Fischione AD, Shilian R, et al. Tolerance of rib raising among hospitalized patients: a pilot study. *J Am Osteopath Med.* 2019;119(1):19–23.
4. Dal Farra F, Risio RG, Vismara L, Bergna A. Effectiveness of osteopathic interventions in chronic non-specific low back pain: A systematic review and meta-analysis. *Complement Ther Med.* 2021;56:102616.
5. Durrand J, Singh SJ, Danjoux G. Prehabilitation. *Clin Med (Lond).* 2019; 19(6):458–464.
6. Shakya P, Poudel S. Prehabilitation in patients before major surgery: a review article. *JNMA J Nepal Med Assoc.* 2022;60(254):909–915.
7. Yang J, Wang HP, Zhou L, Xu CF. Effect of dietary fiber on constipation: a meta analysis. *World J Gastroenterol.* 2012;18(48):7378–7383.
8. CODA Collaborative; Flum DR, Davidson GH, Monsell SE, et al. A randomized trial comparing antibiotics with appendectomy for appendicitis. *N Engl J Med.* 2020;383:1907–1919.
9. Bilski J. A refresher course in patient positioning. association of perioperative registered nurses. outpatient surgery magazine. Published March 6, 2023. Accessed 2023. https://www.aorn.org/outpatient-surgery/the-magazine/article/a-refresher-course-in-patient-positioning?
10. Wirth P. Treating work-related musculoskeletal injures in surgeons. General Surgery News. Pulished July 26, 2022. Accessed January 23, 2025. https://www.generalsurgerynews.com/Video/Article/07-22/Surgeon-Injuries/67577
11. Velanovich V, Rider P, Deck K, et al. Safety and efficacy of bupivacaine HCl collagen-matrix implant (INL-001) in open inguinal hernia repair: results from two randomized controlled trials. *Adv Ther.* 2019;36(1):200–216.
12. Bagul A, Taha R, Metcalfe MS, Brook NR, Nicholson ML. Pre-incision infiltration of local anesthetic reduces postoperative pain with no effects on bruising and wound cosmesis after thyroid surgery. *Thyroid.* 2005; 15(11):1245–1248.
13. Long JN. Principles of good soft-tissue technique. *Musculoskeletal Key.* Accessed 2023. https://musculoskeletalkey.com/1-principles-of-good-soft-tissue-technique/
14. Padilla, PL, Khoo KH, Ho T, Cole EL, Sirvent Ramón Z, Phillips LG. Chapter 69. In: Townsend Jr. C et al., eds. *Sabiston Textbook of Surgery.* 21st ed. Elsevier; 2021:1916–1944.

15. Lanfranco AR, Castellanos AE, Desai JP, Meyers WC. Robotic surgery: a current perspective. *Ann Surg*. 2004;239(1):14–21.
16. Melnyk M, Casey RG, Black P, Koupparis AJ. Enhanced recovery after surgery (ERAS) protocols: Time to change practice? *Can Urol Assoc J*. 2011;5(5):342–348.
17. Knight PH, Kramme KE, Sawyer RG. Chapter 3: The inflammatory response. In: Townsend Jr. C, ed. *Sabiston Textbook of Surgery*. 21st ed. Elsevier; 2021:26–43.
18. Moore JE Jr, Bertram CD. Lymphatic system flows. *Annu Rev Fluid Mech*. 2018;50:459–482.
19. Nelson, K., Sergueef,N. *Osteopathy for the Over 50s: Maintaining Function and Treating Dysfunction*. Handspring Publishing; 2014:306.
20. Peña N, Prieto H, Pierce-Talsma S. OMT for cancer patients after bowel resection. *J Am Osteopath Assoc*. 2018;118(1):e1.
21. Baltazar GA, Betler MP, Akella K, Khatri R, Asaro R, Chendrasekhar A. Effect of osteopathic manipulative treatment on incidence of postoperative ileus and hospital length of stay in general surgical patients [published correction appears in J Am Osteopath Assoc. 2013 Apr;113(4):271]. *J Am Osteopath Assoc*. 2013;113(3):204–209.
22. Rorris F, Skouteli E, Papakonstantinou K, Kokotsaki L, Skotiniotis E, Kokotsakis J. Osteopathic manipulative treatment in cardiac surgery patients: a systematic review. *Int J Osteopath Med*. 2022;46:29–35.
23. Aliano KA, Boukovalas S, Norbury WB, Phillips LG. Chapter 6: Wound Healing. In: Townsend Jr. C, eds. *Sabiston Textbook of Surgery*. 21st ed. Saunders/Elsevier; 2021:119–149.
24. Tevis SE, Kennedy GD. Postoperative complications and implications on patient-centered outcomes. *J Surg Res*. 2013;181(1):106–113.

87 Osteopathic Considerations in Sports Medicine

PER GUNNAR BROLINSON ▪ ALBERT J. KOZAR ▪ KEVIN D. VALVANO ▪ MOHAMED SHITIA ▪ NATHAN NAKKEN

KEY CONCEPTS

- Sports medicine is a multidisciplinary branch of medicine with both surgical and nonsurgical arms.
- Each member of the athletic medical team has a special role and responsibility.
- Osteopathic medicine has a unique history and role in sports medicine.
- Understanding the pathomechanics of sports- and exercise-related disease and dysfunction is key to making an accurate diagnosis and formulating a successful management plan.
- Diagnosing and treating somatic dysfunction is integrated into the management plan of the injured athlete.
- There are many unique medical challenges associated with athletic event sideline coverage and management.
- The osteopathic physician must develop a rational management plan for injury and illness and understand the factors that must be considered prior to returning the athlete to play.

OVERVIEW

- Sports medicine is a branch of medicine that focuses on physical fitness and the prevention and treatment of sport- and exercise-related injuries.
- Sports medicine has both surgical (American Orthopaedic Society for Sports Medicine) and nonsurgical (American Medical Society for Sports Medicine, American Osteopathic Academy of Sports Medicine) arms within the specialty.
- Sports medicine encompasses a multidisciplinary team composed of:
  - Sports medicine primary care physicians
  - Osteopathic physicians including osteopathic neuromusculoskeletal physicians
  - Orthopedic surgeons
  - Sports cardiologists
  - Emergency medicine physicians
  - Physical medicine and rehabilitation physicians
  - Musculoskeletal radiologists
  - Podiatrists
  - Sports physical therapists
  - Athletic trainers
  - Exercise physiologists
  - Strength and conditioning coaches
  - Personal trainers
  - Nutritionists
  - Paramedics
  - And others
- Each member of this team has a specific role to play within the scope of sports medicine.
- The goal of sports medicine is to help train athletes to prevent injuries and treat them, and restore function as quickly as possible when injury or illness does occur.
- Common office visits include[1]:
  - Concussion
  - Sprained ligaments
  - Strained muscles
  - Fractures
  - Knee, hip, shoulder, and other joint injuries
  - Tendonitis
  - Exercise-induced asthma
  - Heat-related illness
  - Eating disorders
  - Cartilage injuries
  - Overuse syndromes
  - Chronic illnesses that impact athletic performance

THE OSTEOPATHIC PHILOSOPHY

The osteopathic sports medicine physician uses a holistic, comprehensive approach to the prevention, diagnosis, and management of sports- and exercise-related injuries.[1]

- Osteopathic physicians believe that structure and function are interrelated and essential for recovering from injury and maximizing athletic potential.
- They assess the entire scope of an athlete's problem, including:
  - Mechanism of injury
  - Environmental influences
  - Inherent postural and neuromuscular imbalances
  - Inherent impairment of body rhythms
  - Psychological effects of injury and rehabilitation
  - Athlete's safe return to play
- The osteopathic physician's philosophic approach is patient oriented, not disease oriented.

Box 87.1 shows the current state-of-the-art terminology that expands upon the basic osteopathic concept of the reciprocity between structure and function.

THE ROLE OF OSTEOPATHIC MANIPULATIVE TREATMENT IN SPORTS MEDICINE

The role of osteopathic manipulative treatment (OMT) in the field of sports medicine dates back to the days of AT Still.[2] Dr. Still encouraged his students at the American School of Osteopathy to

BOX 87.1 Structure/Function Reciprocity

Structure/function reciprocity has moved beyond "simple" muscle and bone to include:

- BioTensegrity
  - Macro—systemic integration of active and passive fascia
  - Micro—individual cellular structure
  - Nuclear—proteomics and mechanotransduction
- Neuromuscular balance
  - Systemic neuromotor integration of stability
  - Engrams
- Real-world muscle function
  - "Econcentric" contraction
  - Supination/pronation link (spiral power)

join the athletics association,[3] and by 1898, the American School of Osteopathy had their own football team called the Kirksville Osteopaths, or later the "Rams," named after the ram of reason (see Fig. 87.1) which produced several famous players and coaches.[2] One coach, National Football Hall of Famer and former coach of Notre Dame and Missouri Tigers was Patrick O'Dea, an Australian by birth, who was known as "the kangaroo kicker" for a 62-yard field goal he kicked in 1892 and a punt of 110 yards.[4] O'Dea coached the Kirksville Osteopaths in 1903. Dr. Still pioneered the field of osteopathic sports medicine, treating the football team, and other professional athletes at his school, as well as others.[5]

Osteopathic physicians provide unique contributions in treating athletes. These include palpatory, diagnostic skills, a holistic approach to patient care, and hands-on treatment of the musculoskeletal system using OMT. There is a long history of involvement of osteopathic physicians (including the author) providing care (including OMT) at both Summer and Winter Olympics as well as other international multisport games such as the Goodwill Games and the Pan American Games (P. Gunnar Brolinson, DO personal communication).

Osteopathic physicians have also participated in the USOPC sports medicine volunteer programs. (usopc.org) Osteopathic physicians work with national governing bodies such as the United States Track and Field and the United States Ski and Snowboard Association (as well as others) and provide care to Olympic athletes during their respective competitive seasons nationally and internationally.[6] An osteopathic physician, Dr. Rebeccah

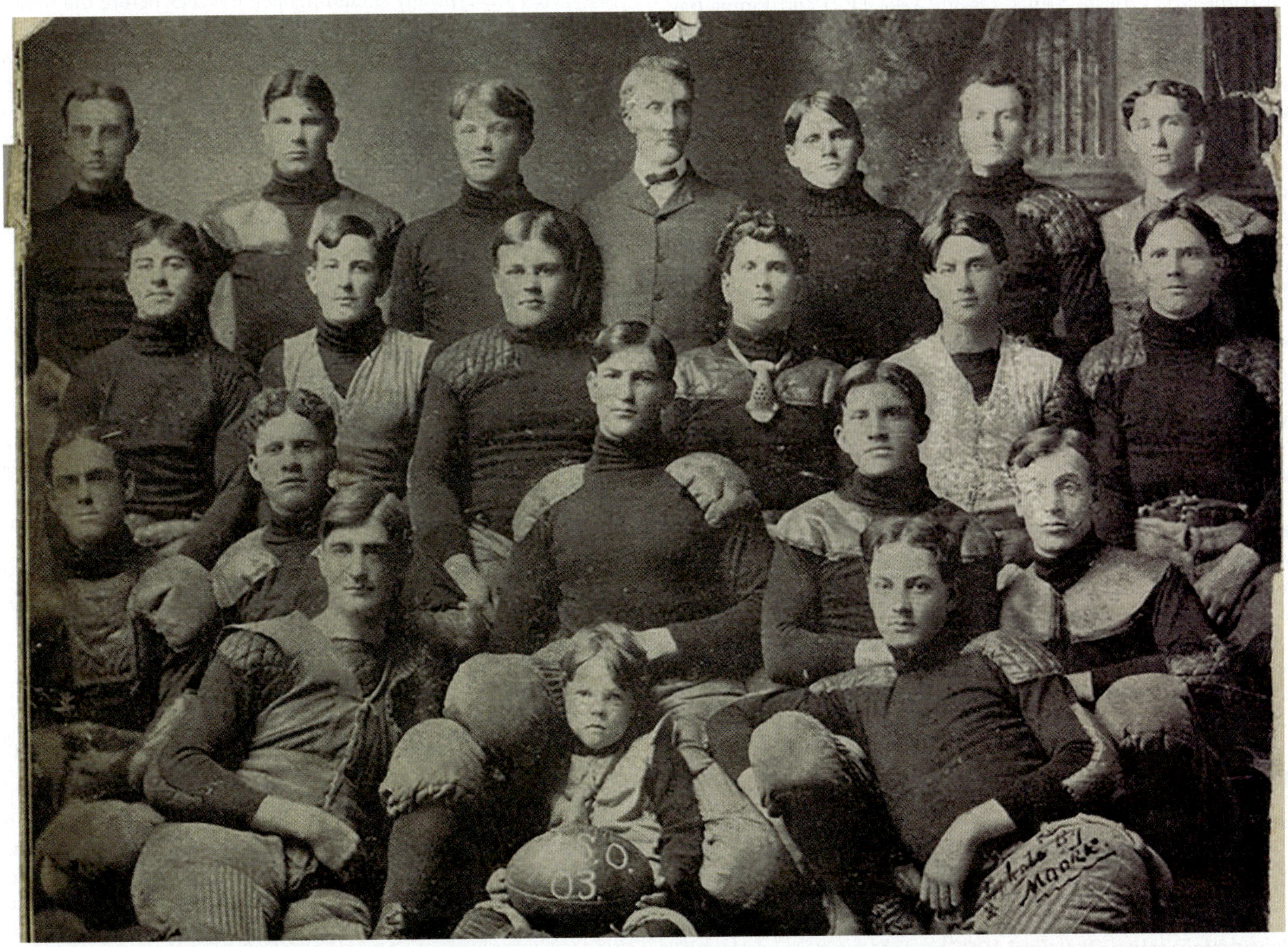

Figure 87.1. The Kirksville Osteopaths in 1903, the college football team of the American School of Osteopathy. The team was comprised of medical students and coached by the legendary "kangaroo kicker," Patrick O'Dea (likely pictured in the center of the back row). (Courtesy of Museum of Osteopathic Medicine, Kirksville, MO. This photo is property of the Museum of Osteopathic Medicine. Catalog number 1982.727.01.11. https://www.atsu.edu/news/quick-facts-on-atsus-college-football-team-the-osteopaths-and-famous-coach-patrick-odea)

BOX 87.2 Osteopathic Pearl: Use of OMT

Osteopathic doctors (DOs) DO NOT rely solely on the prescription pad to relieve pain, decrease edema, or improve performance. Many athletic injuries can be effectively managed using osteopathic evaluation followed by OMT.

Rodriguez Regner serves the USOPC as a Team USA physician and was on the medical staff at the Olympic Training Site in Chula Vista, CA as team physician for 10 years. She also served as the Medical Director for the high-performance center for Team USA (11 sports) at the 2016 Olympics in Rio. She was part of the medical staff as Team USA physician at the 2019 Pan American Games in Lima, Peru.

Outside of the Olympics, osteopathic physicians have a rich history of being involved in the medical care of many professional teams. Some examples from past and present include the Chicago Bears (Robert Kappler, DO), the Detroit Red Wings (John Finley, DO), the New Orleans Saints (David Leslie, DO), and Tampa Bay Buccaneers (Fred Brennan, Jr., DO) (personal communication).

In addition to providing comprehensive medical care, a recent study showed that collegiate athletes who were treated by DO's and received OMT reported general satisfaction in their recovery and return to sports. The study showed that 94.4% reported a decreased need for pain medication, and 83.3% reporting reduced stress and anxiety related to their injury when receiving OMT.[7] Additionally, in the field of sports medicine, the addition of OMT has been shown to be effective in:

- Decreasing the number and severity of symptoms following concussion[8,9]
- Increasing shoulder range of motion (ROM), decreasing posterior shoulder tightness, and decreasing subacromial impingement in overhead athletes like baseball pitchers[10–12]
- Providing significant functional improvement in chronic lateral epicondylitis[13,14]
- Improving short-term physical outcomes in neck pain and back pain[1,7]
- Decreasing pain in runners with patellofemoral pain syndrome[15]
- Decreasing swelling and increasing ROM after ankle sprains[16]
- Providing clinical improvement in plantar fasciitis[17]
- Improving performance among both offensive and defensive football players receiving precompetition OMT[18]
- Improving lactate clearance after exercise[19]
- And many other areas (Box 87.2)

THE SPORTS MEDICINE OFFICE VISIT

- There are two common exams in sports medicine office visits:
  - Preparticipation physical (PPE) exam
  - The injured or ill athlete visit

Preparticipation Physical (PPE)

BACKGROUND

- In the United States, about half of all children and adolescents participate in sports.[20]
- PPE5
  - In 2019, the American Academy of Pediatrics, with representatives from the American Academy of Family Physicians, American College of Sports Medicine, American Medical Society for Sports Medicine, American Orthopaedic Society for Sports Medicine, and American Osteopathic Academy for Sports Medicine, as well as the recommendations of the American Heart Association and European Society of Cardiology, published updated PPE recommendations called the Preparticipation Physical Evaluation (PPE), 5th edition (PPE5).[20] These guidelines establish the evidence-based practice recommendations for sudden cardiac death screening as well as providing medical clearance to play sports.[21]
  - Goals of the PPE
    - According to the guidelines, the general goals of the PPE are to[20–22]:
      - Determine general physical and psychological health.
      - Evaluate for life-threatening or disabling conditions, including risk of sudden cardiac arrest and other conditions that may predispose the athlete to illness or injury.
      - Serve as an entry point into the health care system for those without a medical home or primary care physician.
- Timing and location of the PPE exam
  - The PPE typically should happen 6 weeks before the season starts to allow time for any medical workup.[21,23,24]
  - The frequency of PPE exams is determined by state PPE law, but the PPE5 recommends full evaluation every 2 to 3 years unless symptoms or concerns arise.[21] The guideline recommends that the evaluation take place in the physician's office rather than in a group setting.[21]
- Scope of the PPE
  - As of 2023, all states except Vermont require PPE exams. Vermont leaves it up to the individual schools.[23,24]
- Billing
  - The ICD-10-CM code for sport-related participation evaluation is Z02.5.

PARTS OF THE PPE

- The PPE should include a thorough history, family history, and structured physical examination that focuses on the cardiovascular, musculoskeletal, and neurologic systems.
- Screening for depression, anxiety disorders, and attention-deficit/hyperactivity disorder is also recommended.
- New for the PPE are questions assessing the mental health of the athlete, as well as questions about sleep, sexual abuse, and transgender identity.[23,24]
- The optimal environment for the PPE is in the medical home by a provider familiar with the athlete's medical history. Group physicals should be discouraged but are commonplace.[23,24]
- Additionally, guidelines have been published regarding return to play for athletes who have had COVID-19.[21]
- Evaluation forms
  - The American Academy of Family Physicians, American Academy of Pediatrics,[7] American College of Sports Medicine, American Medical Society for Sports Medicine, American Orthopaedic Society for Sports Medicine, and American Osteopathic Academy of Sports Medicine have endorsed a standardized preparticipation athletic evaluation form that addresses important aspects of the history and examination[25] (see Fig. 87.2).
  - The Preparticipation Physical Evaluation (PPE) Monograph, 5th edition serves as a resource for medical providers to

This form should be placed into the athlete's medical file and should *not* be shared with schools or sports organizations. The Medical Eligibility Form is the only form that should be submitted to a school or sports organization.

Disclaimer: Athletes who have a current Preparticipation Physical Evaluation (per state and local guidance) on file should not need to complete another History Form.

PREPARTICIPATION PHYSICAL EVALUATION (Interim Guidance)

HISTORY FORM

Note: Complete and sign this form (with your parents if younger than 18) before your appointment.

Name: ______________________ Date of birth: ______________

Date of examination: ______________ Sport(s): ______________

Sex assigned at birth (F, M, or intersex): ________ How do you identify your gender? (F, M, non-binary, or another gender): ________

Have you had COVID-19? (check one): ☐ Y ☐ N

Have you been immunized for COVID-19? (check one): ☐ Y ☐ N If yes, have you had: ☐ One shot ☐ Two shots ☐ Three shots ☐ Booster date(s) ______________

List past and current medical conditions. ______________

Have you ever had surgery? If yes, list all past surgical procedures. ______________

Medicines and supplements: List all current prescriptions, over-the-counter medicines, and supplements (herbal and nutritional).

____

Do you have any allergies? If yes, please list all your allergies (ie, medicines, pollens, food, stinging insects).

____

Patient Health Questionnaire Version 4 (PHQ-4)

Over the last 2 weeks, how often have you been bothered by any of the following problems? (Circle response.)

	Not at all	Several days	Over half the days	Nearly every day
Feeling nervous, anxious, or on edge	0	1	2	3
Not being able to stop or control worrying	0	1	2	3
Little interest or pleasure in doing things	0	1	2	3
Feeling down, depressed, or hopeless	0	1	2	3

(A sum of ≥3 is considered positive on either subscale [questions 1 and 2, or questions 3 and 4] for screening purposes.)

GENERAL QUESTIONS (*Explain "Yes" answers at the end of this form. Circle questions if you don't know the answer.*)	Yes	No
1. Do you have any concerns that you would like to discuss with your provider?		
2. Has a provider ever denied or restricted your participation in sports for any reason?		
3. Do you have any ongoing medical issues or recent illness?		
HEART HEALTH QUESTIONS ABOUT YOU	**Yes**	**No**
4. Have you ever passed out or nearly passed out during or after exercise?		
5. Have you ever had discomfort, pain, tightness, or pressure in your chest during exercise?		
6. Does your heart ever race, flutter in your chest, or skip beats (irregular beats) during exercise?		
7. Has a doctor ever told you that you have any heart problems?		
8. Has a doctor ever requested a test for your heart? For example, electrocardiography (ECG) or echocardiography.		

HEART HEALTH QUESTIONS ABOUT YOU (*CONTINUED*)		Yes	No
9. Do you get light-headed or feel shorter of breath than your friends during exercise?			
10. Have you ever had a seizure?			
HEART HEALTH QUESTIONS ABOUT YOUR FAMILY	**Unsure**	**Yes**	**No**
11. Has any family member or relative died of heart problems or had an unexpected or unexplained sudden death before age 35 years (including drowning or unexplained car crash)?			
12. Does anyone in your family have a genetic heart problem such as hypertrophic cardiomyopathy (HCM), Marfan syndrome, arrhythmogenic right ventricular cardiomyopathy (ARVC), long QT syndrome (LQTS), short QT syndrome (SQTS), Brugada syndrome, or catecholaminergic polymorphic ventricular tachycardia (CPVT)?			
13. Has anyone in your family had a pacemaker or an implanted defibrillator before age 35?			

Figure 87.2. Preparticipation physical exam.

BONE AND JOINT QUESTIONS	Yes	No
14. Have you ever had a stress fracture or an injury to a bone, muscle, ligament, joint, or tendon that caused you to miss a practice or game?		
15. Do you have a bone, muscle, ligament, or joint injury that bothers you?		
MEDICAL QUESTIONS	**Yes**	**No**
16. Do you cough, wheeze, or have difficulty breathing during or after exercise?		
17. Are you missing a kidney, an eye, a testicle, your spleen, or any other organ?		
18. Do you have groin or testicle pain or a painful bulge or hernia in the groin area?		
19. Do you have any recurring skin rashes or rashes that come and go, including herpes or methicillin-resistant *Staphylococcus aureus* (MRSA)?		
20. Have you had a concussion or head injury that caused confusion, a prolonged headache, or memory problems?		
21. Have you ever had numbness, had tingling, had weakness in your arms or legs, or been unable to move your arms or legs after being hit or falling?		
22. Have you ever become ill while exercising in the heat?		
23. Do you or does someone in your family have sickle cell trait or disease? Unsure		
24. Have you ever had or do you have any problems with your eyes or vision?		

MEDICAL QUESTIONS (*CONTINUED*)	N/A	Yes	No
25. Do you worry about your weight?			
26. Are you trying to or has anyone recommended that you gain or lose weight?			
27. Are you on a special diet or do you avoid certain types of foods or food groups?			
28. Have you ever had an eating disorder?			
MENSTRUAL QUESTIONS	**N/A**	**Yes**	**No**
29. Have you ever had a menstrual period?			
30. How old were you when you had your first menstrual period?			
31. When was your most recent menstrual period?			
32. How many periods have you had in the past 12 months?			

Explain "Yes" answers here.

____

I hereby state that, to the best of my knowledge, my answers to the questions on this form are complete and correct.

Signature of athlete: ______________________________

Signature of parent or guardian: ______________________________

Date: ______________________________

Figure 87.2. (*Continued*)

keep athletes safe and healthy while participating in sports (Box 87.3).[25]

- Medical and family history
  - A good history "can detect up to 88% of general medical conditions and 67% to 75% of musculoskeletal conditions pertinent to sports participation."[21]
  - Personal and family history
    - This includes a general medical history, current medical conditions, cardiovascular conditions, recent illnesses including COVID-19, history of heat-related illness, current medications, immunizations, injury history (musculoskeletal injuries, concussion, spine injuries), surgeries, loss of any paired organs like an eye, kidney, or testis, and a cardiovascular history, recent weight loss and body image, and for females' menstrual history.
    - The history (including pertinent family history) and review of systems detect approximately 75% of conditions that restrict participation or require further evaluation.[26]
  - Disqualifying conditions:
    - It is important to ask about disqualifying conditions including spinal injuries, brachial plexus injuries, concussions, neurologic disorders, diabetes mellitus, loss of a paired organ, skin conditions, asthma or exercise-induced bronchospasm, hematologic disorders, and musculoskeletal injuries.[21]
  - Cardiovascular history:
    - It is important to obtain a cardiovascular history (HTN, cardiac murmur, high cholesterol, myocarditis, Kawasaki disease, hypertrophic obstructive cardiomyopathy, long QT syndrome).[21]
    - Most important = History of exertional chest pain, family history of premature cardiac conditions or sudden cardiac death for any reason before age 50, excessive exertional and unexplained dyspnea/fatigue or palpitations, associated with exercise.
    - History of abnormal EKG or echocardiogram, syncope, near syncope, angina, palpitations, fatigue, or arrhythmia during exercise that is unexplained should exclude the athlete from sports or strenuous exercise pending a cardiac evaluation.[20]
    - History of chest pain[2]
      - Common complaint in children and is usually benign.
      - More serious if it interrupts sleep, or is associated with exertion, fever, palpitations, syncope, or if true angina (substernal, deep pressure that radiates to the jaw or arm).
    - Family history of sudden death before age 50.[21]

BOX 87.3 Preparticipation Examination

Additional goals and objectives of the preparticipation examination:

- Screen for life-threatening conditions
- Decide eligibility or restriction of play (based on classification of sport: contact, limited contact, noncontact)
- Determine disqualifying medical conditions for sports participation
- Evaluate the function of the musculoskeletal system and prior injuries
- Record a baseline minimental status examination
- Check for communicable diseases
- Counsel/educate on athletic injury prevention and cancer screening examinations based on the population
- Establish rapport with athletes
- Perform functional screening and, when able, sports-specific functional screening, in order to evaluate for risks of injury and areas of performance enhancement
- Educate the athlete on closed head injury, use of ergogenic aids, and proper protective equipment
- *Osteopathic physicians should perform a screening musculoskeletal examination with emphasis on evaluation for the presence of somatic dysfunction that impedes function*

  - Family history of heart disease (hypertrophic cardiomyopathy, Marfan syndrome, arrhythmogenic right ventricular cardiomyopathy, long QT syndrome, short QT syndrome, Brugada syndrome, catecholaminergic polymorphic ventricular tachycardia, pacemakers, defibrillator, unexplained sudden death, drowning, or seizures).[20]
- Other medical conditions:
  - History of unexplained seizure[20]
  - Hematologic disorders
    - History of clotting disorders, sickle cell anemia, enlarged spleen
- Mental health history:
  - PPE5 recommends screening for depression with the Patient Health Questionnaire-9 (PHQ-9) and anxiety with a Generalized Anxiety Disorder-7 (GAD-7).
  - The history should also include questions about mental substance use, and high-risk behavior.[21]
  - Screening for tobacco, vaping/electronic cigarettes, performance-enhancing supplements, alcohol, marijuana, and prescription analgesics should also be performed.[21]

ASSOCIATED SYMPTOMS[20]

- Cardiac (discussed above)
- Respiratory (asthma-induced bronchospasm)
- Musculoskeletal (back, knee, or other joint pain or stiffness)
- Neuro (Concussion-like symptoms—obtain SCAT testing for baseline)

PHYSICAL EXAM[21]

- The PE should include:
  - **General:** vital signs (height, weight, BMI, ideal body weight [IBW], body composition)

BOX 87.4 Cardiovascular Preparticipation Screening of Competitive Athletes

1. A complete medical history, physical examination, and brachial artery blood pressure should be performed before participation in organized high school (grades 9 through 12) and college sports.
2. Screening should be repeated every 2 years; in intervening years, a history should be taken.
3. A national standard for preparticipation examinations should be developed.
4. A health care professional with the training, skills, and background necessary to reliably obtain a detailed cardiovascular history, perform a physical examination, and recognize heart disease should perform athlete screening.

  - **Head, Ears, Eyes, Nose and Throat:** pupils equal, hearing intact, vision testing (visual acuity of 20/40 or better or refer for corrective lenses)
  - **Cardiovascular**[20]: a detailed cardiac exam should be performed including:
    - Resting BP (right arm) and resting heart rate (often <40 bpm in elite athletes).
      - If there is weight loss and the heart rate is <40, may indicate insufficient caloric intake
    - Evaluating for heart murmur, arrhythmias, assess upper extremity and femoral pulses to exclude coarctation, auscultation should be performed with the patient in both the supine and standing positions with provocative maneuvers (i.e., Valsalva maneuver and squat test), specifically to identify murmurs of dynamic left ventricular outflow tract obstruction.
    - Visualize for stigmata of Marfan syndrome (see section on Marfan syndrome below).
    - Consideration may be made for EKG and cardiology referral based on your physical exam findings (Box 87.4).
- **Respiratory:** pain with pressure over the sternum (may indicate costochondritis), auscultate for wheezing.
- **Neurologic:** neurologic screening including DTRs, muscle strength testing, and light touch sensation.
- **Musculoskeletal**[20]: a comprehensive musculoskeletal exam should be conducted including:
  - Any prior on-field joint injuries are assessed as these regions may have sustained a fracture, dislocation, or compromised vital structures (Fig. 87.3).

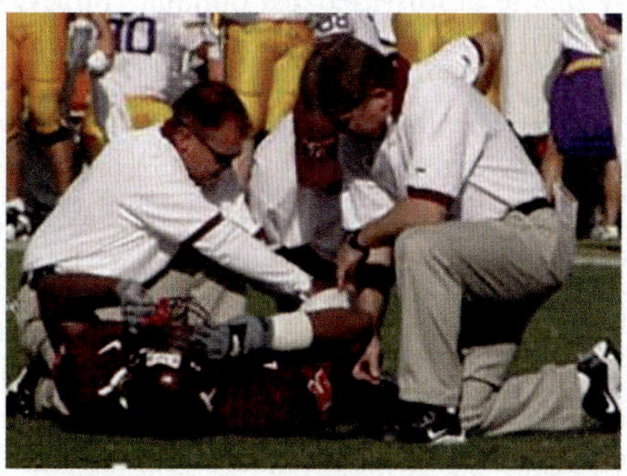

Figure 87.3. Assessment of athletic injury on field. (Photo taken by Delmas Bolin, MD, used with permission.)

- It is also important to perform a whole-body functional screen.
- Evaluation of symptomatic joints and other potentially related kinetic chain dysfunctions.
  - The kinetic chain refers to all the muscles and joints that work together to perform movement.
    - For example, to throw a baseball, the pitcher must have shoulder rotation with good flexibility and strength, the kinetic chain also includes scapulothoracic motion, leg stability, hip rotation, core strength, and the coordinated motion of multiple muscles and joints. In this case, the lower extremity and trunk serve as the main force generator for the kinetic chain.[27]
- Keep in mind direct and indirect anatomic correlations of body connectedness through complex fascial, neurologic, reflexive, and metabolic relationships are essential since athletes rely heavily on cross-body and spiral transfer of energy between different regions of the body through fascial and myofascial-ligamentous connections.

Standing assessment for structural asymmetry

- Head tilt (may indicate cervical spine injury, trapezius, or cervical muscle spasm).
- Prominence and levelness of one acromioclavicular joint (AC joint separation).
- Asymmetric shoulder heights (trapezius or paraspinal strain, neck or shoulder injury, primary spine injury or scoliosis, limb length discrepancy).
- Asymmetric iliac crest heights (scoliosis, short leg, pelvic rotation, or spasm of the lumbar paraspinal muscles).
- Spine
  - Back (scoliosis—only excluded if Cobb angle >40 degrees).
  - Neck ROM (if limited, pain, or weakness excluded from sports until further workup).

Upper extremities

- Shoulder
  - ROM (Apley scratch test)
  - Strength (general screen major muscle groups and Jobes test)
  - Laxity (especially if history of dislocation)
- Elbow and hand
  - ROM
  - Strength (general screen major muscle groups and Jobes test)
- Lower extremities
  - ROM/strength
    - Knee and hip (Duck walk—have them squat placing the buttock on the heel and, while maintaining this position, take four steps forward, then turn around and take four more steps).
  - Atrophy of the vastus medialis obliquus (VMO) (indicates a leg injury that has caused the athlete to avoid normal use of the leg)
  - Prominent, tender tibial tuberosity (Osgood–Schlatter disease)
  - Swelling of any extremity (inflammation or injury)
  - Long limbs relative to the trunk, arachnodactyly, and pectus deformity of the chest (Marfan syndrome)
  - Ankle—have them hop as high as they can on one foot five times; then the other (if unable = instability or unrehabilitated injury)
- **Abdomen:** evaluate for organomegaly (disqualified from sports)
- **Genitourinary (GU):** if only one testicle, may still play sports if they use a cup, if a single kidney—discuss the risks of contact sports and have them discuss with their nephrologist.
- Other parts of the GU exam, such as testing for hernias, are not routinely indicated for clearance for sports; however, it is indicated if done as part of a health care maintenance visit.
- **Skin:** evaluate for any signs of contagious skin infections (i.e., herpes simplex virus, varicella, impetigo, tinea corporis, scabies, molluscum contagiosum, or methicillin-resistant staphylococcus aureus lesions disqualify an athlete from sports until the condition is cleared).
- **Lymph:** further workup is indicated if the athlete has signs of edema or lymphadenopathy.
- **Mental health:** The PPE5 now contains new guidelines relative to the mental health of athletes as already discussed above.[21]

WORKUP[20]

- Labs—in the absence of symptoms, routine blood work is not recommended.
- According to the American Heart Association and the American College of Cardiology, screening EKG and echocardiogram are not necessary unless there is clinical concern.[28,29]

PPE GUIDELINES RELATIVE TO COVID-19

- The COVID-19 pandemic raised questions about the postinfection risks to athletes.
- Exercise volume and intensity, participation in sports, and minimizing the risk of contracting the disease were all topics that were crucial during the pandemic.[30]
- Areas of postinfection risk to athletes that should be addressed include:
  - Cardiovascular[30–34]
    - Myocarditis and rapid-onset heart failure.
    - Arrhythmias—myocarditis can lead to tissue scarring which can cause fatal arrhythmias.
    - HTN—patients with hypertension have an increased risk of poor outcomes after contracting COVID-19. While there is theoretic risk between angiotensin-converting enzyme inhibitors (ACEi) and COVID-19, studies have not confirmed increased risk due to ACEi or angiotensin-II receptor blocker, and these medications should be continued.
  - Pulmonary—COVID-19 has been shown to affect pulmonary vasculature.
- Risks of COVID-19 to the athlete:
  - Patients of any age with the following underlying medical conditions are at increased risk if infected with the COVID-19 virus: chronic kidney disease, chronic obstructive pulmonary disease, immunocompromised state (from solid organ transplant), obesity (body mass index [BMI] > 30), serious heart conditions (such as heart failure, coronary artery disease, or cardiomyopathy), sickle cell disease, and type 2 diabetes mellitus.
  - The centers for disease control recommends people with the following conditions might also be at an increased risk for severe illness from COVID-19: asthma (moderate to severe), cerebrovascular disease, cystic fibrosis, hypertension, immunocompromised state (from bone marrow transplant), immune deficiencies, HIV, use of corticosteroids or use of other immune-weakening medicines, neurologic conditions, liver disease, pregnancy, pulmonary fibrosis, smoking, thalassemia, and type 1 diabetes mellitus.[35,36]
  - Asthma
    - Chronic pulmonary conditions including moderate-to-severe asthma are associated with poor COVID-19 outcomes.

        - Patient should use their medications including steroid inhalers.
        - Worsening asthma in a well-controlled athlete may be a sign of early COVID-19 infection.
    - Obesity
        - Evidence suggests obesity and excessively overweight people are at a higher risk of death or serious outcomes.
        - Lifestyle recommendations are generally recommended.
    - Sickle cell disease
        - Sickle cell disease is an increased risk for poor outcomes in persons with COVID-19.
        - Sickle cell trait is not a risk factor for poor outcomes.
- Guidelines[30]:
    - During active COVID-19 infection, exercising outdoors with physical distancing is relatively safe, especially if there is no sharing of athletic equipment (i.e., towels, clothing, shoes, balls, or sports-specific equipment) and there is no body contact.
    - Currently, infected or recovered athletes may have silent clinical pathology in any organ, including the heart.[30]
    - Cardiac complications may increase the risk of sudden death associated with exercise. COVID-19–related damage to the kidney, lungs, and vascular system has implications for fluid balance, coagulopathy, and heat stroke during exercise.
    - An athlete who reports any recent symptoms should be evaluated and treated based on clinical or laboratory diagnosis of COVID-19. The PPE should be postponed until the athlete is well or symptom free for at least 2 weeks.[25]
    - Group personal protective equipment (PPE) is not recommended. This became even more important with physical distancing during the COVID-19 pandemic.[30]
    - Telemedicine:
        - During the COVID-19 pandemic, telemedicine became a popular way for patients to interact with their physician; however, given the importance of listening to the heart for murmurs, telemedicine should not be the mode for the PPE.[23,24]
        - Virtual care visits for sports preparticipation evaluations are often not covered or reimbursed.[30]
        - They can, however, be a good option for evaluating athletes with symptoms of COVID-19.[30]
    - Athletes with sequelae related to COVID-19 infection may require specialized evaluation and care (cardiac, pulmonary, and renal).
    - COVID-19–positive athletes without symptoms should not exercise or participate in sports for a determined period and remain in self-quarantine while monitoring for symptoms.
        - During the PPE, all parties (providers, patients, and family members) should wear masks and stay 6 feet apart whenever possible.
        - If the athlete is asymptomatic after a given period, exercise and return to sports may be gradually resumed with medical supervision.
        - If symptoms return, restrict exercise and sports play.
    - A 12-lead electrocardiogram should be considered in asymptomatic athletes following COVID-19 infection.[29]
    - PPE5 suggests rescinding medical eligibility, either temporarily or permanently, when medical conditions are discovered (COVID-19 infection is such a condition) after eligibility has been established.
- Evidence-based data specifically addressing the athletes during the COVID-19 pandemic continues to evolve.

CLEARANCE

- After the PPE is performed, there are different levels of clearance[23,24]:
    - Unconditional clearance: cleared for all sports and levels of participation.
    - Cleared with recommendation for follow-up.
    - Not cleared with clearance status to be determined after further evaluation, treatment, or rehabilitation.
    - Not cleared for any sport or level of competition.
- Most children and adolescents with chronic medical conditions can participate in a sport at some level after appropriate evaluation and/or treatment. Sports participation recommendations for specific medical conditions are available through the American Academy of Pediatrics website.[2,25]

STANDING SCREENING/SCANNING EXAMINATION

The standing screening examination of the athlete is performed in the same fashion as for the general population (as detailed in Chapters 30 and 31); however, there are some differences. Awareness of the loads and motions related to a particular sport indicates if specific findings are physiologic adaptations or pathologic (Box 87.5).

Paravertebral humping

- On forward bending, asymmetry of muscle mass in the paraspinal muscles is not uncommon. This paravertebral muscle "humping" or prominence may:
    - be related to idiopathic spinal scoliosis or functional group curve mechanics (see Chapter 30)
    - or occur as a developmental response on the dominant hand side related to sports participation.

Marfan syndrome

- Tall athletes may have an arm span longer than height, arachnodactyly (long, thin fingers), and kyphoscoliosis.
    - This may warn the physician to consider Marfan syndrome.
        - Genetic testing for mutations in fibrillin-1 (FBN1) and other genes has become an important and reliable option to aid in the diagnosis of Marfan syndrome.[37]
    - Because of potential aortic and cardiac structural abnormalities, patients suspected to have Marfan syndrome need a thorough cardiovascular workup prior to competition.

BOX 87.5 Osteopathic Pearls: Muscle Function

- Evaluating and treating muscle imbalances is key to preventing or treating somatic complaints. It is not necessary to wait until an injury has occurred to utilize manual treatments. With osteopathic medicine, it's never too early, nor it is ever too late to initiate treatment.
- Absolute muscle strength is NOT the most important variable in pathology or rehabilitation of functional stability.
- Proper timing and automatic activation of dynamic stabilizers are MORE IMPORTANT for functional stability.
- Deficits of low-threshold muscle recruitment and motor control inefficiency increase the risk of chronic, or recurrence of, musculoskeletal injury.

PALPATORY EXAMINATION

Osteopathic physicians have unique palpatory skills, which can be useful in determining if there is a somatic component to a patient's medical condition or somatic dysfunction (SD) that may be a result of, or lead to, injury.[1,38] This approach allows for the detection of additional structural and functional information (see Chapters 29 and 30 for further information).

Muscle and fascial tissue:

- Healthy muscles and fascia feel smooth, elastic, and homogeneous.
- The palpatory examination can determine the presence and severity of tissue texture abnormalities, as well as the size, shape, and tone of the muscles, tendons, and ligaments.

Neural tissue:

- Flaccid or atrophic muscles may be related to a lower motor neuron lesion.
- Athletes with a herniated disk and radiculopathy may have palpable findings in the affected extremity.

Ligaments:

- Torn ligaments are locally tender and may have a palpable defect.

Bones:

- Palpation of a tender bony step-off may be indicative of a fracture, whereas point tenderness on palpation may be indicative of a stress injury.

Functional palpation:

- This is palpation when the athlete is performing a particular motion.
- Tenderness of muscle during a concentric or eccentric contraction may indicate a muscular strain.
- A defect noted during muscular contraction may be indicative of tear or high-grade strain.
- Tissue that does not actively contract and may be locally tender during functional palpation may indicate scar tissue.

Firing patterns:

- Observation and/or palpation of muscle-firing patterns can also provide useful information.
- Palpation allows the physician to determine if a particular muscle is "turning on" or if it is inhibited. Lack of muscle activation or easy fatigability may indicate impaired muscle-firing sequences.
  - This factor is important to assess to guide therapeutic osteopathic intervention prior to prescribing more advanced therapeutic exercises and appropriate neuromuscular retraining.

MOTION TESTING

Motion testing should include axial and appendicular joints, soft tissues, fascia, and cranial motion.[1]

- Testing is performed in areas that were found to contain significant tissue texture abnormalities upon screening.
- Prior to motion testing, it is important to understand that athletes may have very different ranges and qualities of motion that may still be considered "normal" for their sports, or pathology that may be masked by their physical training.[1]
  - Some athletes have significant flexibility in their ligaments and joints, yet this is not appreciated readily because of the generalized tone of the muscles.
  - Adolescent females may have ligamentous laxity or hypermobility, typically in the knees and shoulders. Hypermobility can be quantified using the Beighton Hypermobility Score (Box 87.6).
  - Other athletes may have a "normal" functional shift of their ROM due to the specific repetitive motion demands of their sport and playing position.

BOX 87.6 Beighton Hypermobility Score[a]

+1 point for each elbow that bends backward
+1 point for each knee that bends backward
+1 point for each thumb that touches the forearm when bent backward
+1 point for each little finger that bends backward beyond 90 degrees
+1 point if while standing forward bending, palms can be placed on the ground with legs straight

Osteopathic Pearls:

- Hypermobility is important to assess in regard to treatment. There are particular osteopathic manipulative treatments in which hypermobility serves as a contraindication or a relative contraindication. Be sure to ask and/or assess prior to treatment.
- Hypermobility may also be a risk factor for poor central body proprioception and stability. This often is seen in association with poor motor firing patterns and recurrent injury.

[a]Max score is 9. Any score ≥6 indicates hypermobility. See Castori M, Tinkle B, Levy H, et al. A framework for the classification of joint hypermobility and related conditions. *Am J Med Genet C Semin Med Genet.* 2017;175(1):148–157 for further discussion.

ARTICULAR MOTION TESTING

Motion testing includes an evaluation of the *quantity* and *quality* of motion (Box 87.7).

- Articular SD typically occurs in the joint's minor motions.
- A significant variable during motion testing is the concept of "end feel." End feel is a qualitative finding of reluctance or resistance to further motion. It is a qualitative descriptor of the restrictive barrier.[1]
  - Microtraumatic injuries (repetitive overuse) may have a firm end feel due to muscle tightness.
  - Macrotraumatic injuries immediately evaluated within the first "golden hour" may produce a loose or sloppy end feel, especially if ligamentous disruption occurred. After this, muscle splinting and swelling of the injured area occurs, and the end feel may become firm.
  - Viscerosomatic reflexes may produce a rubbery end feel in the tissues.

BOX 87.7 Osteopathic Pearl: Diagnosis

An accurate assessment of the type of restriction found during motion testing helps guide the selection of manipulative treatment.

BOX 87.8 Osteopathic Pearl: Kinetic Chain

The most important symptom of disturbed motor function is usually pain. To evaluate and rehabilitate athletic injuries, physicians must think in terms of a functional kinetic chain and/or the concept that living beings are functional biotensegrity units. Understanding the integrated ground reaction force, center of body weight, muscle movements, balance between all compressive and tensile elements in the body, and other external complementary forces will allow successful integration of the involved tissue into the entire kinetic chain system.

THE FUNCTIONAL BIOMECHANICAL EXAMINATION

Sports performance is primarily a function of the neuromusculoskeletal system (Box 87.8).[1,34,36,37] A functional biomechanical examination might include the double-leg squat test, single-leg squat test, and step drop test.

- The athlete is subject to the biomechanical strength and flexibility demands of the particular sport, as well as the gravitational challenges producing the ground reaction forces associated with the loads and motions of their sport.
- When approaching the injured athlete, it is vital to consider functional anatomy, with the understanding that joints are both mechanical and sensory organs producing both proprioceptive and nociceptive information. Assessment should include functional movement tasks related to sports-specific activities.
- Screening both duel and single-leg static and dynamic motion, with both eyes open and eyes closed can give a glimpse into both the presence and location of underlying neuromuscular dysfunction in the periphery or in the central system.
- The purpose is to identify dysfunctional patterns and guide neuromusculoskeletal behavioral patterns that are favorable to health and that are functionally and biomechanically more efficient.

DIAGNOSIS OF SOMATIC DYSFUNCTION AND SPORTS-RELATED INJURIES

The following clinical examples demonstrate the importance of diagnosing and treating SD that accompanies common sports injuries. See Chapters 39, 40, and 91 of this text on OMT procedures and discussions related to upper and lower extremity SD.

Head

HEADACHES

Background

- Headache is the most common neurologic disease.[39–41] The International Headache Society describes 13 categories of headaches and about 150 headache syndromes.
- When evaluating an athletic headache, it is important to rule out other forms of headache, which may be secondary to medication intracranial mass.
- Sinusitis.
- Other medical ailments.

Differential Diagnosis:

Effort headache[42]:

- Mechanism:
  - □ Secondary to increased intracranial pressure associated with athletic effort.
- Incidence:
  - □ Equal in both males and females.
- H+P:
  - □ Rapid onset, described as a frontal or bifrontal type of headache.
  - □ Duration—lasts several minutes to up to 24 hours.
- Diagnosis:
  - □ Usually clinical, may order imaging such as CT angiography (CTA) to rule out vascular causes.
- Treatment:
  - □ Medications such as Indomethacin or Propranolol may be prescribed.
  - □ OMT.

Cervicogenic headache[43]:

- Mechanism:
  - □ Headache related to cervical sprain. This is felt to be secondary to stretching of cervical ligaments and tendons, which results in a reflex muscle contraction or spasm of the paracervical musculature
- Incidence:
  - □ More common in males; associated with combative/whiplash sports
- H+P:
  - □ Pain in the upper cervical, occipital, and/or parietal regions
  - □ Duration: Several days or weeks
- Diagnosis:
  - □ Clinical
  - □ CT or MRI may show disorder in the cervical spine or soft tissues of the neck that can cause headache
- Treatment:
  - □ Physical therapy
  - □ Medications
  - □ Exercises
  - □ Nerve blocks
  - □ OMT

Acute effort migraine:

- Mechanism:
  - □ Likely related to decreased cerebral CO_2 secondary to hyperventilation, which results in vasoconstriction
- H+P:
  - □ Migraine following short, intense activity
  - □ Risk factors:
    - Caffeine use or discontinuance
    - Poor nutrition
    - Dehydration
    - Head load
    - Hypoglycemia
    - Alcohol use
- Diagnosis:
  - □ Clinical
  - □ Imaging may be ordered to rule out other causes
- Treatment:
  - □ Prevention: A gradual warm-up may help in prevention by inducing a "refractory period" with respect to migraine
  - □ Reduce risk factors

- □ Medication
- □ OMT

Trauma-triggered migraine:

- Mechanism:
  - □ Initiated by head trauma
- Incidence:
  - □ More common in athletes with a prior history of migraine headache; more common in contact or collision sports
- Diagnosis:
  - □ Clinical
  - □ Symptoms follow head trauma
- Treatment:
  - □ Typically responds to the patient's migraine treatment plan
  - □ OMT

Post-traumatic headache[44]:

- Mechanism:
  - □ Headache that is also often associated with concussion
- Incidence:
  - □ More common in males who are involved in contact and combative sports
  - □ This is also a common cause of disability in military personnel
- H+P:
  - □ Duration: Hours to weeks
  - □ Note: Intensity of headache may not be related to the severity of trauma
- Diagnosis:
  - □ Clinical diagnosis:
    - Headache with an onset of within 7 days following trauma or injury
    - Headache within 7 days of regaining consciousness, or after the ability to sense and report pain following trauma or injury
    - Some patients may experience symptoms several months to one year after the trauma or injury
    - CT without contrast may be ordered to rule out cerebral hemorrhage
- Treatment:
  - □ Oral medications
  - □ Behavioral therapy
  - □ OMT

CONCUSSION[45]

- One of the biggest issues facing the sports medicine physician is concussion.[46,47]
- Concussion is defined as a complex functional process affecting the brain, induced by traumatic biomechanical forces.
- Mechanism:
  - □ Cause: A direct blow to the head, face, neck, or elsewhere on the body.
  - □ Note that concussion may also result from an impact to the body, transmitted to the head and neck, resulting in a whiplash injury which will result in similar neuromyofascial findings.
  - □ The opposite is true as well. A blow to the head may transmit force to the rest of the body that may result in SD.
  - □ Pathophysiology is complex involving neurochemical and neurometabolic events after an injury to the head resulting in altered neurologic function.
  - □ The exact pathophysiology of concussion has not been described.
  - □ Most physicians and scientists specializing in the field agree that concussion symptoms are the result of neuronal dysfunction that is linked closely with an "energy crisis" and neuroinflammatory response resulting from biomechanical forces applied to the brain.
  - □ A blow to the head will transmit forces to the rest of the body that may result in SD.
  - □ Acceleration, deceleration, or rotation can result in acute axonal injury via disruption of organization of the neurofilaments.
  - □ Release of electrolytes leads to release of neurotransmitters and resultant neurologic dysfunction.
  - □ There are also changes in glucose metabolism and cerebral blood flow.
  - □ There may be mitochondrial dysfunction.
- H+P:
  - □ Rapid onset of short-lived impairment of neurologic function that resolves spontaneously
  - □ Concussion may ultimately result in neuropathologic changes, but the acute clinical symptoms largely reflect a functional disturbance rather than a structural injury[48]
  - □ Irritability, mood changes
  - □ Cognitive changes including confusion, amnesia, mental fogginess, and difficulty concentrating
    - >90% will not have a loss of consciousness
  - □ Headache
  - □ Dizziness
  - □ Difficulty with balance
  - □ Visual changes
  - □ Sleep disturbances including drowsiness or difficulty sleeping
- Diagnosis:
  - □ While the definition of concussion and best practice recommendations remain a subject of ongoing inquiry and debate, international consensus supports clinical diagnosis based on a constellation of signs and symptoms, with a high index of suspicion.[49,50]
  - □ Current mainstays of concussion evaluation include symptom assessment, neurologic examination, and cognitive testing.
  - □ There have been many different clinical tests created to attempt to diagnose concussion.
  - □ There is not yet a simple, specific, definitive diagnostic test. We rely on symptoms, physical examination, and clinically informed concussion assessment protocols.[50]
  - □ May use the SCAT6 tool for assessment of concussion.
  - □ Imaging: Typically, no abnormality on standard structural neuroimaging studies is seen; however, CT may help rule out other pathology such as intracranial bleeding; however, the majority of patients diagnosed with a concussion do not need imaging.
  - □ If symptoms last longer than 7 days, you may consider MRI of the brain.
  - □ There are two serum biomarkers that show promise in the future of diagnosing concussions, ubiquitin C-terminal hydrolase and glial fibrillary acidic protein. These appear to be elevated in the early postinjury phase.
- Treatment[39,51–57]:
  - □ Immediate removal of the athlete from play.
  - □ Treatment and prevention protocols are regularly reexamined and revised when needed to improve long-term outcomes following a concussion. Wearing protective headgear does not prevent concussion (see Fig. 87.4).[58]

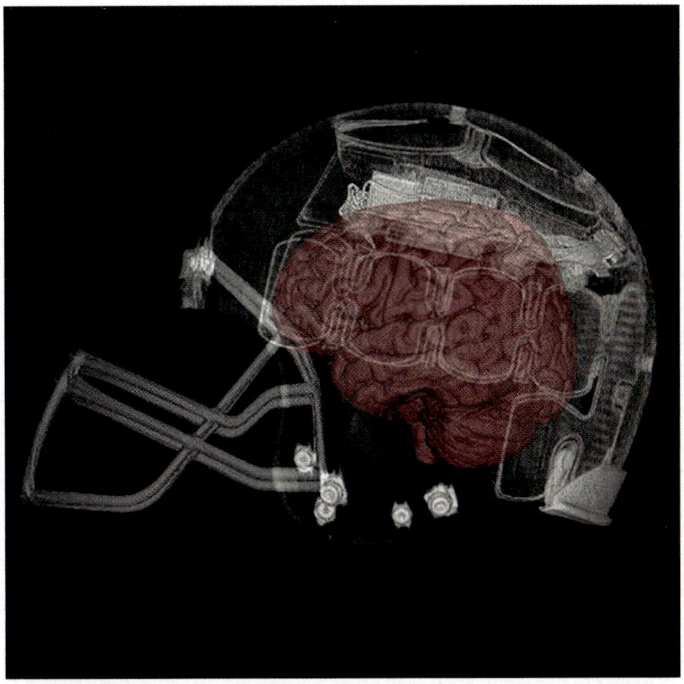

Figure 87.4. Depiction of football helmet protection on an athlete's brain. Concussions may still occur even with proper protection in place.

- Educate on warning signs requiring further work up.
- Initial physical and cognitive rest followed by gradual, stepwise return to previous activity levels. There is no longer a role for prolonged, strict cognitive, and physical rest.
- The long-term health of the athlete and the prevention of secondary neurologic injury guide the return-to-play protocol. Physical and cognitive rest are recommended for the first 24 to 48 hours per the 2022 Consensus Statement Guidelines.[59]
- Relative rest can start as early as 24 hours after injury.
- Early return-to-activities is now recommended if they do not increase their symptom evaluation scores by more than 2 points and do not increase symptoms for longer than 1 hour.[60]
  - Return-to-learn is an important component of this protocol.
- Physical therapy and medications may also be of benefit.
- OMT should be used early (even postgame, if serial exams are stable and not concerning) and often to address the mechanical factors associated with the whiplash injury that has occurred (Box 87.9). These can occur in any part of the peripheral system, neurocranium, or viscerocranium. Manipulation can also help differentiate which presenting symptoms are neurologic versus mechanical in nature.

BOX 87.9 Osteopathic Pearl: Concussion

There is new evidence to suggest cranial, cervical, and sacral manipulation in an acute concussion may help speed up recovery and improve patient symptoms.[29–32] There are currently ongoing studies regarding cranial manipulation for the concussed athlete.

SECOND IMPACT SYNDROME[61]

- Mechanism:
  - Second impact syndrome is when a patient experiences a second concussion before complete recovery from the first head injury.
  - This leads to dysfunctional cerebral blood flow autoregulation, which in turn, causes increased intracranial pressure.
  - This syndrome is often deadly with an approximately 50% mortality rate, and nearly a 100% morbidity rate.[62]
  - Second impact syndrome often results in brain herniation secondary to the increased intracranial pressure.
- Incidence:
  - Unknown, but there were 35 probably cases among American football players between 1980 and 1993.[62]
- H+P:
  - The patient still has symptoms of concussion when a second concussion occurs.
  - The patient will be unlike to be able to give a good history. Information should be gathered from those who witnessed the incident.
  - Inquire if there was any seizure, concussion history, alcohol or drug use, loss of consciousness, resultant weakness or paresthesias, difficulty walking, bladder or bowel incontinence.
- Diagnosis:
  - CT scan
- Treatment:
  - Immediate neurosurgical referral if signs of increased intracranial pressure.
  - There is limited research, but current guidelines suggest relative rest (cognitive and physical), followed by a graded return to play.
  - The athlete should be protected from further sports-related concussions until they fully recover and should not be cleared for return to play until they have completed the full protocol.
  - OMT.
  - Prevention is the best treatment for second impact syndrome.
    - To avoid second impact syndrome, return to contact sports should only be allowed after the athlete is asymptomatic both at rest and with exertion, and has passed all steps in the protocol.[47]
      - Further, repeat concussions generally require a longer period of asymptomatic rest, although the ideal duration is unclear.
      - Several studies have demonstrated that neuropsychiatric testing can detect cognitive impairment after mild traumatic brain injury.[63–67] This testing can be a helpful adjunct in the return-to-play decision-making process.
      - Any athlete with repeat concussions and prolonged symptoms should undergo multidisciplinary evaluation, including neuropsychiatric testing, prior to returning to play.

POSTCONCUSSIVE SYNDROME[68]

Some athletes may develop postconcussive syndrome.[47] This includes a constellation of symptoms including physical, cognitive, behavioral, and/or emotion symptoms.

- Mechanism:
  - Blunt force, nonpenetrating to the head causing mild traumatic brain injury, but concussive symptoms persist longer than 3 months.
  - While the exact cause is unknown, the syndrome is believed to be secondary to post-traumatic altered neurotransmitter function and inflammatory changes in the brain.

- H+P:
  - ☐ Symptoms persist longer than 3 months
  - ☐ This can include:
    - Ongoing headache
    - Headache with exertion
    - Dizziness
    - Fatigue
    - Irritability
    - Impaired memory
    - Decreased concentration
    - Decreased academic and athletic performance
- Diagnosis
  - ☐ Clinical and includes cognitive deficits in attention or memory and at least three of the following:
    - Fatigue
    - Sleep disturbance
    - Headaches
    - Dizziness
    - Irritability
    - Affective disturbance
    - Apathy or personality changes
  - ☐ These symptoms must last longer than 3 months
- Treatment
  - ☐ Reassurance—most patients will improve within 3 months.
  - ☐ Physical and cognitive rest are recommended for the first 24 to 48 hours per the consensus statement guidelines.
    - Relative rest can start as early as 24 hours after injury.
    - Early return-to-activities are now recommended if they do not increase their symptom evaluation scores by more than 2 points and do not increase symptoms for longer than 1 hour.
  - ☐ Medications such as amitriptyline, propranolol, or indomethacin may be helpful for headaches.
  - ☐ Greater occipital nerve block for refractory headaches may be considered.
  - ☐ Education to avoid second concussion.
  - ☐ Active forms of therapy targeting the patient's pain, visual, or balance symptoms such as cervical therapy, vision therapy, or vestibular rehabilitation.
  - ☐ Encourage regular, low-level exercise.
    - Patients with postconcussive syndrome who engage in low-level exercise recover faster.
  - ☐ OMT.

RETURN-TO-PLAY CONSIDERATIONS

Decisions governing the return to sports after head injury often lie with the primary care physician.[47,64]

- There are several published clinical guidelines intended for physicians.
- In 2008, the Zurich Consensus Statement recommended a graded and progressive stepwise approach to concussion rehabilitation prior to returning to play.[28]
- This approach has been modified to include a "return-to-learn" component concurrent with the return-to-play progression (Fig. 87.5).
- In 2022, the 6th International Consensus Conference on Concussion in Sports took place in Amsterdam.[59]
- The following was released from this conference:
  - ☐ The definition of concussion was updated to:
    - A traumatic brain injury caused by a direct blow to the head, neck, or body resulting in an impulsive force

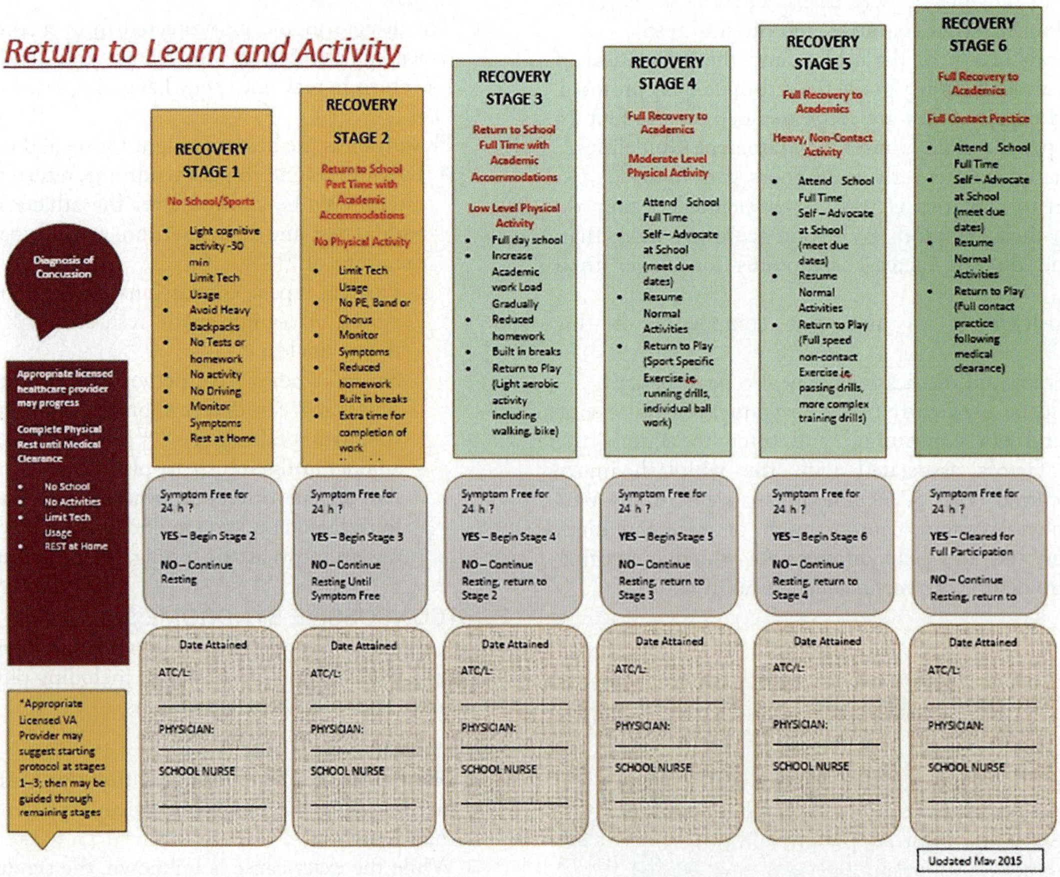
Return to Learn and Activity
Diagnosis of Concussion
Appropriate licensed healthcare provider may progress
Complete Physical Rest until Medical Clearance
• No School • No Activities • Limit Tech Usage • REST at Home
*Appropriate Licensed VA Provider may suggest starting protocol at stages 1–3; then may be guided through remaining stages
RECOVERY STAGE 1
No School/Sports
• Light cognitive activity -30 min • Limit Tech Usage • Avoid Heavy Backpacks • No Tests or homework • No activity • No Driving • Monitor Symptoms • Rest at Home
RECOVERY STAGE 2
Return to School Part Time with Academic Accommodations
No Physical Activity
• Limit Tech Usage • No PE, Band or Chorus • Monitor Symptoms • Reduced homework • Built in breaks • Extra time for completion of work
RECOVERY STAGE 3
Return to School Full Time with Academic Accommodations
Low Level Physical Activity
• Full day school • Increase Academic work Load Gradually • Reduced homework • Built in breaks • Return to Play (Light aerobic activity including walking, bike)
RECOVERY STAGE 4
Full Recovery to Academics
Moderate Level Physical Activity
• Attend School Full Time • Self – Advocate at School (meet due dates) • Resume Normal Activities • Return to Play (Sport Specific Exercise ie, running drills, individual ball work)
RECOVERY STAGE 5
Full Recovery to Academics
Heavy, Non-Contact Activity
• Attend School Full Time • Self – Advocate at School (meet due dates) • Resume Normal Activities • Return to Play (Full speed non-contact Exercise ie, passing drills, more complex training drills)
RECOVERY STAGE 6
Full Recovery to Academics
Full Contact Practice
• Attend School Full Time • Self – Advocate at School (meet due dates) • Resume Normal Activities • Return to Play (Full contact practice following medical clearance)
Symptom Free for 24 h ? YES – Begin Stage 2 NO – Continue Resting
Symptom Free for 24 h ? YES – Begin Stage 3 NO – Continue Resting Until Symptom Free
Symptom Free for 24 h ? YES – Begin Stage 4 NO – Continue Resting, return to Stage 2
Symptom Free for 24 h ? YES – Begin Stage 5 NO – Continue Resting, return to Stage 3
Symptom Free for 24 h ? YES – Begin Stage 6 NO – Continue Resting, return to Stage 4
Symptom Free for 24 h ? YES – Cleared for Full Participation NO – Continue Resting, return to
Date Attained
ATC/L:
PHYSICIAN:
SCHOOL NURSE
Updated May 2015

Figure 87.5. **The return-to-learn method gauges an athlete's ability to return to play following a concussion, based on recovery from symptoms.**

being transmitted to the brain that occurs in sports and exercise-related activities.
  - This initiates a neurotransmitter and metabolic cascade, with possible axonal injury, blood flow change, and inflammation affecting the brain.
  - Symptoms and signs may present immediately, or evolve over minutes or hours, and commonly resolve within days, but may be prolonged.
  - No abnormality is seen on standard structural neuroimaging studies (computed tomography or magnetic resonance imaging T1- and T2-weighted images), but in the research setting, abnormalities may be present on functional, blood flow, or metabolic imaging studies.
  - Sport-related concussion results in a range of clinical symptoms and signs that may or may not involve loss of consciousness.
  - The clinical symptoms and signs of concussion cannot be explained solely by (but may occur concomitantly with) drug, alcohol, or medication use, other injuries (such as cervical injuries, peripheral vestibular dysfunction), or other comorbidities (such as psychological factors or coexisting medical conditions).
- □ They recommended sports-specific strategies for concussion prevention including rule changes to reduce collisions in various sports, neuromuscular training in warm-ups, and mouthguard use in ice hockey, which was shown to reduce concussion rates in hockey by 28%.
- □ They also recommended implementation of optimal concussion management strategies to reduce recurrent concussion rates such as disallowing body checking in child or adolescent ice hockey and limiting the number of contact practices, intensity of contact, and restricting collision time in practice in American football.
- □ Concussion tools were updated including the Concussion Recognition Tool-6 (CRT6), Sport Concussion Assessment Tool-6 (SCAT6), and Child SCAT6 (for patients ages 8–12).[59]
  - These are best used in the first 72 hours (and up to 1 week) following suspected concussion.
  - The player should be removed from the field if there is suspicion of concussion and Maddock questions remain useful for athletes >12 years of age without clear signs of concussion.
  - If there are signs of seizure, loss of conscience, tonic posturing, ataxia, poor balance, confusion, behavioral changes, or amnesia, the patient should be immediately removed from play and should not return to play that day unless evaluated acutely by an experienced HCP with a multimodal assessment showing the symptoms was not related to a concussion (i.e., poor balance due to another musculoskeletal condition).

- Return-to-learn and return-to-sport strategies were also updated. A systematic review showed that 93% of athletes have a full return-to-learning by 10 days.[59] The guidelines recommend a new strategy of no longer recommending complete rest, but rather relative rest even starting 24 hours after injury. Early return-to-activities are now recommended if they do not increase their symptom evaluation scores by more than 2 points and do not increase symptoms for longer than 1 hour. Patients should have a modified school schedule with frequent breaks and limited screen time. Activities should be modified to avoid falls or collisions. The curriculum should be adjusted to allow more time to complete tasks. Tests and quizzes should be delayed, or more time should be allowed for their completion.
- New evidence shows the benefits of physical activity and aerobic exercise treatment as early interventions, where strict bedrest was previously recommended.[59]
  - □ Relative rest (including reduced screen time) is recommended for up to 2 days postinjury.
  - □ Patients may return to light physical activity 24 to 48 hours after a concussion. This includes walking, stationary cycling, or other activities that mitigate the risk of collision or fall.
  - □ They may continue to advance activity duration and intensity as long as there is no more than a 2-point increase in their assessment score versus the pre-exercise value and no more than a 1-hour exacerbation of their concussion-related symptoms.
- Cervico-vestibular rehabilitation is recommended for patients with neck pain, dizziness, headache, and/or balance problems.
- Patients should be reevaluated in office 72 hours to a week postinjury using the Sport Concussion Office Assessment Tool (SCOAT6/Child SCOAT6).[59]
- If symptoms persist >4 weeks, the patient should be evaluated with a multimodal clinical assessment including standardized and validated symptom rating scales.

If completed successfully, without symptoms, each step of the progression will take approximately 24 to 48 hours.

- Recent literature suggests that clinical outcomes are improved with early onset of light aerobic activity rather than complete rest.[59]
- With the new guidelines suggesting improved clinical outcomes with early onset of light aerobic activity rather than complete rest, the duration from the beginning of the "return-to-learn" progression to full game participation may happen gradually over a 5- to 10-day period.
- However, if any symptoms occur during the progression of activities, the athlete will be required to repeat the stage asymptomatically before moving forward.[59]
- To begin the return-to-play progression, an athlete should be assessed by a physician for near or complete resolution of symptoms.
- Baseline testing comparisons can also be utilized to help guide the physician's decision.
- Please see Table 87.1 for current RTP Guidelines.[59]
  - □ Athletes may begin Step 1 (i.e., symptom-limited activity) within 24 hours of injury, with progression through each subsequent step typically taking a minimum of 24 hours.
  - □ If more than mild exacerbation of symptoms (i.e., more than 2 points on a 0–10 scale) occurs during Steps 1–3, the athlete should stop and attempt to exercise the next day.
  - □ Athletes experiencing concussion-related symptoms during Steps 4–6 should return to Step 3 to establish full resolution of symptoms with exertion before engaging in at-risk activities.
  - □ Written determination of readiness to RTS should be provided by an HCP before unrestricted RTS as directed by local laws and/or sporting regulations.

Upper Extremity

ROTATOR CUFF TENDONITIS[69]/IMPINGEMENT SYNDROMES[70]

- Rotator cuff tendonitis and subacromial bursitis are common sports medicine diagnoses.[38,71] Subacromial impingement syndrome is the most common cause of shoulder pain.

TABLE 87.1

Graduated Return-to-Play Protocol

Rehabilitation Stage	Activity	Goal
1. Symptom-limited activity	Daily activities that do not exacerbate symptoms (e.g., walking).	Gradual reintroduction of work/school
2. Aerobic exercise **2A—Light** (up to approximately 55% maxHR) **then** **2B—Moderate** (up to approximately 70% maxHR)	Stationary cycling or walking at slow to medium pace. May start light resistance training that does not result in more than mild and brief exacerbation[a] of concussion symptoms.	Increase HR
3. Sport-specific exercise	Sport-specific training away from the team environment (e.g., running, change of direction and/or individual training drills away from the team environment). No activities at risk of head impact.	Add movement, change of direction
4. Noncontact training drills	Exercise to high intensity including more challenging training drills (e.g., passing drills, multiplayer training) can integrate into a team environment.	Resume usual intensity of exercise, coordination, and increased thinking
5. Full contact practice	Following medical clearance, participate in normal training activities	Restore confidence and assess functional skills by coaching staff
6. Return to play	Normal game play	

Reproduced from Patricios JS, Schneider KJ, Dvorak J, et al. Consensus statement on concussion in sport: the 6th International Conference on Concussion in Sport-Amsterdam, October 2022. *Br J Sports Med.* 2023;57(11):695–711, with permission from BMJ Publishing Group Ltd.

- Mechanism:
  - Shoulder impingement often happens in repetitive overhead activities like baseball pitchers when there is impingement of the supraspinatus against the acromion.
  - Rotator cuff tendinitis is often seen in association with shoulder impingement.
  - It is often due to repetitive overuse injuries, or secondary to direct trauma to the shoulder, poor throwing mechanics in sports like baseball, javelin throwers, or falls on an outstretched arm.
  - Impingement syndromes can occur due to multiple factors.[71]
    - The space between the undersurface of the acromion and humeral head is called the rotator cuff interval.
    - This space narrows with arm abduction (Fig. 87.6).
    - Any condition that functionally or anatomically narrows this space can cause impingement.

External impingement: There is not enough room under the acromion for the supraspinatus tendon to glide freely.[70,71]

- Common causes:
  - An arthritic spur or anatomic variant at the acromion
  - Protracted shoulder position (ventrally tilted, externally rotated, and forward scapulae)
  - Weak or inhibited rotator cuff muscles
  - Humeral head elevation

Internal impingement[70,71]:

- Common causes:
  - Overuse
  - Multidirectional instability
  - Microtrauma
  - A superior glenoid labrum tear (SLAP lesion)
  - A fracture (Bankart lesion)
  - A depression-type fracture of the humeral head (Hill–Sachs deformity)

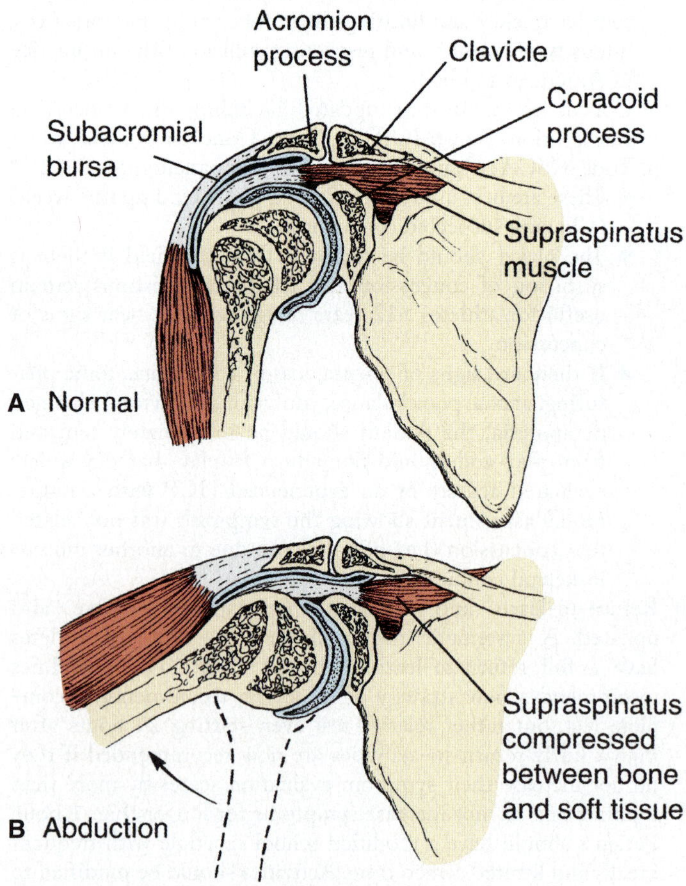

Figure 87.6. A, B. Supraspinatus/impingement. (Reprinted with permission from Anderson MK, Hall SJ. *Fundamentals of Sports Injury Management.* Williams & Wilkins; 1997:405. Figure 11.16.)

- Common age: Less than 35 years of age
- Incidence:
  - Shoulder pain is the third most common musculoskeletal complaint at the physician's office.
  - Most commonly seen in baseball, handball, swimming, volleyball.
  - Incidence rises with age, happening most commonly in people older than 35 years of age, peaking at the sixth decade of life.
- H+P
  - History can help pinpoint the diagnosis of upper extremity complaints.
  - In athletes, these conditions typically result from sport-specific overuse.
  - Risk factors for shoulder impingement include smoking, bearing heavy loads, infection, and fluoroquinolone antibiotics.
  - Pain with lifting the arm, or while lying on the affected side.
  - May have weakness and stiffness secondary to the pain.
  - Onset is usually gradual.
- Diagnosis:
  - Not all shoulder pain is due to rotator cuff pathology. The clinician must also consider referred pain from other nearby structures, such as the cervical spine.
  - Diagnosis is generally clinical. Check shoulder ROM. Hawkins, Neers, and Jobes, and drop arm special tests may help with diagnosis.
  - Radiograph (two views), MRI, or ultrasound (US) may be considered.
- Treatment:
  - Controlled exercise program
  - Physical therapy with focus on the rotator cuff muscles especially the supraspinatus and infraspinatus, as well as the trapezius and serratus anterior to stabilize the scapula.
    - Studies have shown that surgery was not more beneficial than physical therapy in reducing shoulder impingement pain.
    - Surgery may be considered for rotator cuff tears in athletes.
  - Non-steroidal anti-inflammatory drugs (NSAIDs)
  - Rest, activity modification
  - Steroid injection
  - OMT
    - SD plays a major role in the pathogenesis of shoulder pain.
    - Injuries to the glenohumeral joint almost always lead to motion restriction.
    - Consider the entire pectoral girdle, rib cage, and axial spine when assessing these injuries and conditions (Box 87.10).

LATERAL EPICONDYLITIS[72]

- Mechanism:
  - Overuse of the extensor carpi radialis brevis and the common extensor tendon.

> **BOX 87.10 Osteopathic Pearl: Rotator Cuff**
>
> OMT directed at somatic dysfunction of the upper thoracic spine, ribs, and cervical spine, and then to the myofascial structures of the pectoral girdle and arm is an important component of treatment in patients with rotator cuff syndrome.

- Incidence:
  - Common cause of elbow pain affecting men and women equally.
  - Half of all tennis players develop pain around the elbow, 75% of which represent true lateral epicondylitis.
  - More common in people over the age of 40.
  - Smoking, obesity, and repetitive movement for 2 hours per day, as well as loads of over 20 pounds are risk factors.
- H+P:
  - Pain on the lateral elbow 1 cm distal to the lateral epicondyle, typically secondary to repetitive extension of the fingers or supination of the forearm.
- Diagnosis:
  - Positive Maudsley test, if necessary, CT/MRI/US of the elbow.
- Treatment:
  - PRICE, OMT such as SCS of the finger extensors, brace/strap, PT, analgesics, local steroid injection.
  - Spontaneous recovery happens within 1 to 2 years in 80% to 90% of the general population.

MEDIAL EPICONDYLITIS[73]

- Mechanism:
  - Inflammation of the wrist flexors and pronators through repetitive pronation of the forearm or flexion of the wrist.
- Incidence:
  - 7–10 times less common than lateral epicondylitis comprising only 10% of all cases of epicondylitis and may be as low as 0.4%.
- H+P:
  - Pain on the medial elbow 5 mm distal and lateral to the medial epicondyle, typically secondary to repetitive forearm flexion or pronation of the forearm.
  - Risk factors include smoking, diabetes, obesity, repetitive wrist flexion, forearm pronation for at least 2 hours per day.
- Diagnosis:
  - Usually clinical diagnosis, if necessary, CT/MRI/US of the elbow.
- Treatment:
  - PRICE, OMT such as SCS of the forearm flexors, brace/strap, PT, analgesics, local steroid injection. Generally self-limited with full recovery in 1 to 3 years in 80% of patients.

Lumbar Region

BACK PAIN AND SPONDYLOLYSIS

Back pain is commonly seen in adolescent athletes (see Box 87.12). Spondylolysis (Fig. 87.7)[74,75] is a stress fracture of the pars interarticularis of the posterior elements of the vertebrae.

- Mechanism:
  - Repetitive hyperextension stress
  - Macrotrauma
  - Incidence: 4% by age 6, 6% by age 14, and thereafter remains constant throughout adulthood
  - Most commonly affects L5 on S1 > L4 on L5 > L3 on L4
- H+P:
  - Often asymptomatic
  - 10% have insidious onset, low back pain that is exacerbated with activity. Pain is localized, unilateral, or central low back pain, especially with extension and/or extension with rotation of the spine.
  - Pain typically does not radiate into the legs.

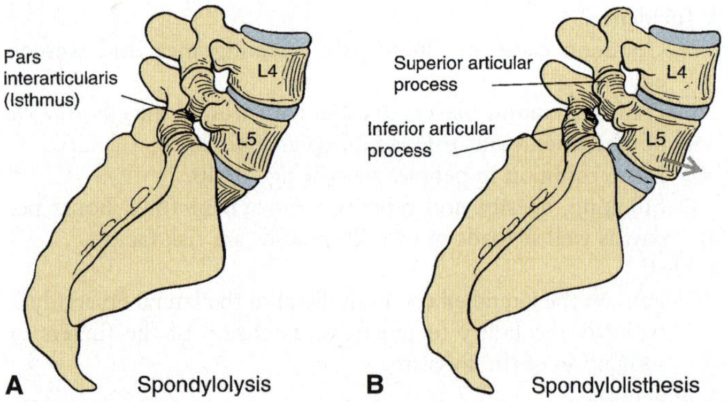

Figure 87.7. A fatigue fracture to the pars interarticularis is called (**A**) spondylolysis. When the fracture occurs laterally, (**B**) spondylolisthesis develops. (Reprinted with permission from Hamill J, Knutzen KM. *Biomechanical Basis of Human Movement*. Williams & Wilkins; 1995:310. Figure 7-22.)

- Neurologic exam will often show increased lumbar lordosis, tight hamstrings, reduced ROM in spinal extension, tenderness to palpation over the pars fracture site.
- Diagnosis:
  - Stork test
  - Special testing:
    - Single-leg hyperextension test (Stork test) provokes low back pain with patient weight bearing on a single leg and backward bending (if this reproduces their symptoms it should be considered spondylolysis until proven otherwise).
  - Imaging (X-rays):
    - A "collar around the Scotty dog's neck" (fracture through the pars interarticularis) on oblique views may be initially negative.
    - A SPECT bone scan helps to confirm the diagnosis and to define severity based on the activity on the scan in relation to the timing of the presenting complaint.
    - Of note, there has been a recent suggestion by some providers to make the diagnosis of spondylolysis using lateral x-ray only, given the increase in radiation dose with oblique views without significant added diagnostic benefit.[76]
    - Treatment: If asymptomatic and discovered incidentally, they may continue current level of activity.
    - If acute symptoms relative spinal bracing with a "soft" lumbar brace ("warm and form") versus a custom-molded neutral lumbar orthosis for 6 to 12 weeks to limit stress on the pars.
      - The patient initially wears the brace all day and is gradually weaned off based on symptomatic improvement. The typical time frame for bracing is about 3 to 4 months.
      - Bracing remains controversial, as limited evidence supports the efficacy of bracing on healing the pars defect over rest or activity modification alone.
      - The choice to brace should be made using the clinician's clinical judgment and experience.
    - Other treatments include activity modification (avoid hyperextension of the spine), physical therapy, ice/heat, NSAIDs, injections, and cognitive-behavioral therapy.
    - Bracing
    - OMT
      - The increased lumbar lordosis and tight hamstrings, stretching the hip flexors, and quadriceps, as well as the gastric soleus complex, and core strengthening may be targets of OMT and PT.

> **BOX 87.11 Osteopathic Pearls: Muscle-Firing Patterns**
>
> Address hip extension muscle-firing pattern. The muscle-firing pattern for hip extension is as follows: hamstrings, gluteus maximus, contralateral lower lumbar erector spinae, and their ipsilateral lower erector spinae.[18] Treatment of the thoracic, lumbar, and pelvic regions with OMT improves activation of these patterns and sets the stage for appropriate rehabilitation to reinforce continued activation.

      - Gentle indirect techniques or muscle energy techniques to relieve SD in the local areas.
      - *Remember, this is a stress fracture, and as such, the use of forceful, direct, articular manipulative techniques to the local area of injury is contraindicated!*
    - Rehabilitation:
      - Initially, emphasize neutral spine positioning. Low load and core stability retraining can begin as pain resolves.
      - Progression through low- and high-load core stability retraining and functional therapeutic exercise are essential prior to sport-specific reintegration (Boxes 87.11 and 87.12).[1,19,44]

Lower Extremity

KNEE INJURIES

ACL Injury[77]

- Mechanism:
  - ACL tears happen as a result of rotational forces on the knee or a direct blow to the knee.
- Incidence:
  - The ACL is the most commonly injured ligament in the knee affecting 1 in every 3,500 people.
  - ACL injury is most common in football, but also affects skiers, soccer, and basketball players.
  - Women appear to be at a slightly increased risk for ACL injury possibly due to weaker hamstrings and preferential use of the quadriceps while decelerating as well as increased valgus angulation of the knee.
- H+P:
  - Athletes often present with a history of sudden changes in the direction of movement, planting a foot and pivoting, sudden deceleration, or a blow to the lateral aspect of the knee.
  - They have a sudden, painful audible "pop."
  - The knee often "gives out."
  - They may have tenderness along the joint line, pain, and swelling.
  - Physical exam includes the anterior drawer test, the pivot shift, and Lachman tests.
    - Positive Lachman test is the most accurate in acute injury.
  - MRI may be ordered.
- H+P:
- Treatment:
  - Protection, Rest, Ice, Compress, Elevate (PRICE), analgesics, bracing, PT, activity modification, OMT, surgical reconstruction if complete tear.
  - The classic O'Donoghue Triad ("unhappy triad") may be seen and includes the following: (1) Rupture of the MCL, (2) Torn medial meniscus, (3) Sprain or rupture of the ACL.

BOX 87.12 Common Areas of Somatic Dysfunction with Spondylolysis

- Psoas spasm (global mobilizer portion of psoas): may present with patient walking in a forward bent position or simply having poor lumbosacral extension.
  - Examination: Beltline low on one side may indicate a psoas spasm or short leg. Pelvic side shift frequently occurs toward the side of the longer leg or opposite to the side of the tighter psoas muscle. A tight psoas resists hip extension. (+) Thomas test.
  - Treatment: With a spondylolysis, decrease psoas hypertonicity. A tight psoas may be associated with a flexed dysfunction in the upper lumbar spine (L1).
- Psoas inhibition (local stabilizer portion of the psoas): Deep third of psoas has segmental innervation and very short fiber length. Therefore, it cannot produce hip flexion momentum but does pull (telescope) the ball of the femur into the socket. This presents as poor lumbosacral extension and anterior pelvic tilt, along with poor single-leg (standing and especially half kneeling) stability/balance. Often, patients will have a component of anterior or lateral hip complaints.
  - Examination: With patient supine, lift heel 3 to 5 in off table, in a loosely packed rotational position; ask the athlete to telescope the leg into the hip socket. Observe and feel for compensatory hip hiking, hip rotation (excessive obliques), and/or knee flexion.
  - Treatment: From same testing position, subtly traction the hip out of socket and ask the athlete to pull it back in. This must be a less than 10% effort with the goal to eliminate excessive superficial abdominal muscle or lower extremity flexor muscle dominance. Correctly treating thoracolumbar junctional and pelvis somatic dysfunction first will help decrease abnormal flexor-dominant neural drive.
- Iliacus dysfunction: Presents as poor lumbosacral extension and anterior pelvic tilt.
  - Examination: (+) iliacus test. Perform Thomas test after first securing the anterior superior iliac spine (ASIS) to the table to prevent anterior innominate rotation that occurs during Thomas test. A tight iliacus also resists hip extension. An athlete can present with a completely normal psoas length but rigid and shortened iliacus.
  - Treatment: one or two clinician iliacus stretch technique. Treat area of somatic dysfunction.
- Flexed upper lumbar dysfunction: Single-level or multiple stacked flexed Fryette type II dysfunction(s) are commonly found in the lower thoracic and/or upper lumbar region.
  - Treatment: Treat the flexed lumbar component followed by stretching the tight psoas and/or iliacus muscle(s). Be careful not to apply excessive forces through the area of spondylolysis in this process.
- Sacroiliac/sacral torsion dysfunction: Types of sacroiliac dysfunction vary.
  1. Extended sacrum: Typically, more painful and harder to treat. It may be related to flexed lumbar dysfunction or AP curve problems.
  2. Bilaterally flexed sacrum: Seen with an increased lumbar lordosis.
     - Treatment: Treating the psoas helps sacroiliac dysfunction. If sacral dysfunction is still present, directly treating the sacrum could be useful.
- Innominate dysfunction: Dysfunction of the innominates or pubes may maintain sacroiliac dysfunction.
  - Do not forget that the ilium is the other half of the sacroiliac joint!

- The triad has subsequently been revisited considering the arthroscopic findings in patients with both ACL and MCL injuries, where a lateral meniscal injury is more common than injury to the medial meniscus. Mechanistically this makes more sense during the pivot shift movement, as the lateral tibiofemoral compartment is compressed, causing failure of the lateral meniscus.[78,79]

Clinical Pearls

- Treat somatic dysfunction and hypertonic flexor dominant muscle groups first prior to attempting facilitation of inhibited local or global stabilizer muscles.
- Remember to assess the lower extremities for dysfunction, pain, and/or instability. The more distant that there is persistent dysfunction, pain, or chronic structural instability in an LE limb, the more it will affect and cause (and potentially prevent correction of) poor central core proprioception and stability and eventually pain or injury.

- The medial meniscus is attached to the MCL and is generally more prone to rupture.
- However, this has been called to question when there is a concomitant ACL injury, as multiple studies showed that the lateral meniscus was more commonly torn with ACL injuries, calling to question the accuracy of the unhappy triad.[80–83]
- Meniscal injuries broadly appear to be of three types: primary acute isolated injury to the meniscus, primary acute combined injury to the ACL and the meniscus, and secondary injury to meniscus following ACL injury after a period of instability.[84]

PCL Injury[85]

- Mechanism:
  - Extreme anterior force applied to the proximal tibia of the knee when flexed such as falling forward onto a flexed knee.
- Incidence:
  - This is most common in soccer-related injuries.
  - Male to female ratio is 2:1.
  - The PCL is 1.3 to 2 times thicker than the ACL, twice as strong, and thus, less prone to injury.

- H+P:
  - Pain and swelling in the popliteal fossa after a direct blow to the front of the knee such as a hard fall onto a bent knee, or hyperextension injury of the knee.
- Diagnosis:
  - Positive posterior drawer test of the knee, MRI.
- Treatment:
  - Same as ACL injury.

Anterior Knee Pain

Anterior knee pain is a common finding in the athletic population. This painful condition is typically related to overuse; however, a traumatic insult may start the process. Overuse may result from training errors or underlying malalignment.[38,86] Causes of anterior knee pain include:

- Chondromalacia patellae
- IT band syndrome
- Osgood–Schlatter disease
- Patellar tendinitis
- Patellofemoral osteoarthritis
- Patellofemoral pain syndrome
- Pes anserine bursitis
- Plica synovialis syndrome
- Prepatellar bursitis
- Quadriceps tendinopathy

Patellofemoral Pain Syndrome ("Runner's Knee")[87]

- Mechanism:
  - Multifactorial and likely due to training practices.
  - Malalignment of the lower extremity or patella or muscle imbalance may contribute.
  - Overload from increased tensions across the patellofemoral joint with resultant inflammation and microinjury.
  - As the process continues, the cartilage on the undersurface of the patella becomes inflamed and damaged.
- Incidence:
  - One of the most common causes of anterior knee pain accounting for 25% to 40% of all knee problems seen in the sports medicine clinic.
  - More common in females (female to male ratio 2:1) due to greater hip adduction angles.
  - Most common in the second and third decades of life.
- H+P:
  - Anterior pain around the patella with a variable amount of local swelling
  - Painful with activity, especially negotiating stairs or hills
  - (+) Theater sign (significant anterior knee pain when standing after prolonged sitting)[86]
- Diagnosis:
  - Patellofemoral pain syndrome is a diagnosis of exclusion. Rule out other intra-articular and peripatellar pathology.
  - Knee examination:
    - Crepitus may be palpated as the knee is flexed and extended.
    - The patella may demonstrate medial and lateral hypermobility.
    - Patellofemoral grind test may be (+) with pain.
    - Swelling may or may not be present depending on injury severity.
    - The remaining knee examination will typically be normal.
  - Functional tests: Lower extremity screening to identify potential contributory kinetic chain dysfunction.
    - Single-leg stance (eyes open and closed—10 seconds each): look for elevation of opposite hip and/or rotation of the pelvis (suggesting poor core stability) and/or (+) Trendelenburg (suggesting poor gluteus medius activity in the stance leg). Also, observe the ankle for motion abnormality.
    - Dual-legged toe raise: look at resting and raised positions of the mid- and hindfoot for varus/valgus deformity and the athlete's ability to correct (or overcorrect) during toe raise. Good endurance is demonstrated by the ability to hold position for 10 seconds.
    - Seated active tibial rotation: Look for compensating foot dorsiflexion, adduction, and inversion suggesting popliteal inhibition (instead of pure tibial rotation—foot should remain flat and parallel to floor).
    - Short foot: look for excessive toe flexion and foot dorsiflexion, which would suggest inhibition of the intrinsic muscles of the foot.
  - Treatment:
    - Rehabilitation and manual therapy to improve firing of the vastus medialis (see Box 87.13).
  - Vastus medialis is primarily a patellar stabilizer. Typically, supine straight leg raises are recommended to strengthen this muscle; however, as the condition improves, one must also include functional dynamic closed-chain therapeutic exercise.
  - Therefore, treatment strategies are additionally directed toward the pelvis, hip, and ankle for:
    - Treatment of identified SD of the hip, pelvis, and lower extremity.
    - Stretching and mobilization of hypertonic dominant flexor muscle groups.
    - Neuromotor retraining of the potentially inhibited gluteus maximus, gluteus medius, vastus medialis, popliteus, foot intrinsics, and other dysfunctional firing patterns.

> **BOX 87.13 Osteopathic Pearl: Palpation**
>
> Palpate for the ability of the vastus medialis oblique muscle to "turn on." Atrophy, flaccidity, or inhibition of this muscle is common in this condition, due to neurologic inhibition, pain, or disuse. Other associated physical findings include the following:
>
> - Increased hamstring tension
> - Fibular motion restriction
> - Interosseous membrane tension
> - Iliotibial band (ITB) tension
> - Restricted lateral fascia of the thigh

Hyperextended Knee[88]

- Mechanism:
  - Forceful hyperextension of the knee
- Incidence:
  - Most common in football players who get tackled by their legs, or basketball players who land awkwardly after a jump
- History and physical:
  - Pain, swelling, and instability of the knee

- Diagnosis
  - Perform anterior/posterior drawer test, Lachman, shift pivot, valgus and varus stress tests to rule out torn ligament
  - May consider radiograph, MRI, or CT
- Treatment:
  - RICE, NSAIDs, OMT, PT
  - If ligament tear, referral for surgery

Inversion Ankle Sprain[89]

- Mechanism:
  - Occur with the ankle in the plantar-flexed position.
  - Plantar flexion decreases the stability of the ankle because the anterior aspect of the talus is no longer wedged between the malleoli.
  - Inversion of the ankle causing stretch or tear, most commonly, of the anterior talofibular ligament and/or the calcaneofibular ligament.
- Incidence:
  - Ankle sprains are the most common athletic injury.[90]
  - They make up:
    - 45% of all injuries in basketball
    - 31% in soccer
    - 25% in volleyball.
  - Inversion-type ankle sprains make up 85% of all ankle sprains.[91]
    - Inversion ankle sprains can be graded as I, II, or III based on degree of ligamentous tear or rupture or by clinical examination criteria (Box 87.14).[92,93]

BOX 87.14 Ankle Sprain Grading

Grading lateral ankle sprains can be made upon physical examination findings as follows[52]:

- Grade I
  - No loss of function
  - No ligamentous laxity (i.e., negative anterior drawer and talar tilt tests)
  - Little or no hemorrhaging
  - No point tenderness
  - Decreased total ankle motion of ≤5 degrees
  - Swelling of ≤0.5 cm
- Grade II
  - Some loss of function
  - Positive anterior drawer test (ATFL involvement)
  - Negative talar tilt test (no CFL involvement)
  - Hemorrhaging
  - Point tenderness
  - Decreased total ankle motion greater than 5 degrees but greater than 10 degrees
  - Swelling greater than 0.5 cm but less than 2.0 cm
- Grade III
  - Near total loss of function
  - Positive anterior drawer and talar tilt tests
  - Hemorrhaging
  - Extreme point tenderness
  - Decreased total ankle motion greater than 10 degrees
  - Swelling greater than 2.0 cm
  - According to stress radiograph results: anterior drawer movement of ≤3 mm can be classified as IIIA and greater than 3 mm of movement IIIB

- H+P:
  - The athlete typically describes coming down wrong on the ankle, stepping on another foot, or rolling the ankle causing inversion of the ankle.
  - Determine if they are able to weight bear.
- Diagnosis:
  - Inspect, and palpate the three lateral ligaments on the anterior, inferior, and posterior aspect of the lateral malleolus.
  - Because fewer than 15% of ankle injuries are found to result in significant fracture, the Ottawa ankle rules were developed to guide clinicians regarding when to obtain a radiograph[91] (Figs. 87.8 and 87.9).
  - Special tests (always compare to the opposite side):
    - Anterior drawer test:
      - Tests anterior talofibular ligament (ATFL)
      - (+) if talus may be moved forward (and into slight internal rotation) ≥4 mm
    - Talar tilt:
      - Tests the calcaneofibular ligament (CFL)
      - Ankle inversion greater than 25 to 30 degrees implies injury or rupture
    - Talar glide:
      - Tests for posterior movement of the talus
      - Almost always restricted after inversion sprains
    - Fibular glide:
      - Tests for proximal fibular head anterior glide and distal fibular head posterior glide during ankle dorsiflexion
      - Almost always restricted after inversion sprains.
    - Tibial rotation:
      - Tests in tibial rotation with the knee flexed at 90 degrees to assess interosseous membrane (IOM) dysfunction
      - Always restricted after ankle and knee sprains
    - Tibial glide:
      - Tests of tibial adduction/abduction distally with the knee flexed at 90 degrees to assess medial or lateral glide restriction in relation to the femur
      - Always restricted after ankle and knee sprains
- Treatment:
  - PRICE protocol (protection, rest, ice, compression, and elevation)
    - Resting the ankle for the first 72 hours then gradual resumption of activity as tolerated.
      - Early weight bearing is associated with quicker return to sports.
    - Crutches if needed for comfort.
    - NSAIDs or acetaminophen if needed for pain.
  - Functional ankle rehabilitation program focused on ROM exercises followed by proprioceptive and neuromuscular training.
  - OMT (Box 87.15).
  - Assess and treat SD throughout the body as part of the kinetic chain.
  - Inversion (supination) ankle sprains stress the lateral ankle ligaments and induce muscle strains throughout the lower extremity, pelvis, and sacrum (Fig. 87.9A,B).
  - Myofascial and indirect techniques are recommended during the acute phases of injury and for fascial and torsional restrictions.
  - Counterstrain points can also be treated in the acute or subacute phases.
  - As the swelling subsides, muscle energy, articulatory, or other direct techniques can be used.

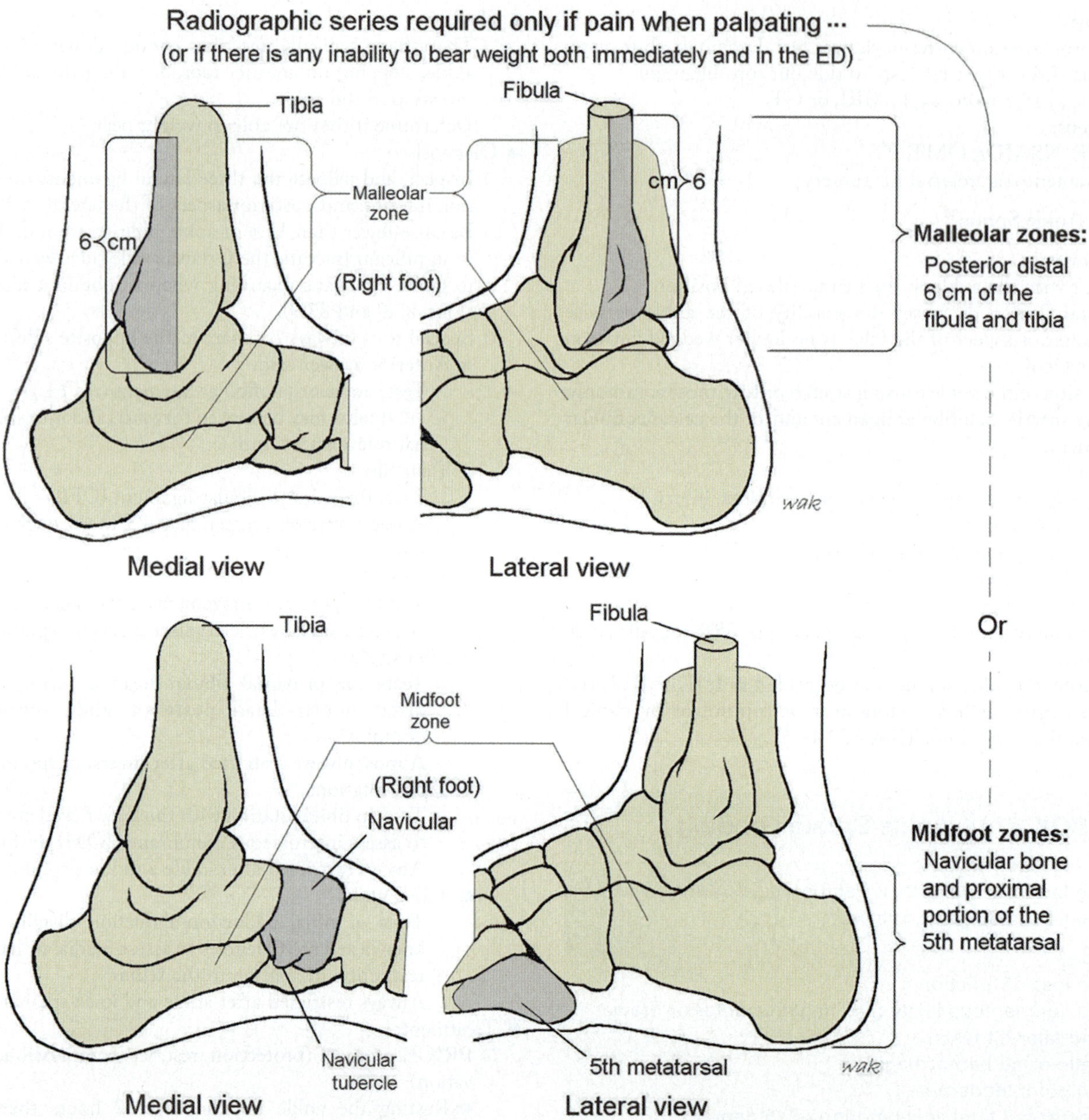

Figure 87.8. Ankle x-ray is recommended when a patient who presents with ankle sprain in the emergency department (ED) has the following signs on physical examination.[21] (Drawing by William A. Kuchera, DO, FAAO, with permission.)

- □ Direct techniques can be used initially in the sagittal plane to mobilize talar and fibular restrictions and avoid further ligamentous injury.
  - For inversion ankle sprains you will often find a posterior fibular head.
- □ Early (as soon as immediately postgame, once fracture is ruled out) and repeated daily treatment of anterior talar SD is critical to advance faster return to play.

Diagnosis of the Somatic Component

It is prudent to include evaluation of the upper thoracic and cervical spine, the costal cage, and internal organs of the chest and abdomen in each patient with an upper extremity problem.[1,38]

- In overhead throwers of any variety, the contralateral stance leg and pelvis should also be screened.
- Even after resolution of upper extremity pathophysiology, persistence of upper extremity pain may be due to referred visceral pain or upper and/or midthoracic viscerosomatic dysfunction.
- Most mechanical neck problems are accompanied by identifiable upper thoracic and upper extremity SD.

Whenever there is dysfunction in any one part of the neuromusculoskeletal system, it is imperative to evaluate the entire kinetic chain as a dynamic unit of function in posture and motion.

- Dysfunction in the upper extremity will also affect scapular position and motion (Fig. 87.10).
  - □ SD of the upper- and midthoracic spine (especially loss of segmental extension) and ribs can affect scapulohumeral rhythm and scapular position.
  - □ Loss of glenohumeral posterior glide (posterior capsule tightness) is common resulting in overuse of scapular motion.

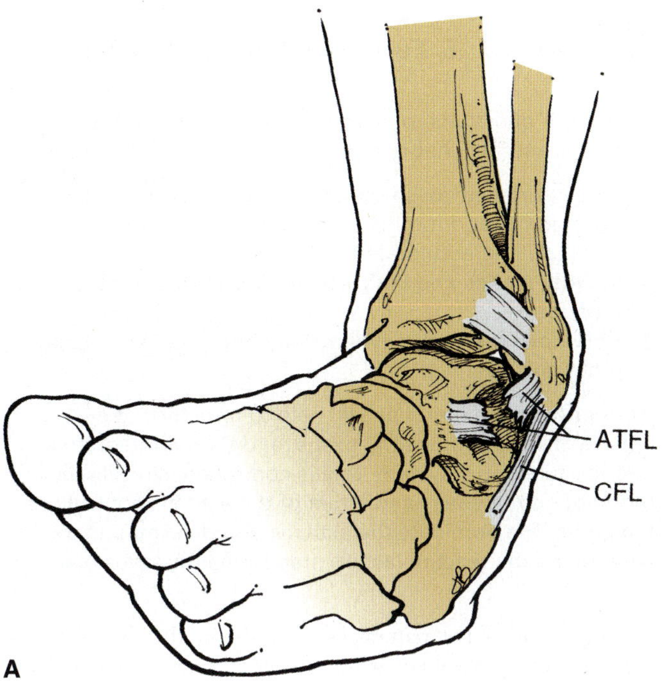

A

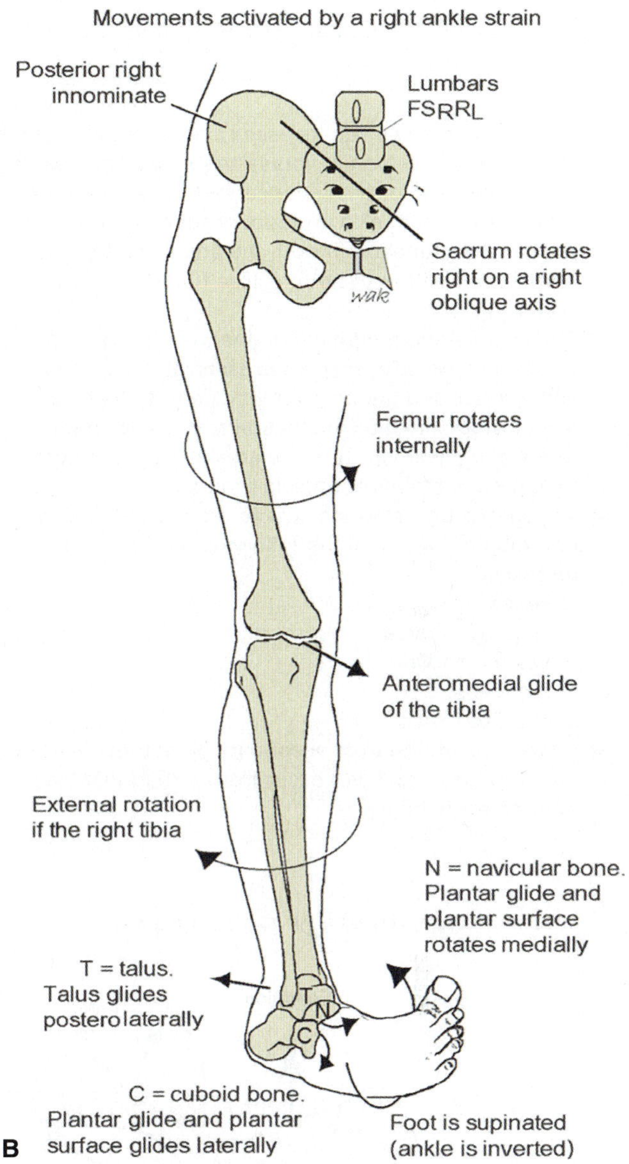

B

Figure 87.9. **A.** Inversion ankle sprain. **B.** Inversion ankle sprain also causes muscle strain in the lower extremity affecting sacral, pelvic, hip, and knee mechanics. (A reprinted with permission from Baker CL Jr., Flandry F, Henderson JM. *The Hughston Clinic Sports Medicine Field Manual*. Williams & Wilkins; 1996:240. Figure 22-1; **B** by William A. Kuchera, DO, FAAO, with permission.)

    - Smooth, efficient movement of the scapula and coordinated strength of the scapular stabilizing muscles are necessary to prevent upper quarter dysfunction, including rotator cuff problems.
- Cervical spine diseases (i.e., herniated disk, osteoarthritis, stenosis) may refer pain to the:
    - Upper thoracic region
    - Shoulder
    - Arm
    - Hand
- SD of the lower cervical and cervical–thoracic junction can produce arm symptoms through three common mechanisms:
    - Direct irritation of segmental levels of somatic cervical spinal nerves
    - Segmental dysfunction of the upper thoracic spine (T1–T4) that provides sympathetic autonomic innervation to the upper extremity
    - Neurovascular compression (thoracic outlet syndromes)
    - Myofascial restrictions resulting in lymphatic obstruction
- See Chapter 39 for further discussion

PRINCIPLE-CENTERED REHABILITATION

Principles are natural laws that, for the most part, are intuitively obvious. The authors of this chapter hope that by introducing principles rather than practices, and describing the principles behind some of the practices, this will better prepare the physician to handle the current challenges of sports medicine rehabilitation, as well as the unknown challenges of the future. The authors hope to prepare the physician to handle each patient and the situations unique to each patient. This approach tends to orient away from a particular treatment protocol, and instead, provides a philosophic approach that will hopefully provide patients with outstanding functional outcomes. See Box 87.16.

In this process, it is essential to:

- Differentiate between "treatment" thinking versus "preventive" thinking.
    - Identify the *root cause* of the injury and orient the rehabilitative process to attack the root cause, rather than simply treating the symptom of the injury.
    - Sports medicine physicians need to avoid falling into the trap of "treating symptoms."

BOX 87.15 Osteopathic Pearls: Ankle Sprains

- Most ankle sprains will be associated with dysfunction of the lateral malleolus, fibular head, interosseous membrane, and/or navicular/cuboid. These restrictions can alter normal ankle and foot motion and produce pain and dysfunction in both the ankle and the knee. A key mobilization to help restore full ROM is the "Talar Tug."
- The venous and lymphatic drainage must travel through myofascial structures associated with the ankle, knee, and hip on their way back to the heart. Addressing somatic dysfunction may assist in the removal of swelling from the area and help restore inhibition of stabilizer muscle groups.
- As rehab progresses, be sure to address retraining of inhibition of any of the following as previously discussed:
  - Psoas
  - Gluteus medius
  - Vastus medialis
  - Popliteus
  - Foot intrinsics.
- It is also useful to treat secondary symptoms (such as low back pain) that can occur from a change in gait after an ankle injury.

MOVEMENTS OF THE SCAPULA

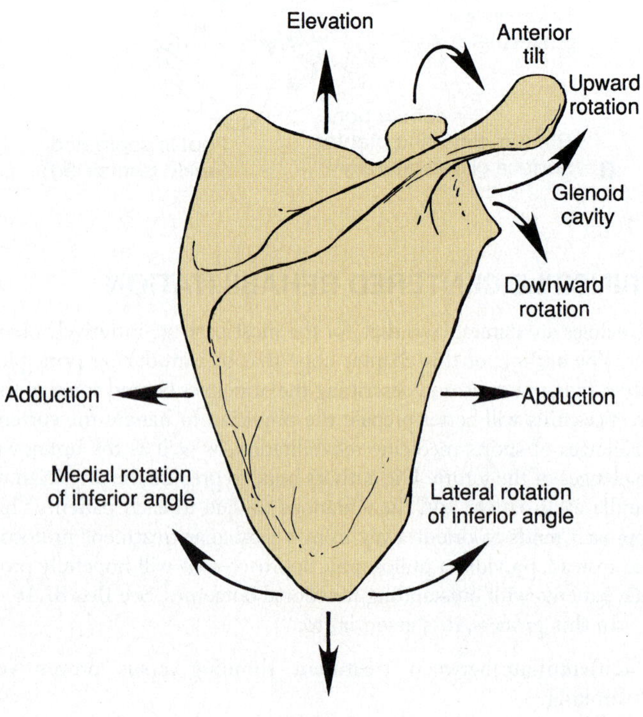

Figure 87.10. Scapular motion. (Reprinted with permission from Kendall FP, McCreary EK, Provance PG. *Muscles: Testing and Function, with Posture and Pain.* 4th ed. Williams & Wilkins; 1993:16.)

BOX 87.16 Functional Rehabilitation

Necessary questions to design an appropriate functional environment for rehabilitation:

1. To what forces does the tissue react?
2. What joints and motions does the tissue decelerate, stabilize, and accelerate?
3. In what planes and with what other tissues does it function?
4. How does the tissue dynamically integrate its isolated function?

Answering these inquiries will help to transform the injured tissues into healthy tissue, and then reintegrate it into the functional system. This is controlled clinically by modulating the stress and strain of the activity, controlling the joints that dominate the activity, and determining in what plane the reaction/action predominantly takes place.

- Be cognizant of the natural laws taught in the disciplines of anatomy and physiology, which include biochemistry and the biomechanics that govern successful (or unsuccessful) function of the neuromusculoskeletal system in the performance of the sport being played.
  - These natural laws usually cannot be violated with impunity, or dysfunction and/or injury will occur.
  - The more physiologically aligned athletes are with these basic principles, the less the opportunity they have for injury, and the greater their chance for success.

Functional Approach

As physicians begin to strategize for the design of a functional rehabilitative process for injured athletes, it is useful to think of the locomotor system as a "kinetic chain."[54]

- Contemporary concepts of fascia and biotensegrity support an understanding of the connectedness and functional integration of the body. Some elements of this chain that help to guide patients in successful athletic activities include, but are not limited to, the:
  - joints
  - muscles
  - bones
  - proprioceptors
- As such, physicians must begin to appreciate that there is a strange relationship between the cause and the cure of injuries

The ultimate goal of rehabilitation is to return the injured athlete back safely to the activity that directly contributed to the injury! Therefore, a vital component of the functional rehabilitative environment will be the causative activity.

- Challenge of rehabilitation: Transform the cause into the cure.
  - The primary aim is to transform the injured tissue into tissue that successfully deals with the loads and motions of the causative activity.
  - In short, reintegrate the injured tissue into a more effective and efficient functional chain reaction system.
- Basis of rehabilitation: Management of a logical progression of clinically controlled techniques that are symptom, and performance, directed.
  - Techniques are based on a strong biomechanical understanding of the kinetic chain and the pathophysiology of injury.

BOX 87.17 Osteopathic Pearl: Compensations

Understanding the potential causes and resultant compensation is based on the biomechanics of function and the timing of function. This understanding allows for more effective treatment of the causes of the injury and the resultant compensations, as well as the symptoms (pain). Pain is a symptom of disturbed motor function. In the face of pain, screening of function throughout the body may be necessary until the cause (dysfunctional area(s)) are found.

The Functional Oxymoron: "Integrated Isolation"

Initially, the physician must isolate the involved tissue to fully understand the site of injury, the extent of injury, and the effect of injury.[54]

- Concurrently, the physician must appreciate the actual function of the involved tissue and how its integration into the functional compensation system allowed for the excessive mechanical loading of the tissue and the resultant injury (Box 87.17).
- The physician must then determine the isolated function and the role of this tissue in the kinetic chain.
- Therefore, the rehabilitative strategy is to design the environment to facilitate the appropriate reaction of the target tissue with functional, progressive exercises and appropriate therapeutic modalities.

Compensations

Compensation occurs in the neuromusculoskeletal system that allows for adaptation to both internal and external stressors. Some compensations can be normal; however, others are abnormal and can be indicative of, or create functional pathology.

Part of the difficulty in determining which compensations are normal and which are abnormal results from the cause-and-effect relationship between functional activity and the resultant compensations.[38]

- Primary drivers for functional compensation:
  - Gravity
  - Ground reaction
  - Momentum
- Extrinsic causes:
  - Footwear
  - Orthotics
  - Equipment
  - Terrain (playing fields, etc.)
- Intrinsic causes:
  - Structural malalignment abnormalities
  - Connective tissue (strength, endurance, and flexibility)
  - Proprioceptive ability
  - Muscle tone

Real-World Muscle Function

In the real world, muscles may function[54]:

- Concentrically at one joint
- Eccentrically or isometrically at another joint
- In another plane at the same joint at the same time

BOX 87.18 Osteopathic Pearl: Econcentric Function

To intelligently rehabilitate injuries, physicians must know not only what the affected tissue is doing during the activity that contributed to its breakdown but also what it does, when it does, and why it does. The concept of "econcentric" muscle function allows physicians to understand the causes and compensations of both acute and overuse injuries and provides them with an enhanced ability to determine the appropriate "econcentric" reaction of the injured tissue to facilitate healing and enhance function. Physicians must also know how the involved tissue is integrated into the entire kinetic chain system.

This occurs within the kinetic chain, reacting with and against gravity, ground reaction, and momentum, in multiple planes of motion. This concept of chain reaction muscle function is best summed up in the phrase "econcentric" which describes the way muscles work in tandem some concentrically contracting while others eccentrically contract allowing three-dimensional motions at the joint. Econcentric is a combination of the words eccentric and concentric (Box 87.18).

- Concentric contraction: A functional shortening of the muscle while it contracts.
- Eccentric contraction: A functional lengthening of the muscle while it contracts.
- Isometric contraction: A stabilizing force during which neither shortening nor lengthening of the muscle occurs.

Additionally, contemporary neuromuscular physiology suggests that many of the individually named muscles often do not have a single limited function. In fact, many individually named muscles have constituent portions with distinct functional roles. For example:

- The gluteus maximus has three distinct portions, each of which functions separately as a global mobilizer, global stabilizer, and local stabilizer.
- The anterior two-thirds of the psoas is a global mobilizer (primarily hip flexion), but the posterior one-third of the psoas is a local stabilizer (primarily telescopes the femoral head into the socket).
- Critical analysis of studies on the same named muscle for differences in the following has led to these discoveries:
  - Fiber orientation
  - Fiber length
  - Innervation pattern
  - Pattern of dysfunction

Osteopathic Manipulative Treatment and Rehabilitation

SD frequently develops in the human neuromusculoskeletal system while adapting to the relentless force of gravity.[1,18,38]

- The athlete's ability to adapt is challenged by the demands of the sport.
- OMT is a vital step to restoring balanced structure and function. It can be provided pregame as well as during and/or after sports activities or competitions (Fig. 87.11).
  - Pregame OMT has been shown to improve athletic performance.[18]

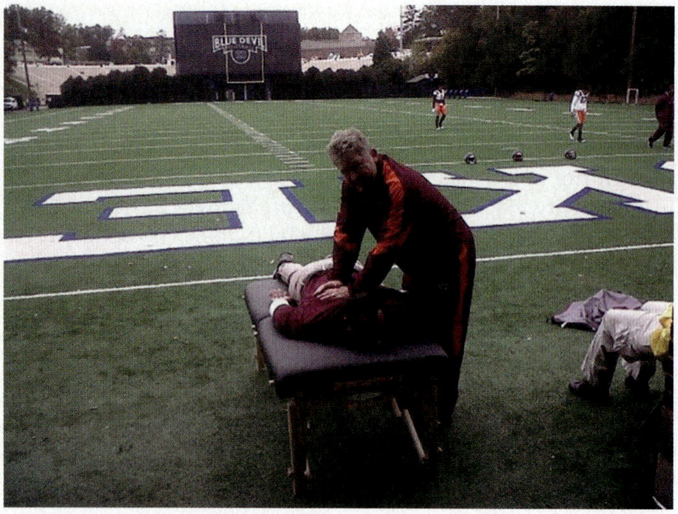

Figure 87.11. **Pregame OMT.**

- Once structure and function have improved, comprehensive neuromuscular retraining can be undertaken, as previously described.

TREATMENT

Prevention of Disease or Injury

BENEFITS OF EXERCISE

Many serious health problems can be controlled, improved, or eliminated through moderate, consistent physical activity.

- Regular exercise, in conjunction with other risk-reducing behaviors, will protect against cardiac events (Box 87.19).
- Improving physical health also improves emotional health.[94]
- Regular exercise is strongly correlated with intellectual function, memory, and improved self-concept.[95–100]
- Regular light-to-moderate exercise is correlated with enhanced functioning of the immune system.[101–103]

PERFORMANCE ENHANCEMENT

Today's athletes are bigger, stronger, and faster than ever before.

- This is accomplished through a holistic approach including advanced functional training and nutritional approaches.
    - ☐ In 2003, Sir Dave Brailsford transformed the British cycling team from a team that had not won the Tour de France in 110 years, and that had only obtained a small handful of gold medals in 100 years of Olympic competitions, into the team that won more gold medals in the 2020 Tokyo Olympics than any other cycling team. He did this by "the aggregation of marginal gains" that entailed making small changes in every aspect of cycling, including equipment, training pattern, kit fabrics, nutrition, and maintenance nuances. His words echo the osteopathic holistic approach to sports medicine when he said, "The whole principle came from the idea that if you broke down everything you could think of that goes into riding a bike, and then improved it by 1 percent, you will get a significant increase when you put them all together."[104]
    - ☐ The osteopathic physician seeks to maximize athlete performance using a holistic approach to every aspect of the athlete's health including nutrition, sleep, mental health, flexibility, strength, and recovery from injury.

BOX 87.19 Benefits of Exercise

- Favorable lipid profile
- Obesity control
- Decreased blood pressure
- Improved glucose tolerance
- Higher bone density
- Improved self-image

BOX 87.20 Osteopathic Pearl: Functional Considerations

Integral components to improved performance that are often overlooked are balance and control of functional movement (functional strength or stability control). Training the body in various neuromuscular patterns that are sport specific is the key to performance enhancement. Improved neuromuscular coordination is achieved through removal of somatic dysfunction and postural and muscle imbalances while repetitively training to improve balance, energy transfer, spiral and fascial torque, and functional strength throughout sport-specific joint motions.

As a team physician, it is important to evaluate those athletes with injuries during the season to be sure they have been maximally rehabilitated during the off-season and are fully recovered (Box 87.20).

- Today's athletes improve performance by working specifically on:
    - ☐ Flexibility
    - ☐ Speed
    - ☐ Strength
    - ☐ Endurance
    - ☐ Nutrition
    - ☐ Psychology

The Use of Performance-Enhancing (Ergogenic) Drugs

Categories of ergogenic aids include:

1. Pharmacologic
2. Nutritional
3. Physiologic, such as blood boosting

There has been increased emphasis on the psychological aspect of sports performance, with many elite athletes using mental imagery and several other relaxation techniques to enhance performance. The following factors best predict athletic success:

- Genes
- Nutrition
- Training techniques
- Mental discipline

With respect to pharmacologic aides, the most used substances include creatine, anabolic steroids, and human growth hormone.[105]

- Anabolic steroids:
    - ☐ Mechanism:
        - Increased protein synthesis

        - Increased red blood cell production
        - Central nervous system effects that include increased aggressiveness.
    - Incidence: Use has been variously reported in the 3% to 12% range.
    - Class of medication: Controlled substance (class III).
    - Side effects: Effects on the cardiovascular, reproductive, and endocrine systems.
- Human growth hormone: Produced using recombinant DNA technology; high cost does in some ways limit its abuse.
    - Mechanism:
        - Increased transport of amino acids into tissue
        - Stimulation of mobilization of fat as an energy source.
    - Incidence: It has been reported that 5% of male American high-school students used or have used hGH as an anabolic agent.[106]
    - Class of medication: naturally occurring peptide hormone secreted by the pituitary gland, however recombinant hGH (rhGH) is developed through genetic engineering.[107]
    - Side effects:
        - Include those mentioned for anabolic steroids, as well as:
            - Acromegaly
            - Diabetes mellitus
            - Heart failure
            - Osteoporosis
            - As with any injectable drug, the risk of infectious disease secondary to needle sharing must also be taken into consideration.
- Amphetamines: Have been used for over 50 years. They were initially used in World War II to prevent "battle fatigue."
    - Mechanism[106–108]:
        - Central nervous system stimulation
        - Speeding of reaction time
        - Masking of symptoms of fatigue
    - Incidence: Currently, 1.2% of people aged 12 to 17 years and 3.1% of people aged 18 to 25 years have nonmedically used stimulants during the past year[108]
    - Class of medication: Stimulants
    - Side effects:
        - Cardiovascular collapse
        - Hypertension
        - Hallucinations
        - Irritability
        - Restlessness
- Caffeine: A special subclass of stimulant that may enhance performance in endurance athletic events. Caffeine is widely considered to be one of the safest, most effective, and extensively studied ergogenic aids.[109]
    - Mechanism:
        - May be related to central nervous system stimulation and enhanced energy utilization
    - Incidence:
        - Approximately 60%, and it is legal for use in low doses (5 to 10 mg/kg). This dose represents about three to four cups of strongly brewed coffee (about a 300-mg dose)
    - Class of medication: Methylxanthine stimulant
    - Side effects:
        - GI intolerance
        - Dehydration
        - Cardiac arrhythmia
        - Tremor
        - Headaches
- Blood doping: A method employed by endurance athletes. Initially, the technique was to donate two units of autologous blood approximately 8 to 12 weeks prior to the athletic event and then reinfuse this blood about 1 week prior to competition. More recently, athletes have used erythropoietin, an injectable medication that stimulates red blood cell production by bone marrow.
    - Mechanism: Increase oxygen-carrying capacity
    - Side effects:
        - Stroke
        - Blood clots
        - Sudden death
        - Transfusion reaction
        - Headache
        - Hypertension

Postural Decompensation and Neuromuscular Imbalance

The physical effects of sports on the different tissues of the body are numerous and complex.[1,38] These include:

- Many athletes, especially at higher levels, compete with injury and can compensate for a certain amount of tissue injury and/or movement dysfunction; however, over time, they progressively decompensate, lose the ability to further compensate, and/or develop significant injury (Box 87.21).
- When assessing athletes, it is important to look not only for the obvious injuries and/or restricted areas of mobility but also specifically for segmental or regional areas of dysfunctional movement patterns.
    - This may initially present as regions of poor movement control, poor neuromotor firing patterns, and poor proprioception.
    - Over time or from additional injury, the local muscular, tendinous, fascial, or ligamentous tissues often develop progressive dysfunction and/or injury.
- Subtle segmental instability can be assessed through careful palpation and by paying attention to quality and range of movement, and end feel.

To help these athletes, treatment cannot be directed toward only one area; rather, a comprehensive management plan must be directed at three key areas:

1. Regenerative treatment for degenerative tissue (muscle, tendon, fascia) and/or ligamentous instability
2. Manual mobilization/OMT of restricted segmental mobility
3. Neuromotor retraining of dysfunctional movement patterns and functional instability from neuromotor imbalance

BOX 87.21 Muscle Imbalances

When should physicians suspect muscle imbalances in athletes?
Abnormal muscle-firing sequences on ROM testing
"Weak" phasic muscles on exam
Easy fatigability of phasic muscles
Poor "core" strength
Poor proprioception (especially with eyes closed) Poor awareness of axial position sense
Need for frequent OMT or recurrent SD/chronic pain
Postural decline
Symptoms of tendinopathy

Clinical Pearl

- Careful and thorough trauma history can often lead the physician to nonpainful areas of the body that need to be assessed for clinical dysfunction (neuromotor and/or structural).

NONOPERATIVE ORTHOBIOLOGIC MEDICAL MANAGEMENT OPTIONS

Prolotherapy

Prolotherapy is a regenerative injection that introduces an exogenous chemical irritant to a degenerated, or painful, region of the body.

- This treatment promotes new collagen fiber formation and the growth of normal cells and tissue, via the body's natural inflammatory cascade.
- Uses:
  - Tendinopathies
  - Osteoarthritis
  - Musculoskeletal pain
  - Joint pain
  - Laxity
- Studies: Currently, there are several supporting the use of prolotherapy for the following indications[105,110–123]:
  - Temporomandibular joint
  - Achilles tendon
  - Lateral epicondylitis
  - Patellar tendinopathy
  - Plantar fasciitis
  - Groin pain
  - Shoulder joint pain
  - Osgood–Schlatter disease
  - Knee OA
  - Hip OA
  - Finger and thumb OA
  - Spinal pain (cervical, thoracic, lumbar)
  - Sacroiliac joint pain
  - Coccygodynia pain
  - Myofascial pain syndrome
  - There are at least four categories of solutions used in prolotherapy:
    - Osmotic shock agents (such as dextrose, the most common proliferant used)
    - Chemotactic agents
    - Particulates
    - Irritants
      - Goal: Restore joint stability by facilitating the proprioception and strengthening of joint stabilizing structures.
      - Many different forms of irritants are available—osmotic agents, neurolytics, direct inflammatory cascade stimulants, and mechanical.
        - Dextrose: Most contain D-glucose, the body's natural form of glucose.
        - Pathophysiology: Dextrose, a hypertonic solution, initiates a change in the osmotic pressure between the extracellular matrix and tendon fibroblasts, causing the inflammatory cascade to release prohealing growth factors and collagen deposition.
          - Dextrose concentrations used in prolotherapy range from 10% to 25%.[124–126]
          - Dextrose is safer and beginners should use dextrose exclusively.
          - Recent studies have found that dextrose (10% and higher)[124–126]:
            - Stimulates the inflammatory response
            - Increases ligament and tendon size
            - Facilitates extracellular matrix and fibroblastic proliferation
            - Repairs articular cartilage defects.
          - A recent study has challenged this concentration and found that the cell viability was decreased in concentrations of more than 5% dextrose and 0.1% lidocaine. They found a lower concentration was still beneficial (1% dextrose and 0.01% lidocaine) which caused a mild proliferation of fibroblasts.[127]
        - P2G (Ongley solution: 25% dextrose, 25% glycerin, and 2.5% phenol): Is always injected at half strength concentration: 12.5% dextrose, 12.5% glycerin, and 1.25% phenol, typically in 0.25% lidocaine or procaine.
          - Solution typically comes prepared at double this dose and is always diluted by half, usually with a local anesthetic.
          - Phenol is neurolytic, and care must be taken with placement of this solution.
        - These additional irritants are sometimes added to the solutions above and/or injected alone:
          - Common—morrhuate sodium
          - Less common—polidocanol, manganese, zinc, human growth hormone, pumice, ozone, glycerin, phenol, or sarapin
        - Occasionally may be mixed with:
          - Platelet-rich plasma (PRP)
          - Bone marrow aspirate
          - Adipose tissue solutions[110]
- See Chapter 89 for further discussion about prolotherapy.

Platelet-Rich Plasma (PRP)

PRP injections are injection solutions prepared by simple same-day, minimal manipulation of autologous whole blood obtained from the patient. The blood is spun down in a centrifuge and the plasma and platelets are removed. The platelets, in addition to providing clotting abilities, are rich in growth factors that help trigger cell reproduction, tissue regeneration, and healing.[128]

- This treatment is predicated on delivering an increased concentration of the patient's own cells with tissue healing potential (i.e., growth factors and cytokines) to improve pain, tissue integrity, and ultimately, function.
- PRP has been rapidly evolving over the last 10 to 20 years as a conservative treatment, via injection, or as an intraoperative add-on procedure.
- There is a significant growing body of evidence on PRP, but due to a large variance in preparation and lack of reporting what was injected, it is difficult to compare results across various preparations and techniques. Currently, there are more than 50 studies supporting the use of PRP for tendinopathy.[129–133]
  - Large-scale research has limited the data to certain body regions; however, anecdotal evidence and many individual case studies reveal possible benefits to muscles, tendons, and ligaments. Sufficiently powered and well-documented clinical studies are needed to determine the full potential and thus therapeutic effects of PRP, in a variety of indications.[128]

- To date, several studies on osteoarthritis of the knee provide the best evidence for PRP, suggesting that the effects are safer, last longer, and are better than corticosteroid and/or viscosupplementation injections.[134–137]

PRP involves the following:

- Mechanism:
  - Activation of the platelet concentrate allows for the secretion of the bioactive molecules in situ.[111]
  - Some physicians use external activators such as calcium chloride or topical thrombin (Recothrom) to cause an immediate or much faster release of growth factors. This method can also be used to create a platelet release that can be applied directly to nerves.
  - Most physicians prefer to allow natural activation from tenocytes (tendon-specific fibroblasts) or synoviocytes (fibroblast-like cells in the synovial joints that produce synovial fluid glycoproteins), which takes place over 3 to 8 days in situ.
  - Autologous nature decreases most side effects and adverse reactions. Other than immediate postprocedural pain, side effects seem to be mild and well-tolerated.
- Uses:
  - Tendinopathies:
    - Lateral epicondylitis[138] and patellar tendon[139] are the most studied, but any tendon with degenerative findings or partial tearing may be a candidate.
  - Ligament partial tears:
    - Cruciate ligaments
    - Knee MCLs
    - Elbow UCLs
    - Ligaments of ankle, wrist, and digits
  - Osteoarthritis (OA):
    - PRP injection was shown to be a valid conservative treatment to reduce pain, improve quality of life and functional scores in a prospective study on 153 patients with knee OA.[140]
  - Nonunion of fractures
    - The current "gold standard" for treatment of nonunion fractures is the use of autologous cancellous bone grafts.[141]
    - One potential alternative, which is gaining popularity in literature, is the use of PRP.
    - The consensus from the literature is that PRP is effective in accelerating the healing of nonunion fractures.[142] However, the success occurs when used in doses from 2.5 to 20 mL, and the nonunion would have to be inherently stable and PRP would ideally be administered within 11 months of injury or initial surgery.[142]
    - Nerve impingement and radiculitis.
    - Published literature now includes randomized studies showing positive benefit to using PRP for:
      - Nerve entrapment
      - Radicular pain
      - Direct injection into lumbar disks
  - Goal: To facilitate the repair of soft tissue, utilizing an autologous solution.
- Injection technique:
  - Several *principles* are important in its application for successful treatment in soft tissue injury:
    - Use of higher concentration (at least 5–6 × concentration) and multiple injections with leukocyte-rich, and RBC-free PRP with adequate volume.
    - US guidance is essential for accurate localization and complete application.
    - Use of *3D Tenotomy* (repeated fenestration of the entire area of injury, injecting slowly with every retraction).
      - Needle feel, in addition to guidance is important in this application.
  - Treatment of the entire *functional unit*
    - This includes not only the local structure, or the end of a structure that is injured, but also the surrounding structures that have been either traumatically injured or repetitively strained due to the primary injury.
    - This is the use of prolotherapy treatment principles in treatment application.
      - For example, chronic anterolateral ankle instability is best treated with 15 to 18 cc total volume applied to, at least, the following structures:
        - Ankle joint and capsule
        - Posterior subtalar joint and capsule
        - Anterior talofibular ligament
        - Anterior inferior talofibular ligament
        - Interosseous membrane
        - Calcaniofibular ligaments
        - Sinus tarsi (for all ligaments here)
        - Spring ligament
        - Additionally, both the posterior tibial and peroneal tendons should be assessed for tendinopathy or tear and treated if present.
- Number of injections:
  - According to researchers, a single injection was as effective as multiple PRP injections in pain improvement; however, multiple injections seemed more effective in joint functionality than a single injection at 6 months.[143]
  - The available evidence is still insufficient, on number of sessions needed, and future research on this specific topic is needed.

Cell Concentrates Containing Stem Cells

- Stem cell therapy is an orthobiologic treatment that begins with harvesting of autologous or allogenic cell concentrates from bone marrow or fat that contain high amounts of stem cells. The goal is to restore tissue functionality by repairing the tissue on a molecular and cellular level.

Stem cell therapies are used to treat neurologic illnesses including cerebral palsy, Alzheimer disease, Parkinson disease, Huntington disease, amyotrophic lateral sclerosis, stroke, spinal cord injuries, autism spectrum disorder, and multiple sclerosis, but are also becoming more readily used for sports injuries.[110,144–147] The traditional types of stem cells used in musculoskeletal medicine are adult mesenchymal signaling cells (MSCs).

Stem cell injections involve the following:

- Mechanism:
  - Emerging evidence strongly supports that injected MSC concentrates primarily stimulate local pericytes (cells with true multilineage differentiation capacity) that line every artery to activate local regenerative and healing pathways.
- MSC tissue sources include mixtures of cell populations from:
  - Adipose stem cells
  - Bone marrow stem cells
  - Peripheral blood progenitor cells
- Uses:
  - Tendinopathies
  - Muscle/tendon tears
  - Joints

- Lateral elbow tendinopathy
- Shoulder (rotator cuff tears)
- Patellar tendinopathy
- Achilles tears
- Meniscal tears
- Cartilage lesions
- Osteoarthritis

- Goal: To facilitate the differentiation and growth of new tissue to improve function.

Ultrasound

The utility of US has grown exponentially over the past 15 years.

- Following advancements in US machine resolution and computer technology leading to faster, yet smaller machines, efficient, portable, tableside US units are commonplace.
- US can now be readily used in the training room and potentially even on the sidelines.
- High-resolution US (HRUS) is a powerful tool that may be used as the first-line imaging modality for the evaluation of many soft tissues. For peripheral nerve pathologies, it has a better confidence level for detecting nerve discontinuity and change in nerve caliber was found to be higher on ultrasonography than magnetic resonance imaging (MRI) (100 vs. 70% and 100 vs. 50%, respectively).[148]
- With increased functionality and practicality, intraoffice US has become the standard of care for the sports medicine physician.
  - US is now being used for both diagnostic and therapeutic purposes.
  - US-guided injections can be completed within the office, with no need for irradiation of the patient as with fluoroscopy.
- US-guided injections are widely used in patients with conditions of the shoulder to improve their accuracy. The use of US over blind injections has been thought to be significantly more accurate and efficacious, as well as causing less pain for the athlete.
- However, a recent randomized control trial determined that the clinical efficacy of US-guided injections compared with blind injections remains controversial.[149]

Diagnostically, US has decreased the need for repetitive CT and MRI imaging.

- A sports medicine physician with a strong knowledge of anatomy can use US at the bedside as an extension of the physical exam.
- Additionally, athletes get real-time visualization of their anatomy, which helps improve the physician–patient relationship.

Additional Ultrasound-Guided Procedures

Because US magnifies the underlying anatomy, lacks iatrogenic radiation exposure, and allows for the observation of motion, new percutaneous US-guided treatments are being developed with significant results. The goal of these treatments is to identify the underlying mechanism thought to contribute to pain production in common orthopedic and sports injuries. One of these key etiologies of pain that is often targeted during US-guided procedures is termed "tendinosis." Tendinosis is commonly defined as an accumulation of microinsults with a failed healing response.[150]

- These microinjuries result in increased local blood flow and neovascularity within the tendon.
- With the neovascular increase, neurogenesis can also occur outside the tendon but in close proximity to these vessels.
- Researchers have recently been studying different techniques that may improve these presentations of tendinopathy.

SCLEROSIS OF NEOVESSELS

- Goal: To decrease the number of neovessels and inhibit neurogenesis within the tendon.
- Procedure: Injection of polidocanol into/around neovessels using US guidance. Injections located outside of the tendon (vs. other types of US-guided injections) require three to five injections, spaced 4 to 8 weeks apart.
- Research: Early results are promising, follow-up studies are less impressive.[111,151]

TENDON SCRAPING

- Goal: To disrupt growth of neovessels and neogenesis around nonsynovial tendons (such as ITB, patellar, and Achilles tendons).
- Procedure: Percutaneous mechanical scraping around tendon with 14 to 21 G needle, using US guidance.
- Research: Anecdotal early positive results. Research is ongoing.[150,151]

HYDRODISSECTION

- Goal: To improve neurovascular mobility by "freeing up" the nerve or "breaking up" the scar tissue within injured fascia or muscle by using the hydrostatic pressure of the injectate to open fascial planes.
- Procedure: Percutaneous injection of saline and or D5W (mild anesthetic) around a nerve to break up adhesions and scar tissue under US guidance[152–154] (Fig. 87.12A–D).
  - D5W appears to affect potassium channels, not sodium channels, affecting repolarization and hyperpolarization. Therefore, it does not affect motor, only sensory, and acts as an excellent diagnostic solution in cases of pain of unclear etiology.
  - D5W also appears to exert direct effect on TRPV1 receptors, those associated with chronic pain, and may help stabilize local glycopenia often associated with the local tissue surrounding entrapment neuropathy.
  - Key technique for nerve hydrodissection includes:
    - US guidance.
    - Letting the fluid do the work.
    - Restoration of the transverse view of the nerve back to a perfectly circular shape. All nerves will assume a perfectly circular shape when there is no tension on them.
    - Restoring this shape over distance.
    - Use of moderate to high volumes of fluid compared to conventional injection.
- Research:
  - Several randomized studies have now popped up on the median nerve in the carpal tunnel along with a few other nerves. However, despite favorable results, many have used too low a volume and simply blocked the nerve (only haloed the nerve and did not restore the nerve to a circular shape over distance) and did not really do a hydrodissection.[154]
  - Several case studies and proof of concept papers have been published to date.

THE ROLE OF SOMATIC DYSFUNCTION AND OMT IN THE ATHLETE

Osteopathic physicians have a unique skillset to offer athletes recovering from injury, illness, or struggles with performance on the field. The clinician must first ask themselves if there is a somatic component to the athlete's injury, illness, or condition. To determine this, a structural and palpatory exam must be part

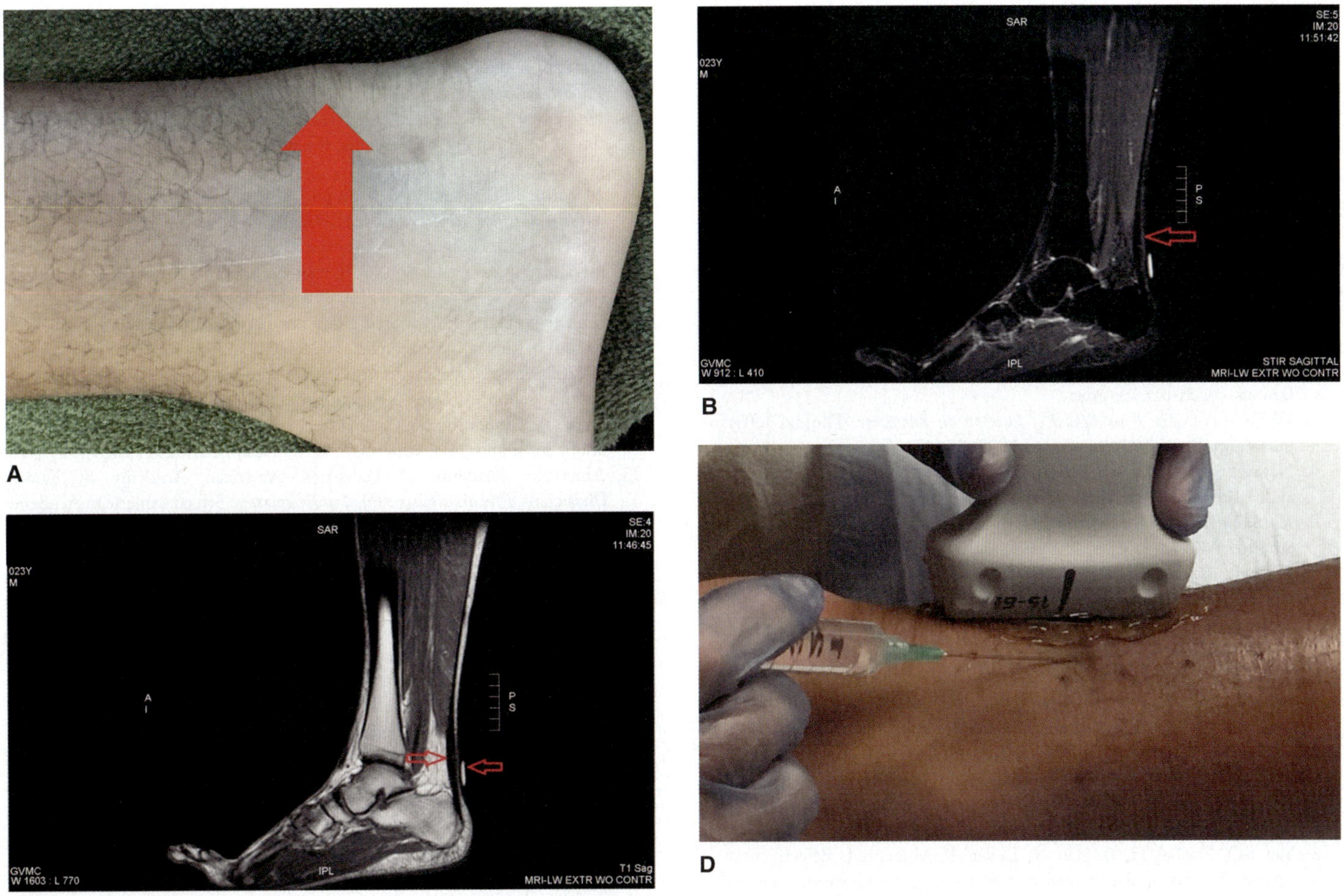

Figure 87.12. Achilles tendinopathy. Diagnosis and treatment. **A.** Haglund deformity on physical exam. **B.** T2, sagittal imaging shows prominent Haglund deformity and fusiform swelling. **C.** T1, sagittal imaging shows prominent Haglund deformity and fusiform swelling. **D.** Lateral view of the hydrodissection of the Achilles tendon with the sural nerve clearly marked. (Photos and x-rays courtesy of Dr. Brolinson, with permission.)

of the PPE, clinical evaluation, or hospital-based assessment. If significant TART changes are present and felt to be related to the medical or structural condition, then SD as a diagnosis has been established. The next step is to determine if, when, and how to treat it. SD can physiologically and anatomically disrupt normal healing mechanisms and the local and distant function of the involved and compensating structures. By resolving SD with OMT and other modalities, the body has a much better chance of healing completely and without unnecessary procedures and surgeries.

Some common examples with their associated SD from this chapter are:

- Concussion
  - ☐ Cranial strain patterns
  - ☐ Cervical type two somatic dysfunctions
  - ☐ Scalene spasm/tenderpoints
- Rotator cuff impingement
  - ☐ AC/sternoclavicular somatic dysfunction
  - ☐ Type two somatic dysfunctions of the thoracic spine
  - ☐ Inhaled/exhaled ribs/first rib dysfunction
- Spondylolysis
  - ☐ Type two upper lumbar dysfunction and psoas hypertonicity
  - ☐ Sacral SD
  - ☐ Innominate dysfunction/iliolumbar ligament pain
- Anterior knee pain
  - ☐ Inhibited VMO from lumbar dysfunction
  - ☐ Hamstring tension and tenderpoints
  - ☐ Fascial restrictions of knee and popliteal space
- Ankle sprain
  - ☐ Posterior fibular head
  - ☐ Talus/calcaneus dysfunction
  - ☐ Tenderpoints foot and ankle

CONCLUSIONS

From its beginnings with AT Still, osteopathic medicine has taken an active role in promoting participation in recreational and competitive athletics as a means to a healthy lifestyle and providing specialized treatment for athletes.[1,19,155]

- Participation in sports is good for the body, mind, and spirit. It provides fitness, confidence, resilience, and essential leadership skills to succeed as adults.
- Osteopathic principles and practice, including the use of manual medicine, have a large role in the treatment of the athlete.
- Each athlete should be evaluated and treated on an individual basis, including a comprehensive evaluation of both structure and function when appropriate.[1,38]
- Participation in sports is an integral part of sports medicine, and preparticipation screening should be encouraged to help prevent injury and allow safe participation.[41]

- Because of the wide variety of potential injuries and medical maladies that can affect the athlete, the sports medicine physician must be comprehensively trained.
- Finally, physicians must always keep the health and safety of the athlete as their primary goal when considering return-to-play decisions.

REFERENCES

1. Brolinson PG, McGinley SMG, Kerger S. Osteopathic manipulative medicine and the athlete. *Curr Sports Med Rep.* 2008;7(1):49–56.
2. A.T. Still University. Quick Facts on ATSU's College Football Team–the Osteopaths–and Famous Coach Patrick O'Dea.https://www.atsu.edu/news/quick-facts-on-atsus-college-football-team-the-osteopaths-and-famous-coach-patrick-odea
3. Walter GW. *The First School of Osteopathic Medicine.* Thomas Jefferson University Press; 1924 (reprinted 1992):39–45.
4. Nauright J. Making an International Legend: The Media, Pat O'Dea and Midwestern Football in the 1890s and 1930s, 45, https://www.researchgate.net/profile/John-Nauright/publication/43491445_Making_an_international_legend_The_media_Pat_O%27Dea_and_midwestern_football_in_the_1890s_and_1930s/links/5657dabb08aefe619b1f351d/Making-an-international-legend-The-media-Pat-ODea-and-midwestern-football-in-the-1890s-and-1930s.pdf
5. Still CE Jr. *Frontier Doctor—Medical Pioneer: The Life and Times of AT Still and His Family.* Thomas Jefferson University Press; 1907 (reprinted 1991, Truman State University Press):180–188, 205–216, 246–247.
6. Civitillo C, DO PT. Osteopathic manipulative treatment and sport: narrative review. *GIOSBE J.* 2018;4(2):1–6.
7. Ofei-Dodoo S, Black JL, Kirkover MA, Lisenby CB, Porter AS, Cleland PM. Collegiate athletes' perceptions of osteopathic manipulative treatment. *Kans J Med.* 2020;13:147–151.
8. Yao SC, Zwibel H, Angelo N, Leder A, Mancini J. Effectiveness of osteopathic manipulative medicine vs concussion education in treating student athletes with acute concussion symptoms. *J Am Osteopath Assoc.* 2020;120(9):607–614.
9. Thomas KD, Lombard ZK, Shadiack AL. Osteopathic manipulative treatment for concussions and postconcussive syndrome in athletes: a literature review. *J Am Osteopath Assoc.* 2023;123(8):395–403.
10. Curcio JE, Grana MJ, England S, et al. Use of the Spencer Technique on collegiate baseball players: effect on physical performance and self-reported measures. *J Am Osteopath Assoc.* 2017;117:166–175.
11. Moore SD, Laudner KG, McLoda TA, Shaffer MA. The immediate effects of muscle energy technique on posterior shoulder tightness: a randomized controlled trial. *J Orthop Sports Phys Ther.* 2011;41:400–407.
12. Bennett S, Macfarlane C, Vaughan B. The use of osteopathic manual therapy and rehabilitation for subacromial impingement syndrome: a case report. *Explore (NY).* 2017;13:339–343.
13. Giulio A, Davide C, Antonella OM, et al. Efficacy of osteopathic manipulative treatment (OMT) vs physiotherapy in chronic lateral epicondylitis. *J Altern Complement Med.* 2022;11(4):1–9.
14. Koh C, Seffinger MA. Muscle energy technique improves chronic lateral epicondylitis. *J Am Osteopath Assoc.* 2016;116(1):58–58.
15. Zago J, Amatuzzi F, Rondinel T, Matheus JP. Osteopathic manipulative treatment versus exercise program in runners with patellofemoral pain syndrome: a randomized controlled trial. *J Sport Rehabil.* 2020;30(4):609–618.
16. Eisenhart AW, Gaeta TJ, Yens DP. Osteopathic manipulative treatment in the emergency department for patients with acute ankle injuries. *J Am Osteopath Assoc.* 2003;103(9):417–421.
17. Wynne MM, Burns JM, Eland DC, Conatser RR, Howell JN Effect of counterstrain on stretch reflexes, Hoffmann reflexes, and clinical outcomes in subjects with plantar fasciitis. *J Am Osteopath Assoc.* 2006;106(9):547–556.
18. Brolinson PG, Smolka M, Rogers M, et al. Precompetition manipulative treatment and performance among Virginia Tech athletes during 2 consecutive football seasons: a preliminary, retrospective report. *J Am Osteopath Assoc.* 2012;112(9):607–615.
19. Akkaş MB, Belviranli M, Okudan N. The effect of osteopathic manipulative treatment on anaerobic performance and lactate clearance in male athletes: a double-blind, randomized, sham-controlled, crossover study. *J Sports Med Phys Fitness.* 2021;62(4):500–507.
20. Hergenroeder AC, Chorley J, Triedman JK, Armsby C. Sports participation in children and adolescents: the preparticipation physical evaluation. UpToDate, Apr 13, 2023.
21. MacDonald J, Schaefer M, Stumph J. The preparticipation physical evaluation. *Am Fam Physician.* 2021;103(9):539–546.
22. Roberts WO, Löllgen H, Matheson GO, et al. Advancing the preparticipation physical evaluation (PPE): an ACSM and FIMS joint consensus statement. *Curr Sports Med Rep.* 2014;13:395–401.
23. Raukar N, Cates J, Moffatt K. The pre-participation evaluation of High School Athletes, MacDonald. 2021;103(9):539–546. Accessed January 25, 2025. https://www.nfhs.org/articles/the-pre-participation-evaluation-of-high-school-athletes/National Federation of High Schools.
24. Smith A. Evaluating policy consistency in preparticipation physical evaluations for high school athletes. *J Pediatr Health Care.* 2023;37(3):315–318.
25. American Academy of Pediatrics, American Academy of Family Physicians. *Preparticipation Physical Evaluation.* 5th ed. American Academy of Pediatrics; 2019. https://www.aap.org/en/patient-care/preparticipation-physical-evaluation/
26. Carek PJ, Mainous AG III. A thorough yet efficient exam identifies most problems in school athletes. *J Fam Pract.* 2003;52:127–134.
27. Seroyer ST, Nho SJ, Bach BR, Bush-Joseph CA, Nicholson GP, Romeo AA. The kinetic chain in overhand pitching: its potential role for performance enhancement and injury prevention. *Sports Health.* 2010;2(2):135–146.
28. Maron BJ, Levine BD, Washington RL, Baggish AL, Kovacs RJ, Maron MS; American Heart Association Electrocardiography and Arrhythmias Committee of Council on Clinical Cardiology, Council on Cardiovascular Disease in Young, Council on Cardiovascular and Stroke Nursing, Council on Functional Genomics and Translational Biology, and American College of Cardiology. Eligibility and disqualification recommendations for competitive athletes with cardiovascular abnormalities: Task Force 2: preparticipation screening for cardiovascular disease in competitive athletes: a scientific statement from the American Heart Association and American College of Cardiology. *Circulation.* 2015;132:e267–272.
29. Maron BJ, Friedman RA, Kligfield P, et al. Assessment of the 12-lead ECG as a screening test for detection of cardiovascular disease in healthy general populations of young people (12-25 years of age): a scientific statement from the American Heart Association and the American College of Cardiology. *Circulation.* 2014;130:1303–1334.
30. Diamond AB, Narducci DM, Roberts WO, et al. Interim guidance on the preparticipation physical examination for athletes during the SARS-CoV-2 pandemic. *Clin J Sport Med.* 2021;31(1):1–6.
31. Dores H, Cardim N. Return to play after COVID-19: a sport cardiologist's view. *Br J Sports Med.* 2020;54:1132–1133.
32. Baggish A, Drezner JA, Kim J, Martinez M, Prutkin JM. Resurgence of sport in the wake of COVID-19: cardiac considerations in competitive athletes. *Br J Sports Med.* 2020;54:1130–1131.
33. Emery MS, Phelan DMJ, Martinez MW. *Exercise and Athletics in the COVID-19 Pandemic Era.* American College of Cardiology; 2020. Accessed June 3, 2020. https://www.acc.org/latest-in-cardiology/articles/2020/05/13/12/53/exercise-and-athletics-in-the-covid-19-pandemic-era
34. Phelan D, Kim JH, Chung EH. A game plan for the resumption of sport and exercise after coronavirus disease 2019 (COVID-19) infection. *JAMA Cardiol.* 2020;5(10):1085–1086.
35. CDC. Underlying Conditions and the Higher Risk for Severe COVID-19. https://www.cdc.gov/coronavirus/2019-ncov/hcp/clinical-care/underlyingconditions.html
36. Rosenthal N, Cao Z, Gundrum J, Sianis J, Safo S. Risk factors associated with in-hospital mortality in a US National Sample of patients with COVID-19. *JAMA Netw Open.* 2020;3(12):e2029058.
37. Milewicz DM, Braverman AC, De Backer J, et al. Marfan syndrome [published correction appears in *Nat Rev Dis Primers.* 2022;8(1):3]. *Nat Rev Dis Primers.* 2021;7(1):64.
38. Brolinson PG, Heinking K, Kozar AJ. An osteopathic approach to sports medicine. In: Ward RC, Jerome JA, Jones JM III, et al., eds. *Foundations*

for Osteopathic Medicine. 2nd ed. Lippincott Williams & Wilkins; 2002:534–550.
39. Guernsey DT, Leder A, Yao S. Resolution of concussion symptoms after osteopathic manipulative treatment: a case report. *J Am Osteopath Assoc*. 2016;116(3):e13–e17.
40. Castillo I, Wolf K, Rakowsky A. Concussions, and osteopathic manipulative treatment: an adolescent case presentation. *J Am Osteopath Assoc*. 2016;116(3):178–181.
41. McCallister A, Brown C, Smith M, Ettlinger H, Baltazar GA. Osteopathic manipulative treatment for somatic dysfunction after acute severe traumatic brain injury. *J Am Osteopath Assoc*. 2016;116(12):810–815.
42. American Migraine Foundation. Primary Exercise Headache. https://americanmigrainefoundation.org/resource-library/primary-exercise-headache/
43. Al Khalili Y, Ly N, Murphy PB. Cervicogenic headache. [Updated 2022 October 3]. In: *StatPearls [Internet]*. StatPearls Publishing; 2023. https://www.ncbi.nlm.nih.gov/books/NBK507862/
44. Tessler J, Horn LJ. Posttraumatic headache. [Updated 2023 January 9]. In: *StatPearls [Internet]*. StatPearls Publishing; 2023. https://www.ncbi.nlm.nih.gov/books/NBK556134/
45. Ferry B, DeCastro A. Concussion. [Updated 2023 January 9]. In: *StatPearls [Internet]*. StatPearls Publishing; 2023. https://www.ncbi.nlm.nih.gov/books/NBK537017/
46. Zhao L, Han W, Steiner C. *Sports Related Concussions, 2008*. Statistical brief no. 114. Agency for Healthcare Research and Quality, Healthcare Cost and Utilization Project; 2011. Accessed September 14, 2018. http://www.hcup-us.ahrq.gov/reports/statbriefs/sb114.jsp
47. Doolan AW, Day DD, Maerlender AC, Goforth M, Brolinson PG. A review of return to play issues and sports-related concussion. *Ann Biomed Eng*. 2011;40(1):106–113.
48. American College of Sports Medicine. *ASCM Handbook for the Team Physician*. Williams & Wilkins; 1996.
49. Eckner JT, Kutcher JS. Concussion symptom scales and sideline assessment tools: a critical literature update. *Curr Sports Med Rep*. 2010;9(1):8–15.
50. Echemendia RJ, Meeuwisse W, McCrory P, et al. The sport concussion assessment tool 5th edition (SCAT5): background and rationale. *Br J Sports Med*. 2017;51:848–850.
51. Baltazar GA, Kolwitz C, Petrone P, Stright A, Joseph D. Osteopathic manipulative treatment relieves post-concussion symptoms in a case of polytrauma. *Cureus*. 2020;12(3):e7317.
52. Wetzler G, Roland M, Fryer-Dietz S, Dettmann-Ahern D. CranioSacral therapy and visceral manipulation: a new treatment intervention for concussion recovery. *Med Acupunct*. 2017;29:239–248.
53. Chappell C, Dodge E, Dogbey GY. Assessing the immediate effect of osteopathic manipulation on sports related concussion symptoms. *Osteopathic Fam Phys*. 2015;7:30–35. https://www.acofp.org/news-and-publications/journal/article-detail/vol-7-no-4-(2015)/assessing-immediate-effect-osteopathic-manipulation-sports-related-concussion-symptoms
54. Brolinson PG. Principle centered rehabilitation. In: Garrett WE, Kirkendall DT, Squire DL, eds. *Principles and Practice of Primary Care Sports Medicine*. Lippincott Williams & Wilkins; 2000:645–652.
55. Maddocks D, Saling M. Neuropsychological deficits following concussion. *Brain Inj*. 1996;10:99–103.
56. Leddy JJ, Haider MN, Ellis MJ, et al. Early subthreshold aerobic exercise for sport-related concussion: a randomized clinical trial. *JAMA Pediatr*. 2019;173(4):319–325.
57. Hitcherich K, Smith K, Cuoco JA, et al. The glymphatic-lymphatic continuum: opportunities for osteopathic manipulative medicine. *J Am Osteopath Assoc*. 2016;116(3):170–177.
58. Rowson S, Brolinson G, Goforth M, Dietter D, Duma SM. Linear and angular head acceleration measurements in collegiate football. *J Biomech Eng*. 2009;131(6):061016.
59. Patricios JS, Schneider KJ, Dvorak J, et al. Consensus statement on concussion in sport: the 6th International Conference on Concussion in Sport–Amsterdam, October 2022. *Br J Sports Med*. 2023;57:695–711.
60. McCrory P, Meeuwisse W, Dvořák J, et al. Consensus statement on concussion in sport-the 5th International Conference on Concussion in Sport held in Berlin, October 2016. *Br J Sports Med*. 2017;51(11):838–847.
61. May T, Foris LA, Donnally CJ III. Second impact syndrome. [Updated 2023 July 3]. In: *StatPearls [Internet]*. StatPearls Publishing; 2023. https://www.ncbi.nlm.nih.gov/books/NBK448119/
62. Cantu RC. Second-impact syndrome. *Clin Sports Med*. 1998;17(1):37–44.
63. American Academy of Neurology. UPDATE: EVALUATION AND MANAGEMENT OF CONCUSSION IN SPORTS. April 30, 2022. Accessed January 23, 2025. https://www.aan.com/Guidelines/home/GetGuidelineContent/583
64. Lovell MR, Iverson GI, Collins MW, McKeag D, Maroon JC. Does loss of consciousness predict neuropsychological decrements after concussion? *Clin J Sport Med*. 1999;9:193–198.
65. Collins MW, Grindel SH, Lovell MR, et al. Relationship between concussion and neuropsychological performance in college football players. *JAMA*. 1999;282:964–970.
66. Echemendia RJ, Putukian M, Mackin RS, Julian L, Shoss N. Neuropsychological test performance prior to and following sports-related mild traumatic brain injury. *Clin J Sport Med*. 2001;11(1):23–31.
67. Jones RD. Neuropsychological assessment of patients with traumatic brain injury: the Iowa-Benton approach. In: Rizzo M, Tranel D, eds. *Head Injury and Postconcussive Syndrome*. Churchill Livingstone; 1996.
68. Permenter CM, Fernández-de Thomas RJ, Sherman AL. Postconcussive syndrome. [Updated 2023 August 28]. In: *StatPearls [Internet]*. StatPearls Publishing; 2023. https://www.ncbi.nlm.nih.gov/books/NBK534786/
69. Varacallo M, El Bitar Y, Mair SD. Rotator cuff tendonitis. [Updated 2023 August 4]. In: *StatPearls [Internet]*. StatPearls Publishing; 2023. https://www.ncbi.nlm.nih.gov/books/NBK532270/
70. Creech JA, Silver S. Shoulder impingement syndrome. [Updated 2023 April 17]. In: *StatPearls [Internet]*. StatPearls Publishing; 2023. https://www.ncbi.nlm.nih.gov/books/NBK554518/
71. Neer CS II. Impingement lesions. *Clin Orthop*. 1983;3:70–77.
72. Buchanan BK, Varacallo M. Lateral epicondylitis (tennis elbow) [Updated 2023 August 4]. In: *StatPearls [Internet]*. StatPearls Publishing; 2023. https://www.ncbi.nlm.nih.gov/books/NBK431092/
73. Reece CL, Susmarski AJ. Medial epicondylitis. [Updated 2023 April 10]. In: *StatPearls [Internet]*. StatPearls Publishing; 2023. https://www.ncbi.nlm.nih.gov/books/NBK557869/
74. McDonald BT, Hanna A, Lucas JA. Spondylolysis. [Updated 2023 August 7.] In: *StatPearls [Internet]*. StatPearls Publishing; 2023. https://www.ncbi.nlm.nih.gov/books/NBK513333/
75. Watkins RG. The spine in sports. Mosby–Yearbook; 1996.
76. Beck NA, Miller R, Baldwin K, et al. Do oblique views add value in the diagnosis of spondylolysis in adolescents? *J Bone Joint Surg Am*. 2013;95(10):e65.
77. Evans J, Nielson JL. Anterior cruciate ligament knee injury. [Updated 2022 May 5.] In: *StatPearls [Internet]*. StatPearls Publishing; 2023. https://www.ncbi.nlm.nih.gov/books/NBK499848/
78. Shelbourne KD, Nitz PA. The O'Donoghue triad revisited. Combined knee injuries involving anterior cruciate and medial collateral ligament tears. *Am J Sports Med*. 1992;19(5):474–477.
79. Gaillard F, Feger J, Iqbal S, et al. O'Donoghue unhappy triad. Accessed on August 17, 2023. https://doi.org/10.53347/rID-1749
80. Shelbourne K, Nitz P. The O'Donoghue triad revisited: combined knee injuries involving anterior cruciate and medial collateral ligament tears. *Am J Sports Med*. 1991;19(5):474–477.
81. Barber FA. What is the terrible triad? *Arthroscopy*. 1992;8(1):19–22.
82. Balmer K, Gunst M, Rüedi T. [The "unhappy triad" (UT): slogan or reality in fresh knee injuries?]. *Helv Chim Acta (in German)*. 1983;49(5):675–677.
83. Staron RB, Haramati N, Feldman F, et al. O'Donoghue's triad: magnetic resonance imaging evidence. *Skeletal Radiol*. 1994;23(8):633–636.
84. Naranje S, Mittal R, Nag H, Sharma R. Arthroscopic and magnetic resonance imaging evaluation of meniscus lesions in the chronic anterior cruciate ligament-deficient knee. *Arthroscopy*. 2008;24(9):1045–1051.
85. Raj MA, Mabrouk A, Varacallo M. Posterior cruciate ligament knee injuries. [Updated 2023 August 8]. In: *StatPearls [Internet]*. StatPearls Publishing; 2023. https://www.ncbi.nlm.nih.gov/books/NBK430726/
86. Post WR. Patellofemoral pain: let the physical exam define treatment. *Phys Sports Med*. 1998;26(1):68–78.

87. Bump JM, Lewis L. Patellofemoral syndrome. [Updated 2023 February 13]. In: *StatPearls [Internet]*. StatPearls Publishing; 2023. https://www.ncbi.nlm.nih.gov/books/NBK557657/
88. Cleveland Clinic. Hyperextended Knee. https://my.clevelandclinic.org/health/diseases/22481-hyperextended-knee
89. Melanson SW, Shuman VL. Acute ankle sprain. [Updated 2023 May 23]. In: *StatPearls [Internet]*. StatPearls Publishing; 2023. https://www.ncbi.nlm.nih.gov/books/NBK459212/
90. Malliaropoulos N, Papacostas E, Papalada A, Maffulli N. Acute lateral ankle sprain in track and field athletes: an expanded classification. *Foot Ankle Clin*. 2006;11:497–507.
91. Trojian TH, McKeag DB. Ankle sprains. *Phys Sports Med*. 1998;26(10): 29–40.
92. Greenman PE. *Principles of Manual Medicine*. 2nd ed. Williams & Wilkins; 1996:452–456.
93. Tandetter HB, Shvartzman P. Acute ankle injuries: clinical decision rules for radiographs. *Am Fam Physician*. 1997;55(8):2721–2728.
94. Sharma A, Madaan V, Petty FD. Exercise for mental health. *Prim Care Companion J Clin Psychiatry*. 2006;8(2):106.
95. Patrick K, Sallis JF, Long B, et al. A new tool for encouraging activity. *Phys Sportsmed*. 1994;22:45–52.
96. Strauss RH. Cardiovascular benefits and risks of exercise: the scientific evidence. In: Wickland EH Jr, ed. *Sports Medicine*. 2nd ed. WB Saunders; 1991:72–80.
97. Scuderi GR, McCann PD, Bruno PJ, et al., eds. *Sports Medicine Principles of Primary Care*. 1st ed. Mosby–Yearbook; 1997.
98. Dailey SM, Oberman A. The athletic heart. *Heart Dis Stroke*. 1993;2: 53–58.
99. Anthony J. Psychologic aspects of exercise. *Clin Sports Med*. 1991;10(1): 171–180.
100. Elia EA. Exercise and the elderly. *Clin Sports Med*. 1991;10(1):141–155.
101. Walsh NP, Gleeson M, Shephard RJ, et al. Position statement. Part one: immune function and exercise. *Exerc Immunol Rev*. 2011;17:6–63.
102. Brolinson PG, Elliott D. Exercise and the immune system. *Clin Sports Med*. 2007;26:311–319.
103. Hojman P, Gehl J, Christensen JF, Pedersen BK. Molecular mechanisms linking exercise to cancer prevention and treatment. *Cell Metab*. 2018;27(1):10–21.
104. Clear J. This coach improved every tiny thing by 1 percent and here's what happened. jamesclear.com/marginal-gains
105. Brolinson PG, et al. Nutritional supplements as ergogenic AIDS. *Prim Care*. 2004;37–45.
106. Rickert VI, Pawlak-Morello C, Sheppard V, Jay MS. Human growth hormone: a new substance of abuse among adolescents? *Clin Pediatr (Phila)*. 1992;31(12):723–726.
107. Saugy M, Robinson N, Saudan C, Baume N, Avois L, Mangin P. Human growth hormone doping in sport. *Br J Sports Med*. 2006;40(Suppl 1): i35–i9.
108. Veliz P, Boyd C, McCabe SE. Adolescent athletic participation and nonmedical Adderall use: an exploratory analysis of a performance-enhancing drug. *J Stud Alcohol Drugs*. 2013;74(5):714–719.
109. Goldstein ER, Ziegenfuss T, Kalman D, et al. International society of sports nutrition position stand: caffeine and performance. *J Int Soc Sports Nutr*. 2010;7:5.
110. Andia I, Maffulli N. Biological therapies in regenerative sports medicine. *Sports Med*. 2016;47(5):807–828.
111. Lackner J, Hauser RA, Steilen-Matias D, Harris DK. A systematic review of dextrose prolotherapy for chronic musculoskeletal pain. *Clin Med Insights Arthritis Musculoskelet Disord*. 2016;9:139–159.
112. Ekwueme EC, Mohiuddin M, Yarborough JA, et al. Prolotherapy induces an inflammatory response in human tenocytes in vitro. *Clin Orthop Relat Res*. 2017;475(8):2117–2127.
113. Empson YM, Ekwueme EC, Hong JK, et al. High elastic modulus nanoparticles: a novel tool for subfailure connective tissue matrix damage. *Transl Res*. 2014;164(3):244–257.
114. Freeman JW, Empson YM, Ekwueme EC, Paynter DM, Brolinson PG. Effect of prolotherapy on cellular proliferation and collagen deposition in MC3T3-E1 and patellar tendon fibroblast populations. *Transl Res*. 2011;158(3):132–139.
115. Hauser RA, Lackner JB, Steilen-Matias D, Harris DK. A systematic review of dextrose prolotherapy for chronic musculoskeletal pain. *Clin Med Insights Arthritis Musculoskelet Disord*. 2016;9:139–159.
116. Wee TC, Neo EJR, Tan YL. Dextrose prolotherapy in knee osteoarthritis: a systematic review and meta-analysis. *J Clin Orthop Trauma*. 2021;19:108–117.
117. Sims SE, Miller K, Elfar JC, Hammert WC. Non-surgical treatment of lateral epicondylitis: a systematic review of randomized controlled trials. *Hand (N Y)*. 2014;9(4):419–446.
118. Rabago D, Nourani B. Prolotherapy for osteoarthritis and tendinopathy: a descriptive review. *Curr Rheumatol Rep*. 2017;19(6):34.
119. Chutumstid T, Susantitaphong P, Koonalinthip N. Effectiveness of dextrose prolotherapy for the treatment of chronic plantar fasciitis: a systematic review and meta-analysis of randomized controlled trials. *PM R*. 2023;15(3):380–391.
120. Rabago D, Best TM, Zgierska AE, Zeisig E, Ryan M, Crane D. A systematic review of four injection therapies for lateral epicondylosis: prolotherapy, polidocanol, whole blood and platelet-rich plasma. *Br J Sports Med*. 2009;43(7):471–481.
121. Sit RW, Chung VCh, Reeves KD, et al. Hypertonic dextrose injections (prolotherapy) in the treatment of symptomatic knee osteoarthritis: a systematic review and meta-analysis [published correction appears in *Sci Rep*. 2017;7:45879]. *Sci Rep*. 2016;6:25247.
122. Bisciotti GN, Chamari K, Cena E, et al. The conservative treatment of longstanding adductor-related groin pain syndrome: a critical and systematic review. *Biol Sport*. 2021;38(1):45–63.
123. Gobbi A, Fishman M. Platelet-rich plasma and bone marrow-derived mesenchymal stem cells in sports medicine. *Sports Med Arthrosc Rev*. 2016;24(2):69–73.
124. Reeves KD, Hassanein KM. Long-term effects of dextrose prolotherapy for anterior cruciate ligament laxity. *Altern Ther Health Med*. 2003;9: 58–62.
125. Topol GA, Reeves KD, Hassanein KM. Efficacy of dextrose prolotherapy in elite male kicking-sport athletes with chronic groin pain. *Arch Phys Med Rehabil*. 2005;86:697–702.
126. Lyftogt J. Subcutaneous prolotherapy treatment of refractory knee, shoulder, and lateral elbow pain. *Australas Musculoskelet Med*. 2007;12:110–112.
127. Woo MS, Park J, Ok SH, et al. The proper concentrations of dextrose and lidocaine in regenerative injection therapy: in vitro study. *Korean J Pain*. 2021;34(1):19–26.
128. Everts P, Onishi K, Jayaram P, Lana JF, Mautner K. Platelet-rich plasma: new performance understandings and therapeutic considerations in 2020. *Int J Mol Sci*. 2020;21(20):7794.
129. Le ADK, Enweze L, DeBaun MR, Dragoo JL. Current clinical recommendations for use of platelet-rich plasma. *Curr Rev Musculoskelet Med*. 2018;11(4):624–634.
130. Barman A, Sinha MK, Sahoo J, et al. Platelet-rich plasma injection in the treatment of patellar tendinopathy: a systematic review and meta-analysis. *Knee Surg Relat Res*. 2022;34(1):22.
131. Li S, Yang G, Zhang H, Li X, Lu Y. A systematic review on the efficacy of different types of platelet-rich plasma in the management of lateral epicondylitis. *J Shoulder Elbow Surg*. 2022;31(7):1533–1544.
132. Arthur Vithran DT, Xie W, Opoku M, Essien AE, He M, Li Y. The efficacy of platelet-rich plasma injection therapy in the treatment of patients with Achilles tendinopathy: a systematic review and meta-analysis. *J Clin Med*. 2023;12(3):995.
133. Masiello F, Pati I, Veropalumbo E, Pupella S, Cruciani M, De Angelis V. Ultrasound-guided injection of platelet-rich plasma for tendinopathies: a systematic review and meta-analysis. *Blood Transfus*. 2022;21(2):119–136.
134. Costa LAV, Lenza M, Irrgang JJ, Fu FH, Ferretti M. How does platelet-rich plasma compare clinically to other therapies in the treatment of knee osteoarthritis? A systematic review and meta-analysis. *Am J Sports Med*. 2023;51(4):1074–1086.
135. Sax OC, Chen Z, Mont MA, Delanois RE. The efficacy of platelet-rich plasma for the treatment of knee osteoarthritis symptoms and structural changes: a systematic review and meta-analysis. *J Arthroplasty*. 2022;37(11):2282–2290.e2.
136. Vilchez-Cavazos F, Blázquez-Saldaña J, Gamboa-Alonso AA, et al. The use of platelet-rich plasma in studies with early knee osteoarthritis versus

advanced stages of the disease: a systematic review and meta-analysis of 31 randomized clinical trials. *Arch Orthop Trauma Surg*. 2023;143(3):1393–1408.

137. Li W, Pan J, Lu Z, Zhu H, Guo J, Xie D. The application of platelet-rich plasma in the treatment of knee osteoarthritis: a literature review. *J Orthop Sci*. 2022;27(2):420–428.
138. Hastie G, Soufi M, Wilson J, Roy B. Platelet rich plasma injections for lateral epicondylitis of the elbow reduce the need for surgical intervention. *J Orthop*. 2018;15(1):239–241.
139. Vetrano M, Castorina A, Vulpiani MC, Baldini R, Pavan A, Ferretti A. Platelet-rich plasma versus focused shock waves in the treatment of jumper's knee in athletes. *Am J Sports Med*. 2013;41(4):795–803.
140. Moretti L, Maccagnano G, Coviello M, et al. Platelet rich plasma injections for knee osteoarthritis treatment: a prospective clinical study. *J Clin Med*. 2022;11(9):2640.
141. Bauer TW, Muschler GF. Bone graft materials. An overview of the basic science. *Clin Orthop Relat Res*. 2000;371:10–27.
142. Andersen C, Wragg NM, Shariatzadeh M, Wilson SL. The use of platelet-rich plasma (PRP) for the management of non-union fractures. *Curr Osteoporos Rep*. 2021;19(1):1–14.
143. Vilchez-Cavazos F, Millán-Alanís JM, Blázquez-Saldaña J, et al. Comparison of the clinical effectiveness of single versus multiple injections of platelet-rich plasma in the treatment of knee osteoarthritis: a systematic review and meta-analysis. *Orthop J Sports Med*. 2019;7(12):2325967119887116.
144. Zumwalt M, Reddy AP. Stem cells for treatment of musculoskeletal conditions–orthopaedic/sports medicine applications. *Biochim Biophys Acta Mol Basis Dis*. 2020;1866(4):165624.
145. Scala P, Rehak L, Giudice V, et al. Stem cell and macrophage roles in skeletal muscle regenerative medicine. *Int J Mol Sci*. 2021;22(19):10867.
146. Yu H, Cheng J, Shi W, et al. Bone marrow mesenchymal stem cell-derived exosomes promote tendon regeneration by facilitating the proliferation and migration of endogenous tendon stem/progenitor cells. *Acta Biomater*. 2020;106:328–341.
147. Ebrahimi A, Ahmadi H, Pourfraidon Ghasrodashti Z, et al. Therapeutic effects of stem cells in different body systems, a novel method that is yet to gain trust: a comprehensive review. *Bosn J Basic Med Sci*. 2021;21(6):672–701.
148. Nischal N, Gupta S, Lal K, Singh JP. Performance evaluation of high-resolution ultrasound versus magnetic resonance imaging in diagnosing peripheral nerve pathologies. *Indian J Radiol Imaging*. 2021;31(1):43–48.
149. Cho CH, Min BW, Bae KC, Lee KJ, Kim DH. A prospective double-blind randomized trial on ultrasound-guided versus blind intra-articular corticosteroid injections for primary frozen shoulder. *Bone Joint J*. 2021;103-B(2):353–359.
150. Alfredson H. Ultrasound and Doppler-guided mini-surgery to treat mid-portion achilles tendinosis: results of a large material and a randomised study comparing two scraping techniques. *Br J Sports Med*. 2011;45(5):407–410.
151. Filardo G, Matteo BD, Kon E, Merli G, Marcacci M. Platelet-rich plasma in tendon-related disorders: results and indications. *Knee Surg Sports Traumatol Arthrosc*. 2018;26(7):1984–1999.
152. Lam KHS, Hung CY, Chiang YP, et al. Ultrasound-guided nerve hydrodissection for pain management: rationale, methods, current literature, and theoretical mechanisms. *J Pain Res*. 2020;13:1957–1968.
153. Lam KHS, Reeves KD, Cheng A. Transition from deep regional blocks toward deep nerve hydrodissection in the upper body and torso: method description and results from a retrospective chart review of the anaglesic effect of 5% dextrose water as the primary hydrodissection injectate to enhance safety. *Biomed Res Int*. 2017:2017:7920438.
154. Buntragulpoontawee M, Chang KV, Vitoonpong T, et al. The effectiveness and safety of commonly used injectates for ultrasound-guided hydrodissection treatment of peripheral nerve entrapment syndromes: a systematic review. *Front Pharmacol*. 2021;11:621150.
155. Kuchera ML, Kuchera WA. *Osteopathic Considerations in Systemic Dysfunction*. 2nd ed. Greyden Press; 1994.

88 An Osteopathic Approach to the Exercise Prescription

NATALIE HYPPOLITE ▪ MALINDA HANSEN

KEY CONCEPTS

- The osteopathic approach to the exercise prescription encompasses the four osteopathic tenants, emphasizes patient education, empowers individuals to take an active role in their health, takes into consideration patient well-being, and tailors the exercise prescription to the individual.
- Exercise is a key component to maintaining good physical and biopsychological health, is beneficial for host immune defense, and is associated with a reduction in abdominal and visceral fat.
- Healthy adults, ages 18 to 65, should participate in a minimum of 30 minutes of exercise 5 days a week, or vigorous intensity aerobic activity for a minimum of 20 minutes per day 3 days per week.
- Types of exercise include aerobic (HIIT, endurance training, resistance, flexibility and stretching, balance and stability exercises, functional training), rehabilitation exercises, group fitness classes, recreational physical activity, and mind–body practices.
- Osteopathic physicians perform osteopathic structural exams and functional assessments to evaluate a patient's movement patterns, flexibility, posture, and musculoskeletal function.
- Building an exercise prescription may include the FITT principle (frequency, intensity, time and type of exercise), engagement and goal-setting to help attain patient buy-in to beginning an exercise program, and should include aerobic physical activity, muscle strengthening, mobility, flexibility exercises, and balance training.
- Exercise prescriptions are most effective when they utilize the principle of progression (the process of gradually advancing the training), and regular follow-up office visits.
- Wearable fitness technology allows patients to monitor and track various aspects of their physical activity and health such as steps taking, distance traveled, heart rate, sleep quality, intensity of activity, and calories burned.
- AI, virtual reality, and gamification of AI exercises have helped promote more regular engagement in exercise.
- There are many online resources and apps that can help encourage physical activity and can be useful in designing an exercise prescription tailored to the specific patient.

INTRODUCTION

When it comes to exercise and physical activity, the osteopathic approach encompasses several key principles:

- Osteopathic physicians view the body as a dynamic and interconnected system, recognizing that structural, biomechanical, and functional factors are interrelated. This holistic perspective considers not only the musculoskeletal system but also the impact of exercise on other systems, such as the cardiovascular, respiratory, and nervous systems.[1]
- Osteopathic physicians assess each patient's unique needs, health status, and medical history when recommending exercise and physical activity. This individualized approach helps tailor exercise programs to address specific health goals, conditions, and limitations.
- Osteopathic physicians often prescribe exercise as a preventive measure to reduce the risk of chronic diseases, improve overall health, and enhance well-being.[1,2]

Exercise is a key component in maintaining good physical and biopsychological health. All exercise is considered physical activity, but the reverse is not always necessarily true. Benefits of any form of exercise or physical activity nearly always outweigh the risks.[3] Some of the better known, evidence-backed benefits of physical activity include, but are not limited to, improved cognitive function and brain health, reducing risk of fall-related injuries, improving quality of life, and decreased risk of mortality.

When considering health care costs, the United States exceeds $100 billion yearly to treat chronic illness that would otherwise be positively affected by reaching the recommended amounts of physical activity.[3] An Osteopathic-minded approach to exercise is uniquely positioned to have a great impact on the way exercise is prescribed by applying the tenets of osteopathy: the person is a unit of body, mind, and spirit, the body is capable of self-healing, structure and function are reciprocally interrelated, and rational treatment, including an exercise prescription, is based on the understanding of the three aforementioned principles (see Table 88.1).[1–3]

HISTORY OF EXERCISE

The original Greek term *gumnazo* (exercise) and *gumnos* (naked or loin-clothed) gave rise to the very word "gymnasium." Taken literally, the word means naked exercise, which, at the time, was a mixture between a university and municipal gym. Participants only could bathe, get massages, exercise, and even attend lectures from philosophy greats such as Plato or Aristotle.[4–7]

There are records in history between the Roman and Persian empires, of gymnasiums and *Zurkhaneh* (Persian meaning "house of strength"), respectively. Since then, worldwide colonization has only expanded the evolution of exercise.

There are innumerable ways to engage the aerobic and anaerobic mechanisms and strengthen the musculoskeletal system. From

TABLE 88.1

Osteopathic Tenets and Their Correlation to Exercise Prescription[5,7,8]

Osteopathic Tenet	Relation to Exercise Prescription
The person is a unit of body, mind, and spirit.	Exercise should involve a combination of movements which challenge all the major components of the neuromusculoskeletal system through aerobic, anaerobic, and strengthening mechanisms.
The body is capable of self-regulation, self-healing, and health maintenance.	Recovery from exercise both during a session and on rest days is important in maintaining a sense of homeostasis and achieving fitness goals.
Structure and function are reciprocally interrelated.	Creating and performing functional movements, while preventing injury is a central aspect of any exercise training program.
Rational treatment is based on the understanding of the connection of the above tenets.	Exercise prescription can be tailored to each individual and adjusted as needed in the event injury arises.

Measel JW Jr. The effect of the lymphatic pump on the immune response: I. Preliminary studies on the antibody response to pneumococcal polysaccharide assayed by bacterial agglutination and passive hemagglutination. *J Am Osteopath Assoc.* 1982;82(1):28–31.

body weight to kettlebells, resistance bands to Olympic lifting, the human system is designed to respond to the demand placed upon it.

The oldest forms of exercise are walking, jogging, and running.[8] The first marathon commemorated the run of a Greek herald, Pheidippides, from a battlefield near the town of Marathon, Greece, to Athens in 490 BC to announce the defeat of the Persians.[8,9] Elite forms of intensive exercise developed into what would later become the Olympic Games where athletes would train for 10 months leading up to the event.[10] The games were overseen by an interdisciplinary team lead by a physician, *gymnaste,* and accompanied by a *paidotribes* and *alepite,* a masseuse and bathing attendant, respectively.[10] This structure laid the framework of the modern-day Sports Medicine team. Herodicus, the father of sports medicine and Hippocrates' mentor and teacher, was the most lauded of the *gymanstes* and is credited for his holistic approach to care of the athletes including incorporation of rehabilitative modalities, diet, and nutrition, paralleling some of the aspects of osteopathic care of patients.[9–11]

After a 25-century hiatus following dissolution in 394 AD, the modern Olympic Games, known as the Athens 1896 Summer Olympics, took place in Athens, Greece, and featured athletes from 14 nations participating in 43 events across nine sports.[10] The Olympics have seen numerous memorable moments, including Jesse Owens' four gold medals in 1936, the Miracle on Ice in ice hockey in 1980, and the return of South Africa to the Olympics in 1992.[10,12]

Olympic creed, coined by Coubertin (the developer of the modern Olympic games), states, "The most important thing in the Olympic Games is not to win but to take part, just as the most important thing in life is not the triumph but the struggle." This quote is also symbolic of the role of exercise prescription in attempt to help patients take part in the journey of improving a component of their well-being through physical activity, regardless of their initial training abilities.

EXERCISE PHYSIOLOGY

Energetics and skeletal muscle metabolism revolve around the making of adenosine triphosphate (ATP) which is generated by the combustion of carbohydrates, fats, and proteins. ATP drives the synthesis of cellular components, muscle contraction, active transport across membranes, glandular secretion, and nerve conduction.[13,14] It is important to understand that the metabolic demand created by activity or exercise acts in a continuum dependent on intensity and duration.

During exercise, the supply of ATP is essential to maintain the ongoing contractile action of muscles. For most vertebrates, there are two ATP generating systems, glycolysis and oxidative phosphorylation. During very intense efforts lasting seconds (throws, jumps, 100 m sprints) or intermittent game activities and field sports, most ATP is obtained from the breakdown of phosphocreatine (PCr) and glycogen to lactate. After the exercise extends beyond approximately 1 to 2 minutes, oxidative phosphorylation is the major ATP-generating pathway, and intramuscular glycogen is the dominant fuel source. In events or activities lasting several minutes to hours, the oxidative metabolism of carbohydrate (CHO) and fat provides almost all the ATP for contracting muscles.[15–21] See Figure 88.1.[22]

ANAEROBIC METABOLISM

Glycolysis does not require oxygen and has lactate (La-) as its byproduct because the equilibrium of the lactate dehydrogenase

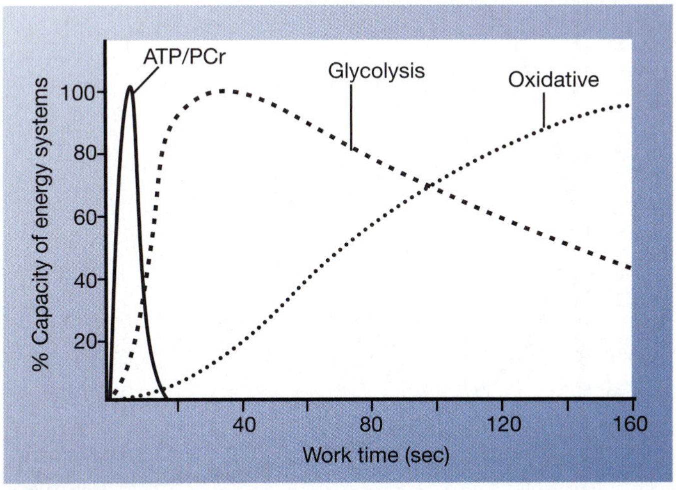

Figure 88.1. Energetics and skeletal muscle metabolism.[1] This figure depicts the actions and interactions of the ATP–PCr, glycolytic, and oxidative metabolic pathways. High-intensity, brief-duration exercise is fueled by the ATP–PCr pathway, whereas high-intensity, short-duration exercise relies on the glycolytic pathway, both of which are anaerobic. The aerobic oxidative pathway provides energy for muscular contraction during prolonged exercise of low to moderate intensity. (Reprinted with permission from O'Connell D, Bezner J. Principles of aerobic conditioning and cardiac rehabilitation. In: Bandy WD, Sanders B, eds. *Therapeutic Exercise for Physical Therapist Assistants.* 3rd ed. Wolters Kluwer Health/Lippincott Williams & Wilkins; 2013:303. Figure 13-1.[19])

reaction is markedly in favor of La-. Lactate is an immediate reservoir supplying pyruvate to mitochondria for complete oxidative combustion. Therefore, lactate stands at the intersection of anaerobic and aerobic metabolism of carbohydrate fuel.[23,24] For years, lactate was thought to be the consequence of oxygen deficiency in contracting skeletal muscle. We now know that the L-enantiomer of the lactate anion is formed under fully aerobic conditions and is utilized continuously in diverse cells, tissues, organs, and at the whole-body level.[24,25] It has been shown that lactate metabolism fulfills at least three functions. It is:

1. A major energy source
2. The major gluconeogenic precursor
3. A signaling molecule with autocrine-, paracrine-, and endocrine-like effects, and is referred to as a "lactormone"[23,25]

Exercise that incorporates anaerobic metabolism can include sprinting, high-intensity interval training, circuit training with or without weights, super-slow resistance training (RT), and any exercise that is at maximal or near-maximal effort.

AEROBIC METABOLISM

In oxidative phosphorylation, the muscles still rely on anaerobic energy for the initial 1 to 2 minutes, but then aerobic metabolism dominates (see Figure 88.2). The respiratory, or electron transport chain in the mitochondria requires reducing the equivalents in the forms of nicotinamide adenine dinucleotide (NADH) and flavin adenine dinucleotide (FADH), free ADP, inorganic phosphate (P_i), and O_2.[13,14,17,26–28] The cardiorespiratory system keeps the delivery of O_2 to contracting muscles, and the by-products of ATP breakdown in the cytoplasm (ADP and P_i) are transported back

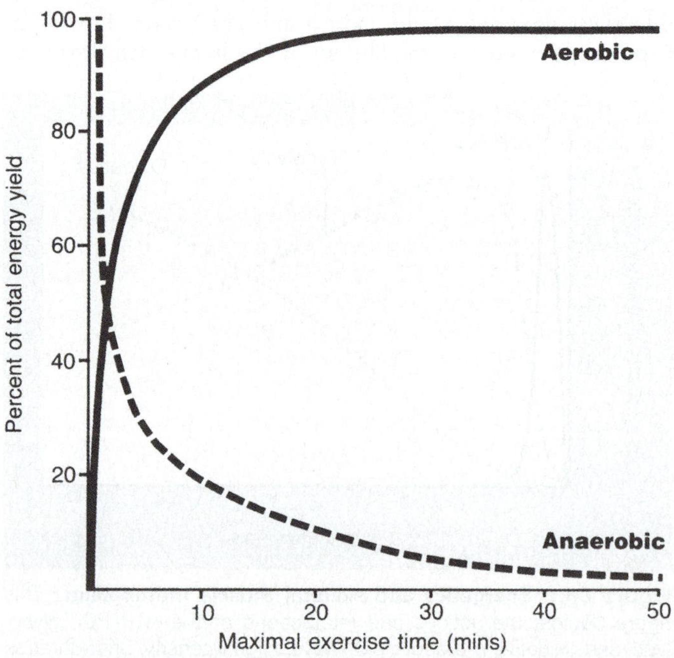

Figure 88.2. Aerobic and anaerobic metabolism.[2] In intense activities lasting 1.5 to 2.0 minutes, the ATP–CP and lactic acid energy systems generate approximately 50% of the energy, and aerobic metabolism supplies the remainder. A distance runner, on the other hand, derives essentially 98% of their energy from aerobic metabolism during a 50-minute training run.[29] (Licciardone JC, Schultz MJ, Amen B. Osteopathic manipulation in the management of chronic pain: current perspectives. *J Pain Res.* 2020;13: 1839–1847.)

TABLE 88.2

ATP Utilization and Resynthesis

ATP utilization	ATP + H_2O → ADP + P_i + H^+ ($\Delta G^{\circ\prime}$ = −6.3 kcal mol^{-1})
ATP resynthesis	**Substrate-level phosphorylation** PCr + ADP + H^+ → + Creatine 2 ADP → ATP + AMP Glycogen$_n$[a] + 3 ADP + 3 P_i a glycogen$_{n-1}$ + 2 lactate + 3 ATP **Oxidative phosphorylation** Glucose + 6 O_2 + 36 ADP → 6 H_2O + 36 ATP[b,c] Palmitate + 23 O_2 + 130 ADP → 16 CO_2 + 16 H_2O + 130 ATP[b,c]

[a] Muscle glycogen is the primary carbohydrate (CHO) source during intense exercise. Glycogen*n* is a glycogen polymer of *n* glucose residues.

[b] The total ATP yield includes that from substrate-level phosphorylation in glycolysis and the TCA cycle.

[c] ATP yields reported are based on the traditionally used value of 3 ATP per NADH, but if the more contemporary values of 2 or 3 ATP per NADH were used, the actual ATP yields would be lower; however, the relative contributions of glucose and palmitate to overall ATP generation remain the same.[9]

into the mitochondria for ATP resynthesis (see Table 88.2). Inside the mitochondria, the tricarboxylic acid (TCA) cycle produces the reducing equivalents and accepts acetyl-CoA, mainly from carbohydrates and fats.[13,14,28] Once inside the mitochondria, fat enters the β-oxidation pathway which produces acetyl-CoA and reducing equivalents NADH and FADH. The long-chain nature of fatty acids result is in generation of large amounts of ATP.[13,14,17,26,28,29] See Figure 88.3.[29]

HOW TO CALCULATE EXERCISE INTENSITY

According the 2018 exercise recommendations from the American College of Sports Medicine (ACSM) and the Centers for Disease Control (CDC), all healthy adults aged 18 to 65 should participate in moderate-intensity aerobic physical activity for a minimum of 30 minutes on 5 days per week or vigorous intensity aerobic activity for a minimum of 20 minutes on 3 days per week (see Table 88.3).[3] The BORG scale of perceived exertion is a useful and popular tool for patients to calculate their exercise efforts.[31] More detailed information per age group and medical categorization can be found in Table 88.4[3,33] below. The CDC and ACSM also encourage adults to perform activities that maintain or increase muscular strength and endurance for a minimum of 2 days per week.[3] In 2016, the CDC gathered data that showed that less than 30% of American adults and 20% of adolescents meet the criteria of achieving weekly recommended aerobic activity and muscle-strengthening exercise.[3] More recently, vigorous intermittent lifestyle physical activity (VILPA) was shown to decrease all cause and cancer mortality by 38% to 40% and 48% to 49% reduction in CVD mortality risk in as little as 1 to 2 minutes of vigorous exercise per day.[32] See Figure 88.4.[31]

Intensity and Metabolic Equivalents of Energy (METs)[3,33]

- Light = <3 METs of energy—"non-sedentary, waking behavior" (i.e., walking <2 mph, light chores such as washing dishes or vacuuming)
- Moderate = Three <6 METs—walking 2.5 mph up to 4 mph, chores like raking yard

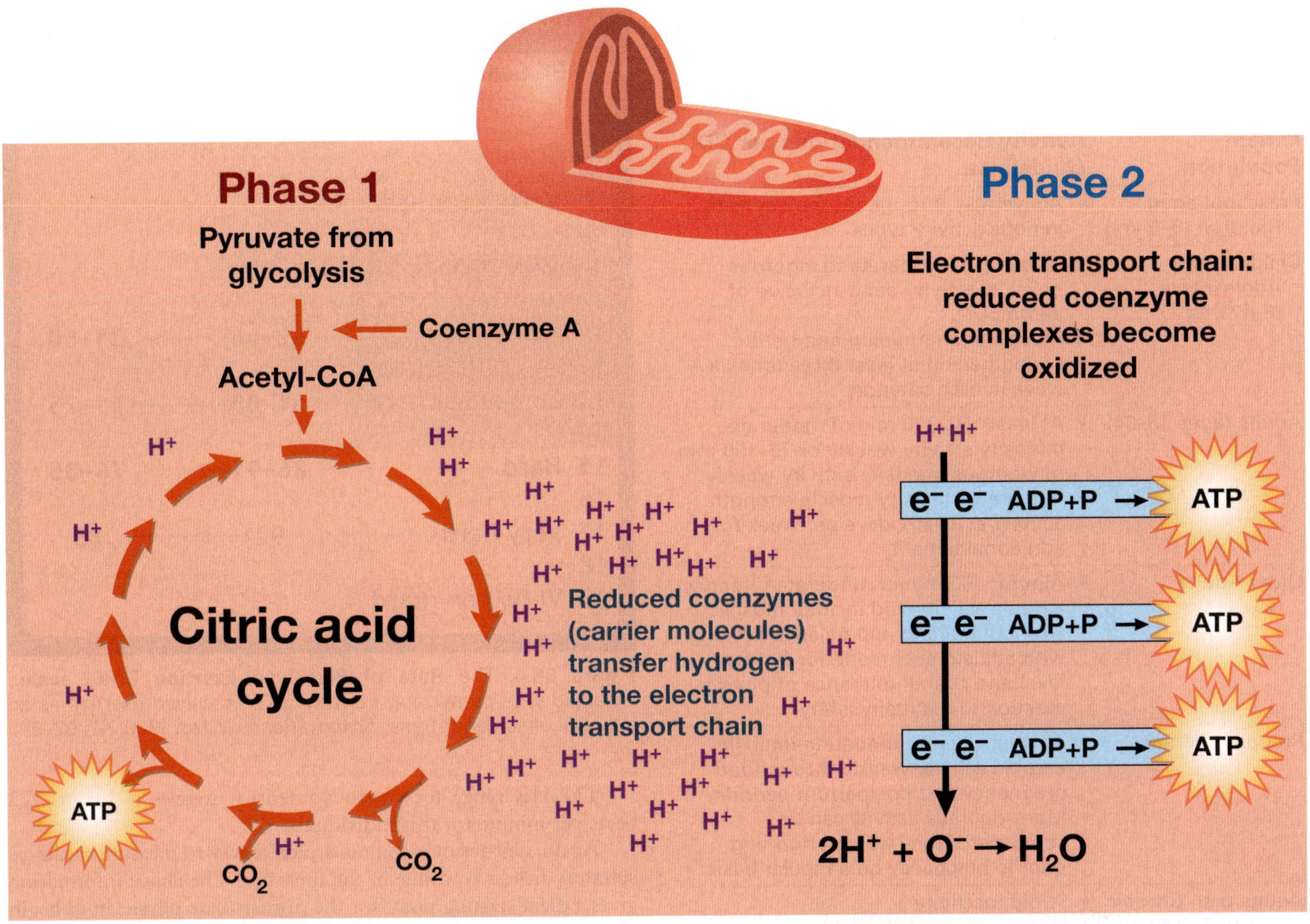

Figure 88.3. Energy metabolism in skeletal muscle.[3] Phase 1: In the mitochondria, the citric acid cycle generates hydrogen atoms during acetyl-CoA breakdown. Phase 2: Significant quantities of ATP regenerate when these hydrogen atoms oxidize via the aerobic process of electron transport–oxidative phosphorylation (electron transport chain).[30] (Reprinted with permission from McArdle WD, Katch FI, Katch VL. *Sports and Exercise Nutrition*. 4th ed. Wolters Kluwer Health/Lippincott Williams & Wilkins; 2013.)

- Vigorous = 6 METs+—jogging, running, carrying heavy groceries upstairs, snow shoveling, high-intensity interval training (HIIT) fitness class

Calculating the correct intensity for an individual has been a source of research and debate for decades. Safety considerations should include a discussion explaining potential risks given the patient's health status. Gradual increases of exercise will build a foundational tolerance versus accelerating a program too quickly which may lead to injury. If an activity or sport requires certain

TABLE 88.3

Exercise Intensities and Their Respective Fuel Sources[2]

Low intensity	≤50% VO_2 max utilizes fat oxidation
Moderate intensity	50–75% VO_2 max utilizes a combination of fat and CHO
Highly aerobic	75–100% VO_2 max utilizes CHO
Anaerobic	Considered % VO_2 max above 100% utilizes CHO

Licciardone JC, Schultz MJ, Amen B. Osteopathic manipulation in the management of chronic pain: current perspectives. *J Pain Res.* 2020;13:1839–1847.

equipment or gear, knowing how to properly use the gear, as well as understanding the key rules and regulation of that sport, will contribute to making the activity safer, as a form of exercise.

The ACSM has done research since the 1990s on cardiorespiratory fitness. They have created an equivalency between VO_2 max and maximal heart rate (HR) values.[29] The gold standard is a comprehensive VO_2 max test. These formulas are also very helpful for exercise prescription for an individual wanting to improve their health. There are several equations for determining maximum heart rate (HR max), some of which are more precise and aimed toward elite performing individuals. For most patients, HR max determined from the CDC's recommended equation will suffice in creating an exercise prescription.

The average primary care physician's office or group practice does not have the equipment or training in exercise physiology to perform a test for maximal oxygen consumption (i.e., VO_2 max testing). If needed, patients may be referred to a Primary Care Sports Medicine Specialist or Sports Performance Academic Center for VO_2 max testing, or physicians may use ACSM target HR zone calculations as shown in Table 88.5.[29]

ACSM TARGET HEART RATES CALCULATION

Swain et al. equation: % HR max = 0.64 × % VO_2 max + 37[34]
Miller et al. formula: HR max = 217 – (0.85 × age)[35]

TABLE 88.4

CDC Exercise Recommendations for Specific Populations

Patient Population	Activity Recommendations per CDC Guidelines
Preschool-aged Children (3–5 yrs)	• Active play throughout the day with various activity types
Children and Adolescents (6–17 yrs)	• 60 min + of moderate to vigorous physical activity daily inclusive of aerobic • Muscle-strengthening and bone-strengthening at least three times a week in each category
Adults (ages 18–64)	• At least 150–300 min of moderate-intensity activity weekly or 75–150 min of vigorous intensity activity weekly • Moderate-intensity muscle strength activity at least 2 days per week for additional benefit
Older Adults (65+ yrs)	• Aim for 150 min of moderate-intensity aerobic activity and include muscle strength training and balance training with adjustments made for fitness level and overall tolerance of physical exertion to maintain safety
Pregnant Persons	• At least 150 min moderate-intensity aerobic activity weekly throughout pregnancy and postpartum periods • More vigorous activity can be conducted if they were performing prior to pregnancy on a regular basis
Adults with Chronic Health Condition and/or Disabilities	• Avoid inactivity • If able, at least 150–300 min of moderate intensity, or 75–150 min of vigorous intensity, or a combination of the two if able • If able, include 2 or more days of muscle-strengthening a week

The CDC uses the following guidelines to calculate target HRs[36]:

- Moderate physical activity has a target HR range of 64% to 76% of HR max.
- Vigorous physical activity has a target HR range of 77% to 93% of HR max.

HR max = 220 – age[36]
Example for a 50-year-old individual:

220 - 50 = 170 beats per minute max HR
64% level: 170 × 0.64 = 109 beats per minute
76% level: 170 × 0.76 = 129 beats per minute

So, the HR range for this individual for moderate-intensity exercise is 109 to 129 beats per minute.

The application of the same equation for vigorous activity is as follows.

Example for a 35-year-old individual:

Max HR = 220 - 35 = 185 beats per minute
185 × 0.77 = 142 beats per minute
185 × 0.93 = 172 beats per minute

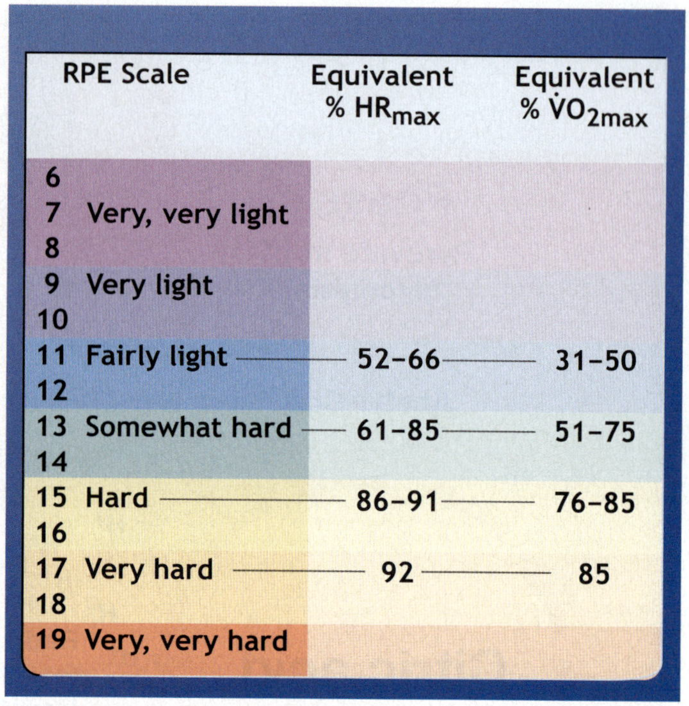

Figure 88.4. The Rate of Perceived Exertion (RPE) scale.[4] (Adapted with permission from Borg G. Perceived exertion as an indicator of somatic stress. *Scand J Rehabil Med.* 1970;2(2):92–98.)

The HR range for vigorous intensity exercise is 142 to 172 beats per minute for this individual.

Again, debates over the most precise way to measure cardiorespiratory fitness continue in the literature. The above information gives a great starting point for the primary care physician to begin the prescription of exercise.

EPIGENETICS

Epigenetics is the study of changes in genome function by any factor.[37,38] The adaptations are extremely complex, heritable, reversible, and influenced by genetic and environmental factors.[37,38] These include processes that influence gene expression without altering the DNA base sequence; specifically:

1. DNA methylation
2. Posttranslational modifications of histone proteins
3. Regulation of gene expression via specific mRNAs[37–40]

At the most basic level, it is the reason for phenotypic differences in otherwise genotypically related individuals and describes

TABLE 88.5

ACSM Target Heart Rate Zones[2]

Target intensity for health benefits	40% VO_2 max = 63% HR max
Target intensity for aerobic fitness	60–80% VO_2 max = 75–88% HR max
Target intensity for elite training	>85% VO_2 max = >92% HR max

Licciardone JC, Schultz MJ, Amen B. Osteopathic manipulation in the management of chronic pain: current perspectives. *J Pain Res.* 2020;13:1839–1847.

various phenomena in medical genetics including the explanation silencing of gene expression leading to genomic imprinting in conditions such as Prader–Willi syndrome and carcinogenesis.[39,40]

Exercise continually challenges whole-body homeostasis, leading to a variety of improvements in performance, cognitive function, immune health, and other health benefits.[41–45] Epigenetic factors regulate gene expression in a tissue-specific manner and represent a link between genotype and the environment.[38,46] It is also responsible for individual responses to different exercise training regimens and is one of the reasons why exercise prescription should be tailored to an individual.[41] Considerable research is being done to elucidate a better understanding of the "epigenetic response" to specific training stimuli.[47]

IMMUNOLOGIC EFFECTS OF EXERCISE

Exercise is known to exhibit anti-inflammatory effects with a single session leading to increases in IL-6 (anti-inflammatory myokine), without an increase in the proinflammatory cytokines TNF-α and IL-1β.[48] Regular bouts of short-lasting (up to 45 minutes) moderate-intensity exercise is beneficial for host immune defense, particularly in older individuals and people with chronic diseases.[49] Training is also associated with reduced activation of toll-like receptors (TLR) signaling and reductions in the abdominal and visceral fat, which can both lead to lower inflammation.[26,50] While a single session of exercise may represent a challenge for cell homeostasis, repeated physical exercise will improve immunosurveillance and immunocompetence.[51] Also, immune cells from the central nervous system will acquire an anti-inflammatory phenotype, protecting central functions from age-induced cognitive decline.[48,51,52] Regular exercise could reduce the risk of chronic metabolic and cardiorespiratory diseases. However, when in exercise is used in excess and without cycles of rest, these anti-inflammatory effects are also likely to be responsible for the suppressed immunity that makes our bodies more susceptible to infections.[49,51] Such intense and prolonged activities can include marathon running and extreme endurance events. Infection burden is reported to be higher among high-performance athletes and is one of the leading causes of lost training days in preparation for major sporting event, second only to injury; although currently this is a theory that is being challenged by researchers.[49,53] There is a key point of agreement, that infection susceptibility has a multifactorial underpinning, although the empirical research is lacking for full understanding of exercise immunology.

Recent studies have shown that acute exercise could reduce side effects from the flu vaccine in adults, especially in older populations, and lead to enhanced antibody responses in this population as well.[54,55] Physical activity has been shown to move lymphatics, and this corresponds well to osteopathic research showing improved antibody response secondary to lymphatic treatment.[56,57] Although there is more research to be completed in this regard, similar results have also been found in studies for the COVID-19 vaccine with moderate-intensity exercise.[58,59]

Other well-studied immunologic benefits of exercise include stress reduction, mood regulation through endorphin release.[60] Studies have shown mood improvements can be achieved with 10 to 30 minutes of moderate anaerobic exercise sessions mainly through the concept of neuroplasticity.[61] As a result of the above, it is important to balance exercise regimens with adequate periods of rest and recovery. With exercise prescriptions, this can be achieved by individualizing each prescription and training regimen to not chronically stress and overwhelm the body's homeostatic mechanisms, and by beginning with the patient's current state of physical health in mind.[61,62]

TYPES OF EXERCISE

Aerobic

A. **High-Intensity Intervals and Interval Training (HIIT)**

Interval training is not new and was studied extensively in the 1970s. It was demonstrated that the improvement of oxygen uptake after HIIT performed 2 days per week is not different from results achieved by training with the same interval regimen performed 4 days per week.[63]

In the early 2000s there was considerable research being done on the physiologic effects of HIIT. Many terms in the literature have been used for this type of intense exercise, such as "vigorous," "all out," "near exhaustion," or "supramaximal efforts." Essentially, HIIT incorporates short bursts of maximal effort exercise that can last from 20 to 240 seconds.[64] There has been no consensus on the exact parameters to define HIIT although exercise intensities are generally higher than 75% of the VO_2 max or peak power output (PPO).[65]

HIIT has been shown to have benefits in cardiorespiratory fitness, improve markers of vascular function in metabolic disorders, improve fasting glucose levels, reducing blood pressure in overweight or obese individuals, increase maximal oxygen uptake, increase mitochondrial biogenesis, angiogenesis, and an increased capacity for glucose and fatty acid oxidation.[18,66–70] HIIT also increases the activity of mitochondrial enzymes, aerobic exercise capacity, and is a time-efficient strategy to improve cardiorespiratory and metabolic health.[14,50,71,72] The aerobic improvements from HIIT are equal to that of traditional endurance exercise, but with the added benefit of improved muscle performance.[27]

Tabata training is one of the most energetically effective high-intensity intermittent training methods. It is training at the intensity that exhausts subjects during the seventh or eighth sets of 20 seconds exercise bouts with a 10-seconds rest between the exercise bouts.[73]

B. **Moderate-Intensity (MOD) Training**

MOD has also been researched and shown to be effective in reducing blood glucose levels, improved exercise capacity in heart failure with reduced ejection fraction (HFrEF), improved body composition in overweight adults, and improved cardiorespiratory fitness among children and adolescents.[63,66–70] Moderate-intensity continuous training is generally considered to be between 50% and 75% of VO_2 max or PPO.[67,74]

Given that both types of training have myriad benefits to the human system, HIIT training has been gaining popularity across the world for the comparable efficacy in a more time-efficient manner. There are many options available for programming including personal training sessions, small group classes, online instruction, and artificial intelligence (AI)–driven home exercise equipment, to name a few.

C. **Endurance Training**

Endurance training has been shown to have the greatest increases in VO_2 max compared to other forms of exercise and have also been shown to be a predictor of all-cause mortality and chronic disease.[75,76] However, varied responses between extent of VO_2 max increase in individuals participating in endurance training have been observed in the literature with the major contributing factor in this variability attributed to genetics and epigenetics, more specifically.[75] Activities which can be classified in this category of aerobic training include running, jogging, walking, dancing, biking, swimming, and jump roping to name a few. In the research realm, "trainability" is a term that has been used to describe variation on an individual level to gauge adaptative responses in endurance training.[75,77,78] When prescribing exercise with "trainability" in mind, there are certain modifiable and nonmodifiable factors to consider. Examples of modifiable factors that will aide in the individualization of a training program include activity type, intensity, and volume while adjusting for the nonmodifiable factors of age, genetics, and sex of an individual.

Anaerobic

A. **Resistance Training**

RT is a type of strength training that uses the resistance of free weights, body weight, resistance bands, machine weights, or any means which must be overcome by voluntary muscular effort.[79] Depending on the muscle contraction type, RT can be:

1. Concentric (muscle shortening)
2. Eccentric (muscle lengthening
3. Isometric (same length)[80]

The variables that govern RT are:

1. Exercise intensity
2. The number of repetitions and the number of sets
3. The duration of rest breaks between sets and repetitions[80,81]

RT has clear benefit in increasing muscle strength, function, and health parameters. There is much data on the benefits of RT in children, adolescents, adults, the elderly, postmenopausal women, poststroke, type 2 diabetes, and for increasing bone density.[82–91]

The overload principle of RT states that the load, intensity, type, or time of a workout must progressively increase to continue to make adaptations.[92] Considering Henneman's size principle, that during muscle contraction, motor units are recruited from smallest to largest in force production, studies have reinforced the overload principle repeatedly.[15,92–94] When sets are performed until volitional failure, neuromuscular fatigue necessitates increasing percentage recruitment of the motor unit pool, and through this mechanism, RT produces a meaningful drive for muscle strength and hypertrophy.[79,92,93,95,96]

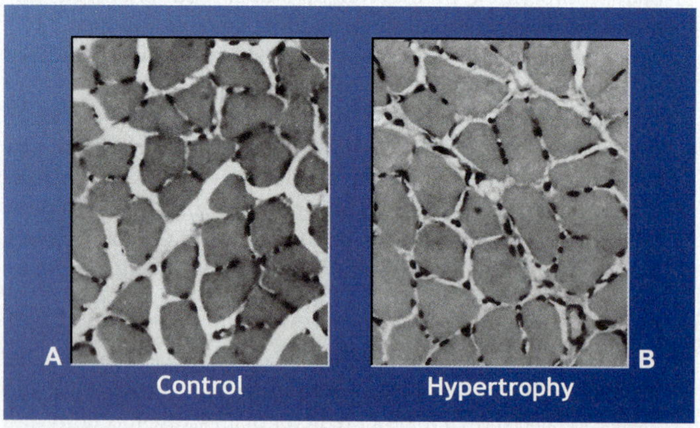

Figure 88.5. Muscle hypertrophy from resistance training.[4] Cross-sections of control and hypertrophied rat soleus muscles: (**A**) control (**left**) and (**B**) hypertrophied (**right**). The average diameter for 50 fibers of the hypertrophied muscle was 24% to 34% greater than for controls; the average number of nuclei in hypertrophied muscle averaged 40% to 52% greater than controls. (Reprinted with permission from Goldberg AL, Etlinger JD, Goldspink DF, Jablecki C. Mechanism of work-induced hypertrophy of skeletal muscle. *Med Sci Sports.* 1975;7(3):185–198. Copyright © 1975 The American College of Sports Medicine.)

TABLE 88.6

Examples of Types of Resistance Training[10–15]

Free weightlifting
Olympic weightlifting/power weightlifting
Machine weightlifting
Kettlebell weightlifting
Body weightlifting
Pilates
Yoga (muscle building style)
"Boot camp" style classes
Barre classes
Suspension training
Aquatic classes/training

As expected, untrained individuals have a greater window for adaptation than highly trained individuals and athletes.[97] See Figure 88.5.[31]

Examples of different types of RT (see Table 88.6)[81,88–90,95,98]

Examples of different types of RT equipment (see Table 88.7)[99]

B. **Flexibility and Stretching**

Flexibility exercises have been shown to maintain and improve joint range of motion in the general population, especially in the elderly.[100,101] When incorporated after aerobic activity or RT, they tend to be more effective, including dynamic stretching exercises.[102] Joint range of motion has been shown to improve after regular stretching or flexibility exercises when done two to three times per week for a period of 3 to 4 weeks.[100,101,103] Stretching can be incorporated in an active or passive manner depending on patient need and access to, or availability of, another individual such as a personal trainer for assistance. Many studies have looked at stretching on the hamstring group as it is one of the most injured areas of the body and has great implications on overall body posture, mobility and task performance.[102] One study showed improvement in sit and reach and popliteal angle testing in young adult recreational tennis players across all stretching groups which included static, ballistic, and contract-relax.[104] Generally, static stretching has been recommended to improve flexibility and seems to enhance performance, while dynamic stretching is recommended during warm up activities.[105]

C. **Balance and Stability Exercises**

In those at risk of falling, balance exercises have been shown to reduce falls and improve functional outcomes, especially in the elderly population.[100,106,107] These exercises should be closely

TABLE 88.7

Examples of Resistance Training Equipment[16]

Dumbbells
Barbells
Kettlebells
Weighted plates (iron or rubber)
Leg press/fixed squat rack (Smith machine)
Medicine balls
Rubber tubing/Exercise bands
Cables and pulley systems
Heavy ropes
Machine weights
Tires/sandbags
Body weight

Dashty M. A quick look at biochemistry: carbohydrate metabolism. *Clin Biochem.* 2013;46(15):1339–1352.

supervised at first, particularly in the untrained, or those at increased fall risk. Focus should also be placed on proprioception with the goal of maintaining a smaller base of support for a particular task while maintaining body control and minimizing excess movement[100,103]

Functional Training

Functional training is a form of physical activity that involves coordinated and multijoint movement patterns to improve overall mobility, functionality, and performance as it pertains to activities of daily living (ADLs).[108] ADLs include transferring, ambulation/mobility, bathing, dressing, toileting, and grooming. Typically, these movement patterns revolve around bending/hinging, squatting, pushing, pulling, and twisting movements. From a strength and RT perspective, these are executed in the form of bench press, deadlift, squat, shoulder press, and pull-up or lat pull down, otherwise known as the "Big 5."[108] Functional training has been shown to be beneficial in improving quality of life and mobility in older adults as well as those with COPD.[109] Gradually building upon different functional movement patterns that utilize bodyweight, and progress to weighted activities as capable, are key in obtaining maximal benefit regarding ADL efficiency.

Rehabilitation Exercises

It is a reasonable for patients with functional and mobility limitations, such as with ADLs, to partake in formalized physical therapy prior to beginning an individualized exercise prescription that incorporates other forms of physical activity.[100,103] Those also recovering from injuries or known neuromuscular imbalances could also benefit from incorporation of rehabilitative exercises as part of their physical activity regimen.

Group Fitness Classes

Group fitness classes come in many varieties and can focus on one form of physical activity such as yoga or be one of combined types of physical activities such as aerobic, HITT-style classes combined with TRX or another strength or RT modality. Most are also targeted for certain levels of physical fitness and can range from beginner to advanced. Prescribing group fitness should keep in mind some of the core components of exercise prescription including patient engagement and motivation, access, financial resources, current fitness level to name a few. Group exercise has been shown to decrease anxiety in a study of college-aged individuals.[110] Group classes also serve as a main point of socialization for many including the elderly. One study during the COVID-19 pandemic showed that real-time online physical exercise classes did not improve physical fitness among the elderly but did maintain overall physical fitness.[111]

Recreational Physical Activity

Recreational sports/physical activities have known, positive social, psychological, and physical impacts on those who partake.[112] They can also serve as stress reducers and mitigate risk of disease development. Finding activities of interest to patients may help in their motivation toward increasing physical activity and help them build a supportive network outside of their traditional environments and routines. Potential challenges that may arise in incorporating new, or consistent recreational physical activity are that often recreational activities require more perceived time than a patient may feel that they have, the activity of interest may not be available in their area or supported by geographic climate (i.e., mountain skiing in Florida), or there are financial constraints for the patient's activities of interest.

Mind–Body Practices

The concept of mindfulness incorporates three main components: intention, attention, and attitude. It allows the conscious to focus or be aware and acknowledge many aspects of existence including feelings, thoughts, and bodily sensations.[113] The act of mindfulness can be applied to many mind–body practices including different forms of meditation, guided imagery, stress reduction, and movement therapies. Mind–body practices can serve as a valuable adjunct to the exercise prescription particularly in the realms of stress reduction, pain reduction, and improvement of quality of life. Mindful movement is an umbrella for any combination of physical activity with a mindfulness practice, breath work, spiritual, or energy-generating practice.[114] Of the movement-based therapies, Tai chi, yoga, and Pilates are the most known and studied.

Tai chi is a martial art form with several subtypes that involve a series of slow movements coordinated with patterned or deep breathing. The ultimate goal is to promote unity and balance of the mind and body which is complementary of the osteopathic tenets. Studies have shown Tai chi's benefit in several common conditions including those of HTN, COPD, osteoarthritis, Parkinson disease, mental health disorders including depression and anxiety.[114–117] In osteoarthritis, Tai chi has been found to improve arthritic pain symptoms, stiffness, and decrease pain, while in Parkinson it has been shown to prevent falls, improve motor planning, and increase overall mobility.[114–116]

Yoga is a form of mindful movement that has also been around for centuries and incorporates a blend of balance, postural, strengthening, and stretching poses in combination with breath and meditative exercises. Like Tai chi and Pilates there are multiple subtypes. Yoga has been shown to have many positive effects on the autonomic nervous system with the resultant benefits of stress reduction, improved spinal mobility, pain reduction, and improved quality of life in many populations including those with cardiovascular disease.[114] Hatha, Yin, and Restorative style yoga are all relatively beginner-friendly and have a role in rehabilitative exercise and modalities for certain conditions such as low back pain in addition to serving as a good starting point for balance, flexibility, and stretching component of the exercise prescription.[114]

Pilates as mindful movement has a strong focus on core strengthening, control, and neuromuscular re-education which improves overall posture and body mechanics. Of the mind–body practices discussed, this form can include more specialized equipment compared to Tai chi and Yoga which both require an exercise mat at most. This is an important factor to take into consideration when prescribing exercise that goes beyond the mat. Studies have shown Pilates to be beneficial in decreasing fall risk, improving lung function, and exercise tolerance.[114,118]

Osteopathic Functional Assessment

Osteopathic physicians may perform structural exams and functional assessments to evaluate a patient's movement patterns, flexibility, posture, and musculoskeletal function. These assessments help identify areas of dysfunction or imbalance that may benefit from targeted exercise interventions.[1]

Osteopathic physicians determine if somatic dysfunction is present and, if significant, alter their recommendations of an exercise program, progression, gear, and rehabilitation accordingly. They can also incorporate OMT into their practice, which involves using the hands to diagnose, treat, and prevent musculoskeletal conditions. OMT may be used in conjunction with exercise to improve musculoskeletal function, reduce pain, and optimize mobility.[1]

BUILDING AN EXERCISE PRESCRIPTION

To date, much of the evidence surrounding individualized exercise prescription for musculoskeletal conditions has focused on one element of the process versus a more comprehensive evidence set that could better guide physicians and other clinicians in clinical practice.[119]

FITT Principle

FITT is a commonly used mnemonic for frequency, intensity, time, and type of exercise and is used to help design exercise prescriptions. The FITT principle is a fundamental framework used in physical fitness training and exercise science to create effective and personalized exercise programs.[103,120]

ENGAGEMENT, ASSESSMENT, AND GOAL SETTING

Patient engagement is critical to the success of any prescription, especially as it pertains to exercise which will require more motivational factors and effort than other traditional prescriptive modalities. It has even been recommended to add patient enjoyment within the framework of the FITT principle to allow for more ease of adherence by individuals.[120] Other factors to consider when prescribing exercise include age, health conditions, safety, including physical environment in which activity is to take place, cost, equipment, or other resources needed (i.e., gym membership, special shoes, or eyewear).

Some key questions to engage patients in discussion include:

- What are their specific goals (i.e., performance, weight loss, appearance, general health)?
- What is their past medical history (including injuries) and surgical history?
- How much time daily, or weekly, would they be able to carve out for exercise on a regular basis?
- Are there any activities they are currently, or previously, engaged in that they did, or did not, enjoy?
- What type of environmental resources do they have available to them (i.e., safe place to walk/jog/run, gym membership, personal trainer, home equipment, pool access)?

After attaining patient buy-in to beginning an exercise program, their baseline level of fitness needs to be well understood. One place to start is to gauge how close to achieving recommended guideline levels of activity for their age group and medical conditions, if present, they are as well as focusing on activities they are already able to perform.[103] Below are general categorizations suggested by the CDC that can be used to do so[3,33]:

- **Inactive**—Does not get any activity beyond basic daily life activities
- **Insufficiently active**—Doing some moderate-to-vigorous activity but not meeting the recommended guidelines
- **Active**—Gets the equivalent of the recommended activity guidelines
- **Highly active**—Exceeds the 300 minutes of moderate-intensity activity each week

A thorough exercise prescription will include aerobic physical activity, muscle-strengthening activity, mobility, and balance training. Each will take into consideration the current level of physical activity and build gradually from there. This will be inclusive of delineating the amount of time, intensity, frequency, sets, and repetitions dedicated to each respective component. The prescription plan should start off simple to ensure maximum health benefits, safety, and patient compliance.

Sample weekly exercise prescription for an adult individual with no significant co-morbidities who is insufficiently active (see Table 88.8)[3,29,33]:

TABLE 88.8

Weekly Training Program Example for Insufficiently Active Person[2,5,6]

Day 1	Day 2	Day 3	Day 4	Day 5
Flexibility: Shoulder ROM—10 min	**Flexibility:** Hip ROM—10 min and foam rolling bilateral lower extremities	**Flexibility:** Total body yoga stretches—15 min	**Flexibility:** Cervical and Thoracic spine ROM—20 min	**Flexibility:** Lumbar spine ROM—15 min
Aerobic: 35 min walk (2.5–4 mph pace)	**Aerobic:** 20 min cycling on stationary bike or road bike	**Aerobic:** 40 min walk (2.5–4 mph pace)	**Aerobic** 30 min elliptical machine (level 1–2)	**Aerobic:** 30 min fitness class
Strength: Small arm circles—90 s each direction Dumbbell lateral raises—3 sets of 10* Dumbbell chest press—3 sets of 10*	**Strength:** Resistance band leg extensions—3 sets of 10 each leg Body weight squats—3 sets of 10	**Strength:** 1 min plank hold 20 abdominal crunches 20 jumping jacks	**Strength:** Small arm circles—90 s each direction Dumbbell lateral raises—3 sets of 10* Dumbbell chest press—3 sets of 10*	**Strength:** Resistance band clam shells—2 sets of 12 each leg Body weight calf raises—3 sets of 12

*Using light 3–8 lb weights depending on experience with resistance training.

Note: Days 6 and 7 would be rest days which do not have to be consecutive.[3,29,33]

Licciardone JC, Schultz MJ, Amen B. Osteopathic manipulation in the management of chronic pain: current perspectives. *J Pain Res.* 2020;13: 1839–1847.

Desai P, Williams AG Jr, Prajapati P, Downey HF. Lymph flow in instrumented dogs varies with exercise intensity. *Lymphat Res Biol.* 2010;8(3): 143–148.

Progression

Progression is considered a core principle of exercise prescription and is used to gradually advance the training stimulus to overload a specific target for further training benefits or to take place.[119] Cardiac rehabilitation is an area where aerobic exercise progression is well established based on certain cardiorespiratory performance metrics, particularly in an outpatient setting.[121,122] In the general population, the decision to progress will be based part on patient feedback and part with different assessment tools and techniques. Examples of such, include the DeLorme and Oxford techniques in RT progression. Both aim to improve strength at a 10-repetition maximum, with the DeLorme escalating the weight amount until 10 reps achieved and Oxford decreasing the weight amount starting at the 10-repetition maximum.[119,123] In the literature, progression has also referred to progression of motor learning principles of cognitive, associative, and autonomous stages which also correlate to muscular adaptations within the novice, advanced, and expert stages of executing a particular task or exercise type.[119]

MONITORING AND EVALUATION

Individualized exercise prescription should include a plan for follow-up and monitoring of progress. The follow-up plan after first initiating a new exercise prescription may occur in shorter intervals in the beginning (i.e., every 8 weeks), especially for beginners and then space out as the patient progresses and is able to tolerate higher levels of activity. There is no specific guideline on how or what intervals this should be carried out in the current literature. It may be possible to use combined methods to achieve this including periodic log reviews of patient activities, dedicated office-based appointments, virtual appointments, and review of mobile app physical activity tracker data.

Patients should be educated on safety and form as it pertains to the type of activity they will be engaging in at the start of the exercise prescription. This topic should be revisited as they progress. They should also receive education on signs of increased stress or overuse so that potential injuries can be avoided or addressed early on.

ADAPTATIONS FOR MEDICAL CONDITIONS

Lee et al. have outlined recommendations for specific medical conditions in adults based off evidence support. These are summarized in Table 88.9.[100]

TABLE 88.9

Exercise Recommendations for Specific Medical Conditions

Medical Condition	Evidence-Backed Activity Recommendations
Cardiovascular Disease	• Stress testing only recommended prior to participation in vigorous activity in those with known CVD • Exercise to pain tolerance in those with peripheral vascular disease
Diabetes Mellitus	• Moderate–vigorous aerobic training at least 3 times per week (nonconsecutive days) and resistance training at least 2 times per week (nonconsecutive days) • Decrease insulin dosage pre-exercise when glucose levels are less than 100 mg/dL
Musculoskeletal conditions including arthritis	• Aquatic or land based aerobic activity 3–5 times per week • Resistance training 2–3 times per week
Obesity	• Aerobic exercise that increases energy expenditure • Resistance training to maintain bone health and lean muscle
Osteoporosis	• Balance training for fall prevention • Resistance training • Can incorporate HIIT type aerobic exercise
Pulmonary Disease	• Pulmonary rehabilitation exercise training program for 6–12 wk

Adapted from Lee PG, Jackson EA, Richardson CR. Exercise prescriptions in older adults. *Am Fam Physician*. 2017;95(7):425–432.[100]

Utilizing Technology for Exercise

A. **Wearable Fitness Technology**

Wearable fitness technology, often referred to as fitness wearables, or simply wearables, refers to electronic devices and accessories that individuals can wear to monitor and track various aspects of their physical activity, health, and wellness including steps taken, distance traveled on foot, sleep quality, HR, HR variability, ECG monitoring, intensity of activity, calories burned during physical activity, body temperature monitoring, ovulation, and other aspects of the menstrual cycle. Globally, the use of wearable activity-trackers has increased tremendously in the past decade. This market, reported to be approximately $2.8 billion in 2020, has been incorporated into the medical community as helpful technology.[124] Activity trackers appear to be effective at increasing physical activity in a variety of age groups and clinical and nonclinical populations. The benefit is clinically important especially when sustained over time. Wearable devices, such as Apple Watch, Fitbit, and Whoop band, to name a few, have been studied more than home AI programs. Based on the studies evaluated, there is sufficient evidence to recommend the use of activity trackers.[125] Most studies available have focused on validation of HR sensors, ECG monitoring, and exercise intensities while wearing such devices. The mechanism of such monitoring is conducted via photoplethysmography which is a noninvasive method of continuous vital sign tracking. The Oura Ring, Apple Watch, and Fitbit all use this technology to obtain an individual's health metrics and some studies have shown promising work in validating the accuracy of HR, HRV, and other nocturnal sleep metrics in the Oura ring, in particular.[126] Several studies have found the Apple Watch HR monitoring to be most valid with walking with decreases noted with jogging and running.[127–129] Similar decreases in the validity of HR and ECG measurements (as measured by FitBit) were noted with increased physical activity intensity.[127] Exercise intensity measurement by wearables have also been shown to be overestimated at moderate and high intensities in certain studies of general population and cardiac subpopulations.[129–131]

Using wearable technology overall has been shown to be beneficial for knowing the general parameters of training goals and target zones for exercise.[125,132] There is also evidence to support that use of wearables or other technology that integrates into an app increases exercise adherence of home-based programs in a manner that is feasible and user friendly in the general population, elderly, and certain medical conditions such as osteoarthritis.[133–136] A modern-day application of smartphone integration with wearables for objective physical health monitoring are through wellness programs sponsored by employers or a patient's insurance company.[137] Many of these programs are incentivized in some way (i.e., time-off accrual, cash prizes, lowered premiums) and also typically involve monitoring of patient biometric studies such as lipid panels and hemoglobin A1c. Research in this area is still in its relative infancy and more is needed in order to be able to make recommendations for specific wearables both at an individual level and specific medical condition subpopulations. Patient preference, budget, and data of interest should be taken into consideration when discussing wearables as a possible tool to utilize in their exercise prescription.

B. **Artificial Intelligence and Home Exercise Systems**

AI has increasingly been integrated into home exercise and fitness programs which was especially notable during the COVID-19 pandemic. It has allowed for the enhancement of effective and personalized workouts. Examples of popular AI home systems include: Fiture, Tempo Move, OxeFit, YogiFi Smart Mat, JRNY, Carol, Tonal, Exer, FORME, and Hydrow, just to name a few. The data is limited as some of this technology was introduced to the market in 2020–2021. AI chat-boxes have also been used as AI tools for exercise technology and have shown to be beneficial by helping write personalized exercise prescriptions that are tailored to the likes and interests of the individual.[138,139]

AI technology has allowed for the development of many complex algorithmic features which can help individuals progress through a training program gradually and safely according to their goals while enhancing exercise volume.[140] Some popular features that exist across various AI platforms include personalization of workouts with adaptations made over time based on performance; form correction and feedback which can help avoid injuries by identifying and correcting improper movements or suggesting modifications; detailed progress tracking over time; voice assistants and/or virtual coaches which mimic aspects of personal training such as motivation, guidance, and encouragement; and integration of AI powered fitness apps with nutrition trackers; building of community and social network through sharing progress on platforms such as Facebook, X, and Instagram.[141–143] Such features as form correction feedback and modifications could also be leveraged to also aide in rehabilitative efforts in the case of injury recuperation.[144]

Virtual reality and gamification of AI exercise systems have helped promote more regular engagement in exercise programming through providing a more immersive experience.

One study compared AI-based gesture recognition video games for obese adolescents and demonstrated efficacy in improving cardiopulmonary function and calorie consumption.[139] Another evaluated workers with neck/shoulder pain using AI chatbot exercise instructions at fixed times daily. They found that daily, short-interval exercise improved both neck and shoulder pain in 12 weeks.[138]

As of this writing, there are no data on the home AI systems, specifically. There are clear benefits of accessibility in a home, as well as challenges of accessibility to individuals with low socioeconomic status as many of the current home AI programs on the market are costly. Wearables are a more widely available and accessible option compared to home AI programs.

C. **Online Resources**

There are myriad ways to engage in exercise; with access to resources online, the opportunities are nearly limitless. From engaging individuals with morbid obesity to elite athletes, there are many options. Below is a short-list of some reputable apps and websites by accredited organizations that can be accessed.

- □ ACSM 7-minute workout (https://www.youtube.com/watch?v=nN-gJJHv874)
- □ ACSM (https://www.youtube.com/watch?v=K4Yc-Os-eyk)
- □ NSCA (https://www.nsca.com/education/nsca-videos/)
- □ AHA (https://www.youtube.com/watch?v=1wi2U2pc8XY)
- □ ACE (https://www.acefitness.org/resources/everyone/exercise-library/video/)
- □ ACE (obesity specific) (https://www.acefitness.org/resources/pros/expert-articles/5296/exercises-for-obese-clients-training-progressions-to-try/)
- □ NCEF (https://www.youtube.com/user/NCEF2829/videos)
- □ American Academy of Orthopaedic Surgeons: https://orthoinfo.aaos.org/en/recovery/ for rehab exercises based on specific conditions
- □ HEP2go.com is a resource for physicians to create home exercise programs for patients.

These can include and be modified to incorporate intervals of any kind, RT, and recovery, and be inclusive of widely diverse populations.

CONCLUSION

Osteopathic medicine recognizes the mind-body-spirit connection and the impact of mental health on physical well-being. Exercise is often recommended as part of a holistic approach to provide comprehensive care. Underlying the exercise prescription are a series of complex physiologic processes and concepts such as epigenetics which are key drivers in a patient's ability to achieve certain adaptations brought on by physical activity. Osteopathic physicians prescribe exercise regimens tailored to a patient's needs and goals. A balanced exercise prescription incorporates a combination of aerobic, resistive, balance, flexibility exercises in the general population. In those with special medical conditions, further modifications are made to ensure patients are receiving maximum benefit while maintaining safety parameters adjusted for their abilities and conditions. Mind–body practices, such as tai chi and yoga as well as group fitness classes and recreational activities can be used as complementary modalities to enhance the patient's experience and relationship with increased physical activity. Osteopathic physicians emphasize patient education, empowering individuals to take an active role in their health and well-being. This interdisciplinary approach ensures that exercise programs are well-rounded and take into consideration all aspects of a patient's health. Technology, such as wearables or AI programs can be used to further enhance the patient experience in adhering to an exercise program, where available and appropriate.

ACKNOWLEDGMENTS

The editor of this chapter would like to acknowledge the contributions of student Cameron Braz.

REFERENCES

1. Seffinger MA. *Foundations of Osteopathic Medicine: Philosophy, Science, Clinical Applications, and Research*. Wolters Kluwer; 2019. https://books.google.com/books?id=bsoDvgAACAAJ

2. Licciardone JC, Schultz MJ, Amen B. Osteopathic manipulation in the management of chronic pain: current perspectives. *J Pain Res.* 2020: 1839–1847.
3. Piercy KL, Troiano RP, Ballard RM, et al. The physical activity guidelines for Americans. *JAMA.* 2018;320(19):2020–2028.
4. McIntosh PC. Hieronymus mercurialis "De arte gymnastica": classification and dogma in physical education in the sixteenth century. *Br J Sports Hist.* 1984;1(1):73–84.
5. Jashemski WF, Gleason KL, Hartswick KJ, Malek A. *Gardens of the Roman Empire.* Cambridge University Press; 2017.
6. Forbes CA. Expanded uses of the Greek gymnasium. *Classical Philology.* 1945;40(1):32–42.
7. St Clair K. *The Golden Thread: How Fabric Changed History.* Liveright Publishing; 2019.
8. Tipton CM. The history of "Exercise is medicine" in ancient civilizations. *Adv Physiol Educ.* 2014;38(2):109–117.
9. Hornblower S, Pelling C. *Herodotus: Histories.* Cambridge University Press; 2017
10. Ryan AJ. A medical history of the olympic games. *JAMA.* 1968; 205(11):715–720.
11. Georgoulis AD, Kiapidou I, Velogianni L, Stergiou N, Boland A. Herodicus, the father of sports medicine. *Knee Surg Sports Traumatol Arthrosc.* 2007;15:315–318.
12. Toohey K, Veal AJ. *The Olympic Games: A Social Science Perspective.* Cabi; 2007.
13. Hall JE, Hall ME. *Guyton and Hall textbook of medical physiology e-Book.* Elsevier Health Sciences; 2020.
14. Hargreaves M, Spriet LL. Skeletal muscle energy metabolism during exercise. *Nat Metab.* 2020;2(9):817–828.
15. Sweeney HL, Hammers DW. Muscle contraction. *Cold Spring Harb Perspect Biol.* 2018;10(2):a023200.
16. Dashty M. A quick look at biochemistry: carbohydrate metabolism. *Clin Biochem.* 2013;46(15):1339–1352.
17. Hargreaves M, Spriet LL. Exercise metabolism: fuels for the fire. *Cold Spring Harb Perspect Med.* 2018;8(8):a029744.
18. Li J, Li Y, Atakan MM, et al. The molecular adaptive responses of skeletal muscle to high-intensity exercise/training and hypoxia. *Antioxidants (Basel).* 2020;9(8):656.
19. Hall Carrie M, Thein Brody L. *Therapeutic Exercise: Moving Toward Function. Lippincott Williams & Wilkins*; 2005:255–263.
20. Hawley JA, Leckey JJ. Carbohydrate dependence during prolonged, intense endurance exercise. *Sports Med.* 2015;45:5–12.
21. O'Brien MJ, Viguie CA, Mazzeo RS, Brooks GA. Carbohydrate dependence during marathon running. *Med Sci Sports Exerc.* 1993;25(9):1009–1017.
22. Hall CM, Brody LT, eds. Therapeutic exercise: Moving toward function. Lippincott-Williams & Wilkins; 1999:707.
23. Brooks GA. Lactate as a fulcrum of metabolism. *Redox Biol.* 2020; 35:101454.
24. Brooks GA. The science and translation of lactate shuttle theory. *Cell Metab.* 2018;27(4):757–785.
25. Ferguson BS, Rogatzki MJ, Goodwin ML, Kane DA, Rightmire Z, Gladden LB. Lactate metabolism: Historical context, prior misinterpretations, and current understanding. *Eur J Appl Physiol.* 2018;118:691–728.
26. Yarizadeh H, Eftekhar R, Anjom-Shoae J, Speakman JR, Djafarian K. The effect of aerobic and resistance training and combined exercise modalities on subcutaneous abdominal fat: a systematic review and meta-analysis of randomized clinical trials. *Adv Nutr.* 2021;12(1):179–196.
27. Schumann M, Feuerbacher JF, Sünkeler M, et al. Compatibility of concurrent aerobic and strength training for skeletal muscle size and function: an updated systematic review and meta-analysis. *Sports Med.* 2022:1–12.
28. Seals DR, Nagy EE, Moreau KL. Aerobic exercise training and vascular function with ageing in healthy men and women. *J Physiol.* 2019;597(19): 4901–4914.
29. American College of Sports Medicine. *ACSM's Resource Manual for Guidelines for Exercise Testing and Prescription.* Lippincott Williams & Wilkins; 2012.
30. McArdle WD, Katch FL, Katch VL. *Sports and Exercise Nutrition.* Lippincott Williams & Wilkins; 2018.
31. McArdle WD, Katch FI, Katch VL. *Essentials of Exercise Physiology.* Lippincott Williams & Wilkins; 2006.
32. Stamatakis E, Ahmadi MN, Gill JM, et al. Association of wearable device-measured vigorous intermittent lifestyle physical activity with mortality. *Nat Med.* 2022;28(12):2521–2529.
33. US Department of Health and Human Services. 2018 Physical Activity Guidelines Advisory Committee Scientific Report. 2018. Accessed October 31, 2023. https://odphp.health.gov/our-work/nutrition-physical-activity/physical-activity-guidelines/current-guidelines/scientific-report
34. Swain DP, Abernathy KS, Smith CS, Lee SJ, Bunn SA. Target heart rates for the development of cardiorespiratory fitness. *Med Sci Sports Exerc.* 1994;26(1):112–116.
35. Miller WC, Wallace JP, Eggert KE. Predicting max HR and the HR-VO2 relationship for exercise prescription in obesity. *Med Sci Sports Exerc.* 1993;25(9):1077–1081.
36. Target Heart Rate and Estimated Maximum Heart Rate. Accessed November 1, 2023. https://www.cdc.gov/physical-activity-basics/about/index.html?CDC_AAref_Val=https://www.cdc.gov/physicalactivity/basics/measuring/heartrate.htm
37. Maloy S, Hughes K, ed. *Brenner's Encyclopedia of Genetics.* Academic Press; 2013.
38. Tollefsbol TO, ed. *Handbook of Epigenetics: The New Molecular and Medical Genetics.* Academic Press; 2017.
39. Thakker RV, Whyte MP, Eisman J, Igarashi T. *Genetics of Bone Biology and Skeletal Disease.* Academic Press; 2017.
40. McManus LM, Mitchell RN, ed. *Pathobiology of human disease: a dynamic encyclopedia of disease mechanisms.* Elsevier; 2014.
41. McGee SL, Hargreaves M. Epigenetics and exercise. *Trends Endocrinol Metab.* 2019;30(9):636–645.
42. Richter EA, Sylow L, Hargreaves M. Interactions between insulin and exercise. *Biochem J.* 2021;478(21):3827–3846.
43. Carapeto PV, Aguayo-Mazzucato C. Effects of exercise on cellular and tissue aging. *Aging (Albany NY).* 2021;13(10):14522.
44. Green DJ, Smith KJ. Effects of exercise on vascular function, structure, and health in humans. *Cold Spring Harb Perspect Med.* 2018;8(4): a029819.
45. Jacques M, Hiam D, Craig J, Barrès R, Eynon N, Voisin S. Epigenetic changes in healthy human skeletal muscle following exercise—a systematic review. *Epigenetics.* 2019;14(7):633–648.
46. Widmann M, Nieß AM, Munz B. Physical exercise and epigenetic modifications in skeletal muscle. *Sports Med.* 2019;49(4):509–523.
47. Plaza-Diaz J, Izquierdo D, Torres-Martos Á, Baig AT, Aguilera CM, Ruiz-Ojeda FJ. Impact of physical activity and exercise on the epigenome in skeletal muscle and effects on systemic metabolism. *Biomedicines.* 2022;10(1):126.
48. da Luz Scheffer D, Latini A. Exercise-induced immune system response: Anti-inflammatory status on peripheral and central organs. *Biochim Biophys Acta Mol Basis Dis.* 2020;1866(10):165823.
49. Simpson RJ, Campbell JP, Gleeson M, et al. Can exercise affect immune function to increase susceptibility to infection? *Exerc Immunol Rev.* 2020;26: 8–22.
50. Mengeste AM, Rustan AC, Lund J. Skeletal muscle energy metabolism in obesity. *Obesity (Silver Spring).* 2021;29(10):1582–1595.
51. Wang J, Liu S, Li G, Xiao J. Exercise regulates the immune system. *Physical Exercise for Human Health.* 2020:395–408.
52. Eckstrom E, Neukam S, Kalin L, Wright J. Physical activity and healthy aging. *Clin Geriatr Med.* 2020;36(4):671–683.
53. Drew MK, Vlahovich N, Hughes D, et al. A multifactorial evaluation of illness risk factors in athletes preparing for the summer olympic games. *J Sci Med Sport.* 2017;20(8):745–750.
54. Bohn-Goldbaum E, Pascoe A, Singh MF, et al. Acute exercise decreases vaccine reactions following influenza vaccination among older adults. *Brain Behav Immun Health.* 2020;1:100009. https://www.sciencedirect.com/science/article/pii/S2666354619300092
55. Bohn-Goldbaum E, Owen KB, Lee VY, Booy R, Edwards KM. Physical activity and acute exercise benefit influenza vaccination response: a systematic review with individual participant data meta-analysis. *PLoS One.* 2022;17(6):e0268625.
56. Desai P, Williams Jr AG, Prajapati P, Downey HF. Lymph flow in instrumented dogs varies with exercise intensity. *Lymphat Res Biol.* 2010;8(3):143–148.

57. Measel JW Jr. The effect of the lymphatic pump on the immune response: I. Preliminary studies on the antibody response to pneumococcal polysaccharide assayed by bacterial agglutination and passive hemagglutination. *J Am Osteopath Assoc.* 1982;82(9):205–208.
58. Hallam J, Jones T, Alley J, Kohut ML. Exercise after influenza or COVID-19 vaccination increases serum antibody without an increase in side effects. *Brain Behav Immun.* 2022;102:1–10.
59. Barni L, Carrasco-Vega E, Olivieri M, et al. Does physical exercise enhance the immune response after vaccination? A systematic review for clinical indications of COVID-19 vaccine. *Int J Environ Res Public Health.* 2023;20(6):5183.
60. Gilani SRM, Feizabad AK. The effects of aerobic exercise training on mental health and self-esteem of type 2 diabetes mellitus patients. *Health Psychol Res.* 2019;7(1).
61. Smith PJ, Merwin RM. The role of exercise in management of mental health disorders: an integrative review. *Annu Rev Med.* 2021;72:45–62.
62. Gronwald T, Törpel A, Herold F, Budde H. Perspective of dose and response for individualized physical exercise and training prescription. *J Funct Morphol Kinesiol.* 2020;5(3):48.
63. Wu Z-J, Wang Z-Y, Gao H-E, Zhou X-F, Li F-H. Impact of high-intensity interval training on cardiorespiratory fitness, body composition, physical fitness, and metabolic parameters in older adults: A meta-analysis of randomized controlled trials. *Exp Gerontol.* 2021;150:111345.
64. Gibala M. Molecular responses to high-intensity interval exercise. *Appl Physiol Nutr Metab.* 2009;34(3):428–432.
65. Menz V, Marterer N, Amin SB, Faulhaber M, Hansen AB, Lawley JS. Functional vs. running low-volume high-intensity interval training: effects on VO_{2max} and muscular endurance. *J Sports Sci Med.* 2019;18(3):497–504.
66. Mendes R, Sousa N, Themudo-Barata JL, Reis VM. High-intensity interval training versus moderate-intensity continuous training in middle-aged and older patients with type 2 diabetes: a randomized controlled crossover trial of the acute effects of treadmill walking on glycemic control. *Int J Environ Res Public Health.* 2019;16(21):4163.
67. Steele J, Plotkin D, Van Every D, et al. Slow and steady, or hard and fast? A systematic review and meta-analysis of studies comparing body composition changes between interval training and moderate intensity continuous training. *Sports.* 2021;9(11):155.
68. Cao M, Quan M, Zhuang J. Effect of high-intensity interval training versus moderate-intensity continuous training on cardiorespiratory fitness in children and adolescents: a meta-analysis. *Int J Environ Res Public Health.* 2019;16(9):1533.
69. Gomes-Neto M, Durães AR, Reis HFCd, Neves VR, Martinez BP, Carvalho VO. High-intensity interval training versus moderate-intensity continuous training on exercise capacity and quality of life in patients with coronary artery disease: A systematic review and meta-analysis. *Eur J Prev Cardiol.* 2017;24(16):1696–1707.
70. Wewege M, Van Den Berg R, Ward RE, Keech A. The effects of high-intensity interval training vs. moderate-intensity continuous training on body composition in overweight and obese adults: A systematic review and meta-analysis. *Obes Rev.* 2017;18(6):635–646.
71. Merz KE, Thurmond DC. Role of skeletal muscle in insulin resistance and glucose uptake. *Compr Physiol.* 2011;10(3):785–809.
72. Callahan MJ, Parr EB, Hawley JA, Camera DM. Can high-intensity interval training promote skeletal muscle anabolism? *Sports Med.* 2021; 51(3):405–421.
73. Tabata I. Tabata training: One of the most energetically effective high-intensity intermittent training methods. *J Physiol Sci.* 2019;69(4):559–572.
74. Richards CT, Meah VL, James PE, Rees DA, Lord RN. HIIT'ing or MISS'ing the optimal management of polycystic ovary syndrome: a systematic review and meta-analysis of high-versus moderate-intensity exercise prescription. *Front Physiol.* 2021:1259.
75. Meyler S, Bottoms L, Muniz-Pumares D. Biological and methodological factors affecting response variability to endurance training and the influence of exercise intensity prescription. *Exp Physiol.* 2021;106(7): 1410–1424.
76. Williams CJ, Williams MG, Eynon N, et al. Genes to predict VO_{2max} trainability: a systematic review. *BMC Genomics* 2017;18(8):831.
77. Hoppeler H. Deciphering $\dot{V}O_{2,max}$: limits of the genetic approach. *J Exp Biol.* 2018;221(21):jeb164327.
78. Ross LM, Slentz CA, Kraus WE. Evaluating individual level responses to exercise for health outcomes in overweight or obese adults. *Front Physiol.* 2019;10:1401.
79. Lopez P, Radaelli R, Taaffe DR, et al. Resistance training load effects on muscle hypertrophy and strength gain: systematic review and network meta-analysis. *Med Sci Sports Exerc.* 2021;53(6):1206.
80. Lim C, Nunes EA, Currier BS, Mcleod JC, Thomas AC, Phillips SM. An evidence-based narrative review of mechanisms of resistance exercise–induced human skeletal muscle hypertrophy. *Med Sci Sports Exerc.* 2022;54(9):1546.
81. Grgic J, Schoenfeld BJ, Mikulic P. Effects of plyometric vs. resistance training on skeletal muscle hypertrophy: a review. *J Sport Health Sci.* 2021;10(5):530–536.
82. Kistler-Fischbacher M, Weeks BK, Beck BR. The effect of exercise intensity on bone in postmenopausal women (part 2): a meta-analysis. *Bone.* 2021;143:115697.
83. Kemmler W, Shojaa M, Kohl M, von Stengel S. Effects of different types of exercise on bone mineral density in postmenopausal women: a systematic review and meta-analysis. *Calcif Tissue Int.* 2020;107:409–439.
84. Shojaa M, Von Stengel S, Kohl M, Schoene D, Kemmler W. Effects of dynamic resistance exercise on bone mineral density in postmenopausal women: A systematic review and meta-analysis with special emphasis on exercise parameters. *Osteoporosis Int.* 2020;31:1427–1444.
85. Veldema J, Jansen P. Resistance training in stroke rehabilitation: systematic review and meta-analysis. *Clin Rehabil.* 2020;34(9):1173–1197.
86. Carcelén-Fraile MdC, Aibar-Almazán A, Martínez-Amat A, et al. Effects of physical exercise on sexual function and quality of sexual life related to menopausal symptoms in peri-and postmenopausal women: A systematic review. *Int J Environ Res Public Health.* 2020;17(8):2680.
87. Loaiza-Betancur AF, Chulvi-Medrano I, Díaz-López VA, Gómez-Tomás C. The effect of exercise training on blood pressure in menopause and postmenopausal women: A systematic review of randomized controlled trials. *Maturitas.* 2021;149:40–55.
88. Thomas E, Gentile A, Lakicevic N, et al. The effect of resistance training programs on lean body mass in postmenopausal and elderly women: A meta-analysis of observational studies. *Aging Clin Exp Res.* 2021;33(11):2941–5952.
89. Lopez P, Pinto RS, Radaelli R, et al. Benefits of resistance training in physically frail elderly: a systematic review. *Aging Clin Exp Res.* 2018;30:889–899.
90. Stricker PR, Faigenbaum AD, McCambridge TM; COUNCIL ON SPORTS MEDICINE AND FITNESS. Resistance training for children and adolescents. *Pediatrics.* 2020;145(6).
91. Nery C, De Moraes SRA, Novaes KA, Bezerra MA, Silveira PVDC, Lemos A. Effectiveness of resistance exercise compared to aerobic exercise without insulin therapy in patients with type 2 diabetes mellitus: a meta-analysis. *Braz J Phys Ther.* 2017;21(6):400–415.
92. Peterson MD, Pistilli E, Haff GG, Hoffman EP, Gordon PM. Progression of volume load and muscular adaptation during resistance exercise. *Eur J Appl Physiol.* 2011;111:1063–1071.
93. Henneman E, Clamann HP, Gillies JD, Skinner RD. Rank order of motoneurons within a pool: Law of combination. *J Neurophysiol.* 1974; 37(6):1338–1349.
94. Del Vecchio A, Casolo A, Negro F, et al. The increase in muscle force after 4 weeks of strength training is mediated by adaptations in motor unit recruitment and rate coding. *J Physiol.* 2019;597(7):1873–1887.
95. Kraemer WJ, Ratamess NA. Fundamentals of resistance training: progression and exercise prescription. *Med Sci Sports Exercise.* 2004;36(4):674–688.
96. Krzysztofik M, Wilk M, Wojdała G, Gołaś A. Maximizing muscle hypertrophy: a systematic review of advanced resistance training techniques and methods. *Int J Environ Res Public Health.* 2019;16(24):4897.
97. Coffey VG, Hawley JA. Concurrent exercise training: do opposites distract? *J Physiol (Lond).* 2017;595(9):2883–2896.
98. Fragala MS, Cadore EL, Dorgo S, et al. Resistance training for older adults: Position statement from the national strength and conditioning association. *J Strength Cond Res.* 2019;33(8):2019–2052.
99. Sanchez-Sanchez J, Rodríguez-Fernández A. Equipment and training devices. *Resistance Training Methods: From Theory to Practice.* 2022:67–79.
100. Lee PG, Jackson EA, Richardson CR. Exercise prescriptions in older adults. *Am Fam Physician.* 2017;95(7):425–432.

101. Garber CE, Blissmer B, Deschenes MR, et al. American College of Sports Medicine position stand. Quantity and quality of exercise for developing and maintaining cardiorespiratory, musculoskeletal, and neuromotor fitness in apparently healthy adults: guidance for prescribing exercise. *Med Sci Sports Exerc.* 2011;43(7):1334–1359.
102. Opplert J, Babault N. Acute effects of dynamic stretching on muscle flexibility and performance: an analysis of the current literature. *Sports Med.* 2018;48:299–325.
103. Seth A. Exercise prescription: what does it mean for primary care? *Br J Gen Pract.* 2014;64(618):12–13.
104. Shaha S, Sharath UR. Comparing the effect of static, ballistic and contract-relax stretching on hamstring muscles flexibility in young individuals. *Int J Phys Educ Sports Health.* 2021;8(1):9–15.
105. Lima CD, Ruas CV, Behm DG, Brown LE. Acute effects of stretching on flexibility and performance: a narrative review. *Journal of Science in Sport and Exercise.* 2019;1:29–37.
106. Sherrington C, Michaleff ZA, Fairhall N, et al. Exercise to prevent falls in older adults: An updated systematic review and meta-analysis. *Br J Sports Med.* 2017;51(24):1750–1758.
107. Shier V, Trieu E, Ganz DA. Implementing exercise programs to prevent falls: Systematic descriptive review. *Inj Epidemiol.* 2016;3(1):1–18.
108. Liu C, Shiroy DM, Jones LY, Clark DO. Systematic review of functional training on muscle strength, physical functioning, and activities of daily living in older adults. *Eur Rev Aging Phys Act.* 2014;11:95–106.
109. De Lima FF, Camillo CA, Grigoletto I, et al. Effects of combining functional exercises with exercise training on daily physical activities and functionality in patients with COPD: a protocol for a randomized clinical trial. *Trials.* 2019;20:1–9.
110. Patterson MS, Gagnon LR, Vukelich A, Brown SE, Nelon JL, Prochnow T. Social networks, group exercise, and anxiety among college students. *J Am Coll Health.* 2021;69(4):361–369.
111. Carrapatoso SM, Abdalla PP, Cadete CM, Carvalho JM, Santos MPM, Bohn L. Does real-time online physical exercise improve physical fitness in seniors? *Act Adapt Aging.* 2022;46(4):286–302.
112. Eather N, Wade L, Pankowiak A, Eime R. The impact of sports participation on mental health and social outcomes in adults: a systematic review and the 'Mental health through sport' conceptual model. *Syst Rev.* 2023;12(1):102.
113. Stevenson, A. *Oxford dictionary of English.* Oxford University Press; 2010.
114. Cifu, DX. *Braddom's physical medicine and rehabilitation E-book.* Elsevier Health Sciences; 2020.
115. Schleicher MM, Wedam L, Wu G. Review of Tai Chi as an effective exercise on falls prevention in elderly. *Res Sports Med.* 2012;20(1):37–58.
116. Yan J, Gu W, Sun J, Zhang W, Li B, Pan L. Efficacy of Tai Chi on pain, stiffness and function in patients with osteoarthritis: a meta-analysis. *PLoS One.* 2013;8(4):e61672.
117. Easwaran K, Gopalasingam Y, Green DD, et al. Effectiveness of Tai Chi for health promotion for adults with health conditions: a scoping review of meta-analyses. *Disabil Rehabil.* 2021;43(21):2978–2989.
118. Alvarenga GMd, Charkovski SA, Santos LKd, da Silva MAB, Tomaz GO, Gamba HR. The influence of inspiratory muscle training combined with the pilates method on lung function in elderly women: A randomized controlled trial. *Clinics (Sao Paulo).* 2018;73.
119. Smith SS, Osmotherly PG, Rivett DA. What elements of the exercise prescription process should clinicians consider when prescribing exercise for musculoskeletal rehabilitation in a one on one setting? A review of the literature and primer for exercise prescription. *Phys Ther Rev.* 2022;27(6):453–463.
120. Burnet K, Kelsch E, Zieff G, Moore JB, Stoner L. How fitting is FITT?: a perspective on a transition from the sole use of frequency, intensity, time, and type in exercise prescription. *Physiol Behav.* 2019;199:33–34.
121. Squires RW, Kaminsky LA, Porcari JP, Ruff JE, Savage PD, Williams MA. Progression of exercise training in early outpatient cardiac rehabilitation. *J Cardiopulm Rehabil Prev.* 2018;38(3):139–146.
122. Amorim H, Cadilha R, Parada F, Rocha A. Progression of aerobic exercise intensity in a cardiac rehabilitation program. *Rev Port Cardiol (Engl Ed).* 2019;38(4):281–286.
123. Fish DE, Krabak BJ, Johnson-Greene D, DeLateur BJ. Optimal resistance training: comparison of DeLorme with oxford techniques. *Am J Phys Med Rehabil.* 2003;82(12):903–909.
124. IDC. Wearable devices market share. Accessed December 21, 2022. https://www.idc.com/promo/wearablevendor
125. Ferguson T, Olds T, Curtis R, et al. Effectiveness of wearable activity trackers to increase physical activity and improve health: a systematic review of systematic reviews and meta-analyses. *Lancet Digit Health.* 2022;4(8):e615–e626.
126. Cao R, Azimi I, Sarhaddi F, et al. Accuracy assessment of Oura Ring nocturnal heart rate and heart rate variability in comparison with electrocardiography in time and frequency domains: Comprehensive analysis. *J Med Internet Res.* 2022;24(1):e27487.
127. Thomson EA, Nuss K, Comstock A, et al. Heart rate measures from the apple watch, fitbit charge HR 2, and electrocardiogram across different exercise intensities. *J Sports Sci.* 2019;37(12):1411–1419.
128. Khushhal A, Nichols S, Evans W, et al. Validity and reliability of the apple watch for measuring heart rate during exercise. *Sports Med Int Open.* 2017;1(06):E206–E211.
129. Bai Y, Hibbing P, Mantis C, Welk GJ. Comparative evaluation of heart rate-based monitors: Apple Watch vs Fitbit Charge HR. *J Sports Sci.* 2018;36(15):1734–1741.
130. Abt G, Bray J, Benson AC. Measuring moderate-intensity exercise with the apple watch: validation study. *JMIR Cardio.* 2018;2(1):e8574.
131. Falter M, Budts W, Goetschalckx K, Cornelissen V, Buys R. Accuracy of apple watch measurements for heart rate and energy expenditure in patients with cardiovascular disease: Cross-sectional study. *JMIR Mhealth and Uhealth.* 2019;7(3):e11889.
132. Germini F, Noronha N, Borg Debono V, et al. Accuracy and acceptability of wrist-wearable activity-tracking devices: systematic review of the literature. *J Med Internet Res.* 2022;24(1):e30791.
133. Daly RM, Gianoudis J, Hall T, Mundell NL, Maddison R. Feasibility, usability, and enjoyment of a home-based exercise program delivered via an exercise app for musculoskeletal health in community-dwelling older adults: short-term prospective pilot study. *JMIR Mhealth and Uhealth.* 2021;9(1):e21094.
134. Lee M, Lee H, Kim Y, et al. Mobile app-based health promotion programs: a systematic review of the literature. *Int J Environ Res Public Health.* 2018;15(12):2838.
135. Alasfour M, Almarwani M. The effect of innovative smartphone application on adherence to a home-based exercise programs for female older adults with knee osteoarthritis in Saudi Arabia: a randomized controlled trial. *Disabil Rehabil.* 2022;44(11):2420–2427.
136. Lambert TE, Harvey LA, Avdalis C, et al. An app with remote support achieves better adherence to home exercise programs than paper handouts in people with musculoskeletal conditions: a randomised trial. *J Physiother.* 2017;63(3):161–167.
137. Higgins JP. Smartphone applications for patients' health and fitness. *Am J Med.* 2016;129(1):11–19.
138. Anan T, Kajiki S, Oka H, et al. Effects of an artificial intelligence–assisted health program on workers with neck/shoulder pain/stiffness and low back pain: Randomized controlled trial. *JMIR Mhealth and Uhealth.* 2021;9(9):e27535.
139. Oh W, An Y, Min S, Park C. Comparative effectiveness of artificial intelligence-based interactive home exercise applications in adolescents with obesity. *Sensors (Basel).* 2022;22(19):7352.
140. Mohan S, Venkatakrishnan A, Hartzler AL. Designing an AI health coach and studying its utility in promoting regular aerobic exercise. *ACM Transactions on Interactive Intelligent Systems (TiiS).* 2020;10(2):1–30.
141. Arai R, Ohsuga M. Development of Exercise Promotion System Using Smartphone and AI Speaker. In: *2020 IEEE 2nd International Conference on Artificial Intelligence in Engineering and Technology (IICAIET)2020IEEE*; 2020:1–4.
142. Johnston C, Davis WE. Motivating exercise through social media: is a picture always worth a thousand words? *Psychol Sport Exerc.* 2019;41:119–126.
143. Kashian N, Liu Y. Posting exercise activity on social media for self-efficacy and well-being. *Southern Communication Journal.* 2020;85(2):73–84.
144. Ekambaram D, Ponnusamy V. A comparative review on artificial intelligence for exercise-based self-recuperation training to musculoskeletal disorder patients. In: *AIP Conference Proceedings 2023. AIP Publishing*; 2023.

89 Prolotherapy for Knee Pain with Enthesopathy

BOBBY B. NOURANI

KEY CONCEPTS

- Prolotherapy may be considered in cases of recurring or refractory pain, enthesopathy, or tissue laxity.
- Clinical evidence suggests that prolotherapy for enthesopathy and ligament laxity is effective.
- Randomized controlled trials and meta-analysis support prolotherapy for knee osteoarthritis.
- Prolotherapy for selected conditions is safe, provides long-term benefit, and can be performed in outpatient settings by trained primary care physicians.

WHAT IS PROLOTHERAPY?

Historically known as sclerotherapy, prolotherapy is an injection-based procedure with a proposed mechanism of action of inducing regeneration of damaged soft tissue. Prolotherapy has been used for over 90 years for the treatment of chronic pain and disability (Box 89.1). There are reports as early as 1923 of successfully treating hernias with injected irritants to stimulate tissue repair.[1] In 1937, Earl Gedney, DO published one of the earliest articles reflecting modern-day prolotherapy targeting weak ligaments and tendons.[2] That same year, the *Journal of the American Medical Association* published an article by Louis Schultz, DDS, MD who used injections to repair temporomandibular joint subluxations.[3] George Hackett, MD built upon these principles to treat enthesopathy, by safely and effectively directing his injections at the enthesis, the site where the muscle tendon or ligament attaches to bone.[4] Weak or dysfunctional ligaments and tendons are commonly tender to palpation at the enthesis. Prolotherapy has been used for a variety of chronic musculoskeletal conditions including knee pain with enthesopathy and symptomatic knee osteoarthritis.[5]

CASE VIGNETTE

CHIEF COMPLAINT

Knee pain

HISTORY OF CHIEF COMPLAINT

A 55-year-old, healthy, athletic male was referred to a neuromusculoskeletal medicine (NMM) and osteopathic manual medicine (OMM) specialty clinic by his primary care physician (PCP) due to 8 months of refractory, left lateral knee pain.

- The PCP treated somatic dysfunctions, including a pelvic rotation, left posterior fibular head, and left talocalcaneal restriction with osteopathic manipulative treatment (OMT) on the first visit.
- Knee x-rays were positive for moderate medial joint space narrowing and small medial and posterior osteophyte—consistent with Grade 2–3 knee (Box 89.2) osteoarthritis based on the Kellgren–Lawrence grading scale.[6]
- The patient was referred to physical therapy for strengthening exercises to balance his muscle tone, which helped his ankle feel stronger, but he continued to have left knee pain even after eight visits over the next 2.5 months. On his second visit to his PCP, he was again treated with OMT for a recurrent left posterior fibular head somatic dysfunction.
  - ☐ MRI of the left knee showed no meniscal, soft tissue defects, or abnormal findings.
  - ☐ The patient received an intra-articular corticosteroid injection followed by a second set of physical therapy appointments.
  - ☐ His condition improved temporarily but the pain returned 3 weeks later.

A review of systems revealed that the onset of his knee symptoms began during recovery from an ankle sprain.

- Ten weeks prior to the onset of knee pain, the patient had a left inversion ankle sprain during a hiking trip that involved traversing numerous uneven planes.

BOX 89.1 What is Prolotherapy?

- Prolotherapy is named for its potential benefit of proliferating soft tissue structures.
- It is an injection procedure used in cases of pain associated with ligament laxity, soft tissue tears, and osteoarthritis.

BOX 89.2 Kellgren–Lawrence Grading Scale for Knee Osteoarthritis on Plain Radiograph

- Grade 0: No radiographic evidence of osteoarthritic changes
- Grade 1: Doubtful joint space narrowing and possible osteophytes
- Grade 2: Definite osteophytes, possible joint space narrowing
- Grade 3: Multiple osteophytes, definite joint space narrowing, sclerosis, and possible bony deformity
- Grade 4: Large osteophytes, definite joint space narrowing, severe sclerosis, and definite bony deformity

- Two days after the ankle injury, he visited an urgent care center due to continued pain and swelling.
  - □ Ankle x-rays showed soft tissue swelling but were otherwise unremarkable.
  - □ He was prescribed ibuprofen (600 mg 3 times daily × 10 days with food) for pain and swelling.
  - □ He was advised to rest, ice, elevate, and apply compression to his ankle.
- After 3 weeks of relative rest and high adherence to recommended care, he gradually returned to swimming and then biking.
- Six weeks post ankle injury he attempted a light jog.
  - □ His ankle felt stable, but after 1/2 mile he experienced sharp anterior and lateral knee pain with each step.
  - □ He stopped a 1/4 mile later to return home and ice his knee.
- Despite repeated rest and ice, he experienced consistent knee pain every time he returned to jogging.

Prior to his ankle sprain and lateral knee pain, the patient had a high level of physical fitness and exercise. He completed multiple marathons and four Ironman triathlons, including an Ironman at the age of 40 and a full marathon at age 45. He has completed a dozen 5k and 10k races in his 50s, most recently 3 months prior to the start of his symptoms. Until 8 months ago, he jogged 5 to 6 miles per week and swam 3 miles weekly.

He denies any history of his left knee "giving out," "buckling," or "locking." He has had no major illnesses, hospitalizations, or surgeries. He takes no prescription medications. NSAIDs were only taken 10 days after his urgent care evaluation.

PHYSICAL EXAM

Vital Signs

Height: 5′10″; weight: 170 lb; BP: 135/80; P: 86; R: 14; T: 98.8°F

Musculoskeletal Osteopathic Structural Exam

The patient is evaluated in the standing, seated, supine, and prone positions. Range of motion of bilateral hips, knees, and ankles are within normal limits. Muscle strength is 5/5 for bilateral hips, knees, and ankles. Sensation is equal bilaterally. Patellar and Achilles deep tendon reflexes are 2/4 bilaterally. Hips are level. There is no scoliosis or short leg. Lumbar lordosis is normal. Neurologic exam is normal.

Bilateral knee exam is negative for joint line tenderness, effusion, erythema, anterior drawer, posterior drawer, Lachman, patellar grind, and Apley compression and traction.

McMurray test of the left knee is negative for valgus stress, but positive for tenderness with varus stress. Further varus testing reveals good stability with a hard end feel indicating the lateral collateral ligament is intact. McMurray testing of the right knee is normal for both varus and valgus stress.

Compared to the asymptomatic right knee, there is left knee tenderness to palpation of the:

- Patellar attachments of the medial and lateral patellar retinaculum
- Anterior proximal tibiofibular ligament attachments
- Pes anserinus attachments
- Lateral collateral ligament origin, midsubstance and insertion

Bilateral ankle exam is negative for anterior drawer, talar tilt, and inversion stress tests. Tenderness to palpation is found along the left.

- Anterior talofibular ligament (ATFL)
- Anterior inferior tibiofibular ligament (AITFL)

ASSESSMENT

Left knee pain with enthesopathy and osteoarthritis
Anterior proximal tibiofibular ligament laxity
History of left ankle sprain with current tenderness of ankle ligaments
Somatic dysfunction of the lower extremity region

Discussion of Findings

This patient's original ankle injury likely affected his knee. Compensatory mechanisms may have caused his concomitant knee strain.[7] Forces transmitted through the talus, tibia, and fibula may have compromised the structural integrity of his lateral collateral ligament; anterior proximal and AITFLs; and other surrounding soft tissue structures (see Fig. 89.1). Laxity or partial tears of these structures may cause flares of pain when structurally stressed. The recurrent posterior fibular head somatic dysfunction, despite multiple osteopathic treatments, in addition to pain induced by palpation along the stabilizing anterior proximal tibiofibular ligament of the knee and AITFL of the ankle, likely indicate laxity of these ligamentous

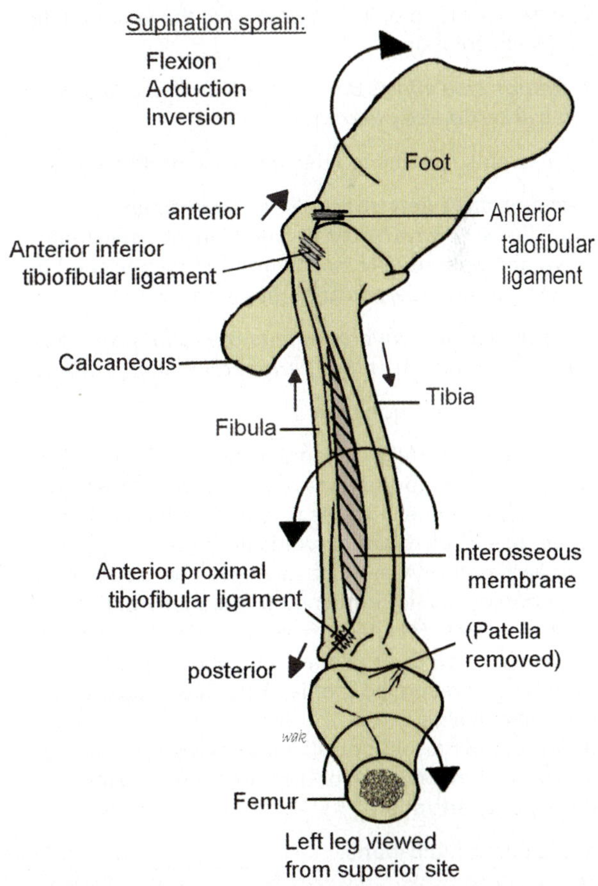

Figure 89.1. Left lower extremity, supination sprain mechanics. Supination ankle sprain about the tibiotalar joint resulting in plantar flexion, adduction, and inversion stress the anterior talofibular ligament. Transmitting forces cause the distal fibula to move anteriorly stressing the anterior inferior tibiofibular ligament. This induces a posterior fibular head stressing the anterior proximal tibiofibular ligament. (Drawing by William A. Kuchera, DO, FAAO, with permission.)

structures. The ATFL is the most commonly sprained ligament of the foot and ankle. Pain with palpation and laxity of the AITFL is often produced with high ankle sprains.[8]

PLAN

This patient is refractory to conservative measures, including rest, analgesics, physical therapy, and corticosteroid injections. After a review of the literature, the patient's history, symptoms, previous failed therapeutic responses, and clinical exam, we determined that he is a good candidate for prolotherapy.

BOX 89.3 Side Effects, Adverse Events, and Contraindications

Common side effects:

- Pain from needling
- Minor bleeding and bruising from needle punctures
- Temporary numbness at the site of injection due to local anesthetic
- Postinjection pain for the first 72 hours due to localized inflammation
- Fullness sensation of local tissue from the volume effect of injected solution

Common side effects are often self-limited and respond well to a short course of acetaminophen.

Adverse events specific to knee dextrose prolotherapy:

- Infections are safety concerns for all injection procedures. Always apply universal safety precautions.
- Nerve damage—due to needle trauma may occur. Limit risk with proper identification of anatomy.

Side effects and adverse events of prolotherapy are no more likely than for other peripheral joint injections.[9]

Relative contraindications:

- Recent use of NSAIDs—theoretically NSAIDs may limit the proinflammatory effects of prolotherapy thereby interrupting the healing cascade and native healing.
- Recent use of steroids—steroids limit the proinflammatory healing suspected to be induced by prolotherapy. It should be noted that many patients on chronic steroids for rheumatoid arthritis, polymyalgia rheumatica, COPD, or similar, still have a good prolotherapy response that is likely due to adaptation to chronic dosing.
- Supra-therapeutic INR or bleeding disorders—alert the patient to increased risk of bleeding and bruising.
- Acute gouty arthritis

Absolute contraindications:

- Patient refusal
- Acute skin or joint infection
- Active rheumatological flare
- Allergic reaction to injection agents: lidocaine or dextrose
- Avoid dextrose injections for patients with corn allergies

BOX 89.4 Injection Solutions

The injection solutions are prepared as follows with standard aseptic technique[10]:

- Extra-articular 15% dextrose solution: In a 10-mL syringe, add 3 mL of 50% dextrose, 2 mL of 1% lidocaine without epinephrine, and 5 mL of 0.9% sodium chloride
- Intra-articular 25% dextrose solution: In a 5-mL syringe, add 2.5 mL of 50% dextrose, 1 mL of 1% lidocaine without epinephrine, 1.5 mL of 0.9% sodium chloride
- Superficial anesthetic 1% lidocaine: In a 5-mL syringe, add 1% lidocaine without epinephrine (buffered or unbuffered)

Risks and benefits of prolotherapy were discussed with the patient, including alternative treatments. The patient has no contraindications to dextrose prolotherapy (see Box 89.3). He has not taken any anti-inflammatory medications in the last 2 weeks. Both the patient and practitioner agree to proceed with a trial of prolotherapy (Box 89.4 and Fig. 89.2).

What is the cause of this patient's pain? Why treat with prolotherapy?

Intra-articular cartilage, bone, and synovium are targets of the degenerative mechanisms in knee osteoarthritis.[10] However, evidence suggests that pain and subsequent functional disability have a more complex etiology and are likely to be outcomes of an interaction between intra- and extra-articular structures in the context of genetic, psychosocial, and other factors. No conventional treatments address all of the potential anatomical pain generators of the symptomatic arthritic knee; however, prolotherapy, which simultaneously treats both peri- and intra-articular structures, is a good option to address the knee in its entirety and is a unique approach to the management of this chronic disease.[11]

Knee pain, whether due to degenerative arthritis, trauma, or overuse, has been one of the most common complaints treated by prolotherapists for the last 60 years.[4,10] Recent research supports

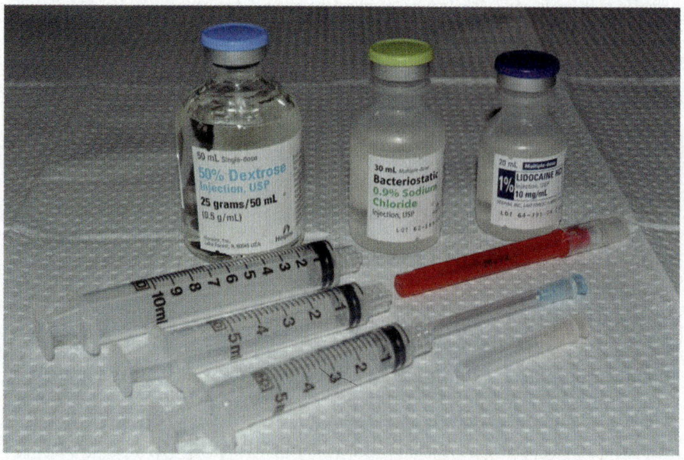

Figure 89.2. Dextrose prolotherapy injection supplies. (Photo courtesy of Dr. Nourani.)

BOX 89.5 Injection Procedure

Points and anatomic structures tender to palpation are identified and marked.

- The knee is cleansed again with chlorhexidine.
- Small amounts of lidocaine are injected intra-dermally at points of tenderness creating skin wheals so deeper injections are less painful.
- Injections of dextrose solutions are performed through the skin wheal with the needle tip contacting bone.
- Solution is injected in a peppering fashion approximately 0.25 to 1.5 mL per square centimeter.

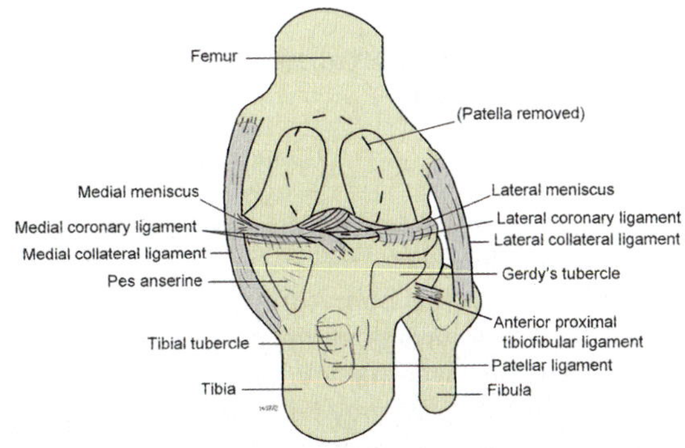

Figure 89.4. Left knee, soft tissue structures. Common soft tissue structures evaluate and treated with prolotherapy. (Drawing by William A. Kuchera, DO, FAAO, with permission.)

its long-term benefits for knee pain and osteoarthritis.[12] The injection protocol directly addresses the current understanding of symptomatic knee osteoarthritis as a product of pain signals from multiple tissues inside and outside the joint capsule. Prolotherapy exposes all intra- and extra-capsular pain-generating structures to therapeutic injection. Because each potential pain generator is treated, prolotherapy is consistent with the current "whole joint" model of knee osteoarthritis and, as such, is ideally suited to address the multifactorial pathology of symptomatic knee osteoarthritis.[11]

- Anatomic sites may be injected in the order of the clinician's preference (Box 89.5). Intra-articular injections are performed first (see Fig. 89.3). The patient has pain along the following structures and is injected accordingly (see Fig. 89.4):
  - □ Lateral coronary ligament
  - □ Lateral collateral ligament
  - □ Anterior proximal tibiofibular ligament
  - □ Medial and lateral patellar retinaculum
  - □ Pes anserinus
  - □ AITFL (ankle)
  - □ ATFL (ankle)
- Most injections are done on or near bone in a peppering fashion (see Fig. 89.5 and Box 89.6).

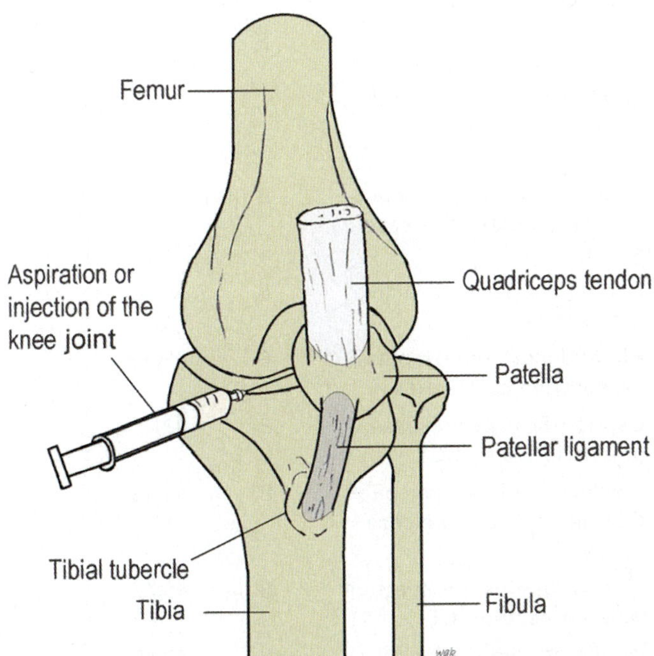

Figure 89.3. Left knee mediolateral view, intra-articular injection. (Drawing by William A. Kuchera, DO, FAAO, with permission.)

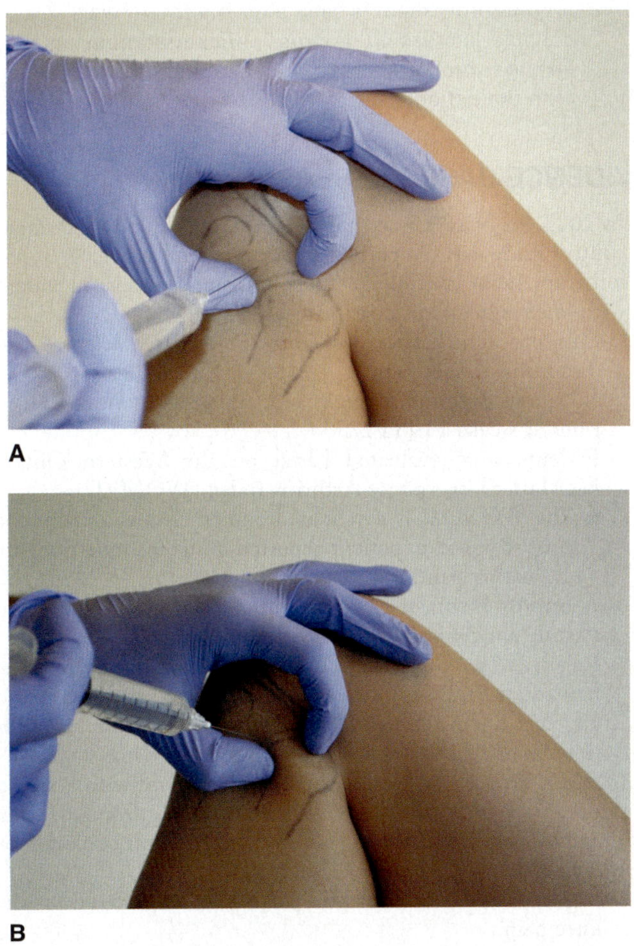

Figure 89.5. Injection of anterior proximal tibiofibular ligament. A. "Tib inj": Injection of tibial attachment. **B.** "Fibula inj": Injection of fibular attachment. (Photo courtesy of Dr. Nourani, with permission.)

BOX 89.6 Postprocedure Instructions and Follow-up

- Postprocedure
  - Most patients experience achiness from the volume effect of the solution
  - It is common to feel pain from the inflammatory effect for 1 to 4 days postinjection—this is often controlled with over-the-counter acetaminophen
  - Occasional narcotics may be used for up to 3 days if patients experience severe pain
  - NSAIDs are anecdotally avoided for 5 to 20 days to limit any impedance of the healing inflammatory cascade
  - Similarly, ice is avoided for 1 to 2 weeks
  - Heat may be applied as needed
  - Avoid activity/overuse during the first few days until the injection-induced pain subsides
  - Gradually increase activity, avoiding strenuous activity for 1 to 2 weeks
- Follow-up
  - Prolotherapy treatments are often spaced 3 to 6 weeks apart
  - Most patients experience benefit by the fourth visit
  - Five to seven treatments are common as the benefit builds upon itself until it plateaus
  - If no improvement is seen after the fourth visit, consider increasing dextrose concentration using a stronger proliferent, and/or evaluating other options with the patient

EVIDENCE-BASED RESEARCH

- In 2013, an NIH-funded three-arm double-blind randomized control study with 90 participants compared the effects of prolotherapy, saline control injections, and home exercise in patients with knee pain and osteoarthritis on x-ray.[10]
  - Subjects were between 40 and 76 years old with at least 3 months of knee pain.
  - Injections occurred at weeks 1, 5, and 9, with optional injections at weeks 13 and 17.
  - Patients were evaluated based on the Western Ontario McMaster Universities Arthritis Index (WOMAC).
    - The WOMAC is a validated outcome measurement tool consisting of a patient-reported outcome questionnaire evaluating pain, stiffness, and function.[13]
    - Improvements of 12 points out of a normalized 100-point scale are clinically and statistically significant.
  - Relative to the control injection group, the prolotherapy group had a statistically significant WOMAC score improvement of 13.9 ± 3.2 points at week 9 and achieved maximum benefit by week 26. At 52 weeks, WOMAC scores were maintained.[10]
- In 2015, Rabago et al. published another study with a similar prolotherapy protocol with 65 subjects suffering from knee pain and osteoarthritis. This study followed participant outcomes for 120 weeks postinjection.[12]
  - Eighty-six percent (56/65) of participants reported decreased knee pain.
  - Sixty-two percent (40/65) had WOMAC score improvements greater than 12 points.
  - Fourteen percent (9/65) of participants reported no improvement.

Other authors have published prolotherapy studies and systematic reviews with meta-analysis that indicate positive results for treating knee pain.[5,11,14,15]

Current prolotherapy research is most extensive for knee pain and osteoarthritis.[5,11] Research for other body regions is less robust. Based on empirical clinical outcomes over the last 70 years, other body regions treated with prolotherapy yield good results in appropriately identified patients with ligament laxity or enthesopathy (see Box 89.7). The box reflects the level of evidence based on the body area.

BOX 89.7 SORT (Strength of Recommendation Taxonomy) Grading of Prolotherapy Relative to Body Region

Body Region	Evidence Rating[16]	References
Knee osteoarthritis: Effective for Knee OA based on two strong RCTs; one systematic review, and one systematic review with meta-analysis. Continued good outcome at 120 weeks	A	5,10–12,14,15, 17–19
Lateral epicondylosis: one large and two small RCTs reflecting strong positive data	A	20–23
Hand and finger OA: one RCT	A	24
Temporomandibular joint dysfunction: prospective study, small RCTs, three systematic reviews and two with meta-analysis,	A	25–31
Nonspecific low back pain: mixed, generally positive results in several systematic reviews and RCTs	B	32–36
Sacroiliac joint dysfunction: RCT and prospective case series	B	37,38
Coccygodynia: prospective case series	B	39,40
Hip adductor; hip dysplasia: prospective case series	B	41,42
Osgood-Schlatter disease: one high-quality RCT	B	43
Achilles tendinopathy: pilot RCT and prospective case series	B	44,45
Plantar fasciitis: prospective case series and RCT	B	46,47
Patellar tendinopathy: prospective case series and systematic review	B	48,49

PROLOTHERAPY SOLUTIONS

Dextrose is the most common proliferent and has been proven safe and effective.[10] Dextrose is approved for invasive use by the US Food and Drug Agency (FDA). Other proliferents include:

- Polidocanol: a fish oil derivative[50]
- Pumice: less used do to its potentially scarring effects[51]
- P2G (phenol–glycerol–glucose)[52]
- Testosterone: anabolic properties to increase regeneration of lax and torn soft tissue and muscles[53]
- Human growth hormone: potential influence on protein synthesis[53]

MECHANISM OF ACTION

Clinical research studying the basic science mechanism of dextrose prolotherapy is lacking. A favored, proposed mechanism of action is that hypertonic properties of dextrose induce an osmolar gradient that causes localized cell lysis initiating the inflammatory and healing cascade.[54] Dextrose-mediated release of potential growth factors healing soft tissue structures and increasing ligamentous cross-sectional area and tensile strength has also been suggested.[55–57] There is more recent evidence that dextrose may play a role in treating neurogenic inflammation.[58–61]

MUSCULOSKELETAL INJECTIONS: PRESENT AND FUTURE

Prolotherapy is one of three major therapies under a broader category of injections, called regenerative injections. The other two are platelet-rich plasma (PRP) and stem cell therapy.[62]

Platelet-Rich Plasma

PRP and stem cell therapy are newer modalities supported by research and clinical outcomes showing benefits. PRP is the injection of autologous plasma with a concentration of platelets with the goal of increasing growth factor response at the local injection site.

Stem Cell Therapy

Autologous stem cell therapy for musculoskeletal pain is the addition of mesenchymal stem cells that are derived from bone marrow and/or adipose tissue. The differentiation of mesenchymal cells may increase healing and regenerate soft tissue structures. These agents are discussed outside of this section. The FDA continues to review the use of autologous and allogeneic stem cell therapy and has published statements regarding their use for musculoskeletal disorders. The reader should refer to the FDA for the most recent approved stem cell therapies and indications.

Improvements in ultrasound imaging and access in ambulatory clinics are improving the diagnostic evaluations of soft tissue tears and needle guidance for regenerative injections. As this field continues to advance, real-time imaging and identification of soft tissue defects will corroborate physical exam findings and allow more precise localization of regenerative injection treatments.

MEDICAL TRAINING

Despite prolotherapy injection procedures and protocols not being taught routinely within medical schools or residency curriculum, there are an increasing number of prolotherapy practitioners within family medicine, sports medicine, physical medicine and rehabilitation, orthopedic medicine, neurology, and anesthesiology as evidenced by the participants at such CME courses. This is likely due to growing research, clinical benefits, and patient- and physician-driven interests in nonsurgical therapies for chronic pain in an era of an opioid use epidemic. Resources for training and research include the Hackett–Hemwall–Patterson Foundation, University of Wisconsin Prolotherapy Education and Research Lab (UW PEARL), International Association for Regenerative Therapy, American Osteopathic Association of Prolotherapy Regenerative Medicine, the American Association of Orthopaedic Medicine, and NMM/OMM training programs.

CONCLUSION

Prolotherapy is a safe and effective treatment for common cases of soft tissue laxity with enthesopathy, such as the one presented above. Patients who are treated with prolotherapy often fail conservative therapy, including rest, NSAIDs, and physical therapy. Research on the use of prolotherapy for knee pain has often included a diagnosis of osteoarthritis.

REFERENCES

1. Donna A. A history of the American College of Osteopathic Sclerotherapeutic Pain Management, the oldest prolotherapy organization. *Journal of Prolotherapy.* 2009;1(4):200–204.
2. EH G. Special technique: Hypermobile joint: a preliminary report. *Osteopathic Profession.* 1937;4(9):30–31.
3. Schultz LW. A treatment for subluxation of the temporomandibular joint. *JAMA.* 1937;109(13):1032–1035.
4. Hackett GS, Hemwall GA, Montgomery GA. *Ligament and Tendon Relaxation Treated by Prolotherapy.* 5th ed. Gustav A. Hemwall; 1993.
5. Nourani B, Rabago D. Prolotherapy for knee osteoarthritis: a descriptive review [journal article]. *Curr Phys Med Rehab Rep.* 2016;4(1):42–49.
6. Kellgren JHJM, Ball J. The epidemiology of chronic rheumatism. In: *Atlas of Standard Radiographs of Arthritis.* Blackwell Scientific Publications; 1963.
7. Scott R, Kuchera M, Patterson J. Orthopedics. In: Ward R, ed. *Foundations for Osteopathic Medicine.* 2nd ed. Lippincott Williams & Wilkins; 2003: 477–499.
8. Brostroem L. Sprained ankles, I: anatomic lesions in recent sprains. *Acta Chir Scand.* 1964;128(0001-5482 (Print)):483–495.
9. Dagenais S, Ogunseitan O, Haldeman S, Wooley JR, Newcomb RL. Side effects and adverse events related to intraligamentous injection of sclerosing solutions (prolotherapy) for back and neck pain: A survey of practitioners. *Arch Phys Med Rehabil.* 2006;87(7):909–913.
10. Rabago D, Patterson JJ, Mundt M, et al. Dextrose prolotherapy for knee osteoarthritis: a randomized controlled trial. *Ann Fam Med.* 2013; 11(3):229–237.
11. Sit RW, Chung V, Reeves KD, et al. Hypertonic dextrose injections (prolotherapy) in the treatment of symptomatic knee osteoarthritis: a systematic review and meta-analysis. *Sci Rep.* 2016;6:25247.
12. Rabago D, Mundt M, Zgierska A, Grettie J. Hypertonic dextrose injection (prolotherapy) for knee osteoarthritis: long term outcomes. *Complement Ther Med.* 2015;23(3):388–395.
13. Bellamy N, Buchanan WW, Goldsmith CH, Campbell J, Stitt LW. Validation study of WOMAC: a health status instrument for measuring clinically important patient relevant outcomes to antirheumatic drug therapy in patients with osteoarthritis of the hip or knee. *J Rheumatol.* 1988;15(12):1833–1840.
14. Reeves KD, Hassanein K. Randomized prospective double-blind placebo-controlled study of dextrose prolotherapy for knee osteoarthritis with or without ACL laxity. *Altern Ther Health Med.* 2000;6(2):68–74, 77–80.
15. Dumais R, Benoit C, Dumais A, et al. Effect of regenerative injection therapy on function and pain in patients with knee osteoarthritis: a randomized crossover study. *Pain Med.* 2012;13(8):990–999.

16. Ebell MH, Siwek J, Weiss BD, et al. Strength of recommendation taxonomy (SORT): a patient-centered approach to grading evidence in the medical literature. *Am Fam Physician.* 2004;69(3):548–556.
17. Rabago D, Zgierska A, Fortney L, et al. Hypertonic dextrose injections (prolotherapy) for knee osteoarthritis: results of a single-arm uncontrolled study with 1-year follow-up. *J Altern Complement Med.* 2012;18(4): 408–414.
18. Rabago D, Patterson JJ, Mundt M, et al. Dextrose and morrhuate sodium injections (prolotherapy) for knee osteoarthritis: a prospective open-label trial. *J Altern Complement Med.* 2014;20(5):383–391.
19. Rabago D, Patterson JJ. Prolotherapy: an effective adjunctive therapy for knee osteoarthritis. *J Am Osteopath Assoc.* 2013;113(2):122–123.
20. Scarpone M, Rabago DP, Zgierska A, Arbogast G, Snell E. The efficacy of prolotherapy for lateral epicondylosis: a pilot study. *Clin J Sport Med.* 2008;18(3):248–254.
21. Rabago D, Lee KS, Ryan M, et al. Hypertonic dextrose and morrhuate sodium injections (prolotherapy) for lateral epicondylosis (tennis elbow): results of a single-blind, pilot-level, randomized controlled trial. *Am J Phys Med Rehabil.* 2013;92(7):587–596.
22. Carayannopoulos A, Borg-Stein J, Sokolof J, Meleger A, Rosenberg D. Prolotherapy versus corticosteroid injections for the treatment of lateral epicondylosis: a randomized controlled trial. *PM R.* 2011;3(8):706–715.
23. Yelland M, Rabago D, Ryan M, et al. Prolotherapy injections and physiotherapy used singly and in combination for lateral epicondylalgia: A single-blinded randomised clinical trial. *BMC Musculoskeletal Disorders.* 2019;20:509.
24. Reeves KD, Hassanein K. Randomized, prospective, placebo-controlled double-blind study of dextrose prolotherapy for osteoarthritic thumb and finger (DIP, PIP, and trapeziometacarpal) joints: evidence of clinical efficacy. *J Altern Complement Med.* 2000;6(4):311–320.
25. Zarate MA, Frusso RD, Reeves KD, Cheng AL, Rabago D. dextrose prolotherapy versus lidocaine injection for temporomandibular dysfunction: a pragmatic randomized controlled trial. *J Altern Complement Med.* 2020;26(11):1064–1073.
26. Louw WF, Reeves KD, Lam SKH, Cheng AL, Rabago D. Treatment of temporomandibular dysfunction with hypertonic dextrose injection (prolotherapy): a randomized controlled trial with long-term partial crossover. *Mayo Clin Proc.* 2019;94(5):820–832.
27. Sit RW-S, Reeves KD, Zhong CC, et al. Efficacy of hypertonic dextrose injection (prolotherapy) in temporomandibular joint dysfunction: a systematic review and meta-analysis. *Sci Rep.* 2021;11(1):14638.
28. Nagori SA, Jose A, Gopalakrishnan V, Roy ID, Chattopadhyay PK, Roychoudhury A. The efficacy of dextrose prolotherapy over placebo for temporomandibular joint hypermobility: A systematic review and meta-analysis. *J Oral Rehab.* 2018;45(12):998–1006.
29. Bahgat MM, Abdel-Hamid AM. Is dextrose prolotherapy beneficial in the management of temporomandibular joint internal derangement? A systematic review. *CRANIO®.* 2023;25:1–9.
30. Refai H. Long-term therapeutic effects of dextrose prolotherapy in patients with hypermobility of the temporomandibular joint: a single-arm study with 1-4 years' follow up. *Br J Oral Maxillofac Surg.* 2017;55(5): 465–470.
31. Priyadarshini S, Gnanam A, Sasikala B, et al. Evaluation of prolotherapy in comparison with occlusal splints in treating internal derangement of the temporomandibular joint – A randomized controlled trial. *J Craniomaxillofac Surg.* 2021;49(1):24–28.
32. Dechow E, Davies RK, Carr AJ, Thompson PW. A randomized, double-blind, placebo-controlled trial of sclerosing injections in patients with chronic low back pain. *Rheumatology (Oxford).* 1999;38(12):1255–1259.
33. Ongley MJ, Klein RG, Dorman TA, Eck BC, Hubert LJ. A new approach to the treatment of chronic low back pain. *Lancet.* 1987;2(8551):143–146.
34. Klein RG, Eek BC, DeLong WB, Mooney V. A randomized double-blind trial of dextrose-glycerine-phenol injections for chronic, low back pain. *J Spinal Disord.* 1993;6(1):23–33.
35. Yelland MJ, Del Mar C, Pirozzo S, Schoene ML. Prolotherapy injections for chronic low back pain: a systematic review. *Spine (Phila Pa 1976).* 2004;29(19):2126–2133.
36. Yelland MJ, Glasziou PP, Bogduk N, Schluter PJ, McKernon M. Prolotherapy injections, saline injections, and exercises for chronic low-back pain: a randomized trial. *Spine (Phila Pa 1976).* 2004;29(1):9–16; discussion 16.
37. Cusi M, Saunders J, Hungerford B, Wisbey-Roth T, Lucas P, Wilson S. The use of prolotherapy in the sacroiliac joint. *Br J Sports Med.* 2010; 44(2):100–104.
38. Hoffman MD, Agnish V. Functional outcome from sacroiliac joint prolotherapy in patients with sacroiliac joint instability. *Complementary Ther Med.* 2018;37:64–68.
39. Khan SA, Kumar A, Varshney MK, Trikha V, Yadav CS. Dextrose prolotherapy for recalcitrant coccygodynia. *J Orthop Surg (Hong Kong).* 2008; 16(1):27–29.
40. Hadhoud M, Elzawawi M, Yasser S, Elshafi A, Shams A. Radiological and Magnetic Resonance Imaging of Idiopathic Coccydynia and Study of the Effect of Prolotherapy Running Head: Radiological and Magnetic Resonance Imaging of Idiopathic Coccydynia and Study of the Effect of Prolotherapy. 2020.
41. Topol GA, Reeves KD, Hassanein KM. Efficacy of dextrose prolotherapy in elite male kicking-sport athletes with chronic groin pain. *Arch Phys Med Rehabil.* 2005;86(4):697–702.
42. Gül D, Orsçelik A, Akpancar S. Treatment of osteoarthritis secondary to developmental dysplasia of the hip with prolotherapy injection versus a supervised progressive exercise control. *Med Sci Monit.* 2020;26:e919166.
43. Topol GA, Podesta LA, Reeves KD, Raya MF, Fullerton BD, Yeh HW. Hyperosmolar dextrose injection for recalcitrant Osgood-Schlatter disease. *Pediatrics.* 2011;128(5):e1121–e1128.
44. Yelland MJ, Sweeting KR, Lyftogt JA, Ng SK, Scuffham PA, Evans KA. Prolotherapy injections and eccentric loading exercises for painful Achilles tendinosis: a randomised trial. *Br J Sports Med.* 2011;45(5):421–428.
45. Maxwell NJ, Ryan MB, Taunton JE, Gillies JH, Wong AD. Sonographically guided intratendinous injection of hyperosmolar dextrose to treat chronic tendinosis of the Achilles tendon: a pilot study. *AJR Am J Roentgenol.* 2007; 189(4):W215–W220.
46. Ryan MB, Wong AD, Gillies JH, Wong J, Taunton JE. Sonographically guided intratendinous injections of hyperosmolar dextrose/lidocaine: a pilot study for the treatment of chronic plantar fasciitis. *Br J Sports Med.* 2009;43:303–306.
47. Kim E, Lee JH. Autologous platelet-rich plasma versus dextrose prolotherapy for the treatment of chronic recalcitrant plantar fasciitis. *PM R.* 2014;6(2):152–158.
48. Ryan M, Wong A, Rabago D, Lee K, Taunton J. Ultrasound-guided injections of hyperosmolar dextrose for overuse patellar tendinopathy: a pilot study. *Br J Sports Med.* 2011;45(12):972–977.
49. Morath O, Beck M, Taeymans J, Hirschmüller A. Sclerotherapy and prolotherapy for chronic patellar tendinopathies - a promising therapy with limited available evidence, a systematic review. *J Exp Orthop.* 2020;7(1):89.
50. Rabago D, Best TM, Zgierska AE, Zeisig E, Ryan M, Crane D. A systematic review of four injection therapies for lateral epicondylosis: prolotherapy, polidocanol, whole blood and platelet-rich plasma. *Br J Sports Med.* 2009;43(7):471–481.
51. Dagenais S, Yelland MJ, Del Mar C, Schoene ML. Prolotherapy injections for chronic low-back pain. *Cochrane Database Syst Rev.* 2007; 2007(2):CD004059.
52. Johnston E, Emani C, Kochan A, et al. Prolotherapy agent P2G is associated with upregulation of fibroblast growth factor-2 genetic expression in vitro. *J Exp Orthop.* 2020;7(1):97.
53. Dubick MN, Ravin TH, Michel Y, Morrisette DC. Use of localized human growth hormone and testosterone injections in addition to manual therapy and exercise for lower back pain: a case series with 12-month follow-up. *J Pain Res.* 2015;8:295–302.
54. Banks A. A rationale for prolotherapy. *J Orthop Med.* 1991;13(3):54–59.
55. Jensen KT, Rabago DP, Best TM, Patterson JJ, Vanderby R, Jr. Early inflammatory response of knee ligaments to prolotherapy in a rat model. *J Orthop Res.* 2008;26(6):816–823.
56. Jensen KT, Rabago D, Best TM, Patterson JJ, Vanderby R. Longer term response of knee ligaments to prolotherapy in a rat injury model. *Am J Sports Med.* 2008;36:1347–1357.
57. Yoshi T, Zhao C, Schmelzer JD, Low PA, An K, Amadio A. The effects of hypertonic dextrose injection on connective tissue and nerve conduction through the rabbit carpal tunnel. *Arch Phys Med Rehabil.* 2009;90:333–339.

58. Rabago D, Kijowski R, Woods M, et al. Association between disease-specific quality of life and magnetic resonance imaging outcomes in a clinical trial of prolotherapy for knee osteoarthritis. *Arch Phys Med Rehabil.* 2013;94(11):2075–2082.
59. Lyftogt J. Pain conundrums: Which hypothesis? Central nervous system sensitization versus peripheral nervous system autonomy. *Australasian Musculoskeletal Medicine.* 2008;13:72–74.
60. Donaldson LF. Neurogenic mechanisms in arthritis. In: Jancso G, ed. *Neurogenic Inflammation in Health and Disease.* Vol 8. Elsevier; 2009:211–241.
61. Nagy I, Paule CC, White JPM. Molecular mechanisms of TRPV1-mediated pain. *Neuroimmune Biol.* 2009;8:75–99.
62. DeChellis DM, Cortazzo MH. Regenerative medicine in the field of pain medicine: Prolotherapy, platelet-rich plasma therapy, and stem cell therapy-Theory and evidence. *Tech Reg Anesth Pain Manag.* 2011;15(2):74–80.

90 Performing Arts Medicine

SAJID A. SURVE ▪ YEIN LEE ▪ JAMES S. ASTON

KEY CONCEPTS

- Performing artists have high injury rates, which are directly tied to what they do.
- Dancer's bodies are subject to high forces and repetitive stress injuries and have internal and external pressures to maintain that physique, potentially leading to body image issues, eating disorders, substance abuse, or malnutrition.
- Dancers often suffer injuries to the lower limb such as tendonitis, bursitis, ligamentous sprains, hypermobility, knee meniscus, or hip labrum injuries.
- Muscle imbalances including anterior pelvic tilt or weakness of the gluteus muscles[1] are common in dancers.
- Body dysmorphia, eating disorders, and malnutrition are common among dancers.
- Common health problems observed in musicians are musculoskeletal disorders, voice problems, hearing loss, and mental health issues.
- Musicians start playing early in life and practice for a few hours per day throughout their childhood leading to unique somatic dysfunction considerations.
- Anxieties, including performance anxiety, depression, and substance use issues are widespread among musicians.[2]
- Musicians often lack health insurance and financial stability, a major social determinant of health among this population.
- Osteopathic physicians are well-suited to working with dancers and musicians, as problems are often multifactorial, due directly to their art, and neuromusculoskeletal in nature.
- Treatment plan for musicians should include counseling, home exercise programs, bracing, rest, and return to play, if necessary.
- Problems specific to musicians include upper limb pathology, facial injuries, playing-related musculoskeletal disorder (PRMD), overuse injuries, tendon injuries, compression neuropathies, hypermobility, focal dystonia, and mental health concerns.[3]
- The osteopathic physician can make significant contributions to the health and well-being of performing artists by applying osteopathic tenets.

INTRODUCTION

Performing artists, as a special population, first came under major scrutiny by the medical community in the late 1980s, when Fishbein et al. surveyed members of the International Conference of Symphony and Orchestra Musicians (ICSOM) inquiring about the medical problems of its musicians. The results surprisingly revealed that 82% of orchestral musicians had at least one medical problem in the past year, and 76% had a problem that severely impacted their ability to play their instrument.[4] Since that time, a small, but dedicated, group of professionals have been studying, advocating for, and providing medical care to performing artists, including dancers, instrumentalists, vocalists, and actors.

When considering the performing artist and their medical needs, a common parallel is often drawn to sports medicine.[5] On its face, the two groups seem to have much in common. Both participants spend years perfecting their craft and are highly specialized. They have high injury rates, which are directly tied to what they do and require care from a team of medical professionals who have an intimate understanding of the tasks involved. Both athletes and artists are expected to perform at optimum levels under extreme pressure and public scrutiny and do so primarily for an audience's entertainment. They suffer from depression and anxiety—specifically performance-related anxiety—at higher levels than the general population. Despite their similarities, key differences separate these two populations. The most significant of these differences is medical and research infrastructure. Sports medicine, sports science, sports psychology, sports engineering, etc. are all well-established industries with robust training programs, ongoing research, and in many cases, policies requiring their presence to support athletes at the professional and collegiate levels. Similar infrastructure for professional or collegiate dance or music programs are scant to nonexistent, leaving their participants without adequate resources, knowledge base, or even awareness of the potential risks from their activities. In addition, athletes are accustomed to regular exercise and are in better cardiovascular health than their performing arts counterparts, whose engagement with physical activity is more variable. Finally, access to funding is different between these two groups. Athletics, especially at the professional level, are revenue-generating institutions, with ticket sales, sponsorships, merchandise, and more to help create financial stability. The performing arts are less financially stable, with many groups, even at the professional level, being supported through philanthropy or grants, rather than being self-sufficient. This lack of financial resources makes addressing the other disparities mentioned above even more difficult to overcome.

In this chapter, an overview of the medical problems of performing artists will be presented, subdivided into dance and music. Each section will provide essential elements for physicians seeking to obtain an occupational history from a performing artist, problems specific to that group that may not be common in the general population, and tips to approach treating the performing artist in that group.

DANCE MEDICINE

Dancers are more closely tied to athletics and have a better understanding of the physicality of their craft, but there are still several factors that play a critical role in understanding this population. Although dancers are often associated with a lithe physique, their bodies are subject to high forces and repetitive stress, which may lead to injury. They also have internal and external pressures to maintain that physique, potentially leading to body image issues, eating disorders, substance abuse, or malnutrition. Because of physical demands, professional dancers have a limited timeframe when they can be employed and will, almost certainly, need to change careers as they age. This financial pressure creates additional stress on the dancer. Below is a summary of points that physicians will need to understand when working with a dancer:

1. Most dancers begin their training extremely early, often at age 3 or 4. Early dance training often starts with ballet, which serves as the foundation for most Western dance traditions. As dancers get older, they will branch out and learn new styles such as jazz, contemporary, modern, tap, or hip hop. In Eastern dance traditions, movements are highly specialized and associated with the culture of that dance's origin, with less branching outward into other dance styles.
2. Start from the ground up. Dancers often wear specialized footwear and may dance on different flooring surfaces such as wood or plastic over rubberized matting (known as sprung flooring) during practice or performance. Asking about changes or problems with footwear or flooring may offer important insight into the problem at hand.
3. As noted above, dancers have pressure to maintain a certain physique, and their job security is tied to their appearance. Asking about diet, exercise regimen, and use of supplements and substances is critical to understanding their risks.
4. Even full-time professional dancers are often hired as independent contractors and are not offered health insurance, and their pay is historically very low. Dancers struggle with financial stressors and may work several jobs to make ends meet. Inquiring about their full occupational history beyond dance may provide a clearer picture of their activity.

OCCUPATIONAL HISTORY FOR DANCERS

Osteopathic physicians are well-suited to working with the dancer population, as problems are often multifactorial and require close patient communication and trust to make significant progress. Dancers, as a community, have a deep distrust of health care professionals, as they often feel misunderstood or are afraid that they might be told they cannot dance anymore.[6] The physician needs to tread carefully when establishing an initial relationship with dancers. When obtaining an occupational history, adding the factors below into a standard history will provide useful information.

1. The most important opening question is to establish what type(s) of dance are practiced and performed, where practice and performances occur, and how much time is spent on each.
2. For each dance setting, inquire about footwear, flooring, costuming, and any other considerations that might affect the chief complaint. Another point to ask about is any recent changes to these areas, such as new shoes or different venues.
3. Take time when understanding social history. Important details can be found in diet, exercise, sleep history, sources of financial or emotional stress, substance use history, and trauma-informed care.
4. Although they are not medical professionals, college-trained dancers are required to receive education on rudimentary anatomy and kinesiology by the National Association of Schools of Dance and have excellent internal awareness of their body. Dancers will often explain their musculoskeletal problems with great specificity and are usually correct. Working with them and taking their knowledge into account can expedite a workup greatly.

PHYSICAL EXAM FOR DANCERS

Physical and structural examination should be carried out as expected, but one factor to consider is that dancers are often hypermobile and have ranges of motion well beyond the general population.[7] Assessing a full range of motion may require deviation from typical methods of assessment to account for this flexibility. In addition, just because a dancer has full strength and range of motion does not mean that they are able to move their body as required for gainful employment. If a dancer is stating that their movement is impaired, then they require further investigation even if a physical examination is normal by conventional standards.

TIPS TO TREATING DANCERS

When putting together a treatment plan for a dancer, taking the opportunity to counsel about lifestyle modification is imperative if any concerns arise during the history. Referrals to mental health professionals, dieticians, trainers, or physical therapists may help with a more comprehensive approach to care. Because of their propensity for musculoskeletal problems and exceptional internal awareness, dancers are also excellent candidates for osteopathic manipulative treatment where appropriate.

PROBLEMS SPECIFIC TO DANCERS

Lower Limb Disorders

Because of the movements and forces involved, most dancer injuries affect the lower limb. Foot and ankle overuse injuries such as tendonitis, bursitis, and ligamentous sprains are exceptionally common. Similarly, knee and hip problems can occur including instability due to hypermobility, knee meniscus or hip labrum injuries, or other acute traumas from falls or incorrect landings.[8] Conducting an appropriate orthopedic examination and managing accordingly will address many lower limb disorders.

Muscle Imbalances

Most dancers are hypermobile by design, and the movements they perform are highly specific. As a result, lower body muscle imbalances are common, including anterior pelvic tilt or weakness of the gluteus muscles.[1] These types of setups can make dancers prone to hyperextension injuries to the spine such as pars defects or spondylolisthesis,[9] and patients will often require imaging to fully evaluate any back injuries. Management of these problems focuses on correcting imbalance through targeted exercise and relative rest and/or bracing for any bony pathology.

Body Issues

As noted above, dancers are overrepresented in cases of body dysmorphia, eating disorders, and malnutrition.[10] Working with the dancer on lifestyle modification can be a good start for mild cases, but many patients will require the help of a mental health professional, preferably one that has special training on treating body issues. In addition, assessing the amount of external pressure a dancer is facing may be required, along with advocacy on the patient's behalf. If a dance company requires that dancers maintain a certain weight or body fat percentage, or threatens termination due to body issues, the dancer may not be able to make requisite changes to improve their health. In these cases, providing a note or contacting the company may be required.

In conclusion, the osteopathic physician has an ideal skillset and disposition to work with dancers. Through targeted questioning and an understanding of the unique needs of this population, physicians can make a significant positive impact on the dance community and help break down barriers to care for future generations.

MUSIC MEDICINE

Musicians experience extraordinary physical and psychological demands and suffer from unique health issues directly caused by their occupations. Common health problems observed in musicians are musculoskeletal disorders, voice problems, hearing loss, and mental health issues.[3] Such pathologies, combined with the unique biopsychosocial environment where musicians live, work, and play, make managing musicians' health issues challenging. Therefore, the osteopathic physicians' distinctive perspectives and training in osteopathic manipulative medicine greatly benefit this unique group of patients.

Before discussing the specifics of the osteopathic approach to managing musicians' health issues, there are a few factors to understand about musicians. The following summary may be helpful when osteopathic physicians encounter musicians.

1. Musicians start playing early, even at 3 or 4 years old. As osteopathic physicians, this is essential information to consider when performing an osteopathic structural exam. Instrumentalists often play their chosen instrument a few hours per day throughout their childhood, leading to unique somatic dysfunction considerations.
2. Music is often a musician's identity. They will play through pain and injuries and will not seek help if they think their playing will be compromised.[11]
3. The music world is highly competitive. Musicians are constantly auditioning and competing and facing harsh criticism. Anxiety, depression, and substance use issues are widespread among musicians, and many struggle with performance anxiety.[12]
4. Many musicians are freelancers. In these instances, they may have multiple venues where they play, none of which provide any health insurance or assurances of a steady income. If musicians do not perform, they do not have any income. Stopping a musician from performing also creates a ripple effect, not just to them, but to all the different groups that must now scramble to provide coverage for their absence.

OCCUPATIONAL HISTORY FOR MUSICIANS

Osteopathic physicians are ideally suited to help musicians as many of their health issues are directly caused by their art form and are neuromusculoskeletal in nature. The osteopathic perspective provides the expertise that musicians seek and need. Osteopathic physicians can manage complex neuromusculoskeletal issues involving the whole person, not just the disease process but also other contributing factors including environmental, psychosocial, financial, and others. A comprehensive evaluation of a musician is not any different than other medical visits; it starts with a thorough history and physical exam, including an osteopathic exam; however, collecting specific information related to playing music, in addition to the usual history, is helpful. The following should be considered:

1. For instrumentalists, it is vital to ask about their instrument(s). If the physician is unfamiliar with the musical instrument, it is essential to ask the patient. Often, musicians are happy to share a video of their performances or even play for the physician live.
2. Ask about recent changes in playing time, intensity, repertoire, upcoming performances, ensemble types (new position), and instruments.
3. For voice users, ask about the types of voice usage. For example, how do they use their voice? Are they singers? Are they actors?
4. Ask about their playing hours (rehearsal hours and practice hours), frequency of breaks, and performance settings (temperature, lighting, size, noise level).
5. It may provide more understanding if musicians are asked about recent stressors (including the current injury or the illnesses), performance anxiety, financial dependency on performances, exercise frequency, fitness level, diet, sleep, and substance use.

PHYSICAL EXAM FOR MUSICIANS

The physical examination also should be like the usual comprehensive exam focused on the chief complaint. However, including a more detailed postural exam, hypermobility exam, and osteopathic structural evaluation with and without play can reveal incredible insights related to their chief complaints. Observe their playing position and note any areas that might be under increased physical stress or be contributing to their problem.

TIPS TO TREATING MUSICIANS

The treatment plan for musicians should include counseling for home exercise programs, bracing, rest, and return to play, if necessary. In addition, the patient should be provided with appropriate prescriptions, referrals to other health care providers (physical therapy [PT], occupational therapy [OT], speech language pathology [SLP], audiology etc.), and procedures such as osteopathic manipulative treatments.

PROBLEMS SPECIFIC TO MUSICIANS

Neuromusculoskeletal Pathologies

Musicians' neuromusculoskeletal pathologies, especially instrumentalists, present as upper limb and face injuries due to repetitive motions and asymmetric and unnatural postures while playing.[13] Any pain and weakness, numbness, tingling, or other symptoms that interfere with the ability to play instruments at the level musicians are often called PRMD or playing-related musculoskeletal disorder.[14] PRMD is usually diagnosed when pain and somatic dysfunctions are present without other specific diagnoses.[14] Overuse injuries are likely the most common significant neuromusculoskeletal pathology observed among instrumentalists.[14] Tendon injuries and compression neuropathies, such as later and medial epicondylitis, carpal tunnel syndrome, and De Quervain tenosynovitis, are common examples of overuse injuries.[14]

Hypermobility

Hypermobility occurs in up to 20% of the musician population.[15] It is more common in the upper limb, especially fingers and wrists. Hypermobility problems are more common in younger and female musicians.[15] The joint laxity could be inherited (such as Ehlers–Danlos, hypermobility, or Marfan syndromes), but many patients have acquired localized joint laxity due to chronic ligamentous stress from repetitive motion. Musicians with hand and arm pain have been shown to have a high correlation with the presence of significant joint laxity.[15]

Musician's Focal Dystonia

Musician's focal dystonia is a painless movement disorder with an incidence as high as 1% among professional musicians.[16] This condition falls under the category of task-specific dystonia, meaning that it only occurs during play.[16] This diagnosis is terrifying to musicians as it will often mark the end of a professional career. At early stages, patients will often complain of slight loss of control in the hands or mouth in situations requiring fast or precise movements, such as trills, fingers sticking on keys or strings (if they're a string or keyboard player), or rapid tonguing in wind instrumentalists. Focal dystonia overwhelmingly affects classical musicians compared to jazz musicians.[16] Many musicians think their problem is due to flaws in technique or lack of practice, resulting in them intensifying their efforts to practice more to try to fix this problem, which often exacerbates their symptoms. Many patients are male, with the onset of symptoms in the late 20s and early 30s.[16]

Mental Health

Musicians experience intimate, intense, long-term relationships with their specific art form. Their art form is tied to their identity. Performance is the center of their function, and they live for the performances. Musicians often work in hostile environments, and their finances are poor, intensifying existing depression and anxiety. Looking for signs of performance anxiety and generalized anxiety, depression, and substance abuse is essential when evaluating a musician.[17]

Older Musicians

Musicians have long careers compared to other disciplines in performing arts. With aging humans experience the following[18]:

1. Changes in skeletal muscle function as above (speed, strength, stability, tone, etc.)
2. Joint disease in multiple regions of the body (not just upper limb/hands, fingers but neck and back)
3. Changes in neurologic systems (coordination of movements, memory, problem-solving, etc.)
4. Declining respiratory function
5. Declining cardiovascular systems
6. Hearing and vision changes
7. Females (effects of menopause)–changes in the mucous membranes, hot flashes

From studying older athletes,[19] it is crucial to consider that older musicians also could experience:

8. Increasing rate of fatigue and recovery time
9. Increased amount of damage and fatigue, as well as the impaired rate of repair
    a. Increasing exercise-induced skeletal muscle damage (as well as the decreased repair ability) is exceptionally well-known
10. Possible decrease of adaptive mechanisms (neuromusculoskeletal)

Therefore, older musicians will need help with the efficiency of play. For example, an older horn player may have efficiency issues due to the type of embouchure contact (use of the lips, facial muscles, tongue, and teeth in playing wind instruments).[20] They will also have increasing problems with strength and endurance, creating more problems for instrumentalists with bigger instruments. If they are woodwind or horn players, they may struggle with cardiovascular and pulmonary capacity issues. Here are a few more areas of consideration for older musicians[18]:

11. Hearing and vision loss
12. Increasing difficulty with sight reading, learning new music, and memory for those who start to have cognitive challenges
13. Pain caused by degenerative joint disease, myofascial pain, entrapment neuropathies, tendinopathies, and other chronic musculoskeletal disorders accumulated over a career

Voice Problems

Voice problems commonly occur in singers and other voice users. Patients present with complaints of voice fatigue, sound changes, hoarseness, and voice strain.[21] However, if the musician patient present after otolaryngologists, speech–language pathologists, and voice coaches' evaluations, and are found to be without any vocal cord pathologies, osteopathic evaluation and treatment can be a powerful addition in resolving their voice problems.[22] For example, somatic dysfunctions in the cranium, temporomandibular joint, muscles of mastication, and cervical and thoracic regions can easily alter voice quality.[23] In these cases, the osteopathic manipulative treatment can be life-altering for musicians with voice problems.

OSTEOPATHIC TREATMENT PRINCIPLES FOR PERFORMING ARTISTS

When approaching a performing artist from a treatment standpoint, the four osteopathic tenets must always be considered. Performers are more than a collection of symptoms and operate in a system that, in many cases, may be directly contributing to their injury or illness. Building a rational treatment plan will likely involve more people than just the performer themself.

Body, Mind, and Spirit

As mentioned above, performing artists define themselves by their identity as an artist. Being unable to perform due to injury has a profound effect on the patient's psyche above and beyond any pain or discomfort. Physicians, caring for this population, must treat performing artist complaints with the utmost care and concern, reflecting the impact that patients are experiencing. Taking a moment to acknowledge the impact that a problem must be having on the performer will help to establish rapport and mend the historical rifts between performers and health care professionals.

Similarly, inquiring about performance anxiety and depression may help to start a conversation that a performer would not necessarily initiate on their own. Beta blockers are commonly used among performers to treat the physical symptoms of performance anxiety, that is, sweating, palpitations, shakiness, or nausea, but physicians must ensure that patients are good candidates for this medication before prescribing.[24] Also, medication will not help with the psychological aspects of performance anxiety such as catastrophizing or overgeneralization. These factors must be addressed through activities like meditation, mindfulness, guided imagery, biofeedback, or referral for counseling.

Self-Healing, Self-Regulation, and Health Maintenance

Performing artists are masters of their craft. They spend countless hours honing, practicing, and perfecting their technique. As a community, they are driven and meticulous. When problems arise that affect their ability to perform, barriers are created for the patient not just in their health but their career. As osteopathic physicians, our charge is to find these barriers and work with the patient to eliminate them so that the patient can return to their state of "health," which is practicing and performing as their career demands.

Structure and Function

Given the physicality of performance, addressing postural and structural concerns among performing artists is a mainstay of treatment. Treating associated somatic dysfunctions with osteopathic manipulative treatment can be an outstanding tool to help restore structure and function for a performer.[22] As discussed above briefly, during the osteopathic exam, it is important to evaluate the artist in performance. This can be done by providing an environment where the performers can demonstrate live in the clinic settings, or they can bring videos and/or pictures of their performers to you.

In dancers, as discussed above, much of the forces are concentrated in the lower limb. Therefore, somatic dysfunctions of the lower limb will be common to observe and often, these somatic dysfunctions are caused by their repertoire, costumes, and/or footwear. Assessing and treating the foot and ankle with direct techniques like articulatory or muscle energy can be helpful. Dancers present often with lower limb pain that can be addressed by diagnosing and treating common tender points in the flexor hallucis longus, tibialis posterior, and gastrocnemius.[25] Structurally, ensuring that the tibia is well centered under the femur and the muscles surrounding the hip joint, namely the piriformis, gluteus medius and minimus, obturators and gemelli, will reduce mechanical loads and improve mobility and allow the dancers to perform optimally.

For instrumental musicians, the structural findings are more commonly concentrated in the upper limb.[26] As stated above, observing and understanding the artists' performance can reveal the causes of the somatic dysfunctions that occur commonly. Addressing the wrist and forearms, including the interosseous membrane with techniques such as balanced tension or myofascial release may help provide more facility of technique. Performing Spencer technique to the shoulder can similarly improve shoulder functionality. Finally, standard assessment of the cervical, thoracic, and lumbar spine in sitting musicians will find expected dysfunction patterns that may be addressed with several models.

Once treated, the critical next step is to empower patients to maintain and/or rehabilitate their own posture and structure either through targeted exercise, therapy referral, or use of adaptive equipment such as bracing or instrument modification where appropriate.

Rational Treatment

An interdisciplinary team is necessary when managing the medical problems of performing artists. Many medical specialties could be involved in this multidisciplinary team, including physiatry, primary care, otolaryngology, and orthopedic surgery. Allied health care professionals such as physical and occupational therapy, speech–language pathology, audiology, voice coaches, nutrition, and psychology may contribute as well in certain circumstances. Finally, the performing arts medicine team should also include the artists' personal instructors, coaches, and family, especially for younger artists. A treatment plan may involve scaling back rehearsals, practice, and performance time, changing instrument setup, changing footwear or costumes, and switching repertoire or technique. These tasks cannot happen without the instructors, coaches, teachers, and family on board with the plan.

Musculoskeletal pathology is the primary medical issue that stops artists from performing.[27] Therefore, the first critical step is to control symptoms and help the artist back into performing as soon as possible. Osteopathic physicians can utilize OMT and other musculoskeletal procedures necessary to achieve this. Acupuncture and/or functional dry needling can also be an effective procedure to manage musculoskeletal pathology without huge risk to the performers.[28] Although there is anecdotal evidence that OMT and needling can be combined for increased synergy of the procedures; the use of acupuncture and dry needling is increasingly popular among osteopathic physicians and clinicians.[29] With appropriate counseling in mechanics, a rehabilitation plan with physical and/or occupational therapy, and meaningful home exercise plan to increase strength, endurance, and body awareness, the artists will be able to stay on stage safely for the long term.[30]

Performing artists are often placed in situations where they are not in control of their bodies. For example, an orchestra or choir rehearsal operates at the pace of the conductor, who instructs musicians when to perform. Similarly, a dancer is often performing choreography that another person created, and subject to the person running a rehearsal. If the performer is unable to meet the demands of their overseers, they may lose their standing or their job. Very few positions are subject to collective bargaining or protections, and employers may use this setup to mistreat their employees, either with or without intention. When performing artists present to physicians seeking care for their medical problems, sometimes the best recourse is advocacy on behalf of the patients. A note or conversation with one conductor may positively impact not just the patient, but the dozens of other performers this conductor supervises.

CONCLUSION

In conclusion, performing artists represent a medically underserved population with specific needs. This group of professionals suffers a disproportionately high rate of injury directly tied to their occupation, and proper treatment of these injures requires specialized knowledge about the activities, settings, and stressors that performing artists face. Armed with information and a willingness to meet performing artists where they are, the osteopathic physician can make significant contributions to the holistic care of this population.

REFERENCES

1. Elam T, Mowen S, Jonas C. Occupational injuries in musicians: a literature review. *Mil Med.* 2022;187(5–6):e619–e623.
2. Middlestadt SE, Fishbein M. Health and occupational correlates of perceived occupational stress in symphony orchestra musicians. *J Occup Med.* 1988;30(9):687–692.
3. Alimena S, Air ME. Trust, satisfaction, and confidence in health care providers among student and professional dancers in France. *Med Probl Perform Art.* 2016;31(3):166–173.
4. Bird HA, Foley EC. Hypermobility in dancers. *Rheumatology (Oxford).* 2013;52(4):585–586.
5. Surve S. Performing arts medicine: an underserved population with unique demands. *Maryland Med.* 2018;18(4):12–13.
6. Khan K, Brown J, Way S, et al. Overuse injuries in classical ballet. *Sports Med.* 1995;19(5):341–357.
7. Gottschlich LM, Young CC. Spine injuries in dancers. *Curr Sports Med Rep.* 2011;10(1):40–44.
8. Langdon SW, Petracca G. Tiny dancer: body image and dancer identity in female modern dancers. *Body Image.* 2010;7(4):360–363.
9. Zuhdi N, Chesky K, Surve S, Lee Y. Occupational health problems of classical guitarists. *Med Probl Perform Art.* 2020;35(3):167–179.

10. Gómez-López B, Sánchez-Cabrero R. Current trends in music performance anxiety intervention. *Behav Sci (Basel)*. 2023;13(9):720.
11. Yang N, Fufa DT, Wolff AL. A musician-centered approach to management of performance-related upper musculoskeletal injuries. *J Hand Ther*. 2021;34(2):208–216.
12. Grahame R. Joint hypermobility and the performing musician. *N Engl J Med*. 1993;329(15):1120–1121.
13. Lockwood AH. Medical problems of musicians. *N Engl J Med*. 1989; 320(4):221–227.
14. Altenmuller E, Jabusch H-C. Focal dystonia in musicians: phenomenology, pathophysiology, triggering factors, and treatment. *Med Probl Perform Art*. 2010;25(1):3–9
15. Schneider E, Chesky K. Social support and performance anxiety of college music students. *Med Probl Perform Art*. 2011;26(3):157–163.
16. Dziechciaż M, Filip R. Biological psychological and social determinants of old age: bio-psycho-social aspects of human aging. *Ann Agric Environ Med*. 2014;21(4):835–838.
17. Catapano M, Ahmed M, Breslow RG, Borg-Stein J. The aging athlete. *PM R*. 2022;14(5):643–651.
18. Franco RA, Andrus JG. Common diagnoses and treatments in professional voice users. *Otolaryngol Clin North Am*. 2007;40(5):1025–1061, vii.
19. Kiepe MS, Fernholz I, Schmidt T, et al. Effects of osteopathic manipulative treatment on musicians: a systematic review. *Med Probl Perform Art*. 2020;35(2):110–115.
20. Chesky K, Devroop K, Ford J III. Medical problems of brass instrumentalists: prevalence rates for trumpet, trombone, French horn, and low brass. *Med Probl Perform Art*. 2002;17(2):92–98.
21. Marszałek S, Niebudek-Bogusz E, Woźnicka E, Malińska J, Golusiński W, Śliwińska-Kowalska M. Assessment of the influence of osteopathic myofascial techniques on normalization of the vocal tract functions in patients with occupational dysphonia. *Int J Occup Med Environ Health*. 2012;25(3):225–235.
22. Fernholz I, Mumm JLM, Plag J, et al. Performance anxiety in professional musicians: a systematic review on prevalence, risk factors and clinical treatment effects. *Psychol Med*. 2019;49(14):2287–2306.
23. Dobson R. Eight in ten dancers have an injury each year, survey shows. *BMJ*. 2005;331(7517):594.
24. Brandfonbrener AG. Joint laxity and arm pain in large clinical sample of musicians. *Med Probl Perform Art*. 2002;17(3):1.
25. Jacobs CL, Cassidy JD, Côté P, et al. Musculoskeletal injury in professional dancers: prevalence and associated factors: an international cross-sectional study. *Clin J Sport Med*. 2017;27(2):153–160.
26. Blackmon AM, Elson L. Dry needling and acupuncture in treatment of dance-related injuries, MD, and PT perspectives. *Phys Med Rehabil Clin N Am*. 2021;32(1):169–183.
27. Rickards LD. Therapeutic needling in osteopathic practice: an evidence-informed perspective. *Int J Osteopath Med*. 2009;12:2–13.
28. Ackermann BJ. Making health care worth it: increasing value and awareness in performing arts medicine. *Med Probl Perform Art*. 2018;33(2): 146.
29. Bird HA. Overuse syndrome in musicians. *Clin Rheumatol*. 2013;32(4): 475–479.
30. Elson LE. *Performing Arts Medicine*. 1st ed. Elsevier; 2018.

91 Osteopathic Approach to Diagnosing and Treating Somatic Dysfunction in the Extremities

KURT P. HEINKING ▪ KRISTA LUND ▪ MICHAEL L. KUCHERA

KEY CONCEPTS

- Somatic dysfunction in the extremities can have both regional and systemic relevance.
- The five models of osteopathic care are useful for organizing information, developing a differential diagnosis of extremity problems, and designing a management plan, including the application of osteopathic manipulative treatment (OMT).
- Knowledge of functional anatomy and the restrictions that lead to somatic dysfunction within specific extremity regions is required for accurate physical examination and development of differential diagnoses.
- Proper assessment of somatic dysfunction within the extremities is needed to formulate an osteopathic management plan that includes OMT.
- OMT of somatic dysfunction in the extremities is commonly used for patients who suffer from sports- or activity-related injuries and traumas.
- OMT can also improve function and reduce pain for other clinical conditions affecting the extremities.

INTRODUCTION

The extremities are vital to performing activities of daily living. Even minor injuries may produce disabilities that significantly affect overall function. A thorough knowledge of functional anatomy of the upper and lower extremities is needed to accurately perform an assessment and develop a treatment plan for any given extremity symptom. Diagnosing the location, etiology, and the significance of the axial somatic components proximal to the affected extremity is as critical as examining the extremity. Somatic dysfunction in the axial body can cause symptoms in the extremities; just as extremity dysfunction can have axial effects.

The clinical screening evaluation, regardless of the chief complaint should include an initial static postural examination, gait observation, and regional range-of-motion testing. In addition to the osteopathic structural examination, standardized tests for ligamentous laxity, orthopedic injuries, and nerve entrapment can help pinpoint the diagnosis. Osteopathic manipulative treatment (OMT) of associated somatic dysfunctions in the spinal regions and in the extremities supports restoration of the patient's maximal health potential.

The following chapters may need to be referred to for more detailed information related to the functional anatomy and diagnostic examination (Section V).

- Upper Extremity region (Chapter 39)
- Lower Extremity region (Chapter 40)
- Osteopathic Structural Examination (Chapters 30) and Osteopathic Segmental Examination (Chapter 31) provide details for identifying somatic dysfunction throughout the body.

The following chapters may be referred to for more detailed information related to the application of osteopathic principles in clinical conditions of the extremities.

- Osteopathic Considerations in Orthopedics (Chapter 84) subsection Specific Orthopedic Tests (Organized by Chief Complaint) provides detailed descriptions of many of the commonly used extremity Orthopedic tests.
- Osteopathic Considerations in Sports Medicine (Chapter 87) discusses specific upper and lower extremity injuries in athletes.
- Postural Considerations in Osteopathic Diagnosis and Treatment (Chapter 92) provides information on the integration of the function of the lower extremities in gait, posture and balance.
- Osteopathic Considerations in Neurology (Chapter 73) describes the specific tests for various neurologic symptoms related to the extremities.

This chapter is divided into sections for easier navigation to specific extremity regions. First, the five models of osteopathic care approach to evaluating and treating the extremities is discussed. After that, each joint region of the upper extremities and lower extremities is divided into individual sections. The motion and nomenclature for somatic dysfunction as well as brief discussions of some osteopathic manipulative methods for those somatic dysfunctions are described first. Then specific clinical conditions related to that region and the osteopathic care approach to those conditions is discussed to varying levels of detail.

Systemic Relevance

The regional structure and the function of the upper and lower extremities are inexorably linked to systemic clinical issues. Several systemic disorders manifest with signs and symptoms in the upper or lower extremities and must be differentiated from alternative local diagnoses. The five models of osteopathic care can be applied to the extremities to organize information obtained during a history and physical examination and develop a management plan that adheres to the osteopathic philosophy and its tenets.

In clinical practice, the osteopathic practitioner seeks to ensure and enhance the structure–function relationships that are important to the biomechanical, neurologic, respiratory–circulatory, metabolic–energetic, and biopsychosocial functions of the extremities. Clinical goals include

- Promotion of energy-efficient, painless motion
- Maintenance of optimal stability–flexibility balance in and around the joints
- Reduction of mechanical stress on somatic (skeletal, arthrodial, myofascial) structures
- Motor, sensory, proprioceptive, and autonomic neural balance
- Elimination of nociceptive drive
- Elimination of afferent referral from associated viscera
- Elimination of entrapment phenomena and compartment syndromes
- Effective venous and lymphatic return

Regional Relevance

Regardless of the systemic implications, the basic examination of the extremity should include an understanding of the functional anatomy and the following regional relationships:

1. Skeletal, arthrodial, ligamentous, and myofascial structure and function
2. Neuromuscular structure and function
3. Vascular and lymphatic structure and function

Throughout this chapter, these relationships will be linked to several regional clinical considerations and some associated osteopathic manipulation techniques.

The Clinical Evaluation

When evaluating extremity discomfort, or other relevant symptoms, the clinician must determine the exact nature of the chief complaint and its duration, location, severity, and associated symptoms. The presenting complaint may be pain; however, it may also be weakness, swelling, or stiffness. Upper or lower extremity discomfort cannot always be attributed to orthopedic conditions or somatic dysfunction in this area. The clinician must obtain as much information as possible in a time-efficient manner to determine whether the discomfort is primarily caused by musculoskeletal dysfunction, a medical diagnosis, or referred from another area.

If the cause of somatic dysfunction lies in the extremity itself, there is generally restricted motion. Flaccidity, severe weakness, or atrophy are signs of nerve entrapment or damage. Hypermobility is usually related to ligamentous laxity, a partial tear, or rupture. Pain is usually localized to specific dermatomes and may be described as acute, sharp, or severe. Discomfort is usually improved by rest, is frequently reproduced by motion, and may lead to the perception of strength loss.

If the discomfort is referred from another area (e.g., the lungs, diaphragm, heart, abdominal viscera, or spine), passive motion does not appear to be restricted. The pain is diffuse and poorly localized. It may be described as nagging, achy, or dull and it is usually worse at night. It is frequently related to symptoms in other areas (difficulty breathing, chest pain, cough, gastrointestinal upset) and may not be reproduced by motion. Motion is generally good but decreased strength or muscle atrophy is possible (e.g., disk herniation).

Pain is not the only presenting complaint. The patient may relate stiffness, swelling, and weakness as well. Specific information in the history may indicate the diagnosis. For example, pain radiating into the deltoid insertion at night and an inability to lie on the involved shoulder correlate with a rotator cuff tear. Pain or numbness radiating down the leg, relieved with lying down, may indicate lumbar radiculopathy. Any patient presenting with extremity discomfort should receive a thorough osteopathic examination. Focused visual observation for asymmetry or restriction of motion and palpation for tissue texture change or tenderness needs to include bilateral extremities, as well as the associated proximal structures.

- For an upper extremity complaint, include evaluation of the cervical and thoracic spine, the ribs, clavicles, and scapula.
- For a lower extremity complaint, include evaluation of the thoracic and lumbar spine, the sacrum, and innominates.

All muscles affecting the extremity from those regions should be palpated, especially those that the history indicates are likely involved. Fascia needs to be assessed both grossly and locally for dysfunction. Common areas of fascial restriction in the upper extremities include the thoracic inlet, pectorals, latissimus dorsi, and interosseous membrane of the forearms. Fascial restrictions within the thoracolumbar, lumbosacral, and sacroiliac junctions as well as the pelvic diaphragm my affect the lower extremities. There are also many special tests of the extremity that are useful to determine if orthopedic, neurologic, or vascular compromise is present. (See Chapter 84 Osteopathic Considerations in Orthopedics section Specific Orthopedic Tests [Organized by Chief Complaint] and Chapter 73 Osteopathic Considerations in Neurology.)

Osteopathic techniques can be applied to the areas of somatic dysfunction. The models described below of structure–function relationships guide the osteopathic practitioner's approach to diagnosis and treatment. The five structure function models provide a framework for integrating objective and subjective clinical findings with osteopathic structural exam findings.

FIVE-MODEL APPROACH TO EVALUATING AND TREATING THE EXTREMITIES

Biomechanical Model

The extremities are susceptible to many common mechanical injuries:

- Bone fractures
- Joint dislocations
- Ligamentous and capsular sprains
- Muscle and tendon strains
- Bursitis
- Skin abrasions, cuts, and bruises
- Somatic dysfunction

Injuries, repetitive overuse, postural strain, muscle imbalance, and scoliosis can all contribute to or be the etiologic factor in upper or lower extremity complaints. Evaluation for a biomechanical axial component of the extremity complaint involves palpation for single type II dysfunctions in key areas, as well as diagnosing group spinal mechanics. Postural considerations such as leg length inequality, flattening or exaggeration of the AP curves, forward head position, and scoliosis, are important biomechanical considerations. The Biomechanical model also considers the myofascial system which interconnects the segmented spinal column to the trunk and extremities. A fascial restriction in area of the body can and frequently does influence motion characteristics of local and distant structures. (See Chapter 52 Myofascial Release.)

When considering the Biomechanical model, the clinician should view the totality of somatic structures as a "kinetic chain."[1,2] A kinetic chain is described as a sequencing of individual body segments and joints to accomplish a task. It generally functions from a base of support proximally and then proceeds distally, but this is entirely dependent on the task at hand. The complexity of the anatomic and biomechanical interactions as well as neuromuscular control issues can make evaluation and accurate diagnosis clinically challenging.

Disruption of the kinetic chain, and its associated somatic dysfunction, if left unidentified and untreated, may lead to altered muscle-firing patterns resulting in overload to connective tissues (capsular laxity and instability, labral tears) or the joint itself (osteoarthritis, etc.). While the patient may complain of pain due to one traumatic event, most mechanical extremity problems result from repetitive overuse of the osteoarticular system and related neural, soft tissue, and muscular elements. One example of this is in overhead athletes, as they try to transmit the ground reactive force from their pelvis and trunk through their upper extremity.[1,2]

Normal sagittal spine–pelvis–lower extremity alignment is crucial for maintaining an ergonomic upright standing posture.[3] To keep upright, the body slightly sways over its base of support using the ankles and hips to counter imbalance. Sway is primarily caused by actions of the ankle musculature attempting to keep the center of mass over the base of support during minor disturbances in balance. Major balance disturbances are managed by the hips and trunk musculature bringing postural center of mass over the base of support. In more extreme circumstances, the upper extremities will move, or the body will step in the opposite direction of the disturbance to shift the base of support and prevent a fall.[4] For these reasons, OMT and rehabilitation (including orthotics, exercises, and other adjunctive strategies) are used to address local, regional issues—such as a pronated foot or an anatomically shortened femur—to affect the more systemic postural issues. (See Chapter 92 Postural Considerations in Osteopathic Diagnosis and Treatment for further discussion of postural considerations.)

Extremity joint function should be examined and treated while recognizing that each joint has both major and minor motions that are distinct to the structure and function of that joint. Each joint is adapted for an optimal balance between flexibility and stability. Major motions of the joints are best recognized by the patient; minor joint motions are glides that are often not able to be produced voluntarily in isolation and that are typically assessed with palpation focused on end-feel. Failure to address the minor motion of a joint with OMT may lead to incomplete restoration of normal joint motion.[5] The pattern of major and minor joint motions helps in the differential diagnosis of each joint.

In addition, joint capsules are subject to pathologic and inflammatory processes. Such processes result in *capsular patterns* of restricted motion in which all or most passive movements of the joint prove painful and limited.[6] A capsular pattern due to inflammation or pathology is palpably different from the patterns of tenderness and restricted motion assessed in somatic dysfunction. Palpation of the capsular pattern is also dramatically different from the laxity assessed in ligamentous sprains. Thus, palpation of the end-feel provides significant information about the differential diagnosis of a painful or improperly functioning joint. Many rheumatologic diagnoses present with deep-seated, toothache-like, sclerotomal pain and a capsular palpatory pattern.

LIGAMENTOUS SPRAIN CLASSIFICATION

In the diagnosis of ligamentous sprains, the joint line and stabilizing ligaments should be directly palpated for tenderness followed by end-feel assessment for arthrodial motion or laxity. The greater the structural damage due to ligamentous spraining, the greater the laxity that results in a loss of normal end-feel and stability. Palpation of joint play and end-feel are, therefore, useful in classification of traumatic and orthopedic conditions such as sprains and in differentiating these from somatic dysfunction.

Ligamentous sprains are traditionally classified from grades I to III[7]:

- Grade I (or first-degree) sprains consist of minor intraligamentous tears with pain but no instability.
  - While tender to specific palpation and painful when stressed, these sprains are generally stable to most orthopedic ligamentous tests. There is little to no swelling, no hemorrhaging, and no significant loss of function.
  - Patients with Grade I sprains commonly respond well to conservative osteopathic care focusing on functional strategies and might even return to activity within days of the injury.[7,8] With proper care, such sprains typically recover with normal function and no ligamentous laxity.
- Grade II (or second-degree) sprains are incomplete tears with pain and mild to moderate instability.
  - The increase in fiber damage of grade II sprains although partial can range in severity and ligament laxity. There is usually some loss of function, swelling, and hemorrhaging.
  - Second-degree sprains do not usually require surgical repair if they are immobilized for a duration that is appropriate to stabilize the amount of structural damage. Prolotherapy[9] or certain rehabilitative procedures may be employed to restore a component of the laxity and lost joint stability. (See Chapter 89 Prolotherapy for Knee Pain with Enthesopathy for more information on Prolotherapy.)
- Grade III (or third-degree) sprains are the most severe with complete ligamentous rupture.
  - These sprains are the most disabling, with no remaining tensile strength and a "sloppy" end-feel of complete instability during orthopedic testing. There is usually significant or total loss of function, swelling, and hemorrhaging.
  - Proper splinting and early surgery may offer the best prognosis when dealing with Grade III ligamentous sprains around the structurally unstable knee. With ligaments of the inherently more stable ankle joint, surgery may be delayed or unnecessary to reestablish stability; recovery can take up to 6 months.[8]

Respiratory–Circulatory Model

The health and function of the extremities requires maintenance of extra- and intracellular environments through the unimpeded delivery of oxygen and nutrients and removal of cellular waste products. For example, proximal arterial compression may produce ischemic symptoms in the distal aspects of the extremities and fascial restrictions can affect the lymphatic drainage of the extremities. Osteopathic manipulation may be used to improve blood flow to the area of injury and remove edema, which may assist in pain reduction, healing, and improved mobility.

Regardless of whether the patient presents with an upper extremity or lower extremity complaint, both diagnosis and treatment of the extremity should begin proximally and move distally. It is important to consider the anatomical structures that could impede vasculature and lymphatic flow throughout the entire drainage system. At the most proximal end, the subclavian vein passes over the first rib and below the clavicle, crossing over the anterior scalene muscle's insertion on the first rib. The left brachiocephalic vein passes posterior to the left sternoclavicular joint (SCJ) and then crosses the midline. Somatic dysfunction involving the anterior and middle scalenes, upper thoracic vertebrae, upper ribs, clavicles, and the fascia of the upper extremity may affect arterial supply and venous return throughout the body. If left untreated, somatic dysfunction may also affect lymphatic drainage, thereby producing congestion in the upper and lower extremities. The right subclavian lymphatic trunk drains into the right lymphatic duct. The thoracic duct, sometimes called the left lymphatic duct, is the

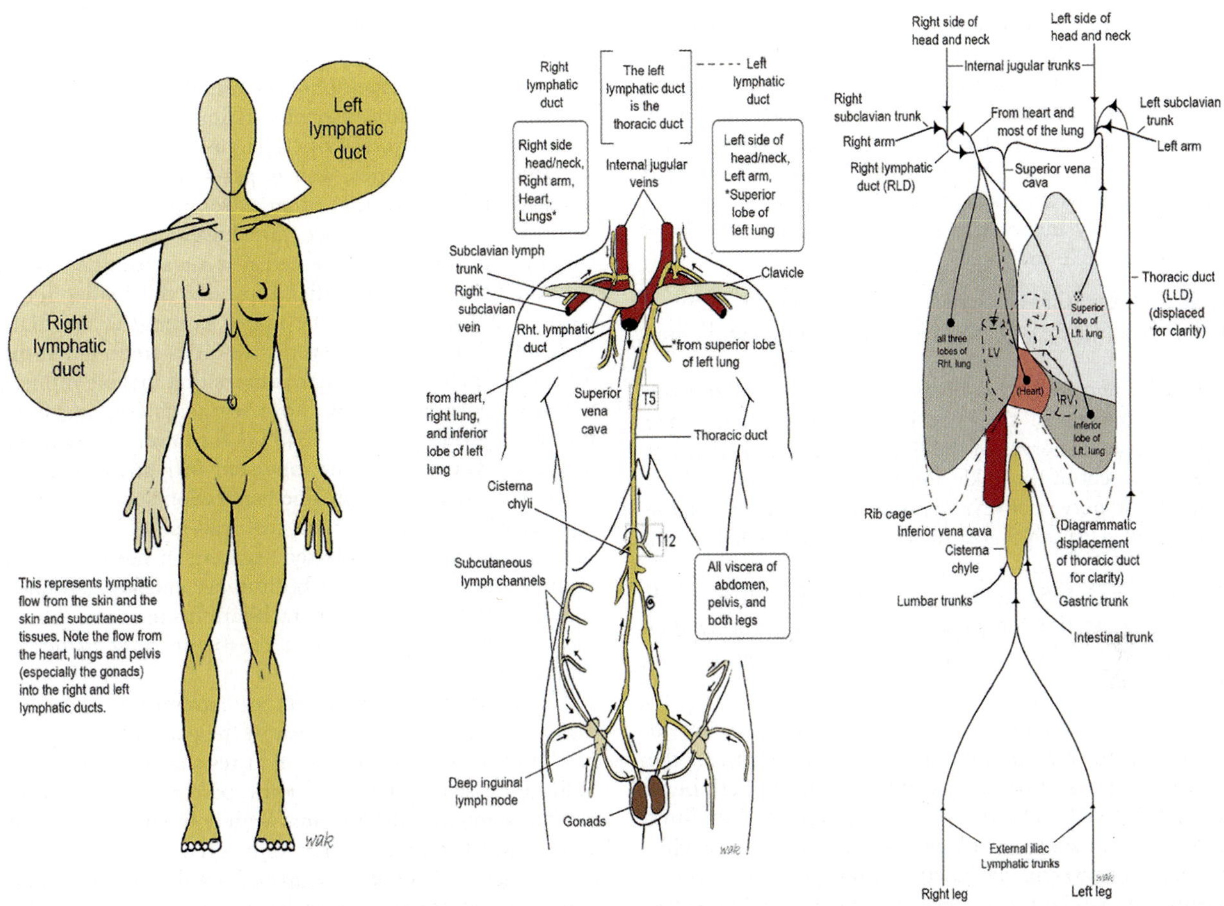

Figure 91.1. Lymphatic drainage of the body. (Illustration by William A. Kuchera, DO, FAAO, with permission.)

final terminal drainage site for the left subclavian lymphatic trunk and bilateral inguinal trunks (Fig. 91.1). Fascial restrictions of the right thoracic inlet and pectoral fascia can cause lymphatic stasis of the right head, neck, chest, and right upper extremity. Fascial restrictions of the left thoracic inlet and pectoral fascia can cause lymphatic stasis of the left head, neck, chest, left upper extremity, and rest of the body.

After addressing thoracic inlet restrictions, improving motion in the lower ribs, lower thoracic, and upper lumbar regions will help the function of the thoracoabdominal diaphragm from a mechanical perspective. Improving motion in the cervical region will help the function of the diaphragm from a neurologic perspective. Both regional approaches restore normal thoracoabdominal diaphragmatic motion, which is the primary driving force to move lymph. Attention may then be directed more specifically to the upper or lower extremities. The sequence of treatments will still address proximal restrictions before moving to more distal restrictions.

For the upper extremity, the removal of pectoral and axillary restrictions is the next step. Originally, Spencer's technique was described as a lymphatic technique for the upper extremity.[10] Over the years, its clinical utility has broadened, and it is often modified to address other musculoskeletal dysfunctions of the upper extremity. Treatment of the distal arm, forearm, and hand may be necessary as well, if indicated.

For the lower extremities, addressing any pelvic diaphragm restrictions should be employed prior to lymphatic treatment of the legs and feet. Terminal lymphatic drainage sites are located just inferior to the inguinal ligament in the femoral triangle, and as severity increases, the congestion extends to fullness in the popliteal region and eventually to the tissues around the Achilles tendon. In addition to fullness or bogginess, dysfunctional drainage results in tissues that are tight, tender, or ticklish. Should one of these peripheral sites be congested without the more proximal site(s), this would indicate a localized trauma rather than a problem involving the entire extremity.

In addition, the very act of locomotion plays an important role in lymphatic and venous return. Use of the lower extremity muscles in walking and running moves these fluids through one-way valves back toward the central vascular system. OMT to open fascial pathways can improve venous and lymphatic drainage of the extremities. Drainage can also be enhanced using a variety of lymphatic pump techniques such as those performed on the chest cage to maximize pressure gradients between the thorax and abdomen or directly through the lower extremities with the pedal pump (Dalrymple) technique (each is described more fully in Chapter 50 Lymphatic Drainage Procedures).

Neurologic Model

Another important objective when addressing extremity complaints is to normalize neurologic input to the extremity. The upper extremities possess motor, sensory, and autonomic innervations that extend from the cervical and upper thoracic region while the lower extremities have innervations that extend from the lower thoracic region to the sacrum.

Pain within the extremities can be directly related to injury and inflammation of the region's anatomical structures. Alternatively, pain may be referred from other skeletal, arthrodial, ligamentous, and myofascial structures as well as from a variety of neural, vascular, and visceral structures that share axial innervation levels.

Upper motor neuron disorders are characterized by hyperreflexia and associated pathologic reflexes such as Hoffman sign in the upper extremity or ankle clonus and/or the Babinski (upgoing toe) reflex in the lower extremity. Upper motor neuron lesions may demonstrate spasticity or rigidity of the muscles. Lower motor neuron disorders are generally characterized by hyporeflexia with accompanying muscle weakness, flaccidity, or atrophy.

Motor and sensory innervation to the extremities arise from specific spinal level nerve root plexus[11]:

- The brachial plexus (C5–T1) innervates the upper extremity.
- The lumbar plexus (L2–L4) gives rise to the femoral and obturator nerves.
  - The femoral nerve conveys fibers to the flexors of the hip joint and extensors of the knee joint, along with multiple anterior cutaneous nerves of the thigh, the anteromedial leg, and medial aspect of the ankle and foot.
  - The obturator nerve conveys fibers to the adductors of the hip joint and a variable area of skin on the medial thigh, above the knee.
- The sacral plexus (L4–S3) gives rise to the sciatic nerve which descends in the posterior compartment of the thigh and further separates into the tibial and common fibular nerve components proximal to the knee.

Axial or sacral dysfunction at any of these levels may impair the function of the nerve roots and thus the specific plexus. As the nerve roots traverse the soft tissues, proximal (axial) and peripheral articular and myofascial restrictions should be removed to limit compression of the neurovascular bundles supplying the specific extremity region. Improving dysfunctional position and motion can help resolve the fascial restrictions, relieve compression to the neurovascular bundle, and improve axoplasmic flow, enhancing the nerves' trophic function.

Dermatomal patterns of pain and/or dysesthesia associated with radicular (nerve root) problems in the extremities follow general patterns as depicted in Figure 91.2. It is also important to differentiate pain descriptions and patterns associated with a dermatomal pattern from pain associated with sclerotomal and myotomal distributions. Sclerotomal referral is a deep, achy sensation that is toothache-like in quality, while myotomal pain referral often results in a sensation described as a *charley horse* or a crampy sensation that *reaches out and grabs* with a particular movement. Often, the pain quality and patterns are mixed.

Myofascial somatic dysfunction in the extremities can also lead to several patient symptoms including pain, weakness, limited range of motion, and/or altered joint function. Myofascial trigger points (MTrPs) as described by Travell and Simons also have predictable referral patterns not associated with dermatomes.[12] See Chapter 43 Clinical Assessment: Viscerosomatic, Somatosomatic, Somatovisceral Reflexes; Counterstrain Points, Myofascial Trigger Points, and Chapman Reflexes for more information about trigger points (TrPs). A synopsis of representative TrPs associated with the lower extremities is illustrated in Figure 40.21 *Travell MTrP patterns in the lower extremity.* These points are a form of somatic dysfunction. They represent impaired or altered function of myofascial tissues with effects also in related neural, vascular, and lymphatic elements. TrPs respond to a wide range of treatment techniques: counterstrain, muscle energy, vapocoolant spray and stretch, dry needling, and procaine injection to name but a few. It is important, however, to identify any precipitating or perpetuating factors including coexistent lumbosacral radiculopathy, muscle imbalance, or poor ergonomics used in a repetitive manner.

Sympathetic stimulation causes peripheral vasoconstriction in the extremities. Patients who have increased sympathetic tone to the extremity can have nondermatomal paresthesia, pain, muscular tension/irritability, vasoconstriction, vascular reactivity, edema, and sweat gland overactivity. Diagnosing somatic dysfunction of the thoracic spine, ribs, and upper lumbar spine is an important step in the evaluation of an extremity complaint. In addition, somatic dysfunction of the mid-lower cervical spine (C4–C7) should be diagnosed and treated as it can affect the function of the cervical sympathetic ganglia. Typically, cell bodies for the sympathetic nerve supply to the upper extremities are found at the levels of T2–T7 and the lower extremities are found at the level of T11–L2. There are also some sources that include influences from vertebra above and below those segments (varying from T1–T9 for upper extremities and T10–L3 for lower extremities)[11,13–16] as increased sympathetic tone can occur with any thoracic or lumbar facilitated spinal segment. The facilitation/sensitization seen with segmental spinal dysfunction can traverse up or down the spine several segments. A facilitated segment in the thoracic spine can even produce symptoms in both upper and lower limbs.[17] Longstanding dysfunctions with facilitation/sensitization of the segmental spinal cord can affect the organs and tissues served by these levels (Fig. 91.3).[18–20]

The quality of pain within an extremity can also assist with making a presumptive diagnosis of the pathophysiologic condition of a joint. Pain occurring prior to resistance of movement might indicate an acutely inflamed joint, pain that is synchronous with resistance might indicate a less acutely inflamed joint and delayed asymmetrical joint pain that only occurs after resistive exercise might suggest a joint predisposed to developing inflammation. Pain upon active motion that disappears when the joint is passively moved might reflect that the pain generator lies in muscles around the joint rather than within the joint itself.

Understanding the difference between various symptoms and palpatory findings will allow the clinician to differentiate suspected diagnoses and treatments. Failure to appreciate the distinction of findings may lead a practitioner to ineffectively treat symptoms rather than causes or to incorrectly consider a patient with legitimate symptoms as a malingerer.

Therapeutic application of OMT within this model focuses on the reduction of mechanical stresses, balance of neural inputs, reduction of pain with elimination of nociceptive drive, and coordination of processes in gait.

Metabolic–Energy (Nutritional) Model

Treatment of somatic dysfunction is postulated to improve blood delivery to the extremities by reducing mechanical restrictions and by reducing vasoconstriction from hypersympathetic activity. This is important for the nutritional status of the tissues and benefits the delivery of medications such as nonsteroidal anti-inflammatory drugs (NSAIDs) to target tissues in the extremities where pharmacologic effectiveness is proportionate to tissue or synovial concentration of the drug.

Efficient transfer of energy is vital to extremity function and performance. The metabolic processes manifest grossly in the biomechanical, cardiac, respiratory, neurologic, and psychological systems. One analogy is to envision the body as a large machine. The cardiovascular system is the engine that drives the metabolic system. This diverse system can adapt quickly to changing needs. When needed, the system shifts from the homeostatic life-sustaining mode to a supercharged state for athletic activity. This is mediated at the cellular level as cell depolarization, resulting in

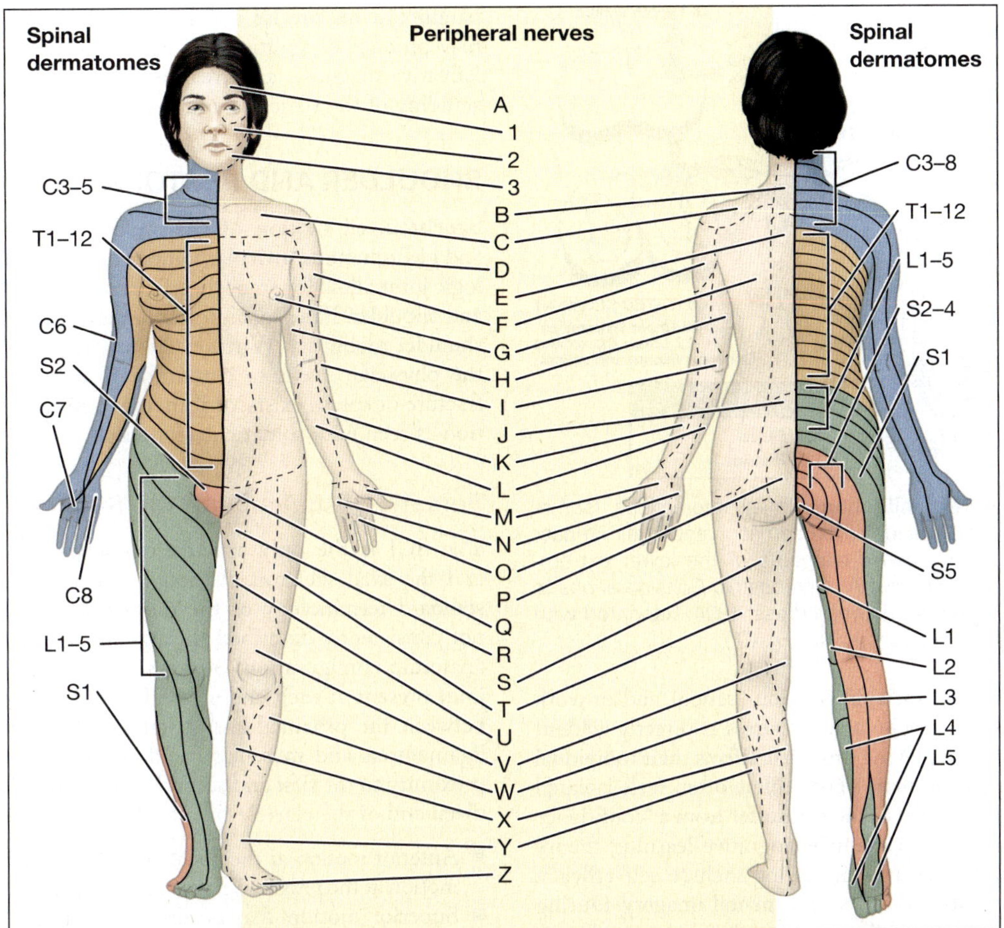

A Divisions of trigeminal 1 Ophthalmic 2 Maxillary 3 Mandibular B Posterior cervical rami C Branches from cervical plexus D Anterior thoracic rami E Posterior thoracic rami F Axillary G Lateral thoracic rami H Branches from medial cord of brachial plexus I Radial J Posterior lumbar rami K Lateral antebrachial cutaneous	L Median antebrachial cutaneous M Radial N Ulnar O Median P Posterior sacral rami Q Iliohypogastric R Ilioinguinal S Posterior femoral cutaneous T Lateral femoral cutaneous U Obturator V Anterior femoral cutaneous W Common peroneal X Saphenous Y Superficial peroneal Z Deep peroneal

Figure 91.2. Cutaneous sensation. The cutaneous sensation patterns of spinal nerve dermatomes differ from the patterns innervated by the peripheral nerves. (Reprinted with permission from Anderson MK, Barnum M. *Foundations of Athletic Training: Prevention, Assessment, and Management.* 7th ed. Wolters Kluwer; 2022:253. Figure 11-7.)

measurable changes in cardiac output that enable the patient to meet the demands placed upon them by activity. The "fuel" that drives this system is supplied by the pulmonary system via the gas exchange that occurs at the level of the pulmonary capillaries. This oxygen-rich blood is transported through the larger pulmonary veins and eventually to the left atrium. This fuel is then supplied to the neuromusculoskeletal system and throughout the rest of the body. Occasionally, these systems function together with perfect harmony and precision. The integration of these processes combined with the influence of psychological factors leads to an efficiently functioning machine. Under these ideal circumstances, there is an optimal balance between energy expenditure and energy intake. Disruption in any of these metabolic processes, as in an injury or illness, shifts the balance and leads to an inefficient system.[21]

Behavioral (Biopsychosocial) Model

Limitations to the normal function of the extremities can affect a person's mood and impact psychosocial, cultural, behavioral, and spiritual elements. As osteopathic physicians who consider the balance of body, mind, and spirit, the psychological impact of extremity conditions and potential for disability can influence

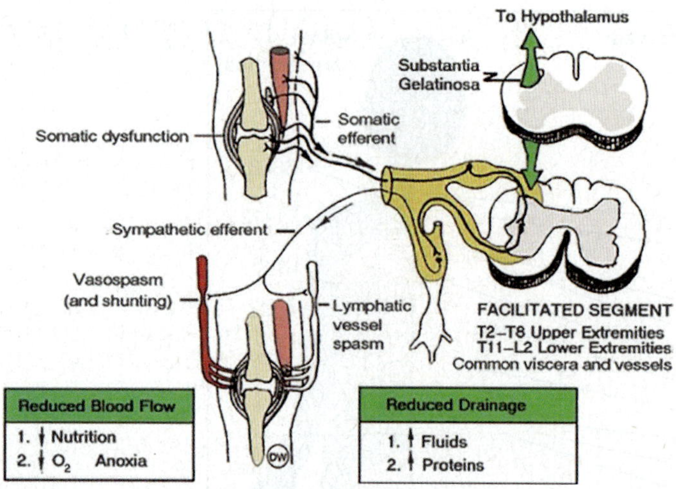

Figure 91.3. Segmental facilitation. Reflex interactions (somatosomatic, somatovisceral, and viscerosomatic) and their impact on normal vascular and lymphatic elements of the lower extremity. (From Kuchera ML, Kuchera WA. *Osteopathic Considerations in Systemic Dysfunction.* 2nd ed. Greyden Press; 1994. Reprinted with permission from Michael L. Kuchera, DO, FAAO.)

interpersonal relationships, social interactions, school, and/or work performance. In athletes, psychological distress is directly evident by the missed practice and playing time that affects their individual season as well as their teammates. The athlete often feels isolated from the team during treatments and can suffer from a "confidence crisis." Using an athlete as an example, cognitive learning theory and skills that apply to the athletic setting include self-efficacy, arousal regulation, attentional focus, and mental imagery. During periods of injury, the athlete's ability to access this system is altered, which can have significant psychosocial and emotional impact. Enhancing an athlete's self-efficacy promotes decision-making skills and problem-solving ability through practice and role playing to deal with disease-related issues.[22]

Among the general population, musculoskeletal injury or orthopedic trauma has a large influence on the psychological well-being of those affected. A Norwegian study demonstrated that patients recovering from orthopedic trauma had lower mental health scores compared to the healthy population.[23] One-third of these patients were diagnosed with PTSD that was still present 2 years following the initial injury.[23] Depression is one of the most common comorbidities seen with PTSD, and the interaction between the two can lead to increased distress levels and functional impairment.[24] In orthopedic trauma patients, the prevalence of depression is high and can be present right after the initial injury and linger for years following injury recovery.[24] Depression itself can increase the risk of subsequent injury 2 years after the initial injury.[25] This is why it is essential for clinicians to make sure they are screening patients for these conditions and treating accordingly. Anxiety was also found to be elevated in trauma cohorts of all ethnic backgrounds.[26] Patients with anxiety following injury have reported lower quality of life scores than their counterparts.[24] Osteopathic physicians should be mindful of the different psychological implications in individuals during rehabilitation for extremity injury and are encouraged to utilize appropriate methods for treatment and further management.

THE UPPER EXTREMITIES

The upper extremities are vital to performing activities of daily living. Coordination and mobility of the upper extremity joints is paramount for precise and fluid movement. Even minor injuries may produce disabilities that significantly affect overall function. Effective diagnosis and treatment necessitate a thorough understanding of the structure and function within this region.

SHOULDER AND PECTORAL GIRDLE

Synchronized motion of the sternoclavicular, acromioclavicular, and glenohumeral articular joints, and the scapulothoracic physiologic joint allow for smooth, efficient motion of the pectoral girdle and shoulder. Functional defects in any of these joints can impair shoulder mobility.[11] When evaluating upper extremity limitations, the physician needs to determine if an orthopedic injury like a fracture or sprain exists, or if there is a more subtle motion restriction as seen with somatic dysfunction.

Somatic Dysfunction of the Sternoclavicular Joint

The SCJ is the only articulation between the upper extremity and the axial skeleton. Although clavicle motion is understood, standard terminology of the motion and somatic dysfunction is not consistently described throughout osteopathic literature. The anatomic configuration, S-like shape of the bone, and types of joint present at each end of the bone allow for reciprocal motion between the proximal and distal ends of the bone. The various ligamentous and muscular (tendon) attachments, along with the proximity to the first and second ribs, allow for more motion at the distal end of the clavicle than at the proximal end.

- Anterior motion at the distal end of the bone results in posterior motion at the proximal end. Occurs about a theoretical vertical axis.
- Superior motion that occurs at the distal end of the clavicle results in inferior motion at the proximal end. Occurs about a theoretical AP axis.
- Rotation (anterior or posterior) of the entire clavicle occurs about a theoretical transverse axis.

Motion of the clavicle is also important during respiration where it must remain mobile during each phase of respiration, as it is related to the mechanics of the first rib. When there is dysfunction of the first or second rib, assessment of the clavicle is important.

Motions at the SCJ are palpated at the proximal end of the clavicle. The proximal clavicle moves/glides within the clavicular notch of the sternum as the shoulder and arm move. Small gliding motions can also be directly introduced manually, feeling for restriction (or freedom) of motion. The two primary dysfunctions of the SCJ are superior displacement and anterior displacement; however, the opposite dysfunctions within those planes may occur. Clavicular rotation often occurs in combination with the other gliding motions (Table 91.1). Assessing for signs of compression as well as for hypermobility is also important.

Clavicle somatic dysfunctions may be treated with a variety of osteopathic techniques including balanced ligamentous tension (BLT), myofascial release (MFR), muscle energy techniques (MET), high-velocity low-amplitude (HVLA), or Still technique.

Somatic Dysfunction of the Scapulothoracic Joint

The scapulothoracic joint is a physiologic joint as there are no boney articulations between the scapula and the posterior thorax. However, the 17 muscles attaching to the scapula and those acting on the pectoral girdle allow for significant scapular mobility on the thoracic wall (Fig. 91.4).

TABLE 91.1

Sternoclavicular Joint (SCJ) Somatic Dysfunction

Sternoclavicular Joint (SCJ) Motion (Proximal Clavicle Moving on Sternum)[11]	Freedom of Motion	Motion Restriction[a]	SCJ Somatic Dysfunction Nomenclature
Elevation	Proximal head of clavicle glides superiorly (elevates) within the SCJ as the distal clavicle descends. This occurs with scapular depression or arm adduction.	Proximal head of clavicle maintains an elevated (superior or cephalad) position when there is restricted inferior glide within the SCJ. This occurs when the distal end of the clavicle and scapula have limited superior motion during shoulder shrugging and/or arm abduction.	• Superior clavicle[16,27] • Upward displacement[14] • Adduction dysfunction[14,16] • Restricted abduction[14,16,28] • Elevated clavicle[16] • Medial clavicle, superior[29,b]
Depression	Proximal clavicle freely glides inferiorly (caudad) within the SCJ as distal clavicle elevates. This occurs when shoulders shrug or arm abducts.	Proximal clavicle remains inferior (caudad) within the SCJ when there is restriction of superior glide proximally as shoulder drops or arm adducts.	• Inferior clavicle[27] • Restricted adduction • Abducted clavicle dysfunction • Medial clavicle, inferior[29,b]
Anterior	Proximal clavicle glides anteriorly within the SCJ as distal clavicle moves posteriorly during scapula retraction.	Proximal clavicle stays anterior within the SCJ when there is restricted posterior glide during scapula protraction or arm horizontal flexion.	• Anterior displacement[14] • Medial clavicle, anterior[29,b] • Anterior clavicle[27] • Restricted horizontal flexion[14,28] • Restricted flexion[16] • Extension dysfunction[16]
Posterior	Proximal clavicle glides posteriorly within the SCJ as distal clavicle moves anteriorly during shoulder protraction (flexed arm reaching toward ceiling when supine)	Proximal clavicle stays posterior within the SCJ when there is restricted anterior glide of proximal clavicle as scapula retracts.	• Posterior clavicle[27] • Horizontal flexion dysfunction
Anteriorly rotated	Entire clavicle rotates anteriorly within the SCJ as arm internally rotates or fully extends	Clavicle remains anteriorly rotated within the SCJ when there is restricted posterior rotation, limiting arm external rotation and flexion.	• Anterior rotation[14] • Clavicle, anteriorly rotated[29,b]
Posteriorly rotated	Clavicle rotates posteriorly within the SCJ as arm externally rotates or fully flexes	Restricted anterior rotation within the SCJ will restrict arm internal rotation and extension.	• Posterior rotation

[a]In addition to the articular joint motion restrictions and asymmetry described above, the physician should also evaluate for the presence of other possible somatic dysfunction manifestations, such as myofascial restrictions (see Chapter 52), counterstrain tender points (see Chapter 47), trigger points and Chapman reflex points (see Chapter 43) within this region.

[b]During production of this table, it was noted that there was an incongruency in the titles and descriptions. The incongruent nomenclature titles cited in this table have been moved to the description of motion, so they match the other sources' description.

Scapular position and motion on the thoracic wall, independent of glenohumeral motion, is dependent on several of the muscles attaching the scapula to the spine and ribs as well as influences from gravity and the inferior sternocostal head of the pectoralis major[11]:

1. Elevation
   a. Trapezius—descending part
   b. Levator scapula
   c. Rhomboids
2. Depression
   a. Gravity
   b. Pectoralis major—inferior sternocostal head
   c. Latissimus dorsi
   d. Trapezius—ascending part
   e. Serratus anterior—inferior part
   f. Pectoralis minor
3. Protraction (abduction)
   a. Serratus anterior
   b. Pectoralis major
   c. Pectoralis minor
4. Retraction (adduction)
   a. Trapezius—middle part
   b. Rhomboids
   c. Latissimus dorsi

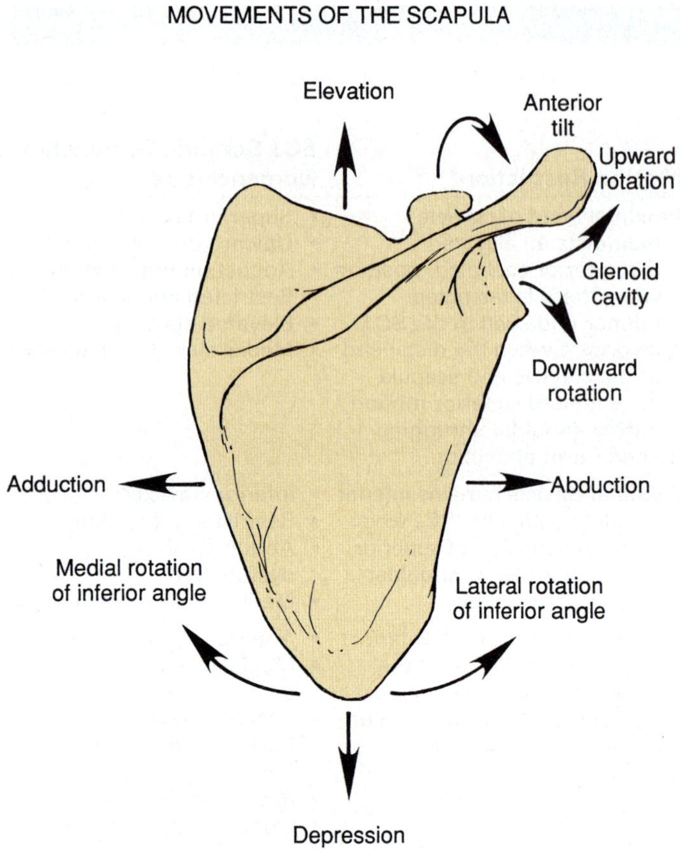

Figure 91.4. Scapular motion. (Reprinted with permission from Kendall FP, McCreary EK, Provance PG. *Muscles: Testing and Function, with Posture and Pain.* 4th ed. Williams & Wilkins; 1993:16.)

5. Upward rotation (lateral rotation of inferior angle)
   a. Trapezius—descending part
   b. Serratus anterior—inferior part
   c. Trapezius—ascending part
6. Downward rotation (medial rotation of inferior angle)
   a. Latissimus dorsi
   b. Levator scapulae
   c. Rhomboids
   d. Pectoralis minor
   e. Pectoralis major—inferior sternocostal head

Muscular and myofascial restrictions in this region can significantly affect overall shoulder motion. Scapulothoracic MFR, soft tissue, and counterstrain techniques can be performed to address the restricted planes of motion and mobilize the scapula. MET that address the restricted scapular and humeral motions have historically been named as acromioclavicular somatic dysfunction. Their motion and nomenclature are described below.

Somatic Dysfunction of the AC Joint

Somatic dysfunction diagnosed at the AC joint occurs when the acromion of the scapula is restricted from rotating on the distal end of the clavicle (about a long axis). This can restrict or be restricted by the motions at the physiologic scapulothoracic joint. No muscles connect the articulating acromion and clavicle; however, its motion is limited by ligaments. The axio-appendicular muscles that attach to and move the scapula cause the acromion to move on the clavicle.[5] This subtle motion can be palpated with one finger on the acromion and a second on the distal end of the clavicle (Table 91.2).

The osteopathic muscle energy treatment approach for these AC restrictions uses the humerus as a lever. Adducting/abducting, flexing/extending, or internally/externally rotating the arm transmits force to the acromion and then through the AC joint. If the arm exhibits restriction of motion, engage the barrier, hold, and have the patient contract against an equal counterforce using principles of MET.

Somatic Dysfunction of the Glenohumeral Joint

Somatic dysfunction of the glenohumeral joint occurs in the minor motions of the joint. Restrictions of translatory motions in many directions may occur due to the ball-and-socket nature of the glenohumeral joint. Some authors call this "joint play," "translation," or "glide." These gliding dysfunctions of the shoulder joint are active or passive exaggerations of its cardinal movements. The humeral head tends to glide more anteriorly during extension and external rotation, posteriorly during flexion (up to 90 degrees) and internal rotation, superiorly with adduction, and inferiorly with abduction and flexion (from 90 to 180 degrees).[32] These gliding restrictions may be evaluated with each plane of motion and treated using principles of MET or articulatory techniques.

In addition to articular restrictions, there are fascial restrictions that traverse the shoulder joint that can limit shoulder motion. Jones strain–counterstrain points and Simon–Travell myofascial tender points occur in the muscles controlling the glenohumeral joint. Dysfunctions elsewhere in the body can produce symptoms referable to the shoulder joint. For example, an AC joint dysfunction can cause deltoid muscle tension, just as a sacroiliac dysfunction can cause latissimus dorsi tightening. Both situations will produce shoulder pain.

The Spencer Technique was developed to provide a series of movements that evaluate and treat the separate ranges of motion and articular glides of the shoulder. This direct technique may be performed as a series of articulatory and/or MET to address each muscular restriction that is found during the examination of the shoulder ranges of motion. The technique was originally described in 1916 by Charles H. Spencer, DO.[10] Conventionally, the evaluation and treatment had a series of seven shoulder ranges of motions.[14,16,28,29,32] However, through the evolution of the technique some osteopathic resources have added an eighth stage of Adduction and External Rotation to occur just before or just after stage 5, Abduction.[33] These two stages are typically labeled stages 5A and 5B but the order of the two stages vary between sources.[14,29]

- Stage 1: Extension (elbow bent)
- Stage 2: Flexion (elbow straight)
- Stage 3: Circumduction with compression (elbow bent)
- Stage 4: Circumduction with traction (elbow straight)
- Stage 5A: Abduction
- Stage 5B: Adduction and External Rotation
- Stage 6: Internal Rotation
- Stage 7: Traction with Inferior Glide[14]

Stage 7 has also been titled Traction Stretch,[16] Distraction in Abduction,[29] and Joint Pump[32] in some sources. Note that the motion described is the same, regardless of the title. See Chapter 57 Articulatory Procedures for full description of technique and notice 5A and 5B are interchangeable in their order.

COMMON SHOULDER CONDITIONS AND THE OSTEOPATHIC APPROACH

The differential diagnosis of shoulder pain is broad. Some of these conditions are included in Table 91.3. Thoracic outlet syndrome

TABLE 91.2

Acromioclavicular Joint Somatic Dysfunction

Acromioclavicular (AC) Motion	Freedom of Motion	Motion Restriction[a]	Somatic Dysfunction Nomenclature
Adduction	As the humerus adducts and externally rotates, the glenoid cavity moves anteroinferior causing scapular downward rotation. The AC ligament drives the distal clavicle to depress and posteriorly rotate. This is palpated as a small gapping motion at the AC joint.	A restriction of palpable AC motion compared to the contralateral side when performing humerus abduction, scapula upward rotation, and distal clavicle elevation and anterior rotation.	• Adduction dysfunction[29] • Restricted abduction[14,28]
Abduction	As the humerus abducts and internally rotates, the glenoid cavity moves posterosuperior causing scapular upward rotation and distal clavicle elevation and anterior rotation. A gapping motion can be palpated at the AC joint.	A restriction of palpable AC motion compared to the contralateral side when performing humerus adduction, scapula downward rotation, and distal clavicle depression and anterior rotation.	• Adduction dysfunction[29] • Restricted adduction[14,28]
Internal rotation	When the humerus internally rotates at 90-degree abduction or when the humerus fully extends the glenoid cavity, acromion and clavicle rotate anteriorly.	Restriction of humeral external rotation or flexion is related to an anteriorly rotated clavicle dysfunction. In this situation, the supraclavicular space feels wider, and the associated fascia is tense.	• Internal rotation dysfunction[29] • Restricted external rotation[14,28] • Anteriorly rotated distal clavicle[30] • Humoral extension dysfunction[31] • Humoral restricted flexion[31]
External rotation	When the humerus externally rotates at 90-degree abduction or when the humerus fully flexes the glenoid cavity, acromion and clavicle rotate posteriorly.	Restriction of humeral internal rotation or extension is related to a posteriorly rotated clavicle dysfunction. In this situation, the supraclavicular space feels narrower, and the associated fascia is less tense.	• External rotation dysfunction[29] • Restricted internal rotation[14,28] • Posteriorly rotated distal clavicle[14] • Humoral flexion dysfunction[31] • Humoral restricted extension[31]
Elevated distal clavicle	Distal clavicle palpably elevated relative to acromion (occurs after a fall on to side or outstretched arm sprains the AC ligament).	Restricted inferior motion of distal clavicle relative to acromion when caudad pressure applied.	• Distal clavicle, elevated[29]
Inferior (depressed) distal clavicle	Not a documented AC dysfunction. The coracoid process and ligaments prevent inferior distal clavicle displacement from the acromion.[11] The treatment that would have an opposite vector than the above dysfunction addresses an elevated SC dysfunction.[29]		

[a]In addition to the articular joint motion restrictions and asymmetry described above, the physician should also evaluate for the presence of other possible somatic dysfunction manifestations, such as myofascial restrictions (see Chapter 52), counterstrain tender points (see Chapter 47), trigger points and Chapman reflex points within this region (see Chapter 43).

(TOS), rotator cuff disease and impingement syndromes, and adhesive capsulitis are described in more detail in this section.

Thoracic Outlet Syndrome

This section provides a brief overview of TOS.

TOS results from compression of the neurovascular bundle (subclavian artery, subclavian vein, and brachial plexus) as it courses through the thoracic outlet. The thoracic outlet is an anatomic region bounded by the clavicle anteriorly, the first thoracic rib posteriorly, the sternum medially, and the insertion of the pectoralis minor muscle onto the coracoid process of the scapula laterally.[34] There are neurogenic, venous, and arterial forms as well as three sites of compression. Each one of these subgroups can be related to either congenital, traumatic, or functionally acquired causes. The three sites of compression include between the anterior and middle scalenes (interscalene triangle), between the first rib and clavicle (costoclavicular space), and under the pectoralis minor (sub coracoid space). Listed below are the structures that pass through each space[35,36]:

- Interscalene triangle: Brachial plexus and subclavian artery
- Costoclavicular space: Brachial plexus, subclavian artery, and subclavian vein

TABLE 91.3

Differential Diagnosis of Shoulder Pain

Muscular/Tendinous	• Rotator cuff tendonitis • Rotator cuff tear • Biceps brachii (long head) tendonitis • Deltoid muscle strain • Trapezius muscle strain • Rhomboid muscle strain
Osseous	• Osteoarthritis • Humeral stress fracture
Capsular	• Shoulder laxity/instability • Adhesive capsulitis • Labral tear • Pigmented villonodular synovitis
Biomechanical	• Impingement syndrome • Subacromial bursitis • Scapular dyskinesis • Acromioclavicular dysfunction • Somatic dysfunction • Neuromuscular inhibition with abnormal muscle-firing patterns
Neurovascular	• Thoracic outlet syndrome • Cervical radiculopathy or radiculitis
Referred Pain Pattern	• Diaphragm, liver, gallbladder • Pancoast tumor or pulmonary pathology

- Subcoracoid space: Brachial plexus, subclavian artery, and vein continue through it as the axillary artery and vein

Neurogenic TOS being the most prevalent, accounting for over 90% of all cases, is caused by compression of the C5 through T1 brachial plexus nerve roots. It may involve the upper or lower brachial plexus. As the nerve roots exit the spinal cord and form the brachial plexus trunks, they travel through the scalene triangle, posterior to the subclavian artery and anterior to the middle scalene muscle, split into anterior and posterior divisions, and exit through the costoclavicular space alongside the subclavian artery.[34]

Causes of TOS include poor posture and sleeping positions, somatic dysfunction, several anatomical abnormalities (cervical ribs, fibrous bands), trauma (whiplash, clavicular fracture) and space-occupying lesions (Pancoast tumors).

CLINICAL PRESENTATION

Patients present with a wide range of symptoms, from minor complaints to debilitating conditions. Neurogenic TOS is the most common and presents with paresthesia (98%), neck pain (88%), trapezius pain (92%),[35] and if prolonged, atrophy of the intrinsic muscles of the hand can occur, along with weakness in the hand and neurologic sensory deficits. Venous TOS, also referred to as Paget–von Schroetter syndrome, comprises 10% to 15% of cases, and is caused by subclavian compression within the costoclavicular space and can present with upper extremity swelling, venous distention, and pain ranging from the hand to the forearm.[35] Arterial TOS is rarely observed, occurring in only 2% to 5% of TOS cases.[35] The arterial variant of TOS can appear with color changes in the upper extremity and diminished pulses and when severe produce ischemia, claudication, and gangrene. Some upper extremity paresthesia is associated with sympathetic autonomic dysfunction, with palpatory findings in the upper thoracic or rib area.

PHYSICAL EXAMINATION

Physical examination begins with observation looking for postural effects, cyanosis, edema of the hands, paleness, and atrophy. It is important to check active and passive range of motion of the cervical spine, shoulders, arms, and hands.

Perform a bilateral complete neurologic exam, assessing the tone, strength, reflexes, and sensation of the affected limb in comparison with the contralateral limb. The distribution of weakness, numbness, and paresthesia may be variable. Upper brachial plexus (C5–C7) involvement is suggested by sensory disturbance of the arm and weakness and atrophy of the deltoid, biceps, and brachialis muscles. Lower plexus (C8–T1) involvement is suspected by weakness in the small muscles of the hand and weakness of wrist and finger flexion.[36]

A vascular exam of both upper extremities should be performed as well as a cardio-pulmonary exam, and palpatory exam for somatic dysfunction. Provocative tests can add weight to a suspected diagnosis of TOS, but alone, their utility has been criticized for leading to a high number of false positives.[36] Therefore, clinicians should use more than one test as this has been shown to raise the specificity.[37]

Provocative maneuvers include[36,37]:

- Spurling Test
  - The patient's head is extended and sidebent toward the affected side. Then the examiner provides axial compression. This test is to rule out cervical radiculopathy.
- Adson Test
  - The affected arm is abducted 30 degrees at the shoulder and maximally extended. Then the patient extends the neck, turns head toward ipsilateral shoulder, and inhales deeply, holding their breath in for a few seconds.
  - Positive: Decrease or absence of ipsilateral radial pulse or reproduction of symptoms
- Upper limb tension test (ULTT) (Elvey test)
  - Hold the affected arm outstretched with the shoulder abducted to 90 degrees and the elbow flexed to 90 degrees, then extend the wrist and start straitening the elbow while the patient tilts the head and neck away from the limb being tested.
  - The ULTT is designed to assess peripheral nerve mobility and recreation of symptoms from stretching the brachial plexus. (Similar to a strait leg raise for the lower extremity.)
  - The test is positive if it reproduces the patient's symptoms and indicates brachial plexus involvement. A negative test suggests against brachial plexus compression. A positive ULTT should be followed up with an elevated arm stress test (EAST) to further support the diagnosis.
- EAST (Roos Test)
  - Arms are placed in the surrender position with shoulders abducted to 90 degrees and in external rotation, with elbows flexed to 90 degrees. This position narrows the scalene triangle. Patient slowly opens and closes hand for 3 minutes.
  - Positive: Precipitates pain, paresthesia, heaviness, or weakness.
  - If both the EAST and ULTT test are positive, this indicates neurologic TOS
- Hyperabduction Test (Wright Test)
  - Monitor the radial pulse in the affected arm as it is moved into hyperabduction and external rotation, and the patient's head is turned in the opposite direction.

- □ Positive: Decreased radial pulse, precipitates pain, paresthesia, heaviness, or weakness

Diagnosing of somatic dysfunction is important as it might be causative, contributory, or an effect of another underlying cause. Several somatic dysfunctions may contribute to compression of the neurovascular bundle and patient symptoms. Palpatory diagnosis should be directed toward dysfunction in the:

- Cervical region somatic dysfunction (articular, fascial, tenderpoints)
- Excessive tension in the anterior and middle scalene muscles
- Dysfunction of the clavicles and the clavipectoral fascia
- Elevated first rib dysfunction
- Upper thoracic region somatic dysfunction (articular, fascial, tenderpoints)
- Tenderness and tension of the pectoralis minor muscle

IMAGING/DIAGNOSTICS

Since the diagnosis is both anatomic and functional based upon positioning, additional studies may or may not be helpful. Initial diagnostic studies include plain radiographs. Electrodiagnostic studies (EMS) are difficult because neurogenic TOS is often transient.[35] If vascular causes are suspected, duplex ultrasound, arteriography, hemodynamic testing (finger plethysmography) at rest and with symptom-producing maneuvers, as well as CT and MR angiography may be ordered.[35] Ongoing developments in the diagnosis of TOS include dynamic CT angiography, and MR neurography.[35]

TREATMENT

There are conservative and surgical treatments. The mainstay of conservative treatment includes OMT and PT addressing somatic dysfunction and postural imbalance. Even in patients with severe symptoms or issues from the condition, conservative management is still the recommended first-line treatment.[38] Patients should avoid positions that aggravate symptoms and have periodic OMT/PT to maintain their improvement. Surgical intervention is for patients who have failed conservative measures for 4 to 6 months. Surgery is considered when there is severe compromise of the vasculature with resultant atrophy of intrinsic muscles of the hand. The surgery of choice is a first rib resection aimed at brachial plexus decompression, in addition to a scalenectomy or scalenotomy.[37]

Rotator Cuff Disease and Impingement Syndromes

Rotator cuff disease and impingement syndromes are commonly seen disorders in occupational, athletic, and traumatically injured patients. They are also common in the aging athletic or active patient, who becomes more sedentary. Rotator cuff disease can be caused by repetitive overuse (microtrauma), a single traumatic event (macrotrauma), instability of the glenohumeral joint, or degeneration and musculotendinous fiber failure. Most rotator cuff problems are muscular and result from degenerative tendinopathy due to intrinsic muscular fatigue. The muscles that constitute the rotator cuff include the supraspinatus, infraspinatus, teres minor, and subscapularis. Supraspinatus muscle tears is the most common rotator cuff injury.[39] Each cuff muscle plays a unique and important role in stabilizing the shoulder.

Shoulder impingement syndromes are biomechanical causes of, or the effect of, rotator cuff disease. Impingement syndromes can be described according to either the location of the impingement, characterized as external or internal, and/or the underlying cause of the impingement, referred to as primary or secondary impingement.[40]

PATHOPHYSIOLOGY

The classic concept of impingement involves external ("outlet") impingement between the greater tuberosity and the acromion. Narrowing of this subacromial space produces soft tissue encroachment, with resultant inflammation, irritation, and degeneration of the anatomic structures within the subacromial space.[40] External impingement may be caused by both anatomic and functional causes as both can decrease the subacromial space and compress the rotator cuff tendons under the subacromial arch. In younger athletes, this type of impingement can occur due to ligamentous laxity and muscle imbalance. Neer classified impingement and rotator cuff disease into three stages: inflammation and edema (I), fibrosis and tendonitis (II), and partial or complete tearing (III).[41]

Another form of impingement exists, primarily in throwing athletes. It is called internal impingement; it involves impingement of the surface of the rotator cuff under the posterosuperior glenoid rim.[41] It is a pathologic condition characterized by excessive or repetitive contact of the greater tuberosity of the humeral head with the posterosuperior aspect of the glenoid rim when the arm is abducted and externally rotated (Fig. 91.5).[42]

Internal impingement occurs secondary to a repetitive impingement in overhead throwers (or laborers) and causes articular-sided rotator cuff pathology, and superior labrum anterior posterior (SLAP) tears.[40]

Either condition, external impingement or internal impingement, can occur due to somatic dysfunction and kinetic chain imbalances. From an osteopathic biomechanical standpoint, these conditions can be due to long-standing maladaptive biomechanical factors and resultant somatic dysfunction. These factors include

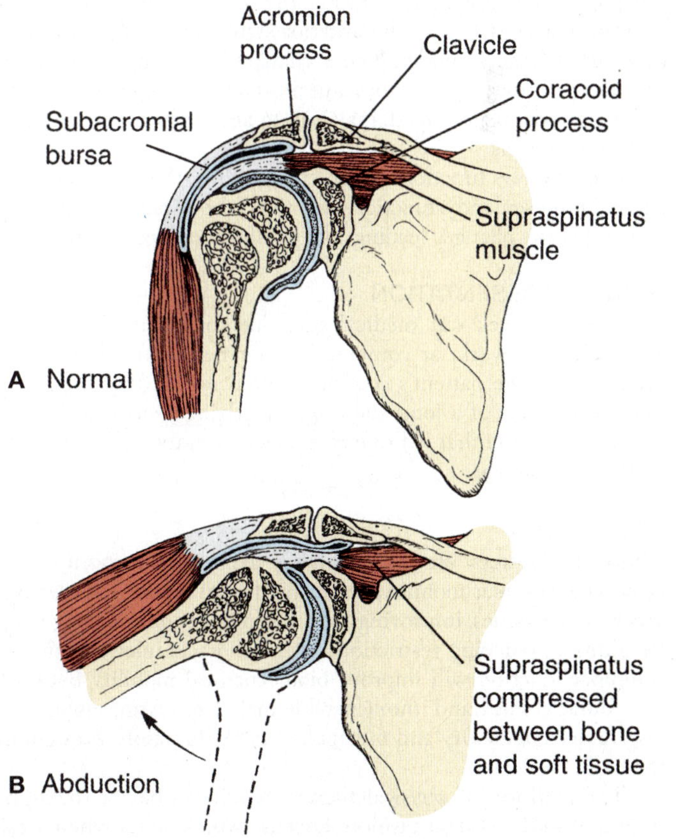

Figure 91.5. Supraspinatus impingement in the subacromial space. (Reprinted with permission from Anderson MK, Hall SJ. *Fundamentals of Sports Injury Management.* Williams & Wilkins; 1997:405. Figure 11.16.)

weakness of the abdominals, gluteus, and scapular stabilizers, with subsequent tightness of the psoas, hamstrings, latissimus dorsi, and upper trapezius muscles. Posture, core muscle strength, and anatomic position of the scapula are critical factors in rotator cuff impingement. It is a total body problem, not an isolated inflammation of local structures. Somatic dysfunction of the upper thoracic spine and ribs contributes to abnormal scapular position,[43] abnormal rotator cuff firing patterns during arm abduction,[28,44] rotator cuff fatigue, and development of Jones tender points or Simon–Travell MTrPs. (Chapter 43 Clinical Assessment: Viscerosomatic, Somatosomatic, Somatovisceral Reflexes; Counterstrain Points, Myofascial Trigger Points, and Chapman Reflexes for more information on these points.) Left untreated, these points perpetuate the problem by maintaining muscle inhibition, tightness, and pain. A forward head position contributes to cervical somatic dysfunction and together they can impair nerve function of the muscles of the rotator cuff, also impairing muscle strength. The forward head position causes tightness of the scalenes, extension in the mid cervical spine, and myofascial strain of the thoracic inlet, clavicles, levator scapulae muscles, and shoulders.

Sacroiliac and lumbar dysfunction can affect the shoulder through tension in the latissimus dorsi muscle. Tension in the latissimus dorsi causes internal rotation and adduction of the humerus, further causing the greater tuberosity of the humerus to impinge upon the glenoid or compress structures in the subacromial space. In addition, sacroiliac and lumbar somatic dysfunction is commonly seen with weakness of the abdominals, and tightness of the iliopsoas and thoracolumbar junction.

Over time, these abnormal biomechanical stresses produce a loosening of the anterior capsule with subsequent tightening of the posterior capsule. As a result, the glenoid fossa's abnormal position places stress on the anterior stabilizers (both static and dynamic) of the shoulder. These changes can lead to abnormal scapular positioning, function, and protraction (scapular dyskinesis) which when prolonged, may lead to abnormal compensations and substitutions.

Form follows function. Given enough time, the biomechanical and neuromuscular dysfunctions described above can result in bony and soft tissue changes leading to a painful shoulder syndrome.

CLINICAL PRESENTATION

Patients may seek out medical care due to a painful shoulder, an inability to work, or compete in their next event. Functional evaluation of the patient's complaint often reveals that the inciting event is part of a long-standing underlying process of kinetic chain dysfunction that led to impingement, rotator cuff pathology, and/or a labral tear.

TREATMENT

Treatment centers around resolving axial spinal dysfunction, improving scapular mobility, decreasing fascial tensions, correcting kinetic chain issues, improving local blood flow, and reducing pain. In addition, reducing restrictions in the thoracic inlet and thoracolumbar junction will improve biomechanical mobility between the thoracic inlet and thoracoabdominal diaphragm, enhancing respiratory/circulatory and metabolic–energy function throughout the body.

The addition of physical therapy is critical, but at the right time, and in the correct fashion. Exercise works better when areas of somatic dysfunction have been improved and inflammation has diminished. Proper strengthening and stretching the correct muscles and retraining firing patterns will decrease the chances of symptoms reoccurring as well.

Failure to assess the functional biomechanical factors related to the shoulder joint complex may lead to less-than-optimal results. For example, after a patient undergoes surgery for a torn rotator cuff, the mainstay of postoperative care is physical therapy. If the therapist and/or clinician fails to recognize dysfunction in the kinetic chain (muscular tightness, weakness, scapular dyskinesis, altered muscle-firing patterns, etc.), the patient's altered biomechanics will place the shoulder and newly repaired cuff under the same abnormal forces as before and result in a suboptimal outcome. The key in any patient with somatic dysfunction is to restore normal structural alignment to allow the kinetic chain to function properly.

Adhesive Capsulitis

Adhesive shoulder capsulitis, or arthrofibrosis, also known as "frozen shoulder," describes a pathologic process in which the body forms excessive scar tissue or adhesions across the glenohumeral joint, leading to pain, stiffness, and somatic dysfunction. It is a debilitating condition that can occur spontaneously or following shoulder surgery or trauma.[45]

Adhesive shoulder capsulitis is a clinical diagnosis made on the basis of medical history and physical examination and is often a diagnosis of exclusion.[45] It has components of both chronic inflammation and fibrosis present. Contracture of the glenohumeral capsule is the hallmark of adhesive capsulitis.[45] It is often regarded as a self-limiting disease that resolves between 1 and 3 years; however, some studies show that between 20% and 50% of patients may develop long-lasting symptoms.[45]

This section will describe some specifics about the clinical presentation, physical examination, and treatment approach with OMT.

CLINICAL PRESENTATION

The clinical presentation is typically a progressive presentation starting with pain prior to restricted motion.[46]

- Phase 1: The painful "Freezing phase" is characterized by diffuse and disabling shoulder pain, initially worse at night, along with increasing stiffness. It can last from 2 to 9 months.
- Phase 2: The "Frozen phase" involves a progressive stiffness and limitation in range of motion in all shoulder planes. The intensity of pain gradually diminishes during this phase. It typically lasts from 4 to 12 months.
- Phase 3: The "Thawing phase" is marked by a gradual return of the range of motion. The recovery of range of motion may take 12 to 24 months for complete restoration.

Symptoms generally are slowly progressive but in some may be more rapid. Pain frequently interferes with sleep. The loss of range of motion usually follows a specific pattern starting with external rotation, followed by abduction, internal rotation, and forward flexion. Pain is generally worse at the extremes of motion when the contracted capsule is stretched.[45]

PHYSICAL EXAMINATION

Pain will often limit a complete and thorough physical exam.[46] The key clinical sign of adhesive capsulitis is a reduction in active and passive range of motion, specifically in forward flexion, abduction, and external and internal rotation. Special tests, such as the Neer and Hawkins tests for impingement and Speed's test for biceps tendinopathy, are often positive.[46] An osteopathic physical examination does not only include the shoulder. Osteopathic structural and palpatory examinations are important as there are often other osteopathic findings throughout the body.

Diagnosing relevant somatic dysfunction is crucial for improved treatment outcomes. Some somatic dysfunction is primary and some secondary due to adaptation/compensation for the condition. Initial findings include an altered arm swing during gait[46] and asymmetric landmarks on a standing structural examination. Based upon clinical experience of the authors, local findings of the involved shoulder typically include an elevated shoulder held in a protracted position. Tissue texture changes often occur in the upper thoracic region and over the posterior rib angles. The thoracic and thoracolumbar regions may exhibit either segmental or group spinal mechanics. The cervical region frequently has muscular tension, segmental dysfunction, and associated anterior and posterior cervical tender points. The levator scapulae muscles, scalenes, and upper trapezius routinely spasm or develop tenderpoints as they compensate for the lack of shoulder abduction. Other common tenderpoints of the shoulder region include the subscapularis, infraspinatus, biceps, pectoralis minor, and anterior or posterior ribs 1–7. Somatic dysfunction of the first rib (typically elevated) is common. Fascial restrictions of the thoracic inlet, anterior and posterior axillary folds, rib cage, and latissimus dorsi are present and asymmetric compared to the other side. Depending on the stage of the condition, tenderness, restriction, and congestion are regularly seen in numerous muscles and tissues.

TREATMENT

Since there are no universal treatment algorithms, and many treatments have controversial support in the literature, treatment should be patient specific. The practitioner must be aware of not only the physical limitations caused by the disease but also the psychological ramifications of the lifestyle changes. Morbidity from this condition has significant individual and societal costs, and disability is always long-lasting, if not permanent. Supportive care, overall treatment guidance, addressing associated dysfunctions, both physically and mentally, and bringing in a consulting orthopedist and physical therapists are all aspects of the team approach.[47]

OMT should be directed to somatic dysfunction often found in the upper thoracic spine, upper ribs, and entire shoulder complex.[7] The objective is to gently improve shoulder mobility, reestablish articular and soft tissue structure and the functional relationships, and restore flow in the arterial, venous, and lymphatic systems to positively affect the inflammatory and fibrotic cascade.[47]

In patients with adhesive capsulitis, it is important to work in a pain-free zone and only progress as fast as the patient can respond. Indirect techniques may be especially effective in the initial treatments.[47] Several different types of treatment approaches may be beneficial, including soft tissue, MFR, MET, strain–counterstrain, lymphatic, articulatory (low-velocity–high-amplitude), HVLA, and TrP treatment, all directed at the specific type of somatic dysfunction diagnosed.[47,48]

The Spencer technique[10] has been performed with good results using a pattern that treats the most pain-free (or best-preserved motion) first, followed by the more restricted motion.[47] Spencer technique may be performed as an articulatory technique or as a muscle energy and articulatory technique. MET has been shown to be effective on functional ability of shoulder in adhesive capsulitis.[48] Similar positive effects have been seen by performing Spencer technique followed by a similar manual manipulation technique using conscious sedation with propofol.[49,50]

Subscapularis TrPs are common in this condition and if left untreated can cause associated TrPs in the surrounding muscles. The activation of subscapular TrPs further restricts abduction of the shoulder, which sensitizes the pectoralis, latissimus dorsi, and triceps.[51] Similarly, a restriction of external rotation leads to sensitization of the anterior deltoid and teres major. Eventually, most, or all the shoulder girdle muscles may be involved, leading to a frozen shoulder. As TrP activity lessens, treatment may be advanced. Initially, passive stretching followed by stabilization exercises, and finally active strengthening exercises, should be incorporated.[47]

Along with OMT and physical therapy, the full patient-specific osteopathic management plan for adhesive capsulitis may include pharmacotherapy, injections, manipulation under anesthesia (MUA), and surgical options.

ELBOW AND FOREARM

The elbow joint consists of three joints within one joint capsule:

1. The humeroulnar joint (ulnohumeral joint)
2. The humeroradial joint (radiohumeral joint)
3. The proximal radioulnar joint

Several principles govern the elbow joint and surrounding area[5]:

1. The primary motions of the elbow are flexion and extension, pronation and supination, and a small amount of abduction–adduction.
2. All three joints participate in elbow function; however, flexion, extension, abduction, and adduction primarily occur at the ulnohumeral joint while pronation and supination are primarily a combined radiohumeral and proximal radioulnar joint movement.
3. Somatic dysfunction of the elbow is found in the minor gliding motions of the joint.
4. Impaired function of any joint of the arm produces compensatory changes in all other joints.
5. If total functional demand overtaxes any one of the other joints, secondary somatic dysfunction is also produced in those joints.

The elbow and wrist joints are functionally linked by the radius' proximal and distal synovial radioulnar joints and the fibrous middle radioulnar joint called the interosseous membrane. The proximal and distal radioulnar joints allow pivot action, permitting supination and pronation of the hand. The interosseous membrane maintains functional symmetry and stability of the forearm.

Patients who repetitively use their forearms may strain the forearm, wrist, or elbow as well as the forearm muscles and interosseous membrane. They may also have increased tension and tenderness in the whole forearm muscular "system." This type of finding may be related to increased sympathetic tone from upper thoracic/rib somatic dysfunction, as well as overuse.

Somatic Dysfunction of the Ulnohumeral Joint

Restriction of the minor medial and lateral gliding motions of the ulnohumeral joint can create somatic dysfunction in ulnar abduction or ulnar adduction (Fig. 91.6). An abduction somatic dysfunction appears as though the arm is more angulated, increasing the carrying angle. In adduction somatic dysfunction, the arm appears straighter, decreasing the carrying angle. Patients may complain of forearm tightness or wrist pain with either dysfunction. Patients occasionally have point tenderness of the lateral or medial epicondyle, confusing this condition with epicondylitis.

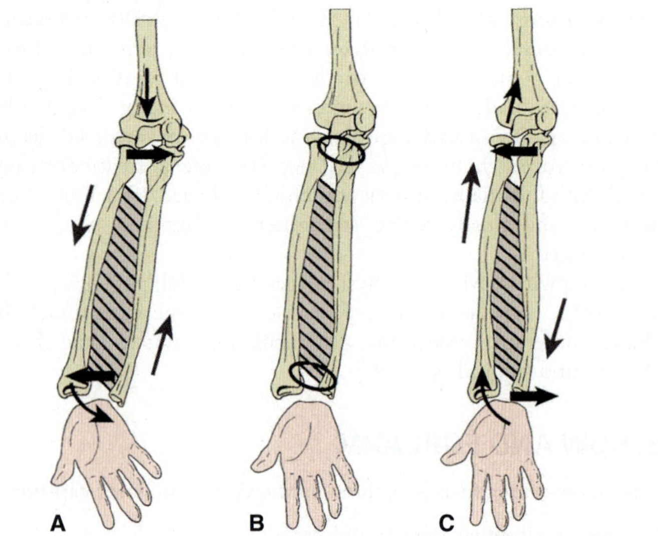

Figure 91.6. Reciprocal motion. A. Ulnar abduction. **B.** Neutral ulna position. **C.** Ulnar adduction. (Illustration by William A. Kuchera, DO, FAAO, with permission.)

Somatic dysfunction of the elbow can also affect full flexion and extension of the elbow. An elbow that does not extend completely may have somatic dysfunction, an orthopedic condition, or both. The "smoothness" or quality of flexion and extension of the elbow may also be affected (Table 91.4).

Reciprocal Motion of Ulnohumeral and Radiocarpal Dysfunction

There is reciprocal motion between the elbow and the wrist. If the elbow prefers abduction, the wrist will prefer adduction and vice versa. The radius and ulna are held in a parallelogram arrangement by the radiocarpal joints (Fig. 91.6). The radius can move more freely than the ulna. With the ulna relatively fixed at the ulnohumeral joint and the radius fairly fixed at the radiocarpal joint (especially with the scaphoid), abduction or adduction of the ulna results in a reciprocal positioning of the hand. During abduction of the ulna, the radius glides distally and pushes the wrist into increased adduction (ulnar deviation). During adduction of the ulna, the radius glides proximally and the wrist is pulled into a more abducted position (radial deviation). If this reciprocal positioning principle of the elbow and the wrist is incorporated in the direct and indirect treatment of ulnar abduction or adduction somatic dysfunctions, these techniques will become more effective and efficient. The parallelogram arrangement of the forearm bones with the action of the proximal and

TABLE 91.4

Ulnohumeral (Elbow) Joint Somatic Dysfunction

Elbow (Ulnohumeral) Motion	Freedom of Motion	Motion Restriction[a]	Somatic Dysfunction Nomenclature
Abduction of ulna	Proximal ulna translates medially as distal ulna moves laterally (increased carrying angle, wrist away from midline)	Proximal ulna is restricted in lateral movement during ulnar adduction	• Restricted adduction[14,28] • Ulnohumeral abduction dysfunction[16,29] • Ulna abducted with medial glide[29,32] • Abduction with medial glide[29,32] • Abduction (pronation) dysfunction[16,b] • Adduction (supination) restriction[16,b]
Adduction of ulna	Proximal ulna translates laterally as distal ulna moves medially (decreased carrying angle, wrist toward midline)	Proximal ulna is restricted in medial movement during ulnar abduction	• Humeroulnar restricted abduction[14,16,28] • Abduction restriction[14,16,28] • Ulnohumeral adduction dysfunction[29] • Ulna adducted with lateral glide[29,32] • Adduction with lateral glide[29,32] • Adduction (supination) dysfunction[16,b] • Abduction (pronation) restriction[16,b]
Extension	Extended elbow position	Restricts full flexion of elbow. Due to tight triceps or to proximal displacement of ulnar olecranon process within the humoral olecranon fossa. Difficult to palpate fossa when elbow extended.	• Restricted flexion[14,16,28] • Ulnohumeral extension dysfunction[29]
Flexion	Flexed elbow position	Restricts full extension of elbow. Due to tight flexor muscles or to distal displacement of ulnar olecranon process within the humeral olecranon fossa.	• Restricted extension[14,16,28] • Ulnohumeral flexion dysfunction[29]

[a]In addition to the articular joint motion restrictions and asymmetry described above, the physician should also evaluate for the presence of other possible somatic dysfunction manifestations, such as myofascial restrictions (see Chapter 52), counterstrain tender points (see Chapter 47), and trigger points within this region (see Chapter 43).

[b]During production of this table, it was noted that one reference describes adduction and abduction as accessory motions of supination and pronation, respectively. This description of diagnosis and muscle energy technique was unique compared to the other referenced Osteopathic sources.

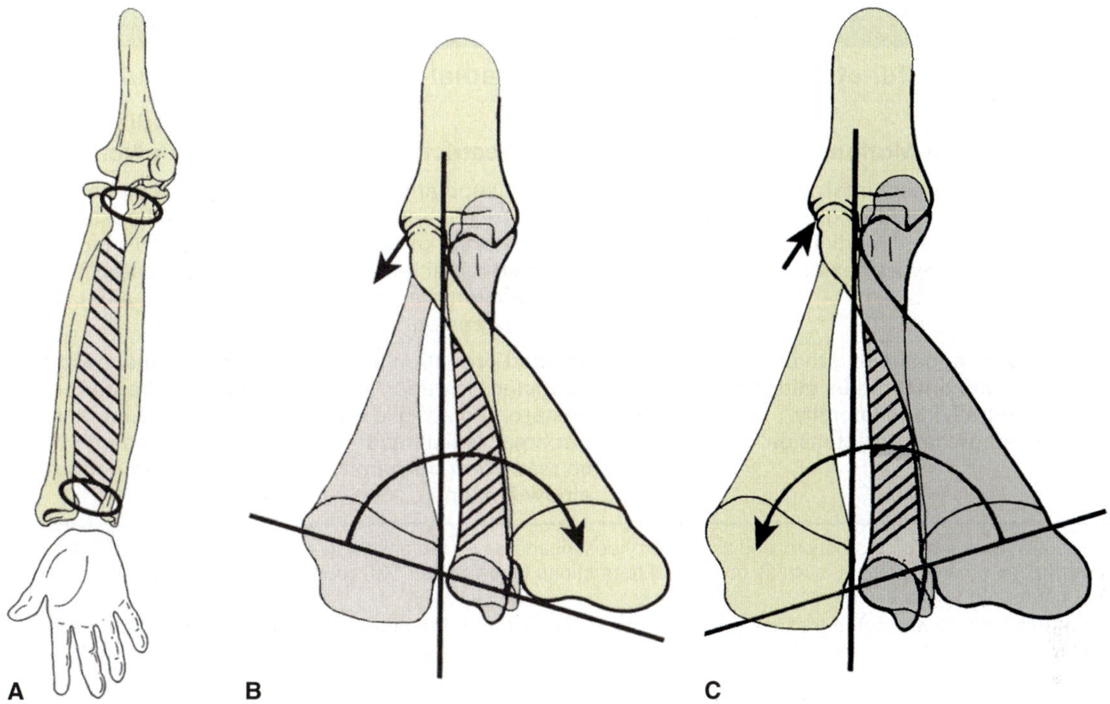

Figure 91.7. Forearm pronation and supination. A. Reciprocal motion occurs at the proximal and distal radioulnar joints during pronation and supination. **B.** During pronation, as the distal radius moves anteriorly, the proximal radial head glides posteriorly. **C.** During supination, as the distal radius moves posteriorly, the proximal radial head glides anteriorly. (Illustration by William A. Kuchera, DO, FAAO, with permission.)

distal radioulnar joints permits forearm/wrist motions. As these motions occur, the interosseous membrane (a radioulnar fibrous joint) provides stability to the forearm and prevents stress of the ligaments and/or bony compression in the forearm or the wrist.

If all ulnohumeral joint somatic dysfunction has been treated, there is no inflammation in the elbow joint, and the elbow still cannot be flexed completely, the problem is most likely one of the radioulnar joints, usually the proximal one. The interosseous membrane may also be involved.

Radial Head Somatic Dysfunction

There is reciprocal motion of the proximal and distal ends of the radius. When the hand is pronated, the distal end of the radius crosses over the ulna as it moves anteriorly and medially. Near the end of full pronation, the head of the radius glides posteriorly, that is, there is reciprocal motion of the radial head relative to the distal radius. Motion in an arc opposite from the position of the pronated hand is called supination. When the forearm is supinated, the distal end of the radius moves posteriorly and the radial head glides anteriorly (Fig. 91.7).

These motions are best palpated near the end of full supination or pronation. They are palpable if the operator's fingers are under the patient's elbow and the thumb of that hand is palpating the radial head while the other hand supinates or pronates the patient's hand. Motion in the symptomatic forearm is compared with motion in the opposite or normal forearm (Table 91.5).

Posterior radial head somatic dysfunction is often produced by a fall **f**orward **o**nto (the palm of) an **o**ut**s**tretched **h**and (FOOSH injury). When a person falls forward, the natural reflex is to pronate the forearm and catch themselves on their outstretched pronated palm. The anterior motion of the distal radius, started by the pronation, is accentuated on impact. The forward vector of the pronated hand and body pushes the distal radius into a more anterior rotation, causing the radial head to move posteriorly (Fig. 91.8).

An anterior radial head somatic dysfunction is likely to result from a fall backward, where the patient extends their supinated arm posteriorly to break the impact of the fall, lands on the palm, and forces the distal end of the radius posteriorly and the radial head anteriorly. In this type of injury, the forearm is in the supinated anatomic position (Fig. 91.9).

There are multiple OMT methods that can be used to address radial head somatic dysfunction. See Chapter 49 High-Velocity Low-Amplitude (HVLA) Thrust for a description of HVLA for a posterior radial head.

Interosseous Membrane Somatic Dysfunction

The fibers of the interosseous membrane extend cephalad from attachment on the ulna to a more proximal attachment on the radius. This arrangement allows the bones of the forearm to share the forces of compression, traction, or torque whether they occur from the hand upward or the shoulder downward. Interosseous membrane dysfunction can perpetuate elbow or wrist disability long after proper orthopedic care and complete healing of strains, sprains, or fractures of the elbow or wrist should have taken place. In some unknown way, the collagen tissues often retain stress patterns of past injury. This means that clinically, it is important to treat forearm dysfunction promptly before these patterns have a chance to develop. In such cases, palpation of the interosseous membrane reveals increased tension and elicits areas of subjective tenderness. Interosseous strains may be treated with direct or indirect fascial treatments.

TABLE 91.5

Radial Head Somatic Dysfunction (Combined Humeroradial and Proximal Radioulnar Joint Motion)

Radial Motion	Freedom of Motion	Motion Restriction[a]	Proximal Radial Head Somatic Dysfunction Nomenclature
Pronation	Forearm appears internally rotated. The proximal radius glides posteriorly (dorsally) and medially. The elbow favors flexion.	Restricted supination and restricted anterior/anterolateral[14] glide of proximal radial head. This restriction may limit elbow extension.[b]	• Posterior radial head[14,16,29,32] • Radial head posterior[14,16,29,32] • Radioulnar pronation dysfunction[16,29] • Radius pronated[16,29] • Restricted supination[14,28]
Supination	Forearm appears externally rotated. The proximal radius glides anteriorly (ventrally) and laterally. The elbow favors extension.	Restricted pronation and restricted posterior/posteromedial[14] glide of proximal radial head. This restriction may limit elbow flexion.[b]	• Anterior radial head[14,16,29,32] • Radial head anterior[14,16,29,32] • Radioulnar supination dysfunction[16,29] • Radius supinated[16,29] • Restricted pronation[14,28]

[a]In addition to the articular joint motion restrictions and asymmetry described above, the physician should also evaluate for the presence of other possible somatic dysfunction manifestations, such as myofascial restrictions (see Chapter 52), counterstrain tender points (see Chapter 47), and trigger points (see Chapter 43) within this region.

[b]During production of this table, it was noted that one reference has an incongruent description of coupling of forearm pronation with elbow extension and forearm supination with flexion. This association was unique to this author compared to the other referenced Osteopathic sources.

COMMON ELBOW CONDITIONS AND THE OSTEOPATHIC APPROACH

Lateral Epicondylitis (Tennis Elbow)

Lateral epicondylitis is a painful condition of the elbow that is typically caused by repetitive overuse. Lateral epicondylitis is caused by repetitive motion leading to microinjury of the wrist extensor muscles that originate from the lateral epicondyle from a common extensor origin. This leads to inflammation and degenerative microtears of the wrist extensor muscles, primarily, the extensor carpi radialis brevis (ERCB). Common activities and occupations requiring repetitive (or loaded) wrist extension may increase risk. Lateral epicondylitis has a tendency for prolonged recovery affecting quality of life. It has been shown to account for significant amounts of lost time from work, recreation time, and frequent work-related disability claims.[52,53]

This section will describe some specifics about the clinical presentation, physical examination, and treatment approach with OMT.

CLINICAL PRESENTATION

The clinical presentation is that of an active patient who has localized pain to the lateral aspect of their elbow, and sometimes the dorsal aspect of their forearm. They may describe a change in the duration and intensity of their athletic activities or changes in their duties or equipment at work.[52]

The pain may be insidious or acute and ranges from mild and annoying to severe and incapacitating. Patients will point to their lateral elbow just distal to the humeral epicondyle and to the forearm when describing their pain. Their pain may be constant or intermittent and worse with activities that involve wrist extension or gripping objects, especially with their elbow extended.

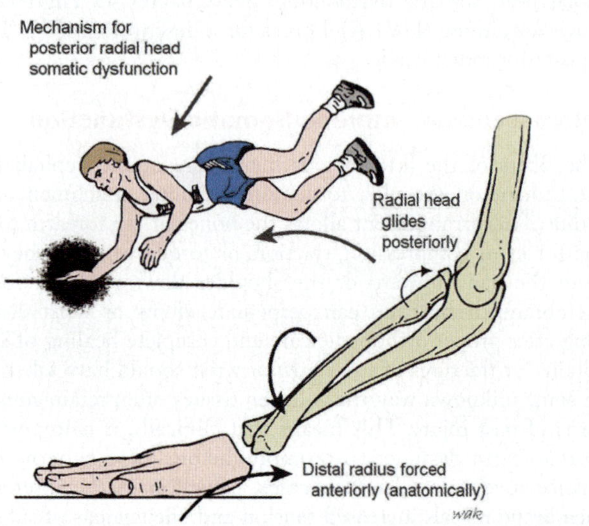

Figure 91.8. Forward fall on an outstretched (pronated) hand. (Illustration by William A. Kuchera, DO, FAAO, with permission.)

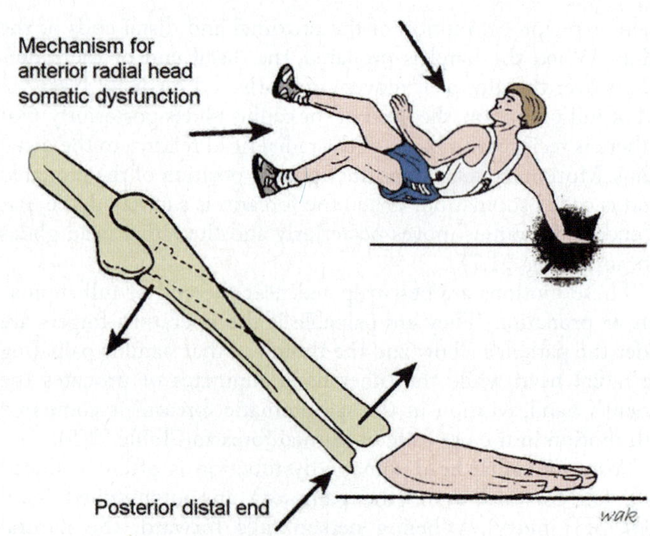

Figure 91.9. Backward fall on an extended (supinated) hand. (Illustration by William A. Kuchera, DO, FAAO, with permission.)

PHYSICAL EXAMINATION

The physical examination should start with a structural examination looking for asymmetries of anatomic landmarks indicating potential deficits in the kinetic chain. It is important to evaluate shoulder and scapular position and motion. The physical examination should also include a neurovascular assessment of the upper extremities, comparing one side to the other.

Palpation for somatic dysfunction should include the upper thoracic spine, ribs, shoulder, thoracic inlet, cervical spine, forearm, wrist, and hand. Segmental somatic dysfunction of the cervical and thoracic spine, rib somatic dysfunction, and their associated tenderpoints all can contribute to this condition. Simon and Travell TrPs of the biceps, triceps, ERCB, wrist extensors, and supinator all can refer pain to the lateral epicondyle.[12,54,55] When palpating the forearm, the origin of the ERCB on the lateral epicondyle may be tender, but classically the tenderness to palpation is just distal to this and is a hallmark finding.[52] Range of motion and muscle strength of the elbow, wrist, and grip should be assessed. There are multiple clinical orthopedic tests to assist in making the clinical diagnosis of lateral epicondylitis. These include the: tennis elbow test, chair test, Thompsen test, Cozen, Mill, and Maudsley tests. All these orthopedic tests are considered positive if they reproduce localized lateral elbow pain. None of the tests are pathognomonic.[52]

OSTEOPATHIC MANIPULATIVE TREATMENT AND PHYSICAL THERAPY

Osteopathic manipulative medicine is useful in the treatment of lateral epicondylitis. MET and joint mobilization techniques have been shown to be more effective than corticosteroid injections.[52,56] In addition to MET for the extensor muscles of the wrist, treatment of radial head somatic dysfunction, joint mobilization, and MFR to the forearm have been found to be effective in improving pain, grip strength, and function.[52,57–59] Common areas of somatic dysfunction include the ipsilateral upper thoracic spine and ribs, the lower cervical spine, the radial head, the ulnohumeral joint, and the pronator teres muscle. In the authors' experience, OMT directed to single segment dysfunction of the upper thoracic spine and counterstrain for the affected ribs will help decrease muscle tension of the forearm as well as tenderness of the lateral epicondyle. Dry needling of myofascial TrPs has been shown to be beneficial.[60,61] Counterstrain for the rotator cuff muscles and wrist extensor tendons is useful as well. Treatment of a radial head dysfunction or an abducted ulna may completely resolve symptoms in patients with lateral epicondyle pain, but not true epicondylitis. As local and regional somatic dysfunction and kinetic chain factors are addressed, physical therapy is also helpful. Physical therapy has been shown to be slightly more efficacious than corticosteroid injections or analgesics.[52,62] Eccentric muscle stretching and exercises have been shown to be beneficial over isometric, concentric, and isokinetic approaches.[52,63]

SUMMARY OF OTHER TREATMENT APPROACHES

Many cases of lateral epicondylitis will improve within 1 to 2 years on their own, even without intervention. However, this lengthy duration of healing is frequently unacceptable for the active patient and or laborer. The treatment of lateral epicondylitis can be divided into conservative, injection, and surgical approaches. There are several nonoperative options for treatment, but a combination of NSAIDs and physical therapy that utilizes eccentric muscle stretching is considered first-line.[52] Each patient has a unique individual management plan depending on where they are in the timeline of healing, and what unique aspects of their lifestyle, occupation, and recreation need to be incorporated into their treatment plan. The concept of relative rest, limiting movements that aggravate the condition, utilization of braces or forearm support, and physical and psychological coping strategies are all important. Patients who have failed conservative treatment for six months to a year may need to be referred to orthopedic surgeons for surgical options.[52]

WRIST AND HAND

The Distal Radioulnar Joint

Distal radioulnar joint motion is primarily supination and pronation. Gliding of the distal radius on the ulna has reciprocal motion to that of the radial head.

- If the distal radius is displaced anteriorly on the ulna, then supination is restricted.
- If the distal radius is displaced posteriorly on the ulna, then pronation is restricted.

Anterior or posterior somatic dysfunction of the distal radioulnar joint may have tissue texture changes at the wrist or in related musculature. Tenderness to palpation may occur over the distal radioulnar joint, the wrist, and/or in the interosseous membrane.[32]

The ulna is not a component of the true wrist joint. It is separated from the wrist joint by a triangular articular disk.[11] However, there is reciprocal motion between the ulnohumeral and radiocarpal joints, as previously described (Fig. 91.6). If the elbow moves freely into abduction, the wrist will move freely into adduction and vice versa. When there is pain in the elbow or wrist, evaluate both. Sometimes, the only sign of elbow somatic dysfunction will be a complaint of wrist pain.

Wrist (Radiocarpal) Joint

The wrist (radiocarpal) joint is formed by the concave distal end of the radius, three convex proximal carpal bones (the scaphoid, lunate, and triquetral bones), and an articular disk.[11] The wrist joint moves around AP and transverse axes, allowing for the movements of flexion, extension, abduction (radial deviation), and adduction (ulnar deviation). Somatic dysfunction is not related to the gross motions of the wrist but instead to dysfunction of the small gliding motions of the proximal carpal bones on the radius as the wrist is moved. The carpals can move slightly anteriorly, posteriorly, medially, or laterally.

Somatic dysfunction of the wrist was conventionally named according to the direction of motion preference. However, documenting the restriction has become increasingly more common. Quality and quantity of wrist motion is most accurately assessed with the patient's arms at their sides and elbows flexed to 90 degrees. When there is restriction of radioulnar pronation and supination, any of the four wrist gliding motions may seem more asymmetric in either supination or pronation. If a wrist can fully extend and is restricted in its full flexion, it may be named an extended somatic dysfunction or restricted wrist flexion (Fig. 91.10). In this extended somatic dysfunction, the three carpal bones glide ventrally, and have motion restriction when gliding dorsally. The opposite is true for a flexed somatic dysfunction of the wrist; similar relationships occur for radial and ulnar deviation (Table 91.6).

Several principles describe somatic dysfunction of the wrist[5]:

1. Observation is important but not specific to somatic dysfunction; swelling of the wrist is an inconsistent sign.
2. Painful compression indicates dysfunction is present but does not diagnose the specific dysfunction that is present.

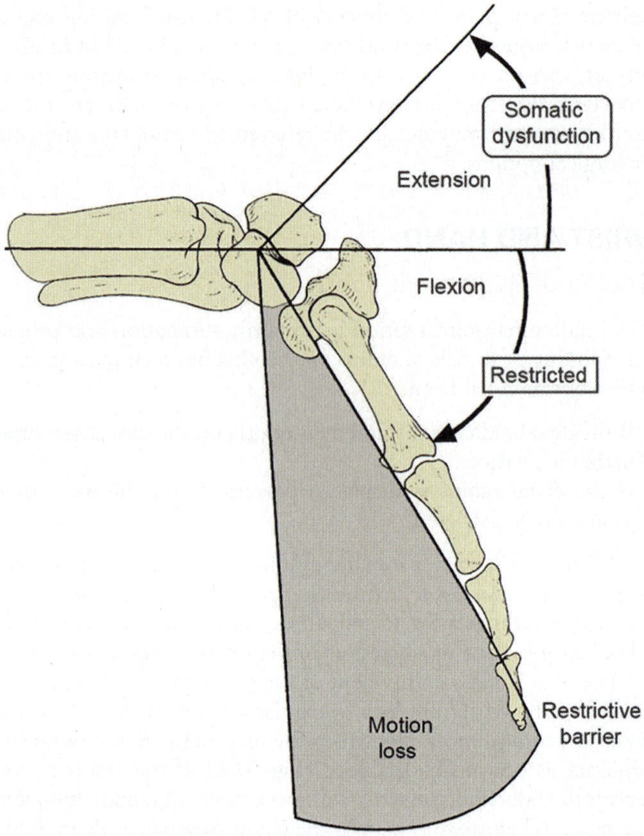

Figure 91.10. Extended wrist somatic dysfunction; restricted wrist flexion. (Illustration by William A. Kuchera, DO, FAAO, with permission.)

3. Radial glide and limited parallelogram motions are not obvious until the opposite motion is attempted and compared bilaterally.
    - □ If there is an adduction somatic dysfunction at the wrist with a distal shift of the radius, the problem may not be evident until abduction of the wrist is tested, and the results are compared with the opposite side.
4. Flexion/extension somatic dysfunction of the wrist is often caused by a trauma that overcomes the ligamentous restraints and opposing muscle pull.
    - □ Restriction of wrist extension is more common than is restriction of wrist flexion.[11]

The prevalence of restricted wrist extension, compared to wrist flexion, is likely due to a more developed and dominant flexor muscle mass. A restriction of wrist extension is typically seen with increased tension of the forearm flexors. Other factors such as osteoarthritis, cartilage tears, or occult fractures can limit wrist motion as well.

RULE OUT SCAPHOID FRACTURE

If the wrist joint is swollen after a trauma, like falling on an outstretched hand, the physician must rule out fracture of the navicular (scaphoid) bone. This is also true if there is pain on pressure over the anatomical snuffbox, or if there is persistent pain and dysfunction after proper conservative care, even if the initial post trauma radiographs showed no evidence of fracture. Sometimes, the scaphoid does not reveal evidence of fracture until the disruption in its blood supply slowly produces degeneration of the bone.

BOX 91.1 Intercarpal Joint Diagnostic Findings

- Tissue texture changes at the wrist or in the related musculature
- Pain with motion or aching at rest
- Tenderness to palpation over the joint lines
- For *flexion with posterior glide:*
    - □ Posterior position of carpal bone
    - □ Flexion with posterior glide is present
    - □ Extension with anterior glide is restricted
- For *extension with anterior glide:*
    - □ Anterior position of carpal bone
    - □ Extension with anterior glide is present
    - □ Flexion with posterior glide is restricted
- For *abduction with medial glide:*
    - □ Abduction with medial glide is present
    - □ Adduction with lateral glide is restricted
- For *adduction with lateral glide:*
    - □ Adduction with lateral glide is present
    - □ Abduction with medial glide is restricted

Midcarpal (Transverse) and Intercarpal Joints

The midcarpal joint is a complex joint between the proximal carpal bones (scaphoid, lunate, and triquetral bones) and the distal row of carpals (the trapezium, trapezoid, capitate, and hamate). The gliding movements between the carpals occur concomitantly with movements at the wrist joint, augmenting them and increasing the overall range of movement. Dysfunction to any one of the carpal bones can affect wrist and hand flexion, extension, abduction, or adduction. Carpal bones can also become displaced anteriorly (ventrally, toward the palm) or posteriorly (dorsally). When this occurs, there is usually some visual and palpatory evidence. Dorsally displaced carpals typically impede wrist extension. Carpals displaced ventrally can impede wrist flexion and can narrow the carpal tunnel (Box 91.1).

Flexion and extension of the hand are initiated at the midcarpal joint. Hand flexion and adduction are greater than hand extension and abduction. Movements at the intercarpal joints are small, with the proximal row being more mobile than the distal row.[11] Intercarpal somatic dysfunction or displacement of individual intercarpal joints often occurs from a fall on an outstretched hand. For this reason, somatic dysfunction in these areas is very likely to have a compression component along with gliding restrictions.

The pisotriquetral joint, formed from the articulation of the pisiform with the palmar surface of the triquetrum can also have a small amount of gliding joint play. Nontraumatic tenderness in this area typically responds well to counterstrain of the flexor carpi ulnaris tendon.

Carpometacarpal (CMC) and Intermetacarpal (IM) Joints

The carpometacarpal (CMC) and intermetacarpal (IM) joints are all classified as plane synovial joints, except the CMC of the thumb, which is a saddle joint. The medial four CMC joints and each of their three IM joints share a common joint cavity. Their gliding motion is primarily anterior and posterior; however, each digit's quantity of motion differs. There is very little movement at the CMC joints of

TABLE 91.6

Radiocarpal (Wrist) Joint Somatic Dysfunction

Radiocarpal Motion	Freedom of Motion	Motion Restriction[a]	Somatic Dysfunction Nomenclature
Extension (dorsiflexion)	The radiocarpal bones (scaphoid, lunate, and triquetral bones) freely glide anteriorly (ventrally) along the distal radius allowing full wrist extension.	Any or all three of the radiocarpal bones are restricted when gliding posteriorly (dorsally) and limit wrist flexion. Restricted palmar motion.	• Restricted flexion[14,16,28,29,64] • Restricted palmar flexion[14,16,28,29] • Extension with anterior glide[32] • Extension dysfunction[29] • Extended wrist[29] • Extended wrist (restricted flexion)[29]
Flexion (palmar flexion)	The radiocarpal bones (scaphoid, lunate, and triquetral bones) freely glide posteriorly (dorsally) along the distal radius allowing full wrist flexion.	Any or all three of the radiocarpal bones are restricted when gliding anteriorly (ventrally) and limit wrist extension. Restricted dorsal movement.	• Restricted extension[14,16,28,29] • Flexion with posterior glide[32] • Radiocarpal flexion dysfunction[29] • Wrist flexed (restricted extension)[29]
Adduction (ulnar deviation)	The radiocarpal bones (scaphoid, lunate, and triquetral bones) freely glide laterally along the distal radius allowing adduction (ulnar deviation).	Any or all three of the radiocarpal bones are restricted when gliding medially and limit abduction (radial deviation). This restriction may occur with the forearm supinated, pronated, or both.	• Restricted abduction[14,16,28] • Restricted pronated radial deviation[14,28] • Restricted supinated radial deviation[14,28] • Adduction dysfunction[14,16] • Adduction with lateral glide[32] • Radiocarpal adduction dysfunction[29] • Wrist adducted with ulnar deviation[29] • Wrist dysfunction in ulnar deviation—wrist restriction in radial deviation[16]
Abduction (radial deviation)	The radiocarpal bones (scaphoid, lunate, and triquetral bones) freely glide medially along the distal radius allowing abduction (radial deviation).	Any or all three of the radiocarpal bones are restricted when gliding laterally and limit adduction (ulnar deviation) This restriction may occur with the forearm supinated, pronated, or both.	• Restricted adduction[14,16,28] • Restricted pronated ulnar deviation[14,28] • Restricted supinated ulnar deviation[14,28] • Abduction with medial glide[32] • Wrist abduction[29] • Wrist abducted with radial deviation[29] • Radiocarpal abduction dysfunction[29] • Wrist dysfunction in radial deviation—wrist restriction in ulnar deviation[16]

[a]In addition to the articular joint motion restrictions and asymmetry described above, the physician should also evaluate for the presence of other possible somatic dysfunction manifestations, such as myofascial restrictions (see Chapter 52), counterstrain tender points (see Chapter 47), and trigger points (see Chapter 43) within this region.

the second and third digits, with slightly more motion at the fourth digit, and moderate motion of the fifth digit with flexion and extension as well as some axial rotation.[11] Palpation at the base of the suspected metacarpal may reveal an abnormal anterior or posterior position in relation to the carpals. Mobility is assessed by moving the metacarpal heads back and forth. Somatic dysfunction of dorsal or ventral glide may be appreciated. A restriction of both motions indicates an impaction or compression type of dysfunction.

The CMC joint of the thumb, as a separate saddle-type joint, has both a concave and a convex articular surface. This configuration permits angular movements in flexion–extension, abduction–adduction, and circumduction, but only a limited amount of axial rotation. Only a ball-and-socket joint has more motion than the CMC joint of the thumb. Because it has very good motion, it is more likely to have compression strain or sprain of the ligaments than to have articular somatic dysfunction.

Metacarpophalangeal (MP) and Interphalangeal (IP) Joints

The metacarpal–phalangeal (MP) joints are condyloid joints permitting flexion–extension and adduction–abduction, while the interphalangeal (IP) joints of the hand are gliding joints that permit gross flexion and extension. The MP and IP joints may develop somatic dysfunction in any one of a combination of six minor gliding motions that cannot be initiated directly by muscle action:

- Anteroposterior glide
- Mediolateral glide
- Internal–external rotational glide

Compression is usually part of MP and IP somatic dysfunctions. IM cramps and pain may be a sign of MP or IP somatic dysfunction. Pain in the metacarpal joints may be referred from an ulnohumeral joint somatic dysfunction. Dysfunction of the fingers typically involves the fascial components. There are usually restrictions of fascial rotation, abduction/adduction, or compression/distraction. These types of problems manifest as impediments in finger flexion, swelling of the digits, or pain. Jones tender points, like the CM1 (thenar point, found in the thenar muscle mass) are commonly found in patients who use their hands repetitively. Techniques like MFR, BLT, articulatory technique, and counterstrain are often used to address hand and finger restrictions.

COMMON WRIST AND HAND CONDITIONS AND THE OSTEOPATHIC APPROACH

Carpal Tunnel Syndrome

Carpal tunnel syndrome (CTS) is characterized as an entrapment neuropathy of the median nerve at the wrist producing a constellation of symptoms including paresthesia and weakness of the hands.

CTS is frequently associated with repeated or sustained activity of the fingers and hands.

This section will describe some specifics about the clinical presentation, physical examination, and treatment approach with OMT.

CLINICAL PRESENTATION

Patients experience numbness or paresthesia on the palmar surface of the thumb, index, and middle fingers and radial half of the ring finger. Numbness and paresthesia of the whole hand may also occur. Pain may be referred to the forearm and, less commonly, to the neck and forearm regions. Pain or tingling of the fingers often occurs at night and is relieved by shaking or exercising the hand.[65] Weakness and atrophy of the thenar muscles usually appears late and can occur without significant sensory symptoms. Some patients have decreased grip strength and inability to use hand tools.

PHYSICAL EXAMINATION

Physical examination for CTS begins with inspection of the hands for signs of osteoarthritis, symmetry, and muscle atrophy.[66] The examination should focus on the distribution of symptoms, rather than just provocative maneuvers to elicit symptoms.[67] The clinician should perform a full upper extremity neurovascular examination to rule out other potential causes. Include an assessment of deep tendon reflexes, sensory and motor testing, and a Spurling sign to rule out cervical radiculopathy. Sensory examination may reveal decreased sensation in the distribution of the median nerve, which includes the palm and the first three and a half fingers.[68] If a physical exam shows sensory and/or thenar weakness, the examiner can use tables in the AMA Guides to rate the disability, combining sensory and motor impairments as appropriate.[69] Specific maneuvers include the Tinel sign, the Flick test, Phalen test, and the carpal compression test (Durkan test). These tests reproduce symptoms when positive.[65,70] The most dependable provocative maneuver, known as the carpal compression test, involves applying steady pressure directly over the carpal tunnel for 30 seconds. A positive test is evident when paresthesia or pain arise within the median nerve distribution during the carpal compression test.[70]

The diagnosis of somatic dysfunction is a key component in patients with CTS. The clinician should evaluate structural asymmetries, repetitive motions, and postures and the patient's ergonomics. These assessments can provide clues to areas of potential somatic dysfunction. Palpation should focus on dysfunction affecting neurologic input to the upper extremity, especially the cervical and upper thoracic spine. Palpation should also focus on the myofascial elements of the scalenes, thoracic inlet, pronator teres, forearm, and hand. Clinicians should check for associated myofascial TrPs of the trapezius and forearm in patients with suspected CTS.[71] A restriction of forearm supination and palpable tension of the pronator teres may indicate a concomitant pronator syndrome. Pronator syndrome is characterized by vague volar forearm pain, with median nerve paresthesia and minimal motor findings.[72]

OSTEOPATHIC MANIPULATIVE TREATMENT AND PHYSICAL/OCCUPATIONAL THERAPY

OMT has been recognized as a management option for CTS, although research on its effectiveness is limited.[73] Osteopathic treatment should address the entire patient with CTS, not just stretching the transverse carpal ligament of the wrist. Using a holistic 5 model approach, the neurologic, vascular/lymphatic, structural, metabolic, and behavioral methodologies should be employed. From a neurologic standpoint, relieving compression to the median nerve is paramount along its entire course. However, it is also important to resolve cervical somatic dysfunction and axillary myofascial restrictions to improve brachial plexus and lymphatic function. Many osteopathic physicians and physical therapists utilize MFR and nerve flossing procedures which incorporate both the neurologic and structural models. Addressing both the vascular and lymphatic systems can be achieved by improving circulation and balancing sympathetic tone to the upper extremity by correcting somatic dysfunction of the upper thoracics, upper ribs, and clavicles.[7] Improving blood flow and reducing congestion through improved lymphatic and venous drainage can be achieved with articulatory techniques like Spencer technique and effleurage. Addressing somatic dysfunction of the elbow, tension of the pronator muscle, and interosseous membrane of the forearm prior to the wrist removes potential sites of additional compression. Finally, increasing space within the carpal tunnel using direct release techniques helps to decrease the pressure within the enclosed carpal tunnel.

Physical or occupational therapy is a key component in the management of CTS. Specific exercises can help reduce pressure on the median nerve at the wrist, which can alleviate symptoms of CTS.[74] These exercises may be combined with other treatment modalities such as bracing and/or splinting, medication, and activity modifications.[74] It is important that these exercises are initially performed under the supervision of a doctor or physical therapist to ensure they are safe and effective for the individual patient.[74]

SUMMARY OF OTHER TREATMENT APPROACHES

Conservative treatment may be offered initially to patients with mild to moderate CTS. Options include splinting, activity modification, osteopathic manipulation, physical therapy, therapeutic ultrasound, and home exercise/stretching programs. NSAIDs and corticosteroids are often also recommended. However, NSAIDs, diuretics, and vitamin B6 have not been shown to be effective therapies.[65] Corticosteroid injections into the carpal tunnel can be used for temporary relief of symptoms.[69] If conservative measures fail to alleviate symptoms or if the patient has severe or rapidly progressive symptoms, surgical intervention may be considered. Surgical treatment, whether open or endoscopic, aims to relieve pressure on the median nerve by cutting the transverse carpal ligament.[75]

LOWER EXTREMITIES

The structure and function of the lower extremities allow them to play significant roles in the body's balance, posture, and locomotion as well as venous and lymphatic fluid return to the central vascular system. The functional condition of an individual's lower extremities is a key factor in designing many exercise protocols that are important for a person's general health. Because of their many roles, structural pathologies and somatic dysfunction in the lower extremities have local, postural, *and* systemic implications.

Differential diagnosis of a given lower extremity symptom begins with a clinical interpretation of the patient's history and a physical examination that integrates the osteopathic screening evaluation and palpatory structural examination.

The clinical screening evaluation of the lower extremities (as a discrete region) typically includes:

- An initial observation of the region standing and during normal walking
- Walking on toes or on heels
- Standing with both eyes open and then both eyes closed
- Squatting
- Bending forward, integrated with a standing flexion test evaluation of PSIS motion

- Active and passive joint range of motion comparison bilaterally of the affected joint as well as the joint above and below
  - This may include lumbosacral, sacroiliac, hip, knee, ankle, and foot joints
- Vascular and lymphatic screening
  - Pulses, skin color, and edema
- Lower extremity motor and sensory screenings (L1–S1)
  - Differentiate dermatomes and myotomes
  - Evaluate patellar and Achilles deep tendon reflexes and assess for ankle clonus
  - Evaluate muscle tone, strength, flexibility, and coordination
- Appropriate orthopedic and neurologic tests
  - Trendelenburg test to assess for pelvic drop on the non–weight-bearing side. This tests the strength of the hip abductor muscles (gluteus medius and minimus) on the stance leg.
  - Straight-leg raising test to assess hamstring muscle tension and/or neuropathy
  - FABER (Patrick) test to assess for hip or sacroiliac pathology
    - The acronym FABER describes the motion of the femur at the hip joint performed during this orthopedic screening test—***F***lexion, ***A***bduction, and ***E***xternal ***R***otation
    - With the patient supine, the hip and knee are passively flexed. Then the femur is abducted and externally rotated. This should result in a "figure 4" position, with the ankle crossed on the opposite distal thigh. The evaluator then stabilizes the opposite anterior superior iliac spine (ASIS) and applies further abduction and external rotation of the femur by applying a gentle downward force on the medial knee.
    - There are some osteopathic sources that also include "extension" as a third plane of motion when the femoral abduction and external rotation is applied toward the table[14,76,77]; however, this aspect of motion is not typically included in orthopedic and physical therapy texts.[78,79]
  - And any other indicated lower extremity orthopedic and neurologic tests, as described in Chapter 84 Osteopathic Considerations in Orthopedics, section Specific Orthopedic Tests (Organized by Chief Complaint) and Chapter 73 Osteopathic Considerations in Neurology.

A positive finding in any of these examinations or an indication from the history warrants the need for further segmental assessment including:

- Palpation to assess tissue texture, tenderness, and any potential entrapment sites
- Assessment of the end-feel during range-of-motion testing of specific joints

When observing posture, it is also important to consider the integrated firing patterns of the lower extremity muscles and how asymmetric postural stresses can lead to somatic dysfunction.

Integrated Firing Patterns

Asymmetric postural stress creates recurrent and predictable patterns of lower extremity muscle somatic dysfunction that are characterized by neuromuscular imbalance or MTrPs. In neuromuscular imbalance, stressed postural (antigravity) muscles exhibit an increased irritability (short and tight), whereas their antagonists demonstrate inhibition (weak and atrophic) (Fig. 91.11).[44]

When stressed, the iliopsoas, piriformis, hamstrings, gastrocnemius–soleus complex, adductor magnus, rectus femoris, and tensor fasciae latae all tend to tighten, while the vasti (especially the vastus medialis), glutei, peroneus, and tibialis anterior all tend to be inhibited and weak.[80] Application of the biomechanical–postural model coupled with an understanding of the myotatic unit, muscle agonists and antagonists, and patterns of use is necessary for efficient diagnostic and therapeutic approaches to the treatment of lower extremity dysfunction that arise from this pattern of neuromuscular dysfunction. Please see Chapter 92 Postural Considerations in Osteopathic Diagnosis and Treatment for more information on this.

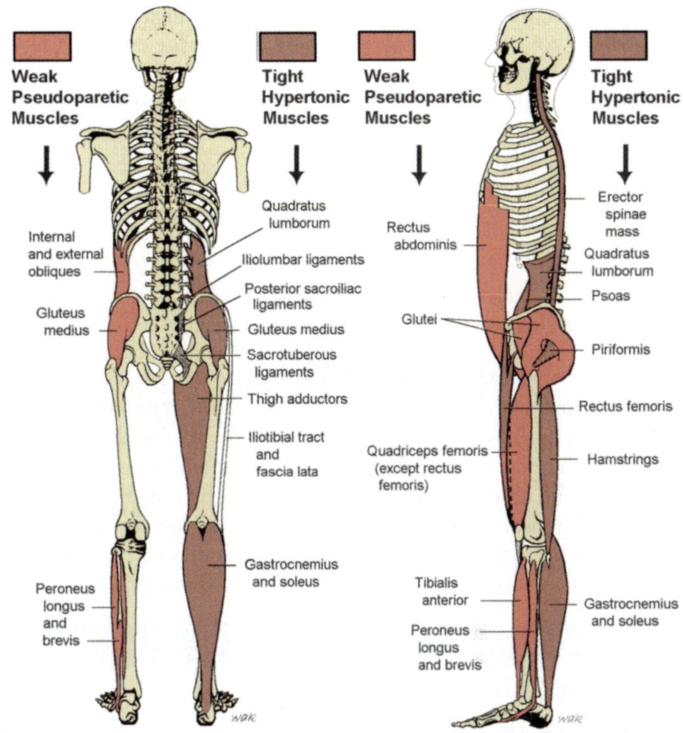

Figure 91.11. Postural pattern of tight (postural) and weak (phasic) muscles. (Illustration by William A. Kuchera, DO, FAAO, with permission.)

HIP

The hip (femoroacetabular) joint forms the connection between the lower extremity and the pelvis. The stable multiaxial ball-and-socket synovial joint allows for weight bearing and motion in flexion, extension, abduction, adduction, internal (medial) rotation, external (lateral) rotation, and circumduction. Average ranges of motion of the hip differ when the knee is flexed or extended. The measurements may also differ between patient populations whose activities require different ligamentous and muscular tensions, as well as sacroiliac and lumbar flexibility.[13,76] For example, expect different averages when testing male collegiate football players compared to teenage female gymnasts.

Average normal measurements for hip motion are as follows[76]:

- Flexion, with knee flexed: 120 to 130 degrees
- Flexion, with knee extended: 90 degrees (limited by hip extensor muscle action)
- Extension, subject prone with opposite leg straight: 20 to 30 degrees
- Extension, subject prone with opposite hip and knee flexed to 90 degrees: 90 to 120 degrees
- Abduction and adduction with hip and knee flexed: 70 to 75 degrees
- Abduction, with hip and knee extended: 40 to 45 degrees

- Adduction, with knee extended and hip only flexed enough to allow leg to cross over anterior aspect of opposite extended leg: 20 to 30 degrees
- Rotation, with hip and knee extended or flexed similarly
  - External rotation: 45 degrees
  - Internal rotation: 35 degrees

Minor joint motions of the hip assessed with end-feel palpation include

- Anterior glide occurring with external rotation
- Posterior glide occurring with internal rotation

Passive hip ranges of motion and assessments of end-feel are usually tested with the patient supine and the pelvis stabilized. Bilateral comparison of both symmetry and the quality of the barrier at the end of motion is often much more important than measuring the absolute number of degrees in the range of motion.

In the presence of asymmetric motion, the quality and pattern of the barriers help to differentiate hypomobility on one side from hypermobility on the other side, and to distinguish somatic dysfunction from pathology. Evaluate both legs for tissue texture changes, tenderness, and strength. The character and pattern of the end-feel of each hip motion may be springy (physiologic) or may suggest loss of joint play, or a capsular, traumatic, or dysfunctional pattern. Subtle differences in somatic dysfunction of myofascial rather than articular origin may also be appreciated by evaluating the quality of the end-feel of the hip joint (Table 91.7).

The muscles and soft tissues of the hip typically limit flexion more than do the ligaments. It is critical to be able to discern between loss of range of motion due to somatic dysfunction, which is amenable to OMT, or to a primary hip pathology that requires medical or surgical care. If the initial findings from the examination of the hip do not follow functional biomechanical principles, they warrant further evaluation. The physical exam can help to clarify this distinction as follows:

- Hip flexion: Straight-leg raising at the hip is limited by the hamstring muscles. When the knee is bent, hamstring influence is removed, and the thigh can be flexed almost to the torso.[13]
  - If significant improvement in hip flexion is not seen after flexing the knee, then somatic dysfunction is unlikely to be the cause.

TABLE 91.7

Hip Joint Somatic Dysfunction

Hip Joint Motion	Freedom of Motion	Motion Restriction[a]	Somatic Dysfunction Nomenclature
Flexion	Symmetric and full flexion of bilateral hip joints when the knee is straight or bent	Affected leg will have limited extension. Hip flexor muscles may feel tight or hypertonic.	• Flexion dysfunction[14,27,29,76,81] • Restricted extension[14,27,29,76,81] • Hypertonicity of hip flexors[14,76] • Psoas or iliopsoas spasm, tension, or hypertonicity[14,29]
Extension	Symmetric and full extension of bilateral hip joints when the knee is straight or bent.	Affected leg will have limited flexion. Hip extensor muscles may feel tight or hypertonic.	• Extension dysfunction[14,27,29,76,81] • Restricted flexion[14,27,29,76,81] • Hypertonicity of hip extensors[14,76] • Hamstring spasm, tension, or hypertonicity[14]
Abduction	Symmetric and full abduction of bilateral hip joints (compare bilaterally with hip and knee flexed or with hip and knee extended).	Affected leg will have limited adduction. Hip abduction muscles may feel tight or hypertonic.	• Abduction dysfunction[14,27,29,76,81] • Restricted adduction[14,27,29,76,81] • Hypertonicity of hip abductors[14,76]
Adduction	Symmetric and full adduction of bilateral hip joints.	Affected leg will have limited abduction. Hip adduction muscles may feel tight or hypertonic.	• Abduction dysfunction[14,27,29,76,81] • Restricted adduction[14,27,29,76,81] • Hypertonicity of hip adductors[14,76]
Internal rotation	Symmetric and full internal rotation of bilateral hip joints. Femur posteriorly glides within the acetabulum at the end-feel of internal rotation.[14,27]	Affected leg will have limited external rotation. A barrier may be palpated with anterior glide of femur during hip external rotation.[14,27] Hip internal rotation muscles may feel tight or hypertonic.	• Femur internal rotation with posterior glide[14,27,32] • Internal rotation dysfunction[14,29,76,81] • Restricted external rotation • Internal rotation lesion of the hip joint[82] • Hypertonicity of hip internal rotators[14,76]
External rotation	Symmetric and full external rotation of bilateral hip joints. The femur anteriorly glides within the acetabulum at the end-feel of external rotation.[14,27]	Affected leg will have limited internal rotation. A barrier may be palpated with posterior glide of femur during hip internal rotation.[14,27] Hip external rotation muscles may feel tight or hypertonic.	• Femur external rotation with anterior glide[14,27,32] • External rotation dysfunction[14,27,29,76,81] • Restricted internal rotation[14,27,29,76,81] • External rotation lesion of the hip joint[82] • Hypertonicity of hip external rotators[14,76] • Piriformis spasm, tension, or hypertonicity[29]

[a]Motion direction and descriptions do not differentiate between articular and myofascial hip dysfunctions. In addition to the articular and muscular joint motion asymmetry described above, the physician should also evaluate for the presence of other possible somatic dysfunction manifestations, such as myofascial restrictions (see Chapter 52), counterstrain tender points (see Chapter 47), trigger points and Chapman reflex points (see Chapter 43) within this region.

- When more pain and limitation of motion coupled with an empty end-feel coincides with bent-knee hip flexion rather than with straight-leg raising, serious conditions including septic bursitis, ischiorectal fossa abscess, osteomyelitis, neoplasm of the upper femur, or other significant pathology of the ilium must be ruled out.[83]
- Hip extension: supine evaluation mimics the Psoas (Thomas) orthopedic test. Prone evaluation can measure as much as 35 degrees extension.
  - Flexing the contralateral hip and knee relaxes some of the muscular restriction to hip extension and should increase the measurement if somatic dysfunction due to muscle tension imbalance is the cause.
- Internal and external rotation: Assess and evaluate the patterns of muscular restriction and the minor motion glides (anterior glide with external rotation and posterior glide with internal rotation).
  - A physiologic end-feel to one motion compared to a barrier in the opposite direction is consistent with a somatic dysfunctional pattern.
  - A capsular pattern of marked limitation to specific directions of motion should raise suspicions of an underlying inflammatory or traumatic process.
- Abduction and adduction: Combine the FABER (Patrick) screening test and FADIR screening test with evaluation for a hip capsular pattern.
  - Arthritic change modifies gliding motions and occurs early in the minor motions of the joint.[83]
  - Hip joint pathology, such as osteoarthritis, will usually create pain in the inguinal region during a FABER test.
  - A positive FABER test that lacks a hip capsular palpatory pattern or has pain limited to the posterior pelvis is more likely to reflect sacroiliac joint pathology.

Arthritic change progresses from functional demand accentuated by biomechanical stress to pathophysiologic response and structural change. For example, the biomechanical stress placed on the hip joint by a short lower extremity results in a higher incidence of greater trochanteric pain syndrome (GTPS) and of osteoarthritis.[84] Somatic dysfunction and arthritic pathology often coexist within this structure–function spectrum; each should be addressed with appropriate therapeutic tools that are integrated into a regimen for total patient treatment.[5]

COMMON HIP CONDITIONS AND THE OSTEOPATHIC APPROACH

Sciatic Neuralgia

The sciatic nerve exits the pelvis through the greater sciatic notch and divides into a tibial and a common peroneal nerve usually prior to the superior angle of the popliteal fossa.[13] In most individuals, it passes under the piriformis muscle; however, in approximately 10% of the population, the common peroneal nerve alone or both the common peroneal nerve and the tibial nerve passes through or above the piriformis muscle.[85] In the buttock or thigh, the sciatic nerve might be affected functionally by the piriformis muscle. Primary causes for such piriformis dysfunction can arise from direct trauma such as a fall onto one buttock or sitting for a prolonged period on a hard surface such as a toilet seat. Secondary dysfunction of the piriformis might be postural in origin or due to articular somatic dysfunctions involving the sacrum (sacral shears in particular) or the hip. Because of the close anatomical relationship between the two, biochemical irritation of the sciatic nerve is possible with irritation of the piriformis. Piriformis structure–function relationships with the sciatic nerve are also addressed in Chapter 73 Osteopathic Considerations in Neurology.

Another source of iatrogenic trauma to the sciatic nerve comes from accidental injection into the nerve. Because the peroneal fibers are more superficial, they are more commonly involved in injection injuries; the resultant side effects include footdrop. Intramuscular injections into the buttocks should be given in the upper outer quadrant to avoid this problem. Injections for piriformis TrPs should avoid steroids to decrease the risk of permanent damage from accidental introduction of the injected contents into the nerve.

Greater Trochanteric Pain Syndrome

GTPS is also known as lateral hip pain, hip periarthritis, gluteal tendinopathy, or trochanteric bursitis.[86,87] Trochanteric bursitis is no longer the preferred term due to the relatively rare occurrence of bursitis on imaging.[87,88] GTPS is a common cause of lateral hip pain and is commonly attributable to both bursitis and tendinopathy as they tend to occur together.[86] GTPS encompasses a range of causes including gluteal medius and minimus tendinopathy/tears, trochanteric bursitis, and external coxa saltans, yet an exact cause remains unknown.[86]

There are many bursae around the hip, however, most individuals have three main ones that may be involved with GTPS. These include[13,86]:

- The gluteus minimus bursa, located anterosuperior to the greater trochanter
- The subgluteus medius bursa, lies deep to the gluteus medius tendon on the superior aspect of the greater trochanter
- The subgluteus maximus bursa (also called the trochanteric bursa) is the largest and lies lateral to the greater trochanter (Fig. 91.12)

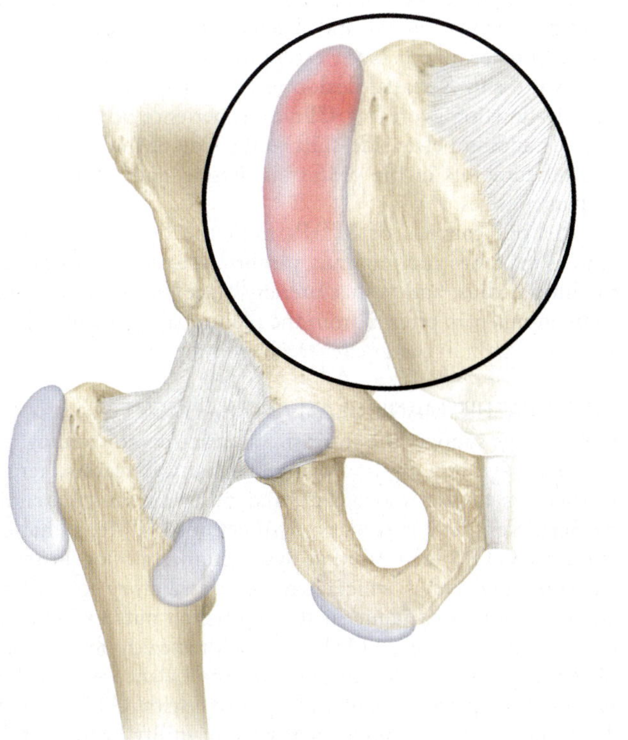

Figure 91.12. Bursa of the hip (anterior view).

The gluteus medius and minimus muscles form part of the abductor mechanism of the hip joint. These muscles and their tendons are also implicated in the pathophysiology of the condition.[86] They are innervated by the superior gluteal nerve, L5, and S1.[13]

This section will describe some specifics about the clinical presentation, physical examination, and treatment approach with OMT.

CLINICAL PRESENTATION

GTPS is a clinical diagnosis commonly defined as pain and tenderness in the region of the greater trochanter, typically reproduced on palpation of the lateral hip, which may radiate down the lateral or posterior part of the thigh.[87] The pain classically increases with walking, especially with stairs, prolonged standing, and rising from a seated position (such as getting out of a car) or lying on the affected side.[87] Patients with tendinopathy clinically present with chronic activity-related pain and impaired performance of the tendon with or without local tendon swelling.[89]

PHYSICAL EXAMINATION

A thorough neurologic and musculoskeletal exam including hip orthopedic testing and straight leg raise should be performed. Clinicians should ascertain the location, quality, and severity of pain. The physical examination may demonstrate a limp or a Trendelenburg gait, and reproduction of the pain on palpation of the greater trochanter. Several clinical tests have been associated with GTPS. Clinicians should perform the FABER, Ober, and Trendelenburg tests. The FABER test appears to be the most clinically useful with 90% specificity and 83% sensitivity.[87,90] Other clinical tests include the external derotation test, which is performed with the hip flexed at 90 degrees and in external rotation, followed by internal rotation against resistance at the ankle; the single leg standing test (for 30 seconds); the resisted abduction test with the patient laying on the contralateral side; and Ober test.[87,90]

The physical examination should determine the location and severity of associated somatic dysfunction. A standing flexion test can help determine if lower extremity or pelvic somatic dysfunction is present. A seated flexion test can help determine if sacroiliac dysfunction is present. Clinical experience of the authors has found standing pelvic side-shift to the side of the GTPS, tension and tenderpoints in the piriformis muscle, and inhibition of the gluteus muscles.

Referral patterns of MTrPs from the quadratus lumborum, gluteus maximus and minimus, piriformis, tensor fasciae latae, vastus intermedius, and vastus lateralis[91] (see Fig. 40.21) as well as ligamentous pain referral from the iliolumbar ligament[92] also have associated pain in the greater trochanter region.

OSTEOPATHIC MANIPULATIVE TREATMENT

OMT helps support the intrinsic mechanisms for healing within the body by way of improving mechanical factors, removing restrictions to free movement, and relieving musculotendinous barriers, identified as somatic dysfunctions.[93] Osteopathic evaluation for GTPS focuses upon dysfunctional motion in the lumbar spine and pelvis which may be contributory to creating an aberrant motion dynamic in the hip which puts excessive strain on the hip abductors.[93] OMT that addresses dysfunctional agonist–antagonist muscles and restores the balance within the hip, sacrum, and pelvis should be a priority with GTPS patients.[93] Techniques such as muscle energy are of utility in this condition. Isometric and isolytic muscle energy treatment of the adductor magnus on the ipsilateral side has a pronounced and immediate effect on greater trochanteric tenderness.[93] Anecdotally, OMT has also shown promise in long term resolution of GTPS, especially when adductor stretching exercises are added to the home exercise regime.[93]

SUMMARY OF OTHER TREATMENT APPROACHES

At present there is no defined treatment protocol for GTPS. There is some evidence to suggest that modifications of daily physical activities to reduce stress on the involved tendons may be beneficial.[86,94–96] Conservative treatment is the gold standard for GTPS with over 90% success rate.[95,96] Treatment in the initial stages encompasses a range of conservative interventions including physiotherapy, OMT, extracorporeal shockwave therapy (ESWT), activity modification, pain-relief and anti-inflammatory medication, weight reduction and if still problematic, local corticosteroid injection, or platelet-rich plasma (PRP) injection.[86,93]

Exercises are intended to address the weakness of the hip abductors and include piriformis stretching, iliotibial band stretching, straight leg raises, wall squats, and gluteal strengthening. Many therapists recommend eccentric strengthening of the abductors, alongside high-level core strengthening and functional training, including sport-specific tasks for the effective management of GTPS.[97]

Some clinical practice guidelines suggest that eccentric-based exercises may not be suitable or tolerated for in-season athletes or at the initial stages of treatment due to the high load it places on the tendon.[98] However, a patient-specific approach utilizing eccentric exercises, while ensuring that exercises are introduced at a suitable stage of rehabilitation, can maximize benefits and minimize risks in the treatment of GTPS.

Most cases respond to initial conservative treatments and injections, with refractory cases potentially requiring surgical intervention.

KNEE AND LEG

The knee is a compound synovial joint consisting of three separate articulations within one joint capsule—the medial and lateral femorotibial articulations and the patellofemoral articulation.[13] The fibula is not considered part of the knee joint. However, dysfunction at the proximal tibiofibular joint, the distal tibiofibular syndesmosis, and the interosseous membrane can also affect knee and ankle mechanics.[99] The functional anatomy of the knee and leg are addressed in Chapter 40.

When examining the knees and legs, all findings are compared bilaterally. Observe the standing patient for signs of *genu valgum*, *genu varum*, or *genu recurvatum* (hyperextended knee) (Fig. 91.13) along with other structural and motion asymmetries.

Femorotibial Articulations

The major motions of the knee joint are flexion and extension. Because of the irregular shape of the joint surfaces, these two motions are combined with some minor involuntary glides, rolling, and rotational motions. Minor motions of the tibial plateau at the knee include:

- Anterior and posterior glides
- Medial and lateral glides
- Internal rotation with posterolateral glide
- External rotation with anteromedial glide

Testing of minor motions of the joint and ligament assessment should be performed with the knee in variable degrees of flexion

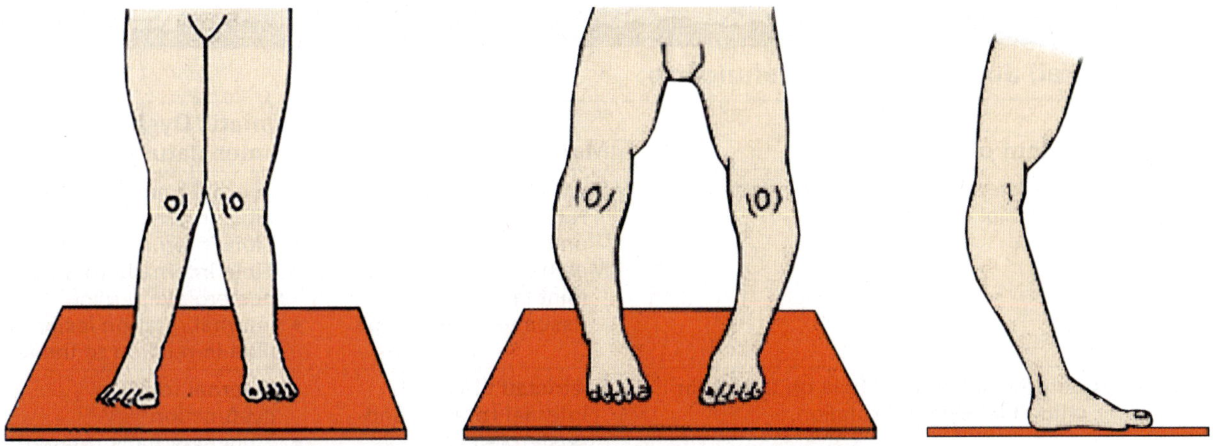

Figure 91.13. Deformities of the knees—anterior and lateral view. From **left** to **right**: *genu valgum, genu varum, genu recurvatum.* (From Department of Neuromusculoskeletal Medicine/Osteopathic Manipulative Medicine at Western University of Health Sciences, College of Osteopathic Medicine of the Pacific. *Osteopathic Principles and Practice: Osteopathic Manipulative Treatment.* 1st ed. Western University of Health Sciences; 2015–2016, with permission.)

because complete extension of the knee creates a bony lock. The osteopathic palpatory examination of the knee incorporates standard knee testing positions and maneuvers while noting the presence and pattern of these findings:

- Gross range of motion
- Restricted gliding minor motions (end-feel)
- Hypermobility and loss of stability (end-feel)

As with other lower extremity joints, all findings are compared bilaterally for asymmetry and the quality of the end-feel motions.

The same testing maneuvers needed to diagnose somatic dysfunction offer orthopedic and rheumatologic information about knee structure. In general, during testing, if the asymmetrical end-feel of the test is too loose, there is an orthopedic diagnosis. If restricted in both directions of a given paired motion (e.g., flexion–extension), there is often a rheumatologic diagnosis. If a pattern of paired motions is assessed to be physiologically free in one direction but ends too abruptly in the other, the diagnosis is typically somatic dysfunction. Thus, interpreting each test for the available dual structure–function information provides twice the diagnostic power in the same amount of time that is usually spent on examining the knee structure alone.

A knee with gross limitation of flexion and slight limitation of extension is consistent with a capsular pattern of that joint. This palpatory finding, correlated with history and other physical findings, leads to an appropriate differential diagnosis of varying types of arthritis and synovitis affecting the knee. The capsular pattern of the knee[80,100] differs significantly from a somatic dysfunction, in which minor motions of the joint are restricted in one aspect of each paired motion and free in the opposite direction (Table 91.8).

The minor motions of the knee joint should be checked for somatic dysfunction by adding an anteromedial glide while inducing external rotation of the tibial plateau and a posterolateral glide while inducing internal rotation of the tibial plateau (Fig. 91.14).

Abduction and adduction of the tibia are passive motions of the knee that typically cannot be voluntarily created by the patient. Examining these motions with valgus and varus stress testing provides information about somatic dysfunction and the stability of the collateral ligaments. Restriction of glide in one direction suggests somatic dysfunction; laxity in one direction suggests ligamentous sprain or tear.

- Valgus stress testing of the knee at 30 degrees of flexion (Fig. 91.15A) induces abduction of the tibia and medial glide of the tibial plateau. Laxity suggests instability of the medial collateral ligament (MCL).
- Varus stress testing at 30 degrees of flexion (Fig. 91.15B) induces adduction of the tibia and lateral glide of the tibial plateau. Laxity suggests instability of the lateral collateral ligament.

Stability of the anterior cruciate ligament (ACL) is checked with an anterior drawer test (knee flexed toward 90 degrees) or, with greater specificity, a *Lachman test* (knee flexed up to 30 degrees). Stability of the posterior cruciate ligament (PCL) is checked with a *posterior drawer test*. These maneuvers also permit assessment of anterior and posterior glide end-feel for dysfunction.

The knee should move into full extension and lock, freely and without restriction. This is tested by grasping the foot of the supine patient with one hand and raising that lower extremity just off the table. The knee is flexed slightly with the other hand and then released, allowing it to extend. A normal knee drops freely into extension and bounces off the ligaments. Structural injuries, especially medial meniscal tears, might result in inability to extend fully or in guarding on extension.

MENISCUS EVALUATION AND OSTEOPATHIC CONSIDERATIONS

It is important to understand that one function of the menisci is to limit extreme knee flexion and extension. In extreme knee extension during the screw-home motion, the menisci are forced anteriorly, and the anterior horns of the menisci block further extension. In full flexion, the posterior horns of the meniscus are driven posteriorly and block knee flexion.[108] Therefore, during meniscus testing like the *McMurray meniscal tests* (see Chapter 40 Lower Extremity), if pain or snapping occurs near maximum knee flexion, the posterior horns are probably involved, and if pain or clunk occurs toward knee extension, the middle to anterior portion of the meniscus is probably involved.

A palpable click accompanied by pain while performing the *McMurray meniscal tests* strongly suggests displacement or a meniscal tear. Palpation of a tender meniscus at the joint line is more sensitive but less specific than the meniscal orthopedic tests.[109] Usually, a combination of maneuvers based upon pain provocation

TABLE 91.8

Knee (Femorotibial) Joint Somatic Dysfunction

Knee Motion	Freedom of Motion	Motion Restriction[a]	Somatic Dysfunction Nomenclature
Internal rotation	Posterolateral glide of the tibia on the femur with tibial internal rotation.	Restricted external rotation and anteromedial glide. May have medial or lateral joint tenderness or tissue texture change.	• Internal rotation dysfunction[101–103] • Tibia internally rotated[81] • Tibia internal rotation[104] • Tibia internally rotated with posterolateral glide[102,105,106] • Internal rotation lesion of the tibia in relation to the femur[82]
External rotation	Anteromedial glide of tibia on the femur with tibial external rotation.	Restricted tibial internal rotation and posterolateral glide. May have medial or lateral joint tenderness or tissue texture change.	• External rotation dysfunction[101,102,103] • Tibia externally rotated[81] • Tibia external rotation[104] • Tibia externally rotated with anteromedial glide[102,105,106] • External rotation lesion of the tibia in relation to the femur[82]
Adduction	Varus stress of tibia on femur where the lateral joint structures are lax, and the medial knee joint approximates.[82] Medial joint approximation causes the distal tibia to be more medial than the proximal tibia (ankle moves toward midline).	Tibial motion on the femur is restricted in medial translatory slide. Tenderness and tissue texture change may be present on the medial or lateral joint.	• Adduction dysfunction[105] • Adduction with lateral glide[106] • Adduction lesion of the knee[82] • Abduction of tibia on femur[b,101]
Abduction	Valgus stress of the tibia on the femur where the medial joint structures are lax, and the lateral knee joint approximates.[82] Lateral joint approximation causes the distal tibia to be more lateral than the proximal tibia (ankle moves away from midline).	Tibial motion on the femur is restricted in lateral translatory slide. May have medial or lateral joint tenderness or tissue texture change.	• Abduction dysfunction[82,105] • Abduction with medial glide[106] • Adduction of tibia on femur[b,101]
Flexion	Anterior glide of tibia on femur with flexion. (This occurs during non–weight-bearing motion testing, open chain kinetics.) ("Movement of the tibia on the femur into flexion is coupled with posterior slide"[101] when weight bearing/closed chain kinetics.)	Restricted extension and posterior movement of tibia on femur. May have anterior or posterior joint tenderness or tissue texture change	• Anterior tibia (posterior distal femur)[102,107] • Tibia flexion with anterior glide[106] • Posterior slide dysfunction[c,101]
Extension	Posterior glide of tibia on femur with extension. (This occurs during non–weight-bearing motion testing, open chain kinetics.) ("Movement of the tibia on the femur into extension is coupled with anterior slide"[101] when weight bearing/closed chain.)	Restricted flexion and anterior movement of tibia on femur. May have anterior or posterior joint tenderness or tissue texture change.	• Posterior tibia (anterior distal femur)[102,107] • Tibia extension with posterior glide[106] • Anterior slide dysfunction[c,101]
The tibia may be driven posteriorly beneath the femur by a fall on the flexed knee, especially if the principal contact is made at the proximal end of the tibia. This can limit knee extension or cause the knee to become "caught" painfully in a position of partial flexion.[82]			• Posterior displacement of the tibia in relation to the femur[82]

[a]In addition to the articular joint motion restrictions and asymmetry described above, the physician should also evaluate for the presence of other possible somatic dysfunction manifestations, such as restrictions of the associated musculature, myofascial restrictions (see Chapter 52), and counterstrain tender points (see Chapter 47), and trigger points (see Chapter 43) within this region.

[b]During production of this table, it was noted that one reference[101] described the identical motions of varus and valgus stress compared to other sources but named the abduction and adduction based on direction of the greater medial or lateral translatory motion at the knee rather than tibial adduction and abduction.[101] Strachan[82] reported both adduction and abduction lesions may occur in combination with either a lateral or medial displacement of the tibia in relation to the femur.[82]

[c]One source[101] had opposite terminology from other sources[102,106,107] for the nomenclature of coupled minor glides with knee flexion and extension. That source may have been describing closed chain mechanics while the other sources were describing open chain mechanics. Strachan[82] did not identify anterior or posterior minor gliding motion with knee flexion or extension. He did report that knee extension may be limited by a posterior displacement of the tibia relative to the femur occurring from a fall on the flexed knee, especially if the principal contact is made at the proximal end of the tibia. Anterior tibial dysfunctions were not described in "Principles of Osteopathic Technic."[82]

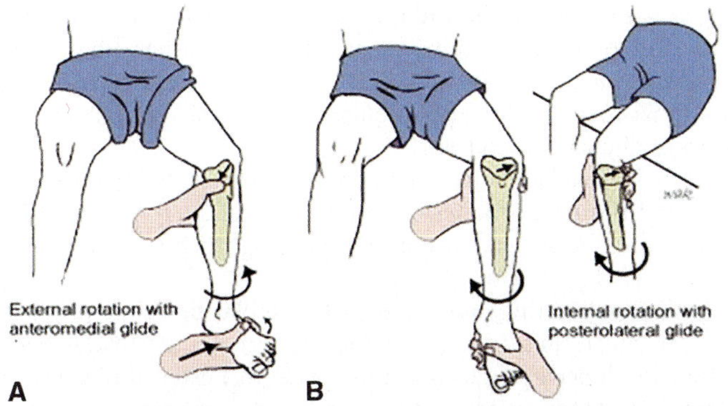

Figure 91.14. Physical examination of minor tibial glides. A. Palpate for anteromedial tibial glide with external rotation. **B.** Palpate for posterolateral tibial glide with internal rotation of the knee. (Illustration by William A. Kuchera, DO, FAAO, with permission.)

with compression, traction, or shear forces is required to confirm the diagnosis.[110]

In addition to pain, patients with a meniscal tear experience swelling, popping, or clicking, limited knee motion, and occasional joint locking during walking. Meniscal tears decrease the shock-absorption properties of the knee joint and can predispose to arthritic change in the joint itself over time.

The vascular supply is very poor to the menisci in the knees. The red zone, along the outer periphery is vascular but toward the central section, the white zone is avascular. The vascularization pattern and nutritional status of a torn meniscus along with the morphologic pattern of the tear are crucial factors determining the success of a meniscus surgery. The healing potential of a torn meniscus is directly dependent on its blood supply.[111]

Minor tears, near the periphery are typically vascular and can often heal with conservative care. They may benefit from OMT or heat to improve blood flow. Lymphatic protocols and MFR in the area are commonly used techniques.

Symptoms of locking due to displacement or medial meniscal tear may be addressed by modifying the McMurray test, starting from the flexed neutral knee position.

- First, gently externally rotate, abduct, and gap the medial side of the knee joint until a slight bulge is felt at the joint line; follow with pressure over the medial meniscus (and the MCL to which all or a fragment of the meniscus may be attached) to reduce the bulge.
- Complete the procedure by holding firm digital pressure over the medial meniscus during knee extension and internal rotation.

This maneuver would be contraindicated in a patient with a more severe or avascular meniscus tear, or when there is laxity and pain of multiple ligaments. The combination of torn ACL and MCL along with a torn medial meniscus occurs predictably from certain traumas featuring valgus stress forces such as a tackle to the outside of the knee with the knee extended fully and the foot fixed. Because this injury causes significant knee instability, historically, many clinicians referred to this constellation as *O'Donoghue triad* or more commonly as the *unhappy (or terrible) triad.*[112,113]

Patellofemoral Joint Dysfunction

The roles of the patella are threefold[114]:

- To increase the moment arm of the quadriceps muscles
- Provide bony protection to the distal joint surfaces of the femoral condyles when the knee is flexed
- Prevent damaging compressive forces on the quadriceps tendon with resisted knee extension

Patellofemoral joint dysfunction and structural change of the patella may each arise from abnormal patella tracking or pressure on the patella. This is often seen when the Q-angle is excessive. An increased Q-angle is referred to as genu valgum (knock-kneed). A decreased Q-angle is referred to as genu varum (bow-legged). (See Chapter 40 Lower Extremity for full description of the Q-Angle.)

Accentuated Q-angles can be associated with symptoms of patellar pain due to ligamentous stress at the knee or through secondary development of muscle imbalance and TrPs. The patella might even sublux laterally with these biomechanical forces, especially with dysfunction or weakness of the vastus medialis muscle. Locking of the patella strongly suggests MTrPs in the vastus

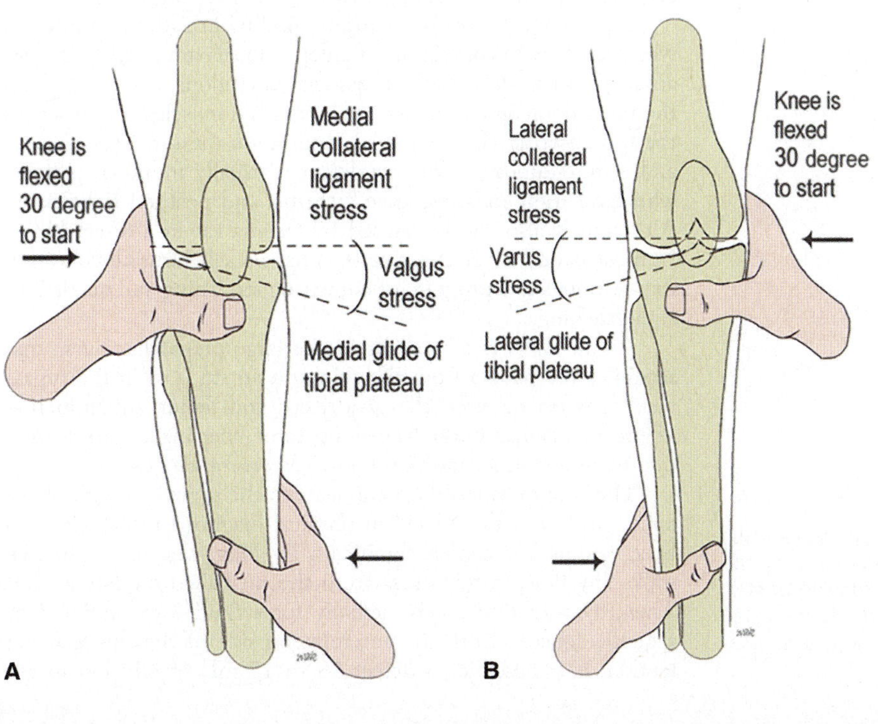

Figure 91.15. Hand placements to assess the integrity of lateral and medial collateral ligaments of a patient's right knee. A. Valgus stress test to assess MCL and medial glide of the tibia. **B.** Varus stress test to assess LCL and lateral glide of the tibia. (Illustration by William A. Kuchera, DO, FAAO, with permission.)

lateralis muscle. Complete locking of the patella immobilizes the knee joint in slight flexion, while partial locking causes difficulty in straightening the knee after sitting in a chair.

Prolonged patellofemoral dysfunction, due to these biomechanical factors, predisposes an individual to structural changes including irregular or accelerated wearing or roughening of the articular surface on the posterior surface of the patella (*chondromalacia patellae*).[115] This coexistence of structural and functional disorders must be considered, appropriately diagnosed, and treated to encourage optimum healing. When the tracking disorder is secondary to muscular imbalance, it is very important to consider neural agonist–antagonist relationships and, therefore, to sufficiently stretch any tight hamstrings prior to trying to strengthen weak quadriceps.[80]

Structural problems of the patella are evaluated, in part, by palpating over and around the patella. Look for subpatellar tenderness, crepitus, grinding, or clicking with compression against the underlying femur (patellar grind test) when gliding the patella medially, laterally, superiorly, or inferiorly. Effusion within the knee joint also strongly suggests structural change. Patellar structural problems also arise from:

- Patellar dislocation
- Chronic or direct patellar trauma
- Fracture of the lower extremity

Postural disorders can create secondary bony alignment and muscular imbalance, causing functional patellar tracking difficulties.

The Fibular Joints and Proximal Fibular Dysfunction

The fibula lies posterolateral to the tibia and is connected by the proximal tibiofibular joint, the distal tibiofibular syndesmosis, and the interosseous membrane between the two shafts. Movement at the superior tibiofibular joint is impossible without movement at the inferior tibiofibular syndesmosis.[13] There is reciprocal anterior–posterior motion between the distal and proximal ends of the fibula. When the distal fibula moves posteriorly, the proximal fibular head moves anteriorly. See Chapter 40 Lower Extremity for a detailed explanation of the tensions and articular angulations that influence the directions of gliding motions of the fibula (Fig. 91.16).

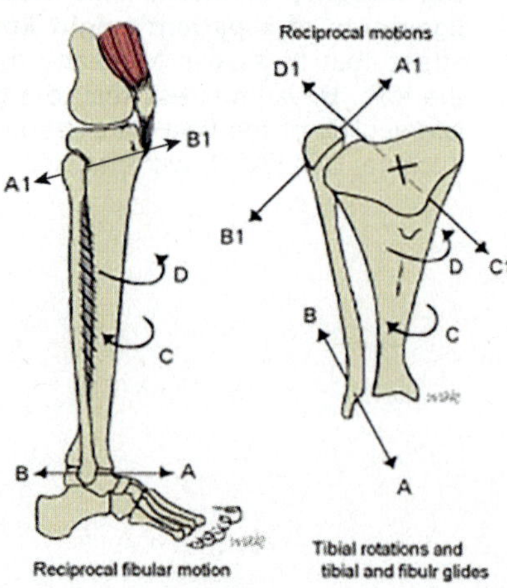

Figure 91.16. Reciprocal fibular motions. Inducing external rotation of the tibia and ankle (*C*) moves the distal fibula posteriorly (*B*) and is reciprocally associated with the fibular head moving anteriorly (*B1*). The opposite is true (*A, A1*) when inducing internal rotation (*D*) of the lower leg. (Illustration by William A. Kuchera, DO, FAAO, with permission.)

This motion can be induced by ankle dorsiflexion and plantarflexion or through translatory motion at either fibular end. Restricted ankle motion warrants examination and treatment of any tibial rotations and tibiofibular syndesmosis tension prior to treating fibular dysfunction.

Fibular head somatic dysfunction is classically named for the preferred position of anterior or posterior glide. It is checked by gliding the fibular head posteriorly (and slightly medial) and anteriorly (and slightly lateral) (Table 91.9).

When evaluating and grasping the fibular head, the physician must take care not to cause undue pressure on the fibular nerve, which lies directly posterior to this structure. Posterior fibular head somatic dysfunction can itself cause symptoms related to entrapment neuropathy or compression of the common fibular nerve. Habitual crossing of one leg over the opposite knee—"crossed leg peroneal palsy"—can also lead to neuropathic symptoms due to prolonged pressure on the nerve against the fibular head. It is especially prevalent in patients with cachexia who have lost significant soft tissue padding in this region.

Fibular head dysfunction often occurs in recurrent ankle sprains and responds well to manipulative procedures.[80,116,117] Treatment of proximal tibiofibular dysfunction, which is almost invariably coexistent with distal fibula dysfunction, will frequently remove the restrictions at the distal joint. If the distal dysfunction persists it may also be treated.[118] (See Ankle and Foot Somatic Dysfunctions section of this chapter.)

Palpation and manipulative treatment of tibiofibular interosseous membrane strain can also help in treating patients who have incurred an ankle sprain as well as other symptoms of leg pain or edema. This can be achieved with ligamentous balancing techniques between the fibula and tibia while palpating at both ends of the fibula.

COMMON KNEE AND LEG CONDITIONS AND THE OSTEOPATHIC APPROACH

Bursitis in the Knee

The knee is a common site for trauma and inflammation to the bursa, which are designed to protect the relatively exposed superficial structures from injury against those underlying them.

Pes anserine bursitis is a common finding in patients or athletes who present with complaints of anterior knee pain (AKP). The pes anserine bursa, along with its associated tendons, is located along the proximomedial aspect of the tibia. The muscles that insert at the pes anserine via a cojoined tendon are the sartorius, gracilis, and semitendinosus. This condition is usually found in patients who have tight muscles, knee arthritis, and postural imbalances. Although it also can be caused by trauma (as in a direct blow). In most patients, pes anserine bursitis is a self-limiting condition that responds to a program of hamstring stretching and quadriceps strengthening.

Patellar bursitis may occur in the large prepatellar bursa that separates the patella from the skin anterior to it or in the suprapatellar bursa between the quadriceps and femur. Inflammation of the prepatellar bursa from long-term kneeling or from other trauma results in a condition known as *housemaid's knee*.

The suprapatellar bursa connects to the synovial cavity of the knee joint and can be used in physical diagnosis to determine if knee trauma has caused significant swelling. The physician first milks any fluid in this bursa from the medial to the lateral side. Then, by palpating anteromedially for a fluid wave initiated by a gentle squeeze from the anterolateral side of the suprapatellar tendon, it is possible to detect 10 to 15 mL of effusion in the

TABLE 91.9 The Proximal Tibiofibular Joint/Fibular Head Somatic Dysfunction

Fibular Head Motion	Freedom of Motion	Motion Restriction[a]	Somatic Dysfunction Nomenclature
Anterior	Anterior (and slightly lateral) glide of proximal fibula (fibular head) on the proximal tibia during translatory motion testing and/or when the foot is dorsiflexed, driving distal fibula posteriorly.	• Posterior (posteromedial) glide is restricted during translatory motion testing or when the foot is plantarflexed. • Lateral malleolus may be held posteriorly and restrict anterior glide. • Talus may be held in external rotation by the lateral malleolus impairing ankle function.[106] • Tenderness and tissue texture change may be present over the fibular head.	• Anterior fibular head dysfunction[81,101,102,104–107] • Anterior lesion of the proximal tibiofibular joint[82]
Posterior	Posterior (and slightly medial) glide of proximal fibula (fibular head) on the proximal tibia during translatory motion testing and/or when the foot is plantarflexed (allowing distal fibula to move anteriorly).	• Anterior (anterolateral) glide is restricted during translatory motion testing or when the foot is dorsiflexed. • Lateral malleolus may be held anterior and restrict posterior glide. • Talus may be held in internal rotation by the lateral malleolus, impairing ankle function.[106] • Tenderness and tissue texture change may be present over the fibular head.	• Posterior fibular head dysfunction[81,101–107] • Posterior lesion of the proximal tibiofibular joint[82]

[a]In addition to the articular joint motion restrictions and asymmetry described above, the physician should also evaluate for the presence of other possible somatic dysfunction manifestations, such as restrictions of the associated musculature, myofascial restrictions (see Chapter 52), and counterstrain tender points (see Chapter 47), and trigger points (see Chapter 43) within this region.

knee. This *bulge test* is used for small effusions (Fig. 91.17A). If the effusion is so large that the tissues become turgid, a fluid pulse might not be able to create a bulge and the test can provide a false-negative result. Large effusions are more accurately diagnosed with a ballottement test (Fig. 91.17B) in which the kneecap is tapped gently (ballotted). A palpable transmission of bony contact is palpated if the effusion is large enough to have distanced the patella from the bone behind it.

The superficial and deep infrapatellar bursae are less often involved in clinical problems.

A *Baker cyst* arises from enlargement of either the semimembranosus bursa or the bursa behind the medial head of the gastrocnemius (Fig. 91.18). The swollen cyst is often painful, especially with flexion of the knee, and the swelling is more prominent in the standing position. Both of these bursae commonly communicate with the synovial cavity of the knee. For this reason,

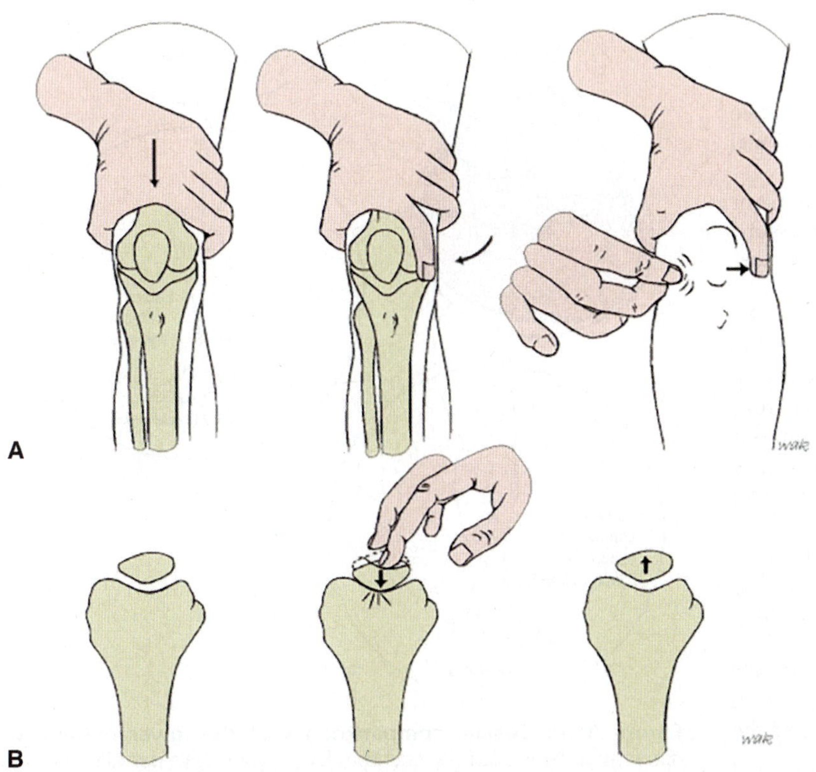

Figure 91.17. Assessing knee effusion. A. Bulge sign. **B.** Ballottement test. (Illustration by William A. Kuchera, DO, FAAO, with permission.)

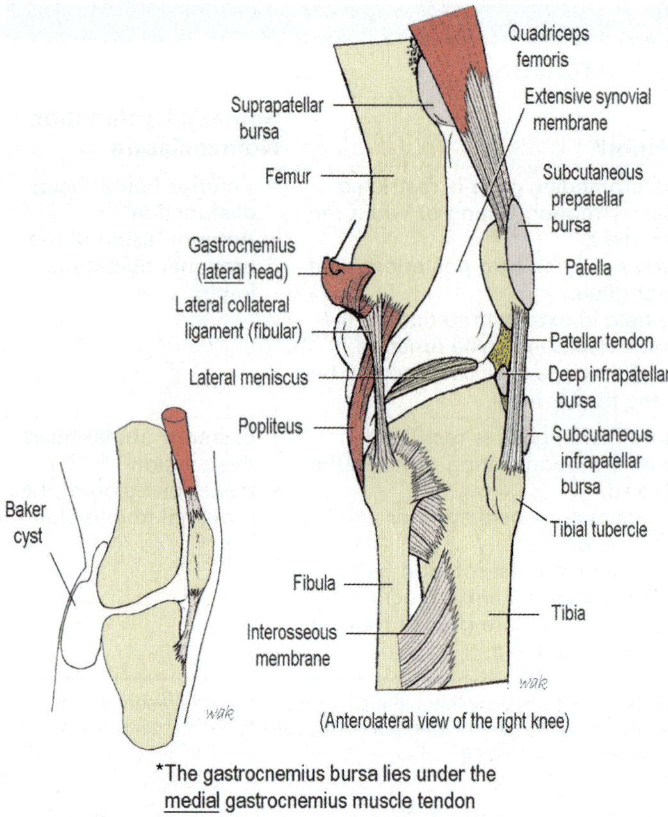

Figure 91.18. Bursae of the knee and Baker cyst. (Illustration by William A. Kuchera, DO, FAAO, with permission.)

knee trauma such as a meniscal tear, or diseases such as rheumatoid arthritis, can initiate the cyst. Rupture of a Baker cyst may be misdiagnosed as thrombophlebitis; extension of a Baker cyst may compress the common peroneal nerve near the fibular head and lead to a footdrop.

Compartment Syndrome

The lower leg is divided into four compartments (Fig. 91.19). See Chapter 40 Lower Extremity for information on the functional anatomy.

Clinically, a compartment syndrome can arise from trauma or vigorous overuse, leading to a rise in intracompartmental pressure. This in turn compromises the circulation, including venous return, within that compartment.

The level of intracompartmental pressure determines the severity of the condition. For example, runners sometimes develop muscle swelling that impairs venous outflow, leading to a rise in intracompartmental pressure. This is most common in the anterior compartment. Palpation may reveal the entire tibialis anterior muscle to be hard and tender. Anterior compartment muscles may exhibit weakness upon testing, and decreased sensation is often present between the first and second toes due to entrapment of the deep peroneal nerve. Peripheral pulses are usually present. Because of the location of the pain on the anterolateral side of the leg, recurrent anterior compartment syndrome is also sometimes called *anterior shin splints*.

In lateral compartment syndrome, pain is located diffusely along the lateral aspect of the lower leg. It recurs in runners with excessive pronation of the foot or might result from rupture of the peroneus longus muscle.

Posterior compartment syndromes typically refer pain anteromedially. While some reserve the term *shin splints* only for periostitis along the line of attachment of a repeatedly overloaded muscle,[119] others include posterior compartment syndrome in the differential diagnosis along with stress fractures of the tibia and chronic periostitis (soleus syndrome). Posterior compartment syndromes are often bilateral and difficult to manage conservatively.

Recurrent mild compartment symptoms are managed with ice and OMT. Ice decreases pain and metabolic demand after activity. OMT also decreases pain and improves venous and lymphatic return. Management of coexisting TrPs can be helpful but not with injections because that would increase pressure in an already tight compartment. Modification of the running surface or the running shoe may be required to prevent recurrent compartment syndromes.

If intracompartmental pressure becomes great enough, arterial circulation is reduced, and ischemia with potential necrosis of muscle in the compartment can occur. An *acute compartment compression* is a surgical emergency requiring fasciotomy. Such a situation is more likely to occur in the anterior compartment than in other divisions of the leg. The acute compartment compression may occur in runners whose symptoms of intense pain develop during the run but do not subside afterward.

Patellofemoral Pain Syndrome

Patellofemoral pain syndrome (PFP) is the most common cause of knee pain in the outpatient setting.[120] With knee pain accounting

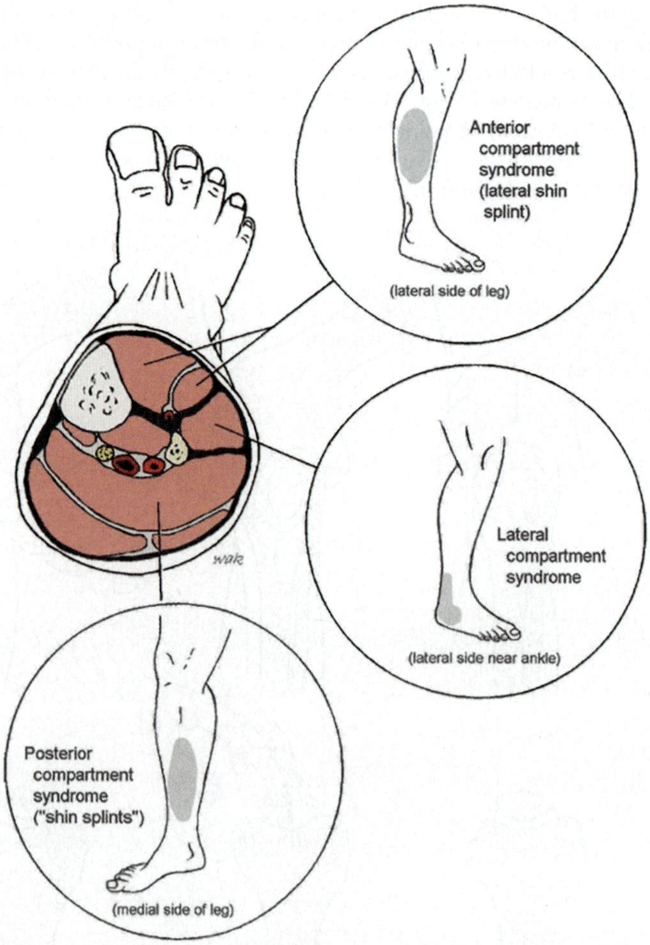

Figure 91.19. Fascial compartments of the lower extremity. (Illustration by William A. Kuchera, DO, FAAO, with permission.)

for almost a third of primary care visits, and 1.9 million visits annually, osteopathic physicians play an important role in improving their patient's overall quality of life.[121]

PFP is a condition that is characterized by the following:

1. Insidious onset of poorly defined pain, localized to the anterior retro patellar and/or peripatellar region of the knee.[114]
2. Reproduction of retro patellar or peripatellar pain with squatting, stair climbing, prolonged sitting, or other functional activities loading the patellofemoral joint in a flexed position
3. Exclusion of all other conditions that may cause AKP, including tibiofemoral pathologies.

The terms "PFP," "PFPS," or "PFS" are often used interchangeably with "anterior knee pain" or "runner's knee."[120] Chondromalacia patellae, a condition in which there is softening of the patellar articular cartilage, occurs in only a subset of patients who have AKP.[122,123]

The risk factors and specifics about the clinical presentation, physical examination, and treatment approach with OMT are described here.

The risk of developing PFP is dependent on the functional anatomy surrounding the joint and the forces placed on the patella, including[114,120,121]:

- Anatomic anomalies (e.g., hypoplasia of the medial patellar facet, patella alta)
- Malalignment and altered biomechanics of the lower extremity (static or dynamic)
- Muscle dysfunction (e.g., quadriceps weakness, improper firing pattern)
- Patellar hypermobility
- Poor quadriceps, hamstring, iliotibial band, or gastrocnemius flexibility
- Previous surgery
- Tight lateral structures (i.e., lateral retinaculum and iliotibial band)
- Training errors or overuse (sports, intense exercise, and/or occupation)
- Trauma

Observational studies concluded that age, body mass, height, and body mass index (BMI) were not risk factors for the development of PFP.[114,124] However, those factors, and gender, race, and genetic predisposition can be risk factors in other causes of AKP, like osteoarthritis.[121,125,126]

CLINICAL PRESENTATION

Patients with patellofemoral pain have variable clinical presentations. The condition is generally associated with exacerbations of AKP when loading the patellofemoral joint. The onset of symptoms can be slow or acutely develop, with a worsening of pain with lower limb loading activities (squatting, participation in sports, stair negotiation, prolonged sitting, running, and walking).[114,127,128] PFP often is related to overuse, and recent changes in activities. The clinician should determine the frequency, duration, and intensity of training, as well as changes to other possible contributors like inappropriate or excessively worn footwear.

Patients with PFP demonstrate some similar clinical characteristics. Swelling of the knee is not characteristic of PFP, although patients may report a sensation of stiffness, especially when the knee is flexed. A "popping" or "catching" sensation may be described. Locking of the joint is not a symptom of PFP and suggests a meniscal tear or loose bodies.

Because PFP is typically a progressive condition with an insidious onset of symptoms, diagnosis is often delayed, and describing the typical clinical course is difficult. Symptoms can restrict participation in physical activity, sports, and work, as well as recur and persist for years.[114]

PHYSICAL EXAMINATION

Physical examination should begin with inspection, palpation, orthopedic testing, and neurologic and vascular examinations. Along with examining both knees, the ipsilateral hip and ankle must be examined to rule out pathology with referred pain to the knee. A standing structural examination can provide clues on alignment and asymmetries of the foot, ankle, knees, hips, and pelvis. Asymmetry of landmarks, uneven iliac crest heights, and greater trochanter levels may direct the clinician to leg length discrepancies, and other functional muscle imbalances.[121]

Patellar alignment should be carefully observed and evaluated for any patella alta/baja, trochlear dysplasia, femoral anteversion, genu valgus, and laterally displaced tibial tuberosity as these can predispose to PFS.[129,130] Some literature noted that Q-angle measurement greater than 16 degrees is a risk factor for PFS; however, it is not a consistent finding.[114,124,130,131]

Palpation of the surrounding musculature and fascia should be performed for any tissue texture changes and tenderpoints.[121] Often, patients report pain with palpation of the distal pole or medial aspect of the patella, the medial plica, and the medial femoral condyle.[114,132] Palpation of the vastus medialis for tone and the ability of the patient to find and contract this muscle is important clinically. The vastus medialis coordination test was designed to assess the mobility of the patella and found to have a reported high specificity.[133] Hamstring and iliotibial band tension should also be assessed.

Diagnosis of regional somatic dysfunction of the pelvis, sacrum, lumbar spine, and lower extremities including the tibia, fibula, ankles, and feet are important and can be integrated into the physical exam. Somatic dysfunctions in proximal regions like the hip can often lead to the body compensating elsewhere to maintain normal gait and posture. This can lead to referred pain in areas like the lower back or the knee.

Specific orthopedic tests can be performed, although there is varying sensitivity and specificity.

- The "J sign" is used to evaluate dynamic patellar tracking. Patients are seated with knees flexed to 90 degrees and then asked to extend the knee into full extension. In a normal examination, the patella will track straight superiorly or slightly superolaterally. Patellar mal tracking will show sudden lateral deviation of the patella at the end of extension due to patellar subluxation out of the trochlear groove.[130,131]
- The patellar glide test is an assessment of medial/lateral mobility of the patella. With the knee flexed to 30 degree, the patella is divided into four quadrants and displaced either medially or laterally. Displacement of three or more quadrants in either direction is indicative of hypermobile patella. This has been correlated to patellofemoral pain.[130,131]
- The patellar tilt test assesses for tightness in the lateral retinaculum. With the knee in a relaxed extended position, the medial aspect of the patella is compressed posteriorly while the lateral edge is raised/tilted anteriorly. If the lateral patella cannot be raised to at least the horizontal plane, this is indicative of a tight lateral retinaculum.[130,131] Haim et al.[134] reported high specificity for the diagnosis of PFP when the patellar tilt test is positive.
- The patellar grind test and Clarke's test are used to mechanically evaluate AKP. In the patellar grind test, the patient's knee is extended and posteriorly directed pressure is applied to the patella. For Clarke's test, a posterior and inferior force is applied

to the superior aspect of the patella, while the patient actively contracts the quadriceps. Both tests produce pain in PFP patients. Unfortunately, they have many false positive findings and have low sensitivity and should not be used.[135]

Clinicians should administer appropriate clinical tests that reproduce pain and assess lower-limb movement coordination, such as squatting, step-downs, single-leg squats, and gait.[136] The most accurate diagnostic clinical test for PFP is pain while performing double leg squats.[130,136,137] These tests can assess a patient's baseline status relative to pain, function, and disability; global knee function; and changes in status throughout the course of treatment.[114] When evaluating a patient with PFP over several months, clinicians may assess body structure and function, including measures of patellar provocation, patellar mobility, foot position, hip and thigh muscle strength, and muscle length.

TREATMENT

Treatment of PFP is based on the history, physical and structural exam findings, and diagnostics. Addressing modifiable risk factors via weight loss, bracing, strengthening exercises, and activity modification is often the initial treatment goal in nontraumatic knee pain presentation.[121]

The mainstay of treatment for PFP is conservative and based upon a comprehensive rehabilitation program. These programs are individualized and tailored to include hip and knee strengthening, especially gluteal, quadriceps, hip abductor, and external rotator strengthening, patellar intramuscular efficacy tapes, and an emphasis on education and activity modification.[138–140] Hip-targeted exercise therapy should target the posterolateral hip musculature. Knee-targeted exercise therapy includes either weight-bearing (resisted squats) or non–weight-bearing (resisted knee extension) exercise.[114] Overall, the combination of hip- and knee-targeted exercises is preferred over solely knee-targeted exercises to optimize outcomes in patients with PFP.[114]

There has been abundant research showing that PFS significantly affects one's quality of life, as patients often forgo recreational activities so as not to experience pain.[130,141] The most frequently cited predictors of poor outcomes are longer duration of symptoms (greater than 6 months) before intervention, overall poorer function, and worse pain.[124] Clinicians should combine physical therapy interventions with other therapies such as patellar taping, knee braces, foot orthoses, dry needling, OMT/manual approaches, and biophysical agents.[114]

OSTEOPATHIC MANIPULATIVE TREATMENT AND OTHER MANUAL APPROACHES

Patients with AKP may have somatic dysfunction anywhere in their body that plays a role in their condition. Key regions for the clinician to diagnose somatic dysfunction would include the lumbar spine, sacrum, pelvis, and lower extremity. Multiple regions can be affected and further contribute to worsening symptoms.

Weakness of the transverse abdominis, multifidus, gluteus, and hip abductors are not uncommon in the clinical evaluation of a knee-pain patient. Likewise, tension of the hamstrings, iliotibial bands, pelvic floor, and gastric/soleus muscles are also commonly seen. This can be due to somatic dysfunction of the abdominal region, pelvis, and lumbar spine impairing the cocontraction of the transverse abdominis and multifidus, and the ability to form an abdominal brace.[142–144] This is necessary for complex movements such as squatting and climbing stairs. Furthermore, lumbar dysfunction can impair the contraction and coordination of the vastus medialis oblique and contribute to tightness of the hamstrings and iliotibial bands.[145] Together these findings alter posture (increased lumbar lordosis) and are commonly seen in the lower crossed syndrome. Lower crossed syndrome is a musculoskeletal condition where patterns of muscle weakness and tightness are seen in regions connecting the dorsal and ventral sides of the body.[146] Patients with PFP may have some components of lower cross syndrome but not all, indicating a functional disturbance rather than an anatomic one.

Manual therapies for the patient with PFP have been shown to be an effective initial approach and can be performed by multiple practitioners including physical therapists, chiropractors, and osteopathic physicians (Fig. 91.20).[147–149] Techniques, such as patellofemoral and talocrural joint mobilization are commonly used to improve joint function, reduce pain and inflammation, and enhance the effectiveness of exercise therapy in those with AKP.[147,148] Manipulations of the spine are thought to deactivate TrPs, leading to improved control and coordination of movement.[147] Treatment aimed at targeting TrPs should be included in the management for a patient with AKP. A systematic review and meta-analysis identified that TrP dry needling, often performed in conjunction with manual therapy or exercise interventions, resulted in moderate short-term improvement in pain and disability for individuals with patellofemoral pain.[148] The combination of manual therapy, dry needling, and physical therapy exercises can reduce pain, enhance muscle activity and performance, postpone the need for surgery, and ultimately reduce healthcare costs.[150–152]

Evidence supports a multimodal approach to knee pain management, which includes osteopathic care. The importance of an osteopathic approach to examination and diagnosis is essential due to the comprehensive care which includes a thorough examination, medication, exercises, nutrition, counseling, and OMT.[121] The role of OMT in managing common causes of knee pain has proven valuable as it has shown pain relief, improved function, postponed surgical intervention, and reduced the need for postoperative opioids.[121] As the body of research grows, OMT may become an increasingly recognized and essential component of multimodal knee pain management strategies.

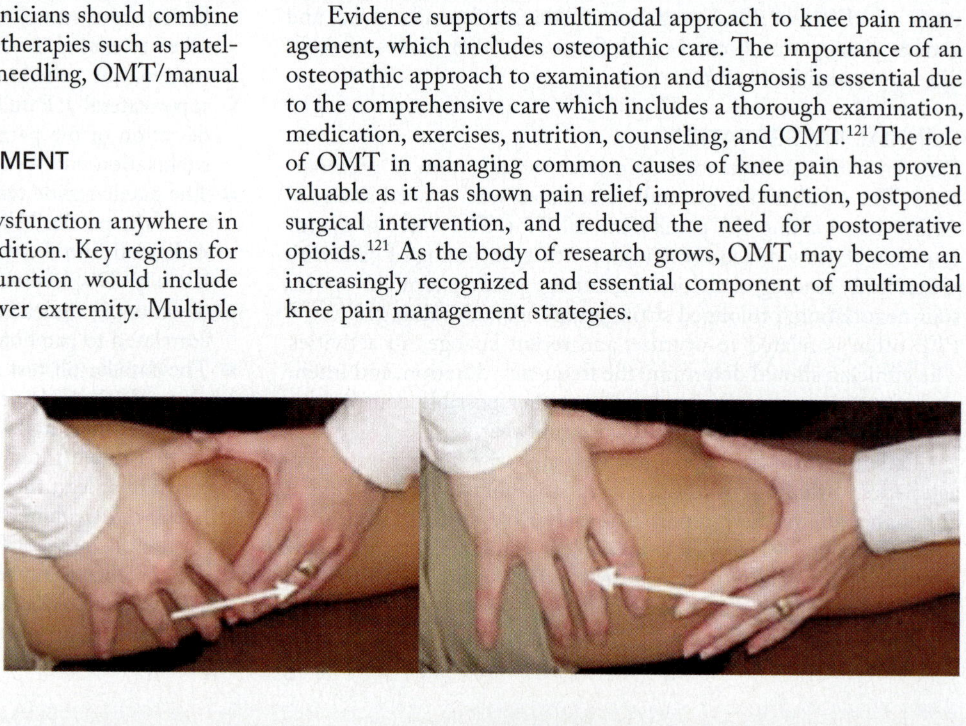

Figure 91.20. Inferior and superior nonthrust manipulations. (Used with permission of Journal of Orthopaedic & Sports Physical Therapy from Lowry CD, Cleland JA, Dyke K. Management of patients with patellofemoral pain syndrome using a multimodal approach: a case series. *J Orthop Sports Phys Ther.* 2008;38(11):691–702; permission conveyed through Copyright Clearance Center, Inc.)

TABLE 91.10

The Distal Tibiofibular Joint/Distal Fibula Somatic Dysfunction

Distal Fibular Motion	Freedom of Motion	Motion Restriction[a]	Somatic Dysfunction Nomenclature
Anterior	Anterior glide of distal fibula (lateral malleolus) during translatory motion testing when the tibia and talus are stabilized.	• Posterior glide is restricted during translatory motion testing. • Tenderness and tissue texture change may be present over the lateral malleolus.	• Anterior distal fibula dysfunction[103] • Anterior distal tibiofibular joint dysfunction[81] • Anterior lesion of the distal end of the fibula[118]
Posterior	Posterior glide of distal fibula (lateral malleolus) during translatory motion testing when the tibia and talus are stabilized.	• Anterior glide is restricted during translatory motion testing. • Tenderness and tissue texture change may be present over the lateral malleolus	• Posterior distal fibula dysfunction[103] • Posterior distal tibiofibular joint dysfunction[81] • Posterior lesion of the distal end of the fibula[118]

[a]In addition to the articular joint motion restrictions and asymmetry described above, the physician should also evaluate for the presence of other possible somatic dysfunction manifestations, such as restrictions of the associated musculature, myofascial restrictions (see Chapter 52), and counterstrain tender points (see Chapter 47), and trigger points (see Chapter 43) within this region.

ANKLE AND FOOT

The ankle joint complex is comprised of the kinetic linkage between the lower leg and the foot. It is comprised of the tibiotalar (talocrural), talocalcaneal (subtalar), and transverse-tarsal (talocalcaneonavicular and calcaneocuboid) joints.[153] The talus has no direct muscular attachments, so its movements are determined by muscle actions on the bones above and below it.[153] The combined proper functions of all the lower extremity joints are needed for mobility and balance.[153,154]

The Distal Tibio–Fibular Joint

The tibiotalar syndesmosis, or high ankle ligaments include the anterior tibiofibular ligament, the posterior tibiofibular ligament, and the interosseous tibiofibular ligament, which continues superiorly with the interosseous membrane. The tibia responds to the foot's pronation and supination with corresponding internal and external rotation. During weight bearing, the motions of the tibia and femur associated with supination and pronation of the foot are as follows[155]:

- During tibial internal rotation, the subtalar joint goes into pronation allowing for a more mobile foot. This is followed by a twist of the forefoot to remain plantigrade.
- During tibial external rotation, the subtalar joint goes into supination, locking the foot and converting it into a rigid lever which is necessary for push off.

The motion of the fibula is tightly coupled with the rotation of the tibia and pronation/supination of the subtalar joint. The typical motions and common somatic dysfunctions of the tibia and the proximal fibula were described previously in the knee section of this chapter (Tables 91.8 and 91.9). Recall there is reciprocal anteroposterior motion of the proximal and distal fibula (Table 91.10).

In common inversion ankle sprains where the foot tends to supinate, the distal fibula is often found to be anterior and the fibular head posterior. In ankle sprains, however, the physician must be sure to check both ends of the fibula, because, with trauma and disruption of the anterior talofibular ligament, the physiologic reciprocal motion described earlier may not occur. BLT between both ends of the fibula can be useful in this situation and is described in Chapter 112 Case Study: Supination Ankle Sprain.

The Tibiotalar Joint (Talocrural Joint)

The tibiotalar joint forms the junction between the distal tibia and fibula of the lower leg and the talus. Dorsiflexion and plantarflexion are the primary motions of the talocrural joint, with an oblique axis of rotation that travels through the medial malleolus, the talar head, and the lateral malleolus.[156,157] The trochlea of the talus fits into the mortise formed from the distal ends of the long bones of the shin. The malleoli of the tibia and fibula act to constrain the talus, such that the joint functions as a hinge joint, and primarily contributes to the plantar- and dorsiflexion motion of the foot. The talus is at its widest anteriorly, meaning the joint is more stable in dorsiflexion. The geometry of the tibiotalar joint contributes to the stability of the joint. Talocrural dorsiflexion/plantarflexion is coupled to fibular translation and rotation in all cardinal planes.[156,158]

For many years, dorsi- and plantarflexion motion was solely attributed to the tibiotalar joint motion, and inversion/eversion was considered to occur only at the subtalar joint.[153] More recently, the complete separation of the motions to each joint has been dismissed; most plantar/dorsiflexion is still considered to occur at the tibiotalar joint but with a few degrees accounted for at the subtalar joint.[159] Somatic dysfunction of ankle plantar/dorsiflexion is typically named in reference to the tibiotalar joint motion (Table 91.11).

Recurrent somatic dysfunction of the ankle at the tibiotalar joint is more commonly found to prefer plantar flexion with anterior glide with a resistant barrier to posterior glide at the end of dorsiflexion. The tibiotalar capsular pattern is, however, restricted in both directions and especially resistant to plantar flexion. Ankle sprains are more likely to occur when the tibiotalar joint is plantar flexed and undergo excessive foot supination and pronation.

Along with plantar flexion and dorsiflexion, the talus has some adduction during subtalar pronation and abduction during subtalar supination. Adduction, toeing-in, and some supination of the foot accompany plantar flexion. This motion carries the lateral malleolus anteriorly. Through reciprocal action of the fibula, the proximal fibular head also glides posteriorly and inferiorly.

Abduction, toeing-out, and some pronation of the foot accompany dorsiflexion. This type of motion carries the lateral malleolus posteriorly and, through reciprocal action, glides the fibular head anteriorly and superiorly. With dorsiflexion, the talus glides posteriorly within the mortise, a more functionally stable position. This

TABLE 91.11

The Tibiotalar/Talocrural Joint (Ankle) Somatic Dysfunction

Talocrural Joint Motion	Freedom of Motion	Motion Restriction[a]	Somatic Dysfunction Nomenclature
Plantar flexion	Anterior glide of talus within the mortise as the ankle plantarflexes, dropping the toes downward about 50 degrees. This places the narrower posterior tragus of talus within the mortise. The anterior aspect of the tragus may be palpable anterior to the distal tibia.	• Posterior glide of the talus and dorsiflexion will be restricted. • Talus may be rotated internally or externally.[106]	• Plantar flexion with anterior glide of the talocrural joint[105] • Talus plantar flexed with anterior glide[106] • Plantar flexed talus[81] • Ankle plantar flexion[162,163] • Restricted dorsiflexion of the talus[81] • Distal tibia posterior[107] • Tibia posterior (talus anterior)[160] • Posterior tibia on talus[107] • Posterior displacement of the tibia in relation to the talus[118] • Anterior talus (relative to tibia)[104]
Dorsiflexion	Posterior glide of talus within the mortise as the ankle dorsiflexes. Normal ankle dorsiflexion is about 20 degrees. Wider anterior portion of tragus of talus is wedged in mortise, providing more stability	Anterior glide of the talus and plantar flexion will be restricted.	• Dorsiflexion and posterior glide of the talocrural joint[105] • Talus dorsiflexed with posterior glide[106,b] • Dorsiflexed talus[81] • Ankle dorsiflexion[161,162] • Distal tibia anterior[107] • Anterior tibia on talus[107] • Anterior displacement of the tibia in relation to the talus[118] • Posterior talus (relative to tibia)[104]

[a]In addition to the articular joint motion restrictions and asymmetry described above, the physician should also evaluate for the presence of other possible somatic dysfunction manifestations, such as restrictions of the associated musculature, myofascial restrictions (see Chapter 52), and counterstrain tender points (see Chapter 47), and trigger points (see Chapter 43) within this region.

[b]Talus Dorsiflexed with Posterior Glide is implied but not actually documented in the source that described Talus Plantar Flexed with Anterior Glide.[106]

stability is the reason taping techniques to treat or prevent ankle sprains usually emphasize a dorsiflexed position.

Subtalar Joint

The subtalar joint is comprised of anterior (talocalcaneonavicular) and posterior (talocalcaneal) articulations that are separated by the tarsal canal.[156] The subtalar joint is often described as a "mitered hinge" and its triplanar orientation allows for the coupling of tibial rotation and hindfoot pronation and supination.[156] The primary motions of the subtalar joint include inversion and eversion around an oblique axis and involve a combination of gliding and rotation within the joint.[153] The axis of rotation is oriented anterior-superomedial to posterior-inferolateral and transects the three cardinal planes.[153,156] During weight bearing, the "forefoot" is fixed by its contact with the ground (closed chain scenario) and the talus is mobile (Fig. 91.21).

The subtalar joint's major motions are inversion and eversion of the ankle and foot, yet it has its own defined distinct pronation and supination. See Chapter 40 Lower Extremity for pertinent anatomy and detailed descriptions of subtalar eversion, inversion, pronation, and supination. The talonavicular relationship is included in the subtalar oblique axis but for simplicity it is customary to use the term "talocalcaneal" when describing the somatic dysfunction in this joint (Table 91.12).[82]

Running is one of the most widespread activities during which overuse injuries of the lower extremity occur and most biomechanical risk factors for such injuries stem from the hindfoot.[165] Subtalar somatic dysfunction is often treated with BLT, articulatory techniques, or counterstrain of associated tender points.

In a supination ankle sprain, inversion of the calcaneus and posterolateral glide of the talus at the talocalcaneal joint occurs. Pronation sprains are less common, but when they occur there is typically eversion of the calcaneus and anteromedial glide at the talocalcaneal joint. Ankle sprains are briefly discussed later in this chapter. Chapter 112 Case Study: Supination Ankle Sprain has a clinical case example and full discussion of the epidemiology, risk factors, causes, mechanisms, physical exam, grading, and patient management including descriptions of specific osteopathic manipulative techniques for some of the common associated somatic dysfunctions of supination ankle sprains.

Transverse Tarsal and Intertarsal Joints

The transverse tarsal joint (Chopart joint) includes the talonavicular and calcaneal cuboid joint. It is considered part of the same functional unit as the subtalar joint because it shares a common axis of motion, also contributing to eversion–inversion motion of the foot.[153,156,166] The cuneiforms, along with the navicular, form part of the medial longitudinal arch. They are supported laterally by the cuboid which forms part of the lateral longitudinal arch. Typically, there should be a small amount of dorsal-to-plantar joint play springing motion with each of the five tarsal bones.

Somatic dysfunction of the tarsal bones (cuboid, navicular, or any of the three cuneiforms) is relatively common (Table 91.13). In middle- and long-distance runners, these bones might even sublux.

- Cuboid somatic dysfunction involves the edge nearest the middle of the foot. This edge glides toward the plantar surface of the foot and rotates laterally around its AP axis (everting or flattening the transverse arch).
- Navicular somatic dysfunction involves the edge nearest the middle of the foot gliding toward the plantar surface and rotating medially around its AP axis (inverting or flattening the transverse arch) (Fig. 91.22).

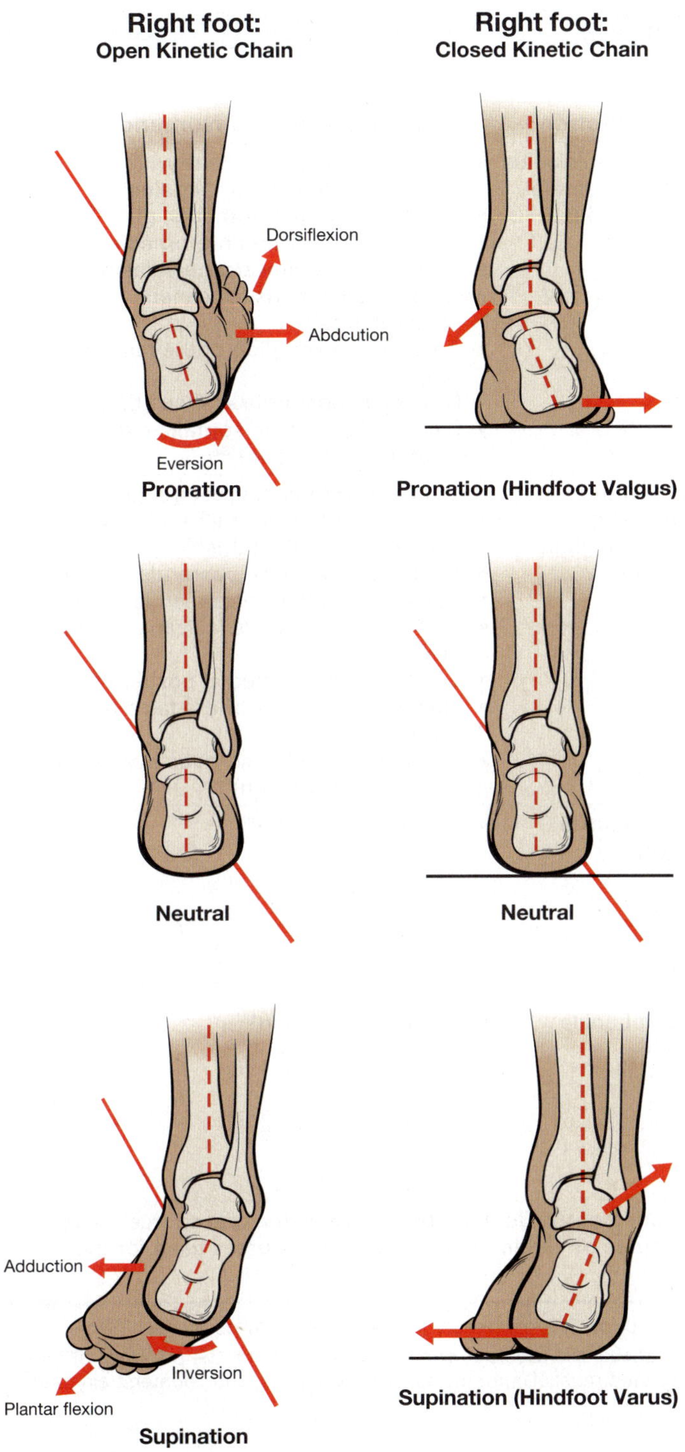

Figure 91.21. Pronation and supination of the right foot. In an open kinetic chain, with the foot off the ground, the foot and ankle move on a fixed tibia at the talocrural and subtalar joints. Pronation is produced by eversion, abduction, and dorsiflexion. Supination is produced by inversion, abduction, and plantar flexion. In a closed kinetic chain, with the foot on the ground, most of the pronation and supination are produced by the weight of the body acting on the talus. In this weight-bearing position, the tibia moves on the talus (talocrural) and the talus moves on the fixed calcaneus (subtalar) to produce pronation and supination. (Adapted with permission from Hamill J, Knutzen K, Derrick TR. *Biomechanical Basis of Human Movement*. 5th ed. Wolters Kluwer; 2022:250. Figure 6-34.)

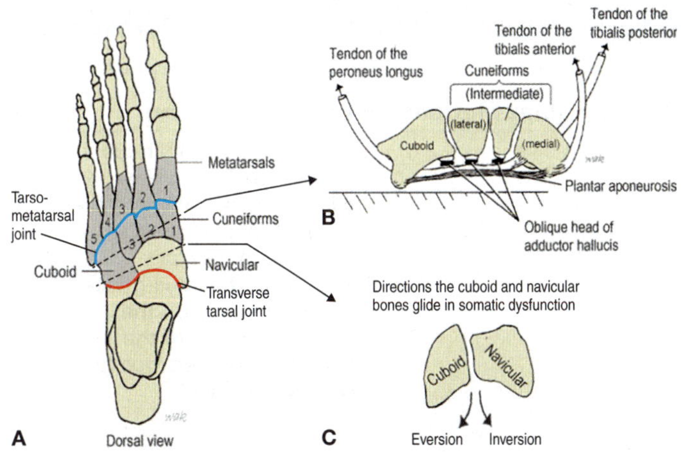

Figure 91.22. Navicular, cuboid, and cuneiform somatic dysfunction; relation to supports of the transverse arch of the foot. A. Foot skeletal anatomy. **B.** Muscle tendons forming the transverse arch of the foot. **C.** Cuboid and navicular somatic dysfunction. (Illustration by William A. Kuchera, DO, FAAO, with permission.)

- Cuneiform somatic dysfunction usually manifests from one of the cuneiforms gliding in the plantar direction (downward). Primary somatic dysfunction of the cuneiform bones is rare, although secondary restrictions following navicular or cuboid somatic dysfunction are common.[82] The second cuneiform is most commonly involved.[5,105,106]

Somatic dysfunction of these tarsal bones can be diagnosed by the combination of tenderness and increased tissue tension over the plantar surface of each of these bones. OMT is effective. Some patients also find orthotics to modify predisposing biomechanical factors useful.

Tarsometatarsal (TMT), Intermetatarsal (IM), Metatarsophalangeal (MP), and Interphalangeal (IP) Joints

The forefoot is composed of the metatarsals and the phalanges. As the forefoot inverts with plantar flexion, the body weight is transferred to the metatarsal articulations for push-off. Foot structure provides two functional axes for push-off: an oblique axis that passes through the heads of the second through fifth metatarsals, and a transverse axis that passes through the heads of the first and second metatarsals.

The first metatarsal head has some up and down gliding and rotates externally and internally. The second to fifth metatarsal heads have limited gliding movement, with the second having the least motion as it is mortised between the first and third cuneiforms. The third to fifth metatarsal heads have sequentially increasing amount of motion.[13,82] Motions may be tested by grasping the shaft of the specific metatarsal and gliding it through the three planes with an arcing circumduction, while the associated tarsals are fixed by the other hand. Similar motion testing may be done between the metatarsals (intermetatarsal [IM] joint). Motion between the metatarsals and phalanges may be tested by stabilizing the proximal bone and moving the distal upon it.

Somatic dysfunction of the tarsometatarsal (TMT), metatarsophalangeal (MP), and IP joints involves their minor motions:

- Plantar or dorsal glide
- Internal or external rotation
- Lateral or medial glide

TABLE 91.12

The Subtalar/Talocalcaneal Joint Somatic Dysfunction

Subtalar Joint Motion[a]	Freedom of Motion	Motion Restriction[b]	Somatic Dysfunction Nomenclature
Eversion	Eversion of the calcaneus rotates the base of the calcaneus laterally and the superior aspect medially—base tilts outward. The base of the talus glides anteromedially on the superior aspect of the calcaneus (valgus position of posterior heel).	Inversion of the calculus and posterior lateral glide of the talus	• Eversion of the calcaneus with anteromedial glide of the talus[106] • Eversion with anteromedial glide[106] • Talus eversion with anteromedial glide[106] • Anteromedial talocalcanean lesion[82] • Anteromedial talus (calcaneus posterolateral)[81] • Anterior medial glide of the talus on the calcaneus[163] • Calcaneus posterolateral position[103] • Calcaneal inversion somatic dysfunction (eversion restriction)[164]
Inversion	Inversion of the calcaneus rotates the base of the calcaneus medially and the superior aspect laterally—base tilts inward. The base of the talus glides posterolaterally on the superior aspect of the calcaneus (varus position).	Eversion of the calcaneus and anteromedial glide of the talus	• Inversion with posterolateral glide[106] • Inversion of the calcaneus with posterior lateral glide of the talus[106] • Talus inversion with posterolateral glide[106] • Posterolateral talocalcanean lesion[82] • Posterior lateral talus (calcaneus anterior medial)[81] • Calcaneus anteromedial position[103] • Posterolateral glide of the talus on the calcaneus[163] • Calcaneal eversion somatic dysfunction (inversion restriction)[164]
Adduction	Anterior aspect of calcaneus deviates medially while tuberosity deviates laterally (in-toeing). Associated with internal rotation of the tibia when non—weight-bearing.	Restriction of ankle abduction	• Subtalar adduction[161]
Abduction	Anterior aspect of calcaneus deviates laterally while tuberosity deviates medially (out-toeing). Associated with external rotation of the tibia when non–weight-bearing.	Restriction of ankle adduction	• Subtalar abduction[161]
"Calcaneus plantar flexion"[160] was also the nomenclature used in a video of the Bootjack technique within one source[160] but was otherwise not described or used in any other section of that source or within other osteopathic sources used for the production of this table.			

[a]The talonavicular relationship is included in the subtalar oblique axis but for simplicity it is customary to use the term "talocalcaneal."[82]

[b]In addition to the articular joint motion restrictions and asymmetry described above, the physician should also evaluate for the presence of other possible somatic dysfunction manifestations, such as restrictions of the associated musculature, myofascial restrictions, and counterstrain tender points within this region.

They may also involve compression or, less commonly, traction.

Restrictions can occur in more than one plane and there may also be associated tissue texture changes and tenderness of the joint.[106] Somatic dysfunction nomenclature may describe the positions of ease or define the restrictions of the specific bone motion in relation to its surrounding bones/joint. Although the nomenclature of motion again varies slightly between sources, the treatments using osteopathic principles to engage or disengage the restriction remain consistent. Some commonly used osteopathic techniques include BLT, MFR, joint play, articulatory technique, and HVLA (thrust) technique.

Variations in nomenclature for the planes of gliding motion include the following:

- *Plantar glide*[81,103,105] may also be called posterior glide[106] or inferior glide[104]
  - A preference for this motion may be called a depressed metatarsal[82]
  - Another example is a plantar dysfunction of the fifth proximal metatarsals (plantar displaced proximal fifth metatarsal or styloid process of fifth metatarsal)[107]
  - If the plantar glide has a tilting component, it will resemble extension[81,107] or dorsiflexion[107,161]

TABLE 91.13

Transverse Tarsal (Talonavicular and Calcaneocuboid) Joint and Intertarsal Joint (Cuneiform Bones) Somatic Dysfunction

Bone	Normal Motion/Position	Somatic Dysfunction	Somatic Dysfunction Nomenclature
Navicular (talonavicular joint)	Navicular typically has an everted (pronated) position to maintain the transverse and medial longitudinal arches.	• Restriction or injury results in the navicular edge nearest the middle of the foot gliding inferiorly toward the plantar surface and rotating medially around its AP axis (inverting). • Dorsal glide is restricted. • Navicular inverts (supinates) and restricts eversion (pronation). • The medial longitudinal arch and transverse arch flattens (flat foot). • There may be tenderness over the plantar aspect of the navicular.	• Downward and medial displacement of the navicular[82] • Navicular pronation restriction[103] • Supinated navicular[103] • Navicular plantar glide and inverted[106] • Dropped navicular (relative to other tarsals)[162,164] • Navicular inversion[104]
	[a]Greenman[81] included both internal and external rotation somatic dysfunction of the navicular bone. However, midline for internal and external rotation was not defined as midline body or middle of foot.		• Navicular internal rotation • Restricted external rotation[81] • Navicular external rotation • Restricted internal rotation[81]
Cuboid (calcaneocuboid joint)	Cuboid typically has an inverted (supinated) position to maintain the transverse and lateral longitudinal arches.	• Restriction or injury results in the cuboid edge nearest the middle of the foot moving inferiorly and rotating laterally around its AP axis (everting). • Dorsal glide is restricted. • Cuboid everts (pronates) and restricts inversion (supination). • The lateral longitudinal arch and transverse arch flatten (flat foot). • There may be tenderness over the plantar aspect of the cuboid.	• Downward displacement of the cuboid on the calcaneus[82] • Dropped cuboid[82,162,164] • Cuboid restricted supination[103] • Pronated cuboid[103] • Cuboid plantar glide and everted[106] • Cuboid pronated (internally rotated)[81] • Restricted supination (external rotation) of the cuboid[81] • Planter displaced cuboid[107] • Cuboid, plantar dysfunction[107] • Cuboid inversion[104]
Cuneiforms[a] (first, second, and third cuneiforms)	The cuneiforms form part of the medial longitudinal arch and are supported laterally by the cuboid. Typically, there should be a small amount of dorsal-to-plantar joint play springing motion.	• Primary somatic dysfunction of the cuneiform bones are rare although secondary restrictions following navicular or cuboid somatic dysfunction are common.[82] • Absence of dorsal to plantar joint play springing motion. • Plantar displacement. • Dorsal glide is restricted. • The medial longitudinal arch flattened (flat foot). • There may be tenderness over the plantar aspect of the cuneiforms.	• Cuneiform resists dorsal motion[103] • Inferior cuneiform[103] • Cuneiform plantar glide[105,106] • Depression of cuneiforms[81] • Restriction of dorsal arching of the cuneiforms[81] • Planter displaced cuneiforms[107] • Planter dysfunction cuneiforms[107] • Dropped cuneiform[107] • Restricted cuneiform motion on the navicular[82,162]

[a]Nomenclature for cuneiform somatic dysfunction will include the specific number of the bone (i.e., plantar dysfunction right second cuneiform).

- Forefoot dorsiflexion,[161] phalangeal dorsiflexion,[161] phalangeal extension dysfunction,[107] great toe dorsiflexion[107]

- *Dorsal glide*[81,103,105,106] may also be called anterior glide[106] or superior glide[104]
  - ☐ A preference for this motion may be called an elevated metatarsal[82]
  - ☐ If the dorsal glide has a tilting component it will resemble flexion[81] or plantarflexion[161]
    - Metatarsal flexion,[160] forefoot plantar flexion,[161] phalangeal plantar flexion[161]
- *Internal rotation*[81,103,105,106] may also be called medial rotation[81]
  - ☐ A preference for this motion may be called an internally rotated metatarsal[82]
- *External rotation*[81,103,105,106] may also be called lateral rotation[81]
  - ☐ A preference for this motion may be called an externally rotated metatarsal[82]
  - ☐ Phalangeal adduction or abduction[161]
- *Lateral glide*[81,103,105,106]
  - ☐ If there is a lateral tilt,[81] it will abduct (i.e., phalangeal abduction[161])

- *Medial glide*[81,103,105,106]
  - If there is a medial tilt,[81] it will adduct (i.e., phalangeal adduction[161])
- *Compression*[103,105] may also be called posterior glide[81,106]
- *Traction*[81,103,105] may also be called anterior glide[81,106]
- Nonspecific restriction/somatic dysfunction:
  - Restriction of joint play at metatarsal heads[81]
  - Metatarsal somatic dysfunction[164]
  - Transtarsal somatic dysfunction[164]
- A joint may be restricted in more than one plane
  - Elevated and externally rotated first metatarsal[82]
  - Depressed and internally rotated first metatarsal[82]

Indirect stacking OMT techniques are especially helpful in jammed toes. A stacking technique is one in which the physician moves a joint in the direction of preference in all its planes, stacking one motion upon the other. Compression or traction is then applied to that combined position. The technique may require holding the position of ease for 90 seconds or until the joint tensions relax. The joint is then slowly returned to a neutral position and rechecked for motion.[105] Diffuse or minimal restriction may be overcome by treating the joints as a group.[82]

COMMON ANKLE AND FOOT CONDITIONS AND THE OSTEOPATHIC APPROACH

Ankle Sprains

Ankle sprains are very common in a primary care or sports medicine practice. In a supination sprain, inversion of the calcaneus and posterolateral glide of the talus at the talocalcaneal joint typically occur. There may also be associated foot, ankle, leg, knee, hip, pelvis, sacrum, and lumbar spine somatic dysfunctions. See Chapter 112 Case Study: Supination Ankle Sprain for a clinical case example and full discussion of epidemiology, risk factors, causes, mechanisms, physical exam, grading, and patient management including descriptions of specific osteopathic manipulative techniques for some of the common associated somatic dysfunctions.

A pure inversion sprain can result in sprain of the calcaneofibular ligament alone. This has occurred in basketball players during rebounding when they land—without any plantar flexion—directly on the lateral aspect of the foot. The anticipated subtalar somatic dysfunction is an inversion of the calcaneus and anteromedial glide at the talocalcaneal joint. However, the deltoid ligament stabilizing the medial side of the ankle is so strong that trauma stressing this structure is more likely to fracture a piece of the medial malleolus than tear the ligament. The Ottawa Ankle Rules for palpatory pain that prompts strong consideration of an ankle radiograph for fracture recognize this. The guidelines states that x-ray studies should be done if one of the following is true[167]:

- Bony tenderness of the lateral malleolus
  - Anywhere along the distal 6 cm of the posterior edge to the malleolar tip
- Bony tenderness of the medial malleolus
  - Anywhere along the distal 6 cm of the posterior edge to the malleolar tip
- Pain or bone tenderness over an area of potential fracture (i.e., lateral malleolus, medial malleolus, base of fifth metatarsal, or navicular bone)
- Inability to bear weight (or take four steps) immediately after the injury and during the physical exam.

Fortunately, pronation sprains are uncommon. This is due both to the strength of the deltoid ligament and the stability imparted by gliding the wide portion of the talus into the tibiotalar joint during dorsiflexion.

Footdrop

There are numerous sites where structural or functional conditions could create weakness in the muscles that help to dorsiflex the foot. The differential diagnosis of footdrop is therefore quite extensive and encompasses systemic conditions such as multiple sclerosis to focal conditions such as L5 radiculopathy.

The most common regional neuromusculoskeletal conditions in the differential diagnosis include from proximal to distal anatomical sites[168]:

- L5 radiculopathy (e.g., secondary to herniated L4 disk)
- Cauda equina lesion (e.g., secondary to spinal adhesions)
- Lumbosacral plexopathy (e.g., secondary to colorectal carcinoma)
- Sciatic nerve injury (e.g., secondary to injection injury)
- Peroneal entrapment neuropathy
  - At piriformis (e.g., due to piriformis syndrome)
  - At fibular head (e.g., due to posterior fibular head somatic dysfunction or Baker cyst)
- Peroneal or tibialis anterior MTrPs (e.g., due to prior severe supination ankle sprain)

The dorsiflexors of the foot are primarily phasic muscles (antagonists to postural muscles); dysfunction or TrPs in these muscles, especially the tibialis anterior, might also lead to weakness and a tendency for mild footdrop symptoms especially after using the muscle(s) for a period of time.[91]

Techniques that remove joint or myofascial somatic dysfunction in the areas discussed above are considered helpful in reducing footdrop symptoms.[91,169] Recommended techniques (depending on the site of entrapment) include:

- Counterstrain for the piriformis muscle after correction of the joints associated with this muscle's bony attachments (sacroiliac and femoroacetabular joints).
- Balanced ligamentous and membranous tension for the fibular head and lower leg interosseous membrane.

Achilles Tendinopathy

Achilles tendon disorders, like Achilles tendinopathy, are quite common among athletes.[170] The Achilles tendon is also notably the most frequently ruptured tendon.[171] It is often associated with "weekend warriors"—individuals who engage in sports requiring agility and speed on a casual basis. Despite the common belief that Achilles injuries only occur in athletes, research has found that only 35% of cases were related to sports activities.[170,172]

The term "tendinopathy" describes the clinical condition characterized by pain, swelling, and impaired tendon function. In contrast, "tendinitis" and "tendinosis" refer to the histopathologic conditions of inflammation of the tissue (tendinitis) and tissue degeneration (tendinosis), typically seen in chronic conditions.[173]

Achilles tendinopathies are categorized based on their location, involving either the midportion or insertional region of the tendon (Fig. 91.23). Midportion Achilles tendinopathy, an overuse injury, causes pain, swelling, and reduced performance. It occurs 2 to 7 cm above the calcaneal attachment.[174] Insertional Achilles tendinopathy (IAT) is a separate less common condition,[175,176] which may present alone or alongside midportion tendinopathy.

IAT is associated with a combination of intrinsic and extrinsic risk factors. Key intrinsic factors include age, chronic comorbidities, and limb alignment defects, while the primary extrinsic risk factor is

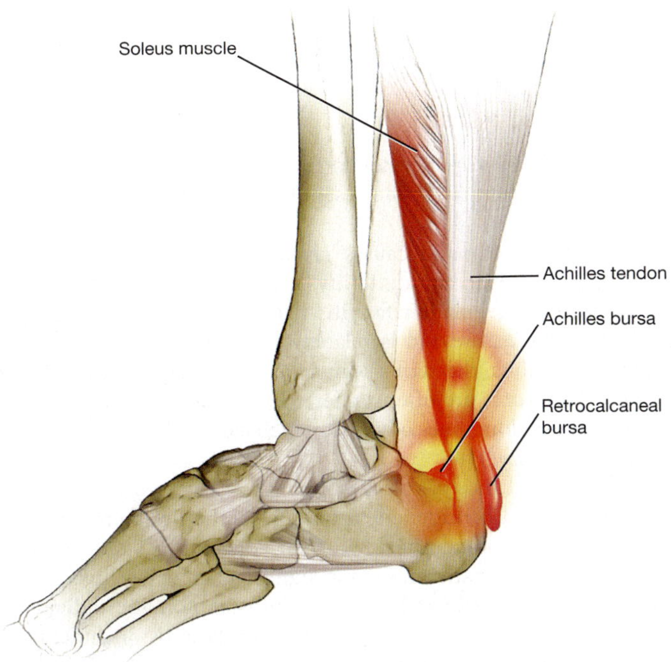

Figure 91.23. Achilles tendinopathy. The Achilles tendon is susceptible to the development of tendonitis at its insertion on the calcaneus as well as its narrowest point ~5 cm above the calcaneal insertion. (Reprinted with permission from Waldman SD. *Comprehensive Atlas of Ultrasound-Guided Pain Management Injection Techniques.* 2nd ed. Wolters Kluwer; 2020:1228. Figure 166.7.)

engaging in unaccustomed activities.[176] IAT specifically affects the enthesis, the critical anatomical and functional interface between tendon and bone, essential for the tendon's viability and biomechanics. This region, where tendon vascularization originates, plays a significant role in both the physiologic and pathologic responses of the tendon to injury. Alterations in ankle biomechanics including lower limb deformities, leg length discrepancies, and limited subtalar joint mobility are predisposing factors for Achilles tendon injuries among active individuals.[172,176] This information makes the osteopathic structural and palpatory exam of the ankle an important element in developing a proper management plan.

Achilles tendinopathy significantly differ histologically, based on location (midportion vs. insertional). Therefore, both the diagnosis and treatment, whether conservative or surgical, should be approached differently for these two conditions.[172]

This section will describe some specifics about the clinical presentation, physical examination, and treatment approach with OMT.

CLINICAL PRESENTATION

The diagnosis of IAT is primarily clinical, characterized by common symptoms such as pain and swelling at the back of the heel, along with impaired function and stiffness. Patients often report that their symptoms worsen at night or during periods of rest, as well as upon resuming activity. The pain typically intensifies with activities like hill running, climbing stairs, and aggressive stretching. Consequently, many patients report a history of increased training intensity, frequency, or duration with stiffness after prolonged rest.[173,177]

A diagnosis of midportion Achilles tendinopathy can be supported by a history of lateral inversion ankle sprain, the location of maximal tenderness approximately 4 cm above the Achilles insertion. Factors such as the patient's age, level of activity, injury mechanism, and morning stiffness also contribute to this diagnosis.[178]

PHYSICAL EXAMINATION

The initial examination for Achilles tendinopathy should encompass observation, active and passive range of motion (AROM and PROM), palpation, and special tests. Observation during a standing structural examination may show heel varus, pes planus, and forefoot deformities.[179] Palpation of the Achilles tendon should check for any lumps, swelling, warmth, thickening, tenderness or Haglund deformity.[179] It is crucial during the examination to compare sides and be aware of any tendinopathy in the patient's opposite Achilles tendon. Following palpation, functional tests should be conducted, including walking on toes and heels, performing the soleus lunge test (ankle dorsiflexion), a painful arc sign,[179] squatting, the Royal London Hospital Test[180] and sports specific movements. Note the patient's feedback of pain experienced during these activities. The osteopathic examination may also include tests for ankle instability, and evaluation for dysfunction of the talus, calcaneus, arches (dropped navicular or cuboid) and fibula.

For IAT, tenderness is typically noted upon palpating the lower part of the tendon, about the last 2 cm.[181] Physical examination typically shows tenderness and thickening at the insertion site and limited dorsiflexion.[173,181]

In cases of midportion tendinopathy, a lump or swelling might be detectable at the muscle-tendon junction, with possible redness and swelling of the overlying skin, and nodularity of the tendon at the midportion or its insertion.[182] If retrocalcaneal bursitis is present, the clinician will find tenderness alongside the medial and lateral aspects of the Achilles tendon insertion.

The Thompson test, also known as the Simmonds–Thompson test or calf squeeze test, is a widely used clinical examination maneuver to assess the integrity of the Achilles tendon. This test is particularly useful for diagnosing a torn or ruptured Achilles tendon, which may not always be apparent through visual inspection or pain assessment due to compensation by other muscles. Squeezing the calf muscle of the affected leg should cause a plantar flexion of the foot. If the foot does not move, this suggests a positive test result, indicative of a potential Achilles tendon rupture.

OSTEOPATHIC MANIPULATIVE TREATMENT

The use of OMT is aimed at alleviating pain, stiffness, and swelling.[183,184] Various techniques can target joint restrictions, tenderpoints, and muscle/fascia tightness resulting from initial injuries and the subsequent compensatory movements.[185] OMT is beneficial early in the treatment process, especially for high-level athletes prone to Achilles tendinopathy, by addressing the root causes of discomfort and facilitating recovery.[186] Recall that limited mobility of the talocrural joint is considered a potential contributing factor to the development of midportion Achilles tendinopathy.[187] Some techniques used for this condition include the following:

- Counterstrain applied to Achilles tendon tenderpoints is effective in reducing the stretch reflex in calf muscles, thereby easing symptoms and promoting healing through decreased muscular tension, facilitating low-pressure drainage and improved muscle function.[188]
- Articulation and springing techniques include gentle, repetitive movements of the talocrural and superior tibiofibular joints, along with subtalar springing, to relieve passive motion restrictions.[76,189,190]
- MET can be used to correct tibial dysfunction and reduce tightness in the gastrocnemius muscle.[191]
- Soft tissue techniques such as cross-fiber stretching and inhibition are employed to treat the plantar fascia and reduce muscle

tightness in the lower leg, including the popliteus and gastrocnemius muscles.[191]

Integrating OMT with an exercise and rehabilitation program is particularly effective for treating acute ankle injuries and improving joint biomechanics. It is important to address the individual's physical limitations that impact daily activities and supports a recovery program aimed at restoring function and promoting independence from ongoing treatment.[172,188] This versatile strategy can be adapted to suit various clinical scenarios, making it an integral part of comprehensive patient care.

SUMMARY OF OTHER CONSERVATIVE TREATMENT APPROACHES

Typically, once other conditions have been excluded, conservative management is the preferred initial strategy for Achilles tendinopathy. Nonsurgical treatment is advised as the primary intervention, with surgery reserved for those who do not benefit from conservative methods.[176]

The RICE protocol (Rest, Immobilization, Compression, and Elevation) is commonly recommended to start. This method aims to minimize activities that could exacerbate the condition and to relieve swelling and pain.[172] The use of NSAIDs should be considered carefully. While they can reduce pain, they may interfere with the healing process. NSAIDs are most appropriate for patients experiencing significant inflammation, especially when surrounding tissues and bursae are affected.[172]

Research on exercise for Achilles tendinopathy often focuses on eccentric exercises, which have been found to improve symptoms and functionality.[192] Combining these exercises with ESWT has been suggested to improve results,[193] by reducing pain and encouraging tissue healing.[193,194]

The efficacy of night splints and orthotics has not been thoroughly investigated, but they may help in reducing tendon tension and preventing stiffness. Heel lifts or wedges can provide temporary pain relief, although their long-term advantages are not well-established.[195]

While there is extensive literature on treatments for the main body of the Achilles tendon,[196] research specifically targeting IAT is limited. A recent systematic review and network meta-analysis regarding the nonsurgical treatment focusing on short-term pain control for IAT found eccentric exercise plus soft tissue therapy was the most effective treatment combination.[181] Integrating established rehabilitation protocols with OMT has been suggested to manage pain and improve functional movement in the ankle and foot.[172]

Plantar Fascia Disorders

The *plantar aponeurosis* extends from the calcaneus to the phalanges and encompasses the sesamoid bones under the great toe (Fig. 91.24).

Functional demand causes chronic stress on this structure, leading to heel pain and disability often termed *plantar fasciitis*.[197] Despite its name, plantar fasciitis has a degenerative rather than inflammatory nature and is related to overuse trauma leading to micro tears; thus, the terms *plantar fasciosis* (degeneration)[198] and *plantar fasciopathy* are often preferred.[197] With time, calcium may be laid down along lines of stress, which can lead to the formation of a *calcaneal heel spur*.

The significance of calcaneal spurs as a cause of plantar fasciitis has received considerable attention in the literature, and currently evidence of calcaneal spurs on conventional radiograph is not considered a pathognomonic sign of plantar fasciitis.[197] Heel spurs are not specific and do occur in asymptomatic individuals. Calcaneal spurs associated with plantar fasciitis include those located within the plantar fascia, which are very uncommon. The most common sight of plantar calcaneal spurs is in the abductor hallucis and flexor digitorum brevis origins, deep to the plantar fascia.

The causes of plantar fasciitis are multifactorial, but most cases result from overuse stress. Biomechanical risk factors include pes planus or pes cavus, excessive pronation or supination, limited ankle dorsiflexion, improper footwear, increased BMI, and activities that involved prolonged standing, walking, running, or jumping.[197,199,200] Medical conditions associated with plantar fasciitis include seronegative spondyloarthropathies and rheumatoid arthritis.[197]

Common symptoms include sharp heel pain and stiffness in the morning or when beginning activity after rest or prolonged sitting. Pain is often sharp at the inferior and medial heel.[197,199] Physical examination may reveal tenderness at the origin of the plantar fascia on the plantar medial calcaneal tubercle, tightness in the gastrocnemius, soleus, and other posterior leg muscles, and limited passive dorsiflexion of the ankle and extension of the toes with associated reproducible pain. Pain reproduced through passive dorsiflexion of the first metatarsal phalangeal joint is referred to as

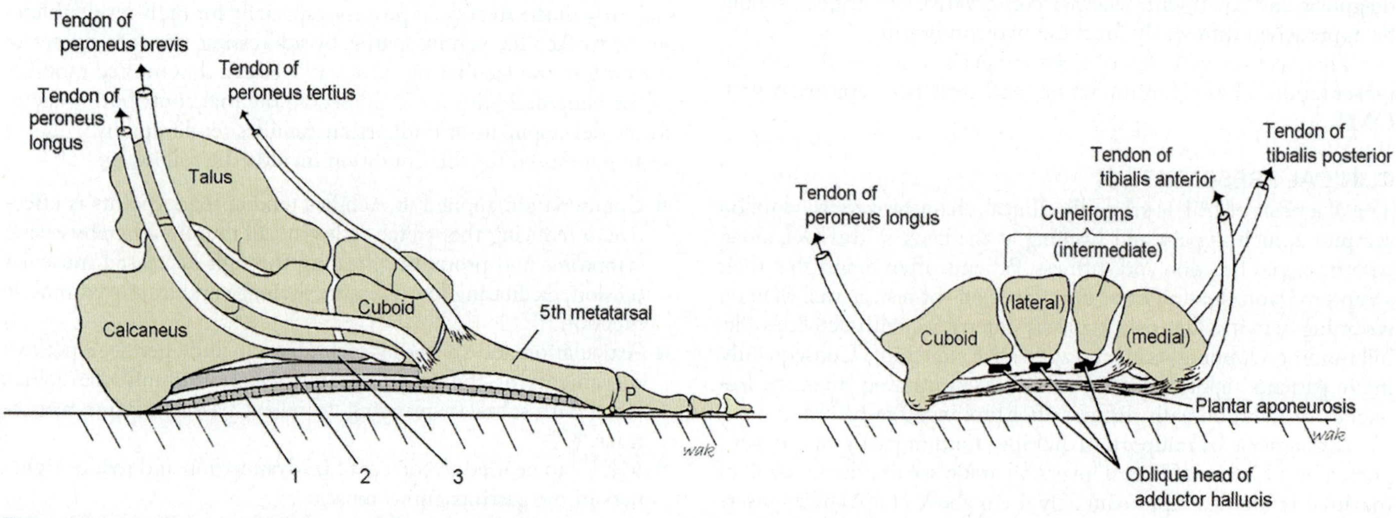

Figure 91.24. Plantar tendons and ligaments supporting the arches of the foot. 1. Plantar aponeurosis. 2. Long plantar ligament. 3. Plantar calcaneocuboid (short plantar) ligament. (Illustration by William A. Kuchera, DO, FAAO, with permission.)

a positive *windlass test*.[199] Imaging can aid in the diagnosis, particularly in recalcitrant cases or may rule out other heel pathology.[197]

MTrPs in the soleus muscle refer pain to the heel and must be considered in the differential diagnosis of heel spurs and plantar fasciitis.[145] Imbalance of strength and flexibility in the supporting musculature of the posterior calf and foot can create a functional deficit in the normal foot biomechanics. Correction of such underlying biomechanical dysfunctions in the foot and calf using manual medicine techniques and devices like supportive shoes, shoe inserts, orthotics, and night splints have been shown to improve symptoms.[199] Manual medicine may include deep friction massage of the arch, counterstrain, MFR, MET and stretching exercises for the plantar fascia, Achilles tendon, gastrocnemius, and soleus. Other conservative treatments including rest, weight reduction when needed, and icing the plantar fascia and heel after activities can also help alleviate pain. Surgery is rarely necessary and the scar from the surgery may even aggravate the condition.[199]

Foot Deformities

Foot deformities are a group of acquired and congenital conditions that affect the functions of the foot. Most people have slightly deformed feet, which does not usually lead to any problems. More severe foot deformities may cause symptoms like pain, calluses, and walking difficulties. Muscular imbalances, structural abnormalities, and abnormal strain on the foot from repetitive activities, abnormal gait patterns, wearing tight shoes, being overweight, and trauma can all play a role in deformities. Other medical risk factors include connective tissue, vascular, and neurologic disorders that affect the supporting structures in the foot.[201]

PES PLANUS AND PES CAVUS

Observing if a foot is pronated (flat), supinated (cavus), or rectus (normal) is part of a structural screening exam; however, observation of the static foot is much less relevant than its dynamic properties.[202]

Persons with *pes planus* (flat foot) have a defect of the foot that eliminates their arch; they have a more horizontal subtalar axis and greater motion in their feet. When standing and walking, most of the foot—from the heel to the ball of the foot—touches the floor.[201] This may lead to abnormal wear on their shoes and some prefer to go barefoot. The condition is most often inherited; however, arches can also fall in adulthood, in which case the condition is sometimes referred to as *posterior tibial tendon dysfunction*.[203] This occurs most often in obese, middle-aged women, but it can occur in anyone.[203] Risk factors for developing pes planus include obesity, diabetes, surgery, injury, rheumatoid arthritis, or use of corticosteroids. It has also been found that habitual footwear use has significant effects on foot-related outcomes in all age groups, such as a reduction in foot arch and hallux angles.[204] Unilateral flat foot can sometimes account for a genu valgus and knee pain or a functional short leg on the same side with secondary postural changes above. It can also be problematic if the foot is unable to supinate during the propulsive phase of gait.

Persons with *pes cavus* (high arch) have a more vertical subtalar axis angle; biomechanically, they have a more rigid foot and a less stable ankle. Therefore, athletes with pes cavus have a greater risk of lateral foot injuries such as stress fractures of the fifth metatarsal and ankle sprain.[153,156]

MORTON FOOT

A *Morton foot* (also called a Morton toe, Greek foot, or Royal toe) is characterized by a short first metatarsal. *Dudley J. Morton* is credited with recognizing a short first metatarsal as being a primary defect of the foot.[205] Structurally, the short first metatarsal is not designed to accept the normal weight-bearing function involved in the push-off portion of gait. Callus forms under the second and third metatarsal heads as they assume the weight-bearing function. Increased functional demand remodels bone. This results in thickening of the second metatarsal; the thickening is evident on x-ray films. Painful walking from this condition may be relieved by treatment of an in-shoe orthotic to add support under the short first metatarsal to modify the structure–function relationships[205] and OMT to permit realignment. This foot configuration has been identified as one of the perpetuating and precipitating factors of Travell MTrPs and muscle imbalance as distant as the temporomandibular joint.[91] Figure 91.25 shows an example of an in-shoe orthotic used to modify structure–function relationships in Morton foot.

HALLUX VALGUS, BUNIONS, AND HAMMER TOES

Hallux valgus and bunions have a significant hereditary component; hammer toes are acquired. Each of these manifest structural changes with associated biomechanical effects and related somatic dysfunction.

Hallux valgus is a structural deformity resulting from the contracture of various periarticular structures of the first MP joint—it is progressive.

Bunion protrusion is accentuated by varus deviation of the first metatarsal. Muscle imbalance aggravates symptoms, but surgical intervention of the structure may be required for symptomatic relief. Applying counterstrain OMT to a tender point on the medial aspect of the great toe often provides symptomatic relief.

Hammer toes are often functional and can be associated with MTrPs in the dorsal interossei. Deformation might disappear after treatment of this particular somatic dysfunction.[91]

Indirect stacking OMT techniques are especially helpful in jammed toes. A stacking technique is one in which the physician

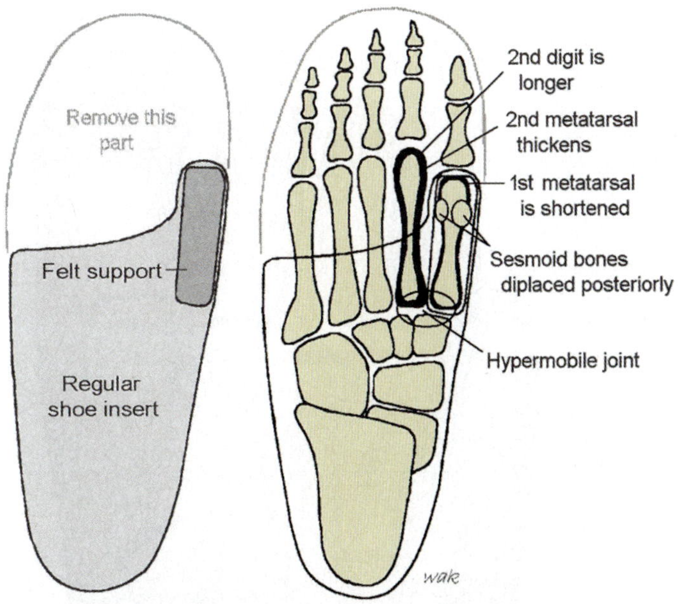

Figure 91.25. Orthotic used to modify structure–function relationships in a Morton foot. The toe portion of the sole insert is removed so support is only under the first metatarsal head. The lateral side of the support must not extend under second metatarsal head. Insert should reach to the distal end of the first metatarsal. (Illustration by William A. Kuchera, DO, FAAO, with permission.)

moves a joint in the direction of preference in all of its planes, stacking one motion upon the other. Compression or traction is then applied to that combined position. The technique may require holding the position of ease for 90 seconds or until the joint tensions relax. The joint is then slowly returned to a neutral position and rechecked for motion.

Morton Neuroma

Morton neuroma is a common pathology affecting the forefoot. It is a fusiform swelling of the common plantar digital nerve in the third IM space (Fig. 91.26).[206,207] It is not a true neuroma, but a fibrosis of the digital nerve. Approximately 17% of patients describe some trauma to the foot resulting in symptoms.[208]

Morton neuroma is caused secondary to pressure or repetitive irritation leading to a thickening of the nerve, which pathologically appears as a fusiform enlargement of a common plantar digital nerve at its bifurcation in the third IM space.[207,208] The exact pathophysiology remains debatable. There are four theories[207]:

- The chronic trauma theory (most widely accepted mechanism)
- The entrapment theory (deep transverse metatarsal ligament compresses the nerve)
- The IM bursitis theory (IM bursitis may cause compression)
- The ischemic theory (plantar digital artery shows ischemic degenerative changes)

This section will describe some specifics about the clinical presentation, physical examination, and treatment approach with OMT.

CLINICAL PRESENTATION

Patients typically have localized forefoot pain, paresthesia, and discomfort mainly on weight bearing.[208] Patients describe the pain as burning in nature, and may describe a feeling of a "pebble in the shoe."[208] The pain is often exacerbated by walking, use of tight or heeled shoes, and is reported by runners due to the increased weight-bearing through the forefoot.[208] Resting the foot or removing the shoe improves pain in most cases. In chronic cases the pain can be constant, and some patients report pain at rest or night.[208]

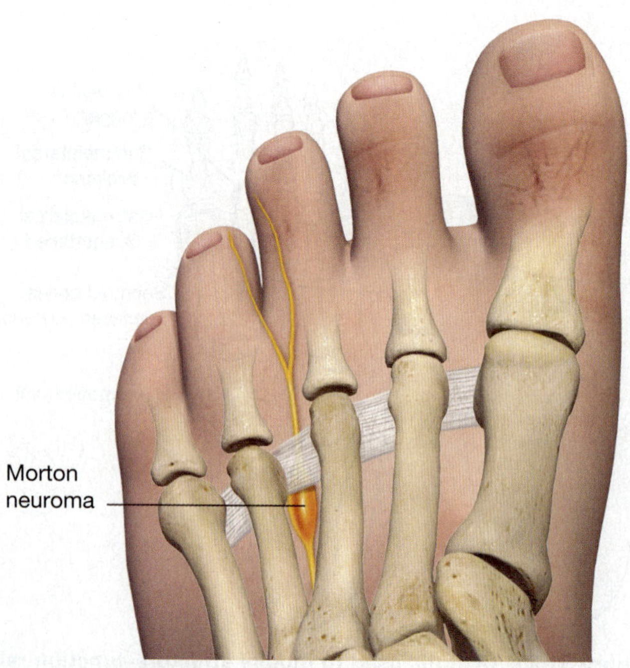

Figure 91.26. Morton neuroma. Fusiform enlargement between the third and fourth metatarsal web space. (Reprinted with permission from Hoppenfeld JD. *Fundamentals of Pain Medicine: How to Diagnose and Treat Your Patients*. Wolters Kluwer Health; 2014:57. Figure 6-8.)

PHYSICAL EXAMINATION

Clinically, there are no visual cues to the presence of a neuroma. However, patients may have forefoot deformities such as hammer toe and hallux valgus. This may contribute to overcrowding of the toes and increased pressure between the metatarsals. It is important to evaluate for plantar callosities around metatarsal heads. These are suggestive of transfer metatarsalgia, synovitis, subluxation, or dislocation of metatarsal–phalangeal joint of second or third toes.[208]

It has been reported that clinical assessment by experienced clinician has up to 98% accuracy as compared to an ultrasound examination. The most sensitive clinical tests for the diagnosis of Morton neuroma are the following[208,209]:

- Thumb and index finger squeeze test
  - The thumb and index finger test is performed by applying pressure in the IM space, to splay apart the toes. The thumb is placed on the dorsal aspect whereas the index finger is kept on the plantar aspect. Positive test results in pain in presence of Morton neuroma.[208,209]
- Mulder click test
  - Mulder click test is performed by dorsiflexing the foot and squeezing the metatarsals. An audible click is suggestive of the presence of Morton neuroma.[208,209]
- Foot squeeze test
  - The foot squeeze test is performed by applying simultaneous medial and lateral pressure on the metatarsals. A positive test cause pain and paresthesia in the involved toes.

OSTEOPATHIC MANIPULATIVE TREATMENT

OMT and manual therapy have been utilized to treat associated somatic dysfunction in patients with many foot conditions, including Morton neuroma. Although robust clinical studies are lacking, a case study on Morton neuroma demonstrated pain improvement with OMT.[210]

Somatic dysfunction of the foot, ankle and lower extremity can alter foot biomechanics and function. Any somatic dysfunction that contributes to a compressive load on the metatarsals, may contribute to the pain and symptomology of Morton neuroma. OMT and other forms of manual therapy may also allow the patient to adapt to prescribed orthotics. Likewise, patients who have Morton neuroma might bear more weight on the uninvolved foot and create somatic dysfunction on either side as a secondary effect. These dysfunctions should be treated to prevent associated ankle, shin, or knee pain, especially if the condition is chronic.

OMT and other forms of manual therapy have been studied in plantar fasciitis.[211–214] Studies have concluded that both MET and MFR were effective in reducing pain and improving lower limb function in patients with this condition.[212] Similarly, addressing any misalignment of the metatarsals may help decrease forefoot pain, because of their ligamentous and muscular attachments within the arches.[215] Providing manual manipulation of the joints affected independently or in conjunction with orthotic therapy may yield more long term and efficacious results than orthotic therapy alone.[216] Postoperative chronic foot pain may also respond to joint mobilization and manipulation.[217]

SUMMARY OF OTHER CONSERVATIVE TREATMENT APPROACHES

The management of neuroma can be split into nonoperative measures or surgical management.

Patient education is very important, and the use of wide toe box shoes can be the simplest method of managing symptoms. The commonest form of treatment (initially) is the metatarsal bar. This insole, made by orthotists, spreads the heads of the metatarsals to relieve pressure on the neuroma and thus improve symptoms. However, this does require the patient to wear broad toe box shoes and use the inserts, so patient compliance is required. There is no evidence to support the use of inversion or eversion insoles, with studies demonstrating no significant improvement in patient-reported outcomes.[218,219] According to Munir,[220] conservative approaches to treatment have shown varying degrees of effectiveness.[221] A systematic review and meta-analysis of nonsurgical approaches were performed and found employing multiple strategies to be effective.[222,223] Also, corticosteroid injections and manipulation/mobilization have the strongest evidence for pain reduction.[222,223] The overall treatment algorithm generally involves nonoperative measures including injection therapy and if these methods fail to improve symptoms, surgical excision is the next option.[224]

SUMMARY

A thorough understanding of the functional anatomy of the extremities, coupled with grounding in osteopathic principles and practice, establishes a foundation for the osteopathic approach to the extremities and their effect on the whole person.

A thorough osteopathic patient assessment is critical, and physicians should use a combination of patient history and physical examinations in conjunction with diagnostic tests to make an accurate diagnosis. The osteopathic clinical examination of the extremities includes the diagnosis of somatic dysfunction integrated into the examination procedure. Palpation assists in differential diagnoses of a wide range of structural and functional disorders in these regions. The relationship between anatomic structure and physiologic function is considered prior to deciding a treatment plan. The osteopathic physician then seeks to balance and improve biomechanical and homeostatic functions to influence a wide range of patient conditions. Osteopathic treatment needs to be individualized and address the specific diagnosis, incorporating the innate ability of the patient to heal given the appropriate environment of improved tissue function. OMT directed at the somatic component of the patient's condition will improve the tissue's function and thus the patient's own ability to heal themselves.

Regardless of clinical specialty, the osteopathic approach to the extremities offers an effective approach to diagnosis, prevention, and treatment.

ACKNOWLEDGMENTS

The authors of this chapter would like to acknowledge the scholarly contributions of Per Gunnar Brolinson, DO, and Thomas A. Goodwin for prior editions of this chapter.

REFERENCES

1. Kibler B, Sciascia A. Kinetic chain contributions to elbow function and dysfunction in sports. *Clin Sports Med.* 2004;23(4):545–552, viii.
2. Chu SK, Jayabalan P, Kibler B, Press J. The kinetic chain revisited: new concepts on throwing mechanics and injury. *PM&R.* 2016; 8(3 Suppl):S69–77.
3. Wang WJ, Liu F, Zhu YW, Sun MH, Qiu Y, Weng WJ. Sagittal alignment of the spine-pelvis-lower extremity axis in patients with severe knee osteoarthritis: a radiographic study. *Bone Jt Res.* 2016;5(5):198–205.
4. Horak FB, Nashner LM, Diener HC. Postural strategies associated with somatosensory and vestibular loss. *Exp Brain Res.* 1990;82(1):167–177.
5. Kuchera WA, Kuchera ML. *Osteopathic Principles in Practice.* Greyden Press LLC; 1994.
6. Cyriax JH. *Cyriax's Illustrated Manual of Orthopaedic Medicine.* Elsevier Science & Technology Books; 1993.
7. Seffinger MA, Hruby RJ. *Evidence-Based Manual Medicine: A Problem-Oriented Approach.* Elsevier Health Sciences; 2007.
8. Halabchi F, Hassabi M. Acute ankle sprain in athletes: clinical aspects and algorithmic approach. *World J Orthop.* 2020;11(12):534–558.
9. Rabago D, Slattengren A, Zgierska A. Prolotherapy in primary care practice. *Prim Care.* 2010;37(1):65–80.
10. Spencer H. Shoulder technique. *J Am Osteopath Assoc.* 1916;15:218–220.
11. Dalley AF II, Agur AMR. Upper extremity. In: *Moore's Clinically Oriented Anatomy.* 9th ed. Lippincott Williams & Wilkins; 2023:142–295.
12. Travell JG, Simons DG. *Myofascial Pain and Dysfunction: The Trigger Point Manual.* Lippincott Williams & Wilkins; 1992.
13. Dalley AF, Agur AM. Lower extremity. In: *Moore's Clinically Oriented Anatomy.* 9th ed. Lippincott Williams & Wilkins; 2023:672–838.
14. Seffinger MA, ed. *Foundations of Osteopathic Medicine: Philosophy, Science, Clinical Applications, and Research.* 4th ed. Wolters Kluwer; 2018.
15. Nelson K, Glonek T, eds. *Somatic Dysfunction in Osteopathic Family Medicine.* 2nd ed. Wolters Kluwer Health; 2015.
16. DiGiovanna E, Amen C, Burns DK. Upper extremity. In: *An Osteopathic Approach to Diagnosis and Treatment.* 4th ed. Wolters Kluwer; 2021:359–396.
17. Larson N. Functional vasomotor hemiparesthesia syndrome. In: *Academy of Applied Osteopathy 1970 Yearbook.* Academy of Applied Osteopathy; 1970.
18. Korr I. Proprioceptors and somatic dysfunction. *J Am Osteopath Assoc.* 1975;74(7):638–650.
19. Denslow J, Korr I, Krems A. Quantitative studies of chronic facilitation in human motoneuron pools. *Am J Physiol.* 1947;150(2):229–238.
20. Bicalho E, Vieira L, Makita DK, Rivas L. Inhibitory tests as assessment tools for somatic dysfunctions: mechanisms and practical applications. *Cureus.* 2020;12(4):e7700.
21. Kerger S. Chapter 10: Exercise principles. In: Karageanes SJ *Principles of Manual Sports Medicine.* Lippincott Williams & Wilkins; 2005:65–76.
22. Allegrante JP, Marks R. Self-efficacy in management of osteoarthritis. *Rheum Dis Clin North Am.* 2003;29(4):747–768, vi-vii.
23. Soberg HL, Bautz-Holter E, Roise O, Finset A. Long-term multidimensional functional consequences of severe multiple injuries two years after trauma: a prospective longitudinal cohort study. *J Trauma.* 2007;62(2):461–470.
24. Vincent HK, Horodyski M, Vincent KR, Brisbane ST, Sadasivan KK. Psychological distress after orthopedic trauma: prevalence in patients and implications for rehabilitation. *PM&R.* 2015;7(9):978–989.
25. van den Berg M, Verdijk NA, Leusink GL, et al. Depression after low-energy fracture in older women predicts future falls: a prospective observational study. *BMC Geriatr.* 2011;11(1):73.
26. Vranceanu AM, Bachoura A, Weening A, Vrahas M, Smith RM, Ring D. Psychological factors predict disability and pain intensity after skeletal trauma. *J Bone Joint Surg Am.* 2014;96(3):e20.
27. Beatty D. *The Pocket Manual of OMT.* 2nd ed. Wolters Kluwer Health/ Lippincott Williams & Wilkins; 2011.
28. DeStefano LA. Chapter 18. In: *Greenman's Principles of Manual Medicine.* 5th ed. Wolters Kluwer; 2017:375–418.
29. Nicholas AS, Nicholas EA. *Atlas of Osteopathic Techniques.* 4th ed. Wolters Kluwer Health/Lippincott Williams & Wilkins; 2022.
30. Seffinger MA. *Evidence-Based Manual Medicine : A Problem-Oriented Approach.* Saunders/Elsevier; 2007. Accessed November 26, 2023. http://archive.org/details/evidencebasedman0000seff
31. Seffinger MA, ed. Chapter 49. In: *Foundations of Osteopathic Medicine: Philosophy, Science, Clinical Applications, and Research.* 4th ed. Wolters Kluwer; 2018:1488–1496.
32. Kimberly PE, Halma K; Kirksville College of Osteopathic Medicine. *Outline of Osteopathic Manipulative Procedures: The Kimberly Manual 2006.* Walsworth Publishing Company; 2008.
33. Patriquin DA. The evolution of osteopathic manipulative technique: the Spencer technique. *J Am Osteopath Assoc.* 1992;92(9):1134–1136, 1139–1146.

34. Connolly MR, Auchincloss HG. Anatomy and embryology of the thoracic outlet. *Thorac Surg Clin*. 2021;31(1):1–10.
35. Jones MR, Prabhakar A, Viswanath O, et al. Thoracic outlet syndrome: a comprehensive review of pathophysiology, diagnosis, and treatment. *Pain Ther*. 2019;8(1):5–18.
36. Povlsen S, Povlsen B. Diagnosing thoracic outlet syndrome: current approaches and future directions. *Diagnostics (Basel)*. 2018;8(1):21.
37. Kuhn JE, Lebus V GF, Bible JE. Thoracic outlet syndrome. *J Am Acad Orthop Surg*. 2015;23(4):222–232.
38. Kaplan J, Kanwal A. Thoracic outlet syndrome. In: *StatPearls*. StatPearls Publishing; 2024. Accessed May 1, 2024. http://www.ncbi.nlm.nih.gov/books/NBK557450/
39. Redondo-Alonso L, Chamorro-Moriana G, Jiménez-Rejano JJ, López-Tarrida P, Ridao-Fernández C. Relationship between chronic pathologies of the supraspinatus tendon and the long head of the biceps tendon: systematic review. *BMC Musculoskelet Disord*. 2014;15:377.
40. Creech JA, Silver S. Shoulder impingement syndrome. In: *StatPearls*. StatPearls Publishing; 2024. Accessed May 1, 2024. http://www.ncbi.nlm.nih.gov/books/NBK554518/
41. Miller MD, Thompson SR, eds. *DeLee & Drez's Orthopaedic Sports Medicine: Principles and Practice*. Saunders; 2003.
42. Heyworth BE, Williams RJ III. Internal impingement of the shoulder. *Am J Sports Med*. 2009;37(5):1024–1037.
43. Kibler WB, Sciascia A, Wilkes T. Scapular dyskinesis and its relation to shoulder injury. *J Am Acad Orthop Surg*. 2012;20(6):364–372.
44. Janda V. Muscle weakness and inhibition (pseudoparesis) in back pain syndromes. In: Grieve GP, ed. *Modern Medicine Therapy of the Vertebral Column*. Churchill Livingstone; 1986:197–200.
45. Le HV, Lee SJ, Nazarian A, Rodriguez EK. Adhesive capsulitis of the shoulder: review of pathophysiology and current clinical treatments. *Shoulder Elb*. 2017;9(2):75–84.
46. St Angelo JM, Taqi M, Fabiano SE. Adhesive capsulitis. In: *StatPearls*. StatPearls Publishing; 2024. Accessed May 1, 2024. http://www.ncbi.nlm.nih.gov/books/NBK532955/
47. D'Amato K, Rogers M. "Frozen shoulder"—a difficult clinical problem. *Osteopath Fam Physician*. 2012;4(3):72–80.
48. Anupama N, Jagga V. Efficacy of muscle energy technique on functional ability of shoulder in adhesive capsulitis. *J Exerc Sci Physiother*. 2014;10(2):72–76.
49. Tafler L, Santanello A, Lysakova Y. The function of osteopathic medicine in the treatment of adhesive capsulitis. *Cureus*. 2022;14(8):e27640.
50. Veera S, Chin J, Kleyn L, Spinelli S, Tafler L. Use of osteopathic manipulation for treatment of chronic shoulder injury related to vaccine administration. *Cureus*. 2020;12(7):e9156.
51. Travell JG, Simons DG. Subscapularis muscle: frozen shoulder. In: *Myofascial Pain and Dysfunction: The Trigger Point Manual*. Lippincott Williams & Wilkins; 1992:410–424.
52. Fleming J, Muller C, Lambert K. Lateral epicondylitis: a common cause of elbow pain in primary care. *Osteopath Fam Physician*. 2021;13(1):34–38.
53. Taylor SA, Hannafin JA. Evaluation and management of elbow tendinopathy. *Sports Health*. 2012;4(5):384–393.
54. Fernández-Carnero J, Fernández-de-Las-Peñas C, de la Llave-Rincón AI, Ge HY, Arendt-Nielsen L. Prevalence of and referred pain from myofascial trigger points in the forearm muscles in patients with lateral epicondylalgia. *Clin J Pain*. 2007;23(4):353–360.
55. Aggarwal A, Daniel J, Palekar TJ. Prevalence of myofascial trigger points in brachioradialis, biceps brachii, triceps brachii, supinator and extensor carpi radialis brevis in lateral epicondylitis. *Indian J Physiother Occup Ther*. 2020;14(1):14–18.
56. Küçükşen S, Yilmaz H, Sallı A, Uğurlu H. Muscle energy technique versus corticosteroid injection for management of chronic lateral epicondylitis: randomized controlled trial with 1-year follow-up. *Arch Phys Med Rehabil*. 2013;94(11):2068–2074.
57. Khuman R. Myofascial release technique in chronic lateral epicondylitis: a randomised controlled study. *Int J Heal Sci Res*. 2013;3(7):45–52.
58. Ajimsha MS, Chithra S, Thulasyammal RP. Effectiveness of myofascial release in the management of lateral epicondylitis in computer professionals. *Arch Phys Med Rehabil*. 2012;93(4):604–609.
59. Lucado AM, Dale RB, Vincent J, Day JM. Do joint mobilizations assist in the recovery of lateral elbow tendinopathy? A systematic review and meta-analysis. *J Hand Ther Off J Am Soc Hand Ther*. 2019;32(2):262–276.e1.
60. McShane JM, Nazarian LN, Harwood MI. Sonographically guided percutaneous needle tenotomy for treatment of common extensor tendinosis in the elbow. *J Ultrasound Med*. 2006;25(10):1281–1289.
61. Kotteeswaran K. Effect of myofascial trigger point release therapy and active stretching on pain among lateral epicondylitis participants. *Int J Res Anal Rev*. 2019;6(2):184–188.
62. Smidt N, van der Windt DAWM, Assendelft WJJ, Devillé WLJM, Korthals-de Bos IBC, Bouter LM. Corticosteroid injections, physiotherapy, or a wait-and-see policy for lateral epicondylitis: a randomised controlled trial. *Lancet Lond Engl*. 2002;359(9307):657–662.
63. Tyler TF, Thomas GC, Nicholas SJ, McHugh MP. Addition of isolated wrist extensor eccentric exercise to standard treatment for chronic lateral epicondylosis: a prospective randomized trial. *J Shoulder Elbow Surg*. 2010;19(6):917–922.
64. Strachan F, Fryette H. Part IV. Appendicular technic. In: *Principles of Osteopathic Technique*. Academy of Applied Osteopathy; 1954:134–199.
65. Wipperman J, Goerl K. Carpal tunnel syndrome: diagnosis and management. *Am Fam Physician*. 2016;94(12):993–999.
66. Padua L, Cuccagna C, Giovannini S, et al. Carpal tunnel syndrome: updated evidence and new questions. *Lancet Neurol*. 2023;22(3):255–267.
67. Keith MW, Masear V, Chung KC, et al; American Academy of Orthopaedic Surgeons. American Academy of Orthopaedic Surgeons Clinical Practice Guideline on the treatment of carpal tunnel syndrome. *J Bone Joint Surg Am*. 2010;92(1):218–219.
68. Werner RA, Andary M. Carpal tunnel syndrome: pathophysiology and clinical neurophysiology. *Clin Neurophysiol Off J Int Fed Clin Neurophysiol*. 2002;113(9):1373–1381.
69. American Medical Association. *Guides to the Evaluation of Permanent Impairment*. 6th ed. American Medical Association; 2008.
70. Sevy JO, Sina RE, Varacallo M. Carpal tunnel syndrome. In: *StatPearls*. StatPearls Publishing; 2024. Accessed May 1, 2024. http://www.ncbi.nlm.nih.gov/books/NBK448179/
71. Azadeh H, Dehghani M, Zarezadeh A. Incidence of trapezius myofascial trigger points in patients with the possible carpal tunnel syndrome. *J Res Med Sci*. 2010;15(5):250–255.
72. Rodner CM, Tinsley BA, O'Malley MP. Pronator syndrome and anterior interosseous nerve syndrome. *J Am Acad Orthop Surg*. 2013;21(5):268–275.
73. Burnham T, Higgins DC, Burnham RS, Heath DM. Effectiveness of osteopathic manipulative treatment for carpal tunnel syndrome: a pilot project. *J Am Osteopath Assoc*. 2015;115(3):138–148.
74. Graham B, Peljovich AE, Afra R, et al. The American Academy of Orthopaedic Surgeons Evidence-Based Clinical Practice Guideline on management of carpal tunnel syndrome. *J Bone Joint Surg Am*. 2016;98(20):1750–1754.
75. Campos-Serna I, Garcia-Espinoza JA, Cahuana-Quispe AI, et al. Diagnosis and treatment of carpal tunnel syndrome in a tertiary care center in Mexico City. *World J Plast Surg*. 2020;9(2):213–218.
76. DiGiovanna E, Amen C, Burns DK. Lower extremity. In: *An Osteopathic Approach to Diagnosis and Treatment*. 4th ed. Wolters Kluwer; 2021:413–463.
77. Krabak BJ, Jarmain SJ, Prather H. Chapter 8: Physical examination of the hip. In: Malanga GA, Nadler SF, eds. *Musculoskeletal Physical Examination: An Evidence-Based Approach*. 4th ed. Hanley & Belfus; 2006:251–278.
78. American Academy of Orthopaedic Surgeons. *AAOS Essentials of Musculoskeletal Care*. 6th ed. Jones & Bartlett Learning; 2021.
79. Lotke PA, Abboud JA, Ende J. *Lippincott's Primary Care Orthopaedics*. Lippincott Williams & Wilkins; 2013.
80. Kuchera M. Chapter 39: Treatment of gravitational strain pathophysiology. In: Vleeming A, Mooney V, Snijders CJ, Dorman TA, Stoeckart R, eds. *Movement, Stability and Low Back Pain: The Essential Role of the Pelvis*. Churchill Livingstone; 1997:477–499.
81. DeStefano LA. Chapter 19. In: *Greenman's Principles of Manual Medicine*. 5th ed. Wolters Kluwer; 2017:419–462.

82. Strachan F, Fryette H. Part IV. Appendicular technic. In: *Principles of Osteopathic Technique*. Academy of Applied Osteopathy; 1954: 200–234.
83. Christman OD. Biomechanical aspects of degenerative joint disease. *Clin Orthop Relat Res*. 1969;64:77–86.
84. Tallroth K, Ristolainen L, Manninen M. Is a long leg a risk for hip or knee osteoarthritis? *Acta Orthop*. 2017;88(5):512–515.
85. Poutoglidou F, Piagkou M, Totlis T, Tzika M, Natsis K. Sciatic nerve variants and the piriformis muscle: a systematic review and meta-analysis. *Cureus*. 12(11):e11531.
86. Reid D. The management of greater trochanteric pain syndrome: a systematic literature review. *J Orthop*. 2016;13(1):15–28.
87. Guemara R, Nissen MJ. The greater trochanteric pain syndrome: clinical presentation, diagnosis, and management. *Curr Treat Options Rheumatol*. 2023;9(4):192–203.
88. Bird PA, Oakley SP, Shnier R, Kirkham BW. Prospective evaluation of magnetic resonance imaging and physical examination findings in patients with greater trochanteric pain syndrome. *Arthritis Rheum*. 2001; 44(9):2138–2145.
89. Kaux JF, Forthomme B, Goff CL, Crielaard JM, Croisier JL. Current opinions on tendinopathy. *J Sports Sci Med*. 2011;10(2):238–253.
90. Fearon AM, Scarvell JM, Neeman T, Cook JL, Cormick W, Smith PN. Greater trochanteric pain syndrome: defining the clinical syndrome. *Br J Sports Med*. 2013;47(10):649–653.
91. Travell JG, Simons DG. *Myofascial Pain and Dysfunction: The Trigger Point Manual: The Lower Extremities*. Vol. 2. 1st ed. Williams & Wilkins; 1992.
92. Hackett GS. *Ligament and Tendon Relaxation*. 3rd ed. Charles C Thomas Pub Ltd; 1958.
93. Torres J, Zipp C. An osteopathic approach to greater trochanteric pain syndrome. *Osteopath Fam Physician*. 2019;11(3):18–21.
94. Ganderton C, Semciw A, Cook J, Moreira E, Pizzari T. Gluteal loading versus sham exercises to improve pain and dysfunction in postmenopausal women with greater trochanteric pain syndrome: a randomized controlled trial. *J Womens Health (Larchmt)*. 2018;27(6):815–829.
95. Brooker AF Jr. The surgical approach to refractory trochanteric bursitis. *Johns Hopkins Med J*. 1979;145(3):98–100.
96. Pretell J, Ortega J, García-Rayo R, Resines C. Distal fascia lata lengthening: an alternative surgical technique for recalcitrant trochanteric bursitis. *Int Orthop*. 2009;33(5):1223–1227.
97. Disantis AE, Martin RL. Classification based treatment of greater trochanteric pain syndrome (gtps) with integration of the movement system. *Int J Sports Phys Ther*. 2022;17(3):508–518.
98. Walters A-M, Sopher RA, Kuczynski JJ. Greater Trochanteric Pain Syndrome. Wexner Medical Center at The Ohio State University. Published July 12, 2017. Accessed February 11, 2025. Available at: "https://nam12.safelinks.protection.outlook.com/?url=https%3A%2F%2Fwexnermedical.osu.edu%2F-%2Fmedia%2Ffiles%2Fwexnermedical%2Fpatient-care%2Fhealthcare-services%2Fsports-medicine%2Feducation%2Fmedical-professionals%2Fhip%2Fgreaterthochantericpainsymdrome.pdf&data=05%7C02%7Clundk%40westernu.edu%7C473f825116bd41de8d0008dd4acaf4a7%7C25a6f4f8d912492a84df376754ba693e%7C0%7C0%7C638748957720595021%7CUnknown%7CTWFpbGZsb3d8eyJFbXB0eU1hcGkiOnRydWUsIlYiOiIwLjAuMDAwMCIsIlAiOiJXaW4zMiIsIkFOIjoiTWFpbCIsIldUIjoyfQ%3D%3D%7C0%7C%7C%7C&sdata=2Z2acgnHjk9D9gQynZFgrgZ9gs74Mhir3sEvIyWbXNM%3D&reserved=0" https://wexnermedical.osu.edu/-/media/files/wexnermedical/patient-care/healthcare-services/sports-medicine/education/medical-professionals/hip/greaterthochantericpainsymdrome.pdf
99. Kingston B. *Understanding Joints: A Practical Guide to Their Structure and Function*. Nelson Thornes; 2000.
100. Ombregt L, Veer H. Disorders of the inert structures: capsular and non-capsular patterns. In: Ombregt L, Bisschop P, ter Veer HJ, Van de Velde T, eds. *A System of Orthopaedic Medicine*. WB Saunders Ltd; 1995:783–800.
101. DiGiovanna E, Amen C, Burns DK. Chapter 94. In: *An Osteopathic Approach to Diagnosis and Treatment*. 4th ed. Wolters Kluwer; 2021.
102. Nicholas AS, Nicholas EA. Chapter 10 MET. In: *Atlas of Osteopathic Techniques*. 4th ed. Wolters Kluwer Health/Lippincott Williams & Wilkins; 2022:347–364.
103. Seffinger MA, ed. Chapter 27. In: *Foundations of Osteopathic Medicine: Philosophy, Science, Clinical Applications, and Research*. 4th ed. Wolters Kluwer; 2018:602–608.
104. Beatty D. Chapter 3. In: *The Pocket Manual of OMT*. 2nd ed. Wolters Kluwer Health/Lippincott Williams & Wilkins; 2011.
105. Seffinger MA, ed. Chapter 49. In: *Foundations of Osteopathic Medicine: Philosophy, Science, Clinical Applications, and Research*. 4th ed. Wolters Kluwer; 2018:1496–1515.
106. Kimberly PE, Halma K; Kirksville College of Osteopathic Medicine Department of Osteopathic Theory and Methods. Chapter 12. In: *Outline of Osteopathic Manipulative Procedures: The Kimberly Manual 2006*. Walsworth Publishing Company; 2008:269–311.
107. Nicholas AS, Nicholas EA. Chapter 11 HVLA. In: *Atlas of Osteopathic Techniques*. 4th ed. Wolters Kluwer Health/Lippincott Williams & Wilkins; 2022:414–430.
108. Jackson JL, O'Malley PG, Kroenke K. Evaluation of acute knee pain in primary care. *Ann Intern Med*. 2003;139(7):575–588.
109. Solomon DH, Simel DL, Bates DW, Katz JN, Schaffer JL. The rational clinical examination. Does this patient have a torn meniscus or ligament of the knee? Value of the physical examination. *JAMA*. 2001;286(13): 1610–1620.
110. Renström P, Johnson RJ. Anatomy and biomechanics of the menisci. *Clin Sports Med*. 1990;9(3):523–538.
111. Pasiński M, Zabrzyńska M, Adamczyk M, et al. A current insight into human knee menisci. *Transl Res Anat*. 2023;32:100259.
112. O'donoghue DH. The unhappy triad: etiology, diagnosis, and treatment. *Am J Orthop*. 1964;6:242–247 PASSIM.
113. Hoveidaei AH, Sattarpour R, Dadgostar H, Razi S, Razi M. Unhappy triad of the knee: What are the current concepts and opinions? *World J Orthop*. 2023;14(5):268–274.
114. Willy RW, Halsey L, Hayek A, Johnson H, Willson JD. Patellofemoral joint and Achilles tendon loads during overground and treadmill running. *J Orthop Sports Phys Ther*. 2016;46(8):664–672.
115. Vinger PF, Hoerner EF. Injuries of the lower extremities. In: *Sports Injuries: The Unthwarted Epidemic*. PSG Publishing Company; 1986:235–249.
116. Blood SD. Treatment of the sprained ankle. *J Am Osteopath Assoc*. 1980; 79(11):680–692.
117. Eisenhart AW, Gaeta TJ, Yens DP. Osteopathic manipulative treatment in the emergency department for patients with acute ankle injuries. *J Am Osteopath Assoc*. 2003;103(9):417–421.
118. Strachan F, Fryette H. Ankle and foot somatic dysfunctions. In: *Principles of Osteopathic Technique*. Academy of Applied Osteopathy; 1954:221.
119. Travell JG, Simons DG. The lower extremities. In: *Myofascial Pain and Dysfunction: The Trigger Point Manual*. Vol. 2. Lippincott Williams & Wilkins; 1992:429–459.
120. Dixit S, Difiori JP, Burton M, Mines B. Management of Patellofemoral Pain Syndrome. *Am Fam Physician*. 2007;75(2):194–202.
121. Datta R, Burina L, Romanelli F, Flaum TB. Knee pain in adults with an osteopathic component. *Osteopath Fam Physician*. 2017;9(1):26–35.
122. Merchant AC. Classification of patellofemoral disorders. *Arthroscopy*. 1988; 4(4):235–240.
123. Cutbill JW, Ladly KO, Bray RC, Thorne P, Verhoef M. Anterior knee pain: a review. *Clin J Sport Med*. 1997;7(1):40–45.
124. Lankhorst NE, Bierma-Zeinstra SMA, van Middelkoop M. Risk factors for patellofemoral pain syndrome: a systematic review. *J Orthop Sports Phys Ther*. 2012;42(2):81–94.
125. Rossignol M, Leclerc A, Allaert F, et al. Primary osteoarthritis of hip, knee, and hand in relation to occupational exposure. *Occup Environ Med*. 2005;62(11):772–777.
126. Felson DT. Risk factors for osteoarthritis: understanding joint vulnerability. *Clin Orthop Relat Res*. 2004;(427 Suppl):S16–S21.
127. Sandow MJ, Goodfellow JW. The natural history of anterior knee pain in adolescents. *J Bone Joint Surg Br*. 1985;67(1):36–38.
128. Post WR. Current concepts: clinical evaluation of patients with patellofemoral disorders. *Arthroscopy*. 1999;15(8):841–851.
129. Gaitonde DY, Ericksen A, Robbins RC. Patellofemoral pain syndrome. *Am Fam Physician*. 2019;99(2):88–94.
130. Walli O, McCay M, Tiu T. Patellofemoral syndrome: a review of diagnosis and treatment. *Curr Phys Med Rehabil Rep*. 2023;11(2):139–143.

131. Collado H, Fredericson M. Patellofemoral pain syndrome. *Clin Sports Med.* 2010;29(3):379–398.
132. Gerbino PG, Griffin ED, d'Hemecourt PA, et al. Patellofemoral pain syndrome: evaluation of location and intensity of pain. *Clin J Pain.* 2006;22(2):154–159.
133. Nijs J, Van Geel C, Van der auwera C, Van de Velde B. Diagnostic value of five clinical tests in patellofemoral pain syndrome. *Man Ther.* 2006;11(1):69–77.
134. Haim A, Yaniv M, Dekel S, Amir H. Patellofemoral pain syndrome: validity of clinical and radiological features. *Clin Orthop.* 2006;451: 223–228.
135. Manske RC, Davies GJ. Examination of the patellofemoral joint. *Int J Sports Phys Ther.* 2016;11(6):831–853.
136. Cook C, Mabry L, Reiman MP, Hegedus EJ. Best tests/clinical findings for screening and diagnosis of patellofemoral pain syndrome: a systematic review. *Physiotherapy.* 2012;98(2):93–100.
137. Nunes GS, Barton CJ, Serrão FV. Hip rate of force development and strength are impaired in females with patellofemoral pain without signs of altered gluteus medius and maximus morphology. *J Sci Med Sport.* 2018;21(2):123–128.
138. Collins NJ, Barton CJ, van Middelkoop M, et al. 2018 Consensus statement on exercise therapy and physical interventions (orthoses, taping and manual therapy) to treat patellofemoral pain: recommendations from the 5th International Patellofemoral Pain Research Retreat, Gold Coast, Australia, 2017. *Br J Sports Med.* 2018;52(18):1170–1178.
139. Barton CJ, De Oliveira Silva D, Morton S, et al. REPORT-PFP: a consensus from the International Patellofemoral Research Network to improve REPORTing of quantitative PatelloFemoral Pain studies. *Br J Sports Med.* 2021;55(20):1135–1143.
140. Sisk D, Fredericson M. Update of risk factors, diagnosis, and management of patellofemoral pain. *Curr Rev Musculoskelet Med.* 2019;12(4): 534–541.
141. Coburn SL, Barton CJ, Filbay SR, Hart HF, Rathleff MS, Crossley KM. Quality of life in individuals with patellofemoral pain: a systematic review including meta-analysis. *Phys Ther Sport.* 2018;33:96–108.
142. Strohl KP, Mead J, Banzett RB, Loring SH, Kosch PC. Regional differences in abdominal muscle activity during various maneuvers in humans. *J Appl Physiol Respir Environ Exerc Physiol.* 1981;51(6):1471–1476.
143. Chevalier AM, Lacôte M, Bleton JP. *Clinical Evaluation of Muscle Function.* Churchill Livingstone; 1987.
144. De Troyer A, Estenne M, Ninane V, Van Gansbeke D, Gorini M. Transversus abdominis muscle function in humans. *J Appl Physiol (1985).* 1990;68(3):1010–1016.
145. Panjabi MM. Clinical spinal instability and low back pain. *J Electromyogr Kinesiol.* 2003;13(4):371–379.
146. Sahu P, Phansopkar P. Screening for lower cross syndrome in asymptomatic individuals. *J Med Pharm Allied Sci.* 2021;10(6):3894–3898.
147. Scafoglieri A, Van den Broeck J, Willems S, et al. Effectiveness of local exercise therapy versus spinal manual therapy in patients with patellofemoral pain syndrome: medium term follow-up results of a randomized controlled trial. *BMC Musculoskelet Disord.* 2021;22(1):446.
148. McClinton SM, Cobian DG, Heiderscheit BC. Physical therapist management of anterior knee pain. *Curr Rev Musculoskelet Med.* 2020; 13(6):776–787.
149. Espí-López GV, Arnal-Gómez A, Balasch-Bernat M, Inglés M. Effectiveness of manual therapy combined with physical therapy in treatment of patellofemoral pain syndrome: systematic review. *J Chiropr Med.* 2017;16(2):139–146.
150. Abbott JH, Robertson MC, McKenzie JE, et al; MOA Trial team. Exercise therapy, manual therapy, or both, for osteoarthritis of the hip or knee: a factorial randomised controlled trial protocol. *Trials.* 2009;10:11.
151. Salamh P, Cook C, Reiman MP, Sheets C. Treatment effectiveness and fidelity of manual therapy to the knee: a systematic review and meta-analysis. *Musculoskeletal Care.* 2017;15(3):238–248.
152. Brantingham JW, Globe G, Pollard H, Hicks M, Korporaal C, Hoskins W. Manipulative therapy for lower extremity conditions: expansion of literature review. *J Manipulative Physiol Ther.* 2009;32(1):53–71.
153. Brockett CL, Chapman GJ. Biomechanics of the ankle. *Orthop Trauma.* 2016;30(3):232–238.
154. Ombregt L, Bisschop P, ter Veer HJ. *A System of Orthopaedic Medicine.* Churchill Livingstone; 2003.
155. Thompson D. *Subtalar Joint Motion (Closed Chain).* University of Oklahoma Health Sciences Center. Published May 4, 2001. Accessed May 3, 2024. https://ouhsc.edu/bserdac/dthompso/web/gait/KNMATICS/STJCLOSE.HTM
156. Fraser JJ, Feger MA, Hertel J. Midfoot and forefoot involvement in lateral ankle sprains and chronic ankle instability. Part 1: anatomy and biomechanics. *Int J Sports Phys Ther.* 2016;11(6):992–1005.
157. Scott SH, Winter DA. Talocrural and talocalcaneal joint kinematics and kinetics during the stance phase of walking. *J Biomech.* 1991;24(8):743–752.
158. Huber T, Schmoelz W, Bölderl A. Motion of the fibula relative to the tibia and its alterations with syndesmosis screws: a cadaver study. *Foot Ankle Surg.* 2012;18(3):203–209.
159. Calhoun JH, Li F, Ledbetter BR, Viegas SF. A comprehensive study of pressure distribution in the ankle joint with inversion and eversion. *Foot Ankle Int.* 1994;15(3):125–133.
160. Nicholas AS, Nicholas EA. Chapter 14 BLT. In: *Atlas of Osteopathic Techniques.* 4th ed. Wolters Kluwer Health/Lippincott Williams & Wilkins; 2022:485–494.
161. DiGiovanna E, Amen C, Burns DK. Chapter 97. In: *An Osteopathic Approach to Diagnosis and Treatment.* 4th ed. Wolters Kluwer; 2021.
162. DiGiovanna E, Amen C, Burns DK. Chapter 96. In: *An Osteopathic Approach to Diagnosis and Treatment.* 4th ed. Wolters Kluwer; 2021.
163. Seffinger MA, ed. Chapter 28. In: *Foundations of Osteopathic Medicine: Philosophy, Science, Clinical Applications, and Research.* 4th ed. Wolters Kluwer; 2018:673–695.
164. DiGiovanna E, Amen C, Burns DK. Chapter 100. In: *An Osteopathic Approach to Diagnosis and Treatment.* 4th ed. Wolters Kluwer; 2021.
165. Hreljac A. Impact and overuse injuries in runners. *Med Sci Sports Exerc.* 2004;36(5):845–849.
166. Ombregt L, Bisschop P, ter Veer HJ. *A System of Orthopaedic Medicine.* 2nd ed. Churchill Livingstone; 2003.
167. Tiemstra JD. Update on acute ankle sprains. *Am Fam Physician.* 2012; 85(12):1170–1176.
168. Steiner C, Staubs C, Ganon M, Buhlinger C. Piriformis syndrome: pathogenesis, diagnosis, and treatment. *J Am Osteopath Assoc.* 1987;87(4):318–323.
169. Oken B, Kuchera M. Chapter 4: Osteopathic considerations in neurology. In: *Complementary Therapies in Neurology: An Evidence-Based Approach.* Parthenon Publishing; 2003:49–90.
170. de Jonge S, van den Berg C, de Vos RJ, et al. Incidence of midportion Achilles tendinopathy in the general population. *Br J Sports Med.* 2011; 45(13):1026–1028.
171. van Dijk CN, van Sterkenburg MN, Wiegerinck JI, Karlsson J, Maffulli N. Terminology for Achilles tendon related disorders. *Knee Surg Sports Traumatol Arthrosc.* 2011;19(5):835–841.
172. Ross G, Macfarlane C, Vaughan B. Combined osteopathy and exercise management of Achilles tendinopathy in an athlete. *J Sports Med Phys Fitness.* 2018;58(1–2):106–112.
173. Krishna Sayana M, Maffulli N. Insertional Achilles tendinopathy. *Foot Ankle Clin.* 2005;10(2):309–320.
174. van Sterkenburg MN, van Dijk CN. Mid-portion Achilles tendinopathy: why painful? An evidence-based philosophy. *Knee Surg Sports Traumatol Arthrosc Off J ESSKA.* 2011;19(8):1367–1375.
175. Clain MR, Baxter DE. Achilles tendinitis. *Foot Ankle.* 1992;13(8): 482–487.
176. Maffulli N, Saxena A, Wagner E, Torre G. Achilles insertional tendinopathy: state of the art. *J ISAKOS.* 2019;4(1):48–57.
177. Chimenti RL, Cychosz CC, Hall MM, Phisitkul P. Current concepts review update: insertional Achilles tendinopathy. *Foot Ankle Int.* 2017;38(10):1160–1169.
178. Kujala UM, Sarna S, Kaprio J. Cumulative incidence of achilles tendon rupture and tendinopathy in male former elite athletes. *Clin J Sport Med.* 2005;15(3):133–135.
179. Achilles tendinopathy. *Physiopedia.* Accessed May 4, 2024. https://www.physio-pedia.com/Achilles_Tendinopathy
180. Martin RL, Chimenti R, Cuddeford T, et al. Achilles pain, stiffness, and muscle power deficits: midportion Achilles tendinopathy revision 2018. *J Orthop Sports Phys Ther.* 2018;48(5):A1–A38.

181. Ko VMC, Cao M, Qiu J, et al. Comparative short-term effectiveness of non-surgical treatments for insertional Achilles tendinopathy: a systematic review and network meta-analysis. *BMC Musculoskelet Disord.* 2023;24(1):102.
182. Pearce CJ, Tan A. Non-insertional Achilles tendinopathy. *EFORT Open Rev.* 2016;1(11):383–390.
183. Whitman JM, Childs JD, Walker V. The use of manipulation in a patient with an ankle sprain injury not responding to conventional management: a case report. *Man Ther.* 2005;10(3):224–231.
184. Howell JN, Cabell KS, Chila AG, Eland DC. Stretch reflex and Hoffmann reflex responses to osteopathic manipulative treatment in subjects with Achilles tendinitis. *J Am Osteopath Assoc.* 2006;106(9):537–545.
185. Hubbard TJ, Hertel J. Anterior positional fault of the fibula after subacute lateral ankle sprains. *Man Ther.* 2008;13(1):63–67.
186. Saini SS, Reb CW, Chapter M, Daniel JN. Achilles tendon disorders. *J Am Osteopath Assoc.* 2015;115(11):670–676.
187. Rabin A, Kozol Z, Finestone AS. Limited ankle dorsiflexion increases the risk for mid-portion Achilles tendinopathy in infantry recruits: a prospective cohort study. *J Foot Ankle Res.* 2014;7:48.
188. Collins CK, Masaracchio M, Cleland JA. The effectiveness of strain counterstrain in the treatment of patients with chronic ankle instability: a randomized clinical trial. *J Man Manip Ther.* 2014;22(3):119–128.
189. Krueger B, Becker L, Leemkuil G, Durall C. Does talocrural joint-thrust manipulation improve outcomes after inversion ankle sprain? *J Sport Rehabil.* 2015;24(3):315–321.
190. Fujii M, Suzuki D, Uchiyama E, et al. Does distal tibiofibular joint mobilization decrease limitation of ankle dorsiflexion? *Man Ther.* 2010; 15(1):117–121.
191. Grieve R, Clark J, Pearson E, Bullock S, Boyer C, Jarrett A. The immediate effect of soleus trigger point pressure release on restricted ankle joint dorsiflexion: a pilot randomised controlled trial. *J Bodyw Mov Ther.* 2011;15(1):42–49.
192. O'Neill S, Watson PJ, Barry S. Why are eccentric exercises effective for achilles tendinopathy? *Int J Sports Phys Ther.* 2015;10(4):552–562.
193. Mansur NSB, Faloppa F, Belloti JC, et al. Shock wave therapy associated with eccentric strengthening versus isolated eccentric strengthening for Achilles insertional tendinopathy treatment: a double-blinded randomised clinical trial protocol. *BMJ Open.* 2017;7(1):e013332.
194. Fan Y, Feng Z, Cao J, Fu W. Efficacy of extracorporeal shock wave therapy for Achilles tendinopathy: a meta-analysis. *Orthop J Sports Med.* 2020;8(2):2325967120903430.
195. Caudell GM. Insertional Achilles tendinopathy. *Clin Podiatr Med Surg.* 2017;34(2):195–205.
196. Maffulli N, Papalia R, D'Adamio S, Diaz Balzani L, Denaro V. Pharmacological interventions for the treatment of Achilles tendinopathy: a systematic review of randomized controlled trials. *Br Med Bull.* 2015;113(1):101–115.
197. Draghi F, Gitto S, Bortolotto C, Draghi AG, Ori Belometti G. Imaging of plantar fascia disorders: findings on plain radiography, ultrasound and magnetic resonance imaging. *Insights Imaging.* 2017;8(1):69–78.
198. Motley T. Plantar fasciitis/fasciosis. *Clin Podiatr Med Surg.* 2021;38(2): 193–200.
199. Buchanan BK, Sina RE, Kushner D. Plantar fasciitis. In: *StatPearls.* StatPearls Publishing; 2024. Accessed May 13, 2024. http://www.ncbi.nlm.nih.gov/books/NBK431073/
200. Mørk M, Soberg HL, Hoksrud AF, Heide M, Groven KS. The struggle to stay physically active-A qualitative study exploring experiences of individuals with persistent plantar fasciopathy. *J Foot Ankle Res.* 2023;16(1):20.
201. In brief: foot deformities. In: *InformedHealth.Org [Internet].* Institute for Quality and Efficiency in Health Care (IQWiG); 2022. Accessed May 13, 2024. https://www.ncbi.nlm.nih.gov/books/NBK513132/
202. Raj MA, Tafti D, Kiel J. Pes planus. In: *StatPearls.* StatPearls Publishing; 2024. Accessed May 13, 2024. http://www.ncbi.nlm.nih.gov/books/NBK430802/
203. Bubra PS, Keighley G, Rateesh S, Carmody D. Posterior tibial tendon dysfunction: an overlooked cause of foot deformity. *J Fam Med Prim Care.* 2015;4(1):26–29.
204. Hollander K, de Villiers JE, Sehner S, et al. Growing-up (habitually) barefoot influences the development of foot and arch morphology in children and adolescents. *Sci Rep.* 2017;7(1):8079.
205. Glasoe WM, Coughlin MJ. A critical analysis of Dudley Morton's concept of disordered foot function. *J Foot Ankle Surg.* 2006;45(3): 147–155.
206. Jain S, Mannan K. The diagnosis and management of Morton's neuroma: a literature review. *Foot Ankle Spec.* 2013;6(4):307–317.
207. Mak MS, Chowdhury R, Johnson R. Morton's neuroma: review of anatomy, pathomechanism, and imaging. *Clin Radiol.* 2021;76(3):235.e15–235.e23.
208. Bhatia M, Thomson L. Morton's neuroma—current concepts review. *J Clin Orthop Trauma.* 2020;11(3):406–409.
209. Mahadevan D, Venkatesan M, Bhatt R, Bhatia M. Diagnostic accuracy of clinical tests for Morton's neuroma compared with ultrasonography. *J Foot Ankle Surg Off Publ Am Coll Foot Ankle Surg.* 2015;54(4):549–553.
210. Sault JD, Morris MV, Jayaseelan DJ, Emerson-Kavchak AJ. Manual therapy in the management of a patient with a symptomatic Morton's neuroma: a case report. *Man Ther.* 2016;21:307–310.
211. Ajimsha MS, Binsu D, Chithra S. Effectiveness of myofascial release in the management of plantar heel pain: a randomized controlled trial. *Foot Edinb Scotl.* 2014;24(2):66–71.
212. Chitara. To compare the effectiveness of muscle energy technique versus myofasial release in pain and lower limb functional activity in subjects having planter fasciitis-a randomized control trial. 2017. Accessed May 4, 2024. https://www.semanticscholar.org/paper/To-Compare-the-Effectiveness-of-Muscle-Energy-in-in-Chitara/93c05fb1a7e590a8d3d7bc2f73f06103ff41a1c9
213. Wynne MM, Burns JM, Eland DC, Conatser RR, Howell JN. Effect of counterstrain on stretch reflexes, hoffmann reflexes, and clinical outcomes in subjects with plantar fasciitis. *J Am Osteopath Assoc.* 2006;106(9): 547–556.
214. Pawar P, Tople R, Yeole U, Gharote G, Panse R, Kulkarni S. A study on effect of strain-counterstrain in plantar fasciitis. *Int J Adv Med.* 2017;4:551.
215. Kanumalla R. Plantar fasciitis: diagnosis and management. Published September 12, 2019. Accessed May 4, 2024. https://www.medcentral.com/pain/foot-ankle/plantar-fasciitis-diagnosis-management
216. Rao A, Mehta S. A literature review of manual medicine for the conservative management of plantar fasciitis. *PNWMSRJ.* Accessed May 4, 2024. https://pnwmsrj.org/review/2020/10/a-literature-review-of-manual-medicine-for-the-conservative-management-of-plantar-fasciitis/
217. Wyatt LH. Conservative chiropractic management of recalcitrant foot pain after fasciotomy: a retrospective case review. *J Manipulative Physiol Ther.* 2006;29(5):398–402.
218. Thomson CE, Gibson JNA, Martin D. Interventions for the treatment of Morton's neuroma. *Cochrane Database Syst Rev.* 2004;(3): CD003118.
219. Kilmartin TE, Wallace WA. Effect of pronation and supination orthosis on Morton's neuroma and lower extremity function. *Foot Ankle Int.* 1994;15(5):256–262.
220. Munir U, Tafti D, Morgan S. Morton neuroma. In: *StatPearls.* StatPearls Publishing; 2024. Accessed May 4, 2024. http://www.ncbi.nlm.nih.gov/books/NBK470249/
221. Rasmussen MR, Kitaoka HB, Patzer GL. Nonoperative treatment of plantar interdigital neuroma with a single corticosteroid injection. *Clin Orthop Relat Res.* 1996;(326):188–193.
222. Saygi B, Yildirim Y, Saygi EK, Kara H, Esemenli T. Morton neuroma: comparative results of two conservative methods. *Foot Ankle Int.* 2005;26(7):556–559.
223. Matthews BG, Hurn SE, Harding MP, Henry RA, Ware RS. The effectiveness of non-surgical interventions for common plantar digital compressive neuropathy (Morton's neuroma): a systematic review and meta-analysis. *J Foot Ankle Res.* 2019;12:12.
224. Bennett GL, Graham CE, Mauldin DM. Morton's interdigital neuroma: A Comprehensive Treatment Protocol. *Foot Ankle Int.* 1995;16(12): 760–763.

92 Postural Considerations in Osteopathic Diagnosis and Treatment

LISA A. DESTEFANO ▪ MICHAEL L. KUCHERA

KEY CONCEPTS

- One of the five major approaches to osteopathic health care, the biomechanical-structural model, also referred to as the postural–biomechanical model, is built on fundamental principles to guide diagnosis and treatment.
- Optimal motor control strategies are key to postural compensation, balance, and structural tensegrity.
- Somatic dysfunction alters motor control and motor programming such that postural decompensation manifests.
- Coronal plane asymmetries can be functional but can also lead to significant structural decompensation.
- Postural decompensation in the sagittal plane, the most common cause of degenerative disk disease (DDD), is primarily due to loss of lumbar lordosis (LL) and pelvic retroversion.
- Radiographic studies and the osteopathic structural examination contribute important insights into static and dynamic postural relationships.
- Patient education is a primary source of initiating a successful, individualized management plan for issues of postural decompensation.

INTRODUCTION

Nearly 2,500 years ago, Hippocrates said, "The regimen I adopt will be for the benefit of my patients according to my abilities and judgment." The guidelines in this chapter lay out principles intended to enhance the ability to understand postural mechanisms as dynamic processes affecting interrelated patient neuromusculoskeletal function. With understanding and practice, the physician's judgment in prescribing individualized postural treatment regimens will evolve and improve.

The osteopathic biomechanical-structural model, also referred to as the postural–biomechanical model is one of five major clinical approaches to implementing osteopathic health care. Within it are important applications evolving from the four foundational osteopathic tenets:

- Body unity: Tensegrity links the physical body together. The attitude of physical posture often reflects (and is reflected in) the nonphysical attitude/aspects of the patient.
- Homeostasis: Postural alignment in a gravitational field and balance and postural compensation processes are largely automatic and self-regulating functions.
- Structure–function interrelationships: Physiologic motions of the musculoskeletal structures are a mainstay in diagnosing and treating somatic dysfunction. Biomechanics, kinesiology, and ergonomics are important foundational fields shaping the postural–biomechanical model.
- Rational osteopathic regimen based upon tenet application: The postural–biomechanical model has broad applicability in conditions involving pain or dysfunction of the locomotor system. Through the full understanding of somatic dysfunction, its role in precipitating or perpetuating neuroautonomic, respiratory–circulatory, and metabolic processes should also be apparent.

Implementing this model begins with a basic understanding of human motor control, movement patterns, and muscle and spinal balance, in addition to an appropriate structural examination, which involves evaluating much more than upright symmetry. This assessment contributes valuable information about the patient's intrinsic capability to resist constant gravitational stress and to adapt to ever-changing situations.

Viewing clinical findings through the "lens" of the postural–biomechanical model provides cogent insights regarding the function and dysfunction of key somatic anatomical, physiologic, and psychological structures. Such insights expand our understanding of both etiology and treatment intervention of a wide range of conditions—especially those related to commonly seen conditions with neuromusculoskeletal problems such as low back pain and headache.

Applying this model, the osteopathic physician strives to maximize function within the patient's structural limitations and prepare their neuromusculoskeletal system to optimally respond to postural balance. This requires accessing and sometimes "reeducating" peripheral and central biomechanically, physiologically, and psychologically linked interactions. This chapter will discuss why it is important to consider the impact of postural balance when evaluating a patient's health status. It will also outline the selection criteria that are clinically relevant for optimal use of this model. Finally, it will describe how to implement this model in planning effective treatment strategies for coronal and sagittal plane decompensation sequelae.

HISTORY AND UNIQUE POSTURAL CONTRIBUTIONS BY THE OSTEOPATHIC PROFESSION

Postural imbalance and radiographic assessment are not exclusive to the osteopathic profession. However, osteopathic physicians were among the first to integrate these two methods to better understand the relationship between the body's structure and function. The discovery of the roentgen ray in 1895 made it possible to visualize structures inside the body. Just 3 years later, the American School of Osteopathy in Kirksville, Missouri had acquired the second machine west of the Mississippi and used it to produce some of the earliest roentgenologic studies.[1] Hoskins and Schwab[2] introduced the standing postural x-ray series in 1921, opening the field for clinical interpretation and integration. Martin Beilke, in 1936, acknowledged the value of the technique by observing, "[t]he osteopathic profession can lay claim to these contributions as being strictly original and especially applicable to our approach in finding etiological factors in a given pathological process and in applying corrective measures."[3]

For many years, the lack of standardization for postural radiographic procedures prevented the profession from combining important multicenter data to develop a common set of guidelines for interpreting postural studies and formulating care. J Stedman Denslow and his coworkers called for such standardization in 1955,[4] although even today, relatively few academic healthcare institutions outside of the osteopathic profession have adopted the recommendation.

Standard protocols provided measurable, accurate, reproducible data correlating with the osteopathic palpatory structural examinations. The osteopathic profession documented the natural history of postural changes and published the consistency of radiographic postural findings in osteopathic literature decades later.[5,6] A compilation of many classic osteopathic articles discussing diagnosis, clinical impact, and treatment of postural subjects can be found in the 1983 Yearbook of the American Academy of Osteopathy, Postural Balance and Imbalance.[5] This compilation, along with a subsequent research study published in the Spine Journal[7] (itself based upon the osteopathic contribution to the importance of postural imbalance), sparked a second renaissance of osteopathic postural research that lasted nearly two decades.

Over the last two decades, osteopathic physicians have gained experience using osteopathic manipulative medicine and found many patients with common structural diagnostic findings, which vary depending on the individual postural–structural balance. Understanding the postural–structural model is essential for understanding somatic dysfunction and its implications in patient care.

BASIC POSTURAL PRINCIPLES AND DEFINITIONS

If we regard posture as the result of the dynamic interaction of two groups of forces—the environmental force of gravity on the one hand and the strength of the individual on the other—then posture is but the formal expression of the balance of power existing at any time between these two groups of forces. Thus, any deterioration of posture indicates that the individual is losing ground in their contest with the environmental force of gravity.[8,9]

It has been observed by many physicians that their patients often exhibit recurring patterns of dysfunction in their musculoskeletal systems.[10–12] Asymmetric functional behavior is commonly found in patients, whereas symmetric function is rarely identified. The universal pattern consists of a cluster of findings:

- pronated right foot
- anteriorly rotated right innominate
- posteriorly rotated left innominate
- right inferior pubis
- left superior pubis
- left-on-left forward sacral torsion
- lower thoracic scoliosis convex to the right
- left lumbar scoliosis
- anterior and inferior right shoulder girdle
- a left cervical scoliosis

Several theories have been postulated to account for this pattern, including the coriolis force of gravity and hand dominance. The dilemma remains a subject for future research. Indeed, this pattern is frequently seen in symptomatic and asymptomatic patients. The question is as follows: What is the clinical significance of this common pattern? Observation shows that if the patient's dysfunctions are out of this pattern, they are more clinically significant. A structural diagnostic finding that does not fit the pattern should alert the osteopathic physician that the presentation is unusual. The presence of the common universal pattern can result in practitioners unwisely treating patients in a cookbook fashion to restore motion to the segments in this universal pattern or treating the pain that is generated from the overuse of the facilitated soft tissues within the pattern. Patients should be viewed from their individual pattern and how it deviates from the more common one.

Analysis of posture provides an enormous amount of information about an individual. If and how the patient compensates or decompensates under gravity's continuous stress speaks volumes about that patient's homeostatic reserves. It offers clinically relevant insight into physical structure–function relationships, such as one's motor control strategies. Observing a patient's posture can give the clinician insight into their emotional, spiritual, and psychological state,[13] as well as potential physical pain and energy depletion that may contribute to nonphysical dysfunctions. The postural model includes various treatment strategies that aim to improve overall health or target the underlying cause of specific issues. These strategies are particularly helpful for managing spinal conditions like scoliosis or spondylolisthesis associated with postural decompensation. Improving posture can also alleviate symptoms of neuromusculoskeletal conditions, as it helps reduce the constant strain of gravity that can lead to myofascial trigger points and other somatic dysfunctions. By reducing nociception and segmental facilitation and supporting the osteopathic respiratory–circulatory model, improving posture can help maintain homeostasis and achieve clinical goals.

Motor Control

In addition to the articular restrictions noted in the universal pattern, there are consistent patterns of asymmetric muscle function, with some muscles becoming tighter and others becoming inhibited and weak.[14] Motor control refers to the complex process by which the central nervous system coordinates and regulates the body's movements. It involves feed forward integration of sensory information, planning and execution of movements, and the continuous adjustment of motor commands based on feedback from the periphery and environment. Motor control encompasses voluntary (conscious) and involuntary (reflexive) movements to efficiently move the body through space or function. Motor control utilizes central somatosensory processing at multiple levels: the spinal cord, the brainstem, the cerebellum, the diencephalon, and the cerebral hemispheres, including the cerebral cortex and basal ganglia. This is combined with feedforward and feedback mechanisms from the visual and vestibular systems. The peripheral somatosensory system comprises muscles, tendons, ligaments, and fascia whose proprioception consists of mechanoreceptors such as free nerve endings (FNE), Ruffini corpuscle (RC), laminated corpuscles (LC), muscle spindles (MS), and Golgi tendon organ (GTO). It is the peripheral somatosensory system that is most vulnerable to injury.[10,15–17]

One's "movement pattern" or "motor program" is the very individualized outcome of one's motor control processes gradually "learned" by the evolving peripheral–CNS interrelationship.[10] Influences begin with forces in utero; then, from birth, throughout the growth process, and into senescence, soft tissue structures, and functions influence and are influenced by the cumulative functional demand placed upon them by postural compensation. Our movement patterns are ingrained and repetitive, becoming unconscious. Like learning to play an instrument, once the senses have developed the pattern of movement required to make the sound, it is no longer obvious to the conscious mind. Motor learning is a physiologic process utilized by the nervous system to improve function and facilitate recovery from injuries.

According to the work of Vladimir Janda and Karel Lewit, any serious, painful disorder at the periphery will cause a central response. The motor program (pattern) will change to spare the painful structure and become permanent even though the painful stimulus is gone. Lewit described this process as a dysfunction in the "locomotor system." He and Janda believed this process could evolve into *muscle imbalance and postural overuse.* The motor program alterations can occur at the motor system's cortical, muscular, or joint level. Whichever it may be, this pathology is typically reflex in nature in a *completely intact nervous system.* Janda defined this pathologic process as *functional impairment* and charged that the pathology of the motor system influenced the function of muscles in a typical consistent pattern throughout the neuromusculoskeletal system.[10, 15–18]

For a better understanding of postural regulation and motor control, it is essential to consider skeletal muscles' unique structure, specialization, and properties. The development of tightness and shortness occurs in muscles with phasic functions, whereas the development of weakness and inhibition occurs in muscles with tonic functions. This imbalance between the two muscle systems can lead to serious consequences. Inner discoordination of muscles can cause overactivity, overuse, or facilitation of some muscle fibers, leading to tendinopathy or enthesopathy.

It is crucial to comprehend muscle function to understand the functional limitations of muscles and their relationship with patients who have neuromusculoskeletal dysfunctions. Therefore, there is a need to expand the classifications of muscle function. Margaret Rood's categorization of stabilizer and mobilizer muscles,[19] which classified them by their function, has been widely accepted:

- Stabilizer muscles are monoarticular or segmental, deep muscles that work eccentrically to control movement and have static holding capacities.
- Mobility muscles are biarticular or multisegmented, superficial muscles that work concentrically with acceleration of movement and produce power.

Bergmark introduced the concept of local and global muscle systems[20]:

- The local system includes muscles that originate or insert at the vertebrae to control the spine curvature and provide mechanical stability.
- The global system involves superficial muscles that link the thorax and pelvis, producing larger torque and force.

Later Mottram and Comerford introduced the local stability, global stability, and global mobility systems for functional classification of muscles.[21]

- The local stability muscles have a particular tonic role in maintaining segmental stability. These muscles do not produce motion as there is little length change with their activity.
- The global stability muscles generate force to control the dynamic range of movement. They work eccentrically to produce movement with stability.
- The global mobility muscles generate torque to produce large ranges of movement. These phasic muscles work concentrically to produce power and speed and work eccentrically to decelerate high loads.

Each classification of muscles exhibits functional impairment. Local stability and global stability muscles experience inhibition and weakness, whereas global mobility muscles consistently demonstrate tightness and facilitation.[21]

Postural Control Strategy

Efficient postural control is achieved through the integration of visual, vestibular, and proprioceptive afferent feedback mechanisms and dynamic feedback mechanisms.[22] Feedforward mechanisms are used for planned or anticipated movements, where the body uses its local and global stabilizers to pretense the system. This allows the global mobilizers to move the body in space efficiently and effectively. Feedback mechanisms, on the other hand, are used for unanticipated postural corrections.[21]

Dynamic Joint Stability

It is fascinating to observe how our movement patterns and somatic dysfunction are related to one another, which often raises questions about which came first and which contributes to the persistence of the other. Joint or muscle dysfunction? Most likely, it is a combination of both. This concept is best exemplified in the spine, particularly at the vertebral level, with the work of Panjabi. He simplified spinal stability into active, passive, and neural subsystems.[23,24]

The *active subsystem* is made up of the muscles controlling the neutral range of motion of the spine. These muscles act as local stabilizers, controlling a single segment within the neutral range of motion with predominately eccentric contraction. They take their cues "arthrogenically" from the articular and joint surface mechanoreceptors.[25] These receptors detect changes in muscle, segmental motion range, joint capsule, or tendon strain. The *passive subsystem* includes bone, the joint capsule, the intervertebral disk, and supporting ligaments. The *neural subsystem* comprises the mechanoreceptors within the passive subsystem and proprioceptors within the active subsystem, providing feedback information to the cord and the active subsystem.

ARTHROGENIC MUSCLE INHIBITION (AMI)

AMI results in changes to motor control, which ultimately lead to joint and clinical instability. Injuries to the peripheral somatosensory system (such as tendons, ligaments, and fascial mechanoreceptors) greatly impair the transmission of information from joint sensory receptors, resulting in impaired spinal reflex excitability and impaired cortical activity. This leaves the joint vulnerable to further injury. Ultimately, joint injury or dysfunction (somatic dysfunction) leads to changes in the feedback control of the joint or vertebral segment due to corrupt neural signaling to the cord, known as deafferentation. The active subsystem or stabilizer muscles become inhibited, and the dynamic stability of the joint is lost. The segmental neutral range of motion then becomes dependent on the passive subsystem, which, over time, can hypertrophy or fail.[12, 26–33]

Clinical instability of the spine begins with joint dysfunction and can result in spondylosis, degenerative disk changes, and/or stenosis. The author believes that all joints follow the same rules as the spine, and that all joint subsystems are interdependent for stabilization. These subsystems function efficiently within a neutral range of stability.

Tensegrity/Biotensegrity

Human tensegrity (biotensegrity) refers to the concept of the human body as a tensegrity structure, which means a structure that maintains its shape and stability through a balance of tension and compression forces. In the context of the human body, biotensegrity describes how bones, muscles, and connective tissues work together to create a stable and flexible structure. The muscles and tendons provide tension, while compression is carried by the bones. This interconnectedness allows the body to distribute forces efficiently, maintain balance, and absorb impact, contributing to strength, resilience, and mobility.[34]

The concept of joint stability and tensegrity is essential in understanding the mechanism of somatic dysfunction. The biotensegrity model also plays a significant role in understanding the effects of postural stress, compensation, adaptation, or decompensation. Introduced by architect Buckminster Fuller in 1929 from the words tension and integrity, tensegrity modeling has been successfully applied to biologic systems.[35] A critical premise behind biotensegrity and dynamic stability is closed kinematic chains (CKCs).[36] CKCs are substantially better than biomechanics in our understanding of biologic movement and dynamic stability of joints. CKCs couple multiple parts into continuous mechanical loops that allow the structure to regulate complex movements and provide an energy-efficient mechanism that optimizes multiple mechanical functions. In humans, CKCs are modular units nested within others at multiple size scales as part of an integrated movement system that, at a macro and micro level, acts in synergy with the nervous system and is evolutionarily designed to respond to specific functional and locomotor needs. Integrating multiple functional units into a more comprehensive movement system is harmonious with the concept of biotensegrity: a structural design principle that recognizes that stability and ease of movement are not due to the strength of individual components but because of the way the entire system is configured to distribute mechanical forces.[37]

This system describes how most of the integrated structure–function arrangements in living systems require little energy for their maintenance (postural integrity). How bony tension elements are held together by connecting elastic elements (ligaments and antigravity muscles) helps create/maintain the balance between stability and strength, and how forces are dispersed through the body diffusely. And the predictable total structural response to tension changes anywhere in the body. The model also helps to explain why certain global or local host factors adversely affect the capability of some individuals to successfully resist the effect of gravity strain or why injury to local sites (e.g., a foot or knee) may lead to secondary symptoms like back pain or headaches. For these reasons, several clinical models cite biotensegrity principles[38–40] when discussing the importance of postural balance and treatment.

Myofascial Force Transformation

Muscular fascia is specialized deep fascia whose mechanics greatly influence skeletal muscle function. Classically the force of muscle contraction is transmitted exclusively to the ends of each muscle fiber onto the myotendinous junction. However, in addition to the myotendinous junction, muscle fibers have fascial connections to each other along their full length, allowing every contraction to transmit force onto fascia arranged in series with the muscle. This muscular force transmission onto the muscle's fascia or the endomysium, perimysium, and epimysium defines a highly mechanoreceptive and proprioceptive, coordinated, functional *myofascial force transmission system.*[41]

Mechanoreceptors and proprioceptors, found within the muscular fascia, report information to the spinal cord and brain on body position and movement, both normal and abnormal. Sophisticated neuromuscular reflexes constantly maintain body posture, and prepare for, initiate, and continue movement patterns. The muscle function is an integrated and highly complex process, motor control through the central nervous system from the premotor cortex through the brainstem, cerebellum, and spinal cord, and finally to the final common pathway, the alpha motor neuron to skeletal muscle.[42] This control system for muscle function is highly complex. It has voluntary and involuntary components highly influenced by afferent impulses from the mechanoreceptors within the articular and fascial systems. Movement patterns are symmetric, coordinated, and free when this central control system works efficiently. When altered, inefficient and uncoordinated movement results.

Line of Gravity, Center of Gravity, and Sagittal Alignment

Posture is defined as the distribution of body mass in relation to gravity over a base of support. As an adult shifts from a standing to a seated posture, this base of support shifts from the feet alone to a base that includes the pelvis. Theoretically, a center of gravity for the entire body could be mathematically approximated using force plates or computer-assisted summation of horizontal cross-sectional measurements for any given posture. However, in a living human, the center of gravity must remain a theoretical point representing the weight center of the body for the given posture; the points about which the body balances in every direction from moment to moment.

Postural balance is best evaluated by measuring the *line of gravity* instead of the center of gravity.[43] This is because the center of gravity changes based on the physical activity and position of the body. In healthy individuals who are asymptomatic, the line of gravity is the outcome of a reaction between the ground and an ideal dynamic chain that connects the trunk, pelvis, and lower limbs.[44] An ideal line of gravity, shown in Figure 92.1, is measured using a force plate. With an anteroposterior view, this vertical line, perpendicular to the ground, passes through the middle of the sacrum. When viewed laterally, it should pass through L3 and slightly posterior to the femoral heads.[43] In order to accurately measure the line of gravity using upright radiographic images, it is necessary to establish pelvic and spinal parameters. This will allow for a more comprehensive evaluation of the overall sagittal alignment of the spine in relation to the pelvis. See Table 92.4.

OPTIMAL POSTURE AND MOVEMENT

As mentioned earlier, the human body's postural control and movement strategies are incredibly complex and involve multiple systems working together to provide balance and stability during everyday activities. The optimal standing posture requires balancing the body's cervical, lumbar, and thoracic curves while standing under the influence of gravity. To better understand how gravity affects one's posture, we can break down the walking cycle and analyze the movement strategies of the shoulders and upper arms separately. It is also essential to consider and observe the stability of the pelvis, trunk, shoulders, and neck while analyzing postural alignment.

Gait and Pelvic Stability

The gait kinetic chain begins during the loading response phase (pronation) of walking. Upon heel strike, the dorsiflexed talocrural joint and inverted subtalar joint rapidly plantar flex and evert, respectively, unlocking the transversal tarsal joint and activating the tibialis anterior and posterior muscles to co-contract in an eccentric effort to decelerate the medial foot as it pronates from heel strike to midstance—the tibialis anterior also co-contracts with the ipsilateral glute medius and TFL in an attempt to stabilize the pelvis in the transverse plane over a relatively fixed femur. The fibularis longus eccentrically controls dorsiflexion of the talus, having transitioned from its role of co-contracting with the tibialis anterior just before the stance phase to stabilize not only the foot

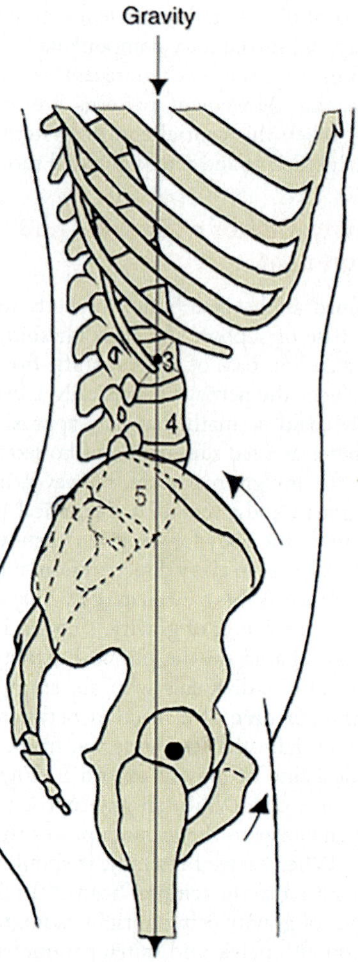

Figure 92.1. The line of gravity. The sagittal vertical axis, corresponding to the "plumb line" in the sagittal plane, is measured as the distance between the line originating in the center of the body of C7 and the posterior-superior corner of the sacrum.

but the knee, as well, as it moves over the foot. Progress from heel strike to midstance requires the tibia and fibula to internally rotate and the fibula to descend, triggering the fibularis longus and biceps femoris muscles to co-contract to stabilize the ipsilateral SI joint via their pull on the ipsilateral sacrotuberous (ST) ligament.[45]

The pelvis is pronating throughout this time as we progress from heel strike to toe-off, which involves the sacrum rotating toward the stance limb on an ipsilateral oblique axis. During stance on the right, the sacrum rotates right about a right oblique axis. Assuming that the lumbar spine is functioning normally when the sacrum rotates to the right and bends to the left, it causes the pelvis on the stance side to adduct (shift right in the frontal plane) and rotate internally (in the transverse plane). In this scenario, if the stance is on the right, the lumbar spine will bend to the right and rotate to the left. As the right foot lifts off the ground, the right innominate bone shifts from posterior to anterior rotation, and the right pubis bone moves superiorly. Meanwhile, the left innominate bone goes through the opposite movement.

Stabilization of the pelvis throughout the gait cycle is critical, and it happens in all three planes, just like all joints involved in the gait cycle. In the frontal plane, the ipsilateral glute medius and glute minimus are the primary stabilizers, with some help from the iliacus. The psoas is a hip flexor AND a strong hip external rotator. As we transition throughout the stance phase, the psoas plays a role in eccentrically controlling the internal rotation of the ipsilateral femur (transverse plane motion). The ipsilateral psoas also works with the contralateral quadratus lumborum to provide "vertical stability" throughout the base of the spine while the abdominals and 4th layer spinal muscles, combined with the thoracolumbar fascia, provide further "corset" stabilization of the trunk. From heel strike to midstance, the fibularis longus co-contracts with the biceps femoris to stabilize the ipsilateral SI joint.[45] After this time, the ipsilateral gluteus maximus takes over to extend the hip and control trunk flexion over the stance femur. The takeover of gluteus maximus should be simultaneous with co-contraction of the contralateral latissimus dorsi, becoming the stabilizer of the stance-side SI joint via the connection of the thoracolumbar fascia.

Thorax Stability

Dynamic stability requires optimal local and global stabilizing system function that ensures that the vertebral load is optimally distributed to all supportive structures. As one better understands the torso's role in force transmission from the thorax and upper extremities, it becomes clear that lumbopelvic stability is a prerequisite for thoracic stability.

Maintaining good posture while sitting or standing is important to have a stable pelvic base and proper abdominal muscle function. This helps distribute load into the lumbodorsal fascia and the torso, the main contributors to myofascial force transmission. The force is transmitted from the spinotransverse muscles (semispinalis, multifidus, and rotatores) to the epaxial fascia or vertebral aponeurosis.[46] This then transmits tension into the serratus posterior superior and inferior, which then lifts the upper four ribs and sternum and lowers the lower ribs, respectively. In response, a force couple is generated between the serratus posterior inferior fascia, external oblique fascia, and the rectus sheath. This load then reconnects to the upward moment of the rib cage and sternum. This simplistic view of thorax stability can only occur when core or torso stability and intra-abdominal pressure are optimized. For this reason, treatment of common clinical problems of the thorax begins with fully optimizing the neuromusculoskeletal function of the lumbopelvic region.

The stability of the thorax is highly dependent on the fascial "passive tension system," derived from the paraspinal muscles, rib cage and intercostal muscles, spinotransverse muscles, vertebral aponeurosis, thoracodorsal fascia, diaphragm, and abdominal musculature. This tension system provides sufficient stability to the spine to match the varying stability demands that arise due to changes in spinal posture and static and dynamic loads.[47] A proprioceptive neural control system, although less defined, is also inherent in this passive tension system and is extremely important.

Scapular Stability and Motion

Deep fascia is made up of axial and appendicular forms. Appendicular deep investing fascia invests the muscles of the extremity and scapula. The appendicular muscles that attach to the thorax and trunk include the pectoralis major and minor, rhomboid major and minor, trapezius, latissimus dorsi, and serratus anterior and serratus posterior.[48] Of these appendicular muscles, the rhomboids, middle and lower trapezius, and serratus posterior superior and inferior all have investing fascia that gains tensile support from the vertebral aponeurosis overlying the epaxial musculature. In addition, the latissimus dorsi muscle fasciae invest into and gain tensile support from the superficial lamina of the thoracolumbar fascia and contralateral gluteal fasciae.

This tensile support for upper extremity function is generated as a part of the proprioceptive role of the lumbodorsal fascia in preparation for upper extremity perturbation.[49,50] In anticipation, the torso muscles contract, transferring tensile force onto the deep and superficial axial fascia and muscles and then to the superficial appendicular fasciae. This force couple simultaneously stabilizes and prepares the thorax for rotatory torque and stabilizes the scapula onto the thorax. This stability optimizes scapulohumeral rhythm or the interaction between the scapula and the humerus.

During arm elevation, the scapula rotates upward, tilts posteriorly, and moves into external rotation. The scapula is dependent on muscle activity for stability as well as activity.[51] As stated above, the trapezius and the rhomboid stabilize the scapula, while the trapezius and serratus anterior provide upward and external rotation.

Cervical Stability

The literature defining the fascial continuum of the deep lamina of the thoracodorsal fascia or vertebral aponeurosis into the cervical shows it blending with the fascia overlying the splenius cervicis and capitis muscles.[52,53] The morphology of the investing fascia of the cervical spine and its impact on cervical passive connective tissue force transmission is not defined in the literature. The majority of the research on the stability of the cervical spine suggests that the postural functions of the deep cervical flexors (longus colli and longus capitis) and posterior cervical muscles (semispinalis cervicis and capitis, splenius cervicis and capitis) work in concert to stabilize the cervical spine in all directions.[54,55] It is conceivable that the posterior cervical muscles are sheathed in the "epaxial fascia" (surrounding those muscles that develop posterior to the transverse processes and receive their innervation by branches of the posterior or dorsal primary ramus) much like the rest of the epaxial muscles. This allows the extensor moment of the posterior cervical muscles to be countered by the deep cervical flexors, creating a stable yet mobile column on which the cranium is supported. Within this construct, the extensor moment of the cervical spine must be generated from the thoracic vertebral aponeurosis and thus rely on a properly stabilized thorax.

In the thoracic region, the epaxial fascia continues as the vertebral aponeurosis. This structure is continuous with the deep lamina of the posterior layer of the thoracolumbar fascia inferiorly.[48] It continues superiorly to attach to the spinous processes of the thoracic vertebra and laterally to the angle of the ribs. It lies superficial to the spinotransverse muscles and, in optimal situations, is passively and actively tensioned by forces derived from the torso onto the deep lamina of the thoracolumbar fascia and contraction of the spinotransverse muscles, respectively. Mechanically, the combined tension of the vertebral aponeurosis acts to extend and lift the anterior rib cage. This lifting of the rib cage is further supported by tensions of the vertebral aponeurosis onto the overlying fasciae of the serratus posterior superior and inferior.

The most superior border of the vertebral aponeurosis lies between the serratus posterior superior and the splenius capitis and cervicis muscles and accompanying fasciae. Adding the medial investing fascia of the rhomboids, this area appears to be a thickened area of the aponeurosis. It is conceivable that this thickened area of the aponeurosis supports the superior thoracic aperture and stabilizes the cervical spine onto the thorax.

POSTURAL ADAPTION AND COMPENSATION

The optimal or ideal posture suggests a perfect distribution of the body mass around the instantaneous line of gravity. The compressive force on spinal disks is balanced by ligamentous tension, and there is minimal energy expenditure from postural muscles.[56] However, structural or functional factors and somatic dysfunction frequently leading to AMI prevent achieving and maintaining optimal or

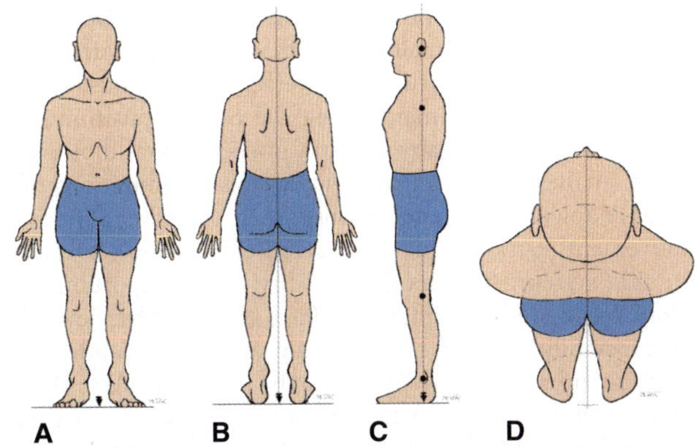

Figure 92.2. A–D. An optimally balanced standing postural alignment in the coronal plane (**A, B**) normally divides the body into two equal parts. The center of gravity line, or "weight-bearing line," runs midway between the feet, through the pubic symphysis, along the midline of the vertebral column, and bisects the center of the suprasternal notch and glabella. Ideally, there would be no rotation in the horizontal plane of any body region (**C**) and no coronal plane side-bending asymmetry. Optimal postural alignment in the sagittal plane (**D**) has been characterized by a weight-bearing line that passes through the lateral malleolus, midknee, femoral head, anterior third of the sacral base, middle of the body of the L3 vertebra, humeral head, and external auditory meatus. (Courtesy of William A. Kuchera, DO, FAAO, with permission.)

ideal posture. When this occurs, postural balance and motor control strategies manifest adaptive and compensatory patterns to provide maximum postural function within the existing structure of the individual,[57] contributing to sagittal or coronal plane imbalance.

Maintaining optimal postural alignment (Fig. 92.2) is crucial for analyzing balance and preventing problems related to spinal imbalance. This alignment is characterized by a line of gravity, which represents the area of reaction with the ground. To improve spinal imbalance, especially in the sagittal plane, it is essential to determine the position of the line of gravity.[43] This line passes through specific points, including the lateral malleolus, midknee, femoral head, anterior third of the sacral base, middle of the body of the L3 vertebra, humeral head, and external auditory meatus. When the body fails to align optimally to its center of gravity, it can cause functional overloading of postural muscles, leading to pain-sensitive soft tissues and joint facets that were not adapted for direct, sustained weight-bearing function.[58]

Multiple factors negatively influence optimal alignment and function and while the degree of influence varies, the accumulation of the factors is certain for symptoms to exist. Somatic dysfunction and sagittal imbalance are two major factors primarily because of their ability to disrupt CKC links and thus alter the critical reflex components of motor control and biotensegrity such as myofascial force transformation, pronation, and the active, passive, and neural subsystem integration. The following are examples of the effects of somatic dysfunction and sagittal imbalance on postural balance and motor control.

The Functional Spinal Unit

The functional spinal unit (FSU) (motion segment or vertebral unit) consists of two adjacent vertebrae, the intervertebral disk (IVD), the facet joints (FJ) and capsules, and adjoining ligaments. It provides passive (intrinsic) stability for that individual unit of motion. Bone, IVD, ligaments, and the facet joint capsule also contain mechanoreceptors that act as transducers, sending a continuous afferent flow of proprioceptive information on the FSU motion, position, and load to the spinal cord that responds with efferent feedback local stabilizer (intertransverse, interspinous, multifidus) muscular action for maintaining the neutral position of the FSU.[59–61] In this fashion, any vertebra in each spinal motion segment, the smallest FSU, can perform various combinations of the main and coupled movements, during which a number of bony and soft movement restraints guarantee stability.[24] The loss of stability within this system, or clinical instability, is an important, often unknown cause of back pain, particularly at the lumbar level. Like stability, instability also lacks a generally accepted definition.[24]

In joint or somatic dysfunction, the joint capsules and the mechanoreceptors they contain generate abnormal afferent transducer signals causing altered or delayed efferent motor response–AMI.[25,27] The altered or delayed efferent motor response increases the likelihood of intrinsic stress/strain on the passive subsystem, which elicits abnormal feedback to the CNS, creating a vicious cycle that may lead to:

- Inflammation with activation of nociceptors.
- Increased global stabilizer muscle overuse and fatigue.
- Increased stiffness or play in the system leading to bone remodeling and spondylosis.

The main purpose of the vertebral column is to enable movement during daily activities and maintain an upright posture while providing optimal dynamic joint stability. In his work, Gracovetsky explains that the synchronized coupled movement of the spine during the gait cycle plays a crucial role in transferring force from the ground to the trunk, which allows for forward momentum of the body. This is essential for proper movement and function of the body during the gait cycle. The combination of coupled side-bending and rotation of the spine, together with spinal lordosis, has been experimentally demonstrated to generate an axial torque estimated to be sufficient to drive the pelvis.[62,63] Type II dysfunctions of the lumbar or thoracic spine and loss of lumbar lordosis (LL) disrupt the transformation of axial torque, causing segmental torque, which is detrimental to the IVD and FJ.

AMI plays a critical role in understanding the impact of joint somatic dysfunction on postural abnormalities. Even minor changes in a single functional vertebral unit can result in significant biomechanical, tensile, and ergonomic alterations elsewhere in the body. For instance, the type-II flexed, side-bent, and rotated (FRS) segment in the lower thoracic region can lead to the inhibition of the lower trapezius, which results in the loss of ipsilateral lower scapular stabilization.[61,64–66]

The Vertebral Column–Osteopathic Construct

Balancing against gravity over an instantaneous base of support is not a passive process. Functional postural demands will also alter the overall structure, usually first at the anatomical transition zones. For example, consider the compensatory response to gravity that begins as soon as an infant attempts to assume an upright position and continues throughout life (Fig. 92.3). To stand upright with the least amount of effort, the infant learns to balance the center of gravity by positioning various segments of the spine over the base of support formed by the region of anatomy immediately underneath. The "toddler" learning to walk exercises postural control to adjust for falling forward as the lower extremity mass is moved forward.[67]

These evolving regional changes typically occur at the anatomical transition zones, which include:

- The lumbopelvic region, where the pelvis joins the lumbar spine.

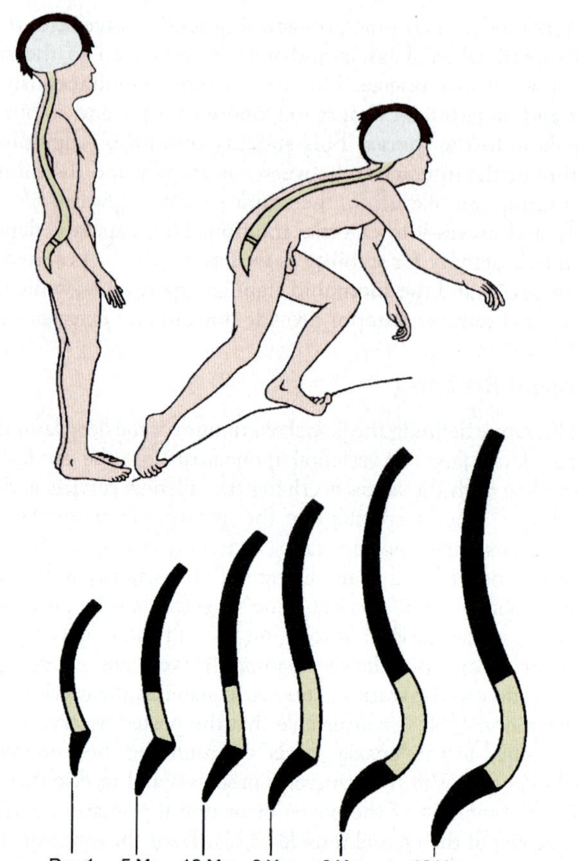

Figure 92.3. Changes in sagittal plane spinal curves from day 1 through age 10 years. (From Kapandji IA. *The Physiology of the Joints*. Vol. 3. Churchill-Livingstone; 1974:17, with permission.)

- The thoracolumbar region (or inferior thoracic outlet), where the lumbar spine joins the thoracic cage.
- The cervicothoracic region (or superior thoracic inlet), where the thoracic cage joins the cervical spine.
- The craniocervical region, where the cervical spine joins the head.

In this fashion, two secondary lordotic group curves normally develop in the cervical and lumbar regions to counterbalance the primary thoracic curve present at birth. Together, these three sagittal spinal curves will increase the resistance to vertical loads much better (up to 17×) than one single sagittal plane curve.[24] They allow a person to function upright yet be flexible enough to allow coordinated compensation in multiple regions and planes.

Most ordinary and compensatory spinal motions involve a group of vertebral segments. In thoracic and lumbar group curves, such spinal motions follow Fryette's first principle of physiologic motion and are necessary to allow for positional changes in the body. This means that when these regions of the spine are in their neutral position (an absence of marked flexion or extension) and side-bending is introduced, the vertebrae rotate into the produced convexity.[68] (Rotation is to the opposite side of side bending.)

Fryette type I dynamic spinal curves may also be produced in the coronal plane by unilateral multisegmental muscle contraction (long restrictor):

- Muscle tension creates a concavity, which results in a lateral curve of three or more segments, and the involved thoracic and/or lumbar vertebrae rotate into the convexity.
- Such type I curves disappear when the muscle relaxes.

- Type I curves become a biomechanical problem when the multisegmental muscle becomes facilitated (long restrictor), and the spine can no longer return to its resting position. This behavior is commonly due to more than one type II dysfunction "stacked" one on the other, common in spinal transition zones.

The total somatic body reaction manifested as postural changes in response to less-than-ideal conditions is better understood by applying knowledge of spinal biomechanics. For example, the bottom-up spinal response to unleveling the sacral base in the coronal plane or an anatomically short lower extremity is guided by spinal biomechanical principles. To keep eye level at the opposite end of the body, the lumbar vertebrae above the sacrum start to side-bend away from the low sacral base, creating a scoliotic curve. As this type I lumbar group curve forms, all other spinal regions capable of adjusting their alignment attempt to accommodate the new postural balance. Similarly, spinal biomechanics largely direct the postural response in a top-down spinal response to certain craniocervical dysfunctions or deformations.

Early postural compensation is associated with developing a longer single lumbar or lumbothoracic scoliotic curve—convex on the side of the low sacral base. In this C-shaped scoliotic curve, the horizontal cephalad planes are typically depressed on the side opposite the depressed pelvic horizontal plane. Later, the compensatory mechanisms redistribute postural responsibilities, forming several lateral curves. In this more chronic postural compensation (an S-shaped scoliotic curve), the shoulders and the greater trochanteric planes are typically depressed on the same side as the depressed sacral base. (The typical biomechanical response to sacral base unleveling is shown in Fig. 92.4.)

Postural terminology applied to group curves is apparent in some situations and requires a thorough understanding of clinical medicine in others.

- Normal postural curves in the sagittal plane are termed kyphotic (forward bending) or lordotic (backward bending) curves; however, when they are pathologic, they are termed kyphosis and lordosis, respectively.
- Similarly, when pathologic, coronal side bending (or scoliotic curves) of more than 5 degrees is termed scoliosis.
- Scoliosis is sometimes called rotoscoliosis because rotation and side bending are inseparably linked. The pathology may be called kyphorotoscoliosis if all three planes are significantly involved.

In postural compensation and adaptation, group curves in each plane typically assume certain patterns. The most common patterns have group curves occurring in one direction in one region and in the opposite direction in the adjacent spinal regions, alternating so that the body can maintain some postural balance. Most

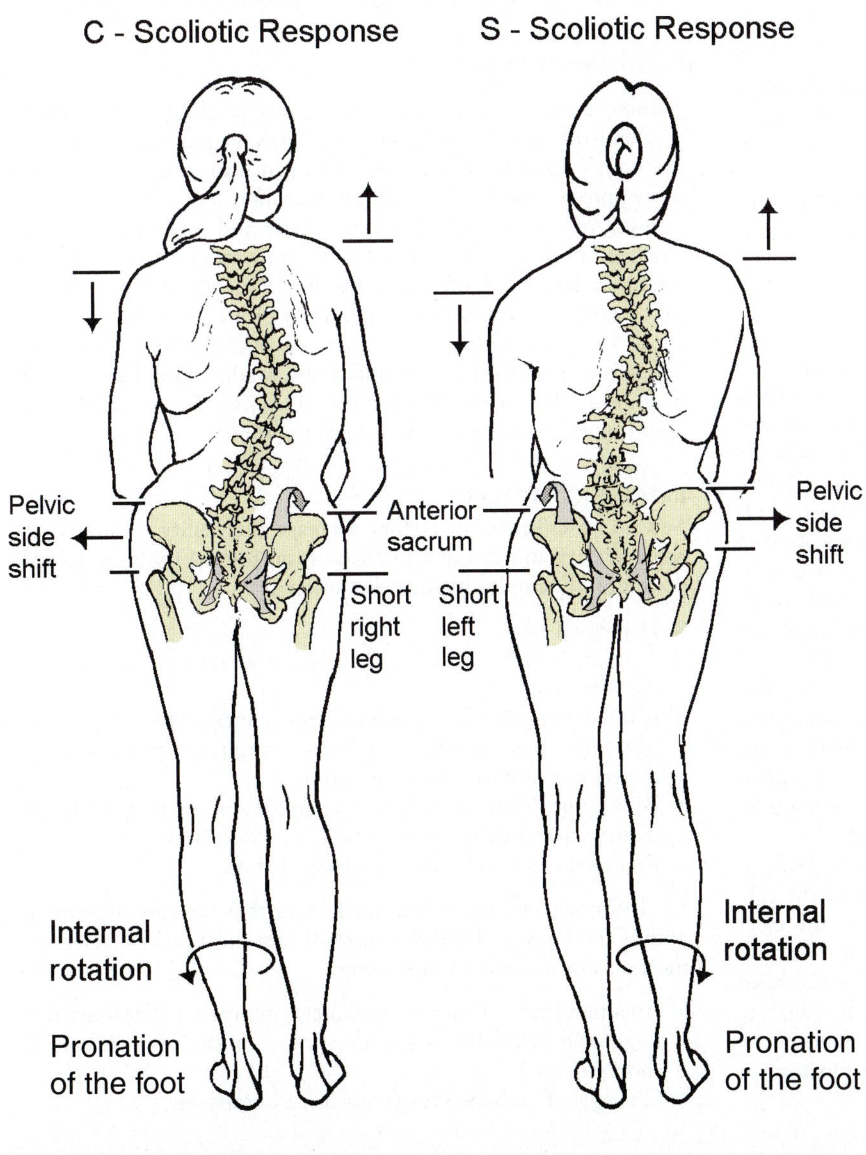

Figure 92.4. Typical postural compensation for short-leg syndrome. (Courtesy of William A. Kuchera, DO, FAAO.)

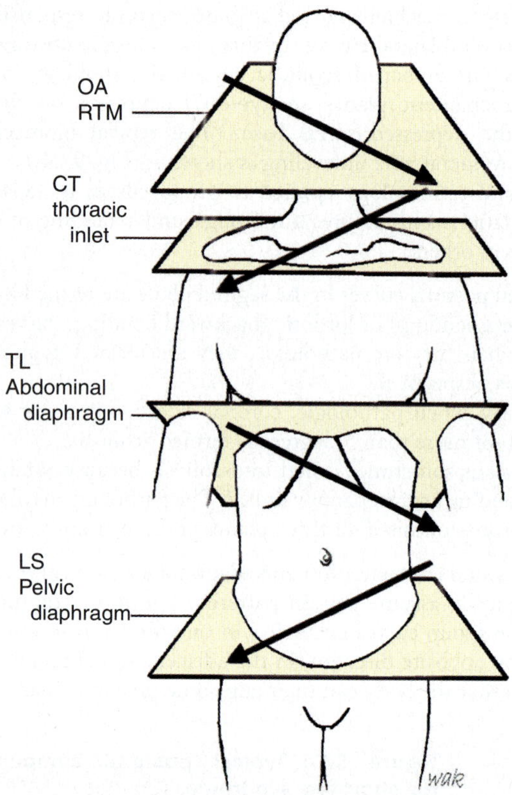

Figure 92.5. Compensation in the horizontal planes: alternating pattern of rotation at transition zones. (Courtesy of William A. Kuchera, DO, FAAO.)

commonly, these changes occur within the so-called transitional regions—areas where anatomic structure changes create the potential for the greatest functional change (Fig. 92.5).

The Vertebral Column–Postural Construct

The ability to stand upright and maintain a horizontal gaze is a unique characteristic of humans. When standing, the human body oscillates within a cone whose apex is situated on the floor between the feet. In the early 1970s, Jean Felix Dubousset described the standing mechanism as the "cone of economy."[69] This system requires several anatomical elements to function properly, including feet with a broad surface area for bearing weight, vertical lower limbs with extended knees, a neutral pelvic position, spinal contours that maintain LL, and the head's center in the same vertical axis as the pelvis ensuring that the axial skeleton is in balance with the feet, lower limbs, and pelvis all the way up to the spinal segments and the cranium. All these components work together, allowing for adaptive motion in all directions on the horizontal plane. Normally, the body maintains balance within a small "cone" with minimal muscle activity. However, in individuals with pathologic lesions of the locomotor system, maintaining a standing posture requires a larger "cone" and greater muscle activity.

When examining a complete skeleton of the human body, it is important to consider the pelvis as the last vertebra of the spinal skeleton. The "pelvic vertebra" plays a crucial role in the erect posture of the human being, as it is interposed between the trunk and lower limbs. Similarly, the "cephalic vertebra," the entire head considered a vertebra, plays a subtle role in the erect skeleton. The head's weight at the other end of the articular chain is the weight of a pendulum, as standing is regarded as the function of an "inverted pendulum."

The "chain of balance"[70] is a system that consists of all the bones and joints in the human body, from the cephalic vertebra to the pelvic vertebra and the skeleton of the lower limbs. This system adapts to provide static and dynamic support, creating a series of curves that allow for mobility and stability. If one element of the chain is affected by a disease or disorder, the other elements in the chain can compensate and adapt to maintain balance.

POSTURAL DECOMPENSATION

The force of gravity is universal and can cause stress to our body systems, affecting our posture. While it affects everyone, some people may have a harder time resisting its effects due to certain intrinsic or extrinsic risk factors that weaken their support mechanisms. Additionally, some individuals may have biomechanical disadvantages that make it difficult to compensate for the force of gravity. Therefore, posture should be considered as a secondary finding based on the impact of gravity on one's body.[71–75]

Chronic attempts to counteract gravity can result in various manifestations of pathophysiology. The most prominent indicators are altered postural alignment and recurring somatic dysfunction. As the body's compensatory mechanisms become increasingly strained, or when the degree of pathologic change is unable to withstand gravitational force, other signs and symptoms of postural decompensation may worsen in frequency and severity.[71,76]

Predisposing Factors

Various conditions can cause stress on postural compensatory mechanisms, whether present since birth, acquired, or related to the body's anatomy. Such conditions can lead to the acceleration of symptoms and postural decompensation. As a result, chronic postural functional demands can initiate and speed up structural changes. This is a classic example of how structure and function are interrelated and affect one another. Patients who have intrinsic or extrinsic factors that make them prone to these conditions are at the highest risk of experiencing postural decompensation. Therefore, it is crucial to identify these predisposing factors while diagnosing the osteopathic postural model by conducting an appropriate history and physical examination.

INTRINSIC FACTORS

Several host (intrinsic) factors decrease the ability to adequately resist gravity and create a predisposition toward postural decompensation. Examples include the following:

- Decreased LL
- Age (intrinsic factors related to muscle weakness, fascial elasticity, bone mass, etc.)
- Altered integrity or response from antigravity soft tissues (systemic hypermobility syndrome, various connective tissue disorders, muscular dystrophy, etc.)
- Poor tissue health (related to poor nutrition, inactivity with subsequent deconditioning, metabolic diseases, etc.)
- Fear avoidance and poor movement habits

Examples of host (intrinsic) factors that increase asymmetry within the body and thereby magnify demands on compensatory mechanisms include the following:

- An altered base of support (unilateral pes planus [flat foot], dysfunctional gait following ankle sprains or strains, anatomically short leg, etc.)
- Changes of body habitus (pregnancy, obesity, etc.)

- Congenital bony asymmetries (scoliosis, small hemipelvis, wedge vertebrae, etc.)
- Ergonomic factors associated with poor sitting or standing habits.
- Strenuous posturing required by certain work environments or recreational activities

EXTRINSIC FACTORS

Traumatic postural decompensation occurs when macrotrauma or recurrent microtraumas disrupt the spine's muscular, ligamentous, or bony stability.

- Such decompensation may occur more frequently in patients with a history of automobile accidents or surgical laminectomies (macrotrauma) or of carrying heavy loads for significant distances or certain high-level sports activities, as exist in gymnastics, weightlifting, golf, or football[75] (microtrauma).
- Fractures of the spine, pelvis, or lower extremity may produce sacral base unleveling or the need for other compensatory changes above the area of the trauma.
- In addition, a few occupations increase extrinsic gravitational stress, such as certain military pilots who experience multiple G-forces.

RESPONSES OF TISSUES

Skeletal–Arthrodial Response

THE VERTEBRAL COLUMN

Initially, when ligaments, disks, and joint capsules of the spine are damaged, they contain mechanoreceptors that generate abnormal transducer signals. These signals are sent to the CNS, resulting in an altered sensorimotor response. This response then increases the mechanical stress of bony and joint spinal components. It also elicits an abnormal feedback response by the FSUs and muscles themselves, thus creating a vicious cycle. This cycle ultimately leads to inflammation, muscle fatigue, and activation of nociceptors that result in acute and chronic pain. If the noxious forces resulting from increased segmental motion due to clinical instability or loss of dynamic stability are not neutralized, bone remodeling will occur, according to Wolff law, over time.[24,77]

The three columns in our spine work together to support our body weight.[78] In the posterior column, the FJ have two essential functions–controlling movement direction and amplitude and distributing loads.[79] Normally, the posterior facets take on anywhere from 0% to 33% of the load, depending on one's posture. However, in cases of hyperlordosis, prolonged weight loading, and disk degeneration, the percentage can increase to 70%. The size of the FJ gradually increases in the sagittal plane to accommodate the increasing functional demand. Eventually, the FJ become remodeled (osteoarthritis) and destabilized, and the posterior ligaments undergo degenerative changes, which can result in degenerative spondylolisthesis.

No FSU would be complete without its IVD composed of superior and inferior cartilaginous endplates, annulus, and nucleus. The IVD has a special structure that helps resist tension and compression. It acts like a ligament and controls the spine's movements in three dimensions. The outer fibers of the annulus are the first to respond to abnormal movement in a healthy spine. The central nucleus acts as a shock absorber for the spine, distributing stress evenly when loads are symmetrical. When loads are asymmetric, the nucleus tends to move toward the area of lower pressure, putting tension on the annulus fibers. Bending movements on the spine cause the outermost layers of the annulus to stretch on the tensile side and compress on the opposing side. Unlike the nucleus, the annulus has high anisotropy in tension due to its laminar architecture of collagen fibers, which requires a significant amount of force to deform. The tensile properties of the annulus are not uniform, with the anterior annulus being stiffer than the posterior annulus and the outer annulus being stiffer than the inner ring. When the pressure in the nucleus of a healthy disk increases, it generates circumferential loads in the annular lamina. As a result, the annular fibers resist stretching and bulging under axial compression. During axial rotation, the annular fibers experience torsional shear stresses, which can eventually lead to delamination[24] and tearing.

The nucleus pulposus experiences hydrostatic pressure due to its high hydration, similar to a pressurized cylinder.[24] Hydrostatic pressure differs from other loading conditions due to the assumption of constant cell and pericellular matrix volumes.[63] Hydrostatic pressure magnitude also varies diurnally in a manner that depends on spinal alignment and physical activity. Hydrostatic pressure magnitude is reduced with aging due to the disk's lower proteoglycan and water content. The nucleus pulposus is the first structure within the disk to show signs of degeneration. During this process, the shear stiffness increases, the pressure decreases, the compression stiffness increases, and the permeability decreases. Subsequently, the nucleus pulposus undergoes a change in composition, transforming from a fluid-like to a solid-like behavior. This, in turn, affects the dynamic viscoelastic properties of the entire disk and triggers a degenerative cascade.[80,81]

Despite the literature, conventional osteopathic wisdom would argue that aging alone cannot explain the etiology of the degenerative disk disease (DDD) cascade.[79] Asymptomatic paraspinal denervation (AMI) may exacerbate, precipitate, or occur in concert with spinal degeneration,[82,83] altering the sensorimotor control of the FSU. Of the three paraspinal muscles innervated by the posterior primary ramus (iliocostalis, longissimus, and multifidi), the multifidi work with the neural arch ligaments to provide compressive forces important for segmental control (see more detail below).[45,84]

Loss of LL[85] and lumbar segmental joint dysfunctions, particularly those that limit extension, lead to non-neutral behavior of the lumbar spine during gait and segmental overload of the FSU.[62,63] More importantly, lumbar segmental dysfunction contributes to a delay in paraspinal muscle firing,[86–88] which is critical for segmental stabilization during function of any sort. The paraspinal muscles work synergistically with the transversus abdominis and internal oblique to transfer tension to the posterior layer of the thoracolumbar fascia, thereby bracing and girdling the paraspinal muscles.[48] Simultaneously, the tension to the posterior layer of the thoracolumbar fascia causes an extensor moment, which lifts each lumbar segment against the vertical load provided by the iliopsoas and the quadratus lumborum muscles. This synergistic system also includes the thoracoabdominal and pelvic diaphragms, which allow for optimized intra-abdominal pressures vital for overall trunk stability and optimized venous and lymphatic flow from below upward into the central circulation.

Unopposed vertical loading from the iliopsoas and quadratus lumborum and loss of segmental control lead to inappropriate segmental compression and torque. With time, the lumbar intervertebral disks can lose height and fluid content. Loss of vertebral height leads to increased segmental movement, which, without segmental control, will eventually lead to IVD derangement, facet, and ligamentum flavum hypertrophy, heralding clinical instability, spondylosis, and spinal stenosis.[89–91]

THE HIP AND KNEE

Degenerative change in the hip occurs when there is accentuated functional demand and asymmetry. Leg length discrepancy (LLD) is mildly correlated with hip and, more significantly, lumbar spine and knee DJD.[92,93]

Structural adaptations in LLD involve torsional changes in pelvic posture. In anatomical LLD, the ilium rotates posteriorly on the longer leg side and anteriorly on the short leg side relative to the contralateral ilium. Additionally, LLD can cause a lateral tilt of the pelvis, leading to functional lumbar rotatory scoliosis, with the convexity usually found on the short leg side. While not universally accepted, some authors believe functional scoliosis can become structural over time.[6,90,94] These adaptations may be responsible for permanent spinal changes, such as asymmetrical facet joint angles, disk degeneration, osteophytic spurs, facet joint OA, disk herniation, muscle imbalance, and scoliosis. A major contributor to the degree of permanent spinal changes is leg length inequality exceeding 10 mm.[95,96]

In addition to LLD, hip degenerative changes often accompany lumbar degenerative changes in patients with a decreased LL (an increased pelvic incidence [PI]).[54,93,97] The pelvic ring acts as the hinge between the spine and the legs, coupling LL with hip extension in the standing position with minimal energy expenditure.[98] Pelvic retroversion and lumbar flattening are the hallmarks of sagittal plane decompensation (see below). Loss of LL leads to degenerative changes in the lower lumbar IVDs and stiffness of the region.[91] Pelvic retroversion leads to acetabular anteversion or coronal and medial-facing orientation, which forces the femoral head upward into extension and external rotation (supination). Loss of LL could negatively impact knee and hip health due to its effect on dynamic pelvic and femoral kinematics essential for healthy hip joint activity.[99–101]

Despite the osteopathic convention that degenerative arthritis of the hip joint often develops on the long leg side, very few studies have actually shown a correlation between the two.[93,95,102]

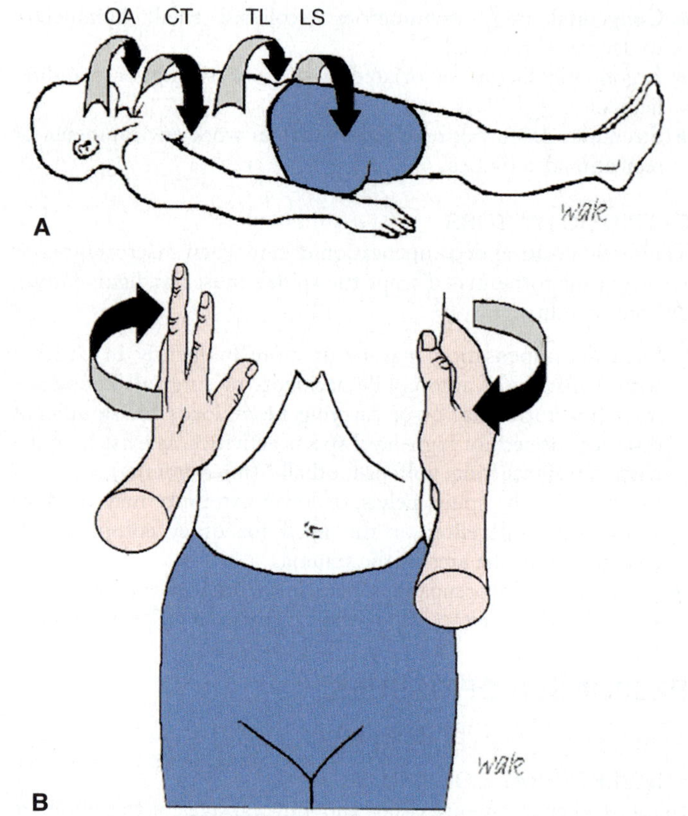

Figure 92.6. **A** and **B.** The interregional compensatory fascial pattern will consist of an alternating directional pattern in one or multiple planes occurring at the transitional regions of the body. When alternating, such patterns typically reflect the impact of long-term upright postural compensation on the fascia. (Courtesy of William A. Kuchera, DO, FAAO.)

Regional (Transitional Zone) Myofascial Response

Postural patterning influences and is influenced by the fasciae and related structures. J Gordon Zink described patterns[37] clinically relevant to diagnosing and treating fascial compensation and decompensation. Based on the palpatory fascial preference to motion, these fascial patterns may be classified as ideal, compensated, or uncompensated (Fig. 92.6 is one of two compensated—meaning directionally alternating—regional patterns). The postural influence on fascial patterning is important for understanding the postural management effect in improving the respiratory–circulatory model.[55] Conversely, fascial preference influences the tissues and skeletal structures of each region.

Fascia plays a crucial role in ensuring optimal muscle function by regulating the transmission of force from the muscle, which allows the tendon to use its elastic energy more effectively at higher frequencies. Fascia can transmit up to 30% to 50% of the longitudinal stress from the muscle to the proximal tendon.[103] Fascia also functions with muscle as an energy reserve, working with the ground-reactive force to absorb, store, and release kinetic energy with every step. Somatic dysfunction or chronic postural changes (motor programming and movement pattern alterations) will cause AMI and can restrict the ability of fascia to transmit force or store energy. This can lead to predictable acute muscle overload or repetitive muscle action that causes fatigue (Fig. 92.7). In such cases, the muscle activity must perform beyond the sustainable capacity of the muscle resulting in persistent or recurrent myofascial trigger point pain syndromes.[104] (See Chapter 43 Clinical Assessment: Viscerosomatic, Somatosomatic, Somatovisceral Reflexes; Counterstrain Points, Myofascial Trigger Points, and Chapman Reflexes for further discussion.)

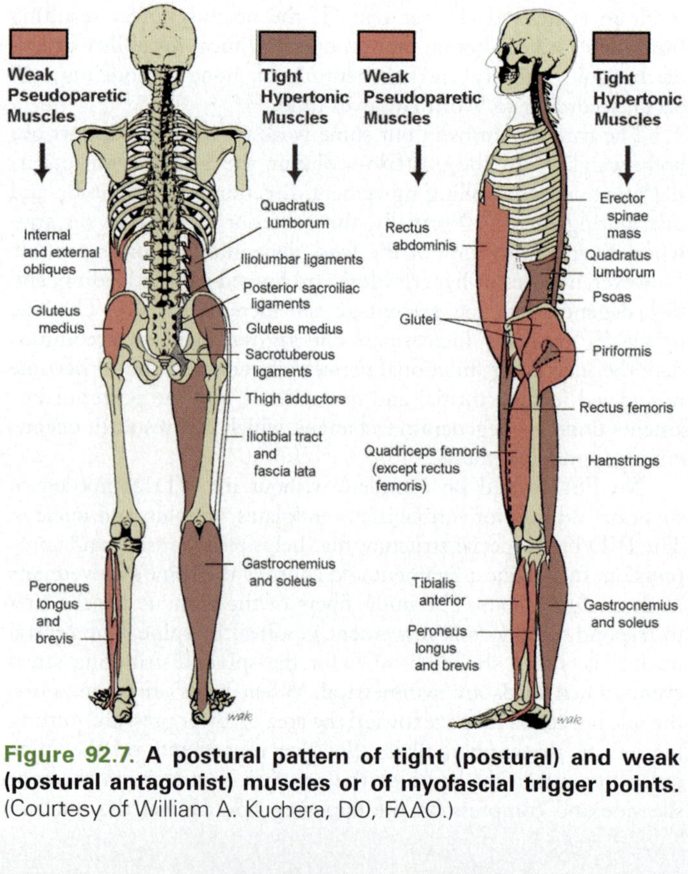

Figure 92.7. **A postural pattern of tight (postural) and weak (postural antagonist) muscles or of myofascial trigger points.** (Courtesy of William A. Kuchera, DO, FAAO.)

TABLE 92.1

Examples of Postural (Hypertonic-Prone) Muscles and Symptoms

Lower Body Muscle(s)	Symptoms
Iliopsoas	Inability to stand straight (psoas posturing); knees flexed; recurrent L1 or L2 NN somatic dysfunction; pain referred to back and anterior groin; positive Thomas test; may falsely increase PI measurements and decrease LS angle unless treated
Quadratus lumborum	Low back pain referred to the groin and hip; may be misdiagnosed as gr. trochanteric bursal disorder; exhalation 12th rib somatic dysfunction; diaphragm restriction
Thoracolumbar erector spinae	Low back pain; recurrent thoracolumbar somatic dysfunction; segmental facilitation
Hamstrings	Pain sitting or walking; pain disturbs sleep; pain referred to posterior thigh; straight leg raising limited mechanically; the combination of tight hamstrings on one side and tight rectus femoris on the other usually suggests postural strain seen with pelvic rotation in the horizontal plane; may cause false-positive straight leg raising test
Rectus femoris	Pain deep inside the knee; the combination of tight hamstrings on one side and tight rectus femoris on the other usually suggests postural strain seen with pelvic rotation in the horizontal plane
Piriformis	Pain down posterior to the thigh; may entrap peroneal portion of the sciatic nerve; perpetuated by (and perpetuates) sacroiliac dysfunction; associated with pelvic floor dysfunction, dyspareunia, or prostatodynia
Thigh adductor (short)	Pain referral to the inguinal ligament, inner thigh, and upper medial knee
Gastrocnemius-soleus complex	Nocturnal leg cramps; pain referral to upper posterior calf, instep, and heel
Upper Body Muscles	**Symptoms**
Upper trapezius	Most likely the muscle in the body to develop TrPs; headache refers to occiput and/or to side of the head near the temple
Sternocleidomastoid	The SCM clavicular head is rich in proprioceptors (informs the CNS where the head is with respect to the body), so dysfunction leads to postural instability and spatial disorientation; may veer off to one side while walking; refers pain to the forehead bilaterally and ear. Sternal head may cause visual and ANS symptoms
Levator scapulae	Stiff neck (especially with rotation); pain to the base of the neck, vertebral border of the scapula, and posterior shoulder
Pectoralis major (upper)	May cause chest wall pain with radiation down the arm in anginal pattern (if on left) and intense nipple hypersensitivity
Pectoralis minor	Prominent in slumped postures with rolled-in shoulders, increased kyphosis, and anterior neck carriage; may entrap brachial nerve and/or axillary artery leading to radially sided dysesthesias and possible loss of the radial pulse
Cervical erector spinae	Headache and neck pain; recurrent cervical somatic dysfunction
Scalenes	The entrappers may entrap neurovascular bundle (especially the lower trunk of the brachial plexus and/or subclavian vein) with dysesthesias to the fifth digit and/or puffy hands; may also reflexly limit thoracic duct return leading to upper extremity swelling; TrPs may cause dysesthesia into the thumb and index finger side of the hand; may lead to recurrent elevated rib 1–2 somatic dysfunction

Recognizing predictable patterns involving multiple muscles (Tables 92.1 and 92.2) should suggest muscle imbalance as a possible underlying cause. In these patients, treatment of somatic dysfunction and dysfunctional postural alignment yield more lasting results than treatment of the secondary recurrent myofascial trigger points or muscle imbalances in isolation.

Ligamentous Response

Stabilizing ligaments are stressed in individuals with sagittal and coronal plane imbalance—in particular, the articular facet joint capsules and neural arch, iliolumbar, sacrotuberous (ST), and long dorsal (posterior) sacroiliac ligaments, each having its own predictable sclerotomal pain pattern.[105] Lumbar articular facet capsule inflammation and joint degeneration are substantial contributors to low back pain. The FJ and neural arch ligaments play a crucial role in load transmission by providing posterior load-bearing support and stabilizing the motion segment during flexion and extension. They also limit axial rotation, contributing to the mechanism of rotational kinematics.[106–108]

The neural arch ligaments consist of the ligamentum flavum, interspinous ligament, supraspinous ligament, and intertransverse ligament (Fig. 92.8). Although all four of the neural arch ligaments are anatomically able to be isolated, as long as the multifidi are functioning properly, they function as a unit.[45] The FJ play a very important role in protecting the IVD from shear forces, axial rotation, and excessive flexion but are not well suited to compressive forces. Postural imbalance[109] and somatic dysfunction play a large role in facet injury, inflammation, and degeneration. Type II somatic dysfunctions limiting lumbar extension will lead to progressive muscle delay (AMI) and possible atrophy of the multifidi muscles causing the neural arch ligamentous (passive subsystem)

TABLE 92.2

Examples of Phasic (Pseudoparesis-Prone) Muscles and Symptoms

Lower Body Muscle(s)	Symptoms
Gluteus minimus	Pain characteristic when arising from chair; pain referral to buttock and lateral and posterior thigh; "pseudosciatica"; antalgic gait; positive Trendelenburg test
Gluteus medius	Pain aggravated by walking; pain referral to posterior iliac crest and sacroiliac joint; positive Trendelenburg test
Gluteus maximus	Restlessness; pain sitting or walking uphill; antalgic gait
Three Vasti (but *not* rectus femoris)	Buckling knee syndrome; weakness going up stairs; thigh and knee pain; patellar tracking imbalance; chondromalacia patellae
Rectus abdominis	Increased lordosis; constipation
Tibialis anterior	Pain referred to great toe and anteromedial ankle; may drag foot or trip when tired
Upper Body Muscle(s)	**Symptoms**
Mid-/lower trapezius	Refers pain and tenderness to the region of the upper trapezius
Latissimus dorsi	Causes chronic midthoracic back pain but with the slack muscle; no particular position offers relief
Rhomboids	Ache between shoulder blades; cracking or scrunching sounds when the shoulder moves
Deep cervical flexors	Longus colli and longus capitis muscles leading to recurrent cervical somatic dysfunction; loss of neck stability

unit to become overloaded, leading to aberrant compressive and shear force onto the disk and facets of the lower lumbar spine.[85,107] Additionally, because the facet capsule is encased in fascia that is continuous dorsally with the ligamentum flavum and ventrally with the investing fascia of the vertebral body,[45] instability may contribute to hypertrophy of these structures.

The iliolumbar ligaments (ILL) are critical for stabilizing the lumbar vertebrae relative to the pelvis[75] and restricting the sagittal motion of the sacrum.[110] They are usually the first structures to be affected by sacral and innominate rotations (Fig. 92.9). The attachments of these ligaments become tender to palpation when stressed. ILL osteophytes may occur with long-standing postural strain because calcium is laid down along the lines of stress (Wolff law). Functional changes include tenderness, edema, and pain referred to the lower extremity (Fig. 92.10).

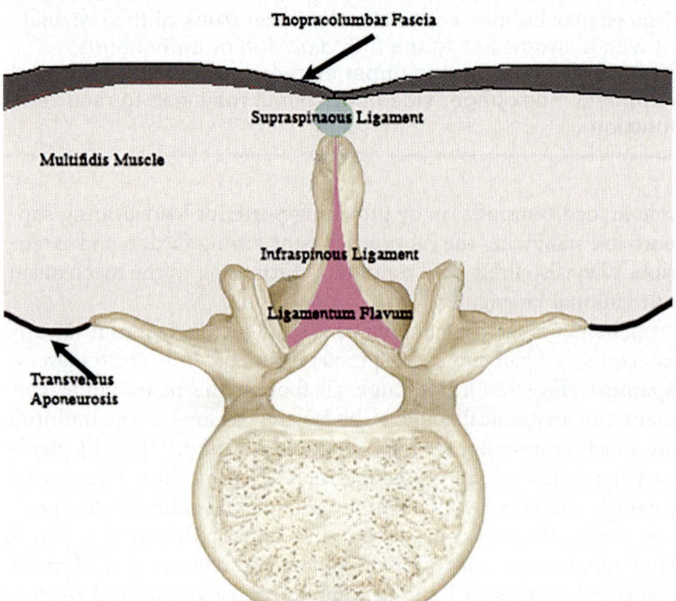

Figure 92.8. Neural arch ligaments.

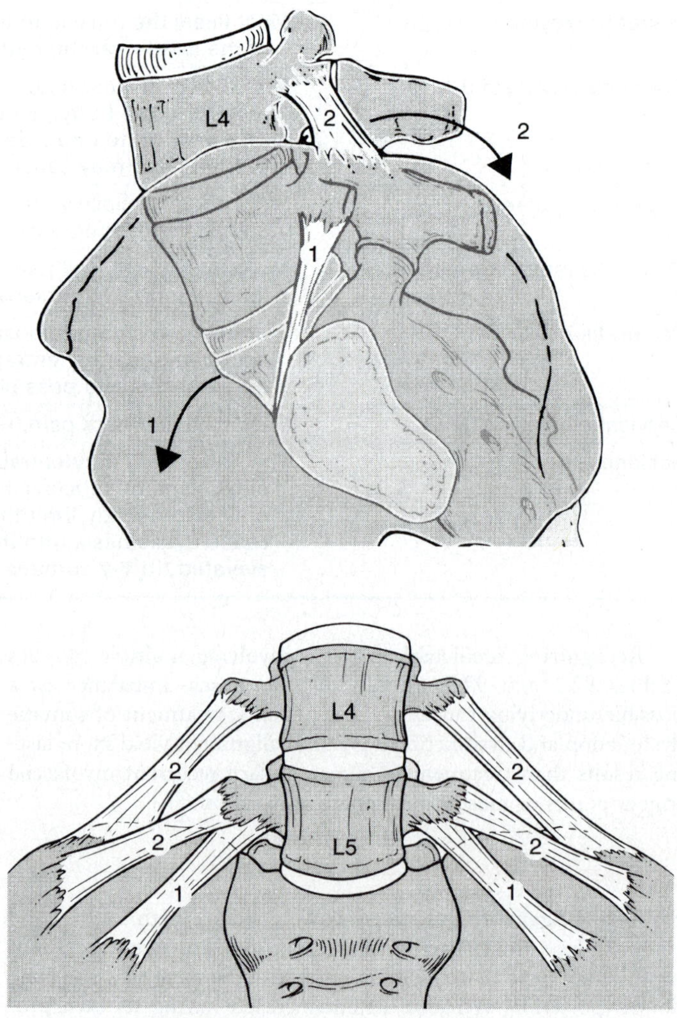

Figure 92.9. Anterior rotation of sacrum bilaterally stresses ligamentous fibers labeled (*1*). Posterior rotation of innominates bilaterally stress ligamentous fibers labeled (*2*).

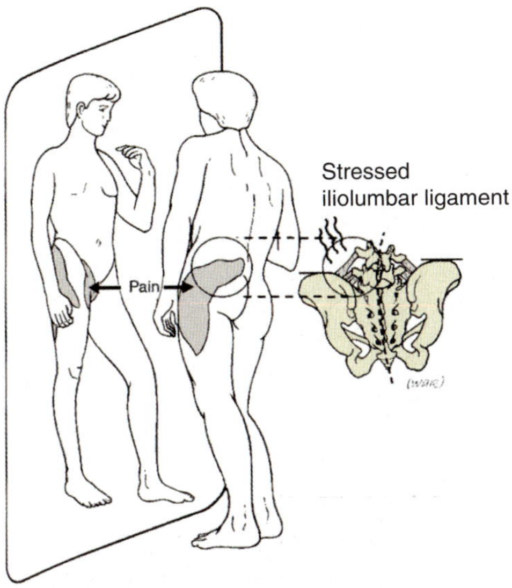

Figure 92.10. Iliolumbar ligament pain pattern from postural imbalance. (Courtesy of William A. Kuchera, DO, FAAO.)

ST ligament and long dorsal sacroiliac (LDSI) ligaments resist anterior and posterior rotation of the sacrum, respectively (Fig. 92.11A, B).[111] The LDSI ligament connects the sacrum and the posterior superior iliac spine (PSIS), whereas the main part of the ST ligament connects the sacrum and ischial tuberosity,[112,113] allowing ground reaction kinetic forces to pass from the biceps femoris to the ST and into the posterior SI ligaments, then through the thoracodorsal fascia to the contralateral latissimus dorsi during gait (force closure of the SIJ).[111] This critical kinetic chain is incumbent on the extension moment provided by sacral nutation, LL, and proper timing of the contraction of the gluteus maximus muscles. Sacral counternutation stresses the LDSI ligaments and causes AMI of the gluteal muscles. This imposes the extensor moment production onto the erector spinae muscles. Erector spinae hypertonicity and unilateral tenderness of the LDSI ligament are thus clinical signs of lumbosacral dysfunction.

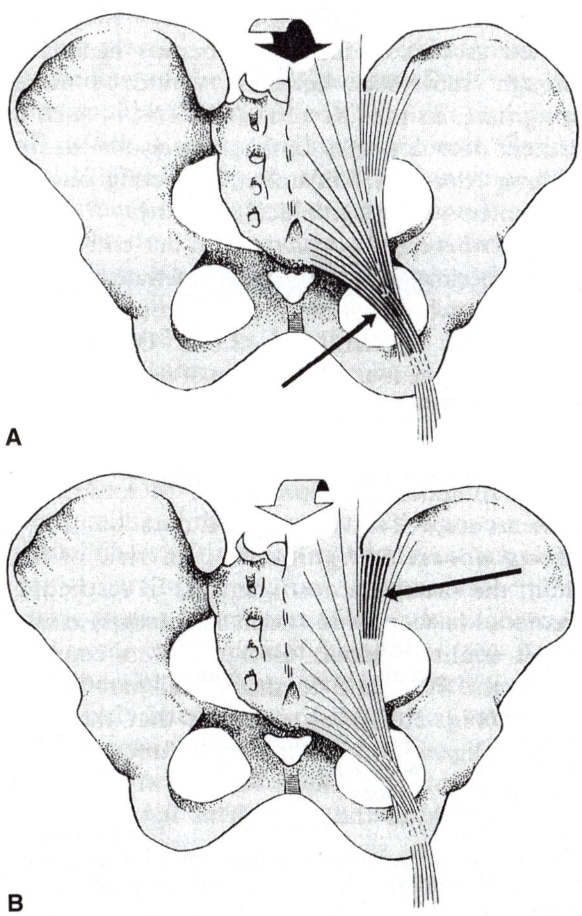

Figure 92.11. A. Anterior sacral rotation winds up ST ligament. **B.** Sacrum rotation posteriorly winds up the LDSI ligament. (From Vleeming A, Mooney V, Dorman T, et al., eds. *Movement, Stability, and Low Back Pain: The Essential Role of the Pelvis.* Churchill-Livingstone; 1997, with permission.)

Response of Related Neural, Vascular, Lymphatic, and Visceral Elements

The postural model overlaps with assessment and treatment considerations related to the respiratory–circulatory, and neurologic models. All three models look to transition zones as key areas for identifying and treating somatic dysfunction. The transition zones are closely linked to transverse diaphragms; dysfunction in these areas influences venous and lymphatic return. Sagittal and coronal imbalance has significant implications for circulatory, cardiac, diaphragmatic, and respiratory functions. Sagittal plane imbalance can also affect autonomic function by causing changes in sensorimotor control, which involves the cervical spine's proprioceptive afferentation from ligaments, muscles, and disks. These components play a significant role in supplying the necessary neurophysiologic information for feed forward and feedback responses through linkages to the central nervous, vestibular, and visual systems.[114]

It has been reported that patients with scoliosis, even as young as adolescence, experience alterations in neurodynamics, manifesting as mechanosensitivity of the nervous system structures (upper and lower limb tension tests), reduced range of motion, or sensory disturbances.[115–117]

POSTURAL RADIOGRAPHS

AP and PA Radiographs

Posture and postural diagnoses involve understanding static (structural) and dynamic (functional) characteristics; x-ray images primarily visualize the static or structural aspect of posture and are used when indicated. Postural x-ray views taken according to a standardized protocol (with precise foot placement, locked knees, and consistent arm positions) can be accurately and consistently measured for static postural information by radiologists. Postural radiographs should be correlated with various dynamic aspects of the clinical examination, including palpation, to uncover relevant structure–function and postural–biomechanical insights. To maximize the interpretation of the static information provided by postural x-rays, the osteopathic postural model also presumes that somatic dysfunction is corrected as much as possible before sending the patient for a postural radiographic series.[118] The somatic dysfunctions that are most likely to create significant transient postural asymmetry on these films are:

- Innominate shear (e.g., superior or up-slipped innominate)
- Iliopsoas muscle spasm[119]
- Quadratus lumborum spasm[120]

Examples of Castellvi classification of lumbosacral transitional vertebral anomalies appear radiographically and have a potentially significant impact when implementing the postural model are depicted in Figure 92.12 and Table 92.3.[121] Several of

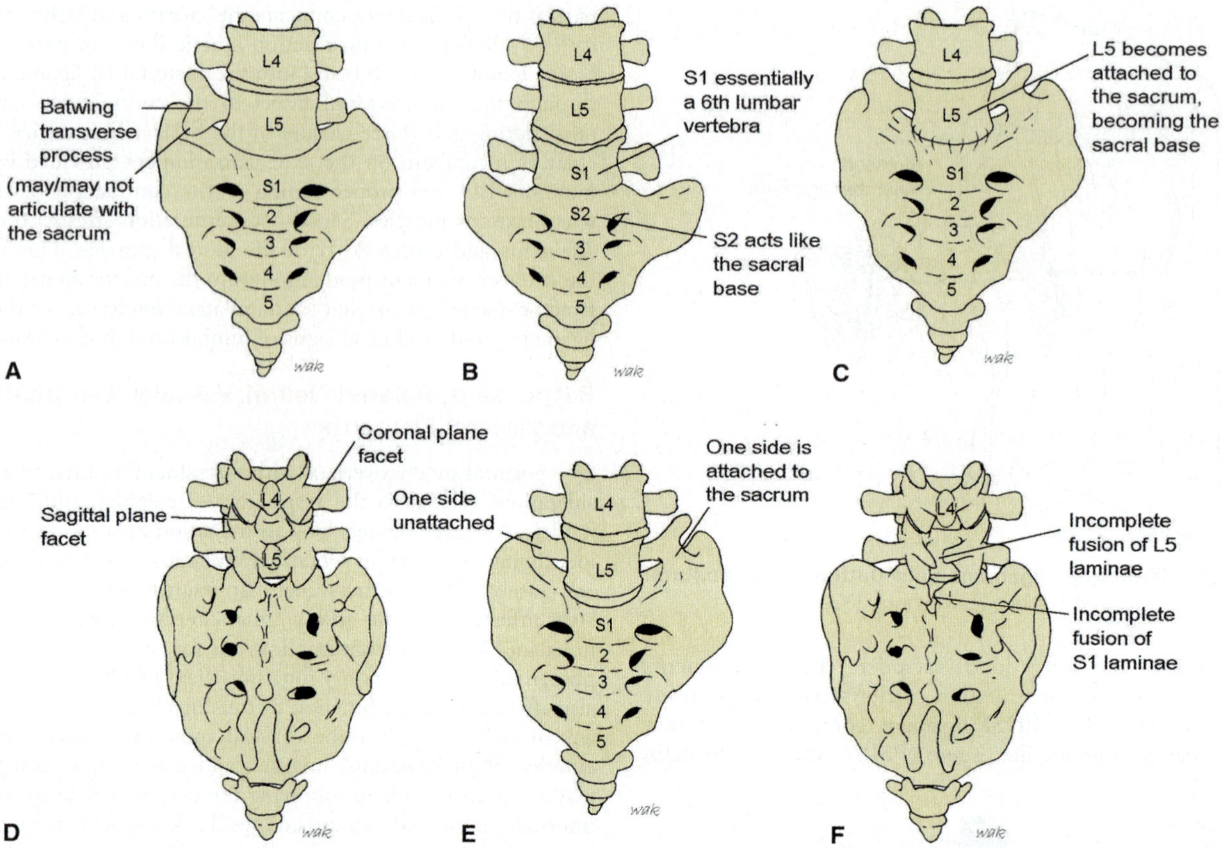

Figure 92.12. Common lumbosacral abnormalities. **A.** Batwing transverse processes of L5. **B.** Lumbarization of S1. **C.** Sacralization of L5. **D.** Facet asymmetry (zygapophyseal tropism) of L4. **E.** Partial sacralization of L5 (Bertolotti). **F.** Spina bifida occulta of both L and of S. (Courtesy of William A. Kuchera, DO, FAAO.)

TABLE 92.3

Radiologic Findings on Postural Films

Radiologic Finding and Appearance	Best X-Ray View	Implications/Comments
Congenital		
Batwing deformity	AP lumbosacral	Clinically: May alter joint mechanics, pain, and inflammation possible if rudimentary L5-iliac joint alters the sacral base level Radiographically: May be unable to accurately measure sacral base unleveling
Sacralization of L5 partial sacralization = Bertolotti syndrome	AP and lateral lumbosacral (both help)	Clinically: Short lumbar curve ($n = 4$) leading to more functional demand per segment and increased likelihood of developing degenerative L4 spondylolisthesis Radiographically: Unable to measure PI or lumbosacral lordotic angle
Lumbarization of S1	AP and lateral lumbosacral (both help)	Clinically: Long lumbar lever arm ($n = 6$) leading to less stability and increased incidence of low back pain Radiographically: Unable to measure PI
Spina bifida occulta	AP lumbosacral	Clinically: May not mean anything; however, may be harbinger of other posterior spinal congenital anomalies; muscles may attach and therefore function differently; often externally small tuft of hair at vertebral site
Facet tropism	AP and lateral lumbosacral (both help visualize)	So common that most radiologists do not even report its presence ("congenital spinal anomaly most commonly occurs"); asymmetric function

TABLE 92.3 (Continued)

Radiologic Findings on Postural Films

Radiologic Finding and Appearance	Best X-Ray View	Implications/Comments
Horizontal L5–S1 facets with listhesis	Lateral lumbosacral	Clinically: Drop-off sign is at level lower than isthmic type because the spine remains attached to its vertebral body as it slides forward. (L5–S1 drop-off)
Small hemipelvis	AP pelvis	Clinically: May be associated with smaller extremity and/or face on same side; may lead to functional scoliosis in seated position (and similar symptoms)
Wedge vertebrae	AP thoracolumbar	Radiographically: Impact on Cobb angle process
Acquired		
Spondylolysis	Oblique lumbosacral	Clinically: May be asymptomatic but usually associated with increased sagittal plane stress and decompensation; called *prespondylolisthesis*
L5–S1 isthmic spondylolisthesis	Lateral and oblique lumbosacral	Clinically: Loss of bony continuity coupled with typical postural anterior weight-bearing mechanics causes stress and strain on posterior support tissues and postural muscles generally; over Meyerding grade II, often very tight hamstrings; drop-off sign at L4–L5 Radiographically: Look also for other signs of calcified show "Scotty dog" deformity at the site of spondylolysis
L4–L5 degenerative spondylolisthesis	Lateral lumbosacral	Clinically: Often very flexible hamstrings; drop-off sign occurs between L4 and L5 spines
(Roto)scoliosis	AP thoracolumbar	Clinically: See text discussion Radiographically: May distort traditional view (e.g., AP view may become spinal oblique view)
Disk thinning	Lateral lumbosacral	Clinically: Decreases homeostatic reserve to swelling in the area of neural foramina and may lead to increased radiculopathy or instability of vertebral unit Radiographically: May wish to do functional flexion-extension to look for low-level secondary degenerative spondylolisthesis or retrolisthesis
Facet arthritis	AP and lateral	Seen especially in posterior weight-bearing mechanics
Unlevel sacral base	AP lumbosacral	Often, a cause of functional scoliotic change above; coronal changes often linked to visual rotational change as well
DJD spurs, figure-of-eight vertebral foraminal changes; calcification of ligaments (e.g., iliolumbar)	Oblique as well as other views	Clinically: Structural signs of long-term functional demand (Wolff law) but themselves may be totally asymptomatic Radiographically: Should raise suspicion of postural stress warranting postural measurements
Fracture(s)	Multiple views; oblique view for optimal view of the pars interarticularis	Clinically: May cause reflect straightening of the spinal curve due to muscle spasm Radiographically: May not be able to accurately assess underlying lordotic angles due to straightening

these anomalies complicate the selection of landmarks used in postural measurements or the interpretation of postural radiographic data. First reported by Bertolotti in 1917, a few are recognized to cause low back pain or lumbar instability.[122] Some incidental insignificant anomalies (such as batwing or sacralized L5) may be considered "risk factors" for local lumbar facet arthropathies.[123,124]

The standing PA film of the cervicocranial junction to the proximal femurs contains qualitative and quantitative information about posture in the coronal and horizontal planes. By noting the relative positions of the two pedicles and the spinous process, thoracic or lumbar vertebral rotation can be qualitatively assessed in AP radiographic views (Fig. 92.13B). Vertebral side bending is easily observed on the AP radiographic view and can be qualitatively reported. Quantitative measurements of group curves are often more formally reported using scoliosis nomenclature. Scoliosis, by convention, is reported in reference to the convexity of the curve. A right scoliosis is side-bent left (convex right). The Cobb method is commonly used to accurately measure scoliotic curves (Fig. 92.13A).[125] Central sacral vertical line and C7 plumb line may be generated to determine sagittal and coronal balance of scoliosis.[126]

The standing AP radiograph of the pelvis contains coronal and horizontal plane postural information.[127] This film is especially

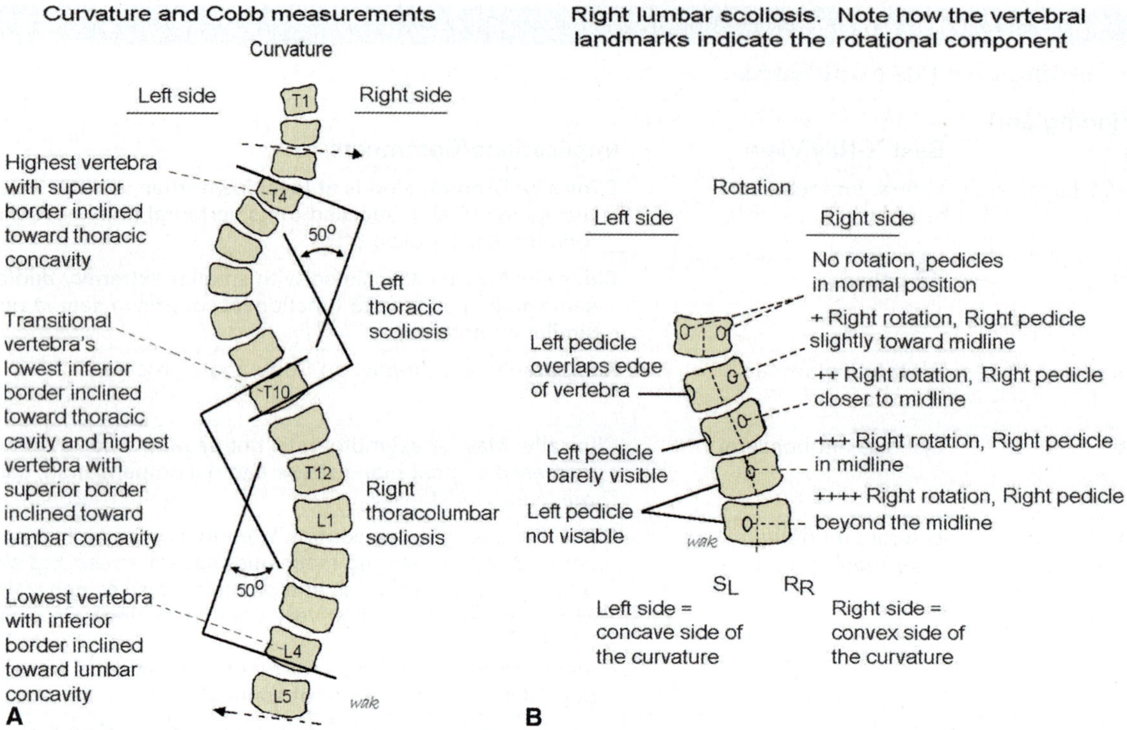

Figure 92.13. A and **B.** Measurement of spinal curvature and rotation by Cobb method. (Courtesy of William A. Kuchera, DO, FAAO.)

important in evaluating the degree of sacral base unleveling, structural leg lengths, and pelvic rotation with the patient in a weight-bearing position, measures that are the central values influencing lift therapy in the osteopathic postural model. The amount of sacral base unleveling is reported as the measured height difference of a line drawn across the top of the sacral base (line of eburnation [see Fig. 92.14] or the juncture of the sacral ala with either the iliac crests or the articular pillars) as extrapolated to its intersection with the femoral head vertical line.

The condition of scoliosis involves a complex three-dimensional deformity of the spine that cannot be accurately evaluated through simple two-dimensional radiographs. However, biplanar x-ray technology allows for standing frontal and lateral radiographs of the spine to be taken with reduced radiation exposure.[128]

Because the osteopathic physician is more interested in leveling the sacral base than in making the leg lengths equal, the standing sacral base palpatory asymmetry (rotation) is usually of more clinical significance than comparing anatomic leg lengths. In the presence of sacral base asymmetry, the direction of the lumbar side-bending component is also clinically relevant. In most cases, the observed iliac crest, femoral head, and sacral base unleveling measurements will be roughly equal. The use of various height shims is invaluable when clinically suspecting LLD.

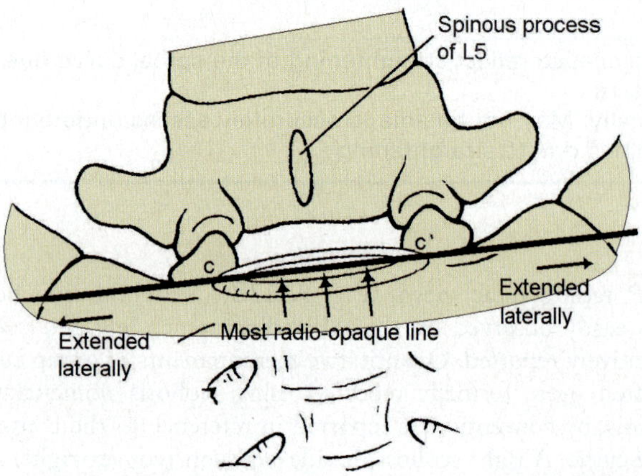

Figure 92.14. Landmark options for measuring sacral base unleveling. (Adapted from Irvin RE. Suboptimal posture: the origin of the majority of idiopathic pain of the musculoskeletal system. In: Vleeming A, Mooney V, Dorman T, et al., eds. *Movement, Stability and Low Back Pain: The Essential Role of the Pelvis.* Churchill-Livingstone; 1997:133–155.)

Lateral Radiographs

In healthy individuals who are asymptomatic, the line of gravity is the outcome of a reaction between the ground and an ideal dynamic chain that connects the trunk, pelvis, and lower limbs. With an anteroposterior view, this vertical line, perpendicular to the ground, passes through the middle of the sacrum. When viewed laterally, it should pass through L3 and slightly posterior to the femoral heads.[43] In order to accurately measure the line of gravity using upright radiographic images, it is necessary to establish spinopelvic (spinal and pelvic) parameters (see Table 92.4). This will allow for a more comprehensive evaluation of the overall sagittal alignment of the spine in relation to the pelvis.[129,130]

Several studies have shown a relationship between spinopelvic parameters, particularly PI, and the organization of the lumbar–thoracic spine. The values and correlations of spinopelvic parameters are well established for symptomatic and asymptomatic individuals. In patients with symptoms, lumbar degenerative changes can impact all the positional spinopelvic parameters and the shape of the pelvis. Therefore, the type of spinopelvic alignment could determine the type of lumbar degenerative disease. For more information, please refer to the section on sagittal plane decompensation later in this chapter.

TABLE 92.4

Spinopelvic (Spinal and Pelvic) Parameters to Measure the Line of Gravity Using Upright Radiographic Images

The Principal Parameters	Name	Value/Range	Description[129,130]	Addendum
Pelvic(s)	Pelvic incidence (PI) angle	Represents the algebraic sum of the sacral slope (SS) and pelvic tilt (PT): PI = SS + PT	The angle between the line from the center of the hip axis to the midpoint of the sacral endplate and a line perpendicular to the sacral endplate	The PI is a morphologic parameter, considered a constant, independent of the spatial orientation of the pelvis (sagittal balance). A small pelvic incidence angle corresponds to a narrow pelvis (small anteroposterior dimension), while a large angle indicates a broad one (large anteroposterior dimension). The sacral slope (SS) corresponds to the angle between the sacral plate and the horizontal plane.
	Pelvic tilt (PT)	The PT corresponds to the angle between the line connecting the midpoint of the sacral plate to the line between the geometric center of both femoral heads and the vertical plane. PT is also a positional parameter.	Both SS and PT are related to pelvis orientation relative to the femurs. This is important because the pelvis can rotate around the axis of the femoral heads. This movement can be forward (anteversion) or backward (retroversion).	**The PT angle increases during retroversion of the pelvis and is important when evaluating sagittal balance compensatory mechanisms (see below).**
	Sacral slope (SS)	The angle between the sacral endplate and a horizontal line	The SS is a positional parameter, varying according to the pelvic positioning. A vertical pelvis implies a low sacral slope, while a horizontal pelvis would have a high slope.	The SS is the important factor in determining the size and shape of lumbar curvature, and the shape and size of the lower lumbar vertebrae are directly affected by the size of the SS.
Lumbar spine	Lumbar lordotic (lordosis) angle (LL)	The LL is measured between L1 and S1 and accounts for only 1/3 of the lumbar lordosis.		A normal LL angle for adults is between 20 and 45 degrees.
Thoracic spine	Thoracic kyphosis (TK)	The TK is measured as the angle between the superior endplate surface of the T1 and the inferior endplate surface of the T12.	This angle tends to increase with aging.	
Cervical spine	C2–C7 angle	This is the angle between the inferior and superior endplates of the C2 and the C7 spine, respectively.	This parameter is used to determine the degree of cervical spine lordosis.	Often used to assess the degree of cervical lordosis in the neck; a larger angle indicates a greater lordosis while a smaller angle indicates a decreased lordosis or potential kyphosis in the cervical spine.
	C7 slope angle	The angle is formed between a horizontal line and the superior endplate surface of the C7.	Positively correlates with cervical lordosis and thoracic kyphosis.	A higher C7 slope angle signifies a more lordotic cervical spine, while a lower angle indicates a flatter or kyphotic curve.
Intrinsic parameters:	The sagittal vertical axis (SVA):	It is measured as the distance from the center of the C7 plumb line to the posterior edge of the upper sacral endplate surface.	The SVA is an important index of the sagittal balance of the spine.	The line should be within 5 mm of the superior–posterior endplate of S1. A high SVA has been linked to pain and lower quality-of-life scores.
	Spinosacral angle (SSA):	The SSA is the angle between the line from the center of the C7 vertebrae to the midpoint of the sacral endplate.	Used to measure the overall kyphosis of the spine.	The SSA is lower in people with diseases like degenerative kyphosis, rheumatoid arthritis, and diskogenic lumbar pain.

CORONAL PLANE DECOMPENSATION

Unleveling of the sacral base or a deformed vertebra, resulting from a fracture or congenital deformation, often leads to compensation that predominantly affects the coronal plane curvatures of the spine. Motion (or lack thereof) in the coronal plane, however, is physiologically linked to that in the horizontal or transverse plane; additionally, abnormal lordosis (sagittal plane) has been specifically implicated as a destabilizing factor in the development and progression of scoliosis.[111]

Compensatory changes in the coronal plane (as occurs with leg length inequality) can also be generalized (Fig. 92.15). The lumbar spine side bends away from and rotates toward the low sacral base. As a unit, the pelvis typically shifts and rotates around a vertical axis toward the long leg side.[131,132] The shifts in lumbar and pelvic tensions typically will encourage the sacrum to rotate to the side of the apparent oblique axis, which is established on the long leg side.[133] The innominate may attempt to compensate for the "short leg" by rotating anteriorly on the short leg side; this functionally lengthens that extremity.[132,134] The innominate on the side of the apparent long leg may rotate posteriorly to functionally shorten that extremity. The foot often assumes a pronated position on the long leg side, and the lower extremity internally rotates. If performed, the pelvic side shift test is to the side of the longer extremity.[133] The lumbosacral angle (LSA) increases by 2 to 3 degrees. The increased LSA, pelvic rotation, and pelvic side shift often mask the presence of an unlevel sacral base.[135] The vertebrae of the most caudal scoliotic curve usually side-bend away from and rotate toward the side of the apparent short leg.

Adaptation or decompensation in the coronal plane as measured in postural radiographic series also correlates with:

- Degenerative osteoarthritis of the hip[136]
- Lumbar osteophytes[131,137]

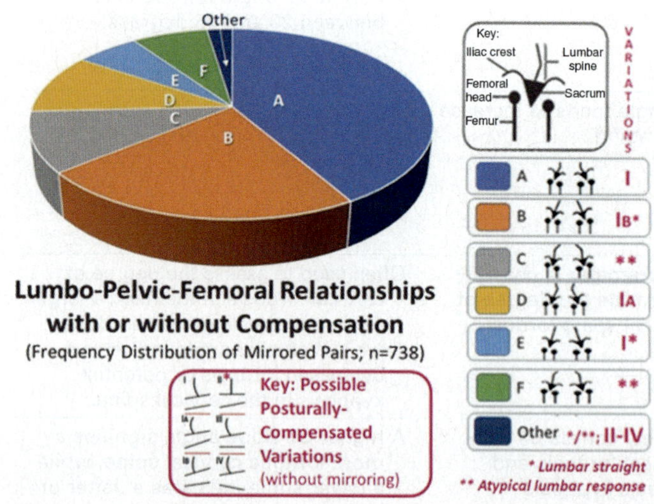

Figure 92.15. Frequency distribution of possible lumbopelvicfemoral relationships to unlevel femoral head heights. Using a common but arbitrary classification system,[116] this pie graph represents 738 general public subjects (children) from a study in Kirksville MO. Similarly, in 365 subjects with low back pain and unlevel femoral heads, the most common sacral base—femoral head relationships were type I and type IB.[138] It should be noted that patients most commonly compensate in the lumbar region with the convexity to their "short leg" side; lack of lumbar compensation may represent compensation elsewhere or other problems; atypical lumbar compensation (concavity to the "short leg" side) in a symptomatic patient may pose a therapeutic dilemma.

- Lumbar vertebral wedging[131]
- Scoliotic patterns (especially where sacral base unleveling measures >10 mm)[138]
- A variety of somatovisceral symptoms[139,140]

Compensatory measures are sometimes so good that any single or paired landmark measurement may fail to provide a true and accurate diagnosis.

- Neither the alignment of spinous processes nor the level of the iliac crests[82] is a good single indicator of sacral base unleveling or short-leg syndrome.
- ASIS or hip-to-ankle measurements using a tape measure are also inaccurate.[70,83,84,86]
- Comparison of the levels of the medial malleoli in the supine position is similarly inaccurate and potentially misleading.[74,75]
- The greater trochanters in the standing position are more helpful clinically but can be an error when unilateral coxa varus or coxa valgus is present.[76]

It has been found that data obtained from radiographic measurements are more accurate in showing postural asymmetry than any clinical estimates. Before proceeding with the x-ray series, it is important to first remove the patient's somatic dysfunction. The resulting x-ray images showcase structural data that depict the best possible homeostatic compensation achieved by the patient at the time. These standardized standing postural x-ray images can accurately measure coronal plane values, including the heights of the iliac crest, femoral heads, and sacral base across the femoral heads. Additionally, the radiographic series provides quantitative measurements of compensatory curvatures in case of scoliosis, along with any congenital or acquired bony anomalies and their degree, location, and type.

Recurrent patterns of somatic dysfunction of the pelvis, spine, cranium, or myofascial structures are the most rational clue that the sacral base is unlevel or that a short leg is present. For a full description of the musculoskeletal pattern of the short-leg syndrome, see Chapter 93 Osteopathic Considerations in the Patient with Low Back Pain.

Before definitive diagnosis of a patient's posture, OMT should be directed to all somatic dysfunction with particular care to correct dysfunctions of the sacrum, innominate, psoas, and quadratus lumborum. After OMT, the demonstration of a standing pelvic side shift test or transverse plane asymmetry of the sacrum should raise the suspicion that lower extremity influences, such as a short lower extremity, are affecting the function of the sacroiliac joint and the patient's posture.[115]

Compensatory changes such as innominate rotations, pelvic rotation, and changes in the LSA might alter the x-ray appearance, which can misrepresent the extent of the patient's actual problem. For these reasons, a leg length difference of less than 5 mm might not be treated unless the patient has other clinically relevant complaints and risk factors. Conversely, the desire to attain "peak physical performance" or to prevent long-term sequelae such as osteoarthritis of the hip that can develop on the long leg side might be an indication to treat the patient.[116]

TREATMENT CONSIDERATIONS

Short-leg syndrome treatment involves lifting the heel of the depressed sacral base side, especially with compensatory curvature bending to the opposite side. Heel lift treatment using the osteopathic postural model is always combined with OMT and is usually not attempted until after an appropriate OMT trial. Harrison Fryette clearly implied the rationale for both: *In the average case,*

I do not attempt a correction until I have mobilized the lumbar joints and established rotation in them; furthermore, if this region cannot be rotated toward the midline, the lift will not do what it is intended of it, for the correction will not take place in the lumbar region—the spine higher up will compensate by increasing its curve and only more trouble will result.[129]

OMT can alleviate functional conditions that appear as short-leg syndrome. OMT prepares somatic tissues for realignment, while lift therapy realigns and reeducates the entire body. Compensation, adaptation, and decompensation can cause soft tissue shortening, bony remodeling, and regional somatic dysfunction. Fryette also remarked: "In the last 15 years, I have added lifts to the short side in many cases under the age of fourteen, and in every case that I have kept under my observation for some time, I have been astonished to find that the legs grew to the same length."[141] Although it is true that compressive force accelerates bone growth, there is no research that supports the osteopathic convention that a shoe or heel lift under a growing child's foot can stimulate growth in the epiphyseal plates of that lower extremity. For a comprehensive review of pediatric and adolescent scoliosis, see Chapter 67 Osteopathic Considerations in Pediatrics.

OSTEOPATHIC HEEL LIFT GUIDELINES

Attempts to formulate specific guidelines to better quantify the amount of lift are best appreciated by studying the writings of David Heilig, DO, FAAO.[142] Heilig discovered that one-third to one-half of the measured sacral base unevenness in certain clinical scenarios was often due to excessive initial lift. He devised a formula (Table 92.5) that took into account the lift amount, which was directly proportional to the measured sacral base unevenness and inversely proportional to host factors such as age, duration of the condition, and amount of compensation or adaptation acquired by the body. Heilig provided examples of patients with a ½-in sacral base unleveling who would receive different initial lifts based on the formula.

Many colleges of osteopathic medicine teach a simple and sensitive protocol that uses a conservative "rule-of-thumb" to avoid unexpected flare-ups of pain or somatic dysfunction during lift therapy. This protocol is designed to be modified by clinical experience and judgment and must be adapted to each individual patient's evaluation and response[143]:

- If lift therapy is required, and if the patient is a "fragile" patient (arthritic, osteoporotic, elderly, having significant acute pain, etc.), begin with a 1/16-in-lift, and lift no farther than 1/16 of an inch every 2 weeks.
- If the spine is flexible, and no more than mild-to-moderate strain is noted in the myofascial system, begin with a 1/8-in lift, and lift at a rate no farther than 1/16 of an inch per week or 1/8 of an inch every 2 weeks.
- If there was a recent and sudden loss of leg length on one side, as might occur following a fracture or a recent hip prosthesis, and the patient had a level sacral base before the fracture or surgery, lift the lost amount.

Guidelines used in lift treatment are not absolute rules. One aspect of the art of medicine is an appreciation of patients' concerns about cost, cosmetic appearance, and convenience. Ideally, the shoe is rebuilt with every increment of lift to prevent alteration of foot mechanics and the introduction of unwanted pelvic rotation. Few patients, however, would agree with this approach. The following guidelines emphasize clinical tolerances and can be pragmatically used in lift treatment. If problems arise, reducing the tolerances or insisting on continuing to the ideal lift may be necessary:

- The true height of a lift is measured from the bottom of the lift to a point where the calcaneal bone strikes the lift; it is not measured at the posterior edge of the lift.
- Up to and including ¼ in of replaceable lift can be used inside of the shoe before the shoe no longer fits well.
- Up to and including a total of a ½-in lift can be placed between the heel of the patient's foot and the floor before foot mechanics are significantly disturbed.
- As a heel is progressively lifted, there is an increased tendency toward pelvic rotation, muscle imbalance, and alteration of foot mechanics.

Application of these principles to change the relative leg length by ½ in may result in:

- ¼-in lift being placed inside the shoe and ¼ in added to the heel of that shoe
- ½ in added to the heel of the shoe
- ¼ in added to one sole and ¼ in removed from the opposite sole[118,144]

These general guidelines allow osteopathic physicians to balance nonphysical factors such as vanity and cost with those related to posture. To maintain a certain normal angle, any increase in height beyond the ½-in heel lift is best added to the heel and anterior half-sole of the shoe (Fig. 92.16). Properly balancing the sacral base with lift therapy to within 1 mm of levelness can result

TABLE 92.5

The Heilig Formula and Patients with Same Sacral Base Unleveling (SBU) but Receiving Different Lifts

The Heilig formula suggests that the initial lift can be calculated as follows:

L < [SBU]/[D + C]

L, lift required; SBU, sacral base unleveling; D, duration; C, compensation

Duration allotted as (D = 1), 0–10 y; (D = 2), 10–30 y; (D = 3), 30+ y. Compensation allotted as (C = 0), none observed; (C = 1), rotation of lumbar vertebrae into convexity of compensatory side bending; (C = 2), wedging of the vertebrae, altered size of facets, horizontal osseous developments from endplates, and/or spurring

Patients with Same Sacral Base Leveling but Receiving Different Lifts

Case 1: Following fracture, minimal duration, no compensatory changes

L = [SBU]/[D + C] = ½ in/[0 + 1] = ½ in

Case 2: Patient age 35, injured in early youth, minimal compensation

L = [SBU]/[D + C] = ½ in/[2 + 1] = ½ in/3 = ⅙ in

Case 3: Patient age 75, injured in youth, spurring, horizontal endplate development, rotation is marked

L = [SBU]/[D + C] = ½ in/[3 + 2] = ½ in/5 = ⅒ in

Case 4: Patient age 26, polio affecting right leg in youth, minimal compensatory change

L = [SBU]/[D + C] = ½ in/[2 + 0] = ½ in/2 = ¼ in

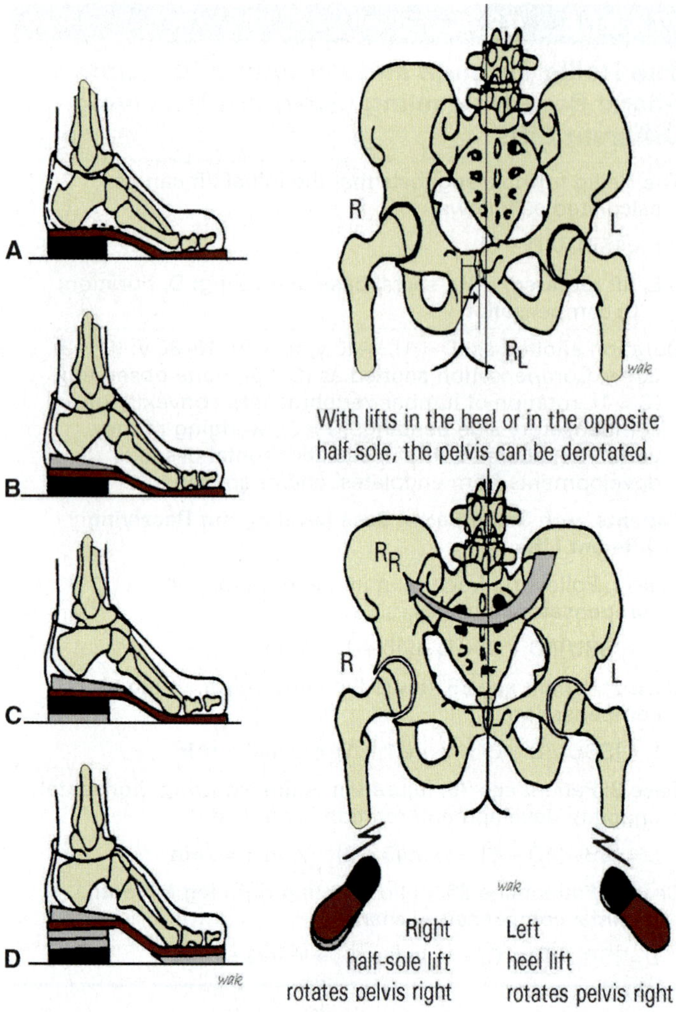

Figure 92.16. Principles of lift therapy. Heel lift measurements made at midcalcaneal line. **A.** Foot in a typical shoe. **B.** Heel lift in place. Maximum lift in shoe is 1/4 in. **C.** If more lift is needed, add to outside heel. **D.** If more than ½ in. is required, or to create minimal disturbance of foot mechanics, the entire sole can be lifted. (Courtesy of William A. Kuchera, DO, FAAO.)

in an 80% reduction in pain and other posture-related symptoms, including functional scoliosis. Balancing the weight of both shoes is also recommended, especially if large lifts are required. To reduce the weight added to one side, cork material can be placed between the shoe and the heel (Box 92.1).

In the spinal mechanical compensatory pattern, changes in each plane of motion in the lumbopelvic region due to postural decompensation are predictable. The typical sagittal plane decompensation begins with a *decrease in lumbar lordosis,* causing the gravity line to shift forward. Regional compensation then occurs in the pelvis as posterior rotation of the pelvis on the femoral heads, defined as *pelvic retroversion*. The spinopelvic parameters involved in pelvic retroversion are an increase in pelvic tilt (PT) and a decrease in sacral slope (SS). Functionally, pelvic retroversion leads to an extension of the hip joints or anterior and lateral glide of the femurs in the acetabulum. This causes the iliopsoas to fire to protect the hips from hyperextension and contributes to upper (proximal) lumbar hyperextension or segmental lordosis to balance against gravity.[146]

Compensation at the thoracic region begins with decreased kyphosis as the erector spinae muscles contract to hold the trunk erect. Similarly, the cervical extensors maintain or increase the cervical lordosis to keep the gaze horizontal. Eventually, this compensation will produce an increase in thoracic kyphosis, lower cervical facet joint derangement, and risk of arthritis with foraminal or central stenosis.

Compensatory knee and ankle flexion are solicited by the decrease in LL and subsequent hip extension during pelvic retroversion. Observed as patellar tracking (patellofemoral syndrome) limitations, meniscal destruction, and knee and hip osteoarthritis, these conditions may be the global effects of sagittal plane decompensation (sagittal imbalance) (Fig. 92.17).[43]

Sagittal plane decompensation (sagittal imbalance) may lead to global compensatory challenges and must be considered when

BOX 92.1 Sagittal Plane Decompensation

"Our spines were developed for the four-footed position and are not yet adapted to the erect, so mechanical weakness at the lumbosacral area is usual rather than exceptional. We must consider the lumbosacral area, not as normal or abnormal, but as mechanically sound or mechanically unsound." —Albert B Ferguson, MD[145]

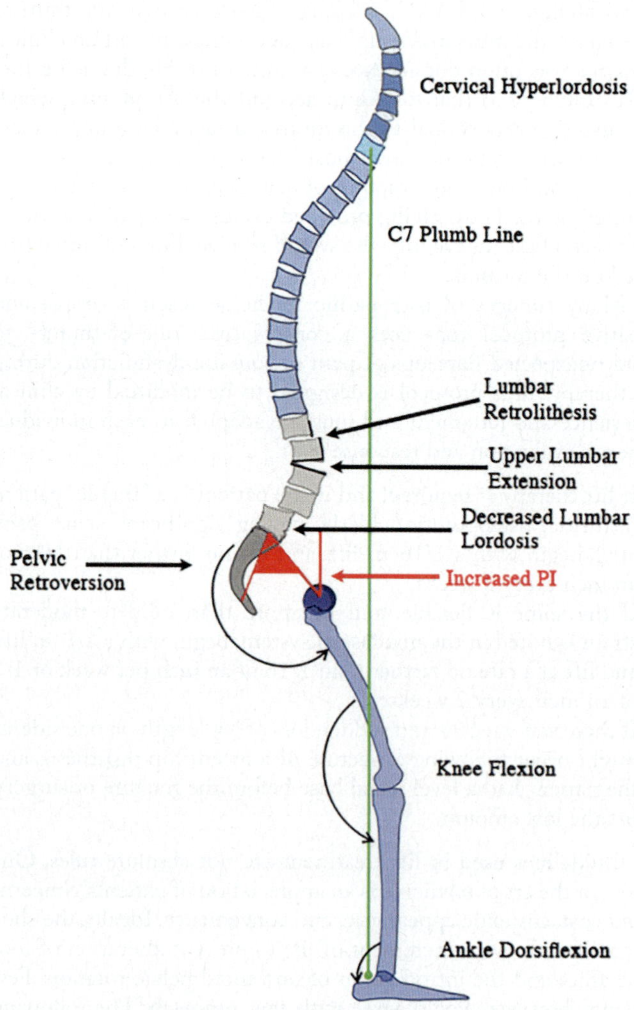

Figure 92.17. Sagittal Plane Decompensation.

addressing any patient with musculoskeletal conditions that limit their locomotor effort. The most common conditions are:

- Degenerative lumbar spondylosis
- Spondylolysis and spondylolisthesis
- Degenerative hip disease (Hip-spine syndrome)
- Cervical degenerative disease
- Knee degenerative disease
- Shoulder degenerative disease (increased kyphosis leads to internal rotation deficit[145]

Clinical Presentation in Sagittal Plane Decompensation

Posture-related disorders in the sagittal plane include:

- Low back pain—general erector spinae overuse
- Facet joint pain—"Baastrup" syndrome
- Sacroiliac joint pain
- Iliopsoas spasm—hip pain arising from a seated position or pain waking from sleep when rolling onto the back.
- Hamstring muscle facilitation
- Patellofemoral syndrome
- Headaches
- Jaw pain (forward head carriage)
- Scapulothoracic syndrome

Sagittal Plane Treatment Strategies

Rational, conservative management of the postural components of patients with certain orthopedic disorders or structural pathology presupposes early and accurate diagnosis and a thorough understanding of the biomechanics involved. While the underlying cause is important for prognosis, central to the treatment design is also the knowledge of static and dynamic effects of sagittal plane imbalance and the pathology on spinal mechanics and the motor strategies required for compensation.

Sagittal plane decompensation is well defined in the spine orthopedic and neurosurgery literature, focusing on spine surgical outcomes. It is not clear from this literature if sagittal plane decompensation is caused by or the result of lumbar degenerative disease. The "lower crossed syndrome" (or "pelvic crossed syndrome") reflects the *pattern* of lower body postural phasic muscles affecting the lower kinetic chain (lumbopelvic hip complex, knee, and ankle). The patient usually presents with posterior PT (pelvic retroversion), decreased LL, and weak abdominals; they usually experience chronic low back pain, piriformis syndrome, and anterior knee pain. This syndrome was popularized by Czech neurologists and manual medicine specialists Vladimir Janda, MD, and Karel Lewit, MD. Janda and Lewit "upper crossed syndrome" reflects the pattern of lower body postural phasic muscles affecting the upper kinetic chain (neck, shoulder, upper chest). The patient usually presents with headaches, upper thoracic pain, and various thoracic outlet syndrome signs and/or symptoms. See Tables 92.1 and 92.2. Patients presenting with symptoms of upper and lower crossed syndromes are likely at risk for sagittal plane imbalance and should be examined and treated from a global muscle balance perspective—hopefully before degenerative changes occur. A good rule of thumb is to first optimize the lumbopelvic region's neuromusculoskeletal function.

OMT

OMT is an integral part of care when implementing the osteopathic postural model. OMT addresses predictable patterns of somatic dysfunction that consistently and recurrently accompany postural problems and helps prepare the soma (muscles, joints, ligaments, and other supportive soft tissues) to better accept the positive postural change sought by postural care regimens. OMT also addresses tensegrity issues by reducing tension and hypomobility that, if left alone, may prevent the reversal of functional group curves or create pain in these sites.[62]

In managing sagittal plane postural decompensation, several considerations exist concerning the treatment of somatic dysfunction with OMT:

- Restore type-I spinal mechanics.
- Treat type-II dysfunctions in the lumbosacral, thoracolumbar, and upper thoracic spine to restore function of the multifidi, lower and middle scapular stabilizers, and intrinsic abdominal musculature.
- Correct pubic symphysis dysfunctions.
- Restore sacroiliac nutation.
- Focus on eliminating/balancing upper and lower crossed syndromes.
- Postural change occurs first at the transition zones. Therefore, these regions should be diagnosed, and dysfunction should be treated when found (Note that the Zink approach that is often used early in the respiratory–circulatory model to diagnose and treat transition zones can be used effectively and efficiently in the postural model.[11])
- The percussion hammer technique (see Chapter 59), taught by Robert Fulford, DO, is clinically helpful in treating some chronic postural problems.

Postural Education and Compliance

Effective postural treatment regimens should emphasize education and compliance, especially in the initial phases of the reeducation program. Compliance is enhanced when the patient understands all of the components of the treatment protocol and their rationale.

In addition to other protocol components, provide the patient with sound biomechanical and ergonomic education emphasizing the following:

- Choice of appropriate footwear and arch support.
- Consider stopping stretches that lead to sacral counternutation and therefore increased sacral instability such as knee-to-chest and forward bending to stretch the erector spinae muscles.
- Limit or correct activities that promote joint and tendon strain and muscle overuse.
- Limit decompensating postures that decrease LL.
- Low inflammatory dietary counseling.
- Rational weight management counseling.
- Avoid heels that exceed ½ in.
- Sleeping on their stomach should be discouraged; sleeping on their sides with a pillow between their knees helps to reduce and relax overused quadratus lumborum muscles.
- Sitting upright with both feet on the floor, directly below their knees.

Postural Exercise

Exercise is an often misunderstood and misused activity. The patient must be given a precise and realistic prescription for the goal, dose, frequency, and duration of physical activities. Other stretches and activities critical for ameliorating sagittal plane imbalance include:

- Using weight training for restoring and maintaining type-I fast-twitch dynamic/phasic muscle mass.

BOX 92.2 Osteopathic Pearl

To intelligently rehabilitate injuries, physicians must understand not only what the affected tissue is doing during the activity that led to its breakdown but also what it does, when it does it, and why it does so. The concept of "econcentric" muscle function enables physicians to grasp the causes and compensations of both acute and overuse injuries, providing them with an improved ability to identify the appropriate "econcentric" response of the injured tissue to promote healing and enhance function. Additionally, physicians need to understand how the involved tissue integrates into the entire kinetic chain system.

- Psoas (hip-flexor) stretches.
- Scalenus (neck flexor) stretches.
- Maintenance of spine mobility using yoga, gyrotonic method, or sport.
- Maintain balance using Thai Chi.
- Proper sleep habits and positions.

(See also Box 92.2 regarding employing an "econocentric" approach to exercise.)

Other Miscellaneous Approaches

When other conservative treatments fail to restore stability, injection techniques using proliferative medication, known as prolotherapy, can be utilized for ligamentous laxity. Prolotherapy involves injecting a proliferant solution at the attachment point of the ligament. Ligamentous laxity can occur when postural strain biomechanically overwhelms structural integrity. To increase stability, a proliferant solution is injected at the ligament's fibro-osseous insertion. Prolotherapy can be an effective and conservative approach to hypermobility and ligamentous laxity when combined with exercise, OMT, and postural realignment to prevent a return of musculoligamentous strain.[147,148] Surgery can be considered a viable option in unstable situations or when conservative care fails.

SUMMARY

The upright posture of human beings, which relies on energy-efficient balance in a gravitational field, is argued to have led to the evolution of several unique aspects of "human-ness." Understanding the principles outlined in this chapter will enable osteopathic physicians to properly consider and effectively apply the postural–biomechanical model to achieve specific clinical goals. This model is one of the five primary approaches that form the basis of osteopathic healthcare and significantly impacts multiple systems, particularly the neurologic–autonomic and respiratory–circulatory models. Its careful consideration and appropriate implementation have been shown to be crucial in successfully managing patients and integrating other osteopathic healthcare approaches.

REFERENCES

1. Smith W. Skiagraphy and the circulation. *J Osteopath.* 1899;3:356–378.
2. Schwab WA. Principles of manipulative treatment: II. Low back problem. *J Am Osteopath Assoc.* 1932;31:216–220.
3. Beilke M. Roentgenological spinal analysis and the technic for taking standing x-ray plates. *J Am Osteopath Assoc.* 1936;35:414–418.
4. Denslow JS, Chace JA, Gutensohn OR, Kumm MG. Methods in taking and interpreting weight-bearing x-ray films. *J Am Osteopath Assoc.* 1955;54:663–670.
5. Peterson B, ed. *Postural Balance and Imbalance (1983 AAO Yearbook).* American Academy of Osteopathy; 1983.
6. Hagen DP. A continuing roentgenographic study of rural school children over a 15 year period. *J Am Osteopath Assoc.* 1964;63:546–557.
7. Friberg O. Clinical symptoms and biomechanics of lumbar spine and hip joint in leg length inequality. *Spine (Phila Pa 1976).* 1983;8(6):643–651.
8. Osoba MY, Rao AK, Agrawal SK, Lalwani AK. Balance and gait in the elderly: a contemporary review. *Laryngoscope Investig Otolaryngol.* 2019;4(1):143–153.
9. Janda V. Muscles: central nervous motor regulation and back problems. In: Korr I, ed. *The Neurobiologic Mechanisms in Manipulative Therapy.* Plenum Publishing; 1977:27–41.
10. Stecco C, Macchi V, Porzionato A, et al. The ankle retinacula: morphological evidence of the proprioceptive role of the fascial system. *Cells Tissues Organs.* 2010;192(3):200–210.
11. Zink JG. Respiratory and circulatory care: the conceptual model. *Osteopath Ann.* 1977;5(3):108–112.
12. Norte G, Rush J, Sherman D. Arthrogenic muscle inhibition: best evidence, mechanisms, and theory for treating the unseen in clinical rehabilitation. *J Sport Rehabil.* 2021;31(6):717–735.
13. Nair S, Sagar M, Sollers J III, Consedine N, Broadbent E. Do slumped and upright postures affect stress responses? A randomized trial. *Health Psychol.* 2015;34(6):632–641.
14. Janda V. Muscle and motor control in cervicogenic disorders: assessment and management. In: Grant R, ed. *Physical Therapy of the Cervical and Thoracic Spine, Clinics in Physical Therapy.* Churchill Livingstone; 1994:195–216.
15. Janda V. Muscle weakness and inhibition (pseudoparesis) in back pain syndromes. In: Grieve GP ed. *Modern Manual Therapy of the Vertebral Column.* Churchill Livingstone; 1986:197–201.
16. Stecco A, Giordani F, Fede C, Pirri C, De Caro R, Stecco C. From Muscle to the Myofascial Unit: Current Evidence and Future Perspectives. *Int J Mol Sci.* 2023;24(5):4527.
17. Janda V. Muscles as a pathogenic factor in back pain. In: *The Treatment of Patients. Proceedings of the 4th Conference on International Federation of Orthopedic Manipulative Therapists.* 1980:1–23.
18. Lewit K. *Manipulative Therapy in Rehabilitation of the Motor System.* 2nd ed. Butterworth; 1991.
19. Goff B. The application of recent advances in neurophysiology to Miss M. Rood's concept of neuromuscular facilitation. *Physiotherapy.* 1972;58(12):409–415.
20. Bergmark A. Stability of the lumbar spine. A study in mechanical engineering. *Acta Orthop Scand Suppl.* 1989;230:1–54.
21. Mottram S, Comerford M. Stability, dysfunction and low back pain. *J Orthop Med.* 1998;20(2):13–18.
22. Shumway-Cook A, Wollacott M. *Motor Control: Translating Research to Practice.* Lippincott Williams and Wilkins; 2016.
23. Panjabi MM. The stabilizing system of the spine. Part I. Function, dysfunction, adaptation, and enhancement. *J Spinal Disord.* 1992;5(4):383–389.
24. Izzo R, Guarnieri G, Guglielmi G, Muto M. Biomechanics of the spine. Part I: spinal stability. *Eur J Radiol.* 2013;82(1):118–126.
25. Cohen LA, Cohen ML. Arthrokinetic reflex of the knee. *Am J Physiol.* 1956;184(2):433–437.
26. Hides JA, Stokes MJ, Saide M, Jull GA, Cooper DH. Evidence of lumbar multifidus muscle wasting ipsilateral to symptoms in patients with acute/subacute low back pain. *Spine (Phila Pa 1976).* 1994;19(2):165–172.
27. Lepley AS, Lepley LK. Mechanisms of arthrogenic muscle inhibition. *J Sport Rehabil.* 2021;31(6):707–716.
28. Rice DA, McNair PJ. Quadriceps arthrogenic muscle inhibition: neural mechanisms and treatment perspectives. *Semin Arthritis Rheum.* 2010;40(3):250–266.
29. Hopkins JT, Ingersoll CD. Arthrogenic muscle inhibition: a limiting factor in joint rehabilitation. *J Sport Rehabil.* 2000;9:135–159.
30. Hopkins J, Ingersoll CD, Edwards J, Klootwyk TE. Cryotherapy and transcutaneous electric neuromuscular stimulation decrease arthrogenic

muscle inhibition of the vastus medialis after knee joint effusion. *J Athl Train.* 2002;37:25–31.
31. Young A. Current issues in arthrogenous inhibition. *Ann Rheum Dis.* 1993;52:829–834.
32. Young A, Stokes M, Iles JF. Effects of joint pathology on muscle. *Clin Orthop Relat Res.* 1987;219:21–27.
33. Stokes M, Young A. The contribution of reflex inhibition to arthrogenous muscle weakness. *Clin Sci (Lond).* 1984;67:7–14.
34. Dictionary.com. "tensegrity." Unabridged. Random House, Inc. Accessed September 3, 2023. http://dictionary.reference.com /browse/tensegrity
35. Ingber DE, Wang N, Stamenovic D. Tensegrity, cellular biophysics, and the mechanics of living systems. *Rep Prog Phys.* 2014;77(4):046603.
36. Levin S, de Solórzano SL, Scarr G. The significance of closed kinematic chains to biological movement and dynamic stability. *J Bodyw Mov Ther.* 2017;21:664–672.
37. Swanson RL II. Biotensegrity: a unifying theory of biological architecture with applications to osteopathic practice, education, and research—a review and analysis. *J Osteopath Med.* 2013;113(1):34–52.
38. Dischiavi SL, Wright AA, Hegedus EJ, Bleakley CM. Biotensegrity and myofascial chains: a global approach to an integrated kinetic chain. *Med Hypotheses.* 2018;110:90–96.
39. Bordoni B, Myers T. A review of the theoretical fascial models: biotensegrity, fascintegrity, and myofascial chains. *Cureus.* 2020;12(2):e7092.
40. Scarr G. A model of the cranial vault as a tensegrity structure, and its significance to normal and abnormal cranial development. *Int J Osteopath Med.* 2008;11(3):80–89.
41. Jaspers R, Huijing P. Myofascial force transmission and molecular pathways involved in adaptation of muscle size: the Tensional Network of the Human Body: the science and clinical applications in manual and movement therapy. In *Fascia: The Tensional Network of the Human Body: The Science and Clinical Applications in Manual and Movement Therapy.* 2nd ed., pp. 688. Elsevier Health Sciences imprint Churchill Livingstone; 2022.
42. Riemann BL, Lephart SM. The sensorimotor system, part ii: the role of proprioception in motor control and functional joint stability. *J Athl Train.* 2002;37(1):80–84.
43. Le Huec JC, Saddiki R, Franke J, Rigal J, Aunoble S. Equilibrium of the human body and the gravity line: the basics. *Eur Spine J.* 2011;20(5): 558–563.
44. Błaszczyk JW, Beck M. Posturographic standards for optimal control of human standing posture. *J Hum Kinet.* 2023;86:7–15.
45. Willard FH. The muscular, ligamentous and neural structure of the low back and its relation to back pain. In: Vleeming A, Mooney V, Dorman T, et al., eds. *Movement, Stability and Low Back Pain: The Essential Role of the Pelvis.* Churchill-Livingstone; 1997:3–35.
46. Loukas M, Shoja MM, Thurston T, Jones VL, Linganna S, Tubbs RS. Anatomy and biomechanics of the vertebral aponeurosis part of the posterior layer of the thoracolumbar fascia. *Surg Radiol Anat.* 2008;30(2): 125–129.
47. Panjabi MM. The stabilizing system of the spine. Part I. Function, dysfunction, adaptation, and enhancement. *J Spinal Disord.* 1992;5(4): 383–397.
48. Willard FH, Vleeming A, Schuenke MD, Danneels L, Schleip R. The thoracolumbar fascia: anatomy, function and clinical considerations. *J Anat.* 2012;221(6):507–536.
49. Claus AP, Hides JA, Moseley GL, Hodges PW. Different ways to balance the spine: subtle changes in sagittal spinal curves affect regional muscle activity. *Spine (Phila Pa 1976).* 2009;34(6):E208–E214.
50. Hodges PW, Cresswell AG, Daggfeldt K, Thorstensson A. Three dimensional preparatory trunk motion precedes asymmetrical upper limb movement. *Gait Posture.* 2000;11(2):92–101.
51. Kibler WB. The role of the scapula in athletic shoulder function. *Am J Sports Med.* 1998;26(2):325–337.
52. Loukas M, Louis RG Jr, Wartmann CT, et al. An anatomic investigation of the serratus posterior superior and serratus posterior inferior muscles. *Surg Radiol Anat.* 2008;30(2):119–123.
53. Barker PJ, Briggs CA. Attachments of the posterior layer of lumbar fascia. *Spine (Phila Pa 1976).* 1999;24(17):1757–1764.
54. Schomacher J, Falla D. Function and structure of the deep cervical extensor muscles in patients with neck pain. *Man Ther.* 2013;18(5):360–366.
55. O'Leary S, Falla D, Elliott JM, Jull G. Muscle dysfunction in cervical spine pain: implications for assessment and management. *J Orthop Sports Phys Ther.* 2009;39(5):324–333.
56. Hasegawa K, Dubousset JF. Cone of economy with the chain of balance-historical perspective and proof of concept. *Spine Surg Relat Res.* 2022;6(4):337–349.
57. Hasegawa K, Okamoto M, Hatsushikano S, et al. Compensation for standing posture by whole-body sagittal alignment in relation to health-related quality of life. *Bone Joint J.* 2020;102-B(10):1359–1367.
58. Iorio JA, Jakoi AM, Singla A. Biomechanics of degenerative spinal disorders. *Asian Spine J.* 2016;10(2):377–384.
59. McLain RF, Pickar JG. Mechanoreceptor endings in human thoracic and lumbar facet joints. *Spine (Phila Pa 1976).* 1998;23(2):168–173.
60. Panjabi MM. Clinical spinal instability and low back pain. *J Electromyogr Kinesiol.* 2003;13:371–379.
61. Riemann BL, Lephart SM. The Sensorimotor system, part II: the role of proprioception in motor control and functional joint stability. *J Athl Train.* 2002;37(1):80–84.
62. Gracovetsky S. Stability or controlled instability? In: *Movement, Stability & Lumbopelvic Pain.* Churchill Livingstone; 2007. pp. 279–294.
63. Gracovetsky SA, Iacono S. Energy transfers in the spinal engine. *J Biomed Eng.* 1987;9(2):99–114.
64. Robinault L, Holobar A, Crémoux S, et al. The effects of spinal manipulation on motor unit behavior. *Brain Sci.* 2021;11(1):105.
65. Liebler EJ, Tufano-Coors L, Douris P, et al. The effect of thoracic spine mobilization on lower trapezius strength testing. *J Man Manip Ther.* 2001;9(4);207–212.
66. Cleland J, Selleck B, Stowell T, et al. Short-term effects of thoracic manipulation on lower trapezius muscle strength. *J Man Manip Ther.* 2004;12(2):82–90.
67. Pope R. The common compensatory pattern: its origin and relationship to the postural model. *Am Acad Osteopath J.* 2003;13.
68. Fryette HH. Physiologic movements of the spine. *J Am Osteopath Assoc.* 1917;18:1–2.
69. Hasegawa K, Dubousset JF. Cone of economy with the chain of balance-historical perspective and proof of concept. *Spine Surg Relat Res.* 2022;6(4):337–349.
70. Dubousset J. The pelvic vertebra, the cephalic vertebra and the concept of the chain of balance. In: Vital J, Cawley D, eds. *Spinal Anatomy.* Springer; 2020.
71. Kuchera ML. Gravitational stress, musculoskeletal strain, and postural alignment. *Spine State Art Rev.* 1995;9(2):463–490.
72. Kuchera ML. Diagnosis and treatment of gravitational strain pathophysiology: research and clinical correlates (parts I & II). In: Vleeming A, ed. *Low Back Pain: The Integrated Function of the Lumbar Spine and Sacroiliac Joints. Proceedings of the 2nd Interdisciplinary World Congress.* University of California (San Diego); 1995:659–693.
73. Cathie AG. Some applied anatomy of postural changes. In: Peterson B, ed. *Postural Balance and Imbalance (1983 AAO Yearbook).* American Academy of Osteopathy; 1983:44–46.
74. Irvin RE. Suboptimal posture: the origin of the majority of idiopathic pain of the musculoskeletal system. In: Vleeming A, Mooney V, Dorman T, et al., eds. *Movement, Stability and Low Back Pain: The Essential Role of the Pelvis.* Churchill-Livingstone; 1997:133–155.
75. Kuchera ML, Bemben MG, Kuchera WA, et al. Athletic functional demand and posture (abstract). *J Am Osteopath Assoc.* 1990;90(9):843–844.
76. Denslow JS, Chase JA. Mechanical stresses in the human lumbar spine and pelvis. In: Peterson B. ed. *Postural Balance and Imbalance (1983 AAO Yearbook).* American Academy of Osteopathy; 1983:76–82.
77. Panjabi MM. The stabilizing system of the spine. Part II. Neutral zone and instability hypothesis. *J Spinal Disord.* 1992;5(4):390–397.
78. Denis F. The three column spine and its significance in the classification of acute thoracolumbar spinal injuries. *Spine (Phila Pa 1976).* 1983;8(8):817–831.
79. Fearing BV, Hernandez PA, Setton LA, Chahine NO. Mechanotransduction and cell biomechanics of the intervertebral disc. *JOR Spine.* 2018;1(3):e1026.
80. Inoue N, Espinoza Orías AA. Biomechanics of intervertebral disk degeneration. *Orthop Clin North Am.* 2011;42(4):487–99, vii.

81. Kirkaldy-Willis WH, Wedge JH, Yong-Hing K, Reilly J. Pathology and pathogenesis of lumbar spondylosis and stenosis. *Spine (Phila Pa 1976)*. 1978;3(4):319–328.
82. Haig AJ. Paraspinal denervation and the spinal degenerative cascade. *Spine J*. 2002;2(5):372–380.
83. Haig AJ, London Z, Sandella DE. Symmetry of paraspinal muscle denervation in clinical lumbar spinal stenosis: support for a hypothesis of posterior primary ramus stretching? *Muscle Nerve*. 2013;48(2):198–203.
84. Matheve T, Hodges P, Danneels L. The role of back muscle dysfunctions in chronic low back pain: state-of-the-art and clinical implications. *J Clin Med*. 2023;12(17):5510.
85. Müller A, Rockenfeller R, Damm N, et al. Load distribution in the lumbar spine during modeled compression depends on lordosis. *Front Bioeng Biotechnol*. 2021;9:661258.
86. Knox MF, Chipchase LS, Schabrun SM, Romero RJ, Marshall PWM. Anticipatory and compensatory postural adjustments in people with low back pain: a systematic review and meta-analysis. *Spine J*. 2018; 18(10):1934–1949.
87. Franklin TC, Granata KP. Role of reflex gain and reflex delay in spinal stability–a dynamic simulation. *J Biomech*. 2007;40(8):1762–1767.
88. Hodges PW, Danneels L. Changes in structure and function of the back muscles in low back pain: different time points, observations, and mechanisms. *J Orthop Sports Phys Ther*. 2019;49(6):464–476.
89. Tsukamoto M, Morimoto T, Kobayashi T, et al. The relationship between traction spurs, Modic change, vacuum phenomenon, and segmental instability of the lumbar spine. *Sci Rep*. 2022;12(1):9939.
90. Barz T, Melloh M, Lord SJ, Kasch R, Merk HR, Staub LP. A conceptual model of compensation/decompensation in lumbar segmental instability. *Med Hypotheses*. 2014;83(3):312–316.
91. Roussouly P, Pinheiro-Franco JL. Biomechanical analysis of the spino-pelvic organization and adaptation in pathology. *Eur Spine J*. 2011;20(5):609–618.
92. Khamis S, Carmeli E. Relationship and significance of gait deviations associated with limb length discrepancy: a systematic review. *Gait Posture*. 2017;57:115–123.
93. Murray KJ, Molyneux T, Le Grande MR, Castro Mendez A, Fuss FK, Azari MF. Association of mild leg length discrepancy and degenerative changes in the hip joint and lumbar spine. *J Manipulative Physiol Ther*. 2017;40(5):320–329.
94. Sarwark JF, Castelein RM, Lam TP, et al. Elucidating the inherent features of IS to better understand idiopathic scoliosis etiology and progression. *J Orthop*. 2021;26:126–129.
95. Raczkowski JW, Daniszewska B, Zolynski K. Functional scoliosis caused by leg length discrepancy. *Arch Med Sci*. 2010;6(3):393–398.
96. Rauh MJ. Leg-length inequality and running-related injury among high school runners. *Int J Sports Phys Ther*. 2018;13(4):643–651.
97. Yoshimoto H, Sato S, Masuda T, et al. Spinopelvic alignment in patients with osteoarthrosis of the hip: a radiographic comparison to patients with low back pain. *Spine (Phila Pa 1976)*. 2005;30(14):1650–1657.
98. Roussouly P, Pinheiro-Franco JL. Sagittal parameters of the spine: biomechanical approach. *Eur Spine J*. 2011;20(5):578–585.
99. Hara D, Nakashima Y, Hamai S, et al. Kinematic analysis of healthy hips during weight-bearing activities by 3D-to-2D model-to-image registration technique. *Biomed Res Int*. 2014;2014:457573.
100. Kobayashi T, Morimoto T, Yoshihara T, Sonohata M, Rivière C, Mawatari M. The significant relationship among the factors of pelvic incidence, standing lumbar lordosis, and lumbar flexibility in Japanese patients with hip osteoarthritis: a descriptive radiographic study. *Orthop Traumatol Surg Res*. 2022;108(2):103123.
101. Fu P, Xu W, Xu P, Huang J, Guo JJ. Relationship between spinal imbalance and knee osteoarthritis by using full-body EOS. *BMC Musculoskelet Disord*. 2023;24(1):402.
102. Gofton JP, Trueman GE. Studies in osteoarthritis of the hip: part II. Osteoarthritis of the hip and leg-length disparity. *Can Med Assoc J*. 1971; 104:791–799.
103. Findley T, Chaudhry H, Dhar S. Transmission of muscle force to fascia during exercise. *J Bodyw Mov Ther*. 2015;19(1):119–123.
104. Gerwin RD. A new unified theory of trigger point formation: failure of pre- and post-synaptic feedback control mechanisms. *Int J Mol Sci*. 2023;24(9):8142.
105. Nicodemus CL, Sikorskii A, Epstein J. Revisiting chronic low back pain: evidence that it is not non-specific. *J Osteopath Med*. 2022;123(3): 143–149.
106. Adams MA, Hutton WC. The mechanical function of the lumbar apophyseal joints. *Spine*. 1983;8(3):327–330.
107. Wang K, Deng Z, Chen X, et al. The role of multifidus in the biomechanics of lumbar spine: a musculoskeletal modeling study. *Bioengineering*. 2023;10(1):67.
108. Jaumard NV, Welch WC, Winkelstein BA. Spinal facet joint biomechanics and mechanotransduction in normal, injury and degenerative conditions. *J Biomech Eng*. 2011;133(7):071010.
109. Soydan Z, Bayramoglu E, Altas O. The impact of spinopelvic alignment on the facet joint degeneration [published online ahead of print, 2023 Mar 9]. *Global Spine J*. 2023;21925682231162813.
110. Pool-Goudzwaard AL, Kleinrensink GJ, Snijders CJ, Entius C, Stoeckart R. The sacroiliac part of the iliolumbar ligament. *J Anat*. 2001;199(Pt 4): 457–463.
111. Vleeming A, Snijders CJ, Stoeckart R, et al. The role of the sacroiliac joints in coupling between spine, pelvis, legs and arms. In: Vleeming A, Mooney V, Dorman T, et al., eds. *Movement, Stability and Low Back Pain: The Central Role of the Pelvis*. Churchill-Livingstone; 1997:53–71.
112. Ashby K, Yilmaz E, Mathkour M, et al. Ligaments stabilizing the sacrum and sacroiliac joint: a comprehensive review. *Neurosurg Rev*. 2022;45(1):357–364.
113. Vleeming A, de Vries HJ, Mens JM, van Wingerden JP. Possible role of the long dorsal sacroiliac ligament in women with peripartum pelvic pain. *Acta Obstet Gynecol Scand*. 2002;81(5):430–436.
114. Moustafa IM, Shousha T, Arumugam A, Harrison DE. Is thoracic kyphosis relevant to pain, autonomic nervous system function, disability, and cervical sensorimotor control in patients with chronic nonspecific neck pain? *J Clin Med*. 2023;12(11):3707.
115. Stępień A, Pałdyna B. Neurodynamic functions and their correlations with postural parameters in adolescents with idiopathic scoliosis. *J Clin Med*. 2022;11(4):1115.
116. Maxwell CM, Lauchlan DT, Dall PM. The effects of spinal manipulative therapy on lower limb neurodynamic test outcomes in adults: a systematic review. *J Man Manip Ther*. 2020;28(1):4–14.
117. Oakley A, Paul IMM, Harrison DE. The influence of sagittal plane spine alignment on neurophysiology and sensorimotor control measures: Optimization of function through structural correction. *Therapy Approaches in Neurological Disorders*. IntechOpen. 2021.
118. Greenman PE. Lift therapy: use and abuse. *J Am Osteopath Assoc*. 1979; 79:238–250.
119. Kuchera ML. Treatment of gravitational strain pathophysiology. In: Vleeming A, Mooney V, Dorman T, et al., eds. *Movement, Stability and Low Back Pain: The Essential Role of the Pelvis*. Churchill-Livingstone; 1997:53–71.
120. Travell JG, Simon DG. *Myofascial Pain and Dysfunction: The Trigger Point Manual*. Vol. II. Williams & Wilkins; 1992:22–88.
121. Nardo L, Alizai H, Virayavanich W, et al. Lumbosacral transitional vertebrae: association with low back pain. *Radiology*. 2012;265(2): 497–503.
122. Fidan F, Balaban M, Hatipoğlu ŞC, et al. Is lumbosacral transitional vertebra associated with lumbar disc herniation in patients with low back pain? *Eur Spine J*. 2022;31:2907–2912.
123. Castellvi AE, Goldstein LA, Chan DP. Lumbosacral transitional vertebrae and their relationship with lumbar extradural defects. *Spine (Phila Pa 1976)*. 1984;9(5):493–495.
124. Hanhivaara J, Määttä JH, Karppinen J, Niinimäki J, Nevalainen MT. The association of lumbosacral transitional vertebrae with low back pain and lumbar degenerative findings in MRI: a large cohort study. *Spine (Phila Pa 1976)*. 2022;47(2):153–162.
125. Langensiepen S, Semler O, Sobottke R, et al. Measuring procedures to determine the Cobb angle in idiopathic scoliosis: a systematic review. *Eur Spine J*. 2013;22(11):2360–2371.
126. Oetgen ME, Matthews AL, Martin BD, Hanway J, Kelly S, Blakemore L. Radiographic resource utilization in the initial referral and evaluation of patients with adolescent idiopathic scoliosis. *J Am Acad Orthop Surg*. 2018;26(12):441–445.

127. Malfair D, Flemming AK, Dvorak MF, et al. Radiographic evaluation of scoliosis: review. *Am J Roentgenol.* 2010;194:3_supplement:S8–S22.
128. Amzallag-Bellenger E, Uyttenhove F, Nectoux É, et al. Idiopathic scoliosis in children and adolescents: assessment with a biplanar X-ray device. *Insights Imaging.2014*;5:571–583.
129. Le Huec JC, Aunoble S, Philippe L, Nicolas P. Pelvic parameters: origin and significance. *Eur Spine J.* 2011;20(5):564–571.
130. Cho Y, Jo DJ, Hyun SJ, Park JH, Yang NR. From the spinopelvic parameters to global alignment and proportion scores in adult spinal deformity. *Neurospine.* 2023;20(2):467–477.
131. Giles LGF, Taylor JR. Lumbar spine structural changes associated with leg length inequality. *Spine (Phila Pa 1976).* 1982;7:159–162.
132. Cooperstein R, Lew M. The relationship between pelvic torsion and anatomical leg length inequality: a review of the literature. *J Chiropr Med.* 2009;8(3):107–118.
133. Nelson KE, Mnabhi AKS. Chapter 36. The patient with back pain: short. In: Nelson KE, Glonek T, eds. *Somatic Dysfunction in Osteopathic Family Medicine.* 2nd ed. Wolters Kluwer Health; 2015:415–431.
134. Menez C, L'Hermette M, Coquart J. Orthotic insoles improve gait symmetry and reduce immediate pain in subjects with mild leg length discrepancy. *Front Sports Act Living.* 2020;2:579152.
135. Kuchera ML, Irvin RE. Biomechanical considerations in postural realignment. *J Am Osteopath Assoc.* 1987;87(11):781–782.
136. Gofton JP, Trueman GE. Studies in osteoarthritis of the hip: part II. Osteoarthritis of the hip and leg-length disparity. *Can Med Assoc J.* 1971; 104:791–799.
137. Morscher E. Etiology and pathophysiology of leg length discrepancies. *Prog Orthop Surg.* 1977;1:9–19.
138. Sheha E, Steinhaus M, Kim H, Cunningham M, Fragomen A, Rozbruch S. Leg-length discrepancy, functional scoliosis, and low back pain. *JBJS Rev.* 2018;6(8):e6.
139. Travell JG, Simons DG. *Myofascial Pain and Dysfunction: A Trigger Point Manual.* Vol. II. Williams & Wilkins; 1992.
140. Kuchera ML, Kuchera WA. *Osteopathic Considerations in Systemic Dysfunction.* 2nd ed. Revised. Greyden Press; 1994.
141. Patriquin DA. Lift therapy: a study of results. In: Peterson B, ed. *Postural Balance and Imbalance (1983 AAO Yearbook).* American Academy of Osteopathy; 1983:119–122.
142. Heilig D. Principles of lift therapy. In: Peterson B, ed. *Postural Balance and Imbalance (1983 AAO Yearbook).* American Academy of Osteopathy; 1983:113–118.
143. Kuchera ML, Kuchera WA. Postural decompensation. In: *Osteopathic Principles in Practice.* 2nd ed. Revised. Greyden Press; 1994.
144. Kuchera WA, Kuchera ML. Postural decompensation. In: *Osteopathic Principles in Practice.* 2nd ed. Revised. Greyden Press; 1994:343–356.
145. Ferguson AB. The clinical and recent roentgenographic interpretation of lumbosacral anomalies. *Radiology.* 1934;22:548–588.
146. Le Huec JC, Charosky S, Barrey C, Rigal J, Aunoble S. Sagittal imbalance cascade for simple degenerative spine and consequences: algorithm of decision for appropriate treatment. *Eur Spine J.* 2011;20(5): 699–703.
147. Hackett GS. *Ligament and Tendon Relaxation Treated by Prolotherapy.* 3rd ed. Charles C Thomas; 1958.
148. Dorman T. Pelvic mechanics and prolotherapy. In: Vleeming A, Mooney V, Dorman T, eds. *Movement, Stability and Low Back Pain: The Essential Role of the Pelvis.* Churchill Livingstone; 1997:501–522.

93

Osteopathic Considerations in the Patient With Low Back Pain

KURT P. HEINKING ▪ MICHAEL LOUGH ▪ MICHAEL L. KUCHERA

KEY CONCEPTS

- Low back pain (LBP) can affect every aspect of a patient's life: difficulty at work, damage to relationships, changing social roles/identity, psycho-emotional problems, and worries about the future.
- Low back pain is the leading cause of productivity loss worldwide and the cost of managing low back pain in the United States is estimated to be $100 billion annually.
- Acute pain is limited to less than 6 weeks, while subacute is defined as LBP lasting beyond the acute-phase and chronic LBP is pain lasting beyond 12 weeks.
- After ruling out emergent causes of LBP, the physician must be confident in diagnosing and treating the patient with an approach conducive to the setting in which they practice.
- It is important to carefully obtain an accurate past medical and surgical history for the clinician to rule out any urgent or emergent conditions that can produce back pain.
- The clinician who evaluates the patient with low back pain needs to understand sensory, motor, and reflex changes and be able to perform the straight leg raising (SLR) test, which is commonly used to assess for lumbar radiculopathy.
- Diagnostic testing in the absence of red flags is not recommended for axial LBP of less than 12 weeks duration.
- There are multiple national and international clinical practice guidelines (CPGs) for clinicians to review regarding the diagnosis and management of patients with lower back pain.
- When making a diagnosis, the osteopathic physician should not only diagnose the medical condition but also address lifestyle and environmental factors, diet and nutrition, and stress.
- In addition to many medical conditions and diseases, somatic dysfunction can cause low back pain and is commonly associated with other orthopedic, visceral, and mechanical causes of low back pain.
- When considering treatment strategies for the patient, first consider how the patient working with the provided medical recommendations can restore wellness which is fostered by self-regulation, self-healing, and health maintenance.
- Successful applications of OMT in patients with low back pain and somatic dysfunction who also have underlying lumbar spinal pathology require special considerations.
- Aerobic exercise is recommended to improve pain, disability, and mental health in patients with nonspecific low back pain.
- Surgical consultation (orthopedic and/or neurologic) and special imaging tests are indicated if red flags are present, or if 6 to 8 weeks of conservative care has not demonstrated steady progress.

INTRODUCTION

One of the most common conditions an osteopathic physician will see in their office, clinic, or hospital will be the patient who is suffering from lower back pain. No matter which setting, osteopathic philosophical principles can and should be utilized. In all settings, the patient should be empathetically evaluated in totality, including body, mind, and spirit. It is commonplace for modern medicine to look primarily at structural/musculoskeletal factors that are involved. Equally important is to ascertain and address the cognitive, emotional, and spiritual concerns the patient may have. Patients with lower back pain, especially if it is chronic, will have distant effects of their condition affecting all aspects of their life including relationships, occupation, and activities. Involving the patient's spouse, family, friends, and children can be useful to providing a supportive environment for the patient. The patient and their care providers need to understand that their body has its own inherent capacity to heal and its own timeline of recovery. The physician's role is to educate and guide the patient and provide care that not only treats the pathologic process but supports the patient's homeostasis and inherent capacity to heal.

During the evaluation, it is important for the physician to determine the interrelationships between the patient's physical structure, emotional state, and current and past functional capacity. Patients are at their best ability to heal when their physical structure is sound, their emotional health is supported, and management of their condition is guided by the physician and health care team involved.

The priority for the physician is to determine if a serious or life-threatening condition is present that needs immediate attention. Following this, obtaining the relevant history, obtaining, and reviewing the past records, and cognitively developing a differential diagnosis are done. Specific aspects of the physical exam should be evaluated for serious conditions and help confirm or exclude specific diagnoses. This baseline information will direct which diagnostic tests, consultations, or treatments are recommended.

Patients with subacute and chronic lower back pain have commonly visited numerous care providers and may not have a diagnosis for their pain. The diagnosis of somatic dysfunction commonly has not been considered or assessed. The patient's emotional health and job satisfaction, two key factors, are often overlooked. The osteopathic approach needs to include these aspects in addition to the patient's structural issues. For structural issues, osteopathic physicians have a unique role because they can clinically evaluate and treat the structural and functional relationships with osteopathic manipulative treatment.

Patients value a physician who actively listens to their concerns, empathizes with them, supports them, and is an advocate for their best interests. Patients desire a physician who will spend the appropriate time, answer questions, and provide clear structured treatment plans. Patients also value a physician who communicates clearly, returns calls and messages promptly, and provides options to the treatment plan that involves their wishes.

Through this framework, osteopathic physicians utilize a comprehensive history, detailed physical examination, accurate differential diagnosis, and appropriate diagnostic modalities/consults, to prescribe a practical and cost-effective treatment plan. To guide their clinical decision making, osteopathic physicians utilize evidence-based recommendations and standard-of-care guidelines. They are also open to the consideration and application of complementary and alternative approaches and approaches that the patient may want to try outside of the traditional medical paradigm.

EPIDEMIOLOGY AND COST

Low back pain (LBP) is the leading cause of productivity loss worldwide.[1] A systematic review of 13 studies on LBP found the prevalence to range between 1.4% and 20.0% and annual incidence to range between 0.024% and 7.0% with the highest incidence reported in the United States. The wide ranges were attributed to variation in lifestyle and occupation among the populations studied.[2] In 2019, a self-reported survey of approximately 32,000 adults in the United States found that 39% had experienced LBP in the last 3 months.[3] The prevalence of LBP increases with age. It is relatively rare in children, with a prevalence of 1.0% and 6.0% in 7- and 10-year-olds, respectively. However, prevalence rapidly increases, to 18.0% in adolescents,[4] with the highest prevalence among females aged 40 to 80 years old.[5]

The socioeconomic costs of LBP include the direct cost of conventional and alternative medical management as well as more difficult-to-quantify costs such as productivity loss, presenteeism, emotional instability, and unmet social expectations. The cost of managing low back pain in the United States is estimated to be $100 billion annually.[6] A cohort study followed 2.5 million patients and analyzed their medical costs in the 12 months after they received a new LBP diagnosis. They concluded that patients who obtain early imaging or receive surgery for LBP without exhausting conservative therapies account for a disproportionate amount of total costs associated with this common condition.[7] Though only 1.2% of patients received surgery, they represented 29.3% of the costs of all patients. Of all patients, 32.3% received imaging within 30 days of LBP diagnosis and 35.3% that received imaging did so prior to a trial of physical therapy. The mean 12-month costs of those patients who had imaging within 30 days of diagnosis were two times greater than in those who did not have imaging ($1,194 vs. $566).

Presenteeism or impaired productivity at work due to a health condition, is a major component of the socioeconomic costs of LBP. A large US healthcare system studied the impact of presenteeism in 7,959 of their employees over a 4-year period and found that the condition with the highest estimated daily productivity loss and annual cost per person was chronic back pain.[8]

Broadening our view and interpreting the impact of LBP within the biopsychosocial model, we recognize that quantitative outcome measures do not capture the total cost. A systematic review that included 42 studies on the qualitative impact of LBP on people's lives found that patients are most concerned with engagement in meaningful activities, but also want to be believed and have their experiences validated. Due to their back pain, they struggle to meet social expectations and obligations. Furthermore, if they do succeed in meeting these expectations the credibility of their pain and disability claims can be jeopardized.[9] LBP can affect every aspect of a patient's life: difficulty at work, damage to relationships, changing social roles/identity, psycho-emotional problems, and worries about the future.

Classification of Low Back Pain

ACUTE PAIN, SUBACUTE, CHRONIC

Acute pain, commonly caused by nociceptors response to proinflammatory cytokines would be limited to less than 6 weeks. Subacute is defined as LBP lasting beyond the acute-phase and chronic LBP is pain lasting beyond 12 weeks. Chronic pain in the above model would be the result of an ineffective reparative response to degeneration which includes vascularization, innervation, neuro inflammation, and sensitization of nociceptors.[10] The chronic LBP can then be further reinforced by maladaptive pain modulation and central sensitization. (Please see Chapter 74 Chronic Pain Management.)

AGE AND EPIDEMIOLOGY RELATING TO ETIOLOGY

Considering age as part of patient epidemiology in LBP is very important. LBP in a patient younger than 20 or older than 50 requires greater evaluation than LBP in a patient 20 to 50 years of age. Younger patients may have congenital or developmental anomalies that should be identified. Older patients are more likely to develop fractures, malignancy, serious infection, and extraspinal pathology such as Paget disease.

SPECIFIC VERSUS NONSPECIFIC

Conventionally LBP has been divided into two categories: specific LBP if the etiology is known, and nonspecific LBP if the etiology is unknown. As noted above, approximately 90% of patients with LBP have been diagnosed with nonspecific LBP.[11] Osteopathic education includes a broad differential of somatic dysfunction and musculoskeletal syndromes which can represent a part or the whole of a patient's nonspecific LBP.

NOCICEPTIVE/NEUROPATHIC/NOCIPLASTIC

LBP can also be classified by the pain type. The pain can be either nociceptive, neuropathic, or nociplastic in nature. Nociceptive pain is the most common type of pain, this is where damage or potential damage to peripheral tissues activates mechano-gated channels in nociceptors resulting in transduction of pain signals. Neuropathic pain is caused by a disease or lesion affecting the somatosensory nervous system responsible for transmission of pain signals. Nociplastic pain refers to pain caused by altered processing of nociceptive pain where there is no actual or potential tissue damage activating the peripheral nociceptors as well as no disease of the somatosensory nervous system such as a neuropathic pain cause. The common endpoint of these three pain types is the signal to the somatosensory cortex resulting in the perception of pain. These pain types exist on a continuum. Over time prolonged nociception can cause neuroinflammation and altered central pain modulation resulting in neuropathic or nociplastic pain, respectively.[12]

ANATOMIC LOCATION

Pain emanating from the lumbar spine can also be divided and classified anatomically into pain coming from the posterior, middle, and anterior spinal elements.[13] This helps organize pain etiology by anatomic location. The anterior elements include the posterior longitudinal ligament, vertebral body, anterior longitudinal ligament, and intervertebral disk. The middle elements include the central spinal canal, meninges, spinal cord, and nerves. The posterior elements include the spinous process, transverse processes, lamina, pedicles, intervertebral joints, ligaments, and joining capsules. LBP most commonly stems from the posterior elements of the spine. In addition, the basic structural element of the spine is the functional spinal unit (FSU). The FSU is the motion segment that consists of two adjacent vertebrae, the intervertebral disk, facet joints, and the connecting ligamentous tissues. For more information on these anatomical divisions of the spine and their clinical implications, please see Chapter 84 Osteopathic Considerations in Orthopedics.

PATHOPHYSIOLOGY AND MECHANISMS

Low back pain is a complex and incompletely understood multifactorial process. A specific cause cannot be found in up to 90% of patients.[11] This leads to frustration for patients and physicians alike. However, osteopathic physicians have the training to diagnose and treat the biomechanical component of the patient's LBP by using their hands to detect the biochemical signs. Palpatory findings such as TART changes signify disturbed local physiology. Some common pathophysiologic processes that occur in back pain patients include spinal degeneration, spinal stenosis and nerve compression, and inflammatory low back pain. In each of these common processes, spinal nociceptors are activated. Nociceptors are found in spinal ligaments, periosteum of the vertebral body, paraspinal muscles, facet joints, and the outer third of the annulus fibrosis, and activation of these causes the majority of LBP.[14]

LBP stemming from the spine itself is typically due to self-limiting degenerative causes that rarely result in neurologic compromise.[15] Terms that describe this condition include lumbago, mechanical LBP, or spondylosis.

The pathophysiology of degeneration of the lumbar disks starts in the nucleus pulposus (see Fig. 93.1). This incompressible structure between vertebral bodies is contained by the annulus fibrosus and supports the anterior spine. The incompressibility of the nucleus pulposus is due to its large water content generated by a matrix of proteoglycans that are synthesized by sparsely present cells within the nucleus pulposus itself. Because the disk is avascular it relies on diffusion of nutrients from capillaries of the adjacent vertebral bodies. The intervertebral disk also lacks scavenger cells, therefore metabolic byproducts accumulate within the disk over time. Insufficient nutrition or increased concentration of proinflammatory mediators causes a decline in the function and population of those sparse cells within the nucleus pulposus. This leaves the disk vulnerable to hereditary conditions and environmental damage.[15] Harm to nucleus pulposus cells causes a reduction in the number of proteoglycans which in turn reduces the hydrostatic pressure and water content within the nucleus pulposus. These changes cause laxity in the nucleus pulposus which exposes the annulus fibrosus to the direct compressive forces of the vertebral bodies, making tearing of the annulus fibrosus more likely. Tears in the annulus fibrosus develop well-vascularized and innervated granulation tissue which releases nerve growth factor, all leading to further worsening of intervertebral disk degeneration and increased nociception via these newly created free nerve endings.[16] These degenerative changes can cause microinstability of the FSU and segmental motion disturbances, which can be determined through palpation/segmental motion testing. However,

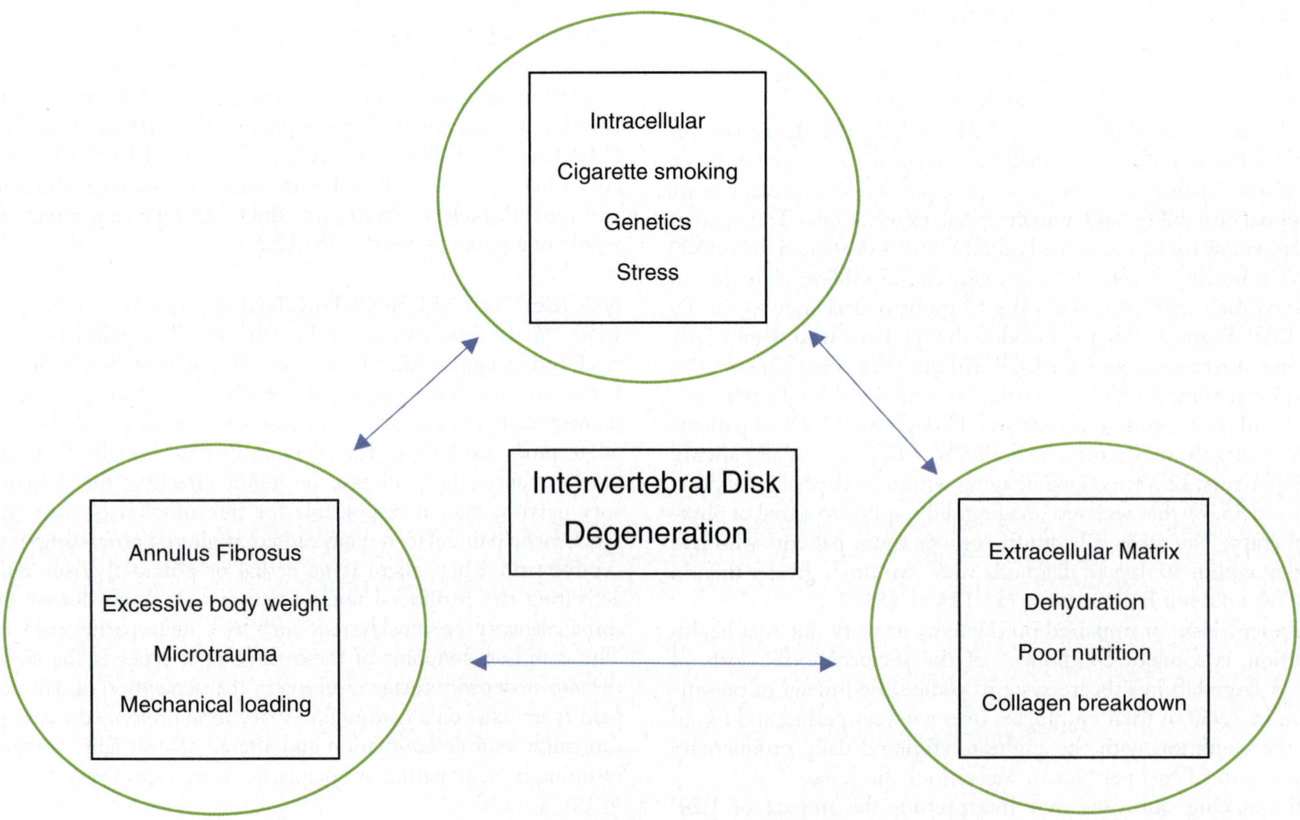

Figure 93.1. Intervertebral disk degeneration. (Adapted from Daly C, Ghosh P, Jenkin G, Oehme D, Goldschlager T. A review of animal models of intervertebral disc degeneration: pathophysiology, regeneration, and translation to the clinic. *Biomed Res Int.* 2016;2016:5952165. http://creativecommons.org/licenses/by/4.0/)

there is also leakage of inflammatory mediators through the annular tear causing inflammation of nearby structures, in particular the spinal nerve root, resulting in radicular pain. The exposure of the nerve root to proinflammatory cytokines can result in inflammatory neuropathy and neuropathic pain.[10] These inflammatory mediators also affect the bone, causing new hypertrophic bone formation and sclerosis at the vertebral body which are visible on imaging as Modic changes.[15] Beyond the chemical radicular pain, annular tears also create the opportunity for disk tissue to herniate through the annular defect resulting in direct compression of the nerve root. In addition to these pathophysiologic causes, there may be causes intrinsic or extrinsic to the spinal canal, disks, and nerve roots. Please see Chapter 84 Osteopathic Considerations in Orthopedics for further discussion on this topic.

Approach to the Patient

INPATIENT, OUTPATIENT, EMERGENCY DEPARTMENT, SPECIALIST

It is imperative that all osteopathic physicians, regardless of setting and specialty, can diagnose and treat LBP because it affects such a broad range of the population. The primary care patient, hospitalized patient, pregnant patient, emergency department patient, rehab patient, and patients presenting to specialists of all types can all present with LBP. Regardless of setting, the initial evaluation must rule out emergent and urgent causes of LBP as covered in the red flag section and further sections on evaluating the patient. After ruling out emergent causes of LBP, the physician must be confident in diagnosing and treating the patient with an approach conducive to the setting in which they practice. Osteopathic physicians have the responsibility to utilize knowledge, skill, and ability from their OMM training to benefit the patient and ease their pain.

CHRONICITY

Establishing the chronicity of LBP determines what diagnostic tests to order, and guides treatment choice, aligning the patient's expectations and recovery. Low back pain chronicity is categorized as acute (lasting less than 6 weeks), subacute (lasting 6 to 12 weeks), and chronic (lasting over 12 weeks). [17] For acute LBP, guidelines recommend nonsteroidal anti-inflammatory medications (NSAIDs) and avoidance of bed rest.[18] While most cases of acute low back pain will resolve without treatment within 6 weeks, approximately 32% of patients will develop chronic LBP.[19] Whereas acute LBP is very common and assumed to resolve spontaneously, chronic LBP is a chronic pain condition with significant risk of recurrence and disability. There is ongoing research into the factors that increase the risk of acute LBP converting to chronic LBP as is discussed further in the "yellow flags" section. For example, to target behaviors that can sustain a chronic pain condition there is a strong recommendation that treatments targeting fear avoidance combined with physical therapy are recommended compared to physical therapy alone in the first 6 months.[17] For example, guidelines strongly recommend cognitive behavioral therapy in combination with physical therapy to improve pain in patients with LBP lasting over 12 months.[17] Medical evidence supports the use of OMT and osteopathic manipulative treatment can reduce pain and improve functional status regardless of LBP duration or setting.[20,21] Physicians should feel confident discussing OMT as an evidence-based recommendation with patients and colleagues.

Obtaining the History

History taking in general is discussed in multiple chapters of the text, and LBP-specific history taking is also discussed in the chapter on orthopedics.

CHIEF COMPLAINT

The chief complaint is preferably documented in the patient's own words. It could simply be "lower back pain," "buttock pain," "hip pain," "backache," and any number of similar complaints. The complaint and documentation may vary based on the patient's age and amount of verbal communication. It may also be obtained from a parent or caregiver.

HISTORY OF PRESENT ILLNESS

During the initial evaluation of a patient with LBP, a detailed history should include asking:

- When the pain began, and if there was an event that coincided with its onset, especially a history of trauma such as a recent motor vehicle collision.
- How the pain has changed over time. Whether it is constant or waxing and waning. If it has been getting gradually better, or worse. There could have been an abrupt event after the initial inciting event that caused the pain to worsen or change dramatically.
- The precise location and radiation of the pain. LBP is notoriously difficult for the patient to pinpoint, nonetheless, it is important to prompt the patient because localization to a particular anatomical location or dermatomal distribution can help immensely in determining etiology.
- Because abnormalities are frequently seen in spine imaging on asymptomatic individuals, pain localization must be obtained to correlate clinically when imaging is ordered.
    - Axial pain: pain focused on or near the spine itself.
    - Radicular pain: pain extending in a dermatomal distribution away from the spine, typically into the lower extremities.
- The quality of the pain, preferably without priming the patient with specific terms—"What does the pain feel like." Quality descriptors such as burning, achy, sharp, tingling, shooting, and pressure can help guide investigating etiology of the pain.
    - Clinicians may utilize a standardized and validated assessment tool that involves the patient's written self-report, such as the McGill Pain Questionnaire [22] for a general assessment of pain, or an assessment of a particular pain type, with the Leeds Assessment of Neuropathic Symptoms and Signs pain scale.[23]
    - The patient may also be asked to write their own self-description/paragraph. It can be addressed to the treating physician or formatted like a diary.
- Activities that make the pain better or worse.
- "Red flags," which include constitutional symptoms (fever, lethargy, weight loss) and neurologic symptoms (numbness, tingling, weakness, incontinence, retention) as well as claudication, morning stiffness, nocturnal pain, and bony tenderness (see Fig. 93.2).
- The treatments the patient has already tried and their respective effectiveness.
- Past medical and surgical history.
- Social history and psychological factors such as "Yellow flags" that may contribute to the patient's pain, affect prognosis, and should be addressed in the treatment plan.
- The way their pain may affect their activities of daily living to gauge disability.
    - A standardized and validated assessment tool such as the Oswestry Low Back Pain Disability Questionnaire.[24]

REVIEW OF SYSTEMS

An essential part of every initial patient encounter is the review of systems (ROS). For more information on the review of systems please see Chapter 27 Osteopathic History and Physical

Sidebar 1: Evaluation for Possible Serious Conditions		
Possible Serious Conditions	**Red Flags (e.g., signs, symptoms, history)**	**Suggested Evaluation[a]**
Cauda equina syndrome or conus medullaris syndrome	• Urinary retention • Urinary or fecal incontinence • Saddle anesthesia • Changes in rectal tone • Severe/progressive lower extremity neurologic deficits	• Emergent MRI[b] (preferred)
Infection	• Fever • Immunosuppression • IV drug use • Recent infection, indwelling catheters (e.g., central line, Foley)	• MRI[c] • ESR and/or CRP
Fracture	• History of osteoporosis • Chronic use of corticosteroids • Older age (≥75 years old) • Recent trauma • Younger patients at risk for stress fracture (e.g., overuse)	• Lumbosacral plain radiography • For inconclusive results, advanced imaging as indicated
Cancer	• History of cancer with new onset of LBP • Unexplained weight loss • Failure of LBP to improve after 1 month • Age >50 years • Multiple risk factors present	• MRI[c] • Lumbosacral plain radiography

[a] Consider specialty consultation

[b] MRI, except where contraindicated (e.g., patients with pacemakers), otherwise CT or CT myelogram

[c] MRI without and with contrast, except where contraindicated (e.g., renal insufficiency)

Abbreviations: CRP: C-reactive protein; CT: computed tomography; ESR: erythrocyte sedimentation rate; IV: intravenous; LBP: low back pain; MRI: magnetic resonance imaging

Figure 93.2. Evaluation of possible serious conditions. (Department of Veterans Affairs, DoD. *VA/DoD clinical practice guideline for the diagnosis and treatment of low back pain.* Ver 3.0. U.S. Government Printing Office; 2022. https://www.healthquality.va.gov/guidelines/Pain/lbp/VADoDLBPCPGFinal508.pdf)

Exam. When assessing LBP, a thorough review of systems is important to identify the common causes of low back pain that are both easy to treat (i.e., rash in shingles) and catastrophic (i.e., constitutional symptoms in malignancy). While questions related to "red flags" will be relevant to nearly all medical specialties, the usefulness of other questions will vary based on patient presentation and clinical context.

- General questions to ask—Have you had weight change, appetite change, generalized weakness, fatigue, fevers, chills, or night sweats?
  - Fever could indicate an infectious cause raising concern of epidural abscess which is why fever is a red flag. Constitutional symptoms such as fever, weight loss, and night sweats could indicate that the LBP is caused by spinal metastasis, this is why constitutional symptoms are a red flag. Constitutional symptoms can also indicate systemic autoimmune diseases such as lupus.
- Cardiovascular questions to ask—Are you experiencing chest pain, abdominal pain, edema, leg weakness with exertion, or discoloration of your limbs?
  - It is important for the clinician to rule out any urgent or emergent conditions that can produce back pain. A dilated, leaking, or ruptured aortic aneurysm is a life-threatening emergency that can present with severe midback pain. Prompt diagnosis and sending the patient to the emergency room is of high importance. Peripheral vascular disease can produce pain and claudication-type symptoms in the lower extremities like the pain referral seen in neuropathy and neurogenic claudication of the lumbar spine. Persistent low back or buttock pain accompanied by claudication, impotence, or decreased pulses should raise concern for Leriche syndrome. Leriche syndrome is caused by severe atherosclerosis of the distal abdominal aorta, iliac arteries, and femoral-popliteal vessels often requiring stenting. Persistent low back pain accompanied by pelvic pain, bowel/bladder symptoms, leg swelling, or leg pain should raise concern for May–Thurner syndrome. May–Thurner syndrome is when the right common iliac artery overlies and compresses the common iliac vein resulting in impaired venous flow and deep venous thrombosis.
- Pulmonary questions to ask—Do you have a cough, shortness of breath, or tire quickly with activity?
  - Lung cancer can metastasize to the spine and can be the etiology of low back pain. It is not uncommon for patients with a chronic cough to develop back pain and diskogenic issues. Long-standing chronic obstructive pulmonary disease (COPD) changes such as a barrel-type chest can affect the function of the AP curves of the spine and diaphragm. Function of the diaphragm can be affected by iliopsoas spasm due to common spinal and myofascial attachments.
- Gastrointestinal questions to ask—Have you had incontinence of stool, constipation, or a bloody bowel movement?
  - Diseases of the gastrointestinal system can produce midback and lower back pain. Patients with Crohn disease, ulcerative colitis, peptic ulcer disease, pancreatitis, colon cancer, cholelithiasis, and irritable bowel syndrome commonly have back pain. This can be multifactorial in nature and involves referred pain, visceral distension and dysfunction, viscerosomatic reflexes, and reflex psoas muscle spasm.
- Genitourinary questions to ask—Have you had incontinence of urine, pain with urination, increased urinary frequency, or flank pain?
  - Renal stones are a common cause of mid- to lower back pain as the kidneys and ureters are retroperitoneal in nature and

stretching of these structures as the stone passes causes reflex thoracolumbar muscle spasm and excruciating back pain. Patients with stones, hydronephrosis, and pyelonephritis can present with back pain, fever, chills, and dysuria.

- Musculoskeletal questions to ask—Have you noticed joint swelling, morning stiffness, back curvature, awakening due to back pain, lower extremity paresthesia, muscle soreness, or weakness?
  - In the younger active population, spondylolysis is more common, especially with repetitive hyperextension stress. In an adolescent, idiopathic scoliosis classically does not cause back pain, however, in adults, degenerative scoliosis can be painful and problematic. In adults, sprains and strains, hip flexor spasms, and somatic dysfunction of the lumbar sacrum and pelvis are very common causes of lower back pain. In the older population, cancer and osteoporosis with subsequent compression fractures may be a cause of thoracolumbar back pain. Osteoarthritis with resultant spondylosis and spinal stenosis are common causes of lower back pain associated with sciatica and leg weakness. It is important to know if the patient has had any manipulative treatment either by a chiropractor, osteopath, or physical therapist (PT) in the past, and the result of such treatment.
- Neurologic questions to ask—Have you experienced numbness, tingling, confusion, tremors, dizziness, or weakness with prolonged walking?
  - Patients with chronic neurologic disease such as Parkinson disease, Alzheimer dementia, and multiple sclerosis, can have postural and mobility issues. Generalized stiffness, a forward-bent posture, and weakness of the core muscles and legs make treatment more challenging especially in the face of concomitant lumbar radiculopathy due to spinal stenosis.
- Integumentary and connective tissue questions to ask—Have you noticed changes in the color or texture of your skin, rashes, itching, or dryness?
  - Patients with low back pain that have a dermatomal unilateral rash may have shingles. Shingles may present with low back pain prior to the development of the rash. Patients who have a history of psoriasis can develop polyarticular arthritis, and commonly have lower back pain. Patients who have hypermobility due to Ehlers–Danlos syndrome or Marfan syndrome may have lower back pain due to many factors. Joint hypermobility and decreased muscle tone in these patients contribute to the development of somatic dysfunction and pain.
- Gynecologic questions to ask—Can you tell me about your menstrual cycles? Have you ever been pregnant before? Have you had pelvic pain, changes in vaginal discharge, dysmenorrhea, genital sores, genital itching, or prior STD exposure and treatment?
  - One of the most common causes of low back pain in gynecologic patients is associated with pregnancy. This pain is multifactorial and not solely related to the hypermobility seen. However, there are many other causes of low back pain in a gynecologic patient such as endometriosis, large uterine fibroids, traumatic delivery, diastasis of the pubic symphysis, etc.
- Hematologic, oncologic, lymphatic questions to ask—Have you noticed unusual bleeding, swelling, bruising easily, or frequent infections?
  - Specific cancers metastasize to the bone more frequently than others. These include lung, colon, breast, and prostate. All these metastatic tumors can cause lower back pain. There are also primary malignancies of the bone such as sarcoma. Multiple myeloma is another condition that frequently presents with back pain.
- Psychiatric questions to ask—Have you experienced sadness, hopelessness, helplessness, or anxiety?
  - Psychiatric conditions such as depression and anxiety are frequent comorbidities with any pain condition, which includes lower back pain. A recent cross-sectional study of 3,478 participants with chronic LBP found that for every one-point increase in the PHQ-4 score for anxiety and depression the odds ratio of high pain intensity increased by 1.25 points.[25] Often management of comorbid psychiatric condition can help manage their LBP with the importance increasing as the pain becomes more chronic.

RED FLAGS IN THE LOW BACK PAIN PATIENT

As discussed above, reviewing the patient's medical history via a systems approach can provide the clinician with useful information to determine what role the patient's medical conditions are playing in the development of their low back pain.

RED FLAGS AND YELLOW FLAGS AND LOW BACK PAIN

A red flag is a clinical finding in the history taking or physical exam that may indicate serious underlying pathology that requires prompt and accurate diagnosis. All LBP management guidelines recommend screening patients for red flags at the initial encounter. A review of guidelines identified 46 discrete red flags in four main categories: malignancy, fracture, cauda equina syndrome (CES), and infection.[26] Red flags warrant further workup, as multiple red flags increase the risk of underlying pathology. For example, LBP following recent trauma carries an 11.4% probability of underlying vertebral fracture, if the patient is >50 years old this probability increases to 13.1%, and if the patient is >70 years old it further increases to 20.5%.[27]

Red flags in patient history[26]

- Cancer
- Physical trauma
- Age >50, greater concern with age >70
- Immunodeficiency
- Immunosuppression
- Osteoporosis
- IV drug use

Red flags in ROS[26]

- Fever >100.4° F
- Pain worsens during rest or at night
- Saddle anesthesia
- Focal leg weakness
- Incontinence of urine or stool
- Urinary retention
- Gait changes
- Unanticipated weight loss
- Night sweats

It is important to know that the sensitivity and specificity of a single red flag are quite low but that combinations of red flags (clusters) significantly increase the probability of having a certain specific pathology. Also, screening red flags only by using questionnaires can lead to false-negative results therefore, a good clinical evaluation remains mandatory.[27,28]

For acute LBP in the absence of red flags or neurologic deficits, guidelines strongly recommend against obtaining imaging.[18] However, a cohort study followed 5,233 patients after their initial presentation to their primary care physician and found that at 6 months 32% had developed chronic LBP.[19] Given the high socioeconomic cost of chronic LBP many clinicians and researchers see it as a serious medical illness with acute LBP as its harbinger. This has spawned a growing interest in secondary prevention of chronic back pain by identifying risk factors for conversion of acute to chronic LBP. It is still important to follow consensus recommendations for acute low back pain, in fact, the same cohort study found that patients exposed to one, two, or three recommendations that were discordant with guidelines within the first 21 days of presentation were 1.39, 1.88, and 2.16 times more likely to develop chronic LBP compared to those with no exposure.[19] It is important for clinicians to educate patients on chronic LBP and help them with lifestyle changes that can decrease this risk.

Whereas red flags screen for serious underlying pathology in LBP, the identified factors that play a critical role in chronic LBP have been categorized as yellow (pain-related behavior), orange (psychiatric symptoms), black (systemic obstacles), or blue (occupational involvement) flags. There are validated screening tools that aim to predict which patients will develop chronic pain and disability after presenting with new LBP such as the Keele STarT back screening,[29] optimal screening for prediction of referral and outcome yellow flag tools,[30] and the National Institute of Health Chronic Pain Criteria.[30] What follows is a simplified list of yellow flags which includes factors from all categories that aims to help physicians recognize patients at higher risk of chronic LBP.

Yellow Flags[31]

- High baseline pain and disability
- Occupation with elevated physical or emotional stress
- Cigarette smoking
- Spinal deformities
- Genetic predisposition
- Peripheral vascular disease
- Obesity
- Sleep problems
- Depression
- Anxiety
- Pain catastrophizing
- Work dissatisfaction
- Poor social support
- Low socioeconomic status
- General health-related (i.e., opioid use and sedentary lifestyle)
- Fear-avoidance beliefs
- Irritability
- Toxic relationships
- Reduced perceived control over one's life

PAST MEDICAL AND SURGICAL HISTORY

It is important to carefully obtain an accurate past medical and surgical history. This is especially true in patients who have had chronic low back pain with extensive evaluations, referrals, surgical procedures, and other pain management procedures. History is the most critical factor in determining the diagnosis. Another important aspect is the age of the patient, and if any red flags are present, leading to more expedited diagnosis and treatment. Obtaining a chronologic history can be beneficial for these patients. Once the diagnostic and management timeline has been determined, the clinician can conclude where the patient is currently in the overall scheme of low back pain management.

Regarding past medical history, it may be important to obtain information from an independent historian such as a spouse or family member. Patients may or may not understand (or remember) what diagnosed medical conditions they have. Reviewing the information that they have put on their history and physical forms and placing an approximate date of diagnosis next to each item can be beneficial. Note what symptoms or issues are currently being worked up yet do not have a formal diagnosis currently.

The past medical history of low back pain patients should always include information on smoking tobacco, job stress, occupational injuries, exercise frequency, and concomitant depression and anxiety. It is very important to elicit a trauma history including slips and falls, motor vehicle accidents, childbirth, fractures, and sports-related injuries.

A detailed surgical history includes type, date, complications, outcome, anesthesia issues, and postoperative course. This information is useful if the patient needs to have surgical consultation regarding their lower back pain.

Medical and surgical history can also be obtained based on body systems. This is in addition to any current symptoms recorded in the review of systems. Many body systems can have relevance in patients with lower back pain.

SOCIAL HISTORY CONSIDERATIONS

Social history considerations in the patient with LBP are made up of three categories of risk factors: biomechanical, psychosocial, and personal. Biomechanical risk factors include activities with increased or asymmetric loading of the lumbar spine. This is described as an occupation or hobby with repetitive spinal loading or repetitive asymmetric tasks, such as working in a shipping warehouse or playing hockey. The psychosocial risk factors include comorbid psychiatric disorders such as generalized anxiety disorder or major depressive disorder but also include psychogenic stress related to job satisfaction, responsibility, and variety. The personal risk factors include previously diagnosed psychiatric disorders as well as obesity, peripheral vascular disease, smoking history, family history, and gender-related risk factors. Please see yellow flags for a comprehensive list of risk factors.

MEDICATIONS AND ALLERGIES

It is important to obtain an accurate history of allergies and/or sensitivities to medications. This is important to know in selecting an appropriate treatment plan. Some patients have multiple drug allergies that are well-defined. Some patients have medication sensitivities, with adverse side effects. Understanding both is important and as is determining if it is due to a specific drug or the entire class of drugs. Sometimes a chronologic history of medication is important to determine the next best step. Patients with multiple drug sensitivities can have pharmacogenomic testing performed. When reviewing the medication history, many patients have tried numerous supplements, herbal compounds, homeopathic remedies, and natural products. Many of these do not exist in the electronic health record, yet still need to be noted.

Obtaining a history of opioid use, side effects, treatment, addiction, and side effects is also important. It has been demonstrated that short-, intermediate-, and long-term opioid use was a predictor of worse back-specific disability, and physical functioning, questioning the utility of opioid therapy for chronic low back pain.[32]

Physical Examination

GENERAL

The osteopathic structural examination is part of the complete physical assessment as detailed in the chapter on the screening and regional osteopathic structural exam. Lumbar, sacral, and pelvic regional anatomy and dysfunction are detailed in the chapters on functional anatomy and diagnosis. Reviewing those chapters in addition to reading this section will be helpful. Some additional items to consider when evaluating the patient with low back pain for somatic dysfunction are as follows:

- A complete physical examination should be performed, with special emphasis on regions that are spotlighted by history, or that have a functional association.
- Examining the part of the body that is painful is best left for the last portion of the evaluation.
- Do not forget to evaluate the vital signs in a patient with low back pain. Vital signs can document the presence of fever associated with an infection or neoplasm.
- Tachycardia may be the sympathetic nervous system's response to the patient's pain.
- Many times, objective physical examination findings do not correlate with a distinct etiology for lower back pain. For example, neurologic examination of the peripheral nerves in the lower extremities lacks sensitivity and specificity for diagnosing lumbar spinal disk herniation and radiculopathy.[33]
- Repeat reexamination is needed to correlate the validity and reproducibility of physical findings with other components of patient evaluation for low back pain.
- There are several active physical tests to evaluate for functional deficits and disabilities in low back pain patients, such as the sit-to-stand test.[34] The following functional assessment questionnaires also evaluate for disabilities:
  - Oswestry disability index
  - Roland-Morris disability questionnaire
  - Hendler 10-minute screening test
- Patients with low back pain often state they cannot sit or stand up straight; however, keep in mind that a slumped posture may also be a sign of depression.
- Clues to thoracic and lumbar somatic dysfunction may be indicated by observing the spacing difference between the arms and the hip/waist on each side of the body with the patient standing at ease. This sign may indicate the presence of scoliosis, strain from sacral base unleveling due to a short leg, or a unilateral muscle spasm.
  - If the protective spasm is unilateral owing to injury of the tissues on one side of the spine, functional scoliosis develops.
  - The spine is tilted to one side because of one-sided muscle spasm.
- If the patient likes to stand in a forward-bent position, consider bilateral psoas muscle spasm or a condition that is putting pressure on lumbar nerves in the intervertebral foramen.
  - If the patient is leaning forward, to one side and has the ipsilateral foot everted when standing or walking, consider a unilateral psoas spasm.
  - If this develops into a severe psoas syndrome on one side, the patient may also complain of pain in the contralateral hip and leg, rarely past the knee.
- When a patient stands very erect and dislikes bending forward, they may be protecting a herniated disk or suffering the effects of spinal stenosis, especially if there are other symptoms, such as muscular weakness, reflex changes, or muscle atrophy.
- Arching the back and increasing the lordosis forces the facet joints together, narrows the foramen through which the nerves exit the spine, and compresses the disk posteriorly.
- Patients with herniated disks have changes in their posture and gait.
- Disk herniation can also cause scoliosis by irritating nerves on one side of the spine. This usually occurs at the L4–L5 level.
- Patients do not like to bear weight on the leg that has sciatica or radicular pain.
- Hip shift during gait and asymmetric pelvic side shift during standing assessment occurs when the lumbar spine cannot side bend to one side as well as the other. This occurs in disk herniation, scoliosis, unlevel sacral base, and lumbosacral somatic dysfunctions.
- Herniation of a nucleus pulposus *lateral* to the corresponding nerve root may cause a sciatic list away from the side of the irritated nerve root.
- Herniation of a nucleus pulposus *medial* to the corresponding nerve root may cause a sciatic list toward the side of the irritated nerve root.

VITALS

The vital signs can indicate that a patient is experiencing pain, specifically tachycardia, hypertension, and tachypnea. These three findings alone or in combination can help validate the patient's subjective experience of pain and can be used to corroborate severity of pain over time. When taking the vital signs, an assessment of the patient's pain is also done using the visual analog scale, or simply asking the patient to rate their pain on a scale of 0 to 10 with 0 being no pain and 10 being the most intense pain imaginable.

GAIT AND STATION

The physical exam begins with observation, this includes how the patient appears in the waiting room, how they walk to the exam room, and their choice of position and activities while waiting in the exam room. As the clinician enters the exam room, they need to assess how the patient is sitting, if they are reading or on the phone, and if they appear comfortable and relaxed. Or are they in obvious discomfort, leaning to one side, and appearing worried?

It is important for the clinician to evaluate the patient's gait and station as their ease with walking can provide clues to their level of functional disability. A high stepping gait may be related to a foot drop and a neurologic source. Hyperextension of one knee while walking may indicate previous injuries to that extremity. Somatic dysfunction of the extremity can cause persistent sacral and pelvic dysfunction which could be key to unraveling their LBP.

GENERAL MEDICAL EXAM—INCLUDING HEENT, HEART, LUNGS, ABDOMEN

Examination of other body systems is imperative to ensure there are no overlooked or underlying visceral diseases related to somatic dysfunction of the lumbar region. Once an underlying disease is diagnosed and managed appropriately, related somatic dysfunction can be addressed at the appropriate time and setting. In the low back pain patient, always evaluate HEENT, heart, lungs, abdomen, and the nervous system on each patient visit for evidence of visceral disease that can refer to pain in the low back. Pertinent examples include the following:

- Auscultate the four quadrants of the abdomen to determine the presence, location, frequency, and pitch of peristaltic waves. An intermittent, low, occasional slow gurgle is normal. Conversely, high-pitched tinkling sounds may denote a developing bowel obstruction.
- Absence of bowel sounds may indicate a paralytic ileus.
- A bruit in the midline of the abdomen between the xiphoid process and the umbilicus could indicate renal stenosis or abdominal aortic aneurysm (AAA) (especially when associated with a pulsating abdominal mass).
- A bruit at the junction between the middle and outer two-thirds of the inguinal region could indicate a significant atherosclerosis of the common iliac or femoral artery.

- A bruit over the umbilical region could indicate saddle thrombosis or severe atherosclerosis at the bifurcation of the abdominal aorta.
- The abdomen is also palpated for masses.
- Palpation is aided by mental visualization of the liver, kidneys, stomach, small intestines, and bifurcation of the aorta at the level of the umbilicus, and the colon.
- The midline region between the xiphoid and umbilicus should be palpated for any pulsating tumor (abdominal aneurysm).
- Anteriorly occurring pulsations are normal, but lateral pulsations of the aorta suggest an aneurysm, especially if it is widened greater than 1 in (a normal adult abdominal aorta should not be wider than 1 in).
- Anterior Chapman points related to organs associated with referred symptoms in the lumbar region are located around the umbilicus and the pelvis and along the iliotibial bands. (Please see the chapter regarding Chapman reflexes for further information.)
- Tender points in these locations may be associated with hypersympathetic activity resulting from viscerosomatic reflexes initiated in an irritated colon or pelvic organ, and the physician should question the patient regarding dysfunction of the organ most likely to be associated with that particular tender point.
- A positive response to specific questioning helps position a somatic clue according to its significance and rank when considering a differential diagnosis.
- If there is an arthritic process or other rheumatologic presentation, the eye examination may reveal the presence of conjunctivitis (reactive arthritis) or iritis (ankylosing spondylitis).
- Examination of the oropharynx may reveal painless (reactive arthritis) or painful (Bechet syndrome) oral ulcers.
- Lymphadenopathy may be associated with neoplastic processes (lymphoma), infectious processes (tuberculosis and subacute bacterial endocarditis), or idiopathic processes (sarcoidosis).

NEUROLOGIC EXAM

It is important to perform a good thorough neurologic examination prior to evaluating the lumbar spinal segments. Attention is paid to the sensory, motor, and deep tendon reflex (DTR) aspects of the neurologic examination. Physicians should be familiar with the neurology of the lower extremity (see Fig. 93.3). It is common practice to evaluate for muscle atrophy (lower motor neuron), dural tension signs and nerve root irritation (radiculopathy), and muscle spasticity with clonus (upper motor neuron). The differentiation of upper motor neuron, nerve root, and peripheral nerve lesions is an important one. The clinician who evaluates the patient with low back pain needs to understand and be able to apply testing for sensory, motor, and reflex changes that can occur at the L1 through S1 levels.

SENSORY EXAM

- The clinician can evaluate gross sensory loss or more specific sensory loss.
- A knowledge of the dermatomal, myotomal, and sclerotomal patterns is important as well as a knowledge of the distribution of the peripheral nerves.
- The best way to evaluate sensation is by two-point discrimination.
- Monofilament testing should be performed on the feet of patients with diabetes and suspected neuropathy.
- Many clinicians use a bent paper clip for this test.
- Testing for hot/cold evaluates the spinothalamic tract.
- Evaluation for balance and proprioception evaluates the dorsal column/medial lemniscus system.

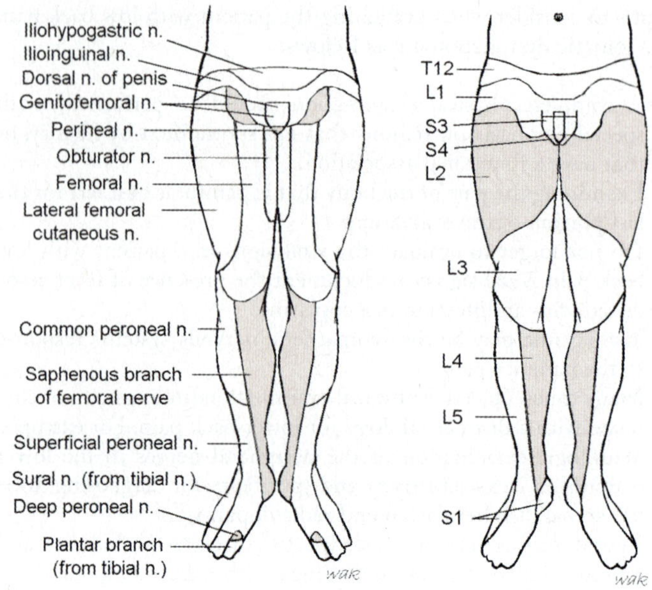

Figure 93.3. A. Peripheral nerve patterns. **B.** Dermatomal or radicular.

MUSCLE STRENGTH EXAM

- Of the possible neurologic abnormalities, true muscle weakness is the most reliable indication of persistent nerve compression with loss of nerve conduction. The following maneuvers help to determine weakness.
  - The patient should perform 10 toe raises on both feet and 10 more on each foot separately.
  - Repeated testing causes fatigue, which accentuates differences in strength in the lower extremities.
  - Patients may also be asked to walk on their heels to test for strength of the dorsiflexors of the foot (L5), or walk on their toes, which test the gastrocnemius/soleus complex (S1).

DEEP TENDON REFLEXES EXAM

- DTRs are monosynaptic. Performing them correctly and symmetrically is important.
- If necessary, have the patient perform the Jendrassik maneuver. The patient attempts to pull apart their locked hands which prevents conscious inhibition of the reflex.
- Unilateral loss of an ankle reflex is a significant neurologic sign, irrespective of age.
- Hyperactive reflexes may indicate an upper motor neuron lesion such as a stroke, spinal cord injury, multiple sclerosis, cerebral palsy, etc. It can be normal if bilateral, but clonus is never a normal finding and requires a workup.
- Certain metabolic conditions can cause hypoactive DTRs (hypothyroidism, hypothermia, calcium or magnesium abnormalities, cerebellar dysfunction, β-blockade).

ADDITIONAL REFLEXES EXAM

- The superficial abdominal reflex is elicited by rubbing a sharp object in a rhomboid shape on the abdomen.
  - A positive abdominal reflex results in the retraction of the umbilicus in the direction of the quadrant stroked.
  - Unilateral absence of the reflex suggests a lesion of an ipsilateral nerve root between T7 and L2, depending on the quadrant affected.

- If a positive Babinski reflex is present, the absence of abdominal reflexes takes on greater significance.
- Palpatory findings of abnormal neurologic activity in the lumbar spine include hyperactive, hypertonic, and irritable lumbar paraspinal muscles.
- The neurologic examination is essential for identifying signs of nerve entrapment, irritation, inflammation, or disease. Further information about the neurologic exam can be found in the chapter on osteopathic considerations in neurology.

STRAIGHT LEG RAISING TEST

The straight leg raising (SLR) test is used to detect radicular pain in patients presenting with LBP by mechanically provoking those irritated nerve roots. Differentiating radicular pain is important because LBP with radiculopathy has a worse prognosis and would benefit from different treatments,[35] such as epidural steroid injections which are discussed later in the chapter. The test is performed with the patient lying supine. A positive test is indicated by eliciting a sharp shooting pain from proximal to distally along the posterior aspect of the thigh, past the knee to the heel and plantar or lateral foot while the supine patient's hip is actively or passively flexed with the knee extended. The degree of hip flexion at which the pain is elicited is noted. Typically, a positive test will be between 30 and 70 degrees (see Fig. 93.4).

A normal sign is no pain, even up to 90 degrees of flexion. Low back pain elicited with the SLR test is also a negative test. A similar test called the slump test, can also be performed with the patient in the seated position, where the physician extends the patient's knee to 180 degrees. There may be hamstring stretching-type pain, which indicates hypertonic hamstring muscles, not radiculopathy.

It is common for the test to provoke pain from irritation of non-neural tissues. The test can be augmented using structural differentiation maneuvers such as neck flexion, ankle dorsiflexion, or hip adduction, all of which are alternative ways to mechanically provoke the irritated nerve. A recent meta-analysis found fair reliability of the test with structural differentiation maneuvers producing at least moderate reliability.[35]

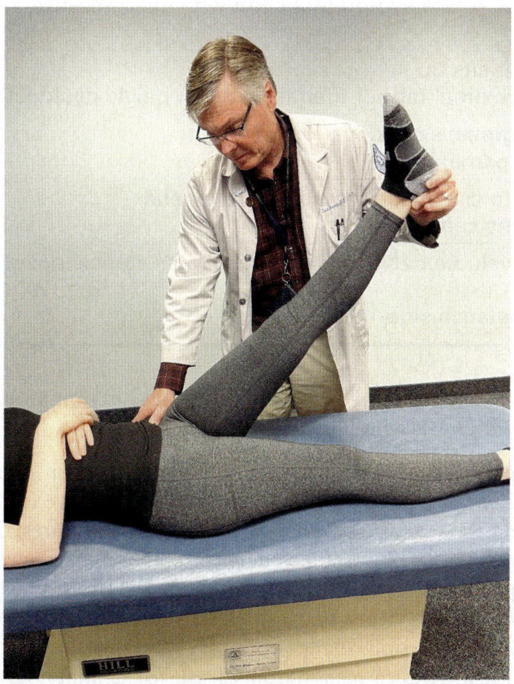

Figure 93.4. The straight leg raising (SLR) test.

PHYSICAL FINDINGS AND CAUDA EQUINA SYNDROME

Although CES affects the lumbosacral region, the physician should perform a complete spine exam. This is because the patient may have compression of the spine at other levels from the same etiology as the lumbosacral compression. The lumbosacral exam for cauda equina involves sensory, motor, and reflex testing. Testing for a dermatomal sensory deficit can be done via pinprick testing at the midanterior thigh (L2), the medial knee (L3), the medial malleolus (L4), the dorsal aspect of the foot (L5), and the lateral edge of the foot (S1). The clinician should evaluate sensation (saddle anesthesia) in the perianal and perineal region to assess the S2–S5 nerve roots and perform a rectal examination for sphincter tone. Testing for lower motor neuron symptoms can be done by evaluating the hip flexors, knee extensors, ankle dorsiflexors/plantar flexors, and great toe extensors for decreased tone and weakness. Assessing lower motor innervation of the bladder can be done indirectly by palpating for a distended bladder and by measuring a postvoid residual volume with sonography. Finally, evaluate lower extremity reflexes at the patellar tendon (L4) and Achilles tendon (S1). If cauda equina has been diagnosed clinically, it is considered a surgical emergency and an MRI should be obtained to confirm the diagnosis and for surgical planning.[36]

ORTHOPEDIC LBP

When evaluating a patient with LBP it is important to rule out contributions from hip or sacroiliac pathology. Hip and SI pathology have nonspecific and overlapping referral patterns (please see the orthopedic chapter) which can make this challenging. There are many orthopedic and physical therapy special tests to help differentiate lumbar spine versus Hip, and SI joint pathology (see Table 93.1). The cause of LBP can become lost in a "series of referrals" between specialists that focus on either the lumbar spine, hip, or SI joint in isolation. It is important that patients have appropriate primary care oversight to coalesce these opinions and guide them with a sustained holistic approach with the goal of a significant, durable benefit.

MOTION TESTING AND SPECIALIZED TESTS

Active motion is motion performed by the patient without assistance. It is always a good idea (especially after an injury) to have the patient actively move (prior to passive testing) to see limitations of motion due to pain. Passive motion testing is performed by the physician with the patient remaining relaxed. It is important that the physician observes and palpates not only the quantity of motion but also the quality of motion. The end feel of any barrier can be found at the end of passive range of motion. Significant viscerosomatic reflexes demonstrate a "reluctance to motion," as contrasted to an absolute restriction. If a visceral source of referred pain to the lumbar region is discovered, it should be addressed before orthopedic referral. Based on the patient's presentation, history and physical the clinician will choose several commonly used manipulative medicine or orthopedic tests to support the suspected diagnosis. There are many nonorthopedic causes of LBP such as the visceral and psychiatric that can make interpretation of the physical exam difficult. Clinicians should consider the nonorthopedic etiologies as well as the more defined anatomic orthopedic conditions the following screening tests can assess. Please see the chapter on orthopedics for a comprehensive list of relevant special tests.

RECTAL AND PELVIC EXAMS

The rectal exam is an important part of the physical examination of a patient with low back pain especially if the clinician is worried about CES or genitourinary dysfunction. The examination

TABLE 93.1

Special Orthopedic and Physical Therapy Tests Performed on the Pelvis

Orthopedic Tests of the SIJs	Characteristics
Ipsilateral prone kinetic test	Prone
Gapping test	Supine, compress/IR both ilia Positive test = SI pain
Approximation test	Supine, or prone, ER both ilia Positive test = SI pain
SI rocking test	Supine, passively flex, and extend sacrum Positive test = SI pain
Squish test	Supine, compress innominates medially Positive test = SI pain
Femoral shear test	Supine, flex hip and knee, compress Positive test = SI pain
Prone springing test	Prone, anterior pressure, springing motion Positive test = pain
Special Tests of the Pelvis	**Characteristics**
Straight leg raising test	Supine, flex hip, knee extended Positive = sciatic nerve radicular pain 30–70 degrees
Prone knee bending test (Nachlas)	Prone, flex knee, extend hip Positive = pain anteriorly along femoral nerve
Gillet test	Standing, flex hip and knee maximally Positive = asymmetry of PSIS, sacral spines
Ipsilateral anterior rotation test	Standing, side lying, passively rotate ilium Positive = pain
Flamingo test	Standing, hip flexed, abducted, ER, knee flexed Positive = pain
Leg length tests	Supine, measure ASIS to medial malleolus Positive = discrepancy
Sign of the buttock	Supine, flex hip with knee extended, then flex knee Positive = knee flexion does not allow further hip flexion
Gaenslen test	Side lying, flex lower hip, hold. Examiner extends top hip Positive = pain in SIJ
Leaguer sign	Supine, flex, abduct, laterally rotate symptomatic hip with overpressure Positive = pain in SIJ
Supine-to-sit (long sitting) test	Supine, legs straight, patient sits up Positive = one leg moves proximal farther than the other = pelvic dysfunction
Yeoman test	Prone, flexes knee to 90 degrees, extend hip Positive = pain anterior SI ligaments
Thomas test	Supine, flex hip, hold knee to chest, allow other leg to extend Positive = unheld hip remains semiflexed
Trendelenburg test	Standing, one leg stance, evaluate pelvic position, evaluates stance leg: gluteus medius strength Positive = hip drops on nonstance side

provides useful information regarding sensation, tone, masses, skin defects (fissures, fistulas), and lower sacral reflexes. It is also important for women to have a pelvic exam to rule out pelvic visceral causes or muscular pelvic floor dysfunction.

STANDING POSTURAL EXAMINATION

The standing postural examination gives useful information prior to evaluating the lumbar spine. There are specific findings to consider from the standing structural exam that will help diagnose somatic dysfunction in the lumbar region. Please see the chapter on structural examination.

Key components of the standing postural examination for the patient with LBP would include the following:

- The presence of paravertebral muscle humping on one side or the other may be indicative of a group lateral curve (scoliosis).
- During the lateral view, changes in the AP curvatures and transition zones can be useful to determine treatment approach.
- Unequal iliac crests, unequal greater trochanters, and asymmetric sacral sulcus depth may indicate a short leg syndrome (SLS) and sacral base unleveling.
- Myofascial pattern recognition, please see Chapter 92 Postural Considerations in Osteopathic Diagnosis and Treatment.

SOMATIC DYSFUNCTION

A knowledge of anatomy and skill in making a regional diagnosis are the critical first steps in helping patients with lower back pain. The reader is referred to the section on functional anatomy and diagnosis in this textbook for reviewing the anatomy and regional diagnosis of the involved body regions discussed below.

GENERAL CONSIDERATIONS

Somatic dysfunction is defined as an altered function of the neural, vascular, lymphatic, and connective tissue elements of the musculoskeletal system.[37] Somatic dysfunction can be mechanical, visceral, reflex, emotional, and/or traumatic in etiology. They should all be considered during palpatory diagnosis. There is a direct relationship between the viscera and the soma through reflexes and the myofascial elements of the body. Somatic dysfunction is defined by four criteria: These include tissue texture change, asymmetry of position, restriction of motion, and tenderness.[37] Somatic dysfunction can adversely affect the patient's homeostasis and ability to heal. Somatic dysfunction can be acute or chronic. Acute findings tend to be locally tender, warm, with increased moisture and a local blush reaction when palpated. Chronic findings tend to be less tender, cool, with decreased skin moisture, and diffuse tissue restriction. The diagnosis of somatic dysfunction typically occurs through palpation of somatic structures, but also includes vascular and connective tissues, reflexes, visceral dysfunction, and dysfunction of the primary respiratory mechanism. If the clinician determines that somatic dysfunction is present and is contributing to low back pain, osteopathic manipulative treatment may be indicated. Clinicians also consider the indications & contraindications of performing OMT, and when OMT is appropriate.

In the lower back pain patient, somatic dysfunction can occur anywhere in the body and have both local and distant effects. This is due to the interconnectedness of the myofascial elements of the human body. Since the body is organized in a biologic tensegrity model, dysfunction of one part may affect the whole structure's integrity. The clinician considers the severity, location, and associated factors of somatic dysfunction. Local and distant somatic dysfunction may be related and are treated based on a clinical objective. It is important to note the response of the somatic dysfunction to OMT and adjust the treatment modality (or treatment plan) based on this response to treatment. With experience, the clinician will start to determine common patterns of somatic dysfunction seen in the lower back pain patient. They also will develop experience in what treatment approach is utilized based on their skill set and the patient. This is unique to each physician and is part of the art of osteopathic medicine.

GROSS POSTURAL AND MYOFASCIAL PATTERNS

Patients with low back pain have predictable postural changes such as an increased lumbar lordosis, thoracic kyphosis, and forward head position. They have poor balance, and many symptoms referable to lumbosacral instability. Such patterning can involve the upper and lower body and has been described, researched, and published by Vladimir Janda, MD, a Czech physiatrist with postpolio syndrome.[38] Janda described a lower crossed syndrome (LCS) in low back pain patients based on an acquired patterning of specific muscle tightness and inhibition/weakness in the lower body. The patterns cross between the dorsal and the ventral sides of the body. This imbalance results in an anterior tilt of the pelvis, increased flexion of the hips, and compensatory hyperlordosis in the lumbar spine. It has been associated with muscle dysfunction and develops into abnormal sequential neuromuscular firing patterns, poor balance, and chronic lower back pain.[38] The change in posture affects joint mechanics and creates somatic dysfunction. When the crossed syndromes are present, they affect the central neuromuscular control, proprioception, gait, and station. Janda's concepts were also published and popularized by Philip Greenman, DO in the book *Principles of Manual Medicine*.[39]

In addition to the upper and LCSs, Gordon Zink, DO developed and taught a common compensatory pattern (CCP)[40] that may be associated with trauma and lower back pain. It is a pattern of somatic dysfunction that can be observed in the spinal transitional zones. It is usually an alternating fascial preference/pattern. With trauma the pattern becomes nonalternating. Zink's pattern can be identified through assessing myofascial and segmental dysfunctions. A retrospective study showed a weak statistically significant correlation between structural and myofascial exam findings, excluding the lumbosacral transition zone.[40] Clinicians utilize both postural/myofascial assessments in their evaluation of the low back pain patient.

SPINAL TYPE II LUMBAR DYSFUNCTIONS

Single-segment spinal somatic dysfunctions (FRS and ERS dysfunctions) are commonly seen in mechanical low back pain. Their presence can produce local and referred pain. The pain generators may be the facets, disks, or connective tissue elements. Type II somatic dysfunctions may occur due to trauma, overuse, postural imbalance, muscular/myofascial restrictions, and reflex causes. Motion characteristics of segmental somatic dysfunctions in the lumbar spine demonstrate side bending and rotation to the same side. They are more commonly FRS dysfunctions but may be ERS dysfunctions as well. Single-segment dysfunction of the L5–S1 vertebral unit causes significant pain at the lumbosacral junction and can refer to the sacroiliac joint (SIJ) and down the leg. The L5 segment commonly has anatomical variations that can alter the spinal mechanics and pain sensitivity. Nociception from L5 can influence and sensitize the sympathetic nervous system contributing to stiffness and tightness of the thoracolumbar junction (personal communication Robert Kappler, DO). Segmental dysfunctions of the lumbar spine can occasionally not follow Fryette's type II mechanics and can sidebend and rotate to opposite sides or be in a neutral position. These atypical presentations of vertebral motion can be related to numerous factors such as underlying orthopedic disease, congenital anomalies, facet arthritis, and trauma. Many experts in osteopathic manipulative medicine feel that type II dysfunctions are not physiologic and are important to be treated first (personal communication Robert Kappler, DO and Fred Mitchell, Jr. DO). Chronic type II dysfunctions may have long term physiologic effects, both locally for that vertebral unit, and associated somatic and visceral structures. Spinal segmental dysfunction also affects muscles and connective tissues in the related dermatome, myotome, or sclerotome. Some muscles innervated by these segments respond by tightness, others by inhibition. Therefore, it is important to treat segmental dysfunction while simultaneously addressing the tightness and weakness of the affiliated muscles.

SPINAL TYPE I LUMBAR CURVES

Patients with lateral curvature of the spine are not only adolescents with idiopathic scoliosis. It is common to see middle-aged patients present with back pain that gets worse as the day goes on. Typically, they will have pain at the apex segment of the curve. Nerve roots on the convex side near the apex can be stretched and painful. Lumbar nerve roots on the concave side might be compressed in narrowed neural foramina. The muscles on the concavity become tight and short, while those on the convexity are stretched and tender.

Type I lumbar curves follow Fryette' s mechanics and occur in neutral with side bending and rotation occurring to opposite sides. These curves may be reflex, structural, or functional in etiology. Structural lumbar curves in older adults may be due to degenerative scoliosis and are frequently painful. They may also be caused by orthopedic issues such as spondylosis, spinal stenosis, herniated disks, and chronic pain.

Functional curves such as those that compensate for postural imbalance are generally related to leg length abnormality, sacral base declination, psoas spasm, muscular imbalances, and fascial tension. In functional curves, single-segment dysfunction of the lumbar spine above or below the curve might also be the cause. Treating the single-segment dysfunction in this scenario can resolve the functional curve. Patients may also have somatic dysfunction of the crossover points and transition zones that contribute to their findings. When the sacral base declination is due to leg length discrepancy with pelvic side shift, heel lift therapy, and OMT can help balance these issues and resolve lower back pain.

Another frequent cause of lumbar group curves is somatic dysfunction of the sacrum such as sacral torsions, unilateral flexions, (Mitchell model), and anterior/posterior (AP) sacrum dysfunctions (Chicago model). Group curves can develop with these dysfunctions as compensation for alterations in the base of support.

Spinal reflexes from visceral disease, referred pain, abdominal surgery, and neurologic causes all can create and maintain a group curve via viscerosomatic and somatosomatic reflexes. These lumbar curves may be painful and persistent. Treatment of these must start with addressing the etiology of the visceral disturbance. A classic example of this scenario is a patient passing a kidney stone. The patient will commonly have diffuse severe spasm and group curve spinal mechanics as the stone passes down the ureter.

Patients with a lumbar group curve may have postural imbalance, a condition that affects the coronal, sagittal, and transverse planes. It is seen frequently in patients with lower back pain. Please see the chapter on postural balance for a detailed explanation.

ANTERIOR/POSTERIOR CURVES

Somatic dysfunction and asymmetry of the anterior and posterior curves predispose patients to significant lower back pain. Changes in the lumbar lordosis may occur with core muscle weakness, genetic factors, postural issues, and occupational stresses. In the case of the increased lumbar lordosis, the sacrum is held in a relatively bilaterally flexed position. This increases shear stress between L5 and the S1 segment (increased pelvic incidence). This anterior-directed force causes lumbosacral instability and reflex tightening of the hamstrings and paraspinal stabilizing muscles. The patient presents with the symptoms of localized lumbosacral pain and intermittent flare-ups of severe back pain. Standing or sitting for prolonged periods of time causes core muscle fatigue and increases symptoms. In the case of decreased lumbar lordosis, this causes loading through the lumbar spinal segments and disks. A straight or kyphotic lumbar spine does not absorb shock like a natural lordosis does. Patients in this situation may also develop spondylolisthesis, retrolisthesis, and chronic pain. Typically, activities with repetitive jarring such as running, football, horseback riding, and water skiing can aggravate this condition. A manipulative medicine and rehabilitative approach should consider what is causing or contributing to the condition. Normalizing iliopsoas tension will improve the position and motion of the upper lumbar segments and the lordosis. Treatment of the lumbosacral junction and prescribed abdominal bracing exercises will help stabilize the lower lumbar spine.

SACROPELVIC DYSFUNCTION

The sacrum is the keystone of the pelvis. LBP of SIJ origin affects innominate and lower lumbar segmental motion. Also, hip abduction and external rotation provokes SIJ pain. Normal sacral position, function, and motion are essential to couple the forces from the lower extremities to the pelvis and spine. (Please review Table 93.2 for examination of the sacrum.) Sacral dysfunction can be caused by trauma/overuse, muscular and fascial tensions, posture, cranial/dural dysfunction, rheumatologic disease, visceral disease viscerosomatic reflexes, and lower extremity and gait issues. Sacral dysfunction, especially the backward sacral torsion, has been associated with chronic lower back pain.[39] It is important for clinicians to determine why the sacrum is restricted in its motion or has an abnormal position. Post treatment with OMT, a negative seated flexion test indicates that the sacral somatic dysfunction is now resolved. Osteopathic manipulation of the SIJ has been shown to improve pain and disability in patients with sacroiliac dysfunction after three weeks of treatment.[41] Please see the section on functional anatomy and diagnosis of the sacrum and pelvis for the anatomy, dysfunctions, and diagnostics of this region.

ILIUM DYSFUNCTION

The ilium can be functionally considered as part of the lower extremity. Its position, motion and function are largely determined by muscular attachments of the legs to the pelvis, ligaments, and gravitational forces. The clinician will check the ASIS compression test as part of the diagnosis (see Fig. 93.5). Since the ilia attaches to the last two lower segments of the lumbar spine,

TABLE 93.2

Examination for Somatic Dysfunction of SI Articulation

Position	Examination	Results
Step 1. Patient standing	Evaluate anatomic landmarks, standing flexion test	A positive standing flexion test indicates dysfunction in the leg and/or pelvis on that side.
Step 2. Patient seated	Perform seated flexion test	Will specifically determine whether there is an SI dysfunction, and if so, which side (but not which arm) of the SIJ is dysfunctional.
Step 3. Patient supine	Positional assessment of ASISs, ASIS compression test, pubic tubercles, and medial malleoli	Helps determine the etiology of the problem and whether it is purely sacral or a "mixed" problem, incorporating iliac and pubic dysfunction.
Step 4. Patient prone	Palpate for depth of sacral sulcus, prominence of ILAs, tissue texture changes, asymmetry and motion testing of the sacrum, motion testing of L5, ligamentous tension testing	Helps the physician discover which axis is involved, find what portion of the SIJ is restricted, determine L5 motion and position, and evaluate pelvic ligamentous tensions.

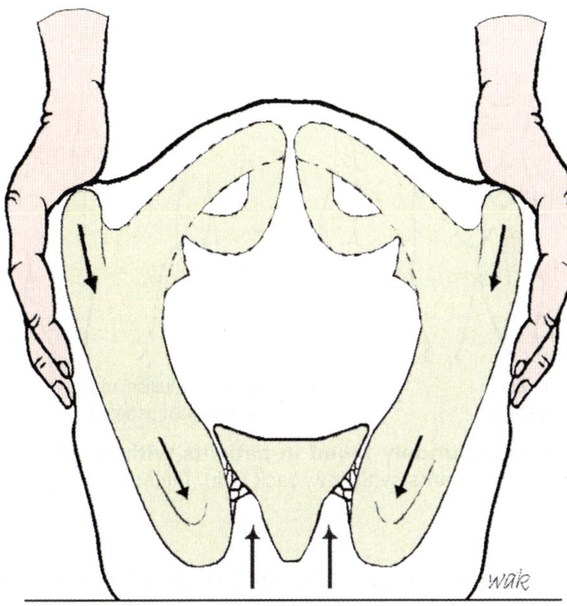

Figure 93.5. ASIS compression test. A positive test is restricted motion and/or pain elicited at either or both SI joints. (Modified by William A. Kuchera, DO, FAAO, from Kuchera WA, Kuchera ML. *Osteopathic Principles in Practice*. 2nd ed. Greyden Press; 1994. Reprinted with permission from Michael L. Kuchera, DO, FAAO.)

through the iliolumbar ligaments, their position and motion are related to the position and motion of L4 and L5. Pelvic obliquity of the ilium is commonly seen and treated in patients with lower back pain.[42] An up-slipped ilium or pelvic shear has also been implicated as a cause for chronic LBP.[39] Muscular and fascial tensions can affect the ilium from above or below. Since the latissimus dorsi and quadratus lumborum muscles attach to the ilium, dysfunction, trigger points, and tension of these muscles can cause lower back pain.

PELVIC SHEAR AND PELVIC FLOOR DYSFUNCTION

Somatic dysfunction of the pubes can be a cause of chronic low back pain, most likely due to maintaining the ilia in an abnormal position. The pelvic obliquity created by this dysfunction can affect the pelvic floor muscles, SIJ s, and lower lumbar spine. Pubic shears are nonphysiologic and can be caused by trauma, pregnancy, childbirth, athletic injuries, or overuse. Pubic somatic dysfunctions have been implicated as an important cause of chronic lower back pain.[39] Please see the chapter on the obstetrical patient for more information on the pelvic floor muscles and their clinical importance.

MUSCULAR/MYOFASCIAL SOMATIC DYSFUNCTION

Myofascial restrictions can cause lower back pain. They may be related to visceral dysfunction, skeletal dysfunction, reflex tender points, cranial dysfunction, and postural patterns. Fascial restrictions may be local or diffuse, can be distant from the area of pain, and affect the body's homeostasis. Myofascial dysfunction may be found in superficial and deep fascial planes and may have many arrangements such as diaphragms, longitudinal cables, sheets, and trigger bands (Specific types of fascial somatic dysfunction, their clinical relevance, and treatment approaches are discussed in the chapters on myofascial release and fascial distortion model). The myofascial and ligamentous system is indivisible from the articular system and both knowledge and skill are required for clinicians to provide lasting results to patients with lower back pain.

PSOAS DYSFUNCTION

One of the most common presentations and postural patterns seen in patients with lower back pain is the flexed forward posture leaning off to one side. This typically indicates a tight hip flexor (iliopsoas) on the side of the lean. Since the iliopsoas originates anteriorly on the upper lumbar segments and inserts on the lesser trochanter of the femur it applies a compressive force to the lumbar spine sacrum and pelvis. During assessment, the clinician will find restricted hip extension on that side and a type II FRS dysfunction in the upper lumbar region rotated to the side of the psoas tightness.[43] Associated findings would include pelvic side shift away from the tight psoas, sacroiliac dysfunction, and hip/ilium dysfunction on the same side. Bilateral iliopsoas dysfunction is also common, and in this scenario the patient has less of a list to one side, is generally more flexed and has severe lumbosacral pain. The lumbar lordosis is decreased, and the hamstrings are tight. The sacrum may be found to have a bilateral extension following the lumbar spine, or possibly a backward torsion or unilateral extension (rare). Treatment is focused on the spinal segments in the upper lumbar spine, tender points of the iliopsoas and iliacus muscles, and myofascial restrictions of the abdominal diaphragm, psoas, and lumbosacral fascia.

QUADRATUS LUMBORUM DYSFUNCTION

Dysfunction of the quadratus lumborum muscle is a common cause of lower back pain.[44] Simon and Travell discuss that trigger points in this muscle are related to lower back pain. Many times, tension of the quadratus lumborum is seen with tenderness of the iliolumbar ligament. Tension of the quadratus lumborum may be seen on the side of pelvic side shift and associated with single-segment or lumbar group curve mechanics. The quadratus lumborum tends to behave like the iliopsoas and becomes reflexively painful and irritated from nephrolithiasis, lower gastrointestinal issues, or other intra-abdominal processes. Since the muscle originates and attaches from the lower rib cage directly it couples somatic dysfunction of the diaphragm and ribs to the ilium, lumbar spine, and pelvis. Treatment should resolve any type II dysfunctions, address any tender points, and level the sacral base. Addressing the myofascial structures laterally including those of the tensor fascial lata and iliotibial band also seems to help.

LIGAMENTOUS SOMATIC DYSFUNCTION

Many ligamentous structures can cause or contribute to lower back pain. Common culprits include the posterior sacroiliac ligaments, the iliolumbar ligaments, the sacrotuberous ligaments, and the posterior longitudinal ligament. Similar and related to the myofascial elements, ligament dysfunction, laxity, and tenderness can be the etiology for many patients with lower back pain. Chronic postural strain, trauma, and repetitive overuse can affect the integrity of the ligaments. There are OMT approaches to treat these dysfunctions, stabilizing approaches through exercises, and regenerative medicine injections (prolotherapy) to decrease laxity. Please see the chapters on balanced ligamentous tension/ligamentous articular strain, and prolotherapy for a more detailed discussion.

VISCERAL SOMATIC DYSFUNCTION

The body's somatic structures are related to the internal organs through neurologic relationships and myofascial attachments. Therefore, viscera dysfunction and disease can cause somatic symptoms and palpatory findings. Each viscus is covered in fascia, so that it can move/glide smoothly during breathing and body movements. The fascia also lines, divides, separates, and supports the viscera. This myofascial mobility can become impaired following

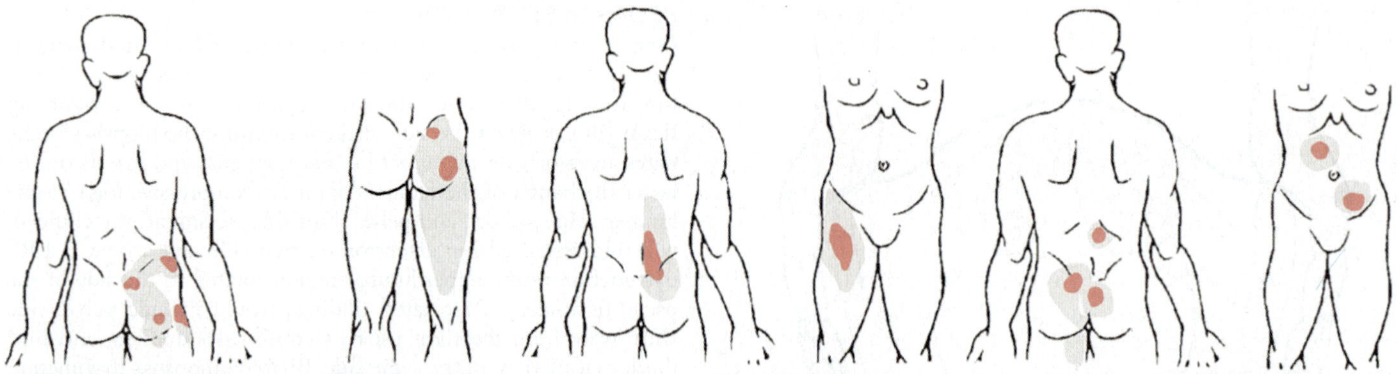

Figure 93.6. Myofascial trigger points and associated pain radiation patterns commonly found in patients with low back pain. Myofascial trigger points and associated pain radiation patterns commonly found in patients with low back pain. (Illustration courtesy of William A. Kuchera, DO, FAAO, with permission.)

surgery, or from disease, distention, and inflammation. Please see the chapters on visceral osteopathy for information regarding visceral dysfunction. Treatment of these visceral mobility restrictions has been beneficial for patients with low back pain.[45] Palpation and treatment of the abdominal viscera occurs through the abdominal wall which also addresses the fascia of the transverse abdominis, and the lumbosacral fascia.

OSTEOPATHIC CRANIAL MANIPULATIVE MEDICINE

Patients with chronic lower back pain have somatic dysfunction throughout their body. Many patients with chronic lower back pain have centralized, neuropathic pain. These patients have neurochemical changes in the brain and spinal cord, abnormal pain processing, and cognitive and emotional effects. They are typically treated with centrally acting medications, cognitive/behavioral therapy, and physical therapy. Since chronic pain involves processes of the CNS, osteopathic cranial manipulative medicine (OCMM) is thought to assist and address these central components. One way this might occur is through OCMM improving relaxation and sleep.[46] It is important for clinicians to diagnose and treat somatic dysfunction of the SBS and PRM in these patients as the anterior myofascial structures are influenced by the sphenoid and the posterior structures are influenced by the occiput. Since the sacrum is attached to the cranial base through the dura, the structures can influence each other, linking the function of the cranial mechanism to the function of the sacrum and pelvis. Many patients with chronic low back pain also have depression. OCMM may provide some relief for those patients with chronic pain and depression.

TENDER POINTS AND TRIGGER POINTS

Patients with lower back pain are commonly found to have dysfunctions of specific muscles, some of which are tight and others that are weak. These factors contribute to segmental spinal dysfunction with their associated anterior and posterior lumbar and pelvic tender points. These tender points tend to be related to spinal segmental dysfunction, the muscle itself, or its neural, vascular, or lymphatic elements. When Jones tender points are appropriately treated, the function of the tissues improves, and back pain diminishes. The lumbar tender points include the anterior L1–L5, posterior L1–L5 spinous process, and L1–L3 transverse process. Tender points in this region are related to spinal somatic dysfunction. In addition, pelvic tender points commonly seen in the low back pain patients include the following: upper pole L5, lower pole L5, high ilium sacroiliac, posterior lateral L3 and L4 (gluteus medius), high ilium outflare/coccygeus, inguinal ligament/pectineus, iliacus, psoas, low ilium/psoas minor, and piriformis points.

Simon and Travell myofascial trigger points are like Jones tender points with some overlap, however by definition, they have a local twitch response, a satellite point or refer to a pain reference zone. They may be treated with counterstrain but classically they are treated with spray and stretch, injection, or inhibition. Specific Simon and Travell myofascial trigger points have been associated with low back pain (see Fig. 93.6).

DIAGNOSTICS, LABS, AND IMAGING STUDIES

When evaluating patients with LBP in the primary care setting, emergent etiology is rare, with about 0.7% of patients having metastatic cancer, 0.01% having spinal infection, and 0.04% having CES.[47] Other conditions that are more prevalent but less urgent include osteoporotic vertebral compression fractures at 4% and inflammatory spine disease at <5%.[47] Diagnostic testing in the absence of red flags is not recommended for axial LBP of less than 12 weeks duration.[18] It is important to avoid ordering imaging indiscriminately when the presentation or chronicity of pain does not justify it, because inappropriate diagnosis and treatment can lead to poor outcomes. This occurs through the costs of testing and potential iatrogenic injury through treatment of the clinically asymptomatic findings that are frequently found. However, it is still important to acknowledge your patient's wishes for a diagnostic workup and explain to them the dangers of unnecessary testing. Many times, the history, physical exam, imaging, and consults correlate and support the diagnosis. However, difficulty in diagnosis arises when the history, physical exam findings, and diagnostics do not correlate with a known diagnosis or suspected diagnosis. This is more commonly seen in patients with chronic nonspecific lower back pain.

Imaging and Diagnostics Based on Differential

Imaging is the most used diagnostic test to evaluate LBP with plain radiography being the most frequent initial test. Diagnostic imaging of the lumbar spine typically reveals abnormal findings in both symptomatic and asymptomatic individuals. Because of the high frequency of lumbar spine abnormalities in patients without LBP, it is important to correlate the history and physical exam with findings on imaging. Good clinical evaluation is the best way of preventing the patient from wasting time and money pursuing treatment of an imaging abnormality that is not the source of their pain. Beyond the diagnostic utility, imaging can also be useful for determining the site of surgical or interventional treatments for LBP.

WHAT IS THE APPROPRIATE IMAGING TO ORDER?

Ideally testing should only be ordered if the result will likely change management or inform the prognosis of the patient's condition. In acute back pain, plain radiographs should be ordered if the clinician strongly suspects a serious condition such as cancer, fracture, or ankylosing spondylitis.[18] If radiography results are inconclusive, then follow-up imaging by MRI with contrast is indicated.[18] In acute back pain, if the clinician strongly suspects infection, or cauda equina as well as herniated nucleus pulposus or spinal stenosis with severe or progressive lower extremity neurologic deficits, then obtaining MRI with contrast is indicated.[18]

PLAIN RADIOGRAPHS

Plain radiographs are used to assess the bony anatomy of the spine. It can detect spinal pathology such as fractures, spondylolysis, spondylolisthesis, transitional vertebra, and bony deformities. When interpreting roentgenograms, an organized and orderly process should be used by the physician to avoid missing subtle findings. It is generally recommended to look at the area of highest interest last. In general, three roentgenographic views are all that are required to assess the lumbosacral spine. An AP view, a lateral view, and spot lateral view to better visualize the lower two interspaces. When a lumbar spine series is ordered, two oblique views are also taken to help identify spondylolysis.

AP VIEW

When looking at an AP radiograph of the lumbar region, the transverse processes will not be located directly lateral to the spinous process of their parent vertebra. The primary soft tissue structure seen in the AP projection is the psoas muscle. The psoas forms a triangular shape with the top at the transverse process of L1 and the base on the iliac crests. Asymmetrical visualization of the psoas muscle indicates clinical pathology in a minority of patients since positioning, muscle contraction, and rotation may affect the definition of the muscle border. The loss of a pedicle ("winking-owl" sign) is frequently seen in patients with metastatic disease to the spine (see Fig. 93.7).[48] Scoliosis is also commonly seen in this view and measurement of the degree of curvature using the Cobb method may be useful.

LATERAL VIEW

The lateral view is useful for identifying spondylolisthesis, an anterior slippage of one vertebra on the spinal segment below. When the vertebrae translate posteriorly, it is termed retrolisthesis. Disk space narrowing, compression fractures, facet joints, vertebral endplate changes, and Schmorl nodes can be seen in this view. It is also possible to measure the amount of lordosis of the lumbar spine using the Cobb method as was done in the AP view. Normal lumbar lordosis ranges from 35 to 50 degrees.

SPOT VIEW

The close-up view (spot view) of the L5–S1 area provides information about the status and alignment of the L5–S1 intervertebral disk space, and the upper portion of the sacrum. The L5–S1 disk space and intervertebral foramina are narrower than the spaces between the other lumbar vertebrae. Another radiographic interpretation is the determination of Ferguson lumbosacral angle. It is a measurement of the degree of lordosis or anterior tilt of the sacral base in relation to the horizontal. It is usually 35 to 45 degrees.

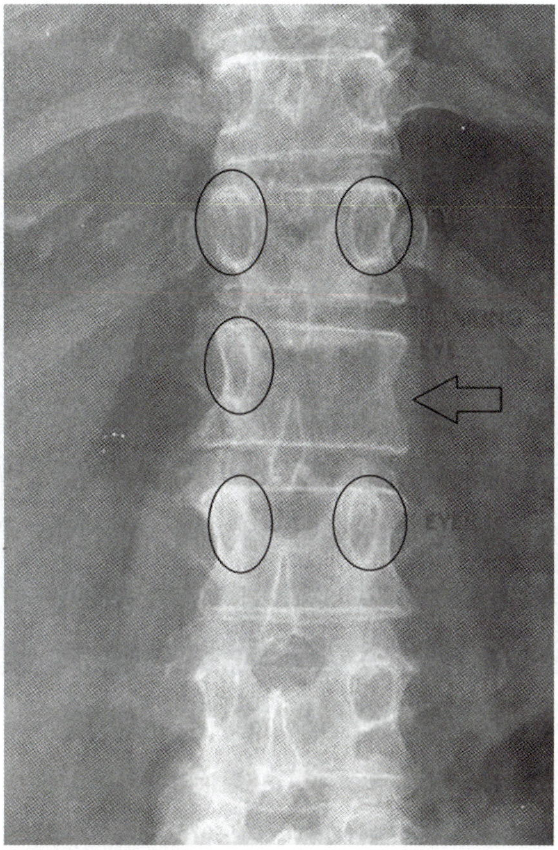

Figure 93.7. Winking owl sign. (Case courtesy of Ian Bickle, Radiopaedia.org, rID: 21937.)

An increased Ferguson lumbosacral angle relates to lumbosacral instability (see Chapter 92 Postural Considerations in Osteopathic Diagnosis and Treatment for further discussion).

OBLIQUE VIEW

The oblique projection is obtained to demonstrate the facet joints and pars interarticularis. In this view, the posterior elements outline a shape that is reminiscent of a "Scotty dog." A collar on the "dog" suggests the presence of spondylolysis, or a stress fracture of the pars interarticularis, an area between the superior and inferior articular facets. The Scotty dog eye is a pedicle, its nose is the transverse process, its front leg is the inferior articular facet, and its hind leg is the spinous process.

MRI of the Lumbar Spine

MRI creates the best distinction between soft tissues of available imaging modalities and is the current gold standard in spinal imaging. Whereas, plain radiography and CT produce clear images of bony structures. MRI produces excellent images of the intervertebral disk, nerve roots, neural foramina, and spinal canal (see Fig. 93.8). The use of contrast with MRI produces better tissue resolution, which aids in diagnosing malignancy or differentiating between scar tissue and recurrent intervertebral disk herniation in patients who have a history of spine surgery. CT uses radiopaque contrast which are iodine or barium based, whereas MRI contrast is gadolinium or manganese based. Although the MRI has the soft tissue resolution to identify pathology if interest in LBP, it is important to avoid obtaining an MRI in acute LBP without red flags or strong suspicion of serious pathology as described earlier in the chapter.

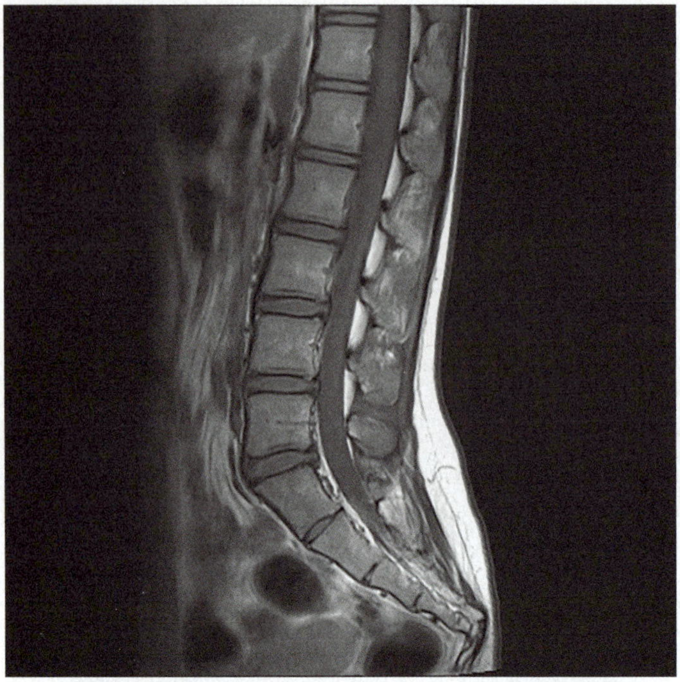

Figure 93.8. Normal lumbar MRI. (Case courtesy of Mohd Radhwan Bin Abidin, Radiopaedia.org, rID: 151544.)

Early MRI, defined as MRI obtained within 4 to 6 weeks of LBP onset, was associated with increased length of disability in patients with acute LBP without red flags at 13.7 days compared to 9.4 days in patients who did not get an early MRI.[49] Another study found that patients who had an early MRI when it was not medically indicated had worse outcomes, which they attributed to the iatrogenic effects of early MRI which included worse disability and increased medical costs and surgery, unrelated to severity of LBP presentation.[50]

MRI does not use radiation and is considered extremely safe when the patient has no implanted metal in their body and is not claustrophobic. The MRI takes considerably more time than a CT scan and can be intolerable for claustrophobic patients. Although it carries additional risk, sedation can be used to improve patient tolerance of MRI. Alternatively, there are "open" MRI scanners which claustrophobic patients can tolerate; however, image quality is significantly reduced compared to conventional MRI. MRI is absolutely contraindicated in patients with ferromagnetic metal implanted in their body. This includes pacemakers, mechanical heart valves, ferromagnetic foreign bodies, leads of many spinal cord stimulators, and intracranial aneurysm clips. This is because the strong magnet may shift the implanted metal resulting in lethal injury.

CT Scan of the Lumbar Spine

CT creates cross-sectional images of the internal structure of the spine at various levels, and, with reformatting, one can also obtain coronal and sagittal sections. The CT scan assesses not only the bony configuration and structure–space relationship but also the soft tissue in graded shadings so that ligaments, nerve roots, free fat, and intervertebral disk protrusions can be evaluated as they relate to their bony environment in a single scan. It is less expensive than MRI.

- CT is the study of choice for delineating the bony detail of the lumbar spine.[51]
- CT is useful in the diagnosis and assessment of trauma, and tumors of the lumbosacral spine.
- CT scan can visualize the medullary portion of the vertebral body and can detect bone destruction before changes are visible on plain roentgenograms.
- Fragments of bone that may not be detectable by plain roentgenograms are localized to the spinal canal by CT techniques.

CT imaging can be augmented with a three-dimensional nuclear medicine imaging technique termed single-photon emission computed tomography (SPECT).[51,52] SPECT scan is useful in the evaluation of vertebral lesions, spondylolysis, stress fractures, facet arthritis, sacroiliitis, pseudoarthrosis, and spinal fusion status. For example, in a patient with a spinal tumor, the activity of that tumor can be localized to specific positions, such as the vertebral body, pedicle, spinous process, or lamina. Lesions that affect the pedicles are a strong indicator of malignancy, whereas lesions in the apophyseal joints are more likely to be benign.

Radionuclide Imaging (Bone Scintigraphy)

Radionuclide imaging is a sensitive yet not specific technique for the detection of bone abnormalities. Any process that disturbs the normal balance of bone production and resorption can produce an abnormality on bone scan. The most used radiopharmaceutical for bone scanning is technetium 99m.

- Increased osteoblastic activity (hot spot) is associated with greater concentration of radionuclide tracer on the bone scan.
- Interruption of the blood flow to the bone results in the absence of tracer on the scan (cold spot).
- A bone scan is used mainly to detect occult fractures, stress fractures, infections, or bony metastases and to differentiate them from degenerative changes.[51]
- Bone scans also can differentiate between an acute versus healed compression fracture because new fractures will appear "hot" and is the test of choice to detect stress fracture of the pars interarticularis or symptomatic spondylolysis.[51]
- A bone scan may remain positive for up to 6 to 9 months after the inciting event in spondylolysis.[52]
- Regarding infections of the bone (osteomyelitis) or disks (diskitis), bone scans are useful because radiographs may not be positive for 10 to 14 days after the onset of the disease, whereas the bone scan may be abnormal within the first day.[52]
- Regarding fractures, trauma to bone, particularly stress fractures, may be difficult to detect by conventional radiography. A normal bone scan virtually excludes the diagnosis of stress fracture.[51] Bone scintigraphy can detect lesions within 3 days of fracture.[52]
- In children, the epiphyseal and metaphyseal growth plates are sites of active bone turnover in the areas of increased radionuclide concentration.[52]
- Other diseases associated with abnormal bone scans include Paget disease, hemoglobinopathies, and aseptic necrosis of bone.[52]
- Patients with sickle cell anemia have positive bone scans.[52]
- In patients with acute infarcts of bone, the bone scan may demonstrate a cold spot.[52]

Electrodiagnostic Studies—Electromyography With Nerve Conduction Velocity Studies

Electromyography (EMG) with nerve conduction velocity is the study of how action potentials propagate to their corresponding muscle fibers. Electrodiagnostic studies are commonly used in the evaluation of diseases affecting the peripheral nervous system and discerning radiculopathy from neuropathy. These studies are extensions of the neurologic examination and provide an objective measure of nerve damage (see Chapters 73 and 76 on osteopathic considerations in neurology and oncology for further information). They can confirm the clinical impression of nerve root compression, define the severity and distribution of involvement, and document or exclude other illnesses of nerves or muscles that could contribute to the patient's symptoms and signs. These studies are also useful in differentiating abnormalities associated with entrapment neuropathies, distal peripheral neuropathies, myopathies, and myelopathies.[52] An abnormal EMG is corroborative evidence of organic disease and helps the surgeon select patients who are candidates for surgery. In many patients, electrical signs of nerve damage do not appear until 21 days after the initial insult. EMG examination done too quickly during events misses the lesion. The test is painful but usually does not require sedation or analgesics. Conduction is measured in the fastest-conducting fibers only. In addition, the extent of EMG abnormalities does not necessarily correlate with the extent of nerve damage. These studies may identify a specific nerve root lesion when clinical symptoms suggest abnormalities at two levels. Electrodiagnostic examination has a degree of accuracy in identifying patients with nerve root compression like that of myelography and clinical examination.

LABORATORY TESTS FOR THE PATIENT WITH LOW BACK PAIN

Most individuals with spinal pain do not require laboratory studies with their initial evaluation. Laboratory tests should be used when a physician has developed a differential diagnosis by means of a history and physical examination for which laboratory data are needed to confirm or reject specific diagnoses. Laboratory test results should never replace a careful history and physical examination in the evaluation of the patient with spinal pain.

Obtaining baseline lab tests does have a role in separating mechanical from systemic diseases. They are also useful in distinguishing metabolic–endocrinologic disorders from those with more inflammatory characteristics. Patients who are candidates for laboratory evaluation include the following:

- A patient who fails to respond to medical therapy
- A patient who develops a significant change in the character of their pain
- A patient with a known or suspected history of infectious or rheumatic condition
- An elderly patient with new-onset spinal pain

The laboratory tests that are important in the study of disorders associated with spinal pain include acute-phase reactants, complete blood counts (CBC), blood chemistries, urinalysis, immunologic studies (cellular and humoral), body fluid analysis, cultures, and tissue biopsy.

ACUTE-PHASE REACTANTS

Acute-phase reactants are a group of plasma proteins that increase or decrease during an inflammatory disorder. The degree of increase is greatest with cancer, severe infections, vasculitis, and burns. However, from a diagnostic or therapeutic orientation, the measurement of inflammatory cytokines does not help identify specific disorders. The most useful test in helping to differentiate medical from mechanical spinal pain is the erythrocyte sedimentation rate (ESR).[52]

ERYTHROCYTE SEDIMENTATION RATE (ESR)

In general, an elevated ESR suggests the presence of inflammation in the body. It can be elevated in response to tissue injury, whatever the source, although it may be normal in patients with systemic diseases, including cancer. It is used to screen for inflammatory disease and to follow the response to therapy. The ESR value must be interpreted according to the sex and age of the patient. The upper limit continues to rise as patients grow older. The change in ESR may be more important than the absolute value when a patient is evaluated by a clinician. A markedly elevated ESR (≥100 mm/h) is most associated with malignancies, particularly those that are metastatic.[52] Other diseases associated with markedly increased ESR include connective tissue disease (polymyalgia rheumatica–temporal arteritis), acute bacterial infection (meningitis), and vertebral osteomyelitis with epidural abscess. The ESR also has utility as a means of following the progression or resolution of an inflammatory disorder. The ESR may remain elevated for up to 3 to 5 weeks after spinal surgery, in the absence of infection.

C-REACTIVE PROTEIN (CRP)

CRP is an acute-phase protein synthesized by hepatocytes which increases within hours of an inflammatory stimulus and reaches a peak in 2 to 3 days and then recedes in 3 to 4 days. CRP is more accurate than ESR in detection of infections after spinal surgery because it returns to baseline more quickly than ESR.[52] Serial determinations of CRP may also be helpful in following the course of acute and chronic inflammatory illnesses.[52] Elevated CRP after disk surgery has been associated with retro diskal infection that has been detected with magnetic resonance (MR) evaluation.[52]

The Complete Blood Count (CBC)

The hemoglobin (Hgb) and hematocrit (Hct) levels are normal in mechanical spinal pain, including herniated nucleus pulposus, spinal stenosis, and muscle strain. A decrease in Hct is a common finding associated with disorders mediated through chronic inflammation, as in anemia of chronic disease. A decreased Hct level should be evaluated with RBC indices, reticulocyte count, serum iron level, total iron-binding capacity, haptoglobin level, and examination of the stool for occult blood.

The white blood cell (WBC) count is normal in mechanical spinal pain. The WBC count is also normal in many forms of medical spinal pain. An elevated WBC (leukocytosis) count suggests the presence of an infection, particularly if early forms of polymorphonuclear leukocytes (band) are present. Increased numbers of WBCs are also seen in malignancies, particularly those of bone marrow or lymphatic origin. Patients on corticosteroids for their lower back pain have an increased WBC count in the 12,000 to 20,000 cells/mm^3 range.

Platelets are normal in mechanical spinal pain and most medical causes as well. In malignancies, platelets are commonly abnormal and may be elevated (thrombocytosis). Platelet levels are frequently decreased in bone marrow and lymphatic tumors.[52]

The Chemistry Panel

Calcium and phosphorus levels are also unaltered in osteoarthritis and mechanical causes of spinal pain. However, malignancies are associated with hypercalcemia. Malignancies with elevated serum calcium levels include those with parathormone activity (parathyroid adenoma and oat cell carcinoma of the lung), bone metastases, and multiple myeloma. In patients with lower back pain potentially related to inflammation, infection, or malignancy (i.e., positive bone scan), indicating osteoblastic activity, one must consider evaluation of alkaline phosphatase (ALP). ALP is produced to the greatest extent by osteoblasts. Any condition that increases osteoblastic activity increases ALP.[52] Disorders associated with ALP elevations include Paget disease, metastatic carcinoma, hyperparathyroidism, osteomalacia, fractures (during healing phase), and hypophosphatemia.

Of the illnesses that cause spinal pain, metastatic tumors and Paget disease cause the greatest increases (2 to 30 times normal). Up to 86% of patients with metastatic prostate carcinoma and 77% with metastatic breast cancer to bone have ALP elevations.[52] Not all elevations of ALP are associated with bone disease. Disease of the hepatobiliary system may be associated with marked increases in ALP activity.

In patients with lower back pain potentially related to chronic inflammation, infection, or malignancy, the total protein may be increased. Patients with increased total protein should be evaluated with a serum protein electrophoresis. A marked increase in total protein associated with elevated globulin levels should raise the possibility of multiple myeloma.

The Urinalysis and Renal Function Tests

Abnormalities detected during a routine urinalysis are most helpful in identifying those individuals with visceral referred lumbar spine pain of genitourinary origin. The presence of proteinuria on a dipstick determination requires further evaluation. Twenty-four-hour urine collections may be helpful in patients with proteinuria to see if they have nephrotic syndrome. If multiple myeloma is suspected, a negative dipstick protein does not rule out the diagnosis because myeloma proteins are not detected by dipstick methods. Elevations in blood urea nitrogen (BUN) and serum creatinine are associated with decreased renal function. Patients with visceral back pain of genitourinary origin may have elevations of these parameters. The drug history is important in a patient with abnormalities of BUN and creatinine.

Rheumatologic Studies

The three tests most ordered are the rheumatoid factor (RF), antinuclear antibody, and uric acid level. The predictive value of these tests is only 35% in a population of individuals with joint disease and an estimated combined prevalence of the three resulting illnesses of 10%.[52]

RFs are a group of autoantibodies to human immunoglobulin G. The classic RF is an IgM antibody. RFs occur in a wide range of autoimmune and chronic infectious diseases. Approximately 80% of patients with rheumatoid arthritis are seropositive for RF. RF in low titer may also be identified in an increasing proportion of normal individuals as they grow older. More than 40% of healthy individuals who are 75 years of age have detectable RF.[52]

CLINICAL PROBLEM SOLVING

Patients with lower back pain can have a wide range of presentations depending on their age, causative factors, chronicity of the problem, past surgeries, and comorbidities. Clinical problem solving may be straightforward and relatively quick in acute situations where the patient may have had a slip and fall, or other uncomplicated minor injury. For patients who have had subacute back pain that should have improved by now but has not, it becomes more complicated as diagnostic studies and consultations are typically involved. For those patients who have had long-standing chronic low back pain despite conservative and/or surgical management the clinical problem solving can be quite complex, as different mechanisms are at play that are contributing or causative of the patient's symptoms. It is important for the clinician to determine if the patient's history is in line with the physical findings and diagnostic studies. It is also important in more complex cases to develop a timeline of diagnostics and treatments and their success or failure. This would include response to medications, injections, therapies, or procedures. It is important to determine if the patient has axial pain, referred pain, or radicular pain.

- Common causes of axial pain include facet joint arthritis, or annular tears in disks.
- Referred pain is dull and poorly localized and is distant from its originating source.
- Radicular pain is sharp or searing and radiates in a dermatome, such as pain from a herniated disk or spinal stenosis.

In addition to the medical aspects of the case, clinical problem solving should also include what factors have been present in the patient's personal life to help them cope with their condition and return to their prior state of health. Problem solving should also include the emotional aspects of the case as these will affect progress in their current treatment plan. Once this is established that the clinician has an idea of what the patient has been through, the emotional support surrounding them, and what has worked and what hasn't, the current physiologic mechanisms should be considered. This is especially true in chronic low back pain cases in which there are multiple mechanisms at play, and they are addressed differently.

In addition to the above concepts, there are clinical practice guidelines (CPGs) that are published to help the clinician and patient make informed decisions based on the medical evidence/research.

Clinical Practice Guidelines (CPGs) and Evidence-Based Medicine (EBM)

There are multiple national and international CPGs for clinicians to review regarding the diagnosis and management of patients with lower back pain. Please see the section "Guidelines to Osteopathic Considerations in the Patient with Low back Pain" at the end of the chapter on CPGs for a summary of each guideline discussed below. When interpreting clinical guidelines, it is important to review that guideline's specific definitions and excluded patients to confirm that the guidelines are applied to the correct type of patient. For example, the North American Spine Society has distinct guidelines for nonspecific low back pain[53] and herniated nucleus pulposus associated back pain.[53] Clinicians should be careful to apply the correct and aligned guideline to their specific patient's condition. An incorrect application of the guideline can lead to inappropriate referral, treatment, and expectations for improvement. When reading guidelines also keep in mind the authors and professional societies that wrote the guidelines. The specialties publishing CPGs naturally perform an extensive review of applicable literature in their field. Some literature of corresponding fields is also included; however, they may apply a limited review of what other specialties can offer, especially when reviewing a nontraditional treatment modality like OMM.

National guidelines in the past 5 years include the 2017 CPGs from The American College of Physicians who provided CPGs for the treatment of lower back pain and provided three recommendations.[54] In 2022, the Department of Veterans Affairs and the Department of Defense published CPGs on lower back pain based on a systematic review of both clinical and epidemiologic evidence. Developed by a panel of multidisciplinary experts, they developed two modules (initial evaluation and management) and 39 recommendations.[55]

An adapted flow chart/algorithm on diagnosis and management from the Department of Veterans Affairs is presented for the reader. The section "Guidelines to Osteopathic Considerations in the Patient with Low back Pain" also contains more detailed recommendations regarding the diagnosis and management of low back pain. Together, the tables, algorithms, and 39 guidelines provide a robust document for best practices in lower back pain. Based on these guidelines please review Figure 93.9 for reference on applying the guidelines from an osteopathic perspective. The authors refer the reader to the following webpage for detailed information.[55]

International guidelines in the past 5 years include: (1) the 2016 NICE guidelines from the United Kingdom, (2) the 2017 CPGs from the Belgian Health Care Knowledge Centre (KCE),[56] and (3) the 2018 CPGs from Denmark.[57] The information below summarizes these guidelines.

In 2017, the Belgian Health Care Knowledge Centre (KCE) published a guideline on lower back and radicular pain. This guideline formed the basis for a national pathway to optimize clinical

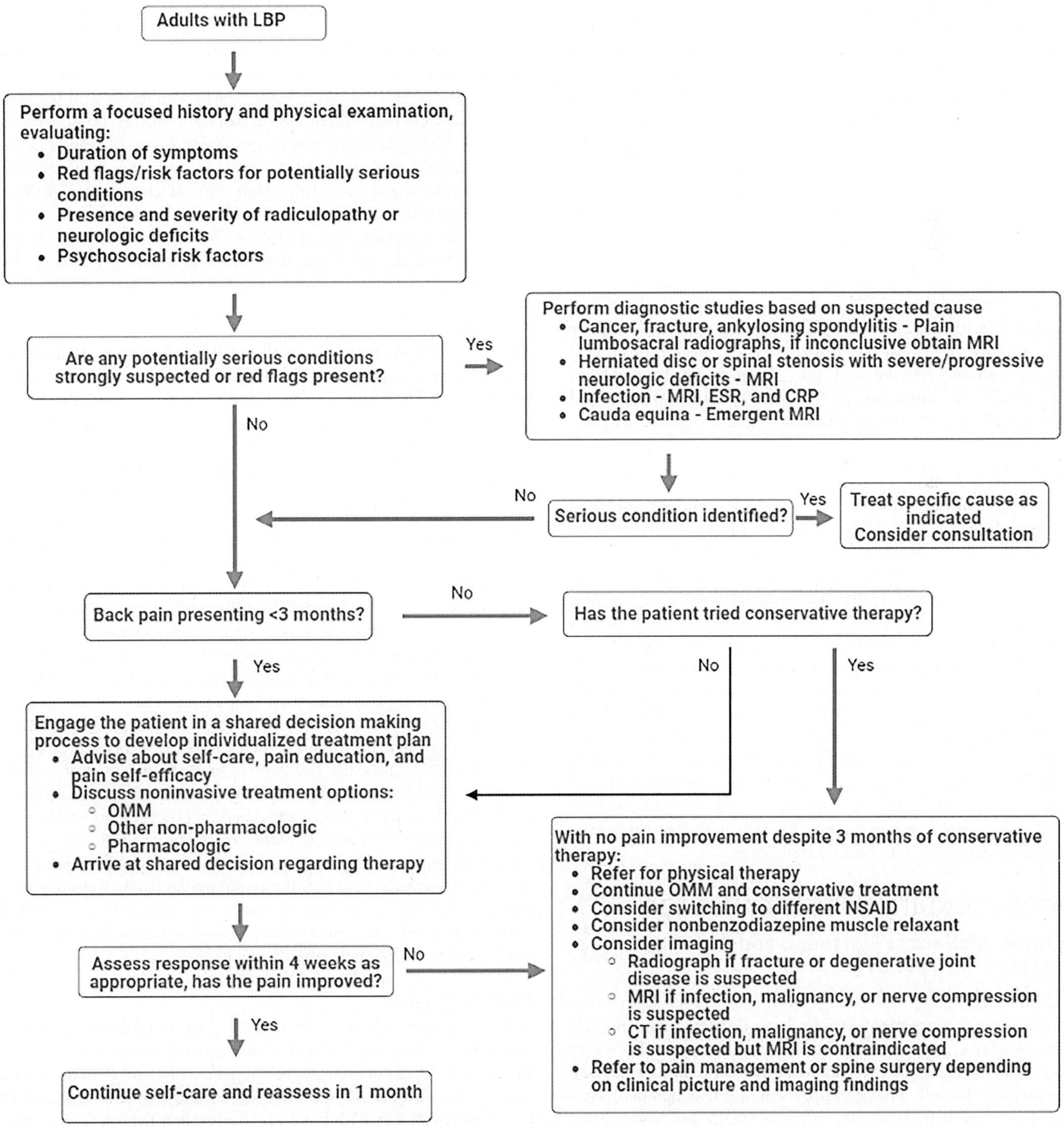

Figure 93.9. **Sample patient management.** (Adapted from the Department of Veterans Affairs, DoD. *VA/DoD Clinical Practice Guideline for the Diagnosis and Treatment of Low Back Pain*. 3rd ed. U.S. Government Printing Office; 2022.)

practice utilizing an interdisciplinary approach. The guideline stressed the importance of a comprehensive clinical assessment and tailored rehabilitation led by physiatrists. Pharmacologic and invasive treatments have a lesser role, and the patient's rehabilitation potential was a central feature.

Most of the guidelines recommend improving function through exercise and nonpharmacologic therapies, including acupuncture, spinal manipulation, Tai Chi, and yoga. Strong focus was also placed on addressing patients' biopsychosocial needs.[58] However, in the United States, despite these recommendations, exercise was prescribed for about 50% of patients with chronic LBP, opioids were prescribed for 61%, and long-term opioid therapy was prescribed for 18%.[58]

Many CPGs recommend the use of a biopsychosocial framework to guide management with initial nonpharmacologic treatment, including education that supports self-management.[59] However, only 12% of patients with LBP and comorbid depression had seen a mental health professional within the past year.[58] The addition of an education program in combination with exercise is effective for preventing LBP.[60,61] For persistent symptoms, the return to normal activities and exercise and psychological support are encouraged to alleviate stress due to their medical condition.

Gaps between the medical evidence and practice exist, with limited use of recommended first-line treatments and inappropriately high use of imaging, rest, opioids, spinal injections, and surgery.[59] The advances with the greatest potential are arguably those that align practice with the evidence and enhance the patient's activity and function, including work participation. A redesign of clinical pathways, with integrated health and occupational interventions to reduce work disability, changes to disability claims policies, and improved public health and prevention strategies are needed.[59]

Making a Diagnosis

An effective clinician will develop a fairly accurate and inclusive differential diagnosis from taking the history alone. The problem-focused physical examination and diagnostic studies are used to support and confirm a presumptive diagnosis and rule out other potentially serious causes. There may be multiple diagnoses at play each contributing to the patient's lower back pain. A treatment plan for each should be recommended. In addition, the patient's lower back pain may be creating another new diagnosis that needs to be addressed. Examples of this include a reactive depression due to chronic pain, or an undiagnosed gastric ulcer from NSAID use. Since the majority of LBP is "nonspecific," a diagnosis may not be able to be determined. However, the clinician and patient working together can determine what is *not* causing the low back pain and narrow in on its etiology. The diagnosis should not only include medical conditions, syndromes, and diseases, but also the social, emotional, nutritional, and cultural influences.

CLINICAL CONDITIONS THAT CAUSE LBP

Iliac Crest, Iliolumbar Ligament, and Thoracolumbar Pain Syndromes

DESCRIPTION

Over the past 30 years many articles have discussed similar conditions associated with localized pain at the posterior iliac crest, related to dysfunction of the thoracolumbar junction (T12–L2). These include the following conditions: iliolumbar ligament syndrome/iliac crest pain syndrome/Maigne syndrome/thoracolumbar junction syndrome/spinal dorsal ramus back pain/and superior cluneal nerve impingement. In all cases, these syndromes tend to be common causes of low back pain yet are rarely considered in the differential diagnosis by practicing physicians. Although some authors consider them distinct, they will be discussed together as they share similar diagnostic and treatment features. The iliolumbar ligament syndrome was discussed and published in the late 1970s as a frequent yet poorly known cause of chronic low back pain and permanent low back disability.[62] In the 1980s, Maigne described the relationship of the thoracolumbar region to pain at the posterior iliac crest (Maigne syndrome).[63] Maigne syndrome is an often unrecognized and treatable cause of low back pain. It has two variants and can be separated into two distinct entities. The central variant is a result of nerve stimulation secondary to changes in facet joint arthropathy at the thoracolumbar junction. The peripheral variant is a result of impingement of the medial branch of the superior cluneal nerve, both result in similar clinical symptoms and signs.[64] Maigne described the thoracolumbar junction syndrome as a condition with typical pain located on the posterior iliac crest and tenderness on palpation of the thoracolumbar junction.[63] Maigne felt it was accompanied by dysfunctions in the spine in about 60% of patients.[63,65] Over the years other authors found that localized pain at the posterior iliac crest was due to syndesmoperiostitis from traction on the posteromedial iliac crest.[66] Due to the insertion and location of localized tenderness on the posterior medial iliac crest, iliolumbar ligament syndrome, also known as iliac crest pain syndrome, was studied, and published.

ANATOMY

The iliolumbar ligament is a small, yet clinically important, ligament that originates from the transverse process of L4 and L5. The superior band inserts at the iliac crest, and the inferior band attaches to the front of the anterior sacroiliac ligament on the pelvic surface of the ilium.[67] Maigne felt that the iliac insertion of the iliolumbar ligament was inaccessible to palpation, being shielded by the iliac crest, yet the dorsal rami of L1 or L2 nerve roots, crossed the crest at 7 cm from the midline, closely correlated with palpable tender points(s).[68] However further anatomic studies confirmed that the location of insertion of the posterior band of the iliolumbar ligament was palpable manually and could lead to the painful syndrome termed iliolumbar syndrome.[69] The posterior (dorsal) rami of the lumbar nerves supply subcutaneous tissue of the upper buttocks and lower waist, while the anterior ramus supplies the lower abdomen and groin, and the lateral cutaneous branch supplies the trochanter.[65,68] Therefore, patients may complain of pseudovisceral pain in the lower abdomen, pseudosciatica, pubic/groin tenderness, and irritable bowel symptoms in addition to low back pain, which can lead to misdiagnosis (see Fig. 93.10).[65,68] Since the ligament is located on both sides of the lower lumbar spine it acts as a stabilizer of the lower spinal segments, restricting the rotational and lateral bending movements at the lumbosacral joint.[67,70,71] It also is influenced by the position and motion of each ilium. In the same region, there is also a palpable trigger point sometimes localized over the iliac crest approximately 7 cm from the midline. This point has been linked to the cutaneous dorsal ramus originating from the thoracolumbar junction rather than from the iliac insertion of the iliolumbar ligament.[68]

EPIDEMIOLOGY

It has been reported that 15% to 25% of pain in patients with pain in the posterior iliac crest area results from injury of the posterior ramus of the T12 thoracic nerve.[65] This may be due to many causes such as facet injury, somatic dysfunction, arthritis, or fracture. In one study of 204 low back pain patients taken from a family practice, occupational health, and a rheumatology clinic, 41% of the cases had iliolumbar ligament syndrome on diagnosis.[72]

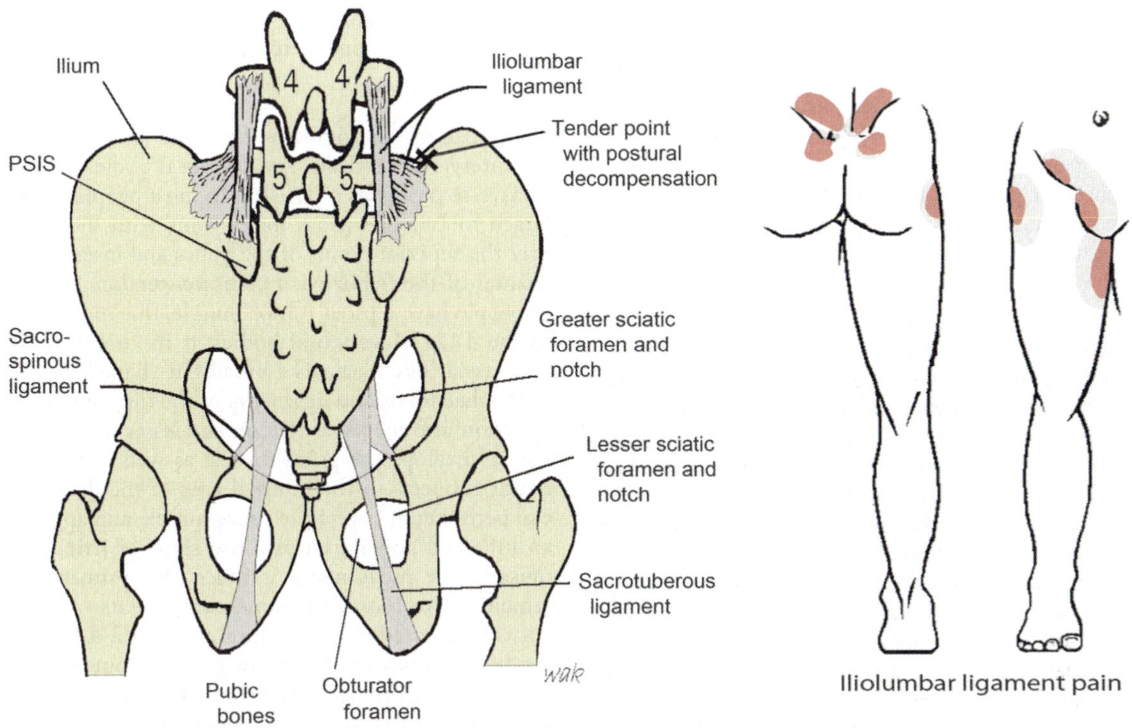

Figure 93.10. The iliolumbar ligament trigger point refers pain to the groin, SI region, and lateral thigh. The iliolumbar ligament trigger point refers pain to the groin, SI region, and lateral thigh. (Illustration courtesy of William A. Kuchera, DO, FAAO, with permission).

CAUSES/RISK FACTORS

Causes include core muscle weakness, aging, arthritis, fracture, somatic dysfunction, and postural imbalance. If this syndrome is severe or exacerbated, it results in instability of the injured lumbar vertebrae, which allows the fourth vertebra to slip and the fifth vertebra to shift. In patients with L5 disk protrusions, instability, or spondylolisthesis, the iliolumbar ligament may become irritated and painful. Repetitive occupational microtrauma, acute strain, and/or poor posture have been postulated as possible etiologies for chronic iliolumbar syndrome. Repetitive overuse can cause pain in the ilio-lumbar ligament due to the development of periostitis of the posterior medial iliac crest.[66] Chronic iliolumbar syndrome has been suggested as a frequent cause of permanent low back disability.[62]

CLINICAL PRESENTATION

Patients with these syndromes commonly have unilateral lumbosacral back pain worse with prolonged sitting and extremes of side bending or rotation of the spine. Clinical symptoms may correlate with the area supplied by the whole spinal nerve or either the posterior or anterior branch. For this reason, patients may report not only low back pain, but also referred pain in the hypogastric area, false sciatic neuralgia, tenderness of the pubic symphysis and abdominal pain.[65,73] They may have pain referred to the groin and may be considered to have a hernia or other causes of groin pain. They may also have pain along the iliac crest, along the SIJ, or lateral aspect of the hip. The pain does not cross the midline.

PHYSICAL FINDINGS

Localized tenderness of the medial posterior iliac crest, near the iliolumbar ligament insertion is common. For unilateral conditions, the L5 vertebral segment is commonly rotated away from the tender ligament. In the standing position, due to postural factors, the patient may have a pelvic side shift toward the side of the iliolumbar ligament. Associated muscular factors include tightness of the thigh adductors and quadratus lumborum on the side of the tender iliolumbar ligament dysfunction. Patients with a marked lumbar lordosis or spondylolisthesis of L5 can have iliolumbar ligament dysfunction bilaterally.

Findings on physical examination include the following:

- Tissue texture change at the iliac insertion of the ligament
- Ipsilateral pelvic side shift
- Ipsilateral adductor muscle is tight
- Tender point on the ipsilateral iliac crest 1 in superior and lateral to the medial edge of the posterior superior iliac spine; it can refer pain to the inguinal region.
- If the patient has a hernia *and* a tender point in the iliolumbar ligament, even successful surgical repair of the hernia, without treating the etiology for the iliolumbar ligament syndrome, may leave the patient with continued symptoms of "the inguinal hernia."

DIAGNOSIS

Diagnosis is a clinical one through specific palpation and evaluation of associated findings listed above. To palpate the insertion of the iliolumbar ligament, with the patient in the prone position, the physician should find the transverse process of L5 and palpate on a slight downward diagonal to the medial inside edge of the ilium. When examining the thoracolumbar junction, the clinician should always specifically diagnose segmental dysfunction between T12 and L2 as well as any associated tender points. Then correlate these findings with tenderness of the posterior iliac crest and diagnosis of the ilium and sacrum for somatic dysfunction. If there is a relationship between the TART findings in the thoracolumbar junction and the posterior iliac crest, treating the segmental T10–L2 dysfunction and their tender points, can resolve the condition confirming the diagnosis. Some authors prefer using ultrasound for the diagnosis of iliolumbar syndrome by detecting a thickened iliolumbar ligament or performing an ultrasound-guided local anesthetic or platelet rich plasma injection into the iliolumbar ligament.[74] One study found that associated clinical features were localized pain (in 73% of patients) and typical pain reproduction by movements of the lumbar spine (64%) or hips (53%), leg raising (37%), and heel-fall test (24%), in contrast to 2% to 12%/sign in patients with LBP without iliac crest pain.[72] Other authors have recommended looking for the presence of a posterior iliac crestal point tenderness and performing a skin rolling test (Kibler fold test) to indicate nerve irritation or sympathetic nervous system involvement.[73]

TREATMENT

Patients with these syndromes respond well to manual manipulative techniques if these are delivered in a technically correct manner and address the appropriate segment.[73] Manipulative techniques for tenderness on or near this ligament primarily include an indirect/counterstrain approach, but direct inhibition and ligamentous articular strain can also be effective. Thoracolumbar junction syndrome is particularly responsive to osteopathic manipulation, and no further treatment is required in most cases if it is performed adequately.[75] In addition to OMT, anti-inflammatories may be needed to manage acute pain, physical therapy for core muscle strengthening, treatment of the LCS, and prolotherapy procedures for ligamentous laxity. Some authors advocate for facet joint steroid injection, but in the case of refractory pain, local anesthesia, and steroid injection directly to the iliac crest can also be used as an alternative strategy.[65]

Psoas Syndrome

DEFINITION

There are multiple biomechanical conditions regarding the iliopsoas that are often combined in discussions. These include: (1) internal snapping hip syndrome, (2) psoas tendonitis, (3) psoas bursitis, (4) psoas spasm, (5) jumper's/dancers' hip, and finally (6) "psoas syndrome." Psoas syndrome is often used interchangeably with the above terms.[76]

In addition, there are a variety of medical, surgical, and traumatic issues that can involve the psoas muscle as well. The definition and categorization depend on who is writing the article. Much of the literature resides in case reports, athletic conditions, and surgical outcomes. Osteopathic literature has been published on the psoas muscle and its clinical relevance for 100 years, since Fryette's seminal paper in 1913.[77] From an osteopathic viewpoint, psoas syndrome is a constellation of postural findings, signs, and symptoms related to a spasm of the iliopsoas muscle.

For clinicians working in an osteopathic primary care, sports medicine, or manipulative medicine clinic, psoas syndrome, and psoas-mediated back pain are relatively common conditions. It also is a frequent cause of groin pain in athletes, especially in kicking sports or adolescent athletes during a growth spurt.[76] Iliopsoas tendonitis can also occur following total arthroscopic hip replacement.[76] However, the literature also states that it is an easily missed diagnosis, and a difficult diagnosis to make, which could be true based on clinical assessment methods.[76,78] It is important to consider this condition as part of the differential diagnosis for patients presenting with low back pain—particularly for osteopathic physicians, because patients may view these practitioners as experts in musculoskeletal conditions.[78]

EPIDEMIOLOGY

The epidemiology of psoas syndrome/psoas tendonitis is higher in athletes where repetitive hip flexion/extension movements occur, such as in plyometrics. The reported prevalence of postoperative iliopsoas syndrome following a total hip arthroplasty is 4.3% in patients.[76] A study of 252 total hip arthroplasty patients showed the incidence of iliopsoas tendonitis to be as high as 24% of cases.[76]

ANATOMY

The psoas major originates from the anterior/lateral margins of the intervertebral disks, and vertebral bodies of T12–L4 and the transverse processes of L1–L5. In most people, the psoas does not attach to L5. The psoas major joins with the iliacus and passes over the superior ramus of the pubes and inserts on the lesser trochanter of the femur via a common tendon. Approximately 40% of people have a psoas minor muscle, this muscle usually attaches to the T12–L1 vertebral bodies at its origin and inserts at the iliac fascia. The iliacus is a broad fan-shaped muscle with origins in the iliac fossa, and ligaments of the hip capsule. It has a diffuse insertion into the psoas tendon and lesser trochanter of the femur. Fascia envelops the psoas muscle as well as the adjacent viscera, and it connects to the internal crus of the diaphragm. The parietal peritoneum covers the psoas muscle and appendix. Therefore, an inflamed appendix can cause signs of irritation of the psoas muscle. The psoas major is innervated primarily by the second lumbar nerve root with some components of L2–L4. The iliacus is innervated by the femoral nerve (L2–L4). Psoas spasm can produce anterior thigh neurologic symptoms because the lumbar plexus passes through the psoas muscle, and muscle spasm can cause nerve irritation. The iliopsoas muscle has a bursa that can get inflamed or infected. Infections such as tuberculosis in the spine can be transferred to the hip through the psoas bursa which is continuous with the hip joint.[77]

FUNCTION

The basic biomechanical function is hip flexion with some internal rotation. Hypertonicity/shortening of the iliopsoas compresses the hip joint, the SI joint, and the lumbar spine. When the psoas muscle is dysfunctional, it may also be weak. Since the psoas is a muscle of postural balance, postural imbalance is a consequence of psoas problems. Spinal flexion, lateral bending, and pelvic side shift occur with psoas tension; contraction of the left psoas produces pelvic side shift right. As the pelvis shifts right, a lumbar curve convex left is produced. Psoas hypertonicity compresses the lumbar spine and sacrum causing restriction of SI motion. If the seated flexion test is positive, in a patient with these findings, the clinician should evaluate the psoas as a possible cause of sacroiliac dysfunction.

CAUSES/RISK FACTORS

The causes and risk factors for a psoas syndrome can be considered from the biomechanical, surgical, and medical domains. The physician must be aware that there are serious organic causes for psoas tension or spasm, and if suspected, these must be ruled out by careful history and/or physical examination and special tests.

BIOMECHANICAL CAUSES

- Somatic dysfunction
- Muscle strain due to repetitive overuse
- Leg length discrepancy
- Postural decompensation
- Inflammatory or degenerative hip arthritis
- Psoas bursitis
- Psoas tendonitis
- Labral tear
- Femoral acetabular impingement
- Disk herniation/degeneration
- Spinal stenosis

SURGICAL/TRAUMATIC CAUSES

- Hip arthroplasty
- Unstable orthopedic prosthesis
- Protruding hardware[76]
- Postsurgical infection/abscess/osteomyelitis
- Postoperative psoas hematoma[76]
- Traumatic muscle strain/tendon rupture

MEDICAL CAUSES

- Cancer of the descending or sigmoid colon
- Nephrolithiasis
- Diverticulitis of the colon
- Ureteral calculi
- Prostatitis
- Salpingitis
- Appendicitis
- Hematoma
- Psoas abscess

CLINICAL PRESENTATION

A patient with psoas syndrome will usually limp into the office flexed forward and listing to one side, complaining of significant central lower back and or flank pain.[78] Pain often occurs with changing positions, moving from a sitting to a standing position, or following prolonged sitting.[76] Psoas syndrome is usually initiated when a person assumes any number of positions that shorten the origin and insertion of the psoas muscle for a significant length of time and then gets up quickly, suddenly lengthening the origin and insertion. Symptoms are made worse with activity, and prolonged sitting, but improve with rest. The location of the pain is described as buttock pain, pelvic pain, lower abdominal pain, or groin pain. The patient may have a feeling of catching in the groin when their knee is flexed to 90 degrees.[76] Radiation of the pain may be down into the sacrum or up the lumbar vertebra. If there is piriformis involvement, patients may also have pain in the gluteal region of the contralateral side with radiation into the contralateral leg. However, this pain classically will not travel below the knee. Severe acute cases may have a hip flexion contracture and an inability of the patient to lie prone. Symptoms of psoas syndrome can often mimic a symptomatic herniated disk of the lumbar region, an inguinal hernia, or appendicitis if on the right side.

PHYSICAL FINDINGS

The physical exam begins as the patient walks into the clinic or hospital to be seen. Acute psoas spasm affects gait and station. The patient may limp or shuffle as they walk, with a forward-bent posture and leaning toward the side of the spasm. They may appear to have a Trendelenburg gait. Their pelvis will be shifted away from the side of the spasm. Sometimes they are wheelchair bound and cannot stand up straight, especially if both psoas muscles are involved. The physical exam can be difficult because of this. Anatomic landmarks will be asymmetric, and compensatory scoliosis may be seen. Side lying is typically tolerated. In this case, the physician can have the patient turn to the lateral recumbent position and attempt to extend the leg at the hip. On exam, hip flexors and the quadriceps are tight on palpation. There may be tenderness to palpation in the groin near the psoas insertion site at the lesser trochanter, and of multiple anterior lumbar counterstrain paints. Separately, the patient may have a decreased range of motion in hip extension.

On the exam, the Ludloff sign may be positive. The examiner directs the patient to sit with their knee in extension, then lift the heel of the affected leg. When pain is reproducible with this maneuver, it is a positive sign.[76] Some clinicians utilize the modified Thomas test for hip extension and psoas assessment. This test is mostly a test of inspection. The patient sits on the end of the exam table, grasps the asymptomatic knee, and lies down. A hip flexion contracture on the symptomatic side will keep the leg elevated from the table. A snapping hip sign may be positive with clunking which may occur on exam as the patient's leg moves from flexion to extension.

For less severe cases, the patient can usually lie prone, and vertebral dysfunction of the lumbar spine and hip extension can both be assessed. Diagnosis of psoas problems involves two separate yet related components (personal communication Robert Kappler, DO).

1. Restriction of hip extension due to hypertonic psoas
2. A flexed type II dysfunction at L1 or L2, rotated and side bent to the side of the hypertonic psoas.

Note: Psoas muscle tension compresses the lumbosacral area and the SIJs. To check psoas tension in the prone patient, grasp the thigh just above the knee, and extend the hip. Compare both sides (see Fig. 93.11). This method of testing provides an excellent "end feel." If the psoas is tight, examination of the upper lumbar spine is essential. The key somatic dysfunction initiating or perpetuating psoas syndrome is believed to be a type II (non-neutral) somatic dysfunction usually occurring in the L1 or L2 vertebral unit. Treatment of the upper lumbar dysfunction by itself will many times resolve the psoas tension and improve hip extension. If this key somatic dysfunction remains, the patient may develop complete psoas syndrome (see Fig. 93.12). The osteopathic profession distinguishes a psoas spasm or a psoas tendonitis from a psoas syndrome by the associated manifestations listed below.

Signs of a psoas "syndrome" include the following:

- Forward-bent posture side bent to the side of the most hypertonic psoas muscle.
- The key dysfunction is a non-neutral (type II) flexed somatic dysfunction at L1 or L2.
- The L1/L2 dysfunction may exist by itself or be part of a group curve and be "out of step" with its neighboring segments.

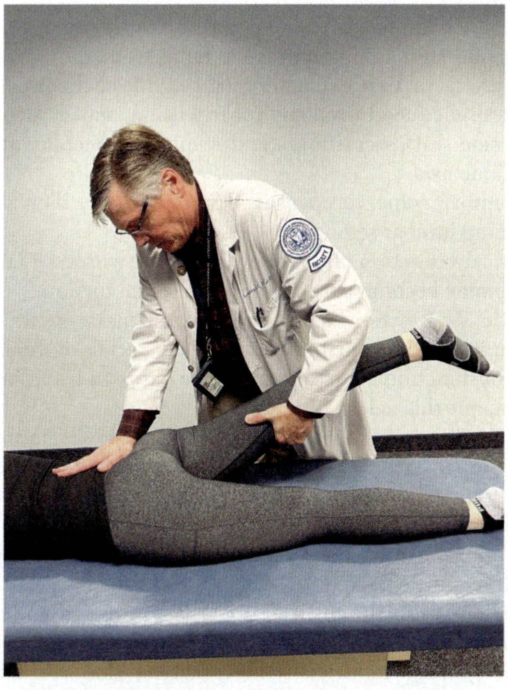

Figure 93.11. Checking prone hip extension for iliopsoas tightness.

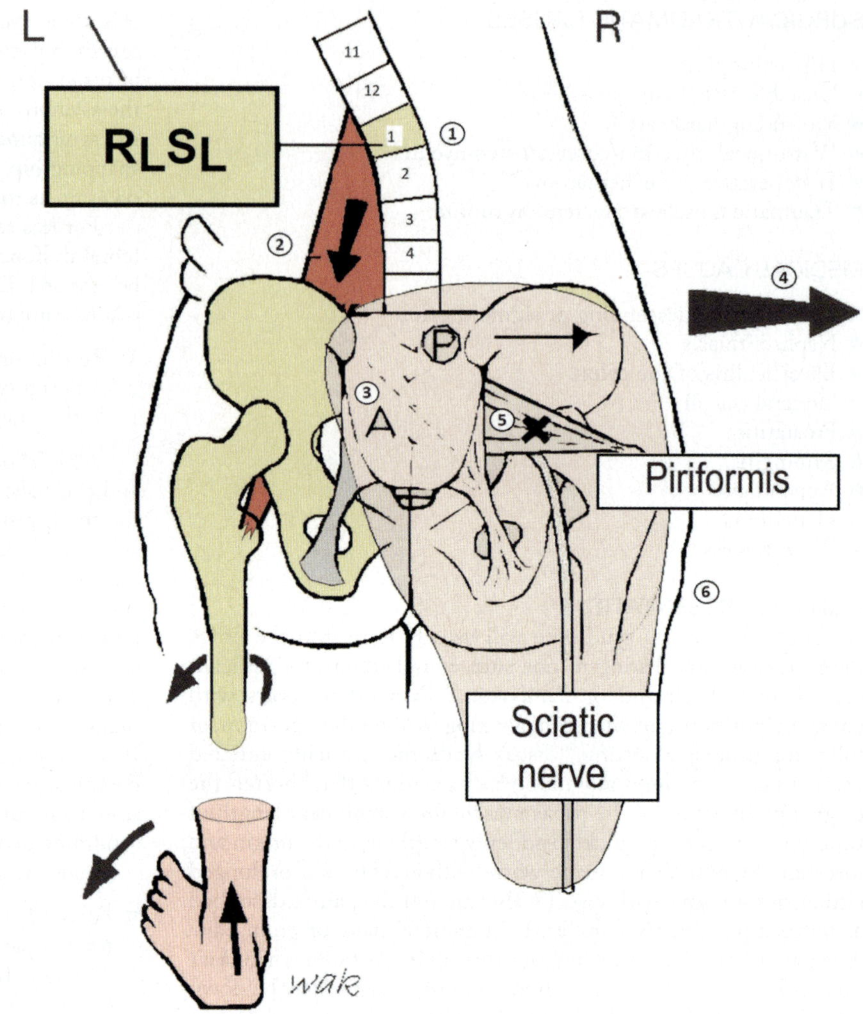

Figure 93.12. Psoas syndrome. As an example, a left-sided psoas syndrome is identified by finding (1) a type II (flexed) L1 or L2 somatic dysfunction rotated and side bent to the left, (2) a hypertonic left psoas muscle, (3) sacral torsion dysfunction (right torsion on a left oblique axis depicted here), (4) a pelvic side shift to the right, (5) a contralateral piriformis trigger point, and (6) sciatic nerve pain above the knee; also depicted is an ipsilateral and externally rotated short left leg. Note that the lumbar group curve has not yet compensated for the pelvic side shift and is still sidebent to the left. As it compensates for the pelvic side shift and shortened left leg, it is often found side bent to the right, that is, convex left (not shown). S, side bent; R, rotated; R, right; L, left. (Illustration courtesy of William A. Kuchera, DO, FAAO, with permission.)

- Initially, the lumbar side bending is ipsilateral to the hypertonic psoas muscle.
- Pelvic side shift occurs to the opposite side of the psoas spasm.
- Pelvic side shift and compressive force from the psoas spasm can cause sacral base declination on the side of the psoas spasm.
- Under applied load from the psoas tension, and influence from pelvic side shift, sacral somatic dysfunction generally occurs on an oblique axis.
- The lumbar spine compensates, first with L5, then with the remaining lumbar segments.
- Somatic dysfunction of L5 may compensate with type I mechanics and may become part of a forward sacral torsion.
- Somatic dysfunction of L5 may compensate with type II mechanics with or without associated sacral dysfunction. If sacral dysfunction is present, it may be part of a backward sacral torsion, but this is less common.
- If the condition is chronic, or significant, the lower lumbar spine then compensates and sidebends to the contralateral side.
- Hypertonicity of the piriformis muscle opposite the side of greatest psoas spasm.
- Radiation of pain to the posterior and lateral thigh not past the knee level on the side of the piriformis spasm.
- Tender points in the ipsilateral iliacus, groin, and contralateral piriformis muscles.
- In the Chicago model, on the ipsilateral side, a triad of the flexed upper lumbar segment, tight psoas, and an anterior sacrum (oblique axis dysfunction) can be seen.
- In the Chicago model, on the contralateral side, a tight/tender piriformis muscle and posterior sacrum (lower SIJ oblique axis dysfunction) contribute to sciatica.
- Both psoas muscles may be hypertonic, but one is more so than the other. One may be very hypertonic and shortened and make the other side hypotonic and weak via antagonistic inhibition.

DIAGNOSIS

The diagnosis of an uncomplicated biomechanical psoas syndrome is made clinically. This includes the history, physical findings from the palpatory and structural exam, and special orthopedic tests. X-rays of the hip are often negative in the case of psoas syndrome and often unwarranted. MRI and US often show enlargement of the bursa as well as thickening of the iliopsoas tendon.[76,79,80]

Psoas impingement syndrome has been described in patients with hip osteoarthritis and following total hip arthroplasty.[81,82] Following surgery, an ultrasound can be helpful in the diagnostic evaluation of intra-articular versus extra-articular origins of hip pain.[83] For psoas syndromes due to postoperative changes, and medically related causes, x-rays, CT of the abdomen with contrast, US, and MRI are all useful in addition to laboratories including inflammatory markers, urinalysis, chemistries, and a CBC.

TREATMENT

Treatment is preceded by ruling out psoas involvement caused by any organic or surgical cause. Organic causes of psoas syndrome, some of which may be serious or life threatening, include AAA, intra-abdominal abscess, appendicitis, diverticulitis, inguinal hernia, prostate or sigmoid colon cancer, prostatitis, salpingitis, ureteral calculi, and Crohn disease.[84] Psoas abscesses may have nonspecific symptoms and are very serious with a 20% mortality rate.[85]

Conservative treatment typically consists of conservative measures such as activity modification, physical therapy, OMT, NSAIDs, dry needling, and corticosteroid injections. OMT is a beneficial treatment option with fewer complications than other proposed nonsurgical measures like corticosteroid injections or pharmaceutical intervention.[86] Osteopathic treatment of the "key" somatic dysfunction (L1 or L2) is essential for the patient's comfort and effective, long-lasting effects of manipulative treatment. Psoas muscle spasm and restricted hip extension often resolves with OMT for the upper lumbar dysfunction. Treatment approaches include high velocity-low amplitude (HVLA) for the segmental dysfunction, counterstrain for any anterior (e.g., psoas) tender points, the Still technique, myofascial release, and muscle energy technique. Isometric stretching of the psoas muscles along with resolution of the lumbar and sacral spine and pelvic somatic dysfunctions generally helps. If an underlying disk protrusion is causing the spasm, the constant rest position, ice, and medications are usually required as well as gentle OMT to control the symptoms and provide some relief to the patient. Using heat in a patient with a psoas problem tends to make it worse rather than better. Involving PT or prescribing exercises needs to be done at the right time. Attempting to exercise an acute psoas major spasm simply compounds the problem. Giving the patient home exercises to gently stretch the psoas may be helpful. Improving the psoas syndrome will allow the clinician to treat other sacral and pelvic dysfunctions more effectively. Clinicians who fail to remove the psoas component and pelvic side shift will find that the lumbosacral and sacroiliac dysfunctions, and low back pain, will recur very quickly (personal communication Robert Kappler, DO). This has been demonstrated in a prospective randomized clinical trial.[87]

Postoperatively psoas muscle tendinitis (syndrome) is difficult to treat and can occur for a variety of reasons ranging from recurrent hematomas in the iliopsoas tendon to protruding surgical screws.[88] In a study by Adib et al., they reported 24% of patients who developed postoperative iliopsoas tendonitis following total hip arthroscopy, 50% of them required a corticosteroid injection to help relieve pain, while 12% required revision.[88] If conservative measures do not relieve symptoms, surgical iliopsoas release can be a consideration.

Anatomic and Functional Leg Length Discrepancy (Short Leg Syndrome, Leg Length Inequality)

DEFINITION

Leg length discrepancy (LLD) is most often divided into two groups: anatomic and functional. Anatomic leg length discrepancy (ALLD) is generally considered to be a structural shortening of the true bony leg length of the lower extremity between the femoral head and the ankle mortise. From an osteopathic perspective, functional leg length discrepancy (FLLD) can be described as lower extremity asymmetry impacting the somatic structures above it. It is essential to discriminate between ALLD and FLLD for proper management and correction. This is most often confirmed by comparing landmark and standing postural x-ray measurements.[89]

FLLD is an appreciable leg length discrepancy often caused by muscle imbalance, muscle spasm, somatic dysfunction, and other soft tissue or postural factors. It can be seen as the result of poor lower limb mechanics, such as excessive foot pronation without any concomitant shortening of the osseous components of the lower limb.[89] While true "short leg syndrome" (SLS) is best literally defined anatomically as ALLD that causes myriad symptoms, it should be noted that colloquially and in much of the past literature, authors have not differentiated well between the FLLD and the ALLD forms of SLS. Symptoms of LLD (and syndromes that might be precipitated or perpetuated by LLD) commonly include LBP but may also include sciatica, commonly in the apparent long leg, as well as pain over the SIJ, hip, outer thigh, groin, knee, shin, ankle, and foot. Taking into consideration its potential role in unleveling the spine's foundational sacral base, the osteopathic profession also perceives systemic impacts on both postural and autonomic balance when discussing LLD and SLS.

BACKGROUND

Anatomic and functional leg length discrepancies are widely recognized across medical specialties. However, many aspects of LLD are poorly understood. There is a lack of interdisciplinary consensus regarding the threshold of LLD considered clinically significant, prevalence of LLD, reliability and validity of measuring methods, and the role of LLD in contributing to low back pain and a variety of neuromusculoskeletal conditions. Some in the orthopedic community have suggested that the medical evidence suggests that, based on the research reviewed, childhood anatomic LLD of less than 15 mm in situations of repeated and/or heavy loading, or less than 20 mm (~¾ in) under normal conditions, are not likely to cause symptoms requiring treatment.[90] However, the osteopathic profession and multiple other clinicians treating neuromusculoskeletal complaints believe that even average leg length discrepancies (approximately 5.2 mm), in the right patient, can cause sacral base declination, frequently becoming symptomatic.[43,84,89,91–96]

PREVALENCE

Leg length discrepancies are common, however, the exact prevalence of LLD is unknown. Studies have estimated a prevalence between 65% and 90% of the general population, with 15% to 20% of individuals exhibiting a difference of >9 mm.[90,97] Providers should remember that 85% of LBP is nonspecific, and a substantial proportion of these patients will likely have a symptomatic anatomic or functional LLD. Therefore, providers should remember to perform adequate structural exams. The mean LLD found in both asymptomatic and symptomatic patients from multiple studies was approximately 5.2 mm.[90] In adult men and women, the right leg is said to be anatomically shorter more often[90] and prior to any OMT when examining the lateral malleoli in the supine position also appears functionally shorter than the left.[98] Friberg and others note that relatively small amounts of anatomic LLD may be clinically significant in patients with prolonged standing and/or repetitive loading.[89,92,98] In a typical population where nearly 90% of people have some degree of LLD, and when 50% of these discrepancies are 5.22 mm or greater, it is prudent for practitioners to keep LLD high on their differential diagnostic list for patients presenting with low back pain.[89]

CAUSES/RISK FACTORS

Anatomic leg length discrepancy (ALLD) may be caused by many factors. Some of these include[99]:

- Lower extremity fracture
- Idiopathic developmental abnormalities
- Arthroplasty
- Trauma to the epiphyseal end plate prior to skeletal maturity
- Degenerative disorders
- Legg–Calvé–Perthes disease
- Cancer or neoplastic changes
- Infections

FLLD may also be caused by many factors. Some of these include[99]:

- Somatic dysfunctions of pelvis/lower extremities/soft tissues (including sacral torsion/obliquity and pelvic shears)
- Lower extremity joint contractures
- Ligamentous laxity
- Axial malalignments (functional group curve, scoliosis)
- Postural imbalance
- Occupational overuse
- Foot biomechanics
- Overpronation
- Collapsed arches

FUNCTIONAL EFFECTS

LLD, no matter the cause, if significant or long standing, can cause gait asymmetries throughout the kinetic chain. There is an increased vertical displacement of the center of mass resulting in increased energy consumption. In running, the vertical oscillation is greater and there is no double support, so weight is not shared between legs.[97,99,100] During walking gait, the stance phase is greater than 50% of the gait cycle. With increasing speeds (e.g., running), the length of the stance phase decreases.[97,99,100] This results in stress on the lower extremity that is three times that of walking.[97,99,100] Compensatory mechanisms for this LLD include rotation of the innominate anterior on the side of the anatomical or functional short leg and posterior rotation contralaterally. With larger amounts of leg length discrepancy, subjects begin to develop pronation of the foot and ankle dorsiflexion on the long leg side. Also seen are knee and/or hip flexion and posterior rotation of the ilium on the long leg side.

From an osteopathic perspective, the functional effect of LLD on spinal posture occurs as the body attempts to establish systemic compensation regarding sacral base unleveling. For this reason, a precise diagnosis and treatment regimen for postural decompensation due to LLD may be suggested by symptomatology and palpatory diagnosis, radiographic diagnosis may be needed (see Chapter 92 Postural Considerations in Osteopathic Diagnosis and Treatment).

CLINICAL PRESENTATION

The first manifestations of symptomatic LLD usually begin in the middle-aged patient with lower back pain that worsens as the day goes on.[43,101] Symptoms are typically precipitated with an injury or significant overuse event and thereafter perpetuated or made worse with excessive standing, walking, or running.[101–103] Occasionally the patient will tell you that they must hem their pants differently or "one shoe wears out." High-demand individuals (e.g., runners, military trainees) who are on their feet most of the day or involved in sports appear more likely to become symptomatic due to LLD than those who are less active.[104] Travell and Simons considered LLD to be one of the most common perpetuating factors in quadratus lumborum trigger points, a somatic dysfunction that they named as "one of the most commonly overlooked musculoskeletal sources of low back pain."[102] Kuchera routinely used findings related to the iliolumbar ligaments to assess for signs of postural decompensation asking patients if their sclerotomal pain pattern referred into the groin and/or greater trochanteric site and palpation for tenderness and tissue texture change over this ligament's origin and insertion.[44] Rannisto found that LLD was associated with low back pain among those who needed to stand while working.[104] In summary, LLD can contribute to extremity, upper and lower back and neck pain, headaches, somatovisceral reflex symptoms, pelvic pain, and fatigue especially in individuals with increased functional demand.[44,96,101]

PHYSICAL FINDINGS

On observation, the clinician might notice an unleveled belt line, a gait that leans to one side, a collapsed arch of the involved foot or a pronation of the foot on the side of the long leg, a surgical scar of the hip or knee, or visible scoliosis. During the structural exam, asymmetric landmarks involving the medial malleoli, anterior superior iliac spines (ASIS), posterior superior iliac spines (PSIS), iliac crests, and lumbar vertebrae almost invariably accompany SLS.[89] Prior to OMT, the following predictable physical exam findings in non–weight-bearing positions are found on the side with the apparently shorter leg: (1) superior medial malleolus, (2) inferior ASIS, (3) superior PSIS, (4) inferior iliac crest, and (5) contralateral side bending and ipsilateral rotation of the lumbar spine.[44,89,96] It is also common in the standing position to find a low iliac crest, a low greater trochanter, and a deep sacral sulcus on the short leg side. Pelvic side shift in the standing position will occur away from the side of the shorter leg. The finding of a deep sacral sulcus on the short leg side with significant tissue texture abnormality and tenderness indicates sacral somatic dysfunction and sacral base declination on that side.[84]

In compensation the innominate on the side of the short LLD rotates anteriorly, thus lengthening the "short leg," while the innominate on the contralateral side of the short LLD rotates posteriorly, shortening the "longer leg." The sacral base tilts toward the side with the short LLD, dropping the iliac crest on the same side.[89] To compensate for the sacral base declination, a lumbar curve convex on the "short leg" side will be seen on the Adams forward bending test with side bending away. (See Chapter 92 Postural Considerations in Osteopathic Diagnosis and Treatment.)

There are multiple methods for clinical evaluation of LLD, but most suffer from poor reliability and validity especially if performed without precise agreement on specific exam protocols.[105] This is compounded by inconsistencies in bony landmark palpation, variable soft tissue coverage, and differences in leg or waist circumference. Using consistent location of the iliac crest heights, PSIS "dimples," and the angle of the lumbar spine ascent from the sacrum, Calliet stated the palpatory, observational measurement of pelvic levelness was accurate to ¼ in (6 mm). In contrast, radiographic measurement of standing sacral base unleveling, which is the gold standard for osteopathic interpretation of FLLD, is <2 mm.[106]

The most widely utilized ALLD method is the tape measure method, in which a tape measure is used to find the distance between two anatomic landmarks (commonly the anterior superior iliac spine and the medial malleolus) while in the supine or standing position (see Fig. 93.13).[104,107] Some clinicians prefer to measure from the floor to the superior aspect of the greater trochanter (see Fig. 93.14). Alternatively, the block method is an indirect clinical measurement of FLLD in which iliac crest height is measured with the patient in a standing position. Lifts are placed on the short leg side to level the pelvis. The final height of the lift required to level the pelvis is the height of the LLD.[108] Hand-held devices such as the palpation meter (PALM) used in the standing position have recently emerged as an alternative measurement of FLLD with studies demonstrating greater reliability than these methods and substantial agreement with gold standard radiographic iliac crest height measurements and LLD.[104,109]

However, from an osteopathic viewpoint, leveling the pelvis may not level the sacral base if significant ligamentous laxity and/or sacral somatic dysfunction is present.[44,84] Providers should also focus on lumbar spinal segment motion testing and the standing flexion test. Treating the somatic dysfunction present first in these regions, and any compensations, prior to clinical measurement of LLD is believed to provide a more accurate measurement.

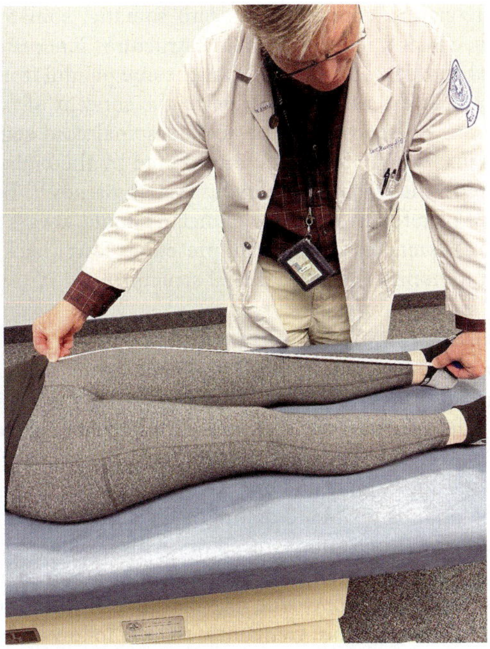

Figure 93.13. Supine leg length measurement.

DIAGNOSIS

It seems reasonable to assume that if providers worldwide knew how to appropriately diagnose LLD, the costs associated with low back pain would be reduced, given the prevalence and magnitude of LLDs in the general population.[89,94] Indeed, based on his research of diagnosis and treatment of patients with LLDs, Irvin claimed that most of the idiopathic and chronic pain of the musculoskeletal system could be alleviated by sufficient improvement of normal posture toward ideal configuration.[94] In addition to the clinical findings, radiography is used as the gold standard for measurement of ALLD.[104] There are multiple radiographic methods available including full limb or pelvic radiographs, postural x-ray series, and CT scanograms.[105,106] The osteopathic postural radiographic series and its interpretation are covered in depth in the postural balance chapter of this textbook; for addressing the impact of LLD, the most important measurement is that of sacral base unleveling.[44,106] Limitations of radiographically assessing patients with LLD include inherent inaccuracy in patients with hip or knee flexion contracture and the technique is subject to a magnification error.[90] Preferences for radiographic analysis methods vary between providers and between specialties.

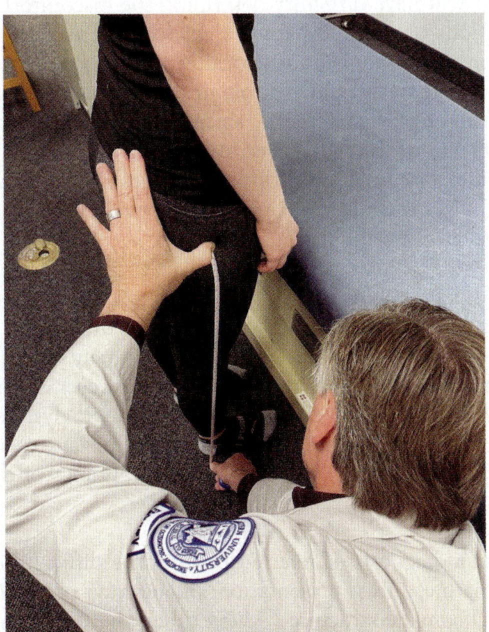

Figure 93.14. Standing leg length measurement.

ASSOCIATED CONDITIONS

Psoas tension may exist in a patient with a symptomatic anatomic short leg. Psoas tension has been linked to low back pain.[84] Depending on which psoas tightens, psoas tension can help compensate for a short leg, or it can exacerbate a short leg problem. Consider the following example:

Given an anatomic short leg left with a chronic sacral dysfunction and pelvic side shift right, tightness of the right psoas will correct the pelvic side shift tendency and improve the patient's postural imbalance. However, tightness of the left psoas will exaggerate the pelvic side shift right worsening the imbalance.

Iliopsoas syndrome has also been reported in the literature as a complication of inappropriate heel lift use.[110]

The piriformis has been found to be dysfunctional on the long leg side. This may contribute to chronic or recurrent sciatic pain and unilateral hip symptoms also on the side of the longer lower extremity.[92]

Regarding osteoarthritis, some authors have found that limbs at least 2 cm shorter are at increased risk of hip OA.[111] Similarly, a cohort study by Harvey et al found an increased risk of knee osteoarthritis on the short limb when leg length discrepancies greater than 1 cm were present.[112] A correlation between LLD and stress fractures has also been found. There is a greater incidence of stress fractures in the tibia, metatarsals, and femur of the longer leg which appears consistent with the greater forces emitted through the longer leg described under hip pain.[92]

TREATMENT

Most people with adequate homeostatic reserves can compensate for a small inequality in leg length. Treatment generally includes a heel lift or building up the patient's shoe. In-shoe heel lifts are generally used for small differences in leg length, while building up the sole of the shoe on the shorter leg side is preferred for larger differences.[44] Clinical indications for heel lift therapy include a symptomatic patient with a low iliac crest, low greater trochanter, ipsilateral deep sacral sulcus with TART changes, TART changes over the iliolumbar ligament and pelvic side shift away from the short leg. The goal of treatment for SLS (LLD) is to level the sacral base and this is often established by measuring a standing anteroposterior osteopathic postural radiograph.[44,95] Treatment of the impact of leg length discrepancy at the sacral base is sought to clinically improve the patient's functional status, gait and station, and pain.

Initial therapeutic heel lift size is also a matter of some debate. Some literature suggests starting with either a 1/16- or 1/8-in lift to level the sacral base depending on the health and age of the patient.[44,89,95,113] Other articles recommend starting out with a heel lift half the size of the FLLD as measured at the sacral base. In either case, a patient typically begins wearing heel lifts smaller than the LLD itself to give the body time to re-compensate. Patients then wear progressively larger heel lifts until the sacral base declination and symptoms improve. When using heel lift therapy, it is agreed upon that a slow, gradual progression of heel lift height should be accompanied by pan-corporeal OMT and/

or at least some form of systemic musculoskeletal therapy such as massage or stretching strategies. Please see Chapter 92 Postural Considerations in Osteopathic Diagnosis and Treatment. For patients with LLD, and especially those with low back pain, the clinician should also strive for improving sacral mobility as LLD and postural imbalance are a cause of SIJ dysfunction.[84]

Manipulative treatment should focus on treating any spinal type II dysfunctions, especially at the crossover points and transition zones. Also important is to improve tensions in the antigravity muscles (especially in the psoas, quadratus lumborum and hamstring muscles), relieve myofascial restrictions and counterstrain points, and improve core muscle function and strength. The status of TART changes at the iliolumbar ligament attachments as well as symmetry of anatomic landmarks including the sacrum, the depth of the sacral sulci, and pelvic side shift can be used clinically to evaluate progress of lift therapy.

Several studies have examined the treatment of low back pain patients with LLD with shoe lifts. Gofton obtained good results: the patients experienced major or complete pain relief that lasted upon follow-up ranging from 3 to 11 years.[114] Helliwell also observed patients whereby 44% experienced complete pain relief, and 45% had moderate or substantial pain relief.[115] Friberg found that 157 (of 211) patients with LBP, treated with shoe lifts, were symptom-free after a mean follow-up of 18 months.[92] Heel-lift customized orthotics with 100% LLD correction are an effective short- and long-term treatment in patients with nonspecific LBP, inducing pain symptom recession and stimulating the improvement of postural parameters without contraindications.[116] Rannisto found that correction of LLD with insoles was an effective intervention among workers with LBP and a standing job.[117] Irvin documented significant and lasting reduction of chronic low back pain by using heel lift orthotics to level the sacral base which also accomplished an overall reduction of ≈70% of many subjects with initial diagnosis of idiopathic multiregional, nonmetabolic chronic pain.[94,95,118]

For pediatric patients, conservative treatment options may include activities that promote epiphyseal growth through compressive stress techniques. Alternatively, surgical interventions can be considered, which may aim to either slow growth by blocking the epiphyseal plates on the longer leg or lengthen the shorter limb using a leg lengthening procedure. Surgical approaches are reserved for severe cases and include techniques such as the Ilizarov distraction method and subtrochanteric femoral shortening osteotomy.[119,120] Surgical limb lengthening in children is generally reserved for LLD greater than 40 to 50 mm as many children simply have transient asymmetric lower extremity epiphyseal growth spurts or will dynamically respond to one or more conservative strategies.

In the adult patient, LLD can be the result of severe long-term degenerative changes of the hip and/or knee.[121] Total hip and knee arthroplasty procedures can help to correct for this loss of height and pan-corporeal OMT is needed to help them recompensate. Conversely, in patients with little to no prior LLD, hip replacement may dramatically create LLD. In these patients who lack prior compensatory or decompensatory change, LLD is best treated with orthotics to totally restore sacral base levelness. Please see Chapter 92 Postural Considerations in Osteopathic Diagnosis and Treatment and Chapter 91 Osteopathic Approach to Diagnosing and Treating Somatic Dysfunction in the Extremities.

Referred Pain

DEFINITION

Referred pain is pain that is perceived at a location other than the site of origin of the painful stimulus.[122] Referred pain is related to the osteopathic concept of viscero-somatic, somato-somatic and somato-visceral reflexes. Somatic structures innervated by the same spinal cord level of a viscera can become painful from visceral dysfunction and disease. This is due to the concept of facilitation (sensitization) of neurons in the related spinal cord segment. In addition, sensory signals may be interpreted by the brain as being experienced in the somatic or nervous system tissues.[123] Because of the concept of referred pain, the clinician should always be aware of "spinal masqueraders" which can present as lower back pain but are related to nonmechanical visceral structures.[122]

CAUSES/RISK FACTORS

The most common causes of referred pain in the lumbar region come from dysfunction in the following structures: spinal segments, SIJ, iliopsoas muscle, abdominal and pelvic viscera, tumors, infections, and the genitourinary system.[124,125] Because of close anatomic relationships, spinal cord and sympathetic nerve sensitization occurs. The brain is unable to distinguish visceral signals from the signals that arise from somatic receptors. This results in pain being interpreted as coming from the somatic regions rather than the viscera.[126] Referred pain follows the distribution of sclerotomes (muscle, fascia, and bone) more frequently than it follows the classical dermatomes. Visceral pain is usually caused by inflammation, distention, or ischemia. The sympathetic nervous system travels along the blood supply to the internal organs and so any of these changes in the wall of the viscera can also affect the blood supply and cause sympathetic nerve irritation and inflammation. There are multiple theories of referred pain, which include: Convergence-projection theory,[127] convergence-facilitation theory,[128] axon-reflex theory,[129] hyperexcitability theory,[130] and the thalamic convergence theory.[127]

There is a significant relationship between the size of local pain and referred pain areas and their related pain intensity ratings.[122,126,131] As an area of large nociceptive input goes to the dorsal horn, or the brainstem neurons, it will cause an expansion of the receptive fields, and potentially the expansion of referred areas that are detected.[126]

CLINICAL PRESENTATION

When there is a referred pain or a visceral pain mechanism present, the patient will have difficulty describing the discomfort. Sensory manifestations of referred pain are experienced as diffuse aching and gnawing pain that is poorly localized. Somatosensory changes do occur, yet there are no neurologic symptoms such as numbness and tingling or paresthesia, since referred pain is not caused by compression of the local nerve roots.[122,131,132] Referred pain can involve wide areas, making it difficult to localize to one anatomic structure.[132] Many times the pain will not be relieved with rest, and it may awaken the patient from sleep.

PHYSICAL FINDINGS

Patients may have pain that is out of proportion to the physical examination findings. For example, the patient may have significant pain in the right hip and sacroiliac region, however all the orthopedic tests and palpatory examination for somatic dysfunction are relatively negative. This should tip off the clinician to consider a referred pain pattern or potentially a visceral etiology of the pain.

DIAGNOSIS

Arriving at a diagnosis of referred pain can be difficult because of the vague nature, diffuse presentation, and negative physical findings of the local somatic structures. Many times, the diagnosis is made through imaging studies demonstrating a visceral, vascular, or neurologic issue that aligns with the patient's history and examination.

TREATMENT

Treatment of referred pain can be difficult as the source needs to be found and addressed. Pain management specialists recommend using ketamine and other NMDA receptor antagonists for this type of pain.[122,124] In one study, applying a mixture of local anesthesia on the skin, just above the referred pain area, reduced the referred pain intensity by 22.7%.[125] A similar result was found after ethyl chloride was sprayed onto a saline-induced referred pain area.[133,134] The pain management literature lists two techniques to block afferents from the referred pain area, by which the referred pain intensity was reduced by 40.2%.[125] These include: (1) Differential nerve blocking with an inflated tourniquet between the site of stimulation and the corresponding distal referred area and (2) intravenous regional analgesia.

There are many other ways to treat referred pain. These may include utilizing a centrally acting medication such as duloxetine, or gabapentin, or utilizing other supportive treatments such as:

1. Osteopathic manual medicine techniques
2. Trigger point Injections[122]
3. Laser therapy[122]
4. Superficial dry needling is the most effective in combination with stretching[123]
5. Acupuncture

Disk Protrusions

DEFINITION

Lumbar disk protrusions are an eccentric bulging of the intervertebral disk with an intact annulus. However, when the annulus is torn and the central nucleus pulposus extrudes, a disk extrusion is present. A disk sequestration or extruded fragment, occurs when the disk material herniates through the annulus and is no longer continuous with the disk space. The disk material can migrate in a proximal or distal direction. Disk protrusions are also characterized by location. These include (1) a central protrusion, (2) a posterolateral protrusion (most common), (3) foraminal or far lateral protrusion, and (4) axillary (less common).[135]

EPIDEMIOLOGY

Disk protrusions are common, with a lifetime prevalence of 10%. However only about 5% become symptomatic and their peak incidence occurs in the fourth and fifth decades. Disk protrusions occur more commonly in males than females and approximately 90% occur at the L5/S1 level. It is the most common level seen, followed by the L4/L5 level.[135]

CAUSES/RISK FACTORS

More than half of disk protrusions are idiopathic in etiology. However, it has been thought that microinstability, and repetitive overuse can result in recurrent torsional strain and tears to the outer annulus leading to herniation of the nucleus pulposus. Spinal flexion and rotation are not well tolerated in the patient who has a herniated disk. The posterior longitudinal ligament is thinner and less robust than the anterior longitudinal ligament allowing disks to protrude to the left or the right. The sinuvertebral nerves provide innervation to the posterior annulus and have been discussed to be one of the causes of vertebral mediated back pain. Although disk herniations can be seen with abrupt spinal trauma, spondylolisthesis, spinal infections, and cancer, the most common cause is idiopathic.

CLINICAL PRESENTATION

Patients with lumbar disk protrusions may present with back pain, sacroiliac pain, and/or leg pain. Occasionally, patients may have bowel or bladder dysfunction possibly indicating CES, which is a medical/surgical emergency. Patients do not tolerate sitting for prolonged periods of time and prefer moving around. When a specific nerve root is involved the leg pain typically follows the dermatome of the irritated nerve root. The pain presentation and physical examination can help the clinician determine which spinal level is involved. However, when there is a more diffuse etiology, or referred pain pattern, the sclerotome or myotome may be involved producing a more diffuse presentation.

PHYSICAL FINDINGS

Patients with a lumbar disk herniation have a difficult time flexing forward due to pain as the disk is loaded. They have limited lumbar range of motion due to the pain and they may have a list away from the side of nerve root irritation to increase the size of the neural foramen. Disk protrusions can cause scoliosis in the lumbar region depending on the size and location of the disk protrusion. Spasms of the paraspinal musculature, segmental somatic dysfunction, tender points, and restricted hip extension (due to psoas spasm) are commonly associated with physical findings. It is also common to see tight hamstrings and sacral/pelvic somatic dysfunction.

On neurologic examination many patients will have a positive SLR test, or a slump test, if there is nerve root involvement. DTR may be diminished due to compression of the involved nerve root. Sensory changes also occur in the dermatomal distribution. Motor weakness is a late finding and typically will involve the gastrocnemius (S1), extensor hallucis longus (L5), and tibialis anterior (L4) nerve roots. Clinicians should check for the ability of the patient to walk on their heels (L4–L5) and their toes (S1) as part of the neurologic exam.

DIAGNOSIS

Diagnosis is made clinically and confirmed with an MRI study of the lumbar spine. Since disk disease is common, and many asymptomatic patients will have disk protrusions on an MRI, clinicians should be selective in imaging and seeking specialist referrals.[136,137]

TREATMENT

Treatment for lumbar disk protrusions is typically conservative in 80% to 90% of cases. Approximately 90% of patients will have improvement of symptoms within 3 months without substantial medical treatment. Conservative management includes physical therapy, osteopathic manipulative treatment, medications, injections, stress management, and patient education. Patients are less likely to improve if still symptomatic after 6 weeks of conservative care and have a greater likelihood of going on to chronic pain.

However, large disk herniations that produce focal neurologic symptoms, changes to bowel, bladder or sexual dysfunction can be causing CES. Its treatment is emergent and microdiskectomy is typically performed within 48 hours (see Fig. 93.15). Elective surgical microdiskectomy is only indicated for severe pain and/or motor deficit that have failed to respond to nonoperative management. It is controversial if surgical treatment is equivalent to nonsurgical treatment in the long term but does provide faster pain relief. In 2020, an orthopedic 10-year follow-up study was performed looking at all levels of evidence. It revealed statistically greater improvement in primary outcomes at 3 months and 2 years in patients who had surgery. In follow-up studies, the 4 year and 8 year as-treated analysis showed both surgical and nonsurgical groups did well, with statistically greater improvements in those patients who were treated surgically.[138]

SOMATIC DYSFUNCTION

Somatic dysfunction is commonly seen in patients with lumbar disk protrusions. Both local and distant dysfunction typically includes

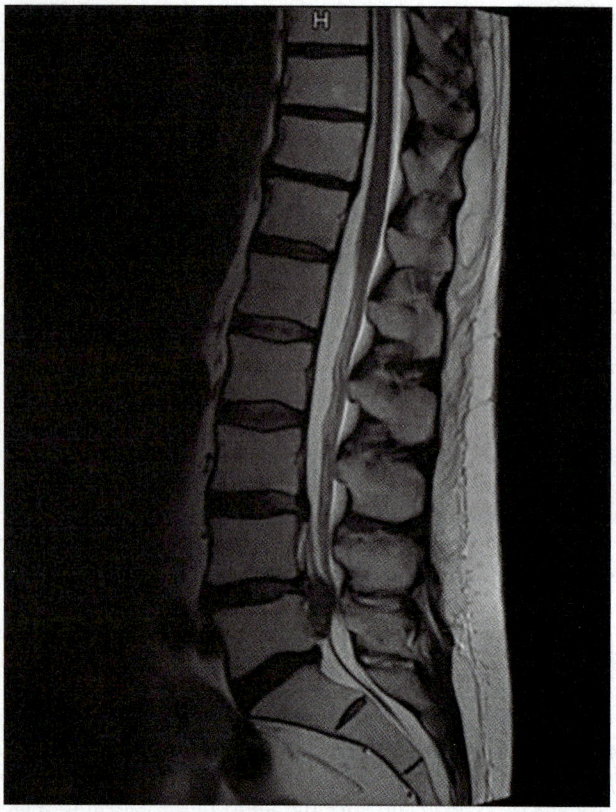

Figure 93.15. Cauda equina syndrome. (Case courtesy of Ian Bickle, Radiopaedia.org, rID: 153884.)

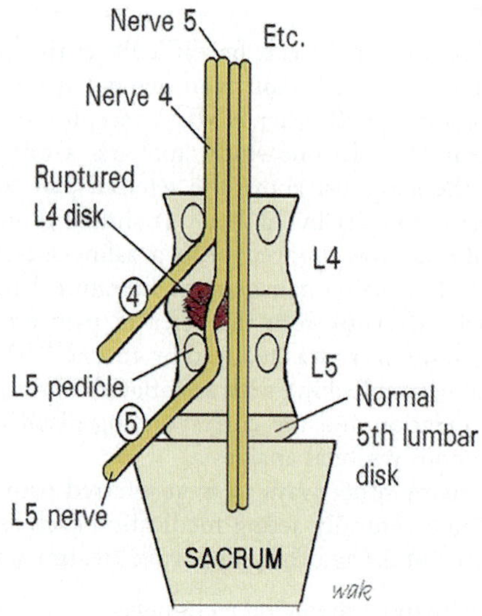

Figure 93.16. Radiculopathy from L4 to L5 disk herniation may impinge upon the L5 nerve root in addition to or rather than the L4 nerve root. (Illustration courtesy of William A. Kuchera, DO, FAAO, with permission.)

single-segment dysfunctions of the lumbar spine and thoracolumbar junction, functional lateral curve of the lumbar spine, spasm of the iliopsoas, hamstrings, rectus femoris, and quadratus lumborum muscles, and inhibition of the gluteal muscles. In addition to these muscular and articular factors, multiple counterstrain points located in the anterior pelvis, posterior lumbar spine, and posterior pelvis are commonly found relating to muscles and spinal segmental dysfunction. Myofascial restrictions of the pelvis and lumbosacral fascia are also common, and the myofascial structures may contain Simon and Travell myofascial trigger points, trigger bands, and other fascial dysfunctions/distortions. Somatic dysfunction of the sacrum may be primary or secondary to the disk protrusion and needs to be treated to improve lumbar/pelvic function during standing and walking.

Lumbar Radiculopathy

DEFINITION

Lumbar radiculopathy is a condition that causes pain or discomfort in the lower back and hip which then radiates down the posterior and/or lateral aspect of the thigh into the leg. It is typically due to compression of the lumbar nerve roots exiting the spine. Patients experience tingling, burning, radiating pain, numbness, and paresthesia. Radiculopathy and radicular pain commonly occur together, but radiculopathy can occur in the absence of pain and radiculopathy can occur in the absence of radiculopathy.[131]

EPIDEMIOLOGY

Lumbar radiculopathy is one of the most common complaints evaluated by a spine surgeon. Its prevalence has been estimated to be 3% to 5% of the population, affecting both men and women.[139] Females have a higher risk, as do specific populations, with physically demanding careers such as service in the military. In the general population, it is more commonly seen in men than women.[140]

CAUSES/RISK FACTORS

Lumbar radiculopathy is caused by compression, irritation, or inflammation of the lumbar nerve root. Degenerative spondyloarthropathies are the primary cause of lumbar radiculopathy.[141] Additional causes include lumbar disk protrusion, foraminal stenosis, arthritis, tumor, abscess, fracture, spondylolisthesis, scar tissue, or hematoma. The characteristic finding is pain in a dermatomal distribution of the lower extremity that corresponds to the level of spinal involvement. The nerve root that gets compressed is the root that exits the foramen below the herniated disk. So, a disk protrusion at L4/L5 will compress the L5 root, and a protrusion at L5/S1 will compress the S1 root (see Fig. 93.16).[142]

CLINICAL PRESENTATION

Patients who have lumbar radiculopathy complain of leg pain greater than low back pain which tends to be clearly described in a dermatomal distribution. Pain may be worse with prolonged sitting and standing and better with rest. Pain will radiate below the knee and into the foot.

PHYSICAL FINDINGS

Physical findings include decreased sensation of the involved dermatome, decreased DTR, corresponding to the nerve root involved, and possible motor weakness of muscles supplied by that nerve root (see Table 93.3). It is not uncommon to see a "sciatic scoliosis" or "trunk list" in compensation for the pain. The pathophysiology of the "sciatic trunk list" is complex, and it may be due to multiple factors, including the compression of a nerve root by herniated disk material.[143] To highlight this point, Kim found that the trunk list was observed even in patients without leg pain/nerve root irritation highlighting the importance of the role of somatic dysfunction.[143] Central disk protrusions produce axial and/or sacral pain, and if large, can compress nerve roots bilaterally. When there is compression of one or multiple nerve roots, the SLR test is frequently positive between 30 and 70 degrees of hip flexion.

DIAGNOSIS

Diagnosis of lumbar radiculopathy is clinical and supported by imaging or electrodiagnostic studies. Plain x-rays are typically

TABLE 93.3

Neurologic Influence of the Lumbar Roots

Root	L1	L2	L3	L4	L5	S1
Sensory dermatome	Back to trochanter	Back	Back	Inner calf to medial portion of foot (first two toes)	Lateral lower leg	Sole
	Groin	Anterior thigh to the level of knee	Upper buttock to anterior thigh		Dorsum of foot	Heel
			Medial lower leg		First two toes	Lateral edge of foot
Innervated muscle(s)	Iliopsoas	Iliopsoas	Iliopsoas	Tibialis anterior	Extensor hallucis	Gastrocnemius
		Sartorius	Quadriceps femoris	Gluteus medius	Tibialis posterior	Gluteus maximus
		Hip adductors (longus, brevis, pectineus, magnus, gracilis)	Sartorius	Gluteus minimus	Hamstrings	Hamstrings
			Hip adductors	Tensor fasciae latae		Peroneus
				Quadratus femoris		
Functional limitation(s)	Hip flexion	Hip flexion	Hip flexion	Knee extension	Toe extension	Ankle plantar flexion
		Hip adduction	Hip adduction		Ankle dorsiflexion	Knee flexion
			Knee extension			
Affected reflex(es)	Cremasteric	Cremasteric	Patellar	Patellar	Tibialis posterior	Ankle
		Adductor		Gluteal	Gluteal?	Hamstring

ordered prior to more advanced imaging such as an MRI. Findings on plain x-rays are most commonly normal, however, they may include spondylolisthesis, spondylolysis, foraminal stenosis, compression fracture, or decreased disk space. A loss of lumbar lordosis is a common finding due to muscle spasm, however, this may indicate an underlying orthopedic or neurologic etiology. A patient who is not improving with conservative care, has red flags, and/or findings on x-ray, may warrant an MRI. The indications for ordering an MRI are pain lasting greater than 1 month and not responding to nonoperative management. The MRI must be correlated with the patient's history and physical examination findings. CT scans and CT myelograms can also be performed. CT scans will define the bony detail and the myelogram will determine if a filling defect of a nerve root is present. However, these are typically utilized for presurgical decision making.

TREATMENT

The treatment of lumbar radiculopathy is initially conservative, unless there are progressive neurologic findings, CES, or red flags. Conservative management includes rest and physical therapy, anti-inflammatory medications, osteopathic manipulative treatment, muscle relaxers, constant rest position, ice, and activity modification. Physical therapy is the usual mainstay of treating this condition. Physical therapy procedures and osteopathic manipulative treatment need to be performed cautiously through the region of nerve root compression, to foster healing and not aggravate the condition. Conservative management can continue if there is no significant motor weakness, CES, or any bowel or bladder dysfunction. Approximately 90% of patients will improve with this approach.

For those with continued pain and failure of medications, a selective nerve root block and corticosteroid injection can be performed typically after 6 weeks. This can lead to lasting improvement in approximately 50% of patients, especially if they have an extruded fragment. Surgical management of lumbar radiculopathy depends on the etiology and if red flags are present. For uncomplicated cases that failed conservative management, whose MRI findings and physical findings correlate, and who have progressive muscle weakness, surgery can be considered. A laminotomy and diskectomy/microdiskectomy can be performed for those with intractable pain greater than 6 weeks' duration. As compared to conservative management surgical management yields faster pain relief, but similar results at 5 years post-treatment.

SOMATIC DYSFUNCTION

Acute disk herniation with radiculopathy is a relative contraindication to direct action techniques at the vertebral level in question. However, OMT, especially indirect methods, myofascial release and soft tissue techniques can be used for associated somatic dysfunction and significantly help decrease pain and improve function.

Degenerative Disk Disease

DEFINITION

Clinicians define and describe degenerative disk disease from imaging studies that reveal disk space narrowing, a loss of central fluid intensity of the disk on T2-weighted MRI and associated degenerative/arthritic changes. However, a study demonstrated that a systematic search of publications using the term degenerative disk disease from 2007 through 2016 showed that the definition of degenerative disk disease is quite broad.[144] Currently there are eight categories of diagnosis, so degenerative disk disease represents an underdeveloped concept, with little consensus or uniformity of the definition.[144]

EPIDEMIOLOGY

The epidemiology and prevalence of disk disease are difficult to find due to the inconsistencies in definition. A review of the epidemiology of disk degeneration reveals wide-ranging prevalence estimates.[145] Despite this, lumbar disk disease carries enormous morbidity leading to disability and a poor quality of life.[145]

CAUSES/RISK FACTORS

It was initially thought that disk degeneration was a result of "wear and tear" from injuries, overuse, and mechanical factors. However, disk degeneration appears to be determined in great part by genetic influences.[146] Although environmental factors also play a role, the cause is not primarily through repetitive physical loading. In addition to genetic influences, disk degeneration is directly correlated with increasing patient age and those with obesity. Men develop this degeneration almost 10 years earlier than women, and women with disk degeneration are likely to suffer more symptoms.[147] The intervertebral disk degeneration leads to facet degeneration and ligamentous laxity. The degenerative changes and ligamentous laxity can lead to microinstability, which over time causes further degeneration and eventual macroinstability and a resultant spondylolisthesis.

CLINICAL PRESENTATION

Patients with degenerative disk disease tend to have axial back pain with inconsistent radiation into the lower extremities. They also tend to have intermittent recurrences of episodic lower back pain which may or may not be related to musculoskeletal overuse or injury. Their pain is usually worse with prolonged sitting or standing. It tends to improve with core strengthening exercises, manipulative medicine approaches, and staying active.

PHYSICAL FINDINGS

Structural examination may demonstrate a decreased lumbar lordosis if significant muscle spasm is present. The gait assessment should look for a Trendelenburg gait, which can reveal an underlying weakness in the gluteus medius muscle. It is also important to assess the patient's ability to arise from the chair and to walk on their heels and toes. A neurologic exam for sensory loss, DTR, and motor strength is then performed followed by an SLR test. The standing and seated flexions are commonly performed as a screening procedure for associated somatic dysfunction of the pelvis and sacrum respectively. It also is important in any evaluation of lower extremity issues to evaluate circulation, as vascular claudication may mirror or mimic the neurogenic issues.[147]

DIAGNOSIS

Evaluation of patients with low back pain typically includes AP and lateral radiographs of the affected area. Some physicians will obtain radiographs of the entire spine. An MRI should not be ordered at the initial presentation of suspected acute disk herniations in patients lacking "red flags." These patients will initially undergo a trial of a 6-week course of physical therapy and OMT with clinical improvement.

Prior to ordering an MRI clinicians should be aware that in a meta-analysis of 20 studies evaluating the magnetic resonance imaging (MRI) of asymptotic individuals, the reported disk abnormalities at any level were[147]:

- 20% to 83% for a reduction in disk signal intensity
- 3% to 56% for disk space narrowing
- 6% to 56% for disks with annular tears

This study supports that disk disease is common and should not necessitate specialist evaluation in the absence of pain or limitations.[147] In addition, the finding of disk disease (degeneration or herniation) on MRI does not correlate with the likelihood of chronic pain or the future need for surgery.[147]

TREATMENT

Conservative management is the initial treatment of choice in the absence of red flags. This includes a course of at least 6 weeks of physical therapy with an emphasis on core strengthening and stretching. Nonsurgical intervention also includes cognitive therapy, lifestyle modification, stress management, and modification of activities. Medications such as NSAIDs are supported by the medical evidence as the first line. Epidural steroid injections may provide moderate, short-term relief of pain due to disk herniations, with radiculopathy, but the literature regarding the usefulness of injections for chronic nonradiating back pain is less certain.[147]

The benefits of spinal surgery for relief of low back and leg pain in patients with degenerative spinal disorders have long been debated. Surgical referrals for patients with disk herniations, as well as degenerative spinal stenosis, should be reserved for those with either neurologic deficits, degenerative spondylolisthesis, or pain-limiting daily functions. Some groups have supported lumbar fusion for patients with chronic LBP refractory to nonsurgical care, as a viable treatment option for reducing pain and improving outcomes.[148] Patients need to understand that while surgical intervention has favorable outcomes for relieving radicular pains, there is a risk of failed back surgical syndrome, and the results are less predictable for nonradiating lower back pain.[147]

SOMATIC DYSFUNCTION

In addition to a decreased lumbar lordosis, tension of the iliopsoas, hamstrings, and rectus femoris is common. Palpatory assessment commonly shows loss of segmental spinal mobility, tender points, and trigger points in the quadratus lumborum, and muscle spasm. When associated instability is found, the patient may have lumbar pain in the prone position with posterior to anterior pressure/glides applied to the involved spinous process.

Spondylolysis

DEFINITION

Spondylolysis is a stress fracture of the posterior elements of the spine, specifically the pars interarticularis. Lumbar spondylolysis typically results from repetitive microtrauma, in a patient who has predisposing anatomical conditions and develops in stages. It represents a continuum of disease, from stress reaction, to fracture, and to potentially a spondylolisthesis.[149]

PREVALENCE/INCIDENCE

The incidence of lumbar spondylolysis in the general population is estimated to be about 6% to 8% but may be much higher in athletes and certain sporting activities.[149]

The incidence of spondylolysis increases with age until adulthood, but not thereafter. Spondylolysis and spondylolisthesis are the most common causes of back pain in children and adolescents over the age of 10 years.[149] There is a higher incidence in Native Americans.[149]

CLINICAL PRESENTATION

Most cases of spondylolysis are completely asymptomatic and represent an incidental radiologic finding. However, spondylolysis can be a cause of spine instability, back pain, and radiculopathy.

CAUSES

The causes of spondylolysis are still debated, but the most accepted theories postulate repetitive microtrauma. The mechanism of injury is usually repetitive extension stress; however, it can be a combination of repetitive flexion, extension, or rotation of the lumbar spine. Spondylolysis diminishes the stabilizing ability of the posterior elements in the spine and may lead to isthmic spondylolisthesis. Spondylolysis primarily involves the L5 vertebra (95% of cases) and the incidence decreases proceeding cephalad.[150] It almost always occurs bilaterally, thus dividing the vertebra into two segments.[150] Although the progression of spondylolysis to spondylolisthesis in skeletally immature individuals is well known, similar progression in adults has been rarely reported.[150] It is classified by the Willse–Newman classification.[149]

CLINICAL PRESENTATION

Patients with symptomatic spondylolysis usually complain of mechanical-type low back pain, which typically is worsened by activity (particularly the repetitive flexion–extension activity of the spine [common to oarsmen, gymnasts, and divers]) and improves with rest.[150] Radicular symptoms are less common in young patients but can occur with more severe grades of slippage.

PHYSICAL FINDINGS

The most common findings on physical examination are hyperlordotic posture and well-localized low back pain with extension of the lumbar spine. Hyperextension of the lumbar spine during a single-limb stance may cause pain. Hamstring tightness is another very common finding in patients with spondylolysis, although the underlying mechanism is unknown.[150] Patients will commonly have bilateral muscle tension in the thoracolumbar junction, and tender points over the iliolumbar ligaments, sacral sulcus, and gluteus medius muscles.

DIAGNOSIS

In the primary care setting, an early diagnosis of spondylolysis is important for treatment considerations. Delayed diagnosis and treatment may progress to a nonunion. This is also crucial in the young athletic patients where chronic nonunion may require surgical intervention. Diagnosis is made initially with plain films as the best initial study. Anteroposterior, lateral, 45 degrees right, and left oblique and lateral views of the spine are usually performed. On the oblique views, a dark line seen at the pars interarticularis, representing a collar on the "Scotty dogs" neck is a helpful visual aid. In the absence of a slip, however, spondylolysis can be a very subtle finding that can be detected only with the use of advanced imaging. CT scan is the most accurate modality for detecting bony defects and may also be used for assessment of healing. However, it is not sensitive for detection of early edematous stress response and exposes the patient to ionizing radiation.[149]

MR imaging should be used as the primary investigation for adolescents with back pain and suspected stress reactions of the lumbar pars interarticularis. MR is the imaging modality of choice for identifying associated disk protrusions, the presence of bone marrow edema, and nerve root compression.[149]

SPECT use is limited by a high rate of false-positive and false-negative results and by considerable ionizing radiation exposure. Technetium 99m methylene diphosphonate bone scintigraphy shows uptake of the isotope in the region of a metabolically active fracture.[149]

It may identify a lesion that is not shown on radiographs because of the orientation, or its early stage in the stress fracture process.[149]

TREATMENT

The treatment for spondylolysis and spondylolisthesis is initially conservative and aims to reduce pain and facilitate healing. Conservative treatment typically requires cessation of aggravating sporting activities and a spinal brace with a thoraco–lumbo–sacral orthosis (TLSO). The duration of wearing the brace is controversial. In one study, athletes returned to play after wearing a TLSO for an average of 5.6 months with the majority having good or excellent results.[151] Others recommend 3 months of full-time wear (more than 20 hours per day) with no sports activities followed by 3 months of full-time wear with sports activities allowed.[150] The goal of bracing is to prevent motion at the stress fracture and allow for osseous healing at the defect. OMT for associated somatic dysfunction is helpful for pain management and functional status. Care must be taken near the fracture site and the clinician may choose to treat other related areas with the patient in the brace. Indirect techniques such as counterstrain and soft tissue/myofascial approaches work well. Treatment of somatic dysfunction that is distant yet functionally related, such as the thoracic spine and ribs, pelvis, and lower extremities can help keep the patient active during their time wearing the brace.

In addition to bracing and careful OMT, an organized physical therapy program including stretching and strengthening exercises, aimed principally at the reduction of lumbar lordosis, as well as at the treatment of the hamstring contracture, is advised.[150] Surgical treatment for spondylolysis is generally reserved for patients who fail to respond to conservative treatment. Patients with more than 6 months of pain despite restriction of activity and bracing are candidates for surgery.

Spondylolisthesis

DEFINITION

Spondylolisthesis is an anterior slippage of one vertebra on the segment below. It may be seen due to trauma, spondylolysis (isthmic), or degenerative in nature.

CLASSIFICATION/CAUSES

Pediatric spondylolysis and spondylolisthesis represent a continuum of disease where there is a fracture of the pars interarticularis (spondylolysis) which may progress to spondylolisthesis. Relatively few patients (5%) with spondylolysis develop spondylolisthesis.[152]

Isthmic spondylolisthesis is most seen at L5/S1 and is caused by a defect in the pars interarticularis. In this situation, an L5 radiculopathy may be present and is usually caused by foraminal stenosis at the L5–S1 level. Degenerative spondylolisthesis is a degenerative condition seen most in females over 40 years of age, at the L4–L5 level. Patients can have L4 nerve root involvement and neurogenic claudication from associated stenosis. Spondylolisthesis is graded depending on the degree of the slip seen on the lateral lumbar radiograph. The slip may be posterior as well and is then called a retrolisthesis.

CLINICAL PRESENTATION

The most common presentation of spondylolisthesis is axial back pain in a patient who has had a long history of intermittent painful episodes of variable intensity and duration. Clinical presentation also includes lumbosacral pain that can wrap around the waist bilaterally. Patients also have buttock and leg pain/discomfort caused by upright walking, relieved by sitting. Associated symptoms include hamstring tightness and pain over the SIJs and into the gluteal region.

PHYSICAL FINDINGS

When spondylolisthesis is present, it can be revealed at the physical examination during palpation of the lumbar spine as a tender step-off of the spinous processes of the involved segment. With palpation of the lumbar spine and sacrum, it is common for patients to have an increased lordosis, tenderness of the iliolumbar ligaments, and a bilaterally flexed sacrum. Lumbosacral pain occurs with posterior to anterior pressure applied to the spinous process of L4 or L5. Patients may also have lumbosacral pain when checking active range of motion in the extremes of spinal flexion or extension.

Depending on the spinal level involved, an L4 or L5 radiculopathy may be present. Patients need to be assessed for the presence of a foot drop. Some patients will go on to develop spinal stenosis and neurogenic claudication which presents as buttock and leg pain that is worse with walking and improves with sitting. Rarely the patient may present with CES if the slip is greater than a grade 2 or an acute traumatic event has occurred. Any patients who have decreased sensation in the perineal region and decreased anal sphincter tone need to be dealt with emergently.

DIAGNOSIS

On x-ray evaluation of the lumbar spine, deformity will be seen in the coronal plane on the lateral view. If spondylolysis is present, a black line will be seen across the pars interarticularis on the oblique view. There will be malalignment of the anterior and posterior margins of one vertebral body compared to the vertebral body below (see Fig. 93.17). On the flexion–extension views, instability is defined as 4 mm of translation, or 10 degrees of angulation of motion compared to adjacent motion segments.

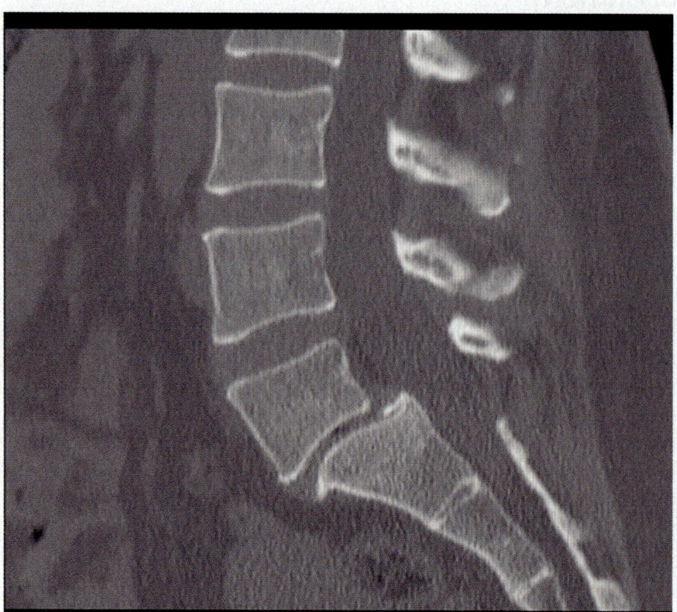

Figure 93.17. Image of spondylolisthesis. (Case courtesy of David Cuete, Radiopaedia.org, rID: 23567.)

TREATMENT

Treatment of the condition depends on the acuity or chronicity of the situation. There are conservative and operative recommendations. The conservative recommendations include activity restriction, NSAIDs, and antilordotic bracing in the acute phase. Somatic dysfunction should be gently treated, especially above and below the area of concern. The involved segment is inherently unstable (especially acutely) and it is a relative contraindication to use direct action manipulative techniques on the level of spondylolisthesis. Spasm of the iliopsoas muscles increases compressive pressure throughout the lumbar spine, worsening the condition. OMT to resolve this spasm is beneficial. Counterstrain for related tender points helps improve local muscle function and pain. Physical therapy is the mainstay of treatment for most cases. For chronic lower back pain due to ligamentous laxity, prolotherapy has been found to be beneficial when combined with spinal manipulation, exercise, and other co-intervention.[153]

Operative treatment includes the L4–S1 decompression with instrumented fusion for patients with progressive neurologic deficit or high-grade spondylolisthesis with persistent and incapacitating pain that has failed 6 months of nonoperative management.[152] In the SPORT study, the intent-to-treat analysis failed to show a significant difference between patients treated surgically for spondylolisthesis as compared to those treated nonoperatively. However, the as-treated analysis revealed statically greater improvements at 6 weeks, 2 years, and 4 years in patients treated surgically.[154]

Spinal Stenosis

DEFINITION

Central spinal stenosis is caused by hypertrophy of the facet joints, ligamentum flavum, disk protrusion, spondylolisthesis, genetic factors, or a combination of these.

ANATOMY/CLASSIFICATION

Lumbar spinal stenosis is defined as the narrowing of the central lumbar canal, the lateral recess, or the intervertebral foramen. The condition is classified as being either congenital, developmental, or acquired. Congenital stenosis is divided additionally into idiopathic and achondroplastic etiologies.[155] Acquired stenosis is subclassified into degenerative, combined congenital and degenerative, spondylotic and spondylolisthetic, iatrogenic, post-traumatic, and metabolic.[155] It may be multilevel or segmental. Stenosis is also the result of bone remodeling following healing of a fracture. Lateral spinal stenosis is a common cause of lumbar radiculopathy. The nerve root canal has been divided into three anatomic zones: the (1) entrance zone, (2) the midzone, and (3) exit zone. The nerve root sleeve contains cerebrospinal fluid and covers the nerve root at the entrance zone. At the midzone, nerve root compression typically occurs from a pars defect.[155] The exit zone corresponds to the intervertebral foramen itself. The minimal height of a normal lateral recess is 5 mm; a height of 3 to 4 mm is suggestive of lateral recess stenosis and a height of 2 mm is considered pathologic.[155] The majority of cases of lateral recess stenosis are produced by posterolateral disk protrusions or hypertrophy of the superior articular process (lateral recess syndrome).[155] The intervertebral foramen height varies from 10 to 23 mm and its width varies from 8 to 10 mm.[155] A foraminal height of less than 15 mm is associated with nerve root compression 80% of the time.[155]

PREVALENCE/INCIDENCE

Degenerative spinal stenosis is seen in 20% to 25% of those >65 years and most commonly occurs at the L4–L5 level. Some of the common causes of spinal stenosis include disk protrusions, arthritic change, degenerative disks, cysts, fractures, and tumors.[144] Approximately 20% of patients with spinal stenosis can have congenital spinal stenosis throughout their spinal canal.[144] Stenosis at multiple levels is more common than at one vertebral segment. In approximately 40% of cases, central stenosis is caused by soft tissue such as disks and hypertrophy of the ligamentum flavum.[144] Central lumbar spinal stenosis and degenerative disk disease have genetic influences.[144]

CAUSES/RISK FACTORS

Central stenosis may be attributable to bone hypertrophy, ligamentous hypertrophy, disk protrusion, spondylolisthesis, or any combination of these elements. Through these factors, in addition to chronic lumbar somatic dysfunction, decreased segmental mobility occurs. One theory is that this loss of mobility in one segment creates abnormal forces and stresses on adjacent spinal segments, which then degenerate at an accelerated pace. The L3–L4, L4–L5 spinal segments seem to be most affected by degenerative stenosis.

CLINICAL PRESENTATION

Lumbar spinal stenosis, when severe, produces symptoms of gait disturbances, radiculopathy, motor or sensory deficits, bowel or bladder dysfunction, and neurogenic claudication. Degenerative spinal stenosis, the most common form of the disease, usually occurs in female > male patients in the sixth or seventh decade of life. Patients describe their symptoms as a discomfort ranging from a heavy feeling in their legs, to leg weakness, and/or pain in the back, buttocks, thighs, and calves. Lower extremity pain is present in approximately 80% of patients and back pain is present in approximately 65% of patients.[155] Central and lateral recess stenosis affects the traversing/descending nerve root and foraminal and extraforaminal stenosis affects the exiting nerve root.[156] A pathognomonic aspect of lumbar stenosis is the relationship between symptoms, structure, and function. Symptoms of neurogenic claudication are common and include back and leg pain with prolonged standing or walking and decrease when the individual sits and rests.[155] The congenital form of spinal stenosis appears in patients in the third or fourth decade of life. The location of the stenosis also contributes to the clinical presentation. Spinal stenosis of the central canal in the thoracic and upper lumbar region, when severe, can cause myelopathy and bladder dysfunction.[155]

PHYSICAL FINDINGS

The classic presentation of a patient with spinal stenosis is preference of a flexed posture and symptoms of the lower limbs after prolonged standing with improvement in sitting.[155] In flexion, the vertebral canal lengthens and the spinal roots stretch. With extension, the canal shortens, increasing the bulging of the ligamentum flavum and intervertebral disks into the spinal canal.[155] On physical examination patients may have a positive Kemp sign with spinal extension.[156] In chronic cases, on structural examination it is not uncommon to see a reversal/flattening of the lumbar lordosis, perhaps as a compensation. A paucity of neurologic findings on physical examination, often despite a history of severe disability, is typical for patients with spinal stenosis. The most common findings are of DTR changes, sensory loss, and muscle weakness. SLR test rarely is positive.[155] Osteoarthrosis of the hips and sacroiliac somatic dysfunction may mimic spinal stenosis because of similar gait disturbance and buttock and referred gluteal/posterior thigh pain.

DIAGNOSIS

Taking a thorough history is key to making the diagnosis. Walking-induced symptoms of neurogenic claudication often disappear when the patient sits or is relieved after a few minutes of rest. In vascular claudication, lower extremity symptoms often decrease or disappear even simply while standing, or walking. On imaging, the clinical diagnosis is confirmed by CT or MRI studies of the lumbar spine. CT diagnostic criteria include <10 mm AP diameter on axial CT.[155] The results of EMG will be abnormal in most patients. EMG is more sensitive than the neurologic examination in these cases. Abnormalities seen on EMG consist of denervation in muscles innervated by lumbosacral nerve roots. EMG findings often are bilateral and in the paraspinal area.[155]

TREATMENT

Treatment is a trial of nonoperative management with NSAIDs, judiciously applied OMT, and physical therapy. Physical therapy focuses on spinal flexion and neutral spine core exercises, glute strengthening, and leg/hip range of motion. OMT and prescribed exercises should limit spinal extension. Treatment of the iliopsoas muscle tension is important as these muscles get overused in the body's attempt to flex the patient forward to open the spinal canal. Long-standing iliopsoas muscle tension flexes the upper lumbar segments reducing the lordosis.

Surgical laminotomy and diskectomy are indicated for progressive disabling pain that has failed nonoperative management, and/or progressive neurologic deficits. However, the best surgical results are achieved when a correlation is established between symptoms and radiographic findings and the decompression appropriately addresses the cause of the symptoms.[155] The SPORT study demonstrated that surgical intervention showed significantly greater improvement in pain and physical function scales from 6 weeks through 4 years. However, the difference between the surgical and nonsurgical groups diminished at 8 years follow-up.[154]

Pregnancy-Related Lower Back Pain

EPIDEMIOLOGY

LBP during pregnancy is a common and important health concern among women worldwide. Low back pain is the most common cause of sick leave after delivery and it may be disabling, limiting everyday activities, impacting productivity, and should not be ignored or left untreated. Low back pain needs to be differentiated from pelvic girdle pain as there are unique aspects to their management.[20] The prevalence of LBP in pregnancy ranges from 24% to 90%, although many authors estimate it to affect 40% to 50% of women.[20,157] The prevalence of LBP in postpartum women increases in the year after delivery. It has been estimated that 67% of women will have low back pain within 12 months of delivery.[157–160]

CAUSES/RISK FACTORS

A history of pelvic trauma, chronic LBP, and low back pain during a previous pregnancy have been suggested as risk factors.[20] However, there is a lack of consensus about the predisposing factors, except for chronic low back pain and LBP in a previous pregnancy which are the most identified risk factors.[161] Severe acute postpartum back pain is also a risk factor for future disability, suggesting that the peripartum period may provide an important opportunity for osteopathic intervention.[162] Early recognition and management may mitigate future disability.[162]

The etiology of low back pain in pregnancy is poorly defined. However mechanical factors, shifting of the body's center of gravity, somatic dysfunction, ligamentous laxity, and weight gain all play a role.[20,163] The association between circulating levels of hormone relaxin and LBP in pregnancy is under debate. Other published risk factors include employment status, parity, baby weight >4 kg, maternal weight, absence of domestic help, and alcohol consumption.[161] Macrosomia has been identified as an independent risk factor for low back pain.[161] Absence of domestic help has been shown to be a modifiable independent risk factor for LBP during pregnancy.[161] Exercise on a regular basis before the pregnancy seems to reduce the risk of suffering from LBP during the pregnancy.

CLINICAL PRESENTATION

Pregnancy-related LBP usually begins between the 20th and the 28th week of gestation, however, it may have an earlier onset. It is most seen in the third trimester due to the rapid growth phase. Most women are affected in their first pregnancy. Low back pain can affect the patient's work, activities, and sleep.

PHYSICAL FINDINGS

Pregnant patients have a characteristic standing and seated posture. This includes an increased lumbar lordosis, external rotation of the hips and legs, decreased arches, and protracted shoulders. It is common to find deep sacral sulci bilaterally and a bilaterally flexed sacrum. These structural changes can cause strain on the pelvic ligaments. The most common tender ligaments seen in the third trimester are the interspinous, iliolumbar, and sacroiliac ligaments. Many pelvic and lumbar muscles develop counterstrain points such as the erector spinae, quadratus lumborum, piriformis, and gluteus medius.

TREATMENT

Conservative management of low back pain is the treatment of choice. This includes exercise, physical therapy, stabilization belts, approved medications, acupuncture, massage, relaxation, and OMT. Since many pain medications are contraindicated in pregnancy, and acetaminophen has limited value in LBP, pain management through other options such as OMT is needed.[163] OMT is efficacious in preventing progressive back-specific dysfunction during the third trimester of pregnancy.[164] The PROMOTE study, a randomized, placebo-controlled trial of 400 women in their third trimester demonstrated that OMT was safe and effective for mitigating pain and functional deterioration compared to the usual care-only group, however, OMT did not differ significantly from placebo ultrasound treatment.[163] Other studies suggest moderate quality evidence that OMT produces clinically relevant benefits for pregnant or postpartum women with LBP. These effects were found to reduce pain and improve functional status in pregnant and postpartum women at 3 months post-treatment.[21,58,165] A recent systematic review was published on the effectiveness of osteopathic care in gynecology and obstetrics.[166] Their findings commented that the osteopathic studies were too heterogeneous to perform quantitative analysis and make clinical recommendations. Nevertheless, they reported that limited evidence suggests that osteopathic care is safe when complementary to traditional gynecologic care.[166] Physical activity including pelvic floor exercises has been shown to be beneficial as a 12-week training program during pregnancy and was effective in the prevention of LBP, at 36 weeks of pregnancy.[167] Education in proper posture, proper lifting techniques and ways to alleviate low back pain provide a rational, evidence-based management plan for pregnant patients.[168,169]

Abdominal Aortic Aneurysm (AAA)

DEFINITION

Abdominal aortic aneurysm (AAA) is an abdominal aortic dilation of 3.0 cm or greater.[170]

EPIDEMIOLOGY

The prevalence of AAA increases with age. It is uncommon in persons younger than 50 years; however, 12.5% of men and 5.2% of women 74 to 84 years of age have AAA.[170] It accounts for approximately 11,000 deaths each year in the United States, with mortality rates from ruptured AAAs reaching up to 90%.[170] The average annual risk of rupture for aneurysms that are 6.0 cm or larger is more than 10%. Between 59% and 83% of patients die before they reach a hospital or have surgery.[171]

CAUSES/RISK FACTORS

Aneurysms develop because of degeneration of the arterial media and elastic tissues.[170] Risk factors are male sex, smoking, age older than 65 years, coronary artery disease, hypertension, first-degree relatives with AAA, history of other vascular aneurysms, previous myocardial infarction, and peripheral arterial disease. Patients with AAA are also at an increased risk of cardiovascular disease and death independent of other factors.[170]

CLINICAL PRESENTATION

AAA is most often clinically silent. When symptoms are present, the classic presentation is characterized by hypotension, shooting abdominal or back pain, and a pulsatile abdominal mass. This triad may be incomplete or absent, and misdiagnosis can occur in up to 60% of cases. Some patients may present with back pain, sciatica, and leg symptoms as well. Therefore, physicians must have a high index of suspicion and be mindful of atypical presentations. Clinicians need to be attentive to new-onset, nonspecific back, or abdominal pain in patients at risk of AAA.[170]

PHYSICAL FINDINGS

Physical examination including abdominal palpation is only moderately sensitive for the detection of AAA. The most common finding is palpation of a pulsatile mass around the level of the umbilicus. The abdominal aorta divides into the common iliac arteries at the level of the umbilicus. Bruits from an AAA are often identified by auscultation near the umbilicus. A bruit from renal artery stenosis can also be auscultated in the midline but more commonly superior and lateral to the umbilicus.

SCREENING/SURVEILLANCE

Screening can improve detection. Ultrasonography has a high sensitivity and specificity (95% and nearly 100%, respectively) for detecting AAA. The US Preventive Services Task Force recommends that men with a history of smoking who are 65 to 75 years of age should undergo one-time AAA screening with ultrasonography (Level B recommendation).[170,171] A history of smoking is defined as at least 100 cigarettes over the individual's lifetime. As aneurysms increase in size, they expand at a greater rate and the risk of rupture increases. Therefore, in persons found to have aneurysms on initial screening, regular surveillance is needed every 6 months to 3 years, depending on aneurysm size.

DIAGNOSIS

Diagnosis of AAA is often made as an incidental finding in imaging studies, such as abdominal ultrasonography or computed tomography. Ultrasound has a sensitivity of 68% and specificity

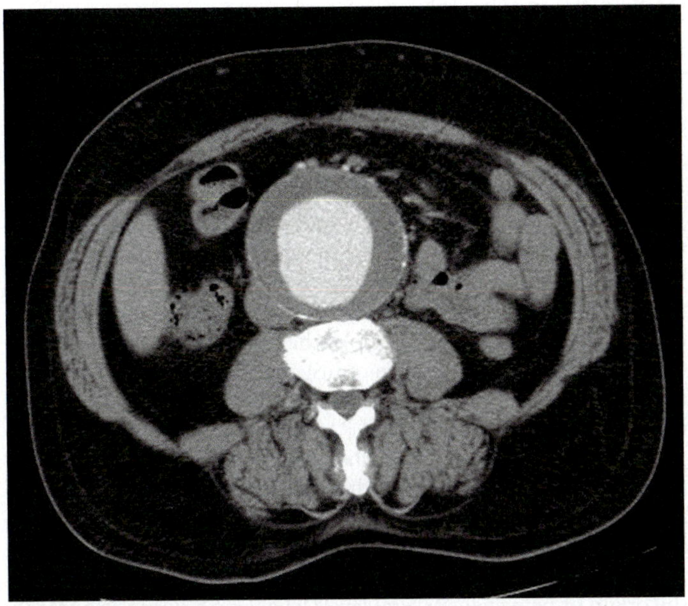

Figure 93.18. Image of AAA. (Case courtesy of The Radswiki, Radiopaedia.org, rID: 11151.)

of 75%.[170] AAA may occasionally be visible on plain radiography if the aneurysm wall is calcified.[170] Abdominal ultrasonography is the preferred modality to screen for AAA because of its cost-effectiveness and lack of exposure to ionizing radiation (see Fig. 93.18). The "classic triad," including hypotension, back pain, and a pulsatile abdominal mass is present in only 50% of those people with ruptured AAAs.[172] One study found that 91% of cases of AAA were accompanied by low back pain, hence its importance of including it as a differential diagnosis.[172]

TREATMENT

A dissecting abdominal aneurysm is a surgical emergency; surgical consultation should be immediately obtained.

NONSURGICAL

Controlling hypertension and smoking cessation are cornerstones of nonsurgical treatment. Smoking causes an incrementally increased growth rate of aneurysms up to 0.4 mm per year.[170] Regarding pharmacologic therapy, statins, antihypertensives, and antibiotics have been studied. Beta-blockers are known to improve perioperative mortality for AAA repair; however, randomized trial results indicate that their effects on AAA enlargement are not significant.[170] Other antihypertensives (e.g., angiotensin-converting enzyme inhibitors) also do not appear to be effective.[170] Statin use is commonly used in nonsurgical management, yet the evidence for reducing AAA growth or rupture has been poor, and better-quality studies do not indicate a direct benefit.[170] Statins do help with cardiovascular risk reduction and do improve all-cause mortality in patients after AAA repair.[170] Roxithromycin (a macrolide antibiotic not available in the United States) and doxycycline have weak evidence for inhibiting AAA growth, due to possible secondary infection in the aortic wall, likely from *Chlamydophila pneumoniae*.[170]

SURGICAL MANAGEMENT

Surgical management, which includes open and endovascular aneurysm repair, is indicated when the aneurysm diameter is 5.5 cm or larger in men and 5.0 cm or larger in women. Surgery is also recommended when it expands by more than 1 cm per year (another risk factor for rupture) or becomes tender or symptomatic.[170] Open and endovascular repair are the two main approaches. Multiple studies have shown that there is no significant difference between the two approaches in terms of overall long-term mortality, yet endovascular repair has a lower 30-day mortality.[170] Many patients (approximately 50%) with ruptured AAAs do not reach the hospital, and those who do survive have a mortality rate as high as 50%.[170] For aneurysms smaller than 5.5 cm, studies suggest that the risks of operative management do not exceed mortality benefits, and that survival is not improved by elective surgery.[170]

Cauda Equina Syndrome (CES)

DESCRIPTION

CES is a rare condition more commonly seen in males that is caused by severe compression of the cauda equina in the thecal sac of the lumbar spine. The proximal aspects of the cauda equina are composed of the L3, L4, L5, and S1 roots. Dysfunction of these roots mainly affects the legs primarily and does not result in what is known as "cauda equina syndrome" which is historically used to describe the results of dysfunction of the nerve roots below S1, namely S2, S3, S4, and S5.[173] To develop CES, compression must occur resulting in lower extremity sensory and motor loss, bowel and bladder dysfunction and perianal anesthesia.[174] There are inconsistencies in the definition, subclassification, and clinical presentation of CES.[173] A comprehensive review of the literature in 2009 proposed the following single definition of CES. For a diagnosis of CES, one or more of the following must be present: (1) bladder and/or bowel dysfunction, (2) reduced sensation in the saddle area, and (3) sexual dysfunction, with possible neurologic deficit in the lower limb (motor/sensory loss, reflex change).[175] The most recent definition (2022) for the condition states:

CES is a clinical diagnosis resulting from dysfunction of one or more of the sacral nerve roots S2 and below. One or more of the following symptoms or signs must be present[173]:

- Bladder and/or bowel dysfunction
- Reduced sensation in the saddle area
- Sexual dysfunction

Back and leg pain, and lower limb motor or sensory changes are often present but are not essential to the diagnosis.

EPIDEMIOLOGY

The incidence of CES is variable, depending on the etiology of the syndrome. Males and females are equally affected. CES is reported as a complication in 0.2% to 1.2% of all lumbar spine operations. These numbers overall correlate with approximately 1% to 3% of every patient who develops an acute lumbar disk herniation and approximately 5 cases per 1,000 surgeries.[174] It is important to note that while acute CES most commonly presents within the first 24 hours after spinal surgery, there have been documented cases occurring as late as 7 days postoperatively.[174]

CAUSES/RISK FACTORS

It is most commonly due to an acute lumbar disk herniation, spinal tumor, epidural abscess, or hematoma.

CLINICAL PRESENTATION

CES symptoms may have sudden onset and evolve rapidly, although sometimes they can be delayed. Each type of CES has different typical signs and symptoms. Low back pain may be the most significant symptom, accompanied by sciatica, lower extremities weakness, saddle or perineal hypoesthesia, sexual impotence, and sphincter dysfunction.[176] If asked, the patient will usually have a history of bladder and/or anal sphincter weakness, because the sphincter is often involved early. Paralysis may develop slowly or occur very rapidly (progressing to complete paralysis of the lower extremities within an hour).

PHYSICAL FINDINGS

Physical findings include significant distress due to low back pain, leg pain, and weakness, and the following signs: urinary retention, diminished or loss of bulbocavernosus reflex, poor rectal tone, saddle anesthesia, and decreased pinprick in the S2–S4 dermatomes.[176] A digital rectal exam is an important part of evaluating the patient with low back pain, especially if these symptoms are present. There will be a diminished or absent bulbocavernosus reflex and a decreased anal wink test.[176]

DIAGNOSIS

Early diagnosis is critical. The diagnosis is made clinically by characteristic symptoms and physical findings. An urgent MRI is performed to confirm the cause.

TREATMENT

Treatment is prompt surgical decompression that should preferably be performed within 24 hours, absolutely within 48 hours. Delays in diagnosis and management can lead to loss of bowel, bladder, or sexual function, and leg weakness. Therefore, immediate surgical consultation and timely emergency surgical decompression of the nerves are mandatory. Although surgery can completely decompress the nerves, if surgery is delayed too long, motor function of the lower extremities and/or sphincters may never return. Motor recovery may occur up to 1 year postop and bladder recovery up to 16 months postop.[176] Regarding the long-term outcomes of CES after decompression, recent literature supporting surgery within 48 hours of the onset of symptoms appears to result in fewer patients with persistent bladder dysfunction.[177] Randomized controlled trials are required to conclusively determine whether early decompression leads to better outcomes.

Failed Back Surgery Syndrome (FBSS)/Chronic Pain After Spinal Surgery (CPSS)/Persistent Spinal Pain Syndrome (PSPS)

DEFINITION

FBSS is an unfortunate occurrence in patients undergoing lumbar spinal decompression laminectomies and fusions for disk herniations, spinal stenosis, spondylolisthesis, and other orthopedic causes. The term FBSS has been fraught with difficulties in orthopedic literature and multiple different studies present changes to the current name. The International Association for the Study of Pain defines FBSS as: *Lumbar spinal pain of unknown origin either persisting despite surgical intervention or appearing after surgical intervention for spinal pain originally in the same topographical location.*[178] The same organization recommended the term chronic pain after spinal surgery (CPSS), as a replacement term and the ICD-11 was being compiled. This term was accepted by the World Health Organization (WHO).[179] Recent recommendations from an international group of experts have proposed the term PSPS emerged as the preferred option of our international group of experts.[179]

EPIDEMIOLOGY

The incidence of lumbar spinal surgery has been markedly increasing from 1998 to the present. It is difficult to assess the prevalence of this condition. However, reviews of the literature state that FBSS is reported to affect approximately 20.6% of patients and probably more.[180] Epidemiology is difficult to determine because of the heterogeneity of the definition, and multiple etiologies.[178] The economic cost is considerable and likely to rise.[179]

CAUSES/RISK FACTORS

There are multiple risk factors leading to FBSS. These risks can be considered as preoperative, intraoperative, and postoperative in nature. The preoperative risks that are associated with this condition include inaccurate diagnosis, poor selection of surgical candidates, anxiety, depression, or other psychiatric comorbidities, obesity, smoking, the presence of litigation or worker's compensation claims, and physical or radiologic findings such as stenosis, fibrosis, and disk herniation.[181–183] Patients who have significant psychosocial factors have been shown to have the strongest association with the development of this condition.[184] Another common risk factor leading to FBSS is undiagnosed lateral recess or foraminal stenosis of the lumbar spine. Intraoperative risk factors include surgery at the wrong spinal level, operating at a single level while the origin of pain spans several levels, choosing a surgical approach that is incorrect for the pathology present, surgical revision in a patient who has had multiple prior lumbar spine surgeries.[185,186] Postoperative risk factors can include patients not following postoperative activity limitations and instructions until complete healing. Many patients are noncompliant with having an evaluation for anxiety, depression, and other psychiatric conditions and need to be encouraged to do this, due to their high comorbidity with FBSS.[178] Smokers had a more regular use of analgesics, worsened walking ability, and inferior overall quality of life 2 years after surgery compared with nonsmokers.[178] Following surgery, some patients will go on to develop epidural fibrosis, increased spinal instability, and redistribution of load to adjacent disk tissue, a phenomenon known as "transition syndrome."[185]

CLINICAL PRESENTATION

Patients who have FBSS present to the clinic with a long history of chronic back pain, and have failed conservative measures, injections, and surgical stabilization. They continue to have persistent lower back pain, pain and sensory disturbances in the legs, and sometimes chronic dysfunction of the bowel and bladder. Many patients are frustrated, discouraged, and have had significant financial and psychosocial impacts on their personal and professional lives. Many of the patients have tried a wide variety of medications and physical treatments without much help, and the quality of their lives is negatively affected.[179]

PHYSICAL FINDINGS

Patients with FBSS need to have a complete history and physical examination. On physical examination, a complete neurologic examination, structural examination, abdominal examination, genitourinary exam, and vascular exam of the legs are all important. Patients who have lumbar spinal stenosis will have a worsening of their pain with spinal extension as this narrows the spinal canal. Pain from recurrent disk herniation will occur with forward bending and leaning to one side such as putting on their shoes. Focal neurologic deficits, such as a positive SLR sign defects in sensation, or muscle weakness require further testing. Some patients may have a psychogenic cause of their lower back pain. Some patients may also have work-related issues and if the clinician has a suspicion of secondary gain/malingering, they may perform Waddell signs.[178]

From an osteopathic perspective, there is a cluster of somatic findings that often underlie the complaints of patients who have

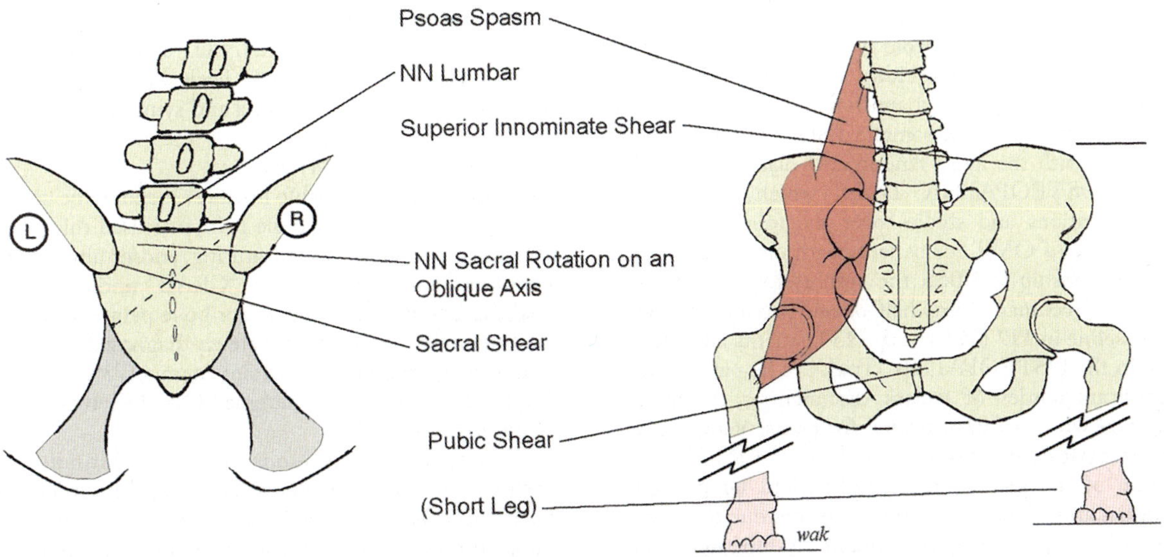

Figure 93.19. The "dirty half-dozen" somatic dysfunctions found commonly in patients seen for persistent low back pain following lumbar spinal surgery. See text for explanation. (Illustration courtesy of William A. Kuchera, DO, FAAO, with permission.)

been diagnosed with "failed low back syndrome" (see Fig. 93.19). Greenman evaluated 183 consecutive patients who had persistent and chronic low back pain after lumbar surgery and found six main types of somatic dysfunction, which he called the "dirty half-dozen."[187] Each patient had between 3 and 6 of these findings. Treatment of these conditions led to significant improvement in about 75% of the patients. The six dysfunctions he found in descending order of prevalence were as follows:

1. Muscular imbalance of the trunk and lower extremity (including psoas syndrome)
2. Non-neutral (type II) lumbar somatic dysfunction
3. Dysfunction of the symphysis pubis (pubic shear)
4. A short leg and pelvic tilt syndrome/sacral base unlevel
5. Restricted flexion (nutation) of the sacral base. This could be either a posterior sacral base or a posterior backward sacral torsion
6. Innominate shear dysfunction

Many patients with the so-called "failed low back syndrome" are also found to have a unilateral sacral flexion (sacral shear). Innominate shears or sacral shears may be asymptomatic at their site, but eventually result in secondary subjective symptoms in the patient's lumbar, upper rib, cervical, suboccipital, or cranial regions. These are regions of increased stress brought about by the body's attempt to compensate for the persistent dysfunction and the pelvic base. Because shears are nonphysiologic, the body is often unable to remove them without outside specific treatment; so, the body tries to compensate for their presence. An ilium upslip (pelvic shear) may even prevent successful manipulative treatment of other somatic dysfunctions. The presence of a shear is also associated with the continuance or return of symptoms shortly after another diagnosed somatic dysfunction has been successfully treated and removed. It is important for the clinician to realize and understand the surgery that took place. If the lumbar spine is fused to the sacrum, this will drastically alter sacroiliac mechanics, and lead to more frequent dysfunction of the pubis and innominate, especially shears. Fusion of the lumbar spine to the sacrum as well as fusion of multiple lumbar spinal segments may lead to chronic SIJ dysfunction and arthritis.[188,189]

DIAGNOSIS/ASSOCIATED CONDITIONS

The diagnosis of FBSS is a clinical one that includes a thorough history and physical examination, diagnostic imaging, and sometimes diagnostic procedures. The patient will have intractable pain and neurosensory symptoms in the lower back, pelvis, and legs following a lumbar decompression/stabilization procedure. The clinician must determine if following the surgical procedure the patient developed an exacerbation of their prior symptoms, developed new symptoms, or both. It is also important to note what symptoms improved from the procedure. This will guide further workup. The diagnosis of FBSS also needs to include the diagnosis of complications/associated conditions from the procedure. The most important complication is to make sure the patient does not have changes to their bowel, bladder, or sexual function indicating CES. Plain lumbar spine x-rays, typically a seven-view series that includes flexion and extension radiographs, are important to determine if the patient has adjacent segment degeneration, spondylolisthesis, compression fracture, spondylolysis, and a stable fusion. It is common to find a loss of lumbar lordosis in these patients, possibly from chronic psoas involvement.[178] To determine recurrent disk herniation, epidural fibrosis, hematoma, abscess, tumor, and occult fractures, CT/myelogram and/or MRI are needed.[178] MRI with and without gadolinium contrast continues to be the gold standard imaging modality for FBSS.[178] However, if the patient has significant artifacts from the metallic implants, a CT myelogram may be preferred. Pain management may be able to perform diagnostic nerve blocks and possible transforaminal epidural steroid injections in these patients. ESR and CRP may be used to evaluate for possible infection, especially in patients with constitutional symptoms or a predisposition toward infection.[190]

TREATMENT

Treatment of the patient with failed back surgical syndrome requires an interprofessional team approach, with cooperation and engagement by the patient, and experienced physicians, therapists and other health care team members.[183] The goal is to improve the patient's day-to-day functional status, decrease pain, and improve quality of life. Initially, it will involve conservative management with physical therapy, active exercise, and OMT for the associated somatic dysfunction. Medication management should be directed at specific symptom control as the evidence is weak for a beneficial effect in this population. Chronic opioid therapy for noncancer pain is associated with an increased morbidity and mortality and does not reliably improve long-term pain and function scores.[191] OMT can be beneficial for the associated somatic dysfunction in this population. Beginning with the large, randomized placebo-controlled clinical trial, the OSTEOPATHIC Trial,[192] which was followed by multiple publications and studies over the following several years on the efficacy of OMT for patients with chronic low back pain.[193–195] In relationship to FBSS, the authors found that psoas syndrome, one of Greenman's "dirty half-dozen" (see Fig. 93.19) to be present at baseline in 117 (51%) of the 230 patients allocated to receive OMT in the OSTEOPATHIC Trial.[194] The patients with the most significant burden of somatic dysfunctions, the highest baseline pain, and who also were treated for psoas syndrome had the best and most lasting response (least relapse) to OMT.[193–195]

Dysfunction of the sacrum, ilium, pubes, and lumbar spine commonly coexist and affect one another, however, due to the centralization of pain in these subjects, somatic dysfunction distant from the sacrum and pelvis may be critical to improving this clinical condition. Physical therapy is the cornerstone of first-line management of FBSS. Physical therapy can help the patient optimize gait and posture and can improve muscle strength and physical function.[196,197] Other conservative measures that may help postoperative back pain involve psychotherapy measures including stress reduction and cognitive behavioral therapy.[198] Finally, noninvasive procedures including acupuncture and scrambler therapy can be used to minimize the pain associated with FBSS.[199–201] Mindfulness-based stress reduction and cognitive-based therapies may also be effective adjuncts.[198] Reoperation generally correlates with inferior outcomes and higher morbidity compared to implantable technologies such as SCS. However, the presence of certain symptoms, such as bowel/bladder impairment, motor weakness, or neural deficit warrants immediate surgical intervention. Interprofessional pain clinics are the gold standard in the setting of treatment for patients with complex chronic pain syndromes such as FBSS.

Multiple Myeloma

DEFINITION

Multiple myeloma is a clonal plasma cell proliferative disorder characterized by the abnormal increase of monoclonal proteins leading to bony lytic lesions and end-organ damage.

EPIDEMIOLOGY

Myeloma occurs predominantly in the geriatric population with a median age at diagnosis of about 70 years and is slightly more commonly seen in males than females (1.4:1).[202] There seems to be an increased incidence in African American and Black populations by as much as twofold compared to Whites.[202]

CAUSES/RISK FACTORS

The exact etiology of multiple myeloma is unknown, yet it is derived from a premalignant, asymptomatic monoclonal gammopathy of undetermined significance (MGUS). There is a relationship between myeloma and promoter genes and other oncogenes. However, frequent alterations and translocations in the promoter genes, especially chromosome 14, are commonly found in multiple myeloma and likely play a role in disease development.[203] In addition, other oncogenes such as neuroblastoma RAS viral oncogene homolog (NRAS), Kirsten rat sarcoma viral oncogene homolog (KRAS), and V-raf murine sarcoma viral oncogene homolog B1 (BRAF) may participate in plasma cell proliferation.[204] Myeloma bone disease is thought to result from overexpression of RANKL by bone marrow stroma. RANKL activates osteoclasts, which resorb bone. Bone breakdown leads to calcium release into the blood, leading to hypercalcemia and symptoms of kidney failure.

CLINICAL PRESENTATION

The presentation is variable however it should be considered in an older adult with back or bone pain, increased thirst and urination, abdominal pain, nausea or vomiting, and/or altered mental status. Symptoms and signs include "CRAB" findings (hypercalcemia, renal dysfunction, anemia, and/or bone pain with lytic lesions). In one study, it was found that in newly diagnosed MM, the following symptoms were seen most often: anemia (73%), bone pain (58%), elevated creatinine (48%), fatigue (32%), hypercalcemia (28%), and weight loss (24%).[205]

Common manifestations and complications of multiple myeloma can include hypercalcemia, renal insufficiency, infection, skeletal lesions, and anemia. Less common complications include venous thromboembolism and hyperviscosity syndrome.[206]

PHYSICAL FINDINGS

On structural examination, patients may present with an increased kyphosis, a loss of height, and bony pain on palpation or percussion. They may have an abnormal neurologic exam, including findings of peripheral neuropathy and/or carpal tunnel syndrome. They may be pale from anemia or have bleeding/bruising of the skin. Bone pain resulting from osteolytic lesions can result in pathologic fractures and vertebral collapse, spinal cord compression, and radicular pain.

DIAGNOSIS

There are several approaches to screening and diagnosis. The presence of any CRAB criteria (hypercalcemia, renal dysfunction, anemia, and/or bone pain with lytic lesions) or any of these additional criteria justifies diagnosis and therapy. The set of diagnostic criteria below is often referred to as SLiM CRAB.[207]

- Renal insufficiency (creatinine greater than 2 mg/dL [greater than 177 micromol/L] or creatinine clearance less than 40 mL per minute)
- Anemia (Hgb less than 10 g/dL or Hgb greater than 2 g/dL below the lower limit of normal)

A skeletal survey (a series of radiographs, performed systematically to cover the entire skeleton) is useful for making the diagnosis of multiple myeloma and also in determining complications (e.g., pathologic fracture). Lytic lesions don't appear until there is substantial bone destruction, thus giving the skeletal survey a high false-negative rate. Whole-body low-dose CT is more accurate than a skeletal survey. MRI is more sensitive in detecting multiple lesions compared to the standard plain film skeletal survey and CT.

One or more osteolytic bone lesions on skeletal radiography, CT, or PET-CT are often described as punched-out, round, radiolucent lesions, with the characteristic "raindrop skull," and endosteal scalloping of the long bones (see Fig. 93.20).

The NCCN guidelines recommend more comprehensive studies including a whole-body PET/CT scan and cytogenetics.[207]

There are several staging systems for multiple myeloma. The two main systems used today are the Durie–Salmon Staging System and the Revised International Staging System (R-ISS).[207]

TREATMENT

Treatment for multiple myeloma is multifactorial and based on clinical presentation, diagnostic studies, imaging, pathology,

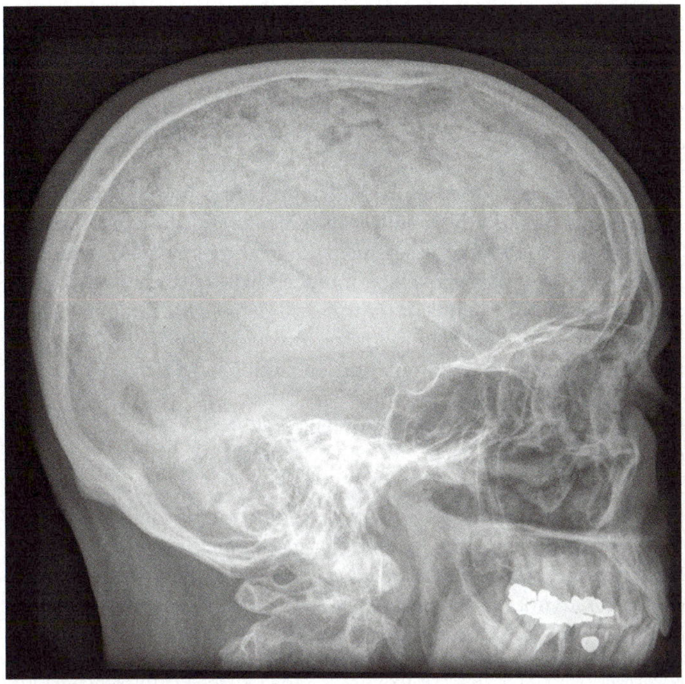

Figure 93.20. Multiple myeloma. (Case courtesy of Frank Gaillard, Radiopaedia.org, rID: 7682.)

comorbidities, and associated symptoms. First, it is important to determine any acute issues that must be stabilized immediately. Once stabilized, the patient's treatment plan is driven by risk stratification and transplant eligibility.[207]

A patient's disease can fall into one of two categories: high or standard-risk MM based on cytogenetics. Patients then are determined to be fit or unfit for autologous stem cell transplant (ASCT). There are treatment algorithms for each of the categories.[208] In addition to hematology/oncology, nephrologists may be required to aid in the management of any new or worsening renal dysfunction. neurosurgery, radiation oncology, or orthopedic surgery consults may be necessary to address any symptomatic bony lesions. Judicious osteopathic manipulative treatment for the associated somatic dysfunction can be performed, however the clinician needs to utilize indirect approaches. The prognosis for multiple myeloma is quite variable, and many factors can affect outcomes. However, perhaps the two main considerations for prognosis would be stage and disease biology.[209] Patient education, a multidisciplinary team, and early diagnosis are crucial in the management of multiple myeloma. The disease itself is complex, and outcomes can be improved if early and appropriate intervention is undertaken.

DEVELOPING A TREATMENT PLAN FOR THE PATIENT WITH LBP

There may be multiple diagnoses, for multiple regions both the acute and chronic pain patient, each having a management plan. It is important to consider the patient as a whole person, and not segmented pieces to rehabilitate. Therefore, the osteopathic management plan should include the patient's overall health, social and cultural factors, diet and exercise, and management of comorbidities.

Developing a management plan for each of the diagnosed medical conditions or suspected diagnoses is important. It is also important to share a written document highlighting your discussion with the patient at the end of the visit which reviews the management recommendations.

As the person ages, and/or with trauma or surgery, lumbar spine mechanics can be altered by anatomical changes in the vertebra or disks and further complicate lumbar biomechanics and reduce the ability of the lumbar spine to compensate for short leg and/or psoas syndromes. Thus, it is imperative to assess above and below the lumbosacral region when a patient complains of low back pain to identify these types of problems and address them appropriately as part of the management plan.

IMMEDIACY

The clinician during the visit needs to determine if there is an emergent, or urgent medical condition that needs to be addressed immediately. If no life-threatening condition exists, is there an urgent medical condition that needs to be addressed, and in what time frame, and by whom? Once these considerations are dealt with the clinician can then start to develop a management plan including a timeline and appropriate follow-up visits.

GOALS AND EXPECTATIONS

It is important that the clinician and the patient discuss and align their goals and expectations for the diagnosis and the management of the patient's condition. Goals can include the tenets of osteopathic medicine such as restoring wellness, fostered by self-regulation, self-healing, and healthy behaviors. The goals can be directed at somatic dysfunction such as to restore postural and mechanical alignment, manage fascial strain, improve tissue texture changes, and encourage the patients innate ability to heal. Goals can be directed toward pain management by decreasing their use of NSAIDs and to find healthy alternatives to decrease their pain. Goals can be functional as well, such as postoperatively to be able to stand for 5 minutes without pain and wash the dishes for 5 to 10 minutes.

GENERAL OSTEOPATHIC TREATMENT RECOMMENDATIONS

When considering treatment strategies for the patient, first consider how the patient working with the provided medical recommendations can restore wellness, that is fostered by self-regulation, self-healing, and health maintenance. This includes their ability to recover from surgery or successfully live with chronic low back pain. The osteopathic approach is to foster a strong doctor–patient relationship, implement the philosophic principles, include OMT to manage somatic dysfunction, and encourage the patient's innate ability to heal. The goal is to assist the patient's internal healing and foster their own homeostatic response.

If the patient is considering conservative or surgical options to manage their lower back pain, it is important that the objective is to remove the causes and influences of the pain, while working within predetermined goals between the physician and the patient. It is important to have aligned goals and expectations to achieve success. It is also important to consider the timeline for healing and utilize a multidisciplinary approach in addressing the patient's body, mind, and spirit. The five models of osteopathic medicine can be used as a framework to help clinicians develop treatment plans that include the biomechanical, neurological, metabolic, respiratory–circulatory, and behavioral aspects (see Chapter 26 The Five Models of Osteopathic Patient Care).

CLINICAL APPLICATION OF THE FIVE MODELS

Clinicians can consider the five osteopathic models in developing a treatment plan. Consider an older diabetic patient with COPD who recently lost her husband. Her past surgical history is significant for a right hip replacement 1 year ago. She is seeing you for mechanical lower back pain after working in the garden.

From a biomechanical standpoint, you address her gait and station and asymmetry of any landmarks on structural examination. From a neurologic standpoint, you perform an accurate neurologic examination of her lower extremities and treat segmental somatic dysfunction that can affect the autonomics in the lumbar and sacral regions. From a metabolic model, you discuss how a diet lower in carbohydrates, and higher in fruits and vegetables can affect her insulin levels, decrease systemic inflammation, as well as protect her kidneys. From a respiratory–circulatory model, you encourage her to exercise 30 minutes a day that can improve her Hgb A1c, preserve her pulmonary function, and strengthen her low back by activating her core muscles. Finally, from a behavioral model, you discuss social support systems with her and how joining community group activities with her park district for her church may help her cope with the loss of her husband and her current medical concerns.

It is important to discuss the patient's emotional health and support system because both conservative care and surgical management can have implications on the patient's ADLs, sleep, family life, community life, and occupation. Treatment of somatic dysfunction supports the body's self-healing mechanisms during recovery from a primary medical or surgical condition. OMT may be indicated prior to surgery and/or following surgery. For the postoperative patient with somatic dysfunction, manipulation is also indicated and makes the patient more comfortable and normalizes local biophysiologic responses.

CONSERVATIVE CARE

The physician should expect that effective conservative treatment of a patient will be accompanied by progressive reduction of subjective and objective signs and symptoms and will be associated with obvious improvement in the patient. The key to good results with conservative treatment is to provide specific forms of acceptable treatment that are indicated by the pathophysiology and functional status of the patient, to monitor progress, to expect steady improvement, and to modify diagnostic procedures and treatment and/or get a consultation as it becomes clinically indicated. Conservative care includes evaluating and reducing modifiable contributing factors. This may include specific treatment of postural imbalance and somatic dysfunction, adequate relief of pain, treatment of contributing medical issues, and reduction of any other mechanical, structural, or psychological stresses. The general approach for nonspecific mechanical lower back pain includes 6 to 8 weeks including patient education, pain management, osteopathic manipulative treatment, physical therapy, medications, and stress management strategies. Conservative care may be carried on longer than 6 to 8 weeks, however low back pain that persists past this has a higher incidence of going on to chronic lower back pain. There are osteopathic published recommendations based on the medical evidence for the conservative management of low back pain.[20]

The increasing use of MRI, opioid prescriptions, epidural steroid injections, and spinal surgery has not improved outcomes or disability rates in patients with chronic LBP.[47] Studies also have demonstrated that osteopathic physicians who practice a holistic approach to medical care offer a lower risk of progression from chronic low back pain to chronic widespread pain, lower widespread pain severity, and lesser deficits in their health-related quality of life score.[210]

OMT

OMT is a distinctive modality commonly used by osteopathic physicians to complement conventional management of musculoskeletal disorders, including those that cause LBP. Osteopathic manipulative treatment is defined in the Glossary of Osteopathic Terminology as *"The therapeutic application of manually guided forces by an osteopathic physician (U.S. Usage) to improve physiologic function and/or support homeostasis that has been altered by somatic dysfunction."*[37] To offer OMT as a treatment for low back pain, it is necessary to establish a diagnosis of somatic dysfunction. Addressing somatic dysfunction in patients with low back pain is done in the context of assessing and treating the whole patient. Most patients with low back pain indeed have somatic dysfunction amenable to OMT. Current national guidelines for nonpharmacologic and nonsurgical treatment for low back pain include manual therapies and spinal manipulation, including OMT.[20,54,57]

INDICATIONS AND CONTRAINDICATIONS OF PERFORMING OMT

Indications for performing OMT include an accurate diagnosis of somatic dysfunction. Somatic dysfunction is defined in the Glossary of Osteopathic Terminology as *"Impaired or altered function of related components of the somatic (body framework) system: skeletal, arthrodial and myofascial structures, and their related vascular, lymphatic, and neural elements. Somatic dysfunction is treatable using osteopathic manipulative treatment."*[37] The diagnostic criteria for the presence of somatic dysfunction include the presence of tissue texture changes, positional asymmetry, restriction of motion, and local tenderness. The clinician must decide from the history, physical, and their clinical experience if the somatic dysfunction present is related to the low back pain and if treatment of that may potentially improve the patient's condition. Contraindications for OMT in low back pain may be relative or absolute. These recommendations are generally based on expert opinion as research is lacking. Absolute contraindications for OMT are centered more around direct action techniques such as HVLA. These would include acute fracture, an unstable patient, ruptured aortic aneurysm, bony metastasis, acute spinal osteomyelitis, and CES. Relative contraindications would include acute herniated nucleus pulposus with active radiculopathy, spondylolisthesis, and spinal stenosis with neurogenic claudication.

GOALS AND EXPECTATIONS

It is important for the clinician to establish an objective for the osteopathic manipulative treatment. It is also important to provide the patient with information and options other than OMT to help facilitate their healing. The patient's goals and expectations of the treatments should also be discussed. Patients with chronic somatic dysfunction will need long-term treatment and OMT is typically combined with physical therapy and other modalities.

REGIONS

Patients with lower back pain may have significant somatic dysfunction in any body region contributing to their presentation and pain. It is the art of osteopathic medicine to determine which areas of somatic dysfunction have the area of greatest restriction (AGR) and/or physiologic effect. This is different for each patient and is based on the unique physiology and comorbid conditions. In general, the lumbar spine sacrum and pelvis work together as a functional unit, especially during gait and station. Treating somatic dysfunction in one of those areas affects the other. However, due to the diffuse interrelated nature of the fascia, restrictions anywhere can create dysfunction and pain in the lower back region. In addition, visceral causes, emotional stress and tension, and repetitive body postures all play a role in creating symptomatic somatic dysfunction.

TECHNIQUE SELECTION

When considering which technique to use, consider what the patient responded to in the past. For new patients, consider starting off with an indirect technique to gauge the patient's response. The technique is also determined by the type of somatic dysfunction present. If articular barrier mechanics are present, then techniques that address these components may be indicated. If myofascial restrictions with positional asymmetry are present perhaps myofascial techniques may be most beneficial. Moderate-quality evidence suggests that MFR is more effective than control treatments in pain reduction and there is very low-quality evidence that MFR is more effective than control interventions in functional improvements.[211] However, an OMT protocol that included abdominal diaphragm techniques, which are primarily myofascial, produced significant and clinically relevant improvements in pain and disability in patients with nonspecific low back pain as compared to the same OMT protocol using sham diaphragm techniques.[212]

If muscle and joint dysfunction with associated pain and tender points predominate, counterstrain may be the best approach. In patients who are anxious and have diffuse problems with myofascial pain and tension, cranial osteopathy may be wise to address initially so that techniques may work better in the periphery.

Technique selection is also determined despite the setting the clinician is working in. There are different techniques and approaches for a hospitalized bedridden patient than an ambulatory healthy outpatient. This is also the case when working in the emergency room, or labor and delivery. The technique must be able to be applied accurately, safely and effectively within the current setting.

Technique selection is determined by this skill and the ability of the clinician. Every clinician has their favorite techniques that they excel at, and others that they do not use routinely. So, it is important for the clinician to choose the appropriate technique for the somatic dysfunction based on the patient, location, and their skill set.

DOSAGE, FREQUENCY, AND DURATION

Patients with chronic disease and the chronic dysfunction associated with it require chronic treatment. This may be performed perhaps one time per month in the outpatient setting, or one time per day in the inpatient setting. If OMT is to be performed more frequently such as once or twice per day in the hospital setting the duration, and dosage is decreased. If an outpatient patient is being seen for an acute condition, it is preferable to follow up within 2 to 3 days. Again, with an acute condition there may be an acute inflammatory response and initial dosage of OMT may be decreased. As the condition resolves the treatment frequency progressively lengthens.

PATIENT AND PHYSICIAN POSITION

The patient and physician position utilized to apply OMT is dependent on multiple variables. This includes the age, height, size, strength of the physician and patient, type of table and setting, and type of technique being executed. It is valuable for a physician to utilize a power table, adjustable stool, and folded towels, or pillows to position the patient in a comfortable manner (see Fig. 93.21). When applying OMT, it is important that both the physician and patient are protected from injury. Some patients have orthopedic conditions, joint replacements, implanted medical devices, spinal rods, etc. that limit the position that is comfortable for them to be treated in. It is also important to maintain the patient's modesty and keep them draped during various procedures.

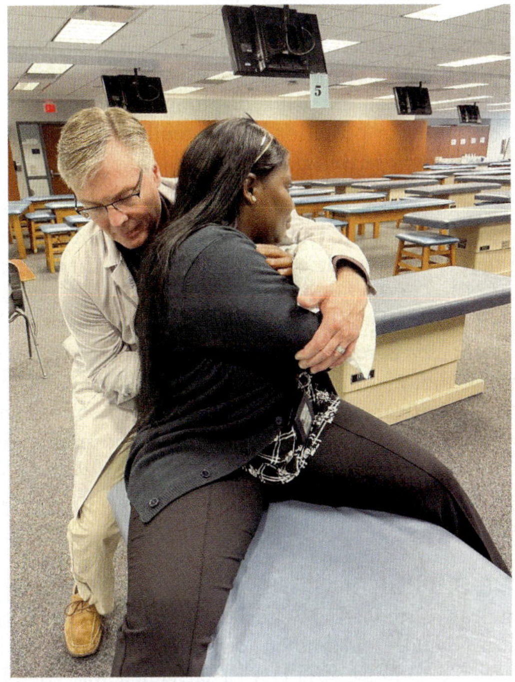

Figure 93.21. Patient comfort. Utilization of the end of the table with patient comfortably seated with arms crossed allowing for physician to maintain localization of applied forces.

SEQUENCING OMT

The sequence of treatment is important; however, it may vary from patient to patient. It is generally accepted (and taught) to treat the lumbar spine, psoas, ilium, and pubes prior to treating the sacrum. However, there is some controversy about this. Starting with the area of greatest restriction (AGR) is appropriate if it was not acutely injured. Since the sacrum and SIJs respond to forces directed from above (due to gravity) and from those coming from below (ground reactive force), leaving it to last in the treatment scheme seems logical.

The muscle energy model bases SI dysfunction on the motion cycle of walking. Dysfunction of the pubes significantly affects this motion cycle, and therefore the sacral–pelvic motion. Because of this, the muscle energy model stresses the importance of treating the pubes first. The muscle energy approach does not consider pelvic side shift. The muscle energy diagnostic approach also does not include tissue texture abnormality. The remainder of the muscle energy model is to treat the pelvis, then the lumbar spine, before the sacrum.

The Chicago Model, as proposed by Kappler insists that the lumbar spine dysfunction and psoas muscle must be treated first, then the pubes and ilium prior to the sacrum.[41] There are several different techniques that can be used for dysfunction of the psoas. Frequently the thoracolumbar area must be treated or included in the process.

The Still technique approach is also very specific that the pelvis and lumbar area must be treated first. If they are treated appropriately, then the Still model of oblique sacrum dysfunction (R, L) and unilateral sacral dysfunction (R, L) is all that remains. (The Still technique model treats innominate upslip as a unique entity.)

Specific technique procedures are beyond the scope of this chapter; however, listed below are goals to accomplish when treating the sacrum and pelvis.

Goals of treatment include the following:

- Treat segmental upper lumbar dysfunctions
- Improve hip extension (iliopsoas tension)
- Improve asymmetry/alignment of the ilia

- Treat any pubic dysfunction
- Level the sacral base
- Improve cranial motion
- Improve abdominal and pelvic diaphragm motion
- Resolve anterior or posterior lumbar tender points
- Obtain a negative seated flexion test

OMT is not just the application of a technique. During treatment, the experienced physician will constantly reassess the "change" that is being made in the tissues and adjust the treatment accordingly. One of the more difficult things to master for students of osteopathy is being able to tell if they made a "change" or not. Another difficulty is regarding dosage and when to say: "enough treatment for today."

OMT is a critical element in returning a patient to health and wellness; however, it is only one aspect of the overall care of the patient. In treating lumbar, sacral, and pelvic problems, corrective exercises for weak inhibited muscles and stretches for tight muscles can be beneficial.

EVIDENCE SUPPORTING THE USE OF OMT FOR LBP

The American Osteopathic Association developed and issued its first clinical practice guideline on low back pain in 2010. This was followed by the OSTEOPATHIC Trial which was completed by the Osteopathic Research Center in 2011. The study assessed the efficacy of osteopathic manipulative treatment in 455 patients with chronic low back pain. Over a dozen publications have reported on the OSTEOPATHIC Trial, including the most recent studies on substantial improvement and recovery from chronic low back pain with osteopathic manipulative treatment.[193–195] A systematic review and meta-analysis were published in 2014 that demonstrated clinically relevant effects of OMT for reducing pain and improving functional status in patients with acute and chronic nonspecific LBP, as well as for LBP in pregnant and postpartum women at 3 months post-treatment.[21] In 2016, the AOA guidelines on low back pain were updated in 2016 stating: *The American Osteopathic Association (AOA) recommends that osteopathic physicians use osteopathic manipulative treatment (OMT) in the care of patients with low back pain. Evidence from systematic reviews and meta-analyses of randomized controlled trials (evidence level 1a) supports this recommendation.*[20] A large randomized controlled trial and a follow-up study 6 years later were conducted to assess the efficacy of OMT for chronic low back pain. It also showed substantial improvement in pain intensity, decreased need for rescue medication for pain, and greater likelihood of recovery in patients with chronic low back pain.[213–215] In addition to these studies, a systematic review and meta-analysis were conducted regarding OMT for chronic low back pain which showed that OMT was more effective than control interventions in pain reduction and in improving functional status.[211] Regarding the cost of OMT, following chronic low back pain patients for 4 months, demonstrated comparable costs between standard of care and standard of care plus OMT groups.[216] In addition, the OMT group in this study had less utilization of opioid analgesics, physical therapy, interventional therapies, radiologic, and diagnostic services for patients, than the standard-of-care group.[216] In the osteopathic research field, there are fewer and smaller studies investigating OMM compared to large multicentered randomized controlled trials, which reflects the economic reality of medical research, not a lack of efficacy.

Pharmacologic Considerations

Analgesic medications can be divided into three categories: nonopioid analgesics, opioid analgesics, and analgesic adjuvants. Analgesics have different durations of effect. Typically, clinicians use a long-acting medication with adequate short acting medication for breakthrough pain. Taking medications on a schedule works far better than taking analgesics intermittently for episodes of pain. For mild to moderate pain, nonopioid analgesics are used. For moderate to severe pain, a combination of nonopioid and opioid analgesics are used.

At initial and/or subsequent visits for LBP pharmacologic management can be offered to the patient. Medications should be chosen based on available evidence demonstrating efficacy for the chronicity and characteristics of the patient's pain. Then consider potential interactions with the patient's other medications and disease as well as the medication's side effect profile and potential harmful adverse events. Although generally safe, acetaminophen has not been shown to significantly control low back pain, and guidelines are mixed on supporting its use.[217] There is variability of recommendations within many medication classes, although oral corticosteroids, benzodiazepines, anticonvulsants, and antibiotics were not recommended by any CPGs for acute or chronic LBP.[218]

Though two medications from the same class may perform similarly when compared in randomized controlled trials, their risk/benefit ratio may still vary from person to person. For example, an antidepressant may be a better choice for a patient with a comorbid mood disorder and NSAIDs should be avoided in a patient with chronic kidney disease. When considering medication choice for an individual patient, keep in mind that the patient could have a better response to one medication than another even within the same class.

NONSTEROIDAL ANTI-INFLAMMATORY DRUGS

NSAIDs are the first-line pharmacologic treatment for low back pain. These medications reversibly inhibit COX-1 and COX-2 enzymes which form prostaglandins. Decreasing prostaglandin formation decreases inflammation which is the mechanism by which these medications improve pain.[219] Nonselective NSAIDs are strongly recommended for acute or chronic LBP,[18] however, there is currently insufficient evidence to recommend selective NSAIDs over nonselective NSAIDs. The COX-2 selective NSAIDs have been shown to have fewer adverse GI events.[220] with similar efficacy to nonselective NSAIDs and should be considered in patients where GI side effects are a concern. NSAIDs are quite safe, however, they should be used with caution in patients susceptible to kidney injury because they decrease production of protective renal prostaglandins.[219] Clinicians should be aware of dosing guidelines, maximum daily dosage, and duration of action of common medications (see Fig. 93.22).

OPIOIDS

A short course of opioids can be considered to treat severe acute LBP or a severe exacerbation of chronic LBP. However, prolonged opioid therapy should be avoided as the risks quickly outweigh the benefits. In chronic LBP, opioids are not more effective than NSAIDs or acetaminophen.[221] When opioid use extends beyond 4 weeks, patients develop opioid tolerance and opioid-induced hyperalgesia making them a very poor choice for long-term treatment.[221] Opioid medication needs monitoring for benefits, tolerance, side effects, and inappropriate use. Pain contracts are commonly used when prescribing opioids. Also, clinicians need to check their state's prescription monitoring program and prescribe through the national prescriber database.

MUSCLE RELAXANTS

Muscle relaxants are a drug class made up of medications with varying chemical structures and mechanisms of action. They include

Dosing for Select Pharmacologic Agents[a,b]

Category	Generic	Starting Dose	Max/Day	Half-life (t½) (hrs)
Muscle Relaxants	Baclofen	5 mg TID	80 mg	~3.75
	Cyclobenzaprine[c]	5 mg TID	30 mg	18
	Metaxalone[c]	800 mg TID	3,200 mg	~9
	Methocarbamol[c]	1.5 gm TID – QID	8 gm (<3 days) 4.5 mg (>3 days)	1 – 2
	Orphenadrine[c]	100 mg BID	200 mg	14 – 16
	Tizanidine	2 – 4 mg TID	36 mg	2.5
Antidepressants	Amitriptyline[c]	10 – 25 mg QHS	150 mg	13 – 36
	Desipramine[c]	10 – 25 mg QHS	150 mg	15 – 24
	Nortriptyline[c]	10 – 25 mg QHS	150 mg	14 – 51
	Duloxetine[c]	20 – 30 mg QD	60 mg	~12
	Venlafaxine ER	37.5 – 75 mg QD	225 mg	~11
NSAIDs[d]	Ibuprofen	400 mg q 4 – 6H	3200 mg	~2
	Indomethacin	25 mg TID	200 mg	2.6 – 11.2
	Ketoprofen	50 mg QID	300 mg	2-4
	Ketorolac[e]	10 mg q 4 – 6H	40 mg	~5
	Nabumetone	1,000 mg QD	2,000 mg	~24
	Naproxen	250 mg BID	1,500 mg	12 – 17
	Diclofenac NA	50 – 75 mg BID	150 – 200 mg	~2
	Piroxicam	20 mg QD	20 mg	50
	Salsalate	1,000 mg TID	3,000 mg	~1
	Sulindac	150 mg BID	400 mg	7.8
	Celecoxib	100 mg BID	400 mg	~11
	Etodolac	200 mg q 6 – 8H	1,000 mg	6.4
	Meloxicam	5 – 7.5 mg QD	15 mg	~15 – 22

Dosing recommendations obtained from the FDA individual product prescribing information.

Listed in order of increased COX-2 selectivity, more selective at the bottom:

More COX 1 Selective   <5-fold COX-2 Selective   5-50 fold COX-2 Selective

[a] Consult full prescribing information for individual drugs; dosing and half-life may be altered by patient age, renal and hepatic function, and product formulation; consider reduced dosing and/or frequency in the elderly.

[b] For those already on long-term opioid therapy, see the VA/DoD Clinical Practice Guideline for the Use of Opioids in the Management of Chronic Pain. Available at: https://www.healthquality.va.gov/.

[c] Use not recommended in patients >65 years of age per American Geriatrics Society 2015 Updated Beers Criteria.

[d] Avoid chronic use in the elderly unless other alternatives are not effective and patient can take a gastroprotective agent (proton pump inhibitor or misoprostol).

Figure 93.22. Dosing for select pharmacologic agents. (Department of Veterans Affairs, DoD. *VA/DoD clinical practice guideline for the diagnosis and treatment of low back pain.* Ver 3.0. U.S. Government Printing Office; 2022. https://www.healthquality.va.gov/guidelines/Pain/lbp/VADoDLBPCPGFinal508.pdf)

baclofen, dantrolene, carisoprodol, chlorzoxazone, cyclobenzaprine, and tizanidine. They can be divided into two subclasses: antispastic and antispasmodic muscle relaxants. The antispastics affect upper motor symptoms by improving exaggerated reflexes and reducing muscle rigidity, and include dantrolene and baclofen. The antispasmodics improve peripheral muscle pain and spasm, while their precise mechanism of action is unknown it is likely related to central nervous system sedation, these include carisoprodol, chlorzoxazone, and cyclobenzaprine.[222] There is moderate-quality evidence to support the use of nonbenzodiazepine muscle relaxants, but only in acute LBP. There is insufficient evidence to support their use in chronic LBP. Muscle relaxants have significant central nervous system side effects that include sedation, headache, dizziness, and nausea.[18]

ANTIDEPRESSANTS

Antidepressants are considered an analgesic adjuvant for the treatment of LBP and can be most useful when the patient has a comorbid mood disorder.[221] The two classes of antidepressants that are commonly prescribed for LBP are serotonin and norepinephrine reuptake inhibitors (SNRIs) and tricyclic antidepressants (TCAs). The SNRI duloxetine has moderate to high-quality evidence that it improves pain and function.[18] Though another SNRI such as venlafaxine is expected to be similarly effective, more studies have been done investigating duloxetine which is why it is the recommended SNRI. TCAs have shown a small improvement in pain severity in older studies, however, a recent systematic review found that TCAs did not benefit pain or function. Therefore, they are currently not recommended for LBP.[18] There is not enough data to make a recommendation on selective serotonin reuptake inhibitors (SSRIs) currently.[18] SNRIs, such as duloxetine, have moderate- to high-quality evidence demonstrating improvements in pain and function. However, they can cause nausea, dizziness, fatigue, insomnia, dry mouth, constipation, hyperhidrosis, somnolence, and sexual side effects.[18]

CORTICOSTEROIDS

Corticosteroids are a medication that is structurally like the naturally occurring hormone cortisol. These medications have frequently been prescribed for low back pain because they have anti-inflammatory and immunosuppressive properties. A recent Cochrane review that included 13 randomized controlled trials found that for radicular low back pain there is moderate-certainty evidence that systemic corticosteroids probably slightly decrease pain compared to placebo at short-term follow-up. However, there was no significant pain improvement in nonradicular or spinal stenosis-related low back pain.[223] The authors conclude that for radicular low back pain, there is a small benefit associated with systemic corticosteroids and few adverse events when given as a single dose or short course, therefore they should be included as an option for patients who desire a short-term improvement in pain and function. They also produce a wide variety of side effects, most commonly difficulty sleeping. They are also associated with serious potential harms that include increased risk of developing sepsis, venous thromboembolism, hyperglycemia, and fracture which make them an inappropriate choice for certain patients.[224]

TRAMADOL

While it is broadly considered a non-narcotic analgesic or a weak opioid, tramadol has a relatively complex pharmacology.[221] It is a serotonin–norepinephrine reuptake inhibitor that is metabolized into O-desmethyltramadol, which is an opioid with a mu-opioid receptor binding affinity less than oxycodone, but more than hydrocodone. Because both tramadol and its metabolite contribute to its pain treatment efficacy it is more useful to view the medication as a combination of an SNRI such as venlafaxine and an opioid precursor such as codeine. Metabolization of tramadol into O-desmethyltramadol is done by the CYP2D6 enzyme, with its activity varying tremendously between individuals with 3% to 10% being poor metabolizers and 2% to 10% being ultrarapid metabolizers.[225] This variability in CYP2D6 genotype makes prescribing tramadol analogous to prescribing venlafaxine and morphine in an unknown ratio. The reliance on metabolic conversion means that drug interactions can reduce its efficacy. The patient may develop opioid withdrawal if they take tramadol on a regular basis for their chronic pain and then start a CYP2D6 inhibitor, such as terbinafine, paroxetine, or even celecoxib. It carries a risk of serotonin syndrome, like other SNRIs, especially when used in conjunction with other serotonergic agents as well as the risks of opioids which include opioid dependence, respiratory depression, and death. Tramadol has been uniquely associated with new-onset seizures[226] and hypoglycemia.[227] Therefore, it should be avoided in patients with a history of seizures or diabetes. Because of its unpredictable pharmacokinetics, and drug interactions, tramadol should only be used if the patient has failed other preferred pharmacologic treatments.

Physical Therapy/Occupational Therapy

Physical and occupational therapy are the mainstay of treatment for patients with nonspecific mechanical lower back pain. The clinician needs to determine the cause(s) of pain, any comorbidities and associated symptoms, the emotional effects, and the functional impact on the patient's daily activities. The aim of physical and occupational therapy is to improve function and prevent disability. Active strategies that involve patient engagement tend to prevent disability, whereas passive strategies are less useful and are discouraged. International guidelines recommend the use of exercise on its own, or in combination with other nonpharmacologic therapies such as Tai Chi, yoga, massage, and spinal manipulation.[228]

PHYSICAL THERAPY

The PT will perform a comprehensive musculoskeletal evaluation and determine the biomechanical factors involved. They can also help confirm a clinician's diagnosis and develop a comprehensive rehabilitation program. It is important for the therapist and the patient to discuss goals and expectations of the therapy and to align these, so that a satisfactory outcome occurs. PT is not only used for patients who have had orthopedic surgery or chronic back pain. It can be used for almost any musculoskeletal condition when functional improvement of the patient is desired. PT may help to reduce pain, control inflammation and swelling, improve gait, improve transfers and balance, guide a general exercise program, rehabilitate specific areas of the body, increase strength, improve range of motion, help patients lose weight, and help patients return to work. PTs have many different approaches to achieve mutually agreed upon goals with each patient. A common one is called the Mckenzie approach and is where the patient's pain is evaluated and through specific movements it is determined what movements centralize, and/or diminish the pain. PTs are also trained in various assistive techniques such as the Graston method and dry needling. Many PT's learn osteopathic manipulative treatment methods such as strain/counterstrain and apply them routinely.

OCCUPATIONAL THERAPY

The occupational therapist (OT) will evaluate and focus on improving the patient's activities of daily living and independent activities of daily living through assessment of their home, work, hobbies, and other activities. OTs work with the patient's environment in order to minimize aggravation of the medical condition during the patient's daily routine. OT's find ways of accomplishing daily tasks in a safe and more efficient way. Some common OT interventions for patients diagnosed with chronic low back pain include medication management, adapting activities, habits, and routines to mitigate pain, coping skills training, sensory reeducation, desensitization training, graded exposure, physical agent modalities, such as ultrasound and transcutaneous electrical nerve stimulation (TENS), and training in self-advocacy.[229] Evidence has shown that OT provides chronic pain self-management interventions that can improve patient's quality of life, increase their self-efficacy, and increase their ability to participate in meaningful activities.[230–232] Chronic low back pain leads to a sense of disempowerment, frustration, and the loss of control to engage in daily activities. As a result, people with CLBP report significant difficulties in their ability to do what they need and want to do, relationships, and life satisfaction.[233] OT's help patients adapt their environment to their condition, helping to decrease their frustration and improve their life satisfaction.

Key Elements of Therapy for Back Pain Patients

Key elements in assessing patients with lower back pain include evaluation of the function of the transverse abdominis muscle, the multifidus muscle group, the pelvic floor muscles, the glutes, and the legs. A thorough evaluation will also include an evaluation of gait and proprioceptive balance.

One of the cornerstones of physical therapy in the patient with lower back pain is to assess and rehabilitate "core" abdominal and pelvic muscles that provide the stability of the lumbar spine and pelvis. The "core" typically includes the following muscles:

- Internal oblique
- External oblique
- Transverse abdominis
- Multifidi
- Pelvic floor muscles
- Abdominal diaphragm
- Hip/gluteal muscles

The core muscles are stabilizers of the lumbar spine and pelvis and assist with transferring forces rather than acting as prime movers. They provide isometric support and limit the degree of rotation of the trunk and spine.[234] This group of muscles acts like a cylinder of compression that influences the spine via intra-abdominal pressure. The transverse abdominis forms the walls of the cylinder while the muscles of the pelvic floor and abdominal diaphragm form its base and lid, respectively. These four muscles are synergistically intact to provide a spinal support mechanism.[235] A common misconception is that strengthening the core includes movements of the spine such as a "sit-up." However, this is not the case. Core stabilization equals *no movement of the spine* as it is done by isometric abdominal bracing maneuvers.[234] There are five different components of core stability: strength, endurance, flexibility, motor control, and function.[236] Motor control is necessary to develop the other components. Treating somatic dysfunction is thought to improve motor control and thus the function of the core muscles to maintain stability and joint integrity. Core muscles must be able to contract before the primary mover muscles activate. In patients with low back pain, the contraction of the transverse abdominis has been shown to be delayed from approximately 50 to 450 ms.[237] A healthy body and spine automatically uses the transverse abdominis to stabilize the spine before initiating any movement of the limbs.[238] Contraction of the transversus abdominis significantly decreases the laxity of the SIJ. This decrease in laxity is larger than that caused by the bracing action using all the lateral abdominal muscles.[239]

Authors have suggested that the midrange of the joint or "neutral zone" is where the contraction of core muscles is most necessary.[240] The transverse abdominis works in synergy with the multifidus and co-contraction of these two muscles is important for spinal stabilization. The co-contraction increases intra-abdominal pressure creating an extension moment at the spine which has been hypothesized to increase the stability or stiffness via connections with the thoracolumbar fascia.[241] This co-contraction and increased stiffness of the lumbar spinal segments do not interfere with trunk movement. With poor core stability, the ligaments are at risk, especially during prolonged specific body postures. This may lead to ligamentous laxity and ligamentous somatic dysfunction.

In addition to the co-contraction of the transverse abdominis and multifidus, it has also been found that inhibition of the gluteus maximus is important.[242–244] The activation of the gluteus maximus is delayed compared to people without lower back pain. In patients with gluteal muscle inhibition, hip extension is initiated by the hamstrings and erector spinae instead of the gluteus maximus. Gluteal inhibition negatively affects performance and lower body strength and is a root cause of many injuries and chronic pain. Therefore, low back pain results in delayed and reduced glute activation with concurrent hamstring and low back compensation. In addition to the gluteus muscles, onset of contraction of the internal obliques, multifidi, and gluteus maximus was delayed on the symptomatic side in patients with sacroiliac pain.[245] If the pain and dysfunction are prolonged, ipsilateral atrophy of multifidus in patients with unilateral LBP can occur.[238]

Rehabilitation begins with three different exercise techniques are used in clinical practice (see Fig. 93.13):

- Drawing-in maneuver
- Abdominal bracing
- Posterior pelvic tilt

The "drawing-in maneuver" is more selective in co-activating the transverse abdominis and multifidus.[239] Greenman recommended a reverse sit-up for training the transverse abdominis muscle.[38] The patient is instructed to hold the contraction for a period and release it. Once mastery of these procedures occurs, then more advanced movements such as planks are performed. From here, advancement might include movements involving the extremities in a coordinated fashion, and activity or sport-specific movements (see Chapter 88 An Osteopathic Approach to the Exercise Prescription for further information).

Evidence for PT

Exercise is one of the main treatments used for CLBP and has been shown to reduce the duration and frequency of back pain.[246,247] In a randomized-controlled trial, the combination of physical therapy methods, exercise, and medical treatment for nonspecific CLBP improved pain and functional status more than just exercise and medical treatment without physical therapy.[248] This improvement was sustained for 3 months after the treatment. CPGs from the NASS provided grade A evidence that aerobic exercise is recommended to improve pain, disability, and mental health in patients with nonspecific low back pain at short-term follow-up. They also found grade B evidence that patients who remained active and used exercise to facilitate recovery had better functional outcomes. Passive therapeutic modalities such as hot packs, ice massages, diathermy, ultrasound therapy, and TENS reduce inflammation, relieve musculoskeletal symptoms, and joint stiffness, thereby, providing symptomatic relief.[249,250]

Psychiatry/Counseling

It is important to discuss with patients how their emotional health has been affected by their pain and medical condition. It is also important to discuss how they feel about their current situation, daily activities, and treatment plan. Screening for depression and anxiety is an important part of management especially in chronic pain patients. Discussions of how the patient deals with stress and tension, job satisfaction, and any recent relationship stressors are important in their overall health and compliance with their treatment plan. Stress reduction and cognitive-behavioral therapy have been shown among adults with chronic low back pain to be beneficial. Patients who underwent either approach resulted in greater improvement in back pain and functional limitations at 26 weeks, compared with usual care.[251]

Pain Management

Pain management is a rapidly evolving field with more than 200 routinely performed interventional procedures, most often by physicians with additional fellowship-level training. These interventions include simple peripheral nerve blocks and epidural injections to more invasive procedures that include implantation of devices. Procedures are generally only considered after conservative management of LBP has failed, typically defined as inadequate pain relief after a 6-week trial of medication, physical therapy, or both. Procedure outcomes are reliant on careful patient selection. Contraindications to interventional spine procedures include active systemic infection, active infection overlying skin at procedure site, anticoagulation, coagulopathy, allergy to injectate, and malignancy at site of injection. Relative contraindications include uncontrolled diabetes, heart failure, pregnancy, and use of an implanted cardiac device in cases of radiofrequency ablation. Complications include infection, systemic glucocorticoid exposure, systemic local anesthetic exposure, and rarely ischemia from vessel occlusion following inadvertent intravascular injection (greater risk with particulate glucocorticoids). A few of the most frequently performed interventions for LBP are described below.

Injection Therapy

The epidural steroid injection is the most frequently performed procedure by pain physicians. Although randomized controlled trials have shown that epidural steroid injections may improve nonspecific LBP (axial LBP), it is widely understood that they are most effective in treating LBP with a radicular component, especially pain secondary to herniated nucleus pulposus.[252] The technique involves delivering an injectate, commonly composed of a local anesthetic and steroid, in the epidural space. When performed blindly, extradural injection can occur in up to 30% of patients, which is why precise needle placement confirmed with fluoroscopy is the standard of care.[253]

The injected volume varies widely depending on the procedure site with medial branch blocks using a volume as little as 0.5 mL and a caudal epidural using a volume of 20 mL or more. The injectate typically includes a local anesthetic such as lidocaine or bupivacaine as well as a steroid, typically methylprednisolone or triamcinolone diacetate. The local anesthetic provides pain relief within minutes with the steroid providing therapeutic efficacy of weeks to months. The steroid dose is usually 40 to 80 mg with a randomized trial comparing 40 mg and 80 mg finding no difference in efficacy.[254]

There are three different approaches to epidural steroid injections: interlaminar (midline or parasagittal), transforaminal, and caudal. The transforaminal approach is more specific, with medication being delivered directly onto the ventral epidural space of the affected nerve root. The interlaminar approach has lower risk, with medication being delivered in the dorsal epidural space at the affected level. The transforaminal approach is used for unilateral symptoms with the needle tip within the intervertebral foramen. The interlaminar approach can be used for unilateral or bilateral symptoms with the needle tip remaining outside of the intervertebral foramen. The caudal approach is considered less effective than the interlaminar or transforaminal approaches, however, it is still used in patients with previous spine surgeries where it may be unsafe or anatomically impossible to use an alternative approach.[255] It involves injecting a relatively large volume, historically 10 to 64 mL through the sacral hiatus.[15] One study found that a 10-mL caudal injection will reach the L3–L4 interspace on most patients, with a 20-mL injection reaching L3 and despite increasing the volume to 50 mL the mean cephalic spread did not surpass L3.[256] Therefore, due to these limitations of spread, the caudal route is not recommended for treatment of disease pathology above L3.[15]

Guidelines recommend that interlaminar and transforaminal epidural injections are likely to benefit patients with LBP and radicular pain originating from disk disease or spinal stenosis as well as chronic LBP after surgical intervention.[255] Caudal epidural injections carry the same recommendation but only in cases where interlaminar or transforaminal approaches are not feasible.[255] In nonspecific LBP there is insufficient evidence to make a recommendation for or against epidural injection.[17]

Facet Interventions

LBP is most often multifactorial, with the muscles, ligaments, intervertebral disks, nerve roots, and facet(zygapophysial) joints all contributing. However, if the facet joint is suspected to be a significant source of the patient's pain, then it can be diagnosed and treated. Image-guided intra-articular facet joint or medial branch nerve blocks are the definitive method for diagnosing facet joint pathology.[15] These diagnostic blocks are used to determine if a patient is a good candidate for denervation procedures such as radiofrequency ablation of the medial branch nerve. Using small volumes during diagnostic blocks helps improve patient selection because there is reduced confounding spread to adjacent structures. Facet joint interventions are the second most performed pain procedure.[15]

The facet joints are paired synovial joints located posterolateral on the vertebral body, with one pair formed from the superior articular process of one vertebra and the inferior articular process of another. The intra-articular volume capacity of the lumbar facet joints is approximately 1 to 1.5 mL.[257] The plane of the joint varies both from L1 to L5 and from patient to patient. The upper lumbar facet joints are more closely oriented in the sagittal plane (26 to 34 degrees), while the lower lumbar facet joints are more closely oriented in the coronal plane.[258]

The sensory innervation of the facet joint is supplied by the medial branch nerves, which are terminal divisions of the posterior ramus, which itself branches off the spinal nerve after it emerges from the intervertebral foramen. Each facet joint is innervated by both the medial branch nerve at the vertebral level of the joint and the level above. For example, the L4–L5 facet joints are innervated by the medial branches from the L3 and L4 spinal nerves.[15] In addition to the facet joint, the medial branch innervates the multifidus muscle, interspinal muscle, interspinal ligament, and periosteum of the neural arch.

If the patient has a satisfactory response following a diagnostic medial branch block, then they are a good candidate for radiofrequency ablation of that medial branch nerve (see Fig. 93.23). This procedure involves introducing the tip of a radiofrequency needle in parallel to the medial branch nerve, at the junction of the transverse process and lateral neck of the superior articular process of the vertebral level of interest.[15] Motor stimulation is used to avoid ablation of motor fibers. Pain relief following successful radiofrequency denervation typically lasts for 6 months to a year. If pain recurs following successful ablation, then the procedure can be performed again and typically provides pain relief comparable to the first procedure.

The most serious and rare complication following medial branch ablation is damage to the ventral nerve root from incorrect needle placement. Motor stimulation is used to help prevent this complication. The most common complication is postdenervation neuritis which typically occurs in less than 10% of procedures and can be reduced further with prophylactic corticosteroid administration.[15] Though recent studies have cast doubt on whether this practice reduces neuritis complications.[259,260] It is likely that prophylactic steroids still have utility in reducing postprocedure pain.[261]

Society guidelines find that intra-articular injection of steroids into the facet joint provides no clinically meaningful improvement at 6 months.[17] There is a strong recommendation that response

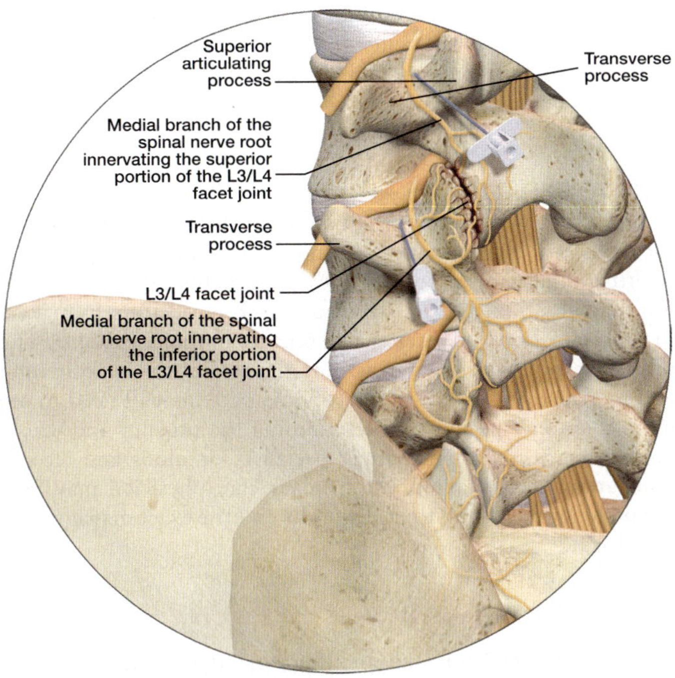

Figure 93.23. Medial branch block. (Reprinted with permission from Hoppenfeld JD. *Fundamentals of Pain Medicine: How to Diagnose and Treat Your Patients*. Wolters Kluwer; 2014. Figure 20-9.)

to diagnostic medial branch block is predictive of response to radiofrequency ablation.[255] Thermal radiofrequency ablation is recommended to treat LBP from zygapophyseal joints with careful patient selection yielding more reliable outcomes. The relief from ablation is durable for at least 6 months following the procedure.[17]

Thermal Radiofrequency Ablation

Thermal radiofrequency ablation is an irreversible denervation technique where focused destruction of the nervous system is used to treat intractable pain. Targets for this procedure include the brain, brain stem, cranial nerves, spinal cord, and peripheral nerves. These techniques have become less commonly used following the invention of intrathecal drug delivery and neurostimulation. However, many ablative procedures are still valuable components of pain treatment.

While destruction of nerves along the pain pathway may seem like the most direct way to treat intractable pain, the outcomes of these procedures are not as plain and direct as the theories behind their use would suggest. This illustrates the complexity of chronic pain and how much is still left to be discovered.

Percutaneous Image-Guided Minimally Invasive Lumbar Decompression (PILD)

PILD is a treatment for lumbar spinal stenosis secondary to ligamentum flavum hypertrophy. The prevalence of lumbar spinal stenosis increases with age, with approximately 10% of people over age 70 suffering from symptoms associated with radiologically confirmed lumbar spinal stenosis.[262] Because conservative measures have limited benefit in this condition,[263] the treatment has been open laminectomy with or without fusion to provide long-term symptom relief. Due to risks of surgery and hospitalization in this elderly population, PILD arose as an alternative, where specially designed instruments are used under fluoroscopic guidance to debulk the ligamentum flavum without direct visualization of the area. Clinical studies have shown that the safety profile of the PILD procedure was equivalent to an epidural steroid injection while having similar efficacy to a decompressive laminectomy.[255] The procedure carries a strong recommendation to treat lumbar spinal stenosis with ligamentum flavum hypertrophy.[255]

Spinal Cord Stimulators

The first spinal cord stimulator was used in 1967, 2 years after the gate control theory of pain was discovered, with the belief that an artificially generated input activating A-beta fibers would prevent transmission of nociceptive signals from A-delta and C fibers. In that first procedure, a patient with neuropathic pain had a monopolar spinal cord stimulator lead placed in the intrathecal space near the dorsal column and they experienced impressive pain relief.[264] Since that first procedure the field has evolved dramatically with a variety of lead types and programming such as conventional, burst, and high-frequency spinal cord stimulators.

Mechanistically, spinal cord stimulators are now hypothesized to also act by suppression of central excitability, vasodilation, and inhibition of sympathetic outflow. However, because technologic advances in stimulator designs have not translated into improved clinical outcomes, it is believed that the mechanism is not completely known and that further research would optimize patient outcomes (see Fig. 93.24).[265]

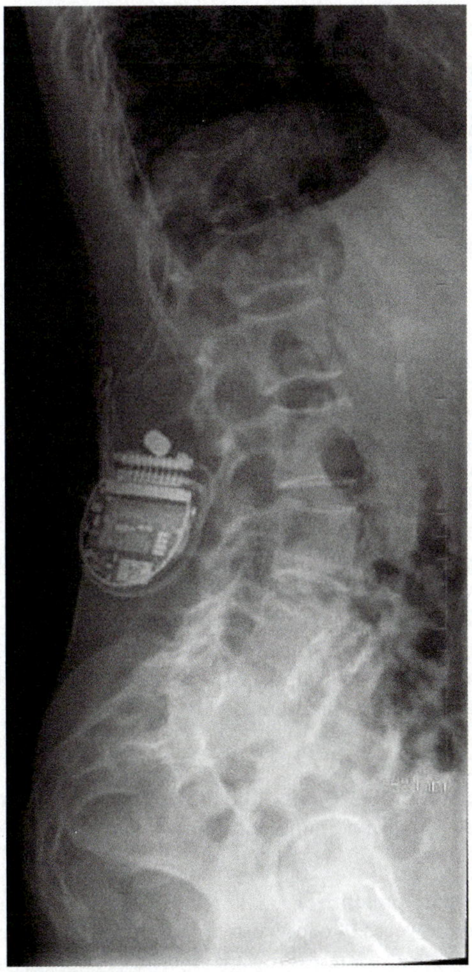

Figure 93.24. Spinal cord stimulator. (Case courtesy of Aneta Kecler-Pietrzyk, Radiopaedia.org, rID: 52468.)

Spinal cord stimulators are currently used to treat neuropathic pain, chronic radicular pain, failed back syndrome, complex regional pain syndrome, peripheral ischemia, intractable axial back pain, and intractable angina.[15] Patient selection is key to more consistent outcomes. The following patient criteria must be met prior to implantation.[15]

- Patient has diagnosis amenable to treatment with spinal cord stimulator
- The patient has failed conservative treatment for at least 6 months
- A major psychological disorder has been ruled out
- No history of illicit drug use
- Spinal cord stimulator trial has demonstrated pain relief

Acupuncture

Acupuncture has been practiced in China for over 3000 years and over that time its use has disseminated across the globe.[266] Over that time many styles and country-specific variations have emerged including: five elements (traditional Chinese acupuncture), Japanese acupuncture, Korean acupuncture, Vietnamese acupuncture, and French acupuncture. Acupuncture treatment focuses on balancing three major principles: Qi, Yin-Yang, and the five elements.[266] In patients with chronic LBP, the addition of acupuncture to usual care is strongly recommended for short-term improvement of pain and function compared to usual care alone.[17] Acupuncture is suggested to be cost-effective when compared to other medical/interventional treatments.[17]

Yoga

In patients with mild chronic LBP, yoga may offer medium-term improvements in pain and function compared to usual care.[17] If the activity is well tolerated by the patient there is a strong recommendation to promote activity and exercise while discouraging bed rest.[17]

Specialist Referral

Specialist referral is an important part of comprehensive healthcare for patients with lower back pain. Prior to referring to a specialist the clinician needs to decide how the specialist's recommendations may affect the current treatment plan. They also need to decide which specialist will provide the most useful information to help the patient improve. Many times, in the workup of chronic lower back pain, other medical conditions are diagnosed and need to be treated prior to continuing the management of the back pain. Sometimes undiagnosed medical conditions arise that take management precedence over the lower back pain. It is important for patients who have multiple specialists assisting with their care of lower back pain to have an effective primary care provider to coordinate diagnostic testing, therapy, surgery, and other recommendations. The patient's goals and expectations should also align with the specialist recommendations.

WHEN TO REFER

Surgical consultation (orthopedic and/or neurologic) and special tests are indicated if certain conditions are present. These include the following:

- Red flags are present
- Six to eight weeks of conservative care that has not been accompanied by steady progress toward reversal of and/or resolution of the symptoms and signs
- Poor clinical response associated with any two or all three of the following: paresthesia, reflex changes, and muscle atrophy
- If the symptoms increase in intensity despite good ongoing conservative care
- Uncertain diagnosis

WHO TO REFER TO

Determining who to refer the patient to depends upon the history, physical findings, and diagnostic modalities. Due to the multifactorial nature of lower back pain many different specialists may be utilized. It is also common for specialists to make a recommendation and refer the patient to another specialist. The primary care physician may assume the role of the coordination and management of this process. Some patients will need to see more than one specialist so determining the urgency and whom to see first is important. Once specialists' opinions and recommendations are obtained, the primary care physician may help the patient understand their diagnosis and the exact management plan for it.

Surgical Decompression/Stabilization

Surgical consultation is indicated for patients who have red flags, progressive neurologic deficits, altered bowel and bladder function, and intractable pain despite conservative measures. Preserving nerve function and ambulation are the primary goals with a secondary goal of relieving back and leg pain. Some patients in this situation have a clearly defined surgical lesion and others do not. Two surgical emergencies that refer pain into the lumbar region include dissecting abdominal aneurysm and CES. Orthopedic conditions that may require surgery include intervertebral disk herniation, spinal stenosis, and degenerative spondylolisthesis. Primary cancers that metastasize to bone (breast, lung, thyroid, kidney, and prostate) may need surgical management (see Chapter 76 Osteopathic Considerations in Oncology for further information). Regarding surgical practice guidelines, the SPORT study was a multicenter, randomized, controlled trial conducted in 11 US states at 13 medical centers with multidisciplinary spine practices. It studied surgical outcomes in lumbar intervertebral disk herniation, spinal stenosis, and spinal stenosis secondary to degenerative spondylolisthesis.[267]

In patients with a herniated disk confirmed by imaging and leg symptoms persisting for at least 6 weeks, surgery was superior to nonoperative treatment in relieving symptoms and improving function. The treatment effect for surgery was seen as early as 6 weeks, appeared to reach a maximum by 6 months, and persisted over 8 years. The nonoperative group also improved significantly, and this improvement persisted with little to no degradation of outcomes in either group (operative and nonoperative) between 4 and 8 years.[268]

In addition to the previous outcomes, the SPORT trial also studied patients with degenerative spondylolisthesis and spinal stenosis. Those treated surgically showed substantially greater improvement in pain and function during a period of 2 years[269] and 4 years than those patients treated nonsurgically.[268,270] The patients receiving nonsurgical treatment, on average, showed moderate improvement in all outcomes. No patients undergoing surgical or nonsurgical treatment had CES. Patients with persistent neurogenic claudication from degenerative spondylolisthesis treated surgically showed substantially greater improvement in pain and function, as well as satisfaction, for 2 years.[270] Carefully selected patients who underwent surgery for a lumbar disk herniation achieved greater improvement than nonoperatively treated patients; there was little to no degradation of outcomes in either group (operative or non-operative) from 4 to 8 years.[271]

TREATING THE PATIENT AS A WHOLE

There are many other ways to treat patients with low back pain in addition to OMT, medications, and exercises. Physical modalities include foot orthotics, heel lift therapy, injections, massage, physical therapy, etc. The patient is a unity of body, mind, and spirit; therefore, the osteopathic approach addresses lifestyle and environmental factors such as proper nutrition, and stress management, including helping the patient remove deleterious habits and activities, such as drug dependency and abuse. Find the best combination for each patient. Consider cost, time required, access to care, and availability.

SUMMARY

LBP is the leading cause of productivity loss worldwide, costs the United States $100 billion annually, and is one of the most common conditions an osteopathic physician will see. It is imperative that all osteopathic physicians, regardless of setting and specialty, can diagnose and treat patients with LBP. The priority for the physician is to determine if a serious or life-threatening condition is present (red flag) that needs immediate attention. Low back pain is a complex and incompletely understood multifactorial process. Patients with lower back pain can have a wide range of presentations depending on their age, causative factors, chronicity of the problem, past surgeries, and comorbidities. LBP can be classified by being specific or nonspecific (most common), or by its location, pathology, chronicity, patient age, and type of pain (nociceptive/neuropathic/nociplastic). Establishing the chronicity of LBP determines what diagnostic tests are ordered and will guide treatment choice.

When obtaining the history, develop a timeline of past diagnostics and treatments and their success or failure. The physical examination needs to include a complete general medical exam with focus on the osteopathic structural and palpatory examination, neurologic examination, abdominal and genitourinary exam, and vascular exam. Somatic dysfunction is a common and globally under-treated cause of nonspecific lower back pain. It must be diagnosed accurately, recorded in the medical record, and treated as the standard of osteopathic care.

Most individuals with spinal pain do not require laboratory studies with their initial evaluation, yet obtaining baseline lab tests does have a role in separating mechanical from systemic diseases. Imaging is the most used diagnostic test to evaluate LBP with plain radiography being the most frequent initial test. Ideally, testing should only be ordered if the result will likely change management or inform the prognosis of the patient's condition. In acute back pain, plain radiographs should be ordered if the clinician strongly suspects a serious condition such as cancer, fracture, or ankylosing spondylitis. Early MRI, defined as MRI obtained within 4 to 6 weeks of LBP onset, was associated with increased length of disability in patients with acute LBP without red flags. Electrodiagnostic studies are commonly used in the evaluation of diseases affecting the peripheral nervous system and discerning radiculopathy from neuropathy.

An appropriate diagnosis/assessment hinges upon an accurate history, and appropriate differential diagnosis, confirming findings with an efficient and accurate physical exam and review of any diagnostics, consults, and laboratory studies.

When planning treatment, it is important that the clinician and the patient discuss and align their goals and expectations. Clinicians should review the CPGs regarding the diagnosis and management of patients with lower back pain. Most of the guidelines recommend improving function through a biopsychosocial framework including exercise and nonpharmacologic therapies, such as acupuncture, spinal manipulation, Tai Chi, and yoga. However, gaps between the medical evidence and practice exist, with limited use of recommended first-line treatments, a lack of screening for depression and anxiety, and inappropriately high use of imaging, rest, opioids, spinal injections, and surgery. Physicians should also consider assisting in the restoration of the patient's wellness, which is fostered by self-regulation, self-healing, and health maintenance. The five models of osteopathic medicine can be used as a framework to help clinicians develop treatment plans.

Conservative care includes evaluating and reducing modifiable contributing factors. Physical and occupational therapy and OMT are the mainstay of treatment for patients with nonspecific mechanical lower back pain. The aim of physical and occupational therapy is to improve function, accomplish daily tasks, and prevent disability. This may include specific treatment of postural imbalance and somatic dysfunction, adequate relief of pain, treatment of contributing medical issues, and improving the patient's mechanical, structural, or psychological issues. OMT and an osteopathic approach, mindfulness, stress reduction, and cognitive behavioral therapy have been shown to provide a greater improvement in back pain and less medication use than usual care.[272] The patient is a unity of body, mind, and spirit; therefore, the osteopathic approach addresses lifestyle and environmental factors, diet and nutrition, and stress.

Specialist referral is an important part of comprehensive healthcare for patients with lower back pain. Prior to referring to a specialist the clinician needs to decide how the specialist's recommendations may affect the current treatment plan. Interventional pain management may range from simple peripheral nerve blocks and epidural injections to more invasive procedures that include implantation of devices. Procedures are generally only considered after conservative management of LBP has failed.

Surgical consultation is indicated for patients who have red flags, progressive neurologic deficits, altered bowel and bladder function, and intractable pain despite failure of conservative means. Preserving nerve function, and ambulation are the primary goals with a secondary goal of relieving back and leg pain. Orthopedic conditions that may require surgery include intervertebral disk herniation, spinal stenosis, and degenerative spondylolisthesis. For these conditions, in properly selected patients, the treatment effect for surgery was seen as early as 6 weeks, appeared to reach a maximum by 6 months, and like conservative management, persisted over 8 years. The appropriate treatment of co-existing somatic dysfunction in these cases fosters the patient's ability to recover.

Patient's value an osteopathic physician who actively listens to their concerns, empathizes with them, supports them, and is an advocate for their best interests. Patient's desire an osteopathic physician who will spend the appropriate time, answer questions, and provide clear structured treatment plans. Patients actively seek out osteopathic physicians to accurately diagnose their condition and then implement osteopathic philosophic principles, and OMT, into a personalized care plan.

FINAL THOUGHTS

Clinical Practice Guidelines

The information below summarizes both national guidelines utilized in the chapter on osteopathic considerations in patients with lower back pain.

American College of Physicians[54]

Recommendation 1: Given that most patients with acute or subacute low back pain improve over time regardless of treatment, clinicians and patients should select nonpharmacologic treatment with superficial heat (moderate-quality evidence), massage, acupuncture, or spinal manipulation (low-quality evidence). If pharmacologic treatment is desired, clinicians and patients should select nonsteroidal anti-inflammatory drugs or skeletal muscle relaxants (moderate-quality evidence) (Grade: strong recommendation).

Recommendation 2: For patients with chronic low back pain, clinicians and patients should initially select nonpharmacologic treatment with exercise, multidisciplinary rehabilitation, acupuncture, mindfulness-based stress reduction (moderate-quality evidence), Tai Chi, yoga, motor control exercise, progressive relaxation, EMG biofeedback, low-level laser therapy, operant therapy, cognitive behavioral therapy, or spinal manipulation (low-quality evidence) (Grade: strong recommendation).

Recommendation 3: In patients with chronic low back pain who have had an inadequate response to nonpharmacologic therapy, clinicians and patients should consider pharmacologic treatment with nonsteroidal anti-inflammatory drugs as first-line therapy, or tramadol or duloxetine as second-line therapy.

Veterans Administration Recommendations[55] (See Tables 93.4 to 93.6)

INTERNATIONAL GUIDELINES

2016 NICE Guidelines from the United Kingdom[273]

In 2016, guidelines for noninvasive treatments for LBP and sciatica were published by The National Institute for Health Care Excellence (NICE) in the United Kingdom. These guidelines addressed patients older than 16 with acute and chronic LBP, with and without sciatica. In 2020, they updated their guidelines to include guidance on opioids for noncancer pain in response to a Public Health England evidence review.[274] Their publication also supports shared decision making and stratified management. Their general recommendations are summarized below:

- Consider alternative diagnoses and use a risk stratification tool.
- Explain to people they may not need imaging unless the result is likely to change management.
- Patients should consider a group exercise program and psychological program, using a cognitive behavioral approach for managing low back pain.
- Do not offer belts or corsets, foot orthotics, acupuncture, ultrasound, TENS, for managing low back pain with or without sciatica.
- Physicians should promote a return to work, normal activities of daily living.
- Consider epidural injections of local anesthetic and steroid in people with acute and severe sciatica.
- Physicians should consider epidural steroid injection, radiofrequency ablation, and spinal decompression for patients with chronic LBP who failed conservative measures.
- Physicians should not offer gabapentinoids, paracetamol, opioids, antiepileptics, oral corticosteroids or benzodiazepines for managing sciatica and chronic LBP.
- Use the lowest effective dose of nonsteroidal anti-inflammatory drugs (NSAIDs) in patients with sciatica.
- Consider oral NSAIDs for managing low back pain yet be aware of the risk of harm and limited evidence of benefit.
- Do not offer spinal fusion for people with low back pain unless as part of a randomized controlled trial.

Brussels: Belgian Health Care Knowledge Centre (KCE) Guidelines[56]

Belgian CPGs include the following:

- The clinician needs to evaluate for signs and or symptoms of possible serious underlying pathology focusing on clusters of red flags.
- Depending on the perceived risk, stratified management should be offered.
- In the absence of red flags, imaging should not be routinely offered and only be prescribed if the results may influence the treatment.
- Paracetamol is no longer the first-line pharmacologic treatment. This is due to the results of the PACE Trial.
- Nonsteroidal anti-inflammatory drugs (NSAIDs) can be considered. However, a systematic review and meta-analysis concluded that although NSAIDs reduced pain and disability in patients with spinal pain, the effects were not clinically significant over placebo.
- Manual therapy and/or a psychological intervention can be added to a supervised exercise program. Multidisciplinary rehabilitation (combination of physical and psychological components) should be reserved for people at high risk for chronicity or persistent impairment.
- Weak opioids can be considered for managing acute LBP or radicular pain if NSAIDs are ineffective, not tolerated, or contraindicated.
- Opioids should not be routinely used for managing chronic LBP or radicular pain.
- Some antidepressants (TCAs or nonselective serotonin–norepinephrine reuptake inhibitors [SNRI]) may be used in the management of chronic pain.
- Anticonvulsants should only be considered if there is a neuropathic pain component.
- Radiofrequency denervation can be considered for chronic LBP with suspected facet joint pain, when evidence-based multimodal noninvasive treatment fails, in the presence of moderate to intense pain, and after a positive response to a diagnostic medial branch block.
- Epidural injections can be considered in acute and subacute (at least 2 to 3 weeks after onset) severe radicular pain.
- Since spinal fusion for LBP does not have a clear advantage compared to other treatments and because of the known risks it should only be offered in very select cases.
- Finally, in case of radicular pain lasting more than 6 to 12 weeks, spinal decompression can be considered when evidence-based multimodal noninvasive treatment did not improve pain or function.

Denmark Guidelines for Low Back Pain (LBP) and Lumbar Radiculopathy (LR)[57]

The group recommended:

- Management should include information about prognosis, warning signs, and encourage physical activity and supervised exercise.

TABLE 93.4

Veterans Administration Recommendations: Evaluation and Diagnostic Approach, Patient Education and Self-Care, Nonpharmacologic and Noninvasive Therapy

Topic	#	Recommendation	Strength[a]	Category[b]
Evaluation and Diagnostic Approach	1.	For patients with low back pain, we recommend the history and physical examination include evaluation for progressive or otherwise serious neurologic deficits and other red flags (e.g., signs, symptoms, history) associated with serious underlying pathology (e.g., malignancy, fracture, infection).	Strong for	Reviewed, Amended
	2.	For patients with low back pain, we recommend diagnostic imaging and appropriate laboratory testing when neurologic deficits are progressive or otherwise serious or when other red flags (e.g., signs, symptoms, history) are present.	Strong for	Reviewed, Amended
	3.	For patients with acute low back pain, without focal neurologic deficits or other red flags (e.g., signs, symptoms, history), we recommend against routinely obtaining imaging studies or performing invasive diagnostic tests.	Strong against	Reviewed, New-replaced
	4.	For patients with low back pain, we suggest assessing psychosocial factors and using predictive screening instruments (e.g., STarT Back and The Orebro Musculoskeletal Pain Screening Questionnaire) to inform treatment planning.	Weak for	Reviewed, New-replaced
	5.	For patients with low back pain, with or without radicular symptoms, there is insufficient evidence to recommend for or against specific physical exam maneuvers to assist in the diagnosis of facet or sacroiliac joint pain, or a lumbar/lumbosacral radiculopathy.	Neither for nor against	Reviewed, New-added
Patient Education and Self-care	6.	For patients with low back pain, there is insufficient evidence to recommend for or against pain neuroscience education, clinician-directed education with patient-led goal setting, or back school.	Neither for nor against	Reviewed, New-replaced
	7.	For the self-management of low back pain, there is insufficient evidence to recommend for or against technology-based modalities.	Neither for nor against	Reviewed, New-added
Nonpharmacologic and Noninvasive Therapy	8.	For patients with chronic low back pain, we suggest cognitive behavioral therapy.	Weak for	Reviewed, New-replaced
	9.	For patients with low back pain, we suggest a structured clinician-directed exercise program (e.g., aerobic, aquatic, mechanical diagnosis and therapy, mobility, motor control, Pilates, strengthening exercises, structured walking program, Tai Chi).	Weak for	Reviewed, New-replaced
	10.	For patients with chronic low back pain, we suggest spinal mobilization/manipulation.	Weak for	Reviewed, New-replaced
	11.	For patients with acute low back pain, there is insufficient evidence to recommend for or against spinal mobilization/manipulation.	Neither for nor against	Reviewed, New-replaced
	12.	For patients with chronic low back pain, there is insufficient evidence to recommend for or against mindfulness-based stress reduction.	Neither for nor against	Reviewed, New-replaced
	13.	For patients with low back pain, there is insufficient evidence to recommend for or against lumbar supports.	Neither for nor against	Reviewed, Amended

[a]For additional information, see Determining Recommendation Strength and Direction.[56]
[b]For additional information, see Recommendation Categorization and Appendix D.[56]

- Physicians should recommend patient education, different types of supervised exercise, and manual therapy.
- For pain relief, manual therapy including joint mobilization and manipulation in addition to usual care was recommended.
- They recommended against the use of pain medication in the form of paracetamol, NSAID, and opioids in addition to usual care.
- Acupuncture was not endorsed.
- Clinicians should not perform routine imaging, that is, x-ray or MRI, in patients presenting with both recent onset LBP and/or lumbar radiculopathy.
- They did not recommend the use of extraforaminal glucocorticoid injections in patients with lumbar radiculopathy.
- Patients with intractable lumbar radiculopathy are referred for surgical consultation within 12 weeks if severe and disabling.

TABLE 93.5

Veterans Administration Recommendations: Nonpharmacologic and Noninvasive Therapy (Cont. from Table 93.4), Pharmacotherapy, Dietary Supplements

Topic	#	Recommendation	Strength[a]	Category[b]
Nonpharmacologic and Noninvasive Therapy (cont.)	14.	For patients with low back pain, with or without radicular symptoms, there is insufficient evidence to recommend for or against mechanical lumbar traction.	Neither for nor against	Reviewed, New-replaced
	15.	For patients with chronic low back pain, there is insufficient evidence to recommend for or against auricular acupressure.	Neither for nor against	Reviewed, New-added
	16.	For patients with low back pain, there is insufficient evidence to recommend for or against yoga or qi gong.	Neither for nor against	Reviewed, New-replaced
	17.	For patients with low back pain, there is insufficient evidence to recommend for or against cupping, laser therapy, transcutaneous electrical nerve stimulation, and ultrasound.	Neither for nor against	Reviewed, New-replaced
Pharmacotherapy	18.	For patients with chronic low back pain, we suggest duloxetine.	Weak for	Reviewed, New-replaced
	19.	For patients with low back pain, we suggest nonsteroidal anti-inflammatory drugs.	Weak for	Reviewed, New-replaced
	20.	For patients with low back pain, with or without radicular symptoms, there is insufficient evidence to recommend for or against gabapentin or pregabalin.	Neither for nor against	Reviewed, Amended
	21.	For patients with low back pain, there is insufficient evidence to recommend for or against tricyclic antidepressants.	Neither for nor against	Reviewed, New-added
	22.	For patients with low back pain, there is insufficient evidence to recommend for or against topical preparations.	Neither for nor against	Reviewed, Amended
	23.	For patients with acute low back pain, there is insufficient evidence to recommend for or against a nonbenzodiazepine muscle relaxant for short-term use.	Neither for nor against	Reviewed, New-replaced
	24.	For patients with chronic low back pain, we suggest against offering a nonbenzodiazepine muscle relaxant.	Weak against	Reviewed, Not changed
	25.	For patients with low back pain, we suggest against acetaminophen.	Weak against	Reviewed, New-replaced
	26.	For patients with low back pain, we suggest against monoclonal antibodies.	Weak against	Reviewed, New-added
	27.	For patients with chronic low back pain, we suggest against opioids. For patients who are already using long-term opioids, see the VA/DoD CPG for the Use of Opioids in the Management of Chronic Pain.[c]	Weak against	Reviewed, New-replaced
	28.	For patients with low back pain, with or without radicular symptoms, we suggest against systemic corticosteroids (oral or intramuscular injection).	Weak against	Not reviewed, Amended
	29.	For patients with low back pain, we recommend against benzodiazepines.	Strong against	Reviewed, Not changed
Dietary Supplements	30.	For patients with low back pain, there is insufficient evidence to recommend for or against any specific diet or nutritional, herbal, or homeopathic supplements (e.g., anti-inflammatory diet, turmeric, vitamin D), cannabis, or cannabinoids.	Neither for nor against	Reviewed, New-replaced

[a]For additional information, see Determining Recommendation Strength and Direction.[56]

[b]For additional information, see Recommendation Categorization and Appendix D.[56]

[c]For additional information, see the VA/DoD Clinical Practice Guideline for the Use of Opioids in the Management of Chronic Pain.[56] Available at: https://www.healthquality.va.gov/.

TABLE 93.6

Veterans Administration Recommendations: Nonsurgical Invasive Therapy, Team Approach (Cont. from Table 93.4)

Topic	#	Recommendation	Strength[a]	Category[b]
Nonsurgical Invasive Therapy	31.	For patients with chronic low back pain, we suggest lumbar medial branch and/or sacral lateral branch radiofrequency ablation.	Weak for	Reviewed, New-replaced
	32.	For patients with low back pain, there is insufficient evidence to recommend for or against sacroiliac joint injections.	Neither for nor against	Reviewed, New-added
	33.	For patients with low back pain, we suggest against the injection of corticosteroids for intra-articular facet joint injections and therapeutic medial branch blocks with steroid.	Weak against	Reviewed, New-replaced
	34.	For patients with chronic low back pain, we suggest acupuncture.	Weak for	Reviewed, Amended
	35.	For patients with acute low back pain, there is insufficient evidence to recommend for or against acupuncture.	Neither for nor against	Reviewed, Amended
	36.	For patients with low back pain, there is insufficient evidence to recommend for or against ortho-biologics (e.g., platelet-rich plasma, stem cells).	Neither for nor against	Reviewed, New-added
	37.	For patients with low back pain, with radicular symptoms, there is insufficient evidence to recommend for or against epidural steroid injections.	Neither for nor against	Reviewed, New-replaced
	38.	For patients with low back pain, we suggest against spinal cord stimulation.	Weak against	Reviewed, New-added
Team Approach	39.	For patients with chronic low back pain, we suggest a multidisciplinary or interdisciplinary program. These programs should include at least one physical component and at least one other component of the biopsychosocial model (psychological, social, and/or occupational) used in an explicitly coordinated manner.	Weak for	Reviewed, Amended

[a]For additional information, see Determining Recommendation Strength and Direction in the full VA/DoD LBP CPG.
[b]For additional information, see Recommendation Categorization and Appendix D in the full VA/DoD LBP CPG.

Clinical Practice Guidelines on Surgery

The National Association of Spine Specialists (NASS) is a global multidisciplinary medical organization dedicated to evidence-based spine care through education, research, and advocacy. Their Clinical Practice Guideline Committee helps develop CPGs regarding the diagnosis and treatment of spinal disorders. In 2020, they, in conjunction with multiple contributing societies, produced CPGs for the diagnosis and management of low back pain.[275] Listed below are some of their more pertinent recommendations. Grade of Recommendation: A = Recommended; B = Suggested; C = May Be Considered; I = Insufficient or Conflicting Evidence

GENERAL RECOMMENDATIONS BASED ON EVIDENCE

- It is recommended that pain severity and functional impairment be used to stratify the risk of conversion from acute to chronic low back pain. Grade of Recommendation: A
- For chronic low back pain; back school is recommended to provide improvements in pain and function when compared with general medical care, modality care, or a simple handout at 6 to 12 months' follow-up. Grade of Recommendation: A

IMAGING STUDIES

- There is insufficient evidence to make a recommendation for or against the cost-effectiveness of the use of routine ordering of lumbar spine radiographs for low back pain lasting greater than 6 weeks in the absence of red flags. Grade of Recommendation: I
- There is insufficient evidence for or against imaging findings correlating with the presence of low back pain. Grade of Recommendation: I
- There is insufficient evidence to determine whether imaging findings contribute to decision making by health care providers to guide treatment. Grade of Recommendation: I

PSYCHOSOCIAL CONSIDERATIONS

- It is recommended that psychosocial factors and workplace factors be assessed when counseling patients regarding the risk of conversion from acute to chronic low back pain. Grade of Recommendation: A
- Cognitive behavioral therapy is recommended in combination with physical therapy, as compared with physical therapy alone, to improve pain levels in patients with low back pain over 12 months. Grade of Recommendation: A

MEDICATIONS

- Antidepressants are not recommended for the treatment of low back pain. Grade of Recommendation: A
- Topical capsicum is recommended as an effective treatment for low back pain on a short-term basis (3 months or less). Grade of Recommendation: Grade of Recommendation: A

- Nonselective NSAIDs are suggested for the treatment of low back pain. Grade of Recommendation: Grade of Recommendation: B
- There is insufficient evidence to make a recommendation for or against the use of lidocaine patch for the treatment of low back pain. Grade of Recommendation: I

COMPLEMENTARY THERAPIES

- Laser acupuncture provides no short-term or medium-term benefit over sham treatment for patients with chronic low back pain. Grade of Recommendation: A
- In patients with subacute or chronic low back pain, traction is not recommended to provide clinically significant improvements in pain or function. Grade of Recommendation: A
- In patients with chronic low back pain, the addition of acupuncture to usual care is recommended for short-term improvement of pain and function compared to usual care alone. Grade of Recommendation: A
- For patients with acute low back pain, spinal manipulative therapy (SMT) results in similar outcomes to no treatment, medication, or modalities. Periodically, short-term improvement is statistically better, but clinical significance is uncertain. Grade of Recommendation: A
- It is suggested that the use of heat for acute low back pain results in short-term improvements in pain. Grade of Recommendation: B
- It is suggested that the combination of laser therapy (low level or high level) with exercise provides better short-term relief of pain than either exercise or laser therapy alone. Grade of Recommendation: B
- It is suggested that, in patients with mild chronic low back pain, yoga may offer medium-term improvements in pain and function compared to usual care. Grade of Recommendation: B
- There is conflicting evidence that bracing results in improvements in pain and function in patients with subacute low back pain. Grade of Recommendation: I

SPINAL MANIPULATIVE THERAPY (SMT)

- It is suggested that the addition of exercise to SMT results in similar outcomes to SMT alone. Grade of Recommendation: B
- For patients with acute or chronic low back pain, SMT is an option to improve pain and function. Grade of Recommendation: C
- For patients with chronic low back pain, there is conflicting evidence that outcomes for SMT are clinically different from no treatment, medication, or modalities. Grade of Recommendation: I
- There is insufficient evidence to make a recommendation for or against the cost-utility of SMT for the treatment of low back pain. I

EXERCISE AND PHYSICAL THERAPY

- Aerobic exercise is recommended to improve pain, disability, and mental health in patients with nonspecific low back pain at short-term follow-up. Grade of Recommendation: A
- It is suggested that a specific stabilization exercise program is equivalent to a general exercise program. Grade of Recommendation: B
- It is suggested that, for patients with acute low back pain, those who exercise more at baseline and use exercise to facilitate recovery are predicted to have better functional outcomes over time than patients who do not exercise. Grade of Recommendation: B
- There is insufficient evidence that outcomes from a home-based exercise program are different than no care. Grade of Recommendation: I
- There is insufficient evidence for or against the use of dry needling as a treatment option for patients with chronic low back pain. Grade of Recommendation: I
- There is insufficient evidence that aerobic exercise improves pain, disability, and mental health in patients with nonspecific low back pain at long-term follow-up. Grade of Recommendation: I
- There is insufficient evidence to make a recommendation for or against lumbar stabilization in patients with chronic low back pain. Grade of Recommendation: I
- There is insufficient evidence that the McKenzie method results in different outcomes when compared to a dynamic strengthening program for the treatment of chronic low back pain. Grade of Recommendation: I

INTERVENTIONAL PROCEDURES

- In patients selected for intra-articular injection of steroids for facet pain, it is suggested that this provides no clinically meaningful improvement at 6 months. Grade of Recommendation: B
- The relief from Thermal radiofrequency ablation is durable for at least 6 months following the procedure. Grade of Recommendation: B
- Intradiskal steroids are suggested to provide short-term improvements in pain and function in patients with Modic changes. Grade of Recommendation: B
- Intradiskal electrothermal annuloplasty is suggested to provide 50% reduction in pain improvement in 40% to 50% of patients for up to 2 years. Grade of Recommendation: B
- Intra-articular steroid joint injections may be considered in patients with suspected SI joint pain. Grade of Recommendation: B
- There is insufficient evidence to make a recommendation for or against the use of interlaminar epidural steroid injections in patients with low back pain. Grade of Recommendation: Grade of Recommendation: I
- There is insufficient evidence to make a recommendation for or against the use of steroid injections into the zygapophyseal joint in patients with chronic back pain and a physical exam suggestive of facet-mediated pain. Grade of Recommendation: I
- There is insufficient evidence to make a recommendation for or against the use of spinal cord stimulation as a treatment for low back pain. Grade of Recommendation: I
- There is insufficient evidence to make a recommendation for or against a particular fusion technique for the treatment of low back pain. Grade of Recommendation: I
- There is insufficient evidence to make a recommendation for or against the cost-utility of surgical therapies versus medical/interventional therapies for low back pain. Grade of Recommendation: I

Academy of Orthopaedic Physical Therapy of the American Physical Therapy Association (2021)[276]

These guidelines updated previous guidelines from 2012 and were linked to the International Classification of Functioning, Disability, and Health. They provided CPGs regarding interventions used by PTs and other clinicians in patients with acute and chronic low back pain.[276] The strength of their evidence was based on levels I and II, and they evaluated four categories: (1) exercise, (2) manual and other-directed therapies, (3) classification systems, and (4) patient education. In distinction to other CPGs presented in this chapter (NASS), these CPGs demonstrate evidence to support the following interventions.

Some pertinent recommendations from there CPGs and their level of evidence include:

- PTs should use exercise training interventions, including trunk muscle strengthening and endurance, multimodal exercise interventions, specific trunk muscle activation exercise, aerobic exercise, aquatic exercise, and general exercise, for patients with chronic LBP. Grade of Recommendation: A
- PTs should use general exercise training to reduce pain and disability in older adults with chronic LBP. Grade of Recommendation: A
- PTs should use thrust or nonthrust joint mobilization to reduce pain and disability in patients with acute LBP Grade of Recommendation: A
- PTs may use thrust or nonthrust joint mobilization to reduce pain and disability in patients with chronic LBP with leg pain. Grade of Recommendation: B
- PTs may use soft tissue mobilization or massage in conjunction with other treatments to reduce pain and disability in the short term for patients with chronic LBP. Grade of Recommendation: B
- PTs may use active education strategies rather than passive strategies (i.e., providing access to educational materials only). Active education strategies include one-on-one education and self-management techniques, such as remaining active, pacing strategies, and back-protection techniques. Grade of Recommendation: B
- PTs may use standard education strategies and pain neuroscience education for patients with chronic LBP, but not as a standalone treatment. Grade of Recommendation: A
- PTs should deliver alongside other physical therapy interventions, such as exercise or manual therapy, to patients with chronic LBP. Grade of Recommendation: A
- PTs may use general education (i.e., postsurgical precautions, exercise, and resuming physical activity) for patients with LBP following lumbar spine surgery. Grade of Recommendation: B

REFERENCES

1. GBD 2017 Disease and Injury Incidence and Prevalence Collaborators. Global, regional, and national incidence, prevalence, and years lived with disability for 354 diseases and injuries for 195 countries and territories, 1990–2017: a systematic analysis for the Global Burden of Disease Study 2017 [published correction appears in Lancet. 2019 June 22;393(10190):e44]. *Lancet*. 2018;392(10159):1789–1858.
2. Fatoye F, Gebrye T, Odeyemi I. Real-world incidence, and prevalence of low back pain using routinely collected data. *Rheumatol Int*. 2019;39(4):619–626.
3. Lucas JW, Connor EM, Bose J. Back, lower limb, and upper limb pain among U.S. adults, 2019. *NCHS Data Brief*. 2021;(415):1–8.
4. Taimela S, Kujala UM, Salminen JJ, Viljanen T. The prevalence of low back pain among children and adolescents. A nationwide, cohort-based questionnaire survey in Finland. *Spine (Phila Pa 1976)*. 1997;22(10):1132–1136.
5. Hoy D, Bain C, Williams G, et al. A systematic review of the global prevalence of low back pain. *Arthritis Rheum*. 2012;64(6):2028–2037.
6. Katz JN. Lumbar disc disorders and low-back pain: socioeconomic factors and consequences. *J Bone Joint Surg Am*. 2006;88(2):21–24.
7. Kim LH, Vail D, Azad TD, et al. Expenditures and health care utilization among adults with newly diagnosed low back and lower extremity pain. *JAMA Netw Open*. 2019;2(5):e193676.
8. Allen D, Hines EW, Pazdernik V, Konecny LT, Breitenbach E. Four-year review of presenteeism data among employees of a large United States health care system: a retrospective prevalence study. *Hum Resour Health*. 2018;16(1):59.
9. Froud R, Patterson S, Eldridge S, et al. A systematic review and meta-synthesis of the impact of low back pain on people's lives. *BMC Musculoskelet Disord*. 2014;15:50.
10. Cosamalón-Gan I, Cosamalón-Gan T, Mattos-Piaggio G, Villar-Suárez V, García-Cosamalón J, Vega-Álvarez JA. Inflammation in the intervertebral disc herniation. Inflamación en la hernia del disco intervertebral. *Neurocirugia (Astur: Engl Ed)*. 2021;32(1):21–35.
11. White AA III, Gordon SL Synopsis: workshop on idiopathic low-back pain. *Spine (Phila Pa 1976)*. 1982;7(2):141–149.
12. Tanaka M, Török N, Tóth F, Szabó Á, Vécsei L Co-players in chronic pain: neuroinflammation and the tryptophan-kynurenine metabolic pathway. *Biomedicines*. 2021;9(8):897.
13. Denis F. The three-column spine and its significance in the classification of acute thoracolumbar spinal injuries. *Spine (Phila Pa 1976)*. 1983;8(8):817–831.
14. Ashton IK, Roberts S, Jaffray DC, Polak JM, Eisenstein SM. Neuropeptides in the human intervertebral disc. *J Orthop Res*. 1994;12(2):186–192.
15. Malik K, Nelson A. Overview of low back pain disorders. In: Benzon HT, Raja SN, Liu SS, Fishman SM, Cohen SP, eds. *Essentials of Pain Medicine*. 4th ed. Elsevier; 2018:193–206.e2.
16. Daly C, Ghosh P, Jenkin G, Oehme D, Goldschlager T. A review of animal models of intervertebral disc degeneration: pathophysiology, regeneration, and translation to the clinic. *Biomed Res Int*. 2016;2016:5952165.
17. Kreiner DS, Matz P, Bono CM, et al. Guideline summary review: an evidence-based clinical guideline for the diagnosis and treatment of low back pain [published correction appears in Spine J. 2021 February 24]. *Spine J*. 2020;20(7):998–1024.
18. Pangarkar SS, Kang DG, Sandbrink F, et al. VA/DoD clinical practice guideline: diagnosis and treatment of low back pain. *J Gen Intern Med*. 2019;34(11):2620–2629.
19. Stevans JM, Delitto A, Khoja SS, et al. Risk factors associated with transition from acute to chronic low back pain in US patients seeking primary care. *JAMA Netw Open*. 2021;4(2):e2037371.
20. Task Force on the Low Back Pain Clinical Practice Guidelines. American Osteopathic Association Guidelines for Osteopathic Manipulative Treatment (OMT) for patients with low back pain. *J Am Osteopath Assoc*. 2016;116(8):536–549.
21. Franke H, Franke JD, Fryer G. Osteopathic manipulative treatment for nonspecific low back pain: a systematic review and meta-analysis. *BMC Musculoskelet Disord*. 2014;15:286.
22. Melzack R. The short-form McGill Pain Questionnaire. *Pain*. 1987;30(2):191–197.
23. Bennett MI, Smith BH, Torrance N, Potter J. The S-LANSS score for identifying pain of predominantly neuropathic origin: validation for use in clinical and postal research. *J Pain*. 2005;6(3):149–158.
24. Fairbank JC, Couper J, Davies JB, O'Brien JP. The Oswestry low back pain disability questionnaire. *Physiotherapy*. 1980;66(8):271–273.
25. Hochheim M, Ramm P, Wunderlich M, Amelung V. Association between chronic low back pain and regular exercise, sedentary behaviour and mental health before and during COVID-19 pandemic: insights from a large-scale cross-sectional study in Germany. *BMC Musculoskelet Disord*. 2022;23(1):860.
26. Verhagen AP, Downie A, Popal N, Maher C, Koes BW. Red flags presented in current low back pain guidelines: a review. *Eur Spine J*. 2016;25(9):2788–2802.
27. Premkumar A, Godfrey W, Gottschalk MB, Boden SD. Red flags for low back pain are not always really red: a prospective evaluation of the clinical utility of commonly used screening questions for low back pain. *J Bone Joint Surg Am*. 2018;100(5):368–374.
28. Wong HK. Should we still use red flags in the diagnosis of low back pain? Commentary on an article by Ajay Premkumar, MD, MPH, et al.: "Red flags for low back pain are not always really red. A prospective evaluation of the clinical utility of commonly used screening questions for low back pain". *J Bone Joint Surg Am*. 2018;100(5):e31.
29. Katzan IL, Thompson NR, George SZ, Passek S, Frost F, Stilphen M. The use of STarT back screening tool to predict functional disability

outcomes in patients receiving physical therapy for low back pain. *Spine J.* 2019;19(4):645–654.

30. Neeley DK, George SZ, Minick K, Snow G, Brennan G. Four variables were sufficient for low back pain: determining which patient-reported tools pain and disability improvements. *J Orthop Sports Phys Ther.* 2022;52(10):685–693.
31. Knezevic NN, Candido KD, Vlaeyen JWS, Van Zundert J, Cohen SP. Low back pain. *Lancet.* 2021;398(10294):78–92.
32. Schultz MJ, Licciardone JC. The effect of long-term opioid use on back-specific disability and health-related quality of life in patients with chronic low back pain. *J Osteopath Med.* 2022;122(9):469–479.
33. Al Nezari NH, Schneiders AG, Hendrick PA. Neurological examination of the peripheral nervous system to diagnose lumbar spinal disc herniation with suspected radiculopathy: a systematic review and meta-analysis. *Spine J.* 2013;13(6):657–674.
34. Denteneer L, Van Daele U, Truijen S, De Hertogh W, Meirte J, Stassijns G. Reliability of physical functioning tests in patients with low back pain: a systematic review. *Spine J.* 2018;18(1):190–207.
35. Nee RJ, Coppieters MW, Boyd BS. Reliability of the straight leg raise test for suspected lumbar radicular pain: a systematic review with meta-analysis. *Musculoskelet Sci Pract.* 2022;59:102529.
36. Kuris EO, McDonald CL, Palumbo MA, Daniels AH. Evaluation and management of cauda equina syndrome. *Am J Med.* 2021;134(12):1483–1489.
37. Seffinger MA. *The Glossary of Osteopathic Terminology, in Foundations of Osteopathic Medicine.* 4th ed. Wolters Kluwer; 2018:1563–1594.
38. Janda V. Va'Vrova'. 1996. Sensory motor stimulation. In Liebenson C, ed. *Rehabilitation of the Spine.* Williams & Wilkins; 319–328.
39. DeStefano L. *Greenman's Principles of Manual Medicine.* 5th ed. Wolters Kluwer; 2017.
40. Sanchez J, Brohard J, Thai R. An exploration of Zink's common compensatory pattern: comparing myofascial restrictions to segmental spinal somatic dysfunctions: a retrospective study. *AAO Journal.* 2018;28(4):16–22.
41. Rodríguez-Pastor JA, Caro-Puértolas B, Caña-Pino A, Sánchez-Preciado AM, Garrido-Ardila EM, Apolo-Arenas MD. Effect of osteopathic manipulation of the sacroiliac joint vs electrotherapy on pain and functional disability in patients with low back pain: a pilot study. *J Back Musculoskelet Rehabil.* 2022;35(6):1219–1226.
42. Kuchera M. *49C Osteopathic Approach to Diagnosing and Treating Somatic Dysfunction in the Extremities, in Foundations of Osteopathic Medicine.* 4th ed. Wolters Kluwer; 2018, 1483–1515.
43. Kappler RE. Role of psoas mechanism in low-back complaints. *J Am Osteopath Assoc.* 1973;72(8):794–801.
44. Yu Q, Huang H, Zhang Z, et al. The association between pelvic asymmetry and non-specific chronic low back pain as assessed by the global postural system. *BMC Musculoskelet Disord.* 2020;21(1):596.
45. Villalta Santos L, Lisboa Córdoba L, Benite Palma Lopes J, et al. Active visceral manipulation associated with conventional physiotherapy in people with chronic low back pain and visceral dysfunction: a preliminary, randomized, controlled, double-blind clinical trial. *J Chiropr Med.* 2019;18(2):79–89.
46. Cutler MJ, Holland BS, Stupski BA, Gamber RG, Smith ML. Cranial manipulation can alter sleep latency and sympathetic nerve activity in humans: a pilot study. *J Altern Complement Med.* 2005;11(1):103–108.
47. Jarvik JG, Deyo RA. Diagnostic evaluation of low back pain with emphasis on imaging. *Ann Intern Med.* 2002;137(7):586–597.
48. Bickle I. Winking owl sign. Case study. *Radiopaedia.org* Accessed July 02, 2023. https://doi.org/10.53347/rID-21937
49. Shraim BA, Shraim MA, Ibrahim AR, Elgamal ME, Al-Omari B, Shraim M. The association between early MRI and length of disability in acute lower back pain: a systematic review and narrative synthesis. *BMC Musculoskelet Disord.* 2021;22(1):983.
50. Webster BS, Cifuentes M. Relationship of early magnetic resonance imaging for work-related acute low back pain with disability and medical utilization outcomes. *J Occup Environ Med.* 2010;52(9):900–907.
51. Lateef H, Patel D. What is the role of imaging in acute low back pain? *Curr Rev Musculoskelet Med.* 2009;2(2):69–73.
52. Borenstein DJ, Wiesel, SW, Bowden, SD. eds. *Low Back and Neck Pain.* WB Saunders; 2004
53. Kreiner DS, Hwang SW, Easa JE, et al. An evidence-based clinical guideline for the diagnosis and treatment of lumbar disc herniation with radiculopathy. *Spine J.* 2014;14(1):180–191.
54. Qaseem A, Wilt TJ, McLean RM, et al. Noninvasive treatments for acute, subacute, and chronic low back pain: a clinical practice guideline from the American College of Physicians. *Ann Intern Med.* 2017;166(7):514–530.
55. Department of Veterans Affairs, DoD. *VA/DoD Clinical Practice Guideline for the Diagnosis and Treatment of Low Back Pain.* 3rd ed. U.S. Government Printing Office; 022. https://www.healthquality.va.gov/guidelines/Pain/lbp/VADoDLBPCPGFinal508.pdf
56. van Wambeke P, Desomer A, Jonckheer P, Depreitere B. The Belgian national guideline on low back pain and radicular pain: key roles for rehabilitation, assessment of rehabilitation potential and the PRM specialist. *Eur J Phys Rehabil Med.* 2020;56(2):220–227.
57. Stochkendahl MJ, Kjaer P, Hartvigsen J, et al. National Clinical Guidelines for non-surgical treatment of patients with recent onset low back pain or lumbar radiculopathy. *Eur Spine J.* 2018;27(1):60–75.
58. Galbraith W, Smith M, Seffinger MA. Treating patients with low back pain: evidence vs practice. *J Am Osteopath Assoc.* 2018;118(7):486–487.
59. Foster NE, Anema JR, Cherkin D, et al. Prevention and treatment of low back pain: evidence, challenges, and promising directions. *Lancet.* 2018;391(10137):2368–2383.
60. Steffens D, Maher CG, Pereira LS, et al. Prevention of low back pain: a systematic review and meta-analysis. *JAMA Intern Med.* 2016;176(2):199–208.
61. Nkhata LA, Brink Y, Ernstzen D, Louw QA. A systematic review on self-management education campaigns for back pain. *S Afr J Physiother.* 2019;75(1):1314.
62. Hirschberg GG, Froetscher L, Naeim F. Iliolumbar syndrome as a common cause of low back pain: diagnosis and prognosis. *Arch Phys Med Rehabil.* 1979;60(9):415–419.
63. Maigne R. Low back pain of thoracolumbar origin. *Arch Phys Med Rehabil.* 1980;61:389–395.
64. Randhawa S, Garvin G, Roth M, Wozniak A, Miller T. Maigne syndrome—a potentially treatable yet underdiagnosed cause of low back pain: a review. *J Back Musculoskelet Rehabil.* 2022;35(1):153–159.
65. Kim SR, Lee MJ, Lee SJ, Suh YS, Kim DH, Hong JH. Thoracolumbar junction syndrome causing pain around posterior iliac crest: a case report. *Korean J Fam Med.* 2013;34(2):152–155.
66. Broudeur P, Larroque CH, Passeron R, Pellegrino J, Le syndrome ilio-lombaire. Une syndesmo-périostite de la crête iliaque. Arguments cliniques, radiologiques, thérapeutiques. Diagnostic avec la lombo-sciatique. 440 observations [Iliolumbar syndrome. A syndesmoperiostitis of the iliac crest. Clinical, radiologic and therapeutic summary. Diagnosis with lumbar sciatica. 440 cases]. *Rev Rhum Mal Osteoartic.* 1982;49(10):693–698.
67. Chaudhry SR, Imonugo O, Jozsa F, Chaudhry K. Anatomy, abdomen and pelvis: ligaments. In: *StatPearls [Internet].* StatPearls Publishing; 2023.
68. Maigne JY, Maigne R. Trigger point of the posterior iliac crest: painful iliolumbar ligament insertion or cutaneous dorsal ramus pain? An anatomical study. *Arch Phys Med Rehabil.* 1991;72(10):734–737.
69. Rucco V, Basadonna PT, Gasparini D. Anatomy of the iliolumbar ligament: a review of its anatomy and a magnetic resonance study. *Am J Phys Med Rehabil.* 1996;75(6):451–455.
70. Maigne R. *Diagnosis and Treatment of Pain of Vertebral Origin: A Manual Medicine Approach.* Williams & Wilkins; 1996.
71. Yamamoto I, Panjabi MM, Oxland TR, Crisco JJ. The role of the iliolumbar ligament in the lumbosacral junction. *Spine (Phila Pa 1976).* 1990;15(11):1138–1141.
72. Collée G, Dijkmans BA, Vandenbroucke JP, Cats A. Iliac crest pain syndrome in low back pain: frequency and features. *J Rheumatol.* 1991;18:1064–1067.
73. Kozera K, Ciszek B, Szaro P. Posterior branches of lumbar spinal nerves—Part III: spinal dorsal ramus mediated back pain—pathomechanism, symptomatology and diagnostic work-up. *Ortop Traumatol Rehabil.* 2017;19(4):315–321.
74. Nayak BK, Singh DK, Kumar N, Jaiswal B. Recovering from nonspecific low back pain despair: ultrasound-guided intervention in iliolumbar syndrome. *Indian J Radiol Imaging.* 2020;30(4):448–452.

75. Maigne R. In: *Diagnosis and Treatment of Pain of Vertebral Origin.* Choi H, trans. Koonja Publishers; 2000.
76. Dydyk AM, Sapra A. Psoas syndrome. [Updated 2022 October 24]. In: *StatPearls [Internet].* StatPearls Publishing; 2022. https://www.ncbi.nlm.nih.gov/books/NBK551701
77. Fryette HH. The psoas muscle. *J Am Osteopath Assoc.* 1937;36(10).
78. Tufo A, Desai GJ, Cox WJ. Psoas syndrome: a frequently missed diagnosis. *J Am Osteopath Assoc.* 2012;112(8):522–528.
79. Laor T. Hip and groin pain in adolescents [published correction appears in Pediatr Radiol. 2010 August;40(8):1461]. *Pediatr Radiol.* 2010;40(4): 461–467.
80. Di Sante L, Paoloni M, De Benedittis S, Tognolo L, Santilli V. Groin pain and iliopsoas bursitis: always a cause-effect relationship? *J Back Musculoskelet Rehabil.* 2014;27(1):103–106.
81. Di Lorenzo L, Jennifer Y, Pappagallo M. Psoas impingement syndrome in hip osteoarthritis. *Joint Bone Spine.* 2009;76(1):98–100.
82. Ala Eddine T, Remy F, Chantelot C, Giraud F, Migaud H, Duquennoy A. Douleur inguinale isolée après prothèse totale de hanche et souffrance de l'ilio-psoas [Anterior iliopsoas impingement after total hip arthroplasty: diagnosis and conservative treatment in 9 cases]. *Rev Chir Orthop Reparatrice Appar Mot.* 2001;87(8):815–819.
83. Yeap PM, Robinson P. Ultrasound diagnostic and therapeutic injections of the hip and groin. *J Belg Soc Radiol.* 2017;101(2):6.
84. Heinking K. *41B Diagnosis and Treatment of Somatic Dysfunction in the Patient with Low Back Pain in Foundations of Osteopathic Medicine.* 4th ed. Wolters Kluwer; 2018, 1040–1081.
85. Moriarty CM, Baker RJ. A pain in the psoas. *Sports Health.* 2016;8(6): 568–572.
86. Eldemire F, Goto KK. Osteopathic manipulative treatment: muscle energy and counterstrain procedure - psoas muscle procedures. In: *StatPearls [Internet].* StatPearls Publishing; 2022.
87. Licciardone JC, Kearns CM, Crow WT. Changes in biomechanical dysfunction and low back pain reduction with osteopathic manual treatment: results from the OSTEOPATHIC Trial. *Man Ther.* 2014;19(4): 324–330.
88. Adib F, Johnson AJ, Hennrikus WL, Nasreddine A, Kocher M, Yen YM. Iliopsoas tendonitis after hip arthroscopy: prevalence, risk factors and treatment algorithm. *J Hip Preserv Surg.* 2018;5(4):362–369.
89. Hensel K, Crapo P. Short leg syndrome: a common cause of low back pain. *Osteopathic Family Physician.* 2016;8(6):1.
90. Knutson GA. Anatomic and functional leg-length inequality: a review and recommendation for clinical decision-making. Part I, anatomic leg-length inequality: prevalence, magnitude, effects and clinical significance. *Chiropr Osteopat.* 2005;13:11.
91. Juhl JH, Ippolito Cremin TM, Russell G. Prevalence of frontal plane pelvic postural asymmetry–part 1 [published correction appears in J Am Osteopath Assoc. 2005 January;105(1):5]. *J Am Osteopath Assoc.* 2004;104(10):411–421.
92. Friberg O. Clinical symptoms and biomechanics of lumbar spine and hip joint in leg length inequality. *Spine (Phila Pa 1976).* 1983;8(6): 643–651.
93. Greenman PE. Lift therapy: use and abuse. *J Am Osteopath Assoc.* 1979; 79(4):238–250.
94. Irvin RE. Reduction of lumbar scoliosis by use of a heel lift to level the sacral base. *J Am Osteopath Assoc.* 1991;91(1):34–44.
95. Irvin RE. 9 Suboptimal posture: the origin of most idiopathic pain of the musculoskeletal system: alleviation of the majority of pain of the musculoskeletal system without known cause by use of orthotics and manual manipulation to optimize normal posture towards an ideal configuration. In Vleeming A, Mooney V, Dorman T, Snijders C, Stoeckart R, eds. *Movement, Stability & Low Back Pain: The Essential Role of the Pelvis.* Churchill-Livingstone; 1997:133–155.
96. Kuchera M *29 Postural considerations in Osteopathic Diagnosis and Treatment, in Foundations of Osteopathic Medicine.* 4th ed. Wolters Kluwer; 2018:696–745.
97. Khamis S, Carmeli E. A new concept for measuring leg length discrepancy. *J Orthop.* 2017;14(2):276–280.
98. Zink GJ, Lawson WB. An osteopathic structural examination and functional interpretation of the soma. *Osteopathic Annals.* 1979;7:12–19.
99. Physiopedia. Leg length discrepancy. https://www.physio-pedia.com/Leg_Length_Discrepancy
100. Novacheck TF. The biomechanics of running. *Gait Posture.* 1998;7(1): 77–95.
101. Nelson KE, Mnahbi, KS. Chpt. 36 The patient with back pain short In: Nelson, KE, Glonek T, eds. *Somatic Dysfunction in Osteopathic Family Practice.* 2nd ed. Wolters Kluwer Health; 2015:415–431.
102. Travell J, Simons D. *Ch 4 Quadratus lumborum. Myofascial Pain and Dysfunction: The Trigger Point Manual.* Williams and Wilkins. 1992;2: 28–88.
103. Gurney B. Leg length discrepancy. *Gait Posture.* 2002;15(2):195–206.
104. Rannisto S, Okuloff A, Uitti J, et al. Leg-length discrepancy is associated with low back pain among those who must stand while working. *BMC Musculoskelet Disord.* 2015;16:110.
105. Alfuth M, Fichter P, Knicker A. Leg length discrepancy: a systematic review on the validity and reliability of clinical assessments and imaging diagnostics used in clinical practice. *PLoS One.* 2021;16(12): e0261457.
106. Kuchera ML, Bemben MG. Comparison of manual and computerized methods of assessing postural radiographs (abstract). *JAOA.* 1990;90(8):714–715.
107. Khamis S, Leisman G, Carmeli E. Detecting the presence of leg length discrepancy based on gait deviations and functional measurement of leg length during walking. *BMJ Case Rep.* 2017;2017:bcr2017219645.
108. Gross MT, Burns CB, Chapman SW, et al. Reliability and validity of rigid lift and pelvic leveling device method in assessing functional leg length inequality. *J Orthop Sports Phys Ther.* 1998;27(4):285–294.
109. Petrone MR, Guinn J, Reddin A, Sutlive TG, Flynn TW, Garber MP. The accuracy of the Palpation Meter (PALM) for measuring pelvic crest height difference and leg length discrepancy. *J Orthop Sports Phys Ther.* 2003;33(6):319–325.
110. Rancont CM. Chronic psoas syndrome caused by the inappropriate use of a heel lift. *J Am Osteopath Assoc.* 2007;107(9):415–418.
111. Kim C, Nevitt M, Guermazi A, et al. Brief report: leg length inequality and hip osteoarthritis in the multicenter osteoarthritis study and the osteoarthritis initiative. *Arthritis Rheumatol.* 2018;70(10):1572–1576.
112. Harvey WF, Yang M, Cooke TD, et al. Association of leg-length inequality with knee osteoarthritis: a cohort study. *Ann Intern Med.* 2010;152(5):287–295.
113. Helig D. Principles of lift therapy. In: Peterson B, ed. *Postural Balance and Imbalance 1983 AAO Yearbook.* American Academy of Osteopathy; 1983:102–112.
114. Gofton JP. Persistent low back pain and leg length disparity. *J Rheumatol.* 1985;12(4):747–750.
115. Helliwell M. Leg length inequality and low back pain. *Practitioner.* 1985;229(1403):483–485.
116. D'Amico M, Kinel E, Roncoletta P. Leg length discrepancy and nonspecific low back pain: 3-d stereophotogrammetric quantitative posture evaluation confirms positive effects of customized heel-lift orthotics. *Front Bioeng Biotechnol.* 2022;9:743132.
117. Rannisto S, Okuloff A, Uitti J, et al. Correction of leg-length discrepancy among meat cutters with low back pain: a randomized controlled trial. *BMC Musculoskelet Disord.* 2019;20(1):105.
118. Irvin R. Disequilibrium of posture as root cause for preponderance of chronic neuromusculoskeletal pain. *Ann Musc Disord.* 2017;1(1):1006.
119. Koczewski P, Shadi M. Lower limb inequality treatment with subtrochanteric femoral shortening osteotomy fixed with intramedullary nail. *Pol Orthop Traumatol.* 2012;77:65–71.
120. Koczewski P, Shadi M, Napiontek M, Marciniak W. Powikłania wydłużania uda za pomoca aparatu Ilizarowa w modyfikacji włoskiej [Problems, obstacles and complications of femoral lengthening with the use of the Italian modification of the Ilizarov device]. *Chir Narzadow Ruchu Ortop Pol.* 2000;65(3):277–286.
121. Kuchera ML. 39 treatment of gravitational strain pathophysiology. In Vleeming A, Mooney V, Dorman T, Snijders C, Stoeckart R, eds. *Movement, Stability & Low Back Pain: The Essential Role of the Pelvis.* Churchill-Livingstone: 1997;477–499.
122. Arendt-Nielsen L, Svensson P. Referred muscle pain: basic and clinical findings. *Clin J Pain.* 2001;17(1):11–19.

123. Urits I, Burshtein A, Sharma M, et al. Low back pain, a comprehensive review: pathophysiology, diagnosis, and treatment. *Curr Pain Headache Rep*. 2019;23(3):23.
124. da Silva JAP, Woolf AD. Inflammatory low back pain. In: *Rheumatology in Practice*. Springer; 2010:241–249. https://doi.org/10.1007/978-1-84882-581-9_24
125. Mehta N, Maloney GE, Scrivani SJ, Bana DS, eds. *Head, Face, and Neck Pain Science, Evaluation, and Management*; John Wiley & Sons; 2011: 534.
126. Silverthorn DU. *Human Physiology: An Integrated Approach*. 5th ed. Pearson; 2010:348.
127. Mense S. Neurobiologische mechanismen der ubertragung von muskelschmerz [Neurobiological mechanisms of muscle pain referral.]. *Schmerz*. 1993;7(4):241–249.
128. Simmons JW Jr, Ricketson R, McMillin JN. Painful lumbosacral sensory distribution patterns: embryogenesis to adulthood. *Orthop Rev*. 1993; 22(10):1110–1118.
129. Yaprak M. The axon reflex. *Neuroanatomy*. 2008;7:17–19.
130. Lidbeck J. Central hyperexcitability in chronic musculoskeletal pain: a conceptual breakthrough with multiple clinical implications. *Pain Res Manag*. 2002;7(2):81–92.
131. Bogduk N. On the definitions and physiology of back pain, referred pain, and radicular pain. *Pain*. 2009;147(1–3):17–19.
132. Klineberg E, Mazanec D, Orr D, Demicco R, Bell G, McLain R. Masquerade: medical causes of back pain. *Cleve Clin J Med*. 2007; 74(12):905–913.
133. Graven-Nielsen T, Arendt-Nielsen L, Svensson P, Jensen TS. Stimulus-response functions in areas with experimentally induced referred muscle pain–a psychophysical study. *Brain Res*. 1997;744(1):121–128.
134. Graven-Nielsen T, Arendt-Nielsen L, Svensson P, Jensen TS. Quantification of local and referred muscle pain in humans after sequential i.m. injections of hypertonic saline. *Pain*. 1997;69(1–2):111–117.
135. Forsthoefel C. Lumbar disc herniation. *OrthoBullets*. www.orthobullets.com/spine/2035/lumbar-disc-herniation
136. Anderson JT, Haas AR, Percy R, Woods ST, Ahn UM, Ahn NU. Lumbar diskography and failed back syndrome in patients receiving workers' compensation. *Orthopedics*. 2015;38(11):e951–e958.
137. Mijiyawa M, Oniankitan O, Kolani B, Koriko T. Low back pain in hospital outpatients in Lomé (Togo). *Joint Bone Spine*. 2000;67(6): 533–538.
138. Oster BA, Kikanloo SR, Levine NL, Lian J, Cho W. Systematic review of outcomes following 10-year mark of spine patient outcomes research trial for intervertebral disc herniation. *Spine (Phila Pa 1976)*. 2020;45(12): 825–831.
139. Berry JA, Elia C, Saini HS, Miulli DE. A review of lumbar radiculopathy, diagnosis, and treatment. *Cureus*. 2019;11(10):e5934.
140. Jordan J, Konstantinou K, O'Dowd J. Herniated lumbar disc. *BMJ Clin Evid*. 2009;2009:1118.
141. Tarulli AW, Raynor EM. Lumbosacral radiculopathy. *Neurol Clin*. 2007;25(2):387–405.
142. Physiopedia. Radiculopathy lumbar. 2022. Accessed February 2, 2025. https://www.physio-pedia.com/Lumbar_Radiculopathy
143. Kim R, Kim RH, Kim CH, et al. The incidence and risk factors for lumbar or sciatic scoliosis in lumbar disc herniation and the outcomes after percutaneous endoscopic discectomy. *Pain Physician*. 2015;18(6):555–564.
144. Battié MC, Ortega-Alonso A, Niemelainen R, et al. Lumbar spinal stenosis is a highly genetic condition partly mediated by disc degeneration. *Arthritis Rheumatol*. 2014;66(12):3505–3510.
145. Battié MC, Videman T. Lumbar disc degeneration: epidemiology and genetics. *J Bone Joint Surg Am*. 2006;88(2):3–9.
146. Battié MC, Videman T, Kaprio J, et al. The Twin Spine Study: contributions to a changing view of disc degeneration. *Spine J*. 2009;9(1): 47–59.
147. Donnally III CJ, Hanna A, Varacallo M. Lumbar degenerative disk disease. [Updated 2023 Jan 15]. In: *StatPearls [Internet]*. StatPearls Publishing; 2023. https://www.ncbi.nlm.nih.gov/books/NBK448134/
148. Phillips FM, Slosar PJ, Youssef JA, Andersson G, Papatheofanis F Lumbar spine fusion for chronic low back pain due to degenerative disc disease: a systematic review. *Spine (Phila Pa 1976)*. 2013;38(7):E409–E422.
149. Skaggs D. Pediatric spondylolysis & spondylolisthesis. *Orthobullets*. Accessed May 10, 2023. https://www.orthobullets.com/spine/2058/pediatric-spondylolysis-and-spondylolisthesis
150. Leone A, Cianfoni A, Cerase A, Magarelli N, Bonomo L. Lumbar spondylolysis: a review. *Skeletal Radiol*. 2011;40(6):683–700.
151. Sutton JH, Guin PD, Theiss SM. Acute lumbar spondylolysis in intercollegiate athletes. *J Spinal Disord Tech*. 2012;25(8):422–425.
152. Moore DW. Degenerative spondylolisthesis. *Orthobullets*. Accessed May 10, 2023. https://www.orthobullets.com/spine/2039/degenerative-spondylolisthesis
153. Dagenais S, Yelland MJ, Del Mar C, Schoene ML. Prolotherapy injections for chronic low-back pain. *Cochrane Database Syst Rev*. 2007; 2007(2):CD004059.
154. Oster BA, Kikanloo SR, Levine NL, Lian J, Cho W. Systematic review of outcomes following 10-year mark of Spine Patient Outcomes Research Trial (SPORT) for degenerative spondylolisthesis. *Spine (Phila Pa 1976)*. 2020;45(12):820–824.
155. Arbit E, Pannullo S. Lumbar stenosis: a clinical review. *Clin Orthop Relat Res*. 2001;(384):137–143.
156. Ahn L, Moore DW. Lumbar spinal stenosis. *Orthobullets*. Accessed May 10, 2023. https://www.orthobullets.com/spine/2037/lumbar-spinal-stenosis
157. Katonis P, Kampouroglou A, Aggelopoulos A, et al. Pregnancy-related low back pain. *Hippokratia*. 2011;15(3):205–210.
158. Brown S, Lumley J. Maternal health after childbirth: results of an Australian population-based survey. *Br J Obstet Gynaecol*. 1998;105(2):156–161.
159. Patel RR, Peters TJ, Murphy DJ. Is operative delivery associated with postnatal back pain at eight weeks and eight months? A cohort study. *Acta Obstet Gynecol Scand*. 2007;86(11):1322–1327.
160. Omoke NI, Amaraegbulam PI, Umeora OUJ, Okafor LC. Prevalence and risk factors for low back pain during pregnancy among women in Abakaliki, Nigeria. *Pan Afr Med J*. 2021;39:70.
161. Zhang M, Cooley C, Ziadni MS, Mackey I, Flood P. Association between history of childbirth and chronic, functionally significant back pain in later life. *BMC Womens Health*. 2023;23(1):4.
162. Hensel KL, Buchanan S, Brown SK, Rodriguez M, Cruser dA. Pregnancy research on osteopathic manipulation optimizing treatment effects: the PROMOTE study. *Am J Obstet Gynecol*. 2015;212(1):108.e1–108.e1089.
163. Licciardone JC, Aryal S. Prevention of progressive back-specific dysfunction during pregnancy: an assessment of osteopathic manual treatment based on Cochrane Back Review Group criteria. *J Am Osteopath Assoc*. 2013;113(10):728–736.
164. Franke H, Franke JD, Belz S, Fryer G. Osteopathic manipulative treatment for low back and pelvic girdle pain during and after pregnancy: a systematic review and meta-analysis. *J Bodyw Mov Ther*. 2017;21(4): 752–762.
165. Ruffini N, D'Alessandro G, Cardinali L, Frondaroli F, Cerritelli F. Osteopathic manipulative treatment in gynecology and obstetrics: a systematic review. *Complement Ther Med*. 2016;26:72–78.
166. Mørkved S, Salvesen KA, Schei B, Lydersen S, Bø K. Does group training during pregnancy prevent lumbopelvic pain? A randomized clinical trial. *Acta Obstet Gynecol Scand*. 2007;86(3):276–282.
167. van Benten E, Pool J, Mens J, Pool-Goudzwaard A. Recommendations for physical therapists on the treatment of lumbopelvic pain during pregnancy: a systematic review. *J Orthop Sports Phys Ther*. 2014;44(7): 464–A15.
168. Licciardone JC, Aryal S. Manual therapy, exercise, and education for low back pain and pelvic pain during pregnancy. *Am J Obstet Gynecol*. 2014;210(6):592–593.
169. Keisler B, Carter C. Abdominal aortic aneurysm. *Am Fam Physician*. 2015;91(8):538–543.
170. Haque K, Bhargava P. Abdominal aortic aneurysm. *Am Fam Physician*. 2022;106(2):165–172.
171. Cates JR. Abdominal aortic aneurysms: clinical diagnosis and management. *J Manipulative Physiol Ther*. 1997;20(8):557–561.
172. García-Macero RA, Balbuena Domínguez JC, Fernández-Castañón Martínez E, Herbello Rodríguez A. Dolor lumbar y aneurisma de aorta abdominal: red flags [Low back pain and abdominal aortic aneurysm: red flags]. *Rehabilitacion (Madr)*. 2022;56(1):74–77.

173. Lavy C, Marks P, Dangas K, Todd N. Cauda equina syndrome-a practical guide to definition and classification. *Int Orthop.* 2022;46(2): 165–169.
174. Bulloch L, Thompson K, Spector L. Cauda equina syndrome. *Orthop Clin North Am.* 2022;53(2):247–254.
175. Fraser S, Roberts L, Murphy E. Cauda equina syndrome: a literature review of its definition and clinical presentation. *Arch Phys Med Rehabil.* 2009;90(11):1964–1968.
176. Forsthoefel C, Moore D. Cauda equina syndrome. *Orthobullets.* Accessed May 10, 2023. https://www.orthobullets.com/spine/2065/cauda-equina-syndrome
177. Kumar V, Baburaj V, Rajnish RK, Dhatt SS. Outcomes of cauda equina syndrome due to lumbar disc herniation after surgical management and the factors affecting it: a systematic review and meta-analysis of 22 studies with 852 cases. *Eur Spine J.* 2022;31(2):353–363.
178. Orhurhu VJ, Chu R, Gill J. Failed back surgery syndrome. In: *StatPearls [Internet].* StatPearls Publishing; 2022.
179. Christelis N, Simpson B, Russo M, et al. Persistent spinal pain syndrome: a proposal for failed back surgery syndrome and ICD-11. *Pain Med.* 2021;22(4):807–818.
180. Inoue S, Kamiya M, Nishihara M, Arai YP, Ikemoto T, Ushida T. Prevalence, characteristics, and burden of failed back surgery syndrome: the influence of various residual symptoms on patient satisfaction and quality of life as assessed by a nationwide Internet survey in Japan. *J Pain Res.* 2017; 10:811–823.
181. Clancy C, Quinn A, Wilson F. The aetiologies of failed back surgery syndrome: a systematic review. *J Back Musculoskelet Rehabil.* 2017;30(3): 395–402.
182. Slipman CW, Shin CH, Patel RK, et al. Etiologies of failed back surgery syndrome. *Pain Med.* 2002;3(3):200–217.
183. Miller B, Gatchel RJ, Lou L, Stowell A, Robinson R, Polatin PB. Interdisciplinary treatment of failed back surgery syndrome (FBSS): a comparison of FBSS and non-FBSS patients. *Pain Pract.* 2005;5(3): 190–202.
184. Carragee EJ, Alamin TF, Miller JL, Carragee JM. Discographic, MRI and psychosocial determinants of low back pain disability and remission: a prospective study in subjects with benign persistent back pain. *Spine J.* 2005;5(1):24–35.
185. Chan CW, Peng P. Failed back surgery syndrome. *Pain Med.* 2011; 12(4):577–606.
186. Daniell JR, Osti OL. Failed back surgery syndrome: a review article. *Asian Spine J.* 2018;12(2):372–379.
187. Greenman PE. Syndromes of the L-spine, pelvis and sacrum. In: Stanton D, ed. *Manual Medicine. Physical Med Rehabil Clin North Am.* WB Saunders; 1996;7(4):733.
188. Bogduk N. Management of chronic low back pain. *Med J Aust.* 2004; 180(2):79–83.
189. Thomson S, Jacques L. Demographic characteristics of patients with severe neuropathic pain secondary to failed back surgery syndrome. *Pain Pract.* 2009;9(3):206–215.
190. Guyer RD, Patterson M, Ohnmeiss DD. Failed back surgery syndrome: diagnostic evaluation. *J Am Acad Orthop Surg.* 2006;14(9):534–543.
191. Amirdelfan K, Webster L, Poree L, Sukul V, McRoberts P. Treatment options for failed back surgery syndrome patients with refractory chronic pain: an evidence based approach. *Spine (Phila Pa 1976).* 2017;42(14):S41–S52.
192. Licciardone JC, King HH, Hensel KL, Williams DG. OSTEOPAThic Health outcomes in chronic low back pain: the OSTEOPATHIC Trial. *Osteopath Med Prim Care.* 2008;2:5.
193. Licciardone JC, Kearns CM, Minotti DE. Outcomes of osteopathic manual treatment for chronic low back according to baseline pain severity: results from the OSTEOPATHIC Trial. *Man Ther.* 2013;18(6): 533–540.
194. Licciardone JC, Aryal S. Clinical response and relapse in patients with chronic low back pain following osteopathic manual treatment: results from the OSTEOPATHIC Trial. *Man Ther.* 2014;19(6):541–548.
195. Licciardone JC, Gatchel RJ, Aryal S. Targeting patient subgroups with chronic low back pain for osteopathic manipulative treatment: responder analyses from a randomized controlled trial. *J Am Osteopath Assoc.* 2016;116(3):156–168.
196. Delitto A, Piva SR, Moore CG, et al. Surgery versus nonsurgical treatment of lumbar spinal stenosis: a randomized trial. *Ann Intern Med.* 2015;162(7):465–473.
197. Keller A, Brox JI, Gunderson R, Holm I, Friis A, Reikerås O. Trunk muscle strength, cross-sectional area, and density in patients with chronic low back pain randomized to lumbar fusion or cognitive intervention and exercises. *Spine (Phila Pa 1976).* 2004;29(1):3–8.
198. Cramer H, Haller H, Lauche R, Dobos G. Mindfulness-based stress reduction for low back pain. A systematic review. *BMC Complement Altern Med.* 2012;12:162.
199. Cho JH, Lee JH, Song KS, et al. Treatment outcomes for patients with failed back surgery. *Pain Physician.* 2017;20(1):E29–E43.
200. Marineo G, Iorno V, Gandini C, Moschini V, Smith TJ. Scrambler therapy may relieve chronic neuropathic pain more effectively than guideline-based drug management: results of a pilot, randomized, controlled trial. *J Pain Symptom Manage.* 2012;43(1):87–95.
201. Byun H, Oh MK, Lee CH. Effects of scrambler therapy in patients with failed back surgery syndromes and factors associated with depression affecting pain before and after the therapy [retracted in: *Pain Res Manag.* 2021 Jan 23;2021:2572391]. *Pain Res Manag.* 2020;2020:9342865.
202. Waxman AJ, Mink PJ, Devesa SS, et al. Racial disparities in incidence and outcome in multiple myeloma: a population-based study. *Blood.* 2010;116(25):5501–5506.
203. Chesi M, Nardini E, Lim RS, Smith KD, Kuehl WM, Bergsagel PL. The t(4;14) translocation in myeloma dysregulates both FGFR3 and a novel gene, MMSET, resulting in IgH/MMSET hybrid transcripts. *Blood.* 1998;92(9):3025–3034.
204. Pasca S, Tomuleasa C, Teodorescu P, et al. KRAS/NRAS/BRAF Mutations as potential targets in multiple myeloma. *Front Oncol.* 2019; 9:1137.
205. Kyle RA, Gertz MA, Witzig TE, et al. Review of 1027 patients with newly diagnosed multiple myeloma. *Mayo Clin Proc.* 2003;78(1):21–33.
206. Terpos E, Kleber M, Engelhardt M, et al. European Myeloma Network guidelines for the management of multiple myeloma-related complications. *Haematologica.* 2015;100(10):1254–1266.
207. Albagoush SA, Shumway C, Azevedo AM. Multiple myeloma. [Updated 2022 February 24]. In: *StatPearls [Internet].* StatPearls Publishing; 2022.
208. Nishimura KK, Barlogie B, van Rhee F, et al. Long-term outcomes after autologous stem cell transplantation for multiple myeloma. *Blood Adv.* 2020;4(2):422–431.
209. Palumbo A, Avet-Loiseau H, Oliva S, et al. Revised international staging system for multiple myeloma: a report from International Myeloma Working Group. *J Clin Oncol.* 2015;33(26):2863–2869.
210. Licciardone JC. Preventing progression from chronic to widespread pain and its impact on health-related quality of life: a historical cohort study of osteopathic medical care. *J Osteopath Med.* 2021;122(1):21–29.
211. Dal Farra F, Risio RG, Vismara L, Bergna A. Effectiveness of osteopathic interventions in chronic non-specific low back pain: a systematic review and meta-analysis. *Complement Ther Med.* 2021;56:102616.
212. Martí-Salvador M, Hidalgo-Moreno L, Doménech-Fernández J, Lisón JF, Arguisuelas MD. Osteopathic manipulative treatment including specific diaphragm techniques improves pain and disability in chronic nonspecific low back pain: a randomized trial. *Arch Phys Med Rehabil.* 2018;99(9):1720–1729.
213. Licciardone JC, Minotti DE, Gatchel RJ, Kearns CM, Singh KP. Osteopathic manual treatment and ultrasound therapy for chronic low back pain: a randomized controlled trial. *Ann Fam Med.* 2013;11(2): 122–129.
214. Licciardone JC. The OSTEOPATHIC trial demonstrates significant improvement in patients with chronic low back pain as manifested by decreased prescription rescue medication use. *J Am Osteopath Assoc.* 2014;114(7):528–529.
215. Licciardone JC, Gatchel RJ. Osteopathic medical care with and without osteopathic manipulative treatment in patients with chronic low back pain: a pain registry-based study. *J Am Osteopath Assoc.* 2020;120(2): 64–73.
216. Cooley D, Bailey J, Jermyn R. Cost comparison of osteopathic manipulative treatment for patients with chronic low back pain. *J Osteopath Med.* 2021;121(7):635–642.

217. Williams CM, Maher CG, Latimer J, et al. Efficacy of paracetamol for acute low-back pain: a doubleblind, randomised controlled trial. *Lancet.* 2014;384:1586–1596.
218. Price MR, Cupler ZA, Hawk C, Bednarz EM, Walters SA, Daniels CJ. Systematic review of guideline-recommended medications prescribed for treatment of low back pain. *Chiropr Man Therap.* 2022;30(1):26.
219. Fitzpatrick FA. Cyclooxygenase enzymes: regulation and function. *Curr Pharm Des.* 2004;10(6):577–588.
220. Chou R, Deyo R, Friedly J, et al. *Noninvasive Treatments for Low Back Pain.* Agency for Healthcare Research and Quality (US); 2016.
221. Berthelot JM, Darrieutort-Lafitte C, Le Goff B, Maugars Y. Strong opioids for noncancer pain due to musculoskeletal diseases: not more effective than acetaminophen or NSAIDs. *Joint Bone Spine.* 2015;82(6): 397–401.
222. Park SC, Kang MS, Yang JH, Kim TH. Assessment and nonsurgical management of low back pain: a narrative review. *Korean J Intern Med.* 2023;38(1):16–26.
223. Chou R, Pinto RZ, Fu R, et al. Systemic corticosteroids for radicular and non-radicular low back pain. *Cochrane Database Syst Rev.* 2022; 10(10):CD012450.
224. Waljee AK, Rogers MA, Lin P, et al. Short term use of oral corticosteroids and related harms among adults in the United States: population based cohort study. *BMJ.* 2017;357:j1415.
225. Stamer UM, Musshoff F, Kobilay M, Madea B, Hoeft A, Stuber F. Concentrations of tramadol and O-desmethyltramadol enantiomers in different CYP2D6 genotypes. *Clin Pharmacol Ther.* 2007;82(1):41–47.
226. Labate A, Newton MR, Vernon GM, Berkovic SF. Tramadol and new-onset seizures. *Med J Aust.* 2005;182(1):42–43.
227. Golightly LK, Simendinger BA, Barber GR, Stolpman NM, Kick SD, McDermott MT. Hypoglycemic effects of tramadol analgesia in hospitalized patients: a case-control study. *J Diabetes Metab Disord.* 2017; 16:30.
228. Shipton EA. Physical therapy approaches in the treatment of low back pain. *Pain Ther.* 2018;7(2):127–137.
229. American Occupational Therapy Association. Role of occupational therapy in pain management. *Am J Occup Ther.* 2022;75(Supplement_3): 7513410010.
230. Uyeshiro Simon A, Collins CER. Lifestyle Redesign® for chronic pain management: a retrospective clinical efficacy study. *Am J Occup Ther.* 2017;71(4):7104190040p1–7104190040p7.
231. Miller J, MacDermid JC, Walton DM, Richardson J. Chronic Pain Self-Management Support with Pain Science Education and Exercise (COMMENCE) for people with chronic pain and multiple comorbidities: a randomized controlled trial. *Arch Phys Med Rehabil.* 2020;101(5): 750–761.
232. Fisher GS, Emerson L, Firpo C, Ptak J, Wonn J, Bartolacci G. Chronic pain and occupation: an exploration of the lived experience. *Am J Occup Ther.* 2007;61(3):290–302.
233. Sahrmann S *Diagnosis and Treatment of Movement Impairment Syndromes.* Mosby; 2002.
234. Hodges PW, van Dieen JH, Cholewicki J. *Spinal Control: The Rehabilitation of Back Pain: State of the Art and Science.* Elsevier Health Sciences; 2013.
235. Waldhelm A. Assessment of core stability: developing practical models. *LSU Doctoral Dissertations.* Louisiana State University and Agricultural & Mechanical College; 2011.
236. Bergmark A. Stability of the lumbar spine. A study in mechanical engineering. *Acta Orthop Scand Suppl.* 1989;230:1–54.
237. Hodges PW, Richardson CA. Contraction of the abdominal muscles associated with movement of the lower limb. *Phys Ther.* 1997;77(2): 132–142.
238. Richardson CA, Snijders CJ, Hides JA, Damen L, Pas MS, Storm J. The relation between the transversus abdominis muscles, sacroiliac joint mechanics, and low back pain. *Spine (Phila Pa 1976).* 2002;27(4): 399–405.
239. Panjabi MM. The stabilizing system of the spine. Part I. Function, dysfunction, adaptation, and enhancement. *J Spinal Disord.* 1992;5(4): 383–397.
240. Urquhart DM, Hodges PW, Allen TJ, Story IH. Abdominal muscle recruitment during a range of voluntary exercises. *Man Ther.* 2005; 10(2):144–153.
241. Nadler SF, Malanga GA, Feinberg JH, Rubanni M, Moley P, Foye P. Functional performance deficits in athletes with previous lower extremity injury. *Clin J Sport Med.* 2002;12(2):73–78.
242. Kankaanpää M, Taimela S, Laaksonen D, Hänninen O, Airaksinen O. Back and hip extensor fatigability in chronic low back pain patients and controls. *Arch Phys Med Rehabil.* 1998;79(4):412–417.
243. Leinonen V, Kankaanpää M, Airaksinen O, Hänninen O. Back and hip extensor activities during trunk flexion/extension: effects of low back pain and rehabilitation. *Arch Phys Med Rehabil.* 2000;81(1):32–37.
244. Hungerford B, Gilleard W, Hodges P. Evidence of altered lumbopelvic muscle recruitment in the presence of sacroiliac joint pain. *Spine (Phila Pa 1976).* 2003;28(14):1593–1600.
245. Barker KL, Shamley DR, Jackson D. Changes in the cross-sectional area of multifidus and psoas in patients with unilateral back pain: the relationship to pain and disability. *Spine (Phila Pa 1976).* 2004;29(22):E515–E519.
246. Liddle SD, Gracey JH, Baxter GD. Advice for the management of low back pain: a systematic review of randomised controlled trials. *Man Ther.* 2007;12(4):310–327.
247. van Middelkoop M, Rubinstein SM, Kuijpers T, et al. A systematic review on the effectiveness of physical and rehabilitation interventions for chronic non-specific low back pain. *Eur Spine J.* 2011;20(1): 19–39.
248. Şahin N, Karahan AY, Albayrak İ. Effectiveness of physical therapy and exercise on pain and functional status in patients with chronic low back pain: a randomized-controlled trial. *Turk J Phys Med Rehabil.* 2017;64(1):52–58.
249. Choi BK, Verbeek JH, Tam WW, Jiang JY. Exercises for prevention of recurrences of low-back pain. *Cochrane Database Syst Rev.* 2010;2010(1):CD006555.
250. Clinical guidelines to address low back pain: using the evidence to guide physical therapist practice. *J Orthop Sports Phys Ther.* 2021;51(11):533–534.
251. Cherkin DC, Sherman KJ, Balderson BH, et al. Effect of mindfulness-based stress reduction vs cognitive behavioral therapy or usual care on back pain and functional limitations in adults with chronic low back pain: a randomized clinical trial. *JAMA.* 2016;315(12):1240–1249.
252. Yang S, Kim W, Kong HH, Do KH, Choi KH. Epidural steroid injection versus conservative treatment for patients with lumbosacral radicular pain: a meta-analysis of randomized controlled trials. *Medicine (Baltimore).* 2020;99(30):e21283.
253. Johnson BA, Schellhas KP, Pollei SR. Epidurography and therapeutic epidural injections: technical considerations and experience with 5334 cases. *AJNR Am J Neuroradiol.* 1999;20(4):697–705.
254. Owlia MB, Salimzadeh A, Alishiri G, Haghighi A. Comparison of two doses of corticosteroid in epidural steroid injection for lumbar radicular pain. *Singapore Med J.* 2007;48(3):241–245.
255. Sayed D, Grider J, Strand N, et al. The American Society of Pain and Neuroscience (ASPN) evidence-based clinical guideline of interventional treatments for low back pain [published correction appears in J Pain Res. 2022 December 24; 15:4075-4076]. *J Pain Res.* 2022;15:3729–3832.
256. Kim KM, Kim HS, Choi KH, Ahn WS. Cephalic spreading levels after volumetric caudal epidural injections in chronic low back pain. *J Korean Med Sci.* 2001;16(2):193–197.
257. Glover JR. Arthrography of the joints of the lumbar vertebral arches. *Orthop Clin North Am.* 1977;8(1):37–42.
258. Masharawi Y, Rothschild B, Dar G, et al. Facet orientation in the thoracolumbar spine: three-dimensional anatomic and biomechanical analysis. *Spine (Phila Pa 1976).* 2004;29(16):1755–1763.
259. Singh JR, Miccio VF Jr, Modi DJ, Sein MT. The impact of local steroid administration on the incidence of neuritis following lumbar facet radiofrequency neurotomy. *Pain Physician.* 2019;22(1):69–74.
260. Fitzpatrick B, Hilton K, Suer M, Poliak-Tunis M, Hetzel S. The impact of local corticosteroid administration on the incidence of post-neurotomy neuritis: a prospective investigation. *Pain Physician.* 2022;25(1):E121–E126.

261. Shustorovich A, AlFarra T, Arel AT, Singh JR, Roemmich RT, Chhatre A. Dexamethasone effectively reduces the incidence of post-neurotomy neuropathic pain: a randomized controlled pilot study. *Pain Physician*. 2021;24(8):517–524.
262. Ishimoto Y, Yoshimura N, Muraki S, et al. Prevalence of symptomatic lumbar spinal stenosis and its association with physical performance in a population-based cohort in Japan: the Wakayama Spine Study. *Osteoarthritis Cartilage*. 2012;20(10):1103–1108.
263. Jain S, Deer T, Sayed D, et al. Minimally invasive lumbar decompression: a review of indications, techniques, efficacy and safety. *Pain Manag*. 2020;10(5):331–348.
264. Shealy CN, Mortimer JT, Reswick JB. Electrical inhibition of pain by stimulation of the dorsal columns: preliminary clinical report. *Anesth Analg*. 1967;46(4):489–491.
265. Jensen MP, Brownstone RM. Mechanisms of spinal cord stimulation for the treatment of pain: still in the dark after 50 years. *Eur J Pain*. 2019;23(4):652–659.
266. Urits I, Wang JK, Yancey K, et al. Acupuncture for the management of low back pain. *Curr Pain Headache Rep*. 2021;25(1):2.
267. Weinstein JN, Tosteson TD, Lurie JD, et al. Surgical vs nonoperative treatment for lumbar disk herniation: the Spine Patient Outcomes Research Trial (SPORT): a randomized trial. *JAMA*. 2006;296(20):2441–2450.
268. Weinstein JN, Lurie JD, Tosteson TD, et al. Surgical versus nonoperative treatment for lumbar disc herniation: four-year results for the Spine Patient Outcomes Research Trial (SPORT). *Spine (Phila Pa 1976)*. 2008;33(25):2789–2800.
269. Weinstein JN, Lurie JD, Tosteson TD, et al. Surgical versus nonsurgical treatment for lumbar degenerative spondylolisthesis. *N Engl J Med*. 2007;356(22):2257–2270.
270. Weinstein JN, Tosteson TD, Lurie JD, et al. Surgical versus nonoperative treatment for lumbar spinal stenosis four-year results of the Spine Patient Outcomes Research Trial. *Spine (Phila Pa 1976)*. 2010;35(14):1329–1338.
271. Lurie JD, Tosteson TD, Tosteson AN, et al. Surgical versus nonoperative treatment for lumbar disc herniation: eight-year results for the spine patient outcomes research trial [published correction appears in Spine (Phila Pa 1976). 2015 January;40(1): E59]. *Spine (Phila Pa 1976)*. 2014;39(1):3–16.
272. Andersson GB, Lucente T, Davis AM, Kappler RE, Lipton JA, Leurgans S. A comparison of osteopathic spinal manipulation with standard care for patients with low back pain. *N Engl J Med*. 1999;341:1426–1431.
273. National Guideline Centre (UK). *Low Back Pain and Sciatica in Over 16s: Assessment and Management*. London: National Institute for Health and Care Excellence (NICE); 2016.
274. Low Back Pain and Sciatica in Over 16s: Assessment and Management. London: National Institute for Health and Care Excellence (NICE); 2020.
275. Shi Y, Guo W, Yu L. [Non-specific low back pain: interpretation of North American Spine Society (NASS) guidelines for evidence-based medicine]. *Zhongguo Xiu Fu Chong Jian Wai Ke Za Zhi*. 2021;35(10):1336–1340.
276. George SZ, Fritz JM, Silfies SP, et al. Interventions for the management of acute and chronic low back pain: revision 2021. *J Orthop Sports Phys Ther*. 2021;51(11):CPG1–CPG60.

PART FIVE

Research Investigating Osteopathic Principles

94 Overview of Methods and Evidence Relating to Osteopathic Manipulative Treatment Research

BRIAN F. DEGENHARDT ▪ KENT P. SIMMONDS ▪ MAUREEN J. SIMMONDS ▪ ANGELA K. TYSON

KEY CONCEPTS

- Humans learn from experiences and observations to predict and influence the future. In the field of medicine, the scientific method is the primary process used to advance knowledge by asking a series of questions about physiologic and pathophysiologic mechanisms, diagnosis, prognosis, management options and related mechanisms of action, and outcomes. Questions may be general questions about a specific disorder, such as "what causes this condition?" or "what are the complications of this condition?" Or they could be very specific questions, such as "what do I do for a patient with this condition to achieve a particular outcome?"
- Astute observations help to provide a framework from which questions or hypotheses are formulated. In some cases, an adequate best-evidence answer to these questions is identified from a critical review and appraisal of the literature. In other cases, scientific evidence has not been established to answer those questions. In these instances, the scientific method provides a way to investigate previously unanswered questions and partially understood phenomena.
- Fundamentally, the scientific process is based on estimations of the probability of event occurrences. These estimates can be used to develop explanatory theories of causal etiology or to predict future events. Such processes consider whether chance alone may have led to the observations made, and research design and statistical interpretations reduce observer bias.
- Basic science explanatory research, which typically has better control of variables than clinical research, may explain potential mechanisms of action and, thereby, provide a foundation for clinical activities. However, translating results from basic science research into clinical practice is limited by the complexity of patients' biopsychosocial systems, which are more difficult to control in clinical studies than in basic science research.
- Clinical research investigating the complex neuromusculoskeletal system and osteopathic manipulative treatment (OMT) is challenging but critically important to:
  - Develop and test explanatory mechanisms of action on the clinical effects of OMT
  - Advance the utilization of OMT to improve outcomes and refine patient care.

"The greatest obstacle to discovery is not ignorance—it is the illusion of knowledge."

—*Daniel J. Boorstin*

Our hope is that this chapter will provide a framework for osteopathic students and clinicians to become more curious, knowledgeable, and motivated; to question what they think they know and how they know it; to identify gaps in knowledge related to osteopathic manipulative medicine (OMM); and to use science to advance patient care in this field. We acknowledge that this chapter could easily fill a book, but we tried to keep the content relevant for novice clinician researchers. In addition to the insights offered in this chapter, we have provided readable and up-to-date references for additional relevant details to support your research activities.

OVERVIEW OF EVIDENCE-BASED MEDICINE

- Evidence-based medicine refers to "the conscientious, explicit, judicious, and reasonable use of modern, best evidence in making decisions about the care of individual patients."[1] This best evidence is then translated into clinical practice and integrated with patient values to produce patient-specific, personalized medical care.[2,3]
- Assessment of best evidence should be a common feature of clinical teaching and practice. Although historically challenging, communication and collaboration between purely practicing clinicians, clinician scientists, and basic scientists should optimize the impact of science. Overcoming this divide is a necessary step to establish bidirectional translation of science for fine-tuning research and efficiently improving the quality of medical care.
- The physician's role in an evidence-based practice is to apply the best scientific approaches in clinical practice to optimize patient outcomes and to actively contribute to scientific activities, thereby participating in updating evidence-based guidelines.[1]

RESEARCH QUESTION: WHERE SCIENCE BEGINS

Osteopathic clinicians need to understand how to identify and develop answerable clinical questions from clinical experiences or in a process by which they seek an answer to a clinical question through review of literature. Critical reviews identify what is known and unknown about a variety of issues related to health. These include the pathophysiology of health conditions, risk factors associated with the development of these conditions, whether it is prevalent, anticipated prognosis and associated complications, and the extent that which various treatments impact expected outcomes to the epidemiology of the community served. Osteopathic physicians are on the front line of clinical care, which makes them well positioned to identify clinically relevant knowledge gaps, refine research questions, and design feasible studies to fill these knowledge gaps. Direct clinical experience enables more efficient translation of shifting real-world clinical practice to optimize care for patients. More perspectives for developing research questions can be found later in this chapter.

CLINICAL RESEARCH PYRAMID AND OSTEOPATHIC MANIPULATIVE MEDICINE RESEARCH

The scientific method is designed to build on itself, insight upon insight. Investigating the quantity, quality, and scope of the observations enables science to build levels of evidence, which are represented by a pyramid (Fig. 94.1). In general, as one moves up the pyramid, the level of rigor of scientific evidence increases. A tool on how to approach what is considered the best evidence-based scientific method on the type of question that is asked can be reviewed through the Oxford Centre for Evidence-Based Medicine 2011 Levels of Evidence (Fig. 94.2).[4]

Individual Observations: The Bedrock of Science

> "*The whole of science is nothing more than a refinement of everyday thinking.*"
>
> **—Albert Einstein**

- Despite their commitment to patient care and the responsibility of making life-altering decisions, few clinicians identify their role as actively contributing to scientific understanding.[5,6] Yet in the 21st century, research has become a multidisciplinary team activity.[7,8] Clinicians need to understand their vital role in the scientific process, developing meaningful questions based on their clinical experience, participating in data collection, identifying outcomes that support and are inconsistent with current understanding, and advocating for a balanced interpretation of outcomes that protects the interest of their individual patients and the population. Recognizing this need, undergraduate and postgraduate training is beginning to incorporate meaningful requirements to equip future physicians with tools to actively contribute to the scientific process.[9] By fulfilling this important role, clinicians will be able to advocate for a scientific process that keeps individual and population well-being their obligation and priority.
- A scientific question may begin with a single observation. Patterns of similar observations over time often lead to conjecture or a question that can be subsequently evaluated through a critical review and appraisal of the literature and, if needed, tested through the scientific method. While true for all aspects of human experience, it is critical to minimize bias in clinical observations and research. Minimizing bias may be particularly relevant in the field of OMM, where clinicians may be conditioned by the educational process to believe certain perspectives are true even though they are based on rational yet hypothetical associations and undocumented causations. This form of bias is known as allegiance bias, when investigators have an allegiance to a specific school of thought, and can result in researchers unconsciously or consciously bringing in additional biases.
- If we think about an observation as a single dot and the information we collect in clinical practice from the history, physical examination, and laboratory and radiologic testing as multiple discrete dots, then osteopathic physicians try to connect the dots to understand complex relationships and see the big picture of what is ailing the patient on a holistic level. However, discrete dots can be connected in different ways to create many different pictures. Although some of the dots of information are relevant and essential for developing an accurate holistic picture, other dots may be incidental and, if used, result in erroneous or unhelpful pictures.
- In recent decades, technologies have enabled humanity to store ever-increasing amounts of data, which has led to the "era of big data." Concurrent advances in computer processing and statistical methods have enabled researchers to utilize this data to improve our understanding by better characterization

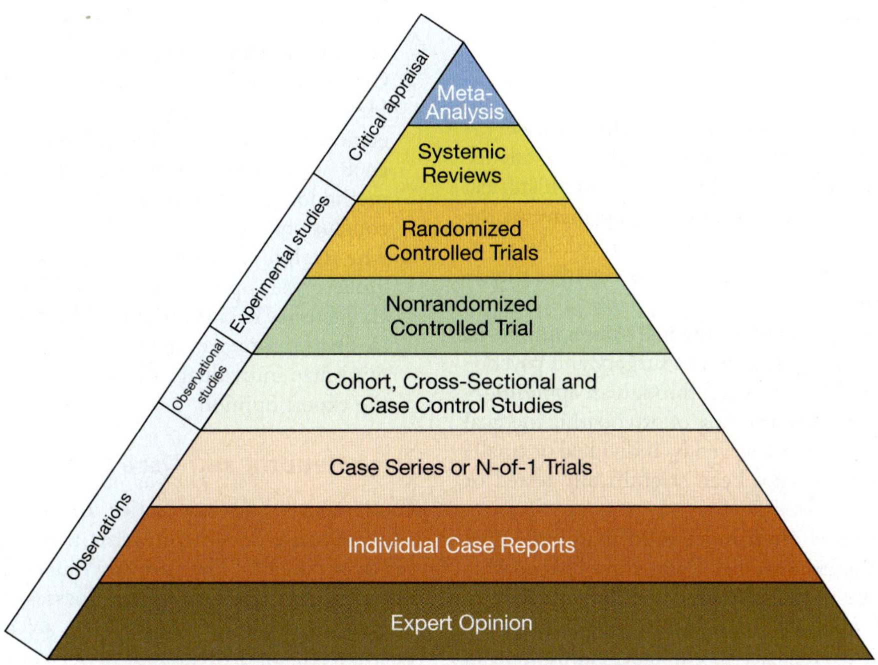

Figure 94.1. The osteopathic clinical research pyramid.

Oxford Centre for Evidence-Based Medicine 2011 Levels of Evidence

Question	Step 1 (Level 1*)	Step 2 (Level 2*)	Step 3 (Level 3*)	Step 4 (Level 4*)	Step 5 (Level 5)
How common is the problem?	Local and current random sample surveys (or censuses)	Systematic review of surveys that allow matching to local circumstances**	Local non-random sample**	Case-series**	n/a
Is this diagnostic or monitoring test accurate? (Diagnosis)	Systematic review of cross sectional studies with consistently applied reference standard and blinding	Individual cross sectional studies with consistently applied reference standard and blinding	Non-consecutive studies, or studies without consistently applied reference standards**	Case-control studies, or "poor or non-independent reference standard**	Mechanism-based reasoning
What will happen if we do not add a therapy? (Prognosis)	Systematic review of inception cohort studies	Inception cohort studies	Cohort study or control arm of randomized trial*	Case-series or case-control studies, or poor quality prognostic cohort study**	n/a
Does this intervention help? (Treatment Benefits)	Systematic review of randomized trials or *n*-of-1 trials	Randomized trial or observational study with dramatic effect	Non-randomized controlled cohort/follow-up study**	Case-series, case-control studies, or historically controlled studies**	Mechanism-based reasoning
What are the COMMON harms? (Treatment Harms)	Systematic review of randomized trials, systematic review of nested case-control studies, *n*-of-1 trial with the patient you are raising the question about, or observational study with dramatic effect	Individual randomized trial or (exceptionally) observational study with dramatic effect	Non-randomized controlled cohort/follow-up study (post-marketing surveillance) provided there are sufficient numbers to rule out a common harm. (For long-term harms the duration of follow-up must be sufficient.)**	Case-series, case-control, or historically controlled studies**	Mechanism-based reasoning
What are the RARE harms? (Treatment Harms)	Systematic review of randomized trials or *n*-of-1 trial	Randomized trial or (exceptionally) observational study with dramatic effect			
Is this (early detection) test worthwhile? (Screening)	Systematic review of randomized trials	Randomized trial	Non-randomized controlled cohort/follow-up study**	Case-series, case-control, or historically controlled studies**	Mechanism-based reasoning

*** Level may be graded down on the basis of study quality, imprecision, indirectness (study PICO does not match questions PICO), because of inconsistency between studies, or because the absolute effect size is very small; Level may be graded up if there is a large or very large effect size.**

**** As always, a systematic review is generally better than an individual study.**

How to cite the Levels of Evidence Table
OCEBM Levels of Evidence Working Group*. "The Oxford 2011 Levels of Evidence".
Oxford Centre for Evidence-Based Medicine. http://www.cebm.net/index.aspx?o=5653
** OCEBM Table of Evidence Working Group = Jeremy Howick, Iain Chalmers (James Lind Library), Paul Glasziou, Trish Greenhalgh, Carl Heneghan, Alessandro Liberati, Ivan Moschetti, Bob Phillips, Hazel Thornton, Olive Goddard and Mary Hodgkinson*

Figure 94.2. Oxford Centre for Evidence-Based Medicine 2011 Levels of Evidence.

of the complex associations, trends, and interactions between variables.[10] The advancement of technologies such as artificial intelligence will supercharge the ability to search for associations in stored data. The role of content experts, such as osteopathic physicians, will become increasingly vital in guiding these technologies to carefully explore relevant associations for interpretation and implementation of the results.

Expert Opinion: The Base of the Pyramid

- Expert opinions usually develop after years of clinical observations and form the base level of the osteopathic clinical evidence pyramid. Partially due to the osteopathic profession's historical focus on providing primary care, the research on many of the foundational concepts of OMM is largely untested. As such, there is a reliance on the expert opinion of osteopathic physicians and their mentors.
- Expert opinion can be based on an individual's observations or on group consensus. As with fields such as surgery and psychotherapy, training in OMM has occurred through an apprenticeship model.[11] Thus, much of the training of osteopathic medical students in OMM remains largely driven by individual or small-group expert opinion that has not been scientifically tested or validated.
- The consensus of a group is often more valid than individual opinions. For decades, the Educational Council on Osteopathic Principles (ECOP) consistently promoted the development of profession-wide expert opinion in OMM, primarily to better standardize educational content across the osteopathic field in the United States.[12]
- However, a primary source of information for ECOP's process has been passed down from generation to generation through the extant historical osteopathic literature and in contemporary publications that promote models consistent with historical perspectives. Historical perspectives are valuable, but if they have never been tested, they may be erroneous or incomplete since they do not incorporate contemporary understanding of mechanisms and clinical outcomes.
- Careful observation is foundational to the progress of science. However, clinical experience cannot differentiate between association and causation. Deducing causation from clinical experience or other nonsystematic observations using proper research methodology leads to bias and premature, potentially erroneous conclusions.
- The Delphi method is a common approach to establishing group expert opinion and is considered the most valid method to characterize expert opinion.[13] This systematic, multistep process involves rigorous evaluation of expert opinions in an attempt to minimize individual influence and potential bias when crafting the expert opinion.

Case Reports and Case Series

Case reports and case series are descriptive study designs that systematically document events that occur in single patients or a series of patients. They provide foundational observations for very rare diseases, newly emerging illnesses, or previously unrecognized conditions and associations. They are also valuable for the diagnostic work-up or treatment of common medical conditions when there are unexpected findings or treatment responses.[14,15]

Case Reports

- These reports refer to a detailed retrospective or prospective case of individual patients who may have interesting or novel symptoms, risk factors, diagnostic findings, or treatment responses. To be useful, case reports should report on an observation considered novel or on rare events in the scientific and clinical literature.
- It is at this level of clinical activity that evidence-based medicine guidelines must be critiqued for quality assurance. For example, because individual responses may vary from the aggregate measure of effect, individual responses should always be validated and considered as part of the application of evidence-based medicine. Further, when cases seem to be consistently falling outside the aggregate measure of effect, those generating guidelines need to be made aware of this pattern of findings.
- Medication side effect profiles and treatment algorithms are formulated based on population-level average responses, which may ignore baseline heterogeneity of treatment effect. Heterogeneity of treatment effect refers to the extent to which there is variability in treatment responses between individuals or subgroups based on differences in baseline risk and propensity to respond.[16] Because less common responses may be underemphasized by practice guidelines and treatment algorithms and underrepresented in the literature, case reports are important to holistically minded practitioners and especially to their patients. The case report allows for astute clinical observation of a given patient's presentation or reaction to an intervention to be disseminated, providing clues for additional investigations.
- Osteopathic physicians are well-positioned to contribute to the movement to make medicine more "personalized" and effective by understanding and remaining attentive to each individual's response. There are many cases in which medicine has been slow to recognize potentially negative side effects. This is the very reason that most treatment recommendations are framed as guidelines and not algorithms.
- Overall, case reports primarily provide evidence for hypothesis or theory generation.
- When used for educational purposes (e.g., as a class assignment), the case study is an important learning experience for the student. However, these assignments are not typically placed in the research hierarchy since they tend to be unique to the presenter but not to the scientific community.

Case Series

- A case series is an extension of a case report and often includes identifying clustered characteristics or treatment responses among a set of patients with common symptoms or illnesses.
- As an example, an early case series involving 121 patients with diabetes mellitus reported clinically relevant reductions in blood glucose within 1 hour of receiving OMT, resulting in completion of a case-control study and subgroup analysis of patients with diabetes mellitus in a randomized controlled trial years later.[17–19]
- Another classic example of a case series included the Centers for Disease Control and Prevention's *Morbidity and Mortality Weekly Report* from June 5, 1981, which reported on five cases of *Pneumocystis carinii* pneumonia among healthy young men in Los Angeles and a cluster of Kaposi sarcoma cases in New York City.[20] These case series led to additional investigations and the eventual identification of HIV.
- Case series provide the foundational observations that begin the process of identifying patterns in data such as symptoms, signs, and tests that are potentially predictive of a disease. They can also help refine and improve the precision of the language used in the biomedical sciences around a particular condition.
- Case presentations are useful in providing a more rigorous experience to those in training for research and scholarly activity than a case study because they provide evidence for stronger hypothesis and theory generation than case reports and the possible need to test these theories with a more rigorous research design (i.e., further up the pyramid).

The N-of-1 Clinical Trial

- Most clinicians at any stage of training or practice want to show that their care is effective. Unfortunately, most of the time research questions related to effectiveness are too broad and require major simplification. Even when the scope of the research question is refined to a researchable question, getting to a final answer often involves several steps in the scientific process and considerable funding. Often, this process is unfeasible for the individual student, resident, or practicing physician.
- An alternative study design for observing effectiveness is called an n-of-1 clinical trial.[21,22] This type of trial uses a specific form of balanced or randomized design and is characterized by periods of active and control (or placebo) treatments with patients periodically crossing over between treatment arms. Even though the crossover design has limitations, challenges, and specific statistical considerations, it also has numerous benefits when appropriately designed and implemented. Because it can be easily developed and managed, it may provide research experience similar to a feasibility study. Data from several related n-of-1 clinical trials can be analyzed as in a meta-analysis, and such outcomes may lead to larger randomized controlled trials (RCTs).

Observational Studies

Observational studies expand on case reports and case series because they enable a comparison between at least two groups. Observational studies can be purely observational of a cohort (nonanalytic studies) or compare naturally occurring phenomena between groups (analytic) that include a reference group and comparison group or groups. The reference group is commonly the standard-of-care group or the group with the largest sample population. For example, in many studies assessing OMT, the reference group may be standard medical care, and the comparison group standard care + OMT.

- Such studies fall into two main categories—retrospective and prospective—depending on the temporal direction of the investigation (Fig. 94.3).
- A key aspect of these studies is that the investigators do not assign patients to a particular treatment group. Instead, the investigators observe and measure differences between naturally occurring treatment groups.
- An attractive feature of observational research is that this study design is far less costly and can be performed more efficiently than an RCT. In addition, there are fewer ethical concerns because treatment groups occur naturally with investigators only observing outcome differences between groups. Performing observational studies can assess the consequences of exposures or interventions that cannot ethically be assigned in a random fashion. Such an example is that of observing consequences of cigarette smoking.
- A disadvantage is that observational studies are subject to several types of bias, which are described later in the chapter.
- Guidelines for reporting observational studies have been developed and are found in the Strengthening the Reporting of Observational Studies in Epidemiology (STROBE) Statement.[23] These guidelines can be helpful during the study design phase to

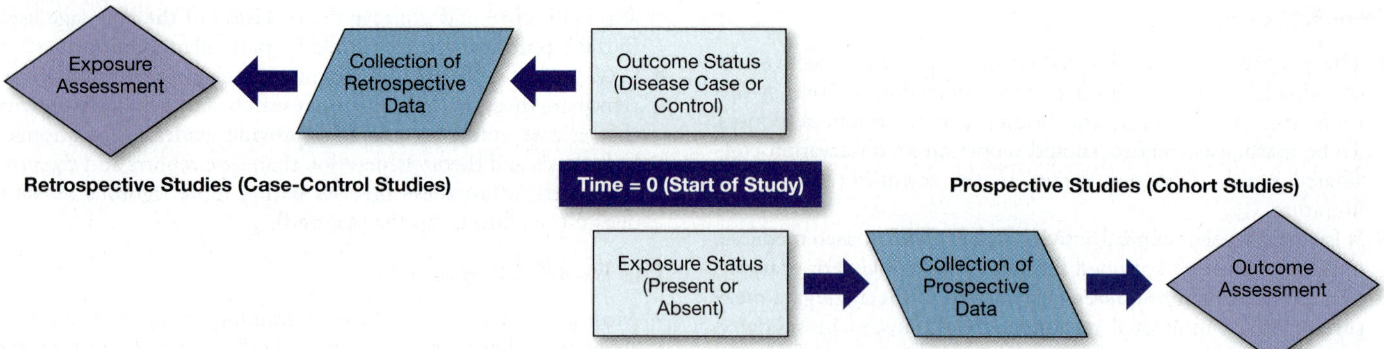

Figure 94.3. Observational study designs.

ensure nothing important is overlooked that may be considered a major flaw at the end of the study.

Case-Control Studies

- The case-control study is a type of retrospective observational design. They are performed more rarely in comparison to other types of studies. These studies look at differences in exposure to different treatments or risk factors are compared between participants with the outcome of interest (cases) and participants without the outcome of interest (controls).
- All case-control studies are considered retrospective by definition since the starting point requires cases (i.e., participants must already have the outcome).
- Case-control studies can be particularly useful to study rare conditions because investigators do not need exceedingly large sample sizes or have to wait for rare outcomes to develop.[24]
  - Cases selection: Cases can be selected from a variety of sources, such as hospitals, clinics, disease registries (e.g., cancer), or public health agencies. The selection of cases has important implications for the generalizability of results. For example, consider a study assessing the effects of physical activity on the development of anginal chest pain. If cases are identified as hospitalized patients admitted for angina, then they likely represent patients with more severe angina when compared with all patients with angina.
  - Control selection: Similar to cases, controls may also be selected from a variety of sources, such as the community, clinics, or hospitals. Community controls may include friends or neighbors or may be selected from existing lists (e.g., school rosters, homeowners association). Hospital or clinic controls may include patients with conditions that are unrelated to cases. For example, if cases are patients hospitalized with anginal chest pain, a hospitalized control may be an orthopedic patient admitted for a leg fracture. Similar to case selection, it is important to consider how controls are representative of the general population.

Cohort Studies

In cohort studies, data for a group (or cohort) of patients is collected over time. An exposure (or treatment) is the starting point for these studies. Cohort studies can be retrospective or prospective.

- Cohorts can be assembled based on a variety of factors, such as birth year, setting, occupation, or even health care provider or health insurer (e.g., Medicare patients).[25]
- Cohort studies are useful for studying the effects of rare exposures because their starting point begins with exposure. For example, a cohort study would be useful to determine the effects of uranium on lung cancer development by following a cohort of uranium miners.

Prospective Cohort Studies

Prospective cohort studies mimic RCTs, except the exposure or treatment occurs naturally and is not randomly assigned by the investigator.

- Prospective cohort studies provide the highest level of evidence from observational data because they are the only observational study design that provides clear evidence of temporality (i.e., the exposure occurred *before* the outcome).[26]
- Famous examples of cohort studies include the British Doctors Study[27] and the Framingham Heart Study.[28] In the British Doctors Study,[27] over 40,000 physicians were followed over 50 years (1951 to 2001) and completed questionnaires about their health and smoking status. The study was among the first to provide strong empirical evidence that linked smoking with increased risks of acute myocardial infarction and lung cancer.
- A more contemporary example of a prospective cohort study in osteopathic medicine involves a cohort study that assessed the risks of adverse outcomes among patients receiving OMT.[29] This study followed 884 patients and reported a 2.5% incidence rate of worsening pain immediately after OMT clinic visits.[29] Pain/discomfort was the most commonly identified type of adverse event, and adverse events were more commonly reported by women.[29]

Retrospective Cohort Studies

Retrospective cohort studies are the most common types of cohort studies because they can capitalize on pre-existing data. In health care, many studies use existing large datasets, such as electronic medical records or administrative data, to assess differences between groups. In these studies, an indexed event is identified as a starting place, and the records can be chronologically reviewed over time until the outcome of interest occurs.[30,31]

Cross-Sectional Studies

In cross-sectional observational studies, data is collected from a cohort at a single moment in time. These tend to be easier studies to perform and are commonly used in public health to evaluate the incidence and prevalence of a condition. However, cross-sectional studies are the weakest form of observational study because they have the greatest risk of bias, especially selection bias (which is covered in greater detail later in the chapter). While the use of the

STROBE checklist was designed to help in the dissemination of an observational study, it is also very helpful in increasing the rigor of an observational study during the design phase, making sure nothing is accidentally overlooked.[32]

Confounding Factors and Limitations of Observational Studies

A major limitation of observational studies is the inability to randomly allocate exposure/treatment groups. These studies are at risk of bias from confounding factors since there may be systematic differences for why participants end up in different groups.

- A confounder is a third variable that is related to the exposure and the outcome of interest. The presence of this third variable distorts the observed association between the exposure and outcome.
- For example, an investigator is interested in assessing the effects of alcohol on the development of lung cancer. A case-control study is conducted, where 100 patients with lung cancer are identified and compared with 100 community controls without lung cancer. Suppose 75 patients with lung cancer reported drinking at least three alcoholic drinks per week, but only 30 patients without lung cancer did. The investigators would likely conclude that people who drink at least three alcoholic drinks per week have 2.5 (75/30) times the odds of developing lung cancer as people who do not drink alcohol. The results of this example are subject to confounding if the investigator does account for the smoking status of the patient because smoking is associated with both alcohol use and lung cancer (Fig. 94.4).
- Confounders can be known or unknown. Known confounders include factors identified from previous studies and clinical experience. Unknown confounders include factors that influence results and were not considered or known by investigators.
- Several methods can be used to control for confounders in observational studies.
  - Restriction: This method involves excluding patients with characteristics that may confound the relationship of interest. For example, patients with a prior smoking history could be excluded.
  - Matching: This method requires patients in the exposure and control groups to be matched on select characteristics (e.g., smoking status). Matching ensures equal balance in select factors to ensure an equal effect between groups. Selection of factors to match are context and study specific but commonly include sociodemographic factors (e.g., age, race/ethnicity, education), clinical factors (e.g., prior comorbidities), or factors related to the setting (e.g., patients from the same hospital).[33]
  - Statistical adjustment: Various statistical methods, such as standardization, stratified analysis, or use of multivariable statistical models, can be used to statistically adjust for potential confounders.

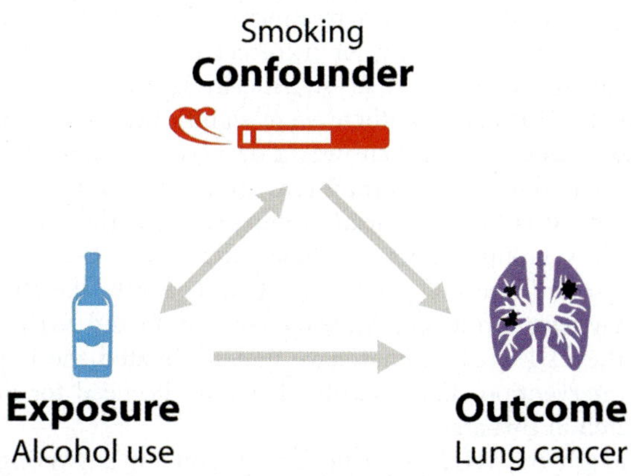

Figure 94.4. Smoking as a confounder in an observational study.

TABLE 94.1

Major Criteria for Assessing Causation between Exposure and Outcome[34]

Criteria	Outcome
Strength of evidence	Evidence from experiments (e.g., randomized controlled trails) is stronger than evidence from observational studies when establishing causation. Prospective studies generally provide stronger evidence than retrospective studies
Strength of association	Causation is more likely as the strength of association between exposure and outcome increases.
Temporality	Causation is more likely if it can be shown that exposure preceded the outcome.
Dose response	Causation is more likely if there is evidence of a dose response between the exposure and outcome (i.e., greater magnitude or longer duration of exposure increases risk of outcome).
Consistency	Causation is more likely if multiple studies involving different investigators and populations demonstrate the criteria for causation.
Biologic plausibility	Causation is more likely if there is a scientific mechanism that explains the relationship between the exposure and outcome.

These are general guidelines; however, causation must be assessed based on the overall evidence that is specific to a given research question.

A common goal in observational and experimental studies is to be able to determine causation between an exposure (i.e., event, illness, treatment) and an outcome. At times research designs can demonstrate association between two features but are unable to determine causation versus those designs that are more likely to demonstrate causation. Specific criteria should be considered when determining the likelihood of causation between the exposure and outcome (Table 94.1).[34]

Experimental Studies

NONRANDOMIZED CONTROLLED TRIALS

Nonrandomized controlled trials (NRCTs) are often overshadowed by what is considered the methodologically superior randomized controlled trials (RCT). Because of the lack of randomization, NRCTs are often classified as quasi-experimental, where interventions are given to different groups to see outcomes, but without randomization and often blinding. Yet all study designs have strengths and limitations, and for RCTs, this will be discussed in the next section. NRCTs are a valuable research design to evaluate research questions in real-world patient populations, those often excluded from RCTs.[35] Nonrandomized controlled trials tend to be more feasible due to ethical and resource issues compared to RCTs. In OMT research, where randomizing interventions and blinding can be challenging if not possible, NRCTs may be the research design of choice.

All study designs have strengths, and all have weaknesses that need to be insightfully managed. NRCTs have an increased risk of several forms of bias without random assignment of participants. But even in RCTs, random assignment only homogenizes a predetermined limited number of factors that may or may not control for all confounders. While some have reported that outcomes from NRCT can produce greater impact (20%) than similar outcomes derived from RCTs, their work also showed very good correlation of outcomes between RCTs and NRCTs.[36] Another analysis has concluded that well performed NRCTs and other observational studies do not overestimate the treatment effect.[37] These issues underscore the importance of sustaining numerous research designs in a particular field to identify consistent outcomes from which generalizations/treatment guidelines can be made.[38]

RANDOMIZED CONTROLLED TRIALS

- Current consensus is that the most effective way to control for or minimize potential confounding factors is to conduct an RCT. This type of experimental study design allows investigators to control the type, amount, and duration of exposure or treatments that participants receive.[39]
- Treatment allocation is determined at random, which theoretically minimizes the likelihood of unequal distribution of all measured and unmeasured confounders. After successful randomization, it is assumed the only difference between the two groups is the treatment of interest. This level of randomization allows investigators to have greater confidence that their results are indicative of a causal relationship between the exposure and outcome.
- For most trials, randomization occurs at the individual level. However, randomization can occur at the group level (e.g., hospitals or community) as seen in clustered RCTs.
- When reporting RCTs, content should conform to updated CONSORT (Consolidated Standards of Reporting Trials) guidelines.[40] Reviewing these guidelines during the development of the research question and study methods can help investigators avoid accidentally overlooking important details early on in a study.
- Preregistration of a protocol and analysis plan for an RCT is considered best practice. Registration of trials can be performed at clinicaltrials.gov.

One of the first notable RCTs of OMT was the Irvine study, which occurred from 1973 to 1979.[41] This study involved randomizing 95 patients with low back pain (LBP) to receive OMT, either high-velocity, low-amplitude (HVLA) or soft tissue massage, in the lumbosacral region.[41] The study reported patients in the OMT group were more likely to report immediate relief after treatment; however, the statistically significant differences between treatment groups were attenuated by discharge.[41]

CHALLENGES WITH RANDOMIZED CONTROLLED TRIALS

- Concealment: This method ensures the randomization process remains unpredictable. Concealment protects against selection bias because participants or investigators cannot select which patients receive which treatment. For example, if treatment selection was determined by randomizing every other patient to a novel treatment or standardized care group, then investigators or clinicians who identified this process could select specific patients for a specific treatment arm.
- Blinding: This method prevents patients, investigators, care providers, or data analysts from knowing which treatment group study participants are in. Blinding is used to protect against measurement bias, performance bias, and several others.
  - An example of measurement bias would be patients in the experimental group reporting higher levels of anxiety because they know they are taking an experimental medication.
  - Alternatively, unblinded health care providers could detect more adverse events among patients in experimental groups because they are more closely examining outcomes out of concern for unknown side effects.
  - For certain treatments, such as OMT, blinding may not be possible or may require specialized processes in the research protocols. For example, in a large RCT, 178 patients with LBP were randomized to receive OMT or usual care.[42] Given the inherent challenge of blinding patients to OMT, patients in the usual care group often received sham OMT.[42] However, research on placebo effects suggests that sham treatments are often not "true" sham because of treatment expectations of the participant and practitioner or conditioning from previous treatments.[43,44]
- In RCTs, it's essential to consider final analysis plans with potentially incomplete data due to some participants not completing their assigned treatment. To account for missing data and potential contamination of treatment and control groups, RCTs may be analyzed under different scenarios (Fig. 94.5).
  - Intention to treat (ITT): Under the ITT framework, all participant data are analyzed under the treatment arm of their original random allocation. Thus, outcomes for participants who switch treatment arms are still analyzed under their original treatment group or they do not complete the study and this would be accounted for in the data analysis plan.
  - Per protocol (PP): Under the PP framework, participants who received care that was inconsistent with their assigned group were dropped from the study. Analysis of the reason for attrition or deviation from the ITT may shed light on the direction of potential bias this may introduce.
  - As treated: Under this framework, outcomes for participants who switched treatments are analyzed under the treatment arm of the treatment they actually received.
- For example, in the Multicenter Osteopathic Pneumonia Study in the Elderly (MOPSE), 378 elderly patients hospitalized with pneumonia were included in the ITT analysis, but 18% were removed from analysis, primarily from the OMT and sham groups, because of missed treatments, delayed onset of treatments, study withdrawal, or incorrect treatments.[45] With the ITT analysis, there were no statistically significant outcomes.[45] With the PP analysis, there were significant changes in outcomes.[45] Specifically, there was a decrease in length of hospitalization, duration of intravenous antibiotics, and incidence of respiratory failure and death compared with the conservative care-only group.[45] Those excluded from the PP analysis had more severe levels of pneumonia. Consequently, the PP analysis may have introduced some contamination and attrition bias, but the ITT analysis may have underestimated the impact of the intervention. These results illustrate the need for ongoing research in this area.
- Although the RCT is particularly useful for answering common questions about treatment effectiveness and safety, these designs require substantial resources and planning, which make

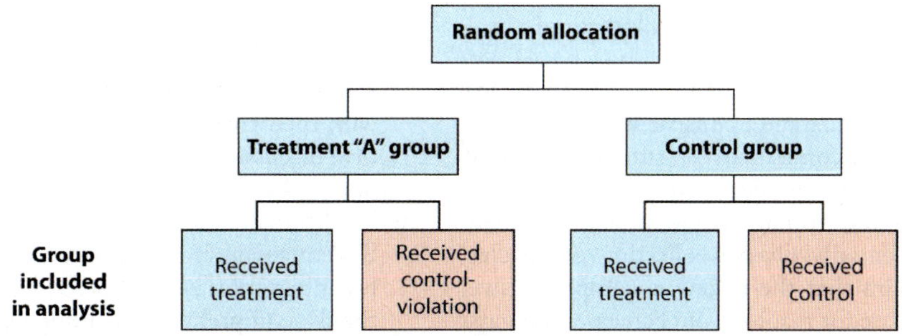

Group included in analysis	Received treatment	Received control-violation	Received treatment	Received control
Intention to treat	Treatment group	Treatment group	Control group	Control group
Per protocol	Treatment group	Ignore	Ignore	Control group
As treated	Treatment group	Control group	Treatment group	Control group

Figure 94.5. Types of analyses for randomized controlled trials.

them difficult for physicians-in-training to design and complete. However, if RCTs are structured to run within residency programs under faculty leadership, they can provide residents with important exposure and experience by contributing to high-level research.

During this century, there has been a remarkable increase in the number of RCTs investigating the impact of OMM on a diverse range of conditions.[46–49] Sustaining this level of research allows the field to continue to build its evidence base and perform more informative systematic reviews and meta-analyses. This trend must continue in an era of evidence-based medicine.

Cumulative Studies: Reviews and Meta-Analysis

Science was designed to be cumulative, and it drives and changes clinical practice based on the totality of evidence rather than individual study findings. There are various forms of reviews to consider when designing a study of this type and developing the research question. Understanding the types of reviews is an important starting point for beginning one's literature appraisal.

Literature Reviews

There are several types of literature reviews. Before starting a study, the types of reviews should be considered to determine the most appropriate one for your research.

- Mapping review: This kind of review provides a high-level overview that maps out and categorizes the complete literature, partially using systematic review methodology.
- Narrative review: This type of review is nonsystematic to present an idea and promote discussion within a field of science.
- Rapid review: This review is a type of scoping review that follows a PICO (population, intervention, comparison, outcome) format.
- Scoping review: This type of review involves a preliminary review that uses some aspects of the systematic literature review process.
- Systematic review: This type of review involves a comprehensive and exhaustive review of the complete literature, following strict criteria.
- Umbrella review: This type of review summarizes evidence from multiple reviews.

Most reviews have structured recommendations that should be followed to avoid bias and enable replication. It is also important to identify systematic standards for assessing review quality for the specific type of review.[50,51] These sources can provide a valuable roadmap for successful completion of a review.

Considerations for Systematic Reviews

- Systematic reviews are a rigorous and comprehensive search, appraisal, and analysis of all existing literature for a specific question of interest.
- Systematic reviews begin with comprehensive and reproducible searches of databases (e.g., PubMed, MEDLINE, Embase). With a focused research question in mind, a list of search terms and a search strategy are developed. During the search, potentially relevant papers are retrieved for review and scored according to preset criteria. In this way, a systematic review and analysis can identify the amount and quality of available evidence that supports a specific question. Further, this review collates empirical evidence from a specific subset of studies related to the research question.
- Systematic reviews are very time consuming for all members of the research team. Early on in the development of the research question, designing such a study and reviewing the literature, searching PROSPERO (https://www.crd.york.ac.uk/PROSPERO/) to identify if another research group has registered a similar study will help to guide your work.[52] Once you have completed the study design, it should be registered with PROSPERO.
- Although systematic reviews are near the top of the research pyramid, they still have weaknesses and are prone to bias. Standardized tools have been developed to improve the rigor of systematic reviews and should be used to direct this type of research. The tool for systematic reviews is called PRISMA (Preferred Reporting Items for Systematic Reviews and Meta-Analyses).[51]
- Prespecifying study factors, such as search terminology and study inclusion criteria, can protect against reviewer bias and prevent cherry-picking of results that support either positive or negative findings.[52]

- Keeping systematic reviews up-to-date is important for progressing science. New designs and technologies such as living reviews may be helpful for ensuring that the biomedical community remains current.[53]
- Performing multiple systematic reviews that use the same general literature source does not guarantee consistent outcomes.[54,55] There can be variability in outcomes between studies because of article selection criteria or interpretation of results.
- Similar to systematic reviews, scoping reviews provide an overview of a large and potentially diverse collection of articles. Although there is no claim that the review is comprehensive, scoping reviews are adequate for mapping out concepts and gaps in current understanding of a topic.

Meta-Analyses

- Meta-analyses are extensions of systematic reviews and involve, when feasible, statistical analyses of pooled data from identified studies to provide a single-point estimate for an estimated effect.
- For example, a 2014 study by Franke et al.[56] assessed the effects of OMT for nonspecific LBP. Seven databases were searched using prespecified search terms, and 307 studies were identified.[56] Of those, 15 studies met the prespecified inclusion criteria.[56]
- Forest plots are commonly used to convey the results of meta-analyses. The forest plot in Figure 94.6 shows the results of each reviewed study and pools the data from 566 patients to provide a single cumulative effect estimate in favor of OMT (mean difference, -12.91; 95% confidence interval [CI], -20.00 to -5.82).[56] This result can be interpreted as the best point estimate of the mean effect of OMT versus control on LBP across the 12 studies for a reduction in pain of 12.91 points on a 0 to 100 visual analog scale. The CI represents the range of uncertainty for the point estimate and indicates there is a 95% chance that the true estimate of the effect of OMT on LBP lies between −20.00 and −5.82 points.
- A limitation and challenge of meta-analyses is there is inherent heterogeneity across studies with respect to their populations, duration, timeline, specific treatments, and outcomes. These differences may result in somewhat subjective decisions regarding which data are similar enough to be pooled.
- Decisions on whether or not to pool data should be based on clinical as well as statistical heterogeneity. Clinical heterogeneity involves a subjective assessment by content experts on whether or not the research question, study population, and methodology are similar enough to pool. Statistical heterogeneity can be estimated using statistical tests such as Cochran's Q, DerSimonian-Laird, or I^2 statistic. In essence, these tests capture the degree of variation in the estimated treatment effect (or risk) estimates with their corresponding 95% CIs across studies. Further statistical discussion of these tests is beyond the scope of this chapter, but further details can be found in the following references.[57–59]
- Traditionally metanalyses have been performed on only RCTs. Recent research by Cameron et al., suggests that the thoughtful integration of both RCTs and NRCS may produce more timely, comprehensive, and generalizable evidence about comparative effectiveness and safety of medical treatments like OMT.[60]
- Variations in OMT-related research provide additional examples of the challenges of pooling data. For example, OMT has been tested in a variety of populations from healthy children to hospitalized adults in the United States to rural patients in developing nations. Further, there may be substantial variations in the specific OMT techniques that practitioners use among similar populations.
- Researchers must be mindful of these differences and decide when pooling data is appropriate. Clinicians should also inform their patients of such limitations when interpreting results.

Clinical Practice Guidelines

- Clinical practice guidelines (CPGs) have been developed by a number of different scientific and professional groups for common conditions. Specifically, CPGs provide summary evidence from systematic reviews of the literature on common clinical conditions.[61]
- These recommendations are intended to assist clinicians with the care of patients using the best available evidence. They are usually developed by a panel of expert researchers and clinicians in the field, and trustworthy guidelines are regularly updated to ensure that they are based on the best currently available evidence. As such, they inform the clinician not only about recommended treatment approaches but also about the level of evidence that supports all treatment approaches.
- CPGs are not fixed protocols and are designed to inform each clinician's treatment decisions. There are excellent databases of CPGs that clinicians can access to help them efficiently evaluate whether their clinical practice is using the best evidence.[62]

Study or Subgroup	Experimental Mean	Experimental SD	Experimental Total	Control Mean	Control SD	Control Total	Weight	Mean Difference IV, Random, 95% CI	Year
Gibson 1985	13	22.5	19	6	22.5	32	7.7%	7.00 [−5.77, 19.77]	1985
Gibson 1985a	13	22.5	19	25	22.5	27	7.5%	−12.00 [−25.21, 1.21]	1985
Andersson 1999	16.2	20	83	18.7	22	72	9.4%	−2.50 [−9.16, 4.16]	1999
Adorjan-Schaumann 1999	−45	23	29	−3	20	28	8.2%	−42.00 [−53.18, −30.82]	1999
Licciardone 2003	31	24.5	18	45.2	20.1	16	7.0%	−14.20 [−29.20, 0.80]	2003
Licciardone 2003a	31	24.5	18	28.5	20.3	19	7.1%	2.50 [−12.04, 17.04]	2003
Heinze 2006	−43	20.6	28	−18	22.2	32	8.3%	−25.00 [−35.83, −14.17]	2006
Chown 2008	−4	19.9	38	−4.8	11.5	33	9.2%	0.80 [−6.64, 8.24]	2008
Mandara 2008	−27	22.9	44	0.3	26.5	50	8.5%	−27.30 [−37.29, −17.31]	2008
Cruser 2012	19.6	14.7	30	37.3	23.9	30	8.5%	−17.70 [−27.74, −7.66]	2012
Vismara 2012	14.1	11.5	10	29.6	8.1	11	8.9%	−15.50 [−24.09, −6.91]	2012
Licciardone 2013	−18	26.1	230	−9	26	225	9.8%	−9.00 [−13.79, −4.21]	2013
Total (95% CI)			566			575	100.0%	−12.91 [−20.00, −5.82]	

Heterogeneity: $Tau^2 = 127.96$; $Chi^2 = 76.67$, df = 11 ($P < 0.00001$); $I^2 = 86\%$
Test for overall effect: Z = 3.57 (P = 0.0004)

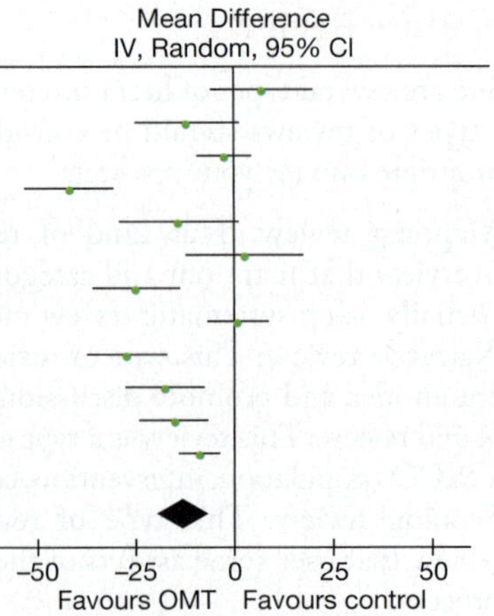

Figure 94.6. Forest plot of reviewed studies from Franke et al.[56] (Reprinted from Franke H, Franke JD, Fryer G. Osteopathic manipulative treatment for nonspecific low back pain: a systematic review and meta-analysis. *BMC Musculoskelet Disord.* 2014; 15:286. http://creativecommons.org/licenses/by/4.0/)

Other Important Considerations when Designing and Performing Clinical Research

- Patient and public involvement (PPI) is a cutting-edge approach to designing any research project just discussed. PPI engages patients and the public in the research process as active partners in research, bringing an important and new form of collaborative and transformative dimensions into the scientific process. PPI improves research by helping researchers focus on issues that are directly relevant to the needs and priorities of society, and builds inclusivity, transparency, and trust needed to have impactful, culturally sensitive, and relevant research that will significantly improve the needs and health of the complex global society.
- Patient registries can also be a valuable source for performing retrospective research and for facilitating prospective research by identifying potential patients who will likely meet the inclusion and exclusion criteria of a study.[63] Searching for registries related to your research question may be quite helpful. Yet you need to make sure you have adequate database and statistical management skills in the research team to perform research with a patient registry dataset.

SPECIAL CONSIDERATIONS WHEN APPRAISING THE SCIENTIFIC LITERATURE

The information in this section and the next are interchangeably relevant. For example, in this section, the presented information provides a view of research from an outsider perspective, so reviewers can learn how to perform research by evaluating how others performed their research. In the next section, the same information is used to build the research from an insider perspective, performing and disseminating research so those outside of the research team can critique and learn from it. Knowing how to critically evaluate the quality of research enables clinicians to continually evolve their practice and provides a strong foundation for creating a research project. The current section provides an overview of key concepts that are critical for all research.[64] Many online resources and citations have also been offered to help clinicians build these skills.

Evaluating for Internal and External Validity

- Internal validity is a construct that refers to the extent to which a study provides an unbiased measure of a true relationship between exposures/treatments and outcomes.
- External validity (or generalizability/representativeness) refers to the extent to which the results of a study may be generalized beyond the study population.

The degree of internal and external validity for studies exists on a spectrum, and while not absolute there is often an inherent trade-off between these two constructs. When considering the internal and external validity of a study, multiple domains should be considered.

- Study participants: Recruitment techniques and inclusion and exclusion criteria have a vital role when considering internal and external validity. Studies with high internal validity generally are methodologically sound in all aspects, with strict enrollment criteria and often utilize restrictive inclusion/exclusion criteria to tightly control for the effect that extraneous factors may have on influencing the relationship between the exposure and outcome. Conversely, studies with high external validity should focus on enrolling much larger, more diverse populations that represent the population to which the results of the study may be applied. Diversity should be considered with respect to various sociodemographic, clinical, and geographic characteristics of the study population.
- Study setting: Several aspects of the study setting should be considered. Studies conducted in settings that enable tight control of research protocols (e.g., basic science laboratories) or have prior experience conducting research (e.g., large academic centers) have stronger internal validity. Conversely, studies conducted in real-world clinical settings are more representative of usual care and thus have stronger external validity. However, internal validity is often reduced because most health care centers are not designed to conduct research and investigators may lack the ability to ensure the research protocols are tightly followed. Other considerations when deciding external validity include factors such as the clinical setting (e.g., intensive care unit vs. ambulatory settings) and geography (e.g., rural vs. urban or country).
- Protocol flexibility: Studies with very rigid and tightly controlled protocols often have high internal validity to better characterize the relationship between the exposure and outcome by controlling for extraneous factors. Studies with the most rigid protocols often include lab-based studies in the basic sciences. However, there is inherent variability in how care is delivered in real-world settings, so studies with more flexible protocols which account for the variation toward how care is delivered in real-world settings tend to have higher external validity.
- Outcome: The selected outcome also has an important impact on internal and external validity. Outcomes with higher internal validity should focus on the extent to which outcomes can be reliably and precisely measured. Alternatively, outcomes with stronger external validity may be easier to measure and should have direct relevance to participants.
- Several factors can underlie which research outcomes do not translate into clinical advances. Understanding these issues is important in interpreting the literature as well as designing and performing research.[65]

Below are examples of two studies related to OMM that have different amounts of internal and external validity.

Example #1: Hicks et al.[66] assessed the effects of dosed myofascial release on human fibroblast preparation, hypertrophy, and cytokine secretions. In this lab-based study,[66] tendons were anchored in a conditioned media and stretched for prespecified interval lengths and set times. Results showed that increased stretching caused increases in several cytokines, including angiotensin, interleukin-3, growth colony-stimulating factor, and chemoattractant cytokines.[66]

Considerations for example #1: The study by Hicks et al.[66] has high internal validity because the investigators were able to tightly control the conditions and accurately measure cytokine release. This study illustrates why studies with high internal validity are good at identifying specific mechanisms. However, this study has poor external validity for several reasons. First, patients are far more complex than tendons in a media. For example, myofascial release may have different effects on a 65-year-old male with a past medical history of hypertension and chronic kidney disease who is taking lisinopril (angiotensin-converting enzyme inhibitor) than a healthy 20-year-old female. Human physiology is dynamic and can be positively and negatively impacted by other physiologic feedback loops, coexisting clinical comorbidities, or pharmacology. Second, reproducing the study's highly specific stretch loads, lengths, and time intervals is unrealistic and unfeasible to implement in real-world clinical practice because of a variety of

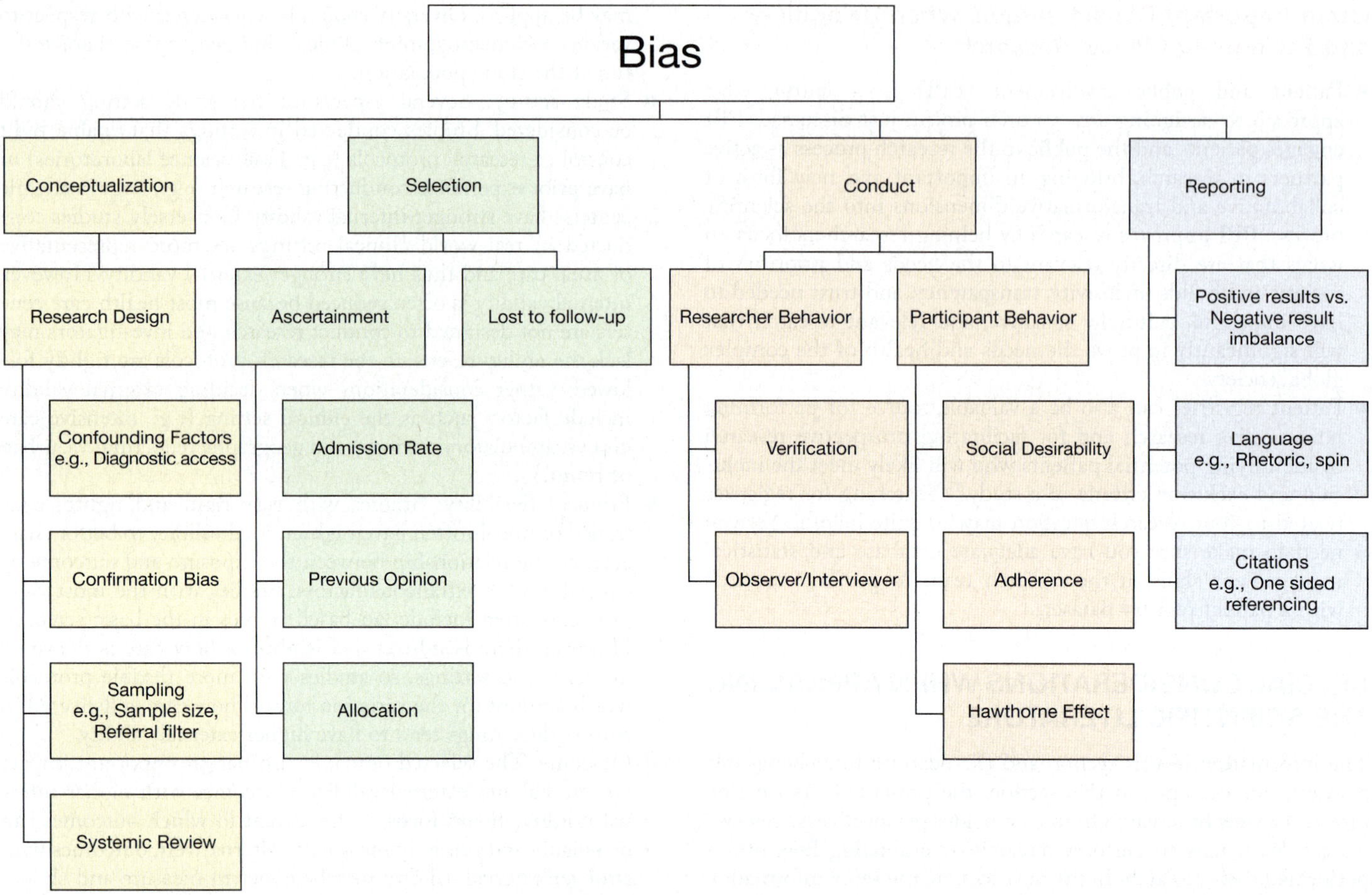

Figure 94.7. **Types of bias.**

patient-specific (e.g., body habitus, muscle mass, degree of somatic dysfunction, age) and provider-specific (e.g., tactile sensation, skill, familiarity with the patient) characteristics.

Example #2: Anderson and McClellan[67] evaluated the effects of spinal manipulation on chronic LBP. In their study, health insurance claims were used to identify a retrospective cohort of 9,948 patients with LBP.[67] After adjusting for age, sex, and a composite risk score for LBP, patients who received OMM as their initial treatment were 33% less likely to require escalated care (defined as additional imaging of the spine, spinal injections, or spinal surgery) than patients who did not receive OMM.[67]

Considerations for example #2: The study by Anderson and McClellan[67] has high external validity because the sample included a large number of real-world patients with LBP. In addition, the selected outcomes have much more clinical relevance to patients than outcomes like cytokines. However, this study has lower internal validity for several reasons. First, it was unable to account for numerous factors, such as severity of back pain, willingness or ability to access medical interventions, or compliance with home exercise programs, that may explain some of the observed differences in outcomes. Second, the data were retrospective claims data; therefore, it was not possible to standardize the force, duration, or even the specific type of OMM performed. Thus, this type of study often lacks the ability to precisely account for all mechanistic factors that may account for observed outcomes.

Identification of Bias

Bias is defined as "any trend or deviation from the truth in data collection, data analysis, interpretation and publication which can lead to false conclusions."[68] In general, clinical studies are designed to compare the effect of a specific factor (i.e., the exposure) on selected outcomes. Bias arises when additional factors beyond the exposure variable of interest affect outcomes. A Catalog of Biases for health care is maintained by the University of Oxford and has documented 49 separate forms of bias that can occur at any stage of the research process.[69] Broadly, these biases can be categorized into four main groups (Fig. 94.7).

- Conceptualization bias is the use of information designed to support an individual's ideas, beliefs, or hypotheses.
- Selection bias is introduced when study participants do not represent the population that the results are ascribed to. Selection bias can be introduced during enrollment of study participants or among participants who have complete data.
- Conduct bias is related to all aspects of performing the study. Examples are poor adherence to the study protocol and unrealistic outcome measures that require study participants to accurately report events or experiences that occurred in the distant past or over a long period.
- Reporting (publication) bias involves choosing to publish a study based on its results. Multiple factors influence publication bias. For example, journal editors are more likely to publish studies with large, significant effects than ones with null effects.

Conceptualization Bias

- This type of bias occurs during the planning phase of a research project. Conceptualization bias generally stems from inadequate review of the relevant literature in a systematic manner before planning a study.

- Conceptualization bias can usually be identified in the introduction, possibly in the discussion section, or in the references of an article.
- The conceptualization phase of a research project is where the scientific process reinitiates, so any bias in the dissemination of previous research projects shapes subsequent projects. Such bias may be identified in the introduction section based on the types and quality of studies used to build the premise for the study.

Selection Bias

Selection bias is present when studies are unable to account for baseline differences between study groups. Selection bias can occur at any point during the study, such as participant enrollment, group assignment, or data analysis. Examples of selection bias are described below.

Ascertainment Bias

- This type of bias typically occurs during participant enrollment and is caused by systematic differences between individuals enrolled in the study and individuals from the target population.
- For example, early volunteers may exhibit exposures or outcomes that are atypical of the target population. Similarly, at the other end of the spectrum, refusers may comprise an atypical component of the target population that is not adequately represented in the study sample. Such individuals may differ in their attitudes or response to the diagnostic procedures or treatments being studied.
- Ascertainment bias can also result from the inclusion and exclusion criteria of studies. For example, consider the earlier example of a case-control study that assessed the effects of physical activity on the development of anginal chest pain. Identifying cases from emergency departments or hospitals skews the results since these patients are typically representative of more severe angina than other patients with angina.
- The use of conservative inclusion and exclusion criteria may result in enrolling participants who do not represent the target population. This limits the study's external validity and may lead to unrepresentative estimates of risk or treatment effect. Often, the restrictive characteristics of the study population are a criticism of RCTs because they limit the real-world clinical application of results.
- If patients are not naive to the experimental treatment, they may be poor candidates for inclusion in clinical trials because they are likely to have specific expectations of the treatment outcome based on previous experiences.

Allocation Bias

This type of bias results when the method used to assign or classify patients to their respective groups causes systematic differences between the respective groups. Observational studies are prone to this type of bias.

- Misclassification bias: This type of bias results from the misclassification of study participants into the wrong group. Participants could be misclassified for a variety of reasons, such as patients forgetting or being unaware of prior exposures and inaccurate or incomplete documentation. For example, in a study evaluating depression, the research team considers head trauma as a confounder and wants to exclude volunteers with depression and previous head trauma. Patients with a remote history of minor head trauma may have forgotten that history, or there may be no documented history in medical records or claims data, particularly if the patient did not seek medical care.
- Loss to follow-up: Despite an investigator's best efforts, all study participants may not complete the study; some may be lost to follow-up. Reasons for loss to follow-up may be related to the allocated treatment. For example, participants may experience adverse events or find the treatment ineffective. Alternatively, participants could be lost to follow-up for reasons unrelated to the study. For example, participants may move or pass away from a condition unrelated to treatment, such as a motor vehicle accident.
- There are a variety of factors to consider when evaluating whether the authors of an article tried to minimize selection bias. For example, did the authors clearly identify the target population and carefully consider the inclusion and exclusion criteria in relation to the target population?
- Randomization is also used to give investigators confidence that selection bias has been eliminated. However, there is always a chance that randomization accidentally clustered certain characteristics in one group versus another, which would bias the outcomes of a study.
- Researchers should also consider whether the study used statistical analyses to minimize the chance of selection bias. Examples of such analyses are multivariable statistical models and matched propensity scores.

Conduct Bias

Conduct bias results from systematic differences in the actions of participants or from differences in how outcomes are measured. Conduct bias is an umbrella term for several types of measurement bias. This type of bias may be identified in the methods section of a study, but it is also important to evaluate whether the authors considered this form of bias in their discussion section. Examples of conduct bias are described below.

Observer Bias

This type of bias results in different responses arising from the participant's awareness of being observed. The Hawthorne effect is a common example of this type of bias. Another example of observer bias is white coat syndrome, which refers to an elevated patient blood pressure when measured in the clinic instead of at home.

Recall Bias

This type of bias results from differences in the probability that participants with and without the outcome of interest can accurately recall previous events. Recall bias is particularly problematic in case-control studies. For example, a case-control study assessing the association between ovarian cancer and talc powder may find that patients with ovarian cancer are more likely to remember using talc powder than healthy women without cancer. In general, patients with poor outcomes are more likely to ruminate over previous exposures.

Expectation Bias

This type of bias arises from differences in how outcomes are measured because of a pre-existing expectation of an uncertain outcome. Using an RCT example provided earlier, a physician taking part in an unblinded trial investigating a new medication may perform closer examinations or spend more time asking participants about side effects of an untested medication than for the standard treatment.

Contamination Bias

This type of bias may occur if patients in the control group inadvertently receive all or part of the experimental intervention, thereby reducing the observed treatment effect. This bias is related to the ITT and PP analyses discussed earlier.

- Contamination bias may also be a factor when developing a hands-on sham treatment for OMT.
- Patients may withdraw from a study because the experimental interventions are not properly delivered, adding potential bias to the data.

Reporting Bias

The issue of publication bias goes beyond the appraisal of an individual article. It is concerned with a broad pattern of publication by a journal or within a field involving numerous journals. Because publications are the basis for future research, biased reporting will misdirect future research efforts. Examples of publication bias follow.

- Scientific or professional societies may publish reports, editorials, or express opinions that do not accurately present controversies or disparate evidence.
- Journal editors may have a predisposition to publish studies with positive results even when the methodologic approaches are questionable. Similarly, they may reject negative studies. Even a systematic review of the literature that highlights negative outcomes may be rejected or never submitted for publication. Although a publication bias, the outcome of this bias then causes conceptualization bias in future research because investigators are unaware of the existing biases.
- Publication bias may lead to inefficiency in the research process by continuing to promote and fund less-than-ideal lines of inquiry.
- Several clinical trial registries have been established to help identify and monitor the results of clinical trials with the goal of minimizing publication bias and its influence on future research planning.
- In the end, investigators should aim to publish in widely circulated journals that cover their research field and provide rapid and fair peer review.
- Journal impact factors and circulation numbers may be used to guide submission decisions. Publishing in journals that are indexed in major bibliographic databases, such as PubMed, or that offer open access ensures study results will be widely disseminated.
  - The *New England Journal of Medicine*, *JAMA*, *JAMA Pediatrics*, and *Annals of Family Medicine* are high-impact general and primary care journals that have published OMT trials.
  - *Spine*, *BMC Musculoskeletal Disorders*, *Manual Therapy*, and *American Journal of Obstetrics and Gynecology* are specialty-oriented journals that have published OMT trials and systematic reviews.
  - The *Journal of Osteopathic Medicine* and the *International Journal of Osteopathic Medicine* publish a wide variety of articles involving all aspects of osteopathic medicine, including basic mechanistic research, clinical studies, and educational research.

Overall Summary

Appraising literature is a skill that needs to be developed throughout one's career. The more the literature is read and critiqued, the more a researcher can identify and appreciate the different types of biases in an easier, quicker, and more insightful manner. A simple starting point is to determine whether the information reported is highly opinionated. For example, do the authors use extreme or one-sided language? Is the study built on unsupported or unsubstantiated claims? Do the claims represent objective outcomes or selected nuances of data that consist of bias or opinion?

MEASURING EXPOSURES AND OUTCOMES

- In clinical practice and research, it is a basic truism that one cannot manage what one does not measure.
- When appraising the methods section of an article, clinicians should consider whether the investigator used valid and reliable data collection tools. This step is critical in all aspects of clinical research. The use of standardized assessment and outcome measures that have been tested in the population of interest and are reliable and valid is essential for the results of any study to have credibility.[65]

Levels of Measurement

- There are four levels of measurement: nominal, ordinal, interval, and ratio.
- For a nominal level of measurement, values are named, and they may or may not have a rank or numerical value. For example, survey questions may be answered as "yes" or "no." Statistical analysis is limited to frequencies or percentages of specific responses.
- For an ordinal level of measurement, characteristics are classified by order or rank. Ordinal measures are frequently used in surveys, where respondents provide an answer on a scale that may have words and numbers. For example, satisfaction or improvement may be rated on a 0 to 5 scale and labeled from "very dissatisfied" through "neutral" to "very satisfied." An important consideration with ordinal measures is that although there is a rank order of numbers and modifier words the distance between each number or word on the scale is not necessarily equal.
- For an interval level of measurement, a scale with numeric values is used, and the distance between each value is equal. Although there may be negative and positive values, there is generally no empirical zero value. For example, a patient and clinician scale that measures the magnitude of change or importance of change between patient visits or over time is an example of an interval scale. Such a scale could have values from −7 ("much worse") through zero ("no change") to +7 ("much improved").
- For a ratio level of measurement, rank values are used, and there are equal distances between values and a zero point. Walking speed or timed repeated sit-to-stand tests of function are examples of a ratio level of measurement.[70] For this type of measurement, collected data can be subjected to more sophisticated statistical analyses.

Properties of Measures

- All measures are associated with some error. Researchers and clinicians need to ensure that the error associated with a specific measurement is minimized and the quantity of error is known. If a clinician wants to document a change in a patient's condition after treatment, it is important to know that the change in measurement reflects a true change in status and not just an error in measurement. Selections of measures that are reliable and valid in the population of interest are of fundamental importance for researchers and clinicians alike.

- There are several forms of reliability and validity. Importantly, reliability and validity are not measured as dichotomous variables, and they often require a series of studies to establish.[70–75] The most common types of reliability and validity are described below.

Test–Retest Reliability

Test–retest reliability or reproducibility is established when the same measurement is taken on two separate occasions, on the same participants, and under the same conditions. The score should be the same. If not, the difference is likely due to measurement error. Interrater (also known as interobserver or interexaminer) reliability relates to the consistency of measurement on the same patient and under the same conditions, except for a different rater or observer. Again, any change in score is attributed to measurement error. In general, test–retest reliability is usually associated with less measurement error than interrater reliability.

Validity

Validity is the ability of a measure to measure what it intends to measure. There are various types of validity.

- Face validity is simple and potentially simplistic. It is established by determining whether the measure appears to measure what it intends to. Other types of validity are generally more desirable to support the use of a specific measure.
- Construct validity is established by determining the degree to which the measure appears to measure a specific and defined construct. For example, the construct of flexibility may be defined by range of motion, but the construct of endurance may be defined by the number of loaded quadriceps contractions or the ability to complete a 6-minute distance walk.
- Concurrent validity can be established by using two instruments that purport to measure the same or a similar construct. Scores on both instruments should be related to establish convergent validity.
- Discriminant validity of a measure is demonstrated when the instrument clearly demonstrates different scores between patients with and without a particular condition.
- Criterion validity reflects the degree to which scores on a specific instrument are related to a reference standard or criterion. For example, a specific OMT spinal examination technique should reflect the reported pathologic findings.
- Predictive validity establishes the extent to which the scores on the measure predict the outcome of a specific condition or treatment. For example, pain intensity or depression in patients with back pain is predictive of relatively poor outcomes.

Responsiveness to Change

In addition to a measure having strong and established levels of reliability and validity, it is also important that the measure is accurate and sensitive enough to measure change. This property is known as responsiveness to change. In general, the more accurate the measure (i.e., less measurement error associated with the specific instrument), the more likely the instrument will be able to measure a change in a patient's status. That change, whether of academic interest or clinical importance, will be judged by the patient, clinician, and researcher. For example, a reduction in pain intensity from a level of 7/10 to 6/10 can be measured and may even be appreciable by the patient. However, this change in pain level may not be clinically meaningful if the patient still needs the same dosage of medication or still has no difference in function. For that change in pain level to be clinically meaningful, a greater level of change (potentially 7/10 to 5/10) is required.

Types of Measures

It is beyond the scope of this chapter to describe and discuss the many different types of assessment and outcome measures that are used across the domains of impairment, performance, function, and disability. However, evaluating the quality and characteristics of these measures is necessary when appraising the literature and designing research.

Analyzing the Data

- Before conducting studies, the specific hypotheses and statistical analyses should be prespecified. These features of good research should be clearly identifiable in the introduction and methods section of a paper. Prespecified analyses are important to protect against data dredging, which refers to conducting multiple, unplanned analyses to look for statistically significant associations among study variables. Data dredging increases the likelihood of identifying false-positive or false-negative associations. Data dredging can occur when using data from patient registries, so it may be necessary to acknowledge this limitation for your outcomes when using this type of study design.
- Such efforts may be suitable for hypothesis generation, but a multiple comparisons statistical adjustment is likely necessary. Conclusions from such a statistical approach are likely invalid.
- Analyzing data for only patients who fully adhere to the research protocol or complete the exit visit may yield biased results. Alternatively, analyzing all data, including incomplete or incorrect application of interventions, likely produces contamination bias. If the ITT analysis shows statistical significance, the intervention is robust enough to overcome the contamination bias, and greater confidence in the outcomes is reasonable. ITT overcomes contamination bias or noncompliance with the assigned treatments, but also the potential bias from drop outs or attrition bias. Yet, interpreting the study when ITT and PP analyses have different outcomes is part of the art of science. It is reasonable to conclude that additional research will be needed to better understand what is happening.
- Clinician researchers should also determine whether statistical methods of imputation were used, when appropriate, to handle missing data. Further, observed outlier data should not be excluded. In those cases, nonparametric statistics should be considered.
- Collapsing measurement scales after data collection tends to obscure significant findings.

SPECIAL CONSIDERATIONS WHEN CONDUCTING RESEARCH IN OSTEOPATHIC MANIPULATIVE MEDICINE

Asking a Clinical Question

- If clinicians are adequately observant and curious, every patient potentially generates clinical questions. The role of the physician is to identify meaningful clinical questions and try to answer them to the best of one's ability. Therefore, research questions should compel and motivate physicians to explore the literature and participate in science to answer questions that are unknown or whose answers are currently inadequate.

- A well-defined clinical question is a critical element in driving evidence-based clinical practice and the scientific process. The question guides the clinician to think carefully and critically about the patient and what the practitioner needs to understand the patient, the condition, diagnostic and treatment methods, and outcomes. A well-defined question should produce an efficient literature search to identify the strength and level of evidence about what is currently known about the question.
- The PICOT (population, intervention, comparison or control, outcome, and time) method is a commonly used framework for asking evidence-based clinical questions. Note, sometimes it is an E for exposure rather than I for intervention in some references. This framework has been shown to improve efficiency in search strategies and when answering clinical questions.[76,77] For example, in patients with chronic back pain (P), does the addition of OMT (I) when compared with standard therapy (C) enhance physical function (O) at 2 weeks (T)?
- Sometimes the question may be similar to an existing study but has not been specifically tested when written as a PICOT question. For example, the comparison treatment or control may differ, the outcome may be physical function rather than pain, or the reassessment time may be different, such as 3 months after treatment instead of immediately after treatment.
- Gaps or fragile foundations in knowledge present opportunities to develop hypotheses and begin a line of inquiry.
    - A strong hypothesis supports a clinical question or idea and compels the investigator to perform the research. A hypothesis is a prediction of the answer to the research question for a specific population or relationship. The hypothesis should not be ambiguous and should be a simple statement.
    - Just because the idea is new to the investigator does not mean that the idea or question is new to the biomedical scientific community. Reviewing the literature is critical for refining the question and learning what nuances of the question have already been determined, what methods have been used to answer other questions related to the question, and what aspects of the question are still unknown.
    - Some important questions to ask when reviewing the literature are presented in Table 94.2.
- Investigators must identify and understand their assumptions, beliefs, and biases related to clinical questions to mitigate their effects on the study. Although the osteopathic profession has a 130-year history of OMM perspectives and practice, actual research in the field has been limited. Often, clinical practice is seen through the colored lens of profession-wide modeling and expert opinion. In research, the goal is to remove all colored lenses and ask simple, direct questions that identify what is instead of what we think or want things to be.
- In the end, a good research question is novel, relevant, important, ethical, interesting to the investigator, and feasible in the allotted time with the available resources.

Mentorship

- Learning to do any new activity is facilitated when someone who has already learned the activity guides the novice.
- A good mentor will inspire the refinement of the research question and study design, help with statistical evaluation and interpretation of data, provide advice on time management and manuscript development, and save the novice a lot of anxiety and time. By providing this assistance, the mentor increases the likelihood that the project will have a meaningful outcome.

TABLE 94.2

How to Evaluate Background Literature for a Clinical Trial

Evaluation of Literature	Question
Background information	Is the literature review thorough and current? Does the content of the literature review relate directly to the research problem? Does the research use a theoretical or conceptual model? Does the model seem appropriate?
Participant selection	Who are the participants? Are the inclusion and exclusion criteria specified? How representative are the participants? Is there a selection bias evident in participant selection?
Design and methods	Is the study design appropriate? How is the research conducted (i.e., the study procedure) and data collected? Are the written methods sufficient to permit replication of the study by another center? Was institutional review board approval obtained?
Data analysis	Are the primary and secondary outcomes defined? If so, are they appropriate? How is the data analyzed? Do the selected statistical tests appear appropriate? Is the study adequately powered?
Research results	What are the findings of the study? Are the results presented in a clear and understandable way? Are the results accurately interpreted as significant or insignificant?
Discussion of results	Do the results support the hypothesis? Do the authors adequately discuss their results in relation to clinical practice? What are the limitations of the study, and do the authors discuss them adequately? How does the study contribute to the extant literature? What additional questions does the study raise? Will the findings of this study change your clinical practice?

- Ideally, a project should have a mentorship team that includes one or more experienced clinician researchers in the field being studied. In a clinical outcome study, it is preferable to have a mentor who is an expert in the condition and another who is an expert in OMM. At least one mentor on the team should be rigorously trained in the scientific method and relatively uninvested in the line of research to minimize bias.
- A statistician is also essential for refining the research question and designing a methodology so that the question can be answered statistically. Statisticians' skills should be used routinely throughout the design and implementation of the study and not just during data analysis. In research, few things are more frustrating than when an investigator completes a study and provides the data to a statistician who then says the research question cannot be answered based on the research design or the

data cannot be used because of assumptions made or a design (fatal) flaw in the study.

- It is not appropriate to provide a dataset to a statistician for analysis without their previous input about the question, design, and data collection and recording process.
- Although certain residency and fellowship training sites have existing mentorship programs, not every program has this infrastructure. To help clinicians without access to such support, the American Academy of Osteopathy's Louisa Burns Osteopathic Research Committee often sponsors a program called the Research Proposal and Mentorship Grand Rounds at their annual Convocation to provide expert mentorship to OMM investigators.

Categories of Osteopathic Manipulative Medicine Research

There are at least four broad categories for OMM research: research specifically related to defining somatic dysfunction, research evaluating how somatic dysfunction is clinically identified, research on the effectiveness and safety of OMT, and research defining the mechanisms of action underlying OMT, including indirect effects associated with the biopsychosocial influences of osteopathic care. While other areas of OMM/OMT research that are also important and needed, such as the research on the incidence, prevalence, prognosis of somatic dysfunction, training OMT skills, and the economic implications of OMM, these research area may be hampered by the vague, imprecise, and irreproducible aspects of defining and identifying somatic dysfunction. A better infrastructure for performing research in OMM is needed to make science in this field meaningful.

RESEARCH DEFINING SOMATIC DYSFUNCTION

- At its origins, somatic dysfunction is a uniquely osteopathic term. As covered previously in this textbook, somatic dysfunction was a 20th-century refinement of the earlier term, osteopathic lesion, and is defined as "impaired or altered function of related components of the body framework system: skeletal, arthrodial, and myofascial structures, and their related vascular, lymphatic and neural elements."[78]
- A definition of a biologic entity should have distinctive biologic features with limiting characteristics for what does and does not belong to the entity. Although the term somatic dysfunction was seen as an advancement of osteopathic nomenclature in the 1950s, the current definition of somatic dysfunction is broad and vague, making it difficult to use or operationalize in biomedical research or to objectively teach.
- In the 21st century, research needs to characterize exactly what somatic dysfunction is or identify multiple distinctive and clearly defined features that are currently poorly defined and understood under the all-encompassing term of somatic dysfunction.
- Somatic dysfunction is identified using four main categories of tests: tissue texture abnormalities, asymmetry, restricted motion, and tenderness (also known as TART).[78] Objective evidence that specifies how these categories of tests are indicators of impaired or altered function and their relationship with the listed anatomical structures is sparse. In addition, evidence indicates inconsistent application and interpretation of these tests.[79–83]
- In the 21st century, new technologies, such as magnetic resonance or ultrasound elastography,[84] are developing with the capability of characterizing various structural and functional aspects of the neuromusculoskeletal system. Further, new initiatives at the National Institutes of Health (NIH) in the area of force-based manipulation have created the opportunity to perform research that critically evaluates what somatic dysfunction is.[85]

HOW SOMATIC DYSFUNCTION IS IDENTIFIED

- Humans are dynamic living organisms and always changing on some level from moment to moment. Because somatic dysfunction is determined by a human on another human, research in OMM needs to evaluate the person being examined and the examiner (i.e., the instrument doing the examination).
- Examiners have differences in tactile sensitivity and use varying levels and directions of force when using their hands to examine for somatic dysfunction. They also have differences in training regarding how to assess and treat patients for somatic dysfunction. This extreme level of variability makes it difficult to produce research whose outcomes can influence future practice.
- Good science requires good observations, consistent use of descriptive terminology to characterize observations, and reproducible descriptions of diagnostic and therapeutic activities of the hand so research outcomes can be reproduced to guide future patient care and research.
- For decades, the ECOP has promoted the development of consistent terminology and expansion of modeling based on historical and current perspectives. Overall, current evidence, although weak, indicates that TART exams have poor reliability.[79–83,86,87]
- It is standard practice in science to calibrate instruments that collect observations so that researchers can assess the comparability of findings produced by the instrument over time. Traditionally, the demonstration of successful calibration has not been part of OMM training, which hampers the progression of science in this field. Only one study showed that the reliability of palpatory skills improves and is sustained with calibration exercises.[88]
- OMM needs an evidence base that shows palpation skills are clearly and consistently definable and reproducible. Currently, this evidence does not exist. Most clinical research and educational programming ignore these issues and, as a result, OMM research outcomes will always be undermined by this lack of fundamental evidence.

RESEARCH ON THE OUTCOMES OF OSTEOPATHIC MANIPULATIVE TREATMENT

- Generally, clinicians are most interested in evaluating the clinical effectiveness of OMT. Although RCTs are considered the gold standard of clinical effectiveness, this design is more complicated and resource intensive than other designs.[89] Even in an ideal situation where the researcher has all the necessary resources and the time to perform an RCT, the rigor of this design is limited by the paucity of research objectively characterizing somatic dysfunction and the lack of adequate reliability between examiners' skills. Even after acknowledging the limitations of defining somatic dysfunction, there are other factors that should also be considered when designing clinical effectiveness research in OMM.
- As previously stated, forming similar cohorts within a study to minimize confounders and bias is critical. This issue is usually addressed by defining inclusion and exclusion criteria and by matching factors such as age, race, gender, and body mass index among participants in the various study groups.
- When performing OMM research, the complexity of forming comparable cohorts is more challenging because of the greater appreciation of the uniqueness of each individual. If the goal is to determine the effectiveness of OMT and if OMT is used, by

definition, to treat somatic dysfunction, should not the presence, absence, or severity of somatic dysfunction in key regions of the body that relate to the research question be used as matching criteria? Therefore, it is critical to try to develop specific, predetermined criteria that can be reliably assessed and used to ensure that study groups are similar regarding the primary focus of the study, that is, somatic dysfunction.

- Another factor worth considering is trauma history. For example, in a LBP study, is it realistic to compare a poorly conditioned participant whose LBP is related to recurrent microtrauma with a well-conditioned person whose LBP is the result of a high-speed motor vehicle accident? Therefore, trauma history may be a reasonable consideration when selecting the study population and is a potential reason for poor reproducibility in outcomes from LBP studies. This factor may also address a previously unrecognized form of patient selection bias.
- From a biopsychosocial perspective, screening or measuring baseline traits related to openness, negative emotionality such as catatrophizing,[90] patient expectations,[91] and the effect of personality traits on placebo/nocebo[92] are also relevant to consider. It is likely that these events and experiences are not exclusive, further representing the complexity of patient selection.
- Clinicians can have biases about intervention effectiveness and expected treatment outcomes based on patient characteristics. For example, an experimental study showed that the very same patients were assessed differently by clinicians and were expected to have a more negative outcome if the clinician believed they were injured at work rather than during recreational activities.[93] In this case, expected outcomes can become actual outcomes through nonspecific (placebo) mechanisms.
- When possible, participants who are naive to OMT should be recruited. When recruiting only naïve participants is not possible, matching between group's research participants who are naive to OMT and those who are regular users of OMT should be considered.
- In addition, researchers evaluating effectiveness of osteopathic interventions need to consider aspects of body unity in participant selection. Questionnaires have been developed that identify characteristics of poor responders to interventions and high-frequency users of health care services. For example, the Pain Catastrophizing Scale[94,95] and the Adverse Childhood Experiences Score[96–98] are two tools worth considering to more holistically identify confounders that may influence outcomes within and between studies or to select more consistent study cohorts.
- Patients and providers may systematically err when measuring and recording treatment outcomes that accord with their expectations but are inconsistent with actual observation. To help overcome this bias, explicit data collection forms should be developed before the study begins and be used consistently throughout the study.
- Repeated measures of somatic dysfunction tests over time are susceptible to intraexaminer and interexaminer variability and to random changes in participants that are unrelated to study factors. Therefore, clinician researchers must consider how to sustain consistency when performing and interpreting procedures. It may be worth having independent examiners and treatment providers to minimize bias.

Treatment Fidelity

Treatment fidelity ensures that the interventions delivered by practitioners in clinical research studies are consistently applied as intended over time and across participating providers and sites.

- Treatment fidelity in OMM research is critical, especially when there is a potential for substantial variation in practitioner skills and their application in research protocols.
- For explanatory research, standardized interventions like those in pharmaceutical research are probably unfeasible for OMT studies. However, such studies involving massage chairs or robots may be possible if location, forces, and force vectors can be preset. Although pure protocol-driven research is possible in OMM research, it is inconsistent with osteopathic philosophy.
- It is reasonable to produce a hybrid OMT protocol based on evidence-based or evidence-informed practice and expert consensus. For example, in the MOPSE study, a standardized portion of the protocol was developed from a century of literature based on physiologic understandings and case reports or case series reporting effectiveness of OMT for people with pneumonia.[99] This protocol also allowed patient-specific treatment for unexpected or unresponsive somatic dysfunctions as long as those treatments were reported on the data collection sheet.[99]
- A similar approach was used in the OSTEOPATHIC Trial,[100] where OMT providers used six common techniques to treat patients with chronic LBP. Providers could also use other optional techniques as time permitted during treatment sessions and if they judged one or more of the designated techniques was contraindicated or ineffective for a particular patient[96] (Fig. 94.8). With this design, it is important to report the variations in treatment for better insight into the specific treatments provided, the effectiveness of such treatments, and the factors that led the provider to provide the specific treatment.
- An important feature of pragmatic research is the clear, consistent, and meticulous reporting of diagnostic findings and treatment procedures. Without such data, the study will be less likely to influence future research or patient care. Replication requires biomechanical details that are generally missing in previous manual therapy research.
- Early on in the development of the study, the investigator needs to decide whether the intervention (OMT) is being performed by one person or multiple people and whether the intervention is a protocol, an algorithm, or pragmatic. There are different requirements for developing and performing these types of studies as outlined in Table 94.3.
- When treatments are based on diagnostic procedures, as in the case of pragmatic studies, then diagnostic fidelity (i.e., making sure the diagnostic process is consistently and reliably performed) is also relevant and important. Providers who are inadequately trained to diagnose somatic dysfunction and deliver treatments will tend to obscure potentially important research findings.
- Reliability and validity in the diagnosis of somatic dysfunction is an inherent requirement for OMT fidelity, especially in pragmatic studies. As stated earlier, research is needed in this area to meet current scientific standards.
- Treatment fidelity has been more thoroughly studied and implemented in other practitioner-based fields that are trying to influence health behavior.
- The Treatment Fidelity Workgroup of the NIH Behavior Change Consortium[101] has identified treatment fidelity goals and strategies that are germane and adaptable to OMT research (Table 94.4).
- Without fidelity training, the interexaminer reliability of osteopathic palpatory findings has generally been unsatisfactory when assessing osteopathic medical students or OMM physicians. Typically, the goal for demonstrating reliability for physical examination research studies equates to a $\kappa \geq 0.40$.[82,102]

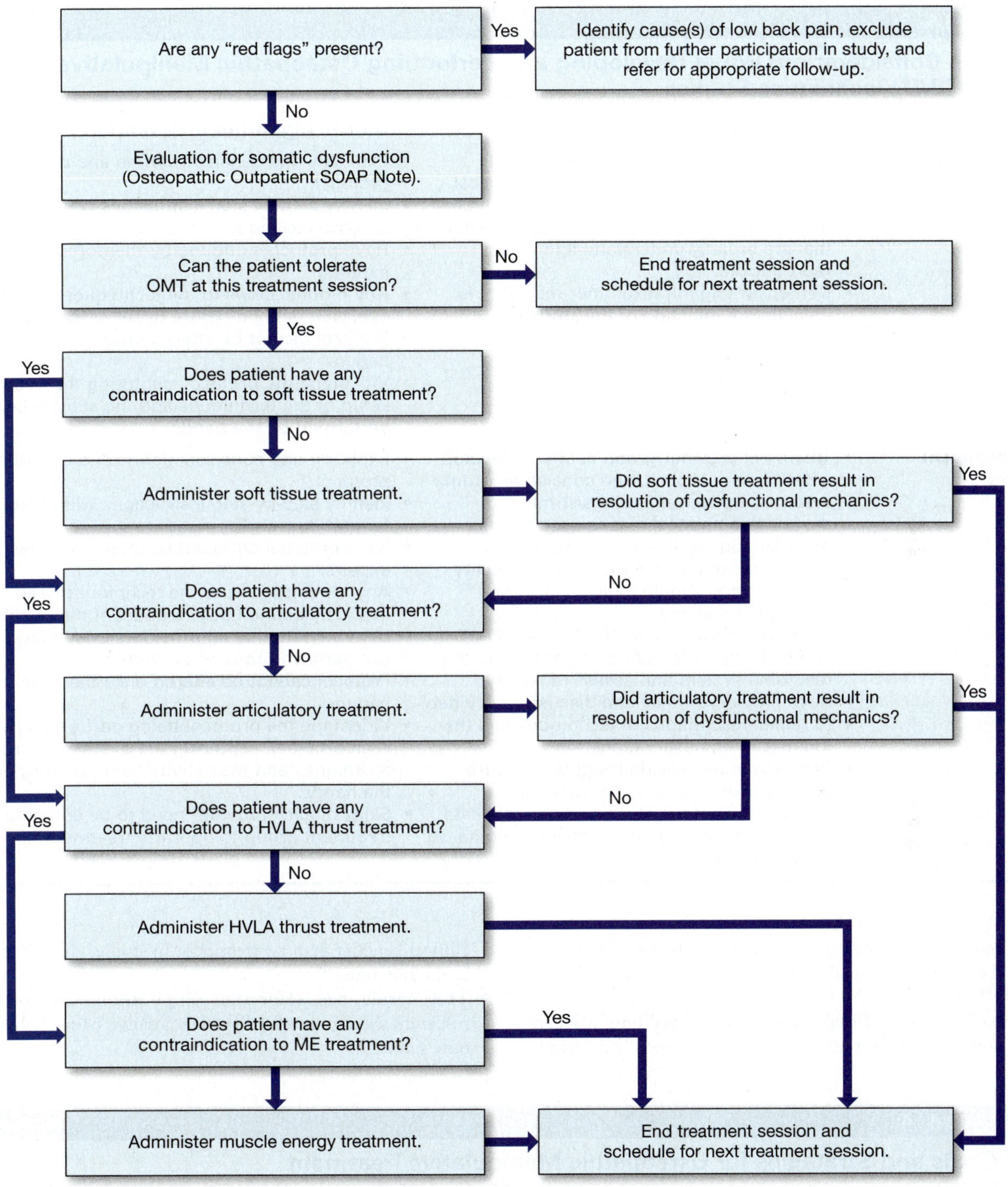

Figure 94.8. Research algorithm for delivering osteopathic manipulative treatment for low back pain.

- When OMM physicians completed 16 to 32 hours of consensus training over 4 months, their interexaminer reliability improved, and κ values achieved satisfactory levels for evaluating asymmetry, tissue texture changes, segmental motion, and tenderness.[102]

Sham Treatment and the Placebo Effect

- A sham is a term for an inert or innocuous intervention, such as a sugar pill or a procedure intended to make the study participant comfortable.[103] A sham treatment allows for the quantification or characterization of the placebo effect.
- The use of shams to evaluate the placebo effect is a gold standard in RCTs evaluating treatments.[104]
- An ideal placebo should be indistinguishable from the experimental intervention and maintain patient blinding. However, this combination is difficult to achieve in trials of complex interventions, such as OMT.
- Important aspects of the placebo effect include credibility of the placebo, expectation of benefit from its use, and adequate blinding of patients with respect to active treatment versus placebo allocation.[105]

TABLE 94.3

Intervention Considerations When Developing and Performing Osteopathic Manipulative Treatment (OMT) Techniques Studies

Number of Providers	Pragmatic Intervention	Protocol/Algorithm Intervention
Single treatment provider	• Need to develop a descriptive, explicit, and concise recording system for physical findings/somatic dysfunction and techniques used during the interventions, using terms that are broadly understandable and reproducible. • Demonstrating intraexaminer reliability is ideal before initiation of the study.	• Explicitly and concisely define and describe the protocol. • Identify step-by-step instructions with references for each technique. • Have protocol critiqued by mentorship team or experts. • Any modifications to the techniques need to be explicitly defined before onset of the study. • Protocol cannot be altered once the study has begun. • Videotape the protocol, capturing the overall setup of the techniques and the activity being performed by the hands.
Multiple treatment providers	• Treatment provider group needs to develop a descriptive, explicit, and concise recording system for physical findings/somatic dysfunction and techniques used by all providers during the interventions. • An assessment of interexaminer reliability is needed and should indicate at least moderate reliability. • Videotape each provider performing OMT and have each member of the team use the recording system and assess reliability. • Have providers watch and discuss each video to refine descriptions of techniques and the tool based on observations. • Research must provide insights so future providers know how to approximate interventions of the study and can replicate outcomes when applied to patients similar to study cohorts.	• Explicitly and concisely define and describe the protocol. • Identify step-by-step instructions with references for each technique. • Have protocol critiqued by mentorship team or experts. • Any modifications to the techniques need to be explicitly defined before onset of the study. • Demonstrate that all providers understand and can perform protocol as written. • Protocol cannot be altered once the study has begun. • Videotape the protocol being performed by each provider, capturing the overall setup of the techniques and the activity being performed by the hands. • Skills of each provider need to be critiqued by the treatment group to optimize treatment fidelity.

- Recent research is uncovering the complex nature of the placebo, and our historically naïve attempt to characterize and control it.[103,106,107]
- A systematic review of clinical trials that included both placebo control and no treatment arms found that placebos had greater clinical benefits than no treatment in studies that involved pain as the outcome.[108]
- This result has important implications for osteopathic research, since many OMT trials involve pain as the primary outcome.

TABLE 94.4

Fidelity Goals and Strategies for Osteopathic Manipulative Treatment

Goal	Strategy
Ensure same treatment dose within and between treatment groups	Adequately describe and monitor the treatment dose (number, frequency, and length of contact) for each participant.
Standardize provider training	Conduct similar training for all treatment providers using a standardized training manual.
Ensure provider skill acquisition	Train treatment providers to well-defined performance criteria using standardized or pilot patients.
Minimize drift in provider skills	Conduct booster training to prevent decay of skills over time.
Ensure adherence to treatment protocol	Have providers complete a checklist of treatment components delivered after each session.
Minimize contamination between comparison groups	Videotape or observe sessions with review and feedback.

- But many placebo-controlled trials evaluating treatments for LBP may yield biased estimates of treatment effect.[109]
- In one systematic review and meta-analysis,[110] 24 clinical trials including 2019 patients evaluated the effectiveness of various forms of manual therapy. Although the studies were of low quality, a sham group was included in all of them. There was no statistically significant improvement for the manual therapy group when compared with the sham treatment group, and there was no difference between the sham treatment group and the control group.[110]
- Sham OMT is most useful in a trial when patients are naive to OMT. If patients are recruited from an osteopathic clinic or practice, they are more likely to deduce that their allocated treatment may be sham OMT rather than active OMT.
- The fidelity of a sham treatment protocol needs to be considered if a sham group is part of the research design. Osteopathic physicians often have difficulty delivering sham OMT because they are accustomed and conditioned to perform active OMT. Many say it is consciously impossible to stop their hands from treating a body, so creating a valid sham treatment is not a simple task.
- At this time, it is reasonable to consider a placebo control design when there are no objective outcome measures. For example, a study that only uses patient-reported outcomes, such as pain, is prone to the placebo response and, thus, a sham group is encouraged.
- If objective measures are being used as an outcome measure, then the need for a sham group is questionable.[108] Instead of trying to create a sham group in a study design with objective measures, researcher efforts should highlight the clinical importance of the study and the relevance of its results (Table 94.3).

DEFINING MECHANISMS OF ACTION UNDERLYING OMT

Typically, clinicians are not involved and generally less interested in engaging in mechanism of action research. However, the amount of mechanistic research in manual therapies has been rapidly growing now that basic scientists have more tools to evaluate the neuromusculoskeletal system. Now is an important time for clinicians to collaborate with basic scientists to ensure research with high levels of internal validity and with designs to improve external validity. New instrumentation and NIH support for this type of research are increasing opportunities and evidence to uncover the mechanisms of action for manual therapies, including OMM. It is important that basic scientists and clinicians in the osteopathic profession actively engage in this level of research.

Practice-Based Research Networks

- Practice-based research networks (PBRNs) originated in the primary care field in the early to mid-20th century and were intended to advance the field of medicine through the experiences of physicians in isolated practices.[111] Networks provide independent practitioners a means to collect comparable data directly from their daily practice using a scientific process.[111] Hypothetically, research from a network has the potential to be easily disseminated and immediately impactful within the network.[111] Although electronic medical records should facilitate PBRN research at the point of care, differences in technologies have hampered the data collection process between systems. Yet with technology-driven data warehouses and artificial intelligence, now is an unprecedented opportunity to become clinician scientists, especially by actively participating in the PBRNs.
- DO-Touch.NET, established in 2010,[112] is the only network specifically designated to evaluate the effectiveness and safety of OMM and OMT. Full members include residents and practitioners worldwide who routinely use OMT.

MOVING TOWARD EVIDENCE-BASED OSTEOPATHIC PRACTICE

Throughout this chapter, we have highlighted numerous factors that need to be addressed to establish an infrastructure to generate meaningful, rigorous OMM research. Everyone within the osteopathic profession should play a role in establishing this infrastructure, especially those who are in or have recently completed training programs and those who provide that training.[113] There are an extensive variety of directions for performing research in OMM. However, fundamental issues need to be addressed before rigorous science can be performed in this field. The amount of variability that exists in what we observe (e.g., TART), in what and how we do our examinations and manipulative techniques (e.g., mechanics), and in how we interpret what we feel must be addressed. These issues underlie and undermine every study performed in OMM, limiting the impact of this research. These issues do not indicate that science is impossible in OMM. Instead, they indicate the importance of research in this field because OMM is not as simple as making a drug to study and then creating a sugar pill that looks identical to a drug.

- Good science is based on good observations. Clinicians need to be careful to avoid letting their interests, beliefs, or hopes influence their interpretation of the results of the literature or research that they design, perform, and report. The goal of the clinician researcher is not to confirm the hypotheses but to answer the research question to advance patient care.

This chapter has provided an overview of the research processes and challenges that must be addressed before acquiring additional evidence on the benefits of OMT in treating patients with LBP and other medical conditions. It is through such efforts that the OMM field will move up the osteopathic clinical research pyramid and that OMM will gain increasing recognition as an evidence-based practice.

ACKNOWLEDGMENTS

The authors and editors of this chapter would like to acknowledge the scholarly contributions of Dr. John Licciardone for prior editions of this chapter.

REFERENCES

1. Masic I, Miokovic M, Muhamedagic B. Evidence based medicine: new approaches and challenges. *Acta Inform Med.* 2008;16(4):219–225.
2. Sackett DL. Evidence-based medicine. *Semin Perinatol.* 1997;21(1): 3–5.
3. Sackett DL, Straus SE, Richardson WS, Rosenberg W, Haynes RB. *Evidence-Based Medicine: How to Practice and Teach EBM.* 2nd ed. Churchill Livingstone; 2000.
4. OCEBM Levels of Evidence Working Group. The Oxford Levels of Evidence 2. Oxford Centre for Evidence-Based Medicine. Accessed October 19, 2023. https://www.cebm.ox.ac.uk/resources/levels-of-evidence/ocebm-levels-of-evidence
5. Ambati BK, Cahoon J. Rejuvenating clinician-scientist training. *Invest Ophthalmol Vis Sci.* 2014;55(3):1853–1855.
6. Eley DS, Jensen C, Thomas R, Benham H. What will it take? Pathways, time and funding: Australian medical students' perspective on clinician-scientist training. *BMC Med Educ.* 2017;17(1):242.

7. Hall KL, Vogel AL, Huang GC, et al. The science of team science: a review of the empirical evidence and research gaps on collaboration in science. *Am Psychol.* 2018;73(4):532–548.
8. Wuchty S, Jones BF, Uzzi B. The increasing dominance of teams in production of knowledge. *Science.* 2007;316(5827):1036–1039.
9. https://www.acgme.org/globalassets/pfassets/programrequirements/275_osteopathicneuromusculoskeletalmedicine_2023.pdf
10. Duan Y, Edwards JS, Dwivedi YK. Artificial intelligence for decision making in the era of big data: evolution, challenges and research agenda. *Int J Inf Manage.* 2019;48:63–71.
11. Lenchus JD. End of the "see one, do one, teach one" era: the next generation of invasive bedside procedural instruction. *J Am Osteopath Assoc.* 2010; 110(6):340–346.
12. Bordoni B, Escher AR Jr. Osteopathic principles: the inspiration of every science is its change. *Cureus.* 2021;13(1):e12478.
13. Thangaratinam S, Redman CWE. The Delphi technique. *Obstet Gynaecol.* 2005;7(2):120–125.
14. Degenhardt BF, Kuchera ML. Osteopathic evaluation and manipulative treatment in reducing the morbidity of otitis media: a pilot study. *J Am Osteopath Assoc.* 2006;106(6):327–334.
15. Origo D, Tarantino AG, Nonis A, Vismara L. Osteopathic manipulative treatment in chronic coccydynia: a case series. *J Bodyw Mov Ther.* 2018; 22(2):261–265.
16. Kent DM, van Klaveren D, Paulus JK, et al. The predictive approaches to treatment effect heterogeneity (PATH) statement: explanation and elaboration. *Ann Intern Med.* 2020;172(1):W1–W25.
17. Bandeen SG. Diabetes: report covering twenty-five years research on stimulation of pancreas, blood chemical changes. *Osteopath Prof.* 1949;17(1): 11–15, 38, 40, 42, 44, 46–47.
18. Licciardone JC, Fulda KG, Stoll ST, Gamber RG, Cage AC. A case-control study of osteopathic palpatory findings in type 2 diabetes mellitus. *Osteopath Med Prim Care.* 2007;1:6.
19. Licciardone JC, Kearns CM, Hodge LM, Minotti DE. Osteopathic manual treatment in patients with diabetes mellitus and comorbid chronic low back pain: subgroup results from the OSTEOPATHIC Trial. *J Am Osteopath Assoc.* 2013;113(6):468–478.
20. Centers for Disease Control and Prevention. Pneumocystis pneumonia: Los Angeles. *MMWR Morb Mortal Wkly Rep.* 1981;30(21):250–252.
21. Lillie EO, Patay B, Diamant J, Issell B, Topol EJ, Schork NJ. The n-of-1 clinical trial: the ultimate strategy for individualizing medicine? *Per Med.* 2011;8(2):161–173.
22. Schork NJ. Personalized medicine: time for one-person trials. *Nature.* 2015;520(7549):609–611.
23. von Elm E, Altman DG, Egger M, Pocock SJ, Gøtzsche PC, Vandenbroucke JP; STROBE Initiative. The Strengthening the Reporting of Observational Studies in Epidemiology (STROBE) statement: guidelines for reporting observational studies. *Lancet.* 2007;370(9596):1453–1457.
24. Kibanga W, Mutagonda RF, Moshiro R, et al. Effectiveness of antenatal dexamethasone in reducing respiratory distress syndrome and mortality in preterm neonates: a nested case control study. *BMC Pediatr.* 2023; 23(1):94.
25. Walker J, Mertens UK, Schmidt CO, Chenot JF. Effect on healthcare utilization and costs of spinal manual therapy for acute low back pain in routine care: a propensity score matched cohort study. *PLoS One.* 2017; 12(5):e0177255.
26. Schafer A, Hall T, Muller G, Briffa K. Outcomes differ between subgroups of patients with low back and leg pain following neural manual therapy: a prospective cohort study. *Eur Spine J.* 2011;20(3):482–490.
27. Stampfer M. New insights from the British Doctors study. *BMJ.* 2004; 328(7455):1507.
28. Mahmood SS, Levy D, Vasan RS, Wang TJ. The Framingham Heart Study and the epidemiology of cardiovascular disease: a historical perspective. *Lancet.* 2014;383(9921):999–1008.
29. Degenhardt BF, Johnson JC, Brooks WJ, Norman L. Characterizing adverse events reported immediately after osteopathic manipulative treatment. *J Am Osteopath Assoc.* 2018;118(3):141–149.
30. Kaiser G, Degenhardt BF, Michael Menke J, Snider KT. Characteristics and treatment of pediatric patients in an osteopathic manipulative medicine clinic. *J Am Osteopath Assoc.* 2020;120(3):153–163.
31. Licciardone JC, Moore S, Fix K, Blair LG, Ta K. Osteopathic manipulative treatment of patients with chronic low back pain in the United States: a retrospective cohort study. *J Osteopath Med.* 2023;123(5):259–267.
32. Knottnerus A, Tugwell P. STROBE: a checklist to strengthen the reporting of observational studies in epidemiology. *J Clin Epidemiol.* 2008; 61(4):323.
33. Simmonds KP, Burke J, Kozlowski AJ, Andary M, Luo Z, Reeves MJ. Emulating 3 clinical trials that compare stroke rehabilitation at inpatient rehabilitation facilities with skilled nursing facilities. *Arch Phys Med Rehabil.* 2022;103(7):1311–1319.
34. Cox LA Jr. Modernizing the Bradford Hill criteria for assessing causal relationships in observational data. *Crit Rev Toxicol.* 2018;48(8): 682–712.
35. Sørensen HT, Lash TL, Rothman KJ. Beyond randomized controlled trials: a critical comparison of trials with nonrandomized studies. *Hepatology.* 2006;44(5):1075–1082.
36. Ioannidis JPA, Haidich A, Pappa M, et al. Comparison of evidence of treatment effects in randomized and nonrandomized studies. *JAMA.* 2001;286(7):821–830.
37. Salcher-Konrad M, Nguyen M, Savović J, Higgins JP, Naci H. Treatment effects in randomized and nonrandomized studies of pharmacological interventions: A meta-analysis. *JAMA Network Open.* 2024;7(9): e2436230.
38. Bosdriesz JR, Stel VS, van Diepen M, Meuleman Y, Dekker FW, Zoccali C, et al. Evidence-based medicine—when observational studies are better than randomized controlled trials. *Nephrology.* 2020;25(10):737–743.
39. Bhide A, Shah PS, Acharya G. A simplified guide to randomized controlled trials. *Acta Obstet Gynecol Scand.* 2018;97(4):380–387.
40. Butcher NJ, Monsour A, Mew EJ, et al. Guidelines for reporting outcomes in trial reports: the CONSORT-Outcomes 2022 extension. *JAMA.* 2022; 328(22):2252–2264.
41. Hoehler FK, Tobis JS, Buerger AA. Spinal manipulation for low back pain. *JAMA.* 1981;245(18):1835–1838.
42. Andersson GB, Lucente T, Davis AM, Kappler RE, Lipton JA, Leurgans S. A comparison of osteopathic spinal manipulation with standard care for patients with low back pain. *N Engl J Med.* 1999;341(19):1426–1431.
43. Benedetti F. Placebo and the new physiology of the doctor-patient relationship. *Physiol Rev.* 2013;93(3):1207–1246.
44. Simmonds MJ. Pain and the placebo in physiotherapy: a benevolent lie? *Physiotherapy.* 2000;86(12):631–637.
45. Noll DR, Degenhardt BF, Morley TF, et al. Efficacy of osteopathic manipulation as an adjunctive treatment for hospitalized patients with pneumonia: a randomized controlled trial. *Osteopath Med Prim Care.* 2010;4:2.
46. Bagagiolo D, Priolo CG, Favre EM, et al. A randomized controlled trial of osteopathic manipulative therapy to reduce cranial asymmetries in young infants with nonsynostotic plagiocephaly. *Am J Perinatol.* 2022; 39(suppl 01):S52–S62.
47. Cerritelli F, Pizzolorusso G, Renzetti C, et al. A multicenter, randomized, controlled trial of osteopathic manipulative treatment on preterms. *PLoS One.* 2015;10(5):e0127370.
48. Hensel KL, Buchanan S, Brown SK, Rodriguez M, Cruser DA. Pregnancy research on osteopathic manipulation optimizing treatment effects: the PROMOTE study. *Am J Obstet Gynecol.* 2015;212(1):108.e1–108.e9.
49. Schwerla F, Rother K, Rother D, Ruetz M, Resch KL. Osteopathic manipulative therapy in women with postpartum low back pain and disability: a pragmatic randomized controlled trial. *J Am Osteopath Assoc.* 2015; 115(7):416–425.
50. Gates M, Gates A, Duarte G, et al. Quality and risk of bias appraisals of systematic reviews are inconsistent across reviewers and centers. *J Clin Epidemiol.* 2020;125:9–15.
51. Tricco AC, Lillie E, Zarin W, et al. PRISMA Extension for Scoping Reviews (PRISMA-ScR): checklist and explanation. *Ann Intern Med.* 2018;169(7):467–473.
52. Systematic review preparation guide. UC San Diego Library. Accessed October 19, 2023. https://library.ucsd.edu/research-and-collections/UCSD-Systematic-Review-Considerations-Checklist.pdf
53. Riley SP, Swanson BT, Shaffer SM, Flowers DW, Cook CE, Brismee JM. Why do 'trustworthy' living systematic reviews matter? *J Man Manip Ther.* 2023;31(4):215–219.

54. Paige NM, Miake-Lye IM, Booth MS, et al. Association of spinal manipulative therapy with clinical benefit and harm for acute low back pain: systematic review and meta-analysis. *JAMA.* 2017;317(14):1451–1460.
55. Rubinstein SM, van Middelkoop M, Assendelft WJ, de Boer MR, van Tulder MW. Spinal manipulative therapy for chronic low-back pain: an update of a Cochrane review. *Spine (Phila Pa 1976).* 2011;36(13): E825–E846.
56. Franke H, Franke JD, Fryer G. Osteopathic manipulative treatment for nonspecific low back pain: a systematic review and meta-analysis. *BMC Musculoskelet Disord.* 2014;15:286.
57. Higgins JPT, Thompson SG, Deeks JJ, Altman DG. Measuring inconsistency in meta-analyses. *BMJ.* 2003;327(7414):557–560.
58. DerSimonian R, Laird N. Meta-analysis in clinical trials revisited. *Contemp Clin Trials.* 2015;45(Pt A):139–145.
59. Gavaghan DJ, Moore AR, McQay HJ. An evaluation of homogeneity tests in meta-analysis in pain using simulations of individual patient data. *Pain.* 2000;85(3):415–424.
60. Cameron C, Fireman B, Hutton B, et al. Network meta-analysis incorporating randomized controlled trials and non-randomized comparative cohort studies for assessing the safety and effectiveness of medical treatments: challenges and opportunities. *Syst Rev.* 2015;4:147. https://doi.org/10.1186/s13643-015-0133-0
61. Beauchemin M, Cohn E, Shelton RC. Implementation of clinical practice guidelines in the health care setting: a concept analysis. *ANS Adv Nurs Sci.* 2019;42(4):307–324.
62. Guideline Central. Guidelines. Accessed July 17, 2023. https://www.guidelinecentral.com/guidelines/
63. Gliklich RE, Dreyer NA, Leavy MB, eds. *Registries for Evaluating Patient Outcomes: A User's Guide.* 3rd ed. Agency for Healthcare Research and Quality; 2014.
64. Morrison K. Dissecting the literature: the importance of critical appraisal. Royal College of Surgeons of England. Accessed July 17, 2023. https://www.rcseng.ac.uk/library-and-publications/library/blog/dissecting-the-literature-the-importance-of-critical-appraisal/
65. Heneghan C, Goldacre B, Mahtani KR. Why clinical trial outcomes fail to translate into benefits for patients. *Trials.* 2017;18(1):122.
66. Hicks MR, Cao TV, Campbell DH, Standley PR. Mechanical strain applied to human fibroblasts differentially regulates skeletal myoblast differentiation. *J Appl Physiol (1985).* 2012;113(3):465–472.
67. Anderson BR, McClellan SW. Three patterns of spinal manipulative therapy for back pain and their association with imaging studies, injection procedures, and surgery: a cohort study of insurance claims. *J Manipulative Physiol Ther.* 2021;44(9):683–689.
68. Simundic AM. Bias in research. *Biochem Med (Zagreb).* 2013;23(1): 12–15.
69. Catalogue of Bias. A taxonomy of biases: progress report. Accessed July 7, 2023. https://catalogofbias.org/2020/02/11/a-taxonomy-of-biases-progress-report/
70. Novy DM, Simmonds MJ, Olson SL, Lee CE, Jones SC. Physical performance: differences in men and women with and without low back pain. *Arch Phys Med Rehabil.* 1999;80(2):195–198.
71. Filho IT, Simmonds MJ, Protas EJ, Jones S. Back pain, physical function, and estimates of aerobic capacity: what are the relationships among methods and measures? *Am J Phys Med Rehabil.* 2002;81(12): 913–920.
72. Lee CE, Simmonds MJ, Novy DM, Jones S. Self-reports and clinician-measured physical function among patients with low back pain: a comparison. *Arch Phys Med Rehabil.* 2001;82(2):227–231.
73. Novy DM, Simmonds MJ, Lee CE. Physical performance tasks: what are the underlying constructs? *Arch Phys Med Rehabil.* 2002;83(1):44–47.
74. Simmonds MJ. Physical function in patients with cancer: psychometric characteristics and clinical usefulness of a physical performance test battery. *J Pain Symptom Manage.* 2002;24(4):404–414.
75. Simmonds MJ, Olson SL, Jones S, et al. Psychometric characteristics and clinical usefulness of physical performance tests in patients with low back pain. *Spine (Phila Pa 1976).* 1998;23(22):2412–2421.
76. da Costa Santos CM, de Mattos Pimenta CA, Nobre MR. The PICO strategy for the research question construction and evidence search. *Rev Lat Am Enfermagem.* 2007;15(3):508–511.
77. Villanueva EV, Burrows EA, Fennessy PA, Rajendran M, Anderson JN. Improving question formulation for use in evidence appraisal in a tertiary care setting: a randomised controlled trial [ISRCTN66375463]. *BMC Med Inform Decis Mak.* 2001;1:4.
78. Educational Council on Osteopathic Principles, American Association of Colleges of Osteopathic Medicine. Glossary of osteopathic terminology. Updated November 2011. Accessed July 17, 2023. https://www.lb7.uscourts.gov/documents/14c42406.pdf
79. Haneline MT, Young M. A review of intraexaminer and interexaminer reliability of static spinal palpation: a literature synthesis. *J Manipulative Physiol Ther.* 2009;32(5):379–386.
80. Lucas N, Macaskill P, Irwig L, Moran R, Bogduk N. Reliability of physical examination for diagnosis of myofascial trigger points: a systematic review of the literature. *Clin J Pain.* 2009;25(1):80–89.
81. Schneider M, Erhard R, Brach J, Tellin W, Imbarlina F, Delitto A. Spinal palpation for lumbar segmental mobility and pain provocation: an interexaminer reliability study. *J Manipulative Physiol Ther.* 2008;31(6):465–473.
82. Seffinger MA, Najm WI, Mishra SI, et al. Reliability of spinal palpation for diagnosis of back and neck pain: a systematic review of the literature. *Spine (Phila Pa 1976).* 2004;29(19):E413–E425.
83. Stolz M, von Piekartz H, Hall T, Schindler A, Ballenberger N. Evidence and recommendations for the use of segmental motion testing for patients with LBP: a systematic review. *Musculoskelet Sci Pract.* 2020;45:102076.
84. Low G, Kruse SA, Lomas DJ. General review of magnetic resonance elastography. *World J Radiol.* 2016;8(1):59–72.
85. Langevin HM. Three new research networks will focus on the neural mechanisms of force-based manipulations. National Center for Complementary and Integrative Health. Accessed July 17, 2023. https://www.nccih.nih.gov/about/offices/od/director/past-messages/three-new-research-networks-will-focus-on-the-neural-mechanisms-of-force-based-manipulations
86. May S, Littlewood C, Bishop A. Reliability of procedures used in the physical examination of non-specific low back pain: a systematic review. *Aust J Physiother.* 2006;52(2):91–102.
87. Seffinger M, Adams A, Najm W, et al. Spinal palpatory diagnostic procedures utilized by practitioners of spinal manipulation: annotated bibliography of content validity and reliability studies. *J Can Chiropr Assoc.* 2003;47(2):93–109.
88. Degenhardt BF, Johnson JC, Snider KT, Snider EJ. Maintenance and improvement of interobserver reliability of osteopathic palpatory tests over a 4-month period. *J Am Osteopath Assoc.* 2010;110(10):579–586.
89. Simmonds KP, Burke J, Kozlowski AJ, Andary M, Luo Z, Reeves MJ. Rationale for a clinical trial that compares acute stroke rehabilitation at inpatient rehabilitation facilities to skilled nursing facilities: challenges and opportunities. *Arch Phys Med Rehabil.* 2022;103(6):1213–1221.
90. Petrini L, Arendt-Nielsen L. Understanding pain catastrophizing: putting pieces together. *Front Psychol.* 2020;11:603420.
91. Mondloch MV, Cole DC, Frank JW. Does how you do depend on how you think you'll do? A systematic review of the evidence for a relation between patients' recovery expectations and health outcomes. *CMAJ.* 2001;165(2):174–179.
92. Kern A, Kramm C, Witt CM, Barth J. The influence of personality traits on the placebo/nocebo response: a systematic review. *J Psychosom Res.* 2020; 128:109866.
93. Simmonds M, Kumar S. Does knowledge of a patient's workers' compensation status influence clinical judgments? *J Occup Rehabil.* 1996;6(2): 93–107.
94. Sullivan MJL, Bishop SR, Pivik J. The Pain Catastrophizing Scale: development and validation. *Psychol Assess.* 1995;7(4):524–532.
95. Wertli MM, Burgstaller JM, Weiser S, Steurer J, Kofmehl R, Held U. Influence of catastrophizing on treatment outcome in patients with nonspecific low back pain: a systematic review. *Spine (Phila Pa 1976).* 2014; 39(3):263–273.
96. Adverse childhood experience questionnaire for adults. Accessed July 7, 2023. https://www.acesaware.org/wp-content/uploads/2022/07/ACE-Questionnaire-for-Adults-Identified-English-rev.7.26.22.pdf
97. Racine N, Killam T, Madigan S. Trauma-informed care as a universal precaution: beyond the adverse childhood experiences questionnaire. *JAMA Pediatr.* 2020;174(1):5–6.

98. Zarse EM, Neff MR, Yoder R, Hulvershorn L, Chambers JE, Chambers RA. The adverse childhood experiences questionnaire: two decades of research on childhood trauma as a primary cause of adult mental illness, addiction, and medical diseases. *Cogent Med.* 2019;6(1):1581447.
99. Noll DR, Degenhardt BF, Fossum C, Hensel K. Clinical and research protocol for osteopathic manipulative treatment of elderly patients with pneumonia. *J Am Osteopath Assoc.* 2008;108(9):508–516.
100. Licciardone JC, Minotti DE, Gatchel RJ, Kearns CM, Singh KP. Osteopathic manual treatment and ultrasound therapy for chronic low back pain: a randomized controlled trial. *Ann Fam Med.* 2013;11(2):122–129.
101. Bellg AJ, Borrelli B, Resnick B, et al; Treatment Fidelity Workgroup of the NIH Behavior Change Consortium. Enhancing treatment fidelity in health behavior change studies: best practices and recommendations from the NIH Behavior Change Consortium. *Health Psychol.* 2004;23(5):443–451.
102. Degenhardt BF, Snider KT, Snider EJ, Johnson JC. Interobserver reliability of osteopathic palpatory diagnostic tests of the lumbar spine: improvements from consensus training. *J Am Osteopath Assoc.* 2005;105(10):465–473.
103. Gupta U, Verma M. Placebo in clinical trials. *Perspect Clin Res.* 2013;4(1):49–52.
104. Simmonds A. Ethics of placebo-controlled trials in developing countries: the search for standards and solutions. *Morningside Rev.* 2011;7:45–51.
105. Licciardone JC, Russo DP. Blinding protocols, treatment credibility, and expectancy: methodologic issues in clinical trials of osteopathic manipulative treatment. *J Am Osteopath Assoc.* 2006;106(8):457–463.
106. Birch S. A review and analysis of placebo treatments, placebo effects, and placebo controls in trials of medical procedures when sham is not inert. *J Altern Complement Med.* 2006;12(3):303–310.
107. Vickers AJ, de Craen AJ. Why use placebos in clinical trials? A narrative review of the methodological literature. *J Clin Epidemiol.* 2000;53(2):157–161.
108. Hrobjartsson A, Gotzsche PC. Is the placebo powerless? An analysis of clinical trials comparing placebo with no treatment. *N Engl J Med.* 2001;344(21):1594–1602.
109. Machado LA, Kamper SJ, Herbert RD, Maher CG, McAuley JH. Imperfect placebos are common in low back pain trials: a systematic review of the literature. *Eur Spine J.* 2008;17(7):889–904.
110. Lavazza C, Galli M, Abenavoli A, Maggiani A. Sham treatment effects in manual therapy trials on back pain patients: a systematic review and pairwise meta-analysis. *BMJ Open.* 2021;11(5):e045106.
111. Green LA, Hickner J. A short history of primary care practice-based research networks: from concept to essential research laboratories. *J Am Board Fam Med.* 2006;19(1):1–10.
112. Degenhardt BF, Johnson JC, Gross SR, Hagan C, Lund G, Curry WJ. Preliminary findings on the use of osteopathic manipulative treatment: outcomes during the formation of the practice-based research network, DO-Touch. NET. *J Am Osteopath Assoc.* 2014;114(3):154–170.
113. Degenhardt BF, Standley PR. 2013–2022 Strategic plan for research: A role for everyone in promoting research in the osteopathic medical profession. *J Am Osteopath Assoc.* 2013;113(9):654–659.

95 Effectiveness and Safety of Osteopathic Manipulative Treatment

KAREN T. SNIDER ▪ ERIC J. SNIDER ▪ ANNA E. ESPARHAM

KEY CONCEPTS

- Research supports the effectiveness of osteopathic manipulative treatment (OMT) for a variety of clinical conditions.
- OMT is considered safe and is well tolerated when applied by appropriately trained clinicians in the absence of contraindications to the techniques used.
- Mild to moderate adverse events can occur with OMT and most commonly include transient post-treatment pain or discomfort.
- Contraindications to OMT are based on an understanding of anatomy and physiology rather than published outcome studies.
- Clinical practice guidelines recommend the inclusion of manual therapies, such as OMT, as part of the management of headaches, low back pain, lymphedema, neck pain, osteoarthritis of the hip and knee, plantar fasciitis, and rotator cuff disorders.
- The decision to perform OMT is a shared decision between the physician and patient and is based on the patient's unique history, physical examination, tolerance to different types of techniques, the physician's technical skill to perform OMT, and a mutual understanding of the risks and benefits.

INTRODUCTION

Manual medicine has been practiced in a variety of forms for millennia[1] and is still practiced worldwide by a variety of clinical professions worldwide. In the United States, some of the professions that use manual medicine include osteopathic medicine, chiropractic, occupational therapy, physical therapy, athletic training, and massage therapy. These professions share many analogous manual therapy techniques even though the names of the techniques may vary by profession.[2–4] For example, the OMT technique known as high-velocity, low-amplitude (HVLA) is called spinal manipulation, thrust technique, or mobilization with impulse by other professions.

Manual medicine is generally considered safe, and its efficacy has been reported in a multitude of studies across professions.[4] When specifically considering OMT, a preponderance of research supports use of OMT in the management of musculoskeletal disorders.[5] But evidence also supports the use of OMT for a variety of visceral, psychiatric, and pediatric conditions. Unfortunately, like most procedural studies, those studies that assess OMT are typically small and methodologically prone to bias because the treating clinician and study participants cannot be blinded to the intervention.[5] Regarding safety, no serious adverse events attributable to OMT have been reported in prospective studies.[5] As such, OMT is generally considered safe, and only nonserious adverse events, such as transient post-treatment pain or discomfort, are most commonly reported.[4–6] The following sections outline the effectiveness and safety of OMT along with contraindications and practice guidelines.

EFFICACY AND EFFECTIVENESS OF MANIPULATION

The effectiveness of manipulation refers to the performance of manual therapy under real-world conditions.[7] Most practice-based research studies and inpatient studies are effectiveness studies, where the manual intervention is compared to treatment as usual in a real clinical setting. Some studies assessing the value of manual medicine are efficacy studies, so conditions are much more highly controlled.[7] Further, the intervention will typically be standardized and compared with a placebo or sham intervention. Many studies are a combination of these two types of study designs. For example, a standardized intervention is performed in a real-world clinical setting and compared with treatment as usual.

There are a large number of studies assessing the efficacy and effectiveness of manual therapies using techniques analogous to those used in osteopathic manipulation, and many new studies are published every year. Because of the similarity of other manual therapies to OMT, providers should consider the wider body of research when contemplating inclusion of OMT as part of the management of a specific condition. However, it is beyond the scope of this chapter to address the entire evidence base for manual medicine. Studies specifically assessing OMT are a small subset of this group and are published by physician and nonphysician osteopathic clinicians worldwide. Table 95.1 summarizes the significant outcomes of OMT interventions assessing the efficacy and effectiveness of OMT in clinical practice. When possible, systematic, scoping, and narrative reviews have been used to summarize these outcomes, but randomized controlled trials, observational, and retrospective studies have also been used. The quality of the evidence as defined by the GRADE approach[8] is not reported in Table 95.1. The quality of evidence and the resulting strength of the recommendations for the use of OMT for a particular condition or population are based, in part, on the number and methodologic design of published studies.[8] With each passing year, more studies assessing the efficacy and effectiveness of OMT, or manual medicine in general, are published, so the grading of that evidence will change over time. Therefore, as the strength of the evidence grows, clinical practice guidelines recommend inclusion of manual therapies, such as OMT, into the management of corresponding conditions.

SAFETY

Manual medicine therapies, such as OMT, are generally considered safe.[4,66] But all procedures carry some level of risk of harm to

TABLE 95.1

Efficacy and Effectiveness of Osteopathic Manipulative Treatment

Condition or Population	Statistically Significant Findings Associated With OMT Intervention	Reference (Study Type)
Achilles tendinitis	Reduced stretch reflex amplitude of soleus, medial, and lateral gastrocnemius; improved symptoms	Howell et al.[9] (NRCT)
Ankle injuries (acute)	Reduced pain; improved edema	Eisenhart et al.[10] (RCT)
Athletes: cardiovascular Autonomic parameters (rugby players)	Increased heart rate variability; reduced mean arterial pressure	Carnevali et al.[11] (RCT)
Athletes: anaerobic performance and lactate clearance (male athletes)	Improved lactate clearance without affecting anaerobic performance	Akkaş et al.[12] (RCT)
Athletes: lower limb function (professional soccer players)	Improved sit and reach test and static balance with open eyes	Thomas et al.[13] (RCT)
Athletes: musculoskeletal complaints and disorders (musicians)	Improved phonation time, voice quality, and voice range in healthy singers; increased cervical ROM in violinists	Kiepe et al.[14] (SR)
Athletes: patellofemoral pain (runners)	Reduced pain; improved function and decreased standing plantar pressure in midfoot; increased posterior thigh flexibility	Zago et al.[15] (RCT)
Athletes: prevention of stress fracture (collegiate cross country athletes)	Decreased annual incidence of stress fractures in male (but not female) athletes	Brumm et al.[16] (PO)
Balance disorders	Positive effect on balance disorders	Tramontano et al.[17] (SR)
Cancer-related symptoms: breast cancer patients (undergoing chemotherapy)	Reduced impact of constipation and diarrhea on quality of life	Lagrange et al.[18] (RCT)
Cancer-related symptoms: geriatric patients (not undergoing chemotherapy)	Reduced pain	Arienti et al.[19] (NRCT)
Carpal tunnel syndrome	Improved symptoms and function; increased transverse carpal ligament length	Burnham et al.[20] (NRCT)
Chronic obstructive pulmonary disease	Improved quality of life and 6 min walk test	Buscemi et al.[21] (RCT)
Depression	Reduced depression using Zung Depression Scale	Plotkin et al.[22] (RCT)
Dizziness (associated with neuro-otologic disorders)	Reduced disability associated with dizziness; reduced dizziness severity and frequency	Rehman et al.[23] (SRMA)
Fibromyalgia	Improved pressure pain threshold, perceived pain, attitude toward treatment, and activities of daily living; reduced chronic pain	Gamber et al.[24] (RCT)
Generalized anxiety disorder	Reduced Hamilton Anxiety Rating Scale score and Intolerance for Uncertainty Scale score	Dixon et al.[25] (NRCT)
Geriatric health (nursing home residents)	Decreased hospitalization rates and medication use	Snider et al.[26] (RCT)
Headaches: migraine	Reduced number of headache days; decreased medication use; reduced headache frequency and severity; improved mental well-being	Cerritelli et al.[27] (SR), Jara Silva et al.[28] (ScR)
Headaches: tension type	Reduced headache frequency and severity	Jara Silva et al.[28] (ScR)
Heart failure	Increased brachial blood flow	Amatuzzi et al.[29] (RCT)
Irritable bowel syndrome (IBS)	Reduced pain and IBS severity index score; decreased rectal sensitivity; reduced abdominal distention	Muller et al.[30] (SR), Lotfi et al.[31] (NR)
Low back pain (acute and chronic)	Reduced pain; improved functional status	Licciardone et al.[32] (SRMA), Franke et al.[33] (SRMA), Dal Farra et al.[34] (SRMA)
Lower urinary tract symptoms (women)	Improved urologic symptom severity level in voiding dysfunction; improved stress and urge incontinence; positive impact on urinary incontinence	Franke and Hoesele[35] (SRMA)
Musculoskeletal pain (chronic noncancer pain)	Reduced pain; improved quality of life; reduced disability	Rehman et al.[36] (SRMA)

TABLE 95.1 (Continued)

Efficacy and Effectiveness of Osteopathic Manipulative Treatment

Condition or Population	Statistically Significant Findings Associated With OMT Intervention	Reference (Study Type)
Neck pain (acute)	Reduced pain	McReynolds and Sheridan[37] (RCT)
Neck pain (chronic and nonspecific)	Reduced pain and disability; improved functional status	Franke et al.[38] (SRMA), Dal Farra et al.[34] (SRMA)
Pancreatitis	Decreased length of hospital stay	Radjieski et al.[39] (RCT)
Parkinson disease	Improved motor function, stride length, and cadence of gait; reduced constipation severity; improved quality of life	Li et al.[40] (NR), Wells et al.[41] (NRCT)
Pediatrics: asthma	Improved peak expiratory flow rate	Guiney et al.[42] (RCT)
Pediatrics: infant colic	Decreased duration of crying; increased duration of sleep	Hayden and Mullinger[43] (RCT)
Pediatrics: newborn and preterm (stable, neonatal ICU)	Decreased hospital length of stay; reduced cost and heart rate, increased SpO2 and weight gain	Lanaro et al.[44] (SRMA), Cicchitti et al.[45] (RO), Manzotti et al.[46] (RCT)
Pediatrics: otitis media	Reduced number of acute otitis media episodes; increased number of surgery-free months; fewer surgical procedures; improved middle ear effusion	Mills et al.[47] (RCT), Steele et al.[48] (RCT)
Pediatrics: plagiocephaly (nonsynostotic)	Reduced cranial asymmetries at 3-mo and 1-y follow-up in young infants	Bagagiolo et al.[49] (RCT)
Plantar fasciitis	Reduced symptom severity; increased peak force and time to reach peak force in calf muscles; reduced plantar fascia thickness	Wynne et al.[50] (RCT), Boucher et al.[51] (PO)
Pneumonia	Decreased hospital length of stay, duration of IV antibiotics, respiratory failure, and death	Noll et al.[52,53] (RCTs)
Pregnancy: hemodynamic control	Improved blood pressure; decreased heart rate during heel raise	Hensel et al.[54] (RCT)
Pregnancy: prenatal care	Decreased frequency of meconium-stained amniotic fluid and occurrence of preterm delivery	King et al.[55] (RO)
Pregnancy: intrapartum care	Decreased duration of labor	Martingano et al.[56] (PO)
Pregnancy: pelvic girdle, low back, and postpartum low back pain	Reduced pain; improved functional status	Franke et al.[57] (SRMA)
Postoperative: cardiac surgery	Reduced postoperative pain; improved respiratory functional capacity; decreased hospital length of stay; improved pulmonary function; increased cardiac index	Rorris et al.[58] (SR)
Postoperative: ileus after abdominal or gastrointestinal surgery	Decreased time to flatus and hospital length of stay; prevention of ileus	Baltazar et al.[59] (RO), Crow and Gorodinsky[60] (RO), Herrmann[61] (RO)
Postoperative: hysterectomy	Improved preoperative and postoperative pain when used as adjunct to morphine analgesia	Goldstein et al.[62] (RCT)
Postoperative: knee replacement surgery	Decreased pain and edema; improved ROM	Zhou et al.[63] (SR)
Shoulder pain	Reduced pain and disability; improved ROM	Schwerla et al.[64] (RCT)
Sleep	Decreased sleep latency	Cutler et al.[65] (RCT)

ICU, intensive care unit; IV, intravenous; NR, narrative review; NRCT, nonrandomized clinical trial; PO, prospective observational study; RCT, randomized clinical trial; RO, retrospective observational study; ROM, range of motion; ScR, scoping review; SpO2, oxygen saturation; SR, systematic review; SRMA, systematic review and meta-analysis.

TABLE 95.2

Common Terminology Criteria for Adverse Events (CTCAE) Grades of Adverse Events[77,78]

Grade	Level	Classification	Description
1	Mild	Nonserious	The event is usually transient, does not typically interfere with activities of daily living, and requires no special treatment or intervention.[79]
2	Moderate	Nonserious	The event impacts usual daily activities but is alleviated with simple noninvasive, therapeutic treatments. Laboratory evaluation indicates injury but without long-term risk or permanent harm.[80]
3	Severe	Nonserious	The event requires intensive therapeutic intervention and interrupts usual daily activities. It may require brief hospitalization or prolong an existing hospitalization but does not result in a persistent or significant disability or incapacity.[81]
4	Life threatening or disabling	Serious	A medically significant event or its immediate sequelae, which places the patient at imminent risk of death or is associated with physical or mental disabilities that affect or limit the ability of a person to perform activities of daily living. The event may result in inpatient hospitalization or prolong an existing hospitalization.[82]
5	Death	Serious	The event is associated with termination of life.[83]

the patient. Developing a culture of safety in osteopathic medicine involves a thorough understanding of clinical medicine, indications, contraindications, risks, and benefits of procedures, such as OMT. The risks of adverse events vary with different types of manual techniques, patient comorbidities, and presenting complaints. By understanding the risks, clinicians can better mitigate those risks and partner with the patient to develop an integrative management plan that leads to the best outcome for the whole patient.[67]

Adverse Events

An adverse event is defined as any unfavorable or unintended disease, sign, symptom, or other medical occurrence (e.g., abnormal laboratory finding) that is temporally associated with a treatment or procedure.[68] However, the adverse event may or may not be related to the treatment or procedure.[68] Temporary pain or discomfort can occur during the physical examination, such as discomfort from palpation of tender points, or during treatment, such as the brief pain that can occur during the initial setup for a manual technique or when the activating force is applied. Pain during the treatment process can vary by technique. For example, trigger-band technique is used to treat taut, tender bands of soft tissue in the fascial distortion model of manual treatment and is associated with brief mild to severe pain during the treatment process.[51,69,70] Adverse events are typically reported after a treatment. As such, a temporal association is not sufficient for determining causality. An adverse event after OMT may be related to a medication, another procedure, or specific activities undertaken by the patient. Thus, an adverse event that occurs after OMT may or may not have been caused by the OMT. An adverse event is not the same as a side effect. A side effect is a secondary, unintended, beneficial, or harmful effect of an intervention.[71] Because the term "side effect" refers to both unintended harm and benefit, its use in reference to adverse events or adverse reactions to an intervention is no longer recommended.[71]

Grades of Adverse Events

Grading the seriousness of adverse events is important for determining risk and guiding recommendations for the use of different types of OMT techniques, especially in the presence of specific clinical conditions or with specific patient populations. The challenge with determining the risk of any intervention is that the terminology used to grade the seriousness of adverse events is not standardized across publications.[72–74] The Common Terminology Criteria for Adverse Events (CTCAE) grades adverse events from 1 to 5 based on the threat to the patient's life or daily functioning. Grades 1 to 3 are described as nonserious,[75] and grades 4 to 5 are described as serious.[76] Nonserious adverse events do not threaten the life of the patient or cause permanent disability, but they can require intensive treatment. Serious events are those that result in death or those that are life threatening or associated with a persistent or significant disability or incapacity.[76] They can also result in inpatient hospitalization or prolong an existing hospitalization.[76] The CTCAE grades are described in Table 95.2. These terms will be used throughout the chapter.

Incidence and Timing of Adverse Events

The incidence of reported adverse events associated with manual therapies varies widely in the literature. Individual outcome studies have reported the incidence of mild to moderate adverse events ranges from 2.5% to 60.9% with no serious adverse events reported.[6,84,85] However, there are concerns that the reporting of adverse events in manual therapy studies is low and complicated by nonstandardized terminology for reporting those events.[73,74,86] This lack of reporting of adverse events has been a particular problem with pediatric studies.[87] Only a few studies have specifically assessed the incidence and timing of adverse events when manual therapies are performed by osteopathically trained providers.[5,6,44,88] Most of the data on the incidence and timing of adverse events comes from studies of the chiropractic profession, which emphasize spinal manipulation.[89–92] Also known as spinal manipulative therapy (SMT), spinal manipulation is a thrusting technique analogous to HVLA and is most commonly used to treat dysfunction of the cervical, thoracic, and lumbar spine and of the sacroiliac joints. Adverse event incidence, types, and timing identified in manual therapy outcome studies are presented in Table 95.3. The data presented is not condition specific and is generalized for patients receiving the specified type of manual therapy.

TABLE 95.3

Adverse Event Incidence, Types, and Timing Associated With Manual Therapies

Study Type	Manual Therapy Type	Incidence of Adverse Events	Types and Timing of Adverse Events	Reference
Systematic review of systematic reviews	Osteopathic (multinational)	Not reported	Timing not reported. Types included mild to moderate transient stiffness, tiredness, and muscle spasticity. No serious adverse events related to OMT were reported.	Bagagiolo et al.[5]
Systematic review of pediatric studies	Nonspecific manual therapy, osteopathic, and chiropractic (multinational)	Not reported	Types included mild to moderate pain lasting up to 24 h, aggravation of presenting symptoms lasting up to 4 d, dizziness, and increased vegetative symptoms in infants (such as vomiting or crying) for up to 48 h. No serious adverse events were reported.	Parnell Prevost et al.[93]
Prospective, practice-based, observational	Osteopathic (multinational)	45 (2.5%) of 1,847 visits with 925 patients	New and established patients reported the following immediately after treatment: mild to moderate pain/discomfort (most frequent), tiredness/fatigue, lightheadedness, nausea/vomiting, headache, numbness/tingling, and stiffness. HVLA techniques had the lowest association with adverse events, while balanced ligamentous tension and ligamentous articular strain techniques had the highest association. No serious adverse events were reported.	Degenhardt et al.[6]
Systematic review of inpatient pediatric studies	Osteopathic (multinational)	Not reported	One of 1,306 preterm infants experienced longer time to full enteral feeding. No serious adverse events were reported.	Lanaro et al.[44]
Systematic review with meta-analysis	Physiotherapy, osteopathic, and chiropractic (multinational)	Pooled estimate based on 42,451 (41%) visits with 22,833 patients	Timing varied by study with the majority of adverse events beginning within 24 h and resolving within 48 h of treatment. Types included mild to moderate local pain and discomfort in the area of treatment, aggravation of presenting complaint, stiffness, headache, pain outside the area of treatment, muscle spasm, radiating pain, tiredness and fatigue, lightheadedness, nausea, vomiting, numbness, and tingling. No serious adverse events were reported.	Carnes et al.[85]
Prospective, practice-based, observational	Physiotherapy, osteopathic, and chiropractic (Belgium)	283 (60.9%) of 465 visits with 465 patients	New and established patients reported the following within 48 h after treatment: headache, stiffness, aggravation of complaints, radiating discomfort, fatigue, muscle spasm, dizziness, and nausea. Approximately 60% of adverse events began within 4 h after manipulation, 64% lasted less than 24 h, and 19% persisted past 48 h. No serious adverse events were reported.	Cagnie et al.[84]
Retrospective, single practice-based, observational	Osteopathic (United States)	35 (8.6%) of 405 patients	Timing not reported. Established patients anonymously reported the following regarding previous visits: mild to moderate pain or soreness (most frequent), headache, nausea, and an unspecified variety of other types. No serious adverse events were reported.	Licciardone et al.[88]

(continued)

TABLE 95.3 (Continued)

Adverse Event Incidence, Types, and Timing Associated With Manual Therapies

Study Type	Manual Therapy Type	Incidence of Adverse Events	Types and Timing of Adverse Events	Reference
Retrospective, practice-based, observational	Chiropractic (Sweden)	274 (44%) of 625 patients with 1858 visits	Established patients reported the following directly to chiropractor regarding previous visit: mild to moderate local reactions in the area of treatment (most frequent), pain outside the area of treatment, fatigue or headache, nausea, and dizziness. After treatment, adverse events began on the same day of treatment (58%), day 2 (33%), or later (4%). Adverse events lasted a few hours (21%), up to 24 h (34%), from 24–48 h (19%), and more than 48 h (19%). Before resolution, 35% of adverse events affected performance of some daily activities. No serious adverse events were reported.	Leboeuf-Yde et al.[89]
Retrospective, practice-based, observational	Chiropractic (Norway)	1,174 (25%) of 4,712 visits with 1,058 patients	Established patients reported the following directly to chiropractor regarding previous visit: local discomfort in the area of treatment (most frequent), headache, tiredness, radiating discomfort, nausea, dizziness, and hot skin. After treatment, adverse events began within 10 min (17%), between 10 min and 4 h (47%), and after 4 h on the day of treatment or the following day (32%). Adverse events resolved during the day of treatment (74%), on day 2 (16%), or on day 3 and later (7%). Before resolution, 11% of adverse events prevented performance of some daily activities. No serious adverse events were reported.	Senstad et al.[90]

HVLA, high-velocity, low-amplitude; OMT, osteopathic manipulative treatment.

Serious Adverse Events Associated with OMT

The International Federation for Manual/Musculoskeletal Medicine (FIMM) estimates the incidence of serious adverse events to be less than 1 in 6 million manipulations.[66] To understand the relative risk of manual therapies, it is important to understand the incidence of serious adverse events in comparison to other commonly used interventions for pain. The incidence of myocardial infarction associated with use of nonsteroidal anti-inflammatory drugs (NSAIDs) is estimated to be 1 in 2,400, and the incidence of gastrointestinal bleed is 1 in 87.[94] Between 1997 and 2008, the estimated mortality from a gastrointestinal bleed associated with NSAID use was 20.9%,[95] which is a grade 5 serious adverse event. Because serious adverse events from OMT are so rare, it is unfeasible to investigate the actual incidence by a prospective randomized, controlled clinical trial.[96] As a result, most serious adverse events are reported as case studies. Further, most reported serious adverse events are associated with SMT of the cervical spine and involve neurovascular accidents, such as cervical artery dissection (CAD) and stroke.[66] The actual incidence of these neurovascular accidents is unknown but estimates range widely from 1 in 20,000 to 1 in 5 million cervical spinal manipulations.[66,97] A retrospective analysis of Medicare claims comparing more than 23 million Medicare beneficiaries aged 65 years and older estimated a lower temporary risk of neurovascular event within 1 week of chiropractic SMT, than within 1 week of a primary care visit without manual therapy (odds ratio of 0.73 for vertebral artery dissection and odds ratio of 0.79 for carotid artery dissection).[98] Based on a review of the safety and efficacy of OMT on the cervical spine, the American Osteopathic Association released a position paper on the use of OMT for the cervical spine, where they specifically stated: "It is the position of the American Osteopathic Association that all modalities of OMT of the cervical spine, including HVLA, should continue to be taught at all levels of education, and that osteopathic physicians should continue to offer this form of treatment to their patients."[99]

Head and neck pain can be a symptom of underlying vascular pathology.[100–102] Currently, it is unknown how often symptomatic vascular pathology masquerades as musculoskeletal pain, which prompts the patient to seek manual therapies.[103,104] According to the National Center for Complementary and Integrative Health, "the available evidence suggests that the incidence of CAD in people getting spinal manipulation is low, and there is disagreement about whether manipulation can actually cause CAD. Nevertheless, patients need to be informed of this potential risk."[105] Because of this potential origin of musculoskeletal pain, it is vital that clinicians understand the signs, symptoms, and risk factors for vascular pathology of the neck and head[94] and perform an appropriate history and physical examination before performing OMT.

Another potentially serious adverse event involves manipulation of the lumbar spine that causes a lumbar disk herniation or cauda equina syndrome.[66,97] The estimated incidence of one of these events occurring is 1 in more than 1,000,000 to 3,720,000 manipulations.[97] A scoping review from 2017, which included published case reports, concluded that the incidence of serious adverse events associated with manual therapies to the spine, including HVLA, was rare.[91] But the study stressed the importance of identifying pre-existing conditions that may represent contraindications by completing a thorough history and appropriate physical examination to best estimate and communicate the risk of the recommended treatment to the patient.[91]

Contraindications to Osteopathic Manipulative Techniques

The decision to recommend OMT is based on an individual patient's unique history and physical examination findings. The clinical indication to perform OMT is the presence of somatic dysfunction found on physical examination and the absence of contraindications to the recommended treatment.[106,107] These contraindications may be absolute and specifically prohibit OMT, or they may be relative contraindications that alter an OMT plan to exclude treatment of specific sites on the patient's body or the use of certain types of techniques.[107] When a contraindication is present for a specific site, OMT can usually be performed in other body areas. When a contraindication is present for a specific type of technique, a different type of technique can be used. The decision to perform OMT is also based on the patient's willingness to receive OMT, their unique tolerance to different types of techniques, and the physician's technical skill to perform OMT. When the physician lacks the skill to perform OMT in general or to perform the type of OMT best suited to the individual patient's circumstances, then the physician should refer to a clinician with the appropriate skill set.[66]

RELATIVE VERSUS ABSOLUTE CONTRAINDICATIONS

There are two classifications of contraindications.[108,109] A relative contraindication means that caution should be used when OMT is performed because there may be a greater-than-usual risk of an adverse event.[108,109] OMT can still be used if the expected benefit outweighs the risk. Absolute contraindication means that OMT carries significant risk of a serious adverse event that exceeds the expected benefit and should not be used.[108,109] Contraindications can be generalized to the patient based on a systemic condition, or they can be site specific based on a localized condition.

Most absolute and relative contraindications to OMT are based on an understanding of anatomy, physiology, and pathophysiology and on the forces applied with a particular type of technique. However, sound judgment suggests OMT should not be used in the following circumstances:

- OMT should not be used when the patient or guardian does not provide verbal or written informed consent for the procedure.
- OMT should not be used in the presence of an unstable condition that involves rapid life-threatening deterioration.
- OMT should not be used if performing OMT will delay definitive diagnosis and treatment of an urgent or emergent condition.
- OMT should not be used without performing an appropriate history and physical evaluation, including evaluation for somatic dysfunction.
- OMT should not be specifically applied to sites of unstable anatomy if the application of forces used with the technique presents a high risk of a deleterious consequence.
- OMT should not be used when the physician's skill level makes it likely they will apply a force that overwhelms the integrity of the tissues.

In 2010, the World Health Organization (WHO) published a list of relative and absolute contraindications to different types of osteopathic manipulative techniques in its *Benchmarks for Training in Osteopathy* report.[107] These contraindications were developed through a consensus within the osteopathic community to promote the safe practice of OMT and minimize the risk of accidents.[107] The list included broad absolute contraindications to direct techniques, such as prolonged bleeding times. As written, they exclude many older patients from receiving relatively gentle direct techniques, such as muscle energy, which involve no more force applied to the tissue than what the patient experiences in ordinary activities of daily living. In 2013, FIMM published its recommendations based on the consensus of a broader group of manual medicine clinicians.[66] In both publications,[66,107] the recommendations were developed by a committee of stakeholders because there is a paucity of published evidence. Therefore, because the patient must be considered as an individual based on their unique history and physical examination, the recommendations should be used as guiding principles with additional consideration of the patient's level of health and tolerance to OMT techniques. Each patient should be informed of the risks and benefits associated with OMT, so that the patient and the physician can decide together whether to proceed with OMT. The contraindications summarized below are based on those published by the WHO[107] and FIMM[66] and are grouped by classification of the technique and condition of the patient. Site-specific contraindications refer to those conditions that should not have OMT applied to the tissues affected by the condition. Patients with site-specific contraindications may receive OMT to other body areas.

CONTRAINDICATIONS TO DIRECT TECHNIQUES

Direct techniques seek to correct somatic dysfunction by applying an activating force with the tissues held at the restrictive barrier.[110] The activating force may use a thrust or impulse like HVLA technique, a muscle contraction like muscle energy technique, fascial loading like direct myofascial release, or passive range of motion like articular technique. Direct techniques can target a local area of tissue or a single joint, or they can be used to affect a larger area of the body and include multiple joints at one time. When a contraindication is present for a direct technique, an indirect technique may be a safe and effective alternative.[107] Absolute and relative contraindications to direct techniques are presented in Table 95.4.

CONTRAINDICATIONS TO INDIRECT, FLUID, AND REFLEX-BASED TECHNIQUES

Indirect techniques seek to correct somatic dysfunction by moving the dysfunctional tissues away from the restrictive barrier.[110] These techniques may include indirect myofascial release techniques that exaggerate the position of ease or balancing techniques, such as balanced ligamentous technique. The contraindications summarized below also refer to fluid techniques, such as lymphatic techniques, and reflex-based techniques, such as rotary stimulation of Chapman reflex points. Both fluid and reflex-based techniques often involve treating one area of the body to influence another area. Indirect techniques can target a local area of tissue or a single joint, or they can be used to affect a larger area of the body and include multiple joints at one time. In general, these techniques do not engage the restrictive barrier. Fluid and reflex-based techniques may also include fascial and soft tissue loading toward the direct barrier as part of the application of the technique.[66,107] Examples include soft tissue inhibition, pedal lymphatic pump, and sphenobasilar compression-decompression techniques. Absolute and

TABLE 95.4

Absolute and Relative Contraindications to Direct Techniques[66,107]

Systemic Conditions: Contraindications to Techniques Applied to Patient

Absolute Contraindications	Relative Contraindications
• Unstable coagulopathies • Conditions with widespread compromised tissue integrity, especially of the soft tissue or joints • Unstable conditions presenting with overt or potential life-threatening deterioration	• Stable coagulopathies • Osteoporosis • Osteopenia • Congenital or acquired connective tissue diseases

Site-Specific Conditions: Contraindications to Techniques Applied at Site

Absolute Contraindications

- Acute inflammatory processes in the abdomen or pelvis with suspected leakage, perforation, or rupture (including cholecystitis, appendicitis, or diverticulitis)
- Spinal pathology with suspected bony compromise or progressive neurologic signs (including osteomyelitis, bony tuberculosis, syringomyelia, and cauda equina syndrome)
- Acutely evolving intracranial processes (including ischemia, bleeding, hydrocephalus, and closed head injury)
- Vascular aneurysms, malformations, or compromise (including vertebral artery stenosis)
- Conditions affecting the structural integrity of the eye (including ocular lens implant in the early postoperative period and uncontrolled glaucoma)
- Localized congenital malformations impairing structural integrity of affected tissues
- In situ or localized malignancy
- Open wounds, skin derangement, or recent surgical incisions

Additional Site-Specific Contraindications to Direct Techniques That Involve Thrust or Impulse[a]

Absolute Contraindications	Relative Contraindications
• Specific technique applied at the site of surgical internal fixation of the joint • Locally compromised bone or joint stability (including fracture, dislocation, metastatic disease, suppurative arthritis, septic arthritis, advanced rheumatoid diseases, or bony tuberculosis) • Bony or intramuscular hematoma or abscess	• Intervertebral disk herniation • Acutely sprained or torn ligaments or muscles • Stable inflammatory arthritis • Stable spinal stenosis, spondylolysis, and spondylolisthesis • Marked hypermobility

[a]Contraindications for direct techniques that involve a trust or impulse force are inclusive of site-specific and systemic contraindications to direct techniques in general.

relative contraindications to indirect, fluid, and reflex-based techniques are presented in Table 95.5.

Prevention of Adverse Events

All procedures have some level of risk. The relative risk of the treatment should be outweighed by the potential benefit. The risks of serious adverse events with OMT are quite small; mild to moderate adverse events, such as transient post-treatment soreness, are most commonly reported.[5,6] Further, the risks associated with OMT can be mitigated by appropriate training in the diagnosis of somatic dysfunction and performance of OMT and by assessing for indications and contraindications as part of performing a history and physical examination. Histories of trauma, joint, and soft tissue diseases (including joint infections, severe rheumatoid arthritis, and connective tissue disease), as well as the presence of malignancies, are major considerations in determining whether OMT should be used or not. The contraindications presented in the previous section are based on an understanding of anatomy, physiology, and pathophysiology rather than on clinical trials of the use of OMT in the presence of the clinical conditions. This understanding is especially important given that clinical trials for manual medicine often include safety-based exclusion criteria. For example, a 2013 study assessing the use of OMT for patients with diabetes mellitus and chronic low back pain excluded any potential participants with "red flag" low back symptoms.[111] Similarly, a 2019 study assessing the use of OMT on the duration of labor in the inpatient obstetrical setting excluded potential participants with severe gestational hypertension or heavy vaginal bleeding.[56]

The choice of OMT technique is also a consideration for reducing the relative risk. If a relative contraindication is present, then special care and consideration of the patient's overall health should be taken before proceeding. If an absolute contraindication is present for a specific type of technique, then an alternative technique can usually be used. If an absolute contraindication is limited to a specific body area, then other areas of the body can usually be treated.[66,107] For example, after a recent surgical procedure, a patient should not have OMT applied to the specific tissues that were surgically manipulated, but OMT can be applied to the tissues near the surgical site with the intent to improve lymphatic drainage as long as the techniques do not place force on the surgical site.

The most commonly reported adverse event to OMT is mild to moderate transient post-treatment pain and discomfort.[5,6] Anecdotally, these symptoms are described as similar to postexercise soreness. The timing of soreness after OMT typically begins within 24 hours and resolves by 48 hours.[84,85,89] Immediate postexercise soreness typically begins during or immediately after exercise, while delayed onset muscle soreness typically begins at 24 hours and resolves within 5 to 7 days.[112] Both immediate- and delayed onset muscle soreness are considered types of muscle strain and are associated with muscle soreness, tenderness, fatigue, and stiffness.[112] There may also be signs of tissue inflammation and muscle fiber damage.[112] Evidence supports massage, stretching, exercise, NSAIDs, heat, and cold to reduce postexercise soreness.[112–114]

TABLE 95.5

Absolute and Relative Contraindications to Indirect, Fluid, and Reflex-Based Techniques[66,107]

Systemic Conditions: Absolute Contraindication to Techniques Applied to Patient	
Absolute Contraindication	
• Unstable conditions presenting with life-threatening deterioration	
Site-Specific Conditions: Contraindications to Techniques Applied at Site	
Absolute Contraindications	**Relative Contraindications**
• Acute inflammatory processes in the abdomen or pelvis with suspected leakage, perforation, or rupture (including cholecystitis, appendicitis, or diverticulitis) • Acutely evolving intracranial processes (including ischemia, bleeding, hydrocephalus, and closed head injury) • Arterial aneurysms and other vascular malformations or compromise (including vertebral artery stenosis) • Conditions affecting the structural integrity of the eye (including ocular lens implant in the early postoperative period and uncontrolled glaucoma) • In situ or localized malignancy • Open wounds, skin derangement, or recent surgical incisions	• Metastatic disease • Closed head injury

Hydration is also recommended because dehydration has been associated with increased muscle soreness symptoms after exercise.[115] It is currently unknown whether pain and discomfort after OMT reflect a similar pathophysiology as postexercise soreness or whether they are an exacerbation of the presenting symptoms. Although there have been no studies assessing the efficacy of these strategies to reduce soreness after OMT, they are commonly recommended.

The skill of the clinician performing the OMT is also important for preventing adverse events. Initial training requires OMT to be practiced under the direct supervision of an experienced clinician in a controlled setting before progressing to supervised practice in a clinical setting.[107,116] This supervised training has been detailed by the WHO for clinicians internationally[107] and by the Commission on Osteopathic College Accreditation in the United States.[116] In addition, in the United States, training should result in attainment of core competencies as defined by the American Association of Colleges of Osteopathic Medicine[117] and the National Board of Osteopathic Medical Examiners (NBOME).[118] Colleges of osteopathic medicine assess competencies related to knowledge, skills, and clinical integration of osteopathic manipulation through hands-on practical examinations, written assessments, and clinical evaluations at the predoctoral levels. In addition, these competencies are evaluated at predoctoral and postdoctoral levels on osteopathic licensure exams. In the United States, these national licensure exams are integrated with osteopathic principles in the context of the full-scope practice of medicine. The content of these exams is detailed in the NBOME COMLEX-USA Master Blueprint[119] and reflect the competencies considered essential for the practice of osteopathic medicine.

The potential risks and benefits should be discussed with the patient to create realistic expectations of outcomes and potential adverse events. If a specific technique is known to cause transient pain or discomfort during the treatment or cause a mild to moderate adverse event after the treatment, then these risks should be communicated to the patient. For example, if a patient presenting with shoulder pain is found to have myofascial dysfunction consistent with a triggerband, the clinician may recommend a manual technique that uses deep soft tissue pressure applied along the band.[51,69] Before proceeding with the recommended technique, the clinician should talk to the patient about the possibility that the treatment may be painful and cause local bruising, and informed consent should be obtained before proceeding with a technique known to cause subcutaneous hematomas.[69] If the patient wishes to proceed, then they do so with appropriate expectations. If they decline, then an alternative technique can be discussed. Patients respond positively to being included as part of decision-making process regarding their treatment.[120] In general, when patients receive OMT from trained clinicians, they perceive OMT to be effective, holistic, patient-centered, and associated with a positive patient–clinician partnership.[120] As a result, patient satisfaction with OMT is generally reported as very good.[88,120–122]

OSTEOPATHIC PRACTICE GUIDELINES

Although the clinical indication to perform OMT is the presence of somatic dysfunction found on physical examination,[106] practice guidelines that recommend treatment with manual therapies should prompt clinicians to specifically assess for somatic dysfunction that may be contributing to the patient's symptoms. Clinical practice guidelines are published by professional organizations and national agencies and reflect the growing body of research that supports the safety, efficacy, and financial cost benefits of manual therapies. By consolidating high-quality systematic reviews and clinical trials, these guidelines inform clinicians how to incorporate manual therapies, including OMT, into patient care. The specific conditions for which manual therapies are recommended are mainly types of musculoskeletal pain, and low back pain has the largest body of evidence for an OMT-specific practice guideline. A systematic review of clinical practice guidelines for the management of musculoskeletal pain found that manual therapy is most often recommended as part of a multimodal management strategy.[123] Further, this strategy should be patient-centered and include an appropriate evaluation for serious pathology and management of psychosocial factors and physical activity.[123] This recommendation for a multimodal strategy is consistent with the holistic osteopathic approach to patient care based on the osteopathic tenets.

Condition-Specific Practice Guidelines for Manual Therapies

Several professional organizations and national agencies have published practice guidelines recommending the inclusion of manual therapies as part of the management of specific conditions or types of musculoskeletal pain. These recommendations are described below.

- Acute pain: The National Academy of Medicine (formerly the Institute of Medicine) recommends that manual therapy be considered as part of a multimodal approach for initial management of acute pain for conditions that are likely to be short in duration.[124]

- Carpal tunnel syndrome: The *Journal of Orthopaedic & Sports Physical Therapy* recommends that manual therapy be included as part of a multimodal approach for treatment of mild to moderate carpal tunnel syndrome that also includes orthoses, home exercise, and ergonomic adjustments.[125]
- Headaches: Clinical practice guidelines published by several countries and by the U.S. Department of Veterans Affairs and the U.S. Department of Defense recommend including manual therapies as part of nonpharmacologic management of headaches.[126,127]
- Low back pain: The American Osteopathic Association published clinical practice guidelines recommending the use of OMT for acute and chronic low back pain, including low back pain in pregnant and postpartum women.[128] In 2007, the American College of Physicians and the American Pain Society recommended nonpharmacologic therapy, including spinal manipulation, for patients with low back pain who have not improved with self-care management.[129] In 2017, the American College of Physicians recommended spinal manipulation for acute and subacute low back pain.[130]
- Lumbar stenosis with neurogenic claudication: The United States Association for the Study of Pain recommends multimodal management of lumbar stenosis with neurogenic claudication that includes education, behavioral changes, manual therapy, home exercise, rehabilitation, and acupuncture.[131]
- Lymphedema associated with breast cancer: The Society for Integrative Oncology identified manual lymph drainage as potentially beneficial for patients being treated for breast cancer lymphedema, especially when used early in the disease process.[132]
- Neck pain: Numerous organizations recommend the use of manual therapy as part of their clinical practice guidelines for neck pain management.[133] In support of the current evidence, the American Osteopathic Association has repeatedly resolved that OMT of the cervical spine, including but not limited to HVLA treatment, is safe and effective for neck pain.[99]
- Osteoarthritis of the knee: The American College of Rheumatology and the American Academy of Orthopaedic Surgeons recommend manual therapy for knee osteoarthritis in conjunction with supervised exercise.[134]
- Osteoarthritis of the hip: The American College of Rheumatology recommends manual therapy for hip osteoarthritis in conjunction with supervised exercise.[134]
- Plantar fasciitis: The American College of Foot and Ankle Surgeons and the Orthopaedic Section of the American Physical Therapy Association recommend manual therapy, such as joint and soft tissue mobilization, to treat lower extremity muscle and joint dysfunction associated with plantar fasciitis.[135,136]
- Shoulder rotator cuff disorders: Several countries and several U.S. states recommend including manual therapies as part of the management of rotator cuff disorders.[137]

CONCLUSION

The body of evidence supporting the integration of manual therapies, such as OMT, into the management of many clinical conditions is steadily expanding. Further, more clinical practice guidelines are being published as the evidence strengthens and provides additional support for a clear benefit-to-risk ratio. These guidelines should encourage clinicians to include an evaluation for any somatic dysfunction that may be influencing the patient's symptoms and to consider OMT as part of patient management. The risk of serious adverse events from OMT is very low. Mild to moderate transient adverse events, such as soreness after OMT, are the most commonly reported. The risks of adverse events can be mitigated by appropriate training in somatic dysfunction diagnosis and OMT techniques; with a thorough understanding of anatomy, physiology, and pathophysiology and of the forces applied during each particular type of technique; and by assessing indications and contraindications for different techniques as part of performing a history and physical examination. Each patient must be assessed individually to determine their level of health and tolerance to different types of OMT techniques. Further, the patient and the physician should partner to develop the best management plan for the patient's unique situation. Osteopathic medicine is distinct among manual medicine professions because OMT is integrated as part of the full-scope practice of medicine. As the health care system shifts toward a more patient-centered approach, the holistic nature of osteopathic medicine aligns well with the evolving paradigm of personalized and integrative care.

REFERENCES

1. Pettman E. A history of manipulative therapy. *J Man Manip Ther.* 2007; 15(3):165–174.
2. Atchison JW, Tolchin RB, Ross BS, Eubanks JE. Manipulation, traction, and massage. In: Cifu DX, ed. *Braddom's Physical Medicine and Rehabilitation.* 6th ed. Elsevier; 2021:316–337.
3. Chiaramonte D, D'Adamo C, Morrison B. Integrative approaches to pain management. In: Benzon HT, Rathmell JP, Wu CL, Turk DC, Argoff CE, Hurley RW, eds. *Practical Management of Pain.* 5th ed. Elsevier; 2014:658–668.
4. Osteopathic International Alliance. Osteopathic healthcare: global review of osteopathic medicine and osteopathy 2020. Accessed August 10, 2023. https://oialliance.org/wp-content/uploads/2021/02/OIA_Report_2020_FINAL.pdf
5. Bagagiolo D, Rosa D, Borrelli F. Efficacy and safety of osteopathic manipulative treatment: an overview of systematic reviews. *BMJ Open.* 2022;12(4):e053468.
6. Degenhardt BF, Johnson JC, Brooks WJ, Norman L. Characterizing adverse events reported immediately after osteopathic manipulative treatment. *J Am Osteopath Assoc.* 2018;118(3):141–149.
7. Singal AG, Higgins PD, Waljee AK. A primer on effectiveness and efficacy trials. *Clin Transl Gastroenterol.* 2014;5(1):e45.
8. Guyatt GH, Oxman AD, Vist GE, et al. GRADE: an emerging consensus on rating quality of evidence and strength of recommendations. *BMJ.* 2008;336(7650):924–926.
9. Howell JN, Cabell KS, Chila AG, Eland DC. Stretch reflex and Hoffmann reflex responses to osteopathic manipulative treatment in subjects with Achilles tendinitis. *J Am Osteopath Assoc.* 2006;106(9):537–545.
10. Eisenhart AW, Gaeta TJ, Yens DP. Osteopathic manipulative treatment in the emergency department for patients with acute ankle injuries. *J Am Osteopath Assoc.* 2003;103(9):417–421.
11. Carnevali L, Cerritelli F, Guolo F, Sgoifo A. Osteopathic manipulative treatment and cardiovascular autonomic parameters in rugby players: a randomized, sham-controlled trial. *J Manipulative Physiol Ther.* 2021; 44(4):319–329.
12. Akkas MB, Belviranli M, Okudan N. The effect of osteopathic manipulative treatment on anaerobic performance and lactate clearance in male athletes: a double-blind, randomized, sham-controlled, crossover study. *J Sports Med Phys Fitness.* 2022;62(4):500–507.
13. Thomas E, Petrucci M, Barretti M, Messina G, Cavallaro AR, Bianco A. Effects of osteopathic manipulative treatment of the pivots on lower limb function in young professional football players. *J Bodyw Mov Ther.* 2022;32:1–6.
14. Kiepe MS, Fernholz I, Schmidt T, et al. Effects of osteopathic manipulative treatment on musicians: a systematic review. *Med Probl Perform Art.* 2020;35(2):110–115.
15. Zago J, Amatuzzi F, Rondinel T, Matheus JP. Osteopathic manipulative treatment versus exercise program in runners with patellofemoral pain

syndrome: a randomized controlled trial. *J Sport Rehabil.* 2020;30(4):609–618.
16. Brumm LF, Janiski C, Balawender JL, Feinstein A. Preventive osteopathic manipulative treatment and stress fracture incidence among collegiate cross-country athletes. *J Am Osteopath Assoc.* 2013;113(12):882–890.
17. Tramontano M, Consorti G, Morone G, Lunghi C. Vertigo and balance disorders—the role of osteopathic manipulative treatment: a systematic review. *Complement Med Res.* 2021;28(4):368–377.
18. Lagrange A, Decoux D, Briot N, et al. Visceral osteopathic manipulative treatment reduces patient reported digestive toxicities induced by adjuvant chemotherapy in breast cancer: a randomized controlled clinical study. *Eur J Obstet Gynecol Reprod Biol.* 2019;241:49–55.
19. Arienti C, Bosisio T, Ratti S, Miglioli R, Negrini S. Osteopathic manipulative treatment effect on pain relief and quality of life in oncology geriatric patients: a nonrandomized controlled clinical trial. *Integr Cancer Ther.* 2018;17(4):1163–1171.
20. Burnham T, Higgins DC, Burnham RS, Heath DM. Effectiveness of osteopathic manipulative treatment for carpal tunnel syndrome: a pilot project. *J Am Osteopath Assoc.* 2015;115(3):138–148.
21. Buscemi A, Pennisi V, Rapisarda A, Pennisi A, Coco M. Efficacy of osteopathic treatment in patients with stable moderate-to-severe chronic obstructive pulmonary disease: a randomized controlled pilot study. *J Complement Integr Med.* 2019;17(1):20180128.
22. Plotkin BJ, Rodos JJ, Kappler R, et al. Adjunctive osteopathic manipulative treatment in women with depression: a pilot study. *J Am Osteopath Assoc.* 2001;101(9):517–523.
23. Rehman Y, Kirsch J, Wang MY, et al. Impact of osteopathic manipulative techniques on the management of dizziness caused by neuro-otologic disorders: systematic review and meta-analysis. *J Osteopath Med.* 2022;123(2):91–101.
24. Gamber RG, Shores JH, Russo DP, Jimenez C, Rubin BR. Osteopathic manipulative treatment in conjunction with medication relieves pain associated with fibromyalgia syndrome: results of a randomized clinical pilot project. *J Am Osteopath Assoc.* 2002;102(6):321–325.
25. Dixon L, Fotinos K, Sherifi E, et al. Effect of osteopathic manipulative therapy on generalized anxiety disorder. *J Am Osteopath Assoc.* 2020; 120(3):133–143.
26. Snider KT, Snider EJ, Johnson JC, Hagan C, Schoenwald C. Preventative osteopathic manipulative treatment and the elderly nursing home resident: a pilot study. *J Am Osteopath Assoc.* 2012;112(8):489–501.
27. Cerritelli F, Lacorte E, Ruffini N, Vanacore N. Osteopathy for primary headache patients: a systematic review. *J Pain Res.* 2017;10:601–611.
28. Jara Silva CE, Joseph AM, Khatib M, et al. Osteopathic manipulative treatment and the management of headaches: a scoping review. *Cureus.* 2022;14(8):e27830.
29. Amatuzzi F, Gervazoni Balbuena de Lima AC, Da Silva ML, et al. Acute and time-course effects of osteopathic manipulative treatment on vascular and autonomic function in patients with heart failure: a randomized trial. *J Manipulative Physiol Ther.* 2021;44(6):455–466.
30. Muller A, Franke H, Resch KL, Fryer G. Effectiveness of osteopathic manipulative therapy for managing symptoms of irritable bowel syndrome: a systematic review. *J Am Osteopath Assoc.* 2014;114(6):470–479.
31. Lotfi C, Blair J, Jumrukovska A, Grubb M, Glidden E, Toldi J. Effectiveness of osteopathic manipulative treatment in treating symptoms of irritable bowel syndrome: a literature review. *Cureus.* 2023;15(7):e42393.
32. Licciardone JC, Brimhall AK, King LN. Osteopathic manipulative treatment for low back pain: a systematic review and meta-analysis of randomized controlled trials. *BMC Musculoskelet Disord.* 2005;6:43.
33. Franke H, Franke JD, Fryer G. Osteopathic manipulative treatment for nonspecific low back pain: a systematic review and meta-analysis. *BMC Musculoskelet Disord.* 2014;15:286.
34. Dal Farra F, Risio RG, Vismara L, Bergna A. Effectiveness of osteopathic interventions in chronic non-specific low back pain: a systematic review and meta-analysis. *Complement Ther Med.* 2021;56:102616.
35. Franke H, Hoesele K. Osteopathic manipulative treatment (OMT) for lower urinary tract symptoms (LUTS) in women. *J Bodyw Mov Ther.* 2013;17(1):11–18.
36. Rehman Y, Ferguson H, Bozek A, Blair J, Allison A, Johnston R. Osteopathic manual treatment for pain severity, functional improvement, and return to work in patients with chronic pain. *J Am Osteopath Assoc.* 2020;120(12):888–906.
37. McReynolds TM, Sheridan BJ. Intramuscular ketorolac versus osteopathic manipulative treatment in the management of acute neck pain in the emergency department: a randomized clinical trial. *J Am Osteopath Assoc.* 2005;105(2):57–68.
38. Franke H, Franke JD, Fryer G. Osteopathic manipulative treatment for chronic nonspecific neck pain: a systematic review and meta-analysis. *Int J Osteopath Med.* 2015;18(4):255–267.
39. Radjieski JM, Lumley MA, Cantieri MS. Effect of osteopathic manipulative treatment of length of stay for pancreatitis: a randomized pilot study. *J Am Osteopath Assoc.* 1998;98(5):264–272.
40. Li R, Jose A, Poon J, Zou C, Istafanos M, Yao SC. Efficacy of osteopathic manipulative treatment in patients with Parkinson's disease: a narrative review. *J Osteopath Med.* 2021;121(12):891–898.
41. Wells MR, Giantinoto S, D'Agate D, et al. Standard osteopathic manipulative treatment acutely improves gait performance in patients with Parkinson's disease. *J Am Osteopath Assoc.* 1999;99(2):92–98.
42. Guiney PA, Chou R, Vianna A, Lovenheim J. Effects of osteopathic manipulative treatment on pediatric patients with asthma: a randomized controlled trial. *J Am Osteopath Assoc.* 2005;105(1):7–12.
43. Hayden C, Mullinger B. A preliminary assessment of the impact of cranial osteopathy for the relief of infantile colic. *Complement Ther Clin Pract.* 2006;12(2):83–90.
44. Lanaro D, Ruffini N, Manzotti A, Lista G. Osteopathic manipulative treatment showed reduction of length of stay and costs in preterm infants: a systematic review and meta-analysis. *Medicine (Baltimore).* 2017; 96(12):e6408.
45. Cicchitti L, Di Lelio A, Barlafante G, et al. Osteopathic manipulative treatment in neonatal intensive care units. *Med Sci (Basel).* 2020;8(2): 24.
46. Manzotti A, Cerritelli F, Lombardi E, et al. Effects of osteopathic treatment versus static touch on heart rate and oxygen saturation in premature babies: a randomized controlled trial. *Complement Ther Clin Pract.* 2020;39:101116.
47. Mills MV, Henley CE, Barnes LLB, Carreiro JE, Degenhardt BF. The use of osteopathic manipulative treatment as adjuvant therapy in children with recurrent acute otitis media. *Arch Pediatr Adolesc Med.* 2003;157(9):861–866.
48. Steele KM, Carreiro JE, Viola JH, Conte JA, Ridpath LC. Effect of osteopathic manipulative treatment on middle ear effusion following acute otitis media in young children: a pilot study. *J Am Osteopath Assoc.* 2014;114(6):436–447.
49. Bagagiolo D, Priolo CG, Favre EM, et al. A randomized controlled trial of osteopathic manipulative therapy to reduce cranial asymmetries in young infants with nonsynostotic plagiocephaly. *Am J Perinatol.* 2022; 39(Suppl 01):S52–S62.
50. Wynne MM, Burns JM, Eland DC, Conatser RR, Howell JN. Effect of counterstrain on stretch reflexes, Hoffmann reflexes, and clinical outcomes in subjects with plantar fasciitis. *J Am Osteopath Assoc.* 2006; 106(9):547–556.
51. Boucher J, Mooney S, Dewey T, Kirtley RG, Walker T, Rabago D. Manual therapy informed by the fascial distortion model for plantar heel pain: results of a single-arm prospective effectiveness study. *J Altern Complement Med.* 2021;27(8):697–705.
52. Noll DR, Degenhardt BF, Morley TF, et al. Efficacy of osteopathic manipulation as an adjunctive treatment for hospitalized patients with pneumonia: a randomized controlled trial. *Osteopath Med Prim Care.* 2010;4:2.
53. Noll DR, Shores JH, Gamber RG, Herron KM, Swift J Jr. Benefits of osteopathic manipulative treatment for hospitalized elderly patients with pneumonia. *J Am Osteopath Assoc.* 2000;100(12):776–782.
54. Hensel KL, Pacchia CF, Smith ML. Acute improvement in hemodynamic control after osteopathic manipulative treatment in the third trimester of pregnancy. *Complement Ther Med.* 2013;21(6):618–626.
55. King HH, Tettambel MA, Lockwood MD, Johnson KH, Arsenault DA, Quist R. Osteopathic manipulative treatment in prenatal care: a retrospective case control design study. *J Am Osteopath Assoc.* 2003;103(12): 577–582.

56. Martingano D, Ho S, Rogoff S, Chang G, Aglialoro GC. Effect of osteopathic obstetrical management on the duration of labor in the inpatient setting: a prospective study and literature review. *J Am Osteopath Assoc.* 2019;119(6):371–378.
57. Franke H, Franke JD, Belz S, Fryer G. Osteopathic manipulative treatment for low back and pelvic girdle pain during and after pregnancy: a systematic review and meta-analysis. *J Bodyw Mov Ther.* 2017;21(4):752–762.
58. Rorris FP, Skouteli EAT, Papakonstantinou K, Kokotsaki L, Skotiniotis E, Kokotsakis J. Osteopathic manipulative treatment in cardiac surgery patients: a systematic review. *Int J Osteopath Med.* 2022;46:29–35.
59. Baltazar GA, Betler MP, Akella K, Khatri R, Asaro R, Chendrasekhar A. Effect of osteopathic manipulative treatment on incidence of postoperative ileus and hospital length of stay in general surgical patients. *J Am Osteopath Assoc.* 2013;113(3):204–209.
60. Crow WT, Gorodinsky L. Does osteopathic manipulative treatment (OMT) improves outcomes in patients who develop postoperative ileus: a retrospective chart review. *Int J Osteopath Med.* 2009;12(1):32–37.
61. Herrmann EP. Postoperative adynamic ileus: its prevention and treatment by osteopathic manipulation. *DO.* 1965;6(2):163–164.
62. Goldstein FJ, Jeck S, Nicholas AS, Berman MJ, Lerario M. Preoperative intravenous morphine sulfate with postoperative osteopathic manipulative treatment reduces patient analgesic use after total abdominal hysterectomy. *J Am Osteopath Assoc.* 2005;105(6):273–279.
63. Zhou Y, Chin J, Evangelista A, Podger B, Wan PJ, Lomiguen CM. Inhibiting the musculoskeletal pathological processes in post-knee replacement surgery with osteopathic manipulative treatment: a systematic review. *Cureus.* 2022;14(1):e21599.
64. Schwerla F, Hinse T, Klosterkamp M, Schmitt T, Rutz M, Resch KL. Osteopathic treatment of patients with shoulder pain. A pragmatic randomized controlled trial. *J Bodyw Mov Ther.* 2020;24(3):21–28.
65. Cutler MJ, Holland BS, Stupski BA, Gamber RG, Smith ML. Cranial manipulation can alter sleep latency and sympathetic nerve activity in humans: a pilot study. *J Altern Complement Med.* 2005;11(1):103–108.
66. International Federation for Manual/Musculoskeletal Medicine. *Guidelines on Basic Training and Safety. Version 3.1.* International Federation for Manual/Musculoskeletal Medicine; 2013.
67. Jonas WB, Rosenbaum E. The case for whole-person integrative care. *Medicina (Kaunas).* 2021;57(7):677.
68. NCI Thesaurus. Adverse event (code C41331). National Cancer Institute. Updated June 26, 2023. Accessed August 10, 2023. https://nciterms.nci.nih.gov/ncitbrowser/ConceptReport.jsp?dictionary=NCI_Thesaurus&ns=ncit&code=C41331
69. Richter D, Karst M, Buhck H, Fink MG. Efficacy of fascial distortion model treatment for acute, nonspecific low-back pain in primary care: a prospective controlled trial. *Altern Ther Health Med.* 2017;23(5):AT5522.
70. Thalhamer C. A fundamental critique of the fascial distortion model and its application in clinical practice. *J Bodyw Mov Ther.* 2018;22(1):112–117.
71. NCI Thesaurus. Side effect (code C2861). National Cancer Institute. Updated June 26, 2023. Accessed August 10, 2023. https://nciterms.nci.nih.gov/ncitbrowser/ConceptReport.jsp?dictionary=NCI_Thesaurus&ns=ncit&code=C2861
72. Funabashi M, Gorrell LM, Pohlman KA, Bergna A, Heneghan NR. Definition and classification for adverse events following spinal and peripheral joint manipulation and mobilization: a scoping review. *PLoS One.* 2022;17(7):e0270671.
73. Gorrell LM, Engel RM, Lystad RP, Brown BT. Assignment of adverse event indexing terms in randomized clinical trials involving spinal manipulative therapy: an audit of records in MEDLINE and EMBASE databases. *BMC Med Res Methodol.* 2017;17(1):41.
74. Ioannidis JPA, Evans SJW, Gotzsche PC, et al; CONSORT Group. Better reporting of harms in randomized trials: an extension of the CONSORT statement. *Ann Intern Med.* 2004;141(10):781–788.
75. NCI Thesaurus. Non-serious adverse event (code C41336). National Cancer Institute. Updated June 26, 2023. Accessed November 11, 2024. https://nciterms.nci.nih.gov/ncitbrowser/ConceptReport.jsp?dictionary=NCI_Thesaurus&ns=ncit&code=C41336
76. NCI Thesaurus. Serious adverse event (code C41335). National Cancer Institute. Updated June 26, 2023. Accessed August 10, 2023. https://nciterms.nci.nih.gov/ncitbrowser/ConceptReport.jsp?dictionary=NCI_Thesaurus&version=23.06d&ns=ncit&code=C41335&key=n1506204425&b=1&n=null
77. Cancer Therapy Evaluation Program (CTEP). Common Terminology Criteria for Adverse Events (CTCAE). National Cancer Institute. Accessed August 10, 2023. https://ctep.cancer.gov/protocoldevelopment/electronic_applications/ctc.htm#ctc_60
78. Common Terminology Criteria for Adverse Events (CTCAE). Version 5.0. National Cancer Institute. Updated November 27, 2017. Accessed August 10, 2023. https://ctep.cancer.gov/protocoldevelopment/electronic_applications/docs/CTCAE_v5_Quick_Reference_8.5x11.pdf
79. NCI Thesaurus. Mild adverse event (code C41338). National Cancer Institute. Updated June 26, 2023. Accessed August 10, 2023. https://nciterms.nci.nih.gov/ncitbrowser/ConceptReport.jsp?dictionary=NCI_Thesaurus&code=C41338
80. NCI Thesaurus. Moderate adverse event (code C41339). National Cancer Institute. Updated June 26, 2023. Accessed August 10, 2023. https://nciterms.nci.nih.gov/ncitbrowser/ConceptReport.jsp?dictionary=NCI_Thesaurus&ns=ncit&code=C41339
81. NCI Thesaurus. Severe adverse event (code C41340). National Cancer Institute. Updated June 26, 2023. Accessed August 10, 2023. https://nciterms.nci.nih.gov/ncitbrowser/ConceptReport.jsp?dictionary=NCI_Thesaurus&ns=ncit&code=C41340
82. NCI Thesaurus. Life threatening or disabling adverse event (code C41337). National Cancer Institute. Updated June 26, 2023. Accessed August 10, 2023. https://nciterms.nci.nih.gov/ncitbrowser/ConceptReport.jsp?dictionary=NCI_Thesaurus&ns=ncit&code=C41337
83. NCI Thesaurus. Death related to adverse event (code C48275). National Cancer Institute. Updated June 26, 2023. Accessed August 10, 2023. https://nciterms.nci.nih.gov/ncitbrowser/ConceptReport.jsp?dictionary=NCI_Thesaurus&ns=ncit&code=C48275
84. Cagnie B, Vinck E, Beernaert A, Cambier D. How common are side effects of spinal manipulation and can these side effects be predicted? *Man Ther.* 2004;9(3):151–156.
85. Carnes D, Mars TS, Mullinger B, Froud R, Underwood M. Adverse events and manual therapy: a systematic review. *Man Ther.* 2010;15(4):355–363.
86. Gorrell LM, Brown BT, Engel R, Lystad RP. Reporting of adverse events associated with spinal manipulation in randomised clinical trials: an updated systematic review. *BMJ Open.* 2023;13(5):e067526.
87. Posadzki P, Kyaw BM, Dziedzic A, Ernst E. Osteopathic manipulative treatment for pediatric conditions: an update of systematic review and meta-analysis. *J Clin Med.* 2022;11(15):4455.
88. Licciardone J, Gamber R, Cardarelli K. Patient satisfaction and clinical outcomes associated with osteopathic manipulative treatment. *J Am Osteopath Assoc.* 2002;102(1):13–20.
89. Leboeuf-Yde C, Hennius B, Rudberg E, Leufvenmark P, Thunman M. Side effects of chiropractic treatment: a prospective study. *J Manipulative Physiol Ther.* 1997;20(8):511–515.
90. Senstad O, Leboeuf-Yde C, Borchgrevink C. Frequency and characteristics of side effects of spinal manipulative therapy. *Spine (Phila Pa 1976).* 1997;22(4):435–440.
91. Swait G, Finch R. What are the risks of manual treatment of the spine? A scoping review for clinicians. *Chiropr Man Therap.* 2017;25:37.
92. Thomas M, Swait G, Finch R. Ten years of online incident reporting and learning using CPiRLS: implications for improved patient safety. *Chiropr Man Therap.* 2023;31(1):9.
93. Parnell Prevost C, Gleberzon B, Carleo B, Anderson K, Cark M, Pohlman KA. Manual therapy for the pediatric population: a systematic review. *BMC Complement Altern Med.* 2019;19(1):60.
94. Rushton A, Carlesso LC, Flynn T, et al. International framework for examination of the cervical region for potential of vascular pathologies of the neck prior to musculoskeletal intervention: International IFOMPT Cervical Framework [erratum appears in *J Orthop Sports Phys Ther.* 2023;53(6):372–374]. *J Orthop Sports Phys Ther.* 2023;*53*(1):7–22.
95. Straube S, Tramer MR, Moore RA, Derry S, McQuay HJ. Mortality with upper gastrointestinal bleeding and perforation: effects of time and NSAID use. *BMC Gastroenterol.* 2009;9:41.
96. Seffinger MA. The safety of osteopathic manipulative treatment (OMT). *J Am Osteopath Assoc.* 2018;118(3):137–138.

97. Nielsen SM, Tarp S, Christensen R, Bliddal H, Klokker L, Henriksen M. The risk associated with spinal manipulation: an overview of reviews. *Syst Rev.* 2017;6(1):64.
98. Whedon JM, Petersen CL, Li Z, Schoelkopf WJ, Haldeman S, MacKenzie TA, Lurie JD. Association between cervical artery dissection and spinal manipulative therapy-a medicare claims analysis. *BMC Geriatr.* 2022;22(1):917.
99. American Osteopathic Association. Osteopathic manipulative treatment (OMT) of the cervical spine: policy statement. Updated 2019. Accessed August 10, 2023. https://osteopathic.org/index.php?aam-media=/wp-content/uploads/policies/Policy_H324-A-19_Osteopathic_Manipulative_Treatment_of_the_Cervical_Spine-2.pdf
100. Carolei A, Sacco S. Headache attributed to stroke, TIA, intracerebral haemorrhage, or vascular malformation. *Handb Clin Neurol.* 2010;97:517–528.
101. Lebedeva ER, Gurary NM, Olesen J. Headache in transient ischemic attacks. *J Headache Pain.* 2018;19(1):60.
102. Pollak L, Shlomo N, Lubetzki IK; National Acute Stroke Israeli Survey Group. Headache in stroke according to National Acute Stroke Israeli Survey. *Acta Neurol Scand.* 2017;135(4):469–475.
103. Cassidy JD, Boyle E, Cote P, et al. Risk of vertebrobasilar stroke and chiropractic care: results of a population-based case-control and case-crossover study. *J Manipulative Physiol Ther.* 2009;32(Suppl 2):S201–S208.
104. Murphy DR. Current understanding of the relationship between cervical manipulation and stroke: what does it mean for the chiropractic profession? *Chiropr Osteopat.* 2010;18:22.
105. Spinal manipulation: what you need to know. National Center for Complementary and Integrative Health. Updated September 2022. Accessed August 10, 2023. https://www.nccih.nih.gov/health/spinal-manipulation-what-you-need-to-know
106. American Medical Association. *CPT Professional 2023.* American Medical Association; 2022.
107. World Health Organization. *Benchmarks for Training in Traditional/Complementary and Alternative Medicine: Benchmarks for Training in Osteopathy.* World Health Organization; 2010.
108. Cook CE. *Orthopedic Manual Therapy: An Evidence-Based Approach.* 2nd ed. Pearson; 2010.
109. Dagenais S, Haldeman S. *Evidence-Based Management of Low Back Pain.* Mosby; 2011.
110. In: Giusti R, ed. *Glossary of Osteopathic Terminology.* 3rd ed. American Association of Colleges of Osteopathic Medicine; 2017.
111. Licciardone JC, Kearns CM, Hodge LM, Minotti DE. Osteopathic manual treatment in patients with diabetes mellitus and comorbid chronic low back pain: subgroup results from the OSTEOPATHIC Trial. *J Am Osteopath Assoc.* 2013;113(6):468–478.
112. Lewis PB, Ruby D, Bush-Joseph CA. Muscle soreness and delayed-onset muscle soreness. *Clin Sports Med.* 2012;31(2):255–262.
113. Nahon RL, Silva Lopes JS, Monteiro de Magalhaes Neto A. Physical therapy interventions for the treatment of delayed onset muscle soreness (DOMS): systematic review and meta-analysis. *Phys Ther Sport.* 2021;52:1–12.
114. Wang Y, Lu H, Li S, et al. Effect of cold and heat therapies on pain relief in patients with delayed onset muscle soreness: a network meta-analysis. *J Rehabil Med.* 2022;54:jrm00258.
115. Cleary MA, Sweeney LA, Kendrick ZV, Sitler MR. Dehydration and symptoms of delayed-onset muscle soreness in hyperthermic males. *J Athl Train.* 2005;40(4):288–297.
116. Commission on Osteopathic College Accreditation. *Accreditation of Colleges of Osteopathic Medicine: COM Continuing Accreditation Standards.* American Osteopathic Association; 2022. Accessed August 10, 2023. https://osteopathic.org/index.php?aam-media=/wp-content/uploads/COCA-2023-COM-Continuing-Standards.pdf
117. American Association of Colleges of Osteopathic Medicine. *Osteopathic Core Competencies for Medical Students.* American Association of Colleges of Osteopathic Medicine; 2012. Accessed August 10, 2023. https://www.aacom.org/docs/default-source/med-ed-documents/corecompetencyreport2012.pdf?sfvrsn=53bed24b_1
118. National Board of Osteopathic Medical Examiners. *Fundamental Osteopathic Medical Competency Domains 2016.* National Board of Osteopathic Medical Examiners; 2016. Accessed August 10, 2023. https://www.nbome.org/Content/Exams/All/FOMCD_2016.pdf
119. National Board of Osteopathic Medical Examiners. COMLEX-USA Master Blueprint. Updated February 2023. Accessed November 11, 2024. https://www.nbome.org/wp-content/uploads/pdf/COMLEX-USA_Master_Blueprint_2024.pdf
120. Lam MT, Banihashem M, Lam HR, Wan AB, Chow E. Patient experience, satisfaction, perception and expectation of osteopathic manipulative treatment: a systematic review. *Int J Osteopath Med.* 2019;32:28–43.
121. Fawkes C, Carnes D. Patient reported outcomes in a large cohort of patients receiving osteopathic care in the United Kingdom. *PLoS One.* 2021;16(4):e0249719.
122. Tramontano M, Cinnera MA, Petracca M, et al. Outpatient satisfaction with osteopathic manipulative treatment in a hospital center: a survey. *Altern Ther Health Med.* 2018;24(5):18–24.
123. Lin I, Wiles L, Waller R, et al. What does best practice care for musculoskeletal pain look like? Eleven consistent recommendations from high-quality clinical practice guidelines: systematic review. *Br J Sports Med.* 2020;54(2):79–86.
124. Institute of Medicine Committee on Advancing Pain Research, Care, and Education. *Relieving Pain in America: A Blueprint for Transforming Prevention, Care, Education, and Research.* National Academies Press; 2011.
125. Carpal tunnel syndrome: a summary of clinical practice guideline recommendations—using the evidence to guide physical therapist practice. *J Orthop Sports Phys Ther.* 2019;49(5):359–360.
126. Ng JY, Hanna C. Headache and migraine clinical practice guidelines: a systematic review and assessment of complementary and alternative medicine recommendations. *BMC Complement Med Ther.* 2021;21(1):236.
127. Sico JJ, Macedo F, Lewis J, et al. The primary care management of headache: synopsis of the 2020 US Department of Veterans Affairs and US Department of Defense clinical practice guideline. *Mil Med.* 2022;187(9-10):e1091–e1102.
128. Task Force on the Low Back Pain Clinical Practice Guidelines. American Osteopathic Association guidelines for osteopathic manipulative treatment (OMT) for patients with low back pain. *J Am Osteopath Assoc.* 2016;116(8):536–549.
129. Chou R, Qaseem A, Snow V, et al; Clinical Efficacy Assessment Subcommittee of the American College of Physicians; American College of Physicians; American Pain Society Low Back Pain Guidelines Panel. Diagnosis and treatment of low back pain: a joint clinical practice guideline from the American College of Physicians and the American Pain Society. *Ann Intern Med.* 2007;147(7):478–491.
130. Qaseem A, Wilt TJ, McLean RM, et al. Noninvasive treatments for acute, subacute, and chronic low back pain: a clinical practice guideline from the American College of Physicians. *Ann Intern Med.* 2017;166(7):514–530.
131. Bussieres A, Cancelliere C, Ammendolia C, et al. Non-surgical interventions for lumbar spinal stenosis leading to neurogenic claudication: a clinical practice guideline. *J Pain.* 2021;22(9):1015–1039.
132. Greenlee H, DuPont-Reyes MJ, Balneaves LG, et al. Clinical practice guidelines on the evidence-based use of integrative therapies during and after breast cancer treatment. *CA Cancer J Clin.* 2017;67(3):194–232.
133. Ng JY, Uppal M, Steen J. Neck pain clinical practice guidelines: a systematic review of the quality and quantity of complementary and alternative medicine recommendations. *Eur Spine J.* 2022;31(10):2650–2663.
134. Hochberg MC, Altman RD, April KT, et al; American College of Rheumatology. American College of Rheumatology 2012 recommendations for the use of nonpharmacologic and pharmacologic therapies in osteoarthritis of the hand, hip, and knee. *Arthritis Care Res (Hoboken).* 2012;64(4):465–474.
135. Martin RL, Davenport TE, Reischl SF, et al. Heel pain—plantar fasciitis: revision 2014. *J Orthop Sports Phys Ther.* 2014;44(11):A1–A33.
136. Schneider HP, Baca JM, Carpenter BB, Dayton PD, Fleischer AE, Sachs BD. American College of Foot and Ankle Surgeons clinical consensus statement: diagnosis and treatment of adult acquired infracalcaneal heel pain. *J Foot Ankle Surg.* 2018;57(2):370–381.
137. Doiron-Cadrin P, Lafrance S, Saulnier M, et al. Shoulder rotator cuff disorders: a systematic review of clinical practice guidelines and semantic analyses of recommendations. *Arch Phys Med Rehabil.* 2020;101(7):1233–1242.

96 Strategic Planning for Research on Osteopathic Principles and Practices

BRIAN F. DEGENHARDT ▪ ANGELA K. TYSON

KEY CONCEPTS

- Research is required to advance our understanding of the causes of and treatments for the body's ailments.
- The osteopathic profession has failed to establish a robust research culture, especially to address its distinctive legacy involving osteopathic principles and practices (OPP).
- The strategic plans of the National Institutes of Health and its Center for Complementary and Integrative Health resonate with osteopathic principles and should help guide and motivate research in OPP.
- A realistic, achievable strategic plan is needed to build a robust research culture/workforce within the osteopathic profession. From a strategic plan perspective, establishing the foundation for such a culture by growing a workforce through our training programs makes sense. Creating the foundation begins with students learning good diagnostic and therapeutic palpatory skills.
- Explicit research training goals and institutional support to deliver training that leads to student proficiency are necessary for osteopathic students to be more competitive in seeking residencies, more effective in generating meaningful research, and sustaining research activities throughout their careers.
- Development of a strategic plan is only as effective as the daily management of that plan.

BACKGROUND

- Feedback from real-world clinical experience is crucial for comparing and improving the use of various interventions (i.e., drugs, manipulation), vaccines, medical devices, and diagnostics for different populations and various circumstances.[1,2] One form of feedback is achieved through research.
- From a societal perspective, medical research is extremely important because it provides important information about functional abilities, disease rates and risk factors, outcomes of treatment or public health interventions, patterns of care across populations, and health care costs.[3]
- A consistent and broad-based research effort seen in biomedical sciences has not occurred in osteopathic principles and practices (OPP).
- A fundamental and defining issue for the osteopathic profession in the 21st century is how today's osteopathic physicians and students contribute to advancing the field of medicine through research.
- A major factor limiting research has been a lack in training and coordination to build a research culture to investigate OPP across the medical specialties.
- Osteopathic medical students (OMS) and residents have a critical role in establishing and ensuring the research capacity and impact of the profession. However, an important question is whether they will receive adequate training and experience to develop the skills to contribute to the scientific process.
- A strategic plan is a roadmap to follow to achieve a goal or vision. The value of a strategic plan is determined by its influence on the daily activities of its stakeholders.

VISION

- The osteopathic profession produces and actively maintains a strategic plan that focuses on the fundamental issues that undermines the profession's ability to contribute to the scientific process—the lack of trained and experienced clinicians who seamlessly perform OPP research in their clinical and academic roles.
- All constituents within the osteopathic profession, staff at colleges, residencies, clinicians, and students, participate in and advance a strategic plan that promotes research in OPP. All constituents have roles that are interdependent and will shape the future practice and influence of osteopathic medicine.
- Osteopathic physicians at all career stages will diligently participate in the implementation of a strategic plan that is designed to establish and sustain a clinician-based research culture and to assess and advance the quality and effectiveness of the care they provide.
- The osteopathic profession succeeds in influencing health care through evidence-based recommendations consistent with many OPP.

This chapter lays out a relevant and feasible strategic plan for research in OPP. It provides specific recommendations to establish training for success in research for undergraduates through postgraduates, thus building a research culture to be sustained throughout one's career and future generations of DOs. Further, the strategic plan will prepare OMS, postgraduate resident physicians, and their trainers for practice in a 21st-century health care system, where physicians in clinical practice participate in research and quality improvement every day to ensure that the practice of medicine is evidence-based, patient-centered, and constantly improving.

Osteopathic Principles and Practices During the Past Century

- During most of the 1900s, OPP isolated the profession. Although this isolation was initially imposed by the allopathic profession, OPP evolved to become a platform that emphasizes the profession's distinctiveness.
- Over the past several decades, the rapid growth of new osteopathic schools has diluted the available workforce for OPP

training. In addition, pressures to expand curricular content has led to a reduction in the number of hours for OPP training, and surveys demonstrate a reduction in the number of clinicians using OMT in practice. In a survey of over 1,600 DO physicians practicing in the United States, over half never use it, over 75% use it on less than 5% of their patients, and less than 5% use it on at least 75% of their patients.[4] Over 40% reported this lack of use was due to lack of confidence of proficiency in the skillset. This data raises the concern that current and future osteopathic practitioners may lack an appropriate depth of understanding and skills in OPP to produce its potential therapeutic outcome.

- As illustrated by web searches, most of the osteopathic tenets have become generally accepted across society and other health care professions,[5–7] so now the tenets offer a foundation for collaboration.
- Mission statements, goals, and values contained in strategic plans from nonosteopathic institutions provide a source of information to compare with osteopathic principles to identify potential collaborators who are interested in or open to holistic health care practices and who have a substantial research capacity currently lacking at most osteopathic institutions.

THE NATIONAL INSTITUTES OF HEALTH (NIH) 2021–2025 STRATEGIC PLAN

- The National Institutes of Health (NIH) is the world's largest source of medical research funding and a major source of advancements in health care.[8]
- The mission of the NIH is "to seek fundamental knowledge about the nature and behavior of living systems and to apply that knowledge to enhance health, lengthen life, and reduce illness and disability."[9(pvii)]
- The NIH's mission and its goal to improve the health of humanity are consistent with osteopathic principles.[9]

Overall, the NIH has three goals for research that are outlined in its 2021–2025 strategic plan.[9]

1. Advancing biomedical and behavioral sciences
   - □ Driving foundational science
   - □ Understanding biologic, behavioral, and social determinants of population health
   - □ Preventing disease and promoting health
   - □ Developing and optimizing treatments, interventions, and cures
   - □ Giving the right treatment to the right patient at the right time
   - □ Catalyzing cell engineering, bioengineering, and regenerative medicine
2. Developing, maintaining, and renewing scientific research capacity
3. Exemplifying and promoting the highest level of scientific integrity, public accountability, and social responsibility in the conduct of science
   - □ The first goal illustrates the complexity of the scope of research that is being prioritized.
   - □ Identifying focused niches for productive members of the osteopathic biomedical community and facilitating their ability to contribute to Goal 1 needs to be an important priority for osteopathic colleges and universities.
   - □ In general, research capacity has been a weakness of the profession. Although several state-funded osteopathic medical schools have established research niches, primarily in basic science research, developing clinical research capacity has been a ubiquitous deficiency and challenge.
   - □ Regarding Goal 2, the NIH has a primary goal that relates to a basic weakness within the osteopathic profession. The profession has struggled throughout its history to develop its scientific research capacity. Although isolated institutions and labs have had periods of success, maintaining that capacity has been difficult and needs to be strategically prioritized. Research capacity is the underpinnings of success for all other goals in a strategic plan.
   - □ Goal 3 is a new strategic goal for NIH and is likely associated with the recent COVID-19 pandemic. Although public opinion regarding the value of science for advancing health care had been well documented, the management of the COVID-19 pandemic highlighted an erosion of trust between many of the public and the corporate/scientific alliance.[10] Physicians and various allied health care providers were and will remain on the front line for management of trust in scientific integrity into the future. As the largest producer of physicians in primary care fields,[11] the osteopathic profession needs to actively participate in reestablishing the public trust in the biomedical sciences.

The National Center for Complementary and Integrative Health

- The National Center for Complementary and Integrative Health (NCCIH) is the primary center at the NIH supporting research related to OPP.
- NCCIH's leadership realizes that evidence-based but currently nonmedical health care approaches should not be considered only as an alternative to standard medical practice but should be integrated into the health care system.
- The center's mission is to "determine, through rigorous scientific investigation, the fundamental science, usefulness, and safety of complementary and integrative health approaches and their roles in improving health and health care."[12,13]
- The outcome of successfully addressing this mission will be a time when scientific evidence informs decision-making by the public, health care professionals, and health policymakers regarding the integrated use of complementary health approaches in a whole person health framework.[12]
- These concepts have been championed by the osteopathic profession throughout its history. Consequently, the profession needs to become an active and consistent contributor supporting the NCCIH mission.

In the 2021–2025 NCCIH strategic plan,[12] five major objectives were identified.

1. Advance fundamental science and methods development.
2. Advance research on the whole person and on the integration of complementary and conventional care.
3. Foster research on health promotion and restoration, resilience, disease prevention, and symptom management.
4. Enhance the complementary and integrative health research workforce.
5. Provide objective evidence-based information on complementary and integrative health interventions.
   - □ As expected, the NCCIH strategic plan[12] has themes that are consistent with the entire NIH.[9] Yet, the NCCIH themes more clearly outline a plan that resonates with OPP. As seen in previous descriptions of this plan in earlier

versions of this chapter, historical concerns about conceptual roadblocks to OPP research at the NCCIH are no longer apparent.

- While the NCCIH has an extensive and broad portfolio of research, a U24 center grant funded in 2022 established three high-priority research networks particularly relevant to OPP: Force.Net, SpineWork, and NeuronS_MATTER. This new initiative is the largest investment by NIH to research in manual therapies. These networks are beginning to address the neural, mechanical, and psychosocial/contextual mechanisms of force-based manipulations, their term for manual therapies, and the factors, such as nomenclature, that inhibit the progress of this work.[14]
- The high-priority research being addressed by each of these networks includes:
  - Terminology and measurement of force-based manipulations
  - Mechanistic multiscale (i.e., molecular, cellular, and circuit) research measuring the physiologic response to force-based manipulations
  - Contextual effects of force-based manipulations
  - Technology and methodology development for mechanistic studies[14]
- This novel initiative will greatly influence the evidence associated with manual medicine/therapies and offers a great opportunity for the osteopathic research community to join these networks and collaborate in this field.

While the osteopathic profession was historically distinctive for its pioneering philosophical approach to holistic and manual medicine, as these approaches continue to become more popular and more commonly practiced, there is a trend toward convergence and cooperation amongst professions practicing manual medicine that DOs should not ignore, but participate in.

An increasing number of practitioners throughout the health care system through the latter half of the 20th century began to share those traditional osteopathic ideals, have incorporated manual therapies into their practices, and are committed to advancing the evidence base of manual therapies. In the current landscape, an important question is whether the osteopathic profession will be an active contributor to the high-priority research area of manual therapy at the NIH. To be an active contributor, the profession has to address the lack of an integrative health research workforce, which is a strategic plan priority for the NCCIH[8] and the NIH[5] and is a consistent area of weakness for the osteopathic profession. Because the osteopathic profession is now a major contributor to the physician pool in the United States, the profession must find ways to directly participate in these goals. As such, a strategic plan for research in OPP needs to prioritize addressing one primary goal: developing and sustaining a skilled integrative health research workforce.

A STRATEGIC PLAN FOR RESEARCH ON OSTEOPATHIC PRINCIPLES AND PRACTICES

- The goal of this proposed strategic plan is to offer meaningful and achievable suggestions that will build the infrastructure and culture of research within the osteopathic profession. It is subdivided into three periods: undergraduate training, postgraduate training, and active practice.
- Undergraduate Training
  - Years 1 and 2: Curricula need to promote the development of fundamental research and examination skills emphasizing accurate palpation of anatomy and differentiating between healthy and unhealthy tissues.
    - Why perform research to investigate outcomes on imprecise, uncalibrated instruments? Why do research with physicians whose skills are imprecise, sloppy, or rudimentary, minimizing the potential of producing therapeutic outcomes? Therefore, each educational program from medical school, residency, and continuing medical education training and the Educational Council on Osteopathic Principles (ECOP) need to emphasize and sustain through all stages of education the development and advancement of precise palpation skills, reinforcing and advancing the accurate localization and identification of anatomy and discriminating between normal and abnormal tissues. These skills translate to almost all forms of clinical practice and so are relevant to all OMS.
    - Appropriate training will ensure that a thorough understanding of functional anatomy, its underlying physiology, and the ability to influence it with the hands will remain distinguishing features of osteopathic physicians.
    - The Commission on Osteopathic College Accreditation (COCA) must hold institutions responsible for providing adequate training to achieve these skills. As the number of osteopathic training programs has increased,[11] the number of skilled faculty able to offer hands-on psychomotor training has not kept pace. Further, the once established faculty-to-student ratio of 8 to 12 students to 1 faculty member has been eliminated from COCA standards.[15] It does not seem feasible that one full-time osteopathic manipulative medicine (OMM) faculty member can teach 90 to 150 students well enough to provide the necessary oversight that will result in physicians with skills representative of the therapeutic potential of the osteopathic model. This level of training is also inadequate for the required research in OPP from which future health care policy will be derived.
    - Current evidence-based features of OPP need to be integrated throughout the DO curriculum. Examples of ideal topics for presentation within an OPP context include current knowledge of mechanisms of action underlying osteopathic manipulative treatment (OMT), neuromotor development and control, pain, stiffness, somesthesis kinesthesis and their association with palpation skills, placebo, and psychosocial responses.
    - Thus, each educational program should continually examine which of the techniques are fundamental and most relevant for use in primary and traditional medical specialty practices and coordinate their rationale within the ECOP to sustain national standards. Those techniques that fall primarily within the specialty of OMM, especially those that require subtler skills with less obvious scientific rationale, should be reserved for more advanced training, especially in residencies where future specialists need to push the boundaries of models, paradigms, and understanding. This strategic rationale is to focus training during the first 2 years of the osteopathic medical curriculum to ensure the development of competent basic palpatory psychomotor skills, both diagnostic and therapeutic, that will be used throughout the students' clinical years of training and throughout their careers. Current evidence indicates that this goal for training and utilization of osteopathic skills is not being achieved.[16,17]

- Research-related skills that need to be part of undergraduate years 1 and 2 include being able to perform the following:
    - critically appraise the literature, focusing on common research designs and fundamental statistics relevant to clinical practice (see Chapter 94);
    - during early clinical experiences, write up a case study and present it; and
    - complete a group project where students go through the process of a systematic review or a research proposal including institutional review board review.
- Years 3 and 4: clinical clerkships
    - Students need to train in an environment that ensures continued use of palpatory skills throughout their clinical rotations. Training programs should identify ways to incentivize clinical faculty to reinforce use of palpatory skills during clinical experiences.
    - Students should participate in a resident-led quality improvement project.
    - As a standard part of the 1- to 4-year curriculum, students should have programming that teaches them how to design a good research question. Ideally, the students should be encouraged to develop research questions related to their residency area of interest and have them critiqued by training staff for refinement.
    - During their clerkship period, students should produce and present a research poster at a university/hospital, regional, or national conference about some aspect of a study they are participating in or an unusual case. A case series is an excellent option if the student has the time.
    - Students need to learn about easy research designs that they could use with research questions they are developing, such as a card study or an n-of-1 study design.[18,19]
- Undergraduate medical training is meant to provide students with the basic tools for success in residency. Because the Accreditation Council for Graduate Medical Education has general requirements for performing quality improvement and research during residency, students need the basic skills outlined above to meet these expectations. Such research skills should be considered in the same light as any other clinical content learned by students during medical school that they are expected to use during their residency.

- Postgraduate training
    - Residency
        - Residency directors and faculty need to acknowledge that establishing a culture of research seamlessly integrated into clinical training is the requirement and responsibility of all residency programs.
        - Not every residency faculty will have the training and experience to mentor research. In these circumstances, collaborating with academic institutions, other residencies with a robust research program, or with a practice-based research network (PBRN) will help to build a research culture within a residency.
        - The research culture is meaningfully established when:
            - directors and residents have clear guidelines, expectations, and resources so that residents do not have to start from scratch when beginning their research. A scenario commonly observed is a resident coming into a residency with no background training for producing research and a residency program with no systematic resources or plan for guidance. Ideally, there should be a well-defined roadmap for developing research in an area of resident interest, which hopefully overlaps with the research area of an experienced resident mentor.
            - research themes that are passed from one year of residents to the next so that a series of related questions are sequentially asked and answered facilitates research. When this occurs, the time to complete clinical and research tasks are optimized.
        - A case presentation should not be considered an adequate project for residency-level research. Only in rare situations, when a case is truly novel, should this be considered acceptable. Instead, case presentations should be an undergraduate expectation as previously discussed that prepares students for a more formal research experience during their residency.
        - Residency programs need to be very comfortable producing simple/manageable but relevant clinical research designs. See Chapter 94 for more details.
        - The American Council for Graduate Medical Education promotes research not only as a requirement for completion, but to develop necessary skills that will be used in clinical practice. The fundamentals for learning how to do research should be an outcome of undergraduate training. For example, graduates entering residencies should have an idea how to construct a good research question. They should not have to start their research from scratch and should instead be able to build on their previous training and the program's experience with performing clinical research.
        - Each residency program needs to provide residents with a standard, explicit timeline that outlines specific deliverables for research when they enter the program.
        - As a starting point for resident research, residency programs should have the ability to extract meaningful data from their electronic medical record (EMR), such as patient profiles of the practice or utilization and practice pattern data. This information should be compared with current evidence-based practice guidelines to evaluate compliance (a good starting point for quality improvement projects) and consistency of outcomes. Any time practice guidelines do not deliver expected outcomes should signal an area deserving of further research.
        - One purpose of EMRs is to be a tool for physicians to glean more insights about their patient population, practice habits, and outcomes. Yet, providing training so residents develop skills to query the database is often overlooked in residency and in practice. Ideally, as a starting point specifically for clinical outcomes research, incoming residents within their first 4 months should have a research question vetted by the residency director/assigned research mentor and use the EMR to be able to extract data relevant to the question when appropriate. Having a clear starting point and defined process for incoming residents facilitates their activities and provides motivation and confidence in the research experience.
        - Residents need to have an assigned research mentor who meets with the resident monthly during the development phase of their research and quality improvement projects and then quarterly to ensure the resident has a successful research experience.
        - Retrospective studies from EMR data are an excellent starting point for establishing a line of research that can be passed on from one set of residents to the next. Outcomes from retrospective studies should lead to relevant prospective research by future residents.

- Residency programs should expect that good resident research will impact the overall clinical practice of the program. If it does not, the management and mentorship of resident research require additional refinement.
- Residency programs should learn how to promote collaboration when performing research. For example, participating in multicenter research across other residencies or within PBRNs is an efficient and effective way of producing higher impact outcomes. This level of experience is crucial for providing residents with the ability to continue performing research that advances OPP within their specialty throughout their careers.
- Practice and research capabilities are rapidly evolving. In recent decades, the advancement of technology and influence of corporations have thrust society into an era of "big data,"[20,21] easily recognized in the health care coding and billing systems and the EMR.
- A new era of artificial intelligence is beginning that will have unprecedented effects and will likely present unforeseeable challenges and opportunities.[22,23]
- In the next decade, it is likely that the design and outcomes of research and their impact on the practice of medicine will substantially change. Yet, these changes will still need to be built upon sound scientific principles and processes, essential skills of osteopathic physicians if the OPP is to survive and thrive for the betterment of society.

- Active practice
  - Career-based OPP research
    - The research experience gained during residency should facilitate continuation of these activities throughout the physician's career.
    - As a result of residency training, practicing clinicians should be able to use their EMR to extract relevant practice-based information for quality assurance purposes and to identify quality improvement programming for their office or clinic.
    - Practicing physicians should be able to use their EMR to help generate and refine research questions.
    - Practicing clinicians should be able to productively contribute to PBRNs in their area of expertise by generating insightful research questions, successfully managing a protocol, and producing and submitting data.
    - Infrastructure to support PBRNs needs to be established through collaborations between specialty colleges and academic institutions. Such collaboration offers clinicians necessary resources that are typically unavailable in clinical practice (e.g., grant writing, methodologic refinement, statistical and scientific writing support).
    - As a concept, vision, and certain forms of technique, OPPs extend well beyond the osteopathic profession. As illustrated by web searches,[4–6] most of the osteopathic tenets have become generally accepted across society and other health care professions, offering a foundation for interdisciplinary and interprofessional research collaboration. The infrastructure for rigorous research and skilled manual therapy among manual therapy professions far exceeds what the osteopathic profession can offer alone. Historical professional isolation impedes the advancement of knowledge and utilization of OPP.
    - Developing collaborations with other professions for research related to OPP/manual therapies is not only an opportunity, but also necessary to advance health care options and the scientific understanding of manual therapies.
    - It is likely that the most successful and impactful research in the 21st century will be collaborative.[24–26]
    - Mission statements, goals, and values contained in strategic plans from nonosteopathic institutions provide a source of information to compare with osteopathic principles to identify potential collaborators who are interested in or open to holistic health care practices and who have a substantial research capacity currently lacking at most osteopathic institutions.
    - It appears that the fourth tenet, how the other tenets are integrated into medical practice, remains uniquely osteopathic but only if the programming of our osteopathic educational programs demonstrates how this is done, remaining true to the profession's heritage and its still visionary principle.

SUMMARY

- Consistent with the current strategic plans of the NIH[9] and the NCCIH,[12] the osteopathic profession needs to build and sustain a research infrastructure to advance health care services prioritizing OPP.
- The rapid growth in the number of osteopathic colleges and training sites indicates that the profession has the potential to influence the type, quality, and impact of research in the practice of medicine.
- The strategic focus for the osteopathic profession at this stage of its development needs to prioritize building and sustaining a research infrastructure, not just at universities but throughout all levels of training and practice. Importantly, all constituents within the osteopathic profession have an opportunity and responsibility to contribute.
- Successful research in the 21st century will be based on the willingness and ability of health care programs to collaborate.
- As a whole, the osteopathic profession and its training programs do not have the experience or infrastructure to be immediately competitive for funding in the national biomedical research enterprise. Yet the profession has important ideologies and resources that may be useful when partnering or collaborating with more research-intensive institutions. It would be strategically wise for osteopathic training programs to participate by performing secondary roles in collaborative research projects with experienced research institutions, demonstrate competency by fulfilling those roles, and eventually pursue greater roles within the biomedical research community after gaining valuable experience. However, this strategy will only be successful if the osteopathic profession has built a strong scientific research capacity through training programs that integrate research education and experience in all phases of clinical training.

REFERENCES

1. Institute of Medicine. *Beyond the HIPAA Privacy Rule: Enhancing Privacy, Improving Health Through Research.* National Academies Press; 2009.
2. National Library of Medicine, National Center for Biotechnology Information. Submission portal. Accessed June 5, 2023. https://submit.ncbi.nlm.nih.gov/
3. Institute of Medicine (US) Committee on Health Research and the Privacy of Health Information: The HIPAA Privacy Rule. 3, The value, importance, and oversight of health research. *In:* Nass SJ, Levit LA, Gostin LO, eds. *Beyond the HIPAA Privacy Rule: Enhancing Privacy, Improving Health Through Research.* National Academies Press (US); 2009.
4. Healy CJ, Brockway MD, Wilde BB. Osteopathic manipulative treatment (OMT) use among osteopathic physicians in the United States. *J Osteopath Med.* 2021;121(1):57–61.

5. https://www.google.com/search?q=mind%2C±body±and±spirit&rlz=1C1GCEU_enUS852US852&oq=mind%2C±body±and±spirit&aqs=chrome..69i57j0i512l9.356798981j0j15&sourceid=chrome&ie=UTF-8–1,190,000,000 sites. Accessed September 12, 2023.
6. https://www.google.com/search?q=body+has+self+healing+and+regulating+properties&sca_esv=564736079&rlz=1C1GCEU_enUS852US852&sxsrf=AB5stBgcXtGRZLDRXxhGiQdXkk7MKsDlxg%3A1694541890615&ei=QqgAZa71JIKxptQPyteYuAc&ved=0ahUKEwiunsm71KWBAxWCmIkEHcorBncQ4dUDCBA&uact=5&oq=body+has+self+healing+and+regulating+properties&gs_lp=Egxnd3Mtd2l6LXNlcnAiL2JvZHkgaGFzIHNlbGYgaGVhbGluZyBhbmQgcmVndWxhdGluZyBwcm9wZXJ0aWVzMgUQIRigAUjdjAFQAFjKiAFwCXgBkAEAmAHAAaABhjeqAQQyLjU0uAEDyAEA-AEBwgIHECMYigUYJ8ICCxAuGIMBGLEDGIoFwgIHEAAYigUYQ8ICCBAuGLEDGIAEwgILEAAYigUYsQMYgwHCAhEQLhiABBixAxiDARjHARjRA8ICBRAAGIAEwgILEAAYgAQYsQMYgwHCAggQABiKBRiRAsICCxAuGIAEGMcBGK8BwgINEAAYgAQYFBiHAhixA8ICCxAuGIAEGLEDGIMBwgIOEC4YxwEYsQMY0QMYgATCAg0QABiABBgUGIcCGMkDwgIIEAAYgAQYkgPCAggQABiABBixA8ICCBAAGIAEGMkDwgIKEAAYgAQYFBiHAsICBhAAGBYYHsICCBAAGBYYHhgPwgIIEAAYFhgeGArCAggQABiKBRiGA8ICBRAhGKsCwgIKECEYFhgeGA8YHcICCBAhGBYYHhgdwgIHECEYoAEYCuIDBBgAIEGIBgE&sclient=gws-wiz-serp –79,100,000 sites. Accessed September 12, 2023.
7. https://www.google.com/search?q=interrelationship+of+structure+and+function&sca_esv=564736079&rlz=1C1GCEU_enUS852US852&sxsrf=AB5stBhBVAlen49_NAkxQfbCMpLGBIsblA%3A1694541982106&ei=nqgAZd2BBpypptQPkoe20A0&ved=0ahUKEwjdyJnn1KWBAxWclIkEHZKDDdoQ4dUDCBA&uact=5&oq=interrelationship+of+structure+and+function&gs_lp=Egxnd3Mtd2l6LXNlcnAiK2ludGVycmVsYXRpb25zaGlwIG9mIHN0cnVjdHVyZSBhbmQgZnVuY3Rpb24yBhAAGBYYHkjuQVAAWKg4cAB4AZABAJgBygGgAYQjqgEHMjEuMjEuMbgBA8gBAPgBAcICBBAjGCfCAgcQIxiKBRgnwgIIEAAYigUYkQLCAg4QABiKBRixAxiDARiRAsICCxAAGIAEGLEDGIMBwgIFEAAYgATCAggQABiABBixA8ICDRAuGIoFGMcBGNEDGCfCAgcQABiKBRhDwgIFEC4YgATCAg0QABiKBRixAxiDARhDwgINEC4YigUYxwEYrwEYQ8ICCxAuGIAEGMcBGK8BwgITEAAYigUYsQMYgwEYkQIYRhj5AcICCxAuGIAEGLEDGIMBwgIqEAAYigUYsQMYgwEYkQIYRhj5ARiXBRiMBRjdBBhGGPQDGPUDGPYD2AEBwgIKEAAYgAQYFBiHAsICEBAAGIAEGLEDGIMBGEYY-QHCAicQABiABBixAxiDARhGGPkBGJcFGIwFGN0EGE. 11,900,000 sites. Accessed September 12, 2023.
8. National Institutes of Health. NIH…turning discovery into health. Accessed June 5, 2023. https://www.nih.gov/about-nih/what-we-do/nih-turning-discovery-into-health
9. National Institutes of Health. NIH-wide strategic plan: fiscal years 2021–2025. Accessed June 5, 2023. https://www.nih.gov/sites/default/files/about-nih/strategic-plan-fy2021-2025-508.pdf
10. Berger ZD, Evans NG, Phelan AL, Silverman RD. Covid-19: control measures must be equitable and inclusive. *BMJ.* 2020;368:m1141.
11. American Osteopathic Association. OMP report: 2023 report tracks increased growth in the osteopathic profession. Accessed June 5, 2023. https://osteopathic.org/about/aoa-statistics/
12. National Center for Complementary and Integrative Health. NCCIH strategic plan FY 2021–2025: mapping a pathway to research on whole person health. Accessed June 5, 2023. https://www.nccih.nih.gov/about/nccih-strategic-plan-2021-2025
13. National Center for Complementary and Integrative Health. Complementary, alternative, or integrative health: what's in a name? Accessed June 5, 2023. https://www.nccih.nih.gov/health/complementary-alternative-or-integrative-health-whats-in-a-name
14. National Center for Complementary and Integrative Health. Neural mechanisms of force-based manipulations: high priority research networks. Accessed June 5, 2023. https://www.nccih.nih.gov/research/neural-mechanisms-of-force-based-manipulations-high-priority-research-networks
15. Snider KT, Seffinger MA, Ferrill HP, Gish EE. Trainer-to-student ratios for teaching psychomotor skills in health care fields, as applied to Osteopathic Manipulative Medicine. *J Osteopath Med.* 2012;112(4):182–187.
16. Sabesan VJ, Schrotenboer A, Habeck J, et al. Musculoskeletal education in medical schools: a survey of allopathic and osteopathic medical students. *J Am Acad Orthop Surg Glob Res Rev.* 2018;2(6):e019.
17. Shannon SC, Teitelbaum HS. The status and future of osteopathic medical education in the United States. *Acad Med.* 2009;84(6):707–711.
18. Lillie EO, Patay B, Diamant J, Issell B, Topol EJ, Schork NJ. The n-of-1 clinical trial: the ultimate strategy for individualizing medicine? *Per Med.* 2011;8(2):161–173.
19. Westfall JM, Zittleman L, Staton EW, et al. Card studies for observational research in practice. *Ann Fam Med.* 2011;9(1):63–68.
20. Batko K, Ślęzak A. The use of Big Data Analytics in healthcare. *J Big Data.* 2022;9(1):3.
21. Tulane University School of Public Health and Tropical Medicine. How big data in health care influences patient outcomes. 2021. Accessed June 5, 2023. https://publichealth.tulane.edu/blog/big-data-in-healthcare/
22. Davenport T, Kalakota R. The potential for artificial intelligence in healthcare. *Future Healthc J.* 2019;6(2):94–98.
23. Johnson KB, Wei WQ, Weeraratne D, et al. Precision medicine, AI, and the future of personalized health care. *Clin Transl Sci.* 2021;14(1):86–93.
24. Research collaborations bring big rewards: the world needs more. *Nature.* 2021;594(7863):301–302.
25. Rahman A. Why do collaborative research. *BMJ.* 2007;335(7614):304.
26. Nyström ME, Karltun J, Keller C, Andersson Gäre B. Collaborative and partnership research for improvement of health and social services: researcher's experiences from 20 projects. *Health Res Policy Sys.* 2018;16(1):46.

97 Case Study: Acute Neck Pain

JESUS SANCHEZ JR ▪ MARCEL P. FRAIX ▪ MICHAEL A. SEFFINGER

KEY CONCEPTS

- The osteopathic approach to patients with neck pain begins with a thorough history and physical examination, including an osteopathic palpatory examination of the neuromusculoskeletal system.
- Differential diagnosis utilizes a structure–function approach in determining whether the pain is due to local pathology, spinal somatic dysfunction of the cervical or upper thoracic region, localized manifestation of a systemic pathophysiologic process, or referred pain from internal organ disease.
- Osteopathic treatment plan includes judicious application of osteopathic manipulative treatment (OMT) to alleviate somatic dysfunction and improve biomechanical, neurologic, metabolic, respiratory/circulatory, and behavioral functions.
- Neck pain due to whiplash-associated disorder (WAD) is a common cause of neck pain in middle-age adults and is considered to involve the whole person, not just the cervical spine.

CASE VIGNETTE

CHIEF COMPLAINT

Neck pain

HISTORY OF PRESENT ILLNESS

A 45-year-old female presents to the ambulatory clinic with a complaint of acute neck pain that began after a motor vehicle accident (MVA) 3 days ago; she requests a note to stay off work. Three days ago, she was sitting in her car at a stoplight in her compact car when it was hit from behind by a pickup truck going about 35 mph. She was wearing her seat belt, hit her head against the headrest, but had no loss of consciousness; however, she did complain of neck pain after she stepped out of her car. She was looking up to the right into her rear-view mirror at the time of impact. She was seen in an emergency room (ER) later that day where a cervical spine x-ray series showed no fractures or dislocations, but loss of cervical lordosis was noted. She was discharged home the same day with a soft cervical collar and given a prescription for an analgesic for pain, a narcotic for severe pain, and a muscle relaxant for muscle spasms.

She still has neck stiffness and pain, rating it an 8/10 on the pain scale. The pain is constant with intermittent sharp and shooting radiating pain to her shoulders and head. She states she feels better lying supine, worse when sitting up. She is unable to look side to side or up and down without pain. It lasts throughout the day and is dulled a little by the analgesics. The neck collar gives her some relief. She has no other medical problems. Currently, she is taking the medications given to her at the ER, which provide some relief, although they make her drowsy and she has been sleeping several times throughout the day. She denies numbness and tingling or loss of strength in her upper extremities bilaterally.

Past Medical History

She has no major medical problems, no hospitalizations.

Past Surgical History

None to date.

Medications

Ibuprofen 800 mg tid prn pain; hydrocodone/acetaminophen 500 mg one every 4 hours prn severe pain; carisoprodol one every 6 hours prn muscle spasms.

Allergies

She has no allergies to medications.

Social History

She works as a secretary at a business office, types, files, and answers phones 8 hours a day, 5 days a week. She is divorced, is sole caregiver for her elderly and frail mother, has two grown children, and has one grandchild. She denies smoking, drinks a glass of wine with dinner nightly, and denies illicit drug use.

REVIEW OF SYSTEMS

General

She denies recent weight loss or gain, fevers, night sweats, or travel.

Cardiovascular

She denies chest pain, shortness of breath, orthopnea, or dyspnea on exertion.

Respiratory

She denies history of tuberculosis, asthma, cough, phlegm, or difficulty breathing.

HEENT

She denies visual, hearing, smell, taste, or phonation problems; no drainage or infections.

GI

She has nausea but no emesis; decreased appetite; constipation; no hematochezia, melena, or hematemesis. She has no history of abdominal pain or distention. No history of ulcers, hepatitis, gallstones, pancreatitis, or colitis.

Neurologic

She gets intermittent dizziness that resolves spontaneously, no history of seizures, stroke, or weakness. Sciatica into the left buttocks.

OB/GYN

She is G2P2. Her last menstrual period was 2 weeks ago, normal flow and regular. She has not been sexually active in the past 2 years. She states that her last Pap and breast examinations were normal 6 months ago.

Psychiatric

She denies fatigue but has had nightmares since the accident. She is anxious, fearing she will not be able to continue her job or take care of her mother. However, she denies a history of anxiety or psychiatric illness or hospitalization. She denies bipolar disease, depression, or schizophrenia. She is frustrated that the narcotics and muscle relaxers make her unable to function. She would like to have another alternative to help her deal with the pain that will allow her to still carry out her responsibilities at home and at work.

Hematologic

She denies history of anemia or bleeding dyscrasias. She sustained a bruise from the seat belt across her neck, but has no history of easy bruising.

Endocrine

She denies heat or cold intolerance; no polydipsia, polyphagia, or polyuria.

MSK

She denies skin lesions or rashes; no swollen joints, hands, or feet; constant bilateral frontal vice-like headaches and low back pain since the accident, with radiation to the left buttocks. She has a history of low back pain treated by a series of visits to chiropractors, osteopathic physicians, and physical therapists off and on for over 10 years since she fell skiing when she was 18. She was told she had scoliosis and a short-left leg for which she wore a ¼ inch lift for 10 years, but stopped using it for the past 17 years. She has not had disabling back or neck pain since then, though on occasion gets a headache or low back pain that resolves with a nonsteroidal anti-inflammatory medication, some stretching exercises for the neck and low back, and a couple of days of rest from strenuous activities.

PHYSICAL EXAMINATION

Vital Signs

Height, 5′6″: weight, 150; BP, 150/88 mmHg; R, 18 breaths/min; P, 86 beats/min; T, 98.6 °F.

General

Although somewhat low energy and anxious in appearance, she is well nourished, well developed, and in obvious pain and discomfort in the seated position with a soft cervical collar around her neck.

Integument

There is a mild abrasion over the left upper shoulder where the seat belt was with slight ecchymosis. No ecchymosis in the other extremities, chest, or abdomen.

HEENT

There are no contusions, lacerations, erythema, discharge, or swelling. Pupils are equal, round, reactive to light and accommodation, and external ocular muscles are intact (pupils are equal, round, reactive to light, and accommodation [PERRLA], extra ocular muscles are intact [EOMI]). There is no thyromegaly or tenderness. No lymphadenopathy.

Heart

Has a regular rhythm without murmurs; no carotid or vertebral bruits.

Lungs

Are clear to auscultation with equal breath sounds bilaterally.

Abdomen

The abdomen is flat; there are bowel sounds present in all four quadrants, nondistended, tympanic, no masses, no hepatosplenomegaly or tenderness. No suprapubic tenderness.

Extremities

No swelling, full ROM of the joints, pulses full, and capillary refill less than 2 seconds in upper and lower extremities.

Neurologic Examination

Alert and oriented to person, place, and time. Gait is normal. Muscle strength is 5+/5+ in all muscles in upper and lower extremities. CNs II to XII are grossly intact. Deep tendon reflexes are 2+/4+ bilaterally, symmetric in the upper and lower extremities. Babinski test elicits bilateral downward going toes. There are no cerebellar or sensory deficits. Straight leg raise is negative bilaterally to 90 degrees. Cognitive examination (minimental status examination) is negative. Spurling maneuver for the cervical spine is negative for eliciting radiating pain.

Osteopathic Structural Examination

Static tests for symmetry of anatomical landmarks: In the standing postural assessment, her head is held anterior to the gravitational line, with loss of cervical lordosis, decreased thoracic kyphosis and lumbar lordosis; the left shoulder is elevated; the left tip of scapula is superior; there is a thoracic scoliosis T5–T11 convex right, apex at T8; there is a lumbar scoliosis L1–L5, convex left with apex at L3; the left posterior superior iliac spine (PSIS), anterior superior iliac spine (ASIS), and sacral base landmarks are lower than the right; the left iliac crest is about 1 cm lower than the right; there is a short left leg approximately ¼ in.

Motion Tests Reveal

Positive standing and seated flexion tests on the left; the sacrum has decreased motion in both flexion and extension and feels compressed into L5; inherent sacral motion is diminished; L1–L5 are neutral, rotated left, side bent right and the sacrum is rotated to the right; T5–T11 are neutral, rotated right, and side bent left; T3 is extended, rotated and side bent right with boggy, edematous, and tender paraspinal soft tissues at that level; T1 and T2 are extended, rotated and side bent left; there are myofascial restrictions of the thoracic inlet; the left first rib is restricted during exhalation; right ribs 3 to 6 are restricted during inhalation; left ribs 6 to 12 are restricted in exhalation; the left diaphragm is restricted during exhalation; there is decreased cervical range of motion (ROM) bilaterally, especially flexion, extension, and side bending; the occipitoatlantal (OA) articulation is extended, side bent left, and rotated right; the atlantoaxial (AA) articulation is rotated right; cranial motion is diminished in amplitude bilaterally with little movement palpable.

Palpation Reveals

Tender anterior cervical muscles; there are bilateral cervical spasms from C3 to C7 making it difficult to assess segmental restrictions; trigger points are present in the trapezius and pectoralis muscles bilaterally; there is a tender L5–S1 interspinous ligament; and Jones tender points are found at the left LPL5, right LC1, right AC1, and right PC2.

ASSESSMENT

1. Neck pain (cervicalgia)
2. WAD
3. Somatic dysfunction: cranium, cervical, thoracic, lumbar, sacrum, pelvis, lower extremity, and rib regions
4. Abrasion
5. Anxiety
6. Contusion
7. Dizziness
8. Muscle spasms
9. Nausea
10. Scoliosis, idiopathic
11. Short left leg

DIFFERENTIAL DIAGNOSIS

Differential diagnosis utilizes a structure–function approach in determining whether the pain is due to local pathology, spinal somatic dysfunction of the cervical or upper thoracic region, localized manifestation of a systemic pathophysiologic process, or referred pain from internal organ disease. Since local neck pain generators may be located in the muscles, fascia, ligaments and joint capsules, periosteum, intervertebral disks, arteries, glands, organs, esophagus, trachea, lung, and dura, all pathologic processes affecting these structures should be considered as possible causes of her pain. These include degenerative, infectious, inflammatory, neoplastic, and congenital diseases; fractures; dislocations; spinal cord and peripheral nerve injuries; and vascular diseases, including arterial dissection. Differential diagnoses of acute neck pain from local pathology are listed in Table 97.1 along with characteristics and diagnostic tests used to confirm each.

In the patient above, gross fracture and dislocation are not likely, but possible, even in light of a negative initial cervical spine x-ray series.[1] The upper cervical somatic dysfunction is symptomatic and likely related to her recent accident, but she has underlying dysfunction in all body regions related to her short leg and scoliosis. Her neck pain could be an exacerbation of her already dysfunctional back and spine.

It is unlikely she has a disease process radiating pain to the neck as her history and physical do not support this theory, so a myocardial infarction, Pancoast lung tumor, esophageal or tracheal tumor or inflammation, thyroiditis or tumor, pulmonary embolus, collapsed lung, pleurisy, vertebral artery dissection, carotid artery dissection, tuberculosis, cancer of the mediastinum, or neck or cervical lymphadenopathy are less likely and can be removed from the differential at this time. However, if her course of recovery does not follow a pattern consistent with a primary musculoskeletal injury, these occult sources of pain might be investigated further.

TABLE 97.1

Differential Diagnosis of Neck Pain from Local Pathology

Diagnosis	Characteristics	Tests
Acute pharyngitis	Erythematous pharynx; exudates	Strep screen
Carotid aneurysm dissection	Tender carotid, bruit on auscultation	Carotid US, angiogram
Carotidynia	Tender carotid	Carotid US
Cervical fracture	Muscle splinting, history of trauma	Cervical spine x-rays
Dental disease	Teeth and/or gingival pain, tenderness, swelling	Dental x-rays
Lymphadenitis	Enlarged, tender lymph nodes	CBC, ESR
Meningitis	Nuchal ligament rigidity, fever, malaise	Spinal tap
Myositis	Very tender muscles	CBC, ESR
Peritonsillar abscess	Tonsil protruding anteriorly and/or medially	Aspiration
Spinal cord injury	Neurologic deficits below neck; if C3–C5: diaphragm paralysis	MRI C-spine
Submandibular gland disease	Tender, mass palpable	US, CT
Temporomandibular joint syndrome	Tender TMJ, deviation of jaw upon opening, decreased movement	CT
Thyroiditis	Palpable thyroid, may be tender	TSH, T4, T3
Torticollis	Contracture of SCM muscle	Cervical x-rays
Tumor of the tongue	Palpable mass	MRI
Vertebral artery dissection	Ophthalmologic and neurologic deficits	US, MRI angiogram

There is no support in the history or physical for an underlying metabolic disease as etiology, for example, osteoarthritis, rheumatoid arthritis, rheumatoid-related diseases (e.g., dermatomyositis, temporal arteritis, Lyme disease, and fibromyalgia), goiter or thyroiditis, soft tissue infections (e.g., cellulitis, cervical disk, lymphangitis), or diet-related calcium or potassium deficits.

Neurologic conditions that cause neck pain need to be considered, such as cervical radiculitis, atypical facial pain, trigeminal and glossopharyngeal neuralgia, complex regional pain syndrome (CRPS), or neurogenic inflammation, but these are less common causes and are unlikely given the history of a recent whiplash injury just before the onset of her pain.

Neck pain from somatic dysfunction that is mechanical in origin is typically amenable to OMT and not only involves the cervical region but also is accompanied by dysfunction in the upper back, ribs, head, and upper extremities.[2] It is characterized by the presence of muscle spasm, decreased ROM, as well as a reduction in the quality of motion; there is pain with movement that improves with rest; and there is no organic pathology that could radiate pain to the region or cause viscerosomatic reflexes.[2]

The incidence of motor vehicle collisions and WAD has increased in Western nations over the past 30 years.[3] Neck pain is the most frequently reported complaint in connection with whiplash (acceleration/deceleration); however, as is the case with low back pain, neck pain, in general, runs an episodic course, and the most significant risk factor predictive of future episodes of neck pain is a previous history of neck pain.[3] The Quebec Task Force on WAD defined whiplash as "an acceleration–deceleration mechanism of energy transferred to the neck that results in soft tissue injury that may lead to a variety of clinical manifestations including neck pain and its associated symptoms."[4] That task force also coined the term "WAD" to describe the clinical entities related to the injury and to distinguish them from the injury mechanism. Though people mostly associate whiplash injury with neck symptoms, osteopathic physicians have long advocated for the perspective of whiplash as a total body, or total person, injury.[5–10] Indeed, along with neck pain, patients also complain of a variety of WAD, including headache, cognitive disturbances, vertigo, visual disturbances, jaw pain, low back pain, and/or interscapular pain.[11,12]

Cervical spine "whiplash" or acceleration/deceleration injury is a mechanism of injury, not a type or extent of injury. There are conflicting theories of the mechanism of the cervical spine component of the injury:

- One is that the body propels forward with the head relatively stationary, followed by hyperextension, which then is followed by hyperflexion of the neck while the head recoils forward (after hitting the headrest), the damage being rapid tissue stretch secondary to traction, hyperextension, and hyperflexion.
- Another theory proposes that compression and concomitant torque at the level of C1 and C7, with a flexion torque at C1 and an extension torque at C7, cause ligamentous and myofascial sprain.[13]

Probably both occur, with hyperextension causing the greatest insult. With hyperextension, if there is no head rest support for the head, the motion far exceeds the physiologic barrier and anterior neck soft tissues can be stretched, strained, and ruptured. However, cervical response is not so simple; it is modified by impact force, awareness, and direction[14]:

- The greater the weight and speed (force) of the impacting vehicle, the more force is transmitted to the person in the car being hit.
- If the person is aware of the impact, muscles will contract in preparation for the collision, stabilizing the spine and diminishing the strain and stretch on the myofascial tissues; an unaware person's muscles and connective tissue would stretch before contracting, likely causing more damage.
- Direction of impact affects the muscles that will be activated in response to the force, and those that will likely be injured by stretch and strain forces.[14]

The patient described above has WAD and somatic dysfunction in several body regions. The dizziness and nausea are likely secondary to the cervical somatic dysfunction as it affects equilibrium and neural afferents involved in the sensation of nausea (CN X). Muscle spasms and tender points are also related to the WAD and associated somatic dysfunctions. The contusion and abrasion are most likely caused by the seat belt restraint. The underlying short leg and scoliosis are chronic problems and, although not directly related to her complaint of neck pain, likely have a significant role in the decreased resilience of the cervical spine to the whiplash motion effect.

OSTEOPATHIC PATIENT MANAGEMENT

Biomechanical Model

The entire postural mechanism needs to be considered even though the patient's primary complaints are in the neck and upper body regions.[5–9] The motion present in the cervical spine is determined by the unique cervical spine articular anatomy (see Chapter 33 Cervical Region) and dynamic interaction of the various muscles attached to the cervical spine that are coordinated in function during head, neck, thoracic, rib, and upper extremity movements.[14] The thoracic spine anchors the origins of muscles that stabilize and extend the cervical spine, such as the splenius cervicis and semispinalis capitis. These are not the muscles often injured in WAD; rather, the muscles most commonly injured, hypertonic, or tender upon palpation include the sternocleidomastoid, splenius capitis, and trapezius.[14]

Assessing the mechanics of any injury is helpful in making a diagnosis and developing a management plan. Mechanical aspects of a whiplash-associated injury affect the degree of injury, treatment options, and prognosis. For example:

- Bracing the hands against the steering wheel reduces anterior translation of the body, thereby reducing cervical injury but increasing the probability of soft tissue injury to the shoulders, ribs, and thoracic region.
- The presence of a headrest on top of the driver's seat reduces the chance of hyperextension and reduces the chance of cervical injury.[15]

The body is a unit mechanism and all parts are deranged in a whiplash injury.[7–9] The prevertebral fascia of the anterior neck is continuous with the mediastinum, which is continuous with the crura of the diaphragm surrounding the psoas major muscle. Thus, hyperextension can lead to strains in fascial patterns and dysfunctions in the thorax, abdomen, pelvis, and even the lower extremities.[9] Comorbidities, in this case, scoliosis and short leg, will decrease the patient's adaptability to the sprained and strained upper body myofascial and ligamentous structures; osteoarthritis, rheumatoid arthritis, and similar soft tissue or joint inflammatory diseases can alter the tissue responses to the acceleration/deceleration injury. In many cases, sacral dysfunctions may prevent the patient from recovering in spite of OMT provided to the cervical and thoracic regions.[5]

Pelvic somatic dysfunction occurs most commonly with the driver planting the foot on the brake in anticipation of, or in attempt to avoid, the accident. The paravertebral muscles of the spine and the latissimus dorsi attach to the iliac crests. Movements of the spine and shoulder girdle operate against the resistance of the stabilized ilium. Patients may exhibit pain and decreased ROM secondary to sacral and ilial dysfunction. Look for iliopsoas strains, strain or sprain of the hip, knee, foot, and ankle.

Hip and pelvic fractures are quite common if the patient's foot was planted at the time of impact. Sacral dysfunction disturbs the body's balance and homeostatic mechanism—thus hindering the healing process.[5] During cervical hyperextension and hyperflexion, the continuity of various muscular, ligamentous, and dural attachments causes the sacrum to be forcibly lifted and dislodged from its floating position between the ilia.[5] Craniosacral restriction may be accompanied by gross lumbosacral and sacroiliac dysfunctions. Becker recommends diagnosing and restoring the primary respiratory (i.e., craniosacral) mechanism before addressing the interaction between the pelvis and the sacrum.[5]

Whiplash injury occurs simultaneously in the cervical and thoracic regions.[6] The continuity of the cervical, thoracic, and lumbar spine that is provided by the ligamentous attachments and paravertebral musculature, along with somatosomatic reflexes, transmits the acute cervical strain to the thoracic and lumbar regions. A significant thoracic extended dysfunction is produced in taller patients, often in the region of the top of the seat. Also, rotation and lateral forces are introduced into the thoracic spine. Last, the intimate relationship of the thoracic and cervical spine with the shoulder girdle makes it especially susceptible to injury.

Usually, the occiput and the sacrum have the same dysfunctions. Asymmetric traction by muscles that attach to the cranium can result in torsions and side bending or rotary dysfunctions; the temporal bones are especially vulnerable to these forces.[7] Strain patterns are usually present if the patient has struck any object.[7] The patient described above has decreased palpable cranial and sacral motion likely because of sphenobasilar compression as well as lumbosacral compression.

An osteopathic approach to this patient would entail helping her to improve her posture, short leg, and scoliosis, as well as to evaluate and improve joint motion with OMT and exercises.

For patients with WAD, even in the 1960s and 1970s, osteopathic physicians advocated for adjunctive therapies in addition to OMT for somatic dysfunctions of the thoracic, lumbar, and sacral areas and any obvious dysfunctions of the cranial and cervical spine[6–8]:

- Acupuncture
- Adequate nutritional support
- Appropriate exercise
- Cervical traction
- Gentler forms of manipulation such as myofascial release and muscle energy (i.e., isometric resistance) techniques
- Heat and cold applications
- Help the patient to effectively address emotional difficulties such as anxiety and depression often associated with WAD
- Muscle relaxants
- Preventative measures including public education regarding whiplash injury and the use of seat belts and appropriately adjusted head restraints while driving
- Treatment of myofascial trigger points with ice massage or ethyl chloride spray and stretch
- Ultrasound
- Various types of neck collars in the acute phase
- Vitamin therapy
- Physical therapy to regain strength and ROM in the cervical muscles

Current evidence-based recommendations emphasize OMT to relieve somatic dysfunction and individualized exercises for rehabilitation[2,16]; cervical collars are still used in the first few days up to a couple of weeks, but evidence has shown that patients who use a soft or firm cervical collar have no measurable benefit in improvement when compared to patients who receive general medical care only.[17]

Respiratory/Circulatory Model

In the respiratory/circulatory model, evaluating and treating patients with neck pain considers the possible respiratory and circulatory relationships involved in the cause as well as in the treatment.

As is common with patients suffering from neck pain, the above-described patient exhibits not only cervical but also thoracic, lumbar, and sacral spinal somatic dysfunctions; costal and diaphragmatic dysfunctions are also present. Respiratory movements are compromised not only at the level of the diaphragm but also in the costal cage and spine. Proper respiratory motion and optimal function rely on normal spinal and costal cage mechanics. The diaphragm attaches to ribs 6 to 10 and to the upper three lumbar vertebrae. Dysfunctions in these joints render the diaphragm less effective. The phrenic nerve, which emanates from cervical spinal nerves C3–C5, controls diaphragm contraction.

Optimal lymph drainage also requires normal costal cage mobility that enables alternating intrathoracic pressure differentials with each breath so that the passive lymphatic channels return lymph from below the diaphragm to the heart via the thoracic duct. Cervical and cranial lymphatics drain into the subclavian veins en route to return to the central circulation via the heart. Cervical somatic dysfunction involving the scalene muscles and anterior cervical fascia can compromise the supraclavicular fascia surrounding the thoracic inlet, thoracic duct, and right lymphatic duct as they empty their contents into the subclavian veins.

The fascial tension can interfere with free flow of the lymphatic drainage, so OMT using, for example, myofascial release will help restore normal motion mechanics to that vital region. Therefore, in addressing the cervical, costal, upper extremity, thoracic, lumbar, and sacral somatic dysfunctions of the patient, consider the goal of restoring normal lymphatic and venous drainage through improved respiratory mechanics. Relieve tense myofascial components of the supraclavicular and thoracic inlet and outlet, the ribs, and the diaphragm. Maximize cervical lymphatic drainage with soft tissue and lymphatic OMT. Relieve somatic dysfunction along the entire spine, including the sacrum and pelvis.

The patient may benefit from a heel lift to relieve strain at the lumbosacral junction due to the unlevel sacral base. Improving sacral motion improves the primary respiratory mechanism function through the core link to the occiput via the spinal dura.

The vertebral artery traverses the cervical spine within the foramen of C6—C1, then makes three 90 degree turns at the C1–occipital joint before entering the foramen magnum to provide blood to the base of the brain and cerebellum via the basilar arteries. Due to the vulnerability of this artery to dissection and occlusion resulting in stroke (cerebral vascular accident and subsequent central nervous system deficits), cervical spine high-velocity low-amplitude (HVLA) procedures, especially those that require extension and rotation at the upper cervical spine to correct somatic dysfunctions, need to be performed with great caution and skill. It is impossible to predict whether a manual procedure will cause vertebral artery compromise; however, if, prior to manipulation of

BOX 97.1 Comorbidities Found in Association with Neck Pain

Comorbid conditions that are found associated most commonly in patients with neck pain include

- Autonomic failure[21]
- Cardiovascular disease[22,23]
- Concentration problems[24]
- Digestive system disease[23,25]
- Dizziness[24]
- Headaches[25,26]
- Low back pain[23,25,26]
- Nausea[24]
- OA osteoarthritis[27]
- Orthostatic hypotension[21]
- Shoulder pain[23,26,28–35]
- TMJ syndrome[36]
- Trapezius muscle ischemia[37]

the upper cervical spine, the patient complains of vertigo or has nystagmus or syncope upon rotation of the head, these could be signs of vertebral artery compromise. If these symptoms or signs are present, performing the HVLA procedure is not recommended. Rather, place the patient's head back on the treatment table and reassess for vertebral artery compromise (auscultate for bruit, and obtain imaging with ultrasound and/or magnetic resonance or computerized axial angiograms to rule out dissection or occlusion) (see Chapter 49 High-Velocity Low-Amplitude [HVLA] Thrust for further information).

Somatic dysfunction in the upper thoracic spine and cervical spine is thought to affect blood flow to the cranium as the sympathetic cervical chain ganglia are situated just anterior to the cervical vertebra bodies. Louisa Burns, DO, demonstrated the effects on cranial blood flow and ears, nose, and throat diseases from experimentally induced thoracic and cervical somatic dysfunction in animal models.[18] Neck pain and its associated somatic dysfunction can have systemic effects. Johnston and Kelso later documented a somatic dysfunction pattern of C6, T2, and T6 in patients with hypertension.[19] In a large retrospective chart review from osteopathic physicians across America in the 1950s, the most common somatic dysfunction related to cardiac symptomatology was OA dysfunction.[20] More recently, many other comorbidities have been found in association with neck pain (Box 97.1).

Neurologic Model

The patient has dizziness from her WAD and somatic dysfunctions. Understanding the upper cervical spine anatomy provides clues to the relationship between the somatic dysfunction found on physical examination and her symptoms. Dizziness is a symptom that occurs when there is disequilibrium. Equilibrium depends on normal vestibular function. The eye and neck movement are coordinated via the tectospinal tract to maintain balance and equilibrium. The temporal bones house the vestibular apparatus that consists of three semicircular canals in three different planes with endolymphatic fluid and cilia that enable us to maintain a sense of where we are in relation to our environment. The posterior suboccipital muscles level the head to the horizon and keep the temporal bones level so we feel balanced. Thus, cervical somatic dysfunction interferes with head position, temporal bone levels, and eye–neck coordination, disturbing equilibrium function. Correcting the cervical somatic dysfunction with OMT should relieve the sense of dizziness if indeed this is the cause of the troublesome symptom. Dizziness could also be a symptom of vertebral artery dissection or occlusion, so the astute osteopathic physician should be aware of this possibility, especially if there are other central neurologic signs of deficit or dysfunction.

The patient also has nausea. Peripherally induced nausea sensation is transmitted to the brain most commonly via the vagus nerve afferents. The inferior nodosal (vagal) ganglia is situated immediately outside the cranial cavity as the vagus nerve exits the jugular foramen between the occiput and temporal bones, before the nerve enters the carotid sheath along with the jugular vein and carotid artery. Osteopathic clinicians believe the vagus nerve is vulnerable to the effects of somatic dysfunction in that vicinity and vice versa; if there is increased vagus nerve activity, that is, from thoracic or abdominal visceral inflammation, the surrounding somatic structures are affected and show signs of somatic dysfunction in the upper cervical spinal joints and surrounding soft tissues. Treatment of the cervical somatic dysfunction with OMT is also intended to restore normal vagal activity and function, including relieving sensation of nausea that is caused by the cervical somatic dysfunction.

The relationship between cervical somatic dysfunction and symptoms of dizziness and nausea and their abolishment by OMT are anecdotal (expert clinical experience) and await animal or human laboratory studies and prospective randomized clinical trials to prove cause and effect. The current trend in osteopathic manual medicine practice, as exemplified by recent articles by osteopathic clinicians, favors treatment of somatic dysfunction not only in the cervical region, but throughout the body for patients with symptoms of dizziness and nausea.[38,39]

The patient has pain and tender points in the cervical as well as pelvic regions. They are likely due to the WAD. However, WAD is not the only cause of acute neck pain. In the United States, almost 85% of neck pain may be attributed to chronic stresses and strains or acute or repetitive neck injuries.[40] In general, somatic dysfunction involving the OA and AA joints usually causes head pain primarily with neck pain secondarily, and somatic dysfunction of C2–C7 joints causes neck pain primarily with head pain and/or shoulder pain secondarily.[41,42]

Cervical facet pain is typically a unilateral, dull aching pain with occasional referral into the occipital or trapezial region, depending on the facet joint involved. C1 and C2 zygapophyseal joints refer pain to the cranium, whereas C3–C7 refer pain to the trapezium and interscapular regions.[40] The pain referral zones for facet pain overlap both myofascial and disk pain patterns making it difficult to ascertain the exact level of the pain generator. In some patients, neck and head pains are associated with trigeminal nerve activity, from dental–facial problems, activation of the cervical branches of the trigeminal nerve, or influence of the trigeminal nerve on the thalamic pain receptor field in the brain.[43] With WAD, myofascial tender points are commonly found in the trapezius, scalene, semispinalis cervicis, semispinalis capitis, and multifidus muscles[10]; the semispinalis capitis muscle seems to be the most likely to develop a painful trigger point.[44]

The most reliable physical examination tests for patients complaining of neck pain are the patient's response to digital pressure on bone or muscle, as is used with assessing for strain/counterstrain tender points; tests for regional ROM; and Spurling maneuver for cervical radiculopathy (extension, side bending, and rotation at the cervical spinal level of suspected spinal nerve root compression, combined with axial compression to limit the size of the intervertebral foramen, to see if pain radiates to the arm

BOX 97.2 Neck Pain and Motor Vehicle Collisions

In a multisite randomized clinical trial comparing the effectiveness of OMT with intramuscular nonsteroidal anti-inflammatory medication (ketorolac tromethamine) for patients with acute neck pain seen in the emergency department, the OMT group had significantly reduced pain intensity and equivalent efficacy at relieving pain assessed at 1 hour post-treatment.[46] More than half of the patients in each group had neck pain because of a motor vehicle collision.

in a dermatomal distribution related to the spinal nerve being assessed).[45] See Box 97.2.

Autonomic effects can accompany cervical somatic dysfunction. Sympathetic innervation to the head and neck regions is derived from preganglionic fibers arising from the lateral horn of the spinal cord from T1 to T6. These fibers proceed cephalad to the sympathetic chain to enter the cervical ganglia and synapse with the postganglionic fibers. The inferior cervical ganglia lie at the superior border of the first ribs, anterior to C7. The inferior cervical ganglia send branches to the heart. The middle cervical ganglia are at the level of the transverse process of C6. The middle cervical ganglia send fibers to the thyroid gland and also to the heart. The superior cervical ganglia are at the level of the AA joint. The superior cervical ganglion postganglionic fibers accompany the internal carotid and ophthalmic arteries into the orbit and to the glands of the head and face. Postganglionic fibers accompany the vertebral arteries and enter the skull to supply the vestibular portion of the ear, some cranial nerves, and the pharynx. In addition, the cervical vertebra bodies and intervertebral disks are entirely surrounded by a network of interlacing nerve fibers.[47] The anterior longitudinal ligament (ALL) receives bilateral contributions from the medioventral small branches of the sympathetic trunk forming a plexus of nerves throughout all levels. The posterior longitudinal ligament (PLL) likewise receives bilateral contributions from the sinuvertebral nerves that form a nerve plexus throughout all levels. There, nerve plexus of both the ALL and the PLL meet through the rami communicantes.[47] Sympathetic symptoms can occur as a result of stimulation of the peripheral nerves as they pierce the soft tissue, stimulation of the sensory elements of C1 and C2, simultaneous compression of the nerve route in its foraminal passage, or compression of the vertebral artery.

Sympathetic symptoms include the following:

- Aural: tinnitus, deafness
- Ocular: blurred vision, retrobulbar pain, and a pupil that dilates when the head is turned and returns to a neutral midline position
- Vestibular: postural dizziness or vertigo

This patient exhibits signs of central and peripheral sensitization or facilitation. OMT would be helpful in decreasing the irritability of the nervous system. It has been demonstrated that cervical spine manipulation alters cortical somatosensory processing and sensorimotor integration; the primary muscle afferents (probably Ia) are the most likely mediators of these effects.[48] Resetting of the muscle spindle afferents with muscle energy OMT increases ROM in cervical spinal joints.[49] In randomized clinical trials, cervical spine manipulation and mobilization provide at least short-term benefits for patients with acute neck pain and headaches.[17]

For this patient, OMT was directed at removing any impingement upon peripheral or central nervous structures, with cervical traction and indirect OMT procedures in the acute phase of recovery; tender points were treated with counterstrain; medications or other adjunct therapies may be needed to modulate neurologic function depending on the patient's response to OMT. Thoracic manipulation has an analgesic effect in patients with mechanical neck pain.[50] OMT for somatic dysfunction in other body regions, especially the thoracic spine and upper ribs, will help relieve the pain and dysfunction of the cervical spine. Relieving somatic dysfunction with OMT to the rest of the body will decrease the somatic burden, relieve pain, and reduce the allopathic load. This will contribute significantly to the restoration of normal neurologic function.

Metabolic Energy Model

The physiologic and metabolic mechanisms, set into motion due to internal or external factors, that are interpreted by the human body as pain are very complex and have yet to be completely elucidated. What is known is that irritation of the tissues through trauma, repetitive/overuse injury patterns, structural abnormalities, infection, or degenerative and systemic disease can lead to the process of nociception and eventually a facilitated spinal cord segment. The inflammatory cascade can lead to a relentless positive-feedback cycle where inflammation can increase the pain that then potentiates the inflammation further.[51] As inflammation and harmful metabolites begin to accumulate, structural changes in the affected tissue begin to occur and can ultimately lead to ischemia of the tissue.[51] If the metabolic and physiologic alternations are not modified and persist for an extended period of time, long-term structural changes occur in the muscles, tendons, or joints and lead to limited functionality and eventual disability. The goal of soft tissue OMT is in part to relieve muscle spasms and assist the lymphatic system in clearing local toxic metabolites.

Some patients present with acute neck pain related to pharyngitis or peritonsillar abscess. Thus, even though there is evidence of somatic dysfunction on palpatory examination, the osteopathic physician should also assess the status of the internal organs capable of causing pain in the cervical region. OMT for somatic dysfunction related to infection or inflammation is directed at improving venous and lymphatic drainage, as in the respiratory–circulatory model. Using antibiotics as an adjunctive therapy is warranted when a bacterial pathogen is identified or highly likely based on the physical examination and course of the signs and symptoms over time.

There are patients with acute neck pain from thyroiditis who need further management with radiation, medication, and/or surgery. In these patients, OMT was employed in the earlier part of the 20th century when no other treatment was available and may be adjunctive in helping to improve lymphatic drainage even today, but in America, OMT is not the standard treatment for this condition in the 21st century. Similarly, neck pain from metastatic cancer in the lymph glands or cervical structures or primary carcinomas in the cervical region is not treated directly with OMT. Patients may benefit from OMT to other body regions with the goal of reducing somatic dysfunction burden and relaxing the nervous system during and after definitive diagnosis and treatment with biopsy, radiation, chemotherapy, and/or surgery.

For this patient, addressing metabolic energy expenditure goals entails applying OMT to relieve muscle spasm and restore normal and efficient spinal motion to decrease the burden of poor posture and motion mechanics on energy expenditure. In addition, ensure proper nutrition using wholesome foods and eliminate fast and fried foods, help the patient to restore normal sleep cycles, and encourage regular exercise. Remove infectious agents and decrease inflammation if present. Restore normal endocrine function if needed.

Behavioral Model

The patient typifies the most common scenario seen in osteopathic primary care practice. Patients with neck pain range in age from the 1st through the 10th decades.[22,23,28,29] However, most patients with neck pain related to motor vehicle collisions are between the ages of 20 and 40.[15] Although neck pain occurs in children and adults of all ages and genders, neck pain is most commonly reported by middle-age females, especially those who experience WAD.[28] In the general population, peak incidence of neck pain is between ages 30 and 59.[22,26] Age and gender standardized annual incidence is 14.6%; however, only less than 1% develop disabling neck pain, so most patients continue to work.[22] The point prevalence of neck pain is 8% to 24%. The lifetime prevalence is 71%.[22,23,28,30] Fifty-four percent of a general population surveyed have experienced neck pain within a 6-month period.[25,52]

Neck pain is a chronic, episodic condition characterized by persistent, recurrent, or fluctuating pain and disability.[22] Only about one-third of patients with neck pain experience complete resolution.[22] About one-half of patients with an acute episode have persistent neck pain at 12 months.[26] After whiplash injury, neck pain along with headache persists for up to 2 years in 29% to 90% of patients (depending on the study), and neck pain alone can persist for 10 years in 74% of patients.[53] Drivers who have sustained a whiplash injury have a nearly threefold risk of neck or shoulder pain 7 years after the collision.[54] Even 17 years after an MVA, 55% still experience neck pain.[11]

Neck pain is one of the most common complaints of patients seen by primary care practitioners worldwide.[31] Mechanical neck disorder is the most common cause of neck pain.[40] Second only to low back pain, neck pain is one of the most common reasons for which patients seek manual medical treatment. Neck pain is the most frequently reported symptom in connection with whiplash injury.[53] Neck pain can result from 66% to 82% of rear-end collisions and 56% of side impact collisions.[53] Seventy percent of patients with neck pain after rear-end traffic collisions are female drivers.[15] For female drivers involved in collisions, neck pain likelihood increases as head restraint height decreases below the head's center of gravity.[15] Reported neck pain decreases for older female drivers, drivers in less severe crashes, and female drivers in heavier cars.[15]

Neck pain accounts for substantial medical consumption, absenteeism from work, and disability.[55] Medical disability can be temporary, but in about 10% of patients, permanent medical disability occurs. Permanent medical disability occurs in about 10% of patients involved in rear-end motor vehicle collisions.[53] Although 79% may return to work within 1 month, 6% are unable to return to work at 1 year.[53] A higher severity of pain at onset and a history of previous attacks seem to be associated with a worse prognosis; however, localization (radiation to the arms/neurologic signs) and radiographic findings (degenerative changes in the disks and joints) are not associated with a worse prognosis.[56] Work-related risk factors for neck pain are listed in Box 97.3. (Compare with non–work-related risk factors in Box 97.4 and risk factors for radicular neck pain in Box 97.5.)

BOX 97.3 Work-Related Risk Factors for Neck Pain

Work-related risk factors for neck pain include

- Hand–arm vibration[57]
- High and low skill[58]
- High quantitative job demands[58]
- Low job control[58]
- Low job satisfaction[58]
- Low social (coworker) support[58]
- Neck flexion (>20 degrees)[58]
- Sitting at work more than 95% of the time[58]
- Sustained arm postures[57]
- Twisting or bending of the trunk[57]
- Use of arm force[57]
- Workplace design not conducive to efficient cervical motion and function[57]

BOX 97.4 Non–Work-Related Risk Factors for Neck Pain

Non–work-related risk factors for neck pain include

- Cycling[26]
- Poor ergonomics with driving[59]
- Female[26,59]
- History of motor vehicle collision[60]
- Older age[26]
- Previous low back pain[26]
- Previous neck injury[26,61]
- Psychological distress[26,35]
- Static postures (children)[62]
- Unemployed[26]
- Very slow or very rapid arm motion speed[63]

BOX 97.5 Characteristics of Patients with Radicular Neck Pain

Characteristics of patients with radicular neck pain include

- Dental–facial problems[43]
- Duration of work with a hand above shoulder level[64]
- Female[64]
- Mental stress[64]
- Middle age[64]
- Other musculoskeletal problems[64]
- Overweight[64]
- Smoking[64,65]

Osteopathic Management of the Case

There is evidence of efficacy for OMT in combination with strengthening exercises for treatment of nonspecific mechanical neck pain for short-term pain relief and increased ROM compared

BOX 97.6 Contraindications and Cautions Regarding Use of OMT for Patients with Acute Neck Pain

Care must be taken in the patient with an unstable cervical spine. Contraindications to HVLA OMT to the cervical spine include the following:

- A history of acute trauma before an assessment for any damage to the anatomy of the region and diagnosis of the origin of the pain
- Acute cervical herniated nucleus pulposus
- Acute cervical vertebra fracture or dislocation
- Carotid or vertebral artery dissection
- Ligamentous laxity
- Metabolic or neoplastic bone disease
- Patient refusal (same as with any medical procedure)
- Primary muscle or joint disease in the cervical spine

to manipulation and/or mobilization alone or in combination.[66] Contraindications and cautions regarding use of OMT for patients with acute neck pain are listed in Box 97.6.

Osteopathic physicians are likely to see many patients with neck pain caused by somatic dysfunction and are amenable to OMT. Neck pain from strain or sprain of the paraspinal soft tissues accounts for the greatest number of primary care visits to an outpatient clinic or ER of all musculoskeletal non–skin laceration soft tissue injuries.[67] Neck somatic dysfunction was the most commonly reported somatic dysfunction in patients seen by 10 osteopathic practitioners board certified in neuromusculoskeletal medicine and osteopathic manipulative medicine over a 6-month period.[68] Somatic dysfunction in the upper back, lower back, and shoulder can also predispose a person to develop cervical somatic dysfunction and pain. Thoracic somatic dysfunction is a significant predictor of neck–shoulder pain and hand weakness symptoms.[50,69–71] This further supports the osteopathic approach to the patient with acute neck pain, which includes assessment and treatment of not only the cervical spine but also the entire musculoskeletal system as an integrated dynamic functional unit.

The human body functions as a unit and typically will respond to trauma, injury, or disease as a unit. This includes the psychological, behavioral, and social response that a person may have to pain and somatic dysfunction. Uncontrolled pain can lead to decreased functional capacity, which then increases the psychological burden of the patient and can lead to increased anxiety, stress, and depression. The increased psychological burden can impair the body's ability to heal and can further exacerbate the pain experienced by the patient. Therefore, it becomes vital for the osteopathic physician to evaluate the patient for comorbidities and mitigating factors that may impede a healthy recovery for the patient. Certainly, anxiety plays a role in this patient's neck pain, but she has no history of chronic anxiety or other psychiatric conditions; her nightmares are related to her anxiety and probably disrupting her sleep patterns, which, along with the muscle spasms, increases her fatigue. She is not an active sports-type person and has a sedentary lifestyle, so her muscles likely lack good tone. Her posture is normally not efficient and does not lend itself to compensation or adaptation to injuries that as she sustained recently.

Better psychological health and greater social support predicted a better outcome in primary care and general population samples with initial neck pain, whereas passive coping predicted a worse outcome.[72] Economically, manual therapy (i.e., spinal mobilization) has been more effective and less costly for treating mechanical neck pain than physiotherapy modalities or care by a general practitioner who doesn't use manipulation.[73]

For patients with neck pain, the osteopathic approach of treating the whole patient and not just the symptoms will help maximize the patient's restorative health potential. Applying the behavioral perspective to this patient, treat her anxiety, work with her to improve her sleep habits and dietary choices and habits, encourage nonsedentary lifestyle, improve posture and exercise habits, and encourage her to stop repetitive work behaviors that aggravate her condition. In patients who are athletes, help them to modify sports or other activities. If there is alcohol, tobacco, and/or drug abuse as part of the clinical picture, encourage and help the patient to eliminate these addictions and abuses as part of the management plan.

Specialist Referral

The patient would be referred to the spine or pain management specialist for further evaluation and management if her neck pain did not improve or progressively worsened in spite of appropriate conservative treatments. If there is progressive or persistent loss of motor or sensory function, or altered sensorium or brain function, certainly, neurologic and surgical referrals are indicated. However, it is less clear if there is only limb paresthesia or radicular pain, which may be indicative of cervical nerve root compression. Nevertheless, it is helpful to utilize screening protocols, such as the Canadian C-spine rules, for patients with a low risk of cervical spine fracture and CT imaging for high-risk patients with blunt trauma to the neck.[74]

In conjunction with the history and physical examination, electromyography (EMG) is relatively sensitive and specific for diagnosing cervical nerve root compression. Often, a neurologist or physiatrist is called upon to utilize the EMG to distinguish neck pain that is radicular versus nonradicular in nature. This distinction, along with an assessment for somatic dysfunction and relevant imaging studies, aids in more clearly identifying the cause of a patient's neck pain and instituting the appropriate treatment.

In general, it appears that the physical examination is more predictive of "ruling out" than "ruling in" a structural lesion, especially when assessing for neurologic compression or significant pathology, such as cervical spine instability.[74] Although MRI is helpful in identifying cervical degenerative changes, these changes are common in asymptomatic subjects and research has failed to demonstrate a correlation between degenerative changes and neck pain symptoms. Similarly, there is no strong evidence supporting the validity of cervical diskography or facet joint injections in diagnosing disk or facet pain, respectively, as the primary cause of neck pain.[74] Evidence supports the use of provocative maneuvers, such as Spurling test or contralateral rotation of the head with arm extension, when evaluating for cervical radiculopathy.[75,76] Other physical examination components that should be incorporated include motor strength and sensory testing and cervical spine ROM evaluation. There is some evidence suggesting that patients with chronic neck pain secondary to WAD have decreased cervical spine ROM when compared to control subjects.[77]

After completing the clinical and diagnostic evaluation and excluding significant pathology, including cervical spine instability or an infectious, neoplastic, or inflammatory process, the physician spine or pain management specialist utilizes a variety of modalities to treat neck pain, including medication, physical therapy, interventional procedures, manual medicine, and referral for surgical consultation. If a patient's neck pain is nonradicular and mechanical in nature, a multitherapeutic approach that incorporates medication, exercise therapy, and manual medicine is a reasonable approach. There is some evidence supporting exercise therapy, either alone or in combination with spinal manipulation, as being positively associated with short-term (6 to 13 weeks) reduction in chronic or recurrent neck pain when compared to spinal manipulation alone or usual care.[17]

Using one's skills as an osteopathic physician is sensible since the evidence supports the use of manual medicine in the treatment of neck pain. Cervical spine manipulation is more effective in reducing neck pain than muscle relaxants or usual care and at least provides short-term benefits for patients with acute neck pain. Furthermore, it appears that the benefits of manual medicine are enhanced when combined with exercise therapy and ergonomic adjustments.[2] There is no evidence supporting the use of epidural or intra-articular corticosteroid injections in the treatment of nonradicular neck pain.[78] In contrast, patients with neck pain secondary to nerve root compression do have short-term improvement of cervical radicular symptoms with epidural or selective nerve root corticosteroid injections.[78] This, however, has not been shown to decrease the overall rate of surgery in patients with significant cervical radiculopathy.[78] The long-term outcomes of treating cervical radiculopathy surgically when compared to nonoperative treatment have not been studied.

Regardless, both anterior cervical diskectomy with fusion and cervical disk arthroplasty seem to offer rapid and substantial relief of pain and impairment in patients with true cervical radiculopathy.[78] As with the clinical evaluation, it is imperative to make the distinction between radicular and nonradicular neck pain when implementing treatment. In doing so, the physician specialist improves the likelihood of successfully treating a patient's neck pain, whether that entails treating radicular pain with injections or mechanical pain with a multimodal approach, including medication, exercise and physical therapy, and manual medicine.

SUMMARY

In summary, the osteopathic approach to the patient with acute neck pain begins with a thorough history and physical examination, including an osteopathic structural examination of the musculoskeletal system. The differential diagnosis considers potential etiologies from local pathology, somatic dysfunction in the cervical as well as other body regions, systemic pathophysiology with cervical manifestations, and referred pain from organs in the vicinity of the cervical region, that is, the lungs and heart. Associated comorbidities are also assessed and treated as appropriate. One of the most common causes of neck pain is a history of whiplash-type injury.

However, though this type of injury affects the cervical spine, its effects are not limited to the cervical region. Understanding the total body response to a traumatic event such as a motor vehicle collision helps to elucidate the application of osteopathic principles in practice. Osteopathic treatment utilizes a health-oriented, patient-centered approach, focusing on improving structure–function interrelationships. This entails applying OMT to alleviate somatic dysfunction and maximize biomechanical, neurologic, metabolic, respiratory/circulatory, and behavioral functions. Patient education, individualized exercise prescription, and close follow-up are important components of the management plan. Referral to a spine or pain specialist is indicated if the patient's pain and/or dysfunction does not improve or progressively worsens with conservative measures.

ACKNOWLEDGMENTS

The authors and editors of this chapter would like to acknowledge the scholarly contributions of student editor Emily Daly.

REFERENCES

1. Greenbaum J, Walters N, Levy PD. An evidenced-based approach to radiographic assessment of cervical spine injuries in the emergency department. *J Emerg Med.* 2009;36(1):64–71.
2. Seffinger MA, Hruby RJ. Mechanical neck and upper back pain. *Evidence-based Manual Medicine: A Problem Oriented Approach.* Saunders/Elsevier; 2007.
3. Holm LW, Carroll LJ, Cassidy JD. The burden and determinants of neck pain in whiplash-associated disorders after traffic collisions. Results of the bone and joint decade 2000–2010 task force on neck pain and its associated disorders. *Spine (Phila Pa 1976).* 2008;33(4S):S39–S51.
4. Spitzer WO, Skovron ML, Salmi LR, et al. Scientific monograph of the Quebec Task Force on whiplash-associated disorders: redefining "whiplash" and its management. *Spine (Phila Pa 1976).* 1995;20(8 Suppl):1S–73S.
5. Becker RE. Whiplash injuries. *Academy of Applied Osteopathy Yearbook.* American Academy of Osteopathy; 1958:65–69;1961: 90–98.
6. Heilig D. "Whiplash" mechanics of injury; management of cervical and dorsal involvement. *J Am Osteopath Assoc.* 1963;63:113–120.
7. Magoun HI Sr. Whiplash injury: a greater lesion complex. *J Am Osteopath Assoc.* 1964;63:524–535.
8. Harakal JH. An osteopathically-integrated approach to the whiplash complex. *J Am Osteopath Assoc.* 1975;74(10):941–956.
9. Cisler TA. Whiplash as a total-body injury. *J Am Osteopath Assoc.* 1994; 94(2):145–148.
10. Nadler S, Cooke P. Myofascial pain in whiplash injuries: diagnosis and treatment. *Spine St Art Rev.* 1998;12(2):357–376.
11. Bunkertorp L, Nordholm L, Carlsson J. A descriptive analysis of disorders in patients 17 years following motor vehicle accidents. *Eur Spine J.* 2002; 11(3):227–234.
12. Ferrari R, Russell AS, Carroll LJ, Cassidy JD. A re-examination of the whiplash associated disorders (WAD) as a systemic illness. *Ann Rheum Dis.* 2005;64(9):1337–1342.
13. Panjabi MM, Pearson AM, Ito S, Ivancic PC, Wang J-L. Cervical spine curvature during simulated whiplash. *Clin Biomech (Bristol, Avon).* 2004;19(1):1–9.
14. Kumar S, Ferrari R, Narayan Y. Kinematic and electromyographic response to whiplash loading in low-velocity whiplash impacts—a review. *Clin Biomech (Bristol, Avon).* 2005;20(4):343–356.
15. Chapline JF, Ferguson SA, Lillis RP, Lund AK, Williams AF. Neck pain and head restraint position relative to the driver's head in rear-end collisions. *Accid Anal Prev.* 2000;32(2):287–297.
16. Gross A, Langevin P, Burnie SJ, et al. Manipulation and mobilisation for neck pain contrasted against an inactive control or another active treatment. *Cochrane Database Syst Rev.* 2015;2015(9):CD004249.
17. Hurwitz EL, Carragee EJ, van der Velde G. Treatment of neck pain: noninvasive interventions. Results of the Bone and Joint Decade 2000–2010 Task Force on Neck Pain and its Associated Disorders. *Spine.* 2008;33(4S): S123–S152.
18. Burns L. *Pathogenesis of Visceral Disease Following Vertebral Lesions.* The American Osteopathic Association; 1948.
19. Kelso AF, Johnston WL. The status of a C6-T2-T6 (CT) pattern of segmental somatic dysfunction in research subjects after 3–7 years. *J Am Osteopath Assoc.* 1989;89(10):1356.
20. Burns L, Treat CL. Incidence of certain etiologic factors in cardiac disorders. *J Am Osteopath Assoc.* 1953;52(7):369–372.
21. Bleasdale-Barr KM, Mathias CJ. Neck and other muscle pains in autonomic failure: their association with orthostatic hypotension. *J R Soc Med.* 1998;91(7):355–359.
22. Côté P, Cassidy DJ, Carroll LJ, Kristman V. The annual incidence and course of neck pain in the general population: a population-based cohort study. *Pain.* 2004;112(3):267–273.
23. Hartvigsen J, Christensen K, Frederiksen H. Back and neck pain exhibit many common features in old age: a population-based study of 4,486 Danish twins 70–102 years of age. *Spine.* 2004;29(5):576–580.

24. Hoving JL, Koes BW, de Vet HCW, et al. Manual therapy, physical therapy, or continued care by a general practitioner for patients with neck pain. A randomized, controlled trial. *Ann Intern Med.* 2002;136(10):713–722.
25. Côté P, Cassidy JD, Carroll L. Is a lifetime history of neck injury in a traffic collision associated with prevalent neck pain, headache and depressive symptomatology? *Accid Anal Prev.* 2000;32(2):151–159.
26. Hill J, Lewis M, Papageorgiou AC, Dziedzic K, Croft P. Predicting persistent neck pain: a 1-year follow-up of a population cohort. *Spine.* 2004; 29(15):1648–1654.
27. Zapletal J, Hekster RE, Straver JS, Wilmink JT, Hermans J. Relationship between atlanto-odontoid osteoarthritis and idiopathic suboccipital neck pain. *Neuroradiology.* 1996;38(1):62–65.
28. Walker-Bone K, Reading I, Coggon D, Cooper C, Palmer KT. The anatomical pattern and determinants of pain in the neck and upper limbs: an epidemiologic study. *Pain.* 2004;109(1–2):45–51.
29. Ståhl M, Mikkelsson M, Kautiainen H, et al. Neck pain in adolescence: a 4-year follow-up of pain-free preadolescents. *Pain.* 2004;110(1–2): 427–431.
30. Vogt MT, Simonsick EM, Harris TB, et al. Neck and shoulder pain in 70- to 79-year-old men and women: findings from the Health, Aging and Body Composition Study. *Spine J.* 2003;3(6):435–441.
31. Bot SDM, van der Waal JM, Terwee CB, et al. Incidence and prevalence of complaints of the neck and upper extremity in general practice. *Ann Rheum Dis.* 2005;64(1):118–123.
32. Andersen JH, Kaergaard A, Mikkelsen S, et al. Risk factors in the onset of neck/shoulder pain in a prospective study of workers in industrial and service companies. *Occup Environ Med.* 2003;60(9):649–654.
33. Borg K, Hensing G, Alexanderson K. Risk factors for disability pension over 11 years in a cohort of young persons initially sick-listed with low back, neck, or shoulder diagnoses. *Scand J Public Health.* 2004;32(4): 272–278.
34. Grooten WJ, Wiktorin C, Norrman L, et al. Seeking care for neck/ shoulder pain: a prospective study of work-related risk factors in a healthy population. *J Occup Environ Med.* 2004;46(2):138–146.
35. Siivola SM, Levoska S, Latvala K, Hoskio E, Vanharanta H, Kainänen-Kiukaanniemi S. Predictive factors for neck and shoulder pain: a longitudinal study in young adults. *Spine.* 2004;29(15):1662–1669.
36. Ciancaglini R, Testa M, Radaelli G. Association of neck pain with symptoms of temporomandibular dysfunction in the general adult population. *Scand J Rehabil Med.* 1999;31(1):17–22.
37. Larsson R, Oberg PA, Larsson SE. Changes of trapezius muscle blood flow and electromyography in chronic neck pain due to trapezius myalgia. *Pain.* 1999;79(1):45–50.
38. Fraix M. Osteopathic manual medicine for vertigo: review of the literature, case report and future research. *Am Acad Osteopath J.* 2009;19(2):25–29.
39. Batchelor K, Gamber R. Migraine and OMT. *Am Acad Osteopath J.* 2008; 18(1):30–33.
40. Narayan P, Haid RW. Treatment of degenerative cervical disc disease. *Neurol Clin.* 2001;19(1):217–229.
41. Lord SM, Barnsley L, Wallis BJ, Bogduk N. Chronic cervical zygapophysial joint pain after whiplash: a placebo-controlled prevalence study. *Spine.* 1996;21(15):1737–1745.
42. Speldewinde GC, Bashford GM, Davidson IR. Diagnostic cervical zygapophyseal joint blocks for chronic cervical pain. *Med J Aust.* 2001; 174(4):174–176.
43. Friedman MH, Nelson AJ Jr. Head and neck pain review: traditional and new perspectives. *J Orthop Sports Phys Ther.* 1996;24(4):268–278.
44. Ettlin T, Schuster C, Stoffel R, Bruderlin A, Kischka U. A distinct pattern of myofascial findings in patients after whiplash injury. *Arch Phys Med Rehabil.* 2008;89(7):1290–1293.
45. Seffinger MA, Najm WI, Mishra SI, et al. Reliability of spinal palpation for diagnosis of back and neck pain: a systematic review of the literature. *Spine.* 2004;29(19):E413–425.
46. McReynolds TM, Sheridan BJ. Intramuscular ketorolac versus osteopathic manipulative treatment in the management of acute neck pain in the emergency department: a randomized clinical trial. *J Am Osteopath Assoc.* 2005; 105(2):57–68.
47. Groen G, Baljet B, Drukker J. Nerve and nerve plexuses of the human vertebral column. *Am J Anat.* 1990;188(3):282–296.
48. Haavik-Taylor H, Murphy B. Cervical spine manipulation alters sensorimotor integration: a somatosensory evoked potential study. *Clin Neurophysiol.* 2007;118(2):391–402.
49. Burns DK, Wells MR. Gross range of motion in the cervical spine: the effects of osteopathic muscle energy technique in asymptomatic subjects. *J Am Osteopath Assoc.* 2006;106(3):137–142.
50. Cleland JA, Childs JD, McRae M, Palmer JA, Stowell T. Immediate effects of thoracic manipulation in patients with neck pain: a randomized clinical trial. *Man Ther.* 2005;10(2):127–135.
51. Howell JN, Willard F. Nociception: new understandings and their possible relation to somatic dysfunction and its treatment. *Ohio Res Clin Rev.* 2005;15.
52. Côté P, Cassidy JD, Carroll L. The factors associated with neck pain and its related disability in the Saskatchewan population. *Spine.* 2000;25(9): 1109–1117.
53. Bilkey WJ Jr. Manual medicine approach to the cervical spine and whiplash injury. *Phys Med Rehabil Clin N Am.* 1996;7(4):749–759.
54. Berglund A, Alfredsson L, Cassidy JD, Jensen I, Nygren A. The association between exposure to a rear-end collision and future neck or shoulder pain: a cohort study. *J Clin Epidemiol.* 2000;53(11):1089–1094.
55. Borghouts JA, Koes BW, Vondeling H, Bouter LM. Cost-of-illness of neck pain in The Netherlands in 1996. *Pain.* 1999;80(3):629–636.
56. Borghouts JA, Koes BW, Bouter LM. The clinical course and prognostic factors of non-specific neck pain: a systematic review. *Pain.* 1998;77(1):1–13.
57. Ariëns GA, van Mechelen W, Bongers PM, Bouter LM, van der Wal G. Physical risk factors for neck pain. *Scand J Work Environ Health.* 2000; 26(1):7–19.
58. Ariëns GA, Bongers PM, Douwes M, et al. Are neck flexion, neck rotation, and sitting at work risk factors for neck pain? Results of a prospective cohort study. *Occup Environ Med.* 2001;58(3):200–207.
59. Krause N, Ragland DR, Greiner BA, Fisher JM, Holman BL, Selvin S. Physical workload and ergonomic factors associated with prevalence of back and neck pain in urban transit operators. *Spine.* 1997;22(18):2117–2126.
60. Bunketorp L, Stener-Victorin E, Carlsson J. Neck pain and disability following motor vehicle accidents—a cohort study. *Eur Spine J.* 2005; 14(1):84–89.
61. Guez M, Hildingsson C, Stegmayr B, Toolanen G. Chronic neck pain of traumatic and non-traumatic origin: a population-based study. *Acta Orthop Scand.* 2003;74(5):576–579.
62. Murphy S, Buckle P, Stubbs D. Classroom posture and self-reported back and neck pain in schoolchildren. *Appl Ergon.* 2004;35(2):113–120.
63. Lauren H, Luoto S, Alaranta H, Taimela S, Hurri H, Heliövaara M. Arm motion speed and risk of neck pain. A preliminary communication. *Spine.* 1997;22(18):2094–2099.
64. Viikari-Juntura E, Martikainen R, Luukkonen R, Mutanen P, Takala EP, Riihimäki H. Longitudinal study on work related and individual risk factors affecting radiating neck pain. *Occup Environ Med.* 2001;58(5):345–352.
65. Hogg-Johnson S, van der Velde G, Carroll LJ, et al. The burden and determinants of neck pain in the general population: results of the Bone and Joint Decade 2000–2010 Task Force on Neck Pain and its Associated Disorders. *Spine.* 2008;33(4S):S39–S51.
66. Cervical and thoracic spine disorders. In: *Occupational Medicine Practice Guidelines: Evaluation and Management of Common Health Problems and Functional Recovery in Workers.* Reed Group, Ltd.; 2016:1–711.
67. United States National Health Survey, 1999–2000, reported Sept. 2004; Ambulatory Care Visits to Practitioner Offices, Hospital Outpatient Departments, and Emergency Departments.
68. Sleszynski SL, Glonek T. Outpatient osteopathic SOAP note form: preliminary results in osteopathic outcomes-based research. *J Am Osteopath Assoc.* 2005;105(4):181–205.
69. Norlander S, Gustavsson BA, Lindell J, Nordgren B. Reduced mobility in the cervico-thoracic motion segment—a risk factor for musculoskeletal neck-shoulder pain: a two-year prospective follow-up study. *Scand J Rehabil Med.* 1997;29(3):167–174.
70. Norlander S, Aste-Norlander U, Nordgren B, Sahlstedt B. Mobility in the cervico-thoracic motion segment: an indicative factor of musculo-skeletal neck-shoulder pain. *Scand J Rehabil Med.* 1996;28(4):183–192.

71. Norlander S, Nordgren B. Clinical symptoms related to musculoskeletal neck-shoulder pain and mobility in the cervico-thoracic spine. *Scand J Rehabil Med.* 1998;30(4):243–251.
72. Caroll LJ, Hogg-Johnson S, van der Velde G. Course and prognostic factors for neck pain in the general population: results of the Bone and Joint Decade 2000–2010 Task Force on Neck Pain and its Associated Disorders. *Spine.* 2008;33(45):S75–S82.
73. Korthalis-de Bos IBC, Hoving JL, van Tulder MW, et al. Cost effectiveness of physiotherapy, manual therapy, and general practitioner care for neck pain: economic evaluation alongside a randomized controlled trial. *BMJ.* 2003;326(7395):911–914.
74. Nordin M, Carragee EJ, Hogg-Johnson S, et al. Assessment of neck pain and its associated disorders. Results of the Bone and Joint Decade 2000–2010 Task Force on Neck Pain and Its Associated Disorders. *Spine.* 2008;33(4 suppl):S101–S122.
75. Rubinstein SM, Pool JJM, van Tulder MW, Riphagen II, de Vet HCW. A systematic review of the diagnostic accuracy of provocative tests of the neck for diagnosing cervical radiculopathy. *Eur Spine J.* 2007;16(3): 307–319.
76. Wainner RS, Fritz JM, Irrgang JJ, et al. Reliability and diagnostic accuracy of the clinical examination and patient self-report measures for cervical radiculopathy. *Spine.* 2003;28(1):52–62.
77. Puglisi F, Ridi R, Cecchi F, Bonelli A, Ferrari R. Segmental vertebral motion in the assessment of neck range of motion in whiplash patients. *Int J Legal Med.* 2004;118(4):235–239.
78. Carragee EJ, Hurwitz EL, Cheng I, et al. Treatment of neck pain: injections and surgical interventions: results of the Bone and Joint Decade 2000–2010 Task Force on Neck Pain and its Associated Disorders. *Spine.* 2008;33(4 suppl):S153–S169.

98 Case Study: Abdominal Pain

PETER ADLER-MICHAELSON ▪ MINDY A. CHILMAN MCCOMB ▪ MICHAEL A. SEFFINGER

KEY CONCEPTS

- Osteopathic evaluation of the patient with abdominal pain considers the five models of osteopathic care: biomechanical/structural, respiratory/circulatory, metabolic/energetic, neurologic, and biopsychosocial/behavioral.
- Differential diagnosis of abdominal pain entails consideration of possible etiologies based on the history and physical using an anatomical and pathophysiologic approach.
- The osteopathic evaluation and treatment of abdominal pain considers the effects of somatovisceral and viscerosomatic reflexes, as well as somatosomatic and viscerovisceral reflexes.
- Somatic dysfunction may be a primary cause or a secondary finding in patients with abdominal pain and/or gastrointestinal (GI) dysfunction.
- Osteopathic management of patients with abdominal pain utilizes the five models of osteopathic patient care.

CASE VIGNETTE

CHIEF COMPLAINT

Right lower quadrant (RLQ) abdominal pain.

HISTORY OF PRESENT ILLNESS

A 28-year-old woman presents to the emergency department (ED) on a weekend with increasingly painful RLQ abdominal pain over the past 8 hours. It is accompanied by slight nausea, but no vomiting. The doctor on call for her primary care physician talked with her on the phone and recommended "she" go to the ED for further evaluation. She was brought by car from home.

The pain initially began 3 weeks prior after traveling to Brazil for her honeymoon. She carried heavy luggage to and from the airport and felt a pull in her right side when yanking it off the conveyor belt. Pain fluctuated daily since then depending on her activities but was usually tolerable with intensity ranging from 2 to 5/10. Today, it rose to 8/10 after lifting groceries out of the trunk of her car. It is now constant and dull in nature though she denies cramping. The pain has been located in the RLQ without radiation since its onset 3 weeks ago. It is worse with standing up after bending over while lifting over 20 lb. The pain abates when she is lying on her side in the fetal (knee to chest) position. Food does not make it worse. Medications such as aspirin, ibuprofen, and acetaminophen have not helped. There is no change in the pain with application of heat or cold. Her menstruation has been regular, normal in amount without clots, and neither exacerbates nor ameliorates the pain. Her pain is such that she cannot tolerate vacuuming, reaching into the cupboard over the kitchen counter, or sexual intercourse. She had right flank pain for 2 days 4 months ago when she passed a kidney stone, but she reports that this pain is different, and she denies having had RLQ pain with that episode.

PAST MEDICAL HISTORY

She has no history of medical illnesses or hospitalizations. Denies prior history of ulcers, gallstones, cholecystitis, gastritis, colitis, appendicitis, pancreatitis, inflammatory bowel disease, sickle cell disease, tuberculosis, diabetes, or lupus erythematosus.

Gynecologic history: G0P0. She is sexually active, has unprotected intercourse with a single male partner (her husband), takes oral contraceptives to prevent pregnancy, and has not missed any periods, which occur every 28 days since she started oral contraception.

PAST SURGICAL HISTORY

Denies past surgical history including dental.

FAMILY HISTORY

Her mother is 54 and had cholelithiasis leading to cholecystectomy, multiple kidney stones throughout the years but no renal failure. Her father is 56 and has hypertension and diabetes. She has two brothers, 34 and 32, and a sister, 26, all well.

SOCIAL HISTORY

The patient is an executive secretary, newly married with no children, working long hours but enjoys her work. She does not smoke and denies any illicit drug use. She rarely drinks alcohol. She is active in sports. She recently traveled to South America with her husband on her honeymoon.

ALLERGIES

No known drug allergies.

MEDICATIONS

Oral contraceptives, multivitamins. No other prescription medications. She takes herbal supplements from a friend who sells them to her for weight maintenance but isn't sure what is in them.

REVIEW OF SYSTEMS

General

She normally sleeps well but has been sleeping poorly due to this pain. She is very health conscious and exercised regularly before this pain started. She describes her nutrition as excellent. She denies fevers, chills, night sweats, or recent weight loss or gain. She has a poor appetite when the pain intensity increases, which is unusual for her.

Skin

Denies rashes, moles, or scaling.

HEENT

Denies head trauma or changes in hearing, vision, smell, taste, or swallowing. Denies sore throat.

Neck

Denies swollen glands.

Breasts

Denies lumps, masses, or discharge.

Cardiovascular

Denies chest pain, shortness of breath, palpitations, or orthopnea.

Respiratory

Denies cough, phlegm, or wheezing.

Gastrointestinal

She has had slight nausea, but denies vomiting, diarrhea, constipation, hematemesis, melena, hematochezia, increased flatulence, or bloating. She has normal daily bowel movements with no change in the color of her stool. Denies intolerance to fatty or fried foods. Denies reflux or heartburn.

Urinary

Passed a kidney stone without sequelae 4 months ago. Denies hematuria, dysuria, or change in color of urine since that episode.

Genital

Periods have been regular without clots, no heavier or lighter than usual. Denies vaginal sores, discharge, or odor. Intercourse has been painful since onset of the RLQ pain 3 weeks ago but she denies prior dyspareunia.

Neurologic

Denies seizures, numbness, weakness, spasms, ticks, or problems with coordination.

Hematologic

Denies easy bruising or bleeding.

Peripheral Vascular

Denies claudication or varicose veins.

Musculoskeletal

Denies fractures, dislocations, joint pains, or swelling. Sprained right ankle while playing tennis 8 years ago. Occasional low back pain which resolves with stretching.

PHYSICAL EXAMINATION

Vital Signs

Pulse: supine, 100 beats per minute; standing, 108 beats per minute. BP: supine, 120/72 mmHg; standing, 124/70 mmHg. Temperature: 37.5°C; RR: 16 breaths per minute. Pulse ox: 98% on room air. Height: 5′8″; Weight: 145 lb.

General

This is a well-developed, well-nourished woman in moderate distress due to abdominal pain, lying comfortably on her right side with knees flexed to chest.

HEENT

Normocephalic, atraumatic. Tympanic membranes intact with normal cone of light and no erythema or discharge. Pupils are equal, round, and reactive to light; external ocular muscles are intact. Nasal septum midline, no erythema or discharge. Mucous membranes slightly dry but without lesions, oropharynx clear without exudate.

Neck

Neck supple; no bruits; no enlarged lymph nodes.

Cardiovascular

Slight tachycardia, with regular rhythm; no extra sounds, murmurs, or rubs.

Thorax and lungs

Thorax expansion symmetric. Clear to auscultation in all fields without adventitious sounds.

Breasts

No masses, erythema, asymmetries, or discharge.

Abdomen

No scars present; no asymmetry to inspection. Bowel sounds normal in all quadrants; no abdominal bruits. Moderate RLQ discomfort to palpation, which is nonradiating; no masses or abnormal pulsations are palpated; no rebound tenderness is elicited. There is no guarding or costovertebral angle tenderness. Negative Rovsing's and Murphy's signs.

Genitalia

Normal external and internal anatomy; no masses palpated; slight referral of pain to the RLQ on bimanual examination; no discharge or unusual odor noted, no cervical motion tenderness.

Rectal

Tone is normal; no masses present; stool is brown, soft, with no gross blood. Guaiac test is negative for occult blood.

Extremities

Normal range of motion in all joints. No swelling is present. No pain is elicited on motion testing; no skin lesions are present. Positive right Thomas test.

Peripheral Vascular

Radial and dorsalis pedis pulse present and equal bilaterally. Capillary refill less than 2 seconds in fingertips. No edema, varicosities, stasis pigmentation, or ulcers.

Neurologic

Cranial nerves II to XII grossly intact; no sensory or motor abnormalities appreciated; DTRs are 2+/4 in biceps, triceps, brachioradialis, patellar, and Achilles tendons bilaterally. Babinski test elicits plantar flexion bilaterally.

Osteopathic Structural Examination

The patient is examined in the standing, seated, prone, and supine positions for evidence of structural landmark asymmetries, altered range or quality of motion, tissue texture abnormalities, tenderness, or temperature variations.

Gait

Gait is not antalgic, cadence is rhythmic with even stride length, but her left lower extremity is slightly externally rotated.

Postural Landmarks

The right shoulder is inferior to the left; the head is held forward of the gravitational line; thoracic kyphosis is diminished as is the lumbar lordosis; the right anterior superior iliac spine is superior, right posterior superior iliac spine is inferior; the right leg appears shorter by 3 mm at the medial malleoli with the patient supine.

Active Motion

Truncal side bending left is restricted. There are positive right standing and seated flexion tests. In the prone position, L5 is rotated left and side bent left and the sacrum is rotated right on a left oblique axis (R/L sacral torsion).

Passive and Inherent Motion

There is an externally rotated right temporal bone; C2 and C3 are flexed, rotated left, side bent left; T1 is extended, rotated right, side bent right; T5 is extended, rotated right, side bent right; T6 is extended, rotated left, side bent left; L1 is flexed, rotated right, side bent right. There is poor compliance of the sacrum to posterior–anterior pressure at L5–S1 (positive spring test). The right thoracic diaphragm is restricted in inhalation. Her axial fascial pattern is rotated left at the craniocervical junction, rotated right at the cervicothoracic junction, rotated right at the thoracolumbar junction, and rotated left at the lumbosacral junction (L/R/R/L). There is restricted internal rotation of the left femur.

Soft Tissue Palpation

There are no abnormal temperature variations over the abdomen or back regions; the superior mesenteric ganglion area is tender to palpation; the right psoas is hypertonic and shortened, and there is a positive right counterstrain tenderpoint for the psoas muscle and a positive left piriformis tenderpoint; there were no Chapman points palpable at the stomach, liver, small intestine, large intestine, kidneys, appendix, and ovarian sites.

DIFFERENTIAL DIAGNOSIS

Regardless of the region of the abdomen in which the patient states she has pain, since the visceral afferents diverge several segments within the spinal cord, the pain is not always an accurate indicator of the precise location of a visceral pathology. The differential diagnosis of subacute RLQ abdominal pain without bowel changes in a woman of childbearing age includes infectious, inflammatory, metabolic, and mechanical pathology.

As an osteopathic emergency physician, the priority is to rule out a life-threatening illness. For example, a ruptured ectopic pregnancy is a true medical/surgical emergency where the patient could bleed profusely from a ruptured fallopian tube and die within minutes, before definitive care can be delivered. The patient must be quickly evaluated, and any emergent treatment measures begun immediately.

Given this patient's presentation, several emergency conditions need to be ruled out. Ectopic pregnancy, appendicitis, infection, internal bleeding, hydronephrosis, hepatitis, pancreatitis, ruptured diverticula, perforated bowel, and bowel obstruction are at the top of this differential. Possible urgent conditions also include pregnancy, placenta previa if pregnant, salpingitis, ovarian cyst, endometriosis, pelvic inflammatory disease, tumor, nephrolithiasis, pyelonephritis, cystitis, and colonic inflammation.

OSTEOPATHIC PATIENT MANAGEMENT

Biomechanical Model

In the ED, whether somatic dysfunction is present or not, it is imperative to first distinguish whether a patient with abdominal pain has pathophysiology requiring solely medical management or surgical management as well. If there is somatic dysfunction present, as in this patient's case, the osteopathic physician should determine if it is due to a musculoskeletal disorder or secondary to internal organ pathophysiology. If the somatic dysfunction is due to a visceral dysfunction, urgency, or emergency, osteopathic manipulative treatment (OMT) may not be the best primary or initial intervention for the patient. However, the osteopathic physician should consider whether osteopathic evaluation and treatment using OMT could help to better diagnose or treat the condition, and/or be useful as an adjunct to the primary treatment, which may be pharmacologic and/or surgical. If the patient has a surgical abdomen, which is typically firm and tender, her soma should display signs of guarding and protecting an obstructed or inflamed internal organ. Related Chapman reflex points would be expected to be identified. Another consideration is whether osteopathic principles or OMT could assist in making the patient a better operative candidate, allow her to better handle the postoperative phase, or assist in the recovery phase.

Conversely, if the somatic dysfunction is determined to be primarily of musculoskeletal origin and there is no evidence of internal organ pathophysiology, then OMT would be the treatment of choice for her problem. Muscle energy treatment to a restricted psoas using isometric contraction against a controlled resistance, followed by the postisometric relaxation phase and passive stretching to lengthen the psoas could be effective. Alleviation of the spinal somatic dysfunctions with high-velocity low-amplitude (HVLA), muscle energy, or other OMT procedures could also be beneficial.

The normal fascial patterns in a healthy patient are either no compensatory alternating rotation (an absence of dysfunction) or a pattern of L/R/L/R or R/L/R/L at the transition zones. Her fascial pattern indicates a loss of compensation and likely an issue of the thoracolumbar region. The pattern of somatic dysfunctions of the ipsilateral respiratory diaphragm and psoas muscle with the contralateral piriformis muscle is a very common pattern with psoas syndrome.

This patient has a positive Thomas test. In a patient with a normal hip joint, a positive test is a good indicator of psoas hypertonicity. The counterstrain tenderpoints for the psoas and iliacus muscles provide further evidence of a primary psoas dysfunction/spasm. The points are palpated and the findings compared left with right. In the case of this patient, both the positive Thomas test and the presence of a counterstrain tenderpoint of the right psoas muscle indicate a somatic dysfunction of the right psoas muscle.

The psoas muscles are attached to the vertebral bodies and the anterior surface of the transverse processes of the lumbar vertebra. They pass along the superior border of the true pelvis, are joined by the iliacus muscles, pass over the superior ramus of the pubic bones, and then turn posteriorly to insert on the lesser trochanter of each femur via common tendons.

Psoas syndrome is usually initiated when a person assumes any number of positions that shorten the origin and insertion of the psoas muscle for a significant length of time and then gets up quickly, suddenly lengthening the origin and insertion, and attempts to assume normal upright activity. The initial positions that might bring about this syndrome include sitting in a soft easy chair or recliner, bending over from the waist for a long period of time, working at a desk, or weeding in the garden. Psoas syndrome can also be precipitated by overuse, such as doing sit-ups with the lower extremities fully extended. Each of these situations creates a neuromuscular imbalance that results in psoas muscle hypertonicity. The subsequent formation of somatic dysfunction then affects the psoas muscle and the lumbar spine. Once a patient realizes that they have been in one of these positions, the possibility of initiating a psoas syndrome can usually be avoided if they *slowly* return to a neutral postural position.

The physician must be aware that there are organic causes for psoas tension or spasm, and if suspected, these must be ruled out by history and/or physical examination and special tests. These include the following:

- Femoral bursitis
- Arthritis of the hip
- Appendicitis
- Diverticulitis of the colon
- Ureteral calculi
- Prostatitis
- Cancer of the descending or sigmoid colon
- Salpingitis
- Psoas abscess

The key somatic dysfunction initiating or perpetuating psoas syndrome is believed to be a type II somatic dysfunction usually occurring in the L1 or L2 vertebral unit. Osteopathic structural examination findings indicative of this syndrome include the following:

- The key type II somatic dysfunction at L1 or L2
- Sacral somatic dysfunction on an oblique axis, usually to the side of lumbar side bending
- Pelvic shift to the opposite side of the greatest psoas spasm
- Hypertonicity of the piriformis muscle contralateral to the side of greatest psoas spasm
- Sciatic nerve irritation on the side of the piriformis spasm
- Gluteal muscular and posterior thigh pain that does not go past the knee, on the side of the piriformis muscle spasm

Manipulative treatment is preceded by ruling out psoas involvement caused by one of the organic etiologies previously listed. Effective treatment of the "key" somatic dysfunction (usually found at L1 or L2) is essential for the patient's comfort and for effective, long-lasting effects of manipulative treatment. Removing somatic dysfunction, wherever it occurs in the body, reduces afferent load to the spinal cord from secondary somatic sources and lessens the segmental activity of the primary facilitated spinal cord segments. This makes the patient more comfortable and supports the body's homeostatic and defense mechanisms, thus hastening recovery.

An iliopsoas or psoas somatic dysfunction with hypertonicity and muscle shortening present for a long enough period of time may create a posterior rotation of the ipsilateral innominate. This is likely due to the superior pull from the muscle leading to a compensatory shift of the innominate to ease tension within the muscle. This often leads to a functional (not anatomic) shortening of the ipsilateral leg, as is demonstrated by this patient.

The L5, sacrum, and innominate dysfunctions are likely compensatory to the initial psoas dysfunction.[1,2]

The C-spine (C3–C5) somatic dysfunction may be related to her diaphragm somatic dysfunction via somatosomatic reflexes. The temporal bone somatic dysfunction is likely secondary to the cervical and sacral somatic dysfunctions. The lack of Chapman points for the foregoing organs lends further weight to the hypothesis that the internal organs are not primarily involved in her case.

Respiratory–Circulatory Model

This patient's respiratory and circulatory functions seem to be unremarkable. On examination, her resting pulse is slightly elevated and mucous membranes are slightly dry. This raises the possibility of her being volume depleted, but orthostatic pulse and blood pressure were within normal limits which suggests only mild volume depletion, if present. With moderate or severe volume depletion, systolic blood pressure would drop more than 20 mmHg and/or diastolic blood pressure would drop more than 10 mmHg, and/or pulse would rise more than 20 beats per minute upon standing. In this case, her elevated heart rate is therefore likely due to pain as opposed to an emergent hemorrhage. She may still have an ectopic pregnancy causing RLQ pain and the resulting tachycardia and a urine pregnancy test should be done.

Pneumoperitoneum is typically discovered on plain upright abdominal x-ray as free air under the diaphragm, and a life-threatening complication of pneumoperitoneum is a gas embolism. Although causing some pain and bloating regardless, the intensity of pain with pneumoperitoneum is piercing if the air transects fascial planes, that is, through the abdominal wall or fascia of the diaphragm, which is contiguous with the pericardium and fascia of the mediastinum. On occasion, air can enter the vaginal canal and find its way through the uterus, fallopian tubes, and into the abdominal cavity. A perforated intestine from ruptured diverticula, cancer, and inflammatory bowel disease can also cause pneumoperitoneum, but there is no evidence in this patient's history or physical examination to suggest this.

The color of the stool is another important finding when assessing a patient with abdominal pain. A finding of bright red blood alerts the physician to consider processes involving the lower gastrointestinal (GI) tract, for example, colon cancer or hemorrhoids. A finding of black tarry stool leads the physician to consider upper GI processes, for example, a bleeding ulcer in the stomach or duodenum. Normal stool color does not rule out GI bleeding; a guaiac test must be done to test for occult blood in the stool. The test is done at the bedside following a rectal examination. If the stool is negative for gross blood and the guaiac test is negative for occult blood, one can be fairly sure that there is no process present involving bleeding within the GI tract. The history along with a normal vascular examination of the abdomen and lower extremities was not suggestive of aortic aneurysm or other vascular problems or bleeding abnormalities in this patient.

An intravenous (IV) line was started with normal saline (NS) at 125 cc/h, as she was kept NPO (*Latin*—nil per os—nothing by mouth) pending further workup. If this patient did have tachycardia due to blood loss or dehydration, she would need greater amounts of IV fluids, usually NS or lactated Ringer's solution.[3] She was started on telemetry monitoring and an EKG was ordered because of tachycardia. Blood was drawn; urine was obtained and sent to the lab.

Neurologic Model

An appreciation of the neuroanatomy of nociception is helpful in discerning the cause of acute abdominal pain. Both somatic (peripheral nervous system) and visceral (autonomic nervous system) innervations are involved. Visceral afferents transmit noxious stimuli, such as stretch, distention, inflammation, and ischemia, to the central nervous system (CNS). However, other tissue-destroying processes, as seen with some intra-abdominal tumors or cancerous growths, or cutting and burning during surgery, cannot be perceived via these visceral afferent nerves and are thus not perceived as pain by the patient.

In the abdomen, sympathetic innervation arrives via the thoracic, lumbar, and pelvic splanchnic nerves, and parasympathetic innervation by the paired vagus nerves arising from the 10th cranial nuclei of the brainstem and the sacral splanchnic nerves arising from S2 to S4 spinal segments. The sympathetic cell bodies are in the intermediolateral cell columns of spinal segments T1–L2 with axons traversing through the ventral roots to the paravertebral ganglia. These paired chains of interconnected ganglia lie along each side of the spinal cord just anterior to the heads of the ribs like a string of pearls. The fibers from the paravertebral sympathetic chain ganglia converge anteriorly to form the sympathetic prevertebral or collateral ganglia: the greater splanchnic nerves from segments T5–T9 form the celiac plexus; the lesser splanchnic nerves from segments T10–T11 form the superior mesenteric plexus, and the least splanchnic nerves from segments T12–L2 form the inferior mesenteric plexus. Postganglionic fibers innervate their target organs.

The parasympathetic innervation structure is more streamlined. Long, preganglionic axons from the vagus nerves extend through the prevertebral ganglia as they pass directly to the viscera. Their short, postganglionic fibers form part of the network in the visceral wall called the enteric nervous system. Both the sympathetic and the parasympathetic nerves exert their effects through the enteric nervous system. This network of fibers is composed of two layers. The outer myenteric plexus (Auerbach) controls GI motility. The inner plexus (Meissner) controls GI secretion and local blood flow. Perception of nociceptive stimuli results in alterations in gut function mediated at this level. For example, marked reduction in gut motility—ileus—commonly occurs in peritonitis via viscerovisceral reflexes.

Specific aspects of this anatomy explain why visceral pain is initially perceived as vague in location and quality. It is generally described as dull, aching, or cramping in nature, rather than sharp or intense. This relates partly to the paucity of visceral afferents compared with the large number of somatic afferents originating in skin and musculoskeletal structures. Equally important is that the transmission of visceral pain occurs via slow nonmyelinated C fibers versus the fast-conducting Aδ-fibers that transmit somatic pain.

Finally, the initial location of pain as regional versus specific relates to the embryologic development of abdominal viscera as midline structures with midline neurovascular supply. They divide into foregut (T6–T9), midgut (T8–T12), and hindgut (T12–L2) areas.[4] Foregut structures include the distal esophagus, stomach, and the proximal duodenum, as well as the liver, biliary tree, and pancreas. Midgut structures include the small intestine, appendix, ascending colon, and proximal two-thirds of the transverse colon. The hindgut includes the distal third of the transverse colon, the descending colon, and the rectosigmoid. They are loosely associated with the celiac, superior mesenteric, and inferior mesenteric ganglia, respectively. Thus, in general, pain from structures innervated at these levels will be perceived as originating in one of the three midline zones of the abdomen (epigastric, midabdominal, or lower abdominal) versus a discrete unilateral location.

The somatic component of acute abdominal pain is caused by the parietal peritonitis that occurs adjacent to the involved viscera as inflammation progresses. Also referred to as the "percutaneous reflex of Morley," it is conducted by Aδ-fibers following the associated dermatome to unilateral spinal segments, which results in the localization and increasing intensity of acute abdominal pain, as well as the increased muscle tone of the abdominal wall associated with guarding and rebound tenderness.

The third component of acute abdominal pain, known as referred pain, is a clear example of how structure interrelates with function. Referred pain is defined as discomfort occurring in a site distant from the diseased organ. The explanation of referred pain lies in the intricacies of the neuroanatomy previously described. The spinothalamic tract is largely nondiscriminatory for visceral versus somatic pain. Because somatic nervous input far exceeds visceral, the CNS is "fooled" and perceives the pain as originating partly in the peripheral structures innervated by the same spinal segments as the diseased viscus. For example, the pain initiated by gallbladder inflammation (T7–T8 visceral afferent innervation) is perceived as occurring in the right subscapular area (T7–T8 somatic afferent innervation).

In a similar manner, visceral afferents synapse on interneurons in the spinal cord that stimulate somatic efferent neurons at the same level. This local reflex activity is referred to as a viscerosomatic reflex. It results in somatosensory changes palpable in a paraspinal location as tissue tenderness, asymmetry, range-of-motion restriction, and tissue texture changes. The finding of specific somatic dysfunction in a patient with acute abdominal pain can provide useful information as to the origin of the pain. The paraspinal location should direct one to consider organs known to have sympathetic innervation at the same level, resulting from the fact that visceral afferents that trigger viscerosomatic reflexes predictably follow the sympathetic efferent pathways.

With this discussion of nociceptive anatomy as a backdrop, consider the more clinical aspects of this patient with acute abdominal pain. The patient does not show signs of peritoneal inflammation or an acute abdomen and her vital signs are mostly within normal limits (with the exception of mild tachycardia). The onset of pain began shortly after strenuous physical activity and was associated with decreased ability to perform activities that required her to extend her hip and trunk. Pain intensity gradually increased over a period of weeks, as opposed to the rapid progression typically seen with an obstructed viscus or acute inflammatory process.

With the patient supine, the sensitivity of the connective tissues surrounding the collateral sympathetic ganglia can be assessed by gently palpating the abdomen overlying these areas. Assessment involves determining the presence of tenderness as well as tissue texture changes in these regions. Positive results will lead to further assessment of structures related to the altered ganglion. In this patient, a tender and noncompliant superior mesenteric ganglion area can be a sign of visceral pathology involving, for example, the small intestine or proximal half of the large intestine, or a kidney; or it can mean an increased afferent input to the segments T10–T11 from another somatic structure, for example, the lower extremity or the respiratory diaphragm. The decreased mobility of the right kidney as compared to the left (which can also be in part due to the respiratory diaphragm somatic dysfunction on the right) may explain the tissue texture changes palpated in the superior mesenteric ganglion area.[5]

A common neurologic problem causing superficial chest or abdominal pain is shingles (herpes zoster), which are vesicular, painful lesions along the path of a cutaneous peripheral nerve, usually the intercostal nerve in the intercostal space, resulting from prior infection as a child (varicella zoster, aka "chickenpox"). However, she denies rashes and her skin has no lesions on exam, so this is less likely.

Certainly, lower thoracic or upper lumbar spinal disease could cause nerve irritation, inflammation, and radiation of pain into the lower abdomen. Although there was spinal somatic dysfunction, there was no history of trauma, cancer, or metastasis, and disk herniation is not common in this patient's age group, so these are unlikely possibilities.

While the diagnostics to rule out emergent and urgent processes are ongoing, treatment involves primarily pain management as well as OMT modalities. OMT to relieve pain is most efficacious when there are palpable signs of somatic dysfunction related to the pain, that is, muscle spasm, fascial restrictions, tissue congestion, or tenderness. Often, visceral OMT relieves pain related to tissue congestion, counterstrain technique relieves counterstrain tenderpoints, and myofascial and articulatory procedures or muscle energy techniques reduce muscle spasms and connective tissue restrictions; HVLA may be indicated for restricted joint motion. For paraspinal muscle spasms and Chapman reflex nodules, inhibition (sustained digital pressure with a slight circular motion) is helpful.

An extremely important issue is whether or not to provide analgesic medication to the patient pending lab and imaging studies or awaiting consultations. Administering a strong analgesic may confuse the clinical picture and presentation, making it more difficult to determine if symptoms are improving or worsening. This patient is uncomfortable enough that she would like medication to treat her pain. Current practice guidelines recommend using an opioid-minimizing approach with the use of acetaminophen or NSAIDs to control the patient's pain while undergoing laboratory and radiographic procedures and waiting for consultants to perform their evaluations.[6]

Metabolic Energy Model

Four of the most common causes of acute abdominal pain that warrant surgical intervention include acute appendicitis, acute cholecystitis, diverticulitis, and small bowel obstruction. In each of these diseases, inflammation and infection are the result of obstruction of normal function of a hollow viscus or duct structure. The obstruction results in luminal distention and stasis of organ contents which causes back pressure against the organ walls. Because venous and lymphatic drainage are passive, low-pressure networks, the increasing back pressure prevents proper drainage of these tissues, resulting in organ wall edema. This progresses to arterial obstruction and ischemia. Ischemia leads to wall gangrene, perforation, and peritonitis.

As the GI tract is colonized with varying levels and types of bacteria, the stasis described above leads to bacterial overgrowth. Transmural infection of the compromised viscus results and contributes to peritonitis caused by gangrene and perforation. Bacterial liberation of endotoxins and the release of inflammatory mediators result in the systemic septic response. Inflammation and infection increase metabolic processes and elicit release of interleukins and other cytokines with subsequent generation of fever. Fatigue ensues. Left untreated, this systemic inflammatory response may lead to multiple organ failure and death.

In considering metabolic pathophysiology as the source of her abdominal pain, recall that she had mild nausea, but she did not have any other signs of GI or genitourinary system dysfunctions, such as vomiting, oral or rectal bleeding, bloating, or fevers. She has a history of a kidney stone, and it is possible she has one again with associated muscle spasm related to a viscerosomatic reflex. A noncontrast, low-dose CT would identify a stone if present however, the absence of urinary symptoms and costovertebral; angle tenderness argues against kidney stone or infection.[7] A urine test is an inexpensive means by which hematuria could be detected if there is a ureteral stone, kidney or bladder inflammation, infection, or hemorrhage. Although she has had regular menstruation cycles and flow, a negative urine pregnancy test will confirm she is not pregnant and also rule out ectopic pregnancy. If necessary, an abdominal ultrasound could detect swelling, enlargement, cysts, or masses in the liver, spleen, pancreas, intestines, kidneys, ovaries, fallopian tubes, or uterus as would an abdominal or pelvic CT.

Although she is afebrile, this does not necessarily rule out an intra-abdominal infection and/or inflammation or other noninfectious pathology. Typically, intra-abdominal inflammation causes inflammation of the peritoneal lining of the intra-abdominal wall. As there was no rebound abdominal tenderness on physical examination, which is a fairly reliable sign of peritonitis, this is unlikely. In addition, the lack of GI symptoms (apart from mild nausea) in the setting of normal bowel sounds, absence of palpable masses and both voluntary and involuntary guarding, and negative Rovsing's and Murphy's signs make it unlikely that she has a significant intra-abdominal pathology.

The right ovary and/or fallopian tube could be inflamed, obstructed, or cystic and cause pain without causing a fever, so these pathologies are possible given her symptoms. The physical examination, including lack of Chapman reflexes, did not localize a pathologic pelvic structure, though pain was felt in the RLQ during the pelvic bimanual examination.

The decision as to which lab tests to order is often a difficult one. Ideally, this is based on having a solid differential diagnosis in mind. Lab test results should not be seen as a definitive "rule-out" but rather as another piece in the larger puzzle of the entire presentation of the patient. For example, with a normal complete blood count (CBC) and unremarkable abdominal ultrasound, one might be inclined to rule out appendicitis in this case.[7] The clinical presentation is always evolving, however, and cases of appendicitis have been identified despite a patient having normal laboratory and radiographic tests. Similarly, with normal liver function studies and a normal abdominal ultrasound examination, the physician might be inclined to rule out gallbladder disease. Transabdominal ultrasound is 96% accurate in detecting gallstones greater than 2 mm, but sole reliance on this modality may miss a diagnosis of small stones or disease that may cause abdominal pain and require surgical treatment.[8] A urine drug screen is also helpful in ruling out confounding metabolic factors as the patient may not divulge this history despite appropriately phrased questions.

Biopsychosocial/Behavioral Model

Biopsychosocial/behavioral factors such as anxiety, depression, or drug abuse, especially opiates, may all cause abdominal pain. A urine drug screen could help determine if drug abuse is a potential cause of her pain. Anxiety and depression are possible but would be less likely to cause the degree of abdominal pain she is experiencing. With somatic dysfunction found in so many regions of the body and now constant abdominal pain causing dyspareunia, anxiety may be present not as the cause, but as a symptom of the underlying condition.

Prolonged sitting at a desk, as may be required of an executive secretary, may be exacerbating this patient's condition. Additional inquiry in a nonemergent setting (and when the patient's pain is better controlled) could be informative for the astute physician. The positive Thomas test on the right suggests a tight psoas muscle, so discussing behavioral modifications (such as frequent standing/walking breaks throughout the workday) or implementing a standing desk to allow for position changes may be considered.

CASE WRAP-UP

OSTEOPATHIC MANAGEMENT

Appropriate laboratory and radiographic workup was ordered following initial patient evaluation. Given her lack of pain relief with acetaminophen, aspirin, and ibuprofen (NSAIDs) prior to presenting to the ED and the goal of minimizing opioids while awaiting test results and potential consultant evaluations, OMT was discussed with the patient and offered as a potential pain-relief measure. She consented and was treated with myofascial release (MFR) technique for the thoracoabdominal diaphragm; visceral techniques for the superior mesenteric ganglion and right kidney; counterstrain and MET for the left piriformis hypertonicity; MFR for the left pelvic floor; HVLA for the right innominate; MET and Still techniques for the sacrum and counterstrain for the right psoas tenderpoint. The patient tolerated OMT well and reported a reduction of pain from 8/10 to 3/10 with resolution of nausea. She did not feel a need for pain medication at that point.

DIAGNOSTIC TEST RESULTS

Regarding blood tests, CBC with differential is within normal limits, as are electrolytes, amylase, lipase, liver function tests, blood urea nitrogen, and creatinine. Urinalysis is negative for white blood cells, red blood cells, and nitrites. Urine drug screen is negative. Stool guaiac is negative for occult blood. Urine and serum pregnancy tests are negative. EKG demonstrates sinus tachycardia but is otherwise unremarkable. Ultrasound study of the abdomen shows no pathology, and follow-up abdominopelvic CT shows no free fluid, no masses, no stones, and no abnormal visceral or vascular structures. The appendix was visualized and appears unremarkable. Thus, a hemorrhagic condition, anemia, electrolyte abnormality, illicit drug use, pregnancy, urinary obstruction, renal failure, urinary tract infection, intra-abdominal, and intrapelvic pathology have been ruled out. If any of these test results were found to be positive or equivocal (unable to discern positive vs. negative test), general surgical and/or gynecologic consults could be ordered for opinions from their perspective (as well as management beyond the ED if the patient requires either hospital admission or ambulatory care follow-up with a surgical specialist).

FINAL DIAGNOSIS

The workup for underlying visceral pathology was negative. The final diagnoses were as follows: RLQ pain most likely due to right psoas muscle spasm or syndrome. Somatic dysfunction of the cranial, cervical, thoracic, lumbar, rib, abdomen, pelvis, sacrum, and lower extremity regions.

DISPOSITION OF THE PATIENT

Based upon the normal workup and improvement following OMT, the patient was relieved to be discharged home to follow-up with a local osteopathic physician skilled in the use of OMT. The patient was instructed to return to the ED or follow-up with her primary care physician if symptoms did not improve or worsened, or if new symptoms developed.

Further Treatment Modality Options

Home exercises and self-help techniques will allow the patient to be proactive in her return to homeostasis. Muscle energy techniques for the psoas and piriformis muscles can be easily learned and applied several times daily for symptomatic relief. Lastly, the patient can perform psoas and piriformis stretches at home to prevent further acute somatic dysfunctions.

REFERENCES

1. Kappler RE. Role of psoas mechanism in low-back complaints. *J Am Osteopath Assoc.* 1973;72(8):794–801.
2. Tufo A, Desai GJ, Cox WJ. Psoas syndrome: a frequently missed diagnosis. *J Am Osteopath Assoc.* 2012;112(8):522–528.
3. Liamis G, Filippatos TD, Elisaf MS. Correction of hypovolemia with crystalloid fluids: individualizing infusion therapy. *Postgrad Med.* 2015;127(4):405–412.
4. Moore KL, Agur AMR, Dalley AF. *Moore's Clinically Oriented Anatomy.* 9th ed. Wolters Kluwer; 2023:538.
5. Patterson MM, Howell JN, eds. *The Central Connection: Somatovisceral/Viscerosomatic Interaction.* American Academy of Osteopathy; 1992.
6. Broder JS, Silva LO, Bellolio F, et al. Guidelines for Reasonable and Appropriate Care in the Emergency Department 2 (GRACE-2): low-risk, recurrent abdominal pain in the emergency department. *Acad Emerg Med.* 2022;29(5):526–560.
7. Expert Panel on Gastrointestinal Imaging, Kambadakone AR, Santillan CS, et al. ACR Appropriateness Criteria® Right Lower Quadrant Pain: 2022 Update. *J Am Coll Radiol.* 2022;19(11S):S445–S461.
8. Expert Panel on Gastrointestinal Imaging, Russo GK, Zaheer A, et al. ACR Appropriateness Criteria® Right Upper Quadrant Pain: 2022 Update. *J Am Coll Radiol.* 2023;20(5S):S211–S223.

99 Case Study: Acute Low Back Pain

MARCEL P. FRAIX ▪ MICHAEL A. SEFFINGER

KEY CONCEPTS

- Osteopathic considerations for patients with low back pain (LBP) entail assessing and treating biomechanical, respiratory–circulatory, metabolic energy, neurologic, and behavioral aspects of the clinical condition.
- Differential diagnosis utilizes a structure–function approach in determining whether the pain is due to spinal or pelvic musculoskeletal somatic dysfunction, localized manifestation of a systemic pathophysiologic process, or referred from internal organ disease.
- Most causes of LBP are musculoskeletal and amenable to osteopathic manipulative treatment (OMT).
- Evidence-based literature and expert consensus guidelines support the utilization of osteopathic manipulative treatment for patients with acute, subacute, and chronic back pain.
- The AOA House of Delegates passed a resolution accepting an evidence-based practice guideline recommending utilization of OMT for patients with LBP.

CASE VIGNETTE

CHIEF COMPLAINT

Low back pain (LBP)

HISTORY OF PRESENT ILLNESS

A 52-year-old male presents to the ambulatory clinic complaining of persistent LBP for the past 3 weeks. The pain started a few days after he hurt his left knee playing tennis. His knee pain has improved, and he is no longer limping, but now he is experiencing dull, achy constant pain in his low back, primarily on the right side. The pain is exacerbated with prolonged sitting and lifting more than 25 lb. It seems to get better with rest and lying down, although he does admit to having difficulty with finding a comfortable position when sleeping and prefers to lie on his side with his knees bent. The pain is sometimes sharp and radiates to the right posterior thigh, but not past the knee or into the foot. In the past, he had LBP that radiated to the lateral foot, causing an intermittent numbness sensation, but it resolved after a week or so with decreased physical activity and stretching. He has also contended with dull and aching back pain periodically throughout the years that also resolved spontaneously after a couple of days. Over-the-counter nonsteroidal anti-inflammatory drugs (NSAIDs) offer some relief and reduce his current acute LBP from an 8/10 to 4/10 in intensity on the pain scale. He is usually relatively active and enjoys playing tennis and golf on the weekends, although he has been unable to do so for the last 3 weeks. He denies loss of strength (LOS) bilaterally in his lower extremities or any problems with bowel or bladder function.

Past Medical History

Hypercholesterolemia, asthma, seasonal allergies, and left tibial stress fracture at age 35 while training to run a marathon, right rotator cuff tendonitis. No hospitalizations. His last physical was 10 months ago. He had a normal baseline prostate evaluation, PSA test, and colonoscopy at age 50. No history of rheumatoid arthritis, direct trauma to the low back, or motor vehicle accidents.

Past Surgical History

Appendectomy at age 16.

Social History

Employed as a software engineer; nonsmoker; occasionally has a glass of wine or beer with dinner; lives at home with his wife and two children aged 16 and 14 who are all well. He denies illicit drug use.

Medications

Atorvastatin 10 mg daily for hypercholesterolemia, loratadine 20 mg daily as needed for allergic rhinitis, and naproxen 500 mg, 1 tablet every 12 hours as needed for pain.

Allergies

Penicillin causes hives.

Review of Systems

General

No fever or weight loss; mild fatigue.

Skin

No rashes or eczema.

HEENT

No history of head trauma and no recent changes in vision, smell, taste, hearing, or swallowing.

Cardiovascular

No chest pain at rest or with exertion; no palpitations; no cyanosis or peripheral edema.

Respiratory

No cough, shortness of breath, or dyspnea; has history of exercise-induced and allergic asthma for which he used to use an inhaler as needed but has not needed it for several months; no history of pneumonia or tuberculosis.

Gastrointestinal

No nausea or vomiting, loss of appetite, or abdominal pain; no bloody stools; no diarrhea or constipation; no history of hepatitis, ulcer, diverticulosis, or gallstones.

Genitourinary

No hematuria, dysuria, incontinence, or urinary retention. He does note that his urinary stream is not as strong as usual; no history of hernia; sexual relations have diminished for the past 3 weeks due to LBP.

Endocrine

No polydipsia, polyphagia, or polyuria. No heat or cold intolerance.

Musculoskeletal

Mild left knee pain; sharp right-sided LBP; history of intermittent LBP that is usually dull and aching in nature; occasional right shoulder pain that is exacerbated with playing tennis.

Neurologic

No history of sciatica neuralgia; no muscle weakness in his upper or lower limbs; no muscle cramping or spasm; no persistent loss of sensation in his feet; occasional headaches characterized by a sensation of bilateral squeezing (tightness), which resolve with rest; no history of seizures or stroke.

Hematologic

No history of anemia, blood dyscrasias, or bleeding tendencies.

Psychiatric

No history of depression, anxiety, mania, hallucinations, or hospitalizations.

Physical Examination

Vital Signs

Height, 5′10″; weight, 170 lb; BP, 135/80; P, 86; R, 14; T, 98.8 °F.

General

Alert and in mild distress due to LBP; appearance is well kept; unable to get comfortable sitting on the treatment table; appears well dressed, clean, and groomed.

Integument

No erythema or increased warmth in lumbar region; no trophic changes in bilateral lower limbs; no malar or other rashes.

HEENT

Head is atraumatic, normocephalic; pupils equal, round, and reactive to light and accommodation; CNs II to XII are grossly intact; external auditory canals are patent and tympanic membranes are intact with good cone of light; nasal mucosa is slightly erythematous and edematous; no sinus pressure tenderness to palpation or percussion; pharynx not injected, no tonsillar hypertrophy, and no erythema or exudates.

Hematologic/Lymphatics

No lymphadenopathy or peripheral edema.

Cardiovascular

Heart has a regular rhythm; no murmurs; lower limbs nonedematous; dorsalis pedis and posterior tibial pulses are palpable bilaterally; no carotid bruits; no abdominal bruits or masses.

Respiratory

Lungs are clear to auscultation bilaterally; no wheezes or rhonchi in the airways; no prolongation of exhalation.

Gastrointestinal

Abdomen is nondistended and bowel sounds are auscultated in all four quadrants without bruits; abdomen is tympanic to percussion and soft and nontender to palpation without rebound tenderness or masses. Normal rectal sphincter tone on digital examination; guaiac stool test is negative for blood.

Genitourinary

The prostate is firm, nontender, and small without nodules. No inguinal hernia.

Neurologic

Full motor strength present in bilateral upper and lower extremities; sensation diminished to light touch and pinprick over dorsal surface of right foot, with remainder of sensory examination normal in the upper and lower limbs; muscle stretch reflexes: bilateral patellar and left Achilles 2+/4+; right Achilles 1+/4+; Babinski tests elicit down going toes bilaterally; straight leg raise tests elicit mild increase in LBP and tingling sensation but no pain in the posterior legs or feet at 80 degrees; bilateral lower limb proprioception intact (negative Romberg test); normal heel and toe walking.

Musculoskeletal

Mildly antalgic gait with decreased loading of left lower limb; increased right-sided lumbar paravertebral muscle tension with moderate tenderness lateral to L5 spinous process, decreased lumbar spine flexion (30 degrees) and extension (10 degrees), and moderate pain with lumbar spine extension and left side bending; limited range of motion of squat test; negative FABERE test bilateral hip joints; medial joint line tenderness of left knee with 5-degree deficit in extension, negative drawer test, and mild pain with McMurray test; no effusion of left or right knee; right bicipital tendon tender to palpation, negative Yergason test; there is a right positive Thomas test for iliopsoas tension.

Osteopathic Structural Examination

Patient is evaluated in the standing, seated, supine, and prone positions.

Cranial

Normocephalic, atraumatic cranium, asymmetrical motion posterior quadrants, primary respiratory mechanism at eight cycles per minute, and restriction of the right occipitomastoid suture.

Cervical

Increased cervical lordosis with head anterior to gravitational line; occipitoatlantal (OA) extended, side bent right, and rotated left; C1 rotated right.

Thoracic

Decreased thoracic kyphosis; T1 extended, rotated right, and side bent right; palpable deep right paraspinal muscle tension (intertransversarii, rotatores, multifidi) at T4–T5 extending out to the 4th intercostal space laterally; T8–T10 neutral side bent left, rotated right; T12–L2 neutral, side bent right, and rotated left; tenderness of the right 12th posterior thoracic counterstrain point.

Costal

Exhalation restriction of the right 1st rib and inhalation restriction of the right 12th rib and thoracic diaphragm.

Lumbar

Decreased lumbar lordosis; L5 flexed, rotated right, and side bent right; tenderness of the 5th posterior lumbar and right piriformis counterstrain points and in the area overlying the right iliolumbar ligament.

Pelvis

Positive left standing flexion test; anterior superior iliac spine (ASIS), posterior superior iliac spine (PSIS), and pubic tubercles are level.

Sacrum

Positive left seated flexion test: positive (poor/decreased) lumbar spring test, and left sacral torsion on a right oblique axis.

Lower Extremities

No gross leg length discrepancy; tenderness of left medial meniscus counterstrain tender point; left ankle decreased quality and range in passive dorsiflexion.

Upper Extremity

Right scapula inferior; full range of motion present in bilaterally upper extremities.

Assessment

- LBP (lumbago)
- Somatic dysfunction (cranial; cervical; thoracic r/o viscerosomatic, lumbar; sacral; lower extremities; rib cage)
- Left medial meniscus injury
- History of hypercholesterolemia, allergic rhinitis, asthma, right bicipital tendonitis

Plan

This patient has acute LBP (<6 weeks' duration) due to somatic dysfunction that is amenable to OMT. A review of the scientific literature supports this diagnosis and management plan.[1–3] Osteopathic manipulative medicine (OMM) methods that can be used to address his somatic dysfunctions include soft tissue, articulatory, muscle energy, strain–counterstrain, high-velocity/low-amplitude (HVLA), osteopathic cranial manipulative medicine, and myofascial release procedures. Lumbar spine range of motion and strengthening exercises, such as the commonly prescribed knee-to-chest and pelvic tilt exercises, 3 cycles of 10 repetitions, once or twice daily, often aid recovery and rehabilitation.[1] Patient-specific exercise prescriptions based on the physical examination findings and goals of treatment are most beneficial.[1,4,5] Physical therapy referral for abdominal, lumbar, and pelvic muscle stabilization exercises and training may be useful if progress is slow with self-directed home exercises.[6]

The American Osteopathic Association recommended parameters for application of OMT for patients with acute somatic dysfunction and low back pain in 1998.[5] The number of regions treated (and type of OMT performed) during any one session is variable and will depend upon the history, examination, and medical decision-making by the clinician. If symptoms and signs are continually improving, OMT should be continued. If symptoms and signs are not improving, or worsening, reassessment of the diagnosis and a new management plan should be initiated.[5] However, this is only a guideline, for, at each visit, the osteopathic physician should determine the medical necessity, frequency, and duration of OMT based on the patient's response to previous treatments, prescribed exercises and ergonomics, and current assessment of the clinical condition.[5]

For patients with acute LBP who do not improve with self-care options, spinal manipulation is the best evidence recommendation.[6] Patients should be educated to stay active and use proper ergonomics[6] (i.e., to pick up something to the side, do not bend over to the side, twisting the lumbar spine, with extended knees, which puts significant strain and stress on the low back; instead, face the object, bend the knees, keep the back extended, and lift the object close to the body). Both acetaminophen and NSAIDs have demonstrated benefits as first-line medications for short-term pain relief.[6]

National evidence-based practice recommendations for patients with subacute (6 to 12 weeks after onset) or chronic LBP (more than 3 months after onset) include spinal manipulation, intensive interdisciplinary rehabilitation, exercise therapy, acupuncture, massage therapy, yoga, tai chi, cognitive–behavioral therapy, or progressive relaxation.[6]

It is not recommended that physicians obtain radiologic or laboratory evaluation routinely on patients with nonspecific (anatomical pathophysiology undefined) acute LBP.[6] This includes patients with somatic dysfunction and no symptoms or signs of radiculopathy below the knee or evidence of organic or spinal pathology. It is recommended to obtain radiologic evaluation (e.g., lumbar spine x-rays, A-P and lateral views, MRI, CT) if the LBP persists beyond 6 weeks, which is the average time frame of resolution of acute symptoms, or if there are signs of radiculopathy or severe or progressive neurologic deficits.[6] Diagnostic imaging is also indicated when serious underlying conditions are suspected based on the history and physical examination.[6] Electromyograms and nerve conduction studies (EMG/NCS) are useful if radiculopathy distal to the knee occurs and persists for longer than 6 to 8 weeks. Referral of patients with persistent radiculopathy below the knee to a pain management specialist for epidural steroid injections, or a surgeon for potential definitive intervention is appropriate.[6] Assess for signs of severe or progressive neurologic deficits, as well as red flags, at each office visit. Refer to a spine surgeon if there are signs of severe or progressive neurologic deficits.[7]

Red flags in ROS[7]:

- Fever >100.4 °F
- Pain worsens during rest or at night
- Saddle anesthesia
- Focal leg weakness
- Incontinence of urine or stool

DIFFERENTIAL DIAGNOSIS

A patient's LBP can be defined as either acute or chronic. In general, acute LBP is self-limiting, and if it lasts longer than 3 months, it can be classified as chronic in nature.[6] While this is a broad generalization, it can be a helpful one, since the diagnosis, prognosis, and treatment of acute versus chronic LBP differ from one another. It is important to keep in mind, however, that up to one-third of patients presenting with LBP will have a recurrent, episodic clinical course over their lifetime.[8]

This patient presents a clinical example of a patient with acute LBP, although he has had episodes of back pain with and without radiculopathy in the past. He currently has no symptoms of pain radiating past his knee, but the physical examination did find dermatome-specific signs of decreased sensation in his foot. This could be residual from previous injury or part of the current clinical picture. Since other neurologic tests, including lower extremity motor, sensory, and reflex examinations, were within normal parameters, continued follow-up examinations at each visit to document improvement, stability, or progression of this sensory deficit are indicated. EMG/NCS and diagnostic imaging will assist in the diagnosis if the deficit persists or progresses.

In developing a differential diagnosis, it is helpful to characterize the patient's LBP as localized or referred. Localized pathophysiology can be categorized as mechanical or nonmechanical. Even though it is oftentimes not possible to define the exact etiology of LBP, up to 97% of LBP is mechanical in nature.[9] Mechanical etiologies can cause pain in the low back region, or the pain may radiate to one or both legs or feet. LBP that is accompanied by radicular symptoms is usually indicative of nerve root irritation or compression. Patients who are experiencing radicular symptoms typically report pain that is "burning" or "shooting" in nature and travels into the leg and below the knee. On the other hand, nonradicular mechanical LBP tends to be characterized as "aching" or "throbbing" in nature and may radiate into the gluteal or upper thigh region, but not usually below the knee. There are also nonmechanical causes of LBP. These include infections, inflammation, and cancer.

Psychological issues may also play a significant role.[6] Last, LBP may be referred from another site. This type of pain can be visceral or retroperitoneal in origin, and although rare, it should not be missed, as it may be indicative of a serious disease process, such as gastrointestinal or renal disease, cancer, or abdominal aortic aneurysm. Other organ systems, aside from musculoskeletal, can serve as sources of back pain with diagnoses such as a ruptured aortic aneurysm, obstructive lung disease, irritable bowel disease, renal stones, shingles, prostate cancer, and multiple myeloma contributing to their pain and dysfunction.

Tables 99.1 and 99.2 categorize the differential diagnosis for LBP and provide a means by which the osteopathic physician can stratify it.

As can be discerned from Tables 99.1 and 99.2, the patient does not have a history or physical findings of any of the pathologic conditions listed; however, the history and physical do support the diagnosis of somatic dysfunction. Thus, the osteopathic physician can be confident in making that diagnosis and provide appropriate OMT as part of the management plan.

TABLE 99.1

Differential Diagnosis of LBP

	Characteristics	Labs/Imaging
Localized LBP—Mechanical Without Radiation Below the Knee		
Nonspecific muscular and ligamentous injury	Localized to low back and buttocks Better with lying down and change of position Worse with activity Cyclic in nature Intact neurologic function	Typically, none
Somatic dysfunction	Asymmetry of structural position Altered range of motion Tissue texture abnormalities Tenderness Resolves with OMT	Typically, none
Degenerative disk disease	Localized to low back and buttocks Better with lying down and change of position Worse with prolonged standing or sitting Chronic > acute	Lumbar films: A/P and lateral views MRI
Degenerative joint disease—facet arthropathy	Localized to low back and buttocks Better with lying down and change of position Worse with spinal extension Chronic > acute	Lumbar films: A/P and lateral views MRI
Fracture: **Vertebral** **Spondylolysis**	Acute > chronic Compression fracture: history of osteoporosis or trauma Pars interarticularis fracture: new-onset LBP in athletically active adolescent or history of trauma	Lumbar films: A/P, lateral and oblique views CT
Localized LBP—Mechanical with Pain Radiation Below the Knee		
Radiculopathy	Leg pain that radiates below the knee Pain with dermatomal distribution Neurologic function may be impaired Lower extremity weakness Diminished reflexes	MRI
Spinal stenosis	Bilateral lower limb pain Neurogenic claudication Neurologic function may be impaired Lower extremity weakness Diminished reflexes	MRI

TABLE 99.1 (Continued)

Differential Diagnosis of LBP

	Characteristics	Labs/Imaging
Cauda equina syndrome	Impaired neurologic function Saddle anesthesia Lower extremity weakness Diminished reflexes Urinary retention	MRI
Localized LBP—Nonmechanical		
Infection: **Osteomyelitis** **Diskitis**	Pain at rest or night Fever Recent skin infection or UTI or IVDA	CBC, blood cultures, MRI
Neoplasm: **Primary: osteosarcoma, osteoid osteoma** **Metastatic: prostrate, breast, lung, kidney** **Multiple myeloma**	Pain at rest or night Weight loss	MRI, CT, PSA, alkaline phosphatase
Inflammation: **Spondyloarthropathy—ankylosing spondylitis reactive arthritis (Reiter disease)** **Rheumatoid arthritis**	Significant morning stiffness Sacroiliac pain Uveitis Urethritis Joint pain and swelling	Lumbar and pelvic films CBC, ESR, CRP, HLA-B27, Rh factor
Referred LBP		
Gastrointestinal disease: **Inflammatory bowel disease** **Diverticulitis** **Pancreatitis**	Abdominal pain, tenderness, distention Hematochezia	Abdominal films, US, CT CBC, amylase/lipase
Renal disease: **Nephrolithiasis pyelonephritis**	Abdominal pain Hematuria	US, CT UA
Gynecologic: **Endometriosis** **Menstrual**	Pelvic pain Cyclical in nature Dysmenorrhea	US
Vascular: **Abdominal aortic aneurysm**	"Ripping" or "tearing"-like abdominal pain Pulsatile abdominal mass	US, CT
Psychological: **Somatoform disorder** **Malingering** **Central sensitization/chronic pain syndrome**	Disproportionate pain	Typically, none

A/P, anterior/posterior; CBC, complete blood count; CRP, C-reactive protein; CT, computerized tomography; ESR, erythrocyte sedimentation rate; HLA-B27, human leukocyte antigen B27; IVDA, intravenous drug abuse; MRI, magnetic resonance imaging; OMT, osteopathic manipulative treatment; PSA, prostatic specific antigen; Rh, rheumatoid; UA, urinalysis; US, ultrasound; UTI, urinary tract infection.

TABLE 99.2

Structure/Function Model of Differential Diagnosis of LBP

	Red Flags: Spinal Pathology (Mechanical)	Somatic Dysfunction (Mechanical, Amenable to OMT)	LBP Work-Related (Behavioral)	LBP Radiating Below the Knee (Neurologic)	Inflammatory Disorder (Metabolic)
History	• Age of presentation <20 or onset >55 • Violent trauma, e.g., fall from height, MVA • Constant, progressive, nonmechanical pain • Thoracic pain • Past history of carcinoma • Systemic corticosteroids • Drug abuse • HIV • Difficulty with micturition • Fecal incontinence	• Aged 20–55 • Pain may be in lumbar and sacral spine, buttocks, and thighs; does not radiate below the knee • Mechanical in nature • Lifting and twisting • Pain varies with physical activity and time	• Postural stress • Whole-body vibration • Monotonous work • Lack of personal control • Low job satisfaction • Smoking	• Unilateral leg pain > back pain • Pain generally radiates to foot or toes • Numbness and paresthesias in the same dermatome distribution	• Gradual onset • Marked morning stiffness • Family history

(continued)

TABLE 99.2 (Continued)

Structure/Function Model of Differential Diagnosis of LBP

	Red Flags: Spinal Pathology (Mechanical)	Somatic Dysfunction (Mechanical, Amenable to OMT)	LBP Work-Related (Behavioral)	LBP Radiating Below the Knee (Neurologic)	Inflammatory Disorder (Metabolic)
Physical	• Systemically unwell • Weight loss • Persisting severe restriction of lumbar flexion • Structural deformity • Loss of anal sphincter tone • Saddle anesthesia around the anus, perineum, or genital • Widespread (greater than one nerve root) or progressive motor weakness in the legs or gait disturbance	• Patient well • Lumbosacral spine and/or pelvis somatic dysfunction present	• Low physical fitness • Inadequate trunk strength	• Nerve root irritation signs • Reduced SLR, which reproduces leg pain • Motor, sensory or reflex change is limited to one nerve root	• Iritis, skin rashes (psoriasis), colitis, urethra discharge • Persisting limitation of spinal movements in all directions • Peripheral joint involvement
Lab and x-ray	• X-ray: look for vertebral collapse or bone destruction • CT or MRI: look for cauda equina compression	• Nondiagnostic	• Nondiagnostic	• Nondiagnostic or MRI: look for disk herniation with compression of peripheral nerve root	• Nondiagnostic or blood tests: look for Rh factor or seronegative arthropathy; ESR > 25 • X-ray shows evidence of arthritis
Course	• If pain not resolved in 6 wk, an ESR and x-ray should be considered	• Prognosis good • 90% recover from acute attack in 6 wk; but most recur throughout life • Manipulation and exercise provide pain relief, improved mobility, and may shorten course	• Usually resolves within 6 wk • Responsive to manipulation and exercise and use of proper posture and ergonomics • Potential for prolonged recovery if there is secondary gain involved	• Prognosis reasonable • 50% recover from acute attack within 6 wk	• Usually resolves with anti-inflammatory medication • Episodic

CT, computerized tomography; ESR, erythrocyte sedimentation rate; MRI, magnetic resonance imaging.

OSTEOPATHIC PATIENT MANAGEMENT

Biomechanical Model

As stated above, the majority of LBP is mechanical in origin. In general, mechanical LBP is improved with rest and exacerbated with activity. Although the etiology of mechanical LBP can at times be identified, such as with degenerative disk and joint disease, much of the time it is not. In the setting of a poorly defined etiology, it is thought that injury of muscular and ligamentous structures play an important role. It likely involves injury of muscle fibers at the musculotendinous junction that is precipitated by physical activity. The musculature of the lumbar spine can be classified as being anterior or posterior.

ANTERIOR MUSCLES

The anterior musculature comprises the abdominal and iliopsoas muscles. Abdominal muscles include the rectus abdominis, external and internal oblique, and transverses abdominis muscles. These muscles act in concert with one another to produce flexion of the lumbar spine. While it is unlikely that they are a source of LBP, these muscles are very important in providing core stability and are of benefit to strengthening in patients with LBP. Iliopsoas is located deep within the abdomen and pelvis, originating along the lateral aspects of the lumbar vertebrae and intervertebral disks and the iliac fossa, and inserting on the lesser trochanter of the femur. It is the primary flexor of the hip joint and can act as a lumbar flexor when the hips are fixed. Because it is a postural muscle, it is prone to shortening in the absence of activity. This leads to decreased hip extension, increased lumbar lordosis, and anterior pelvic tilt, which may predispose a patient to develop lumbar and pelvic somatic dysfunction and LBP.

POSTERIOR MUSCLES

The posterior muscles are subdivided into superficial, intermediate, and deep layers. The superficial layer comprises the lumbodorsal fascia. This expansive layer of connective tissue provides stability for the thoracolumbar and pelvic regions, as well continuity with the upper limb via its connection with the latissimus dorsi muscle. The intermediate layer consists of the iliocostalis, longissimus, and spinalis muscles. These erector spinae muscles function bilaterally to produce extension and unilaterally to produce side bending of the lumbar spine. The deep layer consists of those muscles responsible for localized vertebral movement, including lateral flexion (sidebending) with contralateral rotation. They include multifidi, rotators, and intertransversarii muscles. The deep layer also contains the quadratus lumborum muscle, which connects the pelvis to the spine and produces lumbar extension when contracting bilaterally. If it undergoes overuse due to deconditioning of the erector spinae muscles, it can be a potential source of LBP.

Just as injury to muscle fibers can cause mechanical LBP, so too can injury to ligamentous structures. Like muscle injury, ligamentous injury is characterized by pain that can be either dull and aching or sharp in nature. Two of the most important ligaments are the anterior and posterior longitudinal ligaments, which traverse the respective surfaces of the vertebral bodies and intervertebral disks. They provide stability and, respectively, prevent hyperextension and hyperflexion of the spine. The posterior longitudinal ligament is of particular interest due to its location within the spinal canal. Its position helps prevent posterior displacement of the intervertebral disk. Because it is richly innervated with nociceptors, it can be a source for LBP.[10] It can also succumb to different disease processes, such as ossification, which can cause other disorders of the spine, including spinal stenosis. Like the posterior longitudinal ligament, the ligamentum flavum, which connects the laminae of adjacent vertebrae, is susceptible to ossification. However, since it contains few nociceptors, it is not considered to be an important pain generator. The iliolumbar ligament is another clinically important ligament that originates from the transverse processes of L4/L5 and inserts on the iliac crest. This ligament can be the source of pain locally upon palpation, as well as in other regions such as referred pain to the groin, SI region, and lateral thigh. This phenomenon is commonly termed iliolumbar ligament syndrome and is important to assess when evaluating a patient with LBP.[11]

Because the precise anatomical source of mechanical LBP is not identifiable in most patients, the physical examination is oftentimes used to exclude serious underlying pathology and confirm the diagnosis. In the absence of well-defined spinal pathology and with signs of TART indicative of somatic dysfunction, osteopathic physicians consider somatic dysfunction as the cause of the LBP if its alleviation with OMT relieves the pain and restores normal function.

In addition to assessing the lumbar region for tissue texture changes, asymmetry, increased or decreased range of motion, and tenderness, the physical examination should include an assessment of gait and posture, neurologic function of the lower limbs, and appropriate provocative tests, such as the straight leg raise and FABERE (hip flexion, abduction, external rotation, and extension) tests. Abdominal and rectal examinations may also be indicated if intra-abdominal or pelvic pathology are suspected, or if the patient has signs/symptoms of a cauda equina syndrome. With the continuity that exists between the lower limbs and pelvis and lumbar spine, it is useful to perform an evaluation of gait, as it may give insight into the etiology of the patient's LBP. For example, a patient with a radiculopathy affecting the 5th lumbar nerve root may have weakness of his ankle dorsiflexors that is demonstrated by high steppage gait. Although it is almost always normal in patients with nonradiating mechanical LBP, a neurologic examination is essential when assessing any patient with LBP. It involves assessing motor strength and sensation for the L1–L5 myotomes and dermatomes, as well as the Achilles and patellar muscle stretch reflexes. The straight leg raising test, as well as other nerve stretching maneuvers (e.g., flexing the knee and passively dorsiflexing the ipsilateral ankle, or squeezing the ipsilateral calf along the midline course of the sciatic nerve), is useful for assessing sciatic nerve inflammation or irritation.

SOMATIC DYSFUNCTION

Since up to 70% of mechanical LBP may be due to somatic dysfunction, performing an osteopathic structural examination can be quite useful.[1] As with other regions of the body, lumbar somatic dysfunction is characterized by asymmetry of structural position, altered range of motion, and palpable tissue texture abnormalities and/or tenderness. There are three primary anatomic sites of somatic dysfunction in the lumbosacral–pelvic region that can cause LBP and are amenable to treatment with OMM. Surrounding soft tissues, for example, lumbar myofascial paraspinal tissues and lumbosacral–pelvic ligaments, are often treated along with the specific lumbar, sacral, or pelvic joint somatic dysfunctions. Box 99.1 lists the soft tissue elements often addressed with OMT, and Table 99.3 lists the three types of somatic dysfunction commonly associated with LBP and the types of segmental somatic dysfunction that are typically found with each one.

As with all osteopathic structural examinations, evaluation of the lumbar spine for segmental somatic dysfunction requires proficiency in palpating the appropriate anatomical landmarks and performing a regional and segmental examination.

From a biomechanical perspective, treatment of LBP seeks to address somatic dysfunction and restore posture and balance to allow the musculoskeletal system to operate more efficiently and with less pain. This entails not only addressing lumbar somatic dysfunction, but somatic dysfunction elsewhere in the body, particularly the spine, pelvis, and lower extremities. Because the spine works as a functional unit, treating somatic dysfunction that exists in the thoracic and cervical spine will ideally allow for restoration of

BOX 99.1 Muscles, Fascia, and Ligaments (Soft Tissues) Commonly Associated with Lumbosacral Somatic Dysfunctions in Patients with LBP

Superficial layer:
- Lumbodorsal fascia

Intermediate layer:
- Erector spinae

Deep layer:
- Multifidi
- Rotatores
- Intertransversarii
- Pelvic diaphragm
- Quadratus lumborum

Lower extremities:
- "Hamstrings"
- Piriformis
- Psoas–iliacus
- Gluteal muscles

Ligaments:
- Interspinous
- Iliolumbar
- Sacroiliac
- Sacrotuberous

TABLE 99.3

Somatic Dysfunctions Associated with LBP

Lumbar Vertebral Joint Somatic Dysfunctions	Lumbosacral—Pelvic (Sacroiliac) Dysfunctions	Ilium—Pelvic (Iliosacral and Pubic) Dysfunctions
Type I: • **Neutral, side bent left or right** *Type II:* • **Flexed or extended, rotated and side bent right or left**	• Sacral torsion (L/L; L/R; R/L; R/R) • Bilateral or unilateral sacral flexion or extension • Lumbosacral joint compression • Unlevel sacral base due to anatomic short leg[21]	• Superior or inferior ilial shear • Anterior or posterior rotated ilium • Inflared or outflared ilium • Superior or inferior pubic symphysis shear

normal spinal motion. Likewise, the aim of treating lower extremity somatic dysfunction is to improve posture and balance and allow the body to cope with the forces of gravity more efficiently during sitting, standing, and ambulation. Certain anatomic structures that are known to cause or exacerbate LBP should be considered when formulating an osteopathic treatment plan. These structures, which are amenable to manipulation, include the lumbar intervertebral joints, myofascial paraspinal soft tissues, sacroiliac joints and iliosacral joints, and lumbosacral and lumbopelvic ligaments. Soft tissue and myofascial techniques such as lumbar prone pressure with counter leverage and lumbosacral decompression can be used to address increased tension of the lumbar paraspinal musculature and lack of compliance in the tissues surrounding the lumbosacral junction. Sidelying lumbar articulatory or HVLA technique is useful for treating lumbar segmental dysfunction at L5.

With respect to pelvic dysfunction, muscle energy techniques can be used to treat sacral torsions and counterstrain technique for piriformis somatic dysfunction. Care should also be taken to address somatic dysfunction outside of the lumbar and pelvis regions. This may entail treating dysfunction at the OA joint with HVLA and decompression of the OA joint, as well as treating knee or ankle somatic dysfunction with counterstrain technique. This again will allow the osteopathic physician to address somatic dysfunction that may have predisposed the patient to develop LBP and interfere with structural balance.

DEGENERATIVE DISK AND JOINT DISEASE

Spondylosis is a term that is used to describe degenerative changes of the spine, including degenerative disk and joint disease. It tends to affect the lumbar spine due to its mobile nature and load-bearing responsibilities. There are five lumbar vertebrae, each of which is separated by an intervertebral disk. Each vertebra consists of a body and vertebral arch. The vertebral arch is further composed of a pair of pedicles and laminae and supports several additional structures, including the inferior and superior articular processes, transverse processes, and spinous processes. It forms the intervertebral foramen, through which the spinal nerves exit, and helps protect the spinal cord by forming part of the spinal canal. The vertebrae articulate with one another via the fibrocartilaginous intervertebral disk and synovial facet joints, which exist on the inferior and superior articular processes. The disk consists of an outer fibrocartilaginous ring, the annulus fibrosis, and inner gelatinous mass, the nucleus pulposus. It acts as a dampening mechanism for forces transmitted along the vertebral column while simultaneously allowing for movement between the individual vertebrae. Disease or injury to any of these structures can potentially lead to instability of the lumbar spine and LBP. While injuries such as fracture of the vertebral body or arch tend to result in acute LBP, spondylosis tends to be associated with chronic LBP. In general, it is a natural part of the aging process, and by 49 years of age, 60% of women and 80% of men have osteophytes and other changes indicative of spondylosis.[12] As with acute LBP due to muscular and ligamentous injury, back pain due to degenerative changes is difficult to localize and symptoms and signs tend to be nonspecific. In addition, radiologic findings, both on MRI and plain films, must be interpreted with caution since there is poor correlation between radiographic degenerative changes and LBP. For example, disk herniation on lumbar MRI is a common finding in asymptomatic patients.[13,14]

PIRIFORMIS SYNDROME

Although it is not part of the musculature or ligamentous structures of the lumbar spine, the piriformis muscle should be a consideration in the differential diagnosis of LBP because pain associated with its dysfunction can be interpreted as low back in origin. Typically, piriformis syndrome–type pain is characterized by aching pain in the gluteal region, especially at the attachment sites of the piriformis muscle. Patients complain of increasing pain after sitting for longer than 15 to 20 minutes. In addition, because of the proximity of the piriformis muscle to the sciatic nerve, patients can report paresthesia's that radiate down the posterior aspect of the thigh. Having an appreciation for the anatomy of the piriformis muscle, as well as its surrounding structures, clarifies the possible pathophysiology behind piriformis syndrome and physical examination findings.

The piriformis muscle originates on the anterior surface of the sacrum and passes through the sciatic notch before inserting on the upper aspect of the greater trochanter. It is innervated by the first and second sacral nerves and primarily acts as an external rotator of the hip joint. With the hip flexed to 90 degrees, it acts as an abductor of the hip. It is an important structure since all neurovascular structures that exit from the pelvis via the greater sciatic notch do so either inferior or superior to the piriformis muscle. This includes the inferior and superior gluteal nerve and artery and pudendal and sciatic nerves. Even though the mechanism of sciatica or radicular-type pain in piriformis syndrome is not completely understood, it is thought that the sciatic nerve may become impinged or compressed by the piriformis muscle. This may be secondary to trauma, such as falling on the buttock, or overuse, both of which can result in inflammation of surrounding tissues and spasm of the piriformis muscle. In addition, in some patients, the sciatic nerve may pierce the piriformis muscle, rendering the sciatic nerve more susceptible to entrapment and injury. Regardless of the etiology, piriformis syndrome is usually characterized by tenderness in the region of the greater sciatic foramen. Provocative maneuvers that evaluate for piriformis syndrome attempt to induce radicular-type pain by either active contraction of the piriformis muscle in resistance or passively stretching it.[15] The straight leg raise test may be positive in piriformis syndrome but is nonspecific since it does not localize where the nerve is compressed and is typically more indicative of nerve root compression. In the supine position, a patient may exhibit external rotation of the affected lower limb, and range-of-motion testing may reveal decreased internal rotation of the affected side. The sacrum is typically rotated anteriorly toward the ipsilateral side on a contralateral oblique axis, resulting in compensatory rotation of the lower lumbar vertebrae in the opposite direction.[16]

SACROILIAC JOINT PAIN

Although the sacrum and sacroiliac joints are technically part of the pelvis, they warrant mention here since pain due to dysfunction of these structures can be difficult to distinguish from pain originating in the lumbar spine. In fact, the prevalence of sacroiliac joint pain, as established based on clinical evaluation, varies from 15% to 30% in patients with LBP.[17] The sacrum is a triangular-shaped bone that is formed from the fusion of five sacral vertebrae. It articulates with the ilium bones at the sacroiliac joints and fifth lumbar vertebra via the last lumbar intervertebral disk and facet joints. The sacroiliac joints are L-shaped synovial joints that are stabilized by a combination of bony and strong ligamentous structures, including the anterior and posterior sacroiliac and sacrotuberous ligaments. As with the lumbar spine, injury, inflammation, degeneration, and somatic dysfunction of the sacroiliac joints can result in LBP. Like mechanical LBP, sacroiliac pain can also be nonspecific and refer to a variety of places, including the low back, buttock, groin, and lower extremity.[18]

The International Association for the Study of Pain suggests incorporating at least three selective sacroiliac joint stress tests to diagnose sacroiliac pain more clearly. These provocative tests include compression, distraction, thigh thrust, Gaenslen test, and Patrick sign.

Lastly, performing a pelvic regional and segmental examination is useful in diagnosing sacroiliac and iliosacral somatic dysfunction that may be responsible for a patient's LBP and amenable to treatment with OMM.

COCCYDYNIA

Coccydynia or pain associated with the coccyx (tailbone). The coccyx is located at the terminal end of the spinal column and is specifically attached to the distal sacrum. It usually consists of three to five segments that may or may not be fused. Pain in this area is uncommon. The complaint of pain may follow from sacral trauma (falls onto the buttocks, post childbirth, severe cases of whiplash). Pain is made worse with sitting or having pressure applied to this area and is reduced or relieved with standing or the reduction of pressure to the coccyx. Treatments used to relieve the symptoms depend upon the knowledge base of the practitioner and include OMT to reposition the coccyx to its normal position by using either direct or indirect MFR or an assessment and treatment of the sacrum and pelvis to correct any associated dysfunctions. Strain–counterstrain, balanced ligamentous tension, or a direct pressure applied to the sacrococcygeal ligaments to relieve strains that might be present can be effective. Other techniques utilized include hot packs, ultrasound (US), sitz baths or towels, acupuncture, and injections into the ganglion impar. Strategies used to reduce the pain include the use of pillows or "donuts" to minimize the pressure against the coccyx and the reduction of time spent in the seated position.

PSOAS SYNDROME

A chronic psoas spasm can create a persistent strain across the lumbosacral junction and impede resolution of lumbosacral somatic dysfunction despite OMT and exercises directed at the L–S region. Treatment of the psoas by relieving the thoracolumbar junction and upper lumbar somatic dysfunction and stretching a hypertonic psoas muscle facilitates resolution of a long-standing lumbosacral somatic dysfunction. Commonly, the L1 or L2 vertebra is flexed and rotated to the side of the shortened, hypertonic psoas muscle. In the patient above, the thoracolumbar junction has two type I curves, one superior and the other inferior, to the thoracolumbar junction. This indicates a long-term somatic dysfunction in that region, as type I group dysfunctions are often compensatory changes to a long-standing type II segmental dysfunction. Treating the type I spinal somatic dysfunctions with OMT as well as stretching the tight psoas muscle would be a reasonable approach in this patient (see Figs. 99.1 and 99.2).

SHORT LEG SYNDROME AND LBP

Patients with anatomic short leg syndrome often have sacral base unleveling and sacroiliac and lumbosacral joint dysfunction and pain (see Chapters 92 and 93 for more information regarding leg length inequality and postural imbalance). OMT combined with lift therapy has been shown to relieve LBP in many of these patients.[18–21]

Respiratory/Circulatory Model

From a respiratory/circulatory perspective, maximizing oxygenation and delivery of nutrients facilitate the recovery of tissues that may have been injured or compromised in a patient with LBP. Therefore, patients may benefit from OMM that addresses somatic dysfunction of the thoracic and pelvic diaphragms and costal cage. The upper lumbar vertebral bodies serve as the sites of

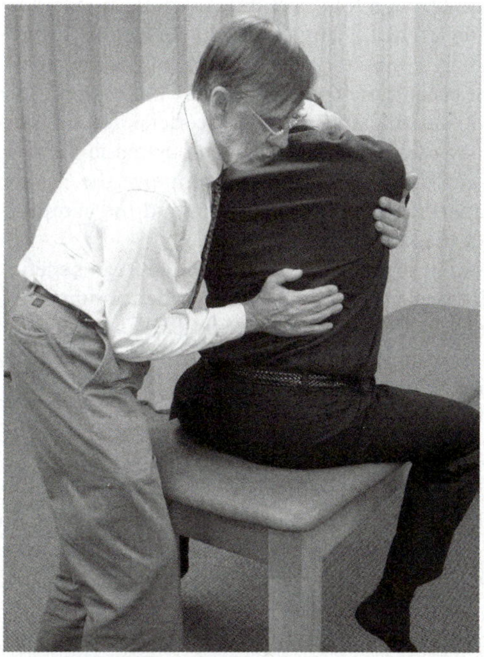

Figure 99.1. Astride table technique (HVLA or MET) to treat Type II somatic dysfunctions. (Reprinted with permission from Nelson KE, Glonek T; American College of Osteopathic Family Physicians. *Somatic Dysfunction in Osteopathic Family Medicine.* Lippincott Williams & Wilkins; 2007. Figure 26.21.)

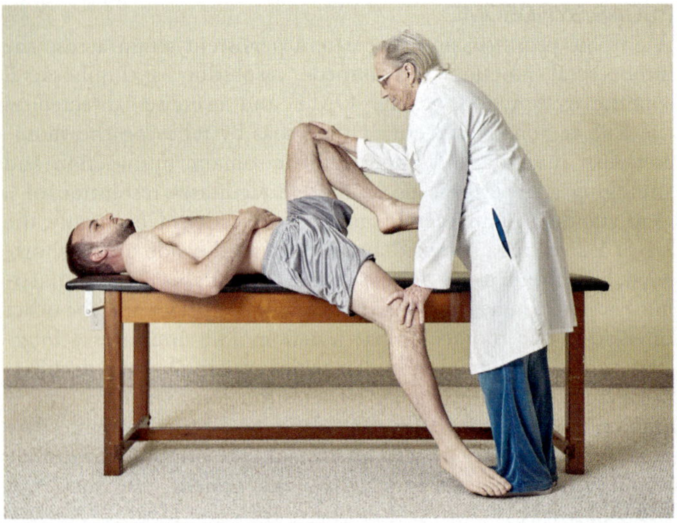

Figure 99.2. MET approach to treat iliopsoas tension. (Reprinted with permission from Schiowitz S, DeRubertis AJ. Exercise therapy. In: DiGiovanna EL, Amen CJ, Burns DK, eds. *An Osteopathic Approach to Diagnosis and Treatment*. 4th ed. Wolters Kluwer; 2021:239. Figure 55-22.)

insertion for the diaphragm. The diaphragm is most efficient when the lumbar spine is in its natural lordosis in the seated or standing positions. An important goal of osteopathic management therefore is to restore lumbar lordosis to maximize diaphragmatic function. As important as the thoracolumbar junction is to diaphragmatic activity, similarly, normal lumbosacral mechanics are key for pelvic diaphragm function. With each breath, the sacrum should be able to oscillate in its articulation with the ilia. The second sacral segment serves as the attachment of the spinal dura, which is also attached firmly to C1, C2, and the occiput at the foramen magnum. Thus, somatic dysfunction of the lumbosacral spine and sacroiliac joints influences mechanics in distal spinal segments as well as in the cranium through this "core link" of spinal dura (see Chapter 53 Osteopathic Cranial Manipulative Medicine for further information). Primary respiratory mechanism motions at the sacrum as well as the occiput are compromised by lumbosacral somatic dysfunction. Evaluating and treating the sacral and occipital somatic dysfunctions using balanced ligamentous tension and osteopathy in the cranial field techniques will improve the motions related to the primary respiratory mechanism and the natural respiratory mobility of the sacrum.

In addition to receiving OMM, patients can benefit from regular cardiovascular exercise. There is evidence supporting the fact that patients with acute, nonspecific LBP who stay active have reduced pain and improvement in function compared to patients who receive bed rest.[22]

Neurologic Model

Neurogenic LBP is characterized by involvement of the nerve roots, cauda equina, or spinal cord. Symptoms include unilateral or bilateral radiation of pain or paresthesia distal to the knee, or muscle weakness, which may include loss of bowel and bladder sphincter control in the case of cauda equine syndrome. It is far less common than mechanical LBP and constitutes approximately 5% to 15% of LBP cases. Because it usually involves compression of a neural structure, it is typically associated with demonstrable pathology, including disk herniation or spondylosis.

The two most common types of neurogenic LBP are lumbar radiculopathy and spinal stenosis. The prevalence of lumbar radiculopathy is approximately 3% to 5%, with L5 and S1 radiculopathies constituting 90% of all lumbosacral radiculopathies.[23] Unlike mechanical LBP, in which pain is mediated by the anterior and posterior rami of the spinal nerves or sinuvertebral nerves, radicular pain is mediated by the proximal spinal nerves. Radicular pain also differs from mechanical LBP in that the symptoms and signs are more specific and tend to point to a diagnosis of lumbar radiculopathy. Patients describe radicular pain as "burning" or "shooting" in nature and traveling into the leg and foot, sometimes following a dermatomal distribution.

Neural tension signs, such as the straight leg test, are helpful in determining if there is compression of a lumbar nerve root. The supine straight leg test has a sensitivity of 91% and specificity of 26%, indicating that when it is negative, a diagnosis of lumbar radiculopathy can be reasonably excluded.[24]

Because spinal pathology is often present, MRI of the lumbar spine is useful. MRI has been shown to have a sensitivity of 83% and specificity of 78% when assessing for compromise of a neural structure in the lumbar spine.[25] However, because it is common to find abnormalities such as bulging or protruding disks in asymptomatic patients, it is important to correlate imaging findings with the history and physical examination.

A detailed neurologic examination is imperative not only to establish a diagnosis, but to also evaluate for serious findings that may warrant immediate intervention. These can include saddle anesthesia, bladder or bowel dysfunction, or progressive neurologic deficits in the lower limbs. These findings must also be kept in mind when evaluating a patient with lumbar spinal stenosis, which is usually the result of spondylosis. Symptomatic lumbar spinal stenosis is characterized by neurogenic claudication, which is defined as aching pain in the lower limbs that is precipitated by walking or standing and alleviated with rest and flexion of the trunk.

Somatic dysfunction is oftentimes present in patients with neurogenic LBP. It may be primary in nature or secondary to compression of lumbar spine nerve roots. In secondary somatic dysfunction, nerve root irritation and its associated spinal pathology may be causing spinal facilitation, which in turn leads to maintenance of the somatic dysfunction.

The neurologic model takes into consideration the integration of central, peripheral, and autonomic nervous systems and how they may be impacted by somatic dysfunction. Since mechanical LBP is often due to somatic dysfunction, it improves with OMT. This, however, does not mean that neurogenic or nonmechanical LBP cannot be helped with OMT. In these situations, it can be helpful in addressing facilitated segments that are due to nonmechanical pathology. OMT can be helpful in providing information regarding the source of the referred pain. Addressing somatic dysfunction in these cases will ideally lead to a reduction in mechanical stress and the nociceptive input associated with it. This in turn will potentially decrease peripheral sensitization and will in turn lead to decreased spinal facilitation and subsequent improvement in lumbar segmental motion. Also, with decreased pain, the patient may perceive less stress and achieve more balanced function of the autonomic nervous system and neuroendocrine immune network. The body will have a decrease in neuroendocrine activation of the hypothalamic–adrenal axis, resulting in decreased cortisol production and sympathetic tone, which will restore autonomic balance. The allostatic load will be diminished, leading to a restoration of homeostasis.

Metabolic Energy Model

The metabolic, energy expenditure, and exchange perspective entails maximizing internal organ functions to support recovery from somatic dysfunction or pathologic conditions causing or related to the LBP. Improving a patient's diet and nutrition can help enhance one's metabolic homeostasis which can help normalize other systems indirectly. Using analgesic medications such as NSAIDs to modulate the pain impulses facilitates healing by decreasing inflammation and allowing the patient to stay active and continue normal daily activities. Bed rest beyond 3 days is not recommended for patients with acute LBP as muscles begin to atrophy and weaken, impeding healing and recovery of normal function. Rheumatologic conditions are primarily managed with medications, though osteopathic manipulation may have an adjunctive role.[26] An inflamed joint, such as the sacroiliac joint (sacroiliitis) found in patients with ankylosing spondylitis, should not be manipulated with direct action OMT as this will aggravate the condition. However, some forms of OMT are designed to improve lymphatic drainage of swollen joints without moving the joint. These techniques are "afferent reduction" type techniques and include functional, balanced ligamentous tension, and strain–counterstrain.

Behavioral Model

The patient evaluated has somatic dysfunction from mechanical LBP. LBP is one of the most common complaints in the outpatient clinic. With a lifetime prevalence of 49% to 70%, most adults will experience an episode of LBP at some point in their life.[27] LBP is the third most reported symptom, the second most frequent cause of worker absenteeism, and the costliest ailment of working-age adults in the United States.[8] It causes more disability among working-age adults than any other disability and is the most common ailment of working-age adults in the United States.[8] Some of the largest components of direct costs include physical therapy, inpatient care, pharmacy, and primary care.[28] The economic burden of LBP, both in terms of direct and indirect costs, is great. The combined direct and indirect costs due to LBP are estimated to be $50 billion.[29] Incorporating OMM may allow the osteopathic physician to manage patients more efficiently with LBP and therefore reduce direct costs. It may also help patients return to work earlier and experience a greater sense of satisfaction with their treatment.[1]

LBP affects males and females of all ages, disabling those in the 35 to 54 years of age, and is found in 30% to 50% of teenagers aged 13 to 18.[1,8] Risk factors for the development of acute LBP include increasing age, demanding physical activity (bending, twisting, and lifting movements and prolonged standing), and psychological factors (work dissatisfaction or monotonous work).[1,8] The strongest known predictor of a future episode of LBP is the history of previous episodes.[8] Fortunately, most acute back pain cases resolve within 6 weeks, but one-third may continue to have intermittent, episodic recurrences.[8] When LBP becomes chronic in nature, typically lasting longer than 6 months in duration, certain risk factors may have a more important role. These include a prior episode of LBP, poor job satisfaction, smoking, and poor coping skills. Comorbid conditions are commonly found in chronic LBP patients, and psychological factors play a greater role than anatomical pathology in predicting persistent LBP.[8,30]

Age is an important consideration when evaluating a patient with LBP. For example, the patient's age in and of itself leads the physician toward a particular diagnosis. Because of the anatomical differences in the adolescent and adult spine, each is susceptible to different spinal pathologies. The adolescent spine is still growing, and its primary and secondary centers of ossification remain active, in the setting of trauma or significant physical activity, this can predispose the adolescent to such spinal disorders as spondylolysis and spondylolisthesis, which can be a significant cause of LBP and instability. On the contrary, an adult spine has a higher likelihood of having spondylosis, which may or may not be related to the LBP. Females over 60 years old, as are those who are postmenopausal, are more prone to osteoporosis-related vertebral fractures as a cause of acute LBP.

The behavioral model also addresses the psychological status of a patient and how health may be affected by stress and environmental and socioeconomic factors. It is particularly important to consider in patients with LBP. Systematic review has found psychological and occupational factors to have the highest reliability among prognostic factors with LBP.[31] These factors are important to consider in patients with acute LBP, as they may predispose a patient to the development of chronic LBP. There is also strong evidence demonstrating that expectation of recovery is a predictor of work outcome in patients with nonspecific LBP.[32] Therefore, it is important to understand not only the life stressors and job satisfaction of patients but also their expectations and goals with respect to recovering from LBP. Encouraging and assisting the patient in restricting abuse of tobacco and alcohol, engaging in regular exercises, and maintaining normal body weight range will aid in restoration of normal low back neuromusculoskeletal function.

PATIENT OUTCOME

After receiving OMT, the patient noted a reduction in his LBP. He was able to walk and sit without pain and no longer required the use of NSAIDs for pain relief. He was also able to sleep comfortably once again on his back and the right lower limb numbness had nearly resolved.

Treatment focused on resolving somatic dysfunction and addressing postural decompensation. Attention was given to restoring postural balance by correcting thoracic, lumbar, and sacral somatic dysfunctions. The patient's sacral torsion and hypertonic piriformis muscle were treated. Physical therapy aimed at restoring the flexibility and strength of the psoas, erector spinae, and abdominal musculature facilitated restoration of the patient's lumbar lordosis, and he reported diminished tenderness around the iliolumbar ligament.

An MRI of the lumbar spine showed a 2-mm broad-based protrusion of the L5–S1 disk with mild right-sided neuroforaminal stenosis at L5. EMG and NCS were normal. Spinal somatic dysfunction improved with OMT, indicating no persistent viscerosomatic reflexes.

Treatment also addressed somatic dysfunction of the thoracic diaphragm and 12th rib, as well as surrounding structures connecting the costal cage with the pelvis, including quadratus lumborum. This assisted in resolving somatic dysfunction within the lumbar region. At the same time, it also helped maximize respiratory and circulatory function and improve the delivery of oxygen and nutrients to and removal of metabolic wastes from the area.

Finally, stressors and ergonomic factors were considered to speed recovery and prevent future episodes of LBP.

SPECIALIST REFERRAL

LBP is one of the most common reasons for a visit to the primary care physician's office. However, even more so than the primary care physician, the spine or pain management specialist routinely evaluates and manages patients with LBP. Fortunately, 90% of acute LBP and 50% of LBP with radicular symptoms resolve within 6 and 4 weeks, respectively.[1] It is typically the patient who does not experience a resolution of his or her LBP who is referred to the physician specialist for further evaluation and management. Regardless of whether it is acute or chronic in nature, diagnosis of LBP is oftentimes complex and requires thorough knowledge of the functional anatomy of the lumbar region and pathophysiology of LBP. This must be integrated with an understanding of the risk factors associated with developing LBP and prognostic factors for recovering from it. For example, the overall health and well-being of a patient are important predictors of back pain.[33] In addition, the risk of developing LBP is approximately double for those with a history of LBP, indicating that it may be less likely to spontaneously resolve and more recurrent in nature than once thought.[34] Therefore, when performing an evaluation, the physician specialist must not only have an appreciation for the complex etiology of LBP, but also for the overall patient and their experiences with it.

When evaluating the patient with LBP, one of the most important factors to consider is age. Because certain age groups are more prone to develop certain lumbar spine pathology than others, it is helpful to stratify a patient by age to simplify the potential causes of the LBP and eliminate more serious conditions, such as fracture, tumor, or infection. This may be particularly true given the fact that a clear diagnosis of LBP cannot be determined in 85% of patients, given the poor association between symptoms, pathologic changes, and imaging results.[35] Although the focus of this chapter is on the evaluation and management of LBP in the adult population, it is important to be able to recognize the primary causes of LBP in the adolescent patient, especially those actively involved in athletics. Unlike adults, it appears that adolescents, particularly those below the age of 12, have an identifiable cause for their LBP 45% to 50% of the time.[36] This is especially true for lumbar spondylolysis, which accounts for 47% of LBP in adolescent athletes versus 5% in adult athletes.[37] When evaluating an adolescent, it is therefore important to have a high index of suspicion for an identifiable cause of LBP and a low threshold for ordering diagnostic imaging studies, including plain films, CT, and MRI.

As with the adolescent patient, it is also useful for the physician, or spine or pain management specialist to identify as best possible the anatomical structure responsible for an adult patient's LBP. This can be quite challenging due to the number of structures that can be involved, including lumbar spine musculature, nerves, disks, and zygapophysial joints. Like other regions of the spine, evaluation should begin with a history and physical examination. This includes defining the duration, location, and quality of the LBP, as well as the factors that alleviate and exacerbate it. As mentioned before, it is valuable to gain an overall sense of the patient, their psychological health, and how they are functioning with their pain since these influence their prognosis for recovery.

As mentioned in the differential diagnosis section, when characterizing pain, it can be particularly helpful to distinguish it as being either mechanical or neuropathic in nature. Mechanical LBP is caused by involvement of the lumbar vertebrae, disks, joints, and myofascial structures, including muscles and ligaments. It is dull and aching in nature, exacerbated with prolonged standing, or sitting, and alleviated with rest. It is also typically associated with lumbar spondylosis and degenerative disease. In contrast, neuropathic pain is shooting and stabbing in nature, radiates into the lower limb and foot, and is indicative of lumbar nerve root irritation or compression. This characterization can be useful, since neuropathic or radicular pain may have a more definable cause, such as a disk herniation, and requires different treatment.[38] When performing the physical examination, the physician can evaluate for lumbar nerve root compression by performing a provocative maneuver such as the straight leg raise test. In fact, in a systematic review, the straight leg raise test was found to be one of the most sensitive tests for radiculopathy.[39] Other important components of the physical examination include motor strength, sensory testing, and lumbar spine range of motion. The osteopathic structural examination evaluates for asymmetry of structural position, altered range of motion, and tissue texture abnormalities or tenderness.

Although it is beyond the scope of this chapter, it is also essential to evaluate the hip and sacroiliac joints since pain in the low back can be referred to from these neighboring structures. After performing a history and physical examination, diagnostic studies may be indicated to further aid in the diagnosis of LBP. The utility of MRI is limited by the high prevalence of lumbar degenerative changes in adults without LBP. Research has shown that approximately 30% of adults without LBP have evidence of a protruded disk and over 50% have bulging or degenerative disks.[40] If the clinical picture is consistent with lumbar spinal stenosis, however, MRI of the lumbar spine can be useful in evaluating for spinal canal narrowing. In general, spinal imaging is typically only indicated if certain conditions are suspected, including fracture, neoplasm, infection, and cauda equina syndrome. Other studies, including lumbar diskography and facet injections, and EMG, can potentially be useful in confirming a diagnosis in patients suspected of having disorders of anatomical structures, such as the intervertebral disk or nerve root. Lumbar provocation diskography is potentially a useful tool in evaluating chronic lumbar diskogenic pain.[41] EMG can be used to assess the physiologic status of the nerves innervating the lower limbs and diagnose lumbar radiculopathy. In addition to the history and physical examination, it can be helpful in distinguishing LBP that is radicular versus nonradicular in nature. This distinction, along with an assessment for somatic dysfunction and relevant imaging studies, aids in more clearly identifying the cause of a patient's LBP and instituting appropriate treatment.

After completing clinical and diagnostic evaluation and excluding significant pathology, including cervical spine instability or an infectious, neoplastic, or inflammatory process, the physician spine or pain management specialist utilizes a variety of modalities to treat LBP, including medication, physical therapy, interventional procedures, manipulative medicine, and referral for surgical consultation. When addressing chronic LBP that is nonradicular in nature, a multidisciplinary plan that combines pharmacologic and nonpharmacologic therapy is reasonable. Nonpharmacologic therapies with evidence of moderate efficacy for chronic or subacute LBP include cognitive–behavioral and other psychotherapies, exercise, spinal manipulation, acupuncture, and interdisciplinary rehabilitation.[42] Because of compelling evidence supporting its use in the treatment of LBP, OMM should be part of most LBP treatment plans.[2] This may entail the physician performing OMM or referring the patient to a neuromusculoskeletal medicine specialist. Meta-analysis of clinical trials examining the efficacy of OMM in the treatment of LBP has demonstrated decreased pain and use of medications when compared to standard medical care.[2] Patients with LBP that is radicular in nature may benefit from lumbar epidural steroid injection. Systematic reviews have demonstrated level II-1 evidence for lumbar transforaminal injections providing short-term relief and level II-2 for long-term improvement in the management of lumbar radicular pain.[43] There is however no evidence supporting the use of these injections in nonspecific LBP. Likewise, there is no strong evidence supporting the use of injections or radiofrequency denervation in the treatment of facet-mediated pain. If conservative treatment and interventional procedures fail, referral to a surgical specialist can be considered. This is especially true if the source of the patient's LBP is clear. For example, in patients with lumbar radiculopathy, surgery can reduce pain and improve function, and in those with disk herniation, it can facilitate a quicker return of function. A favorable outcome appears to be far less likely in those patients with chronic LBP and common lumbar degenerative changes who undergo surgical intervention.[44] Ultimately, it is helpful for the physician to employ specific treatment if the etiology of a patient's LBP is clear and a multidisciplinary approach that incorporates OMM if there is evidence of somatic dysfunction.

In July 2009, the American Osteopathic Association House of Delegates passed a resolution in support of submitting a profession-wide interdisciplinary Guideline for Utilization of OMT for patients with LBP. The guideline was based upon a systematic review and meta-analysis of randomized clinical trials of osteopathic manipulation for patients with LBP,[2] as well as two other clinical practice guidelines developed by interdisciplinary groups of physicians for treatment of patients with LBP developed by the US Department of Defense and Veteran's Administration in 2022.[45] The AOA's evidence-based guideline recommends that osteopathic physicians utilize OMT to treat somatic dysfunction found in patients with LBP. It is posted on the AOA's website, and updated in 2016.[46]

ACKNOWLEDGMENTS

The authors and editors of this chapter would like to acknowledge the scholarly contributions of student editor Reem Darwish.

REFERENCES

1. Seffinger MA, Hruby RJ. *Evidence-Based Manual Medicine: A Problem-Oriented Approach*. Saunders/Elsevier; 2007.
2. Franke H, Franke JD, Fryer G. Osteopathic manipulative treatment for nonspecific low back pain: a systematic review and meta-analysis. *BMC Musculoskelet Disorders*. 2014;15:286.
3. Task Force on the Low Back Pain Clinical Practice Guidelines. American Osteopathic Association Guidelines for Osteopathic Manipulative Treatment (OMT) for patients with low back pain. *J Am Osteopath Assoc*. 2016;116(8):536–549.
4. Greenman PE. *Principles of Manual Medicine*. 3rd ed. Lippincott Williams & Wilkins; 2003.
5. American Osteopathic Association Protocols for Osteopathic Manipulative Treatment. 1998. American Osteopathic Association. Accessed December 5, 2024. https://www.yumpu.com/en/document/read/50780256/aoa-protocols-for-omt-american-academy-of-osteopathy/
6. Chou R, Qaseem A, Snow V, et al. Diagnosis and treatment of low back pain: a joint clinical practice guideline from the American College of Physicians and the American Pain Society. *Ann Intern Med*. 2007;147(7):478–491.
7. Premkumar A, Godfrey W, Gottschalk MB, Boden SD. Red flags for low back pain are not always really red: a prospective evaluation of the clinical utility of commonly used screening questions for low back pain. *J Bone Joint Surg Am*. 2018;100(5):368–374.
8. Hurwitz EL, Shekelle PG. Epidemiology of low back syndromes. In Morris CE, ed. *Low Back Syndromes: Integrated Clinical Management*. McGraw-Hill Publishers; 2006.
9. Deyo RA, Weinstein JN. Low back pain. *N Engl J Med*. 2001;344: 363–370.
10. Groen GJ, Baljet B, Drukker J. Nerves and nerve plexuses of the human vertebral column. *Am J Anat*. 1990;188:282–296.
11. Maigne JY, Maigne R. Trigger point of the posterior iliac crest: painful iliolumbar ligament insertion or cutaneous dorsal ramus pain? An anatomic study. *Arch Phys Med Rehabil*. 1991;72(10):734–737.
12. Devereaux M. Low back pain. *Med Clin North Am*. 2009;93(2):477–501.
13. Jensen MC, Brant-Zawadzki MN, Obuchowski N, Modic MT, Malkasian D, Ross JS. Magnetic resonance imaging of the lumbar spine in people without back pain. *N Engl J Med*. 1994;331:69–73.
14. Boden SD, Davis DO, Dina TS, Patronas NJ, Wiesel SW. Abnormal magnetic-resonance scans of the lumbar spine in asymptomatic subjects: a prospective investigation. *J Bone Joint Surg Am*. 1990;72(3):403–408.
15. Papadopoulos EC, Khan SN. Piriformis syndrome and low back pain: a new classification and review of the literature. *Orthop Clin North Am*. 2004;35(1):65–71.
16. Boyajian-O'Neill LA, McClain RL, Coleman MK, Thomas PP. Diagnosis and management of piriformis syndrome: an osteopathic approach. *J Am Osteopath Assoc*. 2008;108:657–664.
17. Szadek KM, van der Wurff P, van Tulder MW, Zuurmond WWA, Perez RSGM. Diagnostic validity of criteria for sacroiliac joint pain: a systematic review. *J Pain*. 2009;10(4):354–368.
18. Slipman CW, Jackson HB, Lipetz JS, Chan KT, Lenrow D, Vresilovic EJ. Sacroiliac joint pain referral zones. *Arch Phys Med Rehabil*. 2000;81(3): 334–338.
19. Hoffman KS, Hoffman LL. Effects of adding sacral base leveling to osteopathic manipulative treatment of low back pain: a pilot study. *J Am Osteopath Assoc*. 1994;94:217–226.
20. Lipton JA, Brooks JS, Hickey MJ, Drew BG, Eggleston MT, Gemmer CH. Lift treatment in Naval Special Warfare (NSW) personnel: a retrospective study. *Am Acad Osteopath J*. 2000;(spring):31–37.
21. Lipton JA, Flowers-Johnson J, Bunnell MT, Carter L. The use of heel lifts and custom orthotics in reducing self-reported chronic musculoskeletal pain scores. *Am Acad Osteopath J*. 2009;19(1):15–17,19–20.
22. Hagen KB, Hilde G, Jamtveldt G, Winnem M. Bed rest for acute low back pain and sciatica. *Cochrane Database Syst Rev*. 2004;(4):CD001254.
23. Tarulli AW, Raynor EM. Lumbosacral radiculopathy. *Neurol Clin*. 2007; 25(2):387–405.
24. Deville WL, van der Windt DA, Dzaferagic A, Bezemer PD, Bouter LM. The test of Lasegue: systematic review of the accuracy in diagnosing herniated discs. *Spine (Phila Pa 1976)*. 2000;25(9):1140–1147.
25. Boos N, Rieder R, Schade V, Spratt KF, Semmer N, Aebi M. 1995 Volvo Award in clinical sciences. The diagnostic accuracy of magnetic resonance imaging, work perception, and psychosocial factors in identifying symptomatic disc herniations. *Spine (Phila Pa 1976)*. 1995;20(24):2613–2625.
26. Fiechtner JJ, Brodeur RR. Manual and manipulation techniques for rheumatic disease. *Rheum Dis Clin North Am*. 2000;26(1):83–96.
27. Koes BW, van Tulder MW, Thomas S. Diagnosis, and treatment of low back pain. *BMJ*. 2006;332:1430–1433.
28. Dagenais S, Caro J, Haldeman S. A systematic review of low back pain cost of illness studies in the United States and internationally. *Spine J*. 2008;8(1):8–20.
29. National Research Council and the Institute of Medicine. *Panel on Musculoskeletal Disorders and the Workplace, Commission on Behavioral and Social Sciences and Education*. National Academy Press; 2001.
30. Pincus T, Burton AK, Vogel S, Field AP. A systematic review of psychological factors as predictors of chronicity/disability in prospective cohorts of low back pain. *Spine (Phila Pa 1976)*. 2002;27:E109–E120.
31. Melloh M, Elfering A, Egli Presland C, et al. Identification of prognostic factors for chronicity in patients with low back pain: a review of screening instruments. *Int Orthop*. 2009;33(2):301–313.
32. Iles RA, Davidson M, Taylor NF. Psychosocial predictors of failure to return to work in non-chronic non-specific low back pain: a systematic review. *Occup Environ Med*. 2008;65(8):507–517.
33. Kopec JA, Sayre EC, Esdaile JM. Predictors of back pain in a general population cohort. *Spine (Phila Pa 1976)*. 2004;29(1):70–77.
34. Hestbaek L, Leboeuf-Yde C, Manniche C. Low back pain: what is the long-term course? A review of studies of general patient populations. *Eur Spine J*. 2003;12(2):149–165.
35. Deyo R, Cherkin D, Conrad D, Volinn E. Cost, controversy, crisis: low back pain and the health of the public. *Annu Rev Public Health*. 1992;12:141–155.
36. Burton AK, Clarke RD, McClune TD, Tillotson KM. The natural history of low back pain in adolescents. *Spine (Phila Pa 1976)*. 1996;21(20):2323–2328.
37. Bono CM. Current concepts review: low-back pain in athletes. *J Bone Joint Surg*. 2004;86-A:382–396.
38. Freynhagen R, Baron R, Gockel U, Tölle TR. PainDETECT: a new screening questionnaire to identify neuropathic components in patients with back pain. *Curr Med Res Opin*. 2006;22(10):1911–1920.
39. Rubinstein SM, van Tulder M. A best-evidence review of diagnostic procedures for neck and low-back pain. *Best Pract Res Clin Rheumatol*. 2008;22(3):471–482.

40. Jarvik JG, Deyo RA. Diagnostic evaluation of low back pain with emphasis on imaging. *Ann Intern Med.* 2002;137(7):586–597.
41. Manchikanti L, Glaser SE, Wolfer L, Derby R, Cohen SP. Systematic review of lumbar discography as a diagnostic test for chronic low back pain. *Pain Physician.* 2009;12(3):541–559.
42. Chou R, Deyo R, Friedly J, et al. Nonpharmacologic therapies for low back pain: a systematic review for an American College of Physicians clinical practice guideline. *Ann Intern Med.* 2017;166(7):493–505.
43. Buenaventura RM, Datta S, Abdi S, Smith HS. Systematic review of therapeutic lumbar transforaminal epidural steroid injections. *Pain Physician.* 2009;12(1):233–251.
44. Cohen SP, Argoff CE, Carragee EJ. Management of low back pain. *BMJ.* 2008;337:a2718.
45. Department of Veterans Affairs, DoD. *Va/DoD Clinical Practice Guideline for the Diagnosis and Treatment of Low Back Pain.* 3rd ed. U.S. Government Printing Office; 2022. https://www.healthquality.va.gov/guidelines/Pain/lbp/VADoDLBPCPGFinal508.pdf
46. Task Force on the Low Back Pain Clinical Practice Guidelines. American Osteopathic Association Guidelines for Osteopathic Manipulative Treatment for Patients With Low Back Pain. *J Am Osteopath Assoc.* 2016;116(8):536–549.

100 Case Study: Child with Ear Pain

MEAGHAN C. NELSEN ▪ KAREN M. STEELE ▪ MIRIAM V. MILLS

KEY CONCEPTS

- Pediatric ear pain can be caused by diseases and processes both within the ear structure and referred to the ear from distant structures.
- Structural, environmental, genetic, ethnic, and other factors predispose some children to be "otitis prone."
- Osteopathic manipulative treatment (OMT) has been shown clinically to be complementary to routine medical care of pediatric ear pain, including acute otitis media (AOM).
- Suggested OMT protocols include the treatment of biomechanical, respiratory–circulatory, neurologic, behavioral, and metabolic-energy model aspects of the pediatric patient.
- The application of OMT differs in pediatric vs. adult patients with otalgia.

CASE VIGNETTE

DW is a 2-year-old Native American female with a history of three prior ear infections in the last 12 months, who presents with irritability, pulling at her right ear, and fever of 102°F for the past day. Her appetite and usual activity level have both decreased. She had a mild upper respiratory infection the previous week, which was getting better until these symptoms presented. Her most recent ear infection, which responded to azithromycin, was 2 months prior, and was followed by documented normal tympanograms.

PAST MEDICAL HISTORY

Her first ear infection was at 6 months of age, soon after she began attending daycare. She has had no other serious illnesses or hospitalizations.

BIRTH HISTORY

She was delivered via vacuum-assisted vaginal delivery at 40 weeks gestational age to a primigravida mother. She attempted direct breastfeeding for only a week, and due to poor sucking, converted to formula feeds, requiring several formula changes during her first few months of life because of frequent vomiting. Also, during her first few months of life, she had episodes of unexplained irritability lasting up to 3 hours, usually in the evening, which resolved by 4 months of age.

DEVELOPMENTAL HISTORY

Her development has been appropriate for her age. Immunizations are up to date.

ALLERGIES

She has no known allergies to medications or food.

SOCIAL HISTORY

She lives at home with her mother who is single and works at the daycare center where the child attends. Mother smokes, but states she does not smoke around the child.

FAMILY HISTORY

There are no contributory inherited diseases, except that the mother has a history of frequent ear infections as a child, requiring placement of myringotomy/tympanostomy tubes.

REVIEW OF SYSTEMS

General

The child's mother states that "she just hasn't been herself." She is more irritable than usual and has trouble sleeping.

Respiratory

She has been congested for about a week with alternating stuffy and runny nose. There has been no coughing, wheezing, or perioral/digital cyanosis.

Gastrointestinal

Her appetite has been decreased since she became congested although she is taking fluids appropriately. There has been no diarrhea.

PHYSICAL EXAMINATION

Vital Signs

Temperature 102°F, respirations 30 per minute, and pulse 105 beats per minute.

General

The child is well hydrated but is irritable and crying.

HEENT

There is no evidence of tenderness with movement of either pinna or palpation over her jaw or face bilaterally. Her right tympanic membrane (TM) is dull and inflamed, with a fluid level of yellow pus visualized behind the TM. The left TM is retracted but pearly, and neither TM moves. There is minimal white-yellow nasal drainage, and her throat shows mild redness, but no exudates. Her 2-year molars are erupting. Neck is supple, with mild anterior cervical lymphadenopathy.

Lungs

Chest is clear to auscultation, and breathing is unlabored.

Heart

Heart is normal sinus rhythm without murmur or gallop.

Abdomen

Abdomen is soft and without organomegaly or masses.

Musculoskeletal

Extremities show no cyanosis, clubbing, or edema, and pulses are normal.

Neurologic

Neurologic exam is intact for cranial nerves (CNs), strength, reflexes, and sensation.

Osteopathic Structural Examination

Head: SBS compression, right temporal bone internally rotated, right occipitomastoid suture compression, suboccipital muscular tension noted bilaterally
Cervical: OA extended, sidebent left, and rotated right
Thoracic: thoracic inlet is flexed, sidebent, and rotated right
Lumbar: no somatic dysfunctions noted
Sacral: right SI joint somatic dysfunction
Pelvic: no somatic dysfunctions noted
Lower extremity: no somatic dysfunctions noted
Upper extremity: right internally rotated clavicle
Rib cage: right ribs 6 to 10 exhalation somatic dysfunction
Abdomen: thoracoabdominal diaphragm is flexed, sidebent right, and rotated left

LABORATORY

Rapid strep test is negative.

DIFFERENTIAL DIAGNOSIS

The causes of ear pain in children are more numerous than many would imagine. Ear pain can arise from the ear structures themselves (*primary etiology*), including the external, middle, or inner components, or from a nonotogenic origin (*secondary, or referred otalgia*), usually resulting from the complex sensory afferent innervation of the ear, which also provides innervation to a wide variety of other structures, many noncontiguous to the ear.

Primary Otalgia

Primary otalgia can arise from structural, behavioral, or metabolic/inflammatory/infectious etiologies in the external ear (otitis externa or mastoiditis) or middle ear (otitis media). Inner ear disease usually does not result in otalgia, due to the nature of its innervation (see discussion of Neurologic Model below).

Biomechanical Model

FOREIGN BODIES IN EXTERNAL AUDITORY CANAL (EAC)

Foreign bodies in the EAC in children are commonly seen in the primary care clinic and emergency department. Most can be removed under direct visualization and without general anesthesia. Impacted cerumen has also been associated with pediatric ear pain. Impacted cerumen may need a few days of softening with an over-the-counter agent prior to in-office removal with a curette or lavage.

Behavioral Model

BAROTRAUMA

Barotrauma is due to rapidly changing pressures against the TM that cannot be adequately accommodated, leading to ear pain. This is most commonly seen in descent when flying in airplanes, when the dysfunctional eustachian tube (ET) is not able to open spontaneously or with yawning or swallowing, to equilibrate the relative negative middle ear pressure. Crying commonly opens the ET, via pull of the tensor veli palatini muscle. Persistent barotitis may result in high negative middle ear pressures and development of effusion.

Metabolic-Energy Model

OTITIS EXTERNA

External ear pain is usually from one of two causes: otitis externa or a foreign body in the ear. Otitis externa can be subdivided into six distinct subgroups:

1. Acute diffuse bacterial (swimmer's ear)
2. Acute localized (furunculosis)
3. Chronic
4. Eczematous
5. Necrotizing
6. Fungal

All of these causes can give rise to exquisite ear pain, and treatment is based on the underlying cause.

OTITIS MEDIA

Of all of the causes of pain originating from the middle ear, otitis media is by far the most common. AOM is the inflammation or infection of the air-filled middle ear space. The middle ear is an air-filled space that transmits sound vibrations from the TM to the inner ear, where sound is recognized. AOM is usually accompanied by development of fluid (effusion) in the middle ear during the inflammatory process. When the middle ear space is filled with fluid, the ability of the TM to vibrate and transmit sound is impaired. Resolution of the middle ear effusion (MEE) can be from 2 to 4 weeks. Persistent MEE is the sequela of AOM for which there is as yet no widely accepted medical treatment supported by the literature.

AOM is more prevalent in children with the following demographics[1]:

- Age lesser than 3 years old
- Non-Hispanic Caucasian (this is not the same as Native American, which is the race of patient in case)
- Male gender
- Siblings
- Atopy
- Family history of recurrent ear infections
- Attendance in day care
- Not being breastfed (at least 50% of the time up to 6 months of age)

Mastoiditis is a rare, but serious, complication of bacterial AOM. Since the mastoid air space is continuous with the middle ear through the aditus ad antrum mastoideum, infection in the middle ear can spread to the mastoid air cells and, if untreated, can further spread into the brain.

SECONDARY OTALGIA

Secondary causes of otalgia in children include

- Tonsillitis (most common) (Metabolic-Energy Model)
- Foreign body in the pharynx or nose (Biomechanical Model)

- Upper respiratory congestion (Respiratory–Circulatory Model)
- Referred pain, for example, from teething (Neurologic Model)
- Dental problems, including temporomandibular disorder (TMD) (Biomechanical Model)
- Gastroesophageal reflux disorder (GERD) (Metabolic-Energy Model)

Rare reports of unusual causes of otalgia include but are not limited to the following pathologies: facial hair in the oropharynx, branchial cleft cysts, dermoid cysts, thyroglossal duct cysts, fibromyalgia, migraine cephalgia, CN neuropathies, ascariasis, thyroiditis, eccrine spiradenoma, malignancy, subdural hematoma, and Munchausen syndrome.[2]

When a child with ear pain has a normal exam of the TM, the practitioner must take into consideration the neuroanatomy of the extensive sensory innervation of the ear arising from six nerve roots, which share common neuronal pathways with many other structures in the head, neck, and thorax (see Chapter 32 Head Region for more details).

In general, young children may not verbalize or localize pain very accurately and will frequently point to the ear when experiencing teething pain, if they have experienced ear pain in the past. If a complete examination of the external and middle ear structures and careful history relating to hearing and balance functions do not point to an etiology relating to the ear structures themselves, it is important to consider the more common etiologies of referred pain, with particular attention to the more rare but insidious presentations of malignancy. A complete head and neck exam should include the nose and nasal cavities, oral cavity, pharynx (particularly teeth and tonsils), temporomandibular joint, and nasopharynx and larynx, which may require fiber-optic endoscopy. Dental appliances should be removed, if possible, to allow for a complete examination, keeping in mind that the appliances themselves may be causing nerve irritation resulting in referred pain. Ultrasound or radiologic imaging may be necessary to rule out abscess or tumor.

Many common infections of the head and neck structures refer pain in the ear in children. These include bacterial, viral, yeast, and fungal infections. Medications are useful to help decrease the amount and virulence of the offending agent to help the host recover. Of note is the viral infection herpes zoster, which may be accompanied by vesicles on the auricle, but intense otalgia may present weeks before they erupt. When this is associated with facial nerve palsy, it is called Ramsay Hunt syndrome and may also involve hearing loss and vertigo. The ear pain may persist for weeks after the vesicles resolve.

The muscles that frequently refer pain in the ear include the lateral pterygoid, the deep masseter, the clavicular sternocleidomastoid, the medial pterygoid, and the suboccipital muscles.

GASTROESOPHAGEAL REFLUX DISORDER

GERD as a potential etiology of recurrent otalgia in children has received much attention in the literature. Children presenting with otalgia secondary to gastroesophageal reflux may be fretful and irritable. Irritation of the respiratory epithelium of the larynx and pharynx by gastric acid stimulates CNs IX and X. Other symptoms may include hoarseness, dysphagia, a sensation of a lump in the throat, chronic cough, or overt intermittent wheezing. It can occur in the absence of typical symptoms of gastroesophageal reflux such as heartburn and regurgitation. Direct irritation of the opening of the ET can cause swelling and contribute to middle ear pathology. Endoscopy may demonstrate evidence of inflammation, and pH monitoring is considered the gold standard for diagnosis. In 60% to 90% of children with OME, gastric pepsin or pepsinogen can be found in middle ear fluid. This in itself may theoretically be a cause of ear pain as well as a contributor to recurrent middle ear infection; however, treatment with antacids and antireflux medication have not been successful at limiting recurrent OME in these children. This indicates that further research is needed to better define the relationship between otitis media, pepsin/pepsinogen, and GERD.[3]

Diagnosis

The diagnosis in this case is AOM, either from a viral or bacterial etiology. This child demonstrates an increased susceptibility to ear infections due to numerous factors:

1. Age and ethnicity-related anatomical and physiologic functioning of the middle ear and auditory canal or ET (Biomechanical Model)
2. A history of stress on the fetal head during delivery (Biomechanical Model)
3. Exposure to other children at the daycare and exposure to passive cigarette smoke at home (Behavioral Model)
4. Presence of somatic dysfunction of the head, neck, and torso impairing clearing of the middle ear excretions (Respiratory–Circulatory Model)
5. Presence of somatic dysfunction of the cranial base, causing pain in the head area, and compression of CNs controlling the feeding process leading to autonomic dysfunction (Neurologic Model)

OSTEOPATHIC PATIENT MANAGEMENT

DW has a history of feeding difficulties and presumed colic, which would lead the osteopathic physician to conclude that the somatic dysfunction diagnosed today has been present since birth and has contributed to feeding disorders and a long-standing impairment of middle ear functioning. In addition to the standard medical care of this child, the addition of OMT to her care is provided with the goal of hastening recovery and reducing the chance of recurrence of middle ear infection.

Dr. Viola Frymann[4] wisely notes that "...the identification of otitis media...is only the beginning. A comprehensive diagnosis of the child who suffers from the disease is essential if the etiologic factors...are to be recognized and addressed."

AOM is the most common condition treated with antibiotics, and the incidence of antibiotic-resistant bacterial strains is increasing.[1] The most common bacterial strains isolated from infected middle ears by tympanocentesis are still *S. pneumoniae*, *H. influenza*, and *M. catarrhalis*, though penicillin-resistant strains are becoming more prominent.[1] Children who have their first ear infection before 12 months old tend to have recurrent infections.[1] Racial differences in the incidence of otitis may be related to variations in cranial base morphology (see biomechanical considerations below; cranial base). It is unclear if secondhand smoke exposure is still to be considered as a risk factor as previously identified.[1]

The Clinical Practice Guideline from the American Academy of Pediatrics (AAP) on diagnosis and treatment of AOM in children published in 2013 is as follows[5]:

- AOM should be diagnosed when there is moderate to severe TM bulging or new-onset otorrhea not caused by acute otitis externa.

- AOM may be diagnosed for mild TM bulging and ear pain for less than 48 hours or for intense TM erythema. In a nonverbal child, ear holding, tugging, or rubbing suggests ear pain.
- AOM should not be diagnosed when pneumatic otoscopy and/or tympanometry does not show MEE.
- AOM management should include pain evaluation and treatment.
- Antibiotics should be prescribed for bilateral or unilateral AOM in children aged at least 6 months with severe signs or symptoms (moderate or severe otalgia or otalgia for 48 hours or longer or temperature 39 °C or higher) and for nonsevere, bilateral AOM in children aged 6 to 23 months.
- On the basis of joint decision making with the parents, unilateral, nonsevere AOM in children aged 6 to 23 months or nonsevere AOM in older children may be managed either with antibiotics or with close follow-up and withholding antibiotics unless the child worsens or does not improve within 48 to 72 hours of symptom onset.
- Amoxicillin is the antibiotic of choice unless the child received it within the past 30 days, has concurrent purulent conjunctivitis, or is allergic to penicillin. In these cases, clinicians should prescribe an antibiotic with additional β-lactamase coverage.
- Clinicians should reevaluate a child whose symptoms have worsened or not responded to the initial antibiotic treatment within 48 to 72 hours and change treatment if indicated.
- In children with recurrent AOM, tympanostomy tubes, but not prophylactic antibiotics, may be indicated to reduce the frequency of AOM episodes.
- Clinicians should recommend pneumococcal conjugate vaccine and annual influenza vaccine to all children according to updated schedules.
- Clinicians should encourage exclusive breastfeeding for 6 months or longer.

The management recommendations in this Clinical Practice Guideline are not to be applied to children with recurrent AOM within 30 days of antibiotic treatment or otitis media with effusion (OME), or children with any underlying condition that may alter the natural course of AOM, such as cleft palate, genetic conditions such as Down syndrome, immunodeficiencies, and presence of cochlear implants.

In essence, antimicrobial treatment is therefore indicated in all children who[6]:

- Are under 2 years of age as well as in children ≥2 years of age who have a temperature ≥39°C
- Are toxic looking
- Have otalgia for more than 48 hours
- Have bilateral otitis media or otorrhea
- Have craniofacial abnormalities
- Are immunocompromised
- Have uncertain access to follow-up

Observation without antibiotics is an option in immunocompetent children ≥2 years of age who have an acute uncomplicated otitis media and nonsevere illness if appropriate follow-up can be arranged.[5,6]

Osteopathic physicians have long reported favorable clinical outcomes in children treated with OMT in addition to standard medical care.[7,8] In 1928, Galbreath reported on the application of manipulation to the jaw for the treatment of "catarrh" (congestion) of the ear.[9] Various case reports, textbooks, and practice recommendations using osteopathic philosophy and principles advocating the use of OMT for the treatment of otitis media have been published in the osteopathic literature since that time, many within the last 30 years.[10–22] Four clinical trials assessing the effectiveness of OMT for children with AOM have been published.[23–26] There were no adverse events reported in these trials.

Mills et al.[23] enrolled 57 patients 6 months to 6 years old, with a history of three episodes of AOM in the previous 6 months or 4 in the previous year, who were not already surgical candidates. It was a prospective, randomized, blinded, controlled, multicenter clinical trial with two study groups: standard care plus OMT and standard care alone. Those participants who received standard pediatric medical care plus OMT demonstrated the following significant findings in comparison to standard medical care alone at 6-month follow-up:

1. Fewer episodes of AOM ($p = .04$)
2. Fewer ENT surgeries ($p = .03$)
3. More surgery-free months ($p = .01$)
4. More normal tympanograms over 6 months ($p = .02$)

Degenhardt and Kuchera[24] administered OMT weekly for 3 weeks to eight children, ages 7 to 35 months, with a history of recurrent otitis media, and then followed these subjects for 1 year. Their results showed that five subjects (62.5%) had no recurrence of symptoms during the year follow-up, one had a bulging TM, one had four episodes of otitis media, and one had surgery after AOM recurrence at 6 weeks post treatment. In addition to reduction of recurrence of otitis media, OMT has also been observed to provide immediate improvement in middle ear functioning in children as measured by tympanograms before and immediately after OMT.

Wahl et al.[25] reported on a randomized, placebo-controlled, two-by-two factorial trial with a 6-month follow-up, on participants aged 12 to 60 months with recurrent otitis media, defined as three or more separate episodes of AOM within 6 months or at least four episodes in 1 year. Ninety children (44% white non-Hispanic, 39% Hispanic, 57% male) were enrolled while well to determine if two different treatment interventions would serve to prevent recurrence of AOM. Eighty-four had follow-up for at least 3 months. Children were randomly assigned to one of four groups: double placebo, echinacea plus sham OMT, true OMT (including cranial manipulation) plus placebo echinacea, or true echinacea plus OMT. An alcohol extract of *Echinacea purpurea* roots and seeds (or placebo) was administered for 10 days at the first sign of each common cold. Five OMT visits (or sham treatments) were offered over 3 months. OMT did not significantly affect risk of getting AOM compared to sham (44% vs. 61%; relative risk, 0.72; 95% CI, 0.48, 1.10).

Steele et al.[26] reported on a dual-site, prospective, randomized, blinded, controlled clinical trial comparing osteopathic manipulative medicine (OMM) plus standard care to standard care only for MEE after an episode of AOM. Standard care consisted of antibiotics and surgery. Participants were children aged 6 to 24 months with abnormal tympanograms indicative of MEE. Forty-three participants completed the study. Participants were between 6 and 24 months old and had 5 weekly study visits, although those in the intervention group received OMM on visits 1 through 3. Patients received weekly tympanogram and acoustic reflectometer (AR) readings as well as daily at-home AR readings for 30 days. Tympanogram data demonstrated a statistically significant improvement in MEE at visit 3 in patients in the standard care plus OMM group (odds ratio, 2.98; 95% CI, 1.16, 7.62; χ^2 test for independence, $p = .02$). The AR data analysis also showed statistically significant improvement at visit 3 for the standard care plus OMM group ($z = 2.05$; $p = .02$).

OMT in children with AOM is directed toward structural impediments to optimum functioning (Biomechanical Model), improvement of middle ear drainage (Respiratory–Circulatory Model), reduction of compression neuropathies affecting functioning of the oropharynx and upper gastrointestinal system and causing pain (Neurologic Model), improvement of the environment in which the child lives (Behavioral Model), and reducing the stress of infection and hearing impairment so the child can exist in their environment with greater functionality and contentment (Behavioral Model) (for a discussion of specific osteopathic techniques for each of these goals, please see the discussion of each model below).

OMT targeted to dysfunctions of the head and neck area as well as postural treatment and education are commonly helpful (Biomechanical Model). OMT without postural realignment and reeducation will generally not provide long-term relief.

If the parent has been trained in the Galbreath mandibular drainage OMT procedure, doing this procedure during descent when flying in an airplane may assist the child in equilibrating the middle ear pressure and hence reduce the pain. Treatment of the underlying ET dysfunction is the recommended means of preventing barotitis. Anatomical and functional changes during maturation of the cranial base and ET make barotitis less likely as the child ages (for a discussion of the rationale for osteopathic treatment to improve ET functioning, please see "The Cranial Base and the Eustachian Tube" section below).

OMT for infections of the head and neck region is used to improve lymphatic circulation and respiratory chest wall excursion (Respiratory–Circulatory Model); reduce pain and dysfunction by relieving compression or irritation of central, autonomic, or peripheral nerves (Neurologic Model); and improve cranial bone and reciprocal tension membrane compliance and reduce muscle spasm of the cervical area that exacerbates pain and reduces mobility (Biomechanical Model). However, direct treatment of the infected areas of the head and neck area should not be performed until the infection is under control with medical management. For example, the addition of OMT in the treatment of mastoiditis should be limited to treatment designed to improve the functioning of the lymphatic system, and no direct treatment of the head and neck should be performed until the mastoid infection is under control. Such a treatment could include myofascial release of the thoracic inlet and abdominal diaphragm and rib raising (Respiratory–Circulatory Model) (see Chapter 83 Osteopathic Considerations in Patients with Head, Eyes, Ears, Nose, and Throat Disorders for further discussion of OMT approaches to head and neck dysfunctions).

TMD often responds to OMT, especially when it relates to orthodontic treatment. In a child with a clear-cut recent history of minor head trauma involving the temporal bone such as a whiplash or fall on the chin, a brief trial of OMT might be warranted and may clear the symptoms completely. The OMT for TMD secondary to dental intervention or head trauma is specific for the somatic dysfunction(s) found and commonly requires treatment of the head using osteopathic cranial manipulative medicine techniques. Examination and treatment of the child's entire body are necessary following trauma in order to remove somatic dysfunction in areas distant to the head that are causing strain and impaired functioning of the TMD (Biomechanical Model).

Compression of the cranial base is a common osteopathic finding seen in children with GERD. From the osteopathic perspective, this compression leads to impingement of the vagus nerve resulting in ineffective closure of the lower esophageal sphincter and reflux of stomach contents.[19] OMT is often helpful in reducing the severity of the reflux, using the whole-body approach. Impaired gastric emptying may occur from spasm of the abdominal diaphragm and can be treated with indirect and direct myofascial techniques (Biomechanical Model). Soft tissue techniques to the upper cervical area reduce impingement of cervical nerves 3 to 5 innervating the diaphragm, and occipital decompression techniques reduce compression on the vagus nerve as it exits the jugular foramen, resulting in improved lower esophageal sphincter functioning and reduction of pain mediated via the vagus nerve (Neurologic Model).

The following discussion will review the biomechanical factors affecting middle ear function and the appropriate use of OMT in the treatment of middle ear disease in children.

Biomechanical Model

THE CRANIAL BASE AND THE EUSTACHIAN TUBE

Middle ear disease is most commonly related to ET dysfunction.[27–29] Under normal conditions, the ET fluctuates between a patent and closed position. Middle ear pressure is equilibrated with atmospheric pressure through the periodic openings of the ET that occur with swallowing and other activities. In children, middle ear pressures are slightly negative compared to adults, and most children, even those without middle ear disease, have difficulty in maintaining appropriate pressures. The ability to maintain appropriate pressures appears to be related to the stiffness and diameter of the ET. If the ET is too compliant or narrow, the resulting negative pressure may promote insufflation, aspiration, or reflux of nasopharyngeal secretions into the middle ear. ET in children with chronic otitis media has been found to be associated with smaller diameter of the ET in the affected ear(s),[27] horizontal level of the ET that inhibits drainage of the middle ear by gravitational forces and patterns and rate of cranial development.[28,29]

Within the Biomechanical Model, ET dysfunction is thought to be influenced by mechanical dysfunctions of the cranial base or the surrounding tissues. The child's cranial base and ET differ anatomically and physiologically from those of the adult in ways that make them more vulnerable to otitis media. At birth, the temporal bone is in three parts: the squamous portion, the petrous portion, and the tympanic ring, joined by cartilage.[21] The ET travels through the petrous portion of the temporal bone, emerging into a cartilaginous sheath, closely adherent to the base of the skull, nestled between the greater wing of the sphenoid and the petrous portion of the temporal bone, emerging into the posterior pharynx at the posterior edge of the medial pterygoid plate of the sphenoid. The juncture, between the osseous and the cartilaginous portions, resembles two "truncated cones," narrower than both portions of the adjacent tube. The tube is lined with pseudostratified columnar epithelium of the ciliated type, continuous with the lining of the tympanic cavity and nasopharynx at each end. It is also tethered at each end by fibrous attachments, at the posterior end extending into the osseous portion by approximately 3 mm, and at the anteromedial end, the cartilage protrudes into the nasopharynx with fibrous bands attaching it to a tubercle on the posterior edge of the medial pterygoid plate.[30]

It is noteworthy that the timing of the decline in frequency of ear infections, about 6 years of age, seems to coincide with the maturation of the cranial base and adjacent structures.[28] The relationship of the tube to other contiguous structures, particularly the tensor veli palatini, the levator veli palatini, and the salpingopharyngeus muscles, and the difference between the characteristics of the cartilage between children and adults may contribute to biomechanical forces acting upon the ET in young children.[21] The medial bundle of the tensor veli palatini muscle lies immediately adjacent to the lateral membranous wall of the ET and, when contracted, opens the tube. This muscle curves around the hamulus of the medial pterygoid plate of the sphenoid and attaches to the posterior margin of the hard palate. In children with cleft palate, its function is less than optimal. In infants, the angle of this muscle to the tube is more acute, placing it closer to the middle ear. When contracted, the tensor veli palatini may actually distort the ET rather than effectively open it.[30] Spasm of this muscle, which is comparatively large compared to the tube in infants, may conversely cause the tube to be patulous, leaving it vulnerable to influx of pharyngeal organisms. Carreiro[21] also suggests a possible contribution of the medial pterygoid muscle, which is comparatively bulkier in the infant, to extrinsic compression on the ET in contraction. Figures 100.1, 100.2, and 100.3A,B demonstrate the relationship of these structures.

Other differences between the adult and the pediatric ET include the fact that the infant's tube is more compliant (and therefore more floppy), smaller in diameter, and shorter in length. There is also a difference in the relationship of the ET as it enters the posterior pharyngeal wall. In the infant, the cartilaginous tube lies at a 10- to 30-degree angle from the horizontal in relation to the osseous portion, although, in adults, it is increased to 45 to 50 degrees.[21,28,30] At the same time, the posterior pharyngeal tissues are relatively more anterior and superior in the child. These differences are due to changes in the shape of the cranial base and the growth of the lower facial bones. The smaller angulation may act to narrow the junction between the two components of the ET, while the position of the posterior pharynx may narrow the orifice of the tube.

The articulation between the temporal and sphenoid changes angle at the point that the ET emerges from the temporal bone. The Biomechanical Model suggests that via its myofascial structures, neck and jaw movements may contribute to passive pumping actions on the ET, "milking" it and helping clear it of secretions.

Skull base configuration is also implicated in explaining the clustering of otitis in certain families and in individuals with skull base malformations such as Down syndrome, Apert syndrome,

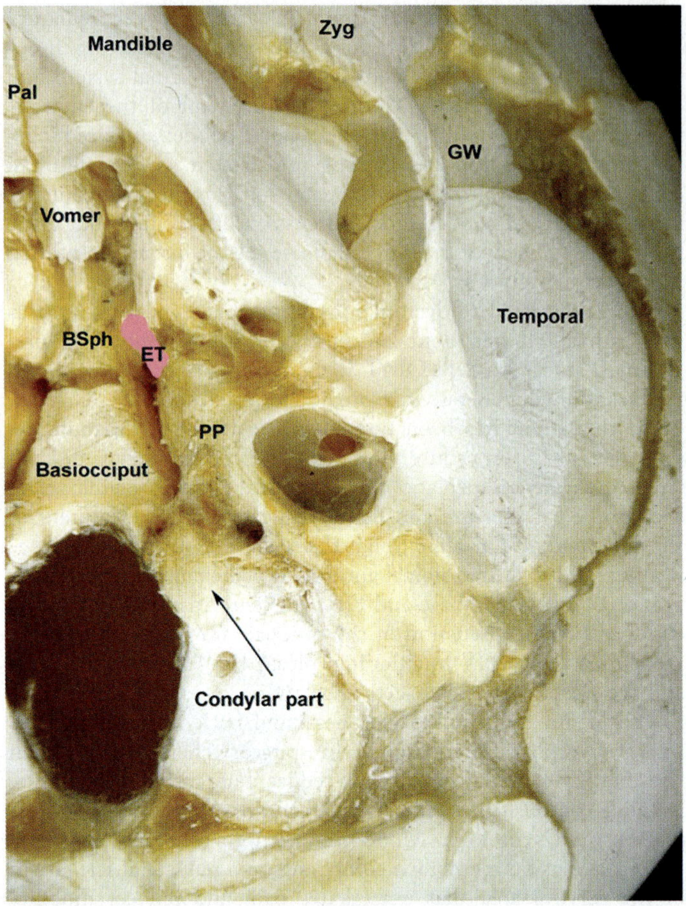

Figure 100.1. Photograph showing location of ET between petrous portion of the temporal bone and the basisphenoid. GW, greater wing of the sphenoid; PP, petrous portion of the temporal bone; Et, eustachian tube; BSph, basisphenoid. (Used with permission from the Willard/Carreiro Collection, University of New England.)

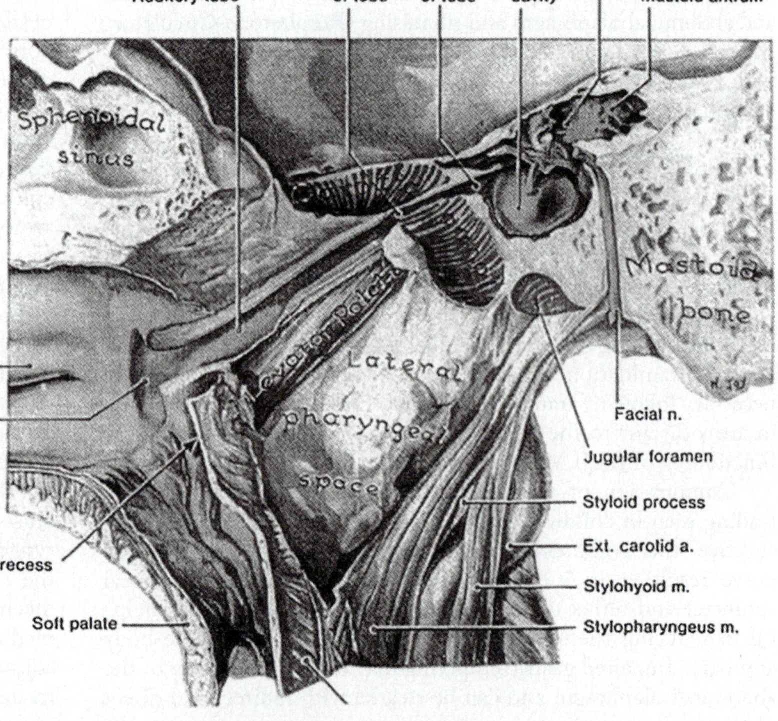

Figure 100.2. Interior view of relationship of ET to adjacent structures in the adult. (From Centers S, Morelli MA, Vallad-Hix C, Seffinger MA. General pediatrics. In: Ward RC, ed. *Foundations for Osteopathic Medicine.* 2nd ed. Lippincott Williams & Wilkins; 2003:315–316.)

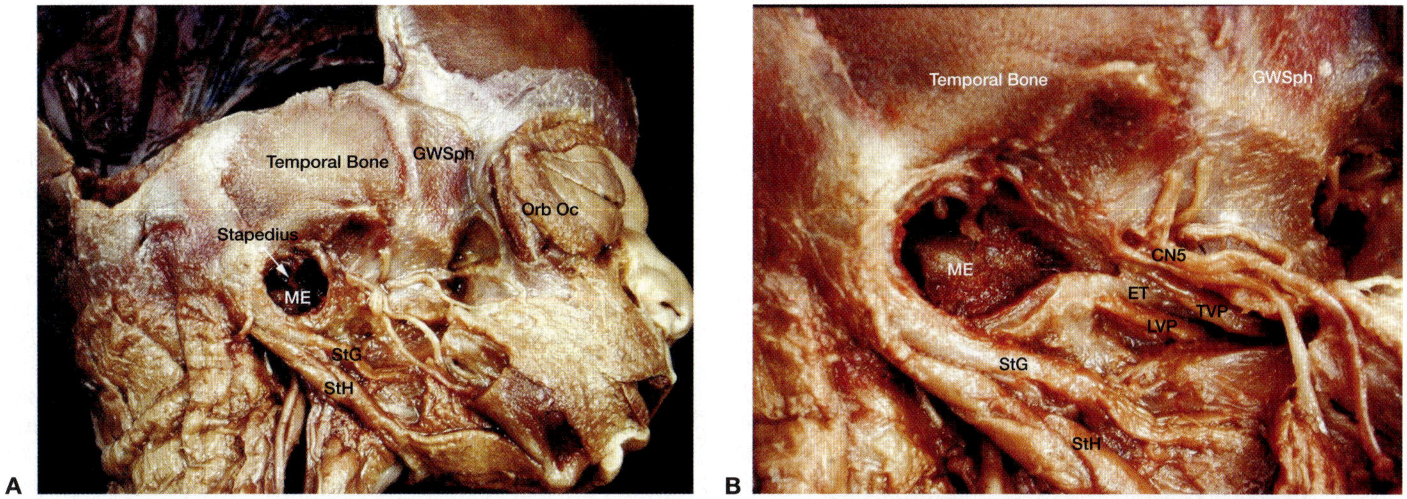

Figure 100.3. **A.** Lateral view of neonatal dissection. The mandible and zygoma bones have been cut and the muscles of mastication removed. The TM has collapsed, revealing the middle ear (ME) and malleus. The styloglossus (StG) and stylohyoid (StH), orbicularis oculi (ORbOc), mandibular branch of the trigeminal (V3), and greater wing of the sphenoid (GWSph) are labeled. **B.** Close-up of area indicated by the arrow in (**A**). The lateral aspect of the temporal bone has been drilled away to reveal the ET surrounded by the tensor veli palatine (TVP) and levator veli palatini (LVP) muscles. Note the relative size of the muscles as compared to the ET. The middle ear (ME), styloglossus (StG), stylohyoid (StH), greater wing of the sphenoid (GWSph), and ophthalmic branch of the trigeminal nerve (V3) are labeled. (**A** and **B**, used with permission from the Willard/Carreiro Collection, University of New England.)

Crouzon syndrome, Treacher Collins syndrome, Hurler–Hunter syndrome, and Turner syndrome.[30] There is a difference in the frequency of ear infections racially, with decreased incidence described by some in African Americans and Chinese and increased in Native American, Canadian, and Alaskan Native children.

According to Sutherland model, the base of the cranium undergoes rhythmic changes that can be palpated.[11] This phasic change is basic to the concept of osteopathic cranial manipulative medicine. Understanding this model allows the osteopathic practitioner to predict the potential effects of palpated strains on middle ear functioning. According to this model, the cranial base and temporal bone are vulnerable to both compressive and tensile mechanical stress. Furthermore, tissue strains of the cranial base and the contiguous soft tissue may influence ET function, as well as potentially all structures above, below, or penetrating the cranial base.[11] For most children, the process of birth is the most profound force their head experiences.

Carreiro has hypothesized that mechanical strains may contribute to edema of the tissues surrounding the ET.[21] This in turn may influence intravascular fluid exchange in the middle ear, drainage of the tube, and fluid flow through its lymphatic and venous channels. In the newborn, the structures of the cranial base are somewhat malleable, allowing for passage through the birth canal and for the rapid growth (doubling in size) of the head in the first year of life. This same malleability makes the cranial base vulnerable to compression or distortion during delivery.

Pilot studies suggest that OMM, and specifically OCMM, may be relevant in treating patients with otitis media and serous otitis media.[23,24] Figure 100.4 shows a child receiving OMT in the form of OCMM, for treatment of AOM, with the parent nearby.

Using chart analysis, Carreiro[21] describes somatic dysfunction of the vault often associated with biomechanical strains in the cranial base and venous sinus system. She hypothesizes that the vault findings are probably secondary and recommends normalizing the base mechanics first. Magoun[11] describes a number of techniques that may be used in infants and children to facilitate function of the ET and the surrounding tissues. These techniques are used to promote more physiologic functioning of lymph, blood, and nerves in the head. The gentle techniques recommended for OMT in children[16] have been shown to be well tolerated, with few side effects and no serious adverse events reported.[31]

Respiratory–Circulatory Model

It is important to have perfect drainage, for without it, the good results from a treatment cannot be expected to follow the osteopathic physician's efforts to relieve diseases above the neck.[7]

The middle ear is continuous with the posterior pharynx via the ET and with the mastoid air cells via the narrow aditus and antrum. Ideally, it is filled only with air and serves to transmit sound waves from the TM to the fenestra vestibuli and the eighth CN. Because of various factors, primarily associated with ET dysfunction, the middle ear may become filled with fluid. If the fluid is not drained naturally, surgery may be considered. OMT may provide a means of facilitating the natural drainage of the middle ear, thereby potentially averting recurrence of infection, antimicrobial resistance, and even surgery.[23]

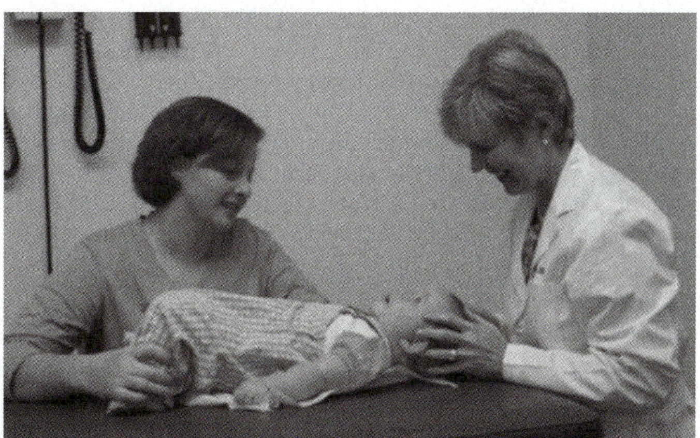

Figure 100.4. Child receiving osteopathic manipulative treatment for AOM with parent nearby, utilizing OCF technique. (Photo courtesy of Dr. Steele.)

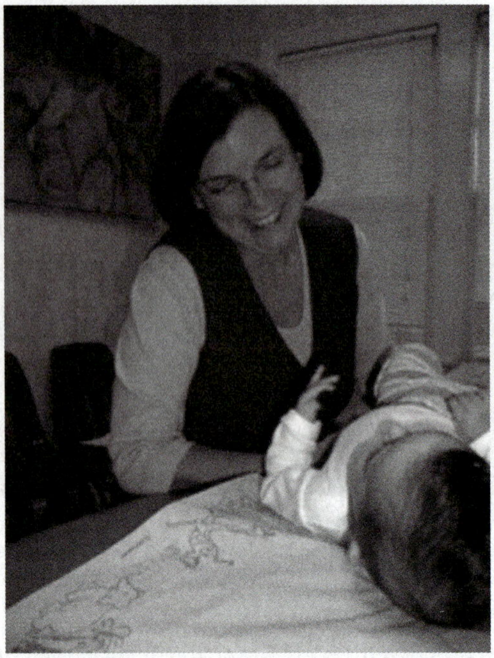

Figure 100.5. Child receiving OMT of the pelvis to assist with function of middle ear drainage. (Photo courtesy of Dr. Mills.)

The body has many natural mechanisms to ensure drainage of the middle ear, so that an air-filled space can be maintained. These include a dense lymphatic and venous network and the natural pumping mechanisms associated with sucking and swallowing. William Sutherland, DO,[10] described another mechanism, a rhythmic motion in the tissues of the cranium occurring 10 to 14 times/min. He hypothesized that this rhythmic motion in the cranial tissues acted to facilitate ET functioning. Some osteopaths have reported an association between impairments in this "cranial rhythmic motion" and otitis media.[23,32,33]

Within the Respiratory–Circulatory Model, chewing, crying, and sucking influence venous and lymphatic structures in the head and neck facilitating tissue perfusion and drainage. In addition, neck movements are thought to provide intermittent tensile forces on the ET and surrounding structures influencing fluid movement through the low-pressure circulatory system.

The Respiratory–Circulatory Model recognizes that breathing and crying alter intrathoracic pressures and contribute to fluid drainage from the head and neck. Within the concept of this model, crawling and walking may affect the circulatory system by generating intermittent tensions on the thoracic outlet via the myofascial attachments of the upper extremities and shoulder girdle, as well as the abdominal diaphragm and lower ribs via the myofascial attachments of the iliocostalis and the crura of the diaphragm. Figure 100.5 demonstrates a child receiving OMT for treatment of pelvic somatic dysfunction, with the goal of improving function of the respiratory–circulatory system and indirectly influencing middle ear drainage.

Neurologic Model

An appreciation of the complex sensory innervations of the structures surrounding the ear and the interaction of these same nerves with other, sometimes more distant, structures may facilitate understanding of the many potentially confusing possible etiologies of otalgia. The ear structures are provided sensory innervation by CNs V, VII, IX, and X and by cervical nerves 2 and 3.

It is important to keep in mind that there is considerable variability among individuals. Though there is no role of the CN VIII in carrying pain fibers from the inner ear, resulting in the observation that significant inner ear pathology can develop without otalgia, sensation mediated by this nerve can be felt by the patient as a "fullness" in the ear, such as is seen in Ménière disease.[34] Clinically, areas innervated by CN IX may refer an intense pain deep in the ear. There is no evidence of referral of pain from ear pathology to the distal structures.[35]

These complex interrelationships are the result of embryologic development, stemming from the otic vesicle coming to lie between the branchial arches 1, 2, 3, and 4, giving rise to CNs V, VII, IX, and X, respectively.[35] The autonomic nerve supply to the upper respiratory tract including the middle ear and sinuses consists of parasympathetic stimulation via the CN VII and sympathetic stimulation via T1–T4.

It is useful to be aware of the location and pathways of these nerves and their ganglia, as somatic dysfunction along the way may contribute to otalgia, and relief of those strain patterns might benefit the patient, even if no underlying cause is found for the ear pain.

There are complex immunohistochemical changes associated with ear pain that may contribute to the pathophysiology of otitis media. Nagaraj and Linthicum[36] described the presence of catecholaminergic nerve fibers in the human middle ear mucus membrane that may play an important role in the pathogenesis of MEEs. Animal studies of the role of substance P in osteoclastogenesis, a common finding in otitis media, and the effect of capsaicin (substance P inhibitor) pretreatment on the neurogenic inflammatory component of otitis media[37,38] led researchers to investigate the role of substance P in AOM and MEE in children. Indeed, Eyigor et al. found high levels of substance P in children with MEE, more so in those 2 to 3 years of age.[39] Although Teodorczyk-Injeyan[40] found that spinal manipulation may reduce inflammatory cytokines but not substance P production in normal subjects, it is unknown whether OMT has an effect on substance P levels in children with AOM and MEE. These findings suggest potential objective markers for monitoring the potential downregulation of neurogenic and inflammatory responses to manipulation. Whether these findings can explain the improvement of pain in patients receiving OMT for AOM and MEE remains to be determined.

The fact that our case child had a difficult delivery and problems sucking does not surprise the osteopathically oriented physician. The history of colic and spitting up may be related to the patient's somatic dysfunction. Frymann's classic study of 1,250 newborns correlated specific areas of somatic dysfunction on osteopathic examination with distinct symptomatology in the newborn.[32] Carreiro[21] postulates that babies with compression dysfunction at the cranial base may also develop symptoms as they start to develop head control, adding more muscle tension to an area already irritated, thereby exacerbating pre-existing somatic dysfunction.

It is the experience of osteopathic practitioners worldwide, and over many years of observation, that there is an association between recurrent AOM and a difficult or rapid delivery.[10,19,21] These same authors also report that children with recurrent AOM are often firstborn and frequently have a concomitant history of colic, dacryostenosis, feeding difficulties, or gastroesophageal reflux in the newborn period. There may also be an association with GERD in DW, which is thought to either be a vagal–vagal reflex or have an inflammatory component. From an osteopathic perspective, gastrointestinal motility and function of the gastroesophageal junction may be influenced by somatic dysfunction in the cranial base via vagal input or thoracolumbar somatic dysfunction influencing the diaphragmatic contribution to the gastroesophageal sphincter. Children who are "otitis prone" also have more episodes of bronchopulmonary, gastrointestinal, and urinary tract infections, as well as more visits to the orthopedic clinic than control subjects.[30] This might lead one to suggest that somatic dysfunction may be a common denominator of these problems.

Metabolic-Energy Model

Good nutrition is a staple of good health. Children, who are undernourished or poorly nourished, may be at greater risk for infectious diseases such as otitis media and less able to respond to therapy. Nutritional supplements have gained favor in some communities, as has an emphasis on eating organic and locally grown foods. See Chapter 22 Energy Balance: Nutrition, Exercise, and the Metabolic Model for further information on dietary requirements for health.

Treatment and Outcome

DW was treated with ibuprofen to achieve pain control and given a prescription for amoxicillin–clavulanate, to be filled if DW's symptoms were not resolved in 48 hours. She was also treated with OMT, consisting of Galbreath mandibular drainage; temporal decompression; occipitomastoid decompression; myofascial release of the upper cervical musculature, thoracic outlet, and abdominal diaphragm; and rib-raising techniques. DW tolerated the procedure very well. Mother was advised to quit smoking and was taught to do the Galbreath mandibular drainage, rib-raising, and lymphatic pump techniques and advised to do them twice daily until recheck. At recheck 2 weeks later, the ear examination was normal and tympanograms were normal.

Behavioral Model

ENVIRONMENTAL AND COMPLEMENTARY MEASURES FOR MIDDLE EAR DISEASE

As previously discussed, socioeconomic and environmental factors have been shown to influence the occurrence of otitis media. For children who are unable to control their surroundings, it falls to the physician to encourage healthy habits in the family that might reduce the risk of recurrence. Considering the particulars of the patient and their home situation, the physician needs to encourage mom to breastfeed, avoid bottle-feeding when supine, avoid exposure to smoke and other environmental toxins and allergens, avoid crowded settings and early child care,[1] and teach hygiene, hand washing, and avoidance of sharing cups among family members. The physician also needs to consider the role of comorbidities such as gastroesophageal reflux, which may predispose to recurrent otitis media. In order to prevent possible bacterial contamination, or oral yeast infection, it is helpful to educate the parent to AVOID doing the following:

- Mix bottles of milk for prolonged room-temperature storage
- Store pacifiers in airtight containers
- Store milk bottles with nipples attached in the refrigerator
- Reuse unconsumed formula after a particular feeding

Parents should also be informed of the most current recommendations of the Center for Disease Control (CDC) for administration of vaccines, such as pneumococcal and *Haemophilus influenzae* type b, in infants and children, which have been shown to reduce the incidence and transmission of respiratory disease, and its secondary AOM.

Physicians need to be aware that some parents may choose to treat their children without prior examination by a health care professional. For the sake of the child, it is very important that the physician maintain a relationship with these parents and not alienate them. Physicians should educate parents as to the warning signs of worsening infection, sepsis, meningitis, and other serious complications of untreated infection. The practitioner should also be aware that a systematic review of serious adverse effects of unconventional therapies for children and adolescents revealed the greatest number of adverse events to occur secondary to herbal medicines.[41]

Parents often feel helpless when their child is ill. This can exacerbate their anxiety and influence their response to the sick child and perhaps even the child's perception of own illness. Interventions that empower the parent without risk to the child may prove beneficial to both on many levels. It is sometimes comforting to apply mild heat to the outer ear, in the form of warm washcloth, heating pad, or hair dryer. A common folk remedy for otalgia is warmed sweet oil, garlic oil, mineral oil, or olive oil instilled in the ear canal. There is no evidence of efficacy, but these pose no threat to the child as long as the eardrum is intact.

In addition, parents may also be taught simple osteopathic techniques such as lymphatic pump, rib raising, or Galbreath mandibular drainage, which can be administered at the first signs of an upper respiratory tract infection. Schmidt's classic study of 100 patients with upper, middle, and pararespiratory illnesses, 63%, who were treated within day 1 of their illness, compared with 34%, who received OMT greater than 2 days after onset of symptoms, showed more rapid resolution of symptoms, fewer complications, and fewer recurrences in the early-treated group.[12] Given that busy medical practices (and busy parent schedules) may not accommodate same-day appointments for patients with very early respiratory symptoms, the possibility of involving parents early in the child's illness may prove beneficial.

NOTES ON TREATING CHILDREN WITH OMT

Treating children with OMT presents some unique challenges, but the practitioner should not be daunted, as the benefits can be enormously rewarding. Children are not just small adults. Their bodies are more flexible, more resilient, and less complex than adults. Their somatic dysfunction is easier to fix, and doing so can be life changing. Parents can be taught many activities of daily living that can improve somatic dysfunction in children. The normal squirming of a child, though it may be distracting to the practitioner, may actually help in the treatment. Treating children takes flexibility and time to develop trust, using positions familiar to the child, face-on first, such as with changing a diaper, or allowing the child to sit in the parent's lap. Toys, books, and frequent changes in position are often necessary to keep the child engaged. In some children, particularly 2-year-olds, brief gentle restraint may be necessary during the treatment.

CONCLUSION

The treatment of a child with ear pain begins with a history and physical to determine the cause of the pain. Working within the osteopathic paradigm, an evaluation for predisposing dysfunction of the entire body is a part of the physical examination. The diagnosis includes consideration of the anatomical and functional differences in the child's head and neck, as compared to the adult.

Treatment is directed to the identified cause of the pain, as well as removing predisposing factors in the child's body with the use of OMT, when appropriate. Factors in the environment that are modifiable are addressed to improve the overall health of the child.

REFERENCES

1. Kaur R, Morris M, Pichichero ME. Epidemiology of acute otitis media in the postpneumococcal conjugate vaccine era. *Pediatrics.* 2017;140(3): pii.e20170181.
2. Steele KM, Mills MV. Child with ear pain. In: Chila AG, Ex. ed. *Foundations of Osteopathic Medicine.* 3rd ed. Wolters Kluwer, LWW; 2010.
3. Miura MS, Mascaro M, Rosenfield RM. Association between otitis media and gastroesophageal reflux. *Otolaryngol Head Neck Surg.* 2012;146(3): 345–352.
4. King HH, ed. *The Collected Papers of Viola M. Frymann, DO.* Legacy of Osteopathy to Children. American Academy of Osteopathy; 1998.
5. Lieberthal AS, Carroll AE, Chonmaitree T, et al. The diagnosis and management of acute otitis media. From the American Academy of Pediatrics Clinical Practice Guideline. *Pediatrics.* 2013;131:e964–e999.
6. Leung AK, Wong AHC. Acute otitis media in children. *Recent Pat Inflamm Allergy Drug Discov.* 2017;11(1):32–40.
7. Still AT. *Philosophy of Osteopathy.* A. T. Still publisher; 1899.
8. Still AT. *Osteopathy: Research and Practice.* Eastland Press; 1910.
9. Galbreath WO. Chronic catarrhal otitis media. *J Am Osteopath Assoc.* 1928;639.
10. Woods R. Osteopathic care of neonates and children. *Osteopath Ann.* 1976;34(4):512–515.
11. Magoun HI. *Osteopathy in the Cranial Field.* 3rd ed. Journal Printing Co.; 1976.
12. Schmidt I. Osteopathic manipulative therapy as a primary factor in the management of upper, middle, and pararespiratory infections. *J Am Osteopath Assoc.* 1982;81(6):382–388.
13. Schmidt MA. *Childhood Ear Infections: What Every Parent and Physician Should Know About Prevention, Home Care, and Alternative Treatment.* North Atlantic Books; 1990.
14. Pintal WJ, Kurtz ME. An integrated osteopathic approach in acute otitis media. *J Am Osteopath Assoc.* 1989;89(9):1139–1141.
15. Heatherington JS. Manipulation of the eustachian tube. *AAO J.* 1995;5: 27–28.
16. Bezilla TA. Acute otitis media: an osteopathic approach. *J POMA.* 1997; 8–12.
17. Pratt-Harrington D. Galbreath technique: a manipulative treatment for otitis media revisited. *J Am Osteopath Assoc.* 2000;100:635–639.
18. Centers S, Morelli MA, Vallad-Hix C, et al. General pediatrics. In: Ward R, ed. *Foundations for Osteopathic Medicine.* 2nd ed. Lippincott Williams & Wilkins; 2003:315–316.
19. Sergueef N. *Cranial Osteopathy for Infants, Children and Adolescents.* Churchill Livingstone Elsevier; 2007.
20. Channell MK. Modified Muncie technique: osteopathic manipulation for eustachian tube dysfunction and illustrative report of case. *J Am Osteopath Assoc.* 2008;108:260–263.
21. Carreiro JA. *An Osteopathic Approach to Children.* 2nd ed. Churchill Livingstone. Elsevier Science Limited; 2009.
22. Carreiro JE. *Pediatric Manual Medicine. An Osteopathic Approach.* Churchill Livingstone. Elsevier Science Limited; 2009.
23. Mills MV, Henley CE, Barnes LLB, Carreiro JE, Degenhardt BF. The use of osteopathic manipulative treatment as adjuvant therapy in children with recurrent acute otitis media. *Arch Pediatr Adolesc Med.* 2003;157: 861–866.
24. Degenhardt BJ, Kuchera ML. Osteopathic evaluation and manipulative treatment in reducing the morbidity of otitis media: a pilot study. *J Am Osteopath Assoc.* 2006:106(6);327–334.
25. Wahl RA, Aldous MB, Worden KA, Grant KL. *Echinacea purpurea* and osteopathic manipulative treatment in children with recurrent otitis media: a randomized controlled trial. *BMC Complement Altern Med.* 2008;8(56):56.
26. Steele KM, Carreiro JE, Viola JH, Conte JA, Ridpath LC. Effect of osteopathic manipulative treatment on middle ear effusion following acute otitis media in young children: a pilot study. *J Am Osteopath Assoc.* 2014;114(6):436–447.
27. Paltura C, Can TS, Yilmaz BK, Dinç ME, Develioğlu ÖN, Külekçi M. Eustachian tube diameter: is it associated with chronic otitis media development? *Am J Otolaryngol.* 2017;38(4):414–416.
28. Pagano AS, Wang E, Yuan D, et al. Cranial indicators identified for peak incidence of otitis media. *Anat Rec (Hoboken).* 2017;300(10):1721–1740.
29. Han WG, Yoo J, Rah YC, et al. Analysis of Eustachian tube dysfunction by dynamic slow motion video endoscopy and Eustachian tube dysfunction questionnaire in chronic otitis media. *Clin Exp Otorhinolaryngol.* 2017;10(4):315–320.
30. Bluestone CD, Simons JP, Healy GB. *Bluestone and Stool's Pediatric Otolaryngology.* 5th ed. Vol. 1. Saunders, Elsevier Science; 2014.
31. Hayes NM, Bezilla TA. Incidence of iatrogenesis associated with osteopathic manipulative treatment of pediatric patients. *J Am Osteopath Assoc.* 2006;106(10):605–608.
32. Frymann VM. Relation of disturbance of craniosacral mechanism to symptomatology of the newborn: study of 1,250 infants. *J Am Osteopath Assoc.* 1966;65:1059–1075.
33. Degenhardt BF, Kuchera ML. The prevalence of cranial dysfunction in children with a history of otitis media from kindergarten to third grade. *J Am Osteopathic Assoc.* 1994;94:754.
34. Shah RK, Blevins NH. Otalgia. *Otolaryngol Clin N Am.* 2003;36(6): 1137–1151.
35. Scarbrough TJ, Day TA, Williams TE, Hardin JH, Aguero EG, Thomas CR Jr. Referred otalgia in head and neck cancer: a unifying schema. *Am J Clin Oncol.* 2003;26(5):e157–e161.
36. Nagaraj BS, Linthicum FH. Autonomic innervation of the human middle ear: an immunohistochemical study. *Am J Otolaryngol.* 1998;19(2):75–82.
37. Basak S, Dikicioglu E, Turkutanit S, Sarierler M. Early and late effects of capsaicin pretreatment in otitis media with effusion. *Otol Neurotol.* 2005;26(3):344–350.
38. Sohn SJ. Substance P upregulates osteoclastogenesis by activating nuclear factor kappa B in osteoclast precursors. *Acta Otolaryngol.* 2005;125(2): 130–133.
39. Eyigor H, Osma U, Yilmaz MD, Eyigor M, Gultekin M, Erin N. Substance P and vasoactive intestinal peptide levels in middle ear effusions of children. *Acta Otolaryngol.* 2012;132(10):1036–1041.
40. Teodorczyk-Injeyan JA, Injeyan HS, Ruegg R. Spinal manipulative therapy reduces inflammatory cytokines but not substance P production in normal subjects. *J Manipulative Physiol Ther.* 2006;29(1):14–21.
41. Ernst E. Serious adverse effects of unconventional therapies for children and adolescents: a systematic review of recent evidence. *Eur J Pediatr.* 2003;162:72–80.

101 Case Study: Uncontrolled Asthma

ROBERT G. LUCAS

KEY CONCEPTS

- Asthma is an obstructive pulmonary disease with an inflammatory component.
- The dynamic balance between sympathetic and parasympathetic influences in the lungs is distorted in asthma.
- Anatomical and physiologic immaturity in young children with asthma results in vulnerability to respiratory muscle fatigue, inefficiency of diaphragmatic mechanics, and ineffectiveness of tissue recoil.
- Biomechanical, respiratory–circulatory, metabolic, and neurologic influences need to be considered in managing a child with asthma.
- Osteopathic manipulative medicine used with standard care may reduce the severity of asthma symptoms and decrease the need for pharmaceutical management.

CASE VIGNETTE

CHIEF COMPLAINT

A 9-year-old female patient with a history of asthma was brought from school to the outpatient clinic by her mother. This patient was well known to the clinic, as she has been seen two to three times per week for her symptoms. She has often come to the clinic during school hours.

HISTORY OF PRESENT ILLNESS

The patient has been inconsistent with her medication usage in the past. On this particular visit, the patient ran out of her albuterol metered dose inhaler (MDI) and was having an asthma attack. The clinic staff approached the patient somewhat dismissively, stating that the patient was only trying to get out of school.

Past Medical History

She has had recurrent upper respiratory tract infections with exacerbation of wheezing and cough. The patient has been hospitalized four times because of asthma exacerbations but has never been ventilated. Her last hospitalization was 2 years ago. She has had many emergency room visits because of her asthma. As an infant, she had acid reflux and recurrent ear infections.

Past Surgical History

Positive for tympanoplasty and tympanostomy tubes at 8 months of age and 2 years.

Family History

Her father is 36 with anxiety/depressive disorder and hypertension. Her mother is 34 with irritable bowel syndrome. Both parents smoked until 2 years ago. She has one elder sister with scoliosis and two younger sisters in good health except for ear infections as infants.

Social History

The patient lives at home with her parents and three sisters. The family is economically challenged, and there is some concern regarding her and her family's ability to comprehend and adhere to medical instructions regarding her asthma therapy.

Medications

Albuterol MDI—two puffs q.i.d. Beclomethasone inhaler—two puffs q4 to 6h as needed.

Immunizations

Up to date.

REVIEW OF SYSTEMS

General

She admits to fatigue but denies fever, chills, and sweats.

HEENT

She denies headache, visual changes, sneezing, and sore throat; she admits to nasal congestion.

Lungs

She admits to "trouble breathing" and feeling "chest tightness" and "out of breath." She admits to having a nonproductive cough. She admits to wheezing.

Cardiovascular

She denies weakness.

GI

She denies nausea, vomiting, stomach pain, diarrhea, and burning chest pain.

Orthopedic

She denies myalgias and arthralgias.

PHYSICAL EXAMINATION

Vital Signs

HR, 98 beats/min; RR, 24 breaths/min; BP, 126/88 mmHg; and pulse oximetry O_2 saturation, 93% while breathing room air. The patient was afebrile.

General

She appears mildly ill and has occasional paroxysms of coughing.

HEENT

Normal.

Heart

Heart rate is regular. No murmur or gallop is auscultated.

Lungs

Diffuse expiratory wheezing with full breath sounds noted bilaterally. Moderate accessory respiratory muscle use without paradoxical thoracoabdominal breathing is present.

Abdomen

Soft and nontender abdomen without hepatosplenomegaly on palpation. Normal bowel sounds.

Osteopathic Structural Examination

There is a mild right rib hump in the middle and lower thorax that is present with forward bending and is 50% reducible with passive side bending to the right. T12–L5 is side bent right and rotated left. The pelvis is rotated right. There is decreased rib compliance and reduced excursion during the exhalation phase of respiration especially involving ribs 3 to 5 on the left with bilateral paraspinal muscle hypertonicity at these levels. T2 is flexed, rotated right, and sidebent right while T3–T5 is neutral, rotated right, and sidebent left. C3 is flexed, rotated left, and sidebent left. There is compression of the cranial base and occipitomastoid area on the right.

DIFFERENTIAL DIAGNOSIS

The symptoms of diffuse expiratory wheezes, tachycardia, and respiratory distress in a patient with a known history of asthma lead to a differential diagnosis that may include uncontrolled asthma, respiratory infection, vocal cord dysfunction, foreign body inhalation, panic disorder, and heart failure. In this case, the diagnosis of asthma exacerbation was a clinical diagnosis based on the patient's history and physical exam, and the staff was notified to begin a nebulized albuterol treatment.

The most common symptoms of asthma include wheezing, shortness of breath, chest tightness, and cough. Although wheezing is a characteristic breath sound in asthma, it may not be heard in the most severe cases in which all breath sounds will be markedly reduced. In cough variant asthma, a dry cough may be the only presenting symptom. In a patient with suspected asthma exacerbation, look for the following additional signs and symptoms when examining the patient: use of accessory muscles of respiration, posturing to enhance respiratory muscle mechanics, flaring of the nostrils, a prolonged exhalation phase of breathing, increased heart rate, and acrocyanosis. In addition to the auscultated wheezes, this patient shows moderate accessory muscle use and a slightly increased heart rate. The severity of asthma should never be underestimated, and if it is not treated adequately, death may result.[1–3]

An asthma diagnosis requires recurring symptoms of airflow obstruction or airway hyperresponsiveness that show partial or complete reversibility for which other diagnoses have been ruled out. In addition to a detailed medical history and physical examination, spirometry is recommended to establish the diagnosis of asthma in patients over 5 years of age. Increases in forced expiratory volume in 1 second (FEV_1) greater than 12% above baseline and increases in FEV_1 greater than 10% of predicted after inhalation of a short-acting beta2-agonist (SABA) are indicative of reversible airway obstruction.[4] When asthma is suspected but the diagnosis is not yet certain, fractional exhaled nitric oxide testing may be useful in patients over the age of 5.[5]

Asthma is classified as intermittent or persistent, with persistent asthma being further divided into mild persistent, moderate persistent, and severe persistent. Classification is determined by five criteria including spirometry and weekly frequency of symptoms, nighttime awakenings, SABA use for symptom control, and interference with normal activity. Generally, symptoms requiring SABA rescue inhaler use more than 2 days per week indicate a need to move a step up in pharmaceutical treatment.[4]

Asthma continues to be one of the most common chronic diseases of children and adolescents.[6] Frequently described asthma endotypes include early-onset allergic, late-onset eosinophilic, exercise-induced, obesity-related, cough-variant, steroid-resistant, and neutrophilic asthma.[1,7] Allergic asthma develops most often during the second decade of life and is more likely to persist into adulthood.[8] Frequent lower respiratory infections early in life are associated with the development of asthma.[1,9]

In the age of targeted therapeutics, an increased understanding of genomics and endotyping has elucidated various molecular mechanisms that underlie asthma. Broadly speaking, bronchial hyperreactivity and inflammation lead to asthma symptoms. Bronchial hyperreactivity is mediated by parasympathetic and sympathetic nervous inputs, leukotrienes, prostaglandins, cytokines, and histamine. The inflammatory pathways in atopic and nonatopic asthma subtypes have some differences, but in general, inflammation is influenced by the cell-mediated pathway via either T-helper 2 or 17 cells. Inflammation and bronchoconstriction in allergic asthma, and some nonallergic asthma subtypes, are also heavily influenced by the antibody-mediated pathway wherein IgE antibodies produced by B cells lead to activation and degranulation of mast cells, basophils, eosinophils, and other airway cells. This leads to the well-known process of histamine release and the inflammatory response. Symptoms in allergic asthma are heavily impacted by allergens to which patients have become sensitized. Common asthma triggers in both extrinsic and intrinsic asthma include viral infections, weather conditions, exercise, emotional stress, mold, gastroesophageal reflux, inhaled irritants such as tobacco smoke or pollution, and medications such as aspirin, NSAIDS, and beta blockers.[1,10–12] Mechanical injuries, for example, to the head or sacrum, may also cause an asthma attack.[13]

Based upon this patient's history and physical examination, she appears to have mild persistent asthma; her symptoms are reportedly occurring more than two times per week, but she does not appear to have nighttime symptoms. The guidelines for asthma management and prevention from the National Asthma Education and Prevention Program (NAEPP) recommend pharmaceutical treatment specific to the severity of asthma. According to these guidelines, this child is probably not receiving optimal medical therapy and her medication regimen may need to be adjusted to include a regular preventative dose of low-dose inhaled corticosteroids (ICS) rather than the as-needed dose she is currently prescribed (Table 101.1). A SABA is more effective for rescue treatment during symptom exacerbation rather than regular control.[5,14] Inhaled corticosteroids are effective at controlling asthma symptoms in most children and may be combined with long-acting beta-agonists for good symptom management in moderate and severe persistent asthma.[2,5]

OSTEOPATHIC PATIENT MANAGEMENT

Biomechanical Model

There are key anatomic considerations when using osteopathic manipulative treatment (OMT) in asthmatic patients (Box 101.1). Depending upon the degree of accessory muscle involvement needed

TABLE 101.1

NAEPP-Preferred Management of Asthma in Pediatric Patients

Age (years)	Intermittent Asthma	Persistent Asthma				
		Mild	Moderate		Severe	
	STEP 1	STEP 2	STEP 3	STEP 4	STEP 5	STEP 6
0–4	PRN SABA and At the start of RTI: Add short course daily ICS	Daily low-dose ICS and PRN SABA	Daily medium-dose ICS and PRN SABA	Daily medium-dose ICS-LABA and PRN SABA	Daily high-dose ICS-LABA and PRN SABA	Daily high-dose ICS-LABA + oral systemic corticosteroid and PRN SABA
5–11	PRN SABA	Daily low-dose ICS and PRN SABA	Daily and PRN combination low-dose ICS-formoterol	Daily and PRN combination medium-dose ICS-formoterol	Daily high-dose ICS-LABA and PRN SABA	ICS-LABA + oral systemic corticosteroid and PRN SABA
12+	PRN SABA	Daily low-dose ICS and PRN SABA or PRN concomitant ICS and SABA	Daily and PRN combination low-dose ICS-formoterol	Daily and PRN combination medium-dose ICS-formoterol	Daily medium-high dose ICS LABA + LAMA and PRN SABA	Daily high-dose ICS-LABA + oral systemic corticosteroids + PRN SABA

Alternatives to long-acting beta-agonists (LABA) include leukotriene receptor antagonists, long-acting muscarinic antagonists (LAMA), mast cell stabilizers, and Zileuton, and vary depending on age, severity, and type of asthma. Immunotherapies and asthma biologics are also used in certain cases. See guidelines available at https://www.nhlbi.nih.gov/health-topics/asthma-management-guidelines-2020-updates

Adapted from National Asthma Education and Prevention Program (NAEPP) Coordinating Committee Expert Panel Working Group Guidelines.[5]

during labored breathing, the muscles engaged in respiration can extend from the cranial base to the pelvis. The thoracic cage is the center of all this activity. It includes the 12 thoracic vertebrae and ribs, costal cartilage, and the sternum, and it houses some of the most vital organs in the human body, namely, the heart, lungs, and great vessels. The thorax is one of the most intricate and dynamic regions of the body, with an orchestrated movement of over 146 joints.[15,16]

The restriction of airflow in asthma increases the work of breathing, which can have significant consequences in pediatric patients due to children's anatomical and physiologic immaturity.

BOX 101.1 Factors that Affect Breathing Difficulties

From an osteopathic perspective, the following areas may contribute to or exacerbate the patient's breathing difficulties.

1. Upper thoracic vertebrae, ribs, sternum
2. T1–T6 because of sympathetic innervation to the lungs
3. Occipitoatlantal junction and the course of the vagus nerve that supplies parasympathetic input to the pulmonary tree
4. Accessory muscles of respiration
5. Anterior cervical fascia
6. Thoracic diaphragm (the diaphragm is enervated by the phrenic nerve from the cervical plexus [C3–C5], and its mobility is influenced by the lower six ribs, L1–L2 and the sternum.)
7. Chapman reflexes for the lungs, sinuses, and adrenal glands
8. The cranial–sacral mechanism
9. T10–L2 and the lower ribs

There is evidence that the immature innervation patterns in respiratory muscles of children more than 3 years old result in uncoordinated and random contraction sequences that become exacerbated during times of increased demand.[17] Additionally, when compared with adults, the mechanical effectiveness of the diaphragm and rib cage is compromised in children less than 10 years old. This is because the rib cage is more flexible and laterally splayed, and the dome of the diaphragm is flatter than in an adult (Figs. 101.1 and 101.2). As a result, diaphragmatic excursion is shallower, intrathoracic respiratory pressures are less negative, and there is less tissue recoil during exhalation.[18] During times of increased demand, children will compensate by increasing the rate and decreasing the depth of respiration. The increased workload of breathing also increases oxygen demand and cellular waste production, which alter pH and change the cellular milieu, which stresses the cardiopulmonary system. Optimizing the mechanical function of the structures involved with breathing may help to decrease the overall workload placed on the child's cardiopulmonary system. Another biomechanical factor to consider is lung overinflation through a process known as "air trapping," especially in individuals who die in status asthmaticus. Mucous plugs, made of mucus, serum proteins, inflammatory cells, and debris, can compromise the medium- and small-sized bronchi and bronchioles. Microscopic pathologic features include both goblet cell hyperplasia and submucosal gland hypertrophy. One study reported up to a threefold increase of both goblet and mucin cells in asthmatic patients versus controls.[19]

Respiratory–Circulatory Model

The primary muscle of respiration is the diaphragm. With average respiratory rates between 12 and 18 breaths/min, the adult diaphragm will contract over 20,000 times in a day. Young children may breathe at nearly twice this rate, and infants breathe upward of three times this amount daily.[20] The diaphragm is intimately

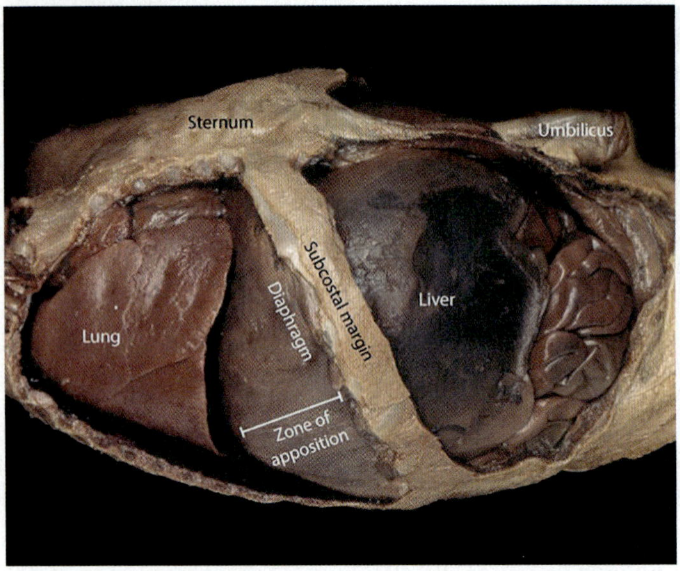

Figure 101.1. Dissection of term infant, right lateral view. The ribs 1 through 9 have been removed as has the right lateral abdominal wall to reveal the dome of the diaphragm draping the superior surface of the liver. The zone of apposition lies between the dome of the diaphragm and its inferior attachment and represents the length of inferior excursion possible during inhalation. (Used with permission from the Willard/Carreiro Collection, University of New England.)

connected to the cardiac and pulmonary pleura above and the hepatic and gastric pleura below. The movement of the diaphragm not only changes the intrathoracic and intra-abdominal pressures but also alters the circulation and lymphatic flow in these respective cavities. The removal of cellular waste products, inflammatory mediators, the maintenance of tissue pH, and the reentry of fluids into the circulatory cycle are influenced by diaphragmatic function. Fluid movement through the vena cava system is dependent upon effective diaphragmatic excursion. Lymphatic fluids and deoxygenated blood reenter the cardiac system through the pressure changes generated by the diaphragm and respiratory muscles. Extravascular fluids in the abdominal compartment are absorbed by lymphatic lacunae situated on the abdominal surface of the diaphragm in response to mechanical changes in the diaphragmatic fascia.[21,22]

Neurologic Model

An important consideration in children with asthma is the dynamic interplay between the sympathetic and parasympathetic

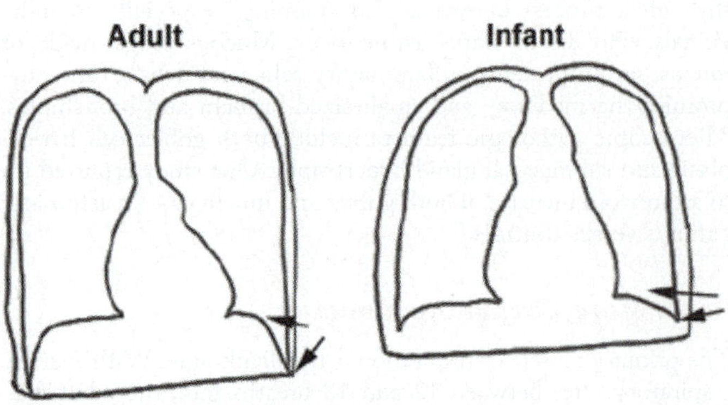

Figure 101.2. Schematic diagram comparing zone of apposition in the infant with that of the adult. The flattened diaphragm and widened thoracic cage contribute to the decreased zone.

components of the autonomic nervous system. Parasympathetic fibers travel within the vagus nerve as they exit the jugular foramen of the cranial vault and traverse down the cervical region and through the thoracic inlet where they then splay onto the lungs. Bronchial smooth muscle is innervated by the bronchial branches of the vagus nerve (CN X) and vasovagal reflexes can cause bronchoconstriction. Bronchial secretions are influenced by vagal input. The reported association between gastroesophageal reflux and asthma may in part be due to an esophagobronchial vagal reflex as well as the microaspiration of gastric acid.[23–25] The sympathetic nerve fibers of the lungs typically arise from the sympathetic chain ganglion at the level of T1–T6. Somatovisceral reflexes associated with asthma have been found in the paraspinal muscles between T1 and T6 in adults.[26] Somatic innervation to the diaphragm comes via the phrenic nerve, which originates from the C3–C5 nerve roots.

The osteopathic physician may attempt to influence sympathetic activity by treating the upper thoracic area and parasympathetic activity by addressing somatic dysfunction in the cervical region, including the craniocervical junction and cranial base.

The bronchodilators, corticosteroids, and anticholinergics used to treat asthma do so by influencing neuronal control and inflammatory mechanisms in the lower airways. Other medications such as leukotriene receptor antagonists, immunotherapies, and mast cell stabilizers are also used to control related allergy symptoms. OMT used in conjunction with these medications may help to reduce the necessary dosage of medication required to control symptoms.

Behavioral Model

The clinician must consider the psychosocioeconomic implications that patients face. There is a documented correlation between asthma and increased risk for anxiety and depression in adolescents.[27] In turn, these psychological factors often exacerbate asthma symptoms both by triggering asthmatic symptoms and potentiating the symptoms of other asthma triggers.[28,29] In older children and adults, breathing exercises may help strengthen peripheral and accessory muscles that aid breathing and positively influence the emotional and stress components of asthma.[30] As with many diseases, obesity increases the risk of developing asthma, frequency and severity of asthma symptoms, and poor responsiveness to therapeutics, highlighting another potentially modifiable aspect of the asthma disease process.[31]

In 2014, the first systematic review analyzing compliance with medical treatment and severe asthma exacerbations highlighted that as patient asthma controller medication compliance increases, severe exacerbations decrease.[32] Some patients prefer to use rescue inhalers when symptoms occur rather than consistently using asthma controller medications such as ICS. Repetitive episodes of inflammation lead to the production of matrix proteins and growth factors that may cause airway remodeling. While patients may be concerned about side effects of regular steroid use, they may not be aware of the airway remodeling that occurs with unmitigated chronic airway inflammation, highlighting an opportunity for patient education.[10,31,33] Three systematic reviews reported improvements in some asthma parameters after self-management education, and one small systematic review reported improvement after family therapy.[34–37] According to the hygiene hypothesis, there is a correlation between allergic asthma and urban environments that stems from immune development through environmental interaction.[12] Some patients develop asthma through exposure to sensitizing or irritating agents in the workplace. Irritants such as smoke and chemical exposure, and allergens such as animal dander, mold, and dust are aspects of the environment that may be modifiable depending on patient circumstances.[10,38]

The national and global difficulty in providing accessible health care for impoverished patients is a concern of all health care providers. Even if patients are able to utilize the necessary medications, their response to these medications is dependent on multifactorial elements ranging from genetics to the environment. In short, one must approach the patient as an individual and treat the person, not the disease.

Metabolic Energy Model

There is no one-size-fits-all diet approach to asthma, especially due to its multifactorial nature. In general, a diet that emphasizes fruits, vegetables, and whole grains and de-emphasizes excess dairy, processed foods, and both sugar and artificial sweeteners may be beneficial for asthma management.[39] Allergies and sensitivities to food and food modifiers can contribute to asthma symptoms and should be part of a wide differential. There is evidence that asthmatics are more likely to have antioxidant imbalances, but studies establishing a clear and generalizable relationship between specific antioxidant supplementation regimens and improvements in asthma are lacking currently.[40] In the acute setting, intravenous magnesium has been shown to have a positive effect on respiratory function and hospital stays in children with asthma.[41] In the outpatient setting, oral magnesium supplementation has shown some potential in decreasing asthma symptom frequency and bronchodilator usage in some pediatric populations.[42] There is evidence that breastfeeding infants not only decreases the risk of developing reactive airway disease but also the risk of respiratory infections.[10,43,44]

While ICS have a far lower side effect profile than systemic steroids, some of the dry powder inhaled steroids are swallowed and pass through the gastrointestinal (GI) tract, affecting GI flora. For this reason, esophageal candidiasis is a commonly reported side effect, and patients are encouraged to gargle and spit water after inhalation of corticosteroids.[45] There is some evidence that chronic ICS use may slow growth rate in children. There are also increased risks of reduced bone mineral density and cataracts associated with their use, but these two risks are more likely to be seen in doses higher than those used in treating asthma.[46–48]

OMT FOR THE ASTHMATIC PATIENT

There are many ways OMT can benefit an asthmatic patient. It is important to address the thoracic cage and diaphragm restrictions and restore optimal diaphragmatic motion. Restrictions to any one of the twelve ribs can impact respiratory quality and should be assessed and treated if found. Rib-raising techniques, among others, help to mobilize the thoracic cage as well as stimulate the sympathetic chain ganglion, and improve sympathetic outflow to the lungs. Treating dysfunctions of the cervical and suboccipital regions should improve parasympathetic input to the lungs. Often accessory muscles are heavily taxed during effortful breathing, and dysfunctions of scalenes, sternocleidomastoids, trapezius, abdominal, and serratus muscles may manifest.[7] Lymphatic restrictions, including the thoracic inlet and abdominal diaphragm, should not be overlooked. Osteopathic cranial manipulative medicine should be considered, especially considering the cases of patients who have suffered a hard fall with mechanical injuries to the head or sacrum that have triggered an asthma attack.[49]

The goal of using OMT in the treatment of a child with asthma is to remove mechanical restrictions that adversely affect respiratory mechanics, optimize the dynamic balance between parasympathetic and sympathetic input to the pulmonary system, and decrease the workload of breathing.

Bockenhauer et al.[50] compared OMT to sham treatment in a pilot study of adults with chronic asthma using a crossover design. Upper thoracic and lower thoracic forced respiratory excursion were statistically increased after osteopathic manipulative procedures compared with sham procedures, although there were no significant changes in peak expiratory flow rates. However, in a randomized controlled trial Guiney et al.[51] reported a statistically significant improvement in peak expiratory flow measures in asthmatic children after treatment with OMT. It was the experience of the previous authors of this chapter that osteopathic modalities applied to asthmatic patients prior to and during the administration of medication contribute to an improvement in symptoms.

SUMMARY

Given its multifactorial nature, asthma is challenging to treat and requires a comprehensive evaluation on the part of the clinician. A multifaceted approach, including diet, allergen prevention, medication, and complementary modalities such as OMT, may work synergistically to control the symptoms of an asthmatic patient and potentially lessen the severity of the disease.[52]

ACKNOWLEDGMENTS

The author and editors of this chapter would like to acknowledge the scholarly contributions of Mary Anne Morelli Haskell and Jesus Sanchez Jr. for prior editions of this chapter.

REFERENCES

1. Mims JW. Asthma: definitions and pathophysiology. *Int Forum Allergy Rhinol.* 2015;5(Suppl 1):S2–S6.
2. Colice G. Asthma severity categorization methods. *Clin Med Res.* 2004;3: 155–163.
3. Uryasjev MO, Ponomareva IV, Bhar M, Glotov SI. The cough variant asthma. *Ter Arkh.* 2020;92(3):98–101.
4. National Asthma Education and Prevention Program, Third Expert Panel on the Diagnosis and Management of Asthma. *Expert Panel Report 3: Guidelines for the Diagnosis and Management of Asthma.* National Heart, Lung, and Blood Institute (US); 2007. https://www.ncbi.nlm.nih.gov/books/NBK7232/
5. Expert Panel Working Group of the National Heart, Lung, and Blood Institute (NHLBI) administered and coordinated National Asthma Education and Prevention Program Coordinating Committee (NAEPPCC), Cloutier MM, Baptist AP, et al. 2020 Focused Updates to the Asthma Management Guidelines: A Report from the National Asthma Education and Prevention Program Coordinating Committee Expert Panel Working Group [published correction appears in *J Allergy Clin Immunol.* 2021 Apr;147(4):1528–1530]. *J Allergy Clin Immunol.* 2020;146(6):1217–1270.
6. Miller GF, Coffield E, Leroy Z, Wallin R. Prevalence and costs of five chronic conditions in children. *J Sch Nurs.* 2016;32(5):357–364.
7. Schend J, Rowane M, Sanan N, Hostoffer SR. An osteopathic modular approach to asthma: a narrative review. *J Am Osteopath Assoc.* 2020;120(11): 774–782.
8. Reed C. The natural history of asthma. *J Allergy Clin Immunol.* 2006; 118:543–550.
9. Carroll KN, Hartert TV. The impact of respiratory viral infection on wheezing illnesses and asthma exacerbations. *Immunol Allergy Clin N Am.* 2008;28:539–561, viii.
10. Cevhertas L, Ogulur I, Maurer DJ, et al. Advances and recent developments in asthma in 2020. *Allergy.* 2020;75(12):3124–3146.
11. Eder W, Ege M, Von Mutius E. The asthma epidemic. *N Engl J Med.* 2006;355:2226–2235.

12. Chiu CJ, Huang MT. Asthma in the precision medicine era: biologics and probiotics. *Int J Mol Sci*. 2021;22(9):4528.
13. King H, ed. *The Collected Papers of Viola M.* Legacy of Osteopathy to Children; American Academy of Osteopathy; 1998.
14. Hong SH, Sanders BH, West D. Inappropriate use of inhaled short acting beta-agonists and its association with patient health status. *Curr Med Res Opin*. 2006;22(1):33–40.
15. Kuchera ML, Kuchera WA. Osteopathic considerations in systemic dysfunction. *Rev. 2nd ed.* 1994:33–56.
16. Moore KL, Dalley AF. *Clinically Oriented Anatomy. UPDATE: 19.* 7th ed. Wolters-Kluwer, Lippincott, Williams & Wilkins; 2014.
17. Haddad GG, Perez Fontain JJ. Development of the respiratory system. In: Behrman RE, Kliegman RM, Jenson HB, eds. *Nelson's Textbook of Pediatrics*. WB Saunders; 1996.
18. Openshaw P, Edwards S, Helms P. Changes in rib cage geometry in childhood. *Thorax*. 1984;39:624–627.
19. Ordonez CL, Khashayar R, Wong HH, et al. Mild and moderate asthma is associated with airway goblet cell hyperplasia and abnormalities in mucin gene expression. *Am J Respir Crit Care Med*. 2001;163:517–523.
20. Fleming S, Thompson M, Stevens R, et al. Normal ranges of heart rate and respiratory rate in children from birth to 18 years of age: a systematic review of observational studies. *Lancet*. 2011;377(9770):1011–1018.
21. Negrini D. Morphological, mechanical and hydrodynamic aspects of diaphragmatic lymphatics. *Biology (Basel)*. 2022;11(12):1803.
22. Shinohara H, Kominami R, Taniguchi Y, Yasutaka S. The distribution and morphology of lymphatic vessels on the peritoneal surface of the adult human diaphragm, as revealed by an ink-absorption method. *Okajimas Folia Anat Jpn*. 2003;79:175–183.
23. Kase JS, Pici M, Visintainer P. Risks for common medical conditions experienced by former preterm infants during toddler years. *J Perinat Med*. 2009;37:103–108.
24. Yoshida Y, Kameda M, Nishikido T, Takamatsu I, Matsumoto T, Doi S. Very short gastroesophageal acid reflux during the upright position could be associated with asthma in children. *Allergol Int*. 2009;58:395–401.
25. Wright RA, Miller SA, Corsello BF. Acid-induced esophagobronchial-cardiac reflexes in humans. *Gastroenterology*. 1990;99(1):71–73.
26. Beal MC, Morlock JW, Somatic dysfunction associated with pulmonary disease. *J Am Osteopath Assoc*. 1984;84:179–183.
27. Katon W, Lozano P, Russo J, McCauley E, Richardson L, Bush T. The prevalence of DSM-IV anxiety and depressive disorders in youth with asthma compared with controls. *J Adolesc Health*. 2007;41(5):455–463.
28. Shankar M, Fagnano M, Blaakman SW, Rhee H, Halterman JS. Depressive symptoms among urban adolescents with asthma: a focus for providers. *Acad Pediatr*. 2019;19(6):608–614.
29. Wood BL, Lim J, Miller BD, et al. Family emotional climate, depression, emotional triggering of asthma, and disease severity in pediatric asthma: examination of pathways of effect. *J Pediatr Psychol*. 2007;32(5):542–551.
30. Chiang LC, Ma WF, Huang JL, Tseng LF, Hsueh KC. Effect of relaxation-breathing training on anxiety and asthma signs/symptoms of children with moderate-to-severe asthma: a randomized controlled trial. *Int J Nurs Stud*. 2009;46(8):1061–1070.
31. Peters U, Dixon AE, Forno E. Obesity and asthma. *J Allergy Clin Immunol*. 2018;141(4):1169–1179.
32. Engelkes M, Janssens HM, de Jongste JC, Sturkenboom MC, Verhamme KM. Medication adherence and the risk of severe asthma exacerbations: a systematic review. *Eur Respir J*. 2015;45(2):396–407.
33. Fehrenbach H, Wagner C, Wegmann M. Airway remodeling in asthma: what really matters. *Cell Tissue Res*. 2017;367(3):551–569.
34. Panton J, Barley EA. Family therapy for asthma in children. *Cochrane Database Syst Rev*. 2005;(2):CD000089.
35. Wolf FM, Guevara JP, Grum CM, Clark NM, Cates CJ. Educational interventions for asthma in children. *Cochrane Database Syst Rev. UPDATE, Add to 32*. 2003;(1):CD000326.
36. Hodkinson A, Bower P, Grigoroglou C, et al. Self-management interventions to reduce healthcare use and improve quality of life among patients with asthma: systematic review and network meta-analysis [published correction appears in *BMJ*. 2023 Jul 27; 382: p. 1743]. *BMJ*. 2020;370:m2521.
37. Harris K, Kneale D, Lasserson TJ, McDonald VM, Grigg J, Thomas J. School-based self-management interventions for asthma in children and adolescents: a mixed methods systematic review. *Cochrane Database Syst Rev*. 2019;1(1):CD011651.
38. Tarlo SM, Lemiere C. Occupational asthma. *N Engl J Med*. 2014;370(7): 640–649.
39. Guilleminault L, Williams EJ, Scott HA, Berthon BS, Jensen M, Wood LG. Diet and asthma: is it time to adapt our message? *Nutrients*. 2017;9(11):1227.
40. Barrera-Mendoza CC, Ayala-Mata F, Cortés-Rojo C, García-Pérez ME, Rodríguez-Orozco AR. Vitaminas antioxidantes en asma [Antioxidant vitamins in asthma]. *Rev Alerg Mex*. 2018;65(1):61–77.
41. Mohammed S, Goodacre S. Intravenous and nebulised magnesium sulphate for acute asthma: systematic review and meta-analysis. *Emerg Med J*. 2007;24:823–830.
42. Bede O, Nagy D, Surányi A, Horváth I, Szlávik M, Gyurkovits K. Effects of magnesium supplementation on the glutathione redox system in atopic asthmatic children. *Inflamm Res*. 2008;57:279–286.
43. Scholtens S, Wijga AH, Brunekreef B, et al. Breast feeding, parental allergy and asthma in children followed for 8 years. The PIAMA birth cohort study. *Thorax*. 2009;64:604–609.
44. Oddy WH. Breastfeeding, childhood asthma, and allergic disease. *Ann Nutr Metab*. 2017;70(Suppl 2):26–36.
45. van Boven JF, de Jong-van den Berg LT, Vegter S. Inhaled corticosteroids and the occurrence of oral candidiasis: a prescription sequence symmetry analysis. *Drug Saf*. 2013;36(4):231–236.
46. Kelly HW, Sternberg AL, Lescher R, et al. Effect of inhaled glucocorticoids in childhood on adult height. *N Engl J Med*. 2012;367(10): 904–912.
47. Weatherall M, Clay J, James K, Perrin K, Shirtcliffe P, Beasley R. Dose-response relationship of inhaled corticosteroids and cataracts: a systematic review and meta-analysis. *Respirol*. 2009;14(7):983–990.
48. Dahl R. Systemic side effects of inhaled corticosteroids in patients with asthma. *Respir Med*. 2006;100(8):1307–1317.
49. Centers S, Morelli MA, Seffinger MA. Pediatrics. In: Ward RC, Ex. ed. *Foundations of Osteopathic Medicine*. 2nd ed. Lippincott, Williams & Wilkins; 2003:305–337.
50. Bockenhauer SE, Julliard KN, Lo KS, Huang E, Sheth AM. Quantifiable effects of osteopathic manipulative techniques on patients with chronic asthma. *J Am Osteopath Assoc*. 2002;102:371–375.
51. Guiney PA, Chou R, Vianna A, Lovenheim J. Effects of osteopathic manipulative treatment on pediatric patients with asthma: a randomized controlled trial. *J Am Osteopath Assoc*. 2005;105:7–12.
52. Rowane WA, Rowane MP. An osteopathic approach to asthma. *J Am Osteopath Assoc*. 1999;99:259–264.

102 Case Study: Adult with Chronic Cardiovascular Disease

BRIAN E. KAUFMAN ▪ AMANDA BERNETT ▪ ALYSSA KAMPEN

KEY CONCEPTS

- Heart failure is a clinical syndrome characterized by fluid overload.
- Fatigue and dyspnea are characteristic symptoms of heart failure.
- Heart failure can be both acute and chronic.
- Patients with both acute and chronic heart failure exhibit changes in the musculoskeletal system.
- These musculoskeletal changes can be addressed using five distinct pathophysiologic models, which provide an osteopathic interpretation of heart failure.
- The osteopathic physician can utilize these models to plan a rationale for treatment of patients with heart failure that includes pharmacologic therapy, lifestyle changes, and osteopathic manipulative treatment (OMT).
- There are biologic and physiologic data to support this approach.

CASE VIGNETTE

CHIEF COMPLAINT

A 79-year-old female comes to the office complaining of shortness of breath and worsening fatigue for 1 week.

History of Present Illness

The patient has a complicated medical history, which is significant for coronary artery disease (CAD), heart failure with a left ventricular (LV) ejection fraction of 45% (Heart failure with mid-range ejection fraction–HFmrEF), hypertension (HTN), hyperlipidemia (HLD), diabetes mellitus type 2 (TIIDM), and osteoporosis.

The patient reports that over the last week, she has had increasing fatigue and worsening shortness of breath from baseline symptoms, which has progressed to shortness of breath at rest over the last 24 hours. This dyspnea is accompanied by nonproductive cough and wheezing and increased lower extremity swelling over the past week. She also states that last night, she slept in a recliner in order to breathe and experienced episodes of chest pressure that improved transiently with nitroglycerin.

Prior to this recent episode, the patient has been feeling depressed due to the recent loss of her husband. She admits her mood has increased her appetite for salty foods and resulted in her missing doses of her medications.

Past Medical History

CAD diagnosed after non–ST elevation myocardial infarction (MI). Mild mitral regurgitation, mild aortic stenosis, and HFmrEF (45% with moderate diastolic dysfunction) evaluated by echocardiogram (ECHO) last year. TIIDM. HLD. Osteoporosis.

Past Surgical History

Appendectomy at 52 years old. Total abdominal hysterectomy with bilateral salpingo-oopherectomy at 63 years old. Coronary artery bypass graft (CABG) at 77 years old with left leg saphenous vein harvesting.

Allergies

No known drug allergies.

Adverse reactions: angiotensin-converting enzyme (ACE) inhibitor caused cough.

Medications

Carvedilol: 12.5 mg twice daily. Valsartan: 320 mg daily. Aspirin: 81 mg daily. Furosemide: 40 mg daily. Amlodipine: 10 mg daily. Atorvastatin: 10 mg daily. Calcium: 600 mg. Vitamin D: 600 IU taken twice daily. Metformin: 1,000 mg twice daily.

Social History

Patient is a retired schoolteacher. Patient lives alone in an assisted living complex. Patient's husband is recently deceased. Patient has two adult children nearby who are active in her life.

Family History

Father deceased at age 57 of MI. Mother deceased at age 80 with no significant medical history. Brother with atrial fibrillation and CAD. Sister with HTN, HLD, and CAD. No family history of diabetes, cancer, or blood disorders.

REVIEW OF SYSTEMS

General

No constitutional symptoms of fever, chills, or night sweats. Admits to fatigue and 12-lb weight gain over the last 2 weeks.

Head

Denies headache or head injuries.

Eyes

Denies diplopia, change in vision, or eye pain.

ENT

Denies change in hearing, earache, or tinnitus. No sinus tenderness or nasal discharge. No voice changes, hoarseness, or sore throat.

Neck

No neck stiffness, tenderness, swelling, or masses.

Cardiovascular

Admits to chest pressure with increased need for nitrate use, shortness of breath, and dyspnea on exertion. Three-pillow orthopnea (dyspnea when lying flat, requiring three pillows to relieve dyspnea). Denies palpitations.

Respiratory

Admits to nonproductive cough and wheezes. Denies hemoptysis or pleuritic chest pain.

GI

Admits to appetite changes and some abdominal fullness. Denies nausea, vomiting, heartburn, abdominal pain, diarrhea, rectal bleeding, or change in bowel habits. No change in stool color or caliber.

GU

No dysuria, hematuria, polyuria, urinary retention, or incontinence. No increased frequency.

CNS

No disturbance of smell, dizziness, vertigo, weakness, convulsions, gait disturbance, or involuntary movement.

Extremity

Admits to recent worsening bilateral lower extremity swelling. Denies cyanosis.

Vascular

No history of claudication but recent complaints of exertional leg pains.

Integument

No rashes, change in moles, pigmentation, or pruritus noted by the patient.

Endocrine

No increased hunger, thirst, or urination. No hot or cold intolerance.

Hematology

No history of bleeding or clotting disorders. No easy bruising/bleeding or active bleeding.

Musculoskeletal

No significant joint pain, stiffness, myalgias, or deformities.

Psychiatric

Admits to feelings of depression. No changes in personality or memory. No suicidal or homicidal ideation.

PHYSICAL EXAMINATION

Vital Signs

Temp: 99 °F; BP: 150/88 mm Hg in right arm; Pulse: 104 bpm; RR: 22 rpm and shallow; Height: 63 in.; Weight: 149 lb; BMI: 26.4.

General

Patient is alert, attentive, and oriented. She appears extremely deconditioned.

Head

Normocephalic and atraumatic.

Eyes

Pupils equal, round, reactive to light and accommodation (PERRLA), extraocular movements intact (EOMI), sclera is anicteric, conjunctivae are pink, and no xanthelasma is appreciated.

ENT

Bilateral tympanic membranes are normal. Pharynx is clear without erythema or exudate.

Neck

Neck is supple, trachea is midline, and no carotid bruit is appreciated. Jugular vein distention (JVD) is noted with neck veins slightly distended at 45 degrees.

Cardiovascular

Faint S1 and prominent S2; rhythm is regular with tachycardic rate; 2/6 systolic ejection murmur at the right upper sternal border (RUSB) without radiation is appreciated; S3 gallop is appreciated.

Pulmonary

Decreased air entry bilaterally with crackles (rales) noted at the lung bases bilaterally extending midway up lower lung fields and wheezes throughout all lung fields.

Abdomen

Abdomen slightly distended but soft and nontender, without guarding or rigidity. Bowel sounds are present and positive hepatojugular reflux is elicited. No palpable fluid wave.

Extremities

Bilateral lower extremities reveal atrophy and warmth to palpation, 3+ pitting edema in left lower extremity, 2+ pitting edema in right lower extremity.

OSTEOPATHIC STRUCTURAL EXAMINATION

Cranial

OA extended, rotated left, and side bent right. Suboccipital tissues are boggy.

Cervical

C2 is flexed, rotated, and side bent to the right, C5 is extended, rotated, and side bent to the left.

Thoracic

Increased kyphosis. T1 is in a neutral position rotated to the right and side bent to the left; T3 and T4 are both extended, rotated, and side bent to the left. Skin was warm and boggy T1–T5. T12 is flexed, rotated, and side bent to the right. Sternum with fascial restriction and poor mobility. Decreased diaphragmatic excursion bilaterally. Chapman point was noted in anterior left 2nd intercostal space.

Ribs

Bilateral ribs 10 to 12 are exhaled.

Lumbar

Psoas hypertonicity on right. Slightly increased lumbar lordosis.

Sacrum

Bilateral sacral extension

Pelvis

Right anteriorly rotated innominate

UE

Left elevated clavicle, internally rotated humerus.

LE

Right internally rotated femur. Left externally rotated femur. Femoral triangle congestion bilaterally.

DIFFERENTIAL DIAGNOSIS AND DISCUSSION

The patient is a 79-year-old female patient with multiple chronic medical problems presenting with acute or chronic dyspnea, nonproductive cough, wheezing, lower extremity edema, and worsening fatigue. She also admits to several episodes of chest pressure which were improved by nitroglycerin. Although this is a complicated case, the patient's complaints can be categorized into those that are potentially life threatening and those related to her chronic disease. With this constellation of symptoms, several systems must be considered, including respiratory, cardiovascular, neuromuscular, psychogenic, and other systemic illnesses. Thus, the differential diagnosis includes but is not limited to, exacerbation of HFmrEF, first episode of exacerbation of chronic obstructive pulmonary disease, acute bronchitis with exacerbation of HFmrEF, pneumonia, nonischemic cardiomyopathy, acute ischemic heart disease, psychogenic dyspnea, and acute renal failure.

To help narrow the differential and arrive at an accurate diagnosis, it is reasonable to check basic laboratory studies. Current guidelines recommend a thorough history and physical examination, including assessment of volume status.[8] Laboratory evaluations should include complete blood count (CBC), serum electrolytes (including sodium, potassium, calcium, and magnesium), blood urea nitrogen (BUN), serum creatinine, urinalysis (UA), glucose, fasting lipid profile, liver function tests (LFTs), iron studies (serum iron, ferritin, transferrin saturation), and thyroid-stimulating hormone (TSH) level. Other tests to consider for patients presenting with dyspnea, history of heart failure, or are at risk for developing heart failure, include B-type natriuretic peptide (BNP) or N-terminal prohormone of B-type natriuretic peptide (NT-proBNP) to corroborate suspicions of heart failure (Box 102.1).[8]

In terms of diagnostic imaging and functional testing, an electrocardiogram (EKG) is included to evaluate for acute changes consistent with cardiac ischemia and arrhythmias. If possible, the EKG should be compared with a previous EKG to evaluate for changes. A hemoglobin oxygen saturation level is used to evaluate the patient's oxygenation status, and if this is abnormal, ABG analysis is a reasonable next step. A chest x-ray (CXR) (Fig. 102.1) can provide evidence of congestive heart failure, such as cardiomegaly, bilateral pleural effusions, alveolar infiltrates, vascular prominence, Kerley B lines, or bilateral pleural effusions.

BOX 102.1 Initial Evaluation of Heart Failure

- History and physical
- CBC
- Basic metabolic panel
- Calcium
- Magnesium
- Iron studies
- Lipid profile
- LFTs
- TSH
- UA
- Cardiac enzymes and BNP
- Oxygen saturation level and arterial blood gas (ABG), if needed
- ECG
- chest x-ray (CXR)
- ECHO, if indicated
- Genetic screening and counseling in first-degree relatives of those with genetic or inherited cardiomyopathies

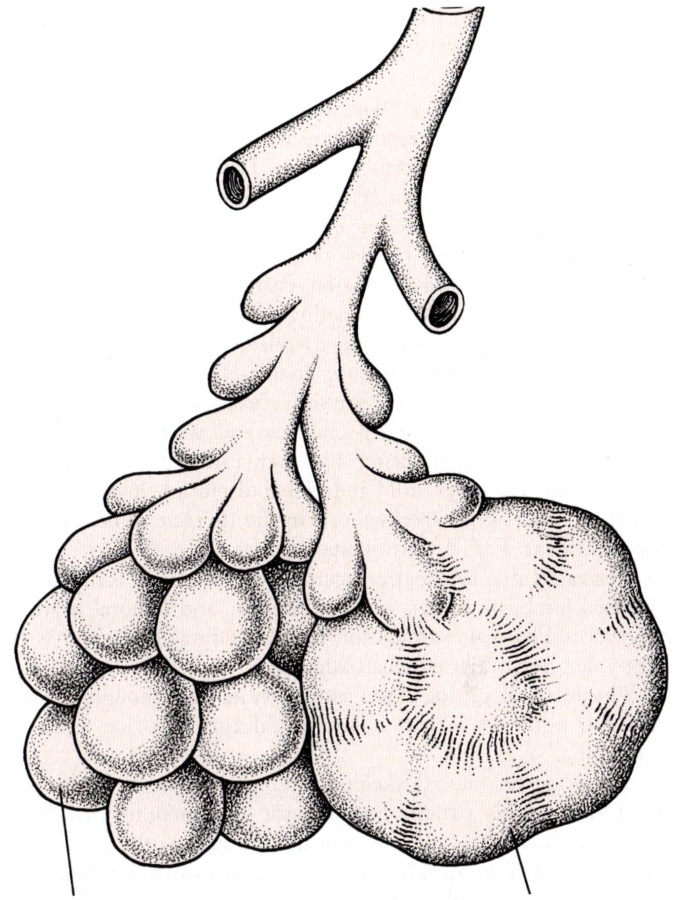

Figure 102.1. Typical heart failure CXR.

Once we have decided on the most likely diagnosis, corroborative tests may be used for confirmation. An echocardiogram is recommended to assess LV function and look for the presence of critical valvular disease.

Ultimately, making an accurate diagnosis is a combination of patient presentation, pattern recognition, test results, and clinical judgment.

In this case, the following laboratory and diagnostic test results were obtained:

Na±: 130 mmol/L
K±: 3.0 mmol/L
Bun/Cr: 66/2.4 mg/dL
Estimated glomerular filtration rate (eGFR): 12 mL/min/1.73 m^2
Magnesium: 1.9 mg/dL
Troponin I: 1.5 ng/mL
BNP: 10,000 pg/mL
AST/ALT: 90/120 units/L
TSH: 1.25 mLU/L
UA: Specific gravity of 1.035, pH of 5.5, no cells or casts seen.
Oxygen saturation: 87% on room air.
EKG: Sinus rhythm at 105 bpm. Left bundle branch block pattern. No changes compared with previous EKG from 1 year ago.
CXR: Cardiomegaly noted. Cephalization of vessels noted. Bilateral infiltrates. Small bilateral pleural effusions.

ECHO: Ejection fraction 35%. Moderate diastolic dysfunction. Mild mitral regurgitation, moderate aortic stenosis.

In summary, this is a 79-year-old female with previous history of CAD, ischemic heart disease with ischemic cardiomyopathy, moderate diastolic dysfunction, now HFrEF (ejection fraction 35% from 45% one year prior) with previous exacerbations who complains of progressive dyspnea, fatigue, chest pressure, increased nitrate use, and a recent history of dietary indiscretion, medication noncompliance, and depression. Past medical history—CAD, HFmrEF, ischemic cardiomyopathy, and diastolic dysfunction. Review of systems—progressive dyspnea, nonproductive cough, wheezing, fatigue, chest pressure, increased nitrate use, dietary changes, and depression. Physical examination—tachypnea, shallow breathing, pulmonary crackles and wheezes bilaterally, increased jugular venous distension, tachycardia, S3 gallop, positive hepatojugular reflex, mild abdominal distention, lower extremity edema bilaterally, hyperkyphosis in the thoracic spine, somatic dysfunction at T3/T4 with tissue texture changes from T1 to T7, decreased diaphragmatic excursion and thoracic compliance, increased lumbar lordosis, sacral restriction, and femoral triangle congestion. Physical examination reveals findings consistent with right-sided heart failure exacerbation.

The bilateral pitting lower extremity edema, though consistent with right-sided heart failure, could also be a side effect of amlodipine.[1]

There are no musculoskeletal findings specific to heart failure; however, this patient had somatic dysfunctions that have been associated with cardiovascular disease such as the changes at occipital–atlantal joint, C2, and the thoracic area (warm, boggy at T3–T4 region).[2] In addition, the changes in thoracic compliance, decreased diaphragmatic excursion, and changes at the lumbar, sacrum, and pelvis while not specific for either heart disease or cardiac disease are common in patients with pulmonary and cardiovascular disease and could have been impacting this patient's presentation.[3] Congestion in the femoral triangle could be seen in any condition of increased lower extremity edema as in this case.

The patient's troponin and BNP are both elevated, which suggests acute cardiac ischemia and heart failure. This is consistent with the patient's complaints of chest pressure that responded to nitrate use. It should be noted, however, that often in cases such as this, it may initially be unclear whether an acute ischemic event has triggered an exacerbation of heart failure or an exacerbation of heart failure has triggered acute cardiac ischemia. Furthermore, this patient has significantly decreased renal function (as shown by elevated BUN and creatinine). The elevated troponin level in the setting of decreased renal function may represent a decrease in clearance of troponins from the blood; however, studies have indicated that mechanisms other than renal clearance play a large role. It is likely that inflammation and fibrosis associated with chronic myocardial injury from chronic disease are also significant etiologies.[4]

The hyponatremia (sodium 130) seen in this patient may be from diuretic use, pulmonary pathology, or pain. It could also result from increased antidiuretic hormone (ADH) secretion and the absorption of free water.[5] Her hyponatremia with an elevated specific gravity of urine indicates increased ADH secretion. This could be from intravascular fluid depletion (dehydration) or decreased effective circulating volume (fluid overload state and increased BUN) due to fluid movement into interstitial spaces.

This patient also has renal failure. Her baseline creatinine was 1.1, and baseline creatinine clearance was approximately 45 mL/min. When she arrived at the hospital, her creatinine clearance had decreased to approximately 20 mL/min. Although this is a complicated topic on its own, it can be explained by a combination of factors.

- In heart failure, there is a decrease in effective circulating volume due to decreased cardiac output. This ultimately causes a decrease in renal blood flow leading to renal demise, a condition known as cardiorenal syndrome.
- In addition, this patient is on a diuretic agent (furosemide), which may have contributed to intravascular depletion and decreased renal blood flow.
- She is also taking an angiotensin 2 receptor blocker. Angiotensin 2 constricts the efferent arteriole in the kidney and acts to increase filtration by raising intraglomerular pressure. Angiotensin 2 receptor blockers remove the ability to constrict the efferent arteriole and effectively reduce intraglomerular pressure and glomerular filtration.
- Although there may be other factors to account for the renal findings, there is sufficient evidence that these factors are all prerenal and would act to reduce renal blood flows.
- The rise in serum creatinine indicates a decrease in glomerular filtration rate.[6]

Hyponatremia, renal failure, increased specific gravity in UA, and elevated BNP in a patient who appears to be clinically volume overloaded help support the diagnosis of acute decompensated heart failure. The diagnosis is further supported by the patient's CXR and echocardiographic findings, both of which are consistent with acute decompensated heart failure.

HOSPITAL COURSE

The patient was admitted to the hospital and placed on a telemetry unit. Therapeutic guidelines for managing acute decompensated heart failure, include the use of vasodilators, diuretics, oxygen, and calcitropes (inotropes that alter myocardial calcium transients to improve cardiac function).[7] Therefore, the patient was started on nitrates to decrease preload and help decrease pulmonary pressures. Intravenous diuretic treatment was instituted to remove excess fluid. Supplemental oxygen raised her oxygen saturation levels to ≥95%. If this had not helped, noninvasive ventilation (NIV) modalities would have been used (e.g., continuous positive airway pressure (CPAP) or bilevel positive airway pressure (BiPap).[8]

On the second day the patient underwent musculoskeletal and osteopathic evaluation. Osteopathic diagnosis determined areas of somatic dysfunction and gentle OMT was instituted as an adjunct to conventional medical treatment.[9] Serial cardiac enzyme testing was performed, which showed a trend of decreasing enzyme levels (troponin). Fluid inputs and outputs were tracked, and daily weights were recorded. She had excellent response to IV diuresis, and over the course of 3 days, lost 5 lb. She showed good improvement in oxygen levels and experienced relief of dyspnea and orthopnea. She was able to be removed from supplemental oxygen. Because of the patient's renal failure, her angiotensin receptor blocker was held. Her Metformin was also discontinued due to advanced age and renal failure, as her eGFR was less than 30.[10] Her diabetes was managed with an insulin regimen during hospitalization.

Over the next 3 days, her laboratory results demonstrated normalization of her renal function, sodium level, and the remainder of her electrolytes. Serial EKGs showed no changes. As serial ECHO evaluations are no longer recommended to assess changes in ejection fraction in stable patients, they were not performed.[11] The patient was eventually restarted on her regular medications. In addition, she received counseling from social work while in the hospital, was started on an antidepressant, and provided information for outpatient counseling resources. This patient was discharged to her home at the assisted living facility with outpatient follow-up arranged with her primary care physician. A visiting nurse was arranged to monitor the patient at home and do serial weight and vital sign checks.[12,13] The patient was referred to a supervised cardiac rehabilitation center to begin a comprehensive rehabilitation course. In the outpatient setting, the patient continued to receive osteopathic evaluation and manipulative treatment as an adjunct to her conventional medical management.[14]

OSTEOPATHIC PATIENT MANAGEMENT

The principles that underlie the models of osteopathic manipulative medicine can apply to many different cardiovascular patients, including this patient and her case of heart failure. The remainder of the chapter will discuss the patient and the topic of heart failure through the osteopathic lens as it relates to musculoskeletal medicine and the osteopathic perspective.

The five pathophysiologic models of osteopathic care are as follows:

1. Biomechanical model
2. Respiratory–circulatory model
3. Neurologic model
4. Metabolic energy model
5. Behavioral model

By understanding these principles, one can understand the role of musculoskeletal medicine in this patient and construct a rationale for the application of OMT to assist in the restoration of homeostasis in this and other patients with cardiovascular disease. At all times, attempts will be made to cite biologic, physiologic, pathophysiologic, and clinical data to support an osteopathic approach; however, randomized clinical trials that meet the rigor of current practices of evidence-based medicine in this field are limited, and further research is warranted. Because of this, one must often rely on biologic and pathophysiologic plausibility to support this approach.

Biomechanical Model

When there is a change in structure, functional changes follow. This is one of the basic osteopathic tenets. Structural changes can lead to changes in physiology and pathology.[15] The heart is a muscular structure that resides in the mediastinum, encased in the pericardium that is anchored to the thoracic diaphragm below, and blends and encases the great vessels above. The pericardial sac is continuous with the deep cervical fascia. The left ventricle pumps blood into the systemic circulation via the aorta, which in turn transmits blood into branching vessels. The arterial system accepts blood via the aorta and distributes it throughout the body. The circulatory system provides nourishment and oxygen for the cells, and via the venous system provides a waste removal and blood return mechanism.[16] The structural model views all of these components as providing support and stability to our system. Structural elements are those of bone, muscle, fascia, and all connective tissues. Alterations in these can affect cardiovascular function. An extreme example is the effect of a pronounced thoracic kyphoscoliosis on cardiopulmonary function.[17] Less obvious examples are the effect of small alterations in posture affecting the efficiency of the body's ability to regulate venous return to the heart and lymphatic flow to return into the systemic circulation.[18] Yet another example is the development of compartment syndrome in an extremity after a trauma.[19]

The heart undergoes remodeling and structural changes after MI and because of heart failure. These changes occur through neurohormonal activation as well as other processes. The structural alterations that remodel cardiac geometry and architecture, in addition to the biochemical and biologic changes that occur, are deleterious. Dilation of the LV, thinning of its wall, change in its shape from elliptical to more spherical, and mitral valve incompetence can all occur. These changes create mechanical factors that worsen function. The progression to a more spherical configuration of the LV creates an increase in end-diastolic wall stress and further dilation, which results in increased LV work and oxygen usage. This is one component of the cascade of events that result in biochemical and other biophysical changes in the myocardium.[20]

The venous and lymphatic systems are low-pressure systems, and as such, are much more susceptible to structural changes.[21] The venous system is assisted by muscular contractions to assist in the return of blood from the periphery into the abdomen. Once in the abdomen, diaphragmatic contractions and pressure differentials created by diaphragmatic contractions help return venous blood to the right atrium where it is then propelled by cardiac contraction to the lungs.[22]

The lymphatic system is also a low-pressure system and depends on several factors for return into the systemic circulation. Though myocardial contraction is the primary force driving lymphatic transport, another driving component is the intrinsic rapid/phasic contractions of lymphatic muscle.[23] The endothelium of lymphatic vessel walls is also anchored firmly to the surrounding tissues by filaments, creating a system that changes in response to surrounding physical mechanics and conditions of the tissues.[23] Movement of the extremities, or structural responses of the vessels to the motion of surrounding tissue, will create pressure changes in the lymph vessel. Muscle contractions contributing to these pressure changes assist in propulsion of fluid away from the extremities, help draw extravascular proteins and fluids into the lymphatic system, and propel lymph toward the larger collecting ducts like the thoracic duct and right lymphatic duct. Valves within the lymphatic vessels help prevent back flow. Once in the abdomen, pressure changes generated by the diaphragm will draw lymph into the cisterna chyli, and eventually return fluid to the venous circulation.[24]

The changes in skeletal muscle tone and volume found in a deconditioned state, combined with decreased physical activity and immobility, can compromise musculoskeletal forces needed to assist in venous and lymphatic return from the periphery. Thoracic mechanics and diaphragmatic action will also greatly influence fluid movement and, if altered, can lead to stasis and edema formation.[25]

In this patient's surgical history, we note that she has had a CABG, which required a midline sternotomy and rib retraction. This can alter the motion of the ribs and fascia poststernotomy.[26] Recent research suggests that fascia has active contractile properties.[27] CABG requires cutting through the pericardium, which may change the fascial relations in the mediastinum and fascial attachments.[28]

The patient's bypass vessels were harvested from her lower left leg. This often predisposes patients to the development of lower extremity edema. This patient had worse pitting edema on the left, and this is a likely contributing factor.[29]

The somatic dysfunction in this patient's pelvis and lower extremities also impacts venous and lymphatic drainage.[30] This is evidenced by the increased congestion in the femoral triangle, which serves as a drainage point for the lower extremities into the pelvis.[31] When considering systemic circulation, drainage is further hampered by decreased diaphragmatic excursion and decreased rib motion as found on osteopathic examination. This diminishes the range of pressure differentials generated with each breath; pressure gradients necessary to promote the movement of lymph. The patient also has somatic dysfunction at the thoracic–lumbar junction and an increased kyphosis which can also decrease pressure changes and pumping action of the thoracoabdominal cylinder. Her somatic dysfunction at T1, T3, and T4, with warm, boggy tissue texture change from T1 to T5, requires consideration of viscerosomatic reflexes relating to heart and lung pathology. The left T2 Chapman point, an important diagnostic aid related to viscerosomatic reflexes, is consistent with the other somatic findings and her clinical presentation.[32]

After informed consent was discussed and signed, this patient underwent osteopathic treatment at the hospital bedside. Gentle osteopathic technique was utilized throughout her treatment course. Osteopathic manipulative modalities used included a combination of soft tissue (ST), balanced ligamentous tension (BLT), myofascial release (MFR), muscle energy (ME), and articulatory (ART) techniques.

The goals were to improve motion restrictions and tissue texture changes noted along the spine, decrease fascial restrictions, and help improve musculoskeletal structural relationships to assist the body in restoring homeostasis.

Respiratory–Circulatory Model

The respiratory–circulatory model is a way of viewing fluid movement throughout the body and maintaining the intracellular and extracellular environments. From the macroscopic perspective, we consider the movement of blood and lymph throughout the body. From a microscopic view, we focus on the exchange of oxygen and nutrients, and removal of metabolic waste products at a cellular level. There are many scenarios where circulation at the macroscopic level appears intact, yet at the microscopic level, the needs of end-organ tissues and cells are not met.[33] If there are inadequate end tissue oxygen levels, the cells shift from aerobic to anaerobic metabolism.[34] This causes the production of lactic acid. If there is inadequate drainage from these regions, then there is accumulation of lactic acid. This is usually a local phenomenon but, in severe cases, can be systemic. These severe cases of lactic acidosis can occur in heart failure, acute cardiac ischemia, and other pathophysiologic states such as sepsis.[35] To prevent this, proper tissue functioning is essential and relies on adequate nutrient, oxygen supply, and waste removal. As already stated, efficient venous and lymphatic drainage from the extremities requires musculoskeletal assistance. Muscle tone and fascial relationships influence this. Neurologic tone influences vascular smooth muscle diameter, which influences arterial, venous, and lymphatic outflow from tissues. Increased sympathetic tone raises blood pressure, which can promote movement of fluids into interstitial spaces and inhibit drainage. It can also increase heart rate, contractility, and respiratory rate, which is an adaptive response to restore homeostasis by providing more flow through the system.

Thoracic cage mechanics and diaphragmatic action are important in moving lymph and venous blood from the abdomen and thorax back into circulation.[25] The thoracic diaphragm acts as the "heart" of the lymphatic and venous system and as such contributes to preload. It anchors the heart within the pericardium and flattens the spinal curves with each contraction. Estimating 12 breaths per minute yields 17,280 breaths per day. Each healthy diaphragmatic contraction causes a profound change in pressure differentials. This contributes to preload, draws air into the lungs, assists in lymphatic flow, flattens the spinal curves, and may contribute to passive diffusion processes throughout the body.[36]

Heart failure is characterized by fluid overload. Fluid overload states are characterized by the movement of body fluids from the intravascular space to the extravascular space. Pulmonary edema is a frequent and potentially life-threatening consequence of decompensated heart failure. This occurs when there is an acute rise in the pulmonary capillary pressure, which overwhelms the ability of the pulmonary lymphatic system to drain the excess fluid.[37]

The lymphatic system removes waste and products of inflammation and relieves congestion. The peripheral lymphatic ducts contain valves that help move the lymph in one direction (Fig. 102.2). The lymphatic system utilizes mechanical advantage as much as possible, and as such, lymphatic vessels travel with the arteries and are usually contained in a sheath. With each pulse bringing arterial blood to the extremities, the lymphatics get a mechanical boost back to the central circulation. Once in the central circulation, lymphatic flow is assisted by the diaphragm—as previously discussed—creating pressure differentials and directly influencing the cisterna chyli.[25]

The patient had pleural effusions documented by CXR and peripheral edema seen on exam. She also had mild abdominal complaints and abdominal distension on examination along with

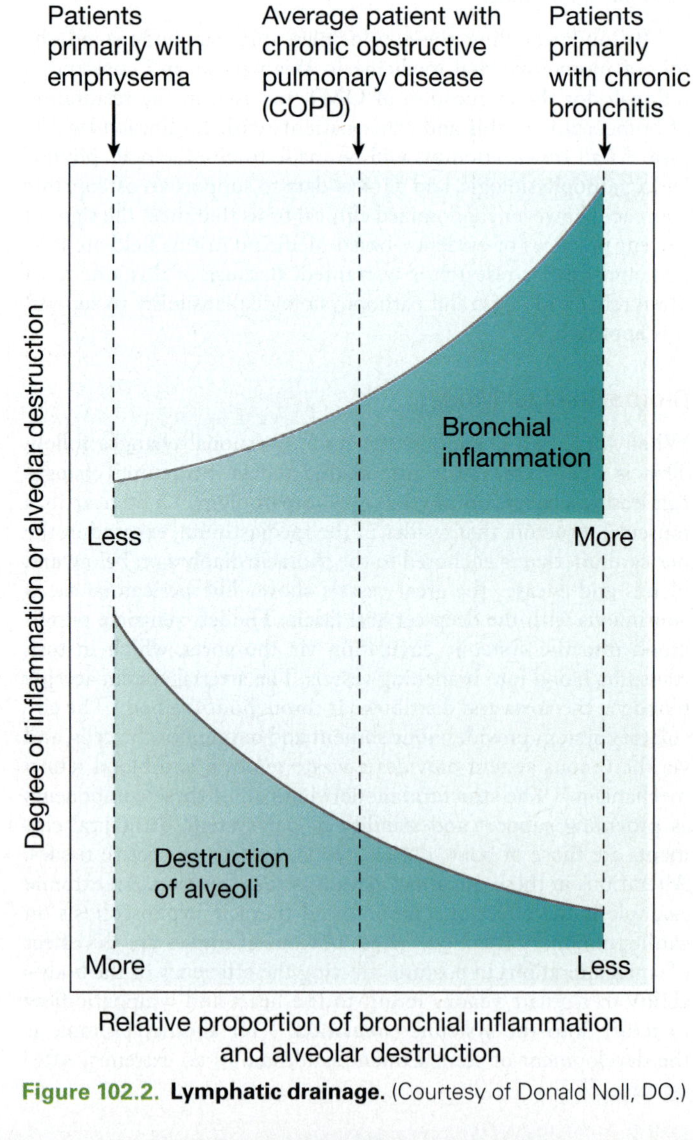

Figure 102.2. Lymphatic drainage. (Courtesy of Donald Noll, DO.)

elevated liver function enzymes in her blood testing. This pattern is consistent with abdominal third spacing and passive hepatic congestion.

In viewing our patient from this respiratory–circulatory perspective, there is evidence of many of the above concepts. This patient had cardiomyopathy with depressed ejection fraction and diastolic dysfunction, which makes her more susceptible to fluid balance disturbances. This patient was taking rapid shallow breaths with poor diaphragmatic and thoracic excursion. In addition, her thoracic mechanics were compromised by poor compliance and an increased kyphosis. This resulted in decreased thoracoabdominal pressure changes. She was quite deconditioned and along with increased lumbar lordosis and sacral nutation had limited musculoskeletal efficiency. She had increased sympathetic activity as evidenced by increased blood pressure, heart rate, and respiratory rate. This is also evidence of vasoconstriction that would affect fluid flow throughout the body.

One of the principles of osteopathic medicine is the ability of the body to self-regulate.[38] It is the osteopathic physician's job to assist the body in this capacity. There are few randomized controlled trials (RCT) addressing heart failure with OMT; however, one such study noted that use of OMT in heart failure patients improved brachial blood flow and increased vagal stimulation.[39] Considering this patient's clinical state and the results of this RCT, a rational treatment approach included osteopathic manipulative intervention to improve this patient's physiology.

In terms of the respiratory–circulatory model, OMT intervention was implemented to augment the pharmacologic and respiratory treatments that were initiated, by aiming to enhance venous and lymphatic drainage to assist in the ability to reabsorb fluids that had been third spaced. This improves the removal of metabolic wastes and, as end-tissue pressures are decreased, helps improve oxygen, nutrient, and possibly medication delivery.

Once the patient in this case had stabilized, OMT was provided to address peripheral drainage by using MR targeting the fascia of the thoracic inlet to improve mechanics of the T1/rib 1/manubrium complex. This was done to optimize thoracic duct drainage. To further induce drainage, a gentle thoracic lymphatic pump technique was used.[40,41] BLT applied to the thoracic and lumbar spine, as well as ART rib raising to the rib cage, were used to improve compliance and pliability of the thorax and decrease the spinal curvature.[42] ME techniques were used to address the bilateral exhaled ribs, likely originating from the patients' nonproductive cough, with the goal of improving thoracic cage movement during inhalation.[39] The diaphragm was redomed to improve efficiency of the thoracoabdominal–pelvic cylinder pump in order to improve flow through the central circulation.[40] The goal of this was to increase pressure changes throughout the thoracoabdominal–pelvic cylinder. Last, lymphatic pedal pump technique was employed to assist drainage from the peripheral tissues to more central lymphatic ducts. As body fluids were mobilized by these procedures from extravascular spaces, and returned to the systemic circulation, cautious observation of the patient's physiologic parameters ensured her heart's ability to adequately move the fluids to the lungs and throughout the body.[42] The patient was not compromised at any point.

In summary, the respiratory–circulatory model deals with fluid movement. The patient had decreased intravascular volume but increased extravascular fluid volume. She was treated with a combination of diuretics (furosemide), preload reduction agents (nitrates), and OMT to assist in restoration of physiologic somatic relationships, venous and lymphatic drainage, and mobilization of the body to ultimately remove excess fluids.

TABLE 102.1

Neurologic Model Considerations

Sympathetic	• Increased catecholamines • Increased chronotropy/ionotropy • Increased BP • Increased oxygen demand • Decreased CBF • Decreased time for diastole • Cardiac remodeling • Impaired lymph drainage • Typical VSR
Parasympathetic	• Vagal • Decreased ionotropy (in some cases increased) • Decreased chronotropy • Decreased BP • Increased CBF • Improved lymph drainage • Myocardial stabilizing • C1/2 segments • No typical musculoskeletal reflex activity

Neurologic Model

The cardiovascular system is under constant influence from the nervous system. The autonomic nervous system (ANS) regulates heart rate, force of cardiac contraction, vascular tone, and blood pressure. The preferred homeostatic state of the cardiovascular system is under parasympathetic dominance. In decompensated heart failure and many chronic cases of heart failure, there are increased levels of catecholamines and hypersympathicotonia.[43]

Under states of increased sympathetic tone, the body experiences increased heart rate (chronotropy), increased force of contraction (inotropy), vasoconstriction, and elevated blood pressure. This, in turn, leads to increased myocardial oxygen demand, which is coupled with decreased coronary blood flow (CBF) from vasoconstriction and decreased time of diastole. These outcomes can lead to cardiac ischemia. Sympathetic and parasympathetic considerations are outlined in Table 102.1.

LV remodeling is recognized in both cardiac ischemia and in the setting of heart failure. Remodeling occurs in response to complex events at the cellular and molecular level, and includes myocyte hypertrophy; changes in myocyte contractility; progressive increases in myocyte death via necrosis, apoptosis, and autophagy; β-adrenergic desensitization; irregular myocardial metabolism and energetics; and decline of the supportive structural matrix of collagen that surrounds myocytes.[44] The resulting decrease in cardiac output leads to activation of neurohormonal systems, such as an increase in efferent sympathetic tone, through "unloading" of peripheral baroreceptors which usually maintain inhibitory parasympathetic tone.[44] Unfortunately, chronic activation of this heightened sympathetic state, along with other neurohumoral influences, produces body compensations that are ineffective and inefficient.[45] There are other pathologic structural changes that occur in the myocardium under these conditions, such as dilation of the left ventricle and valve incompetency, discussed in the preceding section. This is part of the basis of providing beta-blockade and has been shown to modify the remodeling process and improve survival.[46–50] Also, adding ACE inhibitors or angiotensin receptor blockers has also been found to prevent and reverse some of the pathologic remodeling that occurs and also improves mortality.[51–55] Current guideline-directed medical therapy for heart failure patients shows that the best clinical outcomes occur when the following four drug groups are used in conjunction: renin–angiotensin system inhibitors, evidence-based β-blockers, mineralocorticoid inhibitors, and sodium–glucose cotransporter 2 inhibitors.[56]

This patient had LV dysfunction/cardiomyopathy from her ischemic heart disease and resultant heart failure. This is a common remodeling pattern. On presentation, she had signs of heightened sympathetic tone with elevated heart rate and blood pressure.

The sympathetic outflow to the heart is from spinal levels T1–T6.[57] The outflow nerves relay through the middle cervical ganglia and the stellate ganglion. They then join up with the cardiac plexus and ultimately synapse on and innervate the myocardium. Cardiac nociceptors are very sensitive to ischemia and inflammation and relay information to afferent nerves.[58] Afferent nerves from both visceral and somatic structures synapse in the spinal cord onto the same lamina and facilitate viscerosomatic reflex–associated somatic dysfunctions.[59,60]

The palpatory findings associated with viscerosomatic reflexes (due to segmental facilitation) are characterized by warmth, muscle spasm, tissue texture change, tenderness, and moisture. These are explained by the physiologic processes of vasodilation, reflex stimulation of alpha motoneurons in the deep back musculature, activation of the inflammatory cascade, and inflammatory mediators such as substance P. These are the basic findings that characterize viscerally mediated somatic dysfunctions. Several studies have been performed that demonstrate this, consistent with the presentation of our patient.[61,62]

In 1983, Cox et al. published a paper entitled "Palpable musculoskeletal findings in CAD: results of a double-blind study." During this study, 97 patients with cardiac symptoms had a blinded musculoskeletal assessment for somatic dysfunction. All patients went on for cardiac catheterization. The authors concluded that there was a high correlation of changes at T4 in patients with significant cardiac disease in men and women.[63]

Nicholas published a similar study in the *British Medical Journal* in 1985 entitled "A somatic component to myocardial infarction." The authors concluded there was a significantly higher incidence of somatic dysfunction confined almost entirely to the upper thoracic levels in patients experiencing MI. The authors then went on to conduct a 3-year follow-up published in the *British Medical Journal* in 1991 whereby they reassessed patients who had had MI in the previous study, after 3 years post-MI. They found a significant decrease in palpable somatic dysfunctions in these patients who had survived and were treated.[64,65]

Although it has been written about in the osteopathic literature, and there are experimental data in animal models demonstrating somatovisceral reflex activity,[66] there are few select human clinical trials that have investigated the impact of somatic dysfunction and, in particular, somatovisceral reflexes on the development or worsening of visceral disease.[39] This is, however, an intriguing concept that indicates need for further study.[67,68]

This patient had changes in her upper thoracic region that correlate with cardiovascular viscerosomatic reflexes. In addition to the findings of acute viscerosomatic reflexes, such as the warm and boggy tissue texture changes from T1 to T5. Treatment was directed to this area; however, any acute viscerosomatic reflexes were treated with extreme care because of the potential to induce somatovisceral input on an already pathologic area.[42] During outpatient follow-up, treatment was focused on this region to reduce the long-term potential of somatovisceral reflexes to influence her cardiac physiology.

Parasympathetic outflow occurs through the right and left vagus nerves. The vagus nerve exits through the jugular foramen at the occipitomastoid suture and enters the cardiac plexus.[69] Parasympathetic activity slows the heart rate, lowers the blood pressure, and has a myocardial stabilizing effect that is antiarrhythmic. In the decompensated heart, such as a patient with heart failure, restoring autonomic balance by increasing parasympathetic activity can increase inotropy by moving the cardiac physiology to a more favorable portion of the Frank–Starling curve.[70,71]

There are well-described "vagal reflexes" in osteopathic literature that tend to involve the C2 segment. These have been described by osteopaths in both cardiac and pulmonary conditions.[42,61] Along with the C2 segment, the occipital–atlantal junction and occipitomastoid region have been written about in osteopathic literature to influence autonomic tone.[72] There has been research to support that targeted OMT to these regions, such as myofascial cervical techniques, can modulate the ANS and increase vagal stimulation.[73] Some experimental animal data also suggests that vagal afferent activity is mediated through the C1 and C2 spinal segments.[74,75] There is evidence that vagal cardiac afferent activity is inhibitory and decreases muscular spasms and cardiac sympathetic activity generated by noxious cardiac stimulation.[76–79]

The patient did have changes at C2, which may indicate that there are changes in vagal tone. If treating C2 and the other areas of vagal outflow (jugular foramen, occipital mastoid suture, occipital–atlantal joints) could change the autonomic balance toward a parasympathetic predominating state, then this could have a positive influence on our patient.

In addition to the changes suggested above that take place, there are endocrine changes in the decompensated heart failure patient. These include a cascade of events that lead to heart failure. Our patient admits to eating salty foods and skipping some of her medications. Noncompliance to medications and recommended lifestyle changes is quite common for heart failure patients.[80] With increased salt load, there is increased retention of fluids. With increased fluids, there is increased pressure in the vasculature. If cardiac function cannot compensate for this increase in pressure, blood flow actually decreases, referred to as a decrease in effective circulating volume. A reduced effective circulating volume can cause substantial vasoconstriction and venous congestion, further resulting in reduced renal blood flow.[81] This is sensed by the kidneys, which leads to activation of the renin–angiotensin–aldosterone system (RAAS). RAAS activation attempts to preserve fluid volume by salt and fluid reabsorption. ADH secretion from the hypothalamus also acts to reabsorb free water and can contribute to the development of hyponatremia. These changes can lead to heart failure, exacerbation of pre-existing heart failure, peripheral edema, and lymphatic stasis.

In summary, along with appropriate medical treatment (renin–angiotensin system inhibitors, β-blockers, mineralocorticoid inhibitors, and sodium–glucose cotransporter 2 inhibitors) to improve neurohumoral balance and prevent or reverse cardiac remodeling, we also utilize osteopathic treatment. Our osteopathic treatment aims to identify somatic dysfunction that may have contributed to our patient's pathology, mitigate facilitated viscerosomatic reflexes, and assist the body in restoring parasympathetic dominance to the autonomic nervous system.

Metabolic Energy Model

Fatigue and dyspnea are common complaints in heart failure patients, and this is illustrated in our own patient's chief complaints. Exercise capacity is the ability to perform activity, or the endurance of an individual. Exercise intolerance is when an individual is unable to exercise at the expected level. This is a concomitant feature of heart failure.[82]

BOX 102.2 Changes Occurring in Heart Failure

- Downregulation of beta receptors
- Increased diastolic dysfunction
- Increased wedge pressure
- Impaired pulmonary diffusion
- Muscle changes
- Myocyte apoptosis
- Reduced capillary density
- Change from fatigue resistant to fatigable
- Change to anaerobic activity and increased lactic add
- Enhanced ergoreceptors and mechanoreceptors
- Diaphragm change from type 2 to type 1 fibers

Exercise capacity depends on the ability of the cardiovascular system to deliver oxygen to exercising skeletal muscle, as well as the ability of that muscle to extract oxygen from the blood. This is based on cardiovascular dynamics, the ability of pulmonary gas exchange, and skeletal muscle metabolism.[82] Peak exercise capacity is defined as the maximum of this capacity, and maximal oxygen uptake (VO_{2max}) has a strong linear correlation with cardiac output and skeletal muscle blood flow.[83]

Heart failure patients have a reduced capacity to increase cardiac output, and therefore have marked exercised intolerance associated with reduced quality of life.[84,85] Several factors may contribute to the inability of heart failure patients to have sufficient response to exercise (Box 102.2). There is downregulation of beta receptors in the setting of chronically elevated catecholamine levels, and this result in a reduced ionotropic and chronotropic response.[86,87] There is an increase in diastolic dysfunction that may impair cardiac output. There is a demonstrated abnormal increase in pulmonary wedge pressure that can exacerbate pulmonary congestion, causing dyspnea and limiting exercise capacity. There can also be impaired pulmonary diffusion even in the absence of pulmonary congestion.

Previously, it was thought that poor exercise capacity was solely due to depressed cardiac output and decreased oxygen delivery, and that treatment with positive inotropes would improve symptoms and exercise capacity. Several studies investigated the impact of inotropes and vasodilators on exercise tolerance and found that although there were measurable increases in both cardiac output and peripheral blood flow, which would also increase oxygen delivery to exercising muscles; there were no significant increases in exercise capacity.[88] The researchers were able to demonstrate that these interventions had limited impact on maximal oxygen consumption (VO_{2max}) and concluded that this may have been from decreased oxygen extraction by the muscle. Subsequently, it became recognized that there were intrinsic skeletal muscle changes, "noncardiac" factors, which were present in heart failure patients that had a substantial role in exercise tolerance.[89] This became known as the muscle hypothesis.[90] Though limited, research shows consistent evidence that multiple skeletal muscle abnormalities are associated with heart failure and that exercise training induces favorable adaptations that contribute to improvements in exercise tolerance.[89]

There are several contributing factors in the development of skeletal muscle abnormalities. Physical deconditioning and inactivity are thought to be one factor. Another factor may be chronic hypoperfusion of skeletal muscle secondary to an inadequate response to exercise and a shift from aerobic to anaerobic metabolism.[91,92] Myocyte apoptosis has also been identified in heart failure patients and correlates with the degree of limitation in exercise capacity.[93] Capillary density is reduced in heart failure patients compared with controls and has an inverse relationship with oxygen consumption.[94] Biochemical abnormalities have been found that include changes in the types of muscle fibers from fatigue resistant to more fatigable types.[92,95] Other studies have found lower intracellular pH, indicating increased lactic acid buildup secondary to anaerobic metabolism, evidence of more rapid depletion, and, less efficient utilization of high-energy phosphates both in the presence of preserved blood flow.[96]

In addition to structural changes, functional abnormalities have been found in patients with heart failure. One example lies in the enhancement of ergoreceptors and metaboreceptors which may partially explain the increased ventilatory response and dyspnea in heart failure.[97–100] Respiratory muscles undergo the above changes in heart failure patients and may also be contributing to the symptom complex by early fatigue.[101] The diaphragm undergoes change from type 2 (fast twitch, glycolytic, fatigue susceptible) fibers to type 1 (slow twitch, oxidative, fatigue resistant) fibers, which is thought to be from the increased work of breathing.[102] These are similar changes to those that occur with endurance training.[103]

Exercise training and cardiac rehabilitation have been studied and have been shown to have many benefits:

- Improved peak VO_2, improved muscle energetics, more efficient oxygen utilization, and improved symptoms of fatigue and dyspnea.[104,105]
- Reduced sympathetic tone and increased vagal tone at rest, decreased systemic vascular resistance, reduced neurohumoral activity, and decreased levels of angiotensin, aldosterone, and BNP have also been demonstrated.[106–109]
- Reversal of skeletal muscle abnormalities such as mitochondrial density and a shift from type 2 to type 1 muscle fibers are seen.[110]
- Improvements in VO_{2peak} can be seen, and this translates to improved symptoms, exercise capacity, and ability to perform activities of daily living and maintain independence.
- Improvement in New York Heart Association (NYHA) class and 6-minute walk distance as well as reduction in hospitalization rates has been noted.[108–114]
- One meta-analysis concluded there were reduced mortality and rate of hospitalization in patients who participated in a supervised exercise program for 8 weeks at 2 years of follow-up.[115]

Thus, exercise training has a class 1 recommendation from the American College of Cardiology and American Heart Association (ACC/AHA) for heart failure patients with preserved and reduced systolic function.[116]

Due to the patient's deconditioned state, she was recommended exercise-based cardiac rehabilitation. To improve efficacy of her rehabilitation, osteopathic treatment focused on improving her stiffened thorax, function of her abdominal diaphragm, legs, and pelvis.

The combined effect of her cardiac rehabilitation and OMT for musculoskeletal dysfunction aimed to improve her work of breathing and oxygen utilization.

One of the tenets of osteopathic medicine is the reciprocal nature of structure and function.[38] Many of the above changes in cardiac and skeletal muscle function illustrate this relationship. This is demonstrated clearly by the diaphragm, which changes structure on the microscopic level to accommodate functional changes on a macroscopic level.

There are very limited studies looking at the impact of osteopathic manipulation on energy utilization or documenting changes in the structure of skeletal, respiratory, or diaphragmatic muscle or the types of biophysical and biochemical changes listed previously in heart failure patients; however, by evaluating and treating somatic dysfunctions, we addressed our patient's structure in the expectation there would be a positive change in her function and functional status.

To summarize, the patient had complaints of dyspnea and fatigue at baseline exacerbated at presentation. Once her acute symptoms were treated and she had clinical improvement, she was appropriately referred for a supervised cardiac rehabilitation program. She continued to undergo outpatient osteopathic diagnosis and treatment with a goal of reducing the work of breathing by improved pulmonary and chest wall compliance and improving her overall functional status through enhanced musculoskeletal relationships and decreased somatic dysfunction severity.

Behavioral Model

In osteopathic medicine, we are trained to look at the person as a whole. One of the basic tenets of osteopathic medicine is that the person is a unity of body, mind, and spirit.[38] When we review the history of this patient, it is important to note some of the behavioral aspects that have a direct impact on this patient's life and well-being. She has recently lost her spouse of many years. Our patient reports feeling depressed after the death of her husband, which has been exacerbated by the recent change in her living arrangement. She went from living independently with her spouse to living interdependently alone in an assisted living apartment and has therefore been grieving these losses. This can cause substantial emotional and personal suffering and a large impact on immediate and long-term health. She admits to eating foods that she knows are deleterious for her. In addition, she is skipping her medications at times. These two factors alone could precipitate her present condition and are more likely to result from behavioral influences rather than medical conditions. This highlights the importance of addressing these concerns.

It has long been suspected that there is an increase in the incidence of depression in patients with heart failure.[117,118] There have been several studies looking at this relationship. It is becoming clear that not only is depression common in heart failure patients, but that it is associated with increased mortality and rehospitalization.[116–121] The findings of depression and social isolation worsen mortality.[122] Anxiety, although also common in this population, has had conflicting data in regard to whether it is associated with increased mortality.[122]

In 2008, an interesting trial was published that looked at treating heart failure patients with an antidepressant, sertraline, for a period of 12 weeks. All patients in the trial received nursing intervention and one arm of the trial received sertraline.[123,124] The trial showed no significant difference in patients treated with the antidepressant versus patients who had just nursing intervention. Ultimately, this lack of appreciable difference found in the sertraline against depression and heart disease in chronic heart failure (SADHART)-CHF study among depressed patients with heart failure who received nursing care versus those who received nursing care and selective serotonin reuptake inhibitors, indicated that nursing intervention was so successful the effects of sertraline alone were masked.[123] Although the study was not powered to look at hospitalization rates, there was a trend toward decreased hospitalization rates in the treatment group.[123] This may indicate that nursing intervention could be a preferred treatment for these patients. Although the extent to which antidepressants may benefit mood in heart failure patients is not certain, they may have the potential to help depressed heart failure patients by the restoration of normal autonomic function, which may improve immune and inflammatory factors.[124]

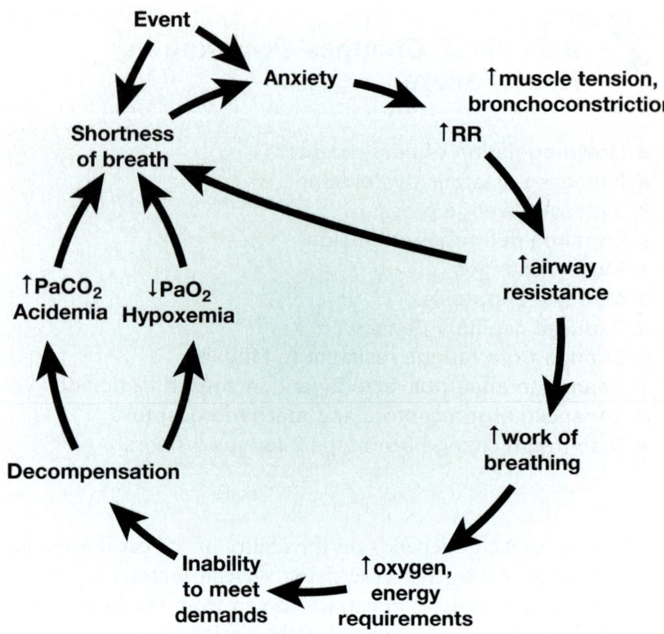

Figure 102.3. Allostatic load.

There are not many controlled trials looking at the treatment of mood disorders with manipulation. The studies that have been performed do not readily translate to the typical heart failure patients.[125,126] These studies have not found any somatic dysfunction pattern that was "typical" for the patient with depression. Despite the lack of applicable randomized control trials, these studies do offer some evidence in favor of osteopathic manipulation as an intervention for patients with depression. The etiology of this benefit is less clear.

One possible explanation may be found in the concept of allostatic load. The term allostatic load was coined by Dr. Bruce McEwen and refers to the physiologic costs of chronic exposure to neuroendocrine immune stress responses. It is used to explain how frequent activation of the body's stress response, an essential tool for managing acute threats, can in fact damage the body in the long run through activation of the hypothalamic–pituitary axis.[127] The nervous system integrates information from the somatic, visceral, and psychological sources, and these can summate to achieve a stress response (Fig. 102.3). It is possible that by treating underlying somatic dysfunction there may be a decrease in the overall allostatic load of these patients.[68,128] Although somatic dysfunction seemingly related to cardiovascular disease has been described,[63,129,130] alleviation of these findings by OMT, or alteration of these findings throughout the course of illness, have yet to be studied in prospective, randomized, controlled clinical trials. The potential benefit of OMT in this patient population also awaits elucidation by further research.

In this patient's case, it was important to discuss her living arrangements and behaviors associated with her current state. To further address these factors, the patient received social work evaluation during her hospitalization and then outpatient follow-up from visiting nurse services and social work after she returned home. In addition, to address her depression, she was given the option of pharmacologic treatment, which she chose to begin. An antidepressant was started during her hospitalization and continued for outpatient treatment. The patient was receiving osteopathic treatment in the hospital as part of a comprehensive plan of acute management for heart failure, and this was also continued after her hospitalization. Over time, this patient's mood did improve, and she demonstrated a renewed interest in her health and well-being.

In osteopathic medicine, one looks at the person as a whole, a unity of body, mind, and spirit.[38] This is demonstrated in the connection between depression, anxiety, social isolation, and outcomes in heart failure referenced above. One intervention we can offer as physicians is to recognize the connection between heart failure and depression and take corrective steps to address this. Frequent outpatient physician visits, visiting nurse services, counseling, or mobilization of support services may provide improved care. Another component of intervention is to include osteopathic diagnosis and treatment in our approach to these patients to treat the somatic dysfunction we find with the intention of decreasing any somatic contribution to the overall allostatic load.

To summarize, there is an established connection between heart failure and depression. This has been demonstrated in several studies and should be in our minds when evaluating patients with either acute or chronic heart failure. It is reasonable to institute appropriate osteopathic interventions in the belief that these will positively impact our patients' health, and although no large RCTs demonstrate this, the suggested evidence of smaller trials and pathophysiologic rationale supports the use of OMT as a possible intervention in this patient population.

SUMMARY

Heart failure is a complicated diagnosis, which has many causes that can lead to changes in the structure of the heart and vasculature (remodeling), neurohumoral changes, and endocrinologic changes throughout the body. There are changes in the skeletal muscle that have a large contribution to two of the hallmark symptoms of heart failure: dyspnea and fatigue. There are medications that have been shown to improve mortality and morbidity and decrease hospitalization rates.[56] Despite the available medical treatments, there are patients who will remain symptomatic, and we must look at other impacting factors, such as skeletal muscle changes. There is a recognized correlation with depression, which should be recognized, evaluated, and will need to be treated in some patients. Cardiovascular disease introduces detrimental somatic changes throughout the body, impairing optimal functioning through diaphragmatic restriction, lymphatic stasis, inflammatory viscerosomatic reflexes, and other systems as mentioned throughout the case. Although few sufficient RCTs have been conducted to examine the role of OMT in heart failure, there are supporting data in the form of physiologic and pathophysiologic plausibility for the use of adjunctive osteopathic diagnosis and treatments.[39] This patient case showed many classic findings and complaints consistent with heart failure and has served to illustrate the principles in the evaluation and treatment of heart failure patients.

REFERENCES

1. Elliott WJ, Ram CVS. Calcium channel blockers. *J Clin Hypertens (Greenwich)*. 2011;13(9):687–689.
2. Prieto H, Pena N, Shubrook JH, Talsma J. Hypertension: an osteopathic perspective. *The AAO Journal*. 2020;30(2):27–34.
3. Beal MC, Morlock JW. Somatic dysfunction associated with pulmonary disease. *J Am Osteopath Assoc*. 1984;84(2):179–183.
4. Banerjee D, Perrett C, Banerjee A. Troponins, acute coronary syndrome and renal disease: from acute kidney injury through end-stage kidney disease. *Eur Cardiol*. 2019;14(3):187–190.
5. Pillai BP, Unnikrishnan AG, Pavithran PV. Syndrome of inappropriate antidiuretic hormone secretion: revisiting a classical endocrine disorder. *Indian J Endocrinol Metab*. 2011;15(Suppl3):S208–S215.
6. Skorecki K, Chertow GM, Marsden PA, et al. *Brenner and Rector's the Kidney*. 10th ed. Elsevier; 2016.
7. Njoroge JN, Teerlink JR. Pathophysiology and therapeutic approaches to acute decompensated heart failure. *Circ Res*. 2021;128(10):1468–1486.
8. Masip J, Peacock WF, Price S, et al. Indications and practical approach to non-invasive ventilation in acute heart failure. *Eur Heart J*. 2018;39(1):17–25.
9. Fitzgerald M, Stiles E. Osteopathic hospital's solution to DRG's may be OMT. *In The DO*. 1984:97–101.
10. Hur KY, Kim MK, Ko SH, et al. Metformin treatment for patients with diabetes and chronic kidney disease: a Korean Diabetes Association and Korean Society of Nephrology Consensus Statement. *Diabetes Metab J*. 2020;44(1):3–10.
11. Heidenreich PA, Bozkurt B, Aguilar D, et al. 2022 AHA/ACC/HFSA guideline for the management of heart failure: a report of the American College of Cardiology/American Heart Association Joint Committee on Clinical Practice Guidelines [published correction appears in *Circulation*. 2022 May 3;145(18):e1033] [published correction appears in *Circulation*. 2022 Sep 27;146(13):e185] [published correction appears in *Circulation*. 2023 Apr 4;147(14):e674]. *Circulation*. 2022;145(18):e895–e1032.
12. Young B, Purden M, Sauvé N, Dufour L, Common C. A "basket of care" for heart failure patients managing at home: evaluating a community-based nursing intervention from a patient's perspective. *Can J Cardiovasc Nurs*. 2008;18(4):10–19.
13. Staples P, Earle W. The nature of telephone nursing interventions in a heart failure clinic setting. *Can J Cardiovasc Nurs*. 2008;18(4):27–33.
14. Seffinger MA. Osteopathic philosophy. In: Ward RC, Ex. ed. *Foundations for Osteopathic Medicine*. William & Wilkins; 1997:4–6.
15. Seo DY, Kwak HB, Kim AH, et al. Cardiac adaptation to exercise training in health and disease. *Pflugers Arch*. 2020;472(2):155–168.
16. Rosse C. *Hollinshead's Textbook of Anatomy. The Thorax, the Pericardium, the Heart, the Great Vessels*. Lippincott-Raven Publishers; 1997:70–82.
17. Thomas MA, Wang Y. Scoliosis and kyphosis. In: Frontera WR, Silver JK, Rizzo TD Jr, eds. *Essentials of Physical Medicine and Rehabilitation: Musculoskeletal Disorders, Pain, and Rehabilitation*. 2nd ed. Saunders/Elsevier; 2008.
18. Wang H, Gao X, Shi Y, Wu D, Li C, Wang W. Effects of trunk posture on cardiovascular and autonomic nervous systems: a pilot study. *Front Physiol*. 2022;13:1009806.
19. Amos T, Yeung M, Gooi J, Fitzgerald M. Survival following traumatic thoracic compartment syndrome managed with VV-ECMO. *Trauma Case Rep*. 2019;24:100249.
20. Burchfield JS, Xie M, Hill JA. Pathological ventricular remodeling: mechanisms: part 1 of 2. *Circulation*. 2013;128(4):388–400.
21. Zhou Y, Huang C, Hu Y, Xu Q, Hu X. Lymphatics in cardiovascular disease. *Arterioscler Thromb Vasc Biol*. 2020;40(11):e275–e283.
22. Magder S. Volume and its relationship to cardiac output and venous return. *Crit Care*. 2016;20(1):271.
23. Zawieja DC. Contractile physiology of lymphatics. *Lymphat Res Biol*. 2009;7(2):87–96.
24. Goswami AK, Khaja MS, Downing T, Kokabi N, Saad WE, Majdalany BS. Lymphatic anatomy and physiology. *Semin Intervent Radiol*. 2020;37(3):227–236.
25. Cahalin LP. Pulmonary evaluation. In: DeTurk WE, Cahalin LP, eds. *Cardiovascular and Pulmonary Physical Therapy: An Evidence-Based Approach*. 3rd ed. McGraw-Hill Education; 2017.
26. Kenyon CM, Pedley TJ, Higenbottam TW. Adaptive modeling of the human rib cage in median sternotomy. *J Appl Physiol*. 1991;70(5):2287–2302.
27. Schleip R, Gabbiani G, Wilke J, et al. Fascia is able to actively contract and may thereby influence musculoskeletal dynamics: a histochemical and mechanographic investigation. *Front Physiol*. 2019;10:336.
28. Bordoni B, Escher A. Pericardial adhesion and chronic non-specific neck pain following thoracentesis: an osteopathic approach. *Clinics and Practice*. 2023;13(6):1313–1318.
29. Heitink MV, Schurink GW, de Pont CD, van Kroonenburgh MJ, Veraart JC. Lymphedema after greater saphenous vein surgery. *EJVES Extra*. 2009;18(4):41–43.
30. Buskirk RLV. Nociceptive reflexes and the somatic dysfunction: a model. *J Am Osteopath Assoc*. 1990;90(9):792–809.

31. Rosse C. The free lower limb. In: *Hollinshead's Textbook of Anatomy*. Lippincott-Raven Publishers; 1997:354.
32. Bath M, Owens J. Physiology, viscerosomatic reflexes. [Updated 2023 May 1]. In: *StatPearls [Internet]*. StatPearls Publishing; 2024.
33. Marino PL. *The ICU Book*. 2nd ed. Lippincott Williams & Wilkins, a Wolters Kluwer business; 188.
34. Loscalzo J. The cellular response to hypoxia: tuning the system with microRNAs. *J Clin Invest*. 2010;120(11):3815–3817.
35. Hotchkiss RS, Karl IE. Reevaluation of the role of cellular hypoxia and bioenergetic failure in sepsis. *JAMA*. 1992;267(11):1503–1510.
36. Bordoni B, Zanier E. Anatomic connections of the diaphragm: influence of respiration on the body system. *J Multidiscip Healthc*. 2013;6: 281–291.
37. Acute pulmonary edema. In: Jameson J, Fauci AS, Kasper DL, Hauser SL, Longo DL, Loscalzo J. eds. *Harrison's Manual of Medicine*, 20e. McGraw-Hill Education; 2020.
38. Bordoni B, Escher AR Jr. Osteopathic principles: the inspiration of every science is its change. *Cureus*. 2021;13(1):e12478. Published 2021 Jan 4.
39. Amatuzzi F, de Lima AC, Da Silva ML, et al. Acute and time-course effects of osteopathic manipulative treatment on vascular and autonomic function in patients with heart failure: a randomized trial. *J Manipulative Physiol Ther*. 2021;44(6):455–466.
40. Zink JG. Respiratory and circulatory care: the conceptual model. *Osteopath Ann*. 1977;1:108–112.
41. Knott EM, Tune JD, Stoll ST, Downey HF. Increased lymphatic flow in the thoracic duct during manipulative intervention. *J Am Osteopath Assoc*. 2005;105(10):447–456.
42. Ettlinger H. Treatment of the acutely ill hospitalized patient. In: Ward RC, Ex. ed. *Foundations of Osteopathic Medicine*. 2nd ed. William & Wilkins; 2003:1115–1135; Chapter 71.
43. Francis GS, Benedict C, Johnstone DE, et al. Comparison of neuroendocrine activation in patients with left ventricular dysfunction with and without congestive heart failure. A substudy of the Studies of Left Ventricular Dysfunction (SOLVD). *Circulation*. 1990;82(5):1724–1729.
44. Mann DL, Chakinala M. Heart failure: pathophysiology and diagnosis. In: Jameson J, Fauci AS, Kasper DL, Hauser SL, Longo DL, Loscalzo J. eds. *Harrison's Principles of Internal Medicine*. 20th ed. McGraw-Hill Education; 2018.
45. Hartupee J, Mann DL. Neurohormonal activation in heart failure with reduced ejection fraction. *Nat Rev Cardiol*. 2017;14(1):30–38.
46. Doughty RN, Whalley GA, Gamble G, MacMahon S, Sharpe N. Left ventricular remodeling with carvedilol in patients with congestive heart failure due to ischemic heart disease. Australia-New Zealand Heart Failure Research Collaborative Group. *J Am Coll Cardiol*. 1997;29(5):1060–1066.
47. Groenning BA, Nilsson JC, Sondergaard L, Fritz-Hansen T, Larsson HB, Hildebrandt PR. Antiremodeling effects on the left ventricle during beta-blockade with metoprolol in the treatment of chronic heart failure. *J Am Coll Cardiol*. 2000;36(7):2072–2080.
48. Bellenger NG, Rajappan K, Rahman SL, et al. Effects of carvedilol on left ventricular remodelling in chronic stable heart failure: a cardiovascular magnetic resonance study. *Heart*. 2004;90(7):760–764.
49. Effect of metoprolol CR/XL in chronic heart failure: metoprolol CR/XL Randomised Intervention Trial in Congestive Heart Failure (MERIT-HF). *Lancet*. 1999;353(9169):2001–2007.
50. Hjalmarson A, Goldstein S, Fagerberg B, et al. Effects of controlled-release metoprolol on total mortality, hospitalizations, and well-being in patients with heart failure: the Metoprolol CR/XL Randomized Intervention Trial in congestive heart failure (MERIT-HF). MERIT-HF Study Group. *JAMA*. 2000;283(10):1295–1302.
51. The CONSENSUS Trial Study Group. Effects of enalapril on mortality in severe congestive heart failure. Results of the Cooperative North Scandinavian Enalapril Survival Study (CONSENSUS). *N Engl J Med*. 1987;316(23):1429–1435.
52. The SOLVD Investigators; Yusuf S, Pitt B, Davis CE, Hood WB, Cohn JN. Effect of enalapril on survival in patients with reduced left ventricular ejection fractions and congestive heart failure. *N Engl J Med*. 1991;325(5):293–302.
53. Granger CB, McMurray JJV, Yusuf S, et al. Effects of candesartan in patients with chronic heart failure and reduced left-ventricular systolic function intolerant to angiotensin-converting-enzyme inhibitors: the CHARM-Alternative trial. *Lancet*. 2003;362(9386):772–776.
54. Erhardt L, MacLean A, Ilgenfritz J, Gelperin K, Blumenthal M. Fosinopril attenuates clinical deterioration and improves exercise tolerance in patients with heart failure. Fosinopril Efficacy/Safety Trial (FEST) Study Group. *Eur Heart J*. 1995;16(12):1892–1899.
55. Pfeffer MA, McMurray JJ, Velazquez EJ, et al. Valsartan, captopril, or both in myocardial infarction complicated by heart failure, left ventricular dysfunction, or both. *N Engl J Med*. 2003;349(20):1893–1906.
56. Patel J, Rassekh N, Fonarow GC, et al. Guideline-directed medical therapy for the treatment of heart failure with reduced ejection fraction. *Drugs*. 2023;83(9):747–759.
57. Rosse C. *The Thorax, the Pericardium, the Heart, the Great Vessels Hollinshead's Textbook of Anatomy*. Lippincott-Raven Publishers; 1997: 481–484.
58. Premkumar LS, Raisinghani M. Nociceptors in cardiovascular functions: complex interplay as a result of cyclooxygenase inhibition. *Mol Pain*. 2006; 2:26.
59. Patterson MM, Wurster RD. Somatic dysfunction, spinal facilitation, and viscerosomatic integration. In: Ward EC, ed. *Foundations of Osteopathic Medicine*. 4th ed. Philadelphia, PA: Lippincott Williams & Wilkins; 2018:300–317.
60. Van Buskirk RL. Nociceptive reflexes and the somatic dysfunction: a model. *J Am Osteopath Assoc*. 1990;90(9):792–809.
61. Beal MC. Palpatory testing for somatic dysfunction in patients with cardiovascular disease. *J Am Osteopath Assoc*. 1983;82(11):822–831.
62. Sato A, Schmidt RF. Reflex modulation of visceral functions by somatic afferent activity. In: Patterson MM, Howell JN, eds. *The Central Connection: Somatovisceral/Viscerosomatic Interaction. 1989 International Symposium*. American Academy of Osteopathy; 1989:53–76.
63. Cox JM, Gorbis S, Dick LM, Rogers JC, Rogers FJ. Palpable musculoskeletal findings in coronary artery disease: results of a double-blind study. *J Am Osteopath Assoc*. 1983;82(11):832–836.
64. Nicholas AS, DeBias DA, Ehrenfeuchter W, et al. A somatic component to myocardial infarction. *Br Med J (Clin Res Ed)*. 1985;291(6487):13–17.
65. Nicholas AS, DeBias DA, Greene CH. Somatic component to myocardial infarction: three year follow up. *BMJ*. 1991;302(6792):1581.
66. Sato A. Somatovisceral reflexes. *J Manipulative Physiol Ther*. 1995;18(9): 597–602.
67. Patterson MM, Wurster RD. Neurophysiological mechanisms of integration and disintegration. In: Ward RC, Ex. ed. *Foundations for Osteopathic Medicine*. 2nd ed. William & Wilkins; 2003:121–134; Chapter 7.
68. Willard F. Nociception, the neuroendocrine immune system and osteopathic medicine. In: Ward RC, Ex. ed. *Foundations for Osteopathic Medicine*. 2nd ed. William & Wilkins; 2003:138–154; Chapter 8.
69. Rosse C. *Hollinshead's Textbook of Anatomy*. Lippincott-Raven Publishers; 1997:481–484.
70. Zile MR, Lindenfeld J, Weaver FA, et al. Baroreflex activation therapy in patients with heart failure with reduced ejection fraction. *J Am Coll Cardiol*. 2020;76(1):1–13.
71. Braunwald E, Bonow RO, Mann DL, Zipes DP, Libby P. *Heart Disease: A Textbook of Cardiovascular Medicine*. 6th ed. Philadelphia, PA: W.B. Saunders Company; 2001:660–694.
72. Magoun HI. *Osteopathy in the Cranial Field*. 3rd ed. 108–115, 268.
73. Carnevali L, Lombardi L, Fornari M, Sgoifo A. Exploring the effects of osteopathic manipulative treatment on autonomic function through the lens of heart rate variability. *Front Neurosci*. 2020;14:579365.
74. Ding X, Hua F, Sutherly K, Ardell JL, Williams CA. C2 spinal cord stimulation induces dynorphin release from rat T4 spinal cord: potential modulation of myocardial ischemia-sensitive neurons. *Am J Physiol Regul Integr Comp Physiol*. 2008;295(5):R1519–R1528.
75. Qin C, Chandler MJ, Jou CJ, Foreman RD. Responses and afferent pathways of C1-C2 spinal neurons to cervical and thoracic esophageal stimulation in rats. *J Neurophysiol*. 2004;91(5):2227–2235.
76. Jou CJ, Farber JP, Foreman FD. Afferent pathways for cardiac-somatic motor reflexes in rats. *Am J Physiol Regul Integr Comp Physiol*. 2001; 281(6):R2096–R2102.
77. Ding X, Ardell JL, Hua F. Modulation of cardiac ischemia-sensitive afferent neuron signaling by preemptive C2 spinal cord stimulation: effect on

substance P release from rat spinal cord. *Am J Physiol Regul Integr Comp Physiol.* 2008;294(1):R93–R101.

78. Ammons WS, Blair RW, Foreman RD. Vagal afferent inhibition of spinothalamic cell responses to sympathetic afferents and bradykinin in the monkey. *Circ Res.* 1983;53(5):603–612.
79. Burton AR, Fazalbhoy A, Macefield VG. Sympathetic responses to noxious stimulation of muscle and skin. *Front Neurol.* 2016;7:109.
80. Van der Wal MH, Jaarsma T, van Veldhuisen DJ. Non-compliance in patients with heart failure; how can we manage it? *Eur J Heart Fail.* 2005;7(1):5–17.
81. Waldum B, Westheim AS, Sandvik L, et al. Renal function in outpatients with chronic heart failure. *J Card Fail.* 2010;16(5):374–380.
82. Del Buono MG, Arena R, Borlaug BA, et al. Exercise intolerance in patients with heart failure: JACC State-of-the-Art Review. *J Am Coll Cardiol.* 2019;73(17):2209–2225.
83. Reddy HK, Weber KT, Janicki JS, McElroy PA. Hemodynamic, ventilatory and metabolic effects of light isometric exercise in patients with chronic heart failure. *J Am Coll Cardiol.* 1988;12(2):353–358.
84. Haykowsky MJ, Tomczak CR, Scott JM, Paterson DI, Kitzman DW. Determinants of exercise intolerance in patients with heart failure and reduced or preserved ejection fraction. *J Appl Physiol.* 2015;119(6):739–744.
85. Kitzman DW, Little WC, Brubaker PH, et al. Pathophysiological characterization of isolated diastolic heart failure in comparison to systolic heart failure. *JAMA.* 2002;288(17):2144–2150.
86. Colucci WS. In vivo studies of myocardial beta-adrenergic receptor pharmacology in patients with congestive heart failure. *Circulation.* 1990;82(2 suppl):144–151.
87. Bristow MR, Minobe WA, Raynolds MV, et al. Reduced beta 1 receptor messenger RNA abundance in the failing human heart. *J Clin Invest.* 1993;92(6):2737–2745.
88. Wilson JR, Martin JL, Ferraro N. Impaired skeletal muscle nutritive flow during exercise in patients with congestive heart failure: role of cardiac pump dysfunction as determined by the effect of dobutamine. *Am J Cardiol.* 1984;53(9):1308–1315.
89. Tucker WJ, Haykowsky MJ, Seo Y, Stehling E, Forman DE. Impaired exercise tolerance in heart failure: role of skeletal muscle morphology and function. *Curr Heart Fail Rep.* 2018;15(6):323–331.
90. Clark AL, Poole-Wilson PA, Coats AJ. Exercise limitation in chronic heart failure: central role of the periphery. *J Am Coll Cardiol.* 1996;28(5):1092–1102.
91. Belardinelli R, Barstow TJ, Nguyen P, Wasserman K. Skeletal muscle oxygenation and oxygen uptake kinetics following constant work rate exercise in chronic congestive heart failure. *Am J Cardiol.* 1997;80(10):1319–1324.
92. Zizola C, Schulze PC. Metabolic and structural impairment of skeletal muscle in heart failure. *Heart Fail Rev.* 2013;18(5):623–630.
93. Vescovo G, Volterrani M, Zennaro R, et al. Apoptosis in the skeletal muscle of patients with heart failure: investigation of clinical and biochemical changes. *Heart.* 2000;84(4):431–437.
94. Duscha BD, Kraus WE, Keteyian SJ, et al. Capillary density of skeletal muscle: a contributing mechanism for exercise intolerance in class II-III chronic heart failure independent of other peripheral alterations. *J Am Coll Cardiol.* 1999;33(7):1956–1963.
95. Mancini DM, Coyle E, Coggan A, et al. Contribution of intrinsic skeletal muscle changes to 31P NMR skeletal muscle metabolic abnormalities in patients with chronic heart failure. *Circulation.* 1989;80(5):1338–1346.
96. Massie B, Conway M, Yonge R, et al. Skeletal muscle metabolism in patients with congestive heart failure: relation to clinical severity and blood flow. *Circulation.* 1987;76(5):1009–1019.
97. Scott AC, Francis DP, Davies LC, Ponikowski P, Coats AJ, Piepoli MF. Contribution of skeletal muscle 'ergoreceptors' in the human leg to respiratory control in chronic heart failure. *J Physiol.* 2000;529 Pt 3(Pt 3):863–870.
98. Chua TP, Ponikowski PP, Harrington D, Chambers J, Coats AJ. Contribution of peripheral chemoreceptors to ventilation and the effects of their suppression on exercise tolerance in chronic heart failure. *Heart.* 1996;76(6):483–489.
99. Ponikowski PP, Chua TP, Francis DP, Capucci A, Coats A, Piepoli MF. Muscle ergoreceptor overactivity reflects deterioration in clinical status and cardiorespiratory reflex control in chronic heart failure. *Circulation.* 2001;104(19):2324–2330.
100. Piepoli M, Clark AL, Volterrani M, Adamopoulos S, Sleight P, Coats AJ. Contribution of muscle afferents to the hemodynamic, autonomic, and ventilatory responses to exercise in patients with chronic heart failure: effects of physical training. *Circulation.* 1996;93(5):940–952.
101. Meyer FJ, Borst MM, Zugck C, et al. Respiratory muscle dysfunction in congestive heart failure: clinical correlation and prognostic significance. *Circulation.* 2001;103(17):2153–2158.
102. Tikunov B, Levine S, Mancini D. Chronic congestive heart failure elicits adaptations of endurance exercise in diaphragmatic muscle. *Circulation.* 1997;95(4):910–916.
103. Plotkin DL, Roberts MD, Haun CT, Schoenfeld BJ. Muscle fiber type transitions with exercise training: shifting perspectives. *Sports (Basel).* 2021;9(9):127.
104. Belardinelli R, Georgiou D, Cianci G, Purcaro A. Effects of exercise training on left ventricular filling at rest and during exercise in patients with ischemic cardiomyopathy and severe left ventricular systolic dysfunction. *Am Heart J.* 1996;132(1 pt 1):61–70.
105. McKelvie RS, Teo KK, McCartney N, Humen D, Montague T, Yusuf S. Effects of exercise training in patients with congestive heart failure: a critical review. *J Am Coll Cardiol.* 1995;25(3):789–796.
106. Coats AJ. Exercise rehabilitation in chronic heart failure. *J Am Coll Cardiol.* 1993;22(4 suppl A):172A–177A.
107. Liu JL, Irvine S, Reid IA, Patel KP, Zucker IH. Chronic exercise reduces sympathetic nerve activity in rabbits with pacing-induced heart failure: a role for angiotensin II. *Circulation.* 2000;102(15):1854–1862.
108. Braith RW, Welsch MA, Feigenbaum MS, Kluess HA, Pepine CJ. Neuroendocrine activation in heart failure is modified by endurance exercise training. *J Am Coll Cardiol.* 1999;34(4):1170–1175.
109. Passino C, Severino S, Poletti R, et al. Aerobic training decreases B-type natriuretic peptide expression and adrenergic activation in patients with heart failure. *J Am Coll Cardiol.* 2006;47(9):1835–1839.
110. Hambrecht R, Fiehn E, Yu J, et al. Effects of endurance training on mitochondrial ultrastructure and fiber type distribution in skeletal muscle of patients with stable chronic heart failure. *J Am Coll Cardiol.* 1997;29(5):1067–1073.
111. Tyni-Lenne R, Gordon A, Jansson E, Bermann G, Sylvén C. Skeletal muscle endurance training improves peripheral oxidative capacity, exercise tolerance, and health-related quality of life in women with chronic congestive heart failure secondary to either ischemic cardiomyopathy or idiopathic dilated cardiomyopathy. *Am J Cardiol.* 1997;80(8):1025–1029.
112. Sullivan MJ, Higginbotham MB, Cobb FR. Exercise training in patients with severe left ventricular dysfunction. Hemodynamic and metabolic effects. *Circulation.* 1988;78(3):506–515.
113. Hambrecht R, Niebauer J, Fiehn E, et al. Physical training in patients with stable chronic heart failure: effects on cardiorespiratory fitness and ultrastructural abnormalities of leg muscles. *J Am Coll Cardiol.* 1995;25(6):1239–1249.
114. Meyer K, Schwaibold M, Westbrook S, et al. Effects of exercise training and activity restriction on 6-minute walking test performance in patients with chronic heart failure. *Am Heart J.* 1997;133(4):447–453.
115. ExTraMATCH Collaborative; Piepoli MF, Davos C, Francis DP, Coats AJS. Exercise training meta-analysis of trials in patients with chronic heart failure. *BMJ.* 2004;328(7433):189–195.
116. Sachdev V, Sharma K, Keteyian SJ, et al. Supervised exercise training for chronic heart failure with preserved ejection fraction: a scientific statement from the American Heart Association and American College of Cardiology. *Circulation.* 2023;147(16):e699–e715.
117. Celano CM, Villegas AC, Albanese AM, Gaggin HK, Huffman JC. Depression and anxiety in heart failure: a review. *Harv Rev Psychiatry.* 2018;26(4):175–184.
118. Williams SA, Kasl SV, Heiat A, Abramson JL, Krumholz HM, Vaccarino V. Depression and risk of heart failure among the elderly: a prospective community-based study. *Psychosom Med.* 2002;64(1):6–12.
119. Jiang W, Alexander J, Christopher E, et al. Relationship of depression to increased risk of mortality and rehospitalization in patients with congestive heart failure. *Arch Intern Med.* 2001;161(15):1849–1856.

120. Jiang W, Kuchibhatla M, Clary GL, et al. Relationship between depressive symptoms and long-term mortality in patients with heart failure. *Am Heart J.* 2007;154(1):102–108.
121. Rutledge T, Reis VA, Linke SE, Greenberg BH, Mills PJ. Depression in heart failure a meta-analytic review of prevalence, intervention effects, and associations with clinical outcomes. *J Am Coll Cardiol.* 2006;48(8): 1527–1537.
122. Friedmann E, Thomas SA, Liu F, et al. Relationship of depression, anxiety, and social isolation to chronic heart failure outpatient mortality. *Am Heart J.* 2006;152(5):940.e1–940.e8.
123. O'Connor CM, Jiang W, Kuchibhatla M, et al. Safety and efficacy of sertraline for depression in patients with congestive heart failure (SADHART-CHF). *Heart Failure Society of America 2008 Scientific Meeting.* Late Breaking Clinical Trials I; 2008.
124. Plotkin BJ, Rodos JJ, Kappler R, et al. Adjunctive osteopathic manipulative treatment in women with depression: a pilot study. *J Am Osteopath Assoc.* 2001;101(9):517–523.
125. Gamber RG, Shores JH, Russo DP, Jimenez C, Rubin BR. Osteopathic manipulative treatment in conjunction with medication relieves pain associated with fibromyalgia syndrome: results of a randomized clinical pilot project. *J Am Osteopath Assoc.* 2002;102(6):321–325.
126. Gans ROB. The metabolic syndrome, depression, and cardiovascular disease: interrelated conditions that share pathophysiologic mechanisms. *Med Clin N Am.* 2006;90(4):573–591.
127. Karlamangla AS, Singer BH, McEwen BS, Rowe JW, Seeman TE. Allostatic load as a predictor of functional decline. MacArthur studies of successful aging. *J Clin Epidemiol.* 2002;55(7):696–710.
128. Logan JG, Barksdale DJ. Allostasis and allostatic load: expanding the discourse on stress and cardiovascular disease. *J Clin Nurs.* 2008;17(7B): 201–208.
129. Beal MC, Kleiber GE. Somatic dysfunction as a predictor of coronary artery disease. *J Am Osteopath Assoc.* 1985;85(5):302–307.
130. Beal MC. Viscerosomatic reflexes: a review. *J Am Osteopath Assoc.* 1985;85(12):786–801.

103 Case Study: Elderly Patient with Dementia (aka Neurocognitive Disorder)

JEFFREY TSAI ▪ REBECCA E. GIUSTI

KEY CONCEPTS

- Nonreversible causes of dementia include Alzheimer disease, frontotemporal dementia, Lewy body dementia, vascular dementia, primary progressive aphasia, and mixed dementia.[1]
- Standard medical evaluation tends to miss some of the most prevalent health issues experienced by older adults; these tend to include the five I's of geriatrics: (a) impaired homeostasis (in some literature this is substituted for instability); (b) impaired cognition, incompetence, or intellectual impairment; (c) iatrogenesis; (d) immobility; and (e) incontinence.[2]
- There has also been a movement to address five items in older adults termed the "Geriatric 5Ms" which include mind, mobility, medications, multicomplexity, matters most.[3]
- Dementia is difficult to diagnose due to the potential multifactorial causes.
- There are no pharmacologic agents that can cure dementia; however, medications may be helpful in slowing the progression of the disease.
- The overall goal in older adult patient care is to maximize the patient's residual functional capacity to meet patient-centered goals for care for an optimal quality of life.

CASE VIGNETTE

CHIEF COMPLAINT

Mr. S, a 77-year-old man, is brought to the office by his daughter for a second opinion due to her concerns regarding his walking and his mood and behavior changes.

HISTORY OF PRESENT ILLNESS

The daughter, who usually lives out of state, notes that Mr. S has had a gradual progression of difficulty walking and he is getting "just mean." The daughter is concerned that he will really hurt himself someday if he falls. He is using a cane at her request, but he is adamant that he does not need it.

She is unsure of the onset of his instability since she lives out of state but relates that he has had memory difficulties for years and was on donepezil for this. His wife had cared for him until her recent passing due to a stroke. The daughter admits that her father had trouble walking for some time and maybe for years, but it has been particularly worrisome to her since he was placed on carbidopa/levodopa for Parkinson disease a few months ago. He has declined since then without the stabilizing influence of his wife.

The patient denies any difficulty and states that he uses the cane only because the daughter insists. Mr. S states that he is forced to use a cane by "those people who are trying to put me away" and wishes "they would stop their incessant talking because they just confuse me." He is unable to identify who "they" are but claims he sees them "when they want to be seen." Mr. S has not actually fallen but admits that he is slowed down by what he feels is arthritis. He complains of generalized stiffness which he attributes to arthritis from his early life of physical labor. The daughter is also concerned about his driving due to slow reaction times from apparent stiffness. Mr. S refuses to give up the car keys and states, "They want to take my car away. How am I supposed to get around?" He has been increasingly frustrated, short tempered, and easily agitated, which he attributes to his daughter's nagging, but the daughter believes his agitation and "weird thoughts" are due to the recent passing of his wife. She notes that he makes accusations about people taking things from him and talks to people who are not there. He no longer enjoys walking or caring for the dog. He now bathes infrequently and will not accept assistance to clean the house. He believes his children want him out of the way and want him in a nursing home.

PAST MEDICAL HISTORY

He has been diagnosed with: hypertension at age 45, dyslipidemia at age 45, osteoarthritis at age 70, Alzheimer disease (AD) at age 75, and Parkinson disease at age 76.

PAST SURGICAL HISTORY

Appendectomy at age 22; left total knee replacement secondary to osteoarthritis at age 68.

SOCIAL HISTORY

He is an ex-smoker (quit 20 years ago) but smoked a pack a day from age 15 until then (42-pack-year history); he drinks a couple of beers on the weekend while watching sports; denies illicit drug use; was married 50 years; has two adult children—alive and well. Daughter lives in another state 4 hours away, son lives overseas and is estranged from the family. Mr. S has been relatively socially isolated due to his illness and his wife's illness. He has not resumed previous activities of reading books or participating in the Rotary Club since his wife's passing.

FAMILY HISTORY

He is the youngest of four siblings. A sister is deceased from renal failure and diabetes at age 84. Still living are a brother aged 83 and a sister aged 80. Both have high blood pressure and live independently. His father died at age 90 of natural causes and his mother died at age 87 from pneumonia.

CURRENT MEDICATIONS

Metoprolol: 50 mg PO BID
Simvastatin: 40 mg PO nightly
OTC: Naproxen sodium 220 mg PO once or twice a day as needed for knee or back pain (average 5 pills/wk)

Chondroitin sulfate from the health food store—dose unknown

Donepezil: 10 mg PO nightly
Carbidopa/levodopa: 10/100 mg PO TID

IMMUNIZATIONS

Flu vaccine last fall. Pneumococcal vaccines at age 65 and 66. Last PPD or tetanus unknown.

REVIEW OF SYSTEMS

Head

Denies headaches; no change in vision, hearing, smell, or taste. He wears bifocals with a new prescription nearly a year ago. He denies syncope, near syncope, or dizziness.

Heart

Denies chest pain or palpitations. He has no cardiac history except as noted in past history without claudication, angina, or history of MI.

Lungs

He denies shortness of breath, wheezing, coughing, dyspnea on exertion, or orthopnea. No history of occupational exposure or TB.

GI

Denies food intolerance, dysphasia, odynophagia, acid reflux, appetite changes, nausea, vomiting, diarrhea, constipation, changes in character of bowel movements, or weight loss, although the daughter believes he looks thinner.

GU

Denies frequency of urination, hematuria, or dysuria. He admits to nocturia once or twice per night. He states his stiffness makes him unable to get to the bathroom when he needs to, which causes occasional urinary incontinence.

Musculoskeletal

He admits to general stiffness usually without pain. He takes naproxen occasionally for what he says is arthritis in his back and left knee. He believes this has caused a slowness of ambulation with gait changes. He denies tics, twitches, convulsions, paresthesias, or paralysis.

Psychiatric History

He has had no psychiatric evaluations or hospitalizations. He claims to be satisfied with his life if people would just leave him alone. He denies feeling sad, hopeless, or worthless. He denies suicidal or homicidal ideation but jokes that he might change his mind if they keep pushing him. Despite reporting seeing people who are not there, he denies delusions, hallucinations, anxiety, or depression. The daughter reports social withdrawal, a short temper, and accusatory language and notes her father gets easily agitated and has difficulty with daily routines. He is not compliant with usual daily routines or medications since his wife died.

Activities of Daily Living

The daughter reports that he dresses himself but would put on the same clothes day after day if she did not lay out the clothes for him. Likewise, he feeds himself but only after she prepares the meals and sets them up. He ambulates with a cane as previously noted. He toilets himself, but the daughter notes occasional urinary incontinence, and his underwear is sometimes soiled as if he does not clean himself well. He frequently has to be reminded to shower, and at those times, the daughter is afraid he will fall, but he refuses her help and refuses to use the shower chair.

Instrumental Activities of Daily Living

Mr. S is able to answer his cell phone but does not make phone calls. He does not go shopping or do housework. His daughter has been shopping, preparing meals, and handling finances for him, which his wife had done for the last 2 or 3 years of her life. Mr. S needs assistance with travel and is unable to plan a trip or describe how to get from his house to places with which he was previously familiar, yet he insists he can drive.

PHYSICAL EXAMINATION

Vital Signs

BP: 119/72 mm Hg; pulse: 64 beats/min; respiratory rate: 14 breaths/min; O_2 Sat: 95%.

General

Mr. S is alert, well hydrated, and well nourished, although there are signs of weight loss as his clothes are ill-fitting. He appears his stated age. He is in no acute distress, but he is obviously displeased at being at the doctor's office.

HEENT

Head is atraumatic and normocephalic. Facies have a paucity of expression. Pupils are equal, round, and reactive to light. Funduscopic examination reveals no papilledema, AV nicking, exudates, or hemorrhages. Pharynx is without erythema or masses. There is no evidence of cervical or submandibular lymphadenopathy. The thyroid is palpated without tenderness, masses, or nodularity.

Heart

Heart rate is regular without murmur, gallop, or rub. The point of maximal impulse is nondisplaced. No jugular venous distention or carotid bruit is appreciated.

Lungs

The lungs are clear to auscultation and percussion with good respiratory excursion bilaterally.

Abdomen

The abdomen is flat and soft without hepatosplenomegaly, masses, tenderness, rigidity, or rebound. Bowel sounds are present. A lower right quadrant scar is present consistent with his history of appendectomy.

Extremities

There is no evidence of digital clubbing, ulceration, or cyanosis. The left knee has a well-healed scar consistent with previous arthroplasty. Degenerative changes of both knees are evident. Dorsalis pedis and tibialis posterior pulses are present and equal bilaterally. The knees are slightly flexed at rest, as are the hips. He sits comfortably on the examination table, uses his arms to rise to the standing position, and sways slightly upon rising. He uses a cane to walk and has a slight hesitation upon initiation of walking, and steps are unequal. He prefers to stand with a widened stance. His attempts to turn are noted to be irregular and discontinuous, and he "plops" into the chair when asked to sit down.

Neurologic

Deep tendon reflexes are +2/4 at knee, elbow, and forearm but 0/4 at the Achilles bilaterally. Strength is 5/5 proximal and distal in upper and lower extremities. Cranial nerves II to XII are intact bilaterally. Facies are flat without droop. Speech is articulate but slow. No tremor or cogwheel rigidity is noted, but joint stiffness is appreciable on range-of-motion testing. Handwriting demonstrates micrographia. No clonus is noted and plantar response (Babinski) is downgoing.

Psychiatric

He is oriented to place and person but believes it is 10 years ago and that it is fall when it is actually winter. He is able to spell "WORLD" forward but not backward. He is able to repeat 3/3 objects immediately but only able to recall 1 of 3 after 5 minutes despite cueing. He follows a two-step command but has trouble with a three-step command. He refuses to draw a clock. He writes a three-word sentence that is difficult to read due to its small size. The patient is cordial and responds to questions although he is not happy about being in the physician's office. He believes his daughter wants him declared incompetent to prevent him from driving and to place him in a nursing home. He relates that he has heard voices telling him she wants him "put away." He has a core of 8 on the Cornell Scale for Depression in Dementia.

Osteopathic Structural Examination

There is slight flexion posturing of the knees and hips with a generalized increase in paraspinal muscle tone in the thoracic and lumbar areas. There is flattening of the lumbar lordosis and a mild accentuation of the thoracic kyphosis. Periarticular changes of the knees and fingers are present.

DIFFERENTIAL DIAGNOSIS

The medical evaluation of older adults differs from standard medical evaluation in three general ways:

1. It focuses on older individuals with complex issues.
2. It emphasizes functional status and quality of life.
3. It frequently takes advantage of an interdisciplinary team of providers.

Quite often, standard medical evaluation will tend to miss some of the most prevalent health issues experienced by older adults. These include the *five I's of geriatrics*[4]:

1. Impaired homeostasis—otherwise referred to as "*homeostenosis*"
2. Incompetence or intellectual impairment
3. Iatrogenesis
4. Immobility
5. Incontinence

These conditions are often considered to be the "giants" in geriatrics because they can lead to significant mortality and morbidity and contribute to the complexity of treating geriatric patients.[2] They are also common and do not occur in isolation.

The geriatric assessment effectively addresses these as well as other areas of older adult care in order to prevent disease and disability while successfully providing care interventions.

It is fitting to review these "giants" in relation to Mr. S and within the context of the osteopathic approach along with the "Geriatric 5Ms": mind, mobility, medications, multicomplexity, and matters most. Considerations and questions that may come to mind for the physician as the geriatric assessment include the following:

Impaired Homeostasis

It appears that aging involves a significant decline in adaptive homeostasis capacity. This is best considered as part of the metabolic model of osteopathic care.

As described by Davies, "adaptive homeostasis is the transient expansion or contraction of the homeostatic range for any given physiological parameter in response to exposure to sub-toxic, non-damaging, signaling molecules or events, or the removal or cessation of such molecules or events."[5] A static homeostatic set-point does not exist; rather there is continual fluctuation arising from internal or environmentally derived stresses, including oxidative stress, heat stress, exercise-induced stress, caloric restriction/fasting, hypoxia, mechanical stress, osmotic stress, and behavioral stress, which can all impact transcriptional and translational changes, with the beneficial effect of increased protection from excessive damage.[6]

Homeostenosis is a well-established geriatric concept referring to the characteristic and progressive reduction of homeostatic reserve that occurs with aging in organ systems.[7]

Homeostenosis manifests as an impaired ability to compensate in the face of internal or external challenges, restricting an individual's ability to successfully respond to stressors in biologic, psychological, and social systems. Frail older adults who experience homeostenosis are unable to regain a steady state after experiencing a stressor such as an infection, malnutrition, hospitalization, or surgery,[8] in contrast to the usual ability to recover homeostasis. Unable to recover equilibrium, these individuals may spiral into further decline and disability.[9]

Is there evidence that this patient's situation is due to homeostenosis? Has there been a change that has interfered with the body's inherent capacity to self-regulate? Does the loss of his caregiver support evidence that a social homeostasis has been lost?

Mind/Impaired Cognition/Intellectual Impairment/Incompetence

With respect to the biopsychosocial/behavioral model, the physician must consider the patient's mentation as well as evaluate for the presence of delirium, dementia, and depression. Delirium is an acute medical emergency while dementia is a chronic cognitive impairment that has generally been present for over 6 months.

Does his mental status examination suggest that he may have intellectual impairment? If so, it is important to determine in what realms and to what degree. Is the impairment quantifiable? Is it due to a metabolic, vascular, psychiatric, or other source, or perhaps a combination?

Per the Diagnostic and Statistical Manual of Mental Disorders, 5th edition (DSM-5), the definition of dementia or a major neurocognitive deficit is classified along a continuum from mild to severe. If function is preserved, the condition is termed mild cognitive impairment. The DSM-5 criteria for major neurocognitive disorder is found in Box 103.2.[2]

Physicians may determine capacity to function, use cognition, perform activities of daily living (ADLs), or meet executive abilities such as planning insight and judgment, but it is the courts

BOX 103.1 Competency Evaluation

Due to psychiatric illness, mental retardation, delirium, or dementia, older adult patients may in some situations be incapable of making decisions that safeguard their own self-interests. Although the MMSE provides useful information regarding a patient's global cognitive function, it is important to assess, by way of an interview, their competency in at least two areas: medical and financial decision-making. Following are questions to consider in the evaluation of a person's competency to make decisions directly affecting their health and financial security:

- Is the patient aware they have a mental illness (as listed above)?
- Does the patient understand the nature of the proposed treatment?
- Does the patient understand the need for treatment and the implications of refusing treatment?
- Does the mental illness interfere with judgment and reasoning so much that it accounts for refusal of treatment?
- Does the patient have knowledge of their current assets?
- Does the patient have knowledge of their monthly expenses and bills?
- Does the patient know where their assets are located and being managed?
- Can the patient complete simple calculations?
- Is the person's judgment so affected that their finances would be in jeopardy?

that decide competence. Therefore, physicians need to be aware of how the courts refer to and define *incompetence*. Box 103.1 presents questions to consider in the evaluation of a person's competency to make decisions directly affecting their health and financial security.

Medications/Iatrogenesis

As part of both the metabolic and biopsychosocial/behavioral model, the physician should determine if iatrogenesis is occurring.

Adverse drug events (ADEs), injury resulting from the use of a drug at its normal dose, account for the majority of iatrogenic injuries. Older adults tend to be more susceptible to polypharmacy, the use of five or more medications, or the use of more drugs than is indicated medically.[2] Polypharmacy is causally implicated in the other geriatric giants and leads to an increase in hospitalization, drug–drug interactions, decreased compliance, and functional decline.[10]

Physicians may use two tools to help avoid ADE, inappropriate drug prescription and polypharmacy; the Beers Criteria and the STOPP/START criteria.[11,12] At each visit, medications should be reviewed and if possible discontinued if they are not beneficial. Prior to prescribing a new medication, the patient's current medications should be carefully reviewed to determine whether they may be causing the problem at hand and to avoid drug–drug interactions.

The physician should consider the following questions. Has a previous diagnosis been in error? Has a treatment been instituted or not instituted that has created or exacerbated the current situation? Has treatment been started that is based on a symptom rather than a cause? Is there a possibility of polypharmacy with drug–drug interactions?

Mobility versus Immobility

While mobility may be considered a strong component of the biomechanical model, this factor spans all the models of osteopathic care. Immobility is not a normal part of aging. It is especially problematic as it is associated with functional decline, disability, dependence, and mortality.[13,14] Immobility negatively impacts almost every organ system and may result in loss of muscle mass, deep vein thrombosis, atelectasis and pneumonia, constipation, and pressure ulcers.[15] Factors that may lead to immobility and thus further instability include joint pathology such as osteoarthritis of the hips and knees, foot pathologies, cognitive impairment, vestibular disorders, muscle weakness and sarcopenia, visual impairment, an unsafe environment, and fear of falling.[2] Being aware of these factors can help guide the clinician in asking the appropriate questions and attempting to mitigate these factors with an appropriate treatment plan before they lead to poor outcomes for the patient.

Is Mr. S's apparent immobility his central and most important problem? Does this put him at risk for a cascade of disasters as his daughter fears? Although it is the chief complaint, is immobility the root cause or the symptom of something significant?

Multicomplexity and Incontinence

Multicomplexity involves comorbidities and complex biopsychosocial situations. It includes the following: health equity, transition of care, hazards of hospitalization, atypical presentation, aging physiology, frailty (assess the patient along the spectrum from fit to frail using a validated screening tool), prognosis, individualized recommendations, sensory impairment (screen for hearing, vision, and oral health concerns that may impact cognition, function, social isolation, and health outcomes and collaborate with other health care fields such as audiology, optometry, and dentistry to optimize care), pressure injuries, and urinary incontinence.[16]

Mr. S has an incontinence issue.

According to the Centers for Disease Control and Prevention, the prevalence of incontinence is 43.8% for noninstitutionalized Americans ages 65 and older, and 70.3% of long-term care residents were reported to have experienced urinary leakage.[17,18] Urinary incontinence is associated with complications such as pressure ulcers, urinary tract infections, falls with fractures, and depression, which negatively impact quality of life, social well-being, and overall health.[19] The patient often experiences anxiety and embarrassment surrounding incontinence leading to distress and social isolation.[20]

The physician needs to determine the etiology of the incontinence: is it stress, urge, overflow (due to a large prostate or neuropathy), functional (no structural abnormalities but unable to reach the toilet due to physical or cognitive impairment)?[2] Perhaps it is not an intrinsic problem unto itself but rather it is the manifestation of another problem.

Matters Most

This is described as each individual's own meaningful health outcome goals and care preferences. It incorporates patient priorities (elicit what matters most to an older adult and work with them and the team to honor these priorities), psychosocial and spiritual needs, symptom assessment (reduce suffering through nonpharmacologic and pharmacologic treatments, based on the patient's

BOX 103.2 DSM-5-TR (2022) Diagnostic Criteria for Major Neurocognitive Disorder

A. Evidence of significant cognitive decline from a previous level of performance in one or more cognitive domains (complex attention, executive function, learning and memory, language, perceptual-motor, or social cognition) based on:
   1. Concern of the individual, a knowledgeable informant, or the clinician that there has been a significant decline in cognitive function; and
   2. A substantial impairment in cognitive performance, preferably documented by standardized neuropsychological testing or, in its absence, another quantified clinical assessment.
B. The cognitive deficits interfere with independence in everyday activities (i.e., at minimum, requiring assistance with complex instrumental activities of daily living such as paying bills or managing medications).
C. The cognitive deficits do not occur exclusively in the context of a delirium.
D. The cognitive deficits are not better explained by another mental disorder (e.g., major depressive disorder, schizophrenia).

BOX 103.3 Potential Reversible Causes for the Dementia

- Brain tumor
- Head injury
- Subdural hematoma
- Normal pressure hydrocephalus
- Postconcussion syndromes
- Sleep deprivation
- Thyroid dysfunction
- Adrenal and pituitary gland diseases
- Insulinoma
- Other metabolic disorders
- Nutritional deficiencies (e.g., vitamin B12, folate, niacin, thiamin)
- Toxins (e.g., alcohol abuse, drugs, medications)
- Autoimmune diseases (e.g., lupus, multiple sclerosis, vasculitis, sarcoidosis)
- Infectious diseases (e.g., meningitis, Lyme disease, AIDS, neurosyphilis)
- Psychiatric diseases (e.g., depression, late-onset schizophrenia)

From Bello VME, Schultz RR. Prevalence of treatable and reversible dementias: a study in a dementia outpatient clinic. *Dement Neuropsychol.* 2011;5(1):44–47. http://creativecommons.org/licenses/by/3.0/

goals of care and safe prescribing principles), communication, and advance care planning.[16]

Assessment for Major Neurocognitive Disorder

This patient's history and physical examination are strongly suggestive of dementia, and although it was not the presenting complaint, his cognitive function has the greatest clinical implication for his long-term health. The physician must determine if the patient meets diagnostic criteria for dementia. The DSM-5 introduced the terms major and minor neurocognitive disorder and lists criteria for diagnosis of dementia (Box 103.2). The diagnostic criteria and text from the DSM-5 publication in 2013 concerning major neurocognitive disorders remain unchanged. However, in 2022, diagnostic entities including Prolonged Grief Disorder, Unspecified Mood Disorder, and Stimulant-Induced Mild Neurocognitive Disorder were added to the DSM-5-TR.[21] Concerning Mr. S, one needs only to apply the findings of short-term and long-term memory decline with the patient's functional capacity in ADLs to recognize that he meets the diagnostic criteria for dementia.

The differential diagnosis of dementia can be divided into two broad classifications—those that are reversible (Box 103.3) and those that are not. The first responsibility of the physician is to distinguish between these two categories, and much of the workup is aimed at precisely this distinction. Failure to identify reversible causes, if they exist, results in unnecessary treatment and stress for the patient and the family.

The initial evaluation for reversible causes of dementia always begins with a thorough history and physical examination. For the osteopathic physician, the history is central to the diagnosis and its impact on the patient and the patient's support system. The physical examination should be thorough in order to identify signs of potentially reversible causes of dementia and will typically emphasize the neurologic and cardiovascular systems. Because the definitive diagnosis of dementia can only be proven by tissue sample from a brain biopsy, the diagnosis is one of exclusion. One must evaluate the patient for other reasonable causes of their symptoms, and when that fails to identify the diagnosis, the physician is left with the likely diagnosis of dementia. Likewise, once it has been determined that dementia is present, it is the constellation of signs and symptoms of the whole person that steers the physician in determining the type of dementia.

The laboratory and imaging evaluations may include the following:

1. Laboratory Evaluation:
   - Complete blood count (CBC)
   - Comprehensive metabolic profile
     - Glucose
     - Renal functions—BUN, creatinine
     - Electrolytes—sodium, potassium, chloride
     - Liver function—AST, ALT
     - Calcium and phosphorus
   - Urinalysis
   - Thyroid function tests
   - Hemoglobin A1c
   - Vitamin B12 and folate
   - Serologic test for syphilis and HIV
   - If appropriate, evaluate erythrocyte sedimentation rate, lumbar puncture, heavy metal screen, ceruplasmin levels, Lyme disease titer, and serum protein electrophoresis.
2. Neuroimaging should be ordered to exclude other intracranial abnormalities, especially if the age of onset is relatively early, atypical, or symptoms are progressing rapidly.
   - Brain MRI without contrast is often the initial test ordered to assess for signs of vascular or ischemic disease and local or global atrophy.

- □ A DaTscan uses a radiotracer to highlight dopamine transporter proteins in a SPECT scan on the presynaptic dopaminergic neurons. This scan can aid in differentiating pathologies that involve loss of the striatal dopaminergic pathway, including Parkinson disease, multiple system atrophy, progressive nuclear palsy, cortical-basal degeneration, and Lewy body dementia from other syndromes.[22]
- □ Functional brain imaging with PET, SPECT, and fMRI can help in the early diagnosis and monitoring of patients with dementia, especially AD, and with the differentiation of etiology of dementia. However, these are primarily used in clinical trial settings and are cost prohibitive and therefore not indicated for routine use in clinical practice.[23]

3. Selected patients may need autoimmune studies and neuropsychological testing.
4. While new CSF and blood tests are being researched to help identify AD and evaluate concentrations of amyloid and phosphorylated tau proteins as well as markers of neurodegeneration, including neurofilament light chain and glial fibrillar acidic proteins, these are not yet ready for regular clinical use.[24]
5. Genetic testing for the apolipoprotein E4 allele is not routinely recommended at this time, though adult children of patients with AD may choose to be tested themselves. Referral for genetic testing should also be considered in patients with several family members diagnosed with AD at a young age in an autosomal dominant pattern, as there are additional genes that may be identified in familial cases.[25]

It is also important to quantify the degree of impairment, both to assist with diagnosis and to provide a baseline for future assessments to determine the effectiveness of interventions. All domains of cognition must be assessed. Multiple cognitive evaluation tools are available for use in the clinical setting to provide a picture of the severity of deficit within specific cognitive domains and can be repeated to assess progression of decline. They should not be used in isolation to diagnose major neurocognitive disorder. These include[26]:

- Mini-mental status examination (MMSE) (also called Folstein Test)
  - □ Takes about 10 minutes to administer.
  - □ The most common tool for assessing severity of AD or other related dementia, easy to use and may be administered at home.
- Montreal Cognitive Assessment (MoCA)
  - □ Takes approximately 10 to 15 minutes to administer.
  - □ Better suited for detecting mild cognitive impairment in addition to major neurocognitive disorder.
- Saint Louis University Mental Status (SLUMS)
  - □ Takes about 7 minutes to administer.
  - □ Known for its brevity and sensitivity for mild cognitive impairment.
- Addenbrooke's Cognitive Examination–Revised (ACE-R)
  - □ Demonstrates good clinical utility for differentiating Lewy body dementia from AD.[27]
- The modified mini-mental state examination, Mini-Cog
  - □ Takes approximately 3 minutes to administer.
  - □ Predominantly used to screen for major neurocognitive disorder.
- Rowland Universal Dementia Assessment Scale (RUDAS)
  - □ Useful in cross-cultural evaluations.
  - □ Can be administered in conjunction with an interpreter if needed.[26]

Screening for depression using tests such as the Geriatric Depression Scale may be helpful as well as a functional assessment of ADLs using the ADLs Scale or the Instrumental ADL (IADL) Scale. Many of these tests are easy to administer and can be done in the office by trained personnel.

Common subtypes of nonreversible dementia include AD, frontotemporal dementia, Lewy body dementia, vascular dementia, primary progressive aphasia, and dementia resulting from a combination of factors, termed mixed dementia. AD is the most common cause of dementia, playing a role in 70% to 80% of all cases.[28] Vascular (previously called multi-infarct) dementia contributes to another 15%; risk factors include hypercholesterolemia, diabetes mellitus, hypertension, and smoking.[29] Lewy body dementia contributes to about 5% of cases but is likely underreported.[30] Parkinson disease plays a role in 10% of cases.[30] Frontotemporal dementia contributes to 25% of dementia cases in patients older than 65 years of age. It is, however, the second most common cause of dementia in patients younger than 65 years.[31] Creutzfeldt–Jakob disease is rare and occurs in about one to two cases per million per year globally.[32] Mixed dementia occurs when a patient has more than one type of dementia. AD with vascular dementia is the most common.[33] When a patient has dementia with detailed hallucinations, parkinsonian signs, and alterations in alertness and attention, one might suspect dementia with Lewy bodies.

Vascular dementias are predominantly caused by circulatory interruption to the brain. Often, they are related to infarcts (strokes). They can be progressive as the patient experiences recurrent infarcts and hence were previously referred to as multi-infarct dementias. Many of these strokes happen at the subcortical level and are too small to cause permanent residual neurologic deficits in the motor or sensory systems. The key characteristic that distinguishes a classic vascular dementia is the typical stepwise decline. Unlike AD which usually shows a steady downward course, vascular dementias show a new decline with each new vascular insult followed by a period of stability and then another decline with the next event.

Mr. S presents with a past history of Parkinson disease and AD with a recent decline in cognition that is slowly getting worse over the previous few months and has been exacerbated since the death of his wife. In treating the whole person, consideration must be given to his previous diagnosis of AD, the recent initiation of anti-Parkinson drugs, and the loss of his primary caregiver whose support may have masked the significance of his cognitive decline.

The physician is left with the quandary of a potential multifactorial cause for the patient's current presentation. This is especially true when one remembers that the body is an integrated sum of its parts and that care of the presenting disease must include considerations by the physician for not only the patient's physical body but also their emotional, social, and spiritual health. The challenge is that there are no algorithms for such considerations; rather, these cases call upon the skill of the physician to consider these factors at every stage of the diagnostic and treatment process. The differential diagnosis of subacute, progressive cognitive decline, and gait and behavioral changes in a 77-year-old man with a history of hypertension, dyslipidemia, AD, and Parkinson disease can be viewed in Table 103.1.

In considering the whole context of Mr. S' presentation, the Parkinson disease diagnosis can be confirmed as illustrated by his handwriting, his gait, and his paucity of facial expressions, among other characteristics. However, the fact that his dementia was exacerbated by the initiation of anti-Parkinson medication and

TABLE 103.1

Differential Diagnosis Chart

Differential Diagnosis	Consideration
Vascular	Vascular dementia
Inflammatory	Unlikely
Neoplasia	Unlikely
Degenerative	Alzheimer disease Lewy body dementia Pick disease
Iatrogenic idiopathic	Adverse medication effect
Congenital	Unlikely
Autoimmune	Unlikely
Trauma/toxins	Unlikely
Endocrine/metabolic	Hypothyroidism
Psychological	Depression, delirium

the presence of delusions and psychotic overlay is suggestive of Lewy body dementia. Lewy bodies are rounded eosinophilic intracytoplasmic neuronal inclusions that contain the protein α-synuclein; they are characteristic of dementia with Lewy bodies and of Parkinson disease. In dementia with Lewy bodies, these inclusions occur in the cerebral cortex and other areas of the brain. In Parkinson disease, Lewy bodies occur in selected subcortical structures, most notably the substantia nigra. Dementia with Lewy bodies, Parkinson disease, and AD overlap considerably. For example, patients who have Parkinson disease may develop dementia with Lewy bodies; patients who have AD may have a modest number of Lewy bodies, and patients who have dementia with Lewy bodies may have neuritic plaques and neurofibrillary tangles, both hallmarks of AD. Further research is needed to clarify the relationships among these disorders.[34–37]

However, in the case of Mr. S, AD is unlikely to be accompanied by the degree of psychotic symptoms displayed by Mr. S. Pseudodementia in the form of depression may also be considered, but his presentation is not convincing for depression based on the DSM criteria for depression or his depression scale score. Vascular dementia usually has a more abrupt onset with a gradual stepwise decline as more vascular events occur and impact brain function.

OSTEOPATHIC PATIENT MANAGEMENT

The osteopathic approach to patient care dovetails well with the field of geriatric medicine, which stresses the care of the individual as much as the care of the disease state. This dynamic interplay is paramount in older adult health care. The physician is tasked with helping the patient achieve maximal residual function. It cannot be stressed enough that the majority of older adults age successfully. As of 2016, nearly 15,600 US nursing homes containing 1.7 million beds cared for over 1.3 million residents.[38] The remainder of older adults are cared for in the community with an increasingly limited number of physicians trained in geriatrics and with limited funding to offset costs of health care. Despite these challenges, it is the physician's responsibility to work with older adult patients and their caregivers to facilitate successful aging well before the onset of a health crisis. Implementing preventive actions at younger ages includes primary and secondary disease prevention and health promotion activities such as proper nutrition, physical exercise, cognitive exercise, and the careful exploration of psychosocial dimensions. These activities can be implemented with patients of all ages and health conditions. Suffice to say, it is never too late to make changes to augment health.

The overall goal is to maximize the patient's residual functional capacity to meet patient-centered goals for care for an optimal quality of life. A variety of measures are useful for the well-being of patients with dementia and their families. These interventions range from the assessment and potential alteration of the physical living environment to education on the use of specific strategies of care in providing information and counseling services or referrals. It is important to remember that this is best accomplished with the involvement of a multiprofessional team. It is incumbent upon the physician to recognize the patient's needs and initiate and follow the coordination of appropriate resources. The management of patients is best done in the least restrictive environment possible. The preparation for changes in level of care must always be anticipated, as dementia is a progressive disease. Support for the family and caregivers is crucial to this effort. Guilt and feelings of being overwhelmed and underprepared are common. The physician should proactively assess the family for signs of physical, emotional, and financial stresses that will impact the care of the patient and thus advocate for strategies that minimize those stresses. Services, such as those from Area Agencies on Aging, the Alzheimer's Association, the Lewy Body Dementia Association, and the Dementia Society of America may be of value. Local agencies and chapters may provide helpful resources and valuable support for patients and their families as well.

Biomechanical Model

While there are no biomechanical changes specific to the diagnosis of dementia, there are certain prevailing tendencies for the older adult population. It should also be emphasized that many healthy older adults often practiced good health habits in their younger years.

However, regardless of past health practices, older adults tend to experience alterations in biomechanical functions such as an increased incidence of protein cross-linking in the soft tissues and a loss of elastin that leads to a generalized stiffening and slowness of reaction. There is a loss of subcutaneous fat and subcutaneous tissues making patients vulnerable to trauma and ecchymoses. Bony joints are subject to the development of degenerative conditions such as arthritis due to longevity and wear and tear. Thus, TART—tissue texture abnormality, asymmetry, restriction of motion, tenderness—findings must be interpreted in the context of usual aging. One can expect that the older adult will have tissue texture abnormalities based on elastin loss and changes in tone and turgor. Asymmetry and motion restrictions tend to be found even in the absence of trauma. Tenderness may be a useful guide to the onset of new conditions for consideration. The older adult patient loses height while preserving span due to the loss of hydration in the intervertebral disks and the prevalence of osteoporosis. The typical older adult will demonstrate a "flexion posture." The knees and hips may not fully extend and forward bending at the lumbar spine may be restricted. There is typically flattening of the usual lumbar lordosis and accentuating of the thoracic kyphosis and/or cervical lordosis. Cranial sutures calcify with age, and cranial motion abnormalities and their interpretation may be difficult to detect in some older adults. A history of concussions from closed-head trauma helps to interpret findings of chronic cranial and cervical somatic dysfunctions.

Osteopathic manipulative treatment (OMT) can be applied in cases where there is degenerative neurologic disease especially in which dopaminergic synapses in the corpus stratum deteriorate leading to tremor, bradykinesis, and muscular rigidity. Muscle energy techniques may be helpful in addressing these symptoms. Relative contraindications to using HVLA technique exist in the form of osteoporosis and/or osteopenia, present in many geriatric patients. A combination of OMT, physical therapy, and strength training, especially in the earlier phases of Lewy body dementia, may improve head and neck posture, increase stride length, increase hip, knee, and ankle flexion, increase foot lift from floor, and decrease incidence of falls and depression, thereby improving quality of life.[39]

Respiratory Circulatory Model

Vascular dementia may develop following a major event such as a stroke, but it can also be caused by the changes in blood flow brought on by aging. Arteries may narrow, slowing capillary flow. This may affect the intrinsic function of the brain. The failure to clear waste also contributes to the accumulation of waste products and toxic β-amyloid, leading to a chemical imbalance and impacting the ability of neurons to function.[40] In the aging brain, reduction in the pulsation of cerebral vasculature and fluid circulation causes impairment in the fluid exchange between different compartments, laying a foundation for neuroinflammation that contributes to AD. The glymphatic system of the central nervous system plays a role in the clearance of brain-derived metabolic waste products, providing an opportunity for osteopathic physicians to facilitate the clearance of macromolecules such as amyloid β proteins. To date, there is no pharmacologic mechanism that can increase fluid circulation in the aging brain, but osteopathic manipulative medicine may have a role. Tobey et al. demonstrated that an osteopathic cranial manipulative medicine technique, compression of the fourth ventricle (CV4), significantly improved spatial memory, reduced amyloid β levels, activated astrocytes, and improved neurotransmission on live animal positron emission tomographic imaging and immunoassays in the naturally aged rat model of AD.[41]

Neurologic Model

Dementia results from a confluence of numerous influences. Some, such as parkinsonian dementia and AD, are rooted in genetic, environmental, and systemic factors that lead to the accumulation of abnormal proteins or reduced oxygen flow to tissues resulting in toxic processes. These toxic processes then lead to observable manifestations. These early symptoms depend on the area of the brain affected but can include tremor, memory loss, executive function losses of planning, insight, and judgment, gait and movement disorders, hallucinations, delusions, and rigidity.

The two hallmarks of AD are plaques and neurofibrillary tangles found in brain tissue. Plaque formation involves the production and deposition of β-amyloid. Tau is the protein that is the chief component of the tangles. These tangles are also commonly found in the frontotemporal dementias such as those associated with Parkinson disease and may be a cause of dementia.

Despite aggressive research,[42] the pathogenesis of AD remains elusive. The greatest risk factor for AD is age. At age 65, the likelihood of having AD is about 3%, rising to over 30% by age 85.[43]

AD can be classified by when the disease manifests, early or late onset, and whether it is inherited. Early-onset AD (EOAD) occurs before age 65, whereas late-onset AD (LOAD), age 65 and beyond, accounts for over 95% of cases.[44] Nearly all EOAD cases are familial and are due to mutations in APP, PSEN1, or PSEN2, and the majority of LOAD cases are sporadic.

Aβ precursor protein (APP) was the first gene shown to have autosomal dominant mutations causing AD. As the precursor of the aggregated peptide in amyloid plaques, this discovery led to the "amyloid hypothesis," which states that the toxic build-up of Aβ starts a cascade of events, leading to neuronal death and disease.[45,46] Over 50 APP mutations have now been identified and account for about 10% of familial cases. Presenilin mutations cause autosomal dominant AD and contribute to around 30% to 50% of familial EOAD cases.[47,48] Other genetic risk factors exist that predispose an individual to AD including an allele of apolipoprotein E (APOE), a protein involved in fat metabolism. Its E4 allele is the most common genetic risk factor for AD.[49]

Sporadic AD often results from a combination of genetic and environmental risk factors, with cerebral hypoperfusion[50] and inflammation[51] being among the most common. AD patients often have higher levels of certain inflammatory markers and activated microglia and astrocytes in the brain, which tend to surround plaques and tangles.[52,53]

A strong component of the care of patients with dementia is pharmacologic therapy which addresses the neurologic pathology and sequelae of the condition. The pharmacotherapeutics fall into three broad categories: drugs that (a) enhance cognition and function, (b) treat coexisting depression, and (c) treat complications of dementia. None of the medications in these categories cure the disease but they may slow progression, adding functional time and delaying further decline of the patient's quality of life. They may also be useful in managing comorbid conditions associated with dementia. Medications currently available to enhance cognition include the cholinesterase inhibitors such as donepezil (Aricept), rivastigmine (Exelon), and galantamine (Razadyne). These drugs work by slowing down the action of acetylcholinesterase to maintain higher levels of the acetylcholine neurotransmitter in the brain. Memantine (Namenda) affects another neurotransmitter, glutamine. Like the cholinesterase inhibitors, this agent will not stop or reverse the dementia, and it may be necessary to use these agents in combination.[54] One of the newest medications approved for the treatment of mild AD is aducanumab. Aducanumab is a human immunoglobulin gamma 1 (IgG1) monoclonal antibody that targets aggregated soluble and insoluble forms of amyloid β. Despite its approval, aducanumab remains controversial due to uncertainty regarding whether patients with AD benefit clinically from the drug. Long-term safety and tolerability of aducanumab are still being studied in a multinational phase 3b clinical trial in patients with early AD.[55,56]

As with all medications, there are risks and benefits, and drug treatment should be instituted with the mantra of "start low, go slow, but go." Low dosages are instituted and gradually adjusted upward, slowly but deliberately. Consequently, repeated assessments and adjustments of medication over time are needed. The astute physician must recognize and counsel the patient and family on these risks and benefits. For many patients and their families, an ethical struggle may eventually ensue around the discontinuation of medications when they no longer serve to meet a patient-centered goal related to quality of life.

In considering which pharmacologic agents to institute, one must also consider which agents the patient may already be taking that can exacerbate symptoms or are incompatible with those planned to be instituted. Reversible causes of dementia may include iatrogenic etiologies, including prescription medications and other treatments.

Mr. S should stop his anti-Parkinson medication as it can exacerbate the psychoses of Lewy body dementia. Antipsychotic medications may be instituted with caution. Donepezil is approved for AD of all stages and this medication should likely be continued. The physician may consider adding memantine due to its potential neuroprotective benefits (it serves as an uncompetitive antagonist of the NMDA receptor and can prevent neurotoxic and excessive influx of calcium to the neuron).[57] However, this should be weighed against cost, the fact that it has shown only modest benefit, and the risks of polypharmacy.

Biopsychosocial/Behavioral Model

Establishing healthy habits at a younger age can provide a foundation for patients to age well. If the osteopathic physician is to see the results of healthy aging, then the interventions such as good nutrition, immunizations, smoking cessation, lipid management, and exercising the mind and body must begin well in advance of the diagnosis of disease.

Exercise and proper nutrition play a large role in healthy aging in general and this may hold true for dementia prevention as well. These seem to reduce concomitant risk factors such as obesity, elevated lipid levels, and high blood pressure. Pursuing intellectual activities and active social contacts are contributors to healthy aging.[58]

In a society with fewer extended families, the psychosocial aspects of dementia can be paramount in care management. In terms of the whole patient, the cultural and spiritual foundations of the patient and the family of caregivers will influence care decisions, the context in which they are suggested by the physician, and the manner in which they are accepted by the patient and caregivers. Autonomy is prized as an ethical precept and should be honored when possible in a patient with decision-making capacity. As dementia progresses, practitioners must increasingly rely on secondary sources of information to determine values and wishes of the patient. It is therefore important to try to determine these preferences as early in the disease process as possible.

The psychosocial elements of dementia are complex, including the emotional response to the diagnosis, stressors from coping with the ongoing management of the individual, and honoring the individual's beliefs and values. Honoring the patient's previously stated wishes may cause dissonance among caregivers who want to honor those wishes but find it difficult to do so. Role reversal as children assume care for their parents is stressful. Practical matters of advanced directives, aggressiveness of interventions, preferences for religious support, and guardianship or power of attorney should be discussed early on in the management. In dementia, the "mind is robbed before the body," and patients and their families may experience a divide between the apparent abilities of the older adult and their actual abilities. Issues of time alone, driving, and financial management may become obstacles and create a dynamic tension in the patient and in intrafamily relationships.[59]

The osteopathic philosophy makes very clear the distinction between treating disease in patients and treating patients who have disease.[60] It is the latter that must dominate the osteopathic approach. Clarity of goals of care, honoring the culture and belief systems of families and individuals, and adequate support systems for patients and families must all be sought. Care must be tailored to the needs of the individual and their families, not institutions.

For the physician, the issue involves more than just managing the disease that is dementia; it is imperative to help the patient make the most of their remaining time and assist the caregivers to prevent burnout.[61]

Most patients with dementia express the desire to remain in their homes. However, the patient's loss of ADL abilities, the increased concern for safety in the home, provision of care, and the need for continual supervision may render this impossible. Caregivers often have considerable guilt and feelings of inadequacy when this is no longer possible. Home health agencies can be of assistance but are often limited as to duration and depth of service availability. Further complicating care for older adults with dementia, the financial costs can be considerable. Regardless of the skill and availability of such care, it is often difficult to secure, even for those with the means to pay out of pocket. The financial burden of care can be significant and must be taken into consideration when generating a plan for the patient.

Metabolic Energy Model

The single most identifying characteristic of the aging process is a narrowing of the homeostatic window. With aging, processes come into play that impact the individual's response to physical, biologic, or psychological insults, leading to homeostenosis. The ability of the body to self-regulate and to marshal resources to heal is challenged in older adults. For example, cardiac reserve is lessened as cardiac output diminishes and the heart is less responsive to a catecholamine stimulus. Similarly, the endocrine system is less responsive to the stimulating hormones. There may be reduced receptor responsiveness to endogenous and exogenous stimuli, immune responses may be blunted, and osmoreceptors are less sensitive to changes in fluid and electrolytes. With less ability for older adults to tolerate physiologic stress, the line between health and disease narrows. Further, a person with dementia may find it difficult to actualize the psychological and social resources to cope with illness. This homeostenosis makes older adults prone to a cascade of disasters. An example of this could be as follows: dementia leads to less mobility, the immobility leads to instability, the instability leads to a fall, the fall leads to a fracture, the fracture leads to further immobility that leads to respiratory stasis and atelectasis, which leads to pneumonia, and so forth. However, it must be stressed that this characteristic of aging does not apply universally. Individuals age individually; meaning that aging itself is not a disease and patients must be approached individually.

Metabolic and lifestyle risk factors for developing vascular diseases, including poor diet, obesity, high cholesterol, and sedentary lifestyle, are also risk factors for dementia.[62,63] Poor diet and high cholesterol can produce metabolic changes that alter oxygen levels both systemically and within the brain.[64] In addition, type 2 diabetes approximately doubles the risk for dementia.[65–67]

The Mediterranean-DASH Intervention for Neurodegenerative Delay (MIND) diet has shown promise in slowing cognitive decline in the aging population,[68] especially following a stroke.[69] However, a large randomized, controlled trial studied an overweight population with a family history of dementia but without cognitive impairment. Subjects following the MIND diet with mild caloric restriction and subjects following a control diet with mild caloric restriction demonstrated similar improvements in global cognition scores after 3 years and similar amounts of weight loss.[70]

In addition to a healthy diet, antioxidants and folate have been of interest to research related to AD. Mega doses of vitamin B and the use of herbal medications and antioxidants have been proposed. Ginkgo biloba has been the leading herbal medication promoted for memory improvement. Vitamin E has like-

BOX 103.4 Principles in Managing Dementia

1. Optimize function
   - Investigate and treat reversible and comorbid medical conditions
   - Avoid unnecessary medications especially anticholinergic and sedating medications
   - Provide appropriate assistive devices such as walkers, hearing aids, or eyeglasses
   - Modify the environment such as widening doors, the addition of grab bars, ramps, elevated toilet seats, and the removal of scatter rugs
   - Prepare patient and family for changes in location and time to adapt to new placements
   - Emphasize nutrition and exercise
2. Identify and manage complications
   - Behavioral disorders
   - Depression
   - Loss of insight and judgment (wandering, driving, planning)
   - Psychoses
   - Incontinence
   - Team-based care with nursing, occupational and physical therapists, social work, home health agencies, and others
3. Information management for patient and family
   - Nature of disease with regular updates of progression and prognosis
   - Social service agency resources such as the Alzheimer's Association
   - Advanced directives
   - Respite service options
4. Family/caregiver counseling
   - Identify supportive services
   - Identify and resolve family conflicts
   - Handle feelings of guilt anger and despair
   - Legal concerns
   - Financial concerns
   - Ethical concerns
   - End-of-life care

Source: Kane R, Ouslander J, Abrass I. *Essentials of Clinical Geriatrics*. 5th ed. McGraw Hill; 2004.
Diagnosis and Management of Dementia: A Review—PMC (nih.gov).

wise had its advocates. Anti-inflammatory medications such as ibuprofen have been recommended for their anti-inflammatory abilities. Despite the fervor of some, none of these has proven more effective than a balanced diet and exercise of the mind and body.[71–74]

The key principles of managing dementia can be found in Box 103.4.[75]

SUMMARY

The management of an older adult with dementia begins with a history and physical examination to determine the current impact of the condition. Applying osteopathic practices and principles includes an evaluation of predisposing dysfunction of the body as part of the physical examination. The diagnosis includes considerations of two broad classifications of dementia—those that are potentially reversible and those that are not. The history, physical examination, labs, and imaging collectively allow the physician to distinguish between these two categories so that potentially reversible causes of dementia are not overlooked.

Treatment is directed toward optimizing function and quality of life of the patient as a whole and includes managing any identified cause(s) of dementia. OMT may be utilized when appropriate to improve physical and cognitive function with a goal of improving quality of life. The patient's environment must also be considered and determining methods to modify the environment to improve overall health, safety, and quality of life is essential.

ACKNOWLEDGMENTS

The authors and editors of this chapter would like to acknowledge the scholarly contributions of Drs. Bruce Bates and Marilyn R. Gugliucci for prior editions of this chapter.

REFERENCES

1. Centers for Disease Control and Prevention. What is Dementia? Alzheimer's Disease and Dementia. Updated October 26, 2022. Accessed December 24, 2024. https://www.cdc.gov/alzheimers-dementia/about/?CDC_AAref_Val
2. Greenstein L, Abraham A, Tipping B. Treating complexity in the older adult—the role of the geriatric giants. *S Afr Fam Pract.* 2019;61(6):10–14.
3. Molnar F, Frank CC. Optimizing geriatric care with the GERIATRIC 5Ms. *Can Fam Physician.* 2019;65(1):39.
4. Wagner EH, Austin BT, Von Korff M. Organizing care for patients with chronic illness. *Milbank Q.* 1996;74:511–544.
5. Davies KJ. Adaptive homeostasis. *Mol Aspects Med.* 2016;49:1–7.
6. Pomatto LCD, Davies KJA. The role of declining adaptive homeostasis in ageing. *J Physiol.* 2017;595(24):7275–7309.
7. Guerriero F, Reid MC. Linking persistent pain and frailty in older adults. *Pain Med.* 2020;21(1):61–66.
8. Makary MA, Segev DL, Pronovost PJ, et al. Frailty as a predictor of surgical outcomes in older patients. *J Am Coll Surg.* 2010;210(6):901–908.
9. Xue QL. The frailty syndrome: definition and natural history. *Clin Geriatr Med.* 2011;27(1):1–15.
10. Maher RL, Hanlon J, Hajjar ER. Clinical consequences of polypharmacy in elderly. *Expert Opin Drug Saf.* 2014;13(1):57–65.
11. O'Mahony D, O'Sullivan D, Byrne S, O'Connor MN, Ryan C, Gallagher P. Corrigendum: STOPP/START criteria for potentially inappropriate prescribing in older people: version 2. *Age Ageing.* 2015;44(2):213–218. Erratum in: *Age Ageing.* 2018 May 1;47(3):489.
12. By the 2023 American Geriatrics Society Beers Criteria® Update Expert Panel. American Geriatrics Society 2023 updated AGS Beers Criteria® for potentially inappropriate medication use in older adults. *J Am Geriatr Soc.* 2023;71(7):2052–2081.
13. Hirvensalo M, Rantanen T, Heikkinen E. Mobility difficulties and physical activity as predictors of mortality and loss of independence in the community-living older population. *J Am Geriatr Soc.* 2000;48(5):493–498.
14. Tan TL, Ding YY, Lee A. Impaired mobility in older persons attending a geriatric assessment clinic: causes and management. *Singapore Med J.* 2001;42(2):68–72.
15. Corcoran PJ. Use it or lose it–the hazards of bed rest and inactivity. *West J Med.* 1991;154(5):536–538.
16. American Geriatrics Society. AGS Geriatric 5Ms. Minimum competencies in geriatrics for medical students. Accessed May 28, 2024. https://adgap.americangeriatrics.org/sites/default/files/media/files/AGS%20Geriatric%205Ms%20Competencies%20for%20Medical%20Students.pdf
17. Davis NJ, Wyman JF, Gubitosa S, Pretty L. Urinary incontinence in older adults. *Am J Nurs.* 2020;120(1):57–62.

18. Gorina Y, Schappert S, Bercovitz A, Elgaddal N, Kramarow E. Prevalence of incontinence among older Americans. *Vital Health Stat 3*. 2014;(36):1–33.
19. Coyne KS, Wein A, Nicholson S, Kvasz M, Chen C-I, Milsom I. Comorbidities and personal burden of urgency urinary incontinence: a systematic review. *Int J Clin Pract*. 2013;67(10):1015–1033.
20. Thakar R, Stanton S. Regular review: management of urinary incontinence in women. *BMJ*. 2000;321(7272):1326–1331.
21. First MB, Yousif LH, Clarke DE, Wang PS, Gogtay N, Appelbaum PS. DSM-5-TR: overview of what's new and what's changed. *World Psychiatry*. 2022;21(2):218–219.
22. Akdemir ÜÖ, Bora Tokçaer A, Atay LÖ. Dopamine transporter SPECT imaging in Parkinson's disease and parkinsonian disorders. *Turk J Med Sci*. 2021;51(2):400–410.
23. Brooks DJ. Future imaging in dementia. *Semin Nucl Med*. 2021;51(3):303–308.
24. Teunissen CE, Verberk IMW, Thijssen EH, et al. Blood-based biomarkers for Alzheimer's disease: towards clinical implementation. *Lancet Neurol*. 2022;21(1):66–77.
25. Falk N, Cole A, Meredith TJ. Evaluation of suspected dementia. *Am Fam Physician*. 2018;97(6):398–405.
26. Emmady PD, School C, Tadi P. Major neurocognitive disorder (dementia). In: *StatPearls*. StatPearls Publishing; 2023. Updated Nov 12, 2022. Accessed May 28, 2024. https://www.ncbi.nlm.nih.gov/books/NBK557444/
27. Prats-Sedano MA, Savulich G, Surendranathan A, et al. The revised Addenbrooke's Cognitive Examination can facilitate differentiation of dementia with Lewy bodies from Alzheimer's disease. *Int J Geriatr Psychiatry*. 2021;36(6):831–838.
28. Schachter AS, Davis KL. Alzheimer's disease. *Dialogues Clin Neurosci*. 2000;2(2):91–100.
29. O'Brien JT, Thomas A. Vascular dementia. *Lancet*. 2015;386(10004):1698–1706.
30. Kane JPM, Surendranathan A, Bentley A, et al. Clinical prevalence of Lewy body dementia. *Alzheimers Res Ther*. 2018;10(1):19.
31. Young JJ, Lavakumar M, Tampi D, Balachandran S, Tampi RR. Frontotemporal dementia: latest evidence and clinical implications. *Ther Adv Psychopharmacol*. 2018;8(1):33–48.
32. Uttley L, Carroll C, Wong R, Hilton DA, Stevenson M. Creutzfeldt-Jakob disease: a systematic review of global incidence, prevalence, infectivity, and incubation. *Lancet Infect Dis*. 2020;20(1):e2–e10.
33. Custodio N, Montesinos R, Lira D, Herrera-Pérez E, Bardales Y, Valeriano-Lorenzo L. Mixed dementia: a review of the evidence. *Dement Neuropsychol*. 2017;11(4):364–370.
34. Aarsland D, Ballard CG, Halliday G. Are Parkinson's disease with dementia and dementia with Lewy bodies the same entity? *J Geriatr Psychiatry Neurol*. 2004;17(3):137–145.
35. Hurtig HI, Trojanowski JQ, Galvin J, et al. Alpha-synuclein cortical Lewy bodies correlate with dementia in Parkinson's disease. *Neurology*. 2000;54(10):1916–1921.
36. Merdes AR, Hansen LA, Jeste DV, et al. Influence of Alzheimer pathology on clinical diagnostic accuracy in dementia with Lewy bodies. *Neurology*. 2003;60(10):1586–1590.
37. Tsuboi Y, Dickson DW. Dementia with Lewy bodies and Parkinson's disease with dementia: are they different? *Parkinsonism Relat Disord*. 2005;11(Suppl 1):S47–S51.
38. Centers for Disease Control and Prevention. Nursing Home Care. Updated Nov 5, 2023. Accessed May 28, 2024. https://www.cdc.gov/nchs/fastats/nursing-home-care.htm
39. DiGiovanna EL, Rowante M. Neurological considerations. In: DiGiovanna EL, Schiowitz S, Dowling DJ. *An Osteopathic Approach to Diagnosis and Treatment*. 3rd ed. Lippincott Williams & Wilkins; 2005.
40. National Institute on Aging. Alzheimer's Disease Fact Sheet. Updated May 16, 2017. Accessed May 28, 2024. https://www.nia.nih.gov/health/alzheimers-disease-fact-sheet
41. Tobey H, Lucas T, Bledsoe D, et al. Effect of osteopathic cranial manipulative medicine on an aged rat model of Alzheimer disease. *J Am Osteopath Assoc*. 2019:10.7556/jaoa.2019.121.
42. Ahmed RM, Devenney EM, Irish M, et al. Neuronal network disintegration: common pathways linking neurodegenerative diseases. *J Neurol Neurosurg Psychiatry*. 2016;87(11):1234–1241.
43. Hebert LE, Weuve J, Scherr PA, Evans DA. Alzheimer disease in the United States (2010–2050) estimated using the 2010 census. *Neurology*. 2013;80(19):1778–1783.
44. Masters CL, Bateman R, Blennow K, Rowe CC, Sperling RA, Cummings JL. Alzheimer's disease. *Nat Rev Dis Primers*. 2015;1:15056.
45. Hardy JA, Higgins GA. Alzheimer's disease: the amyloid cascade hypothesis. *Science*. 1992;256(5054):184–185.
46. Hardy J, Allsop D. Amyloid deposition as the central event in the aetiology of Alzheimer's disease. *Trends Pharmacol Sci*. 1991;12(10):383–388.
47. Singleton AB, Hall R, Ballard CG, et al. Pathology of early-onset Alzheimer's disease cases bearing the Thr113-114ins presenilin-1 mutation. *Brain*. 2000;123(Pt 12):2467–2474.
48. Cruts M, van Duijn CM, Backhovens H, et al. Estimation of the genetic contribution of presenilin-1 and -2 mutations in a population-based study of presenile Alzheimer disease. *Hum Mol Genet*. 1998;7(1):43–51.
49. Liu CC, Liu CC, Kanekiyo T, Xu H, Bu G. Apolipoprotein E and Alzheimer disease: risk, mechanisms and therapy. *Nat Rev Neurol*. 2013;9(2):106–118.
50. Duncombe J, Kitamura A, Hase Y, Ihara M, Kalaria RN, Horsburgh K. Chronic cerebral hypoperfusion: a key mechanism leading to vascular cognitive impairment and dementia. Closing the translational gap between rodent models and human vascular cognitive impairment and dementia. *Clin Sci (Lond)*. 2017;131(19):2451–2468.
51. Kinney JW, Bemiller SM, Murtishaw AS, Leisgang AM, Salazar AM, Lamb BT. Inflammation as a central mechanism in Alzheimer's disease. *Alzheimers Dement (N Y)*. 2018;4:575–590.
52. Beach TG, Walker R, McGeer EG. Patterns of gliosis in Alzheimer's disease and aging cerebrum. *Glia*. 1989;2(6):420–436.
53. Navarro V, Sanchez-Mejias E, Jimenez S, et al. Microglia in Alzheimer's disease: activated, dysfunctional or degenerative. *Front Aging Neurosci*. 2018;10:140.
54. Qaseem A, Snow V, Cross JT Jr, et al; American College of Physicians/American Academy of Family Physicians Panel on Dementia. Current pharmacologic treatment of dementia: a clinical practice guideline from the American College of Physicians and the American Academy of Family Physicians. *Ann Intern Med*. 2008;148(5):370–378.
55. Dhillon S. Aducanumab: first approval. *Drugs*. 2021;81(12):1437–1443. Erratum in: *Drugs*. 2021 Sep;81(14):1701.
56. Rabinovici GD. Controversy and progress in Alzheimer's disease—FDA approval of Aducanumab. *N Engl J Med*. 2021;385(9):771–774.
57. Robinson DM, Keating GM. Memantine: a review of its use in Alzheimer's disease. *Drugs*. 2006;66(11):1515–1534.
58. Snowdon DA; Nun Study. Healthy aging and dementia: findings from the Nun Study. *Ann Intern Med*. 2003;139(5 Pt 2):450–454.
59. Family Caregiver Alliance. Is This Dementia and What Does It Mean? Updated March 2, 2022. Accessed May 29, 2024. https://www.caregiver.org/resource/is-this-dementia-what-does-it-mean/
60. Still AT. *The Philosophy and Mechanical Principles of Osteopathy*. Hudson-Kimberly; 1892.
61. Rabin BS. Social networks and dementia. *Lancet*. 2000;356(9223):76–77.
62. Akbaraly TN, Singh-Manoux A, Dugravot A, Brunner EJ, Kivimäki M, Sabia S. Association of midlife diet with subsequent risk for dementia. *JAMA*. 2019;321(10):957–968.
63. de Bruijn RFAG, Ikram MA. Cardiovascular risk factors and future risk of Alzheimer's disease. *BMC Med*. 2014;12:130.
64. Uranga RM, Keller JN. Diet and age interactions with regards to cholesterol regulation and brain pathogenesis. *Curr Gerontol Geriatr Res*. 2010;2010:219683.
65. Ott A, Stolk RP, van Harskamp F, Pols HA, Hofman A, Breteler MM. Diabetes mellitus and the risk of dementia: the Rotterdam Study. *Neurology*. 1999;53(9):1937–1942.
66. Biessels GJ, Staekenborg S, Brunner E, Brayne C, Scheltens P. Risk of dementia in diabetes mellitus: a systematic review. *Lancet Neurol*. 2006;5(1):64–74. Erratum in: *Lancet Neurol*. 2006 Feb;5(2):113.
67. Butterfield DA, Di Domenico F, Barone E. Elevated risk of type 2 diabetes for development of Alzheimer disease: a key role for oxidative stress in brain. *Biochim Biophys Acta*. 2014;1842(9):1693–1706.
68. Morris MC, Tangney CC, Wang Y, et al. MIND diet slows cognitive decline with aging. *Alzheimers Dement*. 2015;11(9):1015–1022.

69. Cherian L, Wang Y, Fakuda K, Leurgans S, Aggarwal N, Morris M. Mediterranean-Dash Intervention for Neurodegenerative Delay (MIND) diet slows cognitive decline after stroke. *J Prev Alzheimers Dis.* 2019;6(4): 267–273.
70. Barnes LL, Dhana K, Liu X, et al. Trial of the MIND diet for prevention of cognitive decline in older persons. *N Engl J Med.* 2023;389(7): 602–611.
71. Engelhart MJ, Geerlings MI, Ruitenberg A, et al. Diet and risk of dementia: does fat matter?: The Rotterdam Study. *Neurology.* 2002;59(12):1915–1921.
72. Kryscio RJ, Abner EL, Caban-Holt A, et al. Association of antioxidant supplement use and dementia in the Prevention of Alzheimer's Disease by Vitamin E and Selenium Trial (PREADViSE). *JAMA Neurol.* 2017;74(5):567–573.
73. Heyn P, Abreu BC, Ottenbacher KJ. The effects of exercise training on elderly persons with cognitive impairment and dementia: a meta-analysis. *Arch Phys Med Rehabil.* 2004;85(10):1694–1704.
74. Mazza M, Capuano A, Bria P, Mazza S. Ginkgo biloba and donepezil: a comparison in the treatment of Alzheimer's dementia in a randomized placebo-controlled double-blind study. *Eur J Neurol.* 2006;13(9): 981–985.
75. Arvanitakis Z, Shah RC, Bennett DA. Diagnosis and management of dementia: review. *JAMA.* 2019;322(16):1589–1599.

104 Case Study: Adult with Myalgias

J. MICHAEL WIETING ▪ WILLIAM FOLEY ▪ CAMERON BRAZ ▪ KURT P. HEINKING

KEY CONCEPTS

- The differential diagnosis of myalgia is extensive and should encompass common, easily diagnosed, conditions as well as others that are less well-recognized.
- Fibromyalgia (FM) is a condition encompassing chronic, relapsing, diffuse aching pain and tenderness, which can be intermittent and nondermatomal.
- Other features of FM include hyperesthesia, allodynia, severe fatigue, insomnia, depression, anxiety, cognitive difficulty (specifically, issues with motivation, concentration, and organization), exercise intolerance, and nonrestorative sleep.
- Approximately 2% of US and Canadian citizens have FM.
- Current pathophysiologic theories include atypical sensory processing in the central nervous system (i.e., central sensitization), dysfunction of skeletal muscle nociception, and dysfunction of the hypothalamic–pituitary–adrenal axis.
- Treatment for FM should include OMT, patient education, and aerobic exercise.

CASE VIGNETTE

A 31-year-old woman reports muscle pain "all over my body" with the most intense pain in the neck, back, shoulders, and thighs. The pain started 2 years ago in her lower back after a minor car accident. The back pain at that time was mild, and plain x-rays were negative. Since then, the pain has gradually spread to her entire body and has become a constant ache that waxes and wanes in intensity. Over-the-counter medications such as ibuprofen and acetaminophen have been somewhat helpful, but only on a temporary basis. She has not used narcotics since they made her nauseated when she took them after a previous surgery.

She describes her pain as a 6/10 currently, but it can range from 4 to 8 on a scale of 1 to 10. About a year ago, she completed 6 weeks of physical therapy that she feels was beneficial, but she did not keep up with her prescribed home exercises due to excessive pain. She reports no known tick or other insect exposures or bites. Her biggest complaint is that she can no longer work due to the pain and that she is having a hard time caring for her two small children. She feels like "a prisoner to her pain." Six months after the car accident, she began experiencing new fatigue, insomnia, and abdominal bloating; she denies abdominal pain, diarrhea, or constipation. Her fatigue is now most pronounced after increased or sustained activity. She can feel exhausted after simple events such as going to the mall or cleaning the house. At night, she falls asleep easily, but awakens two to three times per night and finds it difficult to fall back asleep.

PAST MEDICAL HISTORY

Her past medical history is significant only for seasonal allergies.

PAST SURGICAL HISTORY

Positive for uncomplicated Cesarean sections × 2.

MEDICATIONS

She is currently taking loratadine 10 mg as needed for her allergies and a daily multivitamin.

ALLERGIES

She has no known drug allergies.

SOCIAL HISTORY

She does not smoke or use illicit drugs. She drinks one glass of wine daily. She reports that she is happily married for 6 years.

REVIEW OF SYSTEMS

HEENT

Her vision and hearing are normal.

Cardiovascular

She has no chest pain, palpitations, or shortness of breath.

Respiratory

She denies shortness of breath, wheezing, and cough.

Gastrointestinal

She denies stomach pain, nausea, vomiting, diarrhea, and change in stools. She admits to bloating.

Skin

She has no skin rash.

Musculoskeletal

She denies joint swelling and joint pain although she admits to muscle pain as described above.

Neurologic

She denies paresthesia, weakness, loss of consciousness, tics, twitches, and seizures.

Psychiatric

She complains of difficulty with concentration, organization of tasks, motivation, and a shortened attention span. Due to her condition, she reports feeling progressively more depressed and also hopeless at times.

Endocrine

She denies chills, fever, and weight change. She admits to fatigue and sleeping difficulties as previously described.

PHYSICAL EXAMINATION

Vital Signs

In the office, her heart rate is 68 beats per minute, respiratory rate is 16 beats per minute, blood pressure is 112/70, and she is afebrile.

General

She appears in no acute distress.

Eyes

Extraocular muscles are intact, and pupils are equally round and reactive to light.

ENT

Her oral mucosa is moist. Her neck is supple with no lymphadenopathy or thyromegaly.

Heart

Her heart has a regular rate and rhythm without murmurs.

Lungs

Breath sounds are full and clear to auscultation.

Abdomen

The abdomen is soft and nontender.

Skin

She has no rash.

Neurologic

Reflexes are +2 and equal in both the upper and lower extremities. Sensation is intact to light touch and pin prick. Muscle strength is 5/5 globally.

Musculoskeletal/Osteopathic Structural

She has no muscle atrophy or visible deformities. Curvatures of cervical, thoracic, and lumbar spine are within normal limits, but both shoulders are protracted. There are no joint effusions or tenderness. No synovitis is palpable. Palpation of spinous processes is nontender. Palpation of cervical, thoracic, and lumbar paraspinal muscles is tender and hypertonic. Multiple tender points are present bilaterally in the following regions: anterior neck at the C5–C7 intertransverse spaces, posterior head at the insertions of the suboccipital muscles, upper thoracic at the midtrapezius and the supraspinatus above the medial scapular spine, upper extremities just distal to the lateral epicondyles, lower lumbar at the upper outer quadrant of the buttocks, and finally in the lower extremities at the medial knees and posterior to the greater trochanter prominences. There are multiple regions of somatic dysfunction found on examination. There is a sphenobasilar synchondrosis compression. The occipitoatlantal junction is extended, side bent right, and rotated left. The atlantoaxial junction is rotated right. The thoracolumbar junction is side bent left and rotated right. The lumbosacral junction is side bent right and rotated left. The right innominate is rotated posteriorly, and there is bilateral sacroiliac restriction.

DIFFERENTIAL DIAGNOSIS

Diffuse myalgia associated with fatigue is a common complaint in the primary care setting. The differential diagnosis of myalgia is extensive and should encompass common, easily diagnosed, conditions as well as others that are less well-recognized, but can present with similar manifestations and may also coexist with FM. Careful history taking and a methodical physical examination can assist in narrowing down the possibilities. The differential (Table 104.1) includes very common conditions such as bursitis, tendonitis or synovitis, and hypothyroidism. Somewhat less common, but deserving of consideration, are infectious conditions, such as Lyme disease and hepatitis C, and inflammatory conditions, such as polymyalgia rheumatica, polymyositis, dermatomyositis, rheumatoid arthritis, systemic lupus erythematosus, and scleroderma.

Degenerative/structural problems, such as cervical stenosis, may present as myalgias. However, this patient's neck pain will typically have associated dysesthesia, numbness, and myelopathic symptoms (if involving the central canal). Myelopathic symptoms include extremity spasms, bowel and bladder dysfunction, unsteady gait, lower limb weakness and numbness, abnormal reflexes, muscle atrophy, and decreased muscle tone. Certain metabolic processes can be associated with myalgias; the most common include thyroid disease and vitamin B_{12} deficiency. Rarely, toxicities or side effects of some lipid-lowering agents and antiviral medications can contribute to myalgias. Frequent concomitant conditions that need to be considered are depression, chronic fatigue, FM, and myofascial pain.

The presence of fatigue, insomnia, or other constitutional symptoms in a patient with diffuse myalgia tends to focus the differential on systemic or chronic conditions. Often, lab work (such as complete blood count [CBC], liver and kidney functions, creatinine phosphokinase [CPK], erythrocyte sedimentation rate [ESR], C-reactive protein [CRP], and thyroid functions) may be needed to rule out diffuse or systemic pathology.

In this case, the patient's pain and constitutional symptoms seem to be temporally related to a motor vehicle accident, suggesting myofascial pain because of trauma rather than a systemic condition. However, some inflammatory diseases such as rheumatoid arthritis and systemic lupus erythematosus can initially present in similar fashion with myalgia as the initial complaint followed by fatigue and other systemic signs. Consequently, a careful review of all systems and laboratory studies is necessary to determine the diagnosis. Also, myofascial disease can coexist with other disorders of defined structural pathology, such as rheumatoid arthritis, FM, and chronic fatigue syndrome. Some conditions such as FM and chronic fatigue syndrome are diagnoses of exclusion, necessitating other causes of diffuse muscle pain be first ruled out.

Workup and Interpretation

This patient's chronic and diffuse clinical temporal profile helps to rule out most infectious processes. However, an elevated white blood cell count could indicate chronic infection or an inflammatory disease. An elevated CRP and ESR are also indicators of inflammation. If either is elevated, further studies would be necessary to identify the etiology of the inflammation. Elevated CPK levels suggest an inflammation of the muscle. Liver and renal function tests can be elevated in hepatitis C, myositis, lupus, rheumatoid arthritis, and other autoimmune diseases. Thyroid disease can present with muscle pain or weakness, depression, fatigue, and insomnia; a thyroid-stimulating hormone (TSH) level is usually sufficient to rule out this as a cause.

Other tests that could be considered in the workup of diffuse myalgia include vitamin B_{12} level, hepatitis C screen, and a Lyme

TABLE 104.1

Differential Diagnosis of Myalgias

Mechanical/Degenerative Conditions	
Bursitis	Involves only one joint or limb
Tendonitis or synovitis	Usually has a single focus and is associated with tendon motion
Cervical stenosis	Neck pain associated with dysesthesia, numbness, and, if involving the central canal, myelopathic symptoms of extremity spasm, bowel and bladder dysfunction, unsteady gait, lower limb weakness and numbness, abnormal reflexes, muscle atrophy, and decreased muscle tone
Infectious Conditions	
Lyme disease	A characteristic erythema migrans, usually only one to two joints are involved, one of which is often the knee and associated neuropathy and nephropathy and frequent facial nerve involvement
Hepatitis C	Need characteristic lab findings
Inflammatory Conditions	
Polymyalgia rheumatica	Features symmetric, proximal weakness, normal CPK, neuropathic pain, and hyperesthesia
Polymyositis and dermatomyositis	Present with severe, symmetric proximal weakness, and high CPK
Rheumatoid arthritis	Morning stiffness that may last for several hours, joint swelling and pain, symmetric polyarthritis, joint warmth and effusion, multiple elevated serum immune complexes, and complement consumption
Systemic lupus erythematosis	Characteristic malar or discoid rash, vasculitis, lymphadenopathy, thrombocytopenia, and nephritis associated dark urine and peripheral edema along with elevated antinuclear antibody
Scleroderma	Features skin and multiorgan fibrosis
Metabolic Processes	
Hypothyroidism	Can be assessed via a TSH level
Thyroid disease	Can be assessed with imaging
Vitamin B_{12} deficiency	A simple blood test can measure B_{12}
Toxicities or side effects of some lipid-lowering agents	This is a diagnosis based upon clinical presentation and exclusion of other etiologies
Toxicities or side effects of antiviral medications	This is a diagnosis based upon clinical presentation and exclusion of other etiologies

titer. Vitamin B_{12} deficiency would be high on the differential if the patient has a history of a small bowel resection, excessive alcohol intake, malnourishment, or followed a vegan diet low in B vitamins. Generally, this information can be obtained from the history and, unless there is suspicion, lab testing is not necessary. In the same way, a hepatitis C screen should be performed if hepatitis C is suspected or if there is a history of blood transfusion, multiple sexual contacts, intravenous drug use, or a prior accidental needle stick. Screening for Lyme disease should be performed if the patient has a history of tick bites, a characteristic rash, or reported migratory joint pains. Even though there was no objective muscle weakness found in this patient, weakness should be assessed by an electrodiagnostic study if it presents after initial workup with an unknown etiology or if there is concern for possible radiculopathy, myopathy, or nerve entrapment. If any of these tests are abnormal, then a muscle biopsy or further testing for immunologic or other systemic disorders may be warranted.

CASE VIGNETTE (CONTINUED)

Lab tests performed during the initial visit with this patient included a CBC, renal and liver functions, CRP, ESR, CPK, and TSH levels. The initial lab work was negative. The history and physical exam, in conjunction with lab results, indicate that her pain is likely myofascial in origin. This patient was diagnosed with FM.

DIAGNOSIS

The three most common causes of myofascial pain are myofascial pain syndrome, chronic fatigue syndrome, and FM. FM is differentiated from myofascial pain syndrome in that it usually has multiple tender points in predictable bilateral locations, chronic widespread pain, a 10:1 prevalence in females, fatigue, and sleep disturbance. On the other hand, myofascial pain syndrome has trigger points, more regionalized pain, a 1:1 ratio of males and females, and rarely has systemic features.

FM may be distinguished from chronic fatigue syndrome by the fact that chronic fatigue syndrome is usually preceded by a viral illness. While fatigue of more than 6 months duration is a characteristic of both diseases, chronic fatigue syndrome also has at least four of the following symptoms: decreased memory or concentration, sore throat, tender cervical or axillary nodes, multifocal joint pain, new headache, postexertional malaise, nonrestorative sleep, and muscle pain. FM is more distinctive of a chronic syndrome, predominantly in women, with generalized chronic pain, multiple well-defined tender points, fatigue, and sleep disturbance. It can be triggered or aggravated by physical or emotional trauma.

The chief complaint in a FM patient is described as a chronic, relapsing, diffuse aching pain, not just tenderness, which can be intermittent and nondermatomal. Patients may complain of hyperesthesia and allodynia. The pain often presents bilaterally in muscles and at muscle–tendon junctions, especially in the neck, shoulders, second ribs, elbows, hips, buttocks, and knees. Other features of FM include severe fatigue, insomnia, depression, anxiety, cognitive difficulty (specifically, issues with motivation, concentration, and organization), exercise intolerance, and nonrestorative sleep. FM patients may have concomitant migraine headaches, temporomandibular joint disorder, urinary frequency, paresthesia in the hands and feet, or irritable bowel syndrome.

The exact cause of FM is not fully understood, but it is believed to involve a combination of genetic, environmental, and psychological factors. To date, no definitive pathology has been found in the muscles of FM patients. The pathophysiologic factors of FM being studied seem to have determined it as a central sensitivity syndrome, triggered by excess excitatory (nociceptive) neurotransmitters (e.g., substance P and glutamate), which concentrate in the insula of the brain.[1] Other anomalies observed are dopamine dysregulation and altered activity of endogenous cerebral opioids, dopamine dysregulation, and autonomic dysfunction.[1]

Evidence has found that patients with FM have a generalized decreased pain perception threshold, excess excitatory (nociceptive) neurotransmitters (e.g., substance P and glutamate), low levels of inhibitory neurotransmitters (such as serotonin and norepinephrine), enhanced temporal summation of pain, altered endogenous opioid analgesic activity, dopamine dysregulation, and autonomic dysfunction.[1] Central sensitization occurs with a long-term potentiation of pain signals associated with *N*-methyl-D-aspartic acid (NMDA) receptor activation and with the induction of specific genes.[2] There is also increasing evidence that indicates that neurogenic-derived inflammatory processes occurring in the peripheral tissues, spinal cord, and brain are also responsible for the pathophysiology of FM.[3–5]

Psychosocial factors seem to play a large role in the development of the disease. According to several studies, the prevalence of psychiatric comorbidities, such as anxiety disorders and depression, reaches 60% in patients with FM.[6] The efficacy of serotonin-norepinephrine reuptake inhibitors (SNRIs) and other double-acting antidepressants, such as mirtazapine, suggests that neurotransmission dysfunction of both serotonin and norepinephrine exists in FM.[7] While the precise risk factors for developing FM are not definitively established, several factors are commonly associated with an increased risk of developing this condition. These include gender, age, genetic predisposition, physical or emotional trauma, infections, rheumatologic conditions, stress, environmental influences, obesity/sedentary lifestyle, and psychosocial change.[1]

OSTEOPATHIC PATIENT MANAGEMENT

Biomechanical Model

This patient has many somatic dysfunctions that are likely to contribute to biomechanical stress and increased nociception. Since 2 years have passed after the suspected inciting insult, treating the original, now chronic, somatic dysfunction in the low back will likely not be sufficient due to local and central sensitization. Therefore, it is important to initially treat all areas of somatic dysfunction in this patient, especially concentrating on the areas of greatest functional compromise. Decreasing biomechanical stress is key to avoiding continued local and central sensitization. Aerobic exercise should combat deconditioning by placing focus on stretching and strengthening the musculature. Core strengthening is also beneficial in treating deconditioned abdominal and paraspinal muscles that are either weak or inordinately tight.

In treating FM, it is important to remember that this is not a localized condition. Treating myofascial trigger points, for example, may help in the short term but has not been shown as effective long-term treatment. An osteopathic treatment approach should address the whole patient.

Respiratory–Circulatory Model

Somatic dysfunction can alter the musculoskeletal system's contribution to tissue perfusion. The venous and lymphatic systems are low-pressure circuits, dependent upon external forces and sympathetic control for proper function. Pain may result in muscle splinting and altered movement mechanics in the thoracic tissues and respiratory muscles. Altered tissue tone and restrictions can directly impede tissue perfusion. Resolution of somatic dysfunction may improve circulation to injured or damaged muscles and nerves.

Neurologic Model

Clinical investigations have suggested that FM is a central sensitivity syndrome that has both a peripheral and central neurophysiologic base. In this patient, pain started locally in the back and then spread. If the original injury to the back did not resolve, it may have continued sending acute nociceptive signals to the spinal cord, which in turn signaled the brain. Chronically sustained insults to a nerve can lead to local sensitization and phenomena known as "facilitation" and "windup," where short-term potentiation of pain signals occurs that is associated with repeated C-fiber stimulation.[8] Afferent pain signals from hypersensitive spinal nerves can affect related muscles and joints. Hyperesthesia, allodynia, and pain may then result in innervated structures. Hypersensitive proprioceptors can cause structural alterations that lead to somatic dysfunctions, such as ligamentous articular strains, muscle spasm, fascial strains, and myofascial trigger points. Any of these can lead to increased or sustained pain.

Peripheral and Central Sensitization

Patients with FM present with a lower pain threshold that generates a condition of diffuse hyperalgesia and/or allodynia. This indicates that there may be a problem with the amplification of pain or with sensory processing in the CNS. These FM phenomena have been confirmed in clinical studies that used functional neuroimaging.[1] However, sensitization is not a unitary phenomenon and a distinction must be made between central, peripheral, and cognitive–emotional sensitization.[1]

Chronic nerve impingement can lead to dorsal horn sensitization of its nerve roots.[2] When central sensitization occurs, it can affect two segments above and below the innervating site. Therefore, multiple spinal levels can become painful and dysfunctional, as is seen in this patient. As a result, pain from a local injury can appear to spread to other regions of the body. Sustained increase of cytokines and chemokines in the CNS also promotes chronic widespread pain that affects multiple body sites. Thus, neuroinflammation drives widespread chronic pain via central sensitization.[9] Nociceptive signals from the spinal cord can be consolidated in the brain causing further sensitization in the central nervous system.[10] In this patient, central sensitization may account for her depression, fatigue, insomnia, and cognitive impairment.[1]

The patient was treated pharmacologically with duloxetine and later pregabalin. The FDA has approved three drugs for the treatment of FM: pregabalin (gamma-aminobutyric acid [GABA] agonist), duloxetine (SNRI), and milnacipran (SNRI). They act on the central nervous system and are likely able to lessen FM symptoms by modulating neurotransmitters and affecting central sensitization. Tricyclic antidepressants have shown benefit with pain and sleep.[11] When using this class of medication, it should be remembered that nortriptyline has a lesser side effect profile (i.e., dry mouth, constipation, fluid retention, weight gain, and decreased concentration). Successful management recommendations include combination drug therapy, cognitive behavioral therapy, as well as education regarding sleep hygiene and exercise.[12] The literature does not support the effectiveness of nonsteroid anti-inflammatory drugs or steroids for the disease, but they can be useful in management if there is a coexisting inflammatory process.[1]

Pharmacologic treatment alone is inadequate for most patients who suffer from FM syndrome. Given the different mechanisms of pain sensitivity, treatments will continue to involve multidisciplinary programs that target the peripheral, central, cognitive–emotional, and interpersonal contributions to the chronic pain that characterizes FM pathophysiology.

Some clinicians are using botulinum neurotoxin (Botox), produced by the anaerobic bacterium *Clostridium botulinum*, which is one of the several neurotoxins that have been shown to inhibit the release of neurotransmitters involved in pain transmission (such as substance P and glutamate) in animal studies; it also reduces signs of pain and local edema. This neurotoxin appears to act only upon motor nerve endings, thereby sparing sensory nerve fibers. By targeting central and peripheral nerve endings, Botox blocks the release of acetylcholine here, hence decreasing muscle spasm at trigger points.[13] Studies on the efficacy of botulinum toxin in reducing myofascial pain and trigger points/tenderpoints are mixed.[14]

Metabolic Energy Model

Finally, it is important to consider the metabolic energy model when planning long-term treatment for a patient with FM. Diet (especially addressing potential deficiencies like 25-hydroxyvitamin D), graded aerobic exercise, lifestyle modifications, and decreased somatic dysfunction load are all important in reducing or eliminating future exacerbations of FM. A clinical study found that women with FM had a lower qualitative and quantitative dietary intake than control subjects.[15] Vitamin D deficiency and FM have also been found to be associated. However, its role in FM pathophysiology and therefore its clinical relevance of identification and treatment requires further clarification. Only vitamin E appears to be related to quality of life and pain sensation.[15–17]

In comparison to the healthy population, FM patients produce higher levels of harmful free radicals and have a decreased antioxidant ability, both of which contribute to more oxidative stress. The central nervous system is highly susceptible to free radicals because of its high lipid content.[1,18] The progression of fibromyalgia may be dependent on increased reactive oxygen species. Treatment with antioxidants and vitamins, in addition to antidepressants and structural analogs of GABA, was able to improve symptoms of FM patients.[1,19] Many FM patients utilize complementary and alternative therapies including herbals and topicals.[20] Bioactive compounds derived from medicinal plants have also demonstrated analgesic activity and antioxidant properties with respect to FM.[1]

Behavioral Model

Empathetic listening, acknowledgment of the legitimacy of the patient's pain, assessing possible perpetuating or concomitant factors, relaxation training, activity pacing, and exercise are useful initial strategies that can be supplemented with other approaches as needed.

Psychological components are often prominent in FM. Not only does the patient report a depressed mood, but also the worry and anxiety about her family and work. While this may be partially emotional, somatic dysfunctions may contribute to the sensitization of the brain's emotional center, the limbic system. Gold and Goodwin[21,22] first reported depression and other "psychological" symptoms in patients with chronic pain. Since that time, the association between depression and pain has become widespread.[23] Recent evidence suggests that, in patients with FM, pain may adversely affect overall health via its contribution to allostatic load.[24]

CASE VIGNETTE (CONTINUED)

PATIENT OUTCOME

Information about FM was provided to the patient through patient–physician discussion and patient handouts from the American Pain Society. OMT was performed, starting on the first visit. Initially, gentle techniques including myofascial release, balanced ligamentous tension, and cranial osteopathy were performed due to the patient's sensitivity even to light touch. As she progressed with treatments, other techniques were added. This treatment effect is in alignment with a systematic review and meta-analysis which found low-quality evidence suggesting that strain–counterstrain (SCS) may reduce tenderpoint palpation pain.[25] She also started an exercise program that consisted of gradually increasing aerobic workouts to reach a goal of 30 minutes of daily exercise. Most authorities agree on the value of patient education and aerobic exercise. Education should be centered on reassurance that the illness is real and that FM is neither progressive nor life threatening.

The patient returned every 4 weeks for reevaluation and OMT. At each visit, continued aerobic exercise was encouraged and medications were adjusted as needed. Counseling to improve diet and decrease stress was also provided at each visit. From the osteopathic perspective, it is important for patients to be as healthy as possible to heal. This includes modifications in diet, habits, exercise, and stress. In this patient's case, diet was not an issue and remained unchanged, but she did start a weekly meditation and yoga class. In other patients, discussion of whole foods, proper water intake, and smoking cessation may need to be addressed. A referral to a nutritionist or psychologist also may be helpful to some patients.

By the fifth treatment, the patient was 75% improved. Follow-up visits progressed to every 3 months where she has been stable for 3 years. While her FM has not completely resolved, she is now able to do work and take care of her family and is not restricted by her disease.

SUMMARY

Using the osteopathic models of patient management, the physician can approach the patient with FM from a whole-person perspective, addressing all the various factors that may contribute to this multifaceted condition.

REFERENCES

1. Siracusa R, Paola RD, Cuzzocrea S, Impellizzeri D. Fibromyalgia: pathogenesis, mechanisms, diagnosis and treatment options update. *Int J Mol Sci.* 2021;22(8):3891.
2. Latremoliere A, Woolf CJ. Central sensitization: a generator of pain hypersensitivity by central neural plasticity. *J Pain.* 2009;10(9):895–926.

3. Slade GD, Conrad MS, Diatchenko L, et al. Cytokine biomarkers and chronic pain: association of genes, transcription, and circulating proteins with temporomandibular disorders and widespread palpation tenderness. *Pain.* 2011;152(12):2802–2812.
4. Sturgill J, McGee E, Menzies V. Unique cytokine signature in the plasma of patients with fibromyalgia. *J Immunol Res.* 2014;2014:938576.
5. Mendieta D, De la Cruz-Aguilera DL, Barrera-Villalpando MI, et al. IL-8 and IL-6 primarily mediate the inflammatory response in fibromyalgia patients. *J Neuroimmunol.* 2016;290:22–25.
6. Epstein SA, Kay G, Clauw D, et al. Psychiatric disorders in patients with fibromyalgia. A multicenter investigation. *Psychosomatics.* 1999;40(1):57–63.
7. Moret C, Briley M. Antidepressants in the treatment of fibromyalgia. *Neuropsychiatr Dis Treat.* 2006;2(4):537–548.
8. Gary J. Neural basis of pain. In: Ballantyne J, ed. *Massachusetts General Hospital Handbook of Pain Management.* 2nd ed. Lippincott Williams & Wilkins; 2002:12.
9. Ji RR, Nackley A, Huh Y, Terrando N, Maixner W. Neuroinflammation and central sensitization in chronic and widespread pain. *Anesthesiology.* 2018;129(2):343–366.
10. Dydyk AM, Givler A. Central pain syndrome. In: *StatPearls [Internet].* StatPearls Publishing; 2023. Updated February 19, 2023. https://www.ncbi.nlm.nih.gov/books/NBK553027
11. Sadreddini S, Molaeefard M, Noshad H, Ardalan M, Asadi A. Efficacy of Raloxifen in treatment of fibromyalgia in menopausal women. *Eur J Intern Med.* 2008;19(5):350–355.
12. Goldenberg DL. Initial treatment of fibromyalgia in adults. Accessed October 26, 2017. https://www-uptodate-com.proxy.westernu.edu/contents/initial-treatment-of-fibromyalgia-in-adults?source=see_link#H5
13. Jabbari B. Botulinum toxin treatment of myofascial pain syndrome and fibromyalgia. In: *Botulinum Toxin Treatment of Pain Disorders.* Springer, Cham; 2022.
14. Borg-Stein J, Iaccarino MA. Myofascial pain syndrome treatments. *Phys Med Rehabil Clin N Am.* 2014;25(2):357–374.
15. Batista ED, Andretta A, de Miranda RC, Nehring J, Dos Santos Paiva E, Schieferdecker ME. Food intake assessment and quality of life in women with fibromyalgia. *Rev Bras Reumatol Engl Ed.* 2016;56(2):105–110.
16. Joustra ML, Minovic I, Janssens KAM, Bakker SJL, Rosmalen JGM. Vitamin and mineral status in chronic fatigue syndrome and fibromyalgia syndrome: a systematic review and meta-analysis. *PLoS ONE.* 2017;12(4):e0176631.
17. Ellis SD, Kelly ST, Shurlock JH, Hepburn ALN. The role of vitamin D testing and replacement in fibromyalgia: a systematic literature review. *BMC Rheumatol.* 2018;2:28.
18. Bagis S, Tamer L, Sahin G, et al. Free radicals and antioxidants in primary fibromyalgia: an oxidative stress disorder? *Rheumatol Int.* 2005;25(3):188–190.
19. Miranda-Díaz AG, Rodríguez-Lara SQ. The role of oxidants/antioxidants, mitochondrial dysfunction, and autophagy in fibromyalgia. In: Wilke WS, ed. *Discussions of Unusual Topics in Fibromyalgia.* Inthech; 2018.
20. Casanueva B, Rodero B, Quintial C, Llorca J, Gonzalez-Gay MA. Short-term efficacy of topical capsaicin therapy in severely affected fibromyalgia patients. *Rheumatol Int.* 2013;33(10):2665–2670.
21. Gold PW, Goodwin FK, Chrousos GP. Clinical and biochemical manifestations of depression. Relation to the neurobiology of stress: part I. *NEJM.* 1988;319(6):348–353.
22. Gold PW, Goodwin FK, Chrousos GP. Clinical and biochemical manifestations of depression: relation to the neurobiology of stress. Part II. *NEJM.* 1988;319(7):413–420.
23. Robinson MJ, Edwards SE, Iyengar S, Bymaster F, Clark M, Katon W. Depression and pain. *Front Biosci.* 2009;14(13):5031–5051.
24. Martinez-Lavin M, Vargas A. Complex adaptive systems allostasis in fibromyalgia. *Rheum Dis Clin North Am.* 2009;35(2):285–298
25. Wong CK, Abraham T, Karimi P, Ow-Wing C. Strain counterstrain technique to decrease tender point palpation pain compared to control conditions: a systematic review with meta-analysis. *J Bodyw Mov Ther.* 2014;18(2):165–173.

105 Case Study: Multiple Small Joint Diseases in an Elderly Patient

STEPHEN FUNG

KEY CONCEPTS

- Hand pain and stiffness are common complaints in the elderly patient, and a thorough history and physical exam need to be done to rule out an inflammatory condition.
- Chronic hand pain and stiffness can adversely affect daily living activities and contribute to depression and a loss of personal motivation in an otherwise healthy individual.
- An integrated approach to the management of the patient with hand pain and stiffness, including pharmacotherapeutics, osteopathic manipulation, and behavioral modification, can provide relief and improved function.

CASE VIGNETTE

Ms. Anderson is a 62-year-old Caucasian female who seeks medical care for chronic severe worsening hand stiffness and pain.

CHIEF COMPLAINT

A 3-month history of chronic aching pain in bilateral hands with associated morning stiffness lasting over 1 hour, as well as chronic daily headaches for the past year.

HISTORY OF PRESENT ILLNESS

The patient denies any recent traumas. The pain has been affecting her in daily activities as well as in employment. Over the past 3 months, Ms. Anderson missed a significant amount of time at work, and she lost her job. She worked at a health food store and had difficulty stocking the shelves. She is concerned about the ongoing discomfort in her hands, as well as having daily headaches. She attributes both to a multilevel cervical fusion 6 years ago. Her hand pain has a severity of 7/10 when opening jars or performing repetitive tasks. She describes symmetrical joint stiffness in her hands, worse in the morning upon awakening, often lasting over 1 hour. She further relates difficulty sleeping at night secondary to pain, predominantly in her neck. She notes that she has significant discomfort when hooking her bra, undoing buttons, or knitting a sweater. She has taken naproxen sodium 200 mg twice daily with minimal improvement. She used a heating pad for her neck, and "arthritis cream" for her hands, but has not used ice for pain relief. She has not had any prior workup or imaging. She denies having numbness, weakness, or paresthesia involving her hands. She denies chest pain, fever, shortness of breath, cough, or stomach upset.

PAST MEDICAL HISTORY

Osteopenia, osteoarthritis (OA) of the cervical spine, knees, hips, gastroesophageal reflux disease (GERD) (acid reflux disease), chronic daily tension headaches, hyperlipidemia, postmenopausal, last colonoscopy 1 year ago normal.

PAST SURGICAL HISTORY

Cervical fusion C5–C7 at age 52, cervical fusion C2–C5 at age 54, right knee replacement at age 59, appendectomy at age 18, tonsillectomy and adenoidectomy at age 6, C-section at age 29.

PAST TRAUMA HISTORY

Motor vehicle accident 1982, minor concussion, whiplash injury

FAMILY MEDICAL HISTORY

Father: deceased secondary to alcohol-induced cirrhosis at age 58; siblings: one brother aged 59, healthy, no family history of rheumatologic disorders other than OA.

GYNECOLOGIC HISTORY

G2 P 1011, last menstrual period (LMP) 12 years ago, last mammogram 2 years ago (normal), last pap and pelvic, rectal exam 2 years ago (normal), last DEXA bone scan 2 years ago osteopenia.

SOCIAL HISTORY

Widowed (husband, John, passed 10 years ago), 1 son (Marty, 29, healthy), positive tobacco use (1 pack per day intermittent for 35 years), denies illicit drug use, and occasional alcohol (holidays). Patient was an employee of a large nutrition store. She does not exercise regularly.

CHILDHOOD ILLNESSES

Chickenpox and possible measles

MEDICATIONS

Alendronate sodium, 70 mg week; atorvastatin calcium, 40 mg daily; esomeprazole magnesium, 40 mg daily; naproxen sodium, 220 mg twice daily; acetaminophen, 500 mg 4 times daily prn; conjugated estrogens/medroxyprogesterone acetate tablets, 0.625 mg daily.

REVIEW OF SYSTEMS

General

She complains of fatigue and daily tension headaches. She denies fever, chills, change in appetite, or weight change.

Cardiopulmonary

She denies chest pain, palpitations, and shortness of breath.

Neurologic

She denies numbness, weakness, and paresthesia of the extremities. She further denies any visual changes.

Musculoskeletal

She admits to neck stiffness, bilateral hand pain and stiffness, and daily tension headaches in the suboccipital and frontal region described as a tight sensation. She denies shoulder and hip discomfort and jaw claudication.

PHYSICAL EXAMINATION

Vital Signs

Temp: 97.6 F; Heart rate: 78 regular; RR: 16; BP: 150/82 mmHg; height: 5′4″; weight: 138 lb.

General

Alert, oriented, cooperative, affect somewhat flat, and a good historian. She appears her stated age.

HEENT

PERRLA EOMI, normal visual acuity. No xerophthalmia or xerostomia. Pharynx without erythema, no adenopathy, no thyromegaly, TMs good cone of light without erythema, no nasal erythema, no sinus tenderness, no tenderness over the temporal arteries or scalp.

Neck

Supple, no jugular venous distention (JVD) or bruits. Some discomfort noted with full range of motion (ROM).

Skin

No rashes, no abnormal appearing moles, multiple seborrheic keratoses (back), dry hair and nails. No petechiae, purpura, livedo reticularis, telangiectasias, or evidence of Raynaud phenomenon.

Breast

No breast masses, nipples everted, no discharge, no axillary adenopathy.

Cardiovascular

Regular rhythm and rate (RRR) without S3 and S4 murmur, no clubbing, cyanosis, or peripheral edema. Equal pulses bilaterally.

Lungs

Clear to auscultation (CTA) without rales, rhonchi, wheezes.

Abdomen

BS × four quadrants without rigidity, rebound, guarding, negative costovertebral angle (CVA) tenderness pain, no masses appreciated. No right upper quadrant (RUQ) discomfort on palpation, negative Murphy sign.

Neurologic

Cranial nerves (CNs) 2 to 12 intact, deep tendon reflexes (DTRs) 2/4 bilateral, no sensory deficits, 5/5 motor strength bilateral.

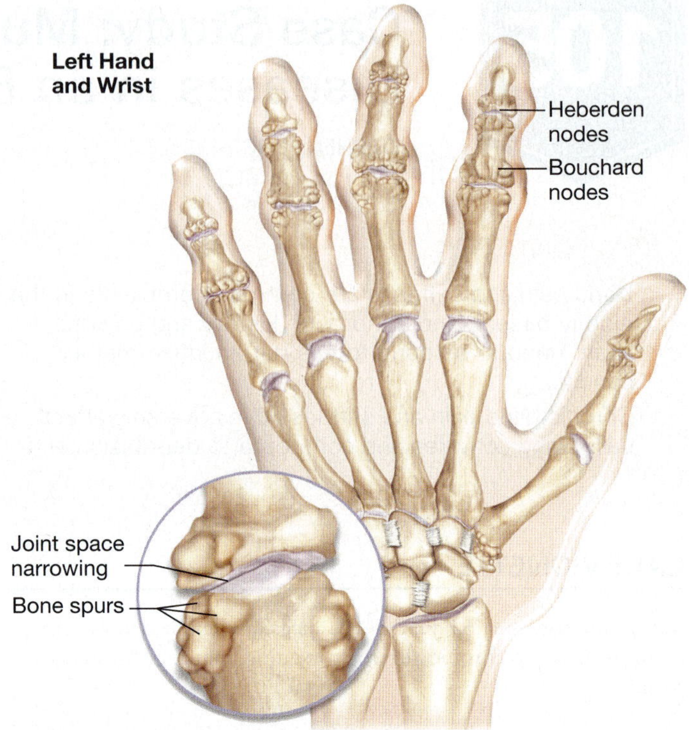

Figure 105.1. Heberden and Bouchard nodes in a patient with osteoarthritis. (From *Anatomical Chart Company: Understanding Arthritis.* Lippincott Williams & Wilkins; 2004.)

Musculoskeletal

Upper extremities: active and passive adduction, flexion, extension, and internal rotation of the shoulders full and pain free. Slightly decreased full extension of both elbows, but no nodules palpated or frank contractures noted. Tenderness over both lateral and medial epicondyles bilaterally. Tenderness and synovitis were noted over the second and third metacarpal phalangeal joints and proximal interphalangeal joints (PIPs) bilaterally, with evidence of underlying bony swelling consistent with Bouchard nodes on multiple PIPs. Several Heberden nodes were also noted (Fig. 105.1). No ulnar deviation was appreciated. Nails appear brittle with ridges, but no pitting is observed. No cyanosis, clubbing, or edema. Pulses equal bilaterally, brisk capillary refill noted. Negative Tinel and Phalen sign. No thenar atrophy. Normal nail fold capillaroscopy.

Lower extremities: full hip, knee, ankle active and passive ranges of motion (AROM, PROM), negative Lachman test, negative joint line pain, negative McMurray and Apley tests, negative Patellar grind, mild crepitus noted in the left knee. Negative hip compression test. Positive bunion deformity of both great toes with tenderness of the metatarsal phalangeal joints bilaterally, without synovitis. No cyanosis, clubbing, or edema. Mild onychomycosis of the toenails. Pulses equal bilaterally, good capillary refill.

Osteopathic Structural Exam

Sphenobasilar compression with a right lateral strain, bilateral occipitomastoid compression. C2 rotated left, occiput rotated right and side bent right, T4 extended rotated and side bent right, increased paraspinal muscle tension bilaterally at T10–T12 and T12–L3 side bent left and rotated right, sacrum has a left-on-left forward torsion, right sternoclavicular joint is superior

TABLE 105.1

Differential Diagnosis for Symmetric Hand Stiffness and Pain in an Elderly Patient

Mechanical	1. Extensor tendonitis 2. Repetitive overuse 3. Thoracic outlet syndrome 4. Compartment syndrome 5. Osteoarthritis of the hands 6. Cervical spondylosis 7. Hemochromatosis
Inflammatory	1. Rheumatoid arthritis 2. Psoriatic arthritis 3. Calcium pyrophosphate dihydrate deposition disease (CPPD or pseudogout) 4. Systemic lupus erythematosus 5. Seronegative spondyloarthropathies 6. Scleroderma 7. Polymyalgia rheumatica 8. Polyarticular gout 9. Behçet syndrome 10. Reactive arthritis 11. Infectious arthritis
Neurologic	1. Peripheral neuropathy 2. Bilateral carpal tunnel syndrome 3. Cervical stenosis/radiculopathy 4. Syringomyelia/myelopathy

with fascial restriction bilaterally in the upper extremities, short right leg, ribs 4 and 5 on the right have an inhalation dysfunction, and first rib on the right is elevated.

DIFFERENTIAL DIAGNOSIS

The most common pathophysiologic processes that need to be considered in the differential diagnosis of bilateral hand pain and stiffness are mechanical, inflammatory, and neurologic processes (Table 105.1).

WORKUP AND INTERPRETATION

Cervical spine and bilateral hand x-rays were obtained. The 4-view (anterior-posterior [AP], lateral, oblique, and open-mouth) cervical spine films showed the following: There is a reversal of the normal cervical lordosis. There is no fracture or subluxation. There is a stable appearing cervical fusion from C2 to C7. Diffuse degenerative changes are seen from C4 to C7. Facet hypertrophy is seen at the C5–C7 levels. Degenerative changes are seen from C0 to C2 suggesting an arthritic process. No evidence of atlantoaxial instability, but full cervical spine series with flexion and extension views are needed to adequately evaluate. Clinical correlation advised.

AP and lateral views of the hands were obtained. There are no fractures or subluxations appreciated. Periarticular soft tissue swelling with a fusiform appearance and juxta-articular osteopenia were noted in interphalangeal joints. Suggestion of small marginal erosions along second and third metacarpophalangeal joints. Some diffuse joint space narrowing was noted. Sclerosis and osteophyte formation predominantly involve distal interphalangeal joints bilaterally, with limited PIP involvement.

DIAGNOSIS

The patient's diagnoses based on the clinical history, examination, and diagnostic imaging were as follows:

1. Rheumatoid arthritis (RA)
2. OA of the cervical spine, knees, and hands
3. Somatic dysfunction: cervical, thoracic, rib, lumbar, sacrum, pelvis, and upper extremity and lower extremity
4. Osteopenia
5. Multilevel cervical fusion C2–C5, C5–C7
6. GERD (acid reflux disease) controlled currently
7. Hyperlipidemia
8. Tobacco abuse

RELEVANT FUNCTIONAL ANATOMY

In a patient with a bilateral upper extremity complaint, a functional anatomy review should cover the thoracic spine and ribs, the cervical spine, the thoracic inlet, and finally the forearm, wrist, and hand. This is because from a biomechanical standpoint, each of these areas can produce, intensify, or be related to the symptoms in this patient. Osteopathic manipulative treatment (OMT) of these anatomic areas may also improve the patient's symptoms; therefore, a prior knowledge of the anatomy is necessary to carry out these procedures (review Chapters 3, 7, 11, 33, 34, 35, 39, 70, 74, and 91 for relevant functional anatomy and discussion regarding somatic dysfunction related to the upper extremities).

The upper extremity is innervated by the sympathetic ganglia that arise from the upper thoracic spinal cord (segments T1–T4). The sympathetic ganglia lie anterior to the rib head, in the fascia common to both structures. Dysfunction in the upper thoracic spine and ribs may increase sympathetic tone to the upper extremity and produce altered motion, nerve dysfunction, and lymphatic and venous congestion.[1] Increased sympathetic tone is accompanied by palpatory findings in the upper thoracic/rib area and increased sensitivity to painful stimulus. Restricted motion or position of the ribs and abnormal position of the costovertebral joints can apply fascial tension to the sympathetic chain ganglia. The upper thoracic spine and ribs are the origin of the scapular stabilizing muscles. These muscles include the rhomboids, serratus anterior, trapezius, and pectoralis minor. Dysfunction in these muscles alters the position of the scapula, which in turn alters the position of the upper extremity. Trigger points in these muscles can refer pain to the upper extremity.

Due to degeneration from aging, genetic factors, trauma, postural effects, and repetitive overuse, the anatomy of the cervical spine may be far from optimal. The cervical vertebrae from C2 to C7 are saddle shaped and contain a specialized set of synovial joints on the lateral surface of the vertebral bodies. These are known as uncovertebral joints (uncinate) or joints of Luschka and provide stability to the cervical spine. They may also decrease the likelihood of herniated nucleus pulposus in the cervical region. The joints of Luschka are not synovial in nature; thus, inflammatory arthropathies would spare these areas. However, the facet joints and atlantoaxial joint have synovial membrane that could be involved in inflammatory arthropathies.

At the base of the skull, the tectorial membrane (occipital–axial ligament) is a strong continuation of the posterior longitudinal ligament that lies immediately behind the body of the axis. The alar ligaments are short, strong bundles of fibrous tissue directed obliquely upward and laterally from either side of the upper part of the odontoid process to the medial aspect of the occipital condyles.[2] They are often referred to as the "check" ligaments. The transverse ligament of the atlas is a broad strong triangular ligament arching across the ring of the atlas and firmly anchored on each side to a tubercle in the medial surface of the lateral masses of the atlas. The transverse ligament has two fascicles layered in a crosswise fashion, which gives it a cruciate configuration. The transverse ligament portion of the cruciate ligament complex supports the atlas in rotating about the dens. The anterior surface of the spinal cord lies immediately posterior to the transverse ligament. Rupture of this ligament (or laxity, which may occur with RA) creates the possibility of the dens contacting the spinal cord and causing catastrophic neurologic damage. The cervical spinal canal is wider at the atlantoaxial level and narrows maximally at the C6 level. The cervical cord itself is wider from C3–T2, corresponding to the increase in nerves supplying the upper extremities.[2]

In the cervical spine, the disks are thicker anteriorly than posteriorly and are entirely responsible for the normal cervical lordosis. Each disk is situated between the cartilaginous endplates of two vertebrae. Successive layers of these fibers slant in alternate directions so that they cross each other at different angles depending on the intradiskal pressure of the nucleus pulposus. Positions of the cervical spine affect intradiskal pressure. Intradiskal pressure is least in the supine position, and extension of the cervical spine results in the greatest intradiskal pressure.[3] After 50 years of age, the nucleus pulposus becomes a fibrocartilaginous mass that has characteristics similar to those of the inner zone of the annulus fibrosis.[3]

The thoracic inlet is anatomically defined as the area above the clavicles; between the sternum, the first thoracic segment (T1), and the first rib. The brachial plexus and the subclavian artery travel through this area. The subclavian artery traverses between the first rib and clavicle (a potential site of compression) and then between the anterior and middle scalene muscles. The brachial plexus also travels between the anterior and middle scalene muscles. The thoracic outlet is the area where the neurovascular bundle travels between the clavicle and first rib, exiting between the anterior and middle scalene muscles. The subclavian vein passes over the first rib anterior to the anterior scalene muscle, so it is not involved in compression.[2] Moving toward the arm, the subclavian artery becomes the axillary artery at the lateral border of the first rib. The axillary artery passes posterior to the pectoralis minor muscle and becomes the brachial artery at the inferior border of the teres major muscle. Branches from the axillary and brachial arteries supply the structures of the shoulder, arm, forearm, and hand.

Lymphatic compression can also occur, usually due to myofascial restrictions. The major lymph nodes of the upper extremities are found in the fibrofatty connective tissue of the axilla. They are arranged in five groups, four of which lie inferior to the pectoralis minor tendon, and one lies superior to it. The thoracic duct is on the left and drains into the brachiocephalic trunk.

The three main peripheral nerves of the upper extremity include the median nerve, the ulnar nerve, and the radial nerve. Understanding the innervation of each nerve and site of potential compression is important. Compression of the median nerve in the carpal tunnel (carpal tunnel syndrome) typically causes sensory symptoms such as night pain, paresthesia, and numbness in the hand in the radial three and one-half digits. Symptoms may be referred proximally from the hand toward the forearm and even the elbow and may be reproduced or elicited by Phalen maneuver or Tinel sign. Thenar muscle weakness and atrophy represent advanced disease. Moving down into the hand, the *scaphoid*, *lunate*, and the *triquetral* bones articulate with the greater multangular (Trapezium) and lesser multangular (trapezoid), the capitate, and hamate where motion between these rows of bones is freer in flexion.

If bony point tenderness is present subsequent to a hand trauma, always x-ray the hand to evaluate the anatomic snuffbox for a scaphoid fracture. If the initial x-ray is negative for a fracture, a repeat x-ray after 2 weeks of the incident is recommended, as it can take time for the fracture to be visible on imaging. The first carpometacarpal articulation is cavo-convex and classified as a saddle-shaped joint. It is freely movable in two planes and rarely subject to dysfunction. The second to fifth carpometacarpal joints are gliding joints. The fifth is the most mobile, and then the fourth, the second, and the third are fairly restricted in motion.[4] Patients with arthritis of the wrists and hands can develop bony encroachment or irritation of tendons, blood vessels, and nerves. This may lead to comorbid conditions such as carpal tunnel syndrome in a patient with wrist OA or de Quervain tenosynovitis in a patient with thumb arthritis and instability of the first carpometacarpal joint.

Motion, Posture, and Biomechanics

The cervical spine is better suited for mobility and is not required to transmit heavy loads. Precise control of head position and unrestricted movement is essential for normal functioning of the special senses. The saddle shape of each cervical vertebra provides mobility and stability. The anterior column composed of the vertebral body, longitudinal ligaments, and intervertebral disk provides some weight-bearing capacity, shock absorption, and a flexible structure. The posterior elements composed of the osseous canal, the zygapophyseal joints, and the erector spinae muscles protect the neural elements and act as a fulcrum, to guide movement for the functional unit.

Alterations in the degree of curvature in one area of the spine result in reciprocal alterations in curvature in other areas of the spinal column to preserve the orientation of the body over the center of gravity. For example, an increase in lumbar lordosis results in increased cervical lordosis.

PHYSIOLOGY

Small joints, in particular those of the hand, are made up of a number of structures that allow for smooth motion, specificity of function, and strength of purpose. The small joint structure includes articular cartilage and subchondral bone forming articulating surfaces in an attempt to work in concert with the musculoskeletal system making demands upon joint structure and function as a whole. Normally, articular cartilage is produced, and functioning bone is maintained, through cellular metabolism, circulation, respiration, synthesis, and remodeling. Homeostasis is a physiologic process by the organism to preserve form and function, an effort that declines in effectiveness as the organism ages.

MANIFESTATIONS OF JOINT DISEASE

Joint disease in general can be monoarticular or polyarticular in nature.[5]

- Monoarticular joint symptoms may be caused by many diseases, including infectious, traumatic, and crystal deposition diseases as well as noninflammatory conditions, such as OA or avascular necrosis.
  - Some inflammatory polyarticular diseases may occasionally present with monoarticular symptoms as well, such as early RA, psoriatic arthritis, viral arthritis, or reactive arthritis.

- Monoarticular joint disease by chronology can be:
  - Transient (intermittent hydrarthrosis)
  - Acute (septic arthritis, trauma, gout)
  - Subacute/chronic (pseudogout, neuropathic Charcot, tumor, infectious granuloma, tuberculosis [TB], or OA)
- Polyarticular joint disease in inflammatory arthritis often presents with symmetric, small joint involvement in diseases such as RA, systemic lupus erythematosus (SLE), psoriatic arthritis, and viral hepatitis.
  - Polyarticular diseases with acute presentations include infectious arthritis, such as gonococcal, meningococcal, viral, Lyme disease, acute rheumatic fever, and bacterial endocarditis.
  - Inflammatory polyarthritis that may be either acute or chronic in nature includes diseases such as RA, juvenile idiopathic arthritis, SLE, reactive arthritis, polyarticular gout, psoriatic arthritis, and arthritis associated with sarcoidosis.
  - Noninflammatory polyarticular symptoms commonly arise from OA, calcium pyrophosphate deposition disease (CPPD), fibromyalgia, benign hypermobility syndrome, and hemochromatosis.

In this case, we will focus on both OA and RA.

PATHOPHYSIOLOGY

Osteoarthritis

OA is a disease process that characteristically includes degeneration of articular cartilage, subchondral sclerosis, hypertrophy of bone at joint margins (osteophytes), and multiple alterations in the synovial membrane as well as the joint capsule itself. There are multifactorial considerations germane to a discussion of the pathogenesis of OA, including biomechanical influences (isolated macrotrauma or repeated microtrauma), genetic alterations, and the relationship to aging, particularly with regard to morphologic changes in cartilage matrix composition and structure.

- While aging is considered the most significant risk factor for the development of OA, obesity, mineral deposition, and systemic hormones all impart a higher risk for OA.
- Morphologic, biochemical, and metabolic changes occur in OA.
- In early OA, irregularity of the surface of articular cartilage and changes in proteoglycan distribution occurs, followed by eventual ulceration of cartilage with exposure of the bone, resulting in attempts at self-repair. Local repair involves increased chondrocyte concentration and new bone formation in the form of osteophytes.
- Biochemical changes vary during the stages of OA, with increased water content of articular cartilage in early OA, and increased collagen and diminished proteoglycan concentrations later in the disease.
- Early degeneration of the cartilage is likely related to matrix metalloproteinases whose enzymes degrade both collagen and proteoglycans.[6]
- The initial stages of OA are thus marked by a complex interplay of multiple factors, including increased cell proliferation and synthesis of matrix proteins, proteinases, growth factors, cytokines, and other inflammatory mediators by chondrocytes.
- The disease process ultimately affects the joint structure in its entirety, including the cartilage, synovium, ligaments, and subchondral bone.

One central problem with OA is that an adult articular chondrocyte has a limited capacity to regenerate damaged original cartilage matrix architecture.

- Indeed, an age-related reduction in chondrocyte function has been shown with the end result of morphologic and structural changes in aging articular cartilage, such as thinning of the articular surface, decreased size of matrix proteoglycans, and diminished strength and stiffness of the matrix.[6]
- The chondrocyte may attempt to regenerate the matrix by mimicking early stages of cartilage development, but original cartilage cannot be replicated.
- Current pharmacologic interventions do not include a proven structure-modifying approach.[7] Current meta-analyses and systematic reviews for viscosupplementation injections with hyaluronic acid have been inconsistent, either beneficial or equivocal to placebo, due to bias and low-quality evidence.
- Cartilage tissue engineering (with or without replacement) or gene therapy is a possible approach in the future.
- Animal models of OA have yet to reproduce the human condition, perhaps in part because they often represent secondary rather than primary OA.[8]

Rheumatoid Arthritis

RA is a chronic systemic inflammatory disease characterized predominantly by persistent, symmetric inflammation of multiple joints, although extra-articular manifestations may also occur.[9]

- It is the most common inflammatory arthritis, affecting approximately 1% of the population.
- The primary target in RA is the synovium, in which infiltration of mononuclear cells, such as T cells and macrophages, synovial intimal lining hyperplasia, and angiogenesis occur.
- A complex interplay between synoviocytes, T cells, B cells, and inflammatory mediators eventually leads to aggressive cartilage destruction and progressive bony erosions.
- Untreated, RA often leads to progressive joint destruction, disability, and premature death.

Although extensive research has been conducted with regard to the pathogenesis of RA, the exact etiology remains elusive.

- Roles of multiple inflammatory mediators, including cytokines, chemokines, growth factors, adhesion molecules, and matrix metalloproteinases, have been defined thus far.
- It is known that these mediators are responsible for both attracting and activating cells in the peripheral blood, in addition to local activation and proliferation of synoviocytes.[9]
- Susceptibility to RA is likely resultant from a combination of environmental and genetic factors.
  - One of the most significant genetic risk factors uncovered thus far involves the major histocompatibility complex class II (MHC-II) haplotype of an individual.
  - Certain HLA-DR molecules are more commonly found in patients with RA (e.g., HLA-DR4), and consistency in a particular amino acid sequence in the third hypervariable region of the beta chain of MHC-susceptible alleles led to the "shared-epitope" hypothesis. This hypothesis postulates that presumed antigens bind to this particular site, resulting in the cascade of inflammation in RA.[10]
  - Polymorphism of human leukocyte antigens (HLA) class II genes determines the predisposition to rheumatoid/inflammatory arthritis, and the epistatic interactions between HLA-DQ and HLA-DR molecules dictate the severity, progression, and modulation of the disease.[11]
  - All DRB1 SE (shared-epitope) alleles strongly interact with smoking in conferring an increased risk of anticitrullinated protein antibody (ACPA)-positive RA.[12]

RA is also closely mimicked by transient arthritic conditions provoked by several microbial pathogens, leading to the consideration of infectious etiologies in the pathogenesis of RA. A role of infection in the development of RA has long been postulated, including potential bacterial and viral pathogens, but it has not yet been proven. Other potential antigens include heat-shock proteins, MHC molecules themselves, and certain epitopes within type II collagen.[10]

A complex array of constituents in the immune system interact to cause the initiation and perpetuation of inflammation found in RA.[10]

- Memory T cells, B cells, plasma cells, cytokines, macrophages, vascular endothelium, and rheumatoid factor all play important roles.
- Just a few of the memory T-cell functions include enhanced T-cell, macrophage, and antigen-presenting cell activation, while macrophages act as effectors, producing multiple proinflammatory cytokines, such as IL-1, IL-6, and tumor necrosis factor (TNF), among others.
- Rheumatoid factors of multiple isotypes form immune complexes that not only fix complement but also activate neutrophils. B cells are also found within the rheumatoid synovium, and although the exact mechanisms involved in pathogenesis are yet unknown, the therapeutic use of rituximab, and a chimeric anti-CD20 (B-cell) monoclonal antibody, has produced significant responses in patients with RA.
- Multiple cytokines exist within the rheumatoid synovium, exhibiting complex roles, including mononuclear cell migration, cell activation, and direct damage to articular cartilage and bone.
- Tumor necrosis factor-α (TNF-α) is an important proinflammatory cytokine, and TNF-blocking therapies (adalimumab, etanercept, and infliximab) have been successful in the treatment of RA.
- Newer therapies focused on cytokines are continually being developed.

OSTEOPATHIC PATIENT MANAGEMENT

For any patient presenting with pain in the hands, a thorough osteopathic examination, using the five-point structure function model, is essential. Osteopathic techniques can be applied to the areas of somatic dysfunction in patients presenting with arthritic-type pathology. The models of structure–function relationships described below guide the osteopathic practitioner's approach to diagnosis and treatment. These models provide a framework for integrating objective and subjective clinical findings with osteopathic structural exam findings.

Biomechanical Model

Short-leg mechanics can lead to a worsening of a patient's arthritic upper extremity symptoms by adding postural stress to the upper extremity with resultant aches and pains. There is an anatomical–biomechanical relationship between sacral base unleveling from short-leg mechanics, subsequent iliac crest unleveling, and the postural tension created in the shoulders through the latissimus dorsi muscle via the thoracolumbar fascia.[13] Altered shoulder biomechanics can strain muscles and increase intrinsic pressure on the intra-articular tissues, both of which may exacerbate joint pain.

Another biomechanical consequence of postural imbalance is concomitant changes in the AP curves. With a forward head position and protracted shoulders, the rotator cuff muscles, levator scapulae, and serratus posterior superior become tight and develop myofascial trigger points. Trigger points in these muscles refer to the upper extremity.[14] Scalene tension can cause neurovascular compression as can elevation of the first rib, narrowing the space between itself and the clavicle. All these factors can biomechanically be related to painful syndromes in the upper extremity, including the hands.

Respiratory–Circulatory Model

Another objective of osteopathic treatment is improvement of local blood flow to the area of arthritis in the hands as well as removal of edema to assist in pain reduction and improve mobility. This is done by addressing the areas of somatic dysfunction that may influence arterial, venous, or lymphatic flow. Our patient has dysfunction in the lower thoracic and thoracolumbar areas, both of which may influence diaphragm function. Improving motion in the lower thoracic region will help the function of the diaphragm from a mechanical prospective. Improving motion in the cervical region may help the function of the diaphragm from a neurologic perspective. Treating both regions will aid in restoring normal diaphragmatic motion, which is the primary driving force to move lymph and venous blood. This treatment should follow thoracic inlet release, which removes any proximal restrictions to lymphatic flow coming from the upper extremities. In the patient described in the case, treatment of the right sternoclavicular restriction will further aid in this process by normalizing fascial tensions of the thoracic inlet. Then, attention can be moved distally to remove pectoral and axillary restrictions and then on to the elbow, wrist, and hand for the same purpose. Abnormal interosseous membrane tension of the forearm may contribute to lymphatic and venous stasis by altering the mechanics of the radius and ulnar and their role in generating intracompartmental pressures. This is especially true in patients who repetitively use their forearms, as their muscles and fascias become tight. Peripheral fascial restrictions in the distal arms may affect the vascular structures traveling through them. Restrictions in the scalene muscles, first rib, or thoracic inlet, may impede fluid movement through the vascular bundle supplying the upper extremity. Treatment of these areas may improve lymphatic and venous drainage and arterial flow.

Neurologic Model

The sacrum is the base of support of the spinal column; unleveling of the sacrum results in adaptive or compensatory curves in the vertebral column. No matter if there is an "S"-shaped or a "C"-shaped adaptive group curve, there will be crossover points of the curve. A crossover point is where the curve changes direction. This vertebral unit is commonly found to have type II dysfunction. These segments can become facilitated and act as an "irritable focus" of neuronal activity (see Chapter 13 Somatic Dysfunction, Spinal Facilitation, and Viscerosomatic Integration for further information). If the crossover point is between T1 and T4, as it is in this patient, the upper extremities may be affected. Increased activity in somatic fibers between T1 and T4 can be referred to the upper extremity via a somatosomatic reflex. Dorsal root reflexes may activate primary afferent fibers in the peripheral area served by the upper thorax resulting in the secretion of proinflammatory substances that may exacerbate arthritic symptoms. Increased nociceptive activity at the level of T1–T4 has the potential to activate fibers in the adjacent lateral horn. As the sympathetic neurons become facilitated, the abnormal sympathetic drive affects vascular tone and peristalsis resulting in venous and lymphatic stasis in the upper extremities. Increased vascular tone can also make muscles stiff and noncompliant. Sympathetic overactivity will alter the secretory activity of sweat glands and sensitize nociceptors and mechanoreceptors (see Chapter 6 Autonomic Nervous System and Chapter 11 Nociception and Pain as well as Chapter 12 The Role of Inflammation in Healing and Homeostasis for further information).

One objective of osteopathic management is to normalize neurologic input from and output to the upper extremity. As stated above, increased sympathetic tone to the upper extremity can cause vasoconstriction, edema, sensitivity of the nerves, irritability of the muscles, and sweat gland overactivity. Therefore, treatment of the upper thoracic and the associated rib dysfunctions may normalize sympathetic chain ganglion output to the upper extremity to improve these pathophysiologic findings.

Peripheral fascial restrictions may affect somatic nerves, in addition to the aforementioned vascular structures. Tension in the anterior scalenes and the thoracic inlet can compress the neurovascular bundle, impairing nerve transmission and vascular supply to the rotator cuff and scapular stabilizing muscles. Removal of the fascial restrictions and resultant compression to the neurovascular bundle will facilitate axoplasmic flow, enhancing the nerves' trophic function. Tension of the pronator teres muscle in the forearm can compress the median nerve (pronator syndrome) producing hand symptoms as well.[15] Stiffness of the joints of the hands and elbows can cause overuse of the forearm muscles to make up the motion lost. Pain in the joints of the hands can lead to disuse and eventually atrophy of the intrinsic hand muscles. Stiffness, swelling, enlargement, and ulnar deviation of the digits can affect the small nerves in the hands. If these nerves are already sensitized from spinal facilitation, they will report increased levels of pain.

Metabolic Energy Model

Patients who have painful musculoskeletal conditions can require increased energy expenditure to function when compared to a healthy patient of the same age. Increased oxygen demand can cause fatigue if they have to ambulate a long distance with arthritic knees, hips, ankles, or feet. For those who repetitively use their hands, as in typing, upper extremity stiffness and pain can be problematic. They can become fatigued, make errors, and become frustrated. Both the working environment and the recreational environment may become affected, changing the patient's ability to cope in comparison to their premorbid condition. Osteopathic patient management must address the factors that may contribute to energy demand and production.

If the clinician's objective is to improve the patient's energy flow and metabolic activity, then removing barriers to the proper function of physiologic mechanisms is important. Osteopathic cranial manipulative medicine recognizes the primary respiratory mechanism as a fundamental component of health (see Chapter 53). According to this approach, patients who have a significant sphenobasilar synchondrosis compression do not have optimal function of the primary respiratory mechanism and therefore suboptimal recuperative capacity. Compression of the fourth ventricle, a cranial technique, has been hypothesized to assist in the normalization of cerebrospinal fluid flow and other components of the primary respiratory mechanism.[16]

Behavioral Model

The emotional component of the patient's condition needs to be evaluated and addressed as small joint disease. Depression is highly prevalent in patient with RA (38.8%) and OA (20%). The patient may develop anxiety and/or depression due to chronic pain and change in functional status, such as increased assistance with activities of daily living (ADLs), and difficulties engaging in occupational responsibilities or hobbies.[17,18] In addition, there are socio-economic considerations such as financial constraints, insurance coverage, and personal reasons that may result in delayed progress/healing. For those patients with small joint disease, simple tasks such as opening a jar of pickles can present a constant reminder of declining capabilities. The challenge in caring for these patients is to provide alternative coping skills for the maintenance of spirit. When met with challenges, many people turn to prayer or spirituality to guide and strengthen their efforts to lead meaningful lives in the larger sense and to accomplish ADLs on a much smaller scale. Support groups may be of value, especially if the patient has expressed feelings of isolation with regard to his or her disease. Patient education can assist in the preservation of self-worth, and educational materials for patients with RA may be obtained from the Arthritis Foundation, the American College of Rheumatology (ACR), and the National Institutes of Health. Encouragement and highlighting ways to overcome pain and limited function in patients with small joint disease can help them maintain spiritual and behavioral satisfaction. The goal is to restore function to a premorbid level or preserve the current functional status, though this may not always be achievable. With proper treatment, patients can maintain their self-image and societal perception of their overall functioning. The osteopathic physician is well-positioned to offer physical care, medication, education, and emotional support to help patients achieve shared goals.

Outcomes Studies and Best Evidence for Manual Treatment

Both OA and RA are common problems and can be chronic disabling conditions. For many patients, conventional therapies are not completely effective and are limited by side effects. This can lead to ongoing pain and frustration. Complementary and alternative medical (CAM) therapies are defined as being outside scientific mainstream medicine. These nonpharmaceutical treatments are generally unproven in efficacy but perceived as safe. The ACR believes practitioners should be informed about CAM therapies and be able to discuss them knowledgably with patients. Meanwhile, scientific studies are underway to test the efficacy of these modalities. OMT may be considered a CAM therapy by some clinicians, while others feel it is an integral part of osteopathic patient care.

Conservative treatment for patients with hand arthritis (both RA and OA) may include (but is not limited to) the following: medications, diet, heat or cold therapy, physical or occupational therapy, modalities, tens, braces and splints, injections, osteopathic manipulation, chiropractic manipulation, manual therapy, massage therapy, and acupuncture.

OMT Considerations

OMT has been shown to be beneficial to decrease pain and increase patient's function in a variety of clinical situations. Manipulative techniques for upper extremity complaints have been taught in the osteopathic schools' curriculum since its inception. OMT is part of the osteopathic physician's overall treatment armamentarium, and the use should follow from the careful consideration of osteopathic principles and practice used in the evaluation of every patient. The use of OMT is frequently based on the physician's ability, the patient's presentation and responses, and the type of dysfunction found. OMT can be tailored to fit almost any practice model.

In patients with RA of the occipitoatlantal and atlantal–axial articulations, caution must be applied to the choice of technique used to treat the somatic dysfunction present. RA of the upper cervical spine is an absolute contradiction to thrust (high velocity low amplitude [HVLA])-type manipulation. This is thought to be due to the relative laxity and instability in this region due to the inflammatory process. In this patient, with a fused cervical spine and degenerative vertebral joint and disk disease, direct action OMT would be contraindicated. However, soft tissue, counterstrain, myofascial release, functional positional release and other indirect treatment approaches can be used to help relieve pain.

Physical therapy joint mobilization manipulative techniques have been employed and studied in the treatment of injuries and OA of the fingers and hand.[19] Efficacy is enhanced when combined with other modalities, such as exercise.[20] Currently, there are no randomized controlled trials assessing effectiveness of OMT in patients with hand manifestations of RA or OA.

Pharmacologic Treatment

While the body has the innate ability to self-heal, therapies with pharmacologic treatments are often essential in the treatment of an inflammatory arthritis such as RA. Disease-modifying antirheumatic drugs (DMARDs), either alone or in combination, as well as biologic therapies (e.g., TNF-α blockers), and nonsteroidal anti-inflammatory drugs (NSAIDs) are often the cornerstone of treatment therapies. Early and aggressive interventions may result in lower morbidity and mortality, as evidenced by slower radiographic progression, less disability, and fewer surgical interventions.[21] Cardioprotective effects of the anti-inflammatory actions of these medications have been documented.[22,23] Patients who do not respond solely to methotrexate often benefit from combined medical therapy.[24] Even in the most skilled hands, most patients require a combined approach with the appropriate use of other treatment modalities including medications or local injections of corticosteroids to reduce inflammation.

Physical and Occupational Therapy

The role of physical and occupational therapy is also of great importance, especially in the early treatment of an inflammatory arthritis such as RA but may also be beneficial in OA as well. Physical therapy usually addresses gross motor skills, mobility, and strength, while occupational therapy focuses on fine motor skills, assessing functional abilities within home-work environments. Patients should be evaluated for cardiovascular endurance and assistance in ADLs, mobility, transfers, and ambulation. Therapists can provide an evaluation of assistive devices, such as a platform walker to offload the weight from the wrist to the forearms and a jar opener with a lever to compensate for weak hand grip. Treatment modalities may then be fashioned to preserve joint function as well as joint protection, and steps may be taken to potentially prevent contractures or deformities.[10] Joint protection interventions have been studied in patients with RA, and home hand exercises have resulted in improved grip strength as well as diminished morning stiffness.[25–29]

Another study evaluating joint protection and home hand exercises for patients with hand OA also showed increased hand strength and global hand function, underscoring the importance of nonpharmacologic interventions in the treatment of both RA and OA.[30] Whole-body strength training and gripper exercises have also been shown to improve dynamic and static grip strength while decreasing pain in older patients with hand OA.[31] These therapeutic modalities have no side effects, are generally readily acceptable, and can be performed easily, making them useful adjunctive treatments in both of these chronic diseases. Other useful nonpharmacologic interventions include adaptive devices that may be customized to improve independence in daily activities, such as opening jars and car doors, self-care, grooming, and dressing.

Evidence supports early intervention in RA, as functional health status tends to decline early in the disease, mortality rates rise over the course of the disease, and radiographic changes occur much earlier in the disease process than previously thought. Work disability increases from approximately 25% at 6.4 years to 50% at 20.9 years after onset of disease.[32] Mortality rates also rise over the course of the disease, with rates as high as 35% by 20 years.[33]

All of these factors have to be taken into consideration, coupled with the need to individualize each case based on patient desire, functional status, and long-term goals. In addition, due to patient desire, medical conditions, and/or other factors, the patient may not be a candidate for certain treatment modalities, such as surgical joint replacement, forcing a conservative approach. More than 70% of patients with RA have some form of hand disability, often crippling hand deformities if the disease has been long standing.[34]

Surgical Intervention

The role of surgical intervention in the treatment of RA remains somewhat controversial, and it should be determined by both the level of pain and the functional status of the individual. Many practitioners will not recommend surgical intervention unless pain disrupts sleep, and meaningful functional gain has to be rigorously assessed. Likewise, nonoperative treatments for OA should be employed, such as medications, intra-articular steroid injections, hand therapies, and splinting prior to consideration of surgical interventions.[35] If a surgical approach is required, the specifics of the procedure should be considered. If two different procedures are being considered, how would each of these different procedures change the duration of healing and required physical therapy postoperatively? How would any or each of these procedures affect the presence of somatic dysfunction in the cervical, thoracic, or lumbar spine? OMT can be a helpful adjunctive therapy postoperatively. Postoperative patients who develop cervical spasm, rib restrictions, atelectasis, or sacral malpositioning, for example, may benefit from OMT for relief of cervical, thoracic, lumbar, or sacral somatic dysfunction. Postoperatively, activity modification, work restrictions, and lifestyle changes are important aspects to address to assist patients in their recovery and to enhance the healing process.

Treatment Sequence

A general principle for the practitioner is to assess how acute the area to be treated actually has become. There are many reflexes active in the body, and generally, the more normal relationships that can be established distant from an acute area the easier it will be to address that remaining acute area for a response. Suppose a patient has an elevated first rib that is causing distal arm pain, but the patient's main complaint is radial head dysfunction felt at the elbow. Advantage can be gained in relaxing to as normal a state the facilitated irritation being generated by the elevated first rib, which can reasonably be expected to increase tone in distal musculature. By following this approach, when the time comes to move the radial head, there may be that much less resistance to movement encountered by muscles attached to the radius. Similarly, with small joint disease, working to release the carpal tunnel from undue pressure via the opponens roll technique may decrease pain perceived distally in the small joints of the fingers.[36]

SUMMARY

In conclusion, it is through the use of multiple modalities that we as osteopathic physicians can provide the most comprehensive and therapeutic treatment strategies for patients with both RA and OA as it involves small joints of the hands. The combination of state-of-the-art pharmacologic interventions, physical and occupational therapies, and osteopathic principles and practice enables osteopathic physicians to uniquely enhance the lives of individuals affected by these debilitating and potentially devastating diseases.

ACKNOWLEDGMENTS

The author and editors of this chapter would like to acknowledge the scholarly contributions of Kurt P. Heinking, James A. Lipton, and Beth A. Valashinas for prior editions of this chapter.

REFERENCES

1. Nelson KE, Glonek T. *Somatic Dysfunction in Osteopathic Family Practice, ACOFP*. Lippincott Williams & Wilkins; 2007:345–349.
2. Moore KL. *Clinically Oriented Anatomy*. 3rd ed. Williams & Wilkins; 1992:528.
3. DeLee JC, Drez D. *Orthopaedic Sports Medicine Principles and Practice*. 2nd ed. Saunders; 2003;2:1065–1095.
4. Fryette HH. *Principles of Osteopathic Technique*. Academy of Applied Osteopathy; 1954:190–202.
5. Hawkins RA. Approach to the patient with monoarticular symptoms. In: *Rheumatology Secrets*. 2nd ed. Elsevier; 2002:88–100.
6. Cesare PE, Abramson SB. Pathogenesis of osteoarthritis. In: Harris ED Jr, Budd RC, Firestein GS, et al., eds. *Kelley's Textbook of Rheumatology*. 7th ed. Saunders; 2004:1493–1537.
7. Peck J, Slovek A, Miro P, et al. A comprehensive review of viscosupplementation in osteoarthritis of the knee. *Orthop Rev (Pavia)*. 2021;13(2):25549.
8. Goldring MB, Goldring SR. Osteoarthritis. *J Cell Physiol*. 2007;13(3):626–634.
9. Firestein GS. Etiology and pathogenesis of rheumatoid arthritis. In: *Kelley's Textbook of Rheumatology*. 7th ed. Saunders; 2004:996–1014.
10. Cush JJ, Kavanaugh A, Stein MC. Rheumatoid arthritis in RhrumaKnowledgy online textbook. 2015; Accessed October 27, 2017. http://www.rheumaknowledgy.com/rheumatoid-arthritis/
11. Taneja V, David CS. Role of HLA class II genes in susceptibility/resistance to inflammatory arthritis: studies with humanized mice. *Immunol Rev*. 2010;233(1):62–78.
12. Lundström E, Källberg H, Alfredsson L, Klareskog L, Padyukov L. Gene–environment interaction between the DRB1 shared epitope and smoking in the risk of anti–citrullinated protein antibody–positive rheumatoid arthritis: all alleles are important. *Arthritis Rheumatol*. 2009;60(6):1597–1603.
13. Vleeming A, Pool-Goudzwaard AL, Stoeckart R, van Wingerden JP, Snijders CJ. The posterior layer of the thoracolumbar fascia: its function in load transfer from spine to legs. *Spine*. 1995;20(7):753–758.
14. Travell JG, Simons DG. *Myofascial Pain and Dysfunction, The Triggerpoint Manual*. Williams & Wilkins; 1983:377–382, 614–618.
15. Rehak DC. Pronator syndrome. *Clin Sports Med*. 2001;20(3):531–540.
16. Magoun HI. *Osteopathy in the Cranial Field*. The Cranial Academy; 1976:336.
17. Matcham F, Rayner L, Steer S, Hotopf M. The prevalence of depression in rheumatoid arthritis: a systematic review and meta-analysis. *Rheumatol*. 2013;52(12):2136–2148.
18. Wang ST, Ni GX. Depression in osteoarthritis: Current understanding. *Neuropsychiatr Dis Treat*. 2022;18(1):375–389.
19. Villafañe JH, Silva GB, Fernandez-Carnero J. Effect of thumb joint mobilization on pressure pain threshold in elderly patients with thumb carpometacarpal osteoarthritis. *J Manipulative Physiol Ther*. 2012;35(2):110–120.
20. Seffinger MA, Hruby RJ. Evidence-based manual medicine. In: Kuchera WA, ed. *Problem Oriented Approach*. Saunders Elsevier; 2007:221–272.
21. da Silva E, Doran MF, Crowson CS, O'Fallon WM, Matteson EL. Declining use of orthopedic surgery in patients with rheumatoid arthritis? Results of a long-term, population-based assessment. *Arthritis Rheum*. 2003;49(2):216–220.
22. Choi HK, Hernán MA, Seeger JD, Robins JM, Wolfe F. Methotrexate and mortality in patients with rheumatoid arthritis: a prospective study. *Lancet*. 2002;359(9313):1173–1177.
23. Jackobsson LT, Turesson C, Gülfe A, et al. Treatment with tumor necrosis factor blockers is associated with a lower incidence of first cardiovascular events in patients with rheumatoid arthritis. *J Rheumatol*. 2005;32(7):1213–1218.
24. Castrejón I, Gibson KA, Pincus T. Efficacy and safety of methotrexate in combination with other non-biologic disease-modifying antirheumatic drugs (DMARDs) in treatment of rheumatoid arthritis. *Bull Hosp Jt Dis*. 2013;71(1):S20–S28.
25. Hammond A, Lincoln N, Sutcliffe L. A crossover trial evaluating an educational-behavioral joint protection program for people with rheumatoid arthritis. *Patient Educ Couns*. 1999;37(1):19–32.
26. Hoenig H, Groff G, Pratt K, Goldberg E, Franck W. A randomized controlled trial of home exercise on the rheumatoid hand. *J Rheumatol*. 1993;20(5):785–789.
27. Hawkes J, Care G, Dixon JS, Bird HA, Wright V. A comparison of three different physiotherapy treatments for rheumatoid arthritis of the hands. *Physiother Theory Pract*. 1986;2:155–160.
28. Shaufler J, Sverdlik SS, Baker A, Krewer SE. "Hand gym" for patients with arthritic hand disabilities: preliminary report. *Arch Phys Med Rehabil*. 1978;59(5):221–226.
29. Castillo BA, el Sallab RA, Scott JT. Physical activity, cystic erosions, and osteoporosis in rheumatoid arthritis. *Ann Rheum Dis*. 1965;24(6):522–527.
30. Stamm TA, Machold KP, Smolen JS, et al. Joint protection and home hand exercises improve hand function in patients with hand osteoarthritis: a randomized controlled trial. *Arthritis Rheum*. 2002;47(1):44–49.
31. Rogers MW, Wilder FV. The effects of strength training among persons with hand osteoarthritis: a two-year follow-up study. *J Hand Ther*. 2007;20(3):244–249.
32. Wolfe F, Hawley DJ. The longterm outcomes of rheumatoid arthritis: work disability: a prospective 18 year study of 823 patients. *J Rheumatol*. 1998;25(11):2108–2117.
33. Scott DL, Symmons DP, Coulton BL, Popert AJ. Long-term outcome of treating rheumatoid arthritis: results after 20 years. *Lancet*. 1987;1(8542):1108–1111.
34. De la Mata Llord J, Palacios Carvajal J. Rheumatoid arthritis: are outcomes better with medical or surgical management? *Orthopedics*. 1998;21(10):1085–1086.
35. Palmieri TJ, Grand FM, Hay EL, Burke C. Treatment of hand OA in the hand and wrist: non-operative treatment. *Clin Rheum Dis*. 1985;11(2):433–445.
36. Sucher BM, Hinrichs BM, Welcher RIL, Quiroz LD, St Laurent BF, Morrison BJ. Manipulative treatment of carpal tunnel syndrome: biomechanical and osteopathic intervention to increase the length of the transverse carpal ligament: part 2. Effect of sex differences and manipulative "priming." *J Am Osteopath Assoc*. 2005;105(3):135–143.

106 Case Study: Difficulty in Breathing

RAMEY ALFARRA

KEY CONCEPTS

- Most acute exacerbations of chronic obstructive pulmonary disease (COPD) are preceded by an infection, either viral or bacterial. The patient typically reports worsening cough and chest congestion, increased sputum production, and dyspnea.
- Obstructive diseases such as COPD require the patients to alter their mechanics of breathing by engaging accessory muscles causing hypertrophy, which alters biomechanics that creates somatic dysfunction.
- Patients with obstructive diseases such as asthma and COPD have restricted movement of the thoracic tissues during the exhalation phase of respiration, potentially reducing local drainage of the lymph from the small airways and central lymph drainage through the thoracic duct.
- Bronchospasm and mucous production, the two main pathophysiologic events of asthma and COPD, are mediated through the vagus nerve.
- Smoking cessation is essential for respiratory health.
- Regular osteopathic manipulative treatment (OMT) visits focused on facilitating normal posture and function may assist in reducing metabolic energy requirements.

CASE VIGNETTE

CHIEF COMPLAINT

A 71-year-old man presents to an ambulatory care clinic with a 3-day history of shortness of breath, fever, wheezing, chest congestion, and a nonproductive cough, requiring more than usual inhaled albuterol to help his breathing.

HISTORY OF PRESENT ILLNESS

He inhales tiotropium every morning and fluticasone and salmeterol every 12 hours each day and usually is comfortable from a pulmonary standpoint. He has never required home oxygen therapy. However, over the last few days, his symptoms have worsened, and he currently feels out of breath while doing routine activities. He denies chest pain and diaphoresis. Just 3 months ago, he was admitted to the hospital for an exacerbation of his COPD.

PAST MEDICAL/SURGICAL HISTORY

Stable angina pectoris, gastroesophageal reflux disease, essential hypertension, and a left inguinal herniorrhaphy 20 years ago.

MEDICATIONS

Albuterol 2 inhalations every 4 hours as needed for dyspnea, tiotropium bromide 18 μg 2 inhalations daily, fluticasone-salmeterol 250/50 mcg 1 inhalation every 12 hours, omeprazole 20 mg daily, amlodipine 10 mg daily, and lisinopril 10 mg daily.

ALLERGIES

None

SOCIAL HISTORY

Divorced, lives alone, retired engineer, three children, all living in another state. He has a 100 pack-year history of tobacco use, presently one-half pack of cigarettes each day. He admits to rarely drinking alcohol, and he has never used illicit drugs.

PHYSICAL EXAM

Vital Signs

HR, 100 beats/min; RR, 24 breaths/min; BP, 180/90 mm Hg; and pulse oximetry O_2 saturation, 89% while breathing room air.

General

Mildly ill and has frequent paroxysm of coughing. He does not have lower extremity edema.

HEENT

Normal. There is no thrush.

Heart

Heart rate tachycardic and cardiac rhythm is regular. No murmur or gallop is auscultated. Jugular vein distension was not found.

Lungs

Diffuse bilateral expiratory wheezing, decreased breath sounds, and poor air movement. Significant accessory muscle use with respiration without paradoxical thoracoabdominal breathing was noted. Mild lower intercostal space muscle retractions were seen.

Abdomen

Soft and nontender without hepatosplenomegaly. Bowel sounds are normal.

Osteopathic Structural Exam

Reveals left ilium posterior, left SI restriction, general decrease in side bending and rotation throughout the lumbar spine with L1 to L3 flattening of normal lordosis. The thoracic spine has a significantly reduced range of motion during side bending and rotation especially between T5 and T10. T10 is flexed, side bent, and rotated to the right. T5 is extended, side bent, and rotated to the right. T2 is also extended but side bent and rotated to the left. There is decreased rib compliance throughout the rib cage with reduced excursion during the exhalation phase of respiration. Chest is barrel shaped. C7 is flexed, side bent, and rotated to the left. C2 is extended, side bent, and rotated to the right. The right occipitoatlantal articulation has restricted motion mechanics. The sternocleidomastoid and scalene muscles are tense and hypertrophied bilaterally. Diaphragm excursion is decreased during inhalation by percussion, and there is decreased motion in the lower ribs.

DIFFERENTIAL DIAGNOSIS

The differential diagnosis of dyspnea with hypoxemia for this patient (Box 106.1) includes COPD, bronchiectasis, pulmonary embolism, pneumonia, and congestive heart failure. Less frequent considerations include pneumothorax, pleural effusion, and myocardial infarction (with or without arrhythmias such as atrial fibrillation/flutter). It is possible that more than one condition is present.[1]

Any patient presenting with dyspnea must be stabilized from both a respiratory and hemodynamic standpoint before more thorough history and examination are conducted. This patient uses accessory respiratory muscles at rest, clearly demonstrating that he is working very hard to breathe.

The patient was immediately placed on nasal cannula O_2, and pulse oximetry was used to carefully monitor an improvement in oxygenation. The use of O_2 in a patient with COPD should be monitored closely because of the risk of CO_2 retention or hypercapnia. An electrocardiogram (EKG) was done, which showed sinus tachycardia. The EKG showed low voltage but no ischemic abnormalities. At this point, the patient was transferred by ambulance to the closest emergency department where he was placed on telemetry. The supplemental O_2 via nasal cannula was continued, and nebulized bronchodilator therapy was initiated.

The initial workup for the complaint of dyspnea should include a chest x-ray (posteroanterior and lateral views), EKG, and several blood studies including complete blood count with differential, serum electrolytes, creatinine, blood urea nitrogen, D-dimer, N-terminal pro B-type natriuretic peptide, brain natriuretic peptide, troponin, and arterial blood gas. In addition, CT angiography and echocardiography can be ordered. This initial workup will determine if the cause is cardiac, pulmonary, metabolic, or due to anemia. With these data, a more focused, in-depth workup can be pursued (Box 106.2).

BOX 106.1 Differential Diagnosis for Dyspnea with Hypoxemia in an Elderly Male with a History of COPD and Cardiovascular Disease

Exacerbation of COPD
Bronchiectasis
Pulmonary embolism
Pneumonia
Congestive heart failure
Pneumothorax
Pleural effusion
Myocardial infarction

BOX 106.2 Initial Workup for Patient with Dyspnea and Hypoxemia (Once They Are Stabilized)

Chest x-ray (posteroanterior and lateral views)
EKG
Complete blood count with differential
Serum electrolytes
Creatinine
Blood urea nitrogen
D-dimer
N-terminal pro B-type natriuretic peptide
Brain natriuretic peptide
Troponin
Arterial blood gas
CT angiography
Echocardiography

The patient's chest x-ray revealed hyperinflated lungs without a lung infiltrate (Fig. 106.1). His hemoglobin and hematocrit were normal, but there was leukocytosis (14,000) without band forms. No metabolic derangement was identified. Arterial blood gas results showed normal acid base balance and moderate hypoxemia, without hypercapnia (Fig. 106.2). These results were used to reduce the initial differential diagnosis to the most likely diagnosis of COPD exacerbation.

The 2023 Global Initiative for Chronic Obstructive Lung Disease (GOLD) report defines a COPD exacerbation as an event characterized by increased dyspnea and/or cough and sputum that worsens in less than 14 days.[1] This event may be accompanied by tachypnea and/or tachycardia and is associated with increased local and systemic inflammation (often caused by some insult to the airways such as an infection or pollution). Based on the 2023 GOLD report's ABE assessment scheme of disease pattern and severity, this patient would be categorized within Group E (≥2 moderate exacerbations per year or ≥1 exacerbation per year leading to hospitalization).[1] Such patients have a high risk of future exacerbations and pharmacologic therapy should include a short-acting beta agonist, a long-acting beta agonist and a long-acting anticholinergic. An inhaled corticosteroid can also be added, particularly if the blood eosinophil count is greater than or equal to 300 cells per microliter. Medications were begun and included a nebulized combination of ipratropium 0.5 mg and albuterol 2.5 mg every hour for the first 3 doses then every 2 to 4 hours as needed, methylprednisolone 60 mg i.v. every 6 hours and ceftriaxone 1 g i.v. daily. An additional albuterol treatment could be given every 2 hours for breathing distress. Supplemental oxygen was continued with a SpO_2 target of 88% to 92% or PaO_2 of 60 to 70 mm Hg to minimize the risk of worsening hypercapnia with excess supplemental oxygen. Roflumilast can be added particularly in patients with an FEV <50% and chronic bronchitis. Azithromycin can also be added, particularly in former smokers, although consideration should be given to the development of resistant organisms. Antiviral therapy such as oral oseltamivir may be appropriate for exacerbations triggered by influenza virus (depending on timing and susceptibility), however zanamivir is contraindicated in COPD patients due to the risk of airway reactivity. Patients

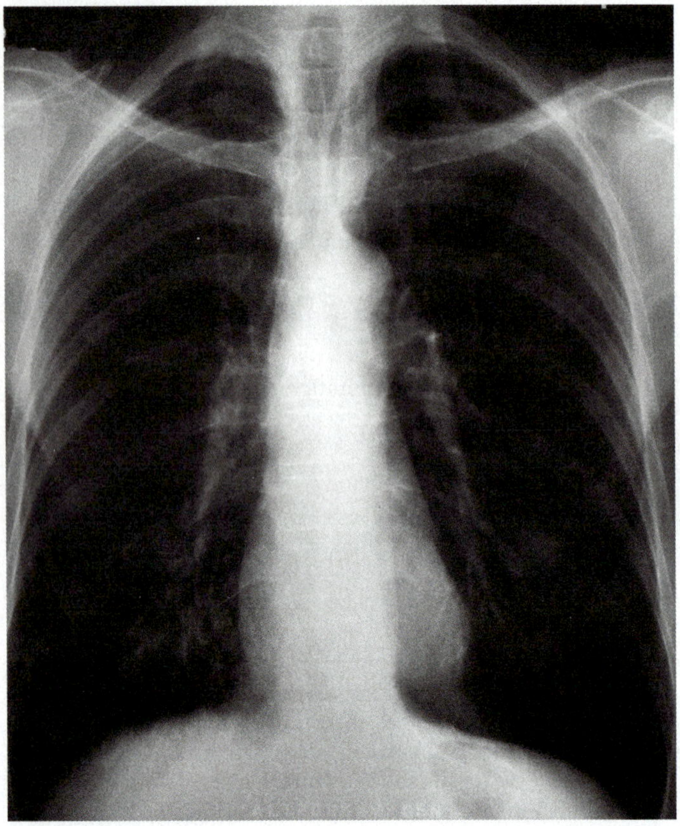

Figure 106.1. COPD. Frontal radiograph shows lung hyperinflation with depressed diaphragm. Note the vertical and floating appearance of the heart, which is compressed by the overinflated lungs.

with COPD that test positive for SARS-CoV-2 are likely to be candidates for Covid-19 therapy and should be closely observed for deterioration. Withdrawal of inhaled corticosteroids can be considered in the case of pneumonia; however this is more likely to be associated with exacerbations particularly if the eosinophils are ≥300 cells per microliter.[1]

Arterial Blood Gas Interpretation Reference			
Normal range: pH 7.35–7.45, $PaCO_2$ 35–45 mm Hg, PaO_2 80–100 mm Hg, HCO_3 22–26 mEq/L			
Disorder	**pH**	**Primary disturbance**	**Compensation**
Respiratory acidosis	↓	↑PCO_2	↑HCO_3
Respiratory alkalosis	↑	↓PCO_2	↓HCO_3
Metabolic acidosis	↓	↓HCO_3	↓PCO_2
Metabolic alkalosis	↑	↑HCO_3	↑PCO_2

Figure 106.2. Arterial blood gas interpretation.

Most acute exacerbations of COPD are preceded by an infection, either viral or bacterial. The patient typically reports worsening cough and wheeze, chest congestion, increased sputum production and purulence, and dyspnea. Tachypnea and hypoxemia are common findings. The chest radiograph may show signs of infiltrate (concomitant community-acquired pneumonia or bronchiectasis), and often there are findings consistent with lung hyperinflation (flat diaphragm, hyperlucent lungs, and increased retrosternal air space). Sputum cultures and computed tomography (CT) of the chest may be necessary if the clinical picture remains unclear. Keep in mind that patients with COPD are at increased risk of other acute events such as decompensated heart failure, pneumonia, and pulmonary embolism that may mimic or aggravate an exacerbation of COPD. Therefore, worsening respiratory symptoms (particularly dyspnea without the other typical characteristics of COPD exacerbation) should prompt careful consideration of the conditions included in the differential diagnosis as they may act as potential contributors to the clinical presentation.[1]

Long-term prognosis following hospitalization for COPD exacerbation is poor. The 5-year mortality rate is roughly 50%. Factors independently associated with poor outcomes include older age, lower BMI, a history of hospitalizations for COPD exacerbations, the need for long-term oxygen therapy at discharge and other comorbidities (such as cardiovascular disease or lung cancer) to name a few. Cold weather spells increase mortality. Patient characteristics such as poorer quality of life, worse lung function, lower exercise capacity, and lower lung density also place them at increased mortality risk following acute COPD exacerbations.[1]

COPD patients often have substantial musculoskeletal findings on examination, and they can benefit from a carefully planned osteopathic treatment program that involves both pharmacologic and nonpharmacologic interventions. Walking tests, such as the paced shuttle walk test or the self-paced 6-minute walk test, can be useful for assessing disability and risk of mortality. These are currently used to assess the effectiveness of pulmonary rehabilitation. Likewise, they can potentially be useful in objectively assessing the impact of osteopathic intervention.[1]

OSTEOPATHIC PATIENT MANAGEMENT

Biomechanical Model

Breathing is in large part a mechanical process. As discussed previously in Chapters 15 and 78:

- Changes in intrathoracic pressures involve contraction and relaxation of skeletal musculature that are attached to the spine and bony thorax.
- These motions, during inspiration and expiration, produce pressure gradients within the thorax and between the thoracic and abdominal cavities.
- This process is critical for respiration and the movement of fluids throughout the body (see Chapters 15 and 78 for further details).
- Although OMT can decrease the somatic burden of the regional dysfunctions, care must be exerted in potentially increasing air trapping.[2]

The physical action of producing a negative intrathoracic pressure requires a definable amount of energy, referred to as the work of breathing. This patient obviously has expended his reserve energy to meet the demands of the effort to breathe and is heading toward respiratory failure.

- This patient can progress to respiratory failure due to an inability to maintain adequate ventilation and oxygenation because of respiratory muscle fatigue and eventual exhaustion.
- He is at risk for impending failure of the thoracic pump due to severe airflow obstruction and thoracic hyperinflation, both of which develop as a result of obstructive air trapping within the lung.
  - Thoracic hyperinflation places the entire pump at a mechanical disadvantage increasing muscle workload and the potential for muscle fatigue.
  - The goal of medical management, which includes the use of OMT, is to improve airflow, reduce hyperinflation, and delay or prevent the onset of muscle fatigue and respiratory failure.

The mechanical process of breathing involves tissue compliance and recoil.

- Compliance is the ease with which tissues are stretched during inhalation.
  - Respiratory system compliance has at least two components, lung tissue and chest wall, that make up the total thoracic compliance.
  - Lung tissue compliance is reduced in disease processes that are infiltrative or restrictive such as pneumonias or effusions.
  - Treating his pneumonia with antibiotics and intravenous fluids will help to increase his lung tissue compliance.
  - OMT should be directed at increasing the compliance of the chest wall.
- Recoil involves the elastic ability of the lung parenchyma to passively contract during exhalation.
  - Lung recoil is affected by the structure of the lung parenchyma.
  - Conditions that destroy or alter the structure of the parenchyma can affect recoil and interfere with the ability of the lung tissue to expel air.
  - The patient's lung structure has been altered by years of tobacco use; stopping this habit is an essential component of the management plan in order to prevent the lung from further decrease in recoil ability.

In COPD, the ability of the lung to expel air is compromised. The increased residual volume and decreased O_2 levels damage the delicate alveoli wall. Adjacent alveoli sacs coalesce forming larger tertiary spaces; as a result, the surface area of the lung is decreased, and there is less area available for gas exchange.

- This condition is called emphysema, which is what this patient has (Fig. 106.3).
- The damage to the parenchyma increases the compliance but decreases the elastic recoil properties of the lung.
- The subsequent tendency for air trapping increases the workload of both expiratory and inspiratory muscles; expiratory muscles are engaged in an attempt to decrease residual lung volumes, while inspiratory muscles must now work against the increased residual alveoli volume.
- Consequently, there is an overall increase in the work of breathing.

This patient has altered mechanics of breathing as he is utilizing his accessory muscles. Respiratory muscle hypertrophy develops in response to the increased breathing workload.

- Muscle hypertrophy alters biomechanics and creates somatic dysfunction.

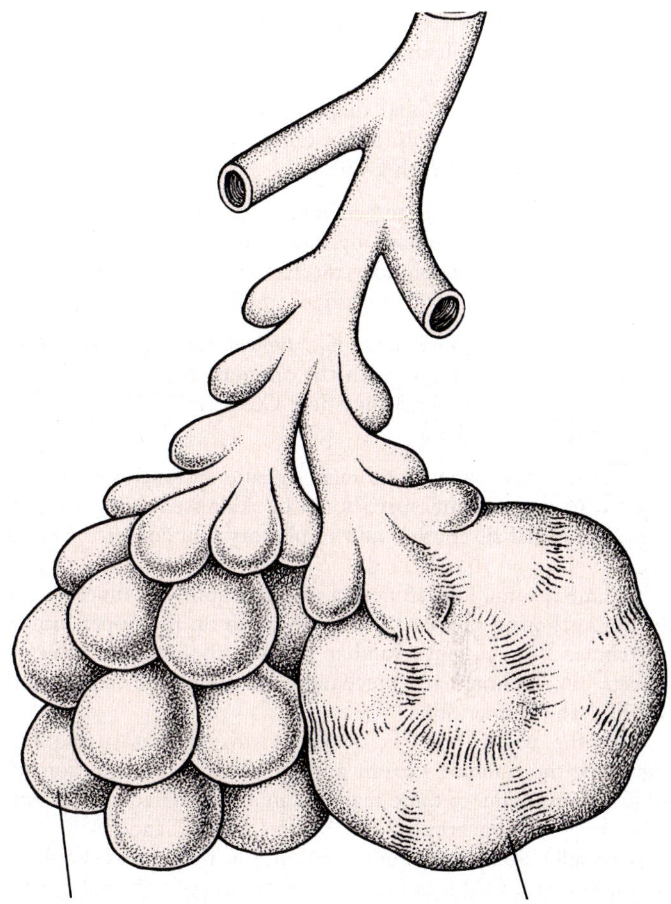

Figure 106.3. Schematic diagram depicting normal alveoli and alveoli in COPD.

- Somatic dysfunction can reduce the compliance of the cervical spine and thoracic spine and costal cage, alter respiratory biomechanics, and further increase the work of breathing.
- Thus, a vicious cycle has been created in which this patient is now compromised in his ability to meet his respiratory demands.
- See Chapter 15 for more information about the anatomy and physiology of the respiratory muscles in patients with COPD.
- OMT should be directed at decreasing the chronic tension in the primary and secondary muscles of respiration in order to allow them to recover from overuse and fatigue.

Somatic dysfunction of the ribs and thoracic spine was found in this patient. The shape of his thorax is related to his emphysema with hyperinflation (barrel chest), which can produce dramatic changes in chest wall compliance. In addition to the specific dysfunctions noted in association with pulmonary disease, this altered chest wall compliance may contribute to the patient's respiratory dysfunction.

- Several osteopathic manipulative techniques may be used to address these thoracic compliance issues, in combination with more specific techniques for individual somatic dysfunctions (see Sections 8 and 9 for OMT procedures and Chapter 78 Osteopathic Considerations and Approaches in the Acutely Ill or Hospitalized Patient for special procedures used with patients in respiratory distress).
- OMT to improve the compliance of the patient's thorax may not necessarily directly alter the parenchymal pathology. However,

it should improve the comfort and work of his breathing and perhaps exercise tolerance, which would ultimately enhance his functional capacity.

- Pursed lip breathing and diaphragmatic breathing have been shown to improve pulmonary function and increase exercise capacity in patients with COPD.[1]

As noted, in addition to general changes in compliance of the bony thorax, specific somatic dysfunctions may have an effect on the function of the respiratory mechanism that goes beyond the changes in compliance they invariably produce.

- Recall that the movement of a typical rib during breathing operates in conjunction with the orientation of its costotransverse and costovertebral joints (see Chapters 34, 35, and 78 for an anatomical review).

Thus, as this patient's thoracic somatic dysfunction adversely affects his rib mechanics; it should be addressed with OMT to support normal rib motion and respiratory function of the costal cage.

Lumbar somatic dysfunction affects diaphragm function due to the anchoring of the diaphragm's crura on the upper lumbar vertebrae. This patient's lumbar somatic dysfunction adversely affects his diaphragmatic mechanics and should be treated with OMT (see Chapter 36).

As the whole body is involved with respiratory motions, including the cranium, sacrum, and the pelvic diaphragm, somatic dysfunction in any of these regions can affect thoracic respiratory mechanics and function (see Chapters 32, 37, and 38 for further details). Somatic dysfunction found in these areas should be addressed with OMT to facilitate restoration of maximal breathing mechanics and function.

OMT can improve the function and efficiency of the respiratory musculature (see Chapter 15 for detailed discussion and specific techniques). It is used in conjunction with the general medical management of the patient. Improvements in mechanical function and thoracic compliance may decrease the need for bronchodilators and steroids. As the patient's respiratory function improves, the ability to clear mucous by coughing may also improve, eliminating the need for expectorants and potentially decreasing airway resistance. Incorporating manipulative treatment into the care of a patient with COPD may allow the physician to decrease the need for pharmaceutical interventions and the risks and complications associated with the use of these agents.

For this patient, the goals of treatment in the biomechanical care model include optimizing the mechanics of breathing, including the work of breathing; the compliance of the thoracic cage and spine, both specifically and generally; and the function and efficiency of the primary respiratory and accessory musculature.

Respiratory–Circulatory Model

Traditionally, the osteopathic concept has viewed the cervicothoracic, thoracolumbar, and pelvic diaphragms as working together to maintain pressure gradients in the pelvis, abdomen, and thorax.[3–6] These gradients aid in fluid movement through the venous and lymphatic systems, often referred to as the low-pressure circulatory system. The patient has somatic dysfunction of his thoracic inlet, diaphragm, thoracic spine and costal cage, and lumbar spinal regions. These should be treated with OMT to improve venous and lymphatic drainage (see Chapters 14 and 50 for further discussion).

The clinical significance of the respiratory–circulatory concept in pulmonary disease is likely very important and underestimated.

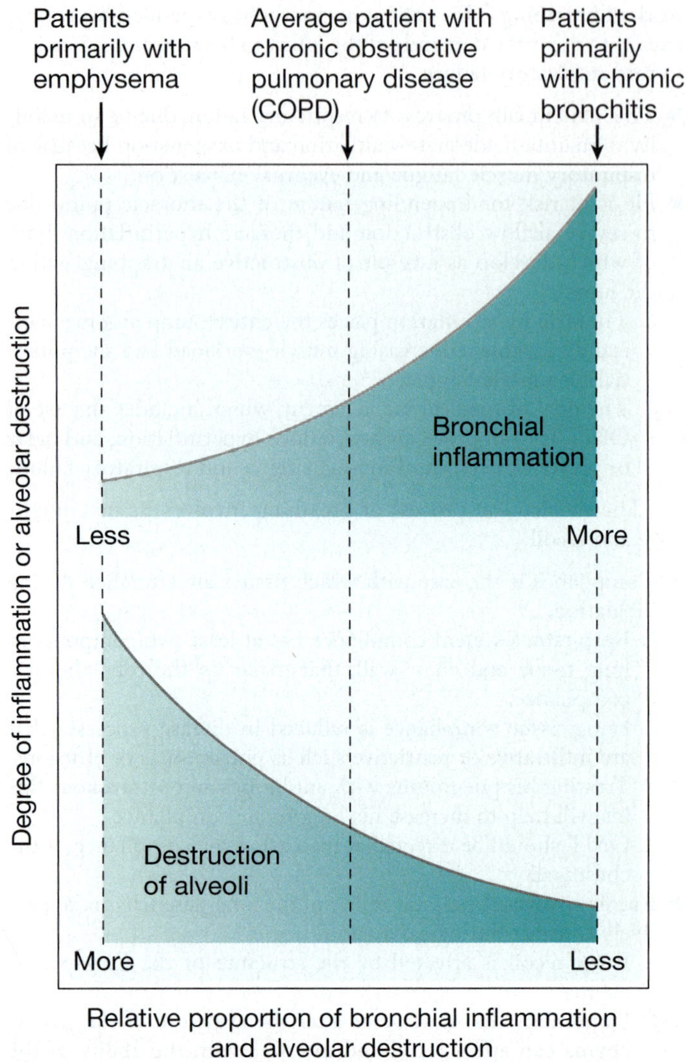

Figure 106.4. The relationship between emphysema and chronic bronchitis. Most patients with COPD have a mixture of bronchial inflammation and alveolar destruction.

Obstructive lung diseases are associated with inflammation of various pulmonary tissues (Fig. 106.4).

This patient has an overall restriction of thoracic movement during the exhalation phase of respiration, reducing both local drainage of lymph from the small airways and central lymph drainage through the thoracic duct.

- During the obstructive exacerbation, initiated by lobar pneumonia or acute bronchitis, there is an intrapulmonary inflammatory process that has produced an increased demand on the regional lymphatic circulation.
- The excursion of the thorax, however, is consistently and significantly reduced by the exacerbation.
- This restriction in movement leads to a reduction in local drainage of exudates, a decrease in the delivery of antigen to regional lymph nodes, and perhaps impairment in both the cellular immunologic response and the transport of antibiotics to the affected areas since lung interstitial pressure rises and shunts blood away from the area.
- Restoring a greater excursion of the thorax will improve his body's ability to move the lymph in this situation; specific OMT lymph pump techniques are also indicated (see Chapter 50 Lymphatic Drainage Procedures for details).

Neurologic Model

Autonomic nervous system influences are important in a variety of lung diseases. Vagal activity is involved in the bronchospasm and mucous production in the pathophysiology of asthma and COPD.[7] This patient has upper cervical spine somatic dysfunction, which is thought to be related to vagal nerve activity. His T2 somatic dysfunction is likely related to his underlying coronary artery disease and his bronchopulmonary disease (see Chapters 6, 13, and 43 for further details).

Chest pain in this patient could occur either from his coronary artery disease or from costochondritis as well as pectoralis tender points that can develop from chronic cough. Osteopathic manipulation to the ribs, sternum, thoracic vertebrae, and chest musculature can resolve myofascial and ligamentous articular strains, thereby decreasing pain.

Metabolic Energy Model

This patient has many metabolic challenges; for example, protein–calorie malnutrition, weight loss or cachexia, and inability to tolerate exercise lead to heart deconditioning and muscle wasting. High caloric supplements or appetite stimulants can be considered but have not shown long-term benefits. Any alteration or restriction in his gait will further increase his oxygen demand. Regular OMT visits focused on facilitating normal posture and function may assist in reducing metabolic energy requirements. Once the patient is stable, comprehensive pulmonary rehabilitation should be considered to improve quality of life and exercise capacity.

Behavioral Model

Shortness of breath caused by lung disease is a major source of anxiety (Fig. 106.5). Increased sympathetic tone may exacerbate vasoconstriction and bronchial constriction. Stress and anxiety may be higher in patients of lower socioeconomic status. Physicians should have appropriate knowledge of their patients' ability to pay for their medications and meet other financial obligations that impact their health status. Smoking cessation and promoting a smoke-free environment are essential for all patients and paramount for

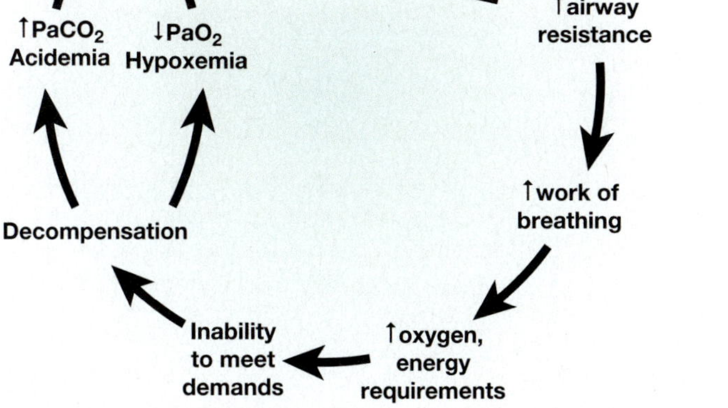

Figure 106.5. The cycle of anxiety and COPD symptoms.

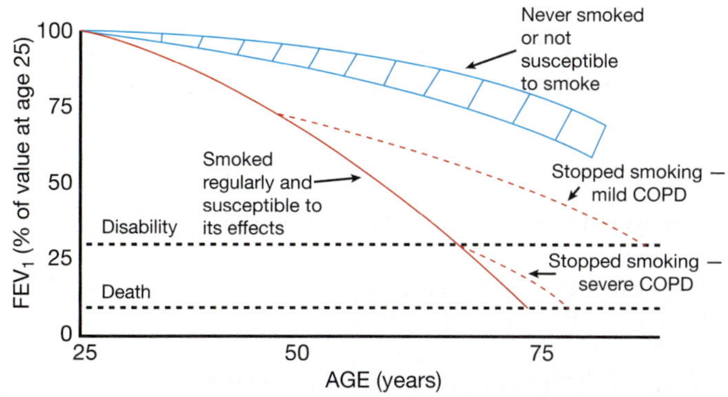

Figure 106.6. Effect of risk factors from smoking on loss of lung function. *Upper curves* are derived from subjects who do not smoke or are not exposed to the effects of smoking. They lose lung function gradually throughout adult life (15 to 30 mL/year). *Lower curves* show accelerated loss to lung function in subjects who are exposed to the effects of cigarette smoke. At age 65 years, there is respiratory disability because FEV1 has decreased from 25% to 30% of predicted (1 to 1.2 L), and further functional deterioration eventually will cause death because of complications of respiratory insufficiency. If the subject stops smoking, life may be prolonged, but a respiratory death still eventually will result. If intervention is initiated earlier in life (between the ages of 40 and 50 years) when COPD is mild, accelerated loss of lung function is reversible and a respiratory death will be prevented. Although this figure illustrates theoretical loss of FEV1 for an adult cigarette smoker, susceptible smokers will lose lung function at different rates, thereby becoming disabled at different ages. (Modified from Fletcher C, Peto R. The natural history of chronic airflow obstruction. *Br Med J.* 1977;1(6077):1645–1648, with permission from BMJ Publishing Group Ltd.)

patients with COPD (Fig. 106.6). The best results are seen when counseling and medication therapy are combined.[8] Checking and empowering the patient's adherence to all prescribed medications (including having patients demonstrate their inhaler technique) is strongly encouraged. Consider prescribing a combination single inhaler as it may be more convenient and effective than multiple inhalers. Promote adequate sleep, a healthy diet and physical activity. Prevention of infection with the proper use of vaccines (such as the pneumococcal, influenza, pertussis, Covid-19, and shingles vaccines) should be discussed with the patient annually.[1]

CASE VIGNETTE (CONTINUED)

PATIENT OUTCOME

The next day the patient had improved. He was now hemodynamically stable. Systemic steroid therapy and nebulized bronchodilator treatments were tapered over the next 7 days. Long-acting anticholinergic and beta-adrenergic inhalers and inhaled corticosteroid therapy were continued, and pulmonary rehabilitation was recommended. Rib-raising and diaphragm-doming techniques (see Chapter 78 for detailed descriptions) were continued daily throughout his hospital stay. As he progressed, more focus was given to the cervical and lumbar areas using indirect, balancing, and soft tissue techniques. The thoracic outlet was also treated to improve lymphatic flow through the thoracic duct. Both thoracic and pedal pumps were initiated and performed 2 to 3 times daily. After discharge from the hospital, the patient followed up for monthly OMT to maintain compliance of his thorax.

BOX 106.3 Suggested OMT Protocol for Treating Patients with COPD

Soft tissue to the paraspinal muscles
Rib raising
Redoming the abdominal diaphragm (indirect myofascial release)
Suboccipital decompression
Thoracic inlet myofascial release
Pectoral traction
Thoracic lymphatic pump without activation

Adapted from Noll DR, Degenhardt BF, Johnson JC, Burt SA. Immediate effects of osteopathic manipulative treatment in elderly patients with chronic obstructive pulmonary disease. *J Am Osteopath Assoc.* 2008;108(5):251–259.

Suggested protocol for using OMT in the acute stage of a COPD exacerbation: Focus the OMT on the ribs, thoracic spine, and diaphragm to reduce mechanical restrictions. Next, incorporate treatments that target the autonomic nervous system (Box 106.3). Start with indirect treatments such as myofascial release, balanced ligamentous tension, osteopathic cranial manipulative medicine, counterstrain, facilitated positional release, and functional technique. As the exacerbation improves, more direct techniques such as high-velocity, low-amplitude (HVLA), and muscle energy are appropriate if no contraindications. This patient may benefit from monthly OMT to prevent further acute exacerbations. The time interval for OMT is individualized and will depend on the patient, but generally speaking follow-up is usually every 1 to 4 months.

In addition to OMT, the osteopathic physician should consult up-to-date national guidelines as appropriate for each patient.[9]

ACKNOWLEDGMENTS

The author and editors of this chapter would like to acknowledge the scholarly contributions of William Foley, Hugh Ettlinger, Gilbert E. D'alonzo Jr, and Jane E. Carreiro for prior editions of this chapter.

REFERENCES

1. Global Initiative for Chronic Obstructive Lung Disease (GOLD). Global strategy for the diagnosis, management, and prevention of chronic obstructive pulmonary disease; 2023. http://www.goldcopd.org
2. Noll DR, Degenhardt BF, Johnson JC, Burt SA. Immediate effects of osteopathic manipulative treatment in elderly patients with chronic obstructive pulmonary disease. *J Am Osteopath Assoc.* 2008;108(5):251–259.
3. Frymann VM. The core-link and the three diaphragms. In: *Year Book of Selected Osteopathic Papers.* American Academy of Osteopathy; 1968: 13–19.
4. Johnson K. An integrated approach for treating the OB patient: treating the five diaphragms of the body, part I. *AAO J Publ Am Acad Osteopath.* 1991; 1(pt 4 winter):6–9.
5. Johnson K. An integrated approach for treating the OB patient: treating the five diaphragms of the body, part II. *AAO J Publ Am Acad Osteopath.* 1992;2(pt 1, spring):10–16.
6. Zink JG, Lawson WB. Pressure gradients in the osteopathic manipulative management of the obstetric patient. *Osteopath Ann.* 1979;7(pt 5): 208–214.
7. Szekely JI, Pataki A. Recent findings on the pathogenesis of bronchial asthma. Part I. Asthma as a neurohumoral disorder, a pathological vago-vagal axon reflex. *Acta Physiol Hung.* 2009;96(1):1–17.
8. Sadr Azodi O, Lindström D, Adami J, et al. The efficacy of a smoking cessation programme in patients undergoing elective surgery: a randomised clinical trial. *Anaesthesia.* 2009;64(3):259–265.
9. Gentry S, Gentry B. Chronic obstructive pulmonary disease: diagnosis and management. *Am Fam Phys.* 2017;95(7):433–441.

107 Case Study: Cervicogenic Headache

RAYMOND J. HRUBY ▪ MARCEL P. FRAIX ▪ REBECCA E. GIUSTI

KEY CONCEPTS

- Osteopathic evaluation of the patient with cervicogenic headache considers the five models of osteopathic care: biomechanical/structural, respiratory/circulatory, metabolic/energetic, neurologic, and biopsychosocial/behavioral.
- The pathophysiology of cervicogenic headache is discussed.
- Differential diagnosis of cervicogenic headache entails consideration of possible etiologies based on the history and physical using an anatomical and pathophysiologic approach.
- Somatic dysfunction may be a primary cause or a secondary finding in patients with cervicogenic headache.
- Osteopathic management of patients with cervicogenic headache utilizes the five models of osteopathic patient care.
- Cervicogenic headache may be amenable to OMT.

CASE VIGNETTE

A 32-year-old right-hand–dominant Caucasian female presents to an ambulatory clinic complaining of episodic headache-type pain for the past 2 months. The pain has a pressure-like quality and is located in the bilateral occipital and frontal regions of the head. It lasts for approximately 30 minutes and primarily occurs in the morning. The headaches occur two to three times per week and appear to be more frequent when the patient experiences increased stress at work or lack of sleep. The patient was involved in a motor vehicle accident 3 years prior as a restrained passenger and sustained a whiplash type of injury. She does not have a history of head trauma and currently denies experiencing photophobia, visual changes, or nausea.

PAST MEDICAL HISTORY

Seasonal allergies

Past Surgical History

Tonsillectomy at age 5 years, wisdom teeth extracted at age 26 years.

Family History

Her mother is 58 years old, and her father is 59 years old with a history of asthma. She has no siblings. There is no family history of migraine headaches.

Social History

She is single, sexually active in a monogamous relationship for 3 years. She is employed as an administrative assistant. She does not use tobacco or illicit drugs and uses coffee and alcohol only occasionally.

Medications

She takes acetaminophen, two tablets every 2 to 4 hours as needed for pain, uses an antihistamine as needed for seasonal allergies, and takes oral contraceptive pills for birth control.

Allergies

No history of drug or food allergies

REVIEW OF SYSTEMS

General

She is in good health, exercises two times per week, and reports no recent change in appetite or weight and no fever or night sweats.

HEENT

No sore throat or dysphagia, no sinusitis, no auditory changes, tinnitus or vertigo, seasonal allergies

Respiratory

No cough or dyspnea

Cardiovascular

No chest pain or palpitations

Nervous

No sensory changes or motor weakness, no ataxia

Musculoskeletal

Intermittent neck and upper back pain that occurs with prolonged sitting at work, no joint pain or swelling

PHYSICAL EXAM

Vital Signs

Temperature 37°C, pulse 82/min and regular, respirations 12/min, blood pressure 128/84 mmHg

General

Well-nourished woman in no acute distress, alert and oriented to person, place, and time

HEENT

No signs of trauma, sclera clear, fundoscopic examination demonstrate sharp disk margins without papilledema, visual acuity is 20/20, auditory canals are clear, and tympanic membranes are intact. No nasal drainage is noted and the nasal septum is midline. The oropharynx reveals no exudates or erythema.

Lungs

No wheezes, rhonchi, or rales

Heart

Regular rate and without murmurs

Neurologic

Cranial nerves II to XII are grossly intact, motor strength is 5/5, and reflexes are 2+/4+ bilaterally in upper and lower limbs. Sensation is intact to light touch and pinprick, and coordination is intact. Gait is nonantalgic and balanced.

Extremities

No cyanosis, clubbing, or edema

Skin

No rashes or ecchymoses

Osteopathic Structural Exam

Cranial: restricted movement of the right occipitomastoid suture.

Cervical spine: decreased active and passive ranges of motion in all planes, somewhat worse with right side bending and rotation. The cervical paravertebral and upper trapezius musculature demonstrate increased tone with mild tenderness to palpation. Specific joint motion restrictions include OA extended, rotated right and sidebent left, AA rotated right, and C2–C3 extended, rotated and sidebent left.

Thoracic spine: T1–T3 neutral, rotated right and sidebent left, T4–T5 extended, rotated and sidebent left.

Costal cage: left diaphragm inhalation restriction

Sacrum: left on left sacral torsion

DIFFERENTIAL DIAGNOSIS

The differential diagnosis of headache includes cervical pathophysiology as well as cranial and systemic etiologies. Using the five models, possible diagnoses can be categorized as follows:

Neurologic Model

- Cervicogenic headache (CGH)
- Occipital neuralgia
- Migraine and tension-type headache

A particularly difficult diagnostic challenge is distinguishing CGH from migraine without aura and tension-type headache. CGH must also be distinguished from other causes of headache that are more serious and potentially life threatening. These include the following:

Respiratory–Circulatory Model

- Arteriovenous malformation
- Cerebral aneurysm
- Epidural, subdural, or subarachnoid hemorrhage
- Chiari malformation
- Glaucoma
- Pseudotumor cerebri
- Vertebral artery dissection

Metabolic Model

- Meningitis
- Posterior fossa tumors
- Vasculitis, such as temporal arteritis
- Herpes zoster (shingles)
- Rheumatoid arthritis

Biopsychosocial/Behavioral Model

- Caffeine or drug related
- Sleep deprived
- Depression
- Stress

Biomechanical Model

- Cervical spondylosis
- Herniated cervical disk
- Somatic dysfunction
- Head and/or neck trauma

The absence of systemic signs such as fever, chills, etc. decreases the likelihood of infection pathology. Normal vital signs and the absence of neurologic signs make tumor, pseudotumor, vertebral artery dissection, arteriovenous malformation, vasculitis, and cerebral aneurysm less likely. There are no visual changes, but intraocular pressures can be assessed to rule out glaucoma. There is a low probability of underlying cervical spine or systemic disease as there are no history or physical signs indicating their existence. However, cervical spine radiographs, computed tomography (CT) magnetic resonance imaging (MRI), and blood tests would help to rule out any suspected underlying conditions.

The most likely differential diagnosis in this patient includes cervicogenic, migraine, or tension-type headache. These three entities are differentiated primarily by patient history. As described below, the most likely diagnosis for this patient is CGH. She also has cranial, cervical, thoracic, costal cage, and sacral somatic dysfunctions, stressful work, and sleep deprivation that factor into the clinical presentation.

OVERVIEW OF CERVICOGENIC HEADACHE

CGH may be defined as pain referred to the head region, typically unilaterally, from cervical musculoskeletal dysfunction. It is characterized by the presence of cervical somatic dysfunction as exhibited by muscle spasm, decreased range of motion, and pain upon digital provocation. It is usually worse with movement and better with rest. It can be associated with tendonitis in any of the cervical muscles, trigger points or tender points in the cervical or head region, and/or inflammation of the cervical spinal joints.[1,2]

Epidemiology

Patients of all ages can be affected by this condition, with the mean age being 42.9 years.[3] CGH is four times more common in females than males and accounts for 14% to 18% of all chronic and recurrent headaches.[4–6] It is a common symptom following neck trauma (54% to 66% of patients with whiplash-associated disorder complain of headache). It should be noted that 54.8% of patients seen by pain specialists have CGH or CGH in combination with other types of headache.[7] The prevalence of CGH in the general population is estimated to be 0.4% to 4.1%.[3,8]

CGHs often lack a regular pattern. They are often episodic and recurrent, lasting hours to days per episode, and can seriously affect the patient's quality of life.[9] Some patients develop CGH after trauma, such as a whiplash injury.[10] These headaches often resolve within a year. However, previous traumas or pre-existing headache and neck pain may lead to chronic CGH after whiplash injury.[11]

The effect of CGH on society is also significant. In a US survey totaling 13,343 respondents, 9.4% reported missing work more than rarely because of headache, 31% reported that their work level was reduced more than rarely by headache, and 9.2% reported that their work level was reduced more than 50% by headaches during work.[12] On average, individuals lost the equivalent of 4.2 d/y because of headache. Subjects with migraine headache were much more likely (57%) to report actual lost workdays because of headache, whereas tension-type and other headache types accounted for a large proportion (64%) of decreased work effectiveness because of headache. Headache type, headache severity, and education level were each independent predictors of workplace impact of headache.

In a 2001 to 2002 random sample telephone survey of over 28,900 American workers, 13% of the total workforce experienced a loss in productive time during a 2-week period due to a common pain condition.[13] Headache was the most common pain condition resulting in lost productive time, accounting for a mean loss of 3.5 hours in productive time per week. Among active workers, lost productive time from common pain conditions (i.e., headache, back pain, arthritis) costs an estimated $61.2 billion per year, with $20 billion due to headache. The majority (76.6%) of the lost productive time was not due to an absence from work but was explained by reduced performance while at work.

Risk factors for developing CGH include the following:

- Head or neck traumatic injuries can predispose a patient to CGH symptoms.
- Sustained neck postures or movements may precipitate CGH.
- Primary or significant compensatory cervical somatic dysfunctions.

Pathophysiology

Cervical somatic dysfunction refers pain to the head and face via the trigeminal nerve (CN V). This same nerve innervates cranial and facial structures, including the cerebral blood vessels and dura mater, and sends its sensory information to the pons in the midbrain and then to the thalamus and somatosensory cortex. The trigeminal nerve also has tracts that descend into the spine. For example, the upper cervical spinal cord contains the trigeminal nucleus caudalis (TNC). The TNC descends as low as C4 and is contiguous with the spinal gray matter in the substantia gelatinosa in lamina II of the dorsal horn.[14–16]

The first three cervical spinal nerves innervate the zygapophyseal joints, the uncovertebral joints, the intervertebral disks, the cervical muscles and ligaments, the vertebral artery, the cervical spinal dura, the posterior scalp, and even the lower layer of the tentorium cerebelli. Afferent fibers from these structures converge with the TNC within the spinal cord. As a result, pain signals from the neck can be referred to the same receptive field in the thalamus as that of the head and face, giving the patient the sensation that the pain is emanating from the head or face when in fact it is coming from the cervical spine.

Nociceptive stimuli from the C5–C7 nerves can also refer pain to the head and face through the TNC since afferent nociceptive information can ascend between one and three levels before entering the dorsal horn and interacting with interneurons that connect with the TNC.

Nociceptive input originating from cervical structures can therefore be perceived as head pain in the regions innervated by the trigeminal nerve.[17,18]

The superior and inferior vagal ganglia lie superior and inferior to the jugular foramina, respectively. The vagus (CN X) is a mixed nerve with motor, sensory, and parasympathetic components. Of interest in CGH is the fact that nociceptive or inflammatory stimuli from the larynx and pharynx, as well as the thoracic and abdominal viscera, are transmitted by the vagus and converge with upper cervical afferents.[19] The increased afferent activity converging in the upper cervical region is thought to increase the efferent discharge of cervical spinal motor neurons accounting for the palpable increase in myofascial tissue tension in the upper cervical spine, thus constituting a viscerosomatic reflex. In addition, primary sensory axons from the superior vagal ganglia terminate in the TNC and convey general sensation from the external auditory meatus, external surface of the tympanic membrane, and the skin of the ear to the trigeminal receptive field in the thalamus. The spinal accessory nerve (CN XI), which sends motor efferents to the trapezius and sternocleidomastoid muscles, also has some sensory afferents that may converge with the TNC.[17,18]

With respect to the sympathetic nervous system, sympathetic nerve fibers are dense in the basal region of the occipital dura mater and alongside as well as independent from blood vessels.[20] The superior cervical ganglia are positioned anterior to the articular pillars of C2. They have postganglionic fibers that innervate the vasculature, mucous membranes of the head region, including the middle ear, the lacrimal glands, and pupils of the eyes. Their preganglionic cell bodies emanate from the spinal cord at levels T1–T4.

Within the peripheral nervous system, a number of structures may be involved with CGH. The greater and lesser occipital nerves originate from roots at C1–C3; the medial branches of the dorsal rami of C2 and C3 form the greater occipital nerve and the third occipital nerve. The greater and lesser occipital nerves innervate the posterior scalp. Occipital neuralgia may arise from entrapment or trauma to these nerves, the upper cervical zygapophyseal joints, or the C2 spinal root. The suboccipital (C1) nerve innervates the occipitoatlantal joint and may be involved with somatic dysfunction that can refer pain to the occipital region. The AA joint and C2–C3 are innervated by the C2 spinal nerve. Neuralgia arising from C2 can result in a deep or dull pain that usually radiates from the occipital to the parietal, temporal, frontal, and periorbital regions. A paroxysmal sharp pain may be superimposed over the constant pain. Lacrimation and conjunctival injection of the eye on the affected side are common associated signs. The third occipital nerve, arising from the dorsal ramus of C3, innervates the joints at C2 and C3. Somatic dysfunction of these joints may be involved in referring pain to the frontotemporal and periorbital regions.[18]

Typical Patient Presentation

Patients may describe the pain of CGH as moderate to severe in intensity, deep, nonthrobbing, and nonlancinating. Certain precipitating factors may be involved, such as certain neck movements or particular sustained head positions. There may be a history of whiplash or other head or neck injury prior to onset of symptoms. It should be noted, however, that patients frequently have difficulty identifying factors that precipitate, aggravate, or alleviate their headaches.

In CGH, the location of the head pain may be in the frontal, posterior, or lateral part of the head, at the vertex, or behind the orbit. The pain is typically unilateral, although it may occasionally be bilateral.[1] The pain may radiate along the ipsilateral side of the head, to the neck and/or shoulder, and occasionally into the arm.[1] There may also be scalp paresthesias or dysesthesia. Other characteristics include headache episodes of varying duration and lack of response to medications that are usually helpful in alleviating other types of headache. Associated symptoms may include nausea, phonophobia, photophobia, dizziness, ipsilateral blurred vision, difficulties with swallowing, and ipsilateral periorbital edema. Coughing or sneezing may also trigger the pain.

Physical Examination of the Patient with Headache

The physical examination of the patient with headache should include vital signs; a screening cardiovascular, neurologic, and musculoskeletal examination; and a regional evaluation of the head and neck. Normal vital signs help to rule out endocrine, cardiovascular, and infectious processes. The screening neurologic examination is used to rule out focal deficits suggesting intracranial mass or event and peripheral etiology such as peripheral nerve impingement with radiculopathy or spinal cord impingement from a herniated cervical disk.

The screening musculoskeletal exam evaluates large and small joints for systemic inflammatory conditions such as rheumatoid arthritis, which may present with headache. The head and neck should be examined for pharyngeal and tonsillar inflammation, glandular hypertrophy and/or tenderness, or lymphadenopathy that would alert the practitioner to internal organic problems that can also be an underlying cause of headache. The carotid arteries should be auscultated for any bruits.

The osteopathic physician performs a general osteopathic structural screening exam of the musculoskeletal system, followed by a regional exam and then a segmental exam. The main areas of focus will likely be the head and cervical spine, but as noted above, other body regions may reveal somatic dysfunction related to the patient's symptoms.

Asymmetry of musculoskeletal structural landmarks, altered quantity or quality of active or passive neck motion, tissue texture abnormalities, and tenderness lead the practitioner to consider mechanical neck disorder or somatic dysfunction diagnosis.

It is also possible that somatic dysfunction of more distant body regions, such as the lumbar spine and pelvis, may be contributing factors in the patient with CGH. Restriction of motion of the AA (C1–C2) joint is a very common finding in patients with CGH.[19] There may be asymmetrical neck and head position in relation to the shoulders. Head pain can often be reproduced by digital pressure over the upper cervical or occipital region on the symptomatic side. Restriction of active and passive neck range of motion, particularly in the upper three cervical joints, is a common finding. Presence of cervical muscle stiffness and trigger points in the lower cervical or shoulder muscles may refer pain to the ipsilateral head region (Fig. 107.1). Identification of clinically significant somatic dysfunction indicates the use of osteopathic manipulative treatment (OMT).

Laboratory and Radiologic Findings

Lab work and imaging are not typically necessary if the history and physical examination is consistent with mild sprain or strain of the neck musculoskeletal tissues. In acute whiplash or other traumas, however, it may be necessary to obtain cervical radiographs to rule out vertebral fracture or dislocation. Patients with chronic mechanical neck pain refractory to OMT and appropriate stretches may require further diagnostic imaging to rule out less common causes underlying persistent neck pain. Blood tests for systemic pathology are typically negative, and any cervical disk herniation seen on MRI or CT scan is usually nonspecific.[20]

FIVE MODELS OF OSTEOPATHIC CARE FOR THE PATIENT WITH CERVICOGENIC HEADACHE

A comprehensive management plan can be developed using the five models of osteopathic care as delineated in Chapters 1 and 26, including the application of OMT.

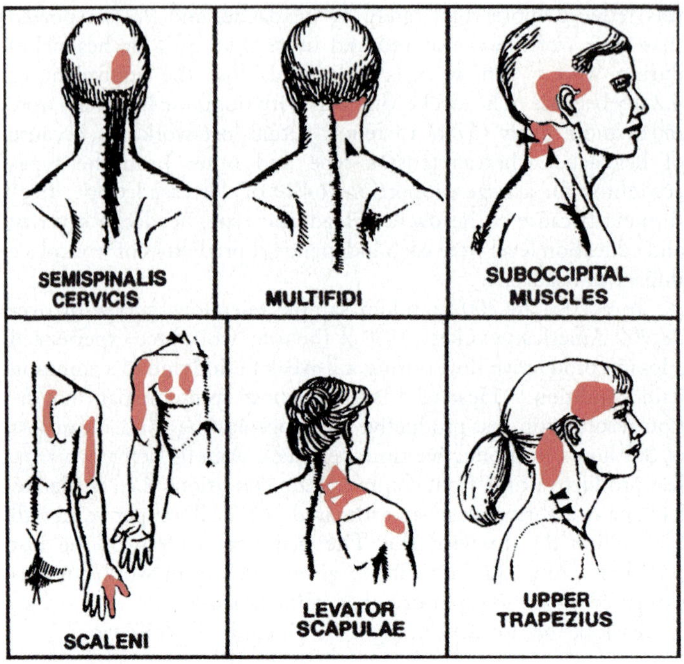

Figure 107.1. Myofascial trigger points in the head, neck, and upper extremity regions. (Illustration adapted from Travell JG, Simons DG. *Myofascial Pain and Dysfunction: The Trigger Point Manual.* Williams & Wilkins; 1983 by William A. Kuchera, DO, FAAO, with permission.)

Biomechanical Model

The case patient has cranial, cervical, thoracic, and sacral somatic dysfunctions that contribute to the overall allostatic load. OMT will likely alleviate these dysfunctions, restore motion, relieve pain, and address biomechanical components of her condition.

Respiratory–Circulatory Model

The patient's somatic dysfunctions of the cranium, cervical, thoracic, costal cage, and sacral regions may impair respiratory mechanics and can adversely affect circulatory functions, including lymphatic and venous drainage. Alleviating these somatic dysfunctions with OMT will restore efficient respiratory mechanics and improve circulatory function.

Neurologic Model

Alleviating her somatic dysfunctions will relieve pain and help her control her headache symptoms. The cranial cephalgia is likely referred from the cervical spine region somatic dysfunction and should be ameliorated when the cervical spine mechanics are restored to normal. A headache pain diary is useful to track progress in controlling or alleviating her symptoms. Essential components include intensity, duration, and frequency of headaches, notation of any associated factors throughout each day, and a daily log of medication utilization.

Metabolic Energy Model

Improving spinal and costal cage motion with OMT facilitates restoration of energy-efficient posture and motion throughout the day. Nutritional support, an exercise program, and stress management will improve her overall energy balance.

Biopsychosocial/Behavioral Model

The treatment goals for this model include optimizing the psychological and social components of the patient's overall health. Some of these components include the patient's spiritual outlook, social support system, ability to cope with stress, and ability to make healthy lifestyle choices. In particular, stress is a well-known cause or contributor to headache, including CGH. Thus, reduction of stress factors can contribute to the ultimate control of CGH in some patients. This might include teaching the patient strategies for stress reduction, helping the patient improve their abilities for constructive social interactions, and helping the patient improve their spiritual outlook. OMT is not commonly a part of the treatment approach in this model, although some osteopathic physicians advocate the use of OMT to improve autonomic balance for these patients, thus secondarily helping to relieve stress on the body and facilitate improved and restorative sleep. The addition of an exercise regimen to her daily routine, eating a nutritious diet, which may include supplementary vitamins and essential nutrients, and drinking plenty of water, will help her maintain her health and prevent recurrence of her headaches (see Chapter 21 Lifestyle Medicine—Osteopathic Perspectives for further information). Poor posture can contribute to somatic dysfunction in the upper thoracic spine.

Many people who work at a desk or computer develop a kyphotic posture where the scapulas are protracted and the shoulders are rolled forward. The upper neck backward bends and the suboccipital muscles tighten. The pectoralis minor muscle subsequently tightens. Workstation problems need to be addressed. Computer screens may need to be raised to the eye level and chair height may need to be altered to promote good posture. The patient may benefit from performing daily postural exercises, scapular stabilization exercises, pectoralis minor stretches, and scalene stretches. Patients with hypermobility affecting the neck may respond to cervical isotonic exercises.

BIOLOGIC BASIS FOR THE USE OF OMT (BEST EVIDENCE)

Although referred pain from visceral organs can elicit pain and increased muscle tone in the cervical region, and cause headache,[21,22] CGH is most commonly related to somatic dysfunction of the OA and AA joints and neck pain most often related to C2–C7 somatic dysfunction. Up to 50% of whiplash patients with chronic neck pain and dominant headache symptoms have C2–C3 zygapophyseal joint pain that can be abolished with nerve blocks.[23,24] Nerve blocks of the greater occipital nerve and lower cervical segments have also abolished headache symptoms, implying that these structures may become sensitized and thus involved in producing CGH.[25,26]

Cervical somatic dysfunction has been thought to involve the trigeminal and spinal accessory cranial nerves, which innervate structures in both cervical and head regions. It is theorized that the TNC in the upper cervical spinal cord interacts with upper cervical peripheral afferents and the spinal accessory nerve (CN XI) to account for the bidirectional referral of painful sensations between the neck and the trigeminal receptive sensory fields of the face and head.[18]

Muscle hypertonicity in the upper cervical and occipital regions may induce tension transmitted through the myodural connective tissue and elicit head pain. The facet joints between C1 and C2 produce pain in the posterior auricular area in the distribution of the greater occipital nerve. Diseases of the structures innervated by the vagus nerve may produce sensitization of upper cervical spinal segments and predispose the patient to upper cervical somatic dysfunction, leading to CGH.[27] Cervicogenic pain has also been abolished with cervical myofascial trigger point and botulinum toxin injections, indicating that peripheral sensitization in the soft tissues plays a role in CGH genesis as well. It has also been shown that increased levels of proinflammatory cytokines and nitric oxide are higher in patients with CGH compared with patients with migraine headaches and likely promote hyperalgesia.[28] However, the lack of calcitonin gene-related peptide in symptomatic CGH patients indicates that the trigeminovascular system is not activated by this condition as it is in migraine patients.[29]

Osteopathic physicians theorize that cervical mobilization and manipulation procedures decrease the afferent stimulus into the spinal cord from cervical joint receptors by relaxing the paraspinal muscles and releasing strain on the connective tissues and joints, thus relieving the pain of CGH. OMT and physical conditioning exercises for moderate to severe pain of any duration are effective for patients of all ages or gender.[30–33] Ongoing exercise and physical conditioning programs can be beneficial for long-term prevention and control of symptoms.[32,33]

Although OMT is a highly safe procedure, there are potential risks associated with its use. The primary risk identified in the literature is hyperextension coupled with rotation of the upper cervical spine due to concern regarding potential occlusion of the vertebral artery. Caution should also be exercised with patients with primary or secondary bone, neural, or muscular disease as is true in any body region. Commonly accepted contraindications to manual medical treatment of the cervical spine include the following:

- Vertebral or carotid artery dissection
- Acute fracture of cervical vertebra or vertebrae
- Metabolic or neoplastic bone disease in the cervical spine
- Acute trauma to the head or neck without established diagnosis
- Certain primary muscle or joint diseases
- Patient refusal of treatment is a medicolegal contraindication for any form of treatment and is not specific to OMT to the cervical spine.

Certain clinical conditions do not necessarily contraindicate the use of OMT but do require caution on the part of the osteopathic physician. For example, patients with congenital anomalies, such as those with Down syndrome, may have deformities of the upper cervical spine that will alter the biomechanics in that region. Caution is also warranted in treating patients with rheumatoid arthritis as there may be laxity of the odontoid ligament and hypermobility of the AA joint.

The benefits of OMT for CGH include decreased pain frequency, intensity, and duration[34]; improved ability to perform activities of daily living and work activities; and decreased reliance on analgesic and other medications that can have unwanted side effects and complications. The consensus among most practitioners is that CGH should be treated with a combination of manual treatment, exercise, locally injected and oral medications, stress reduction counseling, and education. Surgery is reserved for refractory conditions.

Physical Medicine and Rehabilitation Perspective

In spite of additional knowledge and experience in managing cervical spine disorders, the physician spine specialist oftentimes still finds the diagnosis of CGH to be quite challenging. Although various anatomical structures, including the cervical spine musculature, nerves, disks, and zygapophyseal joints, have been implicated in the pathophysiology of CGH, there is limited evidence that supports any of these structures as clearly causing CGH. Most research regarding this issue has focused on examining patient symptomology in response to structure-directed treatment, including facet and trigger point injection and cervical diskectomy and fusion. Diagnosing the cause of CGH is also made more challenging by the fact that it is oftentimes difficult to differentiate between cervicogenic, migraine, and tension-type headaches. Given these challenges, it is helpful to use an approach, such as the five osteopathic conceptual models, that addresses the various structures and pathologic processes that may be concomitantly causing CGH.

One reason why it may be difficult to diagnose and define the cause of CGH is that the upper cervical nerve roots innervate many of the structures typically suspected of causing CGH. These nerve roots converge with trigeminal nerve fibers in the upper cervical spinal cord, potentially explaining why nociceptive input from cervical spine structures may cause pain in the head and face. Diagnosis is also difficult because there is no diagnostic or clinical finding that is specific to CGH. Historically, radiologic abnormalities of the cervical spine have been used as diagnostic criteria for CGH.[2] Even though radiographic abnormalities such as cervical spondylosis may be present when evaluating a patient with CGH, there is limited evidence demonstrating that these abnormalities are specific to CGH.[35] In addition, studies examining the cervical MRI studies of patients with CGH failed to demonstrate a difference between control subjects and those with CGH when evaluating for MRI abnormalities such as cervical disk bulging.[20] While laboratory results may be abnormal in the presence of systemic disease, such as rheumatoid arthritis, there is also no laboratory marker that is specific for patients with CGH. Some research, however, has demonstrated that proinflammatory mediators may be higher in patients with mechanically induced CGH than those patients with migraine headache.[36] Due to the equivocal nature of these diagnostic findings, it is important that the spine specialist performs a detailed history and physical examination when evaluating a patient for CGH. This is helpful in identifying cervical spine disease, including cervical spondylosis and nerve root compression, as well as excluding more serious conditions such as tumor or infection.[37] Important components of the clinical evaluation include cervical range of motion, motor and sensory testing, and provocative testing for nerve root compression. Clinical evaluation can also be helpful in differentiating CGH from migraine headache. These are often difficult to discern from one another due to the overlap in diagnostic criteria, including photophobia and nausea. It appears that the most significant criterion in distinguishing CGH from migraine headache is the precipitation of headaches with movement of the neck or application of pressure to the neck.[38] Given the fact that the etiology of CGH may be multifaceted and that its diagnosis requires assessment of multiple structures and physiologic processes, it again may be useful to use the five osteopathic models of care when evaluating a patient with CGH.

Because of its multifaceted nature, management of CGH often entails a combination of treatments, including osteopathic manipulative medicine (OMM), medication, injections, and surgery. As an expert in spinal disorders, the spine specialist is interested in better understanding the potential pain-generating source of CGH, so as to potentially render more effective treatment. One way in which this is accomplished is through the use of cervical injection techniques, which can be helpful in both diagnosing and treating the pain-generating structures causing CGH. These include cervical zygapophyseal joint and medial branch blockade for facet disease, epidural for degenerative disk disease and nerve root compression; occipital and cervical nerve blockade; and trigger point or botulinum toxin injection for muscle spasm. Although there is limited evidence supporting the efficacy of these techniques, it does appear that patients may experience some degree of pain relief if their CGH is secondary to a well-defined disease process. The idea that CGH may be due to abnormal muscle tension is potentially supported by a study, which found that injection of botulinum toxin into the cervical paraspinal muscles significantly reduced pain and increased cervical range of motion.[39] Surgical techniques such as anterior diskectomy and fusion are typically reserved for refractory cases that demonstrate clear cervical spine pathology, including cervical radiculopathy and degenerative disk disease. Some studies have suggested that such surgical techniques are effective in treating CGH when it is associated with specific cervical spine pathology.[40] Like much of the research examining the efficacy of injection techniques, however, they are of limited value given their small sample sizes and suboptimal outcome measures.

Interestingly, it appears that manual spinal manipulation is the means of treatment most supported by a reasonable body of literature.[3,41–48] This includes a randomized controlled trial demonstrating that cervical manipulation utilizing high-velocity, low-amplitude technique resulted in reduced CGH intensity and frequency and analgesic use when compared to deep friction massage.[41] This is an important point to consider when integrating osteopathic manual medicine into the treatment plan, whether that entails the physician performing OMM or referring a patient to a neuromusculoskeletal medicine/OMM specialist. Exercise and mind-based therapies have also shown to be an effective adjunct to the management plan.[48]

Summary

CGH is a common medical problem affecting a significant percentage of the population. A holistic, patient-centered approach, consistent with osteopathic philosophy, principles, and practice, provides a strategy for optimal control of this condition in patients. Osteopathic physicians can use the tenets and organizing principles of osteopathic medicine, a five-model approach to patient care, and their distinctive OMT modalities to achieve a high degree of success in helping patients with this condition.

REFERENCES

1. Sjaastad O, Fredriksen TA, Pfaffenrath V. Cervicogenic headache: diagnostic criteria. The Cervicogenic Headache International Study Group. *Headache*. 1998;38(6):442–445.
2. Headache Classification Committee of the International Headache Society (IHS). The International Classification of Headache Disorders, 3rd edition (beta version). *Cephalalgia*. 2013;33(9):629–808.
3. Haldeman S, Dagenais S. Cervicogenic headaches: a critical review. *Spine J*. 2001;1(1):31–46.
4. Pöllmann W, Keidel M, Pfaffenrath V. Headache and the cervical spine: a critical review. *Cephalalgia*. 1997;17(8):801–816.
5. Pfaffenrath V, Kaube H. Diagnostics of cervicogenic headache. *Funct Neurol*. 1990;5(2):159–164.
6. Nilsson N. The prevalence of cervicogenic headache in a random population sample of 20–59 year olds. *Spine*. 1995;20(17):1884–1888.
7. Skovron ML. Epidemiology of whiplash. In: Gunzbrug R, Szpalski M, eds. *Whiplash Injuries: Current Concepts In Prevention, Diagnosis, and Treatment of the Cervical Whiplash Syndrome*. Lippincott-Raven; 1998.
8. Sjaastad O. Cervicogenic headache: comparison with migraine without aura; Vågå study. *Cephalalgia*. 2008;28(Suppl 1):18–20.
9. van Suijlekom HA, Lame I, Stomp-van den Berg SG, Kessels AGH, Weber WEJ. Quality of life of patients with cervicogenic headache: a comparison with control subjects and patients with migraine or tension-type headache. *Headache*. 2003;43(10):1034–1041.

10. Drottning M, Staff PH, Sjaastad O. Cervicogenic headache after whiplash injury. *Cephalalgia*. 1997;17:288–289.
11. Drottning M, Staff PH, Sjaastad O. Cervicogenic headache (CEH) after whiplash injury. *Cephalalgia*. 2002;22(3):165–171.
12. Schwartz BS, Stewart WF, Lipton RB. Lost workdays and decreased work effectiveness associated with headache in the workplace. *J Occup Environ Med*. 1997;39(4):320–327.
13. Stewart WF, Ricci JA, Chee E, Morganstein D, Lipton R. Lost productive time and cost due to common pain conditions in the U.S. workforce. *JAMA*. 2003;290(18):2443–2454.
14. Strandring S, Editor-in-Chief. *Gray's Anatomy. The Anatomical Basis of Clinical Practice*. Elsevier Churchill Livingstone; 2005.
15. Hack GD, Koritzer RT, Robinson WL, Hallgren RC, Greenman PE. Anatomic relation between the rectus capitis posterior minor muscle and the dura mater. *Spine*. 1995;20(23):2484–2486.
16. Nash L, Nicholson H, Lee ASJ, Johnson GM, Zhang M. Configuration of the connective tissue in the posterior atlanto-occipital interspace: a sheet plastination and confocal microscopy study. *Spine*. 2005;30(12):1359–1366.
17. Biondi DM. Cervicogenic headache: mechanisms, evaluation, and treatment strategies. *J Am Osteopath Assoc*. 2000;100(9 suppl):S7–S14.
18. Biondi DM. Cervicogenic headache: a review of diagnostic and treatment strategies. *J Am Osteopath Assoc*. 2005;105(4 suppl 2):S16–S22.
19. Hall T, Robinson K. The flexion-rotation test and active cervical mobility—a comparative measurement study in cervicogenic headache. *Man Ther*. 2004;9(4):197–202.
20. Coskun O, Ucler S, Karakurum B, et al. Magnetic resonance imaging of patients with cervicogenic headache. *Cephalalgia*. 2003;23(8):842–845.
21. Foreman RD. Integration of viscerosomatic sensory input at the spinal level. *Prog Brain Res*. 2000;122:209–221.
22. Artico M, Cavallotti C. Catecholaminergic and acetylcholine esterase containing nerves of cranial and spinal dura mater in humans and rodents. *Microsc Res Tech*. 2001;53(3):212–220.
23. Lord SM, Barnsley L, Wallis BJ, Bogduk N. Third occipital nerve headache: a prevalence study. *J Neurol Neurosurg Psychiatry*. 1994;57(10):1187–1190.
24. Lord SM, Barnsley L, Wallis BJ, Bogduk N. Chronic cervical zygapophysial joint pain after whiplash. A placebo-controlled prevalence study. *Spine*. 1996;21(15):1737–1744.
25. Bovim G, Berg R, Dale LG. Cervicogenic headache: anesthetic blockades of cervical nerves (C2–C5) and facet joint (C2/C3). *Pain*. 1992;49(3):315–320.
26. Bovim G, Sand T. Cervicogenic headache, migraine without aura and tension-type headache. Diagnostic blockade of greater occipital and supra-orbital nerves. *Pain*. 1992;51(1):43–48.
27. Kuchera ML. Osteopathic principles and practice/osteopathic manipulative treatment considerations in cephalgia. *J Am Osteopath Assoc*. 1998;98(4):S14–S19.
28. Martelletti P, van Suijlekom H. Cervicogenic headache: practical approaches to therapy. *CNS Drugs*. 2004;18(12):793–805.
29. Frese A, Schilgen M, Edvinsson L, Frandsen E, Evers S. Calcitonin gene-related peptide in cervicogenic headache. *Cephalalgia*. 2005;25(9):700–703.
30. Jull GA, Trott P, Potter H, et al. A randomized controlled trial of exercise and manipulative therapy for cervicogenic headache. *Spine*. 2002;27(17):1835–1843.
31. Jull GA, Stanton WR. Predictors of responsiveness to physiotherapy management of cervicogenic headache. *Cephalalgia*. 2005;25(2):101–108.
32. Bronfort G, Nilsson N, Haas M, et al. Non-invasive physical treatments for chronic/recurrent headache. *Cochrane Database Syst Rev*. 2004;(3):CD001878.
33. Biondi DM. Physical treatments for headache: a structured review. *Headache*. 2005;45(6):738–746.
34. Mandara A, Ceriani A, Guzzetti G, Gulisano V, Fusaro A, Bado F. Osteopathic manipulative treatment for chronic neck pain: a randomized placebo controlled trial on the effect on pain and disability. *Int J Osteopath Med*. 2010;13(3):104.
35. Fredriksen TA, Fougner R, Tangerud A, Sjaastad O. Cervicogenic headache. Radiological investigations concerning head/neck. *Cephalalgia*. 1989;9(2):139–146.
36. Martelletti P, Stirparo G, Giacovazzo M. Proinflammatory cytokines in cervicogenic headache. *Funct Neurol*. 1999;14(3):159–162.
37. Nordin M, Carragee EJ, Hogg-Johnson S, et al. Assessment of neck pain and its associated disorders: results of the bone and joint decade 2000–2010 task force on neck pain and its associated disorders. *Spine*. 2008;33(4 suppl):S101–S122.
38. Sjaastad O, Bovim G. Cervicogenic headache. The differentiation from common migraine. An overview. *Funct Neurol*. 1991;6(2):93–100.
39. Freund BJ, Schwartz M. Treatment of chronic cervical-associated headache with botulinum toxin A: a pilot study. *Headache*. 2000;40(3):231–236.
40. Schofferman J, Garges K, Goldthwaite N, Koestler M, Libby E. Upper cervical anterior diskectomy and fusion improves discogenic cervical headaches. *Spine*. 2002;27(20):2240–2244.
41. Nilsson N, Christensen HW, Hartvigsen J. The effect of spinal manipulation in the treatment of cervicogenic headache. *J Manipul Physiol Ther*. 1997;20(5):326–330.
42. Gross A, Langevin P, Burnie SJ, et al. Manipulation and mobilisation for neck pain contrasted against an inactive control or another active treatment. *Cochrane Database Syst Rev*. 2015;2015(9):CD004249.
43. Huisman PA, Speksnijder CM, de Wijer A. The effect of thoracic spine manipulation on pain and disability in patients with non-specific neck pain: a systematic review. *Disabil Rehabil*. 2013;35(20):1677–1685.
44. Cross KM, Kuenze C, Grindstaff TL, Hertel J. Thoracic spine thrust manipulation improves pain, range of motion, and self-reported function in patients with mechanical neck pain: a systematic review. *J Orthop Sports Phys Ther*. 2011;41(9):633–642.
45. Young JL, Walker D, Snyder S, Daly K. Thoracic manipulation versus mobilization in patients with mechanical neck pain: a systematic review. *J Man Manip Ther*. 2014;22(3):141–153.
46. Franke H, Franke JD, Fryer G. Osteopathic manipulative treatment for chronic nonspecific neck pain: a systematic review and meta-analysis. *Int J Osteopath Med*. 2015;18:255–267.
47. Varatharajan S, Ferguson B, Chrobak K, et al. Are non-invasive interventions effective for the management of headaches associated with neck pain? An update of the bone and joint decade task force on neck pain and its associated disorders by the Ontario Protocol for Traffic Injury Management (OPTIMa) Collaboration. *Eur Spine J*. 2016;25(7):1971–1999.
48. Wong JJ, Shearer HM, Mior S, et al. Are manual therapies, passive physical modalities, or acupuncture effective for the management of patients with whiplash-associated disorders or neck pain and associated disorders? An update of the bone and joint decade task force on neck pain and its associated disorders by the OPTIMa collaboration. *Spine J*. 2016;16(12):1598–1630.

108 COVID-19

STEPHANIE Z. BROWN

KEY CONCEPTS

- COVID-19 induces a systemic disease process that involves multiple body systems including the respiratory, vascular, lymphatic, and endocrine systems.
- In the COVID-19 patient, consideration should be given to evaluating and treating the lymphatics, vasculature, autonomic nervous system including viscerosomatic reflexes, neuroendocrine structures, thoracic and mediastinal viscera, and the cranium.
- The five models of osteopathy can guide COVID-19 treatment to improve respiration, circulation, innervation, metabolism, and impact of disease.

HISTORY OF PRESENT ILLNESS

T.M. is a 58-year-old hospitalized male with a history of diabetes mellitus type 2 (DMII), chronic kidney disease II (CKD), hypertension, and morbid obesity who presents to the hospital with shortness of breath, cough, and exposure to COVID-19.

The patient presents to the hospital in respiratory distress. He states that he has a known contact at home who is sick with COVID-19. He started feeling ill 2 days ago and has progressively been feeling worse. He was trying to self-treat at home with acetaminophen and hydration, but presented to the hospital when he could not think straight and could not catch his breath. He admits to dry cough, dyspnea at rest, fatigue, body aches, feeling feverish, and loss of appetite.

PAST MEDICAL HISTORY

DMII diagnosed 15 years ago. Hypertension diagnosed 18 years ago. CKD stage II that developed within the last 3 years. Morbid obesity.

PAST SURGICAL HISTORY

Cholecystectomy at age 45

SOCIAL HISTORY

Patient is a factory worker. Patient is divorced and lives at home with two teenage daughters.

FAMILY HISTORY

Father deceased at age 67 from MI. Mother still living with history of DMII and chronic obstructive pulmonary disease (COPD). Two siblings still alive, one with DMII.

MEDICATIONS

Metformin 500 mg BID, Lantus 20 units QHS, lisinopril 5 mg daily

IMMUNIZATIONS

Childhood vaccinations completed, tetanus unknown, flu 2 years ago, no COVID vaccination.

ALLERGIES

No known drug allergies.

REVIEW OF SYSTEMS

General: Admits fever, chills, fatigue, and body aches.
Head: Admits headache and loss of taste and smell. Denies blurred vision.
Cardiovascular: Admits palpitations. Denies chest pressure.
Respiratory: Admits shortness of breath, nonproductive cough. Denies wheezing, hemoptysis, or pleuritic pain.
Gastrointestinal: Admits decreased appetite, loose stools, nausea. Denies constipation.
Musculoskeletal: Denies joint or muscle injury.
Neurologic: Denies numbness, tingling, or muscle weakness.

PHYSICAL EXAMINATION

Vitals on arrival were Temp: 104 °F, BP: 147/92, Pulse 103 bpm, RR: 22, Height: 74 in, Weight: 348 lb. Oxygen saturation at the time of arrival was 89%.
General: Pale, ill-appearing, somnolent, oriented, obese male, appearing stated age.
HEENT: Normocephalic, atraumatic, PERRLA.
Cardiovascular: Tachycardic, regular rhythm, no murmur, rub, or gallop.
Respiratory: Basilar rhonchi, expiratory wheezes from upper lobes, conversational dyspnea, and accessory muscle use.
Gastrointestinal: Obese abdomen, bowel sounds decreased but present, no tenderness to palpation.
Extremities: No edema, 2+ pedal pulses, no bruising or rashes.
Neurologic: CN grossly intact, 5/5 muscle strength of C5–7 and L3–S1 nerve roots, sensation intact of C5–8 and L1–S1 dermatomes.

OSTEOPATHIC STRUCTURAL EXAMINATION

Cranial: Superior SBS strain, OA ESlRr, boggy suboccipital tissues
Cervical: C2 FRS right, C7 FRS left
Thoracic: T1 FRS right, T5 FRS right, boggy tissue texture changes from T3-7, tension of pulmonary arteries and aortic arch, mediastinal fascial and visceral tension
Ribs: Bilateral ribs 7–12 inhaled with pleural tension
Abdomen: Diaphragm inhaled bilaterally

Lumbar: L1–3 NSlRr
Pelvis: Posterior left innominate rotation
Sacrum: Right on left sacral torsion
UE: Elevated left clavicle, left protracted scapula
LE: Externally rotated left femur

RELEVANT LAB TESTS AND IMAGING

WBC: 7,162
PLT: 230,859
ESR: 31.42
CRP: 29.86
Serum ferritin: 543.3
Oxygen saturation: 89%
Blood gas:
  pCO_2: 45
  pO_2: 30
COVID-19 rapid: positive
CXR: Diffuse lung consolidations

DIFFERENTIAL DIAGNOSIS

Given patient exposure and presenting symptoms, a COVID-19 rapid test was performed upon arrival to the emergency department (ED). This patient tested positive for COVID-19, ruling in the diagnosis of COVID-19 pneumonitis. The patient's oxygen saturation on arrival at 89% and blood gas levels are concerning for hypoxemia and acute respiratory distress syndrome (ARDS).[1] In addition, the patient meets sepsis criteria given abnormal vitals including heart rate >90 bmp, respiratory rate >20, temperature >100.4 °F, and suspected infection.[2]

HOSPITAL COURSE

The patient was admitted to the hospital due to ARDS and COVID-19 pneumonitis. After failing high-flow nasal cannula, the patient was transferred to the ICU and placed on mechanical ventilation. Medications recommended by the National Institute of Health for mechanically ventilated patients with COVID-19 were provided. First, immunomodulators including dexamethasone plus tocilizumab (interleukin [IL]-6 inhibitor) and/or baricitinib (Janus kinase [JAK] inhibitor) have been shown to reduce the mortality rate of COVID-19 hospitalized patients.[3] Second, the patient was started on remdesivir, a broad-spectrum antiviral medication. Remdesivir has been found to be effective in treating COVID-19 in patients who have presented early in the course of disease who are at high risk for developing severe COVID-19, or for COVID-19 patients requiring high-flow nasal cannula oxygen.[3] Remdesivir is not recommended for COVID-19 patients who are not at risk of developing severe COVID-19 or for patients requiring mechanical ventilation or extracorporeal membrane oxygenation (ECMO).[3] Since T.M. started remdesivir before failing high-flow nasal cannula oxygenation, his course of remdesivir was continued to completion. Finally, the patient was started on prophylactic heparin for anticoagulation therapy given increased risk for thrombotic event.[3]

During the patient's hospital course, he was consulted to the osteopathic neuromusculoskeletal manipulative medicine (ONMM) service that provided 3 to 5 weekly osteopathic manipulative treatments (OMT).

T.M. required mechanical ventilation for 15 days. He remained in the hospital for an additional 9 days to normalize body function and regain strength. After 24 days in the hospital, he was discharged home with rehabilitation resources.

OMT APPROACHES TO THE COVID-19 HOSPITALIZED PATIENT

The OMT approach to the COVID-19 hospitalized patient is like most inpatient OMT, with a few applications of OMT specific to COVID-19 manifestations. Inflammation should be addressed by treatments to the lymphatic and vascular systems. As circulatory structures such as the aorta, vena cava, and lymphatic duct pass through diaphragms, lymphatic and diaphragm treatments are essential to promote optimal flow of fluids, nutrition, and metabolites in the body. Myofascial release or other OMT modalities to the pelvic, respiratory, and thoracic inlet diaphragms should be considered. Lymphatic pumps such as the pedal pump should be considered to stimulate lymphatic circulation.[4]

The autonomic nervous system and any segmental facilitation should also be addressed in the COVID-19 hospitalized patient. Given the propensity for lung involvement in the disease process, there are likely to be viscerosomatic reflexes in the upper thoracic spine (T2–T5). Attention should be given along the sympathetic chain of T1–L2 for multiorgan involvement. In addition, parasympathetic effects should be investigated at the occipito-atlanto joint and the sacrum.[5]

For the COVID-19 hospitalized patient, neuroendocrine immune considerations should be investigated within the hypothalamic–pituitary–adrenal axis. The hypothalamus monitors information throughout the body including information about immunity and inflammation. Through a hormonal cascade, information is propagated through the pituitary and adrenal glands to support homeostasis. By utilizing osteopathic cranial manipulative medicine (OCMM) such as balanced membranous tension (BMT) or sphenobasilar synchondrosis (SBS) decompression, the sphenoid can be treated to affect homeostasis through important local structures such as the diaphragma sella, pituitary gland, and venous portal circulation.[4]

The thorax is of significant concern when treating the COVID-19 hospitalized patient with OMT. Given the involvement of the lungs in pneumonitis, the rib cage and surrounding structures should be treated. Rib raising or rib balanced ligamentous tension (BLT) are two such treatments that are beneficial in mobilizing the rib cage. The functioning of the respiratory diaphragm should be insured with a diaphragm treatment such as re-doming of the diaphragm.[4]

More specifically to COVID-19, restriction of mediastinal structures such as the pleura of the lungs and heart should be investigated. Visceral techniques are beneficial in improving the inherent motion of these organs which may optimize organ function and improve lymphatic drainage. In addition, the cranium should be palpated for SBS strain and addressed with BMT or SBS decompression to enhance primary respiration, neurologic function and cerebrospinal fluid (CSF) circulation.[4]

OSTEOPATHIC MANAGEMENT

Biomechanical Model

The biomechanical approach to the COVID-19 hospitalized patient involves the understanding of anatomical infrastructure and inherent motions of the body.

Awake prone positioning is a postural consideration for non-mechanically ventilated patients with ARDS on high-flow nasal cannula. Use of prone positioning involves the patient lying on their stomach for as many hours as is tolerated in the day with a typical average of 5 hours. This change in gross positioning has been found to improve oxygenation and reduce the risk of progression to mechanical ventilation.[6]

The COVID-19 hospitalized patient should be assessed for somatic dysfunction which may compromise biomechanical function of the body. When addressing a COVID-19 hospitalized patient with an osteopathic structural exam and OMT, consideration should be given to the lymphatic system, diaphragms, autonomic nervous system, thorax, and cranium which contribute to the overall function and health of the body.[4]

Respiratory–Circulatory Model

The respiratory–circulatory model is perhaps the most impactful model for the COVID-19 hospitalized patient, as the disease process so heavily burdens the respiratory and circulatory systems. Moderate COVID-19 is diagnosed in patients with evidence of lower respiratory disease with an oxygen saturation ≥94% on room air at sea level. Severe COVID-19 is diagnosed in patients with an oxygen saturation <94%, respiratory rate >30 breaths/min, or lung infiltration >50%.[7]

COVID-19 pneumonitis has grave effects on the body's capacity to facilitate breathing and oxygenation. With infectious processes taking place in the alveoli, inflammation assaults the lungs. The activation of inflammatory cascades involving bradykinin, leukotrienes, and macrophages cause leaky capillaries which worsen the fluid burden in the alveoli.[8] In addition, it is difficult for oxygen to reach capillary membranes and enter pulmonary circulation. This results in compromised cellular respiration and the hypoxemic findings common on pulse oximetry and blood gas readings. As the body fails to oxygenate, it recruits accessory muscles such as the rectus abdominus, intercostals, and scalenes to aid in the mechanical breathing process.[9] This recruitment has deleterious and exhausting impacts on the body, because involvement of more muscle groups demands more oxygen, of which there is a shortage.

When a patient is on a mechanical ventilator, the rate and volume of the machine overrides the inherent motion of the lungs and rib cage. The external stimulation of thoracic motion compromises the function of numerous structures in the thoracic cavity including the diaphragm, lymphatic vessels, and thoracic viscera. Effects on the diaphragm will influence not just breathing, but the gastrointestinal tract. The loss of pressure gradients derived from sporadic inspiration and expiration will diminish the lymphatic return to the terminal drainage site at the thoracic duct. Overriding the inherent motion of the lungs may lead to somatic dysfunction of the rib cage and thoracic spine as well as other fascial strains of the pulmonary and cardiac pleura.[9]

COVID-19 hospitalized patients are at risk for thrombosis. The elevation in inflammatory markers is associated with this increased risk.[10]

Neurologic Model

A large component of the neurologic model in the context of the COVID-19 hospitalized patient is the autonomic nervous system and how it is implicated in the organs most affected by COVID-19. The most affected organ are the lungs, though there may be systemic effects to other organs including the heart, gastrointestinal tract, and kidneys.

Viscerosomatic reflexes may be impacted by the sympathetic nervous system. For the lungs, viscerosomatic reflexes are likely to occur from T2 to T5. Findings for the heart are likely to occur at T4 to T5. Findings for the gastrointestinal tract are likely to occur from T5 to L2. Findings for the kidneys are likely to occur from T11 to L1.[11]

Viscerosomatic reflexes may also occur at parasympathetically innervated sites. The upper viscera including the lungs, heart, and upper gastrointestinal tract (before the splenic flexure of the colon) will be impacted by the vagus nerve. Viscerosomatic reflexes may manifest at the occipito-atlanto joint where the vagus nerve courses. Lower structures including the lower gastrointestinal tract (past the splenic flexure of the colon) will be influenced by the pelvic splanchnic nerves.[11]

Metabolic Energy Model

Within the metabolic energy model, inflammation is a strong component of the disease process in a COVID-19 hospitalized patient. Hospitalized COVID-19 patients requiring oxygen were found to have improved mortality rates when treated with corticosteroids such as dexamethasone. It is thought that the treatment reduces the systemic inflammatory process incited by COVID-19 infection that leads to lung injury and systemic multisystem organ dysfunction.[12]

Another aspect of the inflammatory process of COVID-19 is the activation of IL-6 which is a proinflammatory cytokine produced by numerous cells such as lymphocytes, monocytes, endothelial cells, and fibroblasts. When the body encounters foreign antigens via toll-like receptors (TLRs), signaling cascades produce IL-6. IL-6 propagates the signal by inducing liver production of proinflammatory molecules such as C-reactive protein.[8] One of the FDA-approved medications for immunomodulation in the COVID-19 hospitalized patient is tocilizumab, an IL-6 inhibitor.[13]

Similarly, Janus kinase (JAK) is an enzyme involved in the inflammatory cascade by catalyzing phosphorylation of the signal transducer and activator of cellular transcription (STAT) proteins. This enzyme is signaled by inflammatory cytokines such as IL-6 and contributes to immune activation and inflammation. This process is easily targeted by medications such as tofacitinib, a JAK inhibitor, to reduce inflammation in the COVID-19 hospitalized patient requiring oxygenation.[14]

Metabolic health of any individual is influenced by diet including vitamins and minerals. Vitamin C, vitamin D, and zinc may benefit a COVID-19 patient. However, current clinical trials on the effects of vitamin C, vitamin D, and zinc are limited by study design or population size. Vitamin C is a water-soluble vitamin that is an antioxidant, giving it anti-inflammatory properties. It promotes cellular immunity and vascular health.[15] Vitamin D is a fat-soluble vitamin involved in bone mineralization. White blood cells including B cells and T cells express vitamin D receptors and metabolize vitamin D,[16] which may indicate that vitamin D has immunomodulatory properties which may benefit COVID-19 patients. Zinc is a mineral which has been found to impair the replication of numerous RNA viruses.[17] The impact of zinc on COVID-19 is under investigation.

Behavioral Model

Human behavior is highly implicated in the prevention and contraction of COVID-19. SARs-CoV-2, the virus responsible for COVID-19, is spread via respiratory droplets that are inhaled, or contaminated hands that touch and infect mucous membranes. Current vaccination series are recommended for eligible patients age ≥6 months.[18]

The concept of addressing the patient as a triad of mind, body, and spirit is prominent for the COVID-19 hospitalized patient. As these patients are facing a life-threatening illness, addressing the spiritual aspect of their life may be welcome.[19]

SUMMARY

COVID-19 in the hospitalized patient is a complicated disease process involving pneumonitis and systemic inflammation. There are guidelines which are helpful in identifying severity and providing appropriate medications and oxygenation that improve mortality and morbidity. Research and clinical trials are ongoing at the time of this publication.

While research on OMT and the COVID-19 hospitalized patient is limited, there are sources supporting the role of OMT in the hospitalized patient. An osteopathic approach to a COVID-19 hospitalized patient should be targeted at improving lymphatic and vascular circulation, respiratory biomechanics, neurologic communication, metabolic turnover, and disease prevention.

REFERENCES

1. MDCalc. Horwitz index for lung function (P/F Ration). 2005–2023. Accessed May 31, 2023. https://www.mdcalc.com/calc/4062/horowitz-index-lung-function-p-f-ratio
2. MDCalc. SIRS, sepsis, and septic shock criteria. 2005–2023. Accessed May 22, 2023. https://www.mdcalc.com/calc/1096/sirs-sepsis-septic-shock-criteria
3. National Institute of Health. Therapeutic management of hospitalized adults with COVID-19. Updated April 20, 2023. Accessed May 22, 2023. https://www.covid19treatmentguidelines.nih.gov/management/clinical-management-of-adults/hospitalized-adults–therapeutic-management
4. Ettlinger H. Additional osteopathic manipulative treatment approaches: acutely ill or hospitalized patient: osteopathic considerations and approaches using OMT. In: Seffinger MA, ex. ed. *Foundations of Osteopathic Medicine.* 4th ed. Wolters Kluwer; 2018:923–944; chapter 40A.
5. Kuchera ML, Ettlinger H, Seffinger MA. Assessing viscerosomatic reflexes and somatosomatic reflexes, jones tender points, trigger points, and chapman reflexes. In: Seffinger MA, ed. *Foundations of Osteopathic Medicine.* 4th ed. Wolters Kluwer; 2018:767; chapter 31.
6. National Institute of Health. Oxygenation and ventilation for adults. Updated April 20, 2023. Accessed May 22, 2023. https://www.covid19treatmentguidelines.nih.gov/management/critical-care-for-adults/oxygenation-and-ventilation-for-adults
7. National Institute of Health. Clinical spectrum of SARS-CoV-2 infection. Updated March 6, 2023. Accessed May 22,2023. https://www.covid19treatmentguidelines.nih.gov/overview/clinical-spectrum
8. Thrush GR. The role of inflammation in healing and homeostasis. In: Seffinger MA, ed. *Foundations of Osteopathic Medicine.* 4th ed. Wolters Kluwer; 2018:350–361; chapter 15.
9. Willard FH, D'Alonzo GE Jr, Krachman SL. Anatomy, mechanics, and physiology of pulmonary respiration. In: Seffinger MA, ed. *Foundations of Osteopathic Medicine.* 4th ed. Wolters Kluwer; 2018:196–197; chapter 9.
10. Al-Samkari H, Karp Leaf RS, Dzik, WH, et al. COVID-19 and coagulation: bleeding and thrombotic manifestations of SARS-Co-V-2 infection. *Blood.* 2020;136(4):489–500.
11. Willard FH, Kuchera WA. Autonomic nervous system. In: Seffinger MA, ed. *Foundations of Osteopathic Medicine.* 4th ed. Wolters Kluwer; 2018: 224–225; chapter 10.
12. National Institute of Health. Corticosteroids. Updated April 20, 2023. Accessed May 23, 2023. https://www.covid19treatmentguidelines.nih.gov/therapies/immunomodulators/corticosteroids
13. National Institute of Health. Interleukin-6 inhibitors. Updated April 20, 2023. Accessed May 23, 2023. https://www.covid19treatmentguidelines.nih.gov/therapies/immunomodulators/interleukin-6-inhibitors
14. National Institute of Health. Janus kinase inhibitors. Updated April 20, 2023. Accessed May 23, 2023. https://www.covid19treatmentguidelines.nih.gov/therapies/immunomodulators/janus-kinase-inhibitors
15. National Institute of Health. Vitamin C. Updated September 26, 2022. Accessed May 23, 2023. https://www.covid19treatmentguidelines.nih.gov/therapies/supplements/vitamin-c
16. National Institute of Health. Vitamin D. Updated September 26, 2022. Accessed May 23, 2023. https://www.covid19treatmentguidelines.nih.gov/therapies/supplements/vitamin-d
17. National Institute of Health. Zinc. Updated March 6, 2023. Accessed May 23, 2023. https://www.covid19treatmentguidelines.nih.gov/therapies/supplements/zinc/.
18. National Institute of Health. Prevention of SARS-Co-V-2 infection. Updated March 6, 2023. Accessed May 23, 2023. https://www.covid19treatmentguidelines.nih.gov/overview/prevention-of-sars-cov-2
19. Fernandez-Sweeny Y, Rogers FJ. Behavioral medicine: spirituality and healthcare. In: Seffinger MA, ed. *Foundations of Osteopathic Medicine.* 4th ed. Wolters Kluwer; 2018:432–435; chapter 19C.

109 Case Study: Rhinosinusitis

SHAN SHAN WU ▪ ROBERT W. HOSTOFFER

KEY CONCEPTS

- The five models of osteopathic care can be utilized as a framework for the treatment of acute rhinosinusitis.
- OMT is used to improve the physiologic function of the sinuses including improving fluid drainage, decrease pain and viscerosomatic and somatovisceral reflexes, and alter mucous viscosity.
- Pharmacotherapy, adjunctive therapies, and surgical intervention may be indicated in selected individuals.

CASE VIGNETTE

HISTORY OF PRESENT ILLNESS

JP is a 42-year-old woman who presents to the family practice clinic complaining of headache, fever, and a scratchy throat for the past 3 days. This has been accompanied by a sensation of "fullness" in her face, pressure behind her eyes, nasal congestion, sensitivity of her nose, pain in her upper teeth, and fatigue. At times, she is sensitive to light and sounds and has a decreased sense of smell. A week earlier, she had a "cold" for which she took an over-the-counter "cold and sinus" preparation. She has a history of similar symptoms 2 to 3 years ago and was treated with antibiotics.

PAST MEDICAL HISTORY

She was hospitalized for uncomplicated vaginal delivery at age 29. Her most recent mammogram was 18 months ago and was reported as normal.

PAST SURGICAL HISTORY

She had a tonsillectomy at age 5, for which she was not hospitalized. She has had no other surgeries.

ALLERGIES

She has no known allergies to medications or food.

MEDICATIONS

Over-the-counter cold and sinus preparation. No prescription medications.

FAMILY HISTORY

Father has hypertension. Mother, sister, and brother are all healthy. No family history of heart disease (other than the father's hypertension), diabetes, stroke, or asthma.

SOCIAL HISTORY

She smokes half a pack of cigarettes per day, has an occasional glass of wine, and she denies illicit drug use. She is married with one child. She lives with two indoor dogs. She works part time as a dental hygienist.

REVIEW OF SYSTEMS

HEENT

She reports having watery, itchy eyes in the spring. She denies any blurred vision, diplopia, or eye pain. Other symptoms as noted in the HPI.

Respiratory

She reports occasional morning cough and gets "colds" several times a year. She denies difficulty breathing or wheezing.

Cardiovascular

She denies chest pain, syncope, shortness of breath, irregular heartbeats, palpitations, or edema of the extremities.

Gastrointestinal

She denies nausea, vomiting, abdominal pain, diarrhea, constipation, or changes in bowel habits.

Genitourinary

G1P1. She denies hematuria, frequency, urgency, or pelvic pain.

Musculoskeletal

She reports frequent neck and upper back stiffness and aching. She denies weakness, muscle cramping, or other areas of back pain.

Neurologic

She denies vertigo, unsteadiness, numbness, tingling, or radiating pain.

Psychological

She denies depression, anxiety, hallucinations, or alterations in consciousness. She reports normal sleep.

Endocrine

She denies intolerance to heat or cold, rashes, or changes in skin or hair.

Hematologic/Lymphatic

She denies swelling or abnormal bruising or bleeding.

PHYSICAL EXAMINATION

Vital Signs

Temperature 101.6°F, respirations 14/min, pulse 90 bpm, blood pressure 134/80, height 5′6″, weight 140 lb.

General

The patient is well-nourished, appears stated age, and is in no acute distress. She appears fatigued.

HEENT

Head is normocephalic and atraumatic. No conjunctival injection. Pupils are equal and reactive to light. Funduscopic evaluation is normal. Erythema and congestion of the nasal mucosa is noted. Mucopurulent drainage is noted with mild to moderate septal deviation caudally to the left. Posterior pharynx is inflamed with mucopurulent drainage. Tympanic membranes are dull with a questionable cone of light but have an adequate response to insufflation. Thyroid is not enlarged. Tenderness is noted over the bridge of the nose and over the maxillae and zygoma. Percussion over the maxilla intensifies the tenderness.

Lungs

Lungs are clear to auscultation in all fields. No wheezing noted and breathing is unlabored.

Heart

The heart has regular rate and rhythm with no murmurs auscultated. Capillary refill is less than 2 seconds. Nail beds and digits appear normal.

Abdomen

The abdomen is soft, nontender, and nondistended with no masses palpated. Bowel sounds are auscultated in all four quadrants.

Musculoskeletal

Extremities show no cyanosis, clubbing, or edema, and pulses are normal.

Neurologic

Patient is oriented to time and place and responds appropriately to questions. Cranial nerves II to XII are intact bilaterally. Deep tendon reflexes of upper and lower extremities are equally responsive. Sensation is intact to light touch and is intact of bilateral upper and lower extremities.

Lymphatic

There is no lymphadenopathy palpated in the cervical or supraclavicular areas bilaterally.

Skin

Skin color is normal. No rashes, plaques, or excoriations noted.

Osteopathic Structural Examination

Tenderness is palpated in the upper cervical, upper thoracic, and right supraclavicular areas. Further evaluation reveals the following somatic dysfunctions; C2 FSR_R, T2 FSR_L, and right rib 1 inhalation somatic dysfunction. Tenderness associated with slight nodularity is palpated anteriorly in the first intercostal space on the right and posteriorly between the spinous and the transverse process of C2 on the right. The suboccipital tissues are hypertonic and tender. There is decreased amplitude of the cranial rhythmic impulse, but the rate is normal.

DIFFERENTIAL DIAGNOSIS

Trigeminal neuralgia, migraine, dental abscess, and craniofacial neoplasm may be present with head and face pain and need to be considered as part of the differential diagnoses. Many patients use the term "sinus headache" without a specific diagnosis of sinus disease. It is the physician's responsibility, using clinical diagnostic skills, to differentiate the various causes of the patient's headache.[1,2]

Upper respiratory infections, nasal polyposis, nasal mass, and nasal foreign body are also possible. Additionally, inflammatory conditions in the nose and paranasal sinuses including allergic rhinitis and nonallergic rhinitis (vasomotor rhinitis) should be considered. JP has a history, symptoms, and examination findings supportive of a diagnosis of rhinosinusitis, with underlying allergic rhinitis or nonallergic rhinitis, both of which are characterized by nasal obstruction, increased secretions, and decreased olfaction.

- In allergic rhinitis, IgE-sensitized mast cells release allergic mediators, including histamine and leukotrienes, leading to a type I hypersensitivity reaction.
- In nonallergic rhinitis, irritants cause inflammation of the nasal mucosa.
- Inflammatory changes cause a hyperreactive nasal mucosa, with exaggerated neural response to all stimuli.
- Autonomic nervous system (ANS) dysfunction (hyperactive parasympathetic nervous system) has been demonstrated in nonallergic rhinitis.[3,4]
- Exposure to fungi is a possibility, but whether this is of consequence in JP's case is controversial.
    - Patients with chronic rhinosinusitis have been shown to exhibit exaggerated humoral and cellular responses to common airborne fungi, particularly Alternaria.[5]
    - On the contrary, Orlandi showed in a prospective in vitro study that IL-5 responses to Alternaria extract were not predictive of the presence of chronic rhinosinusitis.[6]
- The role of atopy in rhinosinusitis remains unclear. Allergy may serve as a contributing factor to rhinosinusitis, with an increased prevalence of allergic rhinitis in patients with chronic rhinosinusitis.[7,8]
- Lymphocytes, plasma cells, and eosinophils are present in the inflammatory infiltrate, similar to that of asthma.
- In a retrospective review of patients with allergic rhinitis without chronic rhinosinusitis, sinonasal anatomical variants, infraorbital cells, frontal intersinus cells, and asthma were found to be associated with faster development of chronic rhinosinusitis in patients with allergic rhinitis.[9]

JP was diagnosed with acute rhinosinusitis with nasopharyngitis. She has underlying structural abnormalities (deviated septum), and her tonsils have been surgically removed possibly due to recurrent infections throughout childhood. She likely has underlying allergic rhinitis with environmental exposures to tobacco smoke and dog dander.

PATIENT MANAGEMENT

The osteopathic physician can use the five models of osteopathic care as a framework to approach the patient suffering from acute rhinosinusitis to provide comprehensive treatment. One may focus on a single model or, as often happens, combine several models in a treatment plan.

Neurologic Model

- As mentioned earlier in this chapter, the ANS plays a crucial role in the physiologic function of the nose and paranasal sinuses.[10,11] The ANS plays a major role in regulating nasal airflow and at least some role in mucociliary transport mechanisms.[11] Proper balance of the sympathetic and parasympathetic systems and appropriate response of the sensory nerves are necessary for optimal function. Disease of the nose and paranasal sinuses results when these factors are dysfunctional, poorly balanced, and in the presence of inflammation.[12] Afferent nerves also provide protective reflexes.
- The parasympathetic effect of vasodilation is much less significant than the glandular effect of nasal secretion.[11]
- Several neuropeptides are associated with the nasal parasympathetic system[12]:
  - Acetylcholine
  - Vasoactive intestinal peptide
  - Neuropeptide Y (inhibitory agonist on parasympathetically induced ciliary beating nerves)
  - Nitric oxide (NO)
  - Enkephalin
  - Somatostatin
- Nitric oxide is thought to be an activator of ciliary beat frequency.[13]
  - Low levels of nasal NO with decreased nitric oxide synthase expression are found in primary ciliary dyskinesia[14]; thus nasal NO can be used as a screening tool for primary ciliary dyskinesia.[15]
  - Low levels of nasal NO are also found in cystic fibrosis. In other upper airway disorders including rhinosinusitis, the use of NO remains to be established.[15]
- Vasoconstriction, caused by the release of norepinephrine and neuropeptide Y, is the primary effect of the sympathetic nerves on the nasal and paranasal sinus mucosa.[12]
- Stimulation of sympathetic nerves has minimal effect on nasal mucus secretion.[12]
- Afferent nerves of the nose and paranasal sinuses have critical roles in maintaining and restoring homeostasis:
  - Afferent nerves that supply the nose are derived from the olfactory nerve and ophthalmic and maxillary branches of cranial nerve V.
  - These nerves provide protective reflexes. For example, exposing the nasal mucosa to mechanical irritation, allergens, or cold air elicits a response of sneezing, coughing, apnea, or avoidance behavior. This occurs through an axonal reflex.
  - They also recruit systemic autonomic reflexes and mediate vascular, glandular, and inflammatory defenses.
  - Stimulation of these afferent nerves leads to the release of neuropeptides such as:
    - Calcitonin gene-related peptide
    - Gastrin-releasing peptide
    - Substance P
    - Neurokinin A

Increase in these sensory neuropeptides along with reduction of their catabolism leads to the process of neurogenic inflammation.[16] Symptoms resulting from nasal neurogenic inflammation are those common to rhinosinusitis—nasal obstruction, rhinorrhea, and headache. Interestingly, similar symptoms accompany migraine and may also implicate neuropeptides in the causal relationship.[17]

Autonomic influence on lymphatic contractility suggests a role for osteopathic manipulative techniques to improve lymphatic circulation not only for its impact on muscle tone but also on autonomic tone.[18]

Osteopathic manipulation's impact on somatovisceral and viscerosomatic reflexes offers a mechanism to improve autonomic balance to the upper respiratory mucosa. If, for instance, somatic dysfunction in the upper thoracic or upper cervical area is inhibiting sympathetic tone or if parasympathetic tone is facilitated by dysfunction of the sphenoid and palatine areas, the nasal mucosa would be congested and/or produce excessive mucus.

- Irritation of the sensory nerves in the nose and sinuses clearly adds to neurogenic inflammation by way of antidromic stimulation and release of neuropeptides.[10,11]
  - Addressing factors, such as pain and mechanical irritation, which excessively stimulate those reflexes in the nose, can offer an opportunity to reduce inflammation of the nasal mucosa.[12]

Metabolic Energy Model

Rhinitis usually precedes sinusitis, sinusitis without rhinitis is rare, and the mucosa of the nose continues into the sinuses.[19] Rhinosinusitis is the inflammation of at least one paranasal sinus and nasal cavity. The 2018 US National Health Interview Survey data conducted by the Centers for Disease Control and Prevention estimated 28.9 million adults diagnosed with sinusitis in the 12 months before the survey.[20]

DIAGNOSTIC ISSUES

- Acute rhinosinusitis: symptoms greater than 10 days and resolves within 12 weeks.
  - "Acute" may also be defined as symptoms greater than 10 days and less than 4 weeks and "subacute" with symptoms between 4 and 12 weeks.[21]
- Recurrent acute rhinosinusitis: at least three episodes of acute rhinosinusitis annually, each episode lasting ≥7 days interspersed with symptom-free intervals.
- Chronic rhinosinusitis: symptoms greater than 12 weeks.
  - Chronic rhinosinusitis is further divided into chronic rhinosinusitis without nasal polyps and chronic rhinosinusitis with nasal polyps.
  - Chronic rhinosinusitis differs in histopathology, prognosis, and management from acute rhinosinusitis.

Predisposing factors to rhinosinusitis include allergy, upper respiratory infections, anatomic abnormalities, ciliary dyskinesia, cystic fibrosis, immune deficiencies, and environmental factors. The patient's medical history, symptoms, physical examination, and at times, labs and/or imaging help guide the physician in the diagnosis and treatment of rhinosinusitis. Often, acute bacterial rhinosinusitis is diagnosed in patients with symptoms of upper respiratory infection persisting longer than 10 to 14 days in addition to dental pain.

JP exhibits classical findings of acute rhinosinusitis. Although transillumination of the sinuses is a valuable diagnostic tool for some practitioners, it has been found to be unreliable for definitive diagnosis.[22]

Acute rhinosinusitis does not usually warrant radiographic diagnosis. Plain film radiographs, ultrasonography, computerized tomography (CT), and magnetic resonant imaging (MRI) of the sinuses should be avoided in the diagnosis of acute rhinosinusitis and reserved for patients at risk for complications. Radiographs and CTs have high false-positive rates for acute rhinosinusitis, and radiography is not cost-effective compared to the use of clinical criteria with indicated treatment regimens.[23]

DIAGNOSIS OF RECURRENT ACUTE RHINOSINUSITIS

Patients with recurrent acute rhinosinusitis exhibit similar symptoms and physical findings as that of acute rhinosinusitis. Patients usually remain asymptomatic or have mild rhinitis symptoms between active episodes. Culture of the sinus secretions can be used to select the appropriate antibiotic therapy. This can be done by aspiration of the maxillary sinus or resection of the middle meatus during endoscopy.

DIAGNOSIS OF CHRONIC RHINOSINUSITIS

Gram-positive aerobes such as coagulase negative *Staphylococcus* and *Staphylococcus aureus* and gram-negative aerobes such as *Haemophilus influenzae* and *Pseudomonas aeruginosa* are commonly found in endoscopically derived bacterial cultures from chronic sinusitis patients. Common anaerobes found include *Peptostreptococcus*, *Bacteroides*, and *Prevotella species*.[24,25] The clinical manifestations of chronic rhinosinusitis are similar to acute rhinosinusitis with more subtle symptoms such as milder pain. In contrast to the acute phase, nasal congestion and olfactory disturbances are more common in chronic rhinosinusitis. On physical examination, the findings are similar to that of acute rhinosinusitis plus possible finding of middle ear effusion. CT of the sinus is the imaging modality of choice as it shows the structures of the ostiomeatal complex and the sinus cavities. CT of the sinus is recommended to be performed 4 to 6 weeks after initiation of medical therapy. Abnormal findings on endoscopy or on a sinus CT scan can be used to confirm the diagnosis.

Evaluation for recurrent acute rhinosinusitis and chronic rhinosinusitis should include testing for predisposing factors, such as aeroallergen testing.

AIRWAY PATENCY AND MUCOCILIARY TRANSPORT

Metabolic-related processes are dependent upon airway patency (respiratory model) and mucociliary transport mechanisms (neurologic–metabolic models) which are in turn affected by biomechanical/structural, neurologic, circulatory, metabolic, and behavioral influences.

Factors Influencing Airway Patency

1. Anatomic structures can compromise airway patency such as:
   - □ Collapsed nasal valve
   - □ Deviated nasal septum
   - □ Nasal polyps
   - □ Turbinate hypertrophy
2. Neural dysfunctions are also associated with upper airway disorders.
   - □ Loehrl suggests that hypoactive sympathetic influence leads to increased nasal airway resistance.[26]
   - □ Vasodilatation, due to increased activity of sensory neuropeptides, occurs in patients with hyperactive nasal mucosa characteristic of allergic and nonallergic rhinitis, as well as chronic rhinosinusitis.[12]
3. Lymphatic congestion due to a variety of causes may add to edema of the mucosa and poor nasal airflow.
4. Infectious processes, especially viral upper respiratory infection, can cause swelling and decreased airway patency.
   - □ Overuse of topical nasal decongestants leads to "rhinitis medicamentosa," or rebound nasal congestion, and loss of responsiveness to topical decongestants.[27,28]

Factors Influencing Mucociliary Transport

The viscosity of mucus and the ciliary beat frequency are two of the main determinants in the quality of mucociliary clearance. Primary ciliary dyskinesia is an intrinsic disorder that reduces the ciliary beat frequency.

Factors affecting viscosity of mucus include:

- Anticholinergic antihistamines
- Poor hydration
- Dairy products
- Cystic fibrosis
  - □ A hereditary disease caused by mutation of the cystic fibrosis transmembrane conductance regular (CFTR) gene, causing thick, abundant respiratory secretions and chronic infections.[29]

Other factors reducing mucociliary clearance include:

- Decreased number of cilia or changes in the mucus in cigarette smokers.[30–32]
- Inflammatory conditions of the nose, sinuses, and airways (allergic and nonallergic rhinitis, rhinosinusitis, and bronchiectasis).[33–35]
- Chronic inflammatory conditions, as seen in patients with chronic infection and in diabetics.

TREATMENT/MANAGEMENT FROM THE PERSPECTIVE OF THE METABOLIC ENERGY MODEL

When evaluating a patient with rhinosinusitis, attention needs to be paid to the factors that decrease airway patency, air flow, and effective mucociliary transport. Treatment can then be directed toward the specific factors influencing each patient's problem.

- An exposure to an allergen might predispose the atopic patient to the development of rhinosinusitis.[7–9,23] Allergic signs and symptoms, such as sneezing, itchy or watery eyes, clear rhinorrhea, and nasal itching, should be noted and their treatment should be integrated into patient care. Furthermore, proper management of chronic rhinosinusitis often results in the improvement of concomitant asthma.
- Fatigue is a complaint that often accompanies rhinosinusitis. Working from a bioenergetic perspective, the physician would consider the impact of somatic dysfunction on body efficiency and energy expenditure. Though not totally explained, there also seems to be therapeutic effect related to the energetic interaction of various hands-on treatment modalities. An awareness of how osteopathic manipulation may impact the patient's feeling of well-being as well as their ability to function more efficiently is consistent with the bioenergetic model.

Biomechanical Model

Osteopathic manipulative treatment (OMT) offers a nonpharmacologic approach to rhinosinusitis. Attention to the possibility of dysfunction in the cranial base and facial bones should be part of the evaluation of any patient with rhinosinusitis.

- Manipulative treatment specific to any identified cranial dysfunction is part of addressing the biomechanical issues of both acute and chronic rhinosinusitis.
- Sutherland describes rhythmic movement of the facial bones (zygoma, maxilla, palatines, and vomer) acting like a "plunger" on the sphenoid and maxillary sinuses to promote air exchange.[36,37] The vomer, forming part of the nasal septum, is important in directing airflow. The location of the sphenopalatine ganglion, as noted above, surrounded by the palatine, sphenoid, and maxillary bones, puts it at risk for mechanical compromise if there is history of facial trauma or cranial somatic dysfunction.
- Many patients with nasal and sinus congestion have tenderness over the area of the ethmoid notch of the frontal bone and respond to release of compression in that area.[38]

- There are also mechanical considerations in the obstruction of venous and lymphatic flow from the head and neck. For example, a variation where the ethmoid cells pneumatize into the middle turbinate, "concha bullosa," leads to enlargement of the turbinates and subsequent narrowing of the ostiomeatal complex.

Respiratory–Circulatory Model

Engorgement of the nasal mucosa, which occurs during sleeping, causes sinus-related pain to be worse in the morning, improving after the patient is upright for a time. Adequate lymphatic and venous circulations are vital to reducing swelling in any part of the body, and the tissues of the upper respiratory system are without exception. Removing metabolic waste products and inflammatory mediators that have accumulated in the tissues is another function of the lymphatic system. It has already been noted that the neuropeptides released from the sensory nerves, when stimulated in the nasal and paranasal mucosa, explain some of the symptoms of rhinosinusitis. OMT focused on removing impediments to venous and lymphatic circulation and stimulating flow when appropriate would aid in decreasing swelling and inflammation in the nasal region.

Impediment to flow often presents in the form of myofascial tightness or constriction. Of particular interest is the anatomical area through which the lymph vessels, the thoracic duct, and right lymphatic duct must course to join the venous system. Working within the respiratory/circulatory model would include releasing myofascial tensions in the neck and upper thorax, particularly in the areas of the trapezius and sternocleidomastoid muscles, clavicle, and first rib.

- Superficial lymphatic drainage techniques such as effleurage to the face are directed at lymphatic flow as it leaves the nose and enters the lymphatics of the skin.[38–40]
- Inhalation/exhalation motion of the ribs and diaphragm excursion also create a pump-like action for venous and lymphatic circulation with alternating negative and positive pressure in the thoracic cavity. Treating somatic dysfunction of the ribs, diaphragm, and their attachments promotes optimal venous and lymphatic circulation via this mechanism.[41]
- There are also lymphatic pump and effleurage techniques intended to increase lymphatic circulation once the impediments to flow are removed, including:
  - ☐ Thoracic pump[42]
  - ☐ Pedal pump[42]
  - ☐ Galbreath technique for mandibular drainage[43]

Arterial vasomotor tone is controlled by the sympathetic nervous system and may be influenced by somatic dysfunction of the upper neck as the origin for sympathetic nerves supplying the head and neck is primarily located within the superior cervical ganglion as well as the T1–T3 region. Lymphatic contractility in the head and neck is also mediated by these sympathetic nerves.[18]

Biopsychosocial/Behavioral Model

From an osteopathic point of view, educating patients as to behaviors that assist the body's innate healing can go hand in hand with OMT.

Lifestyle modifications are important aspects in the treatment of rhinosinusitis, for example:

- Smoking cessation
- Allergen avoidance
- Adequate hydration
- Efficient breathing mechanics
- Stress relief

Educating patients on the appropriate use of all pharmacologic agents and symptomatic treatment options will generally improve patient compliance and satisfaction.

Palpation and identification of the structural and biomechanical dysfunctions associated with their condition can give patients confidence and trust in the treating physician. Patients with chronic rhinosinusitis often experience frustration and difficulty with treatment options. The ability to give them symptomatic relief with manipulative techniques at the same office visit relieves some of the anxiety and stress that accompanies any disease.

Osteopathic Research Related to Sinusitis

Osteopathic literature is replete with studies describing the use of OMT to treat upper respiratory conditions including sinusitis. Primarily considered biomechanical treatment approaches, OMT is used to improve physiologic function in each of the five domains of osteopathic care. Thus, it has been used to improve fluid drainage from the sinuses (respiratory–circulatory model), decrease pain and viscerosomatic and somatovisceral reflexes, and alter mucus viscosity (neurologic, circulatory, and metabolic models). Examples include the following:

- Sphenopalatine ganglion stimulation of the parasympathetic system results in thinning of the mucus secretion as well as alleviating referred pain from maxillary sinuses.[44,45]
- In the 1930s, articles in "The Osteopathic Profession" describe osteopathic manipulative approaches to address lymphatic drainage, normalize circulation, and balance viscerosomatic relationships for patients with sinusitis.[46,47]
- L.M. Bush, DO, at the 1942 American Osteopathic Association meeting in Chicago presented, "How the 'Old Doctor' treated nose and throat conditions," stressing "correction of spinal lesions and lesions of the clavicle."[48]
- In each of the following decades, case reports, promoting the use of OMT for sinusitis, appear in the literature. Shrum et al. describe the integration of pharmacologic agents and OMT (occipitoatlantal decompression, rib raising, lymphatic pump, myofascial release to the cervical, thoracic and lumbar areas, and mandibular drainage technique) into the treatment of sinusitis in children.[49]
- Opinions expressed in letters to the editor of the *Journal of the American Osteopathic Association* in recent years advocated for the use of OMT in the treatment of sinusitis.[50,51]
- The physiologic studies of Sato and Schmidt showed that various types of mechanical, thermal, and chemical stimulation of the skin, muscles, and joints at various spinal levels produce reflex responses in visceral organs,[52] that somatic afferent nerve stimulation can reflexively regulate various visceral functions and gives credence to the practice of relieving somatic dysfunction in the upper thoracic and cervical spine to improve function of the upper respiratory mucosa.
- Beal reviewed the specific somatic manifestations of visceral disease. Correlation of palpatory findings with visceral diagnoses suggests that an osteopathic structural examination makes a valuable contribution to clinical diagnosis.[53]
- Data gathered by the survey responses of 955 osteopathic physicians indicated that 2.49% of the respondents used OMT to treat sinusitis.[54]
- A report on the use of OMT in the emergency department suggests that symptoms of sinusitis (as well as several other complaints) could be ameliorated or eliminated with OMT.[55]
- When students were surveyed regarding which conditions they anticipated using OMT as part of their treatment plan, 20% included sinusitis.[56]

Recommended Pharmacotherapy

Osteopathic care based on the above five models will remove obstructions to the patient's innate ability to self-heal and self-regulate and help restore optimum structure and function. Pharmacotherapy is another important component of the osteopathic tenets and may include the following when indicated.

Antibiotics

- Amoxicillin–clavulanate or amoxicillin is recommended as the first-line therapy in patients with rhinosinusitis who require antibiotics and do not have risk factors for resistance.[57]
- Alternatives such as doxycycline, levofloxacin, and moxifloxacin should only be used for patients allergic to both first-line drugs.
- Additionally, for penicillin-allergic patients who can tolerate cephalosporins, a third-generation oral cephalosporin (cefixime 400 mg daily or cefpodoxime 200 mg twice daily) prescribed with or without clindamycin (300 mg every 6 hours) is another option. Monotherapy with a third-generation cephalosporin is likely adequate for most patients, particularly those without risk factors for resistance.
- Macrolides and trimethoprim-sulfamethoxazole are no longer recommended for empiric treatment of acute bacterial rhinosinusitis due to emerging resistance.[57]
- Avoid fluoroquinolones and doxycycline in children.

Intranasal corticosteroids (INS)

- Intranasal corticosteroids can be used for the treatment of acute rhinosinusitis as monotherapy or with antibiotics.
- They are indicated also for chronic rhinosinusitis and nasal polyps.
- They decrease the inflammatory response and are more effective if used after an intranasal decongestant.

Systemic corticosteroids

- In the past, a short course of oral corticosteroids was recommended in conjunction with antibiotics for the treatment of chronic rhinosinusitis during an acute exacerbation.[19] However, the literature now suggests avoiding the use of systemic glucocorticoids in the treatment of acute bacterial rhinosinusitis. It appears that, when given in addition to antibiotics, oral glucocorticoids may shorten the time to symptom resolution or improvement, but the benefits are small and pose a potential risk for side effects that outweigh the clinical benefits.[58]

Since many cases of acute rhinosinusitis are due to viral infections and do not require antibiotics, treatment is targeted toward symptomatic management and inherent healing mechanisms. There still remains insufficient evidence for the benefit of adjunctive therapies such as decongestants and antihistamines. However, they are included in the list below for the sake of completeness.

ADJUNCTIVE THERAPIES

Decongestants

- Improve airflow and allow for better mucociliary transport and clearing of contaminants from the sinuses by targeting the hypoactive sympathetic response contributing to vasodilation of the nasal mucosa.
- Guidelines recommend limiting use within 3 days to prevent rebound congestion and decrease risk of adverse effects such as hypertension and cardiac arrhythmias, among others.
- Examples: sympathomimetics (phenylephrine) and alpha-receptor agonists (oxymetazoline, naphazoline).

Mucolytics

- Mucolytics are used to thin secretions.
- Guaifenesin has been associated with improvement of nasal congestion and thickened nasal secretions.
- Studies so far have been unable to demonstrate changes in mucociliary transport or ciliary beat frequency, so the mode of action is unclear.[59]

Antihistamines

- Antihistamines may be used if a patient has a history of atopy, such as seasonal allergic rhinitis.
- Since many patients have already used over-the-counter antihistamines to treat the symptoms of an upper respiratory infection, overdrying of the mucosa and thickening of the mucus may have occurred.
- First-generation antihistamines have sedative effects.
- Second-generation antihistamines are usually recommended given less CNS depression and mucosal drying.

Cysteinyl leukotriene blockers

- These agents such as montelukast and cromolyn have been indicated in the treatment of asthma and allergic rhinitis to decrease the inflammatory response.
- They are not recommended as first-line agents for rhinosinusitis and are not efficacious when used alone.

Considering the underlying pathophysiologic process can direct decision-making in recommendation of these therapies.

Promoting mucociliary clearance is essential to the overall treatment of rhinosinusitis and prevention of complication.

- Patients may be instructed to drink warm, clear fluids to hydrate the mucous membranes and refrain from drinking milk.
- Saline nasal irrigation may relieve symptoms and is a low-cost option.
- If the patient history is suggestive of an allergic component, such as perennial allergy symptoms, further allergy testing, and immunotherapy should be offered to reduce nasal inflammation. Patient education is essential in addressing the avoidance of allergens or irritants.
- Smoking cessation and avoidance of second-hand smoke and other chemical irritants are important for reducing inflammation and improving health of the mucous membranes.

COMPLICATIONS

Serious complications of acute bacterial sinusitis are rare, but patients with new ophthalmic (visual changes, abnormal extraocular movements, proptosis, periorbital inflammation) or neurologic signs and symptoms require a more in-depth workup and should be referred appropriately.

Local extension of infection can cause:

- Orbital or periorbital cellulitis
- Osteitis

Infection spread beyond the paranasal sinuses can cause:

- Meningitis
- Brain abscess
- Venous sinuses infection

CT is appropriate if any of the above complications are suspected.

Most patients with acute viral rhinosinusitis improve without antibiotics. However, a 7- to 14-day course of empiric antibiotics is recommended for patients who experience symptoms for more than 10 to 14 days, which is suggestive of acute bacterial rhinosinusitis, and for those with more severe symptoms including fever with purulent nasal discharge, facial pain/tenderness, and periorbital swelling.[19]

For partial resolution, the antibiotics can be continued for another 10 to 14 days or switched to an alternative antibiotic. If there is no improvement or worsening of symptoms within 3 to 5 days, consider broadening the microbial coverage or changing to an antibiotic that covers resistant pathogens.[19] Patient education regarding the incidence of antibiotic-resistant infections is important, whether antibiotic therapy is prescribed or not. Antimicrobial resistance information is available online at https://www.cdc.gov/drugresistance/[60]

CONSULTATION AND SURGICAL INTERVENTION

Consultation and referral to an otolaryngologist should be considered for patients who do not respond to treatment of acute rhinosinusitis, who have multiple recurrences, or who have polyps or other nasal structural problems contributing to chronic rhinosinusitis.

- Patients with chronic rhinosinusitis may require surgical intervention to remove polyps, correct a deviated septum, reduce the size of hypertrophied nasal turbinates, or address the patency of the sinus ostia.
- Of course, signs of potential complications such as periorbital edema, double vision, ophthalmoplegia, severe, unrelenting frontal headache, or focal neurologic signs require immediate referral.[19]

CONCLUSION

Experience, coupled with anatomic and physiologic principles, strongly suggests that diagnosing and treating sinusitis, like so many other conditions, can be enhanced by the utilization of osteopathic principles. This includes patient education and preventative care, musculoskeletal considerations for venous and lymphatic drainage and autonomic balance, and the use of other medical interventions that acknowledge the patient's self-healing mechanisms and respect their psychosocial milieu.

REFERENCES

1. Levine HL, Setzen M, Cady RK, et al. An otolaryngology, neurology, allergy, and primary care consensus on diagnosis and treatment of sinus headache. *Otolaryngol Head Neck Surg*. 2006;134(3):516–523.
2. Patel ZM, Setzen M, Poetker DM, DelGaudio JM. Evaluation and management of "sinus headache" in the otolaryngology practice. *Otolaryngol Clin North Am*. 2014;47(2):269–287.
3. Jaradeh SS, Smith TL, Torrico L, et al. Autonomic nervous system evaluation of patients with vasomotor rhinitis. *Laryngoscope*. 2000;110(11):1828–1831.
4. Vayisoglu Y, Ozcan C, Pekdemir H, Gorur K, Pata YS, Camsari A. Autonomic nervous system evaluation using heart rate variability parameters in vasomotor rhinitis patients. *J Otolaryngol*. 2006;35(5):338–342.
5. Shin SH, Ponikau JU, Sherris DA, et al. Chronic rhinosinusitis: an enhanced immune response to ubiquitous airborne fungi. *J Allergy Clin Immunol*. 2004;114(6):1369–1375.
6. Orlandi RR, Marple BF, Georgelas A, Durtschi D, Barr L. Immunologic response to fungus is not universally associated with rhinosinusitis. *Otolaryngol Head Neck Surg*. 2009;141(6):750.e1-2–756.e1-2.
7. Karlsson G, Holmberg K. Does allergic rhinitis predispose to sinusitis? *Acta Otolaryngol Suppl*. 1994;515:26–28.
8. Fokkens WJ, Lund VJ, Mullol J, et al. European position paper on rhinosinusitis and nasal polyps 2012. *Rhinol Suppl*. 2012;23:1–298.
9. Sedaghat AR, Gray ST, Chambers KJ, Wilke CO, Caradonna DS. Sinonasal anatomic variants and asthma are associated with faster development of chronic rhinosinusitis in patients with allergic rhinitis. *Int Forum Allergy Rhinol*. 2013;3(9):755–761.
10. Loehrl TA. Autonomic function and dysfunction of the nose and sinuses. *Otolaryngol Clin North Am*. 2005;38(6):1155–1161.
11. Yao A, Wilson JA, Ball SL. Autonomic nervous system dysfunction and sinonasal symptoms. *Allergy Rhinol (Providence)*. 2018;9:2152656718764233.
12. Lacroix JS. Chronic rhinosinusitis and neuropeptides. *Swiss Med Wkly*. 2003;113(41–42):560–562.
13. Landis BN, Beghetti M, Morel DR, Giger R, Rimensberger PC, Lacroix JS. Somato-sympathetic vasoconstriction to intranasal fluid administration with consecutive decrease in nasal nitric oxide. *Acta Physiol Scand*. 2003;177(4):507–515.
14. Pifferi M, Bush A, Maggi F, et al. Nasal nitric oxide and nitric oxide synthase expression in primary ciliary dyskinesia. *Eur Respir J*. 2011;37(3):572–527.
15. Manna A, Montella S, Maniscalco M. Clinical application of nasal nitric oxide measurement in pediatric airway disease. *Pediatr Pulmonol*. 2015;50(1):85–89.
16. Lacroix JS, Coignard RA. Neurogenic inflammation and chronic rhinosinusitis. *Rev Med Suisse*. 2005;1(37):2392–2395.
17. Bellamy JL, Cady RK, Durham PL. Salivary levels of CGRP and VIP in rhinosinusitis and migraine patients. *Headache*. 2006;46(1):24–33.
18. Degenhardt BF, Kuchera ML. Update on osteopathic medical concepts and the lymphatic system. *J Am Osteopath Assoc*. 1996;96(2):97–100.
19. Peters AT, Spector S, Hsu J, et al; Joint Task Force on Practice Parameters, representing the American Academy of Allergy, Asthma and Immunology, the American College of Allergy, Asthma and Immunology, and the Joint Council of Allergy, Asthma and Immunology. Diagnosis and management of rhinosinusitis: a practice parameter update. *Ann Allergy Asthma Immunol*. 2014;113(4):347–385.
20. Villarroel MA, Blackwell DL, Jen A. *Tables of Summary Health Statistics for U.S. Adults: 2018 National Health Interview Survey*. National Center for Health Statistics; 2019. Accessed January 3, 2023. http://www.cdc.gov/nchs/nhis/SHS/tables.htm
21. Rosenfeld RM. Clinical practice. Acute sinusitis in adults. *N Engl J Med*. 2016;375(10):962–970.
22. Otten FW, Grote JJ. The diagnostic value of transillumination of maxillary sinusitis in children. *Int J Pediatr Otorhinolaryngol*. 1989;18(1):9–11.
23. Fokkens W, Lund V, Bachert C, et al; EAACI. EAACI position paper of rhinosinusitis and nasal polyps executive summary. *Allergy*. 2005;60(5):583–601.
24. Finegold SM, Flynn MJ, Rose FV, et al. Bacteriologic findings associated with chronic bacterial maxillary sinusitis in adults. *Clin Infect Dis*. 2002;35(4):428–433.
25. Thanasumpun T, Batra PS. Endoscopically-derived bacterial cultures in chronic rhinosinusitis: A systematic review. *Am J Otolaryngol*. 2015;36(5):686–691.
26. Loehrl TA. Autonomic dysfunction, allergy and the upper airway. *Curr Opin Otolaryngol Head Neck Surg*. 2007;15(4):264–267.
27. Lin CY, Cheng PH, Fang SY. Mucosal changes in rhinitis medicamentosa. *Ann Otol Rhinol Laryngol*. 2004;113(2):147–151.
28. Knipping S, Holzhausen HJ, Goetze G, Riederer A, Bloching MB. Rhinitis medicamentosa: electron microscopic changes of human nasal mucosa. *Otolaryngol Head Neck Surg*. 2007;136(1):57–61.
29. Armengot M, Escribano A, Carda C, Sánchez C, Romero C, Basterra J. Nasal mucociliary transport and ciliary ultrastructure in cystic fibrosis: a comparative study with healthy volunteers. *Int J Pediatr Otorhinolaryngol*. 1997;40(1):27–44.
30. Stanley PJ, Wilson R, Greenstone MA, MacWilliam L, Cole PJ. Effect of cigarette smoking on nasal mucociliary clearance and ciliary beat frequency. *Thorax*. 1986;41(7):519–523.
31. Mahakit P, Pumhirun PA. A preliminary study of nasal mucociliary clearance in smokers, sinusitis and allergic rhinitis patients. *Asian Pac J Allergy Immunol*. 1995;13(2):119–121.
32. Cikojević D, Krnić M, Marčina S. Influence of smoking on the nasal mucosa mucociliary transport. *Acta Med Croatica*. 2014;68(3):247–251.
33. Schuhl JF. Nasal mucociliary clearance in perennial rhinitis. *J Investig Allergol Clin Immunol*. 1995;5(6):333–336.

34. Stanley PJ, Wilson R, Greenstone MA, Mackay IS, Cole PJ. Abnormal nasal mucociliary clearance in patients with rhinitis and its relationship to concomitant chest disease. *Br J Dis Chest.* 1985;79(1):77–82.
35. Awotedu AA, Babalola OO, Lawani EO, Hart PD. Abnormal mucociliary action in asthma and bronchiectasis. *Afr J Med Med Sci.* 1990;19(3):153–156.
36. Brooks RE. *Life in Motion: The Osteopathic Vision of Rollin E. Becker, D.O.* Rudra Press; 1997.
37. Sutherland WG. *Teachings in the Science of Osteopathy.* 1st ed. Rudra Press; 1990.
38. Careirro J. *An Osteopathic Approach to Children.* Churchill; 2003.
39. Moser RJ. Sinusitis, the effective osteopathic manipulative procedures in the management thereof. *Yearbook Acad Appl Osteopath.* 1953:15–16.
40. Schmidt IC. Osteopathic manipulative therapy as a primary factor in the management of upper, middle, and pararespiratory infections. *J Am Osteopath Assoc.* 1982;81(6):382–388.
41. Stiles EG. Osteopathic manipulation in a hospital environment. *Yearbook Am Acad Osteopath.* 1977:17–32.
42. Chikly BJ. Manual techniques addressing the lymphatic system: origins and development. *J Am Osteopath Assoc.* 2005;105(10):457–464.
43. Galbreath W. Manipulative structural adjustive treatment in middle ear deafness. *J Am Osteopath Assoc.* 1925;24:741.
44. Hoyt WH III. Current concepts in management of sinus disease. *J Am Osteopath Assoc.* 1990;90(10):913–919.
45. Travell JG, Simons DG. *Myofascial Pain and Dysfunction: A Trigger Point Manual.* Lippincott Williams & Wilkins; 1983.
46. Deason WJ. Specific circulatory results: in the field of Otolaryngology conditions. *Osteopath Prof.* 1935;2(9):7–11, 44, 46, 48.
47. Schoelles GJ. Treatment of Sinusitis: a technique for normalizing circulation in acute cases. *Osteopath Prof.* 1937;4(7):11–13.
48. Bush LM. How the old doctor treated nose and throat conditions. Selected papers from the sections of Technic and Manipulative Therapy. American Osteopathic Association. 1942:3–5.
49. Shrum KM, Grogg SE, Barton P, Shaw HH, Dyer RR. Sinusitis in children: the importance of diagnosis and treatment. *J Am Osteopath Assoc.* 2001;101(5 suppl):S8–S13.
50. Abend DS. Revisiting the role of osteopathic manipulation in primary care. *J Am Osteopath Assoc.* 1999;99(2):88–89.
51. Dudley G. Sinusitis supplement missing osteopathic component. *J Am Osteopath Assoc.* 1998;98(10):539–540.
52. Sato A, Schmidt RF. Reflex modulation of visceral functions by somatic afferent activity. *The central connection: somatovisceral/viscerosomatic interaction. Am Acad Osteopath Symp*; 1989:53–72.
53. Beal MC. Viscerosomatic reflexes: a review. *J Am Osteopath Assoc.* 1985;85(12):786–801.
54. Johnson SM, Kurtz ME. Conditions and diagnosis for which osteopathic primary care physicians and specialists use osteopathic manipulative treatment. *J Am Osteopath Assoc.* 2002;102(10):527–532, 537–540.
55. Paul F, Buser BR. Osteopathic manipulative treatment applications for the emergency department patient. *J Am Osteopath Assoc.* 1996;96(7):403–409.
56. Chamberlain NR, Yates HA. A prospective study of osteopathic medical students' attitudes toward use of osteopathic manipulative treatment in caring for patients. *J Am Osteopath Assoc.* 2003;103(10):470–478.
57. Chow AW, Benninger MS, Brook I, et al; Infectious Diseases Society of America. IDSA clinical practice guideline for acute bacterial rhinosinusitis in children and adults. *Clin Infect Dis.* 2012;54(8):e72–e112.
58. Liu D, Ahmet A, Ward L, et al. A practical guide to the monitoring and management of the complications of systemic corticosteroid therapy. *Allergy Asthma Clin Immunol.* 2013;9(1):30.
59. Sisson JH, Yonkers AJ, Waldman RH. Effects of guaifenesin on nasal mucociliary clearance and ciliary beat frequency in healthy volunteers. *Chest.* 1995;107(3):747–751.
60. Centers for Disease Control and Prevention. *Antibiotic/Antimicrobial Resistance.* 2021. Accessed February 3, 2023. https://www.cdc.gov/drugresistance

110 Dizziness

CHRISTOPHER MEDINA

KEY CONCEPTS

- Balance depends on the intricate interaction of sensory input (vestibular, visual, and proprioceptive), central processing (vestibular nuclear complex and cerebellum), and motor response (eyes and postural muscles).
- Disturbance in the cervical proprioceptive input to the vestibular nuclear complex and cerebellum is suggested as a cause for dizziness without hearing loss (cervicogenic vertigo), following neck injury.
- Benign paroxysmal positional vertigo, a common and well-described form of vertigo, is effectively treated with particle repositioning maneuvers, aimed at the return of displaced otoconia to the vestibule.
- Looking for the root cause of dizziness is paramount, since dizziness is a symptom that can be associated with a multitude of conditions and diseases.
- Vestibular sedating drugs such as meclizine and diazepam impair the process of central compensation by decreasing sensory input. These drugs should be avoided in most cases of dizziness or limited to a short course.
- Because of its effect on proprioceptive input and its ability to help patients stay more active, osteopathic manipulative treatment has an important role in the treatment of many forms of dizziness.

CASE VIGNETTE

HISTORY OF PRESENT ILLNESS

HH is a 72-year-old male who presents to an outpatient clinic complaining of dizziness. He reports a sensation of whirling and unsteadiness, which occurs daily and lasts from several seconds to 2 hours, aggravated by head and neck movement. These symptoms began 1 month ago shortly following a motor vehicle accident in which he was the driver. He was stopped at a red light, and was struck from behind by a car going 35 mi/h. Although he was wearing a seat belt, he experienced rapid flexion and extension of his neck, with subsequent neck pain that was diagnosed as cervical strain.

PAST MEDICAL HISTORY

He has type II diabetes controlled with diet and exercise, mild osteoarthritis of bilateral knees, and hypertension controlled with medication, diet, and exercise.

PAST SURGICAL HISTORY

He had a right medial meniscectomy 20 years ago.

ALLERGIES

He has no known allergies to medications or food.

MEDICATIONS

Chlorothiazide 500 mg daily for control of hypertension; ibuprofen 200 mg b.i.d. to t.i.d. as needed for joint pain and stiffness.

FAMILY HISTORY

Mother had hypertension and died of a myocardial infarction at age 92. Father died of colon cancer at age 80. Two younger siblings are living with no apparent health problems. There is no family history of vertigo or neurologic diseases.

SOCIAL HISTORY

He denies smoking, admits to drinking 4 to 5 beers a week, and denies use of recreational drugs. He is a retired engineer, married with grown children.

REVIEW OF SYSTEMS

Constitutional

He denies fever, fatigue, malaise, unintended weight loss or weight gain.

HEENT

The patient's vision is corrected with glasses. He reports no blurred vision, diplopia, or eye pain. He has dizziness. He denies hearing loss, tinnitus, earaches, sore throat, rhinorrhea, and epistaxis.

Respiratory

He denies difficulty breathing, wheezing, and cough.

Cardiovascular

He was diagnosed with hypertension 5 years ago. He denies chest pain, fainting, shortness of breath, irregular heartbeats, and palpitations: reports no edema in extremities.

Gastrointestinal

He denies nausea and vomiting, abdominal pain, diarrhea, and constipation. He had a normal colonoscopy 1 year ago.

Genitourinary

He has no complaint of dysuria, hesitancy, or frequency. His last prostate examination, 6 months ago, revealed mild hypertrophy with no masses.

Musculoskeletal

He complains of neck pain and stiffness worse on the right side in the upper neck. Ibuprofen offers some relief. He has low back and bilateral knee pain with prolonged standing, also helped by ibuprofen. He denies muscle weakness.

Neurologic

He has vertigo as noted and denies tremors, seizures, headaches, numbness, or tingling in the extremities. He has no difficulty with gait other than the unsteadiness associated with his dizziness. He denies memory loss and difficulty with speech or coordination.

Psychological

He denies anxiety, unwarranted sense of panic, or depression. He reports no disturbance of sleep.

Endocrine

He denies fatigue, skin and hair changes, and intolerance to heat or cold.

Hematologic/lymphatic

He reports no abdominal swelling, bruising, or bleeding; denies fatigue and feeling faint.

PHYSICAL EXAMINATION

Vital Signs

Temperature 98.6 °F, respirations 14/min, pulse 74 bpm, blood pressure 130/74 with no significant change from supine to upright, height 6′1″, weight 204 lb.

General

The patient is well-nourished, elderly male, appears as stated age, and is alert and communicative. He ambulates with a normal gait.

HEENT

Head is normocephalic without signs of trauma. Pupils are equal and reactive to light and accommodation; the conjunctiva is clear. Funduscopic examination is normal. With the patient looking straight ahead (seated on a swivel stool), nystagmus is noted during rotation of the body. ENT examination is within normal limits. Mild, high-frequency, bilateral hearing loss is identified. There are no bruits auscultated over the carotids, and no lymphadenopathy or masses are noted in the neck.

Lungs

Lungs are clear to auscultation, and breathing is unlabored.

Heart

The heart is regular rate and rhythm with no murmurs auscultated.

Abdomen

The abdomen is soft, nontender, and nondistended with no masses palpated. Bowel sounds are heard in all four quadrants.

Musculoskeletal

There is tenderness and hypertonicity in the suboccipital and right upper cervical muscles, the lumbar paraspinal muscles are hypertonic on the right.

Extremities

Extremities show no cyanosis, clubbing, or edema, and pulses are normal.

Neurologic

Neurologic examination reveals cranial nerves II to XII are intact and deep tendon reflexes are equally responsive bilaterally in upper and lower extremities. No atrophy, spasticity, clonus, or tremors are noted. The patient can perform finger-to-nose, heel-to-shin, and Romberg tests. Sensation and two-point discrimination are intact.

Osteopathic Structural Examination

Head: Left occipitomastoid suture restriction, left temporal internally rotated, right sphenobasilar side-bending rotation, OA FS_LR_R
Cervical spine: C3 FRS_L
Thoracic spine: T1 ER_LS_L, T2–T4 NR_RS_L
Lumbar spine: L5 FR_LS_L
Sacrum: Right on left sacral torsion
Pelvis: Right superior innominate shear
Lower extremity: Right anterior talus (posterior tibia on talus)
Upper extremity: Right scapula elevated. Right levator scapulae tender point
Rib cage: No somatic dysfunction noted
Abdomen/Other: No somatic dysfunction noted

DIFFERENTIAL DIAGNOSIS

Dizziness may be due to disease in almost any of the body systems and often presents a perplexing challenge for diagnosis and treatment. Severe dizziness can be disabling, and although it seldom represents a life-threatening condition, urgent and emergent conditions need to be included in the differentials to avoid complications leading to morbidity and mortality.

- An accurate history and physical will often differentiate dizziness-like symptoms that are related to:
  - Anemia
  - Cardiac irregularities
  - Orthostatic hypotension
  - Transient ischemic attacks
  - Stroke
- The association with vascular headaches may identify dizziness as a component of migraine.
- Neurologic signs could suggest a central nervous system lesion and require imaging for further diagnosis.
- Dizziness is identified in the *Physicians' Desk Reference* as a side effect to numerous medications, and an accurate drug history in relation to the patient's symptoms may indicate a pharmacologic cause.
- Furthermore, lightheadedness, giddiness, and faintness can be associated with hyperventilation, anxiety, and panic disorder, making a history of phobias, apprehension, worry, and insomnia helpful in diagnosis.

The assessment of vertigo, or a "room spinning" sensation while the body remains stationary, depends on an understanding of the body's systems of balance. Dysfunction in any of the components can cause a patient to complain of dizziness or vertigo. Familiarity with the pertinent anatomy and physiology is important in interpreting any presentation of dizziness.

Although it is possible this patient is suffering from the effects of a stroke due to hypertension, his symptoms along with the physical findings of somatic dysfunction and lack of other neurologic deficits support the diagnosis of cervicogenic vertigo. Ménière's disease is another possibility as he has hearing loss, but it is consistent with age-related loss and not necessarily related to his vertigo. His tympanic membranes did not show signs of otitis media with effusion (OME), and he had no history of recent upper respiratory tract illnesses, so this is less likely. HH was diagnosed with cervicogenic dizziness and treated with OMT.

Cervicogenic Vertigo

Disturbance in the cervical proprioceptive input to the vestibular nuclear complex and cerebellum has been suggested as the probable cause:

- De Jong and De Jong[1] produced ataxia and nystagmus by injection of local anesthetic into the neck.
- Studies based on posturography data showed patients with cervicobrachial pain had poorer postural control than normal subjects.[2]
- Prolonged contraction of the posterior cervical muscles, bilaterally, can alter balance control.[3]
- Montfoort et al.[4] observed increased cervico-ocular reflex (COR) gain in patients with Whiplash-associated disorder (WAD), seemingly linked to reduced neck mobility, and offering a possible explanation for the vertigo reported by these patients.

Various studies have shown different types of manual manipulation to be successful in improving symptoms of dizziness.[5–9] In addition, numerous case reports in osteopathic literature discuss the success of osteopathic manipulation in treating dizziness and vertigo. Still, controversy remains as to whether cervicogenic vertigo is a distinct diagnosis.

Patients with mechanical neck pain or neck pain from WAD both respond to manual approaches and exercises, although patients with WAD initially have higher levels of central sensitization.[10] Li and Peng[11] recommend manual therapy for the treatment of proprioceptive cervical vertigo.

Ménière Disease

Ménière's disease is a consideration in this patient. Some cautions about treating this condition before other more likely diagnoses are ruled out include the following:

- Although salt restriction and diuretics have been used as treatment, there is no consensus on their effectiveness.
- Betahistine, a strong histamine-3 antagonist and a weak histamine-1 agonist, is thought to increase cochlear blood flow, increases histamine turnover in the central nervous and vestibular system, and decreases vestibular input in the peripheral vestibular system.[12] It has been used for prophylaxis with some effectiveness.[13]
- In a multicenter, double-blind, randomized, placebo-controlled, dose-defining superiority trial, the primary outcome revealed that placebo had the same reduction of attack rates over a 9-month treatment period as betahistine.[12]
- Other vestibular suppressants should only be used during acute attacks and not on a chronic basis. Many patients require psychological support in coping with the ramifications of the disease.

OSTEOPATHIC PATIENT MANAGEMENT

As dizziness is a symptom that can be associated with a multitude of conditions and diseases, looking for the root cause is paramount. Somatic dysfunction may be present in any of these cases as an associated finding or, as some suggest, a significant etiologic factor. Somatic manifestations of vestibular disease could appear in the cervical area by way of shared neural reflex pathways (vestibulospinal reflex [VSR] and vestibulocollic reflex [VCR]).

Certainly, any identified underlying cause of dizziness needs to be treated. Often, a cause is not identified, or available treatment is only symptomatic. Addressing the management from a multifaceted approach is usually the most successful.

Biomechanical Model

Trauma seems to play a role in some types of dizziness.

- Patients with WAD frequently complain of dizziness[14,15]
- Lockhart[16] reported on two cases of Ménière's syndrome resulting from multiple traumatic brain injuries.
- Treleaven et al.[17] showed WAD patients with dizziness showed significant error in returning their head to natural posture (joint position error), compared to controls and WAD patients without dizziness.

OMT can alleviate dizziness related to somatic dysfunction and is useful in the management of patients with balance disorders in that it:

- Normalizes proprioceptive input
- Improves range of motion
- Promotes venous and lymphatic circulation
- Balances neurologic reflexes
  1. OMT targeting cervical somatic dysfunctions:
     - Proprioceptors in the neck supply important information to the balance system of the central nervous system.
     - Inappropriate signals due to cervical somatic dysfunction may be responsible for some forms, or exacerbation of dizziness due to other causes.
     - Cervical Jones counterstrain tender points may play a crucial role in diagnosis and treatment of eustachian tube dysfunction.[18]
     - Some studies demonstrate decreased range of motion in the cervical spine causes increased activity in the cervico-vestibulo-ocular reflex[4] and may partially explain the improvement in dizziness reported with manual manipulation.[5–8,19]
  2. OMT targeting feet and ankles somatic dysfunction:
     - Other areas of the body also provide proprioceptive input to help regulate balance and must respond when postural adjustments need to be made.
     - Somatic dysfunction in any of these areas, particularly the feet and ankles, may impact balance and the individual's ability to compensate for imbalance.
     - Range of motion in the extremities is important for balance rehabilitation training.
     - OMT to improve extremity motion can be beneficial in rehabilitation for those patients suffering from dizziness.
  3. OMT targeting temporal bone dysfunction:
     - Magoun states, "vertigo often follows trauma to the ear or the neck."[20]
     - Considering the location of the paired labyrinth organs on the petrous portions of the temporal bones bilaterally, and the importance of coordinated input from the two sides, dysfunction of the temporal bone may be responsible for disturbance of equilibrium.
     - For those skilled in the cranial approach, addressing restriction of the occipitomastoid sutures as well as gently realigning the temporal bones to their proper orientation and motion will normalize the inner ear mechanisms.

BOX 110.1 Patient Education: Self-Treatment of Dizziness from BPPV

- These instructions accompany the illustrations in Figure 83.7 in Chapter 83, Osteopathic Considerations in Patients with HEENT Disorders. Refer to these diagrams while reading these instructions.
- These exercises can be best done with the help of an assistant.
- If on initial attempt of these exercises the response is too severe to continue, the prescribed medication may be used.

Identification of Problem Ear

The first step in the self-treatment of dizziness is to identify the side of the poorly functioning ear. This is done as follows:

1. Identify the position on a firm bed where you can lie back without hitting anything.
2. Identify where your shoulders will lie when you lie back in the bed.
3. Place a midsized pillow on the bed where your shoulders will land when you lie back in the bed.
4. Position yourself in the bed as above.
5. Lower yourself with your shoulders contacting the pillow and your head contacting the bed and your head turned to the left.
6. Remain in that position for 2 minutes, and record your feelings.
7. Repeat the above maneuver in No. 5; however, this time turns your head to the right.
8. Again remain in that position for 2 minutes, and record your feelings.
9. Identify the side your head is turned to, which produced the most uncomfortable feelings whether they be dizziness, anxiety, or fear.
10. Record this side that produced the most uncomfortable feelings.

Treatment of the Dizziness

1. Sit on the bed positioned as above and with the pillow positioned as above.
2. Turn your head 45 degrees as illustrated in Figure 83.7 in Chapter 83 (Letter A).
   - If your head turned to the right produced the most uncomfortable feelings, turn to the right before doing the maneuver described in No. 5 above.
   - If your head turned to the left produced the most uncomfortable feelings, turn to the left before doing the maneuver described in No. 5 above (Letter B).
3. Rapidly lie down in the bed turning your head to the above position, as described in No. 5 above, with your shoulders positioned on the pillow and your head touching the bed.
4. Remain in that position for 1 minute.
5. Turn your head 90 degrees toward the opposite side (45 degree angle but to the other side) without raising your head, as depicted in Letter C.
6. Remain in that position for 1 minute.
7. Turn your head 90 degrees further in the direction you are presently turned (so you will be looking down at an angle), and move your body as necessary, as depicted in Letter D.
8. Hold this position for 1 minute.
9. Sit up in this manner:
   - Keep facing the direction your head was turned as depicted in Letter E.
   - Hang your feet off the bed in preparation to stand up.
   - Place your chin on your chest, and slowly sit up, keeping your chin on your chest throughout the sitting up motion.
10. Remain in that sitting position for 1 minute.
11. Do not lie flat for 24 hours. A semirecumbent position is best (recliner position).
12. Assume normal activity after 24 hours.

BPPV is a common and well-described form of vertigo, most effectively treated with particle repositioning maneuvers (Box 110.1).[21] The goal of the maneuvers is the return of displaced otoconia to the vestibule. Vestibular sedating drugs such as meclizine and diazepam are not effective and usually not recommended for these patients.

Good structural diagnosis can help direct appropriate musculoskeletal treatment and home exercises. Lower extremity strength, range of motion, and coordination have important roles in the rehabilitation of vertiginous conditions. OMT for somatic dysfunction in the neck, cranium, and extremities can offer relief to many patients suffering from dizziness. For those with cervicogenic vertigo, resolution of involved somatic dysfunction is the treatment of choice.

Respiratory–Circulatory Model

Congestion in the middle and inner ear, while not a major recognized cause of vertigo, is a component to some diseases (e.g., Ménière's and OME) and may be associated with lightheadedness and imbalance.

1. OMT aimed at improving venous and lymphatic circulation from the head and neck may offer symptomatic relief in those cases.
   - The vestibular system is particularly susceptible to vascular compromise.
   - Awareness of postures and maneuvers that may impede blood flow through the vertebrobasilar system is important for patient education and when applying any type of manipulation.

- Avoidance of hyperextended positions of the upper cervical spine is recommended. Treat any underlying structural or functional nasopharyngeal condition that may be associated with eustachian tube dysfunction.
- Channell documented successful use of the "modified Muncie technique" to treat a dysfunctional eustachian tube in a patient with a history of serous otitis media secondary to seasonal allergies. The patient was complaining of intermittent subjective vertigo. A gloved finger was applied to the palatine tonsil, and a lateral force was applied while creating circular traction. Traction near the opening of the eustachian tube is thought to break up adhesions and equalize pressure, which may result in improved drainage. Two modified Muncie treatments combined with HVLA to the patient's cervical dysfunction were applied, and the patient experienced resolution of symptoms within 2 weeks.[22]
- The Galbreath technique may be implemented to drain fluid effectively by using "pumping motion" in opening and closing the eustachian tube.
- Antihistamines may be indicated when atopy is associated with eustachian tube dysfunction.[18]
- Steele et al. compared standard care only and standard care plus OMT in evaluating the efficacy of an OMT protocol on middle ear effusion resolution following an episode of acute otitis media and found that standard care plus OMT may result in faster resolution of middle ear effusion following acute otitis media than standard care alone.[23]
- Severe sinusitis, especially inflammation of the sphenoid sinus, may cause dizziness.[18] OMT targeting the autonomic system, such as enhancing the parasympathetic response by applying sphenopalatine ganglion stimulation, promotes thinning and drainage of secretions[24] and may reduce associated dizziness.

2. Cranial treatment to improve cranial bone motion has been used with some success to reduce the symptoms of Ménière's disease.
   - The endolymphatic space of the labyrinth does not directly communicate with the subarachnoid space.
   - However, fluid movement in the inner ear may be augmented by cranial movement.

Diuretics and salt restriction diets have been used with varying success in the treatment of Meniere's to decrease the inner ear fluid volume.

Neurologic Model

When one aspect of the sensory input to the brain stem and cerebellum balance system is absent or in a state of dysfunction, the brain compensates by using information from the other systems. The more disinformation or lack of information, the more difficult is the compensation process.

Rehabilitating patients with vertigo and balance disorders includes retraining the coordination of eye movement with head, neck, and body movements through exercises. Enhancing the intact sensory inputs may entail sharpening proprioceptive input from the neck or extremities through exercises, encouraging activities and OMT.

For example:

- Manipulative techniques contributing to a decrease in afferent load (e.g., counterstrain, indirect myofascial) could help balance the involved neural reflexes.
- Corrective lenses, when needed, can improve the accuracy of sensory input from the eyes.
- Dural tension around the internal auditory meatus has been suggested to impair proper function of the nerves coursing there (vestibular, cochlear, and facial).
- Osteopathic Cranial Manipulative Medicine addresses bony relationships and dural tensions in the head, thereby impacting function of the vestibular nerve.
- Relieving tension in the upper cervical spine and around the jugular foramen (occipitomastoid suture) may also reduce symptoms of nausea and vomiting by effecting vagal tone.
- Myofascial trigger points (MTrPs) (see Chapter 43 for further information) in the sternocleidomastoid muscle may refer pain to the eye and may be associated with balance abnormalities. Motor vehicle accidents, especially from the rear, may produce MTrPs in the sternocleidomastoid, splenius cervicis, and trapezius muscles. Treating these may help to reduce imbalance and pain symptoms.[24]

Using manual manipulation for subjective dizziness and vestibular dysfunction is not a new concept in medicine. Though some classic techniques such as the Epley maneuver and Brandt–Daroff maneuver are known to be effective and taught widely, a large Dutch survey of general practitioners found that they are widely underutilized.[25]

Survey results from Van Vugt et al. discovered the most common reason Epley maneuver, vestibular rehabilitation, and Brandt–Daroff exercise were not performed was a lack of skill or knowledge. Physicians were also more likely to use the techniques if they were trainers themselves, while a small percent did not use the techniques due to perceived lack of efficacy. This illustrates the value of disseminating knowledge and practicing manual skills, as well as continuing to investigate effectiveness of OMT for dizziness.[25]

Medication use must be carefully considered, as vestibular sedatives, such as meclizine, impair the process of central compensation by decreasing the sensory input. If needed to control severe dizziness, these drugs should be limited to a short course (usually two to three doses). Anticholinergic (e.g., scopolamine) and antidopaminergic (e.g., prochlorperazine) drugs may also offer some relief. Combination therapy can be beneficial when a single drug regimen fails. Again, the sedating effects can be counterproductive to rehabilitation.

Behavioral Model

Patients with dizziness who succumb to a sedentary lifestyle have worse outcomes. Persistent vertigo can be very disruptive to a patient's life, and many patients become frustrated, even depressed. In addition, some antidepressant medications have dizziness as a side effect. Psychological disorders may also manifest symptoms of dizziness. It is the second most common symptom reported by people with panic disorder.

Behavioral recommendations:

- Encourage mobility and increase activity.
- Seek psychological support.
- Monitor pharmacologic treatments carefully, especially antidepressants.
- Patient education on self-treatment options for dizziness from BPPV is self-empowering (Box 110.1).

Metabolic Energy Model

Postural considerations are especially important in the management of dizziness and balance disorder, and proper treatment can play an integral part in the resolution of dizziness and unsteadiness.

Evaluation and treatment of postural imbalance include assessing for

- Sacral base unlevelness
- Muscle tone problems
- Postural strains

Drugs with potential for ototoxicity must be considered as a cause of vertigo. A few drugs such as the aminoglycoside antibiotics and some antineoplastic drugs cause irreversible damage. Others such as aspirin, when stopped, will result in resolution of symptoms.

In a nonrandomized pilot study, Fraix showed that OMT was well tolerated in 18 patients with vertigo. Interventions included using muscle energy, counterstrain, and myofascial release technique to treat somatic dysfunction of the cervical, thoracic, and lumbar spine; ribs; sacrum; and upper and lower extremities and a balanced ligamentous tension technique to treat cranial somatic dysfunction. The treatment effectiveness was measured with the use of a self-assessment inventory, the Dizziness Handicap Inventory (DHI).[26]

In a prospective study of 16 participants, Fraix et al. utilized a validated instrument (SMART Balance, NeuroCom) to evaluate the effectiveness of OMT for dizziness greater than 3 months. The researchers reported significant quantitative and qualitative improvements after OMT. Though the sample size was small and not randomized, the study represents the first reported use of computerized dynamic posturography and SMART Balance to quantitatively study effectiveness of various OMT techniques in subjective dizziness.[27]

Using the same validated instrument, in a randomized, controlled, comparative feasibility study of 23 patients, Fraix et al. showed a significant reduction in vertigo and improvement in balance 3 months after combined treatment with OMT and vestibular rehabilitation therapy.[9]

Papa et al.[28] designed a randomized controlled study using a sham control group, doubled the sample size, and used a stabilometer platform along with the DHI to assess effect of osteopathic manipulative therapy (OMTh) on balance and quality of life in patients with BPPV.

- Thirty-one patients with BPPV were randomly assigned into two groups that both received four weekly sessions: 19 patients received OMTh and 12 patients received sham therapy.
- Significant improvements favored the OMTh group on both DHI and stabilometer measures ($P < .03$).

CONCLUSION

Since dizziness is used to describe a variety of sensations and may result from a variety of problems, an approach to a patient complaining of dizziness must start with an in-depth history. Description of the patient's sensation must be specific as to whether it is disorientation, a sense of moving, being off-balance, difficulty walking, impending faint, lightheadedness, motion sickness, panic, trouble focusing, or spinning.

The history of present illness should include the timing and nature of the first episode and subsequent episodes, along with the frequency and duration of the spells, and the timing of the spells. Precipitating factors and associated symptoms need to be considered. Other contributory information is found in medication history, allergy history, family history, social history, and review of systems.

Appreciation of the sensorineural integration involved in balance helps in diagnosis and treatment of dizziness. Always consider the three major components in achieving good balance—sensing the environment, central processing of information, and musculoskeletal response. Also consider the three dominant sensory inputs to this system—vestibular (inner ear), visual, and somatosensory (joint proprioception).

Comprehensive history and understanding of the involved anatomy and physiology will make the evaluation and treatment of patients with dizziness much more satisfying.

ACKNOWLEDGMENTS

The author and editors of this chapter would like to acknowledge the scholarly contributions of Shan Shan Wu, Robert W. Hostoffer, Kathleen Gibbons, Harriet H. Shaw, and Michael B. Shaw for prior editions of this chapter.

REFERENCES

1. de Jong P, de Jong M, Cohen B, Jongkees LB. Ataxia and nystagmus induced by injection of local anesthetic in the neck. *Ann Neurol.* 1977;1(3):240–246.
2. Karlberg M, Persson L, Magnusson M. Impaired postural control in patients with cervicobrachial pain. *Acta Otolaryngol Suppl.* 1995;520(2):440–442.
3. Schieppati M, Nardone A, Schmid M. Neck muscle fatigue affects postural control in man. *Neuroscience.* 2003;121(2):277–285.
4. Montfoort I, Van Der Geest J, Slijper HP, De Zeeuw CI, Frens MA. Adaptation of the cervico- and vestibulo-ocular reflex in whiplash injury patients. *J Neurotrauma.* 2008;25(6):687–693.
5. Reid SA, Rivett DA. Manual therapy treatment of cervicogenic dizziness: a systematic review. *Man Ther.* 2005;10(1):4–13.
6. Galm R, Rittmeister M, Schmitt E. Vertigo in patients with cervical spine dysfunction. *Eur Spine J.* 1998;7(1):55–58.
7. Malmström EM, Karlberg M, Melander A, Magnusson M, Moritz U. Cervicogenic dizziness-musculoskeletal findings before and after treatment and long-term outcome. *Disabil Rehabil.* 2007;29(15):1193–1205.
8. Heikkila H, Johansson M, Wenngren BI. Effects of acupuncture, cervical manipulation and NSAID therapy on dizziness and impaired head repositioning of suspected cervical origin: a pilot study. *Man Ther.* 2000;5(3):151–157.
9. Fraix M, Badran S, Graham V, et al. Osteopathic manipulative treatment in individuals with vertigo and somatic dysfunction: a randomized, controlled, comparative feasibility study. *J Osteopath Med.* 2021;121(1):71–83.
10. Castaldo M, Catena A, Chiarotto A, Fernández-de-Las-Peñas C, Arendt-Nielsen L. Do subjects with whiplash-associated disorders respond differently in the short-term to manual therapy and exercise than those with mechanical neck pain? *Pain Med.* 2017;18(4):791–803.
11. Li Y, Peng B. Pathogenesis, diagnosis, and treatment of cervical vertigo. *Pain Physician.* 2015;18(4):E585–E595.
12. Adrion C, Fischer CS, Wagner J, et al. Efficacy and safety of betahistine treatment in patients with Meniere's disease: primary results of a long term, multicentre, double blind, randomised, placebo controlled, dose defining trial (BEMED trial). *BMJ.* 2016;352:h6816.
13. Meyer ED. [Treatment of Meniere disease with betahistin-dimesilate (Aequamen)—a double-blind, placebo controlled study versus placebo (crossover)]. *Laryngol Rhinol Otol.* 1985;64(5):269–272.
14. Oka H, Matsudaira K, Fujii T, et al. Risk factors for prolonged treatment of whiplash-associated disorder. *PLoS One.* 2015;10(7):e0132191.
15. Spritzer WO, Skovron ML, Salmi LR, et al. Scientific monograph of the Quebec Task Force on Whiplash-Associated Disorders: redefining "whiplash" and its management. *Spine (Phila Pa 1976).* 1995;20(8 suppl):1S–73S.
16. Lockhart W. Meniere's syndrome resulting from multiple traumatic brain injury: two case studies. *Am Acad Osteopath J.* 1999;9(3):21–24.
17. Treleaven J, Jull G, Sterling M. Dizziness and unsteadiness following whiplash injury: characteristic features and relationship with cervical joint position error. *J Rehabil Med.* 2003;35(1):36–43.
18. Kuchera ML, Kuchera WA. *Part I Systemic Disorders Related to Head & Neck: Chapter 1. Osteopathic Considerations in Head, Eyes, Ears, Nose, Throat Disorders.* Greyden Press, LLC; 2012:50.

19. Williams NH. Prevalence and treatment of dizziness. *Lett Br J Gen Pract.* 1998;48(431):1344.
20. Magoun HI Sr. The temporal bone: trouble maker in the head. *J Am Osteopath Assoc.* 1974;73(10):825–835.
21. Brooks JG, Abidin MR. Repositioning maneuver for benign paroxysmal positional vertigo (BPPV). *J Am Osteopath Assoc.* 1997;97(5):277–279.
22. Channell MK. Modified Muncie technique: osteopathic manipulation for eustachian tube dysfunction and illustrative report of case. *J Am Osteopath Assoc.* 2008;108(5):260–263.
23. Steele KM, Carreiro JE, Viola JH, Conte JA, Ridpath LC. Effect of osteopathic manipulative treatment on middle ear effusion following acute otitis media in young children: a pilot study. *J Am Osteopath Assoc.* 2014;114(6):436–447.
24. Travell J, Simons D. *Myofascial Pain and Dysfunction: A Trigger Point Manual.* Lippincott Williams & Wilkins; 1983:263.
25. van Vugt VA, Diaz Nerio PM, van der Wouden JC, van der Horst HE, Maarsingh OR. Use of canalith repositioning manoeuvres and vestibular rehabilitation: a GP survey. *Scand J Prim Health Care.* 2017;35(1):19–26.
26. Fraix M. Osteopathic manipulative treatment and vertigo: a pilot study. *PMR.* 2010;2(7):612–618.
27. Fraix M, Gordon A, Graham V, Hurwitz E, Seffinger MA. Use of the SMART Balance Master to quantify the effects of osteopathic manipulative treatment in patients with dizziness. *J Am Osteopath Assoc.* 2013;113(5):394–403.
28. Papa L, Amodio A, Biffi F, Mandara A. Impact of osteopathic therapy on proprioceptive balance and quality of life in patients with dizziness. *J Bodyw Mov Ther.* 2017;21(4):866–872.

111 Case Study: Upper Extremity

KURT P. HEINKING ▪ CAMERON BRAZ

KEY CONCEPTS

- The five models of osteopathic care provide a framework for integrating objective clinical findings into an osteopathic management plan.
- The shoulder girdle has complex movements and neuromuscular control and due to this it requires a comprehensive examination to narrow the differential.
- Disruption of the kinetic chain, if left unidentified, may lead to altered muscle-firing patterns resulting in overload to connective tissues and related joints.
- A major goal in the treatment of acute shoulder pain is the control of inflammation while maintaining motion.
- Manipulative treatment for the shoulder girdle, in addition to standard medical care, can accelerate recovery from shoulder symptoms and reduce their severity.

CASE VIGNETTE

Ms. Jones is a 52-year-old Caucasian right-hand dominant high-level recreational tennis player who seeks medical care following an injury to her right shoulder.

CHIEF COMPLAINT

Acute exacerbation of chronic aching pain in her anterior/lateral right shoulder for the past 6 weeks, after participating in the Regional United States Tennis Association (USTA) event.

HISTORY OF PRESENT ILLNESS

The pain has been present for the past 6 weeks. The pain began after participating in the USTA regional event where her team qualified for the state tournament. She noted that the pain began while playing in a doubles match during which she hit multiple overhead strokes in addition to normal serving in the closely contested match. Just prior to the regional event, she purchased a new racquet with "all of the latest technology." She states that the pain has not improved despite taking 1 week off from playing, and now she is developing stiffness in the right shoulder. She is concerned about the ongoing discomfort as she wants to prepare for the State tournament with her team. She describes her pain as being a constant 5/10 in intensity and having a burning/aching quality. When she attempts to reach overhead, the pain increases to a 7/10 in intensity. When asked where the pain radiates, she points to the right medial scapular border and also down the biceps muscle anteriorly. Her pain makes sleeping on her right side difficult as she develops pain in the region of the deltoid insertion. Activities of daily living (ADLs) like hooking her bra or putting a sweater on overhead have also been causing her significant discomfort. She denies having significant neck pain but does endorse some stiffness in turning left and right. She denies having numbness or weakness involving her right hand. In the past, her right shoulder pain has resolved with home treatment. This time, she has taken naproxen sodium 220 mg twice daily without improvement. She also used ice on the shoulder for the first 2 days but has not used any ice or heat since then. There has not been other workup or imaging performed as of this time.

Past Medical History

Positive for gastroesophageal reflux disease, hyperlipidemia, and menopause.

Past Surgical History

Appendectomy at age 18, tonsillectomy and adenoidectomy at age 6.

Past Trauma History

Motor vehicle accident in 1982 during which she sustained a minor concussion and whiplash.

ORTHOPEDIC TESTING

Family Medical History

Mother (age 75) with hypertension and type II diabetes; father is deceased (aged 58 with cirrhosis of the liver); one brother (age 49) who is healthy.

Gynecologic History

G2 P2002; last menstrual period was 2 years ago; last mammogram was 1 year ago with normal results; last Pap smear, pelvic, and rectal examination was 1 year ago and reported as normal.

Social History

Married for 22 years to husband Roger; has two children, Mary (21 healthy) and Grace (19 healthy); denies tobacco and illicit drugs; drinks alcohol occasionally; works as office manager for medical group; plays tennis 4 to 5 times weekly.

Childhood Illnesses

Chickenpox, possible measles, mononucleosis at age 18.

REVIEW OF SYSTEMS

General

She denies fever, chills, and malaise.

HEENT

She admits to occasional tension headaches, which have not changed since the onset of the shoulder pain. She denies dizziness.

Cardiovascular

She denies chest pain, shortness of breath, and fatigue.

Pulmonary

She denies cough, wheezing, and pain with breathing.

Gastrointestinal

She denies abdominal pain, nausea, vomiting, intolerance to fatty foods, excessive alcohol use, change in stools, and change in appetite.

Musculoskeletal

She denies pain, swelling, and stiffness in other joints; although she does admit to episodes of mid and upper back pain.

Neurologic

She denies generalized weakness and numbness.

Endocrine

She denies weight change; she admits to occasional hot flashes. She is menopausal.

PHYSICAL EXAMINATION

Vital Signs

T: 97.6; P: 78; R: 16; BP: 140/82; height: 5′6″; weight: 148 lb.

General

Alert, oriented, cooperative, neatly groomed, and an excellent historian. She appears younger than her stated age.

Skin

No rashes, no abnormal-appearing moles, normal hair and nails.

HEENT

Pupils are equal, round, and reactive to light and accomodation, extraocular eye movements intact, pharynx without erythema, no adenopathy, tympanic membranes visible with good cone of light without erythema, no nasal erythema, no sinus tenderness.

Cardiovascular

Regular rate and rhythm without S3 S4 murmurs, no clubbing, cyanosis, or peripheral edema. Equal pulses bilaterally.

Lungs

Lungs are clear to auscultation bilaterally without rales, rhonchi, or wheezes.

Breast

No breast masses, nipples everted, no discharge, no axillary adenopathy.

Abdomen

Normal and active bowel sounds × 4 quadrants, soft and nontender in all quadrants including right upper quadrant without rigidity, rebound, or guarding, no masses appreciated. Negative costovertebral angle pain, negative Murphy sign.

Neurologic

Cranial nerves 2 to 12 intact, bilateral upper extremities (UEs) and lower extremities (LEs) grossly had no sensory deficits, 2+/4 deep tendon reflexes, and 5/5 strength.

Musculoskeletal

Upper Extremities

Range of Motion

Active range of motion (AROM) is full and pain free in her left shoulder. AROM and passive range of motion (PROM) of her right shoulder both demonstrate a painful arc from 50 degrees to full abduction. External rotation is also limited to 20 degrees secondary to pain. AROM and PROM are full and pain free in adduction, flexion, extension, and internal rotation.

ORTHOPEDIC TESTING

The right shoulder has a positive supraspinatus test (Jobe aka empty/full can test); positive impingement tests (Hawkin sign and Neer test), negative Speed test, negative drop arm test, positive acromioclavicular (AC) tenderness, negative subscapularis test (lift-off/Napoleon's), negative labral test (O'Brien's), negative thoracic outlet syndrome test (Adson and Roos tests). There was no gross scapular winging, although observation of active scapular motion reveals right scapula dyskinetic in early abduction coupled with flexion.

Scapular Assessment

Upon standing evaluation of landmarks, her right shoulder is protracted, and the medial border of her right scapula is held in a more lateral position than her left in relation to the spine. There is also mild winging of the inferior border of her right scapula. When watching her demonstrate her backhand, she hikes her right shoulder during follow through.

Vascular Examination

No cyanosis, clubbing, or edema. Pulses equal bilaterally, brisk capillary refill.

Lower Extremities

AROM and PROM are full in all major actions of bilateral hips, knees, and ankles. Negative joint line pain, negative anterior cruciate ligament instability (Lachman test), negative meniscal injury (McMurray and Apley tests); negative patellofemoral pain (grind test), negative hip comp. No cyanosis, clubbing, or edema. Pulses equal bilateral, brisk capillary refill.

Osteopathic Structural Examination

Cervical: C5 is flexed, rotated, and side bent right.
Thoracic: T4 is extended, side bent, and rotated right.
Lumbar: L1 is flexed, rotated, and side bent right.
Sacrum: Left on left sacral torsion.
Pelvis: Right anterior innominate.
Lower extremity: Right psoas hypertonic and tight.
Upper extremity: Superior right sternoclavicular joint.
Ribs: Exhalation dysfunction involving rib 10 on the right.

DIFFERENTIAL DIAGNOSIS

Table 111.1 outlines the differential diagnoses for shoulder pain.

WORKUP AND INTERPRETATION

Four-view right shoulder x-rays were obtained, including an AP view, axillary view, scapular Y-view, and outlet view. The x-rays demonstrated a type III acromion with cystic changes at the acromioclavicular joint. The humeral head was without osteoarthritis, fracture, or subluxation. The remainder of the osseous anatomy was normal. An MR-arthrogram of the shoulder was also obtained. AC joint findings were demonstrated again in addition to a full-thickness tear of the supraspinatus tendon with retraction. A small amount of fluid was seen in the subacromial bursa. The humeral head was without osteoarthritis, fracture, or subluxation. The glenoid labrum showed some possible degenerative changes but no discrete superior labral tear (Fig. 111.1).

TABLE 111.1

Differential Diagnosis of Shoulder Pain

Muscular/ Tendinous	Osseous	Capsular	Biomechanical	Neurovascular	Referred Pain Pattern
Rotator cuff tendonitis	Osteoarthritis	Shoulder laxity/ instability	Impingement syndrome	Thoracic outlet syndrome	Diaphragm, liver, gallbladder
Rotator cuff tear	Humeral stress fracture	Adhesive capsulitis	Scapular dyskinesis	Cervical radiculopathy radiculitis	Pancoast tumor or pulmonary pathology
Subacromial bursitis		Labral tear	Acromioclavicular dysfunction		
Biceps brachii (long head) tendonitis		Pigmented villonodular synovitis	Somatic dysfunction		
Deltoid muscle strain			Neuromuscular inhibition with abnormal muscle-firing patterns		
Trapezius muscle strain					
Rhomboid muscle strain					

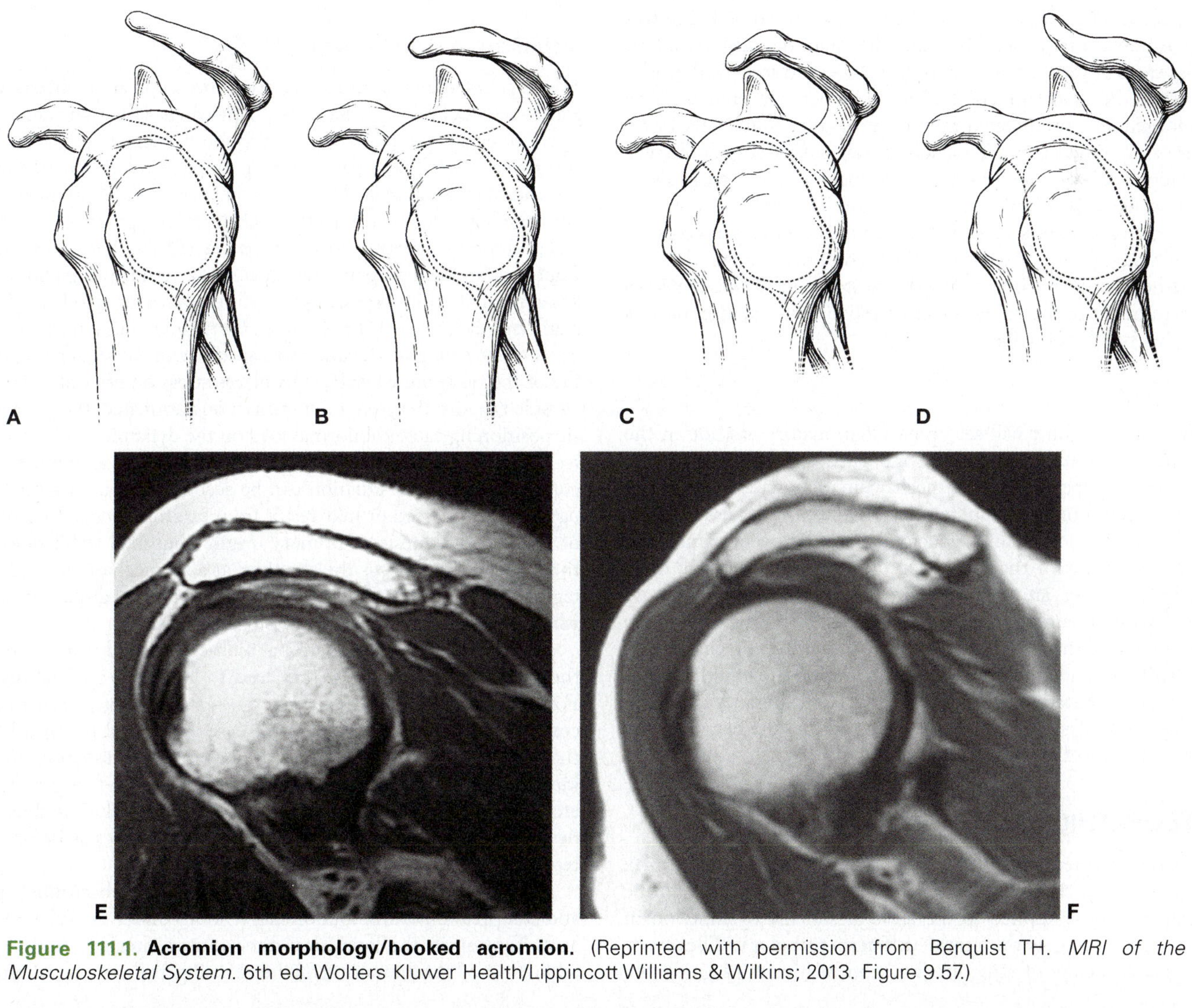

Figure 111.1. Acromion morphology/hooked acromion. (Reprinted with permission from Berquist TH. *MRI of the Musculoskeletal System*. 6th ed. Wolters Kluwer Health/Lippincott Williams & Wilkins; 2013. Figure 9.57.)

Diagnosis

The patient's diagnosis based on the clinical history, examination, and diagnostic imaging was as follows:

1. Full-thickness rotator cuff tear with retraction of supraspinatus tendon
2. Type III acromion osteoarthrosis of the acromioclavicular joint
3. Somatic dysfunction: Cervical, thoracic, rib, lumbar, sacrum, pelvis, and lower and upper extremities
4. Scapular dyskinesis
5. Kinetic chain dysfunction
6. GERD (acid reflux disease)—controlled currently

Relevant Functional Anatomy

The shoulder complex is a loosely constructed highly mobile complex of bones, muscles, and ligaments. It is designed for increased mobility to the upper extremity with stability sufficient to provide a proper foundation for muscular function that is vital for the performance of sports or ADLs. The shoulder complex includes both static and dynamic stabilizers. The static stabilizers are glenoid, glenoid labrum, capsule, ligaments, and joint cohesion. The static stabilizers are intact in this patient; however, the dynamic stabilizers are not. The dynamic stabilizers are the rotator cuff muscles along with the long head of the biceps. She has a large supraspinatus tear that significantly affects dynamic joint stability. In addition, she is showing signs of "sick scapula syndrome" or scapular dyskinesia, a functional disorder of the kinetic chain. The scapulothoracic stabilizers are the rhomboids, trapezius, serratus anterior, and the pectoralis minor muscles. Weakness and tightness of these muscles, and their associated somatic dysfunction, affect the global function of the shoulder. Movement of the shoulder requires coordinated movement of three joints (sternoclavicular, acromioclavicular, and glenohumeral) and the scapulothoracic articulation. All four components work together in a synchronous fashion to allow an extensive range of motion (circumduction). In any given arm position, the scapula aligns itself to allow the glenoid cavity to be in the best position to receive the head of the humerus. For our patient, her shoulder was elevating due to weakness of these muscles and recruitment of the upper trapezius and levator scapulae muscles during her backhand swing.

Physiology

Injury to a large joint will set up an inflammatory cascade in the structures involved. The severity, intensity, and location of the inflammation depend upon the mechanism of injury and the structures involved. For the shoulder, many times, the issue is repetitive overuse. Tendonitis and subacromial bursitis occur commonly, as does tendonitis of the long head of the biceps. Because most shoulder problems are soft tissue in nature, pain, tightness, and stiffness with impaired mobility are concerns. Pain is usually due to impingement of the soft tissue structures under the coracoacromial arch. Stiffness and decreased range of motion are multifactorial and can be mediated anatomically, biomechanically, and/or neurologically. Loss of strength may indicate rotator cuff tear but may also be related to the factors described above.

OSTEOPATHIC PATIENT MANAGEMENT

Any patient presenting with pain in the shoulder joint complex should receive a thorough osteopathic examination. Osteopathic techniques can be applied to the areas of somatic dysfunction in patients presenting with rotator cuff tear pathology. The models described below of structure–function relationships guide the osteopathic practitioner's approach to diagnosis and treatment. The five models of osteopathic care provide a framework for integrating objective and subjective clinical findings with osteopathic structural exam findings.

Biomechanical Model

A kinetic chain is described as a sequencing of individual body segments and joints to accomplish a task. It generally functions from a base of support proximally and then proceeds distally, but this is entirely dependent on the task at hand. Because of the tremendous demands that overhead sporting activities place on the spine and the shoulder joint complex, the ability to recognize kinetic chain disorders related to the upper extremity and their interactions with related components of the musculoskeletal system is important for athletic medical practitioners. Due to the complexity of the anatomic and biomechanical interactions as well as neuromuscular control issues, evaluation and accurate diagnosis are clinically challenging.

Disruption of the kinetic chain, if left unidentified, may lead to altered muscle-firing patterns resulting in overload to connective tissues (capsular laxity and instability, labral tears) or the joint itself (osteoarthritis, etc.). While the patient may complain of pain due to a traumatic event, most shoulder problems result from repetitive overuse of the osteoarticular system and related neural, soft tissue, and muscular elements. This is especially true in overhead athletes, as they try to transmit the ground reactive force from their pelvis and trunk through their upper extremity.

Impingement Syndrome

Weakness of the abdominals, gluteus, and scapular stabilizers with subsequent tightness of the psoas, hamstrings, latissimus dorsi, and upper trapezius produces the substitution patterns that begin at the myofascial level. These patterns may result in outlet obstruction at the coracoacromial arch. This situation is known as "impingement." Impingement syndrome results in part from suboptimal biomechanical position manifesting grossly as protracted shoulders, weak lower trapezius, and tight upper trapezius. As a result, the glenoid fossa's abnormal position places stress on the anterior stabilizers (both static and dynamic) of the shoulder. Over time, this abnormal stress leads to loosening of the anterior capsule with subsequent tightening of the posterior capsule. This places stress on not only the joint capsule but also the glenoid labrum. If left untreated, the asymmetric positioning causes abnormal load on the dynamic stabilizers (the rotator cuff muscles) that may eventually manifest as frank rotator cuff pathology. This situation can be secondary to internal pathology as just discussed or may result from external causes. In the case of scapular dyskinesis of primary origin, abnormal stabilization of the scapula again places the shoulder at a biomechanical disadvantage. This leads to abnormal scapular positioning as discussed above, which may lead to the same pathologic conditions.

Failure to assess the functional biomechanical factors related to the shoulder joint complex may lead to less-than-optimal results. For example, after a patient undergoes surgery for a torn rotator cuff, the mainstay of postoperative care is physical therapy. If the therapist and/or clinician fails to recognize dysfunction in the kinetic chain (scapular dyskinesis, altered muscle-firing patterns, etc.), the patient's altered biomechanics will place the shoulder and newly repaired cuff under the same abnormal forces as before and result in a suboptimal outcome.

Impingement is caused by a decrease in the subacromial space and compression of the rotator cuff tendons under the subacromial arch. Tension in the latissimus dorsi causes internal rotation and adduction of the humerus, further causing the greater tuberosity of the humerus to impinge upon the acromion. Weak abdominals cause an increase in the lumbar lordosis, an increase in the thoracic kyphosis, a slumped posture, and a forward head. The forward head position causes tightness of the scalene muscles and myofascial strain of the thoracic inlet, clavicles, and shoulders. The clinical biomechanical summation of the above results in a "functional thoracic kyphosis" characterized by rotator cuff impingement resulting from scapular dyskinesis (protracted scapula) and may ultimately lead to rotator cuff muscle fiber failure.

Form follows function. Given enough time, the biomechanical and neuromuscular dysfunctions described above can result in bony and soft tissue changes leading to a painful shoulder syndrome for which the patient seeks medical attention. Functional evaluation of this patient's complaint often reveals that the inciting event is part of a long-standing underlying process of kinetic chain dysfunction.

The key in any patient with somatic dysfunction is to restore normal structural alignment to allow the kinetic chain to function properly (form follows function). In this patient, when considering the biomechanical model, the physician needs to address the flexed lumbar dysfunction and the psoas tension. By treating these, normal sacral motion should be restored, which will allow the ground reactive force to be efficiently transmitted up the kinetic chain. Osteopathic treatment will also restore functional mobility to the thoracolumbar junction. This will improve diaphragm motion and decrease latissimus tension. Treatment of the upper thoracic dysfunction should correct scapular dyskinesis. The result will be restoration of normal postural alignment and kinetic chain function.

Respiratory/Circulatory Model

Osteopathic manipulation may be used to improve blood flow to the area of injury and remove edema, which may assist in pain reduction and improve mobility. The axillary vein receives tributaries that correspond to the branches of the axillary artery. The subclavian vein passes over the first rib and below the clavicle, crossing over the anterior scalene muscles' insertion on the first rib. The left brachiocephalic vein passes posterior to the left sternoclavicular joint and then crosses the midline. The right subclavian lymphatic trunk drains into the right lymphatic duct. The left subclavian lymphatic trunk drains into the thoracic duct. Somatic dysfunction affecting the venous system may also affect lymphatic drainage, thereby producing congestion in the upper extremity. Fascial restriction of the thoracic inlet and pectoral fascia can also cause lymphatic stasis of the upper extremity (Fig. 111.2).

Improving motion in the lower thoracic region will help the function of the diaphragm from a mechanical perspective. Improving motion in the cervical region will help the function of the diaphragm from a neurologic perspective. Both restore normal diaphragmatic motion, which is the primary driving force to move lymph. This treatment should follow thoracic inlet release, which removes any proximal restrictions to lymphatic flow. In this patient, treatment of the right sternoclavicular restriction will further aid in this process by normalizing fascial tensions of the thoracic inlet. Then, attention is moved distally to remove pectoral and axillary restrictions. Originally, Spencer technique was described as a lymphatic technique for the upper extremity. Over the years, its clinical utility has broadened, and it is often modified to address other musculoskeletal dysfunctions of the upper extremity. It may be used in this case as an adjunctive treatment. Treatment of the distal arm and hand may be necessary as well if indicated.

In addition, somatic dysfunction involving any of the following structures may affect arterial supply and venous return: anterior and middle scalene muscles, upper thoracic vertebrae, upper ribs, clavicles, and the fascia of the upper extremity.

Neurologic Model

Another objective is to normalize neurologic input to the upper extremity. Sympathetic innervation to the shoulder joint complex is mediated through treatment of the T4 dysfunction and the

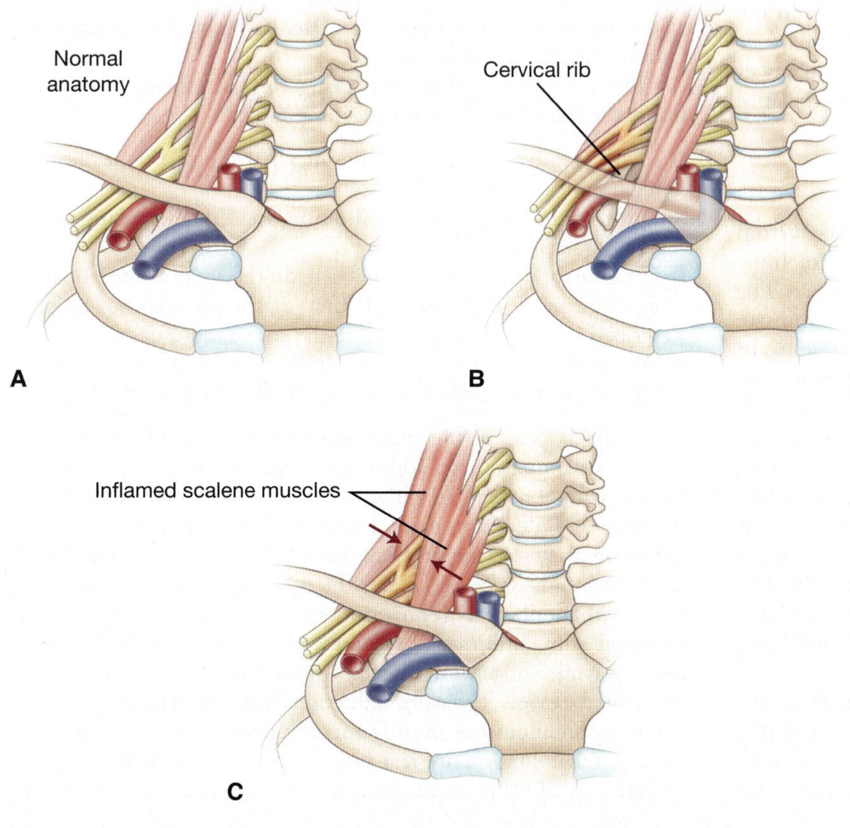

Figure 111.2. Abnormalities in thoracic outlet syndrome. A. Normal anatomy of the thoracic outlet. **B.** The presence of a first cervical rib can lead to compression of the subclavian artery and/or the brachial plexus (*red-shaded region*) between the cervical rib and the clavicle. **C.** Hypertrophy of the anterior and middle scalene muscles following trauma can lead to compression (*arrows*) of the subclavian artery and/or the brachial plexus. (Reprinted with permission from Johansen K, Chung TT, Thomas GI. Pain due to thoracic outlet syndrome. In: Ballantyne JC, Fishman SM, Rathmell JP, eds. *Bonica's Management of Pain*. 5th ed. Wolters Kluwer; 2019:575. Figure 39.1.)

associated ribs. Increased sympathetic tone to the upper extremity can cause vasoconstriction, edema, sensitivity of the nerves, irritability of the muscles, and sweat gland overactivity. OMT in this region can improve those related pathophysiologic findings.

Also, proximal (axial) and peripheral fascial restrictions are removed to limit compression of nerves supplying the region. Tension in the anterior scalene muscles and the thoracic inlet can compress the neurovascular bundle, impairing nerve transmission and vascular supply to the rotator cuff and scapular stabilizing muscles. Removal of the fascial restrictions and resultant compression to the neurovascular bundle will facilitate axoplasmic flow, enhancing the nerves' trophic function.

Metabolic-Energy Model

Efficient transfer of energy in the overhead athlete is vital to performance. While the biomechanical implications of this have been discussed, metabolic processes are also responsible. These manifest grossly in the cardiac, respiratory, neurologic, and psychological systems. One analogy is to envision the body as a large machine. The cardiovascular system is the engine that drives the metabolic system. This diverse system can adapt quickly to changing needs. When needed, the system shifts from the homeostatic life-sustaining mode to supercharged state for athletic activity. This is mediated at the cellular level as cell depolarization that results in measurable changes in cardiac output that enable the athlete to meet the demands placed upon him or her by athletic activity. The "fuel" that drives this system is supplied by the pulmonary system via the gas exchange that occurs at the level of the pulmonary capillaries. This oxygen-rich blood is transported through the larger pulmonary veins and eventually to the left atrium. This fuel is then supplied to the neuromusculoskeletal system and throughout the rest of the body. Occasionally, these systems function together with perfect harmony and precision. The integration of these processes combined with the influence of psychological factors leads to an efficiently functioning machine that some have referred to as the "quantum athlete." Some believe this balance is responsible for an athlete's "court sense" or "being in the zone." Under these ideal circumstances, there is an optimal balance between energy expenditure and energy intake. Disruption in any of these metabolic processes, as in an injured athlete, shifts the balance and leads to an inefficient system.[1]

Behavioral Model

An athlete's mood is affected whenever he or she is restricted from practice and competition. Often an athlete's perception of himself or herself is intimately tied to their athletic performance. The effects of an athlete's injury can manifest in many ways and can impact psychosocial, cultural, behavioral, and spiritual elements. In an affected athlete, this can influence interpersonal relationships, social interactions, school, and/or work performance.

Cognitive learning theory and skills that apply to the athletic setting include self-efficacy, arousal regulation, attentional focus, and mental imagery. During periods of injury, the athlete's ability to access this system is altered, which can have significant psychosocial and emotional impact. For the athlete, this is directly evident by the missed practice and playing time that affects their individual season as well as their teammates. The athlete often feels isolated from the team during treatments and can suffer from a "confidence crisis."

Self-efficacy allows the athlete to actively participate in the rehabilitative process and regain confidence in his or her ability to get better and return to competitive athletics. Enhanced self-efficacy predicts psychological well-being, adherence to prescribed treatments, and pain-coping mechanisms. Poor self-efficacy produces mood fluctuations, reduction in functional ability, and a feeling of helplessness that frustrates both the patient and the clinician if not understood.[2] Enhancing self-efficacy promotes decision-making skills and problem-solving ability through practice and role playing to deal with disease-related issues.[3]

Integrative Treatment Approach

Osteopathic physicians use OMT, which can be a powerful treatment tool for musculoskeletal complaints. Application of osteopathic principles is an important component in the treatment of musculoskeletal complaints. As has been discussed previously, restoration of proper function of the shoulder requires reestablishment of normal structure. For this reason, barring contraindications, OMT should be performed in all patients with shoulder complaints, as indicated. The type of treatment is based on the physician's ability; the patient's response and presentation, the type of dysfunction found, and time limitations of the practice.

While the body has the innate ability to self-heal, adjunctive therapies may be required; most patients will require a comprehensive approach including the appropriate use of other treatment modalities such as medications, injections, physical/occupational therapy, activity modification, dietary changes, occupational changes, and counseling (or emotional support as discussed above) if necessary. In a patient with a full-thickness rotator cuff tear and pain in the shoulder joint complex, the decision between a surgical or conservative approach may not always be straightforward. Each case should be individualized based on patient desire, activity level, and long-term goals. A patient who wished for nothing more than pain relief would be treated differently than a patient who desired high-level physical activity. A detailed discussion of surgical options is beyond the scope of this chapter. If a surgical approach is elected, an informed consent discussion with the patient on the specifics of the procedure should be the first step. For the patients who undergo surgery, OMT can be used as an adjunctive therapy postoperatively (see Chapter 84 Osteopathic Considerations in Orthopedics).

The osteopathic physician caring for the athlete often confronts the following clinical decision points:

- If conservative treatment is chosen, what should be the chronologic sequence of rehabilitation?
- During these stages of rehabilitation, are different manipulative techniques required?
- If conservative treatment is chosen, do the areas of somatic dysfunction need to be removed first, or should exercises be prescribed initially to help alleviate the somatic dysfunction?
- Where should treatment start—in the involved extremity, at the area of greatest restriction, or at a site distant from the injury?

A major goal in the treatment of acute shoulder pain is to control inflammation. In addition to cryotherapy (icing), systemic therapy with nonsteroidal anti-inflammatory drugs will help resolve swelling and decrease pain. Local anti-inflammatory measures (with corticosteroid medication or NSAIDs) can also be employed. Corticosteroids or NSAIDs may be used topically by iontophoresis and phonophoresis (enhancement of topical drug delivery via electrical stimulation or ultrasound, respectively) during physical therapy, while subacromial bursal corticosteroid injections may be performed as well. Typically, reduction of inflammation is accompanied by simultaneous improvement in range of motion. The next steps in rehabilitation are restoring proprioception, flexibility, and strength. In addition, some patients may require narcotic analgesic for short-term use. Muscle spasticity may need to be treated with muscle relaxers or benzodiazepines.

Shoulder manipulation has been shown to be effective in improving mobility and reducing pain.[4] Activity modifications, work restrictions, and lifestyle changes are important aspects of the rehabilitative process. Here, the physician needs to stress and specify relative rest versus absolute rest. If the patient restricts certain ranges of motion too much, eventually the shoulder capsule will adapt to this decreased range of motion and fibrous adhesive capsulitis will result. Many times, Codman pendulum exercises and wall walking exercises are prescribed to maintain mobility in the setting of an immobilized shoulder. Overhead movements can exacerbate impingement and should be modified. In the case of fractures, dislocations, and surgeries, shoulder immobilizers such as casts, splints, or braces are usually required for short periods of time.

Risks and Benefits of Manipulative Treatment for the Shoulder

Complications or adverse events occurring after manipulation of the shoulder have not been reported in the literature.[4] None of the clinical trials evaluating this modality have reported any complications or adverse events in patients with shoulder somatic dysfunction.

Risks of increasing shoulder pain, dislocation, and disability may occur if proper diagnosis is not made. For example, if the practitioner manipulates a hypermobile shoulder that is already unstable due to loss of integrity (i.e., tear) of the rotator cuff, labrum, or other primary shoulder structure, a poor outcome may result.

OMT can be used to treat shoulder pain related to somatic dysfunction. Manual procedures can increase motion, strengthen weak muscles, lyse adhesions, and decrease pain. As described above, manipulative treatment for the shoulder girdle in addition to standard medical care by a primary care practitioner can accelerate recovery from shoulder symptoms and reduce their severity.[4]

ACKNOWLEDGMENTS

The authors and editors of this chapter would like to acknowledge the scholarly contributions of Per Gunnar Brolinon and Thomas A. Goodwin for prior editions of this chapter.

REFERENCES

1. Kerger S. Exercise principles. Ch. 10. In: Karageanes SJ, ed. *Principles of Manual Sports Medicine*. Lippincott, Williams & Wilkins; 2005:65–76.
2. Strecher VJ, DeVellis BM, Becker MH, Rosenstock IM. The role of self-efficacy in achieving health behavior change. *Health Educ Q*. 1986;13(1):73–92.
3. Allegrante JP, Marks R. Self-efficacy in management of osteoarthritis. *Rheum Dis Clin North Am*. 2003;29(4):747–768.
4. Seffinger MA, Hruby RJ. *Evidence Based Manual Medicine: A Problem Oriented Approach*. Saunders/Elsevier; 2007.

112 Case Study: Supination Ankle Sprain

MICHAEL L. KUCHERA ▪ KURT P. HEINKING ▪ JASON VO

KEY CONCEPTS

- Important risk factors in evaluating a patient with an ankle sprain include previous history of an ankle sprain, being overweight, ankle joint laxity, and impaired balance.
- A careful physical exam including provocative tests is important to rule out both local and distant injuries.
- The Ottawa Ankle Rules have been shown to be one of the most accurate guidelines for excluding fractures in the event of an acute ankle injury.
- Conservative treatment including the PRICEM principle has been shown to effectively manage pain and functional recovery of mild–moderate ankle sprains.
- Clinical Practice Guidelines (CPG) recommend manual therapy for improving recovery of ankle injuries in both the short and long term.
- A multidisciplinary approach to ankle sprains including osteopathic manipulative treatment (OMT) and physical therapy (PT) can optimize recovery while reducing the risk of functional ankle instability.

CASE VIGNETTE

A 22-year-old amateur soccer player presents with acute swelling and right lateral ankle pain after twisting his right ankle by stepping in a small pothole in the playing field 48 hours earlier. He describes the mechanism of his injury as plantar flexion with inversion. His pain level is 5/10 in intensity, located at the lateral ankle and described as sharp with certain movements. He has his right ankle wrapped with an over-the-counter elastic bandage using a figure-of-eight pattern extending from metatarsals to midcalf. He can bear weight gingerly but prefers to use a set of crutches due to discomfort. The patient has been taking ibuprofen for the pain as well as icing and elevating the leg, all which seems to help. He has associated edema and bruising along the lateral aspect. He denies having associated knee, hip, or back pain.

PAST MEDICAL HISTORY

- Seasonal allergies
- Past right ankle sprain (1 year ago, right side)

PAST SURGICAL HISTORY

- Tonsillectomy at age 5 years
- Appendectomy at age 12 years
- Wisdom teeth extracted at age 18 years

FAMILY HISTORY

His mother is 58 years old with a history of asthma, and his father is 59 years old with a history of diabetes mellitus, hypertension, and hyperlipidemia. He has no siblings. There is no family history of orthopedic issues.

SOCIAL HISTORY

He is single, sexually active in a monogamous relationship for 2 years. He is employed as a web page developer. He does not use tobacco or illicit drugs. He drinks coffee and alcohol only occasionally.

MEDICATIONS

He takes two tablets of OTC ibuprofen every 4 hours as needed for pain. He uses loratadine as needed for his allergies.

ALLERGIES

- No history of drug or food allergies

REVIEW OF SYSTEMS

General

- No fever, no chills, no fatigue, no recent weight loss

HEENT

- No sore throat or dysphagia, no sinusitis, no auditory changes, tinnitus or vertigo, no nose bleeds, no loss of smell
- Some nasal stuffiness and itchy eyes

Respiratory

- No cough, no shortness of breath, no wheezing, no hemoptysis, no dyspnea on exertion

Cardiovascular

- No chest pain, no palpitations

Neurologic

- No sensory changes or motor weakness, no ataxia, no dizziness, no lightheadedness, no headache

Musculoskeletal

- Pain and swelling of lateral right ankle, states weight bearing causes discomfort

Skin

- Reports some bruising of his foot, no rash, no pruritus

PHYSICAL EXAM

Vital Signs

- Temperature 37 °C, pulse 82/min and regular, respirations 12/min, blood pressure 120/74

General

- Well-developed, well-nourished male in no acute distress, alert and oriented to person, place, and time.

HEENT

- No signs of trauma, sclera clear, auditory canals are clear, and tympanic membranes are intact. No nasal drainage is noted, some edema of the turbinate's, the nasal septum is midline. The oropharynx reveals no exudates or erythema.

Lungs

- Clear to auscultation bilaterally, no wheezes, no rhonchi, no rales

Cardiovascular

- Regular rate and rhythm, no murmurs
- Peripheral pulses intact and equal

Abdomen

- Bowel sounds present, nontender, no guarding, no rigidity, no rebound, and soft

Neurologic

- Cranial nerves II to XII are grossly intact, motor strength is 5/5, and reflexes are 2+/4+ bilaterally in upper and lower limbs. Sensation is intact to light touch and pinprick, and coordination is intact. Gait is antalgic, favors injured ankle.

Extremities

- Moderate swelling and mild bruising of the right lateral ankle.
- Able to walk without crutches 30 ft and back, with some discomfort.
- No bony tenderness of the lateral or medial malleolus of the distal 6 cm.
- Tenderness to palpation over the right anterolateral aspect of the foot just anterior and distal to the fibula over the anterior talofibular ligament (ATFL) and some tenderness over the calcaneofibular ligament (CFL).
- Limited dorsiflexion 5 to 10 degrees, and inversion due to pain, positive right ankle anterior drawer test (ADT) with moderate laxity, negative talar tilt test, compared to the left, negative squeeze test.
- There was approximately 1 cm of swelling of the lateral right ankle.
- The left ankle had a pain free normal range of motion, with no swelling.
- No pain to palpation of the proximal fibula
- The right knee was normal in appearance without swelling, bruising or deformity. The Lachman's test, sag sign, and valgus varus stress tests were negative. There was no joint line pain or patellar grinding. The right hamstring and calf were hypertonic.
- There was pain free passive range of motion of the right hip.

Skin

- No rashes, purple bruising lateral aspect right foot

OSTEOPATHIC STRUCTURAL EXAM

Standing Landmarks

- Positive right seated flexion test
- Positive right standing flexion test
- Group curve convex left lumbar spine
- Slightly diminished right arch
- Level iliac crests

Lumbar Spine

- L1–5 N SB right Rot left
- L5 F SB right rotated left

Sacrum

- Right on right forward sacral torsion

Pelvis

- Right posterior innominate

Lower Extremity

- Right anterior lateral malleolus
- Right posterior fibular head
- Posterior tibia on talus dysfunction (restricted dorsiflexion)
- Posterolateral talocalcaneal dysfunction
- Externally rotated tibia with anterior medial glide
- Fibularis longus and tibialis anterior tender points (see Box 112.1)

> **BOX 112.1 Inversion/Supination Ankle Injury (Rt.)**
>
> - Plantar flexion is free
> - Talus has a posterolateral dysfunction (to calcaneus)
> - Calcaneus inverts (tilts inward)
> - Distal talofibular joint glides anterior
> - Fibular head glides posteriorly
> - Tibia rotates externally
> - Femur rotates internally in relation to tibia
> - Ipsilateral ilium is posterior
> - Sacrum rotates R on R
> - Fibularis longus and tibialis anterior tender points

DIAGNOSTICS/IMAGING

Ankle x-rays are not indicated initially due to the Ottawa Ankle Rules. The guidelines state that x-ray studies should be done if one of the following is true[1]:

- Bony tenderness distal 6 cm at the posterior edge of the lateral malleolus
- Bony tenderness distal 6 cm at the posterior edge of the medial malleolus
- Patient is unable to bear weight (or take four steps) immediately after the injury and during the physical exam.
- Pain or bone tenderness over an area of potential fracture (i.e., lateral malleolus, medial malleolus, base of fifth metatarsal, or navicular bone)

The Ottawa Ankle Rules have been shown to be one of the most accurate guidelines for excluding fractures in the event of an acute ankle injury.[1,2]

However, if imaging was needed, the preferred initial imaging is anteroposterior (AP), "mortise view" (AP with 10 to 20 degrees internal rotation) and lateral views (see Fig. 112.1) should be obtained.[3,4] In a skeletally immature patient, Salter–Harris type 1 fracture should not be overlooked, when there is tenderness over the distal growth-plate of the tibia or fibula.[5] For very small fractures, a computed tomography (CT) scan can be performed. For a suspected syndesmotic injury, a

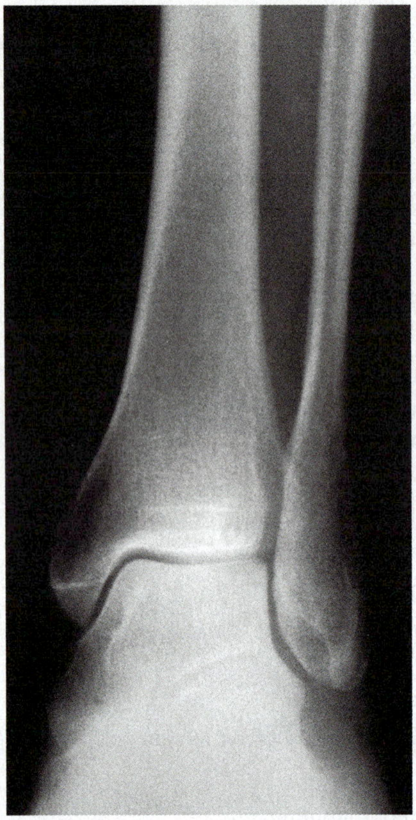

Figure 112.1. Ankle mortise x-ray. (Reprinted with permission from Baron RL, Strugielski CF, Christman RA. Positioning techniques and terminology. In: Christman RA, ed. *Foot and Ankle Radiology*. 2nd ed. Wolters Kluwer; 2015:58. Figure 4.17B.)

weight-bearing cone-beam CT can be performed.[3] An advantage of this type of CT scan is that it can evaluate the stability of the distal tibiofibular joint under compression which can become unstable after an ankle injury.[3] MRI can be obtained but it is not typically done for simple ankle sprains. MRI can be helpful in the situation of severe trauma, extreme clinical findings, suspicion of syndesmotic injury, persistent complaints, and surgical planning.[3]

DIFFERENTIAL DIAGNOSIS

Differential includes but is not limited to:

- Ankle sprain
- Peroneal (fibularis) tendon strain
- Ankle fracture
- Lisfranc joint injury
- Tendon rupture
- Tendon subluxation
- Chondral/osteochondral injury
- Maisonneuve fracture
- Peroneal nerve injury
- Somatic dysfunction, ankle, fibula

IMPRESSION/DIAGNOSIS

- Supination ankle sprain, grade II
- Somatic dysfunction of the lower extremity (foot, leg, knee), pelvic region, sacrum, and lumbar region

DISCUSSION

Epidemiology

Acute ankle sprain is one of the most common reasons for primary care office and emergency department visits in the United States, with an overall incidence of 2.15 per 1,000 person-years.[6] Reportedly ankle sprains account for 12% of all injuries seen in emergency departments and up to 30% of all sports injuries.[7,8] Likewise, 29% of all injuries to the lower extremities in soccer affect this joint, 75% of them to the lateral ligaments.[9] According to a systematic review by Fong et al.[10] the ankle was the second most common injured body site after the knee, and ankle sprain was the most common type of ankle injury. In athletes the incidence of ankle injury and ankle sprain was high in court games and team sports, such as rugby, soccer, volleyball, handball, and basketball.[10]

Ankle sprains cause pain and restricted range of motion; and can lead to functional deficits, post-traumatic osteoarthritis, and chronic ankle instability.[8] One-fourth of all individuals who have experienced a significant ankle sprain will continue to have pain, instability, and sprain recurrence.[11] These signs can appear in 44% of patients with a sprain 1 year after the injury.[8,12]

Risk Factors, Causes, Mechanisms

Previous history of an ankle sprain is the most important risk factor, as well as other considerations such as being overweight, ankle joint laxity, and impaired balance.[4] Taking the time to do a thorough history and physical will allow the physician to accurately diagnose ankle injuries and create a plan for recovery. If the injury is not appropriately treated, it can potentially result in chronic ankle instability.[13] According to a recent study, Dolan et al.[14] found 12 variables to be associated with increased incidence of ankle sprain. To reduce the risk of ankle sprain, BMI, ankle plantar and dorsiflexion strength, hip strength, and single leg landing performance should be determined and incorporated in athlete assessment and subsequent program design. Mechanisms in soccer include catching the lateral side of the foot on the ground, an awkward landing on the opponent's foot, or contacting an opponent's supporting leg during a slide tackle.[4] There are different theories on why ankle sprains occur describing intrinsic and extrinsic mechanisms. One theory describes mechanical instability due to damaged support structures including ligaments and muscle, while another theory identifies functional instability owing to dysfunctional neural-proprioceptive pathways that inaccurately report ankle position.[15] Most sprains affect the lateral collateral ligament complex, which is injured in 85% of the ankle sprains.[4] The ATFL ruptures first, then the CFL, and PTFL ruptures usually only occur after ankle dislocation.[3] Medial collateral ligaments injuries are far less frequent than lateral collateral ligaments and occur in 5% to 15% of ankle sprains.[3]

Physical Exam and Grading

Diagnosis typically involves a physical examination beginning with inspection, observing gait and station, with an assessment of the patient's neurovascular status. This includes light touch sensation, capillary refilling, and dorsal pedal pulses.[4] Next, looking for a fracture by careful palpation of the critical anatomic checkpoints (especially lateral and medial malleoli, the base of the fifth metatarsal and navicular bones), ecchymosis, edema, point tenderness, ROM, ligamentous laxity, and muscle strength should be carefully evaluated in all suspected ankle sprains.[4] Localized tenderness over the ATFL and CFL are common findings and usually the point of maximal tenderness.[16]

The provocative tests are also important. The ADT and talar tilt (inversion stress) tests are utilized to evaluate lateral ankle

TABLE 112.1

Grading of Ankle Sprains[19]

	Grade I	Grade II	Grade III
Loss of Function	None	Some	Significant
Laxity	None	Some	Significant
Ortho Tests	Negative	Positive anterior drawer test, negative tilt test	Positive anterior drawer and tilt test
Point Tenderness	None	Yes	Yes
Decreased Ankle Motion	Yes, <5 degrees	Yes, 5–10 degrees	Yes, >10 degrees
Hemorrhaging	None	Yes	Yes
Swelling	<0.5 cm	Yes, 0.5–2 cm	Yes, >2 cm

instability. These tests should be performed in comparison with the uninjured ankle. Tests are regarded as positive in cases of increased laxity. A positive test for ATFL laxity is 10 mm of displacement in the injured ankle or more than 3 to 4 mm of difference in translation compared with the healthy side.[4,17] The talar tilt test evaluates the integrity of the CFL. In this test, the angle between the talar dome and the tibial plafond is measured during forced heel inversion while the tibiotalar joint is in the neutral position. If there is more than 5 degrees of difference with the normal side, the test is considered positive.[4,17] If possible, patients should be examined again 3 to 5 days later.[18] To rule out less common syndesmotic injuries, provocative tests are helpful. These tests including the squeeze test (lower leg squeeze at midcalf), external rotation stress test (concurrent external rotation and dorsiflexion), and Cotton test (applying a medial and lateral translation force to the foot) to stress the syndesmosis and elicit pain above the ankle joint.[1]

Lateral ankle sprains are characteristically classified as grade I, II, or III, based on the severity of injury to the lateral ligaments (see Table 112.1).[19] Mild swelling, tenderness, and minimal difficulty in ROM are usually seen in lower grades. However, diffuse swelling, ecchymosis, tenderness, positive provocative tests, and inability of weight bearing are associated with substantial instability in a grade III injury.[17] According to a systematic review, 96% of patients with all four findings of swelling, ecchymosis, tenderness, and a positive ADT have a lateral ligament rupture in contrast to only 14% of individuals without all these findings.[20]

PATIENT MANAGEMENT

Osteopathic patient management should start with the patient not the ankle. Consideration of the biopsychosocial model is part of the osteopathic approach. In determining a holistic management plan, the osteopathic physician should determine the effect of the injury on the patient, what their goals, expectations, concerns, and fears are; and what they can and cannot do. Evaluating the social determinants of their treatment including any barriers to healing is important. Consideration of the patient's rehabilitation timeline, motivation, activity level, social support, and financial constraints will determine their treatment plan. Each patient with an ankle sprain is unique, even though there are clinical practice guidelines to help direct care.

According to Ruiz-Sánchez et al.[8] who evaluated current clinical practice guidelines (CPGs) and their level of evidence, clinicians should utilize the following treatments in clinical practice.

- Cryotherapy
- Functional supports
- Early ambulation
- Short term NSAIDs
- Manual therapy
- Rehabilitation

PRICEM principle

Together the use of cryotherapy, functional supports, elevation, and medication is known as the PRICEM principle. PRICEM = protection, rest, ice, compression, elevation, mobility/medication. Clinical practice guidelines suggest the application of cryotherapy for the first 3 to 7 days to reduce pain and swelling, combined with the use of functional supports such as air stirrup braces or lace-up supports to facilitate early mobilization.[8] The application of ice in the acute phase of an ankle sprain considerably reduces pain compared to the use of analgesic drugs.[8] However, studies show low effectiveness of cryotherapy in the recovery phase, indicating that it should be applied only to acute ankle sprains to reduce pain, minimize swelling, and avoid secondary injuries.[21] The use of functional support for 4 to 6 weeks has been shown to be preferable to immobilization or elastic bandage/Kinesio tape.[8,22] However, there is some recent evidence to support Kinesio Taping such as a stabilizing effect with significant improvement in gait functions, reduction in inversion and eversion range of motion, a decrease in muscle activation and postural sway.[23] In a large review, Ortega-Avila et al.[24] included 20 studies, involving 2,236 subjects, to demonstrate that conservative treatment (e.g., RICE, cryotherapy, exercise, and manual therapy) effectively manages pain and functional recovery.[25]

For severe (grade III) ankle sprains, a cast may be used to manage pain and swelling. However, the cast should be worn for no more than 10 days.[26] After this period, remove the cast and begin functional treatment, which includes exercises and activities to restore mobility and strength. In addition, short-term use of NSAIDs and rehabilitation exercises are advised to aid recovery and prevent chronic ankle instability.[8] NSAIDs in the acute phase of the injury is highly recommended, being considered a safe procedure; however, their long-term use is not recommended.[22] Specifically, naproxen taken for a week after an ankle injury has been shown to help decrease pain and swelling with weight bearing and at rest.[27]

In acute injuries, following these recommendations have been shown to help people recover quicker.[28] Protection is important to prevent reinjuring an ankle during the recovery process. Rest, ice, compression, and elevation help provide better conditions for pain relief and recovery of the joint. Early mobility and ambulation have been shown to improve ankle function when compared to more immobile recovery.[29]

Manual Therapy/OMT

Osteopathic manipulative treatment (OMT) has been identified as a beneficial therapeutic approach for patients experiencing ankle pain or sprains. Clinical studies have demonstrated that OMT can lead to statistically significant improvements in edema and pain for acute ankle sprains when applied in emergency department settings.[30] OMT in the early stages of an ankle injury can aid the recovery progress faster due to addressing somatic dysfunction associated with the injury. In addition, OMT techniques such as muscle energy and counterstrain have been shown to increase the range of motion while decreasing pain and edema in patients with first-degree ankle sprains.[31] The efficacy of OMT in the management of acute ankle injuries is supported by data indicating that even a single session targeting patient-specific somatic dysfunction, can provide immediate improvement in pain, edema, and range of ankle motion and can significantly affect the treatment outcomes.[31,32] Clinical Practice Guidelines (CPGs) strongly recommend manual therapy for improving ankle injury recovery. This recommendation is based on high-quality scientific evidence and applies to both short-term and long-term recovery periods.[8] A single session was associated with an improvement in edema and pain in individuals with acute ankle sprains.[22,26,33] Likewise, passive mobilizations should be used to increase ankle dorsiflexion and improve its function.[8]

Inversion ankle sprain also causes muscle strain in the lower extremity affecting sacral, pelvic, hip, and knee mechanics (see Fig. 112.2). Indirect OMT plays an important role in initial management as patient tolerance to OMT needs to be considered. Subsequently, as the initial phase resolves, strategies shift to effective rehabilitation including early mobilization, and correction of somatic dysfunctions that could limit shock absorption, ankle range of motion (especially dorsiflexion), and muscle-proprioceptive imbalance.

OMT may be utilized based on the clinical applications of the five models of osteopathic care. Considering the biomechanical–postural model, diagnosing and treating somatic dysfunction of the tibia and talus is useful to improve ankle dorsiflexion. Research studies have shown that patients with an 11 degrees loss of ankle dorsiflexion have nearly five times the risk of ankle sprain of compared to people with average flexibility.[34] Considering the neurologic model, improving pain, and resolving somatic dysfunction in joints and muscles known to impair proprioceptive balance mechanisms is also beneficial in ankle healing.[35] Furthermore, osteopathic treatment utilizing the respiratory–circulatory model opening restricted myofascial pathways to provide reduction of swelling, loss of function, and residual dysfunction seen in acute ankle trauma.[32] Outcomes associated with the use of manual treatment suggest more rapid resolution of pain, swelling, and dysfunction and it also might reduce the risk of reinjury.[32,36–39] Patient education and exercise (strengthening, range of motion,

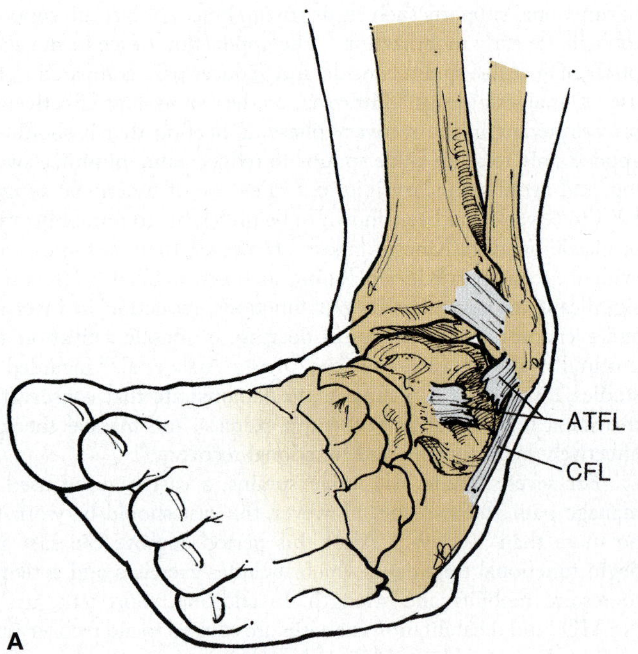

A

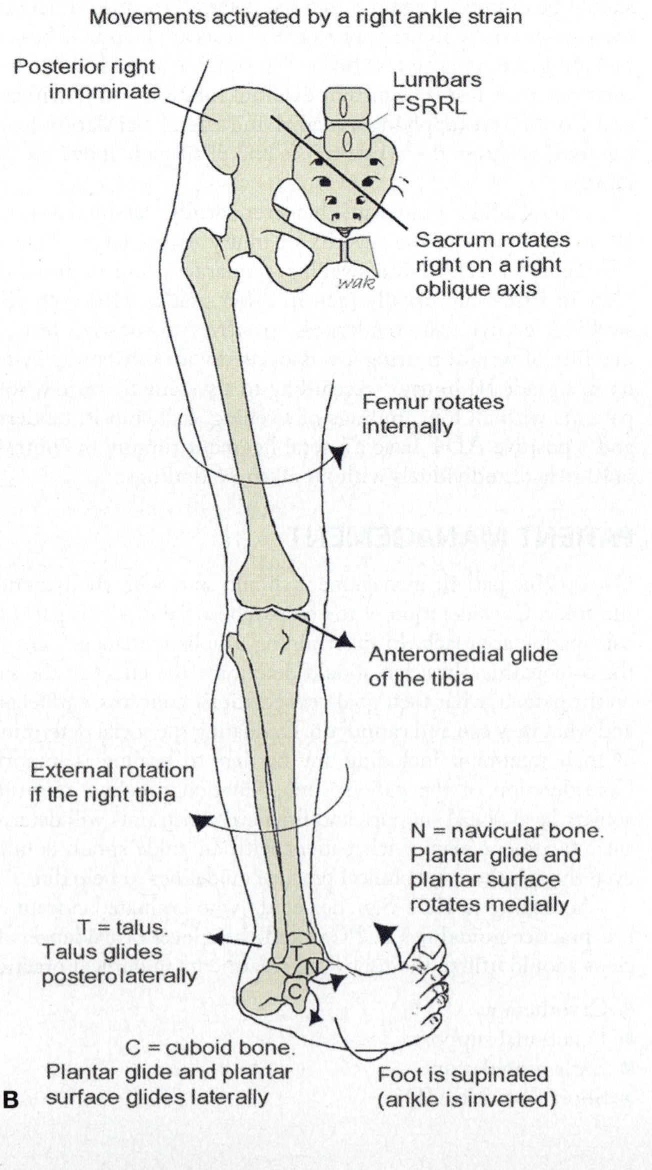

B

Figure 112.2. Inversion/supination ankle sprain. A. Inversion ankle sprain. **B.** Inversion ankle sprain also causes muscle strain in the lower extremity affecting sacral, pelvic, hip, and knee mechanics. (**A,** Reprinted with permission from Baker CL Jr., Flandry F, Henderson JM. *The Hughston Clinic Sports Medicine Field Manual.* Williams & Wilkins; 1996:240. Figure 22-1; **B** by William A. Kuchera, DO, FAAO, with permission.)

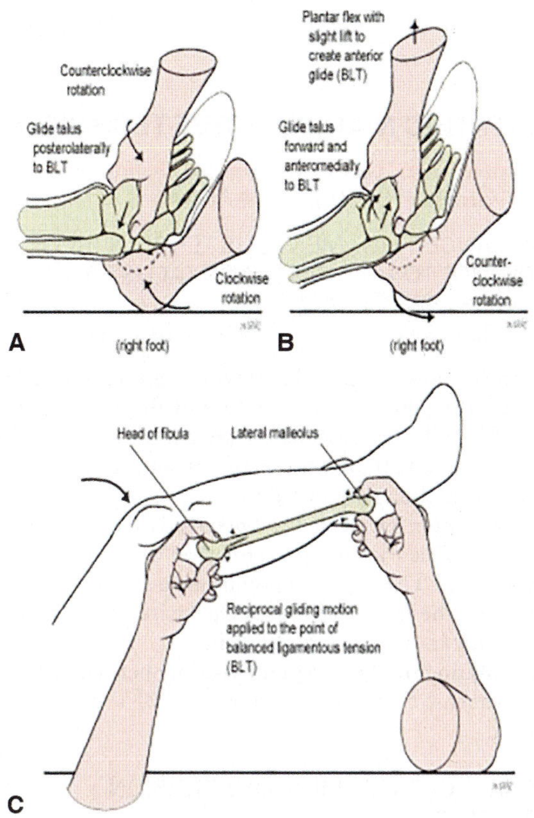

Figure 112.3. A–C. BLT/BMT OMT for patients with supination sprain (**A**) posterolateral talocalcaneal SD; (**B**) plantar flexion with anterior glide talotibial SD; (**C**) fibular head SD with interosseous strain. (Illustration by William A. Kuchera, DO, FAAO, with permission.)

and proprioceptive) often play a role in this stage for full return of function and prevention of recurrence.[40]

Osteopathic Technique Application

This chapter contains an effective combination of osteopathic techniques used in ankle sprain patients (see technique section). The balanced ligamentous and balanced membranous techniques (BLT/BMT) are appropriate even immediately after a sprain. With experience the clinician can transition from the tibiotalar joint into the subtalar joint (see Fig. 112.3A) and from that point of balance, carry the indirect fascial unwinding technique up through the ATFL into the interosseous membrane (see Fig. 112.3B). These techniques with practice can be done seamlessly without changing hand positions around the talocalcaneal joint. In addition, a BLT technique for the fibula is depicted in Figure 112.3C. Fascial unwinding may be performed from the foot–ankle up and from the hip down, making a time-effective approach to this injury. For more chronic conditions, or after the initial injury has healed, direct action technique may be utilized if necessary. These generally include muscle energy technique, HVLA, articulatory and soft tissue (see technique section).

In chronic conditions (or when the swelling recedes in a recent ankle sprain), gentle direct-action techniques such as popliteal spread may be performed (see Fig. 112.4).

For articular dysfunction, muscle energy technique or HVLA may be added if needed. Direct OMT procedures include those for the talocrural joint, tarsal bones, and proximal fibula. Some examples of these techniques can be seen in the technique section (see Figs. 112.5 and 112.6).

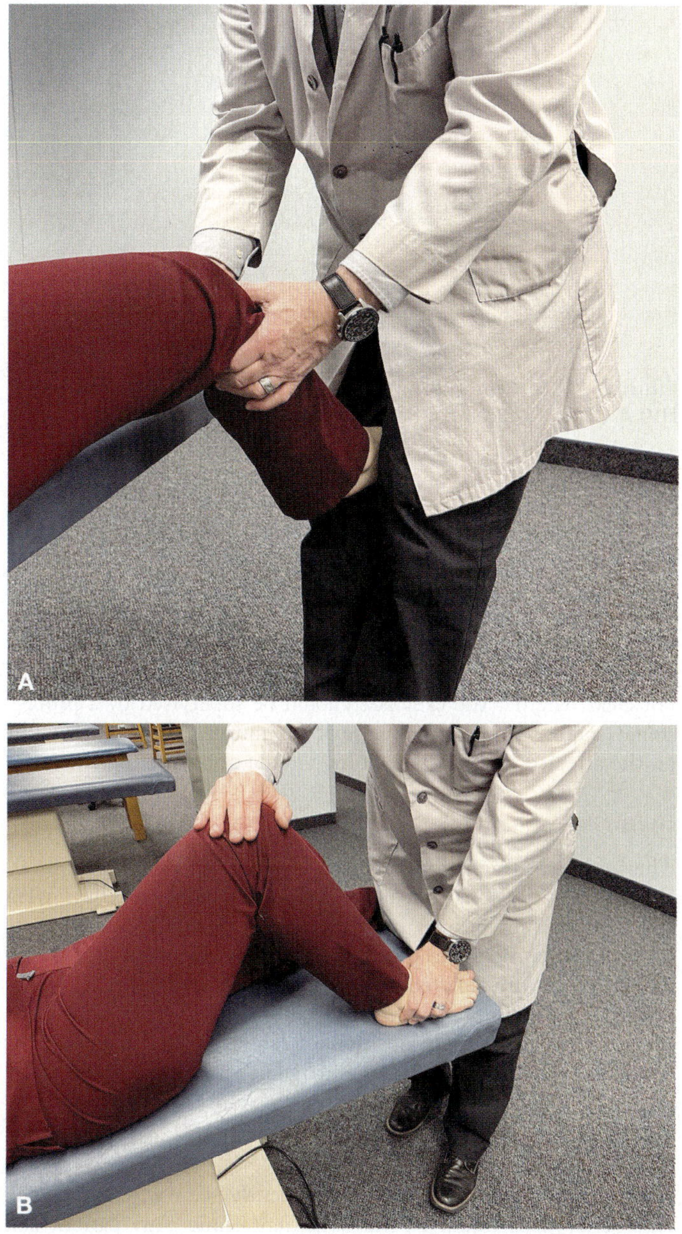

Figure 112.4. A. Popliteal spread, fascial unwinding. **B.** Lateral fluctuation.

The involvement of OMT as a supplement to the patient's rehabilitation can help improve movement and decrease pain during the recovery period. Together OMT and PT can address damaged support structures as well as dysfunctional proprioceptive pathways contributing to ankle instability.

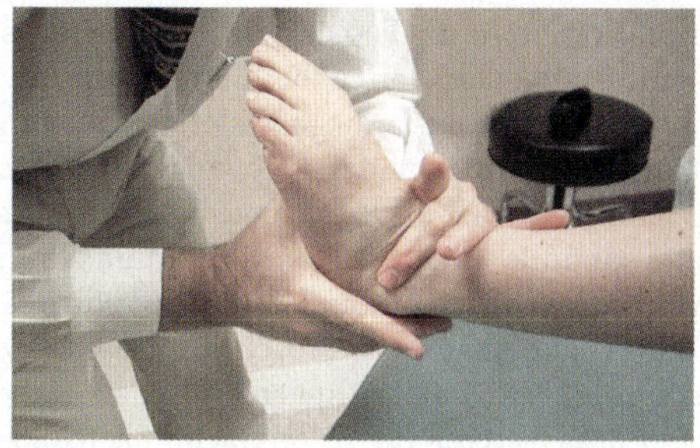

Figure 112.5. Correction of talocrural dysfunction using HVLA OMT. (Courtesy of Per Gunnar Brolinson, DO.)

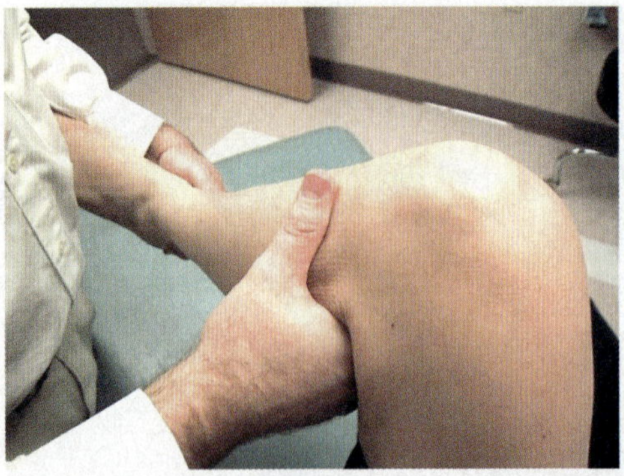

Figure 112.6. Correction of fibular head dysfunction using HVLA OMT. (Courtesy of Per Gunnar Brolinson, DO.)

Rehabilitation/PT

An exercise program should be comprehensive and progressive including the range of motion, stretching, strengthening, neuromuscular, proprioceptive, and sport-specific exercises.[4] Regarding rehabilitation, physical exercise has a high grade of recommendation to reduce the risk of functional ankle instability and optimizes a better recovery of joint function of the ankle.[21,22] Although it is not clear whether the exercises should be supervised by a professional or not.[22] In the acute phase of the injury; walk or bear weight on the affected limb also had a high grade of recommendation.

Referral and Surgical Management

The initial treatment for fractures, ligament and tendon injuries, osteochondral lesions and nerve lesions should be PRICE with strictly no weight-bearing on the affected foot and specialty referral to a sports medicine physician or orthopedic surgeon.[31] High level athletes with isolated total rupture of the collateral ligaments and severe instability may be treated surgically.[41] Other indications for surgery include interposition of lateral collateral ligaments, (osteo)chondral lesions, impingement, and dislocated fractures.[41]

SUMMARY

Patients with ankle injuries are frequently seen whether in the emergency department or the outpatient clinic. Any patient can have an ankle injury, but athletes are more susceptible to ankle injuries due to the sport that they play. When it comes to evaluating joint injuries, it is very important to solicit a thorough history and perform a detailed physical to make an accurate diagnosis. The strongest risk factor for an ankle sprain is a previous ankle sprain. Clinicians should assess one joint above and one joint below the injured structure(s). Diagnosis of associated somatic dysfunction is important for patient management. Imaging of the ankle is indicated if the patient has bony tenderness to palpation over the medial or lateral malleolus or if the patient is unable to walk four steps immediately after the injury or during the physical evaluation. After making a diagnosis of an acute ankle sprain, the patient management includes following the PRICE recommendations along with NSAIDs for acute pain relief. Each patient with an ankle sprain is unique, so an osteopathic clinician should address any personal concerns, social issues, and barriers to healing that exist. OMT and manual approaches for associated somatic dysfunction are supported by the literature. Rehabilitation of ankle sprains is critical, as patients can go on to chronic pain and disability. Implementing conservative management using the PRICEM principles, physical therapy, and OMT can help improve swelling, mobility, strength, and balance returning the patient to their active lifestyle.

OSTEOPATHIC MANIPULATIVE TECHNIQUES

OMT Procedures Using Indirect Activating Forces (Away From the Restrictive Barrier)

OMT: BALANCED LIGAMENTOUS TENSION (BLT) OF FOREFOOT TO HIND FOOT AND TALUS TO CALCANEUS (SEE FIG. 112.3A)

Diagnosis: Posterolateral talocalcaneal dysfunction

1. The doctor uses the right hand with the thumb and first digit pinching the talus of the right foot of the supine patient; the remainder of the fingers hold the arch of the patient's right foot. The left hand stabilizes the patient's right calcaneus between the fingers and thenar eminence.
2. Using a motion between the two hands like "wringing out a wet cloth," glide the talus posterolateral on the calcaneus to the point of BLT. The right hand will move slightly counterclockwise, while the left hand moves clockwise; the right hand will also slightly increase the foot's arch.
3. Concentrating on the persistent yielding between the talus and the calcaneus, continuously adjust the BLT until a release is palpated.

OMT: BALANCED LIGAMENTOUS TENSION (SEE FIG. 112.3B)

Diagnosis: Plantar flexion with anterior glide of the talocrural joint.

1. Maintaining the same hand hold as above, gently lift the lower extremity off the table to create a gentle anterior glide of the talus in the ankle mortise and add just enough plantar flexion (and additional anterior glide) to feel BLT between the talus and the rest of the lower leg at the ankle.
2. Concentrating on the persistent yielding between the talus in the mortise, continuously adjust the BLT until a release is palpated.
3. If the doctor wishes a slight shift of focus can be made at this point to gently pull in an anteromedial direction through the ATFL into the distal fibula and the interosseous membrane.

OMT: BLT OF FIBULA AND BMT OF THE INTEROSSEOUS MEMBRANE (SEE FIG. 112.3C)

Diagnosis: Fibular head dysfunction (usually posterior) with strain of interosseous membrane.

1. The doctor's left thumb pad contacts the right fibula just posterior to the fibular head; the right thumb pad is placed just posterior to the lateral malleolus. The supine patient's hip and knee on that side are bent so that the lower extremity sits comfortably on the doctor's thumbs. The weight is adjusted to avoid compression over these thumbs. (The doctor may use fingers or even a forehead to help take weight off of the thumbs.)
2. The lower extremity is adjusted by modifying the hip and knee bend (and perhaps a bit of external rotation at the hip) so that the fibula at both ends feels as if the same slight weight is resting on each thumb. (The doctor will typically have both elbows resting on the table.)
3. The fibula is then balanced (to BLT) with either a slight amount of inferosuperior glide from the lateral malleolus thumb to move the fibular head posterior to balance—OR—with a slight amount of superoanterior pressure from the fibular head thumb to glide the fibular head anterior to balance.

4. Final fine-tuning usually consists of an inferior longitudinal balancing force through both thumbs along the long axis of the fibula that often also needs slight medial glide of the distal fibula (in the direction of the sprained ATFL) to the point of BMT.
5. Concentrating on the persistent yielding of the fibular head in the direction it first preferred, and along the interosseous membrane between the tibia and fibula, adjust the BLT/BMT until a release is palpated.

OMT: POPLITEAL SPREAD, FASCIAL UNWINDING, AND LATERAL FLUCTUATION OF THE LOWER EXTREMITY TO ENHANCE HOMEOSTASIS TO HANDLE INFLAMMATION AND EDEMA (FIG. 112.4A,B)

Diagnosis: Edema, inflammation, and fascial torsion in lower extremity.

1. The patient is supine with leg slightly flexed and abducted to allow the doctor (standing at the end of the table) to place the patient's ankle/foot between his or her lower thighs to help control the patient's leg.
2. Using the fingers of both hands, the doctor contacts the medial and lateral edges of the hamstring muscle tendons and gently spreads these away from the midline of the popliteal region. ("Popliteal spread technique").
3. Abduct/adduct, flex/extend, and internally/externally rotate at the hip to the point of BLT.
4. Maintain hip but stack major and minor motions at the knee (flex/extend, abduct/adduct, and externally/internally rotate with anteromedial or posterolateral glides, respectively).
5. Maintain hip and knee balanced tensions and now add an approximation of pronation/supination of the foot.
6. Add a little traction or compression along the longitudinal axis of the lower extremity again to BLT.
7. As "fascial unwinding" is performed, ask where the patient feels warmth. It should progress from thigh to knee to calf to foot to toes over a period of a minute or less. (If the progression stops, it indicates a site of significant somatic dysfunction that may require specific OMT.)
8. Now, for the lateral fluctuation component, place the patient's feet flat on the table with knee flexed to 90 degrees and hip flexed to 45 degrees (see Fig. 112.4B).
9. The doctor's caudad hand holds the dorsum of the patient's foot and ankle and the cephalad hand rests on top of the patient's knee.
10. The patient's knee is moved medial and lateral at the knee to find the position of greatest ligamentous balance.
11. From that point of balance, the doctor institutes a small rhythmic medial to lateral excursion that is maintained until treatment is finished.

OMT Procedures Using Direct Activating Forces (Toward the Restrictive Barrier)

These procedures are most safely used after the sprained ankle has healed and yet somatic dysfunction persists. They can be used alongside the indirect BLT and BMT OMT procedures above or afterward if the latter has not shown to be effective enough to restore normal motion and mechanics. Sometimes, the patient presents for care long after the ankle sprain has healed, and the direct-action procedures below are used initially to restore normal joint mechanics. The BLT and BMT OMT procedures can be used before or after the direct action OMT procedures at the same office visit.

Talocrural/Talotibial Dysfunction

OMT: MOBILIZATION WITH IMPULSE

Diagnosis: An ankle sprained with a supination mechanism results in restriction of eversion, dorsiflexion, and posterior glide of the talocrural joint.

1. The patient is supine on the table, while the physician stands at foot of table facing the patient (Fig. 112.5).
2. The physician grasps the dorsum of the involved foot at the talocrural junction.
3. The physician lifts, everts, and dorsiflexes the foot with enough posterior glide to reach the end point of motion.
4. Gentle traction is applied to remove "slack" in joint space and soft tissue structures, followed by a quick "mobilization with impulse" longitudinal tug.
5. This restores functional motion to the talocrural joint.

Fibular Head Dysfunction

OMT: MOBILIZATION WITH IMPULSE

Diagnosis: Following a supination ankle sprain, the fibular head frequently is found in a posteriorly displaced position.

1. The patient is supine; the physician stands alongside and facing the patient's involved extremity (Fig. 112.6).
2. Using the hand closest to the patient's foot, the physician grasps the patient's heel and lifts it off the table, passively flexing the leg at the knee.
3. The physician places the first metacarpal phalangeal (MCP) joint of the other hand behind the fibular head.
4. To encourage the distal fibula to move posteriorly, the subject's leg is externally rotated and flexed further until the proximal fibular head contacts the MCP joint.
5. Flexion of the hip and knee is continued to end point of motion.
6. A "mobilization with impulse" (HVLA) is delivered into further flexion at the knee causing the fibular head to contact the physician's MCP joint and be driven anteriorly (pry technique), thereby restoring normal motion and function.

Fibularis Longus and Brevis Contraction

OMT: SOFT TISSUE TECHNIQUE

Diagnosis: With an ankle sprain, the fibularis longus and brevis muscles, which attach laterally to the fibula and wrap under the lateral aspect of the foot, are strained, resulting in reflex spasm, hypertonicity, or possible creation of myofascial trigger points.

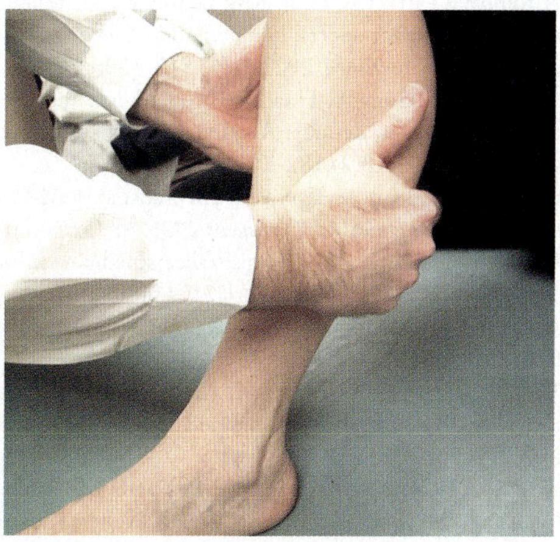

Figure 112.7. Treating fibularis longus and brevis with soft tissue OMT. (Courtesy of Per Gunnar Brolinson, DO.)

1. The patient is supine with the involved leg flexed to 90 degrees and the foot resting flat on the table; the physician stands to the side or end of the table near the patient's affected leg (Fig. 112.7).
2. The involved fibularis muscles are manually massaged and kneaded to release the spasm and hypertonicity and to help milk out any edema.

ACKNOWLEDGMENTS

The authors and editors of this chapter would like to acknowledge the scholarly contributions of Per Gunnar Brolinon and Thomas A. Goodwin for prior editions of this chapter.

REFERENCES

1. Tiemstra JD. *Am Fam Physician.* 2012;85(12):1170–1176.
2. Barelds I, Krijnen WP, van de Leur JP, van der Schans CP, Goddard RJ. Diagnostic accuracy of clinical decision rules to exclude fractures in acute ankle injuries: systematic review and meta-analysis. *J Emerg Med.* 2017;53(3):353–368.
3. Jungmann PM, Lange T, Wenning M, Baumann FA, Bamberg F, Jung M. Ankle sprains in athletes: current epidemiological, clinical and imaging trends. *Open Access J Sports Med.* 2023;14:29–46.
4. Halabchi F, Hassabi M. Acute ankle sprain in athletes: clinical aspects and algorithmic approach. *World J Orthop.* 2020;11(12):534–558.
5. Dubin JC, Comeau D, McClelland RI, Dubin RA, Ferrel E. Lateral and syndesmotic ankle sprain injuries: a narrative literature review. *J Chiropr Med.* 2011;10(3):204–219.
6. Waterman BR, Owens BD, Davey S, Zacchilli MA, Belmont PJ Jr. The epidemiology of ankle sprains in the United States. *J Bone Joint Surg Am.* 2010;92(13):2279–2284.
7. Nielsen AB, Yde J. Epidemiology and traumatology of injuries in soccer. *Am J Sports Med.* 1989;17:803–807.
8. Ruiz-Sánchez FJ, Ruiz-Muñoz M, Martín-Martín J, et al. Management and treatment of ankle sprain according to clinical practice guidelines: A PRISMA systematic review. *Medicine (Baltimore).* 2022;101(42):e31087.
9. Medina McKeon JM, Bush HM, Reed A, Whittington A, Uhl TL, McKeon PO. Return-to-play probabilities following new versus recurrent ankle sprains in high school athletes. *J Sci Med Sport.* 2014;17(1):23–28.
10. Fong DTP, Hong Y, Chan LK, Yung PSH, Chan KM. A systematic review on ankle injury and ankle sprain in sports. *Sports Med.* 2007;37(1):73–94.
11. Kibler WB. *Coiegio Norteamericano de Medieina Deportiva: Manual A.C.S.M. dc Medieina Depotiiva*, 1st ed. Editorial I'aidotribo; 1998.
12. Richie DH Jr. Functional instability of the ankle and the role of neuromuscular control: a comprehensive review. *J Foot Ankle Surg.* 2001;40(4):240–251.
13. Doherty C, Delahunt E, Caulfield B, Hertel J, Ryan J, Bleakley C. The incidence and prevalence of ankle sprain injury: a systematic review and meta-analysis of prospective epidemiological studies. *Sports Med.* 2014;44(1):123–140.
14. Dolan P, Kenny I, Glynn L, et al. Risk factors for acute ankle sprains in field-based, team contact sports: a systematic review of prospective etiological studies. *Phys Sportsmed.* 2023;51(6):517–530.
15. Xue X, Ma T, Li Q, Song Y, Hua Y. Chronic ankle instability is associated with proprioception deficits: A systematic review and meta-analysis. *J Sport Health Sci.* 2021;10(2):182–191.
16. Ankle Sprains, Inversion & Eversion. In: Papadakis MA, McPhee SJ., eds. *Quick Medical Diagnosis & Treatment 2023.* McGraw-Hill Education; 2023. Accessed April 21, 2024. https://accessmedicine.mhmedical.com/content.aspx?bookid=3241&sectionid=271741488
17. Aslan A, Sofu H, Kirdemir V. Ankle ligament injury: current concept. *OA Orthop.* 2014;2:5–10.
18. van Dijk CN, Lim LS, Bossuyt PM, Marti RK. Physical examination is sufficient for the diagnosis of sprained ankles. *J Bone Joint Surg Br.* 1996;78(6):958–962.
19. Brolinson PG. An Osteopathic Approach to Sports Medicine. In: Seffinger M, ed. *Foundations of Osteopathic Medicine*, 4th ed. Wolters Kluwer; 2018: 1464.
20. Ivins D. Acute ankle sprain: an update. *Am Fam Physician.* 2006;74(10): 1714–1720.
21. Kaminski TW, Hertel J, Amendola N, et al. National Athletic Trainers' Association position statement: conservative management and prevention of ankle sprains in athletes. *J Athl Train.* 2013;48(4):528–545.
22. Vuurberg G, Hoorntje A, Wink LM, et al. Diagnosis, treatment, and prevention of ankle sprains: update of an evidence-based clinical guideline. *Br J Sports Med.* 2018;52(15):956.
23. Biz C, Nicoletti P, Tomasin M, Bragazzi NL, Di Rubbo G, Ruggieri P. Is kinesio taping effective for sport performance and ankle function of athletes with Chronic Ankle Instability (CAI)? A systematic review and meta-analysis. *Medicina (Kaunas).* 2022;58(5):620.
24. Ortega-Avila AB, Cervera-Garvi P, Marchena-Rodriguez A, et al. Conservative treatment for acute ankle sprain: a systematic review. *J Clin Med.* 2020;9(10):3128.
25. Gaddi D, Mosca A, Piatti M, et al. Acute ankle sprain management: an umbrella review of systematic reviews. *Front Med (Lausanne).* 2022;9:868474. Published 2022 Jul 7.
26. Kerkhoffs GM, van den Bekerom M, Elders LAM, et al. Diagnosis, treatment and prevention of ankle sprains: an evidence-based clinical guideline. *Br J Sports Med.* 2012;46(12):854–860.
27. Hajimaghsoudi M, Jalili M, Mokhtari M, Nejati A, Mesbahi J, Paydary K. Naproxen twice daily versus as needed (PRN) dosing: efficacy and tolerability for treatment of acute ankle sprain, a randomized clinical trial. *Asian J Sports Med.* 2013;4(4):249–255.
28. Bleakley C, Davison G. Management of acute soft tissue injury using Protection Rest Ice Compression and Elevation: Recommendations from the Association of Chartered Physiotherapists in Sports and Exercise Medicine (ACPSM) [Executive Summary]; 2010. Accessed January 26, 2024. https://www.semanticscholar.org/paper/Management-of-acute-soft-tissue-injury-using-Rest-Bleakley-Davison/642528ac5f107f730ed3484 90f414fda1142ad74
29. Bleakley CM, O'Connor SR, Tully MA, et al. Effect of accelerated rehabilitation on function after ankle sprain: randomised controlled trial. *BMJ.* 2010;340:c1964.
30. Roberge RJ, Roberge MR. Overcoming barriers to the use of osteopathic manipulation techniques in the emergency department. *West J Emerg Med.* 2009;10(3):184–189.
31. Daniel JN, Reb CW, Ronald Torrance II, Stout AM. Evidenced-based clinical review: laterally based ankle and hindfoot pain. *Osteopath Fam Physician.* 2014;6(5):28–32.
32. Eisenhart AW, Gaeta TJ, Yens DP. Osteopathic manipulative treatment in the emergency department for patients with acute ankle injuries. *J Am Osteopath Assoc.* 2003;103(9):417–421.
33. Martin RL, Davenport TE, Paulseth S, Wukich DK, Godges JJ. Orthopaedic Section American Physical Therapy Association. Ankle stability and movement coordination impairments: ankle ligament sprains. *J Orthop Sports Phys Ther.* 2013;43(9):A1–40.
34. de Noronha M, Refshauge KM, Herbert RD, Kilbreath SL, Hertel J. Do voluntary strength, proprioception, range of motion, or postural sway predict occurrence of lateral ankle sprain? *Br J Sports Med.* 2006;40(10): 824–828, discussion 828.
35. Travell JG, Simons DG. Myofascial pain and dysfunction: The trigger point manual. *The Lower Extremities.* Vol. II. Williams & Wilkins; 1992:429–459.
36. Blood SD. Treatment of the sprained ankle. *J Am Osteopath Assoc.* 1980; 79(11):680–692.
37. Pellow JE, Brantingham JW. The efficacy of adjusting the ankle in the treatment of subacute and chronic grade I and grade II ankle inversion sprains. *J Manipulative Physiol Ther.* 2001;24(1):17–24.
38. Lopez-Rodriguez S, Fernandez de-Las-Penas C, Alburquerque-Sendin F, Rodriguez-Blanco C, Palomeque-del-Cerro L. Immediate effects of manipulation of the talocrural joint on stabilometry and baropodometry in patients with ankle sprain. *J Manipulative Physiol Ther.* 2007;30(3):186–192.
39. Bleakley CM, McDonough SM, MacAuley DC. Some conservative strategies are effective when added to controlled mobilisation with external support after acute ankle sprain: a systematic review. *Aust J Physiother.* 2008;54(1):7–20.
40. Higgins R. The ankle joint. In: Hutson M, Ellis R, eds. *Textbook of Musculoskeletal Medicine.* Oxford University Press; 2006:331–337.
41. Michels F, Pereira H, Calder J, et al. Searching for consensus in the approach to patients with chronic lateral ankle instability: ask the expert. *Knee Surg Sports Traumatol Arthrosc.* 2018;26(7):2095–2102.

113 Case Study: Endocrinology

REEM DARWISH ▪ KURT P. HEINKING

KEY CONCEPTS

- The osteopathic approach to the patient with fatigue includes a thorough history and physical examination which includes an osteopathic assessment.
- Differential diagnosis should consider different etiologies from a variety of body systems as well as must "not miss" diagnoses. These help to organize a work-up and management plan for the patient.
- Osteopathic treatment plan includes application of osteopathic manipulative treatment (OMT) to alleviate somatic dysfunction resulting from visceral pathology, as well as improving biomechanical, respiratory–circulatory, metabolic, neurologic, and behavioral functions.
- Autoimmune hypothyroidism is a common cause of fatigue in middle-aged females and can present with a variety of symptoms.

CASE VIGNETTE

CHIEF COMPLAINT

Increased fatigue

HISTORY OF PRESENT ILLNESS

A 48-year-old female presents to clinic with complaints of worsening fatigue beginning 4 months ago. She states that she is a professor at a university and initially attributed her fatigue to the winter season and work-related stress. She noticed she was generally tired throughout the day despite a full night's rest and reduced workload. The patient denies any problems falling asleep or staying asleep and can obtain approximately 7 to 8 hours of rest per night. She reports her fatigue has worsened over the months, as well as some increased difficulty concentrating while grading her students' assignments, oftentimes needing to repeat the same tasks multiple times. Approximately 1 month ago, she additionally noticed some wrist discomfort that worsened with her computer activity. She denies any pain but does admit to some numbness and tingling in her fingers. She reports that the sensation does come back and improves with less computer work, which is difficult to avoid due to her work responsibilities. To combat the fatigue she is experiencing, she has decreased the number and size of her meals per day, as she usually is more lethargic following food intake. She has also increased her caffeine usage but states she does not want to rely on energy drinks "to feel normal." Medication use and wrist wrapping have minimally improved her wrist discomfort on long workdays. The patient reports feeling depressed, as nothing she has done has helped improve her symptoms. She also comments that she has noticed some hair loss, weight gain, and increased sleep which she attributes to her worsening mental health. The patient has no other diagnosed medical conditions.

PAST MEDICAL HISTORY

Obesity, Vitamin D deficiency, and iron-deficiency anemia.

PAST SURGICAL HISTORY

None to date.

MEDICATIONS

Over-the-counter acetaminophen 325 mg two tablets as needed for pain. Daily multivitamin gummies. Patient denies any use of oral contraceptive pills or other forms of birth control.

ALLERGIES

None reported.

SOCIAL HISTORY

She works as an English professor at the local university where she lectures 5 d/wk and utilizes her computer almost every day for 7 to 10 hours. She is single, never married. She does not have any children. She has never smoked, and drinks one to two beers about once per month. She denies any illicit drug use.

REVIEW OF SYSTEMS

General

Patient reports a 30-lb weight gain over the past year. She denies any fevers, headaches, night sweats, or recent travels.

Cardiovascular

She denies any chest pain, shortness of breath, or dyspnea on exertion. She does admit to occasional palpitations that she relates to her caffeine intake.

Respiratory

She denies a history of asthma, cough, tuberculosis, or difficulty breathing.

HEENT

She denies any changes in vision, hearing, smell, or taste. She reports no recent infections, runny nose, sore throat, or difficulty swallowing.

GI/GU

She notes decreased appetite, increased bloating, and constipation with occasional crampy abdominal pain. She denies nausea, vomiting, dysuria, other changes in bowel movement, or blood in the urine or stools.

Neurologic

She reports occasional numbness and tingling in her index and middle fingers bilaterally. She denies any weakness or pain. Patient has no history of stroke, seizures, or dizziness.

OB/GYN

Patient is G0P0. Her last menstrual period was 3 months ago, light in flow (patient describes it more as spotting), and lasted 3 days. Patient states that for the last 6 months, her period has been irregular in time, length, and flow. One year ago she had her menstrual period every 30 days and it was regular in flow and lasted 6 days. She has been sexually active within the past year with one partner utilizing condoms as protection. Patient's last breast and pap examination done 10 months ago were normal.

Psychiatric

Patient admits to fatigue, tiredness, difficulty concentrating, anxiousness, and depressed mood over the past 4 months. She notes increased hair loss. She denies any history of anxiety, depression, or other psychiatric illnesses or hospitalizations. Patient denies any thoughts of self-harm, suicidal, or homicidal ideation.

Dermatologic

She reports increased dry skin with it being the worst in her hands and feet. She denies any pruritis, rashes, or lesions elsewhere. Patient states her acne has worsened with increased breakouts over her face. She also notes her nails being more fragile and brittle with them breaking easily.

Hematologic

She denies excess bruising or bleeding. Patient denies history of anemia.

Endocrine

The patient denies any heat or cold intolerance. She notes that usually she layers up and keeps the heater on due to the cold weather in the Midwest.

MSK

She admits to a "discomfort" in her wrists that occasionally has some numbness and tingling in her fingers but denies any associated weakness or pain. She reports her fingers are larger so she can no longer wear some of her rings, but attributes this to her weight gain. She denies any swollen joints, lesions, or rashes. The patient does report some pain and stiffness in her midback. She rates it as a 3/10 and states that it comes and goes. It is worse with sitting at her desk.

PHYSICAL EXAMINATION

Vital Signs

Height, 5′5″, Weight 210 lb, BMI 34.90, BP 138/87, RR 17 breaths/min, Pulse 83 bpm, Temperature 98.4 °F.

General

Patient seems to be anxious and in low spirits. She appears well developed and well nourished, in no obvious pain or discomfort.

Integument

No rashes, erythema, or ecchymosis. Patient's skin appears dull with evidence of xerosis. Patient has flaking skin on the dorsum of her hands, around her knuckles, and spanning circumferentially around her medial and lateral malleoli. Patient does have multiple pustules along her forehead, cheeks, and mandible. Scalp appears to have widespread thinning of hair with normal appearing scalp and hair shafts.

HEENT

Pupils are equal, round, reactive to light and accommodation (PERRLA), external ocular muscles are intact (EOMI), no scleral icterus, and no evidence of swelling surrounding the eyes or exophthalmos. Ear canals are clear with visual of the tympanic membrane with no evidence of effusion or erythema. Nares are patent bilaterally, septum midline, nasal mucosa pink, no evidence of discharge. Uvula midline, oral mucosa pink, poor periodontal health, altered tooth morphology, enlarged tongue, and small hypopharynx. No evidence of exudates or adenopathy. Nontender supple neck with mild nontender thyromegaly. No cervical, suboccipital, submandibular, or submental lymphadenopathy.

Heart

Has a regular rate and rhythm (RRR) without murmurs, rubs, or gallops. No S3, S4, carotid or vertebral bruits.

Lungs

Clear to auscultation bilaterally (CTAB) with no rales, rhonchi, or wheezes.

Abdomen

The abdomen is distended with bowel sounds present in all four quadrants. There is tenderness in the left lower quadrant. No evidence of masses, hepatosplenomegaly, or suprapubic tenderness. No rebound tenderness, rigidity, or guarding.

Extremities

No edema, full range of motion of the joints, pulses full and even bilaterally, and capillary refill less than 2 seconds in upper and lower extremities. Positive Phalen & Tinel tests over the median nerve bilaterally. Negative Finkelstein test. Nails are short with rigid edges with evidence of onycholysis.

Neurologic Examination

Alert and oriented to person, place, and time. Gait is normal. CN II to XII intact. Muscle strength 5/5. Deep tendon reflexes are 1/4 bilaterally in both upper and lower extremities. Babinski test is negative. No sensory defects to pinprick, vibration, or fine touch.

Osteopathic Structural Examination

Standing Osteopathic Examination

- There is loss of cervical lordosis and decreased thoracic kyphosis.
- Her right acromion and inferior scapular angle are superior compared to the left.
- Her left mastoid process, iliac crest, and greater trochanters are elevated compared to the right.
- Positive Adam's forward bending test showing paravertebral humping around the right upper thoracic region.
- Positive standing and seated flexion tests on the left.
- Pelvic side shift even in both directions.

Cranial

Left posterior occiput with restricted left occipitomastoid suture. Cranial rhythmic impulse (CRI) diminished in amplitude, rate around 4 cycles per minute.

Cervical

TART changes in the suboccipital region with myofascial tension and restriction bilaterally. Posterior right atlas. C3 flexed rotated left side bent left. C5 flexed rotated right side bent right. Tender anterior cervical muscles with a Jones tender point found at the left AC1.

Thoracic

T1 extended rotated right side bent right. Slight group curve from T2–T5, neutral rotated right side bent left. There are myofascial restrictions of the thoracic inlet. Increased paraspinal hypertonicity bilaterally from T1–T4 and from T10–L1 on the right side. Chapman point palpated lateral to the T2 spinous process on the right. Right diaphragm restriction during exhalation.

Ribs

Elevated left first rib. Anterior rib two tenderpoint on the left. Ribs 3 to 7 on the left are exhaled. Prominent Chapman points palpated in the right anterior second intercostal space near the sternum.

Lumbar

L1 flexed rotated right side bent right. L2–L5 are neutral, rotated left and side bent right. Increased left-sided paraspinal hypertonicity from L1–L3. AL1 Jones tender point palpated at the right medial side of the anterior superior iliac spine (ASIS).

Sacrum

Sacrum is rotated right on a right oblique axis, with a posterior right inferior lateral angle and a deep left sacral sulcus. Sacral base is level.

Pelvis

Superior left pubic tubercle and ASIS. Inferior left posterior superior iliac spine. Posterior left ilium.

DIFFERENTIAL DIAGNOSIS

1. Hypothyroidism
2. Pregnancy
3. Obstructive sleep apnea (OSA)
4. Anemia
5. Somatic dysfunction: cranium, cervical, thoracic, ribs, lumbar, sacrum, and pelvic regions.
6. Constipation
7. Major depressive disorder
8. Carpal tunnel syndrome (CTS)
9. Chronic fatigue syndrome
10. Obesity (mild to moderate)
11. Generalized anxiety disorder

DIFFERENTIAL DIAGNOSIS DISCUSSION

Physicians oftentimes create a list of differential diagnoses which are a broad array of diagnoses that relate to the patient's presentation representing different body systems and types of pathology responsible for one's symptomatology. Since fatigue alone can be a symptom of endocrine, autoimmune, hematologic, metabolic, cardiovascular, pulmonary, neoplastic, infectious, psychogenic, or many other etiologies, it is important to consider them all as underlying causes of her current presentation. There is no support in the history or physical for etiologies such as an underlying infectious cause (Lyme disease, pneumonia, mononucleosis, etc.), cardiovascular cause (congestive heart failure, arrhythmias, coronary artery disease), or pulmonary cause (chronic obstructive pulmonary disease, asthma, interstitial lung disease).

In the patient above, she complains of fatigue, decreased appetite, weight gain, hair loss, brittle nails, restless sleep, constipation, decreased concentration, hand symptoms, and a lack of menses over the last 3 months. At this point, it is important to assess for pregnancy in our patient. Her presentation can be characteristic of what is seen during pregnancy which includes CTS.[1] Those with excessive gestational weight gain and a BMI over 30 are at increased risk of developing CTS during pregnancy.[2] An initial workup can include a urinary pregnancy test which detects levels of human chorionic gonadotropin (hCG). Urinary hCG tests can be positive in 95% of those who are pregnant, meaning that a negative does not rule out pregnancy.[3] Low levels of hCG seen early in pregnancy can result in a false negative due to the concentration of hCG being below testing threshold. If pregnancy is suspected in a patient, a repeated serum hCG is taken after 48 hours to evaluate for a doubling in levels indicating gestation.[4] After urinary and repeat serum hCG testing, results indicated that our patient is not pregnant.

OSA should also be worked up in our patient due to her excessive fatigue, weight gain, and trouble concentrating. Obesity puts her at increased risk of having OSA. Due to her living home alone, the patient is not sure if she snores at night or has any pauses in her breathing. It is possible that the constipation, hair loss, and brittle nails are due to an ongoing concurrent issue separate from OSA. Definitive testing includes a sleep study that can either be done at home or in a facility.[5,6] Our patient's sleep study indicated no evidence of OSA.

Anemia can contribute to our patient's fatigue, lack of concentration, menstrual irregularities, palpitations, as well as her hair and nail changes. Although, with anemia other symptoms such as muscle weakness, dizziness, shortness of breath, low blood pressure, and pale or yellowing conjunctiva and skin are often present.[7] It is unlikely that anemia is contributing to her loss of appetite, weight gain, and constipation. Obtaining a complete blood count with differential, iron studies, vitamin B9 (folate) and B12 levels, reticulocyte count, and peripheral blood smear can help with initial assessment of anemia.[8] Anemia itself can be a symptom of underlying disease and pathology elsewhere in the body (such as malignancy, autoimmune processes, and infections); so although laboratory studies can help assess the presence of anemia, other etiologies should be ruled out as causes to the patient's presentation.[9]

In this case, our patient's symptoms align with the classic presentation of hypothyroidism. In some patients with hypothyroidism, they can exhibit CTS due to weight gain and increased pressure from fatty tissue that compresses the median nerve within the carpal tunnel.[10] In addition, it has been found that in those with hypothyroidism there is increased deposition of mucinous substance and mucopolysaccharides on the median nerve itself.[10,11] Hypothyroidism can lead to amenorrhea due to its impact on the hypothalamic–pituitary–ovarian (HPO) axis. Initially, there is an increase in thyrotropin-releasing hormone (TRH) from the hypothalamus in response to low T3/T4 levels, which stimulates prolactin secretion from the anterior pituitary, which then suppresses the release of follicle-stimulating hormone (FSH) and luteinizing hormone (LH) in the ovaries which impedes the menstrual cycle.[12] Initial assessment of hypothyroidism should include obtaining levels of thyroid-stimulating hormone (TSH), total thyroxine (T4), and free T4. If these are abnormal or there is a high index of suspicion for thyroid-etiology, other labs can include levels of triiodothyronine (T3); reverse T3, presence of thyroid antibodies, radioactive iodine uptake (RIU), and ultrasound imaging.[13] Further work-up in our patient resulted in her diagnosis of an autoimmune hypothyroidism known as Hashimoto thyroiditis.

LABORATORY RESULTS

- TSH: 6.8 μU/mL (normal: 0.5–5.0 μU/mL)[14]
- Total thyroxin (T4): 3.0 mcg/dL (normal: 5.4–11.5 mcg/dL)[15]
- Free thyroxine (free T4): 0.4 (normal: 0.7–1.8 ng/dL)[15]
- Triiodothyronine (T3): 35 ng/dL (normal: 70–205 ng/dL)[16]
- Reverse T3: 13 ng/dL (normal: 10–24 ng/dL)[16]
- Thyroid antibodies:
  - Thyroid peroxidase (TPO) antibody: positive (normal: negative)
  - Thyroglobulin (TG) antibody: positive (normal: negative)
  - TSH receptor antibody: negative (normal: negative)

OSTEOPATHIC PATIENT MANAGEMENT

Biomechanical Model

The musculoskeletal system is primarily involved in the physiologic function of posture and motion. Our patient likely has somatic manifestations that are indicative of her underlying medical condition/visceral disease. There is musculoskeletal evidence of thyroid dysfunction as seen in her Chapman points located at the right second intercostal space anteriorly and lateral to the T2 spinous process on the right posteriorly, as well as a viscerosomatic reflex found from T1 to T4.[17] The patient also has viscerosomatic reflexes (VSRs) from T10 to L3 which could be due to her constipation. The other somatic dysfunctions seen on physical examination could further contribute to her signs and symptoms of hypothyroidism. Dysfunctions of the musculoskeletal system affect endocrine function, and endocrine disorders affect the musculoskeletal structures and their functions. Sitting at her computer for long hours can increase muscle tension in her upper thoracic region with subsequent somatic dysfunction. Likewise, typing on the keyboard for 7 hours a day can result in an overuse of the wrist flexors, whose tendons traverse the carpal tunnel. Further explanations of how treatment of these areas of musculoskeletal dysfunction can help improve the patient's Hashimoto's are discussed in the other models of osteopathic medicine.

Respiratory–Circulatory Model

Improving oxygenation and increasing the delivery of nutrients can help with the recovery of tissues that have been compromised and normalize endocrine function in patients who have had alterations in their hypothalamic–pituitary axis. From this respiratory–circulatory perspective, patients receiving OMT can benefit by improving lymph flow and blood return to the heart. For example, occipito-atlantal decompression was found to improve blood flow to the brain through increased diastolic flow after 1 week of treatment.[18] Osteopathic cranial manipulative medicines as well as other applications of OMT are thought to promote blood flow throughout the body.

According to Andrew T. Still, malposition of the cervical spine, upper thoracic vertebrae, first and second ribs, and myofascial restrictions in the thoracic outlet region can result in a backup of lymph and blood in the thyroid resulting in inflammation and thyroiditis.[19] Improvement in blood flow is essential in our patient to help remove any further irritation of the thyroid and ultimately helps normalize some of her symptoms. Before targeting each of these areas, it is important to open up all five diaphragms first to allow for uninterrupted flow, improve venous drainage, and increase lymphatic absorption.[20–22]

Recent research discusses the five diaphragms: the respiratory diaphragm, pelvic diaphragm, thoracic outlet, tentorium cerebelli, and the tongue.[23–25] These areas function together and are connected through a myofascial network. During inhalation, both the respiratory and pelvic diaphragm descend (this has been verified with MRI imaging).[25,26] The five diaphragms are intertwined both anatomically and functionally. For example, the posterolateral portion of the five diaphragms connects with one another at the thoracolumbar fascia.[23] Due to these fascial connections, a restriction in any one of the five diaphragms can have downstream effects in all the five diaphragms. To maximize respiration, it is important to address each one of these regions during treatment.

The patient has a slow primary respiratory mechanism indicating restricted motion in the skull and potentially the tentorium cerebelli. Keep in mind anatomically; the diaphragma sellae is a sheet of dura that is right above the pituitary gland with attachments to the tentorium cerebelli.[27] The endocrine functions and fascial restrictions of this area can worsen the symptoms that have been exhibited in our patient.

Cervical, thoracic, and upper rib dysfunctions can lead to restrictions of the thoracic outlet, impairing lymphatic drainage and thoracic diaphragm motion. Somatic dysfunction in the lumbar, sacral, and pelvic regions can affect tension, tone, and movement of the pelvic diaphragm. Four of the five diaphragms have been impeded through osteopathic evaluation and diagnosis. The fifth diaphragm, the tongue, can be impacted through any restrictions of the vagus nerve or tentorium cerebelli. The vagus nerve's relationship with the trigeminal nucleus through afferent connections has downstream impact on the floor of the mouth and tongue.[25,28–30] The tentorium cerebelli is innervated by a tentorial branch of the ophthalmic division of the trigeminal nerve (the nervus tentorii).[31] Therefore, any dysfunction of the vagus nerve or tentorium cerebelli can affect the tongue.[25,32] One particular reason why the tongue is of interest, in this case, is due to the thyroid's embryonic origin from it. The thyroid gland originates from the foramen cecum found at the posterior third of the tongue.[33] As one continues to develop, the thyroid descends caudally along the pharynx. The thyroglossal duct (made from the descent) is what maintains the connection between the tongue and the thyroid.[34,35] In hypothyroidism, thickening of the tongue (macroglossia) is due to increased accumulation of subcutaneous mucopolysaccharides.[36] Treating the somatic dysfunction of these five diaphragms may help to normalize the mechanics of the axial-vertebrae, fascial elements, and both cellular exchange and pulmonary respiration. It is recommended to treat with the patient supine or prone to eliminate any tension created from musculature involved in posture control.[25]

Metabolic Energy Model

Resting metabolic rate (RMR) is the amount of energy one's body uses to function at rest. These functions include cellular metabolism and the utilization of nutrients to produce ATP for baseline function.[37] Research has shown that thyroid hormones impact metabolic rate due to its role in thermogenesis, lipid and glucose metabolism, fat oxidation, and food intake.[38] Higher levels of thyroid hormone result in a greater metabolic rate whereas a lower levels result in a lower metabolic rate.[39,40] In hypothyroidism, the RMR is lowered in the entire body slowing all metabolic functions resulting in fatigue, weight gain, and cold intolerance.[41] Weight gain is commonly seen in hypothyroidism due to a decrease in RMR, resulting in less fat used as energy. It is important to note that not all weight gain in those with hypothyroidism is from hypothyroidism itself; behavioral and social factors as well as other underlying health issues can contribute to weight changes.[38]

Improving thyroid function, increasing fluid circulation, and exercise are all methods that can increase metabolic rate. AT Still describes milking of the thyroid gland toward the thoracic outlet to help improve activity of the gland and encourage fluid movement.[17] In those with autoimmune processes, there is a buildup of immune cells, inflammatory cytokines, and enzymes in the area targeted by the autoantibody contributing to a worsening irritation, inflammation, and overall disease process.[42] Utilizing techniques to help improve blood flow, lymph flow, and overall circulation can help to remove some of these irritants from the thyroid and facilitate healing. An improvement in flow can also help the patient participate in physical activity by dampening musculoskeletal pain. Oftentimes in those with hypothyroidism, exercise is not performed due to low energy levels and body pains. The utilization of OMT in those with hypothyroidism can help combat pain experienced from a workout; techniques can help prevent tissue injury by removing metabolites and lowering edema which improves circulation to the area resulting in increased oxygen and nutrient delivery to the active tissue.[43–45] Once a patient can endure exercise, they may be able to increase their RMR to help combat their fatigue as well as other symptoms.

Neurologic Model

The nervous system can be impacted by hypothyroidism in several modalities whether it be through autonomic tone, nerve compression syndromes, or reflex arcs with somatic manifestations. There are multiple ways to treat any neurologic dysfunction given its connections to certain anatomical regions, each of which will be discussed in further detail.

For example, the phrenic nerve originates at the roots of C3–C5 and runs inferiorly through the thoracic outlet, and traverses the mediastinum to contact the respiratory diaphragm. The vagus nerve anastomoses with the phrenic nerve through the crural region of the diaphragm.[25,28,29] This is important to note as it shows how diaphragmatic innervation is in direct contact with the parasympathetic nervous system, and therefore any restrictions of the cervical region impacting the phrenic nerve can have a further downstream effect on the actions of the parasympathetic nervous system through the vagus nerve. In our patient, there is a notable decrease in parasympathetic tone as seen in her complaints of constipation.

Constipation is commonly seen in those with hypothyroidism due to low metabolic rates that reduce the activity of the gastrointestinal system.[46,47] One way to combat this is through the utilization of the central autonomic nervous system: while the sympathetic nervous system originates in the thoracic and lumbar regions and slows down the GI tract when stimulated, the parasympathetic nervous system has origins in the cranial, upper cervical, and sacral regions and promotes activity of the GI tract when stimulated.[48] Targeting occipito-atlantal and atlanto-axial regions with OMT can result in enhanced vagal tone which stimulates the gastrointestinal tract and reduces symptoms of constipation.[17] Treating cervical dysfunction can contribute to the normalization of parasympathetic tone by eliminating any restrictions of the phrenic nerve that have interfered with the vagus nerve itself due to their connection at the diaphragm.[25,28,29] Release of the celiac, superior mesenteric, and inferior mesenteric ganglions can enhance venous and lymphatic drainage as well as normalize any excessive sympathetic tone as these are postsynaptic ganglion of the sympathetic nervous system.[49] "Colonic milking" and mesenteric lift procedures can encourage GI motility and reduce the need for laxative or medicinal intervention for constipation.[50]

Nerve compression syndromes such as CTS are commonly seen in those with hypothyroidism. The carpal tunnel is a narrow space formed by the flexor retinaculum and carpal bones. In this space runs the median nerve which supplies motor and sensory innervation to the palm and the first 3.5 digits of the hand.[51] Oftentimes CTS is due to a reduction of available space due to obesity, pregnancy, or extension/flexion of the wrist for long periods of time which interferes with the normal function of the median nerve. In the case of hypothyroidism, CTS often is a result of deposited mucinous substances and mucopolysaccharides directly onto the median nerve.[10] In our patient it is not clear whether her CTS is due to Hashimoto disease or her frequent computer use resulting in hyperextension of her wrist for hours at a time. The patient stated that her symptoms of numbness and tingling improved when she spent less time at her desk doing work which favors the hypothesis that hand position is the most likely cause. The utilization of OMT can help alleviate some of the fascial restrictions in the area and help relax any tight musculature that is worsening wrist positioning.[52] Studies have shown that following OMT utilizing myofascial release, muscle energy, articulation, and high-velocity low-amplitude, participants were found to have increased wrist mobility, absent or fewer carpal tunnel symptoms, increased dimensions of the carpal tunnel on magnetic resonance imaging, and improvement in nerve conduction studies.[52–54]

Osteopathic medicine has thoroughly explored relationships between visceral systems and somatic presentations known as VSRs. Stress on viscera can have a physical manifestation at a site distant from the affected organ. The location of these sites is related segmentally to the body through origins in embryonic development. The identification of these somatic manifestations can help with further diagnosis and treatment of underlying visceral disease. Chapman points are a type of VSR that result in pea-sized, gangliform, palpable nodules in distinct areas anteriorly and posteriorly. Treatment is aimed to interrupt the reflex arc created by the affected viscera which results in somatic manifestation at the corresponding vertebral segment.[55] The T1–T4 and T10–L3 VSRs can be treated with myofascial release, soft tissue, and articulation techniques which will help dampen stimulation of the neurons and normalize sympathetic tone in the area.[56] The Chapman points are treated with circular pressure over the designated areas until the palpable mass is no longer present. The utilization of OMT can help alleviate stimulation of neurons in reflex pathways, normalize autonomic tone, and improve visceral functioning.

Behavioral Model

Addressing and treating a patient's mental health is essential in maintaining a holistic approach to one's management. Behavioral problems can feed into a patient's current disease and impact their recovery. Interestingly, the osteopathic profession has a long history of treating patients with mental health concerns with OMT due to the core belief of the person being a unit with a dynamic interaction of the body, mind, and spirit.[57,58] Modern studies have found that the rate of CRI can be decreased in those with stress, mental depression, and other psychiatric conditions.[59] This contributes to the concept that abnormalities in mental health can exhibit physical manifestations. There has been debate about whether CRI can be utilized to help guide management in those with psychiatric conditions, and further research is needed to evaluate its role in behavioral medicine. For our patient her mental health has been affected from multiple aspects. Due to her sleep, trouble concentrating, low mood, and change in appetite over the course of 4 months, screening was performed in the office (PHQ-9) and our patient fits the criteria for having major depressive disorder. Ultimately, OMT can minimize some of the symptoms our patient has been suffering from as well as improve symptoms and potentially the severity of her autoimmune thyroid disease.

Anxiety and depression signs have been found to be more intense in those with hyper- and hypothyroid compared to the general population.[60] Multiple studies have demonstrated the comorbidity of depression and hypothyroidism at approximately 60%.[61–65] Oftentimes, those with neuropsychiatric disorders recover mentally once their underlying hypothyroidism was treated.[66] Those with less education about their diagnosis had more severe symptoms of anxiety and depression compared to those who were more educated about their autoimmune disease and prognosis.[60] OMT can be utilized to help ease some of the symptoms from hypothyroidism including fatigue, pain, constipation, and improve metabolism and circulation. A reduction in symptoms can improve the quality of life in those with Hashimoto's and improve their mental health as a result. Further improvements can consist of simply educating the patient about their diagnosis so they are aware that their presentation is due to an underlying process that can be managed with hormone replacement to eliminate worsening symptoms and improve energy levels.[67]

Specialist Referral

The primary treatment for a patient with hypothyroidism is hormone replacement therapy utilizing medication such as levothyroxine. With the diagnosis of Hashimoto's, a patient may be managed by their primary care physician or an endocrinologist until their T3/T4/TSH reaches stable levels. Changes in medication dosage are made slowly due to thyroid function tests being checked every 6 to 8 weeks in newly diagnosed patients until adequate levels are achieved.[68,69] Following appropriate dosage, patients can have their thyroid levels checked as soon as every 3 months if needed.[69] If untreated, severe hypothyroidism can result in myxedema coma (considered a medical emergency) and present as worsening mental status, hypothermia, and a variety of symptoms indicating decreased function of organs.[70] If the patient is exhibiting these signs, they should go to the emergency room as soon as possible. Similarly, if the patient's hypothyroidism is overcorrected with medication, they can exhibit symptoms such as difficulty sleeping, heat intolerance, weight loss, and diarrhea. The managing physician needs to make sure the dose is altered correctly and utilizes the patient's clinical presentation as well as thyroid function lab tests to manage accordingly.

In addition, due to the autoimmune nature of this disease, a rheumatologist may be consulted for further evaluation of other potential autoimmune processes since oftentimes there is increased incidence in coexistent autoimmunity seen in those with existent autoimmune disease.[71,72] Due to the impact on her mental health, a psychiatrist and/or clinical psychologist should be included on the care management team for the patient. Physical therapy or occupational therapy can also be utilized to help strengthen muscles, build endurance, and assist in the management of her CTS. The skills of an osteopathic physician in addition to the care team listed above can help with minimizing symptoms and reducing the number of visitations needed for specialists, which can cut down the costs for the patient.

SUMMARY

In summary, the osteopathic approach to the patient with fatigue includes a thorough history and physical examination which includes an osteopathic assessment. The differential diagnosis should consider different etiologies from a variety of body systems. Autoimmune thyroiditis is common in middle-aged women and can manifest as fatigue, weight gain, difficulty concentrating, cold intolerance, constipation, CTS, hair loss, and nail changes. Understanding the pathophysiology of this autoimmune disease can help explain the application of osteopathic medicine to an underlying visceral disease. Patient education, medication management, and follow up with the health care team are important to the management plan. Further referral to other specialists can be indicated if there is no improvement in symptoms. Worsening of symptoms or medication noncompliance can result in myxedema coma which is a medical emergency that needs treatment as soon as possible.

REFERENCES

1. de Oliveira GAD, Bernardes JM, de Souza Santos E, Dias A. Carpal tunnel syndrome during the third trimester of pregnancy: prevalence and risk factors. *Arch Gynecol Obstet*. 2019;300(3):623–631.
2. Wright C, Smith B, Wright S, Weiner M, Wright K, Rubin D. Who develops carpal tunnel syndrome during pregnancy: an analysis of obesity, gestational weight gain, and parity. *Obstet Med*. 2014;7(2):90–94.
3. Gnoth C, Johnson S. Strips of hope: accuracy of home pregnancy tests and new developments. *Geburtshilfe Frauenheilkd*. 2014;74(7):661–669.
4. Guha S, Ayim F, Ludlow J, et al. Triaging pregnancies of unknown location: the performance of protocols based on single serum progesterone or repeated serum hCG levels. *Hum Reprod*. 2014;29(5):938–945.
5. Gottlieb DJ, Punjabi NM. Diagnosis and management of obstructive sleep apnea: a review. *JAMA*. 2020;323(14):1389–1400.
6. Semelka M, Wilson J, Floyd R. Diagnosis and treatment of obstructive sleep apnea in adults. *Am Fam Physician*. 2016;94(5):355–360.
7. Anemia - Symptoms and causes. Mayo Clinic. Accessed January 6, 2024. https://www.mayoclinic.org/diseases-conditions/anemia/symptoms-causes/syc-20351360
8. Cascio MJ, DeLoughery TG. Anemia: evaluation and diagnostic tests. *Med Clin North Am*. 2017;101(2):263–284.
9. Fraenkel PG. Understanding anemia of chronic disease. *Hematology*. 2015; 2015(1):14–18.
10. Karne SS, Bhalerao NS. Carpal tunnel syndrome in hypothyroidism. *J Clin Diagn Res*. 2016;10(2):OC36–OC38.
11. Duncan SFM, Bhate O, Mustaly H. Pathophysiology of carpal tunnel syndrome. In: Duncan SFM, Kakinoki R, eds. *Carpal Tunnel Syndrome and Related Median Neuropathies: Challenges and Complications*. Springer International Publishing; 2017:13–29.
12. Shufelt CL, Torbati T, Dutra E. Hypothalamic amenorrhea and the long-term health consequences. *Semin Reprod Med*. 2017;35(3):256–262.
13. So M, MacIsaac RJ, Grossmann M. Hypothyroidism: investigation and management. *Aust Fam Physician*. 2020;41(8):556–562.
14. Cappola AR. The thyrotropin reference range should be changed in older patients. *JAMA*. 2019;322(20):1961–1962.
15. Fischbach FT, Dunning MB. *A Manual of Laboratory and Diagnostic Tests*. Lippincott Williams & Wilkins; 2009.
16. Pagana KD, Pagana TJ, Pagana TN. *Mosby's Diagnostic and Laboratory Test Reference-E-Book: Mosby's Diagnostic and Laboratory Test Reference-E-Book*. Elsevier Health Sciences; 2018.
17. DiGiovanna EL, Amen C, Burns D. *An Osteopathic Approach to Diagnosis and Treatment*. Lippincott Williams & Wilkins; 2020.
18. Roberts B, Makar AE, Canaan R, Pazdernik V, Kondrashova T. Effect of occipitoatlantal decompression on cerebral blood flow dynamics as evaluated by Doppler ultrasonography. *J Osteopath Med*. 2021;121(2):171–179.
19. Still AT. *Osteopathy, Research and Practice*. CreateSpace Independent Publishing Platform; 1924.

20. Sagrillo LM, Frigo LF. The respiratory diaphragm in osteopathic vision: a literature review. Manual Therapy, Posturology & Rehabilitation Journal. Published online December 27, 2016:1–6.
21. Byeon K, Choi JO, Yang JH, et al. The response of the vena cava to abdominal breathing. *J Altern Complementary Med.* 2012;18(2):153–157.
22. Abu-Hijleh MF, Habbal OA, Moqattash ST. The role of the diaphragm in lymphatic absorption from the peritoneal cavity. *J Anat.* 1995;186(Pt 3):453–467.
23. Bordoni B. The five diaphragms in osteopathic manipulative medicine: myofascial relationships, part 1. *Cureus.* 12(4):e7794.
24. Bordoni B. The five diaphragms in osteopathic manipulative medicine: neurological relationships, part 2. *Cureus.* 2020;12(6):e8713.
25. Bordoni B, Zanier E. The continuity of the body: hypothesis of treatment of the five diaphragms. *J Altern Complementary Med.* 2015;21(4):237–242.
26. Talasz H, Kremser C, Kofler M, Kalchschmid E, Lechleitner M, Rudisch A. Phase-locked parallel movement of diaphragm and pelvic floor during breathing and coughing-a dynamic MRI investigation in healthy females. *Int Urogynecol J.* 2011;22(1):61–68.
27. Gittinger J. Tumors of the pituitary gland. In: *Management of Pituitary Tumors; The Clinician's Practical Guide,* Second Edition.; 2005:1531–1536. Accessed November 26, 2023. https://www.scribd.com/document/340304979/985
28. Drake RL, Vogl W, Mitchell AWM, Gray H. *Gray's Anatomy for Students.* Churchill Livingstone/Elsevier; 2010.
29. Pickering M, Jones JFX. The diaphragm: two physiological muscles in one. *J Anat.* 2002;201(4):305-312.
30. Messlinger K, Fischer MJM, Lennerz JK. Neuropeptide effects in the trigeminal system: pathophysiology and clinical relevance in migraine. *Keio J Med.* 2011;60(3):82–89.
31. Lee SH, Shin KJ, Koh KS, Song WC. Visualization of the tentorial innervation of human dura mater. *J Anat.* 2017;231(5):683–689.
32. Kemp WJ, Tubbs RS, Cohen-Gadol AA. The innervation of the cranial dura mater: neurosurgical case correlates and a review of the literature. *World Neurosurg.* 2012;78(5):505–510.
33. Allen E, Fingeret A. Anatomy, head and neck, thyroid. In: *StatPearls.* StatPearls Publishing; 2024. Accessed January 28, 2024. http://www.ncbi.nlm.nih.gov/books/NBK470452/
34. Fancy T, Gallagher D III, Hornig JD. Surgical anatomy of the thyroid and parathyroid glands. *Otolaryngol Clin North Am.* 2010;43(2):221–227.
35. Organ GM, Organ CH Jr. Thyroid gland and surgery of the thyroglossal duct: exercise in applied embryology. *World J Surg.* 2000;24(8):886–890.
36. Chandna S, Bathla M. Oral manifestations of thyroid disorders and its management. *Indian J Endocrinol Metab.* 2011;15(Suppl2):S113–S116.
37. Speakman JR, Selman C. Physical activity and resting metabolic rate. *Proc Nutr Soc.* 2003;62(3):621–634.
38. Sanyal D, Raychaudhuri M. Hypothyroidism and obesity: an intriguing link. *Indian J Endocrinol Metab.* 2016;20(4):554–557.
39. Mullur R, Liu YY, Brent GA. Thyroid hormone regulation of metabolism. *Physiol Rev.* 2014;94(2):355–382.
40. Connors JM, Devito WJ, Hedge GA. The effects of the duration of severe hypothyroidism and aging on the metabolic clearance rate of thyrotropin (TSH) and the pituitary TSH response to TSH-releasing hormone. *Endocrinology.* 1984;114(5):1930–1937.
41. El-Haddad B, Bizri IE, Kallail KJ, Zackula RE, Hoffman JM. Fatigue and TSH levels in hypothyroid patients. *Kans J Med.* 2012;5(2):51–57.
42. Teng X, Cornaby C, Li W, Morel L. Metabolic regulation of pathogenic autoimmunity: therapeutic targeting. *Curr Opin Immunol.* 2019;61:10–16.
43. Sonberg M, Mullinger B, Rajendran D. Can osteopathy help women with a history of hypothyroidism and musculoskeletal complaints? Outcome of a preliminary, prospective, open investigation. *International Journal of Osteopathic Medicine.* 2010;13(1):11–16.
44. King HH, Jänig W, Patterson MM. *The Science and Clinical Application of Manual Therapy.* Elsevier Health Sciences; 2010.
45. Stone C. *Science in the Art of Osteopathy: Osteopathic Principles and Practice.* Nelson Thornes; 1999.
46. Chang YJ, Hwu CM, Yeh CC, Wang PS, Wang SW. Effects of subacute hypothyroidism on metabolism and growth-related molecules. *Molecules.* 2014;19(8):11178–11195.
47. Brown TR. The effect of hypothyroidism on gastric and intestinal function. *J Am Med Assoc.* 1931;97(8):511–513.
48. Browning KN, Travagli RA. Central nervous system control of gastrointestinal motility and secretion and modulation of gastrointestinal functions. *Compr Physiol.* 2014;4(4):1339–1368.
49. Agustina K, Margiani NN, Anandasari PPY, Mahastuti NM. Constipation that needs attention: late Hirschsprung disease. *Intisari Sains Medis.* 2021;12(1):64–67.
50. Modlin SE, Borofka K, Franzini D, Klene-Bowns AC, Nuño VA. OMT for the prevention and management of chronic constipation and distal intestinal obstructive syndrome in cystic fibrosis: a pilot study. *J Am Osteopath Assoc.* 2019;119(7):e31–e35.
51. Padua L, Cuccagna C, Giovannini S, et al. Carpal tunnel syndrome: updated evidence and new questions. *Lancet Neurol.* 2023;22(3):255–267.
52. Siu G, Jaffe JD, Rafique M, Weinik MM. Osteopathic manipulative medicine for carpal tunnel syndrome. *J Osteopath Med.* 2012;112(3):127–139.
53. Sucher BM. Myofascial manipulative release of carpal tunnel syndrome: documentation with magnetic resonance imaging. *J Am Osteopath Assoc.* 1993;93(12):1273–1278.
54. Sucher BM, Hinrichs RN, Welcher RL, Quiroz LD, St Laurent BF, Morrison BJ. Manipulative treatment of carpal tunnel syndrome: biomechanical and osteopathic intervention to increase the length of the transverse carpal ligament: part 2. Effect of sex differences and manipulative "priming." *J Am Osteopath Assoc.* 2005;105(3):135–143.
55. Beal MC. Viscerosomatic reflexes: a review. *J Am Osteopath Assoc.* 1985;85(12):786–801.
56. Bath M, Owens J. Physiology, viscerosomatic reflexes. In: *StatPearls.* StatPearls Publishing; 2023. Accessed November 26, 2023. http://www.ncbi.nlm.nih.gov/books/NBK559218/
57. Zegarra-Parodi R, Esteves JE, Lunghi C, Baroni F, Draper-Rodi J, Cerritelli F. The legacy and implications of the body-mind-spirit osteopathic tenet: a discussion paper evaluating its clinical relevance in contemporary osteopathic care. *International Journal of Osteopathic Medicine.* 2021;41:57–65.
58. Fahlgren E, Nima AA, Archer T, Garcia D. Person-centered osteopathic practice: patients' personality (body, mind, and soul) and health (ill-being and well-being). *PeerJ.* 2015;3:e1349.
59. Kovanur Sampath K, Roy DE. Management of mood disorders by osteopaths in New Zealand: a survey of current clinical practice. *International Journal of Osteopathic Medicine.* 2015;18(3):161–170.
60. Gulseren S, Gulseren L, Hekimsoy Z, Cetinay P, Ozen C, Tokatlioglu B. Depression, anxiety, health-related quality of life, and disability in patients with overt and subclinical thyroid dysfunction. *Arch Med Res.* 2006;37(1):133–139.
61. Bathla M, Singh M, Relan P. Prevalence of anxiety and depressive symptoms among patients with hypothyroidism. *Indian J Endocrinol Metab.* 2016;20(4):468–474.
62. Kvetny J, Ellervik C, Bech P. Is suppressed thyroid-stimulating hormone (TSH) associated with subclinical depression in the Danish General Suburban Population Study? *Nord J Psychiatry.* 2015;69(4):282–286.
63. Ittermann T, Völzke H, Baumeister SE, Appel K, Grabe HJ. Diagnosed thyroid disorders are associated with depression and anxiety. *Soc Psychiatry Psychiatr Epidemiol.* 2015;50(9):1417–1425.
64. Cosci F, Fava GA, Sonino N. Mood and anxiety disorders as early manifestations of medical illness: a systematic review. *Psychother Psychosom.* 2015;84(1):22–29.
65. Blum MR, Wijsman LW, Virgini VS, et al. Subclinical thyroid dysfunction and depressive symptoms among the elderly: a prospective cohort study. *Neuroendocrinology.* 2016;103(3-4):291–299.
66. Samuels MH. Psychiatric and cognitive manifestations of hypothyroidism. *Curr Opin Endocrinol Diabetes Obes.* 2014;21(5):377–383.
67. Rakhshan M, Ghanbari A, Rahimi A, Mostafavi I. A comparison between the quality of life and mental health of patients with hypothyroidism and normal people referred to Motahari Clinic of Shiraz University of Medical Sciences. *Int J Community Based Nurs Midwifery.* 2017;5(1):30–37.
68. Kiel S, Ittermann T, Völzke H, Chenot JF, Angelow A. Frequency of thyroid function tests and examinations in participants of a population-based study. *BMC Health Serv Res.* 2020;20(1):70.

69. National Guideline Centre (UK). *Monitoring Thyroid Disease: Thyroid Disease: Assessment and Management: Evidence Review F.* National Institute for Health and Care Excellence (NICE); 2019. Accessed January 28, 2024. http://www.ncbi.nlm.nih.gov/books/NBK577227/
70. Wartofsky L, Klubo-Gwiezdzinska J. Myxedema coma. In: Luster M, Duntas LH, Wartofsky L, eds. *The Thyroid and Its Diseases: A Comprehensive Guide for the Clinician.* Springer International Publishing; 2019:281–292.
71. Fallahi P, Ferrari SM, Ruffilli I, et al. The association of other autoimmune diseases in patients with autoimmune thyroiditis: review of the literature and report of a large series of patients. *Autoimmun Rev.* 2016;15(12): 1125–1128.
72. Boelaert K, Newby PR, Simmonds MJ, et al. Prevalence and relative risk of other autoimmune diseases in subjects with autoimmune thyroid disease. *Am J Med.* 2010;123(2):183.e1–183.e9.

GLOSSARY OF OSTEOPATHIC TERMINOLOGY

INTRODUCTION

The Educational Council on Osteopathic Principles (ECOP) was formed in 1969 by the Chairs of the Osteopathic Principles and Practice Departments of the six osteopathic schools of the time. They charged themselves with developing national standardized terminology for the profession, a textbook for the profession, and a national core curriculum. In 1974, they joined the American Association of Colleges of Osteopathic Medicine (AACOM) as one of their councils. AACOM is the leading voice for the education and training of physicians who practice osteopathic medicine and plays an important role in establishing standards of excellence for medical education at the accredited colleges of osteopathic medicine in the United States, and in graduate medical education through internships and residencies at US medical centers, hospitals, clinics, and health systems.

The result of many years' work by members of the ECOP, the *Glossary of Osteopathic Terminology* (Glossary), was first published in the *Journal of the American Osteopathic Association* April 1981 (No. 80, pp. 552–567). It has been included as an appendix in each edition of the *Foundations of Osteopathic Medicine* textbook: first edition (1997, pp. 1126–1140); second edition (2003, pp. 1229–1253); and third edition (2011, pp. 1087–1110); and fourth edition (2018, pp. 1563–1594). The revision process for the Glossary is ongoing, conducted by members of the ECOP Glossary Review Committee. The most current and revised version is available on two websites: AACOM in PDF format at www.aacom.org and the American Osteopathic Association (AOA) at www.osteopathic.org.

CONTRIBUTING MEMBERS

Rebecca Giusti (Chair of Glossary of Osteopathic Terminology committee)

Regina Fleming, DO (Chair)
Gregory Stevens, DO (Vice Chair)
Crystal Martin, DO (Secretary)
Kevin Treffer, DO (Sergeant-at-Arms)
John Garlitz, DO (Historian)
Rance McClain, DO (AACOM ECOP Liaison)
Kendi Hensel, DO, PhD
Steven Ma, DO
Jeff Johns, DO
Tom Fotopoulos, DO
Jason Sneed, DO
Eric Snider, DO
Melchiorra Mangiracina, DO
Tracy Middleton, DO
John Biery, DO
Victoria Chang, DO
Jan Pryor, DO
Adrienne Kania, DO, FAAO
Tom Motyka, DO
Adrian Woolley, DO
Brianne Wehner, DO
Tanisha Denning, DO
Kelley Joy, DO
Nicole Myers, DO
Teanna Moore, DO
Douglas Westin, DO
Greg Heller, DO
J'Aimee Lippert, DO
Nathan Nakken, DO
Sheldon Yao, DO, FAAO
Michael Terzella, DO
Shawn Kerger, DO
Jean Rettos, DO
Jennifer Wilson, DO
Don Allison, DO
David Fuller, DO, FAAO
Ravi Yarid, DO
Kristie Petree, DO
Danielle Cooley, DO
Christopher LaFontano, DO
Kristin Putnam, DO
Mischa Coleman, DO
Juanita Brown, DO
Dennis Rau, DO
Nicole Pena, DO
Melissa Pearce, DO
Carol Browne, DO
Bethany Powers, DO
Ethan Worthington, DO
To Shan Li, DO
Angela Branda, DO
Susan Miliani, DO
Victoria Troncoso, DO
David Eland, DO, FAAO
Laura Griffin, DO, FAAO
Deborah Schmidt, DO
Kevin Hayes, DO
David Harden, DO
Kurt Heinking, DO, FAAO
Jan Hendryx, DO, FAAO
James Kribs, DO
Paul Rennie, DO, FAAO

ECOP acknowledges all previous and current members and especially Walter Ehrenfeuchter, DO, FAAODist, for their contribution to the development of the current and past versions of Glossary of Osteopathic Terminology.

PURPOSE

The purpose of this osteopathic glossary is to present important and frequently used words, terms, and phrases that are unique or with special significance to the osteopathic profession. It is not meant to replace a dictionary. The glossary offers the consensus of a large segment of the osteopathic profession and serves to standardize terminology. The ECOP Glossary Review Committee specifically seeks to include those definitions that are uniquely osteopathic in their origin or common usage, distinctive in the osteopathic usage of a common word, and/or important in describing osteopathic principles and practice (OPP), philosophy, and osteopathic manipulative treatment (OMT). The Glossary is expected to be useful to students and practitioners of osteopathic medicine and helpful to authors and other professionals in understanding and making proper use of osteopathic vocabulary.

Osteopathic treatment methods are a group of techniques that apply a set of distinct unifying principles that guide individualized treatment including high velocity, low amplitude (HVLA), muscle energy, osteopathic cranial manipulative medicine, counterstrain, myofascial release, and soft tissue. "Methods" are described as being direct, indirect, or combined.

The five models used in discussion of osteopathic patient care are as follows:

1. Respiratory–circulatory
2. Biomechanical–structural
3. Metabolic–nutritional
4. Neurologic
5. Behavioral–biopsychosocial

A

accessory joint motions *See* secondary joint motion.

accessory movements Movements used to potentiate, accentuate, or compensate for an impairment in a physiologic motion (e.g., the movements needed to move a paralyzed limb).

accommodation A self-reversing and nonpersistent adaptation.

active motion *See* motion, active.

activating force A force which initiates, enhances, or facilitates any osteopathic treatment method. Typical examples of extrinsic activating forces include breathing, compression, traction, and muscle movements. Typical examples of intrinsic/inherent activating forces include primary respiratory mechanism (PRM), fluid movement, and motility.

acute somatic dysfunction *See* somatic dysfunction, acute.

adaptation A responsive alteration or adjustment in the reciprocal relationship between structure and function, by which an individual is able to better accommodate changes in their environment.

allopathy A therapeutic system in which a disease is treated by producing a second condition that is incompatible with or antagonistic to the first. *(Dorland's) See also* allopath, allopathic physician.

allopath, allopathic physician

1. A term originated by Samuel Hahnemann, MD, to distinguish homeopaths from physicians practicing traditional/orthodox medicine.
2. In common usage, a general term used to differentiate MDs (medical doctors) from other schools of medicine.

anatomical barrier *See* barrier, motion.

angle

Ferguson angle *See* angle, lumbosacral.

lumbolumbar lordotic angle An objective quantification of lumbar lordosis typically determined by measuring the angle between the superior surface of the second lumbar vertebra and the inferior surface of the fifth lumbar vertebra; best measured from a standing lateral x-ray film (Fig. 1).

lumbosacral angle *Also called* Ferguson angle. Represents the angle of the lumbosacral junction as measured by the inclination of the superior surface of the first sacral vertebra to the horizontal (this is actually a sacral angle); usually measured from standing lateral x-ray films (Fig. 2).

lumbosacral lordotic angle An objective quantification of lumbar lordosis typically determined by measuring the angle between the superior surface of the second lumbar vertebra and the superior surface of the first sacral segment; best measured from a standing lateral x-ray film (Fig. 3).

anterior component A positional descriptor used to identify the side of reference when rotation of a vertebra has occurred; in a condition of right rotation, the left side is the anterior component; usually refers to the less prominent transverse process. *See also* posterior component.

anterior compression test *See* anterior superior iliac spine compression test.

anterior iliac rotation *See* innominate somatic dysfunction of, anterior innominate rotation.

anterior nutation *See* nutation.

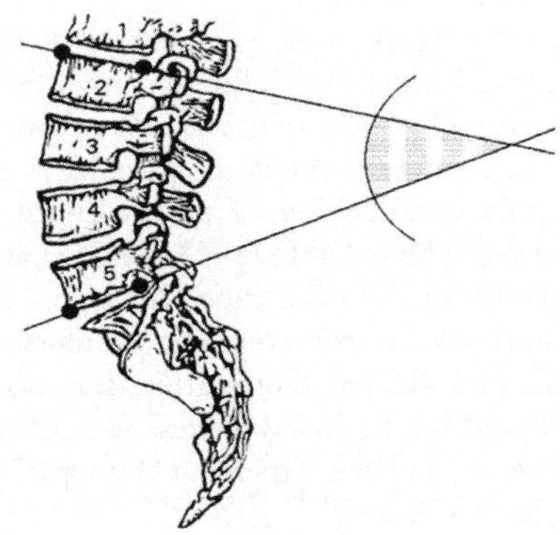

Figure 1. Lumbolumbar angle (L2–L5).

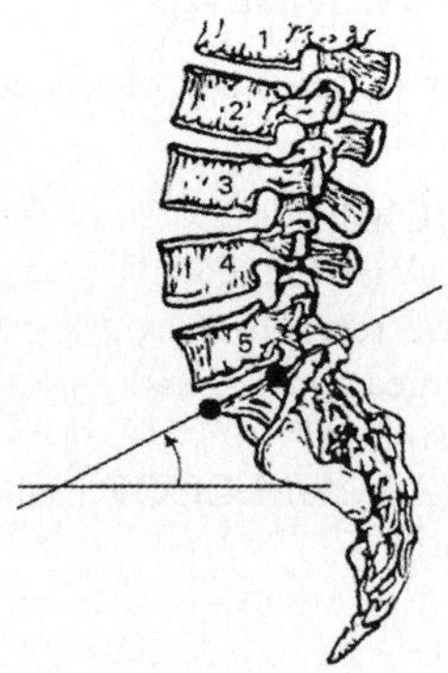

Figure 2. Lumbosacral angle (S1-horizon) (Ferguson angle).

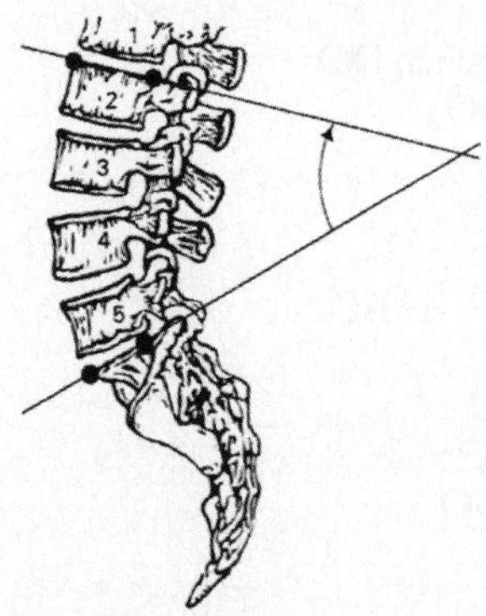

Figure 3. Lumbosacral lordotic angle.

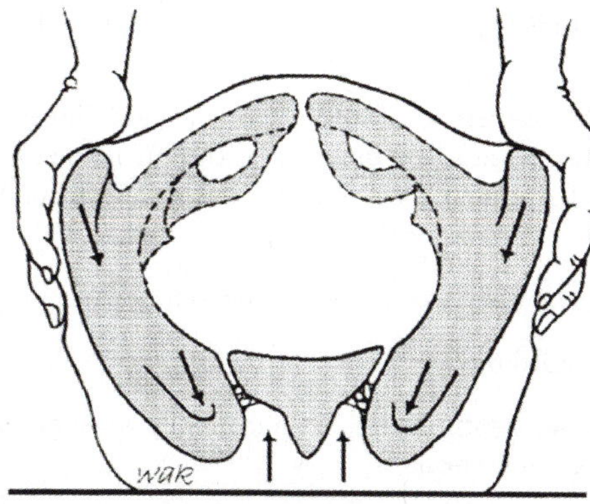

Figure 4. ASIS compression test.

anterior rib *See* rib somatic dysfunction; inhaled rib somatic dysfunction.

anterior superior iliac spine (ASIS) compression test *Also called* ASIS ilial compression test. A test for lateralization of somatic dysfunction of the sacrum, innominate, or pubic symphysis. Application of a force through the ASIS into one of the pelvic axes to assess the mechanics of the pelvis. *See also* sacral motion, axis of (Fig. 4).

articular pillar

1. Refers to the columnar arrangement of the articular portions of the cervical vertebrae.
2. Those parts of the lateral arches of the cervical vertebrae that contain a superior and inferior articular facet.

articulation

1. The place of union or junction between two or more bones of the skeleton.
2. The active or passive process of moving a joint through its permitted anatomic range of motion. *See also* osteopathic manipulative treatment method, articulatory.

articulatory pop The sound made when cavitation occurs in a joint. *See also* cavitation.

ART *See* osteopathic manipulative treatment, articulatory.

articulation *See* osteopathic manipulative treatment, articulatory method (ART).

ASIS compression test *See* anterior superior iliac spine compression test.

asymmetry Absence of symmetry of position or motion; dissimilarity in corresponding parts or organs on opposite sides of the body that are normally alike; of particular use when describing position or motion alteration resulting from somatic dysfunction. This term is part of the *TART* acronym for an osteopathic somatic dysfunction.

axis

1. An imaginary line about which motion occurs.
2. The second cervical vertebra.
3. One component of an axis system.

axis of rib motion *See* rib motion, axis of rib motion.

axis of sacral motion *See* sacral movement axis.

axoplasmic flow *See* axoplasmic transport.

axoplasmic transport The antegrade movement of substances from the nerve cell along the axon toward the terminals toward the nerve cell.

B

backward bending Opposite of forward bending. *See also* extension.

backward bending test (Sphinx test)

1. This test discriminates between forward and backward sacral torsion/rotation.
2. This test discriminates between unilateral sacral flexion and unilateral sacral extension.

backward torsion *See* sacrum, somatic dysfunctions of, backward torsions.

balance point The position at which the tension within the tissues is symmetrically distributed. *See* neutral.

balanced ligamentous tension (BLT)

1. The precise physiologic point in which the proprioceptive information provided by the ligaments allows the body to equalize the stresses exerted on an articulation in all directions.
2. A treatment method that is a regional interpretation based on the article "Osteopathic Technique of William G. Sutherland," published in the *1949 Year Book of Academy of Applied Osteopathy*. The method involves the minimization of periarticular tissue load and the placement of the affected ligaments in a position of equal tension in all appropriate planes so that the body's inherent forces can resolve the somatic dysfunction.
3. Evolved from Anne Wales, DO and the New England study group. See also ligamentous articular strain. See also osteopathic manipulative treatment, balanced ligamentous tension (BLT).

balanced membranous tension (BMT) The precise physiologic point in which the proprioceptive information provided by the dural membranes and sutures allows the body to equalize the stresses exerted on those structures in all directions. *See also* osteopathic manipulative treatment, balanced membranous tension. *See also* osteopathic cranial manipulative medicine (OCMM).

barrier (motion barrier) The limit to motion; in defining barriers, these palpatory end-feel characteristics are useful (Fig. 5).

anatomic(al) barrier The limit of motion imposed by anatomic structure; the limit of passive motion.

elastic barrier The range between the physiologic and anatomic barrier of motion in which passive ligamentous stretching occurs before tissue disruption.

pathologic barrier A restriction of joint motion associated with pathologic change of tissues (e.g., osteophytes). *See also* barrier, restrictive barrier.

physiologic barrier The limit of active motion.

restrictive barrier A functional limit that abnormally diminishes the normal physiologic range.

batwing deformity *See* transitional vertebrae, sacralization.

bind Palpable resistance to motion of an articulation or tissue. Synonym: resistance. Antonyms: ease, compliance, resilience.

biomechanics Mechanical principles applied to the study of biologic functions; the application of mechanical laws to living structures; the study and knowledge of biologic function from an application of mechanical principles.

BLT *See* balanced ligamentous tension.

BMT *See* balanced membranous tension.

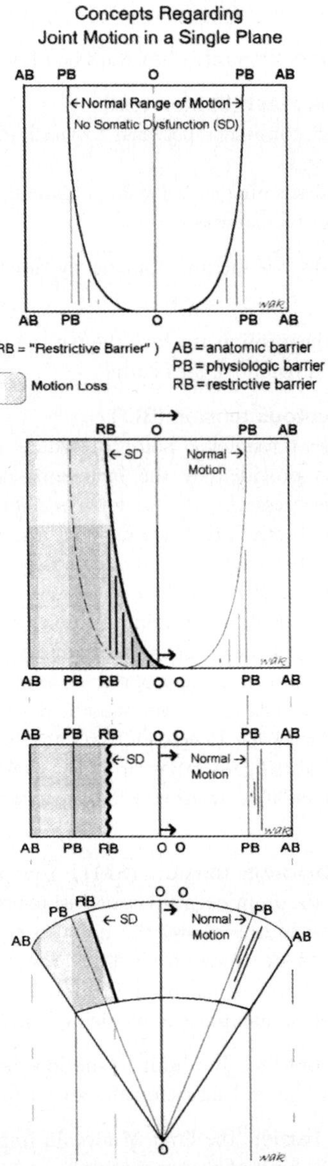

Figure 5. Somatic dysfunction in a single plane: three methods illustrating the "restrictive barrier" (the restrainer): AB, anatomic barrier; PB, physiologic barrier; RB, restrictive barrier; SD, somatic dysfunction. (From Scott RA, Kuchera ML, Patterson JJ. Orthopedics. In: Ward RC, Jerome JA, eds. *Foundations for Osteopathic Medicine.* Williams & Wilkins; 1997:484.)

body unity One of the basic tenets of the osteopathic philosophy; the human being is a dynamic unit of function; the person is a unit of body, mind, and spirit. *See also* osteopathic philosophy.

bogginess A tissue texture abnormality characterized principally by a palpable sense of sponginess in the tissue, interpreted as resulting from congestion due to increased fluid content.

bucket-handle rib motion *See* rib motion, bucket handle.

C

caliper rib motion *See* rib motion, caliper rib motion.

caudad Toward the tail or inferiorly.

caught in exhalation *See* rib somatic dysfunction, exhaled rib dysfunction.

caught in inhalation *See* rib somatic dysfunction, inhaled rib dysfunction.

cavitation The formation of small vapor and gas bubbles within fluid caused by local reduction in pressure. This phenomenon is believed to produce an audible "pop" in certain forms of osteopathic medical treatment.

CCP *See* fascial patterns, common compensatory pattern.

cephalad Toward the head.

cephalad pubic dysfunction *See* pubic bone, somatic dysfunctions of, superior pubic shear.

cerebrospinal fluid, fluctuation of A description of the hypothesized action of cerebrospinal fluid with regard to the craniosacral mechanism.

Certification in Neuromusculoskeletal Medicine and Osteopathic Manipulative Medicine (C-NMM/OMM) Certification is granted by the American Osteopathic Association (AOA) through the American Osteopathic Board of Neuromusculoskeletal Medicine (AOBNMM). First granted in 1999. *See also* Neuromusculoskeletal Medicine (NMM).

Certification in Special Proficiency in Osteopathic Manipulative Medicine (C-SPOMM) Specialty board certification in Osteopathic Manipulative Medicine prior to 1999. A certification granted by the American Osteopathic Association through the American Osteopathic Board of Special Proficiency in OMM. Replaced by C-NMM/OMM in that year. *See also* C-NMM/OMM.

cervicolumbar reflex *See* reflex, cervicolumbar.

Chapman reflex
1. A group of palpable points occurring in predictable locations on the anterior and posterior surfaces of the body that are considered to be reflections of visceral dysfunction or disease.
2. Originally used by Frank Chapman, DO, and described by Charles Owens, DO.

chronic somatic dysfunction *See* somatic dysfunction, chronic somatic dysfunction.

circumduction
1. The circular movement of a limb.
2. The rotary movement by which a structure is made to describe a cone, the apex of the cone being a fixed point (e.g., the circular movement of the shoulder).

C-NMM/OMM *See* Certification in Neuromusculoskeletal Medicine and Osteopathic Manipulative Medicine.

combined technique *See* osteopathic manipulative treatment, combined treatment method.

common compensatory pattern *See* fascial patterns, common compensatory pattern.

compensation A process in which there is an adaptive response to any alteration of structure or function in an attempt to optimize health.

complete motor asymmetry Asymmetry of palpatory responses to all regional motion inputs including rotation, translation, and active respiration.

compliance
1. The ease with which a tissue may be deformed.
2. Direction of ease in motion testing.

compression
1. Somatic dysfunction in which two structures are forced together.
2. A force that approximates two structures.

compression of the fourth ventricle (CV-4) *See* osteopathic manipulative treatment (CV-4). *See also* osteopathic cranial manipulative medicine.

conditioned reflex *See* reflex, conditioned.

contraction Shortening and/or development of tension in muscle.

concentric contraction Contraction of muscle resulting in approximation of attachments.

eccentric contraction Lengthening of muscle during contraction due to an external force.

isokinetic contraction
1. A concentric contraction against resistance in which the angular change of joint motion is at the same rate.
2. The counterforce is less than the patient force.

isolytic contraction
1. A form of eccentric contraction designed to break adhesions using an operator-induced force to lengthen the muscle.
2. The counterforce is greater than the patient force.

isometric contraction
1. Change in the tension of a muscle without approximation of muscle origin and insertion.
2. Operator force equal to patient force.

isotonic contraction
1. A form of concentric contraction in which a constant force is applied.
2. Operator force less than patient force.

contracted muscle The physiologic response to a neuromuscular excitation. *See also* contractured muscle.

contractured muscle Histologic change substituting noncontractile tissue for muscle tissue, which prevents the muscle from reaching normal relaxed length. *See also* contracted muscle.

core link The connection of the spinal dura mater from the occiput at the foramen magnum to the sacrum. It coordinates the synchronous motion of these two structures.

coronal plane *See* plane, coronal plane.

costal dysfunction *See* rib, somatic dysfunction.

counternutation Posterior movement of the sacral base around a transverse axis in relation to the ilia. *See also* nutation.

counterstrain technique *See* osteopathic manipulative treatment, counterstrain.

counterstrain point
1. A discrete area of tissue texture abnormality, which often exhibits tenderness and responds to a positional release technique.
2. Points used in counterstrain technique developed by Lawrence Jones, DO. *See also* tender points. *See also* osteopathic manipulative treatment, counterstrain.

cranial manipulation *See* osteopathic cranial manipulative medicine. *See also* osteopathic manipulative treatment method, osteopathic cranial manipulative medicine.

cranial rhythmic impulse *Also called* CRI.
1. A rhythmic fluctuation palpable throughout the entire body believed to be synchronous with the primary respiratory mechanism.
2. Term coined by John Woods, DO, and Rachel Woods, DO.

cranial technique *See* osteopathic manipulative treatment, osteopathic cranial manipulative medicine. *See also* primary respiratory mechanism.

craniosacral manipulation *See* osteopathic manipulative treatment, osteopathic cranial manipulative medicine.

craniosacral mechanism
1. A term used to refer to the anatomical connection between the occiput and the sacrum by the spinal dura mater.
2. A term coined by William G. Sutherland, DO. *See* extension, sacral. *See also* flexion, sacral. *See also* primary respiratory mechanism.

creep The capacity of fascia and other tissue to lengthen when subjected to a constant tension load resulting in less resistance to a second load application.

C-SPOMM *See* Certification in Special Proficiency in Osteopathic Manipulative Medicine.

CV-4 *See* osteopathic manipulative treatment, compression of the fourth ventricle (CV-4).

D

Dalrymple treatment *See* osteopathic manipulative treatment, pedal pump.

decompensation A dysfunctional, persistent pattern, in some cases reversible, resulting when homeostatic mechanisms are partially or totally overwhelmed.

deformation

plastic deformation A nonrecoverable deformation. *See also* elastic deformation.

elastic deformation Any recoverable deformation. *See also* plastic deformation.

depressed rib *See* rib somatic dysfunction, exhalation rib dysfunction. *See also* exhaled rib dysfunction.

dermatome
1. The area of skin supplied by cutaneous branches from a single spinal nerve (neighboring dermatomes may overlap).
2. Cutis plate; the dorsolateral part of an embryonic somite (Figs. 6 and 7).

diagnostic palpation *See* palpatory diagnosis.

diagonal axis *See* sacral movement axis, oblique axis (diagonal).

direct method (technique) *See* osteopathic manipulative treatment, direct treatment.

DO
1. Doctor of Osteopathy (graduate of a school accredited by the American Osteopathic Association Commission on Osteopathic College Accreditation [COCA]).
2. Doctor of Osteopathic Medicine (graduate of a school accredited by the American Osteopathic Association-COCA).
3. Diplomate in Osteopathy (the first degree granted by American School of Osteopathy).
4. Diplomate of Osteopathy, a degree granted by some schools of osteopathy outside the United States (not accredited by the American Osteopathic Association-COCA).

Doctor of Osteopathic Medicine (DO), United States An osteopathic physician who has graduated from a COCA-accredited institution and is a fully qualified physician, educated within the context of a distinct patient-centered, health-oriented philosophy, trained to combine specialized diagnostic and therapeutic hands-on skills (Osteopathic Manipulative Treatment) with the latest advances in the science and practice of medicine to offer comprehensive healthcare to patients. (Approved by AOA House of Delegates 2025.)

E

ease Relative palpable freedom of motion of an articulation or tissue. Synonyms. compliance, resilience. Antonyms. bind, resistance.

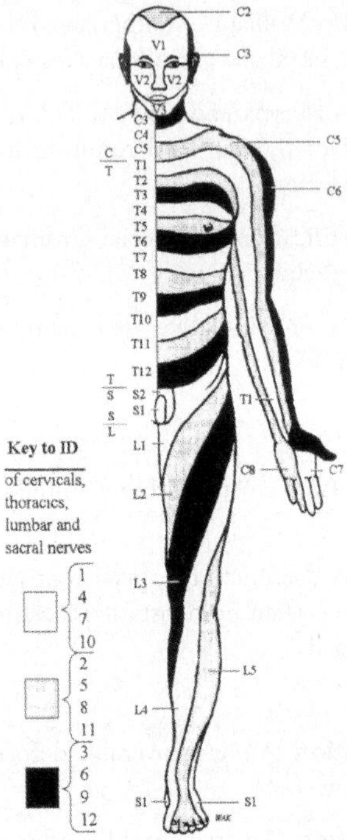

Figure 6. Dermatomal map (anterior). (Modified with permission from Agur AMR. *Grant's Atlas of Anatomy.* 9th ed. Williams & Wilkins; 1991:37.)

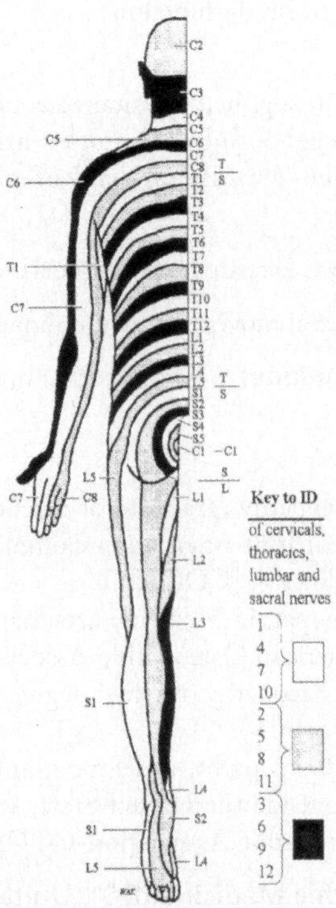

Figure 7. Dermatomal map (posterior). (Modified with permission from Agur AMR. *Grant's Atlas of Anatomy.* 9th ed. Williams & Wilkins; 1991:38.)

easy normal *See* neutral, definition #2.

-ed A suffix describing status, position, or condition (e.g., extended, flexed, rotated, restricted).

ECOP *See* Educational Council on Osteopathic Principles.

Educational Council on Osteopathic Principles (ECOP) A component group of the American Association of Colleges of Osteopathic Medicine (AACOM). The council is composed of one representative from each osteopathic medical school who oversees the teaching of osteopathic principles and practice, including osteopathic manipulative treatment at each institution.

effleurage Stroking movement used to move fluids.

elastic deformation *See* deformation, elastic.

elasticity Ability of a strained body or tissue to recover its original shape after deformation. *See also* plasticity; viscosity.

elevated rib *See* rib somatic dysfunction, inhalation rib dysfunction. *See also* rib motion, exhalation rib restriction.

end feel Perceived quality of motion as an anatomic or physiologic restrictive barrier is approached.

enthesitis

1. Traumatic disease occurring at the insertion of muscles where recurring concentration of muscle stress provokes inflammation with a strong tendency toward fibrosis and calcification.
2. Inflammation of the muscular or tendinous attachment to bone.

ERS A descriptor of spinal somatic dysfunction used to denote a vertebral position that is extended (E), rotated (R), and side bent (S).

ERS left Somatic dysfunction in which the vertebral unit is extended, rotated, and side bent left; usually preceded by a designation of the vertebral unit(s) involved (e.g., T5 ERS left or T5 ERLSL).

ERS right Somatic dysfunction in which the vertebral unit is extended, rotated, and sidebent right; usually preceded by a designation of the vertebral unit(s) involved (e.g., C3–C5 ERS right or C3–C5 ERRSR).

exaggeration treatment method *See* osteopathic manipulative treatment, exaggeration.

exaggeration technique *See* osteopathic manipulative treatment, exaggeration technique.

exhalation rib dysfunction *See* rib somatic dysfunction, exhalation rib dysfunction.

exhalation rib restriction *See* rib somatic dysfunction, inhaled rib dysfunction.

exhaled rib Historic term, using positional (static) diagnosis. *See* rib somatic dysfunction, inhaled somatic dysfunction.

extension

1. Accepted universal term for backward/posterior motion of the spine in the sagittal plane about a transverse axis; in a vertebral unit when the superior part moves backward/posteriorly.
2. In extremities, it is the straightening of a curve or angle (biomechanics).
3. Historic term, separation of the ends of a curve in a spinal region.

regional extension *Also called* Fryette regional extension (Fig. 8). Historically, the straightening in the sagittal plane of a spinal region.

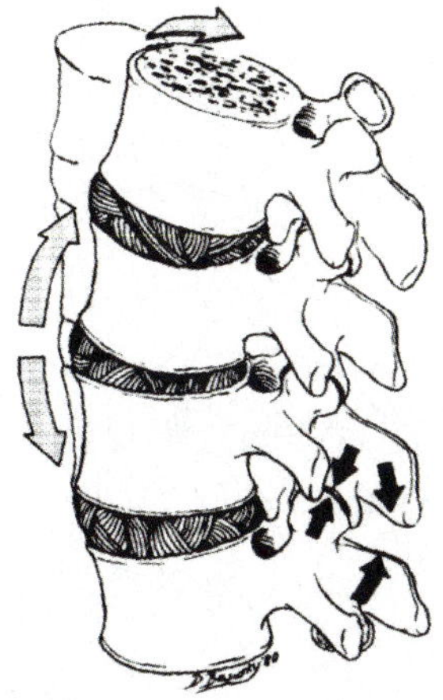

Figure 8. Regional extension.

sacral extension

1. Posterior movement of the base of the sacrum in relation to the ilia (Fig. 9). *See also* flexion, sacral; counternutation and nutation.
2. In osteopathic cranial manipulative medicine, extension is said to occur when the sacral base moves anteroinferiorly as the sphenobasilar synchondrosis (SBS) descends and flattens during the exhalation phase of the primary respiratory mechanism (Fig. 10).

extrinsic corrective forces Treatment forces external to the patient that may include operator effort, effect of gravity, mechanical tables, etc. *See also* intrinsic corrective forces.

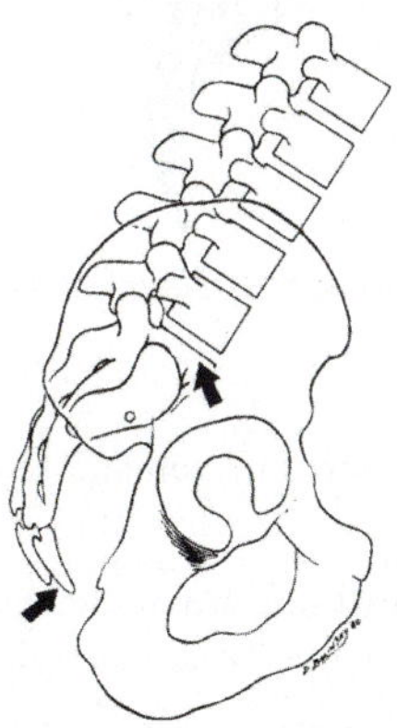

Figure 9. Sacral Extension or Counternutation.

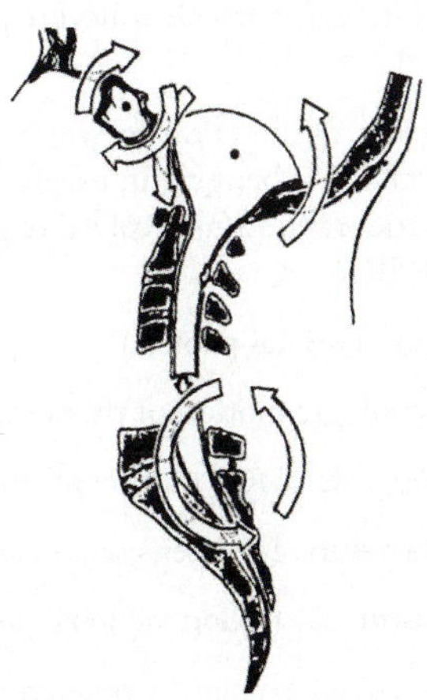

Figure 10. Sacral Extension during the exhalation phase of the primary respiratory mechanism.

F

FAAO *See* Fellow of American Academy of Osteopathy.

facet asymmetry Configuration in which the structure, position, and/or motion of the facets are not equal bilaterally. *See also* facet symmetry; tropism, facet.

facet symmetry Configuration in which the structure, position, and/or motion of the facets are equal bilaterally. *See also* facet asymmetry; symmetry.

facilitated positional release *See* osteopathic manipulative treatment, facilitated positional release.

facilitated segment *See* spinal facilitation.

facilitation *See* spinal facilitation.

fascial patterns

1. Systems for classifying and recording the preferred directions of fascial motion throughout the body.
2. Based on the observations of J. Gordon Zink, DO, and W. Neidner, DO.

common compensatory pattern (CCP) The specific finding of alternating fascial motion preference at transitional regions of the body described by Zink and Neidner (Fig. 11).

uncommon compensatory pattern The finding of alternating fascial motion preference in the direction opposite that of the common compensatory pattern described by Zink and Neidner (Fig. 12).

uncompensated fascial pattern The finding of fascial preferences that do not demonstrate alternating patterns of findings at transitional regions. Clinically, this generally occurs following postural stress or trauma and is frequently associated with development of symptomatology.

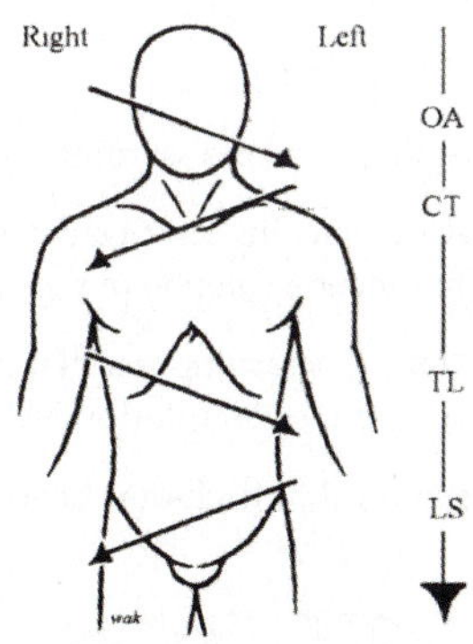

Figure 11. Common compensatory fascial pattern (Zink).

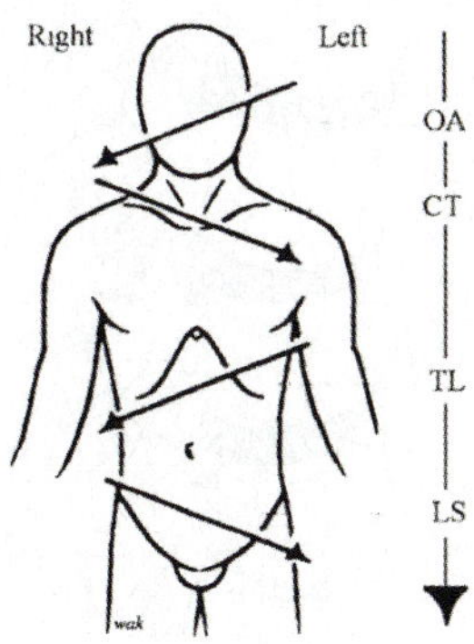

Figure 12. Uncommon compensatory fascial pattern (Zink).

fascial release technique *See* osteopathic manipulative treatment, myofascial release.

fascial unwinding *See* osteopathic manipulative treatment, fascial unwinding.

Fellow of American Academy of Osteopathy (FAAO) This earned postdoctoral fellowship is conferred by the American Academy of Osteopathy. Those who earn the FAAO must demonstrate their commitment to osteopathic principles and practice through teaching, writing, and service, performed at the highest level of professional and ethical standards.

Ferguson angle *See* angle, lumbosacral.

flexion

1. Accepted universal term for forward/anterior motion of the spine, in its sagittal plane about a transverse axis; in a vertebral unit when the superior part moves forward/anteriorly.
2. In the extremities, it is the approximation of a curve or angle (biomechanics).
3. Approximation of the ends of a curve in a spinal region. *See* flexion, regional flexion.

regional flexion *Also called Fryette regional flexion.* Historically, is the approximation of the ends of a curve in the sagittal plane of the spine (Fig. 13). *See* flexion.

sacral flexion

1. Anterior movement of sacral base in relation to the ilia (Fig. 14). *See also* extension, sacral extension; nutation, and counternutation.
2. In osteopathic cranial manipulative medicine, sacral flexion is said to occur when the sacral base moves posterosuperiorly as the sphenobasilar synchondrosis (SBS) ascends and angulates during the inhalation phase of the primary respiratory mechanism (Fig. 15).

flexion left *See* side bending.

flexion right *See* side bending.

flexion tests Tests for iliosacral and sacroiliac somatic dysfunction.

seated flexion test A screening test that determines the side of sacroiliac somatic dysfunction (motion of the sacrum on the ilium).

standing flexion test A screening test that determines the side of iliosacral somatic dysfunction (motion of ilium on the sacrum).

forward bending Reciprocal of backward bending. *See also* flexion.

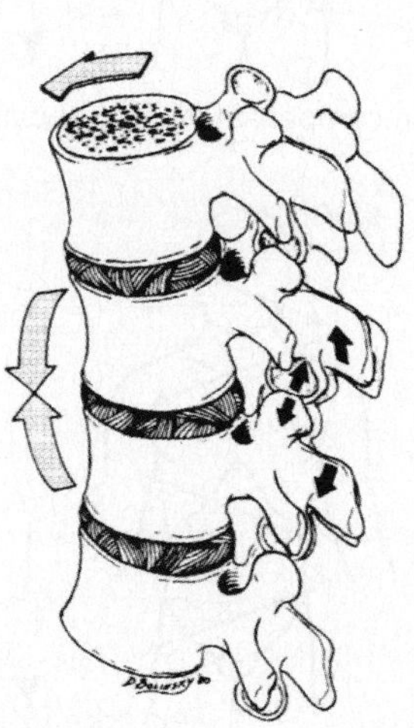

Figure 13. Regional flexion.

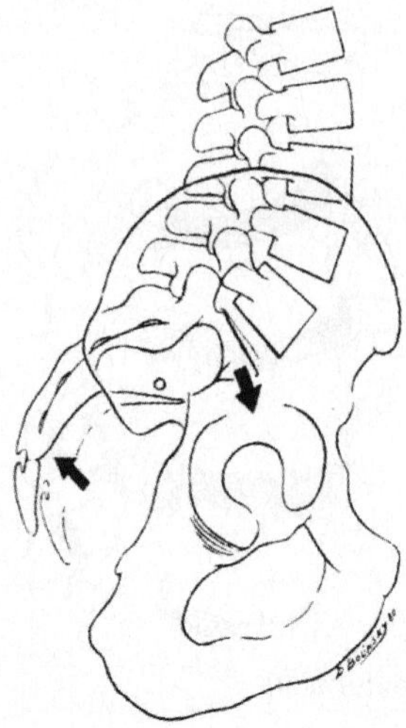

Figure 14. Sacral flexion or nutation.

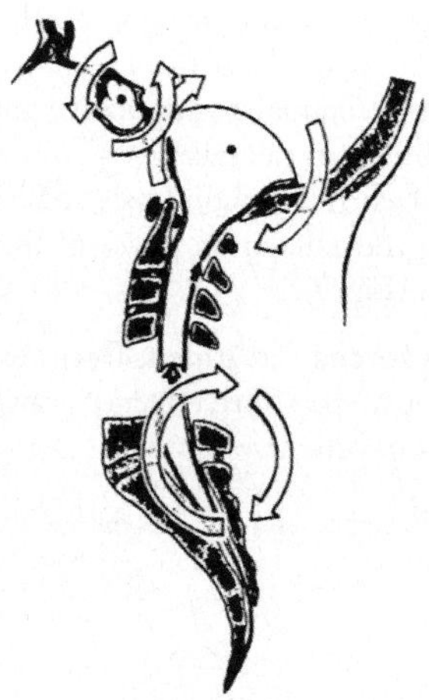

Figure 15. Sacral flexion during the inhalation phase of the primary respiratory mechanism.

forward torsions *See* sacrum, somatic dysfunctions of, forward torsions.

FRS A descriptor of spinal somatic dysfunction used to denote a vertebral position that is flexed (F), rotated (R), and side bent (S).

FRS left A somatic dysfunction in which the vertebral unit is flexed, rotated, and sidebent left; usually preceded by a designation of the vertebral unit(s) involved (e.g., T5 FRS left or T5 FRLSL).

FRS right A somatic dysfunction in which the vertebral unit is flexed, rotated, and side bent right; usually preceded by a designation of the vertebral unit(s) involved (e.g., C3–C5 FRS right or C3–C5 FRRSR).

frontal plane *See* plane, coronal plane.

Fryette laws *See* physiologic motion of the spine.

Fryette principles *See* physiologic motion of the spine.

Fryette regional extension *See* extension, regional extension.

Fryette regional flexion *See* flexion, regional flexion.

FSR A descriptor of spinal somatic dysfunction used to denote a vertebral position that is flexed (F), side bent (S), and rotated (R). *See* FRS.

functional treatment method *See* osteopathic manipulative treatment, functional treatment.

functional technique *See* osteopathic manipulative treatment, functional treatment method.

G

gait A forward translation of the body's center of gravity by bipedal locomotion.

Galbreath treatment technique *See* osteopathic manipulative treatment, mandibular drainage.

glymphatic system A network of channels formed by glia in the central nervous system, which seem to function as a waste clearance pathway for cerebrospinal fluid, interstitial fluid, and interstitial solutes.

gravitational line Viewing the patient from the side, an imaginary line in a coronal plane which, in the theoretical ideal posture, starts slightly anterior to the lateral malleolus, passes across the lateral condyle of the knee, the greater trochanter, through the lateral head of the humerus at the tip of the shoulder to the external auditory meatus; if this were a plane through the body, it would intersect the middle of the third lumbar vertebra and the anterior one third of the sacrum. It is used to evaluate the A-P (anteroposterior) curves of the spine. *See also* mid-malleolar line (Fig. 16).

H

habituation Decreased physiologic response to repeated stimulation.

health Adaptive and optimal attainment of physical, mental, emotional, spiritual, and environmental well-being.

hepatic pump *See* osteopathic manipulative treatment, hepatic pump.

high-velocity low-amplitude treatment method (HVLA) *See* osteopathic manipulative treatment, high velocity low amplitude.

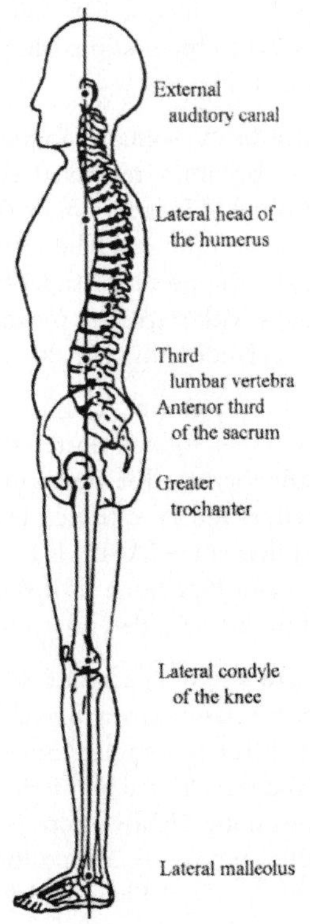

Figure 16. Gravitational line.

hip bone *See* innominate. *See also* innominate, somatic dysfunctions of.

homeostasis Maintenance of static or constant conditions in the internal environment. The level of well-being of an individual maintained by internal physiologic harmony that is the result of a relatively stable state or equilibrium among the interdependent body functions.

homeostatic mechanism A system of control activated by negative feedback.

Hoover technique *See* osteopathic manipulative treatment, Hoover technique.

hysteresis During the loading and unloading of connective tissue, the restoration of the final length of the tissue occurs at a rate and to an extent less than during deformation (loading). These differences represent energy loss in the connective tissue system. This difference in viscoelastic behavior (and energy loss) is known as hysteresis (or "stress–strain").

hypertonicity A condition of excessive resting tone of skeletal muscle characterized by increased resistance of the muscle to passive stretching.

HVLA High velocity low amplitude. *See* osteopathic manipulative treatment, high velocity low amplitude.

I

I/IND Indirect method. *See* osteopathic manipulative treatment, indirect method.

ILA Inferior lateral angle of the sacrum. *See* sacrum, inferior lateral angle of.

ilia The plural of ilium. *See* ilium.

ilial compression test *See* anterior superior iliac spine (ASIS) compression test.

ilial rocking test *See* anterior superior iliac spine (ASIS) compression test.

iliosacral motion Motion of one innominate (ilium) with respect to the sacrum. Iliosacral motion is part of pelvic motion during the gait cycle.

iliosacral dysfunction *See* innominate somatic dysfunctions.

ilium The expansive superior portion of the innominate (hip bone or os coxa). *See also* innominate.

indirect method *See* osteopathic manipulative treatment, indirect method.

inferior ilium *See* innominate, somatic dysfunctions of, inferior innominate shear.

inferior lateral angle of the sacrum (ILA) *See* sacrum, inferior lateral angle.

inferior pubis *See* pubic bone, somatic dysfunctions of, inferior pubic shear.

inferior transverse axis *See* sacral movement axis, inferior transverse axis.

inhalation rib *See* rib somatic dysfunction, inhalation rib dysfunction.

inhalation rib restriction *See* rib somatic dysfunction, exhalation rib dysfunction.

inhibition *See* osteopathic manipulative treatment, inhibitory pressure.

inhibitory pressure technique *See* osteopathic manipulative treatment, inhibitory pressure.

innominate *Also called* the os coxa, hip bone, or pelvic bone. One of two large, irregularly shaped bones of the pelvis. Each consists of three parts: ilium, ischium, and pubis.

innominate rotation Rotational motion of one innominate bone relative to the sacrum about the inferior transverse axis.

innominate somatic dysfunctions

anterior innominate rotation A somatic dysfunction in which the innominate bone is rotated anteriorly about a transverse axis relative to the sacrum. The innominate moves more freely in anterior rotation and is restricted in posterior rotation. The anterior superior iliac spine (ASIS) is positioned inferiorly and the posterior superior iliac spine (PSIS) is positioned superiorly when compared to the contralateral landmarks (Fig. 17).

downslipped innominate *See* inferior innominate shear.

inferior innominate shear A somatic dysfunction in which the innominate bone translates inferiorly relative to the sacrum and becomes restricted. The innominate moves more freely in inferior translation and is restricted in superior translation. The anterior superior iliac spine (ASIS), posterior superior iliac spine (PSIS), and ischial tuberosity are positioned inferiorly when compared to the contralateral landmarks (Fig. 18).

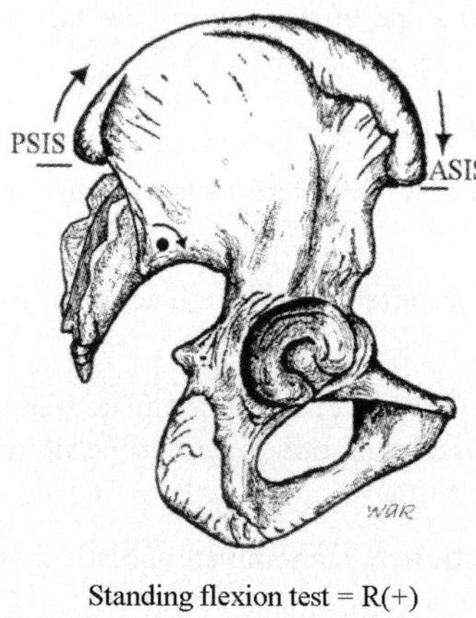

Figure 17. Anterior right innominate rotation.

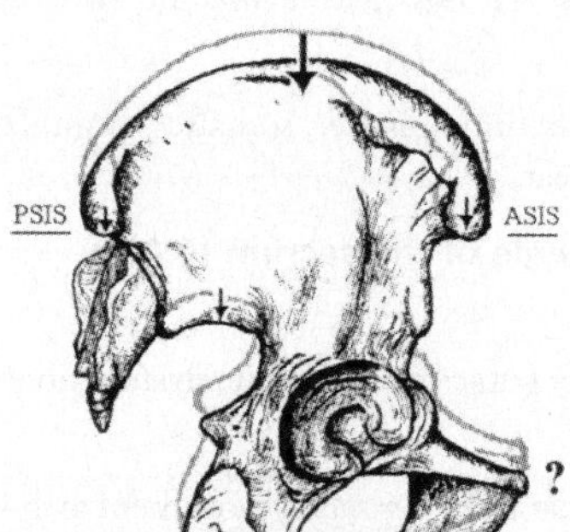

Figure 18. Right inferior innominate shear.

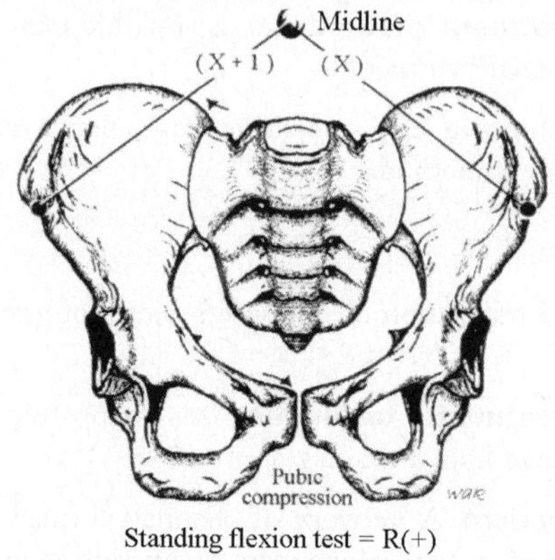

Figure 19. Inflared right innominate.

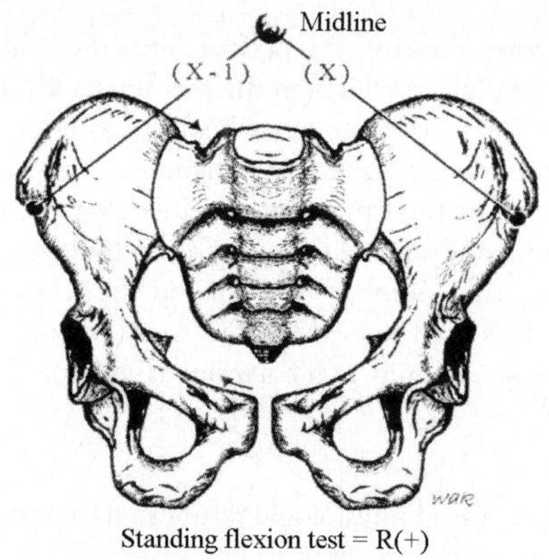

Figure 20. Outflared right innominate.

inflared innominate A somatic dysfunction in which the innominate bone becomes restricted such that the anterior superior iliac spine (ASIS) moves more freely in a medial direction and is restricted in the lateral direction. The ASIS is positioned medially and the posterior superior iliac spine (PSIS) is positioned laterally with respect to the midline when compared to the contralateral landmarks (Fig. 19).

outflared innominate A somatic dysfunction in which the innominate bone becomes restricted such that the anterior superior iliac spine (ASIS) moves more freely in a lateral direction and is restricted in the medial direction. The ASIS is positioned laterally and the posterior superior iliac spine (PSIS) is positioned medially with respect to the midline when compared to the contralateral landmarks (Fig. 20).

posterior innominate rotation A somatic dysfunction in which the innominate bone is rotated posteriorly around a transverse axis relative to the sacrum. The innominate moves more freely in posterior rotation and is restricted in anterior rotation. The anterior superior iliac spine (ASIS) is positioned superiorly and the posterior superior iliac spine (PSIS) is positioned inferiorly when compared to the contralateral landmarks (Fig. 21).

superior innominate shear A somatic dysfunction in which the innominate bone translates superiorly relative to the sacrum and becomes restricted. The innominate moves more freely in superior translation and is restricted in inferior translation. The anterior superior iliac spine (ASIS), posterior superior iliac spine (PSIS), and ischial tuberosity are positioned superiorly when compared to the contralateral landmarks (Fig. 22).

upslipped innominate *See* superior innominate shear.

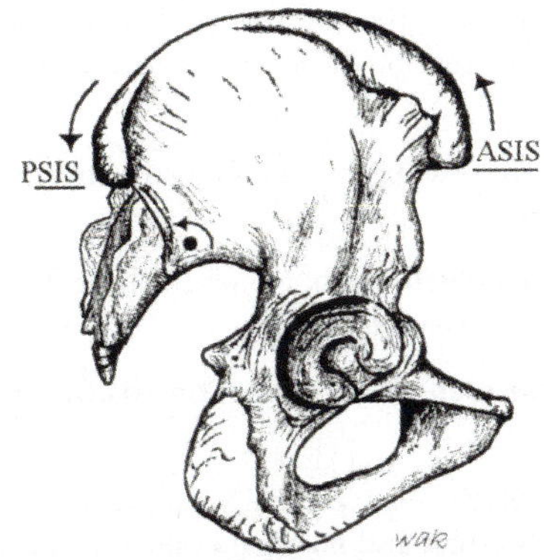

Standing flexion test = R(+)

Figure 21. Posterior right innominate rotation.

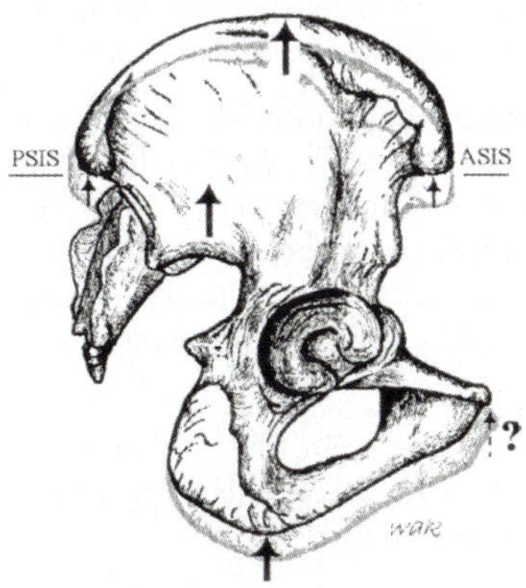

Seated flexion test = R(+)

Figure 22. Superior right innominate shear.

integrated neuromusculoskeletal release *See* osteopathic manipulative treatment, integrated neuromusculoskeletal release.

intersegmental motion Designates relative motion taking place between two adjacent vertebral segments or within a vertebral unit that is described as the upper vertebral segment moving on the lower.

intrinsic corrective forces Voluntary or involuntary forces from within the patient that assist in the manipulative treatment process. *See also* extrinsic corrective forces.

isokinetic exercise Exercise using a constant speed of movement of the body part.

isolytic contraction *See* contraction, isolytic.

isometric contraction *See* contraction, isometric.

isotonic contraction *See* contraction, isotonic.

J

Jones technique *See* osteopathic manipulative treatment, counterstrain.

junctional region *See* transitional region.

K

key lesion *See* somatic dysfunction, primary.

kinesthesia The sense by which muscular motion, weight, position, etc. are perceived.

kinesthetic Pertaining to kinesthesia.

kinetics The body of knowledge that deals with the effects of forces that produce or modify body motion.

klapping Striking the skin with cupped palms to produce vibrations with the intention of loosening material in the lumen of hollow tubes or sacs within the body, particularly the lungs.

kneading A soft tissue technique that utilizes an intermittent force applied perpendicular to the long axis of the muscle.

kyphoscoliosis A spinal curve pattern combining kyphosis and scoliosis. *See also* kyphosis; scoliosis.

kyphosis The exaggerated (pathologic) or normal A-P (anteroposterior) curve of the thoracic spine with concavity anteriorly. Abnormally increased convexity in the curvature of the thoracic spine in the lateral view.

kyphotic Pertaining to or characterized by kyphosis. *See also* kyphosis.

L

lateral flexed vertebral body *See* side bent.

lateral flexion *Also called* lateroflexion. *See* side bending.

lateral masses (of the atlas) The bulkiest and solid parts of the atlas that support the weight of the head.

lateroflexion *See* sidebending.

law

Fryette law of motion *See* physiologic motion of the spine.

Head law When a painful stimulus is applied to a body part of low sensitivity (e.g., viscus) that is in close central connection with a point of higher sensitivity (e.g., soma), the pain is felt at the point of higher sensitivity rather than at the point where the stimulus was applied.

Sherrington law

1. Every posterior spinal nerve root supplies a specific region of the skin, although fibers from adjacent spinal segments may invade such a region.
2. When a muscle receives a nerve impulse to contract, its antagonist receives, simultaneously, an impulse to relax. These are only two of Sherrington's contributions to neurophysiology; these are the ones most relevant to osteopathic principles.

Wolff law Every change in form and function of a bone, or in its function alone, is followed by certain definite changes in its internal architecture, and secondary alterations in its external conformations (e.g., bone is laid down along lines of stress) (*Stedman's*).

lesion (osteopathic) Historic term used to describe somatic dysfunction. *See* somatic dysfunction.

ligamentous

ligamentous articular strain (LAS) Any somatic dysfunction resulting in abnormal ligamentous tension or strain. *See also* osteopathic manipulative treatment, ligamentous articular strain technique.

ligamentous articular strain technique (LAS) *See* osteopathic manipulative treatment, ligamentous articular strain technique.

strain ligamentous Motion and/or positional asymmetry associated with elastic deformation of connective tissue (fascia, ligament, membrane). *See* strain; ligamentous articular strain.

line of gravity *See* gravitational line.

linkage A somatic dysfunctional segmental behavior where a single vertebra and an adjacent rib respond to the same regional motion tests with identical asymmetric behaviors (rather than opposing behaviors). This suggests visceral reflex inputs.

liver pump *See* osteopathic manipulative treatment, hepatic pump technique.

load The application of a biomechanical force (compression, distraction, or torsion) by the osteopathic physician directed to a specific anatomic structure or tissue.

localization

1. In manipulative technique, the precise positioning of the patient and vector application of forces required to produce a desired result.
2. The reference of a sensation to a particular locality in the body.

longitudinal axis *See* sacral motion axis, longitudinal axis.

lordosis The anterior convexity in the curvature of the lumbar and cervical spine as viewed from the lateral view. The term is used to refer to both an abnormally increased curvature (also called hollow back, saddle back, sway back) and to the normal curvature (normal lordosis).

lordotic Pertaining to or characterized by lordosis.

lumbarization *See* transitional vertebrae, lumbarization.

lumbolumbar lordotic angle *See* angle, lumbolumbar lordotic.

lumbosacral angle *See* angle, lumbosacral.

lumbosacral lordotic angle *See* angle, lumbosacral lordotic.

lumbosacral spring test *See* spring test.

lymphatic pumps *See* osteopathic manipulative treatment, lymphatic pump. *See also* osteopathic manipulative treatment, pedal pump. *See also* osteopathic manipulative treatment, thoracic pump technique.

lymphatic treatment *See* osteopathic manipulative treatment, lymphatic technique.

M

mandibular drainage technique *See* osteopathic manipulative treatment, mandibular drainage technique.

manipulation Therapeutic application of manual force. *See also* technique; osteopathic manipulative treatment.

manual medicine

1. The skillful use of the hands to diagnose and treat structural and functional abnormalities in various tissues and organs throughout the body, including bones, joints, muscles, and other soft tissues as an integral part of complete medical care.
2. This term originated from the German Manuelle Medizin (manual medicine) and has been used interchangeably with the term manipulation.
3. This term is not identical to manual therapy, which has been used by nonphysician practitioners (e.g., physical therapists).

massage Therapeutic friction, stroking, and kneading of the body. *See also* osteopathic manipulative treatment, soft tissue treatment method.

membranous articular strain Any cranial somatic dysfunction resulting in abnormal dural membrane tensions.

membranous balance The ideal physiologic state of harmonious equilibrium in the tension of the dura mater of the brain and spinal cord.

mesenteric lift *See* osteopathic manipulative treatment, mesenteric release technique.

mesenteric release technique *See* osteopathic manipulative treatment, mesenteric release technique.

middle transverse axis *See* sacral motion axis, middle transverse axis (postural).

mid-heel line A vertical line used as a reference in standing anteroposterior (A-P) x-rays and postural evaluation, passing equidistant between the heels.

mid-gravitational line *See* gravitational line.

mid-malleolar line A vertical line passing through the lateral malleolus, used as a point of reference in standing lateral x-rays and postural evaluation. *See also* gravitational line.

mirror-image motion asymmetries A grouping of primary and secondary sites of somatic dysfunction describing a three-segment complex fundamental to dysfunction in a mobile system. Each adjacent segment, above and below the primary locus, demonstrates opposing asymmetries to that locus. For example, if the primary locus resists rotation right, the segments above and below resist rotation left.

mobile point In counterstrain, the final position of treatment at which tenderness is no longer elicited by palpation of the tender point. *See also* counterstrain.

mobile segment A term in functional methods to describe a bony structure with its articular surfaces and adnexal tissues (neuromuscular and connective) for segmental motion, which affects movement, stabilizes position, and allows coordinated participation in passive movement.

mobile system An osteopathic construct associated with functional methods in which the body as a whole is viewed as a centrally integrated system in which all of the individual elements (e.g., mobile segments) have coordinated and specific motion characteristics. *See also* osteopathic manipulative treatment, functional method.

mobile unit *See* mobile segment.

models of osteopathic care Five models that articulate how an osteopathic physician seeks to influence a patient's physiologic processes.

behavioral-biopsychosocial model The goal of this model is to improve the biologic, psychological, and social components of the health spectrum. This includes emotional balancing and compensatory mechanisms. Reproductive processes and behavioral adaption are also included under this model.

biomechanical-structural model The goal of the structural model is biomechanical adjustment and the mobilization of joints. This model also seeks to address problems in the myofascial connective tissues, as well as in the bony and soft tissues, to remove restrictive forces and enhance motion. This is accomplished by the use of a wide range of osteopathic manipulative techniques such as high velocity low amplitude, muscle energy, counterstrain, myofascial release, ligamentous articular techniques, and functional techniques.

metabolic-nutritional model The goal of this model is to enhance the self-regulatory and self-healing mechanisms, to foster energy conservation by balancing the body's energy expenditure and exchange, and to enhance immune system function, endocrine function, and organ function. Lymphatic pump techniques are examples of osteopathic manipulative treatment that influence this area of patient health. Nutritional counseling, diet, and exercise advice are the most common approaches to balancing the body through this model.

neurologic model The goal of the neurologic model is to attain autonomic balance and address neural reflex activity, remove facilitated segments, decrease afferent nerve signals, and relieve pain. The osteopathic manipulative techniques most used to influence this area of patient health include counterstrain and Chapman reflex points.

respiratory–circulatory model The goal of the respiratory–circulatory model is to improve all of the diaphragm restrictions in the body. Diaphragms are considered to be "transverse restrictors" of motion, venous and lymphatic drainage, and cerebrospinal fluid. The osteopathic manipulative techniques most used to influence this area of patient health are osteopathic cranial manipulative medicine, ligamentous articular strain, myofascial release, and lymphatic pump techniques.

motion

1. A change of position (rotation and/or translation) with respect to a fixed system.
2. An act or process of a body changing position in terms of direction, course, and velocity.

active motion Movement produced voluntarily by the patient.

inherent motion Spontaneous motion of every cell, organ, system, and their component units within the body.

passive motion Motion induced by the osteopathic physician while the patient remains passive or relaxed.

physiologic motion Changes in position of body structures within the normal range. *See also* physiologic motion of the spine.

MFR *See* osteopathic manipulative treatment, myofascial release.

muscle energy technique *See* osteopathic manipulative treatment, muscle energy.

myofascial release technique *See* osteopathic manipulative treatment, myofascial release.

myofascial technique *See* osteopathic manipulative treatment, myofascial release, myofascial technique.

myofascial trigger point *See* trigger point, myofascial.

myogenic tonus

1. Tonic contraction of muscle dependent on some property of the muscle itself or of its intrinsic nerve cells.
2. Contraction of a muscle caused by intrinsic properties of the muscle or by its intrinsic innervation (*Stedman's*).

myotome

1. All muscles derived from one somite and innervated by one segmental spinal nerve (*Stedman's*).
2. That part of the somite that develops into skeletal muscle.

N

Neuromusculoskeletal Medicine (NMM) The specialty within osteopathic medicine that emphasizes the incorporation of osteopathic manual diagnosis and osteopathic manipulative treatment into the evaluation and treatment of the nervous, muscular, and skeletal systems in their relationships to other systems of the body as well as the whole person. *See also* Certification in Neuromusculoskeletal Medicine. *See also* Osteopathic Neuromusculoskeletal Medicine (ONMM).

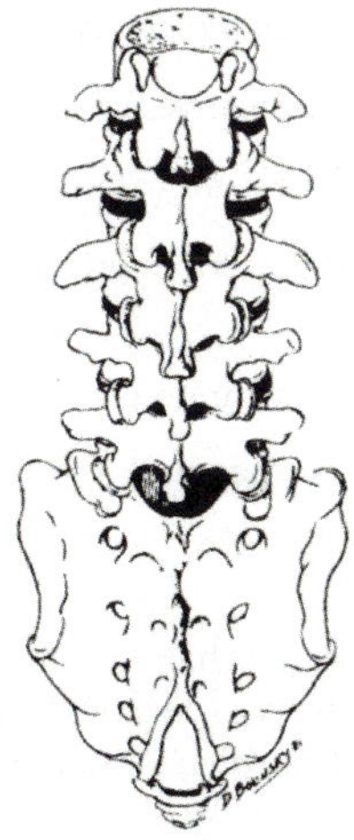

Figure 23. Neutral spinal position.

neurotrophicity *See* neurotrophy.

neurotrophy The nutrition and maintenance of tissues as regulated by direct innervation.

neutral

1. The range of sagittal plane spinal positioning in which the first principle of physiologic motion of the spine applies.
2. A point of tissue or articular balance from which all motions physiologic to that structure may take place. *See also* physiologic motion of the spine (Fig. 23).

NMM *See* Neuromusculoskeletal Medicine. *See also* Osteopathic Neuromusculoskeletal Medicine.

NMM-OMM Neuromusculoskeletal Medicine-Osteopathic Manipulative Medicine. *See* Osteopathic Neuromusculoskeletal Medicine.

nonneutral The range of sagittal plane spinal positioning in which the second principle of physiologic motion of the spine applies. *See also* extension. *See also* flexion. *See also* physiologic motion of the spine.

nonallopathic lesion Historic term used to describe somatic dysfunction. *See* somatic dysfunction.

normalization The therapeutic use of anatomic and physiologic mechanisms to facilitate the body's response toward homeostasis and improved health.

NSR A descriptor of spinal somatic dysfunction used to denote a vertebral position that is neutral (N), side bent (S), and rotated (R) vertebral position; similar descriptors may involve flexed (F) and extended (E) position.

nutation Nodding forward; anterior movement of the sacral base around a transverse axis in relation to the ilia.

O

oblique axis *See* sacral motion axis, oblique axis (diagonal).

OCMM *See* osteopathic manipulative treatment, osteopathic cranial manipulative medicine.

OMM *See* osteopathic manipulative medicine.

OMT *See* osteopathic manipulative treatment.

OMTh *See* osteopathic manipulative therapy.

ONMM *See* Osteopathic Neuromusculoskeletal Medicine.

OP&P Historic term for osteopathic principles and practice. *See also* osteopathic philosophy.

OPP Osteopathic principles and practice. *See also* osteopathic philosophy.

os coxa *See* innominate.

osteopath

1. A person who has achieved the nationally recognized academic and professional standards within their country to independently practice diagnosis and treatment based upon the principles of osteopathic philosophy. Individual countries establish the national academic and professional standards for osteopaths practicing within their countries (international usage).
2. Considered by the American Osteopathic Association (AOA) to be an historic term when applied to graduates of US schools. *See also* DO.

osteopathic lesion (complex) *Also called* nonallopathic lesion. Historic term used to describe somatic dysfunction. *See* somatic dysfunction.

osteopathic manipulative medicine (OMM) The application of osteopathic philosophy, structural diagnosis, and use of osteopathic manipulative treatment (OMT) in the diagnosis and management of the patient. *See also* osteopathic manipulative treatment (OMT).

osteopathic manipulative therapy (OMTh) The therapeutic application of manually guided forces by an osteopath (nonphysician) to improve physiologic function and homeostasis that has been altered by somatic dysfunction.

osteopathic manipulative treatment (OMT) The therapeutic application of manually guided forces by an osteopathic physician (US usage) to improve physiologic function and/or support homeostasis that has been altered by somatic dysfunction.

active method Any technique in which the patient voluntarily performs an osteopathic physician-directed motion.

articulatory treatment Historic term. *See* osteopathic manipulative treatment, articulatory.

articulatory A direct treatment method employing a low velocity/moderate to high amplitude force applied to a dysfunctional joint. The osteopathic physician can choose to employ a repetitive springing motion or a single movement of the joint through the restrictive barrier.

balanced ligamentous tension (BLT)

1. A treatment method that is a regional interpretation based on the article "Osteopathic Technique of William G. Sutherland," published in the *1949 Year Book of Academy of Applied Osteopathy*. The method involves the minimization of periarticular tissue load and the placement of the affected ligaments in a position of equal tension in all appropriate planes so that the body's inherent forces can resolve the somatic dysfunction.
2. Evolved from Anne Wales, DO and the New England study group. See also ligamentous articular strain. See also balanced ligamentous tension (BLT).

balanced membranous tension (BMT) Any OCMM method in which the goal of treatment is to achieve a state in which the affected craniosacral structures are equalized in all appropriate planes. *See also* balanced membranous tension (BMT). *See also* osteopathic cranial manipulative medicine (OCMM).

Chapman reflex treatment A treatment method in which either classic rotatory motion or other methods used to address soft tissue dysfunction are applied to Chapman reflex points. *See* Chapman reflex.

combined treatment method

1. A treatment strategy where the initial movements are indirect; as the technique is completed, the movements change to direct forces.
2. A manipulative sequence involving two or more different osteopathic manipulative treatment method (e.g., Spencer technique combined with muscle energy technique).
3. A concept described by Paul Kimberly, DO.

combined treatment Historic term. *See* osteopathic manipulative treatment, combined treatment method.

compression of the fourth ventricle (CV-4) A cranial technique in which the lateral angles of the occipital squama are manually approximated slightly exaggerating the posterior convexity of the occiput and taking the cranium into sustained extension. *See also* osteopathic cranial manipulative medicine (OCMM).

counterstrain (CS)

1. An osteopathic method of diagnosis and indirect treatment in which the patient's somatic dysfunction, diagnosed by an associated myofascial tender point, is treated by using a position of spontaneous tissue release while simultaneously monitoring the tender point.
2. Developed by Lawrence Jones, DO, FAAO, in 1955 (originally termed "spontaneous release by positioning," then "strain–counterstrain," and "counterstrain").

cranial treatment (CR) *See* osteopathic cranial manipulative medicine (OCMM). *See also* primary respiratory mechanism.

CV-4 *See* compression of the fourth ventricle. *See also* osteopathic cranial manipulative medicine (OCMM).

Dalrymple technique *See also* osteopathic manipulative treatment, pedal pump.

direct method (technique) An osteopathic treatment in which the restrictive barrier is engaged and a final activating force is applied to correct somatic dysfunction.

exaggeration An osteopathic treatment method in which the body part is moved slightly farther toward the direction of dysfunction so that the body's inherent forces can correct the somatic dysfunction.

exaggeration technique An indirect procedure that involves carrying the dysfunctional part away from the restrictive barrier, then applying a high-velocity low-amplitude force in the same direction.

facilitated oscillatory release (FOR)

1. A treatment method intended to normalize neuromuscular function by applying a manual oscillatory force, which may be combined with any other ligamentous or myofascial technique.
2. A refinement of a long-standing use of oscillatory force in osteopathic diagnosis and treatment as published in early osteopathic literature.
3. A technique developed by Zachary Comeaux, DO, as an extension of his work with Robert Fulford, DO.

facilitated positional release (FPR)
1. An osteopathic treatment method in which a dysfunctional body region or structure is addressed with a combination of neutral positioning, application of an activating force (e.g., compression, distraction, or torsion), and placement into position of ease.
2. A technique developed by Stanley Schiowitz, DO, FAAO.

fascial distortion model (FDM)
1. A method of diagnosis and treatment of one or more of six specific types of somatic dysfunction referred to as fascial distortions. Each of the six types of fascial distortions has a unique set of symptoms and findings, along with a specific method of treatment.
2. Originally developed by Stephen Typaldos, DO.

fascial release treatment *See* osteopathic manipulative treatment, myofascial release.

fascial or myofascial unwinding An osteopathic treatment method in which the dysfunctional fascial tissues are engaged in a dynamic continuous process in response to palpatory feedback of ease and/or bind.

functional method An indirect treatment utilizing passive regional motion input in multiple directions to encourage optimal ease of the somatic dysfunction. The osteopathic physician guides the manipulative procedure while the dysfunctional area is being monitored in order to obtain a continuous feedback of the neurophysiologic response to increased ease of motion.

Galbreath technique *See* osteopathic manipulative treatment, mandibular drainage.

hepatic pump technique Rhythmic compression applied over the liver for purposes of increasing blood flow through the liver and enhancing bile and lymphatic drainage from the liver.

high velocity low amplitude (HVLA) *Also called* thrust treatment method. An osteopathic method in which the restrictive barrier is engaged in one or more planes of motion and then a rapid, therapeutic force of brief duration traveling a short distance is applied within the anatomic range of motion.

Hoover technique
1. A form of functional method.
2. Developed by H.V. Hoover, DO. *See also* osteopathic manipulative treatment, functional method.

indirect method (I/IND) A manipulative treatment in which the restrictive barrier is disengaged and the dysfunctional body part is moved away from the restrictive barrier.

inhibitory pressure A treatment method in which steady pressure is applied to soft tissues to reduce reflex activity and promote tissue relaxation.

integrated neuromusculoskeletal release (INR) A treatment method in which indirect, direct, and/or release-enhancing maneuvers are applied to reflexively influence the biomechanics of the musculoskeletal system and respective peripheral and central neural control mechanisms.

Jones technique *See* osteopathic manipulative treatment, counterstrain.

ligamentous articular strain (LAS)
1. An osteopathic treatment method that involves disengagement, exaggeration, and taking the dysfunctional opposing ligaments to a point of balance. Ligamentous articular strain (LAS) is similar to balanced ligamentous tension (BLT).
2. Any somatic dysfunction resulting in abnormal ligamentous tension or strain. See also osteopathic manipulative treatment, ligamentous articular strain technique. See balanced ligamentous tension.
3. Evolved by Rollin Becker based on his interpretation of his work with Dr. WG Sutherland and his interpretation of the article "Osteopathic Technique of William G. Sutherland," published in the *1949 Year Book of Academy of Applied Osteopathy*.

liver pump *See* osteopathic manipulative treatment, hepatic pump technique.

lymphatic technique A diverse group of osteopathic treatment methods and techniques designed to promote and augment the flow of interstitial fluid and lymph and/or decrease impediments to lymphatic circulation.

lymphatic pumps A group of osteopathic techniques employing rhythmic motion to promote a change in pressure gradients and to influence lymphatic flow.

mandibular drainage technique
1. Soft tissue manipulative technique using passively induced jaw motion to improve drainage of middle ear structures via the eustachian tube and lymphatics.
2. A technique first described by William Otis Galbreath, DO.

mesenteric release technique (mesenteric lift) A technique in which the double layer of peritoneum that invests the intestines and its associated vascular, neural, and lymphatic structures is relieved of tension from the attachments to the posterior wall of the abdomen, which include the root of the mesentery, hepatic and splenic flexures, and ascending and descending colon.

muscle energy technique (MET)
1. A direct osteopathic treatment method in which a patient, on request, actively uses their muscles from a controlled position and in a specific direction against a distinct counterforce. The basic concepts of MET involve using isometric, isotonic, and isolytic muscular contractions to achieve a variety of effects on the targeted structures.
2. First described in 1948 by Fred Mitchell, Sr, DO.

myofascial release (MFR)
1. An osteopathic treatment method that alleviates restriction of somatic dysfunction through its related fascia and musculature by utilizing continual palpatory feedback and engagement of the involved tissues. Activating forces may be used to facilitate the treatment process for both direct and indirect myofascial release. *See also* direct myofascial release; indirect myofascial release.
2. Technique first described by Andrew Taylor Still, DO, and his early students.

direct myofascial release The myofascial tissues are engaged with a dynamic force into the direction of the restrictive barrier(s) until motion is improved.

indirect myofascial release The myofascial tissues are engaged with a dynamic force into the direction(s) of ease until motion is improved.

myofascial technique Any technique directed at the muscles and fascia. *See also* osteopathic manipulative treatment, myofascial release. *See also* osteopathic manipulative treatment, soft tissue method.

osteopathy in the cranial field (OCF) Historic term.
1. Refers to the system of diagnosis and treatment first described by William G. Sutherland, DO.
2. Title of reference work by Harold Magoun, Sr, DO. *See* Osteopathic Cranial Manipulative Medicine.

osteopathic cranial manipulative medicine (OCMM) (Cranial Osteopathy) A system of diagnosis and treatment that utilizes the primary respiratory mechanism with a focus on the skull, sacrum, membranes, fluids and their related structures. *See also* primary respiratory mechanism. See also balanced membranous tension. *See also* osteopathy in the cranial field (OCF).

passive method Any technique in which the patient is instructed to refrain from voluntary muscle contraction.

pedal pump *Also called* the pedal fascial pump; Dalrymple treatment. A venous and lymphatic drainage technique applied through the lower extremities.

percussion vibrator method

1. A treatment method involving the specific application of mechanical vibratory force to treat somatic dysfunction.
2. An osteopathic manipulative technique developed by Robert Fulford, DO.

progressive inhibition of neuromuscular structures (PINS)

1. A method of diagnosis and treatment in which the osteopathic physician localizes sensitive points and sequentially applies inhibitory pressure along a predictable pathway to this series of related points.
2. Developed by Dennis Dowling, DO, MA, FAAO.

soft tissue method (ST) A group of direct techniques that usually involve lateral stretching, linear stretching, deep pressure, traction and/or separation of muscle origin, and insertion while monitoring tissue response and motion changes by palpation. Historically considered a form of myofascial treatment.

Spencer technique A series of direct manipulative procedures to prevent or decrease soft tissue and articular motion restrictions about the shoulder. *See also* osteopathic manipulative treatment, articulatory treatment (ART).

splenic pump technique Rhythmic compression applied over the spleen for the purpose of enhancing the patient's immune response. *See also* osteopathic manipulative treatment, lymphatic pump.

spontaneous release by positioning *See* osteopathic manipulative treatment, counterstrain.

springing A low-velocity/moderate-to-high amplitude activating force using pressure and motion applied repeatedly against the restrictive barrier of a dysfunctional structure. *See also* osteopathic manipulative treatment, articulatory.

strain–counterstain *See* osteopathic manipulative treatment, counterstrain.

Still technique

1. A combined manipulative method utilizing both indirect and direct components. The dysfunctional region is first placed in an indirect position, a force vector (compression, traction, torsion) is added and then used to carry the region directly past neutral toward or through its restrictive barrier.
2. Attributed to Andrew Taylor Still, DO.
3. Title of reference work by Richard Van Buskirk, DO, PhD, FAAO.

thoracic pump technique

1. A technique that consists of intermittent compression of the thoracic cage.
2. Developed by C. Earl Miller, DO.

thrust technique *See* osteopathic manipulative treatment, high-velocity low-amplitude technique (HVLA).

traction technique A procedure in which the parts are stretched or separated along a longitudinal axis with continuous or intermittent force.

v-spread Technique using forces transmitted across the diameter of the cranium to improve sutural motion.

ventral technique *See* osteopathic manipulative treatment, visceral manipulation.

visceral approach/manipulation (VIS) An osteopathic method of diagnosis and treatment applied to the viscera and/or the supportive structures to improve physiologic function. Historically called ventral techniques

osteopathic manipulative treatment method A group of techniques that apply to a set of distinct unifying principles that guide individualized treatment.

osteopathic manipulative treatment technique A specific therapeutic manual procedure, e.g., Dalrymple pedal pump, Galbreath mandibular drainage, pectoral traction, CV-4.

osteopathic medicine The preferred term for a complete system of medical care practiced by physicians with an unlimited license that is represented by a philosophy that combines the needs of the patient with the current practice of medicine, surgery, and obstetrics. Emphasizes the interrelationship between structure and function and has an appreciation of the body's ability to heal itself.

osteopathic musculoskeletal evaluation The osteopathic musculoskeletal evaluation provides information regarding the health of the patient. Utilizing the concepts of body unity, self-regulation, and structure–function interrelationships, the osteopathic physician uses data from the musculoskeletal evaluation to assess the patient's status and develop a treatment plan. (*AOA House of Delegates.*)

Osteopathic Neuromusculoskeletal Medicine (ONMM) The osteopathic neuromusculoskeletal medicine residency program is a primary residency disciplined in the neuromusculoskeletal system, its comprehensive relationship to other organ systems, and its dynamic function of locomotion. The principle focus of the discipline is osteopathic and patient centered; specifically, it embodies structural and functional interrelation, body unity, self-healing, and self-maintenance. *See also* Certification in Neuromusculoskeletal Medicine and Osteopathic Manipulative Medicine (C-NMM/OMM). *See also* Neuromusculoskeletal Medicine (NMM).

osteopathic philosophy A concept of health care supported by expanding scientific knowledge that embraces the concept of the unity of the living organism's structure (anatomy) and function (physiology). Emphasizes the following principles:

1. The body is a unit; the person is a unit of body, mind, and spirit.
2. The body is capable of self-regulation, self-healing, and health maintenance.
3. Structure and function are reciprocally interrelated.
4. Rational treatment is based upon an understanding of the basic principles of body unity, self-regulation, and the interrelationship of structure and function.

osteopathic physician A person with full unlimited medical practice rights who has achieved the nationally recognized academic and professional standards within their country to practice diagnosis and treatment based upon the principles of osteopathic philosophy. Individual countries establish the national academic and professional standards for osteopathic physicians practicing within their countries.

osteopathic postural examination The part of the osteopathic structural examination that focuses on the static and dynamic responses of the body to gravity while in the erect position.

osteopathic practitioner Refers to an osteopath, an osteopathic physician, or an allopathic physician who has been trained in osteopathic principles, practices, and philosophy.

osteopathic principles *See* osteopathic philosophy.

osteopathic principles and practice (OPP) The application of the philosophy of osteopathy in healthcare, framed in the models of osteopathic care, which may include osteopathic manipulative treatment (OMT).

osteopathic structural examination The examination of a patient by an osteopathic physician with emphasis on the neuromusculoskeletal system as it reflects and interacts with other body systems in the context of total patient care. This is accomplished primarily via inspection, motion testing, and palpation with the goal of determining the cause of the patient's complaint and any somatic dysfunction that may be associated with it. Using the concepts of body unity, self-regulation, and structure–function interrelationships, the findings of the structural examination guide the osteopathic physician to the appropriate choice of treatment.

osteopathic tenets Express the underlying philosophy of osteopathic medicine:

1. The body is a unit; the person is a unit of body, mind, and spirit.
2. The body is capable of self-regulation, self-healing, and health maintenance.
3. Structure and function are reciprocally interrelated.
4. Rational treatment is based upon an understanding of the basic principles of body unity, self-regulation, and the interrelationship of structure and function. *(approved by the AOA House of Delegates)*

osteopathy Historic term. No longer a preferred term in the United States. *See* osteopathic medicine.

P

palpation The application of the fingers to the surface of the skin or other tissues, using varying amounts of pressure, to selectively determine the condition of the parts beneath.

palpatory diagnosis A term used by osteopathic practitioners to denote the process of palpating the patient to evaluate the structure and function of the neuromusculoskeletal and visceral systems.

palpatory skills Sensory skills used in performing palpatory diagnosis and osteopathic manipulative treatment.

passive method *See* osteopathic manipulative treatment, passive method.

passive motion *See* motion, passive motion.

patient cooperation Voluntary movement by the patient (on instruction from the osteopathic physician) to assist in the palpatory diagnosis and treatment process.

pedal pump *See* osteopathic manipulative treatment, pedal pump.

pelvic bone *See* innominate.

pelvic declination (pelvic unleveling) Pelvic rotation about an anteroposterior (A-P) axis.

pelvic girdle dysfunction *See* somatic dysfunction, pelvic.

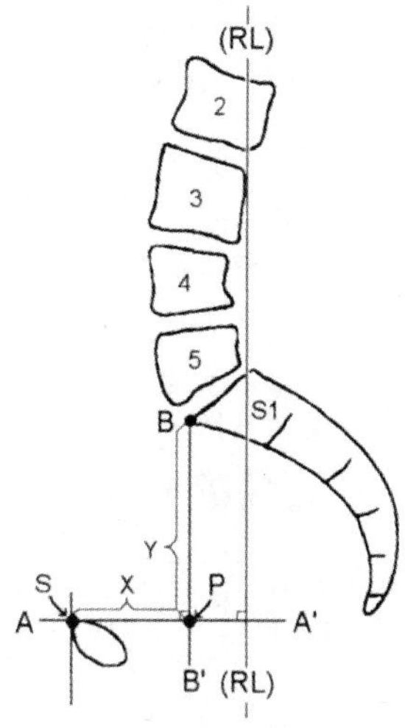

Figure 24. Pelvic index (PI). (Modified from Kuchera WA, Kuchera ML. *Osteopathic Principles in Practice.* 2nd ed. Greyden Press; 1994: 263. Reprinted with permission from Michael L. Kuchera, DO, FAAO.)

pelvic index (PI) Represents a ratio of the measurements determined from postural radiograph. One (y) beginning from a vertical line originating at the sacral promontory to the intersection with the horizontal line from the anterosuperior position of the pubic bone. The second measurement (x) is along this same horizontal line. Normal values are age related and increase in subjects with sagittal plane postural decompensation. Pelvic index (PI) equals x/y (Fig. 24).

pelvic rotation Movement of the entire pelvis in a relatively horizontal plane about a vertical (longitudinal) axis.

pelvic sideshift Deviation of the pelvis to the right or left of the central vertical axis as translation occurs along the horizontal (z) axis. Usually observed in the standing position.

pelvic somatic dysfunctions A group of somatic dysfunctions involving the sacrum and innominate. *See* somatic dysfunction. *See* somatic dysfunction, innominate.

pelvic tilt Pelvic rotation about a transverse (horizontal) axis (forward or backward tilt) or about an anteroposterior axis (right or left side tilt).

pelvis Within the context of structural diagnosis, the pelvis is made up of the right and left innominates (hip bones or os coxae), the sacrum, and the coccyx.

percussion vibrator technique *See* osteopathic manipulative treatment, percussion vibrator technique.

pétrissage Deep kneading or squeezing action to express swelling.

physiologic barrier *See* barrier, physiologic barrier.

physiologic motion *See* motion, physiologic motion.

physiologic motion of the spine The three major principles of physiologic motion are as follows:

I. When the thoracic and lumbar spine are in a neutral position (easy normal), the coupled motions of side bending and rotation for a group of vertebrae are such that side bending and rotation occur in opposite directions (with rotation occurring toward the convexity) (Fig. 25). *See* somatic dysfunction, type I somatic dysfunction.

II. When the thoracic and lumbar spine are sufficiently forward or backward bent (nonneutral), the coupled motions of side bending and rotation in a single vertebral unit occur in the

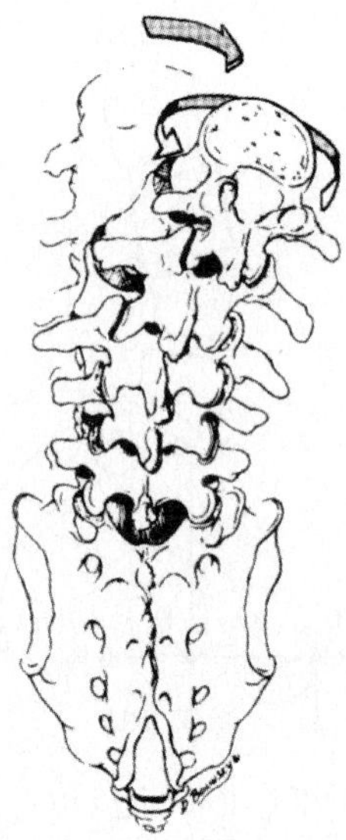

Figure 25. Physiologic motion of the thoracic or lumbar spine resulting from a neutral spinal position (Type I motion).

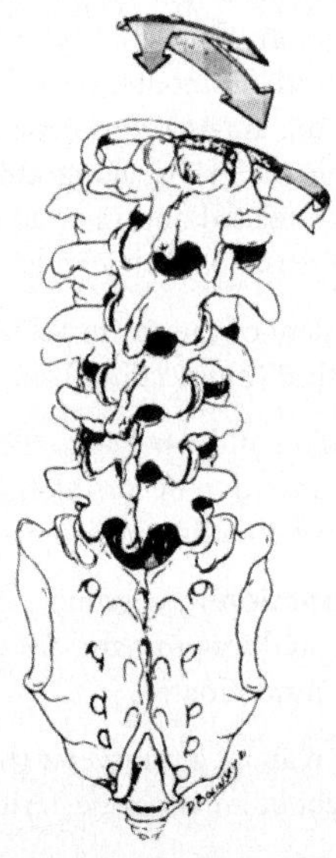

Figure 26. Physiologic motion of the thoracic or lumbar spine resulting from a nonneutral spinal position (type II motion).

same direction (Fig. 26). *See* somatic dysfunction, type II, somatic dysfunction.

III. Initiating motion of a vertebral segment in any plane of motion will modify the movement of that segment in other planes of motion.

Principles I and II of thoracic and lumbar spinal motion were described by Harrison H. Fryette, DO (1918); Principle III was described by C.R. Nelson, DO (1948). *See* rotation. *See also* rotation of vertebra.

PINS *See* progressive inhibition of neuromuscular structures (PINS).

plane A flat surface determined by the position of three points in space. Any of a number of imaginary surfaces passing through the body and dividing it into segments (Fig. 27).

AP plane *See* plane, sagittal plane.

coronal plane (frontal plane) A plane passing longitudinally through the body from one side to the other, and dividing the body into anterior and posterior portions.

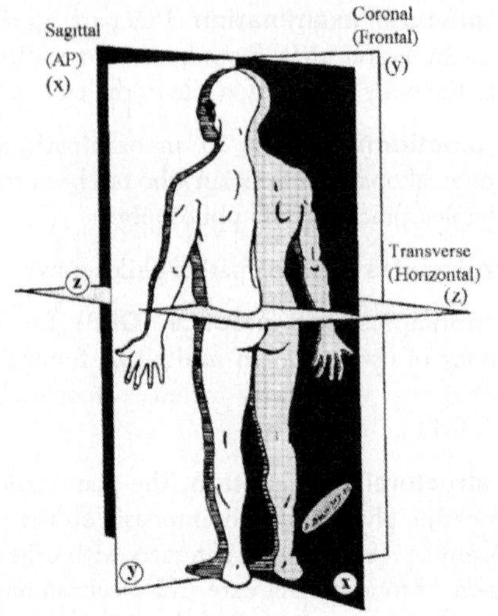

Figure 27. Planes of the body.

frontal plane *See* plane, coronal plane.

horizontal plane *See* plane, transverse plane.

sagittal plane A plane passing longitudinally through the body from front to back and dividing it into right and left portions. The median or midsagittal plane divides the body into approximately equal right and left portions.

transverse plane (horizontal plane) A plane passing horizontally through the body perpendicular to the sagittal and frontal planes, dividing the body into upper and lower portions.

plastic deformation A nonrecoverable deformation. *See also* elastic deformation.

plasticity Ability to retain a shape attained by deformation. *See also* elasticity. *See also* viscosity.

posterior component A positional descriptor used to identify the side of reference when rotation of a vertebral segment has occurred. In a condition of right rotation, the right side is the posterior component. It usually refers to a prominent vertebral transverse process. *See also* anterior component.

posterior nutation *See* counternutation.

postisometric relaxation Immediately following an isometric contraction, the neuromuscular apparatus is in a refractory state during which enhanced passive stretching may be performed. The osteopathic physician may take up the myofascial slack during the relaxed refractory period.

postural axis *See* sacral motion axis, postural axis.

postural balance A condition of optimal distribution of body mass in relation to gravity.

postural decompensation Distribution of body mass away from ideal when postural homeostatic mechanisms are overwhelmed. It occurs in all cardinal planes but is classified by the major plane(s) affected. *See* plane (Fig. 27).

coronal plane postural decompensation Causes scoliotic changes.

horizontal plane postural decompensation May cause postural changes where part or all of the body rotates to the right or left. When viewed from the right or left sides, alignment appears asymmetrical.

sagittal plane postural decompensation Causes kyphotic and/or lordotic changes.

postural imbalance A condition in which ideal body mass distribution is not achieved.

primary machinery of life

1. The neuromusculoskeletal system. A term used to denote that body parts act together to transmit and modify force and motion through which the person acts out their life. This integration is achieved via the central nervous system acting in response to continued sensory input from the internal and external environment.
2. A term coined by I.M. Korr, PhD.

primary respiratory mechanism

(1) A conceptual model that describes a process involving five interactive, involuntary functions.

1. The inherent motility of the brain and spinal cord.
2. Fluctuation of the cerebrospinal fluid.
3. Mobility of the intracranial and intraspinal membranes.
4. Articular mobility of the cranial bones.
5. Mobility of the sacrum between the ilia (pelvic bones) that is interdependent with the motion at the sphenobasilar synchondrosis.

The mechanism refers to the presumed inherent (primordial) driving mechanism of internal respiration as opposed to the cycle of diaphragmatic respiration (inhalation and exhalation). It further refers to the innate interconnected movement of every tissue and structure of the body. Optimal health promotes optimal function, and the inherent function of this interdependent movement can be negatively altered by trauma, disease states, or other pathology.

(2) This mechanism was first described by William G. Sutherland, DO, in 1939 in "The Cranial Bowl," published by the Western Osteopath journal. The mechanism is thought to affect cellular respiration and other body processes. In the original definition, the following descriptions were given:

primary Because it is directly concerned with the internal tissue respiration of the central nervous system.

respiratory Because it further concerns the physiologic function of the interchange of fluids necessary for normal metabolism and biochemistry, not only of the central nervous system but also of all body cells.

mechanism Because all the constituent parts work together as a unit carrying out this fundamental physiology. *See also* osteopathic manipulative treatment; osteopathic cranial manipulative medicine (OCMM).

prime mover A muscle primarily responsible for causing a specific joint action.

progressive inhibition of neuromuscular structures (PINS) *See* osteopathic manipulative treatment, progressive inhibition of neuromuscular structures.

prolotherapy *See* sclerotherapy.

pronation In relation to the anatomical position, as applied to the hand, rotation of the forearm in such a way that the palmar surface turns backward (internal rotation) in relationship to the anatomical position. Applied to the foot: a combination of eversion and abduction movements taking place in the tarsal and metatarsal joints, resulting in lowering of the medial margin of the foot. *See also* supination.

prone Lying face downward (*Stedman's*).

psoas syndrome A painful low back condition characterized by hypertonicity of psoas musculature. The syndrome consists of a constellation of typically related signs and symptoms.

typical associated somatic dysfunctions As a long restrictor muscle, psoas hypertonicity is frequently associated with flexed dysfunctions of the upper lumbar vertebrae, extended dysfunction of L5, and variable sacral and innominate dysfunctions. Tender points typically are found in the ipsilateral iliacus and contralateral piriformis muscles.

typical gait Trendelenburg gait.

typical pain pattern Low back pain frequently accompanied by pain on the lateral aspect of the lower extremity extending no lower than the knee.

typical posture Flexion at the hip and side bending of the lumbar spine to the side of the most hypertonic psoas muscle.

pubic bone, somatic dysfunctions of

anterior pubic shear A somatic dysfunction in which one pubic bone is displaced anteriorly as compared to the normal contralateral pubic bone.

inferior pubic shear A somatic dysfunction in which one pubic bone is displaced inferiorly as compared to the normal contralateral pubic bone (Fig. 28).

posterior pubic shear A somatic dysfunction in which one pubic bone is displaced posteriorly as compared to the normal contralateral pubic bone.

superior pubic shear A somatic dysfunction in which one pubic bone is displaced superiorly as compared to the normal contralateral pubic bone (Fig. 29).

pubic abduction *See* pubic gapping.

pubic adduction *See* pubic compression.

pubic compression *Also called* pubic adduction. A somatic dysfunction in which the pubic bones are forced toward each other at the pubic symphysis. This dysfunction is characterized by tenderness to palpation over the pubic symphysis, lack of apparent asymmetry, but associated with restricted motion of the pelvic ring (Fig. 30).

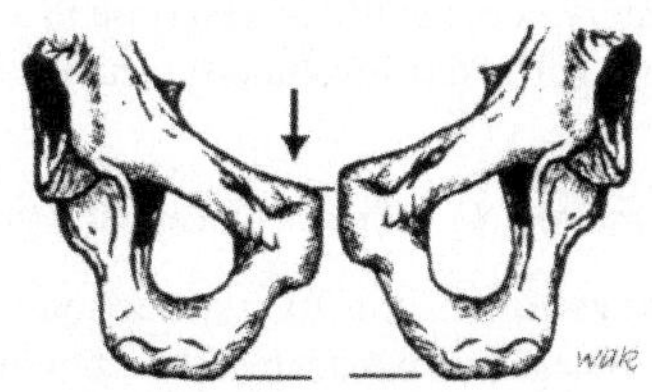

Standing flexion test = R(+)

Figure 28. Right inferior pubic shear.

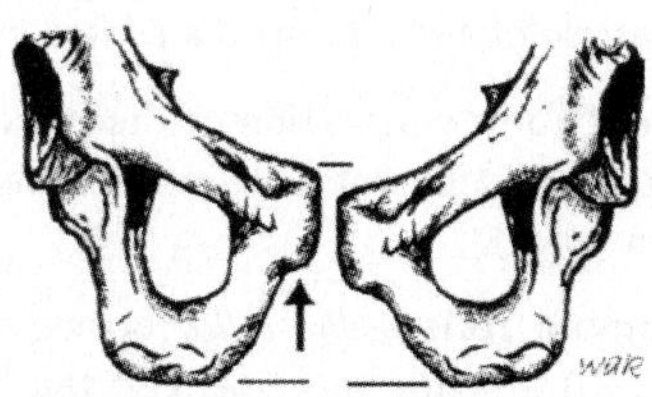

Standing flexion test = R(+)

Figure 29. Right superior pubic shear.

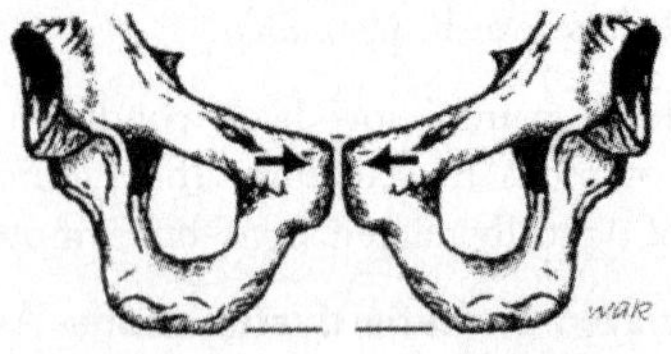

Standing flexion test = Bilaterally(+)
(False negative)

Figure 30. Pubic compression.

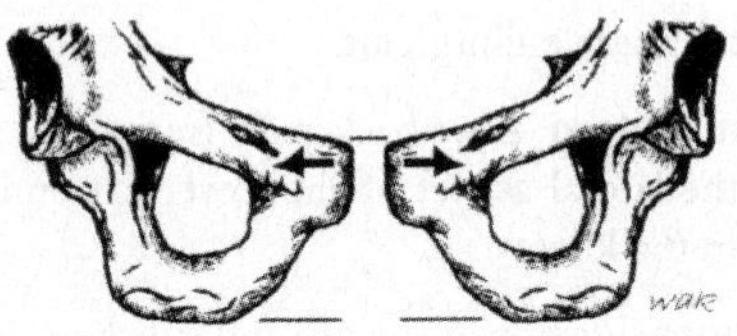

Standing flexion test = Bilaterally(+)
(False negative)

Figure 31. Pubic gapping (pubic abduction).

pubic gapping *Also called* pubic abduction. A somatic dysfunction in which the pubic bones are pulled away from each other at the pubic symphysis. This dysfunction is frequently seen in women following childbirth (Fig. 31).

pubic symphysis, somatic dysfunctions of *See* pubic bone, somatic dysfunctions of.

pump handle rib motion *See* rib motion, pump handle motion.

Q

No q terms.

R

reciprocal inhibition The inhibition of antagonist muscles when the agonist is stimulated. *See also* law, Sherrington.

reciprocal tension membrane The intracranial and spinal dural membrane including the falx cerebri, falx cerebelli, tentorium cerebelli, and spinal dura.

red reflex *See* reflex, red.

reflex An involuntary nervous system response to a sensory input. The sum total of any particular involuntary activity. *See also* Chapman reflexes.

cephalogyric reflex *See* reflex, oculocephalogyric.

cervicolumbar reflex Automatic contraction of the lumbar paravertebral muscles in response to contraction of postural muscles in the neck.

conditioned reflex One that does not occur naturally in the organism or system, but that is developed by regular association of some physiologic function with a related outside event.

myotatic reflex Tonic contraction of the muscles in response to a stretching force due to stimulation of muscle receptors (e.g., deep tendon reflex).

oculocephalogyric reflex *Also called* oculogyric reflex; cephalogyric reflex. Automatic movement of the head that leads or accompanies movement of the eyes.

oculogyric reflex *See* oculocephalogyric reflex.

red reflex

1. The erythematous biochemical reaction (reactive hyperemia) of the skin in an area that has been stimulated mechanically by friction. The reflex is greater in degree and duration in an area of acute somatic dysfunction as compared to an area of chronic somatic dysfunction. It is a reflection of the segmentally related sympathicotonia commonly observed in the paraspinal area.
2. A red glow reflected from the fundus of the eye when a light is cast upon the retina.

somatosomatic reflex Localized somatic stimuli producing patterns of reflex response in segmentally related somatic structures.

somatovisceral reflex Localized somatic stimuli producing patterns of reflex response in segmentally related visceral structures.

viscerosomatic reflex Localized visceral stimuli producing patterns of reflex response in segmentally related somatic structures.

viscerovisceral reflex viscerovisceral reflex: Localized visceral stimuli producing patterns of reflex response in related visceral structures. (Also referred to as cross-organ reflex)

regenerative injection therapy (RIT) *See* sclerotherapy.

region

1. An anatomical division of the body defined by natural, functional, or arbitrary boundaries.
2. Body areas for the diagnosis and coding of somatic dysfunction as defined in the International Classification of Diseases (At time of print, ICD-10 CM) using the codes. *See also* transitional region.

M99.00 Segmental and somatic dysfunction of head region
M99.01 Segmental and somatic dysfunction of cervical region
M99.02 Segmental and somatic dysfunction of thoracic region
M99.03 Segmental and somatic dysfunction of lumbar region
M99.04 Segmental and somatic dysfunction of sacral region
M99.05 Segmental and somatic dysfunction of pelvic region
M99.06 Segmental and somatic dysfunction of lower extremity
M99.07 Segmental and somatic dysfunction of upper extremity
M99.08 Segmental and somatic dysfunction of rib cage
M99.09 Segmental and somatic dysfunction of abdomen and other regions

regional extension *See* extension, regional extension.

regional motor inputs Motion initiated by an osteopathic physician through body contact and vector input that produces a specific response at each segment in the mobile system.

release The palpable change toward normalization of abnormal tissue texture, joint motion, or inherent motion perceived during or following an osteopathic manipulative treatment.

resilience Property of returning to the former shape or size after mechanical distortion. *See also* elasticity. *See also* plasticity.

respiratory axis of the sacrum *See* sacral motion axis, superior transverse axis.

respiratory cooperation An osteopathic physician–directed inhalation and/or exhalation by the patient to assist the manipulative treatment process.

restriction A resistance or impediment to movement.

joint restriction This term is part of the TART acronym for an osteopathic somatic dysfunction. *See* barrier (motion barrier). *See also* TART.

retrolisthesis Posterior displacement of one vertebra relative to the one immediately below.

rib lesion Historic term. *See* rib, somatic dysfunction of.

rib motion

axis of rib motion A hypothetical functional line through the costotransverse and the costovertebral articulations of the rib.

anteroposterior rib axis *See also* rib motion, bucket-handle motion (Fig. 32).

bucket-handle motion Movement of the ribs during respiration such that with inhalation, the lateral aspect of the rib moves cephalad resulting in an increase of transverse diameter of the thorax. This type of rib motion is predominantly found in lower ribs, increasing in motion from the upper to the lower ribs (Fig. 33). *See also* rib motion, axis of. *See also* rib motion, pump handle.

caliper rib motion Motion of ribs 11 and 12 characterized by single joint motion; analogous to internal and external rotation.

exhalation rib restriction Involves a rib or group of ribs that first stops moving during exhalation. The key rib is generally found at the inferior aspect or bottom of the group. *See also* rib somatic dysfunction, inhalation rib dysfunction.

inhalation rib restriction Involves a rib or group of ribs that first stops moving during inhalation. The key rib is generally found at the superior aspect or the top of the group. *See also* rib somatic dysfunction, exhalation rib dysfunction.

pump handle motion Movement of the ribs during respiration such that with inhalation the anterior aspect of the rib moves cephalad and causes an increase in the anteroposterior diameter of the thorax. This type of rib motion is found predominantly in the upper ribs, decreasing in motion from the upper to the lower ribs (Fig. 34). *See* rib motion, axis of. *See also* rib motion, bucket-handle motion.

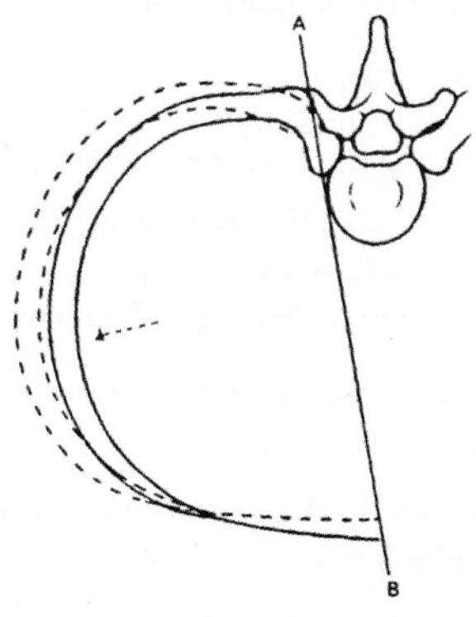

Figure 32. The functional anterior–posterior rib axis for bucket handle rib motion.

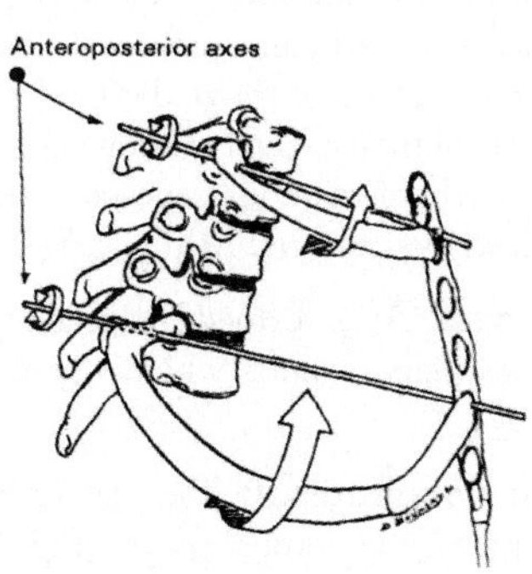

Figure 33. Bucket handle rib motion.

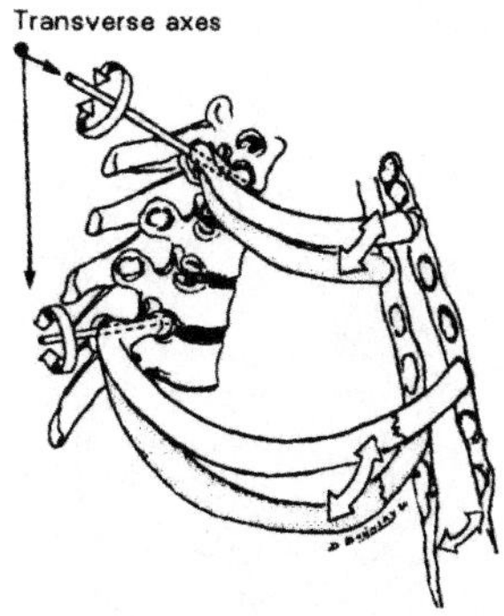

Figure 34. Pump handle rib motion.

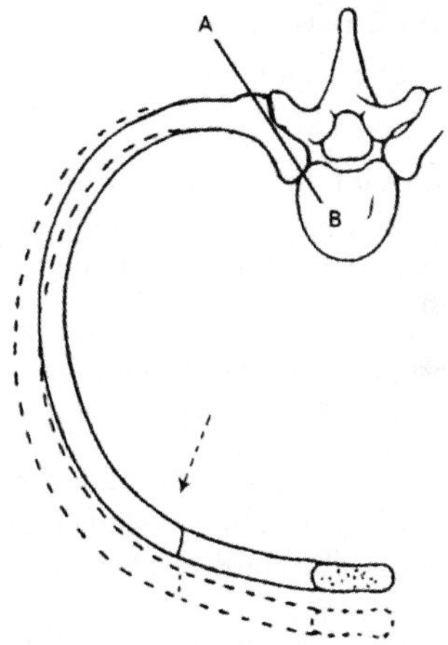

Figure 35. The functional transverse rib axis for pump handle rib motion.

transverse rib axis *See* rib motion, bucket handle rib motion inhalation. *See also* rib motion, inhalation rib restriction. *See also* rib motion, exhalation rib restriction (Fig. 35).

rib, somatic dysfunction of A somatic dysfunction in which movement or position of one or several ribs is altered or disrupted. For example, an elevated rib is one held in a position of inhalation such that motion toward inhalation is freer, and motion toward exhalation is restricted. A depressed rib is one held in a position of exhalation such that motion toward exhalation is freer and there is a restriction in inhalation. *See also* rib motion, inhalation rib restriction. *See also* rib motion, exhalation rib restriction.

exhaled rib dysfunction

1. Somatic dysfunction characterized by a rib being held in a position of exhalation such that motion toward exhalation is more free and motion toward inhalation is restricted. Synonyms: caught in exhalation, exhalation rib dysfunction, inhalation rib restriction, depressed rib.
2. An anterior rib tender point in counterstrain. *See also* rib motion, inhalation rib restriction.

inhaled rib dysfunction A somatic dysfunction characterized by a rib being held in a position of inhalation such that motion toward inhalation is more free and motion toward exhalation is restricted. Synonyms: caught in inhalation, inhalation rib dysfunction, exhalation rib restriction, elevated rib.

RIT *See* regenerative injection therapy (RIT). *See* sclerotherapy.

ropiness A tissue texture abnormality characterized by a cord-like feeling. *See also* tissue texture abnormality.

rotation Motion about an axis.

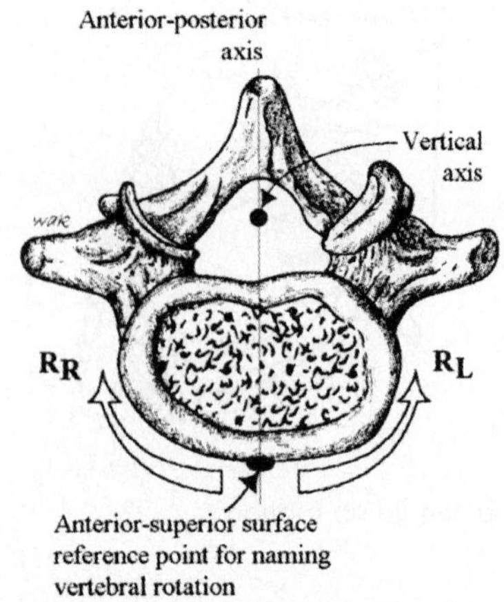

Figure 36. Rotation of a vertebra (lumbar).

rotation dysfunction of the sacrum Movement of the sacrum about a vertical (*y* axis) usually in relation to the innominate bones. *See* sacrum, somatic dysfunctions of, rotation of sacrum.

rotation of vertebra Movement about the anatomical vertical axis (*y* axis) of a vertebra; named by the motion of a midpoint on the anterosuperior surface of the vertebral body (Fig. 36).

rule of threes A method to locate the approximate position of the transverse process (TP) of a thoracic segment by using the location of the spinous process (SP) of that same vertebra. The relationship is as follows:
T1 to T3, TP is at the same level as tip of the SP.
T4 to T6, TP is one-half vertebral level above the tip of the SP.
T7 to T9, TP is one full vertebral level above the tip of the SP.
T10, TP is one full vertebral level above the tip of the SP.
T11, TP is one-half vertebral level above the tip of the SP.
T12, TP is at the same level as tip of the SP.

S

sacral base In osteopathic palpation, the uppermost posterior portion of the sacrum. The most superior or cephalad portion of the first sacral segment.

sacral base anterior *See* sacrum, somatic dysfunctions of, bilateral sacral flexion.

sacral base declination (unleveling) With the patient in a standing or seated position, any deviation of the sacral base from the horizontal in a coronal plane. Generally, the rotation of the sacrum about an anteroposterior (A-P) axis.

sacral base posterior *See* sacrum, somatic dysfunctions of, bilateral sacral extension.

sacral base unleveling *See* sacral base declination (unleveling).

sacralization *See* transitional vertebrae, sacralization.

sacral movement axis

anteroposterior (A-P) (*x*) axis Axis formed at the line of intersection of a sagittal and transverse plane.

inferior transverse axis (innominate)

1. The hypothetical functional axis of sacral motion that passes from side to side on a line through the inferior auricular surface of the sacrum and ilia and represents the axis for movement of the ilia on the sacrum.
2. A term described by Fred Mitchell, Sr, DO (Fig. 37).

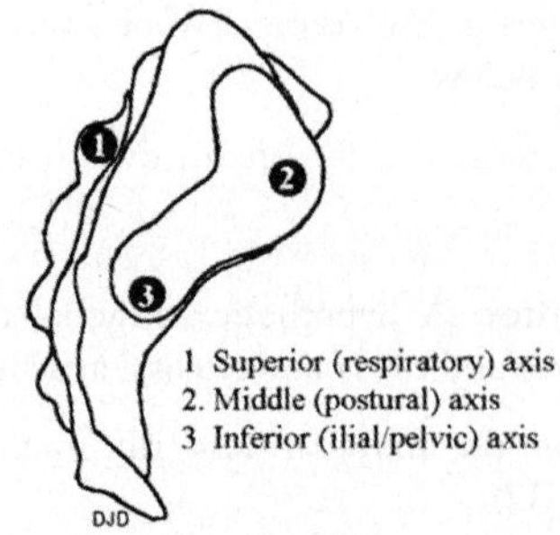

Figure 37. Sacral transverse axes (lateral view).

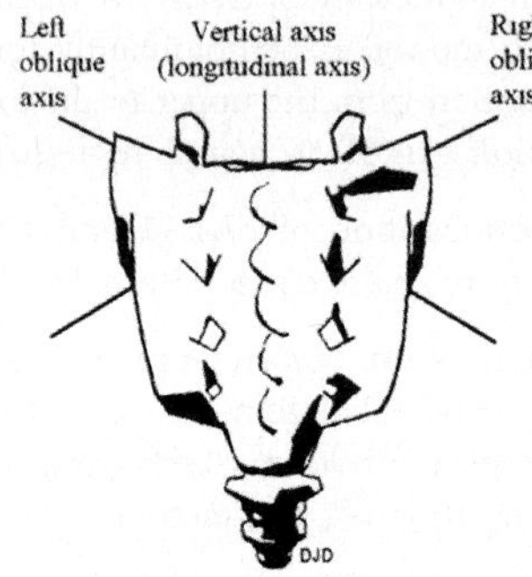

Figure 38. Axes of sacral motion (posterior view).

longitudinal axis The hypothetical axis formed at the line of intersection of the midsagittal plane and a coronal plane, *See* sacral motion axis, vertical (*y*) axis longitudinal (Fig. 38).

middle transverse axis (postural)

1. The hypothetical functional axis of sacral nutation/counternutation in the standing position, passing horizontally through the anterior aspect of the sacrum at the level of the second sacral segment.
2. A term described by Fred Mitchell, Sr, DO (Fig. 37).

oblique axis (diagonal)

1. A hypothetical functional axis from the superior area of a sacroiliac articulation to the contralateral inferior sacroiliac articulation. It is designated as right or left relevant to its superior point of origin.
2. A term described by Fred Mitchell, Sr, DO (Fig. 38).

postural axis *See* sacral movement axis, middle transverse axis (postural) (Fig. 37).

respiratory axis *See* sacral movement axis, superior transverse axis (respiratory) (Fig. 37).

superior transverse axis (respiratory)

1. The hypothetical transverse axis about which the sacrum moves during the respiratory cycle. It passes from side to side through the articular processes posterior to the point of attachment of the dura at the level of the second sacral segment. Involuntary sacral motion occurs as part of the craniosacral mechanism and is believed to occur about this axis.
2. A term described by Fred Mitchell, Sr, DO (Fig. 37).

transverse (*z*) axes Axes formed by intersection of the coronal and transverse planes about which nutation/counternutation occurs (Fig. 37).

vertical (*y*) axis (longitudinal) The axis formed by the intersection of the sagittal and coronal planes (Fig. 38).

sacral somatic dysfunction *See* sacrum, somatic dysfunctions of.

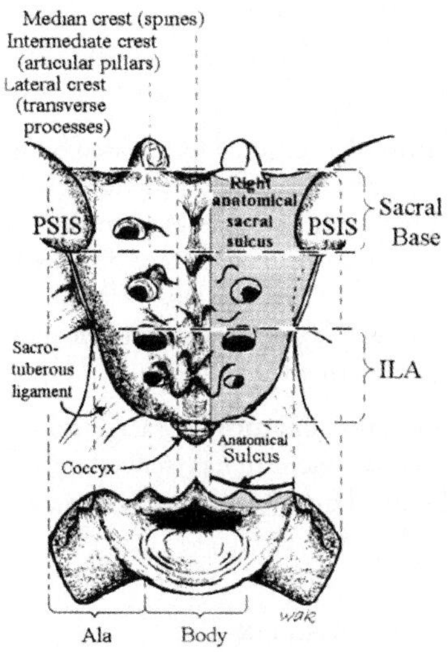

Figure 39. Anatomical sacral divisions.

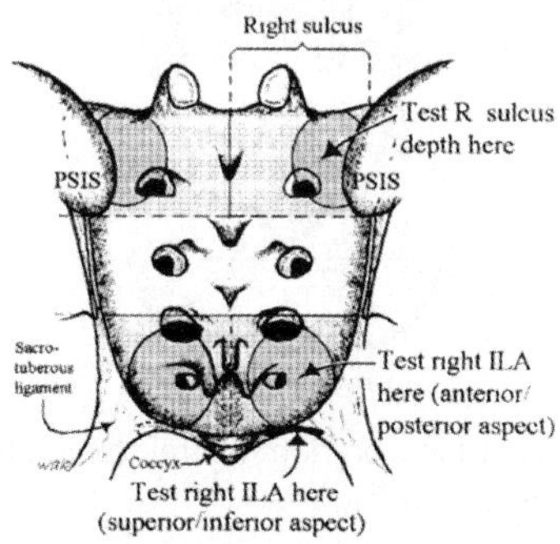

Figure 40. Clinical sacral divisions: sacral sulcus at the base, and inferior lateral angles (ILA).

sacral sulcus A depression just medial to the posterior superior iliac spine (PSIS) as a result of the spatial relationship of the PSIS to the dorsal aspect of the sacrum (Figs. 39 and 40).

sacral torsion

1. A physiologic function occurring in the sacrum during ambulation and forward bending.
2. A sacral somatic dysfunction referring to motion at the lumbosacral junction where the sacrum and L5 are rotating in opposite directions. Rotation of the sacrum is motion about an oblique or diagonal axis. Sacral torsions include a relationship between the sacrum and the ilium.
3. If the L5 does not rotate opposite to the sacrum, L5 is termed maladapted. Other terms for this maladaptation include rotations about an oblique axis, anterior or posterior sacrum, and a torsion with a noncompensated L5, a historic use. *See also* sacrum, somatic dysfunctions of.

sacroiliac motion Motion of the sacrum in relationship to the innominate(s) (ilium/ilia).

sacrum, inferior lateral angle (ILA) of The point on the lateral surface of the sacrum where it curves medially to the body of the fifth sacral vertebrae (Figs. 39 and 40).

sacrum, somatic dysfunctions of *See also* somatic dysfunction of sacrum.

anterior sacrum A positional term based on the Strachan model referring to sacral somatic dysfunction in which the sacral base has rotated anterior and side bent to the side opposite the rotation. The upper limb (pole) of the SI joint has restricted motion and is named for the side on which forward rotation had occurred. Tissue texture changes are found at the deep sulcus. The motion characteristics of L5 are not described (Fig. 41).

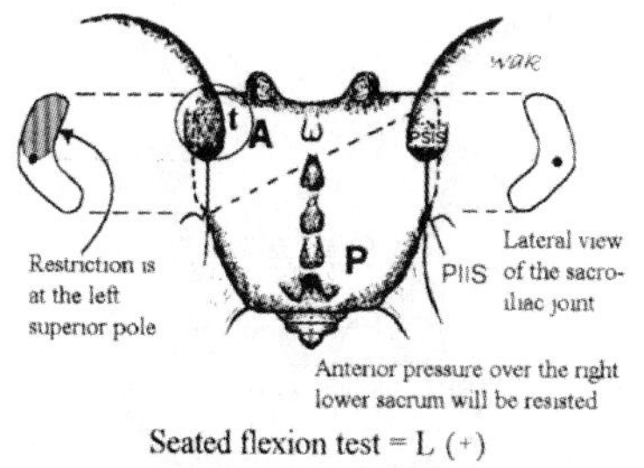

Figure 41. Anterior sacrum left. Motion of L5 is not described. There is tissue texture change (t) over the left sacral base. The superior pole of the left sacroiliac joint is affected and the left sacral base will not move posteriorly when an anterior test pressure is applied over the right lower sacrum.

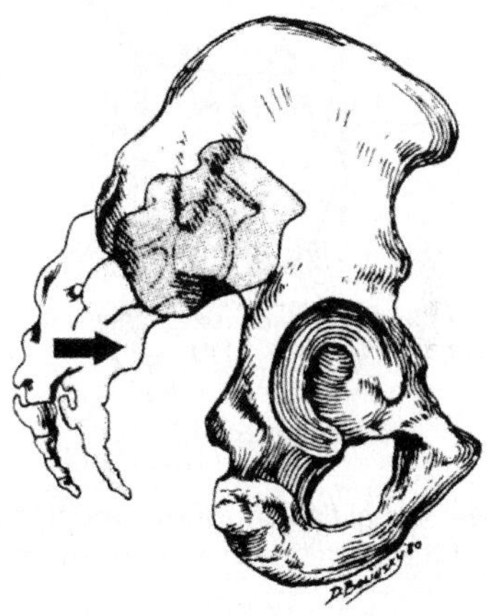

Figure 42. Anterior translated sacrum.

anterior translated sacrum A sacral somatic dysfunction in which the entire sacrum has moved anteriorly (forward) between the ilia. Anterior motion is freer, and the posterior motion is restricted (Fig. 42).

backward torsions *Also called* nonneutral sacral somatic dysfunctions, a historic use.

1. A backward sacral torsion is a physiologic rotation of the sacrum around an oblique axis such that the side of the sacral base contralateral to the named axis rotates posteriorly. L5 rotates in the direction opposite to the rotation of the sacral base.
2. A term by Fred Mitchell, Sr, DO, that describes the backward torsion as being nonphysiologic in terms of the walking cycle.

bilateral sacral extension (sacral base posterior)

1. A sacral somatic dysfunction that involves rotation of the sacrum about a middle transverse axis such that the sacral base has moved posteriorly relative to the pelvic bones. Posterior movement of the sacral base is freer, anterior movement is restricted, and both sides of the sacral sulcus are shallow.
2. The reverse of bilateral sacral flexion (Fig. 43).

bilateral sacral flexion (sacral base anterior)

1. A sacral somatic dysfunction that involves rotation of the sacrum about a middle transverse axis such that the sacral base has moved anteriorly between the pelvic bones. Anterior movement of the sacral base is freer, posterior movement is restricted, and both sides of the sacral sulcus are deep.
2. The reverse of bilateral sacral extension (Fig. 44).

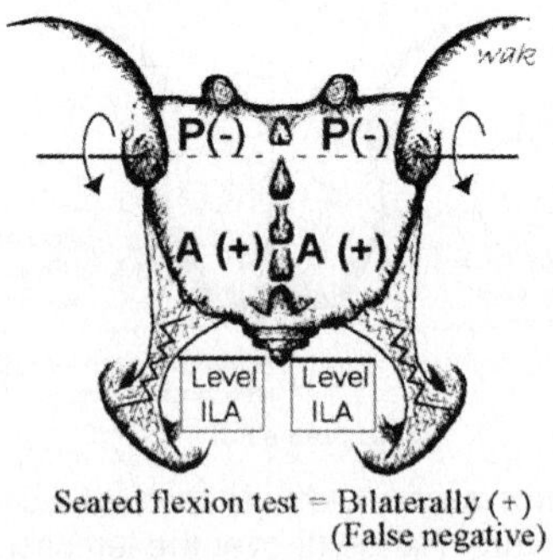

Figure 43. Bilateral sacral extension. The seated flexion test is considered equivocal and the sacral base is relatively posterior.

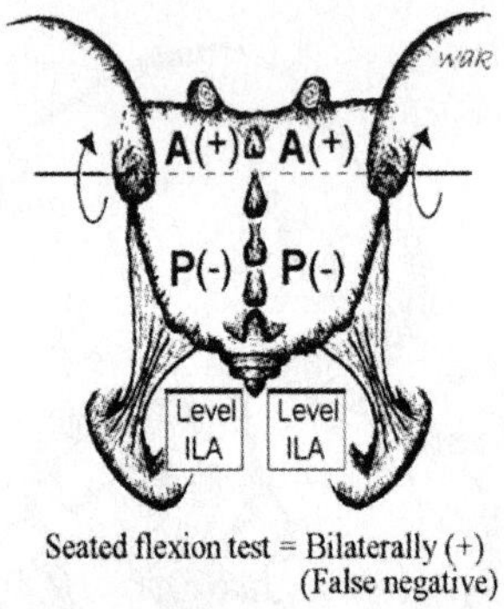

Figure 44. Bilateral sacral flexion. The seated flexion test is considered equivocal and the sacral base is relatively anterior.

forward torsions *Also called* neutral sacral somatic dysfunctions, a historic term.

1. Forward torsion is a physiologic rotation of the sacrum around an oblique axis such that the side of the sacral base contralateral to the named axis glides anteriorly and produces a deep sulcus. L5 rotates in the direction opposite to the rotation of the sacral base.
2. A group of somatic dysfunctions described by Fred Mitchell, Sr, DO, based on the motion cycle of walking.

left on left (forward) sacral torsion Refers to left sacral rotation about a left oblique axis. Findings: There is a positive seated flexion test on the right. The right sacral sulcus is deep or anterior and the left ILA is posterior/inferior. L5 is neutral SLRR. The lumbosacral spring test is negative and the backward bending test is symmetric (Fig. 45). *See also* sacral torsion.

left on right (backward) sacral torsion Refers to left sacral rotation about a right oblique axis. Findings: There is a positive seated flexion test on the left. The left sacral sulcus is posterior or shallow, and the right ILA is anterior or deep. L5 is nonneutral SRRR. Left superior sacral sulcus will be restricted when springing. The lumbosacral spring test is positive, and the backward bending test is asymmetric (Fig. 46). *See* sacral torsion.

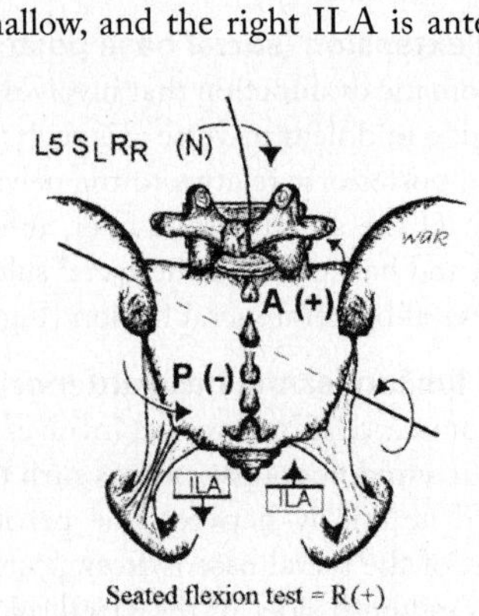

Figure 45. Left on left sacral torsion (left on left forward torsion).

posterior sacrum A positional term based on the Strachan model referring to a sacral somatic dysfunction in which the sacral base has rotated posterior and side bent to the side opposite to the rotation. The dysfunction is named for the side on which the posterior rotation occurs. The tissue texture changes are found at the lower pole on the side of rotation. The motion characteristics of L5 are not described (Fig. 47).

posterior translated sacrum A sacral somatic dysfunction in which the entire sacrum has moved posteriorly (backward) between the ilia. Posterior motion is freer, and anterior motion is restricted (Fig. 48).

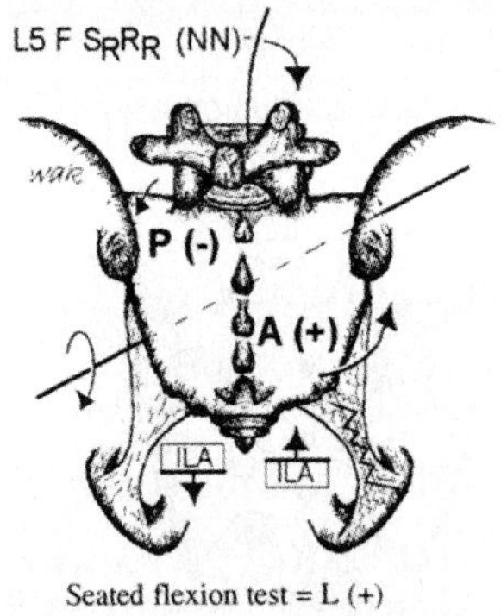

Figure 46. Example of left on right sacral torsion (left on right backward torsion).

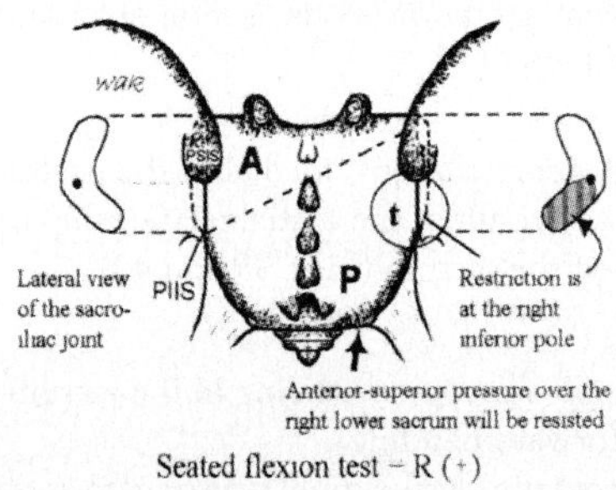

Figure 47. Posterior sacrum right. Motion of L5 is not described. There is tissue texture change (t) over the right sacroiliac joint (SI). The inferior pole of the right SI joint is affected. During motion testing, there is resistance to an anterior/superior test pressure applied over the right lower sacrum.

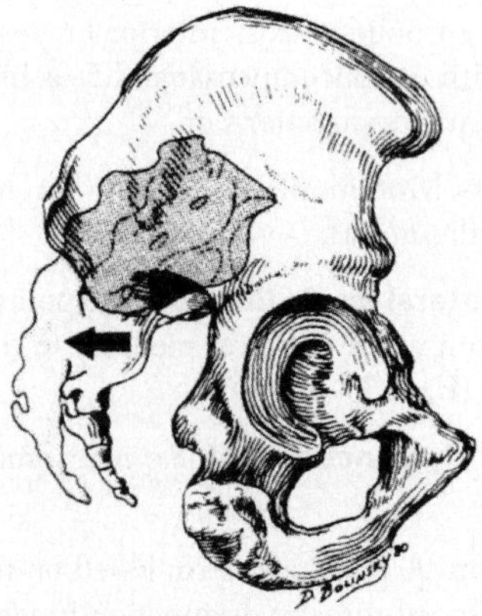

Figure 48. Posterior translated sacrum.

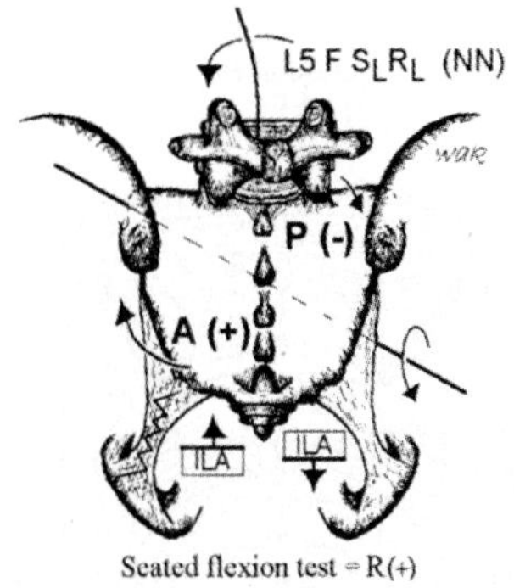

Figure 49. Example of right on left sacral torsion (right on left backward torsion).

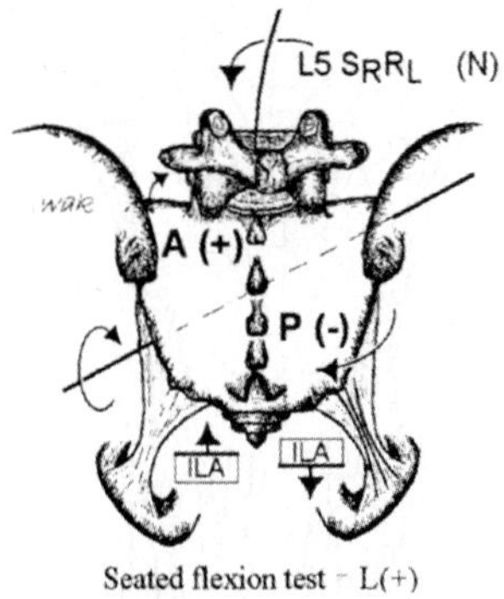

Figure 50. Right on right forward torsion.

right on left (backward) sacral torsion Refers to right rotation on a left oblique axis. Findings: The seated flexion test is positive on the right. The right sacral sulcus is posterior or shallow, and the left ILA is anterior or deep. L5 is nonneutral SLRL. The right superior sacral sulcus is restricted when springing. The lumbosacral spring test is positive. The backward bending test is asymmetric (Fig. 49). *See* sacral torsion.

right on right (forward) torsion Refers to a right sacral rotation about a right oblique axis. Findings: There is a positive seated flexion test on the left. The left sacral sulcus is deep or anterior and the right ILA is posterior/ inferior. L5 is neutral SRRL. The lumbosacral spring test is negative and the backward bending test is symmetric (Fig. 50). *See* sacral torsion.

rotated dysfunction of the sacrum A sacral somatic dysfunction in which the sacrum has rotated about an axis approximating the longitudinal (*y*) axis. Motion is freer in the direction that rotation has occurred and is restricted in the opposite direction (Fig. 51).

sacral shear A sacral somatic dysfunction in which the sacrum appears to have slipped anteriorly or posteriorly around a transverse axis allowing it to shift within the auricular L- or C-shaped sacroiliac joint. This anterior slippage is equivalent to a unilateral sacral flexion and extension. *See also* sacrum, somatic dysfunctions of, unilateral sacral flexion. *See also* sacrum, somatic dysfunctions of, unilateral sacral extension.

unilateral sacral extension

1. A sacral somatic dysfunction in which the dysfunctional side of the sacral base is posterior (the sacral sulcus of that side is shallow) in relation to the ilia and the ipsilateral ILA is anterior.
2. First described by Fred Mitchell, SR, DO (Fig. 52).

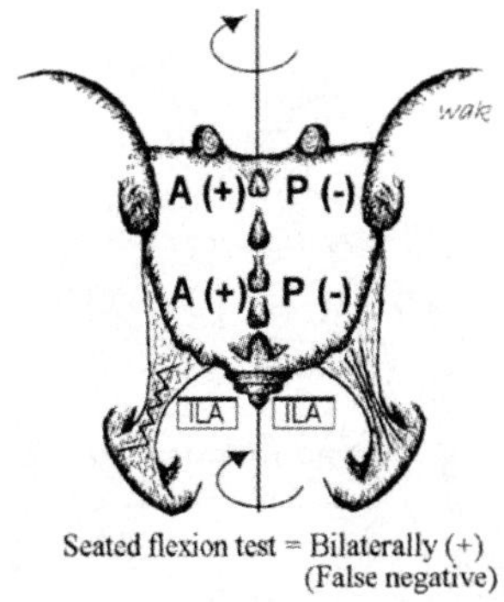

Figure 51. Right rotated dysfunction of the sacrum (right rotation about a vertical axis).

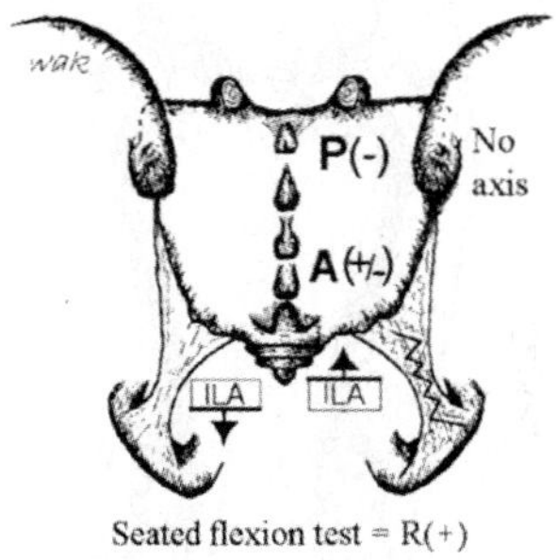

Figure 52. Right unilateral sacral extension (right superior sacral shear).

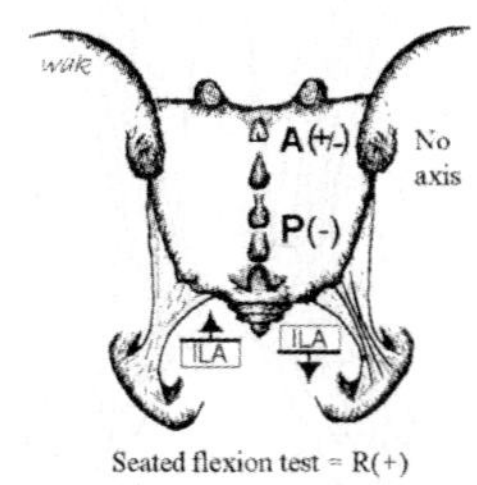

Figure 53. Right unilateral sacral flexion (right inferior sacral shear).

unilateral sacral flexion

1. A sacral somatic dysfunction in which the dysfunctional sacral base is anterior (the sacral sulcus of that side is deep) in relation to the ilia and the ipsilateral ILA is posterior.
2. First described by Fred Mitchell, Sr, DO (Fig. 53).

sagittal plane *See* plane, sagittal plane.

SBS *See* sphenobasilar synchondrosis.

scan An intermediate detailed examination of specific body regions that have been identified by findings emerging from the initial examination.

scaphocephaly *Also called* scaphoid head or hatchet head. It is a transverse compression of the cranium with a resultant midsagittal ridge.

scaphoid head *See also* scaphocephaly.

sclerotherapy

1. Treatment involving injection of a proliferant solution at the osseous–ligamentous junction.
2. Treatment involving injection of irritating substances into weakened connective tissue areas such as fascia, varicose veins, hemorrhoids, esophageal varices, or weakened ligaments. The intended body's response to the irritant is fibrous proliferation with shortening/strengthening of the tissues injected.

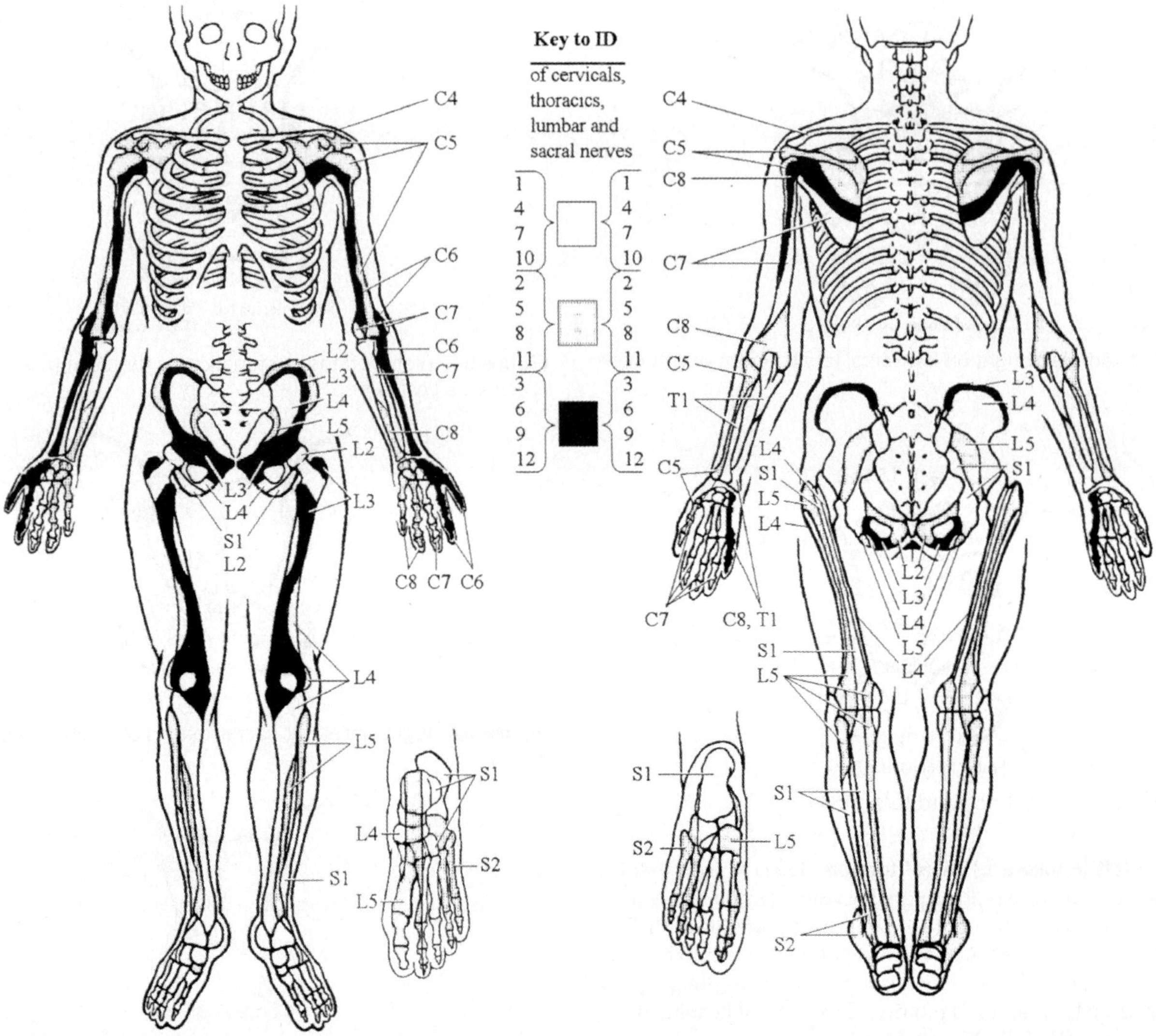

Figure 54. Anterior and posterior sclerotomal innervations. (Modified from Kuchera WA, Kappler RE. Musculoskeletal examination for somatic dysfunction. In: Ward RC, Jerome JA, eds. *Foundations for Osteopathic Medicine*. Williams & Wilkins; 1997:644.)

sclerotome

1. The pattern of innervation of structures derived from embryonal mesenchyme (joint capsule, ligament, and bone).
2. The area of bone innervated by a single spinal segment.
3. The group of mesenchymal cells emerging from the ventromedial part of a mesodermal somite and migrating toward the notochord. Sclerotomal cells from adjacent somites become merged in intersomatically located masses that are the primordia of the centra of the vertebrae (Fig. 54).

sclerotomal pain Deep, dull achy pain associated with tissues derived from a common sclerotome (Fig. 54).

scoliosis

1. Pathologic or functional lateral curvature of the spine.
2. An appreciable lateral deviation in the normally straight vertical line of the spine (Fig. 55).

screen The initial general somatic examination to determine signs of somatic dysfunction in various regions of the body. *See also* scan.

secondary joint motion *Also called* accessory joint motion. Involuntary or passive motion of a joint.

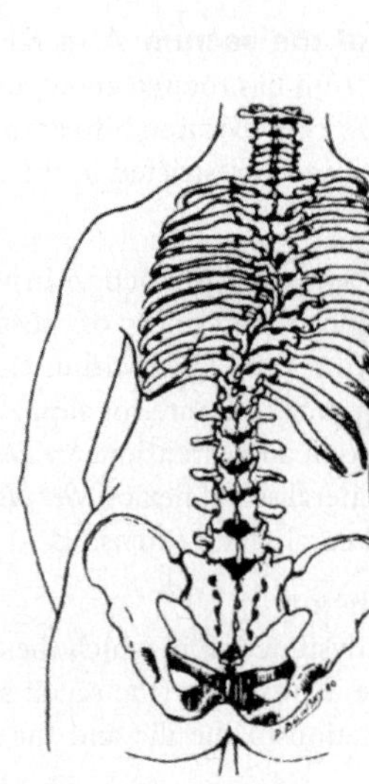

Figure 55. Scoliosis.

segment
1. A portion of a larger body or structure set off by natural or arbitrarily established boundaries, often equated with spinal segment.
2. To describe a single vertebra or a vertebral segment corresponding to the sites of origin of rootlets of individual spinal nerves.
3. A portion of the spinal cord.

segmental diagnosis The final stage of the spinal somatic examination in which the nature of the somatic dysfunction is detailed at a segmental level. *See also* scan. *See also* screen.

segmental dysfunction Dysfunction in a mobile system located at explicit segmental mobile units. Palpable characteristics of a dysfunctional segment are those associated with somatic dysfunction. Responses to regional motor inputs at the dysfunctional segment support the concepts of complete motor asymmetry and mirror-image motion asymmetries. *See also* STAR. *See also* TART.

segmental mobile unit A unit of the human movement system consisting of a bone, with articular surfaces for movement, as well as the adnexal tissues that create movement, allow movement, and establish position under motor control.

segmental motion Movement within a vertebral unit described by central nervous system (CNS) response to repeated sensory stimulation that generally follows habituation.

sensitization Hypothetically, a short-lived (minutes or hours) increase in central nervous system (CNS) response to repeated sensory stimulation that generally follows habituation.

shear An action or force causing or tending to cause two contiguous parts of an articulation to slide relative to each other in a direction parallel to their plane of contact. *See also* pubic bone, somatic dysfunctions of. *See also* innominates, somatic dysfunctions of, inferior innominate shear. *See also* innominates, somatic dysfunction of, superior innominate shear. *See also* sacrum, somatic dysfunctions of, sacral shear.

Sherrington law *See* law, Sherrington.

sidebent The position of any one or several vertebral bodies after side bending has occurred (Fig. 56). *See also* side bending.

sidebending *Also called* lateral flexion, lateroflexion, or flexion right (or left). Movement in a coronal (frontal) plane about an anteroposterior (*x*) axis.

skin drag Sense of resistance to light traction applied to the skin. Related to the degree of moisture and degree of sympathetic nervous system activity.

soft tissue (ST) *See* osteopathic manipulative treatment, soft tissue method.

soft tissue technique *See* osteopathic manipulative treatment, soft tissue method.

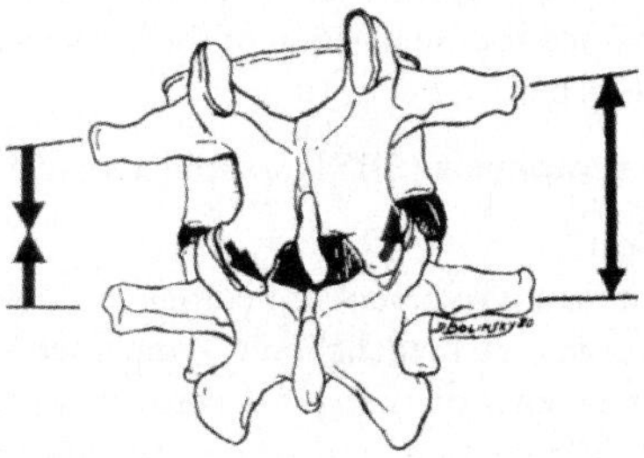

Figure 56. Sidebent.

somatic dysfunction Impaired or altered function of related components of the body framework system: skeletal, arthrodial, and myofascial structures, and their related vascular, lymphatic, and neural elements. It is characterized by positional asymmetry, restricted range of motion, tissue texture abnormalities, and/or tenderness. The positional and motion aspects of somatic dysfunction are generally described by:
1. The position of a body part as determined by palpation and referenced to its defined adjacent structure.
2. The directions in which motion is freer.
3. The directions in which motion is restricted.

Somatic dysfunction is treatable using osteopathic manipulative treatment.

acute somatic dysfunction Impairment or altered function of related components of the body framework system that is characterized in early stages by one or more of the following: pain, erythema, a palpable sense of relative warmth, moisture and bogginess, vasodilation, edema, tenderness, and tissue contraction. Identified by TART. *See also* TART.

chronic somatic dysfunction Impairment or altered function of long-standing duration of related components of the body framework system characterized by one or more of the following: itching, paresthesias, a palpable sense of tissue dryness, coolness, tissue contracture, fibrosis, tenderness, and pallor.

somatic dysfunction of

pubic bone *See* pubic bone, somatic dysfunctions of.

pubic symphysis *See* pubic bone, somatic dysfunctions of.

sacrum *See* sacrum, somatic dysfunctions of.

abdominal A somatic dysfunction of the abdomen and other regions.

cranial A somatic dysfunction of the head and the occipitoatlantal region.

cervical A somatic dysfunction of the cervical region and the cervicothoracic region.

lower extremity A somatic dysfunction of the lower extremity region and the femoral–acetabular region.

lumbar A somatic dysfunction of the lumbar region and lumbosacral region.

pelvic A somatic dysfunction of the pelvic (iliosacral) region, pubic region, and hip region.

rib A somatic dysfunction of rib cage, costochondral, costovertebral, sternal, and sternochondral regions.

sacral A somatic dysfunction of the sacral region, sacroiliac joint, and sacrococcygeal region.

thoracic A somatic dysfunction of the thoracic region and thoracolumbar region.

upper extremity A somatic dysfunction of the upper extremity region, and the scapulathoracic, acromioclavicular, sternoclavicular, and glenohumeral regions.

primary somatic dysfunction
1. The initial or first somatic dysfunction to appear temporally.
2. The somatic dysfunction that maintains a total pattern of dysfunction, including secondary somatic dysfunction.

secondary somatic dysfunction
1. Somatic dysfunction arising in response from a primary somatic dysfunction.
2. Somatic dysfunction arising as a consequence of other etiology.

type I somatic dysfunction A group dysfunction of the thoracic and lumbar vertebrae. These vertebrae are neutral relative to the sagittal plane and demonstrate a preference for side bending and rotation in opposite directions (e.g., side bent right and rotated left or side bent left and rotated right).

type II somatic dysfunction A single segmental dysfunction of the thoracic or lumbar vertebrae. This vertebra is significantly flexed or extended and demonstrates a preference for side bending and rotation in the same direction (e.g., rotated right and side bent right or side bent left, and rotated left).

somatogenic That which is produced by activity, reaction, and change originating in the musculoskeletal system.

somatosomatic reflex *See* reflex, somatosomatic reflex.

somatovisceral reflex *See* reflex, somatovisceral reflex.

spasm A sudden, violent, involuntary contraction of a muscle or group of muscles, attended by pain and interference with function, producing involuntary movement and distortion (compare with hypertonicity) (*Dorland's*).

Spencer technique *See* osteopathic manipulative treatment, Spencer technique.

sphenobasilar synchondrosis (SBS) *Also called* sphenobasilar symphysis. The cartilaginous junction between the basilar portion of the sphenoid and the basilar portion of the occiput.

somatic dysfunctions of SBS Any of a group of somatic dysfunctions involving primarily the interrelationship between the basilar portion of the sphenoid (basisphenoid) and the basilar portion of the occiput (basiocciput).

SBS compression Somatic dysfunction in which the basisphenoid and basiocciput are held forced together significantly limiting SBS motion.

SBS extension Sphenoid and occiput have rotated in opposite directions around parallel transverse axes; the basiocciput and basisphenoid are both inferior in SBS extension with a decrease in the dorsal convexity between these two bones (Fig. 57).

SBS flexion Sphenoid and occiput have rotated in opposite directions around parallel transverse axes; the basiocciput and basisphenoid are both superior in SBS flexion with an increase in the dorsal convexity between these two bones (Fig. 58).

lateral strain Sphenoid and occiput have rotated in the same direction around parallel vertical axes. Lateral strains of the SBS are named for the position of the basisphenoid, right or left (Fig. 59).

side bending–rotation Sphenoid and occiput have rotated in opposite directions around parallel vertical axes and rotate in the same direction around an anteroposterior (A-P) axis. SBS side bending–rotations are named for the convexity, right or left (Fig. 60).

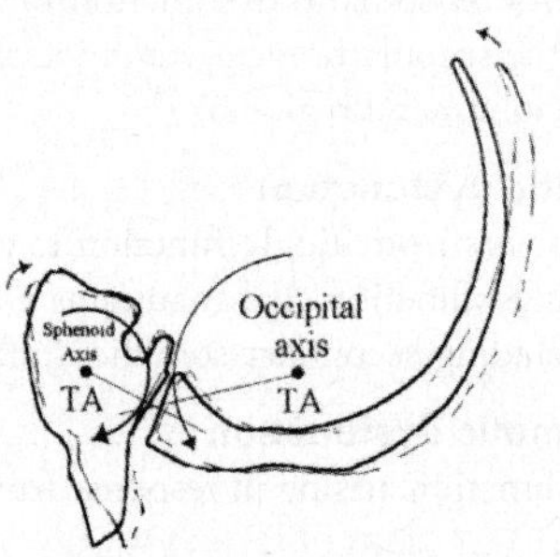

Figure 57. SBS extension. (TA, transverse axis)

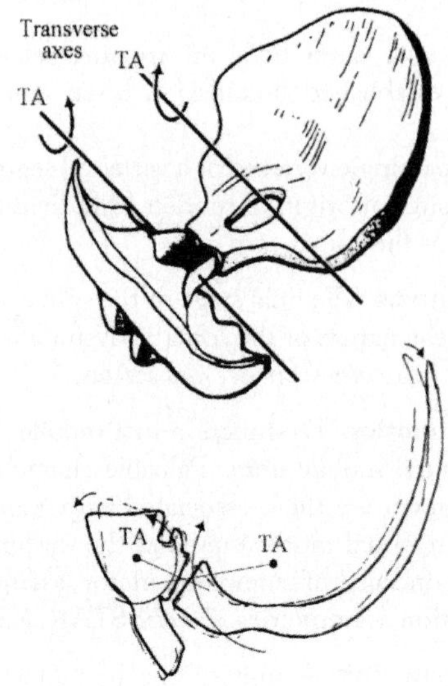

Figure 58. SBS flexion.

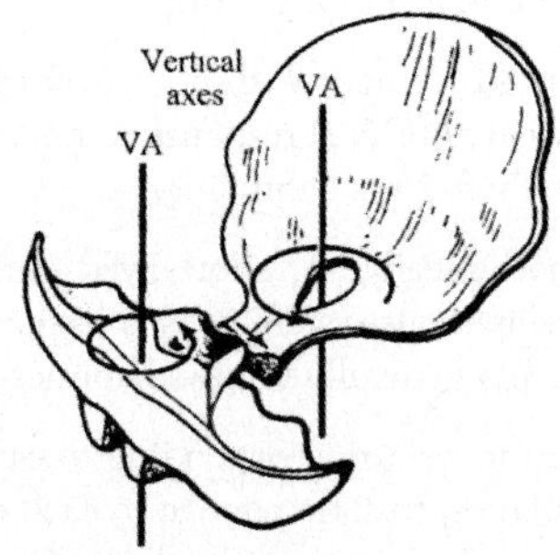

Figure 59. Right lateral strain (SBS).

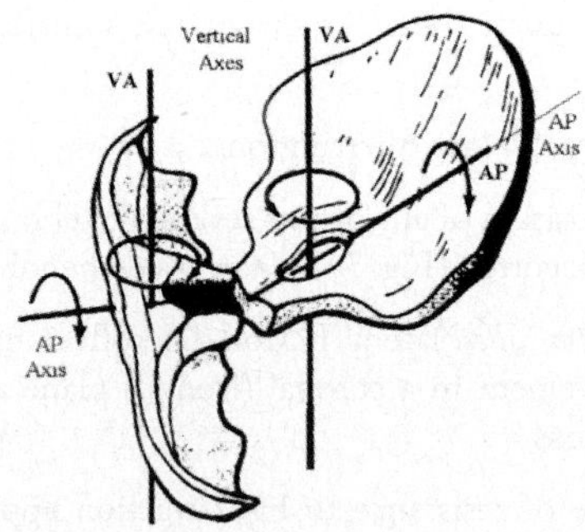

Figure 60. Left sidebending/rotation (SBS).

torsion Sphenoid and occiput have rotated in opposite directions around an anteroposterior (A-P) axis. SBS torsions are named for the high greater wing of the sphenoid, right or left (Fig. 61).

vertical strain Sphenoid and occiput have rotated in the same direction around parallel transverse axes. Vertical strains of the SBS are named for the position of the basisphenoid, superior or inferior (Fig. 62).

sphenobasilar symphysis (SBS) *See* sphenobasilar synchondrosis.

spinal facilitation

1. The maintenance of a pool of neurons (e.g., premotor neurons, motor neurons, or preganglionic sympathetic neurons in one or more segments of the spinal cord) in a state of partial or subthreshold excitation; in this state, less afferent stimulation is required to trigger the discharge of impulses.

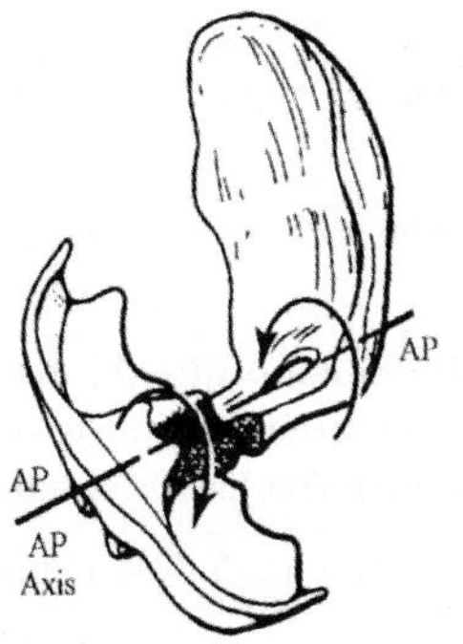

Figure 61. Right torsion (SBS).

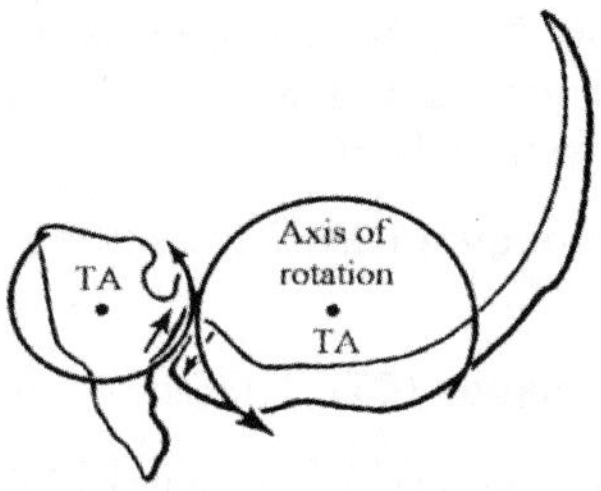

Figure 62. Superior vertical strain (SBS).

2. A theory regarding the neurophysiologic mechanisms underlying the neuronal activity associated with somatic dysfunction.
3. Facilitation may be due to sustained increase in afferent input, aberrant patterns of afferent input, or changes within the affected neurons themselves or their chemical environment. Once established, facilitation can be sustained by normal central nervous system (CNS) activity.

splenic pump technique *See* osteopathic manipulative treatment, splenic pump technique.

spontaneous release by positioning *See* osteopathic manipulative treatment, counterstrain.

sprain Stretching injuries of ligamentous tissue (compare with strain).

first degree: Microtrauma.

second degree: Partial tear.

third degree: Complete disruption.

springing technique *See* osteopathic manipulative treatment, springing technique; osteopathic manipulative treatment, articulatory.

sphinx test *See* backward bending test.

spring test
1. A test used to differentiate between backward or forward sacral torsions/rotations.
2. A test used to differentiate bilateral sacral extension and bilateral sacral flexion.
3. A test used to differentiate unilateral sacral extension and unilateral sacral flexion. *See also* lumbosacral spring test.

STAR An acronym for four diagnostic criteria of somatic dysfunction: sensitivity changes, tissue texture abnormality, asymmetry, and alteration of the quality and quantity of range of motion.

static contraction *See* contraction, isometric contraction.

Still, DO, Andrew Taylor Physician and surgeon who founded osteopathic medicine; 1828–1917. First announced the tenets of osteopathic medicine on June 22, 1874; established the American School of Osteopathy in 1892 at Kirksville, MO.

still point
1. A term used to identify and describe the temporary cessation of the rhythmic motion of the primary respiratory mechanism. It may occur during osteopathic manipulative treatment when a point of balanced membranous or ligamentous tension is achieved.
2. A term used by William G. Sutherland, DO.

Still Technique *See* osteopathic manipulative treatment, Still Technique.

strain
1. Stretching injuries of muscle tissue.
2. Distortion with deformation of tissue. *See also* ligamentous strain.

strain–counterstrain *See* osteopathic manipulative treatment, counterstrain.

Strachan model *See* sacrum, somatic dysfunctions of, anterior sacrum. *See also* sacrum, somatic dysfunctions of, posterior sacrum.

stretching Separation of the origin and insertion of a muscle and/or attachments of fascia and ligaments.

stringiness A palpable tissue texture abnormality characterized by fine or string-like myofascial structures.

structural examination *See* osteopathic structural examination.

subluxation
1. A partial or incomplete dislocation.
2. A term describing an abnormal anatomical position of a joint that exceeds the normal physiologic limit but does not exceed the joint's anatomical limit.

superior (upslipped) innominate *See* innominate, somatic dysfunctions of, superior innominate shear.

superior pubic shear *See* pubic bone, somatic dysfunctions of. *See also* symphyseal shear (Fig. 29).

superior transverse axis *See* sacral motion axis, superior transverse axis (respiratory); sacral motion axis, transverse (*z*) axis.

supination
1. Beginning in anatomical position, applied to the hand, the act of turning the palm forward (anteriorly) or upward, performed by lateral external rotation of the forearm.
2. Applied to the foot, it generally applies to movements (adduction and inversion) resulting in raising of the medial margin of the foot, hence of the longitudinal arch. A compound motion of plantar flexion, adduction, and inversion. *See also* pronation.

supine Lying with the face upward.

symmetry The similar arrangement in form and relationships of parts around a common axis, or on each side of a plane of the body.

Sutherland fulcrum A shifting suspension fulcrum of the reciprocal tension membrane located along the straight sinus at the junction of the falx cerebri and tentorium cerebelli. *See also* reciprocal tension membrane; osteopathic manipulative treatment, osteopathic cranial manipulative medicine (OCMM).

symphyseal shear The result of an action or force causing or tending to cause the two parts of the symphysis to slide relative to each other in a direction parallel to their plane of contact. It is usually found in an inferior/superior direction but is occasionally found to be in an anterior/posterior direction (Figs. 28 and 29).

T

tapotement Striking the belly of a muscle with the hypothenar edge of the open hand in rapid succession in an attempt to increase its tone and arterial perfusion.

TART An acronym for four diagnostic criteria of somatic dysfunction: tissue texture abnormality, asymmetry, restriction of motion, and tenderness.

technique Methods, procedures, and details of a mechanical process or surgical operation. *See also* osteopathic manipulative treatment.

tenderness
1. Discomfort or pain elicited by an osteopathic physician through palpation.
2. A state of heightened sensitivity to touch or pressure.

tender points Small, hypersensitive points in the myofascial tissues of the body that do not have a pattern of pain radiation. These points are a manifestation of somatic dysfunction and are used as diagnostic criteria and for monitoring treatment. *See also* tenderpoints. *See also* trigger point.

tenderpoints A system of myofascial tender points used for the counterstrain system for the diagnosis and treatment of somatic dysfunction originally described by Lawrence Jones, DO, FAAO. *See also* osteopathic manipulative treatment, counterstrain.

thoracic aperture (superior) *See* thoracic inlet.

thoracic inlet
1. The functional thoracic inlet consists of T1–4 vertebrae, ribs 1 and 2 plus their costal cartilages, and the manubrium of the sternum.
2. The anatomical thoracic inlet consists of T1 vertebra, the first ribs and their costal cartilages, and the superior end of the manubrium. *See* fascial patterns.

thoracic pump *See* osteopathic manipulative treatment, thoracic pump technique.

thrust technique *See* osteopathic manipulative treatment, thrust technique. *See also* osteopathic manipulative treatment, high-velocity low-amplitude technique (HVLA).

tissue texture abnormality (TTA) A palpable change in the tissues of the body away from their normal state. Common findings include bogginess, thickness, ropiness, stringiness, firmness, and changes in temperature or moisture. This term is part of the "TART" acronym for the diagnostic criteria of somatic dysfunction. *See also* TART.

tonus A normal physiologic state in which there is a slight continuous tension of muscle tissue, which in skeletal muscles, aids in the maintenance of posture and facilitates a response to stimulation.

torsion A motion or state where one end of a part is twisted about a longitudinal axis while the opposite end is held fast or turned in the opposite direction.

torsion, sacral *See* sacral torsion. *See also* sacrum, somatic dysfunctions of.

torsion, sphenobasilar synchondrosis A physiologic motion pattern about an anteroposterior axis of the sphenobasilar symphysis/synchondrosis. *See also* sphenobasilar synchondrosis (SBS), torsion.

traction A linear force acting to draw structures apart.

traction technique *See* osteopathic manipulative treatment, traction technique.

transitional region Areas of the axial skeleton where structure changes significantly lead to functional changes; transitional areas commonly include the following:

occipitocervical region (OA) Typically the OA-AA-C2 region is described.

cervicothoracic region (CT) Typically C7–T1.

thoracolumbar region (TL) Typically T10–L1.

lumbosacral region (LS) Typically L5–S1.

transitional vertebrae A congenital anomaly of a vertebra in which it develops characteristic(s) of the adjoining structure or region.

lumbarization A transitional segment in which the first sacral segment becomes like an additional lumbar vertebra articulating with the second sacral segment.

sacralization
1. Incomplete separation and differentiation of the fifth lumbar vertebra (L5) such that it takes on characteristics of a sacral vertebra.
2. When transverse processes of the fifth lumbar (L5) are atypically large, causing pseudoarthrosis with the sacrum and/or ilia(um), referred to as batwing deformity, if bilateral.

translation Motion along an axis.

translatory motion *See* motion, translatory motion.

transverse axis of sacrum *See* sacral, sacral movement axis, transverse (*z*) axis (Fig. 37).

transverse process Projects laterally from the region of each pedicle. The pedicle connects the posterior elements to the vertebral body (Fig. 63).

transverse rib axis *See also* rib motion, pump handle rib motion (Fig. 34).

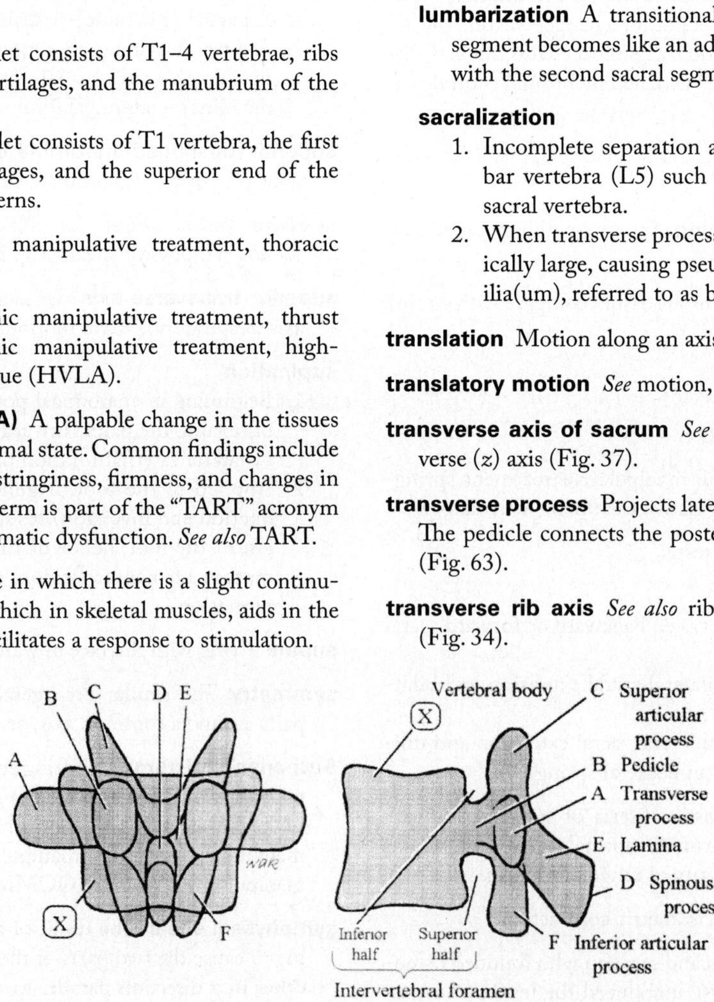

Figure 63. The pedicle (*B*) is the key structure from which other vertebral parts can be identified. (Modified from Kuchera WA. Lumbar region. In: Ward RC, ed. *Foundations for Osteopathic Medicine*. 2nd ed. Lippincott Williams & Wilkins; 2003:730.)

Traube–Hering–Mayer wave An oscillation that has been measured in association with blood pressure, heart rate, cardiac contractility, pulmonary blood flow, cerebral blood flow and movement of the cerebrospinal fluid, and peripheral blood flow including venous volume and thermal regulation. This whole-body phenomenon, which exhibits a rate typically slightly less than and independent of respiration, bears a striking resemblance to the primary respiratory mechanism.

Travell trigger point *See* trigger point.

treatment, active A historical term. *See* osteopathic manipulative treatment, active method.

treatment, osteopathic manipulative techniques *See* osteopathic manipulative treatment.

Trendelenburg test A test performed to assess for hip dysfunction, primarily weakness of the hip abductors such as the gluteus medius and gluteus minimus. The patient, with back to the examiner, is told to lift first one foot and then the other. The position and movements of the gluteal fold are observed. When standing on the affected limb, the gluteal fold on the sound side falls instead of rising. Seen in conditions including poliomyelitis, ununited fracture of the femoral neck, coxa vara, and congenital dislocations.

trigger point (myofascial trigger point)

1. A small hypersensitive site that, when stimulated, consistently produces a reflex mechanism that gives rise to referred pain and/or other manifestations in a consistent reference zone that is consistent from person to person.
2. These points were most extensively and systematically documented by Janet Travell, MD, and David Simons, MD.

trophic Pertaining to nutrition, especially in the cellular environment (e.g., trophic function—a nutritional function).

trophicity

1. A nutritional function or relation.
2. The natural tendency to replenish the body stores that have been depleted.

trophotropic Concerned with or pertaining to the natural tendency for maintenance and/or restoration of nutritional stores.

tropic A word termination denoting turning toward, changing, or tendency to change.

tropism, facet Unequal size and/or facing of the zygapophyseal joints of a vertebra. *See also* facet asymmetry.

type I somatic dysfunction *See* somatic dysfunction, type I somatic dysfunction. *See also* physiologic motion of the spine.

type II somatic dysfunction *See* somatic dysfunction, type II somatic dysfunction. *See also* physiologic motion of the spine.

U

uncommon compensatory pattern *See* fascial patterns, uncommon compensatory pattern.

uncompensated fascial pattern *See* fascial patterns, uncompensated fascial pattern.

V

v-spread *See* osteopathic manipulative treatment, v-spread.

velocity The instantaneous rate of motion in a given direction.

ventral technique *See* osteopathic manipulative treatment, visceral manipulation.

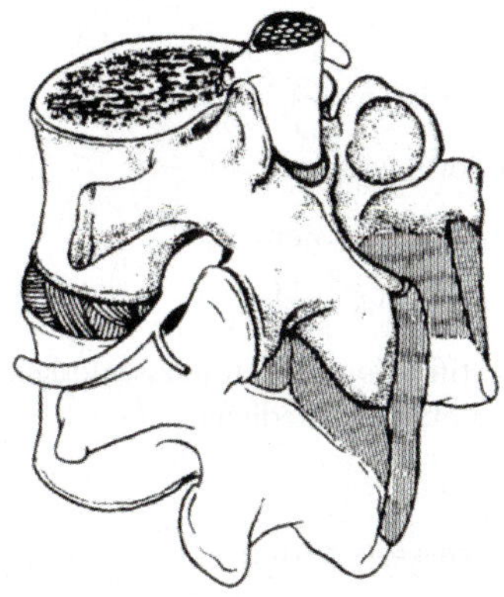

Figure 64. Vertebral unit.

vertebral unit Two adjacent vertebrae with their associated intervertebral disk, arthrodial, ligamentous, muscular, vascular, lymphatic and neural elements (Fig. 64).

vertical axis *See* sacral motion axis, vertical (y) axis (longitudinal).

visceral dysfunction Impaired or altered mobility or motility of the visceral system and related fascial, neurologic, vascular, skeletal, and lymphatic elements.

visceral manipulation *See* osteopathic manipulative treatment, visceral manipulation.

viscerosomatic dysfunction Somatic dysfunction related to a viscerosomatic reflex. *See* reflex, viscerosomatic.

viscerosomatic reflex *See* reflex, viscerosomatic reflex.

viscerovisceral reflex *See* reflex, viscerovisceral reflex.

viscosity

1. A measurement of the rate of deformation of any material under load.
2. The capability possessed by a solid of yielding continually under stress. *See also* elasticity; plasticity.

W

weight-bearing line of L3 *See* gravitational line (Fig. 16).

X

No x terms.

Y

No y terms.

Z

No z terms.

Abbreviations

AA atlantoaxial

AACOM American Association of Colleges of Osteopathic Medicine

AAO American Academy of Osteopathy

AOA American Osteopathic Association

AOBNMM American Osteopathic Board of Neuromusculoskeletal Medicine

A-P anteroposterior

ART articulatory

AIIS anterior inferior iliac spines

ASIS anterior superior iliac spines

BLT balanced ligamentous tension

BMT balanced membranous tension

C-NMM/OMM Certification in Neuromusculoskeletal Medicine/ Osteopathic Manipulative Medicine

C cervical

CCP common compensatory pattern

CNS central nervous system

CO coccygeal

COCA Association Commission on Osteopathic College Accreditation

CR cranial

CRI cranial rhythmic impulse

CS counterstrain treatment

CT cervicothoracic

CV-4 compression of the 4th ventricle technique

D direct treatment

DIR direct treatment

DO Doctor of Osteopathic Medicine or Diplomat in Osteopathy

E extended

ECOP Educational Council on Osteopathic Principles

ERS extended/rotated/sidebent

F flexed

FAAO Fellow of the American Academy of Osteopathy

FOR facilitated oscillatory release treatment

FPR facilitated positional release treatment

FRS flexed/rotated/side bent

HVLA high-velocity low-amplitude treatment

I indirect treatment

ILA inferior lateral angle

IND indirect treatment

I/IND indirect method

INR integrated neuromusculoskeletal release treatment

JTP Jones tender point

L left or lumbar

LAS ligamentous articular strain treatment

LS lumbosacral

ME muscle energy treatment

MFR myofascial release treatment

MTrP myofascial trigger point

N neutral

NBOME National Board of Osteopathic Medical Examiners

NMM-OMM neuromusculoskeletal medicine–osteopathic manipulative medicine

NRS neutral/rotated/side bent

OA occipitoatlantal

OCF osteopathy in the cranial field (historical)

OCMM osteopathic cranial manipulative medicine

OMM osteopathic manipulative medicine

OMT osteopathic manipulative treatment

OMTh osteopathic manipulative therapy

ONMM osteopathic neuromusculoskeletal medicine

OPP osteopathic principles and practice

PINS progressive inhibition of neuromuscular structures

PSIS posterior superior iliac spines

R right or rotated or rib

RIT regenerative injection therapy

S side bent or sacrum

SBS sphenobasilar synchondrosis

SD somatic dysfunction

ST soft tissue

STAR sensitivity/tissue texture changes/asymmetry/restriction of motion

T thoracic

TART tenderness/asymmetry/restriction of motion/tissue texture change

TL thoracolumbar

TP tender point

TrP Travell trigger point

TTA tissue texture abnormality

VIS visceral manipulative treatment

INDEX

Note: Page numbers followed by '*f*' indicate figures, page numbers followed by '*t*' indicate tables, and page numbers followed by '*b*' indicate boxes.

A

C

D

E

G

H

J

K

M

O

S